INDEX-CATALOGUE

OF

THE LIBRARY

OF THE

SURGEON-GENERAL'S OFFICE,

UNITED STATES ARMY.

AUTHORS AND SUBJECTS.

VOL. IX.

MEDICINE (Popular)—NYWELT.

WASHINGTON:
GOVERNMENT PRINTING OFFICE.
1888.

WAR DEPARTMENT, SURGEON-GENERAL'S OFFICE,
MEDICAL MUSEUM AND LIBRARY DIVISION,
Washington, D. C., June 26, 1888.

General JOHN MOORE,
Surgeon-General, U. S. Army:

GENERAL: I have the honor to present herewith the ninth volume of the Index-Catalogue of the Library of this Office.

This volume includes 13,151 author-titles, representing 6,834 volumes and 12,818 pamphlets. It also includes 9,999 subject-titles of separate books and pamphlets, and 29,120 titles of articles in periodicals.

The following table shows the number of titles in the Index-Catalogue, as far as published:

Volumes.	AUTHOR-TITLES.			SUBJECT-TITLES.		Portraits.
	Titles.	Volumes.	Pamphlets.	Book titles.	Journal articles.	
I	9,090	8,031	6,398	9,000	34,604	....
II	12,496	4,934	9,810	11,550	37,310	....
III	9,043	10,076	7,386	8,572	28,846	4,335
IV	4,802	1,926	3,885	12,361	48,977	....
V	15,555	5,755	12,596	8,069	34,127	....
VI	7,900	2,543	7,250	14,590	35,290	....
VII	14,688	5,987	12,372	6,371	34,903	....
VIII	13,405	5,307	13,205	12,642	24,174	....
IX	13,151	6,834	12,818	9,999	29,120	....
Total	100,130	51,393	85,720	93,154	307,351	4,335

Very respectfully,
Your obedient servant,

JOHN S. BILLINGS,
Surgeon, U. S. Army.

III

SECOND ADDITION

TO THE

ALPHABETICAL LIST

OF

ABBREVIATIONS OF TITLES

OF

MEDICAL PERIODICALS

EMPLOYED IN THE

INDEX-CATALOGUE,

PUBLISHED IN THE SEVENTH VOLUME.

☞ For explanations, see the Alphabetical Lists of Abbreviations of Titles, etc., in Vol. I, p. [1], Vol. VII, p. [1], and Vol. VIII, p. [1].

A.

Abhandl. d. math.-phys. Cl. d. k. sächs. Gesellsch. d. Wissensch., Leipz.
Abhandlungen der mathematisch-physischen Classe der königl. sächsischen Gesellschaft der Wissenschaften. Leipzig. No. 2, v. 14, 1887. 8°.

Academia de Esculapio. Madrid. [*See* Eco de la med., Madrid.]

Académie royale de chirurgie. Paris. [*See* Obs. surg. dis. head & neck. Select. Mem. Roy. Acad. Surg. of France, Lond.]

Actes Cong. internat. d'anthrop. crim., Rome.
Actes du premier Congrès international d'anthropologie criminelle. Biologie et sociologie. (Rome, novembre 1885.) Turin, Rome, Florence. 1 v., 1886-7. 8°.

Actes Cong. pénitent. internat. de Rome.
Actes du Congrès pénitentiaire international de Rome. Novembre 1885. Rome. v. 1-2, 1887-8. 8°.

Aerztl. Centr.-Anz. f. Deutschl., Hamb.
Aerztlicher Central-Anzeiger für Deutschland. Organ für die wirthschaftlichen und materiellen Interessen des practischen Arztes. Hamburg. v. 3, 1888. fol.

Akushersko-ginekologicheski Obshestvo v Kieve. [*See* Protok. zasaid. akush.-ginek. Obsh. v Kieve.]

Alumnæ Association of the Woman's Medical College of Pennsylvania. [*See* Rep. Proc. Alumnæ Ass. Woman's M. Coll. Penn., Phila.]

Am. Ann. Deaf, Wash.
American Annals of the Deaf. Washington, D. C. v. 31-32, 1886-7. 8°. [Continuation, after 1885, of: Am. Ann. Deaf & Dumb.]

Am. Anthrop., Wash.
American (The) Anthropologist. Published under the auspices of the Anthropological Society of Washington. Washington, D. C. v. 1, 1888. 8°. [Continuation of: Tr. Anthrop. Soc. Wash.]

American Climatological Association. [*See* Tr. Am. Climat. Ass.]

Am. J. Psychol., Balt.	American (The) Journal of Psychology. Baltimore. v. 1, 1887–8. 8°.
	American Society for Psychical Research. [*See* Proc. Am. Soc. Psych. Research, Bost.]
An. d. Mus. nac. de México.	Anales del Museo nacional de México. México. v. 1–4, 1877–87. fol.
Anat. Anz., Jena.	Anatomischer Anzeiger. Centralbl. für die gesamte wissenschaftliche Anatomie. Amtliches. Organ der anatomischen Gesellschaft. Jena. v. 1–3, 1886–8. 8°.
	Anatomical Society of Great Britain and Ireland. [*See* Proc. Anat. Soc. Gr. Brit. & Ireland, Lond.]
	Anatomische Gesellschaft [Jena]. [*See* Anat. Anz., Jena.]
Ann. clin. d. Osp. d. incur. in Napoli.	Annali (Gli) clinici dell' Ospedale degl' incurabili in Napoli. Giornale di medicina e chirurgia. Napoli. 1887. 8°.
Ann. Gynæc., Bost.	Annals of Gynæcology. A monthly review of gynæcology, obstetrics, and abdominal surgery. Boston. v. 1, 1887–8. 8°.
Ann. d'orthop. et de chir. prat., Par.	Annales d'orthopédie et de chirurgie pratique. Journal bi-mensuel. Paris. v. 1–2, 1887–8. 8°.
Ann. d. Univ. libera di Perugia. Fac. di med. e chir.	Annali dell' Università libera di Perugia. Anno 1º, 1885–6. v. 1. Facoltà di medicina e chirurgia. Perugia. roy. 8°.
Annual J. Ill. Dent. Soc., Chicago.	Annual (The) Journal of the Illinois State Dental Society. Transactions. Chicago. For the years 1870–82, 1884–7, 1870–87. 8°.
	Anthropological Society of Bombay. [*See* J. Anthrop. Soc. Bombay.]
	Anthropological Society of Washington. [*See* Am. Anthrop., Wash.]
Arb. a. d. chir. Univ.-Poliklin. zu Leipz.	Arbeiten aus der chirurgischen Universitäts-Poliklinik zu Leipzig. Hrsg. von Benno Schmidt. Leipzig. Hft. 1, 1888. 8°.
Arb. d. pharmakol. Inst. zu Dorpat, Stuttg.	Arbeiten des pharmakologischen Institutes zu Dorpat. Stuttgart. v. 1, 1888. 8°.
Arch. de hist. da med. portugueza, Porto.	Archivos de historia da medicina portugueza. Porto. v. 1, 1886. 8°.
Arch. de laryngol., de rhinol. [etc.], Par.	Archives de laryngologie, de rhinologie et des maladies des premières voies respiratoires et digestives. Paris. v. 1, 1887–8. 8°.
Arch. de méd. et chir. prat., Brux.	Archives de médecine et de chirurgie pratiques. Bruxelles. v. 2, 1887–8. 8°. [Continuation of the following.]
Arch. mens. de méd. et chir. prat., Brux.	Archives mensuelles de médecine et de chirurgie pratiques. Bruxelles. v. 1, 1886–7. sm. 8°. [Continued in v. 2 as the preceding.]
Arch. de obst. y ginec., Madrid.	Archivos de obstetricia y de ginecología. Continuación de los "Anales de obstetricia, ginecología y pediatria" y de los "Anales de la Sociedad ginecológica española". Órgano oficial de la misma. Madrid. v. 12, 1888. 8°.
Arch. roum. de méd. et chir., Par.	Archives roumaines de médecine et de chirurgie. Paris. v. 1, 1887–8. 8°.
Atti d. Cong. farm. ital.	Atti del primo Congresso farmaceutico italiano tenutosi in Torino dal 4 all' 8 ottobre 1886. Torino. 1 v., 1887. roy. 8°.
Aula méd., Vallad.	Aula (El) médica. Revista decenal de medicina. Valladolid. Nos. 14–15, March 20–30, año 2, 1888. 8°.

B.

Beitr. z. exper. Path. u. Physiol., Berl.	Beiträge zur experimentellen Pathologie und Physiologie, hrsg. von Dr. L. Traube. Berlin. 1 v., 1846. 8°.
Beitr. z. klin. Chir., Tübing.	Beiträge zur klinischen Chirurgie. Mittheilungen aus der chirurgischen Klinik zu Tübingen. Hrsg. von Paul Bruns. Tübingen. v. 2–3, 1886–7. 8°. [Continuation of: Mitth. a. d. chir. Klin. zu Tübing.]
Beitr. z. path. Anat., exper. Path. [etc.], Leipz.	Beiträge zur pathologischen Anatomie, experimentellen Pathologie und praktischen Medicin. Herrn Dr. F. A. von Zenker, zur Feier seines 25jähr. Professoren-Jubiläums gewidmet von seinen Freunden und Schülern. Leipzig. 1 v., 1887. roy. 8°.

Beitr. z. path. Anat. u. klin. Med., Leipz.	Beiträge zur pathologischen Anatomie und klinischen Medicin. Ernst Leberecht Wagner zum 20. December 1887, dem 25jährigen Gedenktage seiner Ernennung zum ordentlichen Professor gewidmet von seinen Schülern. Leipzig. 1 v., 1887. roy. 8°.
Beitr. z. path. Anat. u. Physiol., Jena.	Beiträge zur pathologischen Anatomie und Physiologie. Hrsg. von E. Ziegler und C. Nauwerck. Jena. v. 1–2, 1886–7. 8°.
Ber. a. d. Baudeputat. zu Frankf. a. M. . . . d. Schulbänke [etc.]	Bericht an die Baudeputation zu Frankfurt am Main zur Beantwortung der Frage über die zweckmässigste Einrichtung der Schulbänke und Schultische. Frankfurt a. M. 1 v., 1871. 4°.
Ber. d. Kinderheilanst. zu Leipz.	Bericht der Kinderheilanstalt zu Leipzig, zugleich als Bericht über deren und der damit verbundenen Frauenstation fünfundzwanzigjähriges Bestehen. Leipzig. 1 v., 1880. 4°.
Ber. d. naturf. Gesellsch. zu Freib. i. Br.	Berichte der naturforschenden Gesellschaft zu Freiburg i. Br. Freiburg i. Br. v. 2, 1887. 8°.
Bisturí, Toledo.	Bisturí (El). Revista mensual de cirujía práctica por el Doctor D. Pedro Gallardo. Toledo. Nos. 1–3, v. 1, 1888. 8°.
Bol. de san., Madrid.	Boletin de sanidad. Publicado por la Dirección general de beneficencia y sanidad. Madrid. Nos. 1–3, año 1, 1888. roy. 8°.
Bol. de saude e hyg. municip. de Lisb.	Boletim de saude e hygiene municipal de Lisboa. Lisboa. v. 1, 1887. roy. 8°.
Boll. d. Osp. di S. Casa di Loreto, Loreto.	Bollettino dell' Ospedale di S. Casa di Loreto. Monitore medico marchigiano. Loreto. v. 1, 1887–8. 8°. [Title of No. 1 reads· Bollettino trimestrale, etc. The subtitle "Monitore", etc., appeared first in No. 3.]
Brooklyn M. J.	Brooklyn (The) Medical Journal. Published monthly by the Medical Society of the County of Kings. Brooklyn, N. Y. v. 1, 1888. 8°.
	Buletinul Societăţei de medici şi naturalişti din Iaşi. [See Bull. Soc. d. méd. et nat. de Jassy.]
Bull. et mém. Soc. de méd. prat. de Par.	Bulletins et mémoires de la Société de médecine pratique de Paris, fondée en 1808. Paris. 1 v., 1888. 8°.
Bull. Soc. centr. de méd. vét., Par.	Bulletin de la Société centrale de médecine vétérinaire. Paris. N. s., v. 5–6, 1887–8. 8°. [Continuation, in 1887, of: Bull. et mém. Soc. centr. de méd. vét., Par.]
Bull. Soc. méd. d. hôp. de Par.	Bulletin de la Société médicale des hôpitaux de Paris. Paris. v. 1, 2, 4, 5 (1849–52 to 1861–4), 1849–64. 8°. [Reprint from: Union méd., Par.]
Bull. Soc. d. méd. et nat. de Jassy.	Bulletin de la Société des médecins et naturalistes de Jassy. Buletinul Societăţei de medici şi naturalişti din Iaşi. Jassy. Nos. 1–4, v. 1, 1887. 4°. [Text Roumanian and French.]
Bull. U. S. Fish Com., Wash.	Bulletin of the United States Fish Commission. Washington. v. 2, 5, 6 (1882–6), 1883–7. 8°.

C.

Canad. Rec. Sc., Montreal.	Canadian (The) Record of Science, including the Proceedings of the Natural History Society of Montreal, and replacing The Canadian Naturalist. Montreal. v. 2, 1887. 8°.
Centralbl. f. Physiol., Leipz. u. Wien.	Centralblatt für Physiologie. Unter Mitwirkung der physiologischen Gesellschaft zu Berlin hrsg. von S. Exner und J. Gad. Leipzig und Wien. v. 1, 1887–8. 8°.
	Chirurgische Klinik zu Kiel. [See Mitth. a. d. chir. Klin. zu Kiel.]
	Chirurgische Universitäts-Poliklinik zu Leipzig. [See Arb. a. d. chir. Univ.-Poliklin. zu Leipz.]
Clin. chir. di Siena.	Clinica chirurgica di Siena, diretta dal prof. dott. G. F. Novaro. Rendiconto dal gennaio al luglio 1886 redatto dall' aiuto dott. Vittorio Remedi. Siena. 1 v., 1887. 8°.
Clin. Reporter, St. Louis.	Clinical (The) Reporter. A journal of homœopathic medicine and surgery. Edited by the Faculty of the Homœopathic Medical College of Missouri. St. Louis, Mo. v. 1, 1888. 8°.
	Colegio médico-farmacéutico. Palma de Mallorca. [See Rev. balear de cien. méd., Palma de Mallorca.]
Coll. Mass. Hist. Soc., Bost.	Collections of the Massachusetts Historical Society. Boston. v. 9 (1804), 1857. 8°.

Comunicaz. batteriol., Napoli.	Comunicazioni batteriologiche. Lavori dei signori A. Cantani, E. De Blasi [*et al.*]. Napoli. Anno 1, 1886. 1887. 8°.
	Congrès international d'anthropologie criminelle. Biologie et sociologie. [*See* Actes Cong. internat. d'anthrop. crim., Rome.]
Cong. internat. de bienfaisance.	Congrès international de bienfaisance. Sessions: 1° de 1856 (à Bruxelles), 2 v.; 2° de 1857 (à Francfort-sur-le-Mein), 2 v. 4 v., 1857–8. 8°.
Cong. internat. d'hydrol. et de climatol. Compt. rend., Par.	Congrès international d'hydrologie et de climatologie. Compte rendu de la première session. Biarritz, 1886. Paris. 1 v., 1887. 8°.
	Congrès pénitentiaire international de Rome. [*See* Actes Cong. pénitent. internat. de Rome.]
	Congresso farmaceutico italiano. [*See* Atti d. Cong. farm. ital.]
	Connecticut Eclectic Medical Association. [*See* Tr. Connect. Eclect. M. Ass., Bridgeport.]
	Conseil d'hygiène publique et de salubrité du département du Rhône. [*See* Hyg. de Lyon. Compt. rend. Cons. d'hyg. pub. du Rhône, Lyon.]
	Consiglio di sanità di Napoli. [*See* Gior. di clin., terap. e med. pubb., Napoli.]
	Convention of Physicians of Ohio. [*See* Proc. M. Convent. Ohio.]

D.

Denkschr. z. Feier ihres 50jähr. Besteh. hrsg. v. d. schles. Gesellsch. f. vaterl. Kult., Bresl.	Denkschrift zur Feier ihres fünfzigjährigen Bestehens herausgegeben von der schlesischen Gesellschaft für vaterländische Kultur. Breslau. 1 v., 1853. 4°.
	Dermatologische Klinik des königlichen Charité-Krankenh. zu Berl. [*See* Mitth. a. d. dermat. Klin. d. k. Char.-Krankenh. zu Berl.]
	Deutsche Gesellschaft für angewandte Chemie. [*See* Ztschr. f. ang. Chem., Berl.]
	Deutsche Gesellschaft für Natur- und Völkerkunde Ostasiens. [*See* Mitth. d. deutsch. Gesellsch. f. Nat.- u. Völkerk. Ostasiens, Yokahama.]
	Deutsche Vereinigung in Amerika graduirter Doctoren der Zahnheilkunde. [*See* J. f. Zahnh., Bresl.]
	Deutscher Verein gegen den Missbrauch geistiger Getränke. [*See* Wissensch. Beitr. z. Kampf gegen d. Alkoholismus, Bonn.]

E.

Écho méd., Toulouse.	Écho (L') médical. Toulouse. 2. s., v. 2, 1888. 8°.
Eco de la med., Madrid.	Eco (El) de la medicina. Periódico de la Academia de Esculapio. Madrid. v. 1, Oct. 5, 1848, to Dec. 30, 1849. 4°.
Électrothérapie, Par.	Électrothérapie (L'). Journal d'électricité médicale. Paris. v. 1, 1888. 8°.
	Elisha Mitchell Scientific Society. [*See* J. Elisha Mitchell Sc. Soc., Raleigh.]
Engin. & Build. Rec., N. Y.	Engineering (The) & Building Record and the Sanitary Engineer. [Continuation of: The Sanitary Engineer.] New York. v. 16–17, 1887–8. fol. [Continuation, after No. 18, v. 16, 1887, of: San. Engin., N. Y.]
Especialista, Madrid.	Especialista (El). Revista quincenal de sifiliografía, oftalmología, affecciones de la piel y del aparato génito-urinario. Madrid. v. 1–2, 1859–60. fol.

F.

Festschr. z. Feier d. 300jähr. Besteh. d. Julius-Maximilians-Univ. zu Würzb., Basel.	Festschrift zur Feier des 300jährigen Bestehens der Julius-Maximilians-Universität zu Würzburg gewidmet von der Universität Basel. Basel. 1882. 4°.
Fraternidad méd. - farm., Alicante.	Fraternidad (La) médico-farmacéutica. Revista quincenal de medicina, cirugía y farmacia, consagrada á defender los intereses de la clase médico-farmacéutica. Alicante. v. 1–2, 1886–8. 8°.

G.

Gaz. d. hôp. de l'empire ottoman, Constant.	Gazette des hôpitaux civils et militaires de l'empire ottoman. Constantinople. v. 1, 1887–8. 4°.
Gaz. d. hôp. de Toulouse.	Gazette des hôpitaux de Toulouse. Journal hebdomadaire. Toulouse. Années 1–2, 1887–8. 4°.
Gen.-Ber. ü. d. öff. Gsndhtsw. im Rgrngsbz. Königsb.	General-Bericht über das öffentliche Gesundheitswesen im Regierungsbezirk Königsberg für die Jahre 1883 bis 1885, erstattet von Dr. R. Naht. Königsberg i. Pr. 1 v., 1887. 8°.
Gen.-Ber. ü. d. San.- u. Med.-Wes. im Rgrngsbz. Liegnitz.	General-Bericht über das Sanitäts- und Medicinal-Wesen im Regierungs-Bezirke Liegnitz mit besonderer Berücksichtigung der Jahre 1883, 1884 und 1885, von Dr. Philipp. Liegnitz. 1 v., 1886. 8°.
Gior. di clin., terap. e med. pubb., Napoli.	Giornale di clinica, terapia e medicina pubblica. Organo ufficiale per gli atti del Consiglio di sanità di Napoli. Napoli. v. 19, 1888. 8°. [Continuation, after 1887, of: Gazz. di med. pubb., Napoli.]
Gior. spec. di farm. sper. e chim. clin., Napoli.	Giornale speciale di farmacia sperimentale e chimica clinica. Napoli. v. 1–2, 1887–8. 8°.

H.

	Hahnemann Medical College (Institute of the), Philadelphia, Pa. [See Med. Inst., Phila.]
	Harvard Medical School. [See Med. Pub. Harv. M. Sch., [Bost.].]
	Homœopathic Medical College of Missouri (Faculty of the). [See Clin. Reporter, St. Louis.]
Honvédorvos, Budapest.	Honvédorvos a hazai katonaorvosi intézmény tudományos és társadalmi érdekeinek közlönye. A m. kir. honvédministerium rendeleteivel. A Gyógyászat melléklete. [The army surgeon, a guide for military surgeons and communications of interest to civilians. By order of ministry for the army. Supplement to Gyógyászat.] Budapest. v. 1, 1888. 8°.
Hosp. Gaz., Lond.	Hospital (The) Gazette. A weekly review of medicine and surgery, and chronicle of hospital practice and college news. London. v. 16, 1888. 4°. [A continuation of: Hosp. Gaz. & Students' J., Lond.]
Hyg. de Lyon. Compt. rend. Cons. d'hyg. pub. du Rhône, Lyon.	Hygiène de Lyon. Compte rendu des travaux du Conseil d'hygiène publique et de salubrité du département du Rhône (du 1er janvier 1860 au 31 décembre 1885). Première partie par A. Lacassagne. Lyon. 1 v., 1887. 8°.

I.

	Illinois State Dental Society. [See Annual J. Ill. Dent. Soc., Chicago.]
	Industrial Education Association. [See Monog. Indust. Educat. Ass., N. Y.]
	Institute of the Hahnemann Medical College, Philadelphia, Pa. [See Med. Inst., Phila.]

	Intercolonial Medical Congress of Australasia. [*See* Tr. Intercolon. M. Cong. Australas.]
Internat. J. Surg. & Antisept., N. Y.	International Journal of Surgery and Antiseptics. Devoted exclusively to surgery and Listerism. New York. v. 1, 1888. 4°.
Internat. klin. Rundschau,Wien.	Internationale klinische Rundschau. Centralblatt für die gesammte praktische Heilkunde, sowie für die Gesammtinteressen des ärztlichen Standes. Wien. v. 2, 1888. fol.
Internat. M. Cong. Rep. Collect. Invest. Com. Norweg. M. Ass., Christiania.	International Medical Congress. Report by Collective Investigation Committee of the Norwegian Medical Association. Christiania. 1 v., 1887. 8°.
Internat. M. & S. Synopsis, St. Louis.	International (The) Medical and Surgical Synopsis. St. Louis, Mo. v. 1, 1887-8. 8°.

J.

J. Anthrop. Soc. Bombay.	Journal (The) of the Anthropological Society of Bombay. Bombay. v. 1, 1886-7. 8°.
J. Dietet.	Journal (The) of Dietetics. Published quarterly. Devoted to investigations into the physiology and pathology of digestion and nutrition, and the relations of regimen to practical medicine. Cleveland, Ohio; Fremont, Ohio. v. 1-2, 1887-8. 8°.
J. Elisha Mitchell Sc. Soc., Raleigh.	Journal of the Elisha Mitchell Scientific Society. Raleigh, N. C. v. 1-4, 1883-7. 8°.
J. f. Gasbeleucht. u. Wasserversorg., München u. Leipz.	Journal für Gasbeleuchtung und Wasserversorgung. Organ des deutschen Vereins von Gas- und Wasserfachmännern. München u. Leipzig. v. 30-31, 1887-8. 8°. [Title on covers: Schilling's Journal, etc.]
J. Morphol., Bost.	Journal of Morphology. Boston. v. 1, 1887. 8°.
J. N. E. Virg. M. Soc., Warrenton.	Journal (The) of the N[orth] E[ast] V[irgini]a Medical Society. Warrenton, Va. v. 1, 1888. 8°.
	Journal of the Proceedings of a Convention of Physicians of Ohio. 1835. [*See* Proc. M. Convent. Ohio.]
	Journal of the Proceedings of the Medical Convention of Ohio. 1838-9. [*See* Proc. M. Convent. Ohio.]
J. f. Zahnh., Bresl.	Journal für Zahnheilkunde. Vereins-Organ der deutschen Vereinigung in Amerika graduirter Doctoren der Zahnheilkunde. Breslau. v. 1-2, 1887-8. fol.
	Julius-Maximilians-Universität zu Würzburg. [*See* Festschr. z. Feier d. 300jähr. Besteh. d. Julius-Maximilians-Univ. zu Würzb., Basel.]

K.

K. Vetensk. Acad. n. Handl., Stockholm.	Kongl. Vetenskaps Academiens nya Handlingar. Stockholm. v. 1-17, 1780-96. 8°.
	Kaiserlich königliche Gesellschaft der Aerzte in Wien. [*See* Wien. klin. Wchnschr.]
	Kaiserlich-japanische Universität (Medicinische Facultät). [*See* Mitth. a. d. med. Fac. d. k.-jap. Univ., Tokio.]
Kal. u. statist. Jahrb. f. d. Königr. Sachs., Dresd.	Kalender und statistisches Jahrbuch für das Königreich Sachsen . . . auf die Jahre 1871-88. Hrsg. vom statistischen Bureau des königl. sächs. Ministerium des Innern. Dresden. 1871-88. 8°.
Klin. Stud. a. d. hydriat. Abth. d. allg. Poliklin. in Wien, Leipz. u. Wien.	Klinische Studien aus der hydriatischen Abtheilung der allgemeinen Poliklinik in Wien. Leipzig u. Wien. v. 1, 1887. 8°.
Klin. voordr. en akad. lessen o. geneesk., Rotterd.	Klinische voordrachten en akademische lessen over geneeskunde. Rotterdam. Nos. 2-4, 1869-70. 8°.
	Königlich sächsische Gesellschaft der Wissenschaften. [*See* Abhandl. d. math.-phys. Cl. d. k. sächs. Gesellsch. d. Wissensch., Leipz.]
	Königliches Charité-Krankenhaus zu Berlin (Dermatologische Klinik). [*See* Mitth. a. d. dermat. Klin. d. k. Char.-Krankenh. zu Berl.]

L.

Lavori accad. d. r. Ist. d' incorag. a. sc. nat. . . . di Napoli.	Lavori (De') accademici del r. Istituto d' incoraggiamento alle scienze naturali economiche e tecnologiche di Napoli. Napoli. 6 nos., 1869–79. 1870–80. 4°.
	Lehigh Valley Medical Association. [*See* Tr. Lehigh Valley M. Ass., Easton, Pa.]
Lond. M. Recorder.	London (The) Medical Recorder. A monthly review of the progress of the medical sciences at home and abroad. London. N. s., v. 1, 1888. 8°. [A continuation, in 1888, of: Lond. M. Rec.]
Lond. Physiol. J.	London (The) Physiological Journal; or monthly record of observations on animal and vegetable anatomy and physiology, chiefly made by the aid of the microscope. London. Nos. 1–5 (Oct., 1843, to Feb., 1844), v. 1. 1843–4. 8°.
Lucine franç., Par.	Lucine française, ou: Recueil d'observations médicales, chirurgicales, pharmaceutiques, historiques, critiques et littéraires, relatives à la science des accouchemens. Par le docteur Sacombe. Paris. v. 1–3, an XI–XIII [1803–5]. 8°.

M.

Manitoba, Northwest & Brit. Columbia Lancet, Winnipeg.	Manitoba, Northwest and British Columbia Lancet. Winnipeg. v. 1, 1887–8. 8°.
	Massachusetts Historical Society. [*See* Coll. Mass. Hist. Soc., Bost.]
Med. besieda, Voronej.	Meditsinskaja besieda. Journal populjarnoi meditsiny i gigieny. Voronej. v. 1–2, 1887–8. 8°.
	Medical Convention of Ohio, 1841, 1842, 1850. [*See* Proc. M. Convent. Ohio.]
Med. Inst., Phila.	Medical (The) Institute. A journal of homœopathy, published monthly during the college year by the Institute of the Hahnemann Medical College, Philadelphia, Pa., U. S. A. Philadelphia. v. 1–3, 1886–8. 8°.
Med. Pub. Harv. M. Sch., [Bost.]	Medical Publications. Harvard Medical School. [Boston.] 1 v., 1887. 8°.
Med. Reg. N. York.	Medical (The) Register of New York, New Jersey and Connecticut. Published under the supervision of the New York Medico-Historical Society. New York. v. 1–17; v. 19; v. 21–25, 1862–87. 12°.
	Medical Society of the County of Kings. [*See* Brooklyn M. J.]
Med. Waif, Lafayette, Ind.	Medical (The) Waif. A practical monthly medical journal, devoted to diseases of children, women, rectum, and anus. Lafayette, Ind. v. 1, 1887–8. 8°.
	Medicinische Facultät der kaiserlich-japanischen Universität. [*See* Mitth. a. d. med. Fac. d. k.-jap. Univ., Tokio.]
Mém. Soc. de méd. de Par.	Mémoires de la Société de médecine de Paris, séante à l'Hôtel-de-Ville. Paris. 1 v., 1817. 8°.
Memphis M. Month.	Memphis Medical Monthly; or, Mississippi Valley Medical Monthly. Memphis. v. 8, 1888. 8°. [Title, after January, 1888, of: Mississippi Valley M. Month., Memphis.]
	Michigan State Pharmaceutical Association. [*See* Proc. Mich. Pharm. Ass.]
Middlesex Hosp. Rep., Lond.	Middlesex (The) Hospital. Reports of the medical, surgical, and pathological registrars for the years 1869–76 and 1878–86. London. 1870–87. 8°.
Minnesota M. Month., Minneap.	Minnesota (The) Medical Monthly. Minneapolis, Minn. v. 1–3, 1886–8. 8°.
Mitth. a. d. chir. Klin. zu Kiel.	Mittheilungen aus der chirurgischen Klinik zu Kiel. Hrsg. von Friedrich von Esmarch. Kiel. 1 v., 1883–8. 8°.
Mitth. a. d. dermat. Klin. d. k. Char.-Krankenh. zu Berl.	Mittheilungen aus der dermatologischen Klinik des königlichen Charité-Krankenhauses zu Berlin. Berlin. 1 v., 1887–8. 8°.

Mitth. d. deutsch. Gesellsch. f. Nat.- u. Völkerk. Ostasiens, Yokahama.
Mittheilungen der deutschen Gesellschaft für Natur- und Völkerkunde Ostasiens. Yokahama. v. 1–4, 1873–6 to 1884–7. 4°.

Mitth. a. d. med. Fac. d. k.-jap. Univ., Tokio.
Mittheilungen aus der medicinischen Facultät der kaiserlich-japanischen Universität. Tokio. No. 1, v. 1, 1887. 4°.

Mitth. a. d. St. Petersb. Augen-Heilanst.
Mittheilungen aus der St. Petersburger Augen-Heilanstalt. St. Petersburg. Hft. 1, 1887. 8°.

Mitth. a. d. zool. Station zu Neapel, Leipz.
Mittheilungen aus der zoologischen Station zu Neapel; zugleich ein Repertorium für Mittelmeerkunde. Leipzig. Hft. 1–2, v. 1, 1878–9. 8°.

Monitore medico marchigiano. Loreto. [See Boll. d. Osp. di S. Casa di Loreto, Loreto.]

Monog. Indust. Educat. Ass., N. Y.
Monographs of the Industrial Education Association. New York. v. 1, 1888. 8°.

Month. San. Rec., Columbus.
Monthly (The) Sanitary Record. The official publication of the Ohio State Board of Health. Columbus, O. v. 1, 1888. 8°.

Museo nacional de México. [See An. d. Mus. nac. de México.]

N.

N. iconog. de la Salpêtrière, Par.
Nouvelle iconographie de la Salpêtrière; clinique des maladies du système nerveux. Paris. v. 1, 1888. 8°.

Nashville M. News.
Nashville (The) Medical News. A semi-monthly journal. Nashville. v. 1, 1887. 8°.

Natural History Society of Montreal. [See Canad. Rec. Sc., Montreal.]

Naturforschende Gesellschaft zu Freiburg i. Br. [See Ber. d. naturf. Gesellsch. zu Freib. i. Br.]

Nauch. Besedy vrach. Zakavkazsk. Povival. Inst., Tiflis.
Nauchnyja Besedy vrachei Zakavkazskago Povivalnago Instituta, sostojashago pod avgusteishim pokrovitelstvom Eja Imperatorskago Vysochestva Gosudaryni Velikoi Knjagini Olgi Feodorovny. [Scientific papers of the Transcaucasian Obstetric Institute [etc.].] Tiflis. v. 1–2, 1886–7. 8°.

New York Medico-Historical Society. [See Med. Reg. N. York.]

New York Post-Graduate Medical School and Hospital. [See Post-Graduate, N. Y.]

New York State Pharmaceutical Association. [See Proc. N. York Pharm. Ass.]

North-East Virginia Medical Society. [See J. N. E. Virg. M. Soc., Warrenton.]

Norwegian Medical Association. [See Internat. M. Cong. Rep. Collect. Invest. Com. Norweg. M. Ass., Christiania.]

Novosti med., St. Petersb.
Novosti meditsiny za 1887 g. (Izdanie Ejem. jour. prakt. med.) [Medical news.] St. Petersburg, 1887. 8°.

O.

Obs. surg. dis. head & neck. Select. Mem. Roy. Acad. Surg. of France, Lond.
Observations on surgical diseases of the head and neck. Selected from the Memoirs of the Royal Academy of Surgery of France. Translated and edited by Drewry Ottley. London. 1 v., 1848. 8°.

Obshestvo vrachei Volhynskoi gubernii. [See Protok. Obsh. vrach. Volhynskoi guber., Zhitomeer.]

Ohio J. Dent. Sc., Toledo.
Ohio (The) Journal of Dental Science. Toledo, Ohio. v. 7–8, 1887–8. 8°. [Continuation, after 1886, of: Ohio State J. Dent. Sc., Toledo.]

Ohio Medical Convention. [See Proc. M. Convent. Ohio.]

Otechestvennyi psichiatria. [See Trudi perv. siezda otechest. psichiat., St. Petersb.]

P.

Papers & Proc. Roy. Soc. Tasmania.
Papers and Proceedings of the Royal Society of Tasmania. Tasmania. 1 v. (1886), 1887. 8°.

Path. Suppl. 32. Rep. Gov. Hosp. Insane, Wash.
Pathological supplement to the thirty-second annual report of the Government Hospital for the Insane to the Secretary of the Interior. 1886-7. Washington. 1 v., 1887. 8°.

Pharmakologisches Institut zu Dorpat. [*See* Arb. d. pharmakol. Inst. zu Dorpat, Stuttg.]

Phila. Photog.
Philadelphia (The) Photographer. An illustrated semi-monthly journal, devoted to photography. Philadelphia; New York. v. 1-25, 1864-88. 8°. ["Monthly" before 1886.]

Physiologische Gesellschaft zu Berlin. [*See* Centralbl. f. Physiol., Leipz. u. Wien.]

Physiologisches Laboratorium der Züricher Hochschule. [*See* Untersuch. a. d. physiol. Lab. d. Zürich. Hochsch., Wien.]

Post-Graduate, N. Y.
Post-Graduate (The). The Journal of the New York Post-Graduate Medical School and Hospital. New York. v. 3, 1887-8. 8°. [Title, after No. 3, v. 2, 1886-7, of: Quart. Bull. Clin. Soc. N. Y. Post Grad. M. School & Hosp., N. Y.]

Prix Soc. de méd. de Par.
Prix de la Société de médecine de Paris, séante à l'Hôtel-de-Ville. Paris. 1 v., 1817. 8°.

Proc. Am. Soc. Psych. Research, Bost.
Proceedings of the American Society for Psychical Research. Boston. Nos. 1-3 (July, 1885, to Dec., 1887), v. 1, 1885-7. 8°.

Proc. Anat. Soc. Gr. Brit. & Ireland, Lond.
Proceedings of the Anatomical Society of Great Britain and Ireland. [Issued with: J. Anat. & Physiol., Lond., 1887-8, xxii.] London. 1887-8. 8°.

Proc. Convent. Off. Wisconsin Nat. Guard, Madison.
Proceedings of the Seventh Annual Convention of Officers of the Wisconsin National Guard, held at Madison, March 8-9, 1888, under the auspices of the National Guard Association of the State of Wisconsin. Madison, Wis. 1888. 8°.

Proc. M. Convent. Ohio.
Proceedings of the Medical Convention of Ohio. V. p. 1835-50. 8°. [Title in 1835: Journal of the Proceedings of a Convention of Physicians of Ohio; in 1838 and 1839: Journal of the Proceedings of the Medical Convention of Ohio; in 1841 and 1842: Proceedings of the Medical Convention of Ohio; 1845-49: Proceedings of the Ohio Medical Convention; in 1850: Proceedings of the Medical Convention of Ohio.]

Proc. Mich. Pharm. Ass.
Proceedings of the Michigan State Pharmaceutical Association. V. p. 2.-5., 1884-7. 8°.

Proc. N. York Pharm. Ass.
Proceedings of the New York State Pharmaceutical Association. V. p. 2.-9., 1880-87. 8°.

Proceedings of the Ohio Medical Convention. 1845-9. [*See* Proc. M. Convent. Ohio.]

Proc. Pub. Health Confer., Frankf., Ky.
Proceedings, addresses, and discussions of a Public Health Conference, held at Louisville, Kentucky, May 24 and 25, 1887, under the auspices of the State Board of Health. Frankfort, Ky. 1 v., 1887. 8°.

Proc. San. Convent. Kalamazoo, Mich., Lansing.
Proceedings and addresses at the Sanitary Convention held at Kalamazoo, Mich., June 1 and 2, 1886, under the direction of a committee of the State Board of Health and a committee of citizens of Kalamazoo. [Supplement to the Annual Report of the Michigan State Board of Health for the year 1886.] Lansing. 1886. 8°.

Progresso med., Napoli.
Progresso (Il) medico. Periodico quindicinale di science mediche e naturali e di veterinaria. Organo ufficiale dei laboratorii e gabinetti scientifici della Facoltà medico-chirurgica e di scienze naturali della Università di Napoli. Napoli. v. 1-2, 1887. 8°.

Protok. Obsh. vrach. Volhynskoi guber., Zhitomeer.
Protokoli Obshestva vrachei Volhynskoi gubernii. [Minutes of Association of Physicians of Volhynski Government.] Zhitomeer. 1874-9; 1885-6. 8°.

Protok. Russk. sif. i dermat. Obsh., St. Petersb.
Protokoli Russkago sifilidologicheskago i dermatologicheskago Obshestva za 1885-86 gg. St. Petersburg. v. 1, 1887. 8°.

Protok. zasaid. akush.-ginek. Obsh. v Kieve.
Protokoli zasaidanii akushersko-ginekologicheskago Obshestva v Kieve. Kieff. v. 1, 1887. 8°.

Protok. zasaid. guber. zemsk. vrach. soveta . . . Kursk.	Protokoli zasaidanii gubernskago zemskago vrachebnago soveta ·i soveta vrachei gubernskoi zemskoi bolnitsy za vtorujou polovinu 1885 g. (Jul.–Dek.) [3. year]. [Transactions at meetings of Government provincial medical council and council of Government physicians for provincial hospitals for the second half year 1885 (July to Dec.).] Kursk. 1 v., 1886. 8°. Public Health Conference, held at Louisville, Kentucky, May 24 and 25, 1887. [*See* Proc. Pub. Health Confer., Frankf., Ky.]

Q.

Quart. J. Econom., Bost.	Quarterly (The) Journal of Economics. Boston. Nos. 1–2, v. 2, 1887–8. 8°.

R.

	R. Istituto d' incoraggiamento alle science naturali economiche e tecnologiche di Napoli. [*See* Lavori accad. d. r. Ist. d' incorag. a. sc. nat. . . . di Napoli.]
Ref. Handb. M. Sc., N. Y.	Reference (A) Handbook of the Medical Sciences, embracing the entire range of scientific and practical medicine and allied science by various writers, illustrated by chromo-lithographs and fine wood engravings. Edited by Albert H. Buck. New York. 4 v., 1886–7. 4°.
Rep. Bd. Health Ohio, Columbus.	Reports (Annual) of the State Board of Health of the State of Ohio. Columbus. 1., 1885–6. 1887. 8°.
Rep. Bureau Statist. Labor, Bost.	Reports (Annual) of the Bureau of Statistics of Labor. 1.–17., 1869–70 to 1885–6. Boston. 1870–86. 8°.
Rep. Dep. Health Brooklyn.	Reports (Annual) of the Department of Health of the City of Brooklyn. 1884–6. Brooklyn. 1885–7. 8°.
Rep. Proc. Alumnæ Ass. Woman's M. Coll. Penn., Phila.	Report of Proceedings of the Alumnæ Association of the Woman's Medical College of Pennsylvania. Philadelphia. 1.–12., 1876–87. 8°.
Rep. Roy. Com. on Hist. Manus., Lond.	Report of the Royal Commission on Historical Manuscripts. Report and appendix. (Pt. I.) London. v. 8, 1881. fol.
Rep. Sapporo Agric. Coll., Japan.	Report (Annual) of Sapporo Agricultural College, Japan. Sapporo. v. 5 (1880), 1881. 8°.
Rep. State Com. Lunacy Penn., Harrisb.	Reports of the State Committee on Lunacy of the Commonwealth of Pennsylvania. 1.–5., 1882–3 to 1886–7. Harrisburg. 1884–8. 8°.
Répert. de thérap. dosimét.	Répertoire de thérapeutique dosimétrique basée sur la physiologie et l'expérimentation clinique. Par le Dr. Burggraeve, avec la collaboration libre des médecins de tous les pays. Paris, Gand. 2.–5. année, 1874–7. 8°. [Continuation of: Répert. de méd. dosimét. Continued as: Répert. univ. de méd. dosimét., Par.]
Répert. univ. d'obst. et gynéc., Par.	Répertoire universel d'obstétrique et de gynécologie. [Supplément aux: Nouvelles Archives d'obstétrique et de gynécologie.] Paris. v. 1–3, 1886–8. 8°.
Rev. balear de cien. méd., Palma de Mallorca.	Revista balear de ciencias médicas. (Medicina, farmacia y veterinaria.) Órgano del Colegio médico-farmacéutico. Palma de Mallorca. v. 4, 1888. 8°. [Continuation, after 1887, of: Rev. balear de med., farm. y vet., Palma de Mallorca.]
Rev. internat. scient. et pop. d. falsific. d. denrées aliment., Amst.	Revue internationale scientifique et populaire des falsifications des denrées alimentaires. Amsterdam. v. 1, 1887–8. 4°.
Rev. de med., ciruj. y farm., Barcel.	Revista de medicina, cirujía y farmacia. Barcelona. v. 1–2, 1887–8. 8°.
Rev. de med. mil., Porto.	Revista de medicina militar. Porto. v. 1–2, 1886–7. 8°.
Rev. méd.-pharm., Constant.	Revue médico-pharmaceutique autorisée par iradé impérial. Constantinople. v. 1, 1888. fol.
Rev. prat. d'obst. et d'hyg. de l'enf., Par.	Revue pratique d'obstétrique et d'hygiène de l'enfance. Paris. v. 1, 1888. 8°.

Rev. de san. mil., Madrid.	Revista de sanidad militar. Publicación consagrada á los intereses científicos y profesionales del Cuerpo de sanidad militar español. Madrid. v. 1-2, 1887-8. 8°.
Rev. d. sc. hypnot., Par.	Revue des sciences hypnotiques. Paris. v. 1, 1887-8. 8°.
	Royal Academy of Surgery of France. [*See* Obs. surg. dis. head & neck. Select. Mem. Roy. Acad. Surg. of France, Lond.]
	Royal Commission on Historical Manuscripts. [*See* Rep. Roy. Com. on Hist. Manus., Lond.]
	Royal Society of Tasmania. [*See* Papers & Proc. Roy. Soc. Tasmania.]
	Russkii Obshestvo ochranenija narodnye zdravija. [*See* Trudi Russk. Obsh. ochran. narod. zdravija (Protok.), St. Petersb.]
	Russkii sifilidologicheskii i dermatologicheskii Obshestvo. [*See* Protok. Russk. sif. i dermat. Obsh., St. Petersb.]
Russk. Slepetz, St. Petersb.	Russkii Slepetz. Journal dlja obsujdenija voprosov, kasajoushichsja uluchshenija polojenija slepych. Vychodit ejemesjachno. [Monthly.] [Russian Blind. Journal devoted to examination of the question how to ameliorate the condition of the blind.] St. Petersburg. v. 2-3, 1887-8. 8°.

S.

Salute pubb., Perugia.	Salute (La) pubblica. Giornale mensile d' igiene pubblica e privata. Perugia. v. 1, 1888. 8°.
Samml. auserl. Abhandl. z. Gebr. prakt. Aerzte, Leipz.	Sammlung auserlesener Abhandlungen zum Gebrauche praktischer Aerzte. Leipzig. v. 1-41, 1774-1835. 8°.
	Sanitary Convention held at Kalamazoo, Mich., June 1 and 2, 1886. [*See* Proc. San. Convent. Kalamazoo, Mich., Lansing.]
	Sapporo Agricultural College, Japan. [*See* Rep. Sapporo Agric. Coll., Japan.]
Sborn. rabot. hyg. lab. Moskov. Univ., Mosk.	Sbornik rabot hygienicheskoi laboratorii Moskovskago Universiteta. Pod redaktsiei ord. prof. F. F. Erismana. Moskva. Vypusk 1. 1886. 8°.
	Schilling's Journal für Gasbeleuchtung und Wasserversorgung. München und Leipzig. [*See* J. f. Gasbeleucht. u. Wasserversorg., München u. Leipz.]
	Schlesische Gesellschaft für vaterländische Kultur. [*See* Denkschr. z. Feier ihres 50jähr. Besteh. hrsg. v. d. schles. Gesellsch. f. vaterl. Kult., Bresl.]
	Siebenbürgischer Verein für Naturwissenschaften in Hermannstadt. [*See* Verh. u. Mitth. d. siebenbürg. Ver. f. Naturw. in Hermannstadt.]
	Sociedad ginecológica española. [*See* Arch. de obst. y ginec., Madrid.]
	Société centrale de médecine vétérinaire. [*See* Bull. Soc. centr. de méd. vét., Par.]
	Société de médecine de Paris. [*See* Mém. Soc. de méd. de Par. *Also:* Prix Soc. de méd. de Par.]
	Société de médecine pratique de Paris, fondée en 1808. [*See* Bull· et mém. Soc. de méd. prat. de Par.]
	Société des médecins et naturalistes de Jassy. [*See* Bull. Soc. d. méd. et nat. de Jassy.]
	Société médicale des hôpitaux de Paris. [*See* Bull. Soc. méd. d. hôp. de Par.]
	St. Petersburger Augen-Heilanstalt. [*See* Mitth. a. d. St. Petersb. Augen-Heilanst.]
Sundh.- Coll. berät. om Med.- Verk. i riket, Stockholm.	Sundhets-Collegii underdåniga berättelse om Medicinalverket i riket. [1851-9.] Stockholm, 1853-60. 8°.
Svens. Läk.-Sällsk. Handl., Stockholm.	Svenska Läkare-Sällskapets Handlingar. Stockholm. v. 1-12, 1817-33. 8°. [1. & 2. Häftet, v. 1, are 2. ed.; 3. Hft., 1813.]

T.

Terap. mod., Napoli.	Terapia (La) moderna. Giornale mensile di farmacologia, terapia sperimentale e clinica, chimica medica e farmaceutica e igiene. Napoli. v. 1–2, 1887–8. 8°.
Thiermed. Rundschau, Halle a. S.	Thiermedicinische Rundschau mit besonderer Berücksichtigung der vergleichenden Pathologie und des gesammten Veterinär-Medicinalwesens. Gleichzeitig Organ zur Vertretung der Interessen des thierärztlichen Standes. Neue Folge der im Jahre 1885 begründeten "Rundschau auf dem Gebiete der Thiermedicin". Halle a. S. v. 2, 1887–8. 4°.
Toulouse-méd.	Toulouse-médical. Bulletin hebdomadaire de médecine et de pharmacie. Toulouse. v. 1, 1887–8. 8°.
Tr. Am. Climat. Ass.	Transactions of the American Climatological Association. V. p. v. 1–4, 1884–7. 8°.
Tr. Connect. Eclect. M. Ass., Bridgeport.	Transactions of the Connecticut Eclectic Medical Association, for the years 1886–7. Bridgeport, Conn. v. 1, 1886–7. 8°.
Tr. Intercolon. M. Cong. Australas.	Transactions of the Intercolonial Medical Congress of Australasia, first session held in Adelaide, South Australia, August–September, 1887. Adelaide. 1 v., 1888. 8°.
Tr. Lehigh Valley M. Ass., Easton, Pa.	Transactions of the Lehigh Valley Medical Association. Seventh annual meeting, August 17, 1887. Easton, Pa. v. 1, pt. 1, 1887. 8°.
Transl. For. Biol. Mem., Oxford.	Translations of Foreign Biological Memoirs. 1. Memoirs of the physiology of nerve, of muscle, and of the electrical organ. Edited by J. Burdon-Sanderson. Oxford. 1 v., 1887. 8°.
Trudi perv. siezda otechest. psichiat., St. Petersb.	Trudi pervago siezda otechestvennych psichiatrov, proizchodivshago v Moskve s 5 po 11 Jan. 1887 g. [Memoirs of first session of national psychiatrists.] St. Petersburg. v. 1, 1887. 8°.
Trudi Russk. Obsh. ochran. narod. zdravija (Protok.), St. Petersb.	Trudi vysochaishe utverjdennago Russkago Obshestva ochranenija narodnago zdravija, sostojachago pod pokrovitelstvom Ego Imperatorskago Vysochestva Velikago Knjazja Pavla Alexandrovicha. [Transactions of the Russian Association for Promotion of National Health; organized under the protection of the Grand Duke Paul Alexandrovich.] St. Petersburg. v. 1–4 (Protok.); v. 2–3 (Balneol. i Klimat.). 1886. 8°.
Trudi voyenno-san. Obsh. v S.-Peterb.	Trudi voyenno-sanitarnago Obshestva v S.-Peterburgie. [Memoirs of the military-sanitary association in St. Petersburg. 1. number.] St. Petersburg. Vypusk 1. 1887. 8°.

U.

	United States Fish Commission. [See Bull. U. S. Fish Com., Wash.]
	Università libera di Perugia. Facoltà di medicina e chirurgia. [See Ann. d. Univ. libera di Perugia. Fac. di med. e chir.]
	Università di Napoli (Facoltà medico-chirurgica e di scienze naturali della). [See Progresso med., Napoli.]
	Universität Basel. [See Festschr. z. Feier d. 300jähr. Besteh. d. Julius-Maximilians-Univ. zu Würzb., Basel.]
Untersuch. a. d. physiol. Lab. d. Zürich. Hochsch., Wien.	Untersuchungen aus dem physiologischen Laboratorium der Züricher Hochschule. Hrsg. von Adolf Fick. Wien. 1. Hft., 1869. 8°.

V.

Verh. u. Mitth. d. siebenbürg. Ver. f. Naturw. in Hermannstadt.	Verhandlungen und Mittheilungen des siebenbürgischen Vereins für Naturwissenschaften in Hermannstadt. Jahrgang 25 (1874)–34 (1883). Hermannstadt, 1875–84. 8°.
	Voyenno-sanitarnoe Obshestvo v S.-Peterburgie. [See Trudi voyenno-san. Obsh. v S.-Peterb.]

W.

West. Dent. J., Kansas City.	Western (The) Dental Journal. Kansas City, Mo. v. 1–2, 1887–8. 8°.
Wien. klin. Wchnschr.	Wiener klinische Wochenschrift. Organ der k. k. Gesellschaft der Aerzte in Wien. Wien. v. 1, 1888. fol.
Wissensch. Beitr. z. Kampf gegen d. Alkoholismus, Bonn.	Wissenschaftliche Beiträge zum Kampf gegen den Alkoholismus, im Aufrage des Vorstandes des deutschen Vereins gegen den Missbrauch geistiger Getränke in Verbindung mit San.-Rath Dr. Baer [*et al.*], hrsg. von P. Pieper. Bonn. Hft. 1–6, 1885–7. 8°.

Z.

	Zakavkazski Povivalnyi Institut. [*See* Nauch. Besedy vrach. Zakavkazsk. Povival. Inst., Tiflis.]
Ztschr. f. ang. Chem., Berl.	Zeitschrift für angewandte Chemie. Organ der deutschen Gesellschaft für angewandte Chemie. Berlin. v. 1, 1888. 8°. [Continuation of: Zeitschrift für die chemische Industrie, and: Repert. f. anal. Chem., consolidated.]
Ztschr. f. Med.-Beamte, Berl.	Zeitschrift für Medicinalbeamte. Berlin. v. 1, 1888. 8°.
	Zoologische Station zu Neapel. [*See* Mitth. a. d. zool. Station zu Neapel, Leipz.]

CATALOGUE.

Medicine (*Popular*) [*including works of charlatans*].

See, also, **Accidents**; **Bone-setters**; **Botany** (*Medical*); **Brandy** *and salt*; **Children** (*Hygiene, etc., of*); **Formulæ**, *etc.*; **Generation**, *etc.* (*Popular treatises on*); **Genitals** (*Diseases of*); **Homœopathy** (*Popular treatises on*); **Hydropathy**; **Hygiene**; **Medicine** (*Botanic, etc.*); **Medicine-chests**; **Medicines** (*Patent, etc.*); **Nurses**, *etc.*; **Obstetrics** (*Systems, etc., of*) *for midwives, etc.*; **Physiology** (*Popular*); **Venereal** *diseases* (*Popular treatises on*); **Women** (*Diseases, etc, of, Popular treatises on*).

ABELIUS (H. C.) Lang-gewünschter medicinischer Gewissens-Spiegel, vorstellend I. Gerechte Klagen über so vieler tausend Menschen frühzeitigen Tod, nebst dessen Ursachen. II. Nachdrückliche Vorschläge, diesem mörderischen Ubel zu steuren, um so viel Menschen beym Leben und beständiger Gesundheit zu erhalten. III. Heilsame Ermahnungen bey Curirung der Kranckheiten, zur Rettung des Gewissens und Erhaltung des Lebens. Mit schönem lehrreichen Theolog. 16°. *Franckfurt a. M.*, 1720.

ABERCROMBIE (R.) New medical system. Consumption, diseases of the heart, bronchitis, asthma, dropsy, tumors, coughs, etc., curable by a peculiar solvent process, [etc.] 22. ed. 12°. *London*, 1877.

ABERNETHIAN (The) code of health and longevity . . . 8°. *New York*, 1831.

ALBERT (L') moderne, ou nouveaux secrets et procédés, utiles ou curieux, pour l'entretien de la beauté et de la santé, la guérison des maux et maladies, la conservation et les diverses préparations des alimens et des boissons, les diverses parties de l'économie, tant civile que rurale, les arts et métiers des villes et des campagnes. 4. éd., augmentée de conseils et avis pour apprécier ces secrets, et d'un troisième volume. 3 v. 12°. *Paris*, 1793.

ALMANACH de la santé et de l'hygiène, à l'usage des familles et des communautés religieuses, par un docteur en médecine. Pour l'année 1881. 12°. *Avignon*, [1881].

AMERICAN (The) gentleman's medical pocketbook and health adviser. By the author of: The lady's medical pocket-book. 16°. *Philadelphia*, [*n. d.*]

ANDRIEU. Avis aux citoyens, sur les causes, les divers caractères et les vrais remèdes de l'aveuglement, de la surdité et des principaux accidens vénériens, [etc.] 8°. *Paris*, 1780.

APOLLINARIS. Ein ausserlesen schön Artzney- und Kräuter-Buch, von mancherley bewehrten Experimenten und Artzneyen, dadurch dem menschlichen Cörper, in zutragenden Fällen, da man die Medicos nicht haben kan, von Häupte an biss auff die Füsse mag Rath schaffen. Je-

Medicine (*Popular*).

dermenniglichen zu Dienst in drey Bücher abgetheilet, unter welchen das letzte absonderlich von Pestilentz-Kräutern handelt. Erstlich durch den . . . Dr. . . . bewehrt befunden und zusammen getragen, jetztundt aber von neuen übersehen, und mit lebendiger Abcontrafactur der fürnemsten Kräuter, neben Beschreibung der Krafft, deren daraus gebrandten Wasser, gebessert und vermehret. 4°. *Erffurdt*, 1629.

ARCHER (J.) Every man his own doctor, compleated with an herbal: shewing first, how every one may know his own constitution and complection by certain signs, also the nature and faculties of all food, as well meats as drinks, whereby every man and woman may understand what is good or hurtful to them. Treating also of air, passions of mind, exercise of body, sleep, the use of tobaco, a new hot bath. Venery, with an infallible secret to prevent the pox. Of the senses, proving six in number, his elixir proprietatis, and its use. The second part shews the full knowledge and cure of the pox, running of the reins, gout, dropsie, scurvy, consumption and obstructions, agues, shewing their causes and signs, and cure. The second edition, with additions, viz: A treatise of melancholly and distraction, with government in cure. Also a compendious herbal, discovering the physical vertue of all herbs in this kingdom, and what planet rules each herb, and how to gather them in their planetary hours. 12°. *London*, 1673.

——. Secrets disclosed; of consumptions, shewing how to distinguish between the scurvy and venereal disease; also how to prevent and cure the fistula by chymical drops, without cutting; also piles, hemorrhoids, and other diseases. 8°. *London*, 1684.

[ARZNEIBUCH (Ein). Deutsche Handschrift aus dem 15. Jahrh. Enthält miraculöse Blutstillungen, Pflaster, Salben, Kräuterkuren, Wundermittel.] MS. 4°. [*n. p., n. d.*]

ARTZNEI-BÜCHLEIN für mancherlei Gebrechen zu gebrauchen. MS. 16°. [*n. p. n. d.*]

ARZNEYBÜCHLEIN von mancherley bewärthen und erfahrnen Arzneyen, für allerley Zufälle und Krankheiten des menschlichen Leibs dienstlich. MS. 16°. [*n. p.*], 1671.

ARZT und Patient. Winke für Beide. 8°. *Stuttgart*, 1884.

ASSEGA (C.) Manuale pratico patologico-terapeutico di medicina semplice ad uso dei seminarii, delle scuole elementari, tecniche e femminili ed anche dei comuni agricoli e delle famiglii in generale. 16°. *Torino*, 1886.

D'AUBRY DE MONTPELLIER (J.) Le triomphe de l'archée, et la merveille du monde, ou la médecine universelle et véritable pour toutes sortes de maladies, les plus désespérées, qu'elle guérit par

Medicine (Popular).

les sueurs ou les transpirations insensibles, en rafraichissant, sans aucune incommodité ny vomissement et sans ayde de l'art magique comme l'on s'estoit persuadé, nouvellement découverte . . . Dédiée à la reine des anges. Augmentée de l'apologie de l'autheur, etc., et de plusieurs remerciemens des cures, etc., et de beaucoup de consultations faites et envoyées en diverses langues au sieur . . . [etc.] 4. éd. 4°. *Paris*, [1661]. .

AUSFÜHRLICHER Bericht von der Artzney, Essentia dulcis genannt, durch welche unter dem Seegen Gottes, allerley schwere Kranckheiten, Gicht, Epilepsie, Stein, allerley Gebrechen an Augen, auch wenn sich Felle angesetzet, Mangel am Gehör, Contractur, u. d. gl. bissher curiret worden, zum drittenmal und verbessert in Druck gegeben. 4°. *Halle*, 1703.

[AZZOGUIDO.] La spezieria domestica. Operetta utile a tutte quelle persone, che bramano di vivere lungamente, e necessaria a quelli che si trovano lontani dal medico o dallo speziale, come per lo più accade a chi vive nella campagna, nei chiostri, collegi, etc., e a chi intraprende viaggi di terra, e principalmente di mare. 16°. *Venezia*, 1784.

B. (M.) Dienstlich en de ghenuchelijck tytverdrijf voor siecken, om ghesont te worden, en voor ghesonde om niet sieck te zijn ; handelende van alle die menschen de welcke in een sieckhuijs van noode sijn, namentlijcke de sieck-maerten, ofte die hun dienen en bijstaen. Tot troost en onderwijs van den krancken beschreven in vloeyende reden, en tot lichter onthouden, en vermaeck van deselve, met veel fraeye kortbondighe spreuken, geschiedenissen en dichtiens doorvlochte. 12°. *v'Antwerpen*, 1654.

BABBITT (E. D.) The health guide ; aiming at a higher science of life and the life forces ; giving nature's simple and beautiful laws of cure ; the science of magnetic manipulation, bathing, electricity, food, sleep, exercise, marriage, and the treatment for one hundred diseases ; thus constituting a home doctor far superior to drugs. 12°. *New York*, [1874].

BALMER-RINCK (T.) Die Gesundheit. Ein Wort an Gesunde und Kranke. Von einem bewährten Arzte geprüft und zur Beherzigung empfohlen. Den Arbeiterfamilien gewidmet. 8°. *Basel*, 1885.

BANNING (E. P.) A peep into the house you live in ; an essay on the causes of some of the ailments to which flesh is heir, and on the value of mechanical appliances in their treatment. 12°. *New York*, 1872.

BAPST (M.) den Eltern. Wunderbarliches Leib und Wund-Artzneybuch. Darinnen neben vielen Denckwirdigen, nützlichen und heilsamen Dingen, Geschichten, Kunststücken, unnd Experimenten, vornemlich von dem schweren Gebrechen, oder hinfallenden Kranckheit, und derselben Cura, aussfürlicher Bericht zu befinden, etc. Aus vieler hochgelarter Ertzte Bücher, und eigener Erfahrunge mit allem Fleiss, den gemeinen Haussvätern, zu nutz und heilsamen Unterricht, zusammen getragen unnd beschrieben. 2 Th. 4° *Eissleben*, 1596–7.

BARONYAY (J.) * Generalia popularis medicinæ principia. 8°. *Pestini*, 1834.

BARRIER (E.) Hygiène et médecine des familles ; lettre à M. le président de l'Académie de médecine de Paris. 8°. *Paris*, 1882.

BARTHOLINUS (T.) De medicina Danorum domestica. Dissertationes x cum ejusdem vindiciis et additamentis. 12°. *Hafniæ*, 1666.

BECKER (G. W.) Kurze, jedoch gründlich Anleitung wie man gesund bleiben, sich und die

Medicine (Popular).

seinigen vor Krankheiten bewahren, davon heilen, und zu einem frohen Alter gelangen kann. Für den gebildeten Bürger und Landmann 12°. *Leipzig*, 1817.

――――. The same. Neue Aufl. 8°. *Leipzig*, 1831.

BELLIOL. Radicale Heilung der Scropheln, Flechten und galanten Krankheiten, sowie aller chronischen Krankheiten des Kopfes, der Brust und des Unterleibes. Nebst Rathschlägen über die körperliche und geistige Erziehung der Kinder und über die Lebensweise der Greise. Nach der siebenten Auflage aus dem Französischen übersetzt. 8°. *Quedlinburg u. Leipzig*, 1839.

――――. The same. Tratado sobre la naturaleza y curacion de las enfermedades crónicas, herpéticas, escrofulosas, y sifilíticas, por un nuevo tratamiento vegetal depurativo y refrescante. Traducido de la octava edicion francesa por F. Vinader y Domenech. 16°. *Barcelona*, 1841.

BERGER (P.) Leefregel voor mageren. Over de oorzaken, de verschijnselen en de behandeling van magerheid, naar het Duitsche populair-medische geschrift. Bewerkt door J. Bartolotti Rijnders. 8°. *Gravenhage*, 1887.

BÉRILLON (E.) Nouveau manuel de la garde-malade, à l'usage des mères de famille, des institutrices, des infirmières, etc. ; art de soigner les malades et les convalescents, règles spéciales aux enfants, préparation des médicaments, accidents, règles spéciales en cas d'épidémie ; pharmacie domestique. 8°. *Paris* 1885.

BESSER (L.) Den deutschen Müttern und Vätern. Ein Buch über das Werden und Wachsen ihrer Kinder als Schlüssel zu deren gesünderer Erziehung. 12°. *Frankfurt a. M.*, 1858.

BEYNON (É.) jeune. Suitte du Samaritain charitable. Où il se trouve toutes sortes de médicaments et remèdes éprouvés par diverses personnes qui s'en sont très-bien trouvées . . . Mis au jour en charité christienne. Traduit d'alleman en françois par Louis France. 12°. *Genève*, 1673.

――――. Barmhertziger Samariter, oder freundbrüderlicher Rath, allerhand Kranckheiten und Gebrechen des menschlichen Leibs, innerlich und äusserlich zu heilen . . . Auch einem sehr nützlichen Unterricht vor die Heb-Ammen in allen zustossenden Fällen. Nebst einem neuen Anhang von der Pest, wie man sich in solcher Zeit verhalten soll. Anjetzo aufs neu übersehen, und von vielen Druck-Fehlern gereiniget. 16°. *Sultzbach*, 1685.

――――. The same. 18°. *Basel*, 1686.

――――. The same. 12°. *Nürnberg*, 1691.

――――. The same. 12°. *Nürnberg*, 1696.

BLACK (W. G.) Folk-medicine ; a chapter in the history of culture. 8°. *London*, 1883.

BLANCHARD (V. W.) Lectures and essays (food-cure system). 8°. *New York*, [1878].

BLOOD (C. L.) A century of life, health, and happiness ; a cyclopedia of medical information for home life and domestic economy. 8°. *Boston*, [n. d.]

BOCK (C. E.) Supplement-Band zu allen Ausgaben von . . . Buch vom gesunden und kranken Menschen. Der Garten-Laube entnommen. 2. Aufl. 12°. *Leipzig*, 1866.

BÖNNEKEN (J. W. F.) Kurtze jedoch auf Vernunfft und Erfahrung gegründete Abhandlung von denen erdhaften Mitteln, welche sehr häuffig von vielen Medicis und auch ohne diss fast von Jedermann in allen und jeden Zufällen des Leibes gebrauchet werden, denen Arztney Unkundigen und dem gemeinen Mann zur selbst eigenen Prüfung vorgeleget. 24°. *Wertheim*, 1742.

Medicine (*Popular*).

[BONORA.] Provvedimenti alle più comuni malattie dei polli. 8°. [*n. p., n. d.*]

BOORDE (A.) The breviarie of health; wherein doth folow remedies for all maner of sicknesses and diseases, the which may be in man or woman. In 2 pts. 8°. *London*, 1575.
Black-letter.

——. The fyrst boke of the introduction of knowledge made by . . . A compendious regyment or a dyetary of helth, made in Mountpellier, compiled by . . . Barnes in the defence of the berde; a treatyse made answerynge the treatyse of Doctor Borde upon berdes. Edited, with a life of Andrew Boorde and large extracts from his brevyary, by F. J. Furnivall. 8°. *London*, 1870.

DAL BOSCO (F.) La prattica dell' infermiero. Nella quale con osservationi fondate nell' uso di moltissimi anni s' addottrina l' assistente, e caritativo infermiere per ben conoscere, e ne' casi repentini applicar li rimedij proportionati a' mali dei suoi infermi. Di nuovo ristampato. 16°. *Milano*, 1670.

BRAND (J. H.) Sorgfältiger und gewissenhafter Land- und Bauren-Doctor; welcher Gott zu ehren, dem armen dürftigen Nächsten zu Nutz und denen nothleidenden Kranken mit guten Arzeneyen mehrentheils geringen Haus-Mitteln, in allen vorfallenden Krankheiten getreulich an Handen gehet. 12°. *Franckfurt u. Leipzig*, 1753.

BRETT (W.) Indigestion, rheumatism, gout, and nervous diseases. 3. ed. 12°. *London*, 1860.

BROBERG (J. V.) Bidrag från vår folkmedicins vidskepelser till kännedomen om våra äldsta tider. Förra afdelningen. 8°. *Stockholm*, 1878.

——. Olai Martini läkiare book efter en i Karolinska Mediko-Kirurgiska Institutets Bibliotek befintlig handskrift utgifven med inledning och anmärkningar. 8°. *Stockholm*, 1879.

BRODUM (W.) A guide to old age, or a cure for the indiscretions of youth. 2 v. in 1. 8°. *London*, 1797.
v. 1 is 5. ed. and v. 2 is 4. ed.

BROWN (O. P.) The complete herbalist; or, the people their own physicians by the use of nature's remedies; showing the great curative properties of all herbs, gums, balsams, barks, flowers, and roots . . . and a new and plain system of hygienic principles. 8°. *Jersey City, N. J.*, 1870.

——. The same. The complete herbalist; or, the people their own physicians by the use of nature's remedies. 8°. *Jersey City*, 1872.

——. The same. 8° *London*, 1876.

BROWN (*Mrs.* W. G.) Metaphysical pamphlet. A synopsis of metaphysics; cause, cure, and prevention of disease, life lengthened, disease kept at bay. 8°. *New York*, [1871?]

BRAUNSCHWEIG (H.) Thesaurus pauperum. Hauss-Apoteck, guter gebräuchlicher Artzney, zu jeden Leibes Gebrechen. Für das arme Landvolck und gemeynen Man an Tag geben. 32°. *Franckf. a. M.*, 1573.

——. The same. 24°. *Franckf. a. M.*, 1579.

——. The same. 16°. *Franckf. a. M.*, 1590.

——. The same. sm. 8°. *Franckf. a. M.*, 1598.

——. The same. 4°. [*Augspurg, n. d.*]

——. Hauss-Artzneybüchlein. Gute gebreuchliche und bewerte Artzneyen, zu allerhand Gebrechen des gantzen Leibs, ausswendig und inwendig, von dem Haupt biss auf die Füss, für den gemeinen Mann insonderheit, so die Apotecken nicht erreychen, oder die Artzte zu ersuchen, am Gut nicht vermag, gestellt und

Medicine (*Popular*).

mit sonderm Fleiss zusammen getragen durch . . . jetzt aber durch einen Liebhabern der Artzney erfarnen, von newen durchsehen, und an vielen Orten gemehrt und gebessert. Zusampt angehenckten Tractätlin von allerley gebranten Wassern, welcher Mass man dieselbigen brauchen und nützen sol, zu Erhaltung und Fristung menschlicher Gesundtheit, etc. 16°. *Frankf. a. M.*, 1580.

——. & SCHRICK (M.) Apoteck für den gemeynen Man, der die Ertzte zu ersuchen am Gut nicht vermugens odder sonst ynn der Not allwege nicht erreychen kan. 4°. *Wittemberg*, 1529.

BRYAN (L. H.) Great medical discovery. The blood poison, its origin and nature, and how it acts upon the system to cause the many and varied diseases that afflict mankind. 8°. *Philadelphia*, 1872.

BUCHHEIM (E.) Volkswohlstand und Volksgesundheit. 8°. *Wien*, 1885.

BUC'HOZ (J.-P.) Remèdes éprouvés avec succès contre la teigne, le scorbut, les vers, même le solitaire, les fleurs blanches des femmes, les pâles couleurs, l'inflammation des yeux, [etc.] Second opuscule concernant le genre humain et la médecine. 12°. *Paris*, 1806.

BÜRING (J.) Neue und sichere Einleitung zu der Artzney-Kunst, und Anschaffung dienlicher und heilsamer Hülffs-Mittel, wider alle sich an des Menschen Leib ereignende heilbare Kranckheiten und Beschwerungen, da dann insonderheit einer jeden Kranckheit würckende Ursach erst kürtzlich untersucht, die dagegen zu gebrauchende geringe Hauss-, Feld- und Reise-Mittel getreulich angewiesen, vornehmlich aber in der Praxi bewährt-befundene Arcana entdecket und mitgetheilet werden . . . Vermehret von Paul Jacob Marberger. 16°. *Frankfurt u. Leipzig*, 1711.

BULLEIN [*or* BULLEYN] (W.) Bulwarke of defence againste sicknes, sornes, and woundes, that dooe daily assaulte mankinde, whiche bulwarke is kepte with Hillarius the gardiner, Health the physician, with their chyrurgian, to helpe the wounded soldiors. Gathered and practised from the moste worthie learned, bothe old and newe; to the greate comforte of mankinde. fol. *London*, 1562.

——. The same. fol. *London*, 1579.

BUNO (G. W.) Medicus philoscepus, oder der eine gehörige Bedeckung des Leibes, beydes, für Gesunde als Krancke, anweisende, kluge und sorgfältige Artzt; wie eigentlich dazu eine gute Policey-Hauss- und Kleider-Ordnung, auch rechtmässige Krancken-Pflege nothwendig erfordert werde. 4°. *Celle*, 1720.

BUTLER (C.) Butler's medicine chest directory and family catalogue of drugs, chemicals, and medicinal compounds, with the properties and doses of such as are more generally used in domestic medicine. 4. ed. 8°. *Dublin*, 1837.

BYRN (M. L.) The mystery of medicine explained; a family physician and household companion; prepared for the use of families, plantations, ships, travelers, [etc.] 8°. *New York*, 1869.

——. The same. 8°. *New York*, 1872.

C. (J.) De wonderlijcke en wel geoeffende genees- en heelmeester, leerende alerley sieckten, gebreken, accidenten, wonden, soo inwendigh als uytwendig oude en nieuwe wel te kennen en te genesen; handelende mede van pestilentie en swangere vrouwen. 8°. *Amsterdam*, 1663.

CALKINS (M.) Diseases of the lungs, heart, and blood, scrofula, consumption, bronchitis; their causes, prevention, and cure; with the

Medicine (*Popular*).

posthumous writings of Calvin Newton. 8°. *Philadelphia*, 1860.

[CAM (J.)] A miscellaneous essay on the rheumatism, gout, and stone, in which the causes of those diseases are proved to arise from the same origin; their cures and prevention are fully and regularly stated, and some peculiar and sure methods and medicines are recommended to the publick. 12°. *London*, 1722.

CARPENTER (R.) The sick man's companion, or a short note on fever and a new method of cure; together with an enumeration of the symptoms which usually attend a number of diseases, and a mode of treatment prescribed with medicine, the production of our own country. 12°. *Johnstown*, 1812.

CARRICHTER (B.) Practica, auss den fürnehmsten. Secretis. I. Von allerhandt Leibskranckheiten. II. Von Ursprung der offnen Schäden, und ihrer Heylung. Jetzt von newem corrigirt ausgegangen. 16°. *Strassburg*, 1577.

——. The same. 16°. *Strassburg*, 1600.

CARTER (R.) Valuable vegetable medical prescriptions, for the cure of all nervous and putrid disorders. 12°. *Frankfort*, 1813.

——. The same. 12°. *Cincinnati*, 1830.

——. A short sketch of the author's life, and adventures from his youth until 1818, in the first part. In part the second, a valuable vegetable medical prescription, with a table of detergent and corroborant medicines to suit the treatment of the different certificates. 4°. *Versailles, Ky.*, 1825.

CHANTRY (*Mrs.* A. W.) Receipts for family medicines that will cure all ills that flesh is heir to. 8°. *Philadelphia*, 1866.

CHEAP (A), sure, and ready guide to health; or, a cure for a disease call'd the doctor. Instructing how to prevent being cheated and destroyed by the exactions and unmerciful usage of ignorant and oppressive physicians and apothecaries; and to prepare at home the proper medicines for usual distempers; with their prices to save nineteen shillings in twenty, and expend little more than a penny a dose. Likewise a new account of the connection of distempers, key to all physic, and to know any disease. Set forth by the benefaction of a very worthy private gentleman, to contain more than any book of the kind, at the lowest rate, as necessary for all families and all persons. 12°. *London*, 1742.

CHOICE and profitable secrets, both physical and chirurgical, formerly concealed, by the deceased Dutchess of Lenox, and now published for the use and benefit of such as live far from physicians and chirurgions; being approved of by eminent doctors, and published by their charitable advice for the publique good. Whereunto is annexed a discovery of the natures and properties of all such herbs which are most commonly known and grown in countrey gardens. 16°. *London*, 1658.

CHRISTIANI (B. G.) * De cura per domestica; von Hauss-Mitteln. sm. 4°. *Halæ Magdeb.*, [1727].

CHURCH (J.) Important information to the afflicted with . . . most disorders incident to human nature. 16°. *New York*, 1800.

CLARIDGE (R. T.) Every man his own doctor. The cold water, tepid water, and friction cure, as applicable to every disease to which the human frame is subject. And also to the cure of disease in horses and cattle. 8°. *New York*, 1849.

CLERC. Histoire naturelle de l'homme considéré dans l'état de maladie, ou la médecine rappellée à sa première simplicité. 2 v. 16°. *Paris*, 1767,

Medicine (*Popular*).

CLOSET (A) for ladies and gentlewomen, or the art of preserving, conserving, and candying. With the manner how to make divers kindes of sirups and all kinde of banqueting stuffes. Also divers soveraigne medicines and salves for sundry diseases. 16°. *London*, 1632.

DE CLOSMADEUC (G.) Esquisse sur la médecine et la chirurgie populaires dans le département du Morbihan. 8°. *Vannes*, 1861.

CLUM (F. D.) Men and women; their structure and function, and how to supply their wants, direct their powers, avoid their afflictions, and sustain their lives. 8°. *Boston*, [1882].

COGAN (T.) The haven of health; chiefly made for the comfort of students, and consequently for all those that have a care of their health, amplified uppon five wordes of Hippocrates, written Epid. 6. Labour, meate, drinke, sleepe, Venus. Hereunto is added a preservation from the pestilence; with a short censure of the late sicknesse at Oxford. sm. 4°. *London*, 1589.

——. The same. 4. ed. sm. 4°. *London*, 1636.

COHEN (G.) The tree of life; its growth and decay; or, light and darkness. With illustrated plate, by Fritz Braun. 12°. *London & Manchester*, 1883.

COLBATCH (J.) Dr. Colbatch's legacy, or the family physician. 12°. *London*, 1733.

COMET (C.-J.-B.) Méthode curative externe des douleurs rhumatismales, goutteuses, nerveuses; des maladies lymphatiques, et des viscéralgies, [etc.] 8. éd. 8°. *Paris*, 1842.

CONTINUATION of the confidential communication, intended for the general benefit of the afflicted, and especially for the service of those of them who apply to the enemy of human diseases, being informed thereby of the cause that has compelled the new condition of their admittance, to which is prefixed various information, and also, the result of the experience acquired on one's frame, concerning the fatal consequences of being exposed to breathe the unsalubrious air of diseased human beings; and in general, the contagious danger of their common intercourse, and the baleful one of the distemper's destructive influence. 8°. *Providence*, 1815.

COOPER (T.) A treatise of domestic medicine, intended for families, in which the treatment of common disorders are alphabetically enumerated. To which is added, a practical system of domestic cookery. Also, the art of preserving all kinds of animal and vegetable substances for many years by M. Appert. 8°. *Reading*, 1824.

COUCH (R.) Praxis catholica; or, the countryman's universal remedy; wherein is plainly and briefly laid down the nature, matter, manner, place, and cure of most diseases incident to the body of man, not hitherto discovered, whereby any one of an ordinary capacity may apprehend the true cause of his distempers; wherein his cure consists, and the means to effect it; together with rules how to order children in that most violent disease of vomiting and looseness, etc., useful likewise for seamen and travellers. Also, an account of an incomparable powder for wounds or hurts which cure any ordinary ones at once dressing, now published with divers useful additions (for public benefit) by Chr. Pack. 24°. *London*, 1680.

Cox's companion to the family medicine chest and compendium of domestic medicine; particularly adapted for heads of families, ship-captains, missionaries, and colonists, with plain rules for

Medicine (*Popular*).

taking the medicines; to which are added a plain description of the treatment of fractures and dislocations, and a concise account of Asiatic or spasmodic cholera. 48. ed. 18°. *London*, 1887.

CRAIG (J.) & MAULE (W.) Medical tracts for the times. 12°. *Edinburgh*, 1886.

CRELL (A. F.) & WALLACE (W. M.) The family oracle of health, economy, medicine, and good living; adapted to all ranks of society, from the palace to the cottage. 4 v. 8°. *London*, 1824-7.

CRÜGENERUS (L. M.) Materia perlata. Das ist: Edle und bewehrte Artzeney, wider Malum hypochondriacum, Miltz-Kranckheit, oder windige Melancholey genannt, etc. Darinn der rechte Gebrauch wider obgedacht und andere Kranckheiten, absonderlich für das Podagra, Zahn-Schmertz, Fraiss, schweere Noth oder hinfallende Seuche. 16°. *Regenspurg*, 1676.

——. XXV medicinisch-historische Episteln, oder: Auffgezeichnete Curen, so durch göttlichen Segen, mit Hülff der edlen Artzney Materia perlata wunderbarer Weise verrichtet, den Liebhabern zu ihrer Gesundheit, und zu Ehren der wahren Medicin den dürftigen nothleidenden Patienten zum Beweiss auffgezeichnet. 16°. *Regenspurg*, 1679.

——. Continuation seiner medicinischen Episteln, [etc.] 16°. *Regenspurg*, 1680.

CULPEPER (N.) Culpeper's school of physick; or, the experimental practice of the whole art ... The narrative of the author's life is prefixed, with his nativity calculated; together with the testimony of his late wife. The general contents of this work are in the next page, with two perfect tables very useful to the reader. 12°. *London*, 1659.

——. The same. 2. ed. 8°. *London*, 1678.

——. Medicaments for the poor; or, the physick for the common people. Containing excellent remedies for most common diseases incident to man's body; made of such things as are common to be had in almost every country in the world, and are made with little art and small charge. Hereunto is added an excellent book called: Health for the rich and poor, by diet without physick. 2. ed. [1656]. 12°. *London*, 1662.

——. Culpeper's last legacy, left and bequeathed to his dearest wife, for the publick good. Being the choycest and most profitable of those secrets which while he lived were lockt up in his breast, and resolved never to be publisht till after his death. Containing sundry admirable experiences in several sciences, more especially in chyrurgery and physick, viz: compounding of medicines, making of waters, syrups, oyles, electuaries, conserves, salts, pills, purges, and trochischs. With two particular treatises; the one of feavers, the other of pestilence; as also rare and choyce aphorismes and receipts, fitted to the understanding of the meanest capacities. The fourth impression. 12°. *London*, 1668.

——. The English physician enlarged, with three hundred sixty-nine medicines, made of English herbs, that were not in any impression until this; being an astrologo-physical discourse of the vulgar herbs of this nation; containing a complete method of physick, whereby a man may preserve his body in health, or cure himself, being sick, for three pence charge, with such things only as grow in England, they being most fit for English bodies. 12°. *London*, 1681.

——. The same. 12°. *London*, 1799.

——. The same. To which is added the family physician, and a present for the ladies, containing the best remedies for every disease

Medicine (*Popular*).

incident to the human body. By Dr. Parkins. 12°. *London*, 1810.

——. The same. (Crosby's improved ed.) 8°. *London*, 1814.

——. The same. 12°. *London*, [*n. d.*]

CULVERWELL (R. J.) Guide to health and long life; to which is added a popular exposition of Liebig's theory of life, health, and disease. 8°. *New York*, 1848.

——. The same. 8°. *New York*, 1850.

——. The same. 8°. *Cincinnati*, [*n. d.*]

——. Diseases of winter. On consumption, coughs, [etc.] 8°. *New York*, 1849.

DAVIES (N. E.) One thousand medical maxims and surgical hints. 12°. *London*, 1883.

DEFRENNE (J. J.) Beschrijving der geneesmiddelen. Benevens een kort begrip van deszelfs genees-wijze in de onderscheidene zicktens, waar in het gebruik der gemelde genees-middelen dienstig is. 8°. *Amsterdam*, 1786.

DE LA HAYE. Le médecin sincère, qui enseigne par une méthode aisée à connoître, à guérir, à soulager et à prévenir les maladies par des remèdes doux et faciles à composer. Il traite aussi des vertus des plantes, des animaux, des métaux et des eaux minérales. Ouvrage utile et très-instructif pour les estudians en médecine, pour les camps et armées, pour les curez de campagne et pour les pères de famille. 2. éd. 8°. *Lyon*, 1697.

DELFRAYSSE DE FRAYSSES (E.-G.) Nouveau guide pratique de la médecine populaire positive basée sur l'action physiologique de médicaments complexes, d'après leur finalité thérapeutique et divisés en spécifiques pour chaque maladie selon les méthodes des Drs. Belloti et Finella. 12°. *Bruxelles*, 1886.

DE SAINT-VINCENT (A.-C.) Nouvelle médecine des familles à la ville et à la campagne, à l'usage des familles, des maisons d'éducation, des écoles communales, des curés, des sœurs hospitalières, des dames de charité, et de toutes les personnes bienfaisantes qui se dévouent au soulagement des malades. 8. éd. 12°. *Paris*, 1886.

DESCHAMPS (L.) The science of medicine reduced to its simplest form. Important philanthropic discovery by means of which every one can be his own physician and druggist, [etc.] 8°. *Williamsburg*, 1850.

DICTIONNAIRE de médecine usuelle, à l'usage des gens du monde, des chefs de famille et de grands établissements, des administrateurs, des magistrats et des officiers de police judiciaire ... Le docteur J.-P. Beaude, chargé de la direction. [With supplement.] 2 v. roy.8°. *Paris*, 1849.

DIXON (E. H.) Back-bone; photographed from "The Scalpel". 8°. *New York*, [*n. d.*]

DOCTOR (The) at home. Illustrated. Treating the disease of man and the horse. 8°. *Enosburgh Falls, Vt.*, 1884.

DODS (J. B.) The philosophy of electrical psychology; in a course of twelve lectures. Stereotype ed. 8°. *New York*, 1852.

DOPPET (F.-A.) Le médecin philosophe; ouvrage utile à tout citoyen, dans lequel on trouve une nouvelle manière de guérir, puisée dans les affections de l'âme, et la gymnastique. 8°. *Turin*, 1787.

DORFDOKTOR (Der). Volkskalender für das Jahr 1886. 12°. *Flensburg*, 1885.

DOVER (T.) The ancient physician's legacy to his country. Being what he has collected himself in forty-nine years' practice ... Designed for the use of all private families. The fourth edition ... With some remarks on the author of: The use and abuse of mercury. 8°. *London*, 1733.

——. The same. 8°. *London*, 1742.

Medicine (*Popular*).

——. The same. 7. ed. 8°. *London*, 1762.

DRAGE (W.) A physical nosonomy; or, a new and true description of the law of God (called nature) in the body of man; confuting, by manifest and manifold experiences of many learned men, as well as the author's, the rules and methods concerning sicknesses and changes in man's body delivered by the antient physicians, and moderns that followed them . . . set forth, I. In a monitory proœmium; wherein be reasons for, and experiences in the stars, influencing upon, and altering our bodies. II. In a tractate of the diseases of the head. III. In a tractate of the diseases of the lungs. IV. In a tractate of dropsies. Also, in the second part of this book is a practice of physick, drawn from the best of moderns, and compleatly treating of those diseases specified in the table, to which is added a treatise of diseases from witchcraft. sm. 4°. *London*, 1665.

DRYANDER [EICHMANN] (J.) Ein new Artzney und Practicyr Büchlein von allerley Kranckheiten, wie man die erkent, und geheylet werden söllen. Aus den berümptesten und erfarnesten, zu unsernn Zeyten lebenden Medicis mit hohem treuem Fleyss, in eyn kurtze Summa zusamengezogen. 12°. *Colonie*, 1527.

——. Der gantzen Artzenei gemeynes Inhalt, wes einem Artzt, bede in der Theorie und Practic zusteht. Mit Anzeyge, bewerter Artzneienn, zu allen leiblichen Gebrechenn, durch natürliche Mittel, hierbei beneben des Menschen Cörpers Anatomei, warhafft contrafeyt und beschriben. Allen Artzten, und eim jeden zu sein selbs, und seins nehsten Noturfft dienlich, wol zu haben und zu wissen. fol. *Franckf. a. M.*, 1542.

——. Artzenei-Spiegel gemeyner Inhalt derselbigen, wesbede einem Leib unnd Wundtartzt, in der Theorie, Pratic, unnd Chirurgie züsteht. Mit Anzeyge bewerter Artzneien, zu allen leiblichen Gebrechen, durch natürliche Mittel, hiebei beneben des Menschen Cörpers Anatomei und chirurgischen Instrumenten, warhafft contrafeyt und beschriben. Allen Artzten, und einem jeden zü sein selbs, und seins nehsten notturfft dienlich, wol zu haben und zu wissen. fol. *Franckf. a. M.*, [1547].

DYES (A.) Verhütung von Augentrübung und Blindheit, sowie Anleitung zur Heilung des chronischen Stockschnupfens. 2. Aufl. 8°. *Berlin*, 1886.

EISENBERG (F. L.) * Initia medicinæ extemporaneæ et domesticæ cum adversariis quibusdam chemicis. sm. 4°. *Erlangæ*, [1780].

ELDER (G.) A series of lectures upon "health", delivered during the winter of 1872–3, at the Mechanics' Institute, Nottingham. 8°. *Nottingham*, [*n. d.*]

[ELEONORA (*Herzogin von Troppau und Jägerndorf*).] Sechs Bücher, ausserlesene Artzney und Kunst Stück, fast vor alle dess menschlichen Leibes Gebrechen und Kranckheiten, auss vielen beschriebenen Artzneybüchern, so bey Fürstlichen unnd andern hohen Personen verwahret werden, mit sonderm Fleiss zusammen getragen, und in solche richtige Ordnung bracht, dass ein jeder, was zu fürfallender Schwacheit dienlich, ohne besondere Mühe darinnen finden kan. fol. *Torgaw*, 1600.

——. The same. 4°. *Leipzig*, 1713.

——. The same. sm. 4°. *Nürnberg*, 1733.

——. The same. 4°. *Wienn*, 1752.

ELIAS DE MOLINS (R.) Tratado de patología rural, o sea la descripcion de las enfermedades mas comunes y el modo de curarlas por medicamentos especialmente vegetales. Segundo y úl-

Medicine (*Popular*).

timo volumen del Tratado de medicina rural. 8°. *Madrid*, [1886].

ELYOT (T.) The castell of helth corrected and in some places augmented, by the first author thereof. 16°. *London*, 1534.

——. The same. 16°. *London*, 1541.

——. The same. And now newly imprinted. 16°. *London*, 1580.

——. The same. 4°. *London*, 1610.

VAN ENGELEN (F. V.) Genees- natuur- en huishoud-kundig kabinet, of uitgezogte verzameling van de nieuwste en nuttigste verhandelingen, proeven en waarneemingen, uit de voornaamste buitenlandsche akademien en genootschappen, en de beroemste in- en uit-landsche schrijveren, ten nutte onzer landsgenooten bijeen vergaderd door eenige liefhebberen dezer weetenschappen. 3 v. 8°. *Leyden*, 1779.

EVERETT (G. H.) Health fragment, or steps toward a true life, embracing health, digestion, disease, and the science of the reproductive organs. Part I. 2. ed. 8°. *New York*, 1878.

[Part II.] Embracing dress, heredity, child training, kitchen and dining-room ethics, by Susan Everett.

EYGEL (A.) Nieuwe Genees-Konst, of Mantissa medicaminum. Dat is, Toegift van medicamenten, tegen de sieckten, aengewesen zijnde door 't menschelick water in sijn drie voorgaende werken, dienende meerendeels voor menschen van 15 of 16 jaren tot 60 of 70. 12°. *Amsterdam*, 1673.

FALGER (F.) Der Priester am Krankenbette. Eine fassliche Belehrung über die wichtigsten Krankheiten und Zufälle des Menschen, sowie die dem Seelsorger dabei zugewiesene Wirksamkeit, mit besonderer Rücksicht auf die neueren Forschungen. sm. 8°. *Münster*, 1867.

FALLOPPIUS (G.) Secreti diversi et miracolosi; ne' quali si mostra la via facile di risanare tutte le infirmità del corpo humano; et etiandio s' insegna il modo di fare molte altre cose, che à ciascuno sono veramente necessarie. 12°. *Venetia*, 1563.

——. The same. Raccolti e approbati da altri medici di gran fama. Novamente ristampati, e à commun beneficio di ciascuno, distinti in tre libri. Nel primo de' quali si contiene il modo di fare diversi olii, ceroti, onguenti, ontioni, electuarii, pillole e infiniti altri medicamenti. Nel secondo, s' insegna à fare diverse sorti di vini e acque molto salutifere. Nel terzo si contengono alcuni importantissimi secreti di alchimia e altri secreti dilettevoli. 16°. *Venezia*, 1578.

——. Kunstbuch, von mancherley nutzlichen, bissher verborgnen, und lustigen Künsten: erstlich welsch durch in beschriben sampt einem andern Buchlin vor etlichen Jaren in frantzösischer Sprach, durch Christophorum Landrinum aussgangen, darinn etliche fürtreffliche bewerte Artzneyen, zu mancherley Leibsgebrechen dienstlich, und doch auss gar schlechten Dingen zubereytet, begriffen seind, jetzt aber beyde in teütsche Sprach verfertiget durch Hieremiam Martium. 16°. *Augspurg*, 1573.

——. The same. Kunstbüch: dess hocherfarnen, und weytberhümpten Herrn . . . der Artzney Doctorn, von mancherley nutzlichen, bissher verborgnen, und lustigen Künsten: erstlich welsch durch ihn beschriben, sampt einem andern Büchlin, vor etlichen Jaren in frantzösischer Sprach, durch Christophorum Landrinum aussgangen, darinn etliche fürtreffliche bewerte Artzneyen, zu mancherley Leibs-Gebrechen dienstlich, und doch auss gar schlechten Dingen zubereytet, begriffen seind, jetzt aber beyde in teütsche Sprach verfertiget, durch: Hieremiam Martium. 12°. [*Augspurg*], 1588.

Medicine (*Popular*).

———. The same. 16°. *Augspurg*, 1597.

FAMILIES' (The) new guide to health, giving a description of the diseases to which families are subject, and their treatment . . . together with an exposition of the Thomsonian preparations of medicine, as given in the N. York M. & Phys. J., v. 1, n. s., 144. 8°. *Baltimore*, 1833.

FAMILY (The) physician, consumptive's guide to health, and lady's medical companion. Compiled chiefly from the works of Benjamin Rush. Edited by A. H. Flanders. 16°. *Lowell*, [1864].

FAULKNER (T.) Each person his own physician! The doctor at home; or the unfailing medical instructor, filled with the proven facts of medical science, and family experience, showing in the plainest manner how to retain health, kill disease, lengthen life, and wonderfully increase mental and physical vigor, in man, woman, or child. 8°. *New York*, [1881].

FAWCETT (B) Lecture on the science of medicine, and the doctrine of disease; or health and how to preserve it, and, if lost or injured, how to restore it. 12°. *Sydney*, 1873.

FELTHAM (J.) A popular view of the structure and economy of the human body . . . To which is annexed an explanation of difficult terms. 12°. *London*, 1803.

FERMIN (P.) Istruzioni importanti al popolo sull' economia animale, che contengono le differenti malattie croniche alle quali è soggetto il corpo umano, con i rimedj più proprj per curarle; per servir di seguito all' Avviso al popolo del sig. Tissot. Opera del . . . Tradotta dal francese, e di note illustrata. v. 1. 8°. *Venezia*, 1717.

FISCHER (A. F.) Heil- und Verhaltungsregeln bei jenen Krankheiten, die sich Jünglinge und Männer durch geheime Vergehungen und durch Ausschweifungen in der physischen Liebe zugezogen haben. 12°. *Leipzig*, 1834.

FITCH (S. S.) Six lectures on the uses of the lungs; and causes, prevention, and cure of pulmonary consumption, asthma, and diseases of the heart; on the laws of longevity, and on the mode of preserving male and female health to an hundred years. 12°. *New York*, 1847.

———. A popular treatise upon diseases of the heart, apoplexy, dyspepsia, and other chronic diseases, with proofs of their curability, [etc.] 8°. *New York*, 1859.

———. The same. A treatise on the causes and curability of diseases of the heart, stomach, liver, bowels, kidneys, etc., and on the treatment of disease in middle-aged and elderly people. 8°. *London*, 1861.

———. Family physician. 8°. *Boston*, 1866.

———. The same. 8°. *New York*, 1868.

FLAMANT [*or* FLAMENT]. Le véritable médecin, ou le moyen de se conserver la santé; contenant plusieurs pratiques de médecine, pharmacie et chirurgie; avec plusieurs remèdes simples, expérimentez et approuvez; ouvrage très-utile au public. 12°. *Paris*, 1699.

———. The same. Die Kunst, sein eigner Medicus zu seyn, oder: Sich durch Beobachtung seines natürlichen Triebs gesund zu erhalten. 2 pts. 18°. *Franckenhausen*, 1721.

FLORINSKY (V. M.) Domashniaja meditsina. Lechebnike dlja narodnago upotreblenija. Izdanie trete, ispravlennoe. [Domestic medicine. A medical book for the use of the people. Third improved edition.] 8°. *St. Petersburg*, 1887.

FORMULA of prescriptions, and various instructions, for the service and guidance of those who have applied, are applying, or shall apply, to the enemy of human disease; to which is prefixed, a vindication, concerning the dietical ab-

Medicine (*Popular*).

stinence, detecting the dangerous tendency of several articles forbidden as pernicious to the human body, in which are included tobacco, salt and salted food, spirituous liquors, all sorts of spices, and coffee. By Sylvan. 8°. *Providence*, 1812.

FORT (T.) A dissertation on the practice of medicine; containing an account of the causes, symptoms, and treatment of diseases; and adapted to the use of physicians and families. 8°. *Milledgeville*, 1849.

FOSSEL (V.) Volksmedicin und medicinischer Aberglaube in Steiermark. Ein Beitrag zur Landeskunde. 8°. *Graz*, 1885.

DE FOUQUET (*Madame*). Recueil des remèdes faciles et domestiques choisis, expérimentez, et très-aprouvez pour toutes sortes de maladies internes et externes, et difficiles à guérir. 2. éd. 2. pt. 24°. *Dijon*, 1679.

———. The same. Augmentée dans cette dernière édition de quantité de secrets qu'on a mis à la fin. Très-utile et nécessaires dans toutes les familles, pouvant faire les remèdes soy-même et à peu de frais. Avec un régime de vie pour chaque complexion et pour chaque maladie; et un traité du lait. Le tout par ordre alphabétique. 2 v. 16°. *Dijon*, 1701.

———. The same. 5. éd. 8°. [*n. p., n. d.*]

———. The same. Sehr nützliches Artzney-Buch, welches auff alle inn- und euserliche Zufälle, so wohl vor Manns- als Weibs-Personen die allerleichtesten und bewährtesten Medicamenta, meistentheils Hauss-Mittel in sich hält . . . samt einem Tractat von der Milch-Cur; aus dem Frantzösischen ins Deutsche übersetzt. 12°. *Dresden*, 1708.

———. The same. Obras médico-quirúrgicas. Economía de la salud del cuerpo humano. Prontario de secretos caseros, fáciles y seguros, sacados y comprados de los médicos y cirujanos mas famosos de toda la Europa, [etc.] Traducidas conforme á la impresion correcta y añadida que se hizo en Lion, en 1739, del francés á la lengua castellana por Francisco Monroi y Olaso. Aumentadas con esquisitas recetas misceláneas, igualmente fáciles y seguras. Nueva ed. 2 v. 8°. *Valencia*, 1872.

FRANKLIN (E. Z.) Illustrated domestic medical counsellor. Laws and science of life, health and self-preservation. Materia medica and pharmacy, [etc.] 12°. *Boston*, 1884.

FRANTZ (J. G.) De opvoeding van den geneeshe r als mensch en als geleerde beschouwd in betrekking tot de familie, den staat en de maatschappij, opgedragen aan de Nederlandsche volksvertegenwoordiging. 8°. *Amsterdam*, 1861.

FREESE (J. R.) General treatise, pt. i. The physician's hand-book and family guide to health. . . . Special treatise, pt. ii. A practical treatise on the diseases peculiar to the genital organs of the male sex. Special treatise, pt. iii. A practical treatise on the diseases peculiar to the genital organs of the female sex, [etc.] 8°. *Cincinnati*, 1856.

FRIEDEL (D.) Expediter und bewährter Medicus, welcher wieder alle, sowohl inn- als äusserliche Kranckheiten, Schäden und Gebrechen des menschlichen Leibes, genugsame und bewährte Artzney-Mittel besitzet, und auff jeden Fall vernünfftig anwendet, auch über dieses seinem Nächsten ziemlicher Anzahl communiciret; das meiste aus eigener Erfahrung und vielfältiger Approbation, mit kurtzen, doch nöthigen Anmerckungen, samt vielen Observationibus und sinnreichen Erzehlungen illustriret, insonderheit denen neu angehenden Medicis, und ihrem Nächsten, geschwind und Gewissenhafft zu rathen;

Medicine (*Popular*).

ingleichen denen Chirurgis, Apotheckern, etc., auch dem gemeinen Menschen zum Nutzen, herausgegeben. 4°. *Leipzig u. Rostock*, 1726.

FRIEDRICH (E.) Gesundheitspflege für das Volk. Rathschläge zur Erhaltung der Gesundheit. 8°. *Berlin*, 1864.

FRIES [*or* PHRIES] (L.) Spiegl der Artzny, desgleichen nie von keinem Doctor in tütsch ausgangen ist, nützlich unnd gutt allen denen, so der Artz Radt begerent, auch den gestreiffelten Leyen, welche sich underwinden mit Artznei umbzegon. In welchem du findest Bericht aller Hendel der Artznei, gezogen aus den fürnemsten Büchern der alten, mit schönen bewärten Stücken unnd kurtzwyligen Reden. fol. *Strassburg*, 1509.

GÄBELE (J.) [Des Wund-Artzney Buches.] 12°. *Memmingen*, [*n. d.*]

GÄBELKHOUER (O.) Artzneibuch, darinnen vast für alle, des meuschlichen Leibs, Anligen unnd Gebrechen, ausserlesene unnd bewehrt Artzneyen, gemeinem Vatterland teutscher Nation zu Gutem auss vilen hohen und niders Stands-Personen geschribnen Artzneybüchern zusameu getragen, unnd in den Truck verfertiget sind. 2 v. in 1. 4°. *Tübingen*, 1594.

——. The same. 4°. *Tübingen*, 1595.

——. The same. The boock of physicke, wherin throughe commanndement of the most illustrious and renoumned duke and lorde, Lorde Lodewijcke, Duke of Wirtenberghe and of Teck, Earle of Mompelgart, etc. Most of them selected and approved remedyes, for all corporall diseases and sicknesses, which out of manye highe and common persons written physick-boockes, are compacted, and united together. Faithfullye translated out of High-Duche by the right worshipfull Mr. Dr. Charles Battus. And now nuelye translated out of Low-Duche into Englishe by A. M. 4°. *Dorte*, 1599.

GALLAHER (F. M.) Lessons in domestic science. 8°. *Dublin*, 1885.

GALTIER-BOISSIÈRE. Bibliothèque scientifique et médicale des gens du monde. Les moyens de se préserver de toutes les maladies épidémiques, contagieuses ou parasitaires, suivis des mesures à prendre contre les empoisonnements, les asphyxies et les piqûres venimeuses. 8°. *Paris*, 1886 [1885].

GARDINER (J.) Observations on the animal œconomy, and on the causes and cure of diseases. 8°. *Edinburgh*, 1784.

GART der Gesuntheit; zu Latin ortus sanitatis, von allerley Thieren, Vöglen, Vischen oder Mörwundern und edlem Gstein, daruss gezogen von den natürlichen Meistern, was dem Menschen zu seiner Gesundtheit dienet, mit höchstem Fleisss durchsucht, corrigiret, und gebessert. fol. [*Strassburg*, 1529.]

GAUTIER (J.) Secours d'urgence dans les maladies subites et dans les maladies par accidents. 12°. *Paris*, 1886.

VON GEHEMA (J. A.) Der qualificirte Leib-Medicus. 16°. [*n. p.*, 1690.]

GEHRIG (L. C.) Ægrotans ipse Medicus: der sich selbsten curirende Patient, oder kurtze, doch deutliche, Methode, nach welcher ein jeder Patient D. b. sich selbsten am allerglücklichsten curiren, [etc.] 4°. *Schneeberg*, 1712.

GENEESKUNDIGE (De) raadsman voor ieder die geneeskundige hulp moet outberen. Vraagbaak op zeereizen, in de tropen enz. Vrij naar het Hoogduitsch door A. Arn. J. Quanjer en J. A. Lodewijks. 12°. *Gouda*, 1884.

GENESUNG (Zur)! Ein lustiges Handbuch für Aerzte und Patienten beiderlei Geschlechtes und sonst Jederman. Hrsg. von einer Masse Mediciner. 3. Aufl. 8°. *München*, [1883?]

Medicine (*Popular*).

DE GIAXA (V.) Piccola enciclopedia di medicina ed igiene ad uso delle famiglie. 2. ed. 2 v. 8°. *Trieste*, 1885.

GIRAUDEAU-DE-SAINT-GERVAIS. Le médecin sans médecine. Conseils aux gens du monde pour gúerir soi-même les dartres, et toutes les maladies provenant de l'âcreté du sang et des humeurs en détruisant leur principe par la methode végétale. 12°. *Paris*, [*n. d.*]

GLEASON (C. W.) Everybody's own physician; or, how to acquire and preserve health. Seventh thousand. 8°. *Philadelphia*, [1874].

GÖZE (C.) * Diss. sistens medicum sui ipsius. 4°. *Halæ Magdeb.*, [1704].

——. The same. 4°. *Halæ Magdeb.*, 1707.

——. The same. 4°. *Halæ Magdeb.*, 1740.

GOLDEN (The) treasure; or, a choice selection of well-tried domestic, experimental, and medical receipts. 1. Am. ed. 8°. *New York*, 1835.

GOLDHAMMER (J.) Compendieuser, aber doch sehr offenhertzige Weiber- und Kinder-Artzt, bey welchem unter göttlichen Seegen, Schwangere, Gebährende, Wöchnerin, Ammen und Kinder nützliche Hauss und bewehrte Artzeneymittel, wieder die vornehmesten und gefährlichsten Zufälle und Krauckheiten finden können. Alles auf das Deutlichste durch Fragen aus denen probatesten Autoribus und eigener Experienz, dem nechsten zu Liebe zum Druck befördert von . . . 16°. *Mühlhausen*, 1717.

——. Chrysologia medico-theologica, das ist: Medicinische und theologische Universal- oder Gold-Arzneyen, wodurch nicht allein der Vermögende, sondern auch der ärmeste Mann sein Lebens-Ziel verlängern, seine hochschätzbare Gesundheit erhalten, und ohne Verletzung seiner Seelen, ein gutes Auskommen erlangen, und dann auch seelig sterben könne. 4°. *Stolberg*, [1735].

——. Kurtzer Bericht von einem Dutzend meiner bewährtesten und mit Fleiss zubereiteten Artzneyen, wie solche zu Erhaltung der hochschätzbaren Gesundheit, und Abwendung vielerley Arten Kranckheiten mit dem grösten Nutzen, nach ihrer Krafft, Tugend und sonderbarer Würckung können genommen und gebrauchet werden: auch wer sein Hauss- und Reise-Apotheckgen darmit anfüllet, dass selbiger um bedürftigenfals nicht allemahl von mir schrifftlichen Unterricht verlangen und hohlen lassen dürffe. 4°. *Stolberg*, [1736].

GORDON (G. A.) The complete English physician; or, a universal library of family medicines. 8°. *London*, 1779.

——. The same. A new ed. 8°. *London*, [*n. d.*]

GOUERNAYLE (The) of helthe: with the medecyne of yᵉ stomacke. Reprinted [fac-simile] from Caxton's edition (*circa* mcccxci). With introductory remarks and notes by William Blades. 8°. *London*, 1858.

GRAHAM (J.) The guardian of health, long life, and happiness; or, Dr. Graham's general directions as to regimen, etc. For the cure or alleviation of all nervous, scorbutic, scrophulous, bilious, gouty, and rheumatic diseases, for the preservation of health, for the happy prolongation of life, for the improvement and preservation of youth and beauty, and for the enjoyment of temporal peace and of eternal felicity; affectionately addressed to every reasonable and candid person who wishes to be healthy, respectable, and truly happy both here and hereafter. To which are added, the Christian's universal, being a paraphrase on our Lord's prayer; and a complete and infallible guide to everlasting blessedness in Heaven. 8°. *Newcastle-upon-Tyne*, 1790.

Medicine (*Popular*).

——. The guardian Goddess of Health; or, the whole art of preventing and curing diseases . . . To which is added, an account of the composition, preparation, and properties of the three great medicines prepared and dispensed at the Temple of Health, Adelphi, and at the Temple of Hymen, Pall-Mall, London, [etc.] 8°. *London*, [n. d.]

GRAHAM (S.) Lectures on the science of human life. 2 v. 8°. *Boston*, 1839.

GRAHAM (T. J.) Modern domestic medicine; or, a popular treatise illustrating the character, symptoms, causes, distinction and correct treatment of all diseases incident to the human frame . . . To which are added a domestic materia medica, a description of the virtues and correct manner of using the different mineral waters of Europe, and the cold, warm, and vapour baths, [etc.] 4. ed. 8°. *London*, 1829.

[GROSCHUFF (F.)] Der curiöse Patiente, oder Erörterung derjenigen Sachen, welche ein Krancker offtmahls zu wissen begehret, und auch wissen soll, nebst einem verständigen Kräuter-Männgen und denen vornehmsten Diäts- und Gesundheits-Regeln, welche ein jeder, der gute Gesundheit erhalten, ingleichen anspinnenden Beschwerungen, bey Zeiten vorbauen will, in Acht zu nehmen hat, sowohl Krancken, als Gesunden nützlich und unterrichtlich zu lesen, eröffnet von Hiatrophilo. sm. 8°. *Leipzig*, 1702.

GRYSSELIUS (J.) * Medicus sui ipsius.
In: LINNÆUS. Amœnitates acad. [etc.] 8°. *Erlangæ*, 1785, viii, 13–25.

GUFER (J.) Tabulæ medicæ seu medicina domestica, euporista ac facile parabilia experientia atque authoritate comprobata medicamenta continens; das ist: Kleine Hauss-Apotheck, darinnen allerhand schöne Experimenta oder Artzneyen, auch von den geringsten und verächtlichsten Sachen beschrieben, und den armen Krancken zu Nutzen an Tag gegeben worden. 16°. *Augspurg*, 1679.

——. The same. 16°. *Augspurg*, 1670.

GUIBERT (P.) Le médecin charitable, enseignant la manière de faire et préparer en la maison, avec facilité et peu de frais, les remèdes propres à toutes maladies, selon l'advis du médecin ordinaire. Augmentée d'un singulier préservatif contre la peste. 8°. *Paris*, 1638.

——. The same. 12°. *Paris*, 1639.

——. The same. 16°. *Troyes*, 1645.

——. The same. The charitable physitian with the charitable apothecary . . . Now faithfully translated into English for the benefit of this kingdome, by I. W. sm. 4°. *London*, 1639.

——. L'apotiquaire charitable, enseignant à faire en la maison les médicamens composez, avec grande facilité à peu de frais, et peu de temps. 16°. *Troyes*, 1646.

——. Toutes les œuvres charitables de . . . sçavoir: Le médecin charitable. Le prix et valeur des médicamens. L'apothicaire charitable. Le choix des médicamens. Le traicté du séné. La manière de faire toutes sortes de gelées. La manière de faire diverses confitures. La conservation de santé. Le discours de la peste. Le traicté de la saignée [par Galien]. La méthode agréable et facile pour se purger doucement et sans aucun dégoust. La manière d'embaumer les corps morts. Revuës, corrigées et augmentées en cette dernière édition par l'autheur. 8°. *Paris*, 1647.
Bound with his: Le médecin charitable, [etc.] 16°. *Troyes*, 1645.

Medicine (*Popular*).

GUYON *Dolois* (L.) Le cours de médecine en françois, contenant Le miroir de beautie et santé corporelle. 2 v. in 1. 4°. *Lyon*, 1664.

——. The same. 4°. *Lyon*, 1678.

GUNN (J. C.) Domestic medicine; or, poor man's friend in the hours of affliction, pain, and sickness. 8°. *Louisville*, 1840.

——. The same. First revised ed., enlarged in 1840. 8°. *Philadelphia*, 1844.

——. The same. New family physician; or, home-book of health. 100. ed.! 8°. *Cincinnati*, 1870.

GUSTER (G.) 101 Winke und Wünsche für Gesundheit. 8°. *Buchs*, 1885.

H. (J.) The pearle of practise, or practiser's pearle for phisicke and chirurgerie, found out, by . . . (a spagericke or distiller). sm. 4°. *London*, 1594.

HAGIUS (J.) Den lust-hof der medecijnen: inhoudende den gront van alle cranckheden ende gebreken daer de menschen mede moghen overvallen worden van den hoofde af tot den voeten toe: haer oorsaken, teeckenen ende remedien om die te genesin niet alleene voor medecijns, chirurgijns ende vroede-vrouwen: maer oock voor alle huijsvaders ende besonder voor de gene die ter plaetsen wonen daer geen medecijns en zijn te becomen, welcx ghelijcken noijt voor desen in onse Nederduytsche tale en is uijtghegaen . . . ende nu eerst int licht ghebracht door zijnen sone Matthijs Haghens. fol. *Dordrecht*, 1616.

HAHN (E.) · Die wichtigsten der bis jetzt bekannten Geheimmittel und Specialitäten, mit Angabe ihrer Zusammensetzung und ihres Werthes. 2. Aufl. 8°. *Berlin*, 1874.

HAHN (T.) Praktisches Handbuch der naturgemässen Heilweise. 3. Aufl., 1. Lfg. 8°. *Berlin*, 1870.

HALL (A. G.) Views of the new theory of disease and of treatment and cure, based upon the nutritive principle, illustrative of the science of fluid physiology and the chemical properties of the blood. For the people. 4 pts. in 1 v. 8°. *Washington, D. C.*, 1852.

HALL (W. W.) The nature, causes, symptoms, and cure of diseases of the throat and lungs. 8°. *Cincinnati*, 1850.

——. Throat-ail, bronchitis, consumption; their causes, symptoms, and cure, in language adapted to common readers. 6. ed. 8°. *New York*, 1851.

HALLIN (O. F.) Handbox i helso- och sjuk-vårdslära populärt framstäld. 8°. *Stockholm*, [1886].
Forsta bandet. Helsolära. Andra bandet. Sjukvårds-och sjukdomslära.

HAMILTON (J.) Culpeper's English family physician, or medical herbal, enlarged . . . with several hundred additional plants, principally from Sir John Hill. Medicinally and astrologically arranged after the manner of Culpeper. And a new dispensatory from the Ms. of the late Dr. Saunders. 2 v. 8°. *London*, 1792.

HAMMACK (E. B.) The family physician and guide to health; a system of domestic medicine, including a treatise on midwifery and the diseases peculiar to women. 8°. *St. Louis*, 1869.

HAND (W. M.) The house surgeon and physician, designed to assist heads of families. 2. ed. 12°. *New Haven*, 1820.

HARDINGE (B.) First elements of vital power: how they were originally generated, and why those original elements are still indispensable to the production and reproduction of vitality in the human economy. An entirely original and startling exposé of important mistakes that

Medicine (*Popular*).

underlie the teachings of medical science (so called), etc. 8°. *New York*, 1870.

HAUSZ-APOTECK oder ein gemein nützliches Hauszartzney-Büchlein, darinnen allerhand Artzneyen für den gemeinen Mann, der in der Eil die Apotecken nicht haben kan oder sonsten dieselbigen zu ersuchen, vermögens nicht were, und also hiemit ihm selbsten mit geringem Unkosten zu Hülffe kommen kan. sm. 4°. *Wittenberg*, 1613.

HEALTH bulletin, and first annual announcement of the "First Medical College of the American Health Society." The official organ of the rational system of medical practice. 8°. *Boston*, 1883.

HEALTH without physic, and no expense. By a friend of the people. 16°. *London*, 1852.

HEILKRAFT (Die) gewisser Bewegungen des Körpers bis in die spätern Lebensjahre zur gänzlichen Vertreibung hartnäckiger Hypochondrie, Gicht, Rheumatismus, Brustbeschwerden, Magenschwäche, Hämorrhoiden und mehrerer anderer Krankheiten, nebst Angabe der durch fünfzigjährige Erfahrung bewährten einfachen und naturgemässen Mittel dagegen. Zur Beförderung des körperlichen Wohles fasslich dargestellt von einem Nichtarzte. 5. Aufl. 8°. *Leipzig*, 1852.

HEINEN (H.) Gesundheits-Schatzkammer, oder kurze, deutliche und richtige Anweisung zur Erhaltung der Gesundheit und Abwendung mancher Krankheiten; sowie auch gute und sichere Mittel zur Wiederherstellung der verlornen Gesundheit. Für Deutsche ganz deutlich und fasslich eingerichtet und denselben zum nützlichen Gebrauch wohlmeinend anempfohlen und gewidmet. 12°. *Lancaster*, [*Pa.*], 1831.

HELLWIG (C.) Curieuses Reise- und Hauss-Apotheckchen, worinnen zwar wenige, jedoch bewährte Artzeneyen zu finden, somit leichter Mühe und Kosten, ein jeder selbst präpariren ... kan ... Nebst einer Zugabe derer zweyen weltberühmten Medicamenten, dem Theriac und Mithridat, deren herrlichen Nutzen, Zubereitung und Gebrauch mit sonderbahrem Fleiss eingerichtet. 16°. *Frankfurth u. Leipzig*, 1711.

HEMLÄKAREN. Populär ordbok i sjukvård och helsolära enligt nutidens medicinska åsigter. En rådgifvare, innan läkarehjelp kan erhållas särskildt för hemmen på landet och för sjöfarande. Efter Prof. A. Thornam's Sundhedslexicon, m. fl. kallor bearbetad af Wilh. Uhrström. Med. förord af Professor P. H. Malmsten. 8°. *Stockholm*, [1881].

VAN DER HEYDEN (H.) Speedy help for rich and poor; or, certain physicall discourses touching the vertue of whey in the cure of the griping flux of the belly, and of the dysentery. Of cold water in the cure of the gout and greenwounds. Of wine-vineger in the preservation from and cure of the plague and other pestilential diseases; as also in the prevention of hydrophobia, or dread of water, caused by the biting of a mad dog, etc. 18°. *London*, 1653.

HILL (J.) Virtues of British herbs. With the history, description, and figures of the several kinds; an account of the diseases they will cure; the family methods of giving them; and the management of the patients in each disease; containing cures of head-achs by feverfew tea ... of consumptions by coltsfoot tea, of hectic fevers by the daisy, colics by leaves of chamomile, and agues by its flowers. A recommendation of the Bidens cernua to supply the place of the Ceylon acmella, so celebrated in the gravel ... and a case of the hooping-cough cured by a tea of the fresh root of elecampane. The

Medicine (*Popular*).

whole illustrating that important truth, that the plants of our own country will cure all its diseases. To which are added cautions against the two othonnas, destructive of sheep. A work intended to be useful to the sick and to their friends, [etc.] 4. ed. 8°. *London*, 1771.

HOFFMANN (F.) Gründliche Anweisung, wie ein Mensch vor dem frühzeitigen Tod und allerhand Arten Krankheiten durch ordentliche Lebens-Art sich verwahren könne. 8°. *Halle i. Magdeb.*, 1715.

HOFFMANN (F.) The popular health almanac for 1877. 12°. *New York*, 1877.

HOFMANN (A.) Encyclopädie der Diätetik, oder allgemeines Gesundheits-Lexicon. Ein vollständiges Real-Wörterbuch des geistigen und körperlichen Verhaltens im gesunden und kranken Zustande für Jedermann, jedes Alter, Geschlecht, Temperament, jeden Stand und alle Verhältnisse des Lebens. Ein Volks- und Hülfsbuch zum augenblicklichen Nachschlagen und zur steten Belehrung, wie man Gesundheit und Leben bis zum spätesten Alter erhalten und bewahren, Krankheiten vorbeugen, sie mildern und heben kann. Beendet von Dr. Jonathan Braun. 8°. *Leipzig*, 1834–42.

HOLBROOK (M. L.) Hygiene of the brain and nerves and the cure of nervousness. With twenty-eight original letters from leading thinkers and writers concerning their physical and intellectual habits. 8°. *New York*, 1878.

——. The same. 8°. *New York*, 1879.

HOLLICK (F.) The family physician; or, the true art of healing the sick in all diseases whatever. 16°. *Philadelphia*, [1851].

HORLACHER (C.) Theatrum arcanorum divinæ sapientiæ, oder gnadenreicher Schauplatz der Göttlichen Weissheit und unerschöpfflichen Barmhertzigkeit, welche erhellet in und auss denen vielfachen Wunder-Geheimnüssen der wahren Medicin, als nemlich der ungemeinen und in diesen letzten Zeiten durch den Göttlichen Gnaden-Geist kundt gemacht, oder geheirten Erörter- und Eröffnung der sichern, ohnschmertzlichen, und nicht kostbaren Wassersuchts, Podagrischer Kranckheit ob Zipperleins, der Fieber, Pest, Ruhr und Hals-Bräune, wie auch der Krätze, und Luis Venere oder so genannten Frantzosen-Cur und Heilungs-Art. In viererley Classes und Gattung abgetheilet, auch christmitleidigst vorgezeiget, und Pflickmässig vorgestellet. 12°. *Franckf. a. M.*, 1699.

HORSCHT (J.) Ein Vorwarnung der Krancken vor ihren selbs eigenen Schaden und Vorseumnuss. Darinn der Artzneyen Ursprung, Anfang, Zunemen, und kegenwertiger Zustandt, sampt vielen wunderbarlichen Geheymnnussen der Natur, kürtzlich und deutlich gelehret wird. 4°. *Görlitz*, 1574.

HORSELL (W.) Das Buch der Gesundheit. Eine volksthümliche Belehrung über die wahren Universal-Mittel zur Erhaltung der Gesundheit, sowie zur Heilung der Krankheiten des menschlichen Körpers. 8°. *Schwelm u. Leipzig*, 1872.

HULME (N.) Anzeige eines sichern und leichten Mittels wider den Blasen- und Nierenstein, den Scorbut, das Podagra, wider auszehrende Fieber und die Würmer. Durch verschiedene Erfahrungen erläutert. Nebst einer Anweisung, Wasser und andere flüssige Körper sehr geschwind, durch eine sehr einfache Mischung, ohne Hülfe einiger Geräthschaft, oder einer zusammengesetzten Maschine, mit fixer Luft anzuschwängern. Aus dem Englischen übersetzt. 18°. *Leipzig*, 1778.

Medicine (*Popular*).

HUNTER (J.) Domestic medicine; or, the herbalist's vade-mecum; containing directions for making tinctures, syrups, etc., the method of compounding medicines, with the nature, use, and various properties of the herbs used in medicine. Their application to the various diseases of the human frame, together with many valuable recipes by which the assistance of the doctor is often rendered unnecessary. The whole forming a complete family physician. 8°. *London*, [*n. d.*]

HUTCHINGS (T. G.) The medical pilot; or, new system; being a family medical companion, and compendium of medicine on a totally new plan, and by which all diseases can be treated successfully without minerals, or any poisons whatever, [etc.] 8°. *New York*, 1855.

INSTRUCTIONS how to possess good health and buoyant animal spirits. To which are now for the first time added instructions how to act in cases of fractures, dislocations, wounds, poison, the bites of rabid animals, suspended animation, [etc.] By a village doctor. 8°. *London*, 1842.

ISRAEL (T.) * De præstantia remediorum domesticorum. 4°. *Halæ Magdeb.*, [1718].

J. (W.) A choice manuall, or rare and select secrets in physick and chirurgery. Collected and practised by the Right Honourable the Countesse of Kent, late deceased. Whereto are added several experiments of the virtues of Gascon pouder, and lapis contra yervam, by a professor of physick, [etc.] 4. ed. 24°. *London*, 1654.

JACOBI (A.) Volksmedicin. Vortrag gehalten vor dem deutschen gesellig-wissenschaftlichen Verein von New York am 11. März 1885. 8°. *New York*, 1885.

JACOBI (H.) Schat der armen, ofte een medecijn boecxken, dienstelijck voor alle menschen: Inhoudende hoe men zijn gesontheydt onderhouden sal: daer by veelerhande simpele remedien ende medicamenten, omme veelerhande steckten, met kleyne kosten, geheel lichtelijcken te genesen. 16°. *Haerlem*, 1661.

[——.] Den kleynen herbarius ofte kruydtboecxken, inhoudende de kracht, ende operatie van alle de ghemeene kruyderen ende bekende vruchten, die men dagelicx gebruyckt, waer deur men met Gods hulpe een yder zijne ghesondtheydt kan onderhouden ende veelderhande siecktken te genesen. Van nieus oversien, en op veel plaetien verbetert, ende vermeerdert. 18°. *Dordrecht*, 1637.

[——.] The same. 18°. *Amsterdam*, 1683.

JÄGER (H.) Der Apothekergarten. Anleitung zur Kultur und Behandlung der in Deutschland zu ziehenden medicinischen Pflanzen. Für Apotheker und Gärtner, Land- und Gartenbesitzer. 8°. *Leipzig*, 1859.

JAHN (F.) Versuch eines Handbuchs der populären Arzneikunde. 12°. *Jena*, 1790.

——. Die Naturheilkraft. Vorarbeit zu einer zeitgemässen Umgestaltung der Heilkunde. 8°. *Eisenbach*, 1831.

JAMES (F.) Disease; its cause and cure; with plain directions for the home treatment of all kinds of complaint. 7. ed. 16°. *Nottingham*, 1883.

JENNINGS (I.) The tree of life; or, human degeneracy; its nature and remedy, as based on the elevating principle of orthopathy. 8°. *New York*, 1867.

JEWETT (M.) Jewett's family physician. The iatroleptic practice of medicine, or the curing of diseases principally by external application and friction. 8°. *Columbus*, 1838.

Medicine (*Popular*).

JOHNSON (R. W.) The nurse's guide, and family assistant, containing friendly cautions to those who are in health; with ample directions to nurses and others, who attend the sick, women in child-bed, etc. 2. Am. ed. 12°. *Philadelphia*, 1819.

JONES (P. B.) Pearls of wisdom, gems of knowledge for all. Common-sense prescriptions and practical information; a systematic treatment in the domestic practice of medicine. 8°. *Kansas City*, 1880.

KADNER (P.) Gelehrte und ungelehrte Heilkunst. Aufklärungen in populären Briefen dem gebildeten nichtärztlichen Publikum . . . gegeben. 12°. *Leipzig*, 1855.

KAISER (J. A.) * De medicina populari. 12°. *Landishuti*, 1816.

KEATING (J. M.) Maternity, infancy, childhood. Hygiene of pregnancy; nursing and weaning of infants; the care of children in health and disease, adapted especially to the use of mothers or those intrusted with the bringing up of infants and children, and training schools for nurses, as an aid to the teaching of the nursing of women and children. 12°. *Philadelphia*, 1887.

KECK (J. E.) Die Hausmutter am Krankenbette, eine gemeinnützige Schrift für alle Stände. 8°. *Berlin*, 1784.

KELLEY (J. C.) Key to medical science. 12°. *New York*, 1842.

——. The same. 8°. *New York*, 1842.
The cover of this book marked "Second uniform edition, New York, J. W. Kelley, 1844".

KEMP (T. L.) The medical guide to the preservation of health and the knowledge of disease . . . Designed for popular use. 8°. *London, Edinburgh, & Dublin*, 1853.

KERN der ganzen Medicin, worinnen auf die allerkürzeste Art die Arzney-Mittel, so bey den vornehmsten medicinischen und chirurgischen Krankheiten wesentlich nothwendig sind, in geringen Recepten so deutlich angegeben und erkläret werden, dass ein Jeder, in benöthigtem Fall, sein eigener Arzt seyn könne. Auf Befehl seiner königlichen Hoheit, des Herzogs von Cumberland, zum Gebrauch des Kriegs-Hospitals, von den königlichen Leib-Aerzten, Wund-Aerzten, dem Ober-Wund-Arzte und Ober-Apotheker zusammen getragen. Aus dem Englischen übersetzt. 16°. *Hamburg*, 1748.

——. The same. 16°. *Rudolstadt*, 1752.

KIESEWETTER (F.) Die Krankenpflege in der Familie. 8°. *Troppau*, 1885.

KLENCKE (P. F. H.) Die physische Lebenskunst, oder praktische Anwendung der Naturwissenschaften auf Förderung des persönlichen Daseins. Ein Familienbuch. 8°. *Leipzig*, 1864.

KLES (F.) Anleitung zur Behandlung und Heilung aller Krankheiten durch die diätetische Heilmethode. Im Interesse der leidenden Menschheit. 8°. *Dresden*, [188 ?]

KNIGHT (W.) & KNIGHT (E.) The patient's vade mecum; or, how to benefit by medical advice and treatment. 12°. *London*, 1884.

KOCH (K. A.) Die Erkältungskrankheiten, oder gründliche Anleitung für Jedermann, sich vor Schnupfen, Husten, Durchfällen, Rheumatismen u. s. w. zu verwahren [etc.] 3. Aufl. 12°. *Leipzig*, [*n. d.*]

KRAMER (C. S.) * De medicina populari. 8°. *Halæ*, [1783].

KRANKE (Der) Mensch, oder Ursache und Heilung der Krankheiten. Belehrungen, wie man die Gesundheit bewahren und Krankheiten durch ein sicheres, angenehmes und Jedermann zugängliches Mittel heilen kann. 8°. *Berlin*, 1873.

Medicine (*Popular*).

KREBEL (R.) Volksmedicin und Volksmittel verschiedner Völkerstämme Russlands. 8°. *Leipzig u. Heidelberg*, 1858.

KUHNE (L.) Bin ich gesund oder krank? Ein Prüfstein und Ratgeber für Jedermann. 8°. *Leipzig*, 1884.

KURTZ-VERFASTES Land- und Haus-Artzney-Büchlein, in welchem allerhand heilsame, an vielen Personen versucht- und bewehrt-befundene Artzney-Mittel dem armen Burger und Landmann, der in der Eil einen bewehrt und erfahrnen Artzt zu erreichen, oder kostbare Mittel zu bezahlen nicht vermag, zum besten, aus christlicher Lieb, vorgestellet. 16°. [*n. p., n. d.*]

L. (C. M.) Der aufrichtige und sichere Arzt, das ist: wahre und umständliche Nachricht von denen vornehmsten, und meist jährlich im Schwange gehenden Kranckheiten, wie man selbige mit leichten, sichern und offt erfahrnen Medicamenten in aller kürtze behutsam begegnen, und nechst Gott curiren könne, dabey denen erst anfangenden Practicanten, und so sich auf dem Lande, in Ermangelung eines erfahrnen Medici, dieses Arztes bedienen wollen. Zur mehrern Erläuterung, eine jede Kranckheit mit einem besondern wahrhafften Casu, und vielmahl gut befundenen sichern Hülfs-Mitteln versehen. 12°. *Quedlimburg u. Aschersleben*, 1717.

LANDRINUS (C.) Haussartzney, in welcher vil schöne, bewerte Künsten, auss geringen, unnd bey menigklich verechtlichen Dingen, zu mancherley Leibsgebrechen dienstlich, zubereytet, begriffen, unnd leichtlich zu bekommen seind, vor etlichen Jahren in französischer Sprach; nun aber dem gemainen Mann zu guttem Teutsch gemacht, durch Hieremiam Martium. 16°. *Augspurg*, 1571.

——. The same. 16°. *Augspurg*, 1573.
——. The same. 12°. [*Augspurg*], 1588.

LAZARUS (M. E.) Passional hygiene and natural medicine; embracing the harmonies of man with his planet. 16°. *New York*, 1852.

VON LEBENWALDT (A.) Land-Stadt-Hauss-Artzney-Buch, in welchem angezeigt und erwiesen wird, wie man denjenigen Kranckheiten, welche ein gantzes Land oder mehr Oerther anstecken, so dann durch Contagion und Anklebung anderweitig fortgepflantzt und ausgebreitet werden, als da seyn: die Pest, Pestilenzial- und petechialische Fieber, ungarische Kranckheit, rothe Ruhr, Kinds-Blattern, etc. Mit Gottes Gnad und Hülff so wohl durch geringe als kostbare Mittel Widerstand thun könne. Samt einer Chronick aller denckwürdigen Pesten, samt einer Information, was zu solcher Contagions-Zeit . . . zu thun haben; dabey eine fünfffache Cur zu finden. fol. *Nürnberg*, 1695.

LEHAMAU (P.-J.-L.) Plantes, remèdes et maladies, ou la médecine simple et facile à la portée de tous. Ouvrage donnant la description complète de plus de 250 plantes médicinales, la plupart représentées et coloriées comme elles existent dans la nature. Les symptômes des maladies et leur traitement, [etc.] 8°. *Gommegnies*, 1887.

LEIBARZT (Der), oder 500 der besten Hausarzneimittel gegen 145 Krankheiten der Menschen . . . Dazu die Kunst ein hundertjähriges Alter zu erreichen, wie auch 20 Gesundheits-Regeln. Ueber die Wunderkräfte des kalten Wassers und Dr. Hufeland's Haus- und Reise-Apotheke. 17. Aufl. 8°. *Quedlinburg u. Leipzig*, 1884.

LEIB- UND LAND-MEDICUS (Der) armer Leute, wie dieselbigen bei diesen verarmeten Zeiten,

Medicine (*Popular*).

mit lauter bewährten und probirten Hauss-Mitteln ohne sonderliche Kosten ihr Leben und Gesundheit erhalten können. sowol auf ansteckende, als auf andere innerliche und äusserliche Kranckheiten gerichtet, von einem alten erfahrnem fürstl. Leib-Medico zusammen getragen, und aus dessen verlassenen Manuscriptis ausgesuchet und in Druck befördert durch Ignatium Regnantem, einen Freund haussarmer Leute. 12°. *Merseburg*, 1682.

LESCURE (F.) La santé à tout le monde; la médecine du peuple, indispensable pour conserver la santé, se préserver et guérir des maladies et pour vivre longtemps; mise à la portée de tout le monde et de toutes les bourses. sm. 8°. *Auch*, 1884.

LETTER (A) to clergymen on the preservation of health and the use of Peruvian syrup, or protected solution of protoxide of iron combined, as a medicinal agent. 8°. *Boston*, [1859].

LEVENS (P.) A right profitable booke for all diseases, called the path-way to health; wherein are to bee found most excellent and approved medicines of great vertue; as also notable potions and drinks, and for the distilling of divers precious waters, and making of oyles, and other comfortable receits for the health of the body, never before imprinted; first gathered and now newly corrected and augmented. sm. 4°. *London*, 1632.

LEVOY (H.) Lebens-Elixir für Jünglinge. Schutz gegen jeden Jugendtaumel. Heilung der Gebrechen und Schwächen nach begangenen Jugendsünden. Gewæhrleistung für Glück und Zufriedenheit in Beruf und Ehe. 16°. *Wien*, 1851.

LIBERALI (C.) Hygienic-medical hand-book for travellers in Italy, with some general notions on the climate of the principal cities of Italy, and more especially on that of Rome. (English translation by D. V. L. son.) 16°. *Rome*, 1878.

LIEBAUT *Dijonnois* (J.) Quatre livres des secrets de médecine, et de la philosophie chymique. Faicts françois par . . . Esquels sont descrits plusieurs remèdes singuliers pour toutes maladies, tant intérieures qu'extérieures du corps humain; traictées bien amplement les manières de destiller eaux, huyles et quinte essences de toute sorte de matières, etc. sm. 8°. *Lyon*, 1593.

LINTON (M. L.) Medicine for the million. A lecture introductory to the session, 1860-61, of the St. Louis Medical College. 8°. *St. Louis*, 1860.

LOBB (T.) The good Samaritan; or complete English physician. Containing observations on the most frequent diseases of men and women, infants and children; with directions for the management of the sick, and a collection of the most approved receipts for making and preparing cheap, easy, safe, and efficacious medicines for their recovery. Likewise directions concerning bleeding . . . with infallible remedies for the bite of a mad dog or any other animal. Likewise, preservations from infections, etc. 12°. *London*, [*n. d.*]

LOBSTEIN (J. T. D.) Dialogues between patients and the physician, on the several principal diseases in this country; with the physician's advice, including a collection of over two hundred domestic remedies; a work useful to families. 8°. *New York*, 1839.

LOCHMANN (J. J.) Sympathetischer Wunder-Doktor in vielen bewährten Heilmitteln gegen viele gefährlichen und schmerzvollen äusserlichen und innerlichen Krankheiten der Menschen

Medicine (*Popular*).

und Thiere. Nebst einer Sammlung der besten und bewährtesten natürlichen Mittel und Recepte für alle Vorkommnisse des menschlichen Lebens. 16°. *Baltimore*, [*n. d.*]

LOH (A.) Lehrbuch der praktischen Naturheilkunde nach Steinbacher's kombinirter Naturheilmethode und achtzehnjährigen eigenen Erfahrungen. 8°. *Berlin*, 1874.

LUTHERITZ (C. F.) Slagfluss och lamheter, eller anwisning att skydda sig för dessa och att bota dem. För både läkare och andre. Öfwersättning af G. Engström. 8°. *Jönköping*, 1829.

MANNINGHAM (*Sir* K.) The use and abuse of physic, with the certain method, to know the disease; leading to the most successful ways of curing all those distempers which are curable; and of relieving all those which are incurable. 2. ed. 8°. *London*, 1754.

MANUAL (The) for invalids. 8°. *Boston*, 1830.

MARBACH (G. B.) Abhandlung der Frühlings- und Herbstcuren. 12°. *Bresslau*, 1753.

MARIE DE SAINT-URSIN (P.-J.) Manuel populaire de santé, à l'usage des personnes intelligentes vivant à la campagne; ou instructions sommaires sur les maladies qui règnent le plus souvent, et les moyens les plus simples de les traiter; suivies de notions chirurgicales et pharmaceutiques. 8°. *Paris*, 1808.

DE MARQUE (J.) Le guide du malade, ouvrage de médecine, philosophique et moral. 12°. *Paris*, 1779.

MARSCHALL (H. G.) Geneeskundig volksboek, ter onderregtinge voor ongehuwde dochters, zwangere vrouwen, moeders, en allen, die met de zorge over jonge kinderen belast zijn; leerende, op eene duidelijke en tevens voorzigtige wijze, wat dezelven tot behoud van derzelver welvaart, vruchbaarheid en gezonheid in agt te neemen hebben: benevens eene aanwijzing van de beste hulpmiddelen in derzelver bizondere ziekten en toevallen. Volgens den tweeden verbeterden en vermeederden Hoogduitschen druck vertaald. 8°. *Dordrecht*, 1792.

MASSINI (V.) Alcune norme indispensabili da servire di scorta alla madri e alle balie nell' allevamento dei bambini. 16°. *Genova*, 1887.

MATECKI. Rady i nauki starego lekarza dla nielekarzy napisal. [Advice by an old physician for the use of non-physicians.] 16°. *Poznań*, 1867.

MATTHEWS (W.) A treatise on domestic medicine and kindred subjects; embracing anatomical and physiological sketches of the human body. 8°. *Indianapolis*, 1848.

MAYOR. Volks-heelkunde, of eenvoudige raadgevingen bij plotselinge ongelukken, gevaarlijke toevallen, vergiftigingen, enz. Bij afwezigheid van een bekwamen heelmeester. Nar het Fransch met aanteekeningen en aanzienlijke bijvoegselen door Thomas Cutler. Uit het Engelsch vertaald door Dr. H. H. Hageman, jr. sm. 8°. *Amsterdam*, 1842.

MEDICINISCHE Arcana zu Herstellung aller Gebrechen des menschlichen Körpers und Erhaltung eines langen Lebens aber Alles nach dem Willen Gottes Seiner Gnade und Barmherzigkeit. 4°. [*n. p., n. d.*]

MERLIN (L.) The treasure of health, or a wonderful collection of the most valuable secrets in medicine, for the cure of all diseases, wounds, and other accidents to which the human body is subject . . . also, the best preservatives against the plague, pestilential fevers, small-pox, [etc.] 12°. *Philadelphia*, 1819.

MEYER (B.) Führer durch die Literatur der Gesundheitspflege, Naturheilkunde, Vegetaris-

Medicine (*Popular*).

mus, Seelendiätetik für Freunde einer naturgemässen Lebensweise, in Verbindung mit solchen herausgegeben. 2. Aufl. 16°. *Rudolstadt i. Th.*, [1884].

MEYRICK (W.) The new family herbal; or, domestic physician; enumerating, with accurate descriptions, all the known vegetables which are any way remarkable for medical efficacy; with an account of their virtues in the several diseases incident to the human frame. 4°. *Birmingham*, 1790.

MICHEL (*Madame*). Les remèdes de bonnes femmes, ou moyens de prévenir, soigner et guérir toutes les maladies. Rédigés et mis en ordre alphabétique. 32°. *Paris*, 1827.

MITCHELL (W.) A family medical companion; a new medical work, devoted to the symptoms and remedies of one hundred and fifty diseases, embracing diseases of women and children. 8°. *Philadelphia*, 1835.

MÖLLER (F.) Die Heilkraft gewisser Bewegungen des Körpers bis in die spätern Lebensjahre zur gänzlichen Vertreibung hartnäckiger Hämorrhoiden, Gicht, Rheumatismus, Hypochondrie, Schwindel, Nervenschwäche, Brustbeschwerden und mehrerer anderer, durch sitzende oder unregelmässige Lebensweise entstandenen Krankheiten, nebst Angabe der bewährten einfachen und naturgemässen Mittel dagegen. Nach fünfzigjährigen Erfahrungen fasslich dargestellt von einem Nichtarzte. 10. Aufl. 8°. *Leipzig*, 1870.

MONCRIEF (J.) The poor man's physician, or the receipts of the famous John Moncrief, of.Tippermalloch; being a choice collection of simple and easy remedies for most distempers, very useful for all persons, especially those of a poorer condition. To which is added the method of curing the small-pox and scurvy, by the eminent Dr. Archbald Pitcairn. 2. ed. 12°. *Edinburgh*, 1716.

———. The same. 3. ed. 12°. *Edinburgh*, 1731.

———. Tippermalluch's receipts. Being a collection of many useful and easy remedies for most distempers. 2. ed. 16°. *Leith*, 1775.

DO MONTE (J. P. X.) O homem medico de si mesmo, ou sciencia e arte nova de conservar cada hum a si proprio a saude, e destruir a sua doença, dirigida ao bem commum. 12°. *Lisboa*, 1760.

DU MONTVERT (R.) Les fleurs et secretz de médecine, lequel traictans de plusieurs remèdes, receptes, et conservatoires pour le corps humain contre toutes maladies comme de peste, fiebvres, pleurésies, enfleures, caterres, gravelles, et plusieurs aultres. Compilé par . . . puis traduict de latin en françois; lequel livre Ypocras envoya à Julius lequel estoit malade de plusieurs maladies tant extérieures qu'intérieures. Nouvellement imprimé. 24°. *Paris*, [1500?]

———. The same. 24°. *Poitiers*, [*n. d.*]

MORGAN (S.) The text book for domestic practice; being plain and concise directions for the administration of homœopathic medicines, in simple ailments. 24°. *New York*, [*n. d.*]

MORISON (J.) Morisoniana; or, family adviser of the British College of Health. With an appendix. 3. ed. 8°. *London*, 1831.

———. The same. 4. ed. 2. v. 8°. *London*, 1833-4.

———. Third edition of the practical proofs of the soundness of the hygeian system of physiology, giving incontrovertible testimony to the afflicted, of the inestimable value of Morison's vegetable universal medicines, [etc.] 12°. *New York*, 1832,

Medicine (*Popular*).

MORISONIANA; ó consejos á las familias del Colejio Británico de la Salud. La causa verdadera de las enfermedades y modo de curarlas . . . [Traducida del inglés por A. Eusberg.] 12°. *Barcelona*, 1844.

VON MURALT (J.) Hippocrates Helveticus; oder der getreu- sichere- und wohl-bewährte Eydgnössische Stadt-Land- und Hauss-Artzt in welchem eine klare und wahrhaffte Beschreibung innerlicher Gebrechen und Kranckheiten des menschlichen Leibs und aller dessen Gliederen, nach den besten Grund-Sätzen der Heil-Kunst enthalten: sammt Entdeckung der gewissesten, kräfftigsten, wohl-befundenen und bewährtesten Artzney-Mitteln, welche wider dieselbigen heilsamlich können gebraucht werden: zu Nutz und Frommen der Eydgnössischen Einwohneren und anderen der Preiss-würdigen Artzney-Kunst Liebhabern, an das Tagliecht gegeben, und zu unausssprechlicher Bequemlichkeit dem Alphabet nach vorgestellet. 8°. *Basel*, 1692.

MURE. Le médecin du peuple; enseignement mettant à la portée des hommes de conscience et de bon vouloir les procédés les plus parfaits et les récentes découvertes de l'art de guérir, indiquant les moyens pratiques de traiter toutes les maladies de l'homme et des animaux selon les principes de l'homœopathie. Revu, augmenté et mis en meilleur ordre par Sophie Liet. 12°. *Paris*, 1883.

MURINO (A.) Lezioni di medicina popolare e preventiva. 12°. *Roma*, 1875.

NAPIER (D.) Neurotonics; the art of strengthening the nerves. A new view of health and disease in relation to the nervous system, the influence of mental emotions upon the body and the origin of chronic diseases, with numerous cases and instructions for cure. 32. ed. 8°. *London*, 1854.

NEUMANN (C. E. O.) Der Männerarzt; ein Ratgeber für junge und alte Männer. Naturgemässe Behandlung der Männerkrankheiten. 8°. *Leipzig*, [n. d.]

NEUMANN (K. G.) Der allgemeine Hausarzt, oder Belehrung für Jedermann, wie er seine Gesundheit erhalten und in Krankheiten und Unfällen sich benehmen solle. 12°. *Aachen*, 1837.

NEW (The) family physician, and guide to health and long life; with a variety of valuable tables on medical statistics; to which is now added an appendix, containing recipes for preparing the most celebrated patent medicines; with rational observations on longevity, founded on the principles of the late John Abernethy. 12°. *London*, [n. d.]

NEWCASTLE (*Duchess of*). The world's olio. fol. *London*, 1655.

NEWTON (R. C.) The doctor's corner. 8°. *London*, 1884.
Repr. from: Newcastle Weekly Chronicle.

NICOLAUS *Prepositas*. Prepositas his practise, a worke very necessary to be used for the better preservation of the health of man. Wherein are not onely most excellent and approved medicines, receiptes, and ointmentes of great vertue, but also most pretious waters, against many infirmities of the body. The way how to make every the said severall medicines, receiptes, and ointmentes. With a table for the ready finding out of every the diseases, and the remedies for the same. Translated out of Latin into English, by L. M. 12°. *London*, 1588.

NORTH (S.) The family physician and guide to health; together with some remarks on surgery; containing a familiar and accurate description of the symptoms of most diseases incident to mankind; together with their gradual pro-

Medicine (*Popular*).

gress, and method of cure; and tables of preparation, with a medical herbal. The whole selected and compiled from the writings of various authors in Europe and America. 8°. *Waterloo, N. Y.*, 1830.

OEHME (J. A.) Extract der medicinischen Fama, wie die Schwindsucht, Scorbut, Podagra und befleckte Venus, auch andere langwierige und fast incurable Kranckheiten zu curiren seyn. 6. Aufl. 8°. [*Dresden*], 1747.

OLSTADIUS (P.) Laetum philosophorum, von Heimlichkeit der Natur, das ist, wie man nicht allein aus Wein sonder auch aus allen Metallen, Fruchten, Fleisch, Eyern, Wurtzlen, Kreutern und aus viel anderen Dingen mehr sol distilliern Aquam vite zu Erhaltung der Gesundheit menschliches Cörpers. Item, Marsilii Vicini Regiment des Lebens, mit Essen, Trincken, [etc.] Dadurch mit der Hilff Gottes sein Leben gesterckt und in Gesundheit behalten biss er alt worden C und VVI. Darbey viel guten Recept für aller handt Kranckheiten dem gemeinem Mann ein wolffeyle und gar nützliche Apoteck. fol. *Franckf. a. M.*, 1551.

OSIANDER (J. F.) Volksgeneeskunde, of eenvoudige middelen en raadgevingen tegen de kwalen en krankheden der menschen. Naar den tweeden druk uit het Hoogduitsch op nieuw nagezien, meer bijzonder ingerigt, [etc.], door J. A. van Oort. 4. ed. 8°. *Leeuwarden*, 1851.

OVERKAMP (H.) Œconomia animalis, oder gründlicher Unterricht, von der Geburt, Nahrung und Wachsthum des Menschen, worbey unterschiedene über Speiss und Tranck, auch andere zum Leben, nöthige Dinge, vorfallende curieuse Fragen nach den Lehrsätzen Renatus des Cartes erörtert werden. Erstlich durch . . . im Holländischen beschrieben; jetzo ins Hochdeutsche zusammen gezogen von Johann Schreyern. 12°. *Leipzig*, 1690.

PAINE (W.) New school treatment reduced to a science, with rules and directions so plain that all who can read understandingly may treat disease with far better success than physicians of the sectarian schools of physic. 16°. *Philadelphia*, 1875.

PAIRMAN (R.) The great sulphur cure brought to the test; and workings of the new curative machine proposed for human lungs and wind pipes. Preface by the Rev. J. Christison. 8. ed. 8°. *Edinburgh*, 1867.

PALMER (S.) Popular illustrations of medicine. 8°. *London*, 1829.

PANAX der biblische Wunder-Medicus, oder von den Grundursachen der Krankheiten und deren sicherer Heilung nach klaren und geheimnissvollen Anweisungen in der heiligen Schrift. Von einem, der die Wunder solcher Arzneien bei gläubigem Gebete selbst erfahren und an andern gesehen. Wortgetreu nach der Ausgabe von 1787. 16°. *Stuttgart*, 1853.

PANSA (M.) Güldenes Kleinod menschlicher Gesundheit; darinnen die Lehr von des Menschen Gesundheit, als welche unter andern Gütern und Kleinödien dieser Welt das allerfürtrefflichste ist, weitleufftig erkläret, und erstlich der Mensch als eine kleine Welt, mit der grossen Welt verglichen wird, und sonderlich mit dem Bergwerck. Dessgleichen was dem Menschen an seiner Gesundheit und langem Leben hinderlich sey, wie und warumb er allmehlig ins Abnehmen gerathe; Item, wie er in Erwehlung und Correction der mancherley Speisen und des Geträncks gute Discretion halten, und durch alle vier Zeiten des Jahrs in der Diät, Purgation, Schweiss, Aderlässe, Schrepffen, und Stärckungen gute Vorsichtigkeit gebrauchen . . .

Medicine (*Popular*).

Auch wie sich sonderlich die alten Leute mit guten Speisen, Labsal und ausserlesenen Artzneyen wol versehen, oder sonsten in Acht nehmen sollen. 4°. *Leipzig*, 1626.

PARACELSUS (T.) 't gasthuys-boeck. Tot nut ende oirboor van alle ghebreckelijcke ende krancke menschen. Over-geset uyten Hoochduytschen in onse Nederlantsche Duytsche sprake. Door M. Everaert. 12°. *Utrecht*, 1567.

PARKINSON (J.) The villager's friend and physician; or a familiar address on the preservation of health, and the removal of disease on its first appearance; supposed to be delivered by a village apothecary, with cursory observations on the treatment of children, on sobriety, industry, etc. 12°. *London*, 1800.

PASCOLI (A.) Il corpo umano, o breve storia dove con nuovo metodo si descrivono in compendio tutti gli organi suoi, e i loro principali uffizi, per istruire a bene intendere, secondo il nuovo sistema, la teorica e pratica medicinale. 4°. *Venezia*. 1750.

PAULINI (K. F.) Flagellum salutis, das ist: Curieuse Erzählung wie mit Schlägen allerhand schwere langweilige und fast unheylbare Kranckheiten offt bald und wohl curiret worden; durch und durch mit allerly annehmlichen und lustigen Historien, selbsteignen Anmerkungen auch andern feinen Merckwürdigkeiten. 12°. *Franckf. a. M.*, 1698.

——. Neu-vermehrte heilsame Dreck-Apotheke, wie nemlich mit Koth und Urin fast alle, ja auch die schwerste, gifftigste Kranckheiten und bezauberte Schaden vom Haupt biss zu Füssen, inn- und ausserlich, glücklich curiret worden; durch und durch mit allerhand curieusen, so nütz- als ergetzlichen Historien und Anmerckungen, auch andern feinen Denckwürdigkeiten, abermals bewahrt und nun zum dritten Mal um ein merckliches vermehrt und verbessert. 8°. *Franckf. a. M.*, 1699.

——. Kleine, doch curiöse und vermehrte Bauren-Physic, von Neuen mit unterschiedlichen Stücken vermehret und verbessert. 3. Auffl. 12°. *Franckfurt u. Leipzig*, 1719.

——. Flagellum salutis, oder Heilung durch Schläge in allerhand schweren Krankheiten. (Nach der Ausgabe von 1698.) Wunderbare Kuren durch Musik, von F. E. Neidten. Lebensverlängerung bis auf 115 Jahre durch den Hauch junger Mädchen, von F. H. Cohausen. 12°. *Stuttgart*, 1847.

PEEP (A) into the house you live in. An essay on the causes of some of the ailments to which flesh is heir, and on the value of mechanical appliances in their treatment. 16°. [*New York*, 1872.]

PEOPLE'S (The) doctor, containing the treatment and cure of the principal diseases of the human system in plain and simple language, including the history and various modes of treatment of the cholera. Revised by H. P. Gatchell. To which is added facts in domestic matters; being a complete family book. 12°. *Cincinnati*, 1849.

PEOPLE'S (The) doctors; a review, by The people's friend. 8°. *Cincinnati*, 1830.

PETRUS *Hispanus* [*Pope John XXI*]. Thesaurus pauperum viri cujuspiam de medica materia quamoptime meriti. 16°. *Lugduni*, 1530.

——. The same. Thesaurus pauperum de mendendis morbis humani corporis liber; experimenta particularia per simplicia medicamenta ex probatissimis autoribus, et propriis observationibus collecta; nunc primum opera et studio Guilielmi Adolphi Scribonii Marpurgensis in lucem editus. 12°. *Francof. a. M.*, 1576.

Medicine (*Popular*).

PHILIATRUS (E.) Schatz. Ein köstlicher, theürer Schatz, darinn behalten sind vil heimlicher gütter Stuck der Artzni, fürnemlich ab r die Art und Eigenschafft der gebzantnen Wasseren und Oelen, wie man dieselbigen bereiten sölle; dessgleichen jeder Wasseren und Oelen Art und Eigenschafft, Nutz und Brauch. Item, wie man mancherlei Wein bereiten sölle, auch den abgestandnen durch Hilff der gebzannten Wasseren, Gewürtzen unnd anderlei Mat· ri, widerumb helffen möge. Alles mit schönen lieblichen Figürlinen angezeigt unnd für die Augen gestellt, gantz lustig, nutzlich und güt allen Alchimisten, hausshalten, insonders den Balbiereren, Apoteckeren, und allen Liebhaberen der Arzni. Erstlich in Latin, und neüwlich verteütscht durch Joannem Rüdolphum Landenberger. 8°. *Zürich*, 1555.

PICTORIUS (G.) Von Zernichten Artzten. Clarer Bericht ob die Christen von den jüdischen Artzten vertrewlich Artznei gebrauchen mögen. Und wie die jetzleuffig Artzney des Weschens erstlich erdacht, unnd was die für Nutz bringe. Sampt einer Declaration des Betriegens so die Marckt Artzt, und die Heiligen-Schender, die von den Büssen tadlen an allen Orten sich gebrauchen. 12°. [*n. p.*, 1557.]

PIERCE (R. V.) The people's common-sense medical adviser in plain English, or medicine simplified. 8°. *Buffalo*, 1883.

PONS (G.) Triunfo de la medicina, en un méthodo racional, y eficacissimo, para curar radicalmente las enfermedades internas, y externas del cuerpo humano, que el vulgo llama incurables . . . sin molestia del paciente, y sin sangrias, ni remedios irritantes, sí bien con especificos medicamentos, gratos, seguros, y eficacissimos, que, para beneficio del público, se dán de gracia, y de limosna. 4°. *Madrid*, 1753.

DU PORT (F.) La décade de médecine, ou le médecin des riches et des pauvres. Expliquant les signes, les causes, et les remèdes des maladies. Composé en vers latins. Nouvellement mis en vers françois par M. du Four. 12°. *Paris*, 1694.
Title-page and text in Latin and French.

POSNER (E. W.) Medicina pastoralis et ruralis. Ein Hand- und Hülfsbuch für Seelsorger, Aerzte, Lehrer und Menschenfreunde. Nach dem neuesten Standpunkte der Wissenschaft und Erfahrung nach den besten Quellen bearbeitet. 12°. *Glogau*, 1844.

PRÆVOTIUS (J.) Medicina pauperum mira serie continens remedia ad ægrotos cujuscunque generis persanandos aptissima, facile parabilia, extemporanea, et nullius, vel perexigui sumptus. Huic pauperum thesauro adjungitur ejusdem auctoris libellus aureus de venenis. 32°. *Mediolani*, 1646.

——. The same. 24°. *Lugduni*, 1660.

PROBLÈMES (Les) d'Aristote. Œuvre fort agréable et utile aux chirurgiens, et à tous ceux qui veulent aprendre les admirables secrets de la nature. 16°. *Rouen*, 1683.

PUJO (J.-O.) *Considérations contre les doutes et les préjugés du monde relatifs à la médecine. 4°. *Paris*, 1834.

QUEEN'S (The) closet opened. Incomparable secrets in physick, chyrurgery, preserving and candying, etc., which were presented to the queen by the most experienced persons of the times; many whereof were had in esteem when she pleased to descend to private recreations. Corrected and revived. 16°. *London*, 1683.

R. (A.) Most excellent and approved medicines and remedies for most diseases and maladies incident to man's body, lately compiled and extracted out of the originals of the most famous

Medicine (*Popular*).

and best experienced physicians both in England and other countries. 16°. *London*, 1652.

RAITH (J.) Der Mensch und seine Gesundheit. Ein praktisches Familienbuch umfassend: I. Das Urmenschengeschlecht. II. Die Gesundheitslehre und Diätetik der organischen Lebensapparate. III. Degeneration der immunen menschlichen Gesundheitsanlage. IV. Die Regeneration und Regenerationscuren. 8°. *Wien*, 1885.

RALPH (J.) A domestic guide to medicine, by which individuals, both male and female, are enabled to treat their own complaints with perfect safety. To this is prefixed a familiar treatise on the genuine hygeian vegetable pills, or universal remedy of Dr. Ralph, [etc.] 8°. *New York*, 1834.

RAPA (G.) Ricordi igienici sul matrimonio, gravidanza, infanzia offerti alle popolazioni del Cremonese. 8°. *Cremona*, 1873.

RASPAIL (F.-V.) Histoire naturelle de la santé et de la maladie chez les végétaux et chez les animaux en général et en particulier chez l'homme; suivie du formulaire pour une nouvelle méthode de traitement hygiénique et curatif. 8°. *Paris*, 1843.

——. Manuel annuaire de la santé, ou médecine et pharmacie domestiques. 8°. *Paris*, 1845.

——. The same. Manuel annuaire de la santé pour 1883. 12°. *Paris*, 1883.

——. The same. Manuel annuaire de la santé pour 1886. Continué par ses fils. 41e année ou 40e éd., considérablement augmentée. 16°. *Paris & Bruxelles*, 1886.

——. The same. Annual diary of health; or, family physician and druggist. Transl. from the Paris ed. of 1846 by A. Fortier, M. T. A. 8°. *New Orleans*, 1846.

——. The same. Neues Heilverfahren, oder theoretische und praktische Anweisung zur Selbstbehandlung der meisten heilbaren Krankheiten und zur Selbstbereitung der einfachen, billigen und bewahrten Heilmittel der neuen Schule. Hrsg. von J. Müller. 8°. *Bern*, [1885].

RATHGEBER für alle Diejenigen, welche an Verschleimung des Halses, der Lungen und der Verdauungswerkzeuge leiden. Nebst Angabe der Mittel, wodurch diese Krankheiten, selbst wenn sie eingewurzelt sind, sicher geheilt werden können. 5. Aufl. 12°. *Quedlinburg u. Leipzig*, 1827.

REECE (R.) A practical dictionary of domestic medicine, comprising the latest discoveries relating to the causes, treatment, and prevention of diseases. With a popular description of anatomy, casualties, chemistry, cloathing, dietetics, pharmacy, physiology, surgery, midwifery, therapeutics, etc. 8°. *London*, 1808.

——. The Reecean pandect of medicine, containing a new nosological arrangement of diseases, and a new system of physic and medical surgery, founded on anatomy, animal chemistry, and surgery. roy. 8°. *London*, 1812.

——. The medical guide, for the use of the clergy, heads of families, and practitioners in medicine and surgery; comprising a practical dispensatory, and treatise on the symptoms, causes, prevention, and cure of the diseases incident to the human frame; with the latest discoveries in medicine. 10. ed., considerably enlarged and improved. 8°. *London*, 1813.

——. The same. 16. ed. 8°. *London*, 1833.

REMEDI boeexken. Inhoudende hoe men met cleyne kosten ooc met bekende slechte remedien, allerhande krancheden ende sieckten sal ghene-

Medicine (*Popular*).

sen, nut ende profijtelijck zijnde voor een peghelijck. 12°. *Amsterdam*, [*n. d.*]

REMER (F.) Ein sehr sehr nützlichs und heilsams wolgegründets Handtbuchlein, gemeiner Practick aller innerlicher und eusserlicher Ertzney, so wider die abscheuliche Kranckheyt der Frantzosen und Lemung, auch für all ander seuchten so auss diesen Kranckheyten erfolgen, wie die erkennt, und zu gründtlicher Cur mögen gebracht werden. Jetzt aber widerumb von newen obersehen, augirt und gebessert, mit sonderem besten Fleiss. 4°. [*Luningen*], 1571.

RICHTER (C. F.) Höchst-nöthige Erkenntniss des Menschen sonderlich nach dem Leibe und natürlichem Leben, oder ein deutlicher Unterricht; von der Gesundheit und deren Erhaltung; auch von den Ursachen, Kennzeichen und Nahmen der Kranckheiten, und bewährten Mitteln gegen dieselben ... Zum zwölfftenmahl nebst einer Vorrede herausgegeben von dessen Sohne, Christian Friedr. Richtern. 12°. *Leipzig*, 1741.

RIDGE (B.) Ourselves, our food, and our physic. (An entirely new ed.) 8°. *London*, 1884.

ROBINSON (L.) Every patient his own doctor; or, the sick man's triumph over death and the grave. Containing the most approved methods of curing every disease incident to the human body, internal or external ... Also, the methods used by the Humane Society for the recovery of persons apparently drowned or suffocated; a certain cure for the bite of a mad dog, viper, adder, etc.; an infallible remedy against the goal distemper, plague, or any other pestilential disorder, etc. sm. 8°. *London*, [1780].

ROOT (H. K.) The people's medical lighthouse; a series of popular and scientific essays on the nature, uses, and diseases of the lungs, heart, etc. 13. ed. 8°. *New York*, 1856.

ROSCH (D.) Chronic diseases, especially the nervous diseases of women. Translated from the German by Charles Dummig. 8°. *New York*, 1850.

ROSENBERG (C.) Androgynik. Beweis für ein neues naturgemässes Heilverfahren zur Verhütung und Ausrottung aller geheimen Krankheiten und deren Folgeübel und zur Wiederherstellung der Mannheit. In Verbindung mit einem Preservativ gegen Infection. 8°. *London*, [1853].

ROSENSTENGEL (J. J.) Myrothecium privatum parvum et compendiosum, seu methodus medendi generalis, remedia domestica euporista et polychresta sisteus ad omnes corporis humani affectus e triplici naturæ regno ad normam et ductum Danielis Ludovici Med. Duc. Saxo-Gothan. selecta, cum dispensatorio Ludoviciano nec non myrothecia privato parvo et compendioso et sufficientissimo in lucem publicam missa. 4°. *Francof. a. M.*, 1717.

ROUVIÈRE (A.) La médecine sans médecin, ou manuel de santé, ouvrage destiné à soulager les infirmités, à prévenir les maladies aiguës, à guérir les maladies chroniques sans le secours d'une main étrangère. 7. éd. 8°. *Paris*, 1826.

——. The same. 12. éd. 8°. *Paris*, 1829.

ROYER (P.-J.-F.) Le suppléant du chirurgien, ou la médecine et la chirurgie pratiques, mises à la portée du peuple, ouvrage d'un genre neuf, et tout différent de Tissot, etc. Édition corrigée. 4 v. in 2. 8°. *Paris, an X* [1802].

RUCCO (J.) Recherches sur la prolongation de la vie humaine, et sur les moyens de donner à chaque individu une règle sûre pour se guider en état de santé ou de maladie; contenant les principes de la pathologie moderne; l'esquisse d'une nouvelle doctrine et la recette d'une liqueur appelée vitale, à cause de son influence dans la diathèse asthénique, sur les vieillards et dans les

Medicine (*Popular*).

fièvres qu'on remarque principalement dans les armées et les hôpitaux. 8°. *Paris*, 1813.

——. La médecine de la nature protectrice de la vie humaine, à l'usage des praticiens et des gens du monde désireux de suivre le progrès de la médecine rationnelle dans la cure des maladies chroniques opiniâtres aux moyens ordinaires. 8°. *Paris*, [*n. d.*]

RYFF (G.) Confectbuch unnd Hauss-Apotek, kunstlich zu berreiten, einmachen und gebrauchen, wer in ordentlichen Apotecken und Hausshaltungen zur Arznei täglicher Notturffe, unnd auch zum Lust, dienlich unnd nüss, trewliche und Errichtung. So wie dem gemeinem Man nötig, in acht Theyl kürzlich abgeheylt. 18°. [*Frankf. a. M.*], 1570.

RYMER (J.) A treatise upon indigestion and the hypochondriac disease; and upon the inflammatory and atonic gout; with the methods of cure, [etc.] 5. ed. 8°. *London*, 1789.

S. (M. R. C.) Home doctoring; a guide to domestic medicine and surgery. 12°. *London*, [*n. d.*]

SAGGIO sopra le malattie più comuni alla gente di campagna e sopra il metodo di medicarle. Opera utile, e necessaria a qualunque genere di persone. 4°. *Milano*, 1784.

SALMON (W.) Iatrica: seu praxis medendi. The practice of curing; being a medicinal history of above three thousand famous observations in the cure of diseases, performed by the author hereof. Together with several of the choicest observations of other famous men; taken from Crato, Forestus, Hildanus, Skenkius, Rulandus, Zacutus, Platerus, Riverius, Willis, and several others, which are falln into the author's hands in manuscript. 4°. *London*, 1681.

——. A compendium of physick, chirurgery, and anatomy. In iv books. Shewing the signs, causes, judgments, and various ways of curing all diseases, whether external or internal, happing to the bodies of humane kind. Perform'd astrologically, Galenically, and chymically. Illustrated with celestial observations; the judgments of urines and pulses ... and a compleat anatomical idea of the whole body of man. 2. ed. 12°. *London*, 1681.

——. Παραληρήματα; or select physical and chyrurgical observations; containing divers remarkable histories of cures, done by several famous physicians. And above seven hundred eminent cures, in the most usual diseases happening to humane bodies, performed by the author hereof; with useful tables for the whole work, as also large and plain directions for the use of every instrument. 12°. *London*, 1687.

——. Medicina practica; or practical physick, shewing the method of curing the most usual diseases happening to humane bodies ... with the preparation of the præcipiolum, or universal medicine of Paracelsus. To which is added the philosophic works of Hermes Trismegistus, Kalid Persicus, Geber Arabs, Artesius Longævus, Nicholas Flammel, Roger Bachon, and George Ripley. All translated out of the best Latin editions into English ... Together with a singular comment upon the first book of Hermes, the most ancient of philosophers. The whole compleated in three books. 8°. *London*, 1692.

——. Iatrica; seu praxis medendi. The practice of curing diseases. Being a medicinal history of near two hundred famous observations in the cure of diseases, performed by the author hereof ... [v. 1.] 4°. *London*, 1694.

——. Collectanea medica, the country physician; or, a choice collection of physick, fitted for vulgar use. Containing: I. A collection of

Medicine (*Popular*).

choice medicaments of all kinds, Galenical and chymical, excerpted out of the most approved authors. II. Historical observations of famous cures, gathered and selected out of the works of several modern physicians. III. Phylaxæ medicinæ pars prima; or, the first part of the cabinet of specifick, select, and practical chymical preparations made use of by the author. IV. Phylaxæ medicinæ pars secunda; the second part of the same cabinet, long since promised to the world, now made publick, for the general good of mankind. 8°. *London*, 1703.

SAMBIN (J.) Le médecin philanthrope, ou lettres sur la médecine, adressées au clergé des campagnes et à toutes les personnes qui, par bienfaisance, se livrent au traitement des maladies. 8°. *Paris*, 1827.

SAUERMANN (E. F.) * De medicina populari. 4°. *Vratislaviæ*, 1825.

SAVORY (J.) A compendium of domestic medicine, and companion to the medicine chest. 10. ed. 12°. *London*, 1886.

SAWA KOKUKEI. Bioka Suchi. [Valuable information for the sick chamber. A cyclopædia of domestic surgery, obstetrics, and pharmacy, illustrated. A mélange of old Chinese, native Japanese, and Dutch methods.] 8 v. 8°. *Yedo*, 1-23.

SCHAT der armen, of huismedicijn boekje van veelerhande medicamenten, om met kleine kosten zijn eigen doctor te zijn, en velerleije ziektens te genezen. Benevens eene aanwijzing, hoe men de gezondheid lang bewaren kan. Derde druk. 12°. *Rotterdam*, 1749.

SCHMIDT (H.) Dr. H. Schmidt's praktiske Lægebog, med Anvisning for Enhver til at kjende og behandle de hyppigst forekommende Sygdomme og Lidelser. Ved Dr. Rupricht. Samt et Tillæg med Anvisning til sikker Helbredelse af hemmelige Synder og Sygdomme og deres Følger. 16°. *Kjøbenhavn*, [*n. d.*]

SCHÖNER (J.) Ein nutzlichs buchlein, viler bewerter Artzney, launge zeyt versamlet und zusammen bracht. Von allerley Kranckhaiten so einem menschen begegnen mögen, mit einem nützlichen unterricht, zu welchen zeyten solche und andere artzney dem Krancken zu gut zu gericht und geraicht sollen werdenn, nach dem lauffe unnd mansion des Mons, [etc.] 4°. [*Nürmberg*, 1528.]

——. The same. sm. 4°. *Franckf. a. M.*, 1649.

SCHOOL (The) of arts; or, the fountain of knowledge, containing among a variety of other information: I. How to diet our bodies ... II. To beautify the face or skin ... Also, the royal physician, being a general collection of most approved recipes for every distemper incident in the human body. 12°. *London*, [*n. d.*]

SCHOONDERMARK (J.), jr. Een boekje voor menschen die ver van een arts verwijderd wonen. 16°. *'s Hertogenbosch*, 1885.

——. Een boekje voor maag- en buiklijders (aambeien). 16°. *'s Hertogenbosch*, [1885].

SCHORDANN (S.) * De medicina populari. 8°. *Pestini*, [1817].

SCHORER (C.) Medicina peregrinantium, oder: Artzney der Raisenden, worinnen begriffen, wie sich die Raisenden in Essen und Trincken, etc., verhalten, und zugleich allerlei Krankheiten begegnen sollen. Zwar nicht nur den Raisenden allein, sondern auch allen Liebhabern der Natur und Gesundheit nützlich zu lesen. 12°. *Ulm*, 1663.

SCHREGER (C. H. T.) Handbuch der Pastoral-Medicin für christliche Seelsorgen. 8°. *Halle*, 1823.

2

Medicine (*Popular*).

SCHRÖDTERN (C.) Wohlerfahrner englischer und jetzo ins Teutsche übersetzte Haus-Artzt in sich haltend die aller raresten und nützlichsten Curen der Menschen, in unterschiedlichen Theilen, [etc.] 8°. *Franckfurdt u. Leipzig*, 1719.

SCOT (J.) Histories of gouty, bilious, and nervous cases, with the safe and easy means by which they were remedied, related by the patients themselves in sundry letters to . . . 8°. *London*, 1780.

SCOTT (G.) Friendly counsels on health; hints for the household; rules for the sick chamber in fever and other infectious cases; how to avoid infection. 8°. *Glasgow*, [*n. d.*]

SCOTT (J. W.) The university guide to health; explaining the causes, symptoms, and treatment of various diseases, hygiene, and the administration of the university medicines. 32°. *New York*, [*n. d.*]

SCUDDER (J. M.) A familiar treatise on medicine. 10. ed. 2 v. in 1. 8°. *Cincinnati*, 1869.

SEARLE (C.) The why and the wherefore; or, the philosophy of life, health, and disease; new and original views explanatory of their nature, causes, and connexion . . . of the treatment of disease upon a few general principles, based upon the laws of nature and common sense; with observations on certain means of renovation of the system. 8°. *London*, 1846.

SEE (J.) Family medicine; or, a treatise on the prevention and cure of fevers, dysentery, and several other diseases. 8°. *New York*, 1833.

SEELIG (G. A.) Des freywillig aufgesprungenen Grenat-Apffels des christlichen Samariters anderer Theil: oder aus christlicher Liebe des nächsten eröffnete Geheimnüsse vieler vortreflicher bewährter Artzneyen, worinnen enthalten die sicherste und beste Methode, die meisten Kranckheiten, Gebrechen und Schwachheiten des menschlichen Leibes, durch die Gnade Gottes sicher und geschwind zu heilen. Dem gemeinen Man zu sonderbaren Nutzen auf Begehren gründlich und deutlich beschrieben. 4. Aufl. 4°. *Wien*, 1753.

SHANNON (R.) Practical observations on the operation . . . of certain medicines in . . . diseases . . . in hot climates . . . written in a familiar style . . . to which are added plain directions for private use in the absence of a physician, [etc.] 8°. *London*, 1794.

SHELTON'S American medicine; or, improvement in uniting his new steam system, and the old practice of medicine; in which doctors' terms are explained, and the complaints of men, women, and children are treated of in a satisfactory manner; and remedies suited to all climates, constitutions, and circumstances of the American people. The valuable practice and preparations of Dr. Isaac Wright, of Tennessee, are fully developed in this work. 8°. *Madisonville, Tenn.*, 1834.

SHERWOOD (H. H.) The motive power of the human system, with the symptoms and treatment of chronic diseases. 8°. *New York*, 1841.
——. The same. 10. ed. 8°. *New York*, 1847.

SIBLY (E.) Medizinischer Spiegel. Oder über die Befruchtung des weiblichen Menschen, den Ursprung der Krankheiten und die Ursachen des Lebens und des Todes. Aus dem Englischen übersezt. 16°. *Leipzig*, 1796.

SIGISMUND (J.) An Herrn D. Andream Petermann, wegen eines Corallarii, multæ hactenus insolitæ laudatæ enchireses in libro, cui titulus est: Die Chur-Brandenburgische Hof-Wehe-Mutter, nituntur vana speculatione; in praxi enim sunt absurdæ. Hinc jure miramur; quo-

Medicine (*Popular*).

modo liber sustinere potuerit censuram totius Collegii medici. Zu Deutsch also lautend: Viele bisshero ungewöhnliche gepriesene Handgriffe in dem Buch, die Chur-Brandenb. Hof-Wehe-Mutter benennet, bestehen auf eine eitele Speculation; dann in der Ubung seyn sie ungereimt. Darum wundern wir uns billig, wie dieses Buch die Censur eines gantzen Collegii medici habe ausdauern können. So in der Disputation de gonorrhæa unter seinem Præsidio zu Leipzig gehalten 1690, d. 5. Dec. Abgelossenes Send-Schreiben. 4°. *Cölln an der Spree*, 1692.

SKELTON (J.) Family medical adviser. 8°. *Leeds*, 1852.
——. The same. 8. ed. 12°. *London*, 1866.

SMID (H.) En skøn nyttelig Lægebog indeholdendis mange atskillige skøne oc forfarne Lægedomme, hvilcke som tiene Bartskerrerne, oc dem som ville lage ferske og gamle Saar. 4°. *Kiøbenhaffn*, 1577.

SMITH (E.) The American physician and family assistant. In five parts, containing: 1. A general description of vegetable medicines. 2. The manner of preparing them for use. 3. Description of diseases and manner of curing them. 4. A description of mineral and vegetable poisons, given by those called regular doctors, under the name of medicines. 3. ed. sm. 8°. *Boston*, 1832.
——. The same. In five parts . . . 5. Health variously illustrated. 4. ed. 12°. *Boston*, 1837.
——. An address to the citizens of Boston, and the people of the United States, on poison, health, disease, vegetable medicine, and manner of curing the sick. 12°. *Boston*, 1836.

SMITH (H.) Formulæ medicamentorum; or, a compendium of the modern practice of physic. To which is prefixed an essay on the effects and uses of blood-letting. 4. ed. 12°. *London*, 1781.
——. The family physician; being a collection of useful family remedies . . . And a short account of those cases in which bleeding and blisters are really serviceable. 9. ed. 4°. *London*, [*n. d.*]

SMITH (J.) Udkast til en "Medicina ruralis" eller medicinsk Haandbog for Landmanden. 12°. *Kiøbenhavn*, 1794.

SMITH (L. L.) The means of prolonging life and avoiding diseases. With which is incorporated, "How to get fat and thin". 12°. *Melbourne*, 1870.
——. Medical household sketches; or, popular treatises, for parlour and bush-hut, on the diseases prevalent in Australasia. 12°. [*Melbourne, n. d.*]
——. The same. No. 2. 12°. [*Melbourne, n. d.*]

SMITH (W.) Nature studied with a view to preserve and restore health . . . with an account of a most powerful and safe deobstruent medicine, [etc.] 8°. *London*, 1774.

SMYTHSON (H.) The compleat family physician, or universal medical repository, containing the causes, symptoms, prevention, and cures of all the various maladies to which human nature is liable, with an account of every celebrated spa, British and foreign, and strictures on quackery; the compleat British herbal; observations on tea, coffee, tobacco, and snuff; and a great variety of most extraordinary cases in physic and surgery; the whole forming a compleat body of domestic medicine, calculated as well to assist gentlemen of the faculty as for the use of private families. 4°. *London*, 1785.

SOCIETY for the Diffusion of Useful Knowledge. The workingman's companion. The physician: I. The cholera. 16°. *London*, 1832.

Medicine (*Popular*).

SOLOMON (S.) A guide to health; or, advice to both sexes, in nervous and consumptive complaints, [etc.] 54. ed. 8°. *New York*, [*n. d.*]

SQUIRRELL (R.) Maxims of health; or, an abridgment of an essay on indigestion; containing advice to persons afflicted with indigestion, nervous, bilious, and gouty disorders; headach, female complaints, worms, etc.; also remarks on sea and cold bathing, the effects of sea air, [etc.] 12°. *London*, 1798.

STATMION (C.) Ein kürtzer doch volkümlicher Bericht, wie man sich in Sterbensleufften halten sol, jedermeniglichen zu gut, Beden denen so von Ampts oder Berüffs wegen nicht gebüret und auch denen so Armut uñ not halben nicht müglich ist zu weichen, sehr nützs unnd gantz tröstlich. 4°. *Cobürgk*, 1551.

STEINHAUSER (G.) Einfache Mittel gegen Unterleibs-Anschoppungen, schwere Verdauung und Blähungs-Beschwerden, nebst einem Anhange über die gebräuchlichsten und besten magenstärkenden und blähungtreibenden Mittel, und Angabe der schwer und der leicht verdaulichen, dabei viel oder wenig nährenden Nahrungsmittel. 8°. *Wien*, 1844.

STEWARD (W.) The first edition of . . . healing art, corrected and improved by the original hand . . . To which he has added, a concise herbal, containing a full description of herbs, roots, barks, and plants, both in their simple and compound use; with a description of their soils and the countries where they are generally found. 12°. *Saco, Maine*, 1827.

[STEWART (A.)] Some account of the life of the author, together with many observations on various diseases of the human frame. With full and copious directions for combining and using his compound vegetable and other pills. 8°. *Roxbury*, 1834.

STÖCKHLIN (Anna Maria). Artzney Buech; worinnen vill un erschidlich guete Hausmitl zu finden. MS. fol. [*n. p., 16th century.*]

STRAUSS (G.) Die Heilkraft der Natur, ihre Erkenntniss im Allgemeinen, und in Beziehung auf die Grundsätze der Zoochirurgie insbesondere dargestellt für Aerzte und Thierärzte. 8°. *Wien*, 1829.

STRONG (S. S.) Lung, female, and chronic diseases. 16°. *New York*, 1866.

STROTHERS (E.) Euodia; or, a discourse on causes and cures. In 2 pts. 8°. *London*, 1718.

STRÜPP (J.) Hochnötiger unterricht geistlicher und leiblicher Artzney in jetzigen Leufften widerumb auffs new gemehret, sampt einem trewhertzigen Consilio medico wie es sonsten auch jederzeit allenthalben nützlich und löblich zu halten. 16°. *Franckfort*, 1567.

STRUVE (C. A.) Krankenbuch. Ueber die Erhaltung des menschlichen Lebens, Verhütung und zweckmässige Behandlung der Krankheiten. 2 v. 12°. *Breslau, Hirschberg u. Lissa in Südpreussen*, 1798–9.

SUNDERLAND (L.) Theory of nutrition. The treatment of disease, and philosophy of healing without medicine. 8°. *Boston*, 1855.

SYMPATHETISCHE (Der) Hausarzt, oder die enthüllten Zauberkräfte der Natur. Eine Sammlung der von den Mysterien des Alterthums, Theophrastus Paracelsus, Albertus Magnus, etc., bis auf die neueste Zeit bewährtesten sympathetischen und magnetischen Curarten, und vieler hundert der wunderbarsten mit dem glänzendsten Erfolg gekrönten und vielfach erprobten Heilmittel gegen die schwersten, bis jetzt für unheilbar gehaltenen Krankheiten und Gebrechen. 2. Aufl. 16°. *Reutlingen*, [1856?]

Medicine (*Popular*).

TANNER (J.) The hidden treasures of the art of physick fully discovered. In four books, containing: I. A physical description of man. II. The causes, signs and cures of all diseases incident to the body. III. The general cure of wounds, tumors, and ulcers. IV. A general rule for making all kinds of medicines; with the use and nature of distilled waters, juyces, decoctions, conserves, powders, electuaries, plasters, etc. To which is added three necessary tables: I. Sheweth the contents of the four books. II. Explaineth all the terms of art which are used in physick and chyrurgery. III. Explaining the nature and use of simples; what they are and where they grow. A work whereby the diligent reader may, without the help of other authors, attain to the knowledge of the art above named. 3. ed. 12°. *London*, 1672.

TAYLER (P.) Tayler's ready doctor; or, cures suitable for most distempers incident to the human body . . . To which is added a treatise on bleeding. 8°. *Falkirk*, 1785.

TAYLOR (T. K.) The medical pocket companion, or domestic adviser; designed for both married and single; containing a brief description of the causes, symptoms, and treatment of the most common and obstinate diseases which affect humanity; together with many valuable hints upon the preservation of health and the proper management of infancy and childhood. New stereotype ed. 12°. *Boston*, 1858.

TEGETMEIER (W. B.) A manual of domestic economy; with hints on domestic medicine and surgery. 5 ed., revised and enlarged. 16°. *London*, 1860.

THEOBALD (J.) Every man his own physician. Being a complete collection of efficacious and approved remedies for every disease incident to the human body; with plain instructions for their common use, necessary to be had in all families, particularly those residing in the country. Compiled at the command of his royal highness the Duke of Cumberland. 8°. *London*, 1764.

———. The same. A new ed., improved. 8°. *London*, 1766.

———. The same. 8°. *London*, 1770.

THOMAS (W.) The safety-valve of life. How to prevent disease and promote health. Vaccination and its results. Why have fevers and smallpox? The soul and brain-startling ideas. Brain fever and the ice-pad treatment. Cholera and hydrophobia. Facts from personal experience, showing how life and health was restored, [etc.] 8°. *London*, 1885.

THOMSON (A.) The family physician; or, domestic medical friend. 8°. *New York*, 1802.

TILKE (S. W.) An autobiographical memoir, with remarks on the various incidents which have occurred during forty-five years of his life, and a full description of his mode of treating diseases, with reasons explanatory of his system. 8°. *London*, 1840.

TOLLAT (I.) Margarita medicinæ, ein meysterlichs ausserlesens Büchlein der Artzney. Für mancherley Kranckheyt und Siechtagen der Menschen. Gemacht der weit berühmten Universitet zu Wien bey dem aller erfarnisten Mann der Artzney Doctor Schwick. 4°. *Nürnberg*, 1516.

TOWN (The) and country friend and physician; or, an affectionate address on the preservation of health and the removal of disease on its first appearance, supposed to be delivered by a country physician to the circle of his friends and patients on his retiring from business; with cursory observations on the treatment of children, etc. In-

Medicine (*Popular*).

tended for the promotion of domestic happiness. In 2 pts. 12°. *Philadelphia*, 1803.

TRALL (R. T.) Die wahre vernunftgemässe Heilkunde im Gegensatze zur Medicin-Heilkunde. 8°. *Berlin*, 1868.

——. Die Kehl- und Lungen-Krankheiten. 8°. *Berlin*, 1870.

——. Die Arzneimittel, ihre Natur, ihre Folgen und Wirkungen. Eine populäre Darlegung der falschen Lehren, auf welche ihre Anwendung sich stützt. 8°. *Berlin*, 1871.

——. The hygienic system. 12°. *Battle Creek, Mich.*, 1872.

TREATISE (A) of diseases of the head, brain, and nerves. More especially of the palsy, apoplexy, lethargy, epilepsy, convulsions, frenzy, vertigo, megrim, inveterate headache, etc., with directions for their thorough cure, and how these and many other deplorable nervous distempers may be prevented as well as cured, and consequently many lives saved by the medicines herein, in English, prescribed without the least reserve. To which is subjoined a discourse on the nature, real cause, and certain cure of melancholy in men and vapours in women; instructing persons how to cure themselves absolutely of those perplexing and pernicious disorders with safety, ease, and expedition. By a physician. 5. ed. 8°. *London*, 1727.

TREATISE (A) on the diseases most prevalent in the United States, with directions for medicine chests. Designed for the use of families. 8°. *Philadelphia*, 1821.

TROOST (Den) der armen, behelzende lighte en souvereijne remedien, tegen verscheijde ziekten, wonden, gezwellen en andere kwaelen des menschens lichaem. sm. 8°. *Gend*, [1712].

TSUDA GENSEN. Rioji Sadan. [Tea-table talks on medicine.] 10 v. 8°. *Yedo*, 1770. Japanese text.

UNIVERSALLY (The) experienced family physitian; or every man and woman their own doctor and chirurgeon. Setting forth the nature, causes, signs, and cure of disease, pains, and griefs incident to men, women, and children, as also how to preserve health, and prevent sickness, to know by various symptoms and dispositions of the body when diseases are approaching, and what remedies are proper to antidote them by almost a never-failing method . . . To which is added a brief herbal, shewing the nature and virtue of herbs, and their physical use; how to prevent miscarriages and abortion, also the pica or immoderate longings of women with child, and many other useful things never before made publick. 16°. *London*, 1720.

VAIDEN (T. J.) The commencement of a practical system of medicine to meet the premonitions of disease, and to secure on rational principles more uniform popular benefit, on the immediate and absolute requirements of nature, through her earliest co-operation, with permanent and satisfactory pledges as to the medicine used in all the departments of fevers of general character. 8°. *Mobile*, 1845.

[VANDERMONDE (C.-A.)] Dictionnaire portatif de santé . . . Le tout recueilli des ouvrages, tant anciens que modernes, des médecins les plus fameux, et augmenté d'une infinité de recettes particulières, et de spécifiques pour toutes sortes de maladies, par M. L. . . . et M. de B. . . . 3 v. 12°. *Paris*, 1760-71.

VAUSSARD (G.) L'opérateur des pauvres, ou la fleur d'opération nécessaire aux pauvres pour conserver leur santé et soy guérir à peu de frais. Où se monstre un discours de opérateurs, avec les remèdes de purgation, le prix que coustent

Medicine (*Popular*).

les drogues, et les moyens de les appliquer. Ensemble le secret du baulme policreston, sa vertu, et autres secrets admirables. 16°. *Troyes*, 1645.

VICARY (T.) The Englishman's treasure; with the true anatomie of man's bodie. Whereunto are annexed many secrets appertaining to chirurgerie, with divers excellent approved remedies for all diseases the which are in man or woman; with emplasters of speciall cure; with other potions and drinkes approved in phisicke. Also the rare treasure of the English bathes. Written by William Turner. Gathered and set forth for the benefit of his friends and countrymen in England, by William Bremer. 8°. *London*, 1599.

——. The same. . . . With divers excellent approved remedies for all captaines and souldiers, that travell eyther by water or land; and likewise for all diseases which are eyther in man or woman . . . and now eighthly augmented and enlarged, with almost a thousand approved waters and medicines, meet and necessarie for physicke and chirurgie; as also oyntment and plaisters; with especiall and approved remedies for the plage, and pestilent fever; by W. B. 8°. *London*, 1633.

VINDEVOGEL (J.) Le guide du poitrinaire, ou méthode à suivre pour prévenir et guérir les maladies du sang et de la poitrine ainsi que la débilité constitutionnelle. 24°. *Bruxelles*, 1881.

——. Recueil clinique, ou répertoire des traitements nouveaux. 24°. *Bruxelles*, 1881.

VITTER (J. C.) Artznei Büchlein, angefangen den 29. Octobris A. 1656. MS. 4°. [*n. p., n. d.*]

VOGEL (S. G.) Kleine Schriften zur populairen Medizin für gebildete Leser, die der Arzneiwissenschaft unkundig sind. 3 v. in 1. 16°. *Berlin*, 1814-17.

VOGTER (B.) Ein nutzlich und nothwendigs Artzney Büchlein für den gemaynen Menschenn, [etc.] 4°. [*Augspurg*, 1533.]

——. Wie man alle Gebresten und Kranckheiten des menschlichen Leibs, ausswendig und ynnwendig, von dem Haupt an biss auf die Füss, ärtzneyen und vertreyben soll, mit ausssepranten Wassern. sm. 4°. *Augspurg*, 1533.

——. The same. 4°. *Franckf. a. M.*, 1550.

VOISIN (B.) Le médecin familier et sincère; qui apprend à un chacun à se guérir soi-même de toutes les maladies vénériennes de même que de la goutte nouvelle, et de calmer les douleurs de celle qui est invétérée, et d'en retarder les attaques des années entières et même plus et de guérir plusieurs autres différentes espèces de maladies avec son secret qu'il a du dépuratif du sang, et de sa panacée végétale. 16°. *Turin*, 1761.

VOUGHT (J. G.) Treatise on bowel complaints; intended for the use of physicians, families, parents, masters of vessels, etc., in the United States. 16°. *Rochester, N. Y.*, 1823.

W. (G.) A rich storehouse or treasurie for the diseased, wherein are many approved medicines for divers and sundry diseases, which have been long hidden and not come to light before this time. First set foorth for the benefit and comfort of the poorer sort of people, that are not of ability to goe to the phisitions. And now sixtly augmented and inlarged by A. T., practitioner in physicke and chirurgerie. sm. 4°. *London*, 1616.

——. The same. 8°. *London*, 1630.

——. The same. 8°. *London*, 1631.

——. The same. The 8. ed., enlarged by D. B. 4°. *London*, 1650.

WALKER (B. B.) The Indian practice of medicine; being a treatise, divested of professional

Medicine (*Popular*).

terms, on the nature, causes, symptoms, and treatment of the diseases of men, women, and children; with appropriate prescriptions, in English. By Benjamin B. Walker, student of Dr. Richard Carter, jr., of Kentucky. 12°. *Louisville*, 1847.
Wants pp 111–119.

WALLACE (*Mrs.* C. L. H.) Physianthrophy; or, the home cure and eradication of disease. sm. 8°. *London*, [*n. d.*]

WALLIS (G.) The art of preventing diseases and restoring health, founded on rational principles, and adapted to persons of every capacity. 8°. *London*, 1793.

WALWYN (W.) Physick for families; or the new, safe, and powerful way of physick, upon constant proof established, enabling every one, at sea or land, by the medicines herein mentioned, to cure themselves, their friends, and relations, in all distempers and diseases. Without any [of] the trouble, hazzard, pain, or danger of purgers, vomiters, bleedings, issues, glisters, blisters, opium, antimony, and quicksilver, so full of perplexity in sickness. 16°. *London*, 1696.

WEICKER (G.) Die Natur heilt, oder das Wasser und die Pflanzenkost in ihrer Beziehung zur Lebens- und Heilkraft in gesunden und kranken Tagen. 8°. *Leipzig*, [1884].

——. Die Natur heilt, oder die Wasser- und Diätkur in ihrer Beziehung zur Heilkraft des menschlichen Körpers. Ein Beitrag zur Frage: Was giebt Lebenskraft? Zugleich Wegweiser in der arzneilosen Heilkunde und volksverständlichen Gesundheitspflege. Mit Heilerfolgen aus der Praxis versehen. 2. Aufl. 8°. *Auerbach*, [*n. d.*]

[WESLEY (J.)] Primitive physick, or an easy and natural method of curing most diseases. 8°. *London*, 1747.

——. The same. 22. ed. 8°. *Philadelphia*, 1791.

——. The same. 23. ed. 12°. *Philadelphia*, 1793.

——. The same. 24. ed. Revised and enlarged by W. M. Cornell. 12°. *Boston*, 1858.

——. The same. 26. ed., corrected. 12°. *New York*, 1804.

——. The same. 27. ed., corrected. 16°. *New York*, 1814.

——. The same. Wesley's family physician, revised, and Ware's medical adviser. A book of receipts, with directions for the use of Dr. Samuel Thomson's medicine and bath. For the benefit of families, clergymen, philanthropists, and reformers. By T. E. Ware. 27. ed. of the Primitive physic. 12°. *Salem, N. J.*, 1839.

WHITNEY (D. H.) The family physician, or every man his own doctor; in three parts. Together with the history, causes, symptoms, and treatment of Asiatic cholera; a glossary, explaining the most difficult words that occur in medical science, and a copious index and appendix. 8°. *New York*, 1834.

CONTENTS.

Part I. Contains the theory and practice of physic.
Part II. Diseases of women and children, and the botanic practice.
Part III. Dispensatory, anatomy, and the practice of surgery.

WILKES (F. C.) A manual of practice for the diseases of Texas. 2. ed. 8°. *Chappell Hill, Tex.*, 1867.

WILKINS (H.) The family adviser, or a plain and modern practice of physic, calculated for

Medicine (*Popular*).

the use of private families, and accommodated to the diseases of America. To which is annexed Mr. Wesley's Primitive physic, revised. 12°. *Philadelphia*, 1793.

——. The same. 4. ed., corrected. 12°. *New York*, 1804.

——. The same. 5. ed. 16°. *New York*, 1814.

WILLEMIER (G. A. F. Q.) Handleiding der bijzondere natuurkunde van den zieken mensch en der geneeskundige behandelingswijze der ziekten. Ten gebruike bij het onderwijs aan 's Rijks kweekschool voor militaire geneeskundigen. 2. deel. 8°. *Utrecht*, 1852.

WILLIAMS (J.) Last legacy, and useful family guide. 8°. *New York*, 1826.

WILSON. Der kranke Mensch, oder Ursache und Heilung der Krankheiten. Belehrungen, wie man die Gesundheit bewahren und Krankheiten durch ein sicheres, wissenschaftliches, angenehmes, wirksames und Jedermann zugängliches Mittel heilen kann. 8°. *Berlin*, 1873.

WINKLER (T. C.) Dokter en patiënt. 12°. *'s-Hertogenbosch*, [1880].

WITTICH (J.) Præservator sanitatis. Ein nützlicher Bericht von den sechs unvermeidlichen Dingen, zur Gesundheit gantz erspriesslichen, wie man sich in denselben beydes zu Hause, und auch über Land verhalten sol. Alles auf die deutsche übliche Kost, Speise und Tranck gerichtet, und mit Sententiosis versibus, alten Rythmis, und guten Ertzneymitteln gezieret. Dabey auch ein Verzeichnis oder Teffelein einer Reise-Apotecken, denjenigen sehr nützlich, so stets über Land reisen müssen, solcher in vorfallenden Nöten zu gebrauchen. Zu Ehren und günstigem Gefallen allen Liebhabern der Gesundheit gestalt. 12°. *Leipzig*, 1590.

——. Arcula itineraria. Das ist: Reisekästlein, für allerhand zukünfftigen Kranckheiten, von vielen nützlichen und probierten Stücken, so in fürfallenden Nöhten kräfftig können gebraucht werden, mit höchstem Fleiss zusammen getragen. Darzu ein kurtzer und hochnötiger Bericht, von den Extractionibus, so man jetziger Zeit auch mit grossem Nutz zu gebrauchen pfleget. Item, von des Theriacæ Andromachi und Mithridati Damocratis rechtem Gebrauch in allerhand Kranckheiten. 12°. *Leipzig*, 1590.

——. The same. Jetzo auffs Newe übersehen, corrigirt, vermehrt und in Druck gegeben. 12°. [*n. p.*], 1607.

——. Vade mecum, das ist: Ein künstlich new Artzneybuch, so man stets bey sich haben und führen kan, in fürfallender Not sich Hülff daraus zu erholen, wider allerhand Kranckheit des menschlichen Leibes, vom Heupt an bis auff die Fussohlen. In gewisse Capitel unnd richtige Ordnung gebracht, und mit guten, heilsamen, schlechten, einfeltigen und zusammen gesetsten Mitteln, aus vieler hochgelährter Leute Bücher, gezieret. Auch zum Anfang ein Unterricht gesatzt, wie man durchs gantze Jahr, gute Gesundheit erhalten möge. Sampt eines vornemen erfarnen Münchs Experimentlein, welcher zu Zeit Fridirici, des ersten Churfürsten zu Sachsen, gelebet, und in sehr grossem Beruff gewesen. Allen Haussvätern, hohes und niedern Standes Personen gantz nützlich. Dergleichen zuvor niemals also in Druck kommen. sm. 4°. *Leipzig*, 1595.

WOLBEWÄHRTE (Der) Kräuter-Artzt, welcher in allerhand Kranckheiten, Wunden und Schäden, so wol bey erwachsenen Manns- und Weibs-Personen, als auch bey kleinen Kindern; des-

Medicine (*Popular*).

gleichen bey Schwangern, Kreisenden, Sechs-wöchnerinnen und Säugenden, durch geringe und sichere Mittel, baldige Hülffe und erwünschte Genesung verschaffen kan. Allen Nothleiden-den zum besten an das Licht gestellet von G. C. W. 16°. *Franckfurt u. Leipzig,* 1725.

WOLFIUS (H.) Tractatus und kurtzer Be-richt, wie man sich vermittelst Göttlicher Hülff, vor der jetzo anfahenden, regierenden Seuche der gifftigen, Pestilentz præserviren, verhalten, dienlichen Mitteln verwahren, und was teglich, so wol ad præservationem, als dann auch cura-tionem, nötig Gebrauch werden könne. Allen den jenigen, da diese Seuche angefangen zu grassiren (oder welches Gott der Allmechtige gnediglich abwenden wolle), inkünfftigen regie-ren möchte. Insonderheit aber denen nothlei-denden Mitchristen, und gemeinem Mann in Vi-cinia, welche der Herren Doctoren und Medico-rum consilia nicht gebrauchen und erreichen können. Aus fürnehmer Herren Doctoren Scrip-tis und Consiliis zu Nutz und Gut colligiret, zusammen gebracht, auch auff begehren wol-meynendlich in Druck verfertiget. sm. 4°. *Gosslar,* 1625.

WOODMAN (P.) Medicus novissimus; or, the modern physician; shewing the principal sigus, causes, and most material prognosticks; to-gether with the true method of curing all the principal and curable diseases incident to man-kind, according to the most modern and best method of practice now in use, [etc.] sm. 8°. *London,* 1712.

[WRIGHT (J.)] The treasurie of hidden se-crets; commonly called the good-huswive's closet of provision for the health of her houshold. Gath-ered out of sundry experiments lately practised by men of great knowledge, and now newly en-larged, with divers necessary physicke helpes, and knowledge of the names and naturall dis-position of diseases that most commonly happen to men and women. Not impertinent for every good huswife to use in her house, amongst her owne familie. sm. 4°. *London,* 1627.

YOUTH'S (The) health-book. 18°. *New York,* 1878.

ZAÁR (L. G.) Nödhjelpare, eller ordbok till anvisning af förnuftsenliga, på säker erfarenhet grundade och minst kostsamma huskurer med allmänt tillgängliga medel, för mindre bemed-lade och fattiga samt i allmänhet dem, som nödgas sakna nog skyndsamt läkare-biträde i de allmännaste sjukdoms-faror; jemte erinringar om de angelägnaste fall, då läkares särskildta råd och hjelp ovilkorligen äro af nöden. [An aid, or phrase-book, for instruction in a rational manner as to cures, with plain, easy remedies, etc.] 8°. *Götheborg,* 1840.

ZIMPEL (C. F.) Der medizinische Haus-Schatz. Neue und alte Heilmittel für Jedermann. Mit besonderer Rücksicht auf die Ars spagyrica, und deren Anwendung zur Bereitung von ausseror-dentlichen medizinischen Geheimmitteln, nebst einigen Bemerkungen über die Universalmedi-zin der Hermetik. 8°. *Bern,* 1870.

ZIPPERLEN (J. B.) Hülfsbüchlein zur Ge-sundheitslehre für alle Stände. Eine gemein-nützige Anleitung zum wirksammen Gebrauch des kalten Wassers in Verbindung mit Bewe-gung in freier Luft und Mässigkeit als der ein-fachsten Mittel zur Förderung des körperlichen Wohlseyns wie zum Schutze gegen Krankheiten. 12°. *Stuttgart,* 1844.

ZWINGER (T.) Sicherer und geschwinder Artzte, oder neues Artzney-Buch, worinnen alle und jede Kranckheiten des menschlichen Leibs,

Medicine (*Popular*).

nach Ordnung des Alphabeths gründlich und deutlich beschrieben; und wie sie gantz sicher und geschwind durch die Gnad Gottes zu heilen, so wol auss eigener, als auss vieler welt-berühm-ten Aertzten langwiriger Erfahrung kurtzlich an den Tag geleget wird. Denen auff dem Land wohnenden, von Aertzen abgelegenen nothlei-denden Leuten, wie auch anderen Liebhabern der edlen Artzneykunst vielfältigem Nutzen. 4. Aufl. 12°. *Basel,* 1703.

——. Die Gestalt eines fürsichtigen Freundes in der Noth. Das ist: Der mitleidige und gewis-senhaffte Apothecker, wie derselbe seine Officin nach einem bey allen verständigen Medicis nun-mehro angenommenen rationalen Medendi me-thodo einrichten und dieser wol fürstehen, als auch die Artzneyen präpariren und nach denen Grund-Regeln der heutigen Distillir-Kunst zu-bereiten, hernach die bewahrtesten Mittel recom-mendiren und mittheilen soll. Neue Aufl. 12°. *Nürnberg,* 1721.

Bartlett (W. R.) Doctors; or, the science of medical thought among the people. Sanitarian, N. Y., 1879, vii, 112-121.—**Beach** (S.) Remarks on popularizing medical truth. Proc. Connect. M. Soc., Hartford, 1853, 61-73.—**Bolschwing.** Volksmedicin der Letten. Repert. f. d. ges. Med., Jena, 1843, vii, 1-5.—**Bondeson** (A.) Om folkets läkekonst i mellersta Halland. Upsala Läkaref. Förh., 1880-81, xvi, 214-221.—**Cohen** (J. S.) Kitchen med-icine. Phila. M. Times, 1873-4, iv, 146.—**Corre** (A.) La médecine populaire au Mexique; analyse et fragments du Trésor de médecine, du R. P. Grégoire Lopez. Gaz. hebd. de méd., Par., 1869, 2. s., vi, 478-480.—**Diday.** Rédiger pour les ouvriers lyonnais un opuscule où ils puissent trou-ver les notions qu'il leur importe le plus de posséder sur leurs intérêts hygiéniques et sanitaires. [Rap. sur les Mé-moires.] Gaz. méd. de Lyon, 1856, viii, 85-91.—**van Dis-sel** (J. A.) Behandeling van ziekten door de Doekoens (inlandsche volks-geneeskundigen) met inlandsche genees-middelen. Nederl. Tijdschr. v. Geneesk., Amst., 1867, 2. R., iii, Afd. 1, 407. — **Domashniaja** apteka. [House apothecary.] Zdorovje, St. Petersb., 1885, xii, nos. 1-6 — **Domestic** quackery. Med. & Phys. J., Lond., 1802, vii, 392-396.—**Heller** (A.) Ueber Volks- und Geheimmittel. Schrift. d. naturw. Ver. f. Schlesw.-Holst., Kiel, 1878, iii, 1-21.—**Hendley** (T. H.) The "Umrit Sagur". Indian M. Gaz., Calcutta, 1874, ix, 6; 91; 119; 171; 234; 291.—**Hof-mann.** Anklage wegen unbefugten Verkaufs eines Ge-heimmittels. Ztschr. f. d. Staatsarznk., Erlang., 1863, lxxxvi, 343-358.—**Kirschleger** (F.) La médecine popu-laire et les herboristes à Strasbourg. Gaz. méd. de Strasb., 1856, xvi.73; 121; 128.—**Medicina** domestica, ossia notizie scientifico-popolari intorno ad alcune piante o prodotti ve-getabili più volgari. Salute, Genova, 1869, iv, 609; 625; 641; 657; 737; 753.—**Meneses** (J. R.) Algunas observaciones sobre los inconvenientes de los libros de medicina en mano del vulgo. An. Univ. de Chile, Santiago, 1867, xxix, 203-213.—**Molleson** (I.) Ocherk narodnoi meditsini v Rossii. [Popular medicine in Russia.] Arch. sudebnoi med., St. Pe-tersb., 1869, v, pt. 3, no. 4, 1-19.—**Muirhead** (C.) Minor ailments and their treatment. Edinb. Health Soc. Health Lect., 1882-3, 3. s., 151-174. — **von Nussbaum** (J. W.) Welche Hilfe kann der Laie bei plötzlichen Erkrankun-gen und Unglücksfällen leisten? Deutsche Rev., Bresl. u. Leipz., 1885, x, 49-58.—**Pantynkhoff** (I.) O narodnoe meditsinae tuzemtsev Rionskoi dolinui. [On popular medi-cine as practised in the valley of Rion (in Mingrelia).] Med. Sbornik, Tiflis, 1869, no. 6, pt. 2, 1-33.—**Rittmann.** Die vorhellenische Heilkunst und die Volkskrankheiten. Allg. Wien. med. Ztg., 1867, xii, 65-68. ——. Die Volks-medizin bei den heidnischen Germanen und Slaven. *Ibid.,* 291-293.—**Röbbelen** (A. H.) Ueber Volksmittel und Volksgebräuche in Krankheiten. Deutsche Klinik, Berl., 1861, xiii, 191; 207; 325; 349.—**Schmitt** (A.) Ueber die Sitten, Gebräuche und Volksmittel in der Rhön. Aerztl. Int.-Bl., München, 1880, xxvii, 361-364. — **Schtschukin** (R. S.) Zur Volksmedicin der Jakuten. [*From:* Journ. M. V. D.] Med. Ztg. Russlands, St. Petersb., 1854, xi, 383.—**Schütte** (D.) Volks-Heilmittel in mehreren Dis-trikten am linken Ufer des Niederrhein und vom West-phalen. N. Jahrb. d. teutsch. Med. u. Chir., Hamm, 1825, x, 1. St., 55-71.—**Strohl** (E.) Une pharmacopée domes-tique des années 1591 et 1593. Mém. Soc. de méd. de Strasb., 1886, xxiii, 257-271.—**Suty** (C.) De la médecine chez les littérateurs. Union méd., Par., 1865, 2. s., xxv, 497; xxviii, 17.—**Visochki** (N.) Ocherki Russkoi narod-noi meditsini. [Sketch of Russian popular medicine.] Zdorovje, St. Petersb., 1876, ii, no. 31, 19-22.—**Vulgari-sation** (Die) der Wissenschaften und besonders der Me-dicin. Ber. d. k. k. Krankenh. Wieden 1863, Wien, 1864, 346-350.

Medicine (*Popular, Journals on*).

See, also, **Hygiene** (*Journals on*).

ABERDEEN (The) Sanitary Reformer and Family Guide to Health. By A. Munro. v. 1–2, 1861–2. 8°. *Aberdeen.*

AERZTLICHE (Der) Hausfreund. Von R. Froriep. v. 1–2, 1833–8. 8°. *Weimar u. Erlangen.*

AERZTLICHE (Der) Hausfreund. Von A. Moschkau. Nos. 1–5, v. 4, 1876. 4°. *Dresden.*

ALLGEMEINE (Der) Volksarzt. Von C. F. Lutheritz. v. 1–2, 1820–21. 8°. *Leipzig.*

ALMANACCO della famiglia. Red.: A. Longhena. v. 1–3, 1873–5. 12°. *Milano.*

ALMANACCO igienico popolare del dott. P. Mantegazza. v. 20, 1885. 12°. *Milano.*

AMERICAN Journal of Health and Medicine. "New series." March to June, 1874. 8°. *New York, Hall's Health Pub. Co.*

AMERICAN (The) Vegetarian and Health Journal. Published by the American Vegetarian Society and edited by W. A. Alcott, T. L. Nichols, and Wm. Metcalfe. [Monthly.] v. 1–4, Nov., 1850, to Oct., 1854. 8°. *Philadelphia.*

ANNALS of Health and Long Life. By Joseph Taylor. 1 v. 8°. *London, 1818.*

BISTOURY (The). A quarterly medical journal, devoted to the exposition of charlatanism in medicine, and the education of the people upon medical subjects. Edited by T. S. Up de Graff. New series. v. 5–21, April, 1869, to July, 1885. 8°. *Elmira, N. Y.*

BLÄTTER für Gesundheitspflege. Red. von Oskar Wysz. v. 5–14, 1876–85. 8°. *Zürich.*

BOSTON (The) Domestic Journal of Medicine. B. F. Hatch, editor and proprietor. [Monthly.] v. 1; No. 1, v. 2, 1852–3. 8°. *Boston, Bazin & Chandler.*

BOSTON Guide to Health, and Journal of Arts and Sciences. Edited by Dr. J. S. Spear. [Semimonthly.] Nos. 1, 6, 9, v. 1, July 25, 1843, April 15, 1844, June 1, 1844. 8°. *Boston, Dow & Jackson.*

BOSTWICK's Medical and Surgical Journal. By Homer Bostwick. Nos. 1–2, v. 1, Jan. to Feb., 1871. 8°. *New York.*

CANADA (The) Health Journal. Edited by Cl. T. Campbell. Nos. 1–5, v. 1, Jan. to May, 1870. 8°. *London, Ontario, J. Cameron & Brother.*

CANADA (The) Health Journal. By E. Playter. Nos. 1–8, v. 5, 1880–82; v. 8–9, 1886–7. 8°. *Toronto & Ottawa.*

CHICAGO (The) Journal of Health. Edited by B. Philips Reynolds. [Monthly.] No. 1, v. 1, July, 1869. 8°. *Chicago.*

CINCINNATI Herald of Health. J. King, J. C. Thomas, editors and publishers. [Quarterly.] No. 1, v. 1, Jan., 1854. 8°. *Cincinnati.*

CINCINNATI (The) Journal of Health. Devoted to instructions in anatomy and physiology and the means of preserving health. Edited by Leonidas M. Lawson. [Monthly.] Nos. 1–3, v. 1, Jan. to March, 1844. 8°. *Cincinnati.*

CLARK's Quarterly Clarion of Health. Uriah Clark, editor. No. 1, v. 1, April, 1866. 8°. *Boston.*

CLEVELAND (The) Health Journal. By E. E. Riopel. Nos. 1–5, v. 1, Jan. to May, 1877. 8°. *Cleveland, Ohio.*

CONSERVATORE (Il) della salute. Red.: C. Cioccari. v. 1–3, 1872–5. 8°. *Napoli.*

CONSULTOR (El) de los padres de familia [etc.] Director: A. G. Collejo. Nos. 1–4, v. 1, 1879. fol. *Madrid.*

Medicine (*Popular, Journals on*).

DISSECTOR (The). A quarterly journal of health and physical culture, devoted to an exposition of the laws of hygiene, abuse of drugs, and social life. Edited by G. Gallatin Lyon. No. 4, v. 1, April, 1867. 8°. *Jerseyville, Ill.*

DOCTOR (The): adapted for the use of families, nurses, etc. v. 1–5, 1832–7. 4°. *London.*

DOCTOR (The). A popular paper for physicians and their friends. C. A. Welles, editor. v. 1, 1886–7. 4°. *New York.*

ESCULAPIAN (The). A medical paper for the people. By C. D. Griswold. Nos. 2–5, Feb. to May, 1853. 4°. *New York.*

FAMILY (The) Doctor. Edited by a physician. v. 1–2, 1881–2. 4°. *London.*

FAMILY (The) Doctor and People's Medical Adviser. v. 1–6, 1885–7. 4°. *London.*

FAMILY (The) Guide to Health and Happiness. No. 1, v. 1, Feb., [1855]. 8°. [*Cincinnati.*]

FAMILY (The) Journal of Health. Edited by John M. Scudder. [Monthly.] Nos. 1–5, v. 1, 1860. 8°. *Cincinnati.*

FAMILY (The) Oracle of Health. By A. F. Crell and W. M. Wallace. [Monthly.] v. 1–4, 1823–7. 8°. *London, J. Walker.*

FEUILLES d'hygiène et de police sanitaire. Par le Dr. Guillaume. v. 3–6, 1877–80. 4°. *Neuchâtel.*

FLEMING's Southern Hygienic Journal; devoted exclusively to human health. Edited by Newton Randolph Fleming. [Monthly.] No. 1, v. 1, Aug., 1855. 8°. *Atlanta, Ga.*

FOOD and Health. By Amelia Lewis. v. 1–2; Nos. 1–3, v. 3, Jan. 29, 1881, to Jan. 1, 1882. fol. *New York.*

FOOTE's (Dr.) Health Monthly. v. 2–12, 1877–87. 8°. *New York.*

GAZETTE de santé. Hrsg. von J. H. Rahn. v. 1, 1782; v. 3, 1784. 8°. *Zürich.*

GENEESKUNDIGE Courant voor het Koningrijk der Nederlanden. v. 1–41, 1847–87. fol. *Tiel.*

GESUNDHEITSTEMPEL der Deutschen. Hrsg. von J. C. Fleck. v. 1–2, 1835–6. 4°. *Weimar u. Ilmenau.*

GESUNDHEITSWACHT. Hrsg. von A. Moschkau. v. 1-2, 1876–8. fol. *Leipzig.*

GESUNDHEITSWÄCHTER (Der). Von E. Krüger. v. 1–6, 1853–9. 8°. *Hamburg.*

GESUNDHEITSZEITUNG. Hrsg. von E. F. W. Streit. v. 1–3, 1828–30. 8°. *Greitz.*

GOOD Health. A popular annual on the laws of correct living, as developed by medical science, etc. [Monthly.] v. 1–3; Nos. 1–6, v. 4, June, 1869, to Nov., 1872. 8°. *Boston, A. Moore.*

GOSPEL (The) of-Health and Journal of the True Healing Art. Edited by R. T. Trall. [Monthly.] Nos. 8, 10, 12, v. 2, 1867–8. 8°. *New York.*

GRAHAM (The) Journal of Health and Longevity. Edited by David Campbell. [Weekly.] v. 1–3, April 4, 1837–9. 8°. *Boston.*

GUARDIAN (The) of Health. A monthly journal of domestic hygiene. Edited by T. E. Bond and C. A. Harris. Nos. 1–3, v. 1, Sept. to Nov., 1841. 8°. *Baltimore, Knight & Colburn.*

GUARDIAN (The) of Health. Edited by W. M. Cornell. [Monthly.] v. 7–8, Jan., 1868, to Dec., 1869. 8°. *Boston.*

GUARDIAN (The) of Health. A bi-monthly journal on the principles of hygiene, showing the English and native way of treating diseases. v. 1–10 [1878–87]. 8°. *Lahore.*
Urdoo text (except title).

Medicine (*Popular, Journals on*).

GUIA (El) de la salud. Red.: J. Fernandez-Ballesteros. v. 1–5, 1881–5. fol. *Sevilla.*

GUIA (O) da saude. Editor: J. B. Birra. v. 1, 1886–7. fol. *Porto.*

GUIDE (Le) sanitaire; journal d'hygiène pratique. No. 1, v. 1, Nov., 1874. 8°. *Montréal.*

HALL's Journal of Health. Edited by W. W. Hall. v. 1–34, 1854–86. 8°. *New York.*

HALL's Medical Adviser. By W. W. Hall. Feb., 1875. 8°. *New York.*

HAUSARZT (Der). Hrsg. von Th. Hahn. v. 1–2, 1876–7. 8°. *St. Gallen.*

HAUSARZT (Der). Hrsg. von O. Reyher. v. 1, 1880–81. 4°. *Leipzig.*

HEALING (The) Voice. By Anna J. Johnson. v. 1, 1884. 8°. *New York.*

HEALTH. By R. Walter [*et al.*]. v. 4–7, 1831–5. 8°. *Wernersville, Pa.*

HEALTH. By A. Wilson. v. 1–6, 1883–6. 4°. *London.*

HEALTH and Home. A journal of sanitary science and home hygiene. Nos. 1–3, v. 1, Feb. to April, 1884. 8°. *Montreal.*

HEALTH and Home. By W. H. Hale. No. 4, v. 11, March, 1884. fol. *Port Chester, N. Y., and Washington, D. C.*
An advertisement.

HEALTH (The) Journal. v. 1–5, 1883–7. 4°. *Manchester, F. Scott.*

HEALTH (The) Journal and Independent Magazine. [Monthly.] No. 1, v. 1, Feb., 1843. 8°. *Boston, J. A. Whitmarsh.*

HEALTH and Life. Published by Drs. Starkey and Palen. v. 1–3, 1880–82. 4°. *Philadelphia.*
An advertisement of the "Compound oxygen treatment".

HEALTH (The) Record. By M. S. Purdy. v. 1–2, 1887. 8°. *Corning, N. Y.*

HEALTH (The) Reformer. Edited by H. S. Lay. [Monthly.] v. 1–13, 1866–78. 8°. *Battle Creek, Mich.*

HEALTH Science Magazine and Laws of Health. By R. Walter. v. 9, 1886. 8°. *Wernersville, Pa.*

HEALTHSIDE (The). By Wm. H. Cook. No. 1, v. 52, July, 1884. 8°. *Cincinnati, O.*

HELSOVÄNNEN. Tidskrift för allmän och enskild helsovård. Utgifvare: Dr. E. W. Wretland. v. 1–2, 1886–7. 8°. *Göteborg.*

HERALD (The) of Health; a monthly health magazine, devoted to hygiene, medication, bodily development, and the laws of life. By R. T. Trall. v. 35–72, 1863–87. 8°. *New York.*

HERALD (The) of Health; a journal of sanitary and social science. Published by T. L. Nichols. v. 1–3, 1875–8. 4° & 8°. *London.*

HERALD (The) of Health. By T. L. Nichols. Nos. 13–96, 1879–85. 4°. *London.*

HERALD (The) of Health. By E. W. Gray. v. 1–2, 1878–80. 8°. *Bloomington, Ill.*

HERALD (The) of Health, and Journal of Happiness. By D. L. Mallison. v. 1, 1842–3. 8°. *New York.*

HIGIENE (La). Semanario científico popular. Director: B. Avilés. v. 1–5, 1882–6. 4°. *Madrid.*

HIGIENE (La) para todos. Director: E. Gelabert. v. 1–7, 1881–7. fol. *Barcelona.*

HOME Health; or the popular science of hygiene. By R. J. Curtiss. v. 1, 1883. 8°. *Peoria, Ill.*

HOME and Health; a monthly magazine, devoted to health and the home circle. Nos. 2–5, v. 1, 1871. 8°. *New York.*

HOME (The) Medical Journal. Nos. 1–2, v. 1, Aug. to Sept., 1879. 4°. *Boston, G. L. Austin & Co.*

How to Live and Breathe. Moses Brown, editor. Nos. 1–3, v. 1, 1860. 8°. *Boston.*

Medicine (*Popular, Journals on*).

HYGEA. Populäre medicinische Zeitung [etc.] Hrsg. von Karsch. v. 1–6, July 1, 1857, to Dec. 31, 1862. 8°. *Münster.*

HYGEIAN (The) Record and Family Adviser. Conducted by an association of hygeists. [Monthly.] v. 4, Dec. 19, 1835, to Dec. 1, 1836; n. s., No. 6, v. 1, 1845. 12°. *New York.*

HYGEIST (The). Nos. 1–50, v. 1–2, 1842–5. 4°. *London.*

HYGEIST (The). Devoted to the preservation and perfection of the human race by teaching the natural, organic, dietetic, intellectual, moral, and social laws of man; with the causes of disease, crime, and misery, their cure and prevention. Edited by Silas Brown and Wm. A. Alcott. [Monthly.] No. 1, v. 1, Jan., 1857. 8°. *Boston.*

HYGIENE; an exponent of sanitary science, preventive medicine, physical culture. Nos. 1–2, Jan., Feb., 1873. 8°. *New York, the Health-Lift Co.*

HYGIENE. A popular journal of sanitary science. [Edited by Frank W. Reilly.] Published fortnightly. Nos. 2–6, v. 1, March 1 to April 26, 1873. 8°. *New York, G. P. Putnam's Sons.*

HYGIÈNE (L') pour tous. Rédacteur: F. Brémond. v. 5–8, 1880–83. fol. *Paris.*

HYGIÈNE (L') pratique. Gérant: Paul Lhotte. v. 1–6, 1882–7. 4°. *Paris.*

HYGIENE Reporter. No. 1, v. 1, Jan., 1881. 12 pp. 4°. *Boston, published by the Hygiene League.*

HYGIENIC Family Almanac, 1875. 8°. *Battle Creek, Mich.*

HYGIENIC (The) and Literary Magazine. M. A. Malsby, editor and proprietor; V. H. Taliaferro, asst. editor. [Monthly.] Nos. 1–4, v. 1, 1860. 8°. *Atlanta, Ga.*

HYGIENIC (The) Monitor; a monthly journal for invalids on therapeutics. Edited by A. G. Hall. v. 1, 1859. 8°. *Boston.*

HYGIENISCHES Familienblatt. v. 1, 1885. 4°. *Bunzlau u. Leipzig.*

IGEA (L'). Giornale d' igiene e medicina preventiva. Red.: P. Mantegazza. v. 1–10, 1862–72. 8°. *Milano.*

INDIANA (The) Scalpel. Devoted to hygiene and rational medicine, etc. Edited by G. O. Glavis. N. s., No. 1, v. 2, Jan., 1860. 8°. *Princeton.*

JAEGER's (Prof. Dr. G.) Monatsblatt. Organ für Gesundheitspflege und Lebenslehre. v. 2–6, 1882–7. 8°. *Stuttgart.*

JOURNAL für Gesundheitspflege. Von D. Bisenz. v. 5–8, 1881–4. 4°. *Wien.*

JOURNAL (The) of Health. Conducted by an association of physicians. [Semi-monthly.] v. 1–4, Sept. 9, 1829, to Aug., 1833. 8°. *Philadelphia, S. C. Atkinson.*

JOURNAL of Health. Conducted by the physicians of the Cincinnati Dispensary and Vaccine Institution. Edited by Vattier, Stuart, and Warder. [Monthly.] N. s., v. 1, 1844–5. 8°. *Cincinnati, O.*

JOURNAL (The) of Health. v. 1, Aug., 1848, to July, 1849. 8°. *London, Ward & Co.*

———. The same. N. s., v. 2–3, Aug., 1852–4. 8°. *London.*

JOURNAL (The) of Health. By J. W. Blackburn. Nos. 1–3, v. 1, Jan. to May, 1874. 8°. *Saint Joseph, Mo.*

JOURNAL of Health of the Metropolitan Medical College. Edited by H. M. Sweet, Geo. Newby, and H. P. Herdman. [Monthly.] Nos. 1–6, 9, v. 1, 1859–60. 8°. *New York, G. Gross.*

JOURNAL (The) of Health and Monthly Miscellany. Edited by W. M. Cornell. v. 1–3, Jan., 1846, to Dec., 1848. 8°. *Boston.*

Medicine (*Popular, Journals on*).

JOURNAL d'hygiène populaire. v. 1–4, May 15, 1884–7. 8°. *Montréal.*

JOURNAL für öffentliche Gesundheitspflege. Von D. Bisenz. v. 4, 1880. 4°. *Wien.*

JOURNAL de santé, par une société de médecins. Nos. 110, 125 (v. 3), 1835–6. 4°. *Paris.*

JOURNAL de santé, spécialement hygiénique, par P.-L. Labbée. No. 2, v. 1, Feb. 1, 1832. 8°. *Reims.*

LANDARZT (Der), oder Archiv für das Landvolk bei allen Ereignissen, welche sowohl das körperliche als auch landwirthschaftliche Wohl und Weh des Bauernstandes betreffen, sich selbst rathen und helfen zu können. (Von J. G. Essig.) v. 1, 1794. 8°. *Augsburg.*

LAWS (The) of Health. By R. Walter. v. 1–3, 1878–81. 4°. *Wernersville, Pa.*

LAWS (The) of Life. Edited by Miss Harriet N. Austin and Jas. C. Jackson. [Monthly.] v. 3–8, 11–30, 1860–87. 4° & 8°. *Dansville, N. Y.*

LEKARZ domowy. Pismo poświęcone dla uzytku domowego. Red.: Dr. M. P. Kossakowski. v. 1, 1886–7. 8°. *Chicago.*

LIBRARY (The) of Health and Teacher on the Human Constitution. Edited by Wm. A. Alcott. [Monthly.] v. 1–6, 1837–42. 12°. *Boston.*

LIFE Crystals. A California health journal. By Mrs. C. F. Young. Nos. 1–8, v. 1, 1882. 4°. *Oakland, Cal.*

MÉDECIN (Le) de la famille. Par A. Festraerts. v. 20–30, 1875–85. 8°. *Liége.*

MÉDECIN (Le) de la maison. Par Dr. Reinvillier. v. 1–6, 1850–56. 4°. *Paris.*

MÉDECINE (La) sans médicaments. Par le Dr. Luce. v. 1–6, 1882–7. 18°. *Paris.*

MEDICAL (The) Adviser and Guide to Health and Long Life. Edited by Alex. Burnett. [Weekly.] v. 1–3, Dec. 6, 1823, to June 4, 1825. 8°. *London, Knight & Lacey.*

MEDICAL (The) Adviser and Complete Guide to Health and Long Life, [etc.] By A. Burnett, Mr. Maginn, and other medical gentlemen. v. 1–2, 1825. 8°. *London.*

MEDICAL (The) Friend of the People. By A. Hunn. No. 7, v. 1, Sept., 1829. 8°. *Harrodsburg, Ky.*

MEDICAL (The) Independent. Devoted to domestic medicine, physiology, hygiene, science, arts, and information for the people. Edited by Wm. Paine. [Weekly.] v. 1–3; Nos. 2–3, v. 4, June 1, 1870–72. fol. *Philadelphia.*

MEDICAL (The) Independent. Devoted to medicine, surgery, physiology, hygiene, art, science, and general information for the people. Edited by R. H. Kline and A. H. Lindley. [Semimonthly.] Nos. 1, 3, 5, 9, v. 1, May 1 to Sept. 17, 1872. fol. *Philadelphia.*

MEDICINA (La) communale. Giornale popolare di scienze mediche, [etc.] Red.: L. Ripa. v. 1–3, 1863–5; v. 12–22, 1873–83. 8°. *Seregno.*

MEDICINISCHE (Der) Hausfreund. Von Th. Köhler. v. 1–2, 1880–82. 4°. *Cassel.*

MEDICO (Il) di casa. Giornale di igiene e medicina popolare, diretto dal professore Paolo Mantegazza. v. 1–9, 1873–81. 8°. *Milano.*

MEDICO-LITERARY (The) Journal. Mrs. M. P. Sawtelle, editor. v. 1–5, 1878–83. 8°. *San Francisco, Cal.*

MEDITSINSKAJA besieda. Journal populjarnoi meditsiny i gigieny. Tom. 1, 1887. 8°. *Voronej.*

MESSENGER (The) of Health. Nos. 1–6, v. 1, June to Nov., 1883. 8°. *Buffalo, N. Y.*

MODERN (The) Physician and Family Adviser. By G. Lade and E. B. Shuldham. v. 2, 1880. 8°. *London.*

MONITEUR d'hygiène et de salubrité publique. Par A. Chevallier fils. v. 1–4, 1866–9. 8°. *Paris.*

Medicine (*Popular, Journals on*).

MONITOR (El) de la salud de las familias y de la salubridad de los pueblos. Red.: P. F. Monlau. v. 1–7, 1858–64. 8°. *Madrid.*

MONITOR (El) de la salud. Red : C. Ronquillo. v. 1–5, 1880–84. 4°. *Barcelona.*

MONTHLY (The) Gazette of Health. Edited by Richard Reece. v. 1–16, 1816–31. 8°. *London.*

MONTHLY (A) Journal of Popular Medicine; explaining the nature, causes, and prevention of diseases, the immediate management of accidents, and the means of preserving health. Conducted by Charles Thomas Haden. v. 1–2, March, 1821, to Feb., 1822. 8°. *London, Simkin & Marshall.*

MONTHLY (The) Monitor and People's Health Journal. Conducted by Calvin M. Fitch and John W. Sykes. No. 1, v. 1, Sept., 1858. 8°. *Pittsburgh, Pa.*

MORAL (The) Reformer and Teacher on the Human Constitution. Wm. A. Alcott, editor. [Monthly.] v. 1–2, Jan., 1835, to Dec., 1836. 8°. *Boston, Light & Horton.*

NATIONAL (The) Independent. Edited by W. Y. Leader and Wm. Paine. [Weekly.] Nos. 4–7, v. 4, 1872. fol. *Philadelphia.*

NATION'S (The) Journal of Health. Published by Dr. S. Van Meter & Co. [Monthly.] No. 181, v. 28, new series, 1873. fol. *Charleston, Ill.* An advertisement.

NATURARZT (Der). Correspondenzblatt für Freunde naturgemässer Heilmethoden. Hrsg. von W. Meinert. v. 2–8, 15–25, 1863–9; 1876–86. 4° & 8°. *Dresden u. Berlin.*

NEW (The) Doctor; a family journal of health. v. 1, 1836–7. 8°. *London, B. Steill.*

ONTARIO (The) Journal of Health. By J. F. Latimer. No. 1, v. 1, April, 1877. fol. *London, Ontario.*

PAINE'S Journal of Domestic Medicine. [Monthly.] v. 1, April, 1873, to March, 1874. 8°. *Philadelphia, W. Paine.*

PARK'S (Dr.) Reform Medical and Family Journal, etc. By W. T. Park. [Monthly.] No. 1, v. 1, March, 1853. 24 pp. 8°. *Lumpkin, Ga.* An advertisement.

PEABODY (The) Journal of Health. A. H. Hayes, editor. [Monthly.] Nos. 1–3, v. 1, Feb., April, 1869. fol. *Boston.* An advertisement.

PENNY (The) Herald of Health. By T. L. Nichols. v. 1, 1878. 4°. *London.*

PEOPLE'S (The) Health Journal of Chicago. By L. D. and S. Ida Wright Rogers. v. 1–2, 1885–6. 8°. *Chicago.*

PEOPLE'S (The) Medical Adviser. [Weekly.] Nos. 1–36. 1 v. 284 pp. 4°. *London, G. Croker,* [*n. d.*]

PEOPLE'S (The) Medical Gazette. By John Davis. Nos. 2–4, v. 1, Oct., 1853, to Jan., 1854. 8°. *Abbeville C. H., S. C.*

PEOPLE'S (The) Medical Journal and Family Physician. Edited by Thomas Harrison Yeoman. [Weekly.] v. 1–3, Jan. 5, 1850, to June 28, 1851. 4°. *London, G. Vickers.*

PEOPLE'S (The) Medical Journal and Home Doctor. By F. Hollick. v. 1–2, July, 1853, to Dec., 1854. 8°. *New York.*

PETIT (Le) journal de la santé. Directeur: Marc de Rossiény. v. 1–3, 1884–6. fol. *Paris.*

PETIT (Le) médecin des familles. v. 1–2, 1887. fol. *Paris.*

PETIT (Le) moniteur de la santé. v. 1–3, 1885–7. 8°. *Paris.*

PHILOSOPHICAL (The) Medical Journal, or Family Physician. Devoted to chemistry, botany, and analytical practice of medicine. Edited by J. Clawson Kelley and J. King. [Month-

Medicine (*Popular, Journals on*).

ly.] v. 1, 1844; Nos. 1–10, v. 2, 1847–8. 8°. *New York.*

PHYSIOLOGIST (The). A popular domestic journal, designed to explain and illustrate the laws of physical culture, [etc.] By C. W. Gleason and A. O'Leary. No. for Nov. 1, 1869. fol. *Louisville, Ky.*
An advertisement.

PHYSIOLOGIST (The) and Family Physician. By Sara B. Chase. v. 1–4, 1878–81. fol. *New York.*

POPULÄRE österreichische Gesundheits-Zeitung zur Warnung für Nichtkranke und zum Troste für Leidende. Hrsg. und redigirt von A. D. Bastler. v. 3, 1832. 4°. *Wien.*

———. Neue Folge. Hrsg. von H. H. Beer. v. 1–4, 1837–40. 8°. *Wien.*

POPULAR (The) Journal of Physical and Mental Hygiene. Edited by Thomas H. Helsby and Thos. J. Mays. [Monthly.] v. 1, April to Dec., 1873. 8°. *Williamsport, Pa.*

PORTER'S Health Almanac for 1832. sm. 4°. *Philadelphia.*

PRACTICAL (The) Physician. By J. J. Rivera. Nos. 1–3, v. 1, March to Sept., 1886. fol. *New York.*

PREVENTIVA (La). Red.: D. Franco. v. 1–4, 1884–7. 8°. *Napoli.*

PROPUGNATORE (Il) della salute. Red.: A. Spatuzzi. v. 1, 1883. 8°. *Napoli.*

PUGET SOUND (The) Sanitarian and Prohibitionist. v. 1, 1885. 8°. *Seattle, W. T.*

PULSE (The) of Health. Frank W. Reilly, edtor. Nos. 1–3, v. 1, Nov., Dec., 1871; Sept., 1872. 4°. *New York, the Health Lift Co.*

RHODE ISLAND (The) Medical Reformer. A family journal for the promotion of health and longevity. Edited by B. Franklin Clark. [Semimonthly.] v. 1, 1843. 8°. *Providence.*

RUSH'S Almanac and Guide to Health. 1882. 12°. *New York, A. H. Flanders.*

SALUD (La). Semanario popular. Director: J. de Letamendi. v. 1, 1877. 8°. *Barcelona.*

SALUTE (La). Red.: G. Du Jardin. v. 1–14, 1865–80. 8°. *Genova.*

SALUTE (La). v. 1, 1886. fol. *Trapani,*

SANITARIUM Journal. Published quarterly. No. 1, v. 1, May, 1874. fol. *Cincinnati.*
An advertisement.

SANITARY (The) Monitor. By J. F. Winn. v. 1–2, May, 1885, to July, 1886. 4°. *Richmond, Va.*

SANTÉ (La) publique. Hygiène et médecine populaires. Réd.: P. Garnier. Nouv. série, v. 1–4, 1872–6. fol. *Paris.*

SANTÉ (La) universelle. Par Jules Massé. [Monthly.] No. 3, v. 1, Dec., 1851. 8°. *Paris.*

SCALPEL (The). A journal of health, adapted to popular and professional reading and the exposure of quackery. Edited by Edward H. Dixon. [Quarterly.] v. 1–12, Jan., 1849–61. 8°. *New York.*

SCHAT der Gezondheid. Een tijdschrift voor alle standen, tot bevordering van volkswelvaart, door verspreiding van eenvoudige beginselen van gezondheidsregeling en hunne toepassing op het individueel en maatschappelijk leven. Onder redactie van Dr. D. Lubach en Dr. L. J. Egeling. Jaargang 1–9, 1858–66. 8°. *Haarlem, C. Zwaardemaker; Amsterdam, 1864; Gorinchem, 1865–6.*

SCHWEIZERISCHE Blätter für Gesundheitspflege. Neue Folge, v. 1–2, 1886–7. 8°. *Zürich.*

SCIENCE and Health. By G. G. Groff. v. 1, 1881–2. 8°. *Lewisburgh, Pa.*

SCIENCE (The) of Health. By S. R. Wells. v. 1–8, 1872–6. 8°. *New York.*

Medicine (*Popular, Journals on*).

SCOTT'S Journal of Health. C. W. Scott, jr., editor. Nos. 1, 5, v. 3; No. 11, v. 4, 1874. 8°. *Boston.*
An advertisement.

SCOTT'S Journal of Medical Information for the People. Edited by J. Walter Scott. [Quarterly.] No. 1, v. 1, Jan., 1870. 8°. *New York.*

SFERZA (La). Giornale popolare [etc.] Red.: T. ed U. Santopadre. Nos. 1–2, v. 1, Sept., 1874. fol. *Bologna.*

SOUTHERN (The) Journal of Health. By H. P. Gatchell. v. 1, 1885. 8°. *Asheville, N. C.; Atlanta, Ga.*

TEACHER (The) of Health and the Laws of the Human Constitution. W. A. Alcott, editor. v. 1, 1843. 12°. *Boston.*

TIJDSCHRIFT voor Gezondheidsleer. Red.: C. P. Pous Koolhaas. v. 1–5, 1867–72. 8°. *'s Gravenhage.*

UNIVERSITY (The) Journal of Health; a common-sense medical magazine for the profession and the people. Edited by J. Walter Scott. [Monthly.] Nos. 1–2, v. 1, 1866. 8°. *New York.*

VITA (La). Periodico popolare. Red.: D. Sbardolini. v. 2–4, 1883–5. fol. *Brescia.*

VOLKSARZT (Der). Von C. Winde und C. B. Griesbach. v. 1–6, 1869–74. 8°. *Leipzig.*

VOLKSARZT (Der). Von Dr. Schulze. v. 2–4, 1885–7. 8°. *Berlin.*

WESTERN (The) Health Journal. Devoted to physiology, hygiene, physical culture. Published by Drs. Jones, Woodbury & Co. [Monthly.] No. 1, v. 1, Dec. 1, 1862. 8°. *Wabash, Ind.*

WHEATLEY'S Journal of Health. By J. B. Wheatley. fol.
An advertisement.

WILSON'S Herald of Health and Atlanta Business Review. Edited by Jno. Stainback Wilson, M. D. [Quarterly.] v. 1, May, 1873–4. 8°. *Atlanta, Ga.*

WILSON'S Herald of Health and Farm and Household Help.
Title of No. 3 *et seq.*, v. 1, **Wilson's** Herald of Health [etc.]

ZDOROVJE nauchno-popularnii gigienicheskii jurnal. v. 1–10, 1874–85. 4°. *St. Petersburg.*

ZEITSCHRIFT des deutschen Vereins für volksverständliche Gesundheitspflege, [etc.] Hrsg. von H. Canitz. v. 11–14, 1883–6. 8°. *Berlin.*

Medicine (*Popular, Manuals of*).

ABERNETHY (J.) The new family physician, and guide to health and long life. 8°. *London,* [*n. d.*]

ABERNETHY'S family physician . . . 2. Am. ed., revised and enlarged by H. Bostwick. 12°. *New York, 1849.*

ANDREW (T.) A cyclopedia of domestic medicine and surgery, being an alphabetical account of the various diseases incident to the human frame . . . With contributions by several members of the Royal College of Surgeons, Edinburgh. roy. 8°. *Glasgow, 1865.*

BEARD (G. M.) Our home physician; a new and popular guide to the art of preserving health and treating disease. 8°. *New York, 1869.*

BEVEROVICIUS [VAN BEVERWYCK] (J.) Schat der ongesontheyt ofte genees-konste van de sieckten. Verçiert met historyen, als oock met verssen van Jacob Cats. 12°. *Dordrecht, 1642.*

———. The same. fol. *Amsterdam, 1656.*

———. Schatz der Ungesundheit, das ist, kurtzer Begrif der algemeinen Artzneikunst; dadurch der schwache, und in Ungesundheit oder Seuchen gefallene Mensch wieder zu volständiger Gesundheit gelangen kan; dem gantzen menschlichen Geschlechte, so wohl den Gesunden als Kranken,

Medicine (*Popular, Manuals of*).

zum nothwendigen Gebrauche beschrieben, und mit allerhand Kupferstükken, wie auch ahrtigen Reimen des . . . Jakob Katsens, gezieret. Aus dem Niederdeutschen, dem Hochdeutschen Liebhaber zum besten, übergetragen, und nach desselben Landesahrt hier und dar eingerichtet. fol. [*Amsterdam*, 1671.]

BOERHAAVE (H.) Aphorismi de cognoscendis et curandis morbis in usum doctrinæ domesticæ digesti. 8°. *Norimbergæ*, 1747.

BOOK (The) of health; a compendium of domestic medicine deduced from the experience of the most eminent modern practitioners; entirely divested of technicalities and rendered familiar to the general reader . . . 1. Am. from the 2. Lond. ed., revised and conformed to the practice of the United States, with additions by a fellow of the Massachusetts Medical Society. 8°. *Boston*, 1830.

BOUDIER. La médecine et la santé mises à la portée de tous; manuel de médecine des familles [etc.] 12°. *Paris*, [1886?]

BOYD (J.) Family medical adviser, giving such information on the practice of physic, and the diseases of women and children, as may prove useful in families when regular physicians can not readily be procured . . . to which is annexed anatomy, surgery, materia medica, and many valuable prescriptions, being a useful companion and guide for intelligent heads of families, overseers of plantations and manufactories, masters of vessels, and travellers. 8°. *Philadelphia*, 1845.

BOYLE (R.) Medical experiments; or a collection of choice and safe remedies, for the most part simple and easily prepared; very useful in families, and fitted for the service of country people. 3 v. in 1. 16°. *London*, 1703.

BUCHAN (W.) Domestic medicine; or a treatise on the prevention and cure of diseases by regimen and simple medicines. 2. ed. 8°. *London*, 1772.

——. The same. With an appendix containing a dispensatory for the use of private practitioners. 3. ed. 8°. *London*, 1774.

——. The same. 7. ed. 8°. *London*, 1781.

——. The same. A new ed. With remarks on vaccination, electricity, galvanism, bathing, [etc.] 18°. *London*, [*n. d.*]

——. The same. 8°. *Philadelphia*, [1771?]

——. The same. 20. ed. 8°. *Waterford*, 1797.

——. The same. 2. Am. ed. 8°. *Philadelphia*, 1774.

——. The same. 3. Am. ed. 12°. *Norwich*, 1778.

——. The same. Revised and adapted to the diseases and climate of the United States of America, by Samuel Powel Griffitts. 8°. *Philadelphia*, 1795.

——. The same. 8°. *Philadelphia*, 1797.

——. The same. Adapted to the climate and diseases of America, by Isaac Cathrall. 8°. *Philadelphia*, 1799. Incomplete.

——. The same. A new ed., revised and amended, by John G. Coffin, M. D. 8°. *Boston*, 1825.

——. The same. Medicina domestica, o sia trattato completo di mezzi semplici per conservarsi in salute impedire e risanare le malattie; opera utile e adattata all' intelligenza di ciascuno. Trad. dall' inglese e arricchita di molte aggiunte ed annotazioni dal sig. Duplanil. 2. Ital. ed. 5 v. 8°. *Padova*, 1789.

——. The same. Médecine domestique, ou traité complet des moyens de se conserver en

Medicine (*Popular, Manuals of*).

santé, [etc.] Trad. de l'anglois par J.-D. Duplanil. 4. éd. 4 v. 8°. *Paris*, 1792.

——. The same. Medicina doméstica, ó tratado completo sobre los medios de conservar la salud, [etc.] Traducida por D. Pedro Sinnot. 2. ed. v. 1. 4°. *Madrid*, 1792.

——. Every man his own doctor; or, a treatise on the prevention and cure of diseases, by regimen and simple medicines. To which is added a treatise on the materia medica, in which the medicinal qualities of indigenous plants are given and adapted to common practice, with an appendix, containing a complete treatise on the art of farriery, [etc.] 8°. *New Haven*, 1816.

BURDETT (H. C.) Hints in sickness, where to go, and what to do. 8°. *London*, 1883.

[CHAMNEY (R. M.)] The Dublin handbook of medicine and surgery; a popular treatise for the million. 5. ed., greatly enlarged and improved. 8°. *Dublin*, 1872.

CHANN (M.) Cours de médecine populaire. 2. série. 8°. *Paris*, 1863.

CHARLOUIS (M.) Genees-, heel- en verloskunde in tijd van nood door leeken in praktijk te brengen. 8°. *Samarang*, 1886.

CHASE (A. W.) Dr. Chase's family physician, farrier, bee-keeper, and second receipt book; being an entirely new and complete treatise, including the diseases of women and children, [etc.] 8°. *Toledo, Ohio*, 1883.

CHURCHILL (T. F.) The new practical family physician; or, improved domestic medical guide. Containing a very plain account of the causes, symptoms, and method of curing every disease incident to the human body, [etc.] 8°. *London*, 1808.

COALES (R.) Popular medicine; or, family adviser; consisting of outlines of anatomy, physiology, and hygiene, with such hints on the practice of physic, surgery, and the diseases of women and children as may prove useful in families when regular physicians cannot be procured. 8°. *Philadelphia*, 1838.

COURVOISIER (L. G.) Die häusliche Krankenpflege. 8°. *Basel*, 1876.

DANCER (T.) The medical assistant; or, Jamaica practice of physic. Designed chiefly for the use of families and plantations. 4°. *Kingston (Jamaica)*, 1801.

——. The same. 2. ed. 4°. *St. Jago de la Vega*, 1809.

DIEPERINK (A. J.) Handboek voor zeevarenden, ter herkenning en genezing van de meest aan boord voorkomende ziekten en gebreken. 8°. *Amsterdam*, 1862.

DÖBEREINER (K.) Medicinisch-diätetisches Lexicon. Die Krankheiten des Menschen, deren Erkennen, sowie alle dem Wohlbefinden dienenden Mittel und Anleitungen. In populärer Darstellung. 8°. *Hamburg*, [1885].

DOMESTIC medicines; their uses and doses . . . Poisons and their antidotes. 32°. *London*, [1866].

DURANTE *da Gualdo* (C.) Il tesoro della sanità. Nel quale s' insegna il modo di conservar la sanità, prolungar la vita, e si tratta della natura de' cibi, e de' rimedij de' nocumenti loro. Con la tavola delle cose notabili. 8°. *Venetia*, 1588.

——. The same. 12°. *Venetia*, 1600.

——. The same. 8°. *Venetia*, 1601.

——. The same. 8°. *Venetia*, 1646.

——. Hortulus sanitatis, dast ist, ein heylsam und nützliches Gährtlin der Gesundtheit. In welchem alle fürnehme Kräutter, die so wol in den beyderley Indien, als an allen andern Orten der Welt zu finden, in einer wunderbaren Kürtze werden beschrieben. In italianischer

Medicine (*Popular, Manuals of*).

Sprach verfertigt, unmehr aber in unsere hoch teutsche Sprach versetzt. Durch Petrum Uffenbachium. 4°. *Franckf. a. M.*, 1609.

DWINELLE (J.) Domestic practice of medicine; an entirely new and original work, containing a minute and faithful description of the causes, symptoms, and treatment of diseases, and designed for the use of heads of families, planters, emigrants, sailors, and all others who are deprived of the immediate services of a physician. 8°. *Syracuse*, 1861.

[ETTNER (J. C.)] Des getreuen Eckharts unwürdiger Doctor, in welchem wie ein Medicus, der rechtschaffen handeln will, beschaffen seyn soll, [etc.] 18°. *Augspurg u. Leipzig*, 1697.

EVERY man his own doctor; or, the poor planter's physician. Prescribing plain and easy means for persons to cure themselves of all or most of the distempers incident to this climate, and with very little charge, the medicines being chiefly of the growth and production of this country. 3. ed. 12°. *Philadelphia*, 1734.

EWELL (T.) American family physician, detailing important means of preserving health, from infancy to old age; the offices women should perform to each other at births, and the diseases peculiar to the sex; with those of children and of adults, with an appendix containing hints respecting the treatment of domestic animals, and the best means of preserving fish and meat. 8°. *Georgetown, D. C.*, 1824.

FAMILIENARZT (Der). Ein Hausbuch zur richtigen Erkenntniss der im menschlichen Leben am häufigsten vorkommenden Krankheiten, mit Angabe der Ursachen, Behandlung, des Verlaufs und der Mittel zur Heilung derselben sowie auch mit Franzbranntwein und Salz. Hrsg. von Dr. J. Müller. 8°. *Bern*, [1885?]

FRASER (J.) The emigrant's medical guide. 12°. *Glasgow*, 1853.

FRISBEE (J.) Family physician; designed to assist heads of families, travellers, and sea-faring people in discerning, distinguishing, and curing diseases; with directions for the preparation and use of a numerous collection of the best American remedies, [etc.] 8°. *Boston*, 1847.

GOODLETT (A. G.) The family physician, or every man's companion; being a compilation from the most approved medical authors, adapted to the southern and western climates. To which is added an account of herbs, roots, and plants, used for medical purposes . . . With an appendix, containing a new and successful mode of treating Asiatic cholera, by the compiler. 8°. *Nashville, Tenn.*, 1838.

DE GORTER (J.) Medicinæ compendium, in usum exercitationis domesticæ. Pars prima. 4°. *Lugd. Bat.*, 1731.

———. The same. Partes prima et secunda in 1 v. 4°. *Venetiis*, 1751.

GROFF (G. G.) A manual of accidents and emergencies . . . With notes on the preservation of health, including the care of the sick, foods for the sick, [etc.] 8°. *Lewisburg, Pa.*, 1881.

HANDY book of medical information and advice; containing a brief account of the nature and treatment of common diseases; also hints to be followed in emergencies . . . By a physician. 8°. *London*, [*n. d.*]

HAYDEN (J.) Dictionary of popular medicine and hygiene . . . Edited by Edwin Lankester. 8°. *London*, 1874.

HEADLAND (F. W.) A medical handbook, comprehending such information on medical and sanitary subjects as is desirable in educated persons. With hints to clergymen and visitors of the poor. 16°. *London*, 1861.

Medicine (*Popular, Manuals of*).

HECQUET (P.) Arzney und Chirurgie der Armen. Aus dem Französischen übersetzt. 2. Aufl. 8°. *Augsburg*, 1781.

HOGG (J.) The domestic medical guide, for families, clergymen, emigrants, and sea captains; giving the best advice in the absence of a physician or surgeon, in cases of accident or sudden illness, [etc.] 4. ed. 12°. *London*, 1857.

HOPE (G. H.) Till the doctor comes, and how to help him. Revised, with additions, by a New York physician. 8°. *New York*, 1871.

HOUSE (The) surgeon and physician; designed to assist heads of families, travellers, and seafaring people in discerning, distinguishing, and curing diseases. With concise directions for the preparation and use of a numerous collection of the best American remedies; together with many of the most approved, from the shop of the apothecary. All in plain English. 16°. *Hartford*, 1818.

HUNT (E. M.) The patients' and physicians' aid; or how to preserve health; what to do in sudden attacks, or until the doctor comes; and how best to profit by his directions when given. 12°. *New York*, 1860.

HUNTER (G. Y.) A new and complete domestic medicine for home and abroad, containing practical hints on hygiene. 12°. *London*, 1879.

IMRAY (K.) A popular cyclopedia of modern domestic medicine . . . 1. Am. ed. To which are prefixed by the editor, popular treatises upon anatomy, physiology, surgery, dietetics, and the management of the sick. 8°. *New York*, 1849.

J[ACOBSZ] (H.) Den kleynen herbarius, ofte kruyt-boecxken, inhoudende de kracht, ende operatie van alle de gemeene kruyden, ende bekende vruchten, die men dagelijer gehebruyckt, waer deur men met Gods hulpe een yder zyne ghesontheyt kan onderhouden ende veelderhande sieckten genesen. Dan nieus obersien, en op veel plaetse verbetert ende vermeerdert. 18°. *Dordrecht*, 1637.

JAHN (M.) Häusliche Krankenpflege. 12°. *Stuttgart*, 1887.

JAMESON (H. G.) The American domestick medicine; or, medical admonisher, [etc.] 2. ed. 8°. *Baltimore*, 1818.

JEFFERSON (R.) The family doctor. A dictionary of domestic medicine and surgery, especially adapted for family use. 15. ed. 12°. *Philadelphia*, 1869.

JENKINS (W. H.) The family medical index, or what to do in cases of emergency; written expressly for the colonies. 8°. *Melbourne*, 1874.

KITTOE (W. H.) The domestic medical pocket book, or family vade necum; containing a concise account of diseases incident to the human frame, with formulas to meet the exigence of the moment, where medical aid is distant or not to be procured; remarks on some of the diseases of women and children, accidents, wounds, etc., poisons, bathing, climate, settlers in distant lands, sea voyages, etc. 8°. *Southampton & London*, 1837.

———. The same. 3. ed. 8°. *London*, 1844.

KNÖRLEIN (J. A.) Die Pflege der Kranken und Verwundeten und die sichersten Schutzmittel zur Zeit herschender Epidemien, [etc.] 12°. *Linz*, 1849.

KRANKENPFLEGE (Die) in der Familie. Zur Aufklärung und Unterstützung in der häuslichen Krankenpflege und als Lectüre für Jedermann herausgegeben von F. Kiesewetter. 8°. *Trappau*, 1885.

LANG (M.) Der vollständige Haus-Doktor. 600 hewährte Hausarzneimittel gegen die meist vorkommenden Krankheiten des Menschen. 30. Aufl. 16°. *Reutlingen*, [*n. d.*]

Medicine (*Popular, Manuals of*).

LITTRÉ (É.) Atlas populaire de médecine, de chirurgie, de pharmacie, de l'art vétérinaire et des sciences qui s'y rapportent pouvant servir de complément à tous les dictionnaires de médecine. 8°. *Paris*, 1885.

MACAULEY (A.) A dictionary of medicine, designed for popular use. 8. ed. 8°. *Edinburgh*, [1828].

——. The same. 10. ed. 8°. *Edinburgh*, 1849.

——. The same. 11. ed. 8°. *Edinburgh*, 1852.

MÉDECINE (La) et la chirurgie des pauvres, qui contiennent des remèdes choisis, faciles à préparer, et sans dépense, pour la plupart des maladies internes et externes qui attaquent le corps humain. Nouv. éd. 16°. *Paris*, 1771.

MEDICAL hints, designed for the use of clergymen and others in places where professional advice cannot be immediately procured. By a medical practitioner retired from business. 8°. *London*, 1820.

MERCKLEIN (G. A.) Neu aussgefertigtes historisch-medicinisches Thier-Buch in vier Theilen verabfasset; deren handelt: I. Von vierfüssigen Thieren, die zur Arzney dienen können. II. Von Vögeln und denen davon entnehmlichen Artzneyen. III. Von Fischen und denen davon in der Medicin brauchbaren Dingen. IV. Von alerley Ungezieffer, oder Gewürm, und kleinen zerkerbten Thierlein, so in Medicin zu gebrauchen seyn. Enthaltende wider fast alle Kranckheiten und Leibes-Zufälle so wohl fremde als eigene verschiedene heilsame Secreta, und bewerte Genessmittel. Durch und durch mit schönen an der Zahl ccxxv Kupfern gezieret. Auf freundliches Begehren zusammen getragen in diese Form gebracht, mit aussführlichen Register versehen und herausgegeben. 16°. *Nürnberg*, 1696.

MILLOT (A.) Médecine perfective, ou code des bonnes mères. 2 v. 8°. *Paris*, 1809.

MOORE (W. J.) A manual of family medicine for India. 8°. *London*, 1874.

MÜHSAM (S.) & BOGINSKY (A.) Die Hausapotheke, enthaltend die unentbehrlichen Hausmittel. 8°. *Berlin*, [*n. d.*]

PARKINSON (J.) Medical admonitions to families, respecting the preservation of health and the treatment of the sick. Also, a table of symptoms, serving to point out the degree of danger, and to distinguish one disease from another; with observations on the improper indulgence of children, etc. 1. Am., from 4. English, ed. 8°. *Portsmouth*, 1803.

READY remedies for common complaints. A manual of domestic and household surgery. 12°. *London*, [*n. d.*]

REYHER (O.) Aerztlicher Rathgeber, oder Belehrungen über Wesen und erste Behandlung der häufigeren Krankheiten. 12°. *Reudnitz-Leipzig*, 1885.

RIKLI (A.) Lehrbuch der Naturheilkunde. 1. Theil: Die Fieberkrankheiten, mit besonderer Berücksichtigung der Blattern. Volksverständliche Abhandlung speziell den schweizerischen Kantonsräthen sowie dem gesammten Lehrerstande Deutschlands und der Schweiz gewidmet. 8°. *Leipzig*, 1886.

RYFFEN (W.) Practicierbuchlin bewerter Leibartzeney, in allen Kranckheiten, und Leibs gebrächen. Erneuwert und gebessert. 16°. *Franckf. a. M.*, 1583.

DE SAINT-VINCENT (A.-C.) Nouvelle médecine des familles à la ville et à la campagne. A l'usage des familles, des maisons d'éducation, des écoles communales, des curés, des sœurs hospitalières, des dames de charité et de toutes les personnes

Medicine (*Popular, Manuals of*).

bienfaisantes qui se dévouent au soulagement des malades. 3. éd. 8°. *Paris*, 1874.

SANKEY (F. F.) Familiar instructions in medicine and surgery, with observations on the means of maintaining the health of men on ship board, or when employed in unhealthy localities. Intended for the use of the merchant navy, commanders of yachts, travellers, [etc.] 8°. *Malta*, 1846.

SIMONS (J. H.) The planter's guide and family book of medicine; for the instruction and use of planters, families, country people, and all others who may be out of the reach of physicians or unable to employ them. With particular directions respecting Asiatic cholera, by a Charleston physician. 8°. *Charleston*, [1848].

SOUTH (J. F.) Household surgery, or hints on emergencies. 12°. *London*, 1847.

STARK (A.) Die Heilung aller Krankheiten ohne Arzt und Apotheke durch Wasser und Diät. Ein unentbehrliches Hausbüchlein für Jedermann. Nach den besten Schriften über die Wasserheilmethode und nach eigenen Erfahrungen einfach und kurz zusammengestellt. 16°. *Reutlingen*, [*n. d.*]

THOMAS (A.) Der Hausarzt. Bewährte Hausarzneimittel gegen die meist vorkommenden Krankheiten des Menschen. Unentbehrlich für Stadt und Land. 16°. *Reutlingen*, [*n. d.*]

THOMAS (R.) The way to preserve good health, invigorate a delicate constitution, and attain an advanced age; together with a treatise on domestic medicine . . . This work is principally intended for the use of the clergy, and other heads of families and seminaries, managers of plantations and factories in the English colonies, and captains of ships having no surgeon on board, but may also prove useful to medical students and young practitioners. 8°. *London*, 1822.

——. The same. 1. Am. ed. Revised by David Hosack. 8°. *New York*, 1822.

THOMSON (S.) A dictionary of domestic medicine and household surgery. 1. Am., from the last Lond. ed., revised, with additions, by Henry H. Smith. 8°. *Philadelphia*, 1859.

TISSOT (S.-A.) Avis au peuple sur sa santé, ou traité des maladies les plus fréquentes. Nouvelle édition, augmentée de la description et de la cure de plusieurs maladies, et principalement de celles qui demandent de prompts secours. Ouvrage composé en faveur des habitants de la campagne, du peuple des villes, et de tous ceux qui ne peuvent avoir facilement les conseils des médecins. 12°. *Liége*, 1763.

——. The same. Advice to the people in general, with regard to their health. But more particularly calculated for those who, by their distance from regular physicians, or other very experienced practitioners, are the most unlikely to be seasonably provided with the best advice and assistance, in acute diseases, or upon any sudden inward or outward accident. With a table of the most cheap, yet effectual, remedies, and the plainest directions for preparing them readily. Transl. from the French edition of Dr. Tissot's: Avis au peuple, by J. Kirkpatrick. 8°. *London*, 1765.

——. The same. 2. ed. 8°. *London*, 1766.

——. The same. To which is added the art of preserving health; containing the most important rules recommended by physicians and philosophers for the preservation of health in the several periods and circumstances of life; together with the reasons on which these rules are founded. By J. Mackenzie. v. 1. 12°. *London*, 1767.

Medicine (*Popular, Manuals of*).

——. The same. With all the notes in the two former English editions, and few additional ones. By J. Kirkpatrick 3. ed. 8°. *London*, 1768.

——. The same. Transl. from the French ed., printed at Lyons; with all the notes in the two former English editions, and a few aditional ones. By J. Kirkpatrick. 4. ed. 8°. *London*, 1771.

——. The same. 9. ed. 12°. *Edinburgh*, 1778.

TROOST (Den) der armen; behelsende lichte ende souvereijne remedien tegen verscheijde siekten, wonden, gezwellen, en andere qualen des lichaems van den mensch, door de ondervindinge goet gekeurt, tot grooten dienst en de troost van vele behoeftige menschen, welker qualen ongeneselijk schijnen te wesen. Seer dienstig in alle familien en hospitalen. Desen laesten druk vermeerdert met eenige nieuwe remedien voor peirden ende horenbeesten, mitsgaders een tafel derselve. 18°. *Gendt*, [1712].

TURNER (D. W.) Hints and remedies for the treatment of common accident and diseases and rules of simple hygiene. The two parts complete. From the 8. Eng. ed. 16°. *New York*, 1882.

UNIVERSAL (The) family physician and surgeon; containing a familiar and accurate description of the symptoms of every disorder incident to mankind; together with their gradual progress and method of cure . . . The whole compiled from Smythson, Tissot, Buchan, Cornwell, [etc.] 8°. *Blackburn*, 1800.

VOGTER (B.) Ein nützlich und notwenndigs Artzney Büchlin für den gemeynenn Menschen, darinnen vonn allen Kranckhaitenn allerlay Art, so dem Menschenn zü stehen mögenn, die zu vetreibenn, mit vil bewertenn Stückenn, Kreijtern, Salbenn, Pflaster unnd Recepten. Durch den weyt berümbtenn Mayster . . . bey dem hochwirdigen . . . Herrn, Herrn Cristoffen, Bischoff zu Augspurg, newlich beschriben und in Truck gegeben. sm. 4°. [*Augspurg*, 1536.]

WARREN (I.) The household physician; for the use of families, planters, seamen, and travellers. Being a brief description, in plain language, of all the diseases of men, women, and children, with the newest and most approved methods of curing them. 8°. *Boston*, 1859.

WOOD'S household practice of medicine, hygiene and surgery. A practical treatise for the use of families, travelers, seamen, miners, and others. Edited by Frederick A. Castle. 2 v. 8°. *New York*, 1880.

WOYTS (J. J.) Gazophylacium medico-physicum, oder Schatz-Kammer medicinisch und natürlicher Dinge, in welcher alle medicinische Künst-Wörter, inn- und äusserliche Kranckheiten, nebst dererselben Genesmitteln, alle Mineralien, Metalle, Ertzte, Erden, zur Medicin gehörige fremde und einheimische Thiere, Kräuter, Blumen, Saamen, Säfte, Oele, Härtze, etc., alle rare Specereyen und Materialien, in einer richtigen lateinischen Alphabet-Ordnung auf das deutlichste erkläret, vorgestellet, und mit einem nöthigen Register versehen sind. 4. Aufl. 4°. *Leipzig*, 1755.

Medicine (*Popular errors in*).

BACHOT (G.) Erreurs populaires touchant la médecine et régime de santé. Œuvre nouvelle, désirée de plusieurs, et promise par feu M. Laurens Joubert. 8°. *Lyon*, 1626.

BEAUSSIER (J.-C.-J.) * De metuendissimis erroribus popularibus in medicina, in hygiene, in therapeutica. 4°. *Parisiis*, 1831.

Medicine (*Popular errors in*).

BEHR (J. C. L.) * De noxis medicinæ popularis. 4°. *Jenæ*, 1791.

BERNHARDI (A.) Ueber die verschiedenen ärztlichen Richtungen. Ein Wort zur gemeinverständlichen Beantwortung der Frage: Welche Aerzte sind die besten? 8°. *Eilenburg*, 1856.

BESSIÈRES (A.-F.-E.) Étude sur les erreurs et les préjugés populaires en médecine. 4°. *Paris*, 1860.

BORIANNE (J.) * Essai sur les erreurs en médecine répandues dans le département de la Haute-Vienne et sur leurs dangers. 4°. *Paris*, 1831.

COLON (P.-P.) * Essai sur la médecine populaire et ses dangers. 4°. *Paris*, 1824.

FÜRSTENAU (J. H.) [Pr.] de præjudiciis in artis exercitio salutaris vulgaribus sedulo vitandis. 4°. *Rintelii*, [1750].

HAWES (W.) An examination of the Rev. Mr. John Wesley's Primitive physic, shewing that a great number of the prescriptions therein contained are founded on ignorance of the medical art and of the power and operation of medicines, and that it is a publication calculated to do essential injury to the health of those persons who may place confidence in it. Interspersed with medical remarks and practical observations. 2. ed. 8°. *London*, 1780.

HOPPE (I.) Ist es erlaubt, dass Nicht-Aerzte Kranke heilen? Eine medicinisch-volkswirthschaftliche Untersuchung. 8°. *Leipzig*, 1864.

D'IHARCE. Erreurs populaires sur la médecine; ouvrage composé pour l'instruction de ceux qui ne professent pas cette science, avec l'explication des termes de l'art dont on n'a pu se dispenser de se servir. 8°. *Paris*, 1783.

JOUBERT (L.) Erreurs populaires et propos vulgaires touchant la médecine et le régime de santé. Revue et augmentée presque de la moitié, etc. 8°. *Bourdeaux*, 1579.

——. The same. La prima parte degli Errori popolari dell' Lorenzo Gioberti . . . Tradotta di franzese in lingua toscana del Mag. M. Alberto Luchi da Colle. 4°. *Fiorenza*, 1592.

LAIB (J. G.) * Perversa judicia de medicis et medicina. 4°. *Halæ Magdeb.*, [1712].

LICHTENBERG (C. F.) * De nonnullis vulgi præjudicatis opinionibus medicæ arti obsistentibus. sm. 8°. *Berolini*, [1822].

MURRAY (J. A.) De limitanda laude librorum medicorum practicorum usu populari destinatorum. sm. 4°. *Gottingæ*, [1779].

PIORRY (P.-A.) * Dissertation sur le danger de la lecture des livres de médecine par les gens du monde. 4°. *Paris*, 1816.

——. La médecine du bon sens. De l'emploi des petits moyens en médecine et en thérapeutique. 2. éd. 8°. *Paris*, 1867.

PRIMROSE (J.) De vulgi erroribus in medicina. Libri iv. 16°. *Amstelodami*, 1639.

——. The same. Popular errours, or the errours of the people in physick, first written in Latin. Divided into four bookes: 1. The first treating concerning physicians. 2. The second of the errours about some diseases, and the knowledge of them. 3. The third of the errours about the diet, as well of the sound as of the sick. 4. The fourth of the errours of the people about the use of remedies. To which is added by the same authour his verdict concerning the antimoniall cuppe. Translated into English by Robert Wittie. 16°. *London*, 1651.

——. The same. Traité de Primerose sur les erreurs vulgaires de la médecine, avec des additions de M. de Rostagny. 12°. *Lyon*, 1689.

RICHARD (M.-J.-M.) * Dissertation sur les erreurs populaires relatives à la médecine, et leurs dangers. 4°. *Paris*, 1833.

Medicine (*Popular errors in*).

RICHERAND (A.) Des erreurs populaires relatives à la médecine. 8°. *Paris*, 1810.

——. The same. Ueber medicinische Volksirrethümer. 8°. *Leipzig*, 1811.

TRIPLER (C. S.) The duties of physicians in relation to popular medical delusions. An address. 8°. *Covington, Ky.*, 1859.

Alpago-Novello (L.) Dei pregiudizi popolari medici. Indipendente, Torino, 1879, xxx, 745; 769.—**Amadeo** (G.) Sulla utilità della opinione, massime pregiudicata del popolo, in medicina. Ann. univ. di med., Milano, 1838, lxxxviii, 410-441.—**Klose** (C. L.) Ueber medicinische Volksschriften, Anpreisung von Heilmitteln und Urtheile über Curmethoden in öffentlichen politischen Blättern. Ztschr. f. d. Staatsarznk., Erlang., 1843, xlv, 52-57.—**Lichtenstädt.** Ueber diejenigen Irrthümer der Volksheilkunde, welche aus der gelehrten Heilkunde entstanden sind. Allg. med. Ann., Leipz., 1828, 145-162.—**Majer** (C. F.) Ueber Volksmedizin und medizinischen Volksaberglauben, besonders in Franken. Deutsche Ztschr. f. d. Staatsarznk., Erlang., 1864, n. F., xxii, 3-24.—**Piorry** (P.-A.) Livres de médecine (lecture de ces livres par les gens du monde). Dict. d. sc. méd., Par., 1818, xxviii, 489-509.—**Washburn** (T. D.) Are the public competent to judge what system of medicine is most desirable, or what practice they should adopt? Buffalo M. & S. J., 1872-3, xii, 241-250.

Medicine (*Preventive*).

See Hygiene.

Medicine (*Psychological*).

See Insanity; Psychology (*Medical*).

Medicine (*Public*).

See Medicine (*State*).

Medicine (*Sacred*).

See Bible (*Medicine of the*).

Medicine (*Spagyric*).

See Medicine (*Magical, etc.*)

Medicine (*State*).

See, also, Charities (*Medical, etc.*); Education (*Medical*), etc.; Evidence (*Medical*); Hygiene (*Public, Laws, etc., of*); Jurisprudence (*Medical*); Medicine (*Legislation relating to*); Night medical service; Prostitution; Quarantine; *and under names of countries, states, and cities.*

ACKERMANN (J. C. H.) Polizeylich-medizinische Miszellen. 8°. *Posen u. Leipzig*, 1806.

AITON (G.) * De politeia medica. 8°. *Edinburgi*, 1820.

ALDERSON (F. H.) Medical attendance for the sick poor, not paupers. 12°. [*London*, 1887.] *Repr. from:* Prov. M. J., Leicester, 1887, vi.

BALK (D. G.) * De artis medicæ relationibus ad rempublicam. 4°. [*Dorpat*], 1802.

BAUMER (J. W.) Fundamenta politiæ medicæ. 8°. *Francofurti et Lipsiæ*, 1777.

BEITRÄGE zur exacten Forschung auf dem Gebiete der Sanitäts-Polizei. Hrsg. von Louis Pappenheim. 1.-4. Hft. 8°. *Berlin*, 1860-62.

VON BENE (F.) Elementa politiæ medicæ. 8°. *Budæ*, 1807.

BERNCASTEL (L.) * De artis medicæ exercitio imperitis in republica bene constituta non permittendo. sm. 4°. *Jenæ*, [1797].

BISCHOFF (C. H. E.) Beiträge zur Staats-Arzneiwissenschaft und Kunst. 12°. *Erlangen*, 1824.

BRITISH Medical Association. Annual meeting, Brighton, 1886. Public medicine section. 8°. *Brighton*, [1886].

BUFALINI (B.) Sull' assistenza sanitaria nelle città e nelle campagne, sugli studj medico-chirurgici e sul servizio medico-chirurgico ospitaliero. Con un' appendice contenente altre due lettere intorno alla statistica sanitaria municipale. 12°. *Siena*, 1876.

CHAILLÉ (S. E.) Address on state medicine and medical organization. With the recommen-

Medicine (*State*).

dations in reference to state medicine of the Louisiana State Medical Society and of the Orleans Parish Medical Society to the Louisiana constitutional convention of 1879. 8°. *New Orleans*, 1879.

CHOULANT (J. L.) Gutachten und Aufsätze im Gebiete der Staatsarzneikunde. 8°. *Leipzig*, 1847.

DANILEVSKY (J. L.) * De magistratu, medico felicissimo. *Gottingæ*, 1784.

In: FRANK (J. P.) Delect. opusc. med. 8°. *Ticini*, 1788, v, 70-120.

DESMARTIS (T.-P.) Lettre à M. le maire de la ville de Bordeaux. 8°. *Bordeaux*, 1860.

DMITRIEFF (I.) Prilojenie k otchetu S.-Peterburgskom gubernskoi upravy za 1885g. Zemsko-meditsinskaja pomotsh v. S.-Peterburgskoi gubernii v trechletie 1883, 4 i 5 gg. Vypusk I. Uezdy: Gdovskii, Lugskii i Schlüsselburgskii. [Annex to report of St. Petersburg government board of assistance for 1885. Provincial medical aid of St. Petersburg government for the triennium 1883-5. 1. pt. Districts: Gdov, Luga, Schlüsselburg.] 8°. *St. Petersburg*, 1886.

DOBSCHA (F.) Specimen qua fragmenta quædam ad politiam medicam spectantia, [etc]. 8°. *Jenæ*, 1707.

VON EHRHART (G.) Entwurf eines physikalisch-medizinischen Polizei-Gesetzbuches und eines gerichtlichen Medizinal-Codex. 4 v. 8°. *Augsburg u. Leipzig*, [*n. d.*]

ELLIOTSON (J.) The introductory lecture of a course upon state-medicine, delivered in Mr. Grainger's theatre, Southwark, on November the first. 8°. *London*, 1821.

EMSMANN (G. A.) * De medicina politica. 4°. *Jenæ*, [1804].

FRANK (J. P.) System einer vollständigen medicinischen Polizey. 13 v. in 6. 12°. *Frankenthal*, 1791-4.

——. The same. Neue Aufl. 6 Bde. in 8 Th. 8°. *Mannheim, Tübingen u. Wien*, 1788-1819.

——. The same. Supplement-Bände zur medicinischen Polizey, oder Sammlung verschiedener, in diese Wissenschaft einschlagender, eigener Aufsätze. 3 v. 8°. *Tübingen u. Leipzig*, 1812-27.

GAINES (E. P.) Address before the Medical Association of the State of Alabama. 8°. *Mobile*, 1880.

GEORGE (C.) Duty of the state towards the medical profession. 8°. *Ann Arbor, Mich.*, [1885].

VAN GEUNS (M.) Oratio, qua an expediat reipublicæ medicinam facientium opera expenditur. 4°. *Hardervici*, [1776].

——. De staatkundige handhaving van der ingezetenen gezondheid en leven aangepreezen, en in eenige proeven voorgedragen; uit het Latijn vertaald door H. A. Bake. 8°. *Amsterdam*, 1801.

HOGG (W.-D.) La médecine publique en Angleterre. 8°. *Paris*, 1883.

HOLLAND. Verzameling van stukken betreffende het geneeskundig staatstoezicht in Nederland. (Uitgegeven door de inspecteurs en adjunct-inspecteurs voor het geneeskundig staatstoezicht.) In de jaaren 1865-83. 18 v. 8°. *'s Gravenhage*, 1867-83.

——. Geneeskundige hulp in Nederland. Kaart aantoonenden het aantal inrichtingen tot verpleging van zieken, dat der geneeskundigen en der vroevrouwen in elke gemeente des rijks in het jaar 1886. broadside, 36 x 40 in. *'s Gravenhage*, [1887].

Medicine (*State*).

Houze de l'Aulnoit (A.) De l'assistance publique à Lille. L'hôpital Saint-Sauveur. 8°. *Lille*, 1866.
Repr. from: Mém. Soc. d. imp. sc., de l'agric. et d. arts de Lille.

Hussty (Z. G.) Diskurs über die medizinische Polizei. 2 v. 8°. *Pressburg u. Leipzig*, 1786.

Lacassagne (A.) Les actes de l'état civil; étude médico-légale de la naissance, du mariage, de la mort. 12°. *Lyon*, 1887.

Lion (A.) sen. Handbuch der Medicinal- und Sanitätspolizei. Nach eignen Erfahrungen und nach dem neuesten Standpunkt der Wissenschaft und der Gesetzgebung für Aerzte, Apotheker und Verwaltungsbeamte. 3 v. in 2. 8°. *Iserlohn*, 1862–75.

——. Compendium der Sanitäts-Polizei und gerichtlichen Medicin. Ein Repetitorium für die Physikats - Prüfung, für Physiker, Juristen und Apotheker. 8°. *Berlin*, 1867.

Loder (J. C.) Anfangsgründe der medicinischen Anthropologie und der Stats-Arzneykunde. 2. Aufl. 8°. *Weimar*, 1793.

Ludwig (C. F.) [Pr.] adversaria ad medicinam publicam. i–iv. 4°. *Lipsiæ*, 1814–18.

Lundy (C. J.) The relations of the state and the medical profession. An address. 8°. *Ann Arbor*, 1886.

de Macedo Pinto (J. F.) Medicina administrativa e legislativa; obra destinada para servir de texto no ensino d'esta sciencia, e para elucidar os facultativos civis e militares, os pharmaceuticos, os engenheiros, os magistrados administrativos, os directores de estabelecimentos de industria e de educação litteraria, etc., nas questões de hygiene pública e policia medica e sanitaria. Hygiene pública. 2 v. 8°. *Coimbra*, 1862–3.

Markus (M.-F.-C.) Essai sur la médecine dans ses rapports avec l'état. 8°. *St.-Pétersbourg*, 1847.

Martini (L.) Elementi di polizia medica. 5 v. 8°. *Torino*, 1824–5.

Michaelis (G. P.) * Diss. exhibens usum et abusum medicinæ in re publica. 4°. *Marburgi*, [1738].

Monatsschrift für exacte Forschung auf dem Gebiete der Sanitäts-Polizei. Hrsg. von L. Pappenheim. Jahrg. 1–2, 1859–62. 8°. *Berlin*.

Monti (B.) Della igiene pubblica della polizia medica della medicina legale e della loro coordinazione sintetica e del principio unitivo nel quale si congiungono. Prolusione letta nella R. Università di Bologna. 8°. *Bologna*, 1860.
Also [Rev.], *in:* Raccoglitore med. di Fano, 1861, 2. s., xxiii, 140–147.

Most (G. F.) Ausführliche Encyklopädie der gesammten Staatsarzneykunde. Im Vereine mit mehreren Doctoren der Rechtsgelahrtheit, der Philosophie, der Medicin und Chirurgie, mit praktischen Civil-, Militair- und Gerichtsärzten und Chemikern bearbeitet und herausgegeben. Für Gesetzgeber, Rechtsgelehrte, Policeibeamte, Militairärzte, gerichtliche Aerzte, Wundärzte, Apotheker und Veterinärärzte. 2 v. 8°. *Leipzig*, 1838–40.

Niemann (J. F.) Taschenbuch der Civil-Medicinal-Polizei für Aerzte und Wundärzte, Medicinal- und Sanitätsbeamte. 12°. *Leipzig*, 1828.

Protokoli zasaidanii gubernskago zemskago vrachelnago soveta i soveta vrachei gubernskoi zemskoi bolnitsy za vtorujun polovinu 1885 g. (Jul. – Dek.) [3. year.] [Transactions of meetings of government provincial medical council and council of government physicians for provincial hospitals for the second half year, 1885 (July-Dec.).] 8°. *Kursk*, 1886.

Medicine (*State*).

Puxeddu (G.) Delle attinenze e de' rapporti dell' igiene della polizia medica, e della medicina legale, col progressivo incivilimento de' popoli; discorso accademico. 8°. [*Torino*, 1859.]

Richter (A. L.) Anleitung zur Vermeidung der Arznei - Verschwendung und zur Wahrnehmung des Staatsinteresses bei der Behandlung von Kranken auf öffentliche Kosten, besonders für Militairärzte. 8°. *Berlin*, 1839.

Rumsey (H. W.) Essays on state medicine. 8°. *London*, 1856.

Sauvaget (P.) * Nécessité d'organiser la médecine publique. 4°. *Paris*, 1883.

Scheidnagel (L.) Apuntes acerca del servicio sanitario en campaña, en relacion con el servicio de ingenieros. 8°. *Madrid*, 1875.

[Schöpff (J. D.)] Ueber den Einfluss des Medizinalwesens auf den Staat und über die Vernachlässigung desselben in den meisten deutschen Staaten. 12°. [*Hof*], 1799.

Schraud (F.) Aphorismi de politia medica. 12°. *Pestini*, 1795.

Schürmayer (J. H.) Handbuch der medicinischen Policei. Nach den Grundsätzen des Rechtsstaates, zu academischen Vorlesungen und zum Selbstunterrichte für Aerzte und Juristen. 8°. *Erlangen*, 1848.

——. The same. 2. Aufl. 8°. *Erlangen*, 1856.

——. The same. Handboek der geneeskundige police; volgens de grondregels van den constitutionelen staat . . . naar het Hoogduitsch, met aanteekeningen en toelechtingen voorzien, door G. Rombouts. 8°. *Tiel*, 1849.

de Sousa Pinto (A. J.) Medicina politica, ou principios necessarios tanto aos professores como uteis aos enfermos. 8°. *Lisboa*, 1822.

Stütz (W. A.) Ueber Medicin und Chirurgie in Beziehung auf den Staat. Nebst einem Anhang, eine Skizze der Medicinalpolizei enthaltend. 8°. *Stuttgart*, 1803.

Tyrrell (G. G.) Annual address delivered before the Medical Society of California. 8°. *Sacramento*, 1882.

Uden. Medizinische Politik. 8°. *Leipzig*, 1783.

Vogel (C.) Das staatsärztliche Verfahren; für Aerzte, Chirurgen, Apotheker, Thierärzte und für Rechtsgelehrte. Nebst einem Anhange, Formularien zu staatsärztlichen Geschäftsschriften enthaltend. 8°. *Jena*, 1836.

——. Die medicinische Polizeiwissenschaft. 8°. *Jena*, 1853.

Wildberg (C. F. L.) Von den polizeylich-medizinischen Geschäften der-Physiker.
Forms 1. Th. of his: Praktisches Handbuch für Physiker. 8°. *Erfurt*, 1823.

Wistrand (A. T.) Afhandlingar i statsmedicinen. 2 pts. sm. 8°. *Stockholm*, 1842–60.

Yeld (H. J.) State medicine in relation to education. 8°. *Sunderland*, 1875.
Also, in: Pub. Health, Lond., 1875, iii, 497–499.

Albert. Bemerkungen und Erfahrungen über einige Gegenstände der medicinischen Polizei. Ztschr. f. d. Staatsarznk., Erlang., 1832, xxiii, 76 ; 279. — **Allen** (N.) State medicine and its relations to insanity and public charity. J. Psych. M., Lond., 1875, n. s., i, 248–266.—**Armaingaud.** Sur les moyens de faire aboutir les projets d'organisation de la médecine publique. Rev. d'hyg., Par., 1881, iii, 147–157. — **Bailogolovi** (I.) O gubernskikh meditsinskikh obshchestvakh. [On governmental medical societies.] Med. Vestnik, St. Petersb., 1867, vii, 9 ; 17.—**Bencke.** Nachricht über den Verein für gemeinschaftliche Arbeiten zur Förderung der wissenschaftlichen Heilkunde. Amtl. Ber. ü. d. Versamml. deutsch. Naturf. u. Aerzte 1856, Wien, 1858, 255–261. — **Bernt** (J.) Auszüge aus des Herrn . . . Beiträgen zur gerichtlichen Arzneikunde, nebst Bemerkungen. Von Joseph Schneider. Ver. deutsche Ztschr. f. d. Staats-Arznk., Freib. i.

Medicine (*State*).

Br., 1851, n. F., ix, 317-342.—**Betrachtungen** über die rechte Stellung der Physiker im Staate als das erste und nothwendigste Mittel, den möglichst grössten Nutzen für das allgemeine Gesundheitswohl durch dieselben zu erreichen. Jahrb. d. ges. Staatsarznk., Leipz., 1835, i, 4. Hft., 16-24. — **Betrachtungen** über die medicinische Polizei, als ein wesentliches Erforderniss eines jeden wohlgeordneten Staats. *Ibid.*, 1837, ii, 205-214.—**Billings** (F. S.) State medicine. J. Am. M. Ass., Chicago, 1885, v, 309-315.—**Blosfeld** (G. J.) Zur medicinischen Statistik und medicinischen Polizei. Med. Ztg. Russlands, St. Petersb., 1844, i, 69.—**Braun.** Die beste Medicinalverfassung. Jahrb. d. phil.-med. Gesellsch. zu Würzb., 1828, i, 2. Hft., 116-134. — **Brefeld.** Uebersicht der Fortschritte, Entdeckungen und Veränderungen in der Staatsarzneikunde in den Jahren 1823-6. Ztschr. f. d. Staatsarznk., Erlang., 1829, 10. Ergnzngshft., 163-328.—**Brock** (H. W.) Report on state medicine and public hygiene. Tr. M. Soc. W. Virg., Wheeling, 1877, 258-266. — **Cabanis.** Quelques principes et quelques vues sur les secours publics. *In his:* Œuvres complètes, 8°, Par., 1823, ii, 185-306.—**Carroll** (A. L.) An address on state medicine. Tr. N. York M. Ass. (1885), 1886, ii, 42-55. — **Chaillé** (S. E.) State medicine and state medical societies. Tr. Am. M. Ass., Phila., 1879, xxx, 299-320. *Also*, Reprint. ——. Annual report for 1881 of the committee on state medicine of the Louisiana State Medical Society. N. Orl. M. & S. J., 1880-81, n. s., viii, 1062-1088.—**Chaudé** (A.) De l'assistance médicale dans les campagnes. Ann. d'hyg., Par., 1881, 3. s., v, 138-155. *Also*, Reprint. — **Chipman** (M. M.) Report of the committee on public hygiene and state medicine. Tr. M. Soc. Calif., Sacramento, 1880, 48-57. *Also*, Reprint. — **Comegys** (C. G.) On the importance of the establishment of legal medical councils of state and medical politics. Tr. Am. M. Ass., Phila., 1877, xxviii, 499-503. — **Condotte** (Le) mediche nei comuni rurali della Sicilia. [Edit.] Ingrassia, Palermo, 1885, i, 281-291.—**Conn** (G. P.) State medicine. Tr. N. Hampshire M. Soc., Concord, 1881, 13-30. *Also*, Reprint.—**Covernton** (C. W.) State medicine, ancient, mediæval, and modern. Rep. Prov. Bd. Health Ontario 1883, Toronto, 1884, ii, 359-371.—**Diday** (P.) La police des mœurs. Lyon méd., 1881, xxxvi, 618-624.—**E.** Het ontwerp van wet regelende het geneeskundig staatstoezigt. Schat d. Gesondh., Haarlem, 1862, v, 321-328.—**Einige** Worte zur Beantwortung der Frage: Woher kommt es, dass in so vielen Ländern die medicinische Polizei so schlecht verwaltet wird, und wie ist eine bessere Verwaltung derselben auf eine leichte Weise zu erreichen? Jahrb. d. ges. Staatsarznk., Leipz., 1835, i, 70-75.—**Eisner.** Bemerkungen aus dem Gebiete der Staatsarzneikunde. Ztschr. f. d. Staatsarznk., Erlang., 1828, 9. Ergnzngshft., 119-158, 1 tab.—**Elsberg** (L.) The domain of medical police. Am. M. Month., N. Y., 1862, xvii, 321-337. *Also*, Reprint.—**Erdmann** (F.) Ueber die Heilkunst in Verhältnisse zum Staate. Ztschr. f. d. Staatsarznk., Erlang., 1841, 29. Ergnzngshft. 28-46.—**Erinnerung** an einige Gegenstände der medicinischen Polizei, welche ungeachtet ihrer Wichtigkeit für Gesundheit und Leben der Landeseinwohner doch an manchen Orten ganz unberücksichtiget gelassen werden. Jahrb. d. ges. Staatsarznk., Leipz., 1835, i, 48-61.—**Fodéré** (F.-E.) Police médicale. Dict. d. sc. méd., Par., 1820, xliv, 42-91.—**Gardner** (J.) On the mutual duties of the state and the citizen, and the relations that exist between both and the physician. Indiana M. Reporter, Evansville, 1880, i, 365-371.—**Gatch** (J. D.) Harmony and associated action in connection with state medicine. Tr. Indiana M. Soc., Indianap., 1880, xxx, 153-161. — **Gianelli** (G. L.) Proposta di ordinata collezione e rivista dei casi ed argomenti di medicina pubblica del prof. ... Gazz. med. ital. lomb., Milano, 1848, 2. s., i, 8-10.—**Gleitsmann.** Darstellung der Fortschritte der Staatsarzneikunde im letzten Decennium und des gegenwärtigen Standes derselben. Arch. f. d. ges. Med., Jena, 1843, v, 177-226.—**Gray** (J. P.) Relations of the State to medical science. Tr. N. York M. Ass. (1885), 1886, ii, 32-41.—**Grimshaw** (T. W.) Address in state medicine. Dublin J. M. Sc., 1884, 3. s., lxxvii, 198-226. ——. The State in its relation to the medical profession. Brit. M. J., Lond., 1887, i, 189-192.—**Grundsätze** für die Organisirung der öffentlichen Medizinal-Verwaltung. Wien. med. Presse, 1869, x, 131-135.—**Häussler** (F.) Kurze Bemerkungen über medicinische Polizei. Ztschr. f. d. Staatsarznk., Erlang., 1830, 13. Ergnzngshft., 302-311.—**Hedrich.** Ideen zur Feststellung periodischer medicinisch-polizeilicher Revisionen durch Landphysiker. *Ibid.*, 1827, xiv. 247-255.—**Heije** (J. P.) Over geneeskundige staatsregeling. Arch. v. Geneesk., Amst., 1843, iii, 1-64.—**Helm** (J. H.) President's address. Tr. Indiana M. Soc., Indianap., 1876, xxvi, 1-13.—**History** of the joint committee on state medicine of the British Medical and Social Science Associations. Brit. M. J., Lond., 1882, i, 921-923.—**Innhauser** (F.) Zur Organisirung des Wiener Stadtphysikates. Wien. med. Bl., 1883, vi, 1389; 1420; 1453.—**Janikowski** (S.) Uwagi o wykładzie medycyny publicznéj szczególniéj zaś sądowéj w uniwersytecie Paryzkim i mektorych Niemieckich. [Medical police and jurisprudence as

3

Medicine (*State*)

taught in the University of Paris and in Germany.] Pam. Towarz. Lek. Warszaw., 1861, xlvi, 153-187.—**Julius.** Nachweis indischer Medicinal-Polizei vor länger als zwei Jahrtausenden. Ztschr. f. d. ges. Med., Hamb., 1839, xii, 425-427.—**Knauer** (R.) Vorschläge zu einer zweckmässigeren Einrichtung in Betreff der Medicinalanstalten; allen Staatsmännern und Aerzten zur Prüfung vorgelegt. Ztschr. f. d. Staatsarznk., Erlang., 1833, 18. Ergnzngshft., 1-47.—**Knolz** (J. J.) Vortrag über den dermaligen Zustand der Staatsarzneikunde in den europäischen Staaten, ihre theilweisen Mängel und die Mittel zu ihrer Vervollkommnung. Deutsche Ztschr. f. d. Staatsarznk., Erlang., 1853, i, 7.—**Kopf.** Notizen und Reflexionen über verschiedene Gegenstände der Staatsarzneikunde. Ztschr. f. d. Staatsarznk., Erlang., 1823, v, 379-396. ——. Notizen über verschiedene, die Staatsarzneikunde berührende Gegenstände. *Ibid.*, 1826, 5. Ergnzngshft., 238-249. ——. Notizen und Miscellen, die Staatsarzneikunde betreffend. *Ibid.*, 1831, xxi, 396-408. — **Kopp** (J. H.) Bemerkungen über das System der Staatsarzneikunde in Hinsicht auf Eintheilung und Bezeichnung. Jahrb. d. Staatsarznk., Frankf. a. M., 1809, ii, 3-17. — **Kuborn.** Communication au sujet de l'organisation d'un service officieux de médecine publique dans le royaume. Bull. Acad. roy. de méd. de Belg., Brux., 1877, 3. s., xi, 292-302.—**Laycock** (T.) Letters on political medicine. Dublin M. Press, 1841, v, 167; 202; 235; 265; 315; 369; 420: vi, 43. — **Lefort** (L.) L'assistance publique et la réorganisation des services d'accouchement. Rev. scient., Par., 1881, 3. s., i, 346; 404.—**Lehre** (Zur) von den Vergehen gegen die Sicherheit des Lebens und der physischen und psychischen Gesundheit. Bl. f. gerichtl. Anthrop., Nürnb., 1857, viii, 5. Hft., 28-61.—**Lehrkanzel** (Die) der Staatsarzneikunde. Mitth. d. badisch. aerztl. Ver., Karlsruhe, 1848, ii, 25-27.—**Linzbauer** (D.) Allseitige Vereinigung zur Anbahnung einer pragmatischen Geschichte der Staatsarznei. Amtl. Ber. ü. d. Versamml. deutsch. Naturf. u. Aerzte 1856, Wien, 1858, xxxii, 238-243.—**Lorentz.** Kurze Untersuchungen der Frage: Darf es von einer guten medicinischen Polizei gestattet werden, dass Aerzte und Chirurgen sich auch mit Hebung natürlicher Geburten abgeben? Jahrb. d. ges. Staatsarznk., Leipz., 1835, i, 4. Hft., 25-28.—**Lundy** (C. J.) State regulation of medical practice. J. Am. M. Ass., Chicago, 1887, viii, 57-60.—**Marc.** Politique (médecine). Dict. de méd., 2. éd., Par., 1842, xxv, 513-534.—**Marcus** (A. F.) Beyträge zu einer Medizinalverfassung. Mag. f. spec. Therap. u. Klin., Jena, 1805-6, ii, 203-271.—**Marinus** (J.-R.) Discours sur la médecine judiciaire et la médecine politique, au point de vue de la science. Bull. Acad. roy. de méd. de Belg., Brux., 1847-8, vii, 769-788. *Also*—Mém. Acad. roy. de méd. de Belg., Brux., 1849, ii, 26-42.—**Mende.** Wie kann das Medizinalwesen für Flecken und Dörfer oder für das platte Land am besten eingerichtet werden? Ἀσκληπίειον, Berl., 1811, i, 721; 737; 785; 865; 935.—**Merrem.** Die Verwaltung der Medizinalpolizei im General-Gouvernement vom Nieder- und Mittelrhein. Jahrb. d. Staatsarznk., Frankf. a. M., 1816, ix, 3-19.—**Michael** (W. H.) An address delivered at the opening of the section of public medicine. At the annual meeting of the British Medical Association in Norwich. Brit. M. J., Lond., 1874, ii, 225; 227. — **Ministerio** de la gobernacion del reino. Direccion de sanidad; circulares. Eco de la med., Madrid, 1848-9, i, 188-191. ——. Direccion general de beneficencia y sanidad; estadistica; circular. Especialista, Madrid, 1860, ii, 155-160.—**Moore** (J. W.) The present and the future of state medicine. Dublin J. M. Sc., 1887, 3. s., lxxxiii, 235-253.—**Munford** (S. E.) A question in state medicine. Tr. Indiana M. Soc., Indianap., 1884, xxxiv, 1-16. *Also*, Reprint. *Also:* Am. Pract., Louisville, 1884, xxx, 129-141. *Also:* Fort Wayne J. M. Sc., 1884-5, iv, 126-137.—**Nederlandsche** Maatschappij tot Bevordering der Geneeskunst. Rapport der commissie belast met het onderzoek naar de werking en de resultaten der wet van 4 Dec. 1872. Staatsblad No. 134 en naar de wenschelijkheid van wettelijke regeling der prostitutie in Nederland. Nederl. Tijdschr. v. Geneesk., Amst., 1879, 2. R., xv, 321-336.—**Nusser** (E.) Ueber die Bedeutung der sanitäts-polizeilichen Obduction und die Möglichkeit, ihre Vornahme zu beschränken. Oesterr. Ztschr. f. prakt. Heilk., Wien, 1868, xiv, 893; 909; 929; 949.—**Orton** (E.) The relation of the state to public health. Tr. Ohio M. Soc., Columbus, 1882, xxxvii, 91-108. *Also*, Reprint.—**Penn** (J.) Geneeskundige staatsregeling. Nederl. Weekbl. v. Geneesk., Amst., 1855, v, 481: 1856, vi, 475; 485; 495; 505. —**Pfeufer** (C.) Ueber die Gränzen der Staatsgewalt in Bezug auf medizinische Systeme. Jahrb. d. ärztl. Ver. zu München, 1835, i, 122-134.—**Prussia.** Reorganisation der Medizinal-Verwaltung, speziell Stellung der Kreisphysici. Haus der Abgeordneten. Med.-Gesetzgeb., Berl., 1886, 36; 43.—**Puccinotti** (F.) Delle relazioni della medicina con la economia politica. Ann. univ. di med., Milano, 1837, lxxxiii, 227-250.—**Rapport** pour l'organisation d'un service médico-rural. Ann. de Cons. centr. de salub. pub. de Brux., 1849-50, v, 39-49. — **Review** (A) of "The domain of medical police. By Louis Elsberg". Brit. & For. M.-

Medicine (State).

Chir. Rev., Lond., 1863, xxxii, 323-328. *Also*, Reprint. — **Roberts** (D. J.) Address in state medicine. J. Am. M. Ass., Chicago, 1884, iii, 1-6. — **Rohé** (G. H.) Address in state medicine; recent advances in preventive medicine. J. Am. M. Ass., Chicago, 1887, ix, 1-11. *Also*, Reprint. — **Roosa** (D. B. St. J.) The relations of the medical profession to the state; anniversary address. Tr. M. Soc. N. Y., Syracuse, 1879, 49-72. *Also, in his:* A doctor's suggestions, etc., 12°, N. Y., 1880, 173-214. *Also* [Abstr.]: Sanitarian, N. Y., 1879, vii, 145-154. — **Rumsey** (H. W.) The public relations of medicine. Brit. M. J., Lond., 1870, ii, 214-218. — **Russell** (J. B.) An address delivered at the opening of the section of public medicine, at the annual meeting of the British Medical Association. *Ibid.*, 1876, ii, 206-211. *Also:* Med. Times & Gaz., Lond., 1876, ii, 193-197. — **von Samson-Himmelstiern** (G.) Mittheilungen aus dem practischen Wirkungskreise des Professors der Staatsarzneikunde au der kaiserlichen Universität Dorpat. Beitr. z. Heilk., Riga, 1849-51, i, 135: 1855, iii, 195. — **Serrano** (M. N.) Discurso [sobre las relaciones de las academias con las ciencias á que corresponden, de sus funciones en la administracion pública y del influjo de la medicina en la ciencia del gobierno]. Mem. r. Acad. méd. de Madrid, 1862, ii, pt. 1, 1-15. — **Smith** (S.) On the reciprocal relations of an efficient public health service and the highest educational qualifications of the medical profession. Am. Pub. Health Ass. Rep. 1874-5, N. Y., 1876, ii, 187-200. *Also*, Reprint. — **Snijders** (C. J.) De gemeentewet en de armenartsen. Nederl. Tijdschr. v Geneesk., Amst., 1887, xxiii, 661-678. — **Société** (La) belge de médecine publique. Tribune méd., Par., 1879, xi, 220; 245; 282; 306. — **Sonderegger.** Aerztliche Antworten auf politische Fragen. Cor.-Bl. f. schweiz. Aerzte, Basel, 1883, xiii, 289-296. — **Sporer** (G. M.) Grundbegriffe über die Staats-Arzneykunde und ihre ersten Verzweigungen. Med. Jahrb. d. k. k. österr. Staates, Wien, 1835, xvii, 96-132. — ——. Das öffentliche Medicinalwesen und seine Tendenzen zur festern Begründung des Gemeinwohls. Ztschr. d. k. k. Gesellsch. d. Aerzte zu Wien, 1844, ii, 205-216. — **State** medicine in Great Britain. J. Pub. Health & San. Rev., Lond., 1856-7, ii, 105-113. — **Stephenson** (F. B.) Duty of the state in public health. N. York M. J., 1887, xlv, 705-707. *Also*, Reprint. — **Stevens** (T. M.) Address on state medicine. Cincin. Lancet & Clinic, 1879, n. s., iii, 527-533. — ——. Report of committee on state medicine. Tr. Indiana M. Soc., Indianap., 1884, xxxiv, 35-39. *Also*, Reprint. — **Stokes** (W.) A discourse on state medicine. Brit. M. J., Lond., 1872, i, 385-389. *Also:* Med. Times & Gaz., Lond., 1872, i. 440-442. — **von Sybel** (H.) Ueber die Wirksamkeit der Staatsgewalt in socialen und ökonomischen Fragen. Cor.-Bl. d. nied.-rhein. Ver. f. öff. Gsndhtspflg., Köln, 1871-2, i, 229-233. — **Symonds** (J. A.) On medical evidence in relation to state medicine. *In his:* Misc., 8°, Lond., 1871, 372-381. — **Thayer** (S. W.) State medicine. Tr. Vermont M. Soc. 1880, Montpelier, 1881, 11-22. — **Thierfelder** sen. Beleuchtung einiger Mängel in der Verwaltung der Medicinalpolizei der Staaten, ihrer Ursachen und der Mittel ihnen abzuhelfen. Deutsche Ztschr. f. d. Staatsarznk., Erlang., 1866, n. F., xxiv, 3-13. — **Verhältniss** (Ueber das) der Aerzte zum Staate und zu den Leidenden; von einem Physicatsarzte. Ztschr. f. d. Staatsarznk., Erlang., 1829, xvii, 47-62. — **Vermischte** Bemerkungen über verschiedene Gegenstände der medizinischen Polizei. Allg. med. Ann., Altenb., 1805, 45; 59; 143; 182. — **Vetter.** Ueber die Grenzen zwischen medicinischen Polizei und anderen auf Sicherheit des Lebens und der Gesundheit abzweckenden Staatseinrichtungen, namentlich der Sicherheits-Polizei überhaupt. J. d. pract. Heilk., Berl., 1819, lxxxix, 1. St., 76-83. — **Virchow** (R.) Der Staat und die Aerzte. Med. Reform, Berl., 1848-9, 213; 217; 221; 225; 228. *Also, in his:* Ges. Abhandl. a. d. Geb. d. öff. Med., 8°, Berl., 1879, i, 50-71. — **Wardner** (H.) State medicine. Indiana M. Reporter, Evansville, 1880, i, 529-539. — **von Wedekind** (G. F.) Ideen zur Polizei der Heilkunde. Jahrb. d. Staatsarznk., Frankf. a. M., 1813, vi, 3: 1814, vii, 3: 1815, viii, 3: 1816, ix, 20: 1817, x, 3. — ——. Noch ein Paar Worte über die Stellung des Arztes im Staate. Ztschr. f. d. Staatsarznk., Erlang., 1829, xvii, 155-162. — **Weigel** (L. A.) State control of medicine. Med. Press West. N. York, Buffalo, 1887, ii, 291-301. — **Wie** kann man auf eine leichte, und nicht allzukostspielige Art, den Wundärzten, denen das Landvolk anvertrauet ist, und die der leidenden Menschheit oft mehr schädlich, als nützlich sind, einen bessern und zweckmässigern Unterricht beybringen? Eine Preisschrift. Arch. f. d. allg. Heilk., Berl., 1792, ii, 501-531. — **Wildberg** (C. F. L.) Erinnerungen an verschiedene zur Verbesserung der Verwaltung der medizinischen Polizei nothwendige Punkte. Jahrb. d. ges. Staatsarznk., Leipz., 1839, v, 469-479. — **Wistrand** (A. T.) Om statsmedicinens tillstånd i Sverige, des brister, dess förhoppningar. Hygiea, Stockholm, 1840, ii, 539-554. — **Wistrand** (A. H.) Kort framställning af statsmedicinens uppkomst och utveckling inom Sverige. *Ibid.*, 1849, xi, 517: 1850, xii, 3; 129; 379; 520: 1851, xiii, 3; 65. — **Yeaman** (G. H.) State medicine. Public Health, N. Y., 1879-80, i, 4.

Medicine (Veterinary).

See, also, **Animals** (*Diseases of*); **Auscultation** *in animals*; **Epizootic** *diseases*; **Hospitals, Veterinary, Jurisprudence, Obstetrics, Surgery,** *Veterinary; also under names of animals, as:* **Birds, Cattle, Dogs, Horses,** etc.; *also under names of diseases, as:* **Eye** (*Diseases of*) *in animals*; **Insanity** *in animals, etc*

ADAMOVICZ (A. F.) *Diss. inaug. morborum inter animalia domestica observatorum indicem singulorumque constantissima signa exhibens; adnexa synonymia Germanica, Gallica, Rossica et Polonica. 8°. *Vilnæ*, [1824].

AMMON (C. W.) Allgemeines Hausvieharzneibuch, oder vollständiger Unterricht, wie man die Krankheiten der Pferde, des Rindviehes, der Schafe, Schweine, Hunde, Katzen und des Federviehes auf die leichteste und wohlfeilste Art selbst heilen kann. 6. Aufl. 8°. *Berlin*, [1873].

BLAINE [D.] Outlines of the veterinary art; or, a treatise on the anatomy, physiology, and curative treatment of the diseases of the horse, and subordinately of those of neat cattle and sheep. 7. ed. By Charles Steel. 8°. *London*, 1865.

——. The same. Notions fondamentales de l'art vétérinaire, ou principes de médecine appliqués à la connaissance de la structure des fonctions et de l'économie du cheval, du bœuf, de la brebis et du chien, avec la manière de traiter leurs maladies. Trad. de l'anglais. 3 v. 8°. *Paris, an XI* [1803].

BLASCO (A.) Manuale del veterinario, ossia trattato sulle malattie del cavallo e sui rimedi necessari per guarirlo a norma delle recenti scoperte della scienza. 8°. *Milano*, 1886.

BOUCHARDAT (A.) Formulaire vétérinaire, contenant le mode d'action, l'emploi et les doses des médicaments simples et composés prescrits aux animaux domestiques par les médecins vétérinaires français et étrangers, suivi d'un mémorial thérapeutique. 2. éd. 12°. *Paris*, 1862.

BOULEY (H.) & REYNAL. Nouveau dictionnaire pratique de médecine, de chirurgie et d'hygiène vétérinaires, publié avec la collaboration d'une société de professeurs vétérinaires praticiens. [A–Jar.] v. 1-10. 8°. *Paris*, 1856-74.

BOURGELAT. Élémens de l'art vétérinaire. Essai sur les appareils et sur les bandages propres aux quadrupèdes, à l'usage des élèves des écoles royales vétérinaires. 8°. *Paris*, 1770.

——. Élémens de l'art vétérinaire; matière médicale raisonnée, ou précis des médicamens considérés dans leurs effets; à l'usage des élèves des écoles vétérinaires, avec les formules médicinales et officinales des mêmes écoles. 3. éd. v. 1. 8°. *Paris, an IV* [1796].

BRACKEN (H.) The gentleman's pocket farrier, with large additions and remarks. 3. ed. 16°. *London*, 1735.

——. Farriery improv'd; or, a compleat treatise upon the art of farriery, [etc.] 4. ed. 2 v. (v. 1), 1742; (v. 2), 1749. 12°. *London*.

——. The same. 2 v. v. 1, 6. ed. (1749); v. 2, 2. ed. (1740). 8°. *London*.

[BUCHAN (W.)] A complete treatise on the art of farriery, wherein are fully explained the nature and structure of that useful creature, a horse; with the diseases and accidents he is liable to, and the methods of cure. Likewise, rules for breeding and training of colts; practical receipts for the cure of common distempers incident to oxen, cows, calves, sheep, lambs, hogs, etc. To which is prefixed ten minutes' advice to the purchasers of horses. 8°. *New Haven*, 1816.

BUCHMÜLLER (A. L.) Allgemeine Pathologie und Therapie der Hausthiere. 8°. *Wien*, 1840.

Medicine (*Veterinary*).

Buc'hoz. Médecine des animaux domestiques, renfermant les différens remèdes qui conviennent pour les maladies des chevaux, des vaches, des brebis, des cochons, de la volaille, des oiseaux de fauconnerie, des petits oiseaux, etc. 2 v. in 1. 16°. *Paris*, 1785.

Bull (B.) A compendious system of veterinary instruction by question and answer. 8°. *London*, 1835.

Busch (J. D.) System der theoretischen und practischen Thierheilkunde. Zum Behuf akademischer Vorlesungen. 4 v. 12°. *Marburg*, 1806–16.

Clark (B.) Pharmacopœia equina; or, new pharmacopœia for horses. 4°. *London*, 1833.

——. Hippiatria; or, the surgery and medicine of horses. 4°. *London*, 1838.

——. Supplementary matter to the Pharmacopœia equina. 4°. [*n. p., n. d.*]

Clater (F.) Every man his own cattle doctor; containing the causes, symptoms, and treatment of all the diseases incident to oxen, sheep, swine, poultry, and rabbits, by Edward Mayhew. New ed. 8°. *London*, 1868.

——. The same. Entirely re-written to the present date by George Armatage. 8°. *London*, 1870.

——. The same. Le vétérinaire domestique, ou l'art de guérir soi-même ses chevaux; traduit de l'anglais sur la 21e éd., par P.-L. Prétot. 8°. *Paris*, 1822.

Comparolo (P.) Il servizio veterinario nel comune di Sondria. Relazione. 8°. *Sondrio*, 1884.

Complete (The) grazier; or, gentleman and farmer's directory. Containing the best instructions for buying, breeding, and feeding cattle, sheep, and hogs, and for suckling lambs. A description of the particular symptoms commonly attending the various distempers to which cattle, sheep, and hogs are subject; with the most approved remedies . . . With several other useful and curious particulars. Written by a country gentleman, and originally designed for private use. 16°. *London*, 1767.

Conferencias agrícolas sobre diferentes temas: Discursos pronunciados por catedráticos de la Escuela veterinaria de Madrid. 8°. *Madrid*, 1877.

Corsaletti (G.) L' empirismo in veterinaria. 12°. *Fano*, 1886.

Courtenay (E.) The practice of veterinary medicine and surgery. 12°. *London*, 1887.

Cressy (N.) Reports of a course of lectures on veterinary science. 8°. [*Burlington*, 1877?]

Delafond (O.) Traité de pathologie générale comparée des animaux domestiques. 2. éd. 8°. *Paris*, 1855.

Delwart (L.-V.) Pathologie spéciale ou descriptive des principaux animaux domestiques. 8°. *Bruxelles*, 1837.

Desmarest (M.-E.) Remarques sur plusieurs cas de pathologie observés chez des animaux. 8°. *Paris*, [1849].
Repr. from. Rev. et mag. de zool., 1849.

Dick (W.) Occasional papers on veterinary subjects. With a memoir by R. O. Pringle. roy. 8°. *Edinburgh & London*, 1869.

Dun (F.) Veterinary medicines; their actions and uses. With an appendix on the diseases of the domesticated animals. 8°. *Edinburgh*, 1864.

——. The same. 4. ed. 8°. *New York*, 1874.

Encyklopädie der gesammten Thierheilkunde und Thierzucht mit Inbegriff aller einschlägigen Disciplinen und der speciellen Etymologie. Handwörterbuch für praktische Thierärzte, Thierzüchter, Landwirthe und Thierbesitzer

Medicine (*Veterinary*).

überhaupt. Hrsg. von Alois Koch. 4 v. [A–Nyrus.] 8°. *Wien u. Leipzig*, 1885–6.
In course of publication.

Ercolani (G. B.) Nuovi elementi teorico-pratici di medicina veterinaria. 8°. *Bologna*, 1859.

Espejo y del Rosal (R.) Diccionario general de veterinaria. Contiene: la definicion de todas las voces de este arte, explicacion de las enfermedades de los animales domésticos y modo de curarlas. Seguido de un formulario completo para recetar, con explicacion de los medicamentos y determinacion de dósis en que deben administrarse. 3 v. 8°. *Madrid*, 1877–83.

Falke (I. E. L.) Universal-Lexicon der Thierarzneikunde. 2 v. 8°. *Weimar*, 1842–3.

——. Die thierärztliche Receptirkunde. 8°. *Leipzig*, 1849.

——. Lehrbuch der gesammten Thierarzneiwissenschaft. 2. Ausg. 3 v. 8°. *Leipzig*, 1855.

Fearnley (W.) The veterinarian's clinical note book. 8°. *Edinburgh*, [*n. d.*]

Félizet (L.) Dictionnaire vétérinaire, à l'usage des cultivateurs et des gens du monde. Précédé d'une introduction par J.-A. Barbal. 16°. *Paris*, 1870.

Fernandez é Isamendi (E.) Tratado de patología especial y terapéutica veterinaria. v. 1. 8°. *Madrid*, 1883.
Imperfect.

Field (J.) Posthumous extracts from the veterinary records, edited by his brother, William Field. 8°. *London*, 1843.

Foringer (E.) Die Ophthalmoskopie in der Veterinär-Medicin. 8°. *Jena*, 1881.

Foster (L.) Recept-Taschenbuch für Thierärzte. 12°. *Wien*, 1873.

Frenzel (J. T. G.) Praktisches Handbuch für Thierärzte und Oekonomen, nach alphabetischer Ordnung, in zwei Theilen. 3 v. 12°. *Leipzig*, 1794–7.

Friedberger (F.) & Fröhner (E.) Lehrbuch der speciellen Pathologie und Therapie der Hausthiere. Für Thierärzte, Aerzte und Studirende. 8°. *Stuttgart*, 1885.

Friedreich. Gerichtliche Veterinärkunde. Ein Separatabdruck aus dessen Handbuch der gerichtsärztlichen Praxis. Zum Drucke befördert und mit Zusätzen versehen von S. Landmann. 8°. *Regensburg*, 1846.

Gamgee (J.) On the study of veterinary medicine; inaugural address. 8°. *Edinburgh*, 1857.

——. Our domestic animals in health and disease. Illustrated. 2 v. 8°. *Edinburgh*, 1863–4.

——. The veterinarian's vade-mecum. 2. ed. 8°. *London*, 1868.

Gibson (W.) The farrier's new guide. Containing: First. The anatomy of a horse, being an exact and compendious discription of all his parts, with their actions and uses. Secondly. An account of all the diseases incident to horses, with their signs, causes, and methods of cure; wherein many defects in the farrier's practice are now carefully supply'd, their errors expos'd and amended, and the art greatly improv'd and advanc'd, according to the latest discoveries. The whole interspers'd with many curious and useful observations concerning feeding and exercise, etc. 2 v. in 1. 8°. *London*, 1720.

——. The same. 3. ed. 8°. *London*, 1722.

——. The same. 5. ed. 8°. *London*, 1727.

——. The farrier's dispensatory in three parts. 8°. *London*, 1721.

——. The same. 4. ed., corrected. 8°. *London*, 1734.

Medicine (*Veterinary*).

——. The same. 5. ed. 8°. *London*, 1741.

——. The true method of dieting horses. Containing many curious and useful observations concerning their marks, colour, and external shape; their temper and instinct; and how they are to be governed, so as to prevent accidents and diseases. The proper method of feeding suited to their age, strength, and constitution; wherein the pernicious customs, which have obtain'd among many ignorant grooms and other pretenders to horsemanship, are exposed, and their errors carefully amended. Under which is likewise contain'd the right and proper exercise necessary, not only in the above-mentioned respects, but apply'd to the most usual services required of horses, whether those for travelling and labour, those for the manage, or those for pleasure. As also observations concerning the right ordering of troop horses, with a discourse of breeding, founded on the Duke of Newcastle's short method; very necessary for the improving of our breed, and raising a beautiful and useful race of horses. 3. ed. 8°. *London*, 1731.

GIRARD (J.) Notice sur le vomissement dans les principaux quadrupèdes domestiques. 8°. *Paris*, 1841.

GLEISBERG (J. P.) Lehrbuch der vergleichenden Pathologie. 8°. *Leipzig*, 1865.

GRESSWELL (G.) & GRESSWELL (C.) The veterinary pharmacopœia, materia medica, and therapeutics. With descriptions of the physiological action of medicines, by Albert Gresswell. 12°. *London*, [1886].

GRESSWELL (J. B.) Veterinary pharmacology and therapeutics. 16°. *London*, 1885.

——. The same. 16°. *New York*, 1885.

—— & GRESSWELL (A.) A manual of the theory and practice of equine medicine. 12°. *London*, 1885.

GSELL (G.) Traité des injections hypodermiques dans la thérapeutique vétérinaire. 8°. *Paris*, 1886.

GURLT (E. F.) Lehrbuch der pathologischen Anatomie der Haus-Säugethiere. Nebst einem Anhange, welcher die Beschreibung der bei den Haus-Säugethieren vorkommenden Eingeweidewürmer enthält. 2 v. 8°. Atlas, fol. *Berlin*, 1832.

HASELBACH (H.) Praktisches Thierarzneibuch, enthaltend die Krankheiten unserer Hausthiere, ihre Ursachen, Kennzeichen und Heilung, nebst einer Anleitung zur Geburtshülfe, den gebräuchlichsten Operationen, zur Errichtung einer Hausapotheke u. a. m. sowie das bestehende Viehseuche-Gesetz. Neu bearbeitet für Landwirthe und Viehbesitzer. 2. Aufl. 8°. *Berlin*, 1885.

HEATLEY (G. S.) Practical veterinary remedies. A useful hand-book on medicine. 12°. *Edinburgh*, 1885.

——. Every man his own vet.: a practical manual of the diseases of domestic animals, with their remedies. 12°. *Edinburgh*, 1886.

HERING (E.) Specielle Pathologie und Therapie für Thierärzte. 3. Aufl. 8°. *Stuttgart*, 1858.

HERING (E.) jun. Etymologisches Wörterbuch für Thierärzte. Enthaltend die Abstammung und eine kurze Erklärung der in der Thierheilkunde und ihren Hülfswissenschaften häufig gebrauchten Fremdwörter. Mit einer Vorrede von Dr. v. Hering. 12°. *Stuttgart*, 1871.

HEUSINGER (C.-F.) Recherches de pathologie comparée. 2 v. 4°. *Cassel*, 1853.

HICKS (H. C.) The gentleman's, farmer's, and traveller's pocket companion; containing many

Medicine (*Veterinary*).

valuable preventatives incident to horses, cattle, and sheep. Also many receipts for the cure of the same when diseased. 16°. *Baltimore*, 1811.

DE HOOG (G.) *De analogia, nexu et reciprocæ applicationis utilitate medicinæ humanæ et animalium rustico-domesticorum, sive veterinariæ artis, non neganda. 4°. *Lugd. Bat.*, 1811.

HURTREL D'ARBOVAL (L.-H.-J.) Dictionnaire de médecine et de chirurgie vétérinaires. 3 v. 8°. *Paris*, 1826-7.

——. The same. 4 v. 8°. *Paris*, 1827-8.

——. The same. 2. éd. 6 v. 8°. *Paris*, 1838-9.

——. The same. Éd. entièrement refondue . . . par A. Zundel. 3 v. 8°. *Paris*, 1874-7.

HUZARD (J.-B.) fils. Élève des animaux domestiques. Sur les mots croisement, métissage, appareillement, appatronnement et appariement, et les faits que ces mots désignent. 8°. *Paris*, 1840.

KAUFMANN (M.) Précis de thérapeutique vétérinaire, avec données scientifiques spéciales sur les effets des alcaloïdes. 12°. *Paris*, 1886.

KNOWLSON (J. C.) The complete farrier or horse-doctor; being the art of farriery made plain and easy; explaining the nature of the disorders to which a horse is subject, and the best methods of preventing or curing them. With an introduction, containing the best directions for chusing horses of all kinds; also instructions how to ride, and how to treat a horse on a journey. With a collection of the best recipes, from practice alone. The whole written in so plain and intelligible a manner that by attending to it those who have horses may manage them and cure the disorders to which they are subject, without the assistance of a farrier. To which is added a catalogue of drugs. 8°. *Otley*, 1820.

——. The Yorkshire cattle-doctor and farrier; a treatise on the diseases of horned cattle, calves, and horses. Written in plain language, which those who can read may easily understand. The whole being the result of seventy years' extensive practice of the author. The twenty-sixth thousand. Revised and corrected. Many of the receipts in this book are worth ten guineas each, and the whole are new to the world. 8°. *London & Otley*, [*n. d.*]

KÖHNE (H. W.) Handbuch der allgemeinen Pathologie für Thierärzte. 8°. *Berlin*, 1871.

KREUTZER (J. M.) Grundriss der gesammten Veterinärmedizin, mit ausführlicher Darstellung aller in sanitäts- und veterinärpolizeilicher, gerichtlicher, praktischer und komparativ-wissenschaftlicher Hinsicht besonders wichtigen Krankheiten. 8°. *Erlangen*, 1853.

LANGGUTH (G. A.) [Pr.] de utilitate atque dignitate artis veterinariæ. 4°. [*Wittembergæ*, 1753.]

——. [Pr.] de recuperanda medicinæ veterinariæ prima dignitate. 4°. [*Wittembergæ*, 1765.]

LAW (J.) The farmer's veterinary adviser; a guide to the prevention and treatment of disease in domestic animals. 12°. *Edinburgh*, [1887].

LEBLANC (U.) & TROUSSEAU (A.) Anatomie chirurgicale des principaux animaux domestiques, ou recueil de trente planches [etc.] [Atlas pour servir de suite au dictionnaire de médecine et de chirurgie vétérinaires de M. Hurtrel d'Arboval.] fol. *Paris*, 1828.

LEONTOVITCH (I.) *Razsujdenie o boliezni, take nazivaemoi puchlinie u loshadei. [Dissertation on pain, called talpa (mal de taupe) in domestic animals.] 8°. *St. Petersburg*, 1870.

Medicine (*Veterinary*).

LOMPAGIEU LAPOLE (J.) Observations relatives à la santé des animaux, ou essai sur leurs maladies. 2 pts. in 1 v. 8°. *Paris*, 1785.

LUDWIG (C. F.) [Pr.] de mulomedicina in civitate regenda. 4°. *Lipsiæ*, [1807].

LUX (J. J. G.) & BENEDICT (T. G. G.) * Disquisitiones politico-œconomicæ et veterinariæ. 4°. *Lipsiæ*, [1806].

MCCLURE (R.) Diseases in the American stable, field, and farm-yard. roy. 8°. *Philadelphia*, 1866.

M'KENDRICK (J. G.) Introductory lecture . . . Edinburgh Royal Veterinary College. 8°. *Edinburgh*, 1875.

MALATS (S.) Elementos de veterinaria que se han de enseñar á los alumnos del Real collegio de veterinaria de Madrid. [Anatomía.] 4 v. 8°. *Madrid*, 1793-4.

—— . The same. [Materia medica.] 2 v. 8°. *Madrid*, 1796.

—— . The same. [Patología.] 3 v. 8°. *Madrid*, 1797-1800.

MÜLLER (G. A.) Veterinär-Receptir- und Dispensirkunde. Auf Grundlage der Pharmacopœa germanica. Ed. altera. 12°. *Berlin*, 1885.

NORTON (W. J. T.) A manual of pharmacy for the student of veterinary medicine; containing the substances employed at the Royal Veterinary College, with an attempt at their classification, and the pharmacopœia of that institution. 7. ed. 12°. *London*, 1868.

OESTERLEN (J. F.) * De hernia interna bobus vectariis familiari. 12°. *Tubingæ*, 1810.

OLALLA (J. M.) Nosología veterinaria. Enfermedades de las fosas nasales. 8°. *Madrid*, 1862.

ORESTE (P.) Lezioni di patologia sperimentale veterinaria. 3 v. 8°. *Milano*, 1871-4.

OSTAPENK (A. P.) Veterinaruaja diagnostika. 8°. *Charkow*, 1885.

PATENTS for inventions. Abridgments of specifications relating to farriery; including the medical and surgical treatment of animals, A. D. 1719-1866. 12°. *London*, 1872.

—— . The same. Pt. 2. A. D. 1867-76. 12°. *London*, 1880.

PEUCH (F.) Précis de police sanitaire vétérinaire, ou exposé des mesures sanitaires applicables aux animaux, en France et en Algérie. 12°. *Paris*, 1884.

PILGER (F.) Systematisches Handbuch der theoretisch-praktischen Veterinär-Wissenschaft. 2 v. 16°. *Giessen*, 1801-2.

PRINGLE (R. O.) The diseases of horses, cattle, sheep, swine, dogs, and poultry; their causes, symptoms, and treatment; corrected and arranged from the best authorities. sm. 8°. *Dublin*, 1871.

PRINZ (C. G.) Quædam de excolenda medicina veterinaria. 4°. *Dresdæ*, 1776.

PROBSTMAYR (W.) Etymologisches Wörterbuch der Veterinär-Medicin und ihrer Hilfswissenschaften. 8°. *München*, 1863.

PÜTZ (H.) Die Stellung der Thiermedicin zu den übrigen Zweigen der Naturwissenschaften. 8°. *Leipzig*, 1880.

—— . Compendium der practischen Thierheilkunde. 1. 8°. *Stuttgart*, 1885.

RATZEBURG (C.) Handbuch der Zoopharmakologie für Thierärzte. Vorzüglich zum Gebrauch bei Vorlesungen in den königlichen Thierarzneischule zu Berlin. 1. Th. 8°. *Berlin*, 1801.

VON REEKEN (C. G.) Volksvoeding-Veeartsenijkunde. Was staat de veeartsenijkunde in Nederland wachten? Eene vraag, ook van gewigt voor onze volksvoeding. 8°. *Utrecht*, 1856.

—— . De geneeskunde der dieren in verband met staats- en volksbelang. 8°. [*n. p., n. d.*]

Medicine (*Veterinary*).

REICHARDT (G.) Der Hausthier-Arzt, oder zweckmässige Wartung und Pflege der Hausthiere in allen Krankheitsfällen. 12°. *Reutlingen*, [*n. d.*]

REYNDERS (J.) & Co. Catalogue of veterinary instruments manufactured and imported. 12°. *New York*, [*n. d.*]

RICHARDSON (J.) The New-England farrier and family physician; containing, firstly, Paul Jewett's farriery, in four parts, wherein most of the diseases which horses, neat cattle, sheep, and swine are liable to are treated of, in 41 pages; secondly, a collection of brutal receipts, many of which are valuable, 23 pages; thirdly, a very valuable collection of receipts for human diseases, 90 pages; fourthly, receipts by a very learned, skilful, and pious English author, 100 pages; fifthly, an extraordinary English author, of great experience and information on neat cattle, sheep, swine, asses, mules, dogs, etc., 82 pages; sixthly, a large number of valuable receipts from Capt. Joseph Smith, of Exeter, and others, on different creatures, but especially horses; seventhly, a very large number of miscellaneous receipts, on various subjects, useful for farmers and mechanics; last of all, Doct. J. Williams' family physician; this man was two years with the Indians, and was assisted in that time by a young Indian educated at one of our best medical colleges. 8°. *Exeter*, 1828.

RIGONI (S.) Trattato di patologia speciale veterinaria. 2. ed. 8°. *Firenze*, 1860.

RÖLL (M. F.) Lehrbuch der Pathologie und Therapie der Hausthiere. 2. Aufl. roy. 8°. *Wien*, 1860.

RUDOLPHI (K. A.) Bemerkungen aus dem Gebiet der Naturgeschichte, Medicin und Thierarzneykunde, auf einer Reise durch einen Theil von Deutschland, Holland und Frankreich gesammelt. 8°. *Berlin*, 1804-5.

RYCHNER (J. J.) Naturgeschichte des krankhaften Zustandes der Hausthiere, oder Grundlagen zu einer naturgerechten, allgemeinen Pathologie und Therapie derselben. 2. Ausg. 8°. *Bern*, 1843.

RYDING (W.) Patologia veterinaria, o sia vademecum del cavaliere, contenente un trattato sulle cagioni e i progressi delle malattie del cavallo, con una narrazione dei metodi i più atti a prevenirle e a medicarle. [Transl. from the English.] 8°. *Firenze*, 1831.

RYSS (A.) * Etwas über Veterinär-Medicin. 4°. *Würzburg*, 1810.

DE SAINBEL (C. V.) Elements of the veterinary art, containing an essay on the proportions of the celebrated Eclipse; six lectures on farriery, or the art of horse shoeing, and on the diseases of the foot. An essay on the grease, which obtained the prize given by the Royal Society of Medicine; an essay on the glanders; and observations on the gripes. 3. ed. 4°. *London*, 1797.

SAXONY. Bericht über das Veterinärwesen im Königreiche Sachsen. Hrsg. von der königl. Commission für das Veterinärwesen durch G. C. Haubner. 30., 1885. 8°. *Dresden*, 1868-86.

SCHLAMPP (K. W.) Das Dispensirrecht der Thierärzte, nebst den für Thierärzte wissenswerthen Abschnitten der Apotheken-Gesetzgebung für Studirende der Thiermedicin, Thierärzte, Apotheker und Beamte. Mit einem Vorwort von J. Feser. 8°. *Wiesbaden*, 1886.

SCHREGER (C. H. T.) [Pr.] insunt: quædam de fatis artis veterinariæ. 4°. *Vitebergæ*, [1813].

SCHURINK (H.) Volledig handboek der veeartsenijkunde voor elken landbouwer, alsmede voor liefhebbers van paarden- en vee-bezitters in

Medicine (*Veterinary*).

het algemeen, met bijzondere beschouwing over verloskunde en operatiën door drie praktische veeartsen omgewerkt en aan 23jarige ondervinding getoetst. 8°. *Zwolle*, 1859.

SCHWAB (K. L.) Katechismus der Hufbeschlagkunst, oder theoretisch-praktischer Unterricht über den Beschlag der Hufe und Klauen im gesunden und kranken Zustande. Neu bearbeitet von Konrad Schreiber. 13. Aufl. 8°. *Stuttgart*, 1863.

SIEDAMGROTZTY (O.) G. C. Haubner's landwirthschaftliche Thierheilkunde. 9. Aufl. 8°. *Berlin*, 1884.

SIGNOL (J.) Aide-mémoire du vétérinaire; médecine, chirurgie, obstétrique, formules, police sanitaire et jurisprudence commerciale. 12°. *Paris*, 1884.

SKEAVINGTON (G.) The modern system of farriery; comprehending the present entire improved mode of practice, according to the rules laid down at the Royal Veterinary College . . . 4°. *London & New York*, [n. d.]

SMALL (M.) Every man his own cattle doctor; or a treatise on the diseases of horses, cattle, dogs, sheep, and swine; with their causes, symptoms, and cure, [etc.] 12°. *Philadelphia*, [n. d.]

——. Veterinary tablet; being a synopsis of the diseases of horses, cattle, and dogs; with their cause, symptoms, and cure. 6. ed. 1 large sheet, in case. *Glasgow*, [n. d.]

SMITH (H. J.) A plea for veterinary surgery; to which is appended a report on epizootic, pleuro-pneumonia, and hog cholera. 8°. *Harrisburg*, 1879.
Repr. from: Rep. Penn. Bd. Agric., 1877.

SPINOLA (W. T. J.) Handbuch der speciellen Pathologie und Therapie für Thierärzte. 2 v. 8°. *Berlin*, 1858.

SPRENGEL (C.) * De Apsyrto Bithynio, hippiatro. 4°. *Halis*, [1832].

STREBEL (V.) & REICHERTER (E.) Neues illustriertes Haus-Tierarzneibuch . . . Ein Handbuch für Landwirte, Tierärzte und Huffschmiede, sowie ein Lehrbuch zum Gebrauch an landwirtschaftlichen Schulen nach dem neuesten Stand der Wissenschaft populär bearbeitet. Hft. 1–8. 8°. *Reutlingen*, 1885.

SWEDEN. Svensk veterinär-farmacopé. 3. uppl., änyo utgifven. 8°. *Stockholm*, 1880.

TABOURIN (M.-F.) Nouveau traité de matière médicale, de thérapeutique et de pharmacie vétérinaires, suivi 1° d'un formulaire raisonné, magistral et officinal; 2° d'une pharmacie légale, ou analyse des dispositions législatives concernant l'exercice de la pharmacie vétérinaire; 3° d'un tableau du prix approximatif des médicaments à Paris, Lyon et Toulouse. 8°. *Paris*, 1853.

TELLOR (L. V.) The diseases of live stock, and their most efficient remedies; including horses, cattle, sheep, and swine. Being a popular treatise, [etc.] 8°. *Philadelphia*, 1879.

THOMAS. Allgemeines Vieharzneibuch, oder des alten Schäfer, Thomas, aus Bunzlau in Schlesien, seine Kuren an Pferden, Rindvieh, Schafen, Schweinen, Ziegen und den übrigen Hausthieren, sowie seine Kenntnisse, Erfahrungen und Hilfsleistungen bei den Geburten der Pferde. Von ihm selbst in seiner Mund- und Schreibart beschrieben und zum Nutzen seiner Nebenmenschen herausgegeben von seinem Sohne, dem Schäfer Thomas in Weissenborn. 8. Aufl. 8°. *Glogau*, 1834.

TINDALL (J.) Tindall's Yorkshire farriery, being a treatise on the diseases of horses, with a statement of cases, and applicable recipes, never before published, whereby gentlemen, sports-

Medicine (*Veterinary*).

men, farmers, and others having the management of horses, are enabled to apply remedies to the diseases incidental thereto. 8°. *London*, 1814.

TOLNAY (A.) Von der Nothwendigkeit und dem Nutzen der Thierarzney besonders für Ungarn. Eine akademische Rede bei Antritt seines Lehramtes gehalten. 8°. *Pest*, 1787.

TOPHAM (T.) A new compendious system on several diseases incident to cattle . . . There is also annexed an essay on the diseases incident to calves, and their curative indications. In the course of this work will be found several observations on the diseases peculiar to horses, and their proper method of treatment. 8°. *York*, 1787.

TURKEY. Instruction aux vétérinaires inspecteurs. 8°. *Constantinople*, [n. d.]

TUSCON (R. V.) A pharmacopœia, including the outlines of materia medica and therapeutics, for the use of practitioners and students of veterinary medicine. 4. ed. 8°. *London*, 1886.

VEGETIUS RENATUS (P.) Artis veterinariæ, sive mulomedicinæ libri quatuor, jam primum typis in lucem æditi. Opus sane in rebus medicis minime aspernandum. sm. 4°. *Basileæ*, 1528.

——. The same. Mulomedicina. Ex trib. vetustiss. codd. varietate adjecta; unde infiniti loci addi et expurgari a quovis poterunt, uso magno publico. Opera Joan Sambuci. 8°. *Basileæ*, 1574.

——. The same. Curante Jo. Matthia Gesnero. 12°. *Mannhemii*, 1781.

——. The same. Flavii Vegetii Renati ain Büchlein, vonn rechter unnd warhaffter Kunst der Artzney, allerlay Kranckheyten, ynnwendigen und ausswendigen aller Thyer, so etwas zyehen oder tragen mügen, als Pferd, Esel, Maulthyer, Ochsen, und anderer, auch wie man allerlay Kranckhayten art uñ gepresten erkeñen soll, die mit Getrencken, Salbungen, Prenungen, Laͤsen, und ander Artzneyen, etc., zu vertreyben, vormals durch Vegetiuͤ Renatuͤ in Latein beschriben, yetzunder inn teütsche Sprach verwendt, allen Vichärtzten, Marstallern, Schmiden, Reyttern, Burgern unnd Pawren, auch allen denen die mit gemelten Vich umbgeend, ganz nutzlich und notwendig zü geprauchen. sm. 4°. [*Augspurg*, 1532.]
It is probable that Flavius Vegetius Renatus, the writer on military art, was not the author of the foregoing work. The Augsburg edition, evidently translated from the editio princeps of 1528, ascribes the work to him, probably on the strength of a passage in the dedication of the latter. The edition by Sambucus, in 1574, which has Publius on the title-page, speaks of the edition of 1528 as being mutilated and corrupt.

VEITH (J. E.) Handbuch der Veterinärkunde für Physiker, Thierärzte und Oekonomen. Vierte Auflage versehen und zeitgemäss vervollständigt von Joh. Elias Veith. 2 v. in 3. 8°. *Wien*, 1840–42.

VENTURINI (A.) Le medicine che da tutte gl' animali si può cavare à beneficio dell' huomo; altre volte intitolato: Il zomista, e secretario degl' animali. Hora accresciuto d' importanti secreti da Francesco Pignocatti, e di un' indice di tutte le infermità per trovar à medicamenti da risolverle. 8. ed. 24°. *Venezia*, 1704.

VETERINARNYI kalendar na 1887 g. od. Spravochnaja klinika dlja veterinarnych vrachei vsiech vedomstve. Izdanie J. M. Schmulevicha. [Veterinary calendar for 1887. Clinical inquiries for veterinary surgeons, with list of names. Issued by J. M. Schmulevich.] 12°. *St. Petersburg*, 1887.

VILLBOURG (C.-A.) Médecine vétérinaire, ou instruction au laboureur, sur la manière de connoître et de guérir les maladies de son bétail

Medicine (*Veterinary*).

à cornes, et de ses brebis; traduite de l'allemand de . . . avec un abrégé de matière médicale, et les noms des remèdes, tant simples que composés; par George Moschard. 12°. *Berne*, 1785.

VINCENZO (G.) Trattato di patologia veterinaria. 2 v. 8°. *Padova*, 1838.

VORTRÄGE für Thierärzte. Redigirt von Prof. Dr. J. G. Pflug. Series 1–7; Hfte. 1–4, Series 8. 8°. *Leipzig*, 1878–86.

WALLEY (T.) Thoughts on the action of medicines, and on veterinary medical politics; with addenda and a defence of science. 8°. *Manchester*, [1871].

WHITE (J.) A treatise of veterinary medicine, in 2 v. v. 2. Containing the materia medica and pharmacopœia. A new ed. 12°. *London*, 1808.

——. The same. In 2 v. v. 1. Containing a compendium of the veterinary art. Or, an accurate description of the diseases of the horse, and their mode of treatment; the anatomy and physiology of the foot; and the principles and practice of shoeing. With observations on stable management, feeding, exercise, and condition. 9. ed. 12°. *London*, 1809.

——. The same. In 4 v. 12°. *London*, 1817–20.

WILLIAMS (W.) * The principles and practice of veterinary medicine. 8°. *Edinburgh*, 1874.

——. The same. 4. ed. 8°. *Edinburgh & Glasgow*, 1884.

——. The same. 8°. *New York*, 1875.

WINTER (G. S.) Hippiater expertus, seu medicina equorum absolutissima, tribus libris comprehensa: Quorum I. agit de equorum temperamentis, ætate cognoscenda, morbis omnibus internis capitis, oculorum, aurium, narium, linguæ, dentium, oris, aliisque his similibus. II. De affectibus internis thoracis et abdominis nempe pulmonum et cordis, itemque hepatis, lienis, ventriculi, intestinorum, renum, vesicæ, nec non de purgatione equorum et pabulatione per gramen, de clysteribus, suppositoriis, de febribus et de peste. III. De omnis generis unguentis; oleis; balsamis et emplastris in genere; item de quibuscunque morbis ac symptomatibus externis; ut: tumoribus, ulceribus et vulneribus cujuscunque generis; ungularum etiam vitiis; fractura et luxatione ossium; medicamentorum ad horum morborum curationem necessariorum variis formulis; de venæsectione; de affectibus nervorum, etc. fol. *Norimbergæ*, 1678.

Title-page and text in Latin and German.

WÜRTH (L.) * De influxu zoojatriæ in anthropojatriam. 8°. *Pestini*, 1828.

YOUATT (W.) & CLATER (F.) Cattle doctor; containing all necessary directions in respect to the diseases, and their cure, of cattle, sheep, and swine. Also, the best method of raising and fattening. 16°. *New York*, 1851.

ZIPF (S.) Lehrbuch der Krankheiten der Thiere, und besonders der Pferde. 1. u. 2. Theil. 12°. *Mannheim*, 1807–8.

Billings (F. S.) A national veterinary police code; with State execution of the laws, and a national institute for the study of comparative pathology and the education of scientifically qualified veterinarians. *Newspaper cutting:* Turf, Field, and Farm, N. Y., Sept. 5, 1879.—**Black** (W. S.) Horse and cattle sickness at the Cape. Med. Times & Gaz., Lond., 1872, i, 173.—**Blumberg** (K.) O znachenii patolog. zootomii v veterinarii. [Importance of pathological zootomy.] Arch. vet. nauk., St. Petersb., 1882, xii, pt. 3, 167–191.—**Buehler** (A.) Esquisse statistique des maladies des animaux domestiques aux Verrières, Suisses, et dans les environs pendant les années 1855–61. Écho méd., Neuchát., 1861, v, 521; 570.—**Cadiot.** Application de l'éssérine à la thérapeutique vétérinaire. Arch. vét., Par., 1884, ix, 681–690.—**Congresso** veterinario. Rapporto sulle deliberazioni del . . . tenutosi in Milano dal 10 al 15 aprile 1865. Ann. univ. di med., Mi-

Medicine (*Veterinary*).

lano, 1865, cxcii, 189.—**Duchesne** & **Michel** (E.) L'hygiène professionnelle des vétérinaires. Bull. Soc. de méd. prat. de Par. (1882), 1883, 28–31.—**Garcia** (M.) Estudio sobre la ranilla en los animales. Observador méd., México, 1872–4, ii, 283–288.—**Geffcken** (E.) Versuch einer Pharmacopœa veterinaria germanica. Arch. d. Pharm., Hannover, 1856, 2. R., lxxxvi, 337: lxxxvii, 93. *Also,* Reprint.—**Gérard.** Observations de médecine vétérinaire. Arch. méd. belges, Brux., 1866, 2. s., iii, 243–251.—**Gsell.** Traité des injections hypodermiques dans la thérapeutique vétérinaire. Bull. et mém. Soc. centr. de méd. vét., Par., 1886, n. s., iv, 419–615. — **Heyfelder.** Thierärztliche Notiz. Med. Ann., Heidelb., 1833, iv, 259. — **Inter-relations** (On the) of human and veterinary medicine. [Edit.] Quart. J. Vet. Sc. in India, Madras, 1883–4, ii, 308–321.—**Koch** (A.) Die Bedeutung der Veterinär-Medecin für den Staat. Tagebl. d. Versamml. deutsch. Naturf. u. Aerzte, Salzb., 1881, liv, pt. 2, 91–95.—**Levi** (G.) Esame critico delle formule più accreditate fra gl' ippiatri in Inghilterra. Gior. di anat., fisiol. e patol. d. animali, Pisa, 1873, v, 74; 220.—**Maiz.** De la medicina veterinaria y de su importancia para el progresso de la agricultura. Gac. méd. de Lima, 1862–3, vii, 30; 46.—**Möller.** Zur Anwendung des Pilocarpins und Physostigmins in der Tierheilkunde. Tagebl. d. Versamml. deutsch. Naturf. u. Aerzte, Eisenach, 1882, lv, 226–228. — **Müller.** Bericht über die königl. Thierarzneischule zu Berlin 1885–6. Arch. f. wissensch. u. prakt. Thierh., Berl., 1886, xii, 313–331.—**Pütz.** Ueber die Stellung der Veterinärmedicin zu den anderen Zweigen der Naturwissenschaften. Tagebl. d. Versamml. deutsch. Naturf. u. Aerzte, Baden-Baden, 1879, lii, 237–244.—**Satterthwaite** (T. E.) The study of comparative pathology; introductory lecture. J. Comp. M. & S., N. Y., 1882, iii, 1–13.—**Schlegel** (J. H. G.) Beobachtungen und Erfahrungen eines Thierarztes über Starrkrampf, Brustwassersucht, Harnruhr, Saamenstrangfisteln, Aderlassfisteln, die Wirkung des Opii puri und der Tinctura opii an verschiedenen Hausthieren. Mat. f. d. Staatsarzneiw. u. prakt. Heilk., Meiningen, 1824, iii, 239–280.—**Schlosser** (M.) Beiträge zur Kenntniss der Stammesgeschichte der Hufthiere und Versuch einer Systematik der Paar- und Unpaarhufer. Morphol. Jahrb., Leipz., 1886–7, xii, 1–136, 6 pl.—**Shufeldt** (R. W.) The veterinary service of the United States Army. J. Comp. M. & S., Phila., 1887, viii, 138–143.—**Vogel.** Das Clystieren nach heutigen Grundsätzen. Repert. d. Thierh., Stuttg., 1885, xlvi, 1–25.

Medicine (*Veterinary, Education in and schools for*).

ALBERT (The) Veterinary College, limited, Queen's Road, Bayswater. Rules and regulations of the . . . 1865. 8°. *London*, [1865].

AMERICAN Veterinary College, New York City. Annual announcements for the sessions of 1876–7 (2.); 1878–9 to 1885–6 (4.–11.); 1887–8 (13.). 12° & 8°. *New York*, 1876–87.

BARANSKI (A.) Veterinarnaja politsija dlja vrachei i studentov. Perevod N. P. Vasīleva, pod redaktsiei P. A. Gordeva. Prilojenie k journalou "Veter. Vestnik". [Veterinary police for physicians and students. Transl. by N. P. Vasileff, under editorship of P. N. Gordeff. Supplement to Vet. Vestnik.] 8°. *Charkoff*, 1887.

BELGIUM. *Ministre de l'intérieur*. École de médecine vétérinaire et d'agriculture de l'état. Rapport de M. le ministre de l'intérieur . . . Chambre des représentants. Séance du 16 mai 1846 (No. 226). fol. [*Bruxelles*, 1846.]

——. École de médecine vétérinaire de l'état. Programmes des cours qui se donnent à l' . . . à Cureghem, Lez-Bruxelles. 8°. *Bruxelles*, 1862.

——. Examen pour les grades de candidat et de médecine vétérinaire. 8°. [*Bruxelles*, 1883.]

BOSTON Veterinary Institute. Prospectus and regulations for the session of 1855–6 (1.). 8°. *Boston*, 1855.

BUMM (K.) Die Prüfungsvorschriften für Thierärzte, mit besonderer Rücksicht auf Bayern, zusammengestellt und erläutert. 24°. *Augsburg u. Leipzig*, 1884.

CHIRURGISCH-MEDICINISCHE Akademie und die Thierarznei-Schule zu Dresden. Nachricht über die Wirksamkeit während des ersten Jahr-

Medicine (*Veterinary, Education in and schools for*).

zehnds nach ihrer Erweiterung, von D. Burkhard Wilhelm Seiler. 4°. *Dresden*, 1828.

COLUMBIA Veterinary College and School of Comparative Medicine, New York City. Annual catalogues and announcements for the sessions of 1879–80 (2.); 1880–81 (3.). 8°. *New York*, 1879–80.

GAMGEE (J.) Veterinary education. 8°. *London*, 1855.

——. On the study of veterinary medicine; inaugural address. 8°. *Edinburgh*, 1857.

HARVARD University. *School of Veterinary Medicine.* Circular announcing its establishment, April 16, 1883. 4°. [*Boston*, 1883.]

——. Annual announcement for the years 1884–5 (2.); 1886–7 (4.). 12°. *Cambridge*, 1884–6.

——. [Circular of the faculty, May 26, 1885.] 4°. [*Boston*, 1885.]

INSTITUTO agronómico-veterinario de la provincia de Buenos Aires en Santa Catalina. Anales del . . . 1. año, Nos. 1–17, 20 Aug., 1886, to 20 April, 1887. 8°. *Buenos Aires*, 1886–7.

KÖNIGLICHE Central - Thierarzneischule in München. Jahresberichte 1.–7., 1876–7, to 1882–3; 9., 1884–5; 10., 1885–6. 8°. *Leipzig*, 1878–87.

KÖNIGLICHE Thierarzneischule zu Hannover. Jahresberichte von dem Lehrer-Collegium, redigirt von dem Director. 1., 1868; 2., 1869; 4.–17., 1871–1884–5. 8°. *Hannover*, 1869–85.

KÖNIGLICH - UNGARISCHE Veterinär - Lehranstalt in Budapest. Bericht für das Schuljahr 1880–81. Veröffentlicht vom Director Béla Tormay. 8°. *Budapest*, 1882.

MONTREAL Veterinary College. Annual announcement for the session of 1883–4 (17.). 8°. *Montreal*, 1883.

NEW YORK College of Veterinary Surgeons and School of Comparative Medicine. Annual announcements for the sessions of 1867-8 (3.); 1877-8 (13.); 1886–7 (22.); 1887–8 (23.). 8°. *New York*, 1867–87.

——. Rules and regulations, with lists of subscribers. 8°. *New York*, 1868.

——. The same. 8°. *New York*, 1870.

——. The same. 8°. *New York*, 1874.

——. Circular of. [With tariff of charges.] 8°. *New York*, [*n. d.*]

PERRONCITO (E.) Breve cenno sulle conferenze tenute alla R. scuola di medicina veterinaria di Torino sulle malattie carbonchiose. 8°. *Torino*, 1887.

PROGRAMME des conditions d'admission aux écoles nationales vétérinaires. 12°. *Paris*, [1880].

PRUSSIA. Reglement für die Prüfung der Thierärzte vom 25. September 1869. 8°. *Berlin*, 1869.

REALE scuola superiore di medicina veterinaria di Milano. Storia e ordinamento programmi degl' insegnamenti istituti scientifici. roy. 8°. *Milano*, 1884.

——. Annuario per l' anno scolastico 1885–6. 8°. *Milano*, 1886.

RIVOLTA (S.) Sulla convenienza del riordinamento delle scuole veterinarie nazionali. 8°. *Torino*, 1885.

RUEFF. Die königlich - württembergische Thier-Arzneischule zu Stuttgart nach ihrem fünfzigjährigen Bestehen. Hrsg. von . . . 8°. *Stuttgart*, 1871.

SELLERS (C.) An appeal to the citizens of Pennsylvania for the foundation of a veterinary department in the University of Pennsylvania. 8°. *Philadelphia*, 1879.

——. Address on the need of a veterinary school in Pennsylvania. 8°. *Philadelphia*, 1879.

Medicine (*Veterinary, Education in and schools for*).

VETERINARY College, London. To the public. [A short statement of its views and objects.] 4°. [*London*, 1814.]

BERICHT über das Wiener k. k. Thierarznei-Institut für die Studienjahre 1858–83. Oesterr. Vrtljschr. f. wissensch. Veterinärk., Wien, 1859, xiii, 91: 1861, xv, 89: xvi, 34: 1862, xvii, 85: xviii, 1: 1863, xix, 88: xx, 128: 1864, xxi, 20: xxii, 21: 18 5, xxiii, 35: xxiv, 87: 1866, xxv, 71: 1867, xxvii, 62: xxviii, 21: 1868, xxix, 28: xxx, 155: 1869, xxxi, 130: 1870, xxxiii, 62: xxxiv, 1: 1871, xxxv, 51: xxxvi, 12: 1872, xxxvii, 147: xxxviii, 29: 1873, xl, 77: 1874, xli, 138: xlii, 65: 1875, xliii, 56: 1876, xlv, 89: xlvi, 1: 1877, xlvii, 149: xlviii, 129: 1878, l, 1: 1879, lii, 75: 1880, liii, 37: 1881, lv, 89: 1882, lvii, 23: 1883, lix, 1: 1884, lxi, 1.—**Chiappero** (F.) Le attuali condizioni per l' ammessione alle scuole veterinarie. Medico vet., Torino, 1876, 4. s., v, 522–539.—**Cothenius.** Considérations sur la nécessité d'une école vétérinaire, avec des projets sur la manière de l'établir, dressés à la réquisition du grand directoire royal, et soumis à l'examen de l'Académie. Trad. du latin. Mém. Acad. roy. de Prusse, Avignon et Par., 1774, ix, pt. 1, 289–343. *Also* [Trad. de l'allemand. *From:* Mém. Acad. roy. d. sc. de Berl.]: Collect. acad. d. mém., etc., Par., 1774, xii, 287–306.— **Decret** portant organisation des écoles vétérinaires. Rec. de méd. vét., Par., 1882, 6. s., ix, 1141–1149.—**Falke** (J. E. L.) Die Thierarzneikunde in Bezug zur Anthropoiatrik, und die Universitäten und Thierarzneischulen als Bildungsanstalten für Thierärzte. Med. Argos, Leipz., 1842, iv, 285–296.—**L'école** vétérinaire d'Alfort. Gaz. d. hôp., Par., 1874, xlvii, 189–191.—**Legrain** (J.-B.) Étude sur l'enseignement de la médecine vétérinaire en Belgique. Ann. de méd. vét., 3. éd., Brux., 1864, xiii, 444; 563. *Also*, Reprint.—**McEuchran** (D.) Veterinary education. Am. Vet. Rev., N. Y., 1877-8, i, 12; 45; 85; 113.—**Neue** organische Bestimmungen für die Thierarzneischule in Stuttgart. Med. Cor.-Bl. d. württemb. ärztl. Ver., Stuttg., 1868, xxxviii, 183–186.—**Plan** zur Organisirung und Erweiterung des k. k. Thierarznei-Institutes zu Wien. Med. Jahrb. d. k. k. österr. Staates, Wien, 1824, n. F., ii, 162: 323.—**Prinz** (C. G.) Bericht über die Thierheilanstalt bei der königl. Thierarzneischule zu Dresden und ihre Leistungen im Jahre 1833. Beitr. z. prakt. Heilk., Leipz., 1834, i, 134–150.—**Quivogne** (F.) Réforme de l'enseignement de la médecine vétérinaire. Congrès méd. de France (Lyon, 1872), Par., 1873, iv, 492–494.—**R.** Università di Pisa. Regolamento provvisorio per le scuole di zoojatria e d' agraria. Gior. di anat., fisiol. e patol. d. animali, Pisa, 1871, iii, 206–221.—**Roloff** (F.) Bericht über die k. Thierarzneischule zu Berlin (1879–82). Arch. f. wissensch. u. prakt. Thierh., Berl., 1881, vii, 1: 1882, viii, 1; 381. — **Verein** deutscher Aerzte in Prag. Petition betreffend die Errichtung einer höheren Thierarzneischule in Prag. Aerztl. Cor.-Bl. f. Böhmen, Prag, 1874, ii, 332–341.—**Veterinärväsendet.** [1851–74.] Sundh.-Coll. Berättelse, Stockholm, 1864–76, *passim*.—**Withington** (C. F.) The school of veterinary medicine of Harvard University. Boston M. & S. J., 1883, cix, 241–244.

Medicine (*Veterinary, History, condition, and legislation of*).

See, also, **Medicine** (*Veterinary, Education, etc., for*).

ADAM (T.) Die Veterinär-Polizei, mit Berücksichtigung der neuesten Gesetzgebungen. 8°. *München*, 1862.

——. Sammlung der veterinär-sanitätspolizeilichen Verordnungen für das Königreich Bayern. Mit allerhöchster Genehmigung herausgegeben. 8°. *München*, 1863.

AMERICAN Veterinary Hospital. Annual report of the . . . 8., 1882–3. 8°. *New York*, 1883.

AUSTRIA. *K. k. Ministerium des Innern.* Veterinär-Berichte für die Jahre 1880–83 . . . Bearbeitet von Dr. M. F. Röll. 8°. *Wien*, 1882–5.

BADEN. Amtliche Bekanntmachungen, betreffend das Veterinärwesen im Grossherzogthum Baden. 11. Jahrg., No. 111, März 1882. 8°. *Karlsruhe* [*Baden*, 1882].

BARAŃSKI (A.) Handbuch sämmtlicher Veterinärgesetze und Verordnungen, die in Oesterreich-Ungarn und Bosnien giltig sind. 8°. *Wien*, 1884.

——. Geschichte der Thierzucht und Thiermedicin im Alterthum. 8°. *Wien*, [1886].

BIERLICH (E.) Der preussische Militair-Rossarzt. Eine Sammlung von Verordnungen, welche

Medicine (*Veterinary, History, condition, and legislation of*).

über die Rossärzte der preussischen Armee entweder direct erlassen worden sind, oder auf dieselben Anwendung finden. 8°. *Berlin*, 1869.

BÜCHTING (A.) Bibliotheca veterinaria, oder Verzeichniss der seit Mitte 1842 bis Ende 1866 im deutschen Buchhandel erschienenen Bücher und Zeitschriften über alle Theile der Thierarzneikunde; im genauen Anschluss an die Wilhelm Engelmann'sche Bibliotheca veterinaria bis zur Mitte des Jahres 1842. Nebst einem vollständigen Materien-Register. 8°. *Nordhausen*, 1867.

COSTA (A.) Sul servizio veterinario militare in Italia. 8°. *Conegliano*, 1884.

CHOMEL (C.) Histoire du corps des vétérinaires militaires en France. 8°. *Paris*, 1887.

EICHBAUM (F.) Grundriss der Geschichte der Thierheilkunde. 8°. *Berlin*, 1885.

ENSLIN (T. C. F.) Bibliotheca veterinaria, oder Verzeichniss der in älterer und neuerer Zeit bis zur Mitte des Jahres 1842 in Deutschland erschienenen Bücher über alle Theile der Thierarzneikunde . . . von neuem gänzlich umgearbeitet von Wilhelm Engelmann. 2. Aufl. 8°. *Leipzig*, 1843.

ERCOLANI (G. B.) Ricerche storico-analitiche sugli scrittori di veterinaria. 2 v. 12°. *Torino*, 1851-4.
Also [Rev.], *in:* Gior. d. r. Accad. med.-chir. di Torino, 1852, 2. s., xiii, 271-275.

FALKE (J. E. L.) Propädeutik und encyklopädische Uebersicht der Thierheilkunde, nebst ihrer neuern bessern Literatur. 2. vermehrte Ausg. 8°. *Leipzig*, 1855.

FESER (J.) Die Nothwendigkeit der Reform des thierärztlichen Unterrichts in Deutschland, bewiesen durch die Geschichte der Münchener Thierarzneischule. Vortrag. 8°. *Berlin*, 1873.

GREAT BRITAIN. *Privy Council Office.* Annual reports of the veterinary department of the Privy Council Office, with appendices. For the years 1872–82. fol. & 8°. *London*, 1873-83.

HENZEN (J. C. G.) Entwurf eines Verzeichnisses veterinärischer Bücher und einzelner Abhandlungen die zur theoretischen und practischen Kenntniss von Pferden, Eseln, Mauleseln, Rindvieh, Schaafen, Ziegen und Schweinen, den Vieharzneykundigen nützen können. 8°. *Göttingen u. Stendal*, 1781.

HIPPOCRATES. Trattati di mascalcia attribuiti ad Ippocrate. Tradotti dall' arabo in latino da maestro Moisè da Palermo volgarizzati nel secolo xiii. Messi in luce per cura di Pietro Delprato, corredati di due posteriori compilazioni in latino e in toscano e di note filologiche per cura di Luigi Barbieri. 8°. *Bologna*, 1865.

HOLLAND. Verslag aan den koning van de bevindingen en handelingen van het veeartsenijkundig staatstoezigt in het jaaren 1871, 1873-7. roy. 8°. & 4°. *'s Gravenhage*, 1872-8.

HUGUES (J.) Le vétérinaire en Belgique et sa déontologie. 8°. *Louvain*, 1880.

NEW YORK (*State*). An act to amend chapter 313 of the laws of 1886, entitled: "An act to regulate the practice of veterinary medicine and surgery in the State of New York". In assembly. No. 201. Feb. 1, 1887. Introd. by Mr. Ingersoll. fol. [*Albany*, 1887.]

NORWAY. Veterinair-Medicinal-Taxt for Norge, som ifölge kongelig Placat af 6te Juli 1861 er gjældende fra 1ste September 1861 indtil videre. 8°. *Christiania*, 1861.

———. Tillæg til Veterinair-Medicinal-Taxten for Norge, udfærdiget af den Kongelige Norske

Medicine (*Veterinary, History, condition, and legislation of*).

Regjerings Departement for det Indre i Henhold til kongelig Resolution af 6te Juli 1861. 8°. *Christiania*, 1862.

———. Andet Tillæg til Veterinair-Medicinal-Taxten for Norge, udfærdiget af den Kongelige Norske Regjerings Departement for det Indre i Henhold til kongelig Resolution af 6te Juli 1861. 8°. *Christiania*, 1863.

———. Tredie Tillæg til Veterinair-Medicinal-Taxten for Norge, udfærdiget af den Kongelige Norske Regjerings Departement for det Indre i Henhold til kongelig Resolution af 6te Juli 1861. 8°. *Christiania*, 1864.

———. Veterinair-Medicinal-Taxt for Norge, ifölge naadigst Bemyndigelse, udfærdiget af den Kongelige Norske Regjerings Departement for det Indre os gjældende fra 1ste Januar 1866 indtil videre. 8°. *Christiania*, 1865.

PADUA (*Province of*). Regolamento pel servizio veterinario nella provincia di Padova. 8°. *Padova*, 1879.

———. Il servizio veterinario nella provincia di Padova nell' anno 1882. Relazione della commissione veterinaria permanente. fol. *Padova*, 1885.

POTTERAT (D.) Bericht an das schweizerische Landwirthschaftsdepartement über den thierärztlichen Unterricht in der Schweiz und die Mittel zur Hebung desselben. 8°. *Bern*, 1885.

PRUSSIA. Jahresberichte der königl. technischen Deputation für das Veterinärwesen über die Verbreitung ansteckender Thierkrankheiten in Preussen. 2.–8., 1877-8 to 1883-4. 8°. *Berlin*, 1879-84.
Suppl. in: Arch. f. wissensch. u. prakt. Thierh., Berl., 1879-84, v-x.

[RUELLIUS (J.)] Zwey nützliche sehr gute Bücher von allerley Gebrechen und Kranckheiten, damit die Rosse, Maulesel, und andere vier füssige Thier, welche etwas schwer tragen, oder ziehen, geplaget, darinnen eigentlich beschrieben. Die Ursach davon sie entspringen, und durch welche Zeychen man dieselb erkennen, und von einander unterscheyden möcht. Desgleichen durch was Mittel und Artzney inen zu helffen und Rath zuschaffen. Vormals in deutscher Sprach niemals gesehen noch gelesen worden. [Uebersetzt von Gregorius Zechendorfer.] fol. *Eger*, 1571.

RUSSIA. *Medical Department.* Otchet med. depart. po veterinarnomu otdieleniu za 1882 g. 8°. *St. Petersburg*, 1885.

RYSS (A.) *Ueber die Organisation des Veterinär-Institutes zu Würzburg. 8°. *Würzburg*, 1808.

———. *Ueber Verhältniss und Einfluss der Thier-Arzneikunde auf die gesammte Haus- und Landwirthschaft. 8°. *Würzburg*, 1815.

SAXONY. Berichte über das Veterinärwesen im Königreiche Sachsen. Herausgegeben von der königl. Commission für das Veterinärwesen durch G. C. Haubner. 1.–13., 1856-68; 22.–29., 1877-84. 8°. *Dresden*, 1857-85.

SCHRADER (G. W.) Biographisch-literarisches Lexicon der Thierärzte aller Zeiten und Länder, sowie der um die Thierheilkunde verdienten Naturforscher, Aerzte, Landwirthe, Stallmeister, etc. roy. 8°. *Stuttgart*, 1863.

TANGUY (H.-M.) Union vétérinaire et agronomique du Nord-Finistère. Assemblée de Landivisiau, le 1er février 1882. De l'inspection sanitaire des foires et marchés dans la première conscription du service départemental des épizooties, et de l'application de la loi du 21 juillet

Medicine (*Veterinary, History, condition, and legislation of*).

1881 relative à la police sanitaire des animaux domestiques, dans le Finistère. 8°. *Angers*, 1882.

VALLADA. Considerazioni zooiatriche sul progetto di legge per un nuovo codice sanitario presentato al senato da S. E. il Ministro dell' Interno nella tornata delli 22 dicembre 1876. 8°. [*n. p., n. d.*]

Repr. from: Veterinaria, Parma.

VERSLAG aan den koning van de bevindingen en handelingen van het veeartsenijkundig staatstoezigt in het jaar 1871. 8°. *Gravenhage*, 1872.

WEISSE (F. D.) The imperative demands for the cultivation of veterinary medicine in the United States. Introductory address. 8°. *New York*, 1867.

ZÜNDEL (A.) Der Gesundheitszustand der Hausthiere in Elsass-Lothringen während der beiden Berichtsjahre vom 1. April 1882 bis Ende März 1884; nach den amtlichen Berichten der Kreisthierärzte und anderer beamteten Thierärzte. 8°. *Strassburg*, 1885.

Baldinger (E. G.) Etwas Litteratur für Thier-Aerzte. N. Mag. f. Aerzte, Leipz., 1796, xviii, 426–434.— **Barański** (A.) Die Thiermedicin im Alterthum. Oesterr. Vrtljschr. f. wissensch. Veterinärk., Wien, 1884, lxii, 71; 165: 1885, lxiii, 125.—**Bayern.** Königl. allerhöchste Verordnung, die Reorganisation des Veterinärwesens betreffend. Arch. d. deutsch. Med.-Gesetzgeb. u. öff. Gsndhtspflg., Erlang., 1858, ii, 345; 353; 410.—**Bonzom** (E.) La médecine vétérinaire en Algérie. Gaz. méd. de l'Algérie, Alger, 1870, xv, 55; 62; 91; 108.—**Corlies** (J. C.) Veterinary report. Rep. Bd. Health N. Jersey, Trenton, 1878, ii, 149–163.—**Csokor** (J.) Ueber das Wiener k. k. Thierarznei-Institut für das Studienjahr 1881–2. d. Die pathologisch-anatomische Anstalt. Oesterr. Vrtljschr. f. wissensch. Veterinärk., Wien, 1883, lix, 93–122. ———. Jahresbericht der pathologisch-anatomischen Anstalt am k. k. Militär-Thierarznei-Institute, pro 1882–83. *Ibid.*, 1884, lxii, 1–28.—**Eckel** (G. F.) Bericht über die im Militär-Jahre 1837 im k. k. Thierarzney-Institute zu Wien behandelten und untersuchten Thiere. Med. Jahrb. d. k. k. österr. Staates, Wien, 1838, xxvi, 82–93. ———. Bericht über die Ergebnisse am k. k. Thierarzney-Institute in Wien im Militärjahre 1839. *Ibid.*, 1841, xxxiii, 434; 597.— **Eletti** (G.) Breve rendiconto sopra cio che riguarda la zoojatria durante lo scorso anno 1853. Gazz. med. ital. lomb., Milano, 1854, 3. s., v, 293–295.—**Erlassene** Sanitäts-Normalien für die Provinz Niederösterreich. Vergütung für die bei der Viehbeschau intervenirenden Individuen. Hofkanzleidecret vom 11. December 1840, Z. 37, 391. Regierungsverordnung vom 22. December 1840, Z. 72, 484. Med. Jahrb. d. k. k. österr. Staates, Wien, 1841, xxxv, 225–227.—**Falke** (E.) Berichte über die Leistungen auf dem Gebiete der Thierarzneiwissenschaft in den Jahren 1856–74. Schmidt's Jahrb., Leipz., 1858–75, xcvii–clxvii, *passim.*—**Falke** (J. E. L.) Thierärztliche Bedenken und Wünsche. Deutsche Ztschr. f. d. Staatsarznk., Erlang., 1861, n. F., xvii, 183–193, 1 pl. ———. Die Entwicklungsgeschichte der vergleichenden Medicin. Thierärztl. Jahrb., Leipz., 1878, i, 1–16. *Also, transl.:* Am. Vet. Rev., N. Y., 1878–9, ii, 504–515.—**Fransk** Lov af 21. Juli 1881 angaende det veterinære Sundhedspoliti. [*From:* Barrals, J. de l'agric., 6. Aug., 1881, 212.] Tidsskr. f. Vet., Kjøbenh., 1882, 2. R., xii, 52–60.—**Hack.** Zur Frage über die Organisation des Veterinärweseus und die Stellung der Thierärzte im Grossherzogthum Baden. Aerztl. Mitth. a. Baden, Karlsruhe, 1863, xvii, 65–80.—**Hamont.** Aperçu général sur l'état actuel de la médecine vétérinaire en France. Bull. Acad. de méd., Par., 1844–5, x, 650–676. ———. Sur l'exercice de la médecine vétérinaire. Union méd., Par., 1847, i, 75.—**Histoire** de la médecine vétérinaire en Angleterre. [*From:* Écho vét.] Abeille méd., Par., 1886, xliii, 201; 241.—**Holcombe** (A. A.) Army veterinary medicine; its history; the present condition of the army veterinary surgeon; his rights as a representative of a scientific profession, and what is required by the Government to establish an efficient veterinary department. Am. Vet. Rev., N. Y., 1881–2. v, 288; 335; 401.—**Hugues.** Rapport sanitaire vétérinaire de la garnison de Liége pendant le second semestre 1868. Arch. méd. belges, Brux., 1869, 2. s., ix, 177; 253.—**Huzard.** [Tableau de l'origine et de l'histoire de l'art vétérinaire en France. Éloge d'. . . par Pariset.] J. d. conn. méd.-chir., Par., 1841–2, ix, pt. 2, 232–240.—**Improvement** in veterinary practice in New York. Med. Reposit., N. Y., 1809–10, xiii, 201.—**Jennings** (R.) The early history of

Medicine (*Veterinary, History, condition, and legislation of*).

veterinary medicine in the United States. J. Comp. M. & S., N. Y., 1883, iv, 42: 1884, v, 25. — **Jessen** (P.) Mit welcher Mission ist der Veterinairarzt in dem Staatshaushalte der civilisirten Nationen betraut? Med. Ztg. Ru-lands, St. Petersb., 1852, ix, 249–254. — **Jonsson** (S.) Husdyrhold og Husdyrsygdomme i Island. [Domestic animals and their diseases in Iceland.] Tidsskr. f. Vet., Kjøbenh., 1879, 2. R., ix, 137–178.—**Königl.** technische Deputation für das Veterinärwesen. Neunter Jahresbericht . . . über die Verbreitung ansteckender Thierkrankheiten in Preussen. Berichtsjahr vom 1. April 1884 bis 31. März 1885, 8°, Berlin, 1885. Arch. f. wissensch. u. prakt. Thierh., Berl., 1885, xi, 1–126, Suppl. *Also*, Reprint.—**Komitet** ab uluchshenii veterinarnoi chaste v' Rossii i o masrakh k' prekrashcheniyu skotskikh padezhei v' imperii. [Commission on the improvement of the veterinary profession in Russia, and on measures for preventing infectious diseases among animals.] Med. Vestnik, St. Petersb., 1861, i, 39.—**Krabbe** (H.) Dyrlægevæsnet i Island. [Veterinary art in Iceland.] Tidsskr. f. Vet., Kjøbenh., 1879, ix, 178–182.— **Küchler.** Ueber die Zuziehung von Menschenärzten zu den Prüfungen der Thierärzte. Deutsche Ztschr. f. d. Staatsarznk., Erlang., 1868, n. F., xxvi, 59–65.—**Lanzilotti-Buonsanti** (N.) La questione della medicina veterinaria in Italia; discorso inaugurale. Arch. di med. vet., Milano, 1877, ii, 401–425.—**Leblanc** (C.) Revue vétérinaire de 1874. Arch. gén. de méd., Par., 1875, i, 578–596.—**Liautard** (A.) History and progress of veterinary medicine in the United States. Am. Vet. Rev., N. Y., 1877–8, i, 5–19.—**Lidl** (J.) Uebersicht der in dem k.-k. Thierarzeney-Institute zu Wien in den Militär-Jahren 1827–32 behandelten kranken, und der untersuchten wüthenden oder wuthverdächtigen Thiere. Med. Jahrb. d. k. k. österr. Staates, Wien, 1832, xi, 450; 617: xii, 150; 275; 437: 1833, xiii, 605.—**Magne** (J.-H.) Rapport sur les progrès de la médecine vétérinaire. Gaz. méd. de Par., 1869, 3. s., xxiv, 180.—**Moroni** (E.) La scienza veterinaria e l'arte zootecnica professate. Atti Accad. fis.-med.-statist. di Milano, 1870, xxvi, 28–44.—**National** (A) veterinary bureau. [Edit.] Med. Rec., N. Y., 1880, xvii, 319–321. — **New York.** An act to incorporate State and judicial district veterinary societies for the purpose of improving the practice of veterinary medicine in the State of New York. Am. Vet. Rev., N. Y., 1878–9, ii, 519–521. ———. [Acts proposed] to regulate the practice of veterinary medicine and surgery in the State of New York. *Ibid.*, 1885–6, ix, 480–485.—**Otchet** Med. Departementa po veterin. otdielenijou za 1881 g. Arch. vet. nauk, St. Petersb., 1884, xiv.—**Patellani.** Sullo studio veterinario. Gazz. med. ital. lomb., Milano, 1849. 2. s., ii, 32–34.—**Plank.** Ueber die Fort- und Rückschritte der Thierarzneiwissenschaft in gegenwärtiger Zeit. Ztschr. f. d. Staatsarznk., Erlang., 1828, xv, 209–223.—**Popoff** (P. S.) Iz zoochirurg. klin. Kazan. Vet. Inst. Uchen. zapiski Kazan. Vet. Inst., 1885, ii, 189–197.—**Prinz** (C. G.) Bericht über die Thierheilanstalt bei der königl. Thierarzneischule zu Dresden und ihre Leistungen in den Jahren 1833–6. Beitr. z. prakt. Heilk., Leipz., 1834, i, 134: 1836, ii, 75: iii, 113: 1837, iv, 209.—**Quivogne** (F.) La candidature de M. Chauveau à l'inspection générale des écoles vétérinaires. Écho d. soc. et ass. vét. de France, Lyon, 1885, vii, 574; 619. — **Röll.** Das k.-k. Militär-Thierarznei-Institut in Wien während des ersten Jahrhundertes seines Bestehens. Oesterr. Vrtljschr. f. wissensch. Veterinärk., Wien, 1877, xlviii, 1–128, 1 pl.—**Sadun** (B.) Uffici della medicina veterinaria. Gior. di anat., fisiol. e patol. d. animali, Pisa, 1869, i, 271–279 [331–339].—**Seiler** (B. W.) Ueber die Organisation des Veterinär-Medicinalwesens, mit besonderer Rücksicht auf das Königreich Sachsen. Ztschr. f. d. Staatsarznk., Erlang., 1833, 18. Ergnzngshft., 156–228.— **Steel** (J. H.) On the progress and present state of veterinary science in America. Veterinarian, Lond., 1880, 4. s., liii, 1–18.—**Taxt** for veterinaire Lægemidler; med Indenrigsministeriets Autorisation fastsat af det veterinære Sundhedsraad, gældende fra 30. April 1879 til 30. April 1880. [Suppl.] Tidsskr. f. Vet., Kjøbenh., 1879, ix, 1–16.—**Taxt** for veterinaire Lægemidler; med Indenrigsministeriets Autorisation fastsat af det veterinære Sundhedsraad. [Suppl.] *Ibid.*, 1883, xiii, (2. H.).—**Tombari** (T.) Le sorti della veterinaria nel regno d' Italia. Gior. di anat., fisiol. e patol. d. animali, Pisa, 1874, vi, 193–201. — **Tomilin** (I. J.) Kratkii ocherk istorii veterinarii. [History of veterinary art.] Arch. vet. nauk, St. Petersb., 1886, xvi, pt. 6, 61; 83.— **Ulrich** (C.) Denkschrift über die Verhältnisse der Militär-Thierärzte und über das gesammte Veterinär-Wesen in der pr ussischen Armee. Preuss. mil.-ärztl. Ztg., Berl., 1862, 229; 241; 253; 265.— **Verheyen** (S.) Des doctrines médicales et de leur influence sur le développement de la médecine vétérinaire. Arch. belges de méd. mil., Brux., 1859, xxiii, 177; 273; 389: xxiv, 91; 193; 257; 321. ———. Rapport sur la question de médecine vétérinaire. Bull. Acad. roy. de méd. de Belge, Brux., 1861, 2. s., iv, 69–98.—**Zucchi** (C.) Sull' esercizio della veterinaria. Gazz. med. ital. lomb., Milano, 1866, 5. s., v, 126–129.

Medicine (*Veterinary, Homœopathic*).

BÖHM (C. L.) Kurze praktische Anleitung für alle Viehbesitzer, welche ihren Hausthieren in den am häufigsten vorkommenden Erkrankungsfällen, durch sorgfältige Auffassung der sämmtlichen sinnlich wahrnehmbaren Krankheitserscheinungen mit den dagegen erprobten homöopathischen Heilmitteln auf die einfachste ganz naturgemässe und wenigst kostspielige Weise selbst Hilfe leisten wollen. 12°. *Leipzig*, 1873.

GÜNTHER (F. A.) Der homöopathische Thierarzt. Die Krankheiten des Pferdes und ihre homöopathische Heilung. 9. Aufl. 8°. *Sondershausen*, 1857.

———. Der kleine homöopathische Thierarzt. Ein für Jedermann verständliches Buch . . . Als Auszug aus den 3 Bänden von Dr. Günther's homöopathischem Thierarzt, bearbeitet und herausgegeben von . . . 12°. *Langensalza*, 1884.

HAYCOCK (W.) Elements of veterinary homœopathy, embracing hints on the application of hydropathy; or, a treatise on the diseases of the horse and cow, with remarks on the general management and principal diseases incidental to the sheep and dog. 8°. *London*, 1852.

HÜBNER (G.) Der homöopathische Hausthierarzt. 8°. *Berlin*, 1864.

HUMPHREYS (F.) Manual of veterinary specific homœopathy, comprising diseases of horses, cattle, sheep, hogs, and dogs, and their specific homœopathic treatment. 12°. *New York*, 1860.

MANUAL (A) of homœopathic veterinary practice, designed for horses, all kinds of domestic animals and fowls. 8°. *New York*, 1873.

MARZO (M.) Examen crítico comparativo de las doctrinas médicas, veterinaria homeopática y alopática, con un apendice del tifus en el caballo. 16°. *Madrid*, 1855.

MÖLLER (J. G.) Hydro-homöopathisches Taschenbuch der Thierheilkunde, oder die Krankheiten der Hausthiere und deren Heilung durch kaltes Wasser, vorzüglich aber durch homöopathische Mittel. Ein neues, alphabetisch bearbeitetes Noth- und Hülfsbuch für jeden Thierarzt und Viehbesitzer. Durchgesehen vom Mag. Lux. 8°. *Leipzig*, 1839.

MOORE (J.) Outlines of veterinary homœopathy; comprising horse, cow, dog, sheep, and hog diseases, and their homœopathic treatment. 7. ed. 12°. *London*, 1874.

———. The same. 9. ed. 12°. *London & Leamington*, 1882.

PERRUSSEL. L'homœopathie, ou la médecine de l'analogie devant la commission d'hygiène hippique au ministère de la guerre (séance officielle du 26 avril 1861). Proposition d'une réforme fondamentale de la médecine vétérinaire, suivie d'un parallèle entre les deux médecines. 8°. *Paris*, 1862.

RUSH (J.) The hand-book to veterinary homœopathy; or, the homœopathic treatment of the horse, the ox, the sheep, the dog, and the swine. From the London edition, with numerous additions translated from the 7th German edition of Dr. F. E. Guenther's Homœopathic veterinary, by Jacob F. Sheek. 16°. *Philadelphia*, 1854.

SCHAEFER (J. C.) New manual of homœopathic veterinary medicine. Translated from the German, with numerous additions from other veterinary manuals, by Charles J. Hempel. 8°. *Philadelphia*, 1871.

SCHWABE (W.) Illustrirter Hausthierarzt. Die innerlichen und äusserlichen Krankheiten der Pferde, Rinder, Schafe, Ziegen, Schweine, Hunde und des Federviehes, die Verhütung und Behandlung derselben, nach den Grundsätzen

Medicine (*Veterinary, Homœopathic*).

der homöopathischen Heilmethode bearbeitet von anerkannt tüchtigen homöopathischen Thierärzten im Verein mit erfahrenen Landwirthen. 3. Aufl. 8°. *Leipzig*, 1873.

Medicine (*Veterinary, Journals and transactions of societies relating to*).

ALIANZA (La) veterinaria. v. 3–4, 1884–5. fol. *Játiva*.

AMERICAN (The) Veterinary Journal; devoted to the diffusion of veterinary knowledge. Edited by George H. Dadd. [Monthly.] Nos. 1, 3, 5, 8, 10–12, v. 1, Sept., 1851, to Aug., 1852.

———. The same. [New series.] v. 1–3; Nos. 1–3, v. 4; Oct., 1855, to March, 1859. 8°. *Boston*.

AMERICAN Veterinary Review. A. Liautard, editor. v. 1–11, 1877–87. 8°. *New York*.

ANNALES de médecine vétérinaire. Par Delwart et Thiernesse. v. 1–36, 1852–87. 8°. *Bruxelles*.

ANNALES de zootechnie et de médecine vétérinaire. Par E. Darbot [*et al.*]. v. 1–2, 1874–5. 8°. *Langres*.

ARCHIV für Thierheilkunde. Hrsg. von der Gesellschaft schweizerischer Thierärzte. Neue Folge. v. 1, 1838–9. 8°. *Zürich*.

ARCHIV veterinarnich nauk. v. 12–17, 1882–7. 8°. *St. Petersburg*.

ARCHIV für wissenschaftliche und practische Thierheilkunde. Hrsg. von C. F. Müller und J. W. Schütz. v. 1–13, 1875–87. 8°. *Berlin*.

ARCHIVES vétérinaires. Publiées à l'école d'Alfort. v. 1–9, 1876–84. 8°. *Paris*.

ARCHIVIO di medicina veterinaria. v. 1–3, 1876–8. 8°. *Milano*.

AUSTRALASIAN (The) Veterinary Journal. By G. Mitchell [*et al.*]. v. 1, 1882. 8°. *Melbourne*.

BAYERISCHE Thierärzte. Bericht über die Versammlung . . . in Nürnberg am 11. Juni 1863. 8°. *Augsburg*, [1863].

Repr. from: Wchnschr. f. Thierh. u. Viehzucht, Augsburg.

BOLETIN de veterinaria. v. 2–3 (Nos. 25–68), 1846–7. 8°. *Madrid*.

BULLETTINO veterinario. Red.: P. Oreste [*et al.*]. v. 1, 1880. 8°. *Napoli*.

CENTRALBLATT für Thiermedicin. Hrsg. von H. Pütz. v. 1, 1884. 8°. *Stuttgart*.

CENTRALBLATT für Veterinärwissenschaften. Red. von H. Pütz. v. 1–4, 1882–6. 8°. *Leipzig*.

CENTRALZEITUNG für die gesammte Veterinärmedicin und ihre Hilfswissenschaften, mit vergleichender Bezugnahme auf die Menschenheilwissenschaft. Hrsg. von Johann Martin Kreutzer. v. 1–5, 1851–5. 4°. *Erlangen*.

CLINICA (La) veterinaria. Red.: N. Lanzilotti-Buonsanti. v. 2, 1879; v. 7–9, 1884–6. 8°. *Milano*.

CONGRÈS national de médecine vétérinaire tenu du 8 au 11 juillet 1880 sous le haut patronage de S. M. Léopold II, roi des Belges. roy. 8°. *Louvain*, 1881.

DEUTSCHE Zeitschrift für die gesammte Thierkeilkunde. Hrsg. von J. D. Busch. v. 1–3, 1830–33. 8°. *Marburg*.

DEUTSCHE Zeitschrift für Thiermedicin und vergleichende Pathologie. Von O. Bollinger und L. Franck. v. 1–13, 1875–87. 8°. *Leipzig*.

ÉCHO (L') des societés et associations vétérinaires de France. F. Quivogne, rédacteur. v. 1–9, 1879–87. 8°. *Lyon*.

EDINBURGH Veterinary Review and Annals of Comparative Pathology. v. 1–6, 1858–64. 8°. *Edinburgh*.

GACETA médico-veterinaria. Director: R. Espejo y del Rosal. v. 2–10, 1880–87. 8°. *Madrid*.

Medicine (*Veterinary, Journals and transactions of societies relating to*).

GAZZETTA medico-veterinaria. Red.: P. Oreste [*et al.*]. v. 1–6, 1871–8. 8°. *Milano & Napoli.*

GIORNALE di anatomia, fisiologia e patologia degli animali. Compilato da L. Lombardini e P. Oreste con l' aiuto dei professori A. Cristin, S. Falconio, G. Generali. v. 1–19, 1869–87. 8°. *Pisa.*

GIORNALE di medicina veterinaria pratica e di zootecnia della Società reale e nazionale veterinaria. v. 5–6, 1856–7; v. 23–36, 1874–87. 8°. *Torino.*

GIORNALE delle razze degli animali utili e di medicina veterinaria. Red.: S. Falconio [*et al.*]. 3. serie. v. 3, 1874. 8°. *Napoli.*

GIORNALE di veterinaria. v. 1–4, 1852–5. 8°. *Torino.*

JAHRBUCH der praktisch-polizeilichen und gerichtlichen Thierheilkunde von und für Bayern. In Verbindung mit vielen Hrn. Gerichts-, Militair- und Civil-Veterinairärzten herausgegeben von der Litteratur-Commission des Industrie- und Cultur-Vereins zu Nürnberg, dirigirt von Dr. Jac. J. Weidenkeller. v. 1–3, 1830–33. 8°. *Nürnberg.*

JAHRESBERICHT der königl. technischen Deputation für das Veterinairwesen über die Verbreitung ansteckender Thierkrankheiten in Preussen. v. 2–6, 8–9, 1877–85. 8°. *Berlin.*

JAHRESBERICHT über die Leistungen auf dem Gebiete der Veterinär-Medicin. Von Dr. Ellenberger und Dr. Schütz. v. 1–6, 1881–6. 8°. *Berlin*, 1882–7.

JOURNAL de médecine vétérinaire militaire. A. Goux, rédacteur. v. 1–14, 1862–77. 8°. *Paris.*

JOURNAL de médecine vétérinaire pratique et de zootechnie. Par J. Pelletan [*et al.*]. Nos. 5–6, v. 2, Jan. to Feb., 1880. 8°. *Paris.*

JOURNAL de médecine vétérinaire théorique et pratique, publié par MM. Bracey-Clark [*et al.*]. May, 1830. 8°. *Paris.*

JOURNAL de médecine vétérinaire et de zootechnie. Rédacteur: F. Peuch. 3. série. v. 1–12, 1876–87. 8°. *Lyon.*

MAGAZIN für die gesammte Thierheilkunde. Hrsg. von E. F. Gurlt und C. H. Hertwig. v. 1–40, 1835–74. 8°. *Berlin.*

MEDICINA (La) veterinaria. Red.: E. F. Isasmendi. v. 4–5, 1887. 8°. *Madrid.*

MEDICO (Il) veterinario. 1861–7; 1871–86. 8°. *Torino.*

MITTHEILUNGEN aus der thierärztlichen Praxis im preussischen Staate. Von C. Müller und F. Roloff. Neue Folge. v. 1–8, 1874–82. 8°. *Berlin*, 1876–83.

NORDDEUTSCHE Thierärzte. Bericht über die am 18. und 19. Mai 1868 in Berlin abgehaltene Versammlung . . . und über die am 20. Mai stattgefundene Jubelfeier des Herrn . . . Gurlt. Hrsg. von den Vorständen des Berliner, schlesischen und rheinprenssischen thierärztlichen Vereins. 8°. *Berlin*, 1868.

NOVOSTI veterinarnoe literaturi otchestvennoi i inostrannoi. v. 2–3, 1885–6. 8°. *St. Petersburg.*

OESTERREICHISCHE Monatsschrift für Thierheilkunde. Von A. Koch. v. 1–11, 1877–87. 4°. *Wien.*

OESTERREICHISCHE Vierteljahrsschrift für wissenschaftliche Veterinärkunde. Red.: Dr. Müller und Dr. Röll. v. 19–64, 1863–85. 8°. *Wien.*

OESTERREICHISCHE Zeitschrift für wissenschaftliche Veterinärkunde. Hrsg. von J. Bayer und St. Polansky. v. 1, 1887. 8°. *Wien.*

PORVENIR (El) de la veterinaria. Dirigido por E. F. Isasmendi. v. 2–4, 1884–6. 8°. *Madrid.*

PRESSE (La) vétérinaire. Par J. Biot [*et al.*]. v. 1–7, 1881–7. 8°. *Paris.*

Medicine (*Veterinary, Journals and transactions of societies relating to*).

QUARTERLY (The) Journal of Veterinary Science in India, and Army Medical Management. By C. Steel [*et al.*]. v. 1–5, 1882–7. 8°. *Madras.*

RECUEIL de médecine vétérinaire. (Nouvelle bibliothèque médicale, 2. série.) v. 1–8, 1824–31; 2. série, v. 1–12, 1832–43; 3. série, v. 1–10, 1844–53; 4. série, v. 1–10, 1854–63; 5. série, v. 1–7, 9–10, 1864–70, 1872–3; 6. série, v. 1–10, 1874–83; 7. série, v. 1–4, 1884–7. 8°. *Paris.*

RECUEIL de mémoires et observations sur l'hygiène et la médecine vétérinaires militaires. v. 1–19, 1847–71; 2. série, v. 2–6, Nov., 1875, to Dec., 1879. 8°. *Paris.*

REPERTORIUM der Thierheilkunde nach homöopathischen Grundsätzen [etc.] v. 1, 1836. 8°. *Leipzig, L. Schumann.*

REPERTORIUM der Thierheilkunde. Von E. Hering. v. 1–48, 1840–87. 8°. *Stuttgart.*

REVUE für Thierheilkunde und Thierzucht. Von A. Koch. v. 1–10, 1878–87. 8°. *Wien.*

RUNDSCHAU auf dem Gebiete der Thiermedicin und vergleichenden Pathologie. Von G. Schneidemühl. v. 1–3, 1885–7. fol. *Osterwick im Harz.*

SCHWEIZER-ARCHIV für Thierheilkunde. Redigirt von A. Guillebeau und E. Zschokke. v. 25–29, 1883–7. 8°. *Zürich.*

SCHWEIZERISCHES Archiv für Thierheilkunde und Thierzucht. Hrsg. von D. v. Niederhæusern [*et al.*]. v. 1–5, 1879–83. 8°. *Bern.*

STUDENTE (Lo) veterinario. Red.: E. Ardenghi. v. 1–3, 1875–8. 4°. *Parma.*

THIERÄRZTLICHE Jahrbücher. Von J. E. L. Falke. v. 1–4, 1878–81. 8°. *Leipzig u. Jena.*

THIERÄRZTLICHE Mittheilungen. Von A. Lydtin. v. 11–22, 1876–87. 8°. *Karlsruhe.*

THIERÄRZTLICHER Verein der Provinz Brandenburg. Bericht über die fünfte Versammlung . . . am 5. October 1872. 8°. *Berlin*, 1872.

THIERÄRZTLICHES Wochenblatt. Von G. Niclas. v. 1–8, 1849–56. 4°. *Neu-Ulm.*

THIERARZT (Der). Von W. Schumacher. v. 2, 1863; v. 15–26, 1876–87. 8°. *Wetzlar.*

THIERFREUND (Der). Von F. A. Zürn. v. 1, 1879. 4°. *Leipzig.*

TIDSSKRIFT for Veterinærer, redigeret af H. Bagge og H. Krabbe. 2. Række, v. 3–17, 1873–87. 8°. *Kjøbenhavn.*

TIJDSCHRIFT voor veeartsenijkunde en veeteelt. Red.: J. J. Hinze [*et al.*]. v. 10–13, 1879–86. 8°. *Amsterdam.*

UCHENIJA zapiski Kazanskago Veterinarnago Instituta. v. 2–4, 1885–7. 8°. *Kazan.*

UNITED STATES (The) Veterinary Journal. v. 1–2, 1882–4. fol. *Chicago.*

VETERINÄR-KALENDER. Von A. Koch. v. 8–9, 1885–6. 12°. *Leipzig u. Wien.*

VETERINARIA (La). Red.: E. Ardenghi e G. Fogliata. v. 1–2, 1880–81. 8°. *Parma.*

VETERINARIA (La) española. Director: S. F. Gallego. v. 20–21, 1876–7; v. 28–30, 1884–7. fol. *Madrid.*

VETERINARIAN (The); or monthly journal of veterinary science. Edited by W. Dick, W. F. Karkeek, W. Percivall, W. Youatt, M. U. Leblanc, Profs. Morton, Simonds, Varnell, Tuson, and Brown. v. 1–60, 1828–87. 8°. *London.*

VETERINARNII Vestnik, journal nauchnoi i prakticheskoi zoojatrii. Red.: E. M. Zemmerom i P. A. Gordiev. v. 3–7, 1884–7. 8°. *Charkoff.*

VETERINARNOE dielo. Red.: A. I. Alexiev. v. 3–5, 1885–7. 8°. *St. Petersburg.*

VETERINARY (The) Gazette. By C. A. Meyer [*et al.*]. v. 1–2, 1880–82. 8°. *New York.*

Medicine (*Veterinary, Journals and transactions of societies relating to*).

VETERINARY (The) Journal and Annals of Comparative Pathology. By G. Fleming. v. 1–25, 1875–87. 8°. *London.*

VETERINARY (The) Record, [etc.] Edited by Professors Spooner, Simonds, and Morton. v. 1–6, 1845–50. 8°. *London.*

VIERTELJAHRSSCHRIFT für wissenschaftliche Veterinärkunde. Herausgegeben von den Mitgliedern des Wiener kaiserlich-königlichen Thierarznei-Institutes. Redacteure : Prof. Dr. Müller, Prof. Dr. Röll. v. 1–18, 1851–62. 8°. *Wien.*

WOCHENSCHRIFT für Thierheilkunde und Viehzucht. Von Th. Adam. v. 20–31, 1876–87. 8°. *Augsburg.*

ZEITSCHRIFT für praktische Veterinair-Wissenschaften. Redigirt von H. Pütz. v. 4–5, 1876–7. 8°. *Bern u. Berlin.*

ZOOTECNICO (Il). Diretta dal Prof. A. de Silvestri. No. 1., v. 1, Jan. 7, 1875. 8°. *Torino.*

Ableitner (K.) Die thierärztlichen Vereine in Deutschland, ihr Entstehen, ihre Entwicklung und Verbreitung, ihre Leistungen innerhalb des letzten halben Jahrhundertes; im Auszuge aus den deutschen Zeitschriften von Kreuzer, Nicklas, Hering, Adam mitgetheilt. Oester. Vrtljschr. f. wissensch. Veterinärk., Wien, 1880, liv, 71–133.

Medicine *and religion.*

See, also, **Baptism** ; **Bible** (*Medicine of the*); **Cæsarean** *section post mortem* ; **Chorea** ; **Convulsions** (*Epidemic*) ; **Ecstacy** ; **Insanity** (*Religious*) ; **Labor** (*Accelerated or forced in the dying*) ; **Materialism** ; **Medicine** (*Magical, etc.*); **Philosophy** (*Medical*) ; **Revivals** ; **Sacred** *embryology* ; **Sacrifices** (*Human*) ; **Superstition.**

ALBERTI (M.) * De medicinæ et doctrinæ moralis nexu. Respondens A. Ajtai. 4°. *Halæ Magdeb.*, [1714].

——. Specimen medicinæ theologicæ, selectiora quædam themata ad scientiam et experientiam medicam præcipue pertinentia cum s. theologia tamen propius firmiusque connexa multis particularibus observationibus necnon casibus conscientiæ illustrata commendans in medicinæ et theologiæ usum directum. Cum præfatione J. M. Langii. sm. 8°. *Halæ Magdeb.*, 1726.

BAITHER (J. G.) *De noxis neoterismi in medicina, et constituendo tribunali medico-catholico. 4°. *Tubingæ*, [1806].

BALDIT (M.) Speculum sacro-medicum octogonum, in quo medicina octo ex angulis, veluti totidem fontibus a primo et in primum salientibus, sacra repræsentatur. Præfixa appendice gemina, tamquam vita speculum æquilibraliter suspensura. 12°. *Lugduni*, 1666.

BOWDITCH (H. I.) An apology for the medical profession, as a means of developing the whole nature of man. A valedictory address . . . Harvard University, March 11, 1863. With additional remarks on a topic of importance at the present hour. 8°. *Boston*, 1863.

BRIGHAM (A.) Remarks on the influence of mental cultivation and mental excitement upon health. 12°. *Philadelphia*, 1833.

——. The same. 3. ed. 12°. *Philadelphia*, 1845.

——. Observations on the influence of religion upon the health and physical welfare of mankind. 8°. *Boston*, 1835.

[BRODIE (*Sir* B. C.)] The healing art the right hand of the Church ; or practical medicine an essential element in the Christian system. By Therapeutes. 8°. *Edinburgh*, 1859.

BROESIKE (J. F.) * De religione medici. 4°. *Halæ Magdeb.*, [1722].

BROWNE (*Sir* T.) Religio medici, cum annotationibus. 16°. *Argentorati*, 1677.

Medicine *and religion.*

——. The same. With annotations never before published, upon all the obscure passages therein. Also observations by Sir Kenelm Digby, now newly added. 8. ed. 18°. *London*, 1682.

CHEVERRY. * De la médecine morale. 4°. *Paris*, 1820.

COMBE (G.) Answer to the attack on " The constitution of man", contained in " Nature and revelation harmonious", etc., by the Rev. C. J. Kennedy, Paisley. 8°. *Edinburgh*, 1848.
See, also, infra.

CONNOR (B.) Evangelium medici, seu medicina mystica ; de suspensis naturæ legibus, sive de miraculis ; reliquisque ἐν τοῖς βιβλίοις memoratis, quæ medicæ indagini subjici possunt. 12°. *Londini*, 1697.

COURAGEOT (A.) * Réflexions sur la médecine morale, et les qualités physiques et morales du médecin. 4°. *Paris*, 1832.

COWLING (R. O.) The relations of medicine to modern unbelief. A valedictory address . . . commencement of the University of Louisville. 8°. *Louisville*, 1876.

CRÜGER (J.) Epicrisis xii, curiosa theologico-medico-chimica, de menstrui obstructione. Et epicrisis xiii, curiosa medico-chimica, de ephialte infantum. 4°. [*n. p.*], 1712.

DALE (J. W.) Essay upon the question : " Is medical science favourable to scepticism?" 8°. *Philadelphia*, 1839.

DEBREYNE (P.-J.-C.) Essai sur la théologie morale, considérée dans ses rapports avec la physiologie et la médecine. Ouvrage spécialement destiné au clergé. 2. éd. 8°. *Paris*, 1843.

DECLARATION (The) of students of the natural and physical sciences. [That it is impossible for the word of God, as written in the book of nature, and God's word written in the holy scripture, to contradict one another.] 8°. *London*, [*n. d.*]

DENKEL. * Ueber die religiöse Seite in der Medizin. 8°. *München*, 1844.

DIFENBACH (J. P.) * Diss. medico-forensis qua rationibus theologicis legalibus et medicis ostenditur fœtum ex utero matris mortuæ mature exscindendum esse et simul singularis observatio de ruptura uteri in partu exhibetur. sm. 4°. *Altorfii*, [1720].

DRAPER (J. W.) History of the conflict between religion and science. 8°. *New York*, 1875.

DRELINCURTIUS [DRELINCOURT] (C.) Oratio doctoralis Monspessula, qua medicos, jugi Dei operum consideratione atque contemplatione permotos, cæteris hominibus religioni astrictiores esse demonstratur ; atque adeo, impietatis crimen in ipsos jactatum diluitur atque propulsatur. *In his:* Opusc. med. 8°. *Hagæ Comitum*, 1727, 57–75.

DÜRFELD (E. A.) * Diss. inaug. commentationem theologico medicam in Jur. Canonic. decreti part. iii. de consecrat. distinct. v, c. xxi, contraria studiose sunt divinæ cognitioni præcepta medicinæ, a jejuniis revocant, lucubrare non sinunt, ab omni intentione meditationis abducunt, itaque qui se medicis dederit, seipsum sibi abnegat, exhibens. 4°. *Halæ Magdeb.*, [1739].

FERDAS (R.) Études de physiologie théologique. Accouplement des sexes et mariage ; accouchement et embryologie selon les théologiens. 8°. *Paris*, 1880.

FIGATELLI (G.) Medico sacro che si piglia pensiero de gl' incurabili ; e pratica rimedij preservativi, curativi, e comfortativi ; quando appunto l' huomo, dovendo far passagio all' eternità dell' altra vita, ò per corso naturale, ò di morte violenta per mano della giustitia, [etc.] 18°. *Venetia*, 1677.

Medicine *and religion.*

GOHL (J. D.) Exarans epistolam gratulatoriam ad Gothofred. Mich. Cortum: in ea expendit obiter hæresin medicam in comparatione cum theologica. sm. 4°.   *Francof. ad Viadr.*, [1724].

HARTWIG (F. G.) Epistola, qua de usu scientiæ medicæ in theologicis breviter disserit. 4°. *Lipsiæ*, [1763].

HOFFMANN (F.) Opuscula theologico-physicomedica, seu scripta selectiora antea diversis temporibus edita, nunc revisa, correcta et aucta. 4°. *Halæ*, 1740.

HOFMANN (J. J. C.) *De verbi divini ministro ad ægrotorum lectulos commorante. 4°. *Vitebergæ*, [1806].

HOPE (M. B.) A discourse designed to show that physiological inquiries are not unfriendly to religious sentiment. 8°. *Philadelphia*, 1845.

JOULIN (J.-D.) Au feu les libres penseurs!!! 3. éd., contenant, outre les trois premières lettres à Mgr. Dupanloup, deux nouvelles lettres à Mgr. de Bonnechose, suivies d'une lettre à son ami Giraud, par le docteur Flavius. 8°. *Paris*, 1868.

KÄHLER (L. A.) Einiges über die Verwandtschaft der Medizin und der Theologie. 4°. *Kottbus*, [1818].

LETTRES intéressantes pour les médecins de profession, utiles aux ecclésiastiques qui veulent s'appliquer à la médecine, et curieuses pour tout lecteur. 2 v. in 1. 12°. *Avignon*, 1759.

LIVRES (Les) secrets des confesseurs, [etc.] 8°. *Paris*, [1884].

MACGOWAN (D. J.) Claims of the missionary enterprise on the medical profession; an address delivered before the temperance society of the College of Physicians and Surgeons of the University of the State of New York, Oct. 28, 1842. 8°. *New York*, 1842.

MEIER (F. A.) *Ueber das Verhältniss der Religion zur Heilkunst. 8°. *München*, 1840.

MEZLER (F. X.) Ueber den Einfluss der Heilkunst auf die praktische Theologie. Ein Beytrag zur Pastoralmedizin. 2 v. 12°. *Ulm*, 1806.

PROUT (W.) Chemistry, meteorology, and the function of digestion considered with reference to natural theology. 8°. *London*, 1834.

ROTHE (J. A.) *De convenientia medicinæ cum theologia practica. 4°. *Halæ Magdeb.*, [1732].

SCOTTI (A. A.) Catechismo medico, ossia sviluppo delle dottrine che conciliano la religione colla medicina. 8°. *Venezia*, 1826.

——. The same. 8°. *Roma*, 1850.

SEBIZIUS (M.) Dissertatio περὶ θείον, de divino, quod Hippocrates in morbis considerandum in prognosticorum suorum vestibulo præcepit. sm. 4°. *Argentorati*, 1643.

SENTIDO (El) católico en las ciencias médicas. Revista médico práctica. v. 1–9, 1879–87. 4° & 8°. *Barcelona*, 1879–87.

SIJBRANDI (N. D.) *De necessitudine, quæ fuit apud veteres inter religionem et medicinam. 8°. *Amstelodami*, 1841.

SPINCKES (N.) The sick man visited, and furnished with instructions, meditations, and prayers for putting him in mind of his change; for supporting him under his distemper, and for preparing him for, and carrying him through, his last conflict with death. 6. ed. 8°. *London*, 1775.

STEVENS (W. B.) The religious teachings of medical science. A sermon. 8°. *Philadelphia*, 1858.

STONHOUSE (J.) Friendly advice to a patient; calculated more particularly for the use of the sick belonging to the infirmaries, as well the out

Medicine *and religion.*

patients as those within the house. 10. ed. 12°. *London*, [1748].

——. Spiritual directions for the uninstructed; not less proper for the use of infirmary patients than for the uninstructed in all conditions. 10. ed. 12°. *London*, [n. d.]

THOMPSON (L. P.) The study and practice of medicine not unfavorable to the cultivation of a religious character. A sermon. 8°. *Buffalo*, 1852.

WEIGAND (J. E.) *De morbis ex concionibus prolixis et impetuosis metuendis. 4°. [*Erfordiæ*, 1778.]

WINDRIF (É.-A.) *Essai sur l'influence des moyens religieux en médecine. 4°. *Paris*, 1840.

ZEITLER (J. B.) *De nexu, qui est inter medicinam et religionem. 8°. *Monachii*, 1834.

Acland (H. W.) The influence of social and sanitary conditions on religion. Med. Press & Circ., Lond., 1874, xviii, 327–329.—**B.** (L.) Medicina e religione. Indipendente, Torino, 1875, xxvi, 241–246.—**Bataillard** (P.) Sur la religion, la morale et l'art au point de vue anthropologique. Bull. Soc. d'anthrop. de Par., 1867, 2. s., ii, 491–570.—**Benavente.** La religion y la medicina. Siglo méd., Madrid, 1856, iii, 257.—**Bernstein** (M.) Betrachtungen über das Verhältniss der Religion zur Medicin. Deutsches Arch. f. Gesch. d. Med. u. med. Geog., Leipz., 1881, iv, 107; 201; 297.—**Bertulus** (E.) El ateísmo del siglo xix en presencia de la historia, la filosofia médica y la humanidad. Siglo méd., Madrid, 1868, xv, 740; 777; 795. ——. De la théophobie scientifique et médicale. Rev. de thérap. méd.-chir., Par., 1872, xxxix, 136–140.—**C. y A.** (J.) Deontología médica; necesidad que tiene el médico de ser católico. Sentido catól., Barcel., 1879, i, 66; 83; 169.—**Combe** (G.) [Review of] Nature and revelation harmonious; a defence of scripture truths assailed in Mr. George Combe's work on the Constitution of man, etc. By J. C. Kennedy, Paisley. Published under the sanction of the Scottish Association for Opposing Prevalent Errors. Edinburgh. W. Oliphant & Sons, 1846, 32mo, pp. 147. Phrenol. J., Edinb., 1847, xx, 425–435. [*See, also, supra.*]—**Coudereau.** Sur la religiosité comme caractéristique. Bull. Soc. d'anthrop. de Par., 1866, 2. s., i, 329–340.—**Denham** (J. F.) On the connexion between morbid physical and religious phenomena. J. Psych. M., Lond., 1856, ix, 39; 385.—**Dimon** (T.) The influence of medical studies upon religious belief. Buffalo M. & S. J., 1875–6, xv, 54–59.—**Fabre** (A.) De la philosophie chrétienne et de son intervention en médecine. Marseille méd., 1872, ix, 506; 553.—**Fränkel** (H.) Die Medizin und die Religion. Med. Alm., Berl., 1829, 50–79.—**Glas** (O.) Tal hället vid Upsala Läkareförenings högtidsdag den 17. September 1875. [Oration delivered at a festival of the Upsala Medical Association.] Upsala Läkaref. Förh., 1875–6, xi, 1–61.—**Hirsch** (A.) Ueber den Zusammenhang der wissenschaftlichen und religiösen Naturanschauung. Amtl. Ber. ü. d. Versamml. deutsch. Naturf. u. Aerzte 1860, Königsb., 1861, xxxv, 28–32.—**Hitchcock** (A.) Organic and parallel relation of some of the truths and errors of christianity and medical science, 1869. Med. Communicat. Mass. M. Soc., Bost., 1866–74, xi, 93–127.—**Letourneau.** De la religiosité et des religions au point de vue anthropologique. Bull. Soc. d'anthrop. de Par., 1865, vi, 581–604.—**Lichtenstädt.** Ueber theologische Ansichten in der Natur- und Heilkunde. Allg. med. Ann., Leipz., 1827, 1–8.—**Martin de Moussy.** La religiosité est-elle un des caractères spéciaux du genre humain? Bull. Soc. d'anthrop. de Par., 1866, 2. s., i, 105–121.—**Martinez** (M.) Discurso phísico sobre si las vivoras deban reputarse por carne, ó pescado, en el sentido en que nuestra madre la Iglesia nos veda las carnes en dias de abstinencia. Repuesta á una consulta, que hicieron los RR. Padres Cartujanos, para en vista de la resolucion poder usar las vivoras á lo menos como medicamento, lo qual en caso de reputarse por carne, les seria vedado, segun su laudable costumbre. *In his:* Noches anatómicas, 4°, Madrid, 1750, 205–222.—**Mestre y Marzal** (C.) El ateísmo y los médicos. Siglo méd., Madrid, 1860, vii, 333; 366; 782.—**Meyn.** Die Feier des Abendmahls, beurtheilt aus staatsarzneilichem Gesichtspunkte. Ztschr. f. d. Staatsarznk., Erlang., 1825, ix, 331–361.—**Moore** (T. V.) Religion and medicine. Maryland & Virg. M. J., Richmond, 1860, xiv, 89–99.—**O'Dea** (J. J.) The development of religious ideas. J. Psych. M., N. Y., 1872, vi, 76–101. *Also*, Reprint.—**Palmer** (B. M.) The pious physician, or the claims of religion upon the medical profession; a discourse delivered upon the occasion of the death of the late John M. W. Picton, Dec. 26, 1858, in New Orleans. N. Orl. M. News & Hosp. Gaz., 1858–9, v, 737–750.—**Polk** (W. M.) Religion and medicine. N. York M. J., 1885, xlii, 421–424.—**Reccupito** (F.) L' igiene sociale e la religione. Riv. ital. di terap. ed ig.,

Medicine *and religion.*

Piacenza, 1887, vii, 90-93.—[**Review** of] The work and the counter work; or the religious revival in Belfast. With an explanation of the physical phenomena. By Edward A. Stopford. 6. ed. Dublin, Hodges, Smith & Co., 1859. J. Ment. Sc., Lond., 1859-60, vi, 167-178.—**Rittmann.** Die Fachmedizin der Alexandriner und die religiöse Heilkunst der Römer. Allg. Wien. med. Ztg., 1867, xii, 223.—**Rougier.** Des dangers de la science moderne, positive ou de l'athéisme. Marseille méd., 1872, ix, 653-663.—**Scotti** (A. A.) Catecismo médico ó armonías entre la medicina y la religión. Sentido catól., Barcel.,1884, vi, 637; 653; 685: 701; 717; 733: 1885, vii, 17: 33; 146; 161; 177; 193; 225.—**Shuttleworth** (J. K.) The moral aspect of the medical art Med. Times & Gaz., Lond., 1857, n. s., xiv, 557; 585.—**Turner** (G.) Diseases of the saints. India J. M. & Phys. Sc., Calcutta, 1842, n. s., vii, 341-345.—**Werner** (M.) Religion und Medicin; aphoristische Studie. Deutsches Arch. f. Gesch. d. Med. u. med. Geog., Leipz., 1885, viii, 97-107.—**Winslow** (F.) On morbid religious thought. Lancet, Lond., 1867, i, 662; 760.

Medicine *as a science.*

See Medicine.

Medicine *and surgery (Relations of).*

See, also, **Medicine** (*History, etc., of*), *by nations — France*; **Physicians** (*Controversies of*) *with surgeons.*

BALLAND (J.-G.) * Dissertation sur l'utilité de l'union de la médecine et de la chirurgie. 4°. *Paris*, 1815.

BISCHOFF (C. H. E.) Ueber das Verhältniss der Medicin zur Chirurgie und die Dreiheit im heilenden Stande zur Verwahrung jeder betreffenden Staats-Anordnung. 8°. *Bonn*, 1842.

COMPARAÇÃO entre os conhecimentos scientificos do cirurgião medico e os do medico. Por em alumno da Eschola medico-cirurgica de Lisboa. 8°. *Lisboa*, 1844.

DE B. Examen impartial des contestations des médecins et des chirurgiens, considérées par rapport à l'intérêt public. 12°. [*n. p.*], 1748.

ECKERMANN (A.) * An et quatenus studium et exercitium medicinæ et chirurgiæ necessario jungenda sint? sm. 4°. *Gottingæ.* [1801].

HERTEL (J. G.) * De officio medici circa casus chirurgicos dictos. 4°. *Halæ Magdeb.*, [1710].

HESSERT (F.-F.-L.) * Essai sur l'utilité de la réunion de la médecine et de la chirurgie. 4°. *Strasbourg*, 1804.

KIRKLAND (T.) An enquiry into the present state of medical surgery; including the analogy betwixt external and internal disorders, and the inseparability of these branches of the same profession. v. 2. 8°. *London*, 1783-6.

MARTIN (R.) Tal om de gränsor, som naturlig billig het synes hafva utstakat imellan medecine och chirurgie. 8°. *Stockholm*, 1757.

MENDEZ ÁLVARO (F.) Defensa de la clase médica contra las pretensiones de cirujanos y practicantes; exámen crítico de la proposicion de ley que los señores diputados Herrera y Ortiz de Zárate han presentado al Congreso, empeñados en realizar la prevaricada metamórfosis de los cirujanos en médicos, y de los ministrantes y practicantes en lo mismo. 8°. *Madrid*, 1866.

PEITHNER (F. E.) * Ueber die Vereinigung der Medicin und Chirurgie. 8°. *Prag*, 1819.

QUESTION de médecine où il s'agit de savoir si le médecin est plus certain que le chirurgien. 12°. [*Paris*], 1739.

Text in Latin and French.

RESPOSTA a carta da despedida que fez a medicina, quando se ausentou deste reino de Portugal, queixando-se das affrontas, e calúmnias, que recebêra dos Portuguezes, dando preferencia aos cirurgiões no curativo das suas enfermidades. Acceita-se-lhe a despedide, fazendo-se ver que a tal ausencia não será sensivel, pois a cirurgia pódo muito bem supprir a s a falta. 8°. *Lisboa*, 1781.

Medicine *and surgery (Relations of).*

RÖSCHLAUB (A.) Ueber Medizin, ihr Verhältniss zur Chirurgie, nebst Materialien zu einem Entwurfe der Polizei der Medizin. 8°. *Frankf. a. M.*, 1802.

SCHWEIZER (G. G.) * De medicinæ et chirurgiæ perpetuo nexu. 4°. *Halæ Magdeb.*, [1705].

DA SILVA PEREIRA (M. M.) Dissertação ácerca da indissoluvel connexão, que existe entre a cirurgia e a medicina, apresentada e defendida na Escola medico-cirurgica do Porto. 8°. *Porto*, 1845.

VON WALTHER (P. F.) Ueber das Verhältniss der Medicin zur Chirurgie und die Duplicität im ärztlichen Stande; eine historische Untersuchung mit dem Endresultat für die betreffende Staatseinrichtung. 8°. *Carlsruhe u. Freiburg*, 1841.

Biermann. Die Gränzen der Medicin und Chirurgie. Ein medicinal-polizeilicher Versuch zur Feststellung des praktischen Verhältnisses zwischen beiden Disciplinen. Ztschr. f. d. Staatsarznk., Erlang., 1834, xxvii, 1-10.—**Daremberg** (C.) Lettre à M. le docteur Salvatore de Renzi sur un passage de Celse relatif à la division de la médecine. Gaz. méd. de Par., 1852, 3. s., vii, 169-177. *Also,* Reprint.—**Fischer** (A. F.) Lässt sich von der zur Norm gewordenen gleichmässigen Ausübung der innern und äussern Heilkunde ein wahrhafter Gewinn für das so erforderliche Fortbilden der wissenschaftlichen Medicin erwarten? Wchnschr. f. d. ges. Heilk,, Berl., 1839, 17-29.—**Frank** (J. P.) De chirurgo medicis auxiliis indigente. *In his:* Delect. opusc. med., 8°. Ticini, 1787, iv, 304-327. *Also, in his:* Opusc. med., 8°. Lipsiæ, 1790, 136-153.—**Gr.** Ueber die Vereinigung der Chirurgie mit der Medizin. Allg. med. Ann., Altenb., 1809, 839; 951; 1039.—**Hensel** (J.) Wo ist die Grenze zwischen Medicin und Chirurgie, oder welches sind innere, welches sind äussere Krankheiten? Org. f. d. ges. Heilk. Berl., 1859, viii, 29-32.—**Mayor** (M.) Des caractères différentiels de la médecine et de la chirurgie, et de la nécessité de les tracer nettement. J. d. conn. méd.-chir., Par., 1842-3, x, pt. 1, 144; 221.—**Nähere** Bestimmung der Sphären der Medizin und der Chirurgie, zufolge der Walther'schen Schrift: Die Chirurgie in ihrer Trennung von der Medizin. Allg. med. Ann., Altenb., 1808, 159-176.—**Nöldeke** (G. J. F.) Ueber die Möglichkeit und Nothwendigkeit, die Medicin und Chirurgie in ihrer Erlernung und Ausübung zu verbinden; in einem Sendschreiben an einen die Heilkunde studierenden Freund. J. d. prakt. Heilk., Berl., 1811, xxxii, 2. St., 87-114.

Medicine-chests.

See, also, **Medicine** (*Naval*).

CARPENTER (G. W.) Carpenter's family medicine chest dispensatory, containing a select catalogue of drugs, chemicals, and family medicines, with the properties and doses of each article most approved of in domestic medicine; to which is appended a concise description of diseases, with directions for the treatment of such as are unattended with serious consequences; showing also, the best immediate measures to be adopted in those disorders and accidents which are destructive to life, when the physician is not at hand, or until his assistance can be procured. 8°. *Philadelphia*, 1835.

CATALOGUE des remèdes dont on peut s'approvisionner pour avoir une cassette de pharmacie bien fournie. L'on y a joint quelques remèdes particuliers connus comme spécifiques, et quelques compositions de pur agrément. Chaque particulier peut réduire sa petite cassette à ce qui est absolument nécessaire dans une maison de campagne, pour une famille et un domestique plus ou moins considérable. 12°. *Paris*, 1765.

COMPANION (A) to the medicine chest, or plain directions for the employment of various medicines and utensils contained in it, and for the treatment of diseases. By a medical practitioner. 12°. *London*, 1802.

DIRECTIONS for the medicine chest. 8°. *North Shields*, 1795.

DIRECTIONS, etc. [for medicine chests]. 12°. [*n. p., n. d.*]

Medicine-chests.

HEERMANN (L.) Directions for the medicine chest. 8°. *New Orleans,* 1811.

INDEX to the portable dispensary, containing directions for the proper application of the medicines usually contained therein. 12°. *London,* 1801.

UNITED STATES. *War Department. Engineers' Office.* [Yarrow (H. C.) & Rothrock (J. T.)] Geographical surveys west of the 100th meridian. Circular containing suggestions for the use of remedies furnished to field-parties. 12°. *Washington,* 1875.

———. The same. 12°. *Washington,* 1878.

———. *War Department. Surgeon-General's Office.* International Exhibition of 1876. Hospital of the Medical Department of the United States Army. No. 5. Description of Perot & Co.'s improved U. S. A. medicine wagon and of Perot & Co.'s U. S. A. mess chest. 8°. *Philadelphia,* 1876.

Novel (A) form of medicine glass. Med. Rec., N. Y., 1880, xvii, 680.

Medicine-holder *and medicine-spoons (Collection of patents relating to).*

Baker (T. M.) Medicine-spoon. No. 233185. Oct. 12, 1880.—**Clayton** (H.) Medical and nursery spoon. No. 244551. July 19, 1881.—**Dorr** (C. S.) Medicine-spoon. No. 353055. Nov. 23, 1886.—**Force** (J. W.) Nursery and medical spoons. No. 212677. Feb. 25, 1879.—**Guion** (E.) Medicine spoon. No. 358197. Feb. 22, 1887.—**Moffitt** (J.) Medicine-spoon. No. 285054. Sept. 18, 1883.—**Noe** (W. R.) Medicine-spoon. No. 350499. Oct. 12, 1886. — **Pelkey** (Sophia). Medicine-spoon and vial-holder. No. 277924. May 22, 1883.—**Sherwin** (B.) Medicine-spoon. No. 339221. April 6, 1886. — **Stittheimer** (J. R.) Veterinary medicine-spoon. No. 291950. Jan. 15, 1884.—**Trueblood** (B. T.) Medicine-spoon. No. 222549. Dec. 9, 1879.—**Welsh** (W. H.) Medical spoon. No. 343510. June 8, 1886. — **Wyeth** (F. H.) Medicine-holder. No. 350406. Oct. 5, 1886.

Medicines.

See, also, **Materia** *medica;* **Pharmacy; Poisons; Therapeutics.**

ABERCROMBY (D.) Nova medicinæ tum practicæ, tum speculativæ clavis; sive ars explorandi medicas plantarum, ac corporum quorumcumque facultates ex solo sapore. 12°. *Londini,* 1685.

———. The same. 8°. *Parisiis,* 1740.

ALBERTI (M.) Disquis. med. de medicamentorum modo operandi in corpore vivo . . . [Præmissa præfatione introductoria de commercio animæ, sive naturæ incorporeæ, cum mediis et remediis corporeis.] 4°. *Halæ Magdeb.,* 1720.

AMAGAT (A.-L.) *Étude sur les différentes voies d'absorption des médicaments. 4°. *Paris,* 1873.

BAUDUS (J. G.) *De acrium natura, usu et abusu. sm. 4°. *Jenæ,* [1696].

BOERHAAVE (H.) Tractatus de viribus medicamentorum. Accesserunt epistolæ duæ. 12°. *Parisiis,* 1723.

———. The same. Ed. nov. Recensuit Benedictus Boudon. 12°. *Parisiis,* 1740.

———. The same. Traité de la vertu des médicamens. Trad. par M. de Vaux. 12°. *Paris,* 1729.

———. The same. De viribus medicamentorum; or, a treatise of the virtue and energy of medicines. 12°. *London,* 1720.

———. The same. A treatise on the powers of medicines. Transl. by John Martin. 8°. *London,* 1740.

BOHN (J.) & PHILIPPI (J. A.) *Diss. med. de medicamentorum chymicorum et galenicorum præpollentia dubia. sm. 4°. *Lipsiæ,* [1706].

BUSHNAN (J. S.) On the classification, administration, modus operandi, and combination of medicines. 8°. *London,* 1834.

Medicines.

CAELS (T. P.) *De viribus medicamentorum. *In:* LOUVAIN Diss. 8°. *Lovanii,* 1795, i, 9-23.

CAMPER (P.) De remediorum specialium requisitis, genuina historia, actione, et optima administrandi methodo; necnon de morbis quorum speciales curationes desiderantur. *In his:* Diss. decem. 8°. *Lingæ,* 1800, ii, 1-126.

CAPUA [*or* DI CAPOA] (L.) Ragionamenti intorno alla incertezza de' medicamenti. 4°. *Napoli,* 1689.

CRAUSIUS (R. W.) [Pr.] commendans studium inquirendi facultates medicamentorum, modumque eorum agendi. sm. 4°. *Jenæ,* 1702.

DETHARDING (G.) Scrutatio physico-medica de operationibus medicamentorum reficientium et adjuvantium, nominatim cordialium, anodinorum, specificorum, [etc.] Resp. Sam. Ernesto Crügner. sm. 4°. *Hafniæ,* [1735].

FAGRÆUS (J. T.) Medicamenta graveolentia. sm. 4°. *Upsaliæ,* 1758.

FOCK (H. C. A. L.) *De quæstione, num pharmaca ante absorptionem effectus specificos præstare possint. 8°. *Traj. ad Rhenum,* 1835.

GEDDY (J. C.) *Experimental essay on the absorption of medicines. 8°. *Philadelphia,* 1802.

GEORGI (F.) *De medicamentis inspissantibus eorumque modo operandi. 4°. *Halæ Magdeb.,* [1745].

GÉRARD (J.) *Contribution à l'étude de la durée de l'élimination des médicaments. 4°. *Paris,* 1880.

GOSKY (C. F.) De cognoscenda corporis humani natura ex effectu remediorum, oder: Wie man die Naturen derer Menschen, aus der Wirckung derer Artzney-Mittel erkennen könne? 4°. *Halæ Magdeb.,* 1732.

HEADLAND (F. W.) An essay on the action of medicines in the system; or, "on the mode in which therapeutic agents introduced into the stomach produce their peculiar effects on the animal economy". 8°. *London,* 1852.

———. The same. 8°. *Philadelphia,* 1853.

———. The same. 3. ed. 8°. *Philadelphia,* 1859.

———. The same. From the 4. Lond. ed. 8°. *Philadelphia,* 1868.

HENGSTMANN (J.-B.) Dissertation sur l'inutilité des médicamens étrangers. *In:* CHIRAC (P.) & SILVA (J.-B.) Dissertations et consultations médicinales. 12°. *Paris,* 1744, i, 61-158.

HENRY (T.) Experiments and observations on the following subjects: 1. On the preparation, calcination, and medicinal uses of magnesia alba. 2. On the solvent qualities of calcined magnesia. 3. On the variety in the solvent powers of quicklime, when used in different quantities. 4. On various absorbents, as promoting or retarding putrefaction. 5. On the comparative antiseptic powers of vegetable infusions prepared with lime, etc. 6. On the sweetening properties of fixed air. 8°. *London,* 1773.

HERMANN (J. G.) De modo operandi remediorum physico-mechanico. 4°. *Halæ Magdeb.,* [1718].

HEZEL (J. L. L.) *De medicamentorum masticatoriorum usu et præstantia. 4°. *Erlangæ,* [1766].

HODGE (B. G.) *Experiments and observations on the absorption of active medicines into the circulation. 8°. *Philadelphia,* 1801.

———. The same. 8°. *Philadelphia,* 1806.

HUBO (C. G.) De medicamentorum effectibus in corpore humano sano. 8°. *Gottingæ,* 1839.

Medicines.

HULSE (I.) * De medicamentorum operationibus. 8°. *Nova-Aurelia*, 1845.

KENENS (H.) * Diss. sistens cogitationes varias circa modum agendi medicamentorum in genere. sm. 4°. *Argentorati*, 1763.

A KHITTEL (C.) * Doctrinæ de viribus medicaminum fata. 8°. *Halæ Magdeb.*, [1792].

KNOLL (J. C. G.) * De medicamentis traumaticis eorumque usu legitimo. sm. 4°. *Halæ Magdeb.*, [1746].

DE KOCK (Y.) jun. * De potioribus vires medicamentorum indagandi subsidiis rationalibus, deque vindicando vero analogiæ botanicæ in hac re usu. 4°. *Traj. ad Rhenum*, [1806].

KORNACHER (J. C.) * De modo agendi medicamentorum in corpore vivo animali. 4°. *Altorfii*, [1798].

KOTTMANN (A.) Die Arzneimittel. 8°. *Basel*, 1884.

KRANICHFELD (F. G. G.) & HILDEBRAND (C. A.) Dissertatio medica de dignitate medicaminibus nonnullis restituenda. 4°. *Berolini*, 1827.

KÜHNE (F. O. E.) * De causis salutarem medicamentorum effectum impedientibus. 4°. *Halæ Magdeb.*, [1763].

LANGEWAGEN (N.) * De medicamentorum operationibus in genere. 4°. *Lugd. Bat.*, 1691.

LANGUTH (J. H. G.) * De inexspectato medicamentorum effectu. sm. 4°. *Halæ Magdeb.*, [1739].

LAVATER (J.) * De æquivalentibus quæ surrogata vulgo dicuntur. 4°. *Gottingæ*, [1811].

LAVERAN & MILLON. Mémoire sur le passage de quelques médicaments dans l'économie animale et sur les modifications qu'ils y subissent. 8°. [*n. p., n. d.*]
Repr. from: Rev. scient. et industr., Par.
Also [Abstr.], *in:* Compt. rend. Acad. d. sc., Par., 1844, xix, 347–350.

LEHMANN (J. G.) * De minus generosis generosorum medicamentorum effectibus. sm. 4°. *Vitembergæ*, [1745].

LHÉRITIER (S.-D.) * Considérations sur quelques-unes des causes qui peuvent faire varier l'action des médicamens. 4°. *Paris*, 1834.

LINEKOGEL (S. F.) * De medicamentorum efficientia generatim determinanda. 4°. *Gottingæ*, [1736].

LYSTHENIUS (G. P. A.) * Principia ad modum operandi medicamentorum intelligendum. 4°. *Halæ Magdeb.*, [1756].

LYSTHENIUS (J. A.) * De medicamentorum modo operandi in corpore vivo specimen tertium. 4°. *Halæ Magdeb.*, [1720].

MARCELLUS ["*Empiricus*"]. De medicamentis.
In: MEDICI antiqui omnes qui latinis [etc.] 4°. *Venetiis*, 1547, 83–141.

——. The same.
In: MEDICI artis principes. fol. [*Francofurti*], 1567, ii, pt. 3, 239–414.

MAURY (C.) * De l'action des médicamens sur l'économie animale. 8°. *Paris, an XI* [1803].

MAYER (J.) * De novorum medicamentorum receptione. 8°. *Monachii*, 1834.

MEISNER (C. B.) * De ignobili nobilium quorundam medicaminum indole atque virtute. sm. 4°. *Francof. ad Viadr.*, [1748].

MELICHIO (G.) Avertimenti nelle composizioni de' medicamenti per uso della spetiaria. Con una diligente esaminazione di molti simplici tratta da più degni auttori. Aggiuntovi un trattato delle mirabili virtù della theriaca, dell' Oratio Guarguanti. sm. 4°. *Venetia*, 1605.

MERINDOLUS (A.) An sint aliquæ medicamentorum facultates occultæ.
In his: Ars medica. fol. *Aquis-Sextiis*, 1633, 405–411.

Medicines.

MOEHRLEN (J.-P.) * Comparaison des médicaments et de leurs principes actifs. 4°. *Strasbourg*, 1863.

MÜLLER (G. W.) * De mechanica operandi ratione medicamentorum sic dictorum alterantium. 4°. *Halæ*, [1698].

MYLIUS (A. C.) * De medicamentis selectioribus. 4°. *Halæ Magdeb.*, 1713.

NELIGAN (J. M.) Medicines, their uses and mode of administration ; including a complete conspectus of the British pharmacopœias, [etc.] 5. ed. 8°. *Dublin*, 1858.

——. The same. With notes and additions conforming it to the Pharmacopœia of the United States, by D. M. Reese. 8°. *New York*, 1844.

——. The same. 3. ed. 8°. *New York*, 1851.

NEUHOF (T. B.) * De virium medicamentorum maxime probabili partitione. 4°. *Lipsiæ*, 1797.

NIMPTSCH (U. S.) * De differenti medicamentorum operatione secundum diversam corporis humani idiosyncrasiam. Von der verschiedenen Würckung derer Artzeneyen nach der verschiedenen Beschaffenheit des menschlichen Cörpers. 4°. *Halæ Magdeb.*, [1731].

O'REILLY (J.) What is the modus operandi of medicines ? Do they produce their effects by their action on the blood as taught by all modern physiologists, or do they produce their effects by their action on the organic nervous system through the agency of the blood ? The latter question considered and affirmatively answered. 8°. *New York*, 1863.

OTT (I.) The action of medicines. 8°. *Philadelphia*, 1878.

PERCIVAL (T.) A physical inquiry into the powers and operation of medicines. 8°. *Manchester*, 1786.

QUELLMALTZ (C. S.) * De medicamentorum delectu. sm. 4°. *Lipsiæ*, [1694].

QUISTORP (J. B.) * Scrutinium operationis medicamentorum evacuantium, nominatim vomitoriorum, purgantium, enematum, suppositoriorum, diaphoreticorum, diureticorum, errhinorum, apophlegmatisantium, salivantium, emmenagogorum, vesicatoriorum, aphrodisiacorum. sm. 4°. *Rostochii*, [1713].

RICHTER (J. G.) De medicamentorum modo operandi in corpore vivo. 4°. *Halæ*, [1719].

RIDIGER (A.) * De veritate virtutis medicamentorum.
In: HALLER. Disp. ad morb. [etc.] 4°. *Lausannæ*, 1760, vii, 79–110.

ROBINSON (B.) Observations on the virtues and operations of medicines. 12°. *Dublin*, 1752.

ROUSSEL (J.-N.) * Considérations sur la nécessité de connaître exactement la nature des médicamens que l'on emploie. 4°. *Paris*, 1832.

DE ROY (H.) * De differentia actionis medicamentorum medicæ et physicæ. 4°. *Halæ Magdeb.*, [1754].

SAUVAGEON (G.) Traicté chymique contenant les préparations, usages, facultez et doses des plus célèbres et usitez médicamens chymiques. 18°. *Rouen*, 1644.

DE SAUVAGES (F. B.) * De medicamentis, quæ certas quasdam partes corporis humani præ aliis afficiunt, atque de causa hujus effectus. [Ex gallico in latinum sermonem translata.] 4°. *Lipsiæ*, [1755].

SAVATIER (C.) * Essai sur les moyens de déterminer le mode d'action des médicamens. 4°. *Paris*, 1824.

4

Medicines.

SCHACHT (C. P.) * De modo quo agant medicamenta adstringentia præcipue martialia in corpus animale. 4°. *Hardervici*, [1789].

SCHAEFFER (J. G.) * De causis cur alimenta et medicamenta alium sæpe effectum edant in hominibus sanis quam in ægrotis. sm. 4°. *Altorfii Noricorum*, [1745].

SCHALTENBRAND (J. F.) * Cogitationes nonnullæ circa efficaciam medicamentorum physicam, vitalem et medicam, cum propositionibus quibusdam chemicis. 4°. *Erlangæ*, 1784.

SCHECHNER (J.) * De efficientia medicaminum in corpore humano ægrotante. 8°. *Passaviæ*, 1829.

SCHOEPFF (J. D.) * De medicamentorum mutatione in corpore humano præcipue a fluidis. 4°. *Erlangæ*, [1776].

SEYLER (D. G.) * De præstantia medicamentorum simplicium et Galenicorum præ chymicis. sm. 4°. *Erfordiæ*, [1713].

SOUQUES (A.-L.) * Propositions sur l'action et les effets des médicamens. 4°. *Paris*, 1821.

STROHL (E.) * De l'action sympathique des médicaments. 4°. *Strasbourg*, 1838.

STRUVE (C. G. F.) * De medicamentorum effectuum similitudine et æqualitate. 4°. *Jenæ*, [1752].

THIERSCH (K.) * Zur Lehre von der Arznei-Wirkung. 8°. *München*, 1846.

THOMAS (C.) * Diss. medicamenta lapidosa ἐν σκιαγραφία sistens. 4°. *Erfordiæ*, [1721].

VAN TOULON (G. W.) * De principii oxygenetici, sive elementi acidifici, eximia et amplissima in corpus humanum efficacitate. 4°. *Trajecti ad Rhenum*, [1801].

TRILLER (D. W.) & KLUNGE (J. J.) * De remediorum sic dictorum specificorum dubia fide et ambiguo effectu.
In: HALLER. Disp. ad morb. [etc.] 4°. *Lausannæ*, 1760, vii, 111–126.

TRINKS (C. F. G.) * De primariis quibusdam in medicamentorum viribus recte estimandis dijudicandisque impedimentis ac difficultatibus. 4°. *Lipsiæ*, [1823].

TUCHSCHERER (A.) * De medicamentorum modo operandi in corpore vivo. 4°. *Halæ Magdeb.*, [1720].

VALENTINI (M. B.) * Continuatio declamationum panegyricarum quarum i. de medicamento optimo, ii. de medicamentorum noxa et officioso medicorum homicidio, iii, de incrementis, etc. . . . habebantur. 4°. *Francof. a. M.*, 1711.

VAN DYKE (R.) Introductory lecture . . . Philadelphia College of Medicine. 8°. *Philadelphia*, 1848.

VEIELIUS (S.) * De medicamentorum proprietatibus. 4°. *Lipsiæ*, [1692].

VENEL (G. F.) * De medicamentis compositis prælectiones. 4°. *Monspelii*, 1761.

WÅHLIN (A.) * Odores medicamentorum.
In: LINNÆUS. Amœnitates acad. [etc.] 8°. *Lugd. Bat.*, 1756, iii, 183–201.

WALMSLEY (T.) * An essay on glandular appetency, or the absorption of medicines. 8°. *Philadelphia*, 1803.

WEDELIUS (G. W.) De medicamentorum facultatibus cognoscendis et applicandis libri duo. 2. ed. 4°. *Jenæ*, 1696.

WENDLER (C.) * De præsentissimarum medicamentis virium. sm. 4°. *Vitembergæ*, [1744].

WILLE (J. H.) * De modo agendi medicamentorum in genere. 4°. *Jenæ*, [1744].

WILLIS (T.) Pharmaceutice rationalis sive diatriba de medicamentorum operationibus in hu-

Medicines.

mano corpore. Pt. I. 24°. *Hagæ-Comitis*, 1674.

——. The same. [2 pts. in 1 v.] 4°. [*Oxoniæ*], 1674–5.

——. The same. 4°. *Lugduni*, 1681.

——. The same. 4°. *Genevæ*, 1694.

——. The same. Pharmaceutice rationalis; or, an exercitation of the operations of medicines in humane bodies, shewing the signs, causes, and cures of most distempers incident thereunto, in two parts. As also a treatise of the scurvy, and the several sorts thereof, with their symptoms, causes, and cure. fol. *London*, 1679.

WÜRTZ (G. C.) * De affinitatibus virtutum medicatarum. 4°. *Argentorati*, [1777].

YEMA, Sinkei. Yakubutsu Koyo Ron. [On the action of medicines.] 5 v. 12°. *Tokio*, 1883. Japanese text.

ZENIUS (L.) * Aphorismorum de viribus medicaminum prolegomena. sm. 4°. *Upsaliæ*, [1793].

Abraham (J.) Short notes on drugs and pharmaceutical preparations of recent introduction. Liverpool M. & S. Rep., 1871, v, 115–119.—**Anglada** (C.) Des rapports de la chimie avec l'action des médicaments. J. Soc. de méd.-prat. de Montpel., 1842, v, 421–444.—**Bambaren** (C.) Penetracion de los medicamentos en el organismo. Gac. méd., Lima, 1875, i, 197; 205; 213; 221; 229; 253; 261; 269.—**Barnes** (J.) Remarks on certain objects of the materia medica, in reply to a paper on the same subject, by Professor Coxe. Am. M. Recorder, Phila., 1822, v, 100–108.—**Barrett** (R. F.) Notes of lectures on the modus operandi of medicines, with letter from the author. Missouri M. & S. J., St. Louis, 1845, i, 33; 56.—**Beck** (J. B.) On the modus operandi of medicines. Am. J. M. Sc., Phila., 1844, n. s., vii, 27–43.—**Blake** (J.) On the action of medicines St. Louis M. & S. J., 1847–8, v, 209; 313.—**Bordier** (A.) De l'élimination des médicaments. Bull. gén. de thérap., etc., Par., 1873, lxxxiv, 49–60.—**Bouvier.** Quelques mots de réponse à un point du travail de M. Haelewyck intitulé: De l'action locale des médicaments. Arch. belges de méd. mil. Brux., 1862, xxx, 73–78.—**Brunton** (T. L.) & **Cash** (J. T.) Why do medicines sometimes fail to act? St. Barth. Hosp. Rep., Lond., 1884, xx, 213–224.—**Cáldwell** (C.) Thoughts on the modus operandi of medicines. Transylv. J. M., Lexington, Ky., 1835, viii, 169–206.—**Chapman** (N.) On the modus operandi of medicines. Phila. J. M. & Phys. Sc., 1821, ii, 295–313.—**Cogswell** (C.) On the endosmotic action of medicines. Lond. J. M., 1852, iv, 205–214.—**Coletti** (F.) Diversità di azione de' farmachi e de' veleni negli animali bruti e nell' uomo. Gazz. med. ital., prov. venete, Padova, 1874, xvii, 11. — **Comendador** (A. S.) Relacion que existe entre las virtudes medicinales de los materiales farmacéuticos procedentes de los reinos animal y vegetal y su organizacion. Restaurador farm., Barcel., 1877, xxxiii, 97–113.—**Corrochano y Casanova** (M. M.) ¿Qué es medicamento? Discurso leido en el paraninfo de la Universidad central el dia 18 de octubre de 1874, en el acto solemne de recibir la investidura de doctor en la Facultad de medicina y cirugía. Pabellon méd., Madrid, 1874, xiv, 500; 547; 559.—**Cumming** (C. F. G.) Strange medicines. Nineteenth Cent., Lond., 1887, xxi, 901–918.—**Davis** (N. S.) What are medicines; what the distinctions between food and medicines; their classification for therapeutic purposes; ætiology. Med. Exam., Chicago, 1875, xvi, 117–126.—**Day** (J.) An attempt to explain the curative action of certain remedies in general use. Austral. Pract., Sydney, 1877–8, i, 223–229.—**Debionne** (J.) De l'histoire du médicament. Gaz. méd. de Picardie, Amiens, 1884, ii (suppl.), 1–8.—**Demarquay.** Recherches sur l'absorption des médicaments faites sur l'homme sain. Union méd., Par., 1867, 3. s, i, 19; 35; 54. *Also, transl.*: South. J. M. Sc., N. Orl., 1867, ii, 225–242.—**Drake** (D.) Observations on the modus operandi and effects of medicines. West. M. & Phys. J., Cincin., 1827–8, i, 249–362.—**Eve** (J. A.) Essay on the modus operandi of medicines. South. M. & S. J., Augusta, 1836–7, i, 449–457.—**Falck** (F. A.) Ueber den Einfluss des Alters auf die Wirkung der Arzneimittel. Arch. f. d. ges. Physiol., Bonn, 1884, xxxiv, 525–529.—**Fonssagrives.** Médicament. (Bibliographie.) Dict. encycl. d. sc. méd., Par., 1873, 2. s., vi, 240–316.—**G.** (N.) Sur quelques propriétés physiologiques et thérapeutiques du butyl-chloral; sur le Gelseminum sempervirens; sur la présence de la dextrine dans l'urine, et sur une indication à apporter au procédé de dosage de la glucose, par la liqueur de Fehling. Union méd., Par., 1876, 3. s., xxi, 977–981.—**Gaston** (J. M'F.) The unknown factor in the equation of the nervous system; the action of medicine on the cure of diseases. Med. & Surg. Reporter, Phila., 1884, l, 359; 385; 417.—**Green** (W. S.) Modus operandi of medicines. West. & South. M. Recorder, Lexington, Ky., 1841–2, i, 259–264, 1 pl.—**Haelewyck.** Idées générales sur l'action locale des

Medicines.

agents thérapeutiques. Arch. belges de méd. mil., Brux., 1862, xxix, 273; 292; 401; 433.—**Hahnemann** (S.) Versuch über ein neues Prinzip zur Auffindung der Heilkräfte der Arzneisubstanzen, nebst einigen Blicken auf die bisherigen. J. d. pract. Arznk. u. Wundarznk., Jena, 1796, ii, 3. St., 391; 4. St., 465.—**Hauff.** Etwas über die Wirkung und Gabe der Arzneistoffe. Med. Cor.-Bl. d. württemb. ärztl. Ver., Stuttg., 1834, iii, 195-198.—**Hecker** (J. F. C.) Allgemeine Lehrsätze über die inneren Wirkungen der Arzneimittel. J. d. Chir. u. Augenh., Berl., 1823, v, 373-390.—**Henschel** (A. W.) Kritische Bemerkungen über die neueren Theorien die Kraft der Arzneimittel betreffend. Mag. f. d. ges. Heilk., Berl., 1828, xxvii, 340-374.—**Hill** (W. N.) Medical economics from the standpoint of the general practitioner. Maryland M. J., Balt., 1884-5, xii, 154-156.—**Hirtz.** Médicament; médication. N. dict. de méd. et chir. prat., Par., 1876, xxii, 10-33.—**Inman** (T.) The duration of the influence of medicines, etc. Liverpool & Manchester M. & S. Rep., 1875, iii, 190-198.—**Johnstone** (J.) A lecture on the accumulative action of medicines, with some remarks on slow poison. Prov. M. & S. J., Lond., 1847, 561-565.—**Jones** (H. B.) Appendix to a course of lectures on the relationship of chemical and mechanical diseases, being a sketch of the action of medicines. Med. Times & Gaz., Lond., 1866, ii, 245; 333.—**Keidel** (G.) On the action of medicine. Balt. J. M., 1861, i, 233-262.—**Laycock** (T.) On observing and judging as to the effects of remedies. Med. Times & Gaz., Lond., 1863, i, 365-368.—**Maddox** (C. C.) A thesis on the action of remedies. Atlanta M. & S. J., 1880-81, xviii, 1-6.—**Nelson** (D.) On the action of medicines singly or combined. Assoc. M. J., Lond., 1863, i, 617-619.—**Nolde** (A. F.) Erinnerung an einige zur kritischen Würdigung der Arzneymittel sehr nothwendige Bedingungen. J. d. pract. Arznk. u. Wundarznk., Jena, 1799, viii, 1. St., 47; 2. St., 75.—**von Nussbaum** (J. N.) Ueber Hausmittel. Deutsche Rev., Bresl. u. Berl., 1886, xi, 174-194.—**Percival** (T.) A physical inquiry into the powers and operation of medicines. Lond. M. J., 1790. xi, 287-308. Also, in his: Works, literary, moral, and medical, 8°, Lond., 1807, iv, 301-320.—**Plugge** (P. C.) Samenstelling en werking van geneesmiddelen. Nederl. Tijdschr. v. Geneesk., Amst., 1884, 2. R., xx, 769-778.—**Pool** (W. H.) Modus operandi of medicines. [Thesis.] Savannah J. M., 1860-61 iii, 77-88.—**Powell** (R. H.) An inquiry into the modus operandi of therapeutic agents upon the human frame. Lond. J. M., 1852, iv, 543; 626.—**Quincke** (H.) Ueber die Ausscheidung von Arzneistoffen durch die Darmschleimhaut. Arch. f. Anat., Physiol. u. wissensch. Med., Leipz., 1868, 150-164.—**Quincy** (J.) The operation of medicines. Phil. Tr., Lond., 1719-33, vii, 586-591.—**Richardson** (B. W.) On the physiological action of the organic hydrides. Med. Times & Gaz., Lond., 1871, ii, 371-375.—**Richter** (A. G.) Läst sich aus der chemischen Zerlegung der Arzneymittel ein sicherer Schluss auf ihre Arzneykräfte machen? In his: Med. u. chir. Bemerk., etc., Berl., 1813, ii, 160-178.—**Rodgers** (M. M.) The modus operandi of medicines. Boston M. & S. J., 1854-5, li, 209-215.—**Sales-Girons.** De l'action des médicaments dans l'organisme vivant. Rev. méd. franç. et étrang., Par., 1860, ii, 5; 68; 129.—**Savary** (A.-C.) Considérations sur l'action des médicamens. J. de méd., chir., pharm., etc., Par., 1811, xxii, 35-46.—**de Savignac** (D.) Des caractères physiques et organoleptiques des médicaments dans leurs rapports avec l'action thérapeutique. Bull. gén. de thérap., etc., Par., 1860, lviii, 337-352.—**Schubarth** (E. L.) Beiträge zur näheren Kenntniss der Wirkungsart der Arzneimittel und Gifte. Arch. f. med. Erfahr., Berl., 1824, i, 53-92.—**Seitz** (F.) Ueber das Verhältniss der Aequivalentzahlen der Arzneikörper zu ihrer Wirkung. Deutsche Klinik, Berl. 1861, xiii, 427; 439; 457; 479.—**Semmola** (M.) Della eliminazione dei farmachi. Riforma med., Napoli, 1886, ii, 574; 580.—**Sgarzi** (G.) Intorno all' azione dei medicamenti. Mem. Soc. med.-chir. di Bologna, 1857, 2. s., v, 169-227.—**Shaw** (W. H.) On the connection of other departments of science with medicine, embracing an investigation of their influence on the existing doctrines in regard to the modus operandi of medicine. Phila. J. M. & Phys. Sc., 1826, xiii, 273-289.—**Spalding** (V. M.) The active properties of plants considered as a feature of relationship. Therap. Gaz., Detroit, 1880, n. s., i, 316-318.—**Spender** (J. K.) Notes on the action of medicines, old and new. Brit. M. J., Lond., 1872, i, 635: 1873, ii, 373: 1875, ii, 99: 1878, i, 285.—**Van Bastalaer** (D. A.) Faut-il étendre l'emploi médical des principes immédiats chimiquement définis et en multiplier les préparations dans les pharmacopées? Cong. périod. internat. d. sc. méd. Compt. rend. 1875, Brux., 1876, iv, 755-765. [Discussion], 777-786. Also, Reprint.—**Watson** (Sir W.) The virtues of drugs. Ibid., 1869, i, 44.—**Zarlenga** (R.) Sulla azione dei rimedii o sulla jamatologia. Filiatre-sebezio, Napoli, 1842, xxiv, 275-281.

Medicines (Action of).

See **Endosmosis**, etc.; **Medicines**; **Medicines** (Physiological action, etc., of); **Therapeutics.**

Medicines (Administration and doses of).

See, also, **Dosimetric** medicine; **Endermic** method; **Formulæ**; **Homœopathy**; **Hypodermic** injections, etc.; **Iatraleptic** method; **Nurses**, etc.; **Therapeutics.**

ALCHINDUS. In suum de medicinarum compositarum gradibus investigandis libellum, præfatio.

In: DOSIBUS (De) seu de justa quantitate [etc.] 12°. Venetiis, 1579, 102-123. Also, in: OPUSC. illust. med. de dosibus. 16°. Lugduni, 1584, 232-283.

ALVARENGA (F. P. da Costa). Apontamentos sobre os pontos d'applicação ou vias d'absorpção dos medicamentos. 8°. Lisboa, 1882.

BAUDOT (E.) *Voies d'introduction des médicaments; applications thérapeutiques. 8°. Paris, 1866.

BERLIOZ (F.) Nagljadnija tablitsi pharmaklicheskago dieistvija niekotorich lekarstvennich vetshestve. Perevod s Frantsuzskago. [Tables indicating the effect of doses. Transl. from the French.] 8°. St. Petersburg, 1882.

CHEVREUL (E.) Considérations sur l'histoire de la partie de la médecine qui concerne la prescription des remèdes, à propos d'une communication faite à l'Académie des sciences, dans sa séance du 29 d'août 1864, par M. Claude Bernard, sur les propriétés organoleptiques de six principes immédiats de l'opium, précédées d'un examen des Archidoxia de Paracelse et du livre de Phytognomonica de J. B. Porta. 4°. Paris, 1865.

CHRESTIEN (A.-T.) *Déterminer l'action des médicaments administrés à haute dose, et les cas dans lesquels ils doivent être préférés. 4°. Montpellier, 1848.

CONAN. Thérapeutique générale. Faut-il ne donner qu'un seul médicament à la fois ou faut-il en donner plusieurs? etc. 12°. Paris, 1886.

CORTI (M.) Ad tyrunculos dosandi methodus.

In: ILLUSTRIUM in re medica [etc.] 12°. Patavii, 1556, 1-18ᵇ. Also, in: DOSIBUS (De) seu de justa quantitate [etc.] 12°. Venetiis, 1579, 1-22.

DOSIBUS (De) seu de justa quantitate, et proportione medicamentorum; opuscula illustrium medicorum [etc.] 12°. Venetiis, 1579.

EULENBURG (A.) Epidermic, endermic, and hypodermic administration of medicines. Transl. by Matthew Hay.

In: HANDB. of gen. therap. [von Ziemssen]. 8°. London, 1885, ii, 367-488.

EXTON (J. A.) The superiority of small and frequent doses in the treatment of disease. 8°. [Arlington, N. J., n. d.]

Read before the Hudson County Medical Society.

FAVENTINUS (B. V.) Compendium breve de dosibus medicinarum.

In: ILLUST. in re med. virorum. 12°. Patavii, 1556, 21-26.

GAUBIUS (H. D.) Libellus de methodo concinnandi formulas medicamentorum. 12°. Lugd. Bat., 1739.

———. The same. 2. ed. 8°. Lugd. Bat., 1752.

———. The same. 3. ed. 8°. Lugd. Bat., 1767.

With which are bound 28 leaves of MS. notes and formulæ.

GEBAUER (J. C.) *De dosibus refractis medicamentorum. 4°. Erlangæ, [1765].

GENTILIS DE FULGINEO. De proportionibus medicinarum. [Fol. 1 begins:] Gracia lucidioris habitus quem Mesue denotat in modis et propositionibus medicinarum [etc.] [Fol. 10 ends:] Explicit tractatus Gentilis de Fulgineo de proportionibus medicinarum et de modo investigandi complexiones earum, et ad sciendum con-

Medicines (*Administration and doses of*).
venientem dosim cuilibet medicinæ, etc. 4°.
[*n. p., n. d.*]
Also, in: DOSIBUS (De) seu de justa quantitate [etc.]
12°. *Venetiis,* 1579. 61–78. *Also, in:* OPUSC. illust. med.
de dosibus. 16°. *Lugduni,* 1584, 138–178.
GERRISH (F. H.) Prescription writing. Designed for the use of medical students who have
never studied Latin. 16°. *Portland, Me.,* 1878.
——. The same. 3. ed. With an appendix
on the metric system in prescriptions. 12°.
Portland, Me., 1880.
GORRÆUS (P.) Formulæ remediorum quibus
vulgo medici utuntur.
In: DOSIBUS (De) seu de justa quantitate [etc.] 12°.
Venetiis, 1579, 189–231.
GRIFFITHS (W. H.) Posological tables; being
a classification of the doses of all officinal substances. 1 sheet fol. *Dublin,* [1873?]
——. Lessons on prescriptions and the art
of prescribing. 12°. *London,* 1875.
——. The same. New ed. 18°. *London,* 1880.
GRUNER (C. G.) Via et ratio formulas medicas conscribendi. 8°. *Halæ,* 1778.
HENRY (A.) Posological and therapeutic
tables, containing the doses, actions, and uses
of the medicines in the British Pharmacopœia,
with poisons. 18°. *Edinburgh,* 1875.
HERSTELLE (D. A.) *De medicamentorum
vehiculis. 4°. *Helmstadii,* [1701].
HORČIČKA (G.) *Diss. sistens artem formulas
medicas concinnandi. 8°. *Pragæ,* 1842.
ILLUSTRIUM in re medica vivorum [opuscula,
id est:] Matthæi Curtii ad tyrunculos dosandi
methodus. Bartholomæi Montagnanæ conclusiones de compositione et dosi medicamentorum.
Benedicti Victorii Faventini breve compendium
de dosibus medicinarum. Gulielmi Rondoleti
de materia medicinali et compositione medicamentorum brevis methodus. 12°. *Patavii,* 1556.
INCE (J.) The Latin grammar of pharmacy.
For the use of medical and pharmaceutical students; with an essay on the reading of Latin
prescriptions. 8°. *London,* 1882.
LANGENBECK (M.) Die Impfung der Arzneikörper. 8°. *Hannover,* 1856.
LEMAIRE (F.-J.) *Est-il utile d'associer les
médicaments? 4°. *Paris,* 1843.
——. The same. 8°. *Paris,* 1843.
LEONARD (C. H.) The multum in parvo reference and dose book. 3. ed. 12°. *Detroit,* 1879.
LUND (A.) Valg af de bekjendteste virksomme Lægemidler til lettere Priser. 8°. *Kjøbenharn,* 1813.
MARTINI (N.) *De prudenti virium medicamenti exploratione. 4°. *Halæ,* 1703.
MEADOWS (A.) The prescriber's companion.
32°. *London,* 1864.
——. The same. 3. ed. 24°. *London,* 1874.
——. The same. 5. ed. With the addition
of new remedies up to the present date, including those of the British Pharmacopœia of 1885.
24°. *London,* 1886.
MERCKELL (J. M.) *Exercit. med. sistens
ideam præscribendarum formularum. 4°. *Lipsiæ,* 1682.
MERRICK (C. H.) The decimal system in writing prescriptions. 18°. *Portland, Oreg.,* [*n. d.*]
MIRUS (S. G.) *De forma medicaminum pro
curandis morbis apte et utiliter exhibenda. sm.
4°. *Lipsiæ,* 1749.
MONTAGNANA (B.) Conclusiones de compositione, et dosi medicamentorum, etiam omnium
fere simplicium.
In: ILLUSTRIUM in re medica [etc.] 12°. *Patavii,* 1556,
27.
——. Tabula dosium communium tam simplicium quam compositorum extantium in usu.
In: ILLUSTRIUM in re medica [etc.] 12°. *Patavii,* 1556, 30.

Medicines (*Administration and doses of*).
——. Tractatus de modo componendi medicinas, et de dosi earum.
In: DOSIBUS (De) seu de justa quantitate [etc.] 12°.
Venetiis, 1579, 23–60. *Also, in:* OPUSC. illust. med. de dosibus. 16°. *Lugduni,* 1584, 50–137.
MORELLUS (P.) Methodus præscribendi formulas remediorum, cum adjuncto materiæ medicæ, systemate. Aucta. variisque modis illustrata,
nunc pro secunda editione recensita a Gerardo
Blasio. 18°. *Amstelodami,* 1665.
——. The same. 24°. *Amsterodami,* 1680.
MÜLLER (F. W.) Der Arzneischatz des praktischen Arztes. Charakteristik, Dosirung, Anwendungsweise und Anwendungsfall aller wichtigen Arzneimittel, unter Berücksichtigung der
einschlägigen Indicationen und Methoden. 8°.
Stuttgart, 1877.
NICOLAI (E. A.) Methodus concinnandi formulas medicamentorum exemplis ad medici
quondam illustris Friderici Hoffmanni mentem
accommodatis illustrata. 16°. *Halæ Magdeb.,*
1747.
OLDBERG (O.) The metric system in medicine, containing an account of the metric system of weights and measures, Americanized and
simplified; a comprehensive dose table, and
three hundred practical illustrations of metric
prescription writing, selected from recipes in actual use in hospital and out-door practice. 8°.
Philadelphia, 1881.
OPWIJRDA (R. J.) Algemeene en bijzondere
recepteerkunst. (Ars formulas medicas præscribendi et præparandi.) Ten dienste van artsen en apothekers, naar onderscheidene bronnen
en in verband met het grammengewicht. 12°.
Amsterdam, 1871.
PALMER (B. W.) Favorite prescriptions of
distinguished practitioners, with notes on treatment. 2. ed. 12°. *New York & London,* 1884.
——. A practical treatise on palatable prescribing, containing the favorite formulary of
the most eminent medical and surgical authorities, collated from their published writings and
private records, and embracing a résumé of the
most eligible prescriptions for the administration of recent additions to the materia medica.
2. ed. 12°. *Detroit,* 1885.
PARENTUS (P. A.) De dosibus medicamentorum liber singularis in ordinem alphabeti digestus... Editio altera, cum præfatione H. D.
Gaubii. 8°. *Lugd. Bat.,* 1751.
PARIS (J. A.) Pharmacologia; comprehending the art of prescribing upon fixed and scientific principles; together with the history of
medicinal substances. 5. ed. 2 v. 8°. *London,*
1822.
——. The same. Pharmacologia; or the
history of medicinal substances, with a view to
establish the art of prescribing [etc.] From
the last Lond. ed., with a general English index.
8°. *New York,* 1822.
——. The same. Pharmacologia; comprehending the art of prescribing upon fixed and
scientific principles, [etc.] 2. Am. from the 5.
[enlarged] Lond. ed., with additions and illustrations of the materia medica of the United
States, by Ansel W. Ives. 2 v. 8°. *New York,*
1823–4.
——. The same. 3. Am. from the 6. Lond.
ed. 8°. *New York,* 1825.
——. The same. 3. Am. from the 6. Lond.
ed., embracing a history of the most important
medicinal substances of the United States, by
Ansel W. Ives. 2 v. 8°. *New York,* 1825.
——. The same. Pharmacologia; being an
extended inquiry into the operations of medicinal bodies, upon which are founded the theory

Medicines (*Administration and doses of*).

and art of prescribing. From the 9. Lond. ed., rewritten in order to incorporate the latest discoveries in physiology, chemistry, and materia medica, with notes by Charles A. Lee. 8°. *New York*, 1846.

——. Appendix to the eighth edition of the Pharmacologia; with some remarks on various criticisms upon the London Pharmacopœia of 1836. 8°. *London*, 1838.

PAULLINI (C. F.) Simplex medicina (aliquando) optima.

In his: Obs. med.-phys. 12°. *Lipsiæ*, 1706, 229–241.

PELLETAN DE KINKELIN (J.) * Essai sur les différentes voies d'introduction des médicamens dans l'économie animale. 4°. *Paris*, 1831.

PHOEBUS (P.) Zur Vereinfachung der Arznei-Verordnungen. 8°. *Giessen*, 1856.

PICHLER (J. F. C.) Methodus formulas medicas conscribendi in usum prælectionum academicarum. 12°. *Argentorati*, 1785.

PLOHN (L.) * De arte formulas concinnandi. 8°. *Pesthini*, 1833.

RECEPTEERKUNDE voor genees- en heelkundigen, naar het tegenwoordige standpunt der schei- en geneeskunde, en hoofdzakelijk met inachtneming van eenvoudigheid en goedkoopte der voorschriften, kritisch bewerkt door een hoogleeraar en prakt. geneesheer. Naar het Hoogduitsch. sm. 4°. *Amersfoort*, 1846.

RONDELETIUS (G.) De materia medicinali et compositione medicamentorum luculentus et brevis methodus.

In: ILLUSTRIUM in re medica [etc.] 12°. *Patavii*, 1556, 40–102.

——. De ponderibus, sive de justa quantitate, et proportione medicamentorum.

In: DOSIBUS (De) seu de justa quantitate [etc.] 12°. *Venetiis*, 1579, 124–188.

RUDBERG (J.) * Diss. sistens saporem medicamentorum. sm. 4°. *Holmiæ*, [1751].

Also, in: LINNÆUS. Amœnitates acad. [etc.] 2. ed. 8°. *Lugd. Bat.*, 1764, ii, 335–355.

RUIZ (P. A.) Tarifa farmacéutica arreglada al sistema métrico decimal. 8°. *Madrid*, 1872.

RULANDUS (M.) Appendix de dosibus, seu justa quantitate ac proportione medicamentorum compositorum omnium, quæ hodie officinis parata extant. 18°. *Argentorati*, 1567.

SAUCEROTTE (A.-A.-F.) * Considérations pratiques sur la posologie. 4°. *Paris*, 1852.

SCHAEBEL (F.) Vejledning i Recept-Læsning. Med. tillhørende Glossarium. Udarbejdet till Brug for Farmacevter og Apotéks-Disciple. 8°. *Kjøbenhavn*, 1884.

SCHAUER (J.) * De vehiculis medicamentorum adpropriatis. 4°. *Erfordiæ*, 1721.

SCHEFFEL (C. S.) [Pr.] de methodo quorundam medicorum tentativa disserit. 4°. *Gryphiswaldiæ*, [1747].

SCHÖMAN (X.) Lehrbuch der Receptirkunst für Aerzte, als Leitfaden zu academischen Vorlesungen und zum Selbststudium. 8°. *Jena*, 1854.

STEWART (M.), jr. Pocket therapeutics and dose book, with classification and explanation of the action of medicines, [etc.] 18°. *Detroit, Mich.*, 1878.

——. The same. 2. ed. 24°. *Detroit*, 1878.

STRUMPF (F. L.) Die Normalgaben der Arzneien nach dem Unzen- und Grammengewicht, zugleich als Repetitorium der Arzneimittellehre. 8°. *Leipzig u. Heidelberg*, 1862.

THOMAS DE GARBO. Tractatus de reductione medicinarum ad actum.

In: DOSIBUS (De) seu de justa quantitate [etc.] 12°. *Venetiis*, 1579, 78–90.

——. Tractatus de gradibus medicinarum.

In: DOSIBUS (De) seu de justa quantitate [etc.] 12°. *Venetiis*, 1579, 91–101.

Medicines (*Administration and doses of*).

TROUSSEAU & REVEIL. The prescriber's complete handbook, comprising the principles of the art of prescribing. A materia medica . . . and a concise sketch of toxicology. Edited, with notes, by J. Birkbeck Nevins. 8°. *London*, 1852.

VARA (F.) * De variis viis ad excipienda medicamenta. 8°. *Monachii*, 1835.

VICTORIUS (B.) *Faventinus.* De dosibus medicinarum.

In: ILLUSTRIUM in re medica. 12°. *Patavii*, 1556, 21.

Also, in: DOSIBUS (De) seu de justa quantitate [etc.] 12°. *Venetiis*, 1579, 18–22.

WYTHE (J. H.) The physician's dose and symptom book, containing the doses and uses of all the principal articles of the materia medica and official preparations, arranged in alphabetical order. Also, table of weights and measures, rules to proportion the doses of medicine, common abbreviations used in writing prescriptions, alphabetical list of materia medica, preparations and modes of administration, list of incompatibles, hints on prescription-writing, table of poisons and antidotes, hints on treatment, table of symptoms. 17. ed. 18°. *Philadelphia*, 1887.

ZABITSANOS (G. N.) Συνταγολογία ἤτοι περὶ τῆς κατ' ἐπιστήμην ἀναγραφῆς καὶ ἐκτελέσεως τῶν συνταγῶν. 8°. *Ἀθήνῃσι*, 1879.

[**Accion** terapéutica especial de algunos medicamentos administrados á dósis elevadas.] Siglo méd., Madrid, 1873, xx, 204; 236; 251; 269; 283; 299; 313; 331; 365; 382; 746; 763; 777; 794; 810.—**Act** (An) to require physicians and others to write the names of medicines in the English language on their recipes; introduced before the Pennsylvania legislature. Med. & Surg. Reporter, Phila., 1-81, xliv, 250.—**Acton** (W.) On best means of disguising the taste of nauseous medicines. Pharm. J. & Tr., Lond., 1846, v, 502-505. *Also*, Reprint.—**Allen** (R. N.) A table for the regulation of doses. Maryland M. Recorder, Balt., 1829, i, 399.—**Austee** (F. E.) On the doses of remedies recommended in the pharmacopœia. Practitioner, Lond., 1873, xi, 259-262.—**Armstrong** (J. A.) Medical latin. Med. Rec., N. Y., 1882, xxii, 566-568; 1883, xxiii, 138. [*See, also, infra*, Rice (C.)]—**Audhoui** (V.) Quelques observations sur l'art de formuler. Thérap. contemp., Par., 1881, i, 561-563.—**Before** or after meals? [Taking medicine] Med. News, Phila., 1883, xliii, 11.—**Black** (J. R.) The comparative value of large and small doses, and long and short intervals, in the administration of medicines. *Ibid.*, 1882, xli, 142-144.—**Bonsieur** (J. P.) The simplification of the present method of prescribing. Clinic, Cincin., 1872, iii, 122.—**Bouilhon.** Moyen pratique de préserver du goût des substances amères. Bull. gén. de thérap., etc., Par., 1870, lxxix, 80-82.—**Bree** (C. R.) On the doses of active medicines. Med. Times & Gaz , Lond., 1866, i, 264. ——. The doses of medicines. *Ibid.*, 379.—**Bruen** (E. T.) Therapeutic dosage in connection with the use of certain medicines as alteratives. Phila. M. Times, 1881-2, xii, 745-749. *Also*: Proc. Phila. Co. M. Soc. 1881-2, Phila., 1882, iv, 196-201.—**Burton** (H.) On the use of different forms of the same medicine in equivalent doses. Lond. M. Gaz., 1841-2, n. s., xxix, 40-44.—**Ceresoli** (F.) Nuovo e più opportuno veicolo per l' applicazione esterna di talune sostanze medicamentose. Gazz. med. ital., prov. venete, Padova, 1879, xxii, 199.—**Chapman** (W. B.) On the uncertainty of the composition of pharmaceutical preparations, and the most eligible form of medicines for administration. Tr. Ohio M. Soc., Dayton, 1853, viii, app., 44-48.—**Chirac** (P.) Doses des remèdes, tant simples que composés. *In:* Chirac & Silva. Diss. et consult. méd., 12°, Par., 1755, iii, 317-322.—**Clarke** (E. H.) A new rule for doses. Boston M. & S. J., 1872-3, lxxxvii, 209. ——. The continued and the frequent dose. *Ibid.*, 1875, xciii, 147 - 152. — **Cockburn** (W.) A problem of finding the true doses of vomiting and purging medicines. Phil. Tr. 1700-20, Lond., 1731, v, 394-404.—**Compton** (J. W.) Solution and absorption of medicines; or, the best means of securing the good effects of medicines in the cure of disease. Am. M. Bi-Weekly, Louisville, 1877, vi, 197 - 203. *Also*, Reprint. — **Cook** (S. A.) Latin prescriptions. Boston M. & S. J., 1846, xxxiv, 48-52.—**Cornaz** (E.) Quelques mots sur les maxima des médicaments très actifs. Écho méd., Neuchât., 1859, iii, 15-22. *Also*, Reprint. — **Coudereau.** Note sur l'intensité d'action des médicaments, proportionnelle à l'augmentation ou à la diminution de poids de l'animal, à propos d'expériences sur l'action physiologique du menthe-chloral. Compt. rend. Soc. de biol. 1874, Par., 1875, 6. s., i, 407 - 410. — **Créquy.** Sur la nécessité d'employer des compte-gouttes identiques. Bull. gén. de thérap., etc.,

Medicines (*Administration and doses of*).

Par., 1877, xcii, 360-362.—**Crummer** (B. F.) Some general considerations in drug prescribing. Tr. Illinois M. Soc., Chicago, 1884, xxxiv, 253-258.—**Culbertson** (H.) Medicinal doses and therapeutic effects. Detroit Lancet, 1880-81, iv, 56-60. *Also*, Reprint.—**Dale** (W.) On the taste of medicines. Lancet, Lond., 1869, ii, 530.—**Dalton** (R. H.) Practical remarks on the doses of medicines. Pacific M. & S. J., San Fran., 1877-8, xx, 347-352.— **D'Ans.** Les doses maxima, pour une prise et pour les vingt-quatre heures, des médicaments énergiques. Arch. belges de méd. mil., Brux., 1862, xxix, 135-138.—**Davis** (J. L.) Palatable prescriptions. Cincin. Lancet & Clinic, 1884, xii, 550-554. ———. Small doses frequently repeated. *Ibid.*, 636-639.—**Dessau** (S. H.) The value of small and frequently repeated doses. Med. Rec., N. Y., 1877, xii, 465-469.—**Deutsch** (W.) Die neue Receptur. Allg. Wien. med. Ztg., 1875, xx, 129.—**Duchesne.** Note sur les médicaments explosibles. Bull. Soc. méd.-prat. de Par. (1884-5), 1886, n. s., i, 242-249.—**Fabre** (A.) Étude sur les effets opposés des agents médicinaux suivant leurs doses et leurs divers modes d'administration. Gaz. hebd. de méd., Par., 1856, iii, 885; 1857, iv, 3; 59.—**Farquharson** (R.) On defects in the domestic measurement of doses. Brit. M. J., Lond., 1876, i, 255. ———. On official dosage, with some remarks on homœopathic tinctures. Practitioner, Lond., 1876, xvi, 369-380. *Also:* Proc. M. Soc. Lond., 1875, iii, 47-52.—**Farre.** Pereira's materia medica; the doses of medicines. Med. Times & Gaz., Lond., 1866. i, 319.—**Fernandez** (A. M.) La influencia del tamaño de las dósis en su accion terapéutica. Repert. méd., N. Y., 1883, i, 70; 97.—**de Fleury** (A.) Des quantités médicatrices en thérapeutique. Gaz. hebd. d. sc. méd. de Bordeaux, 1884, iv, 156; 170; 180.—**Fordyce** (G.) Some observations upon the combination of medicines. Tr. Soc. Improve. M. & Chir. Knowl., Loud., 1800, ii, 314-343.—**Forget.** Quelques réflexions sur l'abus des médicaments, ou polypharmacie; rappel à la simplicité des formules. Bull. gén. de thérap., etc., Par., 1842, xxiii, 241-251.—**Fouquier.** Considérations générales sur le mode d'administration des médicaments; et observations sur l'usage interne de l'acétate de plomb. Bull. Fac. de méd. de Par., 1820-21, vii, 207-238.—**Franklin** (G. S.) What is the nature and office of a medical prescription, and to whom does it belong? Tr. Ohio M. Soc., Columbus, 1880, xxxv, 103-108.—**Frédault.** Les aggravations produites par les médicaments sont-elles la raison des doses infinitésimales? Les doses massives. Rev. de thérap. méd.-chir., Par., 1872, xxxix, 170-181.—**French** (M. S.) An unobjectionable form for the administration of medicines. Med. & Surg. Reporter, Phila., 1884, l, 388-390.—**Fuller** (H. W.) On drugs; their action and their doses. Brit. M. J., Lond., 1868, i, 191-193.—**Gassot** (A.) Les doses. Concours méd., Par., 1883, v, 232; 254.—**Gottschalk** (A.) Die zusammenziehenden Arzneimischungen. Ztschr. f. d. ges. Med., Hamb., 1843, xxiii, 137: 1844, xxv, 160.—**Grasset** (J.) L'art de prescrire. Montpel. méd., 1882, xlix, 197; 316.—**Grayson** (W. H.) The importance of liquefaction in the successful administration of medicines. St. Louis Eclect. M. J., 1879, vi, 309-315.—**Griffiths** (W. H.) Lessons on prescription and the art of prescribing. Med. Press & Circ., Lond., 1874, n. s., xvii, 154; 276; 426; 465; 1874, n. s., xviii, 265; 341; 375.—**Guichard.** Essai sur la posologie des médicaments composés. J. de chim. méd., etc., Par., 1873, xlvii, 220-224.—**Guilliermond** (A.) De l'emploi des granules pour l'administration de l'acide arsénieux et des toxiques en général. Gaz. méd. de Lyon, 1850, ii, 235.— **Hale** (J.) On prescriptions. Am. Pract., Louisville, 1871, iv, 257-262.—**Hecker.** Von der Schwierigkeit, die Dosen einiger wirksamen Arzneymittel genau zu bestimmen. J. d. pract. Arznk. u. Wundarzuk., Jena, 1800, ix, 2. St., 59-86.—**Hemenway** (H. B.) Influence of dose on the action of remedies. Med. Rec., N. Y., 1882, xxii, 623.— **Höglauer.** Kurze Bemerkungen über die Anwendung progressiv erhöhter Arzneidosen in mehreren chronischen Krankheiten. Med. Cor.-Bl. bayer. Aerzte, Erlang., 1841, ii, 689-704.—**Hoppe** (J.) Die Begründung der Dosenlehre und der Lehre von der Wiederholung der Arzneien auf das Verhalten der thierischen Thätigkeiten. Memorabilien, Heilbr., 1860, v, 109; 129.—**Howison** (W.) On various circumstances important to be attended to in prescribing medicines. Lancet, Lond., 1831-2, i, 909-914.—**Hudson** (J.) Medicines; their modes of administration, etc. Physician & Surg. Ann Arbor, Mich., 1879, i, 152-159.—**Hughes** (C. H.) Note on the value of adequate doses repeated at judiciously lengthened intervals, especially in nervous affections. N. Eng. M. Month., Sandy Hook, Conn., 1883-4, iii, 254-256.—**Jacquez.** Mémoire en réponse à la question: Quels sont les meilleurs procédés à suivre dans l'administration des médicaments qui répugnent au goût des malades? Ann. Soc. de méd. de Gand, 1849, xxiii, 101-144.—**Jeannel** (J.) & **Moncel** (L.) Formules magistrales pour l'administration des corps gras et du copahu. J. de méd. de B rdeaux, 1858, 2. s., iii, 37-39. — [**Joy** (W. B.)] Preliminary remarks on the art of prescribing; with extemporaneous formulæ. Syst. Pract. M. (Tweedie), Phila., 1841, v, 388-477.—**Keene** (J. W.) Cacoëpy in medicine. Buffalo M. & S. J., 1879-80, xix, 277-

Medicines (*Administration and doses of*).

285.—**Kennedy** (H.) A few general remarks on the modes of administering medicines. Dublin M. Press, 1861, xlv, 137-139.—**Kinglake.** Maximum doses of medicine. Med. & Phys. J., Lond., 1822, xlvii, 89-94.—**Lagneau** (G.) fils. Recherches sur le moyen de faire parvenir des médicaments dans l'intestin grêle, en les préservant de l'action du suc pancréatique. Gaz. hebd. de méd., Par., 1857, iv, 558.—**Lauret.** De l'introduction des substances médicamenteuses dans le corps humain par l'influence de l'électricité. Gaz. hebd. d. sc. méd. de Montpel., 1884, vi, 73-76.—**Leffmann** (H.) Criticisms, from a chemical point of view, on some favorite prescriptions. Tr. Coll. Phys. Phila., 1884, 3. s., vii, 157-162. *Also:* Boston M. & S. J., 1884, cx, 411. *Also:* N. Orl. M. & S. J., 1883-4, n. s., xi, 920-924. *Also:* N. York M. J., 1884, xxxix, 536. *Also:* Maryland M. J., Balt., 1884-5, xi, 4. *Also* [Abstr.]: Polyclinic, Phila., 1883-4, i, 161.—**Logan** (W. M.) A new method of prescribing and administering medicines. Clinic, Cincin., 1878, xiv, 74.—**Luxer.** Du danger de doser certaines substances végétales, d'après la quantité de principe actif qu'elles renferment. Exposé d. trav. de la Soc. d. sc. méd. de la Moselle, Metz, 1853, 165-168.— **Markbreiter** (P.) Zur Vermittlung der Extreme in der Dosenlehre. Wien. Med.-Halle, 1860, i, 37; 60; 98.— **Martin** (F. H.) Palatable therapeutics. Therap. Gaz., Detroit, 1886, 3. s., ii, 11-14.—**Maurin** (S. E.) Cuadro general de posología, segun el doctor S. E. Maurin. Encicl. méd.-farm., Barcel., 1882, vi, 598; 615; 629; 647; 662; 676; 693; 708; 724; 739; 756; 771.—**Mays** (T. J.) On the elective action and small doses of medicines, with illustrative cases. N. York M. J., 1879, xxix, 251-267.—**Milligan** (E.) On the doses of the ancient physicians. Edinb. M. & S. J., 1820, xvi, 186-198.—**Morris** (J.) Effects of medicine in small doses. Med. & Surg. Reporter, Phila., 1878, xxxix, 199-204.—**Netwald** (J.) Ueber die Anwendung neuer Heilmittel im allgemeinen und insbesondere chemischer. Verhandl. d. k. k. Gesellsch. d. Aerzte zu Wien, 1843, ii, 161-177.—**O'Reilly** (J.) On the art of prescribing; an introductory address. Am. Pract., Louisville, 1872, v, 209-214. *Also*, Reprint.—**Overton** (J.) Of the modus agendi of remedial and noxious agents upon the living body; and of its diffrent surfaces suitable for their application and necessary for the exercise of their respective properties. South. J. M. & Phys. Sc., Knoxville, 1857, vi, 79-97.—**Parrish** (E.) Thoughts on prescribing. Med. & Surg. Reporter, Phila., 1863, x, 112; 145.—**Pleischl** (A.) Mittel, den unangenehmen, bittern und scharfen Geschmack einiger Salze, und zwar: des Bittersalzes, des Duplicatsalzes, des Glaubersalzes, des Salmiaks und des Salpeters, zu verhüllen. Oesterr. med. Wchnschr., Wien, 1848, 65-71.—**Pooley** (J. H.) The art of prescribing. Cincin. Lancet & Clinic, 1886, xvii, 5-10.— **Potain.** Du choix du médicament et de son dosage. Tribune méd., Par., 1880, xii, 5; 15: 77.—**Professional** ollapodrida. Atlanta M. & S. J., 1858-9, 709: 1859-60, v, 1.—**Quincke** (H.) Ueber Dosirung und Anfertigung flüssiger Arzneien. Deutsche med. Wchnschr., Berl., 1881, vi, 121.—**R.** Einige Bemerkungen über das Receptschreiben. Allg. med. Ann., Altenb., 1807, 275-282.—**Ramsey** (F. A.) Thoughts upon prescribing. South. M. Rec., Atlanta, 1874, iv, 190-205.—**Restelli & Strambio** (G.) Expériences sur l'action comparative de certains médicaments administrés par l'estomac et par le rectum. Gaz. méd. de Par., 1847, 3. s., ii, 128.—**Réveil.** Posologie des liquides médicamenteux à propos du compte-goutte Salleron. Bull. gén. de thérap., etc., Par., 1863, lxiv, 262-271.—**Rice** (C.) Medical Latin: a rejoinder [to J. A. Armstrong's article]. Med. Rec., N. Y., 1882, xxii, 637.— **Rosenthal.** Presse zur Compression voluminöser Arzneimittel. Sitzungsb. d. phys.-med. Soc. zu Erlang., 1873-4, vi, 147-154.—**Sandras.** De l'influence de la dose sur la médication. Expérience, Par., 1838, ii, 167-170.— **Schmidt** (W.) Vorschläge zur Verminderung der Arzneikosten. J. d. pract. Heilk., Berl., 1837, lxxxiv, 5. St., 24-48.—**Schmidtmann.** Einige Bemerkungen über das Verfassen der Arznei-Formeln. *Ibid.*, 1827, lxv, 3. St., 50-62.—**Schmitt** (E.) De la posologie des toxiques. J. d. sc. méd. de Lille, 1882, iv, 508-513.—**Schwalbe.** Ueber den Werth des Alkohols und der Jodtinctur für subcutane und parenchymatöse Injectionen. Tagebl. d. Versamml. deutsch. Naturf. u. Aerzte, Salzb., 1881, liv, pt. 2, 158.—**Sheardown** (T. W.) Physicians' prescriptions analyzed. Northwest. Lancet, St. Paul, 1884-5, iv, 217-223.—**Simon** (J.) Essai sur le dosage des médicaments chez les enfants. Mouvement méd., Par., 1876, xiv, 211; 228.—**Smith** (A. A.) A lecture on the frequent repetition of doses. N. York M. J., 1883, xxxvii, 145-148.—**Smith** (W. H.) Doses of certain preparations that are not given in Stewart's dose-book. Physician & Surg., Ann Arbor, Mich., 1882, iv, 4-18.—**Snijders** (C. J.) Heroïca. [Heroic doses.] Nederl. Tijdschr. v. Gen esk., Amst., 1883, xix, 453-466.—**Spender** (J. K.) The administration of medicines in comparatively small and frequent doses. Brit. & For. M.-Chir. Rev., Lond., 1872, xlix, 209-236.—**Squibb** (E. R.) The proper method of writing prescriptions. Bull. N. York Acad. M., 1860-62, i, 116-124.—**Stillwell** (W. C.) Overdosing and giving disagreeable medicines

Medicines (*Administration and doses of*).
unnecessarily. Phila. M. Times, 1880-81, xi, 524.—**Sturges** (O.) On the sanctions with which drugs are administered. Lancet, Lond., 1872, i, 711-714.—**Vandenburg** (M. W.) Small and frequent doses. N. York M. J., 1883, xxxvii, 277.—**Vée.** De la nécessité de mieux assurer, à Paris, l'authenticité des prescriptions médicales. Union méd., Par., 1849, iii, 573.—**Walker** (R.) A table of the proportionate doses of medicine, from one grain to one ounce, etc., for every different age. Med. & Phys. J., Lond., 1816, xxxvi, 104-108. — **Wall** (O A.) On the administration of medicines. St. Louis Cour. Med., 1882, viii, 297-307.—**Wardrop.** On the benefits that may be derived from placing medicinal substances upon the tongue instead of into the stomach. Lancet, Lond., 1852, i, 80.—**Warner** (F.) The frequent repetition of doses. Lancet & Clinic, 1884, n. s., xii, 505.—**Wickersham** (S.) The selection of remedies and the art of prescribing them. Chicago M. Exam., 1863, iv, 139-149.—**Woodworth** (J. M.) Eligible pharmaceutical forms for the administration of medicines; an inaugural thesis. *Ibid.*, 1862, iii, 145-152.

Medicines (*Adulterations and inspection of*).
See, also, **Apothecaries**; **Drugs** (*Adulteration of*); **Pharmacy** (*Legislation in relation to*).

Aschoff (E. F.) Anvisning till läkemedlens pröfning, jemte en praktisk handledning vid anställandet af apotheks-visitationer; för läkare och apothekare. 8°. *Norrköping*, 1831.

Ebermayer (C.) Manuel des pharmaciens et des droguistes, ou traité des caractères distinctifs, des altérations et sophistications des médicamens simples et composés, traduit en français sur la dernière édition de l'ouvrage allemand de . . . et approprié à la nouvelle pharmacopée française par J.-B. Kapeler et J.-B. Caventou. 2 v. 8°. *Paris*, 1821.

Ernst (F.) Die Visitation der Apotheken, oder Anleitung zur gründlichen Untersuchung sämmtlicher bis jetzt bekannter Arzneimittel auf ihre Aechtheit, Güte und Verfälschung. 8°. *Ulm*, 1840.

Gay (F.) *Altérations dites spontanées des médicaments chimiques. Causes et phénomènes. Moyens de conservation. 4°. *Paris*, 1884.

Henkel (J. B.) Die Merkmale der Aechtheit und Güte der Arzneistoffe des Pflanzen- und Thierreichs, nebst Anleitung zur Prüfung derselben auf ihren Gehalt an wirksamen Bestandtheilen. Zugleich ein Leitfaden bei Apothekenvisitationen. 8°. *Tübingen*, 1864.

Herbelin (M.-A.) Dosage de l'azote appliqué à l'essai de quelques substances et préparations pharmaceutiques. 8°. [*Nantes*, 1867-76?]

Pekarik (A.) *Examen medicamentorum. 4°. *Budæ*, [1834].

Roloff (J. C. H.) Anleitung zur Prüfung der Arzneykörper bey Apothekenvisitationen für Physiker, Aerzte und Apotheker. 2. Aufl. 4°. *Magdeburg*, 1817.

Von den Sande (J.-B.) La falsification des médicaments dévoillée ; ouvrage dans lequel on enseigne les moyens de découvrir les tromperies mises en usages pour falsifier les médicaments tant simples que composés et où on établit des règles pour s'assurer de leur bonté. 8°. *La Haye*, 1784.

—— & Hahnemann (S.) Die Kennzeichen der Güte und Verfälschung der Arzneimittel. 8°. *Dresden*, 1787.

Spalteholz (J. T.) * De medicamentis præparatis adulteratis. 4°. *Vitebergæ*, [1803].

Wittstein (G. C.) Anleitung zur Darstellung und Prüfung chemischer und pharmaceutischer Präparate . . . Mit einer Vorrede von J. A. Buchner, sen. 2. Aufl. 8°. *München*, 1851.

Wolff (E.) & Hirsch (B.) Die Prüfung der Arzneimittel, nebst Anleitung zur Revision der öffentlichen und Privat-Apotheken, Dispen-

Medicines (*Adulterations and inspection of*).
sir- und Mineralwasser-Anstalten, Droguerie- und Materialwaaren-Handlungen. 8°. *Berlin*, 1866.

Zapp (E.) Anweisung zur Prüfung und Aufbewahrung der Arzneimittel. 8°. *Köln*, 1863.

Binz (C.) Ueber Pilze in arzneilichen Flüssigkeiten. Wien. med. Presse, 1880, xxi, 865 ; 897.—**Black** (H.) Adulterated medicines. Virginia Clin. Rec., Richmond, 1873-4, iii, 481-497.—**Gaughey** (J. B.) Adulterations and impurities of medicines. Northwest. M. & S. J., St. Paul, Minn., 1871-2, ii, 322-328.—**Hiller** (A.) Ueber Arzenei-Pilze. Ztschr. f. klin. Med., Berl., 1881, iii, 221-227.—**Lepage** (P.-H.) Essai sur les caractères physiques, organoleptiques et chimiques que doivent présenter les principales préparations pharmaceutiques officinales ainsi que les médicaments chimiques le plus fréquemment employés. Dép. de l'Eure. Rap. du Cons. centr. d'hyg., etc., Évreux (1864), 1865, 55-158.—**Medical Society** of the State of New York. Report of special committee to devise some means of controlling the use of adulterated and inefficient medicines. Tr. M. Soc. N. Y., Albany, 1861, 201-207.—**Medicines**, their impurities and adulterations. Spiritus ammonia aromaticus. Lancet, Lond., 1863, ii, 661-664.—**Ménière** (C.) Des insectes rongeurs qu'on rencontre dans les racines, les feuilles, les fleurs, les fruits, etc. Répert. de pharm., Par., 1874, n. s, ii, 9 ; 39.—**Murray** (J.) On the adulterations and substitutions of medicines. Dublin M. Press, 1852, xxvii. 177.—**Pemberton** (J. S.) Adulterated medicine. Atlanta M. & S. J., 1877-8, xv, 71-74.—**Rosenthal** (M.) Zur Bildung pflanzlicher Organismen in Arzneien. Wien. med. Presse, 1880, xxi, 932-934.—**Schaarschmidt** (G.) Némely gyógyitó-anyagban és vegyi szerben tenyészö penészekröl. [On the fungi germinating in some remedies and chemical preparations.] Orvosi hetil., Budapest. 1885, xxix, 397-399.—**Schmidt** (J.) Pharmacological change in its relation to therapeutic action. Therap. Gaz., Detroit, 1885, 3. s., i, 369-371.—**Squibb** (E. R.) Simple tests for some important medicinal preparations. N. York J. M., 1858, 3. s., v, 15-21.— **Willard** (A.) Adulterated medicines in the country. *Ibid.*, 1852, [2.], n. s., viii, 361-365.

Medicines (*Antagonism of*).
See, also, **Pharmacy.**

Amiard (F.-T.) Étude sur l'antagonisme de diverses substances toxiques et médicamenteuses. 4°. *Paris*, 1872.

Faliu (M.) * De l'antagonisme entre les médicaments. 4°. *Paris*, 1860.

Valenti (S.) L' antagonismo dei farmaci. 8°. *Catania*, 1886.

Bartholow (R.) On the antagonism between medicines and between remedies and diseases. Being the Cartwright lectures for the year 1880. N. York M. J., 1881, xxxiii, 32 ; 197. *Also*, Reprint. *Also* [Abstr.]: Med. Rec., N. Y., 1880, xviii, 561 ; 589 ; 617 ; 645 ; 673 : 1881, xix, 1. *Also* [Abstr.]: Boston M. & S. J., 1880, ciii, 499 ; 525 ; 533 ; 557 ; 581 ; 629.—**Bennett** (J. H.) Report of the committee of the British Medical Association to investigate the antagonism of medicines. Brit. M. J., Lond., 1874, ii, 436 ; 464, 485 ; 518 ; 547 ; 581 ; 615 ; 674 ; 697 ; 771 ; 805 : 1875, i, 97. *Also*, Reprint.—**Brunton** (T. L.) Veränderte Wirkung zweier Arzneimittel, wenn sie gleichzeitig in den Organismus eingeführt werden. Centralbl. f. d. med. Wissensch., Berl., 1873, xi, 689. — **Chirone.** Antagonismi farmacologici. Gazz. d. osp., Milano, 1883, iv, 153 ; 161 ; 209 ; 217 ; 241 ; 257 ; 281 ; 353 ; 369.—**Fraser** (T. R.) Lectures on the antagonism between the actions of active substances. Brit. M. J., Lond., 1872, ii, 457 ; 485.—**Gubler** (A.) & **Labbée** (E.) De l'antidotisme, ou de l'antagonisme thérapeutique. Bull. gén de thérap., etc., Par., 1873, lxxxiv, 510 ; 556.—**Husemann** (T.) Antagonistische und antidotarische Studien. Arch. f. exper. Path. u. Pharmakol., Leipz., 1876-7, vi, 335 : 1878, ix, 414 : 1878-9, x, 101.—**Leblanc** (F.) De l'antagonisme thérapeutique dans les formules complexes. J. de thérap., Par., 1880, vii, 50-56. *Also, transl.*: Gazz. med. di Roma, 1880, vi, 60-62. *Also, transl.*: Gazz. med. ital., prov. venete, Padova, 1880, xxiii, 85-87.—**Prevost** (J.-L.) Antagonisme physiologique. Cong. périod. internat. d. sc. med. Compt.-rend. 1877, Genève, 1878, v, 716-743. *Also*: Arch. de physiol. norm. et path., Par., 1877, 2. s., iv, 801-839.—**Ringer** (S.) On the antagonism between veratria and potassium salts. Practitioner, Lond., 1883, xxx, 17-19.—**Ringer** (S.) & **Buxton** (D.) An examination of the supposed action exerted by the antagonism between acids and alkalies in modifying the tonicity of the heart and arteries. Lancet, Lond., 1885, i. 6 —**Smith** (W. G.) The antagonism of drugs. Dublin J. M. Sc., 1884, 3. s., lxxvii, 33-39.—**Vertrees** (W. M.) The antagonism of medicine. South. Pract., Nashville, 1885, vii, 397 ; 445 ; 493.

Medicines (*Classification and nomenclature of*).

See, *also*, **Materia** *medica*; **Medicines** (*Prices, etc., of*).

ACLAND (H. W.) Standard medicines, or revision of remedial agents; a paper read at the Social Science Association. 8°. *London*, 1862.

BAUDRIMONT (A.-É.) *Sur la classification des médicamens. 4°. *Paris*, 1831.

BECKER (C. A.) *De medicamentorum acrium vegetabilium classificatione. 8°. *Berolini*, [1819].

BÉRAL (P.-J.) Nomenclature et classification pharmaceutiques, accompagnées d'une nouvelle méthode de formuler, et d'un grand nombre de formules rédigées d'après cette méthode; avec des tableaux représentant d'autres nomenclatures et classifications pharmaceutiques. 4°. *Paris*, 1830.

BOSTOCK (J.) Remarks on the reform of the pharmaceutical nomenclature; and particularly on that adopted by the Edinburgh College. 8°. *Liverpool*, 1807.

CHÉREAU (A.) Nouvelle nomenclature pharmaceutique, avec tableaux, synonymie ancienne et nouvelle et vocabulaire abrégé. 8°. *Paris*, 1825.

FLEMING (A.) On the classification of medicines according to their action on the healthy body. 8°. *Dublin*, 1852.

FOY (F.) *Propositions pharmacologiques et thérapeutiques, suivies d'une nouvelle classification des médicamens. 4°. *Paris*, 1830.

HUFELAND (A.) Addresse à tous les médecins sur la nécessité de conserver le nom officinal des médicamens. 12°. *Berlin*, 1821.

Also, in: N. Jour. de méd., chir., pharm., etc., Par., 1821, xii, 97–109.

KING and Queen's College of Physicians in Ireland. Catalogue of the museum. 8°. *Dublin*, 1864.

KÜSTER (J. E.) *Introductio in akologiam systematicam et rationalem. 8°. *Halæ*, 1795.

LERSCH (B. B.) Beiträge zur Arzneiverordnungslehre und chemischen Nomenklatur. 8°. *Aachen*, 1851.

PIETSCH (J. G.) *Schema novum systematis circa divisionem medicamentorum. 4°. *Helmstadii*, [1747].

PITET (J.-P.-M.-F.) *Histoire de la classification des médicaments. 4°. *Paris*, 1851.

RUDOLPHY (J.) Pharmaceutical directory of all the crude drugs now in general use; their etymology and names in alphabetical order. In 4 pts. 2. ed. 8°. *New York*, 1872.

SCHREGER (C. H. T.) [Pr.] novam medicamentorum divisionem præmittit. sm. 4°. *Vitebergæ*, [1811].

SERAUS (F.) Petitorium seu index medicamentorum simplicium et compositorum, quæ quilibet hujus urbis, regnique pharmacopola in officina sua servare et in regia annuali visitatione exhibere tenetur. Regio jussu correctum, et editum ab almo hujus urbis chemiatrorum collegio. 4°. *Neapoli*, 1780.

TRAGUS (H.) Dissertationes fere quinquaginta, de herbarum quarundam nomenclaturis. *In:* VERA (De) herbarum. fol. *Argentorati*, 1532, 156–165.

WÜRTZ (G. C.) Conamen mappæ generalis medicamentorum simplicium secundum affinitates virium naturalium nova methodo geographica dispositorum. 4°. *Argentorati*, 1778.

Bärwald. Ueber Béral's pharmazeutische Nomenclatur und Classification. J. d. Chir. u. Augenh., Berl., 1837, xxvi, 111–124.—**Bartholow** (R.) The claim of Dr. Z. Collins McElroy to priority in the invention of a certain classification of remedial agents. Clinic, Cincin., 1877, xiii, 40.—**Berlin** (N. J.) Något om läkemedlens benäm-

Medicines (*Classification and nomenclature of*).

ning. [On nomenclature of remedies.] Hygiea, Stockholm, 1841, iii, 550–554.—**Classification** of the materia medica; a review. Dublin Q. J. M. Sc., 1850, ix, 452–464. *Also*, Reprint.—**Elliott** (J. B.) Classification of the materia medica. N. Orl. M. & S. J., 1878-9, n. s., vi, 423–431.—**Falck** (C. P.) Versuch einer Classification der Arzneimittel in den allgemeinsten Umrissen dargestellt. Ztschr. f. rat. Med., Heidelb., 1847, vi, 204–232.—**Fleming** (A.) On the classification of medicines according to their action on the healthy body. Dublin Q. J. M. Sc., 1852, xiv, 278–309.—**Foy** (F.) Un mot sur une classification nouvelle des médicaments. Bull. gén. de thérap., etc., Par., 1842, xxii, 241–246.—**Holt** (T.) Remarks on the nomenclature and constitution of certain pharmaceutical substances. Lond. M. Gaz., 1842, xxx, 886–890. — **Lichtenstädt.** Ueber alte, neue und neueste Nomenclatur der Arzneien. J. d. pract. Heilk., Berl., 1829, lxix (Supplhft.), 3–47.—**Lyall** (R.) Copy of a letter on pharmaceutical nomenclature. Edinb. M. & S. J., 1816, xii, 417–422.—**Matthäi** (K. C.) Einige Ideen über Arzeneimittel und ihre Klassifikazion. Mag. z. Vervollk. d. Heilk., Frankf. a. M., 1800, iv, 63–114. — **Miergues** (A.) Nécessité d'une réforme dans la classification des médicaments. Rev. de thérap. du midi, Montpel., 1854, vii, 206–212.—**Payne** (J. F.) On the classification of medicines, and especially of general remedies. St. Thomas's Hosp. Rep. 1877, Lond., 1878, n. s., viii, 363–384.—**Review** of Dr. Tully's synopsis or classification. Boston M. & S. J., 1865, lxxii, 189; 211; 231; 252.—**Sée** (G.) Définition et classification physiologiques des médicaments. Bull. gén. de thérap., etc., Par., 1878, xcv, 337–343.—**Sprenger** (A.) Arabic terms of materia medica. Tr. M. & Phys. Soc. Calcutta, 1844-5, ix, pt. 1, 52–130. — **Thomson** (W. H.) Classification of medicines, according to the time required for their operation. Bull. N. York Acad. M. (1870–71), 1872, iv, 219–233. *Also:* Med. Rec., N. Y., 1870-71. v, 531–534.

Medicines (*Dispensing of*) *by physicians.*

See **Pharmacy** (*Legislation in relation to*); **Physicians** (*Relations of*) *to pharmacists.*

Medicines (*Doses of*).

See **Medicines** (*Administration, etc., of*).

Medicines (*Effects of*) *on the fœtus.*

See **Fœtus** (*Effects of medicines on*).

Medicines (*Endermic application of*).

See **Endermic** *method.*

Medicines (*Nomenclature of*).

See **Medicine** (*Dictionaries, etc., of*); **Medicines** (*Classification, etc., of*); **Pharmacy.**

Medicines (*Patent, proprietary, quack, and secret*).

See, *also*, **Abortion** (*Criminal, etc.*); **Formulæ**; **James's** *powder*; **Litholysis**, *etc.*; **Medicine** (*Popular*); **Medicines** (*Specific*); **Toxicology** (*Cases, etc., of*); **Venereal** *diseases* (*Popular treatises on*); **Warburg's** *tincture.*

ACADÉMIE de médecine, Paris. Extrait d'un rapport [sur l'examen des remèdes secrets], présenté à S. Exc. Mgr. le ministre secrétaire d'état de l'intérieur. 4°. [*Paris*, 1823.]

ACCOUNT (An) of remarkable cures, performed by the use of Maredant's antiscorbutic drops prepared by John Norton. 12°. *London*, 1774.

ANTHONIE (F.) The apologie, or defence of a verity heretofore published concerning a medicine called aurum potabile, that is, the pure substance of gold, prepared and made potable and medicinable without corrosives, helpefully given for the health of man in most diseases, but especially availeable for the strengthning and comforting of the heart and vitall spirits, the performers of health; as an universall medicine. Together with the plaine and true reasons, manifold and irrefragable testimonies of fact, confirming the universalitie thereof. And lastly, the manner and order of administration or use of this medicine in sundrie infirmities. sm. 4°. *London*, 1616.

D'ARAUJO (A. J.) Agua d'Inglaterra preparada no laboratorio pharmaceutico. 16°. *Porto*, 1856.

Medicines (*Patent, proprietary, quack, and secret*).

BARRETT (C. B.) Directions for the use of Dr. C. B. Barrett's guardian in connection with his medico-electro-galvanometer, for the treatment and removal of certain diseases incidental to woman. 12°. *New York*, 1848.

DE BAVAY (P.-J.) Petit recueil d'observations en médecine sur les vertus de la confection tonique résolutive et diurétique pour toutes les fièvres intermittentes, l'asthme, la toux, l'enroüement, la phthisie au premier degré, la jaunisse et toutes les obstructions, la concrétion et l'inflammation absente. 8°. *Bruxelles*, 1753.

BENOIST. Mémoire pour servir d'avis concernant les propriétés et usages de plusieurs spécifiques. 12°. [*n. p., n. d.*]

BETA (H.) Die Geheimmittel- und Unsittlichkeits-Industrie in der Tagespresse. 8°. *Berlin*, 1872.

BRUINSMA (V.) Onze strijd tegen den geheimmiddelhandel in Nederland. I. De industrie van de firma F. A. Richter & Co. te Nijmegen. 8°. *Leeuwarden*, [*n. d.*]
Repr. from: De Farmaceut.

———. Onze strijd tegen den geheimmiddelhandel in Nederland. II. Wat men deed, wat men doet, en wat men moest doen tegen deze kwakzalverij. 8°. *Leeuwarden*, [*n. d.*]
Repr. from: De Farmaceut.

———. Onze strijd tegen den geheimmiddelhandel in Nederland. III. Nieuwe bijdragen tot de kennis der kwaal. 8°. *Leeuwarden*, [*n. d*]
Repr. from: De Farmaceut.

CASTELLUS (J. P. C.) De diatartari julapii temperamento, qualitatibus, usu et dosi enarratio. 8°. [*n. p., n. d.*]

CLARIN (C. F.) * De laudationibus nimiis medicamentorum arcanorum venalium: was von denen Artzeneyen zu halten, welche als Arcana, mit vielen Lobes-Erhebungen öffentlich feil gebohten werden. sm. 4°. *Rostochii*, [1731].

CLUTTON (J.) A true and candid relation of the good and bad effects of Joshua Ward's pill and drop. Exhibited in sixty-eight cases, [etc.] 12°. *London*, 1736.

COLLECÇÃO de decretos, avisos, e outras ordens regias a favor da verdadeira, e unica agoa de Inglaterra, da composição do doutor Jacob de Castro Sarmento, preparada por José Joaquim de Castro na sua real fabrica em Lisboa. fol. *Lisboa*, 1814.

DAVY's lac-elephantis; or, medicated milk of elephants. An effectual cure for debility, seminal weakness, gleets, impotency, spasmodic stricture, and the venereal disease, in both sexes; with a plain prescription, whereby all persons, afflicted by impure connexion, can radically cure themselves the first day. [Under the caveat of government.] 5. ed. 8°. *London*, 1815.

DOUSSIN-DUBREUIL (J.-L.) De l'emploi du remède contre les glaires, et observations sur ses effets. 8°. *Paris*, [*n. d.*]

DREWRY (G. O.) Consumption and wasting diseases successfully treated by "hydrated oil", with cases showing the immediate increase in weight produced by it. 4. ed. 16°. *London*, [1877].

EDLEBER (J. S.) * De panacæa salutari, sive remedeo panchresto. 4°. *Wirceburgi*, [1735].

EPPERSON (J. P.) A bomb in the camp of the enemy, or an exposure of quackery and "patent medicines". 8°. *Columbia*, 1845.

ETTMÜLLER (M.) De singularibus. 4°. *Lipsiæ*, 1663.

GENERAL treatise on the nature and cause of disease in the human body, together with proofs of the efficacy of Vaughn's vegetable lithontriptic mixture, as a general restorer of the system, and purifier of the blood, with numerous testimonials, [etc.] 8°. *Buffalo*, [1845].

GUSTAFSON (A.) The medicine stamp tax; an oppressive burden on the sick, an encouragement to quackery, a stigma upon legitimate medicine, giving foreign trade unfair advantage over English commerce. 8°. [*London*], 1884.

GYÖNGYÖSSI (P.) * De empiricis remediis. 2. ed. 4°. *Lugd. Bat.*, [1753].
Also, in: HALLER. Disp. ad morb. [etc.] 4°. *Lausannæ*, 1760, vii, 127–140.

[HEIM (A.)] A short treatise on Mathey-Caylus's gluten capsules of pure copaiba and other medicines. Uzac's iodo-phosphated mineral water, the best substitute for cod-liver oil. Mathey-Caylus's injection for the cure of recent and chronic gleets. 8°. *New York*, [1854].

HEINS (A.) Ueber die Ursachen der Krankheiten und deren Heilung, nebst Betrachtungen über medicinische Vorurtheile und Mode-Kuren im Gegensatz gegen eine vernünftige Behandlung der Kranken, bey Gelegenheit eines neuen von dem Verfasser erfundenen Arzney-Mittels, unter dem Namen: Elixirum naturæ completum. 2 Aufl. 12°. *Hamburg*, 1793.

HOYER (E.) Die medizinischen Geheimmittel. Ihr Zweck, ihre Verwerflichkeit und die Mittel zur Beseitigung des damit getriebenen Schwindels. Nebst einer Zusammenstellung von etwa 70 Geheimmittelenthüllungen. 8°. *Hannover*, 1866.

JAPAN. *Home Department.* Notification of the sanitary bureau. April 7, 1879. Changes in method of examining stamps on medicines (revenue). No. 10. sm. 4°. [*Tokio*, 1879.]

JUNGKEN (J. H.) Höchstgemüsigt- und abgenöthigte Defension- und Remonstrations-Schrifft contra der hiesigen Herrn Apothecker unbesonnenes und absurdes Petitum. Mir meiner sonderbahren selbst erfundenen Medicamenten, eigenhändige Elaboration, zu verbiethen, etc., ut intus. 4°. [*Frankfurth*, 1708.]

KEITH (B.) Manual of the active principles of indigenous and foreign medicinal plants, as prepared at the laboratory of B. Keith & Co. 16°. *New York*, 1863.

KEYSER. Réponse à l'auteur anonyme d'un livre intitulé: Traité des tumeurs et ulcères. 12°. [*n. p.*], 1759.

VON KNÖR (L. G.) Truckne Sauerbrunnen-Cur, vermittelst eines, mit dem solarischen Schwefel vereinigten astralischen Gold-Saltzes, samt ausführlicher Anweisung, wie die Cur durch dieses Universal-Saltz, mit höchstem Nutzen, an allen Orthen, zu allen Zeiten, und mit leichter Bequemlichkeit, in denen meisten Kranckheiten, fürnemlich aber den Morbis-Chronicis, zu gebrauchen, darinne man des vielen Wasser-Trinkens überhoben seyn kan, weil eine geringe Dosis dieses Saltzes mehr effectuirt, als viel Kannen des Sauer-Wassers thun mögen. 12°. *Leipzig*, [*n. d.*]

LEGITIMATE medicine and pharmacy *vs.* nostrum venders. 8°. [*Detroit*, 1881.]
Repr. from: Therap. Gaz., Detroit, 1881, n. s., ii.

LEROY (L.) Lettre à M. Pariset [on his secret remedy]. 8°. *Paris*, 1826.

VON MADAI (D. S.) A short account of the effects and use of some approved medicines, which are dispensed in the Orphanhouse at Halle, in the Dutchy of Magdeburg, and by which not only slight, but also hard and difficult diseases by the blessing of God may be successfully cured. Transl. from the German. 8°. *Halle*, [*n. d.*]

Medicines (*Patent, proprietary, quack, and secret*).

MEDICAL (The) Observer. No. 1. On advertised or empirical medicines, etc. 8°. *London*, 1806.

MEDICAL Society of the County of New York. Reports on nostrums or secret medicines. Pt. 1. 8°. *New York*, 1827.

Also [Rev.], *in:* N. York M. & Phys. J., 1827, vi, 426–442.

MEMORIA sobre a excellencia, virtudes, e uso medicinal da verdadeira agua de Inglaterra da invenção do Dr. Jacob de Castro Sarmento, por José Joaquim de Castro. 8°. *Lisboa*, 1845.

———. The same. 4. ed. 8°. *Lisboa*, 1845.

MONROE County Medical Society. Report of a committee on Dr. Lovejoy's alleged new remedies. Published by vote of the . . . Rochester, June 9, 1858. 8°. *Rochester*, 1858.

MORTIMER (C.) An address to the public, containing narratives of the effects of certain chemical remedies in most diseases; particularly exemplified in the histories of various cases, both medical and chirurgical, attested by the patients themselves or by their friends; whereby it appears that these medicines have cured many distempers with single doses, and given great relief in the gout and some disorders usually pronounced incurable. To which is prefixed a preface giving an account of the uses and operations of these particular remedies with practical remarks on some diseases, and a few hints relating to virtues, not commonly known, of some medicines already in use. 8°. *London*, 1714.

NEGRI (L.) * Sul farmaco cerotto-Briziano. Due parole del dottore Luigi Negri al dottor cavaliere Melchiori Giovanni. 8°. *Milano*, 1869.

NORRIS (T.) A short essay on the virtues of Dr. Norris' drops for fevers. 8°. *London*, 1777.

NOTICE sur la médecine électropathique du docteur J.-P. Bachoué de Lostalot, de Vialer (Basses-Pyrénées), approuvée par l'Académie de Paris, sur la loi terpathique organique . . . 8°. [*n. p., n. d.*]

OBSERVATIONS on the baume de vie, first discovered by M. Le Lievre, the king's apothecary at Paris. Wherein all the objections made to it by the ignorant and interested are fully refuted, and its wonderful efficacy in a variety of diseases justified on the most reasonable principles; with letters and attestations in its favour, from people of the first distinction. 8°. *London*, 1765.

PAGE (J.) Receipts for preparing and compounding the principal medicines made use of by the late Mr. Ward. Together with an introduction, [etc.] 8°. *London*, 1763.

PAINE (W.) The medical properties and uses of concentrated medicines. 8°. *Philadelphia*, 1865.

PATENT and public medicines. An essay on the virtues, uses, and effects of some valuable genuine patent and public medicines, invented and prepared by men of science, for the relief and cure of asthma, head ache, indigestion, tooth ache, etc., etc. To which are added some observations respecting public medicines and the conduct of the faculty in general, by a candid physician. 8°. *London*, [*n. d.*]

PHILADELPHIA Medical Society. First report of the committee of the . . . on quack medicines. Read on the 15th Dec., 1827. 8°. *Philadelphia*, 1828.

Also, in: N. Am. M. & S. J., Phila., 1828, v, 149–183.

POSITIVE medical agents, being a treatise on the new alkaloid, resinoid, and concentrated preparations of indigenous and foreign medical plants. By authority of the American Chemical Institute. 8°. *New York*, 1855.

Medicines (*Patent, proprietary, quack, and secret*).

REFLEXÕES criticas do doutor . . . sobre as direcções para o uso da agoa de Inglaterra, composta e manipulada por Antonio José de Sousa Pinto, boticario na cidade de Lisboa, ou exame comparativo da mesma agoa com a verdadeira agoa de Inglaterra do doutor Jacob de Castro Sarmento, manipulada por José Joaquim de Castro na sua real fabrica. 8°. *Lisboa*, 1811.

REMARKS, preliminary to the exhibition of Dr. Phelps' practically established arcanum. 8°. *Boston*, [*n. d.*]

RICHTER (H. E.) Das Geheimmittel-Unwesen; nebst Vorschlägen zu dessen Unterdrückung. 2 v., paged consecutively. 8°. *Leipzig*, 1872–5.

RIDIGER (A.) Observationes et meditationes de veritate virtutis medicamentorum propriæ et methodo hanc explorandi. 4°. *Lipsiæ*, [1750].

SCHMELTZ (J.) Guide pratique pour l'emploi des remèdes dynamiques. 12°. *Nice*, 1885.

SCHMITT (F. L.) * De vanitate remediorum universalium. sm. 4°. *Gottingæ*, [1757].

Also in: VOGEL (R. A.) Opusc. med. selecta, etc. 4°. *Gottingæ*, 1768, 115–146.

SÉGUIN (G.) Vin spécifique fébrifuge et stomachique. 8°. *Paris*, [*n. d.*]

SEMBENINI (G. B.) Manuale pratico di rimedi moderni di segreti analizzati e di altri preparati tecnici e specifici nuovi o migliorati dopo le ultime edizioni delle opere di G. Ruspini e G. Orosi. 8°. *Verona*, 1868

SEMMEDO (J. C.) Compendio dos segredos medicinaes ou remedios curvianos. 16°. *Lisboa*, 1783.

SHORT (A) account of Sir Astley Cooper's vital restorative, the only acknowledged successful remedy for the removal of general, local, and nervous debility, confided to Messrs. Harvey and Co., consulting surgeons. (Registered under the new medical act.) 16°. *London*, 1864.

SIMONS (G.) Den troost der armen, behelsende lichte ende souvereine remedien tegen verscheide siekten, wonden, gezwellen, ende andere qualen des lichaams van den mensch, door de ondervindinge goet gekeurt, tot grooten dienst en troost der behoeftige menschen, welker qualen ongeneselijk schenen te wesen, zeer dienstig in alle familien en hospitalen, xiv. druk, door den autheur vermeerdert, met nieuwe remedien voor menschen en beesten. 12°. *Dordrecht*, [1711].

SOUBEIRAN. Discours sur les remèdes secrets, autorisés par le gouvernement. 8°. *Paris*, [*n. d.*]

DE SOUSA PINTO (A. J.) Direcções sobre o uso da agua d'Inglaterra. 8°. *Lisboa*, 1809.

———. Documentos que authorisão a verdadeira agua de Inglaterra da composição, e manipulação. fol. [*Lisboa*], 1810.

STEWART (F. E.) An old system and a new science. 8°. *Detroit*, [1882].

STRINGEO (M.) Variety of surprising experiments, made of two incomparable medicines: elixir febrifugum martis, and salt of limons; as also of elixir renovans, shewing their virtues, use, and operations; being the peculiar secrets and acquisitions of the author. 12°. *London*, 1707.

SWAIM (W.) A treatise on Swaim's panacea; being a recent discovery, for the cure of scrofula, or king's evil, mercurial disease, deep-seated syphilis, rheumatism, and all disorders arising from a contaminated or impure state of the blood. With cases illustrating its success. 12°. *Philadelphia*, 1822.

———. The same. 8°. *Philadelphia*, 1825.

———. Some remarks upon a publication by the Philadelphia Medical Society concerning Swaim's panacea. 8°. *Philadelphia*, 1828.

Medicines (*Patent, proprietary, quack, and secret*).

———— Cases of cures performed by the use of Swaim's panacea. 12°. *Philadelphia*, 1829.

————. The same. 8°. *Philadelphia*, 1831.

————. A collection of cases, illustrating the restorative and sanative properties of Swaim's panacea in a variety of diseases. 8°. *Philadelphia*, 1832.

————. Plain and practical observations upon diseases resulting from worms; with remarks upon the utility of Swaim's vermifuge in cholera-morbus and in many other diseases originating in debility of the digestive organs. 8°. *Philadelphia*, 1833.

TOSCANELLI (C. M.) Del maraviglioso specifico delle lucertole, o ramarri per la radical cura del cancro, della lebbra, e lue venerea ultimamente scoperto dal signor D. Giuseppe Flores alle di cui sperienze, ed osservazioni si aggiungono le relazioni di varie cure fatte recentemente nel Piemonte, con una distinta ed esatta analisi della lucertola, e del ramarro, volgarmente detta da Piemontesi l'ayeul. 12°. *Torino*, 1784.

UNITED STATES. *Congress. House of Representatives.* Report from the select committee to whom was referred the resolution of the House of Representatives, ordering an inquiry into the expediency of so amending the patent laws as to prevent the patenting of compound medicines. 30. Cong., 2. sess. H. of R. Feb. 6, 1849. Rep. No. 52. [To accompany bill H. R. No. 755.] 8°. [*Washington*, 1849.]

————. A bill repealing the tax on proprietary medicines. 47. Cong., 1. sess., H. R. 2108. In the H. of Reps. Dec. 19, 1881. [Introd. by Mr. Joyce.] roy. 8°. [*Washington*, 1881.]

————. A bill to provide for extension of letters patent for improved medical compound to J. W. Ewing, assignee of M. R. G. Garsam, administrator of the estate of C. H. Mitchell, deceased. 48. Cong., 1. sess. H. R. 7243. June 9, 1884. Introd. by Mr. Halsell. roy. 8°. [*Washington*, 1884.]

VARIGNANE (G.) Secreta sublima ad varios curandos morbos verissimis autoritatibus illustrata; flosculi itemque plurimi in gratiam studiosorum utiliter superadditi, cum marginalibus decorationibus et singulorum capitum tabula. 12°. *Lugduni*, 1539.

WAGNER (J. G.) De medicamento arcano polychresto lacrymæ Jobi dicto in artis salutaris incrementum consignata. 4°. [*n. p.*], 1733.

AM UND VOM WALD (G.) Gemehrter Bericht, wie und was gestalt die new erfundne, unnd nicht allein in teutscher Nation, sonder auch andern weit aussligenden Ländern, von sieben und zweintzig Jaren hero, viel probirte Terra Sigillata am Waldina, wider die Pestilentz zauberisch unnd andere empfangne gifften Fieber, Schlag, Fallendtsucht, Freysz, Schwindel, Wassersucht, Geelsucht, Grimmen, Griesz, Ruhren, Contractur, Podagram, Aussatz, Frantzosen, Rothlauff, und viel andere schwere Kranckheiten mehr, ohn alle Gefahr zu gebrauchen sey. Zu Nutz unnd frommen arm unnd reichen krancken Personen, widerumb an Tag gegeben. 4°. *Stutgart*, 1601.

WARD'S pill dissected and examined, etc. With a full confutation of Mr. Clutton's new hypothesis of arsenick being a part of its composition. By a chemist of London. 8°. *London*, 1736.

Adelon. Sur la concession de brevets d'invention pour remèdes. Ann. d'hyg., Par., 1838, xix, 226–231.—**Bachiller** (J. J. G.) ¡¡Siga la broma!!! Siglo méd., Madrid, 1858, v, 378.—**Barning** (A.) Is de leer der geheimartsen vijandig aan den vooruitgang der geneeskunde? Tijdschr. v. geneesk. ervaring, Tilburg, 1852, i, 377–416.—**Bavaria.** Königl. bayersche Verordnung, den Verkauf von Geheimmitteln betreffend. Med.-chir. Ztg., Innsbruck, 1838, iii,

Medicines (*Patent, proprietary, quack, and secret*).

77.—**Bernhold's** (G.) Algophon. Wien. med. Wchnschr., 1853, iii, 170.—**Biach** (A.) Referat über die vom iv. österr. Aerztevereinstage angeregte Frage der Bekämpfung des Verkaufes von Geheimmitteln. Mitth. d. Ver. d. Aerzte in Nied.-Oest, Wien, 1882, viii, 55–63.—**Bigelow** (H. R.) Trade mark pharmacy. Chicago M. J. & Exam., 1882, xliv, 130.—**Blümlein.** Eine Folge der Anpreisung von Heilmitteln in öffentlichen Blättern, nebst einigen Bemerkungen über das Verhältniss der Sanitätspolizei zu denselben. Vrtljschr. f. gerichtl u. öff. Med., Berl., 1863, xxiv, 327–341.—**Boé** (A.) Du danger des remèdes secrets; empoisonnement par le sirop de Pagliano. Bull. gén. de thérap., etc., Par., 1877, xcii, 267–270.—**Braconnot.** Sur la poudre de Godernaux. J. de chim. méd., etc., Par., 1835, 2. s., i, 406–410.—**Brard.** Restauration de la patente sur les médecins. Proposition de M. . . . représentant du peuple, sur l'établissement d'une taxe professionnelle. Union méd., Par., 1849, iii. 45.—**Broberg** (J. V.) Om "Hjärnes testamente". Hygiea, Stockholm, 1880, xlii, 283–286.—**Brouardel** (P.) Affaire de remède secret; cosmétique Delacour. Ann. d'hyg., Par., 1883, 3. s., ix, 163–180.—**Buignet.** Rapport sur les spécialités pharmaceutiques. Bull. Acad. de méd., Par., 1875, 2. s., iv, 20–24.—**Carey** (St. G.) Nostrums and patent medicines; general consideration of their nature and effects, with a remedy. West. Lancet, Cincin., 1852, xiii, 713.—**Carter.** Notes on the English law as to patent medicines. Liverpool M. Chir. J., 1885, v, 56–59.—**Chester** assizes. Accusation of manslaughter against one of "Graham's Own". Lancet, Lond., 1844, ii, 382.—**Chevallier** (A.) Remède secret; l'eau Brocchieri: tromperie sur la nature de la marchandise vendue. J. de chim. méd., etc., Par., 1855, 4. s., i, 31–34.—**Chittenden** (T. W.) Nostrums. Rep. Bd. Health Wisconsin, Madison, 1882, vii, 164–180. *Also:* Rep. Bd. Health N. Hampshire 1884–5, Conc rd, 1885, iv, 290–304.—**Clerical** quackery; Taylor's specific liniment. Glasgow M. J., 1858–9, [2.] s., vi, 424–433.—**Companions** for "bread-pills". Lancet, Lond., 1839, ii, 351.—**Condie** (D. F.) Report on quack medicines. Tr. M. Soc. Penn., Phila., 1856, n. s., i, 20–24.—**Coventry** (A.) Extracts from addresses on epidemic fevers, patent medicines, etc. Tr. M. Soc. N. Y., Albany, 1859, 343–366.—**Cowley** (R A.) Informe de la comision de remedios nuevos y secretos. An. r. Acad. d. cien. méd. . . . de la Habana, 1869–70, vi, 129; 200; 238.—**Craig** (A. L.) Patent medicine. Chicago M. J. & Exam., 1883, xlvii, 41–46.—**Crosby** (A.) Some of the ev:ls which result from the free and injudicious administration of nostrums to infants and young children. Rep. Bd. Health Mich. 1881, Lansing, 1882, ix, 160–164.—**Death** from Morison's pills; post-mortem appearances. Lond. M. & S. J., 1835–6, viii, 605.—**De-Simoni** (S. B.) Dell' abuso dei remedi segreti e delle specialità medicinali. Atti Cong. gen. d. Ass. med. ital. 1880, Genova, 1882, ix, 724–731.—**Devergie** (A.) Affaire de remède secret (pilules Cronier); jurisprudence du tribunal; inconvénients de cette jurisprudence; définition des spécialités et du remède secret donnée en 1875 par l'Académie de médecine. Ann. d'hyg., Par., 1877, 2. s., xlviii, 151–172. *Also:* Soc. de méd. lég. de France. Bull. 1877–8, Par., 1879, v, 89–110.—**Dorr** (J. A.) Are improvements in medicine and surgery proper subjects for patents? Lancet, Lond., 1847, i. 523.—**Empoisonnement** par le baume de Fioraventi. J. de chim. méd., etc., Par., 1857, 4. s., iii, 656.—**Examen** chimique des pilules dites de Morison. *Ibid.*, 1839, 2. s., v, 20–26.—**Fritschi** (J.) Ueber Kurpfuscherei und ihre Bannerträger; die Geheimmittelfabrikanten und Geheimmittelkrämer. Gesundheit, Elberfeld, 1875–6, i, 299; 314.—**Geheimmittel-Polizei.** (Aus den Acten der Aerzte-Commission.) Cor.-Bl. f. schweiz. Aerzte, Basel, 1877, vii, 249–253.—**Gonzalez** (A. F.) Las medicinas de patente. Voz de Hipócrates, México, 1885, iii, 65–67.—**Guerrier** (L.) Remèdes secrets. Que faut-il entendre par remède secret? Annonces relatives aux remèdes secrets; interdiction aux charlatans, et même aux pharmaciens et docteurs, de vendre des remèdes secrets; pénalités. Union méd., Par., 1871, 3. s., xii, 764–766.—**H.** (K. B.) Vegetable medicines. Nashville J. M. & S., 1877, 2. s., xix, 7–9.—**Hare** (R.) Mercury detected in Swaim's panacea by chemical analysis. Am. J. M. Sc., Phila., 1829, iv, 530.—**History** of panaceas and nostrums. Boston M. & S. J., 1829–30, ii, 577; 593.—**Holloway's** pills and ointment. Med. Circ., Lond., 1853, ii, 45; 67; 86.—**Hubbard** (H. W.) Patent medicines. Macmillan's Mag., Lond., 1883, xlvii, 499–504.—**Inconsistency** (The) of ethical physicians in regard to copyrighted medicines. [Edit.] Therap. Gaz., Detroit, 1881, n. s., ii, 19. *Also, in:* Legitimate medicine, [etc.], 8°. [Detroit, 1881], 5–7.—**Inexpediency** (On the) and invalidity of granting patents for medicines, considered in a medico-legal view. Boston M. & S. J., 1835, xii, 218–221.—**Itard.** Rapport général sur les remèdes secrets. Mém. Acad. de méd., Par., 1833, ii, 24–31.—**Janikowski** (S.) O pokątném leczeniu. [Secret medicines.] Pam. Towarz. Lek. Warszaw., 1864, lii, 161–165.—**Jealous** (A) Watchman and a Religious Herald on quack remedies. [Edit.] Med. Rec., N. Y., 1883, xxiii, 463.—**Jeanjean.** Des re-

Medicines (*Patent, proprietary, quack, and secret*).

mèdes secrets et des spécialités. Gaz. hebd. d. sc. méd. de Montpel., 1880, ii, 351; 374.—**Jeannel.** Sur un cas d'empoisonnement par les pilules de Crosnier. Soc. de méd. lég. de France. Bull., Par., 1875-6, iv, 489-491.—**Keller** (A.) Examen de quelques remèdes secrets, recettes, articles de toilette, etc. Monit. scient., Par., 1865, vii, 1073-1081.—**Klein** (A.) Erfahrungen über die Wirksamkeit des Gleichenberger Brust-Saftes und der Gleichenberger Pastillen. Wien. med. Presse, 1870, xi, 656-658.—**König.** Untersuchung und Gutachten über die einer Kranken von Seite einer Pfuscherin angerathenen sogenannten "privilegirten blutreinigenden Kaiserpillen". Ztschr. f. d. Staatsarznk., Erlang., 1851, lxi, 376-395.—**Lang'sche** Pillen. Wien. med. Wchnschr., 1852, ii, 670. — **Lereboullet**(L.) Les spécialités pharmaceutiques. Gaz. hebd. de méd., Par., 1879, 2. s., xvi, 549; 565.—**Lettre** sur les remèdes secrets. J. gén. de méd., chir. et pharm., Par., 1829, cviii, 161-166.—**Lindsley** (C. A.) Essay. Resolved, That it is demoralizing to the medical profession, and detrimental to the public welfare, to prescribe proprietary medicines for the sick. Proc. Connect. M. Soc., Hartford, 1882, 103-120. *Also*, Reprint. ———. The uncertainties and risks attending the use of proprietary and other ready-made medicines. Rep. Bd. Health Connect. 1882, Hartford, 1883, v, 95 - 99. — **Lissner.** Die Geheimmittel. Deutsche Vrtljschr. f. öff. Gsndhtspflg., Brnschwg., 1870, ii, 214; 220. — **Lobethals** Essentia antiphthysica. Wien. med. Wchnschr., 1853, iii, 12.—**McGraw.** Why clergyman should not recommend quack medicines. Detroit Rev. Med. & Pharm., 1868, iii, 47-51.—**Magnes** fils. Quelques mots sur les remèdes secrets. J. de méd. et chir. de Toulouse, 1844-5, viii, 309-316.—**Malmsten.** Härfärgningsmeder "Hall's hair-renewer". Förh. v. Svens. Läk.-Sällsk. Sammank., Stockholm, 1871, 63-69.—**Mathelin.** Des spécialités pharmaceutiques en médecine publique. Rev. d'hyg., Par., 1880, ii, 486-505.—**Mayet.** Sur l'annonce et la vente des remèdes secrets. Ann. d'hyg., Par., 1879, 3. s., ii, 433-438.—**Mesures** à prendre contre l'annonce et la vente des remèdes secrets. Bull. Soc. méd. de la Suisse Rom., Lausanne, 1877, xi, 171-176.—**Moller** (J.) Etwas über Volksmittel und Sabina. Ztschr. f. Nat.- u. Heilk. in Ungarn, Oedenburg, 1859, x, 35 —**Nielsen's** schwedischer Balsam gegen Frostbeulen. Wien. med. Wchnschr., 1854, iv, 105.—**Nochrasir-**, Kühl- und Glätt-Essenz. *Ibid.*, iii, 1853, 247.—**Nostrum** (The) trade; its influence on health and morals. Boston M. & S. J., 1848-9, xxxix, 129-140.—**Paasch.** Analyse der sogenannten Wiener Kaiserpillen. Wchnschr. f. d. ges. Heilk., Berl., 1846, 304-306.—**Patent** (The) medicine evil; its extent and a few of its many dangers. Canada Health J., Ottawa, 1887, ix, 60-62.—**Patent** (The) medicine stamp question. Midland M. Misc., Leicester, 1884, iii, 290. — **Patentovanniya** zagranichniya laikarstva i mineralniya vodi. [Patent medicines and mineral waters.] Med. Vestnik, St. Petersb., 1861, i, 236.—**Pfeffermann'sche** Zahnpasta. Wien. med. Wchnschr., 1853, iii, 24. — **Pharmacopœia** empirica, or the list of nostrums and empirics. Gent Mag. & Hist. Chron., Lond., 1748, xviii, 348-350.—**Philadelphia** (The) medical profession and copyrighted medicines. [Edit.] Therap. Gaz., Detroit, 1881, n. s., ii, 19. *Also, in:* Legitimate medicine, [etc.], 8°, [Detroit, 1881], 3-5.— **Pierron** (J. J.) Examination of "pain killers". West. Lancet, San Fran., 1877, vi, 39.—**Prescott** (A. B.) Constituents of proprietary remedies for rheumatism. Physician & Surg., Ann Arbor, Mich., 1880, ii, 97-100. ———. Nostrums in their relations to the public health. Rep Bd. Health Mich. 1881, Lansing, 1882, ix, 151-160. *Also:* Physician & Surg., Ann Arbor, Mich., 1881, iii, 213-225. ———. Should proprietary medicines be required to give an account of contents? Tr. M. Soc. Mich., Lansing, 1885, 153-158.—**Professor** Virchow and secret remedies. Lancet, Lond., 1883, i, 1135.— **Quack** medicines, their history, composition, and qualities. Med. Circ., Lond., 1853, ii, 8; 25; 45; 67; 86; 106; 126; 146; 167; 188; 207; 227; 266; 347; 386; 406; 492; 509; 1854, iv, 8; 31; 85; 118.—**Qu'entend-on** par spécialités pharmaceutiques? Quel degré de confiance peut-on leur accorder? Bull. Soc. méd. de la Suisse Rom., Lausanne, 1878. xii, 69-73.—**Ramaer** (J. N.) Over het begrip van specifieke geneesmiddelen. Arch. v. Geneesk., Amst., 1844, iv, 1-76. — **Remarks** on some empirical medicines and modes of treatment. Glasgow M. J., 1859-60, [2.] s., vii, 422-432.—**Remède** secret; Rob Boyveau-Laffecteur; poursuites contre le sieur Giraudeau, dit de Saint-Gervais, prévenu de tromperie sur la nature de la marchandise vendue. Ann. d'hyg., Par., 1848, xxxix, 224-228.—**Remèdes** secrets. *Ibid.*, 1851, xlv, 450-453.— **Robinet.** Note sur le remède secret et sa définition. J. de chim. méd., etc., Par., 1831, vii, 614 - 628. — **St. Jacob's** oil. Ephem. Mat. Med., Brooklyn, 1882, i, 113.—**Schauer's** Augsburger Lebensessenz. Wien. med. Wchnschr., 1852, iv, 497.—**Schneider** (P. J.) Ueber Arcanen-Sucht und medicinische Geheimnisskrämerei; besonders über das Laeyson'sche Augenpulver. Ztschr. f. d. Staatsarznk., Erlang., 1828, xv, 98-143.—**Schuppe** (K.) Patentovan. vrachebnija sredstva. [Patented medicines.]

Medicines (*Patent, proprietary, quack, and secret*).

Vrach, St. Petersb., 1881, i, 319; 743. *Also, transl.:* Pharm. Ztschr. f. Russland, St. Petersb., 1882, xxi, 77; 101.—**Secret** remedies. Med. Times, Lond., 1851. n. s., iii, 208-210. — **Sewall** (J. G.) The pernicious influences of nostrums or secret remedies upon the morals and health of the community. Tr. M. Soc. N. Y., Albany, 1851, 173-185.— **Sobre** la elaboracion y venta de medicamentos secretos y no secretos. Siglo méd., Madrid, 1857, iv, 85. — **Soubeiran** (E.) Discours sur les remèdes secrets qui ont reçu l'autorisation du gouvernement. Gaz. méd. de Lyon. 1853, v, 17; 33.—**Stahl** (G. E.) Anchiater, seu venenum pro remedio venditum, febrifugum nequissimum. *In his:* Obs. chym.-phys.-med. [etc.], 16°, Francof. et Lips., 1697-8, 219-304.—**Stewart** (F. E.) The "therapeutic boom" and unscientific advertising. Med. & Surg. Reporter, Phila, 1880, xliii, 465-468. *Also:* Therap. Gaz., Detroit, 1881, n. s., ii, 23 - 25. *Also, in:* Legitimate medicine [etc.], 8°, [Detroit, 1881], 7-14 —**Swaim's** panacea. Boston M. & S. J., 1828-9, i, 26.— **Tanner** (G. C.) American patent medicine in Belgium. Rep. Consuls U. S. on commerce, etc., Wash., 1882, no. 25, 23. — **Therapeutic** (The) Gazette. No. 3. Supplement: Shall quackery be permitted to triumph? Comments on the last efforts of the trade-mark and patent medicine ring. Therap. Gaz., Detroit, 1882, n. s , iii, suppl.—**Trébuchet.** Des brevets d'invention délivrés pour remèdes secrets. Ann. d'hyg., Par., 1843, xxix, 203-211. — **Tribunal** correctionnel d'Avignon; exercice illégal de la médecine: vente de remèdes secrets; escroquerie. Union méd., Par., 1865, 2. s., xxv, 98-100.—**Use** (The) of proprietary medicines. Med. Rec., N. Y., 1876, xi, 423. — **Van de Warker** (E) The criminal use of proprietary or advertised nostrums. N. York M. J., 1873, xvii, 23-35. *Also*, Reprint. —**Verdale** (H.) La patente des médecins; sa suppression prochaine. Gaz. méd. de Bordeaux, 1877, vi, 25 - 28.—**Vermifuge,** Swaim's. Remède américain patenté. Bull. gén. de thérap., etc., Par., 1850, xxxix, 543.—**Welches** sind die kräftigsten Mittel gegen die herumziehenden Arzneikrämer? Allg. med. Ann., Altenb., 1808, 463-466.—**White'sches** Augenwasser. Wien. med. Wchnschr., 1854, iv, 456.—**Wildberg** (C. F. L) Ueber das öffentliche Anpreisen und den Verkauf von Geheimmitteln. Jahrb. d. ges. Staatsarznk., Leipz., 1840, vi, 178 - 182. —**Wilson** (J. S.) Remarks on the use of empirical remedies; with some suggestions as to the best means of abating the evil. South. M. & S. J., Augusta, 1853, n. s., ix, 76-81.

Medicines (*Physiological action and investigation of*).

See, also, **Heart** (*Effects of drugs on*); **Medicines** (*Antagonism of*).

ALVARENGA (P. F. da C.) Pharmacothermogenese, ou theorias da acção dos medicamentos sobre a temperatura animal. 8°. *Lisboa*, 1880.

BARRIER (G.-B.-J.) * Exposition de nouveaux principes de pharmacologie qui forment de la matière médicale une science nouvelle. 8°. *Paris*, [1803].

BELLINI (R.) Delle azioni simpatiche, invocate a spiegazione di alcuni fenomeni occasionali dalle sostanze medicamentose. [8°. *Firenze*, 1850.]

Repr. from: Gior. ital. di sc. med. e nat. Il Progresso, ii.

BÉNIQUE (P.-J.) * Recherches expérimentales sur l'action de quelques médicamens. 4°. *Paris*, 1835.

BISCHOFF (G. T. H.) * Sciagraphia methodi materiæ medicæ qualitatum æstimationi superstructæ. Pars 2. 12°. [*Tubingæ*, 1793.]

BLAKE (J.) Report on the physiological action of medicines. 8°. *London*, 1844.

Repr. from: Rep. Brit. Ass. Adv. Sc., Lond., 1843.

———. The same. 8°. *London*, 1846.

Repr. from: Rep. Brit. Ass. Adv. Sc., Lond., 1846.

BREIDTHARDT (E.) * Experimenta quædam de vi gummi gutti, jalapæ, elaterii cum in hominibus tum in animalibus instituta. 8°. *Bonnæ*, 1865.

BRUNTON (T. L.) Experimental investigation of the action of medicines. 8°. *London*, 1875.

See, also, infra.

BURNESS (A. G.) & MAVOR (F. J.) The specific action of drugs on the healthy system; an index to their therapeutic value, as reduced from experiments on man and animals. 8°. *London*, 1874.

Medicines (*Physiological action and investigation of*).

CAZENAVE (P.-L.-A.) De l'appréciation des divers moyens qui peuvent être employés pour connaître les propriétés des médicamens. 4°. *Paris*, 1839.

DEBOVE (G.-M.) * L'action physiologique des médicaments, peut-elle devenir la règle de leur emploi thérapeutique? 8°. *Paris*, 1875.

DIEKERHOFF (F.) * De remediorum quorundam vi sanguinem cerebro et meningibus contentum diminuendi. 4°. *Bonnæ*, [1833].

DROOP (J. D.) * Diss. sistens veram in medicamentorum vires inquirendi rationem. 4°. *Gottingæ*, [1793].

ELSNER (C. F.) *Analecta de methodis determinandi medicamentorum virtutes. 4°. *Regiomonti*, [1774].

FABER (G. E.) * Experimenta quædam circa effectus nonnullorum venenorum et medicamentorum vegetabilium in diversis animalibus. sm. 4°. *Tubingæ*, 1813.

FILOMENA (F.) Breve saggio sull' operazione dell' oppio, e dell' aria fissa ed infiammabile negli animali, secondo il sistema dell' elettricità. 8°. *Napoli*, 1781.

FRANK (J. P.) De virtutibus corporum naturalium medicis æquiori modo determinandis. *Ticini*, 1789.

In his: Delect. opusc. med. 8°. *Ticini*, 1789, vii, 189-218. *Also, in his:* Opusc. med. 8°. *Lipsiæ*, 1790, 256-275.

———. Oratio altera de virtutibus corporum naturalium medicis æquiori modo determinandis.

In his: Delect. opusc. med. 8°. *Ticini*, 1790, viii, 175-204.

FRIEDLÁNDER (G.) * De experimento pharmacologico. 8°. [*Dorpat*], 1852.

[GATTENHOFF (G. M.)] Specimen inaugurale medicum de ventriculi et intestinorum ratione habenda, in ordine ad æstimandas medicamentorum vires. [1756.]

In: COLLECTIO diss. [etc.] 8°. *Heidelbergæ*, 1791, i, 29-52.

GUÉRARD (J.-A.) * Des inductions que la thérapeutique peut tirer de l'action physiologique des médicaments. 8°. *Paris*, 1839.

HAGENTORN (W.) * Disquisitiones pharmacologicæ de quarundam convolvulacearum resinis institutæ. 8°. *Dorpati*, 1857.

HANBURY (D.) Science papers, chiefly pharmacological and botanical. Edited, with memoir, by Joseph Ince. 8°. *London*, 1876.

HEADLAND (F. W.) An essay on the action of medicines in the system; or, "on the mode in which therapeutic agents introduced into the stomach produce their peculiar effects on the animal œconomy". Being the prize essay to which the Medical Society of London awarded the Fothergillian gold medal for 1852. 2. ed. 8°. *London*, 1855.

HEBENSTREIT (J. E.) [Pr.] de cognoscendis medicamentorum facultatibus. Spec. xxvi. 4°. [*Lipsiæ*, 1750.]

[HENNICKE (G.) * Panaceas apponet. 4°. *Heidelbergæ*, [1686].

———. The same. De panaceis. Tractatio medico-chymica. Curiosis experimentis ac ratiociniis illustrata. 16°. *Francof. a. M.*, 1689.

HERHOLDT (J. D.) De quæstione medica: Num vires medicamentorum (plantarum verbi gratia) officinalium aut chymica analysi, aut sensium ope, aut consideratione similitudinis in partibus essentialibus rectius cognoscuntur? 8°. *Havniæ et Lipsiæ*, [1792].

———. The same. 12°. *Havniæ*, 1794.

HERMANN (L.) Experimental pharmacology. A hand-book of methods for studying the physiological actions of drugs. Transl., with notes and

Medicines (*Physiological action and investigation of*).

additions, by R. M. Smith. 12°. *Philadelphia*, 1883.

HIORTZBERG (L.) * De methodo investigandi vires medicamentorum chemica. 4°. *Upsaliæ*, [1754].

Also, in: LINNÆUS amoenitates acad. [etc.] 8°. *Erlangæ*, 1785, ix, 23-34.

HIRSCHEL (B.) Rules and examples for the study of pharmacodynamics. Transl. and edited, with additions from the author's writings, by T. Hayle. 8°. *Manchester, Eng.*, 1857.

HOPPE (I.) Anleitung zum Experimentiren mit Arzneimitteln an den thierischen Thätigkeiten. 8°. *Giessen*, 1857.

HOUAT (L.-T.) Des propriétés physiologiques et curatives du Culex pipiens, de l'Hydrocotyle asiatica et pathogénésie nouvelle de Viola odorata. 8°. *Paris*, 1883.

JOUSSET (P.-G.) * De l'expérimentation thérapeutique, et de l'appréciation de la valeur des agens de la matière médicale. 4°. *Paris*, 1829.

KIMMIJSER (W. C.) * Onderzoekingen over de reductie van chloraten in het levend organismus. 8°. *Arnhem*, 1884.

KISSEL (C.) Handbuch der physiologischen Arzneiwirkungslehre. 8°. *Tübingen*, 1856.

KÜRSSNER (J. G. D.) * Diss. sistens cautelas quasdam circa chemicam remediorum explorationem observandas. 4°. *Halæ Magdeb.*, [1753].

LEBOUCHER (A.) * Jusqu'à quel point peut-on conclure de l'action des médicaments sur l'homme sain à leur application thérapeutique? 4°. *Paris*, 1851.

LEINEWEBER (K.) * Ueber Elimination subcutan applicirter Arzneimittel durch die Magenschleimhaut. 8°. *Duderstadt*, 1883.

LICHTENSTEIN (G. R.) Dubia circa chemiæ in virtutibus medicamentorum eruendis præstantiam proponens.

In: WEBER (G. H.) Vollständ. Ausz. a. n. Diss. [etc.] 8°. *Bremen*, 1775, i, 135-140.

LOBO LEITE PEREIRA (J.) *A acção physiologica dos medicamentos será uma base segura para as indicações therapeuticas? 4°. *Rio de Janeiro*, 1880.

LONGO (A.) Pensieri sopra l' azione dei rimedi. 8°. *Palermo*, 1847.

Repr. from: Rivista di scienze mediche, 1847, i.

MARTIN (C.-P.) *Propositions de pharmacologie. 4°. *Paris*, 1819.

MARTINI (N.) * De prudenti virium medicamenti exploratione. 4°. *Halæ*, 1703.

MASIUS (M.) *Experimentelle Untersuchungen über die Wirkungen gewisser Arzneistoffe, insbesondere des Jod und Alkohols, auf die Nieren. 8°. *Breslau*, 1882.

MEYER (C. J.) Pharmakologische Blätter zur Mittheilung und Besprechung des Neuesten und Wissenswerthesten aus dem Gebiete der Arzneimittellehre. 8°. *Güns*, 1840.

MORSHEAD (E. A.) Tables of the physiological action of drugs. 12°. *London*, 1880.

MÜLLER (C.) Die Quellen der Arzneimittellehren. Eine kritische Beleuchtung der herrschenden Ansichten. 8°. *Leipzig*, 1860.

NICOLAI (E. A.) [Pr.] de viribus medicamentorum explorandis. 4°. *Jenæ*, [1770-71].

PIPER (G. O.) * De exploranda medicamentorum natura. 8°. *Lipsiæ*, [1838].

PLAGGE (M. W.) Handbuch der Pharmakodynamik für Aerzte, Wundärzte und Studirende. Nach den neuesten Erfahrungen des In- und Auslandes wie auch nach eigener dreissigjähriger Erfahrung am Krankenbette. 8°. *Braunschweig*, 1847.

Medicines (*Physiological action and investigation of*).

PLAZ (A. G.) [Pr.] de plantarum virtutibus ex ipsarum charactere haud quaquam addiscendis prolusione priore præfatus. 4°. [*Lipsiæ*], 1762.

PLUGGE (P. C.) Overzicht van de wisselende chemische samenstelling en pharmacodynamische waarde van eenige belangrijke geneesmiddelen. 8°. *Amsterdam*, 1885.

RIEMER (G.) * De medicamentorum viribus rite æstimandis. 4°. *Rintelii*, [1751].

SCHREGER (C. H. T.) [Pr.] succinctam pharmacologiæ systematum censuram præmittit. Comment. i–iv. 4°. *Vitebergæ*, [1811].

SIMON (J.) * La méthode expérimentale appliquée à l'étude des substances médicamenteuses et toxiques, les succédanés en thérapeutique. Étude comparative de l'action physiologique des quatre principaux alcaloïdes du quinquina : quinine, cinchonine, cinchonidine, quinidine. 4°. *Paris*, 1883.

SOUBEIRAN (E.) * De l'étude de la pharmacologie. 4°. *Strasbourg*, 1853.

STOLL (O.) * Ueber die Einwirkung einiger Arzneistoffe und Gifte auf die Form der Pulswelle beim Hunde. 8°. *Greifswald*, 1876.

STORR (G. C. C.), BEBEL (F. G.) & BISCHOFF (G. T. H.) Sciagraphia methodi materiæ medicæ qualitatum æstimationi superstructæ. Pars prima et secunda. 12°. *Tubingæ*, 1792–3.

THOMSON (H.) * Ueber die Beeinflussung der peripheren Gefässe durch pharmakologische Agentien. 8°. *Dorpat*, 1886.

VOGT (P. F.) Lehrbuch der Pharmakodynamik. 4. Aufl. 2 v. 8°. *Giessen*, 1838.

WILLEMOES (F.) * Diss. sistens nonnulla ex pharmacologia generali momenta secundum principia theoriæ incitationis. 8°. *Havniæ*, 1803.

WILLIS (T.) Pharmaceutice rationalis, sive diatriba de medicamentorum operationibus in corpore humano. 4°. *Genevæ*, 1676.

——. The same. 4°. *Genevæ*, 1694.

WOOD (H. C.) An investigation into the action of convulsants. 8°. [*n. p., n. d.*]

Aglia anti-spasmodici succedono gli scuotenti, o tetanizzanti, noce vomica, fava di S. Ignazio, stricnina, solfato di stricnina, brucina. Ippocratico, Fano, 1871, 3. s., xix, 121–132. — **Albers.** Isopathische und homöopathische Heilversuche an Thieren. Med. Ztg., Berl., 1834, iii, 63–67. — **Avila y Pezuela** (L. R.) Efectos fisiológicos y terapéuticos que causan algunos medicamentos en la economia humana. ii. Pabellon méd., Madrid, 1875, xv, 400; 447. — **Badia** (S.) Accion fisiológica de algunos medicamentos sobre el higado é intestinos. Encicl. méd.-farm., Barcel., 1884, viii, 322–324. — **Bardeleben** (K.) Die Einwirkung von Kali- und Natronsalzen auf die Muskeln des menschlichen Darmes. Arch. f. path. Anat., etc., Berl., 1882, lxxxix, 190–192. — **Bartholow** (R.) The ophthalmoscope and the sphygmograph in the study of the physiological action of medicines. Tr. Ohio M. Soc., Cincin., 1871, 213–226. *Also:* Clinic, Cincin., 1871, i, 78; 89. — **Bennett** (J. H.) Report of the committee of the British Medical Association to investigate the antagonism of medicines. Brit. M. J., Lond., 1874, ii, 436; 464; 485; 518; 547; 581; 615; 674; 697; 771; 805. [*See, also, infra,* Coyne.] — **Blake** (J.) Observations on the physiological effects of various agents introduced into the circulation, as indicated by the hæmadynamometer. Edinb. M. & S. J., 1839, li, 330–345. *Also,* Reprint. ——. Sur l'action physiologique des sels de lithium, de rubidium et de potassium. [Extr.] Compt. rend. Acad. d. sc., Par., 1886, cii, 128.— **Botkin** (S.) jun. Zur Frage über den Zusammenhang der physiologischen Wirkung mit den chemischen Eigenschaften der Alkalimetalle der ersten Gruppe nach Mendelejeff. Centralbl. f. d. med. Wissensch., Berl., 1885, xxiii, 849–852. — **Brown** (A. C.) & **Fraser** (T. R.) On the changes produced by direct chemical addition on the physiological action of certain poisons. Proc. Roy. Soc. Edinb., 1866–9, vi, 228–232. *Also,* Reprint. ——. On the physiological action of the salts of the ammonium bases derived from atropia and conia. Proc. Roy. Soc. Edinb., 1866–9, vi, 461–464. ——. On the connection between chemical constitution and physiological action ; on the physiological action of the salts of ammonia, of tri-methylamine, and of tetramethylammonium ; of the salts of tro-

Medicines (*Physiological action and investigation of*).

pia, and of the ammonium bases derived from it ; and of tropic, atropic, and isatropic acids and their salts ; with further details on the physiological action of the salts of methyl-strychnium and of ethyl-strichnium. *Ibid.*, 556.

——. On the connection between chemical constitution and physiological action, with special reference to the physiological action of the salts of the ammonium bases derived from strychnia, bruciæ, thebaia, codeia, morphia, and nicotia. J. Anat. & Physiol., Lond., 1868, ii, 224–242. **Brunton** (T. L.) Lectures on the experimental investigation of the action of medicines. Brit. M. J., Lond., 1871, i, 413 ; 439 ; 495 ; 521 ; 581 ; 663 : ii, 659 ; 687 ; 749 : 1875, i, 201. ——. Researches made in the pharmacological laboratory of St. Bartholomew's Hospital. St. Barth. Hosp. Rep., Lond., 1876, xii, 125–134. ——. The Goulstonian lectures on pharmacology and its relation to therapeutics. Brit. M. J., Lond., 1877, i, 251 ; 285 ; 315 ; 345 ; 379 ; 415. — **Brunton** (T. L.) & **Cash** (T.) On the action of various alkaloids on processes of oxidation. St. Barth. Hosp. Rep., Lond., 1882, xviii, 267–270. — **Bufalini** (G.) L' attuale indirizzo nella farmacologia sperimentale. Gior. di clin. e terap., Messina, 1883, ii, 1–19.— **Cameron** (C. A.) On the physiological activity of super-oxidised molecules, especially of those of quinine iodate and bromate. [Abstr.] Lancet, Lond., 1882, i, 1026.—**Cavazzani** (G.) Sull' azione dell' atropina, della digitalina e della chinina associate principalmente sulla circolazione. Ann. univ. di med. e chir., Milano, 1879, ccxlvii, 3–42.—**Chirone** (V.) La farmacologia sperimentale. Arch. med. ital., Torino, 1882, i, 48–73. — **Cléroux** (L.-J.-V.) Considérations générales sur la physiologie du médicament. Union méd. du Canada, Montréal, 1882, xi, 245 ; 327.— **Coyne.** De l'action des médicaments. Recherches du comité de the British Medical Association. Gaz. méd. de Par., 1874, 4. s., iii, 556 ; 570 ; 607. [*See, also, supra,* Bennett (J. H.)] — **Curci** (A.) Azione di alcuni medicamenti sulla circolazione del sangue nel cervello. Sperimentale, Firenze, 1884, liii 248–265.—**Dubois** (R.) Note sur l'action des vapeurs de quelques liquides organiques neutres sur la substance organisée. Compt. rend. Soc. de biol., Par., 1883, 7. s., v, 376–379.— **Fenoglio** (I.) Azione d' alcuni rimedi sulla ricchezza emoglobinica del sangue. Indipendente, Torino, 1881, xxxii, 241–246.— **Field** (H. M.) Six generic drug modifications. Boston M. & S. J., 1884, cx, 601 : cxi, 3. *Also,* Reprint.— **Fleming** (A.) On the classification of medicines according to their action on the healthy body. Dublin Q. J. M. Sc., 1852, xiv, 278–309. *Also,* Reprint. — **Flöel** (O.) Die Wirkung der Kalium- und Natrium-Salze auf die glatte Muskulatur verschiedener Thiere. Arch. f. d. ges. Physiol., Bonn, 1884–5, xxxv, 157–173.—**Fraser** (T. R.) Report on pharmacology. J. Anat. & Physiol., Lond., 1873–4, viii, 217–232.—**Gnoinski** (O.) K' voprosu o materialakh dlya budushchei pharmakodinamiki. [On the data for a science of pharmacodynamics.] Med. Vestnik, St. Petersb., 1864, iv, 497 ; 507. — **Heger** (P.) Notice sur l'absorption des alcaloïdes dans le foie, les poumons et les muscles. J. de méd., chir. et pharmacol., Brux., 1877, lxv, 305–317. *Also,* Reprint.— **Inosemitzeff** (T.) Programm eines wissenschaftlichen therapeutischen Experimentes als des besten Mittels zur richtigen Ausarbeitung einer rationellen Therapie. Berl. klin. Wchnschr., 1864, i, 504.— **Jaworski** (W.) Badania doświadczalne nad zachowaniem się soli leczniczych w żołądku ludzkim. [Influence of medicinal salts upon the stomach.] Przegl. lek., Kraków., 1882, xxi, 529 ; 537 ; 546 ; 581 ; 597 ; 606 ; 619 ; 642 ; 654 ; 667. *Also:* Medycyna, Warszawa, 1882, x, 647 ; 661 ; 675 ; 691. *Also, transl.* [Abstr.]: Ztschr. f. Biol., München, 1883, xix, 397–445, 1 tab.—**Klenke.** Beitrag zur Prüfung gewisser Heilpotenzen in ihrer Wirkung auf sogenannte mikroskopische Krankheitsmonaden. Ztschr. d. k.-k. Gesellsch. d. Aerzte zu Wien, 1844, ii, 253–266.—**Kobert** (E. R.) Ueber den Einfluss verschiedener pharmacologischer Agentien auf die Muskelsubstanz. Arch. f. exper. Path. u. Pharmakol., Leipz., 1881–2, xv, 22–80. ——. Ueber digitalisartig wirkende Arzneimittel. Schmidt's Jahrb., Leipz., 1883, cxcvii, 185–205. — Ueber die Beeinflussung der pheripheren Gefässe durch pharmakologische Agentien. Arch. f. exper. Path. u. Pharmakol., Leipz., 1886–7, xxii, 77–106. — **Laborde** (J.-V.) Du rôle de l'expérimentation dans la recherche et la détermination des succédanés, en thérapeutique. Tribune méd., Par., 1880, xii, 88–92. — **Leech** (D. J.) The relation of pharmacology to therapeutics. *In:* Six introductory lectures, 12°, Manche-ter, 1884, 49–78.—**Lépine** (R.) Sur l'action vaso-motrice de certains médicaments. Semaine méd., Par., 1887, vii, 113.— **Le Thière** (G.) Action physiologique de quelques médicaments sur l'homme sain et leur application en cas de maladie. *In his:* Études méd., 8°, Par., 1869, 70–112.— **Martin** (H. N.) The study of the physiological action of drugs. Tr. M. & Chir. Fac. Maryland, Balt., 1885, 79–92.—**Masoin & Bruylants.** Recherches expérimentales sur l'action physiologique des essences d'aspic, de lavande, de marjolaine et de romarin. Bull. Acad. roy. de méd. de Belg., Brux., 1879, 3. s., xiii, 547–562.—

Medicines (*Physiological action and investigation of*).

Matkevich (F.) O daiistvii alkogolya, strikhnina i opiya. [On the effects of alcohol, strychnia, and opium.] Med. Vestnik, St. Petersb., 1864, iv, 1; 9; 17.—**Mays** (T. J.) The action and antagonism of some drugs on the frog's ventricle. Therap. Gaz., Detroit, 1885, 3. s., i, 73–90. ———. A new and delicate method for determining the local sensory action of drugs. J. Physiol., Lond., 1886, vii, 458–462.—**Mérat** (F.-V.) Pharmacologie. Dict. d. sc. méd., Par., 1820, xli, 246–260.—**Mitscherlich.** Ueber die Einwirkung der Gerbesäure, der Thonerde und des Mangans auf den thierischen Organismus. Med. Ztg., Berl., 1838, vii, 213; 219; 229.—**Monro** (A.) An attempt to determine by experiments how far some of the most powerful medicines, viz, opium, ardent spirits, and essential oils, affect animals, by acting on those nerves to which they are principally applied, and thereby bringing the rest of the nervous system into sufferance by what is called sympathy of nerves; and how far these med cines affect animals, after being taken in by their absorbent veins, and mixed and conveyed with their blood in the course of its circulation; with physiological and practical remarks. Essays & Obs. Phil. Soc. Edinb., 1771, iii, 292–365.—**Moreau** (A.) Analyse de l'action physiologique des sulfates de magnésie et de soude. Compt. rend. Acad. d. sc., Par., 1879, lxxxviii, 737.—**Moretti** (E.) D' alcune sperienze sull' azione fisiologica dell' arsenico, del fosforo, degl i oduri di mercurio, e di altri energici rimedi. Gior. di med. mil., Torino, 1862, x, 436–441.—**Morries** (J. D.) Observations on the chemical and physiological properties of the empyreumatic oils of foxglove, henbane, and tobacco. Edinb. M. & S. J., 1833, xxxix, 377–383. *Also, Reprint.*—**Mosso** (A.) La pharmacologie expé imentale. Rev. scient., Par., 1876, 2. s., x, 523–526.—**Murray** (W.) On the therapeutic and physiological action of remedies. Med. Times & Gaz., Lond., 1865, i, 383. ———. The physical and physiological action of medicines. J. Anat. & Physiol., Lond., 1866–7, i, 319–322.—**Nechaev** (A.) Ob ugnetajoutshem vlijanii na otdelenie jeludochnago soka : atropina, morphija, chlorad-gidrata i razdrajenija chuvstvitelnich nervov. [Depressing action on arteries of atropine, etc.] Arch. klin., etc., St. Petersb., 1883, vii, 325–387.—**Nehrer.** Ueber Arzneiprüfungen an gesunden Menschen. Med. Jahrb. d. k. k. österr. Staates, Wien, 1842, xl, 160; 315.—**Oken.** Idee der Pharmakologie als Wissenschaft. Jahrb. d. Med. als Wissensch., Tübing., 1806–7, ii, 75–94.—**Padioleau.** De la réserve que doit apporter le praticien dans l'appréciation de l'action thérapeutique des médicaments. Bull. gén. de thérap., etc., Par., 1865, lxix, 219–224.—**Petrone** (L. M.) Contribuzione sperimentale sull' azione di certi farmaci sopra la mucosa respiratoria. Sperimentale, Firenze, 1883, li, 614–618. ———. Note di farmacologia sperimentale. Ann univ. di med. e chir., Milano, 1883, cclxiii, 539–556.—**Poiscuille.** Recherches expérimentales sur les médicaments. Compt. rend. Acad. d. sc., Par., 1844, xix, 994–1006.—**Purkinje** (J. E.) Einige Beiträge zur physiologischen Pharmacologie. N. Breslau. Samml. a. d. Geb. d. Heilk. . . . d. schles. Gesellsch. f. vaterl. Kult., Bresl., 1829, i, 423–444.—**Restelli** (A.) & **Strambio** (G.) Recherches et expériences sur cette question: Les médicaments narcotiques et les tétaniques agissent-ils sur le système nerveux directement ou par l'intermédiaire du sang veineux? Gaz. méd. de Par., 1847, 3. s., ii, 196.—**Ringer** (S.) Concerning the influence of season and of temperature on the action and on the antagonisms of drugs. J. Physiol., Lond., 1880–82, iii, 115–124.—**Ringer** (S.) & **Sainsbury** (H.) Concerning the action of salts of potash, soda, and ammonia on the frog's heart. Med.-Chir. Tr, Lond., 1882, lxv, 191–223, 3 diag. ———. On the influence of certain drugs on the period of diminished excitability. J. Physiol., Lond., 1883–4, iv, 350–364, 1 pl.—**Ross** (J.) Lecture on comparative pharmacology and therapeutics. Brit. M. J., Lond., 1875, i, 236–239.—**Rummo** (G.) Prolusione al corso universitario di farmacologia sperimentale e terapia. Med. contemp., Napoli, 1884, i, 297–310.—**Rutherford** (W.) An abstract of an experimental research on the physiological actions of drugs on the secretion of bile. Gaillard's M. J., N. Y., 1879, xxviii, 519–536.—**Sassezky** (N.) Ueber den Einfluss der Temperatur der Arzneien auf die Resorption derselben. St. Petersb. med. Wchnschr., 1880, v, 155.—**Scalzi** (F.) La formola chimica in servizio della farmacodinamia. Gazz. med. di Roma, 1886, xii, 145; 169.—**Schauenstein & Spaeth.** Ueber den Uebergang medicamentöser Stoffe aus dem Kreislaufe der Säugenden in ihre Milch und aus dem Kreislaufe der Schwangeren in ihr Fruchtwasser und ihren Fötus. Jahrb. f. Kinderh., Wien, 1858–9, ii, 13–18.—**Scherzer** (C.) Pharmakologische Skizzen, gesammelt auf einer Reise in Central-Amerika. Wchnbl. d. k.-k. Gesellsch. d. Aerzte zu Wien, 1856, ii, 149–154.—**Schneller.** Die Prüfung der Arzneimittel an Gesunden. Ztschr. d. k.-k. Gesellsch. d. Aerzte zu Wien, 1844, ii, 372–381.—**Scuotenti** o tetanizzanti di azione così detta elettiva. Pulsatilla, Rhus radicans, Rhus toxicodendron, segale cornuta, e ergotina. Ippocratico, Fano, 1871, 3. s., xx, 161–174.—**Shumovski**

Medicines (*Physiological action and investigation of*).

(V.) O pharmakologicheskikh izslaidovanii. [On pharmacological investigations.] Med. Vestnik, St. Petersb., 1863, iii, 437; 445. ———. Daiistvie dvuatomnikh tyazhilikh metallof na krof. [Effect of combinations of heavy metals on the blood, such as mercury, silver, zinc.] *Ibid.*, 1864, iv, 305; 321; 337; 353.—**Smith** (R. M.) Methods of studying the physiological action of drugs. Therap. Gaz., Detroit, 1884, n. s., v, 385; 490.—**Stiles** (R. C.) Action of medicines on the blood-vessels. Tr. M. Soc. County Kings, Brooklyn, Buffalo, 1865, ii, 3–30. *Also, Reprint.*—**Stokvis** (B.-J.) Sur les effets physiologiques des acides salicylique, paraoxybenzoïque, métaoxybenzoïque et orthocrésotinique (d'après des expériences instituées au Laboratoire pathologique d'Amsterdam par C. de Rooy). Cong. périod. internat. d. sc. méd. Compt.-rend., Amst., 1881, vi, pt. 2, 364–369.—**Stuart** (T. P. A.) On the physiological action of large doses of nickel and cobalt. Australas. M. Gaz., Sydney, 1883-4, iii, 9; 32.—**Święcicki** (H.) O wpływie koniny i niektorych przetworów sporyszu na skurcze pochwy. [Effect of conine and some preparations of Secale cornutum on the contraction of the vagina.] Gaz. lek., Warszawa, 1884, 2. s., iv, 463–465.—**Thomas** (H. O.) On the solution of the actions of remedies, and on the existence of nerves of inhibition as exemplified by the action of sedatives and stimulants. Med. Press & Circ., Lond., 1883, n. s., xxxv, 225; 248; 270.—**Verbeck** (W. J. L.) Mededeelingen uit het gebied der pharmacologie. Boerhaave. Tijdschr., etc., Amst., 1847, n. s., vi, 97: Gravenh., 1848, n. s., vii, 94. *Also, transl.:* Ann. méd. de la Flandre occid., Roulers, 1851, v, 441; 510; 536.—**Werneck** (V.) Beiträge zur Pharmakologie. Wchntl. Beitr. z. med. u. chir. Klin., Leipz., 1833-4, iii, 129–140.—**Wood** (H. C.) On the action of drugs upon the motor system of animals. Phila. M. Times. 1876–7, vii, 169–171.—**Wood** (H. C.) & **Reichert** (E. T.) A contribution to our knowledge of the action of certain drugs upon bodily temperature. J. Physiol., Lond., 1880–82, iii, 321–326.—**Zaikovski** (D.) O daiistvii na organizm phosphora, mwishyaka i surmi. [On the effects of phosphorus, arsenic, and antimony.] Med. Vestnik, St. Petersb., 1865, v, 290.

Medicines (*Prices and lists of*).

See, also, **Medicine-chests**; **Pharmacy** (*Legislation in relation to*).

APOTHEKER-TAXE für Kurhessen. 4°. *Cassel*, 1827.

AUGSBURG. Taxa, sive pretium medicamentorum simplicium, et compositorum, in officinis pharmaceuticis Augustanis usualium. fol. [*n. p., n. d.*]

AUSTRIA. Neue Apothecker Tax-Ordnung, oder der Werth und Preiss aller, so wohl einfachen, als zusamm-gesezten, theils chymisch-, theils Galenischen Artzeneyen, welche in denen Hof-Feld- und burgerlichen Stadt Wiennerischen Apothecken bey jetzigen Zeiten gebräuchig seynd; verfasset nach dem neu-aufgelegten Wiennerischen Dispensatorio pharmaceutico, aus allerhöchst königlichen Befehl dem allgemeinen Weesen, und königlichen Ærario, zum besten herausgegeben und publiciret. Mit besonderer königlichen Privilegio. fol. *Wienn*, 1744.

———. The same. fol. *Wien*, 1765.

———. *Ministerium des Innern.* Arznei-Taxe für das Jahr 1884 zur österreichischen Pharmakopöe vom Jahre 1869 und zum Anhange derselben vom Jahre 1878. 8°. *Wien*, 1884.

———. The same. Arznei-Taxe für das Jahr 1885 [etc.] 8°. *Wien*, 1885.

BASEL. Neue Apotheker-Taxe der Stadt Basel. sm. 4°. *Basel*, 1701.

BAVARIA. *Staatsministerium des Innern.* Arznei-Taxe für das Königreich Bayern. Abänderungen nach höchster Entschliessung des königl. Staatsministeriums des Innern vom 11. Dezember 1883. Amtliche Ausgabe. 8°. *München*, 1884.

BAWKER (H. L.) & Co. Price list and descriptive catalogue of extracts, acids, and essential oils, etc. 8°. *Boston*, 1884.

BETÆNKNING og Forslag til Grundsætninger, hvoref er en ny Medicinaltaxt antages at burde forfattes. [Prices for apothecaries.] 8°. *Christiania*, 1855.

Medicines (*Prices and lists of*).

BULLOCK & CRENSHAW. Catalogue of drugs, pharmaceutical preparations, utensils, apparatus, surgical instruments, anatomical preparations, etc. 8°. *Philadelphia*, 1860.

CHENEY & MYRICK. Druggists' hand-book of American and foreign drugs, their common English and botanical names, arranged in alphabetical order. 12°. *Boston*, 1878.

COMISO. Tariffa di medicamenti deliberata dalla Congregazione di Carità di Comiso il 7 febbrajo 1886. 12°. *Comiso*, 1886.

DRUGGIST'S (The) manual; being a price current of drugs . . . with Latin and English synonyms, a German, French, and Spanish catalogue of drugs, tables of specific gravities, etc. Compiled by direction of the Philadelphia College of Pharmacy. 8°. *Philadelphia*, 1826.

ELENCHUS medicamentorum una cum formulis medicinalibus in usum medicorum et pharmacopœorum nosodochia et institutiones publicas regni Bavariæ respicientum. Cura collegii in re medica supremi. 16°. *Monachii*, 1820.

DE LA FUENTE PIEROLA (G.) Tyrocinio pharmacopeo, methodo medico y chimico. En el qual se continen en los canones de Joanes Mesue Damasceno, y su explicacion . . . comprobada con el prohemio de Dioscorides y otras autores . . . añadida la tarifa general de precios de las medicinas simples y compuestas, que ha de aver, y venderse en las boticas. fol. *Pamplona*, 1721.

GUYBERT (P.) Le prix et valeur des médicamens.
In his: Toutes les œuvres charitables. Dernière éd. sm. 8°. *Paris*, 1647, 87–150.

HANSEN (G.) Supplement til Medicinaltaxten for 1885. 8°. *Christiania*, 1885.

HARMONIA et disharmonia taxarum. Das ist, Vergleichung der österreichischen, rheinländischen, ober- und nieder-sächsischen Apotheker-Taxe. Mit kurzen Anmerkungen, warum etliche Misshelligkeiten eingeschlichen. Allen Liebhabern der Medicin, Wund-Artzney und Apotheker-Kunst, wie auch jedem, der eine Familie hat sehr nützlich. sm. 4°. *Hannover u. Wolffenbüttel*, 1700.

HELLWIG (C.) Dreyfacher als Thüringisch-Meissnischer und Niedersächsischer Teutsch- und lateinischer Apotheker-Tax, darinne der Werth aller und jeder sowohl einfachen als zusammen gesetzten Artzneyen zu finden, samt einer nöthigen und aussführlichen Vorrede, wie solches Werck nicht nur alle Liebhaber der Medicin, der Artzney- und Wund-Artzney-Kunst Ergebene, desgleichen die Materialisten, sondern auch jedweder Hauss-Vater und Haus-Mutter in Städten und Dörffern sehr nützlich gebrauchen können. sm. 4°. *Franckfurt u. Leipzig*, 1714.

HESSE. Arzneimittel-Taxe für die Apotheken des Grossherzogthums Hessen. 8°. *Darmstadt*, 1884.

JIMENEZ (M.) Tarifa general farmacéutica, ó método general, fácil y sencillo de tasar recetas, que contien los precios de cuantos medicamentos se usan en el dia por los profesores de la ciencia de curar, y las reglas que deben observar los farmacéuticos para tasar las recetas que despachen en sus boticas, fundado todo en principios fijos y constantes para que haya uniformidad en el valor del honorario científico. 8°. *Madrid*, 1838.

KOCH (C. F.) Beitrag zur Revision der Medicinal-Taxen. 8°. *Merseburg*, 1847.

LEHMANN (M.) Reductions- und Arzneipreistabellen zur leichteren Berechnung der Arzneipreise auf Grund des Gesetzes, betreffend die Einführung eines allgemeinen Landes-Gewichtes vom 17. Mai 1856. 8°. *Schönebeck*, 1858.

Medicines (*Prices and lists of*).

MENIER. Catalogue commercial, ou prix courant général des drogues simples, produits pharmaceutiques et chimiques, plantes médicinales, médicaments spéciaux et homœopathiques, instruments de pharmacie, de chirurgie, de chimie, de physique et tous autres articles et appareils scientifiques et industriels à l'usage de la pharmacie et de la médecine. 5. éd. 8°. *Paris*, 1860.

MÜHLHAUSEN. Erneuert- und verbesserte Medicinal, Apotheker, Chirurgorum, und andere dahin gehörige Ordnungen, etc., samt beygefügt-revidirter Taxa, derer in hiesigen privilegirten Apotheken befindlicher Waaren und Artzneyen, auch selbigen ertheiltes Privilegium, etc. Eines Hoch Edlen und Hochweisen Raths der käyserlichen freyen- und des heiligen Reichs-Stadt Mühlhausen in Thüringen, K. K. Zu jedermanns Wissenschaft und Nachricht von neuem in den Druck gegeben. sm. 4°. *Mülhausen*, 1715.

——. Revidirte und erneuerte Apotheker-Taxa aller Medicamenten, Materialien, Specereyen und Waaren, welche man bey denen privilegirten und geschwornen Apothekern in der käyserlichen Reichs-Stadt Mülhausen zu kauffe findet. sm. 4°. *Mülhausen*, 1715.

NOVA pharmacopœorum taxa, seu ordo ac pretium omnium medicamentorum, tam simplicium quam compositorum, chymicorum, atque Galenicorum, moderno tempore in officinis publicis pharmaceuticis Viennensibus in Austria magis usualium, justa normam dispensatorii pharmaceutici Austriaco-Viennensis formata ac præparata, et ex . . . regio mandato in publici et ærarii emolumentum tradita et publicata. fol. *Viennæ Austriæ*, 1744.
Text Latin and German.

PAVIA. [Enactment regarding price-list for apothecaries, dated Pavia, September 7, 1823.] fol. *Pavia*, 1823.

PONTIN (M.) Anvisning till valet af läkemedel för allmänna sjukvarden, till inrättande af socken-apothek. 8°. *Stockholm*, 1816.

PORTUGAL. Regimento dos preços dos medicamentos simplices, preparados, e compostos, assim como se descrevem na farmacopea geral do reino, feito, e publicado por ordem de sua magestade El-Rei nosso senhor, para governo dos boticarios no reino de Portugal e Algarves. 8°. *Rio de Janeiro*, 1818.

——. Regimento dos preços das drogas medicinaes, e dos medicamentos preparados, simplices, e compostos, feito, e publicado por ordem de S. M. El-Rei nosso senhor, para governo dos boticarios dos reinos de Portugal, Algarves, e seus dominios. oblong 8°. *Lisboa*, 1831.

PRUSSIA. Königliche preussische und churfl. brandenburgische Medicinal-Edict und Ordnung; wie auch erneuerte Apothecker-Taxa, auff seiner königlichen Majestät allergnädigsten Verordnung aufs neue herausgegeben und publiciret, von der Collegio medico. Die 3. Aufl., mit dem französischen und andern Sachen vermehret, wovon die beygefügte Vorrede ausführliche Nachricht ertheilen wird. Mit Ihro königl. Majestät allergnädigsten Privilegio. sm. 4°. *Berlin*, 1715.

——. Revidirte und erneuerte Taxa, aller auf den Apotheken befindlicher Medicamenten. sm. 4°. *Berlin*, 1715.

——. Königlich preussische Arznei-Taxe für 1804; 1832; 1849; 1853; 1857–9; 1861–4; 1866–8; 1870–74; 1875–80; 1883–5. 4° & 8°. *Berlin*, 1804–85.

REGOLATIONE de pretii delle cose medicinali semplici, e composte, che si vendono nelle specia-

Medicines (*Prices and lists of*).

rie della magn. città di Verona. fol. *Verona*, [1696].

REVISED and enlarged manual of the active principles of indigenous and foreign medicinal plants, as prepared at the laboratory of B. Keith & Co., New York. 32°. *Jersey City*, 1882.

SAXONY. E. e. und hochweisen Raths der Stadt Leipzig vor die Apotheken daselbst auffgerichtete und von Churf. Durchl. zu Sachsen gnädigst confirmirte Ordnung und Taxa. sm. 4°. *Leipzig*, [1689].

———. Zweiter Nachtrag zur zehnten Auflage der Arznei-Taxe für das Königreich Sachsen auf das Jahr 1885. 8°. [*Dresden*, 1885.]

———. Zweiter Nachtrag zur fünften Auflage der thierärztlichen Arznei-Taxe für das Königreich Sachsen auf das Jahr 1885. 8°. [*Dresden*, 1885.]

SERVIA. Taksa apotekarska. [Standard prices of drugs.] 4°. *Beogrd*, 1881.

SOCIEDADE pharmaceutica Lusitana. Formulario dos preparados pharmaceuticos a que se refere o regimento dos preços dos medicamentos de 1854, não inseridos no Codigo pharmaceutico Lusitano. 8°. *Lisboa*, 1855.

DE SOUSA FERREIRA (M. J.) Preço corrente da pharmacia. 8°. *Porto*, 1858.

STRASSBURG Apotheker-Tax, oder Verzeichniss und Tax aller Arzneyen, welche sich, auf Befehl eines hochlöblichen Magistrats gedachter Stadt, in den Apotheken zu Strassburg nach der neuesten Verbesserung befinden, und befinden sollen. Dem Publico zum Besten öffentlich angezeiget in lateinisch-, deutsch- und französischer Sprache. 4°. *Strassburg*, 1760.

TASSA delle robbe medicinali tanta semplici quanto composte ad uso di questa illustrissima città di Modana et suo distretto. Dall' illustrissima communità, e dall' eccellentissimo collegio de signori medici con l' intervento delli eletti del collegio de spetiali, con ogni cautezza esattamente revista, et approvata il presente anno 1677. fol. *Modana*, 1677.

TASSA de medicinali semplici, composti, e spagirici, disposta con l' ordine dell' alfabeto e publicata dall' ... Collegio di medicina ed ..., compagnia degli speciali della città di Bologna l' anno mdcci. fol. *Bologna*, 1701.

TAXA anni mdcci, seu prætia Veneta rerum medicinalium, tam simplicium, tam compositarum. fol. [*Venetiis*, 1701.]

TAXA medicamentorum in pharmacopœa Austriaco-Provinciali emendata contentorum pro anno mdccvii. Taxe der in der umgearbeiteten österreichischen Provinzial-Pharmacopöe enthaltenen Arzneyen für das Jahr 1807. 12°. *Wien*, [1807].

TAXA pharmaceutica universalis, oder allgemeine Apothecker-Taxe, bestehend in der Augspurger, Brandenburger, Braunschweiger, Frankfurther, Leipziger, Nürnberger, Prager, Ulmer, Wiener, Würtemberger. Zu bequemen Gebrauch sämtlich neben einander in Tabellen gesetzt, [etc.] fol. *Nürnberg*, 1747.

TAXA seu pretium tam simplicium quam compositorum juxta dispensatorium Wirtenbergicum præparandorum et aliorum in officinis pharmaceuticis usualium medicamentorum mandato. Ducis adornatum et statutum. fol. *Stuttgardiæ*, 1741.

TAXATIO seu valor medicamentorum omnium, tam simplicium, quam compositorum, quæ in officina pharmaceutica Isnacensi præstant. Tax oder Werth aller Arzneyen, sowohl einfachen als zusammengesezten, welche in der Apotheken zu Eisenach zu finden. 8°. *Jena*, 1681.

Medicines (*Prices and lists of*).

TSENY lekarstvennuych vetshestve, nevoshedshich v aptekarskuju taksu, v g. S.-Peterburge, s 1 Jan. 1887 g. [Price-list of medical preparations not included in pharmaceutical tariff, for the city of St. Petersburg, Jan. 1, 1887.] 8°. *St. Petersburg*, 1887.

VALOR sive taxatio medicamentorum tam simplicium quam compositorum, quæ in officinis Francofurtanis prostant. Tax und Werth aller deren Artzneyen, welche in den Apothecken zu Frankfurt anzutreffen und zu finden. 4°. *Franckf. a. M.*, 1628.

VERORDNUNG des Ministers des Innern vom 28. October 1876, betreffend die neue österreichische Arznei-Taxe. 24°. [*Wien*, 1877?]

WEINLIG (C. G.) Index singulorum tam simplicium quam compositorum medicamentorum, quibus officina medicinalis quæ auspiciis serenissimæ principis regiæ et electoralis Dominæ Mariæ Antoniæ Dresdæ jam floret, instructa est, publicæ luci expositus. 4°. *Fridricostadii*, [1761].

WHITE (C.) A catalogue of the materia medica and of pharmaceutical preparations. 16°. *Boston*, 1817.

WITTSTEIN (G. C.) Arznei-Taxe der deutschen Staaten, oder: Vergleichende Uebersicht der neuesten Arznei-Taxen des Kaiserthums Oesterreich, Königreichs Bayern, Königreichs Würtemberg, Grossherzogthums Baden, Kurfürstenthums Hessen, Königreichs Sachsen, Königreichs Hannover und Königreichs Preussen. 4°. *Nürnberg*, 1843.

Act licensing apothecaries and druggists and regulating the sale of drugs. Rep. Bd. Health South Car., Columbia, 1882, iii, 117–120.—**Allerhöchste** Verordnung, die allgemeine Medicinal-Taxe für das Königreich Bayern betreffend. Ztschr. f. d. Staatsarznk., Erlang., 1836, xxxii, 140–156.—**Eisenmann.** Vorschläge zu einer Arznei-Taxe für Deutschland. Med. Argos, Leipz., 1840, iii, 257–260.—**Forhandlingen** af Opium og Morfin fra Apothekerne. [Sale of opium and morphine by apothecaries.] Ugesk. f. Læger, Kjøbenh., 1883, 4. R., viii, 73–77.—**Fristedt** (R. F.) Nyheter från pharmakologiska museum. Upsala Läkaref. Förh., 1869–70, v, 238–245.—**Gyógyszerek** árszabvanya. Taxa medicamentorum. Gyógyászat, Budapest, 1884, xxiii, 81; 97; 115; 130; 145; 165; 196; 232.—**Hjelt** (E. A.) Om handeln med gifter, jemte förslag till dess ordnande i Finland. [Trade in poisons, and proposition regulating the same in Finland.] Finska läk.-sällsk. handl., Helsingfors, 1870, xii, 73–115.—**Lista** de los medicamentos y utensilios que debe tener toda oficina farmacéutica, con determinacion de las cantidades mínimas de cada una, segun resolucion de la Facultad. Gac. méd., Lima, 1877, iii, 132–136.—**Monthly** list of the drugs on sale in the English market, with their prices and several duties. Lond. M. Gaz., 1839–40, xxv, 175.—**Müller** (B.) Ueber Arzneitaxe. Ztschr. f. Nat.- u. Heilk. in Ungarn, Oedenburg, 1859, x, 363; 378; 386; 395; 400: 1860, xi, 209; 249.—**Prix** des produits chimiques et pharmaceutiques. Abeille méd., Par., 1849, vi, 196–198.—**Quarterly** report of prices of substances employed in pharmacy. Lond. M. Reposit., 1817, vii, 174; 526: viii, 270; 544: 1818, ix, 262; 525: x, 262; 526: 1819, xi, 262; 534: xii, 271; 543: 1820, xiii, 279; 542: xiv, 262; 530: 1821, xv, 263; 526: xvi, 260; 526: 1822, xvii, 262; 526: xviii, 274; 542: 1823, xix, 262; 526: xx, 266: 1824, xxii, 526: 1825, xxiii, 526: xxiv, 294; 582: 1826, xxv, 286; 574: xxvi, 278; 562: 1827, xxvii, 278; 566: xxviii, 279.—**Tribunal** supremo de justicia; sentencia absolutoria por expendicion de drogas. Bol. de med. y cirug. de Jaen, 1881–2, iv, 24–28.—**Ulrich.** Bemerkungen über die königliche preussische Arznei-Taxe. Ztschr. f. d. Staatsarznk., Erlang., 1830, xxx, 237–252, 1 tab.—**Verordnung** des Ministeriums des Innern und des Ministeriums des Handels vom 31. December 1875 betreffend die Arzneitaxe mit Rücksicht auf das durch das Gesetz vom 23. Juli 1871, R. G. B. Jahrgang 1872, Nr. 16, eingeführte metrische Gewicht. Med.-chir. Centralbl., Wien, 1876, xi, 15.

Medicines (*Quack*).
See **Medicines** (*Patent, etc.*)

Medicines (*Secret*).
See **Medicines** (*Patent, etc.*)

Medicines (*Specific*).
See, also, **Medicines** (*Patent, etc.*)

BAUER (G. F.) * De specifica quorundam remediorum efficacia. 4°. *Halæ Magdeb.*, [1727].

Medicines (Specific).

BOYLE (R.) De specificorum remediorum cum corpusculari philosophia concordia. Cui accessit dissertatio de varia simplicium medicamentorum utilitate usuque. Ex Anglico . . . trad. D. A. 16°. *Londini*, 1686.

———. Nouveau traité sur la convenance des remèdes spécifiques avec la philosophie des corpuscules, et sur l'usage et les propriétez des médicamens simples. De la traduction de Rostagny. 18°. *Lyon*, 1689.

ECHTE (P. G.) * De specificis. 4°. *Gottingæ*, [1805].

GASTELLIER. Des spécifiques en médecine. 8°. *Paris*, 1783.

HALBMAYER (J. M.) * De cauto specificorum usu et commendatione. 4°. [*Erlangæ*, 1765.]

HENNIG (E. A.) * Adnotationes quædam de medicamentis specificis. 8°. *Halis*, 1847.

DE JONG (P.) * De specificiis. 4°. *Lugd. Bat.*, 1693.

KINDLER (E. E.) * De remediorum specificorum notione. 8°. *Francof. ad Viadr.*, [1804].

KLIMM (J. C.) * De medicamentis specificis, eorumque agendi modo. 4°. [*Halæ Magdeb.*, 1694.]

MAYER (E. R.) Hints towards a better knowledge of some of the methods of, and substances used in, specific medication; a paper read before the Luzerne County Medical Society, at Pittston, Pa., Sept. 13, 1876. 8°. [*Wilkesbarre, Pa.*], 1876.

MILDE (G. G.) * De specificis eorumque operandi modo et usu. 4°. *Halæ*, 1747.

MOLIN (L.-J.-J.) * Des spécifiques en médecine. 4°. *Paris*, 1847.

SCUDDER (J. M.) Specific medication and specific medicines. 8°. *Cincinnati*, 1870.

———. The same. Revised, with an appendix containing the articles published on the subject since the first edition. And a report of cases illustrating specific medication. 4. ed. 8°. *Cincinnati*, 1873.

———. The same. 5. ed. 8°. *Cincinnati*, 1874.

SPEYER (C. F.) * De remediis specificis sic dictis. 4°. *Jenæ*, [1800].

Boisseau (F.-G.) Quelques considérations sur les spécifiques; lues à la Société médicale d'émulation. J. univ. d. sc. méd., Par., 1826, xliii, 276–292. *Also*, Reprint.—**Brefeld.** Warum leisten manche als spezifik empfohlene Mittel nicht immer was von ihren Urhebern gerühmt wird, warum heilt die Sabina nicht immer Gicht? Allg. med. Ann., Altenb., 1803, 39–45.—**Busi** (C.) Del caustico di Canquoin e dello specificismo secreto. Ippocratico, Fano, 1863, 3. s., iii, 148–155.—**Dührsen** (H. C.) Ueber specifische Mittel. Mitth. a. d. Geb. d. Med., Altona, 1836, iv, 11. Hft., 16.—**Fiorito** (G.) Considerazioni sopra i rimedii specifici. Gior. d. sc. med., Torino, 1839, iv, 11–86.—**Frey** (H.) Ueber specifische Heilmittel. Arch. f. physiol. Heilk., Stuttg., 1853–4, xii, 99–111.—**Gedanken** von specifischen Mitteln. Abhandl. u. Beob. v. einer Gesellsch. v. Aerzten in Hamb., 1776, 255–273.—**Gobée** (C.) Specifieke methode en specifieke middelen. Pract. Tijdschr. v. de Geneesk., Gorinchem, 1856, n. s., ii, 513; 592.—**Griesselich** (L.) Die nichtspecifische Heilkunde und die exanthematische Heilmittel. Berl. med. Centr.-Ztg., 1839, viii. 759–765.—**Hecker** (A. F.) Versuche, die eigentliche Würkungsart solcher Mittel zu bestimmen, die oft als spezifische angesehen werden. Arch. f. d. allg. Heilk., Berl., 1790, i, 38–76.—**Mühry** (A.) Die exanthematischen Arzneisymptome und die specifische Heilkunde. Wchnschr. f. d. ges. Heilk., Berl., 1839, 461–472.—**Nye** (E. B.) Specifics. Proc. Connect. M. Soc. 1864–7, N. Haven, 1867, n. s., ii, 120–125. — **d'Orneilas** (A.-E.) Des prétendus spécifiques. J. de thérap., Par., 1879, vi, 292–298.—**Tanchou.** Considérations sur l'existence et sur la nature des spécifiques. Rev. méd. franç. et étrang., Par., 1826, iv, 202–208.—**Vacquié.** Considérations sur l'action réelle des médicamens dits spécifiques d'organes, introduits dans l'économie animale par voie d'absorption. J. compl. du dict. d. sc. méd., Par., 1826, xxv, 332–345.—**Walther** (J. A.) Kritische Bemerkungen über die Behandlung mit Specificis im gewöhnlichen Sinne, hinsichtlich der flechtenartigen und herpetischen Ausschläge insbesondere. Allg. med. Ann., Altenb., 1812, 66–78. — Von dem Begriff der Specifika und ihrer Wahrheit. J. d. pract. Heilk., Berl., 1839, lxxxviii, 5. St., 62–92.

Medicines (Testing of).

See **Medicines** (Adulterations, etc., of); **Medicines** (Physiological action, etc., of).

Medicines (Tolerance of).

See **Therapeutics**.

Medicinisch-chemische Untersuchungen.

Aus dem Laboratorium für angewandte Chemie zu Tübingen, hrsg. von Felix Hoppe-Seyler. Hft. 1–4, May 5, 1866–71. 1 v. 593 pp. 8°. *Berlin, A. Hirschwald.*
Completed.

Medicinisch-chirurgische Aufsätze,

Krankengeschichten und Nachrichten. Eine Fortsetzung des Taschenbuchs für deutsche Wundärzte. Hrsg. von Fr. Aug. Waitz. v. 1, 1791. 8°. *Altenburg.*
v. 2 and 3 wanting.

Medicinisch-chirurgische Bibliothek,

von Johann Clemens Tode. v. 1–10, 1775–87. 8°. *Copenhagen.*
Completed.

Medicinisch-chirurgische Gesellschaft in Hamburg.

Mittheilungen aus dem Gebiete der gesammten Heilkunde. 2 v. xii, 388 pp., 1 l., 2 tab., 1 pl.; 3 p. l., 437 pp. 8°. *Hamburg, Hoffmann u. Campe*, 1830–33.

Medicinisch-chirurgische Gesellschaft des Kantons Zürich.

Denkschrift zur Feier des fünfzigsten Stiftungstages den 7. Mai 1860. 171 pp., 7 pl. 4°. *Zürich, Zurcher u. Furrer*, 1860.

Medicinisch-chirurgische *Josephs-Academie.*

B. Die med.-chirurg. Josephs-Akademie in Wien. Eine historisch-kritische Skizze. Allg. Ztg. f. Mil.-Aerzte, Brnschwg., 1845, iii, 289; 316.—**Flögel** (J.) Aufhebung, Fortbestand oder Umstaltung der medicinisch-chirurgischen Josephs-Academie. Oesterr. med. Wchnschr., Wien, 1848, 966–970. — **Gegenwärtige** Wintervorlesungen in der k. k. Josephinischen Akademie zu Wien. Med. Nat.-Ztg. f. Deutschl., Altenb., 1798, i, 173.—**von Töltenyi.** Aufhebung oder Umstaltung der k. k. medicinisch-chirurgischen Josephs-Academie. Oesterr. med. Wchnschr., Wien, 1848, 673–682.—**Verzeichniss** der in den Schuljahren 1833–40 an der medicinisch-chirurgischen Josephs-Academie graduirten Doctoren der Chirurgie, Magister der Geburtshülfe und Augenheilkunde. Med. Jahrb. d. k. k. österr. Staates, Wien, 1835, n. F., ix, 2: 1837, xiii, 189: 1838, xvii, 104: 1840, xxiii, 167: 1841, xxvii, 89.—**Wort** (Ein) zu seiner Zeit, die k. k. medic. chirurg. Josephinische Akademie zu Wien betreffend. Med.-chir. Ztg., Salzb., 1794, ii, 321–334: iii, 49–75.

Medicinisch-chirurgische Journal-Revue.

Beilage des "Med.-chir. Centralblattes". Hrsg. von Christ. Ludwig Praetorius. Jahrg. 1876–87. 8°. *Wien.*
Current. Want no. 12 in 1878; nos. 4, 15, in 1880; title and index for 1881.

Medicinisch-chirurgische Monatshefte.

Kritisches Sammeljournal für praktische Heilkunde. Hrsg. von Fr. Emil Friedrich und Alfred Vogel in München. [2 v. annually.] v. 1–15, 1857–64. 8°. *Erlangen, F. Enke.*
A continuation of: **Neue** medicinisch-chirurgische Zeitung. In 1860 Vogel dropped and W. Brattler added; in 1861 Brattler dropped; in 1863 O. v. Franque and A. Geigel became editors.

Medicinisch-chirurgische Rundschau.

Monatsschrift für die gesammte praktische Heilkunde des In- und Auslandes. Hrsg. von Ph. Markbreiter und Jo. Schnitzler. v. 3–28, 1862–87. 25 v. 8°. *Wien.*
Current. Want Jan., 1873. See: **Revue** der Wiener Medizinal-Halle for v. 1–2, 1860–61. v. 19 edited by Karl Bettelheim; in 1879 W. F. Loebisch became editor.

Medicinisch-chirurgische Zeitschrift für Landärzte und Chirurgen.

Hrsg. von Franz Andreas Ott. [4 Nos. form 1 v.] v. 2–3, 1832–5. 2 v. 8°. *München.*
Title of v. 1 was: **Zeitschrift** der praktischen Medicin, Chirurgie und Geburtshilfe [etc.]

Medicinisch-chirurgische Zeitung. Hrsg. von J. J. Hartenkeil und F. X. Mezler. [Issued every 4 days; 4 v. annually.] 1790–1839. 200 v. 8°. Nebst 43 Ergänzungsbänden. *Salzburg, F. X. Oberer,* 1790–1820; *Innsbruck,* 1821–39.

In 1794 Mezler dropped; Hartenkeil died June 7, 1808; in 1808 J. N. Ehrhart became editor. Continued as: **Neue** medicinisch-chirurgische Zeitung.

Medicinisch-chirurgisches Centralblatt. Organ der praktischen Aerzte. Redaction von Ch. L. Praetorius. [Weekly.] v. 11–22, 1876–87. 12 v. 4°. *Wien.*

Current. Contains a supplement: **Medicinisch-chirurgische** Journal-Revue.

Medicinisch - chirurgisches Correspondenz-Blatt für deutsch-amerikanische Aerzte. In Verbindung mit Dr. Meisburger [*et al.*] hrsg. und redigirt von Marcell Hartwig. [Monthly.] v. 1–2, 1883, to July, 1884. 8°. *Buffalo, N. Y.*

Completed. No. 19, July, 1884, last published.

Medicinisch-chirurgisches Journal.

Was title of v. 3–5, 1798–1804, of: **Medicinisches** Journal (J. C. Tode).

Medicinisch - chirurgisch - therapeutisches Wörterbuch, oder Repertorium der vorzüglichsten Kurarten, die in dem Zeitraume von 1750 bis 1838, mit Rückblicken auf die ältere und älteste Zeit, von den berühmtesten Aerzten Deutschlands, Englands, Frankreichs und Italiens angewendet und empfohlen worden sind. Hrsg. durch einen Verein von Aerzten. Mit einem Vorworte des Prof. Dr. Barez. 3 v. 8°. *Berlin, A. Duncker,* 1839–40.

Medicinisch - chymisch- und alchemistisches Oraculum, darinnen man nicht nur alle Zeichen und Abkürzungen, welche so wohl in den Recepten und Büchern der Aerzte und Apotheker, als auch in den Schriften der Chemisten und Alchemisten vorkom₁en, findet, sondern dem auch ein sehr rares chymisches Manuscript eines gewissen Reichs . . . beygefüget. Neue Auflage, nebst einem Auszug aus einem Briefe eines grossen Alchemisten an einen Unglaubigen. 2 p. l., 74 pp. 8°. *Ulm,* 1783.

Medicinische Aehrenlese. Eine Zeitschrift für die wissenschaftlich - praktische Gesammtheilkunde. Hrsg. von August Droste. [Monthly.] v. 1–10, 1856–65. 8°. *Osnabrück.*

Completed.

Medicinische Analecten. Wochenschrift für praktische Aerzte. Unter Mitwirkung mehrerer Fachgenossen hrsg. von Hermann Rahn. [Weekly.] Nos. 1–21, 24, Jan. 1 to June, 1870. 88 pp., 44 l. 4°. *Harzgerode, W. Grupe.*

Each no. contains 4 pp., not numbered.

Medicinische Anekdoten; oder Sammlung besonderer Fälle, welche in die Anatomie, Pharmaceutik, Naturgeschichte, etc., einschlagen, nebst einigen merkwürdigen Nachrichten von den berühmtesten Aerzten, aus dem Französischen übersetzt. 2. Th. in 1 v. 19 p. l , 256, 255 pp. 8°. *Frankfurt u. Leipzig,* 1767.

Medicinische Annalen; eine Zeitschrift herausgegeben von den Mitgliedern der grossherzoglich-badischen Sanitäts-Commission in Carlsruhe und den Vorstehern der medicinischen, chirurgischen und geburtshülflichen Anstalten in Heidelberg, F. A. B. Puchelt, M. J. Chelius und F. C. Nägele. v. 1–13, 1835–48. 8°. *Heidelberg, J. C. B. Mohr.*

Continuation of: **Heidelberger** klinische Annalen. Completed.

Medicinische Anordnung wegen der jetzt an vielen Orten grassirenden Fleck-Fieber, wie sich besonders die Leute auf dem Lande dabey zu verhalten haben, die entweder keinen Medicum haben, oder nicht bezahlen können. 28 pp. 4°. *Schneeberg,* 1759.

Medicinische Anweisung wegen der tollen Hundewuth [followed by "Vorschrift für die Wundärzte und Barbierer, besonders auf Dörfern, was sie im ersten Anfang bei den von wüthigen Thieren gebissenen Menschen zu beobachten haben"]. 36, iv pp., 1 pl. 4°. *Stuttgart, C. F. Cotta,* 1782.

Medicinische-Arcana zu Herstellüng aller Gebrechen des menschlichen Körpers und Erhaltung eines langen Lebens; aber Alles nach dem Willen Gottes, seiner Gnade ünd Barmherzigkeit. 18 l. 4°. [*n. p., n. d.*]

Medicinische (Der) Bernhäuter, vorgestellet in einem lustigen Discours, ehe dessen in calenctischer Sprache herausgegeben, auf inständiges Begehren aber anjetzo verteutscht durch Septimus Podagra, M. D. 2 p. l., 120 pp. 12°. [*n. p.*], 1720.

Medicinische Bibel, oder die Gesundheits-Störungen und ihre Ausgleichung. 2 v. iv, 219; 224 pp., 1 l. 8°. *Leipzig, I. Müller,* 1845.

Medicinische Bibliographie und Anzeiger zum Centralblatt für die gesammte Medicin, bearbeitet von Arthur Würzburg. [Weekly.] v. 1–5, March 3, 1883-7. 8°. *Leipzig, Breitkopf u. Härtel.* Current.

Medicinische Bibliothek. Hrsg. von J. F. Blumenbach. v. 1–3, 1783–8. 12°. *Göttingen, Dieterich.*

Medicinische Böcke, von Aerzten, welche sich für infallible Herren über Leben und Tod halten, in der Cholera geschossen. XXXX—weniger I. 24 pp. 4°. *Bocksdorf u. Schussbach, S. Tresser u. Comp.,* [1832, vel subseq.].

Medicinische Briefe. Beobachtungen und Erfahrungen in der Wissenschaft und am Krankenbette. Von I. Hoppe. [Monthly.] Hft. 1, 2, 4, Jahrg. 1, 1854; Jahrg. 2, 1855. 2 v. 8°. *Freiburg im Breisgau, Herder.*

Medicinische und chirurgische Berlinische wöchentliche Nachrichten von D. Samuel Schaarschmidt, nebst einer Vorrede D. Friedrich Hoffmanns. v. 1–3, 1738–40. 4°. *Berlin, J. A. Rüdiger,* 1742.

Medicinische Chronik. Hrsg. von Joseph Eyerel. v. 1–3, 1793–4. 8°. *Wien, Meyer u. Patzowsky.*

v. 3 edited by Eyerel and Sallaba.

Medicinische Denkwürdigkeiten aus der Vergangenheit und Gegenwart für practische Aerzte. In monatlichen Lieferungen hrsg. von Dr. Albert Sachs. v. 1 (Nos. 1–6), July to Dec., 1834. 608 pp. 8°. *Berlin, A. Hirschwald.* Completed.

Medicinische Ephemeriden; nebst einer medicinischen Topographie der Grafschaft Ravensberg. xii, 268 pp., 5 tab. 12°. *Chemnitz, K. G. Hofmann,* 1793.

Medicinische Ephemeriden von Berlin. Hrsg. von Dr. L. Formey, 1. Bd. in 4 Hft., 1799–1800. 12°. *Berlin, Nauck.*

Medicinische Facultät zu Heidelberg. Beleuchtung der von der medicinischen Facultät zu Heidelberg gegen die Errichtung der neuen badischen Irrenanstalt erhobenen Einwürfe. 19 pp. 8°. [*Heidelberg,* 1837.]

Medicinische Fakultät in Würzburg. Herrn Franz von Rinecker ihrem hochverdiensten Senior, bringt zum 31. März 1877, an welchem Tage derselbe vor 40 Jahren seine Lehrthätigkeit als Professor begann, die medicinische Fakultät in Würzburg ihre besten Glückwünsche und ihren aufrichtigen Dank dar. 42 pp., 2 pl. 4°. *Leipzig, W. Engelmann,* 1877.

—— Festschrift zur dritten Säcularfeier der Alma Julia Maximiliana, gewidmet von der . . . 2 v. 2 p. l., 308 pp., 8 pl.; 1 p. l., 305 pp., 9 pl. imp. 4°. *Leipzig, F. C. W. Vogel,* 1882.

Medicinische Geschichte des russisch-türkischen Feldzugs in den Jahren 1828 und 1829 von Seidlitz, Petersenn, Rinck und Witt neu hrsg. und mit kritischen Anmerkungen begleitet von Dr. Friedrich Alexander Simon. 1 p. l., 292 pp., 2 pl. 12°. *Hamburg, Hoffmann u. Campe,* 1854.

Medicinische Gesellschaft zu Leipzig. Verhandlungen. v. 1 (1863–4). xv, iv, 205 pp., 2 l., 159 pp. 8°. *Leipzig, Veit u. Comp.,* 1864.

———. Bericht über die wissenschaftlichen Vorträge der . . . in den Jahren 1875 und 1876. 52 pp. 8°. *Leipzig, F. C. W. Vogel,* 1877.

———. Statuten. 8 pp. 8°. [*n. p., n. d.*]

Medicinische (Der) Hausfreund. Redacteur: Dr. Th. Köhler. [Semi-monthly.] v. 1–2, Dec. 12, 1880, to Dec. 30, 1882. 8° & 4°. *Cassel.*
Title of nos. 1–2, v. 1, was: **Hausfreund** (Der).

Medicinische Jahrbücher. Wien, 1861–87. *See* **Medizinische** Jahrbücher.

Medicinische Jahrbücher für das Herzogthum Nassau. Aus Auftrag der Landes-Regierung. Hrsg. von J. B. von Franque, W. Fritze, P. Thewalt und C. Vogler. Hfte. 1–23, 1843–66. 10 v. 8°. *Wiesbaden, A. Scholz.*
1851–5 also under title: **Mittheilungen** des Vereins nassauischer Aerzte an seine Mitglieder. In 1866, edited by L. C. T. Heydenreich, W. Fritze, and Edward Bickel.

Medicinische Jahrbücher des kaiserlich-königlichen österreichischen Staates. Hrsg. von den Directoren und Professoren des Studiums der Heilkunde an der Universität zu Wien. v. 1–6, 1811–21. Neue Folge, v. 1–3, 1822–6. Neueste Folge, v. 1–57, 1829–48. 66 v. 8°. *Wien, C. F. Beck.*
From 1841 to 1848, also: " **Oesterreichische** medicinische Wochenschrift als Ergänzung der medicinischen Jahrbücher des kaiserlich-königlichen österreichischen Staates". v. 11, 1832, hrsg. von Dr. A. J. Freyherrn von Stifft, und redigirt von Dr. Joh. Nep. Ed. von Raiman; v. 21, 1837, Stifft dropped; v. 23, S. C. Fischer, A. Rosas, and Joh. Wisgrill added; v. 60, 1847, Raiman dropped and Dr. Wil. Ed. v. Well added. In 1829: **Beobachtungen** und Abhandlungen aus dem Gebiete der gesammten praktischen Heilkunde, merged in this journal.

Medicinische Literatur für practische Aerzte. Hrsg. von Joh. Christ. Traugott Schlegel. Theil 1–12, 1781–9. In 9 v. 8°. *Leipzig, C. F. Schneider.*
v. 12 contains index to v. 1–12. Continued as: **Neue** medicinische Literatur [etc.]; also, in 1795–7, as: **Schlegels** Uebersicht der neuesten medicinischen Literatur.

Medicinische Litteratur des Jahres 1794. Hrsg. von Paul Usteri. Erste Hälfte. 1 v. 616 pp. 8°. *Leipzig, P. P. Wolf,* 1795.
A continuation of: **Repertorium** der medicinischen Litteratur, Zürich.

Medicinische Merkwürdigkeiten für Criminalrichter, Aerzte und Prediger. xvi, 352 pp. 8°. *Cassel, Cramer,* 1805.

Medicinische Neuigkeiten; ein Intelligenzblatt für praktische Aerzte. Herausgeber: Dr. Kastner. [Weekly.] v. 1–35, 1851–85. 4°. *Erlangen, J. J. Palm u. Enke.*
In v. 3 A. Wintrich became editor; in v. 35 Aloys Martin editor. In 1870–85, title: **Medicinische** Neuigkeiten für praktische Aerzte.

Medicinische Novitäten. Rundschau auf dem Gebiete der medicinischen Literatur. Hrsg. von O. Reyher. [Semi-monthly.] Nos. 1–12, v. 1, 1884. 8°. *Leipzig, Denicke.*

Medicinische (Die) Praxis der bewährtesten Aerzte unserer Zeit, systematisch dargestellt. Zweite durchaus umgearbeitete und ansehnlich vermehrte Ausgabe. Bartels, Baumgärtner, *et al.* 2 v. in 3. xii, 1115 pp.; xii pp., 1 l., 1408 pp. 8°. *Berlin u. Wien, Veit u. Comp. u. C. Gerold,* 1840–41.

Medicinische Reform. Eine Wochenschrift, erschienen vom 10. Juli 1848 bis zum 29. Juni

Medicinische Reform—continued.
1849. Hrsg. von R. Virchow und R. Leubuscher. 1 v. 276 pp. 4°. *Berlin, G. Reimer.*
Completed.

Medicinische Repetitorien u. Examinatorien. 5. Bd. Repetitorium der Physiologie des Menschen, nebst beigefügtem Examen von Dr. C. Kolb. 16°. *Stuttgart, A. Krabbe,* 1864.

Medicinische Unterhaltungs-Bibliothek, oder Collectiv-Blätter von heiterem und ernstem Colorite für alte und junge Aerzte. v. 1–10, 1838–43. 8°. *Leipzig, W. Engelmann.*
Completed. Continued as: **Medicinisches** u. naturw. Unterhaltungs-Magazin.

Medicinische (Der) Unterricht an der Wiener Hochschule und seine Gebrechen. Von einigen Studirenden. 24 pp. 8°. *Wien, G. J. Manz,* 1869.

Medicinische Zeitung. Hrsg. von dem Verein für Heilkunde in Preussen. [Weekly.] v. 1–26, Sept. 5, 1832, to Dec. 30, 1857. fol. Neue Folge. v. 1–3, 1858–60. fol. & 4°. *Berlin, T. C. F. Enslin.*
In 1858, E. Müller became editor. Continued as: **Preussische** Medicinal-Zeitung.

Medicinische Zeitung des Auslandes. Redigirt von Dr. Kalisch. No. 4, v. 2, Jan. 14, 1834. fol. *Berlin, E. S. Mittler.*

Medicinische Zeitung Russlands, redigirt und hrsg. von den DDrr. M. Heine, R. Krebel und H. Thielmann. [Weekly.] v. 1–17, 1844–60. 16 v. 4°. *St. Petersburg.*
Want v. 2, 1845, and nos. 2, 29 in 1851. Followed, in July, 1861, by: **St. Petersburger** medicinische Zeitschrift.

Medicinischer Almanach für das Jahr 1836. [Also for 1837–84.] 49 v. 8°. *Berlin, C. Heymann.*
v. 2–13 edited by J. J. Sachs. After 1846, title: **Sachs'** medicinischer Almanach. In 1847–8 edited by W. Hoffbauer; in 1849 by Dr. Abarbanell; in 1850 *et seq.* by L. Posner.

Medicinischer Argos. Hrsg. von H. A. Hacker und Hobl. Bde. 1–6 à 3 Hfte., 1839–45. 8°. *Leipzig, O. Wigand.*
Title of v. 6 is: **Argos**: Zeitschrift für Kritik und Anti-Kritik auf dem Gesammtgebiete der Medicin. In v. 4–6 Hacker sole editor.

Medicinischer Briefwechsel von einer Gesellschaft Aerzte hrsg. St. 1–2, 1785–6. 8°. *Halle, J. J. Gebauer.*

Medicinisches Bedencken, wie man bey Infections-Zeiten sich sowohl preservative als curative zu verhalten habe. *See* **Saxony.**

Medicinisches Conversationsblatt. Hrsg. von Dr. Carl Hohnbaum und Dr. Ferdinand Jahn. v. 1–3, 1830–32. 4°. *Hildburghausen.*
Completed.

Medicinisches Conversations- und Correspondenzblatt für die Aerzte im Königreich Hannover. Hrsg.: Dr. Schneemann. [Semi-monthly.] Jahrg. 5, April, 1854, to March, 1855. 1 v. 188 pp. 4°. *Hannover, Helwing.*

Medicinisches Correspondenzblatt. 1801–5.
An appendix to: **Allgemeine** medizinische Annalen.

Medicinisches Correspondenz-Blatt bayerischer Aerzte. Unter Mitwirkung vieler Aerzte hrsg. von Dr. Heinrich Eichhorn. [Weekly.] Jahrg. 1–11, 1840–50. 8°. *Erlangen, F. Enke.*
Completed.

Medicinisches Correspondenz-Blatt rheinischer und westfälischer Aerzte. Hrsg. von F. Nasse und J. F. H. Albers. [Fortnightly.] v. 1–4, 1842–5. 4°. *Bonn, H. B. König.*
Completed.

Medicinisches Correspondenz-Blatt des württembergischen ärztlichen Vereins. Aus Auftrag desselben hrsg. von J. F. Blumhardt [*et al.*]. v. 1–57, March 1, 1832–87. 4°. *Stuttgart, J. B. Metzler.*
Current. v. 47 *et seq.* edited by C. B. Arnold, O. Köstlin and J. Teuffel. 40 nos. form 1 v. Indexes to v. 1–55 accompany.

Medicinisches Jahrbuch. Kurze Darstellung der für die praktischen Aerzte wichtigsten Fortschritte auf dem Gebiete der Medicin. In Verbindung mit zahlreichen Faehmännern hrsg. von Paul Börner. Jahrg. 1, 1877. 8°. *Leipzig, R. E. Kloz,* 1878–9.

Medicinisches Jahrbuch der Thermalquellen von Teplitz-Schönau in Böhmen. Begründet und hrsg. von Franz X. Berthold und Joseph Seiche. Jahrg. 1855. Der ganzen Reihe 4. Hft. 218 pp. 8°. *Leipzig, Meissen u. Riesa.*

Medicinisches Journal. Von E. G. Baldinger. v. 1–9, 1784–96. 8°. *Göttingen, J. C. Dieterich.*
    Continued as: **Neues** medicinisches und physisches Journal.

Medicinisches Journal. Von D. Johann Clemens Tode. v. 1–5, à 4 Hfte., 1793–1804. 8°. *Kopenhagen u. Leipzig, A. Nitschke.*
    Completed. Title of v. 3–5, 1798–1804, was: **Medicinisch-chirurgisches** Journal.

Medicinisches Journal über allerhand in die Arzneywissenschaft und deren Ausübung einschlagende Materien. Hrsg. von Gottwald Schuster. Theil 1–5, 1767–70. 2 v. 8°. *Chemnitz.*

Medicinisches und naturwissenschaftliches Unterhaltungs - Magazin. Eine Monatsschrift von heiterm und ernstem Colorite für alte und junge Aerzte, wie für Freunde der Natur- und Heilkunde überhaupt. [Monthly.] Jahrg. 8–9, Jan., 1845, to Dec., 1846. 2 v. 8°. *Nordhausen u. Leipzig, B. G. H. Schmidt.*
    Title of: Jahrg. 1–6, 1838–43, was: **Medicinische** Unterhaltungs-Bibliothek, [etc.] Jahrg. 7, 1844, wanting.

Medicinisches Reformblatt für Sachsen. Hrsg. von G. B. Günther, Millies, Clotar Müller, Hugo Sonnenkalb und Winter. Organ des Ausschusses der sächsischen Aerzte. v. 1–3, July, 1848–50. 4°. *Leipzig, O. Klemm.*
    Completed. At first published fortnightly; in Oct., 1848, became weekly; in Jan., 1850, became monthly. No. 9, v. 3, 1850, issued March 3, 1851, was the last published.

Medicinisch - klinisches Institut der k. Ludwig-Maximilians-Universität zu München. Arbeiten des . . . hrsg. von Dr. H. v. Ziemssen und Dr. Jos. Bauer. v. 1. 8°. *Leipzig,* 1884.

Medicinisch-physischen (Ueber die) Lehranstalten der ganzen Welt. 2. St., über Wien. 48 pp. 16°. *Wien,* [1796].

Medicinisch-politische Blätter, oder Mittheilungen für die Reformen im Medicinal-Wesen. In zwanglosen Lieferungen. Lieferungen 1–11, June 20 to Nov. 17, 1848. 1 v. 640 pp. 8°. *Nürnberg.*
    Dr. von Jan, editor.

Medicinisch-practische Bibliothek, worin Nachrichten von den neuesten zur Ausübung der Heilkunde gehörigen Schriften und Vorfällen geliefert werden. Von Johann Andreas Murray. v. 1–3, 1774–80. 12°. *Göttingen, J. C. Dieterich.*

Medicinisch - therapeutisches Wörterbuch, etc.
    See **Siegert** (Johann Christoph). 8°. *Berlin,* 1856.

Medicinsk Tidning. [Weekly.] Nos. 1–20. Sept. 3, 1818, to Jan. 28, 1819. 4°. *Stockholm, A. Gadelius.*

Medicinske Selskab i Christiania. Forhandlinger i det medicinske Selskab i Christiania om Forplantelsesmaaden af Cholera. 106 pp., 1 map. 8°. [*Christiania,* 1854.]
    Bound with: Actstykker angaaende Cholera-Epidemien. 8°. *Christiania,* 1854.

Medicinskt Archiv. Utgifvet af läkarne vid Carolinska Institutet i Stockholm, redigeradt af E. A. Key, C. J. Rossander, S. G. Troilius. v. 1–3, 1863, to Aug., 1868. 8°. *Stockholm, Samson & Wallin.*
    In no. 3, v. 1, Troilius dropped and A. Kjellberg added. v. 3 contains, also, "Tillaggshäfte", 170 pp. Continued as: Nordiskt medicinskt Arkiv.

Medicis (De) quos Halberstadiensis, Quedlinburgensis, Wernigerodensis ditio vel genuit vel aluit. viii, 90 pp. 8°. *Halberstadii,* 1840.

del Medico (Giuseppe). Anatomia per uso dei pittori e scultori. 84 pp., 38 pl. fol. *Roma, V. Poggioli,* 1811.

Medico (Il) di Casa. Giornale di igiene e medicina popolare ; diretto dal Professore Paolo Mantegazza. [Semi-monthly.] Anno 1–9, 1873–81. 8°. *Milano.*
    Completed. A continuation of: **Igea** (L').

Medico (El) casero, ó el conservador de la salud. Reglas dirigidas á toda clase de personas acerca de los peligros que les importa evitar para mantener la salud y prolongar largos años la vida. 5 p. l., 13–411 pp., 9 l. 32°. *Barcelona, de el Barcelonés,* 1849.

"Medico Chirurgus" [*pseudon.*]. A letter addressed to the medical profession, on the encroachments on the practice of the surgeon-apothecary by a new set of physicians. 20 pp. 8°. *London, for the author,* 1826.

Médico (El) y cirujano centro-américano. Publicacion mensual de medicina, cirujía y los ramos colaterales. Propietario y editor: Ferd. C. Valentine. [Monthly.] v. 1–2, 1880, to Oct., 1881. 4°. *Guatemala.*

Medico (Il) omeopatico di casa e di viaggio, ossia manuale indispensibile ad ogni persona, ed in particolare a tutti i padri di famiglia che dimorano in campagna lontana dai socorsi del medico, onde potere, senza di essi, ne' casi di subitanea malattia da sè stessi aiutarsi ne' primi momenti del male. Tradotto dal tedesco. 210 pp., 1 l. 8°. *Capolago, tipog. e libreria Elvetica,* 1840. [P., v. 1456.]

Medico (Il) veterinario. Giornale teorico-pratico della Regia scuola di medicina veterinaria di Torino. Redattori: i professori ed assistenti della scuola. [Monthly.] 2. s., v. 2–6, 1861–5; 3. s., v. 1–2, 6, 1866–7, 1871; 4. s., v. 1–6, 1872–7; 5. s., v. 1–6, 1878–83; 6. s., v. 1–4, 1884–7. 24 v. 8°. *Torino.*
    Current.

Medico-Botanical Society of London. Origin and progress of the society, with general proceedings from Oct., 1827, to Jan., 1829, and appendix. 31, 32, 78 pp. 8°. *London,* 1830. [P., v. 32.]

———. By-laws. 28 pp. 8°. *London,* 1831. [P., v. 32.]

Medico-Chirurgical College of Philadelphia. Annual announcements for the sessions of 1881–2 (1.); 1882–3 (2.); 1885–6 (5.). 8° & 12°. *Philadelphia,* 1881–5.
    List of graduates for 1881–2, in : Announcement for subsequent year. 2. is 12°. Opened April 4, 1881.

Medico-Chirurgical (The) Journal; or, London Medical and Surgical Review.
    Was title of v. 2, 1819–20, of : **Medico-Chirurgical** (The) Journal ; or Quarterly Register of Medical and Surgical Science.

Medico-Chirurgical (The) Journal; or Quarterly Register of Medical and Surgical Science ; including memoirs of naval and military medicine. Conducted by James Johnson. Quarterly series. v. 1–2, July, 1818, to April, 1820. 8°. *London.*
    A continuation of: **Medico-Chirurgical** (The) Journal and Review. Title of v. 2, 1819–20, was: **Medico-Chirurgical** (The) Journal ; or London Medical and Surgical Review. Continued as: **Medico-Chirurgical** (The) Review, and Journal of Medical Science.

Medico-Chirurgical (The) Journal and Review. Conducted by William Shearman, James Johnson, and Shirley Palmer. [Monthly ; 2 v. annually.] v. 1–5, Jan., 1816, to June, 1818. 8°. *London.*
    Continued as: **Medico-Chirurgical** (The) Journal ; or Quarterly Register of Medical and Surgical Science.

Medico-Chirurgical (The) Quarterly. Edited by John Butler and George M. Dillow. v. 1; No. 1, v. 2, Oct. 1880, to Oct., 1881. 8°. *New York.*
Completed. A continuation of: **American** (The) Journal of Electrology and Neurology.

Medico-Chirurgical (The) Review. Conducted by associated physicians and surgeons, and superintended by James Johnson. [Quarterly; 2 v. annually.] New series. v. 1–47, June 1, 1824, to Oct., 1847. 8°. *London.*
A continuation, "new series", of: **Medico-Chirurgical** (The) Review, and Journal of Medical Science. In 1824, 1 v. only published, 2 nos., June 1 and Sept. 1. No. 3 dated Jan. 1, 1825. In Jan., 1827, a new series commenced, title: **Medico-Chirurgical** (The) Review and Journal of Practical Medicine. In Jan., 1828, *et seq.*, published by S. Highley. In 1834 H. J. Johnson added as editor. In 1843 James Johnson dropped; died Oct. 10, 1845. In Jan., 1848, consolidated with: **British** (The) and Foreign Medical Review, forming: **British** (The) and Foreign Medico-Chirurgical Review or Quarterly Journal of Practical Medicine and Surgery.

——. The same. General index to the new series of the Medico-Chirurgical Review, v. 1–20, inclusive [from June 1, 1824, to June 1, 1834]. With an appendix, comprising an index to the series of four annual volumes, from June, 1820, to April, 1824. 110 pp. 8°. *London, S. Highley,* 1834.

Medico-Chirurgical (The) Review, and Journal of Medical Science. Exhibiting a comprehensive analytical record of progressive medicine and surgery. Conducted by associated physicians and surgeons, and superintended by James Johnson. (Analytical series.) [Quarterly.] v. 1–4, June 1, 1820, to March 1, 1824. 8°. *London.*
A continuation of: **Medico-Chirurgical** (The) Journal, [etc.] Continued as: **Medico-Chirurgical** (The) Review.

Medico-Chirurgical (The) Review and Journal of Medical Science. Conducted by associated physicians and surgeons, and superintended by James Johnson. [Quarterly.] Analytical series, v. 1–4; new series, v. 1–47, June 1, 1820, to Oct. i, 1847. 8°. Am. reprint. *London, republished in New York, J. V. Seaman and R. & G. S. Wood.*

Medico-Chirurgical (The) Review and Journal of Practical Medicine.
Was title of: **Medico-Chirurgical** (The) Review in 1827–47.

Medico-Chirurgical Society of Edinburgh. Transactions. v. 1–3, 1824–9. 4 v. 8°. *Edinburgh,* 1824–9.

——. Laws. 12 pp. 8°. *Edinburgh, Balfour & Jack,* 1841. [P., v. 1199.]

——. Transactions, sessions 1881–2 to 1885–6. New series, v. 1–5. 8°. *Edinburgh,* 1882–6.

Medico-Legal (The) Journal. Published under the auspices of the Medico-Legal Society of New York. Clark Bell, editor. [Quarterly.] v. 1–5, June, 1883–7. 8°. *New York.*
Current.

Medico-legal report on the medical testimony of the Schoeppe murder trial, presented to the College of Physicians of Philadelphia, and unanimously adopted, Nov. 3, 1869. pp. 77–91. 8°. *Philadelphia, M. Dahlem,* 1869.

Medico-Legal Society of the City of New York. Constitution and by-laws. 11 pp. 12°. *New York, G. A. Francis,* 1869.
Founded in 1866. Incorporated in 1869.

——. Report of the committee on criminal abortion. 15 pp. 8°. *New York, D. Appleton & Co.,* 1872.
Repr. from: N. York M. J., 1872, xv.

——. First annual dinner, March 19, 1873. 45 pp., 1 phot. 8°. *New York, H. E. Thomson & Co.,* 1873.

Medico-Legal Society [etc.]—continued.
——. Constitution, by-laws, and list of officers, members, library contributions, etc. 28 pp. 8°. *New York, C. Levey & Co.,* 1874.
Another copy bound with: BELL (Clark). Inaugural address. 8°. *New York,* 1874.

——. Proceedings, March 26, 1874. Care and safe keeping of lunatics. Medical jurisprudence of the Stokes case. 15 pp. 8°. *New York, Sanitarian publ. office,* 1874.

——. Proceedings, April 23, 1874. Discussion of Prof. W. A. Hammond's paper on morbid impulse. 9 pp. 8°. *New York, Sanitarian publ. office,* 1874.

——. Papers read before the Medico-Legal Society of New York, from its organization. First series. Revised edition. xv, 552 pp. 8°. *New York, McDivitt, Campbell & Co.,* 1874.

——. The same. Second series. Revised edition. vi, 528 pp., 1 l., 4 port., 1 diag. 8°. *New York, W. F. Vanden Houten,* 1882.

——. The same. Third series. Revised edition. 3 p. l., 550 pp., 1 l., 9 port. 8°. *New York, Med.-Leg. Soc.,* 1886.

——. Report of special committee upon school hygiene. 12 pp. 8°. *New York, Terwilliger & Peck,* 1876.

——. Charter, constitution, by-laws, and list of officers and members. 5. ed. 20 pp. 8°. *New York, Terwilliger & Peck,* 1877.

——. Bulletin. (Aug., 1879, to March, 1880.) 256 pp. 8°. *New York,* 1879–80.
Issued with: **Physician** and Pharmacist, N. J., 1879–80, xii–xiii.

——. Bulletin Nos. 1–6, v. 4 (Nov., 1880, to April, 1881). Edited by George W. Wells. 220 pp. 8°. *New York, T. B. Mead,* 1880–81.

——. Charter, constitution, by-laws, and resolution establishing permanent commission. 6. ed. xvi pp. 8°. *New York, T. B. Mead,* 1881.

——. Constitution and by-laws, officers, committees, and members, and list of donors and contributors to the library to December 31, 1882. 40 pp. 8°. [*New York,* 1882.]

——. Report of the permanent commission of the . . . in answer to the senate resolutions of January 4, 1882, in reply to the letter of the attorney-general and State commissioner in lunacy of the State of New York. 16 pp. 8°. [*New York,* 1882.]

——. [Organization, objects, and plans.] List of papers read and of officers for 1872–3. 5 pp., 1 l. 8°. [*n. p., n. d.*]

——. Constitution and by-laws. 6 pp. 8°. [*New York, n. d.*]

——. Constitution, by-laws, and list of members. 14 pp. 8°. *New York, H. E. Thomson & Co.,* [*n. d.*]
See, also, **Wood** (C. S.) The Medico-Legal Society historically considered. Bull. Med.-Leg. Soc. N. Y., 1880–81, iv, 1–31.

Medico-Legal Society of Philadelphia. An act [proposed] to establish a State board of medical examiners and licensers, and to define the duties and power of such board. 4 ff. fol. *Philadelphia, Siddall Bros.,* [1884].

Medico-Literary (The) Journal. A monthly, devoted to the diffusion of medical knowledge among women. Mrs. M. P. Sawtelle, editor and publisher. v. 1–6, Sept., 1878–84. 8°. *San Francisco.*

Medico-Pharmaceutical (The) Abstract and Review. [Monthly.] v. 1, Sept., 1874, to Aug., 1875. 352 pp. 4°. *London, R. Hardwicke & Co.*
In Oct., 1874: **Chemists'** (The) and Druggists' Advocate incorporated with this journal.

Medico-Psychological Association. The memorial of a committee appointed at a meeting

Medico-Psychological Association—cont'd. of the association held at the Royal College of Physicians, London, on the 4th of August, 1868. 3 pp. 8°. [*London*, 1868.]

——. Draft of petition to the lord advocate, to be submitted to the meeting on 1st Nov., 1876. Adopted by the superintendent and other officers of the Scottish district and parochial asylums for the insane, Oct. 31, 1876. 2 pp. fol. [*Edinburgh*, 1876.] [P., v. 1295.]

——. Pensions in British asylums. Extracts from circular issued by the . . . and forwarded to the board of directors of every lunatic asylum in the three kingdoms, Aug. 4, 1879. 1 sheet. 4°. [*London*, 1879.] [P., v. 1295.]

——. Handbook for the instruction of attendants on the insane. Prepared by a subcommittee of the Medico-Psychological Association appointed at a branch meeting held in Glasgow on the 21st February, 1884. 64 pp. 8°. *London, Baillière, Tindall & Cox*, 1885.

——. Rules of. 3 pp. 8°. [*n. p., n. d.*]

"Medico-Psychologicus" [*pseudon.*]. The treatment of lunatics; a reply to the "Lancet" annotation of Saturday, January 22, 1870. 19 pp. 8°. *London, J. Churchill & Sons*, 1870.

Medicorum græcorum opera quæ extant. Editionem curavit Carolus Gottlob Kühn. 28 v. 8°. *Lipsiæ*, 1821–33.
v. 1–20, Galen; 21–23, Hippocrates; 24, Aretæus; 25–26, Dioscorides.

Medicorum Silesiacorum satyræ, quæ varias observationes, casus, experimenta, tentamina ex omni medicinæ ambitu petita exhibent. Spec. i–vi. 6 pts. in 1 v. 8°. *Wratislaviæ et Lipsiæ, imp. J. J. Kornii*, 1736.
Each part has separate title-page and pagination.

Medico-Statistical Association. First report by W. T. Gairdner and J. W. Begbie, secretaries. 14 pp. 8°. *Edinburgh, Sutherland & Knox*, 1852. [P., v. 97.]

Medicus [*pseudon.*]. See [**Pidduck** (Isaac)]. National Medical Establishment [etc.].

"Medicus" [*pseudon.*]. Human frailty; or, physiological researches into the causes and effects of diseases of the generative system, [etc.] vii, 122 pp. 12°. *New York, H. A. Barrow*, [1856].
24 pl. missing.

"Medicus" [*pseudon.*]. A short letter to a noble lord, on the present state of lunatic asylums in Great Britain. 10 pp. 8°. *Edinburgh, A. Neill & Co.*, 1806.

Medicus (Carolus Fridericus Guilielmus). *Ideæ de mammalium systemate. [Munich.] 56 pp., 2 tab. 8°. *Lutrinæ, L. Vatter*, 1847.

Medicus (Carolus Ludovicus) [1810–]. *Nonnulla de morbis pancreaticis. 30 pp., 1 l. 8°. *Berolini, typ. Nietackianis*, [1835].

Medicus (Friedrich). *Geschichtliche Darstellung der unblutigen Steinzerstörungs-Methoden. vi, 7–80 pp. 8°. *Würzburg, F. Bauer*, 1827.

Medicus (Friedrich Casimir) [1736–1808]. Send-Schreiben von der Ausrottung derer Kinder-Blattern. 1 p. l., 121 pp. 12°. *Franckfurth u. Leipzig*, 1763.

——. Geschichte periodischer Krankheiten. 16 p. l., 370 pp., 12 l. 12°. *Carlsruhe, M. Macklot*, 1764.
2 v. in 1, paged consecutively.

——. Geschichte periodehaltender Krankheiten. 2. Aufl. xv pp., 16 p. l., 370 pp. 12°. *Carlsruhe, M. Macklot*, 1792.

——. The same. Traité des maladies périodiques sans fièvre; ou histoire de ces maladies, avec la vraie méthode curative qu'il faut suivre pour les guérir. Trad. de l'allemand, par Lefebvre de Villebrune. xxiv, 380 pp. sm. 8°. *Paris, Maradan & Perlet*, 1790.

Medicus (Friedrich Casimir)—continued.

——. Brief an den Herrn Joh. Georg Zimmermann über einige Erfahrungen aus der Arzenei-Wissenschaft. 52 pp. 16°. *Mannheim*, 1766.

——. Sammlung von Beobachtungen aus der Arzneiwissenschaft. 2 v. 7 p. l., 332 pp.; 335– 882 pp. 12°. *Zürich, Heidegger u. Comp.*, 1766.
2 v. paged consecutively.
For Portrait, see **Collection**—von Kaathoven.

Medicus (Georgius Fridericus). Anacrisis medico-historico diætetica, seu dissertationes quadripartitæ de caffe et chocolate, nec non de herbæ thee ac nicotianæ natura, usu et abusu. 50 l., 4 pl. 4°. [*n. p.*], 1720.

Medicus (Karl). Ueber die Brechweinstein-salbe zur Heilung von Geisteskrankheiten. 84 pp. 8°. *Würzburg, C. W. Becker*, 1824.

Medicus (Ludwig). Sudebno-med. izsledovanie pitshevich i v kusovich sredstve. Perevod s Nemetskago N. Kruzensterna i A. Dobroslavina. [Medico-legal examinations of food and beverages, with means of detecting adulterations.] 133, ii pp. 8°. *St. Petersburg, Med. Biblioteka*, 1881.

Medicus (Max).
See **Kretinen-Heilanstalt** zu Ecksberg bey Mühldorf in Oberbayern. Bericht. 8°. *München*, 1854.

Medicus (Maximilianus Lud. Phil.) * De organismi et rerum externarum actione mutua. vi, 7–23 pp. 8°. *Monachii, J. A. Giesser*, 1834.

Medicus afflictus, oder der wohl-geplagte Medicus, etc. *See* **L.** (C. T. A. S. M.)

Medicus politicus, dat is, onderwijs aan een jonger medicus, wegens de politike steeken, welke in de praktijk der medicijnen ingesloopen zijn. 148 pp., 1 l. 12°. *Amsterdam, N. ten Hoorn*, 1700.

Medicus Romanus servus sexaginta solidis æstimatus. 46 pp. 12°. *Lugd. Bat.*, 1671.
Foot-note on last page says: Recusum 1746.

Médieux (A.) * Essai sur les appareils plâtrés; de leur emploi en chirurgie de guerre. 44 pp. 4°. *Paris, A. Parent*, 1879, No. 136.

Mediko-pedagogicheski Vestnik. Izdanie vrachebno-vospitatelnago zaredenija. Redaktor, I. V. Maljarevski. Nos. 1–2, v. 1, Jan. to Feb., 1885; Nos. 1–3, v. 2, 1886. 8°. *St. Petersburg*, 1885; Nos. 1–3, v. 2, 1886.

Mediko-topographicheskii Sbornik. Izdanie meditzinskago departamenta. v. 1–2, 1870– 71. roy. 8°. *St. Petersburg*.

Medin (Oskar). *Meningitis cerebro-spinalis epidemica infantum. Ett bidrag till kännedomen om sjukdomarna bland de späda barnen på Allm. Barnhuset i Stockholm under åren 1842–76. 80 pp., 1 tab. 8°. *Stockholm, P. A. Norstedt & söner*, 1880.

Medina.

BOURILLET (C.) * Essai de topographie médicale sur le poste de Médine (Sénégal). 4°. *Montpellier*, 1875.

Medina y Gutierrez (Francisco de P.) Tratado de patología quirúrgica general. xvi, 426 pp. 12°. *Cadiz, F. Joly*, 1877.

de Medina é Jsasi (Rafael).
See **Ruiz y Sauroman** (Emilio). Manual del practicante de sanidad, etc. roy. 8°. *Madrid*, 1881.

Meding (C. Th. Bernardus). *Ad naturam glycogenii. 18 pp., 1 l. 8°. *Lipsiæ, typ. L. Schnaussii*, 1860.

Meding (Carolus Henricus) [1791–1851]. * De regeneratione ossium per experimenta illustrata. 40 pp., 1 l., 15 pp. 4°. *Lipsiæ, typ. Hirschfeldianis*, [1823]. [*Also, in:* P., v. 1607.]
For Biography, see **Kuehn** (Carolus Gottlob.)

Meding (Heinrich Ludwig) [1822–65]. * De erroribus et peccatis quibusdam in re obstetricia sæpius occurrentibus. viii, 16 pp. 4°. *Lipsiæ, typ. C. E. Elberti*, [1846].

Meding (Heinrich Ludwig)—continued.
———. Essai sur la topographie médicale de Paris; examen général des conditions de salubrité dans lesquelles cette ville est placée. 4 p. l., 282 pp., 1 ch. 12°. *Paris, J.-B. Baillière,* 1852.
———. Paris médical. Vade-mecum des médecins étrangers. Renseignements historiques, statistiques, administratifs et scientifiques sur les hôpitaux et hospices civils et militaires, l'enseignement de la médecine, les académies et sociétés savantes. Précédés d'une topographie médicale de Paris et suivis d'un précis de bibliographie médicale française et des adresses de tous les médecins de Paris. 2 v. 352, 558 pp., 1 pl. 12°. *Paris, J.-B. Baillière,* 1852–3.
———. The same. Manuel du Paris médical; recueil de renseignements [etc.] 558 pp., 1 ch. 12°. *Paris, J.-B. Baillière,* 1853.
———. Bibliothèque du Paris médical. Enseignement et bibliographie de la médecine. x, 84 pp. 12°. *Paris, V. Masson,* 1855.
———. Congrès international de statistique. Compte rendu critique des travaux sur le cadre nosologique des décès fait à la Société médicale allemande de Paris. 39 pp. 8°. *Paris, V. Masson,* 1856.
See, also, **Verein** deutscher Aerzte in Paris. Fest-Bericht [etc.] 4°. *Paris, Leipzig, Bonn, Breslau,* 1854.

Meding (Henricus Ferdinandus). * Diss. sistens observationem de hydrocephalo interno chronico. vi, 7–32 pp. 4°. *Jenæ, typ. Schreiberi et soc.,* [1819].

Mediterranean (*The*).

See, also, **Fever** (*Malarial, History, etc., of*), *by localities; and under names of islands and bordering countries.*
HENNEN (J.) Sketches of the medical topography of the Mediterranean; comprising an account of Gibraltar, the Ionian Islands, and Malta; to which is prefixed a sketch of a plan for memoirs on medical topography. Edited by his son, J. Hennen. 8°. *London,* 1830.
HORNER (G. R. B.) Medical and topographical observations upon the Mediterranean; and upon Portugal, Spain, and other countries. 8°. *Philadelphia,* 1839.
American Medical Library.
Daremberg (G.) Comparaison des climats d'hiver sur les côtes africaine et française de la Méditerranée. Cong. périod. internat. d. sc. méd. Compt.-rend. 1877. Genève, 1878, v, 606–637.— **Kay** (W. S.) Contributions to the medical topography of the Mediterranean. Med. Times, Lond., 1847, xvi, 290; 413; 470; 1847–8, xvii, 34; 75; 445; 1848, xviii, 123; 236; 266; 1848–9, xix, 73; 215; 529.

Meditsinskaja Biblioteka. Ejemiesjachnii journal. 1881–6. 8° *St. Petersburg.*
Current. Want no. 7, 1881.

Meditsinskii kalendar dlja vrachei vsech vedomstve. Pod red. V. V Svjatlovskago. 1885. 12°. *St. Petersburg,* 1884.

Meditsinskii Sbornik; isdavaemir Kavkaskim meditsinskim obshestvom. Nos. 1–40, Jan., 1866–87. 8°. *Tiflis.*
Current. In nos. 13, 1871, *et seq.,* "imperatorskim" inserted before "Kavkaskim ".

Meditsinskii Vestnik, eshtshenedelnaya gazeta, izdavaemaya N. A. Nikitinuim, pod redaktsiyu Y. A. Chestovitch. [Weekly.] v. 1, 3–9, 16–24, 1861, 1863–9, 1876–87. 17 v. 4°. *St. Petersburg.*
In v. 3-9 Dr. Chestovitch sole editor.

Meditsinskija Novosti. Gazeta dlja vrachei, veterinarov i farmatsevtov. [Weekly.] v. 1–2, 1884–5. fol. *St. Petersburg.*
Completed. No. 29, v. 2, last published.

Meditsinskija pribavlenija k morskomu sborniku. Ejemiesjachnii journal, izdavaemii upra-

Meditsinskija pribavlenija [etc.]—cont'd.
releniem Flota General-Stab-Doktora. [Monthly.] 1882–7. 5 v. 8°. *St. Petersburg.*
Current.

Meditsinskoe Obozrainie, ejemaisjachnii journal. [Monthly; 2 v. annually.] v. 5–26, 1876–87. 22 v. 8°. *Moscow.*
Current. v. 12 contains general index to v. 1–12, 1874–9. In 1884 became semi-monthly. Four supplements issued with this journal.

Mediziner (Der). Berliner Monatsschrift für ärztliche Unterhaltung. v. 1, 1844. 554 pp. 8°. *Berlin, W. Hermes.*

Mediziner (Der). Berliner Wochenblatt für ärztliche Neuigkeiten. Hrsg. von Dr. M. Kalisch. v. 1–3, Jan. 3, 1846, to July 8, 1848. fol. *Berlin, Voss.*
Want nos. 27–52, v. 3 (July to Dec., 1848).

Medizinische Jahrbücher. Zeitschrift der k. k. Gesellschaft der Aerzte in Wien. Redigirt von A. Duchek, J. Klob, A. Schauenstein. [6 Hfte. forming 2 v. annually.] v. 1–20, 1861–70. 8°. *Wien.*
A continuation of: **Zeitschrift** der k.-k. Gesellschaft der Aerzte in Wien. In 1862 Klob dropped and C. Langer added; in 1863 Langer dropped; 1864–70 by Duchek, C. Braun, and L. Schlager. See **Wochenblatt** der Zeitschrift [etc.], a supplement to this journal. Continued as: **Medicinische** Jahrbücher [von Stricker].

Medizinische (Die) Praxis der bewährtesten Aerzte unserer Zeit, systematisch dargestellt. Nach Baumgärtner, Berends, [etc.] 3 v. 8°. *Berlin, Veit u. Comp.,* 1838–9.

Medizinische Jahrbücher. Hrsg. von der kaiserlich-königlichen Gesellschaft der Aerzte. Redigirt von S. Stricker. Jahrgänge 1–16, 1871–87. 8°. *Wien, W. Braumüller.*
Current. A continuation of: **Medicinische** Jahrbücher, 1861–70. No. 1, 1881, edited by R. Heschl; in no. 2, 1881, E. Albert and E. Ludwig became editors; in 1883 H. Kundrat added.

Medizinische Nationalzeitung für Deutschland und die mit selbigem zunächst verbundenen Staaten. v. 1–2, 1798–9. 4°. *Altenberg.*
Continued as: **Allgemeine** medicinische Annalen [etc.]

Medizinische (Die) Polizei und gerichtliche Arzneiwissenschaft in den k. k. Erbländern. Ein unentbehrliches Handbuch für Kreis-Magistratual-Polizei- und Wirthschaftsbeamte, wie auch für Advokaten, Phisiker, Aerzte, Wundärzte, Hebärzte und Hebammen, Apotheker, und alle, die das allgemeine Gesundheitswohl der Menschen und des Viehes, eine gesezmässige Volksarzneikunde, und die Pflichten und Rechten des Arzneipersonals interessirt, bearbeitet von Johann Dionis John. 2 v. 16 ff., 17–486 pp.; 724 pp. 8°. *Prag, J. G. Calve,* 1796–8.
Continuation of: Lexikon der k. k. Medizinalgeseze, 1790–91.

Medizinischer Kalender für Aerzte und Nichtärzte auf das Jahr 1813 [also for 1814]. Mit besonderer Hinsicht auf die Herzogthümer Mecklenburg und Schwedisch-Pommern. Hrsg. von Georg Heinrich Masius. v. 1–2, 1813–14. 8°. *Rostock.*

Medizinisch–Hermeneutische Untersuchung derer in der Bibel vorkommenden Krankengeschichten. 388 pp. 12°. *Leipzig, Meygand,* 1794.

Medjez-el-Bab.

Catrin (L.) Medjez-el-Bab (Tunisie); essai de topographie médicale. Arch. de méd. et pharm. mil., Par., 1883, ii, 301–325.

Medlicott case.

See **Morphine** (*Toxicology of*); **Toxicology** (*Cases, etc., of*).

Medlock. Report on the sulphuretted waters from the wells of Strathpeffer, near Dingwall, N. B., on the estate of the Marchioness of Stafford. 8 pp. 8°. *Edinburgh,* 1861. [P., v. 880.]

Medoc.

CHABANNES (A.) * Essai sur la topographie médicale de cette partie du département de la Gironde, qui portait ci-devant le nom du Médoc. 4°. *Paris, an XIII* [1805].

LE GENDRE (L.-F.-M.) * Sur la topographie médicale du Médoc. 4°. *Paris, 1866.*

Médoc (*Fort*).

Mainvielle. Description topographique du fort Médoc. Rec. de mém. de méd. . . . mil., Par., 1826, xix, 26-39.

Medon. Die Traubenkur and ihre Anwendung. 4. Aufl. 10 pp. 8°. *Grünberg, W. Levysohn,* [*n. d.*]

Medulla.

See Marrow.

Medulla medicinæ universæ, or a new compendious dispensary, wherein is contained in a direct summary way all that is essentially necessary either with respect to physick or surgery to answer every medicinal intention of cure. By the king's physicians and surgeons, the surgeon general and apothecary general of the army. To which is added an English translation with a comment subjoined to every formula, shewing in what specific cases each prescription is peculiarly efficacious; with proper indexes referring to the various maladies incident to the human body and their respective cures, and a preface displaying the design and use of the whole. Calculated equally for the benefit of others as of those of the faculty. iv, 62 pp. 8°. *London, J. Robinson,* 1747.

———. The same. Medulla medicinæ universæ; or a new compendious dispensatory, compiled at the command of his royal highness the duke, for the use of the military hospital abroad, during the late war. 4. ed., with a large additional appendix. 5 p. l., 226 pp. 12°. *London, R. Griffiths,* 1752.

Medulla *oblongata.*

BEISSO (T.) Contributo allo studio della midoila allungata. roy. 8°. *Genova,* 1884.

CAREL (E.) * Esquisse des récents travaux sur l'anatomie normale et pathologique du bulbe rachidien. 4°. *Paris,* 1875.

DEAN (J.) The gray substance of the medulla oblongata and trapezium. 4°. *Washington,* 1864.

———. The same. 4°. *Washington,* 1870.

KELLNER (F. X.) * Zur Physiologie und Pathologie der Medulla oblongata. 8°. *München,* 1867.

SCHROEDER VAN DER KOLK (J. L. C.) Bau und Functionen der Medulla spinalis und oblongata und nächste Ursache und rationelle Behandlung der Epilepsie. Aus dem Holländischen übertragen von Dr. Friedrich Wilhelm Theile. 8°. *Braunschweig,* 1859.

Bechtereff (V.) Ob otpravlenii olivchatich tiel prodolgovatago mozga. [Function of olivary processes of medulla oblongata.] Vrach, St. Petersb., 1882, iii, 566; 586.— **Brown-Séquard** (E.) Recherches sur les causes de mort après l'ablation de la partie de la moelle allongée qui a été nommée point vital. J. de la physiol. de l'homme, Par., 1858, i, 217-233.—**Clarke** (J. L.) Researches on the intimate structure of the brain, human and comparative; first series, on the structure of the medulla oblongata. Phil. Tr., Lond., 1858, cxlviii, 231-259, 6 pl. *Also,* Reprint.—**Claus.** Ein Beitrag zur Lehre von den Pyramidenbahnen. Allg. Ztschr. f. Psychiat., etc., Berl., 1877, xxxiv, 452-471, 1 pl.—**Couty, Guimaes & Niobey.** De l'action des lésions du bulbe rachidien sur les échanges nutritifs. Compt. rend. Acad. d. sc., Par., 1884, xcix, 388-390.—**van Deen** (I.) Vorläufige Beschreibung von einigen an der Medulla oblongata von Rana temporaria (Land-Frosch) gemachten Versuchen. Holländ. Beitr. zu d. anat. u. physiol. Wissen., Düsseld. u. Utrecht, 1846, i, 27-38. *Also, transl.:* N. Arch. v. bin.-en buitenl. Geneesk., Zwolle, 1846, i, 304-319.—**Duchenne.** Recherches icono-photographiques sur la morphologie et sur la structure intime du bulbe humain, leur application à l'étude anatomo-patho-

Medulla *oblongata.*

logique de la paralysie glosso-labio-laryngée. Arch. gén. de méd., Par., 1870, i, 539-517.—**Duret** (H.) Sur la distribution des artères nourricières du bulbe rachidien. Arch. de physiol. norm. et path., Par., 1873, v, 97-114, 2 pl.— **Edinger** (L.) Zur Kenntniss des Verlaufes der Hinterstrangfasern in der Medulla oblongata und im unteren Kleinhirnschenkel. Neurol. Centralbl., Leipz., 1885, iii, 73-76.—**Fabiana** (A.) O mechanizmach w mózgu żaby tamujących odruchy rdzenia. [The mechanism for reflex action of the medulla oblongata in the brain of the frog.] Gaz. lek., Warszawa, 1869, vii, 161-167.—**Farabeuf** (L.-H.) Moelle épinière; moelle allongée, ou bulbe rachidien. Dict. encycl. d. sc. méd., Par., 1873, 2 s., viii. 299-330.— **Hall** (M.) On the reflex function of the medulla oblongata and medulla spinalis. Phil. Tr., Lond., 1833, cxxiii, 635-665.—**Kesteven** (W. H.) The structure and functions of the olivary bodies. St. Barth. Hosp. Rep., Lond., 1877, xiii, 59-61.—**Kilian** (F. M.) Ueber die Beziehungen des Uterus zur Medulla oblongata. N. Ztschr. f. Geburtsk., Berl., 1848, xxv, 65-94.—**Kramsztyk** (Z.) O wpływie korzeni tylnych rdzenia kręgowego na pobudzalność przednich. [Influence of the posterior pyramid of the medulla oblongata in producing motion.] Gaz. lek., Warszawa, 1870, ix, 209; 243.—**Kronecker** (H.) & **Meltzer** (S.) On the propagation of inhibitory excitation in the medulla oblongata. Proc. Roy. Soc. Lond., 1881-2, xxxiii, 27-29.—**Laborde.** Recherches expérimentales sur quelques points de la physiologie du bulbe rachidien. Influence du bulbe: 1° sur les mouvements associés des yeux; 2° sur les phénomènes trophiques et de sensibilité de l'œil, du nez, de l'oreille et de la face en général. Gaz. méd. de Par., 1877, 4. s., vi, 637: 1878, 4. s., vii, 29; 53. *Also:* Tribune méd., Par., 1878, x, 313; 337; 361. *Also:* Compt. rend. Soc. de biol. 1877, Par., 1879, 6. s., iv, pt. 2, 81-96.—**Mislavski** (N. A.) K gistologii prodolgov. mozga. [Histology of medulla oblongata.] Arch. psichiat., etc., Charkov, 1885, vi, no. 2, 50-54, 4 pl.—**Moos.** Zur Diagnose der absoluten Acusticuslähmung; Beitrag zur Pathologie der Medulla oblongata. Arch. f. Augen- u. Ohrenh., Carlsruhe, 1871-2, ii, 115-119.—**Oré.** Recherches expérimentales sur l'influence que la moelle épinière et le bulbe rachidien exercent sur la sensibilité et la motilité. J. de méd. de Bordeaux. 1853, iv, 597-604.—**Ott** (I.) The decussation of the motor fibres in the medulla oblongata. Detroit Lancet, 1879-80, n. s., iii, 402-405. ———. On the path of the inhibitory and sensory fibres in the medulla oblongata. N. York M. J., 1880, xxxi, 6-9.— **Pflueger** (E.) Die psychischen Functionen der Medulla oblongata und spinalis. (Auszug.) Arch. f. Anat., Physiol. u. wissensch. Med., Berl., 1851, 484-494.—**Reid** (J.) On some points in the anatomy of the medulla oblongata. Edinb. M. & S. J., 1841, lv, 12-17, 1 pl.—**Rolando** (L.) Recherches anatomiques sur la moelle allongée. J. de physiol. expér., Par., 1824, iv, 317-354.— **Schiff** (M.) Einfluss des verlängerten Marks auf die Athmung. Arch. f. d. ges. Physiol., Bonn, 1870, iii, 624: 1871, iv, 225.—**Spitzka** (E. C.) Notes on the architecture of the oblongata. N. York M. J., 1881, xxxiv, 233-240, 1 pl.—**Velpeau** (A.) Mémoire sur une altération profonde de la moelle allongée, sans que les fonctions nerveuses aient été troublées. Arch. gén. de méd., Par., 1825, vii, 52-58.—**Vulpian.** Note sur quelques points de l'anatomie du bulbe rachidien et de la protubérance annulaire chez l'homme. Compt. rend. Soc. de biol. 1858, Par., 1859, 2. s., v, 169-176.—**von Wittich.** Ueber die Beziehungen der Medulla oblongata zu den Athembewegungen bei Fröschen. Arch. f. path. Anat., etc., Berl., 1866, xxxvii, 322-345.

Medulla *oblongata* (*Diseases of*).

See, also, Paralysis (*Bulbar, etc.*)

Althaus. Disease of the lateral columns of the medulla; double histrionic spasm and torticollis. Brit. M. J., Lond., 1872, i, 48.—**Benedikt.** Ueber Reflexe bei Affektionen des verlängerten Markes und der Varolsbrücke, nebst Vorstellung zweier Kranken. Wien. med. Wchnschr., 1865, xv, 1874. *Also:* Wien. med. Presse, 1865, vi, 1268.—**Berger.** Acuter halbseitiger Bulbärläsion. Breslau. aerztl. Ztschr., 1882, iv, 258.—**Bourdon** (H.) Étude sur les maladies du bulbe rachidien. Gaz. hebd. de méd., Par., 1872, 2. s., i, 354-357.—**Bruny.** Observation d'un cas de gangrène de l'axe cérébro-rachidien chez une aliénée. J. de méd. de Bordeaux, 1860, 2. s., v, 21-25.—**Cruveilhier.** [Bulbe rachidien atrophié et de dureté presque pierreuse.] Bull. Soc. anat. de Par., 1834, ix, 122.— **Dépéret-Muret.** Apoplexie du mésocéphale. *Ibid,* 1838, xiii, 42-49.—**Dumville.** Paralysis of gullet; inflammatory induration of medulla oblongata. Lond. M. Gaz., 1846, n. s., iii, 848.—**Epifani** (G.) Storia clinica d' un caso di sifilide de midollo oblongata. Morgagni, Napoli, 1877, xix, 515-520.—**Erb** (W. H.) Diseases of the spinal cord and medulla oblongata. Cycl. Pract. M. (Ziemssen), N. Y., 1878, xiii, 1-822.—**Etter** (P.) Zwei Fälle acuter Bulbärmyelitis. Cor.-Bl. f. schweiz. Aerzte, Basel, 1882, xii, 769; 809.—**Fardel** (M.-D.) Note sur deux observations de ramollissement du bulbe rachidien. Gaz. méd. de Par., 1854, 3. s., ix, 521-523.—**Fuller.** Case of pressure of

Medulla *oblongata* (*Diseases of*).

the medulla oblongata complicated by apoplexy. Lancet, Lond., 1870, ii, 404. — **Galliard** (L.) Tubercule volumineux de la protubérance. Bull. Soc. anat. de Par., 1880, lv, 654–658.—**Gentilhomme.** Inflammation diffuse du bulbe rachidien. Bull. Soc. méd. de Reims, 1876–7, xv, 39–48.—**Hamilton** (A. M. L.) A consideration of certain symptoms associated with morbid changes in the medulla oblongata. Tr. N. York Acad. M. (1874–6), 1876, 2. s., ii, 79–109. *Also,* Reprint.—**Hammond** (W. A.) On the cause of Vice-President Wilson's death. Boston M. & S. J., 1875, xciii, 693–704.—**Handyside** (P. D.) On a remarkable diminution of the medulla oblongata, and adjacent portion of the spinal marrow, consequent upon spontaneous dislocation of the processus-dentatus, and ankylosis at the upper part of the spine, yet unattended with any symptom of paralysis. Edinb. M. & S. J., 1840, liii, 376–379, 1 pl.—**Hertz.** Ein Fall von Erweichungsherd in der Medulla oblongata, bedingt durch Hypertrophie und abnorme Stellung des Processus odontoideus epistrophie. Deutsches Arch. f. klin. Med., Leipz., 1874, xiii, 385–402.—**Kesteven** (W. B.) Notes of a peculiar form of "granular degeneration" observed in a medulla oblongata. Brit & For. M.-Chir. Rev., Lond., 1869, xliii, 492–494.—**Lacombe.** Tubercules du bulbe chez un enfant idiot. Bull Soc. anat. de Par., 1869, xliv, 127. — **Larcher** (O.) Mémoire sur un cas de sclérose générale de la protubérance annulaire. Arch. gén. de méd., Par., 1868, i, 702–715 —**Larison** (C. W.) Cases of affection of the medulla oblongata Tr. M. Soc. N. Jersey, Newark, 1875, 203–207.—**von Lenhossék.** Ein anhaltender Druck auf das verlängerte Mark hemmt die Entwickelung des Körpers und die Geschlechtsreife bei einem jungen Menschen. Med. Jahrb. d. k. k. österr St.ates, Wien, 1826, n. F., iii, 96–102.—**Leyden** (E.) & **von Wittich.** Myelitis apoplectica der Med. oblongata; Parese aller Extremitäten mit Schüttellähmung und verlangsamter motorischer Leitung. Arch. f. path. Anat., etc., Berl., 1872, lv, 3–10.—**Lœwenthal** (N.) Dégénérations secondaires ascendantes dans'le bulbe rachidien, dans le pont et dans l'étage supérieur de l'isthme. Rev. méd. de la Suisse Rom., Genève, 1885, v, 511; 572, 1 pl. —**McDowel.** Acute inflammation of the medulla spinalis. Dublin Q. J. M. Sc., 1851, xi, 464–466. — **Mackenzie** (S.) Cases of intracranial disease involving the medulla oblongata. Brit. M. J., Lond., 1883, i, 408–410.—**Möser** (H.) Beitrag zur Diagnostik der Lage und Beschaffenheit von Krankheitsherden der Medulla oblongata. Deutsches Arch. f. klin. Med., Leipz., 1884, xxxv, 418–445.—**Morelli** (C.) Illustrazione fisio-patologica di quattro casi d' affezione del midollo allungato e delle parti superiori della spina. Sperimentale, Firenze, 1877, xxxix, 521; 611.—**Mulvane** (J. K.) Hyperæmia of the medulla oblongata. J. Nerv. & Ment. Dis., N. Y., 1882, n. s., vii, 129–132.—**Nairne** (A.) Alcoholic inflammation of the medulla oblongata. Brit. M. J., Lond., 1879, ii, 1020.— **Putzel** (L.) Diseases of the medulla oblongata. Cycl. Prac. M. (Ziemssen), N. Y., 1881 (suppl.), 560–563.—**Quinquaud.** Anomalie des fibres arciformes du bulbe rachidien. Bull. Soc. anat. de Par., 1867, xlii, 19–21.— **Skobel** (S.) Przypady w rdzeniu przedłużonym u chorego dotkniętago kiłą wczesną. [Symptom of affection in medulla oblongata in a case of syphilis of recent date.] Przegl. lek., Kraków., 1882, xxi, 519; 533.—**Teschemacher.** Verhärtung der Medulla oblongata. Gen.-Ber. d. k. rhein. Med.-Coll. 1844, Koblenz, 1846, 76. *Also:* Wchnschr. f. d. ges Heilk., Berl., 1847, 535.—**Toribio González.** Parálisis sintomática por congestion activa de la médula oblongata. Union méd., Carácas, 1881, i, 131.—**Weber** (H.) Observations d'affections de la moelle allongée. Monit. d. sc. et pharm., Par., 1861, iii, 937.

Medulla *oblongata* (*Hæmorrhage on or into*).

Bouillaud (J.) Cinquante-cinq ans environ; chute; impossibilité de se relever; mouvemens épileptiformes; écume à la bouche; respiration stertoreuse; mort au bout de deux ou trois heures; hémorrhagie dans la partie postérieure de la moelle allongée et dans le quatrième ventricule. J. hebd. de méd., Par., 1829, ii, 56.—**Charrier** (A.) Hémorrhagie du bulbe rachidien; mort subite après le 12e jour des couches; autopsie. Arch. de physiol. norm. et path., Par., 1869, ii, 660.—**Clemens** (T.) Apoplexia medullæ oblongatæ. Deutsche Klinik, Berl., 1850, ii, 503.— **Cotting** (B. E.) Abdominal cancer; supposed by the patient to be pregnancy in third to fourth month; accompanied by apoplexy of the medulla oblongata; death in twenty-four hours after apoplectic attack. Boston M. & S. J., 1866–7, lxxv, 187. *Also:* Extr. Rec. Bost. Soc. M. Improve. (1862–6), 1867, v, 235.—**Jodin** (C.) Observation d'hémorrhagie dans le bulbe rachidien; mort instantanée. J. univ. et hebd. de méd. et chir. prat., Par., 1833, xi, 538–546. — **Mesnet.** Apoplexie du bulbe rachidien dans sa partie supérieure en arrière de la protubérance annulaire. Monit. d. sc. méd. et pharm., Par., 1861, iii, 737. —**Mignot.** [Flux hémorrhoïdal abondant depuis plusieurs années; cessation; trois attaques d'hématémèse; apoplexie de la protubérance.] Bull. Soc. anat. de Par., 1850, xxv,

Medulla *oblongata* (*Hæmorrhage on or into*).

227.—**Oettinger** (J.) Opis przypadku gruźlicy z urazem rdzenia przedłużonego i korzeni nerwów błędnych. [Clots found in the medulla oblongata.] Przegl. lek, Kraków., 1862, i, nos. 21–25. — **Siredey.** [Apoplexie de la protubérance, et, chez le même sujet, des kystes et tumeurs des reins.] Bull. Soc. anat. de Par., 1858, xxxiii, 446.—**Terry.** Apoplexy of the medulla oblongata. Med. Rec, N. Y., 1867–8, ii, 545.—**White** (W. H.) Hyperæmia and hæmorrhages in the medulla oblongata causing sudden death, owing to the implication of the vagal nucleus. Tr. Path. Soc. Lond., 1881–2, xxxiii, 15–19, 1 pl.

Medulla *oblongata* (*Tumors of*).

Charcot. Tumeur du volume d'un œuf de pigeon comprimant le côté droit de la moelle allongée et les nerfs qui en partent. Compt. rend. Soc. de biol. 1851, Par., 1852, iii, 19–23. — **Chevalier** (T. W.) Case of tumor in the medulla oblongata. Lond. M. Gaz., 1834, xiv, 10–15.—**De Venezia** (P.) Sintomatologia dei tumori della protuberanza anulare. Gior. veneto di sc. med., Venezia, 1866, 3. s., iv, 105–108. *Also, transl.:* J. de méd., chir. et pharmacol., Brux., 1866, xliii, 114–116.—**Edwards.** Tumour in the medulla oblongata; phthisis; tubercle and small cavities in the spleen. Brit. M. J., Lond., 1870, i, 131.—**Erichsen** (J.) Zur Casuistik der Tumoren des verlängerten Marks. St. Petersb. med. Ztschr., 1870, n. F., i, 105–114.—**Glynn.** Tumour of medulla oblongata in the neighbourhood of the calamus scriptorius. Liverpool M.-Chir. J., 1887, vii, 428–433.—**Godlee** (R. J.) Melanotic sarcoma in the medulla oblongata secondary to a similar growth situated probably in a lymphatic gland. Tr. Path. Soc. Lond., 1873–4, xxv, '18–23, 1 pl. — **Hasse** (C. E.) Carcinoma medullæ oblongatæ. Deutsche Klinik, Berl., 1855, vii, 310.— **Heydenreich** (A.) Tumeur du bulbe. Bull. Soc. anat. de Par., 1875, 3. s., x, 131–133. — **Hobson** (J. M.) A case of tumour in the medulla oblongata and pons Varolii, with remarkable paralytic symptoms. Brain, Lond., 1881–2, iv, 531–539.—**Johnson** (G.) & **Ferrier.** Tumour of medulla oblongata. Brit. M. J., Lond., 1883, ii, 821. — **de Jonge** (D.) Tumor der Medulla oblongata; Diabetes mellitus. Arch. f. Psychiat , Berl., 1882, xiii, 658–670, 1 pl. — **Macgregor** (A.) Case of tumour of the pons Varolii and medulla oblongata. Lancet, Lond., 1886, ii, 1127.—**Potain.** Paralysie alterne; tumeur du bulbe. Gaz. d. hôp., Par., 1880, liii, 137.—**Riquard.** Kyste séro-purulent développé au devant du bulbe rachidien. J. de méd. de Bordeaux, 1857, 2. s., ii, 669–672. — **Schulz** (R.) Gliomatöse Hypertrophie des Pons und der Medulla oblongata. Neurol. Centralbl., Leipz., 1883, ii, 5–9. — **Steudener** (F.) Fibrome mit Amyloidkörpern. Arch. f. path. Anat., etc., Berl., 1874, lix, 424–426, 1 pl.—**Taylor** (F.) Glioma of the medulla oblongata. Tr. Path. Soc. Lond., 1886, xxxvii, 26–28.

Medulla *oblongata* (*Wounds of*).

Brinton. The appearance of grape sugar in the urine after the operation of M. Claude Bernard, of puncturing the medulla oblongata in the middle line of the floor of the fourth ventricle, or between the roots of the vagus nerves. Tr. Path. Soc. Lond., 1849–50, ii, 280. — **Hendrick** (J.) Cas de piqûre de la moelle allongée à travers l'apophyse basilaire. Gaz. méd. de Par., 1868, xxiii, 635.—**Kendrick** (P. J.) Case of puncture of the medulla oblongata through the basilar process. Med. Times & Gaz., Lond., 1867, i, 585.—**Vix.** Ein Fall von einseitiger Verletzung des verlängerten Markes und seine Folgen; tiefe Störungen der Motilität auf der rechten, der Sensibilität auf der linken Körperhälfte. Cor.-Bl. d. ärztl. Ver. d. Rhein-Prov., Bonn, 1874, No. 14, 66–75.

Medusæ.

BROOKS (W. K.) The life-history of hydromedusæ. A discussion of the origin of medusæ and of the significance of metagenesis. 4°. *Boston,* 1886.

Repr. [with same pagination] *from:* Mem. Bost. Soc. Nat. Hist., 1886, iii, 359–430, 8 pl.

REID (J.) Observations on the development of the medusæ. 8°. [*n. p.,* 1848.]

Repr. from: Ann. & Mag. Nat. Hist., Jan., 1848.

Brooks (W. K.) List of medusæ found at Beaufort, N. C., during the summers of 1880 and 1881. Johns Hopkins Univ. Stud. biol. lab., Balt., 1881–3, ii, 135–146. ——. Notes on the medusæ of Beaufort, N. C. Pt. ii. *Ibid.,* 465–475.—**Colasanti** (G.) Studi sul pigmento blu delle idromeduse. Bull. d. r. Accad. med. di Roma, 1882, viii, 326–328. ——. Il pigmento blu delle idromeduse. Atti Accad. med. di Roma, 1883–6, 2. s., ii, 273–288.—**Ebbesen** (J.) Om Medusa, dens Anvendelse og Virkninger. Norsk Mag. f. Lægevidensk., Christiania, 1850, iv, 601–615.— **Hunnius.** Thierischer Schlamm, oder: die Meduse und ihre medicinische Anwendungsweise in Hapsal. Med. Ztg. Russlands, St. Petersb., 1859, xvi, 43.—**Huxley** (T.

Medusæ.

H.) On the anatomy and the affinities of the family of the medusæ. Phil. Tr., Lond., 1849, 413–434, 2 pl. ———. Observations upon the anatomy and physiology of salpa and pyrosoma, together with remarks upon doliolum and appendicularia. *Ibid.*, 1851, 567–605.—**von Lendenfeld** (R.) The function of nettlecells. Quart. J. Micr. Sc., Lond., 1886–7, n. s., xxvii, 393–399, 1 pl.—**M'Kendrick.** Some observations on the colouring matter of jelly-fishes. J. Anat. & Physiol., Lond., 1880–81, xv, 261–264.—**Romanes** (G. J.) The physiology of the nervous system of medusæ. Notices Proc. Roy. Inst. Gr. Brit. 1875–8, Lond., 1879, viii, 166–177. ———. Observations on the locomotor system of medusæ. Communicated by Prof. Huxley. Phil. Tr., Lond., 1877, clxvi, 269: 1878, clxvii, 659: 1880, clxxi, 161, 4 pl. *Also* [Abstr.]: Proc. Roy. Soc. Lond., 1879, xxviii, 266.—**Schäfer** (E. A.) "Observations on the nervous system of Aurelia aurita." Communicated by W. Sharpey. [Abstr.] Proc. Roy. Soc. Lond., 1878. xxvii, 16.—**de Varenne** (A.) Sur les causes de la formation des gonophores et des méduses chez les hydraires. Compt. rend. Soc. de biol., Par., 1882, 7. s., iv, 8–10.

Medviedski (P.) * K ucheniou o tifie lichoradki pri zabolievanii rogatago skota chumoiou. [Investigation of the rinderpest.] 56 pp., 2 l., 4 tab. 8°. *St. Petersburg*, 1875.

Medycyna. Czasopismo tygodniowe dla lekarzy praktycznych. Redaktor odpowiedzialny : Dr. K. Benni. v. 1–14, 1873–86. 8°. *Warszawa.*
Current. v. 3–9 edited by Dr. J. Rogowicz; in v. 10, 1882, G. Fritsche became editor.

Mee (Isaac). * De nutritione. 37 pp. 8°. *Edinburgi, Balfour, Auld et Smellie,* 1770.

Meebold (Christian). * Chemische Untersuchung des Faserstoffes und des gelben elastischen Gewebes. 19 pp. 8°. *Tübingen, G. Bähr,* 1834.

van Meegen (Antonius Guilielmus). * De morborum origine in graviditate. 4 p. l., 68 pp. 8°. *Lugd. Bat., J. W. van Leeuwen,* 1835.

Meeh (Julius Joseph Ehrenreich). * Sechzehn Kropf-Operationen. iv, 5–25 pp. 8°. *Erlangen, Junge u. Sohn,* 1864.

Meeker (C. H.)
See **Rausse** (J. H.) Errors of physicians and others in the practice of the water-cure [etc.] Transl. by C. H. Meeker. 12°. *New York*, 1855.

Meeker (D.)
Editor of: **Opium** eating, its consequences and cure, Laporte, Ind., 1872–3.

van Meek'ren (Job.) [–1666]. Heel- en geneeskonstige aanmerkkingen. 9 p. l., 495 pp., 6 l. 12°. *Amsterdam, C. Commelijn,* 1668.

———. Rare und wunderbare chirurgisch und geneesskünstige Anmerckungen wie solche vor fünff Jahren und also kurtz nach seinem des Authoris tödtlichen Hintritt auf vielfaltiges Anhalten und Begehren denen Kunstlieben zu Gefallen ans Licht gegeben, nunmehr aber auch der hochteutschen Nation zu Nutz getreulich übersetzt und zum Druck befördert. 6 p. l., 536 pp., 12 l. 12°. *Nürnberg, P. Fürsten,* 1675.

———. The same. Observationes medico-chirurgicæ, ex belgico in latinum translatæ ab Abrahamo Blasio. 6 p. l., 392 pp., 3 l. 8°. *Amstelodami, ex off. H. et vid. T. Boom,* 1682.

Meel (Joh. Christophorus). De sympathia atque antipathia rerum naturalium. 13 l. 4°. *Wittebergæ, lit. M. Henckelii,* 1663.

van Meenen (Adolf). * Beiträge zur Kenntniss der Kohlehydrate des Thierkörpers. 23 pp. 8°. *Würzburg, P. Scheiner,* 1886.

van der Meer (Gerhardus). * Diss. exhibens historias quatuor operationum, in diversis capitis regionibus institutarum. 34 pp., 6 l., 3 pl. 4°. *Groningæ, J. Römelingh,* [1829].

van der Meer (Joh.) * De fame canina. 3 l. 4°. *Lugd. Bat., F. Moyaert,* 1660. [P., v. 1217.]

van der Meer Mohr (Joh. Hubertus). * Casus morborum cerebri. ii, 64 pp. 8°. *Amstelodami, H. A. Frijlink,* 1853.

Meerane.

Geissler. Sterblichkeits- und Krankheitsverhältnisse in Meerane während der Jahre 1835 bis 1869. Deutsche Vrtljschr. f. öff. Gsndhtspflg., Brnschwg., 1871, iii, 34–55.

van Meerbeeck (Philippe-Jacques) [1813–72]. * Considérations sur l'emploi de la compression circulaire permanente amovible dans les maladies chirurgicales. 2 p. l., 120 pp., 1 pl. 8°. *Lovanii, Vanlinthout & Vandenzande,* [1839].

———. Recherches historiques et critiques sur la vie et les ouvrages de Rembert Dodoens (Dodonæus). xiv pp., 1 l., 340 pp., 1 pl. 8°. *Malines, P.-J. Hanicq,* 1841.

———. Coup d'œil sur l'état actuel de l'enseignement médical à Paris comparé à celui qui se donne en Belgique. 1 p. l., ii, 26 pp. 8°. *Bruxelles, F. Vertenuil,* 1842.

———. Rapport sur l'état de l'enseignement médical de l'Université de Berlin, pendant le premier semestre de l'année académique 1841–2. 9 pp. 8°. *Bruxelles, F. Vertenuil,* 1842.
Bound with preceding.

———. Relation d'un voyage médical en Hollande, fait pendant l'année académique 1840–41. vi, 7–39 pp. 8°. *Bruxelles, F. Vertenuil,* 1842.
Bound with preceding.

Meerburg (Petrus Cornelius). * De ætatis et sexus differentiis. 3 p. l., 84 pp., 2 l. 8°. *Lugd. Bat., apud vid. D. du Saar,* 1833.

Meerburg (Samuel. Antonius). * De ovariis necnon ovariorum morbis. 4 p. l., 103 pp. 8°. *Lugd. Bat., G. G. Menzel,* 1839.

van Meerdervoort (Jacobus Pompe). * De locatione et conductione. 23 pp. 4°. *Lugd. Bat., S. Luchtmans,* 1730. [P., v. 987.]

Meerfurth (J. Fr. Adolphus). * De sede morborum psychicorum. 32 pp. 8°. *Gryphiæ, F. G. Kunike,* [1846].

Meerhold (Joh. Gottlieb. Augustus). * De usu ac vi chemiæ hodiernæ ad explicandam corporis animalis ægroti rationem. 30 pp. 4°. *Vitebergæ, lit. C. H. Graessleri,* [1705].
For Biography, see **Vogt** (Traugott Carolus Augustus).

Meermann (Peter).
See **Matthiæ** (Friedrich Christian). Ueber Meermann's auf hiesiger Stadtbibliothek [etc.] 4°. *Frankf. a. M.,* 1821.

Meerovitch (I. J.) K etiologii roji i soputstvujoutshich ee zabolevanii. Bakteriologicheskoe izsledovanie. [Etiology of erysipelas and erysipelatous affections. Bacteriological investigations.] 129 pp. 8°. *St. Petersburg, tipog. N. A. Lebedeva,* 1887.

Meers (*John Daggett*) [1794–1878].
Meers (E. S.) Obituary. Proc. Connect. M. Soc., Hartford, 1878, 208.

van der Meersch (Desideratus Josephus). * De hypochondria. 2 p. l., 13 pp. 4°. *Lugd. Bat., J. W. van Leeuwen,* 1817.

de Meersman (Eduardus). * De præcipuis mediis ad aëris vitia corrigenda aptis. 40 pp. 4°. *Gandavi, H. Vandekerckhove,* [1829]. [P., v. 959.]

Meerstadt (Jan Willem Gerhardus). * Bijdrage tot de casuistiek der chorea minor. 2 p. l., 96 pp. 8°. *Leiden, S. C. Van Doesburgh,* 1882.

van Meerten (Hubertus Elisa). * De morbo strumoso. 1 p. l., 122 pp., 2 l. 4°. *Lugd. Bat., J. Hasebroek [et al.],* 1788.

Meerut.

Murray (J.) On the topography of Meerutt, and the principal diseases which prevailed in the 1st brigade of horse artillery at that place. Printed by order of government. 8°. *Calcutta,* 1839.
Jackson (T.) General and medical topography of Meerut. Tr. M. & Phys. Soc. Calcutta, 1823–5, 1, 292–298.

Mees (Lucas). * Over uitscheiding en omzetting van digestiefermenten. 2 l., 49 pp., iv. 8°. *Groningen, Scholtens & Zoon,* 1885.

Mees (Ludovicus Adrianus Alting). Dissertatio medica, continens quædam de usu chloroformi in operationibus chirurgicis. 4 p. l., 67 pp., 3 l. 8°. *Groningæ, P. W. van Heijningen Bosch,* [1855].

Mees (Willem). * Over de werking van Eucalyptus globulus. 2 p. l., 72, vi pp., 2 l. 8°. *Groningen, R. J. Schierbeek,* 1873.

Mees ten Oever (J.) * Een geval van haematometra in den rudimentairen hoorn van een uterus unicornis. 1 p. l., 53 pp., 1 pl. 8°. *Groningen, P. Noordhoff,* 1879.

de Meester (Petrus). * De sudore. 28 pp., 4 l. 4°. *Lugd. Bat., S. et J. Luchtmans,* 1762. [P., v. 1000; 1473.]

Meesters (Theodorus). * De plethora. 21 pp., 3 l. sm. 4°. *Lugd. Bat., J. Hasebroek,* 1735.

van Meeteren (Gysbertus Nicolaus Westerouen). * De animi pathematibus. 2 p. l., 40 pp. 8°. *Lugd. Bat., J. W. van Leeuwen,* 1819.

Megabacchus (*Joh.*) [1495–1555]. *Portrait in:* **Collection**—van Kaathoven.

Megalomania.
See **Insanity** *with delusions of greatness.*

Megastoma.
See **Parasites,** *etc.*

Mège (Jean-Baptiste) [1787–]. * Sur les objets de toilette qui peuvent nuire à la santé. vi, 7–28 pp. 4°. *Paris,* 1813, No. 74, v. 97.

——. Description d'une fièvre intermittente épidémique, avec une notice topographique et des réflexions sur la nouvelle doctrine des fièvres. viii, 64 pp. 8°. *Paris, Bechet,* 1822. [*Also, in:* P., v. 1618.]

——. Observation d'une fistule aérienne occasionnée par une rougeole rentrée, et guérie par un bandage compressif. 7 pp. 8°. *Paris, C. L. F. Panckoucke,* [1824]. *Repr. from:* J. compl. du dict. d. sc. méd., Par., 1824, xix.

——. Lettre à S. Exc. le grand-maître de l'Université royale de France, au sujet de son exclusion du concours des agrégés près la Faculté de médecine de Paris. 30 pp. 8°. *Paris, Ponthieu,* 1824.

——. Des principes fondamentaux de la phrénologie appliqués à la philosophie. Discours prononcé à la séance annuelle de la Société phrénologique de Paris le 9 février 1845. 24, 4 pp. 8°. *Paris, Guiraudet & Jouaust,* 1845.

Megerlin (Amadeus).
See **Scultetus** (Joannes). Wund-artzneyisches Zeug-Hauss. sm. 4°. *Franckfurt,* 1665.

Megerlin (Christian Albertus). * De diabete hypochondriacorum periodico. 28 pp. 4°. *Tubingæ, typ. G. H. Reisi,* 1696.

Mégevand (Alphonse). * Étude de physiologie expérimentale; action de la digitale et de la digitaline. 84 pp. 4°. *Paris,* 1872, No. 253.

Meggen.
See **Gurnigel.**

Meggenhofen (Carol. August.) * Diss. sistens indagationem lactis muliebris chemicam. 22 pp. 4°. *Francof. a. M., C. Naumann,* 1826.

Meglin (Auguste). *Aperçu historique et pratique sur l'opération de la taille chez l'homme. 1 p. l., 28 pp. 4°. *Strasbourg,* 1822, v. 50.

Mégnin (J.-P.) Mémoire sur l'affection typhique du cheval ou le typhus d'écurie (typhus equilis). 95 pp. 8°. *Paris, Renou,* 1874.

——. Étude sur la diathèse dartreuse (herpétisme), et ses manifestations tégumentaires chez les animaux domestiques. 9? pp. 8°. *Paris, Ves. Renou, Maulde & Cock,* 1875.

Mégnin (J.-P.)—continued.

——. Des conditions de la contagion de la gale des animaux à l'homme. 31 pp. 8°. *Paris, P. Asselin,* 1876. *Repr. from:* Arch. gén. de méd., Par., 1876, 6. s., xxxviii.

——. Les parasites et les maladies parasitaires chez l'homme, les animaux domestiques et les animaux sauvages avec lesquels ils peuvent être en contact. Insectes, arachnides, crustacés. Avec un atlas. 1 p. l., 478 pp., 26 pl. 8°. *Paris, G. Masson,* 1880.

——. Formes extérieures et anatomie élémentaire du cheval. 1 broadside fol. *Paris, P. Asselin,* [n. d.]

——. Tableau de l'âge des animaux domestiques. Âge du cheval, du bœuf, du mouton et du chien. 1 broadside fol. *Paris, P. Asselin,* [n. d.]

——. Tableau de l'anatomie élémentaire des maniements et des coupes de boucherie du bœuf. 1 broadside fol. *Paris, P. Asselin,* [n. d.]

——. Tableau de la ferrure du cheval, du mulet et du bœuf. 1 broadside fol. *Paris, P. Asselin,* [n. d.]

——. Tableau des tares et défectuosités du cheval. 1 broadside fol. *Paris, P. Asselin,* [n. d.]

Megrim.
See **Hemicrania.**

Mehadia.
POPOVICIU (A.) Das Herkulesbad bei Mehadia in Siebenbürgen. 8°. *Wien,* 1885.

SCHWARZOTT (J. G.) Die Hercules-Bäder bei Mehadia. 8°. *Wien,* 1831.

Chorin. Mittheilungen aus den Herculesbädern nächst Mehadia. Wien. med. Presse, 1866, vii, 1131; 1155; 1178; 1235.

Meharry medical department of Central Tennessee College, Nashville. Proceedings of the second annual commencement, held Feb. 22, 1878. 14 pp. 8°. *Nashville, Weekly Pilot print,* 1878.

——. Annual announcements for the sessions of 1879–80 to 1884–5 (4.–9.); 1886–7 (11.). 8°. *Nashville,* 1879–86. List of students and graduates for the years 1878–9 to 1883–4; 1885–6, in announcements for subsequent years. Organized in 1875 for colored students. Opened Oct., 1876.

Méhée (Jean). Traité des plaies d'armes à feu, dans lequel on démontre l'inutilité de l'amputation des membres à la suite des blessures faites par les coups de fusils, et l'inutilité générale de cette opération, dans le plus grand nombre des autres cas. x, 11–268 pp. 8°. *Paris, an VIII* [1800].

——. The same. Abhandlung über die Schusswunden. Aus dem Französichen übersetzt von C. R. W. Wiedemann. xiv, 296 pp. 8°. *Braunschweig, C. Reichard,* 1801.

Méhée de La Touche [Jean]. Traité des lésions de la tête par contre-coup, avec des expériences propres à en éclairer la doctrine. xix, 264 pp. 8°. *Meaux, L.-A. Courtois,* 1773.

Méhes (Samuelis). De respiratione animalium commentatio. 4, 60 pp. 4°. *Heidelbergæ, Pfaehler,* 1810.

Mehler (Hermann). * Das partielle Herzaneurysma. 32 pp. 8°. *Berlin, G. Lange,* [1868].

Mehlhausen (A.) Die Cholera-Epidemie des Jahres 1873 in der Armee des ehemaligen Norddeutschen Bundes. *In:* BERICHTE der Cholera-Kommission für das deutsche Reich. 5. Hft. 4°. *Berlin,* 1877, 1–88.

——. Ueber künstliche Beleuchtung. Vortrag gehalten in der deutschen Gesellschaft für öffentliche Gesundheitspflege zu Berlin am 23. Februar 1885. 23 pp. 8°. *Berlin, E. Grosser,* 1885. *Repr. from:* Deutsche Med.-Ztg., Berl., 51. Hft., 1885, vi. *See, also,* **Charité-Annalen.** 1.–5. Jahrg. (1874–8.) 8°. *Berlin,* 1876–80.

Mehlhausen (Felix). * Ein Fall von Aneurysma der Arteria poplitæa, welches durch Stangendruck geheilt wurde. 14 pp., 1 l. 8°. *Kiel, Schmidt u. Klaunig,* 1884.

Mehlhausen (Frid.) [1792–]. * De asthmate convulsivo. 31 pp. 8°. *Berolini, typ. J. F. Starckii,* [1825].

Mehlhausen (Gustavus Guilelmus) [1823–]. * De meningitide. 29 pp., 1 l. 8°. *Berolini, fratrum Schlesinger.* [1849].

Mehlhose (Christophorus) [1800–]. * De intestinis se intussuscipientibus. 28 pp., 1 pl. 4°. *Berolini, typ. Brueschckianis,* [1827].

Mehlhose (Ludov.) * De tumoribus ovariorum cysticis, adjecta morbi historia. 2 p. l., 57 pp. 8°. *Gryphiæ, F. G. Kunike,* 1856.

Mehlig (Fridericus Ludovicus). * De ferro candente ejusque in arthrophlogosibus usu. 27 pp. 4°. *Lipsiæ, ex off. Sturmii et Koppei,* [1843].

Mehling (Stanislas-Joseph). *Cure radicale de l'hydrocèle par la méthode de l'incision avec les précautions antiseptiques. 134 pp., 1 l. 4°. *Montpellier,* 1883, No. 60.

Mehlis (Car. Frid. Ed.) [1796–1832]. Commentatio de morbis hominis dextri et sinistri. 119 pp. 4°. *Gottingæ, C. Herbst,* 1818.
Also, in : FRANK (J.) Delect. opusc. ad prax. med. spec. 8°. *Novocomi,* 1827, i, 1–222.

Mehlis (Christian). * Die Grundidee des Hermes vom Standpunkte der vergleichenden Mythologie. 64 pp., 1 l., 1 tab. 8°. *Erlangen, E. T. Jacob,* 1875.

Mehlis (Georgius Henr. Conradus). * De excitantium usu in febribus, potissimum putridis. 1 l., 59 pp. 8°. *Gottingæ, J. A. Barmeier,* [1787].

Mehlis (Theodor). * Ueber Heptylsäure aus Oenanthol und einige ihrer Derivate. 30 pp. 8°. *Erlangen, E. T. Jacob,* 1876.

Mehliss (Carl Wilhelm) [1806–]. * Helcographiæ specimen. 40 pp. 8°. *Berolini, typ. A. Petschii,* [1830].

———. Ueber Virilescenz und Rejuvenescenz thierischer Körper. Ein Beitrag zur Lehre von der regelwidrigen Metamorphose organischer Körper. 1 p. l., 114 pp. 8°. *Leipzig, L. Schreck,* 1838.

———. Die Krankheiten des Zwerchfells des Menschen. x, 212 pp., 1 l. 8°. *Eisleben, G. Reichardt,* 1845.

Mehls (Guilielmus Ludovicus). * De tussi convulsiva. 30 pp. 8°. *Regiomonti, typ. Hartungianis,* 1814.

Mehnert (Joannes Gotthelfus).
See **Leonhardi** (Fridericus Gottlob.) & **Mehnertus** (Joannes Gotth.) Symbolæ ad historiam agriculturæ [etc.] 4°. *Lipsiæ,* 1790.

ver Mehr (Joa. Leon. Corn.) * De endosmo et exosmo. 4 p. l., 59 pp., 1 pl. 8°. *Lugd. Bat., Haak et soc.,* 1835.

Mehring (*Abraham Buffington*) [1842–78].
Hewston (G.) Obituary. Tr. M. Soc. Calif. 1878–9, Sacramento, 1879, 249.

Mehrmann (H. B.)
Co-Editor of : **California** Medical Journal, Oakland, 1886.

Méhu (Camille-Jean-Marie). * Recherches pour servir à l'histoire chimique et pharmaceutique de la petite centaurée. 44 pp. 4°. *Paris, Pillet fils aîné,* 1862.
École sup. de pharm. de Par.

———. *Étude chimique et physique sur l'érythrocentaurine et sur la santonine. 38 pp. 4°. *Paris,* 1865, No. 263.

———. Observations pharmaceutiques. 13 pp. 8°. [*Paris,* 1868.]
Repr. from : J. de pharm. et chim., Par., 1868, 4. s., viii.

———. Nouvelles observations sur l'huile phosphorée. 8 pp. 8°. [*Paris,* 1868, *vel subseq.*]
Repr. from : J. de pharm. et chim., Par., 1868, 4. s., viii.

Méhu (Camille-Jean-Marie)—continued.
———. Traité pratique et élémentaire de chimie médicale appliquée aux recherches cliniques. vii, 394 pp. 12°. *Paris, P. Asselin,* 1870.

———. The same. 2. éd. viii, 592 pp. 12°. *Paris, P. Asselin,* 1878.

———. L'urine normale et pathologique. Les calculs urinaires. Histoire médicale, analyse chimique. vi, 391 pp. 8°. *Paris, Asselin & Cie.,* 1880.
Also, Editor of : **Annuaire** de la pharmacie française et étrangère, Paris, 1875-7.—**Annuaire** pharmaceutique, Paris, 1871-4. — **Annales** des maladies des organes génito-urinaires, Paris, 1882.
See, also, **Sestier** (F.) De la foudre, [etc.] 8°. *Paris,* 1866.

Meibomian *glands.*
See **Eyelids.**

Meibomian *glands* (*Diseases of*).
See **Eyelids** (*Diseases of*).

Meibomius (*Brandanus*) [1678–1740].
Portrait in : **Collection**—van Kaathoven.—**Collection** of Portraits of Phys. & Men of Sc., 116.

Meibomius (Daniel. Henricus). *Disputatio de patellæ osse ejusque læsionibus et curatione. 1697.
In : HALLER. Disp. anat. [etc.] 4°. *Groningæ,* 1751, vi, 209–224.

Meibomius (Henricus) [1638–1700]. De incubatione in fanis deorum medicinæ causa olim facta. 19 pp. 4°. *Helmstadi, typ. H. Mulleri,* 1659.

———. Exercitatio medica de observationibus rarioribus in nupero subjecto anatomico. *Groningæ,* 1660.
In : HALLER. Disp. anat. [etc.] 4°. *Groningæ,* 1751, vi, 635–651.

———. De longævis. 30 pp. 4°. *Helmæstadi, typ. H. Mulleri,* 1664.

———. * De vasis palpebrarum novis epistola. 11 l., 1 pl. sm. 4°. *Helmstadi, typ. H. Mulleri,* 1666.

———. De motu sanguinis naturali et præternaturali. *Helmst.,* 1668.
In : HALLER. Disp. anat. [etc.] 4°. *Groningæ,* 1747, ii, 567–593.

———. De medicorum historia scribenda. Epistola ad Georg. Hier. Velschium. 7 l. 4°. *Helmstadii, typ. H. Mulleri,* 1669.

———. Exercitatio anatomico-medica de valvulis seu membranulis vasorum earumque structura et usu. *Helmstadii,* 1682.
In : HALLER. Disp. anat. [etc.] 4°. *Groningæ,* 1747, ii, 49–78.

———. De abscessuum interiorum natura et constitutione. Discursus, in academia Julia e cathedra olim habitus, et nunc a paterna bibliotheca communicatus a J. G. B. med. dr. 120 pp. sm. 4°. *Dresdæ et Lipsiæ, J. J. Wincklero vid.,* 1718.

———. De catheterismo.
In : HALLER. Disp. chir. [etc.] 4°. *Lausannæ,* 1755, iv, 441–456.
See, also, **Cober** (Tobias). Observationum medicarum castrensium Hungaricarum decades tres, [etc.] 4°. *Helmstadii,* 1685.—**Quatuor** luculentorum opusculorum, [etc.] 12°. *Lugd. Bat.,* 1723.
For Portrait, see **Collection**—van Kaathoven.—**Collection** of Portr. of Phys. & Men of Sc., 110.

Meibomius (Henricus Johannes). De methodo præcavendi in consolidandis vulneribus et ulceribus cicatricem. 16 pp. 4°. *Jenæ, lit. Croekerianis.* 1739.

———. * De texturæ solidorum in humano corpore diversitate, ejusque cognitione in diæta ordinanda et medicamentis præscribendis necessaria. 23 pp., 3 l. 4°. *Helmæstadi, typ. P. D. Schnorrii,* [1740].

———. * Diss. sistens casum rarissimum hepatitidem fluxu alvi purulento solutam sicque per-

Meibomius (Henricus Johannes)—continued.
fecte sanatam. 38 pp. 4°. *Helmœstadi, lit.
Drimbornianis*, [1741].

——. Gegründetes Bedencken über einen Gestanck aus dem Munde, benebst der Untersuchung und Widerlegung des darin befindlichen
Visi reperti. Mit Anmerckungen von Paul Gottlieb Werlhof. 64 pp. 4°. *Franckfurt u. Leipzig*, 1743.

Meibomius (Joannes Henricus) [1590–1655].
De flagrorum usu in re veneria, et lumborum
renumque officio. 79 pp. 32°. *Londini*, 1665.

——. Magni Aurelii Cassiodori, formula comitis
archiatrorum; commentario [etc.] 2 p. l., 86 pp.
4°. *Helmestadi, typ. H. Mulleri*, 1668.

——. De cerevisiis potibusque et ebriaminibus
extra vinum aliis commentarius. Accedit Adr.
Turnebi libellus de vino. 96 l. sm. 4°. *Helmestadii, typ. J. Heitmulleri*, 1668.

See, also, **Bartholinus** (Thomas), **Meibomius**
(Joannes Henricus), & **Meibomius** (H.) De uso flagrorum in re veneria. 8°. *Francofurti*, 1670.—**Hippocrates**. "Ορκος, sive jusjurandum [etc.] 4°. *Lugd. Bat.*,
1643.

Meichernerus (Matthias). De formis materialibus. 9 l. 4°. *Wittebergœ, typ. hœred. J. Ha-
ken*, [1654].

Meichinger (J.) *See* **Widman** (Joh.), *dictus*
Meichinger.

Meidinger (Heinrich). Statistische Uebersicht der geistigen und sittlichen Zustände in
Grossbritannien und Ireland. 1 p. l., 144 pp.,
4 l. 8°. *Leipzig, F. Fleischer*, 1851.

Repr. from: Britische (Das) Reich in Europa [ein grös-
seres Werk desselben Verfassers].

Meier (Arnoldus). * De errore loci. 25 pp., 2 l.
sm. 4°. *Lugd. Bat., T. Haak*, 1720.

Meier (Car. Theod. Maxim.) [1810–]. * De
morbis senii nonnulla. 30 pp., 1 l. 8°. *Berolini, typ. Nietackianis*, 1836.

——. Case of carcinoma of the eyelid, cured by
blepharoplastic operation. 4 pp. 8°. *New York,
J. F. Trow*, 1852.

Repr. from: N. York J. M., 1852, n. s., ix.

——. On the formation of an artificial anus.
8 pp. 8°. [*New York*, 1859.]

Repr. from: Am. M. Month., N. Y., 1859, xi.

See, also, **Dieffenbach** (Joh. Fried.) Vorträge in
der chirurgischen Klinik, [etc.] 4°. *Berlin*, 1840.

Meier (Carolus Gottlob.) * De carice arenaria
sive sassaparilla germanica. 40 pp. 4°. *Francof. ad Viadr., typ. J. C. Winteri*, [1772].

For Biography, see **Winkler** (Joan. Henricus).

Meier (Christ. Frid. Guil. Immanuel.) * Diss.
sistens idealem organismi animalis construc-
tionem. 2 p. l., 44 pp., 1 l. 8°. *Halœ, formis
J. C. Hendelii*, [1804].

Meier (Christianus Ernestus) [1773–]. * De
varia sodæ indole et nova eidem medendi methodo. 29 pp. 8°. *Erfordiœ, J. C. Goerling*,
[1792].

Meier (Dan. Edward). Geburtshülfliche Beobachtungen und Ergebnisse, gesammelt in der
obstetricischen Klinik zu Halle, nebst Beschreibung der Niemeyerschen Kopfzange und eines
Kephalopelykometer. xvi, 169 pp., 1 l., 2 pl.
8°. *Bremen, C. Schünemann*, 1838.

——. Die neue Krankenanstalt in Bremen. 2.
Aufl. 72 pp., 3 pl. 8°. *Bremen, C. Schünemann*,
1850.

——. Ueber künstliche Beine. vii, 56 pp. 8°.
Berlin, A. Hirschwald, 1871.

Meier (Franz Andreas). * Ueber das Verhältniss der Religion zur Heilkunst. 30 pp. 8°.
München, J. Deschler, 1840.

Meier (Fridericus Gottlieb.) * De malo hysterico. 28 pp. sm. 4°. *Gottingœ, lit. J. C. L.
Schultzii*, [1741].

For Biography, see **Richter** (Geo. Gottlob).

Meier (Friedrich Gottlieb).

See **Brendel** (Joh. Gothofred.) Medicina legalis sine
forensis, etc. sm. 4°. *Hannover*, 1789.

Meier (Gerhardus). * De diarrhœæ pathologia.
36 pp., 4 l. 4°. *Jenœ, lit. Ritterianis*, [1752].

For Biography, see **Kaltschmied** (Carolus Friedericus.)

Meier (Heinrich) [1860–]. * Die combinierte
Wendung bei Placenta prævia. 47 pp. 8°.
Berlin, O. Francke, [1884].

Meier (Henr. Joan.) * De pneumoniæ diagnosi.
24 pp. 8°. *Herbipoli, ex off. vid. C. Becker*,
1841.

Meier (Henricus Lohalmus). * De animi, ejusque
affectuum quoad valetudinem, impressionibus in
corpus. 7 l. 4°. *Lugd. Bat., A. Elzevier*, 1696.

Meier (J. L. J.)

See **Brera** (Valeriano Luigi). Klinischer Commentar
über die Behandlung der Wasserscheu, [etc.] 8°. *Brandenburg*, 1822.

Meier (Jacobus Ericus). * De usu aquæ diætetico. 1 p. l., 32 pp. 4°. *Gottingœ, H. M.
Grape*, [1789].

——. The same. 32 pp. 4°. *Gottingœ, J. D.
G. Brose*, 1789.

Meier (Joan. Christianus Fridericus Immanuel.)
* De affectibus gravidarum. 57 pp. 4°. *Halœ
Salicæ, œre Hendeliano*, [1779].

Meier (Joannes Ludovicus). * De æthiope vegetabili cum analectis nonnullis de salibus. lxxii
pp. 4°. *Erlangœ, typ. Waltherianis*, 1774.

Meier (Joh. Ludolphus Christianus). * Historia
nuperæ dissectionis feminæ gravidæ. 20 pp.
sm. 4°. *Gottingœ, A. Vandenhoek*, [1739].

Meier (Otto Fridericus). * De dysenteriæ curationibus antiquis. 36 pp. sm. 4°. *Gottingœ,
lit. Schulzianis*, 1765.

Meier (Wilhelm) [1785–1853]. Entwurf einer
Hospital-Ordnung für die Hospitäler oder Krankenhäuser im Grossherzogthum Baden. 3–40 pp.
8°. *Freiburg, F. Wagner*, 1843.

Repr. from: Ann. d. Staatsarznk., Freib., 1843, viii, 4.
Hft.

——. Mittheilungen über die Einrichtung mehrerer badischen Militär-Hospitäler und über den
Stand der Kranken und Verwundeten in denselben während der revolutionären und kriege-
rischen Bewegung des Jahres 1849. 44 pp. 8°.
Erlangen, F. Enke, 1853.

Repr. from: Deutsche Ztschr. f. d. Staatsarznk., Erlang., 1853, n. F., i.

——. Erinnerungen aus den Feldzügen 1806 bis
1815. Aus den hinterlassenen Papieren eines
Militärarztes. viii, 160 pp. 8°. *Karlsruhe, C.
F. Müller*, 1854.

Meierei "Zschadras".

See **Landes-Versorg-Anstalt** zu Colditz. Ueber
die Fortentwickelung der . . . 8°. [*Berlin*, 1872.]

von M[eiern] (C[aroline]). Entdeckung des
Geheimnisses die Cholera-Krankheit im Keime
zu ersticken, und zugleich diejenigen bewährten Schutz- und Heilmittel enthält, welche diese
Krankheit schon früher in Deutschland ausge-
rottet haben, [etc.] 64 pp., 1 l. 8°. *München,
F. S. Hübschmann*, 1831.

Meierott (Henric. Frideric.) * De incremento
corporis animalis. 27 pp. 8°. *Halœ, typ. J. C.
Hendelii*, [1801].

Meierus (Michael). * De epilepsia. 11 l. 8°.
Basileæ, C. Waldkirch, 1596. [P., v. 133.]

Meige (Achille). * De l'application de la galvano-puncture au traitement des anévrysmes.
44 pp. 4°. *Paris*, 1851, No. 253, v. 512.

Meige (Léon). * Étude sur les métastases goutteuses et leurs principales causes. 52 pp. 4°.
Paris, 1862, No. 182.

Meige (Pierre-Ulysse). * Sur la métrite, considérée dans son état aigu et chronique. 23 pp.
4°. *Paris*, 1827, No. 90, v. 207.

Meige (Victor-Pierre) [1856–   ].   *Recherches sur les variations de l'urée du sang dans les différentes maladies et en particulier dans la rétention d'urine. 83 pp., 1 l.   4°.   *Paris*, 1885, No. 109.

Meigs (Arthur V.)   Milk analysis.   4 pp.   8°.   *Philadelphia*, 1882.
   Repr. from : Phila. M. Times, 1881-2, xii.

——.   Memoir of J. Forsyth Meigs.   Read before the College of Physicians of Philadelphia, March 5, 1884.   25 pp.   8°.   *Philadelphia*, 1884.
   Repr. from : Tr. Coll. Phys. Phila., 1884, 3. s., vii.

——.   Milk analysis and infant feeding.   A practical treatise on the examination of human and cows' milk, cream, condensed milk, etc., and directions as to the diet of young infants.   vi, 102 pp.   12°.   *Philadelphia, P. Blakiston, Son & Co.*, 1885.

Meigs (Charles D.) [1792–1869].   An oration delivered before the Philadelphia Medical Society, February 18, 1829.   28 pp.   8°.   *Philadelphia, J. Kay, jr., & Co.*, 1829.   [*Also, in :* P., v. 763.]

——.   The Philadelphia practice of midwifery. xii, 370 pp.   8°.   *Philadelphia, J. Kay, jr., & Bro.*, 1838.

——.   The same.   2. ed.   408 pp., 1 l., 36 pp. 8°.   *Philadelphia, J. Kay, jr., & Bro.*, 1842.

——.   Introductory lecture to a course on obstetrics, delivered in Jefferson Medical College. 18 pp.   8°.   *Philadelphia, Merrihew & Thompson*, 1841.

——.   A lecture introductory to the course of obstetrics in Jefferson Medical College.   31 pp. 8°.   *Philadelphia, Merrihew & Thompson*, 1842.

——.   Lecture introductory to his course of lectures for 1843-4.   31 pp.   8°.   *Philadelphia, Merrihew & Thompson*, 1843.

——.   Introductory lecture.   24 pp., 1 l.   8°. *Philadelphia, Merrihew & Thompson*, 1846.

——.   Lecture on some of the distinctive characteristics of the female.   20 pp.   8°.   *Philadelphia, Collins*, 1847.   [*Also, in :* P., v. 102.]

——.   An introductory lecture.   20 pp.   8°. *Philadelphia, C. Sherman*, 1848.

——.   Females and their diseases; a series of letters to his class.   xii, 17-670 pp.   8°.   *Philadelphia, Lea & Blanchard*, 1848.

——.   The same.   Woman; her diseases and remedies.   A series of letters to his class.   2. ed. xvi, 25-690 pp.   8°.   *Philadelphia, Lea & Blanchard*, 1851.

——.   The same.   3. ed.   xvi, 38-672 pp.   8°. *Philadelphia, Blanchard & Lea*, 1854.

——.   The same.   4. ed.   706 pp.   8°.   *Philadelphia, Blanchard & Lea*, 1859.

——.   Remarks on spasmodic cholera.   68 pp. 8°.   *Philadelphia*, 1849.
   Printed, not published.

——.   Obstetrics: the science and art.   xx, 685 pp.   8°.   *Philadelphia, Lea & Blanchard*, 1849.

——.   The same.   3. ed., revised.   xxiii, 33-758 pp.   8°.   *Philadelphia, Blanchard & Lea*, 1856.

——.   Observations on certain of the diseases of young children.   viii, 17-215 pp.   8°.   *Philadelphia, Lea & Blanchard*, 1850.

——.   Introductory lecture.   20 pp.   8°.   *Philadelphia, T. K. & P. G. Collins*, 1850.

——.   A memoir of Samuel George Morton, M. D., late president of the Academy of Natural Sciences of Philadelphia.   48 pp.   8°.   *Philadelphia, Collins*, 1851.   [*Also, in :* P., v. 161; 848.]

——.   Charge to the graduates of Jefferson Medical College, delivered March 6, 1852.   15 pp.   8°. *Philadelphia, T. K. & P. G. Collins*, 1852.

——.   A biographical notice of Daniel Drake, M. D., of Cincinnati.   Prepared by appointment of the College of Physicians of Philadelphia. 38 pp.   8°.   *Philadelphia, Lippincott, Grambo & Co.*, 1853.

Meigs (Charles D.)—continued.

——.   On the nature, signs, and treatment of childbed fevers, in a series of letters addressed to the students of his class.   xvi, 33-362 pp.   8°. *Philadelphia, Blanchard & Lea*, 1854.

——.   A treatise on acute and chronic diseases of the neck of the uterus.   116 pp., 22 pl.   8°. *Philadelphia, Blanchard & Lea*, 1854.

——.   Introductory lecture to the class of midwifery.   24 pp.   8°.   *Philadelphia, Collins*, 1854.

——.   Charge to the graduating class of Jefferson Medical College.   (With a list of the graduates.)   16 pp.   8°.   *Philadelphia, Collins*, 1858.

——.   Introductory lecture.   21 pp.   8°.   *Philadelphia, J. M. Wilson*, 1859.

——.   A farewell address to his class, Feb. 27, 1861.   16 pp.   8°.   *Philadelphia, Collins*, 1861.
   Also, Co-Editor of: **North American** (The) Medical and Surgical Journal, Philadelphia, 1826-7.
   See, also, **Colombat** (Marc).   A treatise on the diseases and special hygiene of females.   8°.   *Philadelphia*, 1845.—**History** (The), pathology, and treatment of puerperal fever and crural phlebitis.   8°.   *Philadelphia*, 1842.—**Hufeland** (Christoph Wilhelm).   A treatise on the scrofulous disease [etc.]   8°.   *Philadelphia*, 1829.—**Lee** (Robert).   On puerperal fever [etc.]   8°.   *Philadelphia*, 1842.—**Velpeau** (A. A. L. M.)   An elementary treatise on midwifery [etc.]   8°.   *Philadelphia*, 1831.
   For Biography, see Boston M. & S. J., 1849, xl, 313; 333.   *Also :* Proc. Am. Phil. Soc., Phila., 1873, xiii, 170-179 (J. Bell).   *Also :* Tr. Coll. Phys. Phila., 1872, n. s., iv, 417-448 (J. F. Meigs).

Meigs (J. Forsyth) [1818–82].   A practical treatise on the diseases of children.   xv, 24-575 pp.   8°.   *Philadelphia, Lindsay & Blakiston*, 1848.

——.   The same.   2. ed.   xvi, 17-711 pp.   8°. *Philadelphia, Lindsay & Blakiston*, 1853.

——.   The same.   3. ed.   xvi, 17-724 pp.   8°. *Philadelphia, Lindsay & Blakiston*, 1858.
   See, also, infra (MEIGS & PEPPER), for later editions.

——.   Address delivered before the managers, medical staff, and students of the Pennsylvania Hospital, on the occasion of the opening of the new lecture and operating room, Jan. 9, 1869. 35 pp.   sm. 8°.   *Philadelphia, Lindsay & Blakiston*, 1871.

——.   A history of the first quarter of the second century of the Pennsylvania Hospital.   145 pp., 1 pl.   8°.   *Philadelphia*, 1877.

——.   On the internal use of water for the sick, and on thirst.   A clinical lecture.   54 pp.   12°. *Philadelphia, Lindsay & Blakiston*, 1880.

——.   Proceedings of the Alumni Society of the medical department of the University of Pennsylvania for 1880.   With the annual address by . . .   31 pp., 1 pl.   8°.   *Philadelphia, Collins*, 1881.
   See, also, **Sanitary** (The) care and treatment of children, etc.   8°.   *Boston*, 1881.
   For Biography, see **Pepper** (W.)   Memoir of J. F. Meigs.   8°.   [n. p., 1883.]   *Also :* Med. News, Phila., 1882, xli, 724.   *Also :* Tr. Coll. Phys. Phila., 1884, 3. s., vii, pp. lxxi-xciii (A. V. Meigs).   *Also,* Reprint.

—— **& Pepper** (William).   A practical treatise on the diseases of childen.   4. ed. (of Meigs On diseases of children).   xvi, 17-921 pp.   8°.   *Philadelphia, Lindsay & Blakiston*, 1870.
   See, also, supra (MEIGS), for prior editions.

——.   The same.   6. ed.   xv, 16-1012 pp.   8°. *Philadelphia, Lindsay & Blakiston*, 1877.

Meigs (James Aitken) [1829–79].   A brief notice of Dr. Martyn Paine's work on the "Institutes of medicine"; with some remarks on the theory of the correlation of the physical and vital forces. 19 pp.   8°.   [*Philadelphia*, 1853.]
   Repr. from : N. Am. M.-Chir. Rev., Phila., 1853.

——.   Essay on the relation of atomic heat to crystalline form.   32 pp.   4°.   *Philadelphia, Merrihew & Thompson*, 1855.
   Repr. from : Proc. Acad. Nat. Sc. Phila., 1855, iii, pt. 2.

——.   Catalogue of human crania, in the collection of the Academy of Natural Sciences of Philadelphia; based upon the third edition of Dr.

Meigs (James Aitken)—continued.
Morton's Catalogue of skulls, etc. 112 pp. 8°. *Philadelphia*, 1857.

——. Hints to craniographers, upon the importance and feasibility of establishing some uniform system by which the collection and promulgation of craniological statistics and the exchange of duplicate crania may be promoted. 8 pp. 8°. *Philadelphia, Merrihew & Thompson*, 1858. [*Also, in:* P., v. 1492.]
Repr. from: Proc. Acad. Nat. Sc. Phila., 1858.

——. Description of a deformed, fragmentary human skull, found in an ancient quarry-cave at Jerusalem; with an attempt to determine, by its configuration alone, the ethnical type to which it belongs. 262–280 pp. 8°. *Philadelphia, Merrihew & Thompson*, 1859.
Cutting from: Proc. Acad. Sc. Phila., 1859.

——. Some remarks on the methods of studying and teaching physiology. 36 pp. 8°. *Philadelphia, J. B. Lippincott & Co.*, 1859.
Repr. from: N. Am. M.-Chir. Rev., Phila., 1859, iii.

——. Valedictory address to the graduating class of the Philadelphia College of Medicine. 16 pp. 8°. *Philadelphia, Bryson*, 1859.

——. Observations upon the cranial forms of the American aborigines, based upon specimens contained in the collection of the Academy of Natural Sciences of Philadelphia. 39 pp. 8°. *Philadelphia*, [1866].
Repr. from: Proc. Acad. Nat. Sc. Phila., 1866.

——. An inaugural address introductory to the course on institutes of medicine in the Jefferson Medical College. (Correlation of the physical and vital forces.) 32 pp. 8°. *Philadelphia, Medical & Surgical Reporter*, 1868.

——. Valedictory address to the graduating class of Jefferson Medical College. 29 pp. 8°. *Philadelphia, Collins*, 1870.

——. Valedictory address to the graduating class of Jefferson Medical College. 20 pp. 8°. *Philadelphia, Collins*, 1879.
For Biography, see Boston M. & S. J., 1879, ci, 742–744. *Also:* Med. Bull., Phila., 1880, ii, 65; 76; 91; 119; 126: 1881, iii, 33–37. *Also,* Reprint. *Also:* Med. Rec., N. Y., 1879, xvi, 502. *Also:* Phila. M. Times, 1879–80, x, 102–104 (F. W.) *Also:* Tr. Am. Ass., Phila., 1880, xxxi, 1069–1075 (F. Woodbury). *Also:* Tr. Coll. Phys. Phila., 1881, 3. s., v, pp. cxvii–cxxxiii (H. C. Chapman). *Also:* Tr. M. Soc. Penn., Phila., 1880, xiii, pt. 1, 385–400 (G. Hamilton). *Also,* Reprint.

Meihsner (Joann. Gust. Car.) [1814–]. *De Paracelso. 34 pp., 1 l. 8°. *Berolini, typ. fratrum Schlesinger*, [1847].

Meihuizen (Samuel). Invloed van sommige stoffen op de reflexprikkelbaarheid van het ruggemerg. 62 pp. 8°. *Groningen, J. B. Wolters*, 1872.

de Meij (Gulielmus Franciscus). *De gastritide. 1 p. l., 55, iv, 4 pp. 8°. *Groningæ, F. Mekel*, [1825].

de Meijer (Gillis van Overbeek). *See* **van Overbeek de Meijer** (Gillis).

de Meijer (Guilielmus Jacobus). *Diss. contineus colitidis gangrænosæ casus duos. 30 pp. 8°. *Lugd. Bat., D. Noothoven van Goor*, [1855].

Meijers (J.) Handleiding voor de verpleging van zieken aan boord Zr. Ms. schepen. vi, 7–134 pp., 3 l., 1 pl. 12°. *Nieuwediep, J. C. De Buisonjé*, 1880.

Meijers (M.), jr.
See **Ultzmann** (Robert) & **Hoffmann** (Karel Berthold). Handleiding tot het onderzoek der urine, [etc.] 8°. *Amsterdam*, 1873.

Meijlink (B.)
See **Hermann** (R.) Schekundig onderzoek van de uitgebraakte en door stoelgang ontlaste stoffen, etc. 8°. *Deventer*, 1831.—**Tilesius** (W. G.) Iets over de cholera en eenige artsenijen, die eene heilzame werking tegen dezelve oefenen. Uit het Hoogduitsch door B. Meijlink. 8°. *Deventer*, 1831.

Meikle (James). Observations on the rate of mortality of assured lives, as experienced by ten assurance companies in Scotland, from 1815 to 1863. 69 pp., 10 diag. fol. *Edinburgh, W. Blackwood & Sons*, 1872.

Meikleham (D. S.)
Editor of: **New York** (The) Medical Intelligencer, or Eclectic Gazette, 1845.

Meilhac (Geraud). *Sur la goutte. vi, 7–31 pp. 4°. *Paris*, 1826, No. 105, v. 200.

Meilhac (P.) *Recherches sur l'amaurose syphilitique. 55 pp. 4°. *Paris*, 1863, No. 36.

Meilheurat (P.-A.) *Sur l'érysipèle. 30 pp. 4°. *Paris*, 1828, No. 195, v. 218.

Meilhon (Abel-Joseph). *Du suicide dans le délire ou folie des persécutions. 56 pp. 4°. *Bordeaux*, 1886, No. 64, 1885–6.

Meilitz (Davides) [1840–]. *De syphilidis historia et theoria. 30 pp., 1 l. 8°. *Berolini, G. Schade*, [1862].

Meillet (Antoine-Frédéric). *I. Des modifications que le sexe apporte dans le traitement des maladies. II. [etc.] 33 pp. 4°. *Paris*, 1841, No. 177, v. 378.

Meillet [H.] *Des déformations permanentes de la main au point de vue de la séméiologie médicale. 130 pp., 2 pl. 4°. *Paris*, 1874, No. 101.

Meilly (Otto Ludovicus) [1844–]. *Quæ anæsthetica usque ad nostra tempora in arte chirurgica adhibita sint. 32 pp. 8° *Berolini, G. Lange*, [1867].

Meïmaroglu (Panagiotis A.) *Ueber einen Acardiacus. 30 pp., 1 l. 8°. *Halle a. S., Plötz*, 1879.

Meinau (Joannes Everhardus). *De insitione morbillorum. 1 p. l., 10 pp., 1 l. 4°. *Hardervici, J. Moojen*, [1777].

Meinberg.

BRANDES (R.) Die Mineralquellen und Schwefelschlammbäder zu Meinberg, nebst Beiträgen zur Kenntniss der Vegetation und der klimatischen und mineralogisch-geognostischen Beschaffenheit des Fürstenthums Lippe-Detmold. 4°. *Lemgo*, 1832.

TRAMPEL (J. E.) Beschreibung der Meinberger Mineralquellen in der Grafschaft Lippe, nebst einem Sendschreiben des Johann Friederich Zückert, vom Meinberger Mineralwasser zum innerlichen und äusserlichen Gebrauch. 2. Aufl. 8°. *Lemgo*, 1775.

UEBERSICHT über die Curmittel Meinbergs, deren Anwendung und Wirksamkeit. 8°. [*Detmold*, 1862.]

ZÜCKERT (J. F.) Vom Meinberger Mineralwasser in einem Sendschreiben an den Herrn D. Johann Erhard Trampel. 12°. *Lemgo*, 1774.

von dem Busch (G.) Ueber die Heilquellen zu Meinberg, namentlich die dortigen Mineral-Schlammbäder und die neuen Einrichtungen zur Benutzung des kohlensauren Gases. J. d. pract. Heilk., Berl., 1837, lxxxiv, 2. St., 61–94.—**Caspari.** Das Bad Meinberg im Fürstenthum Lippe und seine kohlensauren Gasquellen. Deutsche Klinik, Berl., 1869, xxi, 49–53. ——. Die Cursaison des Jahres 1869 in Meinberg, Lippe. *Ibid.*, 1870, xxii, 133; 143. ——. Bad Meinberg im Fürstenthum Lippe-Detmold. *Ibid.*, 1871, xxiii, 108; 141; 151. ——. Ueber Curerfolge bei Tabes dorsualis und anderen Central-Lähmungen im Bade Meinberg, Fürstenthum Lippe. *Ibid.*, 1872, xxiv, 135; 149. ——. Geschichtliches über Meinberg, besonders Auffindung der kohlensauren Gasquellen daselbst. *Ibid.*, 249–252. ——. Ueber die Curerfolge bei Gicht und Rheumatismus zu Bad Meinberg. [15 cases.] *Ibid.*, 1873, xxv, 34–37. ——. Lage, Umgebung und Einrichtung von Bad Meinberg. *Ibid.*, 153; 161. ——. Meinberg als Curort für Frauenkrankheiten. *Ibid.*, 457; 469. ——. Die Schwefelschlammbäder in Meinberg. Jahrb. f. Balneol., etc., Wien, 1876, ii, 94–102. ——. Die Kursaison des Jahres 1877 in Meinberg. Deutsche med. Wchnschr., Berl., 1878, iv, 145–148.—**Piderit.** Meinberg im Sommer 1836. Jahrv. f. Deutschl. Heilq. u. Seebäder, Berl., 1837, ii, 147–182. ——. Meinberg im Sommer 1837. *Ibid.*, 1838, iii, 439–474.

Meindersma (Sieds). * Iets over resectie van de onderkaak. 2 p. l., 58 pp. 8°. *Utrecht, Kemink & Zoon,* 1882.

Meindl (Josephus). * De osteomalacia. 19 pp. 8°. *Monachii, F. S. Hübschmann,* 1843.

Meinecke (Augustus Henricus) [1808–   ]. * De inguinum bubonibus syphiliticis quædam. 32 pp. 8°. *Berolini, typ. fratrum Unger,* [1830].

———. Das Chloroform und seine schmerzstillende Kraft. 69 pp. 8°. *Hamburg, Hartwig u. Müller,* 1849.
Repr. from: Ztschr. f. d. ges. Med., Hamb., 1849, lx.

Meinecke (Chr. Andr. Davides) [1801–   ]. * De cyanosi. 43 pp. 8°. *Berolini, formis Brüschckianis,* [1825].

Meineke (Albertus Christophorus). * De vera morbi hypochondriaci sede, indole, ac curatione. 36 pp. sm. 4°. *Halæ Magdeb., typ. C. Henckelii,* [1719].

Meineke (Daniel. Christophorus). * De incubo. 13 l. 4°. *Jenæ, typ. vid. S. Krebsii,* 1683.

Meineke (Guilielmus). * Systematis medicorum psychici succinctam historiam . . . publice defendet. 37 pp. 8°. *Halæ, typ. J. C. Hendelii,* [1800].

Meinel (Carl August). Ein Fall von Aetherisation mit lethalem Ausgang, bei Tetan. traumaticus. 32 pp. 8°. *München, J. Rösl,* 1847.

Meinel (Eugen August) [1819–52]. * Ueber Knochentuberkeln. [Munich.] iv, 64 pp. 8°. *Erlangen, F. Junge,* 1842.

Meinel (Friedrich). * Ueber die Erkrankung der Lungen durch Kieselstaubinhalation (Chalicosis pulmonum). 46 pp. 8°. *Erlangen, E. T. Jacob,* 1869.
C.
See, also, **Layet** (A.) Allgemeine und specielle Gewerbe-Pathologie, [etc.] 8°. *Erlangen,* 1877.

Meinel (Joannes Georgius Christophorus). * De difficili vulnerum in nosocomiis militaribus cura ejusque causis. 22 pp. 4°. *Altorfii, lit. J. P. Meyeri,* [1799].

Meinel (Joh. Heinricus). * De cataractæ nova pathologia. Von dem weisen oder grauen Stahr. 11 l. 4°. *Erfordiæ, typ. Groschianis,* 1708.

Meiners (Heinrich). Das städtische Wohnhaus der Zukunft, oder, wie sollen wir bauen und auf welche Weise ventiliren und heizen? Theoretisch-practische Abhandlungen über Bau-Ausführungen vom hygienischen, ökonomischen und staatlichen Standpunkte aus beleuchtet. 2. Aufl. vi pp., 1 l., 136 pp. roy. 8°. *Stuttgart, K. Wittwer,* 1880.

Meinert (August Wilhelm Erich). * Bericht über die Militär-Pockenstation zu Leipzig im Jahre 1871. 37 pp., 1 l., 3 tab. 8°. [*Leipzig,* 1872.]

Meinert (C. A.) Armee- und Volks-Ernährung. Ein Versuch Prof. C. von Voit's Ernährungstheorie für die Praxis zu verwerthen. 1. u. 2. Th. 2 v. 1 p. l., 544 pp., 1 l.; vi, 390 pp., 1 l., 8 pl. 8°. *Berlin, E. S. Mittler u. Sohn,* 1880.

———. Die neueste Ernährungstheorie und deren praktische Verwerthung der der Ernährung der Armee, mit besonderer Berücksichtigung des von Prof. Dr. Med. Franz Hofmann dargestellten und empfohlenen Patent-Fleischpulvers. 1 p. l., 544 pp., 1 l. 8°. *Berlin, E. S. Mittler u. Sohn,* 1880.
Title of 1. pt. of his: Armee- und Volks-Ernährung.

———. Die Kost in staatlichen und kommunalen Anstalten, die Volksküchenkost und die Kost der arbeitenden Klassen, mit besonderer Berücksichtigung des Patent-Fleischpulvers. vi, 390 pp., 1 l., 8 pl. 8°. *Berlin, E. S. Mittler u. Sohn,* 1880.
Title of 2. pt. of his: Armee- und Volksernährung.

———. Wie nährt man sich gut und billig? Ein Beitrag zur Ernährungsfrage. Preisgekrönt durch den Verein "Concordia". 1 p. l., 100 pp., 2 pl. 8°. *Mainz, E. S. Mittler u. Sohn,* [1882].

Meinert (C. A.)—continued.

———. The same. Comment on se nourrit bien et à bon marché; étude de la question alimentaire. Trad. de l'allemand par F. Timmerhans. 2. éd. 111 pp., 2 tab. 8°. *Paris, Le Soudier,* 1883.

———. Ueber Massen-Ernährung. Mit besonderer Berücksichtigung der von Sanitätsrath Dr. Bär, von Dr. Paul Jeserich, und von dem Verfasser, in Plötzensee angestellten Ernährungsversuche. vii, 122 pp., 2 pl. 8°. *Berlin, S. Gerstmann,* 1885.

Meinert (Eugenius Theodorus Hugo) [1833–   ]. * De typhi pathologia et therapia. 31 pp. 8°. *Berolini, G. Schade,* [1859].

Meinert (Fr.) Crustacea isopoda, amphipoda et decapoda Daniæ: Fortegnelse over Danmarks isopode, amphipode og decapode Krebsdyr. pp. 57–248. 8°. *Kjøbenhavn, Thieles,* 1877.
Cutting from: Naturhistorisk Tidsskrift, 3. R., 2. B., 1877.

Meinert (Herrm. Aug.) * De enormitate virium vitalium in organismo humano. 28 pp. 8°. *Budæ, typ. Reg. Scient. Univ. Hung.,* 1835. [P., v. 1327.]

Meinert (W.) Behandeling van de ziekten en verzwakking der mannelijke geslachtsdeelen, uitgaande van het standpunt der natuurgeneesleer. Voorlezingen in de Vereeniging van de natuurgeneesvrienden (Hydro-diätetischen Verein) te Dresden in Februarij 1864. Ook als wederlegging van het over dit onderwerp uitgegeven boek van Doctor La' Mert onder de titels "Zelfbewaring" en "Het zelfbehoud". Vrij vertaald. 71 pp. 8°. *Zutphen, W. J. Thieme & Cie.,* 1864.

Meinert (Wilhelm).
Editor of: **Wasserfreund** (Der), Dresden, 1861-2.— **Naturarzt** (Der), Dresden u. Berlin, 1863-6.—**Physiatrische** Blätter, Dresden, 1867.

Meinesz (Jan Tobias). * Over een geval van schedel- en hersenbeleediging. 34 pp., 3 l. 8°. *Groningen, H. Geertsema,* 1865.

Meinhard (Georgius Christ.) [1798–   ]. * De abortu. 47 pp. 8°. [*Berolini*], *formis Brüschckianis,* [1823].

Meinhard (Victor). * De placenta retardata. 49 pp. 8°. *Herbipoli, C. A. Zürn,* 1838.

Meinhardt (Adolphus Guilelmus) [1812–   ]. * De pemphigo diutino. 32 pp. 8°. *Berolini, typ. Friedlaenderianis,* [1837].

Meinhardt (Eugen). Ueber die Addison'sche Krankheit. 30 pp. 8°. *Wien, J. Löwenthal,* 1866.
Repr. from: Wien. med. Presse, 1866, vii.

Meinhardt (Henricus). * De pyopneumothorace. 25 pp. 8°. *Gryphiswaldiæ, F. G. Kunike,* 1863.
C.

Meinhardt (Volkmar). * Ueber chronische Bleivergiftung. 35 pp. 8°. *Jena, J. G. Schreiber u. S.,* 1864.

Meinhoefer (Carolus Fridericus Gottlob.) * De mictu cruento. 22 pp. sm. 4°. *Vitebergæ, lit. C. H. Græssleri,* [1810].
For Biography, see **Kletten** (Georgius Ernestus.)

Meinhoefer (Joannes Fridericus). * De metritide. 28 pp. 4°. *Vitebergæ, lit. hæredum C. H. Graesleri,* [1815].
For Biography, see **Kletten** (Georgius Ernestus.)

Meinhof. Das preussische Medicinal-Gewicht. 21 pp. 8°. *Berlin, G. Reimer,* 1868.
Repr. from: Deutsche Klinik, Berl., 1867, xix.

Meinhold (Julius) [1844–   ]. * Gleichmässig verengtes Becken mit Exostosen und Ankylose des Os sacrum und Os coccygis. 32 pp. 8°. *Berlin, G. Lange,* [1868].

Meinicke.
See **Marcet** (Alexander). Chemische Untersuchungen [etc.] 8°. *Nürnberg,* 1820.

Meinicke (Joannes Georgius). * De mammarum structura et morbis. 28 pp. 4°. *Vitebergæ, lit. viduæ Tzschiedrichii,* [1805].
For Biography, see **Seiler** (Gulielmus).

Meinieu (Nicolas). * Sur la métrite. 14 pp. 4°.
Paris, 1821, No. 161, v. 167.

Meiningen.

Hermann (R.) Mortalitätsstatistik der Residenz-
stadt Meiningen für das Jahr 1876. Cor.-Bl. d. allg. ärztl.
Ver. v. Thüringen, Leipz., 1878, vii, 25–30. ———. Mor-
talitätsstatistik der Residenzstadt Meiningen für das
Jahr 1880. Veröffentl. d. k. deutsch. Gsndhtsamtes,
Berl., 1881, v, 267.

Meire (Norbertus). * De medicina et ejus objecto.
1788.
In: LOUVAIN Diss. 8°. *Lovanii*, 1796, iv, 144–161.

de Meirelles (Antonio da Cunha Vieira). Memorias de epidemologia portugueza. 251 pp. 8°.
Coimbra, 1866.

de Meirelles (*Joaquim Candido Soares*)
[1777–1868].
Biography. Brazil. Biog. Ann. [Macedo], Rio de
Jan., 1876, iii, 373–378.

de Meirelles Kendall (Henrique Carlos).
Ao illustrissimo e excellentissimo senhor Antonio
Augusto Pereira de Miranda digno membro da
commissão encarregada de rever o regulamento
das quarentenas nameado por decreto de 23 de
Maio de 1872. 30 pp. 8°. *Porto*, 1874. [P., v.
1267.

Meirieu (Auguste-Pierre). * Quelques réflexions
sur l'influence de la civilisation dans les maladies. viii, 9–39 pp. 4°. *Paris*, 1820, No. 8, v. 154.
———. Résumé complet d'hygiène privée, ou exposition des moyens propres à maintenir les
fonctions de nutrition, de relation et de génération dans le meilleur état de santé possible ; précédé d'une introduction historique et suivi d'une
biographie, d'une bibliographie et d'un vocabulaire. Revu par Léon Simon. xii, 268 pp. 32°.
Paris, Bachelier, 1828.
Constitues 1 v. of: **Encyclopédie** portative, etc , par
une société de savans sous la direction de M. C. Bailly de
Merlieux.
———. Compendio completo di chirurgia, seguito
dall' arte obstetrica, e preceduta da un' introduzione storica. [Transl.] xi, 271 pp., 2 pl. 16°.
Milano, A. F. Stella e figli, 1835.

Meisburger (W.)
Editor of: **Nordamericanische**, deutsch' medicinische Zeitschrift für praktische Heilkunde, Buffalo, N. Y.,
1865.

Meischner (Christianus Ernestus). * De præcipuis quibusdam morbis per menses angustum,
septembrem et octobrem anno 1817 Lipsiæ observatis. 1 l., 27 pp. 4°. *Lipsiæ, J. B. Hirschfeld*, [1818].

Meischner (Gustav Friedrich). * Die acute
Phosphorose und einige Reflexionen über die
acute gelbe Leberatrophie und die entzündlichen
Zustände in Leber und Nieren überhaupt. 89
pp., 1 l., 5 tab. 8°. *Leipzig, G. Kreysing*, 1864.

Meisel (Henricus). * De febri puerperali. 31
pp. 8°. *Lipsiæ, typ. C. W. Vollrathii*, 1849. c.

Meiselbach (Jo. Theoph.) * De periostei inflammatione. 36 pp., 1 l. 8°. *Halæ, formis F.
Grunerti*, [1824].

Meisels (Ambros Wilh.) Studien über das Zooid
und Okoid bei verschiedenen Wirbelthier - Abtheilungen. 8 pp., 1 pl. 8°. [*Wien*, 1881.]
Repr. from: Sitzungsb. d. k. Akad. d. Wissensch.
Math.-naturw. Cl., Wien, 1881, lxxxiv.

Meisenburg (Carolus)[1]. * De docimasia pulmonum hydrostatica. 45 pp., 1 l. 4°. *Berolini,
typ. C. F. Brettschneiderii*, [1830]. [*Also, in:* P.
v. 1606.]

Meisenburg (Carolus)[2]. * De diabete mellito.
25 pp., 1 l. 8°. *Bonnæ, typ. F. Kruegeri*, 1865. c.

Meisius (David) jun. De pleuritide. 7 l. 4°.
Jenæ, typ. T. Steinmanni, 1604.

Meisner (Carolus Henricus Augustus) [1811–
]. * De gangræna nosocomiali. 32 pp. 8°.
Berolini, typ. Nauckianis, [1841].

Meisner (Caspar Benjamin). * De ignobili mo-
bilium quorundam medicaminum indole atque
virtute. 32 pp. sm. 4°. *Francof. ad Viadr., ex
off. J. C. Winteri*, [1748].

Meisner (Christianus). * De incurabilibus af-
fectibus. 32 pp. 4°. *Halæ Magdeb., typ. C.
Henckelii*, [1705].
———. The same. 32 pp. 4°. *Halæ Magdeb.*, 1717.
For Biography, see **Stahl** (Geo. Ernst).

Meisner (I.) Rukovodstvo dlja feldscherskich
schkol v dvuch chastjach. Izdanie dvadtsatoe
ispravlennoe i vnov dopolnennoe. [Manual for
army assistant surgeons.] 393, vi pp. 8°. *Vilna,
topogr. A. G. Sirkin*, 1884.

Meisner (Joh. Guilielmus). * De hyemis præter
naturam tepidæ et humidæ noxis earundemque
præcautionibus. 22 pp., 1 l. 4°. *Vittenbergæ,
lit. A. Kobersteinii*, [1722].

Meisner (Joh. Theodorus). * De febre catarrhali. 9 l. sm. 4°. *Traj. ad Rhenum, F. Halma*,
1689.

Meisner (Leonh. Ferdinand.) De caffee, choco-
latæ, herbæ, thee ac nicotianæ natura, usu, et
abusu ; anacrisis medico - historico - diætetica.
124 pp. 12°. *Norimbergæ, sumpt. J. F. Rudigeri*,
1721.

Meisner (Paul). * Ueber einen Fall von Ectopia
vesicæ urinariæ. 30 pp., 1 l., 1 pl. 8°. *Greifswald, F. W. Kunike*, 1873. c.

Meisner ([Paulus] Hugo)[1840–]. * De chorea
St. Viti. 32 pp. 8°. *Berolini, G. Lange*, 1865.

Meissel (Gustavus Fridericus). * De medico
minus duro omnium durissimo. 48 pp. 4°.
Vitembergæ, prelo E. G. Eichsfeldi, [1745].
For Biography, see **Vater** (Abraham).

Meissen.

See **Fever** (*Typhus, History, etc., of*), by localities.
Morbilitätsstatistik des Medicinal-Bezirks Meissen auf die Jahre 1867–72. Jahresb. d. Landes-Med.-Coll.,
etc., 1867, Dresd., 1869, i, 135: (1868), 1871, ii, 125: (1869),
1872, iii, 104: (1870–71), 1874, iv, 124; 127: (1872–3), 1875, v,
242: 1874, Leipz., 1876, vi, 150.

Meissen (Ernst) [1854–]. * Ueber Placenta
prævia und deren Behandlung. 37 pp., 1 l. 8°.
Berlin, G. Schade, [1877].

Meissen (Hugo Ferdinandus) [1825–]. * De
auditus diminutione et abolitione. 38 pp. 8°.
Berolini, formis Brüschckianis, [1825].

Meissen - Falkenstein. Ueber Lungenschwindsucht und deren Behandlung. 35 pp.
8°. *Berlin, E. Grosser*, 1884.
Repr. from: Deutsche Med.-Ztg., Berl., 1884, v.
———. Zur Kenntniss der menschlichen Phthise.
56 pp. 8°. *Berlin*, 1885.
Repr. from: Deutsche Med.-Ztg., Berl., 1885, vi, 59.

Meissner.

Portrait in: **Collection**—van Kaathoven.

Meissner (Æmilius Theodorus). * Nova symbola ad scrophuloseos pathologiam ac therapiam.
vi, 7–24 pp. 4°. *Grimmæ, ex off. Reimeria*, [1837].

Meissner (Alfred). * De helminthiasi intestinorum. 39 pp. 8°. *Pragæ, ex typ. filiorum A.
Haase*, 1846.

Meissner (Alfred). * Ein Fall von Verengerung
der Pfortader durch chronische Peritonitis bei
Gallensteinerkrankung. 24 pp. 8°. *Erlangen,
E. T. Jacob*, 1875.

Meissner (C.) * Beobachtungen über vaccinales
Früherysipel. 28 pp., 1 l. 8°. *Halle a. S.,
Plötz*, 1880.

Meissner (Carolus Henricus). * De hydrocele.
1 p. l., 16 pp., 1 l. 4°. *Vitebergæ, lit. Meinelianis*,
[1808].

Meissner (Carolus Leopoldus). * De præcipuis
corticis Peruviani substitutis, imprimis de æsculo
hippocastano. iv, 5–20 pp. 4°. *Jenæ, ex off.
Goepferdti*, [1810].

Meissner (Edmund Paul). *De ruptura tubæ gravidæ, præmissis duabus morbi historiis recentibus. 20 pp. 8°. *Lipsiæ, Giesecke et Devrient,* 1856. c.

Meissner (Emil). Transport-Bett für Kranke und Verwundete. 6 pp., 1 pl. 8°. *Wien,* 1864.

Meissner (Emil Apollo) [1827-84]. *De cautelis duabus in sectione cæsarea instituenda observandis. Præmissa sunt relata de puerperis duabus, in quibus Lipsiæ nuper hæc operatio peracta. 36 pp. 8°. *Lipsiæ,* 1851. c.

——. Ueber Rheumatismus uteri gravidi. Vortrag. 22 pp. 8°. [*Leipzig, A. T. Engelhardt,* 1860.]
Repr. from: Monatschr. f. Geburtsk. u. Frauenkr., Berl., 1860, viii.

——. Der Keuchhusten und dessen Beziehungen zum Gehörorgane im Besonderen. Vortrag, gehalten in der Sitzung der medizinischen Gesellschaft zu Leipzig am 27. Mai 1862. 30 pp. 8°. *Leipzig, H. Luppe,* 1863.

——. Ueber Cholera infantum.
In: SAMML. klin. Vortr., Leipz., 1878, No. 157 (Innere Med., No. 53), 1363-1390.

Meissner (Frid. Adolphus) [1803-   ]. *De perterebratione cranii quædam; addita historia fracturæ cranii cum depressione, sine trepanatione feliciter sanatæ. 40 pp. 8°. *Berolini, formis Brüschckianis,* [1826].

Meissner (Friedericus). *De naturæ auxilio in sanandis uteri polypis, adjectis duabus de hac re observationibus. 1 p. l., 21 pp., 1 l. 8°. *Vratislaviæ, typ. A. Neumanni,* [1863].

Meissner (Friederich Ludwig) [1796-1860].
*Diss. animadversiones nonnullas ad doctrinam de secundinis ac de superfœtatione continens. vi, 26 pp. 4°. *Lipsiæ, J. C. Werther,* [1819].

——. Ueber die Unfruchtbarkeit des männlichen und weiblichen Geschlechts, ihre Ursachen, Erkenntniss und Heilart. Nebst einem Anhange über Jörgs Perforatorium. xvi, 372 pp. 8°. *Leipzig, C. H. F. Hartmann,* 1820.

——. Die Dislocationen der Gebärmutter und der Mutterscheide von Seiten ihrer Entstehung, ihres Einflusses und ihrer Behandlung. 3 v. 12°. *Leipzig, C. H. F. Hartmann,* 1821-2.
v. 1. Der Vorfall der Gebärmutter und der Mutterscheide, nebst einer geschichtlichen und critischen Beleuchtung der Pessarien.
v. 2. Die Schieflagen und die Zurückbeugung der Gebärmutter, nebst einer Zugabe über die neuerlich bekannt gewordene Umbeugung derselben.
v. 3. Die Umstülpung der Gebärmutter und der Mutterbruch.

——. Was hat das neunzehnte Jahrhundert für die Geburtshülfe gethan? Zeitraum 1801 bis 1832.
1. and 4. Theil of his: Forschungen des neunzehnten Jahrhunderts, etc. 8°. *Leipzig,* 1826-33.

——. Was hat das neunzehnte Jahrhundert für die Erkenntniss und Heilung der Frauenkrankheiten gethan? Zeitraum 1801 bis 1832.
2. and 5. Theil of his: Forschungen des neunzehnten Jahrhunderts, etc. 8°. *Leipzig,* 1826-33.

——. Was hat das neunzehnte Jahrhundert für die Erkenntniss und Heilung der Kinderkrankheiten gethan? Zeitraum 1801 bis 1832.
3. and 6. Theil of his: Forschungen des neunzehnten Jahrhunderts, etc. 8°. *Leipzig,* 1826-33.

——. Forschungen des neunzehnten Jahrhunderts im Gebiete der Geburtshülfe, Frauenzimmer- und Kinderkrankheiten. 6 Theile. 8°. *Leipzig, C. H. F. Hartmann u. A. Lehnhold,* 1826-33.

——. Die Kinderkrankheiten nach den neuesten Ansichten und Erfahrungen zum Unterricht für practische Aerzte und zum Gebrauche für academische Vorlesungen. 2 v. in 1. xvi, 447 pp.; iv, 464 pp. 12°. *Leipzig, A. Fest,* 1828.

Meissner (Friederich Ludwig)—continued.
——. The same. 2 Th. in 1 v. viii, 9-384 pp.; 402 pp. 8°. *Reutlingen, J. N. Ensslin,* 1832.

——. The same. 2. Aufl. 2 v. viii, 540 pp.; vi, 554 pp. 8°. *Leipzig, Fest,* 1838.

——. The same. Erster und zweiter Theil. 3. ganz umgearbeitete und sehr vermehrte Aufl. viii, 595 pp.; iv, 635 pp. 8°. *Leipzig, Fest,* 1844.

——. Ueber schwammige Auswüchse der weiblichen Geschlechtsorgane. Denkschrift zur Feier des 25jährigen Bestehens der Entbindungsanstalt zu Leipzig unter Leitung ihres Stifters und Directors Joerg. 1 p. l., 26 pp., 1 l., 3 pl. 4°. *Leipzig, O. Wigand,* 1835.

——. Die Frauenzimmerkrankheiten nach der neuesten Ansichten und Erfahrungen; zur Unterricht für praktische Aerzte bearbeitet. 4 pts. in 2 v. 8°. *Leipzig, O. Wigand,* 1842-6.

——. The same. De ziekten der vrouwen, naar het standpunt der wetenschap, tot onderrigt voor practiserende geneesheeren. Uit het Hoogduitsch vertaald door M. J. Godefroi en J. E. C. van Campen. 160 pp. 8°. *Gorinchem, A. van der Mast,* 1849.

——. Grundlage der Literatur der Pädiatrik, enthaltend die Monographien über die Kinderkrankheiten. vi, 245 pp. 8°. *Leipzig,* [*E. Polz*], 1850.
See, also, **Bereicherungen** für die Geburtshülfe. v. 1. 8°. *Leipzig,* 1821. — **Encyclopädie** der medicinischen Wissenschaften nach dem Dictionnaire de médecine. 13 v. 8°. *Leipzig,* 1830-35. — **Magendie** (F.) Physiologische und medicinische Untersuchungen über den Harngries, [etc.] 12°. *Leipzig,* 1830.
For Biography, see **Kuchn** (C. G.)
For Portrait, see **Collection**—van Kaathoven.

Meissner (Georg). Beiträge zur Physiologie des Sehorgans. 1 p. l., 121 pp., 4 pl. 8°. *Leipzig, W. Engelmann,* 1854.

——. Ueber die Bewegungen des Auges. Nach neuen Versuchen. 47 pp. 8°. *Leipzig, E. Polz,* 1859.
Repr. from: Ztschr. f. rat. Med., Leipz., 1859, 3. R., viii.

——. Untersuchungen über die elektrische Ozonerzeugung und über die Influenz-Elektricität auf Nicht-Leitern. 109 pp., 2 pl. 4°. *Göttingen, Dieterich,* 1871.
Repr. from: Abhandl. d. k. Gesellsch. zu Götting.
Also, Co-Editor of: **Zeitschrift** für rationelle Medizin, Leipzig u. Heidelberg, 1856-71.

——. & **Shepard** (C. W.) Untersuchungen über das Entstehen der Hippursäure im thierischen Organismus. vi pp., 1 l., 204 pp., 1 pl. 8°. *Hannover, Hahn,* 1866.

Meissner (Gustavus Hermannus). *De sudoris secretione. 20 pp. 8°. *Lipsiæ, typ. A. Edelmanni,* 1859.

Meissner (Henricus Bernardus). *De chlorosi. 35 pp. 8°. *Lipsiæ, typ. Societat. typog.,* [1852].

Meissner (Joannes Carolus Guilielmus). *Anatome physiologia et pathologia ventriculi. 37 pp. 4°. *Vitebergæ, F. I. Seibt,* [1811].
For Biography, see **Schreger** (Christianus Henricus Theodorus).

Meissner (Joh. Theodorus). *De atrophia in genere. 13 l. sm. 4°. *Lipsiæ, typ. Krügerianis,* [1688].

Meissner (Otto Franciscus). *De erysipelate. 4 p. l., 42 pp. 8°. *Gryphiæ, F. G. Kunike,* [1841].

Meissner (P. T.) Die Ventilation und Erwärmung der Kinderstube und des Krankenzimmers. Mit Berücksichtigung der Feuerwirthschaft bei kleinen Haushaltungen und dem Sparherde. vi, 84 pp. 8°. *Wien, L. Forster,* 1852.

——. Beiträge zur Kenntniss der Cholera und zwar Nachweis der Ursache ihres Entstehens, aus den Beobachtungen und Erfahrungen der im Jahre 1830 ausgebrochenen verheerenden Seuche. 48 pp. 8°. *Wien, bei dem Verfasser,* 1864.

Meissner (*Paul Franz*) [1778–   ].
Portrait in: **Portraiten-Gallerie.** 4°. *Wien*, 1838, No. 8.

Meissner (Rudolphus) [1830–   ]. * De hydropathia sive hydrotherapia. 31 pp. 8°. *Berolini, typ. Trowitzschii et filii*, [1853].

Meissner's *corpuscles.*
Fischer (E.) Ueber den Bau der Meissner'schen Tast-Körperchen. Arch. f. mikr. Anat., Bonn, 1876, xii, 364–390, 1 pl.

Meister (Carol. Guil. Rudolph.) [1803–   ]. * De caloris usu externo atque interno. 32 pp. 8°. *Berolini, typ. Brüschckianis*, [1829].

Meister (Franc. Ser.) * De rheumatismo in genere. 30 pp. 12°. *Vindobonæ, J. N. Fridrich*, 1839.

Meister (Jo. Conradus). * De succis herbarum recentium eorumque usu ad morbos præter scorbutum alios.
In: LEIDENFROST (J. G.) Opus. phys.-chem. et med. 12°. *Duisb. ad Rhen.*, 1797, i, 277–320.

Meister (Joannes Jacobus). * Nonnulla de phlebolithis. 24 pp. 8°. *Halæ, formis Ploetzianis*, 1835.

———. * De secundinis arte removendis. 23 pp. 8°. *Turici, typ. Orellii, Fuesslini et soc.*, 1838. [*Also, in*: P., v. 586.]

Meister (Joh. Christian Friedrich). Urtheile und Gutachten in Peinlichen und andern Straffällen. 3 p. l., x–xvi, 530 pp , 2 l. 8°. *Frankf. a. d. Oder*, 1808.

———. Eines T. Lucretius Carus Schauergemälde der Kriegs-Pest in Attika. Original-Text nach der Heinr. Ca. Abr. Eichstädtschen Ausgabe. Vol. 1, Leipzig, 1801. Buch vi, Vers 1089, bis zu Ende. Des Herrn Obristwachtmeisters von Knebel Uebersetzung in Hexametern. Erläuternde Anmerkungen über Sprache, und aus der Geschichte. Fortlaufender arzneiwissenschaftlicher Kommentar. viii, 152 pp. 8°. *Züllichau, Darnmann*, 1816.
For Portrait, see **Collection** of Portr. of Phys. & Men of Sc., 118.—**Jahrb.** d. Staatsarznk., Frankf. a. M, 1816, ix.

Meister (Josephus). * De chlorosi. xvi pp. 8°. *Augustæ Vindel.*, 1842.

Meitl (Maximilian). Sternberg bei Schlan in Böhmen. Ein Taschenbuch für die dortigen Kurgäste. 68 pp. 16°. *Prag, T. Thaber*, 1833.

Meitzen (Theodor. Robertus) [1816–   ]. * De sectione cæsarea. 25 pp., 2 l. 8°. *Berolini, typ. fratrum Schlesinger*, [1843].

Méjan (André).
See **Provençal** (Jean-Michel). Questions de chirurgie, etc. 4°. *Montpellier*, 1811.

Mejansac (J.-M.-Alphonse). * De la pleurésie diaphragmatique. 38 pp. 4°. *Paris*, 1855, No. 246, v. 577.

Méjasson (Henri). * Des blessures de la cornée au point de vue du pronostic et du traitement. 64 pp., 1 l. 4°. *Paris, A. Parent*, 1879, No. 208.

Mejdunarodnaja Klinika. Ejemesjachnii journal, sobranie originalnich i perveodnich lektsii i statei. Redaktor: V. Popoff. [International clinic; a monthly journal containing original and translated articles.] v. 3–6, 1884–7. 3 v. 8°. *St. Petersburg.*

Mejer (Henricus Gerhardus). * De intellectu impuro sectio prior. 30 pp. sm. 4°. *Vitembergæ, lit. vid. Gerdesiæ*, [n. d.]

Mejer (Joh. Martinus). * De morbis ex motu sanguinis circulatorio imminuto oriundis. 1 p. l., 26 pp. sm. 4°. *Basileæ, typ. F. Lüdij*, 1719.

Mejer (Ludovicus). * De aneurismate arteriæ occipitalis. 95 pp. 8°. *Wircibergi, F. E. Nitribitt*, 1804.

Mejia (Demetrio). Estadística de mortalidad en México. Memoria de concurso premiada por

Mejia (Demetrio)—continued.
la Academia de medicina. 32 pp., 4 tab. 8°. *México, I. Escalante*, 1879.

Mekerttschiantz (Minas ter - Gabrielian) [1843–   ]. * Ueber die Ovariotomie und Diagnose der Ovarialcysten. 59 pp. 8°. *Berlin, M. Niethe*, [1872].

Mekus (Jos. Arminius). * De hæmatocele retrovaginali et retrouterina intraperitoneali. 32 pp. 8°. *Regimonti Pr., typ. Dalkowskianis*, 1866. c.

Mel.
See **Honey.**

Mel (Franciscus Petrus). * Mel saccharo præstantius. 20 pp. sm. 4°. *Altdorfi Noric., typ. J. G. Kohlesii*, [1724].

Melæna.
See, *also*, **Amaurosis** (*Causes of*) ; **Fever** (*Malarial, Hæmorrhagic*); **Hæmatemesis** ; **Hæmorrhage** (*Intestinal*); **Infant** (*New-born, Diseases of*).

ANDERS (J.) * Ueber Melæna neonatorum. 8°. *Greifswald*, [1885].

BREVEL (F. G.) * Quædam de morbo nigro Hippocratis. 4°. *Lipsiæ*, [1802].

BRION (J.-J.) * Recherches sur la maladie noire. 4°. *Paris, an XII*, [1804].

BRYAN (O. A.) * De melæna. 8°. *Edinburgi*, 1786.

CHATEL (L.-M.) * Sur le mélæna. 4°. *Strasbourg*, 1806.

DINGELSTEDT (F. G. C.) * De morbo nigro. sm. 8°. *Berolini*, [1820].

FRIEDLEIN (L.) * De melæna. 8°. *Wirceburgi*, 1838.

GASSER (T. M.) * De morbo nigro Hippocratis. 4°. *Argentorati*, [1761].

GENRICH (E.) * Ueber die Melæna neonatorum. 8°. *Berlin*, [1877].

GIESECKEN (C. H.) * De morbo nigro Hippocratis. 8°. *Gottingæ*, [1829].

HALL (H.) * De melæna. 8°. *Edinburgi*, 1782.

HERTIUS (J. C.) * De morbo nigro Hippocratis. 4°. *Halæ*, [1701].

HIMMER (C. W.) De morbo nigro. 4°. *Lipsiæ*, [1811].

HOEHN (A. C. F.) * De morbo nigro Hippocratis, vomitu cruento, et diarrhœa cruenta. 8°. *Jenæ*, [1796].

HOIN (F. J.) * De morbo nigro. 4°. *Vesuntione*, [1769].

KELLER (J. B. M.) * De melæna. 8°. *Monachii*, 1836.

KLING (L.) * Ueber Melæna neonatorum. 8°. *München*, 1875.

KUERSCHNER (T. F.) * De melæna seu morbo nigro Hippocratis. 8°. *Berolini*, [1851].

LANDAU (L.) Ueber Melæna der Neugeborenen, nebst Bemerkungen über die Obliteration der fötalen Wege. 8°. *Breslau*, 1874.

LICHTSCHLAG (J.) * Melænæ Hippocraticæ genuinæ imago, indoles, et diagnosis specialior. 4°. *Bonnæ*, [1828].

LOEWY (A. S.) * De melæna. 8°. *Pragæ*, 1826.

MESTINGH (J. E.) * De melæna. 8°. *Traj. ad Rhenum*, 1843.

MOREL (J.-T.) * Essai sur le mélæna, ou la maladie noire. 4°. *Paris, an XIII* [1805].

NOYER (J.-B.-F.) * Sur le melæna. 4°. *Paris*, 1816.

PASQUIER (R.) * Sur le mélæna. 4°. *Paris*, 1815.

PETIT (J.-J.) * Dissertation sur la nature et les véritables caractères du mélæna. 4°. *Paris*, 1813.

Melæna.

Poma (J. F.) * De melæna. 4°. *Argentorati, an. XI* [1803].

de Rooy (J.) * De morbo nigro Hippocratis. 4°. *Lugd. Bat.*, 1793.

Schoningh (T. J. J.) * De morbo nigro Hippocratis. 4°. [*Groningæ*], 1768.

Stern (G. C.) * Diss. inaug. sistens meletemata de atra bile Hippocratis. 8°. *Isebergæ*, [1794].

Also, in his: Epist. med. pract. 18°. *Lausannæ*, 1770, 1-180.

Tissot (S. A. D.) De morbo nigro, scirrhis viscerum, cephalea, inoculatione, irritabilitate, cum cadaverum sectionibus. 12°. *Loranii*, 1764.

Also, in : Sandifort. Thesaurus diss. [etc.] 4°. *Roterdami*, 1768, i, 65-83.

————. The same. A letter to Dr. Zimmermann on the morbus niger; including some opposite cases equally curious and interesting. The whole illustrated with an account of the morbid appearances of the dissected bodies. Transl. from the French by John Burke. 8°. *London*, 1776.

Also, transl. with additions, in his: Obs. et diss. de méd. prat. 12°. *Lausanne*, 1780, i, 27-145.

Wundram (E. G. L.) * Quædam circa melænam. sm. 4°. *Gottingæ*, 1803.

Zeising (J. E.) * De morbo nigro Hippocratis vomitu cruento et diarrhœa cruenta. 4°. *Jenæ*, [1824].

Auvity fils. Observation sur un méléna fébrile. Bull. Fac. de méd. de Par. (1809-11), 1812, ann. 7, ii, 105.—**Bard.** Quelques recherches sur la nature du mélæna, et sur les moyens curatifs à lui opposer. J. gén. de méd., chir. et pharm., Par., 1815, lii, 269-280.—**Belcombe** (H. S.) Melæna. Lond. M. Gaz., 1829, iv, 109. *Also:* Boston M. & S. J., 1829-30, ii, pt. 2, 455.— **Bennewitz.** Melæna in Folge seltener Veranlassung. J. d. pract. Heilk., Berl., 1839, lxxxix, 1. St., 84-96.—**Berger.** Morbus niger Hippocratis nach Wechselfieber, mit glücklichem Ausgange. Med. Ztg., Berl., 1839, viii, 241.—**Betz** (F.) Zur Aetiologie der Melæna neonatorum. Memorabilien, Heilbr., 1879, xxiv, 549-557.—**Bonté.** Sur la maladie noire. J. de méd., chir., pharm., etc., Par., 1795, viii, 222-241. — **Bouteille** (N.) Observations et réflexions sur la maladie noire. Ann. Soc. de méd.-prat. de Montpel., 1808, xii, 407-444.—**Brieude.** Observations sur la maladie noire, et méthode curative. Rec. périod. Soc. de santé de Par., 1797, i, 441-455.—**Brooke** (W.) Three cases of melæna, in which the most decided good effects appear to have been produced by the exhibition of the oil of turpentine. Tr. Ass. King's & Queen's Coll. Phys. Ireland, Dubl., 1817, i, 124-149. — **Bugnion & Rapin.** Observation d'un cas de melæna. Bull. Soc. méd. de la Suisse Rom., Lausanne, 1880, xiv, 127-130. — **Butler** (A.) Melena fulminante palúdica. Diario méd.-farm., Madrid, 1884, i, nos. 161; 163.—**Campardon.** Sur la maladie noire. J. de méd., chir., pharm., etc., Par., 1760, xii, 298-317. — [**Cases.**] Morbus niger, or vomiting of matter resembling black clotted blood. New Lond. M. J., Lond., 1792, i, 367. — Melæna (μέλαινα νοῦσος s. morbus niger Hippocratis), Hæmatemesis s. vomitus cruentus und Diarrhœa cruenta. Mat. f. d. Staatsarzneiw. u. prakt. Heilk., Jena, 1800, 1. Samml., 105-110.—Vomitus cruentus (morbus niger Hippocrat.). Ann. d. med.-chir. clin. Inst. zu Götting., 1801, i, 94-99.—Melæna. Ann. d. k. klin. Inst. am St. Jakobshosp. in Leipz., 1810, i. 1. Abth., 125-132.— Melæna acuta. Med. Ztg., Berl., 1838, vii, 243.—**Cheyne** (J.) A case of melæna; with observations on the alternate excess of morbid action in the mucous and serous membranes. Dublin Hosp. Rep., 1818, i, 259-271.— **Clemens** (A.) Geheilte Melæna. Würzb. med. Ztschr., 1865, vi, 370-373.—**Clos.** Sur la maladie noire. Ann. Soc. de méd.-prat. de Montpel., 1808, xi, 426-442.—**Courbon-Pérusel.** Observation d'un méléna qui a été mortel, et dont les causes ont été soigneusement recherchées sur le cadavre. Bull. Fac. de méd. de Par., 1821, x, 237-242.—**Crisp** (E.) Cases of melæna; with observations. Lancet, Lond., 1846, i, 155-157. — **Croom** (J. H.) Melæna neonatorum; four cases. Med. Times & Gaz., Lond., 1880, ii, 480-482 — **Crusiz.** Heftige, entzündliche Meläna. Oesterr. med. Wchnschr., Wien, 1844, 1125-1127. —**Dassen** (J.) Jets over den oorsprong van het uitgebraakte bloed in den morbus niger Hippocratis. Pract. Tijdschr. v. de Geneesk., Gorinchem, 1838, xvii, 197-205.— **De Glatigny.** Sur la maladie noire. J. de méd., chir., pharm., etc., Par., 1760, xii, 317-323.—**Dieterlen.** Mélæna des nouveau-nés. Bull. Soc. clin. de Par. (1881), 1882, v, 101-105.—**Fleischmann** (L.) Zur Aetiologie der Melæna vera. Jahrb. f. Kinderh., Leipz., 1869-70, n. F., iii, 211-216. — **Gaude-**

Melæna.

chon. Observation sur une maladie noire (melæna) dans laquelle une femme a rendu environ dix-sept livres de sang noir, coagulé et fétide, guérie avec les astringens, les réfrigérans, les calmans et le repos le plus parfait. J. de méd., chir., pharm., etc., Par., 1805, x, 123-129.—**Gobée** (C.) Intermitterend bloedbraken en bloedige diarrhee. N. Pract. Tijdschr. v. de Geneesk., Gorinchem, 1856, n. s., ii, 637-642. — **Goldie** (G.) Melæna. Cycl. Pract. M. (Tweedie), Phila., 1845, iii, 279-284. — **Gondinet.** Mémoire contenant des observations et remarques sur le melæna atrabiliaire des anciens, et le melæna hémorrhagique des modernes. Ann. clin., Montpel., 1811, xxiv, 315-348.— **Hanius** (M. B.) Melæna in Folge äusserer Gewalt. Jahrb. d. ges. Staatsarznk., Leipz., 1837, ii, 92-114. — **Henoch.** Melæna neonatorum. Berl. klin. Wchnschr., 1883, xx, 334.—**Hesse** (C. G.) Von dem Blutbrechen und der Meläna der Neugebornen. Allg. med. Ann., Leipz., 1825, 721-744. — **Holscher** (G. P.) † Hannov. Ann. f. d. ges. Heilk., 1840, v, 344-349. — **Horn** (E.) Glückliche Heilung eines mit Brustkrämpfen und Zehrung verwickelten Morbus niger Hippocratis. Arch. f. med. Erfahr., Berl., 1811, i, 81-89. —**Hurd** (J.) Melæna. Lond. M. Gaz., 1832, ix, 908-910. — **Jackson** (G.) Case of melæna treated with the oil of turpentine, strongly illustrating the efficacy of that medicine in the disease. Lancet, Lond., 1831-2, i, 818-821. — **Jackson** (W.) † *Ibid.*, 1832, ii, 497-499. — **Jacob.** † Med. Cor.-Bl. d. württemb. ärztl. Ver., Stuttg., 1837, vii, 62-64.—**Larsen** (C.) Melæna neonatorum. Norsk Mag. f. Lægevidensk., Christiania, 1875, v, 198-200. — **Lederer** (J.) Bedeutende Darmblutung bei einem 48 Stunden alten Kinde (Melæna). Wien. med. Wchnschr., 1860, x, 615. ————. Ueber Melæna neonatorum. Allg. Wien. med. Ztg., 1877, xxii, 394.—**Leviseur.** Morbus niger mit intermittirendem Tertiantypus. San.-Ber. d. k. Med.-Coll. zu Posen f. 1830, Posen, 1832, 27.— **Makka** (N.) Περὶ μελαίνης. Γαληνὸς, Ἀθῆναι, 1881, Ε΄, 397; Γ΄, 8.—**Mareschal de Rougeres.** Réflexions sur la maladie noire. J. de méd., chir., pharm., etc., Par., 1772, xxxvii, 217-226. —**Martland** (R.) † With dissections. Edinb. M. & S. J., 1824, xxi, 299-301.—**Mehlhose** (C. G.) Melæna. J. d. pract. Heilk., Berl., 1837, lxxxv, 4. St., 124-128. — **Melion.** Magen- und Darmblutung bei einem neugebornen Kinde. Oesterr. med. Wchnschr., Wien, 1845, 641-643. — **Mémoire** sur la maladie noire. J. de méd. chir., pharm., etc., Par., 1760, xiii, 483-510. — **Mérat.** Mélæna ou mélæna. Dict. d. sc. méd., Par., 1819, xxxii, 189-191. — **Moll.** Melæna bei Neugebornen. Med. Ztg., Berl., 1837, vi, 51.—**Morache** (G.) Mélæna. Dict. encycl. d. sc. méd., Par., 1873, 2. s., vi, 333-343.—**Nicholl** (W.) † Tr. Ass. King's & Queen's Coll. Phys. Ireland, Dubl., 1820, iii, 274-279. — **Nicolais du Saulsay.** Observation sur la maladie noire. J. de méd., chir., pharm., etc., Par., 1765, xxii, 502-513.—**Nückel.** Melæna. Gen.-Ber. d. k. rhein. Med.-Coll. 1840, Koblenz, 1841, 65.—**Portal** (A.) Observations sur la nature et sur le traitement du mélæna, vulgairement maladie noire. Mém. Soc. méd. d'émulat. de Par., an vii [1799], ii, 107-168.—**Rahlf** (G.) De mélæna, calculorum biliosorum ac emeticorum effectu, hujusque mali memorabili exemplo. Acta reg. Soc. med. Havn., 1829, vii, 20-42. — **Rehn** (H.) Zur Genese der Melæna neonatorum. Centr.-Ztg. f. Kinderh., Berl., 1877-8, i, 227. — **Rembold** (S.) Beitrag zur Lehre von der Melæna neonatorum (Ulcus ventriculi sive duodeni neonatorum). Deutsche med. Wchnschr., Berl., 1881, vii, 385.—**Renard.** Sur la maladie noire. J. de méd., chir., pharm., etc., Par., 1765, xxii, 449-455.—**Rillet.** Mémoire sur les hémorrhagies intestinales chez les nouveau-nés (melæna des enfants). Gaz. méd. de Par., 1848, 3. s., iii, 1029-1033. *Also :* Ann. de méd. belge, Brux., 1849, i, 107-131. *Also, transl.* [Abstr.]: Schweiz. Ztschr. f. Med., Chir. u. Geburtsh., Zürich, 1850, vi, 119.—**Ritter** (A.) Zur Casuistik der Melæna vera neonatorum. Aerztl. Mitth. a. Baden, Karlsruhe, 1882, xxxvi, 15-17.—**Rodamel.** Observation sur un méléna. Mém. Soc. méd. d'émulat. de Par., an xiv [1806], vi, 145-149. — **Rouchette.** Melæna s'accompagnant de symptômes très graves; terminaison heureuse. Courrier méd., Par., 1848, xviii, 5. — **Sawtell** (T. H.) Hæmatemesis and melæna in which blood was first vomited twenty-one and a half hours after birth; death within twenty-four hours. Brit. M. J., Lond., 1885, ii, 741. *Also:* Med. Times & Gaz., Lond., 1885, ii, 547. *Also:* Med. Press & Circ., Lond., 1885, n. s., xl, 349.—**Schmid** (H.) Melæna neonatorum. Med. Cor.-Bl. d. württemb. ärztl. Ver., Stuttg., 1884, liv, 193.—**Schmitt** (W. J.) Ueber das Phänomen des blutigen Erbrechens und Stuhlabsetzens neugeborner Kinder. Med. Jahrb. d. k. k. österr. Staates, Wien, 1817-18, iv, 86-101.—**Schupmann.** Sections-Befund bei einem an Morbus niger Hippocr. verstorbenen Manne. J. d. pract. Heilk., Berl., 1832, lxxiv, 4. St., 130-133.—**Silbermann** (O.) Ueber Melæna vera neonatorum. Jahrb. f. Kinderh., Leipz., 1877-8, n. F., xi, 378-384, 1 tab. *Also* [Abstr.]: Jahresb. d. schles. Gesellsch. f. vaterl. Kult. 1877, Bresl., 1878, lv, 205.—**Skorkowski** (A.) Czarna choroba Hippokratesa. Gaz. lek., Warszawa, 1873, xiv, 276-278.—**Sorgoni** (A.) Morbo nero associato a perniciosa apopletica; cura. Raccoglitore, Fano, 1846, xvii, 113-123.—**Stenger** (A.) Eine besondere Form von Blut-

Melæna.

erbrechen und blutigem Stuhlgang bei Säuglingen. Berl. klin. Wchnschr., 1887, xxiv, 457.—**Thomann** (J. N.) Schwarze Krankheit. Ann. d. klin. Anst. in d. Julius-Hosp. zu Würzb., 1801, 320–327.—**Tidd** (C. H.) Melæna neonatorum. Detroit Rev. Med. & Pharm., 1876. xi, 789–792.—**Tissot** (S. A. D.) Dissertatio historica de morbo nigro. Acta Helvet., Basileæ, 1777, viii, 61–67.—**Trousseau.** Leçon sur le mélæna. Gaz. d. hôp., Par., 1854, xxvii, 205.—**Vandermonde.** Observation sur une maladie noire d'une espèce particulière. Rec. périod. d'obs. de méd. de chir. et pharm., Par., 1757, vi, 336–341.—**Varnier.** Observations sur la maladie noire. Ibid., 83–95.—**Veit** (O.) Fall von sogen. Melæna neonatorum. Ztschr. f. klin. Med., Berl., 1882, iv, 471.—**Vicat** (P. R.) Melæna diuturna post lapsum ex alto, gravissima facta, sed lenissimorum laxantium et resolventium ope, multo rarior et tolerabilior quam antea erat, reddita. In his: Delectus obs. pract. ex diario clin., 8°, Vitodurum, 1780, 96–110.—**Walker** (H. V.) † In a newly-born female child; recovery. Med. Times & Gaz., Lond., 1885, ii, 632.—**Watson.** Cause of the black color of the blood in hæmatemesis; intestinal hæmorrhage; hæmorrhage from the urinary organs. Lond. M. Gaz., 1833, x, 465–473.—**Webber** (S.) Case of melæna cruenta. N. York M. & Phys. J., 1827, vi, 73–78.—**Wendrykowski.** Melæna, fluxus lienis s. hepaticus, s. vomitus cruentus. Org. f. d. ges. Heilk., Berl., 1861, x, 331–337.—**White** (J. F.) Vomiting and purging of blood in an infant twenty hours after birth. Cincin. M. Obs., 1857, ii, 298–304.—**Wiggert.** Zur Casuistik der Melæna vera neonatorum. Allg. med. Centr.-Ztg., Berl., 1878, xlvii, 206.—**Woronichin** (N.) Ueber den Nigrismus. Jahrb. f. Kinderh., Leipz., 1877–8, n. F., xi, 385–392.—**Wright** (T. H.) Case of melæna. Am. J. M. Sc., Phila., 1830, vii, 130–133.—**Zacchiroli.** Della melæna, ossia del morbo nero d' Ippocrate. Oss. med.-prat. e chir. di val. clin ital., Imola, 1793, i, 99–141.—**Zarlenga.** Caso di melena. Filiatre-sebezio, Napoli, 1815, xxix, 343–346.

Melaleuca flaviflora.

Martin (S.) Essence de miaouli, son action médicale. Bull. gén. de thérap., etc., Par., 1879, xcvii, 402–404.

Melaleuca Paraguariensis.

Bonpland (A.) Notes sur le Melaleuca Paraguariensis. [Mémoire remis par M. Norbert Wuy.] J. de thérap., Par., 1879, vi, 334–342.

Melampus. De nævis corporis tractatus.

In: MELETIUS. De natura structuraque hominis opus, etc. sm. 4°. Venetiis, 1882, 189–191.

Melampyrus.

See, also, Flour, etc.

Dizé. Expériences sur la coloration du pain par la graine du mélampyre. Mém. Acad. de méd., Par., 1833, iii, 340–349.—**Gaspard** (B.) Mémoire sur la rougette ou mélampire, Melampyrum arvense, L. J. de physiol. expér., Par., 1829, ix, 236–286.—**Henry.** Note à ajouter au mémoire de M. Dizé sur le mélampyre. Mém. Acad. de méd., Par., 1833, iii, 350–353.

Melanæmia.

See, also, Fever (Malarial, Complications, etc., of); Pigment (Abnormities, etc., of).

Benthaus (F.) * Ein Beitrag zur Kenntniss der Melanämie. 8°. Greifswald, 1875.

Armanni (L.) & **Lepidi** (G.) Sovra un caso di melanemia congenita. Morgagni, Napoli, 1871, xiii. 145–153, 1 pl. Also: Movimento, Napoli, 1871, iii, 49–52.—**Ball** (B.) Mélanémie. Dict. encycl. d. sc. méd., Par., 1873, 2. s, vi, 350–359.—**von Basch** (S.) † Med. Jahrb., Wien, 1873, iii, 233–239.—**Beckmann** (O.) † Arch. f. path. Anat., etc., Berl., 1859, xvi, 183–187. — **Cardarelli** (A.) Un caso raro di melanemia acuta. Morgagni, Napoli, 1887, xxix, 193–202. Also [Abstr.], in his: Alcune lez. clin., 12°, Napoli, 1887, 30–37.—**Carter** (H. V.) Melanæmia. Tr. M. & Phys. Soc. Bombay (1885), 1886, n. s., viii, 30–34. 1 pl.—**Charcot** (J.-M.) De la mélanémie, altération du sang par des granules et des corpuscules de pigment. Gaz. hebd. de méd., Par., 1857, iv, 659–665. — **Colin** (L.) Sur la migration du pigment sanguin à travers les parois vasculaires dans la mélanémie palustre. Ibid., 1872, 2. s., x, 35. ———. Des rapports qui existent entre la pigmentation splénique et la pigmentation des autres tissus dans la mélanémie. Bull. et mém. Soc. méd. d. hôp. de Par. (1873), 1874, 2. s., x. 407. Also: Union méd., Par., 1874, xxviii, 38. ———. La mélanémie palustre, considérée comme preuve de la migration des leucocytes à travers les parois des vaisseaux. Compt. rend. Soc. de biol. 1875, Par., 1876, 6. s., ii, 298–300.—**De Keghel.** Observation de mélanémie, suivi de guérison. [Rap. de Van Bambeke.] Bull. Soc. de méd. de Gand, 1869, xxxvi, 9; 95.—**De Martini** (A.) Considerazioni sulla melanemia cutanea, seguita da due storie di siffatta malattia. Rendic. Accad. med.-chir. di Napoli, 1856, x, 66–71, 1 pl. — **Frerichs** (F. T.) Die Melanämie und ihr Einfluss auf die Leber und auf andere

Melanæmia.

Organe. Ztschr. f. klin. Med., Bresl., 1855, vi, 321–338. Also, transl.: Arch. gén. de méd., Par., 1859, i, 513–532.—**Grohe** (F.) Zur Geschichte der Melanämie, nebst Bemerkungen über den normalen Bau der Milz und Lymphdrüsen. Arch. f. path. Anat., etc., Berl., 1861, xx, 306: xxii, 437, 1 pl.—**Hardy.** Mélanhémie. Gaz. d. hôp., Par., 1881, liv, 907.—**Jaccoud** (J.) Sur les maladies bronzées, à propos d'une observation de M. le professeur Fauvel, de Constantinople. Gaz. hebd. de méd., Par., 1864, 2. s., i, 1; 17.—**Karametsas** (G.) Δύω περιπτώσεις μελαναιμίας. Ἀσκληπιός, Ἀθῆναι, 1872–3, xi, 271–279. — **Kartoule** (S.) Περίπτωσις μελαναιμίας. Γαληνὸς, Ἀθῆναι, 1880, Δ´, 65–67.—**Köhler** (H.) Melanæmia; tuberculosis pulmonum; tabes dorsualis. Deutsche Klinik, Berl., 1859, xi, 110.—**Mohedano** (P.) Un caso de melanemia; el ácido acético y el alcohol empleados en su curacion. Andalucía méd., Córdoba, 1881, vi, 25–31. — **Mosler** (F.) Melanämie. Handb. d. spec. Path. u. Therap. (Ziemssen), Leipz., 1875, viii, 2. St., 182–196. ———. Ueber das Vorkommen von Melanämie. Arch. f. path. Anat., etc., Berl., 1877, lxix, 369–379. — **Nesti** (L.) & **Brigidi** (V.) † Sperimentale, Firenze, 1867, xix, 289–307.—**Nyström** (C.) † Upsala Läkaref. Förh., 1872–3, viii, 491; 658. — **Perroud.** Cachexie paludéenne; mélanose du foie et de la rate. Mém. et compt.-rend. Soc. d. sc. méd. de Lyon (1865), 1866, v, 286–289.—**Terzi** (G.) Della melanemia. Ippocratico, Fano, 1864, vi, 295–312.—**Tigri** (A.) Tre casi di cachessia per diatesi melanotica (milza nera), senza alterazione delle cassule soprarenali. Gazz. med. ital. feder. tosc., Firenze, 1857, 3. s., iii, 161. ———. Sulla cachessia melanotico (milza nera) in relazione della malattia descritta dal Addison. Ibid., 317–320. — **Tommasi Crudeli** (C.) Di alcuni effetti delle embolie di pigmento nel corso della melanemia, e specialmente di una tubercolosi polmonale prodotta da esse. Riv. clin. di Bologna, 1873, 2. s., iii, 90–93, 1 pl.—**Töngel** (C.) Melanämie. [5 cases.] Klin. Mitth. v. d. med. Abth. d. allg. Krankenh. in Hamb., 1861, 18–23.—**Wilks** (S.) Melanæmia and discoloration of the tissues arising from intermittent fever. [2 cases.] Guy's Hosp. Rep., Lond., 1859, 3. s., v, 100–108.

Melancholia.

See, also, Criminals (Mental condition, etc., of)— Special cases; Hypochondria; Insanity; Insanity (Periodic, etc.); Insanity (Religious); Insanity (Treatment of); Insanity and suicide; Insanity in women.

ANCEAUME (F.-H.) *De la mélancholie. 4°. Paris, 1818.

ARNOULD (J.) *De melancholia. 8°. Edinburgi, 1808.

BEAUX (J.-J.) * Quelques idées sur la mélancolie; le jugement, la manie, [etc.] 4°. Paris, 1822.

———. * Quelques idées sur la mélancolie. 4°. Paris, 1823.

BERGONIER (L.) * De la mélancolie, considérée comme cause de tuberculisation. 4°. Paris, 1871.

BLACK (A.) * De melancholia. 8°. Edinburgi, 1809.

BOISRAGON (H. C.) * De melancholia. 8°. Edinburgi, 1799.

BOURIENNE (A.) * De la mélancolie. 4°. Paris, 1853.

BOUSCHON (V.) * De melancholia. 8°. Monspelii, 1789.

VAN BRIENEN (N.) * De melancholia. roy. 4°. Lugd. Bat., [1738].

BRIGHT (T.) A treatise of melancholy, containing the causes thereof, and reasons of the strange effects it worketh in our minds and bodies, [etc.] 16°. London, 1613.

BUQUOY (J. A.) * De melancholia. 4°. Lugd. Bat., 1800.

BURTON (R. ["Democritus"]). The anatomy of melancholy, what it is, with all the kinds, causes, symptoms, prognostics, and several cures of it, [etc.] 8. ed. 8°. Philadelphia, 1857.

CAMERARIUS (M. R. J.) * Tensio cordis lipothymiæ causa occasione experimenti pneumatici exposita. sm. 4°. Tubingæ, [1686].

CHARPENTIER (C.-A.-T.) * Essai sur la mélancolie. 8°. Paris, an XI [1803].

CHÉGUT (L.) * De la lypémanie et de ses rapports avec la paralysie générale. 4°. Paris, 1868.

Melancholia.

CHRISTIAN (J.) Étude sur la mélancolie. Des troubles de la sensibilité générale chez les mélancoliques. 8°. *Paris*, 1876.

CHRISTOPHE (C.-A.) * Sur la mélancolie. 4°. *Strasbourg*, 1831.

CLEMENS (J. F.) * De melancholia hysterica. sm. 4°. *Erfordiæ*, [1727].

COBET (J. H.) * De atra bile. 8°. *Marburgi Cattorum*, [1793].

COLIN (L.) De la mélancolie; mémoire couronné. sm. 8°. *Paris*, 1866.

CRELL (J. F.) * De melancholia hysterica. sm. 4°. *Lipsiæ*, [1732].

CRICHTON (A. G.) * De melancholia. 8°. *Edinburgi*, 1810.

CROU (L.) * Essai sur la susceptibilité nerveuse et les affections mélancoliques. 4°. *Paris*, 1814.

DU VIVIER (E.) De la mélancolie. 8°. *Paris*, 1864.

ENGELMANN (J. M.) * De melancholia. 4°. *Argentorati*, [1754].

FREYTAG (G.) * De lypothymia. sm. 4°. *Altdorffi*, 1660.

FREYTAG (J.) Kurtzer Bericht von der Melancholia hypochondriaca. Nebenst zwölff curiosen Fragen und einer Analogia der grossen Welt mit der kleinen. 12°. *Franckfurt a. M.*, 1643.

FRIDERICUS (J. W.) * Diss. sistens melancholiam, vulgo die Schwermüthigkeit. sm. 4°. *Erfordiæ*, 1728.

FUCHS (J. C.) * De melancholia. 4°. *Jenæ*, 1671.

GERARDI (J.) * De tristitia. 4°. *Lugd. Bat.*, 1665.

GERBER (C. G.) De melancholia hypochondriaca. 4°. *Erfordiæ*, [1715].

GRAEBNER (G. L.) * De melancholia vera et simulata. 4°. *Halæ Magdeb.*, [1743].

HALICZKY (A.) * Imago melancholiæ. 8°. *Budæ*, [1833].

HASSE (G.) * Die Melancholie mit Rücksicht auf Aetiologie und Ausgang in Suicidium. 8°. *Greifswald*, 1886.

HEINSIUS (J. S.) * De syncope et lipothymia. 4°. *Jenæ*, [1715].

HERING (H.) Microcosmus melancholicus seu tractatus singularis de melancholia in genere, et affectione hypochondriaca in specie, una cum appendice variorum exemplorum et medicamentorum probatissimorum ex optimis autoribus collectorum. 16°. *Bremæ*, 1638.

HEYDENREICH (J. R.) * Diss. proponens juvenem melancholia laborantem. 4°. *Jenæ*, [1675].

HIRSCHEL (L. E.) * De morbis melancholicomaniacis. 4°. *Halæ Magdeb.*, [1763].

HOFRICHTER (B.) * De locis in melancholia adfectis. 8°. *Halæ*, [1797].

KLEIN (G.) * De melancholia, ex epitome praxeos clinicæ. 4°. *Jenæ*, [1707].

KOKUYT (I.) * De melancholia. 4°. *Lugd. Bat.*, 1685.

VON KRAFFT-EBING (R.) Die Melancholie. Eine klinische Studie. 8°. *Erlangen*, 1874.

KRAUSSOLD (C.) Melancholie und Schuld. Psychologische und psychiatrische Betrachtungen. 8°. *Stuttgart*, 1884.

LANDIS (C.) * De melancholia ex mente. 8°. *Gottingæ*, 1788.

LE FEBURE (J. L.) * De melancholia. 1785. *In:* LOUVAIN Diss. 8°. *Lovanii*, 1796, iii, 243–264.

LETUAL (F.-J.-P.) * Essai sur la mélancolie. 4°. *Strasbourg*, 1810.

LEVIEIL (J.-L.) * Sur la mélancolie. 4°. *Paris*, 1813.

Melancholia.

LORRY (A. C.) De melancholia et morbis melancholicis. 2 v. 8°. *Lutetiæ Parisiorum*, 1765.

MAIRET (A.) De la démence mélancolique. Contribution à l'étude de la périencéphalite chronique localisée et à l'étude des localisations cérébrales d'ordre psychique. 8°. *Paris*, 1883.

MARCADÉ (L.) * Sur la mélancolie. 4°. *Paris*, 1870.

DE MARCQ (E.) * De melancholia. 4°. *Lugd. Bat.*, 1751.

MASSÉNAT (J.-F.) * Sur la mélancolie. 4°. *Paris*, 1820.

MATYUS (S.) * De melancholia universali et hypochondriaca. 4°. *Traj. ad Rhenum*, 1756.

MEYLER (A.) * De melancholia. 8°. *Edinburgi*, 1803.

MULLER (J. B.) * De melancholia. sm. 4°. *Jenæ*, [1727].

MULLER (J. J.) * De melancholia attonita raro litteratorum affectu. 4°. *Jenæ*, [1741].

A MURILLO (T.) Novissima, verifica, et particularis hypochondriacæ melancholiæ curatio, et medela. 16°. *Lugduni*, 1872.

NEERINCX (V.) * De melancholia. sm. 4°. *Lugd. Bat.*, 1727.

NEUSE (J. G.) * De melancholia. sm. 4°. *Jenæ*, [1685].

NICOLAU (J.-B.) * Essai sur la mélancolie ou lypémanie proprement dite. 4°. *Montpellier*, 1824.

OHM (W.) * De melancholiæ specie qua affectæ pro sagis vulgo habentur. 4°. *Heidelbergæ*, [1681].

OLPIUS (J.) * De natura, causis, signis, differentiis et curatione humoris melancholici. sm. 4°. *Marpurgi Cattorum*, 1628.

PEON (A.) De la mélancolie avec délire. 8°. *Paris*, 1874.

PETERA (W.) * De melancholia attonita, adnexis historiis morbi synopticis. 8°. *Pragæ*, 1842.

PICHON (F.) * Essai sur la mélancolie. 4°. *Paris*, 1821.

LE PIPER (J.) * De melancholia. sm. 4°. *Lugd. Bat.*, 1621.

POHL (E.) Die Melancholie nach dem neuesten Standpunkte der Physiologie und auf Grundlage klinischer Beobachtungen bearbeitet. 8°. *Prag*, 1852.

RAESVELT (T. L.) * De melancholia. 4°. *Traj. ad Rhenum*, [1687].

REIGNIER (G.) Traité de mélancholie simple. 8°. *Paris*, 1885.

REINHARDT (F. G.) * Quædam de morbo atrabilario veterum, adjecta morbi historia. 8°. *Berolini*, [1826].

RELACION histórica del extraordinario phenomeno médico, que ha ocurrido en el Hospital general con un enfermo, que entró en él á 22 de enero de este año, y dictámen que sobre el conocimiento pronóstico, y curacion de su enfermedad han dado los médicos de número de los reales hospitales general, y passion de esta corte. sm. 4°. *Madrid*, 1763.

RÉVEILLÉ-PARISE (J.-H.) Mémoire sur l'existence et la cause organique du tempérament mélancolique. 8°. *Paris*, 1831.

REYES Y ZAMORA (A.-W.) * De la stupeur simple et de la stupeur mélancolique. 4°. *Paris*, 1873.

RODRIGUES DE PAYVA (G.) Epicrisis critico-apologetica de affectu atrabilario, mirachiali, sive de morbis cerebri et mentis, qui extra cerebrum originem ducunt. 4°. *Romæ*, 1751.

ROLFINCK (W.) * De melancholia. Resp. Joh. Casp. Horn. 4°. *Jenæ*, 1729.

DE SANTACRUCE (A.) Dignotio et cura affectuum melancholicorum. fol. *Matriti*, 1622.

Melancholia.

SARLUIS (J.) * De differentia inter melancho-liam et melænam, tum secundum veteres tum secundum recentiores. 8°. *Hagæ-Comitis*, 1840.

SCHIRMEYER (L.) * Ueber das melancholische Anfangsstadium der Geistesstörungen. 8°. *Strassburg*, 1886.

SCHÖNLINUS (J. T.) Discursus philosophicus et medicus de melancholia et catarrho, in quo de eorum differentiis, causis, signis, et curandi ratione accurate disseritur. Ex . . . Andreæ Laurentii . . . libello latio adscriptus. 18°. *Augustæ* [*Vindelicorum*], 1620.

SÉBIRE (A.-L.-H.) * De la mélancolie, considérée comme tristesse habituelle sans dérangement de la raison. 4°. *Paris*, 1831.

SIMONNOT (E.-L.) * Essai médico-philosophique sur la mélancolie. 4°. *Strasbourg*, 1827.

DE SMETH (J.) De la mélancolie. Étude médicale. 8°. *Bruxelles*, 1872.

THEOPOLD (H. L.) *Melancholici cujusdam vita ac melancholiæ ejus curatio. 8°. *Jenæ*, [1835].

TOUSSAINT (A.) *Dissertation sur la mélancolie. 4°. *Paris*, 1818.

VENATOR (A.) De triplici melancholia. sm. 4°. *Lugd. Bat* , 1618.

WACHTEL (J. C.) * Diss. exhibens mulierem melancholia hypochondriaca laborantem. sm. 4°. *Jenæ*, 1674.

WILLE (L.) * Ist die Melancholie eine psychische Depressionsform ? 8°. *Erlangen*, 1858.

Adam (J.) A case of melancholy, with stupor and catalepsy. J. Ment. Sc., Lond., 1883-4, xxix, 508-511.—**Adradas** (C. L.) Un caso de lipemania parcial auto-motriz. An. de cien. méd., Madrid, 1876, i, 509-515.—**Andry.** Recherches sur la mélancholie. Hist. Soc. roy. de méd. 1782-3, Par., 1787, v, 97-150.—**Ayres** (S.) Acute melancholia; phimosis; circumcision; recovery. Pittsburgh M. Rev., 1886-7, i, 168.—**Baillarger.** De la mélancolie avec stupeur. Ann. méd.-psych., Par., 1853, 2. s., v, 251-276.—**Ballestero** (A.) Lipemania sintomática de una cloro-anemia. Corresp. méd., Madrid, 1878,.xiii, 67-69.—**Bayles** (G.)· On causes of melancholia. Tr. M. Soc. N. Jersey, Newark, 1883, 88-112. *Also:* N. York M. J., 1883, xxxviii, 171; 202.—**Bifii** (S.) Della melancholia con stupore o melancolia attonita. Gazz. med. ital. lomb., Milano, 1853, 3. s., iv, 421-422.—**Billot** (E.) Du délire mélancolique considéré comme signe précurseur de la paralysie générale. Rev. méd. franç. et étrang., Par., 1860, ii, 399-403.—**Blum** (Z. A.) Melancholia passiva s charakterom psychichesk. virojdenija. [Passive melancholy as a characteristic psychical degeneration.] Med. Sbornik, Tiflis, 1885, no. 39, 75-80.—**Boucher.** Sur un cas de délire panique; épilepsie et mélancolie. Bull. Soc. clin. de Par., 1884, viii, 33-37.—**Bouvier.** Mémoire sur la mélancolie dans les fièvres. Rec. périod. Soc. de méd. de Par., 1792, iv, 343-358.—**Broadbent.** Cases of melancholia. Med. Press & Circ., Dubl., 1868, n. s., iii, 284.—**Brosius.** Melancholia simplex (nebst Bemerkungen über die Genesis dieses Falles und des Irreseins überhaupt). Med. Ztg., Berl., 1857, xxvi, 9; 13; 19.—**Brückmann.** Beobachtung eines Falles von hypochondrischer Melancholie und Wahnwitz. Arch. f. med. Erfah., Berl., 1812, i, 135-138.—**Bücking.** Zu den vielen noch eine besondre Art der Melancholie. N. Mag. f. Aerzte, Leipz., 1785, vii, 47-52.—**Buzzard** (T.) A case of recovery from melancholia, after refusal of food and obstinate silence during four years. Tr. Clin. Soc. Lond., 1875, viii, 31-37.—**Calmeil.** Lypémanie (bibliographie). Dict. encyl. d. sc. méd., Par., 1870, 2. s., iii, 542-575.—**Campbell** (J. A.) Two cases of melancholia presenting similar mental manifestations, evidently the result of visceral lesion. J. Ment. Sc., Lond., 1874-5, xx, 596-600. *Also,* Reprint.—**Caruso** (G.) Contributo allo studio della demenza melancolica. Manicomio, Nocera, 1885, i, 123-148.—**Chometowski** (S.) Szal melancholiczny (raptus melancholicus). Gaz. lek., Warszawa, 1871, x, 737; 757; 774.—**Constantinus** *Africanus.* De melancholia libri duo. *In his:* Opera [etc.], fol., Basileæ, 1536, 280-298.—**Corlieu** (A.) Études sur les causes de la mélancolie. [Rap. de M. de Kergaradec.] Bull. Acad. de méd., Par., 1860-61, xxvi, 479 - 486. ———. Quelques considérations sur la mélancolie. Bull. Soc. méd. du Panthéon de Par., 1865, 16 - 19. ———. Symptomatologie de la mélancolie. Courrier méd., Par., 1871, xxi, 307; 315; 355. ———. Pathologie mentale; diagnostic différentiel de la mélancolie. J. d. conn. med. prat., Par., 1874, xli, 305-308.—**Cotard** (J.) Du délire hypochondriaque dans une forme grave de la mélancolie anxieuse. Ann. méd.-psych., Par., 1880, 6. s., iv, 168-174. *Also,* Reprint. ———. Perte de la vision

mentale dans la mélancolie anxieuse. Arch. de neurol., Par., 1884, vii, 289-295. *Also* [Abstr.]: Progrès méd., Par., 1884, xii, 22.—**Cullerre** (A.) Étude clinique de la lypémanie stupide. [Prix Esquirol.] Ann. méd.-psych., Par., 1873, 5. s., x, 210; 394.—**Dahl** (L.) Psychiatriske Meddelelser. Norsk Mag. f. Lægevidensk., Christiania, 1855, ix, 217; 384; 449.—**Davy** (R. B.) A case of melancholia co-existant with aneurism of the arch of the aorta. South. Clinic, Richmond, 1883, vi, 169-173. *Also:* Cincin. Lancet & Clinic, 1883, n. s., x, 338-340.—**Delasiauve.** Du diagnostic différentiel de la lypémanie. Ann. méd.-psych., Par., 1851, iii, 380-442. *Also,* Reprint. ———. De la mélancolie avec stupeur, de M. Baillarger. Rev. méd. franç. et étrang., Par., 1853, ii, 385-399. ———. Sur la mélancolie avec stupeur. *Ibid.*, 1854, ii, 459-464.—**Douty** (J. H.) Melancholia, in its relations to diminution of the oxygen supply. Lancet, Lond., 1884, ii, 633-635. ———. Senile melancholia; its characters and pathology. Am. J. Insan., Utica, N. Y., 1885-6, xlii, 328-333.—**Dufour.** Réflexions à propos d'un cas de lypémanie compliquée de spasmes, etc. Ann. méd.-psych , Par., 1867, 4. s., x, 468-479.—**Du Laurens** (A.) Des maladies mélancholiques, et du moyen de les guarir. *In his:* Discours de la conservation de la veüe, 12°, Rouen, 1620, ff. 73-146.—**Ellero** (R. B.) Raptus melancholicus; studio psico-patologico e medico-legale. Gazz. med. ital., prov. venete, Padova, 1884, xxvii, 353; 361.—**Erhard.** Ueber die Melancho'ie. Comment. d. n. Arznk., Tübing., 1800, vi, 323-404.—**Erlenmeyer.** Die Melancholia transitoria. Cor.-Bl. d. deutsch. Gesellsch. f. Psychiat., etc., Neuwied, 1859, vi, 113; 129; 145.—**Esquirol.** Mélancolie. Dict. d. sc. méd., Par., 1819, xxxii, 147-183.—**Fischer** (R.) Vesania melancholica, durch Brechweinstein behoben. Med. Jahrb. d. k. k. österr. Staates, Wien, 1842, xxxix, 37-44.—**Ford** (W. E.) The early management of cases of mental depression. Tr. M. Soc. N. Y., Syracuse, 1886, 225-236.—**Foville** (A.) fils. Lypémanie. N. dict. de méd. et chir. prat., Par., 1875, xxi, 105-131.—**French** (E.) Melancholia. Tr. N. Hampshire M. Soc., Manchester, 1885, 105-112.—**Frese** (A. B.) Ueber den physiologischen Unterschied der Melancholie und Manie. Allg. Ztschr. f. Psychiat., etc., Berl., 1871-2, xxviii, 487-502.—**Fritsch** (J.) Zur Kenntniss der Melancholia atonita. Wien. med. Presse, 1878, xix, 1477; 1512; 1574. ———. Zur Differentialdiagnose der Melancholie. Jahrb. f. Psychiat., Wien, 1879, 119-149. ———. Diagnostik und Therapie der melancholischen Krankheitsformen. Ztschr. f. Diagn. u. Therap., Wien, 1882, i, 101; 113; 121.—**Galceran** (A.) Melancolia aguda con delirio ambicioso y accesos de agitacion. Rev. frenopát. barcel., 1881, i, 113-117.—**Gatti** (E. A.) Storia di una melancolia mirachiale stranamente guarita. Gior. anal. di med., Milano, 1830, xiv, 434-447.—**Giacchi** (O.) Melanconia spermatica. Sperimentale, Firenze, 1887, lix, 54-59.—**Giraud** (A.) De la mélancholie dans ses rapports avec la paralysie générale. Mém. et bull. Soc. de méd. et chir. de Bordeaux, 1878, 96-133. *Also:* J. de méd. de Bordeaux. 1878-9, viii, 208-220.—**Greisel** (J. G.) Von einer melancholischen Todsucht. Auserl. med.- chir.- . . . Abhandl. d. röm.-kais. Akad. d. Naturf., Nürnb., 1756, iii, 67-70.—**Gull** (W. W.) Case of melancholia. Tr. Clin. Soc. Lond., 1875, viii, 37-41.—**Gutinkov** (Z. V.) Starcheskaja melancholija. [Melancholia in old age.] Arch. psichiat., etc., Charkov, 1885, vi, no. 2, 92-100.—**Hagen.** Fall einer Melancholie, welcher Aphasie vorhergegangen war. Sitzungsb. d. phys.-med. Soc. zu Erlang., 1870-71, 3. Hft., 37-39.—**Harbinson** (A.) A case of typical melancholia from hereditary predisposition. J. Ment. Sc., Lond., 1877-8, xxiii, 359 - 362. – [**Hausbrand.**] Heilung einer Melancholia attonita. Mag. f. d. ges. Heilk., Berl., 1831, xxxiii, 608-612.—**Heinroth** (J. C. A.) Krankheitsberichte. Ztschr. f. psych. Aerzte, Leipz., 1818, i, 2. Vrtljhrshft., 231-254.—**Hildenbrand.** D'un élément symptomatique secondaire de la mélancolie et de son traitement. Ann. méd.-psych., Par., 1879, 6. s., ii, 387-397.—**Hill** (R. G.) Melancholia. Med. Circ., Lond., 1858, xii, 99.—**Hoffmann** (H.) Melancholie mit starker Aufregung und Gehörs-Illusionen. Jahresb. ü. d. Verwalt. d. Med.-Wes., d. Krar-kenanst. . . . d. Stadt Frankf. (1859), 1861, iii, 266. ———. Opium ein hülfreiches Mittel in Fällen von einfacher Melancholie. *Ibid.* (1862), 1865, vi, 139. ———. Günstig endender Fall von Melancholie cum excitatione et cum stupore. *Ibid.* (1863), 1867, vii, 129. ———. Melancholie mit Hallucinationen des Hautgefühls. *Ibid.* (1864), 1867, viii, 98.—**Hospital.** Observation intéressante de lypémanie. Ann. méd.-psych., Par., 1875, 5. s., xiii, 11-18.—**Hughes** (C. H.) Glycosuria and melancholia. Weekly M. Rev., Chicago, 1883, viii, 312. *Also,* Reprint. — **Hutchinson** (H. A.) Acute melancholia caused by impacted fæces. Am. J. Insan., Utica, N. Y., 1886-7, xliii, 365.—**Jaenichen** (J. G.) Melancholia ex ulcere neglecto. *In his:* Pentas obs. med., 4°, Halæ, 1768, 15.—**Johnstone** (C.) Case of profound and somewhat prolonged suicidal melancholia; diarrhœa with fever; recovery. J. Ment. Sc., Lond., 1885-6, xxxi, 203-205.—**Josselyn** (E. E.) The early recognition of incipient melancholia. Med. News, Phila., 1887, l, 314-318.—**Judée.** Mélancolie avec stupeur. France méd., Par., 1870, xvii, 89.—**Kelp.** Melancholie

Melancholia.

mit völliger Abmagerung und tödtlichen Ausgang bei zwei Geschwistern. Cor.-Bl. d. deutsch. Gesellsch. f. Psychiat., etc., Neuwied, 1855, ii, 17–20. —————. Melancholia cataleptica. *Ibid.*, 1863, x, 353 : 1864, xi, 321. —————. Tod durch Convulsionen bei Melancholie. Irrenfreund, Heilbr., 1875, xvii, 161–164. —————. Melancholie mit tödtlichem Ausgang bei zwei Geschwistern. Memorabilien, Heilbr., 1878, xxiii, 397–404.—**Kelp** (F.) Melancholia activa mit besonders hervortretenden Gemeingefühlsstörungen. Allg. Ztschr. f. Psychiat., etc., Berl., 1873-4, xxx, 461–468.— **Kitchen** (D. H.) Melancholia. Ohio M. & S. J., Columbus, 1877, n. s., ii, 237–256.—**Klein.** Ein Fall von Melancholia attonita. Allg. med. Centr.-Ztg., Berl., 1852, xxi, 525–529.—**Kovalevski** (P.) Sostojanie chuvstva miesta u melancholikov. [Nature of the feeling of grief in melancholia.] Moskov. med. Gaz., 1876, xix, 906; 938; 979; 1014; 1034; 1066; 1098; 1143; 1321; 1353. *Also* [Abstr.] : Med. Vestnik, St. Petersb., 1876, xvi, 385 393; 405; 416; 427; 440 : 451; 461; 477; 489; 500; 509. —————. Ob izmienenijach chuvstvitelinosti koji ü melancholikov. [Diminished sensibility of skin in melancholia.] Voyenno-med. J., St. Petersb., 1877, cxxviii, 53; 165; 238.—**von Krafft-Ebing.** Melancholia sine delirio; Anzünden einer Pulvermühle um aus der Welt oder in's Zuchthaus zu kommen. Irrenfreund, Heilbr., 1883, xxv, 33–37. —————. Melancholie; Selbstbeschuldigungen; fraglicher Werth derselben. Friedreich's Bl. f. gerichtl. Med., Nürnb., 1887, xxxviii, 121–130.—**Kramer.** Geschichte einer komplicirten Melancholie. Arch. f. med. Erfahr., Berl., 1825, ii, 417–431.—**Lagardelle.** Quelques mots sur la lypémanie. J. de méd. ment., Par., 1867, vii. 257–259. —————. Troubles de la sensibilité générale dans le délire mélancolique. Gaz. hebd. d. sc. méd. de Bordeaux, 1880-81, i, 705; 791; 840.—**Lamndrid** (J. J.) A supposed case of melancholia. Proc. M. Soc. County Kings, Brooklyn, 1877, ii, 36–42.—**Lasègue** (C.) La mélancolie perplexe. Arch. gén. de méd., Par., 1880, 6. s., iii, 177; 345. — *Also, in his:* Études méd., 8°. Par., 1884, i, 701–721.—**Leidesdorf** (F.) Melancholie. Allg. Wien. med. Ztg., 1859, iv, 23; 31; 51; 72.—**Leidesdorf** (M.) Ein klinischer Beitrag zur Lehre von der Melancholie. Wien. med. Presse, 1869, x, 289; 313. —————. Zur Lehre der Melancholie. Oesterr. Ztschr. f. prakt. Heilk., Wien, 1871, xvii, 201–206.—**Lichtener.** Krankengeschichte einer Melancholia. Beob. u. Abhandl. . . . v. österr. Aerzten, Wien, 1823, iii, 421–432.—**Lotz.** Fall von Melancholia transitoria. Allg. Ztschr. f. Psychiat., etc., Berl., 1868, xxv, 552–563.—**Mabille** (H.) Étude clinique sur quelques points de la lypémanie. Ann. méd.-psych., Par., 1880, 6. s., iii, 177; 345.—**Macdonald** (A. E.) Clinical lecture on melancholia. Med. Rec., N. Y., 1879, xvi, 481–484.—**Majorfi** (G.) Delirio acuto degli alienati a forma melancolico-stupida. Arch. ital. per le mal. nerv., Milano, 1883, xx, 173–216, 2 diag.—**de Mattos** (J.) Variedades melancolicas. Med. contemp., Lisb., 1884, ii, 33; 60; 67.—**Mauer** (F.) Die Melancholia attonita; eine gekrönte Preisschrift. Ztschr. f. d. Staatsarznk., Erlang., 1858, lxxv, 197–244.—**Meinert.** Melancholia. Vrach. Vaidom., St. Petersb., 1881, vi, 2441; 2504.— **Melanconia** con allucinazioni visive ed uditive. Boll. d. priv. manic. Fleurent, Napoli, 1886, xii, 77. — **Melendez** (L.) Melancolia sin estupor; repugnancia hácia los alimentos; alimentacion forzada; muerte. Rev. méd.-quir., Buenos Aires, 1881-2, xviii, 179–181. —————. Lipemanía simple. *Ibid.*, 1886-7, xxiii, 357. — **Meynert** (T.) Ueber Melancholie. Wien. med. Bl., 1881, iv, 793; 827; 857; 887.—**Michéa.** De la lypémanie, ou folie mélancolique, de ses genres, de ses espèces, de ses variétés, de ses formes. Rev. de thérap. méd.-chir., Par., 1859, xxvi, 535; 564; 622.—**Mickle** (A. F.) Insanity of twins; twins suffering from melancholia. J. Ment. Sc., Lond., 1884, xxx, 67–74.—**Mills** (C. K.) Clinical lecture on stuporous melancholia. Phila. M. Times, 1885-6, xvi, 481–483.—**Moeli.** Ueber Melancholie nach Verrücktheit. Tagebl. d. Versamml. deutsch. Naturf. u. Aerzte, Eisenach, 1882, lv, 310.—**Musso** (G.) Sui movimenti del respiro nell' angoscia precordiale degli stati melancolici. Arch. ital. per le mal. nerv., Milano, 1886, xxiii, 75–86.—**Nagel.** Gedanken über die Melancholia attonita bezüglich ihrer Verwandtschaft mit einem besonderen Krankheitszustande des Rückenmarkes und über den vermeintlichen oder muthmasslichen Sitz derselben daselbst. Ztschr. f. Med., Chir. u. Geburtsh., Magdeb., 1856, x, 112–116. — **Neftel** (W. B.) On periodical melancholia. Med. Rec., N. Y., 1875, x, 545–549. *Also, Reprint.* — **Oka Genkai.** [Epileptic melancholia.] Iji Shinbun, Tokio, 1884, no. 126, July 5. — **Otto.** Melancholia attonita. Cor.-Bl. d. deutsch. Gesellsch. f. Psychiat , etc., Neuwied, 1857, iv, 139–141.—**Paris** (A.) Cas de guérison rapide de lypémanie avec mutilation. Ann. méd.-psych., Par., 1883, 6. s., ix, 219–222.—**Pattou** (A.) Two cases of melancholia. J. Ment. Sc., Lond., 1885-6, xxxi, 499–501. — **Pepper** (W.) Melancholia; malignant disease of the left lobe of the liver. Med. Bull., Phila., 1886, viii, 36–39. — **Petit.** Observation de lypémanie. J. de la sect. de méd. Soc. méd. Loire-Inf., Nantes, 1856, n. s., xxxii, 20–33. — **Petræus** (H.) De melancholia. *In:* Nosol. harmonica dogmat. et hermet., 4°, Marpurgi Cattorum, 1615, i, 55–68. — **Pihl.**

Melancholia.

Föredrag om melancholien. Upsala Läkaref. Förh., 1865-6, i, 111–117.—**Pitts** (G. R.) Hints on melancholy. Am. M. Recorder, Phila., 1823, vi, 596–602. — **Poggi** (C.) Raptus melancholicus; perizia medico-legale sullo stato di mente di P. G. . . . Arch. ital. per le mal. nerv., Milano, 1885, xxii, 469–490. — **Potain.** Mélancolie avec stupeur. Gaz. d. hôp., Par., 1877, l, 825. — **Poterín du Motel** (E.-P.) Études sur la mélancolie et sur le traitement moral de cette maladie. Mém. Acad. de méd., Par., 1857, xxi, 443–527.—**Redi** (F.) Per ulcere in bocca, piaghe nelle gambe, rogna, magrezza, stitichezze e malinconia. *In:* Cons. med. di varii autori, 12°, Venezia, 1839, i, 26–40. — **Reiman** (J. A.) Historia morbi melancholici. Samml. v. Nat.- u. Med.- . . . Gesch. 1717, Bresl., 1718, ii, 297–299 (Latin text).—**Richarz.** Ueber Wesen und Behandlung der Melancholie mit Aufregung (melancholia agitans). Allg. Ztschr. f. Psychiat., etc., Berl., 1858, xv, 28–65.—**Rodriguez y Rodriguez** (A.) Cuatro casos de melancolía en sus diversas formas. Rev. frenopát. barcel., 1885, v, 83–89, 4 pl. — **Rösch.** Melancholie mit Exaltation bei einem 18jährigen Bauernburschen plötzlich entstanden. Med. Cor.-Bl. d. württemb. ärztl. Ver., Stuttg., 1853, xxiii, 133.—**Russell** (I.) Melancholia. Alienist & Neurol., St. Louis, 1881, ii, 195–207. — **Sales-Girons.** Faut-il admettre une troisième espèce de mélancolie dite la mélancolie avec stupeur (de M. Baillarger)? Rev. méd. franç. et étrang., Par., 1853, i, 461–477.—**Sanborn** (B. T.) Acute melancholia. Tr. Maine M. Ass., Portland, 1885, 535–545. — **Sankey** (W. H. C.) On melancholia. J. Ment. Sc., Lond., 1863-4, ix. 173–196.—**Sarget** (J. M.) Hiperfrenia melancólica. Union de l. cien. méd., Cartagena, 1883-4, ii, 229. — **Savage** (G. H.) Melancholia. Guy's Hosp. Gaz., Lond., 1876, 2. s., i, 132; 137. —————. Twins suffering from similar attacks of melancholia. J. Ment. Sc., Lond., 1882-3, xxviii, 539.— **Schlager** (L.) Ueber die sogenannte Melancholia attonita oder stupida. Oesterr. Ztschr. f. prakt. Heilk., Wien, 1857, iii. 417; 441; 461; 480. — **Schmid** (J.) Von der falschen Einbildung einer melancholischen Person. Auserl med.-chir.- . . . Abhandl. d röm.-kais. Akad. d. Naturf., Nürnb., 1761, ix, 72–74.—**Schüle** (H.) Ein interessanter Fall von Melancholia agitata mit Ausgang in Genesung. Irrenfreund, Heilbr., 1883, xxv, 17–23.—**Seglas** (J.) Note sur un cas de melancolie anxieuse. Arch. de neurol., Par., 1884, viii 56–68.—**Semal.** De la sensibilité générale et de ses altérations dans les affections mélancoliques. Ann. méd.-phys., Par., 1875, 5. s., xiii, 323–353.— **Semelaigne.** Du diagnostic et du traitement de la mélancolie. Mém. Acad. de méd., Par., 1861, xxv, 188–296.— **Stahley** (G. D.) Oxaluria in melancholia. Med. News, Phila., 1886, xlviii, 621–623. — **Steenberg.** I Anledning af Prof. Lange's Skrift om periodiske Depressionstilstande. Hosp.-Tid., Kjøbenh., 1886, 3. R., iv, 628–648. — **Steinheim.** Melancholie mit Bewusstsein. Ein Gegenstück zur Mania sine delirio. Wchnschr. f. d. ges. Heilk., Berl., 1834, iii, 297–305. — **Stillings** (F. A.) Melancholia, and its connection with ancient and modern suicides. Tr. N. Hampshire M. Soc., Concord, 1880, 75–87.—**Sutherland** *et al.* Melancholia. Rep. (Further) Com. Lunacy, Lond., 1847, pt. 4, 447–463.—**Taub.** Zwei Fälle von Melancholie mit dem Ausgange in Genesung. Wien. Med.-Halle, 1861, ii, 260; 287; 297.—**Tott** (C. A.) Melancholia autochirica und Wahnsinn. Ztschr. d. deutsch. Chir.-Ver., Magdeb., 1853, vii, 89–94.—**Turnbull** (F. M.) A report of three cases of melancholia, being especially a consideration of the prognosis. Boston M. & S. J., 1886, cxiv. 230.—**Tuttle** (G. T.) Cases of melancholia. *Ibid.*, 1884, cx, 77–80.—**Vauréal** (C.) Recherches sur les causes de la mélancolie. J. de méd. ment., Par., 1867, vii, 234–243. *Also:* France méd., Par., 1867, xvi, 316; 323; 329.—**Voisin** (A.) & **Burlureaux** (C.) De la mélancolie dans ses rapports avec la paralysie générale. Mém. Acad. de méd., Par., 1880, xxxiii, 1–264.—**Voisin** (J.) Note sur un cas de mélancolie avec stupeur à forme cataleptique, avec conservation de l'intelligence, ayant duré six ans. Arch. de neurol., Par., 1887, xiii, 354–366.—**Weber.** Geschichte eines melancholischen Wahnsinnes bey zwey Schwestern. Med. Jahrb. d. k. k. österr. Staates, Wien, 1824, n. F., ii, 79–89.— **Weigel** (C. J.) Fall von Melancholie. Beitr. z. prakt. Heilk., Leipz., 1834, i, 407–414.—**Wiglesworth** (J.) On the pathology of certain cases of melancholia attonita, or acute dementia. J. Ment. Sc., Lond., 1883-4, xxix, 355–372, 1 pl. —————. Four cases of melancholia in one family. *Ibid.*, 1884, xxx, 553–556.—**Wilhelmi** (B.) Zur Casuistik der Melancholia cataleptica. Cor.-Bl. d. deutsch. Gesellsch. f. Psychiat., etc., Neuwied, 1864, 71. —————. Ein Fall von Melancholia transitoria. *Ibid.*, 1873, 177–189.— **Wille** (L.) Melancholie. Deutsche Med.-Ztg., Berl., 1884, ii, 321; 333.—**Wilsey** (O. J.) Report of a case of melancholia, with stupor of five years' duration; recovery; synopsis of patients; asylum experience. Alienist & Neurol., St. Louis, 1886, vii, 209–216. — **Wood** (H. C.) Melancholia. Therap. Gaz., Detroit, 1885, 3. s., i, 793–799.— **Yeguchi** (J.) [Acute melancholia.] Iji Shinbun, Tokio, 1886, no. 194, May 25. — **Zippe** (H.) Melancholie; Verfolgungswahn; Mord. Wien. med. Wchnschr., 1877, xxvii, 1142; 1166; 1193; 1221.

Melancholia (*Treatment of*).

COLOMBIER (J.) * An melancholicis peregrinatio? Præses L. A. Gervaise. 4°. [*Paris*, 1767.]

GOURBELLY (C. A.) * An melancholici leniter purgandi? 4°. [*Paris*, 1771.]

MIDY (J.) * An diluentia, in affectibus melancholicis, purgantibus præferenda? 4°. *Parisiis*, 1737.

SCHRAMM (A.) * Ueber die Wirkungen des Amylnitrits insbesondere bei Melancholie. 8°. *Berlin*, 1874.

Also, in: Arch. f. Psychiat. 1874, Berl., 1875, v, 317-340.

SPIESS (J. C.) Melancholia hypochondriaca salivatione mercuriali cito, tuto ac radicitus exstirpata; quam secundum omnes circumstantias methodumque curandi adhibitam ulteriori philiatrorum disquisitioni exposuit. 12°. [*n. p.*], 1704.

Albers (J. F. H.) Die Temperaturentziehung als Heilmittel in der unruhigen Melancholie. Allg. Ztschr. f. Psychiat., etc.; Berl., 1864, xxi, 235-243.—Blake (J. E.) & Hamilton (A. McL.) A preliminary report upon the use of dilute nitrous oxide gas in the treatment of melancholia and nervous exhaustion. Med. Rec., N. Y., 1880, xvii, 118.—Brierre de Boismont (A.) On the treatment of melancholia, or lypemania. J. Psych. M., Lond., 1875, n. s., i, 21-37.—Chometowski (S.) Nowy sposób leczenia posepnicy z otepieniem (melancholia attonita), za pomaca elektryczności indukcyjnéj (pradow przerywanych). [New method of treating . . . by the electric inductive current.] Gaz. lek., Warszawa, 1866, i, 101; 133.—Clerici (G.) Del vantaggio dell' opio nelle melancolie. Gazz. med. ital. lomb., Milano, 1856, 4. s., i, 369-371.—Courtenay (E. M.) The use of opium in the treatment of melancholia. West Riding Lun. Asyl. Rep., Lond., 1872, ii, 254-277.—Cubitt (W. R.) A case of incipient melancholia, treated by pressure on the nerves of the neck and carotids. Midland M. & S. Reporter, Worcester, 1830-31, ii, 139-146.—Delmas (P.) Traitement hydrothérapique de la lypémanie simple. Bordeaux méd., 1874, iii, 115; 121.—Evers (O. J.) Ein halb Dutzend besonderer Wirkungen von der Belladonna oder gemeinen Wolfskirsche in melancholischen Krankheiten. Berl. Samml. z. Beförd. d. Arzneyw., etc., Berl., 1773, v, 565-583.—Hoestermann (C. E.) Ueber die Anwendung des Amylnitrites bei Melancholie. Wien. med. Wchnschr., 1872, xxii, 1148; 1176; 1201.—Hughes (C. H.) An outline brief in the management of melancholia. Alienist & Neurol., St. Louis, 1886, vii, 217-236.—Leidesdorf. Die Behandlung der Melancholie. Memorabilien. Heilbr., 1859, iv, 60-62.—Lucaszewski (J.) Ein Fall von frischer Melancholie durch Morphiuminjectionen geheilt. Allg. Ztschr. f. Psychiat., etc., Berl., 1884, xli, 173-179.—Marcé (L.-V.) Observation de mélancolie traitée et guérie par l'opium à haute dose. Gaz. d. hôp., Par., 1857, xxx, 103.—Melion. Melancholie, geheilt durch den Gebrauch der versendeten Franzensquelle. Oesterr. med. Wchnschr., Wien, 1848, 353-358.—Mendel (E.) Zur Therapie der Melancholie. Berl. klin. Wchnschr., 1872, ix, 287-301. *Also:* Verhandl. d. Berl. med. Gesellsch. (1871-3), 1874, iv, 1. Theil, 86-99.—Mickle (W. J.) Morphia in melancholia; its influence on temperature, etc. Practitioner, Lond., 1881, xxvi, 430-435.—Moreau. Lypémanie avec stupeur; tendance à la démence; traitement par l'extrait (principe résineux) de cannabis indica; guérison. Gaz. d. hôp., Par., 1857, xxx, 391.—Moulton (A. R.) The treatment of melancholia. Alienist & Neurol., St. Louis, 1887, viii, 69-83.—Muzell (F. H. L.) Von einer Melancholie, bey welcher der tartarus tartarisatus nichts helfen wollen, welche aber durch Bäder im kalten Wasser dennoch curirt worden ist. *In his:* Med. u. chir. Wahrnehm., 12°, Berl., 1764, 2. Samml., 54-60.—Pasta (A.) Cura della melanconia. Gazz. med. ital. lomb., Milano, 1868, 6. s., i, 345.—Polli (G.) Storia di una lipemania guarita principalmente con forti dosi di solfato di chinina. unito ad un po' di oppio. Gazz. med., Milano, 1842, i, 49-51.—Schivardi (P.) Delirio melancolico guarito coll' elettricità. Gazz. med. ital. lomb., Milano, 1867, 5. s., vi, 31-32.—Schubert. Desperatio æternæ salutis durch Opium heilbar. Med. Ztg., Berl., 1857, xxvi, 105.—Seguin (E. C.) The treatment of mild cases of melancholia at home. Am. Clin. Lect., N. Y., 1876, ii, 41-65. *Also, in his:* Op. min.. [etc.], 8°, N. Y., 1884, 655-671.—Tigges. Zur Behandlung der Melancholie mit Opium. Allg. Ztschr. f. Psychiat., etc., Berl., 1864, xxi, 421-444.—Williams (S. W. D.) On the treatment of melancholia attonita with refusal of food, by the continuous current. Lancet, Lond., 1873, i, 127.

Melancholia (De) et morbis melancholicis.

See [Lorry (Annæus Carolus)].

Melanchthon (Philippus) [1497-1560]. Loci

aliquot . . . in libro de anima, de moderatione cibi et potus, item somni et vigiliarum.

In: MORESCOTTI (Alfonso). Compendium medicinæ totius. 16°. *Herbornæ Nassoviorum*, 1604, 391-394.

See, also, Magirus (Joannes). Anthropologia. sm. 8°. *Francofurti*, 1603.—Salernum (School of). De conservanda bona valetudine opusculum scholæ Salernitanæ. 18°. *Parisiis*, 1555. ——. The same. 16°. *Francofurti*, 1556. ——. The same. 12°. *Francoforti*, 1557.

Melandri-Contessi (Girolamo). Nuove ri-

cerche fisico-chimiche ed analisi delle acque minerali di Recoaro e delle acque di Staro e di Civillina. 206 pp , 1 l., 4 pl. 8°. *Padova, tipi della Minerva*, 1830. [P., v. 1213.]

Melanesia.

See, also, Ethnology.

Codrington (R. H.) Religious beliefs and practices in Melanesia. J. Anthrop. Inst., Lond., 1880-81, x, 261-316, 1 map.

Mélanges de chirurgie étrangère, par une so-

ciété de chirurgiens de Genève, composée de J.-P. Maunoir, etc. 2 v. xv, 476 pp., 2 l., 2 pl.; xi, 603 pp., 2 l. 8°. *Genève, J.-J. Paschoud*, 1824-5.

Melanin.

Dressler (W.) Ein weiterer Beitrag zur Kenntniss der im Organismus vorkommenden, Melanin genannten Pigmente. Vrtljschr. f. d. prakt. Heilk., Prag. 1869, ci, 59 - 68. — Miura (M.) Beitrag zur Kenntniss des Melanins. Arch. f. path. Anat., etc., Berl., 1887, cvii, 250-259.—Pribram (A.) Melanin im Harne. Vrtljschr. f. d. prakt. Heilk., Prag, 1865, lxxxviii, 16-22.

Melanoderma.

See Addison's *disease*; Skin (*Discoloration, etc., of*).

Melanosarcoma.

See Melanosis, *etc.*

Melanosis *and melanotic tumors*.

See, also, Choroid, Foot, Groin, *Tumors of*; Liver (*Tumors of, Melanotic*); Lungs (*Melanosis of*).

ASCH (S.) * De melanosi. 8°. *Vratislaviæ*, [1847].

BAUMBACH (H. F.) * De melanosi. 8°. *Berolini*, [1839].

BENZLER (H.) *Die Nævi als Ursprungsstätten melanotischer Geschwülste. 8°. *Berlin*, [1880].

BERDEZ (J.) * Recherches chimiques sur deux pigments pathologiques mélanines. [Bern.] 8°. *Genève*, 1885.

BLINZIG (G.) * Ueber Melanose. 8°. *Tübingen*, [1848].

BRESCHET (G.) Considérations sur une altération organique appelée dégénérescence noire, mélanose, cancer mélané, etc. 8°. *Paris*, 1821.

Also, in: Rev. méd. hist. et phil., Par.. 1821, vi, 304-322. *Also, transl. in:* N. Jahrb. d. teutsch. Med. u. Chir., Elberfeld, 1822, v, 1. St., 87-106.

CÉRALE (É.) * Essai sur la mélanose vraie. 4°. *Montpellier*, 1880.

CLAUZEL (E.) * Du diagnostic de la généralisation des tumeurs mélaniques par l'examen microscopique du sang, des urines et des crachats. 4°. *Paris*, 1874.

——. The same. 8°. *Paris*, 1874.

DRECKER (R.) * De melanosi. 8°. *Berolini*, [1848].

GAUTRET (A.-P.) * De la mélanose. 4°. *Paris*, 1863.

GILLET (A.) * Contributions à l'histoire de la mélanodermie. 4°. *Paris*, 1869.

GROENE (G.) * De carcinomate melanode. 8°. *Gryphiswaldiæ*, 1861.

KAWKA (P.) *Ueber Melanosarcom. 8°. *Berlin*, [1883].

KREBS (E. H.) * De melanoseos anatomia pathologica. 8°. *Halæ*, [1839].

Melanosis *and melanotic tumors.*

LAURENS (M.-L.) * Sur la mélanose. 4°. *Paris*, 1833.

LESCRÖEL DESPREZ (T.-E.) * Sur la mélanose et principalement sur ses caractères anatomiques. 4°. *Paris*, 1831.

MARIUS (C. G. F.) * De melanosi. 8°. *Groningæ*, 1835.

MÖRNER (K. A. H.) * Bidrag till kännedomen om färgämnena i melanotiska svulster. 8°. *Stockholm*, 1886.

NEHSE (A.) * De melanosi. 8°. *Berolini*, 1839.

NIEBERG (C.) * Zur Statistik der melanotischen Geschwülste. 8°. *Würzburg*, 1882.

NOACK (C. A.) * De melanosi cum in hominibus tum in equis obveniente. Specimen pathologiæ comparatæ. 4°. *Lipsiæ*, 1826.

PEULEVÉ (M.-V.) * Contribution à l'étude de la mélanose généralisée. 4°. *Paris*, 1866.

REUSS (A.) * Tentamen anatomico pathologicum de melanosi. 8°. *Pragæ*, 1833.

ROEDERER (J.) * De la mélanose en général et celle de l'œil en particulier. 4°. *Strasbourg*, 1835.

ROEMHILD (J. C. G. L.) * De melanosi. 4°. *Halis*, [1833].

SAINT-LAGER (J.-B.) * De la mélanose. 4°. *Paris*, 1850.

SCHIER (M.) * De morbo quodam maculoso quem melanosin recentiores appellant. 8°. *Berolini*, 1826.

SCHILLING (E.) * De melanosi. 4°. *Francof. a. M.*, 1831.

SCHNEIDER (R.) * Vom melanotischen Krebs. 8°. *Jena*, 1864.

SPERBER (J.) * De melanosi. 8°. *Halæ*, 1843.

THUAU (P.) * Étude sur la mélanose généralisée. 4°. *Paris*, 1876.

VAZEILLE (M.) * Quelques considérations générales sur la mélanose à propos d'un cas de mélano-sarcome de l'œil. 4°. *Paris*, 1879.

WEISSER (P.) * Ueber Melanosarcoma. 8°. *Berlin*, 1876.

ZIMMERMANN (C.) * De melanosi. 8°. *Strasburgi*, [1828].

Albers (J. F. H.) Zur Lehre vom Fungus melanoides. J. d. Chir. u. Augenh., Berl., 1830, xiv, 339–372. — Arnstein. Bemerkungen über Melanämie und Melanose. Arch. f. path. Anat., etc., Berl., 1874, lxi, 494–508, 1 pl.— Bard (L.) De la nature parasitaire de la mélanose et de certaines tumeurs mélaniques. Lyon méd., 1885, xlviii, 407–414.— Bendz (J. C.) Einige Beobachtungen über die Melanose. Aus dem Danischen, nebst Zusätzen, mitgetheilt von Nevermann J. d. Chir. u. Augenh., Berl., 1835, xxiii, 102; 250; 415; 590.— Berdez (J.) & Nencki (M.) Ueber der Farbstoffe der melanotischen Sarkome. Arch. f. exper. Path. u. Pharmokol., Leipz., 1885–6, xx, 346–361.— Berend (H. W.) Ueber Melanosis. Wchnschr. f. d. ges. Heilk., Berl., 1849, 497–509, 1 pl.— Bolotof (T. G.) Melyano-sarkoma u loshadi. [Melano-sarcoma in the horse.] Med. Sbornik, Tiflis, 1876, No. xxii, pt. 5, 29.— Bolze. Zur Harnuntersuchung bei Pigmentkrebs. Vrtljschr. f. d. prakt. Heilk., Prag, 1860, lxvi, 140 – 142.— Bredin (J. N.) Case of melanotic sarcoma. Lancet, Lond., 1887, i, 367.— Carswell (R.) Melanosis. Cycl. Pract. M. (Tweedie), Phila., 1845, iii, 284–303.— Case (A) of melanotic sarcoma. Sei-i-Kwai M. J., Tôkyô, 1887, vi, 160.— Cazenave (A.) Mélanose. Dict de méd., 2. éd., Par., 1839, xix, 324–355.— Contra-indications (The) to the removal of melanotic tumours, derived from the microscopic examination of the blood and the urine. Med. Times & Gaz., Lond., 1874, i, 355.— Cornil (V.) & Trasbot (L.) De la mélanose. Mém. Acad. de méd., Par., 1867–8, xxviii, 319–423. — Cullen (W.) & Carswell (R.) On melanosis. Tr. Med.-Chir. Soc. Edinb., 1824, i, 264–284.— Delpech. Sur la mélanose. Mémor. d. hôp. du midi, Par., 1829, i, 454; 508. — Dieterich (P.) Ein Beitrag zur Statistik und klinischen Bedeutung melanotischer Geschwülste. Arch. f. klin. Chir., Berl., 1887, xxxv, 289–320.— Eberth (C. J.) Ueber die embolische Verbreitung der Melanosarcome. Arch. f. path. Anat., etc., Berl., 1873, lviii, 58–64.— Eiselt (T.) Die Diagnose des Pigment- (melanotischen) Krebses durch den Urin. Vrtljschr. f. d. prakt. Heilk., Prag, 1858, lix, 190–192. ——. Ueber Pigmentkrebs. *Ibid.*, 1861, lxx, 87: 1862, lxxvi, 26. — Fergusson. Melanosis, and the indefinite nature of melanoid

Melanosis *and melanotic tumors.*
tumours. Lancet, Lond., 1855, ii, 439. — Ganghofner (F.) & Přibram (F.) Ueber das Verhalten des Harnes bei Melanosen [etc.] Vrtljschr. f. prakt. Heilk., Leipz., 1876, cxxx, 77–100, 1 tab.— Godlee (R. J.) Melanosis of finger. Tr. Path. Soc. Lond., 1879–80, xxxi, 336.— Goujon (E.) Inoculation de matière mélanique. Compt. rend. Soc. de biol. 1867, Par., 1869, 4. s., iv, 93–98.— Gussenbauer (C.) Ueber die Pigmentbildung in melanotischen Sarcomen und einfachen Melanomen der Haut. Arch. f. path. Anat., etc., Berl., 1875, lxiii, 322–355, 1 pl.— Haushalter (P.) Contribution à l'étude du sarcome mélanique généralisé. Rev. méd. de l'est, Nancy, 1887, xix, 111; 151.— Heurtaux (A.) Mélanose. N. dict. de méd. et chir. prat., Par., 1876, xxii, 43–90.—Hutchinson (J.) Melanosis often not black; melanotic whitlow. Brit. M. J., Lond., 1886, i, 491. ——. Melanotic whitlows. Am. J. M. Sc., Phila., 1886, n. s., xci, 470.—Kolaczek. Zur Lehre von der Melanose der Geschwülste. Deutsche Ztschr. f. Chir., Leipz., 1879, xii, 67–84. *Also, in:* Fischer (H.) Mitth. a. d. k. chir. Klin. zu Bresl., 8°, Leipz., 1880, 67 – 84. — Laennec. Sur les mélanôses. Bull. Fac. de méd. de Par. [1804–8], 1812, i, 2. année, 24–26.— Legg (W.) Melanosis after melanotic sarcoma of the choroid. Brit. M. J., Lond., 1883, ii, 1242. *Also:* Lancet, Lond., 1883, ii, 1128.— Les (M.) Czarny barwnik (melanina) w organizmie zwierzęcym. [Melanosis in the animal organism.] Wiadomości farm., Warszawa, 1885, xii, 265–269.— Little. Melanotic sarcoma. Pathologist, Brooklyn, 1882, ii, 132.— Mauri (F.) Contribution à l'étude de la mélanose. Rev. méd. de Toulouse, 1885, xix, 545–555 [609–619].— Melsens. Recherches chimiques sur la matière des mélanoses. Compt. rend. Acad. d. sc., Par., 1844, xix, 1293–1299.—Mörner (K. A. H.) Zur Kenntniss von den Farbstoffen der melanotischen Geschwülste. Ztschr. f. physiol. Chem., Strassb., 1886–7, xi, 66–141, 2 diag.— Moore (N.) The death of Catherine of Aragon. Athenæum, Lond., 1885, Jan. 31, 152. — Nepveu (G.) Contribution à l'étude des tumeurs mélaniques. Gaz. méd. de Par., 1872, 4. s., i, 325; 385. *Also:* Compt. rend. Soc. de biol. 1872, Par., 1874, 5. s., iv, pt. 2, 3–16. *Also,* Reprint. ——. Contre-indications à l'extirpation des tumeurs mélaniques, tirées de l'examen microscopique du sang et des urines. Gaz. méd. de Par., 1874, 4. s., iii, 59. *Also:* Compt. rend. Soc. de biol. 1874, Par., 1875, 6. s., i. 82–86. — Oppenheimer (O.) Beiträge zur Lehre der Pigmentbildung in melanotischen Geschwülsten. Arch. f. path. Anat., etc., Berl., 1886, cvi, 515–554, 1 pl.— Pamard (P.) Observations opthalmologiques propres à infirmer l'opinion généralement admise sur la nature cancéreuse des mélanoses. Ann. d'ocul., Brux., 1853, xxix, 25 – 31. — Panné. Tumeurs mélaniques de la peau; tumeurs et infiltration mélaniques des divers organes profonds, y compris les capsules surrénales; mélanodermie; autopsie. Progrès méd., Par., 1887, 2. s., v, 527–530: vi, 46–48. — Pemberton (O.) Observations on the history, pathology, and treatment of melanosis. Midland Q. J. M. Sc., Birmingh., 1857, i, 129–166, 4 pl.— Pick (F. J.) Ueber Melanosis lenticularis progressiva. Vrtljschr. f. Dermat., Wien, 1884, xi, 3–32, 4 pl.—Pouchet (G.) Sur la formation du pigment mélanique. Compt. rend. Soc. de biol. 1880, Par., 1881, 7. s., ii, 306. ——. Sur la formation du pigment mélanique. *Ibid.*, Par., 1887, 8. s., iv, 164 – 166. — Ranvier. Les résultats de l'étude histologique d'un fait de mélanose généralisée. J. de l'anat. et physiol., etc., Par., 1868, v, 326–329.— Rindfleisch. Ueber einen Fall von Melanose; mit Demonstration. Sitzungsb. d. phys.-med. Gesellsch. zu Würzb., 1885, 125–127. — Robin (C.) Mélanose. Dict. encycl. d. sc. méd., Par., 1873, 2. s., vi, 374 – 410. — Rundle (H.) Multiple melanotic sarcomata; necropsy. Lancet, Lond., 1886, ii, 1221. — Schultz (C. H.) Ueber Entstehung der Melanosen. Beitr. z. physiol. u. path. Chem. u. Mikr., Berl., 1843–4, i, 574 – 577. — Schwalbe. Experimentelle Melanämie und Melanose. Tagebl. d. Versamml. deutsch. Naturf. u. Aerzte, Magdeb., 1884, lvii, 201. *Also:* Wien. med. Bl., 1884, vii, 1323 - 1325.— Second-Féréol. Mélanose généralisée et compliquée de cancer encéphaloïde. Bull. Soc. anat. de Par., 1858, xxxiii, 350 – 355.— Semmer (E.) Melanosarcomatose und Melanämie bei Schimmeln. Deutsche Ztschr. f. Thiermed., Leipz., 18×3, ix, 89.— Siebold. Ueber den melanotischen Hautausschlag der Cyprinoiden. Amtl. Ber. ü. d. Versamml. deutsch. Naturf. u. Aerzte, Königsb. (1860), 1861, xxxv, 138.— Tavignot. La mélanose est-elle un cancer ? Ann. d'ocul., Brux., 1853, xxix, 279 – 282. — Trousseau & Leblanc. De la mélanose. Arch. gén. de méd., Par., 1828, xvii, 165–188. — Verneuil. Du cancer mélanique. Mouvement méd., Par., 1876, xiv, 87.— White (J. C.) Melanosis lenticularis progressiva. Boston M. & S. J., 1885, cxiii, 645.

Melanosis *and melanotic tumors (Cases of).*

See, also, Arachnoid (*Diseases of*); Eye (*Tumors in*).

ALTMANN (A.) * Einige Fälle von Melanose. 8°. *Erlangen*, 1885.

Melanosis *and melanotic tumors* (*Cases of*).

ANGER (B.) & WORTHINGTON (L.-S.) Mélanomes. 8°. *Paris*, 1866.

FAWDINGTON (T.) A case of melanosis, with general observations on the pathology of this interesting disease. 8°. *London*, 1826.

MATTISSEN (J.) *Ein Fall von multiplem melanotischem Sarkom. 8°. *Bonn*, 1879.

NATORP (C. G.) *Diss. sistens historiam morbi de melanosi, cordis, hepatis totiusque telæ cellulosæ. 8°. *Berolini*, [1836].

TRÖLTSCH (E.) *Ein Fall von Cancer melanodes. [Erlangen.] 8°. *Augsburg*, 1857.

Albers (J.-F.-H.) Observations suivies de réflexions sur le fongus mélanode. J. compl. du dict. d. sc. méd., Par., 1831, xxxix, 354-373 [wrongly paged 338-373].— **Allen.** Melanoid tumours of many organs. Austral. M. J., Melbourne, 1880, n. s., ii, 507.—**Alonzo.** Enorme tumor melánico; operacion; muerte de la enferma. Siglo méd., Madrid, 1860, vii, 355.— **Arnott** (H.) Case of multiple melanotic tumours. Tr. Path. Soc. Lond., 1868-9, xx, 322-324.—**Aubert.** Mélanose de la rate, du foie et des reins; albuminurie et anasarque; état anémique très-avancé; mort. Mém. et compt.-rend. Soc. d. sc. méd. de Lyon (1865), 1866, v, 284-286.—**Béhier.** Diathèse mélanique. Arch. gén. de méd., Par., 1838, 3. s., iii, 286-293.— **Bennett.** Melanosis. Month. J. M. Sc., Lond. & Edinb., 1851, xiii, 189-193.—**de Beurmann.** Mélanose de la face; un traumatisme accidentel; deux interventions chirurgicales; trois récidives avec extension sur place. Bull. Soc. anat. de Par., 1875, 3. s., x, 739-742. *Also:* Progrès méd., Par., 1876, iv, 277. ———. Mélanose généralisée; tumeurs multiples du tissu cellulaire sous-cutané; disparition spontanée de deux de ces tumeurs. Bull. Soc. anat. de Par., 1875, 3. s., x, 742-747. *Also:* Progrès méd., Par., 1876, iv, 278.—**Birkett.** Secondary melanotic cancer of the lumbar glands and omentum; multiple melanotic cancer of the skin. Med. Times & Gaz., Lond., 1854, n. s., ix, 467. ———. Excision of a melanotic tumor from the thigh. *Ibid.*, 1860, ii, 455.—**Black.** Case of melanic cancer in the horse. Tr. Path. Soc. Lond., 1855-6, vii, 400.—**Blasius** (E.) Melanosis. Klin. Ztschr. f. Chir. u. Augenh., Halle, 1836-7, i, 145-159.—**Bonaccioli** (T.) Alcune annotazioni sopra casi di melanosi. Rendic. Accad. med.-chir. di Ferrara, 1853, 37-42.—**Bond** (R.) Melanosis. Tr. Coll. Phys. Phila. (1856-62), 1863, iii, 204-206.—**Bosi** (L.) Caso di melanosi vera diffusa. Rendic. Accad. med.-chir. di Ferrara, Bologna, 1843, 39-47.—**Breschet.** Considérations sur l'altération organique appelée mélanose. J. de physiol. expér., Par., 1821, i, 354-373.—**Broca.** Tumeur mélanique de la racine du nez. J. de méd. et chir. prat., Par., 1877, xlviii, 208.— **Bryant** (T.) Melanotic tumour developed in a mole; excision, and the secondary formation of melanotic tumours in the integuments and nearly every internal organ. Tr. Path. Soc. Lond., 1862-3, xiv, 246. *Also:* Lancet, Lond., 1863, ii, 37. *Also:* Med. Times & Gaz., Lond., 1863, i, 480.— **Bulkley** (L. D.) Case of multiple melano-sarcoma of the skin. Boston M. & S. J., 1880, cii, 218-220.—**Bullock.** Melanosis of the eye, liver, and mesentery. Tr. Path. Soc. Lond., 1853-4, v, 330.—**Casamayor** (J.-A.-L.) Tubercules mélanés; foie du poids de vingt-quatres livres. J. hebd. de méd., Par., 1830, vii, 213-220.—**Cases** of melanosis. Med. Times & Gaz., Lond., 1853, n. s., vi, 523.— **Cattermole** (J.) Case of idiopathic tuberiform melanosis. Canada Lancet, Toronto, 1876-7, ix, 69-71.—**Chomel.** Mélanose du foie, du poumon et du tissu cellulaire de l'orbite droite, compliquée de quelques autres lésions organiques. N. Jour. de méd., chir., pharm., etc., Par., 1818, iii, 41-45.—**Clark** (A.) Disseminated melanosis of the heart, lungs, liver, kidneys, and bones secondary to melanosis of the eye. Tr. Path. Soc. Lond., 1871-2, xxiii, 251-254.—**Clendinning.** Cast and drawing of tubercular melanosis which had pervaded the whole frame. *Ibid.*, 1846-8, i, 42.—**Coats** (J.) On a case of multiple melanotic sarcoma, with remarks on the mode of growth and extension of such tumours. Glasgow M. J., 1885, [4.] s., xxiv, 92-97.—**Collis** (M. H.) Case of melanosis. Dublin Q. J. M. Sc., 1863, xxxv, 241-246.—**Coote** (H.) Instances of melanosis. Lancet, Lond., 1846, ii, 122; 142.—**Crampton** (J.) Case of melanosis. Dublin M. Tr., 1830, n. s., i, 23-28.—**Crucknell** (H. H.) Melanoid disease of liver and supra-renal capsules. Tr. Path. Soc. Lond., 1863-4, xv, 249.—**Davies** (H.) Melanosis of the eye, liver, kidney, and ovaries. *Ibid.*, 1848-9, ii, 128-130.—**De Morgan.** Melanotic sarcoma of femoral glands, secondary to tumour over the heel; sarcomata in spleen and iliac glands. Lancet, Lond., 1875, ii, 449.—**De Saussure** (H. W.) Case of melanosis. South. J. M. & Pharm., Charleston, 1846, i, 129-136.—**Drivon** (J.) Quelques remarques sur la mélanose à propos d'un cas de mélanose généralisée. Mém. et compt.-rend. Soc. d. sc. méd. de Lyon (1868), 1869, viii, 17; 143.—**Duplay.** Mélanose; tumeurs mélaniques

Melanosis *and melanotic tumors* (*Cases of*).

et leur généralisation. France méd., Par., 1876, xxiii, 109.— **Falls** (W. H.) A case of melanosis. Cincin. Lancet & Clinic, 1882, n. s., ix, 479-488, 3 pl.—**Fano.** Mélanose et tumeur mélanique de la conjonctive. Gaz. d. hôp., Par., 1872, xlv, 651. — **Fayrer** (J.) Melanosis. Indian Ann. M. Sc., Calcutta, 1864-5, ix. no. 18, 103-106. — **Ferber** (R. H.) Fall von melanotischem Krebse, mit zahlreichen Ablagerungen in fast allen Organen und Vergrösserung der Nebennieren. Arch. d. Heilk., Leipz., 1863, iv, 565-569. — **Ferguson** (G.-B.) Ablation d'un sarcôme mélanique développé dans la gaine du muscle couturier. France méd., Par., 1876, xxiii, 165.—**Fergusson** (W.) Melanotic tumors in different parts of the trunk. Lancet, Lond., 1852, ii, 176. ———. Melanotic cancer recurring after several operations; curious change in colour of the hair. Med. Times & Gaz., Lond., 1855, n. s., xi, 468. ———. Melanosis recurring in the scar of a previous operation; no signs of constitutional affection. Assoc. M. J., Lond., 1857, ii, 919. ———. Melanosis of the groin. Lancet, Lond., 1857, i, 62. ———. Melanotic tumours of the groin, excised, in a man aged thirty-six, who had a similar growth removed from the great toe five years ago, with recurrence; recovery. *Ibid.*, 1857, i, 289. ———. Melanotic tumour of the left arm, growing from the cicatrix of a mole eradicated by caustics. *Ibid.*, 1861, i, 262. ———. Melanotic deposit in an ulcer inside the lip; extirpation. *Ibid.*, 1862, ii, 617.—**Folet** (H.) Note sur un cas de mélanose généralisée. Bull. méd. du nord, Lille, 1870-71, 2. s., xi, 161-177.— **Folsom** (N. L.) Case of melanosis; false membrane passed per anum. Boston M. & S. J., 1856-7, lv, 203-205. — **Forster** (C.) Melanosis of the toes; partial amputation of the foot by Chopart's operation. Lancet, Lond., 1862, ii, 617.—**Gaillard.** Melanosis of the inguinal glands. South. J. M. & Pharm., Charleston, 1847, ii, 35.—**Gairdner.** Melanotic cancer. Glasgow M. J., 1875, [4. s.], vii, 410-412.—**Gallwey** (M. B.) Two cases of unusual discharge of carbonaceous matter from the nares and intestines. Lancet, Lond., 1859, ii, 387. ———. Discharge of carbonaceous matter from the nares, etc. *Ibid.*, 1860, i, 635.—**Gherini** (A.) †† Gazz. med. ital. lomb., Milano, 1854, 3. s., v, 188-190.—**Gillette.** Plusieurs cas de sarcome mélanique. Union méd., Par., 1874, 3. s., xviii, 625-630.—**Gillkrest.** Extraordinary case of melanosis of the skin in a woman in whom the greater part of the surface became of a dark color. Lond. M. Gaz., 1839, xxiv, 721-723. *Also, transl.:* Bull. Acad. de méd., Par., 1839-40, iv, 493.—**Griscom.** Melanotic tumors of various thoracic and abdominal viscera without external signs of melanosis. Tr. Coll. Phys. Phila. (1856-62), 1863, n. s., iii, 156-158.—**Gross** (S. W.) Case of universal melanosis. Proc. Path. Soc. Phila. (1857-60), 1860, i, 286 ———. Melanosis of the skin and areolar tissue. *Ibid.* (1866-70), 1871, iii, 121. *Also:* Am. J. M. Sc., Phila., 1870, n. s., lix, 121.—**Halliday** (A.) Case of melanosis. Lond. M. R. posit., 1823, xix, 441-443. ———. Case of melanosis. *Ibid.*, xx, 197-204, 1 pl.—**Hayne** (A. P.) Case of scirrho-melanotic tumour of the ovaries, accompanied with melanotic degeneration of several internal organs. Charleston M. J., 1848, iii, 141-151, pl.—**Heath** (C.) Melanosis of the skin of the arm and of an axillary gland; with microscopical examination of the tumour by Mr. Bruce. Tr. Path. Soc. Lond., 1867-8, xix, 365-367.—**Hebb** (R. G.) Melanotic sarcoma. *Ibid.*, 1884-5, xxxvi, 413.—**Hénoque.** Mélanose ganglionnaire. Bull. Soc. anat. de Par., 1868, xliii, 233-236.—**Heurtaux.** Organes provenant d'un homme mort de sarcome mélanique; mélanose de divers organes. J. de méd. de l'ouest, Nantes, 1884, 2. s., viii, 121-123— **Hewett** (P.) Melanosis affecting both groins, as well as other parts of the body; recurrence after removal six years ago; removal a second time. Lancet, Lond., 1856, i, 657. ———, Sequel to a case of recurrent melanosis of both groins and back; the disease reappearing in the brain, heart, pancreas, liver, and other organs. *Ibid.*, 1861 i, 263.—**Hodges.** Melanosis. Boston M. & S. J., 186 , lxiv, 92.—**Hollister.** Melanotic cancer on the arm; metastasis to the liver; autopsy. Chicago M. J. & Exam., 1875, xxxii, 905.—**Hughes** (J. W.) Case of melanosis, with brief history. Tr. M. Soc. Penn., Phila., 1871, 6. s., ii, 337.—**Hutchinson.** Melanotic disease of the great toe, following a whitlow of the nail. Tr. Path. Soc. Lond., 1856-7, viii, 404.—**Jackson** (J. B. S.) Case of melanosis. Am. J. M. Sc., Phila., 1848, n. s., xv, 379-382.—**King** (J. S.) Melanotic cancer. Canada Lancet, 1873-4, vi, 331-333. — **Kirkley** (C. A.) Diffused melanosis. Ohio M. Recorder, Columbus, 1876-7, i, 163-165.— **Kleybolte.** Fall von Melanosis tuberosa. Wchnschr. f. d. ges. Heilk., Berl., 1846, 318-323. — **Knipfer.** Tuberkulöse und melanotische Degeneration. Med. Ztg., Berl., 1854, xxiii, 181.—**Knoblauch** (J. G. A.) † Jahresb. ü. d. Verwalt. d. Med.-Wes., d. Krankenanst. . . . d. Stadt Frankf. (1864), 1867, viii, 104-106.—**Küchler** (H.) Melanose fast des ganzen rechten Unterkiefers; Ausrottung derselben; histologische Untersuchung der Geschwulst; Tod. Deutsche Klinik, Berl., 1861, xiii, 366.—**Kürner.** Relation über eine acute Dyscrasia melanodes nebst Encephaloma.

Melanosis *and melanotic tumors* (*Cases of*).

lacie. Med. Cor.-Bl. d. württemb. ärztl. Ver., Stuttg., 1856, xxvi, 185 ; 193.—**Laboulbène** (A.) Diathèse cancéreuse mélanique. Compt. rend. Soc. de biol. 1854, Par., 1855, 2. s., i, 32-36.—**Lancereaux.** Tumeur pigmentaire et épithéliale de la région malaire ; deux ganglions correspondants atteints de mélanose. *Ibid.* 1860, Par., 1861, 3. s., ii, 19-21.—**Lancereaux & Dubreuil.** Tumeurs mélaniques multiples ; mélanose ayant envahi la plupart du système organique. *Ibid.*, 111-116.— **Landrieux.** Mélanose généralisée ; autopsie. Bull. Soc. anat. de Par., 1867, xlii, 497-509.—**Lawrence.** Subcutaneous melanosis scattered over the trunk and extremities ; the tuberculated sarcoma of Mr. Abernethy. Lancet, Lond., 1864, i, 183 ; 382. *Also :* Med. Times & Gaz., Lond., 1864, i, 225. — **Lazarevich** (I. P.) † Med. Vestnik, St. Petersb., 1876, xvi, 1-4.—**Lobstein** (J. F.) Observation sur des mélanoses disséminées en très grand nombre dans beaucoup de parties du corps et notamment dans la peau. Répert. gén. d'anat. et physiol. path., Par., 1829, vii, 48-51. 2 pl.—**Lücke** (A.) Melanotisches Carcinom der Wange, in die Vene hineingewuchert ; Exstirpation ; Heilung. Berl. klin. Wchnschr., 1868, v, 341. ———. Melanoma [10 cases]. Deutsche Ztschr. f. Chir., Leipz., 1872-3, ii, 242-246.—**M'Clintock.** Melanosis of peritoneum. Dublin Hosp. Gaz., 1856, n. s., iii, 90.—**Markoe** (F. M.) Case of false melanosis. N. York J. M., 1850, n. s. [2.], iv, 332. — **Maupin.** Tumeurs mélaniques ; réflexions sur la mélanose cutanée et sous-cutanée. Rec. de mém. de méd . . . mil., Par., 1859, 3. s., i, 340-349.—**Monneret.** Mélanose des deux poumons, du péritoine, de l'épiploon, du tissu cellulaire sous-péritonéal, des ganglions mésentériques, de l'intestin grêle. Union méd., Par., 1863, n. s., xx, 418-425.—**von Mosengeil** (K.) Ein Fall von verhältnissmässig gutartigem Melanom. Arch. f. klin. Chir., Berl., 1870, xi, 734.—**Nepveu** (J.) Contribution à l'étude des tumeurs mélaniques. Gaz. méd. de Par., 1872, 4. s., i, 335 ; 384. *Also :* Compt. rend. Soc. de biol. 1872, Par., 1874, 5. s., iv, pt. 2, 3-16.—**Norris** (W.) A case of fungoid tumor, succeeded by melanosis. Tr. Prov. M. & S. Ass., Lond., 1835-6, iv, 437-446. ———. Eight cases of melanosis. Midland Q. J. M. Sc., Birmingh., 1857, i, 229-239. ———. Cases of melanosis. St. Andrew's M. Grad. Ass. Tr. 1869, Lond., 1870, iii, 153-161.—**O'Grady** (E. S.) Removal of a melanotic tumour from the left suprascapular region ; recovery. Dublin J. M. Sc., 1875, lx, 39, 2 pl.—**Ozenne.** Mélano-sarcome du pied ; généralisation ; tumeur cérébrale de même nature ; aphasie ; mort. France méd., Par., 1880, xxvii, 233. *Also :* Progrès méd., Par., 1880, viii, 804-806. *Also :* Bull. Soc. clin. de Par. (1880), 1881, iv, 45-50.—**Pamard.** Observations propres à démontrer la nature non cancéreuse des mélanoses. Rev. méd.-chir. de Par., 1852, xii, 334-339.—**Parrish** (I.) Case of melanosis. Am. J. M. Sc., Phila., 1837, xx, 266-268.—**Payne** (J. F.) Melanotic sarcoma occurring in the liver, lungs, and other parts. Tr. Path. Soc. Lond., 1872-3, xxiv, 134-136. — **Petel.** Mélanose généralisée ayant pour origine une tache mélanique congénitale de la joue gauche. Bull. Soc. anat. de Par., 1875, 3. s., x, 833. *Also :* Progrès méd., Par., 1876, iv, 419.— **Petit.** Mélanose affectant à la fois les poumons, les ganglions bronchiques, l'épiploon, le foie, la rate, le pancréas, la capsule surrénale gauche, le rein droit, le tissu cellulaire sous-muqueux de l'intestin grêle, le sous-cutané de l'aisselle et celui des parois de la poitrine du côté gauche. J. hebd. de méd., Par., 1829, ii, 122-124.— **Peulevé.** Mélanose généralisée. Examen microscopique par Cornil. Bull. Soc. anat. de Par., 1865, xl, 341-355.— **Poisson.** Mélanose généralisée. *Ibid.*, 1876, 4. s., i, 108-111. *Also :* Progrès méd., Par., 1876, iv, 399.— **Porter.** True melanosis. Tr. M. Soc. County Albany (1851-70), 1872, ii, 77-80.—**Richet** (C.) Sarcome mélanique ; généralisation. Bull. Soc. anat. de Par., 1873, 5. s., vii, 136.—**Rindfleisch.** Ueber einen Fall von Melanose. Sitzungsb. d. phys.-med. Gesellsch. zu Würzb., 1885, 125-127.—**Robin.** Tumeur cancéreuse mélanotique de la peau. Compt. rend. Soc. de biol. 1849, Par., 1850, i, 91.—**Rollet.** Fall von Melanosis tuberosa. Wien. med. Presse, 1865, vi, 19.—**Rothacker** (W. A.) & **Thompson** (J. A.) A case of melano-sarcoma. Med. News, Phila., 1885, xlvii, 262-265.—**Sanderson.** Melanotic cancer in various organs. Tr. Path. Soc. Lond., 1854-5, vi, 324-328.—**Sava** (R.) Sopra una singolarissima congenita melanosia. Filiatre-sebezio, Napoli, 1843, xxvi, 193-196.—**Scott** (W. E.) Case of melanotic cancer. Canada M. J., Montreal, 1865, i, 224-227.—**Seiler** (C.) A case of general melanosis. Tr. Path. Soc. Phila. (1883-5), 1886, xii, 276-278.—**Spry** (E. J.) History of a case illustrative of specimens of punctiform and tubercular melanosis. Prov. M. & S. J., Lond., 1847, 599. — **Stokes.** Case of melanotic cancer. Irish Hosp. Gaz., Dubl., 1874, ii, 341-343. —**Tennent** (G. P.) On a case of multiple melanotic sarcoma. Glasgow M. J., 1885, [4.] s., xxiv, 81-91, 2 phot.—**Terrillon.** Mélanose généralisée ayant débuté par une petite lèvre de la vulve. Ann. de gynéc., Par., 1886, xxvi, 1-8.— **Thompson** (H.) Subcutaneous malignant tumours containing melanotic matter. Tr. Path. Soc. Lond., 858-9, x, 257. ———.

Melanosis *and melanotic tumors* (*Cases of*).

Melanoid cancer, developed in a common dark mole containing pigment. *Ibid.*, 1860-61, xii, 206.—**Thompson** (M. D.) Melanosis. Lancet, Lond., 1842, ii, 573-575.— **Thompson** (W.) Cases of melanosis. *Ibid.*, 1833, ii, 422.—**Tripier** (L.) Rapport sur un cas de mélanose généralisée. Mém. et compt.-rend. Soc. d. sc. méd. de Lyon (1868), 1869, viii, 143-151.—**Velpeau.** Mélanose développée spécialement dans deux ganglions lymphatiques de la tête. Gaz. d. hôp., Par., 1861, xxxiv, 273.— **Wagner** (E.) Fall von Combination eines Pigmentkrebses mit einer reinen Pigmentgeschwulst. Arch. d. Heilk., Leipz., 1864, v, 280-284.—**Wheeler.** Melanotic carcinoma of thigh. Dublin J. M. Sc., 1880, 3. s., lxx, 160.—**Wilks** (S.) Melanotic tumours of leg. Guy's Hosp. Rep., Lond., 1862, 3. s., viii, 267.—**Williams** (C. J. B.) Melanotic cancer in the spinal canal, orbit, etc. Tr. Path. Soc. Lond., 1846-8, i, 42-44.—**Williams** (D.) Case of melanosis. Tr. Prov. M. & S. Ass., Lond., 1832-3. i, 244-257, 1 pl.—**Wormald.** Melanosis of the skin of the back ; excision ; recovery. Med. Times & Gaz., Lond., 1853, n. s., vi, 553.—**Zeller** (J. A.) Beobachtung eines Morbi nigri. N. Mag. f. Aerzte, Leipz., 1781, iii, 251-255.

Melanthon (Philippus). *See* **Melanchthon** (Philippus).

Melanuria.

See **Urine** (*Coloring matter, etc., of*).

Melardi (Salvatore). * Paralisi ed ipercinesia del nervo faciale. Effeto terapeutico dello stiramento del 7° paio nel tic convulsivo. 89 pp., 1 l., 1 pl. 8°. *Messina,* 1885.

Melart (Carolus Christianus). * De tempore exhibendi emetica in febribus intermittentibus maxime opportuno. 38 pp. sm. 4°. *Gottingæ, J. C. Dieterich,* [1782].

Melasma.

See **Addison's** *disease* ; **Skin** (*Discolorations, etc., of*).

Melays (Marie - Louis). * I. Des rapports qui existent entre la pathologie et l'anatomie pathologique. II. [etc.] 23 pp. 4°. *Paris,* 1840, No. 377, v. 363.

Melber (Georg. Carol. Frid.) [1816 – 73]. * De medulla spinalis erethismo. [Heidelberg.] 80 pp. 8°. *Francof. a. M., typ. Andreæ,* 1838.

Melber (Joannes David.) [1773 – 1824]. * De febre putrida, ex principiis Brunonianis explicata. 48 pp. 8°. *Jenæ, lit. Maukianis,* [1794]. *For Biography, see* **Gruner** (Christ. Goth.)

Melbourne.

See, also, **Children** (*Hospitals, etc., for, Reports, etc., of*) ; **Education** (*Medical*), *etc.,* **Fever** (*Typhoid, History, etc., of*), **Hospitals** (*Descriptions, etc., of*), **Hospitals** (*Management, rules, etc., of*), **Hospitals** (*Maternity, etc.*), *by localities* ; **Inebriates,** *etc.,* (*Asylums for*) ; **Insane** (*Asylums for*).

GIBBONS (S.) Air and water poisoning in Melbourne. 8°. [*Melbourne,* 1869.]
Also [Abstr.], *in :* Austral. M. Gaz., Melbourne, 1869, i, 259.

MELBOURNE International Exhibition, 1880. Opened Oct. 1, 1880. The official catalogue of exhibits, with introductory notices of countries exhibiting. 2. ed. 2 v. 8°. *Melbourne,* 1881.

NEUMAYER (G.) Results of the magnetical, nautical, and meteorological observations made and collected at the "Flagstaff Observatory", Melbourne, and at various stations in the colony of Victoria, March, 1858, to February, 1859. fol. *Melbourne,* [1860].

———. Discussion of the meteorological and magnetical observations made at the "Flagstaff Observatory", Melbourne, during the years 1858-63. 4°. *Mannheim,* 1867.

VICTORIA. Return for the month of November, 1879, showing the estimated population, the number of registered births and deaths of persons, males and females, in the statistical district of Melbourne. fol. [*Melbourne,* 1879.]

Melbourne.

――――. Monthly record of results of observations in meteorology, terrestrial magnetism, etc., taken at the Melbourne Observatory; together with abstracts from meteorological observations obtained at various localities in Victoria. Under the superintendence of R. L. J. Ellery, government astronomer. Jan. to Sept., Nov. and Dec., 1879; March to June, Sept., 1880. 8°. *Melbourne*, 1879–80.

Culcheth (W. W.) The drainage of Melbourne. Tr. & Proc. Roy. Soc. Victoria 1881, Melbourne, 1882, xviii, 60–71.—"**Night-soil**" (The) and "sewage" question in Melbourne. Med. Times & Gaz., Lond., 1872, i, 107.—**Our** sanitary condition. Austral. M. J., Melbourne, 1861, vi, 120–129.—**Robertson** (J.) Vital statistics of the Benevolent Asylum, Melbourne, more particularly in relation to phthisis. *Ibid.*, 203–210.

Melbourne Hospital. Rules. 20 pp. 8°. *Melbourne, Stillwell & Knight*, [1863].

――――. Annual reports of the committee of management to the contributors. 24.–26. (1871–3). 8°. *Melbourne*, 1872–4.

Founded 1846.

Melbourne Lying-In Hospital and Infirmary for Diseases of Women and Children. Annual report of the committee of management to the subscribers. 15., 1871. 23 pp. 8°. *Melbourne, Stillwell & Knight*, 1872.

Melbourne Medical Record. [Weekly.] v. 4–7, Feb. 27, 1875, to Nov. 7, 1877. 4 v. 4°. *Melbourne, R. T. Clarke*.

Ended. Title of v. 1–3. 1861–3, was: **Medical** (The) Record of Australia. In Oct., 1875, became semimonthly. No. 5, v. 7, last published.

Melbourne Observatory. *See* **Victoria**.

Melbourne Retreat for the Cure of Inebriates. Report of the sub-committee on the inebriate question. 36 pp. 12°. *Melbourne, Stillwell & Knight*, 1872.

――――. Annual reports of the committee of management to the subscribers. 1., 1871–3; 2., 1873. 8°. *Melbourne*, 1873–4.

Melcher (Richard). * Ueber Wasserausscheidung durch Lungen und Haut beim normalen und fiebernden Thiere. 30 pp., 1 l. 8°. *Königsberg i. Pr., R. Leupold*, 1883.

Melchert (Hermann). * Beitrag zur Diagnose der subacuten Poliomyelitis und multiplen degenerativen Neuritis. 30 pp., 1 l. 8°. *Greifswald, C. Sell*, 1881.

Melchin (Joh.)

See **Hoffmann** (Christianus). Problema physicum [etc.] Respondente Joh. Melchin. 4°. [n. p.], 1671.

Melchior (Christoph). * Geschichte der Forschungen über den Geburtsmechanismus während des Anfangs des elften Lustrums des achtzehnten Jahrhunderts. 51 pp., 2 l. 8°. *Giessen, G. D. Brühl*, 1857. c.

See, also, **Geschichte** der Forschungen, etc. 8°. Giessen, 1857–9. — **Schrey** (Caspar Heinrich). Thermarum contenta, etc. 12°. *Leipzig*, 1696.

Melchior (Joannes Henricus). * De scirrho tam interno quam externo. 48 pp., 2 l. 4°. *Lugd. Bat., C. Wishoff*, [1729].

Melchior (Nathan Gerson) [1811 – 72]. * De strabismo. Respondente Sally Simon Neukirch. 1 p. l., 75 pp. 8°. *Havniæ, S. Frier*, 1839.

――――. De myotomia oculi. Resp. Ludovico Reumert. 3 p. l., 93 pp. 8°. *Havniæ, ex off. Frieri*, 1841.

Melchior (Paulus). * De morbo castrensi. 50 pp. 4°. *Gissæ Hassorum, typ. F. Kargeri*, 1675.

Melchior (Petrus Jacobus). * De panaritio. 26 pp. 8°. *Duisburgi, typ. vid. Benthonianæ*, [1789].

Melchior (Richardus). * De elongatione uteri. 18 pp. 8°. *Jenæ, typ. Schreiberi et fil.*, [1857]. [P., v. 401.]

Melchior (Robertus). * De structura glandulæ thymus microscopica ejusque degenerationibus. 20 pp., 1 pl. 8°. *Jenæ, typ. Ratii*, 1859.

Melchiori (Giovanni) Di alcune lesioni traumatiche della colonna vertebrale; osservazioni pubblicate nella Gazzetta medica italiana federativa, Stati Sardi. 19 pp. 12°. *Genova, Ferrando*, [1850]. [P., v. 1409.]

Repr. from: Gazz. med. ital. federativa, Stati Sardi, 2. semestre, 1850.

――――. Incrostazione calcare della vaginale del testicolo; tumore fibro-plastico dell' albuginea; fungo del testicolo arrestato nel canale inguinale; strappamento d' ambedue i testicoli operatosi da un pazzo. 10 pp. 8°. [*Milano*, 1852.] [P., v. 1409.]

Repr. from: Gazz. med. ital. lomb., Milano, 1852, 3. s., iii.

――――. Caso di estirpazione di tumore sottopubico assieme a tutta l' uretra in una donna. Lettera al dottor Agostino Bertani. 11 pp. 8°. *Milano, G. Chiusi*, 1854. [P., v. 1409.]

Repr. from: Gazz. med. ital. lomb., Milano, 1854, 3. s., v.

――――. Ritenzione del sangue mestruo per atresia della vagina. Lettera al dottore Agostino Bertani. 15 pp. 8°. *Milano, G. Chiusi*, 1855. [P., v. 1409.]

Repr. from: Gazz. med. ital. lomb., Milano, 1855, 3. s., vi.

――――. Rassegna dei casi più importanti di chirurgia osservati nel civico spedale di S. Giacomo di Novi. 62 pp. 8°. *Genova, tip. del R. I. de' sordo-muti*, [1856]. [P., v. 1409.]

Repr. from: Liguria med., Genova, 1856, i.

――――. Del volvolo dell' S iliaca. 30 pp. 8°. *Milano*, 1859. [P., v. 1409.]

Repr. from: Ann. univ. di med., Milano, 1859, clxx.

――――. Induramento infiammatorio del muscolo sterno-cleido-mastoideo nei neonati. 11 pp. 8°. *Torino, G. Biancardi*, 1861. [P., v. 1409.]

Repr. from: Gazz. med. ital., Prov. Sarde.

――――. Sulla insalubrità delle filature da seta. Memoria premiata dal governo con voto della R. Accademica medico-chirurgica di Torino nella seduta del 17 maggio 1859. 60 pp. 8°. *Milano*, 1861. [P., v. 1409.]

Repr. from: Ann. univ. di med., Milano, 1861, clxxv.

――――. Rovesciamento incompleto dell' utero in seguita a parto ridotto da una successiva gravidanza. 11 pp. 8°. [*Milano*, 1862.] [P., v. 1409.]

Repr. from: Ann. univ. di med., Milano, 1862, clxxx.

――――. Efficacia anafrodisiaca del bromuro di potassio. Lettera al dottore Angelo Scarenzio. 7 pp. 8°. [*Milano*, 1863.] [P., v. 1409.]

Repr. from: Ann. univ. di med., Milano, 1863, clxxxiii.

――――. Della fessura all' ano e più particolarmente della sua eziologia. 21 pp. 8°. *Milano*, 1864. [P., v. 1409.]

Repr. from: Ann. univ. di med., Milano, 1864, clxxxvii.

――――. Memoria sopra una varietà rara e poco conosciuta di ernia inguinale a sacco intravaginale o a doppio sacco; ernia saccata della tonaca vaginale di A. Cooper; del dottore Bourguet d'Aix. (Gaz. hebd. de méd. et de chir., No. 44 e seg., 1844.) Annalisi bibliografica con aggiunta di casi clinici. 24 pp. 8°. [*Milano*, 1865.] [P., v. 1409.]

Repr. from: Ann. univ. di med., Milano, 1865, clxxxxi.

――――. Dell' idrocele della tonaca vaginale, sue varietà, e di altri tumori acquosi del testicolo e del cordone spermatico. Note cliniche. 110 pp. 8°. *Milano*, 1866. [P., v. 1409.]

Repr. from: Ann. univ. di med., Milano, 1866, clxxxxvi.

――――. Caso di amputazione sopracondiloidea del femore col metodo del Dott. Rocco Gritti, cioè con lembo patellare, per ferita da arma da fuoco; preceduto da altri due, in cui fu conservata la

Melchiori (Giovanni)—continued.
rotella, disarticolando il ginocchio ed amputando ai condili femorali. 13 pp. 8°. *Milano*, 1867. [P., v. 417 ; 1409.]
Repr. from: Ann. univ. di med., Milano, 1867, cc.

———. Ferita da arma da fuoco alla regione del toidea del braccio con frattura dell'omero. Disarticolazione scapulo-omerale. 6 pp. 8°. [*Milano*, 1867.]
Repr. from: Ann. univ. di med., Milano, 1867, cc.

———. Delle ferite cagionate dallo scoppio di armi da fuoco. Note cliniche. 61 pp. 8°. *Milano*, 1868. [P., v. 1409.]

———. Del cancro periuretrale nella donna, con processo operativo. 31 pp. 8°. *Milano*, 1869.

———. Dell' emorragia e dell' ematocele da pun tura dell' idrocele della tonaca vaginale nelle aberrazione del testicolo e del cordone spermatico. 54 pp. 8°. *Milano*, 1870. [P., v. 322.]
For Biography, see Ann. univ. di med. e chir., Milano, 1880, ccli, 541-543. *Also:* Gazz. med. ital. lomb., Milano, 1880, 8. s., ii, 99-101 (L. De Maria).

Melchisedech (Joannes) [1837–   ]. * De emphysemate pulmonum. 32 pp. 8°. *Berolini, G. Lange,* [1863].

Melcion (Charles-Élophe). * Sur les fièvres intermittentes pernicieuses. 23 pp. 4°. *Paris*, 1835, No. 134, v. 286.

Melcion (Gustave-Émile). * De quelques complications peu connues de la scarlatine. 1 p. l., 31 pp. 4°. *Nancy*, 1878, 1. s., No. 54.

Melcion (J.-F.-J.) * Considérations sur les luxations en général. 1 p. l., 32 pp. 4°. *Strasbourg*, 1835, v. 67.

Melcombe-Regis.

CLARK (G. T.) Report to the General Board of Health, on a preliminary inquiry into the sewerage, drainage, and supply of water, and the sanitary condition of the inhabitants of the parish of Melcombe-Regis, in the county of Dorset. 8°. *London*, 1849.

———. The same. On a further inquiry as to the boundaries which may be most advantageously adopted for the borough of Melcombe-Regis and Weymouth, in the county of Dorset. 8°. *London*, 1851.

Melcop (Friedrich). * Ueber die diagnostische Verwerthbarkeit localer Temperaturen bei Erkrankungen der Brustorgane. 36 pp. 8°. *Göttingen, W. F. Kästner*, 1880.   c.

Melczer (Joannes). * De pyrola umbellata. 27 pp. 8°. *Pestini, J. Patzko,* [1829], No. 12. [*Also, in :* P., v. 1317.]

Meldon (Austin) [1843–   ]. A treatise on diseases of the skin and its appendages. 8°. *London, Longmans [and others]*, 1872.

———. A treatise on gout, rheumatism, and rheumatic gout. xi, 9-146 pp. 8°. *London, Longmans [and others]*, 1872.

———. The same. 10. ed. xii, 206 pp. 12°. *London, Baillière, Tindall & Cox*, 1886.

Melendez (Antonio). Cólera, su preservacion. 45 pp. 8°. *Madrid, A. Santa Coloma*, 1855.

Melendez (Lucio) & **Coni** (Emilio R.) Consideraciones sobre la estadística de la enagenacion mental en la provincia de Buenos Aires. 38 pp., 3 pl. 8°. *Buenos Aires, P. E. Coni*, 1880.

Melenfeld (J.) * O peptonach volokniny. [Peptonized albuminous bodies.] 27 pp. 8°. *St. Petersburg, J. Treja*, 1872.

Meletius. De natura structuraque hominis opus Polemonis Atheniensis insignis philosophi naturæ signorum interpretationis. Hippocratis de hominis structura. Dioclis ad Antigonem regem de tuenda valetudine epistola. Melampi de nevis corporis tractatus. Omnia hæc non prius edita, Nicolao Petreio Corcyræo interprete. 4 p. l., 191 pp., 17 l. sm. 4°. *Venetiis, ex off. Gryphii*, 1552.

Meletius—continued.
———. The same. Περὶ τῆς τοῦ ἀνθρώπου κατασκευῆς. Tractatus de natura hominis. pp. 1075-1326. fol. [*Rostock*, 1833?]
Greek and Latin text.
Cutting from: Patrol. Gr., lxiv.

Meleux (Augustin-M.-A.) * Des ovaires, de l'utérus, ou quelques considérations anatomiques et physiologiques sur ces organes. 43 pp. 4°. *Paris*, 1860, No. 233.

Melhorn (Bernhardus Fridericus Henricus).
See **Hagen** (Carolus Godofredus). *Stannum*. Pars secunda. 4°. *Regiomonti*, 1776.

Meli (Domenico). Su la condizione patologica delle febbri biliose. Nuovi fatti esposti. 53 pp. 8°. *Milano*, 1824. [P., v. 1350.]

———. Lettere polemiche su l' abuso del salasso e sopra dell' eccezioni fatte al tentativo di conciliare i medici italiani. v. 1. 402 pp., 2 l. 8°. *Pesaro, A. Nobili*, 1827.

———. Risultamenti degli studii fatti a Parigi sul cholera-morbus per ordine di sua santità Papa Gregorio XVI, 1832. xv, 320 pp., 2 pl. 8°. *Roma, stamperia camerale*, 1833.

———. Trattato delle febbri biliose ; nuova edizione, corretta ed arricchita di molte giunte dall' autore ; con un discorso preliminare e varie note del dottore N. M. Sormani. 240 pp., port. 4°. *Milano*, 1837.
See, also, **Soardi** & **Meli** (D.) Analisi medica delle acque minerali di Trescore [etc.] 8°. *Milano*, 1812.

Méli (H.) Du choléra asiatique dans la ville de Marseille en 1849. Rapport fait à la Société nationale de médecine de Marseille. 86 pp. 8°. *Marseille, P. Chauffard*, 1850. [P., v. 461.]

Mélian (O.) * Recherches sur le bacille tuberculeux, surtout au point de vue de sa valeur diagnostique et pronostique dans la phtisie pulmonaire. 49 pp., 1 pl. 4°. *Montpellier*, 1884, No. 73.

Melianah.

See **Medicine** (*Military, History of*)—*Campaigns, etc.*

Melicerta.

Joliet (L.) Développement de l'œuf des mélicertes. Compt. rend. Acad. d. sc., Par., 1881, xciii, 856-858.

Melichar (Joannes). * De dulcamara. 29 pp., 1 l. 8°. *Pragæ, J. Spurny*, 1840.

Melicher (Ludwig Joseph) [1816-71]. * Tractatus de apoplexia. x, 11-212 pp. 8°. *Vindobonæ, C. Ueberreiter*, 1840.

———. Die angebornen Verrenkungen. xiv, 220 pp., 2 pl. 8°. *Wien, C. Gerold*, 1845. [P., v. 879.]

———. Die Wendungs-Krücke und deren Anwendung bei den tiefen Schulterlagen mit vorgefallenem Arme des Kindes. 1 p. l., x, 16-70 pp., 1 l., 1 pl. 8°. *Wien, C. Ueberreuter*, 1846.

———. Erster Bericht über das Institut für schwedische Heilgymnastik und Orthopädie zu Wien, Alservorstadt, No. 59. 44 pp. 4°. *Wien, J. B. Wallishausser*, 1853.

Melichio (Giorgio). Avertimenti nelle compositioni de' medicamenti per uso della spetiaria. Con una diligente esaminatione di molti simplici, tratta da più degni autori antichi et moderni. 15 p. l., 253 pp., 1 l. 4°. *Venetia*, 1575.

———. The same. Aggiuntovi un trattato delle mirabili virtù della theriaca, dell . . . signor Ofatio Guarguanti. 15 p. l., 200 ff. sm. 4°. *Venetia*, 1605.
See, also, **Sgobbis** (Antonio). Universale theatro farmaceutico, etc. fol. *Venetia*, 1682.

Mélier (François) [1798-1866]. * Essai sur le diagnostic médical. 42 pp. 4°. *Paris*, 1823, No. 32. [P., v. 178.]

Mélier (François)—continued.

——. Mémoire et observations sur quelques maladies de l'appendice cœcal. 30 pp. 8°. [*Paris, Crapelet*, 1827.] [*Also, in:* P., v. 1398.]
Repr. from: J. gén. de méd., chir. et pharm., Par., 1827, c.

——. Études sur les subsistances envisagées dans leurs rapports avec les maladies et la mortalité. 5–40 pp. 4°. *Paris, J.-B. Baillière*, 1842.
Repr. from: Mém. Acad. de méd., Par., 1841-3, x.

——. Des affections intermittentes à courte période. 24 pp. 4°. [*Paris*, 1842.]

——. Expériences et observations sur les propriétés toxiques du sulfate de quinine. Mémoire lu à l'Académie royale de médecine. 28 pp. 4°. *Paris, J.-B. Baillière*, 1843.

——. Ouverture du lazaret de Ratoneau. 16 pp. 8°. *Marseille, Barlatier-Feissat & Demonchy*, 1850. [P., v. 468.]
Repr. from: Moniteur universel.

——. Relation de la fièvre janne survenue à Saint-Nazaire en 1861. Lue à l'Académie impériale de médecine dans les séances des 7, 14, 21, et 28 avril 1863. Suivie d'une réponse aux discours prononcés dans le cours de la discussion et de la loi anglaise sur les quarantaines. 276 pp., 3 pl. 4°. *Paris, J.-B. Baillière & fils*, 1863.
For Biography, see **Bardinet** (B.-A.) Éloge de F. Mélier. 8°. *Paris*, 1867. *See, also:* Ann. d'hyg., Par., 1866, 2. s., xxvi, 464-478 (A. Guérard). *Also:* Bull. Acad. de méd., Par., 1865-6, xxxi, 1167-1175 (Bergeron).

Mélik (Léon). *Des indications du raclage de l'utérus dans le cas de fongosités. 69 pp. 4°. *Paris*, 1887, No. 133.

Melikoff (Ivan). *Razbor sposobov iskustvennago uvlajnenija vozducha jilych pomeshenii. [Analysis of air in dwellings.] 28 pp., 1 l. 8°. *St. Petersburg, tipog. N. A. Lebedeva*, 1882.

Melillo (Jeronymo). A parteira na noções necessarias sobre o nascimento do homem. x, 11–93 pp. 8°. *Rio de Janeiro, H. Laemmert & Co.*, 1883.

Melilotus.
Clausen (C. H. E.) Ueber den kamphorartigen Bestandtheil der Herba meliloti. Mitth. a. d. Geb. d. Med., etc., Altona, 1837-8, v, 7.-8. Hft., 77.

Melin (F.-A.-E.) *Diagnostic différentiel des affections aiguës des bronches, du poumon et de la plèvre. 31 pp. 4°. *Paris*, 1835, No. 176. [P., v. 287.]

Melion (Jos. Vinc.) *Diss. sistens conspectum morborum chronicorum in clinico anno 1839 observatorum. 44 pp. 8°. *Pragæ, C. Geržabek*, 1841.

Melipotius (Nicolaus). *De pleuritide. 8 l. 4°. *Lugd. Bat., A. Elzevier*, 1684.

Mélique (P.-M.) *Considérations sur l'ophthalmie. 29 pp. 4°. *Paris*, 1821, No. 52, v. 164.

Melis (Giovanni). Estirpazione della scapola conservando l' arto superiore. Tesi di Laurea. 16 pp. 8°. *Cagliari, tipog. del Corriere*, 1886.
Dalla clinica chirurgica della R. Università di Cagliari diretta dal Prof. Inc. Angelo Roth.

Melissa.
Boyer. Boyer's Carmelite melissa cordial (eau de mélisse des Carmes) of the Barefooted Carmelites of the Rue de Vaugirard. Historical and medical essay. 12°. *New York*, [*n. d.*]
Reuss (G. D.) *De melissa. 4°. *Halæ*, [1739].

Melissa ('H) τῶν 'Αθηνῶν, σύγγραμμα περιοδικὸν ἐκδιδόμενον ἅπαξ τοῦ μηνός. 'Υπὸ Α. Ν. Γούφα. [2. s.] v. 1–2, 1864–5. 8°. 'Εν 'Αθήναις.
A continuation (2. s.) of: **Athenais** ('H ἐν) 'Ιατρικὴ Μέλισσα.

Melissenos (Giulio C. A.) L' igiene omicida e gli odori di Napoli. xxxiv, 132 pp., 1 l. 12°. *Napoli, tipog. dell' Accademia reale delle scienze*, 1882.

Mélisson (Jules-Benjamin-Louis). *Des calculs urinaires développés dans des cavités anormales. 39 pp. 4°. *Paris*, 1873, No. 186.

Melisurgo (Giulio Cesare). Ingegnerie sanitarie ed urbane. xxiii, 240 pp. 8°. *Napoli*, [1880].

Melitagra.
Alibert. Nouvelles observations sur la mélitagre flavescente. J. univ. d. sc. méd., Par., 1829, lvi, 68-72.—**Arnal.** Observations sur la mélitagre flavescente. Ibid., lv, 70-77.

Melitsch (Joh.) [1763–]. Abhandlung von der sogenannten Umbeugung der Gebährmutter, zum Anfange seiner Privatvorlesungen über die Eutbindungskunst, vorgetragen den 21. Herbstmonds, 1789. Nebst einer Nachricht des damit verbundenen praktischen Institutes. 2 p. l., 87 pp. 8°. *Prag, Elsenwanger*, 1790.

Melituria.
See **Diabetes.**

Melizan (Léopold). *Des taches de la cornée et de leur traitement. 63 pp. 4°. *Montpellier*, 1873, No. 43.

Melksham Cottage Hospital. Annual report of the committee to the subscribers. 15., 1882–3. 15 pp. 12°. *Melksham, J. H. Maggs*, 1883.
Established 1868.

de Melle (Christophorus Andreas). *De vi vitali, quoad medicinam et ex illa morbi oriuntes. 62 pp., 2 l. sm. 4°. *Lugd. Bat., J. Bos*, 1761.

a Melle (Franc. Jacobus). *De fortuitis in medicina proficuis. 1 p. l., 44 pp. 4°. *Argentorati, lit. D. Maagii*, 1718.

a Melle (Franciscus Josephus). *Adagiorum medicinalium sylloge. 1 p. l., 24 pp. sm. 4°. *Altorfii Noric., lit. I. G. Kohlesii*, [1717].

Meller (Joannes Henricus) [1828–]. *De tussi convulsiva. 29 pp., 1 l. 8°. *Berolini, typ. fratrum Schlesinger*, [1853].

Meller (Josef). *Beitrag zur Lehre vom Scleroderma adultorum. [Strasburg.] 36 pp. 8°. *Crefeld, G. Kühler*, 1883.

Mellerstadt (Martin). *See* **Pollichius** (Martinus).

Mellet (David-Louis). *Sur le rachitis. 27 pp. 4°. *Paris*, 1823, No. 171, v. 182.

Mellet (François-Louis-Édouard). *Considérations générales sur les déviations des pieds (pieds-bots). viii, 9–32 pp., 2 pl. 4°. *Paris*, 1823, No. 82, v. 179.

——. Manuel pratique d'orthopédie, ou traité élémentaire sur les moyens de prévenir et de guérir toutes les difformités du corps humain. xv, 5–524 pp., 18 pl. 16°. *Paris, J. Rouvier*, 1844.

Mellez (Jacques). *Réflexions relatives à la pourriture d'hôpital. 1 p. l., 12 pp. 4°. *Strasbourg*, 1834, v. 58.

Melli (Sebastiano). La comare levatrice istruita nel suo uffizio secondo le regole più certe, e gli ammaestramenti più moderni. 1 p. l., viii, 448 pp., 19 pl. 4°. *Venezia, C. Palese*, 1766.

Melliar (Jacobus). *De asthmate spasmodico. 1 p. l., 38 pp. 8°. *Edinburgi, Balfour et Smellie*, 1777.

Mellié (Albert-Charles-Jules-Ernest). *Recherches sur le mode d'action du pansement ouaté. 26 pp., 1 l. 4°. *Paris*, 1877, No. 309.

Mellier (Alfred). *Études sur les bossus observés dans les établissements d'aliénés. [Montpellier.] 52 pp., 1 l. 4°. *Avignon, Bonnet et fils*, 1866, No. 104.
c.

Mellier (Frédéric). *Observations pratiques sur quelques dérangements de la menstruation, et principalement sur la difficulté de leur diagnostic. 69 pp. 8°. *Montpellier, J. Martel aîné*, 1836.

Mellin (Christoph Jakob) [1744–1817]. *Frictionum præstantissimus usus in arte salutari

Mellin (Christoph Jakob)—continued.
ostenditur. 32 pp. 4°. *Jenæ, apud G. M. Marggrafii viduam*, [1766].

——. Auszüge aus den besten medicinischen Probeschriften des 16. und 17. Jahrhunderts. 2 v. in 1. viii, 296, 309–312 pp.; ii, 225–316 pp. 12°. *Altenburg, Richter*, 1771–4.
Incomplete; want pp. 1–224 of v. 2.

——. Praktische Materia medica. 2. Ausg. 7 p. l., 303 pp., 16 l. 12°. *Altenburg, Richter*, 1778.
For Biography, see **Kaltschmied** (Car. Frid.)

Mellin (J. J.)
See "**Unterricht** für Personen", etc. 12°. *Frankf. a. M.*, 1796.

Mellinghaus (Henricus) [1808–]. *De noma pathologica quædam. 31 pp. 8°. *Berolini, typ. Nietackianis*, [1833].

Mellinghoff (Gerhardus) [1827–]. *De anthrace. 26 pp., 3 l. 8°. *Berolini, fratrum Schlesinger*, [1852].

Mellis (*John*) [1819–86].
Obituary. Brit. M. J., Lond., 1886, i, 761.

Melliss (D. Ernest). *Contributions to the chemistry of zirconium. 31 pp. 8°. *Göttingen, E. A. Huth*, 1870.
C.

Melliss (John Charles). The sewage question solved; or, how to purify our rivers. 22 pp., 1 l., 1 pl. 8°. *London, E. Wilson*, 1875.
See, also, **Robinson** (H.) Purification of water-carried sewage, [etc.] 8°. *London*, 1877.

de Mello (Carlos Augusto). *Hypoemia intertropical. 4 p. l., 78 pp., 1 l. *Rio de Jan., Santos & C.*, 1883.

de Mello (José Alves). *Molestia de Bright. 34 pp., 1 l. 4°. *Bahia, typog. do Correio da Bahia*, 1871.

——. *Corpos gordurosos, sua constituição é propriedades. 2 p. l., 40 pp. 4°. *Bahia, imp. do Diario*, 1872.
Concurso.

——. *Da synthese em chimica mineral. 2 p. l., 61 pp. 4°. *Bahia, imp. Economica*, 1875.
Concurso.

de Mello Franco (Francisco) [1757–1823]. Elementos de hygiene; ou dictames theoreticos, e practicos para conservar a saude, e prolongar a vida. xiii, 347 pp. 8°. *Lisboa*, 1814.

——. The same. Publicados por ordem da Academia real das sciencias pelo seu socio. 3. ed. vi, xiii, 354 pp. 8°. *Lisboa*, 1823.

de Mello Franco (*Manoel*) [1812–71].
Biography. Brazil. Biogr. Ann. [Macedo], Rio de Jan., 1876, iii, 367–372.

de Mello e Senna (Henrique Augusto). *Dissertação. Cadeira de clinica psychiatrica. Das allucinações, sua importancia no diagnostico da alienação. Proposições tres sobre cada uma das cadeiras da Faculdade. 3 p. l., 85 pp., 1 l. 8°. *Rio de Janeiro, Laemmert & Co.*, 1886.

de Mello de Souza Brandão e Menezez (Luiz). *Considérations sur les propriétés physiologiques et thérapeutiques du nitrate d'argent. 67 pp. 4°. *Paris*, 1856, No. 8, v. 593.

——. *Contribuições para á historia do myosis ou bicheiro das fossas nazaes. 34 pp., 1 l. 4°. *Rio de Janeiro, E. & H. Laemmert*, 1875.

Melloni (Macedonio) [1798–1854]. Nouvel électroscope. 8 pp. 4°. [*Paris, Mallet-Bachelier*, 1854.] [P., v. 796.]
Repr. from: Compt. rend. Acad. d. sc., Par., 1854, xxxix.
For Biography, see **Nobile** (Antonio). Elogio storico di Macedonio Melloni, recitato nella reale Accademia delle scienze di Napoli nella tornata del 1 dicembre 1854. fol. *Napoli*, 1855.

Mellor (Georgius Henricus). *De hepatitide chronica. 1 p. l., 43 pp. 8°. *Edinburgi, C. Stewart*, 1813. [P., v. 864.]
7

Mellwig (Joh. Jos.) *De fluxus menstrualis anomaliis per excessum. 2 p. l., 56 pp. 8°. *Gryphiæ, F. G. Kunike*, [1839].

Melm (Godofredus). *De rhachitide. 1 p. l., 52 pp., 2 pl., 1 l. 4°. *Duisburgi ad Rhenum, J. Sas*, [1730].

Melnotte (Émile). *Contribution à l'étude des perforations intestinales. 70 pp. 4°. *Paris*, 1880, No. 42.

Melocchi (Vincenzo). Considerazioni clinico-scientifiche intorno al reumatismo articolare acuto e cronico, o adenodermopatia reumatica discrasica e sua terapia, in ispecie per gli alcalini, e bagni idropatici e termo-minerali. 90 pp., 1 tab. 8°. *Napoli, P. Androsio*, 1878.

Meloë *proscarabæus.*
Fiedler (R.) Fall einer tödtlichen Vergiftung durch ein aus Meloë proscarabæus bereitetes Pulver. Summ. d. Neuest. u. Wissenswürd. a. d. ges. Med., Leipz., 1838, n. F., viii, 95–99.—**Hoffbauer.** Vergiftung durch ein Pulver von Meloë proscarabæus und M. violaceus. Vitljschr. f. gerichtl. Med., Berl., 1875, n. F., xxiii, 244–264.

Melograno.
Righini (G.) Cenni intorno ad un nuovo principio rinvenuto nella corteccia della radice del melograno silvestre, e sopra alcuni preparati della medesima contenenti lo stesso principio. Bull. d. sc. med. di Bologna, 1843, 3. s., iv, 341–354.

Meloni-Satta (Pietro). Teratologia in genere ed illustrazione di alcuni casi in specie. Conferenze tenute nella R. Università di Cagliari. [Anno 1.] 104 pp., 1 l., 3 pl. 8°. *Sassari, G. Dessi*, 1885.

Melons.
Commaille (A.) Note sur les hydrates de carbone solubles contenus dans les sucs de melon et de pastèque. Rec. de mém. de méd.... mil., Par., 1869, 3. s., xxii, 230–235.—**Nati da Bibbiena** (M. P.) Breve discorso intorno alla natura del popone, e sopra il cattivo uso del ber fresco con la neve. *In:* Rac. d' opusc. scient. e filol., 16°, Venezia, 1730, iv, 373–398.

Melopsittacus *undulatus.*
See **Intestines** (*Comparative anatomy of*).

Melot [–1832].
Cruveilhier. Quelques mots sur Melot. Bull. Soc. anat. de Par., 1832, vii, 167.

Melquiond (C.-E.-J.-A.) *De l'influence de la brusque transition du chaud au froid dans la production des phlegmasies. 36 pp. 4°. *Paris*, 1853, No. 62, v. 545.

Melsens (Louis-Henri-Frédéric) [1814–86]. Recherches sur la persistance des impressions de la rétine. 42 pp. 8°. *Bruxelles*, [1857].
Repr. from: Bull. Acad. roy. d. sc. de Belg., Brux., 1857, 2. s., iii.

——. Mémoire sur l'emploi de l'iodure de potassium pour combattre les affections saturnines, mercurielles, et les accidents consécutifs de la syphilis. 167 pp. 8°. *Bruxelles, M. Hayez*, 1865.

——. Note sur la conservation du vaccin. 4 pp. 8°. [*Bruxelles, H. Manceaux*, 1871.] [P., v. 797.]
Repr. from: J. de méd., chir. et pharmacol., Brux., 1871, liii.

——. Note sur les plaies produites par les armes à feu, sur quelques effets de la pénétration des projectiles dans divers milieux et sur l'impossibilité de la fusion des balles de plomb qui frappent les hommes ou les chevaux. 61 pp. 8°. *Bruxelles, H. Manceaux*, 1872. [P., v. 797.]
Repr. from: J. de méd., chir. et pharmacol., Brux., 1872–3, liv–lv.

——. Sur la congélation des liquides alcooliques. 12 pp. 8°. [*Bruxelles, F. Hayez*, 1873.] [P., v. 801.]
Repr. from: Bull. Acad. roy. de méd. de Belg., Brux., 1873, 2. s., xxxv.

——. Sur les boissons alcooliques glacées portées à des températures très-basses et sur le refroidissement et la congélation des vins ordi-

Melsens (Louis-Henri-Frédéric)—continued. naires ou mousseux. 25 pp. 8°. [*Bruxelles, F. Hayez*, 1873.] [P., v. 801.]
Repr. from: Bull. Acad. roy. de méd. de Belg., Brux., 1873, 2. s., xxxv.

——. Emploi thérapeutique de l'ammoniaque, de ses sels et des composés ou mélanges ammoniacaux complexes dans les affections des organes respiratoires. 8 pp. 8°. *Bruxelles, H. Manceaux,* 1881.
Repr. from: Bull. Acad. roy. de méd. de Belg., Brux., 1881, 3. s., xv.

——. Deuxième note sur les matières albuminoïdes. 48 pp., 1 pl. 8°. *Acad. roy. de Belgique,* [*n. d.*]
Repr. from: Bull. Acad. roy de Belg., Brux., xxiv.
For Biography, see Art méd., Brux., 1886-7, xxii, 109-111.

Melsheimer (Julius). * Ueber die Lehre vom Affect in gerichtlich-medicinischer Beziehung. 20 pp., 2 l. 8°. *Giessen, F. C. Pietsch,* 1862. c.

Meltz (Hermann). *Casuistischer Beitrag zu den Resectionen. 41 pp., 1 l. 8°. *Greifswald, C. Sell,* 1876.

Meltzer (Franz Carl). Abhandlung von dem Keichhusten. 7 p. l., 135 pp. 12°. *St. Petersburg, C. Tornow u. Comp.,* 1790.

Meltzer (H. A.) Flugblatt Nr. 1. Höchst wichtige Mittheilung für Jedermann! 3. Aufl. 16 pp. 12°. *Leipzig, Frankenstein u. Wagner,* [1881].
Repr. from his: Lehrbuch ü. Naturheilk.

Meltzer (S.) [1853–]. *Das Schluckcentrum, seine Irradiationen und die allgemeine Bedeutung derselben. 35 pp. 8°. *Berlin, H. S. Hermann,* [1882].

——. Schluckgeräusche im Scrobiculus cordis und ihre physiologische Bedeutung. 4 pp. 8°. [*Berlin,* 1883.]
Repr. from: Centralbl. f. d. med. Wissensch., Berl., 1883, xxi.
Bound with: Arb. a. d. spec. physiol. Abth. d. physiol. Inst. d. Univ. Berl., 1883, [No. 2].

Melun.
Le Brise-Orgueil. Topographie médicale de Melun. J. de méd., chir., pharm., etc., Par., 1786, lxvi, 8-15.

Melvill (John). Observations on the nature and properties of fixible air, and on the salutary effects of the aqua salubris, in preserving health and preventing diseases; to which are added strictures on the present practice of physic, [etc.] 92 pp. 8°. *London, the author,* [1787].

Melville (Alexander)[1]. *De apoplexia. 2 p. l., 53 pp. 8°. *Edinburgi, R. Allan,* 1797. [*Also, in:* P., v. 6.]

Melville (Alexander)[2]. *De hepatitide. 1 p. l., 35 pp. 8°. *Edinburgi, C. Stewart et soc.,* 1801. [P., v. 19.]

Melville (Henry). The modern treatment of pulmonary consumption and other diseases of the respiratory organs, being suggestions to invalids on the most rational method of cure. 76 pp. 12°. *New York,* 1859.
Also, Co-Editor of: **Hunter's** Medical and Surgical Specialist, New York, 1855-7.—**Upper Canada** (The) Journal of Medical, Surgical, and Physical Science, Toronto, 1851-3.

Melvin (*S. N.*)
Portrait in: **Collection** of Portr. (Libr.)

Melyssyl.
VON PIEVERLING (L.) *Ueber Melissyl-Alcohol und seine Umsetzungsprodukte. 8°. *Erlangen,* 1876.

Melzer (Antonius). Tractatus de diminuendo sub partu fœtus capite. vi, 56 pp., 1 pl. 8°. *Labaci, L. Eger,* 1821.

Melzer (Franciscus Carolus). *De hernia crurali incarcerata. 30 pp. sm. 4°. *Argentorati, typ. J. H. Heitzii,* [1769].
Also [Abstr.], *in:* WEIZ (F. A.) Vollständ. Ausz. [etc.] 12°. Leipzig u. Budissin, 1771, iii, 434-441.

Melzer (Raimund). Studien über die asiatische Brechruhr. 58 pp., 5 pl. 8°. *Erlangen, F. Enke,* 1850.

Melzner (Joannes Jacobus). *De majori frequentia apoplexiæ in eruditis quam alius sortis hominibus observanda. 28 pp., 2 l. sm. 4°. *Halæ Magdeb., typ. J. C. Hendelii,* [1755].

Membrana *tympani.*

See, also, **Chorda** *tympani;* **Ear** (*Ossicles of*); **Tensor** *tympani.*

AEPLI (A. T.) *De membrana tympani. 4°. *Gynopedii,* 1837.

BÜRKNER (K.) Atlas von Beleuchtungsbildern des Trommelfells. 8°. *Jena,* 1886.

CORNELIUS (F.) *De membranæ tympani usu. 8°. [*Dorpat*], 1825.

FICK (A.) Betrachtungen über den Mechanismus des Paukenfelles. 8°. *Würzburg,* 1886.
See, also, infra.

HOME (E.) On the structure and uses of the membrana tympani of the ear. 4°. [*London,* 1799.]

NOLDA (A.) *Phonautographische Studien als Beiträge zur Physiologie der Membrana tympani des Menschen. 8°. *Würzburg,* 1886.

POLITZER (A.) Die Beleuchtungsbilder des Trommelfells im gesunden und kranken Zustande. Klinische Beiträge zur Erkenntniss und Behandlung der Ohren-Krankheiten. 8°. *Wien,* 1865.

——. The same. The membrana tympani in health and disease. Clinical contributions to the diagnosis and treatment of diseases of the ear, with supplement. Transl. by A. Mathewson and H. G. Newton. 8°. *New York,* 1869.

POPPER (M.) *Sosudi i nervi barabannoi pereponki. [Vessels and nerves of membrana tympani.] 8°. *St. Petersburg,* 1869.
Also, transl. in: Monatschr. f. Ohrenh., Berl., 1869, iii, 63; 79.

VERKADE (P.) *Verhandeling over het trommelvlies en de gehoorbeentjes. 8°. *Amsterdam,* 1856.

WALTHER (A. F.) *Diss. anat. de membrana tympani, respondente Caspar Bose. sm. 4°. *Lipsiæ,* [1725].
Also, in: HALLER. Disp. anat. [etc.] 4°. Gottingæ, 1749, iv, 337-354.

WIRTZ (P.) *Ueber das Foramen Rivini und seine Beziehungen zu den Eiterungsprozessen hinter der Membrana flaccida. [Bonn.] 8°. *Oberhausen,* 1886.

Bau (Ueber den) des Annulus tendinosus seu cartilagineus des Trommelfelles. Allg. Wien. med Ztg., 1869, xiv, 43.—**Berthold** (E.) Optische Darstellung der durch Schallleitung durch die Kopfknochen erzeugten Bewegungen des Trommelfells am Lebenden. Monatschr. f. Ohrenh., Berl., 1872, vi, 29-32.—**Bing** (A.) Ueber Bewegungserscheinungen am Trommelfelle. Wien. med. Bl., 1886, ix, 473; 509. — **Blake** (C. J.) The use of the membrana tympani as a phonautograph and logograph. Arch. Ophth. & Otol., N. Y., 1876, v, 108, 1 pl.; 1878, vii, 457. *Also,* Reprint.—. The membrana tympani telephone. Am. J. Otol., N. Y., 1880, ii, 180-183. ——. The progressive growth of the dermoid coat of the membrana tympani. *Ibid.,* 1882, iv, 266-268. — **Burnett** (C. H.) A contribution to the comparative distribution of bloodvessels in the membrana tympani. Am. J. M. Sc., Phila., 1873, lxv, 119-122. *Also,* Reprint. *Also, transl.* [Abstr.]: Monatschr. f. Ohrenh., Berl., 1872, vi, 17. — **Cooper** (A.) Observations on the effects which take place from the destruction of the membrana tympani of the ear. Phil. Tr., Lond., 1800, xc, 151-160. ——. Farther observations on the effects which take place from the destruction of the membrana tympani of the ear: with an account of an operation for the removal of a particular species of deafness. *Ibid.,* 1801, xci, 435-450, 1 pl — **Coyne.** Morphologie de la membrane du tympan au niveau de la portion flaccide dite de Schrapnell. Gaz. hebd. d. sc. méd. de Bordeaux, 1880, i, 147-150.—**Crombie** (J. M.) Function of the membrana flaccida of the tympanic membrane. Nature, Lond., 1882, xxvii, 129-131. ——. On the membrana tympani. J. Anat. & Physiol., Lond., 1882-3. xvii, 523-536.— **Dalby** (W. B.) On the diagnostic value of morbid appearances in the tympanic

Membrana *tympani*.

membrane. Lancet, Lond., 1876, i, 493.—**Dufrane.** De l'exploration de la membrane du tympan. Arch. méd. belges, Brux., 1876, 3. s., ix, 328–347.—**Fick** (A.) Beobachtungen über den Mechanismus des Paukenfelles. Verhandl. d. phys.-med. Gesellsch. zu Würzb., 1887, n. F., xx, 73-83. [*See, also, supra.*]—**Fleischmann.** Einiges über das Wittmannsche Loch im Trommelfelle. Berl. med. Centr.-Ztg., 1836, v, 321. — **Föhrenschwarz** (M.) Die Erkenntniss der Trommelfellbewegungen; Beschreibung einer optischen Vorrichtung für didaktische Zwecke. [Myringoscop.] Allg. Wien. med. Ztg., 1870, xv, 601: 1871, xvi, 36.—**Galton** (J. C.) Notes on the condition of the tympanic membrane in the insane. West Riding Lun. Asyl. Rep., Lond., 1873, iii, 258–272.—**Gellé.** Développement de la partie flaccide de la membrane du tympan. Trav. lab. physiol. Fac. méd. de Par. (1884), 1885, i, 185-191, 1 pl. — **Green** (J. O.) Restoration of the membrana tympani after its almost complete destruction from chronic inflammation. Boston M. & S. J., 1870, lxxxiii, 347-349.—**Gruber** (J.) Beiträge zur Anatomie des Trommelfelles. Allg. Wien. med. Ztg., 1866, xi, 385. *Also:* Wchnbl. d. k. k. Gesellsch. d. Aerzte in Wien. 1867, vii, 1; 169. [*See, also, infra,* Prussak (A.)] ——. Ueber den feineren Bau des Ringwulstes am Trommelfelle. Wien. med. Presse, 1869, x, 178–180. *Also:* Monatschr. f. Ohrenh., Berl., 1869, iii, 17–20. ——. Anatomische Bemerkungen über das Trommelfell. Monatschr. f. Ohrenh., Berl., 1870, iv, 93; 101; 109; 117. ——. Ueber die normalen Spannungsverhältnisse des menschlichen Trommelfells. *Ibid.,* 1877, xi, 67–70. — **Hauff.** Ueber die willkürliche Bewegung des Trommelfells. Med. Cor.-Bl. d. württemb. ärztl. Ver., Stuttg., 1850, xx, 135. — **Home** (E.) The Croonian lecture. On the structure and uses of the membrana tympani. Phil. Tr., Lond., 1800, xc, 1-21. ——. On the difference of structure between the human membrana tympani and that of the elephant. *Ibid.,* 1823, cxiii, 23–26, 3 pl.—**Kessel** (J.) Nerven und Lymphgefässe der menschlichen Trommelfelles. Centralbl. f. d. med. Wissensch., Berl., 1869, vii, 356; 369. — **Kiesselbach** (W.) Ueber partielle Vorwölbung der Membrana tympani bei gleichmässig verstärktem Luftdruck. Monatschr. f. Ohrenh., Berl., 1885, xix, 5.—**Küpper.** Ueber Pulsationen am Trommelfell. Arch. f. Ohrenh., Leipz., 1880, xv, 271.— **Lucae** (A.) Ueber die Respirationsbewegungen des Trommelfells. *Ibid.,* Würzb., 1864, i, 96-106.—**Luschka.** Ueber die willkürliche Bewegung des Trommelfelles. Arch. f. physiol. Heilk., Stuttg., 1850, ix, 80–84. — **Magendie.** Sur les organes qui tendent ou relachent la membrane du tympan et la chaîne des osselets de l'ouïe dans l'homme et les animaux mammifères. J. de physiol. expér., Par., 1821, i, 341-347.—**Martin.** Observations sur la membrane du tympan. J. de méd., chir., pharm., etc., Par., 1769, xxxi, 178-183.—**Michelsen** (F. J.) Een door de natuur gevormd kunstmatig trommelvlies. Nederl. Tijdschr. v. Geneesk., Amst., 1884, xx, 731–733. — **Moldenhauer** (W.) Vergleichende Histologie des Trommelfells. Arch. f. Ohrenh., Leipz., 1878, xiii, 113-162, 4 pl.—**Moos** (S.) Untersuchungen über das Verhalten der Blutgefässe und des Blutgefäss-Kreislaufs des Trommelfells und Hammergriffs. Arch. f. Augen- u. Ohrenh., Wiesb., 1877, vi, 475–500, 2 pl. *Also, transl.:* Arch. Ophth. & Otol., N. Y., 1877–8, vi, 574-602, 2 pl.— **Politzer** (A.) Ueber die willkürlichen Bewegungen des Trommelfells. Wien. Med.-Halle, 1862, iii, 168. ——. Ueber ein Höhlensystem zwischen Trommelfell und Hammerhals. Wien. med. Wchnschr., 1870, xx, 234; 252. ——. Zur Frage über die Innervation des Musc. tensor tympani. Arch. f. path. Anat., etc., Berl., 1876, lxviii, 77-84.—**Potter** (M.) Sosudi i nervi barabannoi pereponki. [Vessels and nerves of membrana tympani.] Voyenno-med. J., St. Petersb., 1869, civ, pt. 2, 49–70, 1 pl.—**Prussak** (A.) Zur Anatomie des Trommelfells. Erwiderung an Herrn Dr. J. Gruber. Wchnbl. d. k. k. Gesellsch. d. Aerzte in Wien, 1867, vii, 209–212. ——. Ueber die anatomischen Verhältnisse des Trommelfells zum Hammer. Centralbl. f. d. med. Wissensch., Berl., 1867, v, 225–227. ——. K' anatomii chelovaicheskoi barabanoi pereponki. [Anatomy of the membrane of the tympanum.] Med. Vestnik, St. Petersb., 1867, vii, 357; 369; 385; 393. *Also, transl.:* Arch. f. Ohrenh., Würzb., 1867, iii, 255–280, 1 pl.— **Ravogli** (A.) Ricerche istologiche sulla membrana del timpano nello stato sano e morboso. Arch. per le sc. med., Torino, 1876, i, 169–174, 1 pl.—**Savart** (F.) Recherches sur les usages de la membrane du tympan et de l'oreille externe. J. de physiol. expér., Par., 1824, iv, 183–219.— **Schoonemark** (J.) Pulsatiën aan het trommelvlies. Geneesk. Courant, Tiel, 1881, xxxv, no. 10. — **Schwabach.** Das Trommelfell am macerirten Schläfenbein. Centralbl. f. d. med. Wissensch., Berl., 1885, xxiii, 673-676.—**Shrapnell** (H. J.) On the form and structure of the membrana tympani. Lond. M. Gaz., 1832, x, 120; 282. — **Stifler** (M.) Ueber Erschlaffung des Trommelfells. Aerztl. Int.-Bl., München, 1876, xxiii, 303; 312.— **Tillaux.** Sur le triangle lumineux et sur sa valeur dans les affections de l'oreille. Bull. Soc. de chir. de Par. (1874), 1875, 3. s., iii, 452. — **Toynbee** (J.) On the structure of the membrana tympani in the human ear. Phil. Tr.,

Membrana *tympani*.

Lond., 1851, 159–168, 1 pl. *Also:* Edinb. M. & S. J., 1852, lxxvii, 320–329. — **Trautmann** (F.) Die Lichtreflexe des Trommelfelles. Arch. f. Ohrenh., Leipz., 1873-4, viii, 1, 1 pl.: 1874-5, ix, 96: 1875-6, x, 10; 87. ——. Der gelbe Fleck am Ende des Hammergriffs. *Ibid.,* 1876, xi, 99 – 112. 2 pl. — **Urbantschitsch** (V.) Ueber eine eigenthümliche Form von Epithelialauflagerung am Trommelfell und im äusseren Gehörgang. *Ibid.,* 1875-6, x, 7-9, 1 pl.—**Vest.** Ueber die Wittmann'sche Trommelfellklappe. Med. Jahrb. d. k. k. österr. Staates, Wien, 1819-20, v, 1. Hft., 123–133.—**Voltolini** (R.) Ueber den Lichtkegel am Trommelfelle. Monatschr. f. Ohrenh., Berl., 1872. vi, 87. ——. Welches Nervenpaar innervirt den Tensor tympani? Physiologische Untersuchungen über diese Frage und über einige hierhergehörige pathologische Erscheinungen. Arch. f. path. Anat., etc., Berl., 1875, lxv, 452-480.—**Weber-Liel.** Die Membrana tympani secundaria. Monatschr. f. Ohrenh., Berl., 1876, x, 7; 53; 72.

Membrana *tympani* (*Abnormities of*).

Bürkner (K.) Zur sogenannten Dehiscenz des Tegmen tympani. Arch. f. Ohrenh., Leipz., 1878, xiii, 185-191 — **Gruber** (J.) Abnorme Verwachsungen des Trommelfells. Aerztl. Ber. d. k. k. allg. Krankenh. zu Wien (1868), 1869, 251-254. ——. Ueber Anomalien in der Spannung des Trommelfells. Monatschr. f. Ohrenh., Berl., 1871, v, 35; 45; 53: 70; 78; 85; 93; 133. ——. Ueber Anomalien in der Verbindung des Hammers mit dem Trommelfell. *Ibid.,* 1874, viii, 45-47. ——. Zur Behandlung der Spannungsanomalien des Trommelfells. *Ibid.,* 1877, xi, 77; 101; 127. — **Zaufal** (E.) Durchlöcherung des rechten und linken Trommelfells bei einem Neugebornen. Wien. med. Wchnschr., 1868, xviii, 445-447.

Membrana *tympani* (*Artificial*).

VON MOSCHZISKER (F. A.) On the use of the artificial membrana tympani in cases of deafness, depending upon perforation or destruction of the natural organ. 8°. *Philadelphia,* 1857.

TOYNBEE (J.) On the use of an artificial membrana tympani in cases of deafness dependent upon perforation or destruction of the natural organ. 8°. *London,* 1853.

——. The same. 3. ed. 8°. *London,* 1855.

——. The same. 4. ed. 8°. *London,* 1855.

——. The same. 6. ed. 8°. *London,* 1857.

Also, transl. in: Wien. med. Wchnschr., 1859, ix, 40; 57: 71; 87; 104.

VEYRAT (E.) *Du tympan artificiel. 4°. Paris,* 1875.

YEARSLEY (J.) Controversy on the artificial tympanum. Reprint from Medical Times and Gazette, with additions. 8°. *London,* 1858.

See, also, infra.

Ayres (W. C.) Artificial drum-heads for the ear. N. Orl. M. & S. J., 1884-5, n. s., xii, 421-434. ——. Further notes on the artificial drum-membrane for the ear; a case of exceeding interest, with remarks. *Ibid,* 1886-7, n. s., xiv, 409-432.—**Bargellini** (D.) Sull' uso della membrana del timpano artificiale in alcuni casi di sordità. Imparziale, Firenze, 1871, xi, 705-708.—**Barr** (T.) Practical observations on the value of the cotton-pellet (Yearsley's artificial tympanic membrane) as an aid to hearing. Brit. M. J., Lond., 1883, ii, 722.—**Barth.** Künstliches Trommelfell. Arch. f. Ohrenh., Leipz., 1885, xxii, 208.— **Buchanan** (T.) On the mode of applying cotton wool as a substitute for the membrana tympani. Med. Times, Lond., 1848, xviii, 203.—**Burnett** (C. H.) Uninterrupted wearing of cotton pellets as artificial drum-heads. Am. J. Otol., N. Y., 1880, ii, 14-21.—**Clark** (J. H.) The elliptical artificial tympanum. Am. M. Month., N. Y., 1859, xi, 261-269.— **Core** (A. S.) Application of cotton pellets in destruction of the membrana tympani; two cases. Arch. Otol., N. Y., 1881, x, 117. *Also, transl.:* Ztschr. f. Ohrenh., Wiesb., 1881-2, xi, 38-40.—**Czarda** (G.) Ein antiseptisches Tympanum artificiale. Illust. Monatschr. d. ärztl. Polytech., Bern, 1882, iv, 85-88.—**Delstanche** (C.) Considérations sur l'emploi du tympan artificiel. Clinique, Brux., 1887, i, 445; 464; 481.—**Erhard.** Der künstliche Tensor tympani, oder Taubheit heilbar durch Druck. Deutsche Klinik, Berl., 1854, vi, 581.—**Field** (G.) On a new form of artificial membrana tympani. Brit. M. J., Lond., 1875, i, 806.—**Giampietro** (E.) Des tympans artificiels. Courrier méd., Par., 1874, xxiv, 106; 114; 122.— **Graf** (F.) Zur Frage vom künstlichen Trommelfell,

Membrana *tympani* (*Artificial*).

insbesondere von Wattekügelchen. Ztschr. f. Ohrenh., Wiesb., 1882, xi, 128–131. *Also, transl.:* Arch. Otol., N. Y., 1882, xi, 109–112.—**Gruber** (J.) Zur Lehre vom künstlichen Trommelfell. Wien. med. Presse, 1874, xv, 929–933. ———. Papier als künstliches Trommelfell. Allg. Wien. med. Ztg., 1882, xxvii, 541.—**Guranowski** (L.) Przyczynek do kazuistyki szczepienia błony z jaja kurzego na przedziurawioną błonę bębenkową. [Introduction of membrane of hen s egg in perforation of membrana tympani.] Medycyna, Warszawa, 1887, xv, 177 ; 20¹ ; 218.—**Hackley** (C. E.) The use of Toynbee's artificial ear-drum. Arch. Otol., N. Y., 1879, viii, 228–230. *Also, transl.:* Ztschr. f. Ohrenh., Wiesb., 1880, ix, 3–5.—**Hartmann** (A.) Ueber eine neue Form des künstlichen Trommelfells. Arch. f. Ohrenh., Leipz., 1876, xi, 167.—**Hassenstein.** Beiträge zur Lehre von der Wirkung des künstlichen Trommelfells. Wien. med. Wchnschr., 1869, xix, 1281–1283.— **Housselle.** Mittheilung über Toynbee's künstliches Trommelfell. Deutsche Klinik, Berl., 1854, vi, 477–480.— **Knapp** (H.) The cotton pellet as an artificial drumhead. Tr. Internat. M. Cong., 7. sess., Lond., 1881, iii, 380–383. *Also:* Arch. Otol., N. Y., 1881, x, 60–69. *Also, transl.:* Ztschr. f. Ohrenh., Wiesb., 1881, x, 262–271.—**Kramer** (W.) Ueber Erhard's künstlichen Tensor tympani. Deutsche Klinik, Berl., 1855, vii, 66.—**Lichtenberg** (K.) Das künstliche Trommelfell. Pest. med.-chir. Presse, Budapest, 1879, xv, 792. *Also:* Wien. med. Presse, 1879, xx, 1186.— **Michael** (T.) Ueber ein flüssiges, künstliches Trommelfell. Tr. Internat. M. Cong., 7. sess., Lond., 1881, iii, 434. *Also:* Wien. med. Bl., 1882, v, 388.—**Modrzejewski** (E.) O sztucznej błonie bębenkowej i jej zastosowaniu. [Artificial membrana tympani and its adaptation.] Gaz. lek., Warszawa, 1884, 2. s., iv, 255; 284.—**Moos** (S.) Ueber die Wirkung des künstlichen Trommelfells. Arch. f. Ohrenh., Würzb., 1864, i, 119–122. *Also:* Verhandl. d. naturh.-med. Ver. zu Heidelb., 1862–5, iii, 147. ———. Alterations of taste and sensibility in the tongue by the application of an artificial tympanum in a case of large perforations in both membranæ tympani. Arch. Ophth. & Otol., N. Y., 1869, i, 140–148. *Also, transl.:* Arch. f. Augen- u. Ohrenh., Carlsruhe, 1869–70, i, 207–216.—**Moos** (S.) & **Steinbrugge** (H.) Ueber die Bildung einer Neomembran in der Paukenhöhle als Theilerscheinung der hämorrhagischen Pachymeningitis. Ztschr. f. Ohrenh., Wiesb., 1881–2, xi, 136–140. *Also, transl.:* Arch. Otol., N. Y., 1882, xi, 97–101.—**Pierce** (F. M.) On the various forms of artificial tympanic membranes. and their comparative value. Brit. M. J., Lond., 1883, ii, 720.—**Politzer** (A.) Ueber das künstliche Trommelfell und seine neueren Modifikationen. Wien. Med.-Halle, 1864, v, 5; 20; 94; 115.—**Pollak** (S.) An artificial membrana tympani made of elastic collodion. St. Louis M. & S. J., 1882, xliii, 372–376.— **Roosa** (D. B. St. J.) Contributions to aural surgery; the use of the artificial membrana tympani. Am. J. M. Sc., Phila., 1866, li, 106–109.—**Spencer** (H. N.) The function and utility of the artificial drum-membrane. Tr. Internat. M. Cong. 1876, Phila., 1877, 974–987.—**Tangeman** (C. W.) Preliminary contributions to the use of new artificial membrana tympani. Med. News, Phila., 1886, xlviii, 314–317.—**Thompson** (B.) A contribution to aural surgery, with a description of a new ear-drum. Med. Rec., N. Y., 1875, x, 294.—**Toynbee** (J.) A case of perforate membrana tympani, treated by the substitution of an artificial membrane. Tr. Path. Soc. Lond., 1852–3, iv, 254–256. ———. On the artificial membrana tympani. Lancet, Lond., 1855, ii, 385. ———. The artificial membrana tympani. Med. Times & Gaz., Lond., 1857, n. s., xv, 614.—**Turnbull** (L.) A new artificial membrana tympani. Med. & Surg. Reporter, Phila., 1876, xxxv, 527–530.—**Valk** (F.) Substitute membrane in the aural canal. Med. Rec., N. Y., 1881, xx, 461.—**Voltolini** (R.) Der Regenschirm als Trommelfell. Monatschr. f. Ohrenh., Berl., 1871, v, 141–143.—**Wagnier.** Du tympan artificiel. Rev. mens. de laryngol., etc., Par., 1887, vii, 313–330.— **Westropp** (T.) On a new form of artificial membrana tympani. Med. Times & Gaz., Lond., 1855, n. s., xi, 390–392. *Also:* Assoc. M. J., Lond., 1855, ii, 932.—**Wiethe** (T.) Ueber das künstliche Trommelfell. Allg. Wien. med. Ztg., 1883, xxviii, 491.—**Yearsley** (J.) On a new mode of treating deafness, attended by loss of the membrana tympani, associated, or not, with discharge from the ear. Lancet, Lond., 1848, ii, 10; 64; 152; 205. *Also, Reprint.* ———. On a new mode of treating deafness. Med. Times, Lond., 1850, xxi, 176. ———. On the artificial tympanum. Lancet, Lond., 1855, ii, 465. ———. The self-adjusting artificial tympanum. Med. Times & Gaz., Lond., 1856, n. s, xiii, 630. ———. On the artificial tympanum. *Ibid.,* 1857, n. s, xv, 575–577. ———. The artificial membrana tympani. *Ibid.,* 640. ———. The history of the artificial tympanum, for the relief of deafness attended by loss or injury of the membrana tympani, and for the cure of discharge from the ear; with a prefatory account of a new and simple mode of applying it. Med. Circ., Lond., 1857. x, 6 ; 28 ; 76. ———. The modus operandi of artificial tympanum. Brit. M. J., Lond., 1858, 723. ———. The artificial tympanum in cases of perforate membrana tympani. Med. Circ., Lond., 1864, xxiv, 17.

Membrana *tympani* (*Artificial*) [*Collections of patents for*].

Culbertson (J. W.) Artificial ear-drum. No. 270284. Jan. 9, 1883. — **Nicholson** (J. H.) Artificial ear-drum. No. 312577. Feb. 17. 1885. With photographic copy. — **Peck** (H. P. K.) Artificial ear-drum. No. 235566. Dec. 14, 1880. ———. Artificial ear-drum. No. 351398. Oct. 26, 1886.—**Wales** (H. A.) Artificial ear-drum. No. 335660. Feb. 9, 1886. — **Williams** (E. A.) Artificial ear-drum. No. 360074. March 29, 1887.

Membrana *tympani* (*Cicatrices of*).

See **Membrana** *tympani* (*Wounds, etc., of*).

Membrana *tympani* (*Diseases of*).

See, also, **Ear** (*Diseases of, Catarrhal, etc.*)

GNIDITSCH (P.) * De morbis membranæ tympani. 4°. *Lipsiæ,* [1780].

JONES (H. M.) Atlas of diseases of the membrana tympani. 8°. *London,* 1878.

NASILOFF (I.) * O vospalenii barabannoi pereponki (myringitis) ve patolog.-anatom. otnoshenii. 8°. *St. Petersburg,* 1867.

Also, transl. [Abstr.] *in:* Centralbl. f. d. med. Wissensch., Berl., 1867, v, 161–163.

ODENTHAL (J.) * Ueber die Entzündungen des Trommelfells. [Bonn.] 8°. *Oberhausen,* 1886.

SCHAPRINGER (A.) Ueber die Contraction des Trommelfellspanners. 8°. [*Wien,* 1870.]

Cutting from: Sitzungsb. d. k. Akad. d. Wissensch. Math.-naturw. Cl., Wien, 1870.

VOGT (H.) * Ueber acute Myringitis. 8°. *München,* 1867.

WANKEL (C. H.) * De morbis membranæ tympani. 8°. *Pragæ,* [1847].

Bezold (F.) Fibrinöses Exsudat auf dem Trommelfell und im Gehörgang. Arch. f. path. Anat., etc., Berl., 1877, lxx, 329–342.—**Bing** (A.) Zur Casuistik der Trommelfellentzündung. Wien. med. Bl., 1880, iii, 967; 995.—**Blake** (C. J.) Acute congestion of the upper portion of the tympanic cavity and membrana tympani. Am. J. Otol., N. Y., 1882, iv, 102–105.—**Boeck** (O.) Ueber Abscesse im Trommelfell. Arch. f. Ohrenh., Würzb., 1867, ii, 135–146.—**Böke** (J.) Die primäre Entzündung des Trommelfells. Wien. med. Presse, 1866, vii, 507; 533.— **Bonnafont.** Maladies de la membrane du tympan. Rev. méd. franç. et étrang., Par., 1860, i, 332–345.— Mémoire sur quelques phénomènes nerveux sympathiques qui se produisent pendant l'inflammation aiguë de la membrane du tympan et souvent même par la simple pression de cette membrane. France méd., Par., 1869, xvi, 593. *Also:* Union méd., Par., 1869, 3. s., viii, 411–415.—**Buck** (A. H.) On painless and only slightly painful ulceration and perforation of the membrana tympani, probably of a tubercular nature. Tr. Am. Otol. Soc., New Bedford, 1882–6, iii, 667–675. *Also:* N. York M. J., 1886, xliv, 208.— **Chimani** (R.) Vollkommen normale Hörschärfe bei hochgradiger Degeneration des Trommelfelles. Arch. f. Ohrenh., Würzb., 1867, ii, 171–173.—**Ciniselli** (G.) Sulla degenerazione calcare dell' anello timpanico. Morgagni, Napoli, 1881, xxiii, 214. — **Coomes** (M. F.) Deafness resulting from relaxation of the drum membrane. Med. Herald, Louisville, 1886–7, viii, 505–508.—**Dalby** (W. B.) The functions of the membrana tympani illustrated by disease. Am. J. M. Sc., Phila., 1886, n. s., xcii, 121–123.— **Fulton** (J. F.) Myringitis. Northwest. Lancet, St. Paul, 1882–3, ii, 182–185. — **Giampietro** (E.) Una diagnosi di sordità per sclerosi della cassa, dimostrata esatta dall' esito della cura. Gazz. di med. pubb., Napoli, 1874, v, 33–39.—**Gottstein.** Sur un cas de myringite aiguë, avec abondante desquamation. Cong. périod. internat. d'otol. Compt.-rend. 1880, Trieste, 1882, ii, 143.—**Gruber** (J.) Ueber Trennungen des Zusammenhanges sowie Substanzverluste im Trommelfelle und deren Behandlung. Allg. Wien. med. Ztg., 1866, xi, 317; 325; 333; 341; 366; 368; 389; 406: 1867, xii, 3; 27; 57; 82; 118; 156; 191. ———. Zur Behandlung der Trommelfell-Entzündung. *Ibid.,* 1869, xiv, 129; 137. ———. Ueber eine eigenthümliche Randtrübung am Trommelfell und deren Bedeutung. Monatschr. f. Ohrenh., Berl., 1878, xii, 106. ———. Schwerhörigkeit und subjective Gehörsempfindungen in Folge von Verwachsung des Trommelfelles mit der inneren Trommelhöhlenwand; secundäre Relaxation des nicht angewachsenen Theiles des Trommelfelles; Trennung der Synechie durch die Luftdouche; Heilung. Allg. Wien. med. Ztg., 1882, xxvii, 173.—**Hermet** (P.) Des épaississements de la membrane du tympan. Union méd., Par., 1882. 3. s., xxxiii, 881; 905.—**Hinton** (J.) Ulceration of the fibrous lamina of the membrana tympani. Tr. Path. Soc. Lond., 1860–61, xii, 201. ———. Clinical remarks on

Membrana *tympani* (*Diseases of*).

perforations and some other morbid conditions of the membrana tympani. Guy's Hosp. Rep., Lond., 1866, 3. s., xii, 617–666.—**Jounia.** Myringite diphthéritique. Rev. de thérap. méd.-chir. de Par., 1883, [xxxi], 291–293.—**Kessel** (J.) Zur Myringitis villosa. Arch. f. Ohrenh., Würzb., 1870, v, 250–253.—**Kramer** (W.) Die acute Entzündung des Trommelfells. Deutsche Klinik, Berl., 1858, x, 211; 223. *Also, transl.:* Gaz. méd. de Par., 1859, 3. s., xiv, 268–272. ———. Die chronische Entzündung des Trommelfells. Deutsche Klinik, Berl., 1858, x, 423; 431. *Also, transl.* [Abstr.] : Gaz. d. hôp., Par., 1859, xxxii, 354. *Also, transl.* [Abstr.] : Gaz. méd. de Par., 1859, 3. s., xiv, 567–571.—**Kun** (Z.) Az idült genyes dobürlob s annak veszélyes befolyása a szervezetre. [Purulent chronic tympanitis and its serious effects upon the organism.] Gyógyászat, Budapest, 1886, xxvi, 921 ; 953.—**Lehrnbecher.** Vier Fälle von Erkrankungen des Trommelfelles. Aerztl. Int.-Bl., München, 1877, xxiv, 119–121. — **Longhi** (G.) Miringite erpetico-desquammativa ambilaterale ; cura; guarigione. Gazz. med. ital. lomb., Milano, 1882, 8. s., iv, 473–475.—**Lucæ** (A.) Aragonitkrystalle in der verdickten Epidermis eines menschlichen Trommelfelles. [Nebst einer Mittheilung des Prof. Gust. Rose.] Arch. f. path. Anat., etc., Berl., 1866, xxxvi, 286–289, 1 pl.—**M'Keown** (W. A.) On a new method of treatment of relaxation of the membrana tympani. Dublin J. M. Sc., 1880, 3. s., lxix, 502 : 1881, 3. s., lxxi, 8.—**Moos** (S.) On the medico-legal significance of atrophy of the tympanum, produced by hardened cerumen. Arch. Ophth. & Otol., N. Y., 1869, i, 321–324. *Also, transl.:* Arch. f. Augen- u. Ohrenh., Carlsruhe, 1869–70, i. 244–246. ———. On the mechanism of chronic purulent myringitis in tuberculous individuals. [Transl. by A. Schapringer.] Arch. Otol., N. Y., 1887, xvi, 31–40, 2 pl.—**Politzer** (A.) Zur pathologischen Anatomie der Trommelfelltrübungen, und deren Bedeutung für die Diagnostik der Gehörkrankheiten. Oesterr. Ztschr. f. prakt. Heilk., Wien, 1862, viii, 777; 793; 817; 879; 977. — **Pope** (B. A.) Relaxation of the membrana tympani. N. Orl. M. & S. J., 1867, xx, 91.— **Roosa** & **Beard.** The appearance of the membrana tympani and fauces in 296 cases of acquired and congenital deaf-mutism. Am. J. M. Sc., Phila., 1867, n. s., liii, 399–402.—**Schlesinger** (Z. V.) A dobhártya sérüléseiröl. [On lesions of the membrana tympani.] Gyógyászat, Budapest, 1885, xxv, 347 ; 366 ; 382 ; 397 ; 414 ; 430 ; 447.—**Schwartze** (H.) Annähernd normale Hörschärfe bei hochgradiger Degeneration beider Trommelfelle. Arch. f. Orenh., Würzb., 1864, i, 142–144. ———. Synechie des Trommelfells mit Promontorium und Steigbügel. *Ibid.*, 1867, ii, 207–210. — **Spear** (E. D.) Remarks about the drum membrane, with cases. Boston M. & S. J., 1887, cxvii, 177–180.—**Swan** (J.) Observations on the tympanum as connected with deafness. Lond. M. Gaz., 1829–30, v, 8.—**Thomas** (L.) On certain abnormal movements in the membrana tympani producing cerebral symptoms. Lancet, Lond., 1877, ii, 837–840.—**Toynbee.** Series of preparations illustrative of the diseases of the membrana tympani. Tr. Path. Soc. Lond., 1849–50, ii, 273–275. ———. Preparations illustrative of hypertrophy in the epidermoid and dermoid laminæ of the membrana tympani. *Ibid.*, 1850–51, iii, 178. ———. Case of ulceration of the fibrous laminæ of the membrana tympani. *Ibid.*, 1852–3, iv, 251.—**von Tscharner.** Ueber die Trommelfellentzündung. Schweiz. Ztschr. f. Med., Chir. u. Geburtsh., Zürich, 1856, xii, 92–105.—**Turnbull** (C. L.) A case of calcareous degeneration of the membrana tympani. Proc. Phila. Co. M. Soc. 1879–80, Phila., 1880, ii, 13.— **Verdós Mauri** (P.) Miringitis parciales crónicas ; un nuevo capítulo para la patología del oido. Gac. méd. catal., Barcel., 1884, vii, 1–7, 1 pl.—**Voltolini** (R.) Die Krankheiten des Trommelfelles. Monatschr. f. Ohrenh., Berl., 1870, iv, 129 ; 137 : 1871, v, 1 ; 17.—**Weber** (F. E.) Bemerkungen über die Hörbeeinträchtigungen bei ganz oder theilweise zerstörtem Trommelfell, resp. defecten Gehörknöchelchen. *Ibid.*, 1868, ii, 9 ; 23. — **Webster** (D.) Case of polypoid granulations of the membrana tympani of ten years' standing cured by four applications of a fortygrain solution of nitrate of silver. Med. Rec., N. Y., 1871–2, vi, 199.—**Westropp** (T.) Case of collapsed membranæ tympanorum. Assoc. M. J., Lond., 1855, ii, 763–765.—**Wette.** Ein Fall von acuter desquamativer Entzündung des Trommelfells. Monatschr. f. Ohrenh., Berl., 1882, xvi, 33–35.

Membrana *tympani* (*Inflammation of*).

See **Ear** (*Diseases of, Catarrhal, etc.*); **Membrana** *tympani* (*Diseases of*).

Membrana *tympani* (*Paracentesis of*).

See **Ear** (*Diseases of, Catarrhal, etc.*); **Ear** (*Surgery of*); **Membrana** *tympani* (*Surgery of*).

Membrana *tympani* (*Perforation of*).

See **Membrana** *tympani* (*Surgery of*); **Membrana** *tympani* (*Wounds, etc., of*).

Membrana *tympani* (*Reproduction of*).

Burnett (C. H.) A rare case of restitution of the membrana tympani after fifteen years of disease. Phila. M. Times, 1872–3, iii, 502.—**Cheatham** (W.) A case of secondary drum membrane. Arch. Otol., N. Y., 1885, xiv, 11.—**Green** (J. O.), jr. Restoration of the membrana tympani after its almost complete destruction from chronic inflammation. Extr. Rec. Bost. Soc. M. Improve. (1866–74), 1876, vi, 158–160.—**Hinton** (J.) Case of restoration of a perforated and collapsed membrana tympani. Med. Press & Circ., Dubl., 1866, ii, 614.—**Richey** (S. O.) Restoration of the membrana tympani. Tr. Illinois M. Soc., Chicago, 1878, xxviii, 218–225. *Also,* Reprint. ———. A case of reproduction of the membrana tympani. Am. J. M. Sc., Phila., 1880, n. s., lxxix, 144–148. *Also,* Reprint.— **Spencer** (H. N.) A case of reproduction of the membrana tympani. Tr. Am. Otol. Soc., Bost., 1871, 39.— **Triquet.** De la reproduction de la membrane du tympan. Gaz. d. hôp., Par., 1865, xxxviii, 418.

Membrana *tympani* (*Rupture of*).

See **Membrana** *tympani* (*Wounds, etc., of*).

Membrana *tympani* (*Surgery of*).

See, also, **Ear** (*Surgery of*); **Membrana** *tympani* (*Artificial*).

BADIN (J.) * Sur la perforation artificielle du tympan. 4°. *Paris*, 1875.

BECK (J. S.) * De tympani perforatione in surditatis cura cautius rariusque adhibenda. 8°. *Erlangæ,* [1806].

Appears, also (with additions), under Harles (C. F.). *See infra.*

BLANCHE (A.-É.-P.) * Dissertation sur l'utilité de la perforation de la membrane du tympan, dans le cas de surdité causée par l'oblitération du conduit guttural. 4°. *Paris,* 1806.

BRUNNER (H. M.) * De tympanectomia. 12°. *Monachii,* 1842.

DELEAU (N.) Mémoire sur la perforation de la membrane du tympan, pratiquée pour rétablir l'ouïe dans plusieurs cas de surdité; avec des observations sur des sourds-muets et quelques considérations sur le développement de l'ouïe et de la parole. 8°. *Paris,* 1822.

FABRIZI (P.) Sopra un nuovo processo di praticare la perforazione della membrana del timpano e sulle malattie che la esigono. Memoria. 8°. *Livorno,* 1827.

Also, transl. in: J. d. progr. d. sc. méd., Par., 1828, vii, 153–166.

FUCHS (J. F.) * Disquisitiones de perforatione membranæ tympani, præcipue de vera hujus operationis indicatione exhibens. 4°. *Jenæ,* [1809].

GRAZZI (V.) Sulle perforazioni della membrana del timpano ; studi clinici e proposte. 8°. *Firenze,* 1884.

GRUBER (J.) Zur Lehre von der künstlichen Perforation des Trommelfelles. 8°. [*Budapest,* 1872.]

Repr. from: Pest. med.-chir. Presse, Budapest, 1872.

KOSEGARTEN (W.) Ueber eine künstliche Gehörsverbesserung bei grossen Trommelfellperforationen. Abhandlung zur Erlangung der Venia legendi. 8°. *Kiel,* 1884.

KÜHNEL (F. M.) * Die Paracentese des Trommelfells. 8°. *Leipzig,* 1868.

MIOT (C.) De la myringodectomie, ou perforation artificielle du tympan. 8°. *Paris,* 1877.

NIEUWENHUIS (L. C.) * Momenta quædam, de surditate per puncturam membranæ tympani curanda. 4°. *Traj. ad Rhenum,* [1807].

PHILIPEAUX (R.) Études sur la surdité. Recherches nouvelles sur la perforation artificielle du tympan. 8°. *Paris,* 1863.

See, also, infra.

SCHWARTZE (H.) Die Paracentese des Trommelfells. Ein Beitrag zur chirurgischen Behandlung der Ohrkrankheiten. 8°. *Halle a. S.,* 1868.

TRUCY (G.-H.) Considérations sur la perforation de la membrane du tympan, dans le cas de surdité causée par l'oblitération de la trompe d'Eustache. 8°. *Paris, an XI* [1802].

Membrana tympani (Surgery of).

Agnew (C. R.) Subacute inflammation of the middle ear, with fluid in the tympanic cavity; puncture of the drum-head; recovery. Arch. Otol., N. Y., 1879, viii, 76. ———. Subacute inflammation of the middle ear, with fluid in the tympanic cavity; relieved by puncture of the drum-head. *Ibid.*, 76.— **von Andrejewskiy.** Ueber die Heilung einer angebornen Taubheit und über ein neues Instrument zum Durchbohren des Trommelfells. J. d. Chir. u. Augenh., Berl., 1830, xiv, 589 - 599. — **Asbury** (J. V.) Strictures, in reply to Mr. Wright's objections to the operation of puncturing the membrana tympani. Med. & Phys. J., Lond., 1819, xli, 281 - 288. — **Balestra** (A. R.) Perforazione chirurgica della membrana del timpano. Boll. d. mal. d' orecchio, d. gola e d. naso, Firenze, 1886, iv, 33. — **Baratoux.** Inflammation chronique des trompes et des caisses avec adhérences multiples des tympans à la grande branche de l' enclume, à l'étrier et aux parties voisines; traitements divers; myringodectomie à gauche; guérison. Mouvement méd., Par., 1877, xv, 248. — **Bartlett** (E. W.) Paracentesis tympani. Tr. Wisconsin M. Soc., Milwaukee, 1876, x, 82-85. — **Berthold** (E.) Ueber Myringoplastik. Wien. med. Bl., 1878, i, 627 - 630. ———. Zwei weitere Fälle von durch seine Methode der Myringoplastik geheilten Trommelfellperforationen. Berl. klin. Wchnschr., 1886, xxiii, 587.— **Bing** (A.) Zur Paracentese des Trommelfells. Allg. Wien. med. Ztg., 1877, xxii, 110; 119; 148.— **Bishop** (S. S.) Operations on the drum-head for impaired hearing; with fourteen cases. J. Am. M. Ass., Chicago, 1886, vii, 232-235. *Also*, Reprint.— **Blake** (C. J.) Acupuncture and drainage in the treatment of serous effusion into the tympanic cavity. Tr. Am. Otol. Soc., Bost., 1875-8, ii, 226-229. ———. Application of paper dressings in treatment of perforations of the membrana tympani. Tr. Internat. Otol. Cong. 1876, N. Y., 1887, i, 125-132. *Also*, Reprint.— **Bonnafont.** Note sur un cas de surdité ancienne rebelle à tous les traitements ordinaires, guérie radicalement par la trépanation de la membrane du tympan pratiquée par un nouveau procédé. Mouvement méd., Par., 1877, xv, 339-341. *Also*: Gaz. d. hôp., Par., 1877, l, 692-694. *Also*: Union méd., Par., 1877, 3. s., xxiv, 113-118. *Also*: Ann. d. mal. de l'oreille et du larynx, Par., 1877, iii, 251-256.— **Brunner** (H. M.) Ueber die Durchbohrung des Paukenfells (Excisio membranæ tympani). Allg. Ztg. f. Chir., München, 1841, i, 131 ; 163.— **Burnett** (C. H.) Tympanic trephine. Tr. Am. Otol. Soc., Bost., 1873, 109.— **Butcher** (R. G. H.) On puncturing the membrane of the tympanum. Dublin M. Press, 1846, xv, 196-198. *Also*: Med. Times, Lond., 1846, xiv, 44.— **Cassells** (J. P.) On parakentesis of the membrana tympani; observations historical and clinical. Glasgow M. J., 1874, [4. s.], vi, 198. [Discussion], 271.— **Chimani** (R.) Ueber die Wirkungsweise der Methode von Dr. A. Politzer zur Behandlung des eitrigen Mittelohrkatarrhs mit Perforation des Trommelfelles. Wien. med. Wchnschr., 1867, xvii, 531; 548.— **Cumberbatch** (A. E.) Paracentesis of the membrana tympani for mucous accumulation in the tympanum. St. Barth. Hosp. Rep., Lond., 1876, xii, 171-174.— **Dalby** (W. B.) Perforations of the membrana tympani. Lancet, Lond., 1870, ii, 251.— **Deleau.** Réponse au mémoire de M. Bonnafont sur la perforation de la membrane du tympan. Union méd., Par., 1877, 3. s., xxiv, 477-479.— **Fabrizj** (P.) Sopra un nuovo processo di praticare la perforazione della membrana del timpano con esportazione di parte. Ann. univ. di med., Milano, 1830, lv, 236 - 283, 1 pl. ———. De la perforation de la membrane du tympan. Gaz. d. hôp., Par., 1839, 2. s., i, 331.— **Giampietro** (E.) Trapanazione della membrana del timpano. Atti. Cong. gen. d. Ass. med. ital. 1878, Pisa, 1879, viii, 434-453. ———. La perforazione del timpano a scopo terapeutico. Salute: Italia med., Genova, 1881, 2. s., xv, 369. ———. Lo speculum perforante nella paracentesi del timpano. Arch. internaz. di otojat., rinojat. ed aeroterap., Napoli, 1885. i, 17-21. ———. Della miringotomia; indicazioni e metodi. Gior. internaz. d. sc. med., Napoli, 1886, n. s., viii, 288-302.— **Giommi** (M.) Della perforazione del timpano nell' otite interna cronica e principalmente della sua cura. Raccoglitore med., Forlì, 1873, xxiii, 225-243.— **Gomez de la Mata** (F.) La perforacion artificial del timpano. Gac. de oftal., otol. y laringol., Madrid, 1886, i, 6; 32. — **Grazzi** (V.) Sur la perforation du tympan, et un nouvel instrument pour la pratiquer. Cong. période. internat. d'otol. Compt.-rend. 1880, Trieste, 1882, ii, 84 - 87. ———. Instruments pour la perforation artificielle du tympan. Bull. de l'arsenal méd.-chir., Par., 1883-4, i, 93.— **Gruber** (J.) Die Myringodectomie als Heilmittel gegen Schwerhörigkeit und Ohrensausen. Allg. Wien. med. Ztg., 1864, ix, 97; 121; 145; 161; 177; 186. ———. Beitrag zur Lehre von der Paracenthese der Trommelhöhle. *Ibid.*, 1871, xvi, 173 ; 181; 200. ———. Die mehrfache Durchschneidung des Trommelfells als Heilmittel gegen primäre oder mit Trübung einhergehende übermässige Spannung desselben. *Ibid.*, 1873, xviii, 2; 17; 33; 49. *Also*: Monatschr. f. Ohrenh., Berl., 1873, vii, 63-66. ———. Beitrag zur Lehre und Casuistik der mehrfachen Durchschneidung des Trommelfells behufs Minderung der abnormen Span-

Membrana tympani (Surgery of).

nung desselben. Allg. Wien. med. Ztg., 1876, xxi, 295; 303 ; 311 ; 319. ———. Ueber Durchschneidung der hinteren Trommelfellfalte zu Heilzwecken. Mitth. d. Wien. med. Doct.-Coll., 1881, vii, 116-119. *Also*: Allg. Wien. med. Ztg., 1881, xxvi, 123; 135.— **Guye.** Paracentesis membr. tympani. Werk. v. h. Genootsch. t. Bevord. d. Nat.-, Genees- en Heelk. te Amst., 1871-2, ii, 23. ———. Paracentese van het trommelvlies. *Ibid.*, 1875, iv, pt. 1, 7-22.— **Harles** (C. F.) De membranæ tympani perforatione in surditatis cura rarius cautiusque adhibenda. *In his:* Opera minora Acad. med. [etc.], 8°, Lips., 1815. i, 189-230.— **Harvey** (W.) On the treatment of perforation of the membrana tympani by operation. Med. Times, Lond., 1850, xxi, 135.— **Heiman** (T.) O przedziurawieniach błony bębenkowej. [On perforation of membrana tympani.] Gaz. lek., Warszawa, 1886, 2. s., vi, 929; 962; 981; 1005; 1030.— **Hewetson** (H. B.) The immediate improvement of hearing following division of cicatrices in the membrana tympani. Brit. M. J., Lond., 1885, ii, 735.— **Hinton** (J.) On accumulation of mucus within the tympanum, and its treatment by incision of the membrana tympani. Guy's Hosp. Rep., Lond., 1869, 3. s., xiv, 149-164.— **van Hoek** (J.) De doorboring van het trommelvlies, als hulpmiddel ter genezing van acuten en chronischen katarrh der trommelholte. Nederl. Tijdschr. v. Heel- en Verlosk., Utrecht, 1866-9, xvi, 376-382.— **Hufeland** (C. W.) Fragmentarische Bemerkungen über die Durchbohrung des Trommelfells zur Kur der Taubheit. J. d. pract. Arznk. u. Wundarznk., Berl., 1806, xxiv, 3. St., 163-169.— **Hunold** (P.) Wiederherstellung des Gehörs mittelst Durchbohrung des Trommelfells, durch zahlreiche Versuche bestätigt. *Ibid.*, 2. St., 172 - 178. — **Kaurin** (E.) Paracentesis membranæ tympani. Norsk Mag. f. Lægevidensk., Christiania, 1876, vi, 583 - 594. — **Kern** (V.) Ueber die Durchbohrung des Trommelfelles. Med. Jahrb. d. k. k. österr. Staates, Wien, 1813-14, ii, 3. pt., 121-132.— **Lévi.** Des divers moyens proposés pour maintenir ouverte une perforation chirurgicale de la membrane du tympan. Ann. d. mal. de l'oreille et du larynx, Par., 1875, i, 349-358.— **Longhi** (G.) Sulla perforazione della membrana del timpano. Gazz. med. ital. lomb., Milano, 1875, 7. s., ii, 65 ; 81.— **M'Keown.** A new method of keeping perforation of the membrana tympani open. Med. Press & Circ.. Lond., 1886, n. s., xli, 215. *Also*: Dublin J. M. Sc., 1886, 3. s., lxxxi, 357-359.— **Maunoir** (J.-P.) Observation sur une maladie de l'organe de l'ouïe, guérie radicalement par la perforation de la membrane du tympan. J. de méd., chir., pharm., etc., Par., 1815, ix, 106 - 110. — **Mercer** (J.) On deafness, caused by hemorrhage into the cavity of the tympanum, successfully treated by perforation of the membrane; with statistic observations on the results of this operation generally. North. J. M., Edinb., 1844, i, 353-361. *Also*, Reprint.— **Millingen** (E.) Sur la perforation artificielle du tympan et le moyen d'assurer sa permanence. Gaz. méd. d'Orient, Constantinople, 1870-71, xiv, 84-87.— **Nasse.** Bemerkungen über A. Cooper's Durchbohrung des Trommelfells. J. d. pract. Arznk. u. Wundarznk., Berl., 1807, xxv, 4. St., 168-190. — **Noyes** (J. F.) Paracentesis membranæ tympani, with an illustrative case. Detroit Rev. Med. & Pharm., 1870, v, 395-400.— **Paquet** (A.) Nouveau procédé de myringodectomie applicable au traitement de l'otite scléreuse. Ann. d. mal. de l'oreille et du larynx, Par., 1881, vii, 187-198. ———. Myringodectomie par formation d'un lambeau à base supérieure adhérente et à sommet inférieur libre. Bull. et mém. Soc. de chir. de Par., 1881, n. s., vii, 332-336.— **Philipeaux** (R.) Mémoire sur la perforation de la membrane du tympan. Ann. Soc. de méd. de Lyon, 1863, 2. s., xi, 152-230. *Also*: Gaz. méd. de Lyon, 1863, xx, 385; 406; 426; 444 ; 468. [*See, also, supra.*]— **Politzer** (A.) Ueber ein Verfahren zum Offenhalten künstlicher Perforationsöffnungen im Trommelfelle. Wien. med. Wchnschr., 1868, xviii, 1567; 1581; 1869, xix, 533. *Also*, Reprint. ——— Plastische Darstellung der Continuitätsstörungen und Wölbungsanomalien des Trommelfelles. Arch. f. Ohrenh., Leipz., 1876, xi, 31-33.— **Pollak** (J.) Ueber den Werth von Operationen, die den Schnitt des Paukenfells erheischen. Allg. Wien. med. Ztg., 1880, xxv, 484 ; 492 ; 505. *Also, transl.*: Med. Press & Circ., Lond., 1881, n. s., xxxi, 114; 489.— **Pomeroy** (O. D.) Cases illustrating some of the results of paracentesis of the membrana tympani, and of the introduction of Politzer's eyelet. Tr. Am. Otol. Soc., Bost., 1873, 92-106. *Also*, Reprint.— **Prout** (J. S.) Paracentesis of the drum-membrane; the conservative, and not "heroic", treatment of severe inflammation of the middle ear. Proc. M. Soc. County Kings, Brooklyn, 1878, iii, 176-178.— **Purves** (W. L.) Trepanation of the membrana tympani. Guy's Hosp. Rep., Lond., 1875, 3. s., xx, 563. ———. One hundred cases of paracentesis of the tympanic membrane, with the results obtained therefrom, and remarks on the methods of operation. Med.-Chir. Tr., Lond., 1878, lxi, 189-200.— **Ribes.** De la perforation de la membrane du tympan. J. de méd., chir., pharm., etc., Par., 1816, xxxv, 222-234.— **Roosa** (D. B. St. J.) On the value of operations in which the membrana tympani is incised. Tr. Am. Otol. Soc., Bost., 1881, ii, pt. 5, 448-463. *Also*: Arch. Otol., N. Y., 1881, x, 181-183. *Also, transl.*: Ztschr. f. Ohrenh.,

Membrana *tympani* (*Surgery of*).

Wiesb., 1881–2, xi, 1–3. [Discussion], 23–25.—**de Salazar** (P.) Memoria sobre la perforacion de la membrana del timpano. Bol. de med., cirug. y farm., Madrid, 1839, vi, 57; 66.—**Sapolini** (G.) Della perforazione della membrana del timpano. Ann. univ. di med., Milano, 1867, cxcix, 298.—**Schurig** (E.) Günstiger Erfolg der künstlichen Ruptur einer Trommelfellnarbe mittelst des Politzer'schen Verfahrens. Wien. med. Presse, 1868, ix, 482. ——. Ueber die Paracentese des Trommelfells. Jahresb. d. Gesellsch. f. Nat.- u. Heilk. in Dresd., 1870, 34–42.— **Schwartze** (H.) La paracentèse du tympan; contribution au traitement chirurgical des affections de l'oreille. J. de méd., chir. et pharmacol., Brux., 1871, lii, 17; 135; 209; 291. *Also*, Reprint. ——. Weitere Erfahrungen und Bemerkungen über die Paracentese des Trommelfells. Arch. f. Ohrenh., Würzb., 1873, vi, 171–199.—**Solera** (G.) Sulla perforazione della membrana del timpano. Ann. univ. di med., Milano, 1830, liii, 81–90.—**Turnbull** (L.) Artificial perforation of the membrana tympani. Med. & Surg. Reporter. Phila., 1877, xxxvii, 361–365. *Also*, Reprint. — **Voltolini** (R.) Die Perforation des Trommelfelles mittelst der Galvanocaustik. Monatschr. f. Ohrenh., Berl., 1867, i, 37–43. ——. De la perforation de la membrane du tympan; énumération des différents procédés employés pour cette opération. J. de méd., chir. et pharmacol., Brux., 1868, xlvii, 201–210. ——. Ueber die Perforation des Trommelfells. Monatschr. f. Ohrenh., Berl., 1870, iv, 140–148. ——. Ueber eine neue Operation am Trommelfelle zur Verbesserung des Gehörvermögens. Berl. klin. Wchnschr., 1873, x, 618. *Also*: Monatschr. f. Ohrenh., Berl., 1874, viii, 12–15. ——. Die ringförmige Canule zum Offenhalten einer künstlichen Perforations-Oeffnung im Trommelfelle. Monatschr. f. Ohrenh., Berl., 1874, viii, 33–38. ——. Etwas zur Perforation des Trommelfelles. *Ibid.*, 74. ——. Hochgradige Schwerhörigkeit, excessive subjective Geräusche, Perforation des Trommelfells; Durchschneidung der Sehne des M. tensor tympani. *Ibid.*, 1876, x, 149–154. ——. Ueber das Offenhalten einer künstlichen Oeffnung im Trommelfelle und die ringförmige Canule. *Ibid.*, 1878, xii, 1–7. — **W.** (A.) Case of deafness effectually cured by puncture of the membrana tympani. Lancet, Lond., 1840, ii, 334–336. — **Weber-Liel** (F. E.) Zur Illustration der von mir vorgeschlagenen Methode, eine persistente Oeffnung im Trommelfell zu erzielen. Monatschr. f. Ohrenh., Berl., 1875, ix, 41–46.—**Yearsley** (J.) Operation of puncturing the membrana tympani in deafness. Lond. M. Gaz., 1841, xxviii, 430–433.

Membrana *tympani* (*Trephining of*).

See **Membrana** *tympani* (*Surgery of*).

Membrana *tympani* (*Tumors of*).

See, also, **Ear** (*Cancer, etc., of*).

Buck (A. H.) Vascular tumors of the membrana tympani. Tr. Am. Otol. Soc., Bost., 1881, ii, pt. 5, 503. *Also*, Reprint. *Also*: Am. J. Otol., N. Y., 1881, iii, 282.— **Moos** (S.) Ueber ein thraumatisches wanderndes Hämatom des Trommelfelles. Ztschr. f. Ohrenh., Wiesb., 1879, viii, 32–36.—**Suñé y Molist** (L.) Pólipo célulo-globular del disco timpánico; utilidad diagnóstica y terapéutica del acido crómico. Sentido catól., Barcel., 1880, ii, 181–184.

Membrana *tympani* (*Wounds and injuries of*).

See, also, **Membrana** *tympani* (*Surgery of*).

Hendriksz (M. A.) * De perforatione membranæ tympani. 4°. *Groningæ*, [1828].

Herz (J.) * Ueber traumatische Rupturen des Trommelfells. 8°. *Würzburg*, 1873.

Kauerz (J. H.) * De perforatione membranæ tympani. 4°. *Argentorati*, 1807.

Neuss (J. H. G.) * De perforatione membranæ tympani. 4°. *Gottingæ*, 1802.

Agnew (C. R.) Acute inflammation of the middle ear apparently caused by rupture of the drum-head while blowing the nose. Arch. Otol., N. Y., 1879, viii, 75. ——. Rupture of the membrana tympani. Med. Rec., N. Y., 1880, xviii, 169–171.—**Agnew** (C. R.) & **Webster** (D.) Double rupture of the membrana tympani from a blow. Arch. Otol., N. Y., 1881, x, 339. *Also, transl.*: Ztschr. f. Ohrenh., Wiesb., 1882, xi, 180.—**Alden** (C. H.) Report of a case of repeated rupture of the membrana tympani by discharges of artillery, with concussion of the auditory nerves and total deafness; result, discharge from service. Rep. Surg.-Gen. Army, Wash., 1885–6, 87. — **Amick** (W. R.) Can a physician recommend a person with a perforated membrana tympani to a life insurance company? Cincin. M. News, 1880, n. s., ix, 793–799. — **Bacon** (G.) Traumatic lesions of the membrana tympani. Med. Rec., N. Y., 1885, xxvii, 403. ——. Injury to the membrana tympani from the twig of a tree. Tr. Am. Otol. Soc., New Bedford, 1882–6, iii, 541. — **Baizeau.** Observation de rupture des deux membranes du tympan, produite par la

Membrana *tympani* (*Wounds and injuries of*).

détonation d'une pièce d'artillerie. Alger méd.; 1873, i, 39. — **Baratoux** (J.) De la perforation du tympan; de ses cicatrices; moyens d'y remédier. Rev. mens. de laryngol., etc., Bordeaux, 1882, iii, 333–343. *Also* [Abstr.]: Rev. de thérap. méd.-chir., Par., 1882, [xxxi], 603. *Also* [Abstr.]: Progrès méd., Par., 1882, x, 944. *Also, transl.* [Abstr.]: Rev. de terap. y farm., Madrid, 1882–3, i, 177. *Also, transl.* [Abstr.]: An. de otol. y laringol., Alcalá de Henares, 1883, i, 37–39.—**Baumgarten** (E.) Beitrag zur Kenntniss der Trommelfellrupturen. Arch. f. Ohrenh., Leipz., 1885–6, xxiii, 31–33. — **Bezold** (F.) Verbrühung des Trommelfells. *Ibid.*, 1881–2, xviii, 49–58. — **Bing** (A.) Zur Perforation des Trommelfelles. Allg. Wien. med. Ztg., 1873, xviii, 484.—**Blake** (C. J.) Ruptured membrana tympani and perception of high tones. Boston M. & S. J., 1873, lxxxviii, 628. ——. A curious result following cicatrix of the membrana tympani. *Ibid.*, 1875, xcii, 692. ——. Treatment of perforations of the membrana tympani. *Ibid.*, 1876, xciv, 42. ——. Application of paper dressings in treatment of perforations of the membrana tympani. Rep. Cong. Internat. Otol. Soc. 1876, N. Y., 1877, 125–132. ——. Manometric cicatrix of the membrana tympani. Arch. Ophth. & Otol., N. Y., 1876, v, 280–282. ——. Manometric cicatrix of the membrana tympani. Am. J. Otol., N. Y., 1880, ii, 201–203. — **Booth** (J. M.) A case of rupture of the tympanum, with paralysis of the face. Brit. M. J., Lond., 1881, i, 922. — **Bos** (A.) Rottura spontanea della membrana del tympano. Imparziale, Firenze, 1866, vi, 231–240. — **Breton.** Observation de perforation par traumatisme de la membrane du tympan; guérison complète et rapide. Rec. de mém. de méd. . . . mil., Par., 1881, xxxvii, 579–581. — **Burnett** (C. H.) Accidental evulsion of the membrana tympani and the ossicles of hearing. Tr. Am. Otol. Soc., Bost., 1872, 50–53. ——. Reflex ulceration in the external auditory canal, with perforation of the membrana tympani, produced by diseased teeth. Am. J. Otol., N. Y., 1880, ii, 285–291. ——. Perforations in the membrana flaccida, the tympanic diseases they accompany, and their treatment. *Ibid.*, 1881, iii, 12–25. — **Casanova** (P.) Perforaciones de la membrana del tímpano. Crón. méd., Valencia, 1879–80, iii, 93; 125; 253; 285; 509. — **Cassellis** (J.) On injuries of the membrana tympani. Glasgow M. J., 1876, [4. s.], viii, 307–323. — **Clarke** (E. H.) Observations on the causes, effects, and treatment of perforation of the membrana tympani. Am. J. M. Sc., Phila., 1858, n. s., xxxv, 13–51. — **Core** (A. S.) Rupture of the drum-head from a box on the ear; recovery complete. Peoria M. Month., 1881–2, ii, 128.—**Cottman** (J. B.) General erethism produced by injury of the membrana tympani. Med. Exam., Phila., 1846, n. s., ii, 521–523.—**Dalby** (W. B.) Perforations of the membrana tympani. Lancet, Lond., 1870, i, 579: ii, 252: 1871, ii, 257; 318. ——. On traumatic rupture of the tympanic membrane. [5 cases.] Tr. Clin. Soc. Lond., 1873, vi, 178–182.—**Demoulin** (A.) Rupture traumatique du tympan par cause indirecte; otite moyenne suppurée consécutive. Gaz. méd. de Par., 1884, 7. s., i, 232.— **Dills** (T. J.) A case of rupture of the drumhead from a box on the ear; rapid and complete recovery. Arch. Otol., N. Y., 1880, ix, 154. *Also, transl.*: Ztschr. f. Ohrenh., Wiesb., 1880, ix, 367–369.—**Field** (G. P.) An analysis of five hundred cases of perforation of the membrana tympani. Med. Press & Circ., Lond., 1880, n. s., xxx, 85; 169; 191.—**Fritsche** (G.) Czy może nastąpić pęknięcie błony bębenkowej skutkiem uderzenia w twarz? [Was the rupture of the membrana tympani caused by a blow on the head?] Medycyna, Warszawa, 1876, iv, 509–511.—**Galligo** (I.) Sulla rottura così detta spontanea della membrana del timpano in generale, ed in ispecie circa una di lei maniera di perforarsi fino ad ora non dimostrata da fatti inconcussi. Gazz. med. ital. feder. tosc., Firenze, 1850–51, 2. s., i, 473; 486.—**Gruber** (J.) Verletzung des Trommelfells. Aerztl. Ber. d. k. k. allg. Krankenh. zu Wien (1867), 1868, 337–345. ——. Ueber eine seltene Form der Continuitätstrennung im Trommelfell. Allg. Wien. med. Ztg., 1868, xiii, 123; 132; 148. ——. Narben des Trommelfelles. Aerztl. Ber. d. k. k. allg. Krankenh. zu Wien (1873), 1874, 255.—**Hallinan** (J. B.) Perforation of the tympanum; deafness; recovery. Boston M. & S.J., 1858, lviii, 93–96.—**Healy** (W.) Rupture of the membrana tympani, the effect of accident. Dublin Hosp. Gaz., 1854, n. s., i, 41.—**Heiman** (T.) Przypadek urazowego potrójnego pęknięcia błony bębenkowej z zejściem śmiertelnem. [Rupture of membrana tympani terminating in death.] Gaz. lek., Warszawa, 1885, 2. s., v, 191; 221. — **Hessler** (H.) Traumatische Ruptur eines in Folge chronischen sklerosirenden Mittelohrkatarrhs verdickten Trommelfells. Arch. f. Ohrenh., Leipz., 1881, xvii, 52. — **Hewetson** (H. B.) A case of rupture of the right membrana tympani during an attack of vomiting. Lancet, Lond., 1875, ii, 417.—**Hinton** (J.) Perforated membrana tympani and the Eustachian tube. *Ibid.*, 1866, i, 481. ——. On the treatment of perforations of the membrana tympani. Guy's Hosp. Rep., Lond., 1871, 3. s., xvi, 241–246.— **Holmes** (E. L.) Perforation of the membrana tympani,

Membrana *tympani* (*Wounds and injuries of*).

with scarcely a symptom of disease. Rep. Cong. Internat. Otol. Soc. 1876, N. Y., 1877, 113.—**Jacob** (G.) Perforation bilatérale du tympan. Mém. et compt.-rend. Soc. d. sc. méd. de Lyon (1883), 1884, xxiii, pt. 2, 103.—**Lichtenberg** (K.) Adatok a dobhártya traumájához. [Upon wounds of the membrana tympani.] Gyógyászat, Budapest, 1881, xxi, 217–222. *Also, transl.:* Pest. med.-chir. Presse, Budapest, 1881, xvii, 437–442.—**Magnus** (A.) Ausgedehnte Zerreissung des Trommelfells mit vollständiger Heilung. Arch. f. Ohrenh., Würzb., 1867, ii, 43–47. ———. Die Zersprengung des Trommelfelles infolge von Schlägen. Allg. Wien. med. Ztg., 1880, xxv, 24.—**Millingen** (E.) Cicatrices of the membrana tympani. Boston M. & S. J., 1871, lxxxiv, 229.—**Moos** (S.) Ueber ein traumatisches wanderndes Hämatom des Trommelfelles. Ztschr. f. Ohrenh. Wiesb., 1879, viii, 32–36. *Also, transl.:* Arch. Otol., N. Y., 1879, viii, 332–335. ———. Rupture des deux tympans, par compression de l'air à la suite d'explosion de l'éther chlorophtalique pendant la préparation de l'éosine. Bull. et mém. Soc. franç. d'otol. et laryngol., Par., 1883–4, i, 208.—**Oppolzer.** Durchbohrung des Paukenfells und Catarrh der Paukenhöhle. Allg. Wien. med. Ztg., 1857, ii, 241.—**Parreidt.** Fall von traumatischer Ruptur des Trommelfells mit Symptomen von Labyrinthreizung. Arch. f. Ohrenh., Leipz., 1874, ix, 179.—**Pflüger.** Zur Casuistik der Trommelfellrupturen; Trommelfellruptur durch Wellenschlag. Monatschr. f. Ohrenh., Berl., 1874, viii, 144. ———. Trommelfellruptur durch Explosion. *Ibid.*, 145.—**Pierce** (F. M.) Two cases of traumatic perforation of the membrana tympani. Specialist, Lond., 1880–81, i, 25.—**Politzer** (A.) Ueber die günstigen Resultate der durch Luftdruck erzeugten Rupturen dünner Trommelfellnarben. Wien. med. Presse, 1868, ix, 6; 39; 94; 116. *Also,* Reprint. ———. Ueber Trommelfellnarben. Wien. med. Wchnschr., 1871, xxi, 9; 33. *Also,* Reprint. *Also, transl.* [Abstr.]: Med. Times & Gaz., Lond., 1871, i, 244. ———. Ueber traumatische Trommelfellrupturen mit besonderer Rücksicht auf die forensische Praxis. Wien. med. Wchnschr., 1872, xxii, 881; 901. *Also,* Reprint.—**Prat.** Perforation traumatique du tympan, datant de deux mois, guérie par une seule irrigation d'eau tiède. Bull. gén. de thérap., etc., Par., 1869, lxxvi, 516. *Also:* Union méd., Par., 1869, 3. s., vii, 775.—**Prout** (J. S.) On the use of adhesive rubber plaster in cases of perforation of the membrana tympani. Tr. Am. Otol. Soc., New Bedford, 1882–6, iii, 686.—**Prussak** (A. F.) Po povodu otverstii v baraban. pereponkie. [Cases of rupture of membrana tympani.] Ejened klin. gaz., St. Petersb., 1886, vi, 53; 76; 102.—**Ravogli** (A.) Rupture of the membrana tympani by an injury of the skull. Cincin. Lancet & Clinic, 1885, n. s., xv, 649–653. *Also* [Abstr.]: Med. & Surg. Reporter, Phila., 1885, liii, 654.—**Ray** (J. M.) Rupture of both membranæ tympani from a fall on the head; escape of blood followed by a watery discharge; fracture of the tympanic portion of both temporal bones. Arch. Otol., N. Y., 1886, xv, 192–194. *Also, transl.:* Ztschr. f. Ohrenh., Wiesb., 1887, xvii, 65–67.—**Reynolds** (L. W.) Case of perforation of membrana tympani from ascaris lumbricoides. Lancet, Lond., 1880, ii, 653.—**Rumbold** (T. F.) The tuning-fork as a means for diagnosing perforation of the membrana tympani. Med. Rec., N. Y., 1874, ix, 174.—**Sajous** (C. É.) Perforating wounds and injuries of the membrana tympani. Med. & Surg. Reporter, Phila., 1879, xl, 161–163.—**Schlesinger** (Z. V.) A dobhártya sérüléseiröl. [Lesions of membrana tympani] Gyógyászat, Budapest, 1885, xxv, 347; 366; 382; 397; 414; 430; 447. *Also, transl.* [Abstr.]: Pest. med.-chir. Presse, Budapest, 1886, xxii, 237–239. — **Schrauth** (C.) Traumatische Trommelfellruptur; Erschütterung des Labyrinthes. Aerztl. Int.-Bl., München, 1882, xxix, 176.— **Schreiber.** Beiträge zur Heilung der Trommelfellperforation. Wien. Med.-Halle, 1864, v, 323; 342.—**Shaw** (H. L.) Three cases of traumatic perforation of the membrana tympani. Boston M. & S. J., 1868–9, lxxix, 257–259. *Also:* Extr. Rec. Bost. Soc. M. Improve. (1866–74), 1878, vi, app., 69–73. ———. Traumatic injuries of the membrana tympani, with cases. Boston M. & S. J., 1870, lxxxii, 269–274.—**Snell** (S.) Case of rupture of the membrana tympani from blows on the ear. Lancet, Lond., 1875, ii, 275.—**Spalding** (J. A.) On the traumatic rupture of the membrana tympani. Tr. Maine M. Ass., Portland, 1881, vii, pt. 2, 358–360.—**Tangeman** (C. W.) Rupture [of the] membranæ tympani. Nashville J. M. & S., 1886, n. s., xxxvii, 59–62.—**Torrance** (R.) Rupture of the membrana tympani, with diffuse myringitis; the result of a snowball. Brit. M. J., Lond., 1881, i, 191.—**Toynbee** (J.) On the treatment of perforate membrana tympani. Lancet, Lond., 1866, i, 309.—**Trautmann.** Ueber die Continuitätstrennungen des Trommelfells. Deutsche mil.-ärztl. Ztschr., Berl., 1873, ii, 422–434.—**Triquet.** Des perforations de la membrane du tympan. Gaz. d. hôp., Par., 1865, xxxviii, 113; 121.—**Turnbull** (C. S.) Perforating wounds and injuries of the membrana tympani. Med. & Surg. Reporter, Phila., 1879, xl, 161–163. *Also,* Reprint. ———. Concerning two cases of perforation of the membrana tympani from

Membrana *tympani* (*Wounds and injuries of*).

ascaris lumbricoides, with remarks upon the curious habits of this human parasite. Med. & Surg. Reporter, Phila., 1881, xlv, 32–37.—**Verdós y Mauri** (P.) De las perforaciones timpánicas. Gac. méd. catal., Barcel., 1884, vii, 421–427, 1 pl.—**Voltolini.** Ueber die Perforation des Trommelfelles. Jahresb. d. schles. Gesellsch. f. vaterl. Kult. 1870, Bresl., 1871, xlviii, 182.—**Weber** (F. E.) On the difficulty of hearing in cases of perforation of the membrana tympani, and on the physiological and therapeutic importance of the tuba Eustachii in such cases. Lancet, Lond., 1866, i, 121; 173.—**Weil.** Einige Fälle von Ruptur des Trommelfells. Memorabilien, Heilbr., 1880, xxv, 486–491.—**Wennerlund** (E.) Några anmärkningar om perforation à membrana tympani. Hygiea, Stockholm, 1863, xxv, 97–101.—**Wilson** (H. A.) Two cases of rupture of the membrana tympani caused by diving. Med. News, Phila., 1882, xli, 173.—**Zaufal** (E.) Casuistische Beiträge zu den traumatischen Verletzungen des Trommelfelles. Arch. f. Ohrenh., Leipz., 1873, vii, 188; 280: 1873-4, viii, 31–49. ———. Ueber Anwendung des Alkohols bei warzenförmigen Trommelfellperforationen. Wien. med. Presse, 1883, xxiv, 1575.

Membrane (*Pupillary*).

See Iris; Pupil (*Membrane of, Persistent*).

Membranes.

See, also, Anatomy (*General, etc.*)

BEREND (J. A. T.) * De mutua cutis et membranarum internarum relatione. 8°. *Halæ,* [1823].

BICHAT (M.-F.-X.) Traité des membranes en général et de diverses membranes en particulier. 8°. *Paris, an VIII* [1800].

———. The same. Nouv. éd. Revue et augmentée par M. Magendie. 8°. *Paris,* 1827.

———. The same. 8°. *Paris,* 1831.

———. The same. A treatise on the membranes in general, and on different membranes in particular. A new edition, enlarged by an historical notice of the life and writings of the author; by M. Husson, Paris, 1802. Transl. by John G. Coffin. 8°. *Boston, Cambridge,* 1813.

See, also, infra.

BONN (A.) * De continuationibus membranarum. 4°. *Lugd. Bat.,* 1763.

Also, in: SANDIFORT. Thesaurus diss. [etc.] 4°. *Roterodami,* 1769, ii, 265–306, 1 pl.

BÜCHNER (G. P.) * De nonnullis notatu dignioribus membranarum mucosarum et serosarum morbis. 4°. *Lugd. Bat.,* 1826.

HIS (W.) Die Häute und Höhlen des Körpers. 4°. *Basel,* 1865.

LUDWIG (C. F.) De membranarum ortu. sm. 4°. *Lipsiæ,* 1778.

Bichat (M.-F.-X.) Dissertation sur les membranes, et sur leurs rapports généraux d'organisation. Mém. Soc. méd. d'émulat. de Par., an vii [1799], ii, 371–385. [*See, also, supra.*]—**Davy** (J.) On the action of vinegar on animal textures. *In his:* Researches, Phys. & Anat., 8°. Lond., 1839, i, 376–383. ———. Experiments and observations on the maceration in water of different textures of the human body. *Ibid.*, ii, 372–412. ———. General remarks on Bichat's theory of membranes in connection with the preceding observations. *Ibid.*, 413–426.—**Gunning** (J. W.) Ueber Imbibition thierischer Membrane. Arch. f. d. holländ. Beitr. z. Nat- u. Heilk., Utrecht, 1860, ii, 245–259.—**Kollmann.** Structurlose Membranen bei Wirbelthieren und Wirbellosen. Sitzungsb. d. math.-phys. Cl. d. k.-bayer. Akad. d. Wissensch. zu München, 1876, vi, 163–192.—**Villermé** (L.-R.) Membranes fibreuses, albugineuses. Dict. d. sc. méd., Par., 1819, xxxii, 230–245.—**Wrisberg** (H. A.) Commentatio de membranarum ac involucrorum corporis humani continuationibus partim dubiis partim veris. *In his:* Comment. med. physiol., etc., 8°, Gottingæ, 1800, i, 343–362.

Membranes (*False*).

See, also, Croup (*Pathology of*); Diphtheria; Diphtheria (*Pathology of*); Intestines (*Concretions, etc., of*); Pleurisy (*Complications, etc., of*); Pleurisy (*Pathology of*); Pseudoplasmata.

NEPPLE (P.-F.) * Dissertation de physiologie pathologique sur les fausses membranes et les adhérences. 4°. *Paris,* 1812.

Membranes (False).

VILLERMÉ (L.-R.) *Essai sur les fausses membranes. 4°. *Paris*, 1814.
See, also, infra.

Balser (H.) Entwicklung quergestreifter Muskelfasern in Pseudomembranen. Ztschr. f. rat. Med., Heidelb., 1846, iv, 17-20. — **Barth.** [Production pseudomembraneuse remarquable, qui a été rejetée par un malade atteint de pleuro-pneumonie.] Bull. Soc. anat. de Par., 1852, xxvii, 103.—**Chomel.** Pseudomembranes. Dict. de méd., 2. éd., Par., 1842, xxvi, 246-262.—**Coxe** (J. R.) On the discharge of various matters from the trachea. Am. J. M. Sc., Phila., 1828, iii, 243.—**Debest de Lacrousille** (A.) Des pseudo-membranes vasculaires ou organisées, des séreuses en général et du péricarde en particulier. France méd., Par., 1865, xii, 441; 450; 457; 466.—**Hallier** (E.) Ueber eine pseudo-diphtheritische Membran. Arch. f. path. Anat., etc., Berl., 1866, xxxvi. 160.—**Klob** (J.) Die Pseudomembranen auf serösen Häuten. Ztschr. d. k.-k. Gesellsch. d. Aerzte zu Wien, 1860, xvi, 561-563. — **Laborde.** [Fausses membranes provenant d'un chien sur lequel on avait essayé de pratiquer la trachéotomie.] Bull. Soc. anat. de Par., 1864, xxxix, 85-87.—**Lassaigne** (J.-L.) Sur la composition des fausses membranes. J. de chim. méd., etc., Par., 1825, i, 68-71. ———. Nouvelles recherches sur la composition chimique des fausses membranes chez l'homme. J. gén. de méd., chir. et pharm., Par., 1826, xciv, 294-299.— **Laugier.** Examen chimique de fausses membranes recueillies sur la plèvre d'une femme décédée à la suite d'une pleuro-pneumonie. J. de chim. méd., etc., Par., 1827, iii, 419-423.—**Law** (R.) Pathological affections and relations of false membranes. Dublin Q. J. M. Sc., 1855, xix, 60-72.— **Leloir** (H.) Contribution à l'étude de la structure et du développement des productions pseudo-membraneuses, sur les muqueuses et sur la peau. Arch. de physiol. norm. et path., Par., 1880, 2. s., vii, 420-458, 1 pl.—**Ozanam** (C.) Mémoire sur les dissolvants et les désagrégeants des produits pseudo-membraneux, et sur l'emploi du brome dans ces maladies. Rev. de thérap. méd.-chir., Par., 1868, xxxv, 5; 484.—**Pigné** (J.-B.) Histoire anatomique et physiologique des pseudo-membranes. Bull. Soc. anat. de Par., 1843, xviii, 349-362. *Also*, Reprint.—**Ramsey** (F. A.) Membranous formations on mucous surfaces. Atlanta M. & S. J., 1872-3, x, 226.—**Roussel** (H.) Nouveau traitement des affections pseudo-membraneuses. Rev. de thérap. méd.-chir., Par., 1876, xliii, 547.—**Shattuck.** False membrane from the pleura, containing a large cavity. Boston M. & S. J., 1865, lxxii, 182.—**Villermé** (L.-R.) Membrane (fausse). Dict. d. sc. méd., Par., 1819, xxxii, 245-269. [*See, also, supra.*]

Membranes (Fœtal).

See Amnion; Chorion; Decidua; Embryology; Labor (*Abnormities of*); Placenta.

Membranes (Mucous).

See, also, Intestines; Mucus; Nose (*Mucous membranes of*); Skin.

AUBERT (L.-R.) *Des muqueuses. 4°. *Paris*, 1833.

BICHAT (M.-F.-X.) A treatise on the anatomy and physiology of the mucous membranes; with illustrative pathological observations; from the French by Jas. Houlton. 8°. *London*, 1821.

DE BORDEU (T.) Recherches sur le tissu muqueux, ou l'organe cellulaire, et sur quelques maladies de la poitrine. Nouv. éd. sm. 8°. *Paris*, 1791.

DE BRANDT (A.) *Nonnulla de anatomia membranarum mucosarum. 8°. *Berolini*, [1835].

CHASSAIGNAC (E.) *Des membranes muqueuses. 8°. *Paris*, 1846.

DEMOULIN (J.-C.) *De quelques productions hétérotopiques de muqueuses à épithélium prismatique cilié. 4°. *Paris*, 1866.
Also [Abstr.], *in:* Bull. Soc. anat. de Par., 1867, xlii, 126-130.

FERRÉ (G.) Les membranes muqueuses. 8°. *Paris*, 1886.

FISCHER (E.) *De imminuta membranarum mucosarum muci secretione. 4°. *Bonnæ*, [1826].

HEIDENHAIN (A.) *Ueber die acinösen Drüsen der Schleimhäute, insbesondere der Nasen-Schleimhaut. 8°. *Breslau*, 1870.

HEMELOT (J.) *Considérations sommaires, physiologiques et pathologiques, relatives au système de la membrane muqueuse. 4°. *Paris*, an XII, [1804].

Membranes (Mucous).

DE MANEE (L. J.) *De membranis mucosis in statu sano et morboso. 8°. *Lugd. Bat.*, 1836.
Czerny. Erfolgreiche Transplantation eines Stückes Epithel der Nasenschleimhaut auf eine granulirende Wundfläche. Allg. Wien. med. Ztg., 1871, xvi, 109.— **Debove.** Sur la couche endothéliale sous-épithéliale des membranes muqueuses. Compt. rend. Acad. d. sc., Par., 1872, lxxv, 1776. ———. Mémoire sur la couche endothéliale sous-épithéliale des membranes muqueuses. Arch. de physiol. norm. et path., Par., 1874, vi, 19-26, 1 pl. — **Droste** (A.) Ueber die Bedeutung der Schleimhäute. J. d. pract. Heilk., Berl., 1841, xcii, 5. St., 94-103. — **Flourens.** Recherches anatomiques sur les structures comparées de la membrane cutanée et de la membrane muqueuse. Compt. rend. Acad. d. sc., Par., 1838, vi, 262-269. *Also:* Gaz. méd. de Par., 1838, 2. s., vi, 145-147. ———. Recherches anatomiques sur la structure des membranes muqueuses. Gaz. méd. de Par., 1841, 2. s., ix, 785-787.— **Hutin** (P.) Recherches d'anatomie physiologique et pathologique sur la membrane muqueuse gastro-intestinale. N. biblioth. méd., Par., 1825, viii, 269; ix, 5; 328. *Also*, Reprint.—**Keber** (F.) Ueber die mikroskopisch nachweisbare Porosität der Gefäss- und Schleimhäute. Arch. f. path. Anat., etc., Berl., 1868, xliii, 19-34. — **List** (J. H.) Ueber Becherzellen und Leydig'sche Zellen (Schleimzellen). Arch. f. mikr. Anat. Bonn, 1885-6, xxvi, 543-552, 1 pl.—**Nathan** (E.) Vom Schleimhautkitzel oder den subjectiven Thätigkeiten der Schleimhaut-Organe. Ztschr. f. d. ges. Med., Hamb., 1840, xv, 293-320.—**Overton** (J.) An essay on the mucous membranes. West. J. M. & S., Louisville, 1845, 2. s., iv, 471-482.—**Posadski St.** Izmaineniya slizistikh obolo_chek. [Modifications of the mucous membranes.] J. dlya normal. i patol. gistologii, St. Petersb., 1876, x, 437-447.— **Robin** (C.) Muqueux (tissu et système); anatomie et physiologie. Dict. encycl. d. sc. méd., Par., 1876, 2. s., x, 406-475.—**Robin** (C.) & **Cadiat.** Sur la structure et les rapports des téguments au niveau de leur jonction dans les régions anale, vulvaire et du col utérin. J. de l'anat. et physiol., etc., Par., 1874, x, 589-620, 1 pl. ———. ———. Sur la constitution des muqueuses de l'utérus male, des canaux déférents et des trompes de Fallope. *Ibid.*, 1875, xi, 83; 105, 3 pl.—**Sebastian** (A. A.) Over de reproductie der slijmvliezen. Tijdschr. v. nat. Geschied. en Physiol., Amst., 1834, i, 223-234, 1 pl.—**Villermé** (L.-R.) Membranes muqueuses, folliculeuses, ou villeuses compliquées. Dict. d. sc. méd., Par., 1819, xxxii, 211-225.—**Voytits.** Beitrag zu den Beobachtungen über die Sensibilitätsverschiedenheit der Schleimhäute. Wien. med. Presse, 1868, ix, 146.—**Zeissl.** Ueber Sensibilitätsverschiedenheit einzelner Schleimhautpartien untereinander und gegenüber der allgemeinen Bedeckung. *Ibid.*, 1867, viii, 1105-1107.

Membranes (Mucous, Diseases of).

BÜCHNER (G. P.) *De nonnullis notatu dignioribus membranarum mucosarum et serosarum morbis. 8°. *Lugd. Bat.*, 1826.

CARNET (J.) *Considérations générales sur l'inflammation des membranes muqueuses. 4°. *Paris*, 1819.

CHAUMAS (J.-B.-V.-O.) *Parallèle entre les phlegmasies aiguës des membranes muqueuses et séreuses. 4°. *Paris*, 1824.

DOUSSIN-DUBREUIL (J.-L.) Des glaires, de leurs causes, de leurs effets, et des indications à remplir pour les combattre, avec les réponses aux questions suivantes: Existe-t-il une humeur considérée comme cause de maladie à laquelle la dénomination de glaires appartienne depuis longtemps? Cette humeur n'est-elle point identique avec celle que secrètent les glandes des membranes dites muqueuses, et n'est-elle pas, par cela même, utile aux fonctions de la vie? 7. éd. 8°. *Paris*, 1813.

GOTTHEIL (L. J.) *Specimen pathologiæ generalis systematis mucosi. 8°. *Berolini*, [1828].

GUEZILLE (C.-M.-J.) *Sur l'inflammation aiguë du système muqueux, ou les affections catarrhales aiguës en général. 4°. *Paris*, 1815.

GUMPERT (S. A. T.) *De inflammatione membranarum mucosarum. 4°. *Francof. ad Viadr.*, [1808].

HAY (E.-C.) *Sur les affections du système muqueux. 8°. *Paris*, an XI [1803].

MAYEUR (M.) *De l'emploi du nitrate d'argent dans la phlegmasie des muqueuses. 4°. *Strasbourg*, 1837.

Membranes (*Mucous, Diseases of*).

MORLET (E.) * I. Établir les différences qui existent entre les inflammations des membranes séreuses et les inflammations des membranes muqueuses, sous le point de vue de l'anatomie pathologique et de la séméiologie. II. [etc.] 4°. *Paris*, 1838.

NEUMANN (A. P. T.) * De inflammatione telæ mucosæ. 8°. *Berolini*, 1820.

PHILIPPE (P.) * De l'influence de l'inflammation sur les sécrétions des membranes muqueuses. 4°. *Paris*, 1833.

ROBIOU DU PONT (L.) * I. De la disposition aux inflammations des membranes muqueuses. II. [etc.] 4°. *Paris*, 1839.

YELLOLY (J.) Observations on vascular appearances of mucous and serous membranes as indicative of inflammation. 8°. *London*, 1836.

Albers (J. F. H.) Ueber Hautausschlägen ähnliche Bildungen auf inneren Häuten. (Die inneren Exantheme.) Mag. f. d. ges. Heilk., Berl., 1832, xxxvii, 452: 1836, xlvi, 403.—**Amard** (L.-V.-F.) Clinique générale interprétative des phénomènes morbides; maladies muqueuses. *In his:* Assoc. intellectuelle, 8°, Par., 1821, ii, 1–72.—**Armor** (S. G.) Catarrhal and croupous inflammation of mucous membranes. N. York M. J., 1871, xiii, 151-163. *Also*, Reprint.—**Arragon** (H.) 1° Étude sur les angiomes des muqueuses. 2° Rapprochement de leurs lésions et de celles du purpura hémorrhagique. Arch. de physiol. norm. et path., Par., 1883, 3. s., ii, 352-366, 3 pl.—**Brown-Séquard.** Simples procédés pour la prévention, dans certaines circonstances, d'affections catarrhales ou d'inflammations de nombre d'organes ou des muqueuses nasales, bucco-pharyngée, laryngée, trachéale ou bronchiale. Compt. rend. Soc. de biol., Par., 1886, 8. s., iii, 109.—**Chamberet.** Maladies muqueuses. Dict. d. sc. méd., Par., 1818, xxx, 291-294.—**Clos** (J.-A.) 1° Quels sont les symptômes caractéristiques de l'inflammation du système muqueux, et quels sont les phénomènes qui résultent de cette inflammation, considérée sous le rapport des organes où elle a lieu? 2° Quelles sont les causes qui déterminent cette inflammation? 3° Comment doit-on traiter cet ordre de phlegmasie, et particulièrement l'inflammation syphilitique de la membrane muqueuse du canal de l'urètre? [Prize essay.] [Premier mémoire.] Actes Soc. de méd. de Brux., 1808, ii, 1–100. *Also:* Actes Soc. de méd., chir. et pharm., Brux., 1808, ii, 1–100.—**Declary** (J. P.) On diseases of the mucous membrane. Transylv. J. M., Lexington, Ky., 1832, v, 461-468.—**Guéneau de Mussy** (N.) Contribution à l'histoire des enanthèmes. France méd., Par., 1884, i, 735-741.—**Guibout.** Étude pathologique comparative des membranes muqueuses et de la peau. Gaz. d. hôp., Par., 1875, xlviii, 386. *Also, transl.:* Tribuna méd., Par., 1875, ii, 85-87.—**Kanonnikoff** (V.) Sluch. mnojest. eksudat. eritemi s porajen. slizist. obolochek. [Erythema multiforme in an affection of the mucous membrane.] Med. Obozr., Mosk., 1885, xxvi, 283-287.—**Liants** (A.) Erythema exsudativum multiforme s porajeniem slizistich obolochek. [Of mucous membranes.] *Ibid.*, xxiii, 927-934.—**Mata** (R.) De los catarros é inflamaciones de las mucosas. Progreso méd., Madrid, 1877, ii, 59-61.—**Mitchell** (J. D.) Exanthematous inflammation of mucous membranes. Indiana J. M., Indianap., 1875, vi, 198-204.—**Quels** sont les symptômes caractéristiques de l'inflammation du système muqueux, et quels sont les phénomènes qui résultent de cette inflammation, considérée sous le rapport des organes où elle a lieu? [etc.] [Troisième mémoire.] Actes Soc. de méd. de Brux., 1808, ii, 169–284.—**Robinson** (B.) On certain morbid alterations of mucous membranes; their influence on speech, and their apparent relations with diseased nerve-structure. N. York M. J., 1875, xxi, 257-267.—**Rose** (A.) Carbonic acid gas as a local application to chronically inflamed mucous surfaces. Ann. Anat. & Surg., Brooklyn, N. Y., 1883, viii, 254-261.—**Sangalli.** Nouveaux faits de succession des tissus pathologiques. Cong. périod. internat. d. sc. méd. Compt.-rend. 1884, Copenh., 1886, i, (sect. de path. gén., etc.), 98-107.—**Socoloff** (N.) Ueber die Bildung der Eiterzellen und die Veränderungen der Membrana propria der Schleimhaut bei Entzündungen der Luftwege. Arch. f. path. Anat., etc., Berl., 1876, lxviii, 611-624.—**Stout** (S. H.) The clinical importance of abnormities of the mucous membrane. Texas Cour.-Rec. Med., Fort Worth, 1883-4, i, no. 4, 5-12.—**Vimont.** 1° Quels sont les symptômes caractéristiques de l'inflammation du système muqueux, et quels sont les phénomènes qui résultent de cette inflammation, considérée sous le rapport des organes où elle a lieu? [etc.] [Deuxième mémoire.] Actes Soc. de méd. de Brux., 1808, ii, 101–168. *Also:* Actes Soc. de méd., chir. et pharm., Brux., 1808, ii, 101-168.

Membranes (*Serous*).

See, also, Arachnoid; Bursæ; Cavities (*Closed*); Membranes (*Synovial*); Pericardium; Peritoneum; Pleura.

BRANTJES (J.) * De membranis serosis. 8°. *Lugd. Bat.*, 1841.

VAN EGMOND (A. S.) * De natura membranarum serosarum in genere, et de anatomia-pathologica pleuræ inflammatæ. [Leyden.] 8°. *Harlemi*, 1835.

FARABEUF (L.-H.) * Le système séreux; anatomie et physiologie. 8°. *Paris*, 1876.

GALVANI (J.) *Quelques considérations sur les membranes séreuses en général au point de vue anatomique, physiologique et pathologique. 4°. *Paris*, 1866.

KOKER (J.) * De subtiliori membranarum serosarum fabrica. 8°. *Traj. ad Rhenum*, [1828].

LUSCHKA (H.) Die Strucktur der serösen Häute des Menschen. 4°. *Tübingen*, 1851.

SCHÜRMAYER (I. H.) * Ueber den Bau und die Verrichtungen der serösen Häute. Als Einleitung zur Lehre von den Krankheiten der Pleura. 8°. *Freiburg*, 1830.

STEFFEN (W.) *Ueber das Verhalten des Endothels der serösen Häute unter verschiedenen pathologischen Ernährungszuständen. 8°. *Freiburg*, 1880.

TAUBE (A.) * De membranis serosis in cavis magnis corporis humani obviis. 8°. [*Dorpat*], 1854.

Altmann (R.) Ueber die Veränderungen des serösen Epithels am blossgelegten Froschmesenterium. Arch. f. mikr. Anat., Bonn, 1878, xvi, 111–117.—**Bizzozero** (G.) Ueber die innere Grenzschicht der menschlichen serösen Häute. Centralbl. f. d. med. Wissensch., Berl., 1874, xii, 210.—**Bizzozero** (G.) & **Salvioli** (G.) Sulla struttura delle membrane sierose e particolarmente del peritoneo diaframmatico. Gior. d. r. Accad. di med. di Torino, 1876, 3. s., xix, 466–470. ——. Studi sulla struttura e sui linfatici delle sierose umane. Arch. per le sc. med., Torino, 1876-7, i, 339, 1 pl.: 1877-8, ii, 247, 1 pl. *Also* [Abstr.]: Gazz. med. ital. lomb., Milano, 1877, 7. s., iv, 401. *Also, transl.* [Abstr.]: Centralbl. f. d. med. Wissensch., Berl., 1877, xv, 754; 769.—**Bourgery.** Sur les nerfs des membranes séreuses. Compt. rend. Acad. d. sc., Par., 1845, xxi, 1380.—**Goodsir** (J.) The structure of the serous membranes. *In his:* Anat. & Path. Obs., 8°. Edinb., 1845, 41-43. *Also, in his:* Anat. Mem., 8°, Edinb., 1868, ii, 436-438.—**Klein** (E.) & **Burdon-Sanderson.** Zur Kenntniss der Anatomie der serösen Häute im normalen und pathologischen Zustande. Centralbl. f. d. med. Wissensch., Berl., 1872, x, 17; 33; 49.—**Knauff.** Zur Anatomie der serösen Häute. Verhandl. d. naturh.-med. Ver. zu Heidelb., 1865-8, iv, 126.—**Lavdowsky** (M.) Einige Bemerkungen, die Beobachtungen von Dr. Klein und Dr. Burdon-Sanderson [Zur Kenntniss der Anatomie der serösen Häute] betreffend. Centralbl. f. d. med. Wissensch., Berl., 1872, x, 257-261.—**Lebert.** Quelques remarques sur les corps étrangers des membranes séreuses. Compt. rend. Soc. de biol. 1852, Par., 1853, iv, 89-96.—**Penzoldt** (F.) Ueber das Verhalten von Blutgefässen in serösen Höhlen. Deutsches Arch. f. klin. Med., Leipz., 1876, xviii, 542-575.—**Robin** (C.) & **Cadiat.** Observations sur quelques points de la texture des séreuses. J. de l'anat. et physiol., etc., Par., 1876, xii, 621-643. ——. Séreux. Dict. encycl. d. sc. méd., Par., 1880, 3. s., xix, 329-351.—**Shumovski** (V.) K' voprosu o razvitii epitelinoi tkani na seroznikh abolochkakh. [On the formation of epithelial tissue on serous membranes.] Med. Vestnik, St. Petersb., 1861, i, 177; 189.—**Tait** (L.) Notices of the abnormalities of serous membranes. Dublin Q. J. M. Sc., 1869, xlvii, 85-90. *Also*, Reprint.—**Tourneux** (F.) Recherches sur l'épithélium des séreuses. J. de l'anat. et physiol., etc., Par., 1874, x, 66-83, 2 pl.—**Villermé** (L.-R.) Membranes séreuses ou villeuses simples. Dict. d. sc. méd., Par., 1819, xxxii, 225-230.—**Willis** (R.) On the import and office of the serous membranes. Lond. M. Gaz., 1845, xxxv, 767.

Membranes (*Serous, Diseases of*).

See, also, Adhesions; Meningitis; Peritonitis; Pleurisy.

BAJARD (A.) * Dissertation sur les phlegmasies des membranes séreuses. 4°. *Paris*, 1818.

CAMBOURNAC (A.-S.) * Dissertation sur les granulations et les tubercules de quelques membranes séreuses. 4°. *Paris*, 1824.

Membranes (Serous, Diseases of).

COLMANT (J.) * Essai sur l'inflammation des membranes séreuses en général. 4°. *Strasbourg*, 1835.

HODGKIN (T.) Lectures on the morbid anatomy of the serous and mucous membranes. 2 v. 8°. *London*, 1836-40.

———. The same. v. 1. 8°. *Philadelphia*, 1838.

KNIEP (T.) * Ueber einige pathologisch-anatomische Veränderungen an den serösen Häuten. 8°. *Rostock*, 1854.

LAHALLE (J.-B.) * Sur l'inflammation du système séreux. 4°. *Paris, an XI* [1802].

LASSERRE (J.-P.-R.-H.) * Des tubercules dans les séreuses. 4°. *Paris*, 1846.

LÜDICKE (A. L. T.) * De serosarum membranarum inflammationibus. 8°. *Halis Sax.*, 1850.

MACQUET (L.-J.) * Recherches cliniques sur l'inflammation des membranes séreuses et synoviales. 4°. *Paris*, 1850.

MARGUERITTE (L.-P.) * Quelques recherches sur les phlegmasies hémorrhagiques de la plèvre, du péricarde, et du péritoine. 4°. *Paris*, 1-62.

MARTIN (A.) * Quelques considérations sur les plaies des membranes séreuses et sur leur mode de cicatrisation. 4°. *Paris*, 1875.

RENOU (E.-F.) * Des séreuses splanchniques et de leur inflammation. 4°. *Paris*, 1860.

SAUVEUR DE LA VILLERAYE (M.-J.-S.) * Essai sur les inflammations du système séreux et du système synovial; recherches et observations pour servir à l'histoire de ces maladies. 4°. *Paris*, 1812.

TEISSIER (C.-J.-A.) * Dissertation sur l'inflammation des membranes séreuses en général et plus particulièrement des membranes séreuses splanchniques. 4°. *Paris*, 1827.

TOUZET (C.) * Considérations générales sur les inflammations du système séreux. 4°. *Paris*, 1824.

Briquet (P.) Du développement simultané de productions hétérologues (tubercules et encéphaloïdes) à la surface de plusieurs membranes séreuses affectées de phlegmasie, et de l'hydropisie qui l'accompagne. Arch. gén. de méd., Par., 1842, 3. s., xv, 174-210. *Also*, Reprint.—**Cohnheim** (J.) Ueber die Entzündung seröser Häute. Arch. f. path. Anat., etc., Berl., 1861, xxii, 516-526, 1 pl.—**Concato** (L.) Sulla poliorromenite scrofolosa, o tisi delle sierose. Gior. internaz. d. sc. med., Napoli, 1881, n. s., iii, 1037-1053.—**Haas** (H.) Ein Fall von Tuberculosis membranarum serosarum. Vrtljschr. f. d. prakt. Heilk., Leipz., 1875, cxxvii, 28-31, 1 tab.—**Hughes** (W. E.) General tuberculosis of serous membranes. Tr. Path. Soc. Phila. (1883-5), 1886, xii, 134.—**Kinnicutt** (F. P.) A case of idiopathic (?) purulent inflammation of the serous membranes of all the great cavities. Med. Rec., N. Y., 1883, xxiii, 427.—**Knauff.** Zur Histologie des Miliartuberkels auf serösen Häuten. Centralbl. f. d. med. Wissensch., Berl., 1867, v, 561-563.—**Koch.** Acute Tuberkulose der serösen Häute. Med. Cor.-Bl. d. württemb. ärztl. Ver., Stuttg., 1869, xxxix, 271.—**Lebert.** Quelques remarques sur les corps étrangers des membranes séreuses. Gaz. méd. de Par., 1852, 3. s., vii, 490-492.—**Liguori** (L.) Intorno ai tubercoli delle membrane sierose. Ateneo, Milano, 1846, i, 221-223. — **Liouville** (H.) Cas de sarcome généralisé des séreuses chez un rat. Arch. de physiol. norm. et path., Par., 1873, v, 206-209. — **Menière** (P.) Mémoire sur la rétraction que subissent les membranes séreuses enflammées. Gaz. méd. de Par., 1857, 3. s., xii, 38-41.—**Perroud.** Observations de tuberculose séreuse généralisée. Gaz. méd. de Lyon, 1867, xix, 511-514. — **Reid** (J.) Case in which accidental cartilages were found in the interior of several of the serous membranes. Edinb. M. & S. J., 1836, xlvi, 61-65.—**Rindfleisch** (E.) Beiträge zur Lehre von den Entzündungen seröser Membranen. Arch. f. path. Anat., etc., Berl., 1862, xxiii, 519-526, 1 pl.—**Robin** (C.) Recherches anatomiques sur l'épithélioma des séreuses. J. de l'anat. et physiol., etc., Par., 1869, vi, 239-288, 2 pl.—**Tait** (L.) Notices of the abnormalities of serous membranes. Dublin Q. J. M. Sc., 1869, xlvii, 85-87.—**Traube** (L.) Ueber den Einfluss starker und anhaltender Diarrhöen auf die Gestaltung peritonitischer Adhäsionen, nebst Bemerkungen über pleuritische Adhäsionen. Berl. klin. Wchnschr., 1874, xi, 36; 49; 63.—**Turner** (W.) On the textural changes which occur in inflammation of serous membranes. Edinb. M. J., 1863-4,

Membranes (Serous, Diseases of).

ix, 908-914. *Also, transl.*: Allg. Wien. med. Ztg., 1864, ix, 217; 227.—**Wilmart** (L.) Curieux spécimen de disposition à l'inflammation des séreuses. Presse méd. belge, Brux., 1881, xxxiii, 3.—**Zink.** Réflexions et observations sur les fongus des membranes séreuses. J. compl. du dict. d. sc. méd., Par., 1825, xxi, 24-37.

Membranes (Synovial).

See, also, **Bursæ**; **Joints**; **Tendons** (*Sheaths of*).

HAGEN-TORN (O.) * Razvitie i stroenie sinovialnych obolochek. [Development and structure of synovial membranes.] 8°. *St. Petersburg*, 1883.

MARC (J.-B.-G.) * Essai sur les synoviales. 4°. *Paris*, 1834.

Landzert. Zur Histologie der Synovialhaut. Centralbl. f. d. med. Wissensch., Berl., 1867, v, 369-371. — **Soubbotine.** Recherches histologiques sur la structure des membranes synoviales. Arch. de physiol. norm. et path., Par., 1880, 2. s., vii, 532-554, 1 pl. — **Tillmanns** (H.) Zur Histologie der Synovialmembranen. Arch. f. klin. Chir., Berl., 1875-6, xix, 693-711. — **Toynbee.** Structure of synovial membrane covering articular cartilage. Tr. Path. Soc. Lond., 1848-9, ii, 101.—**Villermé** (L.-R.) Synoviales (capsules ou membranes). Dict. d. sc. méd., Par., 1821, liv, 97-122.

Membranes (Synovial, Diseases of).

See, also, **Joints** (*Diseases of*).

BRUNARD (J.-P.) * Sur l'inflammation des membranes synoviales. 4°. *Strasbourg*, 1823.

FRÖLICH (T.) * Die Entzündung der Synovialhäute. 8°. *Tübingen*, 1846.

THOMSON (S.) * Quelques considérations pathologiques sur la phlegmasie du tissu synovial. 4°. *Paris*, 1837.

Barton (J. M.) Splint for the treatment of synovitis of the wrist-joint. Tr. Am. Surg. Ass., Phila., 1883, i, 503. — **Barwell** (R.) Three cases illustrating the good effects of pressure in strumous synovitis. Lancet, Lond., 1859, ii, 433.—**Bidder.** Ueber Entstehung fester Körper in den von Synovialhäuten gebildeten Höhlen. Ztschr. f. rat. Med., Heidelb., 1845, iii, 99-109. — **Broca.** [Cas de transformation graisseuse des synoviales tendineuses de l'extenseur commun des doigts.] Bull. Soc. anat. de Par., 1851, xxvi, 23.—**Bruning** (J.) Ontsteking der peesscheeden. N. pract. Tijdschr. v. de Geneesk., Gorinchem, 1856, n. s., ii, 129-139.—**Bulteau** (A.) Inflammation des gaines synoviales de la main; phlegmon de l'avant-bras; albuminurie; mort. Bull. Soc. anat. de Par., 1878, 4. s., iii, 146-148.—**Crocq** (J.) De la formation de matière tuberculeuse à l'intérieur des synoviales. Ann. Soc. méd.-chir. de Bruges, 1853, 2. s., i, 481-492. *Also*: Presse méd. belge, Brux., 1852-3, v, 413-416.—**Gross.** Deux observations de synovite tendineuse tuberculeuse. Mém. Soc. de méd. de Nancy, 1884-5, 14-23.—**Gross** (S D.) Synovitis of the foot. Med. Times, Phila., 1870-71, i, 374.—**Hewitt** (D. B.) Cases of suppuration in and near synovial cavities. Med. Press, Dubl., 1865, 2. s., xi, 438.—**Hicguet.** Synovite à grains riziformes de la bourse séreuse interne ou cubitale; incision; drainage; guérison. J. d'accouch., Liége, 1883, iv, 253.—**Hopkins** (W. B.) Tenosynovitis; its causes, nature, symptoms, and treatment; based upon the analysis of fifteen cases. Boston M. & S. J., 1882, cvii, 81. *Also*: Cincin. Lancet & Clinic, 1882, n. s., ix, 74.—**Lapeyre** (J.) Du phlegmon des gaines synoviales tendineuses des fléchisseurs de la main. Gaz. hebd. d. sc. méd. de Montpel., 1884, vi, 484; 494; 505; 519; 533; 544; 553. — **Lecocq.** Synovite tendineuse; phlegmon chronique; carie des os du carpe; amputation de l'avant-bras. Arch. méd. belges, Brux., 1880, 3. s., xviii, 467-471.—**Lerotas** (J.) Case of synovial effusions complicating hemiplegia. Indian M. Gaz., Calcutta, 1876, xi, 212. — **McClintock** (J. C.) A case of pyaemic synovitis. Kansas City M. Rec., 1884, i, 173.—**McGraw** (T. A.) Two cases of enlarged synovial sacks, containing fibrinous concretions. Detroit Clinic, 1882, i, 185.—**Macnamara** (C.) Clinical lecture on synovitis and granular disease of the synovial membrane; pulpy degeneration; scrofulous synovitis. Indian M. Gaz., Calcutta, 1879, xiv, 213-217.—**Maunder** (C.F.) Clinical lecture on gelatinous disease of synovial membrane. (New operation) Lancet, Lond., 1876, i, 559.—**Mori** (G.) Sul trattamento delle sinoviti acute. Gazz. med. ital. lomb., Milano, 1885, 8. s., vii, 303; 333. — **Nicaise.** Synovite tendineuse à grains riziformes; incision; traitement antiseptique; guérison. Bull. et mém. Soc. de chir. de Par., 1881, n. s., vii, 402-406. *Also*: Gaz. d. hôp., Par., 1881, liv, 916. *Also*: Rev. méd. franç. et étrang., Par., 1881, ii, 479-483. ———. Rapport sur une communication de M. le Dr. Schwartz, intitulée: Synovite à grains riziformes de la gaine carpo-phalangienne interne; incision; drainage sous le pansement de Lister; guérison complète et per-

Membranes (*Synovial, Diseases of*).

sistante. Bull. et mém. Soc. de chir. de Par., 1883, n. s., ix, 470–472.—**Paget** (S.) Synovial cyst of the calf from chronic synovitis of the knee. Tr. Clin. Soc. Lond., 1886, xix. 329.—**Péan.** Affections des synoviales tendineuses. *In his:* Leçons de clin. chir., etc., 8°, Par., 1882, 34–82. **Peculiarity** in treatment of synovitis. Med. Rec., N. Y., 1873, viii, 502.—**Pierce** (J. G.) Synovitis. Tr. Maine M. Ass. Portland, 1883, viii, pt. 1, 69–75.—**Poupon** (H.) Synovite crépitante double du poignet. France méd., Par., 1885, i, 797–799.—**Ramonet.** Épanchement traumatique de sérosité dans la synoviale sous-tricipitale, sans communication avec l'articulation du genou; déductions anatomiques et cliniques. Rec. de mém. de méd. . . . mil., Par., 1880, 3. s., xxxvi, 574–580.—**Reclus** (P.) Synovites fongueuses des gaines des tendons. *In his:* Clin. et crit. chir., 8°, Par., 1884, 259–276.—**Regensburger** (A.) A case of syphilitic synovitis. West. Lancet, San Fran., 1876, v, 413–415.—**Reid** (J. J.) Synovitis of tendons of the wrist. N. York M. J., 1880, xxxi, 49.—**Riedel** (B.) Zur Kenntniss der primären akuten resp. subakuten Synovitis tendinum manus. Centralbl. f. Chir., Leipz., 1883, x, 113–116.—**Rokitansky** (C.) Ueber die dendritischen Vegetationen auf Synovialhäuten. Ztschr. d. k.-k. Gesellsch. d. Aerzte zu Wien, 1851, vii, 2–8.—**Schilling** (C.) Chronic serous synovitis. St. Louis Cour. Med., 1883, ix, 40.—**Shirman** (A.) Sluchai tenosynovitidis, okonchivchiisja polnim vizdorovleniem. [Case of tenosynovitis; perfect recovery.] Voyenno-med. J., St. Petersb., 1877, cxxix, 21–22.—**Terrier** (F.) & **Verchère** (F.) De la synovite tendineuse tuberculeuse et en particulier de la synovite tuberculeuse des gaines du poignet, de la main et des doigts. Rev. de chir., Par., 1882, ii, 543–561.—**Terrillon.** Kyste synovial de la gaine du long fléchisseur du pouce droit; grains riziformes nombreux; fongosités abondantes; ouverture; raclage des fongosités; guérison. Bull. et mém. Soc. de chir. de Par., 1886, n. s., xii, 862–864.—**Thomas** (J. D.) Acute traumatic synovitis. Pittsburgh M. J., 1882, ii, 361–366.—**Torras Pascual.** Sinovitis aguda supurada de la mano. Sentido catól., Barcel., 1881, iii, 316–321.—**Von Donhoff** (E.) Chronic serous synovitis (hydrarthrus). Am. Pract. & News, Louisville, 1887, n. s., iii, 193.

Memel.

See **Cholera** (*Asiatic, History, etc., of*), *by localities.*

Memelsdorf (Alexander). * Zum Coma diabeticum. 32 pp. 8°. *Würzburg, Becker,* 1881.

Memis (John). The midwife's pocket companion; or, a practical treatise of midwifery on a new plan. Containing full and plain directions for the management and delivery of child-bearing women in the different cases, and the cure of the several diseases incident to them and new-born children in the safest manner and according to the best improvements. Adapted to the use of the female as well as the male practitioner in that art. viii, 234 pp., 3 l. 8°. *London, E. & C. Dilly,* 1765.

———. The same. In 3 pts. iv (1 l.), 127 pp., 2 l. sm. 8°. *Aberdeen,* 1786.

Memoir of Baron Larrey [Dominique-Jean], surgeon-in-chief of the grande armée. From the French. 2. ed. xix, 273 pp. 8°. *London, H. Renshaw,* 1862.

Memoir (A) of Charles Hilton Fagge. 7 pp. 8°. [*Philadelphia, P. Blakiston, Son & Co.,* 1886.] Bound with: FAGGE (C. H.) The principles and practice of medicine. v. 2. 8°. *Philadelphia,* 1886.

Memoir of Dr. Thomas Thomson, F. R. S., regius professor of chemistry in the University of Glasgow. 8 pp. 8°. *London, Reeve & Co.,* 1852.

Repr. from: Lit. Gaz.

Memoir of Edward A. Holyoke, M. D., LL. D., prepared in compliance with a vote of the Essex South District Medical Society, and published at their request. 80 pp., 2 port., 1 pl. 8°. *Boston, Perkins & Marvin,* 1829.

Memoir of Élie-Magloire Durand. 10 pp. 8°. [*Philadelphia,* 1873, *vel subseq.*]

Memoir of James Alex. Oswald. 13 pp. 12°. *Edinburgh,* 1818.

Memoir of John Collins Warren. 14 pp., port. 8°. [*Boston,* 1865.]

Repr. from: Historical and Genealogical Register, Jan., 1865.

Memoir of John W. Francis, jr. 3 pp. 8°. [*New York,* 1855.]

Repr. from: N. York M. Times, 1855, iv.

Memoir of the late Alfred Smee, F. R. S., by his daughter, with a selection from his miscellaneous writings. xiv, 422 pp., 1 pl. 8°. *London, G. Bell & Sons,* 1878.

Memoir of the late Henry Park, surgeon, of Liverpool. 38 pp., 1 pl., port. 8°. *Liverpool, D. Marples,* 1840.

Repr. from: Tr. Prov. M. & S. Ass. 1838, Lond., 1839, vii, 459–484.

Memoir and trial of Mrs. [Christina] Gilmour [for poisoning by arsenic]. ix, 97 pp. 8°. [*Edinburgh,* 1844.] [P., v. 1168.]

Memoir of William Clift. 7 pp. 8°. [*London, R. & J. E. Taylor, n. d.*] [P., v. 1563.]

Memoir of William Proctor, jr., late professor of pharmacy in the Philadelphia College of Pharmacy. 27 pp., port. 8°. *Philadelphia, Merrihew & Son,* 1874.

Mémoire sur l'amélioration des biens communaux, le desséchement des marais, le défrichement des terres incultes et la replantation des bois; avec les moyens de procéder à leur partage. 32 pp. 12°. *Paris, imprimerie royale,* 1790.

Mémoire pour Anne Grandjean, connu sous le nom de Jean-Baptiste Grandjean, accusé et appellant, contre monsieur le procureur général, accusateur et intimé. Question: Un hermaphrodite qui a épousé une fille, peut-il être réputé profanateur du sacrement de mariage, quand la nature qui le trompoit, l'appelloit à l'état de mari? 23 pp. 4°. *Paris, L. Cellot,* 1765. [P., v. 630.]

Mémoire sur le bureau de la santé de Marseille, et sur les règles qu'on y observe. 81 pp. 4°. *Marseille, P. Boy,* 1753.

Mémoire sur un cas d'hermaphrodisme masculin. 15 pp. 8°. [*Paris, Grégoire,* 1836?] [*Also, in:* P., v. 450.]

Mémoire à consulter. [Letter from a commission composed of MM. Bigot, Mirault, Dumont, Farge, Daviers, relative to concealment of a supposed case of infanticide.] 10 pp., 1 l. 4°. *Angers, Cosnier & Lachèse,* 1850. [P., v. 479.]

Mémoire à consulter avant de modifier les lois existantes sur la pharmacie. (Recueillis par M. le Dr. Quesneville.) 75 pp. 8°. *Paris, L. Martinet,* 1847. [P., v. 467.]

Repr. from: Rev. scient. et industrielle.

Mémoire à consulter pour M. Jules Guérin, contre MM. Malgaigne, Vidal (de Cassis) et Henroz. iv, 362 pp. 4°. [*Paris, F. Malteste & Cie.*], 1844.

Mémoire sur les dépôts d'engrais désinfectés, système Goux, établissements de deuxième classe. 15 pp. 8°. *Paris, A. Chaix & Cie.,* 1880.

Mémoire sur l'eau de Selters, ou de seltz naturelle. Sa source dans le duché de Nassau; sa supériorité sur l'eau de Selters factice; sa composition chimique; ses vertus curatives et hygiéniques. 75 pp., 1 pl. 8°. *Paris, J.-B. Baillière,* 1841.

Mémoire sur l'emploi de la méthode Künckel, contre les maladies de la peau; par un docteur de la Faculté de Paris. 47 pp. 8°. *Paris, M. Künckel,* 1844.

Mémoire sur l'empoisonnement par l'arsenic. 44 pp. 8°. *Paris, Pagnerre,* 1842. [P., v. 874.]

Mémoire historique sur la vie et les écrits de Abraham Trembley. 88 pp. 8°. *Neuchâtel, S. Fauche,* 1787. [P., v. 516.]

Mémoire sur la maladie qui a attaqué, en différens temps, les femmes en couche, à l'Hôtel-Dieu de Paris . . . Suivi d'un rapport, fait par ordre du gouvernement, sur le même sujet; avec des réflexions sur la nature et le traitement de la fièvre puerpérale. Lu dans la séance de la So-

Mémoire sur la maladie [etc.]—continued.
ciété royale de médecine, tenue au Louvre le 6
septembre 1782. 34 pp. 4°. *Rouen, J.-J. de
Boullenger,* 1783.

Mémoire sur la nécessité de transférer et re-
construire l'Hôtel-Dieu de Paris, suivi d'un projet de translation de cet hôpital, proposé par le
sieur Poyet, architecte et contrôleur des bâtimens de la ville. 44 pp. 4°. [*Paris*], 1785.

Mémoire présenté à son altesse royale Mgr. le
duc d'Orléans, régent de France, concernant la
précieuse plante du gin-seng de Tartarie, découverte en Amérique par le père Joseph-François
Lafitau, de la compagnie de Jésus, missionnaire
des Iroquois du Sault St.-Louis. Nouv. éd., précédée d'une notice biographique, par M. Hospice
Verreau, et accompagnée d'un portrait du père
Lafitau, d'un fac-simile de son autographe et de la
planche représentant le gin-seng. 39 pp., 1 pl.
8°. *Montréal, Sénécal, Daniel & Cie.,* 1858.
Portrait wanting.

Mémoire en réponse à un écrit anonyme, intitulé: Observations présentées au roi, sur la
Faculté de médecine. [Par la Faculté de médecine.] 36 pp. 4°. [*Paris, Didot jeune,* 1815?]
[*Also, in:* P., v. 856.]

Mémoire sur le sirop de pointes d'asperges de
Johnson. 32 pp. 8°. *Paris, Delauny,* 1837.

Mémoire sur les subsistances militaires. 2 v.
MS. 321 pp., 3 l.; 375 pp., 5 l. 4°. [*n. p., n. d.*]

Mémoires de l'Académie impériale des sciences,
arts et belles-lettres de Dijon. 2. s., 1857; v. 12-
16, 1864-70; 3. s., v. 1, 1871; 7-8, 1881-2 to 1883-4.
8°. *Dijon,* 1857-85.

Mémoires de l'Académie impériale des sciences
de St.-Pétersbourg. Sciences mathématiques,
physiques et naturelles. 6 s., livr. 1 & 2, v. 1,
220 pp., 3 pl. 4°. *St.-Pétersbourg, M. Graef,* 1830.

Mémoires de l'Académie impériale des sciences
de St.-Pétersbourg. Sciences politiques, histoire
et philologie. 6 s., livr. 1 & 2, v. 1, 204 pp., 2
pl. 4°. *St-Pétersbourg, M. Graef,* 1830.

Mémoires de l'Académie impériale et royale des
sciences et belles-lettres de Bruxelles. v. 1-5.
8°. *Bruxelles,* 1777-88.

Mémoires de l'Académie de médecine. v. 1-34.
4°. *Paris,* 1828-84.

Mémoires de l'Académie royale de chirurgie.
v. 1-5. 4°. *Paris,* 1743-74.

———. The same. 15 v. 8°. *Paris,* 1771-87.

Mémoires de l'Académie royale de chirurgie.
3 v. 8°. *Paris,* 1838.

Mémoires de l'Académie royale de médecine
de Belgique. v. 1-4, fasc. 1, v. 5. 4°. *Bruxelles,* 1848-69.

Mémoires de l'Académie royale de Prusse. Concernant l'anatomie, la physiologie, la physique,
la minéralogie, etc. 9 v. in 10. 12°. *Avignon
& Paris,* 1768-74.

Mémoires de l'Académie des sciences de l'institut de France. v. 24; 35. 4°. *Paris,* 1854-66.

Mémoires de l'Académie de Stanislas. 1860-
76. 17 v. 8°. *Nancy,* 1861-77.

Mémoires d'un apothicaire sur la guerre d'Espagne, pendant les années 1808 à 1814. 206 pp.
8°. *Philadelphia, Carey, Lea & Blanchard,* 1833.

Mémoires et bulletins de la Société de médecine de Bordeaux. 1869-71. 2 v. 8°. *Bordeaux,*
1869-71.

Mémoires et bulletins de la Société de médecine
et de chirurgie de Bordeaux. 1872-86. 15 v.
8°. *Bordeaux,* 1872-86.

Mémoires et bulletins de la Société médico-
chirurgicale des hôpitaux et hospices de Bordeaux. v. 1-6. 8°. *Bordeaux,* 1866-71.

Mémoires et comptes-rendus de la Société des
sciences médicales de Lyon. v. 1-25. 8°. *Lyon,*
1862-86.

Mémoires des concours et de savants étrangers,
publiés par l'Académie royale de médecine de
Belgique. v. 1-7, fasc. 1, v. 8. 4°. *Bruxelles,*
1847-74.

Mémoires couronnés et autres mémoires publiés par l'Académie royale de médecine de Belgique. v. 1-7, fasc. 1, v. 8. 8°. *Bruxelles,*
1870-86.

Mémoires de la Faculté de médecine de Paris,
et de la société établie dans son sein. 372 pp.,
13 pl. 4°. *Paris,* 1812.

Mémoires sur la guerre [etc.] *See* **M**[aire
d'Olainville].

Mémoires littéraires, critiques, philologiques,
biographiques et bibliographiques, pour servir
à l'histoire ancienne et moderne de la médecine
[par Jean Goulin]. Année 1775. 416 pp. 4°.
Paris, Pyre & Bastien, [1775].

Mémoires et observations de la Société de médecine d'Anvers. 116 pp., 1 pl. 8°. *Anvers,
J.-B. Heirstraeten,* 1836.

Mémoires sur les parties sensibles et irritables
du corps animal; tome troisième, contenant les
expériences de plusieurs anatomistes d'Allemagne, de France, d'Angleterre et d'Italie.
Ouvrage qui sert de suite aux Mémoires de M.
de Haller. 512 pp. 16°. *Lausanne, S. D'Ainay,*
1760.

Mémoires sur les questions proposées par l'Académie impériale et royale des sciences et belles-
lettres de Bruxelles qui ont remporté les prix
en mdcclxxi-mdcclxxxvii. 2 v. 4°. *Bruxelles,
imp. académique,* [1772-88].

Mémoires de la Société d'agriculture, sciences,
belles-lettres et arts d'Orléans. v. 11-25. 8°.
Orléans, 1868-84.

Mémoires de la Société d'anthropologie de Paris. v. 1-3; 2. s., v. 1-2. 8°. *Paris,* 1860-82.

Mémoires de la Société centrale de médecine
vétérinaire. v. 12; 2. s., v. 1-2. 8°. *Paris,*
1882-4.

Mémoires de la Société de chirurgie de Paris.
v. 1-7. 4°. *Paris,* 1847-74.

Mémoires de la Société ethnologique. v. 1-2.
li, 294, 296 pp.; lxiv, 320, 271 pp. 8°. *Paris,*
1841-5.

Mémoires de la Société de médecine d'Anvers.
1838-9. xxx, 21 pp. 4°. *Anvers, J.-B. Heirstraeten,* [*n. d.*]

Mémoires de la Société de médecine de Nancy.
1871-2 to 1885-6. 9 v. 8°. *Nancy,* 1872-86.

Mémoires de la Société de médecine de Paris,
séante à l'Hôtel-de-ville. cxiv, 258 pp. 8°.
Paris, 1817.

Mémoires de la Société de médecine de Strasbourg. v. 1-23, 1850-86. 12 v. 8°. *Strasbourg,*
1850-86.

Mémoires de la Société médicale d'émulation de
Lyon. xlvi, 294 pp. 8°. *Paris & Lyon, J.-B.
Baillière,* 1842.

Mémoires de la Société médicale d'émulation
de Paris. 1798-1826. 9 v. 8°. *Paris,* 1799-
1826.

Mémoires de la Société médicale d'observation. 2 v. 412; 596 pp. 8°. *Paris, F. Masson,*
1837-44.

Mémoires de la Société de physique et d'histoire
naturelle de Genève. v. 5, 19-23. 4°. *Genève,*
1867-73.

Mémoires de la Société des sciences naturelles
de Cherbourg. v. 1-23. 8°. *Cherbourg & Paris,*
1853-80.

Mémoires de la Société des sciences naturelles
et médicales de Seine-et-Oise de 1874 à 1882. v.
12. lxxiv, 480 pp. 8°. *Versailles,* 1883.

Mémoires de la Société des sciences physiques
et naturelles de Bordeaux. v. 5-10, 1867-75; 2.
s., 1-5, 1875-83. 8°. *Bordeaux,* 1867-83.

Mémoires sur les sujets proposés pour les prix de l'Académie royale de chirurgie. 5 v. 8°. *Paris, Menard & Desenne fils*, 1819.

Memoirs.

See **Biography**; *and under individual names.*

Memoirs of the American Academy of Arts and Sciences. v. 1–4, 1785–1818; n. s., v. 1–9, 1833–73; v. 10, pt. 1, 1868. 8° & 4°. *Boston & Cambridge*, 1785–1873.

Memoirs of the Anthropological Society of London. v. 1–3. 8°. *London*, 1863–9.

Memoirs from the biological laboratory of the Johns Hopkins University. Selected morphological monographs. v. 1. 4°. *Baltimore*, 1887.
Repr. from: Phil. Tr., Lond.; Mem. Bost. Soc. Nat. Hist.; and Rep. scient. results of the voyage of H. M. S. Challenger.

Memoirs on diphtheria. From the writings of Bretonneau, Guersant, Trousseau, Bouchut, Empis, and Daviot. Selected and translated by Robert Hunter Semple. With a biographical appendix, by John Chatto. 407 pp. 8°. *London, New Sydenham Society*, 1859.

Memoirs of the Literary and Philosophical Society of Manchester. v. 1–3; 3. s., v. 1–9. 8°. *Warrington*, 1785–90; *Manchester*, 1862–84.

Memoirs of the Medical Society of London. v. 1–2. xxviii, 496 pp., 4. l.; xx, 538 pp., 4 l. 8°. *London*, 1787–9.

Memoirs of the Medical Society of London. 6 v. ·8°. *London, C. Dilly*, 1792–1805.

Memoirs of the National Academy of Sciences. v. 1–2, 1864–5 to 1883; v. 3, pt. 2, 1886. 4°. *Washington*, 1866–86.

Memoirs of the Royal Academy of Surgery of Paris. 3 v. 12°. *London, J. Rivington & J. Fletcher*, 1759.

Memoirs of a stomach. *See* [**Whiting** (Sydney)].

Memoirs of William Hawes. 14 pp. 8°. [*London*, 1802.] [P., v. 517.]
Repr. from: European Mag. & Lond. Rev., June, 1802.

Memorabilien. Hrsg. und redigirt von Friedrich Betz. [Fortnightly.] v. 1–32, 1856–87. v. 1–16, fol.; v. 17 *et seq.*, 8°. *Heilbronn, Güldig.*
Current. In 1858 became monthly; sub-title: "Organ für praktische und wissenschaftliche Mittheilungen rationeller Aerzte". In 1872–80, sub-title: "Monatshefte für rationelle Aerzte". v. 26, 1881, also called v. 1. new series, sub-title: "Zeitschrift für rationelle praktische Aerzte". 9 nos. forming 1 v. Title of v. 1–2, 1856–7, was: **Memorabilien** aus der Praxis.

Memorabilien der Heilkunde, Staatsarzneiwissenschaft und Thierheilkunst. Hrsg. von J. J. Rausch. v. 1–3, 1813–19. 8°. *Züllichau.*

Memorabilien aus der Praxis.
Was title of v. 1–2 of: **Memorabilien.**

Memoranda der Aetiologie. viii, 160 pp. 24°. *Weimar, Landes-Industrie-Comptoir*, 1839.

Memoranda der allgemeinen Anatomie. 1 l., 46 pp. 32°. *Weimar*, 1838.

Memoranda der allgemeinen Pathologie. iv, 82 pp. 32°. *Weimar*, 1838.

Memoranda der allgemeinen Therapie. viii, 87 pp. 32°. *Weimar*, 1840.

Memoranda der Augenheilkunde. xxiv, 440 pp. 24°. *Weimar, Landes-Industrie-Comptoir*, 1840.

Memoranda der Hautkrankheiten. xl, 586 pp. 32°. *Weimar*, 1841.

Memoranda der Ohrenheilkunde. xvi, 266 pp. 32°. *Weimar*, 1841.

Memoranda der Pharmacopöe. iv, 526 pp. 32°. *Weimar*, 1840.

Memoranda der Semiotik. xvi, 536 pp. 32°. *Weimar*, 1839.

Memoranda der speciellen Anatomie des Menschen. viii, 314 pp. 24°. *Weimar, Landes-Industrie-Comptoir*, 1839.

Memoranda der Toxicologie. x, 144 pp. 32°. *Weimar*, 1839.

Memorandum on cholera, adopted by a medical conference held in the bureau of agriculture, in March, 1866. Printed by authority. 34 pp. 12°. [*Ottawa*], *printed by the Bureau of Agriculture and Statistics*, 1866.

Memorandum of facts and considerations relating to the "cruelty to animals bill", by teachers of physiology in England, Scotland, and Ireland. 6 pp. fol. [*London*, 1882.]

Memorandum of facts and considerations relating to the practice of scientific experiments on living animals, commonly called vivisection. Issued by the Association for the Advancement of Medicine by Research. 14 pp. fol. [*London*, 1882.]

Memoria apologetica dos cirurgiões militares portuguezes, offerecida por elles aos dignos pares do reino, e aos senhores deputados da nação. 20 pp. 8°. *Lisboa*, 1835. [P., v. 1264.]

Memoria científico-descriptiva de las aguas minero-medicinales de la Favorita de Carabaña (provincia de Madrid), autorizada por real orden de 11 de diciembre de 1883. 116 pp., 1 l. 12°. *Madrid, tipog. Gutenberg*, 1884.

Memoria histórico-científica sobre la epidemia de fiebre amarilla sufrida en Barcelona en 1870, redactada por una comision especial compuesta de los académicos de número doctores D. Antonio Mendoza, D. Ramon Torent, D. Luis Carreras y Arago, D. Bartolomé Robert y D. Francisco de P. Campá, secretario ponente. Publicase por acuerdo de la corporacion tomado en sesion de 15 de julio de 1872. 222 pp., 2 pl. 8°. *Barcelona, J. Jepús*, 1872.

Memoria histórica del cólera-morbo en la Habana. v, 100 pp. 4°. *Habana*, 1843.
Bound with: REPERT. méd.-habanero, Habana, 1843, following page 348.

Memoria Joannis Nathanaelis Lieberkühnii. x pp. 4°. [*London*, 1757?]

Memoria medica. A medical commonplace book, with an alphabetical index of the most common terms occurring in practice. Carefully selected and arranged by a fellow of the Massachusetts Medical Society. Index 20 pp.; MS., 176 pp. 4°. *Boston, Carter & Hendee*, 1829.

Memoria presentada por el contador. Del orígen de los ingresos y gastos municipales de los que la novísima ley concede á los municipios, de los propiedades del excmo. ayuntamiento y de su estado económico en 30 de setiembre de 1878. 117 pp. 8°. *Habana*, 1878.

Memoria sobre a excellencia, virtudes, e uso medicinal da verdadeira agua de Inglaterra da invenção do Dr. Jacob de Castro Sarmento . . . Actualmente preparada por José Joaquim de Castro, na sua real fabrica. Por decretos de sua alteza real o principe regente n. s. ordenada por M. J. H. de P. 4. ed. x, 56 pp. 8°. *Lisboa*, 1845. [P., v. 1248; 1260.]

Memoria sobre as medidas sanitarias executadas em 1856 contra o commercio maritimo do Porto a pretexto da febre amarella. 101 pp. 8°. *Porto*, 1857. [P., v. 1254.]

Memoria sobre a utilidade da inoculação das bexigas vaccinas. Traduzida do alemão. 48 pp. 16°. *Lisboa*, 1801. [P., v. 1261.]

Memoria sulla pellagra e sulle condizioni della proprietà fondiaria e della classe agricola in Italia. G. Scanzi, relatore. 16 pp. 4°. *Milano, G. Pisola*, 1882.

Memoria, en que se trata del insecto grana ó cochinilla, de su naturaleza y série de su vida, como tambien del método para propagarla y reducirla al estado en que forma uno de los ramos mas útiles de comercio, escrita en 1777 por el autor de esta gazeta. [P., v. 1242.]
Cutting from: Gazeta de literatura, México, 1794, iii, no. 26, 199–259, 3 pl.

Memorial. Ebenezer Alden, M. D. [1788–1881]. [Commemorative sketch by Rev. Increase N. Tarbox. Address at the funeral service, by Rev John C. Larabee. Remarks at the funeral service, by the Hon. Alpheus Hardy.] 24 pp., port. 8°. [*Boston, D. Clapp & Son*, 1881.]

"Memorial" (A) by certain line officers of the navy, intended to re-open a dispute which was settled by Congress in 1871, after full discussion and deliberation. With notes, comments, and an appendix. 39 pp. 8°. [*Washington*], 1879.

Memorial of committee representing the medical profession of the United States, praying for an appropriation to aid in defraying the expenses of the International Congress to be held in Washington, D. C., in 1887. 49. Cong., 2. sess. Sen. Mis. Doc. No. 35. Jan. 24, 1887. 7 pp. 8°. [*Washington*, 1887.]

Memorial Cottage Hospital, Mildmay Park, N. [Report from re-opening of the hospital Sept., 1886, to March 31, 1887.] 10 pp., 4 l. sm. 4°. [*London, Harrison & Sons*, 1887.]

Memorial of Dr. James Monroe Sturdevant. Prepared for private distribution. 44 pp., port. 8°. *New York, T. Holman*, 1874.

Memorial Hospital, Jarrow-on-Tyne. Balance sheet for the year 1882. 2 l. 12°. [*Jarrow-on-Tyne*, 1883.]

Memorial Hospital and Dispensary of Orange, N. J. By-laws. 17 pp. 12°. *Orange, Orange Journal office*, 1873.
Incorporated April, 1873.

Mémorial des hôpitaux du Midi, et de la clinique de Montpellier. Par le Prof. Delpech. v. 1–2; No. 1, v. 3, Jan., 1829, to Jan., 1831. 4°. *Paris, Gabon.*
Completed. A continuation of: **Éphémérides** médicales de Montpellier.

Memorial for John Bell and Charles Bell, members of the Royal College of Surgeons of Edinburgh, against the managers of the Royal Infirmary of Edinburgh. [With an appendix.] 78, 28 pp. 4°. [*Edinburgh*, 1801.] [P., v. 1623.]

Memorial of the life and work of Charles Morehead [1807–1882], edited by Hermann A. Haines. vi pp., 1 l., 125 pp., 1 pl. 12°. *London, W. H. Allen & Co.*, 1884.

Memorial to the lord advocate of Scotland, by medical officers and proprietors of public and private asylums in Scotland. 1 l. fol. [*n. p., n. d.*] [P., v. 1291.]

Memorial for the managers of the Royal Edinburgh Asylum for the Insane. 8 pp. 8°. [*Morningside*, 1848.] [P., v. 1053.]

Memorial or notice on the iodine oil of Mr. J. Personne, approved by the Academy of Medicine of Paris. 8 pp. 8°. *Paris, Labelonye*, 1862. [P., v. 1031.]

Memorial (A) of Paul Joseph Revere and Edward H. R. Revere. 218 pp. 12°. *Boston, W. P. Lunt*, 1874.

[**Memorial** and petition of physicians and surgeons to Senators and Representatives in Congress, requesting their special attention and favorable consideration of an application for a fire-proof building for the Army Medical Museum and Library at Washington, and protesting against the separation of the library from the museum.] 2 l. 4°. [*New York*, 1884?]

[**Memorial** (The) of physicians and superintendents of chartered and private asylums in Scotland unto the lord advocate for Scotland. Considerations upon bill for the amendment of the present lunacy act for Scotland.] 4 pp. 4°. [*Edinburgh, n. d.*] [P., v. 1291.]

Memorial relating to the University of Edinburgh. [Being an appeal to the public for a general subscription to rebuild the institution on

Memorial relating to [etc.]—continued.
a new plan.] 12 pp. 4°. *Edinburgh, Balfour, Auld & Smellie*, 1768. [P., v. 641.]

Memorial (A) of Samuel Conant Foster, obiit April 18, 1873. 14 pp. [*New York*, 1873.]

Memorial de sanidad del ejército y armada. Publicada por una reunion de oficiales de sanidad. Editor responsable. Manuel Alvarez. [Semi-monthly.] v. 1–2, Dec. 1, 1858, to Feb. 1, 1860. 8°. *Madrid.*

Memorial to the senate and house of delegates of the State of West Virginia [for the establishment of a State board of health. By the special committee of the American Medical Association for the State of West Virginia]. 2 l. 8°. [*Wheeling*, 1876.]

Memorial of the surgeons and physicians of the Massachusetts General Hospital, at Boston, and members of the Massachusetts Medical Society, in support of the claim of W. T. G. Morton, for the discovery of etherization. 36–39 pp. 8°. [*Boston*, 1852.] [P., v. 1202.]
Cutting.

[**Memorial** tribute to Dr. Winslow Lewis.] pp. 396–402, port. [8°. *Boston*, 1875.]
Cutting from: N. Eng. Free Mason, [Bost.], 1875, iii.

[**Memorial** tribute to Dr. Winslow Lewis.] vii, 87–386 pp. 8°. *Boston, Rockwell & Churchill*, 1875.
Cutting from: Proc. Grand Lodge of . . . Masons, Bost., 1875, 87 ; 118 ; 322.

Memorial, etc., to the trustees of the University of Pennsylvania. [In relation to the professorship of botany.] 26 pp. 8°. [*Philadelphia*, 1820.]

[**Memorial** to the trustees of the University of Pennsylvania, recommending the appointment of Dr. H. Lenox Hodge, as professor of clinical surgery. Philadelphia, May 26, 1877.] 1 sheet. 8°. [*Philadelphia*, 1877.]

Memorial of upwards of one hundred physicians and surgeons of the city of New York, praying for the incorporation of the Manhattanville College. To the hon. the legislature of the State of New York. In assembly, March 28, 1828. 2 pp. fol. [*Albany*, 1828.]

Memoriale della medicina contemporanea. Opera periodica mensile, diretta dai dottori Adolfo Benvenuti e L. Paolo Farrio. [Monthly; 2 v. annually.] v. 7–13, Jan., 1842, to June, 1845. 7 v. 8°. *Venezia.*
Each year forms a separate series ; 1842 is 4. series. In July, 1850, united with: **Giornale** per servire [etc.], forming: **Giornale** veneto di scienze mediche.

Memoriale presentato da un medico italiano agli eccellentiss. e venerandi collegj ed università medicali d'Italia sopra la necessità ed il modo di guarire la medicina dalla grave malattia dell'impostura. xlii, 222 pp. 8°. [*n. p.*], 1766. [P., v. 1138.]

Memorials of Agnes Elizabeth Jones, by her sister. 7. ed. xxxix, 486 pp., port. 12°. *London, Strahan & Co.*, 1873.

Memorials from Ben Rhydding, concerning the place, its people, its cures. 1 p. l., ix, 249 pp., 1 pl. 8°. *London, C. Gilpin*, 1852.

Memorials of Dr. Calvin Ellis [1826–83]. 14 pp. 8°. *Cambridge, J. Wilson & Son*, 1884.

Memorials in favour of Robert Dundas Thomson, candidate for the chair of chemistry in the University of Glasgow. 26 pp. 8°. [*Glasgow*, 1852.]

Memorials of judges, inspectors, wardens, physicians, and philanthropists, approving the recommendations of the board of public charities, in behalf of the insane in the prisons and poorhouses of Pennsylvania. 8 pp. 8°. *Philadelphia, A. C. Bryson & Co.*, 1874.

Memoriam (In). Dr. Landon Rives Longworth, born December 25, 1846; died January 14, 1879. [By] M. F. F. Edmund Dexter, born September 25, 1835; died March 19, 1879. [By] G. McL. 12 pp. 8°. [*Cincinnati, R. Clarke & Co.,* 1879.]

Memoriam (In). Eli Geddings. 71 pp. 12°. *Charleston, Walker, Evans & Cogswell,* 1878.

Memoriam (In). Francis Asbury Ashford, born September 19, 1841; died May 19, 1883. [Proceedings of directors of Children's Hospital.] 15 pp. 8°. *Washington, D. C., Gibson Brothers,* 1883.

Memoriam (In). Francis Asbury Ashford. [Proceedings of various societies.] 20 pp. 8°. *Washington, D. C., Gibson Brothers,* 1883.

Memoriam (In). Howard Townsend, M. D., died January 16, 1867. 41 pp. 8°. *Albany,* 1867.

Memoriam (In). James Crowdhill Hall, M. D. [By the board of directors of the Children's Hospital of the District of Columbia.] 14 pp. 8°. *Washington, Gibson Bros.,* 1880.

Memoriam (In). Dr. James Crowdhill Hall. [Proceedings of the Medical Society of the District of Columbia, with memoir by Grafton Tyler.] 32 pp. 8°. *Washington, W. H. Moore,* 1881.

Memoriam (In). James Platt White [1811–81]. 33 l., port. 8°. [*n. p., n. d.*]

Memoriam (In). James Warburton Begbie. 12 pp. 8°. *Edinburgh, Oliver & Boyd,* 1876.

Memoriam (In). J[ohn] M[etcalfe] S[mith] [1828–70], founder of the Cookridge Convalescent Hospital, Leeds. Containing also a report for the first six (6) months from the opening, July 12 to Dec. 31, 1869. 43 pp. 4°. *Leeds, E. Baines & Sons,* 1871.

Memoriam (In). John Rose Baillie Cormack [1848–76]. 2 l. 8°. [*n. p., n. d.*]
Repr. from: Med. Times & Gaz., Lond., 1876, i (B. W. R.). Union méd., Par., 1876, xxi (G. Decaisne).

Memoriam (In). The late Dr. Wm. Whelan, chief of Bureau of Medicine and Surgery, Navy Department. Sept. 4, 1865. 1 sheet. 8°. [*Washington,* 1865.]

Memoriam (In). Proposition to erect a hall in memory of Azariah Smith, M. D., in connection with the medical department of the Central Turkey College. 2 l. 8°. [*n. p.,* 1874?]

Memoriam (In). Randle Wilbraham Falconer [1814–81]. 8 pp. 12°. [*Bath,* 1881.]
Repr. from: Bath Herald, May 7 & 14, 1881.

Memoriam (In). Thomas B. Hitchcock [1839–74]. 38 pp., 1 l., phot. 12°. *Boston, G. L. Keyes,* [*n. d.*]

Memoriam (In) viri Antonii Guilielmi Plazii. Oratione anniversaria. xxviii pp. 4°. [*Lipsiæ, ex off. Klaubarthia,* 1785.]

Memoriam (In). William Beverly Drinkard. Born December 7, 1842; died February 13, 1877. 8 pp. 8°. *Washington, D. C., H. L. Rose,* 1877.

Memoriam (In). William Beverly Drinkard. [Proceedings of the Medical Society of the District of Columbia upon the death of . . .] 10 pp. 8°. [*Washington,* 1877.]

Memoriam (In). William P. Johnston [1811–76]. [By the board of directors of the Children's Hospital of the District of Columbia.] 8 pp. 8°. *Washington, D. C., Gibson Bros.,* 1876.

Memorias leidas en la Sociedad anatómica española. 4 v. 8°. *Madrid,* 1873–6.

Memorias premiadas por la real Academia de medicina de Madrid. v. 1. 4°. *Madrid,* 1860.
Date on cover, 1870,

Memorias de la real Academia médica de Madrid. v. 1–4. 4°. *Madrid,* 1797–1877.

Memorias de la Sociedad médico-farmacéutica de Toluca. Comision de publicacion: Juan Rodrigues [*et al.*]. [Monthly.] v. 1; Nos. 1–2, v. 2, Sept. 16, 1875, to Oct. 15, 1876. 4°. *Toluca, P. Martinez.*

Memorie dell' Accademia delle scienze dell' Istituto di Bologna. 2. s., v. 7–10; 3. s., 1–10; 4. s., 1–5. 4°. *Bologna,* 1868–83.

Memorie sul bonificamento delle Maremme Toscane. 4 p. l., 486 pp., 1 tab. 8°. *Firenze, G. Molini,* 1838.

Memorie sul cholera-morbus. Appendice al bullettino delle scienze mediche pubblicato per cura della Società medico-chirurgica di Bologna. 1 p. l., 238 pp., 6 tab. 8°. *Bologna, Nobili e Comp.,* 1836.

Memorie di diverse provisioni, et usi, praticati nella città di Palermo con occasione della peste gl' anni 1624, 1625, 1626. 12, 12 pp. 4°. *Modena, G. Cassiani,* 1630.

Memorie del dottore Leopoldo Biaggi di Padova. Edizione corretta e rifusa. 144 pp., 1 pl. 8°. *Padova, A. Sicca,* 1842.

Memorie di quanto s' e fatto per preservazione dalla peste in Ferrara durante il governo dell' . . . Cardinale Sacchetti Legato, etc., nelli anni 1629, 1630, 1631; fatte ristampare à comune benefizio dagl' . . . Alessandro Roverella . . . e signori conservatori di sanità, sotto la legazione dell' . . . Cardinale d' Elci Legato, etc. In occasione del contaggio di Messina l' anno mdccxliii. 32 pp. 4°. *Ferrara, Barbieri,* 1743.

Memorie della reale Accademia medica di Roma. 120 pp. 4°. *Roma,* 1882.

Memorie del reale Istituto lombardo di scienze e lettere. Classe di lettere e scienze matematiche e naturali. v. 10–16. 4°. *Milano,* 1865–86.

Memorie del reale Istituto lombardo di scienze e lettere. Classe di lettere e scienze morali e politiche. v. 10–13. 4°. *Milano,* 1865–73.

Memorie del reale Istituto veneto di scienze, lettere ed arti. v. 14–22. 4°. *Venezia,* 1869–85.

Memorski (Metrophanes). *O vlijanii mestnych uslovii na kroveobrashenie i o javlenijach diffusii vnutri glaza. [Effect of local conditions on circulation and on phenomena of diffusion within the eye.] 47 pp., 1 l. 8°. *St. Petersburg, tipog. K. Stremmera,* 1863.

Memory.

ARNOLDUS DE VILLA NOVA. Tractatus de bonitate memoriæ. MS. 4°. [*n. p.,* 1480?]

BLONDUS (M. A.) De memoria libellus, in quo non tam dogmata quam et præsidia præstantissima narrantur, cum horis mercurialibus, quibus omnibus servatis, et compressa excitatur, et firma solatur, procul dubio et diuturna servatur memoria prudentium. 16°. *Venetiis,* 1545.

CREIGHTON (C.) Illustrations of unconscious memory in disease, including a theory of alteratives. 8°. *London,* 1886 [1885].

——. The same. 8°. *New York,* 1886.

FAUVEL-GOURAUD (F.) Phreno-mnemotechnic dictionary; being a philosophical classification of all the homophonic words of the English language; containing also separate classifications of geographical, mythological, biographical, scientific, and technical homophonic words, to be used in the application of the phreno-mnemotechnic principles. [Pt. 1.] 8°. *New York,* 1844.

FOREL (A.) Das Gedächtniss und seine Abnormitäten. Rathhausvortrag gehalten am 11. Dezember 1884. 8°. *Zürich,* 1885.

FOWLER (L. N.) Memory; how to secure and retain it. 12°. *London,* [*n. d.*]

Memory.

GRATAROLUS (G.) De memoria reparanda, augenda, conservandaque ac de reminiscentia; tutioria omnimoda remedia, præceptiones optimæ. *In: AB INDAGINE (J.) Introductiones apotelesmaticæ [etc.] 12°. Aug. Treboc., 1563, 129–215. Also, in: RANTZOVIUS (H.) De conservanda valetudine, etc. 24°. Franckofurti, 1596, 193–239. Also, in: ——. The same. 24°. Francofurti, 1604, 193–239.*

HAGEN (J. C.) *De memoria. 4°. Regiomonti, [1709].

MIDDLETON (A. E.) All about mnemonics. 12°. London, 1885.

PIELZ (J. G.) De memoria memorabili. 4°. Lipsiæ, [1699].

RYFF (G. H.) De memoria artificiali quam memorativam artem vocant. Opusculum rarum ac insigne, totius ejus negotii rationem, mira industria et brevitate complectens. Item, de naturali memoria, quomodo medicinæ beneficio excitanda, capitis et cerebri bona contemperatione roborationeque; libellus studiosis omnibus longe utilissimus. 16°. [n. p.], 1541.

SELS (J.) *Memoriæ physiologia et pathologia. 8°. Bonnæ, 1836.

WEGENER (G. F.) *De natura, labe et præsidiis memoriæ humanæ. 4°. Gottingæ, [1752].

WOLFF (C. J.) *De memoria ejusque remediorum natura usu et abusu. 4°. Jenæ, [1696].

VAN ZYL (D.) *De memoria, ejusque vitiis. 4°. Lugd. Bat., 1694.

Davies (W. G.) Memory and the brain. J. Ment. Sc., Lond., 1864–5, x, 34–49. — **Eyselin** (O.) Ueber Erinnerungstäuschungen. Arch. f. Psychiat., Berl., 1874–5, v, 575–577. — **Fauvelle.** Des idées et de la mémoire. Bull. Soc. d'anthrop. de Par., 1885, 3. s., viii, 485–507. — **Henle.** Ueber das Gedächtniss in den Sinnen. Wchnschr. f. d. ges. Heilk., Berl., 1838, 281; 297. — **Jolly.** De la mémoire. Bull. Acad. de méd., Par., 1877, 2. s., vi, 76–86. Also: Union méd., Par., 1877, 3. s., xxiii, 122–126. Also: Rev. méd. franç. et étrang., Par., 1877, i, 129; 161. Also: Moniteur. J. de méd., etc., Par., 1877, ii, 73; 89. — **Kelso** (J. J.) Memory, its influence and importance. Lancet, Lond., 1844, i, 579. ——. On memory; its influence and importance as a source of action in animals. Ibid., 1845, ii, 233; 1846, i, 488. — **Laycock** (T.) A chapter on some organic laws of personal and ancestral memory. J. Ment. Sc., Lond., 1875, xxi, 156–187. Also, Reprint. — **Louyer-Villermay.** Mémoire (physiologie et psychologie). Dict. d. sc. méd., Par., 1819, xxxii, 278–330. — **Mnémotechnie** (La) appliquée à l'art de la médecine. Courrier méd., Par., 1874, xxiv, 281. — **Mortimer-Granville** (J.) Ways of remembering. Lancet, Lond., 1879, ii, 458–460. — **Ross** (A.) Mind and memory. N. South Wales M. Gaz., Sydney, 1871–2, ii, 97–100.

Memory (*Disordered*).

See, also, **Aphasia**; **Consciousness** (*Double*); **Puerperal** convulsions (*Complications, etc., of*).

BLANDET (E.-A.-É.) *De l'hypermnésie, ou de l'exaltation de la mémoire. [Fragment d'une analyse psychologique de l'homme malade.] 4°. Paris, 1840.

RIBOT (T.) Les maladies de la mémoire. 4. éd. 12°. Paris, 1886.

——. The same. Boliezni pamjati. Perevod s Frantsuzskago pod redaktsiejou A. Cheremshanskago. [Diseases of the memory. Transl. from the French.] 8°. St. Petersburg, 1881.

——. The same. The diseases of memory. Transl. from the French, by J. Fitzgerald. 8°. New York, 1882.

——. The same. Transl. from the French, by W. H. Smith. 8°. New York, 1882.

TAVERNIER (A.) *Quelques considérations sur l'amnésie. 4°. Paris, 1825.

WIRSNIZER (G. A.) *De memoriæ læsione. 4°. Altorfii, [1725].

Anjel. Beitrag zum Capitel über Erinnerungstäuschungen. Arch. f. Psychiat., Berl., 1877–8, viii, 57–64. — **Berthier.** Amnésie syphilitique. (Recueillie par M. Fortin.) Gaz. d. hôp., Par., 1868, xli, 346. — **Bitot.** Sur l'efficacité de la cautérisation légère (badigeonnage de

Memory (*Disordered*).

teinture d'iode) de la muqueuse pharyngienne contre certaines névroses coïncidant avec de l'amnésie; rôle présumé du ganglion cervical supérieur dans cette circonstance. Bull. Acad. de méd., Par., 1876, 2. s., v, 1042. — **Bonucci** (F.) Della memoria che la mania lascia di sè medesima, specialmente in relazione alla medicina legale. Arch. ital. per le mal. nerv., Milano, 1864, i, 255–258. — **Bristowe** (J. S.) Right hemiplegia; amnesia; bronchitis; autopsy. Tr. Path. Soc. Lond., 1869–70, xxi, 34–36. — **Calmeil.** Amnésie. Dict. de méd., 2. éd., Par., 1833, ii, 401–410. — **Chailly.** Observation sur une affection cérébrale aiguë, avec diminution considérable de la mémoire, et oubli de la plupart des noms substantifs. J. gén. de méd., chir. et pharm., Par., 1820, lxxiii, 308–316. — **Chamberet.** Perte de la mémoire des noms substantifs, survenue à la suite d'une fièvre intermittente. J. compl. du dict. d. sc. méd., Par., 1818, ii, 364–367. — **Cowling** (R. O.) The influence of shock on memory. Am. Pract., Louisville, 1880, xxi, 1–5. — **Davies** (F. P.) Remarkable case of sudden loss of memory. Am. J. Insan., Utica, N. Y., 1886–7, xliii, 460–472, 1 phot. — **Dickson** (S. H.) Case of amnesia. Am. J. M. Sc., Phila., 1830, vii, 359–361. — **Dobrzycki** (H.) Z dziedziny chorób pamięci. [Hereditary disease of memory.] Medycyna, Warszawa, 1883, xi, 156. — **Drake** (D.) A case of partial amnesia, in which the memory for proper names was lost. West. J. M. & Phys. Sc., Cincin., 1835, viii, 209–212. — **Duval** (E.) Amnésie profonde causée et entretenue chez une jeune dame, par une vie d'entraînement; guérison rapide, sous l'influence de l'hydrothérapie. Méd. contemp., Par., 1877, xix, 13–15. — **Egger** (V.) & **Lereboullet** (L.) Étude psychologique et physiologique de l'amnésie dans certaines névroses. Gaz. hebd. de méd., Par., 1877, 2. s., xiv, 357; 374. — **Falret** (J.) Amnésie. Dict. encycl. d. sc. méd., Par., 1869, iii, 725–742. — **Finzi** (L. M.) Caso di una perdita periodica di memoria. Rendic. Accad. med.-chir. di Ferrara, 1846–9, 171. — **Galcerán** (A.) Mnemopatias. Rev. frenopát. barcel., 1881, i, 445; 1882, ii, 5; 45. — **Guardia** (J.-M.) Les maladies de la mémoire. Rev. scient., Par., 1881, 3. s., i, 738–747. — **Guillemeau.** Observation sur une perte de mémoire singulière, à la suite d'une apoplexie, dans une personne qui n'étoit pas réglée. J. de méd., chir., pharm., etc., Par., 1764, xx, 61. 66. — **Hamilton** (F. H.) Effect of the loss of consciousness upon the memory of preceding events. Sanitarian, N. Y., 1876, iv, 49–59. — **Hun** (T.) A case of amnesia. Am. J. Insan., Utica, 1850–51, vii, 358–363. — **Jackson** (S.) Case of amnesia. Am. J. M. Sc., Phila., 1828, iii, 272–274. Also: Am. M. Recorder, Phila., 1829, xv, 272–274. — **Koempfen.** Observation sur un cas de perte de mémoire. Mém. Acad. de méd., Par., 1835, iv, 489–494. — **Laycock** (T.) On certain organic disorders and defects of memory. Edinb. M. J., 1873–4, xix, 865–879. Also, Reprint. — **Legrand du Saulle.** Les maladies de la mémoire; troubles morbides multiples; conditions pathogéniques et étiologiques; valeur diagnostique et pronostique. Gaz. d. hôp., Par., 1884, lvii, 1105; 1129; 1153; 1177; 1193. — **Littré** (E.) Congestion cérébrale et perte momentanée de la mémoire de quelques mots. J. hebd. de méd., Par., 1828, i, 218. — **Louyer-Villermay.** Essai sur les maladies de la mémoire, suivi d'un tableau synoptique des aliénations. Mém. Soc. de méd. de Par., 1817, 68–96. — **Mills** (C. K.) Some disorders of consciousness and memory. Polyclinic, Phila., 1886–7, iv, 292–298. — **Pelman** (C.) Ueber das Verhalten des Gedächtnisses bei den verschiedenen Formen des Irreseins. Allg. Ztschr. f. Psychiat., etc., Berl., 1864, xxi, 63–121. — **Perassi.** Caso di amnesia parziale con afasia consecutiva a ferita del cranio al disopra della bozza frontale sinistra. Gior. d. r. Accad. di med. di Torino, 1870, 3. s., ix, 164–166. — **Pick** (A.) Zur Casuistik der Erinnerungstäuschungen. Arch. f. Psychiat., Berl., 1875–6, vi, 568–574. ——. Zur Pathologie des Gedächtnisses. Ibid., 1886, xvii, 83–98. — **Pigeolet.** Histoire d'un cas d'amnésie, survenue subitement pendant la convalescence d'une affection exanthématique. J. de méd. chir. et pharmacol., Brux., 1846, iv, 137–142. — **Sacanella** (E.) Anamnésis etiológica; caso clínico que demuestra su gran importancia terapéutica. Sentido catól., Barcel., 1882, iv, 559–562. — **Sander** (W.) Ueber Erinnerungstäuschungen. Arch. f. Psychiat., Berl., 1873–4, iv, 244–253. — **Tenneson.** Amnésie consécutive à une cautérisation par la pâte de Vienne. Union méd., Par., 1868, 3. s., vi, 896–898. Also: Bull. Soc. méd. d'émulat. de Par., 1869, ii, 188–190. — **Tommasi** (T.) Le memorie locali e il Daltonismo. Sperimentale, Firenze, 1884, liii, 64–71. — **Zaborowski.** La mémoire et ses maladies. Bull. Soc. d'anthrop. de Par., 1881, 3. s., iv, 514–516.

Memory (In) of Edwin Channing Larned [1820–84]. 130 pp. 8°. Chicago, A. C. McClurg & Co., 1886.

Memory (In) of Ernst Krackowizer. 68 pp. 8°. New York, G. P. Putnam's Sons, 1875.

Memphis. Report of the chief engineer to the water-works and sewerage commissioners upon

Memphis—continued.

a public water supply and a system of drainage for the city of Memphis. 110 pp. 8°. *Louisville, J. P. Morton & Co.*, 1868.

——. Annual report of the board of education of the city of Memphis. 25. (1875-6.) 8°. *Memphis*, 1877.

——. Biennial report of the president of fire and police commissioners of the taxing district (Memphis), Shelby County, Tennessee, to the governor of the State, for the years 1879-80. 8°. *Memphis*, 1880.

For 22 months ending Nov. 30, 1880.

——. Annual reports of the board of health of the taxing district of Shelby County (city of Memphis). 1.-8., 1879-86. 8°. *Memphis*, 1880-87.

——. [Circular in relation to the Waring system of sewers in Memphis. By Niles Meriwether, engineer in charge.] Dec. 1, 1882. 1 sheet. 4°. [*Memphis*, 1882.]

——. Monthly reports of deaths. Official report of the board of health of the taxing district of Shelby County, Tennessee (city of Memphis). Jan. to Dec., 1882; March, 1883; June, 1883. sm. 4°. [*Memphis*, 1882-3.]

——. Map of the taxing district of Shelby County, showing construction of sewers, 1883. fol. 10 x 16 in. [*Memphis*, 1883.]

——. Water committee. Report on a public water supply for the city of Memphis. Feb. 23, 1886. 72 pp. 8°. *Memphis, S. C. Toof & Co.*, 1886.

——. Water committee. Report on a public water supply for the city of Memphis. Dec., 1886. 60 pp., 3 plans. 8°. *Memphis, S. C. Toof & Co.*, 1887.

Memphis.

See, also, **Cholera; Education** (*Medical*); **Fever** (*Malarial*), **Fever** (*Yellow, History, etc., of*), *by localities.*

[HOLT (J.)] Discussion on the Memphis system of sewerage. A defence of the principles of organized effort in the sanitation of New Orleans. 8°. *New Orleans*, 1881.

HOWARD (The) Association of Memphis. Charter, constitution, and by-laws. 8°. *Memphis*, 1875.

LAVOINNE. Assainissement de Memphis, Tennessee (États-Unis). 8°. *Saint-Germain*, 1881.

Repr. from: Ann. industrielles. 1881.

QUINTARD (C. T.) A report on the health and mortality of the city of Memphis, Tenn., for the year 1852. 8°. *Memphis*, 1853.

SECTION of a human stomach, having been used twelve years in trying to digest Wolf River third-best water, showing cause of dyspepsia. Respectfully dedicated to the original incorporators of the Memphis water-works. By ——, M. S. P. C. A. fol. [*Memphis, n. d.*]

THORNTON (G. B.) The present improved sanitary condition of Memphis. 8°. *Nashville*, [1887].

VANCE (C. F.) Address on Memphis as the Shelby County taxing district, delivered before the Old Folks' Society. 8°. *Memphis*, 1882.

Billings (J. S.) Report on sanitary survey of Memphis, Tenn. Rep. Nat. Bd. Health 1880, Wash., 1882, ii, 416-441.—**Billings** (J. S.) [*et al.*]. Report of the committee charged with making a sanitary survey of Memphis, Tenn. *Ibid.*, 1879, 237-262. ——. The sanitary condition of Memphis. Nat. Bd. Health Bull., Wash., 1879-80, i, 187-189.—**Grant** (G. R.) The vital statistics and sanitary condition of Memphis, Tenn. N. Orl. M. & S. J., 1851-2, viii, 689-705. *Also*, Reprint. ——. The meteorology, sanitary condition, prevailing diseases, and mortuary statistics of Memphis, Tenn., in 1852. Am. J. M. Sc., Phila., 1853, n. s., xxvi, 94-115. ——. The sanitary condition of Memphis, Tenn., in 1853. Memphis M. Recorder, 1854, ii, 285-298.—**Kedzie** (R. C.) "The city of destruction": a paper read before the Sanitary Convention at Detroit, Jan. 8, 1880, with supplemental remarks by

Memphis.

J. S. Billings. Detroit Lancet, 1879-80, iii, 345-353 *Also:* Proc. . . . San. Convent. Detroit, Lansing, 1880, 72-81.—**Maury** (R. B.) Memphis; its sewers and its health. Med. News, Phila., 1882, xl, 168.—**Memphis** and sewer gas. San. Engin., N. Y., 1882-3, vii, 241.—**Memphis** (The) water supply. *Ibid.*, 1883, viii, 399.—**Merrill** (A. P.) Health and mortality of Memphis, Tenn.; a public address delivered by appointment of the Memphis Medical Society, January, 1853. Memphis M. Recorder, 1852-3, i, 81-95. ——. On the health and mortality of Memphis. *Ibid.*, 1885, iii, 193-201.—**Quintard** (C. T.) On the mortuary statistics of Memphis, Tenn. N. Orl. M. & S. J., 1853-4, x, 252. ——. A report on the health and mortality of the city of Memphis, for the year 1853. Memphis M. Recorder, 1854, ii, 193-220. — **Radford** (G. K.) Mr. Waring and the Memphis sewerage. San. Engin., N. Y., 1880-81, iv, 302. — **Report** of the committee charged with making a sanitary survey of Memphis, Tennessee. Nat. Bd. Health Bull., Wash., 1879-80, i (Suppl. no. 3), 1-12.—**"Ro."** Sanitary condition of Memphis. Maryland M. J., Balt., 1878-9, iv, 290-292. — **Shanks.** Report of the mortuary statistics of Memphis, Tenn., for 1851. N. Orl. M. & S J., 1852-3, ix, 12-21.—**Smith** (G. A.) On the sanitary condition of Memphis. *Ibid.*, 1851-2, viii, 706-714. *Also*, Reprint. — **Sormani** (E. B.) La fognatura della città di Memfi nel Tennessee, Stati Uniti d' America. Gior. d. Soc. ital. d'ig., Milano, 1882, iv, 544-548, 1 pl.—**Thornton** (G. B.) Memphis sanitation and quarantine, 1879-1880. Am. Pub. Health Ass. Rep. 1880, Bost., 1881, vi, 189-203. *Also*, Reprint. *Also:* Sanitarian, N. Y., 1881, ix, 59-61. ——. The death rate of Memphis. Mississippi Valley M. Month., Memphis, 1881, i, 297-304. *Also*, Reprint. ——. Negro mortality of Memphis. Mississippi Valley M. Month., Memphis, 1882, ii, 413-426. *Also:* Sanitarian, N. Y., 1882, x, 721-730. *Also:* Am. Pub. Health Ass. Rep. 1882, Bost., 1883, viii. 177-186. *Also* [Abstr.]: San. Engin., N. Y., 1882, vi, 516. ——. Six years' sanitary work in Memphis. Mississippi Valley M. Month., Memphis, 1886, vi, 437-450. — **Waring** (G. E.), jr. The sewerage of Memphis, U. S. A. With an abstract of the discussion upon the paper. Tr. San. Inst. Gr. Brit., Lond., 1880, ii, 291-306, 2 pl. *Also*, Reprint.—**Winn** (W. B.) The sewer system of Memphis, U. S. America. San. Jour., Glasg., 1882-3, n. s., vi, 177-180. *Also*, Reprint.—**Working** and cost of the Memphis sewers. San. Engin., N. Y., 1883-4, ix, 380.—**Wright** (D. F.) The nosology and meteorology of Memphis, Tenn., for the first six months of the year 1857. Memphis M. Recorder, 1858, vi, 26-40. *Also*. Reprint.

Memphis Cotton Exchange. Proceedings with reference to the public health. 13 pp. 8°. *Memphis, Price, Jones & Co.*, 1880.

Memphis Hospital Medical College. Medical department of Southwestern Baptist University. Annual announcements for the sessions of 1881-2 to 1885-6 (2.-6.). 8°. *Memphis*, 1881-5.

List of students and graduates for the sessions of 1880-81 to 1883-4, in announcements for subsequent years.

——. Announcement of the spring course of instruction for 1882. 2 l. 8°. [*Memphis*, 1882.]

Memphis Institute. Catalogue of the officers and professors, with the address of the trustees and the announcement of the faculties respectively [including the medical department (eclectic)], for the session of 1849-50. 16 pp. 8°. *Memphis, Twyman & Tannehill*, 1849.

Memphis (The) Journal of Medicine; devoted to the advancement of reformed medicine. Edited by T. C. Gayle. [Monthly.] Nos. 3-12, v. 1; Nos. 1-7, 10, 12, v. 2; Nos. 1, 2, 5-10, v. 3, March, 1853, to Nov., 1857. 8°. *Memphis, Tenn.*, 1853-6; *Holly Springs, Miss.*, 1857.

R. H. Harrison added as editor in v. 2; v. 3 edited by Harrison and Jerome Cochrane.

Memphis Medical College. (Medical department of Cumberland University.) Annual announcements for the sessions of 1851-2 (4.); 1852-3 (5.); 1854-5 to 1858-9 (7.-11.); 1869-70 to 1872-3 (17.-20.). 8°. *Memphis*, 1851-72.

Organized in 1846: suspended for two years, 1849-50 and 1850-51; reorganized in 1851; again suspended from 1862-3 to 1867-8, and reorganized again, in 1868, and finally ceased to exist in 1873. List of students and graduates for the sessions of 1851-2; 1853-4 to 1857-8; 1870-71; 1871-2.

Memphis (The) Medical Journal of the Progressive Medical and Physical Sciences. Edited by H. J. Hulce. [Monthly.] Nos. 1-2, v. 1, Oct., 1851, May, 1852. 8°. *Memphis, McClanahan & Hutton.*

Memphis Medical Recorder. Published bi-monthly by the Memphis Medical College. Edited by A. P. Merrill and C. T. Quintard. v. 1–6, July, 1852–8. 8°. *Memphis.*

Want no. 6, v. 6 (1858). Title of v. 1, 1852–3, was: **Medical** (The) Recorder. In v. 4–5, 1855–7, Dr. Merrill sole editor; v. 6, 1857–8, edited by Daniel F. Wright.

Memphis Water Company. Annual report of the directors to the stockholders of the ... April 30, 1873. 48 pp., 1 plan. 8°. *Memphis, S. C. Toof,* 1873.

Men *of letters.*
See **Literary** *men.*

Men and woman medical students, and the woman movement. 13 pp. 8°. [*Philadelphia*], 1869.

Men and women medical students. The hospital clinics and the woman movement. No. 2. 20 pp. 8°. *Philadelphia,* 1870.

Mena (Ferdinand). Commentaria in libros Galeni de sanguinis missione et purgatione, quibus additur libellus utilissimus de ratione permiscendi medicamenta, quæ passim in usum veniunt. 2. ed. 8 p. l., 227 ff., 9 l. 12°. *Augustæ Taurinarum, J. B. Benilaquam,* 1587.

Mena (Thomas-Antoine). * I. Dans le traitement des tumeurs érectiles faut-il préférer la cautérisation à l'excision ou à la ligature de la base de la tumeur? Quel traitement doit-on employer contre les tumeurs érectiles des membres? II. [etc.] 36 pp., 1 pl. 4°. *Paris,* 1842, No. 218, v. 393.

Menagé (Auguste). * Étude sur les calculs de la prostate. 72 pp. 8°. *Paris,* 1880, No. 275.

Ménage (M.-A.) * Sur la phthisie pulmonaire. 27 pp. 4°. *Paris,* 1808, No. 8, v. 69.

Menage (Narcisse-A.-T.) * Quelques considérations sur les affections cérébrales qui peuvent donner lieu à la paralysie. 23 pp. 4°. *Paris,* 1830, No. 175, v. 234.

Ménager (Édouard-Louis). * De l'absorption cutanée de l'iode et de quelques accidents consécutifs chez l'enfant. 31 pp. 4°. *Paris,* 1877, No. 168.

Ménager (Émile). * De la mortalité et de la morbidité du premier âge, et des moyens de les combattre. 49 pp. 4°. *Paris,* 1882, No. 300 & 334.

Ménager (Eugène). * De la résection tibio-tarsienne avec conservation de la malléole externe. 1 p. l., 72 pp., 2 pl. 4°. *Paris,* 1885, No. 339.

Menalda (Henricus). * De usu sacchari in curatione scorbuti. 2 p. l., 51, v pp. 8°. *Groningæ, G. Wouters,* [1833].

"Menapius" [*pseudon.*]. Mir nach! Zur Medizinalreform. iv, 55 pp. 8°. *Crefeld, Funcke u. Müller,* 1846.

Menapius *Insulanus* (Gulielmus) [–1561]. De ratione victus salubris. Opus nunc recens natū, et in lucem editum, cum præfatione Paulo Longiore, ad instar justæ declamationis, in qua laus et utilitas quoque diætetices continentur. 9 p. l., lxxvii pp. 8°. *Coloniæ, apud I. Schoensteniū,* 1540.

———. Encomium febris quartanæ; adjecta quoque est ejusdem quartanæ febris curandæ exactissima ratio, ex doctiss. tam Græcorum quam Latinorum atque Arabum monumentis deprompta. 3 p. l., 86 pp., 1 l. 16°. *Basileæ, J. Oporinus,* 1542. [P., v. 951.]

———. The same. L'éloge de la fièvre quarte, où il est doctoralement prouvé: I. Que ceux qui ont le bonheur d'avoir cette fièvre ne peuvent trop s'en féliciter. II. Que ceux qu'elle n'a pas encore honoré de sa visite ne peuvent la souhaiter avec trop d'ardeur. Traduit du latin, par Monsr. Gueudeville. 108 pp. 16°. *Leide, T. Haak,* 1728.

Bound with: COULET (É.) L'éloge de la goute. 16°. *Leide,* 1728.

Menapius *Insulanus* (Gulielmus)—continued.

———. The same. Le fébricitant philosophe, [etc.] Ouvrage très-sérieux comique. 108 pp. 12°. *La Haye & Francfort sur Meyn,* 1743.

Bound with: COULET (É.) Le gouteux en belle-humeur, etc. 12°. *La Haye & Francfort sur Meyn,* 1743.

Ménard (Alfred). * De la pourriture d'hôpital. 38 pp. 4°. *Paris,* 1856, No. 272, v. 593.

Menard (Amand). * Sur le renversement de la matrice. 16 pp. 4°. *Paris,* 1816, No. 10, v. 119.

Menard (Armand). * De la paralysie faciale syphilitique au début des accidents secondaires. 51 pp. 4°. *Montpellier, Boehm & fils,* 1865, No. 53.   C.

Ménard (Auguste-Arsène). * I. Quelle est la valeur séméiologique de la léthargie? II. [etc.] 40 pp. 4°. *Paris,* 1840, No. 308, v. 363.

Ménard (Charles-Auguste). * Étude pour servir à l'histoire de l'invagination intestinale. 48 pp. 4°. *Paris,* 1873, No. 147.

Ménard (Emmanuel). * Essai sur l'indifférence en matière de thérapeutique. 63 pp. 4°. *Paris,* 1877, No. 555.

Ménard (Eugène). * Étude expérimentale sur quelques lésions de l'empoisonnement aigu par le phosphore. 28 pp., 3 l., 1 pl. 4°. *Strasbourg,* 1869, 3. s., No. 150.

Ménard (Gustave). * Étude sur la maladie kystique du testicule. 66 pp., 2 pl., 1 l. 4°. *Montpellier, P. Grollier,* 1865, No. 71.   C.

Ménard (Louis)[1]. * Du rhumatisme articulaire aigu, et de son traitement. 31 pp. 4°. *Paris,* 1852, No. 209, v. 529.

Menard (Louis)[2]. * Essai sur la congestion pulmonaire localisée aux sommets. 52 pp. 4°. *Paris,* 1875, No. 157.

Ménard (Pierre). * De l'otite moyenne purulente. 35 pp. 4°. *Paris,* 1876, No. 156.

Ménard (Saint-Yves). * Contribution à l'étude de la croissance chez l'homme et les animaux. (Physiologie et hygiène comparées.) 119 pp., 2 pl. 4°. *Paris,* 1885, No. 122.

———. The same. 113 pp., 2 ch. 8°. *Paris, Asselin & Houzeau,* 1885.

Ménard (Victor). * Contribution à l'étude des tumeurs blanches et des abcès froids dans leurs rapports avec l'infection tuberculeuse. 134 pp., 1 l. 4°. *Paris,* 1884, No. 91.

Menardus.
See **Stathmion** (Christophorus). De tertiana febri astrologica experientia, [etc.] 16°. *Vitebergæ,* 1556.

Menaut (Jacques). * De la mort subite dans le décours et la convalescence de la fièvre typhoïde. 39 pp. 4°. *Paris,* 1875, No. 360.

Mencelius (Franciscus Wilhelmus). * De structura mammarum. 32 pp. sm. 4°. *Lugd. Bat., J. van der Aa,* [1720].

Also, in: DE OBERKAMP (F. J.) Collect. diss. 4°. *Francof. a. M.,* 1767, i, 525–548.

Mencelius (Joannes). Gründlicher Bericht und Ordnung, wie bey vorstehenden Sterbenssläufften die Gesunden für der abscheulichen Gifft-Seuche sich präserviren, und die Krancken so damit angezündet worden, sich verhalten sollen, damit sie widerumb curiret und geheylet werden mögen. Gestellet vor die volckreiche Gemeine der Stadt Gross Glogaw, und zugehörige Landschafft. 591. sm. 4°. *Gross Glogaw, J. Funck,* 1613.

Menchaca (Anjel).
See **Wilde** (Eduardo). Curso de hijiene pública, etc. 8°. *Buenos Aires,* 1878.

Menche (Hermann). * Ein zusammengesetztes Cystom des Ovarium mit adhärentem Processus vermiformis. 22 pp. 8°. *Göttingen, Hofer,* 1873.

Menche de Loisne. Étude de l'alimentation en eau de la ville de Lille. Rapports de commission. 58 pp., 2 plans. 8°. [*Lille,* 1864.]

Mencke (W.) Das Krankenpflegehaus in Wilster. Seine Entstehung, Einrichtung und ein-

Mencke (W.)—continued.

jährige Thätigkeit. Rechenschaftbericht. 12 pp. 8°. *Wilster*, 1871.

——. Das Krankenhaus der kleinen Städte. Ein Fortschritt auf dem Gebiete der öffentlichen Heilkunst. 92 pp., 6 pl. 8°. *Berlin, T. C. F. Enslin*, 1879.

——. Kriegschirurgische Hülfe unter freiem Himmel. Eine Skizze den Vereinen vom rothen Kreuz gewidmet. 28 pp., 3 pl. 8°. *Berlin. T. C. F. Enslin*, 1884.

Mencke (Wilhelm). * De tumoribus cavernosis. 15 pp. 8°. *Kiliæ, C. F. Mohr*, 1853.

Mencken (Frid. Otto). De vita, moribus, scriptis meritisque . . . Hieronymi Fracastorii Veronensis . . . Commentatio. 229 pp. 4°. *Lipsiæ, Breitkopf*, 1731.

Mencucci (G. B.) Del Manicomio Anconitano nel triennio 1865–7; tavole statistiche illustrate. 32 pp., 23 tab. 4°. *Ancona, G. Cherubini*, 1868.

——. The same. Nel triennio 1868–70. 58 pp., 28 tab. 4°. [*n. p.*], 1871.

Menda (Adolphus Carolus). * De electromagnetismo. 39 pp. 8°. *Pragæ, C. Geržabek*, [1846].

Mendacity.

See **Insanity** (*Diagnosis, etc., of*).

Mende (Henricus Guilielmus). * Nonnulla de venarum inflammatione, præsertim phlebotomiam excipiente. 59 pp. 8°. [*Dorpat*], *typ. J. C. Schünmanni*, 1826, v. 15.

Mende (Ludwig Julius) [1779–1832]. * De exanthemate tutorio quod vulgo variolas vaccinas dicunt, cujus primam partem vaccini morbi descriptionem . . . publice defendet. 43 pp. 8°. *Gottingæ, in off. Barmeieriana*, [1801].

——. Die Krankheiten der Weiber, nosologisch und therapeutisch bearbeitet. 2 v. 2 p. l., 309 pp.; viii, 400 pp. 8°. *Leipzig u. Berlin, C. Salfeld*, 1810–11.

——. Von der Bewegung der Stimmritze beym Athemholen. Eine neue Entdeckung, mit beygefügten Bemerkungen über den Nutzen und die Verrichtung des Kehldeckels. 24 pp., 1 l. 4°. *Greifswald*, 1816. [*Also, in :* P., v. 1581; 1606.]

German and Latin text.

Additional title: De actione glottidis in respiratione novum inventum.

——. Ausführliches Handbuch der gerichtlichen Medizin für Gesetzgeber, Rechtsgelehrte, Aerzte und Wundärzte. 6 Th. in 6 v. 8°. *Leipzig, Dyk*, 1819–32.

6. Theil: Mit einer Vorrede von C. Gottl. Kühn.

——. Die menschliche Frucht, das Fruchtkind, und das Kind kurz vor, in, und gleich nach der Geburt. In gerichtlich-medicinischer Hinsicht dargestellt. 1 p. l., 136 pp. 12°. *Göttingen, Vandenhoek u. Ruprecht*, 1827.

——. Commentatio anatomico-physiologica de hymene seu valvula vaginali. 22 pp., 6 pl. 4°. *Gottingæ, typ. Dieterichianis*, 1827.

——. De partu arte præmaturo, auxiliisque quibus perficitur; cum descriptione et imagine instrumenti ad os uteri gravidi clausum in hunc finem dilatandum. 20 pp., 1 pl. 4°. *Gottingæ, typ. Dieterichianis*, 1831.

——. Die Geschlechtskrankheiten des Weibes, nosologisch und therapeutisch bearbeitet. [Zweiter Theil: Nach dessen Tode fortgesetzt von Dr. Franz Anton Balling.] 2 v. viii, 325, 736 pp., 1 l. 8°. *Göttingen, Dieterich*, 1831–6.

Also, Editor of : **Beobachtungen** und Bemerkungen aus der Geburtshülfe und gerichtlichen Medicin, Göttingen, 1824–6 —**Zeitschrift** für die Geburtshülfe in ihrer Beziehung auf die gerichtliche Medicin, Göttingen, 1827–8. *Also, Co-Editor of :* **Gemeinsame** deutsche Zeitschrift für Geburtskunde, Weimar, 1826–32.

For Biography, see N. Ztschr. f. Geburtsk., Berl., 1834, i, 1. Hft , 1–6.

For Portrait, see **Collection**—van Kaathoven.—**Collection** of Portr. of Phys. & Men of Sc., 26.

Mende (Paul). * Ein entwickelungsgeschichtlich interessanter Fall von frühzeitiger Verwachsung der Mesocola mit dem parietalen Bauchfelle bei gleichzeitigem abnormen Verhalten des Netzes und der Leber. 30 pp., 1 l. 8°. *Breslau, Breslauer Genossenschafts-Buchdruckerei*, 1887.

Mende (Paulus). * De hepate adiposo, addita morbi historia. 2 p. l., 34 pp. 8°. *Gryphiæ, F. G. Kunike*, 1859.

Mende (Paulus Julius). * De hypertrophia cordis. 28 pp., 1 l. 8°. *Turici, ex off. Zürcheri et Furreri*, 1839. [*Also, in :* P., v. 586.]

Mende (R. Theophil). * Beiträge zur Lehre von der Aufsaugung und Absonderung. [Zürich.] 52 pp. 8°. *Winterthur, J. Westfehling*, 1876.

Mende (Stephanus). * De dystociis dynamicis. 3 p. l., 26 pp., 1 l. 8°. *Vratislaviæ, typ. A. Neumanni*, 1865.

c.

Mendel (Albertus) [1834–]. * De bronchotomia ad extrahenda corpora aliena. 31 pp. 8°. *Berolini, G. Schade*, [1859].

Mendel (Emanuel) [1839–]. * De operationibus ad sanandam epilepsiam adhibitis, adjectis duabus observationibus. 34 pp. 8°. *Berolini, G. Lange*, 1860.

——. Die progressive Paralyse der Irren. Eine Monographie. xii, 352 pp., 12 pl. 8°. *Berlin, A. Hirschwald*, 1880.

——. Die Manie. Eine Monographie. viii, 196 pp. 8°. *Wien u. Leipzig, Urban u. Schwarzenberg*, 1881.

Also, Editor of : **Neurologisches** Centralblatt, Leipzig, 1882.

Mendel (Levi). * De suffocatis. 44 pp. 4°. *Argentorati, J. H. Heitz*, 1776.

Mendel (Mauritius Henricus) [1777–1813]. De perinæi cura in partu. Commentatio maxime ad rei obstetriciæ historiam spectans. 39 pp. 4°. *Vratislaviæ, G. T. Korn*, 1811.

——. Versuche und Beiträge geburtshülflichen Inhalts. 1. Hft vi pp., 1 l., 163 pp. 12°. *Breslau, C. F. Barth*, 1812.

——. Lehrbuch der Geburtshilfe für Hebammen. 2. Ausg. Nach dem Tode des Verfassers neu bearbeitet und mit Zusätzen versehen von Dr. Moriz Küstner. xvi, 331 pp. 12°. *Breslau, J. Mar u. Comp.*, 1824.

Mendel (Philippus). * De saccharo. 24 pp. 4°. *Francof. ad Viadr., typ. J. C. Winteri*, [1761].

Mendelson (Walter). On the renal circulation during fever. An experimental research . . . Cartwright prize essay for 1883. 24 pp. 8°. [*n. p.*, 1883.]

Repr. from : Am. J. M. Sc., Phila., 1883, n. s., lxxxvi.

See, also, **Schreiber** (Joseph). A manual of treatment by massage. [etc.] 8°. *Philadelphia*, 1887.

Mendelssohn (Arnoldus) [1817–]. * De porrigine lupinosa. 32 pp. 8°. *Berolini, typ. Friedlaenderianis*, [1841].

——. Der Mechanismus der Respiration und Cirkulation, oder das explicirte Wesen der Lungenhyperämien. 2 p. l., 384 pp., 1 l. 8°. *Berlin, B. Behrs*, 1845.

Mendelssohn (Maurice). * Untersuchungen über die Muskelzuckung bei Erkrankungen des Nerven- und Muskel-Systems. 89 pp., 1 l. 8°. *Dorpat, Schnakenburg*, 1884.

Also, Co-Editor of : **Archives** slaves de biologie, Paris, 1886.

—— **& Richet** (Charles). Revue des travaux slaves de physiologie pour l'année 1885. 71 pp. 8°. *Paris*, 1886.

Repr. from : Arch slaves de biol., Par., 1886, i.

Mendelssohn (Salomon) [1839–]. * Die Mechanik der Gallensecretion. 33 pp. 8°. *Berlin, G. Lange*, [1868].

Mendenhall (George) [1814–74]. Report of the committee on the epidemics of Ohio. 6 pp. 8°. *Philadelphia, Collins*, 1858.

Repr.from : Tr. Am. M. Ass., Phila., 1858, xi.

[———.] Report on the epidemics of Ohio, Indiana, and Michigan, for the years 1852 and 1853. 132 pp., 1 map, 3 diag. 8°. [*Philadelphia*, 1858.]

Repr.from : Tr. Am. M. Ass., Phila., 1858, xi.

———. Introductory address at the opening of the sixth session of the Miami Medical College of Cincinnati, Nov. 1st, 1865, on : Professional success. 24 pp. 8°. *Cincinnati, A. Moore*, 1865.

———. Address delivered before the American Medical Association at its twenty-first annual meeting. 21 pp. 8°. *Philadelphia, Collins*, 1870.

———. The medical student's vade mecum. A compendium of anatomy, physiology, chemistry, poisons, materia medica, pharmacy, surgery, obstetrics, practice of medicine, diseases of the skin, etc. 10. ed. 692 pp. 8°. *Philadelphia, Lindsay & Blakiston*, 1871.

———. Catalogue of the medical library, and surgical instruments, etc., of the late . . . 17 pp. 8°. *Cincinnati, J. Barclay*, [1877].

Also, Co-Editor of : **Western** (The) Lancet, Cincin , 1850–53.—**Cincinnati** (The) Medical Observer, 1856–7.—**Cincinnati** (The) Lancet and Observer, 1858.

For Biography, see Cincin. Lancet & Obs., 1874, xvii, 439–443. *Also :* Tr. Am. M. Ass., Phila., 1875, xxvi, 447–449. *Also :* Tr. Ohio M. Soc., Piqua, 1874, 379–383 (T. W. Gordon). *Also : Ibid.,* Cincin, 1876, 87–89 (B. B. Leonard).

Mendenhall (T. C.) Characteristic curves of composition. 16 pp. 8°. *Terre Haute, Moore & Langen*, 1887.

Mendes (A. Maia).

Editor of : **Saude** (A) publica, Porto, 1884.

Mendès (Catulle).

See **Monin** (E.) L'hygiène de la beauté. 12°. *Paris*, 1886.

Mendes (João Clemente). Estudo sobre a hemeralopia a proposito dos casos observados na guarnição de Lisboa offerecido a Academia real das sciencias de Lisboa. 1 p. l., 80 pp. 8°. *Lisboa*, 1862.

Mendes (José-Pereira). * Du typhus d'Europe, et en particulier de son traitement par les affusions d'eau froide. vi, 7–43 pp. 4°. *Paris*, 1831, No. 136. v. 241.

sá Mendes (M. H. de N.) A questão da ophthalmia do regimento 12, considerada pelo lado scientifico, mormente em referencia ao seu tratamento. iv, 28 pp., 3 ch. 8°. *Lisboa*, 1856. [P. v., 1266.]

Mendes de Leon (M. A.) * Ueber die Zusammensetzung der Frauenmilch. [Heidelberg.] 36 pp. 8°. *München, R. Oldenbourg*, 1881.

Mendeville (Albert). * Quelques considérations sur les tumeurs gommeuses. 42 pp. 4°. *Paris*, 1871, No. 216.

Mendez (Gualberto). * Du phlegmon et des abcès de la paume de la main. 32 pp. 4°. *Paris*, 1857, No. 215, v. 607.

Mendez (Julio). * Esclerodermia (lesion trófica). 72 pp. 8°. *Buenos Aires, impr. de la Nacion*, 1884.

Mendez (Rafael Rodriguez). Prolegómenos de higiene. 79 pp., 1 pl. 8°. *Barcelona, J. Jepus*, 1874.

See, also, **Giné y Partagás** (Juan). Curso elemental de higiene, [etc.] 8°. *Barcelona*, 1874–6.—¿ **Son** antagonistas la caquexia palúdica y la tisis? 8°. *Cartagena*, 1884.

Mendez Álvaro (Francisco) [1806–83]. Defensa de la clase médica contre las pretensions de cirujanos y practicantes ; exámen crítico de la proposicion de ley que los señores diputados Herrera y Ortiz de Zárate han presentade al Congreso, empeñados en realizar la prevaricada metamórfosis de los cirujanos en médicos, y de los

Mendez Álvaro (Francisco)—continued. ministrantes y practicantes en lo mismo. 134 pp., 1 l. 8°. *Madrid, T. Fortanet*, 1866.

See, also, **Masse** (J. N.) Atlas completo, [etc.] 12°. *Madrid*, 1845.

For Biography, see Encicl. méd.-farm., Barcel., 1883, vii, 784–787. *Also :* Gac. d. l. hosp., Valencia, 1883-4, ii, 481–485 (Cantó). *Also :* Higiene, Madrid, 1883, ii, 366, port. *Also :* Siglo méd., Madrid, 1883, xxx, 785–795, port.

Mendheim (Gustavus Albertus) [1842–]. * De signis graviditatis. 31 pp. 8°. *Berolini, G. Schade*, [1866].

Mendiboure (Alexandre) [1858–]. * Contribution à l'étude de l'ictère spasmodique. 43 pp. 4°. *Paris*, 1884, No. 355.

Mendikil.

Polak (E.) Scheikundig onderzoek van water uit de warme bron te Mendikil. Natuurk. Tijdschr. v. Nederl. Indië, Batav., 1867-8, xxx, 371–374.

Mendini (Giuseppe). La fulminazione. 32 pp. 8°. *Milano, E. Sonzogno*, 1887.

Mendiondo (André-Marie-Joseph) [1857–]. * Étude clinique sur deux cas de péricardite hémorrhagique. 51 pp. 4°. *Paris*, 1883, No. 245.

Mendler (Leopoldus). * De capitis dolore, sive cephalodynia. 23 pp. 8°. *Monachii, J. Roesl*, 1836.

de Mendoça (Luys Hurtado). *See* **Hurtado de Mendoça** (Luys).

de Mendonça (Joaquim Jacintho). Boletim do expediente da presidente da provincia de Sergipe contendo medidas e providencias em soccorro da população da mesma provincia affectada do cholera morbus desde 1862 até 1863. 126 pp. 4°. *Sergipe, typ. provincial*, 1863.

Mendousse (Frédéric). * Considérations sur le diagnostic des tumeurs qui peuvent simuler la pleurésie. 68 pp. 4°. *Paris*, 1872, No. 135.

de Mendoza (Manuel Hurtado). *See* **Hurtado de Mendoza** (Manuel).

Mendoza y Rueda (Antonio) [1811–72]. Estudios clínicos de cirujía. Pts. 1 & 2: Comprende las clínicas quirúrgicas general, particular y especiales, conforme al órden de enseñanza establecido y reglamentos vigentes. Pt. 3 : Comprende el diagnóstico quirúrgico, y correspondiente anatomía patológica. Pt. 4: Comprende el formulario y varios preceptos terapéuticos aplicables al tratamiento de las principales afecciones quirúrgicas. 8°. *Barcelona, A. Flexas*, 1850–52.

For Biography, see **Roquer y Torrents** (J.) Bosquejo necrológico del Dr. Antonio Mendoza y Rueda, leido en la Academia de medicina y cirujía de Barcelona . . . el dia 20 de noviembre de 1872. 2. ed. 8°. *Barcelona*, 1879.

Mendrisio.

See **Cholera** (*Asiatic, History, etc., of*), *by localities.*

Mène (Édouard-Edme). * De la névralgie fémoro-poplitée et de son traitement par la cautérisation transcurrente. 40 pp. 4°. *Paris*, 1859, No. 14, v. 634.

See, also, **Mène** (Maurice) & **Mène** (Édouard). Nouvelles recherches sur les causes de la surdité, etc. 8°. *Paris*, 1860.

Mène (Maurice). * Sur la rougeole. 15 pp. 4°. *Paris*, 1828, No. 76, v. 215.

———. De la nature du siége de la migraine (hémicranie), de la surdité accidentelle et leur traitement rationnel. 4. éd. viii (1 l.), 160 pp., 2 pl. 8°. *Paris, chez l'auteur*, 1840. [*Also, in :* P., v. 1245.]

——— & **Mène** (Édouard). Nouvelles recherches sur les causes de la surdité, les bourdonnements, les étourdissements et la migraine, leurs traitements. 8. éd. vii, 8–224 pp., 2 pl. 8°. *Paris, Allouard*, 1860.

Meneboo (Pierre-François-Louis). * Sur l'aménorrhée. 48 pp. 4°. *Paris*, 1819, No. 283, v. 153.

Ménécier (Charles). Notice sur la rage, avec un projet nouveau de police sanitaire sur la race canine, présenté à son excellence M. le ministre de l'agriculture et du commerce. 59 pp., 1 l. 8°. *Paris, A. Delahaye; Marseille, Camoin,* 1864.

——. Enquête générale sur la rage. Rapport à monsieur le maire de Marseille sur les cas de rage canine observés en 1864. 47 pp. 8°. *Paris, A. Delahaye,* 1865.

——. Historique de l'épidémie de choléra à Marseille, 1865. 61 pp., 1 l. 8°. *Paris, A. Delahaye; Marseille, Camoin,* 1866.
Repr. from: Actes du Comité méd. d. Bouches-du-Rhône, Marseille, 1865.

Menees (Thomas) & **Morton** (John W.) Addresses, delivered at the public commencement, Feb. 28th, 1868, medical department, University of Nashville. 30 pp. 8°. *Nashville, W. H. F. Ligon,* 1867.

Menegazzi (Giuseppe). Prospetto d' un piano di riforma dell' arte medica. 260 pp. 8°. *Venezia, G. Gatti,* 1786.

——. Analisi critica del prodromo alla terza parte del trattato dei bagni di Abano, e apologia del libretto intitolato: Della efficacia delle acque termali di S. Elena, ecc. 34 pp. 12°. *Vicenza, B. Paroni,* 1805. [P., v. 940.]

——. Antipiretologia, o nuova idea delle febbri; memoria. 72 pp. 12°. *Padova,* 1807.

Meneghelli (Mario). Note sulla igiene del bambino. 124 pp. 12°. *Verona, H. F. Münster,* 1886.

Meneghini (Joseph). * De axe cephalo-spinali. 1 p. l., 276 pp. 8°. *Patavii,* 1834.

Meneguin (Joseph-Alfred). * Études cliniques sur l'hypertrophie du cœur. 94 pp., 3 l. 4°. *Montpellier,* 1876, No. 4.

Ménestrel (Alexandre - Charles - Ferdinand) [1802–]. * De l'influence du système de Gall sur l'idéologie. 36 pp. 4°. *Paris,* 1836, No. 64, v. 295.

Menestrel (P.-M.) * Des signes de la mort, considérés sous le rapport médico-légal. 53 pp. 4°. *Paris,* 1837, No. 283.
See, also, **Thouvenel** [Pierre]. Éléments d'hygiène, [etc.] 8°. *Paris,* 1840.

Menet (J. Kaspar). Radicale Heilung der Brüche, oder das bewährte Bruchpflaster. 78 pp. 8°. *Teufen, J. J. Brugger,* 1856.

Ménétrez (Alphonse). * Des polypes de l'urèthre chez la femme. 36 pp. 4°. *Paris,* 1874, No. 466.

Menetrier (Pierre-Eugène). * Grippe et pneumonie en 1886. 203 pp. 4°. *Paris,* 1887, No. 110.

Meng (Richard Magendie). * De cataracta. 29 pp., 1 l. 8°. *Lipsiæ, typ. E. Polzii,* 1859.

Mengarduque (Louis). * Des sarcomes aponévrotiques. 59 pp., 1 pl. 4°. *Bordeaux,* 1884, s. 7., No. 7.

Menger (Æmilius) [1840–]. * De operatione rhinoplastica. 32 pp. 8°. *Berolini, G. Lange,* [1864].

Menger (Henry) [1844–]. * Die Nervenendigungen und Epithelien der Geschmackspapillen. 32 pp. 8°. *Berlin, G. Lange,* [1869]. c.

Menger (Rudolph). * Ueber das Adenom der Niere, eine neue Geschwulstform. 16 pp. 8°. *Leipzig, Sturm u. Koppe,* 1875.

Mengering (Heinricus Andreas). Faciem Hippocraticam levi penicillo adumbratam . . . sistit. 13 l. 4°. [*Lipsiæ*], *typ. hæred. T. Honii,* [1651].

——. * De quartana. 18 l. 4°. *Lipsiæ, lit. Q. Bauchi,* [1652].

von Mengershausen (Julius). * Ueber Cystosarcoma ovarii duplex. 31 pp. 8°. *Jena, Hossfeld u. Oetling,* 1876.

Menges (Peter). * Die Ursachen der Speckhautbildung, ein Beitrag zur Lehre der empfindlichen Blutkrasis. 71 pp. 8°. *Würzburg, C. Becker,* 1844.

Menges (Peter)—continued.

——. Statistik der Lebens- und Gesundheits-Verhältnisse in Nassau im Allgemeinen und derjenigen der Aerzte im Besonderen. 143 pp. 4°. *Weilburg, L. E. Lanz,* 1855.
Repr. from: Mitth. d. Ver. nassau. Aerzte, Weilburg, 1854–5.
Also, Co-Editor of: **Correspondenzblatt** des Vereins nassau'scher Aerzte, Weilburg, 1856–67.

von Menghin (Joannes Michael.), *Ritter von Brunenthal* [1738–89]. * Diss. sistens diagnoses morborum ventriculi et intestinorum. 64 pp. 12°. *Viennæ, typ. Ghelenianis,* 1764.

Mengus (Antoine). * I. Des eaux distillées. II. [etc.] 28 pp. 4°. *Strasbourg,* 1839, No. 27, v. 4.

Mengus (Joseph-Jules-Césaire). * Essai sur le lupus. 37 pp. 4°. *Strasbourg,* 1868, 3. s., No. 102.

Menici (Ranieri). Osservazioni sulle aneurisme. 48 pp., 1 pl. 8°. *Pisa, S. Nistri,* 1824.

——. Observations ad clinicam externam pertinentes anno academico 1827. 110 pp., 2 pl. 8°. *Pisa, ex typog. Nistrio,* 1829.

Ménier. Catalogue commercial, ou prix courant général des drogues simples, produits pharmaceutiques et chimiques, plantes médicinales, médicaments spéciaux et homœopathiques, instruments de pharmacie, de chirurgie, de chimie, de physique et tous autres articles et appareils scientifiques et industriels à l'usage de la pharmacie et de la médecine. 5. éd. 672 pp., 7 pl. 8°. *Paris, H. Plon,* 1860.

Ménier (Jean-Frédéric). * Considérations générales sur les fractures et leur traitement. 40 pp. 4°. *Paris, an XIII* [1805], No. 494, v. 57.

Menier (Jules). * De la cure des végétations par l'usage à l'intérieur de la teinture de Thuya occidentalis. 32 pp. 4°. *Paris,* 1879, No. 541.

Ménier (Réné-François). * Des fièvres intermittentes. Anatomie pathologique, causes, traitement. 40 pp. 4°. *Paris,* 1860, No 25.

Ménière (Émile). * Des moyens thérapeutiques employés dans les maladies de l'oreille. 3 p. l., 119 pp., 2 l., 1 pl. 4°. *Paris,* 1868, No. 57.

——. The same. 3 p. l., 119 pp., 1 l., 1 pl. 8°. *Paris, E. Thunot & Cie.,* 1868.

——. Du traitement de l'otorrhée purulente chronique. Quelques considérations sur la maladie de Ménière. Mémoires lus au deuxième congrès otologique international tenu à Milan en septembre 1880. 46 pp. 8°. *Paris, Germer-Baillière,* 1880.

Ménière (Louis-Pierre). * De la vitesse relative d'absorption par les différentes membranes de l'économie et particulièrement de l'absorption cutanée. viii, 47 pp. 4°. *Paris,* 1873, No. 422.

——. Variations de composition et réactions chimiques des humeurs normales et morbides de l'appareil génital de la femme. 29 pp. 8°. *Paris, O. Doin,* 1885.
Also, Editor of: **Gazette** de gynécologie, Paris, 1885.

Ménière (Prosper) [1799–1862]. * Recherches sur la constitution médicale du troisième trimestre de 1826 (juillet, août, septembre). 22 pp. 4°. *Paris,* 1828, No. 28, v. 213.

——. L'Hôtel-Dieu de Paris en juillet et août 1830. Histoire de ce qui s'est passé dans cet hôpital pendant et après les trois grandes journées, suivie de détails sur le nombre, la gravité des blessures et les circonstances qui ont les rendus fatales. 367 pp. 8°. *Paris, C. Heideloff & U. Canel,* 1830.

——. De l'importance des signes fournis par le pouls dans le diagnostic des maladies. 20 pp. 4°. *Paris,* 1832, No. 368.
Concours.

Ménière (Prosper)—continued.
———. De la guérison de la surdi-mutité. De l'instruction des sourds-muets. 14 pp. 8°. *Paris*, 1853. [P., v. 481.]
Repr. from: Moniteur universel.
———. Études médicales sur les poètes latins. vii, 450 pp. 8°. *Paris, Germer-Baillière,* 1858.
———. Cicéron médecin. Étude médico-littéraire. 2 p. l., 376 pp. 8°. *Paris, Germer-Baillière,* 1862.
———. Les consultations de Madame de Sévigné. 145 pp., 1 l. 8°. *Paris, Germer-Baillière,* 1864.

Ménière's *disease.*
See **Vertigo** *from aural disease.*

Meninges.
See, also, **Arachnoid; Dura** *mater;* **Pia** *mater.*
BAUMER (J. W.) *De meningibus. 4°. *Giessæ,* 1775.
ETTMÜLLER (M. E.) [Pr.] de menynges anatome nonnulla. 4°. [*Lipsiæ,* 1721.]
MARTIN-SAINT-ANGE (G.-J.) Recherches anatomiques et physiologiques sur les membranes du cerveau et de la moelle épinière, et sur le liquide cérébro-spinal. 4°. *Paris,* 1829.
Also, in: J. hebd. de méd., Par., 1830, vi, 97–107: vii, 379–388, 1 pl.
Archambault. Méninges. Dict. encycl. d. sc. méd.; Par., 1873, 2. s., vi, 525–632.—**Arnold** (F.) Anatomical remarks on the membranous coverings of the brain and spinal marrow. Lancet, Lond., 1839–40, i, 112–120.—**Betz** (F.) Ueber die Luftinjection der weichen Hirnhäute bei Enthaupteten. Med. Cor.-Bl. d. württemb. ärztl. Ver., Stuttg., 1852, xxii, 385.—**Conti** (A.) De l'épaisseur de l'écorce du cerveau humain. Internat. Monatschr. f. Anat. u. Histol., Berl., 1884, i, 395–403.—**Coote** (H.) The morbid anatomy of the coverings of the brain. J. Psych. M., Lond., 1850, iii, 521–529.—**Jaccoud** (S.) & **Labadie-Lagrave** (F.) Méninges. N. dict. de méd. et chir. prat., Par., 1876, xxii, 92–299.—**Key** (A.) & **Retzius** (G.) Bidrag till kännedomen om hjärn- och ryggmärgshinnorna, med särskildt afseende på de serösa rummen och lymfbanorna jämte deras förbindelser. Nord. med. Ark., Stockholm, 1870, ii, no. 6, 13–18.

Meninges (*Diseases of*).
See, also, **Meningitis.**
MARIN (O.) *De meningum cerebri ossificatione abnormi. 8°. *Lundæ,* 1834.
Anstie (F. E.) Remarkable case of death from meningeal congestion, without inflammation. Tr. Clin. Soc. Lond., 1874, vii, 34–42.—**De Hart** (J. N.) Contribution to the study of ossification of the meninges. J. Nerv. & Ment. Dis., Chicago, 1878, v, 293–296.—**Mosler** (F.) Zur localen Behandlung der Hirnhautaffectionen. Deutsches Arch. f. klin. Med., Leipz., 1879, xxiv, 246–248.—**Quain** (R.) Cartilaginous deposit in the spinal arachnoid. Tr. Path. Soc. Lond., 1848–50, ii, 25.—**Reynolds** (J. P.) & **Webber** (S. G.) Calcareous degeneration of the membranes of the spinal cord; severe spasmodic affection of the muscles of the body generally before death. Boston M. & S. J., 1868–9, lxxix, 247. *Also:* Extr. Rec. Bost. Soc. M. Improve. (1866–74), 1876, vi, 76.—**Wernicke** (R.) Hiperemia de los meninges espinales y cerebrales. An. d. Circ. méd. argent., Buenos Aires, 1880–81, iv, 365–370.—**Wilks.** Bony plates on the spinal arachnoid. Lancet, Lond., 1860, i, 323.—**Zengiruf** (A.) Sluchai organiches-nago porazheniya mozgovoi kori. [Organic affection of the cerebral membranes.] Med. Obozr., Mosk., 1876, vi, 35–39.

Meninges (*Tumors of*).
SABATIÉ. *Étude sur les tumeurs des méninges encéphaliques. 4°. *Paris,* 1873.
Althaus. Case of syphilitic tumours of the cerebral membranes. Med. Press & Circ., Lond., 1883, n. s., xxxvi, 375. *Also:* Med. Times & Gaz., Lond., 1883, ii, 531.—**Cayley** (W.) Sarcoma of the cerebral pia mater. Tr. Path. Soc. Lond., 1874–5, xxvi, 1.—**Coppée** (C.) Cas de fongus de la dure-mère rachidienne. Bull. Soc. de méd. de Gand, 1854, xxi, 101. [Rap. de Meulewaeter], 106.—**Dowse** (T. S.) Fibro nucleated tumor from the dura mater of the cervical portion of the spinal cord. Brit. M. J., Lond., 1875, i, 705.—**Dutard.** Une tumeur des méninges qui repose sur la convexité du cerveau à l'union du tiers postérieur de l'hémisphère gauche. Bull. Soc. anat. de Par., 1850, xxv, 360–362.—**Humbert.** Cancer des côtes; tumeur des méninges comprimant la troisième circonvolution frontale gauche; aphasie. Ibid., 1870, xlv, 335–337.—**Lebert.** Tumeur fibro-plastique des méninges. Ibid., 1850, xxv, 170.—

Meninges (*Tumors of*).
Richter (J.) Ueber einen Fall von multiplem Sarcom der inneren Meningen des Centralnervensystems. Prag. med. Wchnschr., 1886, xi, 213–215.—**Sawyer.** Hydatid cyst in the meninges of the brain. Lancet, Lond., 1873, i, 201.—**Taube** (J.) Lymphangiom der Pia spinalis: Druckmyelitis. Neurol. Centralbl., Leipz., 1887, vi, 247–250.—**Tyson** (J.) Primary sarcoma of the cerebral meninges. Tr. Path. Soc. Phila. (1871–3), 1874, iv, 194. *Also:* Phila. M. Times, 1872–3, iii, 634.

Meningitis.
See, also, **Brain** (*Inflammation of*); **Brain** (*Sinuses of*); **Brain** (*Syphilitic disease of*); **Cranium, Dura** *mater, Diseases of*; **Ear** (*Diseases of, Catarrhal, etc.*); **Ear** (*Diseases of, Complications, etc., of*); **Erysipelas; Erysipelas** (*Facial*), *etc.* ; **Fever** (*Malarial, Masked, etc.*); **Fever** (*Typhoid, Complications, etc., of*); **Head** (*Injuries of*); **Insanity** (*Pathology, etc., of*); **Mastoid** *process* (*Diseases of*); **Mumps, Pneumonia, Smallpox,** *Complications, etc., of.*
BELLEBON (L.) *Essai sur l'inflammation des membranes du cerveau. 4°. *Paris,* 1810.
BIERBAUM (J.) Die Meningitis simplex. 8°. *Leipzig,* 1866.
BOURSE (P.-L.) *De l'inflammation des méninges et du traitement qui lui convient. 4°. *Paris,* 1821.
BRODARD-LEROY (P.-F.) *Essai sur la méningite aiguë. 4°. *Paris,* 1832.
BROUILLET (E.) *Contribution à l'étude de la méningo-encéphalite traumatique. 4°. *Paris,* 1881.
CAILLIOT (E.-A.) *Observations de méningo-périencéphalite, chronique et primitive; considérations sur cette affection. 4°. *Strasbourg,* 1864.
VON CAMPE (H.) *Beiträge zur pathologischen Anatomie der meningitischen und meningo-encephalitischen Processe. 8°. *Tübingen,* 1882.
DEMIANY (P.) *De orrhymenitide psyctica. 8°. *Pestini,* [1835].
DESBIEZ (C.-É.) *De la méningite cérébrale. 4°. *Paris,* 1851.
DESLANDES (L.) *Examen des différentes formes que peut prendre la phlegmasie des méninges. 4°. *Paris,* 1817.
DOURY (C.-J.-H.) *De la méningite aux différents âges. 4°. *Paris,* 1846.
VAN DRIEL (A. H. C.) *Spec. exhibens casum meningitidis suppurantis in nosocomio academico observatum. 8°. *Traj. ad Rhenum,* 1854.
DUBOSCQ (L.) *De la méningite. 4°. *Paris,* 1848.
FERAUD (S.-H.-H.) *Sur l'arachnoïdite. 4°. *Paris,* 1824.
FOUQUES (G.-F.-V.-D.) *Sur la méningite cérébrale aiguë. 4°. *Paris,* 1836.
FOUSEK (J. A.) *De tunica arachnoidea ejusque inflammatione. 4°. *Vindobonæ,* 1831.
FRANKENBERGER (J. N.) *Diss. sistens meningitidem, adnexa morbi historia 'synoptica. 8°. *Pragæ,* 1843.
GARNIER (L.-A.) *Sur l'arachnitis aiguë cérébrale et rachidienne. 4°. *Paris,* 1830.
GASTON (J.-F.) *Sur la méningite. 4°. *Paris,* 1830.
GIGNOUX (I.) *Sur la méningite. 4°. *Paris,* 1835.
HELLEBAUT (L.-F.) *De phrenitide. 4°. *Gandæ,* [1823].
HERPIN (F.) *Meningitis, ou inflammation des membranes de l'encéphale ; précédé de quelques considérations physiologiques sur ces membranes, et suivi de plusieurs observations recueillies à l'armée du Rhin. 8°. *Paris,* [1803].
HILDEBRAND (O.) *Beitrag zur Lehre von der Aetiologie der Meningitis traumatica suppurativa. 8°. *Jena,* 1886.

Meningitis.

HIPPMANN (W. J.) * Diss. sistens tractatum de inflammatione arachnoideæ, adnexa historia morbi synoptica. 8°. *Pragæ*, 1840.

KIECKENS (C. A. A.) * Diss. sistens quasdam observationes medico-practicas de meningitide. 8°. *Lugd. Bat.*, [1849].

KREMJANSKI (J.) * O krovotochivom vospalenii tverdoi mozgovoi obolochki sukazaniem na svjaz ego s pjanstvom i povalnoe pojavlenie v nastojashee vremja v S.-Peterburge. [Pachymeningitis hæmorrhagica interna prevailing epidemically at present time in St. Petersburg.] 8°. *St. Petersburg*, 1865.

LEROUX (H.-A.) * De la méningite aux différents âges. 4°. *Paris*, 1850.

LEROY (A.-L.) * Quelques considérations sur la méningite cérébrale aiguë. 4°. *Paris*, 1869.

LION (J.-B.-M.-É.) * De la méningite cérébrale aiguë. 4°. *Paris*, 1852.

MALAUSSÈNE (M.) * De la méningite cérébrale aiguë simple et de ses diverses variétés étiologiques. 4°. *Montpellier*, 1877.

MARTEL (F.-E.) * De la méningite, ou inflammation des membranes du cerveau. 4°. *Paris*, 1827.

MEHLHAUSEN (G.) * De meningitide. 8°. *Berolini*, [1849].

MONTEIRO (A.-P.-M.) * Sur la nature, les symptômes de l'inflammation de l'arachnoïde, et son rapport avec l'encéphalite. 4°. *Paris*, 1829.

MORLOT (J.-B.) * De la méningite aux différents âges. 4°. *Paris*, 1846.

NEISSER (J.) Die acute Entzündung der serösen Häute des Gehirns und des Rückenmarks. Nach eigenen Beobachtungen am Krankenbett geschrieben. 8°. *Berlin*, 1845.

ODOLENSKI (I.) * Izsliedovanija gnoiniche forme vospalenija mjagkoi mozgovi obolochki u chelovieka i jivotuiche ve patologo-anatom. otnoshenii. [Suppurating meningitis in man and animals.] 8°. *St. Petersburg*, 1868.

PAIRIER (C.) * Sur l'arachnoïdite aiguë. 4°. *Paris*, 1829.

PARENT-DUCHATELET (A.-J.-B.) & MARTINET (L.) Recherches sur l'inflammation de l'arachnoïde cérébrale et spinale, ou histoire théorique et pratique de l'arachnitis. Avec un rapport fait à l'Institut de France, par MM. Portal, Pelletan [*et al.*]. 8°. *Paris*, 1825.

PHELIPPON (F.-A.) * Essai sur la méningite cérébrale des adultes. 4°. *Strasbourg*, 1863.

PHILIBERT (J.-M.) * Propositions médicales sur l'inflammation de l'arachnoïde. 4°. *Paris*, 1823.

POLÁK (F.) * De meningitide, præcedente historia morbi memorata digni, in clinico pro chirurgis medico anno scholastico 1839–40 tractati. 8°. *Pragæ*, 1841.

RAINALDI (R.) Fu una meningitide traumatica? Perizia medico-legale del D. . . . 8°. *Filottrano*, 1885.

RIVET (G.) * Quelques considérations sur la méningite simple aiguë et la méningite tuberculeuse. 4°. *Montpellier*, 1866.

SCHNELL (A.) * De la méningite chronique en général dans la périencéphalite chronique diffuse en particulier. 4°. *Strasbourg*, 1867.

TURQUET (T.) * De la méningite cérébrale aiguë. 4°. *Paris*, 1833.

VIANCIN (C.-E.) * De la méningite aux différents âges. 4°. *Paris*, 1845.

VIGOT (L.-P.) * Sur la méningite aiguë. 4°. *Paris*, 1836.

WEBER (F.) * De meningitide. 8°. *Pragæ*, [1843].

WENETZKI (H.) * De arachnitide. 8°. *Berolini*, [1841].

Meningitis.

Adams. Acute inflammation of the pia mater, with inflammation of the cerebrum. Proc. Path. Soc. Dubl., 1840-49, i, 210-213.—Amati (N.) Meningo-cefalite. Arch. di med., chir. ed ig., Roma, 1871, iv, 38-40.—André. Méningite suppurée extra et intra-ventriculaire. Bull. Soc. anat. de Par., 1851, xxvi, 367. — Bacon (G. M.) A case of cerebral meningitis. J. Ment. Sc., Lond., 1868-9, xiv, 504-506.—Bailly. Observations sur les deux formes principales de la méningite. Clin. d. hôp. d. enf., Par., 1844, iii, 289-308. — Banon. Arachnitis. Dublin Q. J. M. Sc., 1864, xxxviii, 208-210. — Banti (G.) Meningite cerebrale; esame batterioscopico. Sperimentale, Firenze, 1886, lvii, 159-163.—Bareggi (C.) Due casi di meningite curati con esito felice. Gazz. d. osp., Milano, 1880, i, 302-307. — Barron (G. B.) Case of acute cerebral meningitis due to excessive school-work. Liverpool M.-Chir. J., 1885, v, 238-247.—Barth. Deux hommes morts de méningo-encéphalite, dont la cause a été manifestement l'insolation prolongée et intense. Bull. Soc. anat. de Par., 1853, xxviii, 333 - 335. ———. Méningite peut être tuberculeuse? Guérison. France méd., Par., 1877, xxiv, 241-243.—Bayle (A.-L.J.) Observations d'inflammation aiguë des méninges. Rev. méd. franç. et étrang., Par., 1827, ii, 347-374. — Bechtereff (V. M.) Leptomeningitis hæmorrhagica, protekavshaja s javlenijami progressiv. paralicha. Ejened. klin. gaz., St. Petersb., 1881, i, 138 ; 153 ; 170.—Benson (A.) Case of meningitis which had occurred in a girl aged seventeen after enucleation of a shrunken eyeball, the result of secondary purulent inflammation excited in an old blind staphylomatous eye. Lancet, Lond., 1884, i, 803. — Bierbaum (J.) Meningitis simplex. Deutsche Klinik, Berl., 1865, xvii, 427 ; 436 : 1866, xviii, 43. ———. Meningitis simplex. J. f. Kinderkr., Erlang., 1867, xlviii, 65 - 79. ———. Meningitis simplex. Deutsche Klinik, Berl., 1873, xxv, 184 ; 193.—Billet. Relation de quatre cas de méningite. Rec. de mém. de méd. . . . mil., Par., 1882, 3. s., xxxviii, 508-518. — Boucaud. Observation de péritonite et de méningite aiguës ; recherche étiologique ; alcoolisme. Mém. et compt.-rend. Soc. d. sc. méd. de Lyon (1864), 1865, iv, 56-60. — Bournéville. Observation d'un cas de méningite présumée alcoolique ; guérison. Bull. et mém. Soc. méd. d. hôp. de Par., 1869-70, vi, 129-131.—Brinton (W.) Case of cerebral meningitis. Lancet, Lond., 1864, i, 3.—Brown (J. D.) Acute arachnitis induced upon chronic disease of the brain, by riding in a vertical swing at a fair. Med. Times & Gaz., Lond., 1852, n. s., iv, 387.—Brunet (D.) Néo-membranes et extravasations sanguines produites par l'inflammation de l'arachnoïde crânienne pariétale. Gaz. méd. de Par., 1864, 3. s., xix, 34 ; 49 ; 104 ; 120 ; 172 ; 200 ; 216.—Burder. Cerebral meningitis, with formation of pus beneath the arachnoid. Lancet, Lond., 1873, ii, 81. — Burkart (A.) Ein Fall von subacuter Meningitis (arachnitis). Med. Cor.-Bl. d. württemb. ärztl. Ver., Stuttg., 1872, xlii, 17; 25.—Burnet (J. B.) Case of acute meningitis. Med. & Surg. Reporter, Phila., 1868, xviii, 3.—Burns (J. J. D.) Case of meningitis. Brit. M. J., Lond., 1862, i, 600.—Cabini (G. A.) Gastro-enterite acuta ; interessamento congestivo cerebro-spinale ; convalescenza in 11ª giornata ; dopo alcuni giorni, forte contenzione ; encefalite periferica, delirante ; guarigione in 9 giorni ; perfetto ristabilimento verso la 40ª giornata. Gazz. med. di Milano, 1845, iv, 241 ; 249 ; 257.—Caccia (E.) Meningite traumatica, lenta, circoscritta con successivo stravaso intermeningeo. Spallanzani, Modena, 1878, vii, 439-444.—Camerer. Acht Fälle von Meningitis cerebr., wovon einer tödtlich endete. Med. Cor.-Bl. d. württemb. ärztl. Ver., Stuttg., 1860, xxx, 73-77.—Camó (J.) ¿Qué parte toman la médulla y las raices medulares en la meningitis aguda? An. de cien. méd., Madrid, 1876, i, 222-228.—Canstatt (C.) Meningitis. *In his:* Klin. Rückbl. u. Abhandl., 8°, Erlang., 1851, 2. Hft., 11.—Carpentier. Alcoolisme chronique ; épilepsie ; autopsie. Presse méd. belge, Brux., 1873-4, xxvi, 73.—Carroll (A. L.) Remarks on "leptomeningitis infantum". Gaillard's M. J., N. Y., 1886, xlii, 498-505.— [Cases.] Meningitis. Med. Jahresb. v. Peter-Pauls-Hosp. in St. Petersb. (1840), 1843, 72-75.—Tod. Ber. d. k. k. Krankenanst. Rudolph-Stiftung in Wien (1865), 1866, 147.—Bellevue & Char. Hosp. Rep., N. Y., 1870, 327.—Rep. Superv. Surg.-Gen. Mar. Hosp., Wash., 1882, 208-210.—*Ibid.*, 1883, 216-219.—Cauzius (J.-L.-O.) Méningite; autopsie 36 heures après la mort. Ann. de méd. belge, Brux., 1835, iii, 124. — Cavagnis (V.) Contributo alla cognizione dell' eziologia della meningite. Gazz. med. ital. lomb., Milano, 1878, 7. s., v, 101 ; 111 ; 121 ; 271 ; 281. — Centeno (A. M.) Sobre un caso de meningitis traumática. An. d. Circ. méd. argent., Buenos Aires, 1886, ix, 22-27.—Cheadle (W. B.) Meningitis. Brit. M. J., Lond., 1872, ii, 623 ; 647. — Chiari. Meningitis suppurativa veranlasst durch die Ulceration eines in die Nasenhöhle perforirenden Adenoms der Hypophysis cerebri. Prag. med. Wchnschr., 1883, viii, 245.—Chomel. Observation sur une inflammation aiguë des méninges, sans mouvement fébrile. N. Jour. de méd., chir., pharm., etc., Par., 1818, ii, 275-280.—Cock (T. F.) Case of arachnitis. N. York M. Times, 1851-2, i, 199-201.—Colin. Observation de méningite aiguë, récidivant chez le même individu à six ans de distance ; et

Meningitis.

guérie pour la seconde fois. Gaz. méd. de Par., 1832, iii, 62.—**Cornellas y Ruiz** (E.) Meningitis de la cara convexa del cerebro. Génio méd.-quir., Madrid, 1875, xxi, 187.—**Craigie** (D.) Cases of meningitis ; three terminated fatally, and one recovered. Edinb. M. & S. J., 1834, xli, 71-76.—**Crisp** (E.) Meningitis. Tr. Path. Soc. Lond., 1876, xxvii, 28-30.—**Crocq.** Autopsie d'un homme décédé à la suite de méningite. Presse méd. belge, Brux., 1874-5, xxvii, 53.—**Cruveilhier.** Deux cas de méningite terminés par la mort. Quelques réflexions sur les altérations cadavériques et sur le traitement. Gaz. d. hôp., Par., 1843, 2. s., v, 429.—**Danillo** (S.) K kazuistikie meningitov. Med. Vestnik, St. Petersb., 1879, xix, 33.—**Davis** (H. W.) Cerebral meningitis. Virginia Clin. Rec., Richmond, 1872-3, ii, 415-417.—**Decloux.** Sur un cas de méningo-encépha lite. Arch. méd. belges, Brux., 1886, 3. s., xxx, 361-367.—**De Renzi.** Leptomeningite della convessità cerebrale senza delirio. Salute (suppl.), Genova, 1877, iii, 97-99.—**Devay.** Symptômes du début d'une méningite ; médication énergique coupant court aux accidents. Gaz. méd. de Lyon, 1850, ii, 281.—**Discussion** on meningitis. Med. Rec., N. Y., 1866, i, 165.—**Dixon** (A.) Sub-acute meningitis. Indiana M. Reporter, Evansville, 1881, ii, 107.—**van Dommelen.** Arachnitis. N. pract. Tijdschr. v. de Geneesk., Gorinchem, 1855, n. s., i, 197-213.—**Dumas.** Deux cas de méningite aiguë apyrétique ; mort. Gaz. hebd. d. sc. méd. de Montpel., 1885, vii, 325-329.—**Dunglison** (R.) Case of arachnitis cerebelli. Lond. M. Reposit., 1822, xviii, 286-288.—**Durand-Fardel.** L'arachnoïde et la pie-mère une infiltration purulente. Bull. Soc. anat. de Par., 1842, xvii, 342.—**Fallot.** Observation d'inflammation de la substance et des méninges du cerveau et de la moelle spinale. J. compl. du dict. d. sc. méd., Par., 1830, xxxvii, 64-67. ——. Observation d'inflammation des méninges et de la substance cérébrale, terminée par ramollissement, épanchement et abcès. Ibid., xxxvi, 291-293.—**Fau** (D.) [Over de paraphrenitis.] Handel v. h. geneesk. Genootsch., Amst., 1792, xvi, 87-149.—**Filiatrault** (C.-M.) Méningite cérébrale. Union méd. du Canada, Montréal, 1883, xii, 289-292.—**Finger.** † Vrtljschr. f. d. prakt. Heilk., Prag. 1858, lx, 7-9.—**Finzi** (E.) Delle varie forme di meningite curate nello spedale militare di Parma durante il 1° quadrimestre del 1884. Gior. med. d. r. esercito, etc., Roma, 1886, xxxiv, 129 ; 257 ; 385.—**Fishburn** (J. H.) A case of acute idiopathic meningitis ; suspected poisoning ; post-mortem examination. Med. Times, Phila., 1871-2, ii, 225.—**Fitzgerald** (J. P.) † Austral. M. J., Melbourne, 1879, n. s , i, 531-535.—**Foot** (A. W.) Acute meningitis terminating fatally in nineteen hours. Dublin M. Press, 1861, 2. s., iv, 338.—**Forget.** Méningite foudroyante sporadique. Gaz. d. hôp., Par., 1859, xxxii, 489.—**Fragments** historiques, relatifs à l'inflammation des méninges, arachnitis ou méningite des modernes. Rev. méd. franç. et étrang., Par., 1835, iii, 161-178.—**Gardner** (C. K.) Simple meningitis (fatal) ; post-mortem examination. South. Clinic, Richmond, 1883, vi, 163.—**Gargam.** Sur un cas de méningite suppurée traumatique. Union méd. de la Seine-Inf., Rouen, 1884, xxiii, 17-21.—**Garnier.** Méningo-encéphalite chronique ; autopsie. Arch. méd. belges, Brux., 1885, 3. s., xxvii, 173-179.—**Gennades** (G. S.) Ἱστορία ὀξείας μηνιγγίτιδος ἰαθείσης. Ἰατρικὴ Ἐφημ., Ἀθῆναι, 1858-9, i, 154-156.—**Gintrac.** Inflammation du feuillet externe de l'arachnoïde. Bull. Acad. de méd., Par., 1842-3, viii, 851-856.—**Goodhart** (J. F.) Cases of meningitis of obscure origin. Tr. Clin. Soc. Lond., 1886, xix, 131-136.—[**Gordon.**] Acute suppurative meningeal inflammation. Dublin Q. J. M. Sc., 1863, xxxvi, 206-209.—**Gordon** (F. E.) Two cases of meningitis by metastasis. N. Orl. M. & S. J., 1849-50, vi, 211-213.—**Gosselin.** Encéphalo-méningite ; fracture de la rotule. Gaz. d. hôp., Par., 1876, xlix, 521.—**Grabacher.** Meningitis. Med. Jahrb. d. k. k. österr. Staates, Wien, 1846, lv, 68-72.—**Graux.** Méningite cérébrale. Presse méd. belge, Brux., 1857-8, x, 381-383.—**Green** (P. H.) Acute meningitis. Lancet, Lond., 1839, ii, 922-924.—**Greenfield** (W. S.) On simple meningitis. St. Thomas's Hosp. Rep., Lond., 1878, n. s., viii, 143-185.—**Gribling** (J. J.) Een geval van vermeerderde urine-secretie bij meningitis. Nederl. Tijdschr. v. Geneesk., Amst., 1887, xxiii, 107-110.—**Guéneau de Mussy** (N.) Arachnitis avec pseudo-membranes. Bull. Soc. anat. de Par., 1836-7, xi, 286-289.—**Guersant** père. Méningite ; autopsie; des caractères anatomiques de la méningite. Gaz. d. hôp., Par., 1843, 2. s., v, 209.—**Guersent.** Méningite. Dict. de méd., 2. éd., Par., 1839, xix, 387-440.—**Haddon** (J.) Meningitis. Liverpool & Manchester M. & S. Rep., 1876, iv, 74-77. Also, in his: Gleanings from private practice, 8°. [Liverp.], 1876, 3-6, 1 pl.—**Hardy.** Méningo-encéphalite franche aiguë chez un sujet tuberculeux. Gaz. d. hôp., Par., 1882, lv, 705.—**Hartmann** (P. J.) Zergliederung eines Menschen, der an einer Entzündung der Hirnhäute starb. Auserl. med.-chir.-. . Abhandl. d. röm.-kais. Akad. d. Naturf., Nürnb., 1766, xv, 120-127, 1 pl.—**Hartshorne.** Cases of meningitis. Tr. Coll. Phys. Phila. (1853-6), 1856, n. s., ii, 342-351.—**Hay** (W.) Cerebral meningitis (intercurrent). Chicago M. J., 1875, xxxii, 481-485.—**Heaton** (J. E. H.)

Meningitis.

Meningitis in the adult. Brit. M. J., Lond., 1877, ii, 694.—**Hellema** (D.) Encephalo meningitis. Geneesk. Tijdschr. v. de Zeemagt, Gravenh., 1870, viii, 339.—**Hellwig.** Tod durch exsudative Meningitis. Med. Ztg., Berl., 1856, v, 240.—**Hermann & Kober.** Die Meningitisepidemie in Beuthen (Oberschlesien). Berl. klin. Wchnschr., 1887, xxiv, 513-515. — **Hertzka** (H.) Meningitis mit typischem Verlaufe. Wien. med. Presse, 1871, xii, 275-277.—**Hiard** (T.) Méningite aiguë suivie d'épanchement; guérison. Gaz. d. hôp., Par., 1857, 3. s., xxx, 580. Also: Rev. de thérap. méd.-chir., Par., 1857, [xxv], 482-484.—**von Hoffmann.** Ueber einen operativ behandelten Fall von Meningitis mit Eiterung im intravaginalen Raum des Nervus opticus. Arch. f. Psychiat., Berl., 1887, xviii, 292-294.—**Hornung** (A. M.) † Med. Jahrb. d. k. k. österr. Staates, Wien, 1835, xviii, 531.—**Howard** (T. G.) A case of meningitis. Tr. M. Ass. Alabama, Montgomery, 1872, 81-84. — **Huguenin.** Zur Casuistik der Meningitiden. Cor.-Bl. f. schweiz. Aerzte, Basel, 1882, xii, 97 ; 129.—**Huss** (M.) Meningitis cerebralis. Hygiea, Stockholm, 1843, v, 272-274. — **Hutchinson** (J.) Direct traumatic arachnitis. Med. Times & Gaz., Lond., 1875, i, 519; 547.—**Hutchinson** (J. H.) Cerebral meningitis. Hosp. Gaz., N. Y., 1879, vi, 470-472. Also: Chicago M. J. & Exam., 1881, xliii, 225-228. — **Jackson.** Very extensive arachnitis, connected with disease of the temporal bone. Boston M. & S. J., 1863-4, lxix, 140. Also: Extr. Rec. Bost. Soc. M. Improve. (1862-6), 1867, v, 95.—**Jacobi** (A.) Brain; in a case of meningitis. N. York M. J., 1866, ii, 134-136.—**Jansen** (J. H.) Meningitis subarachnoidea cerebralis et spinalis, in verband staande met verettering der dura mater en caries van het rotsbeen, na ostitis interna. Nederl. Lancet, Gravenh., 1849-50, 2. s., v, 408-415.—**Johnson** (W.) An anomalous case of meningitis. Med. & Surg. Reporter, Phila., 1859, n. s., ii, 269-272.—**Jolly.** Observation sur une méningite aiguë. Bull. Soc. de méd. de Poitiers, 1842, no. 6, 106-113.—**Jones** (C. H.) Clinical lecture on cases of meningitis. Med. Press & Circ., Dubl., 1867, n. s., iv, 1-3. ——. Observations on the changes in meningitis in the small vessels. Tr. Path. Soc. Lond., 1886, xxxvii, 203-215.—**Judée.** Des épanchements purulents sous-arachnoïdiens. Gaz. d. hôp., Par., 1862, xxxv, 457.—**Kiemann.** Meningitis; Tod. Ber. d. k. k. Krankenanst. Rudolph-Stiftung in Wien (1883), 1884, 302.—**Klob** (J.) Ueber das Arachnoideal-Epithel und die Eiterbildung bei Meningitis. Wchnbl. d. k. k. Gesellsch. d. Aerzte in Wien, 1861, xvii, 225-228. — **Klynpennink** (J. R.) [Over de paraphrenitis.] Handel. v. h. geneesk. Genootsch., Amst., 1792, 1-83. — **Krämer.** Meningitis cerebralis et spinalis. Med. Cor.-Bl. bayer. Aerzte, Erlang., 1850, xi, 481-485. — **Kremyanski** (N.) Krovetochnom vospalenii tverdoĭ mozgovoĭ obolochki. [Meningitis from internal hæmorrhage.] Med. Vestnik, St. Petersb., 1865, v, 113.—**Lardier.** Méningite a frigore; effet remarquable du tannin; guérison. Bull. méd. d. Vosges, Rambervillers, 1886-7, no. 4, 45-50, 1 diag.—**La Roche** (R.) A case of acute supervening or chronic arachnitis, attended with symptoms of nervous irritation without fever; death in consequence of a fall. N. Am. M. & S. J., Phila., 1830, ix, 176-187. — **de La Tremblaye.** Observation de méningite idiopathique, suivie de guérison. Rec. d. trav. Soc. méd. d'Indre-et-Loire, Tours, 1850, 58-63. — **Lebeau.** Encéphalo-méningite consécutive à la grippe; compression cérébrale; nécroscopie. Arch. belges de méd. mil., Brux., 1858, xxi, 346-351. — **Lees.** Acute meningitis, with softening of substance of brain. Dublin Hosp. Gaz., 1855, ii, 358.—**de Lemos Vianna.** Meningite. Gaz. d. hosp. mil., Lisb., 1879, iii, 126.—**Leroy-Dupré** (M.-A.-H.) Observation de méningite subaiguë, suivie de guérison. Gaz. méd. de Par., 1849, 3. s., iv, 512.—**Lettsom** (J. C.) & **Ware** (J.) History and dissection of a fatal case, attended with a painful affection of the head. Mem. M. Soc. Lond., 1792, iii, 44-57.—**Leubuscher** (R.) Zur Pathologie der Meningitis. Arch. f. path. Anat., etc., Berl., 1856, x, 221-224. — **Leveran** (A.) Méningite. Dict. encycl. d. sc. méd., Par., 1873, 2. s., vi, 632-676.—**Lewisson.** Fall von Meningitis. Berl. klin. Wchnschr., 1865, xxiv, 249.—**Litardière.** Observations de méningite. Bull. Soc. de méd. de Poitiers, 1842, no. 6, 116-122.—**Löwenhard.** Ueber die Entzündung der Schleimhaut des Gehirns. J. d. pract. Heilk., Berl., 1832, lxxv, 3. St., 61-76. — **Luczkiewicz.** Dwa równoczesne wypadki piorunującego zapalenia oslon mózgowych. [Meningitis tonans.] Gaz. lek., Warszawa, 1872, xiii, 769-776.—**McGaughey** (J. D.) Cases of cerebral meningitis. Phila. M. Times, 1872-3, iii, 195; 216.—**M'Kendrick** (J. G.) A case of meningo-cerebritis, caused probably by exposure to the sun. Edinb. M. J., 1868-9, xiv 517-522.—**Maclagan** (D.) Case of meningitis. Edinb. M. & S. J., 1835, xliv, 342-348.—**Martinet** (L.) De quelques cas de guérison d'arachnitis. Rev. méd. franç. et étrang., Par., 1824, i, 76-85.—**Martinet** (L.) & **Parent-Duchatelet.** Résultats de recherches sur l'inflammation de l'arachnoïde. Rev. méd. hist. et phil., Par., 1821, v, 76-86.—**Mead** (R. M.) A case of meningitis. Proc. M. Soc. County Kings, Brooklyn, 1883-4, viii, 231.—**Mendoza** (A.) Rasgos de una aracnoiditis aguda

Meningitis.

con conatos de suicidio. Gac. méd., Madrid, 1849, v, 171; 177.—**Meniggitidos** (Περὶ). Ἰατρικὴ Μέλισσα, Ἀθῆναι, 1857-8, v, 289-324.—**Merbach.** Ueber die Meningitis pseudomembranosa. J. f. Kinderkr., Berl., 1847, ix, 241-253.—**Moore.** Cases of idiopathic and tubercular meningitis. Dublin Q. J. M. Sc., 1862, xxxiv, 169-172.—**Morehead.** [Meningitis with effusion; autopsies.] [2 cases.] Tr. M. & Phys. Soc. Bombay, 1839, ii, 100-102. — **Morton** (T) † † Med. Press & Circ., Lond., 1882, n. s., xxxiii, 395; 415.—**Morton** (T. G.) Meningitis of the convex surface of the brain; tubercular deposit in the lungs. Proc. Path. Soc. Phila., 1857-60, i, 68. — **Murphy** (J. A.) † Death. Cincin. Lancet & Obs., 1866, ix, 355. — **Nacquart.** Opération de gastro-duodénite avec complication d'arachnitis. J. gén. de méd., chir. et pharm., Par., 1826, xciv, 352-360.—**Nash** (J. B.) Cerebro-arachnitis. Northwest. M. & S. J., Chicago, 1851-2, viii, 319-321.—**Netter.** De la méningite due au pneumocoque (avec ou sans pneumonie). Arch. gén. de méd., Par., 1887, i, 257; 434, 1 pl : ii, 28. — **Neve** (E. F.) Case of rapid acute meningitis, with death. Lancet, Lond., 1883, i, 586. ———. Case of simple meningitis; necropsy. *Ibid.*, 1884, ii, 1139.—**Newman** (D.) A brain which was the seat of idiopathic suppurative meningitis. Glasgow M. J., 1885, [4. s.], xxiii, 63.—**Nixon.** Meningitis of the convexity of the brain. Brit. M. J., Lond., 1877, i, 684. — **O'Ferrall.** Sub-arachnoid meningitis of Cruveilhier. Dublin J. M. Sc., 1844, xxv, 496.—**Ogle** (J. W.) Cases illustrating the formation of so-called false membranes, in connection with the immediate coverings of the brain. Arch. Med., Lond., 1857-9, i, 277: 1860-61, ii, 85.—**Ogston** (F.) A case of acute meningitis. Brit. M. J., Lond., 1885, i, 984.—**Onderdonk** (H. U.) Case of disease in the head, with the appearances after death. N. York M. Mag., 1815, i, 326-330.—**Oppolzer** (J.) Meningitis acuta idiopathica; mit besonderer Berücksichtigung der Diagnose und Therapie. [Case.] Deutsche Klinik, Berl., 1859, xi, 399; 410. ———. Ueber Meningitis acuta. Allg. Wien. med. Ztg., 1861, vi, 427; 436. ———. Medizinische Klinik. Meningitis. Spitals-Ztg., Wien, 1864, 367; 373; 381; 389; 397.—**Osborne** (T. C.) A case of meningo-cerebritis. West. J. M. & S., Louisville, 1849, 3. s., iii, 202-204.—**Papabasileios** (B.) Σημειώσεις ἐπιστημονικαὶ ληφθεῖσαι κατὰ τὴν τελευταίαν ἐπιστράτευσιν παρά τισι τῶν ἐν Θεσσαλίᾳ θέραπευτηρίων. Γαληνὸς, Ἀθῆναι, 1886, ΙΣΤ', 153; 165.—**Partridge.** Latent meningitis. Lancet, Lond., 1850, ii, 510.—**Peabody.** Cerebral meningitis. Med. Rec., N. Y., 1883, xxiii, 49.—**Penfold** (O.) Case of arachnitis following a fall on the head; trephining; death. Lancet, Lond., 1869, ii, 119.—**Picirilli** (L.) Caso di meningite cerebrale. N. Liguria med., Genova, 1874, xix, 433-439. —**Pierson** (S. B.) Observations on brain fever. Edinb. M. & S. J., 1813, ix, 326-332. — **Pingault** fils. Observation d'arachnitis (fièvre cérébrale), suite d'une chute sur la partie postérieure de la tête; autopsie. Bull. Soc. de méd. de Poitiers, 1841, v, 46 - 56. — **Plant** (W. T.) A lecture on acute meningitis. N. York M. J., 1883, xxxviii, 677-680. *Also:* North Car. M. J., Wilmington, 1884, xiii, 13-21.—**Popis.** Deux observations de méningite aiguë. J. de méd. et chir. de Toulouse, 1845-6, ix, 36-42. — **Pratbernou.** Observations sur les inflammations des méninges et du cerveau. J. gén. de méd., chir. et pharm., Par., 1823, lxxxii, 74-92.— **Putzel** (L.) Pachymeningitis hæmorrhagica interna. Cycl. Pract. M. (Ziemssen), N. Y., 1881, [suppl., 551-554].—**Ramskill** (J. S.) Simple meningitis. Syst. Med. (Reynolds), 8°, Lond., 1868, ii, 356.—**Rapin** (O.) Relation d'un cas de méningite traumatique. Rev. méd. de la Suisse Rom., Genève, 1881, i, 248-250, 1 pl.—**Reisz** (C.) Leptomeningitis. Hosp.-Tid , Kjøbenh., 1864, vii, 129. — **Rendu.** Méningite aiguë suppurée; mort. Bull. Soc. anat. de Par. (1872), 1874, 2. s., xlvii, 157.—**Reynolds.** Case of meningitis. Med. Times & Gaz., Lond., 1870, i, 665. — **Richter** (S.) Zur Characteristik der Meningitis-Epidemie in Beuthen O.-S., mit einigen allgemeinen Bemerkungen über diese Erkrankungsform. Breslau. aerztl. Ztschr., 1887, ix, 121-125.— **Ritter von Rittershain** (G.) Klinische Betrachtungen über die Cerebral-Meningitis. [16 cases.] Deutsche Klinik, Berl., 1855, vii, 305; 320; 335 ; 343; 355.—**Roger**(H.) Considérations sur la méningite primitive simple et sur la méningite consécutive à l'otite. Abeille méd., Par., 1865, xxii, 394-396.—**Rogers** (A. W.) Case. [Meningitis?] Tr. M. Soc. N. Jersey, Newark, 1879, 304-308.—**Romberg.** Ueber Arachnitis oder Entzündung der Spinnewebenhaut. Arch. f. med. Erfahr., Berl., 1821, ii, 1; 195.—**Rosenstein.** Zur Kenntniss der primären Meningitis cerebri simplex. [6 cases] Berl. klin. Wchnschr., 1872, ix, 345.—**Ross** (G.) Case of acute purulent meningitis, the result of acute otitis ; with report by Dr. Buller. Canada M. & S. J., Montreal, 1879-80, viii, 343-345. — **Rostan.** Quelques mots sur la méningite ; du phlegmon de la fosse iliaque et de son traitement. Union méd., Par., 1847, i, 390.—**Rothamel.** Ueber Hirnfieber. Med. Ann., Heidelb., 1844, x, 387-407.—**Roux.** Méningite. Rev. de lit. méd., Par., 1876, i, 82-84. — **S.** Meningitis, su diagnóstico y tratamiento. Siglo méd., Madrid, 1883, xxx, 727 ; 796 —**Sansen.** Méningite simple aiguë; autopsie. Arch. méd. belges, Brux., 1884, 3. s., xxxvi, 258-261.—**Sauerwald.** Ein schwerer Fall von

Meningitis.

Meningitis simplex. Deutsche med. Wchnschr., Berl., 1878, iv, 242. *Also:* Deutsche Ztschr. f. prakt. Med., Leipz., 1878, v, 465.—**Savard.** Méningite aiguë simple généralisée survenue dans le cours d'une pleuro-pneumonie. Bull. Soc. anat. de Par., 1879, liv, 162-165. *Also:* Progrès méd., Par., 1879, vii, 710.—**Schillinger** (F.) Sehr acute Meningitis mit rascher Genesung. Oesterr. Ztschr. f. prakt. Heilk., Wien, 1855, i, 237.—**Sée** (G.) Méningite de la base; diagnostic; pathogénie physiologique. Praticien, Par., 1878-9, i, 103-105. *Also:* Abeille méd., Par., 1879, xxxvi, 91.—**Semple** (A.) Meningitis; death. Med. Press & Circ., Lond., 1883, n. s., xxxv, 421.—**Semple** (C. E. A.) A case of acute meningitis in which complete recovery took place. Lancet, Lond., 1887, i, 368.—**Sharp** (H. J.) Cerebral meningitis. Northwest. Lancet, St. Paul, 1881-2, i, 186-192. — **Sinclair.** Acute cerebral meningitis; recovery. Lancet, Lond., 1885, i, 13.—**Singleton** (J. N.) A case of arachnitis followed by hydrocephalus; recovery. Nashville J. M. & S., 1867-8, n. s., iii, 115-120.—**Skoda.** Ueber Meningitis cerebralis und spinalis. Allg. Wien. med. Ztg., 1865, x, 49; 59; 81 ; 97; 113 ; 131 ; 137.—**Smith** (L.) Idiopathic meningitis. Med. Rec., N. Y., 1869-70, iv, 521.—**Smith** (W. A. DeW.) Traumatic suppurative meningitis. Canada M. & S. J., Montreal, 1886-7, xv, 594-596.—**Sokolowski** (A.) Przypadek zapalenia osłon mózgowych (meningitis acuta) z przebiegiem bardzo ostrym. Medycyna, Warszawa, 1881, ix, 519-521.—**Solomka** (N. V.) Sluchai meningita vipuklich chastei mozga (meningitis simplex) ot neizvéstnich prichin. Protok. zasaid. Kavkazsk. med. Obsh., Tiflis, 1882-3, xix, 488-496.—**Somma** (G.) Meningite semplice acuta con esito in guarigione in una bambina lattante. Arch. di patol. inf., Napoli, 1886, iv, 80 ; 97.—**Southey** (R.) Case of acute cerebral meningitis. Med. Press & Circ., Lond., 1884, n. s., xxxvii, 180.—**Stäger.** Arachnitis purulenta mit Erweichung und Vereiterung der Gehirnsubstanz. Beitr. z. Heilk., Riga, 1849-51, i, 258-263. — **Steffen** (A.) Zur entzündlichen Erkrankung der Pia mater. Jahrb. f. Kinderh., Leipz., 1877-8, n. F., xii, 105-115.—**Steiner.** Beitrag zur Aetiologie und Casuistik der Meningitis epidemica. Deutsche med. Wchnschr., Leipz., 1887, xiii, 191-193.— **Stewart** (G.) Case of pachymeningitis interna with hæmorrhage, and temporary relief by trephining. Brit. M. J., Lond., 1887, i, 877 —**Stewart** (T.), jr. A case of cerebral meningitis. Tr. M. Soc. Penn., Phila., 1882, xiv, 315-317.—**Stillé** (A.) Simple acute meningitis. Tr. Coll. Phys. Phila. (1863-74), 1874, n. s., iv, 362. *Also:* Am. J. M. Sc., Phila., 1871, n. s., lxi, 418.—**Stub** (A.) Acute leptomeningitis. N. York M. J., 1885, xlii, 469-471.—**Tanquerel des Planches.** Observation de méningo-céphalite, ayant offert des circonstances remarquables. Gaz. méd. de Par., 1838, 2. s., vi, 181-183. *Also:* Ann. de méd. belge, Brux., 1838, ii, 5-8. — **Tant.** Deux cas de méningite suppurée; autopsie. Arch. méd. belges, Brux., 1881, 3. s., xx, 199-204.—**Thirion** (E.) Nouveau fait de méningo-céphalite, consécutive à une gastro-entérite, guérie par le vésicatoire appliqué sur la tête, alors que beaucoup d'autres moyens avaient échoué. J. de méd., chir. et pharmacol., Brux., 1844, ii, 248-252.—**Thomas** (R. H.) Arachnitis, hyperæmia of the brain, etc. Balt. M. & S. J. & Rev., 1833, i, 362-364.—**Ticier.** Observation de méningite aiguë suivie de guérison. J. de méd., chir. et pharm. de Toulouse, 1853, n. s., v, 5-10.—**Tolosa** (L.) Meningitis aguda simple; curación. Consulta, Cádiz, 1882, i, 73-77.—**Tommasi** (S.) Intorno un caso di meningo-cerebrite. Morgagni, Napoli, 1877, xix, 18-25.—**Trastour** (E.) Deux observations de méningo-encéphalite chez des moissonneurs. J. de la sect. de méd. Soc. Acad. Loire-Inf., Nantes, 1854, xxx, 149. *Also:* Monit. d. hôp., Par., 1854, ii, 963-965.—**Trumet.** Fragment d'une étude sur la méningite. J. de méd., chir. et pharm. de Toulouse, 1859, 3. s., iv, 65-79.—**Ulrich** (C.) † † Deutsche Klinik, Berl., 1859, xi, 344.—**Varrentrapp.** Zwei Fälle von Arachnitis. Jahresb. ü. d. Verwalt. d. Med.-Wes., d. Krankenanst. . . . d. Stadt Frankf. (1858), 1860, ii, 94.—**Vines** (C.) Case of meningitis. Lond. M. Gaz., 1843, xxxii, 422-424.—**Vossius** (A.) Geheilte Meningitis nach Enucleation eines nicht an eitriger Panophthalmitis erkrankten Auges. Klin. Monatsbl. f. Augenh., Stuttg., 1883, xxi, 237 – 241.—**Wagner** (P.) Eine mit schnellem Tode geendigte Vereiterung der Spinnewebenhaut im ganzen Umfange des erweichten Gehirnes und Rückenmarkes, ohne bei Lebzeiten wahrnehmbare Krankheitserscheinungen. Ein Beitrag zur Lehre von der Zurechnungsfähigkeit. Oesterr. med. Wchnschr., Wien, 1842, 73-80. *Also, transl.* [Abstr.]: Prov. M. J., Lond., 1842-3, v, 190.—**Waldenström** (J. A.) Purulent meningitis vållad af snufva. Upsala Läkaref. Förh., 1874-5, x, 423-425. *Also, in his:* Tvá fall af dilatatio cum hypertrophia ventriculi, [etc.], 8°, Upsala, 1875, 10 - 19. — **Walsh** (P. D.) Meningitis. Boston M. & S. J., 1864, lxx, 398-400.—**Ward** (S. B.) Subacute meningitis; atheroma of arteries at base of brain. Med. Rec., N. Y., 1874, ix, 242.—**Westmoreland** (J. G.) [Case of meningitis with cerebritis, with discussion in Atlanta Acad. Medicine.] Atlanta M. & S. J., 1873-4, xi, 444.—**Wharry** (R.) † St. Barth. Hosp. Rep., Lond., 1876, xii, 267-271.—**Whitton** (T. B.) Two cases of

Meningitis.

meningitis; acute and chronic, both terminating fatally. Australas. M. Gaz., Sydney, 1886-7, vi, 192 – 194. — **Winner** (W. G.) A case of basilar meningitis. Therap. Gaz., Detroit, 1887. 3. s., iii, 24–27.—**Wirgin** (A. G.) Meningitis cerebralis acuta. Hygiea, Stockholm, 1848, x, 527–530.— **Wise** (J. C.) A case of acute cerebral meningitis. Proc. Naval M. Soc., Wash., 1882–3, i, 102–105.

Meningitis (*Complications and sequelæ of*).

See, also, **Meningitis** (*Diagnosis, etc., of*).

KRAFFT (J.) * De meningitidis cerebralis et spinalis cum hydrocephalo chronico complicatæ rariori casu. 8°. *Berolini*, [1835].

PARINAUD (H.) * Étude sur la névrite optique dans la méningite aiguë de l'enfance. 4°. *Paris*, 1877.

SALVY (B.) * De la coexistence de la méningite suppurée et de la pneumonie au troisième degré. 4°. *Paris*, 1881.

Alexander. Ein Fall von Arachnitis und Transport des Exsudates aus dem Gehirn in den Bulbus. Klin. Monatsbl. f. Augenh., Stuttg., 1874, xii, 354 – 356. — **Annan** (S.) Arachnitis; pleuritis; adhesion of the pericardium to the heart; colitis; softening of the spleen and kidneys. Maryland M. & S. J., Balt., 1839-40, i, 334–337.—**Armangué** (J.) Méningite probablement tuberculeuse; traitement par l'iodure de potassium; guérison; aphasie consécutive. Gaz. hebd. d. sc. méd. de Montpel., 1883, v, 61; 89; 97; 124; 137; 159; 169; 181; 193. — **Baginsky** (A.) Meningitis simplex; käsige Pneumonie; Miliartuberculose; Ileotyphus. Oesterr. Jahrb. f. Paediat. 1877, Wien, 1878, viii, 101–104, 1 pl.—**Barth** (H.) Un cas de méningite suppurée survenue comme complication dans le cours d'une pneumonie. Rev. de méd., Par., 1882, ii, 681–684.— **Bennett** (A. H.) Clinical lecture on a case of chronic cerebral meningitis; chronic abscess of brain; limited peritonitis; obstruction of the portal and splenic veins; and acute cerebro-spinal meningitis. Brit. M. J., Lond., 1882, i, 727–729.—**Berthold** (E.) Zur Kenntniss der nach Meningitis vorkommenden Erkrankungen des Augapfels. Arch. f. Ophth., Berl., 1871, xvii, 1. Abth., 178–185.—**Bierbaum** (J.) Komplizirte Meningitis simplex. J. f. Kinderkr., Erlang., 1861, xxxvii, 188 – 192. — **Boboue** (T.) Caso di meningite acuta con trombosi dei seni cerebrali in seguito ad otite media cronica purulenta. Osservatore, Torino, 1879, xv, 417 – 423. — **Bolton** (J. A.) Fatal case of meningitis, with an encephaloid tumour of velum interpositum. Newcastle & Gateshead Path. Soc. Communicat., Lond., 1851-2, i, 8–11. *Also:* Med. Times & Gaz., Lond., 1852, n. s., v, 249.—**Brigidi** (V.) & **Banti** (G.) Meningite cerebrale con schizomiceti. Sperimentale, Firenze, 1882, xlix, 494–497.—**Broadbent** (W. H.) Dropsy of the sheath of optic nerve in meningitis. Tr. Path. Soc. Lond., 1872, xxiii, 216–218.—**Bush** (J. M.) Case of insidious inflammation of the pia mater, complicated with pleuritis. Transylv. J. M., Lexington, Ky., 1837, x, 39–42.—**Cuignet.** Œdème du nerf optique et de la rétine, par suite de méningite granuleuse. Rec. de mém. de méd. . . . . mil., Par., 1863, 3. s., x, 359–374.—**Dauchez** (H.) Méningite aiguë; kyste du cervelet. Bull. Soc. anat. de Par., 1883, lviii, 501. *Also:* Progrès méd., Par., 1884, xii, 500. — **Da Venezia** (P.) Meningite probabilmente in causa d' insolazione; diminuzione progressiva della vista fino alla cecità; guarigione. Gior. veneto di sc. med., Venezia, 1869, 3. s., xi, 141–145.— **Dickinson.** Meningitis; long continued and extreme retraction of the head and flexion of the limbs; double optic neuritis and loss of vision; bed-sores; recovery with good vision and powers of movement. Brit. M. J., Lond., 1882, ii, 738.—**Dressler.** Ein Fall von geheilter Meningitis mit Hinterlassung von Taubheit. Prag. med. Wchnschr., 1864, 321. — **Duguet.** De la méningite suppurée comme complication de la pneumonie au troisième degré. Paris méd., 1881, vi, 314–317. — **Elleaume.** Méningite aiguë compliquée de catalepsie et d'éclampsie. Bull. Soc. de méd. prat. de Par., 1857, 72 – 76. *Also:* Gaz. d. hôp., Par., 1858, xxxi, 83. — **von Etlinger** (N.) Ein Fall von Meningitis purulenta nebst multiplen Hirnabscessen, wahrscheinlich metastatischen Ursprungs, bei einem Säugling. Berl. klin. Wchnschr., 1880, xvii, 667. — **Fallot.** Céphalalgie; vomissements; symptômes d'apoplexie; mort; adhérence de la dure-mère au cerveau; hypertrophie considérable du foie et de la rate; refoulement du diaphragme; déviation du cœur. J. hebd. d. progr. d. sc. et inst. méd. Par., 1834, iv, 289–297.—**Flint** (A.) Case of circumscribed arachnitis, situated at the base of cerebellum, attended by effusion, terminating fatally, complicated with miliary tuberculosis of the lung. Buffalo M. J., 1848-9, iv, 743–749.—**Geffrier.** Attaques épileptiformes dans le cours d'une méningo-encéphalite chronique. France méd., Par., 1880, xxvii, 449. *Also:* Bull. Soc. clin. de Par. (1880), 1881, iv, 96–100.—**Grossmann** (L.) Verminderte Sehschärfe beider Augen, hochgradige Schwerhörigkeit des linken Ohres in Folge traumatischer Einwirkung auf den Kopf,

Meningitis (*Complications and sequelæ of*).

Basilar- und Covexitäts-Meningitis. Allg. Wien. med. Ztg., 1881, xxvi, 217. — **Hastings** (C.) Cases of meningitis, co-existing with and obscuring the signs of bronchial inflammation. Midland M. & S. Reporter, Worcester, 1831-2, iii, 103 – 117. — **Hayem** (G.) & **Giraudeau** (C.) Contribution à l'étude des lésions du bulbe consécutives à la méningite chronique. Rev. de méd., Par., 1883, iii, 186–193. — **Hood** (A.) Case of meningitis, with gelatiniform softening and perforation of the stomach. Edinb. M. & S. J., 1834, xli, 243–245.—**van Hoof.** Méningite compliquée. Ann. Soc. de méd. prat. de la prov. d'Anvers, Boom, 1848, vii, 20 – 24. — **Hutton.** Effusion of lymph between the petrous portion of the temporal bone and the dura mater; purulent effusion on cerebellum. Dublin Q. J. M. Sc., 1846, i, 511. — **Jacobi** (A.) Acute meningitis, followed by erysipelas, in a rachitical child; recovery. Med. & Surg. Reporter, Phila., 1878, xxxix, 177.—**Lees** (D. B.) Bronchopneumonia, otitis, and meningitis in an infant of six months: recovery. Practitioner, Lond., 1886, xxxvii, 81–88.—**Lester** (T. B.) Relation of neuralgia of the fifth pair to meningitis. St. Louis Cour. Med., 1879, ii, 209–218. — **Mello** (M.) Observation d'une méningite aiguë, compliquée d'une pneumonie. J. univ. et hebd. de méd. et chir. prat., Par., 1832, vi, 379.— **Moos** (S.) Ein äusserst rapid verlaufender Fall von Meningitis bei einem Erwachsenen; rasche Genesung mit Hinterlassung von bleibender Taubheit und schwankendem Gang. Ztschr. f. Ohrenh., Wiesb., 1883, xii, 101.— **Morehead.** [Meningitis complicated with remittent and typhoid fever. 5 cases.] Tr. M. & Phys. Soc. Bombay, 1843, vi, 61–67.—**Mucci** (D.) Meningite cerebrale con essudato localizzato al centro motorio corticale dell' arto inferiore destro. Guglielmo da Saliceto, Piacenza, 1879-80, i, 301–306.—**Namias** (H.) Meningitis, latente Lungentuberculose. Allg. Wien. med. Ztg., 1863, viii, 117.—**Orsi** (F.) Esoftalmia doppia da meningite basilare essudativa suppurativa. Gazz. med. ital. lomb., Milano, 1882, 8. s., iv, 3.— **Papavoine.** Observation de méningo-encéphalite, avec complication de gangrène sur diverses parties du corps, d'anasarque, etc.; deux mois de maladie; guérison. J. univ. et hebd. de méd. et chir. prat., Par., 1833, xii, 40–50.— **Parrot** (J.) De la dislocation des os du crâne dans la méningite chez les enfants. Rev. de méd., Par., 1882, ii, 112 – 116. — **Pereira** (J. A.) Meningite rachidiana; nephrite parenchymatosa; kystos hidaticos dos ventriculos lateraes do cerebro. Rev. med., Rio de Jan., 1877, iv, 239–241.—**von Pommer.** Plötzlicher Tod bei theilweiser Entzündung der Spinnweben- und Gefässhaut des Gehirns, so wie des Herzbeutels und der äussern Oberfläche des Herzens, ohne vorhergegangene Krankheitserscheinungen. Med. Cor.-Bl. d. württemb. ärztl. Ver., Stuttg., 1833, ii, 2; 5.—**Ritter von Rittershain** (G.) Meningitis; icterus; pharyngitis phytoparasitica; entero-catarrhus. Oesterr. Jahrb. f. Paediat., Wien, 1870, i, 62.— **Robert** (B.) Meningitis encéfalo-raquidiana: absceso cerebral. Rev. de med. y cirug. práct., Madrid, 1882, x, 201; 297.—**Roosa** (D. B. St. J.) Cases of deafness following basilar meningitis. Am. J. M. Sc., Phila., 1874, n. s., xlviii, 377 – 400. — **Semple** (A.) Simple cerebral meningitis (?); purulent discharge from right nostril; recovery. Med. Press & Circ., Lond., 1883, n. s., xxxvi, 198.—**Socin** (B.) Beitrag zur Lehre von den Sehstörungen bei Meningitis. Deutsches Arch. f. klin. Med., Leipz., 1870-71, viii, 476–488.—**Todd** (C. A.) The cause of deafness in children after meningitis. St. Louis Cour. Med., 1882, viii, 529–531.—**Tüngel** (C.) Einige Fälle von protrahirter Meningitis cerebralis mit Hydrops ventriculorum. Klin. Mitth. v. d. med. Abth. d. Allg. Krankenh. in Hamb., 1864, 125–153.—**Verhaeghe.** Méningite aiguë; mort prompte; ramollissement et perforation de l'estomac révélés à l'autopsie. Ann. Soc. méd.-chir. de Bruges, 1844, v, 226–228.—**Wallace** (J. K.) Meningitis, associated with local paralysis and gastric ulcer. Indian M. Gaz., Calcutta, 1879, xiv, 200.—**Weeks.** Ein Fall von Augapfelabscess nach Meningitis. Centralbl. f. prakt. Augenh., Leipz., 1885, ix, 129–134.—**Werner.** Entzündlicher Process an den Meningen; embolische (?) Ablagerungen in der rechten, hämorrhagischer Infarct in der linken Lunge. Med. Cor.-Bl. d. württemb. ärztl. Ver., Stuttg., 1882, lii, 225.—**Wilmart.** Une méningite compliquée d'hémorrhagie méningée. Ann. Soc. d'anat. path. de Brux. Bull., 1870, 17–24.—**Wood** (H. C.) Chronic inflammation of the cortex of the brain, following meningitis. N. York M. J., 1883, xxxviii, 706.

Meningitis (*Diagnosis and symptoms of*).

See, also, **Chemosis.**

BADAN (J.) * Sur quelques points du diagnostic des méningites chez les enfants. 4°. *Paris*, 1861.

BAFFREY (J.) * Du diagnose de la méningite tuberculeuse chez les enfants. 4°. *Strasbourg*, 1848.

Meningitis (*Diagnosis and symptoms of*).

BALABAN (S.) Ueber den Gang der Temperatur bei Meningitis tuberculosa basilaris der Kinder und das Verhalten der Pulsfrequenz zu derselben. 8°. *Heidelberg*, 1884.

BERQUET (M.-G.-F.) *Essai critique sur la température dans la méningite. 8°. *Lille*, 1884.

BOUTAN (J.) *Essai sur la température, le pouls et la respiration dans la méningite tuberculeuse des enfants. 4°. *Paris*, 1877.

GUYOT (L.-L.-E.) *Du rapport des symptômes avec les lésions dans la méningite. 4°. *Paris*, 1859.

JENNICKE (A.) *Ueber die Temperaturen bei Meningitis basilaris. 8°. *Jena*, 1877.

KEYZER (Y.) *Diss. exhibens casum meningitidis, febrim biliosam mentitæ. 8°. *Traj. ad Rhenum*, 1849.

LUBBOCK (M.) *Du diagnostic des différentes formes de méningite cérébrale aiguë et tuberculeuse. 4°. *Paris*, 1879.

PARINAUD (H.) Étude sur la névrite optique dans la méningite aiguë de l'enfance, avec vingt observations suivies d'autopsie recueillies à l'Hôpital des enfants. 8°. *Paris*, 1877.

TRIER (M.) *De symptomatologia meningitidis cerebralis acutæ. 8°. *Havniæ*, 1847.

VIEL (B.) *Étude clinique et expérimentale sur les différences que peut présenter la symptomatologie de la méningo-encéphalite de la convexité du cerveau suivant le siège des lésions. 4°. *Paris*, 1878.

Allbutt (T. C.) On the diagnostic value of the opthalmoscope in tubercular meningitis. Lancet, Lond., 1869, i, 596; 632. ———. Acute local meningo-cerebritis with aphasia. *Ibid.*, 1872, ii, 146.—Bailey (F. K.) Reflex phenomena; threatened meningitis. Detroit Rev. Med. & Pharm., 1875, x, 334–336.—Barrier (F.) Mémoire sur le diagnostic de la méningite chez les enfants, ses difficultés et son importance dans la pratique. J. de méd. de Lyon, 1842, ii, 173–209.—Bell (W. W.) Spurious meningitis. Indiana J. M., Indianap., 1871-2, ii, 97–102.—Bierbaum (J.) Semiotisch-diagnostische Analyse der Erscheinungen bei der Meningitis tuberculosa. J. f. Kinderkr., Erlang., 1871, lvi, 323–402. ———. Individuelle Physiognomie der Meningitis tuberculosa. Deutsche Klinik, Berl., 1873, xxv, 310; 318; 333; 343; 353; 358; 372.—Bigelow (H. R.) The opthalmoscopic diagnosis of acute meningitis. Cincin. M. News, 1874, iii, 291–294.—Blasi. De la termometria en la meningitis tubercular de los niños. Gac. méd. de Sevilla, 1883, v, 17; 28; 41.—Bochefontaine & Viel. Méningo-encéphalite déterminée expérimentalement chez les chiens sur la convexité du cerveau; symptômes différents, suivant les points où elle siège. Compt. rend. Soc. de biol. 1877, Par., 1879, 6. s., iv, 447–451. *Also:* Gaz. méd. de Par., 1878, xliv, 7.—Bókai (J.) Meningitis basil. tuberculosa, felette alacsony hömérsékkel. [. . . remarkably low temperature.] Orvosi hetil., Budapest, 1883, xxvii, 1002–1005. *Also, transl.:* Pest. med.-chir. Presse, Budapest, 1883, xix, 904.—Bouchut (E.) La méningite granuleuse étudiée par l'ophthalmoscope. Gaz. d. hôp., Par., 1862, xxxv, 225. *Also, transl.:* J. f. Kinderkr., Erlang., 1862, xxxix, 254–258. ———. De la méningite étudiée à l'ophthalmoscope. Gaz. d. hôp., Par., 1862, xxxv, 469. *Also, transl.:* J. f. Kinderkr., Erlang., 1863, xl, 444–449. ———. Ueber den Gebrauch des Ophthalmoskopes zur Diagnose der Meningitis. Spitals-Ztg., Wien, 1863, 20–22. ———. De l'ophthalmoscopie dans la méningite aiguë. Union méd., Par., 1865, 2. s, xxviii, 356–361. ———. De la dilatation des veines de la rétine et de l'hémorrhagie de la rétine dans les cas de méningite tuberculeuse et de phlébite des sinus de la dure-mère. Compt. rend. Soc. de biol. 1865, Par., 1866, 4. s., ii, 31. ———. Du diagnostic de la méningite avec l'ophthalmoscope. Gaz. méd. de Par., 1868, 3. s., xxxi 30; 76; 105; 148; 473; 627; 641; 693. ———. De la pseudo-méningite. Union méd., Par., 1869, 3. s., viii, 690; 750; 820; 890; 939. ———. Méningite de la convexité de l'hémisphère droit; névrite optique à droite; autopsie. Gaz. d. hôp., Par., 1869, xlii, 173. ———. Du diagnostic des méningites par l'ophthalmoscope. Cong. périod. internat. d. sc. méd. Compt.-rend. 1877, Genève, 1878, v, 865–869. ———. Leçon d'ouverture sur le diagnostic de la méningite par l'ophthalmoscope. Gaz. d. hôp., Par., 1877, l, 1137–1139. *Also, transl.:* Med. Exam., Lond., 1878, iii, 95.—Bourdalé. Sur un cas de méningo-myélite rapide à forme paraplégique contracturante. Gaz. hebd. d. sc. méd. de Bordeaux, 1885, vi, 199–201.—[Case.] Triangular decubitus as a result of tubercular meningitis. Med. Rec., N. Y., 1879, xvi, 155.—Cianciosi (A.) Sulla

Meningitis (*Diagnosis and symptoms of*).

meningite tubercolosa e i suoi caratteri differenziali con la febbre tifoide. Bull. d. sc. med. di Bologna, 1878, 6. s., i, 241–265.—Collins (M.) Tubercular meningitis; aphasia; paralysis of arm, leg, face, and tongue; convulsions; death. Lancet, Lond., 1884, i, 423.—Cruveilhier. Deux cas de méningite suivie de guérison. Gaz. d. hôp., Par., 1843, 2 s., v, 143.—Dobler (A.) Meningitis cum hydrophobia symptomatica. Oesterr. med. Wchnschr., Wien, 1841, 217–219.—Dowse (T. S.) Case of occipito-spinal meningitis, accompanied by double facial and general paralysis. Brit. M. J., Lond., 1874, i, 172.—Duhamel. Méningite aiguë; catalepsie et éclampsie. Bull. Soc. de méd. prat. de Par., 1857, 81.—Dupuy. Méningite sub-aiguë simulant la méningite tuberculeuse; guérison. *Ibid.*, 1867, 55.—Esquerdo (P.) Exposicion de los sintomas y lesiones de un caso de meningitis especial aguda y simple; estudio razonado de los mismos; consideraciones semeióticas y terapéuticas. Rev. de med. y cirng. práct., Madrid, 1878, ii, 388–397. — Fournier (A.) Méningite tuberculeuse; début insidieux; intermittence des symptômes dans la première et la deuxième périodes. J. d. sc. méd. de Lille, 1880, ii, 845–847. — Fränkel (B.) Weitere Beobachtungen von Aderhauttuberkeln. Berl. klin. Wchnschr., 1869, vi, 37 – 39. — Gairdner. Two cases of tubercular meningitis in the adult, with rather remarkable absence of some of the symptoms commonly regarded as characteristic. Glasgow M. J., 1868-9, [4. s.], i, 260–268.—Garcerá (J.) Observaciones al artículo "Diagnóstico comparativo entre la meningitis y la fiebre tifoídea en un caso médico legal". Encicl. méd.-farm., Barcel., 1877, i, 403. [*See, also, infra,* Ponti (G.).] ———. Contestacion al último artículo del Dr. D. Gerónimo Ponti, "Diagnóstico comparativo entre la meningitis y la fiebre tifoídea en un caso médico-legal". *Ibid.*, 462.—Garlick (G.) Observations on the ophthalmoscopic appearances in the tubercular meningitis of children. Med.-Chir. Tr., Lond., 1879, lxii, 441–463. *Also* [Abstr.]: Proc. Roy. M. & Chir. Soc. Lond., 1879, viii, pt. 8, 421. *Also* [Abstr.]: Med. Times & Gaz., Lond., 1879, i, 711.—Gatti. Le forme anomale di meningite tubercolare. Riv. clin. e terap., Napoli, 1885, vii, 295–304.—Gintrac (E.) Mémoire qui a obtenu le prix sur la question suivante, proposée par la Société de médecine de Caen: "Distinguer les signes de la maladie appelée fièvre cérébrale chez les enfans; de ceux que détermine la présence des vers dans les voies digestives; établir comparativement le diagnostic de ces deux cas". J. gén. de méd., chir. et pharm , Par., 1825, xciii, 3–52.—Gnändinger (H.) Drei Fälle von Meningitis tuberculosa mit abnorm niedrigen Körpertemperaturen. Jahrb. f. Kinderh , Leipz., 1880, n. F., xv, 459 – 464. — Graham (C. R.) Analysis of the ophthalmic appearances in tubercular meningitis. Abstr. M. & S. Cases Gen. Hosp. Sick Children 1882, Pendlebury, Manchester, 1883, ii, 100 – 102. — Greffier. Diagnostic de la méningite tuberculeuse au début. France méd., Par., 1882, ii, 805 – 810. — Guaita (R.) Della pseudo-meningite dentale. Gazz. d. osp., Milano, 1883, iv, 27 ; 36 ; 51 ; 68.—Guillery. Meningitis tubercul. mit eigenthümlichen Initialerscheinungen. Deutsche mil.-ärztl. Ztschr., Berl., 1885, xiv, 136. — Henoch. Ueber die Temperaturverhältnisse bei der Meningitis tuberculosa der Kinder. [8 cases.] Charité-Ann. 1877, Berl., 1879, iv, 505 – 516. — Henoch (E.) Meningite o uremia? Arch. di patol. inf., Napoli, 1885, iii, 6-9.—Henrot (W.) Des troubles hémithermiques (hémi-hyperthermie, hémi-hypothermie) dans la méningite. Union méd. et scient. du nord-est, Reims, 1879, iii, 47–54.—Jacobi (Mary P.) Case of tubercular meningitis, with measurements of cranial temperatures. J. Nerv. & Ment. Dis., Chicago, 1880, n. s., v, 51–56. *Also,* Reprint.—Jakovleff (I. M.) Sluchai paresis w sympathiei pri meningo-enceph. chron. Ejened. klin. gaz., St. Petersb., 1881, i, 206.—Kernig (W.) Ueber ein wenig bemerktes Symptom bei acuter Meningitis. Cong. périod. internat. d. sc. méd. Compt.-rend. 1884, Copenh., 1886, ii (Sect. de méd.), 143.—Lasègue. Sur un signe de méningite (douleurs cérébrales des membres). J. de méd. et chir. prat., Par., 1884, lv, 7–9.—Lebron. Diagnostic différentiel de la méningite vermineuse et de la méningite tuberculeuse. France méd., Par., 1864, xi, 242. — Legroux (A.) Du diagnostic entre la méningite tuberculeuse à son début et le torticolis postérieur rhumatismal aigu chez l'enfant. Encéphale, Par., 1885, v. 21–30.—Loeb (M.) Ein Erklärungsversuch der verschiedenartigen Temperaturverhältnisse bei der tuberculösen Basilar-Meningitis. Deutsches Arch. f. klin. Med., Leipz , 1883-4, xxxiv, 443–450.—Longstreth (M.) Autopsy in a case of acute meningitis with diseased heart; remarks on diagnosis. Boston M. & S J., 1882, cvii, 601. — Mader. Meningitis tuberculosa mit ungewöhnlichen Initialsymptomen corticaler Natur; Tod. Ber. d. k. k. Krankenanst. Rudolph-Stiftung in Wien (1881), 1882, 308. *Also:* Wien. med. Bl., 1883, vi, 131. ———. Fibrinös eitrige Meningitis nach Pneumonie; deutliche linksseitige Hemiparesis, anscheinend bedingt durch weitaus stärkere Exsudation über dem motorischen Gyris der rechten Grosshirnrinde; Tod. Ber.

Meningitis (*Diagnosis and symptoms of*).

d. k. k. Krankenanst. Rudolph-Stiftung in Wien (1884), 1885, 328. ———. Tuberculose Meningitis; initiale Aphasie und Schwäche des rechten Armes; dem entsprechend ausgesprochen überwiegende Affection über der 3. Stirnwindung; Tod. *Ibid.*, 329.—**Maes.** Symptômes singuliers de méningite tuberculeuse, se jugeant par l'expulsion d'un tænia. [Rap. de Poirier.] Bull. Soc. de méd. de Gand, 1866, xxxiii. 40-45. [Discussion], 87-97. — **Malherbe.** Observations de méningite tuberculeuse, suivies de réflexions sur le diagnostic de cette maladie. J. de la sect. de méd. Soc. acad. Loire-Inf., Nantes, 1842, xviii, 100-124. *Also,* Reprint.—**Marques** (J. A.) Dor nos joelhos como symptoma da meningite. Escholiaste med., Lisb., 1865, xvi, 55.—**von Maschka.** Rasch und unerwartet eingetretener Tod; Verdacht einer Vergiftung; eitrige Meningitis. Wien. med. Wchnschr., 1887, xxxvii, 781.— **Pagès.** Observation de méningite épileptiforme. Gaz. d. hôp., Par., 1861, xxxiv. 138. — **von Pfungen** (R.) Ueber topische Begründung der Bewegunsstörungen an den Augenmuskeln bei Meningitis. W.en. med. Bl., 1883, vi, 213; 253; 281; 314. — **Pitt** (G. N.) Non-tubercular meningitis; persistent retraction of the head and neck. Med. Times & Gaz., Lond., 1885, ii, 872.—**Pizzamiglio** (A.) Sul valore della febbre nel processo flogistico-suppurativo degli involucri cerebrali. Gazz. med. ital. lomb., Milano, 1861, 4. s., vi, 221. — **Pontí** (G.) Diagnóstico comparativo entre la meningitis y la fiebre tifoidea en un caso médico-legal. [Contestacion á las observaciones de José Garcerá.] Encicl. méd.-farm., Barcel., 1877, i, 65; 423; 496.—**Poulet** (V.) Note sur le diagnostic de la méningite. Concours méd., Par., 1883, v, 76.—**Reynaud.** Note sur un cas de pseudo-méningite hystérique simulant une méningite tuberculeuse. Loire méd., St.-Étienne, 1886, v, 57-60.—**Rilliet** & **Barthez.** Mémoire sur le diagnostic de la méningite tuberculeuse. J. de méd., chir. et pharm. de Toulouse, 1857, 3. s., ii, 161; 193.— **Roosa** (D. B. St. J.) A case of basilar meningitis in which the ophthalmoscope appearances (choked disk) were observed one month before death; with the account of the post-mortem examination. Phila. M. Times, 1874-5, v, 389.—**Rühle.** Ueber den Einfluss, welchen die Combination einer Meningitis basilaris mit allgemeiner Miliartuberculose auf die Diagnose beider Processe habe. Sitzungsb. d. nied.-rhein. Gesellsch. f. Nat.- u. Heilk. zu Bonn, 1879, 397.—**Sänger** (M.) Oculomotorinslähmung bei Meningitis tuberculosa adultorum durch periphere und centrale Blutung. Arch. f. Psychiat., Berl., 1879-80, x, 158-178, 1 pl.—**Santos Gonzalo Lope.** Un caso de meningitis (?). Siglo méd., Madrid, 1881, xxviii, 201-203. — **Satterthwaite.** High temperature with acute cerebral meningitis. Med. Rec., N. Y., 1880, xvii, 519. — **Schnabel.** Ueber einen Fall von Exophthalmie als Symptom von Meningitis. Jahresb. d. schles. Gesellsch. f. vaterl. Kult. 1872, Bresl., 1873, l, 208.—**Sée** (G.) Diagnostic et physiologie de la méningite tuberculeuse. Union méd., Par., 1879, 3. s., xxvii, 790; 813; 889; 909; 945.—**Siredey** (F.) Note sur un caractère du pouls de la méningite. Bull. et mém. Soc. méd. d. hôp. de Par. (1868), 1869, 2. s., v, 210-214. *Also:* Union méd., Par., 1868, 3. s., vi, 216-220.—**Smith** (J. L.) An analysis of the symptoms of twenty-one cases of meningitis in the adult. N. York J. M., 1855, n. s., xiv, 258-263.—**Smith** (W. F.) Case of subacute meningitis of the membranes of the brain and spinal cord, connected with ischæmic papilla; diagnosed by the ophthalmoscope, and verified by post-mortem examination. West. Lancet, San Fran., 1872-3, i, 482-487.—**Turin** (J.) Ueber Temperaturverhältnisse bei der Meningitis tuberculosa der Kinder. Jahrb. f. Kinderh., Leipz., 1880-81, n. F., xvi, 1-34, 2 tab. *Also,* Reprint. — **Vance** (R. A.) The ophthalmoscope as a means of diagnosis in tubercular meningitis and the diseases which simulate it. Canada M. & S. J., Montreal, 1873-4, ii, 13-25.— **Vigla.** Deux cas de méningite avec taches lenticulaires rosées, sans lésions intestinales. Gaz. d. hôp., Par., 1851, 3. s., iii, 233.— **Votteler** (J.) Ueber Puls und Temperatur bei der tuberkulösen Meningitis im Kindesalter. Jahrb. f. Kinderh., Leipz., 1881-2, xvii, 69-87, 1 chart. — **Wilber** (G. D.) The diagnosis of meningitis. Tr, Wisconsin M. Soc. 1874, Milwaukee, 1875, viii, 74-80. — **Willich** (E.) Zur Lehre von den meningitischen Erscheinungen bei croupöser Pneumonie, zugleich ein Beitrag zur Lehre von dem sporadischen Vorkommen der Meningitis cerebrospinalis epidemica. Deutsche med. Wchnschr., Berl., 1879, v. 294; 307; 321. *Also,* Reprint.—**Zepeda** (F.) Diagnóstico diferencial entre la meningitis franca y la meningitis tuberculosa. Observador méd., México, 1869-71, i, 99-107.

Meningitis (*Treatment of*).

See, also, Meningitis (*Tubercular*); Meningitis *in children, etc.*

LEVY (E.) * De l'emploi des affusions froides dans le traitement de la méningite. 4°. *Strasbourg*, 1856.

Armangué (J.) Meningitis probablemente granulosa; tratamiento por el yoduro potásico; curacion; afasia consecutiva; reflexiones sobre la naturaleza de la menin-

Meningitis (*Treatment of*).

gitis granulosa. Rev. de cien. méd., Barcel., 1883, ix, 201; 229; 273; 328; 360; 391; 422; 463; 483; 524.—**Barré.** Observations d'arachnitis, suivies de réflexions sur l'emploi des frictions mercurielles. J. de la sect. de méd. Soc. acad. Loire-Inf., Nantes, 1836, xii, 178-188.—**Bauer.** Ein Fall von Meningitis tuberculosa, geheilt durch Jodoform. Deutsche med. Wchnschr., Berl., 1882, viii, 250.—**Bazin.** Études sur le traitement de la méningite granuleuse. Rec. de mém. de méd. . . . mil., Par., 1857, 2 s , xix, 160-178.— **Benavente.** Apuntes sobre los resultados que produce en la meningitis tuberculosa el tratamiento por el iodure de potasa. Siglo méd., Madrid, 1863, x, 161-163. — **Bierbaum** (J.) Therapie der Meningitis tuberculosa. J. f. Kinderkr., Erlang., 1872, lviii, 133; 330.—**Bonamy.** Sur un cas de guérison de méningite; bons effets de l'iodure de potassium. Bull. gén. de thérap., etc., Par., 1876, xc, 453-455. ———. De l'iodure de potassium dans les méningites. *Ibid.*, 1882, ciii, 366-370. — **Bourrousse de Laffore.** Du traitement de la méningite tuberculeuse par l'iode et les iodures. Monit. d. sc. méd. et pharm., Par., 1861, iii, 498; 509; 514; 530; 539; 556; 566; 570; 580.—**Brodnax** (D. W.) Report of a case of meningitis, with remarks on the use of opium in inflammation of the brain and its meninges. Stethoscope & Virg. M. Gaz., Richmond, 1851, i, 433-439.— **Buch** (M.) O liechenii giperemii mozga i mozgoviche obolochek razdrajenijami koji. [Treatment of meningitis.] Vrach, St. Petersb., 1880, i, 861-865.—**Cadet de Gassicourt.** De la guérison de la méningite. Rev. mens. d. mal. de l'enf., Par., 1884, ii, 145; 209. — **Cersoy.** De la médication arsenicale dans la tuberculos méningitique et péritonéale. Bull. gén. de thérap., etc., Par., 1871, lxxx, 416-419. — **Collins** (L. J.) Hypodermic use of veratrum in meningitis. Clinic. Cincin., 1873, iv, 61.—**Constant** (T.) Note sur l'emploi des cautères et des moxas dans le traitement de la méningite et de l'encéphalite chez les enfans. Bull. gén. de thérap , etc., Par., 1835, ix, 303-307.— **Cross** (J.) Meningitis; recovery under the use of mercury with chalk and iodide of potassium. Brit. M. J., Lond., 1876, ii, 492. — **Cuffer.** Méningite tuberculeuse guérie par l'iodure de potassium. France méd., Par , 1878, xxv, 369. — **Debauge** (H.) De l'emploi du sulfate de quinine dans le traitement de la méningite. Gaz. méd.-chir. de Toulouse, 1874, vi, 73; 81. *Also:* Lyon méd., 1874, xv, 22-36.—**Derasse.** De l'iodure de potassium dans la méningite simple et dans la méningite tuberculeuse. Arch. méd. belges, Brux., 1881, 3. s., xx, 377-380.—**Descrimes.** Observation d'arachnitis, accompagnée de redoublemens, de délire et de convulsions, traitée par le sulfate de quinine, associé à l'opium. Rev. méd. franç. et étrang., Par., 1827, ii, 188-193.—**Dujardin-Beaumetz.** A lecture on the treatment of meningitis. [Transl. by E. P. Hurd.] N. York M. J., 1883, xxxviii, 141-144.—**Fleming** (A.) Tubercular meningitis; use of the iodide of potassium; recovery. Brit. M. J., Lond., 1871, i, 443.—**Fuller** (W.) Treatment of meningitis. Canada M. Rec., Montreal, 1876-7, v, 237-239.—**Garcia de Castro** (L. J.) Meningitis aguda, de su tratamiento y curacion por el bromuro de potasio. Gac. méd. de Sevilla, 1880, ii, 62; 81.— **Gauchet.** Huile de croton en frictions sur le cuir chevelu dans les inflammations des méninges cérébrales. Bull. gén. de thérap., etc., Par., 1869, lxxvii, 470-474.— **Gélineau.** D'un nouveau traitement de la méningite. Rev. de thérap. méd.-chir., Par., 1876, 141; 199; 227; 317; 374; 404.—**Gibbs** (O. C.) On the treatment of tubercular meningitis. Med. Exam., Phila., 1853, n. s., ix, 144-147.— **Gibney** (V. P.) Cure of tubercular meningitis by ergot. Med. Rec., N. Y., 1877, xii, 707-710.—**Green** (W. E.) Tubercular meningitis treated with free phosphorus. Practitioner, Lond., 1884, xxxiii, 438-440.—**Greenway** (H.) Treatment of tubercular meningitis by phosphorus. Brit. M. J., Lond., 1884, i, 1145.—**von Grünewaldt.** Fall von Meningitis serosa, der unter Pilocarpin einen auffallend guten Verlauf genommen hat. St. Petersb. med. Wchnschr., 1881, vi, 78.—**Hasbrouck** (M. C.) Symptoms of cerebral meningitis, recovered from under the influence of the sulphate of morphia. Med. Rec., N. Y., 1869-70, iv, 99.—**Hentz** (C. A.) Meningitis; treatment. Atlanta M. & S. J., 1877-8, xv, 275-277. — **Holt** (R. C.) Iodoform-inunction in meningitis. Practitioner, Lond., 1887, xxxviii, 342-345. — **Jaegerschmits.** Cas de méningite aiguë traité avec succès par les antiphlogistiques et les révulsifs. Bull. gén. de thérap., etc., Par., 1849, xxxvi, 464-466.—**Jelks** (J. T.) Meningitis, and its treatment. Atlanta M. & S. J., 1872-3, x, 159.—**Keetley** (C. B.) A case of severe traumatic meningitis treated in the stage of coma by cold douche for 2½ hours; recovery. Tr. Clin. Soc. Lond., 1879, xii, 145-148. *Also:* Brit. M. J., Lond., 1879, i, 629. *Also:* Lancet, Lond., 1879, i, 478. *Also:* Med. Times & Gaz., Lond., 1879, i, 433.—**Lacroix** (L.) De l'ergotine dans le traitement de la méningite aiguë. Bull. méd. du nord, Lille, 1884, xxiv, 462-481.—**de Larroque** (B.) De l'efficacité de quelques agents thérapeutiques dans le traitement de la méningo-céphalite essentielle et aiguë. Bull. gén. de thérap., etc., Par., 1844, xxvii, 264-275.—**Latour** (A.) De la curabilité de la méningite granuleuse. Union méd., Par., 1856, x, 138-140.—**Liégard.** Note sur le traitement des fièvres

Meningitis (*Treatment of*).

cérébrales par les frictions mercurielles. Rev. méd. franç. et étrang., Par., 1837, i, 68–73.—**Lyman** (F. R.) Report of cases of meningitis treated with iodide of potassium. Am. M. Times, N. Y., 1862, iv, 333.—**McKinney** (J. W.) Some remarks in reference to the necessity of early and free venesection in the treatment of meningitis; with cases. Northwest. M. & S. J., Chicago, 1856-7, xiii, 118–125.—**Martinet** (L.) Du traitement de l'arachnitis cérébrale. Bull. gén. de thérap., etc., Par., 1833, v, 197–203.—**Mazade** (J.) Sur l'emploi des frictions mercurielles à haute dose dans le traitement de la méningite. Rev. méd. franç. et étrang., Par., 1840, iv, 66–82. *Also*, Reprint.—**Mello.** Observation sur une méningite aiguë traitée et guérie par les seuls antiphlogistiques. J. univ. et hebd. de méd. et chir. prat., Par., 1831, iii, 369–372.—**Mescure.** Observation sur une phlegmasie des membranes du cerveau, guérie par la glace. J. gén. de méd., chir. et pharm., Par., 1815, liv, 300–304.—**Meslier.** Sur le traitement de la granulie méningée par l'extrait de noyer. Bull. gén. de thérap., etc., Par., 1876, xc, 416–420.—**Morand** (L.) Observations de méningite; emploi de l'emplâtre stibié; guérison. *In his*: Mém. et obs. clin. [etc.], 2. éd., 8°, Tours, 1844, 51–58.—**Oberlin** (L.) Note sur le traitement de la méningite tuberculeuse par l'iodure et le bromure de potassium. Rev. méd. de l'est, Nancy, 1886, xviii, 79–85.—**Ogle** (J. W.) Tetanoid convulsions overcome for a time by applications of ice to the spine; death; strumous meningitis. Med. Times & Gaz., Lond., 1866. i, 634.—**Papillaod** (L.) Del tratamiento y de la profilaxis de la meningitis tuberculosa. An. r. Acad. de cien. méd. . . . de la Habana, 1871–2, viii, 394–404.—**Peter.** Méningite tuberculeuse guérie par l'iodure de potassium. Bull. Soc. clin. de Par. (1878) 1879, ii, 145–148.—**Philippoff** (N. N.) O dieistvii tallina pri meningitis simplex u dietei. [Effect of thallin in meningitis simplex in children.] Russk. Med., St. Petersb., 1886, iv, 506.—**Quintana** (J.) Meningitis raquidea aguda; evacuaciones sanguineas generales y locales muy repetidas: aplicacion casi continua del hiclo; uso del tintura de digital y del estracto de belladona; curacion. Gac. méd., Madrid, 1850, vi, 321–323.—**Rilliet** (F.) Of the curability of tubercular meningitis. Virginia M. & S. J., Richmond, 1854, ii, 458–465.—**Rodet** (A.) Observation de méningite aiguë traitée par l'iodure de potassium à haute dose; guérison rapide. Ann. Soc. de méd. de Lyon, 1878, 2. s., xxvi, 262–270. *Also*: Lyon méd., 1878, xxix, 611–618.—**Roquer y Torrents** (J.) Efectos de las aplicaciones tópicas del hielo en la fiebre cerebral de la infancia. Gac. méd. de Cataluña, Barcel., 1879, ii, 266–273.—**Rougon.** Observation de méningite traitée par l'iodure de potassium. Union méd., Par., 1881, 3. s., xxxi, 800; 813.—**Schützenberger.** De l'emploi des affusions froides répétées dans les méningites et l'hydrencéphale aigu. Gaz. méd. de Strasb., 1855, xv, 33–41. ——. Méningite aiguë guérie par les affusions froides. *Ibid.*, 1868. xxviii, 7–9. *Also, in his*: Fragments d'études path. et clin., 8°, Par., 1879, 131–137.—**Senlis** (A.) Un mot sur la méningite des enfants, et sur son traitement au moyen d'un cautère placé au sommet de la tête. Bull. gén. de thérap., etc., Par., 1838, xv, 180–183.—**Solles** (E.) Méningite traumatique; traitement révulsif énergique; guérison; perte de la vue consécutive; retour de la méningite avec épanchement; abolition des facultés intellectuelles pendant cinq mois; traitement par l'iodure de potassium; guérison. *In his*: Études de clin. interne, 8°, Par., 1879, 66–73.—**Somma** (L.) Sulla cura della meningite granulosa. Clinica, Napoli, 1876, iii, 189–195.—**Staffhorst.** Ueber die Anwendung des Chinins in grossen Dosen bei Meningitis tuberculosa. Prakt. Arzt, Wetzlar, 1868, ix, 121.—**Thibault.** Fièvre cérébrale chez un garçon de dix ans et demi; friction avec la pommade stibiée sur le cuir chevelu préalablement rasé; guérison. Gaz. d. hôp., Par., 1859, xxxii, 102. ——. Deux cas de méningite chez des enfants, traités avec succès, à la troisième période de la maladie, par des frictions stibiées sur le cuir chevelu préalablement rasé. J. de méd. de l'ouest, Nantes, 1878, xii, 83–116, 1 tab.—**Vovard.** Traitement de la méningite des enfants. J. de méd. de Bordeaux, 1882–3, xii, 131; 143; 166; 178. *Also*, Reprint. *Also*: Quinzaine méd., Par., 1882–3, i, 71; 88; 149.

Meningitis *in children and infants*.

See, also, **Hydrocephalus** (*Acute*); **Meningitis** (*Complications of, etc.*); **Meningitis** (*Diagnosis of, etc.*); **Meningitis** (*Treatment of*); **Meningitis** (*Tubercular*).

BAYLE (P.) * De la méningite des enfants. 4°. *Paris*, 1865.

DANGUY (L. - A.) * Étude de la méningite aiguë franche de l'enfance. 4°. *Paris*, 1880.

DUCHOSAL (J.-H.) * De la méningite aiguë chez les enfants. 4°. *Paris*, 1846.

SIEBER (J.) * Ueber die Meningitis der Kinder. 8°. *Speyer*, 1866.

Meningitis *in children and infants*.

Arnold (B.) Ein Fall von Meningitis cerebralis mit massenhafter, pseudomembranöser Exsudation, ausgezeichnet durch den eigenthümlichen Verlauf, bei einem 1jährigen Kinde beobachtet. Med. Cor.-Bl. d. württemb. ärztl. Ver., Stuttg., 1852, xxii, 174.—**Baginsky.** Ueber Typhus und typhoide Meningitis der Kinder. Verhandl. d. Berl. med. Gesellsch. (1871–3), 1874, iv, 2. Theil, 108–120. — **Bailly.** Ueber die beiden Hauptformen der Meningitis im kindlichen Alter. J. f. Kinderkr., Berl., 1844, ii, 421–432.—**Bierbaum** (J.) Meningitis simplex. *Ibid.*, Erlang., 1866, xlvii, 68.—**Blache** (R.) Réflexions à propos de quelques cas de méningites guéris chez des enfants. Union méd., Par., 1881, 3. s., xxxi, 541; 555; 601.—**Bókai** (J.) Nem-gümös alapi lágy-agyburoklob egy esete. [Meningitis, non-tubercular.] Orvosi hetil., Budapest, 1881, xxv, 917–920.—**Bourneville** & **Wuillamié.** Méningo-encéphalite chronique généralisée chez un enfant; décortication de la substance blanche. Bull. Soc. anat. de Par., 1881, lvi, 638–648. *Also*: Arch. de neurol., Par., 1882, iii, 327–336, 1 pl. *Also*: Progrès méd., Par., 1882, x, 498–501.—**Braun.** Meningit hos ett barn genom hämmad otarrhé; hemiplegi och afasi. Förh. Svens. Läk.-Sällsk., Stockholm, 1871, 210.—**Brockmann.** Meningitis mesencephalica; ein Beitrag zu den Krankheiten des kindlichen Alters. Hannov. Ann. f. d. ges. Heilk., 1842, n. F., ii, 678–707: 1843, n. F., iii, 3–30.—**Carroll** (A. L.) Lepto-meningitis infantum. Boston M. & S. J., 1886, cxv, 428.—[**Case.**] Seul cas de guérison de méningite observé depuis longtemps à l'Hôpital des enfans. Bull. gén. de thérap., etc., Par., 1835, ix, 35–37.—**Cloquet** (H.) Quelques idées sur la fièvre hydrocéphalique, ou cérébrale des enfans. N. Jour. de méd., chir., pharm., etc., Par., 1818, i, 129–138.—**Cullingworth** (C. J.) Purulent non-tubercular meningitis in an infant, three months after injury. Med. Times & Gaz., Lond., 1880, ii, 644. — **Davies** (J.) Remarks on the symptoms and treatment of meningitis in children. Lond. M. Reposit., 1825, xxiii, 15–36. ——. A case of meningitis. *Ibid.*, 290–294. — **Dawson.** Meningitis in children. N. York M. J., 1883, xxxvii, 267. *Also*: Tr. N. York Obst. Soc. (1881–5), 1885, iii, 157.—**Day** (W. H.) Two cases of simple meningitis in children, and the difficulties attending their diagnosis. Med. Press & Circ., Lond., 1886, n. s., xli, 466–469. — **Delcour** (J.) Recherches sur la méningo-encéphalite des enfants. [Rap. de Snellaert, et discussion.] Bull. Soc. de méd. de Gand, 1843, ix, 40; 51. *Also*: Ann. Soc. de méd. de Gand, 1843, xii, 166–472. *Also*, Reprint.—**D'Espine.** Hypertrophie du cerveau avec sclérose bulbaire chez un enfant mort à 2 ans et demi d'une méningite aiguë de la convexité. Rev. méd. de la Suisse Rom., Genève, 1881, i, 489–497. — **Dunn** (R.) Cases of acute arachnitis occurring in children. Lancet, Lond., 1844, i, 718–720.—**Escorihuela.** Meningitis cerebral en los niños; curacion por los revulsivos generales. Génio méd.-quir., Madrid, 1879, xxv, 249. — **Fraser** (W.) A case of lepto-meningitis infantum. Glasgow M. J., 1882, [4. s.], xviii, 355–358.—**Goode** (B. P.) Case of meningitis in a child. Cincin. Lancet & Clinic, 1879, ii, 443.—**Guibert** (T.) Observations de phlegmasies de l'arachnoïde et de la pie-mère chez les enfans, suivies de remarques pratiques sur ces maladies. J. compl. du dict. d. sc. méd., Par., 1828, xxxi, 97: xxxii, 321: 1829, xxxiii, 50.—**Hauff.** Ueber die Meningitis der Kinder. Med. Ann., Heidelb., 1844, x, 241–251. — **Hauner.** De la méningite observée à l'hôpital des enfans de Munich. Union méd., Par., 1855, ix, 342. — **Liouville** (H.) Contribution à l'étude anatomo-pathologique de la méningite cérébro-spinale tuberculeuse. Arch. de physiol. norm. et path., Par., 1870, iii, 490–498. — **Maes.** Quelques mots sur la méningite aiguë des enfants, improprement dite hydrocéphale aiguë, et sur l'emploi du sulfate de quinine dans cette maladie. Ann. Soc. méd.-chir. de Bruges, 1843, iv, 113–123.—**Maillard.** Méningite des enfants. Abeille méd., Par., 1856, xiii, 61.—**Maschka.** Erkrankung und Tod zweier Knaben unter den Erscheinungen einer Coxitis mit secundärer Meningitis nach einer Verletzung. Allg. Wien. med. Ztg., 1862, vii, 133; 141.—**Mazet** (A.) Histoire de deux fièvres cérébrales chez deux enfans, l'un de cinq ans, et l'autre de trois ans. N. Jour. de méd., chir., pharm., etc., Par., 1821, x, 17–25.—**Peacock.** Acute meningitis in an infant; death. Lancet, Lond., 1873, ii, 415.—**Plant** (W. T.) Acute meningitis in children. Obst. Gaz. Cincin., 1883, vi, 561–568.—**Porter** (P. B.) Two cases of meningitis of different character occurring in children. Richmond & Louisville M. J., Louisville, 1877, xxiii, 353–358.—**Rilliet.** De l'inflammation franche des méninges chez les enfants. Arch. gén. de méd., Par., 1846, iii, 385–414: 1847, i, 30; 182: ii, 287–313. *Also*: Ann. de méd. belge, Brux., 1846, iv, 388–407: 1847, i, 378–415: iii, 118–137. *Also, transl.*: J. f. Kinderkr., Berl., 1847, viii, 244; 351: ix, 345; 411. *Also, transl.*: Prov. M. & S. J., Lond., 1847, 151; 181; 234; 516. — **Rouxeau** (C.) Quelques mots sur la méningite des enfants. J. de la sect. de méd. Soc. acad. Loire-Inf., Nantes, 1855, xxxi, 219–246.—**Rufz** (E.) Quelques mots sur les diverses espèces de méningites des enfans. Gaz. méd. de Par., 1841, 2. s., ix, 49–52. — **Seguin** (E. C.) Localized basal meningitis in children. Hosp. Gaz., N. Y., 1878, iii, 101–105. *Also, in his*: Op. min. [etc.], 8°, N. Y.,

Meningitis *in children and infants.*

1884, 251-255.—**Somma** (L.) Le meningiti dei bambini; lezione cliniche. *In his:* Clin. pediat. dell' Osp. dell' Annunz. di Napoli, 8°, Napoli, 1877, 1-50.—**Swift** (L. C.) Report of two cases of simple meningitis, complicating pertussis in infants. Iowa State M. Reporter, Des Moines, 1884-5, ii, 55-58.— **Tubbesing** (J. W.) Krankenge-schichte einer Meningitis exsudativa, wo das erkrankte Kind sieben Wochen lang nie bei klarem Bewusstsein und fast acht Wochen blind gewesen ist. Org. f. d. ges. Heilk, Aachen, 1856, v, 76-90. — **Wilks** (S.) Simple acute meningitis in children. Guy's Hosp. Rep., Lond., 1860, 3. s., vi, 114-117. —. Two cases of simple arachnitis in children. *Ibid.*, 117-120.

Meningitis *in pregnancy and the puerperal state.*

Dreyfous (F.) Méningite cérébro-spinale chez une femme en couches. Progrès méd., Par., 1876, iv, 820.— **Erhardt.** Meningitis puerperalis exsudativa. Aerztl. Mitth. a. Baden, Karlsruhe, 1873, xxvii, 64-66.—**Smoler.** Meningitis in gravida. Oesterr. Ztschr. f. prakt. Heilk., Wien, 1863, ix, 8 ; 20 ; 37.

Meningitis (*Basilar*).

See, also, Meningitis (*Cerebro-spinal*) ; Meningitis (*Diagnosis, etc., of*).

DE JONGH (H. A.) * Een ziektegeval van leptomeningitis basilaris. 8°. *Groningen,* 1873.

KREISSMANN (R.) * Zur Casuistik der Meningitis basilaris tuberculosa der Erwachsenen. 8°. *Jena,* 1876.

LABARRIÈRE (É.) * Essai sur la méningite en plaque, ou scléreuse limitée à la base de l'encéphale. 8°. *Paris,* 1878.

LANGE (G.) * Ueber zwei Fälle von Meningitis basilaris tuberculosa. 8°. *Berlin,* [1875].

RAMAGLIA (P.) Studi intorno alla meningite basilare granulosa. 8°. *Napoli,* 1876.

SCHIAN (R.) * Ueber Meningitis basilaris tuberculosa. 8°. *Würzburg,* 18~0.

ZWICKE (A.) * Beitrag zur Heilung der Meningitis basilaris tuberculosa. 8°. *Bonn,* 1868.

Aphel (F.) Meningite con esito di guarigione. Gazz. med. di Torino, 1885, xxxvi, 830-833.—**Bärwindt.** Meningitis basilaris. Jahresb. ü. d. Verwalt. d. Med.-Wes., d. Krankenanst. . . . d. Stadt Frankf. (1860), 1863, iv, 89.—**Barth** (H.) & **Déjérine** (J.) Note sur un cas de méningite bulbaire, survenue chez un individu atteint de paralysie diphthérique du voile du palais. Arch. de physiol. norm. et path., Par., 1880, 2. s., vii, 673-682. — **Bebczynski** (A.) Przypadek ostrego zapalenia osłony miekkiej na podstawie mozgu (meningitis basilaris acuta). Medycyna, Warszawa, 1877, v, 264-267.—**Bókai** (J.) jun. Ein Fall von Meningitis basilaris non tuberculosa. Jahrb. f. Kinderh., Leipz.. 1882, xviii, 105-109, 1 tab.—**Bouneau.** Méningite de la base du crâne ; délire; mort. Gaz. d. hôp., Par., 1833, vii, 141.—**Cabot.** Case of basilar meningitis. Boston M. & S. J., 1875, xcii, 593. — **Camó** (J.) ¿Qué parte toman la médula y las raices medulares en la meningitis basilar aguda? Án. de cien. méd., Madrid, 1876, i, 269 ; 478. — **Carpentier.** Trois cas de méningite simple de la base du cerveau. J. de méd., chir. et pharmacol., Brux., 1879, lxviii, 406-418.—**Charon.** Un cas de méningite basilaire chronique. Ann. Soc. d'anat. path. de Brux., 1880, 104-108.—**Clark** (A.) Case of acute basilar meningitis (idiopathic). Med. Times & Gaz., Lond., 1881, ii, 9.—**Cross** (T. M. B.) Chronic localized basilar meningitis. Psych. & Med.-Leg. J., N. Y., 1875, ii, 220-240. — **Crous** (J.) Meningitis bulbo-raquidiana crónica y en el primer período ó de escitacion. Rev. de cien. méd., Barcel., 1879, v, 300-305. — **Derblich** (W.) Meningitis basilaris primaria mit raschem lethalen Ausgange. Spitals-Ztg., Wien, 1864, 244-246. — **Englisch.** Mehrfache Knochenentzündung; Basilarmeningitis; Tod. Ber. d. k. k. Krankenanst. Rudolph-Stiftung in Wien (1877), 1878, 445. — **Fleischmann** (L.) Meningitis basilaris. Jahrb. f. Kinderh., Leipz., 1872-3, n. F., vi, 404-411.—**von Franque** (A.) Ein Fall von Meningitis basilaris. Cor.-Bl. d. deutsch. Gesellsch. f. Psychiat., etc., Neuwied, 1863, x, 8-10.—**Gatteschi.** Méningite basilaire non tuberculeuse chez un enfant de 3 ans, suivie de guérison. Gaz. méd. d'Orient, Constantinople, 1867-8, xi, 162-166.—**Green** (J. O.) Basilar meningitis; chronic otorrhœa; carious fistula through the mastoid. Extr. Rec. Bost. Soc. M. Improve. (1874-9), 1880, vii, 75.—**Greenough** (F. B.) Basilar meningitis; chronic otorrhœa; carious fistula through the mastoid. Boston M. & S. J., 1877, xcvi, 377-379.— **Guaita** (R.) Un caso di meningite basilare con esito in guarigione. Arch. di patol. inf., Napoli, 1883, i, 179-185.— **Gysberti Hodenpyl** (L. P.) Een geval van meningitis basilaris met sectieverslag. Nederl. mil. geneesk. Arch., etc., Utrecht, 1882, vi, 26.—**Hammond** (W. A.) On

Meningitis (*Basilar*).

chronic basilar meningitis. Brit. M. J., Lond., 1873, i, 665-667. — **Herz** (M.) Ein Fall von Meningitis basilaris mit Ausgang in Genesung. Arch. f. Kinderh., Stuttg., 1881-2, iii, 156-166. — **Huppert** (M.) Eitrige Meningitis an der Basis und in den Ventrikeln bei allgemeiner Verwirtheit. Arch. d. Heilk., Leipz., 1865, vi, 569.—**Lederer.** Zwei Fälle von Meningitis basilaris. Wien. med. Presse, 1876, xvii, 1064.—**Löbel.** Meningitis basilaris tuberculosa, incipiens cum aphasia ; mors. Ber. d. k. k. Krankenanst. Rudolph-Stiftung in Wien (1866), 1867, 181-183.—**Lyons.** Arachnitis situated at the base of the brain. Med. Press & Circ., Dubl., 1866, n. s., ii, 69. — **Martinet** (L.) Observation d'arachnitis de la base et des ventricules latéraux, compliquée de ramollissement des parties centrales du cerveau. Rev. méd. franç. et étrang., Par., 1829, i, 62-67.—**Mettenheimer** (C.) Ueber die Wirkung der Narcotica in der basilaren Meningitis. Memorabilien, Heilbr., 1867, xii, 105-107.—**Modl** (E.) Ein seltener Fall von Meningitis basilaris. Wien. med. Wchnschr., 1880, xxx, 821.— **Palois.** Observation pour servir à l'histoire de l'arachnitis de la base du crâne et du conduit rachidien ou spinal. J. de la sect. de méd. Soc. acad. Loire-Inf., Nantes, 1827, iii, 95-99.—**Ritter von Rittershain** (G.) Meningitis purulenta basil.; Thrombosis ven. mening., venæ jugul. ext. sin.; Infarcti pulmonum; Tumor lienis acutis; Dermatitis erysipelatosa; Pyophthalmia. Oesterr. Jahrb. f. Paediat.. Wien, 1870, i, 60. ——. Meningitis basilaris. *Ibid.*, 67.—**Rödelheimer.** Ein Fall von Meningitis der Basis. Med. Cor.-Bl. d. württemb. ärztl. Ver., Stuttg., 1867, xxxvii, 108; 113.—**Scholz.** [Meningitis basilaris purulenta ; Hydrocephalus acutus.] Aerztl. Ber. d. k. k. allg. Krankenh. zu Wien (1873), 1874, 49.—**von Schrötter.** Meningitis basilaris; Tod. Ber. d. k. k. Krankenanst. Rudolph-Stiftung in Wien (1879), 1880, 326.—**Schützenberger** (C.) Méningite de la base et de la moelle allongée; mort. Gaz. méd. de Strasb., 1845, v, 196-199.—**Schuh** (L.) Ueber autochthone Hirnarterienthrombose als Ursache halbseitiger Motilitätsstörungen bei Meningitis basilaris tuberculosa. Verhandl. d. phys.-med. Gesellsch. in Würzb., 1875, n. F., viii, 179-204, 1 pl.—**Schultze** (F.) Leptomeningitis acuta tuberculosa cerebrospinalis (vulgo: Meningitis basilaris). Arch. f. path. Anat., etc., Berl., 1876, lxviii, 111-120. ——. Ueber das Verhalten des Rückenmarks und der Rückenmarksnervenwurzeln bei akuter Basilarmeningitis. Berl. klin. Wchnschr., 1876, xiii, 2; 17.—**Sée** (G.) Méningite de la base; diagnostic; pathogénie physiologique. Praticien, Par., 1879, ii, 103-105.—**Süe.** Méningite de la base du cerveau; emphysème général produit par une piqûre de sangsue dans le pharynx; mort. Gaz. d. hôp., Par., 1833, vii, 539—**Teissier** (B.) Méningite partielle et chronique de la base du cerveau; caillot sanguin de forme polypeuse dans le ventricule moyen; céphalalgie intense; contractions douloureuses des muscles de la face; strabisme convergent; amblyopie; dyplopie. Gaz. méd. de Lyon, 1855, vii, 303-307. *Also:* Monit. d. hôp. Par., 1855, iii, 853-855.—**Traube.** Meningitis tuberculosa basilaris. Ann. d. Char.-Krankenh. . . . zu Berl., 1862-3, x, 2. Hft., 166-172.—**Venturini** (E.) Storia di meningite basilare. Riv. clin. di Bologna, 1867, vi, 329-331.—**Williams** (A. C.) Das Verhalten des Rückenmarks und seiner Häute bei tuberculöser und eitriger Basilarmeningitis. Deutsches Arch. f. klin. Med., Leipz., 1879-80, xxv, 292-297.

Meningitis (*Cerebro-spinal*).

See, also, Fever (*Cerebro-spinal*) ; Meningitis (*Spinal*) ; Meningitis (*Tubercular*) ; Puerperal state (*Complications of*).

CLAVERIE (P.) * Méningites cérébro-spinales observées à Rochefort pendant l'hiver 1885-6. 4°. *Bordeaux,* 1886.

CONDORELLI (G. M.) Rapporto medico sulla meningite-cerebro-spinale-epidemica sviluppatasi in Misterbianco li 7 marzo 1883 alla Commissione sanitaria di Catania. 8°. *Catania,* 1884.

DEZON (F.-J.) * De la méningite cérébrospinale épidémique. 4°. *Paris,* 1850.

HERRMANN (R.) * De meningitide cerebrospinali ezorta ex otitide interna. 8°. *Regimonti Pr.,* 1866.

KAEMMERER (K.) * Ein Fall von Doppelempfindung nach Meningitis cerebrospinalis. 8°. *Warburg,* 1882.

MAJER (E. L.) * Ein seltener Fall von Meningitis cerebrospinalis. 8°. *Tübingen,* 1871.

MIREWS (P.) * Des accès pernicieux à forme cérébro-spinale. Diagnostic et traitement. 4°. *Montpellier,* 1882.

OHLSEN (G.) * Beitrag zur Meningitis cerebro-spinalis. 8°. *Würzburg,* 1866.

Meningitis (*Cerebro-spinal*).

SALFELD (A.) * Beitrag zur Symptomatologie der Meningitis cerebro-spinalis. 8°. *Jena*, 1872.

SCHMIDT (L.) * Ein Fall von Meningitis cerebro-spinalis epidemica. 8°. *Greifswald*, 1886.

SIEVERS (R.) * Om meningitis cerebro-spinalis epidemica i Sverige, Norge och Finland. 8°. *Helsingfors*, 1886.

VIVIER (A.) * De la méningite cérébro-spinale épidémique. 4°. *Strasbourg*, 1866.

ZIEMEK (A.) * Zur Kenntniss der Meningitis cerebro-spinalis epidemica. 8°. *Greifswald*, 1885.

Alling. Méningo-encéphalite sur-aiguë cérébro-rachidienne avec symptômes tardifs. Bull. Soc. anat. de Par. (1869), 1870, xliv, 130.—**Andrew.** † Autopsy. Tr. Path. Soc. Lond., 1864-5, xvi, 28-30.—**Andruss.** † Recovery. Tr. M. Soc. N. Jersey, Newark, 1872, 298.—**Armstrong** (G. A.) † † Canada M. & S. J., Montreal, 1882-3, xi, 544.—**Arnell** (D. R.) Observations on the spotted fever, as it appeared in Orange County, State of New York, in 1808 and 1809. N. Med. & Phys. J., Lond., 1810-11, i, 117-120.—**Axe** (J. W.) Facts and observations tending to elucidate the etiology and pathology of cerebro-spinal meningitis. Veterinarian, Lond., 1883, lvi, 521-535.—**Bäumler** (C.) † Med. Times & Gaz., Lond., 1867, ii, 59-62.—**von Bamberger.** Genickkrampf (Meningitis cerebrospinalis epidemica). Ztschr. f. Therap. m. Einbzhng. d. Elect.- u. Hydrotherap., Wien, 1886, iv, 90; 98.—**Banks** (J. T.) Cerebro-spinal meningitis. Dublin Hosp. Gaz.,1855, n. s., ii, 83-85. ——. Cerebro-spinal arachnitis, with paralysis of the right third nerve. Dublin Q. J. M. S., 1866, xli, 448-450. ——. Remarkable case of cerebro-spinal arachnitis. Dublin M. Press & Circ., 1866, n. s., i, 561.—**Barillari** (G.) Méningite cérébro-spinale; purulence des urines. J. de méd. et chir. prat., Par., 1875, xlvi, 501.—**Barth** (H.) Méningite cérébro-spinale prise d'abord pour une fièvre typhoïde. France méd., Par., 1877, xxiv, 162-164.—**Barton.** Cerebro-spinal meningitis. Dublin Q. J. M. Sc., 1867, xliv, 431.—**Baudelocque.** Méningite rachidienne, mésocéphalique et cérébelleuse; tubercules pulmonaires. Gaz. méd. de Par., 1835, 2. s., iii, 73-75.—**Bell** (J.) † [Autopsy.] Canada M. Rec., Montreal, 1872-3, i, 241-244. *Also:* Canada M. & S. J., Montreal, 1872-3, i, 543-547.—**Bernhardt** (M.) Notiz über die mit den Symptomen einer (Cerebro-) Spinalmeningitis einsetzenden Abdominaltyphen. Berl. klin. Wchnschr., 1886, xxiii, 859.—**Bessey** (W. E.) Leeching in the treatment of cerebro-spinal meningitis. Canada M. Rec., Montreal, 1875-6, iv, 122-126. ——. † Fatal in thirty-eight hours. Canada M. & S. J., Montreal, 1872-3, i, 113-115.—**Bézy** (P.) Méningite cérébro-spinale subaiguë rhumatismale; guérison. Gaz. méd.-chir. de Toulouse, 1883, xv, 283.—**Blache.** Méningite cérébro-spinale; érysipèle de la face; guérison. Gaz. d. hôp., Par., 1863, xxxvi, 489.—**Bleything** (G. D.) Cerebro-spinal meningitis. N. York M. J., 1873, xviii, 479-490.—**Blum** (Z. A.) K kazuistikie meningitis cerebro-spinalis non epidemica. Protok. zasaid. Kavkazsk. med. Obsh., Tiflis, 1883-4, xx, 29-37.—**Borland** (J. N.) Cerebro-spinal meningitis. Boston M. & S. J., 1865, lxxii, 309-312. *Also:* Extr. Rec. Bost. Soc. M. Improve. (1862-6), 1867, v (appx.), 185-189. ——. †† Boston M. & S. J., 1872, lxxxvi, 406-408. *Also:* Extr. Rec. Bost. Soc. M. Improve. (1866-74), 1876, vi, 227-231. — **Bramwell** (B.) Case of cerebro-spinal meningitis, and a case of tubercular meningitis, occurring in the same family, at the same time, and simulating epidemic cerebro-spinal meningitis. Lancet. Lond., 1878, i, 9.—**Briquet.** Méningite cerebro-spinale. Gaz. d. hôp., Par., 1860, xxxiii, 133.—**Brown** (N. F.) †† Detroit Rev. Med. & Pharm., 1872, vii, 339-343.—**Bull** (C. S.) Report of three cases of choroiditis following cerebro-spinal meningitis. Am. J. M. Sc., Phila., 1873, n. s., lxv, 99-102.—**Burcht van Lichtenberg** (V. D.) Een geval van meningitis cerebro-spinalis, gevolgd door genezing. Nederl. mil. geneesk. Arch., etc., Utrecht, 1882, vi, 753-758.—**Burrall** (F. A.) † Specimens. Bull. N. York Path. Soc., 1881, 2. s., i, 148-152. *Also:* Med. Rec., N. Y., 1881, xx, 73-75.—**Buttersack** (T.) Acht Fälle von Meningitis cerebro-spinalis epidemica. Memorabilien, Heilbr., 1866, xi, 228.—**Cain** (D. J.) Calabar bean in cerebro-spinal meningitis. Charleston M. J. & Rev., 1876, n. s., iii, 257.—**Canstatt** (C.) Meningitis cerebro-spinalis. *In his:* Klin. Rückbl. u. Abhandl., 8°, Erlang., 1851, pt. 2, 12-20.—**Carpio** (L. H.) & **Poza** (M.) Meningitis cerebro-espinal. Gac. méd. de México, 1866, ii, 44-47.—**Carrington** (R. E.) Cerebro-spinal meningitis; a sporadic case of cerebro-spinal fever? Tr. Path. Soc. Lond., 1881-2, xxxiii, 19-21.—[**Cases.**] Méningite cérébro-spinale; érysipèle intercurrent de la face; guérison. Bull. gén. de thérap., etc., Par., 1863, lxv, 372-375.— Meningitis cerebro-spinalis ex spondylitide; compressio medullæ. Ber. d. k. k. Krankenanst. Rudolph-Stiftung in Wien (1865), 1866, 148.—Aerztl. Ber. d. k. k. allg. Krankenh. zu Wien (1880), 1881, 54-56.—**Ceccherelli** (A.) La pilocarpina in un caso di meningite cerebro-spinale di natura

Meningitis (*Cerebro-spinal*).

sifilitica. Bull. d. sc. med. di Bologna, 1882, 6. s., x, 98-102.—**Chagnon** (J. B.) Hydrate of chloral in cerebro-spinal meningitis. Canada M. J., Montreal, 1870-71, vii, 62-65.—**Chandler** (J. L.) Cerebro-spinal meningitis. Boston M. & S. J., 1864, lxx, 202-206.—**Charcot.** Observation d'un cas de méningite cérébro-spinale chez une vieille femme. Bordeaux méd., 1873, ii, 18-21.—**Chewning** (J.) Salicylic acid in cerebro-spinal meningitis. Med. & Surg. Reporter, Phila., 1884, l, 411.—**Chipley** (W. S.) Spinal meningitis; cerebro-spinal meningitis; méningite rachidienne. West. Lancet, Cincin., 1848, viii, 83-95.—**Chronic** cerebro-spinal meningitis. [Edit.] Med. Exam., Chicago, 1873, xiv, 133.—**Churchill** (A.) Cerebro-spinal meningitis, or spotted fever. Tr. M. Soc. N. Y., Albany, 1867, 143-147.—**Cleveland.** Cerebro-spinal meningitis. Cincin. Lancet & Clinic, 1881, vi, 519-523. ——. Sporadic cerebro-spinal meningitis. Cincin. Lancet-Clinic, 1887, n. s., xix, 343-345.—**Clouston** (T. S.) † J. Ment. Sc., Lond., 1871-2, xvii, 225-230.—**Cole** (T.) On cerebro-spinal meningitis. Brit. M. J., Lond., 1875, ii, 667-670.—**Comby** (J.) Méningite cérébro-spinale à forme foudroyante; mort en trente-six heures. France méd., Par., 1881, ii, 757-760. *Also:* Bull. Soc. clin. de Par. (1881), 1882, v, 237-243.—**Conkling** (J. T.) † Buffalo M. & S. J., 1864-5, iv, 367. *Also:* Tr. M. Soc. County Kings 1858-64, Brooklyn, 1865, i, 323.—**Corlieu.** † Guérison. Bull. Soc. méd.-prat. de Par., 1862, 26-31.—**Cullen** (J. S. D.) † Treated by ergot and chloral; recovery. Virginia Clin. Rec., Richmond, 1871-2, i, 107.—**Currie.** †† Med. Exam., Lond., 1876, i, 482.—**Cutler** (E. G.) † Death on the fourth day. Med. & Surg. Rep. Bost. City Hosp., 1882, 3. s., 379.—**Czapek** (F.) † Prag. med. Wchnschr., 1879, iv, 505.—**Da Costa** (J. M.) Acute cerebro spinal meningitis due to chronic suppurative otitis. Phila. M. Times, 1886-7, xvii, 251-253. — **Davis** (N. S.) Chronic cerebro-spinal meningitis. Tr. Illinois M. Soc., Chicago, 1872, xxii, 219-223.—**Day** (H.) Cerebro-spinal meningitis. *In his:* Clin. Hist., 8°., Lond., 1866, 1-24.—**Decloux.** Quatre nouveaux cas de typhus cérébro-spinal. Arch. méd. belges, Brux., 1886, 3. s., xxx, 289-309.—**Deltenre.** † Guérison. *Ibid.*, 1884, 3. s., xxvi, 261-263. ——. † Sporadique. *Ibid.*, 1886, 3. s., xxix, 99-106.—**Devay.** † Symptômes insidieux; mort. Monit. d. hôp., Par., 1853, i, 1236-1238.—**Dichiara** (F.) Meningite cronica cerebro-spinale curata con la corrente continua. Gazz. clin. di elettroter., Palermo, 1886, iv, 65-67.—**Dickinson.** † Tr. Path. Soc. Lond, 1869, xx, 22.—**Discussion** on cerebro-spinal meningitis. St. Louis M. & S. J., 1865, n. s., ii, 438-451.—**Discussion** (Die) über Meningitis cerebrospinalis in der Section Wien des Vereines der Aerzte in Niederösterreich am 19. Mai 1886. Wien. med. Bl., 1886, ix, 704; 738; 806.—**Donders** (F. C.) Een woord over herkenning van hersenen ruggemergs-verlamming. Nederl. Lancet, Gravenh., 1849-50, 2. s., v, 576-588.—**Dowse** (S.) † With myelitis of the chord. Lancet, Lond., 1872, i, 756. ——. † With cerebral disturbance. *Ibid.*, ii, 9. ——. On basic cerebro-spinal meningitis. Med. Times & Gaz., Lond., 1874, i, 124; 150. ——. Case of cerebro-spinal meningitis, albuminuria, pericarditis and mitral fibroid thrombosis originating in ulcerative endocarditis. *Ibid.*, 1875, i, 59. ——. Basic cerebro-spinal meningitis; acute softening. Med. Press & Circ., Lond., 1877, n. s., xxiii, 278.—**Draper** (W. H.) Cerebro-spinal meningitis. Med. & Surg. Reporter, Phila., 1884, li, 232-234.—**Drasche.** † Tod. Ber. d. k. k. Krankenanst. Rudolph-Stiftung in Wien (1868), 1869, 267.—**Duffield** (G.) Cerebro spinal meningitis. Am. Lancet, Detroit, 1866, n. s., x, 241-245.—**Dupont** (E.) Contribution à l'étude de la méningite cérébro-spinale. Ann. Soc. de méd. d'Anvers, 1887, xlviii, 44-69.—**Durodié** (F.) † Chez une fille de dix ans; guérison. J. de méd. de Bordeaux, 1882-3, xii, 394-397. *Also:* Mém. et bull. Soc. de méd. et chir. de Bordeaux (1883), 1884, 46-54.—**Dutcher** (A. P.) † Terminating in insanity. Cincin. M. Obs., 1857, ii, 251-255.—**Dyer** (G. A.) † South. M. Rec., Atlanta, 1877, vii, 29—**Ellis.** Cerebro-spinal meningitis. Boston M. & S. J., 1864, lxx, 381.—**Evans** (R. F.) †† Tr. M. Soc. Tennessee, Nashville, 1878, 55-57.—**Ewart.** A case of cerebro-spinal meningitis; recovery; remarks. Lancet, Lond., 1887, i, 571.—**Faludi** (A.) † Orvosi hetil., Budapest, 1883, xxvii, 53; 84. *Also, transl.:* Pest. med.-chir. Presse, Budapest, 1883, xix, 173-176.—**Ferguson** (J. G. B.) Cerebro-spinal meningitis. St. Louis M. & S. J., 1865, n.s., ii, 508-510.—**Fergusson** (A. A.) † † Canada M. Rec., Montreal, 1873-4, ii, 1.—**Field** (J. T.) † Texas Cour.-Rec. Med., Fort Worth, 1885-6, iii, 296-299. — **Finlay.** † Med. Times & Gaz., Lond., 1878, ii, 167.—**Fischer** (E) Meningitis cerebro-spinalis. Med.-chir. Centralbl., Wien, 1882, xvii, 424.—**Foà** (P.) & **Bordoni-Uffreduzzi** (G.) Sulla meningite cerebro-spinale epidemica. Gior. d. r. Accad. di med. di Torino, 1886, 3. s., xxxiv, 52. ——. Ueber Bakterienbefunde bei Meningitis cerebrospinalis und die Beziehungen derselben zur Pneumonie. Deutsche med. Wchnschr., Berl., 1886, xii, 249.—**Fort** (W. K.) † N. Orl. M. & S. J., 1876-7, n. s., iv, 510-518.—**Fränkel** (A.) Ueber einen Bacterienbefund bei Meningitis cerebrospinalis, nebst Bemerkungen über die Pneumonie-Micrococchen. Berl. klin. Wchnschr., 1886, xxiii, 366. [Discus-

Meningitis (*Cerebro-spinal*).

sion], 396–398. *Also:* Verhandl. d. Berl. med. Gesellsch. (1885-6), 1887, xvii, 89–100. [Discussion], 101–108. *Also:* Deutsche med. Wchnschr., Berl., 1886, xii, 209–213. — **Frensdorf.** Sporadisches Auftreten der Meningitis cerebro spinalis. Prakt. Arzt, Wetzlar, 1884, xxv, 169–172.— **Fulton** [*et al.*]. Cases of cerebral meningitis. Austral. M. J., Melbourne, 1886, viii, 420–425. — **Gahlberg** (A.) Bericht über die in Mailberg und Umgebung beobachteten Fälle von Meningitis cerebro-spinalis epidemica. Wien. med. Wchnschr., 1886, xxxvi, 821-825. ———. Meningitis cerebro-spinalis. Mitth. d. Ver. d. Aerzte in Nied.-Oest., Wien, 1886, xii, 153; 167.— **Gairdner.** † Glasgow M. J., 1883, [4. s.], xix, 459-461. — **Gallard.** † Chez un alcoolique. Gaz. d. hôp., Par., 1870, xliii, 109. — **Galler.** Meningitis cerebro-medullaris mit dem Ausgange in Kokkygodynie und endliche Heilung. Aerztl. Int.-Bl., München, 1865, xii, 358–360.— **Gasté** (L.-F.) Résumé clinique sur les méningites excéphalo-rachidiennes observées pendant le 1er trimestre 1840. *In his:* Mélanges de méd., 8°, Metz, 1841, 98–130.— **Gaston** (J. McF.) Treatment of a case of cerebro-spinal meningitis. South. M. Rec., Atlanta, 1885, xv, 161; 210.— **Gibbon** (S.) † (Seven days) with purple spots (thirty hours). Med. Times & Gaz., Lond., 1867, ii, 58.— **Giebens.** † Ann. Soc. de méd. d'Anvers, 1851, viii, 32–37. *Also:* Arch de la méd. belge, Brux., 1851, xxxv, 133–136.— **Gifford** (B. D.) Notes on some cases of cerebro-spinal meningitis. Boston M. & S. J., 1873, lxxxix, 277–280.— **Giraux** (H.) Méningite cérébro-spinale chronique. Mouvement méd., Par., 1877, xv. 292–295.— **Goralevitch** (I. A.) † † [Intermittent types.] Protok. zasaid. Kavkazsk. med. Obsh , Tiflis, 1882-3, xix, 147–150.— **Gougenheim** (M.) Méningite cérébro-spinale sous-arachnoïdienne suppurée. Bull. Soc. anat. de Par., 1864, xxxix, 123–125. — **Gray & Tuckwell.** † † Lancet, Lond., 1876, i, 812.— **Greene** (J. S.) † Boston M. & S. J., 1865-6, lxxiii, 356–359. — **Greenwade** (R. H.) † Med. Herald, Louisville, 1879–80, i, 102. — **Grimshaw.** Cerebro-spinal arachnitis. Dublin Q. J. M. Sc., 1868, xlvi, 469–471. ———. Cerebro-spinal meningitis. *Ibid.,* 1870, xlix, 481. ———. † With some peculiar symptoms. Brit. M. J., Lond., 1870, ii, 554. ———. † Cure; autopsy. Irish Hosp. Gaz., Dubl., 1874, ii, 16.— **Gui** (A.) † † Bull. d. Soc. Lancisiana d. osp. di Roma, 1882, ii, 92–98.— **Hadden** (W. B.) † Chronic. Tr. Path. Soc. Lond., 1884–5, xxxvi, 13–15. *Also:* Lancet, Lond., 1885, i, 845.— **Hagiwara** (Sankei). [On epidemic cerebro-spinal meningitis.] Chingai Iji Shinpo, Tokio, 1886, no. 158, Oct. 25.— **Hamilton** (G.) Cerebro-spinal meningitis. St. Louis M. & S J., 1883, xliv, 237–245.— **Hammond** (J. F.) † Georgia Eclect. M. J., Atlanta, 1879–80, i, 319–325. — **Hampeln.** Ueber acute Cerebro-Spinal-Meningitis. Deutsches Arch. f. klin. Med., Leipz., 1875-6, xvii, 300–303.— **Harry** (S. I.) Nitro muriatic acid and strychnia in cerebro-spinal meningitis. Med. & Surg. Reporter, Phila., 1866, xv, 218.— **Hayden.** Cerebro-spinal arachnitis. Med. Press & Circ., Dubl., 1866, n. s., ii, 439.— **Hayes** (R. A.) Case of cerebro-spinal meningitis. Brit. M. J., Lond., 1886, i, 1216. *Also:* Tr. Acad. M. Ireland, Dubl., 1886, iv, 89.— **Hayward** (G.) † Boston M. & S. J., 1864, lxx, 200–202. *Also:* Extr. Rec. Bost. Soc. M. Improve. (1862–6), 1867, v (app.), 93- 95.— **Heffinger** (A. C.) Sporadic cerebro-spinal meningitis. Boston M. & S. J., 1879, ci, 172.— **Heineman** (H. N.) † With acute endocarditis and pericarditis. Bull. N. York Path. Soc., 1881, 2. s., i, 323–325. *Also;* Med. Rec., N. Y., 1881, xx, 746.— **Heller** (A.) Zur anatomischen Begründung der Gehörstörungen bei Meningitis cerebrospinalis. Deutsches Arch. f. klin. Med , Leipz., 1867, iii, 482–487.— **Hemey.** † Chez un alcoolique. Rec. d. trav. Soc. méd. d'obs. de Par., 1866-70, 2. s , ii, 414–420.— **Hendley** (J.) Acute sporadic cerebro-spinal meningitis. Med. Herald, Louisville, 1880–81, ii, 540.— **Henoch** (E.) Zur Pathologie der Meningitis cerebrospinalis. Charité-Ann. 1884, Berl., 1886, xi, 575–586.— **Hérard.** † Guérison. Gaz. d. hôp., Par., 1861, xxxiv, 409; 413.— **Hickman** (J. G.) † † St. Louis M. & S. J., 1872, n. s., ix, 358–360.— **Höchst.** Sporadisches Auftreten der Meningitis cerebro-spinalis. Prakt. Arzt, Wetzlar, 1879, xx, 241; 265.— **Holden** (L.) Sporadic cerebro-spinal meningitis. Austral. M. J., Melbourne, 1884, n. s., vi, 289–291.— **Hollister** (J. H.) † † Med. Exam., Chicago, 1873, xiv, 169–172.— **Homans** (C. D.) † Autopsy. Boston M. & S. J., 1866-7, lxxv, 125.— **Homolle.** Méningite cérébro-spinale suppurée chez un enfant atteint d'endocardite chronique avec anévrysme valvulaire de l'orifice aortique et perforation de la cloison interventriculaire. Bull. Soc. anat. de Par., 1873, xlviii, 840-844. — **Houzé.** Quelques mots sur la méningite cérébro-spinale. Arch. méd. belges, Brux., 1887, 3. s., xxxi, 366–375. — **Hughes** (H. F.) † St. Louis M. & S. J., 1850, viii, 128–130. — **Humphries** (W. F.) † † St. Louis M. & S. J., 1884, xlvi, 219–223.— **Hunt** (J. W.) Case of purulent cerebral and spinal meningitis; no symptoms; sudden death by coma. Brain, Lond., 1879–80, ii, 409–412.— **Hutchinson** (J. H.) † Proc. Path. Soc. Phila. (1860-66), 1867, n. s., 209–211. *Also:* Am. J. M. Sc., Phila., 1866, n. s., lii, 125–127.— **Hutinel.** Méningite cérébro-spinale suppurée. France méd., Par., 1878, xxv, 189.— *Also:* Bull. Soc. clin. de Par. (1878), 1879, ii, 26–29.— **In-**

9

Meningitis (*Cerebro-spinal*).

gals (E. F.) † Marked symptoms treated with Cannabis indica, in large doses ; speedy and almost perfect recovery. Med. Exam., Chicago, 1872, xiii, 132.— **Jacobi.** Taches méningitiques in the diagnosis of cerebro-spinal meningitis. N. York M. J., 1882, xxxv, 524. *Also:* Tr. N. York Obst. Soc. (1881–5), 1885, iii, 56.— **Jacobi** (Mary P.) Cerebro-spinal meningitis; pseudo-membranous croup. Med. Rec., N. Y., 1877, xii, 237.— **Janeway** (E. G.) † Autopsy. N. York M. J., 1880, xxxii, 60.— **Jones** (C. H.) † Autopsy. Med. Times & Gaz., Lond., 1880. i, 657–659.— **Jones** (S. J.) Notes of some recent cases of deafness, following cerebro-spinal meningitis. Chicago J. Nerv. & Ment. Dis., 1874, i, 171–175.— **Junkin** (S. B.) Cerebro-spinal meningitis. Buffalo M. & S. J., 1872–3, xii, 15–17. — **Kalfus** (H. F.) On cerebro-spinal meningitis. Am. Pract , Louisville, 1873, vii, 345–353.— **Keene** (S. S.) † † Boston M. & S. J., 1870, lxxxii, 261–263. — **Kehrer** (F. A.) Ueber Cerebro-spinalmeningitis bei Säuglingen. Oesterr. Jahrb. f. Paediat., Wien, 1873, i, 69–78.— **Kelk** (J. W.) Waarneming eener meningitis cerebro-spinalis subarachnoidea, met zwarte verweeking van den oesophagus. Nederl. Lancet, Gravenh., 1845, 2. s., i, 193–214. *Also,* Reprint.— **Kendall** (J. V.) Cerebro-spinal meningitis, or "the brain fever" of 1857. Tr. M. Soc. N. Y., Albany, 1858, 97–111.— **Kernig** (V. M.) Ob odnom malo izviestnom priznakie vospalenija mjagkoi mozgovoi obolochke. [Diagnosis of cerebro-spinal meningitis.] Vrach, St. Petersb., 1884, v, 427; 446.— **Kiemann.** Meningitis cerebrospinalis serosopurulenta cum hydrocephalo acuto interno; Prostatitis suppurativa; Tod. Ber. d. k. k. Krankenanst. Rudolph-Stiftung in Wien (1880), 1881, 329–332. ———.† Tod. *Ibid.,* 341–343. ———.† Genesung. *Ibid.* (1883), 1884, 303–305.— **Kingsley** (J. P.) Paralysis from cerebro-spinal meningitis, and the humerus out of the glenoid cavity. Proc. St. Louis M. Soc. Missouri (1879), 1880, ii, 209–211. ———. Cerebro-spinal meningitis; a clinical lecture. St. Louis Cour. Med., 1881, v, 489–497.— **Kirchner.** Ueber Meningitis cerebrospinalis und deren Bedeutung für das Gehörorgan. Deutsche med. Wchnschr., Berl., 1884, x, 65–68.— **Knapp** (H.) Two cases of deafness from cerebro-spinal meningitis, the one one-sided, the other double-sided with simultaneous affection of both eyes, ending in recovery in one. Arch. Otol., N. Y., 1884, xiii, 297–300. *Also, transl.:* Ztschr. f. Ohrenh., Wiesb., 1884–5, xiv, 241–244.— **Kornfeld** (H.) Traumatische cerebrospinale Meningitis. Prag. med. Wchnschr., 1883, viii, 325–328.— **Kratschmer.** Ein Beitrag zum Krankheitsbilde der Meningitis cerebrospinalis. Wien. med. Wchnschr., 1872, xxii, 656; 717.— **Krohn** (V.) † † Ugesk. f. Læger, Kjøbenh., 1885, 4. R., xii, 421–425.— **Kuhnt & Schultze.** Méningite cérébro-spinale par suite de sarcome du cervelet et de la moelle épinière ; névro-rétinite; guérison avec paraplégie; épilepsie spinale ; eschares; autopsie ; histologie. Paris méd., 1881, 2. s., vi, 105; 113.— **Kunkler** (G. A.) † Followed by paralysis of the lower extremities. Med. Counsellor, Columbus, 1856, ii, 243.— **Lannelongue.** † Opisthotonos; paralysie de la face; paraplégie; kyste apoplectique des tubercules quadrijumeaux et des pédoncules supérieurs du cervelet. J. de méd. de Bordeaux, 1861, 2. s., vi, 55–63.— **Langer** (A.) † Pest. med.-chir. Presse, Budapest, 1883. xix, 305–309.— **Larrabee** (J. A.) † † Richmond & Louisville M. J., Louisville, 1872, xiv, 764–785.— **Lasègue.** Méningite cérébro spinale à frigore. Arch. gén. de méd., Par., 1876, ii, 88–91.— **Lauschmann** (G.) Meningitis cerebrospinalis egy esete. Gyógyászat, Budapest, 1886, xxvi, 465–468.— **Lawson** (H. M.) Cerebro-spinal meningitis. Med. & Surg. Reporter, Phila., 1866, xv, 141.— **Leonardi** (M.) † Con apparenze di delirium tremens. Bull. d. sc. med. di Bologna, 1846, 3. s., x, 124–133. ———. Gravissima meningite cerebro-spinale con apparenze di delirium tremens. *Ibid.,* 1847, 3. s., xi, 244–246.— **Lespiau.** † Sporadique; guérison. Gaz. d. hôp., Par., 1865, xxxviii, 389.— **Leyden** (E.) Bemerkungen über Cerebrospinalmeningitis und über das Erbrechen in fieberhaften Krankheiten. Ztschr. f. klin. Med., Berl., 1887, xii, 385–400.— **Liegey.** Fièvre dyspnéique méningitique chez un enfant à la mamelle, et méningite cérébro-spinale débutante sous la forme dyspnéique, chez un enfant plus âgé à la suite d'une rougeole anormale. Courrier méd., Par., 1878, xxviii, 21–23.— **Lignerolles.** Méningite cérébro-spinale purulente consécutive à une carie du rocher. Bull. Soc. anat. de Par., 1866, xli, 248–252. ———. Méningite cérébro-spinale suppurée consécutive à une carie du rocher. *Ibid.,* 350.— **Lipari** (G.) Caso di meningite cerebro-spinale senza sintomi. Morgagni, Napoli, 1885, xxvii, 301; 406.— **Little** (J.) A case of cerebro-spinal meningitis, in which hypodermic injections of morphia and atropia were freely used. Dublin J. M. Sc., 1874, lvii, 266–271. *Also* [Abstr.]: Irish Hosp. Gaz., Dubl., 1874, ii, 79.— **Little** (P. C.) Cerebro-spinal arachnitis. Med. Press & Circ., Dubl., 1866, n. s., i, 7–9. ———. Traumatic cerebro-spinal arachnitis. *Ibid.,* 1867, n. s., iii, 243. — **London** (B.) † Wien. med. Presse. 1865, vi, 785–787.— **Longstreth** (M.) † Tr. Path. Soc. Phila. (1871-3), 1874, iv, 195.— **Lorey** (J. B.) † Bei einem 15jährigen Mädchen ; Section. Jahresb. ü. d. Verwalt. d. Med.-Wes., d. Krankenanst. . . . d. Stadt Frankf. (1865), 1869, ix, 33–36.— **Luzzatti.** † Resoc.

Meningitis (*Cerebro-spinal*).

san. d. Osp. civ. di Trieste (1876), 1878, iv, 133.—**Macdonnell** (R. L.) Case of acute cerebro-spinal arachnitis, the patient having presented during his whole life an irregular intermitting and slow pulse. Brit.-Am. J. M. & Phys. Sc., Montreal, 1848-9, iv, 202-206.—**MacLaurin** (H. N.) † N. South Wales M. Gaz., Sydney, 1873-4, iv, 109; 132.—**Mackall** (L.), jr. A case of intermittent cerebro-spinal meningitis. Nat. M. J., Wash., 1871-2, ii, 524-531.—**Mader** (J.) † Ausdehnung sämmtlicher Ventrikel durch massenhaften Eiter (mit secundärer Vereiterung der Gehirnsubstanz); sehr langsamer Verlauf; sehr geringe Affection der Psyche; Tod. Ber. d. k. k. Krankenanst. Rudolph-Stiftung in Wien (1876), 1877, 341-344. ———. Meningitis cerebro-spinalis; epidemica? Wien. med. Bl., 1880, iii, 385; 411. ———. Ausgedehnte Paralysen und Muskelatrophie nach Meningitis cerebrospinalis (Myelitis?); gebessert. Ber. d. k. k. Krankenanst. Rudolph-Stiftung in Wien (1880), 1881, 338. ———. Eitrige (epidemische?) cerebro-spinale Leptomeningitis; eitriger Hydrocephalus; Tod. *Ibid.* (1883), 1884, 305. — **Maier** (E. L.) † Jahrb. f. Kinderh., Leipz., 1871-2, v, 109-116.—**Maixner** (E.) Ein Fall von traumatischer Spinal-Meningitis. Med.-chir. Centralbl., Wien, 1882, xvii, 304.—**Major** (G. W.) † Canada M. & S. J., Montreal, 1881-2, x, 592-594.—**Mann** (E. C.) On the treatment of blindness and deafness resulting from cerebro-spinal meningitis, by the constant current of electricity. Med. Gaz., N. Y., 1880, vii, 687. *Also:* J. Psych. M., Lond., 1881, n. s., vii, 70-73. ———. Cerebro-spinal meningitis. Am. Pract., Louisville, 1885, xxxi, 134.—**Markusy.** Beiderseitige Panophthalmitis in Folge von Meningitis cerebro-spinalis. Centralbl. f. prakt. Augenh., Leipz., 1879, iii, 165-167. —**Martin.** † (Idiopathic.) Med. Times & Gaz., Lond, 1865, i, 465.—**Masferrer** (R.) & **Espuche** (R.) Tifus cerebro-espinal. Gac. méd. catal., Barcel., 1883, vi, 429-434. — **Mason.** Chronic cerebro-spinal meningitis; specimens from the case of a boy aged 11. Brit. M. J., Lond., 1885, i, 944.—**Mason** (A. L.) †† One, of the fulminant type, treated by subcutaneous injections of apomorphia, morphine, and atropine; recovery; one autopsy. Boston M. & S. J., 1884, cx, 121.—**Matheson** (A. R.) Cerebro-spinal meningitis. Michigan Univ. M. J., Ann Arbor, 1872-3, iii, 577-585.—**Maurer** (A.) Croupöse Pneumonie und Meningitis cerebro-spinalis bei Kindern im ersten Lebensjahre. Deutsches Arch. f. klin. Med., Leipz., 1874, xiv, 47-63.—**Mayne.** Acute cerebro-spinal arachnitis; effusion into the subarachnoid tissue. Proc. Path. Soc. Dubl., 1846, i, 375-377.—**Mayne** (R.) Cerebro spinal meningitis. Dublin Hosp. Gaz., 1859, n. s., vi, 259-261.—**Miller** (J. S.) Cerebro-spinal meningitis. Peoria M. Month., 1883-4, iv, 433.—**Mills** (B. L.) Case of epidemic cerebro-spinal meningitis. Edinb. M. J., 1886-7, xxxii, 500-502.—**Moffett** (J.) Cerebro-spinal meningitis. Tr. Indiana M. Soc., Indianap., 1867, xvii, 108-115.— **Monette** (G. N.) †† Am. Pract., Louisville, 1873, vii, 264-266.—**Moore.** † Followed by complete aphasia; recovery. Irish Hosp. Gaz., Dubl., 1874, ii, 228-230.—**Moos** (S.) Eigenthümliche Gehörsstörungen nach Meningitis cerebrospinalis; bedeutende Besserung durch den constanten Strom. Arch. f. Augen- u. Ohrenh., Carlsruhe, 1869-70, i, 1. Abth., 216-222. *Also, transl.:* Arch. Ophth. & Otol., N. Y., 1869, i, 332-340.—**Moreland.** Cerebro-spinal meningitis. Boston M. & S. J., 1866-7, lxxv, 66.—**Morris** (M.) Cerebro-spinal meningitis. Med. Rec., N. Y., 1872, vii, 245.—**Murchison.** † Tr. Path. Soc. Lond., 1866-7, xviii, 14-18. *Also:* Lancet, Lond., 1867, i, 483.—**Murphy** (T. C.) Cerebro-spinal meningitis. Chicago M. J., 1870, xxvii, 202-204.—**Nechacff** (A. A.) K symptomatol. meningitis cerebrospinalis. Ejened. klin. gaz., St. Petersb., 1884, iv, 529-535.—**Neufeld** (J.) † Intermittens quartana. Gaz. lek, Warszawa, 1879, xxvii, 201-203.—**Newhall.** Cerebro-spinal meningitis. Boston M. & S. J., 1873, lxxxviii, 651.—**Niemeier** (G.) Intermittent cerebro-spinal meningitis. Buffalo M & S. J., 1872-3, xii, 6-9.—**Noquet.** Otite moyenne purulente double; ostéite des apophyses mastoïdes et de la région des rochers avoisinant les caisses; pus dans les labyrinthes (pièces pathologiques recueillies sur un sujet mort de méningite cérébro-spinale). Bull. méd. du nord, Lille, 1880, xx, 45-50.—**Oeller** (J. N.) Retinitis und Cyclitis suppurativa bei Cerebrospinalmeningitis. Arch. f. Augenh., Wiesb., 1878-9, viii, 357-378.—**Ohr** (C. H.) Cerebro-spinal meningitis; spotted fever. Tr. M. & Chir. Fac. Maryland, Balt., 1879, lxxxi, 116-121.—**Olivier.** Indigestion; commencement de méningite cérébro-spinale; gastro-entérite; guérison. Clin. d. hôp. d. enf., Par., 1844, iii, 129-133.—**O'Meagher** (W.) †† Am. M. Times, N. Y., 1860, i, 134.—**O'Neill** (E. D.) Simulative cerebro-spinal meningitis, with abnormally high temperature. Med. Press & Circ., Lond., 1879, n. s., xxviii, 131.—**Oreste** (P.) Sulle varie forme di meningite ed in particolare di quella cerebro-spinale negli animali domestici. Arch. ital. per le mal. nerv., Milano, 1873, x, 348-352.—**O'Ryan.** Hysteria progressing to spino-cerebral arachnitis, attended by some unusual symptoms. Dublin M. Press, 1848, xix, 177-179.—**Osgood** (W.) † Recovery. Boston M. & S. J., 1874, xci, 415-417.—**Otte** (R.) † Complicirt mit Noma; Heilung. Allg. med. Centr.-Ztg., Berl., 1866, xxxv, 73-75.—**Oudin.** Pneumonie et mé-

Meningitis (*Cerebro-spinal*).

ningite cérébro-spinale à marche insolite. France méd., Par., 1878, xxv, 378.—**Pätsch.** † Hemiplegia sinistra; Heilung. Charité-Ann. 1879, Berl., 1881, vi, 176-182.—**Parker** (R. W.) † Traumatic; post-mortem. Med. Times & Gaz., Lond., 1881, i, 457-459.—**Parks** (L.), jr. A case of cerebro-spinal meningitis, with remarks. Extr. Rec. Bost. Soc. M. Improve. (1862-6), 1867, v (app.), 73-85.—**Payne** (J. F.) † With disease of the kidneys. Tr. Path. Soc. Lond., 1869-70, xxi, 7-9.—**Peabody** (G. L.) Cerebro-spinal meningitis. Tr. N. York Path. Soc., 1881, 2. s., i, 102.—**Petersen** (A.) Meningitis cerebro-spinalis. Hosp.-Tid. Kjobenh., 1876, 2. R., iii, 177-180.—**Petrini** (G.) † J. Soc. sc. med. d. Bucuresci, 1879, i, 261-268.—**Philip** (D. L.) Cerebro-spinal meningitis. Canada Lancet, Toronto, 1872-3, v, 541-546.—**Potapovoi** (T. A.) K kazuistikie cerebro-spinalnago meningita. Protok. zasaid. Kavkazsk. med. Obsh., Tiflis, 1883-4, xx, 318-327.—**Powell** (T. S.) †† Georgia M. Companion, Atlanta, 1871, i, 101-107.—**Prewitt** (T. F.) Cerebro-spinal meningitis. St. Louis M. & S. J., 1865, n. s., ii, 205-211.—**Pumphrey** (G. W.) † Leavenworth M. Herald, 1869-70, iii, 389.—**Rampold.** Zur Cerebrospinalmeningitis der französischen Aerzte. Med. Cor.-Bl. d. württemb. ärztl. Ver., Stuttg., 1846, xvi, 4-6. ———. Einiges über Herrn Dr. Roger's Bemerkungen zu der von mir mitgetheilten Beobachtung einer Cerebrospinalmeningitis. *Ibid.*, 110-112.—**Ramsey** (D. C.) Salicylic acid in the treatment of cerebro-spinal meningitis. St. Louis Cour. Med., 1884, xi, 97-100.—**Rapisarda** (O.) Due casi di meningite cerebro-spinale guariti col bromuro di potassio ad alte dosi. Arch. clin. ital., Roma, 1884, xiv, 257-259. *Also:* Riv. clin. e terap., Napoli, 1884, vi, 315-318. — **Reignier** (G.) Méningite cérébro-spinale à forme rabique. France méd., Par., 1869, xvi, 394. — **Ricaille.** † Ann. Soc. d'anat. path. de Brux. Bull., 1875, 55-59.—**Richter.** Zur Incubationszeit der Mening. epidemica. Breslau. ärztl. Ztschr., 1887, ix, 161.—**Rickards.** † Brit. M. J., Lond., 1875, ii, 365.—**von Ritter.** Eiterig-faserstoffige Entzündung der Meningen der Hirnbasis und der Rückenmarks. Vrtljschr. f. d. prakt. Heilk., Prag, 1851, xxxiii, 52-56.—**Robinson** (T.) A case of cerebral meningitis. Med. Exam., Lond., 1878, iv, 95. ———. Case of cerebro-spinal meningitis; autopsy. Lancet, Lond., 1880, ii, 612.—**Rodenstein** (C. F.) Papers on "cerebro-spinal meningitis". Med. Rec., N. Y., 1872, vii, 71. ———. Thermometry in cerebro-spinal meningitis. Arch. Scient. & Pract. M. & S., N. Y., 1873, i, 210-222. *Also*, Reprint.—**Roger.** Bemerkungen über die von Herrn Dr. Rampold mitgetheilte Beobachtung von Cerebrospinalmeningitis. Med. Cor.-Bl. d. württemb. ärztl. Ver., Stuttg., 1846, xvi, 85.—**Rollo** (J. B.) Meningite cerebro-espinhal (esporadica). Escholiaste med., Lisb., 1863, xiv, 349-351.—**Roosa** (D. B. St. J.) (Cases of deafness following cerebro-spinal meningitis.) Am. J. M. Sc., Phila., 1874, n. s., lxviii, 377-400.—**Rosenfeld** (A.) Fall von Meningitis cerebrospinalis mit Heilung. Wien. med. Presse, 1886, xxvii, 1078.—**Rosenthal** (M.) Contribuzione allo studio della meningite cerebro-spinale. [Transl. by E. Coen.] Boll. d. clin., Milano, 1887, iv, 162-168.—**Ross** (G.) † Recovery. Canada M. & S. J., Montreal, 1872-3, i, 111-113.—**Sachero** (G.) † Seguita da improvvisa apoplessia capillare, con epicrisi. Gior. . . . d. Soc. med.-chir. di Torino, 1842, xv, 257-268. — **Sanders.** Cerebro-spinal meningitis. Indian M. Gaz., Calcutta, 1886, xxi, 151-154.—**Schenk** (K. A.) Chetire sluchaja tserebrospinalnago meningita. Ejened. klin. gaz., St. Petersb., 1881, i, 213-217.—**Seifert** (O.) Ein Fall von Myelitis nach Meningitis cerebro-spinalis mit Doppelempfindung und deren graphische Darstellung. Wien. med. Wchnschr., 1882, xxxii.785; 821.—**Senator** (H.) Ueber einige Fälle von infectiöser epidemischer Cerebrospinalmeningitis, nebst Bemerkungen über die Diagnose dieser Krankheit. Charité-Ann. 1884, Berl., 1886, xi, 248-264.—**Sensenig** (J. B.) † Practitioner, Lancaster, 1884, ii, 12.—**Shaffner** (C.) A mild case of cerebro-spinal meningitis followed by blindness. Phila. M. Times, 1873-4, iv, 520.—**Shaw** (T. W.) † Pittsburgh M. J., 1880-81, i, 136.—**Sicherer** (P. F.) Die gastrischen Fieber und die Cerebrospinalmeningitis. Med. Cor.-Bl. d. württemb. ärztl. Ver., Stuttg., 1847, xvii, 245-247.—**Silfverskiöld** (P.) Om en epidemi af meningitis cerebrospinalis i Göteborg 1883. Eira, Göteborg, 1886, x, 31; 73; 103, 1 diag., 1 map.—**Silvestrini** (G.) † Gazz. med. ital., prov. venete, Padova, 1876, xix, 137; 145.—**Sinclair.** Acute sporadic cerebro-spinal meningitis; death on the fourth day; necropsy; remarks. Lancet, Lond., 1887, i, 312.—**Skinner** (C. M.) Cerebro-spinal meningitis again. Therap. Gaz., Detroit, 1885, 3. s, i, 139-141.—**Smith** (C. W.) Report of a case of sporadic, malignant cerebro-spinal meningitis, with death in thirty-six hours. Indiana M. J., Indianap., 1886-7, v, 493. — **Smith** (J. H.) Cerebro-spinal meningitis. Tr. Vermont M. Soc. 1874-6, St. Albans, 1877, 457-475.—**Smith** (J. L.) Cerebro-spinal meningitis. Tr. N. York Path. Soc., 1881, 2. s., i, 239-246. *Also:* Cycl. Pract. M. (Ziemssen), N. Y., 1881 (suppl.), 151-163.—**Sokolowski** (A.) † Medycyna, Warszawa, 1882, x, 339-344.—**Southall** (J. H.) Cerebro-spinal meningitis. Richmond & Louisville M. J., Louisville, 1872, xiv, 138-146.—**Spörer.** † St. Petersb. med. Ztschr., 1866, x, 48-50.—**Standthartner.**

Meningitis (*Cerebro-spinal*).

† Aerztl. Ber. d. k. k. allg. Krankenh. zu Wien (1875), 1876, 56.—**Steinbrügge** (H.) Doppelseitige Labyrintherkrankung während einer Cerebrospinal-Meningitis. Ztschr. f. Ohrenh., Wiesb., 1886, xvi, 229-237.—**Steiner** & **Neureutter.** Krankheiten des Rückenmarkes. Vrtljschr. f. d. prakt. Heilk., Prag, 1863, iii, 71-73.—**Stewart.** † Recovery. Edinb. M. J., 1880-81, xxvi, 128-131.—**Stille.** Cerebro-spinal meningitis. Tr. Coll. Phys. Phila. (1856-62), 1863, n. s., iii, 104-106.—**Stoltz.** Méningite cérébrospinale, congénitale, idiopathique. Gaz. d. hôp., Par., 1857, xxx, 395 — **Stone** (J. O.) †† *In his:* Clinical cases, 8°, N. Y., 1878, 73-78.—**Stone** (R. K.) Cerebro-spinal meningitis. Boston M. & S. J., 1849, xl, 297-299.—**Summerell** (J. J.) † (Erysipelatous.) Med. J. N. Car.. Edenton,1858-9, i-ii. 349-354.—**Sutton** (W. H.) † With embolism. Med. Herald, Louisville, 1879-80, i, 393-396.—**Sweringen** (H. V.) † Obst. Gaz., Cincin., 1883, vi, 172.—**Teleky** (H.) Ueber Meningitis cerebrospinalis infectiosa. Wien. med. Bl., 1886, ix, 1535; 1570; 1605.—**Tempini** (G.) Un caso sporadico e fulminante di meningite cerebro-spinale. Gazz. med. ital. lomb., Milano, 1872, 6. s., v, 237-241.—**Thompson** (H.) † Death. Lancet, Lond., 1876, i, 849.—**Thomson** (W. H.) Cerebro-spinal meningitis. Med. Rec., N. Y., 1878, xiv, 329.—**Tilden** (G.) † Idiopathic. Proc. Nebraska M. Soc., Omaha, 1873, 7-9.—**Török** (J.) † Gyógyászat, Budapest, 1880, xx, 289-292.—**Tosquinet.** Méningite cérébro-spinale épidémique. Arch. méd. belges, Brux., 1886, 3. s., xxx, 160-169.—**Traube** (L.) † (Ob tuberculöser Natur?) Ann. d. Char.-Krankenh. . . zu Berl., 1862-3, x, 2. Hft., 172-176. ———. Zur Lehre von der Cerebrospinal-Meningitis mit Bemerkungen über das Verhalten und die diagnostische Wichtigkeit der Temperaturcurve bei dieser Krankheit. Ges. Beitr. z. Path. u. Physiol., Berl., 1878, iii, 565 —**Trenholme** (E. H.) † Canada M. Rec., Montreal, 1873-4, ii, 121.—**Trilesski** (A.) Cerebrospinal. meningit v g. Ismaile. Ejened. klin. gaz., St. Petersb., 1886, vi, 476; 497; 508.—**Troisier.** Méningite cérébro-spinale purulente. Bull. Soc. anat. de Par., 1873, xlviii, 608.—**Turnbull** (L.) Observations on the nature and treatment of the diseases of the eye in cerebro-spinal meningitis. Med. & Surg. Reporter, Phila., 1868, xviii, 205-207.—**Turner** (F.C.) Spinal cords from two cases of cerebro-spinal meningitis. Tr. Path. Soc. Lond., 1883-4, xxxv, 63. — **Upham** (J. B.) † Boston M. & S. J., 1867, lxxvi, 485-489.—**Van Bellinghen.** Méningite cérébro-rachidienne, suite d'accès hystériques; antiphlogistiques; calomel; torsion abdominale; guérison. Presse méd. belge, Brux., 1879, xxxi, 353-355. — **Van Dewalker** (J. G.) Cerebro-spinal meningitis. [Treatment by Calabar bean.] Chicago M. Times, 1872, iv, 54-57.—**Van Houten** (J.A.) Cerebro-spinal meningitis, the result of an abscess opening into the spinal canal. N. York M. J., 1877, xxv, 182.—**Verline.** Méningite cérébro-spinale. Bull. Soc. anat. de Par., 1863, xxxviii, 110-112.—**Vinogradoff** (K.) † Protok. zasaid. Obsh. russk. vrach. v St. Petersb., 1877-8, xliv, 40-54. — **Voronich** (N.) Ob izmienii. mejpozvonoch. chriatsha pri meningitis cerebro-spinalis. [On the changes of the spinal cord in cerebro-spinal meningitis.] Voyenno-med. J., St. Petersb., 1877, cxxix, pt. 2, 25l-266.—**Webber** (S. G.) † Boston M. & S. J. (1872), 1873, lxxxvii, 96. ———. Three cases of cerebral meningitis from different causes. *Ibid.*, 1879, ci, 357-362.—**Weichselbaum** (A.) Gehirnabscesse bei Meningitis cerebro-spinalis. Ber. d. k. k. Krankenanst. Rudolph-Stiftung in Wien (1883), 1884, 381.—**Weiver** (J.B.) Salicylic acid in cerebro-spinal meningitis. Med. & Surg. Reporter, Phila., 1884, l, 410.—**Welch** (S.) Cerebro-spinal meningitis. Med. Herald, Louisville, 1882-3, iv, 443.—**Westmoreland** (J.G.) Cerebro-spinal meningitis; its pathology and treatment. Tr. M. Ass. Georgia, Atlanta, 1873, xxiv, 132-137. ———. Cerebro-spinal meningitis. Atlanta M. & S. J., 1876-7, xiv, 712-714. ———. † *Ibid.*, 1878-9, xvi, 712-714.—**White** (C. A.) Cerebro spinal meningitis. Chicago M. J., 1865, xxii, 529-532. — **Whitehead** (F. P.) Cerebro-spinal meningitis. Richmond & Louisville M. J., Louisville, 1872, xiv, 156.—**Whithall** (S.) Specimen of cerebro-spinal meningitis with history. Med. Rec., N. Y., 1872, vii, 206. ———. †† Hosp. Gaz., N. Y., 1876-7, i, 45.—**Whitmire** (J. S.) Cerebro-spinal arachnitis or paralysis. Northwest. M. & S. J., Chicago, 1851-2, viii, 381-388. — **Whitmore** (B. T.) † St. Louis Cour. Med., 1882, vii, 133-135.—**Widerhofer.** †† Jahrb. f. Kinderh., Leipz., 1885, n. F., xxiii, 429-441. — **Wiebecke.** Meningitis cerebro-spinalis. Allg. Ztschr. f. Psychiat., etc., Berl., 1866, xxiii, 115-119. — **Wilcox** (R. W.) The pulmonic form of cerebro-spinal meningitis. N. York M. J., 1887, xlvi, 262-264.—**Wilkie** (D.) Cerebro-spinal meningitis, pneumonio-pleuritis; acute hydrocele, commencing pericarditis. [Case.] Indian M. Gaz., Calcutta, 1878, xiii, 37-39. ———. † Psoas abscess. *Ibid.*, 39.—**Williams.** Loss of sight and hearing after cerebro-spinal meningitis. Weekly M. Rev., Chicago, 1884, ix, 416.—**Wilson** (A.) A rapid case of acute cerebro-spinal meningitis. Brit. M. J., Lond., 1884, i, 717.—**Wilson** (H.) Diseases of the eye in cerebro-spinal meningitis. Dublin Q. J. M. Sc., 1867, xliii, 302-306. *Also,* Reprint.—**Witter** (G. F.) † Tr. Wisconsin M. Soc., Milwaukee, 1872, vi, 115-117.—**Wood** (G.) † Canada

Meningitis (*Cerebro-spinal*).

M. & S. J., Montreal, 1872-3, i, 152-154. — **Wood** (L. M.) Recovery, under electricity, of a case of hemiplegia, due to cerebro-spinal meningitis. Virginia M. Month., Richmond, 1876-7, iii, 428. — **Woronichin** (N.) Ueber die pathologischen Veränderungen in der Structur der Intervertebralknorpel bei Meningitis cerebro-spinalis. Jahrb. f. Kinderh., Leipz., 1877, n. F., xi, 287-293.—**Worthington** (A.) An account of a case of intermittent epidemic cerebro-spinal meningitis. Canada M. & S. J., Montreal, 1885-6, xiv, 598-604.—**Xella** (F.) † In un uomo dell' età di 52 anni; guarigione perfetta. Raccoglitore med., Forlì, 1876, v, 342-353.—**Young** (R.) †† Am. Pract., Louisville, 1874, ix, 88-92. — **Zeroni.** Meningitis cerebro-spinalis. Aerztl. Mitth. a. Baden, Karlsruhe, 1876, xxv, 166-170.—**Ziemssen** & **Hess** (F.) Klinische Beobachtungen über Meningitis cerebro-spinalis epidemica. Deutsches Arch. f. klin. Med., Leipz., 1865-6, i, 72; 346. - **Zitéke** (J. X.) Acute cerebro-spinal meningitis. Therap. Gaz., Detroit, 1887, 3. s., iii, 452-457.

Meningitis (*Cerebro-spinal*) *in animals.*

Ekkert (N. J.) K kazuist. abortiv. formi enzooticheskago cerebro-spinal. meningita u doshadei. Arch. vet. nauk; St. Petersb., 1884, xiv, pt. 3, 125-135. — **Harms.** Meningitis cerebrospinalis, Genickkrampf, beim Wiederkäuer. Deutsche Zts hr. f. Thiermed., Leipz., 1886-7, xiii, 72-74.—**James** (H. F.) Cerebro-spinal meningitis in the horse. Vet. J. & Ann. Comp. Path., Lond., 1883, xvi, 81-92. *Also:* Am. Vet. Rev., N. Y., 1882-3, vi, 468-479.—**Meningitis** cerebro-spinalis bei Pferden. Ber. ü. d. Veterinärw. im Königr. Sachs., Dresd., 1879, xxiv, 121-129.

Meningitis (*Chronic*).

See, also, Insanity; Meningitis (*Syphilitic*).

Annan (S.) Chronic arachnitis; bronchitis; peritonitis; chronic gastritis; hypertrophy of the bladder and rectum; epilepsy. Maryland M. & S. J., Balt., 1840, i, 323-325. — **Arnoldi** (F. C. T.) Three cases of chronic meningitis. Montreal M. Gaz., 1844, i, 225.—**Ashhurst** (J.), jr. Chronic arachnitis; death from effusion. Proc. Path. Soc. Phila. (1860-66), 1867, ii, 136. *Also:* Am. J. M. Sc., Phila., 1863, n. s., xlvi, 401. — [**Bencke** (F. W.)] Meningitis chronica mit consecutiver Atrophie der Rindensubstanz des Gehirns. Arch. d. Ver. f. gemeinsch. Arb. z. Förd. d. wissensch. Heilk., Götting., 1858, iii, 205.— **Bennett.** Chronic cerebral meningitis; inflammatory induration surrounded by softening of a portion of the left cerebral hemisphere. Month. J. M. Sc., Lond. & Edinb., 1851, xii, 280-282.—**Broadbent.** A case of chronic cerebral meningitis; death. Med. Times & Gaz., Lond., 1880, i, 120.—**Cardoso Teixeira** (J. J.) Meningite chronica. Escholiaste med., Lisb., 1864, xv, 385.—**Charon** (E.) Méningite chronique chez un enfant de quatre ans; pneumonie lobulaire; caséification; autopsie. Presse méd. belge, Brux., 1880, xxxii, 105.—**Chevalier.** Observation de méningo-encéphalite chronique simple. Ann. Soc. de méd. d'Anvers, 1872, xxxiii, 595-604. [Rap. de Kums], 553. *Also:* Arch. méd. belges, Brux., 1873, iii, 156-165.— **Chomel.** Méningite chronique avec hémiplégie légère; symptômes de compression; mort; épanchement séreux considérable dans les ventricules; caractères anatomiques de la méningite. Gaz. d. hôp., Par., 1842, xv, 675.—**Comegys** (C.G.) Case of chronic meningitis, with softening of cerebellum. Cincin. Lancet & Obs., 1874, xvii, 290-292. — **Da Costa** (J. M.) A case of chronic meningitis. Clin. News, Phila., 1880, i, 61-63. — **Davis** (N. S.), jr. Chronic meningitis, with partial paralysis. Chicago M. J. & Exam., 1887, lv, 49-52. — **Font** (R. P.) Observacion de un caso de meninjitis crónica con reblandecimiento del cerebelo. Rev. méd. de Chile, Sant. de Chile, 1873, i, 463-467.—**Gaultier** (E.-M.) Observation sur une inflammation chronique de l'arachnoïde, manifestée seulement peu d'heures avant la mort. J. gén. de méd., chir. et pharm., Par., 1811, xlii, 384-392. — **Guibert** (T.) Observation sur une arachnoïdite chronique, qui a déterminé une céphalalgie opiniâtre. *Ibid.*, 1827, ci, 36-40.—**Hastings** (C.) Remarks on the connection between abdominal diseases and chronic meningitis; and on the application of ice to the head, illustrated by cases. Midland M. & S. J., Worcester, 1831-2, iii, 43-51.—**Hilles** (M. W.) Observations on idiopathic chronic arachnitis, with cases. Lancet, Lond., 1837, i, 806-811.—**Huss** (M.) † Hygiea. Stockholm, 1846, viii, 425-428.—**Lepidi-Chioti** (G.) Meningo-cerebrite cronica. Ann. clin. d. osp. incur., Napoli, 1882, vii, 3; 73. — **Lustgarten** (L.) O niezwykłej chorobie goryczkowéj, obserwowanéj w praktyce prywatnej. [Case of chronic meningitis resulting in atrophy.] Przegl. lek., Kraków, 1880, xix, 121-123.—**Malmsten** (P.) † Förh. v. Svens. Läk.-Sällsk. Sammank. 1860-61, Stockholm, 1862, 188-190.—**Mettenheimer** (C.) Ueber Pachyleptomeningitis chronica. J. f. Kinderkr., Erlang., 1868, l, 96-120.—**Meyer** (L.) Untersuchungen über die Identität der chronischen Meningitis und der allgemeinen progressiven Paralyse mit vergleichenden Beobachtungen über die Körperwärme in Geisteskrankheiten. [19 cases.] Ann. d. Char.-Krankenh. . . . zu Berl., 1857-8, viii, 2. Hft., 44-202.—**Mitchell** (S. W.) Headache; chronic meningitis; opium

Meningitis (Chronic).

habit. Boston M. & S. J., 1879, c, 445–447. — **Pinco** (P.) Chronic meningitis. *Ibid.*, 1858 – 9, lix, 116. — **Rendu.** Idiotie; impotence; symptômes de méningite cérébro-spinale à marche lente; mort. Bull. Soc. anat. de Par. (1872), 1874, xlii, 121–124.—**de Ricci** (H. R.) Chronic subacute arachnitis. Dublin Q. J. M. Sc., 1861, xxxi, 267–273. — **Satchell** (W. M.) Chronic meningitis with osseous development in the dura mater. Lancet, Lond., 1880, i, 622.— **Smythe** (A. G.) † Tr. Mississippi M. Ass., Jackson, 1879, xii, 193–196.—**Taczanowski** (P. B.) Excytacya maniakalne (excicatio maniacalis) zapalenie opon mozgowych (meningitis chronica), śmierć w skutku ostrego obrzęku (œdema cerebri acutum). Pam. Towarz. Lek. Warszaw., 1869, lxi, 178–183. — **Takács** (E.) Meningitis chronica. Orvosi hetil., Budapest, 1878, xxii, 5. — **Vigla.** Méningite chronique. Gaz. d. hôp., Par., 1846, viii, 117. — **Walshe** (W. H.) Chronic meningitis. Lancet, Lond., 1849, i, 58–61.

Meningitis (Intermittent).

Abranches (G.) Meningite aguda do cerebro e do cerebello com fórma intermittente; suppuração abundante na pia mater da face inferior do cerebello e base do cerebro; injecção intensa da pia mater da cenvexidade do hemispherio cerebral dirito; substancia cerebral no estado normal; considerações sobre a fórma intermittente da meningite; factos analogos observados em diversos paizes; difficuldades do seu diagnostico. Gaz. med. de Lisb., 1853-4, i, 164–172. — **Lemoine.** Observation de choléra intermittent et de méningite intermittente. Rev. méd. franç. et étrang. Par., 1835, iv, 223–227. — **Putnam** (S.) A case of remittent subacute meningitis. Tr. Vermont M. Soc. 1871–3, Montpellier, 1874, 386–389. *Also:* Boston M. & S. J., 1877, xcvii, 124–126.

Meningitis (Rheumatic).

See, also, Meningitis (*Spinal*); Rheumatism (*Cerebral, etc.*)

Bussen (F.) *Ueber Rheumatismus articulorum acutus, complicirt durch meningitische Erscheinungen, mit Berücksichtigung eines speziellen Falles. 8°. *Greifswald,* 1872.

Diard (J.-L.-O.) *Essai sur la méningite cérébrale rhumatismale. 4°. *Paris,* 1861.

Flamm (E. O.) *Ueber meningitische Symptome beim Rheumatismus acutus. 8°. *Tübingen,* 1865.

Gintrac (E.) De la méningite rhumatismale 8°. *Bordeaux,* 1865.

Viallaron (A.) *De la méningite cérébrale rhumatismale. 4°. *Paris,* 1874.

Ancell (H.) A case of acute rheumatism, with arachnitis and pericarditis, supervening on chronic rheumatism and a remarkably diseased heart. Month. J. M. Sc., Lond. & Edinb., 1848-9, ix, 446–452.—**Armellini** (G.) Meningite reumatica acutissima. Gazz. med. di Roma, 1877, iii, 157–160.—**Bamford** (W. A.) Case of metastasis of muscular and arthritic rheumatism to the membranes and substance of the brain, constituting meningo-cerebritis. Pacific M. & S. J., San Fran., 1877, xx, 241–246.—**Bergson** (J.) Beobachtung eines acuten Gelenkrheumatismus mit Metastase auf die Gehirnhäute. Deutsche Klinik, Berl., 1860, xii, 49.—**Blake** (J. G.) A case of meningeal rheumatism, simulating cerebro-spinal meningitis. Boston M. & S. J., 1871, vii, 230.—**Bouchut.** De la méningite rhumatismale; sa nature, son diagnostic à l'ophthalmoscope et son traitement. Gaz. d. hôp., Par., 1868, xli, 429. *Also, transl.:* Wien. med. Presse, 1868, ix, 969–972.—**de Boyer** (H.-C.) Note sur un cas de méningite cérébro-spinale aiguë d'origine rhumatismale. Arch. de neurol., Par., 1880–81, i, 373–390. — **Crawford** (J.) Case of rheumatic arachnitis. Brit.-Am. J. M. & Phys. Sc., Montreal, 1846-7, ii, 120–122.—**Dalla Rosa** (E.) Un caso di meningite cerebro-spinale reumatica. Riv. clin. di Bologna, 1868, vii, 75–82.— **Dentler.** Rheumatismus acutus mit darauf folgender Meningitis. Org. f. d. ges. Heilk., Berl., 1861, x, 147–150.—**Dowse** (T. S.) Chronic meningo-myelitis (rheumatic) incipient softening; cure. Med. Press & Circ., Lond., 1877, n. s., xxiv, 61.—**Eisenmann.** Beiträge zur Lehre von der rheumatischen Meningitis und dem Delirium tremens. Med. Cor.-Bl. bayer. Aerzte, Erlang., 1840, 241: 1841, ii, 529.—**Gosset.** Observation d'un cas de méningite rhumatismale; autopsie. Actes Soc. méd. d. hôp. de Par., 1851-2, ii, 79–89. [Rap. de Valleix], 90–104. — **Little.** Rheumatic inflammation of pia mater. Dublin Q. J. M. Sc., 1870, xlix, 491–493.— **Mosler** (F.) Zur localen Behandlung der Gehirnhautaffectionen bei acutem Gelenkrheumatismus. Deutsche med. Wchnschr., Berl., 1878, iv, 292; 303. — **Ross** (G.) Case of acute rheumatism; pericarditis; effusion on the brain and death by coma. Canada M. J., Montreal, 1868, iv, 539–541. — **Scharlau.** Rheumatische Affection der harten Haut des Rückenmarks und Gehirns mit seröser

Meningitis (Rheumatic).

Ueberfüllung der Hirn- und Rückenmarkshöhlcn. Wchnschr. f. d. ges. Heilk., Berl., 1844, 65–73. ———. Rheumatismus der harten Hirnhaut mit gleichzeitig vorhandener Polycholie. *Ibid.*, 85–88.—**Thore** fils. Méningites rhumatismales. Rec. d. proc.-verb. . . . Soc. de méd. prat., Par., 1856, 55–66. *Also:* Gaz. d. hôp., Par., 1856, xxix, 522. *Also:* Gaz. méd. de Par., 1857, 3. s., xii, 68–71. — **Thorp** (H.) Acute rheumatic arthritis; sudden subsidence of articular disease, followed by the symptoms of meningeal inflammation and effusion, rapidly fatal. Dublin Hosp. Gaz., 1858, v, 100.—**Vecchetti** (E.) Meningite lenta reumatica con essudato alla base del cervello. Imparziale, Firenze, 1871, xi, 321–334.

Meningitis (Spinal).

See, also, Meningitis (*Cerebro-spinal*); Meningitis (*Tubercular*); Nerve-stretching; Spina bifida (*Treatment of*); Spine (*Diseases of, Complications, etc., of*).

Burtin (L.) *De la pachyméningite spinale hypertrophique. 4°. *Paris,* 1878.

Clausing (F.-G.) *Essai sur la méningite rachidienne. 4°. *Strasbourg,* 1837.

Joffroy (A.) *De la pachyméningite cervicale hypertrophique (d'origine spontanée). 4°. *Paris,* 1873.

Also [Abstr.], *in:* Bull. Soc. anat. de Par., 1873, xlviii, 194–205.

Köhler (H.) Monographie der Meningitis spinalis nach klinischen Beobachtungen bearbeitet. 8°. *Leipzig u. Heidelberg,* 1861.

Le Bouteiller (R.-A.) *De la méningite spinale tuberculeuse. 4°. *Paris,* 1872.

Noetel (F. G.) *De meningitide spinali. 8°. *Berolini,* [1861].

Smid (P. J.) *De meningitide spinali. 8°. *Groningæ,* [1845].

Weissenberg (D.) *De meningitide spinali. 8°. *Berolini,* [1861].

Adradas (C. L.) Meningomielitis espinal de origen periférico (?). Gac. de sanid. mil., Madrid, 1879, v, 582–584.—**Albers.** Die Entzündung der harten Haut des Rückenmarks (perimeningitis medullæ spinalis). J. d. Chir. u. Augenh., Berl., 1833, xix, 347–362. *Also, transl.:* Gaz. méd. de Par., 1833, 2. s., i, 857–860.—**Arrighi** (G.) Storia di aracnoitide cervicale per la di cui effetti vengono confermata le dottrine del Bellingeri sull'ufficio del midollo, e de' nervi spinali. Ann. univ. di med., Milano, 1830, liii, 526–533.—**Aufrecht.** Salicylsäure bei einem Falle von acuter Spinal-Meningitis. *In his:* Path. Mitt., 8°, Magdeb., 1881, 162.—**Bass** (J. F.) A peculiar case of spinal meningitis, with complications. South. Clinic, Richmond, 1878, i, 81–84.—**Bell.** Spinal meningitis, with general paralysis. N. York J. M., 1860, 3. s., viii, 332–334.—[**Bennett** (J. H.)] Spinalmeningitis. Syst. Pract. M. (Tweedie), Phila., 1840, ii, 304–308.—**Blain des Cormiers.** Moelle épinière atteinte de méningite. Bull. Soc. anat. de Par., 1853, xxviii, 219.—[**Bodine** (J. S.)] † Proc. Path. Soc. Phila., 1871, iii, 67.—**Bonorden.** Arachnitis spinalis der Kinder. Med. Ztg., Berl., 1837, vi, 45. *Also, transl.:* Tidskr. f. Läk. o. Pharm., Stockholm, 1838, vii, 9–12.—**Borland.** Rachidian meningitis. Boston M. & S. J., 1867, lxxvi, 42. *Also:* Extr. Rec. Bost. Soc. M. Improve. (1866–74), 1876, vi, 17–19.—**Bouchut.** De la pachy-méningite spinale et de ses caractères ophthalmoscopiques. Gaz. d. hôp., Par., 1877, l, 625–627.—**Bowditch** (H. I.) Spinal meningitis and latent pleuritic effusion. Am. J. M.-Sc., Phila., 1854, n. s., xxvii, 354. *Also:* Extr. Rec. Bost. Soc. M. Improve., 1854–6, ii, 42.—**Braun** (J.) Bemerkungen über, besonders nach Feldzügen beobachtete, Meningitis spinalis der Offiziere. Deutsche mil.-ärztl. Ztschr., Berl., 1872, i, 116–132.—**Bristowe.** Idiopathic inflammation of the theca vertebralis, with accumulations of pus following the course of the spinal nerves. Tr. Path. Soc. Lond., 1855, vi, 45–48.—**Cagnetta** (F.) Meningite spinale esudativa; guarigione. Ann. clin. d. osp. incur., Napoli, 1877, n. s., ii, 4–12.—**Carleton** (C. M.) Report of a case of spinal meningitis with no cerebral complication. Proc. Connect. M. Soc., Hartford, 1878, 113–116.—**Carpentier.** Méningite spinale aiguë. Presse méd. belge. Brux., 1883, xxxv, 113–115.—**Charcot.** De la pachyméningite cervicale hypertrophique. Progrès méd., Par., 1874, ii, 669–671. *Also* [Abstr.]: Gaz. d. hôp., Par., 1874, xlvii, 98.—**Chvostek** (F.) Ein Fall von Meningitis spinalis chronica mit ausserordentlich grossen Kalkplättchen in der Arachnoidea und Dura mater spinalis, Magencarcinom. Wien. med. Bl., 1878, i, 6–9.—**Clemens** (T.) Hydrorhachis rheumatica. Deutsche Klinik, Berl., 1850, ii, 490–492. — **Collin** (J. G.) Om inflammation i ryggmärgen och dess hinnor hos barn. Hygiea, Stockholm, 1843, v, 637–641. — **Colson** (E.) † Recovery. Lancet, Lond.,

Meningitis (*Spinal*).

1879, ii, 275.—**Concato.** Meningite spinale reumatica diffusa. Riv. clin. di Bologna, 1865, iv, 193-210.—**Cornil** (V.) Anatomie pathologique de la dure-mère dans le mal de Pott; inflammation chronique des vaisseaux lymphatiques de cette membrane. Compt. rend. Soc. de biol. 1873, Par., 1875, 5. s., v, 363-367. ———. Pachyméningite spinale caséeuse; localisation des foyers caséeux dans les espaces lymphatiques Bull. Soc. anat. de Par., 1874, xlix, 605.— **Cotting** (B. E.) A case of abscess in the cerebellum and meningeal disease of the spinal cord. Boston M. & S. J., 1861-2, lxv, 381-385. *Also:* Extr. Rec. Bost. Soc. M. Improve. (1859-61), 1862, iv, 255-259.—**Cowan** (R.) Hydrorachitis. Glasgow M. J., 1830, iii, 326.—**Croskery** (H.) Case of spinal meningitis, treated by quinine and opium, with mercurial inunction; recovery. Dublin Q. J. M. Sc., 1867, xliii, 115-119.—**Day** (W. H.) Spinal meningitis in a child following spinal concussion; recovery. Lancet, Lond., 1883, i, 770.—**Delcour** (J.) Recherches sur la méningo-encéphalite des enfants. Arch. de la méd. belge, Brux., 1844, xiii, 43-49. — **Delmotte.** Méningo-myélite aiguë; absence de désordres fonctionnels. Ann. de méd. belges, Brux., 1837, i, 2-4.—**Dowse** (T. S.) Abridged notes of cases of meningo-myelitis. Lancet, Lond, 1876, i, 168.—**Dumolard.** Méningite cervicale hypertrophique. Gaz. méd. de Par., 1877, 4. s., vi, 333. — **Duncan** (J. F.) Spinal arachnitis; its diagnosis; rarity of the idiopathic form; its epidemic appearance; appropriate treatment. Dublin M. Press, 1848, xix, 369-371.—**Dunlop.** Meningitis caused by penetration of a fish-bone into the spinal canal. Brit. M. J., Lond., 1879, i, 289. *Also:* Glasgow M. J., 1879, xi, 247.—**Elliott** (G. F.) Case of chronic spinal meningitis after a fall; improvement. Lancet, Lond., 1877, ii, 725.— **Esquerdo y Esquerdo** (P.) Meningitis espinal aguda. *In his:* Lecc. de clin. méd., 8°, Barcel., 1879, 5-28. — **Facen** (J.) Meningite rachidea acuta. Gazz. med. ital. lomb., Milano, 1851, 3. s., ii, 29-31.—**Feith.** Pachymeningitis interna cerebro-spinalis; paralytische Geisteskrankheit. Allg. Ztschr. f. Psychiat., etc., Berl., 1864, xxi, 271-278.—**Fieber** (F.) † † Aerztl. Ber. d. k. k. allg. Krankenh. zu Wien (1873), 1874, 238.—**Forrest** (W. H.) Meningitis of the spinal cord. Lond. M. & S. J., 1834, iv, 306.—**Forrester** (W.) Case of acute spinal meningitis. Richmond & Louisville M. J., Louisville, 1874, xvii, 511-517. — **Fox** (E. L.) Cases illustrating some of the lesions included under the term spinal meningitis. Lancet, Lond., 1883, ii, 682-684.—**von Franque** (A.) Ueber Meningitis spinalis. Cor.-Bl. d. Ver. nassau. Aerzte, Weilburg, 1862, 17.— **Gauné.** Épidémie de congestion rachidienne, observée à Niort. Arch. gén. de méd., Par., 1858, 5. s., xi, 1-10. *Also* [Abstr.]: Gaz. d. hôp., Par., 1858, xxxi, 9. — **Gölis.** Beobachtungen über die Entzündung der Rückenmarkshäute der Kinder, und die Zellgewebsverhärtung. Med.-chir. Ztg., Salzb., 1815, iv, 125-128.—**Grosstern** (W.) Peripachymeningitis spinalis. Gaz. lek., Warszawa, 1877, xxiii, 1; 17.—**Gull** (W.) Paraplegic rigidity of the muscles of the upper and lower extremities from limited arachnitis of the cervical portion of the cord; the affection of the upper extremities preceding that of the lower for some months. Guy's Hosp. Rep., Lond., 1856, 3. s., ii, 165-168, 1 pl.—**Hasse** (C. E.) † Deutsche Klinik, Berl., 1855, vii, 309.—**Heck.** Meningitis spinalis thoracica. Wchnschr. f. d. ges. Heilk., 1847, 171-174.—**Helm** (E. C.) Spinal meningitis. Cincin. Lancet & Clinic, 1880, n. s., iv, 512-514.—**Henoch.** Beitrag zur Pathologie der Meningitis spinalis. Wchnschr. f. d. ges. Heilk., Berl., 1845, 661; 677; 697. — **Holcombe** (A. A.) Strychnia in spinal meningitis. Am. Vet. Rev., N. Y., 1880, iii, 428-430.— **Hutinel.** Méningite spinale traitée par le salicylate de soude. Bull. Soc. clin. de Par. (1878), 1879, ii, 29-33. *Also:* France méd., Par., 1878, xxv, 198.—**Jacobs.** Méningite spinale chronique suivie de méningite cérébro-spinale aiguë; autopsie. Presse méd. belge, Brux., 1886, xxxviii, 305.—**Jadelot.** Méningite spinale; guérison. Clin. d. hôp. d. enf., Par., 1841, i, 191-193.—**Jennings** (F. B.) † † Med. Exam., Chicago, 1872, xiii, 211. — **Joffroy** (A.) La pachyméningite cervicale hypertrophique. Arch. gén. de méd., Par., 1876, xxviii, 542-558.—**Kennedy** (H.) † Dublin M. Press, 1848, xix, 17-19.—**Kernig.** † St. Petersb. med. Ztschr., 1872, n. F., iii. 80-82. —**Kreuser.** Meningitis spinalis. Med. Cor.-Bl. d. württemb. ärztl. Ver., Stuttg., 1868, xxxviii, 324.—**Lachowicz** (A.) Zapalenie opon mózgowych gościcowe. [Meningitis spinalis.] Przegl. lek., Krakow., 1877, xvi, 233-235.— **Landenberger.** Ein schwerer Fall von Meningitis spinalis mit Heilung; Anwendung des Curare. Med. Cor.-Bl. d. württemb. ärztl. Ver., Stuttg., 1864, xxxiv, 161-163. — **Laveran.** Observations de méningite spinale, suivie de roideur des extrémités inférieures, d'oblitération des veines crurales et d'œdème des membres inférieurs. Gaz. d. hôp., Par., 1861, xxxiv, 513.—**Lemoine** (G.) & **Lannois** (M.) Périmeningite spinale aiguë. Rev. de méd., Par., 1882, ii, 533-544.—**Lewitzky** (P.) Ein Fall von Peripachymeningitis spinalis. Berl. klin. Wchnschr., 1877, xiv, 227-230. — **Little.** Spinal meningitis. Lancet, Lond. 1860, i, 296. — **Lordereau & Troisier.** Pachyméningite hypertrophique d'origine spontanée de la région dorsolombaire. Bull. Soc. anat. de Par., 1877, lii, 539-541. *Also:*

Meningitis (*Spinal*).

Progrès méd., Par., 1878, vi, 13.—**Lussana** (F.) Meningite spinale; cura antiflogistica; guarigione. Gazz. med. ital. lomb., Milano, 1849, 2. s., ii, 31.—**Mader.** Compressionsmyelitis durch tuberculisirende Meningitis spinalis in Folge von tuberculöser Wirbelcaries; Tod. Ber. d. k. k. Krankenanst. Rudolph-Stiftung in Wien (1885), 1886, 362.—**Maixner** (E.) Ein Fall von traumatischer Spinal-Meningitis. Aerztl. Ber. d. k. k. allg. Krankenh. zu Prag (1879), 1881, 94-97. — **Malmsten.** Meningitis spinalis. Förh. v. Svens. Läk.-Sällsk. Sammank., Stockholm, 1855-6, 26.—**Morf** (J.) Meningitis spinalis durch Curare zur Heilung gebracht. Aerztl. Int.-Bl., München, 1874, xxi, 497.— **Nixon** (C. J.) Spinal meningitis, probably of syphilitic origin. Dublin J. M. Sc., 1874, lviii, 212-215. — **Nourse** (W. E. C.) Case of acute spinal meningitis. Lancet, Lond., 1859, i, 554.—**Observação** de um caso de congestão meningo-spinal. Progresso méd., Rio de Jan., 1877-8, ii, 133-135.—**O'Connor.** Case of spinal meningitis, simulating tetanus. Dublin Q. J. M. Sc., 1860, xxix, 486-488. — **Pavlinoff** (K.) Meningitis spinalis. *In his:* Lektsii, 8°, Moskva, 1879, 21-28. — **Pepper** (W.) Spinal meningitis. Proc. Path. Soc. Phila. (1866-70), 1871, iii, 67. *Also:* Am. J. M. Sc., Phila., 1868, n. s., lvi, 151.— **Peter.** Méningite spinale. J. de méd. et chir. prat., Par., 1875, xlvi, 392-395. — **Piorry.** Sur la méningite rachidienne. Gaz. d. hôp., Par., 1849, xxii, 111.—**Pointer** (S. C.) Spinal meningitis. N. York J. M., 1856, 3. s., i, 81-83.—**Pullino** (T.) Storia di meningo mielite antica. Gior. d. sc. med., Torino, 1838, iii, 44-55. — **Putzel** (L.) A rare case of peripachymeningitis spinalis, with hemiplegia; complete recovery. Med. Rec., N. Y., 1878, xiii, 64-66. — **Rendu.** Pachyméningite spinale antérieure, comprimant le renflement lombaire et les nerfs de la queue de cheval; myélite diffuse, surtout périépendymaire. Bull. Soc. anat. de Par., 1874, xlix, 598-604. — **Robert.** Observations de méningite spinale. Arch. méd. belges, Brux., 1874, 3. s., vi, 382-390. — **Robinson** (E.) Symptoms of spinal meningitis. Lancet, Lond., 1862, i, 237.— **Rodgers** (J. K.) Case of inflammation of the theca vertebralis. N. York M. & Phys. J., 1825, iv, 219-222. — **Schulz.** Ueber einen Fall von Meningitis spinalis. Cor.-Bl. d. ärztl. Ver. d. Rhein-Prov., Bonn, 1876, No. 17, 11-20.—**Seeligmüller** (A.) Lähmung nach Spinalmeningitis im Kindesalter. Arch. f. Kinderh., Stuttg., 1880, i, 133-142.—**Sieffert** (A.) Spinal meningitis. Indiana M. Reporter, Evansville, 1881, ii, 203; 241. — **Smith** (T. C.) Meningitis spinalis. Detroit Rev. Med. & Pharm., 1874, ix, 578-594.—**Spinal** meningitis. [Case.] Statist. Rep. Health Navy 1871, Lond., 1873, 64. — **Steinthal.** Zur Casuistik der Meningitis spinalis. Berl. klin. Wchnschr., 1867, iv, 235.—**Stillé** (A.) Rheumatic spinal meningitis. Richmond & Louisville M. J., Louisville, 1868, vi, 166-175.—**Tamburini** (A.) Sopra alcuni casi di arachnoite spinale ossificante nella paralisi progressiva. Soc. med.-chir. in Modena. Resoc., 1876, 1-4.—**Tatom** (S. Z.) A case of spinal meningitis, treated with large doses of quinine. South. M. & S. J., Augusta, 1854, n. s., x, 161.—**Tessier.** Storie di meningiti spinali tetaniche sanate col metodo antiflogistico. Ann. univ. di med., Milano, 1841, xcviii, 418-429.—**Traube** (L.) Meningitis spinalis; ausgezeichnete Wirkung des Jodkalium zur Entfernung des Exsudats. Ann. d. Char.-Krankenh. . . . zu Berl., 1863, x, 2. Hft., 162-166. ——. Zwei Fälle von Peripachymeningitis spinalis. *In his:* Ges. Beitr. z. Path. u. Physiol., Berl., 8°, 1871, ii, pt. 2, 1039-1043. — **Tungel** (C.) Meningitis spinalis. Klin. Mitth. v. d. med. Abth. d. allg. Krankenh. in Hamb. (1859), 1861, 73. — **Vecchietti** (E.) Storia di un caso di meningite spinale reumatica con paralisi degli arti inferiori, della vesica e del retto. Riv. clin. di Bologna, 1874, iv, 65-69.—**Vogel** (J.) & **Dittmar.** Meningitis spinalis. Deutsche Klinik, Berl., 1851, iii, 243; 251. — **Voisin** (A.) De la méningo-myélite occasionnée par le froid. Gaz. d. hôp., Par., 1865, xxxviii, 97; 101; 111; 118. *Also,* Reprint. — **Weber.** Sur la méningite cérébro-rachidienne et l'apoplexie de la moelle épinière. Gaz. méd. de Strasb., 1851, xi, 298-300. — **Werdmüller** (O.) Meningitis spinalis rheumatica mit Trismus, Tetanus und Opistotonus. Schweiz. Ztschr. f. Med., Chir. u. Geburtsh., Zürich, 1847, 11.—**Westphal.** Sensibilitäts- und Motilitätsstörung im Bereiche des Plexus pudendalis und coccygeus; Autopsie; gummöse Meningitis spinalis sacralis; Compression der Wurzeln des Plexus pudendalis; oberflächliche Caries des Kreuzbeins. Charité-Ann. 1874, Berl., 1876, i, 421-427.— **Wilks.** Chronic inflammation and ossification of the membranes of the spinal cord. Tr. Path. Soc. Lond., 1855-6, vii, 35-37. — **Vecchietti.** † Austral. M. J., Melbourne, 1882, n. s., iv, 125.—**Wyman** (H. C.) † Therap. Gaz., Detroit, 1881, n. s., ii, 453.

Meningitis (*Syphilitic*).

FLECHSIG (P. E.) *Bemerkungen über Meningitis luetica und einen dahin zu stellenden Fall. 8°. Leipzig, 1870.

Blachez & **Luys.** Observation de méningite granuleuse, présumée syphilitique; détails microscopiques. Gaz. hebd. de méd., Par., 1861, viii, 198-201. — **Bru-**

Meningitis (*Syphilitic*).

berger. Ein Fall von Meningitis syphilitica, nebst Bemerkungen über Syphilis der Centralorgane. Arch. f. path. Anat., etc., Berl., 1874, lx, 285 – 298. — **Dreyfous** (F.) De la méningite chronique chez les enfants; ses rapports avec la syphilis héréditaire tardive. Rev. mens. d. mal. de l'enf., Par., 1883, i, 497–511.—**Jeannoel** (V.) Observation de méningite syphilitique, recueillie à l'hôpital de Civita-Vecchia. Rec. de mém. de méd. . . . mil., Par., 1856, 2. s., xviii, 237–239.—**Laucereaux.** De la méningite et de l'encéphalite syphilitiques. Gaz. hebd. de méd., Par., 1873, 2. s., x, 506; 514—**Pick** (J. P.) Chronic meningitis in a case of syphilitic disease of the bones of the skull. Tr. Path. Soc. Lond., 1867 – 8, xix, 34. — **Poncet** (A.) Observation de méningite syphilitique. Ann. de dermat. et syph., Par., 1872, iv, 185–190. — **Quinquaud.** Méningite chronique de la base de l'encéphale probablement d'origine syphilitique. Bull. Soc. clin. de Par., 1877, 32–38. *Also:* France méd., Par., 1877, xxiv, 298.—**Read** (T.) Notes on cases of syphilitic meningitis. Dublin Q. J. M. Sc., 1852, xiii, 53–68.—**Richardson** (B. W.) Case of syphilitic meningitis; osteitis and periostitis. Dublin Hosp. Gaz., 1856, iii, 92.—**Warner** (F.) & **Beach** (F.) Chronic syphilitic meningitis, causing progressive dementia. Lancet, Lond., 1887, i, 878.

Meningitis (*Tubercular*).

See, also, **Brain** (*Tubercle of*); **Ear** (*Diseases of*) *in children*; **Hydrencephaloid** *disease*; **Hydrocephalus** (*Acute*); **Meningitis** (*Basilar*); **Meningitis** (*Cerebro-spinal*); **Meningitis** (*Diagnosis, etc., of*); **Meningitis** (*Treatment of*); **Meningitis** *in children, etc.*; **Phthisis** (*Complications of*).

ADAMS (J. M.) * On tubercle of the brain in children. 8°. *Glasgow*, 1846.

ANSPACH (M. H.) * De meningitide granulosa. 8°. *Jenæ*, 1863.

AUDIFFRED (P.-V.) * De la méningite tuberculeuse chez les enfans. 4°. *Paris*, 1845.

BÉCHET (V.-F.) * De la méningite simple et de la méningite tuberculeuse comparées chez les enfants. 4°. *Paris*, 1852.

DE BECHON (J.-R.) * De la méningite tuberculeuse (forme cérébro - spinale). 4°. *Paris*, 1878.

BECQUEREL (A.) Recherches cliniques sur la méningite des enfants. 8°. *Paris*, 1838.

BERGERHOF (H.) * De meningitide tuberculosa. 8°. *Berolini*, [1860].

BREEN (J.) * De la méningite cérébro-spinale tuberculeuse. 4°. *Paris*, 1870.

BUSCHBECK (G.) * Beitrag zur pathologischen Anatomie von Meningitis tuberculosa. 8°. *Würzburg*, 1877.

CASTANET (A.-M.) * De la méningite tuberculeuse chez l'adulte. 4°. *Paris*, 1866.

CHANTEMESSE (A.) * Sur la méningite tuberculeuse de l'adulte. Les formes anormales en particulier. 4°. *Paris*, 1884.

CHATEAUFORT (L.-A.) *Contribution à l'étude de la méningite spinale tuberculeuse. 4°. *Paris*, 1878.

DESHAYES (V.-M.) * Contribution à l'étude de la méningite tuberculeuse, avec considérations sur la tuberculose, les localisations cérébrales au point de vue du diagnostic de la maladie, de ses symptômes et de ses lésions anatomiques. 4°. *Montpellier*, 1878.

DREYFOUS (F.) * Essai sur les symptômes protubérantiels de la méningite tuberculeuse. 4°. *Paris*, 1879.

FAIVRE (J.-J.-A.-E.) * Des granulations méningiennes. 4°. *Paris*, 1853.

FICHOT (J.-M.-J.) * De la méningite granuleuse chez l'adulte (signes et diagnostic). 4°. *Paris*, 1868.

FLIESS (J.) * De meningitide tuberculosa infantum. 8°. *Berolini*, [1851].

GARDIN (H.) *Observations pour servir à l'histoire de la méningite tuberculeuse chez les adultes. 4°. *Meaux*, 1873.

GAUDIN (G.) * De meningitide tuberculosa. 8°. *Berolini*, [1846].

Meningitis (*Tubercular*).

GERDES (A.) * Ueber Meningitis tuberculosa der Kinder. 8°. *Würzburg*, 1854.

GEZYMATTO (B.) * De meningitide tuberculosa infantum. 8°. *Petropoli*, 1854.

GOULLON (H.) * De meningitide granulosa. 8°. *Jenæ*, 1859.

HAHN (H.) De la méningite tuberculense étudiée au point de vue clinique. Monographie couronnée. 8°. *Paris*, 1853.

Also [Abstr.], *in:* Bull. Soc. de méd. de Gand. 1853, xx, 198–218.

———. The same. Die Meningitis tuberculosa. 8°. *Köln*, 1857.

HEIDEMANN (H. E. R.) * De meningitide tuberculosa infantium acuta. 8°. *Berolini*, [1854].

HESSERT. * Ueber tuberkulöse Meningitis. 8°. *Würzburg*, 1860.

Also, in: Würzb. med. Ztschr., 1860, i, 315–343.

JAKOB (A. R. H.) * De meningitide tuberculosa infantium. 8°. *Berolini*, [1860].

JUVIGNY (A.) * Contribution à l'étude de la méningite tuberculeuse du nouveau-né et de l'adulte. 4°. *Paris*, 1886.

KOTHER (J.) * Ueber Meningitis tuberculosa. 8°. *Bonn*, [1872].

LACOMBE (T.-B.) * De la méningo-encéphalite tuberculeuse des enfants. 4°. *Paris*, 1860.

LE DIBERDER (V.) * Sur l'affection tuberculeuse aiguë de la pie-mère chez les adultes, maladie connue chez les enfants sous les noms d'hydrocéphale aiguë, fièvre cérébrale, méningite, méningo-encéphalite, méningite granuleuse ou tuberculeuse. 4°. *Paris*, 1837.

LE ROUX (J.) * De la méningite tuberculense de l'enfance. 4°. *Paris*, 1877.

MAEDER (G. F. R.) * De meningitide tuberculosa. 8°. *Berolini*, [1863].

MARTIN (J. - B.) * Sur l'anatomie pathologique de la méningite tuberculeuse et sur les diverses phases qu'a parcourues son histoire depuis les premières observations qui en ont été faites jusqu'à nos jours. 4°. *Paris*, 1870.

MAUREL (T.-H.) * De la méningite tuberculeuse, ou fièvre cérébrale chez les enfants. 4°. *Paris*, 1853.

MERGANT (C. - F.) * De la méningite aiguë tuberculense des enfants. 4°. *Strasbourg*, 1844.

MÜHSAM (J.) * Fünf Fälle von Meningitis tuberculosa. 8°. *Berlin*, [1874].

PIEPER (O.) *Fünf Fälle von Meningitis tuberculosa. 8°. *Berlin*, 1872.

PIET (J.-A.) * Sur la méningo-céphalite tuberculeuse des enfants (hydrocéphale aiguë). 4°. *Paris*, 1836.

PIVENT (J.-B.-A.) * De la méningo-encéphalite tuberculeuse (fièvre cérébrale des enfants). 4°. *Paris*, 1852.

PONTIS (J.-B.) * De la méningite tuberculeuse chez les enfants. 4°. *Paris*, 1851.

POTT (R.) Quæstiones de symptomatibus meningitidis tuberculosæ puerorum. 8°. *Halis Sax.*, [1876].

PROUCHET (A.) * Étude de la méningite tuberculeuse. 4°. *Paris*, 1866.

REDIER (J.-M.) * Quelques observations d'affection tuberculeuse aiguë de la pie-mère chez des adultes. 4°. *Paris*, 1871.

RENDU (H.) *Recherches cliniques et anatomiques sur les paralysies liées à la méningite tuberculeuse. 4°. *Paris*, 1873.

———. The same. 8°. *Paris*, 1874.

RÖDELHEIMER (R.) *Ueber Meningitis tuberculosa. 8°. *Tübingen*, 1886.

SAKELLARIO (G.) * De meningitide tuberculosa. 8°. *Berolini*, [1855].

SÄLTIN (F. V.) * Iakttagelser öfver meningitis tuberculosa hos barn. 8°. *Helsingfors*, 1864.

Meningitis (*Tubercular*).

SARLIN (V.-A.) * De la méningite tuberculeuse. 4°. *Paris*, 1848.

SAVOURET (P.) * De l'encéphalo-méningite tuberculeuse, ou fièvre cérébrale des enfants. 4°. *Paris*, 1853.

SCHLÆSINGER (S.) * Observationes circa meningitidem tuberculosam infantum. 8°. *Berolini*, [1850].

SCHUH (L.) * Ueber autochthone Hirnarterienthrombose als Ursache halbseitiger Motilitätsstörungen bei Meningitis basilaris tuberculosa. 8°. *Würzburg*, 1874.

SEITZ (J.) Die Meningitis tuberculosa der Erwachsenen. 8°. *Berlin*, 1874.

SEITZ (P.) * Ueber Meningitis tuberculosa der Kinder. 8°. *Würzburg*, 1864.

SERGIU (D.) * La méningite tuberculeuse des adultes. 4°. *Paris*, 1866.

SICHTING (O.) * De meningitide tuberculosa. sm. 8°. *Berolini*, [1865].

SORNAS (F.-A.) * Contribution à l'étude clinique de la méningite tuberculeuse à forme de delirium tremens. 4°. *Paris*, 1886.

STEINBACH (R.) * Ueber die Ursachen der Meningitis tuberculosa. 8°. *Würzburg*, 1878.

VIARD (L.) Contribution à l'étude de la méningite tuberculeuse chez l'adulte. 4°. *Paris*, 1881.

VIVANT (J.) * Contribution à l'étude de la méningite tuberculeuse chez l'adulte, forme apoplectique. 4°. *Paris*, 1886.

WEISSENFELS (P.) * Meningitis tuberculosa. 8°. *Würzburg*, 1882.

WESSBERGER (G.) * Beitrag zur pathol. Anatomie und Aetiologie von Meningitis tuberculosa infantum. 8°. *Würzburg*, [1880?]

WORTMANN (J.) * Beitrag zur Meningitis tuberculosa und der Gehirntuberculose im Kindesalter. [Strasburg.] 8°. *Leipzig*, 1883.
Also, in: Jahrb. f. Kinderh., Leipz., 1883, n. F., xx, 300-340.

A. Du traitement et de la prophylaxie de la méningite tuberculeuse. Gaz. méd. de Par., 1871, 3. s., xxvi, 412; 420.—**Albers** (J. F. H.) Tuberculosis der Pia mater; Blutmangel des Gehirns; olighämisches Hydrocephaloid. Deutsche Klinik, Berl., 1850, ii, 467-469.—**Arnold** (A.B.) Tubercular meningitis. Med. & Surg. Reporter, Phila., 1867, xvi, 206-209.—**Bandera** (J. M.) Un caso de meningitis tuberculosa. Gac. méd., Méjico, 1886, xxi, 70-73.—**Barrett** (H.) On some cases of tubercular meningitis. St. George's Hosp. Rep. 1879, Lond., 1880, x, 607-626.—**Barth.** Méningite peut-être tuberculeuse? Guérison. Bull. Soc. clin. de Par., 1877, 47-54.—**Bastian** (H. C.) Tubercular meningitis and otorrhœa, with small fibro-cellular growths from the dura mater. Tr. Path. Soc. Lond., 1866-7, xviii, 4. ——. Portions of pia mater from a case of tubercular meningitis. *Ibid.*, 21. ——. On the pathology of tubercular meningitis. Edinb. M. J., 1866-7, xii, 875-901, 1 pl. *Also,* Reprint.—**Baxter** (E. B.) Cerebral fever ending in death; optic neuritis an early symptom; meningeal tuberculosis without meningitis. Brit. M. J., Lond., 1878, i, 295.—**Bergeret.** Fibrome disséminé des méninges; hyperhydrurie. Mém. et compt.-rend. Soc. d. sc. méd. de Lyon (1873), 1874, xiii, pt. 2, 175-178.—**Berneaudeaux.** Méningite tuberculeuse. Gaz. méd. de Nantes, 1883-4, ii, 152-154.—**Bertalot** (A.) Ueber Meningitis tuberculosa bei Kindern. Jahrb. f. Kinderh., Leipz., 1876, ix, 227-258.—**Bierbaum** (J.) Meningitis tuberculosa. [12 cases.] J. f. Kinderkr., Erlang., 1860, xxxv, 62: 1863, xli, 16×: 1866, xlvii, 61: 1868, l, 90. ——. Aetiologie der Meningitis tuberculosa. *Ibid.*, 1871, lvii, 273-371. ——. Die Prognose der Meningitis tuberculosa. Deutsche Klinik, Berl., 1871, xxiii, 102; 110. ——. Geschichtlicher Rückblick auf die Meningitis tuberculosa. *Ibid.*, 221; 233; 244. ——. Pathologische Physiologie der Meningitis tuberculosa. *Ibid.*, 261; 279; 290; 297. ——. Anatomischer Character der Meningitis tuberculosa. *Ibid.*, 1873, xxv, 81-84.—**Bitsare** (A.) Μηνιγγῖτις κοκκώδης ἢ φυματώδης. Ἀσκληπιός, Ἀθῆναι, 1871-2, x, 98-116.—**Blache** (R.) Méningite tuberculeuse; guérison. Tribune méd., Par., 1875, viii, 195-197.—**Blasi** (P.) Caso di meningite tuberculosa al 2° stadio portato a guarigione. Gior. veneto di sc. med., Venezia, 1864, 2. s., xxiii, 599-601. ——. Della termometria nella meningite tuberculose dei bambini. Bull. d. r. Accad. med. di Roma, 1882, viii, 368-389.—**Bock** (K. E.)

Meningitis (*Tubercular*).

Tuberkulose mit Meningitis. Deutsche Klinik, Berl., 1850, ii, 324.—**Bókai** (J.) Granulöse Meningitis mit Hirnhöhlenwassersucht und weisser Gehirnerweichung; lobuläre Pneumonie der rechten Lunge und Pleuropneumonie der linken, mit tuberculöser Infiltration. Jahrb. f. Kinderh., Wien, 1861-2, v, 99-108. — **Booth** (J. M.) Case of tubercular meningitis. Edinb. M. J., 1882-3, xxviii, 690-694.—**Borland** (J. N.) Tubercular meningitis, with general tuberculosis. Boston M. & S. J., 1869, lxxix, 145-148.—**Bouchut** (E.) Tubercules de la choroïde et tuberculose générale; méningite de la base et de la convexité; névro-rétinite; thromboses et varices phlébo-rétiniennes. Bull. et mém. Soc. méd. d. hôp. de Par. (1869), 1870, 2. s., vi, 175-177. *Also:* Gaz. d. hôp., Par., 1869, xlii, 113. ——. Méningite tuberculeuse sans symptômes; diagnostic par la cérébroscopie; névrite optique et tubercules de la choroïde. Gaz. d. hôp., Par., 1874, xlvii, 1018. ——. Méningite tuberculeuse; absence des symptômes caractéristiques; névro-rétinite; tubercule de la choroïde. *Ibid.*, 1876, xlix, 241-243. ——. Méningite tuberculeuse guérie; hydrocéphalie chronique consécutive; autopsie. Paris méd., 1882, vii, 241.—**Bouillaud.** Einige Bemerkungen zur richtigen Beurtheilung der tuberkulösen Meningitis. J. f. Kinderkr., Erlang., 1863, xl, 161-173.—**Bourneville & Pillet.** Imbécillité et hémiplégie droite symptomatique de méningite tuberculeuse; tuberculose généralisée; mal de Pott. Progrès méd., Par., 1886, 2. s., iii, 554-558.—**Bouygues.** Méningite tuberculeuse en plaque, siégeant sur le lobule paracentral et ayant occasionné une monoplégie crurale, avec attaques épileptiformes. Bull. Soc. anat. de Par., 1884, lix, 423-428. *Also:* Progrès méd., Par., 1885, 2. s., i, 232.—**Bristowe** (J. S.) †† Lancet, Lond., 1874, i, 297; 366. ——. †† St. Thomas's Hosp. Rep. 1883, Lond., 1884, n. s., xiii, 97-123.—**Bruck** (L.) Meningitis basilaris tuberculosa; Tod im zweiten Stadium. Wien. med. Presse, 1882, xxiii, 1053.—**Bucquoy & Hanot.** Méningite aiguë au début de la tuberculose. France méd., Par., 1874, xxi. 83.—**Burnet** (J. B.) †† Med. & Surg. Reporter, Phila., 1867, xvii, 335.—**Butler.** † Brit. M.J., Lond., 1875, i, 142.—**Califano** (L.) Memoria intorno ad un caso di tuberculosi meningea, e di cangrena pulmonale. Rendic. Accad. med.-chir. di Napoli, 1858, xii, 25-28.—**Capozzi** (D.) Due casi di meningite tuberculare in persone adulte. Gior. internaz. d. sc. med., Napoli, 1880, ii, 23-35.—**Carter** (W.) Symptoms of meningitis, probably tubercular; recovery. Med. Times & Gaz., Lond., 1881, i, 378.—[**Cases.**] Meningitis tuberculosa. Oesterr. Ztschr. f. Kinderh., Wien, 1856-7, ii, 524. — Aerztl. Ber. a. d. k. k. allg. Krankenh. zu Wien (1857), 1858, 38.—*Ibid.* (1880), 1881, 14-21.—Jahresb. ü. d. med. Abth. d. Spit. zu Basel, 1876, 63.—Rep. Superv. Surg.-Gen. Mar. Hosp., Wash., 1883, 215.—**Caspari.** † Cor.-Bl. f. schweiz. Aerzte, Basel, 1883, xiii, 365-368.—**Cayla** (F.) Aphasie et méningite tuberculeuse chez une fillette de six ans. Gaz. hebd. d. sc. méd. de Bordeaux, 1885, vi, 127-130.—**Cerf** (E.) Ein Fall von circumscripter linksseitiger tuberculöser Convexitätsmeningitis, Lähmung der rechten oberen und unteren Extremität und acuter Miliartuberculose der Lunge bei einem Kinde. Deutsches Arch. f. klin. Med., Leipz., 1882, xxxi, 431-438.—**Chambrelent.** Méningite tuberculeuse. Gaz. hebd. d. sc. méd. de Bordeaux, 1880-81, i, 570-572.—**Champouillon.** Méningite cérébrale tuberculeuse. Gaz. d. hôp., Par., 1853, xxvi, 123.—**Chantemesse.** Méningite tuberculeuse en plaque à l'union du tiers moyen avec le tiers supérieur du sillon de Rolando; monoplégie brachiale. Bull. Soc. anat. de Par., 1884, lix, 338-343. *Also:* Progrès méd., Par., 1885, 2. s., i, 103.—**Charon** (E.) Méningite tuberculeuse compliquée de dothiénentérie; autopsie. Presse méd. belge, Brux., 1876, xxix, 25-27.—**Charrier.** Méningite tuberculeuse; tubercule du nerf optique droit, chez un enfant de onze mois. Bull. Soc. anat. de Par., 1859, xxxiv, 44-47.—**Cheadle** (W. B.) Cerebro-spinal meningitis; opisthotonos; general muscular rigidity and hyperæsthesia; extreme emaciation; treatment by iodide of mercury; recovery; tubercular meningitis three months later; post mortem. Brit. M. J., Lond., 1879, ii, 986.—**Chouppe.** Méningo-encéphalite tuberculeuse; rotation de la tête et déviation conjugée des yeux du côté de la lésion, chez une jeune fille scrofuleuse. Bull. Soc. anat. de Par. (1871), 1873, xlvi, 380-384.—**Choyau.** Méningite tuberculeuse et maladie de Addison. *Ibid.* (1868), 1874, xliii, 272-276.—**Colberg.** Hemiplegie, bedingt durch circumscripten Gehirnödem (Apoplexia serosa) in Verbindung mit circumscripter acuter Tuberculose der Pia mater. Deutsches Arch. f. klin. Med., Leipz., 1869, v, 562-565.—**Corazza** (L.) Tubercolosi migliare della pia meninge cerebrale. Riv. clin. di Bologna, 1867, vi, 43-45.—**Crohn** (M.) Ein Fall von Solitärtuberkel im Pons bei tuberculöser Meningitis. Arch. f. Kinderh., Stuttg., 1882-3, iv, 91-93.—**Cullerre.** Méningite granuleuse. Bull. Soc. méd. de l'Yonne 1878, Auxerre, 1879, xix, 82-87.—**Curran** (W.) Tubercular meningitis. Brit. M. J., Lond., 1860, ii, 974.—**Da Costa.** Tubercular meningitis. Med. & Surg. Reporter, Phila., 1863, x, 86.—**Danforth** (I. N.) A typical case of tubercular meningitis. Am. Q. Micr. J., N. Y., 1879, i, 180-185, 1 pl.—**Danis.** Quelques réflexions au sujet de la méningite

Meningitis (*Tubercular*).

tuberculeuse. Bull. méd. du nord, Lille, 1865, 101–109.—
Davenport (F. H.) Tubercular meningitis. Boston
M. & S. J., 1879, c, 229.—**Dawson** (Y.) Tubercular meningitis in an infant: necropsy. Lancet, Lond., 1884, i,
660.—**Day** (W. H.) On tubercular meningitis and the
mode of treatment. Proc. M. Soc. Lond., 1879–81, v, 339–
348.—**Debove.** Note sur la méningite spinale tuberculeuse. Bull. et mém. Soc. méd. d. hôp. de Par. (1878),
1879, 2. s., xv, 285–288. *Also :* Union méd., Par., 1879, 3.
s., xxvii. 696–699. *Also :* Progrès méd., Par., 1879, vii,
37.—**Delafield** (F.) Tubercular meningitis. Med. Rec.,
N. Y., 1877, xii, 306.—**Delany** (J. J.) Tubercular meningitis; atrophy of the kidney. N. York M. J., 1878,
xxviii, 385–387.—**Deschamps.** De la méningite tuberculeuse ultime simulant l'hémorrhagie corticale ou méningée. France méd., Par., 1877, xxiv, 577; 585.—**Descroizilles.** Méningite tuberculeuse; autopsie. *Ibid.,*
1884, ii, 1155–1161.— **Doutrelepont.** Fall von Meningitis tuberculosa nach Lupus; Tuberkelbacillen im Blute.
Deutsche med. Wchnschr., Berl., 1885, xi, 98.—**Drazic.**
Tuberculosis meningum, pulmonum et glandularum lymphaticarum. Oesterr. med. Wchnschr., Wien, 1843, 1261–
1264.— **Dreyfus.** Tuberculose méningée; autopsie.
Compt. rend. Soc. de biol. 1876, Par., 1877, 6. s., iii, 75.—
Dubar (L.) Méningite cérébro - spinale tuberculeuse.
Bull. Soc. anat. de Par., 1879, 4. s., iv, 240–243. *Also :*
Progrès méd., Par., 1879, vii, 834.—**Du Castel.** Ménin-
gite tuberculeuse du lobule paracentral. Bull. et mém.
Soc. méd. d. hôp. de Par., 1884, 3. s., i, 250–254. *Also :*
Gaz. hebd. de méd., Par., 1884, 2. s., xxi, 450 – 452.—
Dudon. Méningite tuberculeuse; guérison; récidive
trois ans et demi après; guérison; nouvelle récidive six
mois plus tard; mort. Mém. et bull. Soc. de méd. et
chir. de Bordeaux, 1876, 95–98. [Discussion], 98–101.—
Dujardin-Beaumetz. Méningite tuberculeuse; arrêt dans la marche de la maladie; guérison des symptômes.
Bull. et mém. Soc. méd. d. hôp. de Par. (1878). 1879, 2. s.,
xv, 256–264. *Also :* Union méd., Par., 1879, 3. s., xxvii,
469–474.—**Duparcque.** Méningite tuberculeuse. Gaz.
hebd. de méd., Par., 1855, ii, 839–842.—**Earle** (C. W.) Tubercular meningitis. Chicago M. J. & Exam., 1879, xxxix,
11–24, 1 pl.—**Edlefsen** (G.) Ueber Meningitis tuberculosa und Tuberculose im Kindesalter. Mitth. f. d. Ver.
Schlesw.-Holst. Aerzte, Kiel, 1879, 51–62.— **Engel** (H.)
Tubercular meningitis. Med. & Surg. Reporter, Phila.,
1885, liii, 57–61.— **Eskridge** (J. T.) Tubercular cerebro-spinal meningitis. *Ibid.*, 1883, xlix, 9; 40; 65. *Also :*
Tr. Coll. Phys. Phila., 1881–3, 3. s., vi, 307–352. *Also :* J.
Nerv. & Ment. Dis., N. Y., 1883, viii, 275–303.—**Faisans**
(L.) Méningite tuberculeuse; lésion circonscrite du lobule paracentral à droite; hémiplégie gauche. Bull. Soc.
anat. de Par., 1877, lii, 277–279. *Also :* Progrès méd.,
Par., 1877, v, 574.— **Fenwick** (J. C. J.) Three cases
of cerebral disease; with a table of cases of tubercular
meningitis. St. George's Hosp. Rep., Lond., 1875, vii,
29–37, 1 tab.—**Finger.** Tuberculöse Meningitis mit
Hydrocephalus und Gehirnerweichung, plötzlich tödtend.
Vrtljschr. f. d. prakt. Heilk., Prag, 1858, iv, 10.— **Finlayson.** Tubercular meningitis in an adult; progress
of case; post-mortem. Glasgow M. J., 1879, xi, 234–236.—
Finny. † Dublin J. M. Sc., 1877, lxiv, 259–261.— **Fish**
(J. C.) †† St. Barth. Hosp. Rep., Lond., 1867, iii, 402–
408.—**de Fleury** (M.) Méningite tuberculeuse. J. de
méd. de Bordeaux, 1883–4, xiii, 76.— **Foucart** (E.) Méningite probablement tuberculeuse guérie. France méd.,
Par., 1879, xxvi, 466.—**von Franque** (A.) Ueber Meningitis cerebro-spinalis tuberculosa. Cor.-Bl. d. deutsch.
Gesellsch. f. Psychiat., etc., Neuwied, 1864, xi, 97–102.—
Froumüller sen. Meningeal-Tuberkulose. Memorabilien, Heilbr., 1875, xx, 247–249.— **Fuchs** (C. H.) †† *In
his :* Ber. ü. d. med. Klin. zu Götting., 1853–4, 8°, Götting.,
1885. — **Fussell.** Tubercular meningitis in an adult;
difficulties of diagnosis. Brit. M. J., Lond., 1879, i, 13.—
Gairdner. † Instructive difficulties in diagnosis. Glasgow M. J., 1878, x, 151.—**Galliard** (L.) Aphasie, symptôme initial de la méningite tuberculeuse; amas de tubercules au niveau des scissures de Sylvius et de Rolando du
côté gauche, et des circonvolutions avoisinantes, sans
altération de la substance cérébrale. Bull. Soc. anat. de
Par., 1881, lvi, 204–206. *Also :* Progrès méd., Par., 1881,
ix, 703.—**Galliaux.** Méningite tuberculeuse cérébro-
spinale. Bull. Soc. anat. de Par., 1880, lv, 435–437. *Also :*
Progrès méd., Par., 1881, ix, 239.— **Gatti** (F.) Le forme
anomale di meningite tubercolare nell' adulto. Gazz. d.
osp., Milano, 1885, vi, 274 ; 284 ; 290 ; 299 ; 315 ; 323.—**Gaucher** (E.) Méningo-encéphalite tuberculeuse, localisée
autour de l'émergence du nerf facial; hémiplégie faciale
directe et complète. Bull. Soc. anat. de Par., 1879, 4. s.,
iv, 30.—**Gee** (S. J.) Tubercular meningitis. Syst. Med.
(Reynolds), Lond., 1868, ii, 371–396.—**Gelinéau.** Méningite tuberculeuse. Rev. de thérap. méd.-chir., Par.,
1879, xlvi, 64–92.—**Gerhard** (W. W.) On the history of
tuberculous meningitis. Med. Exam., Phila., 1840, iii,
293–295.—**Gibbs** (O. C.) Pathology and treatment of tubercular meningitis. Nelson's North. Lancet, Plattsburg,
N. Y., 1853–4, viii, 23–25. ———. On meningeal tuberculosis. Am. M. Month., N. Y., 1856, v, 1–12.— **Gibson**

Meningitis (*Tubercular*).

(F. W.) † Autopsy. Brit. M. J., Lond., 1869, i, 75.—
Giscaro. † Guérison apparente; rechute dix jours après;
guérison définitive. Rev. méd. de Toulouse, 1879, xiii, 37–
48.—**Godard.** † Tubercules dans les reins, l'utérus, etc.
Bull. Soc. anat. de Par., 1847, xxii, 221–225.—**Grabacher.**
Meningitis tuberculosa cum hydrocephalo subacuto. Med.
Jahrb. d. k. k. österr. Staates, Wien, 1845, li, 63.—**Grasset** (J.) Deux observations de méningite tuberculeuse.
I. Lésions du cervelet; vertige, nystagmus. II. Lésions
de la zone motrice corticale; hémiplégie transitoire. Montpel. méd., 1878, xli, 48–59.—**Green** (P. H.) Observations
on the tubercular meningitis of children, with preliminary
remarks on hydrocephalus. Lancet, Lond., 1835-6, ii, 263–
276. *Also, transl. :* Mag. f. d. ges. Heilk., Berl., 1837,
xlviii, 179–232. ———. †† Lancet, Lond., 1837-8, ii, 536;
1839-40, ii, 183.—**Greenfield** (W. S.) †† *Ibid.*, 1874, i,
833 ; 904.—**Grimes** (G. J.) † Tr. Georgia M. Ass., Atlanta,
1878, xxix, 59–63.—**Guarnieri** (G.) Osservazioni istologiche sulla meningite tubercolare. Bull. d. r. Accad. med.
di Roma, 1882, viii, 129–133. ———. Note istologiche sulla
meningite tubercolare. Arch. per le sc. med., Torino,
1883-4, vii, 59–70, 1 pl.—**Guillaumet.** Méningite cérébro-spinale tuberculeuse; tuberculose généralisée (poumon, plèvres, foie, rein); péricardite adhésive tuberculeuse. Bull. Soc. anat. de Par., 1873, xlviii, 758–764.—
Gussner (C.) Meningitis baseos cerebri et spinalis tuberculosa; myelomalacia; tuberculosis pulmonum retro-
grada. Deutsche Klinik, Berl., 1850, ii, 119–121.—**Guttmann.** Ein Fall von Meningitis tuberculosa (hydrocephalica) mit Erweichung und theilweiser Verhärtung
des grossen und kleinen Gehirn. Med. Cor.-Bl. d. württemb. ärztl. Ver., Stuttg., 1848, xviii, 97–103.—**Hahn.**
Recherches sur la méningite tuberculeuse et sur le traitement de cette maladie. Arch. gén. de méd., Par., 1849, 4.
s., xx, 385 : xxi, 43.—**Halson** (G. J.) Case of tubercular
meningitis, with softening around the ventricles of the
brain, large cavity in the summit of the right lung,
and deposit of gray granulations in the left lung. Med.
Exam., Phila., 1839, ii, 678–680.—**Hayem** (G.) Note
sur deux cas de méningite spinale tuberculeuse liée à la
tuberculose miliaire généralisée. Compt. rend. Soc. de
biol. 1869, Par., 1870, 5. s., i, 287–291.—**Hengst** (D. A.) †
Med. & Surg. Reporter, Phila., 1881, xliv, 150.—**Hennig.** † Deutsche Klinik, Berl., 1849, i, 35.—**Henoch**
(E.) Zur Pathologie der Meningitis tuberculosa der Kinder. Charité-Ann. 1877, Berl., 1879, iv, 517–526. *Also :*
Wien. med. Bl., 1879, ii, 717; 750. ———. Meningitis tuberculosa. Charité-Ann. 1882, Berl., 1884, ix, 596 - 599.
Also, transl. : Arch. di patol. inf., Napoli, 1885, iii, 9–11.—
Hervey. Méningite tuberculeuse. Bull. Soc. anat. de
Par., 1873, xlviii, 498–501.—**Hill** (W. R.) †† Brit. M. J.,
Lond., 1860, ii, 836–838.—**Hirons** (J. B.) Tubercular
meningitis. Nashville J. M. & S., 1886, n. s., xxxvii, 195–
198.—**Hochhaus** (H.) Ein Beitrag zur Diagnose der
eitrigen und tuberculösen Hirnhautentzündung. Berl.
klin. Wchnschr., 1887, xxiv, 10.—**von Höring.** Tuber-
kulose; chronische latente Hirnhautentzündung. Med.
Cor.-Bl. d. württemb. ärztl. Ver., Stuttg., 1861, xxxi, 336.—
Hurd (A.) Tubercular meningitis. Detroit Lancet, 1879,
n. s., ii, 83–95.—**Husson.** Méningite granuleuse; affection organique du cœur; mort. Bull. Soc. anat. de Par.,
1836, xi, 91. [Rap. de Tessier], 98.—**Hutchinson** (J. H.)
Tubercle of the meninges and of the kidney. Proc. Path.
Soc. Phila., 1857-60, i, 231. ———. Tubercular meningitis.
Med. Gaz., N. Y., 1880, vii, 261. ———. Case of tubercular
meningitis suddenly developed in an adult. Phila. M.
Times, 1881–2, xii, 386.— **Hutinel.** Méningite cérébro-
spinale tuberculeuse; tuberculose généralisée. Bull. Soc.
anat. de Par., 1874, xlix, 390–394.—**Jaccoud** (S.) Sur la
méningite tuberculeuse de l'adulte. *In his :* Leçons de clin.
méd., 8°, Par., 1885, 349–363. ———. Méningite cérébro-
spinale tuberculeuse. Gaz. d. hôp., Par., 1887, lx, 250.—
Jackson (J. B. S.) Tubercular meningitis in the adult.
N. Eng. Q. J. M. & S., Bost., 1842-3, i, 211–221. ———. Tubercular meningitis in the adult. Am. J. M. Sc., Phila.,
1853, n. s., xxvi, 366.—**Jadelot.** † Autopsie. Gaz. d. hôp.,
Par., 1843, 2. s., v, 454. *Also, transl. :* J. f. Kinderkr., Berl.,
1844, ii, 53–59.—**Janikowski** (A.) O zapalenia gruzel
howém blon mozgowych u dzieci (meningitis tuberculosa).
Pam. Towarz. Lek. Warszaw., 1838-9, ii, 391–411.—**Jaques**
(H. P.) † Autopsy. Boston M. & S. J., 1885, cxiii, 5 - 7.
Also : Obst. Gaz., Cincin., 1885, viii, 365 - 374. —**Jenner.**
Case of acute tubercular meningitis. Med. Times & Gaz.,
Lond., 1860, ii, 504. ———. Case of chronic tubercular me-
ningitis. *Ibid.*, 505.—**Joffroy & Lepiez.** Méningo-en-
céphalite tuberculeuse localisée; hémorrhagie cérébrale.
Bull. Soc. anat. de Par. (1871), 1873, xlvi, 208–212.—**John-
ston** (W. W.) Tubercular meningitis; caseous mass at
apex of lung; miliary tubercle in pia mater, spleen, etc.
Tr. M. Soc. Dist. Columb., Wash., 1876, iii, 50 – 58.—
Kahler (O.) Ueber Wurzelneuritis bei tuberculöser
Basilarmeningitis. Prag. med. Wchnschr., 1887, xii, 33–
35.—**Kiemann.** Meningitis tuberculosa; Tod. Ber. d.
k. k. Krankenanst. Rudolph-Stiftung in Wien (1880), 1881,
281. ———. Meningitis tuberculosa basilaris; Tod. *Ibid.*,
284. ———. Meningitis basilaris tuberculosa; Tuberculosis
chronica pulmonum et renum; Tod. *Ibid.*, 285–287. ———.

Meningitis (*Tubercular*).

Meningitis tuberculosa chronica in fossa Sylvii sinist. subsequente meningitide basilari recente; Pneumonia lobularis; Tuberculosis chronica pulmonum intestinum et glandularum lymphaticarum; Tod. *Ibid.*, 287. ———. Meningitis basilaris tuberculosa; Tuberculosis vetus apicum pulmonum et glandularum bronchial. ; cystitis incipiens; Tod. *Ibid.*, 289. ———. Meningitis tuberculosa; tuberculosis pulm. ; Tod. *Ibid.* (1882), 1883, 365.—**Knowles** (H.) † Lancet, Lond., 1867, ii, 357.—[**Koller** & **Schmidt.**] Meningitis tuberculosa cum exfoliatione ossium cranii. Jahrb. f. Kinderh., Wien, 1863, vi, 186-189.—**Kreuser.** Meningitis granulosa. Med. Cor.· Bl. d. württemb. ärztl. Ver., Stuttg., 1866, xxxvi, 299.—**Lancereaux.** Méningite tuberculeuse; encéphalite. Gaz. d. hôp., Par., 1870, xliii, 401.—**Landouzy** (L.) Méningite tuberculeuse chez un enfant; absence de symptômes; ganglions axillaires mésentériques et thoraciques caséeux, sans lésion notable des viscères; rapports entre la caséification ganglionnaire et la méningite tuberculeuse. Bull. Soc. anat. de Par., 1873, xlviii, 8-12. ———. Méningite tuberculeuse. Gaz. d. hôp., Par., 1884, lvii, 169.—**Larsen.** Meningitis tuberculosa. Norsk Mag. f. Lægevidensk., Christiania, 1866, xx, 1024-1026.—**Leared** (A.) Cerebral disease, apparently tubercular meningitis; recovery. Med. Times & Gaz., Lond., 1864, i, 121.—**Lederer** (I.) Ein Beitrag zur Meningitis tuberculosa. Jahrb. f. Kinderh., Leipz., 1882, n. F., xix, 179-188.—**Lees.** Tubercular meningitis. Dublin Q. J. M. Sc., 1854, xvii, 448.—**Legendre.** De la méningite tuberculeuse étudiée au point de vue clinique. J. de méd. de Bordeaux, 1852, x, 73; 129; 217; 328; 592; 669. *Also:* Ann. de méd. belge, Brux., 1852, ii, 333: iii, 26; 212: iv, 60.—**Léger** (H.) Convulsions partielles précédées d'une aura et prémonitoires de méningite tuberculeuse. Gaz. méd. de Picardie, Amiens, 1885, iii, 38.—**Leroux** (C.) De la méningite tuberculeuse de l'adulte. J. d. conn. méd. prat., Par., 1884, 3. s., vii, 257.—**Levy** (M.) Mémoire sur trois cas d'affection tuberculeuse aiguë de la pie-mère, chez les adultes. [Rap. de Rochoux.] Bull. Acad. de méd., Par., 1847-8, xiii, 1134-1139.—**Lewis** (M. J.) Tubercular meningitis, with a tubercle granulation on the floor of the fourth ventricle. Tr. Path. Soc. Phila. (1879-81), 1882, x, 172-176.—**Liandier.** Méningite tuberculeuse chez l'adulte. France méd., Par., 1882, i, 726-728. *Also:* Bull. Soc. clin. de Par. (1882), 1883, vi, 131-133.—**Limasset.** Mal de Pott; méningite tuberculeuse. Bull. Soc. méd. de Reims, 1868, No. vi, 75-81.—**Liouville** (H.) Faits de méningites cérébro-spinales tuberculeuses. Compt. rend. Soc. de biol. 1869, Par., 1870, 5. s., i, 296; 347. ———. Méningite cérébro-spinale tuberculeuse. Bull. Soc. anat. de Par., 1873, xlviii, 133.—**Löwenstamm.** Zur Meningitis tuberculosa. Med.-chir. Centralbl., Wien, 1877, xii, 113. ———. † *Ibid.*, 1878, xiii, 124.—**Looten.** Contribution à l'étude de la granulie; caractères qui la distinguent de la méningite tuberculeuse et de la fièvre typhoïde; curabilité de cette affection. Bull. méd. du nord, Lille, 1876, xv, 33-42.—**Lorey** (C.) † Bei einem einjährigen Knaben. Jahresb. ü. d. Verwalt. d. Med.-Wes., d. Krankenanst. . . . d. Stadt Frankf., 1869, xiii, 89.—**Macleod** (G. H. B.) Symptoms of tubercular meningitis in an adult, suddenly developed, during treatment for simple fracture of the thigh. Glasgow M. J., 1871-2, 4. s., iv, 13.—**Macneven** (W. H.) † N. York J. M., 1849, ii, 306-312.—**Mader** (J.) Tuberculosis mening. et corticis cerebri primaria subchronica in regione superiori; Tod. Ber. d. k. k. Krankenanst. Rudolph-Stiftung in Wien (1877), 1878, 282. ———. Meningitis tuberculosa mit ungewöhnlichem Verlauf. *Ibid.* (1878), 1879, 293. ———. Meningitis tuberculosa mit ungewöhnlichem Verlauf. Med.-chir. Centralbl., Wien, 1880, xv, 520. ———. Meningitis tuberculosa; ungewöhnliche Initialerscheinungen; Tod. *Ibid.*, 1886, xxi, 340.—**Magnan.** Note sur une observation de méningite tuberculeuse cérébro-spinale. Compt. rend. Soc. de biol. 1869, Par., 1870, 5. s., i, 284-287.—**Malmsten.** Fall af meningitis tuberculosa cerebro-spinalis cum spondylarthrocace tuberculosa. Förh. v. Svens. Läk.-Sällsk. Sammank. 1850-51, Stockholm, 1852, 78.—**Manouvriez** (A.) Observation de granulie de forme cérébrale. Bull. méd. du nord, Lille, 1876, xvi, 161-166.—**Martel** (E.) Méningite tuberculeuse à la suite du redressement d'une fausse ankylose du genou. Bull. et mém. Soc. de chir. de Par., 1885, n. s., xi, 674. ———. Curabilité de la méningite tuberculeuse. Rev. internat. d. sc. méd., Par., 1886, iii, 287-294.—**Mathieu** (A.-M.) Méningite tuberculeuse cérébro-spinale. France méd., Par., 1882, ii, 793-796.—**Maubrac.** Méningite tuberculeuse; évolution anormale. Gaz. méd. de Par., 1885, 7. s., ii, 315-317.—**Mayr.** † Jahrb. f. Kinderh., Wien, 1859-60, iii, 259-266.—**Medin** (O.) Om meningitis tuberculosa hos späda barn. Nord. med. Ark., Stockholm, 1883, xv, no. 26, 1-30. ———. Den tuberkulösa meningitens behandling med jodoformsalva. Svens. Läk.-Sällsk. n. Handl., Stockholm, 1886, 201-206.—**Michelacci** (M.) Orromenite tubercolare. Sperimentale, Firenze, 1879, xliii, 14.—**Mickle** (W. J.) On meningeal tuberculosis of the cerebral convexity. Med. Times & Gaz., Lond., 1882, i, 377-379.—**Milligan** (W.) † Lancet, Lond., 1883, ii, 900.—**Mills** (C. K.) Localised tubercular meningitis, with cortical softening; involvement of the

Meningitis (*Tubercular*).

centres for the limbs and face. Brain, Lond., 1879-80, ii, 554-560. ———. Localised tubercular meningitis with cortical softening; involvement of oro-lingual centres; internal pachy-meningitis of the opposite hemisphere. *Ibid.*, 560-563. ———. Tubercular meningitis; disseminated miliary tuberculosis. J. Nerv. & Ment. Dis., N. Y., 1887, xiv, 359.—**Mills** (C. K.) & **Ott** (L.) † † Med. & Surg. Reporter, Phila., 1881, xlv, 5-11.—**Mills** (T. W.) † Canad. J. M. Sc., Toronto, 1879, iv, 57-61.—**Minot** (F.) Tubercular meningitis. Syst. Pract. M. (Pepper), Phila., 1886, v, 723-739.—**Money** (A.) A remarkable case of tubercular meningitis. Tr. Clin. Soc. Lond., 1884, xvii, 165-167.—**Monod.** Méningite tuberculeuse; tuberculose granuleuse abdominale; tuberculisation partielle des organes génitaux (trompes) sans tubercules pulmonaires; chez une petite fille de neuf ans; autopsie. Bull. Soc. anat. de Par., 1867, xlii, 686-690.—**Morel-Lavallée.** Méningite tuberculeuse; ramollissement cérébral, étendu à tout l'insula; paralysie avec contracture des membres et du facial inférieur, du côté opposé à la lésion; déviation conjuguée de la tête et des yeux. *Ibid.*, 1884, lix, 656-660. *Also:* Progrès méd., Par., 1885, 2. s., ii, 182.—**Moxon** (W.) Miliary tubercle of spinal dura mater in a case of tubercular meningitis. Tr. Path. Soc. Lond., 1869-70, xxi, 12.—**Murchison.** † Death. Lancet, Lond., 1872, i, 826.—**Musser** (J. H.) † † Phila. M. Times, 1885-6, xvi, 412-414. *Also:* Polyclinic, Phila., 1885-6, iii, 131-133. *Also:* Med. News, Phila., 1886, xlviii, 205-207. *Also,* Reprint.—**Nilsson** (E.) † † Med dödlig utgång, ett fall behandladt med jodoformingnidning; helsa. Hygiea, Stockholm, 1885, xlvii, 393-397. *Also, transl. :* Arch. f. Kinderh., Stuttg., 1885-6, vii, 214-217. *Also, transl. :* N. Yorker med. Presse, 1885-6, i, 217-220.—**Nixon.** Tubercular meningitis, acute tuberculosis. Dublin Q. J. M. Sc., 1873, lvi, 335-337.—**Ogle** (J. W.) Case of scrofulous meningitis, with sarcinæ ventriculi found after death. Tr. Path. Soc. Lond., 1854-5, vi, 16.—**Old** and recent tubercular meningitis. Abstr. M. & S. Cases Gen. Hosp. Sick Children, Pendlebury, Manchester (1885), 1886, v, 77.—**Oppolzer.** Ueber Meningitis tuberculosa. Deutsche Klinik, Berl , 1850, ii, 73. ———. † † Wien. med. Wchnschr., 1851, i, 343. ———. Meningitis tuberculosa, Hydrocephalus acutus und Miliartuberculose sämmtlicher parenchymatösen und serösen Organe. Allg. Wien. med. Ztg., 1856, i, 45. ———. Meningitis tuberculosa. Wien. med. Wchnschr., 1858, viii, 198; 215; 238; 278. ———. Meningitis tuberculosa. Spitals-Ztg., Wien, 1862, 209-211.—**Osler** (W.) Meningeal affection slight; ventricles distended, walls soft; very few miliary tubercles in the organs. Montreal Gen. Hosp. Path. Rep., 1877, i, 81.—**Oxley** (M.) Tubercular meningitis as it occurs in children ; with an appendix of illustrative cases. Liverpool M.-Chir. J., 1885, v, 259-288, 2 pl.—**Papavoine.** Observations d'arachnitis tuberculeuses. J. hebd. de méd , Par., 1830, vi, 113-119.—**Peacock.** † Lancet, Lond., 1874, i, 266.—**Pelvet.** Tuberculisation des organes génitaux chez une femme morte de méningite tuberculeuse. Bull. Soc. anat. de Par., 1863, xxxviii, 285.—**Pepper** (G.) Phthisis pulmonalis; death from tubercular meningitis in an adult. Proc. Path. Soc. Phila. (1860-66), 1867, ii, 221-224.—**Pepper** (W.) Tubercular meningitis in an adult, following disseminated cheesy deposits in the lungs. Phila. M. Times, 1871, i, 216.—**Picot.** Sur un cas de méningite tuberculeuse de la convexité avec suspension presque complète des fonctions cérébrales. Gaz. hebd. d. sc. méd. de Bordeaux, 1886, vii, 199; 257; 438.—**Piet** (A.) Recherches sur la maladie connue sous les noms de méningite, arachnitis, hydrocéphale aiguë des enfants et en particulier sur la méningite granuleuse ou tuberculeuse. Gaz. méd. de Par., 1837, 2. s., v, 273-283. *Also:* Ann. de méd. belge, Brux., 1837, ii, 232-247.—**Porter** (W.) & **Fischel** (W. E.) Tubercular meningitis; dilatation of the pulmonary artery. Proc. St. Louis M. Soc. Missouri, 1878, i, 219.—**Posadski** (S. V.) K kazuist. pervich. bugorchat. vospalen. miatkoi mozgovi obolochki (meningitis tuberculosa). Ejened. klin. gaz., St. Petersb., 1886, vi, 221; 242.—**Prud'homme.** Attaques antérieures de delirium tremens; tuberculitis intim miliaire; maladie de Bright; méningite ultime. Gaz. d. hôp., Par., 1870, xliii, 261.—**Radcliffe.** Case of strumous meningitis of obscure character. Lancet, Lond., 1869, i, 602.—**Rautenberg.** Meningitis tuberculosa ohne Vorhandensein eines käsigen Heerdes. St. Petersb. med. Ztschr., 1869, xvi, 228-231.—**Raymond** (F.) Méningite tuberculeuse de l'adulte. Progrès méd., Par., 1881, ix, 787. *Also:* Gaz. d. hôp., Par., 1881, liv, 883.—**Raymond** (P.) Méningite tuberculeuse de l'adulte; aphasie transitoire. Bull. Soc. anat. de Par., 1885, lx, 84-86. *Also:* Progrès méd., Par., 1885, 2. s., ii, 333.—**Raynaud.** † Bull. Soc. anat. de Par., 1860, xxxv, 167-169.—**Récamier.** Céphalalgie; douleurs des lombes; stupeur; contraction des membres thoraciques suivie de résolution et d'un retour de la rigidité musculaire; arachnitis; tubercules en dehors de la dure-mère rachidienne. Rev. méd. franç. et étrang., Par., 1825, iii, 165-168.—**Reibel.** Méningites tuberculeuses; leur curabilité. Proc.-verb. . . . Soc. de méd. de Strasb., 1880, xiv, 32-37.—**Reimer.** Meningitis tuberculosa. Jahrb. f. Kinderh., Leipz., 1877, xi, 2-10.—**Rendu** (H.) Méningite

Meningitis (*Tubercular*).

tuberculeuse cérébro-spinale; prédominance des symptômes spinaux; lésions confluentes au niveau du renflement lombaire, très peu accentuées sur l'encéphale. Bull. Soc. clin. de Par. (1883), 1884, vii, 2–9. *Also:* France méd., Par., 1883, i, 169; 181.—**Richardson** (J. B.) Tubercular cerebral meningitis. St. Louis M. & S. J., 1880, xxxix, 700–703. ———. Tubercular cerebral meningitis. Louisville M. News, 1885, xix, 225–233.—**Riemslagh.** Observation d'un cas de tuberculose des méninges; autopsie. Arch. méd. belges, Brux., 1880, 3. s , xvii, 237–242.—**Rilliet.** Nouvelles recherches sur la méningite tuberculeuse chez les enfants. Gaz. méd. de Par., 1846, 3. s., i, 4; 22; 872; 894. *Also:* Ann. de méd. belge, Brux., 1846, i, 67; 244: iv, 224; 367. *Also, transl.:* J. f. Kinderkr., Berl., 1846, vi, 255–275. *Also, transl.:* Schweiz. Ztschr. f. Med., Chir. u. Geburtsh., Zürich, 1847, 69: 1848, 372. ———. De la guérison de la méningite tuberculeuse. Arch. gén. de méd., Par., 1853, 5. s., ii, 641–674. ———. De la guérison de la méningite tuberculeuse. Actes Soc. méd. d. hôp. de Par., 1855, iii, 126–159.—**Roger** (G.-H.) † Rev. mens. d. mal. de l'enf., Par., 1886, iv, 14–24, 1 pl.—**Roskoten** (O. J.) † Peoria M. Month., 1884–5, v, 23–25.—**Ross** (G.) Case of acute general tuberculosis, fatal by meningitis. Canada M. & S. J., Montreal, 1876–7, v, 59–61. ———. † *Ibid.*, 258–262. ———. †† *Ibid.*, 1881–2, x, 344–347.—**Rousseau.** Un cas de guérison de méningite granuleuse. Encéphale, Par., 1882, ii, 460–463.—**Rowbotham** (H. C.) † In an adult. Med. Times & Gaz., Lond., 1879, i, 317.—**Sauvage** (R.) † Recovery. N. O. l. M. & S. J., 1882–3, n. s., x, 739–748.—**Scarpari** (S.) La meningite tubercolare primitiva del cervello. Ann. univ. di med. e chir., Milano, 1882, cclxi, 497–518.—**Schlager.** [Residuen einer Meningitis an der Convexität, chronischer Hydrocephalus, Tuberculosis pulm. und ein Fibroma uteri.] Aerztl. Ber. d. k. k. allg. Krankenh. zu Wien (1872), 1873, 364.—**Scholz.** †† *Ibid.* (1879), 1880, 64–66.—**Scholz & Standthartner.** †† *Ibid.* (1875), 1876, 53–56. **Schütz** (E.) Aphasie als Initialsymptom von Meningitis tuberculosa. Prag. med. Wchnschr., 1881, vi, 301; 316.—**Séjournet.** Note sur deux cas de méningite tuberculeuse guérie chez l'adulte. Bull. et mém. Soc. de thérap., Par., 1884, xvi, 118–128.—**Semple** (C. E. A.) † Med. Press & Circ., Lond., 1883, n. s., xxxv, 202. ———. † Death. *Ibid.*, xxxvi, 439. ———. Case of tubercular meningitis with tubercle of the choroid; death. *Ibid.*, 1885, n. s., xxxix, 557.—**Seymour** (C.) A case of acute tubercular meningitis. Phila. M. Times, 1873, iii, 407.—**Silfverberg** (E.) Et Tilfælde af Meningitis granulosa helbredet. Hosp.-Tid., Kjøbenh., 1858, i, 69.—**Silvestrini** (S.) Meningite tuberculosa; rammolimento e tumore al lobo mediano del cervelletto, sintomi agli organi genitali. Arch. ital. per le mal. nerv., Milano, 1873, x, 29–33.—**Simon** (J.) De la méningite tuberculeuse. Praticien, Par., 1887, x, 147–149.—**Simonovitch** (J. M.) Dva sluchaja bugorchatago vospalenija mjagkoi mozgovoi obolochek (meningitis tuberculosa), nachavshiesja afazicjou. Ejened. klin. gaz., St. Petersb., 1882, ii, 449–453. ———. † *Ibid.*, 510–517.—**Skeer** (J. D.) A pathognomonic symptom in the diagnosis of tubercular meningitis. Chicago M. J. & Exam., 1887, liv, 41–46.—**Smith** (L.) Tubercular meningitis. N. York M. J., 1873, xviii, 176–199.—**Smith** (W.) Tubercular meningitis; tubercular tumours in cerebellum. Glasgow M. J., 1879, n. s., xi, 150.—**Smoler.** Akute Miliartuberkulose; meningitis. Memorabilien, Heilbr., 1866, xi, 149.—**Solomki** (N. V.) K kazuistikie meningitis basilaris tuberculosa. Protok. zasiid. Kavkazsk. med. Obsh., Tiflis, 1883, xx, 257–267.—**Southey** (R.) Clinical lecture on tubercular meningitis. Brit. M. J., Lond., 1876, i, 97–99. ———. Tubercular meningitis. *Ibid.*, 1877, ii, 557; 585.—**Stillé.** † Med. Exam., Phila., 1850, n. s., vi, 137–140.—**Storer.** Tubercular meningitis complicated by intercurrent measles. Am. J. M. Sc., Phila., 1853, n. s., xxvi. 354.—**Stunde.** † St. Petersb. med. Ztschr., 1868, xiv, 124–126.—**Surmay.** Mémoire sur la tuberculisation aignë des méninges chez l'adulte. Gaz. méd. de Par., 1855, 3. s., x, 808; 820.—**Szontagh** (F.) Az agy gümökóros megbetegedésének néhány érdekesebb esetéröl. [Some interesting cases of tuberculous meningitis.] Orvosi hetil., Budapest, 1887, xxxi, 869–874.—**Tachard** (E.) Analyse clinique d'un cas de méningite tuberculeuse. Rev. méd. de Toulouse, 1879, xiii, 3–17.—**Talamon** (C.) Méningite tuberculeuse circum-pédonculaire; agitation choréique et mouvement giratoire. Bull. Soc. anat. de Par., 1879, liv, 34–39. *Also:* Progrès méd., Par., 1879, vii, 486.—**Taylor** (J.) Case of tubercular meningitis; tubercles in the lungs; intestines; bronchial and mesenteric glands; post mortem. Lancet, Lond., 1846, i, 24.—**Tosquinet.** † Autopsie. Arch. méd. belges, Brux., 1878, 3. s , iv, 116–118.—**Trastour.** † Guérison. J. de méd. de l'ouest, Nantes, 1882, xvi, 71–76.—**Traube** (L.) †† Ann. d. Char.-Krankenh. . . . zu Berl., 1862–3, x, 2. Hft., 176–185. ———. Alte Lungentuberkulose; Tod durch tuberculöse Meningitis im 2ten Stadium; eigenthümlicher Verlauf derselben mit epileptiformen und tetaniformen Anfällen. *Ibid.*, 198–202. ———. †† *Ibid.*, 1863, xi, 3. Hft., 15–37. ———. Meningitis basilar. tuberculos.; Tod im zweiten Stadium. Berl. klin. Wchnschr., 1864, i, 305. *Also, in his:* Ges. Beitr. z. Path. u.

Meningitis (*Tubercular*).

Physiol., Berl., 1871, ii, pt. 2, 717–722. — **Troisier.** Méningite cérébro-spinale tuberculeuse. Bull. Soc. anat. de Par., 1873, xlviii, 366–368. *Also:* Progrès méd., Par., 1873, i, 56.—**Trousseau.** Méningite granuleuse. Gaz. d. hôp., Par., 1841, 2. s., iii, 271 ; 295.—**Ulrich** (C.) Erscheinungen einer acuten Meningitis ; Tod am 6. Tage ; allgemeine Miliartuberculose ; Infarcte im Gehirn und der Milz ; Caries der linken Tibia. Deutsche Klinik, Berl., 1859, xi, 350.—**Valleix.** Note sur un cas de tuberculisation des méninges, chez un adulte, avec ramollissement et apoplexie capillaire. Arch. gén. de méd., Par., 1846, 4. s., xi, 192–204. *Also:* Ann. de méd. belge, Brux., 1838, i, 102–112.—**Vergely** (P.) Méningite tuberculeuse; symptômes très obscurs au début; paralysie de la vessie; mort rapide; autopsie; tuberculose généralisée. Bordeaux méd., 1877, vi, 289. — **Villar.** † Gac. méd., Lima, 1875, i, 277–279.—**Vogelsang** (F.) Meningitis cerebro-spinalis tubercul. Memorabilien, Heilbr., 1872, xvii, 393–409.—**Vrain** (L.) Méningite tuberculeuse en plaque au niveau du sillon de Rolando, avec épilepsie Jacksonnienne et monoplégie brachiale chez un débile. Encéphale, Par., 1886, vi, 356–361.—**Wardell** (J. R.) Tubercular meningitis. *In his:* Contrib. Path. & Pract. Med., 8°, Lond., 1885, 667–673.—**Warfvinge** (F. W.) Fem fall af tuberkulös meningit med framgaug behandlade med ingnidning af jodoformsalva. Hygiea, Stockholm, 1886, xlviii, 479–491.—**Weber** (H.) On the connection of tubercular meningitis and tuberculosis of the other serous membranes with the presence of caseous deposits in the body. Tr. Path. Soc. Lond., 1869–70, xxi, 14–22. ———. Specimens of the brain, lungs, caseous glands and other organs from a case of tubercular meningitis. *Ibid.*, 23 —**Weeks.** Acute tubercular meningitis. Boston M. & S. J., 1877, xcvi, 318.—**Weir** (J.) † Recovery. Louisville M. News, 1885, xx, 354.—**Wengler.** Ueber eine mit Aphasie complicirte tuberculöse Meningitis. Deutsches Arch. f. klin. Med., Leipz., 1880, xxvi, 179–189.—**Werner** (H.) Acute Miliartuberculose der Hirnhäute. Ber. d. k. k. Krankenh. Wieden 1871, Wien, 1873, 97–93.—**West** (F.) † Med. Exam., Phila., 1851, n. s., vii, 485–489.—**Wilks.** †† In adults; with remarks on the obscurity of the early symptoms. Med. Times & Gaz., Lond., 1863, ii, 274–278.—**Williams.** Tubercular meningitis. Proc. Path. Soc. Phila., 1860–63, 1867, ii, 186–188. *Also:* Am. J. M. Sc., Phila., 1866, n. s., li, 409–411.—**Willshire.** Tubercular meningitis. Lancet, Lond., 1846, i, 467.—**Wise** (J.) Case of tubercular spinal meningitis with deposit of tubercle in the liver and peritoneum. Indian M. Gaz., Calcutta, 1874, ix, 179.—**Woods** (O. T.) Tubercular meningitis in an adult idiot; no tubercle found in lungs. Brit. M. J., Lond., 1874. ii, 32.—**Zaragoza** (L. M.) Meningitis tuberculosa. Estudio, México, 1876, i, 249–252. — **Zinke** (E. G.) † Cincin. Lancet & Clinic, 1881, n. s., vi, 398–401. ———. † *Ibid.*, 1883, n. s., x, 385–389.

Meningocele.

See, also, **Encephalocele: Hydrencephalocele; Spina** *bifida.*

Agnew (D. H.) Meningocele. Phot. Rev. M. & S., Phila., 1870–71, i, 2, 1 pl.—**Bailey** (J. S.) † Am. J. Obst., N. Y., 1873, vi, 265.—**Barcey** (C. J.) † Med. Times & Gaz., Lond., 1873, i, 531.—**Billroth** (T.) Ein Fall von Meningocele spuria cum fistula ventriculi cerebri. Arch. f. klin. Chir., Berl., 1862, iii, 398–412, 1 pl.—[**Case.**] Case of very large meningocele. Bristol M.-Chir. J., 1883, i, 129, 1 pl.—**Chudnovski** (J. V.) Hydromeningocele cerebralis congenitum (s. hernia meningea nasofrontalis). Vrach, St. Petersb., 1886, vii, 782–785. — **Fackler** (G. A.) Meningocele. Cincin. Lancet & Clinic, 1885, n. s., xiv, 293–297. — **Hamilton** (J. A. G.) Meningocele and imperforate anus in the same child; operations; recovery. Proc. South Austral. Branch Brit. M. Ass., Adelaide, 1883–4, 18. *Also:* Australas. M. Gaz., Sydney, 1882–3, ii, 271.—**Hebert** (T.) Remarks and suggestions on meningocele. N. Orl. M. & S. J., 1887–8, n. s., xv, 95–101.—**Hirigoyen** (L.) Présentation d'un enfant atteint de méningocèle. Mém. et bull. Soc. de méd. et chir. de Bordeaux (1884), 1885, 326–329.—**Holmes** (T.) Case of meningocele, in the occipital region, which was injected with iodine without ill consequences, the patient dying of broncho-pneumonia. St. George's Hosp. Rep., Lond., 1866, i, 35–46. — **Kingsley** (J. P.) Meningocele. St. Louis M. & S. J., 1880, xxxviii, 108–112.—**Larger.** Diagnostic de la méningocèle; pathogénie des kystes dermoïdes. Bull. et mém. Soc. de chir. de Par., 1886, n. s., xii, 313–318.—**Lazzari** (A.) Meningocele del cranio; legatura elastica; guarigione. Gazz. med. di Torino, 1885, xxxvi, 124–131.—**Marshall** (L. W.) † Operation; necropsy. Lancet, Lond., 1885, i, 890. — **Nicoladoni** (P. C.) Meningocele falsa, geheilt durch wiederholte Injektion von Jodtinktur. Wien. med. Presse, 1886, xxvii, 41–44. — **Nicoli** (L.) Voluminoso tumore idromeningeo crani de operato mediante la pinzetta enterotoma del Prof. Rizzoli. Bull. d. sc. med. di Bologna, 1876, 5. s., xxi, 125–129.—**Rasori** (E.) † † Gazz. d. osp., Milano, 1882, iii, 338.—**Roddick** (T. G.) A case of occipital meningocele, treated by seton, with antiseptic precautions; death. Montreal Gen. Hosp. Rep., 1880, i, 201–206, 1 pl., 1 l.—**Roy**

Meningocele.

(M. C.) A case of meningocele (congenital) complicated with chronic hydrocephalus. Indian M. Gaz., Calcutta, 1874. ix, 181.—**Smith** (N.) A new plan of operating upon meningocele. Lancet, Lond., 1884, ii, 490.—**Steavenson** (W. E.) † Tr. Clin. Soc. Lond., 1881, xiv, 181, 1 pl.—**Svensson** (A.) Hydromeningocele frontalis. Upsala Läkaref. Förh., 1886-7, xxii, 576-579. — **Viura y Carreras** (J.) Meningocele en la region occipital. Rev. de cien. méd., Barcel., 1882, viii, 590-596. *Also, transl.:* Ann. de gynéc., Par., 1883, xix, 212-216.—**West** (J. F.) Case of meningocele associated with cervical spina bifida, cured by aspiration. Lancet, Lond., 1875, ii, 552.

"Meninto." Gespräche im Reiche der Krancken. II. Entrevue, zwischen einen Podagricum und Calculosum, oder: zwischen einen Podagristen und einen mit Stein beladenen. Darinnen ein jeder von seiner Kranckheit sich gründlich unterredet, und eine jede nach ihrer Beschreibung, Unterschied, Person die es trift, Kennzeichen, Ursachen, was daraus entstehet, Hülfs-Mittel, Diæt und Cantelen aufs deutlichste erkläret und ausführet, und im Eingange die Charlatanerie und übles Bezeigen vieler gewinnsüchtiger Apothecker gegen den Krancken, dargestellet und entworffen wird. 56 pp. 4°. *Franckfurt u. Leipzig,* 1738.

Menis (W. [Gulielmo?]) [1793–]. Saggio di topografia statistico-medica della provincia di Brescia aggiuntevi le notizie storico-statistiche sul cholera epidemico che la desolò nell' anno 1836 dell' I. R. medico provinciale. 2 v. in 1. vii, 9–327, 311 pp. 8°. *Brescia, tipog. della Minerva,* 1837.

Menispermum.

See, also, **Cocculus** *indicus.*

BLOTTIÈRE (R.) *Étude anatomique de la famille des ménispermées. 4°. Paris,* 1886. MAURIN (E.-H.-A.) * Sur la famille des ménispermées. 4°. *Strasbourg,* 1863. **Lacalle** (J.) Nota sobre las propiedades terapéuticas del menispermum rimosum. Gac. de sanid. mil., Madrid, 1877, iii, 258-260.—**Planat** (F.) Des propriétés de la ménispermine. Nice-méd.. 1878-9, iii, 303-308. — **Ram Comol Shen.** Remarks on the native drug called Gulancha. Tr. M. & Phys. Soc. Calcutta, 1826-7, iii, 295-299.

Ménissier (E.-D.) *Considérations générales sur quelques maladies qui affectent les femmes à l'âge critique. 27 pp. 4°. *Paris,* 1808, No. 62, v. 70.

Menissier (Pierre). * Sur l'inflammation en général. 22 pp. 4°. *Paris,* 1815, No. 130, v. 111.

Menjaud (Albert - Louis) [1830-66]. * De la rétraction spontanée et progressive des doigts dans ses rapports avec la goutte et le rhumatisme goutteux. 31 pp. 4°. *Paris,* 1861, No. 148. *See, also,* **Béhier** (Louis-Jules). Conférences de clinique médicale [etc.] 8°. *Paris,* 1864. *For Biography, see* Gaz. hebd. de méd., Par., 1866, 2. s., iii, 288.

Menjot (Antoine) [1615–96]. Febrium malignarum historia et curatio. Accesserunt dissertationes pathologicæ. 322 pp., 2 l. 8°. *Parisiis, G. Meturas,* 1660.

——. The same. Item dissertationes pathologicæ. Editio altera . . . selectisque aliquot dissertationibus . . . adaucta. 3 p. l., 245 pp., 1 l. 4°. *Parisiis, T. Jolly,* 1662.

——. The same. In duas partes divisæ, quarum prior tertium jam editur, sed emendatior multaque commentatione ac meditatione locupletior. Altera nunc primum in lucem prodit. 11 p. l., 775 pp. 4°. *Parisiis, Cramoisy,* 1665. With autograph note of the author, presenting the work to Melchior Sebizius.

Menke (Carolus Theodorus) [–1861]. * De leguminibus veterum. Part. prima. 32 pp. 4°. *Gottingæ, H. Dieterich,* 1814.

——. De nova morbos chronicos ope pastus taraxacini curandi ratione. 13 pp. 4°. *Pyrmonti,* [1833].

Menke (Carolus Theodorus)—continued.

——. Pyrmont und seine Umgebungen, mit besonderer Hinsicht auf seine Mineralquellen; historisch, geographisch, physikalisch und medicinisch. 2. Ausg. xxii, 448 pp., 1 pl., 1 map. 8°. *Pyrmont, G. Uslar,* 1840. *See, also,* **Trampel** (Joh. Erh.) Wie erhält man sein Gehör gut, [etc.] 8°. *Hannover,* 1822.

Menke (Gustav). * Ueber das chronische Magengeschwür. 29 pp. 8°. *Marburg, C. L. Pfeil,* 1862. C.

Menke (Jos. Christoph). * Ueber den Durchbruch des Empyem in die Lunge. 20 pp. 8°. *Würzburg, F. X. Bucher,* 1882.

Menn (Joannes Georgius). Harmonia, subsidia, nexus, et affinitas theorematum medicorum cum disciplinis altioribus demonstrata a Petro Wilhelmo Josepho de Ginetti, Joanne Wilhelmo Heis, Matthia Josepho Meyer, Francisco Stephano Schuirmann Agrippinatibus medicinæ licentiatis. Curante Joanne Georgio Menn. 52 pp. 4°. [*Coloniæ*], *typ. academicis,* [1779].

Menne (Ferdinand). * Ueber Hodgkin'sche Krankheit. 48 pp. 8°. *Würzburg, Becker,* 1878.

Menne (Ferdinandus). * De vomitoriorum effectu et usu medico. 28 pp., 1 l. 4°. *Gottingæ, scriptis Barmerianis,* [1802].

Menne (Janus Hermanus). * De tuberculosi renum. [Leyden.] 2 p. l., 48 pp. 8°. *Amstelodami, Ipenbuur et van Seldam,* 1855.

Mennecy. *Bureau de bienfaisance de Mennecy.* Compte-rendu médico-moral du service de santé du 29 août 1843 au 31 octobre 1845; par Eug. Danzanvilliers. 96 pp. 8°. *Corbeil,* 1846.

Mennehand (Lucien). * De la cautérisation actuelle. 47 pp. 4°. *Strasbourg,* 1868, 3. s., No. 93.

Mennehand (Paul-Henri). * De l'examen chimique des urines. 32 pp. 4°. *Strasbourg,* 1859, No. 502, 2. s., v. 27.

Mennens (Guilielmus) [1525–]. Aurei velleris, sive sacræ philosophiæ vatum selectæ et unicæ, mysteriorumque Dei, naturæ, et artis admirabilium libri tres. *In:* THEATRUM chemicum. 12°. *Argentorati,* 1660, v, 240-428.

Mennesson-l'Héritier (Alfred). * De la métrite aiguë simple. 32 pp. 4°. *Paris,* 1853, No. 130.

Mennicke (Gustav Adolph). * Ueber Angina membranacea. 29 pp, 1 l. 8°. *Halle, W. Plötz,* 1868. C.

Mennicke (Robert). * Vergleichende Versuche über die Wirksamkeit verschiedener Aconitinpräparate. 34 pp., 1 l. 8°. *Halle a. S., Plötz,* 1883.

Mennus (Joh. Henricus). Guldiner Apffel. Von dem Goldbaum dess irrdischen Lebens decerpiret, durch welches Anatomi die geheime und verborgne Universal Medicin, sampt anderen hierzu nöttigen Wissenschafften geoffenbahret. 60 l. 24°. *Tübingen, J. C. Geyssler,* 1635. *Bound with:* JONSTON (Joh.) Idea hygieines recensita. Libri ii. 24°. *Jenæ,* 1661.

Menobranchus.

van der Hoeven (J.) Les globules du sang du menobranchus. Arch. néerl. d. sc. exactes, etc., La Haye, 1867, ii, 288.

Menocal (Francisco de S.) *Du croup des adultes. 50 pp. 4°. *Paris,* 1859, No. 88, v. 634.

Menon (Dominique). L'école de Salerne. Traduite de latin en françois. Où chacun trouvera, conformément à ses humeurs, la manière de vivre, et se conserver long-temps dans une bonne et parfaite santé. 24 pp. 12°. *La Haye, A. Moetjens,* 1695. *Bound with:* HARVEY (G.) Ars curandi morbos expectatione, etc. 12°. *Amstelodami,* 1695.

Menon (Jean-Jacques-Clément). * Sur l'iode, et son emploi en médecine. 26 pp. 4°. *Paris,* 1827, No. 287, v. 212.

Menon (V.) * Sur le spasme de la vessie et de l'urètre. 23 pp. 4°. *Paris,* 1829, No. 79, v. 223.

Menopause.

See **Menstruation** (*Cessation of*).

Menorrhagia.

See, also, **Hemorrhage** (*Uterine*).

APELBAUM (P.) * Menorrhagiæ erroneæ casus singularis. sm. 4°. *Lundæ,* [1781].

ASSELINEAU (B. - A. - A.) * Sur la ménorrhagie, ou flux immodéré des règles. 4°. *Paris,* 1808.

AUSSANDON (J.) * Sur la ménorrhagie. 4°. *Paris,* 1806.

BILLING (J. H. F.) * Menorrhagia seu uteri hæmorrhagia. 4°. *Wirceburgi,* [1799].

BILLOT (J.-A.-E.) * Sur la ménorrhagie, ou le flux immodéré des règles. 4°. *Paris, an XII* [1804].

BOTTLER (J. E.) * De metrorrhagia. 8°. *Monachii,* 1836.

BRISEZ (N.-L.) * Sur la ménorrhagie. 4°. *Paris,* 1813.

BURGERS (H.-J.) * Sur la ménorrhagie. 4°. *Paris,* 1815.

DALY (D.) * De menorrhagia in non gravidis nec puerperis. 8°. *Edinburgi,* 1774.

DUHEM (J.) * Sur la ménorrhagie. 4°. *Paris,* 1819.

DUVERNOY (C.-L.-A.) * Essai sur la ménorrhagie, ou flux immodéré des menstrues. 4°. *Strasbourg,* 1829.

DUVIGNEAUD (J.-B.-C.) * Sur la ménorrhagie, précédée de quelques considérations générales sur la menstruation. 4°. *Paris,* 1808.

ERICH (F. J.) * De mensium fluxu immodico. 4°. *Jenæ,* [1688].

FEILD (R.) * De menorrhagia. 8°. *Edinburgi,* 1790.

FOERTSCH (C. J.) * De fluxu menstruorum nimio. 8°. *Gottingæ,* [1793].

FORRESTER (R.) * De menorrhagia. 8°. *Edinburgi,* 1795.

GRIEFSMAYR (P.) * De catameniorum excessu ejusque cura. 12°. *Viennæ,* 1817.

HARDER (K.) * Ein Fall von menstrueller Verblutung. 8°. *Kiel,* 1885.

HOMMEY (H.) * De l'intervention chirurgicale dans la ménorrhagie grave. 4°. *Paris,* 1865.

KMETI (P.) * De hæmorrhagia uteri non gravidi. 8°. *Pestini,* 1829.

LABERNARDIE (L.) * Sur la ménorrhagie active. 4°. *Paris,* 1811.

LEFRANC (J.-B.) * Sur la ménorrhagie. 4°. *Paris,* 1818.

LENTSCH (D.) * De fluxu mensium nimio. 4°. *Vitembergæ,* [1704].

MÂCÉ (A.-A.) * Sur la ménorrhagie, précédée de considérations générales sur l'utérus et la menstruation. 4°. *Paris,* 1817.

NEUMANN (S.) * De fluxu mensium immodico. 4°. *Jenæ,* 1746.

PERONNEAU (R.) * De menstruorum profluvio immodico. 8°. *Edinburgi,* 1775.

PFENNIGKAUFFER (F.) * De fluxus menstrualis anomaliis per excessum. 8°. *Marburgi,* 1822.

PHENÈ (P.) * De mensium abundantia. 8°. *Edinburgi,* 1802.

PIN (P.) * Étude sur la ménorrhagie au point de vue pathogénique et thérapeutique. 4°. *Montpellier,* 1866.

POTHEAU (A.) * Étude sur la valeur séméiologique de la ménorrhagie, ou exagération du flux menstruel. 4°. *Paris,* 1873.

——. The same. 8°. *Paris,* 1873.

Menorrhagia.

SAYERS (A.) * De menorrhagia. 8°. *Edinburgi,* 1782.

SJÖBORG (A. M.) * De menorrhagia rubra. 4°. *Lundæ,* [1794].

SUCHET (L.) * Sur la ménorrhagie, ou flux immodéré des menstrues. 4°. *Paris,* 1813.

TABOURIER (A.-P.) * Sur la ménorrhagie. 4°. *Paris,* 1818.

WILL (C. A.) * De diagnosi et cura menorrhagiæ. 8°. *Regiomonti Pr.,* [1738].

WURSTSCHMIDT (J. O.) * Hæmorrhagiæ uteri menstruæ prænaturalis, θεωρίαν καὶ θεράπειαν . . . exhibet. 4°. *Jenæ,* 1770.

Andrews (R. H.) Sulphate of bebeeria in the treatment of menorrhagia. Tr. M. Soc. Penn., Phila., 1877, xi, pt. 2, 662.—**Atthill** (L.) On some forms of menorrhagia. Dublin Q. J. M. Sc., 1871, lii, 497-502. *Also:* Brit M. J., Lond., 1871, i, 666-668.—**Aulde** (J.) Rational treatment of menorrhagia. Med. & Surg. Reporter, Phila., 1883, xlviii, 59-62.—**Barker** (B. F.) Climacteric menorrhagia. *Ibid.,* 1867, xvi, 1.—**Battey** (R.) Cinchona in menorrhagia. Atlanta M. & S. J., 1858-9, iv, 734.—**Bernutz.** De la ménorrhagie. Rev. de thérap. méd.-chir., Par., 1880, xlvii, 57; 85.—**Bertrand.** Ein Fall von fulminanter Erblindung nach Menorrhagie. Deutsche Ztschr. f. prakt. Med., Leipz., 1878, 160.—**Black** (J. R.) Bromide of ammonium in catamenial excesses. Cincin. Lancet & Obs., 1874, xvii, 265-267.——. Bromide of ammonia in too frequent menstruation. Ohio M. Recorder, Columbus, 1879, iii, 398.—**Brambilla** (G.) La coprostasi è causa di menorragia. Guglielmo da Saliceto, Piacenza, 1884, vi, 88-91.—**Breslau** (B.) Aeusserst hartnäckige Menorrhagie bei vollständig retroflectirtem Uterus, geheilt durch Einspritzung von Liquor ferri sesquichlorati in die Uterinhöhle. Monatschr. f. Geburtsk. u. Frauenkr., Berl., 1857, x, 274-277.—**Brewer** (W. P.) Menorrhagia treated by plugging the uterus. N. Orl. M. & S. J., 1879-80, vii, 778.—**Brown** (A. S.) Case of menorrhagia successfully treated with cathartics. Transylv. J. M., Lexington, Ky., 1828, i, 556-559.—**Brown** (J.) Cannabis indica; a valuable remedy in menorrhagia. Brit. M. J., Lond., 1883, i, 1002.—**Campä.** De las menorragias sintomáticas de las alteraciones cardíacas. Crón. méd., Valencia, 1879-80, iii, 7-11.—**Carstens** (J. H.) Menorrhagia and metrorrhagia. Obst. Gaz., Cincin., 1882, v, 393-399. *Also, transl.:* Rev. méd.-chir. d. mal. d. femmes, Par., 1882, iv, 680-688.— [**Case.**] Ménorrhagie causée par un polype. Rev. d. hôp. civ. de Metz, 1852, 56-59.—**Chapman** (J.) Menorrhagia and menorrhagic pain treated successfully by the spinal hot-water bag. Med. Mirror, Lond., 1867, iv, 6-9.—**Chapman** (N.) A lecture on menorrhagia. Med. Exam., Phila., 1839, ii, 197; 213.—**Cleveland** (J. L.) The influence of malaria in some cases of metrorrhagia and menorrhagia. Clinic, Cincin., 1876, xi, 217-219.—**Copland** (P.) An account of the good effects of opium, administered in clysters in cases of menorrhagia. Med. Facts & Obs., Lond., 1793, iv, 118-125.—**Crooks** (J.) Creasote in menorrhagia. West. J. M. & S., Louisville, 1853, 3. s., xi, 279-281.—**Crooks** (W. C.) On the application of ice to the spine in menorrhagia or excessive menstruation. Med. & Surg. Reporter, Phila., 1868, xix, 141-144.—**Curran** (J. W.) On menorrhagia. Med. Mirror, Lond., 1870, vii, 4-6.—**Davies** (J. B.) Remarks on menorrhœa, with cases. Stethoscope & Virg. M. Gaz., Richmond, 1851, i. 142-144.—**Ditterich.** Zur Behandlung des übermässigen Monatsflusses. N. med.-chir. Ztg., München, 1845, n. F., iii, 1-4.—**Drysdale** (C.) Menorrhagia treated by sea-tangle tents. Med. Press & Circ., Lond., 1872, xiv, 320.—**Duncan** (J. M.) On simple menorrhagia. Edinb. M. J., 1872, xvii, 769-776. ——. Clinical lecture on menorrhagia. Med. Times & Gaz., Lond., 1880, ii, 145-147.—**Dutcher** (A. P.) Menorrhagia; a case of three years' standing, cured with Trillium pendulum (bethroot) and Scutellaria laterifolia (scullcap). Cincin. Lancet & Obs., 1858, n. s., i, 411-413.—**East** (L. A.) Viburnum prunifolium in menorrhagia. Louisville M. News, 1879, viii, 56.—**Edis** (A. W.) Menorrhagia; granular os and cervix; utero-gestation. Lancet, Lond., 1874, ii, 761. ——. Cases illustrating the diagnosis and treatment of menorrhagia. Brit. M. J., Lond., 1877, ii, 763. ——. The rational treatment of menorrhagia. *Ibid.,* 1882, ii, 409-411. ——. Cases of menorrhagia. Lancet, Lond., 1882, i, 862. ——. On exploration of the uterine cavity in cases of menorrhagia. Brit. M. J., Lond., 1886, i, 115.—**Elmer** (G. E.) † N. Orl. M. Times, 1861, n. s., i, 109.—**Faulcon** (E. W.) Oxide of silver in menorrhagia. Stethoscope & Virg. M. Gaz., Richmond, 1854, iv, 333.—**Fenner** (E. D.) Menorrhagia; extraordinary case; singular mode of recovery. N. Orl. M. News & Hosp. Gaz., 1857-8, iv, 388-390.—**Fifield.** Menorrhagia, with symptoms of purpura; death. Boston M. & S. J., 1872, lxxxvi, 350.—**Gaston** (J. McF.) Treatment of menorrhagia with ergot. Charleston M. J., 1857, xii, 459-466.—**Guthrie** (W. B.) Menorrhagia. Cincin. Lancet & Obs., 1871, n. s., xiv,

Menorrhagia.

322–325.—**Haus.** Einige Worte über heilsame und die nachtheilige Wirkung der Stahlquellen bei den verschiedenen Arten von Gebärmutterblutflüssen. Gem. deutsche Ztschr. f. Geburtsk., Weimar, 1830, v, 400–409.—**Hewitt** (G.) Ergot of rye in menorrhagia. Lancet, Lond., 1862, ii, 646.—**Hicks** (J. B.) Menorrhagia ten months; dilatation of cervix uteri; discovery of polypus; removal; recovery. Med. Times & Gaz., Lond., 1863, i, 109.—**Hime** (T. W.) Transfusion in profuse menorrhagia. Brit. M. J., Lond., 1881, ii, 153.—**Kinney** (H. W.) Menorrhagia produced by mental disturbance; two cases. Detroit Lancet, 1884–5, n. s., viii, 445.—**Lall** (R.) Ergot of rye and Indian hemp in obstinate cases of menorrhagia. Indian M. Gaz., Calcutta, 1866, i, 256.—**Lanyon** (R.) On the utility of the secale cornutum in menorrhagia rubra. Lancet, Lond., 1828–9, ii, 56; 551.—**Lever** (J.C.W.) Menorrhagia. Guy's Hosp. Rep., Lond., 1846, 2. s., iv, 181.—**Locock** (C.) Menorrhagia. Cycl. Pract. M. (Tweedie), Phila., 1845, iii, 303–308.—**Maclure** (W.) Menorrhagia. In his: Collect. Med.-Chir. [etc.], 8°, Lond., 1845, 137–143.—**Malgaigne.** Perte utérine continue et rebelle arrêtée immédiatement par l'abrasion de la surface interne de l'utérus. Rev. méd.-chir. de Par., 1850, vii, 367.—**Mann** (J.) Observations upon menorrhagia and leucorrhœa; and the beneficial employment of blisters, acetate of lead, and the submuriate of mercury in those diseases. Med. Communicat. Mass. M. Soc. 1809–10, Bost., 1813, ii, 274–282.—**Mantle** (A.) The occurrence of menorrhagia or metrorrhagia during the febrile state. Lancet, Lond., 1887, i, 1227–1229.—**Massie** (W.) A case of menorrhagia and treatment. West. J. M., Indianap., 1868, iii, 144–151.—**Massy** (T.) Excessive hæmorrhage during the catamenia. Med. Times, Lond., 1849, xix, 287.—**Meadows** (A.) On ovarian menorrhagia. Brit. M. J., Lond., 1879, ii, 45–47.—**Menorrhagia.** Lancet, Lond., 1867, i, 602.—**Menorrhagia.** Med. & Surg. Reporter, Phila., 1868, xviii, 494–496.—**Merrill** (A. P.) The sulphate of bebeerine in menorrhagia. Memphis M. Recorder, 1856, iv, 88–90.—**Mettauer** (J. P.) Practical observations on menorrhagia, with report of a case of this disease connected with malposition of the uterus, and adhesion of its cervix and os tincæ to the corresponding portions of the vagina. Am. J. M. Sc., Phila., 1842, n. s., iii, 298–306.—**de Meza** jun. De menorrhagia chronica ope radicis ipecacuanhæ sedata. Acta Soc. med. Havn., 1791, ii, 32–34.—**Michelotti** (P. A.) Von einer zu starken monatlichen Reinigung, die durch Umschläge von kaltem Wasser und Essig gehoben wurde. N. Samml. d. auserl. u. n. Abhandl. f. Wundärzte, Leipz., 1783, 3. St., 234–238.—**Mitchell** (T. R.) On the treatment of menorrhagia with Indian hemp. Dublin M. Press, 1847, xviii, 214.—**Moyer** (E. C.) A case of menorrhagia and treatment. Atlanta M. & S J., 1857–8, iii, 16.—**Neumann.** Höchst seltner Fall eines schnellen Todes von innerer Verblutung im Unterleibe ohne Zerreissung, durch unterdrückte monatliche Reinigung. J. d. pract. Heilk., Berl., 1821, lii, 2. St., 114–116.—**Ogden** (W. W.) Menorrhagia, with its treatment by bromide of amonium. Dominion M. J., Toronto, 1869–70, ii, 181–184.—**Osborne** (J.) Observations on the use of emetics of ipecacuan in menorrhagia. Tr. Ass. King's & Queen's Coll. Phys. Ireland, Dubl., 1828, v, 18–27.—**Osiander** (F. B.) Beobachtung des Hervorfliessens des Menstruation-Blutes. Ann. d. Entbind.-Lehranst. a. d. Univ. zu Götting., 1800, i, 1. St., 174–176.—**Pallen** (M. A.) Menorrhagia caused by subinvolution of the uterus after delivery. St. Louis M. Reporter, 1867–8, ii, 225–229.—**Parker** (H.) Fatal menorrhagia. Boston M. & S. J., 1840, xxii, 127.—**Payne** (J. B.) On the use of sulphate of bebeerine in menorrhagia. Memphis M. Recorder, 1856, iv, 346.—**Pulido** (A.) Un caso notable de menorragia. An. Soc. ginec. españ., Madrid, 1877, iii, 112–118.—**Raciborski.** Nouvelles considérations pratiques sur la ménorrhagie et ses rapports avec l'hématocèle péri-utérine. Congrès méd. de France, Par., 1863, i, 124–133.——. De la ménorrhagie et de son traitement. Rev. de thérap. méd.-chir., Par., 1864, 146–148.—**Regius** (H.) Medicatio fœminæ, superfluis mensibus laborantis. In his: Medicinæ libri iv, 2. ed., 4°, Traj. ad Rhenum, 1657, 609–611.—**Rigby** (E.) Reports on uterine diseases. [Observations on menorrhagia.] Med. Times, Lond., 1844, x, 505; 547. Continued in: Med. Times & Gaz., Lond., 1852, n. s., v, 410; 508; 588: 1853, n. s., vi, 33: 1854, n. s., ix, 29; 53; 207; 313; 385; 437; 538.—**Ritter** (H. B.) On the treatment of menorrhagia. Med. Herald, Louisville, 1884–5, vi, 337–341.—**Roché.** Ménorrhagie promptement mortelle, survenue à la troisième menstruation, dans l'état de vacuité de l'utérus, chez une jeune fille de 17 ans, au milieu de la santé la plus florissante. Gaz. d. hôp., Par., 1861, xxxiv, 328.—**Routh** (C. H. F.) Three cases of menorrhagia, two of them depending upon the presence of uterine polypi, successfully treated. Lancet, Lond., 1858, i, 503.——. Four cases of menorrhagia treated by injection, or the removal of the uterine mucous membrane by the gouge, or both means combined. Tr. Obst. Soc. Lond., 1860, ii, 117–134. Also [Abstr.]: Lancet, Lond., 1860, i, 397–399.—**Sarubbi.** Menorragia grave guarita con l' ergotina. Rendic. Accad. med.-chir. di Napoli, 1856, x, 74.—**Savage** (H. N.) On obstinate menorrhagia. Lancet,

Menorrhagia.

Lond., 1857, ii, 570.—**Schott** (A.) Menorrhagieen und chronische Hyperämieen des Uteruskörpers. Samml. klin. Vortr., No. 161, Leipz., 1879 (Gynäkol., No. 47), 1241–1272.—**Silver** (A.) On the value of Indian hemp in mennorrhagia and dysmenorrhœa. Med. Times & Gaz., Lond., 1870, ii, 59–61.—**Smith** (W. R.) Case of menorrhagia, with complications. Nashville J. M. & S., 1859, xvi, 392–397.—**Southworth** (J. W.) Apyretic malarial menorrhagia. Buffalo M. & S. J., 1871–2, xi, 174–177.—**Stevens** (A. D.) A severe case of menorrhagia. Med. Chron., Montreal, 1858, v, 205–207.—**Strother** (C. S.) Carbolic acid in metrorrhagia and menorrhagia. Atlanta M. & S. J., 1872–3, x, 446–448.—**Sutphin** (P. C.) Case of obstinate menorrhagia, successfully treated with injections of acetate of lead. Stethoscope, Richmond, 1855, v, 669–671.—**Tanner** (T. H.) On the use of cinnamon in certain examples of menorrhagia. Lancet, Lond., 1853, ii, 363.—**Thomas** (T. G.) † Am. J. Obst., N. Y., 1872, v, 465–467.——. Menorrhagia and metrorrhagia. Med. Rec., N. Y., 1874, ix, 395–398.—**Thweatt** (J. J.) On the use of the oxide of silver in certain forms of menorrhagia, with cases and remarks. Am. J. M. Sc., Phila., 1849, n. s., xviii, 69–72. Also, transl.: Rev. méd.-chir. de Par., 1850, viii, 17–21. Also: Gaz. d. hôp., Par., 1850, 3. s., ii, 349.—**Tott** (C. A.) Bemerkungen über die mit hysterischen Affectionen verbundenen Blutungen aus dem Uterus im Alter der Decrepidität, nebst Mittheilung eines Falls von Catamenialfluss auf ungewöhnlichem Wege. J. f. Geburtsh., Leipz., 1835, xiv, 105–118.—**Trousseau.** De la digitale à haute dose dans la ménorrhagie. Gaz. d. hôp., Par., 1860, xxxiii, 597.—**Valcárcel Vargas** (L.) Dilatación del cuello uterino en el tratamiento de las menorragias. Correo méd. castellano, Salamanca, 1886, iii, 20–24.—**Valeur** (De la) du chanvre indien dans le traitement de la ménorrhagie et la dysménorrhée. Bull. gén. de thérap., etc., Par., 1870, lxxix, 417–422.—**Vercelli** (M.) Tre casi di menorragia trattati colla divisione del collo dell' utero. [3 cases.] [From: Osservatore, Torino, sett. 1866.] Gazz. med. ital., prov. venete, Padova, 1866, ix, 325–328.—**Vogelsang.** Menorrhagie mit letalem Ausgang. Memorabilien, Heilbr., 1876, xxi, 447–451.—**Waldenström** (J. A.) Om behandlingen af för ymniga menses. Upsala Läkaref. Förh., 1876–7, xii, 435–452.—**Westmoreland** (J. G.) [Carbolic acid in the treatment of menorrhagia.] Atlanta M. & S. J., 1871–2, ix, 330–333.—**Wooster** (D.) Chromic acid in the treatment of menorrhagia and uterine leucorrhœa. Am. J. M. Sc., Phila., 1869, n. s., lviii, 367–370.—**Zuccari** (G.) Cenno sull' efficacia dell' ossisetonato depurato di potassa (nitro V. S.) nella cura della menorragia. Ann. univ. di med., Milano, 1824, xxix, 270–277.

Menou. *Étude critique sur le traitement de la fièvre typhoïde par l'acide phénique. 56 pp. 4°. Paris, 1884, No. 183.

de Menou (Georges-Louis-Auguste). *I. Faire l'histoire de l'anasarque idiopathique. II. [etc.] 23 pp. 4°. Paris, 1842, No. 65, v. 387.

Menouillard (L.) *I. Faire connaître les causes, la marche et les symptômes de la mentagre. II. [etc.] 33 pp. 4°. Paris, 1840, No. 274, v. 363.

Menradus de Vorwaltnern. See de Vorwaltnern.

Mens (Joachimus Guilelmus Sigismundus) [1795–]. *Disquisitio ætiologica in morbum articularem. iv, 38 pp., 1 l. 8°. Berolini, A. Petsch, 1818.

Mensa philosophica. In hoc opusculo tractatur de his quibus utimur in mensa. De naturis rerum, videlicet cibi et potus. De questionibus mensalibus variis ac jocundis quibus in mensa recreamur, deque conditionibus eorum quibus in mensa conversamur phylosophice hilariterque procedit; quare merito appellatur: Mensa philosophica. 51 l. 4°. Colonie, [1500].
Bound with: MAGNINUS Mediolanensis. Regimen sanitatis. 4°. Argentine, 1503.

van der Mensbrugghe (G.) Notice sur J.-A.-F. Plateau. 98 pp., 1 pl. 12°. Bruxelles, F. Hayez, 1884.
Repr. from: Ann. Acad. roy. d. sc. de Belg., Brux., 1885.

Mensch (Der) und der Parasit. Ein fliegendes Blatt für Aerzte und Naturforscher beider Hemisphären von Dr. Supinator Longus. 2. Aufl. vii, 12 pp. 12°. Magdeburg, R. Kretschmann, 1863.
——. The same. 4. ed. 33 pp. 8°. Magdeburg, Kretschmann u. Koltzsch, 1872.

Mensching (August. Ludov.) * De regulis generalioribus in morborum curationibus ubique observandis. 1 p. l., 28 pp. 4°. *Gottingæ, J. C. Dieterich*, [1777].

Mensching (Fridericus David. Wilhelm.) * De operationibus quibusdam chirurgicis temere institutis. 24 pp. sm. 4°. *Rostochii, lit. Adlerianis*, [1756].

Mensching (Joann. Henricus). * De aëris fixi ac dephlogisticati in medicina usu. 1 p. l., 106 pp., 1 l. 12°. *Gottingæ, J. A. Barmeier*, [1787].

Mensert (Henricus Marinus). * De diabete. [Leyden.] 4 p. l., 64 pp., 2 l. 8°. *Amstelodami, C. G. van der Post*, 1841.

Mensert (Wilhelm) [1780–1848]. Verhandeling over de keratonyxis (punctio corneæ, horenvlies-steek). Eene onlangs uitgevondene kunstbewerking, om de blindheid, welke door de cataract ontstaat, te genezen; benevens eenige genomene proeven en waarnemingen aangaande deze nieuwe methode. 1 p. l., viii, 208 pp. 8°. *Amsterdam, L. van Es*, 1816.

———. Geschiedkundige verhandeling over de operatie tot vorming van een kunstigen oogappel (pupilla artificialis), benevens de beschrijving eener nieuwe en zekerder manier, om dezelve door eene tweevoudige of dubble schaar te bewerkstelligen. viii, 56 pp., 2 pl. 8°. *Amsterdam, L. van Es*, 1828.

———. Verhandeling aangaande de uitvinding, het gebruik en het misbruik der brillen, benevens algemeene aanwijzingen, om eenen bril te kiezen, en wat men vooral bij het gebruik van denzelven heeft in acht te nemen. xiv, 199 pp. 8°. *Amsterdam, G. Portielje*, 1831.

———. The same. Nieuwe uitgave. xvi, 199 pp. 8°. *Amsterdam, G. Portielje*, 1846.

———. Wees toch voorzigtig met de oogen, en doe er niet te veel aan! Eene raadgevende waarschuwing, tot behoud en bewaring van het gezigt. xvi, 68 pp., 2 l. 8°. *Amsterdam, S. de Grebber*, 1842.

———. Betoog ter overweging, aangaande eene voorgestelde geheele vereeniging, zoowel als van het doelmatige van de bestaande scheiding, doch slechts in de beoefening der bijzondere vakken van genees- en heelkunst. 34 pp. 8°. *Amsterdam, C. G. Sulpke*, 1842. [P., v. 766.]

———. Beschouwingen en mededeelingen betreffende de oogheelkunde benevens een overzigt aangaande de inrigtingen van onderwijs, met betrekking tot de oogheelkunde in Duitschland, vertaald volgens Beger en met aanmerkingen vermeerderd. xii, 95 pp., 3 pl., 1 l. 8°. *Utrecht, N. van der Monde*, 1843.

———. Hoe men het gezigt, het edelste zintuig van den mensch, het beste tegen de dikwerf ongepaste aanwending van den bril, behoeden en bewaren kan; medegedeeld in eene rede, bij gelegenheid van eene nieuwe uitgave der Verhandeling aangaande de uitvinding, het gebruik en het misbruik der brillen. 18 pp. 8°. *Amsterdam, G. Portielje*, 1846.

Menses (*Retention of*).

See, also, **Hymen** (*Imperforate*); **Vagina** (*Abnormities of*).

BREIDENBACH (E.) * De retentione mensium commentatio, inprimis respiciens ad hæmatometram unius lateris in utero et vagina duplici. 8°. *Bonnæ*, 1866.

DEREUX (A.) * Des accidents consécutifs à l'opération dans les cas de rétention menstruelle. 4°. *Paris*, 1886.

DIETERICI (J. T.) * De tumoribus singularibus a mensium suppressione obortis. 4°. *Vitembergæ*, [1758].

Menses (*Retention of*).

GANSEL (E.) * De hæmatometra ex atresia vaginæ hymenaica orta ejusque operatione. 8°. *Vratislaviæ*, [1864].

HEILBUT (M. S.) * De atresia vaginæ, adjectis duobus casibus atresiæ vaginalis, et analysi chemica sanguinis menstrui ex atresia vaginæ retenti. 4°. *Heidelbergæ*, 1832.

HELENIUS (H. G.) * De retentione mensium. 4°. *Jenæ*, [1736].

HESS (F.) * De hymene clauso, adjunctis de sanguine menstruali retento disquisitionibus. 8°. [*Dorpat*], 1854.

LABADIE DE LALANDE (J.-B.-C.-O.) * De l'occlusion complète du conduit vulvo utérin, et de ses rapports avec la menstruation. 4°. *Paris*, 1856.

MELCHIORI (G.) Ritenzione del sangue mestruo per atresia della vagina; lettera al dottore Agostino Bertani. 8°. *Milano*, 1855.

OSANN (H. W.) * Tributum lunare in virgine retentum. 4°. *Erfordiæ*, [1701].

SALNEUVE (G.-H.-A.) * Essai sur l'ischoménie, ou rétention des menstrues. 4°. *Strasbourg*, 1823.

SMIBERT (W.) * De menstruis retentis. 8°. *Edinburgi*, 1762.

A. (F.) Retencion de meses, producida por el himen imperforado. Gac. méd., Madrid, 1849, v, 74.—**Appley** (W. L.) Obstruction of the vagina, with retention of the menstrual fluid for two years. Med. & Surg. Reporter, Phila., 1870, xxiii, 93.—**Ashwell.** Case of adhesion between the walls of the vagina, occasioning retention of the catamenia. Guy's Hosp. Rep., Lond., 1837, ii, 244–247.—**Bailey** (D. F.) Case of retained menstruation with anomalous symptoms. South. M. & S. J., Augusta, 1838, ii, 93–96.—**Bauer** (A.) Hymen imperforatus: hæmatokolpos; hæmatometra. Wien. med. Wchnschr., 1877, xxvii, 101–103.—**Bayard** (W.) Hydrometra with absence of the vagina. Canada M. & S. J., Montreal, 1878, vi, 289–291.—**Becasseau** (C.) Imperforation du col de la matrice. Ann. Soc. d. sc. méd. et nat. de Brux., 1842, 59–63.—**Bedford** (G. S.) Retention of the menses with hæmatemesis in a girl 17 years of age. Nelson's North. Lancet, Plattsburg, N. Y., 1852–3, vi, 5.—**Bernutz** (G.) Mémoire sur les accidents produits par la rétention du flux menstruel. Arch. gén. de méd., Par., 1848, 4. s., xvii, 129; 433: xviii, 405: 1849, 4. s., xix, 186.—**Bertherand** (A.) Imperforation de l'hymen; accidents graves; incision; réocclusion de l'ouverture; guérison. Gaz. méd. de l'Algérie, Alger, 1874, xix, 139.—**Breinig** (P. B.) Retention of menses, for over three years and a half, from occlusion of os uteri, resulting from adhesive inflammation produced by severe and protracted labor. Tr. M. Soc. Penn., Phila., 1875, x, 703.—**Brincken** (G. T. L.) En fuldkomment imperviabel enorm stor Hymen, og derved fleeraarig forhindret Udløb af Menstrua. Eyr, Christiania, 1834, ix, 97–99.—**Brown** (I. B.) Case of retained menses from imperforate os uteri. Lancet, Lond., 1860, i, 465. ———. Case of retained menses, of two years' duration, caused by atresia vaginæ; puncture of the uterus by the rectum; recovery. Tr. Obst. Soc. Lond. (1862), 1863, iv, 21: (1863), 1864, v, 162. *Also* [Abstr.]: Lancet, Lond., 1862, i, 175.—**Byford** (W. H.) Occlusion with retention of menses. Med. Exam., Chicago, 1874, xv, 535–539. —**Cabaret** (F.-J.) Rétention des règles par imperforation du vagin. Rev. de thérap. méd.-chir., Par., 1854, ii, 340–342.—**Cabaret** (P.-J.) Ménaphragie déterminée par l'imperforation du vagin. J. Soc. de méd.-prat. de Montpel., 1847, xv, 97–103. —**Calvi** (P.) Atresia vaginale incompleta; raccolta di sangue mestruo nel cavo uterino, per antiversione; guarigione perfetta procurata la uscita per la via dell' intestino retto. Gazz. med. ital. lomb., Milano, 1851, 3. s., ii, 245.—**van Camp** (F.-L.) De rétention des règles par imperforation de la membrane hymen. Mém. Soc. de méd. d'Anvers, 1838–9, 17.—**Campbell** (W.) Case of emansio mensium from interception of the vagina by a preter-natural membrane. Edinb. J. M. Sc., 1826, i, 339–342.—**Caraigedue.** Observation sur une tumeur formée par le sang menstruel, et qui avait pour cause la réunion de la membrane dite de l'hymen. J. de méd., chir., pharm., etc., Par., 1803, vi, 420–422.—**Carter** (C. H.) Absence of the vagina; uterus distended by retained menstrual fluid; operation; recovery. Tr. Obst. Soc. Lond. (1880), 1881, xxii, 251–260.—**Carville.** Imperforation du vagin; aménorrhée; hématocèle considérable; opération; rupture des trompes; mort par péritonite latente. Bull. Soc. anat. de Par., 1867, xlii, 306–310.—[**Case.**] Uterus distended with menstrual blood; diagnosis of pregnancy. Med. & Surg. Reporter, Phila., 1876, xxxv, 209.—**de Castella.** Ein Fall von Retentio mensium in Folge von Atresie des Hymens.

Menses (*Retention of*).

Schweiz. Ztschr. f. Med., Chir. u. Geburtsh., Zürich, 1851, 140–144. *Also, transl.*: Gaz. méd. de Par., 1852, 3. s., vii, 295. — **Chapman** (W.) Case of retention of the catamenia for more than two years in a married woman. Tr. Obst. Soc. Lond., 1863, iv, 251 - 255. — **Chavériat** jeune. Imperforation de l'hymen; rétention du sang menstruel; opération; guérison. Gaz. méd. de Lyon, 1851, iii, 159–161. *Also*: Gaz. d. hôp., Par., 1851, 3. s., iii, 410.—**de Chégoin** (H.) Imperforation complète et congéniale de l'utérus, avec absence totale du col, et rétention des règles depuis dix-sept ans, déterminant des douleurs atroces; guérison par une ouverture pratiquée au corps de la matrice et entretenue pendant plusieurs mois. J. hebd. de méd., Par., 1830, vi, 49–55.—**Clarke** (W. M.) On the treatment of retention of the menses from occlusion of the vagina and uterus. Brit. M. J., Lond., 1865, ii, 655–658. — **Cock** (T. F.) Two cases of retention of the menses. N. York M. Times, 1855, iv, 342–346. — **Colvan** (J.) Case of imperforate hymen with retained menses, treated successfully. Lancet, Lond., 1832, i, 695.—**Copeman** (E.) On the treatment of imperforate hymen, with retained menstrual fluid. Tr. Obst. Soc. Lond. (1868), 1869, x, 246–263. *Also* [Abstr.]: Brit. M. J., Lond., 1869, i, 37. — **Coporandy.** Observation de rétention menstruelle par imperforation de l'hymen. Mém. et compt.-rend. Soc. d. sc. méd. de Lyon, 1863-4, iii, pt. 2, 14–18. *Also*: Gaz. méd. de Lyon, 1863, xv, 366 - 368. — **Craddock** (S.) Case of occluded vagina after delivery, with subsequent retention of the menses. Tr. Obst. Soc. Lond. (1871), 1872, xiii, 101.— **Craghead** (W. G.) Case of catamenial retention from imperforated hymen. Stethoscope, Richmond, 1855, v, 191–193. — **Curling.** Menstrual retention from imperforate hymen, with distension of one of the Fallopian tubes. Lancet, Lond., 1864, i, 381.—**Davis** (J. H.) Complete occlusion of the os uteri, with retention of the menses after difficult labour. Tr. Obst. Soc. Lond. (1862), 1863, iv, 91–96.—**Depaul.** Imperforation congéitale du vagin; dilatation considérable de ce conduit avec accumulation de liquide dans son intérieur; estomac situé à droite; rate réduite à un petit tubercule situé dans l'hypochondre droit. Compt. rend. Soc. de biol. 1857, Par., 1859, 2. s., iv, pt. 1, 46–48.—**Desmond** (L. E.) Case of retention of menses from imperforate hymen. Med. Times & Gaz., Lond., 1852, n. s., iv, 353.—**Després.** Rétention des règles dans l'utérus; tumeur ombilicale. Bull. et mém. Soc. de chir. de Par., 1886, n. s. xii. 39–44.—**Downes** (E.) Case of complete congenital occlusion of the os uteri; operation; recovery. Lancet, Lond., 1882, ii, 660. — **Duncan** (J. M.) Clinical lecture on retention of blood. Med. Times & Gaz., Lond., 1880, i, 1–3. ———. Retention of menses. *Ibid.*, 1883, ii, 733–735.—**Eastman** (J. A.) Case of suppression of the menses of ten months' duration, from imperforate os tincæ, complicated with retroversion. Cincin. Lancet & Obs., 1868, n. s., xi, 526. — **Elkington** (F.) Imperforate uterus; retained menses; uterus twice opened by a trocar. Prov. M. & S. J., Lond., 1850, 128.—[**Emmett** (T. A.)] Case of occluded vagina with retained menses; operation. N. York M. J., 1876, xxiii, 404. ———. Congenital absence, and accidental atresia of the vagina; mode of operating. Tr. Am. Gynec. Soc. 1877, Bost., 1878, ii, 437–478.—**Evans** (G. H.) Case of retained menses, with complete atresia of seven years' standing. Nashville J. M. & S., 1869, n. s., v, 16–18.—**Fletcher.** Menstrual fluid confined in the uterus by an imperforate hymen. Prov. M. & S. J., Lond., 1852, 274.—**Fleury.** Imperforation de l'hymen; accumulation de sang dans l'utérus; incision de la membrane; guérison prompte. Gaz. d. hôp., Par., 1864, xxxvii, 147. — **Frankenhäuser.** Ueber Retentionsgeschwülste bei gedoppelten innern Genitalien. Cor.-Bl. f. schweiz. Aerzte, Basel, 1882, xii, 517–522.—**Frerichs** (F. T.) Fälle von Retention des Menstrualblutes. Deutsche Klinik, Berl., 1851, iii, 528–530.—**Frisbie** (J. B. S.) Occlusion of the os uteri in a supposed case of pregnancy. Virginia M. J., Richmond, 1857, ix, 305–307.—**Furtado** (A. G.) Obliteração da vagina; retenção do producto catamenial por mais de sete annos; cura. J. Soc. d. sc. med. de Lisb., 1861, 2. s., xxv, 302–304.— **Galabin** (A. L.) Retention of menstrual fluid in one-half of a double uterus. Tr. Obst. Soc. Lond. (1882), 1883, xxiv, 21–28. *Also*: Brit. M. J., Lond., 1882, i, 344. *Also*: Lancet, Lond., 1882, i, 398. *Also*: Am. J. Obst., N. Y., 1882, xv (Suppl.), 132–134.—**Gantt** (W. H.) Imperforate hymen, presenting symptoms of pregnancy. Nashville J. M. & S., 1854, vi, 6–8. — **Gaudin.** Cloisonnement transversal du vagin; rétention des règles; mort par péritonite, par suite de perforation tubaire. Marseille méd., 1886, xxiii, 432–436. *Also* [Abstr.]: Gaz. de gynéc., Par., 1885-6, ii, 275.—**Genin.** Rétention des menstrues par imperforation de la membrane hymen; accusation d'infanticide. J. de méd. et chir. prat., Par., 1841, xii, 337–339. — **Gilbert** (F. D.) Observations on a case of retention of the menses. Med. Chron., Montreal, 1853-4, i, 286.—**Gillette.** Imperforation de l'hymen; accidents produits par la rétention du flux menstruel et ayant fait croire à un accouchement. Union méd., Par., 1874, xxviii, 120. — **Gimeno** (J.) Occlusion vaginal completa; retencion menstrual durante cuatros años; operacion. Clínica, Zaragoza, 1884, iv, 267.— **Greenhalgh.** Case of atresia of the vagina with reten-

Menses (*Retention of*).

tion of the catamenial fluid. Brit. M. J., Lond., 1874, i, 273.—**Griffin** (E.) A case of retained menstrual matter from occluded os. Atlanta M. & S. J., 1879-80, xvii, 65–67.—**Halbertsma** (T.) Atresia vaginæ met retentio mensium sedert 10 jaren; hæmatometra tot bijna een handbreed boven den navel, gecompliceerd met een tweede tumor (nitgezette tuba Fallopii); punctie met den troisquart explorateur; genezing. Nederl. Tijdschr. v. Geneesk., Amst., 1869, 2. R., v, 1. Afd., 541–544.—**Hamilton** (F. H.) Complete occlusion of the vagina and retention of menses, relieved by an operation through the rectum. Buffalo M. J., 1856-7, xii, 198.—**Hemman** (J. A.) Verhaltung der monatlichen Reinigung wegen Verschliessung der weiblichen Scheide, oder des innern Muttermundes. *In his*: Med.-chir. Aufsätze, [etc.], 8°, Berl., 1778, 41–83.— **Henson** (S.) Retention of the menses from imperforate hymen. Lancet, Lond., 1859, i, 402.—**Hicks** (B.) & **Galabin.** Case of complete occlusion of the vagina and retention of menses, consequent upon an abortion; relief by operation. Obst. J. Gr. Brit., Lond., 1875, iii, 507–509.— **Hicks** (J. B.) Retention of menses from imperforate hymen; operation: recovery. Med. Times & Gaz., Lond., 1861, ii, 163. — **Holdsworth.** Case of occlusion of the vagina following parturition, causing retention of menses; evacuation; cure. Lancet, Lond., 1883, i, 949. — **Hubbard** (T. W.) A case of imperforate hymen: confined secretion entirely fluid. Brit. M. J., Lond., 1877, ii, 292.— **Kennedy** (E.) Case of occlusion of vagina with retention; operation; ultimate rectal menstruation. Proc. Dubl. Obst. Soc., 1874, 10 - 21. — **Larrivé.** Occlusion vaginale consécutive à une parturition; rétention du flux menstruel, sans dilatation de la cavité utérine; opération. Lyon méd., 1880, xxxiv, 236–241. *Also*: Arch. de tocol., Par., 1881, viii, 112–116.—**Latta** (J. F.) Case of imperforate hymen, occasioning retention of the menstrual fluid; division of the membrane, etc. Med. Exam., Phila., 1839, ii, 677.—**Lawrence** (A. E. A.) Notes on a case of retained menstrual discharge. Tr. Bristol Med.-Chir. Soc., Lond., 1874-8, i, 98. *Also*: Obst. J. Gr. Brit., Lond., 1877, v, 108–112.— **Lee** (R.) Imperforate vagina: puncture; peritonitis. Brit. M. J., Lond., 1857, i, 126.— **Lees.** Retained menses from imperforate hymen. Dublin Hosp. Gaz., 1858, v, 345.—**Lees** (L. D.) Obstruction of the bowels from retention of the menses. Med. Times & Gaz., Lond., 1857, xiv, 347.—**Lever** (J. C. W.) Case of retained catamenia. Guy's Hosp. Rep., Lond., 1850–51, 2. s., vii, 150–154.—**Lewis** (E. S.) Case of retention of menstruation with regurgitation in left Fallopian tube. N. Orl. M. & S. J., 1880–81, n. s., viii, 1123–1126.—**Mackenzie** (F. M.) Imperforate hymen: retained menses: puncture; death from peritonitis Clin. Lect. & Rep. Lond. Hosp., 1867-8, iv, 306–308.—**Mallory** (J. B.) A case of occlusion of the vagina, with protracted retention of the catamenia. Richmond & Louisville M. J., 1870, x, 130 - 135.— **Mapleton** (R.) Singular case of imperforate vagina, and vicarious menstruation from the bladder (?) with uninterrupted regularity for 27 years. Lond. M Gaz., 1840, xxvi, 543.—**Marchand** & **Marcé.** Rétention du sang menstruel par imperforation congéniale du vagin; incision de la membrane obturatrice; expulsion d'une énorme quantité de sang; péritonite consécutive, occasionnée par un épanchement sanguin intra-péritonéal, provenant des trompes de Fallope. J. de la sect. de méd. Soc. acad. Loire-Inf., Nantes, 1850, n. s., xxvi, 335–353.—**Maxwell** (T. J.) Atresia vaginæ with retention of the menses. Chicago M. J. & Exam., 1877, xxxv, 269–271.—**Melchiori** (G.) Ritenzione del sangue mestruo per atresia della vagina. Gazz. med. ital. lomb., Milano, 1855, 3. s., vi, 145–150.—**Mörck.** Casus af hämmad menstruation. Förh. v. Svens. Läk.-Sällsk. Sammank. 1844-5, Stockholm, 1846, 63 - 65. — **Monks** (E. H.), sr. Retention of catamenia; pains simulating labour. Brit. M. J., Lond., 1886, i, 201.—**Montgomery** (E. E.) Case of atresia vaginæ with retention of menses. Phila. M. Times, 1884-5, xv, 140.— **Murray** (W.) A case of vaginal atresia and absence of menstruation cured by the use of tangle-tents. Brit. M. J., Lond., 1863, ii, 5.—**Oldham** (H.) Two cases of retention of the menses relieved by puncture through the rectum. Guy's Hosp. Rep., Lond., 1857, 3. s., iii, 244–251. ———. Retained menses from imperforate hymen. Med. Times & Gaz., Lond., 1857, n. s., xv, 628.— **Owen** (J.) Case of imperforate os uteri with retention of the menses. Lancet, Lond., 1837, i, 79.— **Palmer** (W. H.) Menses retained from occlusion of the os uteri; operation. Boston M. & S. J., 1858, lviii, 252. — **Parcet** (J. B.) Retencion de menstruos por oclusion de vagina; error de diagnóstico. Rev. de cien. méd., Barcel., 1878, iv, 219–222.—**Peltier** (H.) Retention of the menses simulating pregnancy. Med. Chron., Montreal, 1853-4, i, 229–232.—**Perrin.** Zwei Beobachtungen über Hymen imperforatum; Retention des Menstrualblutes, und hiedurch bewirkte und verkannte Uterus- und Scheidengeschwülste. Wien. med. Wchnschr., 1866, xvi, 907–909.—**Picard.** Rétention des règles par suite d'une imperforation de la matrice, compliquée d'une imperforation de l'hymen; opération; guérison. Gaz. d. hôp., Par., 1858, xxxi, 254. — **Pincott** (R.) On a case of retention of the menses from congenital occlusion

Menses (*Retention of*).

of the vagina. Austral. M. J., Melbourne. 1872, xvii, 234–236.—**Pirovano** (I.) Atresia puntiforme de la vagina; menstruacion laboriosa; operacion. Rev. méd.-quir., Buenos Aires, 1881–2, xviii, 83.—**Richardson** (E. H.) Report of a case of complete atresia of cervix uteri, with retention of menses, produced by nitric acid, relieved by aspiration and bilateral division of the cervix. Tr. Georgia M. Ass. 1882, Augusta, 1883, xxxiii, 172–176.—**Ringer** (B. S.) Case of imperforate hymen; retention of menses; operation; recovery. Lancet, Lond., 1869, ii, 804.—**Robbins** (H. C.) Case of retained catamenia. Boston M. & S. J., 1866, lxxiv, 420.—**Roberts** (D. L.) Notes of a case of imperforate hymen, with retained menstrual fluid. Brit. M. J., Lond., 1873, ii, 261. ———. Short notes of a case of imperforate hymen, in which upwards of one hundred ounces of retained menstrual fluid were evacuated. *Ibid.*, 456.—**Robinson** (F. C.) Retention of the catamenia from obstruction. Chicago M. J., 1866, xxiii, 252.—**Rossignol.** Diaphragme placé transversalement dans le vagin, et s'opposant à l'écoulement du sang des menstrues. Gaz. d. hôp., Par., 1856, xxix, 142.—**Roziés.** Occlusion complète du vagin chez une fille de 19 ans; accidents produits par la rétention du sang menstruel. J. de méd. et chir. de Toulouse, 1856, 3. s., i, 255–260. *Also:* Monit. d. hôp., Par., 1856, iv, 971–973. *Also:* Union méd., Par., 1857, xi, 30.—**Santesson** (C.) Defekt af moderslidans nedre hälft; atresia af den öfre; retentio mensium; operation; en månad derefter symtomer af trombos i bäckenvenerna på högra sidan, uti vena iliaca og cruralis dextra samt vena cava inferior; sekundär pleuropneumoni; död. Hygiea, Stockholm, 1858, xx, 577–583. *Also, transl.:* Dublin M. Press, 1860, xliii, 42.—**Scarburgh** (G. T.) Case of retention of the menstrua, from occlusion of the os uteri. Virginia M. J., Richmond, 1858, xi, 171–174.—**Schäffer.** Ausgezeichnete Wirkung der Herba Adianthi aurei gegen Retentio mensium. Prov. San.-Ber. d. k. Med.-Coll. v. Pommern 1834, Stettin, 1835, 60–62. — **Schuh.** Verwachsung der Scheide mit Zurückhaltung des Menstrualblutes; Operation; Tod. Wchnbl. d. k. k. Gesellsch. d. Aerzte in Wien, 1857, iii, 497–501.—**Seidler.** Unterleibskrämpfe als Folge eines durch Atresia vaginæ zurückgehaltenen Monatsflusses entstanden und durch die Operation geheilt. Mag. f. d. ges. Heilk., Berl., 1826, xxii, 3<?>8–391.—**Sherwen** (J.) A case of imperforated hymen, attended with uncommon circumstances. Med. Rec. Private M. Ass., Lond., 1798, 279–288.—**Simon** (J.) Angeborene Atresie der linken Scheidenhälfte am Introitus vaginæ bei Duplicität des Uterus und der Scheide; Retention des Menstrualblutes in der verschlossenen Hälfte bei gleichzeitigen Metrorrhagieen aus der offenen Hälfte der Verdoppelung. Monatschr. f. Geburtsk. u. Frauenkr., Berl., 1864, xxiv, 292–298.—**Simons** (T. G.) Atresia vagina; death from tetanus at menstrual period; post-mortem. Tr. South Car. M. Ass., Charleston, 1872, 56–59.—**Swinnerton** (S.) Pent up catamenia from imperforate hymen. Lancet, Lond., 1843–4, i, 68.—**Syme** (J.) Obstructed vagina, with retention of the menstrual discharge. Month. J. M. Sc., Lond. & Edinb., 1850, xi, 147.—**Thomas** (T. G.) Laparotomy performed for the removal of a large quantity of menstrual blood from one horn of a bicornate uterus. Illust. M. & S., N. Y., 1882, i, 19–22. *Also, Reprint. Also* [Abstr.]: N. York M. J., 1882, xxxv, 517–519. *Also:* Tr. N. York Obst. Soc. (1881–5), 1885, iii, 44–46.—**Thompson** (H.) Retention of the menses from malfo<r>mation of the vagina. Dublin Hosp. Gaz., 1856, iii, 150. ———. A case of imperforate hymen, with retained menses. Lancet, Lond., 1867, i, 538.—**Toulmouche** (A.) Observations sur l'occlusion du vagin, suivies de réflexions sur la nature chimique du sang retenu dans ce conduit. Arch. gén. de méd., Par., 1829, xix, 236–242.—**Tourneret** (A.) Imperforation de l'hymen, avec rétention du sang menstruel dans un utérus bicorne; ponction aspiratrice, suivie de l'excision de l'hymen et de la suture; guérison. Gaz. méd. de Strasb., 1874, xxxiii, 125–128.—**Trumet** (A.) Cas de vice de conformation de l'utérus et du col utérin; accidents produits par la rétention du sang des règles; tentatives chirurgicales pour remédier à ce vice de conformation; angine couenneuse; péritonite; autopsie. Gaz. méd. de Par., 1851, 3. s., vi, 341–343.—**Tubbs** (W. J.) Case of occluded vagina; retained menses; operation; cure. Brit. M. J., Lond., 1865, i, 85.—**Tuckwell** (H. M.) Three cases of imperforate hymen with retention of the menstrual fluid. Brit. & For. M.-Chir. Rev., Lond., 1867, xl, 203–210. *Also, Reprint.*—**Valentino** (M.) Ritenzione dei mestrui in utero didelphys con diverso grado di sviluppo dei due uteri, congiunto a vagina unica con atresia. Raccoglitore med., Forli, 1885, 4. s., xxiii, 57–65.—**Verneuil.** Oblitération cicatricielle du vagin; rétention des règles; opération; guérison; fistule vésico-vaginale; guérison spontanée. Bull. Soc. de chir. de Par., 1864, 2. s., iv, 271–282.—**Voisin.** Rétention menstruelle causée par imperforation du vagin; mort. Bull. Soc. anat. de Par., 1856, xxxi, 145.—**Ward** (C. S.) Retained menstrual fluid; method of removal. Am. J. Obst., N. Y., 1880, xiii, 609–611.—**Warren** (J. M.) Cases of occlusion of the vagina, with retention of the catamenia, relieved by an operation. Am. J. M. Sc., Phila., 1851, n. s.,

Menses (*Retention of*).

xxii, 13–22. *Also, Reprint.* ———. Occlusion of vagina; retention of menstrual fluid. Boston M. & S. J.,* 1857, lvi, 298. *Also:* Extr. Rec. Bost. Soc. M. Improve. (1856–8), 1859. iii, 93.—**Weber.** Hymen non perforatum, musculosum; bæmometra. Wien. med. Presse, 1867, viii, 809–811.—**Williams** (E. K.) Atresia of vagina. Mississippi Valley M. Month., Memphis, 1886, vi, 526–529.—**Winsor** (F.) Imperforate hymen with large accumulation of menstrual fluid. Boston M. & S. J., 1877, xcvii, 36–40.—**Wood** (J.) Complete occlusion of the vagina in a patient aged 21; retension of menses for nine months; operation; speedy recovery. Med. Times & Gaz., Lond., 1865, i, 520.

Mensing (Joh.) *Beiträge zur Statistik der Kniegelenksresectionen. 36 pp., 1 a. l. 8°. *Kiel, C. F. Mohr*, 1883.

Mensinga.
Co-Editor of: **Frauenarzt** (Der), Berlin, 1886.

Mensinga (W. P. J.) *Monstri gallinacei bicorporei bicephali descriptio anatomica, una cum disquisitione de ejus ortu. 17 pp., 1 pl. 4°. *Kiliæ, C. F. Mohr*, 1861.
In: SCHRIFT. d. Univ. zu Kiel, viii, 1861, vii, med. iii.

———. Das Pessarium occlusivum und dessen Application. Supplement zu "Ueber facultative Sterilität, etc.". Von Dr. C. Hasse (Pseudonym). 3. Aufl. 15 pp. 8°. *Leipzig u. Neuwied, L. Heuser*, 1883.

Mensonides (Justus Alderts). *De absorptione molecularum solidarum nonnulla. 2 p. l., 44 pp. 8°. *Traj. ad Rhenum, C. Bielevelt*, 1848. [*Also, in:* P., v. 1097.]

Mensonides (Willem Carl). *Over den invloed van actieve hyperaemie op den lymphstroom. 2 p. l., 72 pp. 8°. *Utrecht, Kemink & Zoon*, 1886.

Menssen (Carolus Christianus). *De malignitate variolarum naturalium tempestivo vesicatoriorum usu avertenda. 1 p. l., 22 pp., 3 l. 4°. *Halæ ad Salam, ære Beyeriano*, [1767].

Menstrual blood.

See, also, **Menstruation**; **Gonorrhœa** (*Causes, etc., of*).

CASPAR (J. P.) *De sanguine menstruo. sm. 4°. *Tubingæ*, 1676.

LAUGIER (C.) *Du fluide menstruel, et de la valeur séméiologique des caillots sanguins dans les règles. 4°. *Paris*, 1846.

REMAK (R.) Die abnorme Natur des Menstrualblutflusses erläutert. 8°. *Berlin*, 1842.

Fischer (D.) De sanguine menstruo philtri loco propinato. Acta Acad. nat. curios., 2. ed., Norimb., 1727, i, 300–314.—**Grube.** Ueber das Menstrualblut. Arch. f. Anat., Physiol. u. wissensch. Med., Berl., 1840, 36.—**Haddon** (J.) On menstrual coagula. Edinb. M. J., 1871–2, xvii, 611–614.—**Hennig** (C.) Die weissen Blutkörperchen und die Deciduazellen. Arch. f. Gynaek., Berl., 1874, vi, 508–510.—**Julia de Fontenelle.** Nature du sang menstruel. J. de chim. méd., etc., Par., 1837, 2. s., iii, 587–589.—**Le Canu.** Si le sang menstruel diffère du sang que fait couler l'accouchement. Bull. Acad. de méd., Par., 1845–6, xi, 255–257.—**Letheby** (H.) Microscopical and chemical examination of menstrual fluid which had been retained for some time within the vagina. Lancet, Lond., 1845, ii, 125–127.—**Müller** (H.) Ueber die Blutkörperchen in zurückgehaltenem Menstrualblut. Ztschr. f. rat. Med., Heidelb., 1846, v, 140–142.—**Remak** (R.) Ueber die Schädlichkeiten des Menstrualblutes und über deren wahrscheinliche Ursachen. Med. Ztg., Berl., 1839, viii, 261.—**Supposed** spontaneous combustion of napkins soiled by the menstrual discharge. J. Gynæc. Soc., Bost., 1872, vi, 418.

Menstruation.

See, also, **Corpus** *luteum*; **Generation**; **Hebephrenia**; **Hygiene** (*Female*); **Menstrual** *blood*; **Ovary**; **Ovulation**; **Puberty**; **Sea** *climate, etc.*; **Uterus**.

ALEXANDER (A.) Physiologie der Menstruation. 8°. *Hamburg*, 1841.

ANGERMANN (C. F. L.) *Catameniorum phænomena in muliere sana et ægrotante. 4°. *Lipsiæ*, [1793].

ARLEBOUT (I. G.) *De sanguine menstruo, ejusque suppressione legitima. 4°. *Traj. ad Rhenum*, 1716.

Menstruation.

ARRAGON (M.) *Utrum a mutuo sanguiferorum lactiferorumque uteri vasorum nisu menstrua mulierum purgatio? Præses A. Pepin. 4°. [Paris, 1740.]

BACQUET (N.) *Thèse sur quelques considérations physiologiques et médicales relatives aux différents phénomènes de la menstruation. 4°. Paris, an XIII [1805].

BAGET (H. J.) *An a superflui humoris perspiratorii refluxu, catamenia? Præses J. J. Nollan. 4°. [Paris], 1771.

BARBIER (É.-F.) *De la menstruation. 4°. Paris, 1849.

BAUDIN (A.) *De la menstruation, de ses causes, de ses rapports avec la fécondation. 4°. Paris, 1845.

BEER (H.) *Aperçu sur la menstruation. 4°. Paris, 1813.

BENNETT (P.) *De menstruis. 4°. Edinburgi, 1745.

BERCHER (P.) Quæstio medica, an ab uteri ejusve vasorum perpendiculari situ, menstrua mulierum purgatio? 4°. [Parisiis, 1749.]
In: HALLER. Disp. anat. [etc.] 4°. Gottingæ, 1750, v, 183-196.

BERNARD (C.-P.) *Études sur la menstruation. 4°. Paris, 1848.

BIDOU (A.-C.) *Sur la menstruation; ses altérations et son influence sur l'état physiologique et pathologique de la femme. 4°. Paris, 1828.

BIRDWOOD (R.) *De causis fluxus menstrui. 8°. Edinburgi, 1769.

BLUMENHAGEN (P. G. G. A.) *Menstruatio physiologice et pathologice spectata. 4°. Gottingæ, [1803].

BOHN (J.) & GÜNTHER (C.) *Diss. chym.-phys. vi. de menstruis. sm. 4°. Lipsiæ, [1863].

BONVALOT (H.) *Sur la menstruation, et les soins qu'elle réclame. 4°. Paris, 1831.

BOONAERTS (V. E.) *De fluxu mensium. 1783.
In: LOUVAIN Diss. 8°. Lovanii, 1796, iii, 108-110.

BOYER (É.) *De la menstruation. 4°. Paris, 1852.

BREBIS (J. A. H.) *De initio mensium fine morborum. sm. 4°. Halæ Magdeb., [1727].

BREBISS (J. G.) *De mensium muliebrium fluxu, s. n., et suppressione, p. n. 4°. Halæ, [1694].

——. The same. 4°. Halæ, [1694].

——. The same. 4°. Recusa Halæ Magdeb., 1710.

BRETET (J.) *Dissertation sur la menstruation. 4°. Paris, 1833.

BREWER (A. F.) *De menstruatione sana et morbosa. 8°. Gottingæ, [1809].

BRIERRE-DE-BOISMONT (A.-J.-F.) De la menstruation, considérée dans ses rapports physiologiques et pathologiques. 8°. Paris, 1842.

——. The same. La menstruacion considerada bajo su aspecto fisiológico y patológico. Traducida libremente al castellano. 2 v. 12°. Madrid, 1850.

BUSCH (F. M.) *Physiologica quædam de catameniis. 8°. Berolini, [1844].

CAILLAT (J.-M.) *Essai sur la menstruation. 4°. Paris, 1836.

CASTILLA (J. R.) *Estudio sobre la menstruacion. 8°. Buenos Aires, 1879.

CAVARÉ (F.) *De la menstruation envisagée aux trois périodes de la vie utérine. 4°. Paris, 1837.

CHAMAILLARD (A.) *Sur l'influence de la menstruation et de ses anomalies. 4°. Paris, 1834.

CHARLETON (G.) Inquisitiones medico-physicæ de causis catameniorum, sive fluxus menstrui; necnon uteri rheumatismo, sive fluore albo; in qua etiam nervose probatur sanguinem in animali fermentescere nunquam. 12°. Lugd. Bat., 1686.

CHASLON (M.) *Essai sur la menstruation. 4°. Paris, an XII [1804].

CHATELAIN (J.-V.) *Essai sur la menstruation, considérée dans l'état de santé et dans son influence sur les maladies. 4°. Paris, 1827.

CHÉNEAUX (M.-G.-L.) *De la menstruation et de la ménopause, au point de vue de la physiologie et de l'hygiène. 4°. Paris, 1859.

CHERBONNEAU (J.-H.) *Des causes de la menstruation. 4°. Paris, 1847.

CHEVALLIER (C.-C.) *De la menstruation. 4°. Paris, 1850.

CLARKSON (J.) *De mulierum menstrua consuetudine. 4°. Lugd. Bat., 1765.

COE (T.) *De fluxu muliebri menstruo morbisque inde oriundis. 4°. Lugd. Bat., 1728.

CORBERUS (H. F.) *De menstruis. Exercitatio chimica. sm. 4°. Jenæ, 1674.

COSTE (J.-P.-E.-B.) *Considérations générales sur la menstruation. 4°. Montpellier, 1837.

DE LA COUR (P.) *De naturali catemeniorum fluxu. sm. 4°. Lugd. Bat., 1733.

COURBET (J.-F.-C.) *De la menstruation, dans ses phénomènes physiologiques et pathologiques. 4°. Paris, 1852.

CRAVEN (J.) *De secretione uterina, vel fluxu qui vulgo menstruum dicitur. 8°. Edinburgi, 1787.

DAVIDGE (J. B.) *De causis catameniorum. 8°. Birmingham, 1794.

DAVIER DE BREVILLE (J. P.) An statim a menstruorum effluvio concepti firmioris valetudinis? Præs. Antonius Le Moine. 4°. [Parisiis, 1715.]

DEHN (C. G.) *De causis catameniorum. 8°. Gottingæ, 1829.

DELAGRAVE (A.-C.) *Considérations générales sur la menstruation. 4°. Paris, 1820.

DELORME (R.-B.) *Quelques considérations sur la menstruation. 4°. Paris, 1847.

DE MEZA (S.) *De menstruis. sm. 4°. Traj. ad Rhenum, 1749.

DESBREST (A.) *Essai sur la menstruation. 4°. Paris, 1851.

DIENER (J. C.) *De menstruatione. 8°. Turici, 1846.

DOBSON (M.) *De menstruis. 8°. Edinburghi, 1756.

DOMONT (A.-J.) *Sur la menstruation. 4°. Paris, 1807.

D'ORVILLE (A.) *Causæ menstrui fluxus disquisitio. sm. 4°. Gottingæ, [1748].

DUCLOS (H.-F.) *Considérations générales sur la menstruation. 4°. Paris, 1820.

DUCLUZAUX (J.-J.) *Essai sur la menstruation. 4°. Paris, 1855.

DUPONS (J.-A.) *Réflexions sur quelques points de la menstruation. 4°. Paris, an XIII [1804].

DUSOURD (J.-B.) Traité pratique de la menstruation considérée dans son état physiologique et dans ses divers états pathologiques, suivi d'un essai sur la chlorose et d'un mémoire sur les propriétés médicinales des diverses préparations de fer. 8°. Paris, 1847.

EMETT (R.) Essais de médecine sur le flux menstruel et la curation des maladies de la tête . . . [Trad. du latin par M. Hurtaut.] 12°. Paris, 1754.

ENGLEBIENNE (F.) *De menstruatione. 4°. Leodii, [1828].

EPPS (J.) Affections of women. No. 1. Monthly period. 12°. London, [1840].

Menstruation.

EVERETT (C.) * An inaugural dissertation on the function of menstruation. 12°. *Philadelphia*, 1795.

FARRAN (M.) * Coup d'œil sur la menstruation et quelques maladies propres au sexe. 4°. *Montpellier*, 1837.

FEIGELL (A.) * De menstruatione. 8°. *Berolini*, [1847].

FISCHER (C.) * I. Menstruation und Ovulation. II. Electrolytische Behandlung der Stenosen des Cervicalcanals des Uterus. 8°. *Würzburg*, 1879.

DE FOERE (L.) * De mensibus paucisque morborum ab eorum vitiis pendentium. 4°. *Gandavi*, 1825.

FOERSTER (D. A.) * De menstruo fluxu ejusque suppressione. sm. 4°. *Helmstadii*, [1722].

FRECH (C.-A.) * Les organes génitaux de la femme et la menstruation. 4°. *Paris*, 1864.

FREIND (J.) Emmenologia; in qua fluxus muliebris menstrui phænomena, periodi, vitia, cum medendi methodo, ad rationes mechanicas exiguntur. 8°. *Oxoniæ*, 1703.

———. The same. 3. ed. 8°. *Londini*, 1720.

———. The same. 16°. *Amstælodami*, 1726.

———. The same. Huic editioni accedunt ejusdem authoris prælectiones chymicæ. 12°. *Parisiis*, 1727.

———. The same. 12°. [*n. p., n. d.*]

———. The same. Transl. into English by T. Dale. 2. ed. 8°. *London*, 1752.

GAGNARD (L.) * De la menstruation en physiologie, et dans ses rapports avec la puberté et quelques maladies de cet âge. 4°. *Paris*, 1860.

GARNIER (L.-A.) * Sur la menstruation et ses anomalies. 4°. *Paris*, 1820.

GARTZWEILER (J. T.) * De fluxus menstrui periodo, et medicamentorum uterinorum operatione. sm. 4°. *Lugd. Bat.*, 1707.

GAŸE (C.) * Zur Statistik der Menstruation. 4°. *Kiel*, 1879.

GENET (P.-A.) * Considérations cliniques et physiologiques sur les troubles survenant du côté des amygdales pendant la menstruation. 4°. *Paris*, 1881.

GOUEL (F.) * An quæ statim a menstrua purgatione concipiunt, citius pariunt? Prop. J. Delagrive. 4°. [*Paris*, 1716.]

GOÜOT (C.-B.) * Histoire naturelle et physiologique de la menstruation. 4°. *Strasbourg*, 1810.

GRAVIÈRES-SELLIER (J.-B.) * De la menstruation. 4°. *Paris*, 1848.

GRIFFIOEN (G.) * De fato muliebri. 4°. *Lugd. Bat.*, [1745].

GUÉNOT (Z.) * Etude sur la physiologie de la menstruation et sur ses rapports avec l'arthritisme et la scrofule. 4°. *Paris*, 1881.

Also [Abstr.], *in:* Rev. méd.-chir. d. mal. d. femmes, Par., 1881, iii, 195; 248.

GUERNSEY (W. J.) Menstruation. 12°. [*n. p., n. d.*]

GUINGUE (J.-H.) * Sur la menstruation et ses accidens. 4°. *Paris*, 1834.

HAHN ([H.] A. [C.]) * De fluxu mensium. 8°. *Berolini*, 1847.

HANNOVER (A.) Om Menstruationens Betydning. En physiologisk, pathologisk og forensisk Undersøgelse. 8°. *Kjøbenhavn*, 1851.

Also, transl. in: Lond. M. Gaz., 1851, xlviii, 626; 797; 969.

HARTE (C. T. E.) * De menstruatione. sm. 8°. *Berolini*, [1866].

HENGESBACH (F.) * Ueber Menstruation und ihre Fortdauer während der Schwangerschaft,

mit besonderer Berücksichtigung eines im hiesigen Gebärhause zur Beobachtung gekommenen Falles. 8°. *Würzburg*, 1879.

HEIM (A. G.) * Diss. physiol. sistens nonnulla de menstruatione. 4°. *Gottingæ*, [1812].

HEISEN (J.) * De fluxu mulierum menstruo ejusque suppressione. 4°. *Lugd. Bat.*, 1684.

HENNENHOFER (H. D.) * Valetudinarium virginale. 4°. *Halæ Magdeb.*, [1721].

HEYMANN (A. C.) * De menstruatione. 8°. *Berolini*, 1867.

VAN HEYST (L. G.) * De mensium fluxu. 8°. *Lugd. Bat.*, 1842.

HOEFER (A.) * De catameniorum physiologia. 4°. *Lipsiæ*, [1820].

HOPFE (H. C. L.) * De menstruis eorumque præcipuis vitiis. 4°. *Helmstadii*, [1798].

HUSBANDS (G.) * De mensibus eorumque emansione. 8°. *Edinburgi*, 1805.

JÆHKEL (T. T.) * Ætiologia fluxus menstrui mulierum. 4°. *Lipsiæ*, [1784].

JAYMES (J.) * Considérations générales sur la menstruation. 4°. *Paris*, 1814.

JUBIOT (L.) * Essai historique sur la menstruation et ses rapports avec l'ovulation spontanée. 4°. *Montpellier*, 1878.

KAPPELHOFF (A.) * De catameniis. sm. 4°. *Traj. ad Rhenum*, 1757.

KEMLO (G.) * De mensibus et amenorrhœa. 8°. *Edinburgi*, 1819.

KOCH (A.) * Ueber menstruale Vorgänge. 8°. *Würzburg*, 1862.

KONING (A.) * De mensium fluxu. 4°. *Harderovici*, 1749.

KRIEG (J. F.) Quæstiones emmenologicæ. 4°. *Lipsiæ*, [1837].

KRIEGER (E.) Die Menstruation. Eine gynäkologische Studie. 8°. *Berlin*, 1869.

LACHEVRIE (M.) * Considérations sur la menstruation et ses dérangemens. 4°. *Paris*, 1826.

LACOMBE (J.-A.) * De la menstruation et de l'aménorrhée. 4°. *Paris*, 1824.

LAMBERT (R.) * Quelques considérations sur la menstruation. 4°. *Paris*, 1835.

LATAUD (L.-F.) * Sur la menstruation. 4°. *Strasbourg*, 1809.

LEHRE (G.) * De menstruorum phænomenis, causis et usu. 8°. *Edinburgi*, 1791.

LEONHARDI (J. G.) De nutrice menstruata. 4°. [*Wittebergæ*, 1788.]

LE TELLIER fils. Critical reflections upon the Emmenology of Dr. Freiud. Transl. from the French. 8°. *London*, 1731.

LEVESTAMM (A.) * De fluxu menstruo, adjuncta de ejusdem causis theoria. 8°. *Kiliæ*, 1824.

LION (P.) Disquisitio critica theorematum quæ nunc de menstruatione et fæcundatione obtinent. 8°. *Vratislaviæ*, 1855.

LORBEER (J. B.) * De fluxus menstrui ratione ad ventriculum et intestina. 4°. *Halæ ad Salam*, [1764].

LOSSIER (L. A.) * De menstruatione ejusque anomaliis. 8°. *Berolini*, [1845].

LOWENSTEIN (M. G.) * De menstruatione normali atque parca. 8°. *Dorpati*, 1835.

LULLIES (F. [R.]) * Ueber die Zeit des Eintritts des Menstruations nach Angaben von 3000 Schwangeren in der königl. gynäkologischen Klinik zu Königsberg i. Pr. 8°. *Königsberg*, 1886.

MCDONALD (B.) * De mensibus et naturaliter et immodice fluentibus. 8°. *Edinburgi*, 1786.

MACLAURIN (J. C.) * De fluxus menstrui indole, causisque. 8°. *Edinburgi*, 1788.

Menstruation.

MAHEUT (F.-V.) *De la menstruation. 4°. *Paris*, 1839.

MARCHAND (J.) *De catameniorum fluxu et eorum morbis. 4°. *Harderovici*, 1733.

MÂREAU (A.) *De la menstruation. 4°. *Paris*, 1854.

MASCHEK (A.) *De fluxu menstruo. 8°. *Ticinii Regii*, [1830].

MAUGHS (G. M. B.) Menstruation; or the menstrual flow; an epiphenomenon of ovulation. 8°. *St. Louis*, 1867.

MAURER (G. J.) *De fluxu catamenorium. 8°. *Budæ*, [1835].

MEADE (R. E.) *De mensibus. 8°. *Edinburgi*, 1800.

MEYER (F.) *De menstruatione ejusque anomaliis. 8°. *Berolini*, [1826].

MEYER (J.) *Klinische Untersuchungen über das Verhalten der Ovarien während der Menstruation. 8°. *Dorpat*, 1883.
Also [Abstr.], *in*: Arch. f. Gynaek., Berl., 1883, xxii, 51–56.

MINERVINI (G.) Memorie fisiologiche riguardante la mestruazione. 8°. *Napoli*, 1854.

MUILMAN (G. V.) *An ex celebrata hactenus opinione de plethora universali, vel particulari, vera fluxus menstrui causa explicari possit? 4°. *Leidæ*, 1772.

NEUMANN (C. G.) *De exclusione ovulorum in salacibus absque ullo præregresso coitu. 4°. *Lugd. Bat.*, 1717.

NIEMEYER (L. H. C.) *De menstruationis fine et usu. 12°. *Gottingæ*, [1796].

VAN OSTERZEE (G. J. K.) *De ratione quæ est inter catamenia et morbos feminarum, annexa historia morbi de chlorosi. 8°. *Lugd. Bat.*, 1849.

OUDEMANS (C. A. J. A.) *De fluxu menstruo. 8°. *Hagæ Comitis*, 1847.

OUDINÉ (P.) *Étude sur la congestion rachidienne de cause menstruelle. 4°. *Paris*, 1882.

PARIS (C.) *De l'influence de la menstruation sur le système physique et moral de la femme. 4°. *Strasbourg*, 1837.

PASTA (A.) Dissertazione sopra i mestrui delle donne. 8°. *Bergamo*, 1757.

PATTE (A.) *Essai sur la menstruation et ses anomalies. 4°. *Paris*, 1829.

PEPIN (A.) Quæstio medica: Utrum a mutuo sanguiferorum lactiferorumque uteri vasorum nisu menstrua mulierum purgatio? 4°. 1740.
In: HALLER. Disp. anat. [etc.] 4°. *Gottingæ*, 1750, v, 173–181.

PÉRIER (L.-M.) *Considérations médicales et physiologiques sur la menstruation. 4°. *Paris*, 1819.

PETRASCH (A.) *De menstruatione ejusque de via normali aberrationibus. 8°. *Gryphiæ*, [1833].

PÉTREQUIN (T.-J.-É.) *Recherches sur la menstruation. 4°. *Paris*, 1835.

PFANNENSCHMID (J. H.) *De menstruis naturæ et artis. 4°. *Traj. ad Rhenum*, 1710.

POUMIÈS DE LA SIBOUTIE (F.-L.) *Essai sur la première menstruation. 4°. *Paris*, 1815.

POWER (J.) An essay on the periodical discharge of the human female, with new views of its nature, causes, and influence on disease. To which are added directions for its management in the different stages of life. 8°. *London*, 1832.

PRIGENT-KALLAIN (J.-B.) *Sur la menstruation et les hémorrhagies utérines. 4°. *Paris*, 1815.

PRIME (B. Y.) *De fluxu muliebri menstruo. 4°. [*Lugd. Bat.*, 1764.]

QUAET (I. M.) *De catameniis eorumque usu. 4°. *Lugd. Bat.*, [1749].

Menstruation.

RACIBORSKI (A.) Traité de la menstruation, ses rapports avec l'ovulation, la fécondation, l'hygiène de la puberté et de l'âge critique, son rôle dans les différentes maladies, ses troubles et leur traitement. 8°. *Paris*, 1868.

RANSHOFF (S.) *De catameniis. 4°. *Gottingæ*, 1818.

REMAK (R.) Die abnorme Natur des Menstrualblutflusses erläutert. 8°. *Berlin*, 1842.
Repr. from: N. Ztschr. f. Geburtsk., Berl., 1843, xiii. See, also, *infra*.

RIVELLI (G.) Della priorità dovuta all' Italia sopra al francese professore C. Nègrier d'Anger ed altri insigni autori relativamente alle cause occasionali della menstruazione, anche queste scoperte dal . . . 8°. *Bologna*, 1853.

ROBERT (L.-B.-T.) *Considérations générales sur la menstruation. 4°. *Paris*, 1833.

RUE (A.-J.) *Essai sur la première menstruation, précédé de quelques considérations sur la chlorose. 4°. *Paris*, 1819.

SAULNIER (J.-F.) *Sur la menstruation et l'aménorrhée. 4°. *Paris*, 1832.

SCHLICHTINGIUS (E. G.) *De catameniis. 4°. *Groningæ*, 1730.

SCHOLLMEYER (J.-F.-G.) *De menstruationis natura. 8°. *Berolini*, [1839].

SCHULZ (G.) *De menstruatione. 8°. *Berolini*, 1864.

SENNFT (J. D.) An fœmina sine catameniorum fluxu perfecta frui possit sanitate?
In: LUDWIG (C. G.) Decas quæst. med. 4°. *Lipsiæ*, 1740, 1–4.

SIBILAT (J.-L.) *De la menstruation. 4°. *Paris*, 1853.

DE SILVESTRI (J.) *De menstruatione. 8°. *Ticini Regii*, [1841].

SIMPSON (A. R.) Emmenologia; an inaugural address. 8°. *Edinburgh*, 1876.

S[IMSON] (T.) *De fluxu menstruo. 4°. *Glasguæ*, 1720.

———. The system of the womb, with a particular account of the menses independent of a plethora; to which are subjoined a few observations relating to cold and its effects upon the body. 8°. *Edinburgh*, 1729.

———. The same. 8°. *London*, 1730.

SNYDER (C. L.) *Catamenia. 8°. *Baltimore*, 1812.

SOMMER (J. L. F. H.) *De menstruationis natura et ratione. 4°. *Erlangæ*, 1821.

STAHL (G. E.) [Pr.] de fluxus muliebris, quatenus menstrui, causa. 4°. [*Halæ Magdeb.*, 1707.]

STEINEBACH (H.) *De mensibus eorumque vitiis. 8°. *Berolini*, [1852].

STEINLEIN (J. P.) *De fluxu menstruo ejusque præsertim ætiologia. 12°. *Bamberg*, 1815.

STEINTHAL (M.) *De menstruorum tam normali, quam abnormi decursu. 8°. *Berolini*, [1821].

STINSTRA (G.) *De fluxu mulierum menstruo. sm. 4°. *Franequeræ*, 1731.

STULLER (J.) *De mensibus eorumque vitiis. 8°. *Vratislaviæ*, [1858].

SURUN (P.-A.) Théorie de la menstruation, fondée sur les caractères naturels de la vie des organes, et particulièrement de l'action nerveuse. 8°. *Paris*, 1819.

SWEDENBORG (J. G.) *De mensibus paucisque morborum ab vitiis eorum pendentium. 8°. *Lundæ*, 1840.

SYLVIUS (J.) De mensibus mulierum et hominis generatione. 16°. *Venetiis*, 1556.

VAN TETTRODE (N.) *De fluxu menstruo. sm. 4°. *Lugd. Bat.*, 1735.

Menstruation.

VAN THIEL (M.) * Over de normale menstruatie der vrouw en de decidua menstrualis. 8°. *Amsterdam*, 1866.

THOMANN (I. N.) * De fluxu menstruo ejusque vitiis. [Pr.] I. De fluxu menstruo naturali ejusque retentione. 8°. *Wirceburgi*, 1796.

THOMSON (D.) * De menstruis. 8°. *Edinburgi*, 1765.

TOBLER (T.) Fragmenta observationum de profluvio menstruo. 8°. *Trogæ*, 1840.

TOEL (L.) * Emmenologia practica. 4°. *Gottingæ*, 1777.

VALLET (A.-L.) * De la menstruation (physiologie). 4°. *Paris*, 1849.

VERZYL (J. J.) * De menstruis, illorumque pubertatis tempore proruptione. 8°. *Lugd. Bat.*, 1820.

VETTE (J. G.) * De catameniis. 4°. *Harderovici*, [1711].

VOSS (F.) * De menstruatione. 8°. *Berolini*, 1846.

WAHREN (J.) * De menstruatione. 8°. *Berolini*, [1845].

VAN DE WALL (J. H. F.) * De catameniis in statu sano. 8°. *Lugd. Bat.*, 1833.

WALLIS (J. C.) * De fluxu mensium. 8°. *Berolini*, [1857].

WHITEFORD (H.) * On the catamenia. 8°. *Philadelphia*, 1802.

WIEDEMANN (F.) * De fluxus menstrui natura. 8°. *Berolini*, [1841].

WOLTERBEEK (C. J.) * De fluxu menstruo. 8°. *Amstelædami*, 1834.

ZELLMANN (J. P.) Exercitatio academica ad emmenologiam Freindianam, qua fundamenti loco suppositæ quædam doctrinæ modeste examinantur. 4°. *Halæ Magdeb.*, [1735].

ZIMMERMANN (J. G.) [Entgegnung] an Herrn J. G. Hempel [auf dessen Schreiben, die monatliche Reinigung der Grönländerinnen betreffend]. 8°. *Hannover*, 1778.

Ahlfeld (F.) Die neuen Anschauungen über Zusammenhang von Menstruation, Ovulation und Befruchtung und die practischen Consequenzen derselben. Deutsche med. Wchnschr., Berl., 1880, vi, 449–452. — Alexander. Zusammenstellung einiger neueren Untersuchungen über die Menstruation, nebst Anmerkungen. Ztschr. f. d. ges. Med., Hamb., 1844, xxvii, 457–472.— Alt (O.) Ueber das Vorkommen und die Bedeutung der Menstruation bei den Völkern der alten Welt. Monatschr. f. Geburtsk. u. Frauenkr., Berl., 1855, vi, 161–179. — Antony (M.) On menstruation. South. M. & S. J., Augusta, 1838, ii, 135–156.— Argenti (F.) Nuovi studj sulla causa immediata della mestruazione, e modificazione alla teoria della fecondazione. Ann. univ. di med., Milano, 1843, cv, 311–328. — Atthill (L.) Menstruation as a disintegration process. Med. Press & Circ., Lond., 1875, ii, 473.— Auvard. Menstruation et ovulation. Gaz. hebd. de méd., Par., 1887, 2. s., xxiv, 273; 388.— Barnes (R.) An inquiry into some of the relations between menstruation, conception, and lactation, and the influence of lactation in causing abortion, founded on an analysis of the histories of one hundred women. Lancet, Lond., 1852, ii, 510–514. — Barnsfather (J.) Is the mucous membrane of the uterus thrown off at each menstrual period? If it is, what are its solvents? Cincin. M. News, 1875, viii, 341–351.— Barthel (E.) Ueber das Verhalten der Menstruation und über die Häufigkeit der Pseudomenstruation bei den verschiedenen Typhusformen. St. Petersb. med. Wchnschr., 1881, vi, 15.— Bayie (F.) De causis fluxus menstrui mulierum. *In his*: Diss. med. tres, 18°, Hagæ-Comitis, 1678, 1–34. — Beigel (H.) Ueber das Verhältniss der Menstruation zur Ovulation. Wien. med. Wchnschr., 1873, xxiii, 637; 665; 688; 709. ———. Ueber Ovulation und Menstruation. *Ibid*, 1875, xxv, 692–696.— Bennet (J. H.) On healthy and morbid menstruation. Lancet, Lond., 1852, i, 35; 65; 215; 328; 353.— Bernard (C.) De l'influence des différens organes génitaux sur la menstruation et sur l'apparence extérieure du corps. Union méd., Par., 1850, iv, 513.— Berti (A.) Ricerche statistiche sul fenomeno della mestruazione. Gazz. med. ital. prov. venete, Padova, 1870, xiii, 2; 9.— von Bischoff. Ueber Ovulation und Menstruation. Wien. med. Wchnschr., 1875, xxv, 449; 473; 497; 521.— Bouté. Objections contre le nouveau système de la menstruation, proposé par M. Le Cat. J. de méd., chir., pharm., etc., Par., 1764, xxi, 315–342.— Borel. Nou-

Menstruation.

velles théories de la menstruation. Bull. Soc. d. sc. nat. de Neuchâtel, 1875-6, x, 335–341.— Bousquet (F.) Des causes qui peuvent faire varier l'époque de la réapparition des règles après l'accouchement et après l'avortement. Marseille méd., 1875, xii, 331; 394. — Braun (E.) Zur Physiologie der Menstruation. Wien. med. Presse, 1878, xix, 729; 762; 792; 826; 888.— Brewer (W. P.) On menstruation: 1st. What are the best means of bringing on the retarded menses, when the possibility of pregnancy is out of the question? 2d. Is the period of the menopause really a critical period? N. Orl. M. & S. J., 1874–5, ii, 918–920.— Brierre de Boismont (A.) De la menstruation; faire connaître l'influence que cette fonction exerce sur les maladies et celle qu'elle en reçoit. Mém. Acad. de méd., Par., 1841, ix, 104–233.— Briggs (C. E.) A menstruating virgin uterus. St. Louis M. & S. J., 1880, xxxviii, 265–269. *Also, in:* Proc. St. Louis M. Soc. Missouri, 1881, iii, 67 – 72.— Campa (F. de P.) Contribucion al estudio de la emmenologia. An. de obst., ginecopat. y pediat., Madrid, 1882, 2. ép., ii, 289; 321.— Campbell (R. E.) Observations upon menstruation; its cause, character, and effects upon the female economy. Atlanta M. & S. J., 1856–7, ii, 10–15.— Carpenter (W. M.) Remarks on the periodical maturation and discharge of ova in man, and other mammiferæ; and the practical bearings of this theory. N. Orl. M. & S. J., 1845–6, ii, 563; 699.— Carstens (J. H.) The Lœwenthal theory of menstruation. Detroit Lancet, 1884–5, n. s., viii, 437–442. — Cauchois. Sur l'augmentation de la tension vasculaire dans le système de la circulation générale pendant la période menstruelle. Compt. rend. Soc. de biol. 1872, Par., 1874, 5. s., iv, 144–147. — Chandelux. Note sur la structure des corps jaunes de Dalton. *Ibid.*, 1880, Par., 1881, 7. s., ii, 266–270. *Also:* Gaz. méd. de Par., 1880, 6. s., ii, 427–429.— Chomel et al. Rapport sur les mémoires envoyés au concours de l'Acadénie; la question est celleci: "Faire l'histoire physiologique de la menstruation, faire connaître l'influence que cette fonction exerce sur ies maladies et celle qu'elle en reçoit". Bull. Acad. de méd., Par., 1837–8, ii, 1056–1067.— Clay (C.) On the duration of that part of human life connected with menstruation, with general remarks on that important function. Med. Times, Lond., 1845, xi, 95; 145; 179.— Cocchi (B.) Intorno alla ovulazione della donna. (Nota all' osservazione del Dott. P. Gaddi.) Ann. univ. di med., Milano, 1850, cxxxv, 5–20.— Cochran (J.) On menstruation as a pathological process. Virginia M. Month., Richmond, 1876, ii, 824–826.— Coe (H.) Remarks upon menstruation; physiological and pathological. Atlanta M. & S. J., 1858–9, iv, 470–473.— Cooley (F.) Do women menstruate during gestation? St. Louis M. & S. J., 1854, xii, 59–63.— Cordes (A.) Influence of bromide of potassium upon menstruation. Obs. J. Gr. Brit., Lond., 1874, ii, 11.— Cortejarena (F.) Sur la menstruation. Cong. méd. internat. de Par. (1867), 1868, 219–222. *Also, transl.:* Siglo méd., Madrid, 1867, xiv, 613 – 615. — Denny (T. S.) Physiology of menstruation. Atlanta M. & S. J., 1859–60, v, 18–20.— Depaul & Guéniot. Menstruation. Dict. encycl. d. sc. méd., Par., 1873, 2. s., vi, 678–738.— Désormeaux & Dubois (P.) Menstruation. Dict. de méd., 2. éd., Par., 1839, xix, 440–480.— Devendorf. On the loss of blood during the menstrual period by the human female an abnormity. Detroit Lancet, 1882–3, n. s., vi, 454–456.— Dewees (W. P.) Observations on menstruation. Phila. J. M. & Phys. Sc., 1826, xii, 283–305. — Draper. Extraordinary cardiac excitement before a first menstruation. Boston M. & S. J., 1886, cxv, 547.— Dubois. De l'hémorrhagie cataméniale. Soc. méd. d'Amiens. Bull. (1878-9), 1880, xviii-xix, 163–165.— Du Bois (E) A dissertation of conception, menstruation, and its irregularities. Med. Reposit., N. Y., 1808, v, 25–31.— Edson (B.) A contribution to the resumption of menstruation after parturition. Am. J. Obst., N. Y., 1882, xv, 890 – 892.— Eklund (F.) Notis om menstruationen has lappqvinnorna. Hygiea, Stockholm, 1876, xxxviii, 105.— Evers (J. C. G.) Statistieke opgaven omtrent het begin en ophouden der menstruatie. Nederl. Tijdschr. v. Geneesk., Amst., 1873, 2. R., ix, 1. Afd., 407.— Faye. De la menstruation en Norvége. Cong. méd. internat. de Par., 1868, 191–195.— Feoktistoff (A. E.) Neskolko slov o princhinach i tseli menstrualnago processa. [Some words on the causes and purposes of menstruation.] Voyenno-med. J., St. Petersb., 1885, clii, pt. 2, 125 – 172. *Also, transl.:* Arch. f. Gynaek., Berl., 1885-6, xxvii, 379–418. *Also-transl. and reprint.*— Flesch (M.) Eine Fiage zur Lehre von der Menstruation. Centralbl. f. Gynäk., Leipz., 1886, x, 289–291.— Fothergill (J. M.) The systemic relations of the menstrual week. Am. J. Obst., N. Y., 1881, xiv, 38–47.— Function (On the) of the ovaries in menstruation. Lancet, Lond., 1840–41, i, 294.— Galippe. De la menstruation dans les établissements consacrés à l'éducation des jeunes filles. Bull. Soc. de méd. pub., Par., 1880, iii, 277–280. *Also:* Ann. d'hyg., Par., 1880, 3. s., iv, 165–167. *Also:* Rev. d'hyg., Par., 1880, ii, 605–608.— Gasparini. Dell' influenza dell' elettricità sulla mestruazione e suoi disturbi. N. Liguria med., Genova, 1873, xviii, 531–539.— George (G. A.) The rationale of the menstrual flow. Lancet, Lond., 1878, i, 346. — Giraudet (E.) De la valeur des théories dans l'explication des causes de la menstruation. Gaz. d.

Menstruation.

hôp., Par., 1858, xxxi, 274.—**Girdwood** (G. F.) Theory of menstruation. Lancet, Lond., 1842–3, i, 825–830. ——. On the theory of menstruation. *Ibid.*, 1844, ii, 312; 333.— **Goddard.** Observations relatives à la menstruation. Compt. rend. Soc. de biol. 1854, Par., 1855, 2. s., i, pt. 2, 107–111.—**Goodman** (J.) Menstruation and the law of monthly periodicity. Richmond & Louisville M. J., Louisville, 1875, xx, 553–567. *Also*, Reprint. ——. The menstrual cycle. Tr. Am. Gynec. Soc. 1877, Bost., 1878, ii, 650–662. ——. The clinical theory of menstruation. Am. J. Obst., N. Y., 1878, xi, 673–694.—**Góth** (E.) Untersuchungen über die Menstruationsverhältnisse der in Siebenbürgen wohnenden Völkerstämme. Pest. med.-chir. Presse, Budapest, 1879, xv, 845; 859; 875; 911; 929; 963.—**Greenhow** (E.) Effects of opium on the catamenia. Lond. M. Gaz., 1844. n. s., xxxiv, 117.—**Grimsdale** (T. F.) Final cause of menstruation. Med. Times & Gaz., Lond , 1852, n. s., iv, 299.—**Gusserow** (A.) Ueber Menstruation und Dysmenorrhoe. Samml. klin. Vortr., Leipz., 1875, No. 81 (Gynäk., No. 27), 619–648.— **Harley** (G.) Uterus and its appendages at the catamenial period. Tr. Path. Soc. Lond., 1861–2, xiii, 170–172. ——. The menstrual secretion; including critical remarks on the pathology of retained menstrual fluids in the organs of reproduction. Brit. M. J., Lond., 1878, i, 815.— **Hausmann.** Beiträge zur Lehre der Decidua menstrualis. Verhandl. d. Gesellsch. in Berl., 1868, xx, 140–155.—**Haussmann** (D.) Bemerkungen zu den Sigismundschen Ideen über das Wesen der Menstruation. Deutsche Klinik, Berl., 1872, xxiv, 66.—**Hegar.** Bemerkungen zur Menstruation. Amtl. Ber. ü. d. Versamml. deutsch. Naturf. u. Aerzte 1883, Freib. i. Br , 1884, lvi, 202.—**Henke** (E.) Ovulation and menstruation. Med. & Surg. Reporter, Phila., 1874, xxx, 305–308.—**Hennig** (C.) Temperaturbeobachtungen während der Menstruation. Arch. f. Gynaek., Berl., 1871, ii, 300; 1872. iv, 371. ——. Ueber das Verhalten des Eileiters während der Menstruation. Arch. d. Heilk., Leipz., 1877, xviii, 418–425. ——. Ueber die Temperatur Menstruirender. Memorabilien, Heilbr., 1882, n. F., ii, 214–216.—**Herman** (G. E.) Cases illustrating the relation between uterine and ovarian pain at the menstrual period. Obst. J. Gr. Brit., Lond., 1880, viii, 145–153.—**Hillyer** (E.) An essay on the physiology of menstruation. South. M. & S. J., Augusta, 1858, n. s., xiv, 795–802—**Hodgdon.** Bifid uterus; ovulation independent of menstruation. Extr. Rec. Bost. Soc. M. Improve. (1874–9), 1880, vii, 13.—**Hogg** (F. R.) Notes on menstruation. Med. Times & Gaz., Lond., 1871, ii, 555.— **Iriepar** (A. E.) La menstruacion considerada bajo el punto de vista fisiológico. Siglo méd., Madrid, 1867, xiv, 755; 789; 804; 819.—**Irwin** (J. A.) The influence of sea-voyaging upon the genital functions in women. N. York M. J., 1885, xli, 536.—**Jackson** (A. R.) Non-ovarian menstruation; with cases, and some remarks upon the ovulation theory. Chicago M. J., 1870, xxvii, 583–593. ——. The ovulation theory of menstruation; will it stand? Tr. Illinois M. Soc., Chicago, 1876, xxvii, 128–161. *Also*: Am. J. Obst., N. Y., 1876, ix, 529–560. *Also*, Reprint. ——. A contribution to the relations of ovulation and menstruation. J. Am. M. Ass., Chicago, 1884. iii, 365–372. *Also*, Reprint.—**Jacquemier.** Menstruation. Dict. d. dict. de méd. (suppl.), Par., 1851, 444–453.—**Jaffé** (T.) Ovulation und Menstruation. Memorabilien, Heilbr., 1886, n. F., vi, 255–266.—**Janzer.** Untersuchung der innern Genitalien eines kurz nach der Menstruation ermordeten Mädchens. Med. Ann., Heidelb., 1848, xiii, 601–604.— **Jenks** (E. W.) Menstruation without ovulation; a few thoughts suggested by a case of double ovariotomy. Tr. M. Soc. Mich. 1870, Lansing, 1871, 137–143.—**Jepson** (S. L.) The relation of ovulation to menstruation. Tr. M. Soc. W. Virg., Wheeling, 1877, 275–285.—**Johnstone** (A. W.) The menstrual organ. Brit. Gynæc J., Lond , 1886–7, ii, 292–306, 3 pl.—**Joulin.** Mémoire sur la menstruation. Cong. méd. internat. de Par. (1867), 1868, 178–186.— **Judée** (C.) Des modifications subies par l'utérus à l'époque menstruelle. Gaz. d. hôp., Par., 1855, xxviii, 154.— **Kahleis.** Remarques sur la menstruation. J. compl. du dict. d. sc. méd., Par., 1824, xviii, 252–257. — **Kersch** (S.) Ueber Veränderung der Körpertemperatur durch den Menstruationsprocess. Memorabilien, Heilbr., 1882, n. F., ii, 65–71.—**Kesteven** (W. B.) An examination into the grounds of the ovular theory of menstruation. Lond. M. Gaz., 1849, xliv, 930–935. *Also, transl.*: Arch. gén. de méd., Par., 1850, 4. s., xxii, 438–447. ——. On the final cause of menstruation. Med. Times & Gaz., Lond., 1852, n. s., iv, 171.—**King** (A. F. A.) A new basis for uterine pathology. Am. J. Obst., 1875, viii, 237–256. [*See, also*, Studley (W. H.)]—**Krieg.** Ueber den Monatsfluss und einige denselben befördernde Mittel. Wchnschr. f. d. ges. Heilk., Berl., 1838, 217–226.—**Lagneau** (G.) Recherches comparatives sur la menstruation française. Bull. Soc. d'anthrop. de Par., 1865, vi, 724–740. [Discussion], 740–751. ——. Recherches comparatives sur la menstruation dans les diverses contrées sous le rapport ethnologique. Cong. méd. internat. de Par. (1867), 1868, 170–178. *Also* [Abstr.]: Gaz. hebd. de méd., Par., 1867, 2. s., iv, 613.—**Langheinrich** (G.) Beobachtung enüber

Menstruation.

die Zeit des Wiedereintritts der Menstruation nach vorausgegangenen Entbindungen. Beitr. z. Geburtsk. u. Gynaek., Würzb., 1854, i, 232–246.—**Lebedeff** (A. I.) K vopr. o menstrual. protsesse sviazi s. teoriei W. Löwenthal'a. [The menstrual process according to Löwenthal's theory.] Ejened. klin. gaz., St. Petersb., 1886, vi, 188–191.— **Le Cat.** Nouveau système sur la cause de l'évacuation périodique du sexe. J. de méd., chir., pharm., etc., Par., 1764, xx, 309–334.—**Lee** (R.) On the state of the ovaries during menstruation. Lancet, Lond., 1845, i, 583–585.— **Lee** (R. G.) Menstruation and the functions of the ovaries; a comparison between the false and true corpus luteum; remarks on the physiology of nutrition and circulation in the fœtus. St. George's Hosp. Rep., Lond., 1875, vii, 45.—**Leopold.** Untersuchungen über Menstruation und Ovulation. Arch. f. Gynaek., Berl., 1883, xxi, 347–408, 2 pl.—**Letheby** (H.) An account of two cases in which ovules or their remains were discovered in the Fallopian tubes of unimpregnated women who had died during the period of menstruation. Phil. Tr., Lond., 1852, 57–63, 1 pl.—**Leudet.** Étude sur la menstruation des femmes de la ville de Rouen et du département de la Seine-Inférieure. Cong. méd. internat. de Par., 1868, 162–170.—**Lieven.** Statistique de la menstruation de mille habitants de Saint-Pétersbourg. Cong. méd. internat. de Par. (1867), 1868, 205.—[**Littré.**] Sur les règles des femmes. [*From*: Mém. Acad. roy. d. sc. de Par., 1720.] Collect. acad. d. mém., etc., Par., 1774, v, 277–279.—**Loewenthal** (W.) Eine neue Deutung des Menstruationsprocesses. Arch. f. Gynaek., Berl., 1884, xxiv, 169–261. *Also* [Rev.]: Wien. med. Bl., 1885, viii, 337; 462. *Also, transl.*: Médecin prat., Par., 1884, v, 577–580. *Also*: Semaine méd., Par., 1884, 2. s., iv, 461. ——. Zwei casuistische Beiträge zur Menstruationslehre. Arch. f. Gynaek., Berl., 1885, xxvi, 156–162. ——. Ueber einige Erfahrungen bei künstlicher Unterdrückung des menstruellen Blutflusses. Tagebl. d. Versamml. deutsch. Naturf. u. Aerzte, Strassb., 1885, lviii, 110. *Also*: Allg. Wien. med. Ztg., 1885, xxx, 442. ——. Bemerkungen zu A. E. Feoktistow's "Einige Worte über die Ursachen und den Zweck des Menstrualprocesses". Arch. f. Gynaek., Berl., 1886, xxviii, 158–160.—**Louge** (P.) De l'invariabilité de fréquence du pouls dans les différentes attitudes pendant la période menstruelle. Gaz. d. hôp., Par., 1885, lviii, 1172.—**Lovett** (R. W.) Menstruation in women and animals. Boston M. & S. J., 1884, cxi, 201–205.—"**Lucina.**" À propos de règles; confidences d'une femme. J. de méd. de Par., 1887, xii, 399–407. *Also, transl.*: Cincin. Lancet-Clinic, 1887, n. s., xviii. 705. *Also, transl.*: Nashville M. News, 1887, i, 174–176.—**M'Colgan** (T. J.) The revelations of a woman doctor reviewed. South. Pract., Nashville, 1887, ix, 291–294.—**McLaury** (W. M.) Remarks on the relation of menstruation to the sexual functions. Am. J. Obst., N. Y., 1887, xx, 158–164. *Also*, Reprint.—**Madusooden Gupta.** On menstruation among Hindus. Tr. M. & Phys. Soc. Calcutta, 1843–5, ix, 308–312, 1 pl.—**Mandl** (L.) Résumé des travaux modernes sur la menstruation et la fécondation. Arch. gén. de méd., Par., 1845, 4. s., viii, 66–86.—**Manley** (J. R.) Remarks on menstruation; being an attempt to show that the generally received doctrines on this subject are not only untrue, but inadequate to explain some of the most interesting phenomena connected with that process. N. York M. & Phys. J., 1825, iv, 52–61.—**Maurel** (A.) De l'influence de la grossesse et des menstrues sur les éléments figurés du sang chez les races hindoue et noire. Arch. de tocol., Par., 1883, x, 705–710.— **Mayer** (C.-E.-L.) Exposé statistique de la menstruation dans l'Allemagne septentrionale et centrale. Cong. méd. internat. de Par. (1867), 1868, 206–219. ——. Statistische Beiträge zur Häufigkeit der Menstruation während des Stillens. Beitr. z. Geburtsh. u. Gynäk., Berl., 1872–3, ii, pt. 2, 136–142.—**Maygrier** (J.-P.) Menstruation. Dict. d. sc. méd., Par., 1819, xxxii, 375–396.—**Meadows** (A.) Menstruation and its derangements. [Abstr. report of Harveian lectures for 1881.] Med. Press & Circ., Lond., 1881, n. s., xxxii, 487; 509; 531; 1882, n. s., xxxii, 1; 19.— **Meckel** (H.) Ueber die anatomischen Verhältnisse der Menstruation. Jenische Ann. f. Physiol. u. Med., Jena, 1850, i, 192–205.—**Menstruation** and the curing of meat. Brit. M. J., Lond., 1878, ii, 541; 654; 714.—**Michaelis** (G. A.) Ausnahmen von der Regel. N. Ztschr. f. Geburtsk., Berl., 1836, iv, 361–389.—**Michel** (M.) On the dependence of menstruation upon the development and expulsion of ova, illustrated by a case in which a corpus luteum in process of formation was found coinciding with menstruation. Charleston M. J. & Rev., 1848, iii, 21–27.— **Minot.** Local congestion vicarious with menstruation. Boston M. & S. J., 1878, xcix, 633.—**Modern** theory of menstruation. Med.-Chir. Rev., Lond., 1845, n. s., ii, 523–543.—**Moericke** (R.) Verhalten der Uterusschleimhaut während der Menstruation. Centralbl. f. Gynäk., Leipz., 1880, iv, 289–291. ——. Die Uterusschleimhaut in den verschiedenen Altersperioden und zur Zeit der Menstruation. Ztschr. f. Geburtsh. u. Gynäk., Stuttg., 1881, vii, 84–137.— **Mojou** (B.) Recherches sur la menstruation. Rev. méd. franç. et étrang., Par., 1836, i, 304–320.—**Moran** (J.) Menstruation. St. Louis Cour. Med., 1882, vii, 26–30.—**Moser**

Menstruation.

(A.) Ueber die Bedeutsamkeit der Menstruation und ihr Verhältniss zu der Brunst der Thiere. N. Ztschr. f. Geburtsk., Berl., 1843, xiv, 427-435.—**Naumann** (M. E. A.) Von der Menstruation. Beitr. z. prakt. Heilk., Leipz., 1834, i, 25; 40. ———. Ueber die physiologische und pathologische Bedeutung der Menstruation. Monatschr. f. Med., Augenh. u. Chir., Leipz., 1839, ii, 18-34.—**Nijhoff** (G. C.) Ovulatie en menstruatie. Nederl. Tijdschr. v. Geneesk., Amst., 1886, xxii, 285-300.—**Nunes** (J. C.) jr. Menstruação; theoria de Rouget elucidada. Rev. med., Rio de Jan., 1877, iv, 137.—**Nourse** (A.) Menstruation and its connection with uterogestation. Boston M. & S. J., 1864, lxx, 490-493.—**Oliver** (J.) Menstruation, not a shedding of mucous membrane. Med. Times & Gaz., Lond., 1885, i, 710. ———. Menstruation; its nerve origin; not a shedding of mucous membrane. J. Anat. & Physiol., Lond., 1886-7, xxi, 378-384. *Also:* Med. Rec., N. Y., 1887, xxxii, 69-71.—**Ormières.** De la menstruation après l'ovariotomie et l'hystérectomie. Paris méd., 1880, 2. s., v, 402-404.—**Osterloh.** Ueber Menstruation. Jahresb. d. Gesellsch. f. Nat.- u. Heilk. in Dresd., Leipz., 1879, 40.—**Ott** (D. O.) K utcheniou o phiziologicheskich projavlenijach polovoi jizni i jentchin krestjanok Kalugskoi gubernii. [Sexual function of women; physiological phenomena.] Zdorovje, St. Petersb., 1879, v, 226; 280; 301; 321.—**Panum** (P. L.) Et lille Bidrag til Kundskab om Forholdet imellem Tidspunkterne for Ägløsning, Samleje og Befrugtning. Nord. med. Ark., Stockholm, 1882, xiv, no. 29, 1-3. *Also, Reprint.*—**Parvin** (T.) Is menstruation pathological? Am. Pract., Louisville, 1875, xii, 140-149. ———. A brief study of 100 cases of menstruation. Am. Pract., Louisville, 1877, xvi, 65-69.—**Pavesi** (C.) Della mestruazione e specialmente della applicazione dell' acetato di sesquiossido di ferro dializzato. Indipendente, Torino, 1881, xxxii, 661-663.—**Payne** (R. L.), jr. Probable want of connection between menstruation and ovulation. North Car. M. J., Wilmington, 1886, xviii, 145-148.—**Perroud** (L.) Influence des pyrexies sur les principaux phénomènes de la menstruation. France méd., Par., 1862, ix, 53; 71; 85; 102; 119.—**Pitcarn** (A.) Observationes quædam de fluxu menstruo. *In his:* Diss. med., 4°, Edinburgi, 1713, 161-174. *Also, in his:* Opusc. med., 4°, Roterod., 1714, 145-157. *Also, in his:* Opera omnia medica, ed. nov., 4°, Lugd. Bat., 1737, 305-314. *Also, transl. in his:* Works, 8°, Lond., 1715, 221-237.—**Ponte** (M. M.) Contribuciones á la historia de la menstruacion. Gac. cient. de Venezuela, Carácas, 1878, ii, 41.—**Post** (A. C.) Appearances of the uterus and appendages in a woman who died soon after menstruation. N. York M. Gaz., 1842, ii, 81-86.—**Power** (J.) On the theory of menstruation. Lond. M. Gaz., 1844, n. s., xxxiv, 217-221.—**Puech** (A.) L'expulsion de l'œuf suit-elle ou précède-t-elle les règles? Gaz. obst., Par., 1880, ix, 49-52.—**Purple** (S. S.) Menstruation, its true nature and office, with a review of the evidence of its vesicular origin, with illustrative cases. N. York J. M., 1846, vi, 229-236.—**Queirel** (A.) & **Rouvier** (J.) Recherches statistiques sur la menstruation à Marseille et dans les Bouches-du-Rhône. Assoc. fran:. pour l'avance. d. sc. Compt.-rend. 1879, Par., 1880, viii, 962-968. *Also:* Ann. de gynéc., Par., 1879, xii, 401-410.—**Rabuteau.** Note sur l'influence de la menstruation sur la nutrition, le pouls et la température. Compt. rend. Soc. de biol. 1870, Par., 1872, 5. s., ii, 75-77. ———. De l'influence de la menstruation sur la nutrition. *Ibid.*, 110-114. *Also:* Gaz. hebd. de méd., Par., 1870, 2. s., vii, 402-405.—**Raciborski** (A.) De la ponte périodique spontanée chez la femme et les femelles des mammifères. Expérience, Par., 1843, xii, 274; 292; 307; 321; 343.—**Ramsbotham** (F. H.) On the final cause of menstruation. Med. Times & Gaz., Lond., 1852, n. s., iv, 57; 115; 138; 219.—**Rauschenberg** (C.) Normal ovariotomy; menstrual physiology. Atlanta M. & S. J., 1874-5, xii, 350-352. ———. Ovulation and menstruation, and Dr. R. Battey's operation of normal ovariotomy. *Ibid.*, 1875-6, xiii, 713-727.—**Remak** (R.) Ueber Menstruation und Brunst. N. Ztschr. f. Geburtsk., Berl., 1843, xiii, 175-233. [*See, also, supra.*] *Also, transl.:* Ann. de la chir. franç. et étrang., Par., 1843, viii, 320-362. *Also:* Ann. de méd. belge, Brux., 1843, iii, 222-233.—**Reynolds** (J. J.) Menstruation a pathological process. Detroit Lancet, 1884-5, viii, 52-55.—**Riedel.** Bemerkungen zur Physiologie und Pathologie der Menstruation und zur Therapie gewisser Menstruationsstörungen. Verhandl. d. Gesellsch. f. Geburtsh. in Berl., 1867, xix, 142-145.—**Ritgen.** Ueber die physiologische Bedeutung der Menstruation. Gem. deutsche Ztschr. f. Geburtsk., Weimar, 1828, ii, 464-487.—**Roberton** (J.) An inquiry into the natural history of the menstrual function. Edinb. M. & S. J., 1832, xxxviii, 227-254. *Also, transl.:* N. Ztschr. f. Geburtsk., Berl., 1840, viii, 361-383.—**Roberts.** Menstruation; its natural history and physiology, and its relations to amenorrhœa. Bull. N. York Acad. M., 1869, iii, 332-342.—**Rossetti** (A.) Menstruation et ovulation. Mouvement méd., Par., 1876, xiv, 305-307.—**Rouvier** (J.) Quelques phénomènes supplémentaires des règles. Ann. de gynéc., Par., 1879, xii, 10; 120: 1880, xiii, 115. ———. Recherches sur la menstruation en Syrie. *Ibid.*, 1887,

Menstruation.

xxvii, 178-201.—**Sakaki** (Junjiro). [A study of the statistics of eight hundred cases of menstruation and conception in Japanese women.] Chiugai Iji Shinpo, Tokio, 1886, no. 156, Sept. 25.—**Santorinus** (J. D.) De catameniis. Opusculum iv. *In:* Baglivius (G.) Opera omnia, 4°, Lugduni, 1710, 843-854. *Also, in his:* Opusc. posth., 16°, Rotterod., 1719, 189-216.—**Schauer** (C. H.) Ueber die Menstruation. Verhandl. d. Gesellsch. f. Geburtsh. in Berl., 1853-5, viii, 1; 14. ———. Die Theorien der älteren und neueren Zeit über die Menstruation. Monatschr. f. Geburtsk. u. Frauenkr., Berl., 1855, v, 94-111.—**Schelver** (F. J.) Die Menstruation. J. d. Naturw. u. Med., Frankf. a. M., 1810, i, 228-241.—**Schwarzschild.** Der Zweck der Menstruation. (Aus einem noch ungedruckten Werke: Die Menstruation, historisch-physiologisch betrachtet.) J. f. Geburtsh., Leipz., 1834, 398-446.—**Shannon** (H.) Ovulation without menstruation; conception; albuminuria; dropsy; delivery at full term; good getting up. Tr. M. Soc. N. Jersey, Newark, 1884, 255.—**Sigismund** (R.) Ideen über das Wesen der Menstruation. Berl. klin. Wchnschr., 1871, viii, 624.—**Simpson** (A. R.) Emmenologia. Obst. J. Gr. Brit., Lond., 1876, iii, 675-688. *Also:* Tr. Edinb. Obst. Soc., 1874-7, iv, 176-194. *Also, Reprint.*—**de Sinéty.** Note sur l'indépendance relative qui peut exister entre l'ovulation et la menstruation. Compt. rend. Soc. de biol. 1876, Par., 1877, 6. s., iii, 365-367. *Also:* Gaz. méd. de Par., 1876, 4. s., v, 623. ———. Recherches sur la muqueuse utérine pendant la menstruation. Compt. rend. Soc. de biol. 1881, Par., 1882, 7. s., iii, 99-102. *Also:* Gaz. méd. de Par., 1881, 6. s., iii, 175.—**Smith** (J. McC) Influence of opium upon the catamenial functions. N. York J. M., 1844, ii, 56-58. *Also:* Lond. M. Gaz., 1843-4. xxxiii, 878.—**Stephenson** (W.) On the menstrual wave. Am. J. Obst., N. Y., 1882, xv, 287-294.—**Stoltz** (A.) Menstruation. N. dict. de méd. et chir. prat., Par., 1876, xxid, 299-339.—**Storer** (H.-R.) De la menstruation sans ovaires. Arch. de physiol. norm. et path., Par., 1868, i, 376-378.—**Stricker** (W.) Aufforderung zu gemeinsamen statistischen Ermittelungen über die Verhältnisse der Menstruation. Arch. f. path. Anat., etc., Berl., 1876, lxviii, 295: 1878, lxxii, 281: 1879, lxxvi, 212: lxxviii, 194: 1882, lxxxviii, 379.—**Strohl** (E.) Recherches statistiques sur la relation qui peut exister entre la périodicité de la menstruation et les phases de la lune. Gaz. méd. de Strasb., 1861, 2. s., i, 93-103.—**Studley** (W. H.) Is menstruation a disease? A review of Professor King's article entitled: "A new basis for uterine pathology". Am. J. Obst., N. Y., 1875, viii, 487-512.—**Suggestive** (A) custom in Devonshire. Lancet, Lond., 1878, ii, 205; 244; 279; 427; 498.—**Sylvius** (J.) De mensibus muliebribus liber: in quo etiam obiter diversi feminei affectus explicantur et curantur: quibus adjicitur de generatione hominis, sive de fœcunditatis et sterilitatis causis libellus. *In:* Gynæciorum [etc.], 4°, Basileæ, 1566, 771-850. *Also:* 8°, Basileæ, 1586, i, 304-310. *Also:* fol., Argentinæ, 1597, 148-166.—**Szukits** (F.) Ueber die Menstruation in Oesterreich. Ztschr. d. k.-k. Gesellsch. d. Aerzte zu Wien, 1857, 509-544.—**Tang-uet** (H.) De l'influence de la menstruation sur le système nerveux. Marseille méd., 1879, xvi, 541-552.—**Tait** (L.) Note on the relations of ovulation and menstruation. Med. Times & Gaz., Lond., 1884, i, 619-624.—**Tauszky** (R.) The ovulation and other theories of menstruation; the anomalies of menstruation, their appreciable causes and treatment. Physician & Pharmac., N. Y., 1879, n. s., xi, 275-282.—**Tholander** (F.) Kritik och belysning af några punkter i läran om menstruationen. [Some points and theories of menstruation.] Svens. Läk.-Sällsk. n. Handl., Stockholm, 1871, 2. s., iv, 1-55.—**Tillaux.** De l'ovulation dans ses rapports avec la menstruation. Bull. Acad. de méd., Par., 1880, 2. s., ix, 880.—**Tilt.** De l'influence du climat et de la race sur la menstruation. Cong. méd. internat. de Par. (1867), 1868, 187-190.—**Torres** (G.) Del uso de agentes terapéuticos durante las reglas. Crón. méd., Valencia, 1878-9, ii, 103-108.—**Townsend** (F.) Ovulation and menstruation considered in their physiological relations. Albany M. Ann., 1885, v, 97-112.—**Trousseau.** Ueber Menstruations-Fieber. Allg. Wien. med. Ztg., 1861, vi, 393; 401.—**Underhill** (C. E.) Note on the uterine mucous membrane of a woman who died immediately after menstruation. Tr. Edinb. Obst. Soc., 1878, iv, 129-132.—**Versari** (C.) Esame critico sulla tesi: Menstrui derivano dalla ovoluzione. Rendic. Accad. d. sc. d. Ist. di Bologna, 1873, 120-124. ———. Intorno la ovulazione muliebre diretta a indurne, se ella, come credono i più, sia proprio, o no la efficienza dei mestrui. Raccoglitore med., Forlì, 1874, xxxvii, 489-498.—**Vogel** (C.) Folgen übermässiger Menstruation. Mag. f. d. ges. Heilk., Berl., 1828, xxvi, 325-336.—**Vogt** (H.) Sur la menstruation normale en Norvège. Cong. méd. internat. de Par. (1867), 1868, 196-204. *Also, transl.:* Norsk Mag. f. Lægevidensk., Christiania, 1867, xxi, 23-37.—**Walker** (A. D.) Ovulation and menstruation. Obst. J. Gr. Brit., Lond., 1874, ii, 412-416.—**Warner** (Helen.) Some objections to Løwenthal's theory of menstruation. Detroit Lancet, 1884-5, n. s., viii, 442-444.—**Warwick** (J.) Notes on menstruation. Lond. M. Gaz.,

Menstruation.

1843-4, n. s., i, 863-866.—**Weber** (F.) Ueber die Menstrualverhältnisse der Frauen in St. Petersburg. St. Petersb. med. Wchnschr., 1883, viii, 329; 337; 345.—**Wendt** (E. C.) Uterus and appendages of a woman who died while menstruating; no marked hypertrophy or destruction of mucous membrane. Med. Rec., N. Y., 1882, xxii, 582.—**Wilder** (A.) Menstruation; its use, or its relation to the moral and religious nature. N. York M. Rev., 1873, n. s., i, 17-22. — **Williams** (J.) Additional cases illustrating the changes which occur periodically in the mucous membrane of the uterus. Obst. J. Gr. Brit., Lond., 1877, v, 593-597; 1884, i, 253; 301.—**Wiltshire** (A.) Lectures on the comparative physiology of menstruation. Brit. M. J., Lond., 1883, i, 395; 446; 500. *Also* [Abstr.]: North Car. M. J., Wilmington, 1883, xi, 251-261. *Also:* Vet. J. & Ann. Comp. Path., Lond., 1883, xvi, 257; 349; xvii, 16. *Also:* J. Comp. M. & S., N. Y., 1883, iv, 284: 1884, v, 58; 163; 254.—**Worster** (J.) Observations on the physiology of menstruation, with notes of a case in point. Med. Rec., N. Y., 1876, xi, 683-685. — **Wyder** (T.) Das Verhalten der Mucosa uteri während der Menstruation. Ztschr. f. Geburtsh. u. Gynäk., Stuttg., 1883, ix, 1-37.

Menstruation (*Abnormal and vicarious*).

See, also, **Fallopian** *tube* (*Rupture of*); **Hymen** (*Imperforate*); **Jaundice** (*Causes, etc., of*); **Menses** (*Retention of*); **Menstruation** (*Premature*); **Ovariotomy** (*Sequelæ, etc., of*); **Pregnancy** (*Menstruation during*); **Vagina** (*Imperforate, etc.*)

ABBAL (G.) * Des principaux caractères cliniques de l'hémoptysie et en particulier de l'hémoptysie supplémentaire à la menstruation. 4°. *Montpeller*, 1865.

ARONSON (J.) * De hæmorrhagiæ narium ac gingivarum salubritate loco fluxus menstrui casu quodam comprobata. 4°. *Halæ*, [1772].

BEAUCHAMP (P.) *Essai sur la xénoménie. 4°. *Strasbourg*, 1864.

CLEMENT (F.) Generalis et brevis tractatus de anomaliis menstruorum. 8°. *Vindobonæ*, [*n. d.*]

HEDLUFF (J. E.) * De viis mensium insolitis. 4°. *Jenæ*, [1745].

JÄSCHKE (G. F.) * De mensium insolitis viis. 4°. *Halæ Magdeb.*, 1707.

Also, in: HALLER. Disp. ad morb. [etc.] 4°. *Lausannæ*, 1758, iv, 525-553.

JAMIN (F.) *Essai sur la ménoxénie, ou déviation du flux menstruel. 4°. *Strasbourg*, 1810.

KELLNER (G.) * De menstruatione anomala. 8°. *Halæ*, 1823.

KIRCHNER (A.) * De congestionibus atque hæmorrhagiis menstruationis vicariis. 8°. *Wirceburgi*, 1833.

LESCHE (C. M.) * De ægra hæmorrhagia narium a suppressione mensium laborante. sm. 4°. *Helmstadii*, [1716].

LOREY (G.) * Des vomissements de sang supplémentaires des règles, et pathogénie des hémorrhagies supplémentaires du flux menstruel, en général. 4°. *Paris*, 1875.

MAISONNAVE. * Quelques considérations sur le traitement des hématémèses supplémentaires des règles. 4°. *Paris*, 1877.

MAUDUIT (J.-A.) * Considérations sur la menstruation, ses anomalies en général, et sur l'hémoptysie sympathétique en particulier. 4°. *Paris*, 1825.

MICHAELIS (E.) * Observationes quædam de catameniorum viis insolitis. 8°. *Berolini*, [1830].

PETER (C.) *Diss. sistens historiam rariorem mammæ cancrosæ sanguinem menstruum fundentis, methodo simpliciore sanatæ. 4°. *Tübingæ*, 1763.

Also, in: FRANK (J. P.) Delect. opusc. med. 8°. *Ticini*, 1791, x, 64-94.

DE RAYSSAC (F.) * Étude sur la menstruation dans ses rapports avec les hémorrhagies supplémentaires et complémentaires des règles. 4°. *Paris*, 1875.

Menstruation (*Abnormal and vicarious*).

SCHACHT (C.) *De menstruatione vicaria. 8°. *Berolini*, [1845].

STITZER (H. C.) *De menstruatione vicaria. 8°. *Halis*, [1860].

TIEDEMANN (H.) * Ueber die stellvertretende Menstruation (Menstruatio vicaria). 8°. *Würzburg*, 1842.

TRILLER (D. W.) [Pr.] . . . præmissa nova veraque explicatione loci cujusdam Hippocratici hactenus obscurissimi e lib. vii de morb. epidem. extrem. de mensibus per nares Leonidæ filiæ erumpentibus, ab imprudenti autem medico cum ipsius interitu infeliciter repressis. sm. 4°. *Vitembergæ*, [1758].

WALLENTIN (G.) *Menstruatio præcox. 8°. *Breslau*, [1885].

ZISSY (D. M.) * De anomaliis catameniorum. 8°. *Herbipoli*, 1836.

Adams (F. W.) Case of apparent Fallopian menstrual secretion. Am. J. M. Sc., Phila., 1836, xviii, 38-43.—**Albertus** (M.) De fluxu menstruo per sudorem sanguinis e pedibus. Acad. nat. curios. ephem., Norib., 1715, cent. iii-iv, 241.—**Alibert.** Hémorrhagie auriculaire, survenue à la suite de la suppression des menstrues. J. de méd. et chir. de Toulouse, 1845-6, ix, 244.—**Allbut** (T. C.) Case of premature menstruation. Lancet, Lond., 1866, ii, 11; 85.—**Allport** (W. W.) A case of vicarious catamenial hæmorrhage from the gums, with recession of the gingival margins and alveolar processes, the result of amenorrhœa. J. Am. M. Ass., Chicago, 1885, iv, 147-149.—**d'Andrade** (A. P.) An account of a case in which the menses were apparently substituted by hæmorrhage from the skin. Tr. M. & Phys. Soc. Bombay (1862), 1863, n. s., viii (app.), pp. xx-xxiv.—**Andreae** (D. W.) Menstrua vetulæ. Acta Acad. nat. curios., 2. ed., Norimb., 1727, i, 82.—**Astbury** (J.) Case of menstruation by the hæmorrhoidal vessels for more than two years. Edinb. M. & S. J., 1821, xvii, 307.—**B.** (W. R.) Vicarious menstruation. Boston M. & S. J., 1850, xli, 63.—**Baker** (E. C.) A case of vicarious menstruation from an ulcer on the right mamma. South. J. M. & Pharm., Charleston, 1847, ii, 152-155, 1 pl.—**Bantock** (G. G.) Amenorrhœa and vicarious menstruation. Med. Times & Gaz., Lond., 1884, i, 210.—**Barancy.** Note sur quelques cas de déviations menstruelles. Ann. méd.-chir. franç. et étrang., Par., 1885, i, 54-56.—**Barbee** (W. J.) Cholera morbus occurring monthly in lieu of menstruation. Maryland M. & S. J., Balt., 1840, i, 287.—**Barham** (C.) Periodical purpura vicarious of the catamenia. Prov. M. & S. J., Lond., 1847, 455.—**Barnes** (R.) On vicarious menstruation. Brit. Gynæc. J., Lond., 1886-7, ii, 151-177. [Discussion], 188-207. ———. Clinical paper on vicarious menstruation. Med. Press & Circ., Lond., 1886, n. s., xli, 397; 419.—**Barnes** (T.) Case of vicarious menstruation, with singular discharge from the ear. Edinb. J. M. Sc., 1826-7, ii, 273-283. - **Barrett** (E. C.) Vicarious menstruation per rectum. Virginia M. Month., Richmond, 1883, ii, 671-673.—**Barry** (E. L. H.) A case of vicarious menstruation. Med. Arch., St. Louis, 1873, ix, 78-81.—**Baster** (J.) Fœmina cui menses per ulcus fluebant, filium sanissimum in lucem edit, subsequente ulceris consolidatione. Acta Acad. nat. curios., Norimb., 1748, viii, 93.—**Belinus.** Menstrua per oculos excreta. Zodiacus med.-gall. 1680, Geneva, 1682, ii, 42.—**Bellamy** (W. J. H.) A case of vicarious menstruation(?). Virginia M. Month., Richmond, 1875, ii, 31-33.—**Beniveni** (A.) Menses vomitione projecti. *In:* Dodonaeus (R.) Med. obs. exempla rara, 16°, Coloniæ, 1581, 196.—**Bennett** (R.) Early menstruation; profuse and long-continued hæmoptysis in connection with scanty menstrual flow. Med. Times & Gaz., Lond., 1857, n. s., xiv, 190.—**Beziat.** Observation d'une veuve bien constituée, continuant d'être réglée à l'âge de quatre-vingt-sept ans. Ann. Soc. de méd. prat. de Montpel., 1804, iv, 188-192.—**Bierling** (C. T.) Signum instantis mensium fluxus in facie. *In his:* Adversariorum curiosorum centuria prima, 4°, Jenæ. 1679, 93. — **Billing.** Vicarious menstruation. Lancet, Lond., 1831-2, ii, 520-522. — **Blackburn** (J. C.) Menstruation in an old woman? Nelson's North. Lancet, Plattsburg, N. Y., 1852-3, vi, 191. — **Blair** (H. A.) A case of attempted vicarious menstruation, attended with conjunctivitis and opacity of the cornea. Oglethorpe M. & S. J., Savannah, 1858-9, i, 11-15.—**Blair** (H. R.) Case of vicarious menstruation. Edinb. M. J., 1858-9, iv, 882.—**Boring** (J.) † † Vicarious menstruation. Atlanta M. & S. J., 1855-6, i, 211-214.—**Borrichius** (O.) Menstrua per nares exeuntia. Acta med. et phil. 1677-9, Hafn., 1680, 174-176. *Also, transl.:* Collect. acad. d. mém., etc., Dijon, 1766, vii, 370.—**Bouchereau.** Observation sur un ulcère au sein, à la suite d'une suppression de règles, guérie par les emménagogues. J. de méd., chir., pharm., etc., Par., 1783, lx, 317.—**Boulger** (E.) Case of a discharge which

Menstruation (*Abnormal and vicarious*).

issued at monthly periods from beneath the left mamma. Lancet, Lond., 1840-41, i, 493.—**Brincken** (G. T. L.) En Deviatio menstruationis, hvorved Blodet afsondredes igjennem de undertiden opbrydende Araf et gammelt leprost Saar paa Ryggen. [Flow of blood from cicatrix of a leprous ulcer.] Eyr, Christiania, 1834, ix, 99-102. *Also, transl.:* J. f. Geburtsh., Leipz., 1838, xvii, 622-624.—**Broers** (H. J.) Anomalie der menstruatie met begeleidende verschijnselen in andere organen; asthma uterinum (van Simpson). Nederl. Tijdschr. v. Heel- en Verlosk., Utrecht, 1859-60, x, 230-239.—**Brosse** (P.) Vicarirende Menstruation. Mitth. a. d. Geb. d. Heilk., Leipz., 1845, 207.—**Buchanan** (G.) Case of menstruating ulcer. Obst. J. Gr. Brit., Lond., 1879, vi, 780-782. *Also:* Glasgow M. J., 1879, xi, 304. — **B——w.** Zwey Beobachtungen von einer zweyjährigen Zurückhaltung der monatlichen Reinigung, die durch Geschwüre des Halses ersetzt wurde. N. Mag. f. Aerzte, Leipz., 1787, ix, 20-26.—**Cabadé.** Sur un cas de menstruation précoce. Gaz. méd. de Par., 1883, 6. s , v, 462; 474.—**Calder** (J.) The menstrua regularly evacuated at an ulcer of the ankle. Med. Essays & Obs. Soc. Edinb., 1735, iii, 380-382.—**Campbell** (H. F.) Menstruation after extirpation of the ovaries. Boston M. & S. J., 1883, cix, 320-323.—**Casati** (E.) Mestruazione precoce. Raccoglitore med., Forlì, 1886, ii, 387.—[**Cases.**] Entzündliches Unterleibsübel a causa externa mit merkwürdiger Anomalie der Menstruation. Mag. f. d. ges. Heilk., Berl., 1830, xxxi, 278-282.—Ein Fall von vikariirender Menstruation und Heilung derselben. [*From:* Tygodnik lekarski.] Allg. med. Centr.-Ztg., Berl., 1858, xxvii, 748-750.—Un cas de céphalæmatome des femmes. Compt.-rend. Soc. méd. de Chambéry (1854-8), 1859, 33.—Hemoptisis suplementaria del flujo menstrual. Aspiracion méd., Madrid, 1867-8, i, 286.—**Caso** (S) Vicarious menstruation (from the gums). Med. Rec., N. Y., 1878, xiii, 213. *Also:* Atlanta M. & S. J., 1878-9, xvi, 28-31.—**Cazenave.** Observation au sujet d'une évacuation périodique des règles, par les mammelles et le visage. J. de méd., chir., pharm., etc., Par., 1759, x, 23-26.—**Cecil** (J. G.) Precocious menstruation. Louisville M. News, 1885, xx, 146.—**Celliez.** Observation sur une femme de soixante-quinze ans, parfaitement réglée. J. de méd., chir., pharm., etc., Par., 1762, xvi, 153-155.—**Chancellor** (J. E.) Abnormal menstruation. Tr. M. Soc. Virg., 13. sess., 1882. Richmond, 1883, iii, pt. 4, 489-492.—**Chevers** (N.) Amenorrhœa and vicarious menstruation. Med. Times & Gaz., Lond., 1884, i, 249.—**Clarke.** Vicarious menstruation; death. Lancet, Lond., 1872, ii, 225.—**Clarke** (J. E.) On vicarious menstruation. Detroit Lancet, 1882-3, n. s., vi, 408-411.—**Clésio.** Observation d'une anomalie de la menstruation. J. de la sect. de méd. Soc. acad. Loire-Inf., Nantes, 1826, ii, 230.—**Coles** (W.) Vicarious menstruation. St. Louis M. & S. J., 1879, xxxvii, 9-22.—**de Corral y Oña.** Historia de una meno-xenia, ó desviacion de la regla; muerte subsiguiente á una metro peritonis puerperal. Telégrafo méd., Barcel., 1849, iii, 161-167.—**Cowan** (C.) Vicarious menstruation. Lond. M. Gaz., 1837, xx, 686.—**Craig** (J.) Case of prolonged menstruation. Tr. M. Soc. N. Jersey, Newark, 1877, 209.—**Criado y Aguilar.** Un caso notable de menstruación ectópica. Progreso ginec., Valencia, 1884-5, i, 641; 657.—**Cummins** (A. H.) Hæmorragia menstrua per talum in gravida. Misc. Acad. nat. curios., Lips., 1670, i, 224. *Also, transl.:* Collect. acad. d. mém., etc., Dijon, 1755, iii, 17. ——. De menstruis serotinis, item ante statum naturæ ordinem fluentibus. Misc. Acad. nat. curios. 1672, Francof. et Lips., 1781, iii, 158. *Also, transl.:* Collect. acad. d. mém., etc., Dijon, 1755, iii, 132.—**da Cunha** (J. G.) On vicarious menstruation. Tr. M. & Phys. Soc. Bombay, 1870, x (app.), pp. xiv-xvi.—**Dassier** (A.) Note sur un cas de déviation des règles. J. de méd., chir. et pharm. de Toulouse, 1875, 3. s., iv, 43.—**Dayton** (A. C.) [Metastasis of the menstrual secretion from the uterus to the mouth.] Ohio M. & S. J., Columbus, 1849, ii, 231.—**Decaisne** (E.) Un cas remarquable de déviation des menstrues. Gaz. d. hôp., Par., 1874, xlvii, 3. — **De Muynck.** Retour des règles à un âge très-avancé; guérison d'affections opiniâtres. Bull. Soc. de méd. de Gand, 1844, x, 168-170. — **De Reynel.** Observations sur deux aberrations du flux menstruel. J. univ. d. sc. méd., Par., 1819, xiv, 361-365.—**Droste** (A.) Menstruation aus dem After. Wchnschr. f. d. ges. Heilk., Berl., 1833, ii, 1197.—**Duchesne** (E.) Aménorrhée complète; sang des menstrues remplacé par des sueurs périodiques. Monit. d. hôp. Par., 1856, iv, 661.—**Duncan** (J. M.) Amenorrhœa and vicarious menstruation. Med. Times & Gaz., Lond., 1884, i, 139-141.—**Dupuis** (T. R.) Case of menstruation in a woman aged sixty-four years. Canada Lancet, Toronto, 1871-2, iv, 21.—**Dupuytren.** Brûlure; dénudation de la peau; flux menstruel s'opérant par cette plaie. Gaz. d. hôp., Par., 1828-9, i, 85. *Also, transl.* [Abstr.]: South. M. & S. J., Augusta, 1836-7, i, 228. — **Edwards.** Menstruation at the age of eight; vicarious hæmoptysis. Med. Times & Gaz., Lond., 1857, xiv, 190.—**Elmslie** (W. J.) A case of vicarious menstruation. Indian M. Gaz., Calcutta, 1867, ii, 102. — **Embling** (T.) Infantile men-

Menstruation (*Abnormal and vicarious*).

struation. Lancet, Lond., 1848, i, 137.—**Emmet** (T. A.) A case of persistent menstruation in a lady seventy years of age. Am. J. Obst., N. Y., 1886, xix, 152. — **Falkenbach** (W. A.) Consensuelle Anschwellung eines Brustknotens während der Menstruation. Gen.-Ber. d. k. rhein. Med.-Coll. 1837, Koblenz, 1839, 218.—**Farre.** Examples of vicarious hæmatemesis. Lancet, Lond., 1861, ii, 447.—**Field.** A case of vicarious menstruation from the ear. Med. Press & Circ., Lond., 1882, n. s., xxxiii, 115.—**Fingerhuth.** Vicarirende Menstruation. Wchnschr. f. d. ges. Heilk., Berl., 1836, 87-89. — **Finley** (S. B. R.) Case of menstruation from the mammæ. Carolina J. M. Sc., Charleston, S. C., 1825, i, 203. — **Flechner** (A. E.) Fall einer dreyzehnjährigen Amenorrhœa mit sechs regelmässig verlaufenden Schwangerschaften. Med. Jahrb. d. k. k. österr. Staates, Wien, 1840, n. F., xxi, 531-534.—**Flechsig.** Merkwürdiges Wiederauftreten der Menstruation im 80sten Lebensjahre mit kritischer Bedeutung für ein chronisches Nervenleiden. Wchnschr. f. d. ges. Heilk., Berl., 1843, 429-432.—**Fleischmann.** Menstrualblutung auf ungewöhnlichem Wege. J. d. pract. Heilk., Berl., 1840, 2. St., xc, 108.—**Forel** (F. A.) Cas de menstruation chez un homme. Bull. Soc. méd. de la Suisse Rom., Lausanne, 1869, iii, 53-61.—**Forster** (I. C.) A case of menstrual ulcer on the face. Lond. M. Gaz., 1851, xlvii, 447.—**Foster** (J. W.) Early menstruation. St. Louis M. & S. J., 1880, xxxviii, 300.—**Fouquier.** Menstruation d'une jeune fille par l'estomac; hematemèse symptomatique. Gaz. d. hôp., Par., 1835, ix, 93.—**Gajani** (M.) Menstruazione dall' apertura fatta da uno spillo in un punto della vena salvatella sul dorso di una mano. Bull. d. sc. med. di Bologna, 1836, 2. s., i, 17-19.—**Gardner** (A. K.) Case of supposed consumption; vicarious menstruation dependent upon stricture of cervix uteri cured by incision of the cervix. Bull. N. York Acad. M., 1860-62, i, 134-137.—**Garrigue.** Déviation du flux cataménial; hématurie; guérison. J. de méd. et chir. prat., Par., 1883, liv, 161-164.—**Gaucher** (E.) Arrêt de développement et imperfoxauon de l'utérus, avec absence complète de cavité utérine et imperforation des oviductes, chez une femme de 44 ans, dont les ovaires étaient normaux et couverts de cicatrices menstruelles, et qui n'avait jamais été réglée. Bull. Soc. anat. de Par., 1880, lv, 229-231. *Also:* Progrès méd., Par., 1880, viii, 936.— **Gay.** Vicarious menstruation following an accident to the finger; removal of the finger, etc. Lancet, Lond., 1843-4, i, 574.—**G[aynor** (J. G.)] A case of vicarious menstruation. Physicians' & Surgeons' Invest., Buffalo, 1884, v, 161-164. — **Gibbs** (O. C.) Case of pregnancy in a female, in whom the menstrual function had been for some years suspended. N. Am. M.-Chir. Rev., Phila., 1857, i, 741-743. — **Gillet.** Un cas de déviation de menstrues chez une jeune fille. Bull. Soc. méd. de l'Yonne 1867, Auxerre, 1868, pt. 2, p. viii. *Also:* Bull. gén. de thérap., etc., Par., 1867, lxxii, 30.—**Gloninger** (J. W.) A case of periodical hæmorrhage from the urethra of a male. Am. M. Recorder, Phila., 1819, ii, 371. ——. A case of hæmoptysis, alternating with a discharge of blood from the uterus. N. York M. & Phys. J., 1824, iii, 64.—**Glückselig** (A. M.) Entzündung und Eiterung der rechten Brustdrüse als vicarirendes Leiden bei zurückgetretener Menstruation. Med. Jahrb. d. k. k. österr. Staates, Wien, 1839, n. F., xx, 156.—**Gordon** (J. T.) An unusual case of vicarious menstruation. Am. J. Obst., N. Y., 1882, xv, 343.—**Gould** (A. A.) Vicarious menstruation. Boston M. & S. J., 1856-7, lv, 266. *Also:* Extr. Rec. Bost. Soc. M. Improve. (1856-8), 1859, iii, 28.— **Gray** (G. D.) A case of vicarious menstruation from mammary glands. Am. M. Bi-Weekly, Louisville, Ky., 1877, vii, 146.— **Green** (J. O.) Vicarious menstruation from a sebaceous tumor of the meatus. Am. J. Otol., N. Y., 1881, iii, 133.—**Gregory** (S. T.) Case of a female, the mother of seven children, who had never menstruated. Am. J. M. Sc., Phila., 1853, n. s., xxv, 549. — **Groër.** Czyszczenie miesieczne nieprawidlowe (menstrua anomala). Gaz. lek., Warszawa, 1874, xvi, 17-23. — **Grosskopf** (A.) Anomale Menstruation durch den After. Oesterr. med. Wchnschr., Wien, 1844, 255-257.—**Gubler.** Des épistaxis utérines. Gaz. d. hôp., Par., 1863, xxxvi, 461.—**Guépin.** Hémorrhagie dans la chambre antérieure supplémentaire du flux menstruel. J. de méd. de Bordeaux. 1861, 2. s., vi, 354.—**Gutgesell.** Widernatürliche monatliche Reinigung. J. d. pract. Arznk. u. Wundarznk., 2. Aufl., Berl., 1800, xi, 1. St., 191.—**Hagendorn** (E.) Nonagenaria menstruata. Misc. Acad. nat. curios. 1687, Norimb., 1707, 2. decuria, vi, 305-307. *Also, transl.:* Collect. acad. d. mém., etc., Dijon, 1766, vii. 461.—**Halliburton** (W. D.) A peculiar case. [Menstruation in a male?] Weekly M. Rev., Chicago, 1884, xii (suppl.), 392. — **Hamilton** (R.) History of a case in which an epistaxis occurred vicarious to the menstrual discharge. Med. Comment. 1786, Edinb., 1787, 2. decade, i, 337-342.—**Hamoir** (C.-P.-E.) Déviation des règles se produisant par une vaste plaie de la jambe; guérison. Gaz. d. hôp. Par., 1853, xxvi, 49. — **Hecking & Elfes.** Menstruatio anomala. Gen.-Ber. d. k. rhein. Med.-Coll. 1836, Koblenz,

Menstruation (*Abnormal and vicarious*).

1839, 188.—**Hedrich.** Vicarirende Milchsecretion, statt der Menstruation. N. Ztschr. f. Geburtsk., Berl., 1844, xv, 469.—**Heine.** Wiederkehr der Menstruation. Summ. d. Neuest. u. Wissenswürd. a. d. ges. Med., Leipz., 1835, xii, 418.—**Heitzmann** (J.) Vicariirende Menstruation und Menstrual-Exantheme. Med. Jahrb., Wien, 1884, 9-41.— **Hellwig** (J.) Menstruus fluxus per oculos. *In his:* Obs. phys.-med., 4°, Aug. Vindel., 1680, 381. — **Hennig.** Merkwürdige Verhärtung im Unterleibe und Unordnung in der Menstruation, von Würmern entstanden. J. f. d. Chir., Geburtsh. u. gerichtl. Arznk., Jena, 1806, iv, 531-537. — **Henry.** Observation au sujet d'une femme qui étoit réglée par la bouche, à l'ouverture du cadavre de laquelle on trouva 207 pierres logées dans la vésicule du fiel. Rec. périod. d'obs. de méd., de chir. et pharm., Par., 1757, vii, 384-389.—**Hildebrand.** Für die Menstruation vicariirende Hämorrhagie aus einer Zahnlücke. Med. Ztg., Berl., 1842, xi, 214. — **Himmelscher.** Menstruation durch die Brüste und einzelne Hautstellen. Ann. f. d. ges. Heilk., Karlsruhe, 1831-2, iv, 2. Hft., 135-138. — **Hinton** (R. L.) A case of vicarious menstruation. Memphis M. Recorder, 1857, v, 657.—**von Hönigsberg.** Vicarirende Menstruation. Wien. Med.-Halle, 1862, iii, 198.—**Hofer.** Wiedereintritt der Menstruation bei einer 75jährigen Frau. Med. Cor.-Bl. d. württemb. ärztl. Ver., Stuttg., 1839, ix, 108.—**Holmes** (A. S.) Vicarious menstruation. Mississippi Valley M. Month., Memphis, 1883, iii, 63-65. — **Hooper** (P.) A sloughing ulcer performing a vicarious function. Phila. M. Times. 1882-3, xiii, 433.—**Horrocks** (P.) Amenorrhœa; monthly epistaxis. Guy's Hosp. Rep., Lond., 1883-4, xlii, 173.—**Hottinger** (J. H.) De catameniorum fluxu in muliere octoginta trium annorum. Misc. Acad. nat. curios. 1701-5, Norimb., 1706, 3. decuria, ix-x, 403.— **Hoyer** (J. G.) De fluxu menstruo in vetula [76 years of age]. Acad. nat. curios. ephem., Francof. et Lips., 1712, cent. i-ii, 239. — — De muliere septuagenaria bis menses iterum experta et tandem pro gravida habita. *Ibid.*, 1717, cent. v-vi, 333.—**Jacobson.** Cas de menstruation habituelle par les deux seins. J. compl. du dict. d. sc. méd., Par., 1828, xxxi, 83-85. *Also:* Clin. d. hôp., Par., 1828-9, iii, 3.—**Jouilletton.** Hémorrhagie périodique et régulière par la verge. J. de méd., chir., pharm., etc., Par., 1813, xxvi, 329. — — Cas d'une femme réglée depuis 5 ans par l'oreille droite, à la suite d'une fausse couche. *Ibid.*, 330.—**Kelly** (B.) A case in which menstruation is performed without any direct or apparent communication between the cavity of the vagina and that of the uterus; the latter being ascertained to exist in a rudimentary condition. N. York J. M., 1859, 3. s., vii, 420-422. — **Kennard** (T.) Anomalies of menstruation. Med. Arch., St. Louis, 1871, vi, 74-81.—**Kenworthy** (J.) [Case of vicarious menstruation.] Med. & Phys. J., Lond., 1811, xxv, 24-27. — **Kilpatrick** (J. B.) Anomalous menstruation; quinine idiosyncracy. Texas Cour.-Rec. Med., Fort Worth, 1883-4, i, 29.—**King** (A. F. A.) Hematemesis. Am. J. M. Sc., Phila., 1870, n. s., lix, 420-422.—**King** (V. O.) Case of menstruation in the male. Canada M. J., Montreal, 1867, iii, 472.—**Kirby** (J.) Singular disease; vicarious menstruation; profuse hæmorrhage from the mouth; nervous symptoms; treatment; recovery. Dublin M. Press, 1852, xxviii, 339.—**Kirk** (C. D. R.) Fatal case of vicarious menstruation. Indiana M. J., Indianap., 1881-2, i, 329.—**Knight** (A. W.) Vicarious menstruation. South. M. & S. J., Augusta, 1852, viii, 660. — **Költsch** (H.) Menstruations-Anomalien. Deutsche Klinik, Berl., 1858, x, 333.—**Kratky.** Eine räthselhafte Krankheitsgeschichte. Allg. med. Ann., Altenb., 1815, pt. 2, 57-64.— **Krishaber.** Hémorrhagie linguale à l'époque de la ménopause. Ann. d. mal. de l'oreille et du larynx, Par., 1877, iii, 38-40.—**Lachmund** (F.) Menstruali partium in puella quadam externarum, utpote aurium, narium, digitorum, etc., mortificatione. Misc. Acad. nat. curios. 1673-4, Francof. et Lips., 1676, iv-v, 238. *Also: Ibid.* (1673-4), 1688, iv-v. 224.—**Landis** (H. G.) Vicarious menstruation. Cincin. Lancet & Clinic, 1880, n. s., iv, 187-192. *Also,* Reprint.— **Lebeuf.** Lettre sur un homme qui est réglé par la verge, comme une femme l'est par le vagin. Rec. périod. d'obs. de méd., de chir. et pharm., Par., 1756, v. 280-283. — **Lee** (J. H.) Vicarious menstruation. South. Pract., Nashville, 1884, vi, 109.—**Leonard** (C. H.) Vicarious menstruation. Penins. J. M., Detroit, 1876, i, 559-571. — **Lewis** (J.) Case of apparently vicarious menstrual discharge. N. Eng. J. M. & S., Bost., 1818, vii, 317-319.—**Lieber.** Merkwürdige Folge des Zahnausziehens während der Menstruation. Wchnschr. f. d. ges. Heilk., Berl., 1833, ii, 1031.—**Lucas.** Menses anomalæ. Gen.-Ber. d. k. rhein. Med.-Coll. 1837, Koblenz, 1839, 97.—**Lyncker** (F.) Neue Menstruation im späten Alter. Wchnschr. f. d. ges. Heilk., Berl., 1839, 590.—**McGraw** (T. A.) A case of vicarious menstruation from an ovariotomy scar. Am. J. Obst., N. Y., 1884, xvii, 912-914.—**Mader.** Vicarirende Hæmoptoe by Menstruationsstörung; Heilung. Ber. d. k. k. Krankenanst. Rudolph-Stiftung in Wien (1885), 1886, 379.— **Malgouvré.** Observation sur un cas de règles dévoyées. Ann. Soc. de méd. prat. de Montpel., 1808, xii,

Menstruation (*Abnormal and vicarious*).

358-365.—**Mann** (M. D.) Vicarious menstruation; general peritonitis without characteristic symptoms. N. York M. J., 1881, xxxiv, 180. *Also:* Am. J. Obst., N. Y., 1882, xv (suppl.), 16.—**Marcacci** (G.) Ovulazione periodica senza mestruazione in giovine di venti anni. Arch. med. ital., Torino, 1883, ii, 248-259. — **Marsden** (W.) Case of mismenstruation with sterility. Brit.-Am. M. & Phys. J., Montreal, 1850-51, vi, 205-207.—**Marsset** (A.) Menstruation précoce. Gaz. d. hôp., Par., 1886, lix, 259.— **Meurer.** Vicarirende Menstruationsthätigkeit der Lungen. Gen.-Ber. d. k. rhein. Med.-Coll. 1837, Koblenz, 1839, 97. — — . Menstruation während der Schwangerschaft; Amenorrhöe ausser derselben. *Ibid.* 217.—**Meynet** (P.) Note sur un cas de déviation des règles; hémorrhagies supplémentaires par les mamelles. Mém. et compt.-rend. Soc. d. sc. méd. de Lyon (1872), 1873, xii, pt. 2, 3-5. *Also:* Lyon méd., 1872, ix, 396-398.—**Michelsen** (G.) Vicariirender Monatsfluss durch ein Geschwür auf dem Schienbein. Ztschr. f. d. ges. Med., Hamb., 1846, xxxii, 527.—**Miller** (C. H.) A case of precocious menstruation, with procidentia uteri. South. Clinic, Richmond, 1887, x, 104-106. — **Moehring** (P. H. G.) Pleuripneumonia, a sanguine menstruo, per vomitorium thoracem versus presso, oborta. Acta Acad. nat. curios., Norimb., 1737, iv, 344-348.—**Montagud** (A.) Apuntes para una historia de menstruacion precoz. Actas . . . Cong. region. de cien. méd. 1879, Cádiz, 1882, 533-540.—**Morris** (G. de C.) Vicarious menstruation. Lancet, Lond., 1882, ii, 1013.—**Moses** (I.) Vicarious menstruation from the umbilicus. Am. J. M. Sc., Phila., 1859, n. s., xxxviii, 356. — — . Vicarious menstruation from an ulcer on the head. *Ibid.*, 357.— **Mosler** (F.) Lebensgefährliche Blutung eines varikösen Geschwürs nach Suppressio mensium. Arch. f. path. Anat., etc., Berl., 1861, xxii, 195-197.—**Mossé.** Épithélioma myxoïde de l'ovaire; ponction; épistaxis utérines chez une femme ayant dépassé depuis quinze ans la ménopause. Bull. Soc. anat. de Par., 1877, lii, 772-776.—**Mühlbrand.** Eine Blutblase als Stellvertreter der Catamenien. Mag. f. d. ges. Heilk., Berl., 1826, xxii, 597.—**Müller.** Fehlende Menstruation. Ann. f. d. ges. Heilk., Karlsruhe, 1827-8, iii, 1. Hft., 72-76.—**Neuhold** (J. J.) De hæmorrhagia narium menstrua, in puella sexenni. Acta Acad. nat. curios., Norimb., 1733, iii (app.), 171.—**Nye.** Vicarious menstruation simulating pulmonary disease. J. Gynæc. Soc. Bost., 1870, ii, 75.—**Obermeier** (O.) Ein Fall von menstruellem Nasenbluten. Arch. f. path. Anat., etc., Berl., 1872, liv, 435.—**Oke** (W. S.) Abnormal menstruation. [3 cases.] Assoc. M. J., Lond., 1853, 392-394.—**Oppel.** Menstruationsanomalien. Wien. med. Presse, 1865, vi, 1048.—**d'Outrepont.** Geschichte einer Atrophie des Uterus und der damit verbundenen Menometastasie (Menstruatio aberrans). Wchnschr. f. d. ges. Heilk., Berl., 1842, 497-508.— **Paget** (G. E.) Menorrhagia brought on in old age by emotional disturbance. Brit. M. J., Lond., 1880, ii, 16. *Also:* Lancet, Lond., 1880, ii, 54.—**Panarolus** (D.) Vetula septuagenaria ab adolescentia ejiciens menses per os. *In his:* Iatrologismorum, 4°, Romæ, 1652, 6. — — . Sanguis fontis modo per mammas scaturiens menstruorum loco. *Ibid.*, 234-236.—**Parvin** (T.) An illustration of xenomenia. Tr. Am. Gynec. Soc. 1876, Bost., 1877, i, 135: (1877), 1878, ii, 482, 2 pl.—**Pauli** (F.) Vicariirende Menses. N. Ztschr. f. Geburtsk., Berl., 1839, vii, 261-263. — **Paullini** (C. F.) Menses verminosi. *In his:* Obs. med.-phys., 12°, Lips., 1706, 34.—**du Peyrou de Cheyssiole & Bonhoure.** [Une paysanne âgée de plus de quatre-vingt-onze ans, assujettie aux évacuations ordinaires à son sexe] Collect. acad. d. mém., etc. Partie franç., Par., 1787, xiv, 320.—**Pitcher** (Z.) A case of vicarious menstruation, showing also the morbid relations of the colon and uterus. Penins. J. M., Ann Arbor, Mich., 1856-7, iv, 121-124. — **Plummer-Bates** (J. W.) Vicarious menstruation. Med. & Surg. Reporter, Phila., 1880, xlii, 295.— **Porter** (I. G.) Vicarious menstruation. Am. J. M. Sc., Phila., 1853, n. s., xxv, 135. — **Post** (A. C.) Remarkable œdema of the arm of a female alternating with the state of the menstrual discharge. N. York J. M. & S., 1841, iv, 215. — **Prion.** Menstruation tardive et avortement à l'âge de 72 ans. Bull. Soc. de méd. d'Angers (1864), 1865, n. s., i, 42-45.—**Puech** (A.) À propos d'une déviation des menstrues ayant persisté pendant toute la durée de la vie sexuelle. Gaz. obst., Par., 1877, vi, 2-7.—**Puéjac** (Anna). Des déplacements de la fluxion utérine menstruelle. Gaz. méd. de l'Algérie, Alger, 1887, xxxii, 85.— **Putney** (G. E.) A case of vicarious menstruation. Boston M. & S. J., 1878, xcviii, 628. — **Ranöe** (A. B.) Hæmoptysis a menstruis suppress. Acta reg. Soc. med. Havn. (1782-8), 1791, ii, 110-113.—**Rau** (W. T.) De vetulis menstruatis. Acta Acad. nat. curios., Norimb., 1752, ix, 159-161.—**Raymann** (J. A.) De hæmorrhagia penis periodica. *Ibid.*, 1742, xi, 17-20.—**Revillout** (V.) Hématémèses supplémentaires des règles. Gaz. d. hôp., Par., 1878, li, 617-619.—**Reydellet.** Des métastases, suites de la suppression ou de la répercussion d'évacuations naturelles ou habituelles. Dict. d. sc. méd., Par., 1819, xxxiii, 61-67.—**Richardson** (B. F.) Case of vicarious menstrua-

Menstruation (*Abnormal and vicarious*).

tion. West. Lancet, Cincin., 1850, xi, 369.—**Richardson** (T. G.) Atresia vaginæ with vicarious menstruation. N. Orl. M. & S. J., 1873-4, n. s., i, 74.— **Richardson** (W. L.) Abnormal menstruation, etc. Boston M. & S. J., 1882, cvi, 207.—**Rommelius** (P.) De voluntaria fluxus menstrui retardatione. Misc. Acad. nat. curios. 1686, Norimb., 1687, 2. decuria, v, 48-52. ———. Mensium defectum menstruum alvi profluvium supplens. *Ibid.* (1691), 1692, 2. decuria, x, 374 - 376.—**Rouxeau.** Ménoxénie; jeune fille de 17 ans, réglée par le sein gauche. Gaz. méd. de Nantes, 1883-4, ii, 39.—**Rubini.** Storia di un atresia, e d' una mestruazione straordinaria. Gior. d. Soc. med.-chir. di Parma, 1811, x, 36-42. ———. Osservazioni in risposta al Prof. Termanini. *Ibid.*, 1812, xii, 94-102.—**Samuels** (F. W.) A case of vicarious menstruation successfully treated with the manganese salts. South-West. M. Gaz., Louisville, 1887, i, 163.—**Schlichting** (J. D.) Menstrua protheiformia. Acta Acad. nat. curies., Norimb., 1742, vi, 112. — **Schneider.** Menstruation durch das Zahnfleisch. Wchntl. Beitr. z. med. u. chir. Klin., Leipz., 1833-4, iii, 165.—**Schultzius** (S.) De menstruis per aliena loca fluentibus. Misc. Acad. nat. curios. 1673 - 4, Francof. et Lips., 1676, iv-v, 63. *Also: Ibid.* (1673-4), 1688, iv-v, 59. ———. De singularibus vesiculis post aures menstrua ordinarie et immediate præcedentibus. Misc. Acad. nat. curios. 1675-6, Francof. et Lips., 1688, vi-vii, 341. *Also, transl.*: Collect. acad. d. mém., etc., Dijon, 1755, iii, 318. — **Schwabe** (C.) Menstrual - Geschwür. Wchnschr. f. d. ges. Heilk., Berl, 1843, 141.—**Scolari** (L.) Mania ricorrente per amenorrea o menostasia, cura energica antiflogistica; guarigione dopo tre mesi circa coll' apparire della mestruazione. Gazz. med. ital. lomb., Milano, 1848, 2. s., i, 279-282.—**Seymour** (F.) A case of vicarious menstruation, and singular action of the uterus developed in its treatment. Cincin. Lancet & Obs., 1872, n. s., xv, 65-68.—**Seymour** (R. H. G.) Case of vicarious menstruation simulating hæmoptysis; treatment. Med. & Surg. Reporter, Phila., 1877, xxxvi, 242.—**Simpson.** Case of amennorrheal ulcer. Month. J. M. Sc. Lond. & Edinb., 1855, xx, 347. — **Sirus-Pirondi & Oddo.** (C.) Quelques considérations sur les hémorrhagies dites supplémentaires à propos d'un cas d'hémorrhagie auriculaire survenue à l'occasion des règles. Marseille méd., 1887, xxiv, 129 - 140. — **Sommer** (F.) Monatlich wiederkehrende Blutung aus Mund und Nase während der ganzen Schwangerschaft, vicarirend für die Menstruation, welche bei kurz vorhergehender Lactation anderthalb Jahre gänzlich ausgeblieben war. Med. Ann., Heidelb., 1844, x, 376. — **Stalpart vander Wiel** (C.) Maandstonden door verstoortheijt uijt beyde tepels gelost. [Menstruation from both nipples.] *In his:* Hondert seldzam aanmerk., 12°, Amst., 1682, 259. *Also, transl. in his:* Obs. rariorum med.-anat.-chir., 12°, Lugd. Bat., 1687. 342.—**Stepanoff** (E. M.) Sluchai ushnich krovot., zamienja. menstrualnija. [Hæmorrhage from ear; vicarious menstruation.] Med. Obozr., Mosk., 1885, xxiv, 588-595.—**Stewart** (F. C.) Extraordinary case of vicarious menstruation. N. York J. M., 1844, ii, 327.—**Stössel** (A.) Ueber vicariirende Menstrual- und Hämorrhoidalblutungen. Wien. Med.-Halle, 1863, iv, 125.—**Stone** (A. J.) A case of vicarious menstruation, with details of treatment. Northwest. M. & S. J., St. Paul, 1871, ii, 376-381.—**Strenbel** (C.) Vom Ausbruch derer Mensium unter dem Knie. Samml. v. Nat.- u. Med.-/... Gesch. 1721, Leipz. u. Budissin, 1722, xvi, 551.—**Sutherland.** Reappearance of the catamenia from mental shock seven years after the change of life. Brit. M. J., Lond., 1877, i, 454. ———. Case of remenstruation at fifty-nine, after eight years' cessation. *Ibid.*, 1879, ii, 774. *Also:* Lancet, Lond., 1880, i, 249.—**Tappan** (J. C.) [Vicarious menstruation.] Tr. M. Ass. South. Central N. Y., Binghamton, 1858-61, ii, 37-39.—**Tauszky** (R.) The anomalies of menstruation; their causes and treatment. Physician & Bull. Med.-Leg. Soc., N. Y., 1880, i, 20-24. *Also,* Reprint.—**Taylor** (W. T.) Case of conception before the appearance of the menses. Med. Exam., Phila., 1852, n. s., viii, 581.—**Termanini.** Lettera sopra la sforia d' un' atresia ed' una menstruazione straordinaria, riferita dal Prof. Rubini. Gior. d. Soc. med.-chir. di Parma, 1812, xii, 81-94.—**Teuffard** (F.) Observation d'une seconde menstruation établie à cinquante-six ans par les seins. Union méd., Par., 1872, 3. s., xiv, 845.—**Thomas** (R.) A case of vicarious menstruation simulating pulmonary phthisis; cure. Am. J. Obst., N. Y., 1886, xix, 141-143.—**Thomas** (R. P.) Case of anomalous menstruation. Tr. Col. Phys. Phila., 1853-6, ii, 160. — **Thomas** (W.) Peculiar idiosyncracy in a family as regards the reappearance of the catamenia late in life. Med. Times, Lond., 1852, n. s., v, 148. ———. A case of vicarious menstruation. Austral. M. J., Melbourne, 1885, n. s., vii, 4-6.—**Tott** (C. A.) Erfahrungen über Anomalien der Menstruation bei den Weibern. N. Ztschr. f. Geburtsk., Berl., 1851, xxx, 232-239.—**Tschierschki.** Für Menstruation vicariirendes Blutbrechen. Wchnschr. f. d. ges. Heilk., Berl., 1843, 45-49.—**Upshur** (J. N.) A case of vicarious menstruation. Virginia M. Month.,

Menstruation (*Abnormal and vicarious*).

Richmond, 1875, ii, 432.—**Van Derveer** (A.) A case of infantile menstruation. Am. J. Obst., N. Y., 1883, xvi, 1005.—**Varges** (A. W.) Blutschweiss am Kopfe als Menstruatio vicaria. Ztschr. f. Med., Chir. u. Geburtsh., Leipz., 1861, xv, 171-174.—**Vasser** (E. M.) Gastric hematemesis, vicarious of regular menstruation, produced by malarial causes. South. M. Rec., Atlanta, 1873, iii, 536-538.—**V[ergar]i** (A.) Mestruazione da un polpastrello d' un dito, alternante con quella delle parti muliebri ordinarie a darle. Esculapio napol., Napoli, 1835, xvii, 90-92.—**Vicarious** hæmoptysis. Med. Times & Gaz., Lond., 1857, n. s., xiv, 189.—**de la Vigne.** Menstruation durch die Lungen. Gen.-Ber. d. k. rhein. Med.-Coll. 1831, Koblenz, 1833, 49. — **Wainwright** (W. A. M.) Vicarious menstruation; general peritonitis without characteristic symptoms. N. York M. J., 1881, xxxiv, 180. *Also:* Tr. N. York Obst. Soc. (1881-5), 1885, iii, 2. — **Ware** (C. E.) Vicarious menstruation in the course of nursing. Am. J. M. Sc., Phila., 1850, n. s., xix, 371.—**Watson** (J.) Atresia vaginæ; vicarious menstruation. N. York J. M., 1858, 3. s., v, 235.—**Wedel** (G. W.) Von dem Fluss der monatlichen Reinigung durch den Hintern. Auserl. med.-chir.-... Abhandl. d. röm.-kais. Akad. d. Naturf., Nürnb., 1756, iii, 35. — **Weisse** (J. F.) Aberratio mensium (Hæmatoplania Plouoquet). Verm. Abhandl. . . . v. einer Gesellsch. pract. Aerzte zu St. Petersb., 1842, vi, 250.—**Wells** (D. E.) Vicarious menstruation. Boston M. & S. J., 1878, xcviii, 617. ———. Protracted menstruation. *Ibid.*, 1882, cvii, 39.—**de Wenckh** (J. B.) De duobus viris styriacis fluxum menstrualem sanguinis per penem patientibus. Misc. Acad. nat. curios. 1701-5, Norimb., 1706, decuria 3, ix - x, 258 - 261. — **Wilks.** On vicarious menstruation. Brit. Gynæc. J., Lond., 1886-7, ii, 177-183.—**Wiltshire** (A.) Clinical lecture on vicarious or ectopic menstruation, or menses devii. Lancet, Lond., 1885, ii, 513 - 517.—**Winkler** (D.) Von dem durch die Verstopfung der monatlichen Reinigung erregten Blutbrechen. Auserl. med.- chir.-... Abhandl. d. röm.-kais. Akad. d. Naturf., Nürnb., 1759, vi, 88. — **Wolf** (I.) Tributum lunare per mammas solutum. *In his:* Obs. med.-chir., 4°, Quedlimburg, 1704, 66-69. — **Wood.** Stomatorrhœa vicarious to the menses. Tr. Coll. Phys. Phila. (1856-62), 1863, n. s., iii, 305. — **Wright** (C. O.) Cases of vicarious menstruation. Am. J. Obst., N. Y., 1887, xx, 88-94.—**Wright** (W.) Menstruatio recidiva after 17 years' cessation. Med. Chron., Montreal, 1855, ii, 381-383.—**Wygrzywalski.** Zatrzymanie miesiaczki przez pietnaście miesięcy, guzy w brzuchu, watpliwe vozpoznanie, potwór, zapatrzenie? [Cessation of menstruation during 15 months; doubtful diagnosis.] Gaz. lek., Warszawa, 1872, xiii, 485-489.—**Yonge** (J.) Of a woman who had the menses to 70 years of age. Phil. Tr., Lond., 1700 - 20, v, 352. — **Zangerl.** Menstruatio vicaria. Oesterr. med. Wchnschr., Wien, 1843, 309-311.

Menstruation (*Cessation of*).

See, also, **Climacteric** *years, etc.*; **Insanity** *in women*; **Uterus** (*Cancer of*).

ARMAND (P.) *Considérations sur l'âge critique des femmes, et sur les moyens de prévenir les maladies qui peuvent survenir à cette période de la vie. 4°. *Paris*, 1820.

ASSEGOND (H.) *De la femme considérée à l'âge critique, changemens physiologiques qui s'opèrent dans son état physique et morale, et de l'application des règles de l'hygiène à cette principale époque de sa vie. 4°. *Paris*, 1821.

AULAGNIER. Considérations sur l'âge critique qui amène la suppression absolue du flux périodique; faisant suite aux observations déjà publiées sur les maladies des femmes. 8°. *Paris*, [*n. d.*]

BARDOUT (C.-M.) *Considérations générales sur la cessation du flux menstruel, et sur les précautions à prendre pour en prévenir les accidens ou les maladies. 4°. *Paris*, 1816.

BARIÉ (E.) *Étude sur la ménopause. 4°. *Paris*, 1877.

BARON (J.-S.) *De la ménopause. 4°. *Paris*, 1851.

BÉCLARD. *Essai sur les maladies auxquelles les femmes sont le plus fréquemment exposées à l'époque de la cessation des menstrues. 8°. *Paris, an X* [1802].

BERTIN (É.) *De la ménopause considérée principalement au point de vue de l'hygiène. 4°. *Montpellier*, 1865.

Montpellier thèses, 1865. Concours pour l'agrégation.

Menstruation (*Cessation of*).

BERTRAND (P.-J.-B.) *Dissertation sur l'amé-norrhée définitive ou âge critique des femmes, sur les accidens auxquels elles sont exposées à cette époque, et sur les moyens thérapeutiques, hygiéniques et prophylactiques les plus appro-priés à leur situation. 4°. *Paris*, 1824.

BÖRNER (E.) Die Wechseljahre der Frau. 8°. *Stuttgart*, 1886.

BOURLET (L.) *Étude sur la métrite interne chronique après la ménopause. 4°. *Paris*, 1879.

BUHL (J. C.) *De præservatione morborum post plenariam mensium cessationem. sm. 4°. *Lugd. Bat.*, 1722.

CHAMBON DE MONTAUX (N.) Maladies chro-niques à la cessation des règles. 8°. *Paris, an VII* [1799].
Sub-title of pt. 5 of his Maladies des femmes, 2. éd.

CHANDELUX (L.) *De l'âge critique de la femme (ménopause). 4°. *Paris*, 1850.

CHOUFFE (J.-B.-P.) *Des accidens et des ma-ladies qui surviennent à la cessation de la men-struation. 8°. *Paris, an X* [1802].

COLLINET (M.) *Des modifications des organes génitaux de la femme à l'époque de la méno-pause. 4°. *Paris*, 1887.

DEVERS (J.) *Essai sur la cessation des règles. 4°. *Paris*, 1822.

DOCÉ (L.-H.) *Dissertation sur la cessation des menstrues, vulgairement appelée âge cri-tique, et sur les moyens hygiéniques que réclame la santé de la femme à cette époque. 4°. *Pa-ris*, 1831.

DUMONT (P.-L.-C.) *Dissertation sur la disparition des règles, les accidens auxquels la femme est alors exposée, et les précautions qu'elle doit prendre pour les éviter. 4°. *Paris*, 1833.

FORCE (V.) *Du rhumatisme à la ménopause. 4°. *Paris*, 1877.

FOTHERGILL (J.) Conseils aux femmes de quarante-cinq à cinquante ans, ou conduite à tenir lors de la cessation des règles. Traduit et extrait des observations et recherches de la So-ciété médicale de Londres, et augmenté de notes par le D. Petit-Radel. 2. éd. 8°. *Paris, an VIII* [1800].
For original, see *infra*.

DE GARDANNE (C.-P.-L.) *Sur les avis à don-ner aux femmes qui entrent dans l'âge critique. 4°. *Paris*, 1812.

———. De la ménopause, ou de l'âge critique des femmes; traité dans lequel sont exposés la description anatomique et physiologique de l'uté-rus à la ménopause, les changemens que cette époque opère tant sur le physique que sur le moral de la femme, les moyens hygiéniques qui doivent être alors employés, enfin les maladies qui surviennent ordinairement à l'âge critique. 2. éd. 8°. *Paris*, 1821.

GÉRARD (B.-E.) *De l'âge critique chez la femme, et des maladies qui l'accompagnent. 4°. *Paris*, 1849.

GILLES (J.-F.) *Sur la cessation de l'écoule-ment menstruel. 4°. *Paris*, 1821.

GLINEL (P.-N.) *Sur l'âge critique des femmes. 4°. *Paris*, 1818.

GUILBERT (J.-N.) *Des purgatifs à la cessa-tion des menstrues. 8°. *Paris, an XII* [1803].

GUIMBAIL (H.) *De la folie à la ménopause. 4°. *Paris*, 1884.

HÉBERT (É.-L.) *Sur la cessation des règles, les accidens auxquels la femme est alors exposée, et les précautions qu'elle doit prendre pour les éviter. 4°. *Paris*, 1817.

JACQUEMART (P.) *Contribution à l'étude du rôle étiologique de la ménopause. 4°. *Paris*, 1884.

Menstruation (*Cessation of*).

JALLON (L.-J.-S.) *Essai sur l'âge critique des femmes. 4°. *Paris, an XIII* [1805].

JARDEL (J.) *Sur les phénomènes qui se manifestent à la cessation du flux périodique, et sur les moyens propres à préserver les femmes des maladies qui peuvent les affecter à cette époque. 4°. *Paris*, 1819.

JEANNIN (L.-M.-A.) *Considérations phy-siologiques, pathologiques et hygiéniques sur l'âge de retour des femmes. 4°. *Strasbourg*, 1830.

JUNOD (C.-L.) *De l'époque critique chez les femmes et des précautions à prendre pour en prévenir et combattre quelques accidens ou ma-ladies. 4°. *Paris*, 1822.

LAMAZE (H.) *Sur la cessation du flux men-struel, et sur les moyens propres à prévenir les accidents et les maladies qui peuvent affecter les femmes à cette époque. 4°. *Paris, an XIII* [1805].

LEFÈVRE (J.-P.) *Considérations générales sur la ménopausie, ou cessation naturelle des menstrues. 4°. *Paris*, 1826.

LEMOYNE (N.-N.-F.) *Considérations géné-rales sur les phénomènes qui se manifestent à la cessation du flux menstruel, et sur le régime que doivent adopter les femmes pour franchir heu-reusement cette époque. 4°. *Paris*, 1824.

LESTRADE (J.-N.) *Considérations générales sur l'époque critique des femmes, et sur les mala-dies qui sont attachées à cet âge. 4°. *Paris*, 1815.

LOEWENHARDT (O. A.) *De pathologia an-norum climactericorum. 8°. *Halis*, 1851.

MALADIÈRE-MONTÉCOT (G.-M.) *Considéra-tions générales sur la ménespausie, ou cessation des menstrues, et sur les moyens à employer pour prévenir les accidens et les maladies qui peuvent l'accompagner. 4°. *Paris*, 1818.

MARTIN (A.-F.) *Essai sur l'hygiène des femmes parvenues à l'âge où l'évacuation men-struelle doit cesser. 4°. *Paris*, 1831.

MARVAUD (G.-F.) *Considérations générales sur la cessation des règles, et sur l'âge fausse-ment appelé critique. 4°. *Paris*, 1829.

MAURICE (P.) *De la ménespausie. 4°. *Pa-ris*, 1832.

MAYER (A.) Conseils aux femmes sur l'âge de retour; médecine et hygiène. 8°. *Paris*, 1875.

MÉNISSIER (E.-D.) *Considérations générales sur quelques maladies qui affectent les femmes à l'âge critique. 4°. *Paris*, 1808.

MENVILLE. Conseils aux femmes à l'époque de l'âge de retour, ou de l'âge critique, et des moyens de combattre et prévenir les maladies qui peuvent survenir à cette époque de la vie. 8°. *Paris*, 1839.

———. De l'âge critique chez les femmes, des maladies qui peuvent survenir à cette époque de la vie, et des moyens de les combattre et de les prévenir. 8°. *Paris*, 1840.

NICAISE (A.) *Essai sur l'âge de retour chez la femme. 4°. *Paris*, 1838.

NOSLEY (J.-B.) *Sur l'âge critique. 4°. *Paris*, 1848.

PELOUX (C.-A.-M.) *Essai sur l'époque cri-tique et sur les moyens propres à prévenir les accidens et les maladies qui en dépendent. 4°. *Paris*, 1812.

PLIHON (G.-A.) *De la ménopause. 4°. *Pa-ris*, 1859.

POIRSON (H.-Q.-F.) *Sur la ménespausie. 4°. *Strasbourg*, 1827.

POQUILLON (J.-B.-L.) *De la ménopause, ou de l'âge dit critique chez la femme. 4°. *Paris*, 1846.

Menstruation (*Cessation of*).

Poussié (J.-A.) Réflexions sur l'hygiène qui convient aux femmes arrivées à l'âge de retour. 4°. *Montpellier*, 1813.

Puyo (B.-G.-É.) *De la ménopause. 4°. *Paris*, 1865.

Ramondenc (S.) *Considérations sur l'état de la femme à l'époque de la cessation des règles. 4°. *Montpellier*, 1820.

Regemann (J. L.) *De morbis ex menstruis per ætatem cessantibus. 4°. *Lugd. Bat.*, 1737.

Remarks on the final cessation of the menses, and on a remedy and method of treatment adapted to prevent and remove the evil consequences attending that period, etc. 8°. *London*, 1775.

Ricard (H.) *Étude sur les troubles de la sensibilité génésique à l'époque de la ménopause. 4°. *Paris*, 1879.

Ripeault (C.-A.-D.) *De la ménopause. 4°. *Paris*, 1848.

Rocque (H.-E.) *Essai sur la physiologie et la pathologie de la ménopause. 4°. *Paris*, 1858. *Also* [Abstr.], *in*: Gaz. d. hôp., Par., 1859, xxxii, 38.

Sauvé (P.-L.) *Réflexions sur l'âge critique et particulièrement sur le régime le plus convenable pour préserver les femmes des accidens qui ont coutume de survenir à cette époque de leur vie. 4°. *Strasbourg*, 1826.

Spitta (H. H. L.) *Commentatio physiologico-pathologica mutationes, affectiones et morbos in organismo et œconomia feminarum cessante fluxus menstrui periodo sistens. 4°. *Gottingæ*, 1818.

Thomasi (A.) *Aperçu sur diverses maladies qui peuvent affecter les femmes à l'âge de retour. 4°. *Montpellier*, 1820.

Tilt (E. J.) On the preservation of the health of women at the critical periods of life. 12°. *New York*, 1851.

———. The change of life in health and disease. A practical treatise on the nervous and other affections incidental to women at the decline of life. 3. ed. 8°. *London*, 1870. *Also* [Abstr.], *in*: Lancet, Lond., 1856, n. s., ii, 564; 592; 644.

———. The same. From 3. Lond. ed. 8°. *Philadelphia*, 1871.

———. The same. 4. ed. 8°. *New York*, 1882. *Also, transl. in*: Rev. méd.-chir. d. mal. d. femmes, Par., 1883, v, 301; 426; 486; 548; 606; 665; 1884, vi, 5; 64; 133; 185; 265; 312; 431; 1885, vii, 141; 246; 369; 493; 665.

Titius (S. D.) *De fine mensium initiis morborum variorum opportuno. 4°. *Halæ Magdeb.*, [1710].

Transtour (J.-A.) *Considérations générales sur quelques maladies qui affectent les femmes à l'âge critique. 4°. *Paris*, 1812.

Vanderlinde (F. J.) *Fata ac incommoda ex menstruis naturæ lege tandem cessantibus oriunda. sm. 4°. [*Heidelberg*, 1789.]

Verne (H.-J.) *Essai sur la cessation des menstrues et sur quelques maladies qui attaquent les femmes à cette époque critique. 4°. *Paris*, 1809.

Verpillat (N.-T.) *Sur les affections organiques les plus fréquentes lors de la cessation des menstrues, et le traitement qui leur est applicable. 4°. *Paris*, 1829.

Vizévene (D.) *De feminarum ætate critica sive de periodo climacterica. 8°. *Lugd. Bat.*, 1835.

Willette (T.) *Étude sur les accidents nerveux de la ménopause. 4°. *Paris*, 1877.

Windrif (L.-J.) *Essai sur les phénomènes de l'âge critique chez la femme; sur les principaux accidens que l'on remarque à cette époque,

Menstruation (*Cessation of*).

et sur les moyens de les prévenir. 4°. *Strasbourg*, 1811.

Zalzal (N.) *Troubles cardiaques de la ménopause. 4°. *Lyon*, 1885.

de Alarcon (G.) La menospausia. Corresp. méd., Madrid, 1879, xiv, 90; 98; 114; 130; 138; 146; 154; 162; 178; 186; 202.—**Aphel** (F.) Menopausa. Gazz. med. di Torino, 1885, xxxvi, 724–734.—**Arnold** (A. B.) The menopause. Med. & Surg. Reporter, Phila., 1880, xlii, 486–488.—**Baer** (B. F.) The significance of metrorrhagia recurring about and after the menopause. Am. J. Obst., N. Y., 1884, xvii, 449–464. *Also, Reprint.*—**Barker** (F.) The age of woman when child-bearing ceases. Phila. M. Times. 1874-5. v, 161–164.—**Clément** (E.) Cardiopathie de la ménopause. Lyon méd., 1884, xlvi, 433; 467. *Also*: Rev. de méd., Par., 1885, v. 118–130. *Also*: J. Soc. de méd. et pharm. de l'Isère, Grenoble, 1884–5, ix, 82; 114; 126.—**Cohnstein.** Ueber Menopause. Deutsche Klinik, Berl., 1873, xxv, 45. ———. Zur Physiologie der Menopause. Arch. f. path. Anat., etc., Berl., 1874, lxi, 100–109.—**Fothergill** (J.) Of the management proper at the cessation of the menses. Med. Obs. Soc. Phys. Lond., 1776, v, 160–186. [*See, also, supra.*]—**Franceschi** (G.) Sulla sinfisi del pube muliebre prima e dopo della menopausa. Bull. d. sc. med. di Bologna, 1886, 6. s., xviii, 15–38.—**Francis** (C. R.) Profuse climacteric menorrhagia and sympathetic vomiting cured by opium. Med. Times & Gaz., Lond., 1882, ii, 492.—**Francotte** (X.) Étude sur la ménopause au point de vue pathologique et thérapeutique. Ann. Soc. de méd. d'Anvers, 1881, xlii, 5; 105.—**Gendrin.** Leçon sur l'âge critique. Gaz. d. hôp., Par., 1850, 3. s., ii, 542.—**Gros.** Du rhumatisme coïncidant avec l'âge critique et de son traitement par les eaux de Lamalou - l'Ancien. Nice-méd., 1883–4, viii, 17–22.—**Guéneau de Mussy** (N.) Érotisme de la ménopause. *In his*: Clin. méd., 8°. Par., 1875, ii, 343–352.—**Guy** (W. A.) On the first and last appearance of the menses, and the relation existing between the two periods. Med. Times, Lond., 1845, xii, 363.—**Halford** (H.) On the climacteric disease. *In his*: Essays and orations, 12°, Lond., 1842, 1–14.—**Helfft.** Die Decrepiditäts - Periode und das Verhalten des Arztes während und nach derselben. Monatschr. f. Geburtsk. u. Frauenkr., Berl., 1854, iii, 201; 273.—**Higgens** (C.) Asthenopia occurring in women about the climacteric period. Brit. M. J., Lond., 1878, ii, 557.—**Ivanoff** (N. P.) K kaznistike chrezmernago potenija i jeltuchi v klimaktericheskom periode. [On the great number of cases of dropsy and jaundice during the period of change of life.] Voyenno-med. J., St. Petersb., 1883, cxlvii, pt. 3, 63–92.—**Jaggard** (W. W.) Functional disorders in connection with the menopause. Syst. Pract. M. (Pepper), Phila., 1886, iv, 432–446.—**Kisch** (E. H.) Die nervösen Leiden der Frauen im klimakterischen Alter. Wien. med. Presse, 1876, xvii, 600; 644.—**Liégeois** (C.) Les sueurs de l'âge critique, leur traitement par le sulfate d'atropine. Rev. méd. de l'est, Nancy, 1879, xi, 460–472.—**Mann** (E. C.) A case illustrating the neurotic disturbances incident to the menopause. N. York M. Month , 1886-7, i, 73.—**Marsh** (J. O.) Menorrhagia and metrorrhagia of the climacteric period, with cases. Obst. Gaz., Cincin., 1881, iv, 285–288.—**Merson** (J.) The climacteric period in relation to insanity. West Riding Lun. Asyl. Rep., Lond., 1876, vi, 85–107.—**Mettler** (L. H.) The menopause and some of its disorders. Med. Reg., Phila., 1887, ii, 323–327.—**Mondouis.** Remarques et observations relatives aux phénomènes de la ménopause. J. de méd., chir. et pharm. de Toulouse, 1858, 3. s., iii, 257–261.—**Orr** (G. W.) Inflammation of the fore-arm caused by cessation of menstruation. Physician & Surg., Ann Arbor, Mich., 1881, iii, 19.—**Parrish** (J.) The change of life in women, with remarks on the periods usually called "critical". N. Jersey M. Reporter, Burlington, 1854, vii, 13; 63; 92; 205; 313; 381.—**Pepper** (W.) The change of life in women. Clin. News, Phila., 1880, i, 505.—**Pray** (T. J. W.) Report on gynæcology. Tr. N. Hampshire M. Soc., Concord, 1876, 55–67.—**de Redondo** (A.) Menopáusia, no edad crítica. Fraternidad méd., Vallad., 1880, ii, 640–654.—**Ribell.** Âge critique. Rev. méd. de Toulouse, 1885, xix, 273–278.—**Rodzevitch** (G. I.) Antropologicheskaja ekskursija po Volga. [Anthropological excursion to the Volga. (Statistics of menopause in different nationalities.)] Vrach. Vaidom., St. Petersb., 1882, vii, 3344–3347.—**Roig y Bofill** (E.) Consideraciones generales acerca del influjo patogénico de la menopausia, especialmente en la produccion del cáncer uterino. Gac. méd. de Cataluña, Barcel., 1878, i, 38–45.—**Schmidt** (J. A.) Eine sonderbare Hautkrankheit [welche mit der cessirenden Menstruation in Verbindung zu stehen schien, und durch die wiederholte Anwendung von Brech- und Purgiermitteln geheilt wurde]. N. Arch. f. med. Erfahr., Berl., 1807, iv, 139–157.—**Smedley** (I. G.) The importance of making a physical exploration during the climacteric period. Hahneman. Month., Phila., 1886, viii, 487–489.—**Sorgoni** (A.) Su varii fenomeni straordinarii, che si sviluppano dopo l' epoca della cessazione de' mestrui. Raccoglitore, Fano, 1839, iii, 161–165.—**Stadler.** Ueber

Menstruation (*Cessation of*).

Unterleibs - Wassersucht zufolge cessirender Menstruation. J. f. Geburtsh., Leipz., 1835, xv, 48; 704.— **Sussdorff** (G. E.) On radical treatment of local disease at the menopause. Med. Rec., N. Y.. 1878, xiv, 486; 506.— **Tait** (L.) Climacteric diabetes in women. Practitioner, Lond., 1886, xxxvi, 401-408. — **Tilt** (E. J.) On uterine pathology at the change of life and after the ménopause. Brit. M. J., Lond., 1870, ii, 435. ———. The right understanding of the change of life. Med. Press & Circ , Lond., 1879, n. s., xxvii, 419. ———. Uterine inflammation at the change of life. *Ibid.*, 481. ———. On uterine inflammation after the menopause. *Ibid.*, xxviii, 103; 201.—**Tott** (C. A.) Einige Erfahrungen über Krankheiten zur Zeit, wo bei Weibern die Catamenien cessiren wollen. J. f. Geburtsh., Leipz., 1837, xvi, 591-598.—**Wyman** (H. C.) The menopause; gangliasthenia. Michigan M. News, Detroit, 1882, v, 313.

Menstruation (*Commencement of*).

See, also, **Menstruation** (*Hygiene, etc., of*); **Pregnancy** (*Early*); **Puberty**.

BARBARIN - DURIVAUD (P.) *Considérations générales sur les phénomènes physiologiques et pathologiques de la femme à la première époque de la menstruation. 4°. *Paris*, 1829.

BERLIOZ (L.-J.) *Sur les phénomènes et les maladies que produit la première apparition des règles. 8°. *Paris, an X* [1802].

BEUIL (L.) *Sur la menstruation à l'époque de la puberté. 4°. *Paris*, 1837.

BOUCHARD (J.-P.) *Sur la première éruption des menstrues. 4°. *Paris*, 1819.

BREBISIUS (J. A. H.) *De initio mensium fine morborum. sm. 4°. *Halæ Magdeb.*, [1727].

CÉSAR (A.) *De la première menstruation. 4°. *Paris*, 1845.

CHARBONNIER (T.) *Aperçu sur les phénomènes et les maladies que produit la première apparition des règles. 4°. *Paris*, 1819.

CHESNEL (A.-L.) *De la menstruation à l'époque de la puberté. 4°. *Paris*, 1847.

DIEUDONNÉ (J.-B.) *Considérations générales sur les causes et les moyens préservatifs des maladies des femmes à l'époque de la première menstruation. 4°. *Paris*, 1817.

GAVAUDAN (J.-B.) *Sur le défaut de menstruation à l'époque de la puberté. 4°. *Paris*, 1807.

GUÉNEAU DE MUSSY (F.) *Considérations sur la première éruption des menstrues et principalement sur le régime qui doit y disposer. 8°. *Paris, an XII* [1803].

GUYARD (F.-M.) *Coup d'œil médical sur la première menstruation, suivi de propositions sur l'accouchement contre-nature. 4°. *Paris*, 1833.

LARTIGAU (L.) *Sur la première menstruation. 4°. *Paris*, 1822.

LIBERT (J.-A.-A.-C.) *Sur les accidens que pent occasionner la première menstruation. 4°. *Paris*, 1827.

MARCUSE (S.) *Ueber den Eintritt der Menstruation, nach Angabe von 3,030 Schwangeren in der königl. Universitäts-Entbindungs-Anstalt zu Berlin. 8°. *Berlin*, [1869].

MOUTARD-MARTIN (E.) *Des accidents qui accompagnent l'établissement de la menstruation, de la chlorose en particulier. 4°. *Paris*, 1846.

RUE (A.-J.) *Essai sur la première menstruation, précédé de quelques considérations sur la chlorose. 4°. *Paris*, 1819.

SABATIER (M.) *Considérations sur les principaux phénomènes de la première menstruation, spécialement sur les causes de la rétention du flux menstruel, les moyens de les prévenir et de les combattre. 4°. *Paris*, 1818.

SAHER (S. G.) *De initio mensium initio morborum. sm. 4°. *Halæ Magdeb.*, [1725].

SAINT-ALARY (D.) *Aperçu sur la première menstruation. 4°. *Paris*, 1819.

Menstruation (*Commencement of*).

WESTHOFF (C.) *Ueber die Zeit des Eintritts der Menstruation, nach Angabe von 3,000 Schwangeren in der königl. Universitäts-Entbindungs-Anstalt zu Marburg. 8°. *Marburg*, [1873].

van den **Burg** (C. L.) Jets over den tijd van het ontstaan der menstruatie bij europeesche meisjes in Indië geboren. Geneesk. Tijdschr. v. Nederl. Indië, Batav., 1879, n. s., viii, 121-124.—**Dawosky** (S.) Merkwürdige Gleichheit der Symptome sowohl beim Beginnen, als beim Aufhören der Menses. J. f. Geburtsh., Leipz., 1838, xvii, 304-306.—**Enko** (P.) O vlijanii phizicheskago razvitija na poiavlenie menstruatsii. [Physical influences in the commencement of menstruation.] Protok. zasaid. Obsh. russk. vrach. v St. Petersb., 1877, xliv, 137-141.—**Fayrer** (J.) Tabular statement showing the birthplace, date of birth, and age at which the catamenia first appeared in twenty-seven girls of European lineage, educated and brought up (many born) in India. Med. Times & Gaz., Lond., 1873, i, 545.—**Heinricius** (G.) Ueber das Alter beim Eintritt der Menstruation bei 3,500 Weibern in Finnland. Centralbl. f. Gynäk., Leipz., 1883, vii, 72.—**Husemann** (T.) Normales Verhalten der Menstruation in Norwegen. Monatsbl. f. med. Statist. u. öff. Gsndhtspflg., Berl., 1868, 24-28.—**Lisfranc.** Des écoulements qui ont lieu par les organes génitaux de la femme; première menstruation. J. de méd. et chir. prat., Par., 1841, xii, 254-256.—**Osiander** (F. B.) Resultate von Beobachtungen und Nachrichten über die erste Erscheinung des Monatlichen. *In his:* Denkwrdgktn. f. d. Heilk. u. Geburtsh., 8°, Götting., 1795, ii, 380-388.—**Raciborski** (A.) Des obstacles mécaniques à la première éruption des règles. Expérience, Par., 1843, xii, 242-248.—**Rigden** (W.) Statistics as to the age at which menstruation commences. Tr. Obst. Soc. Lond. (1869), 1870, xi, 243.—**Rodzevich** (G. I.) [Anthropological excursion along the Volga. Comparative statistics of first appearance of menstruation in different nationalities.] Vrach. Vaidom., St. Petersb., 1882, vii, 3376-3379. ———. K statistike nachala polovoi zrelosti. [Statistics of female puberty.] *Ibid.*, 1883, viii, 3950. ———. O nachalie pojavlenija regul u 44,056 jentschin Evropeiskoi Rossii voobtshe. [Commencement of menstruation.] *Ibid.*, 4386-4389.—**Schlichting** (F. X.) Statistisches über den Eintritt der ersten Menstruation und über Schwangerschaftsdauer. Arch. f. Gynaek., Berl., 1880, xvi, 203-232.—**Tilt** (E. J.) Reflections on the causes which advance or retard the appearance of first menstruation in woman, with a synoptical table, showing the mean age of first menstruation in 10,422 women, in hot, temperate, and cold climates. Month. J. M. Sc., Lond. & Edinb., 1850, xi, 289-296.

Menstruation (*Difficult and painful*).

See **Decidua** (*Menstrual*); **Dysmenorrhœa**.

Menstruation (*Disordered, irregular, suppressed, etc.*)

See, also, **Amaurosis** (*Causes of*); **Amenorrhœa**; **Angina** (*Causes of*); **Breast** (*Engorgement of*); **Chlorosis**; **Dysmenorrhœa**; **Erysipelas** (*Causes, etc., of*); **Eye** (*Diseases of, Causation of*); **Goitre** (*Causes of*); **Hæmatemesis**; **Hysteria**; **Hysteria** (*Causes of*); **Insanity** *in women*; **Menorrhagia**; **Menstruation** (*Abnormal, etc.*); **Nervous** *system* (*Diseases of*) *of uterine origin, etc.*; **Paralysis** (*Reflex*); **Pemphigus** (*Cases of*); **Spinal** *cord* (*Congestion of*); **Tetanus** (*Causes of*).

ALLARDT (S. C.) *De emansione mensium. 4°. *Francof. ad Viadr.*, [1723].

APPENRODT (G. A.) *De mensium anomaliis convulsivis. 4°. *Halæ Magdeb.*, 1716.

BARNSTORFF (F. A.) *De mensium fluxu nimio. sm. 4°. *Halæ Magdeb.*, [1723].

BERVEILLER (S.-M.) *Dissertation sur l'aménie. 4°. *Strasbourg*, 1818.

BIDLOO (N.) *De menstruorum suppressione. 4°. *Lugd. Bat.*, 1697.

BIRCH (J.) Considerations on the efficacy of electricity in removing female obstructions. To which is annexed cases, with remarks. 8°. *London*, 1779.

BOUDET (F.-P.-I.) *Des dérangements dans la menstruation. 4°. *Paris*, 1848.

BOUDEWYNSEN (I.) *De sanguinis menstrui suppressione. 4°. *Lugd. Bat.*, 1761.

BRANDT (E. L.) *Disp. exhibens casum de nimio hæmorrhoico mensium fluxu in virgine observato. 4°. *Erfordiæ*, [1710].

Menstruation (*Disordered, irregular, suppressed, etc.*)

BRAUN (S.) *De casu, in quo menses p. n. emanentes per menagoga ciendi non sunt. 4°. *Tubingæ*, 1690.

CALMETTE (F.) *Essai sur l'aménorrhée, précédé de quelques considérations sur la menstruation. 4°. *Paris*, 1854.

CAMIADE (J.-H.) *Étude sur la déviation des menstrues. 4°. *Paris*, 1872.

CASTAING (S.-E.) *Sur les accidens relatifs à la menstruation. 4°. *Paris*, 1821.

CASTERAN (E.-A.-E.) *Considérations sur quelques points relatifs à l'aménorrhée. 4°. *Montpellier*, 1837.

CLEOPHAS (M.) *De suppressione mensium. sm. 4°. *Wittebergæ*, 1664.

COLAS (É.) *Traitement des accidens qu'éprouvent les femmes lors de l'apparition des règles, quand le cours en est interrompu, et lorsqu'elles veulent disparaître. 4°. *Paris*, 1823.

CRÜGER (J.) Epicrisis xii, curiosa theologico-medico-chimica de menstrui obstructione, et epicrisis xiii, curiosa medico-chimica de ephialte infantum. sm. 4°. [*n. p.*], 1712.

DIETERICUS (J. T.) *De tumoribus singularibus a mensium suppressione obortis. sm. 4°. *Vitembergæ*, [1758].

DREYER (D.) *De menstruo fluxu sufflaminato. 4°. *Lugd. Bat.*, 1683.

DUBOILLE (C.-B.) *Sur les irrégularités de la menstruation. 4°. *Paris*, 1814.

DUROUSSEAU-DUGONTIER (É.-F.) *Pathologie de la menstruation. 4°. *Paris*, 1844.

DUSONCHET (J.-M.) *De la menstruation, de ses dérangemens et de leurs traitemens. 4°. *Paris*, 1835.

DUVIGNEAUD (J.-B.-C.) *Dissertation sur la ménorrhagie, précédée de quelques considérations générales sur la menstruation. 4°. *Paris*, 1808.

EFFLER (J. H. D.) *De menstruatione vitiosa. sm. 4°. *Gottingæ*, [1800].

EPPS (J.) Affections of women. No. 1. Monthly period. 12°. *London*, [1840].

FAUCONNEAU-DUFRESNE (V.-A.) De l'emploi de l'apiol dans le traitement de l'aménorrhée et de la dysménorrhée. 4°. *Paris*, 1876.

FEILLÉ-GRANDPRÉ (C.-J.) *Quelques considérations sur la menstruation. De la suppression des règles. 4°. *Paris*, 1856.

FISCHER (C. E.) *De mensibus suppressis. 4°. *Gottingæ*, [1793].

FRIEDRICH (C. G.) *De mensium suppressione. 4°. *Lipsiæ*, [1815].

FRIESE (C. E.) *De nonnullis causis mechanicis ad menstruationem retentam conferentibus. 8°. *Berolini*, [1829].

GALLARD (T.) Pathologie des ovaires. Leçons cliniques sur la menstruation et ses troubles. 8°. *Paris*, 1885.

GRAHAM (D.) Massage in amenorrhœa and dysmenorrhœa. 8°. [*Boston*, 1876.]

GRIESSMAYR (P.) *De catameniorum excessu ejusque cura. sm. 8°. *Viennæ*, [1817].

HARRIS (H.) *De morbis virginum quibusdam a mensium vitiis oriundis. 8°. *Edinburgi*, 1780.

HAUSWALD (C. F.) *De affectibus rheumatico-arthriticis ex emansione mensium. 4°. *Erfordiæ*, [1761].

HEISTERMAN (T.) *De suppressione mensium. sm. 4°. *Lugd. Bat.*, 1680.

HEYDENREICH (S. R.) *De suppressione mensium. 4°. *Jenæ*, 1706.

HIRZEL (J. C.) *De ataxia mensium provide dijudicanda et curanda. 4°. *Erlangæ*, [1772].

Menstruation (*Disordered, irregular, suppressed, etc.*)

HOFFMANN (F. G.) *De fluxu menstruorum nimio. 8°. *Herbipoli*, 1834.

HOLSTER (B. J.) *De amenorrhœa ejusque cura, imprimis per electricitatem, additis observationibus. 8°. *Traj. ad Rhenum*, 1856.

HORN (J. J.) *De menstruorum fluxu nimio. 4°. *Erfordiæ*, [1753].

KAST (J. J.) *Diss. med. qua primarium catameniorum vitium, h. e. suppressio, submittit. sm. 4°. *Argentorati*, [1686].

KNOCKERS VAN OOSTERZEE (G. J.) *De ratione quæ est inter catamenia et morbos feminarum, annexa historia morbi de chlorosi. 8°. *Lugd. Bat.*, 1849.

KOCH (J. E. A.) *De morbis sexus elegantioris ex vitiis mensium. 4°. *Halæ ad Salam*, [1779].

KRÆHE (C. T.) *Nonnulla de pathologia catameniorum. sm. 4°. *Lipsiæ*, [1820].

LAAN (J.) *De suppressione mensium. 4°. *Traj. ad Rhenum*, 1831.

LALLEMANT (J.) *An menstruis morantibus chalybeata? Præses C. L. Liger. [1743.] *In:* SIGWART (G. F.) Quæst. med. Paris. 4°. *Tubingæ*, 1789, i, 233–238.

LATASTE (J.) *Sur la déviation des règles. 4°. *Montpellier, an VI* [1798].

LIOTARD (A.) *Aperçu sur l'aménorrhée, ou suppression morbifique du flux menstruel. 4°. *Montpellier*, 1824.

LOEWENSTEIN (L.) *Ueber den ätiologischen Zusammenhang der Katamenien mit ihrer Anomalien mit den Geistesstörungen. 8°. *Berlin*, [1877].

MANGON (A.-P.) *De l'hématidrose et de ses rapports avec la menstruation. 4°. *Bordeaux*, 1886.

MARESTANG (L.-E.) *De la navigation comme cause de troubles menstruels. 4°. *Montpellier*, 1885.

MARTLEY (J. F.) *De mensibus paucisque morborum ab eorum vitiis pendentium. 8°. *Edinburgi*, 1783.

MELLIER (F.) *Observations pratiques sur quelques dérangements de la menstruation, et principalement sur la difficulté de leur diagnostic. 8°. *Montpellier*, 1836.

MELLWIG (J. J.) *De fluxus menstrualis anomaliis per excessum. 8°. *Gryphiæ*, [1839].

MISTRAL (A.) *Essai clinique sur les troubles de la menstruation. 4°. *Paris*, 1881.

MORIN (E.) *Des maladies et en particulier des affections pulmonaires résultant de la suppression brusque des menstrues. 4°. *Paris*, 1878.
Also, in: Rev. de lit. méd., Par., 1878, iii, 513; 541: 1879, iv, 19; 47; 69; 88; 111; 140; 162; 185.

MOSCHO (S. P.) *De mensium vitiis. 8°. *Halæ*, 1800.

MÜLLER (F.) *De caussis perturbati catameniorum profluvii, et huic pedisequa chlorosi, addita sparsim therapia. 12°. *Pragæ*, 1817.

MUNIER (J. C.) An suppresso et immoderato catameniorum fluxui aperientia? Præs. A. J. Seron.
In: HALLER. Disp. anat. [etc.] 4°. *Gottingæ*, 1750, v, 197–232. *Also, in:* SIGWART (G. F.) Quæst. med. Paris. 4°. *Tubingæ*, 1789, i, 289–326.

MURET (H.) *Sur le traitement des principaux dérangemens des menstrues, considérées dans les différens âges de la femme. 4°. *Paris*, 1826.

NEITHARDUS (P.) *De tributo lunari fœminarum intercepto, in certo quodam casu. 4°. *Altdorfi*, 1681.

Menstruation (*Disordered, irregular, suppressed, etc.*)

NEUHOFER (G.) * De morbosa catameniorum suppressione. 4°. *Lugd. Bat.*, 1750.

NICOLON (J.-J.) * Observations sur la ménorrhagie qui survient à l'approche de l'âge critique, et sur l'aménorrhée par vice de conformation. 4°. *Strasbourg*, 1808.

NIEDT (G. W.) * De vitiis menstrui fluxus perite emendandis. 4°. *Halæ Magdeb.*, [1754].

NORDMANN (J. P.) * De obstructione sanguinis menstrui. sm. 4°. *Jenæ*, [1757].

PACZKOWSKI (S.) * Observationes quædam de menstruationis anomaliis atque exanthematibus. 8°. *Gryphiswaldiæ*, 1865. C.

PAGENSTECHER (H.) * De menstruationis perturbationibus. 8°. *Berolini*, 1846.

VAN PEENE (J.-H.) Dissertation sur l'emménologie et sur les maladies les plus communes des filles pubères, qui ont un rapport plus ou moins spécial avec la menstruation. 8°. *Gand*, 1815.

PET (O.) * De suppressione mensium. sm. 4°. *Traj. ad Rhenum*, 1727.

PETIT (G.) * Des rapports de la paralysie générale chez la femme avec certains troubles de la menstruation. [Paris.] 4°. *Coulommiers*, 1886.

Also [Abstr.], *in:* Arch. de tocol., Par., 1887, xiv, 337–347.

PETRÆUS (H.) * De suppressione et profluvio menstruorum, resp. Andrea Lipio.

In his: Nosologia harmonica dogmat. et hermet. 4°. *Marpurgi Cattorum*, 1616, ii, 370–386.

PRAEGER (J. C. G.) * In menorrhœæ pathologiam inquirens. 4°. *Vitebergæ*, 1801.

RIEMBAULT (A.) * Quelques recherches pour servir à l'étude de la menstruation en pathologie. 4°. *Paris*, 1854.

ROGENHOFER (J. N.) * De menstruatione morbosa. 8°. *Landishuti*, [*n. d.*]

ROUSSEL (C.-F.-C.) * Sur l'épischoménie, ou suppression accidentelle des règles. 4°. *Strasbourg*, 1829.

RUEFF (J. A.) * Diss. sistens casum puellæ post mensium suppressionem epilepticæ et postea sub fluxu eorum difficili hystericæ, cum epicrisi. 4°. *Tubingæ*, [1780].

SAMALENS (G.) * De la suppression brusque de la menstruation. 4°. *Paris*, 1857.

SAURIN (B.) * Essai sur l'aménorrhée, ou la suppression morbifique des règles. 4°. *Montpellier*, 1820.

SCHILL (C. F.) * De mensium defectu cum casu huc pertinente. 8°. *Giesæ*, [1793].

SCHMID (J. G.) * De suppressione mensium. 4°. *Argentorati*, [1782].

SEHRENK (F.) * Ueber Menstrualexanthemum. 8°. *Würzburg*, 1885.

SMIBERT (W.) * De menstruis retentis. 8°. *Edinburgi*, 1762.

SOLIER DE LA ROMILLAIS (B.-M.) *An suppressis menstruis varia, pro variis symptomatibus, instituenda venæ sectio? 4°. [*Paris*, 1770.]

SUTER (J.) *De mensibus retardatis. 8°. *Wirceburgi*, 1820.

THOELE (T. A.) * De pathologia catameniorum. 8°. *Berolini*, [1840].

TORTHE (L.) *D'une forme rare de déviation menstruelle. 4°. *Paris*, 1877.

TOUGES (L.-U.) *De la non apparition des menstrues chez les filles parvenues à l'âge de la puberté. 4°. *Paris*, 1831.

TOURNEUX (L.) *De l'érysipèle cataménial. 4°. *Paris*, 1886.

UPSHUR (J. N.) The disorders of menstruation. A practical treatise. 12°. *New York & London*, 1886.

DE VALLETTI (C.-S.) * De la suppression des règles. 4°. *Paris*, 1826.

Menstruation (*Disordered, irregular, suppressed, etc.*)

VINCENT (J.-F.) *Sur la suppression accidentelle des règles. 4°. *Paris*, 1823.

VROLO (V.) *Tantum non omnes morbos ex mensium suppressione deducens. sm. 4°. *Traj. ad Rhenum*, 1757.

WIENAND (H. G.) * De pathologia catameniorum. 8°. *Gryphiæ*, [1845].

DE WITT (J.) De vera mensium suppressione. sm. 4°. *Lugd. Bat.*, 1721.

ZIEGLER (J. H. E.) * De suppressione menstruorum. 4°. *Rintelii*, 1757.

Adams (C. W.) Menstrual septicæmia. Kansas City M. Index, 1886, vii, 423–428.—**Aldridge** (J.) On the use of iodide of potassium in menstrual suppression. Dublin Hosp. Gaz., 1845, ii, 50.—**Allen** (J.) Remarks on the development and decline of the function of menstruation when not in correspondence with the general system. Med. Times & Gaz., Lond., 1856, n. s., xiii, 567.—**Ancelot.** De la suppression des règles. Rev. de thérap. méd.-chir., Par., 1878, xlv. 113–116.—**Aufrage** [über die Krankheits-Zufälle einer Frau]. N. Arch. f. d. Geburtsh., etc., Jena, 1798–1800, i, 1. St., 58–62.—**Antony** (M.) On menstrual irregularities. South. M. & S. J., Augusta, 1837, i, 711–731.—**Artaud** (F. E.) Amenorrhœa. N. Orl. M. & S. J., 1882, n. s., x, 408–412.—**Ashby** (T. A.) Note on the treatment of amenorrhœa with permanganate of potash. Maryland M. J., Balt., 1887, xvii, 85–88. *Also*, Reprint.—**Austin.** On the effect of electricity in removing obstructions of the menses. Essays & Obs. Phil. Soc. Edinb., 1771, iii, 116–120.—**B.** (P.) Observacion de una gastro-entero-encefalitis aguda, producida por una insolacion y la supresion del flujo menstruo. Décadas de med. y cirug. práct., Madrid, 1828, xviii, 142–146.—**Bardsley** (J. L.) On the medicinal properties of strychnia in amenorrhœa. *In his:* Hosp. Facts & Obs., 8°, Lond., 1830, 51–58.—**Barker** (F.) Permanganate of potassium in the treatment of amenorrhœa. [Abstr.] N. York M. J., 1886, xliii, 238–240. [Discussion], 249.—**Báron** (J.) Teljes szüzhártyazárlat következté ben létrejött hüvely-és méhvérdag (hæmatocolpos et hæmatometra). [Complete atresia vaginæ in a virgin, followed by...] Orvosi hetil., Budapest, 1876, xx, 568; 592.—**Barthez.** Consultation sur des coliques nerveuses déterminées par la suppression des règles. Hist. Soc. de méd.-prat. de Montpel., 1808, v, 94–100.—**Batuaud** (J.) Un cas d'érysipèle cataménial; arrêt brusque du flux menstruel; eczéma des fosses nasales: pharyngite et adénopathie cervicale; érysipèle de la face; acide picrique; guérison. Rev. méd.-chir. d. mal. d. femmes, Par., 1886, viii, 260–265.—**Bayard** (R.) Effects of venesection in abdominal dropsy, supervening on a suppression of the catamenia. N. York M. & Phys. J., 1828, vii, 81–85.—**Bell** (S.) Permanganate of potassium in amenorrhœa. Med. Age, Detroit, 1886, iv, 385–388.—**Beni-Bade.** De l'hydrothérapie dans quelques troubles de la menstruation. Ann. Soc. d'hydrol. méd. de Par., 1873, xix, 64–84.—**Bernutz** (G.) Mémoire sur les accidents produits par la rétention du flux menstruel. Arch. gén. de méd., Par., 1848, 4. s., xvii, 129; 433: xviii, 405: 1849, 4. s., xix, 186. *Also*, Reprint.—**Billington** (C. E.) Permanganate of potassium in amenorrhœa. Med. Rec., N. Y., 1886, xxix, 270–274.—**Bird** (F.) Ueber den Nutzen der Birkenblätter in der Gicht; und der Sabina mit Borax in unterdrückter Menstruation. N. Jahrb. d. teutsch. Med. u. Chir., Hamm, 1824, viii, 2. St., 28–34.—**Blackwood** (W. R. D.) Treatment of amenorrhœa. Med. Bull., Phila., 1881, iii, 7–9.—**Boardman.** Case of menstrual decidua. Boston M. & S. J., 1883, cviii, 466.—**Boldt** (H. J.) Therapeutics of amenorrhœa. Med. Rec., N. Y., 1886, xxix, 623–625. *Also* [Abstr.]: Therap. Gaz., Detroit, 1887, 3. s., iii, 31.—**Bolton** (J.) Case of disordered menstruation. Stethoscope & Virg. M. Gaz., Richmond, 1852, ii, 192–197.—**Bonfils** (J.-F.) Observations sur des déviations menstruelles. J. gén. de méd., chir. et pharm., Par., 1828, cv, 162–167. *Also:* Tr. méd., Par., 1831, vi, 26–34.—**Borel.** Observation sur une tumeur formée par le sang menstruel avec des points gangréneux et rétention d'urine. Ann. Soc. de méd.-prat. de Montpel., 1804, iii, 316.—**Borland** (J. N.) Death following catamenial suppression. Boston M. & S. J., 1865, lxxii, 373.—**Brame** (C.) Sur le traitement de l'aménorrhée et de la dysménorrhée. Bull. et mém. Soc. de thérap., Par., 1884, xvi, 75–78.—**Browne** (B. B.) On the use of electricity in the treatment of amenorrhœa. Maryland M. J., Balt., 1882-3, ix, 49–51.—**Byrn** (M. L.) Remarkable case of suppression of the menses. Nelson's North. Lancet, Plattsburg, N. Y., 1851-2, iv, 137.—**Campá.** Contribucion al estudio de las emmenopatías; fisiología patológica de la menstruacion. Crón. méd., Valencia, 1880–81, iv, 353; 481.—**Carlé** (J.) Acné sebáces, tal vez sucesivo, de la cura, producida y sostenido por desórdenes menstruales. Independ. méd., Barcel., 1872-3, iii, 67.—**Carrasco** (L.) Urticaria febril intensa producida por retropulsion del flujo catamenial. Rev. de med.

Menstruation (*Disordered, irregular, suppressed, etc.*)

y cirug. práct., Madrid, 1877, i, 538–541.—**Carroll** (R. C.) Cases of menstrual derangement in negro women. South. M. & S. J., Augusta, 1860. n. s., xvi, 332–337.—**Carstens** (J. H.) Remarks on the mechanical therapeutics of amenorrhea. Am. J. Obst., N. Y., 1883, xvi, 1143–1146.— **Chéron** (J.) Désordres graves des fonctions biliaires causés par la suppression brusque et la rétention des règles. Rev. méd.-chir. d. mal. d. femmes, Par., 1880, ii, 503–512.—**Chevalier** (P.-J.) Observation d'une suppression subite du flux menstruel, occasionnée par une affection morale, et des suites auxquelles elle a donné lieu. Mém. Soc. méd. d'émulat. de Par. (an v), an vi [1798], i, 62–66. — **Chmelik** (C.) Ueber den Nutzen kalter Sitzbäder bei Anomalien der Menstruation. Oesterr. med. Wchnschr., Wien, 1846, 389–392.—**Christensen.** Synsforstyrrelser ved Menstruationsanomalier. [Disturbance of vision in connection with anomalies of menstruation.] Ugesk. f. Læger, Kjøbenh., 1879, 3. R., xxvii, 270 – 274. — **Christopher** (H.) A case of suppressed menstruation. South. M. Rec., Atlanta, 1886, xvi, 285–287.—**Churchill** (F.) Notes on some of the disorders of menstruation. Edinb. M. & S. J., 1836, xlv, 344 – 358. *Also*, Reprint. — **Cocchi** (A.) Sregolatezza de' mestrui. *In his:* Consulti med., 8°, Milano, 1824, 404–406. — **Coomes** (M. F.) Menstrual amblyopia. Med. Herald, Louisville, 1882–3, iv, 273–276. *Also*, Reprint.—**Cougnet** (J.) L'aménorrhée et la dysménorrhée, doivent-elles être considérées comme maladies à part, ou comme symptômes de plusieurs affections? Nice-méd., 1878–9, iii, 181–184.—**Darling.** Merkwürdige Irregularität in der Menstruation. J. f. d. Chir., Geburtsh. u. gerichtl. Arznk., Jena, 1797, i, 355. — **Deas** (P. M.) Note on the use of permanganate of potash in cases of insanity associated with amenorrhœa. Brit. M. J., Lond., 1885, i, 778.—**De-Pietra-Leone** (E.) Un caso raro tra le anomalie della mestruazione. Arch. clin. ital., Roma, 1882, xii, 286.—**Dittel.** Colica menstrualis ex hyperæmia spinali activa. Oesterr. med. Wchnschr., Wien, 1844, 903.—**Dobrourawow** (W. A.) Siebenjährige Amenorrhöe; Heilung. St. Petersb. med. Wchnschr., 1884, n. F., i, 98.—**Doering** (E. J.) Some remarks on the value of permanganate of potassium in amenorrhœa. Chicago M. J. & Exam., 1885, l, 283–287. *Also*, Reprint.—**Dugas.** Menstruation not appearing for six months. South. M. & S. J., Augusta, 1837, i, 567–573.—**Dumas.** Ventouse emménagogue. Gaz. hebd. d. sc. méd. de Montpel., 1886, viii, 1–3, 16–20. *Also*, Reprint. — **Duncan** (J. M.) On intra-uterine menstrual coagula. Obst. J. Gr. Brit., Lond., 1880, viii, 129–137.—**Egan** (J.) Menorrhagia and metrorrhagia. St. Louis M. J., 1884, xi, 291–299.—**Eller** (J. T.) Observatio de cephalæa atrocissima a mensium obstructione originem trahente, et cariem cranii denique admittente. *In his:* Med. u. chir. Anmerck. . . . d. Charité zu Berl., 12°, Berl., 1730, 26 – 30. — **Ellis** (W. P.) Permanganate of potassium in the treatment of menstrual derangements. Am. Pract. & News, Louisville, 1887, n. s., iii, 5–7.—**Eskridge** (J. T.) Abscess of the liver following arrested menstrual discharge from exposure to cold; pyræmic abscesses of the lungs and spleen; perforation of the bowel; severe heart complications; death during the seventh week. Med. & Surg. Reporter, Phila., 1882, xlvii, 684. *Also:* Phila. M. Times, 1882–3, xiii, 201. *Also:* Med. News, Phila., 1882, xli, 664. *Also:* N. York M. J., 1883, xxxvii, 76–78.—**Fabre** (A.) Du rôle du système nerveux dans les troubles morbides de la menstruation. Marseille méd., 1869, vi, 473 – 482. — **Farlow** (J. W.) Anomalous menstrual symptoms with atrophy of the uterus. Boston M. & S. J., 1883, cix, 296. — **Fauquez** (R.) Deux cas d'aménorrhée traités par l'électricité statique. Rev. méd.-chir. d. mal. d. femmes, Par., 1884, vi, 619–625.—**Fellner** (L.) Beiträge zur Pathologie und Therapie der Menstruationsanomalien. Wien. med. Presse, 1872, xiii, 443 ; 467 ; 506; 555; 579. — **Ferguson** (R.) Disordered menstruation. Syst. Pract. M. (Tweedie), Phila., 1841, iv, 433–457. — **Ferrer** (L.) Menostasia y amenofenia. Correo méd. castellano, Salamanca, 1886, iii, 3–7. — **Fleckles** (L.) Ueber Menstruations-Anomalien; Amenorrhœ und Dysmenorrhœ. Allg. med.Centr.-Ztg., Berl., 1863, xxxii, 113–116.—**Friborg** (N.) Aphonia a suppressis menstruis ortum ducens. Soc. med. Havn. collect., 1775, ii, 183.— **Garcia Quintero** (R.) Dos palabras sobre desarreglos de menstruales. Clinica, Zaragoza, 1881, v, 378. *Also:* An. obst., ginecopat. y pediat., 2. ép., Madrid, 1881. i, 369–372.— **Gee** (S.) Menstrual fever. St. Barth. Hosp. Rep., Lond., 1886, xxii, 93–95. — . Menstrual colic. *Ibid.*, 95.— **Goldthwaite** (H.) Sudden coma during menstruation relieved by venesection. N. York M. J., 1882, xxxvi, 180. *Also:* Tr. N. York Obst. Soc. (1881–5), 1885, iii, 91.— **Good** (R. R.) The continued electro-galvanic current in amenorrhœa. Med. Times & Gaz., Lond., 1880, ii, 562.— **Goodell** (W.) A clinical lecture on amenorrhea and dysmenorrhea. Louisville M. News, 1880, ix, 175–177.— **Graham** (D.) Massage in amenorrhœa and dysmenorrhœa. Boston M. & S. J., 1876, xciv, 146 – 150. *Also*, Reprint.—**Grechen** (M.) Periodischer, zur Zeit der Menses auftretender Pemphigus acutus. Frauenarzt, Berl., 1887,

Menstruation (*Disordered, irregular, suppressed, etc.*)

ii, 195. — **Grollemund** (W.) Accidents cérébraux et pulmonaires réflexes dépendant d'une rétention du flux menstruel. Rev. méd. de l'est, Nancy, 1884, xvi, 392–400.— **Guyénot.** Aménorrhée pseudo-membraneuse avec vaginite épithéliale. Ann. Soc. de méd. de Lyon, 1875, 2. s., xxiii, 76–81.—**Hamersley** (A.) On the combined administration of nauseating and purgative medicines in cases of difficult and suppressed menstruation. N. York M. & Phys. J., 1826, v, 164–176.—**Hammond** (W. A.) Cases of certain menstrual neuroses Med. Gaz., N. Y., 1881, viii, 334.—**Handford** (H.) Menstruation and phthisis. Brit. M. J., Lond., 1887, i, 153. — **Hannemann** (J. L.) Euporiston contra menstrua suppressa. Misc. Acad. nat. curios. 1689, Norimb., 1690, 2. decuria, viii, 366–370.— **Harrison** (R.) A case of interrupted menstruation. Virginia M. & S. J., Richmond, 1855, iv, 215.—**Hennig** (C.) Menstruale Vorboten und Herzfehler. Jahrb. f. Kinderh., Leipz., 1884, n. F., xxii, 225.—**Herman.** Late menstruation; primary dysmenorrhœa; division of vaginal portion; relief. Med. Times & Gaz., Lond., 18·2, i, 637.—**Hester** (A.) Sudden suppression of the menses. N. Orl. M. & S. J., 1857, xiv, 190–192.—**Hidrotorax** é hidropericardias que resultaron de una supresion repentina de los meses. Gac. méd., Madrid, 1845, i, 35.—**Hildebrand.** Suppressio menstruorum mit Geschwulst der Milz. San.-Ber. d. k. Med.-Coll. zu Posen (1830), 1832, pt. 2, 27.—**Hofmann.** Beantwortung der Anfrage über die Krankheitszufälle einer Frau. N. Arch. f. d. Geburtsh., etc., Jena, 1798–1800, i, 3. St., 249–263. [*See, also*, Anfrage, *supra.*]—**Hopper** (H. A.) Menstrual headache. Tr. M. Soc. N. Jersey, Newark, 1881, cxv, 183–190. — **Irvine** (R. H.) On menstruation; the true and the anomalous symptoms of pregnancy, and regarding dysmenorrhœa with fibrinous secretion and more or less head affection. India Reg. M. Sc., Calcutta, 1848, i, 731–756.—**Jacobson** (L.) Acute Erkrankung des schallempfindenden Apparates nach plötzlichem Ausbleiben der Menses; Heilung durch Pilocarpin. Arch. f. Ohrenh., Leipz., 1884, xxi, 280–282.—**Janskowich** (M.) Herzentzündung aus unterdückter Monatsreinigung, beendet durch ein eintägiges Wechselfieber. Med. Jahrb. d. k. k. österr. Staates, Wien, 1836, n. F., xi, 598–603.— **Jauzion.** Toux sympathique guérie par l'application des sangsues à la vulve. Hist. Soc. de méd.-prat. de Montpel., 1808, xvii, 45–48.—**Johnson** (C. R.) Suppressed menses, a cause of convulsions. Tr. Texas M. Ass., Austin, 1886, 475–480. — **Jourdain** (C.) Des troubles de la menstruation. Ann. de gynéc. et pédiat., Brux., 1842, 2. s., ii, 568–571.—**Jugand** (L.) Cas d'aménorrhée complète chez une femme de 35 ans; traitement par l'albuminate de fer; grossesse. Gaz. d. hôp., Par., 1881, liv, 1043. *Also:* Arch. de tocol., Par., 1881, viii, 743. *Also:* Union méd., Par., 1881, 3. s., xxxi, 486. *Also:* Progrès méd., Par., 1881, ix, 222. — . Cas d'aménorrhée chez une femme de trente-cinq ans; traitement par l'albuminate de fer; grossesse. Gaz. d. hôp., Par., 1884, lvii, 268.—**Kearney** (T. J.) Manganese in the treatment of menstrual disorders. Med. Rec., N. Y., 1886, xxx, 225–227.—**Kerr** (A. F.) Ame orrhœa producing septicæmia and dermatitis multiformis. Virginia M. Month., Richmond, 1886–7, xiii, 704 – 711.— **Koch** (T.) Amenorrhœa; dermatochysis vaga et periodica. Med. Ztg. Russlands, St. Petersb., 1850, vii, 33–37.— **Labbé** (L.) Péritonite chronique aiguë à la suite d'un refroidissement et de l'arrêt brusque de l'écoulement menstruel. France méd., Par., 1880, xxvii, 442. *Also:* Rev. méd.-chir. d. mal. d. femmes, Par., 1880, ii, 533 – 538.— **Landesberg** (M.) Augenleiden in Verbindung mit normaler Menstruation. Centralbl. f. prakt. Augenh., Leipz., 1883, vii, 134–138. — **Lechaptois.** Suppression des menstrues; menorrhagie spontanée du ma-entère; mort. [Rap. de Capuron.] Bull. Acad. de méd., Par., 1839–40, iv, 73–75. — **Lecoq** (J.) De l'influence de l'électrisation sur la menstruation. Gaz. d. hôp., Par., 1857, xxx, 295. — **Ledouble.** Infiltration sanguine des membres inférieurs; ecchymoses cutanées, purpura, coïncidant avec une suppression menstruelle. Rec. d. trav. Soc. méd. d'Indre-et-Loire 1877, Tours, 1878, lxxiv, 3–9.—**Leonard** (B. F.) A case of acquired amenorrhœa with complete uterine atresia; atrophy of the uterus; probable atrophy of the ovaries, and absence of molimen. Med. Chron , Balt., 1883–4, ii, 160. — **Le Pileur.** Aménorrhée consécutive à l'avulsion d'une dent pendant la période menstruelle, chez une hystérique. Rev. méd.-chir. d. mal. d. femmes, Par., 1879, i, 401–403. — **Leviseur.** Alalie und Aphonie nach plötzlich zurückgetretener Menstruation. San.-Ber. d. k. Med.-Coll. zu Posen (1830), 1832, pt. 2, 21.—**Lindsley** (H.) Cases of deranged menstruation. Am. J. M. Sc., Phila., 1833–4, xiii, 366–370. — **Lisfranc.** Quelques considérations pratiques sur l'aménorrhée et la dysménorrhée. Bull. clin., Par., 1835–6, i, 145–148. — **Locock** (C.) Menstruation, pathology of. Cycl. Pract. M. (Tweedie), Phila., 1845, iii, 308–312.—**Lothrop** (C. H.) Case of suppressed menstruation. Boston M. & S. J., 1860–61, lxiii, 457.—**Martin** (A.) Observation de coliques hépatiques sous la dépendance de la menstruation et d'un fibrome utérin chez une femme de

Menstruation (*Disordered, irregular, suppressed, etc.*)

45 ans. Union méd., Par., 1886, 3. s., xlii, 1037-1039.— **Martin** (F. H.) Manganese as a stimulant of the menstrual organs and as a remedy in certain forms of amenorrhœa and menorrhagia or metrorrhagia. Med. Rec., N. Y., 1883, xxiv, 344. ———. Manganese as a remedy in menstrual troubles. N. York M. J., 1885, xli, 110.— **Martin** (J. W.) Arrested menstruation; pain and tenderness in the uterine and right ovarian regions; pains down the right thigh, and in the right knee joint; sensation of chills up the spine; headache; insomnia; nervous excitement and restlessness; pyrexia; treatment; recovery. Med. Press & Circ., Lond., 1883, n. s., xxxv, 294.— **Martini.** Zwei Fälle von Menstruations-Störungen (Menostasis) und plötzliche Herstellung der Menses durch psychischen Einfluss. Allg. Ztschr. f. Psychiat., etc., Berl., 1871-2, xxviii, 657-659.— **Meade** (R. H.) Amenorrhœa from over brain-work, followed by atrophy of uterus. Med. Press & Circ., Lond., 1887, n. s., xliii, 98.— **Meissner** (F. L.) Eine Pneumonie und eine Hepatitis in Folge unterdrückter Menstruation. J. f. Geburtsh., Frankf. a. M., 1826, vi, 324-326. — **Menstruationsstörungen** (Die) und ihre Beseitigung durch Tsatsin. Cor.-Bl. d. Aerzte u. Apoth. d. Grossherz. Oldenburg, 1864-5, iii, 158-160.— **Métrorrhagie** (De la) passive chez les jeunes filles, et de son traitement. Bull. gén. de thérap., etc., Par., 1841, xxi, 150-160. *Also:* Ann. de méd. belge, Brux., 1841, iv, 29-33.— **Michaloff** (E.) Sluchai katamenial. roji. [Case of menstrual exanthem.] Med. Obozr., Mosk., 1885, xxiii, 693-697. *Also:* Trudi Obsh. Russk. vrach., Mosk., 1886, 44-49. — **Middleton** (F.) Aplicacion de las corrientes eléctricas continuas al tratamiento de la amenorrea concomitante de las enfermas del pulmon. Bol. de med., Santiago, 1884, i, 60-63.— **Mombert** (M.) Ueber Afterprodukte in Folge des zu frühen Wegbleibens der Menstruation. N. Ztschr. f. Geburtsk., Berl., 1847, xxii, 147-156.— **Moré y Bargit** (M. E.) Vómitos estercoráceos producidos por una falta menstrual. Rev. de cien. méd., Barcel., 1882, viii, 136-141.— **Morse** (W. H.) Delayed menstruation and pelvic contraction. N. York M. J., 1881, xxxiii, 428-434.— **Moses** (I.) Cases of disordered menstruation producing phenomena simulating the symptoms of grave diseases. Am. J. M. Sc., Phila., 1859, n. s., xxxviii, 355.— **Noxon** (Mary W.) Absence of menstruation terminating in Addison's disease. Tr. Homœop. M. Soc. N. Y. 1880-81, Havana, 1882, xvi, 355-358. *Also:* Homœop. J. Obst., N. Y., 1881, iii, 286-292.— **Ortiz de Laredo** (A.) Supresion brusca de la menstruacion; fiebre intermitente, terciana con síntomas gastrorrágicos, abcesos en el triángulo axilar derecho del volúmen de un melon pequeño; curacion. Corresp. méd., Madrid, 1872, vii, 367.— **Panarolus** (D.) Menstrua in virginibus maxima prudentia revocanda. *In his:* Iatrologismorum, 4°, Romæ, 1652, 178.— **Paper** (Ernestina). Due casi di amenorrea guariti colla corrente elettrica. Imparziale, Firenze, 1883, xxiii, 687.— **Parsons** (S. C.) Menstrual leucorrhœa contra indications for vaginal injections. South. M. Rec., Atlanta, 1884, xiv, 201.— **Parvin** (J.) Disorders of menstruation from psychical causes. Am. Pract., Louisville, 1872, vi, 146-158.— **Pauli.** Amenorrhoe, Menstrualerythem und Menstrualerysipel. Berl. klin. Wchnschr., 1880, xvii, 646.— **Penny** (E. J.) Sudden death from hæmorrhage into the abdominal cavity during menstruation. Brit. M. J., Lond., 1886, i, 539.— **Phreze** (A.) Ob otnozhenie nepravilnostie menstruatsii. [On irregular menstruation.] Med. Vestnik, St. Petersb., 1861, i, 97-102.— **Pitcairn** (A.) De mensium suppressione. *In his:* Op. omn., 4°, Lugd. Bat., 1737, 179-183.— **Poilroux.** Histoire d'une suppression menstruelle, suivie d'hydropisie ascíte. Ann. Soc. de méd.-prat. de Montpel., 1807, ix, 46-64. — **Prati** (P.) Un caso di asma, ed un' altro di colica catameniale curati e guariti secondo gl' insegnamenti della restaurazione Ippocratica in Italia. Raccoglitore med. di Fano, 1861, xxiii, 306-310.— **Puech** (A.) De la rétention du flux menstruel. Gaz. d. hôp., Par., 1859, xxxii, 162.— **Regius** (H.) Medicatio virginis a mensium suppressione epilepticæ. *In his:* Medicinæ libri iv, 2. ed., 4°, Traj. ad Rhenum, 1657, 324-330.— **van Rhyn** (H. B.) Menostasia; paralysis; mentis alienatio; status veternosus; gangræna ex decubitu; mors; hydatis ad tubum Falloppii sinistrum; serum limpidum effusum inter medullam spinalem ad nuchas et lumbos. *In his:* Brevis conspectus morborum, etc., 8°, Lugd. Bat., 1840, 36-38.— **Riebe** (J.) Welchen Einfluss üben die Schwangerschaft und die Menstruationsstörungen auf das Zahnfleisch und die Zähne aus? Deutsche Monatschr. f. Zahnh., Leipz., 1885, iii, 527-533.— **Riggs** (C. E.) Neurasthenic amenorrhœa. Northwest. Lancet, St. Paul, 1886-7, vi, 161-167. — **Ringer** (S.) & **Murrell** (W.) On manganese in the treatment of menorrhœa. Lancet, Lond., 1883, i, 7.— **Rockwell** (A. D.) Electricity in the disorders of menstruation. N. Eng. M. Month., Bridgeport, Conn., 1885-6, v, 201-204.— **Röhring.** Ueber den menstruellen Rothlauf. Centralbl. f. Gynäk., Leipz., 1884, viii, 827.— **Romiti** (G.) Della peritonite nelle mestruanti, e riflessioni scientifiche sulla mestruazione. Raccoglitore

Menstruation (*Disordered, irregular, suppressed, etc.*)

med., Forlì, 1875, xxxviii, 193-205. — **Rossetti** (A.) Des divers troubles de la menstruation. Mouvement méd., Par., 1876, xiv, 438; 451.— **Routh** (A.) Santonin in amenorrhœa. Lancet, Lond., 1886, i, 61.— **Rouvier** (J.) Quelques considérations sur les déviations menstruelles. Marseille méd., 1879, xvi, 257; 328. ———. Recherches sur les déviations menstruelles. Compt. rend. Acad. d. sc., Par., 1884, xcviii, 244. ———. Étude sur les déviations menstruelles. Ann. de gynéc., Par., 1885, xxiii, 24; 103; 177. *Also,* Reprint. — **Sainton.** Péritonite chronique aiguë à la suite d'un refroidissement et de l'arrêt brusque de l'écoulement menstruel. France méd., Par., 1880, xxvii, 442. *Also:* Bull. Soc. clin. de Par. (1880), 1881, iv, 73-76.— **Salazar** (M. R.) Menogeniavómica-consecutiva; curacion. Gac. méd., Madrid, 1846, ii, 376.— **Sanctuary** (T.) Concerning the action of certain remedies in "functional" amenorrhœa. Lancet, Lond., 1885, i, 59.— **Schrader.** Beiträge zur Pathologie der Menstruation. *In:* Ahlfeld (F.) Ber. u. Arb. a. d. geburtsh.-gynaek. Klin. zu Marb., 8°, Leipz., 1885, ii, 207-237.— **Schramm.** Zur Casuistik der Menstrual-Exantheme und der Urticaria nach mit Blutegelanwendung am Muttermund. Med.-chir. Centralbl., Wien, 1878, xiii, 556.— **Schroeter** (R.) Ueber das Verhalten der Menstruation bei Psychosen. Beitr. z. Geburtsh. u. Gynäk., Berl., 1874-5, iii, 294-310.— **Schuermans.** Rôle des ovaires dans la dysménorrhée et l'aménorrhée. Presse méd. belge, Brux., 1849, i, 393-395.— **Schulz.** Die Reflex-Wirkungen der Induktions-Elektrizität in allgemeinen und deren Benutzung als Heilmittel, insbesondere gegen Abnormitäten der Menstruation. Wien. med. Wchnschr., 1855, v, 790; 806.— **Seger** (G.) Von unvorsichtiger Stillung eines allzuhäufigen Abgangs der monatlichen Reinigung bey einer vollblütigen Person, und dem dadurch verursachten Tode. Auserl. med.-chir.- . . . Abhandl röm.-kais. Akad. d. Wissensch., Nürnb., 1756, ii, 56-59.— **Semmedo** (J. C.) Quandam ex continenti austeræ religionis vita perpetuæ mensium obstructiones, ex iis autem immanis salsugo et acrimonia, quæ mordacem atque pustulosum creabant pruritum, occuparunt; hanc pluribus et appositissimis auxiliis sic persanavimus, ut abolitis etiam minimis ipsorum reliquiis superstitem reddiderimus. *In his:* Obs. ægritudinum, fol., Ulyssipone Occid., 1718, 22-24.— **Simpson** (J. Y.) Amenorrhœa. *In his:* Works [Dis. of Women], 8°, Edinb., 1871, iii, 604-643.— **Skene** (A. J. C.) Deranged menstruation from imperfect development of the reproductive organs and diseases of the general system. Med. Rec., N. Y., 1874, ix, 451-455. ———. Amenorrhœa. Med. News, Phila., 1885, xlvii, 253-257.— **Sorel.** Documents pour servir à l'histoire d'une donleur hypogastrique intermenstruelle. Gaz. méd. de Picardie, Amiens, 1886, iv, 167-170.— **Stedman** (C. E.) Fetid menstruation relieved. Boston M. & S. J., 1880, ciii, 482.— **Steinberger.** Struma nach Unterdrückung der Menstruation. Gemein. deutsche Ztschr. f. Geburtsk., Weimar, 1831, vi, 249. ———. Eine, durch plötzliche Unterdrückung der Periode entstandene Seelenstörung. *Ibid.,* 250-253.— **Stephen** (J.) Chronic suppression of the menses. Am. J. M. Sc., Phila., 1870, n. s., lix, 429.— **Stevens** (E. B.) The condition of the cervical canal, as affecting the menstrual flow. Obst. Gaz., Cincin., 1879-80, ii, 1-6.— **Tate** (W. H.) Amenorrhœa [treated with potassæ permangana]. Peoria M. Month., 1885-6, vi, 505.— **Terrillon.** Des troubles de la menstruation après les lésions chirurgicales ou traumatiques et après l'ovariotomie. Ann. de gynéc., Par., 1882, xvii, 161-172.— **Thenance** (J.-S.) Observation sur une hémiplégie occasionnée par la suppression des règles, guérie par l'instrument tranchant. Ann. Soc. de méd.-prat. de Montpel., 1806, vii, 351-361.— **Tilt** (E. J.) Treatment of remittent menstruation by sulphate of quinine. Lancet, Lond., 1851, i, 148.— **Tumeurs** (Les) péri-utérines cataméniales de cause hémorrhagique. Gaz. d. hôp., Par., 1881, liv, 714.— **Vance** (R. A.) The effect of menstrual disorders upon the vascularity and nutrition of the intra-ocular structures. Boston M. & S. J., 1872, lxxxvi, 293-295. — **Vicat** (P. R.) Spasmi et dolores varii, post menses ab iracundia suppressos; phthisis funesta malorum scenam claudit. *In his:* Delect. obs. pract. ex diario clin., 8°, Vitodurum, 1780, 212-228.— **Voisin** (A.) Du traitement de l'aménorrhée par la suggestion hypnotique. Ann. méd.-psych., Par., 1887, 7. s., v, 279-283. *Also,* Reprint.— **Watkins** (J. L.) The salts of manganese in functional disorders of menstruation. Therap. Gaz., Detroit, 1886, 3. s., ii, 746-753.— **te Wechel** (W. A.) Deviatio menstruationis. Boerhaave. Tijdschr., etc., Gravenh., 1840, ii, 231-234.— **Whitbeck** (C. E.) Cases of malposition and disease of the uterus in young girls, as a cause of amenorrhœa and dysmenorrhœa. Toledo M. & S. J., 1880, iv, 126-128.— **Whitehead** (W.) Santonin in amenorrhœa. Lancet, Lond., 1885, ii, 430.— **Whitmire** (J. S.) Sudden suppression of the catamenia and amenorrhœa, as belonging to the neuroses. Tr. Illinois M. Soc., Chicago, 1884, xxxiv, 215-224.— **Wilhelm** (L.) Ueber Menstrual-Exantheme. Berl. klin. Wchnschr., 1878, xv, 50.— **Wiltshire** (A.)

11

Menstruation (*Disordered, irregular, suppressed, etc.*)

An offensive catamenia, or bromomenorrhœa. Med. Times & Gaz., Lond., 1882, ii, 551.—**Winter** (M.) Apoplexia e suppressione mensium. Med.-chir. Centralbl., Wien, 1882, xvii, 159.—**Wittke.** Folgen einer plötzlich unterdrückten Menstruation. Mag. f. d. ges. Heilk., Berl., 1826, xxii, 558–565.—**Wortham** (J. W.) Case of interrupted menstruation. Transylv. J. M., Lexington, Ky., 1839, xii, 39–41.—**Yount** (S. T.) The use of indigo as an emmenagogue. Med. Rec., N. Y., 1887, xxxii, 47.—**von Ziemssen.** Peritonitis rheumatica menstrualis. Sommersem. (Ein) in d. Klin. von Ziemssen zu München [1879], 1883, 54–57.

Menstruation (*Excessive*).

See **Menorrhagia**; **Menstruation** (*Disordered, etc.*)

Menstruation (*Hygiene and management of*).

BRASSEUR (F.) * Diss. hygiénique sur la femme considérée sous le rapport de la menstruation. 4°. *Paris*, 1828.

CHAZAL (S.-G.) * De l'hygiène des femmes à l'époque de la cessation des menstrues. 4°. *Paris*, 1826.

CHEVALIER (J. D.) *An quo tempore fluunt catamenia noxia Venus? 4°. [*Paris*, 1716.]

DUPLESSIS (E.) * De l'âge critique, et des soins hygiéniques que réclament les femmes à cette époque. 4°. *Paris*, 1828.

GARNIER (J.-F.) * Considérations sur l'âge critique, et sur l'hygiène des femmes à cette époque. 4°. *Paris*, 1820.

GRAVIS (J.-P.) * Sur la cessation des menstrues, et sur les conseils à donner aux femmes pour les préserver des accidens ou maladies dont elles sont menacées à cette époque. 4°. *Paris*, 1813.

GUBIAN (L.) * Considérations générales sur l'état physiologique de la femme parvenue à l'âge critique, et sur les moyens hygiéniques qui lui conviennent. 4°. *Paris*, 1816.

JACOBI (Mary P.) The question of rest for women during menstruation. Boylston prize essay for 1876. 8°. *New York*, 1877.

Also, transl. [Abstr.] *in:* Rev. méd.-chir. d. mal. d. femmes, Par., 1880, ii, 411; 459; 512; 572.

LAVILLE (J.-C.-A.) * Considérations générales sur les causes et les moyens préservatifs des maladies des femmes à l'époque de la cessation des menstrues. 4°. *Paris*, 1816.

LEVIN (W. E.) * De regimine tempore mensium observando. sm. 4°. *Halæ*, [1742].

OLIVE (A.-A.) * Sur la première menstruation, l'âge critique, et les soins hygiéniques que réclament les femmes à ces deux époques. 4°. *Paris*, 1819.

ROBILLARD (J.) * Considérations générales sur les soins à donner à la première menstruation. 4°. *Paris*, 1829.

Cederström (C.) Om bad under qvinnans menstruation och grossess. Hygiea, Stockholm, 1877, xxxix, 92–96.—**Cotting.** Professional management of menstruation. Boston M. & S. J., 1872, lxxxvi, 350.—**Delmas** (P.) Du traitement hydriatique pendant la menstruation. Bordeaux méd., 1876, v, 74; 290; 385.—**Fürst** (L.) Eine verbesserte Menstruationsbinde. Centralbl. f. Gynäk., Leipz., 1885, ix, 577–581. *Also,* Reprint.—**Levin** (P. A.) Några ord till genmäle af spörjsmålet: Ar en hydriatisk behandling möjlig och lämplig under qvinnans menstruation? Hygiea, Stockholm, 1877, xxxix, 1–6.—**Putnam** (C. G.) The cold bath during menstruation. Boston M. & S. J., 1871, lxxxv, 81.—**Raciborski** (A.) Réflexions sur l'administration des médicaments au moment des règles. Bull. gén. de thérap., etc., Par., 1868, lxxiv, 350–353. *Extr. from his:* Traité de la menstruation, 8°, Par., 1868.—**Stenger** (A.) Die Trikot-Badehose in der Gynäkologie. Centralbl. f. Gynäk., Leipz., 1887, xi, 203.

Menstruation (*Hygiene and management of*). [*Collection of patents.*]

Amia (N.) Catamenial sack. No. 296104. April. 1, 1884.—**Campbell** (Gertrude). Monthly-protector. No. 276770. May 1, 1883.—**Farr** (H. G.) Menstrual receptacle. No. 300770. June 24, 1884.—**Johnston** (G. E.) Catamenial

Menstruation (*Hygiene and management of*).

sacks. No. 182024. Sept. 12, 1876.—**Knabe** (F. A.) Catamenial sack. No. 174540. March 7, 1876.—**Korff** (J.) Catamenial sack. No. 235884. Dec. 28, 1880.—**Lange** (L.) Catamenial sack. No. 282201. July 31, 1883.—**Levy** (C. H.) Catamenial sack. No. 297274. April 22. 1884.—**Meacom** (G.) Improvement in catamenial sacks. No. 168515. Oct. 5, 1875.

Menstruation (*Irregular*).

See **Menstruation** (*Disordered, etc.*)

Menstruation (*Lactation in*).

See **Lactation** *in menstruation, etc.*

Menstruation (*Premature*).

See, also, **Pregnancy** (*Early*); **Puberty** (*Early, etc.*)

Allbutt (T. C.) Case of premature menstruation. Med.-Chir. Tr., Lond., 1865-6, xlix, 161–164. *Also:* Proc. Roy. M. & Chir. Soc. Lond., 1864–7, v, 193.—**Alonzo** (D.) [Una niña de 8 años está menstruando con el órden, regularidad y constancia.] Siglo méd., Madrid, 1857, iv, 224.—**Arnold** (C. D.) Infantile menstruation. Louisville M. News, 1876, ii, 42.—**Berdot** (D. C. E.) Menstruus hæmorrhoidum fluxus in puella trienni. Acta Helvet., Basileæ, 1762, v, 192.—**Bertrand.** Observation sur un enfant de huit ans, réglé depuis l'âge d'un an et demi. J. de méd., chir., pharm., etc., Par., 1762, xvi, 227.—**Berry** (W.) Notes of a case of early menstruation. Med. Press & Circ., Lond., 1882, n. s., xxxiii, 202.—**Betschler** (J. W.) Menstruatio præmatura. Ann. d. klin. Anst. d. Univ. zu Bresl. f. Geburtsh., 1832, i, 198.—**Brebisius** (J. G.) De mensium fluxu præcoci putatitio. Acta Acad. nat. curios.. 2. ed., Norimb., 1727, i, 372.—**Bronson** (J. O.) Case of early menstruation. Am. M. Month., N. Y., 1855, iv, 180–182.—**Buxtorf** (J.) Menstruus fluxus puellæ septem dies natæ. Acta Helvet., Basileæ, 1772, vii, 107.—**Campbell** (E. N.) Infantile menstruation. Peoria M. Month., 1885–6, vi, 75.—**Cazals.** Menstruation précoce. Ann. Soc. de méd.-prat. de Montpel., 1808, xi, 361–364.—**Cortejarena.** Un caso de menstruacion infantil ó precoz. An. r. Acad. de med., Madrid, 1880, ii, 202–205.—**Craig.** A case of precocious menstruation. Tr. M. Soc. N. Jersey, Newark, 1877, 122; 209.—**Davis** (M. M.) A case of early menstruation; dysmenorrhœa. Tr. Wisconsin M. Soc., Milwaukee, 1876, x, 69.—**Descuret.** Note sur une menstruation précoce. N. Jour. de méd., chir., pharm., etc., Par., 1820, vii, 100.—**Drummond** (D.) Case of early womanhood. Brit. M. J., Lond., 1879, ii, 47.—**Duncan.** Sur une fille prématurée. [*From:* J. d. scavans, 1683.] Collect. acad. d. mém., etc., Dijon, 1755, i, 296.—**Eschenbach** (C. E.) Menses præcoces *In his:* Obs. anat.-chir.-med. rariora, 12°, Rostoch., 1769, 210–214.—**Fitch** (G. L.) A singular case of menstrual flooding in a girl nine years old. Pacific M. & S. J., San Fran., 1872, n. s., vi, 394.—**Forman** (W.) Case of periodical discharge of a sanguineous fluid from the vagina of a child six years old. Am. M. Recorder, Phila., 1822, v, 664–666.—**Gautier** (V.) Des hémorragies génitales des petites filles; de la menstruation et de la maturité précoces. Rev. méd. de la Suisse Rom., Genève, 1884, iv, 501; 553; 633, 1 pl.—**Harding** (G. C.) Unusually early menstruation. Lancet, Lond., 1879, ii, 71.—**Harle** (C. E.) Monthly sanguineous discharge in an infant. Brit. M. J., Lond., 1880, i, 848.—**Harris** (T. M.) A case of precocious development. Med. & Surg. Reporter, Phila., 1882, xlvi, 27.—**Lenz.** Menstruation bei einem Kinde. Wchnschr. f. d. ges. Heilk., Berl., 1840, 651.—**Lieber.** Frühzeitige Menstruation. *Ibid.*, 1833, 143.—**Littel** (C. H.) [Menstruation in an infant.] Detroit Lancet, 1880–81, n. s., iv, 350.—**M'Crary** (E. W.) Precocious development. Louisville M. News, 1879, vii, 271.—**Marable** (J. T.) Cases of early catamenia. Memphis M. Recorder, 1858, vi, 1–4.—**Modery.** Menstruus fluxus in puella trienni. Zodiacus med.-gall. 1679, Geneva, 1680, i, 143.—**Müller** (J. M.) De mensium fluxu in puella 7 annorum. Acad. nat. curios. ephem., Noribergæ, 1717, cent. v–vi, 83–85. — **Pechlin** (J. N.) De fluore sanguinis tertio ætatis anno, et circa septenario primo erumpente. Misc. Acad. nat. curios. 1678–9, Norimb., 1693, ix–x, 84. *Also, transl.:* Collect. acad. d. mém., etc., Dijon, 1755, iii, 371.—**Prochownick.** Fall von Menstruatio præcox mit Sectionsbericht. Arch. f. Gynæk., Berl., 1881, xvii, 330–337.—**Reuter** (C. F.) Ueber Präcocität der Menstruation in psychologischer und kranioskopischer Hinsicht. Med. Jahrb. f. d. Herzogth. Nassau, Wiesb., 1846, v, 1–47.—**Robillard.** Case of early menstruation. Canada M. J., Montreal, 1870–71, vii, 409.—**Röbbelen** (A. H.) Menses prematuri. Deutsche Klinik, Berl., 1864, xvi, 269.—**Schönheit.** In typischer Reihenfolge zurückkehrende Menstruation bei einem siebenjährigen Mädchen. Ztschr. f. Nat.- u. Heilk. in Ungarn, Oedenburg, 1856, vii, 74.—**Smith** (J.) Remarkable case of early menstruation and pregnancy. Lond. M. Gaz., 1848, n. s., vii, 751.—**Stalpart van der Wiel** (C.)

Menstruation (*Premature*).

Maand-stonden bij een kint van een jaar. [Menstruation at one year.] *In his:* Hondert seldzame aanmerk., 12°, Amst., 1682, 254–256. — **Stocker** (O.) Ein Fall von Menstruatio præcox. Cor.-Bl. f. schweiz. Aerzte, Basel, 1879, ix, 261–263. — **Treyling** (J. J.) Lac in mammis puellæ vix natæ, et quæ vix trimula menstruata fuit. Acta Acad. nat. curios., Norimb., 1740, v, 442. — **Van Derveer** (A.) A case of infantile menstruation. Am. J. Obst., N. Y., 1883, xvi, 1005. *Also,* Reprint. — **Van Patten** (P.) Early appearance of the catamenia. Iowa M. J., Keokuk, 1853, i, 131. — **Vella.** Mestruazione precoce. Morgagni, Napoli, 1857, i, 123. — **Wachs** (O.) Ein Fall von vorzeitiger Menstruation bei einem dreijährigen Kinde. Ztschr. f. Geburtsh. u. Gynäk., Stuttg., 1877, i, 173–188. — **Wedel** (G. W.) Von einem Mädgen von sechs Jahren, welches schon die monatliche Reinigung bekam. Auserl. med.-chir.-... Abhandl. d. röm.-kais. Akad. d. Naturf., Nürnb., 1766, xv, 197. — **Whitmore** (W. H.) Case of menstruation in an infant, commencing a few days after birth. North. J. M., Edinb., 1845, iii, 70.

Menstruation (*Suppressed*).

See Amenorrhœa; Menstruation (*Disordered, etc.*)

Menstruation (*Vicarious*).

See Menstruation (*Abnormal, etc.*)

Menstruation in animals.

Alt (O.) Ueber die Identität der Menstruation mit der Brunst der Thiere. Monatschr. f. Geburtsk. u. Frauenkr., Berl., 1854, iv, 85–96. — **Gerrard** (J.) Menstruation in the lower animals. Vet. J. & Ann. Comp. Path., Lond., 1877, iv, 323–331. — **Numan** (A.) Over de periodische ontlasting van bloed uit de geslachtsdeelen bij sommige huisdieren, bepaaldelijk bij de koe; en beschouwing van dit verschijnsel, in betrekking tot de menstruatie der vrouw. Tijdschr. v. nat. geschied. en Physiol., Leiden, 1837–8, iv, 334–358. — **Sutton** (J. B.) Menstruation in monkeys. Med. Press & Circ., Lond., 1886, n. s., xlii, 259–261. *Also:* Brit. Gynæc. J., Lond., 1886–7, ii, 285–292. *Also, transl.:* France méd., Par., 1886, ii, 1421–1425. *Also:* Arch. de tocol., Par., 1887, xiv, 260–265.

Menstruation and disease.

See, also, Erysipelas (*Periodic*); Insanity *and menstruation*; Menstruation (*Cessation of*); Menstruation (*Disordered, etc.*); Small-pox (*Diagnosis, etc., of*); Uterus (*Cancer of*).

DANLOS (H.) *Étude sur la menstruation au point de vue de son influence sur les maladies cutanées. 4°. *Paris*, 1874.

FEUGIER (T.) *Influence des maladies sur la menstruation et réciproquement. 4°. *Paris*, 1864.

GLOCKENGIESSER (W. T.) *Diss. sistens casum menstrui fluxus anomali animique pathematibus perturbati. 4°. *Halæ Magdeb.*, [1740].

GODOT (A.) *De l'érysipèle menstruel. 4°. *Paris*, 1883.

D'HEURLE (L.-E.) *Sur l'apparition des menstrues pendant le cours des maladies aiguës. 4°. *Paris*, 1847.

HOLMAN (J.-B.) *Sur la menstruation chez les femmes rhumatisantes. 4°. *Paris*, 1877.

LADMIRAL (E.) *Des altérations du système utérin et particulièrement des règles chez les phthisiques. 4°. *Paris*, 1876.

MICHAUX (E.) *De l'influence menstruelle sur la production d'accidents rhumatismaux. 4°. *Paris*, 1876.

PANZER (F. G.) *De fluxu mensium febribus acutis et malignis superveniente ut plurimum funesto. 4°. *Altorfii*, 1753.

SICHELING (J. S.) *De effectibus mensium morbis supervenientium. sm. 4°. *Halæ Magdeb.*, [1757].

SMITS (P.) *De ratione quæ est inter catamenia et morbos feminarum. 8 *Lugd. Bat.*, 1848.

TAGUET (H.) *De l'influence de la menstruation sur le système nerveux. 4°. *Paris*, 1872.

VRAIN (O.) *La menstruation et la grossesse dans leurs rapports avec quelques manifestations cutanées diathésiques. 4°. *Paris*, 1878.

Menstruation and disease.

WOPRŠÁLEK (T.) *Diss. sistens historias synopticas morborum organicorum ex anomaliis menstruorum prodeuntium in schola medico-chirurgica anno scholast. 1839 tractatorum. 8°. [*n. p.*], 1841.

Bernard des Carriers. Observation sur plusieurs maladies dépendantes de suppression de règles, guéries par une espèce d'eau minérale artificielle. J. de méd., chir., pharm., etc., Par., 1773, xxxix, 416–422. — **Bluff.** Merkwürdige Folge einer plötzlichen Unterdrückung der Menstruation. J. f. Geburtsh., Frankf. a. M., 1834, xiii, 137–140. — **Cerda** (R. O.) Influencia del flujo menstrual sobre la salud i enfermedades de la mujer. Rev. méd. de Chile, Sant. de Chile, 1874, ii, 310; 333. — **Chrestien** (J.-A.) [Observations sur la suppression des règles, accompagnée de fièvre intermittente; l'emploi extérieur de l'opium.] J. d. conn. méd.-chir., Par., 1852, xx, 311. *Also:* Rev. de thérap. méd.-chir., Par., 1853, i, 535. — **Clemens** (T.) Ueber den Einfluss der Menstrual-Ausdünstungen auf den Verlauf verschiedener Infections-Krankheiten. Allg. med. Centr.-Ztg., Berl., 1883, lii, 369. — **Coe** (H. C.) Metrorrhagia at the time of puberty. N. York M. J., 1887, xlvi, 238–241. — **Danillo** (S.) O częstości chorób organów płciowych u kobiet obłąkanych. [Frequency of mental disturbances in women during menstruation.] Pam. Towarz. Lek. Warszaw., 1882, lxxviii, 537–551. — **Daremberg** (G.) Influence de la fonction menstruelle sur la marche de la phthisie pulmonaire. Arch. gén. de méd., Par., 1880, cxlvi, 533; 685. *Also* [Abstr.]: Rev. méd.-chir. d. mal. d. femmes, Par., 1879, i, 493–497. — **Dawosky** (S.) Merkwürdige der Periode vorhergehende Zeichen. J. f. Geburtsh., Leipz., 1837, xvi, 632–634. — **Dor** (A.) Deux cas d'affections oculaires dépendant de troubles de la menstruation. Bull. et mém. Soc. franç. d'opht., Par., 1884, ii, 152–156. — **Duncan** (W. A.) Case of recurrent pemphigus pruriginosus following checking of the menses. Lancet, Lond., 1881, i, 53. — **Dutcher** (A. P.) Menstruation; its condition in pulmonary tuberculosis. Med. & Surg. Reporter, Phila., 1861–2, vii, 30–33. *Also:* Cincin. M. Repert., 1871, iv, 389–399. — **Grellety** (L.) De l'érysipèle lié à la menstruation. Abeille méd., Par., 1878, xxxv, 195–197. — **Hérard** (H.) De l'influence des maladies aiguës fébriles sur les règles et réciproquement. Actes Soc. méd. d. hôp. de Par., 1852, ii, 153–212. [Rap. de Trélat] 213–223. *Also,* Reprint. — **Janovsky & Schwing.** Herpes beider Hände als Menstrualexanthem. Centralbl. f. Gynäk., Leipz., 1882, vi, 257–259. — **Kelly** (W.) Menstruation in small-pox. N. York M. Times, 1852, ii, 167–169. — **Landesberg** (M.) Eye diseases in connection with normal menstruation. Med. Bull., Phila., 1883, v, 203–205. — **Lopez** (J. F.) De la influencia de la menstruacion en la exacerbacion de algunos enfermedades. Siglo méd., Madrid, 1857, iv, 362; 380. — **Metcalfe** (J. T.) Pneumonia of apex of right lung; menstruation; death; appearance of the uterus and ovaries. N. York J. M., 1851, vii, 90. — **Moreno** (L. B. R.) Menofania y clorósis; empleo del protoxalato de hierro del Dr. Girard; curacion. Siglo méd., Madrid, 1879, xxvi, 260. — **Pallen** (M. A.) Menstrual neuroses. J. Nerv. & Ment. Dis., N. Y., 1877, iv, 463–473. — **Perroud** (L.) Influence des pyrexies sur les principaux phénomènes de la menstruation. Mém. et compt.-rend. Soc. d. sc. méd. de Lyon, 1861–2, i, 148–168. *Also:* Gaz. méd. de Lyon, 1862, xiv, 17; 39. ———. Note sur les pseudo-menstruations liées aux pyrexies. [5 obs.] Mém. et compt.-rend. Soc. d. sc. méd. de Lyon (1870), 1871, x, 114–131. [Discussion], pt. 2, 102. *Also:* Lyon méd., 1870, v, 437; 462. — **Piccirilli** (L.) Su l' amministrazione de' rimedi nelle malattie al periodo della mestruazione. N. Liguria med., Genova, 1874, xix, 113–119. — **Raciborski** (A.) De l'influence des affections des organes respiratoires sur la menstruation et de celle que cette évacuation exerce sur la marche de ces affections. (Extrait de l'ouvrage couronné par l'Académie royale de médecine.) Gaz. méd. de Par., 1842, 2. s., x, 401–407. ———. Du rôle de la menstruation dans la pathologie et la thérapeutique; de son influence sur la marche des maladies, et réciproquement. Monit. d. hôp., Par., 1855, iii, 681; 690; 699; 715; 732; 755; 764; 772; 857; 881; 917; 945; 953; 961; 985; 1003; 1081; 1089; 1097. — **Rouvier** (J.) Quelques phénomènes supplémentaires des règles. Ann. de gynéc., Par., 1879, xii, 10; 120: 1880, xiii, 115. — **Santos Fernandez** (J.) Amaurosis congénita curada espontáneamente á la presentacion de la primera erupcion menstrual. Actas... Cong. region. de cien. méd. 1879, Cádiz, 1882, 238–243. — **Schramm** (J.) Zur Casuistik der Menstrual-Exantheme und der Urticaria nach Blutegelanwendung am Muttermund. Berl. klin. Wchnschr., 1878, xv, 626–628. — **Stiller** (B.) Ueber Menstrual-Exantheme. *Ibid.*, 1877, xiv, 731–733. — **Tait** (L.) Menstrual irregularities and their relation to diseases of the nervous system. Obst. J. Gr. Brit., Lond., 1873, i, 94; 173. — **Terrillon.** Troubles de la menstruation après les lésions chirurgicales ou traumatiques. Progrès méd., Par., 1874, ii, 737; 754; 774; 790. — **Tilt** (E. J.) On catamenial diarrhœa. Lond. J. M., 1851, iii, 696–702. *Also* [Abstr.]: Med. Times, Lond., 1851, n. s., ii, 247. — **Tucker** (A. B.) Pathology and treatment of diseases of

Menstruation *and disease.*

menstruation. Savannah J. M., 1860–61, iii, 367–372 [377–382].—**Walther** (J. A.) Regulativ für die Praxis bei den Krankheiten des Weibes nach dem Aufhören der Menstruation überhaupt, insbesondere aber in Hinsicht auf die zu dieser Zeit eintretenden, oft so hartnäckigen Diarrhöen und Hustenzufälle. J. d. pract. Heilk., Berl., 1824, lix, 6. St., 3–19.

Menstruation *in males.*

See **Menstruation** (*Abnormal, etc.*)

Menstruation *in old age.*

See **Menstruation** (*Abnormal, etc.*)

Menstruation *in pregnancy.*

See **Pregnancy** (*Menstruation during*).

Mentagra *and sycosis.*

BERNHARDT (H.) * De sycosi. 8°. *Berolini*, [1862].

CHAUSIT (J.-M.) Sycosis ou mentagre. 8°. *Paris*, 1859.

VALLÉE (J.-P.) * Propositions et observations sur la mentagre et son traitement. 4°. *Paris*, 1831.

WARION (J.-P.-A.) * Du sycosis. 4°. *Strasbourg*, 1861.

Anderson (T. McC.) Pathology of sycosis menti. Edinb. M. J., 1867–8, xiii, 1089–1093, 1 pl.—**Bazin.** Considérations générales sur la mentagre et les teignes de la face. Gaz. d. hôp., Par., 1854, xxvii, 301; 305; 341; 354; 365; 370. *Also*, Reprint. ———. Mentagre; mentagra; sycosis. Dict. encycl. d. sc. méd., Par., 1873, 2. s., vi, 738–767.—**Beicher** (T. W.) Remarks on a case, illustrative of some points of difference between sycosis parasitica and impetigo sycosiformis. Dublin Q. J. M. Sc., 1867, xliv, 316–320.—**Cartaz.** Observation de blépharite mentagreuse. Lyon méd., 1870, iv, 112–116.—**Cazenave** (A.) Sycosis ou mentagre. Dict. de méd., 2. éd., Par., 1844, xxix, 81–90. ———. Observations et réflexions sur le sycosis. Gaz. d. hôp., Par, 1851, 3. s., iii, 457; 465. ———. Leçon sur le sycosis. Monit. d. hôp., Par., 1854, ii, 698–701.—**Chausit** (M.) Des complications du sycosis. *Ibid.*, 514–516. ———. Étude clinique du sycosis, et en particulier du sycosis tuberculeux. Gaz. hebd. de méd. et chir., Par., 1856, iii, 412; 452; 510.—**Cumin** (W.) Sycosis. Cycl. Pract. M. (Tweedie), Phila., 1845, iv, 296–298.—**Dale** (J. Y.) † Sycosis cured by sulphite of soda. Am. J. M. Sc., Phila., 1866, n. s., li, 281.—**Devergie** (A.) Thérapeutique de la mentagre ou sycosis. J. de méd. et chir. prat., Par., 1846, xvii, 123–128. ———. De l'épilation dans le traitement de la mentagre et des divers facteurs de ce traitement. *Ibid.*, 1861. 2. s., xxxii, 304–308.—**Diday** (P.) Traitement de la mentagre en une séance. Cong. méd. de France 1864, Par., 1865, ii, 467. *Also:* Gaz. méd. de Lyon, 1864, xvi, 590.—**Durand.** Sycosis parasitaire. Mém. et compt.-rend. Soc. d. sc. méd. de Lyon, 1867–8, vii, 5–8.—**Fox** (T.) Clinical lecture on tinea sycosis. Lancet, Lond., 1873, ii, 141.—**Gaskoin.** Case of true sycosis. Med. Times & Gaz., Lond., 1873, ii, 89. — **Gintrac** (H.) Observation de mentagre. J. de méd. de Bordeaux, 1859, 2. s., iv, 39–44.—**Godon** (F. W.) Clinical notes on two cases of sycosis. Arch. Dermat., N. Y., 1875, ii, 37–39.—**Haughton** (R. E.) On mentagra, or sycosis. Cincin. Lancet & Obs., 1858, n. s., i, 660–663.—**Hebra.** Sycosis. Allg. Wien. med. Ztg., 1864, ix, 283.—**Hutchinson.** On the true nature of the disease known in England as sycosis or mentagra. Brit. M. J., Lond., 1868, i, 52. — **Janson** (L.) Dartre mentagra pustulosa, guérie par la dépilation. Ann. Soc. de méd. de Gand, 1835, i, 76–79. [Rap. de G. Beydler, 80–82.] *Also:* Ann. de méd. belge, Brux., 1835, ii, 1.—**Köbner** (H.) Ueber Sycosis. Arch. f. path. Anat., etc., Berl., 1861, xxii, 372–411, 2 pl.—**Köbner** (H.) & **Michelson** (P.) Ueber parasitäre Sykosis. Arch. f. Dermat. u. Syph., Prag, 1869, i, 7–17.—**Laycock.** Notes of some cases of sycosis, and of a case of eczema produced by paraffin oil. Med. Times & Gaz., Lond., 1864, ii, 650.—**Le Blus** (C.) Dartre, mentagre guérie par l'emploi de la belladonne unie à l'onguent mercuriel. Ann. Soc. de méd. d'Anvers, 1846, 507. [Rap. de De Maeyer], 508–511.—**Lewin.** Ueber parasitäre Sycosis. Charité-Ann. 1874, Berl., 1876, i, 639–648.—**Löwenstamm.** Zur Sycosis. Med.-chir. Centralbl., Wien, 1878, xiii, 219. — **Lutens** jeune. Dartre mentagra pustulosa, guérie par la dépilation, ou plutôt par la calotte du menton. Ann. Soc. de méd. de Gand, 1835, i, 312–314. *Also:* Ann. de méd. belge, Brux., 1835, iv, 192. *Also* [Abstr.]: Bull. Soc. de med. de Gand, 1835, i, 149. — **Manassei** (C.) Mentagra. Gior. ital. d. mal. ven., Milano, 1877, xi, 212–220.—**Masse** (E.) Sycosis parasitaire; nouveau traitement par la créosote. Montpel. méd., 1864, xiii, 441–446.—**Matson** (S.) Sycosis menti cured by the sulphite of soda. Am. J. M. Sc., Phila., 1866, n. s., lii, 276.—**Santlus.** Eine Frage über die Bartfinne (Mentagra). Deutsche Klinik, Berl., 1854,

Mentagra *and sycosis.*

vi, 377.—**Smith** (A. C.) On sycosis; a clinical study. N. York M. J., 1876, xxiii, 119–124.—**Stark** (G. A.) Case of sycosis, treated by carbolic acid and Canada balsam. Canada M. & S. J., Montreal, 1876–7, v, 97–99.—**Turner** (W. M.) Sycosis, and its treatment. N. Orl. J. M., 1868, xxi, 727–733.—**Veiel.** Sycosis. Deutsche Klinik, Berl., 1855, vii, 221. ———. Ueber die Behandlung der Sykosis in der Heilanstalt zu Cannstatt. Bl. f. Heilwissensch., München, 1873, iv, 81; 89.— **Werner.** Mentagra; Heilung durch Ausziehen der Barthaare und Touchiren der kranken Fläche mit Lapis. Ztschr. f. Wundärzte u. Geburtsh., Stuttg., 1859, xii, 117–119.— **Wertheim** (G.) Ueber Sycosis. Med. Jahrb., Wien, 1861, ii, 87–100. — **Ziemssen** (H.) Sycosis oder Mentagra. Greifswalder med. Beitr., Danzig, 1864, ii, 99–110, 1 pl.

Mental *disease.*

See **Insanity**; **Psychology** (*Medical*).

Mental *effort.*

See **Epilepsy** (*Causation of*); **Mind** (*Overwork of*).

Mental Healing Monthly. Published by Mental Science and Christian Healing Association. Miss M. B. Gage, editor. v. 1–2, August, 1886–7. 8°. *Boston.* Current.

Mental *philosophy.*

See **Psychology**.

Mental *responsibility.*

See **Responsibility**.

Mental Science Magazine and Mind-Cure Journal. A. J. Swarts, editor. [Monthly.] Nos. 4–12, v. 2; v. 3, January, 1886–7. 2 v. 8°. *Chicago, Mental Science University.* Current. Title of prior nos. was: **Mind-Cure** Journal.

Mental *strain.*

See **Mind** (*Overwork of*).

Mente (Christophorus). * De phthisis curatione per lac. 15 l. sm. 4°. *Helmœstadi, typ. G. W. Hammii,* [1687].

Mentel (*Jacques*) [1599–1670].

Corlieu (A.) Jacques Mentel et le réservoir du chyle. France méd., Par., 1874, xxi, 246. ———. Jacques Mentel, docteur régent et professeur à la Faculté de médecine de Paris. *Ibid.*, 1880, xxvii, 345; 361; 377.

Mentha.

See, also, **Puerperal** *fever* (*Treatment of*).

D'HEILLY (C.) * De la menthe poivrée. 4°. *Paris*, 1861.

KNIGGE (T.) De mentha piperitide; commentatio botanico-medica. 4°. *Erlangœ,* [1780].

LAURIN (C. G.) * De menthæ usu. sm. 4°. *Upsaliœ,* [1767].

ROZE (L.) La menthe poivrée, sa culture en France, ses produits, falsifications de l'essence, et moyens de les reconnaître. 12°. *Paris*, 1868.

Coletti. Veneficio per essenza di menta. Gazz. med. ital., prov. venete, Padova, 1864, vii, 426–429. —**Delioux de Savignac.** L'essence de menthe et ses propriétés antalgiques. Bull. et mém. Soc. de thérap. 1871–2, Par., 1875, iv (app.), 41–57. *Also:* Gaz. méd. de Par., 1874, 4. s., iii, 424; 447; 484. *Also:* Union méd., Par., 1874, xxviii, 557; 597; 639.—**Martin** (S.) Un mot sur la menthe poivrée et sur la falsification de son essence. Bull. gén. de thérap., etc., Par., 1867, lxxiii, 317–319. ———. Un mot sur la menthe poivrée cultivée à Gennevilliers. *Ibid.*, 1872, lxxxiii, 224–226.—**Poisoning** from an over-dose of oil of pennyroyal. [Edit.] South. Clinic, Richmond, 1883, vi, 323.—**Starke.** Ueber die verschiedene Qualität des inländischen und englischen Pfeffermünzkrautes und Pfeffermünzöls. J. d. Chir. u. Augenh., Berl., 1835, xxiii, 671–676.—**Viglezzi** (F.) Caso di veneficio per essenza di menta. Gazz. med. ital., prov. venete, Padova, 1864, vii, 425.—**Wilcox** (W. A.) Poisoning by pennyroyal. Boston M. & S. J., 1868, lxxviii, 394.

Menthol.

Cammann (D. M.) Menthol *versus* pain. Med. Rec., N. Y., 1883, xxiii, 458.—**Casper** (L.) On menthol. Med. & Surg. Reporter, Phila., 1885, liii, 489–491.—**Goldscheider.** Ueber die specifische Wirkung des Menthols auf die Temperatur-Nerven. Arch. f. Physiol., Leipz.,

Menthol.

1886, 555–558.—**Macdonald** (A. D.) On a new antiseptic and antineuralgic agent. Edinb. M. J., 1880–81, xxvi, 121–128.—**Rosenberg** (A.) Das Menthol, ein Ersatz des Cocain zur Erzeugung localer Anästhesie in Nase und Pharynx. Berl. klin. Wchnschr., 1885, xxii, 449. ———. Zur Beseitigung der von der Nase ausgelösten Reflexneurosen durch Menthol. *Ibid.*, 788–790. — **Schmitz** (A.) Ueber Menthol und seine Wirkung. Centralbl. f. klin. Med., Leipz., 1885, vi, 537–543.—**Wendt** (E. C.) Note on the use of the menthol cone as an anodyne. N. York M. J., 1884, xxxix, 104. *Also:* Med. News, Phila., 1884, xliv, 111.

Menton et ses environs par un touriste anglais, accompagné du panorama des montagnes de M. Moggridge. 75 pp., 3 l., 1 map. 8°. *Paris*, [*n. d.*]

Mentone.

BENNET (J. H.) Mentone, the Riviera, Corsica, and Biarritz as winter climates. 2. ed. 8°. *London*, 1862.

DRYSDALE (A.) Wintering abroad : Mentone and the Riviera. 12°. *London*, [1884].

FARINA (J. F.) Le climat de Menton, son influence sur le traitement de la phthisie pulmonaire. Étude clinique accompagnée de statistiques et d'observations météorologiques. 12°. *Paris*, 1879.

GENZMER (W.) Mentone und die Riviera. In klimatologisch-medicinischer Darstellung. 8°. *Mainz*, 1865.

MENTON et ses environs par un touriste anglais, accompagné du panorama des montagnes de M. Moggridge. 8°. *Paris*, [*n. d.*]

SIORDET (J. L.) Mentone, in its medical aspect ; being letters addressed to a medical friend. 12°. *London*, 1863.

STIEGE (E.) Mentone und sein Klima. Nach eigenen Beobachtungen. Nebst einer kurzen Abhandlung zur Geologie Mentone's von Dr. H. A. Pagenstecher. 8°. *Berlin*, 1868.

Bennet (J. H.) A winter at Mentone, near Nice. Lancet, Lond., 1860, ii, 2–5. ———. The new drainage of Mentone. *Ibid.*, 1883, ii, 926.—**Cazenave de la Roche**. De l'action physiologique du climat de Menton. France méd., Par., 1880, xxvii, 682.—**De Pascale**. Observations on the climate of Nice, Mentone, and San Remo. Brit. M. J., Lond., 1861, ii, 329.—**Dührssen**. Mentone, sein Clima und seine Bedeutung als südlicher Curort. Deutsche Klinik, Berl., 1869, xxi, 13 ; 33. ———. Einfluss des Clima von Mentone auf kranke Individuen im Allgemeinen. *Ibid.*, 257 ; 279.—**Fenger** (S.) Menton som Vinteropholdssted for Brystsyge. Hosp.-Tid., Kjøbenh., 1878, 2. R., v, 625 ; 641.—**Guiraud**. Notes statistiques et cliniques sur l'action thérapeutique du climat de Menton. Cong. périod. internat. d. sc. méd. Compt.-rend. 1877, Genève, 1878, v, 590–598. *Also:* Gaz. méd.-chir. de Toulouse, 1878, x, 193 ; 201.—**Matvieff** (V. G.) Opit statistich. izsledovanija boleznennosti i smertnosti jitelei Mentona. Voyenno-med. J., St. Petersb., 1885, clii, pt. 7, 11–52, 2 tab. *Also,* Reprint.—**Pagenstecher** (H. A.) Mentone als Kurort. Verhandl. d. naturh.-med. Ver. zu Heidelb., 1862–5, iii, 68–79. *Also,* Reprint.—**Price** (P. S.) Winter climate of Menton. Med. Times & Gaz., Lond., 1862, ii, 53 ; 78. — **Sybrandi** (N. D.) Iets over Mentone en andere zuidelijk gelegene plaatsen, welke als winterverblijf voor borstlijders worden aanbevolen. Nederl. Tijdschr. v. Geneesk., Amst., 1867, 2. R., iii, 2. Afd., 285–307.

[**Mentor.**] Good news for the blind. 2 pp. 8°. [*Philadelphia*, 1834.]
Repr. from: Poulson's Am. Daily Advertiser.

Mentz.

See, also, **Medicine** (*Clinical, Cases of*).

HELWIG (A.) Beiträge zur Mortalitäts-Statistik der Stadt Mainz vom Anfang dieses Jahrhunderts bis incl. 1872. 4°. *Mainz*, 1873.

KUPFERBERG (F.) Ein Beitrag zur Beurtheilung des Gesundheits-Zustandes einer Stadt mit besonderer Berücksichtigung Mainzer Verhältnisse. 8°. *Mainz*, 1877.

RAUTERT (A.) Beiträge zur Wasserleitungs-Frage der Stadt Mainz. 8°. *Mainz*, 1879.
———. The same. 2.Theil. 8°. *Mainz*, 1879.

Jahres-Tabelle der Sterblichkeits- Verhältnisse der Stadt Mainz während des Jahres 1876. Veröffentl. d. k. deutsch. Gsndhtsamtes, Berl., 1877, i, No. 8.—**St.** (J.) Die

Mentz.

Kanalisation der Stadt Mainz. Centralbl. f. allg. Gsndhtspflg., Bonn, 1882, i, 189 ; 261. — **Wittmann**. Ueber stehende Constitution in medicinisch-praktischer Hinsicht. Ferner über die Krankheiten, welche von 1815 bis hieher zu Mainz und in der Provinz Rheinhessen beobachtet wurden. N. Jahrb. d. teutsch. Med. u. Chir., Bonn, 1821, iv, 2. St., 80 – 118. ———. Ueber die Krankheiten, welche von 1815 bis jetzt (1822) zu Mainz und in der Provinz Rheinhessen beobachtet wurden. *Ibid.*, Elberfeld, 1822, v, 3. St., 30–99.

Mentz (Jo. Gabriele). Religionem medicorum esse optimam paucis asserit. 8 pp. 4°. *Longosalissæ, lit. Heergarthianis*, [1755].
See, also, **Vater** (Abraham) & **Mentz** (J. Gabr.) Phosphori loco medicamenti, [etc.] 4°. *Wittenbergæ*, 1751. *In:* HALLER. Disp. ad morb. [etc.] 4°. *Lausannæ*, 1760, vii. 288–301.
For Biography, see **Vater** (Abraham).

Mentz (Joannes Henricus). * De chlorosi. 3 p. l., 46 pp., 1 l. 8°. *Traj. ad Rhenum, C. Bielevelt*, 1845.

Mentzel (C. A.)
See **Handbuch** für den Bau der Feuerungsanlagen, etc. 3. Aufl. 8°. *Halle a. S.*, 1875–6.

Mentzel (*Christian*) [1622–1701].
Portrait in: **Collection**—van Kaathoven.—**Collection** of Portr. of Phys. & Men of Sc., 189.

Mentzel (Christianus Ludovicus). * De sensu vitali. 72 pp. sm. 4°. *Halæ Magdeb., lit. C. Henckelii*, [1716].

Mentzel (Emanuel Gottlob). Exercitationem litterariam de Joannis Langii studiis botanicis publice defendet. 20 pp. 4°. *Traj. ad Viadr., e typog. Winteriano*, [1774].

Mentzel (Georgius Godofredus). * De anthelmicorum convenienti usu et operandi modo. 39 pp. sm. 4°. *Halæ Magdeb., typ. J. G. Kittleri*, [1748].

Mentzel (Jo. Henricus Daniel.) * De mortibus repentinis juvenilibus annis potissimum imputandis. 24 pp. 4°. *Wit enbergæ, lit. C. C. Durrii*, [1772].
For Biography, see **Boehmer** (Geo. Rudolphus).

Mentzel (Joh. Christianus) [–1718]. * De venenis. 24 pp. sm. 4°. *Francof. ad Viadr., lit. C. Zeitleri*, [1682].

Mentzel (Joh. Christophorus). * De diæta principum. 47 pp. 4°. *Halæ Magdeb.*, [1728].

[**Mentzer** (Balthasar).] Das bey strenger Kälte entlarvte Wetter-Glass. 16 pp., 1 pl. 4°. *Hamburg, C. Neumann*, 1709.

Mentzler (Franciscus Jacobus). * De venæsectionis in purpura abusu et usu. 28 pp. sm. 4°. *Argentorati, typ. M. Pauschingeri*, 1744.

Menu (Ferdinand). * De la périostite dans le cours du rhumatisme articulaire aigu. 56 pp. 4°. *Paris*, 1874, No. 105.

Menu (J.-O.) * De la transplantation du sol ciliaire comme méthode de traitement du trichiasis et de l'entropion chroniques. 62 pp. 4°. *Paris*, 1873, No. 472.

Menu (Joannes). * De pleuritide vera. 39 pp., 2 l. 4°. *Lugd. Bat., apud A. Costerum*, 1782.

Menuau (Félix-Charles). * I. Histoire anatomique de l'amaurose. II. [etc.] 46 pp. 4°. *Paris*, 1840, No. 177, v. 363.

Menudier (Adolphe). * I. De la gastro-entérite chronique par empoisonnement. II. [etc.] 36 pp. 4°. *Paris*, 1839, No. 215, v. 346.

Menuret de Chambaud (Jean-Jacques) [1733–1815]. Nouveau traité du pouls. xlvi, 280 pp. 12°. *Paris, Vincent*, 1768.
Another copy bound with: MICHEL. Nouvelles observations sur le pouls. 12°. *Paris*, 1757.

———. Essai sur l'action de l'air dans les maladies contagieuses, qui a remporté le prix proposé par la Société royale de médecine. xxiv, 112 pp., 2 l. 12°. *Paris, Soc. roy. de méd.*, 1781.
Bound with: AIKIN (Jean). Observations sur les hôpitaux [etc.] 12°. *Londres*, 1788.

Menuret de Chambaud (J.-J.)—cont'd.
——. Essais sur l'histoire médico-topographique de Paris; ou lettres à M. D'Aumont, sur le climat de Paris, sur l'état de la médecine, sur le caractère et le traitement des maladies, et particulièrement sur la petite vérole et l'inoculation. xii, 293 pp., 2 l. 12°. *Paris, N.-H. Nyon.* 1786.
Another copy bound with: [TULLY.] Essai sur les maladies de Dunkerque. 12°. *Dunkerque,* 1760.

——. Essais sur les moyens de former de bons médecins; sur les obligations réciproques des médecins et de la Société; partie d'un projet d'éducation nationale, relative à cette profession. xvi, 150 pp. 8°. *Paris, Belin,* 1791.
For Biography, see J. univ. d. sc. méd., Par., 1816, i, 384–380 (F.-P. C.).

Menut (B.) * De la virulence du bubon qui accompagne le chancre mou. 80 pp. 4°. *Paris,* 1885, No. 33.

Menville. De l'âge critique chez les femmes, des maladies qui peuvent survenir à cette époque de la vie, et des moyens de les combattre et de les prévenir. 567 pp. 8°. *Paris, Germer-Baillière,* 1840.

——. Histoire médicale et philosophique de la femme considérée dans toutes les époques principales de sa vie, avec tous les changements qui surviennent dans son physique et son moral, avec l'hygiène applicable à son sexe et toutes les maladies qui peuvent l'atteindre aux différents âges. 3 v. 8°. *Paris, chez l'auteur,* 1845.

——. The same. Histoire philosophique et médicale de la femme considérée dans toutes les époques principales de la vie, avec ses diverses fonctions, avec les changements qui surviennent dans son physique et son moral, avec l'hygiène applicable à son sexe et toutes les maladies qui peuvent l'atteindre aux différents âges. 2. éd. 3 v. 8°. *Paris, J.-B. Baillière & fils,* 1858.

Menville (Ch.) * Sur l'hémorrhagie cérébrale. 22 pp. 4°. *Paris,* 1831, No. 150, v. 242.

Menville (É.) * Étude sur les variations de la température sous l'influence de l'acide phénique. 49 pp., 1 l. 4°. *Paris,* 1880, No. 331.

Menyanthes *trifoliata.*
FRIESE (C. F.) * Trifolium fibrinum, Fieber-Klee. 4°. *Erfordiæ,* [1716].
KAEMPFE (G.) * Ueber die Wirkung einiger Amara beim gesunden Menschen. 8°. *Greifswald,* 1885.
KIELLMAN (C. J.) * De usu menyanthidis trifoliatæ. sm. 4°. *Upsaliæ,* [1797].
Willius (J. V.) Vires trifolii fibrini. Acta med. et phil. 1674–5, Hafn., 1677, iii, 123–132. *Also, transl.:* Collect. acad. d. mém., etc., Dijon, 1766, vii, 279–286.

Menyhért (Fésüs). Ertekezés az ember testineveléséröl. [Dissertation on physical education.] xvi, 64 pp. 8°. *Budán, á magyar Királyi univ. betüivel,* 1829. [P., v. 1317.]

Menz (Carolus Christianus Fridericus). De febre continua remittente putrida. 16 pp. 8°. *Lipsiæ, lit. Sommeri,* [1781].

——. * Quædam de motuum in morbis utilitate ac præstantia. 11 pp. 4°. *Lipsiæ, typ. Waltherianis,* 1783.

——. * Pathologia rheumatismi in morbis puerperarum. 50 pp. 4°. *Lipsiæ, ex off. Solbrigia,* 1788.
See, also, **Pohl** (Joh. Ehrenfried). Diss. de varice interno morborum quorundam caussa. 4°. *Lipsiæ,* 1785.
—— The same. 8°. *Ticini,* 1790.

Menz (G. Fridericus). * De secundinarum retardationibus nonnulla. [Marburg.] viii, 59 pp. 8°. *Cassellis, typ. H. Hotopii,* 1838.

Menz (Otto Fridericus) [1842–]. * De aneurysmate. 32 pp. 8°. *Berolini, G. Lange,* [1865].

Menzel (Abr. Frid. Guilielmus) [1800–]. * De tractu intestinorum ejusque functionibus. 31 pp. 8°. *Berolini, typ. Spæthenianis,* [1824].

Menzel (Arthur) [1844–78]. Ueber die Einwirkung des Urins auf das Zellgewebe. Eine experimentelle Studie über die Urin-Infiltration. 23 pp. 8°. [*Wien, C. Finsterbeck,* 1869.]
Repr. from: Wien. med. Wchnschr., 1869, xix.
For Biography, see Wien. med. Wchnschr., 1878, xxviii, 577 (Brettauer).

Menzel (Carolus). * De fundi oculi morbis ophthalmoscopio cognoscendis. 32 pp. 8°. *Regiomonti Pr., typ. Dalkowskianis,* [1855].

Menzel (Frid. Guilelm.) [1799–]. * De debilitate nervosa. 32 pp. 8°. *Berolini, C. A. G. Schmidt,* [1826].

Menzel (Hugo). * Ueber die in der Breslauer Frauenklinik im Studienjahre 1882–3 operirten 22 Urinfisteln. 1 p. l., 31 pp. 8°. *Leipzig, A. T. Engelhardt,* 1883.

Menzel (Josephus Davides). * De hydrope ovariorum. 2 p. l., 46 pp., 2 l. 8°. *Halæ, formis Plœtzianis,* [1835].

Menzel (Karl). * Die operative Eröffnung der Schädelhöhle. 38 pp. 8°. *Berlin, M. Niethe,* [1881].

Menzer (Joannes Philippus Bodo). * De sellæ obstetriciæ usu et optima ejus forma. 21 pp., 1 pl. 8°. *Gottingæ, ex off. Barmeieriana,* [1802].

Menzies (Alexander). * De dysenteria. 2 p. l., 41 pp. 8°. *Edinburgi, Balfour et Smellie,* 1793.

Menzies (Archibald).
See **Home** (Everard) & **Menzies** (Archibald). A description of the anatomy of the sea-otter. 4°. *London,* 1796. *See, also,* **Smyth** (J. C.) A description of the jail distemper, etc. 8°. *London,* 1800.

Menziès (G.-A.) * Sur quelques cas de diphthérite, avec des réflexions relatives à l'origine commune de la diphthérite, de la fièvre typhoïde et de la méningite cérébro-spinale. 24 pp. 4°. *Paris,* 1881, No. 5.

Menzies (Joannes). * De prostata tumida. 1 p. l., 21 pp. 8°. *Edinburgi, J. Ballantyne et soc.,* 1828. [P., v. 108.]

Menzies (Joh.) * De inflammatione hepatis. 10 pp., 1 l. 4°. *Traj. ad Rhenum, G. Vande Water,* 1709.

Menzies (Robert). * De respiratione. 1 p. l., 59 pp., 1 pl. 8°. *Edinburgi, G. Creech,* 1790. [P., v. 386.]

——. The same. A dissertation on respiration. Transl. from the Latin of . . . with notes by Charles Sugrue. iv, 66 pp., 1 pl. 8°. *Edinburgh, G. Mudie & Son,* 1796. [*Also, in:* P., v. 4; 86; 821; 1521.]

Menzing (Wilhelm). * Beitrag zur Kenntniss der Sputa bei Bronchectasie. 19 pp. 8°. *Erlangen, Junge u. Sohn,* 1878.

Menzius (Frid.) Memoriam Christophori Seyfferti oratione recolendam indicit. 12 pp. 4°. *Lipsiæ, ex off. Langenhemiana,* [1740].

Menzius (Joan. Christianus). * De saliva non temere exspuenda. 3 p. l., 23 pp. 4°. *Lipsiæ, ex off. Langenhemiana,* 1741.

Meola (Felice).
Co-Editor of: **Eco** (L') degli ospedali, Napoli, 1883.

Meola (Gio. Battista). Il vade-mecum degli erniosi, ossia regolamento pratico-popolare onde ridurre prontamente l' ernie incarcerate. 42 pp., 1 l. 8°. *Napoli, G. Nobile,* 1853. [*Also, in:* P., v. 1141.]

Mephitism.
See **Gases** (*Irrespirable*); **Latrines**, *etc.*

Méplain (Firmin). Du café. Étude de thérapeutique physiologique. 104 pp. 4°. *Paris,* 1868, No. 167.

Méplain (J.-B.-Auguste). * Considérations physiologiques sur l'homme moral, ou introduction à l'étude des passions. 39 pp. 4°. *Paris,* 1817, No. 145, v. 134.

Meppel.

See **Cholera** (*Asiatic, History, etc., of*), by localities.

Meppen (N. C.)

See **Kluyskens** (Joseph François). Berigt betrekkelijk de febris inflammatoria, etc. 8°. *Amsterdam*, 1818.

Mequinenza.

See **Fever** (*Yellow, History, etc., of*), by localities.

Meran.

JAROSZYŃSHI (W.) Meran i Arco jako lecznicze stacye klimatyczne. [Meran and Arco as medico-climatic stations.] 8°. *Lwów*, 1885.

MAZEGGER (B.) * Méran-Maïs, station climatérique pendant les saisons d'automne, d'hiver et de printemps. Trad. de l'allemand. 2. éd. 12°. *Méran*, 1887.

PIRCHER (J.) Meran als klimatischer Curort mit Rücksicht auf dessen Molken- und Traubencur-Anstalt. 8°. *Wien*, 1860.

——. The same. 8°. *Wien*, 1862.

——. The same. 3. Aufl. 8°. *Wien*, 1875.

Hausmann (R.) Ueber den Winteraufenthaltsort Meran. Berl. klin. Wchnschr., 1866, iii, 382; 390; 413; 423; 445.—**Helfft.** Meran als Molken-, Trauben- und klimatischer Kurort. Deutsche Klinik, Berl., 1860, xii, 407-411. ——. Ueber Meran und Venedig als Winteraufenthaltsorte für Kranke und die klimatischen Kurorte im Allgemeinen. Berl. klin. Wchnschr., 1864, i, 74; 83.—**Klein** (B.) Meran in Süd-Tyrol als Aufenthaltsort für Leidende. Ztschr. f. klin. Med., Bresl., 1851, ii, 374-384.—**Pircher** (J.) Der Kurort Meran, 1861-62. Deutsche Klinik, Berl., 1862, xiv, 443. ——. Vorzüge von Meran als klimatischer Kurort. *Ibid.*, 1863, xv, 268-270. ——. Meran als klimatischer Kurort. Rückblicke auf die Saison 1864-65. Wchnbl. d. k. k. Gesellsch. d. Aerzte in Wien, 1865, xxi, 277; 288. —**Sigmund.** Bemerkungen über den Kurort Meran. Wien. med. Wchnschr., 1851, i, 357.—**Thomson** (St. C.) Meran in midwinter. Med. Times & Gaz., Lond., 1885, i, 363.

Meran.

Co-Editor of: **Union** (L') médicale de la Gironde, Bordeaux, 1856-7.

Méran (Blaise-Gustave). * Sur l'érysipèle. 27 pp. 4°. *Paris*, 1845, No. 146, v. 435.

Mérandon (Léopold). *Action physiologique et thérapeutique des sels de potasse. 38 pp. 4°. *Paris*, 1868, No. 100.

Mérat (François-Victor) [**Mérat-De-Vaumartoise**] [1780-1851]. * Sur la colique métallique, vulgairement appelée colique des peintres, des plombiers, du plomb, etc. 180 pp. 8°. *Paris, P.-F. Rigot, an XI* [1803]. [*Also, in:* Paris theses, v. 33.]

——. The same. Traité de la colique métallique, vulgairement appelée colique des peintres, des plombiers, de Poitou, etc.; avec une description de la colique végétale, et un mémoire sur le tremblement des doreurs sur métaux. 2. éd. xii, 187 pp. 8°. *Paris, Méquignon-Marvis*, 1812.

——. Du tænia, ou ver solitaire, et de sa cure radicale par l'écorce de racine de grenadier; précédé de la description du tænia et du bothriocéphale, avec l'indication des anciens traitements employés contre ces vers. 164 pp. 8°. *Paris, J.-B. Baillière*, 1832. [P., v. 501.]

See, also, **Bourdon** (Isidore). Mémoire sur le vomissement [etc.] 8°. *Paris*, 1819.—**Morelot** (Simon). Cours élémentaire théorique et pratique de pharmacie-chimique, [etc.] 3 v. 8°. *Paris*, 1814.

——— & **De Lens** (A.-G.) Dictionnaire universel de matière médicale et de thérapeutique générale; contenant l'indication, la description et l'emploi de tous les médicaments connus dans les diverses parties du globe. 4 v. 8°. *Bruxelles, Hanman & Cie.*, 1838.

——. The same. 7 v. 8°. *Paris, J.-B. Baillière*, 1829-46.

Méraut (Camille). * De l'absorption par le tégument externe dans le bain. 35 pp. 4°. *Paris*, 1867, No. 176.

Méray (René). * De l'épistaxis. 18 pp. 4°. *Paris*, 1824, No. 37, v. 184.

Merbach (Curtius Fridericus). * De osse ac callo. 29 pp., 1 l. 8°. *Berolini, typ. Nietackianis*, [1842].

Merbach (Paulus Mauritius). * De sani cordis dimensionibus earumque commutatione in nonnullis morbis chronicis conspicua. 39 pp. 8°. *Lipsiæ, typ. J. H. Nagelii*, [1844].

Merbitzius (Joh. Valentinus). * De varietate faciei humanæ, discursus physicus. Appendicis loco accedunt carmina figurata Rabani Mauri. 7 p. l., 69 pp., viii, 2 l. sm. 4°. *Dresdæ, apud M. G. Hübnerum*, 1676.

——. Biga disputationum physicarum, quarum prima de infantibus supposititiis, vulgo Wechsel-Bälgen, altera de nymphis, Germanis Wassernixen. 26 pp. sm. 4°. [*Lipsiæ*], sumt. J. C. Mithii, [1678].

Mercadal Martín (J.) [–1887].

[**Obituary** by] Rodríguez Méndez. Gac. méd. catal., Barcel., 1887, x, 130, port.

Mercadier (Casimir). * Sur la fréquence, les formes, les causes de la phthisie dans l'armée. 32 pp. 4°. *Paris*, 1855, No. 289, v. 578.

Mercadier (Hippolyte). * De l'hépatite. 22 pp. 4°. *Paris*, 1853, No. 145, v. 545.

Mercadier (Jean-Hippolyte). * Contribution à l'étude de la pectoriloquie aphonique dans la pleurésie. 40 pp. 4°. *Paris*, 1876, No. 335.

Mercado (Luiz) [**Mercatus** (Ludovicus)] [1573–99]. De mulierum affectionibus libri iiii. Primus de communibus mulierum passionibus disserit. Secundus virginum, et viduarum morbos tractat. Tertius sterilium et prægnantium accidentia ad unguem exequitur. Quartus puerperarum et nutricum accidentia ad unguem exequitur. 3 p. l., 528 pp., 8 l. 4°. *Venetiis, apud F. Valgrisium*, 1587.

——. The same. 3 p. l., 567 pp., 8 l. 8°. *Basileæ, C. Waldkirch*, 1588.

Being v. 4 of: GYNÆCIORUM. 8°. *Basileæ*, 1588.

——. The same. De communibus mulierum affectionibus.

In: GYNÆCIORUM, [etc.] fol. *Argentinæ*, 1597, 803-1080.

——. The same. 9 p. l., 475 pp. 4°. *Venetiis, apud Societatem Venetam*, 1602.

——. De communi et peculiari præsidiorum artis medicæ indicatione. Accessit proemii loco methodus universalis in tres classes dissecta: i. affectas partes, ii. affectus ipsos, iii. medendi rationem monstrat. 14 p. l., 952 pp., 31 l. 16°. *Coloniæ, J. B. Ciotti sen.*, 1588.

——. De pulsibus libri duo in quibus tota ars cognoscendi morbos et prognosticandi disertissime tractatur. 9 p. l., 184 ff. 4°. *Patavii, apud P. Meiettum*, 1592.

——. De essentia, causis, signis et curatione febris malignæ, in qua maculæ rubentes similes morsibus pulicum per cutem erumpunt. Cui accessit consilium continens summam totius prædictionis et curationis in eodem affectu. 203 pp., 10 l. 16°. *Basileæ, C. Waldkirch*, 1594.

——. Libro en que se trata con claridad la naturaleza, causas, providencia, y verdadera orden y modo de curar la enfermedad vulgar, y peste que en estos años se ha divulgado por toda España. 1 p. l., 85 ff. 16°. *Madrid*, [*V. de*] *Castro*, 1599.

——. The same. 4 p. l., 128 ff. 16°. *Madrid, C. Sanchez*, 1648.

——. Opera omnia, in quatuor tomos divisa. Sedulo ac accurate relecta, emaculata, brevibus epitomis, ac indice locuplete donata, a Zacharia Palthenio. Cum præfatione ac encomio Joannis Hartmanni Beyeri. 4 v. in 2. 11 p. l., 516, 438 pp., 4 l., 682 pp. fol. *Francofurti*, 1608.

——. Consultationes morborum complicatorum et gravissimorum: cum disputationibus necessa-

Mercado (Luiz)—continued.
riis ad naturam cujusque morborum capessendam, præsagium et curationem, quibus accedunt, I. Tractatus unicus, continens gravissimas atque difficiles abditarum rerum disputationes, magni momenti et usus. II. Libri duo, de puerorum educatione, custodia et providentia, atque de morborum, qui ipsis accidunt, curatione. Operum ejusdem auctoris tomus quintus. 7 p. l., 291 pp., 15 l. fol. *Francofurti, e collegio musarum Paltheniano*, 1614.

——. Opera medica. 3 v. in 2. fol. *Francofurti, sumpt. hæred. Z. Palthenii*, 1619–20.
See, also, **Vidius** (Vidus). De febribus, [etc.] 4°. *Patavii*, 1591. ——. The same. sm. 4°. *Patavii*, 1595.

Mercanti (Ferruccio). Sul muscolo ciliare dei rettili. 8 pp., 1 pl. 4°. *Roma, Salviucci*, 1884.
Repr. from: Atti d. r. Accad. d. Lincei. Cl. di sc. fis., matemat. e nat., Roma, 1883-4, 3. s., xix.

Mercanton. Analyses des eaux minérales de Bex. 32 pp., 1 pl. 8°. *Lausanne, frères Blanchard*, 1824. [P., v. 1398.]

Mercanton (Victor). *Du traitement des plaies de l'estomac. [Strasburg.] 39 pp. 8°. *Lausanne, G. Bridel*, 1875.

Mercat (Edgard). *La fréquence relative de la colique hépatique chez l'enfant. 27 pp., 2 l. 4°. *Paris*, 1884, No. 32.

Mercati (Michele) [1541–93]. Instruttione sopra la peste . . . Aggiuntevi tre altre instruttioni sopra i veleni occultamente ministrati. Podagra et paralisi. 12 p. l., 143 pp. 4°. *Roma, V. Accolto*, 1576.
For Portrait, see **Collection**—van Kaathoven.

Mercatus (Ludovicus). *See* **Mercado** (Luiz).

Mercé (Donatien-Pierre). *I. Peut-on constater la présence d'un sel de brucine longtemps après l'inhumation d'un cadavre? II. [etc.] 25 pp. 4°. *Paris*, 1838, No. 340, v. 331.

——. Manœuvre simplifiée des accouchements artificiels ou contre nature que l'on termine à l'aide de la main et du forceps, précédée du mécanisme raisonné de l'accouchement naturel et suivie d'un article sur la délivrance avec les indications pratiques. viii, 9–328 pp. 8°. *Paris, Vve. Hildebrand*, 1848.

Mercedes, *Queen of Spain.*
Historia clínica de la enfermedad de S. M. la Reina Doña María de las Mercedes de Orleans y Borbon. Rev. de med. y cirug. práct., Madrid, 1878, iii, 152-159. *Also:* An. de cien. méd., Madrid, 1878, vi, 121-128. *Also:* Siglo méd., Madrid, 1878, xxv, 483-487.

Mercelis (Cornelius Petrus). *De morbis convulsivis in genere. 24 pp. 4°. *Gandavi, P. F. de Goesin-Verhaeghe*, [1829].

Mercenarius (Archangelus). Disputatio de putredine. 3 p. l., 31 l. 4°. *Patavii, apud P. Meietum*, 1583.

——. Adversus Erasti responsionem; secunda de putredine disputatio; in qua, præter ea, quæ ad exactam putredinis notitiam spectant, plurima philosophie, medicinæque studiosis necessaria explicantur. 5 p. l., 60 l. 4°. *Patavii, apud P. Meietum*, 1585.
Bound with preceding.

Mercenier (L.-C.-Stanislas). *De l'hydropéritonie. 42 pp. 4°. *Paris*, 1852, No. 201, v. 529.

Mercer (A. Clifford). Myxœdema. 16 pp. 8°. *New York, Trow*, 1881.
Repr. from: Med. Rec., N. Y., 1881, xix.

Mercer (Alfred). The relations of general (scientific medicine) to special and specific modes of medication. 18 pp. 8°. *Buffalo, Baker, Jones & Co.*, 1874.
Repr. from: Buffalo M. & S. J., 1874, xiii.

——. An address, presenting the claims of the medical department, read before a council in the interest of Syracuse University, held at Syracuse,

Mercer (Alfr d)—continued.
N. Y., December 18, 19, 1878. 19 pp. 8°. *Syracuse, N. Y., Masters & Stone*, 1879.

Mercer (Græmius). *De pathematibus animi, eorumque in corpus humanum effectibus. 2 p. l., 45 pp. 8°. *Edinburgi, Balfour et Smellie*, 1784. [*Also, in:* P., v. 18.]

Mercer (James). A probationary essay on the special pathology of the accessory organs of hearing. vii, 133 pp. 8°. *Edinburgh, Neill & Co.*, 1840. [*Also, in:* P., v. 95; 897; 1018; 1165.]

——. Observations on the cavernous sinus; with a description of an additional sinus occasionally found in its external wall. 15 pp. 8°. *Edinburgh, Neill & Co.*, 1840. [*Also, in:* P., v. 897; 1172.]
Repr. from: Lond. M. Gaz., 1840, xxvi.

——. Anatomical observations on the analogous structure and uses of the lingualis and panniculus carnosus muscles. 16 pp. 8°. *Edinburgh, Neill & Co.*, 1841. [P., v. 109; 897; 1051; 1524.]
Repr. from: Lond. M. Gaz., 1841, xxviii.

——. Syllabus of lectures on anatomy and physiology, delivered in the School of Anatomy, Edinburgh. 46 pp. 8°. *Edinburgh, Neill & Co.*, 1841. [*Also, in:* P., v. 95; 918; 1175.]

——. On deafness, caused by hemorrhage into the cavity of the tympanum, successfully treated by perforation of the membrane; with statistic observations on the results of this operation generally. 9 pp. 8°. [*Edinburgh*, 1844.] [P., v. 95; 1020; 1509.]
Repr. from: North. J. M., Edinb., 1844, i.

——. Contributions to acoustic pathology. Pt. 3. 11 pp. 8°. [*Edinburgh, Sutherland & Knox*, 1848.] [P., v. 1175.]
Repr. from: Month. J. M. Sc., Lond. & Edinb., 1847-8, viii.

Mercer (Samuel). *De chorea Sancti Viti. 1 p. l., 28 pp. 8°. *Edinburgi, A. Neill et soc.*, 1805.

Mercer *County.*
See **Illinois**; **Pennsylvania**.

de Mercey (A.-B.) Des lésions traumatiques des vaisseaux rétro-pelviens. 136 pp. 8°. *Paris, L. Leclerc*, 1869.

Merchant Taylors' Company's Convalescent Home, at Bognor, Sussex. The report of the special committee, consisting of the master and Messrs. Bosteker, Fletcher, Fuller, and Davis, appointed by the court of the 11th of January, 1869, to consider and lookout for a site suitable for a convalescent home. 4 pp. fol. [*London*, 1869.]

——. Reports of the committee for conducting the . . . to the court. 1.-4.. 1869-72. 8°. [*London*], 1869-73.
Semi-annual.

——. General rules and regulations of the . . . With rules and regulations for the patients. 10, 7 pp. 12°. [*London, n. d.*]

——. Blank forms of the . . . I. Application for admission. II. Matron's weekly return. fol. [*London, n. d.*]

Merchants.
Alexander (J.) Pathological researches illustrative of the diseases which are more particularly incidental to commercial life. Lancet, Lond., 1835-6, ii, 321; 385.

Merche.
Editor of: **Journal** de médecine vétérinaire militaire, Paris, 1873-7.

Merchie (Z.) Des secours à porter aux blessés sur les champs de bataille. Réponse à M. le Dr. André Uytterhoeven. 42 pp. 8°. *Bruxelles, C. Lelong*, 1855.
Repr. from: Arch. belges de méd. mil., Brux., 1855, xv

——. Appareils modelés, ou nouveau système de déligation pour les fractures des membres

Merchie (Z.)—continued.

précédé d'une histoire analytique et raisonnée des principaux appareils à fractures employés depuis les temps les plus reculés jusqu'à nos jours. xii, 607 pp. 8°. *Paris, J.-B. Baillière,* 1858.

———. Maladies des organes respiratoires. Leçons cliniques professées à l'Hôpital militaire de Bruxelles, année 1863-4. vii, 112, 12 pp. 8°. *Bruxelles, H. Manceaux,* 1864.

———. Manuel pratique des appareils modelés, ou nouveau système de déligation pour les fractures . . . les luxations . . . [etc.] xv, 328 pp., 1 pl. 8°. *Bruxelles, H. Manceaux,* 1872.

———. Guerre de 1870-71. Les secours aux blessés après la bataille de Sédan, avec documents officiels à l'appui. vi, 244 pp. 8°. *Bruxelles, H. Manceaux,* 1876.

See, also, **Goffres** (Joseph-Marie). Appréciation des appareils modelés [etc.] 8°. *Paris,* 1862.

Mercié (Louis). * De l'enchondrôme des os. 59 pp. 4°. *Paris,* 1884, No. 7.

Merciei-Theillet (Emmanuel). * Sur la métrite aiguë. 25 pp. 4°. *Paris,* 1826, No. 167, v. 202.

Mercier.

See **Robin** (Ch.) & **Mercier.** Mémoire sur l'hématoïdine [etc.] 8°. *Paris,* [1855].

Mercier [1857-]. * Contribution à l'étude du hoquet. 41 pp., 1 l. 4°. *Paris,* 1880, No. 451.

Mercier (A.)[1] Anatomie et physiologie de la vessie au point de vue chirurgical. 86 pp. 8°. *Paris, J.-B. Baillière,* 1872.

Mercier (A.)[2] * Considérations cliniques sur quelques cas de fractures comminutives avec plaies. 44 pp., 1 pl., 1 l. 4°. *Paris,* 1874, No. 398.

Mercier (A.-F.-Victorien). * De la bronchite. 76 pp. 4°. *Paris,* 1857, No. 274, v. 607.

Mercier (Amédée). * Sur le traitement du zona, notamment par les applications topiques du perchlorure de fer. 50 pp. 4°. *Paris,* 1877, No. 78.

Mercier (Amédée-Hippolyte). * Sur la chlorose, ou pâles couleurs, chez les jeunes filles. 18 pp. 4°. *Paris,* 1831, No. 197, v. 243.

Mercier (Armand). * De l'étiologie du scorbut dans les prisons. 39 pp. 4°. *Paris,* 1884, No. 246.

Mercier (Auguste). * Des complications des fractures de la clavicule et en particulier de la blessure du poumon. 38 pp., 1 l. 4°. *Paris,* 1881, No. 261.

Mercier (Augustin - Anatole). * Du tabac et particulièrement de l'empoisonnement aigu par le tabac. 46 pp. 4°. *Paris,* 1870, No. 263.

Mercier (Augustin-François). * Étude sur l'arthrite survenue pendant le cours de la grossesse (pseudo rhumatisme de la grossesse.) [Paris.] 55 pp., 2 l. 4°. *Le Mans,* 1883.

Mercier (Benoît). * Précis sur la paralysie, suivi de nouvelles observations sur les effets curatifs de la noix vomique dans cette maladie. 25 pp. 4°. *Paris,* 1818, No. 132, v. 139.

Mercier (Carolus Julius). * De hyspospadia et epispadia. 26 pp., 3 l., 1 pl. 8°. *Berolini, typ. Nietackianis,* [1841].

Mercier (Charles). A national want. [A letter to the editor of "The Globe", July 8, 1873, showing the necessity for such an institution as the Saint John's Hospital for Diseases of the Skin, and appealing to the public for support.] 1 sheet. 4°. [*London,* 1873.]

Repr. from: The Globe, July 14, 1873.

———. The proposed new hospital. [A letter published in "The Echo", April 25, 1873, soliciting support for the erection of a proper hospital

Mercier (Charles)—continued.

for diseases of the skin.] 2 l. 4°. [*London,* 1873.]

Repr. from: The Echo, April 25, 1873.

See, also, **Saint John's** Hospital for Diseases of the Skin, Leicester Square, London. A proposed new hospital. 4°. [*London,* 1873.]

Mercier (E.) Le lait devant les tribunaux. Du galactomètre ou pèse-lait au point de vue des poursuites judiciaires et des pénalités édictées dans les règlements des fromageries. 32 pp. 12°. *Nantua, A. Arêne,* 1882.

Mercier (Élie). * Mélæna et hématémèse des nouveau-nés et leurs rapports avec les gerçures des seins. 92 pp. 4°. *Paris,* 1878, No. 355.

Mercier (Étienne-Julien). * I. Apprécier les caractères anatomiques de l'endocardite. II. [etc.] 35 pp. 4°. *Paris,* 1839, No. 364, v. 346.

Mercier (F.-M.) * Essai sur cette question: Existe-t-il une fièvre puerpérale? 131 pp. 4°. *Paris, an XII* [1804], No. 191, v. 47.

Mercier (Félix - François - Olivier). * Sur l'hémoptysie active. 35 pp. 4°. *Paris,* 1828, No. 162, v. 217.

Mercier (Francis). * De l'embolie artérielle. 39 pp. 4°. *Paris,* 1859, No. 57, v. 634.

Mercier (Gabriel). * De l'expulsion spontanée des calculs de la vessie. 79 pp. 4°. *Paris,* 1881, No. 25.

Mercier (J.) * Sur l'hydrothorax. vi, 7-40 pp. 4°. *Paris,* 1810, No. 63, v. 80.

Mercier (J.-Étienne). * Des inflammations de la paume de la main. 30 pp. 4°. *Paris,* 1859, No. 231, v. 634.

Mercier (J.-J.-C.-Alfred). Oration delivered before the Physico - Medical Society of New Orleans, at their University meeting, held December, 1854. 22 pp. 8°. *New Orleans,* 1854.

———. * De la fièvre typhoïde, dans ses rapports avec la phthisie aiguë. 30 pp. 4°. *Paris,* 1855, No. 211, v. 578.

———. La fièvre jaune; sa manière d'être à l'égard des étrangers à la Nouvelle-Orléans et dans les campagnes. Quelques mots sur son passé et son avenir en Europe. Lettres adressées à la Gazette des hôpitaux de Paris, avec un avant-propos et un appendice. 32 pp. 8°. *Paris, A. Delahaye,* 1860.

Mercier (J.-L.) * Du traitement de la fièvre typhoïde. 66 pp. 4°. *Paris,* 1854, No. 265, v. 563.

———. De l'identité du catarrhe et du rhumatisme. 86 pp., 1 l. 8°. *Genève & Bâle, H. Georg,* 1869.

Mercier (Jean - Baptiste). * Des convulsions chez les enfants. 31 pp. 4°. *Paris,* 1857, No. 129, v. 607.

Mercier (Jean-Gabriel-Alexis). * Sur les bains. vi, 7-38 pp. 4°. *Paris,* 1815, No. 227, v. 115.

Mercier (Jean-Marie). * De l'anatomie chirurgicale de l'œil. 1 p. l., 30 pp. 4°. *Strasbourg,* 1837, v. 70.

Mercier (Jules)[1]. * Des polypes du rectum. 39 pp. 4°. *Paris,* 1857, No. 288, v. 607.

Mercier (Jules)[2]. * De l'emploi thérapeutique du phosphure de zinc. 54 pp. 4°. *Paris,* 1878, No. 215.

Mercier (Jules)[3]. L'homme régénéré par la méthode sommaire: Chapitre I. Affaiblissement. Impuissance. Stérilité. II. Spermatorrhée, ou pertes séminales involontaires . . . Causes, symptômes, marche et complications de ces affections. Leur traitement par la méthode régénératrice. 105 pp. 12°. *Paris, chez l'auteur,* 1885.

Mercier ('Julien) [1857-]. * Des troubles hépatiques dans les affections cardiaques. 71 pp. 4°. *Paris,* 1881, No. 143.

Mercier (Léon). *Contribution à l'étude des rapports de la puerpéralité et de la syphilis et en particulier de la fièvre syphilitique pendant les suites de couches. 37 pp. 4°. *Paris*, 1886, No. 95.

Mercier (Louis-Auguste) [1811–82]. *I. De l'influence que le rétrécissement organique de l'urèthre exerce dans l'application de la lithotritie et de la cystotomie. II. [etc.] 43 pp. 4°. *Paris*, 1839, No. 10, v. 346.

——. Recherches anatomiques, pathologiques et thérapeutiques sur les maladies des organes urinaires et génitaux, considérées spécialement chez les hommes âgés; ouvrage entièrement fondé sur de nouvelles observations. ix, 390 pp., 1 l. 8°. *Paris, Béchet jeune & Labé*, 1841.

——. Résumé analytique des travaux sur les organes génito-urinaires et leurs maladies, présentés à l'Académie royale de médecine, le 21 septembre 1844 pour le prix d'Argenteuil. 16 pp. 8°. *Paris, E. Bautruche*, 1846. [P., v. 454; 464.]

——. Recherches anatomiques, pathologiques et thérapeutiques sur les valvules du col de la vessie, cause fréquente et peu connue de rétention d'urine, et sur leurs rapports avec les inflammations et les rétrécissements de l'urèthre, [etc.] 2. éd. 3 p. l., 480 pp., 1 l. 8°. *Paris, Vve. le Normant*, 1848.

——. Troisième série d'observations et remarques sur le traitement de la rétention d'urine causée par les valvules du col de la vessie. 79 pp. 8°. [*Paris, Vve. le Normant*, 1850.]

——. Mémoire historique sur divers points de la pathologie urinaire. 103 pp. 8°. [*Paris*, 1854.]

——. Lettre à mes confrères, en réponse à une lettre du Dr. J. Leroy, soi-disant d'Étiolles, sur les maladies de la prostate et du col de la vessie. 16 pp. 8°. *Paris, Vve. le Normant*, 1854.

——. Recherches sur le traitement des maladies des organes urinaires considérées spécialement chez les hommes âgés et sur celui des rétrécissements de l'urètre, suivies d'un essai sur la gravelle et la pierre, principalement sur la lithotritie, l'extraction des fragments, et sur celle des autres corps étrangers. viii, 623 pp. 8°. *Paris, Labé*, 1856.

——. Étude sur divers points d'anatomie et de pathologie des organes génito-urinaires faite à propos de quelques ouvrages anglais. 56 pp. 8°. *Paris, V. Masson*, 1860.

Repr. from: Gaz. hebd. de méd., Par., 1860, vii.

——. Traitement préservatif et curatif des sédiments, de la gravelle, de la pierre urinaire et de diverses maladies dépendant de la diathèse urique. viii, 540 pp. 12°. *Paris, A. Delahaye*, 1872.

——. Quelques mots sur la taille périnéale par dilatation et sur la lithotritie périnéale. 14 pp. 8°. *Paris, A. Delahaye*, 1874.

——. Perfectionnements apportés à la lithotritie. 19 pp. 8°. *Paris, V. A. Delahaye & Cie.*, 1879.

See, also, **Sergi** (Paolo). Il metodo di curare le malattie orinarie del dottor Caponato, [etc.] 8°. *Messina*, 1854.

Mercier (Louis - Edmond). *Des phénomènes cutanés dans la fièvre typhoïde. 38 pp. 4°. *Paris*, 1856, No. 46, v. 593.

Mercier(Marie-Placide-Jules-Armand). *I. Décrire le prurigo des parties génitales. Indiquer son diagnostic et son traitement. II. [etc.] 65 pp. 4°. *Paris*, 1841, No. 223, v. 378.

Mercier (Maurice). *De la syphilis cérébrale tertiaire avec accidents comateux sidérants. 44 pp. 4°. *Paris*, 1875, No. 420.

Mercier (N.-M.) *Sur l'opération de la castration. 35 pp. 8°. *Paris, an XI* [1803], v. 36.

Mercier(P -A.-M.) *Sur l'hémoptysie, considérée comme symptôme de la phthisie tuberculeuse et de l'hypertrophie, avec ou sans dilatation du ventricule droit. 22 pp. 4°. *Paris*, 1836, No. 295, v. 302.

Mercier (Pierre-J.) *De la congestion pulmonaire rapide; de l'œdème aigu du poumon avec ou sans expectoration albumineuse, leurs rapports réciproques, leurs rapports avec la pleurésie et son traitement; étude de pathologie clinique, expérimentale et critique. 84 pp., 1 l. 4°. *Paris*, 1876, No. 495.

Also, Co-Editor of: **Revue** mensuelle des maladies de l'enfance, Paris, 1886.

See, also, **de Saint-Germain** (L.-A.) Déviations latérales du rachis. Traitement de la scoliose, [etc.] 8°. *Paris*, 1882. ——. Chirurgie orthopédique. 8°. *Paris*, 1883. ——. Chirurgie des enfants, etc. 8°. *Paris*, 1884.

Mercier (Pierre-Philippe). *Considérations sur les causes de la phthisie pulmonaire, plus particulièrement envisagées chez les femmes. 27 pp. 4°. *Paris*, 1815, No. 20, v. 108.

Mercier (S.-E.) *Sur la gangrène, considérée sous le rapport de la nosologie. 82 pp. 4°. *Paris*, 1824, No. 119, v. 186.

Mercier (T.-S.-D.) *Considérations générales sur quelques complications de la scarlatine. 38 pp. 4°. *Paris*, 1862, No. 11.

Mercier De Sainte-Croix (Pierre-Henri). *Sur l'asthme. 75 pp. 4°. *Paris*, 1847, No. 56, v. 462.

Mercier-Valenton (H.) [1855–]. *Étude sur les tumeurs malignes des os du crâne. 54 pp., 1 l. 4°. *Paris*, 1881, No. 411.

Merck (C. H.) *De anatomia et physiologia lienis ejusque abscessu feliciter curato. 44 pp. 4°. *Giessæ Cattorum, lit. Braunii*, 1784. [P., v. 58.]

Merck (Christian). *Die croupöse Pneumonie. 40 pp. 8°. *München, F. Wild*, 1850.

Merck (E.)

Co-Editor of: **Annalen** der Pharmacie, Lemgo u. Heidelberg, 1836-7.

Merck (J. A.) De comparatione plantarum et animalium. 111 pp. 8°. *Berolini, F. G. Birnstiel*, [1780].

Merck (Wilhelm Ernst) [1860–]. *Ueber Cocaïn. 37 pp., 1 l. 8°. *Kiel, C. F. Mohr*, 1886.

Merck (Wolfgang Christoph). *Der Schwefeläther in seiner Bereitung, Wirkung und Anwendung. 36 pp. 8°. *München, C. Wolf*, 1847.

Merckel (Joannes Gottlob.) *De fluxu hepatico. 31 pp. sm. 4°. *Vitembergæ, ex off. Gerdesianæ viduæ*, [1715].

Merckel (Martinus). *De apoplexia. 181. 4°. *Jenæ, typ. J. Wertheri*, 1668.

——. De minera Martis. 27 pp., 1 l. sm. 4°. *Jenæ, lit. Wertherianis*, [1668].

Merckel (P. F.)

See **Voigtel** (F. G.) Handbuch der pathologischen Anatomie. 3 v. 8°. *Halle*, 1804-5.

Merckell (Joh. Matthæus). *Exercitatio medica sistens ideam præscribendarum formularum. *Lipsiæ, typ. vid. Galli Niemanni*, 1682.

In: ETTMÜLLER (M.) Diss. xiix med. 4°. *Francof. et Lips.*, 1685, 55 ff.

Merckens (H.) Hahnemann en de homoeopathie. Uitgegeven van wege de Vereeniging tot Bevordering der Homoeopathie in Nederland. 40 pp. 8°. *Gravenhage, C. Blommendaal*, 1887.

Mercker (Friedrich Karl Leopold). *Ueber die Anwendung des Meisels bei Schädelverletzungen. 26 pp. 8°. *Marburg, C. L. Pfeil*, 1859.

Mercker (Joh. Christophorus). *De hydrocardia. 16 pp. 4°. *Traj. ad Rhenum, G. van de Water*, 1711.

Mercker(Ludovicus Augustus Ernestus) [1840–]. *De gravidi uteri rupturis. 30 pp. sm. 8°. *Berolini, G. Schade*, [1866].

Mercklin (August).   *Studien über die primäre Verrücktheit. 102 pp., 1 l. 8°. *Dorpat, H. Laakmann,* 1879.

Mercklin (Bartholome). Kurtzer verfasster Underricht wie unnd wassen man sich bey disen so gefährlichen pestilentzischen Zuständen: Zur Verhütung oder Præservation zu halten und zu Curation solcher Seuchen brauchen soll. Auss Befelch eines ehrsamen Rahts der fürstl. pfältzischen Stadt Lauingen gestelt. 9 l. 4°. *Dilingen, E. Lochner,* 1627.

Mercklin (*Georg Abraham*) [1613–84].
Portrait in: **Collection**—van Kaathoven.

Mercklin (Georg Abraham) [1644–1702]. Prodromus palindromiæ. 7 l. 4°. *Altdorphi, typ. vid. J. L. Winterbergeri,* [1670].

——. Tractatio med. curiosa de ortu et occasu transfusionis sanguinis, qua hæc, quæ sit e bruto in brutum, a foro medico penitus eliminatur; illa, quæ e bruto in hominem peragitur, refutatur; et ista, quæ ex homine in hominem exercetur, ad experientiæ examen relegatur. 13 p. l., 112 pp., 2 l. 12°. *Norimbergæ, typ. C. Gerhardi,* 1679.

——. Sylloge physico-medicinalium casuum incantationi vulgo adscribi solitorum, maximeque præ cæteris memorabilium decurias vi. complectens; cum inspersis partim, partim subnexis huc spectantibus judiciis et curationibus. Cui loco mantissæ accesserunt. I. Quæstio solemnis: An monstrosa varia illa excreta revera in corpore fuerint vel extrahantur? an vero præstigiæ dæmonis sint extra saltim talia in corporis superficie ostentantis? II. Helmontii tract. de receptis injectis: de injectis materialibus: de injaculatorum modo intrandi. III. Laevin. Fischer de morbis magice per sagas inductis naturaliter curandis. IV. Bartholom. Carrichteri, ratio medendi morbis ab incantatione dependentibus, nunc primum Latinitate donata. V. Collectanea et secreta Myliana ad morbos magicos, maximam partem e germanica in latinam linguam translata, et nunc primum publicam in lucem emissa. 20 p. l., 254 pp., 6 l. 4°. *Norimbergæ, J. Zieger et G. Lehmann,* 1698.

——. Tractatus physico-medicus de incantamentis, sexaginta casus, maxime præ cæteris memorabiles complectens, cum subnexis eorundem judiciis et curationibus. Cui mantissæ loco accesserunt, varia huc spectantia, partim ex aliis authoribus excerpta, partim nunc primum publicam in lucem emissa. Frontispiece, 21 p. l., 254 pp., 6 l. 4°. *Norimbergæ, J. F. Rudiger,* 1715.
See, also, **Fraundorffer** (Philippus). Tabula smaragdina, etc. 16°. *Norimbergæ,* 1713.—**van der Linden** (Joh. Anton.) Lindenius renovatus sive Johannis Antonidæ van der Linden de scriptis medicis libri duo. 4°. *Norimbergæ,* 1686.—**Malfi** (Tiberio). Neue Anleitung zur Barbier- und Wund-Artzney-Kunst, etc. 12°. *Nürnberg,* 1676.—**Pandolphinus** (Josephus). Tractatus de ventositatis spinæ [etc.]. 18°. *Noribergæ,* 1764.
For Portrait, see **Collection**—van Kaathoven.

Mercklin (Joh. Abrahamus) [1674–1710]. *De hydrope saccato. 24 pp. 4°. *Altdorffi, H. Meyer,* 1695.

——. De feliciori nunc quam olim medicina diascepsis, plurima neotericorum inventa medica breviter complectens. 2 p. l., 32 pp. sm. 4°. *Patarii, S. Spera,* 1696.
For Portrait, see **Collection**—van Kaathoven.

Mercklinghaus (P. F. Ludov.) [1801–]. * De blepharoblennorrhœa neonatorum. 28 pp. 8°. *Berolini, lit. A. Petschii,* [1826].

Mercur (Wm. H.)
See **Rindfleisch** (Edward). The elements [etc.] 8°. *Philadelphia,* 1884.

Mercurialis (Hieronymus) [1530–1606]. Nomothelasmus seu ratio lactandi infantes. 47 pp. 8°. *Patavii,* 1552.
A reprint, probably printed at Treviso in 1778.

Mercurialis (Hieronymus)—continued.
——. Variarum lectionum libri quatuor. In quibus complurium, maximeque medicinæ scriptorum infinita pæne loca vel corrupta restituuntur, vel obscura declarantur. Alexandri Tralliani de lumbricis epistola, ejusdem Mercurialis opera et diligentia græce, et latine nunc primum edita. 18 p. l., 122 ff. 4°. *Venetiis, sumpt. P. et A. Meieti,* 1570.

——. The same. 18 p. l., 122 ff. 4°. *Venetiis, sumpt. P. et A. Meieti frat.,* 1571.

——. The same. 15 p. l., 276 pp., 21 l. 16°. *Basileæ, ex off. P. Pernæ,* 1576.

——. The same. Variarum lectionum in medicinæ scriptoribus et aliis libri sex. Ab auctore hac quoque postrema editione aucti et recogniti. 7 p. l., 145 l., 20 l. 4°. *Venetiis, apud Juntas,* 1598.

——. De peste in universum, præsertim vero de Veneta et Patavina. Item de morbis cutaneis, et omnibus humani corporis excrementis. 7 p. l., 148 pp., 12 l., 421 pp., 14 l. 12°. *Basileæ,* [1577?]

——. De pestilentia . . . lectiones habitæ Patavii mdlxxvii. mense Januarii. In quibus de peste in universum, præsertim vero de Veneta et Patavina, singulari quadam eruditione tractatur A. Hieronymo Zaccho. 3 p. l., 114 pp., 7 l. 4°. *Venetiis, apud P. Meietum,* 1577.

——. The same. Ejusdem tractatus de maculis pestiferis, de hydrophobia, et de venenis ac morbis venenosis. 101 pp., 4 l. fol. [*Venetiis, apud Juntas et Baba,* 1644.]
Bound with his: Opuscula aurea, etc. fol. *Venetiis,* 1644.

——. De puerorum morbis tractatus locupletissimi; varia doctrina referti, nec solum medicis, verum etiam philosophis magnopere utiles; ex ore . . . diligenter excepti, atque in libros tres digesti: Opera Johannis Groscesij. Addita Alexandri Tralliani de lumbricis epistola, cum ejusdem Mercurialis versione. Ejusdem de venenis et morbis venenosis libri ii. seorsim editi. 3 p. l., 468 pp., 14 l.; 3 p. l., 168 pp., 4 l. 12°. *Francofurti, apud heredes Wecheli,* 1584. [*Also, in:* P., v. 134.]
Bound with his: De peste in universum. 12°. *Basileæ,* 1577?

——. The same. Opera Johannis Chrosczieyoioskij. 12 p. l., 116 ff. 4°. *Venetiis, apud Juntas,* 1615.
Bound with his: De arte gymnastica. 4°. *Venetiis,* 1601.

——. Censura operum Hippocratis. 19 l. 4°. *Venetiis, apud Juntas,* 1585.
Another copy, bound with his: De arte gymnastica. 4°. *Venetiis,* 1601.

——. De arte gymnastica libri sex, in quibus exercitationum omnium vetustarum genera, loca, modi, facultates, et quidquid denique ad corporis humani exercitationes pertinet, diligenter explicatur. 3. ed. 6 p. l., 308 pp., 13 l. 4°. *Venetiis, apud Juntas,* 1587.

——. The same. 4. ed. 8 p. l., 308 pp., 13 l. 4°. *Venetiis, apud Juntas,* 1601.

——. The same. Editio novissima . . . Christ. Coriolani emendata. Frontispiece, 5 p. l., 387 pp., 19 l., 7 pl. 4°. *Amstelodami, sumpt. A. Frisii,* 1672.

——. De morbis muliebribus prælectiones ex ore jam dudum a Gaspare Bauhino exceptæ, ac paulo antea inscio autore editæ; nunc vero per Michaelem Columbum, ex collatione plurium exemplarium consensu auctoris locupletiores, et emendatiores factæ; cum indice capitum et rerum locupletissimo. 11 p. l., 197 pp. 4°. *Venetiis, apud F. Valgrisium,* 1587.
Also, in: GYNÆCIORUM, etc. 8°. *Basileæ,* 1586, ii, 1–195.
Also, in: GYNÆCIORUM. fol. *Argentinæ,* 1597, 209–303.

Mercurialis (Hieronymus)—continued.

——. The same. 4. ed. 12 p. l., 236 pp. 4°.
Venetiis, Juntas, 1601.
> Bound with his: De morbis cutaneis. 4°. *Venetiis,* 1601.

——. The same. 5. ed. denuo non solum auctæ.
12 p. l., 236 pp. 4°. *Venetiis, apud Juntas,* 1618.
> Bound with his: De arte gymnastica. 4°. *Venetiis,* 1601.

——. Responsorum et consultationum medicinalium, nunc primum a Michaele Columbo collecta et in lucem edita tomus primus et alter. 2 v. in 1. 9 p. l., 263 pp.; 9 p. l., 262 pp. fol. *Venetiis, apud Jolitos,* 1589.

——. De compositione medicamentorum tractatus, tres libros complectens: I. De compositione medicamentorum. II. De medicamentorum dosi. III. Medicamentorum componendorum rationem et methodum tradit. Ejusdem de oculorum, et aurium affectibus prælectiones seorsim editæ. Omnia primum a Michaele Columbo in lucem edita. 3 p. l., 312 pp. 12°. *Francofurdi, apud J. Wechelum,* 1591.

——. Prælectiones Pisanæ in epidemicas Hippocratis historias, non minus ad theoricam atque practicam medicinam utiles quam ob eruditionem jucundæ. Necnon tractatus: 1. De hominis generatione. 2. De balneis Pisanis. 3. De vino et aqua. 7 p. l., 208, 56, 11 pp., 2 l. fol. *Venetiis, apud Juntas,* 1597.

——. De morbis cutaneis et omnibus corporis humani excrementis tractatus locupletissimi variaque doctrina referti, non solum medicis verum etiam philosophis magnopere utiles, atque in libros quinque digesti, opera Pauli Aicardii. Quibus accessit alius libellus de decoratione ex ejusdem Mercurialis prælectionibus exceptus, et in capita redactus a Julio Mancino. 15 p. l., 210 pp. 4°. *Venetiis, apud Juntas,* 1601.

——. Tractatus de compositione medicamentorum. De morbis oculorum, et aurium. Ipso prælegente olim Patavii diligenter excepti, et nunc primum a Michaele Columbo editi. 7 p. l., 106 ff.; 4 l., 63 ff., 1 l. 4°. *Venetiis, apud Juntas,* 1601.

——. De decoratione liber non solum medicis, et philosophis verum etiam omnium disciplinarum studiosis apprime utilis. 8 p. l., 44 ff. 4°. *Venetiis, apud Juntas,* 1601.
> Bound with his: De arte gymnastica. 4°. *Venetiis,* 1601.

——. Medicina practica, seu de cognoscendis, discernendis et curandis omnibus humani corporis affectibus, earumque causis indagandis, libri v., in Patavino gymnasio, olim ab ipso publice prælecti, et thesauri instar a quibusdam hactenus reconditi, plurimorumque votis et desiderio summe expetiti: nunc autem post obitum autoris, publici boni causa, in lucem editi, studio et opera Petri de Spina. 3 p. l., 594 pp., 20 l. fol. *Francof. a. M., in off. J. T. Schönwetteri,* 1602.

——. Commentarii eruditissimi, in Hippocratis Coi prognostica, prorrhetica, de victus ratione in morbis acutis, et epidemicas historias. Quibus accessere tractatus luculentissimi, de hominis generatione, vino et aqua, balneisque Pisanis. A Marco Cornacchino . . . ex ore ipsius diligentes excepti, nunc primum in lucem editi. 2 p. l., 848 pp., 11 l. fol. *Francofurti, typ. J. Saurii, imp. J. T. Schönwetteri,* 1602.

——. Prælectiones Patavinæ, de cognoscendis, et curandis humani corporis affectibus. In quibus præter alia quæ ad praxim exercendam plurimum conferunt, et præter variam eruditionem, gravissimæ quoque theoriæ enodantur. Nuper inscio, et tanquam mortuo authore editæ, nunc vero, tum ex diversis exemplaribus, eodem

Mercurialis (Hieronymus)—continued.

permittente ac annuente, tum ex ipsiusmet ore præmonstrante atque dictante, recognitæ, emendatæ et tertia parte auctæ, opera ac studio Guglielmi Athenii Bruxellensis. 16 p. l., 656 pp. fol. *Venetiis, apud Juntas,* 1603.

——. The same. De cognoscendis, et curandis humani corporis affectibus. In quibus præter alia quæ partim ad praxim in re medica exercendam, partim ad uberiorem eruditionem comparandam plurimum conferunt, gravissimæ quoque theoriæ difficultates enodantur . . . opera, ac studio Guglielmi Athenii, et hac postrema editione summa cum diligentia correctæ . . . et aliorum principum. 13 p. l., 644 pp. fol. *Venetiis, apud Juntas,* 1627.

——. Tractatus varii de re medica, a variis medicis olim ex ipsius ore excepti, nunc vero, post ejus obitum, in gratiam studiosorum medicinæ evulgati. Horum primus de morbis muliebribus, in quatuor libros distinctus. Secundus de puerorum morbis, cum Tralliani de lumbricis epistola ab eodem auctore in latinum versa, et de venenosis, ac venenis opusculo. Tertius de peste, præsertim de Veneta, et Patavina. Quartus de morbis cutaneis, in tres libros digestus. Quintus demum, de excrementis, in tres libros divisus. 4°. *Lugduni, sumpt. A. Pillehotte,* 1623.

——. In secundum lib. epid. Hipp. prælectiones Bononienses. Opus multiplici eruditione, doctrina, ac fere innumeris problematibus refertum, [etc.] 7 p. l., 314 pp. fol. *Forolivii, apud Cimattios,* 1626.

——. In omnes Hippocratis aphorismos prælectiones Patavinæ, in quibus innumeri pene ipsius Hippocratis obscuriores loci ac sententiæ elucidantur, problemataque permulta abstrusiora facili methodo enodantur. Nunc primum a Maximiliano auctoris filio publici juris factæ, atque in postrema hac editione opera Pancracii Marcellini notis marginalibus ditatæ; denuo summa cum diligentia et labore revisæ et emendatæ. 3 p. l., 770 pp., 22 l. 4°. *Lugduni, sumpt. A. Pillehotte,* 1631.

——. Opuscula aurea, et selectiora. Accedit novum consilium de ratione discendi medicinam aliasque disciplinas hactenus editum. Curante F. Baba. 36 p. l., 492 pp., 4 l. fol. *Venetiis, apud Juntas et Baba,* 1644.
> *See, also,* **Haase** (C. A.) Das Stottern. 8°. *Berlin,* 1846. — **Hippocrates.** Opera. fol. *Venetiis,* 1588. — **Munster** (J.) Discussio eorum, etc. 12°. *Francofurti,* 1603. — **Varolius** (Constantinus). Anatomiæ . . . libri iv. 8°. *Francofurti,* 1591.
> *For Biography, see* **Boerner** (F.) De vita, moribus, meritis et scriptis Hieronymi Mercurialis Foroliviensis commentatio. *In his:* Noctes Guelphicæ. 8°. *Rostochii et Wismariæ,* 1755, 15–59.
> *For Portrait, see* **Collection**—van Kaathoven.—**Collection** of Portr. of Phys. & Men of Sc., 220.

Mercurialis *perennis.*

> **Cases** of poison. Boston M. & S. J., 1830–31, iii, 358.— **Schulz** (H.) Zur Wirkung der Mercurialis perennis L. Arch. f. exper. Path. u. Pharmakol., Leipz., 1886, xxi, 88–96.

Mercuric *ethyl.*

> **Hepp** (P.) Ueber Quecksilberäthyl. Centralbl. f. klin. Med., Leipz., 1885, vi, 665. ———. Ueber Quecksilberäthylverbindungen und über das Verhältniss der Quecksilberäthyl- zur Quecksilbervergiftung. Arch. f. exper. Path. u. Pharmakol., Leipz., 1887, xxiii, 91–128.

Mercuric *methide.*

> **Edwards** (G. N.) Two cases of poisoning by mercuric methide. St. Barth. Hosp. Rep., Lond., 1865, i, 141: 1866, ii, 211.

Mercurin (Paul). * Relation médicale d'un hivernage à l'île Maurice (1866-7). 54 pp., 1 l. 4°. *Montpellier, Boehm & fils,* 1868, No. 51. c.

Mercurio (Geronimo Scipio) [1550-95?]. La commare o riccoglitrice. 19 p. l., 356 pp. 4°. *Venetia, G. B. Ciotti,* 1601.

Mercurio (Geronimo Scipio)—continued.

———. The same. 17 p. l., 363 pp. 8°. *Venetia, G. B. Ciotti,* 1601.

Books 2 and 3 have separate title-pages and are dated 1620. The dedication of this edition is dated at "Milano, xxx ottobre 1604".

———. The same. 17 p. l., 363 pp. 4°. *Venetiis, G. B. Ciotti,* 1621.

———. The same. In questa ultima édittione corretta ed accresciuta di due trattati; uno del colostro, dove si tratta di diversi mali de i bambini con loro cause e rimedj singolari del . . . Ezechiele di Castro. L' altro di un gravissimo auttore, nel quale si risolvono alcuni dubj importanti circa il battesimo de i bambini, e si danno alcuni avisi spirituali molto à proposito per le parturienti. 10 p. l., 327 pp. 4°. *Verona, F. de' Rossi,* 1645.

———. The same. 10 p. l., 350 pp. 4°. *Venetia, G. F. Valuasense,* 1686.

———. The same. Kindermutter. Oder Hebamen Buch, worinnen von dem wunderbaren Werck der Empfängnüss, und Geburth eines Menschen; und was deroselben anhänget; wie sich ein Weib vor der Geburth; in der Geburth; und nach der Geburth zu halten; von dem ampt der Kindermutter, so wohl bey einer Rechten, und Natürlichen; als bey denen Bösen, Unrechten, und schweren Geburthen; von denen Zufällen und Kranckheiten der Sechswöchnerin, so meistentheils auf eine schwere Geburth zu folgen pflegen; ingleichen von den Kinder-Kranckheiten; und wie denenselben, und mit was vor Hauss- und Weiber-Mitteln, bey Entstehung eines Medici, soll, und kan gerathen werden, gehandelt wird. Darbey auch allerhand curiose, und anmuthige Sachen zu finden seynd. Welches auss dem Italiänischen in die Hochteutsche Sprache versetzet, an vielen Orthen vermehret und mit denen Alten, auch etzlichen neuen Kupffern verbessert hat Gottfriedt Welsch. 14 p. l., 844 pp., 23 pl. 4°. *Leipzig, T. Ritzschen,* 1652.

———. The same. 14 p. l., 844 pp., 23 pl. 4°. *Leipzig, T. Ritzschen,* 1653.

The title-page and 1. and 2. leaves of preface are a different imprint from the edition of 1652 by the same publisher.

———. The same. 16 p. l., 844 pp., 22 pl. 4°. *Wittenberg, T. Mevii sel. Erben u. E. Schumacher,* 1671.

———. De gl' errori popolari d' Italia. Libri sette, divisi in due parti. Nella prima si trattano gl' errori, che occorrono in qualunque modo nel governo de gl' infermi, e s' insegna il modo di corregerli. Nella seconda si cõtengono gl' errori quali si commettono nelle cause delle malattie cioè nel modo del vivere, come nell' uso dell' aere, dell' esercitio, e ozio; mangiare, e bere, evacuatione, dormire, e veghiare e passioni dell' animo, con gli suoi rimedj, dove, come in uno horologio della sanità si mostra 'l modo di allungar la vita e viver sano senza medico, e senza medicine. Parte prima. 6 p. l., 592 pp. 4°. *Verona, F. Rossi,* 1645.

Mercurio delle scienze mediche. [Monthly; 2 v. annually.] v. 1–10, Dec., 1823, to Dec., 1828. 8°. *Livorno.*

Continued as: **Nuovo** mercurio delle scienze mediche.

Mercury.

See, also, **Bile**; *and under diseases, as:* **Hipjoint** (*Diseases of, Treatment of*); **Hydrocephalus** (*Acute, Treatment of*); **Intestines** (*Obstruction of, Treatment of*) *by metallic mercury, etc.*; **Syphilis** (*Treatment of*).

ABELE (C. A.) *Diss. sistens experimenta circa præsentiam hydrargyri in sanguine animalium infrictionibus mercurialibus necatorum, et circa quantitatem ferri in sanguine. 4°. *Tubingæ,* [1824].

Mercury.

AMELUNG (C. C. G.) *De mercurio solubili Hahnemanni. 4°. *Jenæ,* [1792].

ARNOTT (J.) An enquiry into the mode in which mercurial ptyalism operates in the cure of acute disease; and whether there exist other remedies of similar action that may be advantageously substituted for it. 8°. *London,* 1824.

AZUM (A.) *Comparer les effets du mercure sur l'homme sain à ceux que produit la syphilis. 4°. *Paris,* 1844.

BAIER (J. G.) *De mercurii in corpus humanum agendi modo secundum leges physicas. sm. 4°. *Altorfi Noric.,* 1739.

BALDINGER (E. G.) [Pr.] historia mercurii et mercurialium medica. Pars i–iv. 4°. *Gottingæ,* 1781.

BAÑARES (G.) Apologia del mercurio; demostracion de la verdadera naturaleza y propiedades de los compuestos que se originan de él, con el método de usarlos con toda seguridad y eficacia, y refutacion de las ideas falsas é infundadas que Laffecteur, Mittié y otros muchos autores han procurio difundir acerca de los efectos del mercurio, ó por no haber conocido su naturaleza y virtudes, ó de intento para ensalzar el rob antisifilítico del primero, y otros secretos empíricos de los extrangeros. 16°. *Madrid,* 1816.

BARULLI (V. N.) Teorie fisico-chimiche ed analisi dimostrative, circa l' unguento mercuriale. 8°. *Napoli,* 1839.

BAUDRIMONT (E.) *Des préparations mercurielles; du mercure et des composés mercuriaux usités en médecine. 4°. *Paris,* 1864.

BAUMANN (C. F. T.) *Diss. inaug. pharm.-med. de hydrargyri natura, viribus et usu medico præsertim interno. 12°. *Marburgi,* [1828].

BAYER (J. A.) *De viribus medicamentosis hydrargyri et inde arte factorum pharmacorum. 4°. *Lipsiæ,* [1783].

BELLOSTE (A.) Esperienze mediche ed osservazioni sopra il mercurio. Tradotto dal francese. 16°. *Venezia,* 1734.

———. The same. Traité du mercure. 12°. [*Paris*], 1738.

———. The same. A treatise on mercury, exhibiting its wonderful powers when taken in a crude state. Translated from the Italian, by an English medical gentleman. With observations in a preface, by R. Carlile. 8°. *London,* [1824?]

———. Traité du mercure. 32°. [*Paris*], 1785.

Although this work is attributed to Belloste on the title-page, it is merely a collection of notices of "Belloste's pills", a specific for syphilis, sold by his widow.

BELLOSTE [M.-A.] Dissertation sur ses pilules mercurielles. 12°. *Paris,* [*n. d.*]

BIELJAEFF (A.) *O vsasivanii rtutnich preparatov jivotnim organizmom. [Absorption of mercurial preparations.] 8°. *St. Petersburg,* 1862.

BLOMBERG (A. G.) *Några ord om qvicksilfrets absorption af organismen. 8°. *Helsingfors,* 1867.

BODENSTEIN (J. C.) *De viribus medicamentosis hydrargyri et inde arte factorum pharmacorum. 4°. *Lipsiæ,* [1773].

BOERHAAVE (H.) De mercurio experimenta, in transactione regiæ soc. Londinensis anni 1733. N. 430 contenta. 4°. *Francofurti et Lipsiæ,* 1736.

BOERNER (C. G.) *De medicamentorum mercurialium varia indole. sm. 4°. *Halæ Sax.,* [1791].

BOLSHESOLSKI (P. K.) *K voprosu o sravnitelnom deistvii dvuiodistoi i dvuchloristoi rtuti kak antisepticheskich sredstve. [Comparative effect of biniodide and bichloride of mercury as antiseptic remedies.] 8°. *St. Petersburg,* 1887.

Mercury.

BOSCHETTUS (B.) Dissertatio de salivatione mercuriali physico-medico-mechanica, in tria capita divisa. Quorum prius continet salivæ naturalis examen, alterum caput ejusdem vitia considerat, tertium salivationem artificialem exhibet. Iis accedunt hystoriæ fœlici, et lethali experimento comprobatæ. sm. 4°. *Venetiis*, 1722.

——. The same. 4°. *Parisiis*, 1732.

Also, in: SYDENHAM (T.) Opera med. fol. *Venetiis,* 1735, 533–574.

BOWLING (W. K.) Mercury and cinchona shown to be therapeutically allied. 8°. *Nashville*, 1868.

BREST (V.) An analytical inquiry into the specific property of mercury relating to the cure of venereal diseases. 8°. *London*, 1724.

——. The same. Dissertation sur l'usage du mercure dans les maladies vénériennes, et autres; et sur la manière de s'en servir avec succès sans salivation. On y a joint une courte relation de l'état de la médecine en Russie, et de quelques cures fort remarquables qu'on y a faites, en suivant la méthode proposée. 8°. *Londres*, 1733.

BURKLIN (P. J.) *De phosphori mercurialis historia, phænomenis, parandi modis, et novis explicationibus. sm. 4°. *Vitembergæ*, 1715.

CABASSUT (M.) *Du mercure et de ses composés au point de vue chimique, pharmacologique et toxicologique. 4°. *Montpellier*, 1885.

CAFFÉ (P.-P.-A.) *Considérations sur les avantages de la méthode des bains mercuriels dans le traitement de la siphilis et de la plupart des affections cutanées. 4°. *Paris*, 1815.

CARNUS (A.) *III. Des préparations pharmacentiques qui ont pour base le mercure. IV. [etc.] 4°. *Paris*, 1839.

CASPAR (J.) *De panacea mercuriali. sm. 4°. *Tubingæ*, 1700.

CHAPUIS (F. X.) *Dissertatio medica sistens hydrargyri usum in quibusdam morbis haud syphiliticis. 4°. *Argentorati*, 1811.

COENEN (J. A. L.) *Over de antifermentatieve werking van calomel in het darmkanaal en het inwendig gebruik van cinnaber als geneesmiddel. 8°. *Amsterdam*, 1887.

COMBES (A.) *IV. Comment peut-on constater la présence de préparations mercurielles longtemps après l'inhumation d'un cadavre? 4°. *Paris*, 1842.

CURRY (J.) Examination of the prejudices commonly entertained against mercury as beneficially applicable to most hepatic complaints, and to various other forms of disease, as well as to syphilis. 8°. *London*, 1809.

——. The same. 2. ed. 8°. *London*, 1810.

DAVIES (D.) An essay on mercury, wherein are presented formulæ for some preparations of this metal, including practical remarks on the safest and most effectual methods of administering them for the cure of liver complaints, dropsies, syphilis, and other formidable diseases incident to the human frame; being the result of long experience and diligent observation. 8°. *London*, 1820.

DESEVEDANG (P.) *IV. Comment reconnaître le bichlorure de mercure dans du vin, dans du café, ou dans la matière des vomissements? 4°. *Paris*, 1840.

DOBROWOLSKI (C.-B.) *IV. Comment peut-on constater la présence d'une préparation mercurielle longtemps après l'inhumation d'un cadavre? 4°. *Paris*, 1842.

DOSE (A. P. J.) Zur Kenntniss der Gesundheitsverhältnisse des Marschlandes. III. Hydrargyrose und Quecksilberwirkung in ihrer Ab-

Mercury.

hängigkeit vòm Chlorgehalt der Luft. 4°. *Leipzig*, 1887.

DOUGLASS (J.) *An experimental essay on mercury. 8°. *Philadelphia*, 1805.

DOWLING (E.) *De hydrargyro. 8°. *Edinburgi*, 1809.

DUCASTEL (W.) *IV. Comment peut-on constater la présence d'une préparation mercurielle longtemps après l'inhumation d'un cadavre? 4°. *Paris*, 1839.

DU FRESNE (C. F.) *Diss. quædam de hydrargyro complectens. 8°. *Edinburgi*, 1814.

ECKMANN (G. G.) *De usu et abusu medicamentorum mercurialium. 4°. *Erfordiæ*, [1705].

EHRMANN (J. F.) *De hydrargyri præparatorum internorum in sanguinem effectibus. sm. 4°. *Argentorati*, 1761.

Also, in: SANDIFORT. Thesaurus diss. [etc.] 4°. *Roterodami,* 1768, i, 539–567. *Also, in:* WITTWER (P. L.) Delect. dis. med. Argent. 8°. *Norimb.,* 1777, i, 175–239.

EISENSTEIN (L. S.) *De hydrargyri actione in corpori animali. 8°. *Halæ*, [1815].

ESCHENBACH (C. G.) [Pr.] de quibusdam auri calcibus et salibus mercurialibus observationes. sm. 4°. *Lipsiæ*, [1785].

FALK (N. D.) A treatise on the medical qualities of mercury, in three parts. I. On the natural properties of mercury, and its operation in the animal œconomy. II. On the principal preparations of mercury. III. On the medical qualities of mercury in various diseases. 12°. *London*, 1776.

FEINLER (G.) *De mercurii in corpore humano agendi modo. sm. 4°. *Erfordiæ*, 1738.

FENWICK (M.) *On mercury. 8°. *Baltimore*, [1813].

FOURTON (F.) *An salutaris sit in medicina facienda, mercurii usus? 12°. *Avenione*, 1713.

FRAEYS (L.) Des préparations mercurielles usitées en médecine. roy. 8°. *Bruxelles*, 1843.

Repr. from: Ann. d. univ. de Belg., Brux., 1841–2, i.

FRANCIS (J. W.) *An inaugural dissertation on mercury, embracing its medical history, curative action, and abuse in certain diseases. 8°. *New York*, 1811.

DE FREITAS SOARES (J. P.) Memorias ácerca do estado, em que se acha o mercurio nos unguentos e outras preparações mercuriaes, feitas por meio da trituração ao a'r livre. 8°. *Lisboa*, 1814.

FRIIS (L. C.) Singulares quasdam observationes circa mercurii usum internum exponit. 4°. *Hafniæ*, [1750].

GNUSCHCKE (J. E.) *De hydrargiri in sanguinem receptione. 8°. *Berolini*, [1827].

GOY (J.) *De virtute mercurii inflammationes resolvente, nec non de modo quo his in morbis agit. 8°. *Moguntiæ*, [1794].

GRIFBERG (I. O.) *De spiritu vini mercuriali. *Upsaliæ*, 1760.

In: SANDIFORT. Thesaurus diss. [etc.] 4°. *Roterodami,* 1769, ii, 307–324. *Also, in:* WEIZ (F. A.) Neue Ausz. [etc.] 12°. *Frankf. u. Leipz.,* 1775, iii, 39–41.

GULDE (C. C.) *De suspectis quibusdam pharmacis salino-mercurialibus. 4°. *Francof. ad Viadr.*, [1759].

HAASE (G. A.) [Pr.] de usu hydrargyri in morbis non syphiliticis. Prol. i–xxxviii. 4°. *Lipsiæ*, 1826–37.

HAICKE (E. F.) *De hydrargyro. 8°. *Halis Sax.*, 1822.

HALLOPEAU (H.) Du mercure; action physiologique et thérapeutique. 8°. *Paris*, 1878.

——. The same. Accion fisiológica y terapéutica del mercurio. Traducido del francés por M. de Riba y Bassols. 8°. *Barcelona*, 1879.

Mercury.

HAMILTON (J.), jr. Observations on the use and abuse of mercurial medicines in various diseases. 8°. *Edinburgh*, 1819.

——. The same. With notes and an appendix by Ansel W. Ives. 8°. *New York*, 1821.

HASSENSTEIN (O.) *Versuche über Quecksilberausscheidung durch die Galle. 8°. *Königsberg i. Pr.*, [1879].

HEGEWISCH (F. H.) De usu hydrargyri in morbis inflammatoriis. 4°. *Kiliæ*, 1810.

HEINRICI (H.) Tela ex pharetra Apollinis a Mercurio in sui securitatem subducta, sive testimonia et argumenta medica pro mercurio militantia, cum contrapugnantibus ex adversariorum præcipue commentariis collecta, inter se collata, [etc.] 4°. *Halæ Magdeb.*, 1713.

HERMANN (J.) Die Nachtheile der Merkurialkur. 8°. *Wien*, 1859.

——. Ueber die Wirkung des Quecksilbers auf den menschlichen Organismus. fol. *Teschen*, 1873.

HEROLD (N. B.) * De usu mercurii phosphorati Schaefferi. 4°. *Jenæ*, [1793].

HERRENSCHWANDT (J. F.) * Diss. sistens historiam mercurii medicam. 4°. *Lugd. Bat.*, [1737].

HOWARD (J.) A treatise on the medical properties of mercury. 8°. *London*, 1782.

DE HOYA (A.) * De variis mercurium sublimatum corrosivum mitigandi et mercurium dulcem parandi modis hujusque genuini notis. 4°. *Gottingæ*, [1791].

HUBER (E.) Mercury and its preparations. A pharmacological and therapeutic study, according to the principles of homœopathy. 8°. [*New York*, 1884.]
Imperfect.

HULLEMAN (J.) * De multiplici usu medicamentorum mercurialium in variis morbis. 4°. *Leidæ*, 1813.

HUNDERTMARK (C. F.) * De mercurii vivi et cum salibus rarie mixti summa in corpus humanum vi atque efficacitate ejusque cum sulphure laxius vel arctius conjuncti virtute in idem nulla. Respondente Friderico Conrado Bergmann. 4°. *Lipsiæ*, [1754].

——. The same. Liber singularis in quo simul varia chemiæ capita illustrantur. 4°. *Lipsiæ*, 1754.

JABLONOWSKI (G.) * Ueber die Einwirkung des Quecksilbers auf den thierischen Organismus. 8°. *Berlin*, [1885].

KARNITSKI (F.) *O vlijanii vlutnoi mazi i sublimata na kolichestvo glikogena ve pecheni. [Effect of mercury on glycogenic function of liver.] 8°. *St. Petersburg*, 1870.

KLATTEN (E. A. A.) * De Louvrierii hydrargyrum adhibendi methodo. 8°. *Berolini*, [1821].

KLITZPERA (F. V.) * De illinitionibus mercurialibus. 8°. [*Pragæ*, 1816.]

KNOPS (F. G.) * De therapia mercuriali in iis, qui vocantur dyscrasiæ chronicæ morbis, imprimis in syphilide. 8°. *Berolini*, [1863].

KORNMESSER (G.) *De hydrargyro. 8°. *Berolini*, [1837].

KOSMANN (C.) * Des préparations mercurielles. Mercure et composés mercuriaux usités en médecine. 4°. *Strasbourg*, 1864.

KRAUSE (R. F. G.) * Diss. analecta quædam de hydrargiro continens. 8°. *Vratislaviæ*, [1821].

KÜNSTEL (J. W.) De salibus metallorum, præsertim auri et mercurii. 2. ed. 4°. *Lipsiæ*, 1711.

——. The same. 3. ed. 4°. *Lipsiæ*, 1760.

KUFNER (J.) *Tentamen sistens rationem qua morbi inter se tam diversi mercurio sanentur. 8°. *Monachii*, 1832.

Mercury.

LANCILOTTI (C.) Il trionfo del mercurio, nel qual si tratta del suo origine, natura e temperamento, dimostrando diverse curiosissime, e utilissime operationi. Con un trattato di diverse acque cosmetiche e medicinali, et altre curiosità estratte da diversi autori. 16°. *Modona*, 1677.

LANGENBECKER (H. G.) *Quædam de mercurii in corpus humanum efficacia. 8°. *Berolini*, [1827].

LAZAREVIĆ (L. K.) * Experimentelle Beiträge zur Wirkung des Quecksilbers. Nebst einem Anhange über den Nachweis des Quecksilbers mittelst Electrolyse. 8°. *Berlin*, [1879].

LEMAIRE (L.) Des effets du mercure et de ses préparations dans les diverses maladies, la syphilis exceptée . . . 1er prix Corvisart. 8°. *Blois*, 1843.

LÖSCH (A.) * Ueber die Einwirkung des Ammoniaks auf Quecksilberoxydulsalze, mit besonderer Berücksichtigung des Hahnemannschen Salzes. 8°. *Dorpat*, 1862.

LOT (C. E.) *Martis cum mercurio conjunctionem usibus practicis commendat. 4°. *Halæ Magdeb.*, [1759].

MACLEAN (C.) A treatise on the action of mercury upon living bodies; and its application for the cure of diseases of indirect debility. 8°. *Philadelphia*, 1797.

MAYWOOD (R.) An essay on the operation of mercury in the human body, in which the manner how salivation is produced by that medicine is attempted to be explained; interspersed with observations on the treatment of the venereal disease. 8°. *London*, 1787.

MITSCHERLICH (C. G.) *Hydrargyri præparata usitatissimi analytice accuratius perscrutata. 8°. *Berolini*, 1829.

MÜLLER (J. C. G.) *De viribus ac usu mercurialium. sm. 4°. *Jenæ*, [1775].

NEGA (J.) * Ein Beitrag zur Frage der Elimination des Mercurs, mit besonderer Berücksichtigung des Glycocollquecksilbers. 8°. *Strassburg*, 1882.

——. Vergleichende Untersuchungen über die Resorption und Wirkung verschiedener zur cutanen Behandlung verwandter Quecksilberpräparate. 8°. *Strassburg*, 1884.

NIETER (A. J. C.) * De vi et effectu hydrargyri in quibusdam morbis non syphiliticis. 8°. *Berolini*, [1818].

NOTTER (J. F.) * De actione mercurii in corpus humanum. sm. 4°. *Argentorati*, [1749].

ŒRIUS (C.) De hydrargyri natura, viribus et usu. 4°. *Basileæ*, [1706].
Also, in: FASCIC. diss. med. select. [etc.] 12°. *Basileæ*, 1710, 222–308.

OSWALD (J. A.) * Quædam de hydrargyro. 8°. *Edinburgi*, 1813.

OTTO (C.) *De actione hydrargyri medica. 2 pts. in 1 v. 8°. *Hafniæ*, 1819.

OWEN (P) *De mercurio. 8°. *Edinburgi*, 1757.
Also, in: SMELLIUS. Thesaurus med. [etc.] 8°. *Edinb. et Lond.*, 1785, ii, 427–451.

PANTELIUS (M.) & VASMARUS (D. P.) Disputatio medico-chymica de mercurio, et ejus in usu medico operandi ratione. sm. 4°. *Regiomonti*, [1698].

PENATUS (B. G.) Quæstiones tres de corporali mercurio.
In: THEATRUM chemicum. 8°. *Argentorati*, 1659, ii, 129–150.

PRÜMERS (H.) * Ueber das Quecksilberäthylchlorid (Aethylsublimat) in physiologischer, chemischer und therapeutischer Beziehung. 8°. *Berlin*, [1870].

Mercury.

Purmann (M. G.) Ausführlicher Unterricht, und Anweisung wie die Salivation-Cur nach allen Umbständen und Vortheilen auffs beste und sicherste vorzunehmen: damit der gebührende Nutzen und gewündschte Hülffe darauf folgen möge. 8°. *Franckfurt u. Leipzig*, 1700.

Quelmalz (S. T.) [Pr.] quod hydrargyri vires a sulphure in c. h. suspensas expendit. 4°. *Lipsiæ*, 1748.
Also, in: Haller. Disp. ad morb. [etc.] 4°. *Lausannæ*, 1757, i, 493–501.

Rambach (J. J.) *Usus mercurii in morbis inflammatoriis. 8°. *Halæ*, [1794].

Rauch (J. G.) *De mercurii usu et abusu. 4°. *Marburgi Cattorum*, [1727].

Robin (É.) *Recherches sur l'influence du traitement mecuriel sur la richesse globulaire du sang. 4°. *Paris*, 1880.

Rolfincius (G.) Non ens chimicum, mercurius metallorum et mineralium. 4°. *Jenæ*, 1570.

Sachs (L. W.) Das Quecksilber. Ein pharmakologisch-therapeutischer Versuch. 8°. *Königsberg*, 1834.

Sartorius (C. F.) *De usu hydrargyri interno. 4°. *Lipsiæ*, 1735.

Schaeffer (J. A. M.) *De mercurialibus quibusdam pharmacis eorumque præcipuis virtutibus. 4°. *Lipsiæ*, 1790.

Schmid (J.) De mercurio in morbis inflammatoriis. 8°. *Monachii*, 1833.

Schmidt (O.) *Ein Beitrag zur Frage der Elimination des Quecksilbers aus dem Körper, mit besonderer Berücksichtigung des Speichels. 8°. *Dorpat*, 1879.

Schulz (J. H.) *Præcipuorum ex hydrargyro remediorum examen chemicum. 8°. *Francof. ad Viadr.*, [1805].

Seeck (J. J.) *Meletema de hydrargyri effectu. 8°. [*Dorpat*], 1859.

Sigmond (G. E.) Mercury, blue pill, and calomel; their use and abuse. 12°. *London*, 1840.

Simon (A.-L.) *Comparer les effects du mercure sur l'homme sain avec ceux que produit la syphilis. 4°. *Paris*, 1847.

Smit (H.) De mercurii usu in quibusdam morbis non venereis. 4°. *Lugd. Bat.*, 1777.

Sommer (C. J.) Cautiones nonnullæ ad liquoris mercurialis Plenkiani usum spectantes. sm. 4°. *Francof. a. M.*, [1769].

Sprengel (C.) [Pr.] hydrargyri antiquitates. 4°. *Halæ*, [1823].

Stang (D. F.) *De usu et abusu mercurii et medicamentorum mercurialium. 4°. *Jenæ*, [1754].

Steuer (G.) *De mercurii in morbis inflammatoriis agendi modo. 8°. *Berolini*, [1819].

Stickel (C.) De evaporatione hydrargyri hujusque ad aquam salsam et corpora organica ratione commentatio chemica, præmio primario ornata. 4°. *Jenæ*, 1837.
Text Latin and German.

Stott (R.) The modern Hermes, or experiments and observations on different methods of combining quicksilver with acids; in supplement of ancient chemistry on mercury. 8°. *Dumfries*, 1811.

Stromeyer (F.) De connubio hydrargyri cum acido acetico. 4°. [*n. p.*, 1809.]

Swainson (I.) Mercury stark naked. A series of letters addressed to Dr. Beddoes, stripping that poisonous mineral of its medical pretentions, and showing that it perpetuates, increases and multiplies all the diseases for which it is administered; and while it may sustain worthless branches of medical practice, the use of it is an opprobrium to the scientific and moral character of the profession. 8°. *London*, 1797.

Mercury.

Swan (J.) An inquiry into the action of mercury on the living body. 8°. *London*, 1822.
———. The same. 8°. *London*, 1847.

Swoboda (A. B.) *De mercurii virtute medicata. 8°. *Pragæ*, 1835.

Tables in the report of the Edinburgh committee on the action of mercury as a cholagogue. fol. [*Edinburgh*, 1868.]
See, also, infra, Bennett (J. H.)

Tissier (M.) Mémoire pour établir la surphosphoresence des corps, par des observations et des expériences sur l'onguent napolitain double, ou mercuriel; sur l'électricité, le galvanisme, etc. 8°. *Lyon*, 1807.

Tóth (J.) *De mercurio juxta recentissima sed moderata principia medica. 8°. *Viennæ*, [1821].

Turnbull (W.) A letter to Mr. Clare, surgeon, on his new and easy method of introducing mercury into the system through the orifices of the absorbent vessels on the inside of the mouth, and recommending it to the consideration of the world in general, and the navy in particular. Also remarks on the same subject by Wm. Turnbull, M. D. 8°. *London*, 1783.
Bound with: Clare (P.) A new and easy method of curing the lues venerea. 8°. *London*, 1780.

Untzerus (M.) Anatomia mercurii spagirica, seu de hydrargyri natura, proprietate, viribus atque usu, libri duo vario doctrinarum genere referti. 4°. *Halæ Sax.*, 1620.

van den Velde (J.) *Specimen medicum solenne de mercuris et medicamentis mercurialibus selectis, ad expugnandos, sine salivatione, morbos corporis humani rebelles. sm. 4°. *Halæ Magdeb.*, [1700].

Wabst (C. X.) De hydrargyro tentamen physico-chemico-medicum. 4°. *Vindobonæ*, 1754.

Walburgerus (D. G.) De mercurio metallorum et mineralium. 4°. *Jenæ*, [1670].

Warren (J.) A view of the mercurial practice in febrile diseases. 8°. *Boston*, 1813.

Wilson (A. P.) Observations on the use and abuse of mercury and on the precautions necessary in its employment. 8°. *Winchester* 1805.

V rcke (V. I. T.) *De Weinholdii hydrargyr n adhibendi methodo. 8°. *Berolini*, [1821].

Wright (W.) Observations on the effects of mercury on the organs of hearing, and the improper use of it in cases of nervous deafness. 8°. *London*, 1822.

Wychgel (D. R.) *De quibusdam hydrargyri præparatis. 8°. *Groningæ*, [1810].

Zwiklitz (P.) *De usu et præparatis mercurii apud veteres, prima historiæ parte libelli a splendidissimo medicorum ordine universitatis Berolinensi præmio ornati. 8°. *Berolini*, 1831.

Allison (J.) On the medicinal properties of mercury and the chlorate of potash. Med. Times, Lond., 1849, xix, 96.—**Armaingaud.** Le mercure engraisse-t-il? Mém. et bull. Soc. de méd. et chir. de Bordeaux, 1874, 480–486. *Also:* Bordeaux méd., 1874, iii, 353. —**Autenrieth & Zeller.** Ueber das Daseyn von Quecksilber, das äusserlich angewendet worden, in der Blutmasse der Thiere. Arch. f. d. Physiol., Halle, 1807–8, viii, 213–263.—**Balzer** (F.) Des accidents locaux déterminés par les injections de calomel et d'oxyde jaune suivant la méthode de Scarenzio. Bull. et mém. Soc. méd. d. hôp. de Par., 1887, 3. s., iv, 213–220. *Also:* Gaz. hebd. de méd., Par., 1887, 2. s., xxiv, 276–278.—**Barbette** (A.) Réflexions sur le mercure, suivies de plusieurs observations de maladies aiguës guéries par ce médicament. Rec. d. trav. Soc. de méd. de Niort, 1837, 7–31.—**Barrallier** (A.) Mercure. N. dict. de méd. et chir. prat., Par., 1876, xxii, 359–407.—**Barry** (E.) On the operation of mercury, in different diseases and constitutions. Med. Tr. Roy. Coll. Phys. Lond.. [3. ed.], 1785, i, 125–164.— **Beck** (J. B.) An account of the origin of the use of mercury in inflammatory diseases. N. York M. Gaz., 1841–2, i, 1–5.—**Beigel** (H.) Notiz zur Lehre vom Quicksilber. Wien. med. Wchnschr., 1856, vi, 232.—**Bell** (A. N.) On the influence of blisters in quickening the effects of mercury upon the system. N. York

Mercury.

J. M., 1858, 3. s., v, 149.—**Bellamy** (W. J. H.) Mode of administering quinine and mercury. North Car. M. J., Wilmington, 1886, xvii, 141-146.—**Bellini** (R.) Dei sali doppi di mercurio. Sperimentale, Firenze, 1871, xxvii, 561-568.—**Bemerkungen** über die Anwendung des Quecksilbers bey Brustentzündungen. J. d. pract. Arznk. u. Wundarznk., Jena, 1800, 2. St., x, 77-119.—**Bennett** (J. H.) Report of the Edinburg committee on the action of mercury on the liver. Brit. M. J., Lond., 1868, ii, 78: 1869, i, 411; 503. [See, also, supra, Tables, etc.] ——. Report of further experiments demonstrating that mercury has no special action on the liver. Ibid., 1871, i, 1.—**Bertini** (J. M. X.) De usu mercurii in medicina tam interno, quam externo dissertatio. In: Astruc (J.) De morbis venereis, 4°, Venetiis, 1760, 455-471.—**Best** (G. P.) The systemic factor in the local use of mercurials. Lancet, Lond., 1879, ii, 463—**Biegański** (W.) Moczopędne działanie przetworów rtęci. [Diuretic action of preparations of mercury.] Gaz. lek., Warszawa, 1887, 2. s., vii, 370; 395; 421; 430.—**Bonfanti** (G.) Osservazioni sull' uso del mercurio. Effem. d. sc. med., Milano, 1840, xv, 5-37.—**Bouilhon** (E.) Formule d'une solution contenant un sel de mercure soluble et sans action sur l s tissus pour emploi hypodermique. Bull. gén. de thérap., etc., Par., 1869, lxxvi, 315.—**Brasse** (L.) Dosage du mercure dans les urines. Compt. rend. Soc. de biol. Par., 1887, 8. s., iv, 297-299.—**Brown** (J. L.) On the action of mercury upon the liver. Tr. M. Soc. N. Y., Albany, 1864, 267-279.—**Brown** (S.) Remarks on Mr. Lee's experiments and observations upon quicksilver. Med. Reposit., N. Y., 1803, vi, 265-271.—**Brückmann.** Ueber die Wiederherstellung des Quecksilbers im menschlichen Körper. N. Arch. f. med. Erfahr., Berl., 1810, xiii, 252-255.—**Brunton** (T. D.) Action of mercury on the liver. Brit. M. J., Lond., 1873, i, 15. Also, Reprint.—**Bürger.** Erfahrungen über die Wirkung von Quecksilbereinreibungen bei sehr weit gediehenen Entzündungen edler Eingeweide. J. d. pract. Heilk., Berl., 1838, lxxxvii, 6. St., 77-85.—**Byasson** (H) Recherches sur l'élimination des sels mercuriels ingérés par l'homme. Au bout de combien de temps un sel mercuriel soluble, introduit chez l'homme, dans l'appareil digestif, apparaît-il dans l'urine, la salive, la sueur? J. de l'anat. et physiol., etc., Par., 1872, viii, 500-505. ——. Note sur quelques instructions pratiques pour la recherche qualitative du mercure dans les liquides de l'économie. Ibid., 397-400.—**Camden** (T. B.) Mercury as an antiphlogistic and cholagogue. Med. & Surg. Reporter, Phila., 1870, xxiii, 313-320.—**Carpenter** (G. W.) On the division or extinction of mercury by trituration; with observations and experiments on the blue mass and other preparations of mercury. Phila. J. M. & Phys. Sc., 1826, xiii, 108-114.—**Chambers** (R.) On the use of mercury in inflammation. Lancet, Lond., 1850, i, 82.—**Chaves** (B.) Salicylate of hydrargirium and its employment in therapeutics. Med. & Surg. Reporter, Phila., 1887. lvi, 519.—**Cholagogue** (On the) action of mercury. Med. Times & Gaz., Lond., 1869, ii, 418.—**Clark** (D.) Mercury as a supersedent. Cincin. Lancet & Obs., 1875, xviii, 140-142.—**Clay** (C.) On the exhibition of small doses of mercury in effecting ptyalism. Lancet, Lond., 1840-41, ii, 751-753.—**Clevenger** (S. V.) Microscopic examination of tissues after the administration of mercury. Am. Month. Micr. J., N. Y., 1880, i, 110; 131. ——. Action of mercury. Inaugural thesis. Chicago M. Gaz., 1880, i, 81-88. Also, Reprint. ——. Mechanical therapeutics, chemistry, and toxicology of mercury. Chicago M. J. & Exam., 1880, xl, 337-353. ——. Mercury; its chemistry and therapeutics. Gaillard's M. J., N. Y., 1883, xxxv, 283-288.—**Coleman** (J. B.) Report on the effects of mercurial preparations on the living animal tissues. 1853. Tr. M. Soc. N. Jersey 1766-1859, Newark, 1875, 560-567.—**Coles** (W.) Remarks on the use of mercury in inflammation. St. Louis M. & S. J., 1869, n. s., vi, 205-215.—**Colson** (A.) Recherches sur l'action du mercure. Arch. gén. de méd., Par., 1826, xii, 68-103. ——. Mémoire sur les effets du mercure sur l'économie animale. Rev. méd. franç. et étrang., Par., 1828, i, 5; 223. ——. De l'influence du traitement mercuriel sur les fonctions de l'utérus. Arch. gén. de méd., Par., 1828, xviii, 24-48.—**Combes-Brassard** (J.-M.) De l'emploi varié du mercure dans un grand nombre de maladies. Mémoir. d. hôp. du midi, Par., 1830, ii, 6; 445; 513; 585.—**Cooper** (W. W.) The uncertain action of mercury and iodide of potassium. Med. Times & Gaz., Lond., 1855, n. s., x, 455; 485.—**Copeman** (E.) Observations on the use of mercury in general, and in certain diseases of the brain in particular. Brit. & For. M.-Chir. Rev., Lond., 1872, xlix, 471-476.—**Currie** (D. A.) The action of mercury. Tr. M. Soc. N. Jersey, Newark, 1876, 168-177.—**Delarue** (E.) De l'onguent mercuriel et de l'influence du vent du nord dans sa préparation. Monit. scient., Par., 1859-60, ii, 563.—**Delhaye** (V.) Constatant l'efficacité des mercuriaux, calomel et onguent mercuriel double, comme antiphlogistique, et spécialement dans l'inflammation des séreuses. Ann. de méd. belge, Brux., 1838, iii, 1-7. ——. Quinze ans d'expérience sur l'emploi des mercuriaux comme agents spéciaux dans beaucoup d'affections irritatives et surtout dans les métro-péritonites graves des femmes en couches. J. de

Mercury.

méd., chir. et pharmacol., Brux., 1855, xx, 434-441. ——. Encore quelques mots sur l'emploi des mercuriaux comme agents spéciaux contre certaines affections. Ibid., xxi, 33-40.—**Desmarest** (J.-L.) Mémoire sur l'extinction du mercure dans l'onguent mercuriel et les préparations analogues. présenté à la Société de pharmacie, le 15 octobre 1828. J. de pharm., Par., 1829, xv, 31-41. Also, Reprint.—**Dobson** (M.) On the benefit of a resuscitated salivation, in the cure of certain anomalous symptoms. Med. Obs. Soc. Phys. Lond., 1784, vi, 174-179.—**Dominguez** (D. S. Y.) Memoria sobre el mercurio y los compuestos que forma con el oxigeno y el azufre. Bibliot. méd.-castr. españ., Madrid, 1852, vi, 303-330.—**Doughty** (W. H.) The therapeutic effects and uses of mercury, as influenced by the report of the Edinburg committee on the action of mercury, podophyllin, and taraxacum on the biliary secretion. Tr. Georgia M. Ass., Atlanta, 1873, xxiv, 95-117. Also: Atlanta M. & S. J., 1873, xi, 265; 325. — **Dumont** (A.) Recherches sur l'action du mercure. Ann. Soc. de méd. de Gand, 1838, iv, 93-142. [Rap. de Lados], 143-156. [Discussion], Bull. Soc. de méd. de Gand, 1838, iv, 37-50.—**Duprat** (A.) De l'action physiologique du salicylate de mercure. Compt. rend. Soc. de biol., Par., 1886, 8. s., iii, 154.—**Eastman** (H. N.) On the action of mercury. Tr. M. Soc. N. Y., Albany, 1877, 281-289. Also: Buffalo M. & S. J., 1869-70, ix, 201-215.—**Eck** (V.) K' vrachebnomu upotreblenyu rtuti. [Medical employment of mercury.] Med. Vestnik, St. Petersb., 1867, vii, 4; 12; 20.—**Effects** of mercury on the constitution of negroes. Boston M. & S. J., 1835, xi, 256.—**Ehrmann** (J. F.) De hydrargyri præparatorum internorum in sanguinem effectibus. In: Weiz (F. A.) Neue Ausz., [etc.], 12°, Frankf. u. Leipz., 1774, ii, 38-52.—**Enderlin** (C.) Ueber das Verhalten der verschiedenen Quecksilber- und verwandter Metall-Salze zu organischen Substanzen im Allgemeinen und zu dem Gallenfarbstoffe insbesondere. N.-Yorker med. Monatschr., 1852, i, 129-137.—**Evans** (J.) Misuse of mercury. Tr. South Car. M. Ass., Charleston, 1882, xxxii, 123-126.—**Farquharson** (R.) The action of mercury. Brit. M.J., Lond., 1873, i, 136.—**Fawcus** (J.) Memorandum on the use of mercury. Indian Ann. M. Sc., Calcutta, 1865, No. xix, 289.—**Ferrari** (P.) & **Asmondo** (G.) Sull' assorbimento del mercurio metallico per la pelle. Gazz. d. osp., Milano, 1886, vii, 643; 651.—**Figuier.** Note sur la préparation de l'onguent mercuriel. Rec. de mém. de méd. ... mil., Par., 1862, 3. s., viii, 310-314.—**Fleischer** (R.) Ueber die Veränderungen verschiedener Quecksilberverbindungen im thierischen Organismus. Deutsche med. Wchnschr., Berl., 1885, xi, 620.—**de Fonseca Henriques** (F.) Tratado unico do uso, e administraçaõ do azo¯gue nos casos, em que he prohibido. In his: Medicina Lusitana, [etc.], fol., Amst., 1731, 799-832. — **Fonssagrives.** Mercure; thérapeutique. Dict. encycl. d. sc. méd., Par., 1873, 2. s., vii, 48-78.—**Francis** (J. W.) Observations on the effects of mercury in its native state, and on its abuse in certain diseases. Med. & Phys. J., Lond., 1813, xxix, 207-226. ——. Observations on mercury; embracing its medical history and its abuse as an article of the materia medica. Am. M. & Phil. Reg., N. Y., 1814, iii, 424-447. ——. Further observations on mercury. Ibid., 1813-14, iv, 476-519. ——. Observations on the natural and medical history of mercury. Am. M. Recorder, Phila , 1822, v, 395-407.—**Fraser** (T. R.) Sketch of the present state of our knowledge respecting the action of mercury on the liver. Edinb. M. J., 1871, xvi, 904-925. Also, Reprint. Also, transl. [Abstr.]: Bull. et mém. Soc. de thérap. 1873, Par., 1875, v, pt. 2, 87-97.—**Fürbringer** (P.) Experimentelle Untersuchungen über die Resorption und Wirkung des regulinischen Quecksilbers der grauen Salbe. Arch. f. path. Anat., etc., Berl., 1880, lxxxii, 491-515. ——. Experimentelle Untersuchungen über die Wirkung des lebenden Blutes auf metallisches Quecksilber. Jenaische Ztschr. f. Naturw., 1881, n. F., vii, 41.—**Gaillard** (L) Action du mercure sur le sang chez les syphilitiques et les anémiques. Compt. rend. Soc. de biol., Par., 1885, 8. s., ii, 395-399. Also: Arch. gén. de méd., Par., 1885, ii, 527-553.—**Garrison** (C. G.) Therapeutics of mercury. Tr. M. Soc. N. Jersey, Newark, 1876, 210-217.—**Gaspard.** Expériences additionnelles sur le mercure. J. de physiol. expér., Par., 1821, i, 142-148. ——. Mémoire sur le mercure. Ibid., 165-189.—**Gibert.** De l'usage thérapeutique de certaines préparations mercurielles employées comme agent spécifique dans les maladies de la peau et dans les maladies vénériennes. Bull. gén. de thérap., etc., Par., 1847, xxxii, 279-287. Also [Rap. de Pâtissier]: Bull. Acad. de méd., Par., 1846-7. xii, 382-391.—**Glover** (J.) Facts and experiments, in answer to some observations on mercury, made by George Lee. Med. Reposit., N. Y., 1803, vi, 241-247.—**Glover** (J. G.) On mercury. Lancet, Lond., 1867, ii, 68.—**Gobley** (T.) [et al.]. Mercure. Dict. encycl. d. sc. méd., Par., 1873, 2. s., vii, 21-89.—**Gray** (D.) On mercury as a curative agent. Lancet, Lond., 1859, ii, 347; 422.—**Greiner.** Bemerkungen über den Gebrauch der Quecksilbermittel. Allg. med. Ann., Altenb., 1803, 111.—**Guelpa.** Des injections hypodermiques des sels insolubles de mercure. Bull. gén. de thérap., etc., Par., 1887, cxii, 289-307. Also: J. de méd. de Par., 1887, xii, 642-644. —

12

Mercury.

Güntz (J. E.) Chemischer Nachweiss von der Ausscheidung des Quecksilbers durch den Harn Quecksilberkranker nach dem Gebrauche der Aachener Kaiserquelle. Vrtljschr. f. Dermat., Wien, 1877, iv, 297–314. ———. Chemischer Nachweiss über die Ausscheidung des Quecksilbers nach dem Gebrauche der Schwefelwässer. Jahresb. d. Gesellsch. f. Nat.- u. Heilk. in Dresd., 1877, 187–206.—**Guersent** & **Cazenave** (A.) Du mercure et des composés mercuriaux envisagés sous le rapport de la thérapeutique. Dict. de méd., 2. éd., Par., 1839, xix, 575–583.—**Haines** (R.) Official reports on preparations of mercury and antimony. Tr. M. & Phys. Soc. Bombay (1855-6), 1857, n. s., iii, 131–139.—**Hamburger** (E. W.) Bemerkungen zur Darstellung des löslichen Quecksilberalbuminats. Wien. med. Wchnschr., 1876, xxvi, 313–316. Untersuchungen über die Ausscheidung von Quecksilber während des Gebrauches von Mercurialcuren. Prag. med. Wchnschr., 1877, ii, 69; 89.—**Hamilton** (J.) Remarks on some of the mercurial compounds. Maryland M. & S. J., Balt., 1842, ii, 166–175.—**Hamilton** (R.) A letter to Dr. Duncan, giving an account of a successful method of treating inflammatory diseases by mercury and opium. Med. Comment., Lond., 1785, ix, 191–205.—**Harden** (J. M. B.) Of mercury and its compounds. South. M. & S. J., Augusta, 1847, iii, 575–597.—**Hayem.** De l'absorption du mercure et de ses effets physiologiques. Gaz. d. hôp., Par., 1880, liii, 1129; 1137.—**Hazeltine** (R.) Observations, and the result, of experiments relating to the preparations of quicksilver. Med. Reposit., N. Y., 1813, n. s., i, 17–28.—**Headland** (F. W.) On mercury, as a study of blood-medicines. Lancet, Lond., 1858, i, 183; 257; 309.—**Hegewisch.** Ueber die Anwendung des Quecksilbers in entzündlichen Krankheiten. J. d. pract. Heilk., Berl., 1809, xxviii, 3. St., 49–108. — **Hennemann** (W.) Eine neue Mercurialseife. Mag. f. d. ges. Heilk., Berl., 1825, xviii, 318–328.—**Holcombe** (W. H.) Physiological and therapeutical action of mercury. West. Lancet, Cincin., 1851, xii, 205–213.—**Holyoke** (E. A.) A letter to Dr. . . . in answer to his queries respecting the introduction of the mercurial practice in the vicinity of Boston, Mass. Med. Reposit., N. Y., 1798, i, 500–503. — **Hufeland** (C. W.) Innerlicher Gebrauch des rothen Quecksilberpräzipitats b i hartnäckigen venerischen und andern Krankheiten. J. d. pract. Arznk. u. Wundarznk., Berl., 1808, xxvii, 4. St., 149–152.—**Hughes** (R.) A few words on mercury; its use and abuse. Brit. M. J., Lond., 1860, ii, 994.—**Inman** (T.) On the action of mercury upon the liver. Ibid., 812–815.—**Ives** (C. L.) Therapeutic value of mercury and its preparations. Proc. Connect. M. Soc. 1864-7, N. Haven, 1867, 2. s., ii, 204–223. Also, Reprint.—**Jacks** (T. M.) Mercurials. Nashville J. M. & S., 1853, v, 145–149.—**Jackson** (S.) On the safety and advantages of mercurial inhalations. Am. J. M. Sc., Phila., 1827, i, 319–332.—**Jaensch** (G. F.) De efficaci mercurialium usu chirurgico. In: Weiz (F. A.) Neue Ausz. [etc.], 12°, Leipz., 1776, iv, 129–132.—**Johnston** (W. W.) On the objections suggested by pathological considerations to the use of mercury in the gastro-intestinal diseases of summer in children. Nat. M. J., Wash., 1871-2, ii, 337–346.—**Keyes** (E. L.) The effect of small doses of mercury in modifying the number of the red blood corpuscles in syphilis: a study of blood-counting with the hématimètre. Am. J. M. Sc., Phila., 1876, n. s., lxxi, 17–37. Also, Reprint.—**Knapp** (M. L.) After-treatment by mercury in grave injuries in life-jeoparding surgical operations. Med. & Surg. Reporter, Phila., 1874, xxx, 353; 377. — **Kopf** (L.) W sprawie chłonienia chlorku rtęciowego z rozczynu wodnego przez skórę. [Absorption by the skin of solution of chloride of mercury.] Przegl. lek., Kraków, 1886, xxv, 533; 545; 559.—**Krupp** (W.) Ueber die Wirkungsart der Quecksilberpräparate. Allg. med. Ann., Altenb. u. Leipz., 1819, 577–584.—**de Lassone** & **Cornette.** Mémoire sur la dissolubilité des précipités mercuriels dans l'eau, et sur la combinaison du mercure avec l'alkali volatil. Hist. Soc. roy. de méd. 1780-81, Par., 1785, iv, pt. 2, 238–247.—**Law** (R.) Observations on the exhibition of mercury in minute doses. Dublin J. M. Sc., 1838-9, xiv, 393–399.—**Lee** (G.) Experiments and observations on mercury. Med. Reposit., N. Y., 1801, iv, 356–364. [See, also, supra, Glover (J.)]—**Lehmann** (V.) Zum Quecksilbernachweis. Ztschr. f. physiol. Chem., Strassb., 1882-3, vii, 362–365.—**Lendrick** (C.) Observations on the use and abuse of mercury. Dublin J. M. Sc., 1837-8, xii, 197–215.—**Lindley** (W.) The action and use of mercury on the animal economy. Cincin. Lancet & Obs., 1875, xxxvi, 264–268.—**Little** (P. W.) Cases illustrative of the use of mercurial ointment in erysipelas, swelled leg, etc. Phila. J. M. & Phys. Sc., 1821, ii, 153–159.—**Lloyd** (F.) The uses and abuses of mercury. Tr. Iowa M. Soc., Davenport, 1871, 111–119.—**Locke** (F. S.) The diuretic action of mercury. Practitioner, Lond., 1886, xxxvii, 170–172.—**Lothrop** (J. R.) An examination of some of the actions of mercury. Buffalo M. & S. J., 1866-7, vi, 369–385.—**Ludwig** (E.) Eine neue Methode zum Nachweis des Quecksilbers in thierischen Substanzen. Med. Jahrb., Wien, 1877, 143–151. ———. Bemerkung zu dem Aufsatze des Herrn Dr. Schuster: Ueber die Ausscheidung des Quecksilbers während und

Mercury.

nach Quecksilberkuren. Vrtljschr. f. Dermat., Wien, 1882, ix, 63. ———. Bemerkung zu der Erwiderung des Hrn. Dr. Schuster. Ibid., 313.—**Lustgarten** (S.) Ein neues Quecksilberpräparat. Wien. med. Wchnschr., 1884, xxxiv, 11; 301; 339; 370; 405.—**Maclean** (C.) A treatise on the action of mercury upon living bodies; and its application for the cure of diseases of indirect debility. In: Yates (W.) & Maclean (C.) A view of the science of life [etc.], 8°, Whitehall (Phila.), 1797, 155–185. Also: Ibid., 8°, Dover, 1801, 121–147. — **Maslieurat.** Mémoire sur l'action du mercure et celle de ses préparations sur l'économie animale. De leurs usages thérapeutiques dans quelques affections des yeux. J. d. conn. méd.-chir., Par., 1841, 133–146. Also: Ann. de méd. belge, Brux., 1841, ii, 98–110.—**Mayençon** & **Bergeret.** Moyen clinique de reconnaître le mercure dans les excrétions et spécialement dans l'urine, et de l'élimination et de l'action physiologique du mercure. J. de l'anat. et physiol., etc., Par., 1873, ix, 81–98. Also [Abstr.]: Marseille méd., 1873, x, 687. Also, transl. [Abstr.]: Riv. di med., di chir. e di terap., Milano, 1873, i, 280.—**Medrano** (N.) Estudios filosóficos sobre el mercurio y sus preparados; y consideraciones prácticas acerca de su aplicacion al tratamiento de varias enfermedades no sifilíticas. Bol. de med., cirug. y farm., Madrid, 1852, 2. s., ii, 108; 156; 163.—**Mercury** (On) as a curative agent. Lancet, Lond., 1859, ii, 274; 399. **– von Mering** (J.) Ueber die Wirkungen des Quecksilbers auf den thierischen Organismus. Arch. f. exper. Path. u. Pharmakol., Leipz., 1880–81, xiii, 86–112. — **Merrill** (A. P.) Observations on the use of mercury. Am. Pract., Louisville, 1871, iii, 262–267. Also, Reprint. — **Michailovski** (J.) O zagriaz. isparen. rtuti bol. i sluch. v otdelen. svtirajou. rtutny. mazjami. [On the absorption of mercury in diseases, and on special cases treated by inunction of mercurial preparations in syphilis.] Mejdunar Klin., St. Petersb., 1886, v, no. 11.—**Most** (C. G. B.) Etwas über den Gebrauch des Quecksilbers bey Entzündungen, besonders bey der häutigen Bräune. J. d. pract. Arznk. u. Wundarznk., Jena, 1799, viii, 3. St., 97–110. — **Mouchon.** Encore un mot sur l'onguent mercuriel. Gaz. méd. de Lyon, 1856, viii, 359–361. — **Mracek** (F.) Die Aufnahme, Umwandlung und Ausscheidung von Quecksilber bei Quecksilberkuren. Wien. med. Presse, 1881, xxii, 823; 859; 913.—**Müller.** Bemerkungen und Erfahrungen über die Mercurialia, als vielfach nützliche Heilmittel Allg. med. Ann., Altenb., 1811, 621–644. — **Müller** (F.) Ueber die Aufnahme von Quecksilber durch Einathmung. Mitth. a. d. med. Klin. zu Würzb., Wiesb., 1886, ii, 355–366. — **Musgrave** (A.) Observations on the unmixed effects of mercury on the syster , with a few practical remarks on some of the most important tropical diseases. Edinb. M. & S. J., 1827, xxviii, 36–61. — **Neumann.** Vergleichung der Louvrierschen und der Weinholdschen Methoden, das Quecksilber anzuwenden. J. f. Chir. u. Augenh., Berl., 1821, ii, 405–433.—**Neumann** (I.) Ueber die Aufnahme des Quecksilbers durch die unverletzte Haut. Wien. med. Wchnschr., 1871, xxi, 1209; 1233; 1255. Also, Reprint. Also [Abstr.]: Allg. Wien. med. Ztg., 1871, xvi, 347. Also: Wien. med. Presse, 1871, xii, 1109. Also, transl. [Abstr.]: Practitioner, Lond., 1871, vii, 279–281.—**Nicol** (W. B.) On the state in which the mercury exists in the hyd. c. creta. and pil. hydrarg. Brit.-Am. J. M. & Phys. Sc., Montreal, 1847, iii, 85–87. — **Oesterlen.** Uebergang des regulinischen Quecksilbers in die Blutmasse und die Organe. Nach Versuchen. Arch. f. phys. Heilk., Stuttg., 1843, ii, 536–543.—**Onsum** (I.) Om Qviksölvforbindelsernes physiologisk - chemiske Forholde. Norsk Mag. f. Lægevidensk., Christiania, 1864, xviii, 242–254.—**Otis** (F. N.) On the mode of elimination of mercury from the system and the time required for its accomplishment. Physician & Surg., Ann Arbor, Mich., 1887, ix, 97–99.—**Padioleau.** Réflexions sur le mercure. J. de la sect. de méd. Soc. acad. Loire-Inf., Nantes, 1836, n. s., xii, 231–240. — **Paschkis** (H.) Ueber den Nachweis des Quecksilbers in thierischen Substanzen. Ztschr. f. physiol. Chem., Strassb., 1882, vi, 495–503.—**von Patruban** (C.) Anatomische Erfahrungen und physiologische Beobachtungen über das Vorkommen von metallischem Quecksilber im menschlichen Organismus. Oesterr. Ztschr. f. prakt. Heilk., Wien, 1859, v, 210–213. — **Peise.** De l'emploi des préparations mercurielles à hautes doses dans les phlegmasies des membranes séreuses de cause externe. Abeille méd., Par., 1855, xii, 341–343.—**Philip** (A. P. W.) On the effects of minute doses of mercury in restoring the vital functions. Lond. M. Gaz., 1831-2, ix, 953–980. Also, Reprint.—**Physick** (P. S.) Some experiments and observations on the mode of operation of mercury on the body. Med. Reposit., N. Y., 1802, v, 288–291.—**Plagge** (T.) Zur Merkurfrage. Memorabilien, Heilbr., 1861, vi, 73–78. — **Plummer** (A.) [On a combination of mercury and antimony.] Med. Essays & Obs. Soc. Edinb., 1733, i, 46–62.—**Polak** (J. E.) Ueber den Gebrauch des Quecksilbers in Persien. Wien. med. Wchnschr., 1860, x, 564–568.—**Polotebnoff** (A.) Materiali k' izucheniyu dai-islviya rtutnikh preparatof. [Effect of mercurial preparations.] Med. Vestnik, St. Petersb., 1863, iii, 389; 405; 421. Also, transl.: Arch. f. path. Anat., etc., Berl., 1864,

Mercury.

xxxi, 35 - 51. — **Potter** (M. G.) Remarks on a new method of determining whether mercury possesses the power of secreting bile or not. Buffalo M. & S. J., 1867-8, vii, 411 - 418. — **Prince** (D.) A paper on the employment of mercury in cholera, dysentery, and diarrhœa, and upon the question of its action upon the liver. St. Louis M. Reporter, 1866-7, i, 577-587.—**Prümers.** Einige Mittheilungen über das Aethylsublimat oder Quecksilberäthylchlorid. Arch. f. path. Anat., etc., Berl., 1872, liv, 259-262.—**Rabuteau.** Die Mercurpräparate. Allg. Wien. med. Ztg., 1872, xvii, 288 ; 306 ; 324 ; 341 ; 354.—**Reale** (N.) Ricerche sulla pomata mercuriale, e proposta d' un nuovo preparato analogo (with rep.). Rendic. Accad. med.-chir. di Napoli, 1866, xx, 24 ; 60.—**Recherche** (Sur la) du mercure dans les analyses chimico-légales. Ann. d'hyg., Par., 1846, xxxv, 206-208. — **Rhades.** Ueber den Uebergang von Quecksilber in das Blut. Deutsches Arch. f. d. Physiol., Halle u. Berl., 1820, vi, 128-135. — **Riedel** (J. C. L.) Bestätigung und Empfehlung der heilsamen Wirkung des Quecksilbers gegen Rheumatismus chronicus et fixus capitis. Allg. med. Ann., Altenb. u. Leipz., 1817, 1369-1371.— **Rindfleisch** (E.) Zur Frage von der Resorption des regulinischen Quecksilbers. Arch. f. Dermat. u. Syph., Prag, 1870, ii, 309-316. — **Robertson** (H.) On the effect of mercury on the living body. Lond. M. Reposit., 1824, n. s., i, 457-464.—**Rogers** (P.) Preparation of mercurial ointment. Am. M. Recorder, Phila., 1819, ii, 331-338.—**Rosenheim** (T.) Zur Keuntniss der diuretischen Wirkung der Quecksilberpräparate. Deutsche med. Wchnschr., Leipz., 1887, xiii, 325 ; 354.—**Ross** (J.) On the action of mercury. Practitioner, Lond., 1870, v, 211-221.—**Saikowsky.** Ueber einige Veränderungen, welche das Quecksilber im thierischen Organismus hervorruft. Arch. f. path. Anat., etc., Berl., 1866, xxxvii, 346-350.—**Schlesinger** (H.) Experimentelle Untersuchungen über die Wirkung lange Zeit fortgegebener kleiner Dosen Quecksilbers auf Thiere. [Gekrönte Preisschrift, 1879.] Arch. f. exper. Path. u. Pharmakol , Leipz., 1880-81, xiii, 317-353.—**Schneider** (F. C.) Ueber die Ausscheidung des Quecksilbers während und nach Mercurialcuren. Med. Jahrb., Wien, 1861, i, 124-138.—**Schuster.** Ueber den Einfluss des schwefelthermalwassers auf die Ausscheidung des Quecksilbers bei und nach Quecksilberkuren. Veröffentl. d. Gesellsch. f. Heilk. in Berl. Balneol. Sect., 1882, vii, 44-58. ——. Ueber die Ausscheidung des Quecksilbers während und nach Quecksilberkuren. Vrtljschr. f. Dermat., Wien, 1882, ix, 51-61. *Also, transl :* J. Cutan. & Ven. Dis., N. Y., 1882-3, i, 353-356. ——. Erwiderung auf die "Bemerkung" des Hrn. E. Ludwig zu meiner Arbeit "Ueber die Ausscheidung des Quecksilbers", nebst weiteren Aufschlüssen über diese Ausscheidung. Vrtljschr. f. Dermat., Wien, 1882, ix, 307-311. ——. [Ausscheidung des Quecksilbers durch den Harn und die Fäces bei und nach Quecksilbercuren.] Ztschr. f. klin. Med., Berl., 1883, vii, 80-82. ——. L'élimination du mercure, introduit dans l'organisme par les voies cutanées. Cong. internat. de méd. d. colonies 1883, Amst., 1884, 369-371. ——. Neue Aufschlüsse über die Ausscheidung des Quecksilbers. Centralbl. f. d. med. Wissensch., Berl., 1884, xxii, 273-275.— ——. Neue Aufschlüsse über die Ausscheidung des Quecksilbers. Deutsche med. Wchnschr., Berl., 1884, x, 278. *Also, transl.:* J. Cutan. & Ven. Dis., N. Y., 1884, ii, 266-268. ——. Die Mercurseife. Allg. Wien. med. Ztg., 1886, xxxi, 86. — **Scivoletto** (P.) Del miglior metodo per constatare la presenza dei sali mercuriali nelle macchie dei tessuti. Movimento, Napoli, 1869, i, 123.—**Scott** (G.) On the influence of mercurial preparations upon the secretion of bile. Arch. Med., Lond., 1859, i, 209-224. *Also,* Reprint.— **Scotti** (G. B.) Pilole detto Dzondi; se convenga sia sottrata la mollica di pane; cautele in proposito. Gazz. med. ital. lomb., Milano, 1855, 3. s., vi, 173.—**Searle** (C.) Mercury; its influence on the system, and the indications for its employment. Med. Times, Lond., 1847, xvi, 153.—**Sichel.** Considérations sur l'usage et l'abus des préparations mercurielles, surtout dans les affections inflammatoires. Rev. méd. franç. et étrang., Par., 1846, n. s., iii, 327-340.—**Siebert.** Notizen über den Gebrauch des versüssten Quecksilbers. Med. Cor.-Bl. bayer. Aerzte, Erlang., 1840, 145-152. ——. Ueber die Wirkung des versüssten Quecksilbers. Amtl. Ber. ü. d. Versamml. deutsch. Naturf. u. Aerzte 1840, Erlang., 1841, 150-152. — **Silva Araujo.** O salicylato de mercurio e suas applicações na syphilis e em algumas dermatoses. J. de med. e pharm., Par., 1877, ii, 12-14.—**Simancas** (E.) Del mercurio. Accion fisiológica y terapéutica. An. de cien. méd., Madrid, 1878, vi, 206-209.—**Simon** jun. Mercurius triumphator. Wchnschr. f. d. ges. Heilk., Berl., 1849, 353 ; 374 ; 389 : 1850, 401; 780: 1851, 449; 476; 491; 505.—**Simon** (J.) Thérapeutique infantile; du mercure. Progrès méd., Par., 1880, viii, 383 ; 419; 447; 485; 531; 577.—**Smith** (H.) Observations on the action of mercury in inflammation, and its effects on the system. Med. Times, Lond., 1847, xvi, 132; 172; 213; 271; 293.—**Snoep** (J.P.) Over het gebruik van het ung. hydrargyri in distorsio en contusio, volgens de methode van Dr. Kerst. Boerhaave. Tijdschr., etc., Amst., 1846, n. s., v, 308-326.—**Soubeiran** (E.) Mercure et mercuriaux (composés). Dict. de méd., 2. éd., Par., 1839, xix,

Mercury.

549-575.—**Spilman** (C. H.) Therapeutic action of mercury. Richmond & Louisville M. J., Louisville, 1873. xvi, 300-312.—**Stephenson** (W.) The action of mercury in children. Edinb. M. J., 1871, xvi, 980-988. *Also,* Reprint.— **Sulzer.** Ueber Merkurial-Präparate, und besonders den Mercuricum phosphoratum. Museum d. Heilk., Zürich, 1797, iv, 178-185.—**Taddei** (T.) Sul modo di attenuare per via di chimici processi le molecole del mercurio, onde renderlo facilmente miscibile con varie sostanze mediante semplici operazioni meccaniche. Gazz. med. ital. feder. tosc., Firenze, 1850 - 51. 2. s., i, 409 - 411.—**Tait** (L.) The action of mercury on the liver. Brit. M. J., Lond., 1869, ii, 132.—**Taylor** (A.S.) Absorption and diffusion of mercury when taken in medicinal doses. Guy's Hosp. Rep., Lond., 1864, 3. s., x, 179.—**Thiry.** De l'absorption et de l'élimination du mercure dans l'organisme humain. Presse méd. belge, Brux., 1887, xxxix, 9-12 — **Thorowgood** (J.C.) On the use of mercury in certain inflammations. Practitioner, Lond., 1878, xx. 336-345.—**Todd** (J. S.) Mercury. Atlanta M. & S. J., 1884, n. s., i, 129-142.— **Tolmatscheff.** Zur Lehre über die Wirkung der Quecksilberpräparate auf den thierischen Organismus. Med.-chem. Untersuch. a. d. Lab. . . . zu Tübing., Berl., 1867, 279-284. *Also,* Reprint.— **Ulmer** (L.) Zur Quecksilberfrage. Wien. Med.-Halle, 1862, iii, 185.—**von Vajda** (L.) & **Paschkis** (H.) Zur Abwehr gegen den Aufsatz von Dr. Schuster: Ueber die Ausscheidung des Quecksilbers während und nach Quecksilberkuren. Vrtljschr. f. Dermat., Wien, 1882, ix, 305. — **Van de Vyvere** (E.) De l'action que l'iodure de potassium exerce sur la pommade mercurielle. Ann. Soc. méd.-chir. de Bruges, 1845, vi, 254-256.— **Vertrees** (W. M.) The action of mercury. South. Pract., Nashville, 1884, vi, 461-464.—**Walker** (J. K.) Some observations on the use of mercury, in acute as well as chronic affections. Midland M. & S. J., Worcester, 1831-2, iii, 17-27.—**Warren** (J.) View of the mercurial practice in febrile diseases. Med. Communicat. Mass. M. Soc. 1809-10, Bost., 1813, ii, 341 - 392.—**Wegg** (W.) Mercury. *In his:* Obs. Relating to the Sc., [etc.], 8°, Lond., 1851, 88 - 123. — **Welander** (E.) Undersökningar om qvicksilfrets absorption af och elimination ur menniskokroppen. Förh. v. Svens. Läk.-Sällsk. Sammank., Stockholm, 1885, 355-363. *Also:* Nord. med. Ark., Stockholm, 1886, xviii, no. 12, 1-56; no. 15, 1-69, 2 tab. *Also, transl.:* Ann. de dermat. et syph., Par., 1886, 2. s., vii, 412-417. — **Westmoreland** (J. G.) An essay on the actions of mercury. Atlanta M. & S. J., 1875, xiii, 104-109.—**Widemann.** Ueber die Anwendung des Quecksilbers in Entzündungskrankheiten. J. d. pract. Arznk. u. Wundarznk., Berl., 1806, xxiv, 3. St., 116-131.— **Wilbouchewitch.** De l'influence des préparations mercurielles sur la richesse du sang en giobules rouges et en globules blancs. Arch. de physiol. norm. et path., Par., 1874, 2. s., i, 509-537.—**Wildhagen.** Om Brugen af Mercur i smaae Doser. Norsk Mag. f. Lægevidensk., Christiania, 1842, v, 34-39.—**Wilson** (J. C.) Note on hydrargyrum formamidatum. Proc. Phila. Co. M. Soc., Phila., 1883-4, vi, 52.—**Winkler.** Ueber die Anwendung der Quecksilbers bei innern Entzündungen. Allg. med. Ann., Altenb.. 1802, 138-143.—**Yandell** (L. P.) An enquiry as to the therapeutic value of mercurials. Nashville J. M. & S., 1867-8, n. s., iii, 1-10.—**Zambrana** (S.) La escrofulosis y los mercuriales. Mem. Soc. méd.-farm. de Toluca, 1876, i, 155-157.—**Zeissl** (H.) Ueber Aufnahme des Merkurs in den Organismus und dessen Ausscheidung aus demselben. Wien. Med.-Halle, 1864, v, 282. ——. Ueber die Theorie der Aufnahme des Mercurs in den Organismus. Oesterr. Ztschr. f. prakt. Heilk., Wien, 1864, 515-519.

Mercury (*Fumigations of*).

See Mercury (*Vapors of*).

Mercury (*Hypodermic use of*).

See, also, Syphilis (*Treatment of*).

BERNARD (H.-U.) * Des injections sous-cutanées de sublimé corrosif dans le traitment de la syphilis. 4°. *Paris,* 1871.

GAILLARD (É.) * Essai sur les injections hypodermiques de peptonate de mercure. 4°. *Paris,* 1880.

MERSCHEIM (A.) * Ueber die hypodermatische Sublimatinjection. 8°. *Bonn,* 1868.

von Bamberger. Ueber hypodermatische Anwendung eines neuen Quecksilber-Präparates. Wien. med. Presse, 1876, xvii, 357-362. — **Bricheteau** (F.) On the application of the hypodermic method to the treatment of syphilis by mercury. Practitioner, Lond., 1869, ii, 141-147.—**Buzzard.** Cases treated by hypodermic injection of mercurialised peptone. Brit. M. J., Lond., 1878, ii, 475. — **Cullingworth** (C. J.) On the subcutaneous injection of mercury. Lancet, Lond., 1874, i, 653; 686.— **Duncan** (J.) Note on the subcutaneous injection of mercury. Edinb. M. J., 1874, xx, 559.—**Engelsted** (S.) Praktiske Meddelelser om Syfilis, behandlet ved Merkur hypodermatisk. Nord. med. Ark., Stockholm, 1871, iii,

Mercury (*Hypodermic use of*).

No. 21, 1–26. — **Gayraud.** Peptonate de mercure en injections hypodermiques. Gaz. hebd. d. sc. méd. de Montpel., 1882, iv, 116. — **Grünfeld** (J.) Ueber hypodermatische Injektionen von löslichem Quecksilber-Albuminat. Wien. med. Presse, 1876, xvii, 1133 ; 1167 ; 1221. — **Gschirhakl.** Ueber die praktische Verwendbarkeit einiger Sublimatpräparate für hypodermatische Injektionen. *Ibid.*, 1638. ———. Ueber Sublimatpräparate für subkutane Injektionen. Wien. med. Wchnschr., 1877, xxvii, 224 ; 267 ; 295 ; 320. — **Hagen.** Zur Kritik der subcutanen Sublimat-Injectionen. [44 cases.] Deutsche Klinik, Berl., 1870, xxii, 149 ; 164 ; 169 ; 184 ; 191 ; 203 ; 212 ; 219. — **Heilborn** (M.) Ueber experimentelle Beiträge zur Wirkung subcutaner Sublimat-Injectionen. Jahresb. d. schles. Gesellsch. f. vaterl. Kult., Bresl., 1878, lv. 219–222. *Also:* Arch. f. exper. Path. u. Pharmakol., Leipz., 1878, viii, 361–374 — **Kaspar** (O.) Note sur la préparation et le titre du peptonate de mercure employé en injections hypodermiques contre la syphilis. Rev. méd. de la Suisse Rom., Genève, 1881, i, 352–357. ———. Note sur les moyens de conserver intact le titre du peptonate de mercure. *Ibid.*, 617–619. — **Kratschmer.** Ueber Sublimatpräparate für subkutane Injection. Wien. med. Wchnschr., 1876, xxvi, 1149 ; 1171. — **Martineau.** Des injections sous-cutanées de peptone mercurique. Siècle méd., Par., 1881, ii, 66. — **Pagello** (P.) Sull' injezione ipodermica del calomelano col metodo del Prof. Scarenzio nella cura dei tumori. Gazz. med. ital. lomb., Milano, 1873, xxxiii. 105. — **Plumert** (A.) Ueber subcutane Injectionen mit Bicyanuretum hydrargiri. Prag. med. Wchnschr., 1880, v, 241–244. — **Rosenbach** (J.) Ueber einige pathologische Veränderungen nach subcutaner Injection von Quecksilberchlorid bei Kaninchen. Ztschr. f. rat. Med., Leipz. u. Heidelb., 1868, xxxiii, 3. R., 36–44. — **von Rothmund.** Ueber subcutane Sublimatinjectionen. Aerztl. Int.-Bl., München, 1873, xx, 1–4. — **Staub.** Chloro-albuminate de mercure pour les injections hypodermiques dans le traitement de la syphilis. Bull. gén. de thérap., etc., Par., 1873, lxxxiv, 257. — **Stefanini** (D.) La injezione sotto cutanea di calomelano quale mezzo diagnostico in un caso dubbio di sifilide. Gior. ital. d. mal. ven., Milano, 1874, ix, 90. — **Stern** (E.) Ueber das Quecksilberchlorid-Chlornatrium und seine subcutane Anwendung. Berl. klin. Wchnschr., 1878, xv, 59–64. ———. Ueber subcutane Quecksilber-Behandlung. Jahresb. d. schles. Gesellsch. f. vaterl. Kult., Bresl., 1878, lv, 213–216. — **von Willebrand** (F.) Till frågan om subkutan-applikation af merkurpreparater. Finska läk. sällsk. handl., Helsingfors, 1870, xii, 116–133.

Mercury (*Inunction of*).

See, also, **Mercury** (*Toxicology of, etc.*)

BROEKER (J.) Iets over unguentum oxydi hydrargyrici. 8°. [*Utrecht,* 1877.]
Repr. from: Haaxman's Tijdschr., July, 1877.

COMBRET (R.) *Notes sur les principales méthodes d'administration du mercure par la peau. 4°. *Paris,* 1882.

RHADES (F. G. F.) *Diss. sistens experimenta quædam circa quæstionem: An hydrargyrum externe applicatum in corpore et præsertim in sanguine reperiatur? 8°. *Halæ,* [1820].

d'Alais (S.) Des frictions mercurielles comme traitement spécial et abortif de l'inflammation aiguë de la peau et du tissu cellulaire qu'elle recouvre. Bull. gén. de thérap., etc., Par., 1832, iii, 5–13. — **B.** (I.) Un mot sur la préparation de l'onguent mercuriel double. Presse méd. belge, Brux., 1852, iv, 371. — **von Basedow.** Heilung entzündlicher Krankheiten der Eingeweide durch Quecksilbersalbe. J. d. pract. Heilk., Berl., 1828, lxvii, 6. St., 82–103 ———. Fernere Beobachtungen über die jatraliptische Anwendung des Merkurs als Antiphlogisticum. *Ibid.*, 1838, lxxxvii, 3. St., 34–84. — **Bouilhon.** Préparation de la pommade mercurielle double. Bull. gén. de thérap., etc., Par., 1872, lxxxiii, 22–25. — **Brachet** (J.-L.) Modifications des frictions mercurielles, d'après la méthode de Clare. J. gén. de méd., chir. et pharm., Par., 1823, lxxxii, 209–237. [Rap. de Lagneau], 289–298. — **Cabaret** (P.-J.) Stomatite mercurielle, déterminée par des frictions avec l'onguent citrin. Rev. de thérap. méd.-chir., Par., 1867, 395–399. — **Cassoni** (E.) Esame critico-analitico di un nuovo processo per preparare l' unguento mercuriale. Bull. d. sc. med. di Bologna, 1857, 4. s., vii, 321–332. — **Centenera** (R.) Consideraciones sobre la pomada mercurial y sus métodos de preparacion. Rev. de sanid. mil. españ., Madrid, 1865, ii, 213. — **Coldefier.** Nouvelle préparation de l'onguent mercuriel. Écho méd., Neuchât., 1857, i, 378. — **Delpech.** Inflammations combattues avec succès par les frictions mercurielles. Rev. méd. franç. et étrang., Par., 1831, ii, 185–216. — **Keber.** Auflösung eines 2 Monate alten Knochencallus durch Einreibung von 3 Drachmen grauer Quecksilbersalbe. Med. Ztg., Berl., 1846, xv, 11. — **Klink** (E.) Untersuchungen über den Nachweis des Quecksilbers in der Frauenmilch

Mercury (*Inunction of*).

während einer Einreibungskur mit grauer Salbe. Vrtljschr. f. Dermat., Wien, 1876, viii, 207. — **Löwenhardt.** Ueber die Anwendung grosser Mercurialfriktionen zur Beseitigung und Abkürzung mehrerer Krankheitszustände, namentlich der Apoplexie, Hepatitis, Febris nervosa gastrica, Pocken, des Kindbettfiebers und des Rheumatismus acutus. *In his:* Beob. u. Erfahr., 8°, Prenzlau, 1838, 13–196. — **Mettauer** (J. P.) Preparation of mercurial ointment. Stethoscope & Virg. M. Gaz., Richmond, 1851, i, 384–386. — **Oberländer.** Die Mercurseife (Sapo mercurialis), ein neues und praktisches Ersatzmittel für die Mercursalbe. Vrtljschr. f. Dermat., Wien, 1882, ix, 709–717. — **Overbeck** (R.) Zur Untersuchung der grauen Quecksilbersalbe. Arch. f. path. Anat., etc., Berl., 1861, xxii, 419. — **Rust** (J. N.) Ueber die Heilkraft der methodischen Quecksilber-Einreibungen in syphilitischen und nicht syphilitischen Krankheiten. Zur Belehrung und Warnung für diejenigen, die sich dieser Heilmethode bedienen wollen. Mag. f. d. ges. Heilk., Berl., 1816, i, 354–451. — **Schuster.** Die Mercurseife (savon napolitain). Vrtljschr. f. Dermat., Wien, 1882, ix, 45–49. — **Serre.** [Les frictions mercurielles.] Gaz. méd. de Montpel., 1841–2, ii, no. 24, 3. — **Sobre** el uso de las fricciones mercuriales para combatir las inflamaciones; o sea, sobre el método de la mercurializacion. Repert. méd. extrang., Madrid, 1833, i, 185–218. — **Stahmann** (F.) Ungewöhnlich rasche Nebenwirkungen des Unguentum neapolitanum. Ztschr. f. Med., Chir. u. Geburtsh., Leipz., 1861, xv, 316–318. — **Strauss** (B.) Zur äussern Anwendung des rothen Quecksilber-Präcipitats. Bl. f. Heilwissensch., München, 1871, ii, 177 ; 184. — **Tomowitz.** Die Durchführung von merkuriellen Friktionskuren unter Zelten. Allg. mil.-ärztl. Ztg., Wien, 1867, viii, 321–323. — **Vergari** (A.) Nuovo metodo sull' uso della pomata mercuriale per applicazione. Esculapio napol., Napoli, 1847, xxv, 705–709. — **Walker** (J. T.) Unguentum hydrargyri oxidi flavi. Phila. M. Times, 1878, viii, 580.

Mercury (*Toxicology of, and accidents from*).

See, also, **Amaurosis** (*Causes of*); **Eczema** (*Mercurial*); **Hat-makers, Looking-glass makers, Diseases of*; **Mercury** (*Ammonio-chloride of*); **Mercury** (*Bichloride of, Toxicology of*); **Mercury** (*Cyanide of*); **Mercury** (*Inunction of*); **Mercury** (*Iodides of*); **Mercury** (*Nitrate of*); **Mercury** (*Sulphur-compounds of*); **Salivation** (*Mercurial*); **Tremor** (*Mercurial, etc.*)

ALLEY (G.) An essay on a peculiar eruptive disease arising from the exhibition of mercury. 8°. *Dublin,* 1804.

BAUER (E.) *Ueber Mercurialismus. [Erlangen.] 8°. *Neustadt,* 1866.

BEAULIES (H.-G.) *Quelques considérations sur la stomatite mercurielle. 4°. *Strasbourg,* 1862.

BECKER (H.) *De erysipelate mercuriali. 12°. *Duisburgi,* 1817.

BLANCHON (C.) *De l'intoxication mercurielle. 4°. *Paris,* 1868.

BONINUS (P.) Consultatio de hydrargyrio. *In:* CIRCAMUNDUS (J. B.) Consult. de hydrarg. 4°. *Maceratæ,* 1618, 17–38.

BRESSON (M.-H.-L.) *De l'intoxication mercurielle. 4°. *Strasbourg,* 1860.

CIRCAMUNDUS (J. B.) Consultatio de hydrargyrio. 4°. *Maceratæ,* 1618.

CORUBOLO (H.) *De morbis a mercurii abusu proficiscentibus. 8°. *Patavii,* 1834.

CRON (C. F.) *De veneficio mercuriali. sm. 8°. *Berolini,* [1817].

DESTAY (A.) *Essai sur la paralysie mercurielle. 4°. *Paris,* 1879.

DIETERICH (G. L.) Die Merkurialkrankheit in allen ihren Formen. 8°. *Leipzig,* 1837.
Also, transl. [Abstr.] *in:* J. d. conn. méd., Par., 1840–41, viii, pt. 1, 12–22.

DROUOT (F.) Des effets pernicieux du mercure (onguent napolitain, calomel, etc.) et de quelques autres agents exclusivement appliqués au traitement des maladies des yeux. 8°. *Paris,* 1849.

DRYSDALE (C.-R.) Traitement de la syphilis et d'autres maladies sans mercure, ou recueil de témoignages tendant à prouver que le mercure

Mercury (*Toxicology of, and accidents from*).

est une canse de maladies, non un remède. Traduit de l'anglais. 12°. *Paris*, 1864.

——. The same. Ueber die Behandlung der Syphilis und anderer Krankheiten ohne Quecksilber. Mit einem Vorworte von Dr. Josef Hermann. 8°. *Wien*, 1868.

DUBELIR (D.) *Eksperimentalnoe izuchenie toksikologicheskago i pharmakologicheskago diestvija rtuti. [Toxicological and pharmacological effects of mercury.] 8°. *St. Petersburg*, 1875.

DUPRÉ (A.-H.) *De l'hydrargyrie. 4°. *Paris*, 1884.

FEINBERG (B.) *Beitrag zur chronischen gewerblichen Quecksilberintoxication. 8°. *Erlangen*, 1878.

FREUND (H.) *De morbis ex hydrargyriasi. 8°. *Berolini*, [1845].

GAUCHERAND (P.) *Des éruptions cutanées causées par l'administration interne du mercure (et en particulier de la forme scarlatineuse). 4°. *Paris*, 1886.

GRAPIN (J.-B.-A.) *De la stomatite mercurielle. 4°. *Paris*, 1846.

GWALTER (E.) *Ein Fall von Quecksilbervergiftung. 8°. *Zürich*, 1877.

HABERSHON (S. O.) On the injurious effects of mercury in the treatment of disease. 8°. *London*, 1860.

HEIM (E. M. A.) *Ueber die Mercurial-Krankheit. 8°. *Erlangen*, 1835.

HERRMANN (J.) Die Mercurial-Krankheiten und deren Verhältniss zur Lustseuche. 8°. *Wien*, 1865.

HERRMANN (O.) Ueber die Merkurialkrankheiten, oder die schrecklichen Folgen, welche ein unzweckmässiger und zu lange fortgesetzter Gebrauch des Quecksilbers bei venerischen Krankheiten nach sich ziehen kann. Zur Warnung und Belehrung für Alle, die vom Quecksilber Gebrauch machen müssen. 12°. *Leipzig*, 1835.

HORN (J. A.) *De noxis in corpus humanum ex abusu mercurialium redundantibus, eorumque remediis. 4°. [*Gryphiswald*, 1728.]

INGRAM (D.) A strict and impartial enquiry into the cause and death of the late William Scawen, esq., of Woodcote-Lodge, in Surry, ascertaining, from the medical evidences against Jane Butterfield, the impossibility of poison having been given him; to which is added an account of accidental poisons, to which families are exposed, with their antidotes, under the following general heads, viz: stings and bites, vegetables, minerals, fumes and vapours. 8°. *London*, 1777.

KALB (O.) *Ein Fall von letalem Mercurialismus. 8°. *Erlangen*, 1876.

KALBÉ (L.) *Quelques observations d'hydrargyrie à la suite de frictions mercurielles. 4°. *Paris*, 1871.

KALBFUS (K.) *Ueber Mercurialkrankheiten hauptsächlich in Bezug auf ihre Aehnlichkeit mit Syphilis, nebst den characteristischen Unterscheidungsmerkmalen von derselben. 8°. *Erlangen*, 1834.

KRAMER (J. A.) *Ueber die Angina mercurialis faucium. 8°. *Erlangen*, [1830].

KUSSMAUL (A.) Untersuchungen über den constitutionellen Mercurialismus und sein Verhältniss zur constitutionellen Syphilis. 8°. *Würzburg*, 1861.

M'MULLIN (J.) *De erythemate mercuriali. 8°. *Edinburgi*, 1805.

MARÉCHAL (P.) *Des troubles nerveux dans l'intoxication mercurielle lente. 4°. *Paris*, 1885.

Mercury (*Toxicology of, and accidents from*).

MASSIE (A.-C.-E.) *Des accidents mercuriels. 4°. *Paris*, 1853.

MATHIAS (A.) The mercurial disease. An inquiry into the history and nature of the disease produced in the human constitution by the use of mercury, with observations on its connexion with the lues venerea. 8°. *London*, 1810.

——. The same. 8°. *Philadelphia*, 1811.

——. The same. 8°. *London*, 1816.

——. The same. Del morbo mercuriale, ossia ricerche sulla storia e natura della malattia prodotta nell' umana costituzione dell' uso del mercurio, con osservazioni intorno alla sua connessione colla lue venerea. Versione italiana del dottore T. Gensana. 8°. *Milano*, 1818.

——. The same. Ueber die Merkurialkrankheit, oder genaue Darstellung der Geschichte und wesentlichen Beschaffenheit aller sich durch Quecksilbermissbrauch im menschlichen Körper erzeugenden Uebelseynsformen, nebst einigen Bemerkungen über die gegenwärtige Behandlungsart der Lustseuche. Nach der 3. engl. Originalausgabe übersetzt und mit vielen praktischen Anmerkungen versehen von Heinrich Robbi. 8°. *Leipzig*, 1822.

MRAOVICH (A.) *De hydrargyrosi. 8°. *Viennæ*, 1825.

NIERMEYER (J. H.) *Akademische proeve, bevattende een door den schrijver waargenomen ziektegeval. [Morbus mercurialis.] 8°. *Leiden*, 1856.

PAULI (H.) *Zur Lehre von der Hydrargyrose und ihrer Therapie. 8°. *Greifswald*, 1874.

RAMBACH (J. J.) *De hydrargyrosi. 8°. *Dorpat*, 1825.

SAMELSOHN (J.) *De hydrargyrosi; adjecta observatione. sm. 8°. *Berolini*, [1864].

SCHMITZ (E. O.) *Ueber Quecksilber-Vergiftung. sm. 8°. *Berlin*, [1869].

SCHREIBER (G. F.) *De morbo mercuriali. 4°. *Erfordiæ*, [1792].

STOLL (J. S. T.) *De mercurii in solidis corporis humani hærentis noxa. 4°. *Argentorati*, [1760].

WARD (D.) An essay on biliary derangement, and the excessive use of calomel, and other mercurials. 8°. *Adrian*, 1848.

WEGLAU (M.) *Das Merkurialgeschwür und seine Behandlung mit Bromwasserstoffsäure. 12°. *Coesfeld*, 1884.

WENDT (J. C. W.) De abusu hydrargyri, jam magis magisque increscente, unde morbi et affectiones morbosæ, syphiliticis persæpe similes, nascuntur. 4°. *Havniæ*, 1823.

WLCŻEK (F. C.) *De hydrargyrosi. 8°. *Vindobonæ*, 1826.

ZANDER (H. A.) *De hydrargyrosi. 8°. *Berolini*, 1849.

ZAWADZINISKI (C.) *De hydrargyrosi. 8°. *Cracoviæ*, 1830.

Acid treatment in mercurial fever. West. M. Reformer, Cincin., 1844, iv, 97–99.—**Aldinger** (H.) Zur Lehre vom Mercurialismus, nach Beobachtungen an Fürther Quecksilberarbeitern. Würzb. med. Ztschr., 1861, ii, 362–375. *Also*, Reprint.—**Alexander.** Ein Fall von acutem universellem Mercurialeczem. Vrtljschr. f. Dermat., Wien, 1884, xi, 105–110.—**Alexandre.** Observation d'hydrargyrie. Gaz. d. hôp., Par., 1835, ix, 46. *Also:* J. hebd. d. progr. d. sc. et inst. méd., Par., 1835, i, 103–108.—**d'Antonio** (G.) Avvelenamento acuto da mercurio per l'uso dell' unguento cedrino come antipsorico. Liguria med., Genova, 1874, xix, 439–442.—**Audhoui.** Intoxication mercurielle; tremblement; ictus apoplectiforme; hémiparésie; hémianesthésie; hémichorée; guérison et rechute. Paris méd., 1885, x, 229–232.—**Axenfeld.** Intoxication mercurielle; pas d'albuminurie; présence du mercure dans la salive et dans les urines; extraction du mercure à l'état métallique sous l'influence de bains électriques. Gaz. d. hôp., Par., 1870, xliii, 97.—**Aynard.** Observation d'un cas de chorée mercurielle. J. de méd.

Mercury (*Toxicology of, and accidents from*).

de Bordeaux, 1863, 2. s., viii, 550–553.—**Baaz** (J.) Beobachtungen über die beim k. k. Quecksilberwerke Idria vorkommenden Erkrankungen an Merkurialismus. Wien. med. Presse, 1886, xxvii, 711; 741; 774; 879; 944; 977; 1010; 1104; 1133. *Also* [Abstr.]: Mitth. d. Ver. d. Aerzte in Steiermark 1886, Graz, 1887, xxiii, 121–126.—**Bacon.** Mercurial poisoning. Am. J. M. Sc., Phila., 1853, n. s., xxvi, 91.—**Baron** (C.) Observations d'hydrargyrie chez des enfans. Gaz. méd. de Par., 1850, 3. s., v, 25; 71. *Also*, Reprint. *Also, transl.:* J. f. Kinderkr., Erlang., 1850, xv, 1–8.—**Bateman** (T.) Some observations in reply to Dr. Edward Percival on the subject of the poison of mercury. Edinb. M. & S. J., 1813, ix, 180–185. ———. Notes of a case of mercurial erethism. Med. Chir. Tr., Lond., 1818, ix, 220–233. — **Bayer.** Beobachtung einer Quecksilber-Vergiftung, entstanden durch Verarbeitung des Quecksilbers in einer Spiegelbelege. Arch. f. med. Erfahr., Berl., 1820, i, 115–127. — **Beaugrand** (E.) Mercure; hygiène professionnelle. Dict. encycl. d. sc. méd., Par., 1873, 2. s., vii, 85–89.—**Belfield** (W. T.) A case of mercurial necrosis, with specimen. Med. Age, Detroit, 1887, v, 368.—**Benham** (R. F.) & **Hendley** (H.) A case of poisoning by ammoniated and red oxide of mercury. Brit. M. J., Lond., 1885, i. 484.—**Bierbaum.** Ein anderer Fall von brandiger Zerstörung der Mundhöhle in Folge des Kalomels, nebst einigen ätiologischen Bemerkungen. Med. Cor.-Bl. rhein. u. westfäl. Aerzte, Bonn, 1845, iv, 6–12.—**Biver.** Observations sur les ulcères mercuriels. Arch. de la méd. belge, Brux., 1843, x, 323–325.—**Blache.** Nouvelles observations sur l'emploi du chlorate de potasse dans le traitement de la stomatite mercurielle. Bull. gén. de thérap., etc., Par., 1855, xlviii, 120–127.—**Blanc.** Observation d'érythème mercuriel scarlatiniforme. Province méd., Lyon, 1887, ii, 393–396.—**Bockhart** (M.) Zur Aetiologie und Behandlung der ulcerösen Merkurial-stomatitis. Monatsh. f. prakt. Dermat., Hamb., 1885, iv, 245–259.—**Bouchard.** Cas d'empoisonnement mercuriel aigu. Compt. rend. Soc. de biol. 1873, Par., 1875, 5. s., v, 227–229. — **Braus** (O.) Exitus lethalis in Folge missbräuchlich gehandhabter Schmiercur. Deutsche med. Wchnschr., Leipz., 1887, xiii, 593. — **Brodbelt** (F. R.) Case of deposition of mercury upon the bones. Mem. M. Soc. Lond., 1799, v, 112–118.—**Brodhurst** (B.) Symptoms resembling syphilis produced by mercury. Med. Times, Lond., 1850, i, 671.—**Buckley** (C.) Chronic mercurial poisoning. Tr. N. York M. Ass. (1884), N. Y., 1885, i, 126–129.—**Burton** (R.) Mercury in the liver of workers in mirror manufactories, an experimental evidence of localization of metallic poisons. Med. Times & Gaz., Lond., 1857, xv, 34.—**Byford** (W. H.) Mercurial muco-enteritis. Am. J. M. Sc., Phila., 1857, n. s., xxxiii, 313–316.—**Cabaret** (P.-J.) Stomatite mercurielle déterminée par des frictions avec l'onguent citrin. Gaz. d. hôp., Par., 1854, xxvii, 119. *Also*: Abeille méd., Par., 1854, xi, 91.—**Canstatt** (C.) Ueber Hydrargyrosis. *In his:* Klin. Rückbl. u. Abhandl., 8°, Erlang, 1848, pt. 1, 91–102.—**Carsten** (B.) Hydrargyrosis na geringe giften calomel. Geneesk. Tijdschr. v. de Zeemagt, Gravenh., 1864, ii, 271–275.—**Cayley.** Case of mercurial tremors and paralysis; unconsciousness: prostration; cured by stimulation. Med. Times & Gaz., Lond., 1881, i, 35. — **de Cérenville.** Note sur l'intoxication mercurielle, suite d'un mode populaire de traitement de la gale. Bull. Soc. méd. de la Suisse Rom., Lausanne, 1873, vii, 163.—**Chandelon** (J.-T.-P.) Description d'un appareil destiné à éviter les dangers d'empoisonnement dans la fabrication de fulminate de mercure. Ann. d'hyg., Par., 1847, xxxvii, 215–217.—**Chapin** (J. B.) Insanity following exposure to fumes of mercury. Am. J. Insan., Utica, N. Y., 1863–4, xx, 335–338.—**Charpentier.** Troubles cérébraux observés dans un cas d'intoxication mercurielle professionnelle. Ann. d'hyg., Par., 1885, 3. s., xiii, 323–330. *Also*: Rev. d'hyg., Par., 1885, vii, 131–137.—**Chevallier.** Sur la santé des ouvriers qui manipulent le fulminate de mercure dans des fabriques d'amorces pour les fusils à percussion. Ann. d'hyg., Par., 1844, xxxii, 322–325.—**Chevallier** [*et al.*]. Rapport médico-légal relatif à des accidens attribués aux émanations mercurielles. *Ibid.*, 1841, xxv, 388–406.—**Chisholm** (C.) Are those diseases attributed to mercurial action on the system of the human body peculiarly and exclusively generated by it? Edinb. M. & S. J., 1812, viii, 291–309.—**Chomel.** Stomatite mercurielle; traitement par les bains de vapeur: guérison. Gaz. d. hôp., Par., 1843, 2. s., v, 53.—**Chronische** Hydrargyrose oder merkurielle Kachexie. Ber. d. k. k. Krankenh. Wieden 1867, Wien, 1868, 189–195, 1 pl.—**Claeys** (G.) Intoxication mercurielle à la suite d'une seule insufflation de poudre de calomel dans le cul-de-sac conjonctival. Livre jubil. publié p. la Soc. de méd. de Gand, etc., Gand, 1884, 287–293.—**Colson** (A.) Coup d'œil général sur les maladies produites par le mercure. J. hebd. de méd., Par., 1830, viii, 497–533.—**Corson** (J. W.) Cases testing the iodide of potassium as an antidote to the injurious effects of mercury, and corroborative of the experiments of M. Melsens. N. York J. M., 1853, n. s., xi, 243–250.—**Cramp-**

Mercury (*Toxicology of, and accidents from*).

ton (J.) Case of fatal result from mercurial ointment. Tr. Ass. King's & Queen's Coll. Phys. Ireland, Dubl., 1824, iv, 91–109.—**Danger & Flandin.** De l'empoisonnement par le mercure. Compt. rend. Acad. d. sc., Par., 1845, xx, 951–954. *Also, transl.:* Med. Times, Lond., 1845, xii, 60–62.—**Darcet.** Sur un moyen de soustraire les ouvriers doreurs aux effets funestes des vapeurs mercurielles. N. Jour. de méd., chir., pharm., etc., Par., 1818, i, 256–258.—**van Deen** (I.) Een merkwaardig geval van hydrargyria maligna. N. Arch. v. bin.- en buitenl. Geneesk., Zwolle, 1848, iii, 1–18.—**Delhaye** (V.) De l'abus des mercuriaux dans les maladies des accouchées. Ann. de gynéc. et pédiat., Brux., 1841, 2. s., i, 116–119.—**Demichelis** (F.) Utilità del joduro di potassio nel morbo mercuriale, e nella stessa lue venerea restia al mercuria. Gior. d. sc. med., Torino, 1842, xiv, 129–140. — **Descroizilles.** Eczéma hydrargyrique, coïncidant avec une stomatite de même nature et observé chez un jeune garçon à la suite de frictions faites avec l'onguent napolitain. France méd., Par., 1885, i, 447–451.—**Deutsch.** Merkurialfieber von Sublimat-Bädern und Typhus. Med. Ztg., Berl., 1856, xxv, 49.—**Dobrzensky** (J. J. W.) Illustrissimi hypochondriaci mors misera ab inunctione mercuriali. Misc. Acad. nat. curios., Lips., 1670, i, 185–196. ———. Von dem auf den äusserlichen Gebrauch einer Mercurialsalbe erfolgten erbärmlichen Tod einer milzsüchtigen gräflichen Person. Auserl. med.- chir.- ... Abhandl. d. röm.-kais. Akad. d. Naturf., Nürnb., 1755, i, 149–165.—**Dowse** (T. S.) Application of mercurial lotion to the scalp. Med. Times & Gaz., Lond., 1871, ii, 425.—**Draper** (W. H.) Mercurial poisoning. N. York M. J., 1880, xxxi, 626–628.—**Droste** (A.) Tod durch zu häufige Wiederholung einer ärztlichen Verordnung. Wchntl. Beitr. z. med. u. chir. Klin., Leipz., 1833–4, iii, 369–371.—**Dubar.** Empoisonnement mercuriel par la pommade au citrate acide de mercure. Gaz. d. hôp., Par., 1867, xl, 493.—**Esser** (C. L.) Einige durch den Missbrauch des Quecksilbers hervorgebrachte Krankheitsfälle. J. d. Chir. u. Augenh., Berl., 1826, ix, 624–638.—**Evers** (J. C. G.) Morbus mercurialis. *In his:* Brevis conspectus morborum [etc.]. 8°, Hagæ-Comitis, 1841, 87–89.—**Falconer** (W.) Reflections on the indiscriminate use of mercurial preparations in medicine. Tr. M. Soc. Lond., 1812, i, 96–114.—**Faucher** (L.) Rapport sur des cas d'intoxication mercurielle par l'usage de capsules au fulminate de mercure. Rev. san. de Bordeaux, 1886, iii, 165–168. *Also*: Rev. d'hyg., Par., 1886, viii, 572–582.—**Fauverge.** Observations sur les mauvais effets de l'emploi du mercure dans quelques cas de maladies scrophuleuses. J. gén. de méd., chir. et pharm., Par., 1809, xxxiv, 172–177.—**Faye.** Schreiben an Prof. Hebra in Angelegenheit der Hermann'schen Hydrargirose. Wien. med. Wchnschr., 1861, xi, 649–651. — **Fernandes.** Del empleo del clorate de potasa en la estomatitis mercurial. Gac. méd., Lima, 1859, iv, no. 75, 340; no. 76, 351; no. 77, 364; no. 78, 377.—**Ferrini** (G.) L' elettro-chimica nella idrargirosi. [6 cases.] Ann. univ. di med., Milano, 1858, clxvi, 252.—**Flügel.** Eine Quecksilberwassersucht. Memorabilien, Heilbr., 1863, viii, 203–205. — **Fournier** (A.) Note sur le chlorate de potasse employé contre la stomatite hydrargyrique avec continuation du traitement mercuriel. Union méd., Par., 1856, x, 397; 401.—**Frank** (J.) Erythema mercuriale. Acta Inst. clin. cæs. Univ. Vilnensis, Lipsiæ, 1812, 22–29.—**Frémy.** Intoxication mercurielle; paralysie diffuse; hémianesthésie. France méd., Par., 1877, xxiv, 65–67. — **Fryer** (C.) Case of caries of hard palate from the abuse of mercury. Med. Press & Circ., Lond., 1870, n. s., ix, 490.—**Gallaher.** Chlorate of potash in mercurial stomatitis. Am. J. M. Sc., Phila., 1857, n. s., xxxiv, 64–66.—**Gallard** (T.) Des maladies causées par le mercure. Union méd., Par., 1867, 3. s., ii, 18; 137; 152. *Also, in his*: Notes et obs. de méd. lég. [ect.]. 8°, Par., 1875, 113–128. *Also, in his:* Clin. méd., 8°, Par., 1877, 577–617.—**Gamberini** (P.) Paralisi tremante degli arti superiori dipendente da idrargirosi. Bull. d. sc. med. di Bologna, 1839, 2. s., vii, 214–216. ———. Del clorato di potassa nella cura della stomatite mercuriale, membranosa ecc., ecc. *Ibid.*, 1856, 4. s., v, 81–93.—**Gintrac.** Stomatite mercurielle guérie rapidement par le chlorate de potasse. J. de méd. de Bordeaux, 1856, 2. s., i, 481.—**Gorup-Besanez.** Quecksilber in der Leiche eines an Mercurial-cachexie verstorbenen Individuums. Jenaische Ann. f. Physiol. u. Med., Jena, 1851, ii, 237–243.—**Gotaas** (J. O.) Misbrug af Mercurius. Norsk Mag. f. Lægevidensk., Christiania, 1852, vi, 35.—**Grattan** (R.) Case of gangrene, occasioned by the use of mercury. Tr. Ass. King's & Queen's Coll. Phys. Ireland, Dubl., 1820, iii, 236–244.—**Günz** (J.) Chemischer Nachweis von der Ausscheidung des Quecksilbers bei Quecksilber-Kranken nach der Anwendung von Salzbädern. Wien. med. Presse, 1877, xviii, 1141; 1476; 1511; 1543.—**Guérin** de Mamers (H.) Observations sur une apoplexie survenue pendant l'administration des frictions mercurielles. Ann. de la méd. physiol., Par., 1824, vi, 24–42.—**Guglielminetti.** Ueber Blei- und Quecksilbervergiftungen. Mitth. d. naturf. Gesellsch. in Bern (1885), 1886, 3. Hft., 131–163.—

Mercury (*Toxicology of, and accidents from*).

Guillery. Cas remarquable d'ulcération au pli de l'aine. Presse méd. belge, Brux., 1852, iv, 269.—**Guldbrand** (J. W.) De angina mercuriali observata. Acta. reg. Soc. med. Havn., 1792, iii, 410-420.—**Hall** (C. R.) Case of hæmorrhage from the mucous surfaces, following the exhibition of mercury, with remarks on the mode of action of mercurials in general. Prov. M. J., Lond., 1843, vi, 169-171.—**Harrison** (J. P.) Cases of mercurial disease, with reflections. West. Med. & Phys. J., Cincin., 1827-8, i, 129-141. ——. Diseases induced by mercury. Proc. M. Convent. Ohio, Columbus, 1841, 9-23.—**van Hasselt** (A. W. M.) Over het vergiftig vermogen van metallisch kwik, vooral in den vloeibaren toestand. Nederl. Lancet, Gravenh., 1849-50, 2. s., v, 81-99. *Also*, Reprint.—**Hebra.** [Einige Bemerkungen in Bezug auf Prof. Faye's Schreiben.] Wien. med. Wchnschr., 1861, xi, 651; 665.—**Hickman** (J. W.) A case of acute hydrargysm. Med. & Surg. Reporter, Phila., 1880, xliii, 424. — **Horn** (E) Bestätigte Wirkungen der Schwefelbäder in einer langwierigen Merkurialkrankheit. Arch. f. med. Erfahr., Berl., 1813, 140. — **Huss** (M.) Hydrargyriasis chronica inauratorum; förgyllaresjukdom. Hygiea, Stockholm, 1840, ii, 345-348. — **Hydrargyrose.** [10 cases.] Ber. d. k. k. Krankenh. Wieden 1870, Wien, 1872, 81-86. — **Indiscreet** (The) use of mercury by physicians. Boston M. & S. J., 1845, xxxii, 118-121.—**Isambert.** De quelques accidents locaux dus aux préparations mercurielles appliquées à la surface de la peau. Bull. et mém. Soc. de thérap. 1867-8, Par., 1868, 18 – 21. *Also:* Bull. gén. de thérap., etc., Par., 1867, lxxii, 488; 561.—**Jackson** (S.) Fever, with death from mercurial irritation. Am. J. M. Sc., Phila., 1828, iii, 289-293.—**Jacquème** (C.) Albumine dans les cas d'empoisonnement mercuriel. Marseille méd., 1874, xi, 660-662.—**Jardon.** Quelques inflexions sur la stomatite mercurielle et sur l'emploi des mercuriaux. J. d. conn. méd.-chir., Par., 1838-9, vi, pt. 2, 56-62.— **Kahleis** (B.) Ueber die Mercurialrose (Erythema mercuriale). J. d. pract. Heilk., Berl., 1823, lvi, 6. St., 49-68.— **Kann** das regulinische Quecksilber in forensischer Beziehung zu den Giften gezählt werden? Bl. f. gerichtl. Anthrop., Nürnb., 1858, ix, 5. Hft., 61-71. — **Keller** (L. J.) Ueber die Erkrankungen in den Spiegelfabriken zu Sophienhütte, Friedrichsthal, Neuhurkenthal und Elisenthal in Böhmen. Wien. med. Wchnschr., 1860, x, 593-596. ——. Zur Frage über den konstitutionellen Merkurialismus. Eine Erklärung an Prof. Kussmaul. *Ibid.*, 1861, xi, 828. – **Kletzinsky** (V.) Die Elektrolyse in der Merkurfrage. *Ibid.*, 1858, viii, 810-812.—**Klob** (J.) Zur pathologischen Anatomie; akute Quecksilber-Vergiftung. Wien. med. Presse, 1868, ix, 641 – 645. — **Kreidmann.** Hydrargyrum-Erysipel. Allg.med. Centr.-Ztg., Berl., 1887, lvi, 957.—**Kussmaul** (A.) In Sachen des chronischen Mercurialismus. Deutsche Klinik, Berl., 1864, xvi, 130.—**Laborde** (J.-V.) De l'emploi du chlorate de potasse comme moyen préservatif et curatif de la stomatite mercurielle. Bull. gén. de thérap., etc., Par., 1858, liv, 10; 115. — **Lamberg** (C. M.) Fall af qvicksilfverförgiftning. Upsala Läkaref. Förh., 1867-8, iii, 681-683.— **Lambron.** La tête d'un chat qui pendant trois mois a pris chaque jour à peu près deux grammes d'onguent mercuriel. Bull. Soc. anat. de Par., 1840, xv, 108.—**Larmande.** Un érythème hydrargyro-atrophique. J. de méd. et chir. prat., Par., 1880, li, 497-499.—**Leiblinger.** Gerichtsärztliche Mittheilung über eine Vergiftung mit Mercurius vivus, in Salbenform in die Haut eingerieben zur Heilung von Scabies. Wien. med. Wchnschr., 1869, xix, 1595-1597.—**Letulle** (M.) Recherches expérimentales sur l'intoxication mercurielle; lésions des nerfs périphériques dans cette intoxication. Compt. rend. Acad. d. sc., Par., 1887, civ, 74-77. *Also:* France méd., Par., 1887, i, 49-51. *Also:* Tribune méd, Par., 1887, xix, 31. *Also, transl.:* Rev. de med. y cirug. práct., Madrid, 1887, xx, 169-172.—**Lolliot.** Stéatose du foie et des reins consécutive à un empoisonnement par le sublimé. Bull. Soc. anat. de Par. (1868), 1874, xliii, 437. [Rap. de Hénocque], 620-623. — **Lorinser** (F. W.) Rachengeschwüre durch chronische Hydrargyrose. Spitals-Ztg., Wien, 1859, 6-9. — **Lowe** (J.) On fatal erethismus mercurialis from inunction. Brit. M. J., Lond., 1882, i, 188.—**Lucas** (J.) [A singular case of mercurialism; from external use of black wash.] Indian M. Gaz., Calcutta, 1886, xxi, 79.—**Ludwig** (E.) Ueber den Nachweis des Quecksilbers in thierischen Substanzen. Med. Jahrb., Wien, 1880, 493-497.—**de Macedo** (L. A) Hidrargiria manifestada generalmente como consecuencia del uso de la pomada mercurial, para combatir la obstruccion esplénica. España méd., Madrid, 1861. vi, 215-217.—**McPherson** (J.) Case of permanent black discoloration of the skin from the effects of cinnabar. Tr. M. & Phys. Soc. Calcutta, 1845, ix, pt. 1, 278. — **M'Mullin** (J.) Essay on erythema mercuriale. Edinb. M. & S. J., 1806, ii, 25-37.—**Mansuroff** (N.) Sluchai merkurialnago zolovo-kruzheniya i drunoti. [Case of mercurial vertigo.] Med. Vestnik, St. Petersb., 1864, iv, 139. — **Mapother** (E. D.) Lecture on mercurial trade disease. Dublin M. Press & Circ., 1866, i, 531-533.—**Marti** (S. B.) Adherencias con-

secutivas á la estomatitis mercurial; incision; recidiva; incision y extirpacion; cicatrizacion aislada de sus extremos por la dilatacion con medios mecánicos; curacion completa. Rev. de cien. méd., Barcel., 1879, v, 113-116.—**Marx** (E.) Observation d'hydrargyrie. J. de méd. de Bordeaux, 1859, 2. s., iv, 169 - 174. ——. Hydrargyrie consécutive à l'emploi de frictions mercurielles. Mém. Soc. méd.-chir. d. hôp. de Bordeaux, 1866, i, 278 - 285. — **Mazade** (*d'Anduze*). Observations sur l'emploi du chlorate de potasse dans le traitement de la stomatite mercurielle et de la stomatite ulcéro-membraneuse. Bull. gén. de thérap., etc., Par., 1856, 1, 337 - 344. — **Melsens.** Mémoire sur l'emploi d'iodure de potassium pour combattre les affections saturnines et mercurielles. Ann. de chim. et phys., Par., 1849, 3. s., xxvi, 215-256. *Also, in:* Brit. & For. M.-Chir. Rev., Lond., 1853, xi, 201 - 224. [*See, also, supra,* Corson.]—**Mercurial** (On) ulcerations. N. Eng. J. M. & S., Bost., 1814, iii, 153-156.—**Merget.** De l'influence qu'il faut attribuer aux vapeurs mercurielles dans l'empoisonnement professionnel par le mercure. Rev. san. de Bordeaux, 1884 – 5, ii, 33. – **Mink & Peklo.** Chronische Quecksilbervergiftung. Ber. d. k. k. Krankenh. Wieden, 1871, Wien, 1873, 144-147.—**Molleson** (J.) Case of immense abscesses and death, resulting from mercury applied in excessive quantity. Tr. Med.-Chir. Soc. Edinb., 1826, ii, 255.—**N . . .** Observation sur un empoisonnement lent produit par la solution de muriate suroxygéné de mercure, connue sous le nom de liqueur de Van-Swieten. J. gén. de méd., chir. et pharm., Par., 1821, lxxv, 313-335.—**Neukirch** (R.) Zwei Fälle von chronischer Quecksilber-Vergiftung. Berl. klin. Wchnschr., 1883, xx, 820-823.—**Nicholson** (J.) Case of erythema mercuriale, accompanied by an affection of the cornea. Edinb. M. & S. J., 1812, viii, 39-41.—**Nicol.** Ein Fall von acuter Vergiftung durch Explosion von Mercurius vivus. Berl. klin. Wchnschr., 1882, xix, 568.—**Nouvelles** observations des effets rapides du chlorate de potasse dans la stomatite mercurielle chez l'adulte. Bull. gén. de thérap., etc., Par., 1855, xlviii, 437-442. — **Observacion** de unas convulsiones mercuriales producidas por los trabajos de las minas de Almaden. Bol. de med., cirug. y farm., Madrid, 1843, 2 s., iv, 203.—**Ollivier** (A.) Contribution à l'histoire de l'empoisonnement mercuriel aigu. Arch. de phys. norm. et path., Par., 1873, v, 547-557.—**Oppolzer.** Stomatitis mercurialis. Spitals-Ztg., Wien, 1862, 200.—**Orfila.** Recherches médico-légales relatives à l'empoisonnement par les composés mercuriels. Dict. de méd., 2. éd., Par., 1839, xix, 587-596. ——. De l'empoisonne ent par les préparations mercurielles, considéré sous un point de vue nouveau. J. de chim. méd., etc., Par., 1830, vi, 289; 321. *Also:* Arch. gén. de méd., Par., 1830, xxiii, 5-35. ——. Mercure; toxicologie. Dict. encycl. d. sc. méd., Par., 1873, 2. s., vii, 78-85.—**Overbeck** (R.) Zur Lehre von der Hydrargyrose. Wien. med. Wchnschr., 1860, x, 198. ——. Regulinisches Quecksilber in menschlichen Knochen. Arch. f. path. Anat., etc., Berl., 1861, xxii, 420. ——. Zur Lehre von der Hydrargyrose beim Menschen. *Ibid.*, 422.—**Passot** (P.) Observation de chloro-anémie mercurielle rapidement guérie par le fer. Gaz. méd. de Lyon, 1852, iv, 119.—**Pedrelli** (M.) Clorato di potassa e mercurio. Bull. d. sc. med. di Bologna, 1876, 5. s., xxi, 424-432. — **Percival** (E.) On the nature of the diseases affecting persons employed in silvering mirrors, described by Dr. Bateman in the report of the Carey Street Dispensary for July, 1812. Edinb. M. & S. J., 1813, ix, 62 – 66. [*see, also, supra,* Bateman.]—**Petithan.** Cas intéressants du mercurialisme. Arch. méd. belges, Brux., 1882, 3. s., xxii, 378 - 381. ——. Iodure intus; mercure extra; myélite grave; guérison. *Ibid.*, 1884, 3. s., xxvi, 73 - 78. — **Piffard** (H. G.) A case of gangrænopsis. North Car. M. J., Wilmington, 1879, iii, 9-11. — **Porta y Vidal** (J.) Estomatitis mercurial; curación por el zumo de Granada. Gac. méd. catal., Barcel., 1883, vi, 120.—**Postei de Franciere.** Lettre sur l'abus des remèdes populaires. J. de méd., chir., pharm., etc., Par., 1761, xv, 426-434.—**Potter** (J. W.) Eighteen grains of blue-pill fatal in an adult. Lancet, Lond., 1838, i, 215.—**Pouchet** (G.) Analyse d'une salive de stomatite mercurielle; salive albumineuse. Ann. de dermat. et syph., Par., 1882, 2. s., iii, 479.—**Prevost** (J.-L.) & **Frutiger** (G.) Étude expérimentale relative à l'intoxication par le mercure; son action sur l'intestin; calcification des reins parallèle à la décalcification des os. Rev. méd. de la Suisse Rom., Genève, 1882, ii, 553; 605, 2 pl.: 1883, iii, 5, 1 diag. *Also* [Abstr.]: Compt. rend. Acad. d. sc., Par., 1883, xcvi, 263-266.—**Probable** or possible poisoning from dentists' amalgams. Cincin. M. & Dent. J., 1885-6, i, 241-247. *Also:* Am. J. Dent. Sc., Balt., 1886-7, 3. s., xx, 65-72.—**Rabuteau.** Mécanisme de l'intoxication aiguë par le mercure; action des sels de ce métal sur le système musculaire. Compt. rend. Soc. de biol. 1873, Par., 1875, 5. s., v, 330 - 334.—**Rambaut.** Case of purpura hæmorrhagica caused by mercury. Dublin Hosp. Gaz., 1845, i, 18-20. — **Ramsay** (A.) Case of erythema mercuriale. Edinb. M. & S. J., 1811, vii, 269 - 274. — **Raymond** (P.)

Mercury (*Toxicology of, and accidents from*).

L'intoxication mercurielle aux mines d'Almaden. Progrès méd., Par., 1884, xii, 1017–1019.— **Reimer.** Mercurialismus. Jahrb. f. Kinderh., Leipz., 1877, xi, 81.— **Reisz.** Zur Lehre von der Hydrargyrose. Allg. Wien. med. Ztg., 1869, xiv, 230.— **Roché** (L.) Stomatite mercurielle, occasionnée par des fumigations faites pour détruire les punaises. Bull. Soc. méd. de l'Yonne, Auxerre, 1869, x, 17–20.— **Rollet** (J.) Mercurielles (maladies). Dict. encycl. d. sc. méd., Par., 1873, 2. s., vii, 96–107.— **Rosner.** Kilka uwag nad znaczeniem przypadów póznéj kily i ich stosunkiem do rtęcicy (hydrargyrosis). Przegl. lek., Krakow., 1868, vii, 49; 57; 65; 96.— **von Russdorf** (E.) Die Mercurialkrankheiten in Russland. Allg. med. Centr.-Ztg., Berl., 1852, xxi, 65; 81; 89; 97; 105.— **Scharlau.** Ueber Mercurialkrankheit. Wchnschr. f. d. ges. Heilk., Berl., 1846, 17–26.— **Scholz.** Stomatitis mercurialis. Aerztl. Ber. d. k. k. allg. Krankenh. zu Wien (1871), 1872. 74.— **Schuster.** Bemerkungen über die Art der Einwirkung der Aachener Schwefelthermen bei Hydrargyrose und bei Syphilis. Berl. klin. Wchnschr., 1872, ix, 164.— **Seguin** (E. C.) Case of desquamation of the kidneys during the administration of mercury and iodide of potassium. Arch. Med., N. Y., 1879, i, 332–334.— **Senné** fils. Observation sur les bons effets de l'opium contre des accidens considérables occasionnés par le mercure. J. de méd., chir., pharm., etc., Par., 1803, vi, 334–339.— **Simon.** Sur la maladie mercurielle. J. compl. du dict. d. sc. méd., Par., 1827, xxviii, 138; 213.— **Simon** jun. Ueber die Merkurial-Krankheit, mit besonderer Beziehung auf den Engländer Mathias. Arch. f. med. Erfahr., Berl., 1826, ii, 441–506.—[**Simplice.**] Mercure est mort!!! Actualité médico-comique en deux tableaux. Union méd., Par., 1867, 3. s., ii, 427–430.— **Smoller** (M.) Vergiftungen mit Quecksilber. Wien. med.-Halle, 1863, iv, 312.— **Snell** (S.) A peculiar idiosyncrasy (induction of pyrexia) as to mercury. Practitioner, Lond., 1882, xxix, 18–21.— **Söderberg.** Mercurialsjukdom hos hornboskap, observerad och i bref beskrifven. Hygiea, Stockholm, 1843, v, 668–670.—**Spens** (T.) Three cases of erythema mercuriale. Edinb. M. & S. J., 1805, i, 7–20.— **Stewart** (C.) Mercurial stomatitis terminating in gangrene and death. N. York J. M., 1846, vii, 19.— **Storrs** (R.) On paralysis from the effects of mercury as a medicine. Prov. M. & S J., Lond., 1847, 398–401.— **Strambio** (G.) Intorno alla mortal malattia di Catterina, Francesca e Giuseppe Terzani; riflessioni medico-legali. Gior. anal. di med., Milano, 1828, x, 143; 363.— **Takács** (A.) Intoxicatio mercurialis chronica. Pest. med.-chir. Presse. Budapest, 1878, xiv, 858. *Also:* Orvosi hetil., Budapest, 1878, 486.— **Thibert** (P. F.) Stomatite mercurielle. Bull. clin., Par., 1835-6, i, 427-429.— **Thomann** (J. N.) Lähmung von genommenem Mercurialgifte. Ann. d. klin. Anst. in d. Julius-Hosp. zu Würzb., 1800, 68–75.— **Toulmonde.** Accidens remarquables à la suite de l'emploi de l'onguent citrin. Union méd., Par., 1849, iii, 539.— **Truyart & Allouel.** Observation sur des accidens graves survenus après l'usage du sublimé-corrosif et de l'eau végéto-minérale à la suite de dartres répercutées. J. de méd., chir., pharm., etc., Par., 1778, l, 344–351.—**Underwood** (A. L.) Mercurial gangrene. Cincin. Lancet & Obs., 1865, n. s., viii, 585–588.— [**de Valle** (A. G.)] O chlorato de potassa na estomatite mercurial. Escholiaste med., Lisb., 1859, x, 193–199. *Also:* J. Soc. d. sc. med. de Lisb., 1860. 2. s., xxiv, 386–397.— **Van-Dekeere.** Observations sur des phlegmasies causées par l'administration du mercure. J. gén. de méd., chir. et pharm., Par., 1829, cvi, 36–66.— **Venot.** Emploi du chlorate de potasse dans le traitement de la stomatite mercurielle. J. de méd. de Bordeaux, 1856, 2. s., 325–332.— **Verdier** (J.) Observation de cachexie mercurielle combattue avantageusement à l'aide des acides végétaux. Rev. de thérap. du midi, Montpel., 1856, x, 107–109.—**Versuch** einer Vergiftung mittelst in Hühnersuppe dargereichten metallische Quecksilbers. Samml. gerichtsärztl. Gutacht. d. Prag. med. Fak , Prag, 1858, 2. F., 215–218.— **Virchow** (R.) Ueber das Vorkommen von Quecksilber in den Knochen. Arch. f. path. Anat., etc., Berl., 1860, xviii, 364–367.— **Vleminckx** (J.-F.) Observation d'une glossite survenue par l'ingestion du mercure. J. de méd., Brux., 1829, i, 31–35.—**Waitz** (F. A. C.) Kurze Schilderung der Hydrargyromanie und Hämatomanie, oder Quecksilber- und Blutwuth unter den Aerzten in Ostindien. Arch. f. med. Erfahr., Berl., 1830, i, 507–566.— **Werbeeck du Chateau.** Beobachtungen über die schädlichen Wirkungen der Quecksilberdünste, und besonders das Zittern der Gliedmassen, welchen die mit jenem Metalle umgehenden Arbeiter unterworfen sind, mit Bemerkungen von Prochaska. Med. Jahrb. d. k. k. österr. Staates, Wien, 1814, ii, 3. St., 95–113.— **Whitley** (G.) Report on the occurrence of mercurial poisoning among persons who work with mercury and its preparations. Rep. Med. Off. Privy Council 1863, Lond., 1864, 358–362.— **Williams** (C. T.) Black deposit in the large intestine from the presence of mercury. Tr. Path. Soc. Lond., 1867, xviii, 111–114.— **Wising** (P. J.) Ett fall af kronisk kvicksilverförgiftning. (C. r. Sur un cas de mercurialisme chronique

Mercury (*Toxicology of, and accidents from*).

simulant la sclérose en plaques, no. 22.) Nord. med. Ark., Stockholm, 1880, xii, no. 17, 1-48, 1 pl.—**Woodman** (W. B.) Cases of chronic mercurial poisoning from the use of pink and red vulcanite in artificial gums, with remarks and experiments. Med. Press & Circ., Lond., 1874, ii, 502–504.—**Zambelli** (V.) Tre casi di mortale infiammazione ventrale avvenuta dietro l' uso esterno di sali metallici e principalmente mercuriali. Gior. anal. di med., Milano, 1828, x, 130–143.—**Zeissl.** Zur Hydrargyrose. Med.-chir. Centralbl., Wien, 1878, xiii, 87. *Also:* Aerztl. Ber. d. k. k. allg. Krankenh. zu Wien (1876), 1877, 238–241.

Mercury (*Vapors of*). [*Includes mercurial fumigations, etc.*]

VON SCHRÖTTER (A. R.) Ueber einen Vorschlag von G. G. Stokes, die schädlichen Wirkungen der Quecksilberdämpfe ganz oder theilweise zu beseitigen, und über das Verhalten von Jod und Schwefel zu diesen Dämpfen. 8°. [*n. p.*, 1872.]

Accidens attribués aux émanations mercurielles. Ann. d'hyg., Par., 1842, xxviii, 227–229.—**Bedford** (J. R.) On mercurial vapour baths. Indian Ann. M. Sc., Calcutta, 1855, ii, 589–597.—**Brame** (C.) Recherches sur la vapeur de mercure. Rec. d. trav. Soc. méd. d'Indre-et-Loire, Tours, 1849, 93–95.— **Burnett** (W.) An account of the effect of mercurial vapors on the crew of his majesty's ship Triumph, in the year 1810. Phil. Tr., Lond., 1823, 402–408. *Also:* Med.-Chir. Rev. & J., Lond., 1823-4, iv, 1010–1014.— **Byrne** (W. S.) Calomel fumigation. Lancet, Lond., 1880, i, 128.—**Clark** (A.) The calomel vapour bath. Brit. M. J., Lond., 1872, i, 211. — **De Lasiauve.** Troubles variés de l'appareil sensitif et moteur, attribués à l'action de la vapeur mercurielle; procès devant la police correctionnelle. Expérience, Par., 1840, vi, 385–389.— **Diffusion** (Sur la) des vapeurs de mercure; théorie et application. Lyon méd., 1872, ix, 72–77. — **Extract** of a letter from Lisbon, giving an account of a singular effect of the fumes of quicksilver in the crews of two ships on that station. Edinb. M. & S. J., 1810, vi, 513.—**Gibson** (A.) Practical observations on mercurial fumigation. Loud. M. & Phys. J., 1825, liv, 12–21.— **Grapin.** Des effets des vapeurs mercurielles sur l'homme; stomatite mercurielle. Arch. gén. de méd., Par., 1845, ii, 327–338.— **Kane** (F. B.) Mercurial fumigation; description of a new apparatus. Dublin J. M. Sc., 1874, lviii, 392–397.—**Lamprey** (J.) On the use of the calomel vapour bath. Med. Times & Gaz., Lond., 1870, i, 507.—**Langlebert** (E.) Note sur un nouveau procédé pour l'emploi des fumigations cinabrées. Arch. belges de méd. mil., Brux., 1856, xvii, 339–341.— **Lee** (H.) The calomel vapor bath. Brit. M. J., Lond., 1862, i, 53; 195. ———. Note on the use of the calomel vapour bath. Lancet, Lond.. 1878, i, 193.— **Ollivier & de l'Orne** (R.) Rapport médico-légal relatif à des accidents attribués aux émanations mercurielles. Expérience, Par., 1841, vii, 1–8.—**Paschkis** (H.) Ueber Quecksilber-Räucherungen. Vrtljschr. f. Dermat., Wien, 1878. v, 415–432. — [**Pollock.**] Improved lamp for calomel fumigation in the treatment of various forms of syphilitic affections. Lancet, Lond., 1857, i, 262.—**Solles** (E.) Résultat de l'absorption des vapeurs de mercure dans l'organisme. J. de méd. de Bordeaux, 1880–81, x, 325; 338.— **Sundelin.** Ueber die durch das Einathmen der Quecksilberdämpfe entstehende Krankheit und ihre Behandlung. Arch. f. med. Erfahr., Berl., 1820, i, 550–558.— **Szabo** (F.) A cinnober-füstölési kuruzs lásnak orvosi megfigyelése. [Cinnabar fumigation by a quack.] Gyógyászat, Budapest, 1883, xxiii, 361–365. *Also, transl.:* Pest. med.-chir. Presse, Budapest, 1883, xix, 671.—**Taylor** (A. S.) Chronic poisoning by mercury through the skin and lungs; death after four years. Guy's Hosp. Rep., Lond., 1864, 3. s., x, 173–179.— **Werneck.** Von der Zinnober-Räucherungskur, oder von der Heilung der Syphilis mittelst auf die äussere Oberfläche geleiteter Zinnober-Dämpfe. J. f. Chir. u. Augenh., Berl., 1830, xiv, 229–234, 1 pl.— **Whistler** (W. MacN.) Local mercurial fumigations. Brit. M. J., Lond., 1880, ii, 881.

Mercury (*Ammonio-chloride of*).

EDHEM-BEY (H.) *Erweiterte Studien über die Umsetzung des Merkur-Ammoniumchlorids. 8°. Bern, 1885.

Cockle. Case of poisoning by ammonio-chloride of mercury. Med. Times & Gaz., Lond., 1882, i, 302.— **Deakin** (S.) Unusual symptoms following applications of unguentum hydrargyri ammoniati. Brit. M. J., Lond., 1883, ii, 1281.— **Giles** (J.) Case of poisoning by white precipitate. Lancet, Lond., 1857, ii, 9.— **Graham** (A. R.) Poisoning by white precipitate. Brit. M. J., Lond., 1869, i, 329.—**Green** (W. E.) Unusual symptoms following the use of unguentum hydrargyri ammoniati. *Ibid.*, 1884, i, 853.—**Hardy** (H. N.) On a case of poisoning by white precipitate. *Ibid.*, 1876, ii, 76.— **Kerner.** Eine tödtliche Vergiftung durch weisses Quecksilberpräcipitat.

Mercury (*Ammonio-chloride of*).

Med. Ann., Heidelb., 1835, i, 479–482.—**Michael** (W. H.) Poisoning by white precipitate. Assoc. M. J., Lond., 1857, ii, 909. — **Moore** (E. H.) Fatal poisoning by white precipitate. Brit. M. J., Lond., 1885, ii, 15.—**Pavy** (F. W.) On the physiological effects of white precipitate on animals. Guy's Hosp. Rep., Lond., 1860, 3. s., vi, 504–510, 1 pl.—**Shout** (A. C.) Case of suspected poisoning by white precipitate. Med. Times & Gaz., Lond., 1860, i, 444. — **Stephens** (E.) Three cases of poisoning by precipitate powder, taken in mistake for milk of sulphur. Brit. M. J., Lond., 1876, i, 781. — **Stevenson** (T.) Poisoning by white precipitate. Guy's Hosp. Rep., Lond., 1874, 3. s., xix, 415. — **Taylor** (A. S.) On poisoning by white precipitate. *Ibid.*, 1860, 3. s., vi, 483–504.

Mercury (*Bichloride, or corrosive chloride, of*).

See, also, **Mercury** (*Hypodermic use of*).

BARBETTE (N.-L.) *Du sublimé corrosif, ou deuto-chlorure de mercure, et de son action sur l'économie animale. 4°. *Paris*, 1826.

BROHM (G. L.) *De balneis hydrargyro muriatico corrosivo medicatis. sm. 8°. *Berolini*, [1836].

HIRSCHEL (L. E.) Betrachtungen über den itzigen innerlichen Gebrauch des Mercuri sublimati corrosivi und des Schierlings in verschiedenen Krankheiten. 2. Aufl. 12°. *Berlin*, 1765.

JACOBI (F.) Descriptio methodi mercurium sublimatum corrosivum tutius copiosiusque exhibendi. 8°. *Monasterii Westphalorum*, 1785.
Also, in: HOFFMANN (C. L.) Opusc. lat. med. arg. 8°. *Monast. Westphal.*, 1789, 243–264.

JOSEPH (G.) *Hydrargyrum bichloratum corrosivum quid in respiratione cordisque actione efficiat? 8°. *Gryphiæ*, 1858.

LAVORT (J.-B.-A.) *Considérations médicales sur le muriate de mercure suroxigéné, ou sublimé corrosif. 8°. *Paris, an X* [1802].

LETTRE de M. Sibuet, adressée à Marie de Saint-Ursin, insérée dans le No. 34 de la Gazette de santé. Réponse de MM. Lajoie, médecin; Marcelot, chirurgien; et Dorez, pharmacien. 4°. [*n. p., n. d.*]

MEURER (F.) *De vitandis in præscribendo mercurio sublimato corrosivo vitiis. 4°. *Lipsiæ*, [1826].

MÜLLER (C. F.) *Diss. de hydrargyro muriatico corrosivo. 4°. *Halæ*, [1825].

PRUD'HON (E.-H.) *Sur le sublimé corrosif, considéré comme agent chimique, toxicologique et thérapeutique. 4°. *Paris*, 1824.

RÜST (J. C. F.) *De mercurii sublimati corrosivi natura et usu. 8°. *Rostochii*, 1829.

STOCKHAUSEN (A. F.) *De mercurii sublimati corrosivi usu medico interno. sm. 4°. *Halæ Magdeb.*, [1758].

Almès (H.) Note sur le sublimé employé comme reconstituant. Union méd., Par., 1869, viii, 158–162.—**Amelang** (F.) Ueber die äusserliche Anwendung des Sublimats in Geschwüren und chronischen Ausschlags-Krankheiten. J. f. Chir. u. Augenh., Berl., 1828, xii, 325–332.—**Barbut.** Observations et remarques sur le sublimé corrosif. J. de méd., chir., pharm., etc., Par., 1776, xlvi, 38–44.— **Baumes.** Observation sur les effets du sublimé corrosif dans les maladies de la lymphe. *Ibid.*, 1778, lvii, 423–430.— **Behrend.** Ueber die Anwendung des Sublimats nach Dzondi. J. d. pract. Heilk., Berl., 1830, lxx, 5. St., 37–49.—**Chantourelle.** Expériences sur l'action du deuto-hydrochlorate de mercure. J. gén. de méd., chir., pharm., etc., Par., 1822, lxxxi, 309–331.—**Coze.** Mémoire sur l'action du sublimé corrosif, sur les fluides du corps humain et sur la réaction de ces mêmes fluides sur le sublimé corrosif. J. de méd., chir., pharm., etc., Par., 1789, lxxx, 29–80.—**D. & P.** Ueber die Bereitung der Sublimat-Verbandstoffe nach der neuen Beilage 5 der Kriegs-Sanitäts-Ordnung. Deutsche mil.-ärztl. Ztschr., Berl., 1887, xvi, 311–321.—**Davy** (J.) Some observations on corrosive sublimate. Phil. Tr., Lond., 1822, 357–366. ———. On the action of corrosive sublimate on the textures of the human body. *In his:* Researches, Phys. & Anat., 8°, Lond., 1839, ii, 279–289.— **Fonssagrives.** Sublimé; pharmacographie. Dict. encycl. d. sc. méd., Par., 1883, 3. s., xii, 480–500.—**Gardiner** (J.) A particular method of giving the corrosive sublimate mercury in small doses as an anthelmintic. Essays & Obs. Phil. Soc. Edinb., 1771, iii, 380–

Mercury (*Bichloride, or corrosive chloride, of*).

394.—**Giacosa** (P.) Sullo siero di latte al sublimato nella medicazione antisettica. Ann. di chim. e di farm., Milano, 1886, 4. s., iii, 152–157. — **Haasbaure.** Beitrag zur Empfehlung der Sublimatbäder bei Flechten und chronischen Fussgeschwüren. J. f. Chir. u. Augenh., Berl., 1831, xv, 144–146.—**Heine** (J.) Ueber die Anwendung des Quecksilbersublimats in einer häufigen Form der Pneumonie und im Hospitalbrande, eingeleitet durch parteiische Betrachtungen über den modernen Typhus und einige Entwicklungsstufen der Humoralpathologie. Ztschr. f. rat. Med., Heidelb., 1844, i, 355–390.—**Heraeus** (W.) Sublimatdämpfe als Desinfectionsmittel. Ztschr. f. Hyg., Leipz., 1886, i, 235–242. — **Hochstetter.** Die Sublimatbäder. Memorabilien, Heilbr., 1858, iii, 24–27.—**Ives** (L.) On the effects of the corrosive sublimate of mercury. Cases & Obs. M. Soc. N.-Haven County, 1788, 42. — **Keraudren.** Des propriétés du sublimé corrosif pour la conservation du bois, et des effets de cette préparation sur la santé des marins. Mém. Acad. de méd., Par., 1835–6, v, 41–63.—**Kreibohm.** Zur Desinfection der Wohnräume mit Sublimatdämpfen. Ztschr. f. Hyg., Leipz., 1886, i, 363–368.—**Marle** (M.) Ueber den Einfluss des Quecksilbersublimats auf die Magenverdauung. Arch. f. exper. Path. u. Pharmakol., Leipz., 1875, iii, 397–411.—**Masserotti** (V.) Intorno all' iodoidrargirato di bicloruro di mercurio. Esculapio napol., Napoli, 1848, xxvi, 54; 108; 167.— **Maut.** Observations sur l'usage intérieur du sublimé-corrosif. J. de méd., chir., pharm. etc., Par., 1777, xlviii, 396–405.—**Meyer** (V.) Versuche über die Haltbarkeit der Sublimatlösungen. Centralbl. f. Chir., Leipz., 1887, xiv, 449–453. — **Pibrac.** Sur l'usage du sublimé corrosif. Mém. Acad. roy. de chir., Par., 1768, iv, 153–163.—**Plummer** (J. T.) Corrosive sublimate as a vesicant. Med. Counsellor, Columbus, 1856, ii, 505–508. — **Pserhofer.** Sublimat. Ztschr. f. Nat.- u. Heilk in Ungarn, Oedenburg, 1856, vii, 1–3.— **Rollet.** Note sur l'emploi thérapeutique du bi-chlorure de mercure dissous dans l'huile d'amandes douces. Gaz. méd. de Lyon, 1858, x, 63.—**von Rothmund** jun. Einige Bemerkungen über die Anwendung des Sublimats. Festschr. d. ärztl. Ver. München, etc., 1883, 296–300.— **Smith** (A. H.) On the tolerance of corrosive sublimate in small and frequent doses. Med. Rec., N. Y., 1884, xxvi, 312.—**Some** observations upon the use of corrosive sublimate. Med. Obs. Soc. Phys. Lond., 1762, ii, 70–87.—**Spender** (J. K.) The function of bichloride of mercury in the treatment of diseases of the skin. J. Cutan. M., Lond., 1870–71, iv, 186–190. — **Theden** (J. C. A.) Vertheidigung des innerlichen Gebrauchs des Sublimats. Med.-chir. Ztg., Salzb., 1791, ii, 373–376. — **Thoulouse** (E.) Des applications de la poudre impalpable de sublimé corrosif. Abeille méd., Par., 1876, xxxiii, 217–221. — **Walter.** Ueber die äusserliche Anwendung des Quecksilbersublimats bei venerischen Geschwüren und Feigwarzen. J. d. Chir. u. Augenh., Berl., 1823, v, 138–141.—**von Wedekind** (F.) Ueber den Gebrauch des Sublimatwassers. J. d. pract. Heilk., Berl., 1822, lv, 2. St., 3; 3. St., 36. — **Wendelstadt.** Bruchstücke aus meiner Erfahrung über die ausgezeichnete Wirksamkeit des ätzenden salzsauren Quecksilbers (Sublimats), nicht nur bei venerischen, sondern auch mancherlei andern Krankheiten. *Ibid.*, 1809, xxviii, 5. St., 69–77.—**van Wy** (J.) Ueber eine besondere Bereitung des ätzenden Sublimats. N. Samml. d. auserl. u. n. Abhandl. f. Wundärzte, Leipz., 1785, 8. St., 246–268.—**Wykissaly** (W.) Diss. med. de mercurii sublimati corrosivi in hylide efficaci tutoque usu. Viennæ, 1780. *In:* Weiz (F. A.) Neue Ausz. [etc.], 12°, Frankf. u. Leipz., 1782, xv, 68–82.

Mercury (*Bichloride of, Antidotes to*).

Azione del ferro sopra del sublimato corrosivo. Esculapio napol., Napoli, 1840, xviii, 302–305.—**Beddow** (G.) Dr. Buckler's proposed antidote to mercurial poisons. Lancet, Lond., 1841–2, i, 643–645.—**Bostock** (J.) Experiments to ascertain how far the presence of albumen and muriatic acid interfere with action of bichloride of mercury and protomuriate of tin upon each other. Edinb. M. & S. J., 1825, xxiii, 65–69.—**Buckler** (T. H.) On the use of gold-dust and iron-filings as a galvanic antidote to corrosive sublimate, and all the other poisonous compounds of mercury. Maryland M. & S. J., Balt., 1840, i, 52–63. *Also:* Lancet, Lond., 1841–2, i, 569–572. — **Dumouceau** & **Planchon.** Observations sur le contrepoison du sublimé corrosif. J. de méd., chir., pharm., etc., Par., 1778, xlix, 36–39.—**Evans** (J.) An account of the good effects of alkaline salts in counteracting the poison of corrosive sublimate. Med. & Phys. J., Lond., 1809, iii, 535.—**Johnston** (C.) On gold dust and iron filings, as an antidote for corrosive sublimate. Am. J. M. Sc. Phila., 1863, n. s., xlv, 339–342.—**Lassaigne** (J.-L.) Recherches sur la nature et les propriétés du composé que forme l'albumine avec le bichlorure de mercure. J. de chim. méd., etc., Par., 1836, 2. s., ii, 458–460; 1837, 2. s., iii, 161; 213.—**Orfila.** Note sur le nouvel antidote du sublimé corrosif proposé par M. Mialhe. [Protosulphuret of iron.] *Ibid.*, 1843, 2. s., ix, 10–12.—**Poumet** (J.-Y.) Recherches et ex-

Mercury (*Bichloride of, Antidotes to*).

périmentations sur le proto-chlorure d'étain, considéré comme contre-poison du deuto-chlorure de mercure. Ann. d'hyg. Par., 1845, xxxiv, 181; 408. *Also*, Reprint.—**Schrader** (L.) Eiweiss und Magnesiahydrat als Antidota bei Sublimatvergiftungen. Deutsche Klinik, Berl., 1854, vi, 87; 399.

Mercury (*Bichloride of, Toxicology of*).

See, also, **Ovariotomy** (*Antiseptic method in*).

BARBÉ (R.-J.) *Sur l'empoisonnement par le sublimé corrosif. 4°. Paris, 1820.

BRAYER (A.-B.) *Sur l'empoisonnement par le subliué corrosif. 4°. Paris, 1814.

CHAUSSIER (F.) Consultations médico-légales sur une accusation d'empoisonnement par le sublimé corrosif. 8°. Paris, 1811.

MANCEL (P.-N.) *De l'empoisonnement par le deuto-chlorure de mercure. 4°. Paris, 1830.

ORLOFF (P. E.) *K voprosu o kolichestvennom opredelenii rtuti v trupach jivotnych otravlennych sulemojou. [Quantitative analysis of mercury in animal body poisoned by corrosive sublimate.] 8°. St. Petersburg, 1880.

PLANCHE(L.-A.) *Essai sur l'action réciproque de quelques sels ammoniacaux et de l'oximuriate de mercure (sublimé corrosif), pour servir à l'histoire de l'empoisonnement par ce sel métallique; précédé d'observations sur un nouveau sel ammoniacal. 4°. Paris, 1815.

Alibert. Eczéma produit par le sublimé corrosif en frictions: dartre squammeuse humide; herpes squammosus madidans de Alibert. Ann. de méd. belge, Brux., 1837, iv, 25.—**Anderseck & Hamberger.** Zwei Fälle von Sublimat - Vergiftung durch Salbe; Obductions - Bericht. Vrtljschr. f. gerichtl. u. öff. Med., Berl., 1864, n. F., i, 187–210.—**Anderson** (C.) Case of severe affection of the stomach, produced by the external application of an alcoholic solution of muriate of mercury. Edinb. M. & S. J., 1811, vii, 437–439.—**Anderson** (H.) Case of poisoning by corrosive sublimate. *Ibid*, 1818, xiv, 474–476.—**Andrew** (J.) Case of poisoning with corrosive sublimate. Month. J. M. Sc., Lond. & Edinb., 1845, v, 102–104.—**Annan** (R.) Fatal periostitis from the incidental external use of corrosive sublimate. Med. Times, Lond., 1846, xiv, 381.—**Arnozan & Vaillard.** Lésions du pancréas chez un lapin empoisonné par du sublimé. J. de méd. de Bordeaux, 1883-4, xiii, 223. *Also:* Bull. Soc. d'anat. et physiol. . . . de Bordeaux, 1883, iv, 31.—**Auer** (L.) Ein Fall von Sublimat-Vergiftung. Aerztl. Int.-Bl., München, 1860, vii, 609.—**Barthélemy.** Empoisonnement accidentel par le deuto-chlorure de mercure. Ann. d'hyg., Par., 1880, 3. s., iv, 337–344. *Also:* Soc. de méd. lég. de France. Bull., Par., 1880-81, vi, 368–375.—**Berthod.** Accouchement normal; huit injections vaginales avec solution de sublimé à 1-2000 pendant les suites de couches; mort. Gaz. méd. de Par., 1887. 7. s., iv, 219.—**Bigham** (J. G.) Sudden death from corrosive sublimate. Am. M. Times, N. Y., 1862, iv, 347.—**Blacklock** (A.) Case of poisoning with corrosive sublimate. Edinb. M. & S. J., 1831, xxxvi, 92–94.—**Boardman** (J.) Report of cases of poisoning by corrosive sublimate. Buffalo M. J., 1858-9, xiv, 196–199.—**Bogg** (T. W.) A case of poisoning by corrosive sublimate. Lancet, Lond., 1878, ii, 877.—**Browne** (H. P.) Case of poisoning from corrosive sublimate and white lead; recovery. Dublin M. Press, 1861, xlv, 121.—**Buchannan** (W.) Case of poisoning by corrosive sublimate. Lond. M. Reposit., 1823, xix, 374–376.—**Budd** (W.) A case of disease produced by taking one ounce of corrosive sublimate; successfully treated. Phila. M. Museum, 1806, ii, 180–183. *Also:* Med. & Phys. J., Lond., 1807, xviii, 347–349.—**Burwell** (B.) Case of poisoning by corrosive sublimate successfully treated. Am. J. M. Sc., Phila., 1841, n. s., ii, 515.—**Butcher** (R. G. H.) On poisoning by corrosive sublimate injected into the vagina. Dublin Q. J. M. Sc., 1856, xxi, 242.—**Butte** (L.) De l'intoxication par le sublimé corrosif employé comme antiseptique. Compt. rend. Soc. de biol., Par., 1886, 8. s., iii, 491–493. *Also:* Ann. d'hyg., Par., 1887, 3. s., xvii, 167.—**Cabot** (S.) Poisoning by corrosive sublimate. Boston M. & S. J., 1861, lxv, 218–220. *Also:* Extr. Rec. Bost. Soc. M. Improve. (1859-61), 1862, iv, 233–235.—**Cadbury** (R.) Salivation from corrosive sublimate dressings. Phila M. Times, 1883-4, xiv, 952.—**Carey** (H. G.) Fatal poisoning from corrosive sublimate. Med. & Surg. Reporter, Burlington, N. J., 1856, ix, 209.—**Case** of death from oxymuriate of mercury. Med. & Phys. J., Lond., 1819, xli, 204–206.—**Caso** di veneficio mortale per sublimato corrosivo. Gazz. med. ital, prov. venete, Padova, 1859, ii, 169–171.—**Cazals.** Observation sur un empoisonnement volontaire par dépit amoureux, contre lequel l'eau à la glace a été employé avec succès. Ann. clin. de Montpel., 1810, xxiii, 337–343.—**Charl-**

Mercury (*Bichloride of, Toxicology of*).

ton (E.) Fatal case of poisoning by corrosive sublimate. Birmingh. M. Rev., 1872, i. 211.—**Charrin & Roger** (G.-H) Des lésions intestinales dues à l'action du sublimé. Compt. rend. Soc. de biol., Par., 1886, 8. s., iii, 359–361.—**Chaussier & Marc.** Gerichtlich-medicinische Untersuchungen über eine zweifelhafte Vergiftung durch Sublimat; nebst einem Vorworte von A. Henke. Ztschr. f. d. Staatsarznk., Erlang., 1824, 3. Ergnzungshft., 1–69.—**C[héron]** (J.) Contributions à l'étude de l'intoxication par le sublimé en obstétrique. Rev. méd.-chir. d mal. d. femmes, Par., 1885, vii, 5–10.—**Chevallier** (A.) Empoisonnement par le sublimé corrosif. J. de chim. méd., etc., Par., 1834, x, 723–727.—**Chevallier & Bastien.** La solution de sublimé corrosif précipite-t-elle l'infusion du thé? *Ibid.*, 1838, 2. s., iv, 516–518.—**Church** (H. M.) On a case of poisoning by corrosive sublimate. Edinb. M. J., 1886-7, xxxii, 795–800.—**Clark** (P. J.) Poisoning from corrosive sublimate in obstetrical practice. Med. Rec., N. Y., 1886, xxx, 345.—**Clevenger** (S. V.) Corrosive sublimate poisoning. Chicago M. Rev., 1880, i, 251. —**Coale** (W. E.) Poisoning by corrosive sublimate; death on the 11th day. Am. J. M. Sc., Phila., 1851, n. s., xxi, 47–49. *Also:* Extr. Rec. Bost. Soc. M. Improve , 1848-53, i, 107–109.—**Coghlan** (J.) Case of poisoning by corrosive sublimate. Med. Times & Gaz., Lond., 1860, i, 162.—**Cummings** (A. I.) Poisoning by bi-chloride of mercury. Boston M. & S. J., 1852, xlvi, 78.—**Da Camin** (F.) Cura di avvelenamento provocato con una dose sorprendente di sublimato corrosivo incojato e condotta felicemente a termine. Gior. per serv. ai progr. d. patol., Venezia, 1837, vi, 84–100.—**Da Costa** (J. M.) Mercurial poisoning from fumes of corrosive sublimate, followed by abscess of the abdominal wall in the hepatic region (supposed to be a sequela of typhoid fever); pleural effusion; death. Hosp. Gaz., N. Y., 1879, vi, 339–341.—**Dahl** (F.) Anatomischer Nachtrag zu dem Sublimatvergiftungsfalle des Prof. Stadfeldt. Centralbl. f. Gynäk., Leipz., 1884, viii, 195.—**Dakin** (W. R.) On mercurialism in lying-in women undergoing sublimate irrigation. Tr. Obst. Soc. Lond. (1886), 1887, xxviii, 281–307.—**Degner** (J. H.) Relatio historica de casu singulari quo per mercurium sublimatum in emplastro adplicatum mors inducta fuit. Acta Acad. nat. curios., Norimb., 1742, vi (app.), 1–36.—**Deutsch.** Vergiftung durch Quecksilber-Sublimat. Med. Ztg. Berl., 1851, xx, 153.—**Devergie** (A.) Observation extraite d'un rapport fait à M. le procureur du roi, sur un empoisonnement par le sublimé corrosif. Arch. gén. de méd., Par., 1825, ix, 461–471. ——. Mémoire sur la valeur des moyens proposés pour reconnaître le sublimé corrosif dans les empoisonnements. Ann. d'hyg., Par., 1834, xi, 411–440. *Also:* J. hebd. d. progr. d. sc. et inst. méd., Par., 1834, i, 205; 245.—**Dimidoff** (A.) Sulema, kak sred., oplotnja. mozge. [Sublimate as a remedy affecting the brain.] Vrach, St. Petersb., 1887, viii, 472–474.—**Doléris & Butte** (L.) Recherches expérimentales sur l'intoxication par le sublimé employé pcur le lavage des muqueuses saines et des plaies. Compt. rend. Soc. de biol., Par., 1886, 8. s., iii, 562–567. *Also:* N. Arch. d'obst. et de gynéc., Par., 1886, i, 739–756.—**Downs** (H. S.) Case of poisoning by corrosive sublimate, and death ensuing in forty hours. Tr. M. Soc. N. Y., Albany, 1861, 69–71.—**Dumm** (A. W.) Poisoning by corrosive sublimate. Ohio M. Recorder, Columbus, 1877, ii, 162–164.—**Durrant** (C. M.) Poisoning by corrosive sublimate; death in four days. Prov. M. & S. J., Lond., 1850, 369.—**Eade.** Case of poisoning with corrosive sublimate. Lancet, Lond., 1870, i, 302.—**Eller.** Gutachten über eine vermuthete Vergiftung. Repert. f. d. öff. u. gerichtl. Arzneyw., Berl., 1789, i, 248–253. —**Elsässer** (M.) Sublimatvergiftung im Wochenbett. Centralbl. f. Gynäk., Leipz., 1884, viii, 449–451.—**Empoisonnement** par le sublimé corrosif. Ann. d'hyg., Par., 1835, xiii, 225–227.—**Empoisonnement** par le sublimé corrosif donné comme calomel. J. de chim. méd., etc., Par., 1855, 4. s., i, 530–535.—**Empoisonnement** par le sublimé corrosif, suivi de mort le 12e jour. Gaz. d. hôp., Par., 1859, xxxii, 445.—**Fiorioli della Lena** (V.) Avvelenamento per biclorur di mercurio. Gazz. med. di Torino, 1885, xxxvi, 457–463.—**Fleischmann** (C.) Tödliche Sublimatvergiftung nach einer zweimaligen Scheidenausspülung. Centralbl. f. Gynäk., Leipz., 1886, x, 761–765. —**Fraenkel** (E.) Ueber toxische Enteritis im Gefolge der Sublimatwundbehandlung. Arch. f. path. Anat., etc., Berl., 1885, xcix, 276–288.—**Fraser.** Case of poisoning with corrosive sublimate. Med. Chron., Montreal, 1857, iv, 163–165.—**Fries.** Fall von Sublimat-Vergiftung. Verhandl. d. Ver. pfälz. Aerzte 1863, Kaiserslautern, 1864, 13.—**Fritsch** (H.) Bemerkung zu dem Aufsatz des Dr. Keller. Centralbl. f. Gynäk., Leipz., 1885. ix, 513.—**Glover** (R. M.) On the absorption of corrosive sublimate in cases of poisoning. Lancet, Lond., 1844, ii, 57.—**Goff** (W. W.) Poisoning with perchloride of mercury. Northwest M. & S. J., Chicago, 1851-2, viii, 405–407.—**Hacker.** Sehr starke Mundaffection nach kleinen Gaben Sublimat. Summ. d. Neuest. u. Wissenswürd. a. d. ges. Med., Leipz., 1836, n. F., ii, 277–280.—**Halla.** Sublimat-Vergiftung. Med.-chir. Centralbl., Wien, 1878, xiii, 441.—**Hastreiter.** Sublimatekzem. Med.-chir. Cor.-Bl. f. deutsch am. Aerzte,

Mercury (*Bichloride of, Toxicology of*).

137.—**Venables** (R.) Fatal cases of poisoning with corrosive sublimate; with the analysis and detection of the poison after incessant vomiting and purging through a survival of eight days. Lond. M. Gaz., 1831, viii, 616–623.—**Vigla.** Empoisonnement volontaire par le sublimé corrosif, suivi de mort le douzième jour. Monit. d. sc. méd. et pharm., Par., 1859, vii, 94–96. *Also:* J. de chim. méd., etc., Par., 1860, 4. s., vi, 15–20.—**Vincent** (E. B.) Poisoning by corrosive sublimate. Clinic, Cincin., 1873, v, 85.—**Vöhtz** (J. C.) Sublimatforgiftning gennem intrauterin Injektion efter Abort. Hosp.-Tid., Kjøbenh., 1884, 3. R., ii, 557–561.—**Wade.** † Lancet, Lond., 1848, i, 500.—**Wanzer** (H.) Poisoning with corrosive sublimate. Chicago M. J., 1866, xxiii, 395.—**Watson** (A.) † Edinb. M. & S. J., 1840, liii, 404.—**Watson** (J.) † Month. J. M. Sc., Lond. & Edinb., 1844, iv, 375–379.—**Wegeler** (J.) Vergiftung durch Sublimat. Gen.-Ber. d. k. rhein. Med.-Coll. 1843, Koblenz, 1845, 112–114. *Also:* Wchnschr. f. d. ges. Heilk., Berl., 1846, 30–32.—**Wesselhoeft** (W.) A case of fatal poisoning by corrosive sublimate. N. Eng. M. Gaz., Bost., 1885, xx, 6–11.—**Westrumb** (A. H. L.) † Mag. f. d. ges. Heilk., Berl., 1834, xlii, 448–463.—**White** (J. C.) Death from corrosive sublimate; was bed-bug poison the preparation employed? Boston M. & S. J., 1861, lxv, 169–175. ——. Death from corrosive sublimate. Extr. Rec. Bost. Soc. M. Improve., 1862, iv (Suppl.), 193–200.—**Williams** (H. W.) Poisoning by corrosive sublimate. Am. J. M. Sc., Phila., 1851, n. s., xxi, 79–83.—**Wood** (A.) Account of a case of poisoning with corrosive sublimate. Edinb. M. & S. J., 1839, li, 114–121. *Also,* Reprint.—**Woodbury** (F.) A case of poisoning by corrosive sublimate. Phila. M. Times, 1872, li, 388.—**Wormley** (T. G.) Notes on some of the chemical reactions of corrosive sublimate. Chem. News, Lond., 1860, ii, 181; 193. *Also:* Columbus Rev. M. & S., 1860–61, i, 73–82.—**Wulfsberg.** Sublimatforgiftning. Forh. Norske med. Selsk. i Kristiania, 1885, 171–176.—**Ziliotto** (P.) & **Namias** (G.) Due casi di veneficio, uno per acidi minerali, l' altro per sublimato corrosivo. Gior. veneto di sc. med., Venezia, 1869, 3. s., x, 66–84.

Mercury (*Bichloride of*) *as a disinfectant.*

See, also, **Antiseptic** *obstetrics*; **Antiseptic** *surgery*; **Wounds** (*Treatment of*).

Cleland (W. L.) Albuminate of corrosive sublimate as a surgical dressing. Australas. M. Gaz., Sydney, 1885–6, v, 65.—**Dubois** (E.) Sur l'emploi du sublimé corrosif comme antiseptique. Livre jubil. publié p la Soc. de méd. de Gand, etc., Gand, 1884, 411–419.—**Kier** (J.) Om Sublimat som antiseptisk Saarbehandlingsmiddel. Hosp.-Tid., Kjøbenh., 1884, 3. R., ii, 577; 601; 627; 649.—**Ognibene** (A.) Il deutocloruro di mercurio nella cura delle piaghe e ferite usato in Italia da oltre venti anni. Gior. di med. mil., Roma, 1884, xxxii, 313–318.—**Olsen** (J.) Sublimat som Desinfektionsmiddel. Norsk Mag. f. Lægevidensk., Christiania, 1884, xiv, 899–901.—**Rudall** (J. T.) On the surgical use of perchloride of mercury as an antiseptic. Austral. M. J., Melbourne, 1887, n. s., ix, 268–272.—**Smith** (C.) Corrosive sublimate as a dressing in minor surgery. Glasgow M. J., 1887, [4.] s., xxvii, 21–25.—**Sternberg** (G. M.) The comparative antiseptic value of the salts and oxides of mercury. Med. News, Phila., 1885, xlvii, 287.—**Szabó** (D.) Sublimat mint fertőztelenítő. [Sublimate as a disinfectant.] Orvosi hetil., Budapest, 1884, xxviii, 1029–1037.—**Taniguchi** (Udzura). [Hydrarg. bichlor. as a surgical dressing.] Chiugai Iji Shinpo, Tokio, 1886, no. 142, Feb. 25.—**Vaughan** (V. C.) Considerations concerning the practical use of mercuric chloride as a disinfectant. Med. News, Phila., 1885, xlvii, 235.

Mercury (*Bromides of*).

Smith (P.) Bromide and bibromide of mercury as therapeutic agents. Brit. M. J., Lond., 1868, ii, 421.—**Werneck.** Therapeutische Versuche über das Brom-Quecksilber. J. f. Chir. u. Augenh., Berl., 1830, xiv, 215–229. *Also, transl.:* J. compl. du dict. d. sc. méd., Par., 1830, xxxviii, 349–358.

Mercury (*Chloride of*).

See, also, **Fever** (*Typhus, Treatment of*); **Mercury** (*Bichloride, etc., of*).

DE BRUIN (S.) * De uso medico muriatis hydrargyri oxydulati in morbo inflammatorio. 8°. *Traj. ad Rhenum,* [1817].

CONTI (G.) Innocuità della miscela degli acidi col mercurio dolce e sue indicazioni. 8°. *Napoli,* 1856.

CRUIKSHANK (W.) Remarks on the absorption of calomel from the internal surface of the mouth; accompanied with a preliminary sketch of the history and principal doctrines of absorp-

Mercury (*Chloride of*).

tion in human bodies. In a letter to Mr. Clare. 8°. *London,* 1779.

EXNER (C.) * De mercurio dulci novaque eum adhibendi methodo. 8°. *Berolini,* [1830].

FUNCKE (C.) * De salubri calomelanos in morbis tubi cibarii inflammatoriis effectu. 8°. *Berolini,* [1832].

HAVIGHORST (J.) * De singulari mercurii dulcis usu in desperatis quibusdam morbis. 4°. *Halæ Magdeb.,* 1724.

——. The same. 4°. *Halæ Magdeb,* 1745. *Also, in:* HALLER. Disp. ad morb. [etc.] 4°. *Lausannæ,* 1760, vii, 181–204.

HÖLZL (A.) * De calomele. 8°. *Vienœ,* [1832].

HOPFENGAERTNER (P. F.) * Diss. exhibens observationes et cogitata circa mercurii cum acido muriatico connubium. 4°. *Stuttgardiæ,* [1792].

HORNEMANN (C. J. E.) * De effectu atque usu majorum dosium calomellis. 8°. *Havniæ,* 1838.

——. * De rationibus dosium calomellis, imprimis majorum, zoochemicis. Resp. S. S. Neukirch. 8°. *Havniæ,* 1839.

——. The same. De viribus et rationibus majorum dosium calomellis. 8°. *Havniæ,* 1839.

INDELICATO (J.) Ensayo sobre el mercurio dulce, y sobre el abuso que se hace de este remedio en la América del Sud. 12°. *Lima,* 1837.

LITTHAUER (H.) * De calomelane modo Mialhiano in sanguinem inducendo. sm. 8°. *Berolini,* [1859].

MEYJES (W. P.) * Kalomel als Diureticum. 8°. *Amsterdam,* 1887.

MIEGE (J.) * De calomele. 8°. *Pragœ,* [1835].

OCKERSE (C. F. R.) * De mercurio dulci ejusque usu in morbis infantum et puerorum. 8°. *Traj. ad Rhenum,* 1823.

AB OETTINGEN (G.) * De ratione, qua calomelas mutetur in tractu intestinali. 8°. [*Dorpat*], 1848.

REBUSCA (A.) * De calomelis virtute pharmaco-dynamica. 8°. *Patavii,* 1834.

STOLLIUS (J. A.) * De mercurio dulci. sm. 4°. *Jenœ,* [1700].

WANNER (F. X.) * Ratio dulcificationis mercurii dulcis hincque pendentes effectus in medicina salutiferi. sm. 4°. *Argentorati,* [1747].

Amelung (F.) Over de nuttigheid van het zoet kwik bij ontstekingachtige ziekten. Pract. Tijdschr. v. de Geneesk., Gorinchem, 1841, xx. 235–262.—**Annesley** (J.) Observations on the use and abuse of calomel. Tr. M. & Phys. Soc. Calcutta, 1825, i, 211–226.—**B.** Saccharated calomel. Atlanta M. & S. J., 1874–5, xii, 75.—**Battey** (R.) Saccharated calomel. *Ibid.,* 1873–4, xi, 261–264.—**Bauwens** (C.) fils. De l'action des acides végétaux sur le calomel. Bull. Soc. de méd. de Gand, 1886, xxiii, 188–190.—**Bayles** (G.) Sedative action of calomel. Med. Rec., N. Y., 1879, xv, 453.—**Bellini** (R.) Contributo alla storia terapeutica del calomelano o proto-cloruro di mercurio. Sperimentale, Firenze, 1873, xxxi, 634–660.—**Blackwell** (E. T.) On calomel as a laxative and local antiphlogistic. Phila. M. Times, 1880, x, 522.—**Calegari** (G.) Sulla formazione del sublimato corrosivo in un miscuglio di calomelano e zucchero. Ann. di chim. applic. a. med., Milano, 1877, lxv, 193–195.—**Calomel** in the army. Chicago M. J., 1863, n. s., vi, 310–320.—**Calomel;** its uses and abuses. Med. & Surg. Reporter, Phila., 1867, xvi, 189.—**Capria** (D. M.) Nota sulle alterazioni del calomelano col sale ammoniaco, e con altri idroclorati. Esculapio napol., Napoli, 1840, xviii, 411–414. — **Cassoni** (E.) Sulla creduta decomposizione del calomelano per mezzo del ribes. Bull. d. sc. med. di Bologna, 1853, 3. s., xxiv, 429–444.—**Cazenave** (A.) Calomelas. Dict. de méd., 2. éd., Par., 1834, vi, 216–236.—**Coe** (H.) Remarks on the modus operandi of calomel. Atlanta M. & S. J., 1859, iv, 533.—**Coletti** (F.) Risposta ad alcuni quesiti sul calomelano e sul clorato di potassa. Gazz. med. ital., prov. venete, Padova, 1870, xiii, 173–175.—**Collins** (F. H.) Calomel as a diuretic. Med. Chron., Manchester, 1886, iv, 310.—**Cross** (J. C.) Note on the sedative action of calomel. West. & South. M. Recorder, Lexington, Ky., 1841–2, i, 193–198. —

Mercury (*Chloride of*).

Curtis (C. R.) Why such quantities of calomel are consumed in the Western States. West. M.-Chir. J., Keokuk, 1852, ii, 231–236.—**Delioux.** De l'incompatibilité du calomel et des émulsions d'amandes. Gaz. hebd. de méd., Par., 1855, ii, 551.— **Depaire** (J.-B.) Sur les variétés de chlorure mercureux employées en médecine; moyen de les distinguer et de reconnaitre les falsifications du calomel à la vapeur. Bull. Acad. roy. de méd. de Belg., Brux., 1853-4, xiii, 220–223.— **Diez** (M. A.) Accion fisiolójica y terapéutica del protocloruro de mercurio. Escuela méd., Carácas, 1874-5, i, 21-24: 1875-6, ii, 58; 105.— **Discussion,** in the College of Physicians and Surgeons of Lexington, on the action of calomel in health and disease. Transylv. J. M., Lexington, Ky , 1837, x, 457 - 475. — **Duckworth** (D.) On the modern neglect of calomel in certain disorders. Practitioner, Lond., 1876, xvii, 1-6. *Also,* Reprint.—**Duclos.** Mémoire sur l'emploi du calomel à doses fractionnées. Bull. gén. de thérap., etc., Par., 1846, xxxi, 10; 85; 166.—**Effects** (On the) of calomel in producing slimy stools in children. Lond. M. & ˚S. J., 1829, ii, 343–346.—**Fonssagrives.** Du rôle du calomel dans la médecine anglaise. Bull. gén. de thérap., etc., Par., 1861, lxi, 481-489. ——. Calomel. Dict. encycl. d. sc. méd., Par., 1870, xi, 714-727.—**Freund** (C. H.) Einiges über die Bereitungsart und Anwendung des Calomels in England. Allg. med. Centr.-Ztg., Berl., 1843, xii, 1-5.—**Gaston** (E.) Cases, illustrative of the sedative and antiemetic effects of calomel in large doses. Tr. Belmont M. Soc., Bridgeport, Ohio, 1849-50,39-51.—**Girin.** Note sur l'emploi du calomel à doses fractionnées. J. de méd. de Lyon, 1847, 2. s., i, 605-613.—**Gisler** (N.) Het nut van de calomel in verscheide ziekten aangetoond. Geneesk. Verhandel. a. de k. Sweed. Acad. (Sandifort), Leiden, 1778, iv, 172-195.—**Graves** (R. J.) On the best method of administering calomel in acute inflammation. Dublin J. M. & Chem. Sc., 1834, vi, 57-61.—**Hatchett** (R. J. H.) Calomel an instantaneous nervous sedative. South. Clinic, Richmond, 1884, vii, 97-103.—**Hauser** (W.) Cases showing the advantage of heroic doses of calomel. Atlanta M. & S. J., 1857-8, iii, 518.—**Herzka** (J.) Das Calomel und seine Stühle. N. - York. med. Monatschr., 1852, i, 106-110.—**Higgins.** Note sur l'emploi thérapeutique du calomel. Union méd., Par., 1847, i, 638.—**Hoyt** (M.) Remarks on calomel. N. York M. & Phys. J., 1826, v, 567-573.— **Jackson** (S.) The use of calomel in the diseases of children. Tr. Coll. Phys. Phila , 1853-6, ii, 131-146. *Also:* Med. Exam., Phila., 1854, x, 129 -139.—**Jacobi** (P.) Provisional report on the sedative dose of calomel. [Proc.] Therap. Soc. N. Y., 1879. 67-89.—**Jeannel.** Théorie de la dissolution du calomel dans l'organisme. Mém. et bull. Soc. méd.-chir. d. hôp. de Bordeaux, 1869, iv, 57-63.— **Jendrássik** (E.) A calomel mint diureticum. Orvosi hetil., Budapest, 1885, xxix, 1301; 1329; 1357. *Also, transl.:* Pest. med.-chir. Presse, Budapest, 1885, xxi, 1017; 1037. *Also, transl.:* Deutsches Arch. f. klin. Med., Leipz., 1885-6, xxxviii, 499-524 —**Johnson** (J. M.) Saccharated calomel. Atlanta M. & S. J., 1874-5, xii, 277-286.—**Jolly.** Note sur l'altérabilité du calomel et sur les précautions à prendre pour son emploi thérapeutique. Bull. Soc. de méd. prat. de Par., 1877, 110-113. *Also:* France méd., Par., 1877, xxiv, 556.—**Joret.** Remarques pratiques sur l'emploi du calomélas en médecine. Arch. gén. de méd., Par., 1835, 2. s., vii, 34-51.—**Lente** (F. D.) On the sedative action of calomel in disease. N. York M. J., 1870, xi, 1-24. *Also,* Reprint.—**Letcher** (S. M.) On the use of calomel as a remedial agent. Transylv. J. M., Lexington, Ky., 1837, x, 648-654.—**Levick** (A. T.) Is calomel a cholagogue? St. Joseph M. Herald, 1883, i, 108-119.— **Limard.** Altération du calomel par l'eau de laurier cerise. J. Soc. de méd. et pharm. de l'Isère, Grenoble, 1879-80, iv, 46-50.—**McElroy** (Z. C.) Case illustrating the action of calomel as a tissue destructive. Cincin. M. Repert., 1869, ii, 69-73.—**McKee** (W. H.) Calomel in large doses as a diuretic in dropsies. Med. Exam., Phila., 1851, n. s., vii, 770-774.—**Mazade** (J.) Nouveaux faits touchant l'emploi thérapeutique du calomel à doses fractionnées. Bull. gén. de thérap., etc., Par., 1846, xxxi, 256-263.—**Means** (A.) Calomel; its chemical characteristics and mineral origin considered in view of its curative claims. South. M. & S. J., Augusta, 1845, i, 97-112.— **Merklein** (F.) Ueber die grünen Stühle, welche nach dem Gebrauche des Calomels im typhösen Fieber entleert werden. Allg. Ztg. f. Chir., etc., Augsb., 1843, iii, 49; 61; 76.—**Michéa.** Le calomel exerce-t-il une influence spéciale sur la sécrétion biliaire? Union méd., Par., 1848, ii, 495; 500.—**Müller** (J.) Weiteres über Quecksilberchlorid-Chlornatrium. Berl. klin. Wchnschr., 1871, viii, 589.—**Munnich** (J.) Beschouwing over de pharmacodynamische werking der kwikmiddelen, in het bijzonder van het calomel. Nat.- en geneesk. Arch. v. Neêrl. Indië, Batav., 1844, i, 563-598.—**Murray.** Experiments illustrative of the physiological effects of calomel on the gastrointestinal mucous membrane of dogs. Tr. M. & Phys. Soc. Bombay, 1841, iv, 3-26. ——. Observations on the good and bad effects of calomel in some of the diseases of India. *Ibid.,* 1842, v, 145-154.—**Orioli** (F.) Di una nuova indicazione terapeutica del calomelano, fondata

Mercury (*Chloride of*).

sulla sua azione diuretica finora non conosciuta. Gazz. med. di Roma, 1887, xiii, 289-295.—**Polk** (C. G.) Saccharated calomel. Phila. M. Times, 1874, iv, 552.—**Provisional** report on the sedative dose of calomel. N. York M. J., 1879, xxix, 639-650: xxx, 78-89.—**Rampold.** Ueber den Gebrauch des Calomel. Med. Ann., Heidelb., 1844, x, 252-281.—**Roucher** (C.) Recherches sur les chlormercurates mercuriques (oxydo-chlorures de mercure). Rec. de mém. de méd. . . . mil., Par., 1850, 2. s., v, 278-295.— **Saccharated** calomel. [Edit.] Atlanta M. & S J., 1874-5, xii, 61.—**Saxon** (W. H.) Saccharated calomel. *Ibid.,* 288.—**Schweich** (H.) Rührt die grüne Farbe der Calomelstühle von der Galle her, oder nicht? Jahrb. f. prakt. Heilk., Tübing., 1845, i, 102.—**Soubeiran** (E.) Calomelano, sua preparazione in polvere impalpabile. Esculapio napol., Napoli, 1843, xxi, 379; 435.—**Stone** (W.) Remarks upon certain pathological conditions of the gastrointestinal mucous membrane, and the effects of calomel. N. Orl. J. M., 1868, xxi, 653-659.—**Terray** (P.) Adatok a calomel húgyhajtó hatásához. [Calomel as a diuretic.] Orvosi hetil., Budapest, 1886, xxx, 805; 894; 912. *Also, transl.:* Pest. med.-chir. Presse, Budapest, 1886, xxii, 785-787.—**Torsellini** (D.) Della influenza della pepsina sulla solubilità del calomelano. Boll. d. Soc. tra i cult. d. sc. med. in Siena, 1886, iv, 5-7. *Also:* Ann. di chim. e di farm., Milano, 1886, 4. s., iv, 105-107.—**Vanoye** (R.) Sur un mode particulier d'administrer le calomel. Ann. Soc. méd. d'émulat. de la Flandre occid., Roulers, 1848, 349-353.—**Wassilieff** (N. P.) Ueber die Wirkung des Calomel auf Gährungsprozesse und das Leben von Mikroorganismen. Ztschr. f. physiol. Chem., Strassb., 1882, vi, 112-134. *Also, transl.:* Ejened. klin. gaz., St. Petersb., 1882, ii, 177; 205; 219. *Also, transl.* [Abstr.]: Brit. M.J., Lond., 1883, ii, 21.— **Weber** (*de Mulhouse*). Note sur l'emploi du calomel dans les affections typhoïdes. Gaz. méd. de Par., 1834, 2. s., ii, 724-726.—**Wedekind.** Einige Bemerkungen über den Gebrauch und den Missbrauch des Calomels in Entzündungskrankheiten. Arch. f. med. Erfahr., Berl., 1827, iv, 610-624.—**Winkler.** Ueber die angebliche Umwandlung des Kalomels in ätzendes Sublimat bei gleichzeitigem Gebrauche von Chlor, Salmiak und Salzsäure, mitgetheilt und bevorwortet von Graff. Ztschr. f. d. Staatsarznk., Erlang., 1848, lvi, 327-339.—**Wolff** (A.) & **Nega** (J.) Ueber die Resorption des Quecksilbers bei Verabreichung des Calomels in laxirender Dosis. Deutsche med. Wchnschr., Berl., 1885, xi, 847.—**Wood** (H. C.) On the use of calomel in functional hepatic diseases. Phila. M. Times, 1874, iv, 375.—**Yeats** (G. D.) Account of the good effects obtained from a combination of calomel and opium in inflammatory diseases; with observations on effects arising from the acetite of copper, and on some other important subjects in the practice of medicine. Ann. Med. 1802, Edinb., 1803, 2. lust., ii, 396-405.—**Zavadzki** (I.) O vlijan. kalomelja na gnienie jelchi i o prichine okraski kalomel. isprajnenii. [Effect of calomel on putrid bile and on the causes of color of calomel evacuations.] Vrach, St. Petersb., 1887, viii, 311; 332.

Mercury (*Chloride of, Toxicology of*).

See, also, **Salivation** (*Mercurial*).

DIALOGO fra li signori P. F. Giaccheri e B. Ciasomigo, autore del manoscritto: Riflessioni critiche intorno la questione se l' unione del mercurio dolce col sale ammoniaco sia venefica. 4°. *Genova,* 1788.

HUDSON (W. N.) An anti - calomel lecture, [etc.] 8°. *Pomeroy, Ohio,* 1854.

KINNIS (J.) * De effectibus muriatis hydrargyri noxiis. 8°. *Edinburgi,* 1814.

Bochardt (L.) Merkwürdige Krankengeschichte einer zufälligen Vergiftung mit vierzehn Drachmen Calomel, auf einmal genommen, mit einem glücklichen Ausgange. Allg. med. Ann., Leipz., 1827, 441-446.—**Bonnewyn** (H.) Empoisonnement par le calomel. Presse méd. belge, Brux., 1851, iii, 368; 405.—**de B[ordes]** (C.) Kwikvergiftiging, waarschijnlijk door calomel-houdende worm-koekjes. Nederl. Tijdschr. v. Geneesk., Amst., 1858, ii, 177-181.—**Brochin** (A.) Un cas d'empoisonnement par le calomel. Bull. Soc. de méd. prat. de Par., 1879, 59-61. *Also:* France méd., Par., 1879, xxvi, 307. *Also:* Art méd., Brux., 1879-80, xv, 130 - 132.—**Campbell** (W.) Premature labour; uterine hæmorrhage; death from an overdose of calomel. Scottish & North of Eng. M. Gaz., Edinb., 1843, i, 199-201.— **Coursserant.** Accidents toxiques survenus pendant l'administration du calomel. Rec. d. proc.-verb. . . . Soc. de méd. prat., Par., 1856, 8-11.—**De Cattanei di Momo** (L. F.) Sunto di alcune sperienze dirette ad avverare se il calomelano si commuta in sublimato corrosivo per i cloruri alcalini, capiti nella scialiva e negli umori che lubricano gli apparati digerenti degli animali, come annunciava il distinto chimico sig. Mialhe. Ann. univ. di med., Milano, 1840, xcvi, 356-377. ——. Nuove sperienze dirette a confermare che il calomelano, nell' economia animale vivente, non si cangia in sublimato corrosivo per l' azione dei

Mercury (Chloride of, Toxicology of).

cloruri alcalini. *Ibid.*, 1841, xcvii, 444–455.—**Engelmann** (F.) Fall von Erythema universale nach Gebrauch von Calomel. Berl. klin. Wchnschr., 1879, xvi, 647.—**Graves** (R.) & **Stokes** (W.) Fatal case of sloughing of the mouth and palate from a small dose of calomel. Dublin Hosp. Rep., 1827, iv, 299.—**Larocque** (A.) Cloruri alcalini, loro azione sul proto-cloruro di mercurio, fatti che servono alla loro storia. Esculapio napol., Napoli, 1843, xxi, 690–700.—**Löwenstein** (M. G.) Calomelvergiftung. Med. Ztg. Russlands, St. Petersb., 1851, viii, 67.—**Mitchell** (T. D.) Calomel considered as a poison. N. Orl. M. J., 1844–5, i, 28–35.—**d'Oliveira** (F. A.) Glosso-stomatite desenvolvida em sequencia a administração d'umas pilulas purgantes com calomelanos; dyscrasia; morte. J. Soc. d. sc. med. de Lisb., 1860, 2. s., xxiv, 45–51.—**Regimbeau.** Observations sur la décomposition du mercure doux par le sel ammoniac et les chlorures de potassium ou de sodium. J. Soc. de méd.-prat. de Montpel., 1840, ii, 73–80, 1 pl —**Rigaccini** (G. B) Un caso di morte per calomelano in un lattante. Arch. di patol. inf., Napoli, 1884, ii, 119–123.—**Robarts** (H. P.) Effects of swallowing nearly an ounce of calomel. Lond. M. Gaz., 1838, xxii, 610–612.—**Ruspini.** Il calomelano introdotto nel corpo umano può venire convertito in sublimato corosivo, in seguito all' uso contemporanco degli acidi vegetali? Bull. d. sc. med. di Bologna, 1863, 4. s., xix, 178–182.—**Spieringshoek** (H. W.) Waarneming eener vergiftiging door de murias hydrargyri. Ἱπποκράτης, Rotterd., 1819, iv, 18–24. — **Verne.** Recherches sur les altérations de calomel par le sucre, le sel marin et les acides. J. Soc. de méd. et pharm. de l'Isère, Grenoble, 1878–9, iii, 118; 213. *Also:* Bull. gén. de thérap., etc., Par., 1880, xcviii, 258–263.—**Visum** repertum über einen durch Selbstvergiftung mit Calomel Umgekommenen. *In:* Bernt (J.) Visa reperta [etc.], 8°, Wien, 1827, i, 374–378.

Mercury (Cyanide of).

Desmartes (T.-P.) De la supériorité du cyanure de mercure sur les autres préparations mercurielles contre la syphilis en général. Rev. de thérap. du midi, Montpel., 1854, vii, 308–317 : 1855, viii, 112–115.—**Moos.** Eine Cyanquecksilbervergiftung. Arch. f. path. Anat., etc., Berl., 1864, xxxi, 117–125. — Note sur l'emploi du cyanure de mercure dans le traitement de la syphilis. Bull. gén. de thérap., etc., Par., 1833, v, 139–144. — **Ollivier** (C.-P.) Mémoire sur l'empoisonnement par le cyanure de mercure. J. de chim. méd., etc., Par., 1825, i, 269–282.—**Tolmatscheff.** Einige Bemerkungen über die Wirkung von Cyanquecksilber auf den thierischen Organismus. Med.chem. Untersuch. a. d. Lab. . . . zu Tübing., Berl., 1867, 285–290. *Also,* Reprint.

Mercury (Iodides of).

See, also, **Acne** (*Treatment of*); **Donovan's** *solution.*

Bellini (R.) Contributo alla storia terapeutica degli ioduri e bromuri di mercurio. Sperimentale, Firenze, 1874, xxxiii, 372–389.—**Bolshesolski** (P. K.) Dvujoud. rtut, kak desinficiens pri laparotomii. [Biniodide of mercury as a disinfectant in laparotomy.] J. akush. i jensk. boliez., St. Petersb., 1887, i, 285–291. — **Bourgoin** (E.) Sur la solubilité de l'iodure mercurique dans l'eau et dans l'alcool. Bull. Acad. de méd., Par., 1884, 2. s., xiii, 1258–1260.—**Cameron** (C. A.) On mercuric iodate; its preparation and reactions. Analyst, Lond., 1876, i, 95–97. — **Carré.** Note sur le protoiodure de mercure contre les artropathies, les orchites, etc. Ann. de la chir. franç. et étrang., Par., 1843, viii, 173–181.—**Dannecy.** Analyse et formule d'une nouvelle combinaison de chlorure et d'iodure de mercure. J. de méd. de Bordeaux, 1858, 2. s., iii, 360–363.——. Nouveau procédé pour la préparation du chloro-iodure mercureux. *Ibid.*, 163–165.—**Döringer** (J.) Zur Pharmakodynamik des Hydrargyrum jodatum flavum. Allg. med. Centr.-Ztg., Berl., 1848, xvii, 705–707.—**Duchesne-Duparc.** Des propriétés physiologiques et thérapeutiques de l'iodochlorure mercureux. Gaz. d. hôp., Par., 1858, xxxi, 290. — **Foot** (A. W.) Paralysis of motion and sensation in the hand and forearm from local contact with cattle blister (red iodide of mercury); recovery. Dublin Q. J. M. Sc., 1873, lvi, 177–197.—**Gibert.** Note sur l'usage thérapeutique du deuto-iodure de mercure et sur un mode spécial d'administrer ce médicament. Bull. gén. de thérap., etc., Par., 1844, xxvi, 412–421. — **Le Canu.** Note pour le protoiodure de mercure. Année méd., Caen, 1877, ii, 9–11.—**Macnamara** (N. C.) Note on the use of biniodide of mercury. Indian Ann. M. Sc., Calcutta, 1862, viii, 184–186.—**Martin-Barbet** (L.) Un dernier mot sur l'iodure de chlorure mercureux. J. de méd. de Bordeaux, 1858, 2. s., iii, 553–558.—**Méhu** (C.) Sur la solubilité du biiodure de mercure dans les corps gras et dans quelques autres dissolvants. Bull. Acad. de méd., Par., 1885, 2. s., xiv, 1118–1124. — **Mialhe.** Réflexions chimico-thérapeutiques sur le composé de chlore, d'iode et de mercure, désigné sous le nom d'iodhydrargirite de chlorure mercureux. Union méd., Par., 1847, i, 63 —**Olioli** (A.) Il proto-ioduro di mercurio nella cura delle malattie veneree sarà tanto più utile, quanto più

Mercury (Iodides of).

verrà dato a dosi ripartite. Ann. univ. di med., Milano, 1875, ccxxxii, 418–420.—**Perrens** (J.) Observations critiques sur la constitution chimique et la préparation de l'iodure de chlorure mercureux. Union méd. de la Gironde, Bordeaux, 1857, ii, 34–38. — **Rieseberg.** Ueber die Wirkungsweise und Heilkraft des Hydrargyrum bijodatum rubrum bei äusserer Anwendung. Med. Ztg., Berl., 1847, xvi, 187.— **Rooney** (M.) The protiodide of mercury. Cincin. Lancet & Obs., 1869, n. s., xii, 1–7. — **Sadler** (M. T.) On the external use of red iodide (biniodide) of mercury in chronic glandular and other tumours. Med. Times & Gaz., Lond., 1864, n. s., i, 447.—**Smeets** (C.) Proto-en deuto-ioduretum hydrargyri, in veronderde syphilitische en scrophuleuse aandoeningen. Pract. Tijdschr. v. de Geneesk., Gorinchem, 1838, xvii, 97–124.—**Taylor** (M. K.) Case of poisoning by biniodide of mercury. Boston M. & S. J., 1870, v, 499–502. *Also,* Reprint.— **Vacher** (L.) De l'iodure double de mercure et de sodium en injections hypodermiques. Gaz. hebd. de méd., Par., 1885, 2. s., xxii, 794.—**Wolff.** Hydrargyrum jodatum flavum. Deutsche Klinik, Berl., 1869, xxi, 383.

Mercury (Metallic).

HARRIS (T.) A treatise on the force and energy of crude mercury, proving the usefulness and innocency of its internal application, by a great variety of experiments and histories of cases, acute and chronick. 2 pts. 8°. *London,* 1734.

HEINRICI (E. G.) * Diss. modum agendi virtutis resolventis mercurii vivi in corpore humano exponens. sm. 4°. *Halæ Magdeb.,* [1748].

KAAU (H.) * De argento vivo. sm. 4°. *Lugd. Bat.,* 1729.

MALLET (J. W.) On the density of solid mercury. 8°. [*n. p.,* 1877.]
Repr. from: Proc. Roy. Soc. Lond., 1877, no. 179.

RÖSELIUS (J. P.) De mercurii crudi usu interno. 4°. *Altdorfi,* [1704].

von Franque (J. B.) Anwendung von Mercurius vivus. Med. Jahrb. f. d. Herzogth. Nassau, Wiesb., 1859, v.-vi. Hft., 750.—**Kirchstein.** Zur Wirkung des Hydrargyrum depuratum. Berl. klin. Wchnschr., 1873, x, 437.—**Löwenhardt.** Ueber die innerliche Anwendung des laufenden Quecksilbers. [5 cases.] Med. Ztg., Berl., 1848, xvii, 53; 57.—**Magaziner** (M.) Das Quecksilber (Hydrargyrum vivum) als Volks- und sympathetisches Heilmittel. Med. Ztg. Russlands, St. Petersb., 1852, ix, 134. — **Maschka** (J.) Beibringung von metallischem Quecksilber im Kaffee bei einem tuberculösen Kinde; Tod; nicht nachweisbarer Zusammenhang; leichte Verletzung. Vrtljschr. f. gerichtl. u. öff. Med., Berl., 1858, xiii, 274–284.—**Möhsen.** Gutachten über e'ne mit rohem Quecksilber versuchte Vergiftung. Repert. f. d. öff. u. gerichtl. Arzneyw., Berl., 1791, i, 233–243.—**Vogler.** Einige Bemerkungen über die innere Anwendung des metallischen Quecksilbers. Deutsche Klinik, Berl., 1856, viii, 442–444. — . Zur inneren Anwendung des metallischen Quecksilbers. Med. Ztg., Berl., 1853, 63.

Mercury (Nitrate of).

See, also, **Hat-makers** (*Diseases of*).

CHAMBÉ (C.) * De l'empoisonnement par le nitrate acide de mercure. 4°. *Strasbourg,* 1857.

CHEVALLIER (A.) * De l'intoxication par l'emploi du nitrate acide de mercure chez les chapelliers. 4°. *Paris,* 1860.

GODART (A.) * De l'emploi du nitrate acide de mercure. 4°. *Paris,* 1826.
Also [Abstr.], *in:* Arch. gén. de méd., Par., 1826, x, 573: xii, 203.

Atthill (B.) On a new form of citrine ointment. Brit. M. J., Lond., 1886, i, 151. — **Bigsley** (J. J.) A case of poisoning by a solution of mercury in nitric acid. Lond. M. Gaz., 1830, vii, 329–331.—**Dymock** (W.) Note on the preparation of unguentum hydrargyri nitratis for use in India and other hot climates. Tr. M. & Phys. Soc. Bombay (1882), 1883, [3.] s., No. ii, 85.— **Empoisonnement** par le nitrate acide de mercure. J. de chim. méd., etc., Par., 1846, 3. s., ii, 734.—**Fauvel.** Observation d'un empoisonnement par le nitrate acide de mercure étendu d'eau. Bull. Soc. anat. de Par., 1837, xii, 175–181.—**Gale** (H. S.) Poisonous symptoms from the use of the acid pernitrate of mercury. Lancet, Lond., 1874, i, 41.—**Gay** (J.) On the external use of the solution of the pernitrate of mercury in epithelial cancer, lupus exedens, and the induration of chancre. Brit. M. J., Lond., 1862, i, 59–61.—**Lyster** (C. E.) Note on the use of acid nitrate of mercury solution. Liverpool M. & S. Rep., 1869, iii, 36–38.—**Ollivier.** Observations et rapport médico-légal sur des accidens déter-

Mercury (*Nitrate of*).

ɪᴢɪnés par l'usage externe du nitrate acide de mercure. Ann. d'hyg., Par., 1842, xxviii, 169–181. — **Scalzi** (F.) Avvelenamento per nitrato acido di mercurio; sintomi; autossia. Gior. med. di Roma, 1867, iii, 14–22, 1 pl. — **Vidal** (E.) Empoisonnement par une application de nitrate acide de mercure sur une large surface de la peau; mort le neuvième jour après l'accident. Compt. rend. Soc. de biol. 1863, Par., 1864, 3. s., v, 193–195. *Also:* France méd., Par., 1864, ii, 565.

Mercury (*Oleate and oleo-stearate of*).

Claiborne (J. H.) The discutient power of oleate of mercury and morphia. Gaillard's M. J., N. Y., 1886, xli, 477–480. — **Hilger.** Ueber ölsaures Quecksilber. Sitzungsb. d. phys.-med. Soc. zu Erlang., 1873-4, vi, 109–112. — **Jeannel** (J.) Combinaisons des oxydes de mercure avec les acides oléique et stéarique, au point de vue chimique pharmacologique. J. de méd. de Bordeaux, 1858, 2. s., iii, 728–740. — **Venot** (J.) Emploi de l'oléo-stéarate de mercure. *Ibid.*, 1857, 2. s., ii, 725–740. ——. Lettre au Dr. Ph. Ricord, sur l'emploi de l'oléo-stéarate de mercure. *Ibid.*, 660–664.

Mercury (*Oxides of*).

Braulik (J. T.) *De mercurio præcipitato rubro, adnexis binis historiis morborum clinicis. 8°. *Pragæ*, 1833.

Giesecke (E. A.) *De hydrargyriis præcipue oxydis. 4°. *Vitebergæ*, [1803].

Müller (M. A.) *De mercurio præcipitato rubro. 4°. *Monachii*, [1835].

Richter (J. T.) *De virtutibus mercurii cinerei Saunderi medicis. 4°. *Wittebergæ*, [1798].

Valli. Lettre à M. Astier, sur la découverte de la vertu antifermentescible de l'oxide rouge de mercure. 8°. [*Paris, n. d.*]

Allison (W.) Poisoning with the red precipitate of mercury. Lancet, Lond., 1836, i, 401. — **Blondeau** (L.) Quel est l'inventeur de la liqueur de van Swieten? Union méd., Par., 1880, 3. s., xxx, 594. — **Duquesnel.** De l'oxyde jaune de mercure obtenu par précipitation; son emploi pour la préparation des pommades opthalmiques. Bull. gén. de thérap., etc., Par., 1871, lxxxi, 73. — **Greiner.** Wirksamkeit des Mercurius præcipitatus ruber beim innerlichen Gebrauch desselben. Allg. med. Ann., Altenb., 1812, 757–759. — **Ibrelisle.** Considérations sur l'oxyde rouge de mercure, employé à l'extérieur, dans plusieurs formes de maladies de la peau. Exposé d. trav. de la Soc. d. sc. méd. de la Moselle, Metz, 1845, 52–64. — **Kennedy** (J.) Account of the phænomena produced by a large quantity of nitric oxide of quicksilver, swallowed by mistake; and of the means employed to counteract its deleterious influence. Med.-Chir. J. & Rev., Lond., 1816, i, 189–196. — **Martin.** Vergiftung mit Mercurius præcip. ruber, gehoben durch schnellen und häufigen Genuss von Milch. Ann. f. d. ges. Heilk., Karlsruhe, 1828, 152. — **Prince** (A.) Two cases of poisoning by the red precipitate powder. Lancet, Lond., 1859, ii, 506. — **Smyth** (F. S.) Poisoning by red precipitate. Brit. M. J., Lond., 1878, ii, 101. — **Stellwag von Carion** (K.) Das gelbe amorphe Quecksilberoxyd. Wien. med. Wchnschr., 1865, xv, 417; 437. — **Torri** (E.) Avvelenamento da deutossido di mercurio. Bull. d. sc. med. di Bologna, 1851, 3. s., xx, 299–302. — **Wecker** (L.) Du bioxyde de mercure hydraté, ou précipité jaune, et de son action thérapeutique dans les cas de conjonctivite pustuleuse et de kératite superficielle. Bull. gén. de thérap., etc., Par., 1862, lxii, 27–31. — **White** (R. P.) Case of poisoning by means of red precipitate. Irish Hosp. Gaz., Dubl., 1873, i, 308.

Mercury (*Peptonate of*).

See **Mercury** (*Hypodermic use of*).

Mercury (*Sulphur compounds of*).

Cadet (S.) *Intorno l' efficacia particolarmente anticolerica del solfuro nero di mercurio detto comunemente etiope minerale. 8°. *Roma*, [1874].

——. Esempj comprovanti l' uso interno del sottosolfato di mercurio ed esempj concorrenti a comprovare l' efficacia antilimica del solfuro nero di esso. Lettera al Erasmo Fabri-Scarpellini. 8°. *Roma*, 1875.

Repr. from: Corrisp. scient. in Roma, 1875, xxvii, no. 27.

——. Ragionamento inteso a comprovare la mirabile efficacia terapeutica del solfuro nero di mercurio detto comunemente etiope minerale in più nature di morbi particolarmente dei pesti-

Mercury (*Sulphur compounds of*).

lenziali e più particolarmente dell' indocolerico. 4°. *Roma*, 1875.

Repr. from: Atti. d. xi. cong. d. sc. ital. tenutosi in Roma nell' ottobre del 1873.

——. Nuovi esempj a comprovare la solenne efficacia antilimica del solfuro nero d' idrargiro. Lettera al Erasmo Fabri-Scarpellini. 8°. *Roma*, 1877.

Clauderus (G.) *De cinnabari nativa hungarica, longa circulatione in majorem efficaciam fixata et exaltata. sm. 4°. *Jenæ*, 1694.

Demetrius (P.) De medicis cinnabaris viribus. 4°. *Lipsiæ*, [1778].

Hilscher (S. P.) [Pr.] I. De æthiope minerali. 4°. *Jenæ*, [1748].

——. The same. II. sm. 4°. *Jenæ*, 1748.

Hofsteier (J. A.) Kurtze Erörterung der Frage: Ob der natürliche und reingewachsene Zinnober, als eine Artzeney in den menschlichen Leib ohne Gefahr gebrauchet werden könne? sm. 4°. *Leipzig*, 1708.

——. Die vortreffliche Güte des natürlichen jedoch reingewachsenen Zinnobers, zur Bewahrung und Wieder-Erlangung menschlicher Gesundheit, entgegengesetzet dem unlängst von Johann Gottfriedt Beckern . . . wider die am Ende beygedruckte Erörterung der Frage: Ob der natürliche und rein-gewachsene Zinnober, [etc.] 4°. *Schlesswig*, 1711.

——. De cinnabari nativa. Resp. Paulo Dons. 4°. *Hafniæ*, [1714].

Lindner (J. C.) *De cinnabaris inertia medica. 4°. *Francof. ad Viadr.*, [1743].

Also, in: Cartheuser (J. F.) Diss. nonn. select. phys.-chym. ac med. 12°. *Francof. ad Viadr.*, 1775, 1-27.

Oetinger (F. C.) *Cinnabaris exul redux in pharmacopolium cum auctore se publico examini sistens. 4°. *Tubingæ*, [1760].

Palm (R.) *Ueber die schwefelbasischen Quecksilbersalze. 8°. *Dorpat*, 1861.

Ponyrka (D.) *De anathymiasi cinnabaris. sm. 4°. *Argentorati*, [1780].

Richter (J. E.) *De medicamentorum mercurialium cum salibus paratorum efficacitate, per adjunctum sulphur ad certos quosdam morbos magis accommodanda. sm. 4°. *Halæ Magdeb.*, [1754].

Schrommius (J. F.) *De æthiope minerali. sm. 4°. [*Altorf*, 1725.]

Stroehlin (J. G.) *De cinnabare factitia vulgari, cinnabari nativæ et antimonii non solum æquiparanda, sed et præferenda. 4°. *Argentorati*, [1749].

Wedelius (G. W.) [Pr.] De minio lunari. 4°. *Jenæ*, [1695].

Divers (E.) & **Shimidzu** (T.) Mercury sulphites, and the constitution of sulphites. J. Chem. Soc., Lond., 1886, xlix, 533–590. — [**Letheby.**] Poisoning by turpeth, or turbith mineral. Tr. Path. Soc. Lond., 1846-8, i, 109–112. — **Love.** Poisoning from sulpho-cyanide of mercury. St. Louis M. & S. J., 1882, xlii, 291–294. — **Lowndes** (H.) A case of poisoning by turbith mineral. Med. Times & Gaz., Lond., 1863, ii, 195. — **McPhedran** (A.) A case of poisoning by turpeth mineral; death. Med. News, Phila., 1883, xliii, 682. — "**Medicus.**" Poisoning by turpeth mineral. Med. & Surg. Reporter, Phila., 1884, l, 93. — **Minnowski** (J.) O siarku rtęci (æthiops mineralis), jako środku lekarskim, skutecznym w cholerze. Gaz. lek., Warszawa, 1871, x, 449-454. — **Murino** (A.) Sull' etiope minerale, o solfuro nero di mercurio. Sperimentale, Firenze, 1873, xxxi, 527. — **Porcher** (F. P.) Use of black sulphuret of mercury (Ethiops mineral) as a means of destroying the effects of contagion, cholera, diphtheria, croup, etc. Results of the recent experience of Italian physicians. Charleston M. J. & Rev., 1875-6, iii, 10–16. — **Randolph** (N. A.) & **Roussel** (A. E.) On certain untoward effects following the administration of turpeth mineral. Med. News, Phila., 1884, xliv, 275. — **Smirnoff** (G. A.) O vlijanii sierovod. na jivotnii organ. s pribavlen. niekotor. dannich k patolog. Cheyne-Stokes dichanija. [Effect of turpeth mineral on the animal organism, and some remarks on Cheyne-Stokes respiration.] Arch.

Mercury (*Sulphur compounds of*).

klin. vnutren. boliez. Botkina, St. Petersb., 1883, ix. pt. 1, 413–558, 2 diag.—**Taylor** (A. S.) Case of poisoning by turpeth mineral; early occurrence of intense salivation; death in eleven days from forty grains. Guy's Hosp. Rep., Lond., 1864, 3. s., x, 180–183.—**Valori** (G.) [Quanto posso dirle intorno al nuovo solfuro nero di mercurio chiamato comunemente Etiope minerale ch' ella, si compiacque osservare nella mia farmacia.] Gior. med. di Roma, 1870, vi, 324–326. *Also*, Reprint.

Mercury (*Tannate of*).

Dornig (J.) Ueber Hydrargyrum tannicum. Wien. med. Wchnschr., 1885, xxxv, 856–860.—**Pauly** (J.) Ueber Hydrargyrum tannicum. Berl. klin. Wchnschr., 1884, xxi, 752.

Mercury *in urine.*

MICHAILOVSKI (J.) *O vidielenii mocheju rtuti pri terapevt. upotreb. eja v forme mazei. [Presence in the urine of mercury during its different applications in the form of ointment.] 8°. *St. Petersburg*, 1886.

MÜLLER (E.) * Untersuchung über die Ausscheidung des Quecksilbers durch den Harn während der Inunctionscur. 8°. *Hameln*, 1879.

SUCHOFF(A.) *O vidielenii mochejou rtuti pri terap. upotreblenii razlich. eja preparat. v forme pod kojnich vprisk. [Mercury in the urine in its different therapeutical preparations, and in the form of subcutaneous injections.] 8°. *St. Petersburg*, 1886.

Also, in: Voyenno-med. J., St. Petersb., 1886, cIvi, pt. 1, 43: clvii. 1: 65.

Alsberg (A.) Ueber den Nachweis von Quecksilber im Harn nach Einstäuben von Calomel in den Bindehautsack. Arch. f. Augenh., Wiesb., 1880, ix, 413–416. — **Borovski** (V.) O vidiel. rtuti mochei. [Proportion of mercury in the urine.] Russk. Med., St. Petersb., 1886, iv, 391.—**Harvey** (E. R.) The influence of mercury upon the urine. Brit. & For. M.-Chir. Rev., Lond., 1862, xxix, 515–520.—**Hayes** (P. S.) Metallic mercury found in the urine following the administration of the green iodide. Chicago M. Gaz., 1880, i, 155.—**Jourda.** Observation sur un malade qui, traité par le muriate suroxygéné de mercure, a rendu avec ses urines du mercure revivifié. J. de méd., chir., pharm., etc., Par., 1813, xxvii, 244–248.—**Mayençon & Bergeret.** Moyen clinique de reconnaître le mercure dans les excrétions et spécialement dans les urines; de l'élimination et de l'action physiologique du mercure. Mém. et compt.-rend. Soc. d. sc. méd. de Lyon (1873), 1874, xiii, pt. 1, 3–21. [Discussion] pt. 2, 15–17. *Also:* Lyon méd., 1873, xii, 82; 164; 383.—**Mayer** (A.) Versuche über den Nachweis des Quecksilbers im Harne. Med. Jahrb., Wien, 1877, 29–38. — **Milutin** (M.) K voprosu ob otkritii rtuti v mochie liechiv. merkuriem. [Detection of quicksilver in the urine in mercurial treatment.] Ejened. klin. gaz., St. Petersb., 1886, vi, 63–68. — **Oberländer.** Versuche über die Quecksilberausscheidungen durch den Harn nach Quecksilberkuren. Vrtljschr. f. Dermat., Wien, 1880, vii, 487–515, 3 tab. — **Shumovski** (V.) O vwidailenie rtutnikh s.edimnii mocheyu. [On mercurial preparations in the urine.] Med. Vestnik, St. Petersb., 1864, iv, 145; 153; 161.—**Spillmann** (P.) De l'élimination du mercure pendant et après le traitement mercuriel et des procédés de recherche du mercure dans les urines, applicables à la clinique. Ann. de dermat. et syph., Par., 1882, 2. s., iii, 721–723. — **Timbal-Lagrave** (A.) De la recherche du mercure dans les urines. Rev. méd. de Toulouse, 1879, xiii, 237; 381.

Mercury seal traps *versus* sewer gas and malaria. 5 l. 8°. *Philadelphia*, 1883.

Mercus Doornik (J. J. F. H. T.) Verslag omtrent de ziekten welke in het jaar 1855 binnen Amsterdam geheerscht hebben. Namens de 6de Commissie (Épidemiologie) van den Geneeskundigen Kring aldaar. 124 pp., 1 plan. 8°. *Amsterdam, Metzler & Basting*, 1856.

de Mercy [François-Christophe-Florimond] [1775–1849]. Σύνοψις πυρετῶν, conspectus febrium, synopsis des fièvres, ou tableaux de plusieurs maladies, tirés des 1er et 111e liv. des épidémies d'Hippocrate, avec le texe grec et les versions interlinéaires française et latine, accompagnés de notes grammaticales et de l'explication des termes de médecine; ouvrage spécialement destiné aux étudians en médecine. xiv, 352 pp. 8°. *Paris, Valade*, 1808.

de Mercy (F.-C.-F.)—continued.

——. De l'enseignement médical, dans ses rapports avec la chimie, considérée comme science accessoire à la théorie de la médecine; suivie d'un nouveau plan d'organisation des sociétés de médecine et de chirurgie et des études médicales, pour le maintien de la chaire d'Hippocrate, fondée aux écoles de médecine de Paris. iv (2 l.), 128 pp., 1 l. 8°. *Paris, J.-M. Eberhart*, 1819.

——. Mémoire de M. le docteur . . . [sur les traductions d'Hippocrate]. 31 pp. 12°. *Paris, V. Renaudière*, 1820.

Bound with: HIPPOCRATES. Nouvelle traduction des aphorismes, etc. 12°. *Paris*, 1821, ii.

——. Demande d'exécution de la loi du 14 frimaire an 3, pour le rétablissement d'une chaire d'Hippocrate fondée aux écoles de médecine de Paris, portée sur le programme des cours et les thèses, et réclamation d'encouragemens pour la continuation de la traduction française et édition grecque complète des œuvres d'Hippocrate. 23 pp. 4°. [*n. p.*, 1820.] [P., v. 858.]

——. Au roi. Considérations sur le rapport de la Faculté de médecine de Paris, pour le maintien de la chaire d'Hippocrate, fondée aux écoles de médecine. [2 memoirs.] 4, 4 pp. 4°. [*Paris*, 1820, *vel subseq.*] [P., v. 858.]

——. Demande du rétablissement d'une chaire d'Hippocrate. Année 1821. Mémoire pour la Commission de l'instruction publique. 46 pp. 12°. *Paris, V. Renaudière*, [*n. d.*]

Bound with: HIPPOCRATES. Nouvelle traduction des aphorismes, etc. 12°. *Paris*, 1821, ii.

——. Traités d'Hippocrate, des préceptes, de la décence, de médecin. Traduits en français, et le texte en regard revu et corrigé sur les manuscrits de la bibliothèque du roi, avec l'analyse de ces traités. ix, 135 pp. 8°. *Paris, J.-M. Eberhart*, 1824.

See, also, **Hippocrates.** Nouvelle traduction des aphorismes d'Hippocrate, etc. 12°. *Paris*, 1817. ——. The same. 2 v. 12°. *Paris*, 1821. ——. Traités de la nature de l'homme, de l'ancienne médecine, des humeurs, de l'art médical. 12°. *Paris*, 1823. ——. Traités de l'ostéologie, du cœur, [etc.] sm. 8°. *Paris*, 1831.—**Tourlet.** Article de [etc.] 8°. *Paris*, 1824.

Merdier (Louis-Charles). * Des symptômes de la goutte irrégulière. II. [etc.] 41 pp. 4°. *Paris*, 1838, No. 192, v. 331.

Mère (La) et l'enfant. Journal illustré d'hygiène de la première et de la seconde enfance. Rédigé sous la direction du Dr. Caradec. [Monthly.] Année 1–2, May, 1885, to May, 1886. fol. *Paris.*

Méreau (Adolphe). * De l'héméralopie, ou cécité nocturne, considérée surtout au point de vue de l'étiologie et du traitement. 34 pp. 4°. *Paris*, 1860, No. 134.

Meredig (Theophilus Daniel.) * De occulta et chronica jecinoris inflammatione. 60 pp. 8°. *Dorpati, lit. M. G. Grenzii*, 1811.

Meredith (Charles). * An inaugural dissertation on phthisis pulmonalis. 28 pp. 8°. *Philadelphia, R. Cochran*, [1802].

Meredith (L. P.) The teeth and how to save them. 271 pp. 8°. *Philadelphia, J. B. Lippincott & Co.*, 1871.

——. Our teeth and their preservation . . . Popular lecture. 43 pp. 12°. *Cincinnati, Hitchcock & Walden*, 1875.

Meredith (W.) *et al.* A comprehensive minute, commemorative of Philip Syng Physick. 14 pp. 8°. *Philadelphia*, 1838.

Meredyth (Adolphus William Leodore Colomiati). On the duality of venereal ulcers. Paper read to the Harveian Society of London, on the 15th March, 1866. iv, 5–19 pp. 8°. *London, R. Hardwicke*, 1866.

Repr. from: Med. Mirror, Lond., 1866, iii.

Meredyth (A. W. L. C.)—continued.
——. On the rational employment of mercury in the treatment of syphilis. iv, 41 pp. 8°. *London, R. Hardwicke*, 1866. [*Also, in :* P., v. 90.]
For Biography, see Med.-Chir. Tr., Lond., 1884, lxvii, 8 (J. Marshall).

Merei (A. Schoepf). On spasms and convulsions of children. 27 pp. 8°. *Edinburgh, Sutherland & Knox*, 1850. [P., v. 41.]
Repr. from : Month. J. M. Sc., Lond. & Edinb., 1850, xi.

——. On the disorders of infantile development, and rickets; preceded by observations on the nature, peculiar influence, and modifying agencies of temperaments. vii, 218 pp. 8°. *London, J. Churchill*, 1855.

—— & **Whitehead** (J.) Children's diseases. First report of the Clinical Hospital for Diseases of Children, Stevenson square, Manchester, containing an account of the results of the first 530 patients there treated. 52 pp. 8°. *Manchester, Bradshaw & Blacklock*, 1856. [P., v. 526.]

Merejkovski (K.) O zadatchach i metodach izsledovanii phizicheskago razvitija dietei. [Recording physical development of children.] 60 pp. 8°. [*n. p., n. d.*]

Merenda (Joannes Petrus). Evacuandi ratio tribus in libris luculenter perstricta. 10 p. l., 203 pp., 23 l. 12°. [*Basileæ, excud. M. Isingrinius*, 1547.]

Mereness (Henry E.) Valedictory address delivered at the commencement exercises of the Albany Medical College, December 22, 1874. 14 pp. 8°. *Albany, N. Y., Van Benthuysen*, 1875.

Merens (Cornelius Gallis). * De dysphagia. 2 p. l., 72 pp., 2 l. 8°. *Lugd. Bat., J. C. Cyfveer*, 1835.

Mérentié (Étienne). * Recherches cliniques et anatomo-pathologiques sur quelques points de l'histoire du typhus (fièvre pétéchiale). 96 pp. 4°. *Paris*, 1857, No. 120, v. 607.

Méresse (Émile-Antoine-Benjamin). * Sur la lithotomie chez la femme. 32 pp. 4°. *Strasbourg*, 1823, v. 52.

Mereu (Giovanni). Brevi riflessi intorno alla prostituzione. 7 pp. 8°. *Cagliari*, 1880.

Mergaut (Charles-François). * De la méningite aiguë tuberculeuse des enfants. 1 p. l., 32 pp. 4°. *Strasbourg*, 1844, No. 124, v. 10.

de Mergeliza (M.) El cólera asiático. Método práctico para su tratamiento. 30 pp. 12°. *Madrid, E. Rubiños*, 1884.

Mergenbaum (Albert). * Der Magen- und Darmcatarrh der Kinder in den ersten Lebensjahren. 26 pp., 1 l. 8°. *Marburg, C. L. Pfeil*, [1870].
c.

Mergentheim.
See, also, **Cholera** (*Asiatic, History, etc., of*), **Fever** (*Typhus, History, etc., of*), *by localities.*
BAUER. Mergentheim und seine Heilquellen. 8°. *Mergentheim*, 1830.
KRAUSS (F.) Beschreibung der Mineralquelle zu Mergentheim im Königreich Württemberg. 12°. *Stuttgart*, 1853.
Herz (J. B.) Ein Wort für Mergentheim. Würzb. med. Ztschr., 1862, iii, 38-43. *Also :* Med. Cor.-Bl. d. württemb. ärztl. Ver., Stuttg., 1862, xxxii, 132–134 —**Höring** sen. Carlsbad bei Mergentheim. Med. Cor.-Bl. d. württemb. ärztl. Ver., Stuttg., 1862, xxxii, 75. ——. Karlsbad bei Mergentheim. Kurzer Bericht über die Badesaison 1865. *Ibid.*, 1866, xxxvi, 127.—**Mergentheimer** (Das) Bad. *Ibid.*, 1837, vii, 272; 281.

Merger (Jules). * Quelques propositions sur l'hygiène des femmes en couches. 21 pp. 4°. *Paris*, 1835, No. 208, v. 288.

Mergiletus (Augustus Fridericus). * De rosa de Jericho, vulgo dicta. 14 pp. sm. 4°. *Argentorati, J. F. Spoor*, [1700].
——. * De pica. 26 pp. sm. 4°. *Argentorati, J. F. Spoor*, 1701.

Mergui.
Waring (E. J.) Medical notes on the Burmese, locality of Mergui. Indian Ann. M. Sc., Calcutta, 1853, i, 93–109.

Merian (Alfons). * Studien an gesteinsbildenden Pyroxenen. [Basel.] pp. 251–315. 8°. *Stuttgart, E. Schweizerbart*, 1884.
Cutting from : N. Jahrb. f. Mineralogie, etc., Beilageband iii.

Merian (Joachimus).
See **Sylvius** (Franciscus Delobe). Opera medica, [etc.] 4°. *Traj. ad Rhenum*, 1695. ——. The same. fol. *Venetiis*, 1707.

Méric (Jules). * Recherches sur l'introduction de l'air et des gaz qui le constituent (oxygène, azote, acide carbonique) dans le système veineux. 44 pp. 4°. *Paris*, 1866, No. 107.

de Méric (Victor) [1811–76]. On prophylactic and curative syphilization. 24 pp. 8°. *London, J. Churchill*, 1853.
Repr. from : Lancet, Lond., 1853, i.

——. Lettsomian lectures on syphilis. Delivered before the Medical Society of London in 1858. 68 pp. 8°. *London, J. Churchill*, 1858.
Repr. from : Lancet, Lond., 1858, ii.

——. Cases of syphilitic affection of the third nerve, producing mydriasis with and without ptosis. Read in the surgical section before the annual meeting of the British Medical Association in Leeds, July, 1869. 9 pp. 8°. *London, T. Richards*, [1869]. [P., v. 1441.]
Repr. from : Brit. M. J., Lond., 1869, ii.
For Biography, see Lancet, Lond., 1876, ii, 413. *Also :* Proc. Roy. M. & Chir. Soc. Lond., 1877, viii, 188.

Mericamp (Jean-Paul). * Contribution à l'étude des arthropathies syphilitiques tertiaires. 94 pp., 1 l. 4°. *Paris*, 1882, No. 321.

Merida.
Dominguez (N.) Observaciones magneto-meteorológicas del Colegio católico de San Ildefonso, en el año de 1876. Emulacion, Mérida, 1877, iii, 50–52.—**Dondé** (J.) La comision nombrada para el análisis de las aguas [de Mérida]. *Ibid.*, 1873-4, i, 29; 41; 53.— **Estado** general de los fallecidos en todo el mes de 1877 con expresion de la causa de su fallecimiento. *Ibid.*, 1878, iii, 111–113.—**Temperatura** media de Mérida, 1873. *Ibid.*, 1873-4, i, 39; 61; 87.—**Villamil** (R.) Memoria sobre las epidemias que han reinado en Mérida desde el año de 1865 hasta el presente. *Ibid.*, i, 47–49.

Meriden. By-laws and city officers, adopted 1876. 29 pp. 8°. [*Meriden*, 1876.]

Meridies (Eugen) [1859–]. * Ein statistischer Beitrag zu den Entbindungen alter Erstgebärender. 51 pp., 1 l. 12°. *Greifswald, C. Sell*, 1883.

Mérielle (Pierre-Hector). * I. Des causes du cancer du foie. II. [etc.] 33 pp. 4°. *Paris*, 1839, No. 354, v. 347.

Merieux (J.-B., *dit* Édouard). * I. Des effets de la foudre sur les corps bruts et sur les animaux. II. [etc.] 26 pp. 4°. *Paris*, 1838, No. 57, v. 331.

Merigot de Treigny (Gabriel-Marie-Auguste). * Étude sur les hernies du gros intestin considérées spécialement dans les régions inguinale et crurale. 181 pp., 1 l. 4°. *Paris*, 1887, No. 143.

Mérijot (Marcel). * De la rupture du tendon rotulien. 50 pp. 4°. *Paris*, 1873, No. 418.

Mérilhon (H.-C.) * Propositions sur les accouchemens; considérations relatives à l'hygiène des femmes nouvellement accouchées. 27 pp. 4°. *Paris*, 1830, No. 160, v. 233.

Merilhou (Louis-Martin). * Sur le scorbut. 18 pp. 4°. *Paris*, 1817, No. 161, v. 134.

Mérille (Adolphe). * Sur les abcès par congestion, provenant de la carie d'une ou de plusieurs vertèbres. 13 pp. 4°. *Paris*, 1834, No. 246, v. 276.

Mérimée (Cézaire-Ernest). * I. Du pronostic des affections tuberculeuses en général. II. [etc.] 22 pp. 4°. *Paris*, 1840, No. 385, v. 363.

Merindolus (Antonius) [1570–1624]. Ars medica in duas partes secta, in qua non solum ea explicantur quæ ad medicinam discendam sunt necessaria; sed multa etiam quæ theologos et philosophos recreare valeant, continentur. Accessit sub finem exercitationum medicinalium decas unica. 14 l., 419 pp., 14 l.; 1 p. l.; 153 pp., 7 l., port. fol. *Aquis-Sextiis, J. Roize*, 1633.

von Mering (Joseph) [1848–]. *Ein Beitrag zur Chemie des Knorpels. 23 pp. 8°. *Cöln, J. S. Steven*, [1873].

Merino (R. Rodriguez). La electricidad y el cólera. 20 pp. 8°. *Madrid, A. J. Alaria*, [1884].

Mériot (Hector) *De la grenouillette sublinguale. 40 pp., 2 l. 4°. *Paris*, 1883, No. 172.

Mériot (Paul). *Des indications et contre-indications de l'ovariotomie et du manuel opératoire. 34 pp. 4°. *Strasbourg*, 1861, No. 554, 2. s., v. 30.

Meriwether (Carolus). *De pneumonia. 2 p. l., 28 pp. 8°. *Edinburgi, Balfour et Smellie*, 1792.

Meriwether (Niles). [Circular in relation to the Waring system of sewers in Memphis. Dec. 1, 1882.] 1 sheet. 4°. [*Memphis*, 1882.]

Merizalde (José Felix).
See **Tourtelle** (Estevan). Epitome de los elementos de higiene [etc.] 8°. *Bogota*, 1828.

Merjeevski (I. P.) Ob uslovijach, blagoprijatstvujoutshich razvitiou dushevnych i nervnych bolieznei v Rossii, i o merach, napravlennych k ich umensheniiou. [On the conditions favoring development of insanity and nervous diseases in Russia, and on the means to diminish them.] 25 pp. 8°. *St. Petersburg, tipog. M. M. Stasoolevitcha*, 1887.

Merjevski (I.) *Klinicheskija izsliedovanija neistovich bolnich (Vesanici). [Clinical researches on insanity.] 59 pp. 8°. *St. Petersburg*, 1865.

Merk (Carl). *Ueber die thierische Bewegung. 2 p. l., 150 pp., 1 l. 8°. *Würzburg, F. E. Nitribitt*, 1818.

Merk (Joannes Matthias). *De curationibus ulcerum difficilium, præsertim in cruribus obviorum. 39 pp., 1 l. sm. 4°. *Gottingæ, F. A. Rosenbusch*, [1776].

Merkel (A. E. Ernestus). *Nonnulla de diabete mellito. 40 pp. 12°. [*Dorpat*], *typ. J. C. Schuenmanni*, 1835.

Merkel (C. F.)
See **Haddock** (Joseph W.) Somnolismus et psycheismus [etc.] 18°. *Leipzig*, 1852.

Merkel (Carl Ludwig) [1812–76]. *De nasi secretionibus specimen i. 28 pp. 4°. *Lipsiæ, typ. Staritzii*, [1838].

——. Anatomie und Physiologie des menschlichen Stimm- und Sprach-Organs (Anthropophonik). Nach eigenen Beobachtungen und Versuchen wissenschaftlich begründet und für studirende und ausübende Aerzte, Physiologen, Akustiker, Sänger, Gesanglehrer, Tonsetzer, öffentliche Redner, Pädagogen und Sprachforscher dargestellt von . . . xxiv, 976 pp. 8°. *Leipzig, A. Abel*, 1857.

——. The same. xxxx, 976 pp. 8°. *Leipzig, A. Abel*, 1863.

——. Die Funktionen des menschlichen Schlund- und Kehlkopfes, besonders beim Schlingen, Brechen, Athmen, Singen und Sprechen. Nach eigenen pharyngo- und laryngoskopischen Untersuchungen. viii, 156 pp., 1 pl. 8°. *Leipzig, O. Wigand*, 1862.

——. Physiologie der menschlichen Sprache (physiologische Laletik). viii, 444 pp. 8°. *Leipzig, O. Wigand*, 1866.

——. Der Kehlkopf, oder die Erkenntniss und Behandlung des menschlichen Stimmorgans im

Merkel (Carl Ludwig)—continued.
gesunden und erkrankten Zustande. xvi, 326 pp. 8°. *Leipzig, J. J. Weber*, 1873.
For Biography, see **Kuehn** (Car. Gott.)

Merkel (Christian Valentin). Wahre Ursachen der jetzt herschenden hitzigen Krankheiten mit der besten Verwahrungsart vor dieselben. Hauptsächlich für den gemeinen Mann und jungen Arzt aufgesetzt. 8 p. l., 88 pp. 12°. *Frankfurt u. Leipzig*, 1776.

——. *Observatio med.-chir. de sarcomate curato et summopere admirando.
In: WEIZ (F. A.) Neue Ausz., [etc.] 12°. *Leipzig*, 1777, vii, 59–64.
For Portrait, see **Collection**—van Kaathoven.

Merkel (Friderich [Sigmund]) [1845–]. *Ueber die Macula lutea des Menschen und die Ora serrata einiger Wirbelthiere. [Erlangen.] 2 p l., 20 pp., 2 pl. 4°. *Leipzig, W. Engelmann*, 1869.

——. The same. 2 p. l., 20 pp., 2 pl. 4°. *Leipzig, W. Engelmann*, 1870.

——. Die Zonula ciliaris. 1 p. l., 23 pp., 2 pl. 8°. *Leipzig, W. Engelmann*, 1870.

——. Die Linea nuchæ suprema, anatomisch und anthropologisch betrachtet. iv, 22 pp., 7 pl. 8°. *Leipzig, W. Engelmann*, 1871.

——. Die Muskulatur der menschlichen Iris. (Gratulationsschrift.) vi, 13 pp., 1 pl. 4°. *Rostock, Stiller*, 1873.

——. Das Mikroskop und seine Anwendung. xii, 324 pp. sm. 8°. *München, R. Oldenbourg*, 1875.

——. Die Anatomie zu Rostock. Vorlesung gehalten am 4. Nov. 1878 bei Beginn der Arbeiten in dem neuen anatomischen Institut. 16 pp. 8°. *Rostock, Stiller*, 1878.

——. Beiträge zur Kenntniss der postembryonalen Entwicklung des menschlichen Schädels. 22 pp., 7 pl. 4°. *Bonn, M. Cohen u. Sohn*, 1882.
Repr. from: Beitr. z. Anat. u. Embryol. J. Henle als Festgabe zum 4. April 1882 dargebracht von seinen Schülern.

——. Die Speichelröhren. iv, 28 pp., 2 pl. roy. 8°. *Leipzig, F. C. W. Vogel*, 1883.

——. Anleitung zur Muskelpräparation im Königsberger Präparirsaal. (Als Manuscript gedruckt.) 28 pp. 8°. *Königsberg i. Br., Gräfe u. Unzer* (*Dreher u. Stürtz*), 1884.

——. Handbuch der topographischen Anatomie. Zum Gebrauch für Aerzte. 1. Bd. 1. u. 2. Lfg. pp. 1–352, 1 tab. 8°. *Braunschweig, F. Vieweg u. Sohn*, 1885.
See, also, **Anatomisches** Institut zu Rostock. 8°. *Rostock*, 1874.

Merkel (G. Hermann). Microscopy in medical practice; its necessity demonstrated in the investigation of disease. 22 pp. 8°. *New York, A. Metz & Co.*, 1881.

——. Ozone, its merits as a disinfectant, antiseptic and anti-zymotic. 19 pp. 12°. *Boston, Rand & Avery*, 1884.
Repr. from: Tr. Am. Eclect. M. Ass., 1883.

Merkel (Gottlieb) [1835–]. *Zur Anatomie, Physiologie und Pathologie der Thränenableitungsorgane. 36 pp. 8°. *Erlangen, A. E. Junge*, 1859.

——. Die Staubinhalations-Krankheiten. 3. Aufl.
In: HANDB. d. Hyg., etc. 8°. *Leipz.*, 1882, 2. Theil, 4. Abth., 131–224.

——. Die neueren Anschauungen über das Wesen der Infektionskrankheiten; ihr Einfluss auf Haus und Gemeinwesen. Vortrag zu Gunsten der evangelischen Mägdeherberge gehalten. 28 pp. 8°. *Nürnberg, Ebner*, 1887.
See, also, **Handbuch** d. spec. Path. (Ziemssen), Leipz. 1874, i: 1875, viii, 2. Hft.—**Cyclopedia** Pract. Med. (Ziemssen), N. Y., 1878, viii.

Merkel (*Heinrich*).
Portrait in: **Collection**—van Kaathoven.

Merkel (J. G.) *Ueber Trepanation im Allgemeinen. 27 pp. 8°. *Würzburg, C. J. Becker,* 1860.

Merkel (Karl). *Beitrag zur Geschichte der Gastromalacie. 20 pp. 8°. *Marburg, C. L. Pfeil,* 1863.

Merkel (Wilhelm). *Beiträge zur pathologischen Entwicklungsgeschichte der weiblichen Genitalien. 36 pp., 1 pl. 8°. *Erlangen, A. E. Junge,* 1856.

Merker (Adolphus) [1817–]. *De vincturis immobilibus. 32 pp. 8°. *Berolini, typ. Nietackianis,* [1840].

Merkius (Henricus Andreas). De ventis incendii tempore orientibus. 9 l. 4°. *Lipsiæ, C. Goezius,* [1587].

Merkius (Michael). *Theses medicæ de venæsectione, ex lib. 2 de meth. med. Joh. Fernelij deductæ, et controversis quæstionibus decadem materia illustratæ. 30 pp. sm. 4°. [*Ulma*], *typ. J. Mederi,* 1622.

Merkl (Joannes Gallus). *De vulnere cum hæmorrhagia arteriosa complicato. 126 pp. sm. 4°. *Monachii, E. A. Fleischmann,* 1826.

Merkle (Max). *Uebersichts-Tabelle der wesentlichen Symptome der Brustfell- und Lungenkrankheiten. 37 pp. 8°. *Tübingen, F. L. Fues,* 1846.

Merklein (Fr.) *Ueber die grünen Stühle, welche nach dem Gebrauche des Calomels im typhösen Fieber entleert werden. 31 pp. 8°. *München, J. Deschler,* 1842.

Merklen (Pierre) [1852–]. *Étude sur l'anurie. 227 pp. 4°. *Paris,* 1881, No. 182.

Merkwürdige Krankengeschichten und seltene praktische Beobachtungen berühmter Aerzte. Ein Auszug aus den Abhandlungen der königlichen medizinischen Societät zu Coppenhagen. Aus dem Lateinischen. 2 p. l., 539 pp., 2 l. 8°. *Halle, Renger,* 1795.

Merland. Singulière affaire de simulation; deux accusés traduits devant trois juridictions; acquittements. 15 pp. 8°. [*Paris, E. Martinet,* 1864.]
Repr. from : Ann. d'hyg., Par., 1864, 2. s., xxii.

Merland (Constant). *Sur le choléra-morbus épidémique. 24 pp. 4°. *Paris,* 1832, No. 215, v. 254.

Merland (Henri). *Des tumeurs du pavillon de l'oreille, chez les aliénés. 36 pp. 4°. *Paris,* 1853, No. 51, v. 545.

Merland (M.-H.-A.) *Sur le diagnostic et le traitement de la pleurésie. viii, 9–39 pp. 4°. *Paris,* 1823, No. 157, v. 182.

Merland (Marie-Hippolyte). *Sur le croup. 34 pp. 4°. *Paris,* 1822, No. 175, v. 175.

Merlande (Jules-Monclésir). *Considérations sur la lactation et l'allaitement. vi, 7–17 pp. 4°. *Paris,* 1828, No. 110, v. 216.

Merlange.

BOURRU (E. C.) *Num chronicis aquæ minerales vulgo de Merlange? 4°. [*Paris,* 1765.]
Examen chymique de l'eau minérale de Merlange. J. de méd., chir., pharm., etc., Par., 1762, xvi, 228–236.

Merlateau (Pierre-Jules). *Des mouvements forcés et de leur emploi en thérapeutique. 46 pp. 4°. *Paris,* 1867, No. 263.

Merle (Adrien-Marie-Camille) [1843–79]. *Étude clinique sur l'accouchement prématuré artificiel. 105 pp., 2 l. 4°. *Montpellier, De Gras,* 1868, No. 88.   C.
For Biography, see Ann. Soc. de méd. de St.-Étienne et de la Loire (1877–80), 1881, 504–514 (Fayet).

Merle (Damien). *Des cicatrices du cou et de leur traitement. 98 pp. 4°. *Paris,* 1869, No. 247.

Merle (Franc. Xaver.) *De matris imaginatione in fœtus formationem efficaci. 51 pp. 8°. *Augustæ Vindelicorum, sumpt. A. Geigeri,* 1810.

Merle (L.-L.) *I. De la nature de l'épilepsie. II. [etc.] 45 pp. 4°. *Paris,* 1842, No. 214, v. 393.

Merle (Octave-Felix-Émiland). *I. De la lithotritie chez les enfants. Faire connaître les dispositions organiques propres à développer des accidents. II. [etc.] 31 pp. 4°. *Paris,* 1839, No. 288, v. 347.

Merle (Thomas-Pierre-Jules). *Du mal vertébral de Pott, ou de la tuberculisation des vertèbres. 39 pp. 4°. *Paris,* 1846, No. 38, v. 447.

Merle-Desisles (C.-R.) *Dissertation médicophilosophique, suivie de propositions de médecine, de chirurgie, et sur les accouchemens. 36 pp. 4°. *Paris,* 1836, No. 233, v. 300.

Merlet (André-Alexandre). *Sur l'usage interne et externe des cantharides en médecine. 21 pp. 4°. *Paris,* 1815, No. 256, v. 116.

Merlet (P.-Ch.-Ferdinand). *Sur la maladie dite fièvre bilieuse essentielle, et sur sa complication adynamique. 27 pp. 4°. *Paris,* 1820, No. 115, v. 157.

Merletta (Vincenzo Frosina). Cenno sopra un nuovo rimedio da servire come mezzo igienico, come profilattico o preservativo e forse come curativo contro il cholera-morbus. 16 pp. 8°. *Catania, E. Coco,* 1866.

———. Appendice al Cenno sul nuovo rimedio contro il cholera-morbus. 15 pp. 8°. *Catania, E. Coco,* 1866.

Merlhiot (L.) *Sur les effets de la saignée, et la préférence qu'on devrait très-souvent donner à celle du pied sur celle du bras. 24 pp. 4°. *Paris, an XIV* [1805], No. 573, v. 59.

Merlin (Lewis). The treasure of health, or a wonderful collection of the most valuable secrets in medicine for the cure of all diseases, wounds, and other accidents to which the human body is subject; with the method of preparing, and instructions for using, the necessary remedies. Also, the best preservatives against the plague, pestilential fevers, small-pox, and other kinds of contagious diseases, discovered, after much research and experience, by the most skilful physicians in Europe, and employed with the greatest success, and unknown till the present time in the United States. Faithfully translated from the French and other foreign languages, and published for the benefit of humanity. 325 pp. 12°. *Philadelphia,* 1819.

Merlin (Louis - Baptiste). *Considérations sur le choléra épidémique qui a sévi au bagne de Toulon en 1863. 53 pp., 1 l. 4°. *Montpellier, L. Cristin & Cie.,* 1866, No. 4.   C.

Merlin-Lemas (A.-M.-H.) *De la colique de plomb. 36 pp. 4°. *Paris,* 1845, No. 114, v. 435.

Merlin Lemas (Armand). *De la réduction des luxations récentes de l'épaule. 42 pp. 4°. *Paris,* 1876, No. 73.

Merling (Fridericus). *Diss. sistens processus vermiformis anatomiam pathologicam. viii, 20 pp., 2 pl. 4°. *Heidelbergæ, J. C. B. Mohr,* [1836].

Merling (H.) *Beiträge zur Casuistik der Tracheotomie bei Croup und Diphtheritis. 43 pp. 8°. *Strassburg, R. Schultz u. Comp.,* 1879.

Merlinja (Petrus). *De hydrope. 26 pp., 4 l. sm. 4°. *Lugd. Bat., C. Wishoff,* 1729. [*Also, in :* P., v. 78.]

Merlit (J.-B.) *Sur les accouchemens, et sur quelques maladies de l'urètre et de la vessie. 19 pp. 4°. *Paris,* 1834, No. 207, v. 275.

Merlo (Ernest). *Ueber Vaginismus. 32 pp., 1 l. 8°. *Bonn, J. F. Carthaus,* [1869].   C.

Merlo (Giuseppe). Del carattere come virtù morale. 13 pp. 8°. *Alessandria, Jacquemod,* 1887.

Merlou. *De l'ovarite aiguë. 89 pp. 4°. *Paris,* 1877, No. 249.

Merly (Jacques-Philippe). *Considérations sur la bronchite herpétique. 40 pp. 4°. *Paris*, 1875, No. 137.

Mermagen (Carl). *Die künstliche Frühgeburt in ihrer Beziehung zum verengten Becken. 34 pp. 8°. *Berlin, G. Lange*, [1868].

Mermann *von Schönberg* (Thomas) [1549–1612]. Consultationes ac responsiones medicæ, a viris doctis hactenus diu multumque desideratissimæ; nunc tand·m opera et studio Francisci Ignatii Thiermairii . . . conquisitæ . . . 16 p. l., 559 pp., 6 l., [port.]. fol. *Ingolstadii, J. P. Zinck*, 1675.
For Portrait, see **Collection**—van Kaathoven. Also: **Collection** of Portr. of Phys. & Men of Sc., 163.

Mermet.
de **Polinière.** Notice biographique de Mermet. Gaz. méd. de Lyon, 1849, i, 53–58.

Mermet (L.-G.) *Du pemphigus dans les névroses. 52 pp. 4°. *Paris*, 1877, No. 323.

Mermet (Louis-Xavier). *Des causes qui peuvent s'opposer à la cicatrisation des plaies et des moyens d'y remédier. 44 pp. 4°. *Paris*, 1845, No. 44, v. 435.

Mermet (Pierre-Marie). *Considérations sur la paralysie en général. 34 pp. 4°. *Paris*, 1833, No. 212, v. 262.

Mermis *aquatilis*.
Bugnion. Note sur les globules sanguins du Mermis aquatilis, Duj., suivie de quelques remarques sur la structure anatomique de cette espèce. Verhandl. d. schweiz. naturf. Gesellsch., Lausanne, 1876-7, lx, 247-255.

Merner (Louis) [1856–]. *De la terminaison par gangrène des corps fibreux intra-utérins; des dangers de leur extirpation partielle. 46 pp., 1 l. 4°. *Paris*, 1883, No. 416.

Merner (Mendheim). *De carcinomate ventriculi. 32 pp. 8°. *Regiomonti Pr., A. Samier*, 1851.
c.

Merocele.
See **Hernia** (*Femoral, etc.*)

Merot (Émile). *Réflexions sur la dyspepsie. 28 pp. 4°. *Paris*, 1822, No. 46, v. 171.

Merrem (Augus·us Carol. Ludov. Blas.) *De tenotomia. 33 pp., 1 l. 8°. *Berolini, typ. Nietackianis.* [1840].

Merrem (Blasius) [1761–1824]. De animalibus Scythicis apud Plinium. 22 pp. 4°. *Gottingæ, H. M. Grape*, [1781].

Merrem (Daniel. Carolus Theodorus) [1790–1859]. *Diss. sistens observationes in Autenriethii methodum tussi convulsivæ medendi. 26 pp., 2 l. 8°. *Marburgi, typ. Kriegeri*, [1810].

——. Animadversiones quædam chirurgicæ experimentis in animalibus factis illustratæ. 46 pp., 1 pl. 12°. *Giessæ, Tasché et Mueller*, 1810.
Bound with: KIEFER (D. G.) Ueber die Natur, Ursachen, Kennzeichen und Heilung, etc. 12°. Göttingen, 1811.

——. Ueber den Cortex adstringens Brasiliensis. iv pp., 1 l., 106 pp. 8°. *Köln am Rhein, J. P. Bachem*, 1828.

Merres (Paul Wilhelm) [1843–]. *Ueber Schenkelhalsbrüche. 32 pp. 8°. *Berlin, G. Lange*, [1867].

Merrett (Christopher) [1614–95]. A collection of acts of Parliament, charters, trials at law, and judges' opinions concerning those grants to the Colledge of Physicians, London, taken from the originals, law-books, and annals. 1 p. l., 135 pp. sm. 4°. [*London*], 1660.

——. A short view of the frauds and abuses committed by apothecaries, as well in relation to patients as physicians, and of the only remedy thereof by physicians making their own medicines. 53 pp. sm. 4°. *London, J. Allestry*, 1669.
Bound with: BELLERS (J.) An essay towards the improvement of physick. sm. 4°. London, 1714.

Merrett (Christopher)—continued.
——. The same. 2. ed. 5, 78 pp. 8°. *London, J. Allestry*, 1670.
See, also, **Boyle** (Robert). New experiments and observations, [etc.] 4°. London, 1683.—**Lex** talionis, etc. 4°. London, 1670.—**Medice** cura teipsum! or the apothecaries plea. 4°. London, 1671.

Merriam (Clinton Hart). The vertebrates of the Adirondack region, Northeastern New York. 1 p. l., 9–106 pp. 8°. [*New York, L. S. Foster*, 1882.]
Repr. from: Tr. Linn. Soc. N. Y., 1882, i.

——. Description of a newly born lynx, Lynx Canadensis (Desm.) Raf. 4 pp., 1 pl. 8°. *Saint John, N. B., J. & A. McMillan*, 1886.
Repr. from: Bull. Nat. Hist. Soc. New Brunswick, 1886, v.

——. Description of a new mouse from New Mexico. Hesperomys (Vesperimus) Anthonyi, sp. nov. 3 pp. 8°. [*Washington*, 1887.]
Repr. from: Proc. Biol. Soc. Wash., 1886-7, iv.

——. Description of a new species of wood-rat from Cerros Island, off Lower California (Neotoma Bryanti, sp. nov.). 2 pp. 8°. *Washington, Gibson Brothers*, [1887].
Repr. from: Am. Naturalist, Wash., 1887, xxi.
See, also, **United States.** Department of Agriculture. Division of Economic Ornithology and Mammalogy. Circulars. 8°. [Washington, 1886.]

Merriam (L[aureston] A[lphonso]) [1843–]. Degeneration the law of disease. 8 pp. 8°. *St. Louis*, 1884.
Repr. from: St. Louis Cour. Med., 1884, xii.

Merrick (C. H.) The decimal system of writing prescriptions. 8 pp. 18°. [*Portland, Oregon, A. G. Walling, n. d.*]

Merrick (Frederick). Introductory lecture delivered to the class of the Starling Medical College. 16 pp. 8°. *Columbus, Legg & Murray*, 1848.

Merrill (A. P.) Medical essays. 24 pp. 8°. *New Orleans, J. Cohn*, 1851.
Repr. from: N. Orl. M. & S. J., 1851-2, viii.

——. A public lecture on medical ethics, and the mutual relations of patients and physician. 18 pp. 8°. *Memphis*, 1857.

——. Lectures on fever. Delivered in the Memphis Medical College, 1853–56. 235 pp. 12°. *New York, Harper & Brothers*, 1865.

——. The cholera pestilence. 27 pp. 8°. *New York*, 1865.

——. Puerperal fever. Chloroform as an internal remedy. 16 pp. 8°. *Louisville, J. P. Morton & Co.*, 1871.
Repr. from: Am. Pract., Louisville, 1871, iv.

——. Uterine diseases. Pneumonia. 16 pp. 8°. *Louisville, J. P. Morton & Co.*, 1871.
Repr. from: Am. Pract., Louisville, 1870-71, ii-iii.

——. Observations on the use of mercury. 8 pp. 8°. *Louisville, J. P. Morton*, 1871.
Repr. from: Am. Pract., Louisville, 1871, iii.

——. The necessity of dentists in the army and navy. 8 pp. 8°. *New York, J. J. Pusey*, 1875.
Also, Co-Editor of: **Memphis** Medical Recorder, 1852-7.

Merrill (Cyrus S.) The introductory address of the course of 1882–3, at the Albany Medical College. 12 pp. 8°. *Albany, J. Munsell*, 1882.

Merrill (*Jesse*) [1794–1860].
Biography. Boston M. & S. J., 1862, lxvi, 291–294.—**Obituary.** Med. Communicat. Mass. M. Soc., Bost., 1866, x, 165.

Merriman (S. William J.) Arguments against the indiscriminate use of chloroform in midwifery. 27 pp. 8°. *London, J. Churchill*, 1848. [P., v. 1204.]

Merriman (Samuel) [1731–1818]. *De conceptu. 18 pp. sm. 4. *Edinburgi, Hamilton, Balfour et Neill*, 1753. [Also, in: P., v. 753.]
Also, in: SMELLIE. Thesaurus med. [etc.] 8°. Edinburgi, 1785, ii, 51-71.

Merriman (Samuel) [1771–1852]. A dissertation on retroversion of the womb, including some observations on extra-uterine gestation. viii, 80 pp. 8°. *London, G. Sidney,* 1810. [P., v. 1062.]

——. A synopsis of the various kinds of difficult parturition; with practical remarks on the management of labours. 2. ed. v pp., 1 p. l., 204 pp. 8°. *London, J. Callow,* 1814.

——. The same. With notes and additions by Thos. C. James. 1. Am. from 2. Lond. ed. viii, 9–297 pp., 5 pl. 8°. *Philadelphia, T. Dobson,* 1816.

——. The same. viii, 80 pp., 2 pl. 8°. *Philadelphia, T. Dobson & Son,* 1817.

——. The same. 3. ed. viii pp., 1 l., 329 pp., 5 pl. 8°. *London, J. Callow,* 1820.

——. The same. New ed. xxxii pp., 1 l., 351 pp., 6 pl. 8°. *London, J. Churchill,* 1838.

——. The same. Die regelwidrigen Geburten und ihre Behandlung. Aus dem Englischen . . . übersetzt von Dr. Herm. Friedr. Kilian. xiv, 354 pp., 5 pl. 8°. *Mannheim, Schwan u. Götz,* 1826.

——. The same. 2. Ausg. xiv, 354 pp., 5 pl. 12°. *Mannheim, F. Götz,* 1845.

See, also, **Lever** (John C. W.) Case of tumour in the pelvis. 8°. *London,* 1840.—**Scott** (P. N.) Case of the separation of the uterus, etc. 8°. *London,* 1821.—**Underwood** (Michael). A treatise on the diseases of children. 8°. *London,* 1827. ——. The same. 8°. *Philadelphia,* 1841. ——. The same. 8°. *Philadelphia,* 1842. *For Biography, see* Lancet, Lond., 1850, n. s., ii, 610–615, port.

Merritt (A. T. B.)
Co-Editor of : **Stethoscope** (The) and Virginia Medical Gazette, Richmond, 1854–5.

Merritt (Emma L.) * Quelques recherches sur le rapport des crevasses du mamelon aux abcès du sein. 52 pp., 2 tab. 4°. *Paris,* 1887, No. 135.

Merruau (Victor-Jérôme). * De la vie considérée à ses diverses époques. x, 11–28 pp. 4°. *Paris,* 1818, No. 156, v. 140.

Merrylees (John). Carlsbad and its environs; with a medical treatise on the use of the waters, by B. London. vii, 199 pp., 14 pl. 12°. *London, S. Low [and others],* 1885.

Merscheim (Anton). * Ueber die hypodermatische Sublimatinjection. 34 pp., 1 l. 8°. *Bonn, F. Krüger,* 1868.

Merschoff (Herm. Anton.) De placentæ solutione artificiali. viii, 20 pp. 8°. *Berolini, typ. J. F. Starckii,* [1817].

Merseburg. Anordnungen, die im Betreff der herannahenden Cholera morbus zu befolgen sind. [*At end :*] Die zu Verhütung der Cholera niedergesetzte Kreis-Commission des Merseburger Kreises. 8 l. fol. [*Merseburg,* 1831.]

——. Berichte über das Medizinal- und Sanitätswesen des Regierungsbezirks Merseburg für die Jahre 1880–82. Erstattet von Dr. E. Wolff. 4°. *Merseburg,* 1881–3.

——. Berichte über das öffentliche Gesundheitswesen des Regierungsbezirk Merseburg für die Jahre 1880–85. Erstattet von Dr. E. Wolff. 4°. *Merseburg,* 1887.

Mersellin (Joannes Wilhelmus). * De vasorum ossificatione et concrescentia ut caussis morborum. 36 pp. 4°. *Halæ Magdeb., lit. Hendelianis,* [1757].

Mersey Steel and Iron Works Sick and Benefit Society. Rules. 7 pp. 12°. *Liverpool, T. Brakell,* 1859.
Established 1835.

de Mersseman (B.-J.) * Essai médico-philosophique sur une question de bromatologie : Quelle est l'action ou l'influence des alimens et des boissons sur l'estomac, et par son intermédiaire sur les autres organes? 1 p. l., 70 pp. 4°. *Strasbourg,* 1828, v. 57.

de Mersseman (Georges). * De l'étiologie de la scrofulose et de sa distribution géographique. 76 pp. 4°. *Paris,* 1878, No. 110.

de Mersseman (Jacobus Oliverius) [1805–53]. * Diss. phys. in qua demonstratur actionem cordis et sanguinis circulationem a systemate nerveo encephalospinali non essentialiter pendere. 55 pp. 4°. *Gandavi, G. de Busscher et fil.,* [1829]. [P., v. 959.]
For Biography, see Ann. Soc. méd.-chir. de Bruges, 1853, 2. s., i, 205–210. *Also :* Mém. Acad. roy. de méd. de Belg., Brux., 1857, iv, 29–32 (D. Sauveur).

de Mersseman (Jacques-Pierre-Marie) [1782–1839]. * Sur le scorbut. 19 pp. 4°. *Paris,* 1819, No. 37, v. 145.

——. The same. * De scorbuto. 15 pp., 1 l., 4°. *Gandari, G. de Busscher et fil.,* [1820]. [P., v. 958.]
For Biography, see Ann. Soc. méd.-chir. de Bruges, 1853, 2. s., i, 33–40, port. (de Meyer).

Merten (Paul). * Ein Beitrag zur Statistik der Gelenkresectionen. 44 pp. 8°. *Greifswald, F. W. Kunike,* 1872.

——. Die Vererbung von Krankheiten und die etwaigen Mittel, derselben Entgegenzuwirken. Eine hygienische Monographie. iv, 43 pp. 8°. *Stuttgart, F. Enke,* 1879.

Mertens (Carolus Henricus). *Anatomiæ batrachiorum prodromus sistens observationes nonnullas in osteologiam batrachiorum nostratium. 2 p. l., 34 pp., 3 l. 16°. *Halæ, F. Grunerti fil.,* [1820]. [P., v. 834.]

von Mertens (Charles) [1737–88]. * Diss. sistens vulnus pectoris complicatum cum vulnere diaphragmatis et arteriæ mesentericæ inferioris. 23 pp. 4°. *Argentorati, typ. J. H. Heitzii,* [1758].

——. Dissertatio exhibens epidemias Viennæ observatas, febris catarrhalis ann. 1762, et dysenteriæ ann. 1763. 21 pp. 8°. *Viennæ, J. T. de Trattnern,* [1766]. [P., v. 909.]

——. Observationes medicæ de febribus putridis, de peste, nonnullisque aliis morbis. 8 p. l., 220 pp., 1 l. 8°. *Vindobonæ, R. Graeffer,* 1778.

——. Traité de la peste, contenant l'histoire de celle qui a régné à Moscou en 1771; ouvrage publié d'abord en latin, actuellement mis en françois et augmenté de plusieurs pièces intéressantes, par l'auteur. xxviii, 142 pp. sm. 4°. *Paris, Didot le jeune; à Vienne & Strasbourg, les frères Gay,* 1784.
The original published in his : Observationes medicæ [etc.] 8°. *Vindobonæ,* 1778.

——. Observationes medicæ de febribus putridis, de peste, nonnullisque aliis morbis. 2 v. in 1. 234 pp. ; 158 pp. 8°. *Ticini, sumpt. B. Comini,* 1791.
v. 1 same as preceding ; v. 2, title : Observationes medicæ.

——. The same. An account of the plague which raged at Moscow in 1771. [Transl. from the French, with notes, by Richard Pearson.] x, 122 pp. 8°. *London, F. & C. Rivington,* 1799.
For Portrait, see **Collection**—van Kaathoven.

Mertens (Christoph Aug. Ludwig) [1812–   ]. * In tegumentis salus. 26 pp., 3 l. 8°. *Berolini, typ. fratrum Schlesinger,* [1839].

——. Zur Physiologie der Anatomie. 86 pp. 8°. *Berlin, T. Trautwein,* 1841.

——. The same. Das Mark. Zweites Bändchen. 111 pp. 8°. *Berlin, A. Hirschwald,* 1845.
See, also, **Lutze** (Arthur). Die Schutzpocken-Impfung [etc.] 8°. *Cöthen,* 1854. ——. The same. 12°. *Cöthen,* 1869.

Mertens (*Franz Carl*) [1764–1831].
Stachow (C. L.) Biographie. Biogr. Skizzen verstorb. Bremisch. Aerzte, Bremen, 1844, 239–392.

Mertens (Joann. Adamus). * De ambustionibus. 2 p. l., 28 pp., 2 l. 8°. *Halæ, typ. H. Ruffii,* [1838].

Mertens (Joh. Wilh. Jos.) *Ueber Ueber-
schwängerung und Ueberfruchtung. 36 pp.
8°. *Giessen, G. D. Brühl*, 1850. c.
Mertens (Karel Hendrik). *Over nitroderi-
vaten van dimethylaniline. 2 p. l., 47 pp., 1
tab. 8°. *Leiden, S. C. van Doesburgh*, 1877.
Merthyr-Tydfil. Annual reports on the sanitary condition of Merthyr-Tydfil, prepared for
the local board of health by their medical officer, T. J. Dyke. 1.–14., 1865–78; 17., 1881; 19.,
1883. 8°. *Merthyr-Tydfil*, 1866–84.
  1.–12. bound in 1 v.
——. Forms for the use of officers of health, by
Thomas Jones Dyke. No. 7. Diary of applications, and visits by medical officers of health.
4°. *Merthyr-Tydfil, Farrant & Frost*, 1873.
Merthyr-Tydfil.
  RAMMELL (T. W.) Report to the General
Board of Health, on a preliminary inquiry into
the sewerage, drainage, and supply of water,
and the sanitary condition of the inhabitants of
the town of Merthyr-Tydfil, in the county of
Glamorgan. 8°. *London*, 1850.
  Dyke (T. J.) The sanitary history of Merthyr-Tydfil.
Brit. M. J., Lond., 1885, ii, 192–196.
Merthyr-Tydfil Union. Report on the sanitary condition of the habitations in the parishes
of Vaynor and Penderyn, and in the hamlet of
Rhigos, part of the district of the rural sanitary
board of the Merthyr-Tydfil Union. Prepared
by their medical officer of health, T. J. Dyke.
1873. 1 p. l., 46 pp., 1 tab. 8°. [*Merthyr-Tydfil*,
1873.]
  Bound with: MERTHYR-TYDFIL. Annual rep. 1.–12.,
1865–76.
——. Annual reports on the sanitary condition
of the rural district of the Merthyr-Tydfil Union,
by T. J. Dyke, to the rural sanitary authority.
1.–6., 1873–8. 8°. *Merthyr-Tydfil*, 1874–9.
  1.–4. *bound with:* MERTHYR-TYDFIL. Annual rep. 1.–
12., 1865–76.
Mertlick (Franciscus Joannes). *De saburra.
18 pp. 4°. *Lipsiæ, ex off. Klaubarthia*, [1786].
  For Biography, see **Platner** (Ernestus).
Mertrud. Hermaphrodite. Dissertation au sujet de la fameuse hermaphrodite qui a paru aux
yeux du public depuis environ trois mois. Laquelle hermaphrodite a été peinte et gravée par
Gautier [d'Agoty]. 1 pl., 1 l. eleph. fol. [*Paris*, 1749.]
  Bound with: GAUTIER D'AGOTY. Essai d'anatomie.
eleph. fol. *Paris*, 1745.
von Mertschinsky (P.) *Beitrag zur Wärme-
Dyspnöe. 21 pp., 2 pl. 8°. *Würzburg, Stahel*,
1881.
  Repr. from: Verhandl. d. phys.-med. Gesellsch. in
Würzb., 1881, xvi.
Mertz (Albert). *Beiträge zur Statistik der Tumoren am Ober-Schenkel. 69 pp. 8°. [*Strassburg*], *G. Schade*, 1882.
Mertz (Jeremias). [*Without title-page; p. 1
begins:*] Von mancherley heimlichen Künsten.
Das erste Buch: In welchem die Art oder Weiss,
mancherley Öll, Pflaster, Salben, Lattwergen,
Pillulen, und unzälbare andere Arztneyen zu
machen begriffen wirdt. Das ander Buch: In
welchem mit schöner Ordnung angezeigt wirdt,
wie man mancherley Wein, und krefftige Wasser
machen soll. Das dritt Buch: In welchem etliche
hochwichtige Heimligkeiten der Arztney, neben
vil anderen kurtzweiligen, und spitzfündigen
verborgnen Künsten begriffen werden. 2 p. l.,
665 pp., 11 l. 16°. *Augspurg, G. Willer*, 1570.
Mertz (Paul). *Zwölf Fälle von Neubildungen
der Vulva. 42 pp., 1 l. 8°. *Breslau, R. Nischkowsky*, 1885.
Mertznich (Joannes Josephus). *De cognitione morborum tracheæ. 48 pp. 8°. *Coloniæ,
typ. Bueschleri sociique*, [1834].

Merulius.
  Göppert. Ueber den Hausschwamm und seine Bekämpfung. Jahresb. d. schles. Gesellsch. f. vaterl. Kult.
1884, Bresl., 1885, lxii, 161–168. — **Poleck.** Ueber gelun-
gene Cultur-Versuche des Hausschwammes (Merulius la-
crimans) aus seinen Sporen. *Ibid.*, 1885, Bresl., 1886, lxiii,
100–111. ——. Ueber die sanitäre Bedeutung des Hausschwammes. *Ibid.*, 73–77.
Merveil (Fortuné). *Considérations sur les
urines albumineuses. 26 pp. 4°. *Strasbourg*,
1861, No. 587, 2. s., v. 31.
Merveilles (Les) de l'homœopathie ou millio-
nisme; discours académique. 24 pp. 8°. *Lyon,
L. Perrin*, 1832. [P., v. 911.]
Merville.
  See **Cholera** (*Asiatic, History, etc., of*), *by localities.*
Mervy (Camille). *Des hémorrhagies dans la
castration, causes et traitement. 40 pp. 4°.
Paris, 1876, No. 39.
Merxhausen.
  See **Hospitals** (*Management, etc., of*), *by local-
ities.*
Méry (César-Auguste). *De quelques accidents
utérins chez les rhumatisantes. 64 pp. 4°. *Pa-
ris*, 1885, No. 196.
—— **& Gentil** (C. J.) Quæstio medico-chirur-
gica an bubo venereus skirrhodes absque cau-
terio curandus? [*Parisiis*, 1751.]
  In: HALLER. Disp. chir. [etc.] 4°. *Lausannæ*, 1755,
iv, 457–461.
Mery (Franciscus).
  See **Roussin de Montabourg** (Joannes Armandus).
An salubrior Sequana? 4°. [*Paris*, 1759.]
Méry (François-Camille). *De la dysenterie des
pays chauds et de son traitement, spécialement
par le sulfate de soude. 31 pp. 4°. *Paris*, 1875,
No. 257.
Mery (J.-Auguste). *Des résorptions purulente
et cancéreuse, de leur théorie, et de la compression comme moyen thérapeutique. 23 pp. 4°.
Paris, 1836, No. 83, v. 296.
Méry (J.-B.-J.) *Sur le goître. 19 pp. 4°. *Paris*, 1826, No. 99, v. 200.
Mery (Jean) [1645–1722]. Observations sur la
manière de tailler dans les deux sexes pour
l'extraction de la pierre, pratiquée par Frère
Jacques. Nouveau système de la circulation du
sang par le trou ovale dans le fœtus humain,
avec les réponses aux objections qui ont été
faites contre cette hypothèse. 9 p. l., ix pp., 7
l., 120 pp.; 6 p. l., ix, 187 pp., 6 pl. 12°. *Paris,
J.-L. Delorme*, 1700.
  The paging of the first treatise is pp. 1–96, followed by
67–90; the total number of pages is 120.
  See, also, **Tauvry** (Daniel). Traité de la génération
etc. 12°. *Paris*, 1700.—**Verheyen** (Philippus). Supple-
mentum anatomicum [etc.]. sm. 4°. *Coloniæ*, 1713.
  For Biography, see **Herpin** (J.-C.) Notice historique
sur la vie et les travaux de Jean Mery. 8°. *Paris*, 1864.
Repr. from: Compt. rend. Soc. du Berry, 1863–4.
  See, also, Collect. acad. d. mém., etc., Par., 1774, v, 388–
390. [*From:* Mém. Acad. roy. d. sc. de Par., 1723.]
  For Portrait, see **Collection**—van Kaathoven.
Merycism.
  See **Rumination** *in man.*
Meryon (Edward). The history of medicine,
comprising a narrative of its progress from the
earliest ages to the present time, and of the delusions incidental to its advance from empiricism
to the dignity of a science. v. 1. viii, 483 pp.
8°. *London, Longman* [*and others*], 1861.
——. Practical and pathological researches on
the various forms of paralysis. vii, 215 pp., 1
pl. 8°. *London, J. Churchill & Sons*, 1864.
——. On the functions of the sympathetic system of nerves, as a physiological basis for a rational system of therapeutics. 68 pp. 8°. *London, J. & A. Churchill*, 1872.

Merz (Carl)[1]. *Ueber das Verhalten des Alloxans zu Asparagin, Malamid, Caffeïn, Chlorbarium und Ammoniak. 29 pp. 8°. *Tübingen, H. Laupp*, 1865. C.

Merz (Carl)[2]. *Ueber Gummata, nebst einer Statistik der in den Jahren 1873-83 vorgekommenen Fälle der hiesigen syphilitischen Abtheilung. 25 pp. 8°. *Würzburg, N. Scamoni*, 1884.

Merz (Christophor. Frider.) *De caricibus quibusdam medicinalibus sarsaparillæ succedaneis. 30 pp., 1 l. 4°. *Erlangæ, stanno Ellrodtiano*, [1784].

Merz (Georges-Hermann). *Du traitement des fièvres pernicieuses. 44 pp., 1 l. 4°. *Paris*, 1877, No. 54.

Merz (Gerardus Joannes Fredericus). *De nephrorrhagia. 1 p. l., 50 pp. 8°. *Lugd. Bat., P. H. van den Heuvell*, 1839.

Merz (Joannes Jacobus). *De digitali purpurea ejusque usu in scrofulis medico. 3 p. l., 16 pp. 4°. *Jenæ, lit. Maukianis*, [1790].

Merz (Paul Constantin) [1856–]. *Ein Fall von Carcinom der männlichen Brustdrüse. 32 pp. 8°. *Berlin, G. Schade*, 1885.

Merz (Victor). *Untersuchungen über das Titan, Silicium und Boron. 38 pp. 8°. *Zürich, Zürcher u. Furrer*, 1864. C.

Merzdorff (J. F. A.)
See **de la Roche.** Zergliederung der Verrichtung des Nervensystems, etc. 8°. *Halle*, 1794-5.

Mesa (Alonso Manuel Sedeño).
See **Hippocrates.** Aforismos de Hypocrates, etc. 12°. *Madrid*, 1789.

Mesch (Casparus). *Cel. Ant. de Hæn, etc. Tom. ii. de morbis humorum, una cum adnexis thesibus medico-practicis. 1 p. l., 64 pp. 8°. *Viennæ, M. A. Schmidt*, [1781].

Mesch (Georg Christoph Michael). *De peripneumonia. 30 pp. 8°. *Erlangæ, typ. Kunstmanni*, [1809].

Meschede (Joannes Franciscus) [1832–]. *De electro-punctura ejusque in sanandis tumoribus cum vasis sanguiferis communicantibus vi et usu. 43 pp. 8°. *Gryphiæ, F. G. Kunike*, 1856. C.

———. Die paralytische Geisteskrankheit und ihre organische Grundlage. 102 pp., 1 pl. 8°. *Berlin, G. Reimer*, [1865].
Repr. from: Arch. f. path. Anat., etc., Berl., 1865, xxxiv.

———. The same. De paralytische waanzinnigheid en hare organische grondslag. Uit het Hoogduitsch door Dr. J. C. van der Voort. viii, 136 pp., 1 pl. 8°. *Utrecht, A. van Dorsten, jr.*, 1867.

———. Bericht über die städtische Krankenanstalt zu Königsberg, Ostpr., für das Jahr 1883-4. 16 pp. 8°. *Königsberg, Hartung*, 1884.

Meschwitz (Johann Jacob). Abhandlung von dem Nutzen der Tobacksblätter in Entzündungen der Augen. 8 pp. sm. 8°. *Kopenhagen, J. R. Thiele*, [1776].

Mesdag (Rein.) *De partu difficili instrumentis secantibus absolvendo. viii, 114, iv pp., 1 l. 8°. *Groningæ, W. Wouters*, 1810.

Mesembryanthemum.

DANNEMANN (J. F.) *Beiträge zur Kenntniss der Anatomie und Entwicklung der Mesembryanthema. 8°. *Halle a. S.*, 1883.

LIEB (J. W. F.) Die Eispflanze als ein fast specifisches Arzneimittel. 8°. *Hof*, 1785.
Wendt. Von den Heilkräften der Eispflanze (Mesembryanthemum crystallinum). J. d. pract. Arznk. u. Wundarznk., Berl., 1801, xi, 3. St., 3-30.

Mesentery.

See, also, **Omentum; Peritoneum.**
DAHLING (G. H.) *De glandulis mesentericis præcipue vero de illarum conjunctione cum arteriis. 4°. *Gottingæ*, [1829].

Mesentery.

EBHARDT (G. S.) *De statu mesenterii naturali et præternaturali. sm. 4°. *Jenæ*, [1755].

ESCHENBACH (C. G.) De glandularum mesaraicarum in chylum actione. 4°. *Lipsiæ*, [1777].

EULER (M. C.) *De mesenterio. 4°. *Argentorati*, [1714].
Also, in: HALLER. Disp. anat. [etc.] 4°. *Gottingæ*, 1750, i, 719-756, 1 pl.

HERTEL (J. H.) *De mesenterio. 4°. *Erfordiæ*, [1767].

RATH (G. S.) *Das Mesenterium, dessen Struktur und höchste Bedeutung. 8°. *Würzburg*, 1823.

RUSH (J.) An inquiry into the use of the omentum. 8°. *Philadelphia*, 1809.
Besnier (E.) Mésentère. Dict. encycl. d. sc. méd., Par., 1873, 2. s., vii, 121-125. ———. Ganglions mésentériques. *Ibid.*, 125-138.—**Fanton** (J.) De mesenterio, vasis chyliferis et lymphaticis. *In his:* Diss. anat., 8°, Taurini, 1745, 165-222.—**Lister** (J.) On the flow of lacteal fluid in the mesentery. Dublin Hosp. Gaz., 1857, iv, 347.—**Reid** (J.) Some observations on the structure of the mesenteric glands in the balænoptera rostrata. Edinb. M. & S. J., 1835, xliii, 9-11. *Also, in his:* Extr. Select Communicat. Edinb. Med.-Chir. Soc., 8°, Edinb., 1835, 1-3.—**Ribes** (F.) Omphalo-mésentériques (vaisseaux). Dict. d. sc. méd., Par., 1819, xxxvii, 305-309, 2 pl.—**Urvich** (B. O.) K vopr. ob otdel. bryjjeiki ot kishki. [On secretions of the mesentery of intestine.] Vrach, St. Petersb., 1886, vii, 921-924.

Mesentery (*Abnormities of*).

See, also, **Intestines** (*Obstructions of*) *by adhesions, etc.;* **Peritoneum** (*Abnormities of*).
Boucaud. Rétrécissement très-ancien du côlon transverse et du côlon descendant; double anomalie de l'épiploon. Mém. et compt.-rend. Soc. d. sc. méd. de Lyon, 1866-7, vi, pt. 2, 13-15. *Also:* Gaz. méd. de Lyon, 1866, xviii, 331.—**Gruber** (W.) Beiträge zu den Bildungshemmungen der Mesenterien. Arch. f. Anat., Physiol. u. wissensch. Med., Leipz., 1862, 588-611, 1 pl.; 588, 1 pl.; 1864, 478, 1 pl. ———. Nachträge zu den Bildungshemmungen der Mesenterien und zu der Hernia interna mesogastrica überhaupt, und Abhandlung eines Falles mit einem Mesenterium commune für den Dünn-Dickdarm, einer beträchtlichen Hernia interna mesogastrica dextra und einer enorm grossen Hernia scrotalis dextra besonders. Arch. f. path. Anat., etc., Berl., 1868, xliv, 215-241, 1 pl. ———. Mesenterium commune für das Colon ascendens und Jejuno-Ileum. *Ibid.*, 1879, lxxvii, 132.—**Heppner** (C. L.) Ein Fall von Bildungshemmung des Mesenterium und Rudiment der Vasa omphaloenterica. St. Petersb. med. Ztschr., 1863, iv, 297-303, 1 pl.

Mesentery (*Abscess of*).

See **Abdomen** (*Abscess, etc., of*); **Mesentery** (*Diseases of*).

Mesentery (*Diseases of*).

See, also, **Fæces** (*Fatty*); **Tabes** *mesenterica*.
AVELLAN (F. W.) *Anmärkningar rörande ett fall af mesenteritis acuta. 8°. *Helsingfors*, [1840].

BARTH (F.) *De glandularum mesaraicarum inflammatione. 8°. *Halæ*, [1821].

BURCHARD (C. M.) [Pr.] de hæmorrhagiis mesenterii culpa ingravescentibus. sm. 4°. *Rostochii*, 1727.

GAYOT (P.) *Recherches sur quelques altérations des ganglions mésentériques chez l'adulte. 4°. *Paris*, 1875.

HEBENSTREIT (J. C. E.) *Diss. sistens casum de scirrho mesenterii exulcerato. 4°. *Halæ Magdeb.*, [1756].

KRAUSE (F. A.) *De glandularum mesaraicarum inflammatione. 8°. *Berolini*, 1834.

MARTINI (M.) De morbis mesenterii abstrusioribus; in scholis medicorum hactenus prætermissis, nec scriptis veterum illustratis. Item affectionum hypochondriacarum priorium quodammodo affinium historia et curatio. 18°. *Lipsiæ*, 1630.

OBERLAENDER (F.) *Ein Fall von Cysticercus cellulosæ im Mesenterium des Menschen. [Greifswald.] 8°. *Leipzig*, [1874].

Mesentery (Diseases of).

RÜCKER (J. D.) *De mensenterio multorum malorum sede. 4°. *Lugd. Bat.*, 1728.

SVINTSOFF. *Material k ucheniou o vospalenii brizjeki. [Inflammation of the mesentery.] 8°. *St. Petersburg*, 1873.

Aeby (C.) Fremde Körper im Mesenterium des Frosches. Ztschr. f. rat. Med., Leipz. u. Heidelb., 1862, 3. R., xiv, 361.—**Bierbaum** (J.) Phthisis mesaraica; Tuberculose der Gekrösdrüsen. Deutsche Klinik, Berl., 1870, xxii, 365; 374.—**Bonnet.** [Ramollissement inflammatoire du mésentère, consécutif à l'inflammation intestinale entretenue par l'abus des purgatifs irritants.] Bull. Soc. anat. de Par., 1847, xxii, 86.—**Booth** (B. S.) Pus in abdominal cavity. Med. Press & Circ., Lond., 1877, n. s., xxiii, 468.—**Bouchut.** De la tuberculose entéromésentérique. Gaz. d. hôp., Par., 1858, xxxi, 237; 246. *Also, transl.:* J. f. Kinderkr., Erlang., 1860, xxxiv, 413-426.—**Boyle** (P. A.) On a case of mesenteric disease with discharge of fæces by the navel. Lancet, Lond., 1849, i, 666.—**Carpentier.** Ganglions mésentériques engorgés et enflammés dont la plupart renferment des noyeaux tuberculeux à l'état caséeux et des foyers purulents. Presse méd. belge, Brux., 1874, xxvi, 127.—[**Case.**] Mesenteric disease; obscure fever. Lancet, Lond., 1858, ii, 577.—**Cholmeley** (W.) Tubercular enlargement and degeneration of the mesenteric glands from an adult male. Tr. Path. Soc. Lond , 1865-6, xvii, 165-167.—**Clebsch.** Mesenterialbrand. Med. Ztg., Berl., 1845, xiv, 7.—**Gull** (W.) Fatty stools from disease of the mesenteric glands. Guy's Hosp. Rep., Lond , 1855, 3. s., i, 369-372.—**Gustin** (J.) Note sur un cas de tuberculisation mésentérique. Ann. Soc. méd.-chir. de Bruges, 1859, 2. s., vii, 23-28. [Rap. de Van Dromme], 118-120. *Also:* Arch. belges de méd. mil., Brux., 1859, xxiv, 108-113.—**Heyfelder.** Degeneration von Mesenterialdrüsen. Med. Ztg., Berl., 1835, iv, 49.—**Johnston** (W.) A case of acute disease of the mesenteric glands. West. Lancet, Cincin., 1842-3, i, 438-441.—**Joninon.** Observation d'une affection squirrheuse des glandes mésentériques; compression exercée par la tumeur sur le canal cholédoque et rendant impossible l'arrivée dans le duodénum de la bile et du suc pancréatique. J. de méd. de Lyon, 1845, viii, 122-125.—**Lederer.** Bauchdrüsen-(Tuberkulose der Mesenterialdrüsen) und Eingeweidewürmer. Wien. med. Wchnschr., 1854, iv, 7; 20.—[**Marques** (J. A.)] Tuberculos mesentericos; massa tuberculosa suppurada; derramamento do pus; morte em poucas horas. Escholiaste med., Lisb., 1854, v, 160.—**Monro** (D.) Case of ossifications in the mesentery. Med. Tr. Roy. Coll. Phys. 1768-71, Lond., 1772, ii, 361-365.—**Nivison** (N.) Case of induration of mesenteric glands successfully treated. N. York J. M., 1856, 3. s , i, 36-42.—**Osler** (W.) Abscesses in the mesentery; suppuration of portal vein; empyema; perforation of appendix; general peritonitis. Montreal Gen. Hosp. Path. Rep., 1877, i, 51.—**Palmer** (S.) [Case of dissection of enlargement and ulceration of the mesentery, complicated with tumefaction of the liver.] Lond. M. Reposit., 1819, xii, 381-387.—**Paulicki.** Carcinom der Mesenterialdrüsen mit Metastasen nach der Leber und den Nieren. Memorabilien, Heilbr., 1869, xiv, 163.—**Pinto Cerqueira** (N. V.) Um caso de completa liquefação de tuberculos mesentericos. Escholiaste med., Lisb., 1856, vii, 269.—**Porter** (C. A.) Case of extensive disease, involving the glands of the mesenterium. U. States M. & S. J., N. Y., 1834-5, i, 171.—**Ribbentrop.** Kann eine tuberkulöse Gekrösdrüsen-Vereiterung sich durch den Nabel entleeren? Med. Ztg., Berl., 1845, xiv, 178.—**Rodinoff** (G.) K patolog. anatomii podjelud. jelezi pri obsh. chron. bolezn. [Pathological anatomy of the mesenteric glands in chronic diseases.] Voyenno-med. J., St. Petersb., 1885, clii, pt. 2, 209-280.—**Romberg.** Peritonitis; Tuberculosis mesenterii. Wchnschr. f. d. ges. Heilk., Berl., 1837, 293.—**Scherb.** Beobachtung einer Verhärtung in dem Gekrös. Museum d. Heilk., Zürich, 1792, i, 137-143.—**Smith** (G.) Case of hæmorrhage into the mesentery. Lancet, Lond., 1881, ii, 1124.—**Southey.** Chronic degeneration of mesenteric glands and marasmus, with cerebral symptoms simulating cerebral tumour, but due to intraventricular pressure. Brit. M. J., Lond., 1878, ii, 518.—[**Thomson** (W.)] Diseases of the mesenteric glands. Syst. Pract. M. (Tweedie), Phila., 1841, iv, 229-238.—**Toel.** Ueber Mesenteritis skrofulöser Kinder. Arch. f. med. Erfahr., Berl., 1824, ii, 467-474.—**Wallach.** Ueber steinige Concremente der Mesenterialdrüsen. Hannov. Ann. f. d. ges. Heilk., 1837, ii, 818-821.—**Wendt** (J. C. G.) De insidiosa mesenterii inflammatione sub ætate puerili. Acta reg. Soc. med. Havn., 1821, vi, 88-99.

Mesentery (Rupture of).

Arnoult. Déchirure du mésentère par violence extérieure; épanchement considérable de sang dans le péritoine. Bull. Soc. anat. de Par., 1845, xx, 46-49.—**Longuet.** Déchirure du mésentère; péritonite suraiguë; mort. *Ibid.*, 1873, xlviii, 767-769.—**Rupture** of mesentery from external violence. Med. Times & Gaz., Lond., 1867, ii, 431.

Mesentery (Tumors of).

AUGAGNEUR (V.) Tumeurs du mésentère. 8°. *Paris*, 1886.

COLLET (F.) *Sur les kistes du mésentère. 4°. *Paris*, 1884.

GRAMBS (J. J.) Anatomische Beschreibung eines monströsen Gewächses, welches in dem Leibe einer Frauen von drey und funfftzig Jahr, an ein gewisses Stück des Mesenterii angewachsen, und achtzehen Pfund schwer ausgewachsen gefunden worden. 4°. *Franckf. a. M.*, 1730.

Allen. Discoid carcinoma of mesentery; cancer involving the semilunar ganglion. Austral. M. J., Melbourne, 1883, n. s., v, 223.—**Arnott** (H.) Spindle-celled sarcomatous tumour in the mesentery, with syphilitic tumours elsewhere. Tr. Path. Soc. Lond., 1868-9, xx, 221-224.—**Bemiss** (J. H.) Encephaloid cancer of mesenteric glands; (pathological report). N. Orl. M. & S. J., 1884-5, n. s., xii, 352.—**Bennett** (J. R.) Cancer of the omentum, mesentery, pleura, etc. Tr. Path. Soc. Lond., 1850-52, iii, 101.—**Beretta** (C.) Di un fungo nel mesenterio simulante un' ipertrofia di milza. Gazz. med. di Milano, 1845, iv, 285-289.—**Berthelot.** Concrétions ostéiformes ayant leur siége dans l'épaisseur du mésentère. Compt. rend. Soc. de biol. 1855, Par., 1856, 2. s., ii, 29.—**Bigelow** (H. J.) Gaseous cysts upon the mesentery and intestine. Extr. Rec. Bost. Soc. M. Improve., 1854-6, ii, 171.—**Bozeman** (N.) Cystic sarcoma of the mesentery and omentum. Med. Rec., N. Y., 1882, xxii, 72.—**Bricheteau** (I.) Observation d'une tumeur fibro-cartilagineuse du mésentère, qui embrassait le duodénum, et comprimait cet intestin au point d'y empêcher le cours des alimens. J. compl. du dict. d. sc. méd., Par., 1824, xx, 205-207.—**Bruschini** (E.) Carcinoma dell' epiploon; coprostasi. Eco d. clin., Napoli, 1887, ii, 129-133.—**Buckner** (P. J.) A very large mesenteric tumour, simulating ovarian disease, successfully extirpated. Am. J. M. Sc., Phila., 1852, n. s., xxiv, 358-365.—**Carter** (C. H.) Large cyst of the mesentery simulating an ovarian cyst; operation; death. Brit. M. J., Lond., 1883, i, 7.—**Church.** Unusually small spleen associated with lymphoma of the mesentery. Tr. Path. Soc. Lond., 1868-9, xx, 375-378.—**Custes** (O.) Καρκίνος τῶν μεσεντερίων ἀδένων, περίσφυγξις τοῦ δωδεκαδακτύλου; θάνατος. Ἰατρικὴ Ἐφημ., Ἀθῆναι, 1858-9, i, 123.—**Dickinson** (W. H.) Mesenteric tumour. Tr. Path. Soc. Lond., 1870-71, xxii, 296-304.—**van Dommelen.** Waarneming van een steatoma mesenterii. Pract. Tijdschr. v. de Geneesk., Gorinchem, 1856, n. s., ii, 73-79.—**Ducasset.** Kyste du mésentère. Bull. Soc. anat. de Par., 1848, xxiii, 67-70.—**Duhamel** (V.) Tumeur du mésentère; cirrhose; ascite; autopsie. Gaz. hebd. de méd., Par., 1863, x, 383-386.—**Eve** (F. S.) Myxo-sarcoma, or so-called colloid or hydatid tumour of the great omentum, and case of tubercle of the great omentum. Tr. Path. Soc. Lond., 1886, xxxvii, 496-499, 1 pl.—**Fraipont** (F.) Un cas de tumeur du mésentère. Ann. Soc. méd.-chir. de Liége, 1886, xxv, 451-459.—**Gallemaerts.** Tumeur de l'épiploon. Presse méd. belge, Brux., 1886, xxxviii, 105-107.—**Garreau.** Tumeur cancéreuse du mésentère. Gaz. méd. de l'Algérie, Alger, 1871, xvi, 25.—**Gooding** (J. C.) Cyst of the great omentum; removal; recovery. Lancet, Lond., 1887, i, 311.—**Gradenwitz.** Krebs der Gekrösdrüsen. Med. Ztg., Berl., 1848, xvii, 103.—**Hahn** (E.) Ueber Mesenterialcysten. Berl. klin. Wchnschr., 1887, xxiv, 408-412.—**Harlan.** Cancer of the mesentery and of the duodenum. Proc. Path. Soc. Phila., 1857-60, i, 271.—**Hayden.** Scirrhus of the mesentery. Irish Hosp. Gaz., Dubl., 1873, i, 43.—**Henry** (F. P.) Myxomatous tumor of mesentery of a hen. Tr. Path. Soc. Phila. (1881-3), 1884, xi, 250.—**Labouibène** (A.) Cancer du mésentère, observé sur une vieille femme. Compt. rend. Soc. de biol. 1854, Par., 1855, 2. s., i, pt. 2, 9-11.—**Ladmiral.** Tumeur fibroplastique très-volumineuse du mésentère, développée probablement dans les ganglions lymphatiques. Bull. Soc. anat. de Par., 1874, xlix, 638-642.—**Lauderdale** (E.) [Tumors of medullary cancer of the mesentery.] Med. Indep., Detroit, 1856, i, 30.—**Leroux.** Observation sur une tumeur carcinomateuse développée dans le mésentère. J. de méd., chir., pharm., etc., Par., 1808, xv, 3-11.—**McKain** (W. J.) Strangulation of the jejunum, produced by an encysted tumour of the mesentery. Charleston M. J., 1848, iii, 276-279.—**McReddie** (G. D.) Case of scirrhus cancer of mesentery. Indian M. Gaz., Calcutta, 1879, xiv, 312.—**Madelung.** Exstirpation eines vom Mesenterium ausgehenden Lipoma œdematosum myxomatodes mit partieller Resection des Dünndarmes; Heilung. Berl. klin. Wchnschr., 1881, xviii, 75; 93.—**Merklen** (P.) Examen histologique d'un kyste du mésentère. Bull. Acad. de méd., Par., 1880, 2. s., ix, 926-930.—**Morris** (T. F.) † Cancer of mesentery. Tr. M. Soc. N. Jersey, Newark, 1875, 181.—**Nasse** (D.) Ein Spindelzellensarkom des Mesenteriums. Arch. f. path. Anat., etc., Berl., 1883, xciv, 473-476.—**Nückel.** † Eigenthümliche Geschwulst zwischen den Platten des Mesenteriums (degenerirte Mesenterial-Drüse?). Med. Ztg., Berl., 1840, ix,

Mesentery (*Tumors of*).

44.—**Rota** (A.) Carcinoma del mesenterio da trauma; peritonite parziale da disordine dietetico; morte. Comment. di med. e chir., Milano, 1874, i, 247.—**Sabourin.** Adéno-lymphocèle du mésentère. Bull. Soc. anat. de Par., 1876, li, 339. *Also:* Progrès méd., Par., 1876, iv, 647.—**Sainsbury** (H.) Primary spindle-celled sarcoma of the mesentery. Tr. Path. Soc. Lond., 1883-4. xxxv, 343-348. ———. Case of malignant disease of the mesentery. Lancet, Lond., 1884, i, 343.—**Sewall** (J. G.) [Tumors, supposed to be cancerous.] N. York M. Times, 1856, v, 387.—**Silcock** (A. Q.) Malignant lymphoma of mesentery. Tr. Path. Soc. Lond., 1883-4, xxxv, 348-350.—**Stobbe** (F.) Ein Myosarcom der Mesenterialdrüsen. Arch. d. Heilk., Leipz., 1876, xvii, 466-468.—**Terrillon.** Lipomes du mésentère. Bull. et mém. Soc. de chir. de Par., 1886, n. s., xii, 23-31. *Also:* Arch. gén. de méd., Par., 1886, i, 257; 434.—**Thornton** (J. K.) Mesenteric and omental cysts. Brit. M. J.. Lond., 1882, ii, 1242.—**Van Bibber** (W. C.) The differential diagnosis of cancer in the mesentery. Maryland M. J., Balt., 1886-7, xvi, 253-258. *Also:* Med. & Surg. Reporter, Phila., 1887, lvi, 193-197.—**Viollet.** Cancer du mésentère; squirrhe atrophique; étranglement interne. Bull. Soc. anat. de Par., 1873, xlviii, 342.—**Voisin.** Tumeurs tuberculeuses ganglionnaires du mésentère accolées aux deux reins; compression de l'artère rénale gauche par l'une d'elles; absence de sécrétion urinaire pendant soixante heures; phénomènes urémiques comateux; mort. *Ibid.*, 1863, xxxviii, 317-324.—**Waldeyer** (W.) Grosses Lipo-Myxom des Mesenteriums mit secundären sarcomatösen Heerden in der Leber und Lunge. Arch. f. path. Anat., etc., Berl., 1865, xxxii, 543.—**Weichselbaum** (A.) Eine seltene Geschwulstform des Mesenteriums (Chylangioma cavernosum). Ein Beitrag zur Lehre von den Gefässgeschwülsten. *Ibid.*, 1875, lxiv, 145-162, 1 pl.—**Wells** (T. S.) Fatty tumour of mesentery removed during life. Tr. Path. Soc. Lond., 1867-8, xix, 243. ——— Note on mesenteric cysts and tumours. Brit. M. J., Lond.. 1882, ii, 1138.—**Woodhouse.** Abdominal tumor. Prov. M. & S. J., Lond., 1850, 693.—**Zinke** (E. G.) Case of round-celled sarcoma of the mesentery, occurring in a boy five years of age. Cincin. Lancet & Clinic. 1884, n. s., xiii, 502-504.

Meseth (Georg). * Vier Fälle von Meningitis cerebro-spinalis epidemica. 28 pp. 8°. *Würzburg, F. E. Thein, 1871.*

Mesinto.

Villa (E.) Topografia e statistica medica dei comuni di Ceriano e Mesinto. Gazz. med. ital. lomb., Milano, 1886, 8. s., viii, 237; 244.

Mesitylene.

Holtmeyer (A.) * Schwefelhaltige Abkömmlinge des Mesitylens. 8°. *Göttingen, 1867.*

Mesko (Joannes). * De camphora. 1 p. l., 32 pp., 1 l. 8°. *Budæ, typ. Reg. Univ. Hung.*, 1830. [P., v. 1318.]

Meslier (Adolphe-Hippolyte). * De la gangrène des poumons. 34 pp. 4°. *Paris, 1857*, No. 252, v. 608.

Meslier (E.-M.-J.) * Sur l'hépatite aiguë. vi, 7-19 pp. 4°. *Paris, 1818*, No. 55, v. 136.

Meslier (Élie). * De la fièvre intermittente simple. 34 pp. 4°. *Paris, 1845*, No. 123, v. 435.

Meslier (James). * Des pleurésies rhumatismales. 44 pp. 4°. *Paris, 1872*, No. 370.

de Meslon (Joannes). * De liene. 24 pp. sm. 4°. *Lugd. Bat., G. Potvliet*, 1738. [P., v. 80.]

Mesly (J.-A.) * Sur les convulsions des enfans, et leurs causes. vi, 7-20 pp. 4°. *Paris, 1819*, No. 235, v. 151.

de Mesmaecker (Joannes Henricus). * De peritonitide puerperali. 20 pp. 4°. *Gandavi, P. F. de Goesin-Verhaeghe*, 1825. [P., v. 957; 1377.]

Mesmer (Friederich Anton) [1733-1815]. Mémoire sur la découverte du magnétisme animal. vi, 85 pp. 12°. *Genève & Paris, P.-F. Didot le jeune*, 1779.
Bound with: D'ESLON. Observations sur le magnétisme animal. 12°. *Londres*, 1780.

———. The same. Abhandlung über die Entdeckung des thierischen Magnetismus. Aus dem Französischen übersetzt. 64 pp. 12°. *Carlsruhe, M. Macklot*, 1781.

———. Précis historique des faits relatifs au magnétisme-animal jusques en avril 1781. Ouvrage

Mesmer (Friederich Anton)—continued.
trad. de l'allemand. 2 p. l., 229 pp., 1 l. 8°. *Londres*, 1781.

———. The same. Kurze Geschichte des thierischen Magnetismus bis April 1781. Aus dem Französischen übersetzt. 1 l., 428 pp. 12°. *Carlsruhe, M. Macklot*, 1783.

———. Lettre de . . . à M. le comte de C . . . [Copie de la requête. À nos seigneurs, nos seigneurs de parlement en la Grand' chambre.] 11 pp. 4°. [*Paris*, 1784.]

———. Lettres de . . . à messieurs les auteurs du Journal de Paris, et à M. Franklin. 16 pp. 16°. [*Paris*, 1784.]

———. Noms des personnes nouvellement admises chez . . . pour être instruites dans sa doctrine. 12 pp. 16°. [*Paris*, 1784.]

———. Mémoire sur la découverte du magnétisme animal. 2 p. l., 7-468 pp., 2 l. 8°. *Paris, an VII* [1799].

———. Lettres sur l'origine de la petite vérole et le moyen de la faire cesser, avec une adresse aux mères. 11, 16, 7 pp. 8°. *Paris, an X* [1802]. [P., v. 1285.]

———. Magnétisme animal. Mémoires et aphorismes, suivis des procédés de d'Eslon. Nouv. éd., avec des notes par J.-J.-A. Ricard. xii, 228 pp. 16°. *Paris, Germer-Baillière & Cie.*, 1846.
See, also, **Bergasse.** Considérations sur le magnétisme animal, [etc.] 12°. *La Haye*, 1784—**Caullet de Veaumorel.** Aphorismes de M. Mesmer [etc.] 2. éd. 8°. *Paris*, 1785.—**Galart de Montjoye.** Lettre sur le magnétisme animal. 8°. *Philadelphie & Paris*, 1784.—**Lettre** d'un médecin de la Faculté de Paris, etc. 16°. *La Haye*, 1781.—**Ricard** (J.-J.-A.) Physiologie et hygiène du magnétiseur. 8°. *Paris*. 1844.—**Théorie** du mesmérisme, etc. 8°. *Paris*, 1817.—**Zender** (J. D. L.) Anthroponomy, or magneto-physiognomico-craniology [etc.] 8°. *New York*, 1863.
For Biography, see **Life** (The) of [Francis Anthony] Mesmer, the discoverer of animal magnetism or mesmerism. By a "Believer". 12°. *London*, 1843.—**Oraison** funèbre du célèbre Mesmer, auteur du magnétisme animal, et président de la Loge de l'Harmonie. 12°. *Grenoble*, 1785.
For Portrait, see **Collection**—van Kaathoven.—**Collection** of Portr. of Phys. & Men of Sc., 201.

Mesmer (Maximilianus). * De mortalitate liberorum. 24 pp. sm. 4°. *Landishuti Bavar., F. S. Storno*, 1826.

Mesmeric Infirmary, London. *See* **London** Mesmeric Infirmary.

Mesmeric (The) Magazine, or Journal of Animal Magnetism. By R. H. Collyer. [Monthly.] No. 1, v. 1, July, 1842. 8°. *Boston, Saxton & Pierce.*

Mesmerism.

See **Hypnotism**; **Magnetism** (*Animal*).

Mesmerism. A reply to a letter addressed by Charlotte Elizabeth [Tonna] to Miss Martineau. 3. ed. 15 pp. 12°. *London, S. Low*, 1845.
In: PURLAND (T.) Collection, v. 4.

Mesmerism. Experiments and inferences. 3 pp. roy. 8°. [*n. p., n. d.*] [P., v. 1565.]

Mesmerism; its pretentions stated, etc. *See* "**Philadelphos**".

Mesmerism in India. Second half-yearly report of the Calcutta Mesmeric Hospital from 1st March to 1st September, 1849, containing accounts of formidable and numerous painless surgical operations, and of the successful administration of mesmerism in insanity and other diseases. To which is added remarks on the conduct of the English medical journalists, and nearly the whole of the medical profession, in reference to the greatest of medical blessings; with some hints to the public on the employment of mesmerism and on mesmerisers. By Dr. Elliotson. 2. ed. 43 pp., 3 pen sketches. 8°. *London, H. Baillière*, 1850.
Repr. from: "Zoist".
In: PURLAND (T.) Collection, v. 4.

Mesmerism in the treatment of insanity. 3 pp. 8°. *London, Walton & Mitchell,* [*n. d.*]
In : PURLAND (T.) Collection, v. 3.

Mesmerist (The). A journal of vital magnetism. [Weekly.] v. 1 (Nos. 1–20), May 13 to Sept. 23, 1843. 1 v. 156 pp. 8°. *London, W. Strange.* Completed.

Mesnage (Edmond). * Des insertions vicieuses du placenta et des hémorrhagies qui en résultent. 54 pp. 4°. *Paris,* 1868, No. 177.

[**Mesnager.**] Sourds et muets. Première et deuxième lettres à M. le docteur Berton. 32 pp. 8°. *Paris, J.-B. Baillière,* [1836].

Mesnard. Discours prononcé... dans la discussion générale du projet de loi relatif à l'enseignement et à l'exercice de la médecine et de la pharmacie. 8 pp. 8°. [*Paris,* 1847.] [P., v. 1676.]
Repr. from : Monit. univ., Par., 1847.

Mesnard (Élise-Marie). * De l'influence de quelques lésions syphilitiques du col de l'utérus sur l'accouchement. [Paris.] 55 pp. 4°. *Rochefort,* 1884, No. 38.

Mesnard (Émile). * Considérations sur la manière dont s'exerce présentement la police de santé dans les campagnes de la Vendée. 39 pp. 4°. *Paris,* 1829, No. 217, v. 227.

Mesnard (Jacques). Le guide des accoucheurs, ou le maistre dans l'art d'accoucher les femmes, et de les soulager dans les maladies et accidens dont elles sont très-souvent attaquées. Ouvrage des plus utiles pour les personnes qui veulent faire une pratique particulière de l'opération des accouchemens. Le tout en forme d'examen. xxxii, 382 pp., 9 l., 15 pl. 8°. *Paris, de Bure l'aîné,* 1743.

———. The same. 2. éd. xxxii, 392 pp. 8°. *Paris, de Bure l'aîné,* 1753.

Mesnard (Léon). * Contribution à l'étude des hémorrhagies utérines dans les pelvi-péritonites. 39 pp. 4°. *Paris,* 1879, No. 411.

Mesnard (Louis) [1853–]. * Du traitement de la pustule maligne. 57 pp., 1 l. 4°. *Paris,* 1881, No. 179.

Mesnard (Pierre-Arsène) [1859–]. * Des exostoses du creux sus-claviculaire. 56 pp. 4°. *Paris,* 1884, No. 350.

Mesner (A.) * Beiträge zur pathologischen Anatomie des Nervensystems. [Strasburg.] 23 pp. 8°. *Stuttgart, J. B. Metzler,* 1881.

Mesnet (Ernest). * Étude des paralysies hystériques. Considérations sur quelques cas d'hémorrhagie traumatique à la partie supérieure de la cuisse, et sur un mode de traitement qui leur est applicable. 114 pp. 4°. *Paris,* 1852, No. 20, v. 529.

———. Étude médico-psychologique sur l'homme dit le sauvage du Var, suivie du rapport de M. le docteur Cerise lu à l'Académie impériale de médecine. 32 pp., 1 pl. 8°. *Paris, J.-B. Baillière & fils,* 1865.
Repr. from : Ann. méd.-psych., Par., 1865, 4. s., v.

———. Choléra 1865; Hôpital Saint-Antoine (service des hommes). 43 pp. 8°. *Paris, P. Asselin,* 1866.
Repr. from : Arch. gén. de méd., Par., 1866, 6. s., vii.

———. De l'automatisme de la mémoire et du souvenir dans le somnambulisme pathologique; considérations médico-légales. 30 pp. 8°. *Paris, F. Malteste & Cie.,* 1874.
Repr. from : Union méd., Par., 1874, 3. s., xviii.

———. De l'hémoglobinurie à frigore. 16 pp. 8°. *Paris, Asselin & Cie.,* 1881.
Repr. from : Arch. gén. de méd., Par., 1881, 7. s., vii.

Mesnet (Raoul). * Des érythèmes blennorrhagiques. (Contribution à l'étude de la blennorrhagie infectieuse.) 49 pp., 1 l. 4°. *Paris,* 1884, No. 345.

Mesnier (Jules-Gabriel). * De l'ergot de seigle, et de son emploi en obstétrique et en médecine. 30 pp. 4°. *Paris,* 1858, No. 205, v. 621.

Mesnier (L. - Jacques - Élie) [1855–]. * Du suicide dans l'armée; étude statistique, étiologique et prophylactique. 126 pp. 4°. *Lyon,* 1881, No. 104.

Mesnil (J.-J.) * Sur la névralgie fémoro-poplitée. 31 pp. 4°. *Paris,* 1819, No. 29, v. 144.

Mesnil (P.) * Relation médicale de onze cas d'empoisonnement par de la viande de conserve altérée, observés au port de Lorient. 50 pp. 4°. *Paris,* 1874, No. 418.

du Mesnil (Theodor). * Ein Beitrag zur Kenntniss der Dermoidcysten. 27 pp. 8°. *Würzburg, Becker,* 1886.

Mesny (A.-M.) * De la diarrhée chronique en Cochinchine et de son traitement par le régime lacté. 51 pp. 4°. *Paris,* 1872, No. 466.

Mesology.
See Environments.

Mesoplodon.
Reinhardt (J.) Mesoplodon bidens, en Tilvæxt til den danske Havfauna. Overs. o. d. k. Danske Vidensk. Selsk. Forh., Kjøbenh., 1880, no. 2, 63–72, 1 pl.—**Turner.** On the form and structure of the teeth of Mesoplodon Layardii and Mesoplodon Sowerbyii. Proc. Roy. Soc. Edinb., 1878–80, x, 250–252.

Mesopodium.
Twining (T.) The mesopodium or saddle-stick. Lancet, Lond., 1851, ii, 107.

Mesopotamia.
See, also, Turkey.
Liétard (G.) Syrie, Mésopotamie et Babylonie. Dict. encycl. d. sc. méd., Par., 1884, 3. s., xiv, 693–758.

Mesquite.
Shumard (G. G.) Gum mesquite as a substitute for gum arabic. West. J. M. & S., Louisville, 1854, 4. s., ii, 437–439.

Mess (Petrus Marinus) [1817–]. * De cephalotribe. [Leyden.] 1 p. l., 48 pp. 8°. *Schoonhoviæ, S. E. van Nooten,* [1839].

———. Handboek over de beenbreuken en ontwrichtingen. En eene voorrede van den hoogleeraar F. W. Krieger. iv pp., 2 l., 406 pp., 1 l. 8°. *Leiden, D. N. van Goor,* 1853.

———. Balneologisch verslag van het badsaisoen 1853. 43 pp. 8°. [*n. p.,* 1853, *vel subseq.*]

———. Balneologischer Bericht über die Bade-Saison des Jahres 1853 in Scheveningen. 36 pp. 8°. *Berlin, G. Reimer,* 1854.
Repr. from : Deutsche Klinik, Berl., 1854, vi.

———. Account of the bathing seasons, 1854 and 1855. 15 pp. 8°. *Edinburgh, Murray & Gibb,* [1856].
Repr. from : Edinb. M. J., 1855–6, i.

———. Brieven over zuidelijk Frankrijk en Italië als verblijf voor borstlijders. 190 pp., 1 l. 8°. *Rotterdam, M. Wijt & Zonen,* 1857.

———. De l'influence sur quelques maladies de l'air et de l'eau de mer, d'après leur degré réciproque de température, avec trois tableaux météorologiques. 30 pp., 1 l., 3 tab. 4°. *La Haye, M. J. Visser,* 1859.

———. Over de toepassing der zeebadkuur bij ziektevormen van menstruatie en zwangerschap. 23 pp. 8°. [*Amsterdam,* 1867.]
Repr. from : Nederl. Tijdschr. v. Geneesk., Amst., 1867, iii.

———. Eene waarschuwing aan het zeestrand. 15 pp. 8°. *'s Gravenhage, M. M. Couvée,* 1873.

Messager (Auguste). * Sur la cataracte. 31 pp. 4°. *Paris,* 1824, No. 233, v. 189.

Messager (P.-E.-C.) * Sur l'érysipèle. 19 pp. 4°. *Paris,* 1815, No. 73, v. 110.

Messand (Henri-Napoléon). * Hygiène des femmes en couches. 38 pp. 4°. *Paris,* 1835, No. 58, v. 283.

Messant (Paul). *Sur la pleuro-pneumonie aiguë. 28 pp. 4°. *Paris*, 1834, No. 128, v. 272.

Messchaert (Nicolaas). *Iets over ovariotomie. viii, 4 pp., li, 5-26 pp. 8°. *Utrecht, J. G. van Terveen & Zoon*, 1863.

Messence (Joannes Jacobus). *An a facili perspiratione, functionum libertas? Præses: Natalis Andræus Joannes Baptista Chesneau. 4 pp. 4°. [*Parisiis, Quillau*, 1747.]
See, also, **de la Noue** (Bartholomæus Petrus). *An acquæ potus omnium saluberrimus? 4°. [*Paris*, 1769.]

Messenger (The) of Health: a monthly journal . . . Edited by the medical and surgical staff of the World's Dispensary and Invalid's Hotel. Nos. 1-6, v. 1, June to Nov., 1883. 74 pp. 8°. *Buffalo, N. Y.*
An advertisement.

Messer (Adam). A probationary essay on amaurosis. 1 p. l., 21 pp. 8°. *Edinburgh, J. Clarke & Co.*, 1826. [*Also, in:* P., v. 1273.]

Messer (Carl). *Beiträge zur colorimetrischen Analyse. 28 pp., 1 l., 1 pl. 8°. *Bonn, C. Georgi*, 1868.
C.

Messer (Hermann). *Ueber Täuschungen des Augenmasses. 34 pp., 1 pl. 8°. *Würzburg, C. J. Becker*, 1875.

Messer (Joh. Frid.) *De cholera morbo. 30 pp., 1 l. sm. 4°. *Halæ Magdeb., lit. C. Henckelii*, [1710].
Also, in: HALLER. Disp. ad morb. [etc.] 4°. *Lausannæ*, 1757, iii, 73-97.

Messer (W. W.)
See **Morse** (E. Malcolm). A treatise on the hot sulphur springs of El Paso de Robles [etc.] 8°. *San Francisco*, 1875.

Messerer (Alexandre). *Des lésions viscérales de l'impaludisme. 99 pp. 4°. *Paris*, 1886, No. 50.

Messerer (Otto). Ueber Elasticität und Festigkeit der menschlichen Knochen. 3 p. l., 103 pp., 16 pl. 4°. *Stuttgart, J. G. Cotta*, 1880.

———. Experimentelle Untersuchungen über Schädelbrüche. 1 p. l., 36 pp., 8 pl. 8°. *München, M. Rieger*, 1884.

Messerschmid (J. Christ.) Antiquitates balneares ex C. Plini. Cæcili secundi epistolis collectas. 28 pp. 4°. *Vitembergæ, typ. J. C. Tzschidrichi*, 1762.

Messerschmidt (Alexander). *Observationes de operationibus chiloplasticis, præsertim in labiis cancrosis. 80 pp. 8°. [*Dorpat*], typ. H. Laakmanni, 1850.

Messerschmidt (Fridericus Gustavus). *De pure et sanie. 4 p. l., 20 pp. 8°. *Lipsiæ, sumt. G. Engelmanni*, [1842].

Messerschmidt (G.) Die Militär-Oeconomie. Handbuch für Militärverwaltungs-Beamte, Militärs und diejenigen, welche sich mit der Militär-Oeconomie vertraut machen wollen. Erster Band: Die Verpflegung der Kriegsheere. xx, 543, 38 pp., 2 pl. 8°. *Berlin, Bahn u. Faudel*, 1854.

Messerschmidt (Georg). *Beiträge zur Aetiologie des Puerperalfiebers. 34 pp. 8°. *Greifswald, F. W. Kunike*, [1872].
C.

Messerschmidt (Gustav). *Ueber Syndactylie. 31 pp. 8°. *Greifswald, C. Sell*, 1885.

Messerschmidt (Heinrich Gottlob) [1776-1842]. *De natura morborum, ipsisque medendi ratione. 37, xiv pp. 4°. *Lipsiæ, ex off. Klaubarthia*, [1805].

———. Beweisführung, dass die Häusersperre als Abwehrungsmittel gegen die Verbreitung der asiatischen Cholera nicht allein nicht nützt, sondern vielmehr schädlich und darum zu unterlassen ist, bei Gelegenheit des Zusammentritts der heutigen Gesundheits-Comité abgefasst. 82 pp. 8°. *Naumburg, Wild*, 1831. [P., v. 739.]
For Biography, see **Ludwig** (Christianus Fridericus).

Messerschmied (Daniel Gottlob) [1685-1735]. *De ratione præside universæ medicinæ. 46 pp., 1 l. sm. 4°. *Halæ Magdeb., typ. C. Henckelii*, [1713].

Messien (Fr.-Omer). Exposé sommaire d'une nouvelle théorie médicale basée sur les fonctions du foie. 2. éd., corrigée et augmentée notamment d'un aperçu sur la respiration pulmonaire. iv, 9-99 pp. 8°. *Tournai, A. Delmée*, 1865.

Messier (Léon). *De la stomatite ulcéro-membraneuse. 34 pp. 4°. *Paris*, 1855, No. 72, v. 578.

Messina. Regolamento di polizia urbana della città di Messina. 86 pp. 12°. *Messina, tip. dell' Operajo*, [1873?]

Messina (Pietro). Mediche osservazioni sopra alcune non ovvie infermità; lette dallo stesso autore all' Accademia Gioenia di Catania nell' ordinaria seduta del dì 30 dicembre 1851. 50 pp. 8°. *Catania, F. Sciuto*, 1851. [P., v. 1115.]
Repr. from: Accademia Gioenia di Catania, 1851, 2. s., viii.

Messina.
See, also, **Cholera** (Asiatic, History, etc., of), **Hospitals** (Ophthalmic, etc.), by localities.
BENIGNI (G.) Fognatura ed igiene pubblica in Messina. 8°. *Messina*, 1884.
TESTA (F.) Relazione istorica della peste che attaccossi a Messina nell' anno mille sette cento quarantatre. Coll' aggiunto degli ordini, editti, istruzioni, ed altri atti pubblici fatti in occasione della medesima. 4°. *Palermo*, 1745.
Costa-Saya (A.) Delle acque potabili in rapporto allo stato sanitario e specialmente di quelle di Messina. Gior. internaz. d. sc. med., Napoli, 1880, n. s., ii, 664; 773; 872. ———. Un' altra parola intorno alla questione dell' acqua potabile di Messina. *Ibid.*, 1881, n. s., iii, 318-322.— **Testa** (B.) Le acque potabili in rapporto allo stato sanitario e specialmente di quelle di Messina. *Ibid.*, 1879, n. s., i, 879-895. ———. Breve risposta al Prof. A. Costa-Saya a proposito della questione delle acque potabili di Messina. *Ibid.*, 1880, ii, 1297-1302.

von Messing (Michael). *Ueber Behandlung der Metrorrhagien Neuentbundener mit Beschreibung eines neuen Verfahrens. 66 pp. 8°. *Würzburg, C. J. Becker*, 1873.

Messing (Wladyslaw). *Anatomische Untersuchungen über den Testikel der Säugethiere, mit besonderer Berücksichtigung des Corpus Highmori. 97 pp., 1 pl. 8°. *Dorpat, C. Mattiesen*, 1877.

Messner. Die chronische Stuhlverstopfung (Hartleibigkeit), mit besonderer Berücksichtigung des Hämorrhoidalleidens und deren Heilung. 37 pp., 1 l. 8°. *Berlin, A. Zimmer*, 1886.

Messner (Heinrich Emil). *Zur Lehre von den epidemischen Entzündungen der Wöchnerinnen. 31 pp. 8°. *Tübingen, L. F. Fues*, 1843.

Messner (Vincentius). *De chorea St. Viti. 38 pp. 8°. *Landishuti, J. Thomann*, [1809].

Messow (Franciscus) [1817-]. *De inflammatione venæ portarum seu pylephlebitide. 56 pp. 8°. *Berolini, typ. Nietackianis*, [1841].

Mestaïer (L.-M.-M.) *Sur la tympanite. 24 pp. 4°. *Paris*, 1820, No. 147, v. 158.

Mestayer (André). *Observations médicales sur plusieurs aphorismes d'Hippocrate; précédées de quelques réflexions sur l'expérience en médecine. 47 pp. 8°. *Paris, an XI* [1803], v. 22.

Mester (Arnoldus). *De prosopalgia. 30 pp. 8°. *Wirceburgi, ex off. vid. C. Becker*, 1847.

Mesterton (Carl Benedict) [1826-]. *Om medfödt hjernbråck. [Congenital cerebral hernia.] 46 pp., 4 pl. 8°. *Stockholm, J. W. Lundberg*, 1855.

———. Studier i bräckläran. 1. Om radicaloperation för ljumskbråck. 100 pp., 1 pl. 8°. *Stockholm, J. & A. Riis*, 1857.

Mesterton (Carl Benedict)—continued.
——. * Om nosocomium academicum och den kliniska undervisningen i Upsala. 35 pp. 4°. *Upsala, E. Berling,* 1869.
——. Ett kejsarsnitt. Inbjudningsskrift till medicine doktorspromotionen i Upsala den 6. September 1877. 1 p. l., 28 pp., 3 pl. 8°. *Upsala, E. Berling,* 1877.

Mestingh (Joannes Eliza). * De melæna. viii, 63 pp. 8°. *Traj. ad Rhenum, Van Dorp et Heringa,* 1843.

Mestivier (Achille-François). * Luxations du bras. vi, 7–19 pp. 4°. *Paris,* 1819, No. 84, v. 146.

Mestivier (E.-A.) * Recherches sur la stérilité considérée dans les deux sexes. 101 pp. 8°. *Paris, an XI* [1803], v. 21.

Mestivier (J.-Léopold). * Des fièvres larvées. 38 pp. 4°. *Paris,* 1863, No. 52.

Mestivier (Jean-Vincent-de-Paule). * De la lèpre. vi, 7–36 pp. 4°. *Paris,* 1820, No. 68, v. 156.

Mestivier (Marcel). * De la saignée des veines ranines dans les maladies du pharynx. 30 pp. 4°. *Paris,* 1856, No. 239, v. 593.

Mestman (Antoine - Herman). * Essai sur la bronchotomie. 1 p. l., 21 pp. 4°. *Strasbourg,* 1828, v. 57.
——. The same. 21 pp. 4°. *Strasbourg, F.-G. Levrault,* 1828.

de Mestral (V.) * De l'opération radicale de la hernie ombilicale. [Basel.] 62 pp. 8°. *Lausanne, G. Bridel,* 1881.

Mestre (Antonio). * Étude sur les vertiges. 50 pp. 4°. *Paris,* 1861, No. 134.
See, also, **Trabajos** de la Comision de medicina legal, etc. 3 v. 8°. *Habana,* 1872–4.
Also, Co-Editor of : **Anales** de la real Academia de ciencias médicas, físicas y naturales de la Habana, 1864–81.

Mestre (J.-A.) * Sur les effets physiologiques immédiats de l'eau, appliquée à la surface du corps, depuis l'état de glace jusqu'à l'état de vapeur sous forme d'ablution, d'immersion, d'affusion, de douche, de bain, etc. 43 pp. 4°. *Paris,* 1824, No. 207, v. 188.

Mestre (J.-F.-G.) Essai sur l'éléphantiasis des Arabes et sur l'éléphantiasis des Grecs observés en Algérie. xii, 13–102 pp., 1 l., 6 pl. 8°. *Montpellier, Boehm,* 1859.
——. The same. x, 11–104 pp., 1 l., 6 pl. 8°. *Montpellier, Boehm & fils,* 1864.
——. Notes et observations sur les causes de l'épidémie qui a sévi contre les habitants de Tunis pendant l'été de 1863. Quel est le traitement que l'on doit opposer à ce genre de maladie? Notice sur les avantages et les inconvénients de la Tunisie. 85 pp. 8°. *Bone, Dagand,* 1864.

Mestre (R.-B.-Baudouin). * Considérations sur les plaies d'armes à feu en général. 36 pp. 4°. *Paris,* 1–37, No. 72, v. 308.

Mestrude (Ferdinand). * Du traitement de la pourriture d'hôpital, et en particulier du traitement par la teinture d'iode. 44 pp. 4°. *Paris,* 1871.

Mestzger (Joh. Caspar). * De naturæ et artis effectu in medendo. 39 pp. 4°. *Halæ Magdeb., lit. C. Henckelii,* 1708.

Mesue *Damascenus* (Joannes) [**Jahja Ben Maseweih Ben Ahmed** (or **Muhammed**) **Ben Ali Ben Abd el-Malik**] [928–1016?]. In nomine Dei misericordis cujus nutu sermo recipit gratiam et doctrina perfectionem, principium verborum Joannis filii Mesue: filii Hamech: filii Hely: filii Abdela regis Damasci. 200 l. fol. [*Ad finem:*] [impressor Clemens pattavinus sacerdos bonus]. *Venetiis,* 1471.
Without signature or catch-words. Illuminated capitals.

Mesue *Damascenus* (Joannes)—continued.
——. The same. [*Ad finem:*] Hoc loci consumantur opera divi Joannis Mesuæ cum complemento et additionibus clarissimi doctoris Francisci de Pedemontium. Ac Nicolao et Servitore. 391 l. fol. *Venetiis, ope et imp. Rainaldi Novimagii,* 1479.
——. The same. [*Ad finem:*] Elaboratum opus faustum et preclarum divi Joannis Mesue omnia opera continens. Cum additionibus Petri Apponi; et Francisci de Pedemontium, ac Nicolai cum Servitore. Emendata accuratissime per eximium artium et medicine doctorem Magistrum Archangelum Senensem. 286 l. fol. *Venetiis, sumpt. et imp. Dionysii de Bertochis de Bononia,* 1484.
Two leaves wanting in signature r.
——. Mesue cum additionibus Francisci de Pedemontium. Et additionibus Petri Aponi. Et cum commento Dini super canones generales. Et cum commento Christophori de Honestis super antidotarium Mesue, Platearius super antidotarium Nicolai, et Saladinus de componendis medicinis. fol. [*Venetiis, P. de Pasqualibus,* 1489–91.

CONTENTS.

F. 2 a (cum sign. a 2). Præclarissimi medici magistri Dini super canones sive de rectificatione medicinarum simplicium solutivarum expositio. F. 1 (cum sign. aa). Joannis Mesuæ Grabadini quod est aggregatio et antidotarium electuariorum et confectionum : et aliarum medicinarum compositarum. F. 1 (cum sign. A et n. 1). Summa secunda hujus Grabadini incipit in qua distinguantur medicinæ appropriatæ ægritudinibus membrorum. F. 223 (cum sign. EE). Incipit antidotarium Nicolai cum expositionibus et glosis clarissimi physici magistri Platearii. F. 293. Incipit liber Servitoris libri xxviii. Bulchasin Benaberazerin translatus a Simone Januensi interprete Abraam Judeo Tortuosiensi. F. 1 (sign. g). F. 14. (cum sign. MM). Domini Saladini de Esculo Serenitatis principis Tarenti phisici principalis aromatariorum compendium feliciter incipit.

——. Mesue cum expositione Mondini super canones universales, ac etiam cum expositione Christophori de Honestis in antidotarium ejusdem. Additiones Petri Apponi. Additiones Francisci de Pedemontium. Antidotarium Nicolai cum expositione Platearii. Tractatus quid pro quo. Tractatus de sinoninis. Libellus Bulcasis sive Servitoris. Compendium aromatariorum Saladini. Joannes de Sancto Amando super antidotarium Nicolai. 332 ff. fol. [*Venetiis, imp. B. Locatellus,* 1495.]
——. The same. 355 ff. fol. *Venetiis,* 1502.
——. The same. 356 l. fol. *Lugduni, imp. V. de Portonariis de Tridino de Monteferrato,* 1510.
——. The same. cccxxvii ff., 6 l. fol. *Lugduni, sumpt. pro et impensis Vincentii de Portonariis de Tridino de Monteferrato,* 1525.
The first folio with title is wanting.
——. [*Incipit:*] In nomine Dei misericordis cujus nutu sermo recipit gratiam et doctrina perfectionem. Principium verborum Joannis filii Mesuæ: filii Hamech, filii Heli: filii Abdelæ regis Damasci. Verbum cecidit inter inquirentes scire quid est quod rememorati sunt quidam de rectificatione medicinarum simplicium solutivarum. Multi sapientes scripserunt. [F. 302:] Hic complentur dicta: et imponitur finis doctrinæ divini Mesuæ: licet imperfecte in de appropriatis, [etc.] [F. 302:] Tabula capitulorum additionum Petri Apponi. [*In fine:*] Petri Apponi . . . in librum Joannis Mesuæ additio feliciter finit. 348 ff. 16°. *Impressum Venetiis, per Jacobum Pentium de Leuco,* 1505.
——. Canones universales divi Mesue de consolatione medicinarum et correctione operationum earundem. Grabadin ejusdem Mesue medicinarum universalium quod antidotarium nuncupat. Liber ejusdem medicinarum particularium. Additio Petri Apponi . . . in librum Joannis Mesue.

Mesue *Damascenus* (Joannes)—continued.

Antidotarium domini Nicolai. Summula Jacobi de partibus per alphabetum super plurimis remediis ex antidotario ipsius Mesue excerptis. 337 l. 16°. *Lugduni, G. de Villiers,* [1511].

Gothic letter, with MS. notes and 31 leaves MS. recipes, etc.

———. The same. 344 l. 16°. [*Lugduni, imp. J. q. F. de Giunta et sociorum Florentini,* 1523.]

———. Generales divi Mesue canones . . . Novissima hac impressione emissi. 32 l. 16°. [*Papie B. de Garaldis,* 1517.]

Bound with: AVICENNA. Ordo novus multiez. 16°. [*Papie,* 1517.]

———. Mesue vulgar. Summario, over collectorio universalissimo extracto da tutti li volumini delli antiquissimi medici Hebrei, Greci, et Arabi, tractanti del rectificar delle medicine, etc. . . . Composto, et con summo artificio compillado per . . . Gioanni Mesue, et altri famosissimi authori . . . el qual collectorio è distincto, e spartito in quattro notabelissimi libri . . . videlicet: De rectificar le medicine, delle medicine simplice, dello antidotario, delle egritudine particulare, etc. Foglio 1. Prohemio. Incomencia el libro della consolatione delle medicine simplice solutive, el quale fece el principe di tutti gli practici Gioanne figliolo di Mesue. Novamente distincto, corretto e diligentemente revisto. 4 p. l., cxiii ff. fol. [*Venetia, C. Arrivabeno,* 1521.]

———. The same. 4 p. l., cxiii ff., 1 l. fol. *Venetia,* 1521.

Another copy bound with: GUY DE CAULIAC. Guidon in cirurgia. fol. *Venetia,* 1521.

———. De consolatione medicinarum simplicium et correctione operationum earum canones cum expositione Mondini de Lentiis feliciter incipiunt. ii–xlii ff. fol. *Lugduni,* 1525.

———. De re medica libri tres, Jacobo Sylvio interprete. 7 p. l., 350 pp. fol. *Paris, ex off. C. Wecheli,* 1544.

———. The same. Index locupletissimus cum capitum, tum omnium quæ scitu digna sunt operi præfixus est: in quo prior numerus, paginam: posterior, lineam indicat. 7 p. l., 495 pp. 16°. *Lugduni, apud G. Rovillium,* 1548.

———. The same. 7 p. l., 421 pp. 12°. *Lugduni, apud G. Rovillium,* 1550.

———. The same. Cum annotationibus et scholiis ejusdem. 248 ff., 4 l. 12°. *Parisiis,* 1553.

———. The same. 7 p. l., 364 pp. 16°. *Lugduni, apud G. Rovillium,* 1566.

———. Mesua et omnia quæ cum eo imprimi consueverunt, pulchrioribus typis reformata, diligentiorique animadversione emendata, et pluribus in locis restituta, atque copiosiori indice, quid in quoque opere contineatur, significante, decorata: quæ in sequenti pagina descripta sunt. Addita est Jacobi Silvii interpretatio canonum universalium simplicium medicinarum, atque antidotarii; in quo et ponderum varietatem in margine annotavimus. Et duo trochisci Mesue, quæ in manuscriptis exemplaribus invenimus, et quædam compositiones ex Galeno, quæ nunc ab aromatariis in usu habentur. 13 p. l., 141 ff., 313 pp. fol. *Venetiis, apud Juntas,* 1549.

———. De morbis internis curandis liber unus. Accessit Petri Aponi ad Mesuen προσθήκη, cum vocum Arabicarum in toto opere contentarum interprætatione, ab Joanne Rænerio adjecta. Omnia ad diversorum exemplarium fidem summa diligentia emendata. 11 p. l., 493 pp. 8°. *Lugduni, apud A. Vincentium,* 1551.

———. Nam purgantium medicamentorum tam universales regulas quam particulariæ exempla descripsit, compositionem etiam cælebrium medicinarum tradidit, ac demum propria cuique membro remedia accommodavit. Ex duplici tralatione, altera quidem antiqua, altera vera

Mesue *Damascenus* (Joannes)—continued.

nova Jacobi Sylvii Medici; item alii omnes, qui cum Mesue imprimi consueverum quorum nomina ac librorum titulos sequens pagina indicat. Adjectæ sunt etiam nunc primum annotationes in eundem Mesue, Joannis Manardi et Jacobi Sylvii. Opus sane divinum medicis aromatariisque omnibus, ne dum utile, sed etiam necessarium, maxima diligentia a doctissimo medico nuperrime castigatum. 20, 172 ff. fol. *Venetiis, apud Juntas,* 1558.

———. Libri dei semplici purgativi e delle medicine composte, nuovamente tradotti in lingua italiana; con la tavola delle cose, che ne' detti libri si contengono, et con la dichiaratione de' vocaboli oscuri. 34 p. l., 331 pp. 16°. *Venetia, appresso gli heredi di B. Costantino,* 1559.

———. Opera quæ extant omnia. Ex duplici translatione: altera quidem antiqua, altera vero nova Jacobi Sylvii. Item authores omnes, qui cum Mesue imprimi consueverunt; quorum nomina, ac librorum titulos sequens pagina indicat. Accesserunt his annotationes in eundem Mesuen Joannis Manardi, et Jacobi Sylvii. Adjectæ sunt etiam nunc recens Andreæ Marini annotationes in simplicia cum imaginibus desideratis. Scholion item ejusdem in olea quædam. Quæ omnia maxima diligentia ab eodem Marino e vetustissimis exemplaribus sunt castigata. 17 p. l., 475 ff. fol. *Venetiis, apud V. Valgrisium,* 1561.

———. Opera a Joanne Costa nunc recognita, et aucta adnotationibus, quibus a recentiorum calumniis divinus hic scriptor vendicatur. Accessere his varia diversorum medicorum opuscula, quæ una cum Mesue imprimi consuevere, ac præterea plantarum de quibus in libro simplicium agitur, legitimæ imagines ad vivum expressæ, in superioribus æditionibus desideratæ. Quibus additus etiam nunc est Cophonis libellus de arte medendi inscriptus, Mesuæ operum veluti correlarium: in quo tractandæ medicæ materiæ ratio atque usus brevissime explicatur. 11 p. l., 204 ff., 314 ff., 12 l. fol. *Venetiis, in off. Juntarum,* 1568.

———. The same. 8 p. l., 258 ff.; 6 l., 277 ff., 11 l. fol. *Venetiis, apud Juntas,* 1589.

———. The same. 252 ff.; 5 l., 278 ff., 10 l. fol. *Venetiis, apud Juntas,* 1602.

———. Opera. De medicamentorum purgantium delectu, castigatione et usu libri duo. Quorum priorem canones universales, posteriorem de simplicibus vocant. Grabadin, hoc est compendii secretorum medicamentorum, libri duo. Quorum prior antidotarium: posterior de appropriatis vulgo inscribitur. Cum Mundini, Honesti, Manardi et Sylvii in tres priores libros observationibus, quæ vulgo cum his ipsis prodire consueverunt. His accessere plantarum in libro simplicium descriptarum imagines ex vivo expressæ. Atque item Joannis Costæi annotationes, tum quas in editione superiori dedimus, tum præterea novæ aliæ in postremas novem antidotarii sectiones, quæ hactenus desiderabantur, [etc.] 7 p. l., 272 ff.; 5 p. l., 277 ff., 12 l. fol. *Venetiis, apud Juntas,* 1581.

In two parts, with separate title-page and pagination. The title of second part reads: Supplementum in secundum librum, etc.

———. The same. 5 p. l., 252 ff.; 5 p. l., 278 ff., 11 l. fol. *Venetiis, apud Juntas,* 1623.

See, also, **Avicenna.** Canticum . . . de medicina [etc.] 12°. *Groningæ,* 1649. — **Campegius** (S.) Officina apothecariorum seu seplasiariorum. sm. 4°. *Lugduni,* 1532. — **Falcutius** (Nicolaus). Audidotarium, etc. fol. [*Argentorati, n. d.*]—**de la Fuente Pierola** (Geronimo). Tyrocinio pharmacopeo, methodo medico y chimico. En el qual se continen los canones de Joanes Mesue Damasceno, y su explicacion . . . fol. *Pamplona,* 1721. — **Hahn** (J. G.) De veris Mesuæ Syri scriptis non deperditis sed sub Jani Damasceni nomine conservatis ad . . . Joannem Albertum Fabricium . . . epistola. 4°. [*Vratislaviæ,* 1733.]—

Mesue *Damascenus* (Joannes)—continued.
Manardus (Joannes Jacobus). Ἰατρολογία ἐπιστολικὴ
sive curia medica, etc. fol. *Hanoviæ,* 1611. — **de Man-
liis** *de Boscho* (Joh. Jacobus.) Luminare majus. fol.
Venetiis, [n. d.] — **Puteanus** (Guil.) Joannis Mesue
aloën aperire ora venarum [etc.] 12°. *Lugduni,* 1537. —
Ranchin (F.) Commentaire sur les théorèmes et canons
généraux de Mesué, dicté à Montpellier aux compagnons
pharmaciens. *In his:* Œuvres pharm. 12°. *Lyon,* 1624,
31–712. — **de Sgobbis** (A.) Universale theatro farmaceutico [etc.] fol. *Venetiis,* 1682. — **Valescus de Tharanta.** Practica Valesci de Tharanta [etc.] 4°. [*Lugduni,* 1401 [1491].

Mesures (Des) prophylactiques et de l'organisation du service d'assistance publique en temps
d'épidémie cholérique. Rapport de MM. Ardouin-
Bey, Brinsenstein, Burlazzi, Chaumery, Sierra et
Valensin, membres de la commission élue par le
corps médical d'Alexandrie 10 juillet 1883. 19
pp. 8°. *Alexandrie, Égypte, E. Debono,* 1883.

Mesureur (P.-J.) * Sur un parallèle des inflammations aiguës de la poitrine. vi, 7–35 pp. 4°.
Paris, 1818, No. 166, v. 141.

Metacarpal *bones.*

CALORI (L.) Di una particolare epifisi del
capitello del primo osso metacarpeo e del primo
metatarseo non che di altra della tuberosità del
quinto. Memoria. 4°. *Bologna,* 1861.
Repr. from: Mem. Accad. d. sc. d. Ist. di Bologna, xi.
Bluff (M. J.) Ueber das sogenannte Os metacarpi pollicis. Arch. f. Anat. u. Physiol., Leipz., 1826, i, 112–116, 1
pl. — **Gruber** (W.) Vorkommen des Processus styloideus
des Metacarpale iii als persistirende und ein neuntes H nd-
wurzelknöchelchen repräsentirende Epiphyse. Arch. f.
Anat., Physiol. u. wissensch. Med., Leipz., 1869, 361–366,
1 pl. ——. Ueber das aus einer persistirenden und den
Processus styloideus des Metacarpale iii repräsentirenden
Epiphyse entwickelte, articulirende, neunte Handwurzel-
knöchelchen. *Ibid.,* 1870, 197–207, 1 pl. ——. Neue Fälle
des Vorkommens eines neunten, den Processus styloideus
des Metacarpale iii, subtituirenden Handwurzelknöchel-
chens beim Menschen. Mélanges biol. Acad. imp. d. sc.
de St.-Pétersb., 1869–71, vii, 635–640. ——. Ueber einen
Fall des Vorkommens des den Processus styloideus des
Metacarpale iii, substituirenden neunten Handwurzelknö-
chelchens beim Menschen, welches mit dem Metacarpale
iii theilweise anchylosirt war. *Ibid.,* 641–648. — **Halford.**
Observations on the metacarpal and metatarsal bones of
the human skeleton. Austral. M. J., Melbourne, 1863, viii,
199–202, 1 pl. — **Hecker.** Widernatürliches Gelenk an dem
Mittelhandknochen des Daumens. Arch. f. physiol. Heilk.,
Stuttg., 1844, iii, 265. — **Retzius** (A.) Om de så kallade
ossa metacarpi pollicis och metatarsi hallucis. Förh. v. de
skandin. Naturf. 1844, Christiania, 1847, 303–305. — **Thomson** (A.) On the difference in the mode of ossification of
the first and other metacarpal and metatarsal bones. J.
Anat. & Physiol., Lond., 1869, iii, 131–146.

Metacarpal *bones (Diseases and in-
juries of).*

See, also, **Excisions** *of wrist;* **Hand** (*Surgery
of*).

B. (W.) Fracture of the metacarpal bones. Boston M.
& S. J., 1843-4, xxix, 459. — **Bennett** (E. H.) Fractures
of the metacarpal bones. Dublin J. M. Sc., 1882, 3. s.,
lxxiii, 72–75, 1 pl. — **Bérenger-Feraud.** Étude sur les
blessures du métacarpe traitées dans la deuxième division
des blessés du Val-de-Grâce pendant le siége de Paris.
Bull. gén. de thérap., etc., Par., 1872, lxxxii, 397–404. —
Birkett. Cancer of the metacarpal bone of the middle
finger of the left hand. Tr. Path. Soc. Lond., 1854–5, vi,
291–295. — **Bouteiller.** Luxation, en arrière, du premier
métacarpien sur le carpe; mécanisme de cette luxation.
Union méd., Rouen, 1874, xiii, 35–37. — **Dean** (H. M.)
Fracture of the metacarpal bones of the right hand. Med.
Bull., Phila , 1881, iii, 201. — **Heath** (C.) Fracture of the
metacarpus. Tr. Path. Soc. Lond., 1867–8, xix, 302, 1 pl. —
Heydenreich. Cas de luxation en avant des quatre
derniers métacarpiens sur le carpe. Rev. méd. de l'est,
Nancy, 1881, xiii, 87. — **Mathieson** (J. H.) Fracture of
the fourth metacarpal bone. Canada M. J., Montreal,
1870–71, vii, 351. — **Maurice** (E.-F.) Luxation du quatrième métacarpien Ann. Soc. de méd. de St.-Étienne et
de la Loire, 1872, iv, 99–101. — **Parker** (R. S.) Caries of the
heads of the metacarpal bones of the right hand. Canada
M. J., Montreal, 1865–6, ii, 11–13. — **Smith** (R. W.) Dislocation of the navicular bone. Dublin Hosp. Gaz., 1855, ii, 76. —
Tuckerman (L. B.) Dislocation of the 5th metacarpal
bone backward, right hand. "The Transactions", Youngstown, Ohio, 1879–8), i, 101. — **Young** (D. S.) The treatment of fractures of the metacarpal bones. Cincin. M.
Repert., 1870, iii 114–117.

Metachloral.

Féréol. Sur l'emploi du métachloral. Bull. gén. de
thérap., etc., Par., 1872, lxxxiii, 123.

Métadier (Paul-Adrien). * Des tumeurs blanches en général. 105 pp., 2 l. 4°. *Montpellier,
J. Martel aîné,* 1864. [P., v. 45.]

Metahæmoglobin.

See **Hæmoglobin.**

Métairie (La), maison de santé. *See* **Maison** de
santé de la Métairie, près Nyon.

Metaisocymol.

KELBE (W.) * Ueber das Metaisocymol.
[Karlsruhe.] 8°. *Giessen,* 1881.

Metalbumin.

Hammarsten (O.) Metalbumin und Paralbumin;
ein Beitrag zur Chemie der Kystomflüssigkeiten. Ztschr.
f. physiol. Chem., Strassb., 1882, vi, 194–226.

Metallic *tinkling.*

See **Auscultation** (*Sounds, etc., in*).

Metallic *tractors.*

See **Tractors** (*Metallic*).

Metalloscopy.

See, also, **Metallotherapy.**
Adler (A. S.) A contribution to the doctrine of bilateral functions, after experiences of metalloscopy. West.
Lancet, San Fran., 1880–81, ix, 536–552. — **Atkins** (R.)
Metalloscopy in hysterical hemianæsthesia. Brit. M. J.
Lond., 1879, ii, 768–770. — **Bernhardt** (M.) Ueber Metalloscopie. Berl. klin. Wchnschr., 1878, xv, 129–131. —
Dumontpallier & **Magnin.** Expériences sur la métalloscopie, l'hypnotisme et la force neurique. Compt.
rend. Soc. de biol. 1881, Par., 1882, 7. s., iii. 359–364. — **El-
vers.** Zur Metalloscopie. Berl. klin. Wchnschr., 1880,
xvii, 52–54. — **Grocco** (P.) Influenza della metalloscopia
sulla linea sfigmica. Gazz. med. ital. lomb., Milano, 1880,
8. s., ii, 189. ——. Studi composti di metalloscopia. *Ibid.,*
319; 340; 351; 360; 379; 409; 429; 439. — **Guitéras** (J.)
Two cases of anæsthesia, with some metalloscopic experiments. Phila. M. Times. 1879, ix, 224–227. — **Mader.** Zur
Lehre von der Metalloskopie. Wien. med. Wchnschr.,
1879, xxix, 681–685. — **Maggiorani.** Alcune sue esperienze di metalloscopia. Atti Accad. med. di Roma, 1878,
iv, fasc. 2, 6; 95. ——. [Sulla metalloscopia.] Bull. d. r.
Accad. med. di Roma, 1880, vi. no. 3, 19–28. *Also, transl.:*
Bull. et mém. Soc. de thérap. 1880, Par., 1881, 2. s., vi, 179–
185. *Also:* Bull. gén. de thérap., etc., Par., 1880, xcix, 100–
106. — **Marzorati** (P.) La metalloscopia. Gazz. med.
ital. lomb., Milano, 1877, 7. s., iv, 211–213. — **Metalloscopy.** Birmingh. M. Rev., 1879, viii, 113–130. — **Meyer**
(A) Zur Metalloscopie. Berl. klin. Wchnschr., 1878, xv,
496. — **Parona** (E.) La metalloscopia studiata in un caso
di acromatopsia bilaterale con emianestesia sinistra ed
amiostenia destra. Ann. univ. di med. e chir., Milano,
1879, ccxlix, 336–366. — **Rumpf** (T.) Ueber den Transfert.
Berl. klin. Wchnschr., 1879, xvi, 533–535. — **Tuke** (D. H.)
Metalloscopy and expectant attention. J. Ment. Sc.,
Lond., 1879, n. s., xxiv, 597–609. — **Vierordt** (H.) Zur
Metalloskopie. Centralbl. f. d. med. Wissensch., Berl.,
1879, xvii, 1–4. — **Westphal** (C.) Ueber Metalloscopie.
Berl. klin. Wchnschr., 1878, xv, 441–446. *Also, transl.*
[Abstr.]: Lond. M. Rec., 1878, vi, 455–458. ——. Ueber
Metalloscopie. Verhandl. d. Berl. med. Gesellsch. (1878–
9). 1880, x, pt. 2, 1–17. [Discussion], pt. 1, 1–3.

Metallotherapy.

See, also, **Chlorosis,** **Hysteria,** *Treatment of;*
Tractors (*Metallic*).

ADLER (A. S.) * Ein Beitrag zur Lehre von
den "bilateralen Functionen" im Anschlusse an
Erfahrungen der Metalloscopie. 8°. *Berlin,*
[1879].

AIGRE (D.) * Étude clinique sur la métalloscopie et la métallothérapie externe dans l'anesthésie. 4°. *Versailles,* 1879.

BURQ (V.) Métallothérapie. Nouveau traitement par les applications métalliques. 8°. *Paris,*
1853.

——. Métallothérapie. Du cuivre contre le
choléra au point de vue prophylactique et curatif. Faits et observations depuis l'épidémie de
1849, [etc.] 8°. *Paris,* 1867.

——. Métallothérapie. Du cuivre contre le
choléra; rapport officiel du Dr. Vernois sur l'immunité cholérique des ouvriers en cuivre. In-

Metallotherapy.

struction pour le traitement préservatif et curatif. 8°. *Paris*, [1871?]

DELHEZ (F.) * Iets over het Burquisme. 8°. *Leiden*, 1881.

INGRIA (V. E.) Metalloterapia e xiloterapia. 8°. *Palermo*, 1885.

JENNINGS (O.) * Comparaison des effets de divers traitements dans l'hystérie, précédée d'une esquisse historique sur la métallothérapie. 4°. *Paris*, 1878.

KÖCHLIN (J. R.) Von den Wirkungen der gebräuchlichen Metalle auf den menschlichen Organismus überhaupt und als Heilmittel und dem Kupfersalmiak-Liquor und andern Kupferpräparaten als solchen insbesondere. 8°. *Zürich*, 1837.

MASOIN & DESGUIN (V.) Le Burquisme, métalloscopie et métallothérapie. [Rapport.] 8°. *Bruxelles*, 1884.
Repr. from: Bull. Acad. roy. de méd. de Belg., Brux., 1883, 3. s., xvii.
See, also, Burq, *infra.*

PETIT (L.-H.) La métallothérapie, ses origines, son histoire et les procédés thérapeutiques qui en dérivent. 2. éd. 12°. *Paris*, 1881.
Repr. from: Bull. gén. de thérap., etc., Par., 1879-80, xcvii-xcviii.
See, also, infra.

RATZLAFF (A.) * Einige Versuche über die bilateralen Functionen nach Application von Hautreizen. 8°. *Greifswald*, 1879.

VOGT (I.) * Ueber hysterische Anästhesie und Metallotherapie. 8°. *Würzburg*, 1880.

Adamkiewicz. Ueber bilaterale Functionen. Arch. f. Physiol., Leipz., 1880, 159-162.—**Adradas** (C. L.) Burquismo; metaloscopia-metaloterapia. Rev. de med. y cirug. práct., Madrid, 1884, xv, 9; 145; 241.—**Allexich** (G.) Sulla metalloterapia. Gazz. med. ital., prov. venete, Padova, 1878, xxi, 113-117.—**Altana** (G.) Caso di iperestesia curata colla metalloterapia. Spallanzani, Modena, 1880, ix, 553-557. *Also:* Arch. ital. per le mal. nerv., Milano, 1881, xviii, 236.—**Bennett** (A. H.) Metalloscopy and metallotherapy. Brain, Lond., 1878, i, 331-339. Notes on a case of hemianæsthesia, treated by metallic and other external applications. Brit. M. J., Lond., 1878, ii, 563. ———. Case of complete anæsthesia of the right and partial anæsthesia of the left side; experiments on metalloscopy and metallotherapy; commentary. *Ibid.,* 759-761.—**Bernheim.** De la magnétothérapie; historique et faits nouveaux. Mém. Soc. de méd. de Nancy (1880-81), 1882, lxii-lxv, pt. 2, 7-49. *Also:* Rev. méd. de l'est, Nancy, 1881, xiii, 305; 547; 579; 620; 654; 688; 728; 1882, xiv, 626; 662.—**Bertran** (E.) Sobre metalloterapia. Encicl. méd.-farm., Barcel., 1877, i, 112-114.—**Bianchi** (L.) Contribuzione clinica alle applicazioni dei metalli, della magnete, e delle leggieri correnti galvaniche. Gior. internaz. d. sc. med., Napoli, 1880, ii, 180-193.—**Bocci** (B.) Nuove ricerche sull' epitelio vibratile e contributo alla metallo-magneto-xiloscopia. Riv. clin. di Bologna, 1882, 3. s., ii, 517-539, 2 diag.—**Bouchaud.** Contribution à l'étude de la métallothérapie; monoplégie avec anesthésie; aphasie, hémiplégie et hémianesthésie; application de pièces d'or; guérison. J. d. sc. méd. de Lille, 1880, ii, 77; 149; 405.—**Bouchut.** La métallothérapie chez les enfants; observation d'hémianesthésie guérie par l'or. Paris méd., 1883, viii, 421-424.—**Boudet de Páris.** Traitement de la douleur par les vibrations mécaniques. Progrès méd., Par., 1881, ix, 93-95.—**Boussi.** Observations de deux cas de paralysie avec anesthésie chez l'homme, guéris par la métallothérapie externe. Bull. Soc. clin. de Par. (1879), 1880, iii, 35-41. *Also:* France méd., Par., 1879, xxvi, 242-244.—**Bouzol.** Note sur deux cas de chorée traités par l'aimant. Lyon méd., 1880, xxx ii, 490-495.—**Briquet.** De la métallothérapie et du traitement des troubles de la sensibilité chez les hystériques par l'électricité. Bull. gén. de thérap., etc., Par., 1880, xcix, 433-444. ———. [À propos de la métallothérapie.] *Ibid.,* 545-548.—**Broadbent** (W. H.) A case of hysterical anæsthesia of both legs below the knee; treatment by metallic bands; cure. Tr. Clin. Soc. Lond., 1877-8, xi, 13-16.—**Burq** (V.) Note pour servir à l'histoire des effets physiologiques et thérapeutiques des armatures métalliques, ou de l'influence de certains métaux sur la paralysie du sentiment. Gaz. méd. de Par., 1850, 3. s., v, 115. *Also,* Reprint. ———. La métallothérapie à l'hôpital Lariboisière. Gaz. méd. de Par., 1877, 4. s., vi, 381; 429; 452; 476. ———. Affection hystérique compliquée d'achromatopsie complète de l'œil droit et partielle de l'œil gauche, guérie par un nouveau procédé de métallothérapie externe. Compt. rend. Soc. de biol.

Metallotherapy.

1878, Par., 1880, 6. s., v, pt. 2, 51-55. *Also:* Gaz. méd. de Par., 1878, 4. s., vii, 613. ———. Conférence sur la métallothérapie. Gaz. d. hôp., Par., 1878, li, 723; 762; 811; 835; 844. ———. Contribution à l'étude comparée des métaux et des aimants au point de vue thérapeutique. *Ibid.*, 1879, lii, 805. ———. De l'action opposée des applications métalliques et des enveloppements isolants (avec soie et ouate) chez les hystériques et les cholériques. Compt. rend. Soc. de biol. 1879, Par., 1880, 7. s , i, 108-110. ———. La métallothérapie à Vichy, de 1873 à 1878, contre le diabète et subsidiairement de l'association des métaux à la médication alcaline, pour en augmenter et corriger les effets. Médecin, Par., 1879, v, no. 49. ———. La métallothérapie; ce que peut la métallothérapie; ce à quoi elle vise et doivent toujours viser les autres moyens, dans le traitement des névroses, quand elle ne peut rien elle-même pourquoi l'hydro-métallothérapie et non point la métallo-hydrothérapie. France méd., Par., 1879, xxvi, 722-724. ———. La métallothérapie en chirurgie. [Rap. de Berger.] Bull. et mém. Soc. de chir. de Par., 1880, n. s., vi, 440-442. ———. À propos de la métallothérapie [with reply by Dr. Briquet]. Bull. gén. de thérap., etc., Par., 1880, xcix, 545-548. ———. La métallothérapie depuis 1850; réponse à MM. Despine et J. Monard, au sujet de la prétendue découverte de la métallothérapie faite par A. Despine dès 1820. Lyon méd., 1880, xxxv, 475; 509; 601: 1881, xxxvi, 52. ———. Les surprises de la métallothérapie; histoire curieuse de 3,000 disques d'acier; enseignements qui en résultent au point de vue de la théorie de "the expectant attention" des Anglais en métalloscopie et de l'action comparée des aimants et des métaux; un mot sur la suggestion mentale dans l'hypnotisme. Compt. rend. Soc. de biol. 1882, Par., 1883, 7. s., iv, 155; 310. ———. Des origines de la métallothérapie. *Ibid.*, 383; 471; pt. 2, 23. *Also:* Gaz. d. hôp., Par., 1882, lv, 525; 635; 891; 908; 916; 933; 1002; 1019; 1075; 1084; 1194: 1883, lvi, 475. ———. Le Perkinisme et le Burquisme; les martiaux et la médication polymétallique dans la chlorose. Compt. rend. Soc. de biol. 1882, Par., 1883, 7. s., iv, 513-518. ———. Les étonnements de la métallothérapie; angine de poitrine chez un bimétallique; guérison rapide par le cuivre extra et l'or intus; action des plaques doubles dans un cas d'hystérie rebelle. *Ibid.*, 541-552. *Also:* Gaz. d. hôp., Par., 1882, lv, 781; 796. ———. Explication des phénomènes métalloscopiques. Compt. rend. Soc. de biol. 1883, Par., 1884, 7. s., v, 173-177. *Also:* Gaz. d. hôp., Par., 1883, lvi, 213. ———. Contribution aux doctrines de M. Pasteur; immunité des ouvriers en cuivre pendant la dernière épidémie de fièvre typhoïde. Compt. rend. Soc. de biol. 1883, Par., 1884, 7. s., v, 298-303. ———. Contribution à la préservation cuprique dans les maladies infectieuses. *Ibid.*, 659-662. ———. Du cuivre contre les maladies infectieuses et de l'innocuité absolue des poussières professionnelles de ce métal. Compt. rend. Acad. d. sc., Par., 1883, xcvii, 1314-1316. ———. Les origines de la métallothérapie. [Rap. de Desguin.] Bull. Acad. roy. de méd. de Belg., Brux., 1883, 3. s., xvii, 1192-1218. [*See, also, supra,* Masoin & Desguin.] ———. Amblyopie hystérique; vomissements incoercibles; anesthésie absolue de tout le côté droit; paralysie complète de la vessie, etc.; traitement par le platine. Gaz. d. hôp., Par., 1883, lvi, 753-755. ———. Enquêtes sur l'immunité cholérique et typhoïque des ouvriers qui travaillent le métal blanc, dit alfénide, et des ouvriers en cuivre. *Ibid.*, 1076; 1178. ———. Contribution à la préservation cuprique dans les maladies infectieuses; enquête de Villedieu. Compt. rend. Soc. de biol., Par., 1884, 8. s., i, 33-36. ———. Un dernier mot sur les antériorités de la métallothérapie et sur la préservation cuprique dans les maladies infectieuses. *Ibid.*, pt. 2, 200-206.—**Burq** (V.) & **Moricourt** (J.) Métallothérapie; hystérie rebelle; aboiement hystérique; hémianesthésie absolue; troubles trophiques de la peau, etc.; guérison rapide par l'aluminium. *Ibid.*, 1883, Par., 1884, 7. s., v, 432-436. *Also:* Gaz. d. hôp., Par., 1883, lvi, 578-580. ———. Ovarie et hyperesthésie mammaire féroces, datant la première de quinze années et la deuxième de huit; disparition immédiate par une application d'argent; un mot sur une malade hypnotique et sur l'aboyeuse de Nevers. Gaz. d. hôp., Par., 1884, lvii, 453.—**Bussy.** Case of anæsthesia induced by the application of metals. Brit. M. J., Lond., 1878, ii, 562.—**Buzzard** (T.) On transfer-phenomena in epilepsy, produced by encircling blisters. *Ibid.*, 1880, ii, 332.—**Caizergues** (R.) Hémianesthésie d'origine cérébrale survenue dans le cours d'un rhumatisme; étude comparée des effets produits par la métallothérapie, les courants continus, les courants induits et le courant téléphonique. Montpel. méd., 1878, xli, 29-47.—**Cartier** (E.) Note sur trois observations d'hémianesthésie hystérique traitée par la métallothérapie. Lyon méd., 1880, xxxiii, 377; 421. [Rap. de J. Tessier], 485-490.—**Cegan** (A.) La metalloterapia in Oriente. Gazz. med. ital., prov. venete, Padova, 1878, xxi, 125-128.—**Charcot.** Remarques sur l'application des métaux dans les anesthésies. Compt. rend. Soc. de biol. 1877, Par., 1879, 6. s., iv, 21-24. De la métalloscopie et la métallothérapie. Gaz. d. hôp., Par., 1878, li, 217; 235; 241. ———. Nouveau procédé de métallothérapie externe. *Ibid.*, 692. ———. Lecture on metalloscopy and metallo-therapy applied to the treatment

Metallotherapy.

of grave hysteria. Lancet, Lond., 1878, i, 81; 158; 302.—
Coriveaud (A.) Hystérie; analgésie du côté gauche, rapidement améliorée par la métallothérapie. Mém. et bull. Soc. de méd. et chir. de Bordeaux, 1878, 137-150. *Also:* Bordeaux méd., 1878, vii, 138; 115. *Also, in his:* Obs. et lect. d'un méd. de campagne, 8°, Par., 1880, 53-62.—**Cullerre.** Emploi de la métallothérapie dans un cas d'hystérie convulsive et vésanique; guérison. Ann. méd.-psych., Par., 1880, 6. s., iv, 349-363. *Also,* Reprint.—**Debove.** Influence curative des aimants sur certaines hémiplégies ou crises gastralgiques avec hématémèses dans l'ataxie. J. de méd. et chir. prat., Par., 1879, l, 532-536. ——. Note sur l'emploi des aimants dans les hémianesthésies liées à une affection cérébrale ou à l'hystérie. Progrès méd., Par., 1879, vii, 973. ——. Note sur diverses variétés de transfert. Bull. et mém. Soc. méd. d. hôp. de Par. (1880) 1881, 2. s., xvii, 8-11. *Also:* Union méd., Par., 1880, 3. s., xxix, 431-433.—**Decraud.** Observation d'hystérie grave compliquée de vaginisme guérie par l'or intus et extra. Abeille méd., Par., 1878, xxxv, 401.—**Desguin** (V.) Étude de métalloscopie et de métallothérapie. Mém. couron. Acad. roy. de méd. de Belg., Brux., 1880, vi, fasc. 1, 1-55. *Also:* Presse méd. belge. Brux., 1880, xxxii, 297; 305; 313; 321.—**Despine**(P.) De l'action des métaux sur les hystériques mises en somnambulisme. Gaz. méd. de Par., 1877, 4. s., vi, 320. *Also:* Marseille méd., 1877, xiv, 317-323.—**Desplats.** Métallothérapie; perte de la sensibilité du membre inférieur gauche; guérison par l'application externe du fer. J. d. sc. méd. de Lille, 1880, ii, 682.—**De Visscher.** Contribution à l'étude de la métallothérapie dans l'hystérie. [Rap. de Verstraeten.] Bull. Soc. de méd. de Gand, 1877, xliv, 489-492. [Discussion], 1878, xlv, 211-213.—**Donkin** (H.) Remarks on metallic and magnetic therapeutics. Brit. M. J., Lond., 1878, ii. 619.—**Dor.** Expériences sur la métallothérapie. Mém. et compt.-rend. Soc. d. sc. méd. de Lyon (1880) 1881, xx, pt. 2, 41-44.—**Dubay** (M.) A fémgyógyászat és fémkémlés. [On metallotherapy and metalloscopy.] Gyógyászat, Budapest, 1878, xviii, 196-199. ——. A metallotherapia és metalloskopia. *Ibid.,* 1881, xxi, 81; 100; 121; 129. ——. Ujabb metallotherapeutikus kóresetek. *Ibid.,* 1883, xxiii, 65; 81; 97; 113; 131; 149; 177; 286. ——. Az uj metalloskopikus készülék. *Ibid.,* 729-731. *Also, transl.:* Pest. med.-chir. Presse, Budapest, 1883, xix, 1089-1091. ——. Ujabb metallotherapikus kóresetek. Gyógyászat, Budapest, 1884, xxiv, 75; 96; 105; 125. *Also, transl.* [Abstr.]: Pest. med.-chir. Presse, Budapest, 1884, xx, 471.—**Dujardin-Beaumetz** & **Abadie** (C.) Cécité hystérique; amélioration par la métallothérapie et les applications d'aimants; disparition complète des troubles visuels sous l'influence de l'électricité statique. Bull. et mém. Soc. méd. d. hôp. de Par. (1879) 1880, 2. s., xvi, 145-149. *Also:* Gaz. d. hôp., Par., 1879, lii, 436; 443. *Also:* Abeille méd., Par., 1879, xxxvi, 185. *Also:* Courrier méd., Par., 1879, xxix, 164.—**Dumontpallier** (A.) Métallothérapie; hémiplégie droite hystérique et achromatopsie. Courrier méd., Par., 1879, xxix, 391. ——. Métalloscopie; métallothérapie. J. de thérap., Par., 1879, vi, 613-616. ——. Sur la métalloscopie. Union méd., Par., 1879, 3. s., xxviii, 333; 381; 421; 457; 473; 657; 673; 726; 771. *Also* [Abstr.]: Rev. de thérap. méd.-chir., Par., 1879, xlvi, 449; 477; 505; 503; 561; 589. *Also, transl.* [Abstr]: Brit. M. J., Lond., 1879, ii, 765-768.—**Dumontpallier** (A.) & **Magnin** (P.) Expériences sur la métalloscopie, l'hypnotisme et la fo ce neurique. Compt. rend. Soc. de biol. 1881, Par., 1882, 7. s., iii, 359-364. *Also:* Gaz. méd. de Par., 1881, 6. s., iii, 741. *Also:* Gaz. d. hôp., Par., 1881, liv, 1140. ——. Étude expérimentale sur la métalloscopie, l'hypnotisme et l'action de divers agents physiques dans l'hystérie. France méd., Par., 1882, i, 76-79.—**Dumontpallier** (A.) *et al.* Rapport fait à la Société de biologie sur la métalloscopie du Dr. Burq. Compt. rend. Soc. de biol. 1877, Par., 1879, 6. s., iv, 1-24. *Also:* Gaz. méd. de Par., 1877, 4. s., 201-207. *Also:* Union méd., Par., 1877, 3. s., xxiii, 812; 833; 941; 993; 1004. ——. Second rapport fait à la Société de biologie sur la métalloscopie et la métallothérapie du docteur Burq. Compt. rend. Soc. de biol. 1878, Par., 1880, 6. s., v, pp. i-xxxii. *Also:* Union méd., Par., 1879, 3. s., xxvii, 98-100. *Also:* Gaz. méd. de Par., 1878, 4. s., vii, 419; 436; 450. *Also, transl.:* Brit. M. J., Lond., 1878, ii, 548-552.—**E.** (A.) Recherches sur le Perkinisme ou de l'influence des tracteurs métalliques, inventés par le docteur Perkins, sur certaines maladies, telles que les douleurs de goutte et de rhumatisme, les tumeurs et l'épilepsie. Ann. clin., Montpel., 1812, xxix, 274-283.—**Engel** (H.) Metalloscopy and metallo-therapeutics, in a case of hysterical hyperæsthesia. Med. & Surg. Reporter, Phila., 1879, xl, 265.—**Eulenburg** (A.) Ueber Metallotherapie. Deutsche med. Wchnschr., Berl., 1878, iv. 315; 327. ——. Metalloskopie und Metallotherapie. Wien. med. Presse, 1879, xx, 1; 41; 109; 137. ——. Ueber Sensibilitäts-Uebertragung. Cong. périod. internat. d. sc. méd. Compt.-rend. 1879, Amst., 1880, vi, 203-205. ——. Metallische Heilwirkungen. Deutsche Rev., Berl., 1881, vi, 258-269.—**Féré** (C.) & **Binet** (A.) Note pour servir à l'histoire du transfert chez les hypnotiques. Compt. rend. Soc. de biol., Par., 1884. 8. s., i, pt. 2, 442-446. *Also:* Progrès méd., Par., 1884, xii, 563. *Also:* Médecin, Par., 1884, x, no. 32-33.—

Metallotherapy.

Firket (C.) Résultats des recherches récentes, entreprises en Allemagne pour l'étude du phénomène de transfert. Ann. Soc. méd.-chir. de Liége, 1879, xviii, 476-479.—**Fournié** (É.) Contribution à l'étude de l'emploi des métaux, de l'électricité et du magnétisme en médecine. Rev. méd. franç. et étrang., Par., 1881, i, 685; 721; 757; 793.—**Fubini** (S.) & **Bono** (G. B.). Uno sguardo alle principali questioni di metalloterapia. Gior. d. r. Accad. di med. di Torino, 1881, 3. s., xxix, 181-226.—**Gajkiewicz.** Metaloterapia (zewnętrzna i wewnętrzna), dzialanie magnesu. Medycyna, Warszawa, 1878, vi, 677; 699.—**Garel** (J.) Note relative à la métallothérapie interne. Mém. et compt.-rend. Soc. d. sc. méd. de Lyon (1880), 1881, xx, pt. 2, 107-112. ——. Contribution à l'étude de la métallothérapie interne. Rev. mens. de méd. et chir., Par., 1880, iv, 432-443. ——. Double mode de combinaison de l'anesthésie provoquée et de l'anesthésie par transfert avec oscillations consécutives. Lyon méd., 1880, xxxiii, 53-55. ——. Traitement de l'hystérie par les feuilles métalliques administrées à l'intérieur. *Ibid.,* 1881, xxxviii, 5; 44; 75.—**Gellé.** La métallothérapie. Tribune méd., Par., 1877, x, 88; 100.—**Georganta** (A. D.) Περὶ μεταλλοσκόπησεως καὶ μεταλλοθεραπευτικῆς. Γαληνός, Ἀθῆναι, 1879, Β΄, 324; 360; 369; 387; 1880, Γ΄, 4; 19; 65; 182; 194; 257; 330; 405.—**Gingeot.** Hémiplégie motrice accompagnée d'hémianesthésie sensitive et sensorielle traitée avec succès par l'emploi des aimants. Bull. et mém. Soc. méd. d. hôp. de Par. (1883), 1884, 2. s., xx, 6-11. *Also:* Union méd., Par., 1883, xxxvi, 37-42. *Also:* Abeille méd., Par., 1883, xl, 258-260.—**Gradle** (H.) Metalloscopy and metallotherapy. J. Nerv. & Ment. Dis., Chicago, 1878, n. s., iii, 715-724.—**Grasset** (J.) Métalloscopie et métallothérapie. Montpel. méd., 1880, xliv, 524-540.—**Guaita** (R.) La metalloterapia e la sua applicazione alle malattie dei bambini. Sperimentale, Firenze, 1878, xli, 400-407. *Also:* Osservatore med.. Palermo, 1878, viii, 356-366.—**Guilland** père. La métallothérapie en 1820. Montpel. méd., 1880, xlv, 159.—**Habermann.** Hysterische Taubheit, Blindheit und Hyperästhesie des Olfactorius bei einem jungen Manne; Metallotherapie; Heilung. Prag. med. Wchnschr., 1880, v, 213; 222.—**Hammond** (W. A.) On metal therapeutics. Med. & Surg. Reporter, Phila., 1878, xxxviii, 383-388.—**Henrot** (H.) Du transfert de l'hémihypothermie. Union méd. et scient. du nord-est, Reims, 1880, iv, 165; 179.—**Horrocks** (P.) Cases of hemianalgesia, illustrating the application of metallotherapy. Brit. M. J., Lond., 1878, ii, 102.—**Hortolès** (C.) De la métalloscopie hystérique; de la métallothérapie interne; observations et réflexions. Montpel. méd., 1882, xlviii, 525-533.—**Houlès** (A.) & **de Pietra-Santa.** Action du cuivre sur l'économie; histoire d'un atelier et d'un village. Compt. rend. Acad. d. sc., Par., 1883, xcvii, 1562.—**Hugues.** Métallothérapie. Nice méd., 1877, i, 402-405.—**Huss** (M.) Öfversigt öfver den metalloterapautiska behandlingsmetoden och denna metods nuvarande ståndpunkt, enligt nedan anförde författare. Hygiea, Stockholm, 1884, xlvi, 354-373.—**Ingria** (V. E.) Metalloterapia in un' caso d' isterismo. Gior. internaz. d. sc. med., Napoli, 1886, n. s., viii, 969-972.—**Johnstone** (A.) Metalloscopy and metallotherapy. Arch. Med., N. Y., 1884, xii, 216-225.—**Kahan** (A. J.) K kazuistike metalloskopii i metalloterapii. Med. Vestnik, St. Petersb., 1882, xxi, 11; 30; 45; 64; 77; 93; 123; 156; 175.—**Kingsley** (J. P.) Treatment by mental impression. St. Louis Clin. Rec., 1878-9, v, 269.—**Köbner** (H.) Zur Casuistik des Transfert. Breslau. aerztl. Ztschr., 1880, ii, 50-52.—**Kratter** (J.) Metalloskopie und Metallotherapie. Oesterr. ärztl. Vereinsztg., Wien, 1879, iii, 2.—**Kraus** (B.) Die hysterische Contractur und der Magnet das merkwürdige Symptom des "Transfert". Allg. Wien. med. Ztg., 1878, xxiii, 507; 515.—**Kun** (T.) A metallotherapiának van-e jövöje? [Has metallotherapy a future?] Gyógyászat, Budapest, 1883, xxiii, 653-657. *Also, transl.:* Pest. med.-chir. Presse, Budapest, 1883, xix, 962.—**Landolt** & **Oulmont** (P.) Du retour de la sensibilité sous l'influence des applications métalliques dans l'hémianesthésie d'origine cérébrale. Progrès méd., Par., 1877, v, 381-383.—**Landouzy.** Relation d'un cas de léthargie provoquée par l'application d'un aimant. Compt. rend. Soc. de biol. 1879, Par., 1880, 7. s., i, pt. 2, 1-9. *Also:* Progrès méd., Par., 1879, vii, 60-62. *Also* [Abstr.]: Gaz. d. hôp., Par., 1879, lii, 45.—**Landowski** (E.) Métalloscopie et métallothérapie. Alger méd., 1879, vii, 353-357.—**Lindh** (A.) Ett försök med den s. k. metalloterapien. Eira, Göteborg, 1879, iii, 748-753.—**Mazzei** (E.) La metaloterapia. Rev. méd. de Chile, Sant. de Chile, 1880-81, ix, 225; 289: 1881-2, x, 44.—**Metallotherapy.** By X. Phila. M. Times, 1878, viii, 327-330.—**Monard** (J.) La métallothérapie en 1820. Lyon méd., 1880, xxxiv, 411; 449; 485.—**Moricourt.** Hystérie; sensibilité au zinc; bons effets de ce métal appliqué extérieurement et administré à l'intérieur. Gaz. d. hôp., Par., 1879, lii, 828. ——. Métallothérapie; vertige mental pris d'abord pour un cas d'alcoolisme, traité avec succès par le chlorure d'or. *Ibid.,* 1881, liv, 716. ——. Contribution à l'étude de l'antisepticité du cuivre contre la fièvre typhoïde. *Ibid.,* 1092. ——. Pied bot varus par contracture, guéri par l'application d'une armature de cuivre pen-

Metallotherapy.

dant une heure; hystérie datant de deux années; disparition des crises par l'argent extra et l'or intus. *Ibid.*, 1885, lviii, 3. ———. Nouveaux procédés métalloscopiques dans les cas d'aptitudes métalliques dissimulées, notamment chez les sujets léthargiques, cataleptiques ou somnambules. Compt. rend. Acad. d. sc., Par., 1885, ci, 95–97. *Also:* Union méd., Par., 1885, 3. s., xl, 663–667.—**Müller** (F.) Metalloskopie und Metallotherapie. Mitth. d. Ver. d. Aerzte in Steiermark 1878, Graz, 1879, xv, 27–46. ———. Vorläufige Mittheilung über Metalloscopie und Metallotherapie. Centralbl. f. Nervenh., Coblenz, 1879, ii, 25–27. ———. Zur Metalloscopie und Magnetwirkung bei hysterischen Lähmungen. Berl. klin. Wchnschr., 1879, xvi, 416; 435.—**Novaro** (D. B.) La metaloscopia y la metaloterapia. An. d. Círc. méd. argent., Buenos Aires, 1880–81, iv, 87; 136.—**Palazzolo** (E.) Contributo alla metallofisiologia; esperienze sopra batraci. Indipendente, Torino, 1881, xxxii, 535–538.—**Peckham** (Grace). Metallotherapy, theoretically and practically considered. Arch. Med., N. Y., 1883, x, 155; 283.—**Petit** (L.-H.) Sur la métallothérapie. Bull. gén. de thérap., etc., Par., 1879, xcvii, 32; 75; 126; 170; 221; 272; 318; 365; 407; 461; 515: 1880, xcviii, 25; 73; 219; 264; 319; 364; 412; 458; 499; 539. *Also:* Rev. internat. d. sc. biol., Par., 1881, viii, 1; 113. [*See, also, supra.*]—**Proust** (A.) & **Ballet** (G.) De l'action des aimants sur quelques troubles nerveux, spécialement sur les anesthésies. Cong. périod. internat. d. sc. méd. Compt.-rend. 1879, Amst., 1880, vi, 304–325.—**Rabuteau.** Perkinisme et métallothérapie; résumé historique et explicatif. Compt. rend. Soc. de biol., Par., 1884, 8. s., i, pt. 2, 84–87.—**Rostan.** Observation remarquable de paralysie musculaire atrophique guérie par les armatures métalliques du docteur Burq. Gaz. d. hôp., Par., 1853, xxvi, 215–217. — **Rumpf.** Ueber den Transfert. Arch. f. Psychiat., Berl., 1879–80, x, 273–275. ———. Ueber Metalloscopie, Metall therapie und Transfert. Memorabilien, Heilbr., 1879, xxiv, 385–400.—**Rusconi** (U.) Studj clinici di metalloscopia e xiloscopia in un caso di emianestesia ed amiostenia isterica con ambliopia ed acromatopsia. Gazz. d. osp., Milano, 1881, ii, 385–387. — **Schiff.** Ueber Metallotherapie. Tagebl. d. Versamml. deutsch. Naturf. u. Aerzte, Baden-Baden, 1879, lii, 148–158. *Also* [Abstr.]: Pest. med.-chir. Presse, Budapest, 1879, xv, 881. *Also:* Centralbl. f. Nervenh., Coblenz, 1879, ii, 464.—**Schiffers.** Hystérie; applications métallothérapiques. Ann. Soc. méd.-chir. de Liége, 1879, xviii, 183–188.—**Sciamanna** (E.) Applicazione dei metalli sulla superficie cutanea (metalloscopia e metalloterapia). Gazz. med. di Roma, 1878, iv, 127.—**Secretan** (L.) Hémianalgésie hystérique; amélioration par la métallothérapie; récidive; guérison par l'électricité statique. Bull. Soc. méd. de la Suisse Rom., Lausanne, 1880, xiv, 213–228.—**Seguin** (E. C.) Hysterical convulsions and hemianæsthesia in an adult male; cure by metallotherapy (gold). Arch. Med., N. Y., 1882, viii, 199–201.—**Singer** (J.) Zur Geschichte der Metallotherapie. Prag. med. Wchnschr., 1880, v, 107.—**Sonin** (D.) Paralich litsevago nerva (ortometalloterapija; vizdorovlenie). [Paralysis of facial nerve.] Arch. vet. nauk. St. Petersb., 1882, i, pt. 3, 76–83.—**Surre.** Cas remarquable de névrose mentale guérie par l'usage du cuivre. Gaz. d. hôp., Par., 18·6, lix, 179. — **T.** (T. T.) Histeria; sensibilidad al zinc; buenos efectos de este metal aplicado tópicamente y administrado al interior. Clinica, Zaragoza, 1879, iii, 301.—**Talko-Hryncewicz** (J.) Magnetyzm zwierzęcy i proby zastosowania go w medycynie (metallotherapia). Gaz. lek., Warszawa, 1880, xxix, 3; 13; 25; 33.—**Teissier** (J.) Pathogénie du transfert dans les phénomènes de métallothérapie. Mém. et compt.-rend. Soc. d. sc. méd. de Lyon (1880), 1881, xx, pt. 2, 100–102. ———. Note sur la pathogénie du transfert dans les phénomènes de métalloscopie. Compt. rend. Soc. de biol. 1881, Par., 1882, 7. s., iii, 210.—**Telnichin** (A.) Sluch. uspesh. primen. metalloterapii pri amblyopia hysterica. [Cure by metallotherapy.] Vestnik oftalmol., Kieff, 1887, iv, 130.—**Thermes** (G.) Des effets de l'excitant thermique (chaleur ou froid) sur l'anesthésie, l'achromatopsie et la contracture des hystériques, leur similitude d'action comparativement à celle des métaux, des aimants artificiels et de l'électricité statique. Gaz. d. hôp., Par., 1878, li, 982. *Also:* Compt. rend. Soc. de biol. 1878, Par., 1880, 6. s., v, 294–299. ———. Note sur un procédé d'hydrométall thérapie externe. Bull. Soc. de méd. prat. de Par., 1879. 165–168. *Also:* France méd., Par., 1879, xxvi, 675.— **Tuke** (D. H.) Metalloscopy and expectant attention. J. Ment. Sc., Lond., 1878-9, xxiv, 589–609. *Also, transl.:* Bull. Soc. de méd. ment. de Belg., Gand, 1879, xiii, 42–59.— **Uspenski** (P. I.) Znachenie musheke i metallove ve terapii nervniche boleznei. [Metallotherapy in nervous disorders.] Ejened. klin. gaz., St. Petersb., 1881, i, 265; 283.—**de Varigny** (H.) La métallothérapie. Rev. scient., Par., 1881, 3. s., i, 769–779.—**Vétault.** De quelques faits ayant trait à l'action des métaux sur les hystériques. Compt. rend. Soc. de biol. 1882, Par., 1883, 7. s., iv, 219.— **de Vicente** (C.) Burquismo (metaloscopia, metaloterapia, agentes estesiógenos). Rev. de med. y cirug. práct., Madrid, 1883, xiii, 289; 337: 388; 481: 1884, xiv, 58. *Also, Reprint.*—**Vigouroux** (R.) Des plaques formées de

Metallotherapy.

plusieurs métaux superposés. Compt. rend. Soc. de biol., 1877, Par., 1879, 6. s., iv, 401–405. ———. Sur un procédé nouveau de métallothérapie externe. *Ibid.* (1878), 1880, 6. s., v, 240–242. *Also:* Progrès méd., Par., 1878, vi, 573. ———. Sur la théorie physique de la métalloscopie. Compt. rend. Soc., de biol. 1878, Par., 1880, 6. s., v, 270–273. *Also:* Gaz. d. hôp., Par., 1877, l, 1059. ———. Métalloscopie, métallothérapie, æsthésiogènes. Arch. de neurol., Par., 1880–82, i, 257; 413; 564: 1881, ii, 92: 1882, iii, 87.—**Wachtel** (D.) Ueber Metallotherapie und deren Anwendung in schmerzhaften Contracturen und in der Chorea. Ztschr. f. Nat. u. Heilk. in Ungarn, Oedenburg, 1860, xi, 97; 105; 113.— **Witthalm** (L.) Ueber Metalloscopie und Metallotherapie. J. f. öff. Gsndhtspflg., Wien, 1880, iv, No. 8, p. 4; No. 9, p. 3.

Metals.

See, also, **Minerals** *in medicine*; **Miners** (*Diseases, etc., of*).

A BERGEN (C. A.) * De gravitate specifica metallorum statice et hydrostatice explorata; resp. J. G. Rammelsberg. 4°. *Francof. ad Viadr.*, [1743].

BOYLE (R.) Observationes de generatione metallorum in minera sua aëri expositorum. 16°. *Londini*, 1676.

CONRAD (H. F.) * De principiis et transmutatione metallorum. sm. 4°. *Jenæ*, [1686].

CRAMER (C.) * De transmutatione metallorum. Resp. J. C. Calckhoff. 4°. *Erfurti*, [1675].

MOLLWEIDE (J. H.) * De modo agendi metallorum in corpore humano. 4°. *Halæ Magdeb.*, 1752.

TIMAEUS (G.) & VIERTEL (J. C.) Disputatio prior, de metallurgia rerum gerendarum nervo. 4°. *Vitembergæ*, [1699].

WEBSTER (J.) Metallographia, or an history of metals. Wherein is declared the signs of ores and minerals both before and after digging; the causes and manner of their generations; their kinds, sorts, and differences; with the description of sundry new metals, or semi-metals, and many other things pertaining to mineral knowledge. As also, the handling and shewing of their vegetability; and the discussion of the most difficult questions belonging to mystical chemistry, as of the philosopher's gold, their mercury, the liquor alkahest, aurum potabile, and such like. Gathered forth of the most approved authors, that have written in Greek, Latine, or High-Dutch; with some observations and discoveries of the author himself. 4°. *London*, 1671.

Béchamp. Sur les métaux qui peuvent exister dans le sang ou les viscères. Ann. d'hyg., Par., 1860, 2. s., xiii, 212–221.—**Chevallier** & **Cottereau.** Essais historiques sur les métaux que l'on rencontre quelquefois dans les corps organisés. *Ibid.*, 1849, xli, 387: xlii, 124.— **Favre** (J.-H.) & **Frantz** (J.-J.) Mémoire sur la transmutation des métaux. France méd., Par., 1866, xiii, 10; 18.—**Huff** (G.) Removal of metals from the system by galvanism. N. York M. Times, 1855, iv, 346–350.—**Jeannel.** Recherches sur le rôle des corps gras dans l'absorption et l'assimilation des oxydes métalliques. Union méd., Par., 1859, 2. s., i, 289–292.—**Kletzinsky** (V.) Ueber die Ausscheidung der Metalle in den Secreten. Wien. med. Wchnschr., 1857, vii, 761; 779; 811: 1858, viii, 20; 101; 116; 355; 718; 901.—**Osius** (C. A.) Ueber die Umwandlung der Metalle im menschlichen Körper; ein Beitrag zur Lehre der Arzneiwirkungen. Med. Ann., Heidelb., 1842, viii, 277–317.—**Robin** (E.) Mode d'action des composés métalliques sur l'économie animale. Gaz. méd. de l'Algérie, Alger, 1875, xx, 55; 62.

Metals (*Toxicology of, and accidents from*).

See, also, **Antimony,** *etc.*, **Arsenic, Bismuth, Copper,** *Toxicology of*; **Iron** (*Sulphate of*); **Lead-poisoning;** **Mercury** (*Toxicology of*); **Occupations,** *etc.* (*Diseases, etc., of*); **Tin** (*Chloride of*); **Zinc-poisoning.**

KOCHLATSCH (S. A.) * De metallicolarum nonnullis morbis. 4°. *Halæ Magdeb.*, [1721].

NEUMANN (J. G.) * De præservandis metallicolarum morbis. 4°. *Halæ Magdeb.*, 1721.

SIEMENS (H. J.) * Metallurgia morbifera. sm. 4°. *Halæ Magdeb.*, 1705.

Metals (*Toxicology of, and accidents from*).

URSINUS (L.) * De morbis metallariorum. 4°. *Lipsiæ*, 1652.

Beaupoil (A.) De l'entéropathie métallique; étude médicale sur les accidents causés vers le tube digestif par la pénétration lente et graduée de certaines substances métalliques dans l'organisme. J. de méd., chir. et pharmacol., Brux., 1854, xviii, 391; 487: xix, 3; 97; 209; 305.—**Bossmann** (H.) Ueber die Einwirkung der Metallstaubinhalation auf die Gesundheit. Friedreich's Bl. f. gerichtl. Med., Nürnb., 1884, xxxv, 348-363.—**Dieudonné** *et al.* Rapport sur l'étamage blanc d'argent du sieur Trannoy. Ann. Cons. centr. de salub. pub. de Brux., 1847, iv, 103-122.—**Dorvault.** Considérations chimiques sur l'emploi de l'iodure de potassium dans les empoisonnements métalliques. Bull. gén. de thérap., etc., Par., 1849, xxxvi, 261-266.—**Girardin** & **Barruel.** Oxides de plomb et de cuivre dans une andouille. Ann. d'hyg., Par., 1833, x, 84-92.—**Guermonprez** (F.) Des corps étrangers spéciaux aux ouvriers de la métallurgie et de quelques accidents qu'ils produisent. Rev. méd. de Toulouse, 1882, xvi, 332; 353. *Also:* Bull. gén. de thérap., etc., Par., 1883, civ, 258-266.—**Jordan.** Die Krankheiten der Arbeiter in den Stahlfabriken. Vrtljschr. f. gerichtl. u. öff. Med., Berl., 1863, xxiii, 136-173.—**Melsens.** Mémoire sur l'emploi de l'iodure de potassium pour combattre les affections saturnines et mercurielles. Ann. de chim. et phys., Par., 1849, 3. s., xxvi, 215-255. *Also, transl.:* Brit. & For. M.-Chir. Rev., Lond., 1853, xi, 201-224.—**Orfila.** Mémoire sur quelques points relatifs à l'empoisonnement produit par les préparations de plomb, de cuivre, d'arsenic et de mercure. Ann. d'hyg., Par., 1847, xxxviii, 163-216.—**Plaseller.** Das Staubfieber der Messing-Hämmerer. Oesterr. med. Wchnschr., Wien, 1844, 1265-1267.—**Richet** (C.) De la toxicité comparée des différents métaux. Compt. rend. Acad. d. sc., Par., 1881, xciii, 649-651.—**Skvortsoff** (I. P.) Gornozavod. promishlen. [Metallurgic industries.] Vestnik sudeb. med., etc., St. Petersb., 1886, i, pt. 3, 1-26: ii, 1-26.

Metamorphopsia.
See **Eye** (*Accommodation, etc., of, Disordered*).

Metamorphosen (Die) des Trigeminus. Comoedia medico-practica in einem Paroxysmus für Aerzte, Apotheker und Naturforscher beider Hemisphären von Dr. Supinator Longus. (Aufgeführt am 17jährigen Stiftungsfeste der medicinischen Gesellschaft zu Magdeburg, den 11. März 1865.) Impressio reiterata. 64 pp. 8°. *Berlin, T. C. F. Enslin* (*A. Enslin*), 1866.

———. The same. 2. Aufl. 64 pp. 8°. *Berlin, T. C. F. Enslin* (*R. Schoetz*), [*n. d.*]

Metamorphosis.
See, also, **Development**; **Embryology**; **Evolution.**

DOBROSLAVIN (A.) * Materiali dlja phiziologii metamorphoza. [Physiological metamorphosis.] 8°. *St. Petersburg*, 1868.

Owen. On metamorphosis and metagenesis. Med. Times, Lond., 1851, n. s., ii, 663-666.

Metaphysician (The). A quarterly magazine. Published by the Metaphysical University. Edited by Mrs. M. G. Brown and her daughter Elizabeth. No. 2, v. 1, Jan., 1875. 8°. *New York.*
An advertisement.

Metaphysics.
See **Mind**; **Philosophy**; **Psychology.**

Metaplasia.
Virchow (R.) Ueber Metaplasie. Arch. f. path. Anat., etc., Berl., 1884, xcvii, 410-430. *Also:* Wien. med. Presse, 1884, xxv, 1205; 1237; 1276; 1307. *Also:* Breslau. aerztl. Ztschr., 1884, vi, 230.

Metastasis.
See, also, **Abscess** (*Metastatic*); **Embolism**; **Gout** (*Complications, etc., of*); **Lochia** (*Physiology, etc., of*); **Menstruation** (*Abnormal, etc.*); **Milk** (*Metastasis of*); **Mumps** (*Complications, etc., of*); **Pyæmia**; **Rheumatism** (*Complications in*).

ALBRECHT (M.) * De metastasibus. 8°. *Berolini*, [1826].

ANDERSEN (L.) Bemerkning om en Metastasis. 12°. *Kjøbenhavn*, [1781].

Metastasis.

VAN BODINCKHUYSEN (A. F.) * De metastasi et consensu. 4°. *Harderovici*, 1745.

BONNAL (P.) * Essai sur les métastases. 4°. *Paris*, 1814.

BRANDIS (J. D.) Versuch über die Metastasen. 8°. *Hannover*, 1798.

BRILLAT-SAVARIN (G.-F.) * Quelques mots sur les métastases. 4°. *Paris*, 1854.

BRÜCKNER (J. C. S.) * De morborum migratione. 4°. *Erfordiæ*, [1755].

CALLENFELS (H. A.) * De metastasi. 4°. *Lugd. Bat.*, 1815.

CHARMEIL (P.-M.-J.) Recherches sur les métastases, suivies de nouvelles expériences sur la régénération des os. 8°. *Metz*, 1821.

DÉLISSALDE (A.) * Considérations générales sur les métastases. 4°. *Paris*, 1822.

EBERSBERGER (K.) * Ueber Metastase. 8°. *Würzburg*, 1843.

GOERLITZ (C. A. E.) * Disquisitiones in vim nervorum ad metastases. 12°. *Tubingæ*, [1819].

HARTOG (F. H.) * De modo et causis quibus fiunt in corpore humano metastases. 4°. *Traj. ad Rhenum*, 1802.

HECKER (C. G.) * De metastasibus sententiæ. sm. 8°. *Berolini*, 1817.

HERZOG (J. T. A.) * De metastasi. 4°. *Jenæ*, [1803].

HILDEBRANDT (H. G.) * Nonnulla de secretionibus vicariis disquisita. 8°. *Berolini*, 1826.

JAHN (C. F.) * De metastasibus. 4°. *Lipsiæ*, [1799].

KRETZSCHMAR (C. T.) * De metastasibus. 4°. *Vitebergæ*, [1810].

LOHR (J. A.) * De febrilibus metastasibus. 4°. *Gottingæ*, [1669].

LORTET (P.) * Sur les métastases en général. 4°. *Paris*, 1819.

MALVIEUX (P. L.) * De metastasi morborum. 4°. *Erlangæ*, [1753].

MANKIEWITZ (E.) * De metastasibus. 8°. *Berolini*, [1843].

MOKE (C. A.) * De metastasi. 4°. *Lugd. Bat.*, 1806.

PAGENSTECHER (H. C. A.) * De metastasi. 8°. *Heidelbergæ*, 1819.

QUINQUAUD (A.) * Des métastases. 4°. *Paris*, 1880.

RODBERG (H. C.) * De metastasi ad viscera venæ portæ. sm. 4°. *Duisburgi ad Rhenum*, 1727.

RUHWANDŁ (D.) * De metastasi. 8°. *Monachii*, 1831.

SCHLEGEL (J. C. T.) * De metastasi in morbis. 4°. *Jenæ*, [1771].

SCHOLTZ (C. C.) * De metastasi febrili. sm. 4°. *Halæ Magdeb.*, [1750].

SONTAG (S.) * De metastasi, sive sede morborum mutata, oder: Wie sich öfters eine Kranckheit in die andere verwandte. 4°. *Halæ Magdeb.*, [1731].

THEISEN (L.) *Adnotationes quædam de metastasibus. 8°. *Halis*, 1847.

TREUNER (T. F. A.) * Diss. inaug. med. sistens morborum migrationes. 4°. *Jenæ*, [1783].

WEGELIN (G. C.) * De metastasi. 4°. *Argentorati*, 1759.

*WINTER (J. L.) * De metastasi morborum. sm. 4°. *Wittebergæ*, [1754].

WYNSTOK (T. C.) * De metastasi atque consensu. 4°. *Harderovici*, 1754.

Ackermann. Einige Bemerkungen über Metastase. Mitth. a. d. Geb. d. Med., etc., Altona, 1837-8, v, 5.-6. Hft., 89-116.—**Adragna** (G.) Saggio sulle metastasi. N. Mercurio d. sc. med., Livorno, 1829, iii, 3-16.—**Albertus** (M.) Transformatio febrium una serie facta. Acta Acad. nat. curios., 2. ed., Norimb., 1727, i, 475-477.—**Allen** (J. A.) Physiology of metastasis. Penins. & Indep. M. J., Detroit, 1858-9, i, 26-30.—**Berlioz** (L.-J.) Observation sur une pleurésie terminée par plusieurs métastases extraordi-

Metastasis.

naires. J. gén. de méd., chir. et pharm., Par., 1822, lxxviii, 34-48.—**Blachez.** Métastase. Dict. encycl. d. sc. méd., Par., 1873, 2. s., vii, 290-299.—**van Calcar** (A.) Comparetur veterum doctrina cum recentiorum theoria de ista affectione pathologica in homine, quæ vocatur metastasis. Indicetur dein quænam ex opinionibus, quas recentiores hac de re protulerunt, maxime probabilis videatur. Ann. Acad. Rheno-Traject. (1821-2), 1823, [no 3], 1-77. — **Caspary** (J.) Zur Lehre von den Metastasen. Vrtljschr. f. Dermat., Wien, 1877, iv, 453-479.—**Cerdó** (R.) ¿Existe la metastasis? Siglo méd., Madrid, 1854, i, 145-147.—**Comes de Goerlitz** (C. A. E.) Untersuchungen über den Einfluss der Nerven auf Versetzungen von Krankheitsstoff. In: Weber (J. S.) Samml. med.-diss. [etc.], 8°, Tübingen, 1820, ii, 63-97.—**Crampton** (J.) Case of conversion of disease. Tr. Ass. King's & Queen's Coll. Phys. Ireland, Dubl., 1824, iv, 69-79.—**Cuynat.** Quelques observations de métastase. Précis d. trav. Soc. méd. de Dijon (1838-41), 1843, 92-97.—**Demaria** (C.) Sulle metastasi. Mem. d. Soc. med.-chir. di Bologna, 1844, 2. s., iii, 343-415. — **Fernet** (C.) Métastase. N. dict. de méd. et chir. prat., Par., 1876, xxii, 410-428.—**Gohlius** (J. D.) De ulcere lumborum, ex translatione hæmorrhoidum fistuloso, per aquam gryseam sanato. Acta Acad. nat. curios., Norimb., 1733, iii, 49-56.—**Goursaud.** Déterminer ce que c'est que la métastase, les maladies chirurgicales où elle arrive, et celles qu'elle produit; les cas où l'on doit l'éviter, et ceux où il faut la procurer; enfin les moyens que l'on doit employer dans l'un et l'autre cas. Mém. . . . pour les prix de l'Acad. roy. de chir., Par., 1819, iii, 1-14.—**Hallock** (L.) Metastasis. Tr. N. York M.-Chir. Soc. (1883), 1884, iii, 129-134.—**Harris** (T.) Observations on metastasis. Am. M. Recorder, Phila., 1822, v, 53-60.—**Heller.** Metastase. Ztschr. f. Wundärzte u. Geburtsh., Stuttg., 1849, ii, 204-207.—**Hornickel.** Zwei Fälle von intervenirenden Metastasen. Org. f. d. ges. Heilk., Berl., 1858, vii, 257-270.—**Hort** (W. P.) Metastasis in disease, illustrated by cases. N. Orl. M. & S. J., 1850-51, vii, 384-387.—**Howship.** Cases of metastasis, or translation of diseased action. Med. & Phys. J., Lond., 1810, xxiv, 178-182.—**Hunt** (T.) On metastasis in its practical bearings. Assoc. M. J., Lond., 1854, i, 390-392.—**Kühlbrand.** Lebensrettung durch höchst merkwürdige Metaschematismen. J. d. pract. Heilk., Berl., 1837, lxxxv, 2. St., 3-12.—**L. de S.** Metastasis de una afeccion interna de la piel del cráneo. Gac. méd., Madrid, 1848, iv, 122.—**Laborde.** Observation sur les métastases singulières dans les maladies. J. de méd., chir., pharm., etc., Par., 1770, xxxiv, 326-335.—**Lichtenstädt** (J. R.) Merkwürdiger Fall von Metastase und Metaschematismus. N. Breslau. Samml. a. d. Geb. d. Heilk. . . . d. schles. Gesellsch. f. vaterl. Kult., Bresl., 1829, i, 288-297.—**Liégey.** Énorme tuméfaction née d'une métastase, d'aspect scorbutique et cancéreux, greffée sur un engorgement ganglionnaire ancien, et développée sous l'influence d'accès névralgiques périodiques; mort; observation précédée d'un coup d'œil sur la constitution médicale de la localité où elle a été recueillie. Ann. méd. de la Flandre occid., Roulers, 1858-60, vi, 481-493. ——. Perturbations cardiaques déterminées principalement par la suspension de sueurs devenues habituelles depuis l'âge critique; métastase rhumatismale sur les extrémités inférieures à l'occasion de bains de pieds sinapisés. Cour. méd., Par., 1877, xxvii, 267; 275.—**Linoli** (O.) Storia di una metastasi. Ann. univ. di med., Milano, 1836, lxxvii, 371-383, 1 pl.—**Lorentz.** Mémoire sur les métastases. J. de méd. mil., Par., 1786, v, 500-528.—**Lugaresi** (V.) Sulle metastasi. Resic. Accad. med.-chir. di Ferrara, 1863, 63-68.—**Nagel** (L.) Einiges über Complicationen verschiedener Krankheitsformen, Metaschematismen und Metastasen. Prakt. Arzt, Wetzlar, 1867, viii, 49; 81.—**Peschier.** Mémoire sur la conversion des maladies. Ann. clin., Montpel., 1810, xxii, 372-382.—**Reil** (J. C.) Von den Versetzungen der Krankheitsmaterien, besonders von den Milchversezungen. J. d. Erfind., etc., Gotha, 1794, ii, 7. St., 55-80.—**Reydellet.** Métastase. Dict. d. sc. méd., Par., 1819, xxxiii, 16-105.—**Scoutetten.** Mémoire sur les métastases considérées d'après les principes de la doctrine physiologique. J. univ. d. sc. méd., Par., 1823, xxx, 129-147.—**Smith** (E. F.) On the metastasis of disease. St. Louis M. & S. J., 1852, x, 308-313.—**Staughton** (J. M.) A case of metastasis. Am. M. Recorder, Phila., 1822, v, 130.—**von Tott** (C. A.) Zwei Fälle von merkwürdigem Metaschematismus bei Epileptischen. J. d. pract. Heilk., Berl., 1838, lxxxvi, 3. St., 117-119. ——. Fälle von Milchmetastase. N. Ztschr. f. Geburtsk., Berl., 1842, xii, 66-70.—**Trumphius** (J. C.) Carbunculi minores, a gutta rosacea retrocedente per metastasin in scroto prorumpentes. Acta Acad. nat. curios., Norimb., 1752, ix, 413.—**Vogler.** Zum Processe der Metastasen. Med. Ztg., Berl., 1850, xix, 79; 83.—**Vose** (J. R. W.) On some vicarious actions of the human body, in health and in disease. Edinb. M. & S. J., 1841, lv, 322-335.—**Walther** (J. A.) Gedrängte geschichtliche Darstellung mehrerer schnell nach einander erfolgter metastatischer Erscheinungen, sammt der allgemeinsten Angabe des Grundes der Metastasen und ihrer Bedeutung überhaupt. J. d. pract. Heilk., Berl., 1811, xxxii, 2. St., 71-86.

Metasyncrisis.

SCHWARZ (X. J.) * De metasyncrisi. 8°. Pragæ, [1843].

Metatarsus (Abnormities, diseases, and injuries of).

See, also, **Foot** (Diseases of); **Foot** (Dislocations of, or in); **Foot** (Surgery of).

MONNIER (P.-P.-M.) * Étude sur une variété de luxation du métatarse, luxation en dehors des métatarsiens. 4°. Paris, 1883.

Delort. Observation d'une luxation des os du métatarse sur ceux du tarse. Bull. Soc. anat. de Par., 2. éd., 1826, i, 184-186.—**Demarquay.** Luxation des 4 premiers métatarsiens; réduction du 1er, subluxation des 2e, 3e et 4e. Bull. Soc. de chir. de Par. (1865), 1866, 2. s., vi, 471-473.—**Gruber** (W.) Ueber die beiden Arten des überzähligen Zwischenknöchelchens am Rücken des Metatarsus (Ossiculum intermetatarseum dorsale Gruber) und über den durch Anchylose eines dieser Knöchelchen entstandenen und eine Exostose am Os cuneiforme i. und Os metatarsale ii. vortäuschenden Fortsatz. Arch. f. path. Anat., etc., Berl., 1877, lxxi, 440-452, 2 pl. ——. Ueber den anomalen Musculus abductor metatarsi quinti, seine Substitution durch einen Sehnenstrang (neu) und sein Auftreten als M. abductor metatarsi quinti circumflexus (neu) beim Menschen sowie über constante Homologien dafür bei Säugethieren. Ibid., 1886, cvi, 489-501, 1 pl.—**Guillet.** Luxation du métatarse en dehors. J. de méd. de l'ouest, Nantes, 1882, xvi, 340.—**Laugier.** Note sur les fractures simples du métatarse, et, en particulier, sur la fracture par arrachement du cinquième métatarsien. France méd., Par., 1882, i, 205-208.—**Machenaud.** Observation de luxation des metatarsiens. Bull. Soc. anat. de Par., 1866, xli, 96.—**Mazet** (C.) Luxation de tous les métatarsiens sur le tarse; amputation; phlébite. Ibid., 1837, xii, 229-242.—**Minonzio** (P.) Caso di lussazione del metatarso sul tarso. Ann. univ. di med., Milano, 1856, clvi, 465.—**Riberi** (A.) Guarigioni di gravi e profonde affezioni cariose e necrotiche del primo osso del metatarso senz' amputazione. In his: Raccolta d. opere minori, etc., 8°, Torino, 1851, ii, 418-432.—**Shaw** (W. C.) Dislocation of metatarsal bone at metatarsotarsal articulation. Pittsburgh M. J., 1882, ii, 301-303.

Metaxa (Luigi) [1778-1842]. L' antrace, i contagi, le intermittenti. Lettere al Paolo Baroni. 199 pp., 1 pl. 8°. Roma, G. Olivieri, 1837.

For Biography, see Gior. . . . d. Soc. med.-chir. di Torino, 1843, xvi, 378-382 (A. Garbiglietti).

Metaxà (Telemaco).

Editor of : **Annali** medico-chirurgici, Roma, 1843-6.

Métaxas (Stavros-Jean). * De l'exploration de la rétine, et des altérations de cette membrane visibles à l'ophthalmoscope. 168 pp., 3 pl. 4°. Paris, 1861, No. 46.

Métaxas (Thémistocle-G.) [1855-   ]. * Des troubles oculaires dans la grossesse et l'accouchement. 96 pp. 4°. Paris, 1882, No. 404.

Metaxas-Zani (Gérasime). * De la cure en deux temps (exérèse - anaplastie) de certaines tumeurs de la face. 190 pp., 1 l. 4°. Paris, 1887, No. 203.

——. The same. Des anaplasties secondaires. Cure en deux temps (exérèse - anaplastie) de certaines tumeurs de la face. 190 pp., 1 l. 8°. Paris, G. Steinheil, 1887.

Metaxylol.

GREWINGK (E.) * Ueber Nitro- und Amidoderivate des Metaxylols. 8°. Dorpat, 1886.

Metazoa.

Bütschli (O.) Ueber eine Hypothese bezüglich der phylogenetischen Herleitung des Blutgefässapparates eines Theils der Metazoën. Morphol. Jahrb., Leipz., 1882, viii, 474-482.

Metcalf (E. C.)

See **Waring** (Geo. E.), jr. Irvington sanitary survey. 8°. New York, 1879.

Metcalf (James W.) Homœopathy and its requirements of the physician; an address delivered before the Homœopathic Medical Society of the State of New York. 24 pp. 8°. New York, Angell, Engel & Hewitt, 1852. [Also, in : P., v. 528.]

See, also, **Pulte** (J. H.) Reply to the article of Dr. J. W. Metcalf, [etc.] 8°. Cincinnati, 1851.

Metcalf (John George). The physiology of the skin. A lecture. 23 pp. 8°. *Boston, Marsh, Capen & Co.*, 1840. [P., v. 751.]

——. The study and practice of midwifery; a discourse read before the Massachusetts Medical Society. 123 pp. 8°. *Boston, J. Wilson & Son*, 1856.

Metcalf (Theodore) & Co. Notes on new remedies, collated from medical and pharmaceutical periodicals, etc. 32 pp. 16°. *Boston*, 1877.

Metcalf (Urbane). The interior of Bethlehem Hospital, humbly addressed to his royal highness the Duke of Sussex, and to the other governors. 16 pp. 8°. *London, the author*, [1818].

Metcalf (*Volney*) [1804–52].
Magoun (C. S.) Biographical sketch of the late Volney Metcalf, M. D., Natchez, Miss. N. Orl. M. & S. J., 1852–3, ix, 484–487.

Metcalfe (Joannes). *De rheumatismo acuto. 2 p. l., 36 pp. 8°. *Edinburgi, A. Smellie*, 1798. [*Also, in :* P., v. 8.]

Metcalfe (John T.)
See **United States** Sanitary Commission. Publications. P. On the subject of the nature and treatment of miasmatic fevers. 8°. *New York*, 1862. ——. The same. Q. On the subject of the nature and treatment of yellow fever. 8°. *New York*, 1862.

Metcalfe (Joseph). Memoir of the Rev. Wm. Metcalfe, M. D. 38 pp. 8°. *Philadelphia, J. L. Capen*, 1866.

Metcalfe (Richard). Medical opinions on the efficacy of hydropathy and the Turkish bath, with Lord Lytton's experiences of the water cure. xxxvi, xvi pp. 8°. *London, R. Metcalfe*, [1869].

——. Sanitas sanitatum et omnia sanitas. v. 1. xx, 334 pp., 1 pl. 8°. *London*, 1877.

Metcalfe (Samuel L.) [1798–1856]. A new theory of terrestrial magnetism. v, 6–158 pp. 8°. *New York, G. & C. & H. Carvill*, 1833.

——. Caloric; its mechanical, chemical and vital agencies in the phenomena of nature. v. 1–2. xxiv, 17–630; viii, 9–481 pp. 8°. *Philadelphia, J. B. Lippincott & Co.*, 1859.

Metcalfe (William) [1788–1862].
Co-Editor of : **American** (The) Vegetarian and Health Journal, Philadelphia, 1850–54.
For Biography, see **Metcalfe** (J.) Memoir of the Rev. Wm. Metcalfe, M. D., [etc.] 8°. *Philadelphia*, 1866.

Metelercamp Cappenberg (Martinus Carolus). *De morbis placentæ universim, et de placuntitide ejusque sequelis in specie. 2 p. l., 36 pp., 21. 8°. *Groningæ, P. van Zweeden*, [1844].

Metelerkamp (Rutger). *De pœnis criminum ingeniis populorum accommodandis. 1 p. l., 55 pp., 3 l. 4°. *Lugd. Bat., S. et J. Luchtmans*, 1792. [P., v. 1012.]

Méténier (Jacques). *Des fièvres intermittentes. 35 pp. 4°. *Paris*, 1857, No. 19, v. 608.

Meteorism.
See **Flatulence**, *etc.*

Meteorology.
See, *also*, **Air; Aurora** *borealis*; **Barometer; Climate; Dew; Hygrometer; Instruments** (*Optical, etc.*); **Ozone.**

ABDILL (D.) A new theory of the weather, and practical views on astronomy. With a description of the constellations from Dick, Barritt, and others. Also a new and important mode of calculating the weather, and a general view of the atmosphere, and formation of clouds, rain, snow, frost, dew, etc., accompanied with a dictionary of philosophical terms. 8°. *Wheeling*, 1842.

ADIE (J.) On meteorological observations. 8°. [*Edinburgh*, 1831.]
Repr. from : Quart. J. Agric., May, 1831.

ARGENTINE REPUBLIC. Anales de la oficina meteorológica argentina por su director, Benja-

Meteorology.
min A. Gould. Tomo II. Climas de Bahia y corrientes. 4°. *Buenos Aires*, 1881.

AUFRUF zur Bildung eines Vereines für landwirthschaftliche Wetterkunde. Gerichtet an die landwirthschaftlichen Vereine der Provinz Sachsen, des Herzogthums Braunschweig, des Herzogthums Anhalt und der sächsischen Herzogthümer. 8°. *Magdeburg*, 1881.

BACON (F.) Historia naturalis et experimentalis de ventis. 16°. *Lugd. Bat.*, 1648.

BARDILI (C. G.) *Diss. philos. continens observatione et explicationes quasdam physicas præsertim meteorologicas. 4°. *Tubingæ*, 1780.

BARTHA (C.) *De meteorologia cosmica. 8°. *Budæ*, [1834].
Hungarian text.

BAUER (J. B.) *De aëris constitutionibus ad formandas indicationes rite æstimandis. 8°. *Landishuti*, 1815.

BECKER (J.) *De grandine. 4°. [*Lipsiæ*, 1659.]

BELOST (S.) *Considérations sur les quatre principaux états de l'atmosphère, ou sur le chaud, le froid, le sec et l'humide. 4°. *Paris, an XII* [1804].

BENKÖ (S.) Ephemerides meteorologico-medicæ, ab ann. 1780 ad ann. 1793. 5 v. 8°. *Vindobonæ*, 1794.

BENT (S.) An address delivered before the St. Louis Historical Society upon the thermometric gateways to the pole, surface currents of the ocean, and the influence of the latter upon the climate of the world. 8°. *St. Louis*, 1869.

BLASIUS (W.) Storms; their nature, classification, and laws. With the means of predicting them by their embodiments, the clouds. 8°. *Philadelphia*, [n. d.]

BRANDIN (A. V.) Observaciones meteorológicas. 8°. [*n. p.*, 1827.]
Repr. from : Anales méd. de Perú, 1827.

BRAUN (J. A.) Oratio academica de atmosphæræ mutationibus præcipuis, earumque præsagiis. 4°. *Petropoli*, 1759.

BRITISH Meteorological Society. Proceedings, 1862–71. Edited by J. Glaisher. 5 v. 8°. *London*, 1863–71.

BRUNING (J. H. L.) *De caussis grandinum nocturnis horis decidentium. 4°. [*Hafniæ*, 1755.]

BUCHAN (A.) A handy book of meteorology. 8°. *Edinburgh & London*, 1867.

——. Introductory text-book of meteorology. 8°. *Edinburgh & London*, 1871.

CANADA. Meteorological service. Monthly Weather Review, for the months of Dec., 1886, Jan., March, 1887. 4°. [*Toronto*, 1887.]

——. Toronto Meteorological Register for the year 1886. 8°. [*Toronto*, 1887.]

CLOUSTON (C.) An explanation of the popular weather prognostics of Scotland on scientific principles. 8°. *Edinburgh*, 1867.

COCK (W.) Meteorologia, oder Witterungs-Lehre, in welcher der rechte Weg, die Veränderungen der Luft und Abwechselungen des Wetters, in unterschiedenen Ländern, vorher zu erkennen. Aus dem Englischen. Von J. M. Glaschke. 4°. *Würzburg*, 1729.

COFFIN (J. H.) Winds of the northern hemisphere. 4°. 1850. Revised 1852. *Washington, D. C.*, 1853.

——. Psychrometrical table, for determining the elastic force of aqueous vapor and the relative humidity of the atmosphere from indications of the wet and dry bulb thermometer. 8°. *Washington*, 1860.

——. The winds of the globe . . . completed . . . by S. J. Coffin; with a discussion and analy-

Meteorology.

sis of the tables and charts by A. Woeikof. 4°. *Washington City*, 1875.

CONGRÈS international de météorologie, tenu à Paris du 24 au 28 août 1878. 8°. *Paris*, 1879.

D'ALEMBERT. Réflexions sur la cause générale des vents. Le même sujet en texte latin : Meditationes de generali ventorum causa. sm. 4°. *Paris*, 1747.

D[ALENCÉ]. Traittez des baromètres, thermomètres, et notiomètres, ou hygromètres. 12°. *Amsterdam*, 1688.

——. The same. Abhandlung dreyer so nothwendig- als nützlichen Instrumenten, nemlich des Barometri, Thermometri und Notiometri oder Hygrometri . . . Ins Teutsche vorgetragen von D. M. H. C. J. sm. 4°. *Mäyntz*, 1688.

DANIELL (J. F.) Meteorological essays and observations. 2. ed. 8°. *London*, 1827.

DAUMIUS (C. L.) De tempestatum varietate et investigandis veris ejusdem rationibus una cum observationibus barometricis et meteorologicis. 4°. *Vittembergæ Saxonum*, [1714].

DAVID (A.) Ursachen und Vorschriften, warum und wie die Witterungs-Beobachtungen anzustellen sind. 8°. *Prag*, 1817.

DAVY (H.-M.) Météorologie. Les mouvements de l'atmosphère et des mers considérés au point de vue de la prévision du temps. 8°. *Paris*, 1866.

DRECHSLER (A.) Das Wetterglas. Vademecum der Witterungskunde. 16°. *Leipzig*, 1867.

DREW (J.) Practical meteorology. Edited by F. Drew. 2. ed. 12°. *London*, 1860.

DU BOULAY (T.) The summer of 1862: founded on the vernal equinox. With observations on the summers of England, coupled with remarks on the locality and meteorology of Great Britain. 8°. *London*, 1862.

——. The summer of 1865: founded on the vernal equinox. 8°. *London*, 1865.

DU CREST (M.) Kleine Schriften von den Thermometern und Barometern. Aus dem Französischen übersetzt und mit einigen Anmerkungen begleitet von J. C. Thenn. 8°. *Augsburg*, 1770.

EISENLOHR (O.) Untersuchungen über den Zusammenhang des Barometerstandes mit der Witterung im Winter. 8°. *Karlsruhe*, 1852.

ESPY (J. P.) The philosophy of storms. 8°. *Boston*, 1841.

——. First report on meteorology made to the Surgeon-General, United States Army. fol. *Washington*, 1843.

——. Second and fourth reports on meteorology made to the Secretary of the Navy. 2 v. 4°. *Washington*, 1850 & 1857.

EXNER (C.) *De pluvia. sm. 4°. *Lipsiæ*, [1648].

FITZROY (R.) The weather book. A manual of practical meteorology. 8°. *London*, 1863.

——. Barometer manual, 1863. 8. ed. 8°. *London*, 1865.

FLUDD [or DE FLUCTIBUS] (R.) Meteorologia cosmica. fol. *Francofurti*, 1626.

DE FONVIELLE (W.) Thunder and lightning. Transl. from the French, and edited by T. L. Phipson. 12°. *London*, 1868.

FORCE (P.) Record of auroral phenomena observed in the higher northern latitudes. (Appendix.) 4°. *Washington, D. C.*, 1856.

FORGET (C.-P.) De l'utilité des observations météorologiques. 8°. [*Paris*, 1854.]

FORRY (S.) The climate of the United States and its endemic influences. Based chiefly on the records of the Medical Department and Adjutant-General's Office, United States Army. 2. ed. 8°. *New York*, 1842.

Meteorology.

FORSTER (T.) Researches about atmospheric phænomena. 3. ed., to which is added the calendar of nature. 8°. *London*, 1823.

FORSTER (T. F.) The pocket encyclopædia of natural phenomena; being a compendium of prognostications of the weather, signs of the seasons . . . compiled principally from the manuscripts and MS. journals of the late T. F. Forster. By T. Forster. 8°. *London*, 1827.

[FRADESSO.] Wiener Meteorologen Congress, 1873. 8°. [*Vienne*, 1873.]

FRITSCH (G.) *De rore microcosmi. sm. 4°. *Lipsiæ*, [1665].

FROBESIUS (J. N.) Nova et antiqua luminis atque auroræ borealis spectacula. Secundum sæculorum atque annorum seriem subnexa mirabilis phænomeni consideratione philosophica. 4°. *Helmstadii*, 1739.

FROELICH (O.) *Ueber den Einfluss der Absorption der Sonnenwärme in der Atmosphäre auf die Temperatur der Erde. 4°. *Königsberg*, [1868].

FROMONDUS (L.) Meteorologicorum libri sex. 4°. *Antverpiæ*, 1627.

FUESS (R.) Neue registrirende meteorologische Apparate. 4°. *Berlin*, 1883.
Repr. from: Ztschr. f. Instrumentenkunde, June, 1883.

FUNCCIUS (C.) De pluvia; aphorismi physici. 4°. *Lipsiæ*, [1647].

FUNCCIUS (J. C.) De coloribus cœli in genere. 4°. *Lipsiæ*, [1705].

GERMANY. Ergebnisse der Beobachtungsstationen an den deutschen Küsten über die physikalischen Eigenschaften der Ostsee und Nordsee und die Fischerei. Veröffentlicht von der Ministerial-Kommission zur Untersuchung der deutschen Meere in Kiel. Hft. 9 u. 10, Sept. u. Oct. 1873. 4°. *Berlin*, 1874.

GIESWALD (H.) Lehre von der Thermometrie, der Pyrometrie, Hygrometrie, Psychometrie und Barometrie in ihrer Gesammtheit dargestellt, und nach den Quellen, namentlich auch zum Gebrauch für Techniker bearbeitet. Nebst einem Anhange mit praktischen Erläuterungen. sm. 8°. *Weimar*, 1861.

GILBY (G. H.) *De mutationibus quas ea quæ e terra gignuntur aëri inferunt. 8°. *Edinburgi*, 1815.

GIRONDE (Département de la). Commission météorologique de la Gironde. Observations pluviométriques et thermométriques faites dans le département de la Gironde de 1883–4 et 1884–5. Notes de M. Rayet. Rapports sur les orages de 1883 et 1884 par M. Lespiault. 8°. *Bordeaux*, 1884–5.

GLAISHER (J.) Hygrometrical tables; containing the temperature of the dew-point, the elastic force and weight of vapour; degree of humidity; weight of air, corresponding to all readings of the dry and wet thermometers, between 10° and 90° of Fahrenheit. 8°. *London*, 1847.

——. Meteorological essays; being cuttings from the Proceedings of the Meteorological Society of London, from 1861 to 1869. 1 v. 8°. [*n. p., n. d.*]

GLAISHER (J.) [*et al.*]. Travels in the air. Edited by J. Glaisher, F. R. S. 8°. *Philadelphia*, 1871.

GLÖCKNER (J. F.) *De pondere nubium. 4°. *Halæ Magdeb.*, [1722].

GREAT BRITAIN. *Army.* Observations made at the magnetical and meteorological observatory at St. Helena, with discussions of the observations at St. Helena, the Cape of Good Hope, the Falkland Islands, Carlton Fort in North America, and Pekin. Printed by order

Meteorology.

of her majesty's government under the superintendence of Major-General Edward Sabine. v. 2, 1844-9. 4°. *London*, 1860.

GUYOT (A.) Tables, meteorological and physical, prepared for the Smithsonian Institution. 3. ed. 8°. *Washington*, 1859.

——. The same. 4. ed., revised and enlarged. Edited by William Libbey, jr. 8°. *Washington*, 1884.

HALLMANN (E.) Die Temperaturverhältnisse der Quellen. Eine meteorologische Untersuchung. 2 v. 8°. *Berlin*, 1854-5.

HANN (J.) Untersuchungen über die Veränderlichkeit der Tagestemperatur. 8°. *Wien*, [1875].
Repr. from: Sitzungsb. d. k. Akad. d. Wissensch. Math.-naturw. Cl., Wien, 1875, lxxi, 2. Abth.

HARE (R.) A verbal communication, respecting some experiments made by . . . to ascertain the comparative heating or cooling influence of changes of density resulting from changes in pressure in dry air, and air replete with aqueous vapour; also, some experiments favourable to the idea that a vacuum has a capacity for caloric. 8°. [*Philadelphia*, 1840.]
Repr. from: Proc. Am. Phil. Soc., Phila., 1840, i.

——. Objections to Mr. Redfield's theory of storms, with some strictures upon his reasoning. 8°. [*New Haven*, 1841?]
Repr. from: Am. J. Sc. & Arts, N. Haven, 1841-2, xlii.

——. Additional objections to Redfield's theory of storms. 8°. [*New Haven, n. d.*]
Cutting from: Am. J. Sc. & Arts, N. Haven.

——. Queries and strictures respecting Espy's meteorological report to the Naval Department. Also, the conclusions arrived at by a committee of the Academy of Sciences of France, agreeably to which tornadoes are caused by heat; while, agreeably to Peltier's report to the same body, certain insurers had been obliged to pay for a tornado as an electrical storm. With abstracts from Peltier's report. 8°. *Philadelphia*, 1852.

HEJSER (J. D.) *De rigidiore, medio ævo in terris borealibus, hyeme. sm. 4°. *Upsaliæ*, 1795.

HEROS (L.) *De ventis. 8°. *Berolini*, [1846].

HOFMANN (J. G.) *De nive. 4°. *Wittebergæ*, [1665].

HOPKINS (T.) On the atmospheric changes which produce rain, wind, storms, and the fluctuations of the barometer. 8°. *London*, 1844.

——. The same. 2. ed. 8°. *London*, 1854.

HOSKINS (S. E.) Tables for the extemporaneous application of corrections for temperature to barometric observations, deduced from the tables published in the report of the committee of physics, Royal Society. 8°. *Guernsey*, 1842.

HUEBLER (C.) *De pluviis prodigiosis. 4°. *Erfurti*, [1695].

HUNTER (F.) *De ætheribus. 8°. *Edinburgi*, 1808.

JAMES (H.) Instructions for taking meteorological observations; with tables for their correction, and notes on meteorological phenomena. Drawn up by order of the secretary of state for war. 8°. *London*, 1861.

JANUS (F. A.) *Diss. hist.-phys. de pluvia prodigiosa. 4°. *Lipsiæ*, [1667].

JENKINS (T. A.) The barometer, thermometer, hygrometer, and atmospheric appearances at sea and on land as aids in foretelling weather, with brief rules for their use, and the practical application of their separate and combined indications as weather guides. 8°. *Washington*, 1869.

JENNER. Signs of rain. Forty reasons for not accepting the invitation of a friend. The

Meteorology.

same in Latin by the late J. Latham. 8°. *London*, [*n. d.*]

JUNCKER (F. C.) De tonitru magno sub pluvio personante et mitescente. 4°. *Halæ Magdeb.*, [1752].

KÄMTZ (L. F.) Vorlesungen über Meteorologie. 8°. *Halle*, 1840.

——. Cours complet de météorologie. Trad. et annoté par C. Martins. 8°. *Paris*, 1843.

——. The same. A complete course of meteorology. With notes by C. Martins; and an appendix, containing the graphic representation of the numerical tables by L. Lalanne. Transl., with notes and additions, by C. V. Walker. 8°. *London*, 1845.

KRAFFT (G. W.) Oratio publica, de insoliti caloris æstivi caussa. 4°. *Tubingæ*, 1750.

KUNZEK (A.) Leichtfassliche Darstellung der Meteorologie. 8°. *Wien*, 1847.

LACHLAN (R.) A paper and resolutions in advocacy of the establishment of a uniform system of meteorological observations throughout the whole American continent. 8°. *Cincinnati*, 1859.

LAMBERT (J. H.) Abhandlung von den Barometerhöhen und ihren Veränderungen. 4°. *München*, [*n. d.*]

LANARCK. Mémoire sur le mode de rédiger et de noter les observations météorologiques, à fin d'en obtenir des résultats utiles, et sur les considérations que l'on doit avoir en vue pour cet objet. 4°. [*n. p., n. d.*]

LANDOLT (H.) Neuerungen an Polaristrobometern 4°. *Berlin*, 1883.
Repr. from: Ztschr. f. Instrumentenkunde, April, 1883.

LATZINA (F.) Sobre meteorolojía. Conferencia popular. 8°. *Córdoba*, 1876.

LEYST (E.) Katalog der meteorologischen Beobachtungen in Russland und Finnland. Vierter Supplementband zum Repertorium für Meteorologie, herausgegeben von der kaiserlichen Academie der Wissenschaften. 4°. *St. Petersburg*, 1887.

LOOMIS (E.) On certain storms in Europe and America. 4°. [*Philadelphia*], 1859.

——. A treatise on meteorology, with a collection of meteorological tables. 8°. *New York*, 1868.

DE LUC (J.-A.) Recherches sur les modifications de l'atmosphère; contenant l'histoire critique du baromètre et du thermomètre, un traité sur la construction de ces instruments, des expériences relatives à leurs usages, et principalement à la mesure des hauteurs et à la correction des réfractions moyennes. 2 v. 4°. *Genève*, 1772.

MERKIUS (H. A.) De ventis, incendi tempore orientibus. 4°. *Lipsiæ*, 1587.

MOHN (H.) Havets Temperatur mellem Island, Skotland og Norge. 8°. [*Christiania*, 1869.]
Repr. from: Særskilt aftrykt af et Foredrag i Vidensk.-Selsk. i Christiania, 1869.

VAN MONS (J. B.) Censura commentarii a Wieglebo nuper editi, cui titulus: De vaporis aquei in aërem conversione. 4°. *Bruxellis*, [*n. d.*]

MORRIS (A. J. T.) A treatise on meteorology; the barometer, thermometer, hygrometer, rain-gauge, and ozonometer; with rules and regulations to be observed for their correct use. To which are appended some of the latest discoveries and theories of scientific men respecting various solar and terrestrial phenomena. Dedicated to the meteorologists of Strathearn. 12°. *Edinburgh*, 1866.

MÜHRY (A.) Untersuchungen über die Theorie und das allgemeine geographische System der

Meteorology.

Winde. Ein Beitrag zur Begründung einer rationellen Lehre von den Luftströmen, für den Gebrauch der Klimatologie und der Nautik. 8°. *Göttingen*, 1869.

MÜLLER (F.) Considérations sur la prévision des tempêtes et spécialement sur celles du 1er au 4 décembre 1863. Supplément aux Annales de l'Observatoire physique central pour l'année 1861. 4°. *St.-Petérsbourg*, 1864.

MÜLLER (J.) Grundriss der Physik und Meteorologie. 5. Aufl. 8°. *Braunschweig*, 1856.

——. The same. Principles of physics and meteorology. 1. Am. ed. 8°. *Philadelphia*, 1848.

NEU-ERFUNDENE mathematische Curiositäten. Enthaltend die wunderbareste Würkungen der Natur und Kunst, worinnen vermittles drey sonderbaren Instrumenten: 1. Die Schwere und Leichte; 2. Die Truckne und Feuchte; 3. Das Ab- und Zunehmen der Hitz und Kälte der Lufft zu beobachten und zu erkennen seynd. Aus dem Frantzösisch in Deutsch übersetzt. 4°. *Mayntz*, 1695.

NEW YORK (City). *Department of Public Parks*. Annual reports of the director of the New York Meteorological Observatory, Central Park, for the years 1870–71; 1873–5; 1877; 1886. 8°. *New York*, 1871–87.

——. Abstract of registers from self-recording instruments. Jan., 1879, to Dec., 1881; July, 1882; Jan. to July, 1886. 4°. [*New York*, 1879–86.]

——. New York Meteorological Observatory, Central Park. Annual tables for the years 1879–81. 4°. *New York*, 1880–82.

NICOLLET (J. N.) Essay on meteorological observations. Printed by order of the War Department. 8°. [*Washington*], 1839.

NOTH (J. T.) *Specimen physicum de pluvia et tonitru quo simul locus Job. xxxviii, 25. 26. 27. explicatur. 4°. *Wittebergœ*, [1787].

NOYES (I. P.) How to be weather-wise. A new view of our weather system. 12°. *New York*, [1882].

OBSERVATORIO-FÍSICO-METEOROLÓGICO de la Habana. [Resúmen. Enero á julio, setiembre á diciembre 1875; enero, marzo á mayo, julio, setiembre, noviembre 1876; julio, agosto 1878.] 4°. [*Habana*, 1875–8.]

——. En la Escuela profesional de la isla de Cuba. Observaciones [diario] desde 1o de enero de 1875 á 30 de noviembre de 1878. 4°. [*Habana*, 1875–8.]

OTAGO (Province of). Geological Survey Office. Meteorological observations. April, Aug., 1863. broadside. [*Duneden*, 1863.]

OLMSTED (D.) On the recent secular period of the aurora borealis. 4°. [*Washington*], 1856.

PEUSCHELIUS (J. F.) De ventis. 4°. *Jenœ*, 1667.

PFAFF (C. H.) Ueber den heissen Sommer von 1811, nebst einigen Bemerkungen über frühere heisse Sommer. Eine academische Gelegenheitsschrift bei Niederlegung seines von Johannis 1810 bis Johannis 1811 geführten Decanats der medicinischen Facultät. 8°. *Kiel*, 1812.

PICKETT (J. C.) Thermopsis. The hot weather. 8°. [*Washington*, 1866.]

PLANERUS (J. A.) *De nive. II. Respondens C. Schmeltzer. 4°. *Vittembergœ*, [1695].

——. The same. III. Respondens W. H. Leubius. 4°. *Vitembergœ*, [1696].

——. The same. IV. Respondens B. Siberus. 4°. *Vitembergœ*, [1696].

POINTER (J.) A rational account of the weather. Shewing the signs of its several changes and alterations, together with the philosophical reasons of them . . . To which are added three essays

Meteorology.

towards accounting for: I. A continued course of wet years. II. The cause of an aurora borealis. III. The cause of the plague. 2. ed. 8°. *London*, 1738.

[PORTUGAL.] Notas explicativas (instrucções) para compor os extractos do Diario nautico conforme o plano approvado e recommendado pela conferencia maritima de Bruxellas. 8°. *Lisboa*, 1854.

——. Notas explicativas para a execução de observações deducções meteorologicas segundo um plano uniforme. 8°. *Lisboa*, 1856.

POUILLET. Éléments de physique expérimentale et de météorologie. 4. éd. roy. 8°. *Bruxelles*, 1840.

——. The same. 4. éd. 2 v. 8°. *Paris*, 1844.

PRAETORIUS (F. C.) & EHRLICH (J. G.) Tentamen physicum de nubium fulminearum genesi. 4°. *Lipsiœ*, 1728.

PRESTEL (M. A. F.) Die jährliche, periodische Aenderung des atmosphärischen Ozons und die ozonoskopische Windrose als Ergebniss der Beobachtungen zu Emden von 1857 bis 1864. 4°. *Dresden*, 1865.

——. Die periodischen und nicht-periodischen Veränderungen des Barometerstandes, so wie die Stürme und das Wetter über der hannoverischen Nordseeküste, als Grundlage der Sturm- und Wetter-Prognose. 4° & fol. *Emden*, 1866.

——. Die Winde über der deutschen Nordseeküste und dem südlichen Theile der Nordsee, nach ihrer periodischen Veränderung im Laufe des Jahres dargestellt. Zugleich als Ergänzung der Seekarten von der Nordseeküste. 4°. *Emden*, 1868.

Repr. from: Kl. Schrift. d. naturf. Gesellsch. zu Emden, xiii.

——. Das Gesetz der Winde abgeleitet aus dem Auftreten derselben über Nordwest-Europa. 4°. *Emden*, 1869.

Repr. from: Kl. Schrift. d. naturf. Gesellsch. zu Emden.

——. Der Sturmwarner und Wetteranzeiger, [etc.] 8°. *Emden u. Aurich*, 1870.

——. Die Temperatur-Verhältnisse und die mit der Höhe zunehmende Temperatur in der Schicht des Luftmeeres, welche die Erdoberfläche unmittelbar berührt. Nach den Beobachtungen auf dem meteorologischen Observatorium zu Emden. 8°. *Emden*, 1871.

PÜSCHEL (C.) De rarefactionis et condensationis aëris effectis in thermometris. 4°. *Servestœ*, [1687].

RAMON DE LA SAGRA. Relacion de los trabajos físicos y meteorológicos hechos por Don Andres Poey tanto en la Habana como en Europa, destinada para servir de introduccion á las futuras tareas del observatorio meteorológico de aquella ciudad; reductada por . . . 8°. *Paris*, 1858.

RAMOND (L.) Mémoires sur la formule barométrique de la mécanique céleste, et les dispositions de l'atmosphère qui en modifient les propriétés; augmentés d'une instruction élémentaire et pratique destinée à servir de guide dans l'application du baromètre à la mesure des hauteurs. 4°. *Clermont-Ferrand*, 1811.

REDFIELD (W. C.) On three several hurricanes of the Atlantic, and their relations to the northers of Mexico and Central America, with notices of other storms. 8°. *New Haven*, 1846.

REID (W.) An attempt to develop the laws of storms by means of facts, arranged according to place and time; and hence to point out a cause for the variable winds with the view to practical use in navigation. 8°. *London*, 1838.

REINZER (F.) Meteorologia philosophico-politica in duodecim dissertationes per quæstiones

Meteorology.

meteorologicas et conclusiones politicas divisa, appositisque symbolis illustrata. fol. *Augustæ Vindelicorum,* 1709.

——. The same. Meteorologia philosophico-politica, das ist: Philosophische und politische Beschreib- und Erklärung der meteorischen, oder in der obern Lufft erzeugten Dinge; in zwölff verschiednen, aus meteorologischen Fragen, und politischen Schlussreden bestehenden, wie auch zugleich mit untermischten schönen Sinn-Bildern gezierten Abtheilungen sonderbaren Fleisses ehedem verfasst durch . . . Anjetzo aber wegen der darinnen enthaltnen raren und anmuthigen Materien, curiosen Gemüthern zu Gefallen, und zu nützlicher Ergötzung, nebst erstgedachten Authoris Vor-Ansprach an den Leser, aus dem Lateinischen in das Teutsche übersetzt. fol. *Augspurg,* 1712.

RETZ. Abhandlung vom Einflusse der Witterung auf die Arzneywissenschaft und den Ackerbau, nebst der Beschreibung eines neuen vergleichbaren Hygrometers. Eine gekrönte Preisschrift. Aus dem Französischen übersetzt und mit einigen Anmerkungen versehen von Christian Friederich Held. 8°. *Greiz,* 1786.

REYE (T.) Die Wirbelstürme, Tornados und Wettersäulen in der Erd-Atmosphäre, mit Berücksichtigung der Stürme in der Sonnen-Atmosphäre dargestellt und wissenschaftlich erklärt. 8°. *Hannover,* 1872.

RITSCHEL (J. A.) The storm. 8°. [*Freyburg in Breisgau,* 1841.]

ROGER (H.) *Des vents ou courants atmosphériques et de leur influence au point de vue de l'hygiène sociale. 4°. *Paris,* 1876.

RUGGLES (D.) Memorial of . . . asking an appropriation, to be expended in developing his system of producing rainfall. 46th Cong., 2. sess. Senate Mis. Doc. No. 39. Feb. 12, 1880. 8°. [*Washington,* 1880.]

RYKATSCHEW (M.) Ueber den Auf- und Zugang der Gewässer des russischen Reiches. Zweiter Supplementband zum Repertorium für Meteorologie, herausgegeben von der kaiserlichen Academie der Wissenschaften. 4°. *St. Petersburg,* 1887.

VAN RYSSELBERGHE (F.) On a universal system of meteorography. 8°. [*n. p., n. d.*]
Repr. from: Quart. J. Meteorol. Soc., July, 1875.

SADLER (J.) Report on temperatures during the winter of 1878-9 at the Royal Botanic Garden, Edinburgh; the effects of the same on open-air vegetation at the Garden, and in other parts of Scotland; with table of dates of flowering of spring plants. 8°. *Edinburgh,* 1880.
Repr. from: Tr. Botanical Soc., Edinb., xiii.

SANNA SOLARO (J.-M.) Recherches sur les causes et les lois des mouvements de l'atmosphère. 8°. *Paris,* 1870.

SAXONY. Monatliche Berichte über die Resultate aus den meteorologischen Beobachtungen angestellt an den königlich sächsischen Stationen in den Jahren 1871-5. Mitgetheilt . . . von Dr. G. Bruhns. 4°. *Dresden,* 1872-6.

SCHERLING (C.) Grundriss der Physik und Meteorologie. Mit besonderer Berücksichtigung der einfacheren Apparate und Instrumente für Gymnasien und Realschulen bearbeitet. 8°. *Leipzig,* 1862.

SCHLÖGL (G.) Tabulæ pro reductione quorumvis statuum barometri ad normalem quemdam caloris gradum publico usui datæ. 4°. *Monachii,* [1787].

SCHMID (E. E.) Allgemeine Encyklopädie der Physik. Band xxi. Lehrbuch der Meteorologie. 8°. *Leipzig,* 1860.

Meteorology.

——. Grundriss der Meteorologie. 8°. *Leipzig,* 1862.

SCHOOCK (I.) De nive, cum rarissimis adhærentibus quæstionibus, de meteoris aqueis. 4°. [*n. p.*], 1673.

SCHOTT (C. A.) Tables, distribution, and variations of the atmospheric temperature in the United States and some adjacent parts of America, collected at the Smithsonian Institution, and discussed under the direction of Joseph Henry, secretary. 4°. *Washington,* 1876.

SIMMONITE (W. J.) The astro-philosopher and meteorologist. 8°. *London,* [*n. d.*]

SIMONS (G.) Commentatio de aquæ vaporibus atmosphæra contentis. 8°. *Traj. ad Rhenum,* 1823.

SMITH (R. A.) Air and rain. The beginnings of a chemical climatology. roy. 8°. *London,* 1872.

SMITHSONIAN Institution. Directions for meteorological observations and the registry of periodical phenomena. 8°. *Washington,* 1860.

SPECH (E.) *De aëre commotione et aqua. 8°. *Vindobonæ,* [1846].

STAHL (G. E.) Einleitung zu der neuen Meteoroscopie, oder Witterungs-Deutung, nach William Cocks Grund-Reguln, und Matthæi Schlüters Curieusen Anmerckungen, wodurch auch jeder gemeiner Mann, ohne einige Schwierigkeit, auss denen in gemeinen Calendern verzeichneten Adspecten von erfolgenden Witterungs-Aenderungen, mit grosser Gewissheit, und zuverlässigen Erfolg, zu urtheilen erlernen kan. 8°. *Halle,* 1716.

STARK (C. A.) Meteorologisches Jahrbuch von 1819 mit Inbegriff der meteorischen und astronomischen Beobachtungen, der Aspecten der Sonne, der Planeten und des Mondes, wie auch der Veränderungen der positiven und negativen atmosphärischen Electricität. 4°. *Augsburg,* 1820.

STEINMETZ (A.) Sunshine and showers; their influences throughout creation. A compendium of popular meteorology. 8°. *London,* 1867.

——. Everybody's weather guide; especially adapted for army and navy officers, medical men and families, farmers and gardeners, [etc.] 8°. *London,* 1867.
Reprinted, with additions, from Colburn's United Service Magazine.

STERNBERGEN (G.) *De ventis. 4°. *Lipsiæ,* [1654].

STRAITS SETTLEMENTS. Annual report on meteorological observations in the Straits Settlements for the year 1886. By principal civil medical officer, Straits Settlements. fol. *Singapore,* 1887.

SWITZERLAND. Instructions pour les observateurs des stations météorologiques de la Suisse. sm. 4°. *Zurich,* 1863.

SYKES. Storm warnings; their importance and practicability. 8°. *London,* [*n. d.*]
Repr. from: Civil Engineering & Architects' J., 1867.

THILO (L.) Ueber eine Methode, die Barometerstände ohne Mitbeobachtung des Thermometers auf eine gewisse Normal-Temperatur zu reduciren. 4°. [*n. p., n. d.*]

THOMSON (D. P.) Introduction to meteorology. 8°. *Edinburgh,* 1849.

TITIUS (J. D.) Impetus ventorum eorumque causas exponit. 4°. *Wittebergæ,* [1782].

—— & HEUN (F. W.) Artis instituendi observationes meteorologicas primæ lineæ. 4°. *Wittebergæ,* [1769].

TYAS (R.) A companion to the weather-glass, designed to record, numerically and graphically, the natural phænomena presented by the barometer, thermometers, rain-gauge, clouds, wind,

Meteorology.

etc.; with blank forms and diagrams, such that the record may be begun at any time in the year. 8°. *London*, [*n. d.*]

——. The same. With a calendar for 1870. 8°. *London*, [1869].

UNITED STATES. *Department of the Interior. Patent Office.* Results of meteorological observations, made under the direction of the United States Patent Office and Smithsonian Institution, from the years 1854 to 1859, inclusive. Being a report of the Commissioner of Patents made at the first session of the Thirty-sixth Congress. v. 1; v. 2, pt. 1. 2 v. 8°. *Washington*, 1861–4.

UNITED STATES. *Navy Department. Naval Observatory.* Astronomical and meteorological observations made at the United States Naval Observatory. Publication authorized by a concurrent resolution of the Forty-eighth Congress. For the years 1851, 1852, 1861–78, 1880–82. 4°. *Washington*, 1863–85.

——. Meteorological observations made at the United States Naval Observatory. Washington observations for the years 1876–82. 4°. *Washington*, 1879–85.

UNITED STATES. *Treasury Department. U. S. Coast Survey.* Methods, discussions, and results. Meteorological researches for the use of the coast pilot. Pt. I. On the mechanics and the general motions of the atmosphere. By Wm. Ferrel. 4°. *Washington*, 1877.

UNITED STATES. *War Department. Signal Office.* Annual reports of the Chief Signal Officer of the Army to the Secretary of War, for the years 1869–70 to 1884–5. 17 v. 8°. *Washington*, 1870–86.

——. Annual reports of the Chief Signal Officer of the Army to the Secretary of War, for the years 1869–70; 1877–8; 1880–81 to 1884–5; 1886–7. 8°. *Washington*, 1870–87.

——. Suggestions as to the practical uses of meteorological reports and weather maps. 12°. *Washington*, 1871.

——. Circular. The practical use of meteorological reports and weather-maps. 8°. *Washington*, 1871.

——. Daily bulletins. Signal Service U. S. Army. Division of telegrams and reports for the benefit of commerce. Meteorological record. Jan. – June, 1871; and Jan., 1872. 3 v. fol. *Washington*, 1871–2.

——. Weather maps, Signal Service U. S. Army. Division of telegrams and reports for the benefit of commerce. Jan., 1871, to July 31, 1872. 6 v. imp. fol. *Washington*, 1871–2.

——. Daily bulletins of weather reports, Signal Service U. S. Army, taken at 7.35 a. m., 4.35 p. m., and 11 p. m., Washington mean time, with the synopses, probabilities, and facts, for the months of Aug., 1872, to Sept., 1875; Jan., 1876, to July, 1877; Jan., 1878, to July, 1879; Sept., 1879; Nov., 1879, to Aug., 1880; Dec., 1880. 8° & 4°. *Washington*, 1872–82.

——. Professional papers of the Signal Service. No. 1. Report on the solar eclipse of July, 1878. By Cleveland Abbe. 4°. *Washington*, 1881.

——. Professional papers of the Signal Service. No. 2. Isothermal lines of United States, 1871–80. By Lieut. A. W. Greely. 4°. *Washington*, 1881.

——. Signal Service notes. No. 3. To foretell frost. By Lieut. James Allen. 8°. *Washington*, 1882.

——. Professional papers of the Signal Service. No. 4. Report of the tornadoes of May 29 and 30, 1879, in Kansas, Nebraska, Missouri, and Iowa, by Sergeant J. P. Finley. 4°. *Washington*, 1881.

Meteorology.

——. Professional papers of the Signal Service. No. 5. Information relative to the construction of time-balls. 4°. *Washington*, 1881.

——. Instructions for voluntary observers of the Signal Service of the United States Army. 8°. *Washington*, 1882.

——. Professional papers of the Signal Service. No. 6. The reduction of air-pressure, to sea-level, at elevated stations west of the Mississippi River. By Henry A. Hazen. 4°. *Washington*, 1882.

——. Professional papers of the Signal Service. No. 8. Recent mathematical papers concerning the motions of the atmosphere. Part I. The motions of fluids and solids on the earth's surface, by W. Ferrel. Reprinted, with notes by Frank Waldo. 4°. *Washington*, 1882.

——. Professional papers of the Signal Service. Report on the character of six hundred tornadoes. By Sergeant J. P. Finley. 4°. *Washington*, 1882.

——. Professional papers of the Signal Service. No. 9. Charts and tables showing geographical distribution of rainfall in the United States. By Lieut. H. H. C. Dunwoody. 4°. *Washington*, 1883.

——. Professional papers of the Signal Service. No. 10. Signal Service tables of rainfall and temperature compared with crop production. By Lieut. H. H. C. Dunwoody. 4°. *Washington*, 1882.

——. Professional papers of the Signal Service. No. 12. Popular essays on the movements of the atmosphere. By W. Ferrel. 4°. *Washington*, 1882.

——. Professional papers of the Signal Service. No. 11. Meteorological and physical observations on the east coast of British America, by O. T. Sherman. 4°. *Washington*, 1883.

——. Professional papers of the Signal Service. No. 13. Temperature of the atmosphere and earth's surface. By W. Ferrel. 4°. *Washington*, 1884.

——. Professional papers of the Signal Service. No. 14. Charts of relative storm frequency for a portion of the northern hemisphere. By Lieut. John P. Finley. 4°. *Washington*, 1884.

——. Professional papers of the Signal Service. No. 15. Researches on solar heat and its absorption by the earth's atmosphere. A report of the Mount Whitney expedition. By S. P. Langley, director of the Allegheny Observatory. 4°. *Washington*, 1884.

——. Professional papers of the Signal Service. No. 16. Tornado studies for 1884. By Lieut. John P. Finley. 4°. *Washington*, 1885.

——. Professional papers of the Signal Service. No. 18. Thermometer exposure. By Henry A. Hazen. 4°. *Washington*, 1885.

——. Extract No. 3, from annual report of the Chief Signal Officer, 1886. Report on State weather services. By authority of the Secretary of War. 8°. *Washington*, 1887.

UNITED STATES. *War Department. Surgeon-General's Office.* Topographico-medical remarks, together with meteorological tables, or diary of the weather, made near the headquarters of the 2d military department, by Benj. Waterhouse, Hosp. Surg. and Director. MS. 4°. 1816.

——. Meteorological register for the years 1822–5, from observations made by the surgeons of the Army, at the military posts of the United States. Prepared under the direction of Joseph Lovell, Surgeon-General of the U. S. Army. 8°. *Washington*, 1826.

——. Meteorological register for the years 1826–30; from observations made by the sur-

Meteorology.

geons of the Army and others at the military posts of the United States. Prepared under the direction of Thomas Lawson, Surg.-Gen. U. S. Army. 8°. *Philadelphia*, 1840.

———. Directions for taking meteorological observations. 8°. *Washington*, 1844.

———. Meteorological register for twelve years, 1831 to 1842, inclusive; compiled from observations made by the officers of the Medical Department of the Army at the military posts of the United States. Prepared under the direction of Thomas Lawson, Surg.-Gen. U. S. Army. 8°. *Washington*, 1851.

———. General meteorological directions, and explanation of barometer in use by the medical department, U. S. Army. 8°. [*Washington*, 1868.]

VEREIN für landwirthschaftliche Wetterkunde für die Provinz Sachsen, die Herzogthümer Anhalt und Braunschweig, die thüringischen Grossherzog-, Herzog- und Fürstenthümer, sowie die Ackermark. Constituirt zu Magdeburg am 2. April 1881. 8°. *Magdeburg*, 1883.

VICTORIA. Results of the magnetical, nautical, and meterological observations made and collected at the Flagstaff Observatory, Melbourne, and at various stations in the colony of Victoria. March, 1858, to Feb., 1859. fol. *Melbourne*, [1860].

———. Monthly record of results of observations in meteorology, terrestrial magnetism, etc., taken at the Melbourne Observatory; together with abstracts from meteorological observations obtained at various localities in Victoria. Under the superintendence of R. L. J. Ellery, government astronomer. Jan. to Sept., Nov. and Dec., 1879; March to June, Sept., 1880. 8°. *Melbourne*, 1879-80.

VOLEGIUS (J.) Theses philosophicæ de pluvia, nive, et grandine. 4°. *Marpurgi Cattorum*, 1595.

VOSSIUS (I.) De motu marium et ventorum liber. 4°. *Hagæ-Comitis*, 1663.

WAHLEN (E.) Wahre Tagesmittel und tägliche Variation der Temperatur an 18 Stationen des russischen Reiches. Dritter Supplementband zum Repertorium für Meteorologie, herausgegeben von der kaiserlichen Academie der Wissenschaften. 4°. *St. Petersburg*, 1887.

VON WALUEW (P. A.) Die Temperatur-Verhältnisse des russischen Reiches. Kritisch bearbeitet von H. Wild. 2. Hlfte. 4°. [With atlas fol.] *St. Petersburg*, 1881.

WALTER (G. F.) Dissertatio physica pluviæ examen sistens. 4°. *Argentorati*, [1710].

WALTON (E.) Clouds; their forms and combinations. 2. ed. 4°. *London*, 1869.

WEDEL (G. W.) [Pr.] de mutationibus aëris. sm. 4°. *Jenæ*, [1719].

WEDEL (J. A.) [Pr.] de aëris frigidi in conclave irruentis accumulatione impedienda. 4°. *Jenæ*, [1720].

WEIHRAUCH (C.) [Meteorologie.] Festrede. 4°. *Dorpat*, 1878.

WEISSMANN (I.) *De etesiis. 4°. *Tubingæ*, [1705].

WERNHER (H. L.) De tonitru hiemali. 4°. *Lipsiæ*, [1705].

———. Ueber Wetterprophezeiung. 4°. *Bern*, 1867.
Repr. from: Ztschr. f. schweiz. Statistik.

WILLIAMSON (R. S.) On the use of the barometer on surveys and reconnaissances. Part I. Meteorology in its connection with hypsometry. Part II. Barometric hypsometry. 4°. *New York*, 1868.

———. Practical tables in meteorology and hypsometry, being the appendix to the paper

Meteorology.

on the use of the barometer on surveys and reconnaissances. 4°. *New York*, 1868.
Bound with the preceding.

WOLFART (J. H.) * De recto instrumentorum alterationibus atmosphæræ cognoscendis inservientium usu. 4°. *Hanoviæ*, 1728.

WUCHERER (J. F.) *Diss. acad. de meteoris igneis et quorundam ficta significatone: von feurigen Lufft-Geschichten. Resp. J. M. Hübschmann. 4°. *Jenæ*, [1724].

ZÜRCHER & MARGOLLÉ. Meteors, aërolites, storms, and atmospheric phenomena. From the French, by W. Lackland. 12°. *New York*, 1870.

Abstract of results of meteorological observations taken at home and foreign stations in the years 1866-83. Army M. Dep. Rep. 1866-83, Lond., 1868-85, viii-xxv. *passim.*—**Atkinson** (J. C.) On the influence of the winds and apparatus employed in meteorological observations. Lancet, Lond., 1849, i, 207; 318; 533: ii, 93.—**Avelloni** (D.) Breve saggio meteorologico intorno i tempi procellosi nell' estate ed intorno l' irregolarità delle presente stagione diviso in due lettere scritte al Vicenzo Miotti. N. rac. d' opusc. scient. et filol., Venezia, 1770, xix, 327-380. ———. Osservazioni meteorologiche ed astrifere da farsi praticamente dagli agricoltori per regolare profittevolmente le loro operazioni campestri all' Giannandrea Crestani. *Ibid.*, 1777, xxxi, 1-109.—**Bérigny.** Historique de la météorologie dans le département de Seine-et-Oise. Mém. Soc. d. sc. nat. et méd. de Seine-et-Oise 1874-82, Versailles, 1883, xii, 322-332.—**Bertherand** (A.) Sur la température *maxima* de quelques points du globe. Gaz. méd. de l'Algérie, Alger, 1873, xviii, 54.—**Blackadder** (H. H.) On the construction of meteorological instruments, so as exactly to determine their indications, during absence, at any given instant or at successive intervals of time. Tr. Roy. Soc. Edinb. (1825), 1886, x, 337-348, 1 pl.—**Blanc** (G.) Narrative of a hurricane; with some reflexions on the effect of commotion in the atmosphere and in the ocean on the economy of nature, and on life and health. *In his:* Select Dissertations, 8°, Lond., 1822, 358-379.—**Bollettino** meteorologico dell' Osservatorio di Venezia. Riassunto delle osservazioni fatte nell' anno meteorologico 1884-5. Atti r. Ist. Veneto di sc., lett. ed arti, 1885-6, 6. s., iv, pp. xcix-cviii.—**Bromby.** Law of weather and storms. Rep. Roy. Soc. Tasmania (1873), 1874, 73-78.—**Buchholtz** (A.) Ergebnisse der meteorologischen Beobachtungen. Cor.-Bl. d. Naturf.-Ver. zu Riga, 1867, xvi, 7; 13; 23; 33.—**Buys Ballot** (C.-H.-D.) Sur la marche annuelle de la température en quelques lieux d'Europe et sur la mesure de sa variabilité Arch. néerl. d. sc. exactes, etc., Harlem, 1880, xv, 75-112.—**Cantoni** (G.) Fisica sperimentale. Su due stromenti meteorologici ideati da Angelo Bellani. R. Ist. Lomb. di sc. e lett. Rendic., Milano, 1877, 2. s., x, 17-23.—**Carruccio** (A.) & **Spagnolini** (A.) Altezza, temperatura, umidità dell' atmosfera terrestre. Spallanzani, Modena, 1878, 2. s., vii, 529-539.—**Casselberry** (I.) A new theory of atmospheric temperature. Cincin. Lancet & Obs., 1860, n. s., iii, 137-145.—**Circulaire** relative aux dispositions à suivre par MM. les médecins chefs de service pour la constatation des observations météorologiques à faire dans les hôpitaux militaires. Rec. de mém. de méd. . . . mil., Par., 1864, 3. s., xi, 1-58, 1 pl.—**Collazo** (J.) Contestacion á las observaciones del D. Pablo Garcia de Mérida, sobre el método ozonométrico adoptado por el observatorio meteorológico central. Emulacion, Mérida, 1878, iii, 133-143.—**la Cour** (P.) Résumé du journal météorologique du célèbre astronome Tycho Brahe, tenu à Uraniborg, de Hveen, pendant les années 1552-97. Overs. o. d. k. Danske Vidensk. Selsk. Forh., Kjøbenh., 1876 (Résumé, etc.), 25-44.—**Denza** (F.) La météorologie en Italie. Inst. san. en Italie, Milan, 1885, 111-129.—**Desbrest.** Lettre sur le froid des hivers 1766 et 1767. J. de méd., chir., pharm., etc., Par., 1767, xxvii, 148-156.—**Dowler** (B.) Researches on meteorology. N. Orl. M. & S. J., 1847-8, iv, 411-434. *Also*, Reprint.—**Faye.** Sur la partie cosmique de la météorologie. Compt. rend. Acad. d. sc., Par., 1877, lxxxv, 247-253.—**Féris.** Contributions à la météorologie; étude sur les climats équatoriaux en général. Arch. de méd. nav., Par., 1879, xxxii, 321-347. *Also*, Reprint.—**Fleury.** Sur les différences entre les maxima et les minima de température diurnes. Rec. de mém. de méd. . . . mil., Par., 1866, 3. s., xvi, 408-411.—[**Gerhard** (J. G.)] Fernere Erläuterung des neuen Cockischen Systematis meteorologici, oder Versuch, ob aus denen von Curiosis bissher geführten Observationibus meteorologicis des Cocks meteorologische Grundsätze nicht etwas zu legitimiren seyn möchten? Samml. v. Nat.- u. Med.- . . . Gesch. 1723. Leipz. u. Budissin, 1724, xxiii. Versuch, 117-120. ———. Von der neuen, oder bissher new-erläuterten Wetter-Astrologie des Hr. W. Cocks. Samml. v. Nat.- u. Med.- . . . Gesch. 1721, Leipz. u. Budissin, 1722, xv. Versuch, 205-213.—**Gottschling** (A.) Uebersicht der Witterungserscheinungen in Hermannstadt

Meteorology.

im Jahre 1883. Verh. u. Mitth. d. siebenbürg. Ver. f. Naturw. in Hermannstadt, 1884, xxxiv, 117–135.—**Grischow** (A.) Beschreibung eines Hyetometers, und desselben sechsjährige hyetometrische Beobachtungen zu Berlin. Phys. u. med. Abhandl. d. k. Acad. d. Wissensch. zu Berl., Gotha, 1781, ii, 19–45.—**Guyot.** Directions for meteorological observations. Rep. Smithson. Inst. 1855, Wash., 1856, 215–244.—**Hasskarl** (J. K.) Meteorologische waarnemingen, gedaan op eene reis van Nederland naar Java, aan boord van het Fregatschip Ambarawa, Kapitein P. E. Karst, gedurende de maanden Junij tot September 1845. Nat.- en Geneesk. Arch. v. Neêrl. Indiê, Batav., 1846, iii, 1–12, 1 tab.—**Hogg** (J.) The importance of uniformity of well constructed instruments in meteorological research. Lancet, Lond., 1856, ii, 189–192.—**Hunt** (S. B.) A sketch of practical meteorology. Buffalo M. J., 1855–6, xi, 76–81.—**Iglesias y Pardo** (L.) Memoria sobre algunos datos atmosferonautológicos de cuatro de nuestros buques de primera clase. Confer. cient. d. Cuerpo de sanid. de la Armada, San Fernando, 1882, i, 58–64.—**King** (T. D.) The science of meteorology, its utility, the necessary instruments and how to use them. Canada M. & S. J., Montreal, 1873, i, 49–56.—**Kluge** (C.) Der Atmosphärograph. Med. Ztg., Berl., 1841, 197; 201.—**Lazerges** (P.) Observations météorologiques faites à Aragnouet (Hautes-Pyrénées) et à Toulouse. Cong. internat. d'hydrol. et de climatol. C. r. 1886, Par., 1887, i, 453–472.—**Ledesma** (J.) Meteorolojía médica; estudio hecho en la ciudad de Buenos Aires. Rev. méd. de Chile, Sant. de Chile, 1885–6, xiv, 305; 353; 401, 3 diag.—**Loewenherz** (L.) Der meteorologische Pavillon und die meteorologischen Instrumente. Ber. ü. d. allg. deutsche Ausst. a. d. Geb. d. Hyg. u. d. Rettungsw. 1882–3, Bresl., 1885, i, 118–140.—**Loomis** (E.) Contributions to meteorology, being results derived from an examination of the observations of the United States Signal Service, and from other sources. Am. J. Sc. & Arts, N. Haven, 1874–9, 3. s., viii–xviii, passim. Continued in: Am. J. Sc., N. Haven, 1880–85, 3. s., xix–xxx, passim. ———. Contributions to meteorology. Mem. Nat. Acad. Sc., Wash., 1886, iii, pt. 2, 5–66, 16 pl.—**Marguet** (J.) Observations météorologiques faites à l'Asile des aveugles de Lausanne. Tableaux mensuels. 2e semestre de l'année 1885. Bull. Soc. vaudoise d. sc. nat., Lausanne, 1886–7, xxii, 97–124.—**Marié-Davy.** Météorologie et physique du globe. Assoc. franç. pour l'avance. d. sc. Compt. - rend. 1872, Par., 1873, i, 462–482. ———. Meteorological registers. [Transl. from: J. de physique, April, 1879.] Nature, Lond., 1879, xx, 320–323.—**Meteorological** register [Edinburgh], 1731–6; [with a description of the instruments used]. Med. Essays & Obs. Soc. Edinb., 1733, i, 7: 1734, ii, 1: 1735, iii, 1: 1737, iv, 1: 1742, v, 1.—**Meteorological** tables; statement furnished by the Chief Signal Officer, U. S. A., showing the mean monthly barometer, reduced to sea-level; temperature; relative humidity; total amount of precipitation in inches and hundredths; prevailing direction of the wind, and the total wind movement, in miles, at the signal stations at Cairo, Chicago, and Springfield, Ills.; Dubuque and Keokuk, Iowa; Indianapolis, Ind.; and St. Louis, Mo., for the year 1885. Rep. Bd. Health Illinois 1885, Springfield, 1886, viii, 79–81.—**Meteorologisches** Tagebuch. In: Reise d. österr. Fregatte Novara [etc.], 4º, Wien, 1862–5, 135–499, 22 maps.—**Morris** (O. W.) Remarks on the quantity of rain at different heights. Rep. Smithson. Inst. 1855, Wash., 1856, 211–214.—**Mozzoni** (G.) Clessidra gastro-cosmica. Gazz. med. ital. lomb., Milano, 1853, 3. s., iv, 145–150.—**Nollet** (F.) Coup d'œil sur l'hygrométrie, thermo-hygromèlre et ses usages. Ann. Soc. d. sc. méd. et nat. de Brux., 1840, 190–194. [Rap. de Leroy], 194–197.—**Noyes** (I. P.) A new view of the weather question. Kansas City Rev. Sc. & Indust., 1878–9, ii, 218; 279. Also, Reprint. ———. Evidence from the weather map. Kansas City Rev. Sc. & Indust., 1879–80, iii, 589–597. Also, Reprint. ———. Tornadoes [prophecy of the weather]. Kansas City Rev. Sc. & Indust., 1880–81, iv, 208–216. Also, Reprint. ———. The storm center and weather prophets. Kansas City Rev. Sc. & Indust., 1880–81, iv, 750–755. ———. The weather map and the official weather indications. Ibid., 1881–2, v, 245–249. Also, Reprint. ———. Meteorological discoveries. Kansas City Rev. Sc. & Indust., 1884–5, viii, 196–204. Also, Reprint.—**Osborne** (J. W.) On a new meteorological instrument. Proc. Am. Ass. Adv. Sc. 1875, Salem, 1876, xxiv, 59–70. Also, Reprint.—**Pauly** (A.) Le rôle des vents dans les climats chauds. Rev. d. deux mondes, Par., 1875, 3. s., ix, 448–463.—**Percival** (T.) On the different quantities of rain which fall, at different heights, over the same spot of ground; with a letter from Benjamin Franklin. Mem. Lit. & Phil. Soc. Manchester, 1785, ii, 106–113.—**Pfaff** (H.) Meteorologische Mittheilungen. Wissensch. Mitth. d. phys.-med. Soc. zu Erlang., 1858, i, 139–164.—**Prestel** (M. A. F.) Ueber die Aenderung der Lage der Achse der thermischen Windrose in der jährlichen Periode. Amtl. Ber. ü. d. Versamml. deutsch. Naturf. u. Aerzte 1862, Karlsbad, 1863, xxvii, 188–190, 1 pl.—**Radau** (R.) Les appareils météorographiques. Monit. scient., Par., 1867, ix, 761–

Meteorology.

776.—**Reissenberger** (L.) Die Witterungserscheinungen des Jahres 1873 in Siebenbürgen. Verh. u. Mitth. d. siebenbürg. Ver. f. Naturw. in Hermannstadt, 1875, xxv, 33–88, 2 tab. ———. Uebersicht der Witterungserscheinungen in Hermannstadt in den Jahren 1879, 1880, 1881, 1882. Ib d., 1881, xxxi, 70: 1883, xxxiii, 117.—**Richardson** (J. G.) Report of the Philadelphia County Medical Society on meteorology and epidemics, for the year 1878. Tr. M. Soc. Penn., Phila., 1879, xii, pt. 2, 814–823. Also, Reprint. ———. Report of the committee on meteorology and epidemics, for the years 1881 and 1882. Tr. Coll. Phys. Phila., 1884, 3. s., vii, 41–63. — **Richter** (H. E.) Meteorologische Schriften. Schmidt's Jahrb., Leipz., 1861, cxi, 115–125. — **Ritter.** Observations météorologiques. Gaz. méd. d'Orient, Constantinople, 1873-4, xvii, 64; 160; 176.—**Roussin** (Z.) Des observations météorologiques. Gaz. méd. de l'Algérie, Alger, 1856, i, 86; 99; 115.—**Scott** (R. H.) Recent progress in weather knowledge. Fortnightly Rev., Lond., 1873, n. s., xiii, 606–617.—**Short** memoirs on meteorological subjects. Transl. by C. Abbe. Rep. Smithson. Inst. 1877, Wash., 1878, 376–478.—**Simonin** (J.-B.) père. Est-il possible de prévoir dix-neuf ans à l'avance la constitution météorologique d'une année? Mém. Acad. de Stanislas 1864, Nancy, 1865, 258–273.—**Sirks** (J.) Nog iets over de "corona" van het noorderlicht. Werk. v. h. Genootsch. t. Bevord. d. Nat.-, Genees- en Heelk. te Amst., 1871-2, ii, 1.—**Soltész** (M.) Zur Meteorologie. Ztschr. f. Nat.- u. Heilk. in Ungarn, Oedenburg, 1858, ix, 2; 9.—**Stewart** (B.) Meteorological research. Nature, Lond., 1876, xiv, 388–390. ———. On the long-period inequality in rainfall. Mem. Lit. & Phil. Soc. Manchester, 1882, 3. s., vii, 161–169. — **Tarry** (H.) Meteorologia. De la prédiction du mouvement des tempêtes et des phénomènes qui les accompagnent. R. Ist. Lomb. di sc. e lett. Rendic., Milano, 1872, 2. s., v, 719–727.—**de Tastes** (F.-M.) La météorologie synoptique et la prévision du temps. Rev. d. deux mondes, Par., 1874, ii, 852–868.—**Trautzsch** (C. F.) Die vorzüglichsten meteorologischen Merkwürdigkeiten des Jahres 1829. Beitr. z. prakt. Heilk., Leipz., 1834, i, 482–524.—**Verelst** (P.-J.) Exposé de la constitution atmosphérique pendant l'année 1844-5. Ann. Soc. de méd. prat. de la prov. d'Anvers, Boom et Malines, 1846, iv, 208–221.—**Wœikof** (A. I.) Meteorology in Russia. Rep. Smithson. Inst. 1872, Wash., 1873, 267–298. Also, Reprint. ———. Études sur l'amplitude diurne de la température et sur l'influence qu'exerce sur elle la position topographique. Bull. Soc. imp. d. nat. de Moscou, 1881, lvi, 81–140, 1 tab.

Meteorology (Medical).

See, also, Acclimation; Air (*Pressure of*); Climate; Cold; Constitutions (*Medical*); Electricity (*Atmospheric*); Fever (*Malarial, Causes of*); Fog; Forests; Heat; Insane (*Influence of night, etc., on*); Neuralgia (*Diagnosis, etc., of*); Ozone; Seasons; Topography (*Medical*); *and under names of countries and places.*

ACKERMANN (H.) Das Wetter und die Krankheiten. 8º. *Kiel,* 1854.

BALLEY (F.) Météorologie et météorographie, pathogénie et nosographie; ou éléments de recherches sur la connexion entre les divers agents météorologiques et la pathogénie civile et militaire à Rome (de 1850 à 1861). Atlas annexé aux nos. 41 et 42 du Recueil de mémoires de médecine, de chirurgie et de pharmacie militaires. 4º. *Paris,* 1863.

BELFRAGE (J.) *De viribus cœli in morbis inducendis. 8º. *Edinburgi,* 1815.

BERT (P.) La pression barométrique; recherches de physiologie expérimentale. 8º. *Paris,* 1878.

FOISSAC (P.) De la météorologie dans ses rapports avec la science de l'homme et principalement avec la médecine et l'hygiène publique. 2 v. 8º. *Paris,* 1854.

———. The same. Meteorologie mit Rücksicht auf die Lehre vom Kosmos, und in ihren Beziehungen zur Medicin und allgemeinen Gesundheitslehre. Deutsch bearbeitet und mit Anmerkungen versehen von Dr. A. H. Emsmann. 8º. *Leipzig,* 1859.

FORSTER (T.) Observations on the casual and periodical influence of particular states of the atmosphere on human health and diseases, particularly insanity. With a table of reference to authors. 8º. *London,* 1817.

Meteorology (*Medical*).

GOUIFFÉS (A.-J.-M.) *Sur l'influence des climats, et de l'atmosphère en particulier. 4°. *Paris, an XII* [1804].

GRABOWSKI (S.-A.) *I. Du baromètre considéré comme instrument d'observation clinique. II. [etc.] 4°. *Paris*, 1838.

GROSSER (G.) *Diss. sistens hominem aërometrum. sm. 4°. *Lipsiæ*, [1694].

GUILLIÉ (É.) *Rapports des maladies avec l'atmosphère. Essai sur l'application de la méthode graphique à leur étude. 4°. *Paris*, 1871.

GUINIER (H.) *Du degré d'importance des études météorologiques pour la connaissance et le traitement des maladies. 4°. *Montpellier*, 1857.

———. Ébauche d'un plan de météorologie médicale. 8°. *Paris*, 1857.

HAVILAND (A.) Climate, weather, and disease. Being a sketch of the opinions of the most celebrated ancient and modern writers with regard to the influence of climate and weather in producing disease. 8°. *London*, 1855.

HOFFMANN (F.) Observationes barometrico-meteorologicæ et epidemicæ Hallenses anni mdcc. Præmissa sunt curiosæ physicæ meditationes in corpora humana ac barometron, etc. 4°. *Halæ Magdeb.*, 1701.

———. De curiosis physicis meditationibus circa ventorum causam, vires et operationes in corpora humana ac barometra.
In his: Diss. phys.-med. [etc.] 8°. *Lugd. Bat.*, 1708, 140–218.

HOPF (C. G.) *Diss. qua instruendæ meteorologiæ medicæ consilia instituuntur. 4°. *Tubingæ*, [1790].

HUNT (S. B.) Report of the committee on the hygrometrical state of the atmosphere in various localities, and its influence on health. 8°. *Philadelphia*, 1855.

HUXHAM (J.) Observationes de aëre et morbis epidemicis, ab anno mdccxxviii ad finem anni mdccxxxvii, Plymuthi factæ. His accedit opusculum de morbo colico Damnoniensi. [v. 1.] 2. ed. 8°. *Londini*, 1752.

———. The same. v. 2. Ab anni nimirum initio 1738 ad exitum usque 1748. 8°. *Londini*, 1757.

———. The same. Observations on the air and epidemical diseases, made at Plymouth from the year mdccxxviii to the end of the year mdccxxxvii. To which is added a short treatise on the Devonshire colick. Transl. from the Latin. v. 1. 8°. *London*, 1758.

———. The same. 8°. *London*, 1759.

———. The same. From the beginning of the year 1738 to the end of the year 1748. v. 2. And now translated from the original, by his son, J. C. Huxham. 8°. *London*, 1767.

LAMPRECHT (J. A. F.) Ætiologia morborum quorundam ex superioris anni constitutione. 4°. *Lipsiæ*, [1786].

LECHAPTOIS (J.) *Sur l'ordre qu'observent les maladies, suivant la température de l'air et des saisons. 4°. *Paris*, 1806.

LEGRAS (L.-P.-J.) *De l'influence des saisons sur l'homme, et dans la production des maladies. 4°. *Paris*, 1817.

LETOURNEUX (J.-B.-P.) *De l'influence des saisons sur le physique et le moral de l'homme. 4°. *Paris*, 1819.

L[I]TT[O]N (E.) Philosophical conjectures on aereal influences, the probable origin of diseases; with an unusual cure in the scurvy. 8°. *London*, 1747.

LYKLAMA Â NYEHOLT (J. E.) *Spec. medicum inaug. ad Hippocratis aphor. v, sect. iii submittit. 4°. *Franequeræ*, 1769.

Meteorology (*Medical*).

MEISNER (J. G.) *De hyemis præter naturam tepidæ et humidæ noxis earundemque præcautionibus. 4°. *Vittenbergæ*, 1722.

OCKEL (C.) *De potentia ventorum in corpus humanum, ubi simul agitur de ascensu et descensu argenti vivi in barometro. 4°. [*Halæ Magdeb.*, 1700.]

PREDIERI (P.) Dei rapporti fra la meteorologia e la medicina, dei progressi che si desiderano e dei vantaggi che si possono attendere discorso preliminare. fol. *Bologna*, 1854.

ROYAL Meteorological Society, London. Meteorology in relation to health. Conferences by the Royal Meteorological Society. 8°. *London*, 1884.

SCALZI (F.) La meteorologia in rapporto alle febbri miasmatiche e pneumoniti nell' anno 1877. Studiate negli ospedali di S. Spirito, di S. Giovanni e nella necrologia della città di Roma. (Lavoro presentato al Congresso meteorologico di Parigi nell' agosto 1878.) roy. 8°. *Roma*, 1878.

SCHULL (P.) *De vi et effectu, quem diversæ tempestates in morbis modificandis exercent. 4°. *Lugd. Bat.*, 1789.

SOELLING (C. H.) *De meteororum actione in corpus humanum. 4°. *Jenæ*, [1746].

SWYGHUISEN (W.) *Diss. exponens magni Hippocratis aphorismum xv, sect. i. 4°. *Groningæ*, 1737.

TONNELIER (A.-D.) *Essai sur les vents. Auquel on a joint plusieurs aphorismes recueillis aux leçons de M. le prof. Corvisart. 8°. *Paris, an XII* [1804].

VIAULD (J.-B.) *Essai sur la constitution de l'hyver de l'an xi, et sur les épidémies catarrhales en général. 8°. *Paris, an XI* [1803].

VIGOUROUX (P.) *De l'influence météorologique sur les manifestations rhumatismales pendant l'hiver 1875. 4°. *Montpellier*, 1875.

WALKER (J.) An essay on the epidemic and pestilential state of the elements, and the principal phenomena of the physical world which have preceded, accompanied, and followed the failure of the potato crop; with observations deduced from the facts stated. 8°. *Ayr*, 1847.

Astegiano (G.) Saggio di meteorologia medica. Gior. di med. mil., Roma, 1883, xxxi, 129; 217; 316; 623. *Also*, Reprint.—**Atkinson** (J. C.) On the effects of different winds on the human constitution. Lancet, Lond., 1849, i, 207; 318; 533: ii, 91. ———. On the connection of meteorological phenomena with cholera, influenza, and other epidemic diseases. *Ibid.*, 1850, i, 240.—**Ballard** (E.) A study of the influence of weather and season upon public health, made upon above 217,000 cases of sickness newly occurring at various institutions for the relief of the sick poor in Islington, during the nine years 1857-65. Med.-Chir. Tr., Lond., 1866-7, l, 189, 7 tab.: 1867-8, li, 277, 1 tab.; 289, 2 tab. *Also* [Abstr.]: Proc. Roy. M. & Chir. Soc. Lond., 1864-7, v; 288: 1867-71, vi, 108. *Also, transl.*: Deutsche Vrtljschr. f. öff. Gsndhtspflg., Brnschwg., 1870, ii, 242-251. ———. On the influence of some of the more important elements of weather upon the absolute amount of sickness. Brit. M. J., Lond., 1869, i, 536-540. ———. On the study of medical meteorology, especially in its relation to epidemic maladies. Tr. Epidemiol. Soc. Lond. (1875-81), 1882, iv, 30-38.—**Baxendell** (J.) On the influence of changes in the character of the seasons upon the rate of mortality. Mem. Lit. & Phil. Soc. Manchester, 1871, 3. s., iv, 303-314.—**Berger.** Zusammenhang zwischen den plötzlichen Todesfällen und den Witterungsverhältnissen. Ztschr. f. Biol., München, 1868, iv, 376-389. *Also* [Abstr.]: Wien. med. Wchnschr., 1869, xix, 679-682.—**Bertulus.** De l'influence réelle ou propre de la chaleur, du froid et de l'humidité sur l'économie animale. Montpel. méd., 1859, ii, 223-251.—**Blasius** (W.) Some remarks on the connection of meteorology with health. Proc. Am. Phil. Soc., Phila., 1875, xiv, 667-673.—**Blodget** (L.) Report upon "non-periodic changes of heat as an element in sanitary climatology". Am. Pub. Health Ass. Rep. 1873, N. Y., 1875, i, 157-163.—**Buchan** (A.) & **Mitchell** (A.) The influence of weather on mortality from different diseases and at different ages. J. Scot. Meteor. Soc., Edinb. & Lond., 1874-5. n. s., iv, 187: 1877, v, 171. *Also* [Abstr.]: Brit. & For. M.-Chir. Rev., Lond., 1876, lviii, 85-105.—**Büchner.**

Meteorology (*Medical*).

Ideen über meteorologisch-medizinische Beobachtungen und deren Nutzen für die gerichtliche Medizin. Ztschr. f. d. Staatsarznk., Erlang., 1851, lxii, 224–230.—**Cagnazzi** (L. de S.) Nota intorno a relazioni osservate nei passato febbraio tra le variazioni barometriche e la salute degli uomini. Esculapio napol., Napoli, 1828, iii, 129–133.— **Campbell** (F. R.) The relation of meteorology to disease. Buffalo M. & S. J., 1885-6, xxv, 193–214. *Also*, Reprint.—**Casper** (J. L.) Der Einfluss der Witterung auf Gesundheit und Leben des Menschen. *In his:* Denkw. z. med. Statist., 8°, Berl., 1846, 3–78, 6 tab. *Also* [Abstr.]: Wchnschr. f. d. ges. Heilk., Berl., 1846, 373; 389.—**Chipman** (M. M.) Report of committee on medical topography, meteorology, endemics, etc.; importance of forest preservation and timber cultivation. Tr. M. Soc. Calif., Sacramento, 1883, 240–281.—**Clarus** (J. C. A.) Versuch einer vergleichenden Uebersicht der merkwürdigsten Witterungs- und Krankheitsereignisse in den Jahren 1833-4. Beitr. z. prakt. Heilk., Leipz., 1834, i, 78; 630.—**Coolidge** (R. H.) Report of the special committee on Government meteorological reports. Tr. Am. M. Ass., Phila., 1859, xii, 63–72. *Also*, Reprint.—**Corden** (G.) On some of the apparent influences of the weather upon the prevalence or otherwise of certain classes of disease. Rep. Cong. San. Inst. Gr. Brit. 1879, Lond., 1880, i, 217–223, 1 tab.—**Davis** (N. S.) *et al.* Report of the committee appointed to confer with the superintendent of the Signal Service Bureau of the U. S. Government relative to the addition of daily observations concerning the electric and ozonic conditions of the atmosphere to the items at present included in the meteorological records made at the several stations in that service; and such other matters as the committee might deem important. Tr. Am. M. Ass., Phila., 1879, xxx, 38–40. ——. Report of the special committee on ozone and other atmospheric conditions in connection with records of the prevalence of diseases, May, 1881. *Ibid.*, 1881, xxxii, 481–490. ——. Report of the standing committee on meteorological conditions and their relations to the prevalence of acute diseases. J. Am. M. Ass., Chicago, 1884, ii, 85; 169.—**Discussion** on the proposed changes in medical meteorology. Bull. N. York Acad. M., 1862, i, 125–133.—**Everett** (J. T.) Studies in relation to the production of pain by weather. Chicago M. J. & Exam., 1879, xxxviii, 253–260. *Also*, Reprint.— **Faulds** (W.) Effects of meteorological influence on health. Tr. M. Soc. N. Y., Albany, 1868, 142–182, 1 ch.— **Fischer.** Das Jahr 1819, meteorologisch-medicinisch dargestellt. J. d. pract. Heilk., Berl., 1825, lxi, 5. St., 74; 6. St., 52: 1826, lxiii, 4. St., 49.—**Forry** (S.) Statistical researches relative to the etiology of pulmonary and rheumatic diseases, illustating the application of the laws of climate to the science of medicine; based on the records of the Medical Department and Adjutant-General's Office. Am. J. M. Sc., Phila., 1841, n. s., i, 13–54.—**Foubert** (H.) État de la météorologie médicale en France dans ses rapports avec la médecine. Arch. gén. de méd., Par., 1866, 6. s., vii, 578; 707. *Also*, Reprint.—**Gaye** (H.) La médecine et la météorologie. Pau méd., 1877, i, 3; 12.—**Gillebert-d'Hercourt.** De l'utilité des observations météorologiques pour la médecine. Ann. Soc. de méd. de Lyon, 1863, 3. s., xi, 295–304. ——. Plan d'études simultanées de météorologie et de statistique médicale proposé à la Société de médecine de Saint-Étienne et de la Loire. Ann. Soc. de méd. de St.-Étienne et de la Loire. Compt.-rend. (1866), 1867, iii, 522–528.—[**Grellois.**] Cours de météorologie professé dans le grand amphithéátre de la Faculté de médecine. Union méd., Par., 1864, 2. s., xxi, 305–311.—**Günther.** Ueber den Gang der Witterung und die Krankheitsconstitution zu Cöln in den Jahren 1823-9. Med.-chir. Ztg., Innsbr., 1824, i, 189: 1825, i, 205; 220: 1826, i, 379: 1827, i, 285; 300: 1828, i, 252; 286: 1829, i, 268; 282: 1830, i, 108; 126.—**Guerry** (A.) Des variations météorologiques comparées aux phénomènes physiologiques. Ann. d'hyg., Par., 1829, i, 228–234.—**Guy** (W. A.) On temperature and its relation to mortality. J. Statist. Soc. Lond., 1881, xliv, 235–262. [Discussion], 262–268. *Also* [Abstr.]: Med. Press & Circ., Lond., 1881, n. s., xxxi, 286; 310; 332. — **Guyot** (J.) Influence de la température de l'air et des instrumens dans les opérations chirurgicales. Ann. de la méd. physiol., Par., 1831, xix, 326–341.—**Harless** (C. F.) Die Meteorologie, in ihrer Anwendung auf die Medicin, und insbesondere auf die Krankheits-Constitutionen und herrschenden wie durchlaufenden Krankheiten; und was ihr Noth thut. Ein historisch-nosologischer Versuch. J. d. pract. Heilk., Berl., 1836, lxxxiii, 1. St., 8; 2. St., 3.— **Haviland** (A.) The iatro-meteorology of Hippocrates. Assoc. M. J., Lond., 1853, 961–964.—**Hewson** (A.) On the influence of the weather over the results of surgical operations, and on the value of the barometer as a guide in the choice of the time for and the prognosis in such operations, as shown by the results of "immediate amputations" during a period of 30 years in the Pennsylvania Hospital. Penn. Hosp. Rep., Phila., 1869, ii, 17–35, 1 ch.— **Hildreth** (E. A.) Synopsis of observations on some of the relations of meteorology and disease. Tr. M. Soc. W. Virg., Wheeling, 1879. 520: 1880, 631: 1882, 783. *Also*, Reprint. of 1879 and 1882.—**Hingeston** (J. A.) The meteorology

Meteorology (*Medical*).

of 1854-8. Assoc. M. J., Lond., 1855, i, 151: 1856, i, 66. *Continued in:* Brit. M. J., Lond., 1858, 85; 163: 1859, 224.— **Hoffmann** (F.) De ventorum generatione ortu, causis ac effectu in corpora humana, et barometron, etc. *In his:* Opusc. theol.-phys.-med., 4°, Halæ, 1740, 169–218.—**Hoppe** (I.) Ueber den Einfluss der Witterung auf die Besserung und Verschlimmerung der Krankheiten, im Gegensatze zu dem Einflusse der angewendeten Arzneien. Memorabilien, Heilbr., 1875, xx, 390–398. — **Hug** (C.) Ueber die Meteorologie als Wissenschaft für den Arzt. Aerztl. Mitth. a. Baden, Karlsruhe, 1866, xx, 65–72.—**Jameson** (H. G.) Diarian observations upon the weather, the seasons, and the diseases of certain seasons. Maryland M. Recorder, Balt., 1829, i, 632–656. — **Ker** (P.) A comparison of the meteorological registers and epidemic diseases at Edinburgh, Rippon, Plymouth, and Nuremberg, from May, 1731, to June, 1736. Med. Essays & Obs. Soc. Edinb., 1742, v, 35–82.—**King** (T.) Notes on meteorology and health. Canada M. & S. J., Montreal, 1873, i, 495–499. —**Ledesma** (J.) Meteorolojía médica; estudio aplicado á la ciudad de Buenos Aires. An. d. Circ. méd. argent., Buenos Aires, 1885, viii, 360; 409. — **Lépine** (R.) De l'influence de la pression barométrique sur les phénomènes vitaux. Gaz. méd. de Par., 1874, 4. s., iii, 285.— **Levy.** Witterung und Krankheiten. Med. Ztg., Berl., 1849, 13; 17.—**von Liebig** (G.) Ueber die Einflüsse der Temperatur und Feuchtigkeit auf die Gesundheit. Berl. klin. Wchnschr., 1870, vii, 245; 256.—**Littel** (S.) On the influence of electrical fluctuations as a cause of disease. N. Am. M.-Chir. Rev., Phila., 1857, i, 390–409. *Also*, Reprint. ——. On the relations which electricity sustains to the causes of disease. Tr. Am. M. Ass., Phila., 1866, xvii, 73–126. *Also*, Reprint.—**Löschner.** Ueber den Einfluss der meteorischen Verhältnisse auf die Entstehung der Kinderkrankheiten. J. f. Kinderkr., Erlang., 1856, xxvii, 7–20.—**Macintyre** (W.) The weather and the more prevalent diseases of the summer of 1846. Lancet, Lond., 1847, i, 85; 111.—**Menges** (P.) Der Einfluss der Witterung in den drei nasskalten Jahren 1829 bis 1831 und in den drei trockenwarmen Jahren 1857-9 auf den allgemeinen Gesundheitszustand in Nassau. Med. Jahrb. f. d. Herzogth. Nassau, Wiesb., 1863, xix-xx, 348–714.—**Meteorologie** (Die) als Hülfswissenschaft zur Medicin. Deutsche Klinik, Berl., 1853, v, 374; 384.—**Minor** (T. C.) Notes on the meteorological medicine of Cincinnati. Cincin. Lancet & Clinic, 1884, n. s., xiii, 544; 562; 630.—**Mitchell** (S. W.) The relations of pain to weather, being a study of the natural history of a case of traumatic neuralgia. Am. J. M. Sc., Phila., 1877, n. s., lxxiii, 305–329. *Also* [continuation of record], *in:* Tr. Coll. Phys. Phila., 1883, 3. s., vi, 411–427, 3 ch. *Also:* Med. News, Phila., 1883, xliii, 46–49.—**Moffat** (T.) On medical meteorology. Assoc. M. J., Lond., 1853, 129.—**Moore** (J. W.) Notes on "mean temperature in its relations to disease and mortality", with special reference to the city of Dublin. Dublin Q. J. M. Sc., 1869, xlviii, 107–122. *Also*, Reprint. ——. On meteorology in its bearing on health and disease. *In:* Lect. on Pub. Health, 8°, Dubl., 1874, 32–61, 5 ch. *Also* [Abstr.]: Lond. M. Rec., 1873, i, 211; 226. *Also* [Abstr.]: Brit. M. J., Lond. 1873, i, 400–402. *Also*, Reprint.—**Morris** (J.) New method of investigating the effect of meteorological changes and conditions on human life. Med. Times & Gaz., Lond., 1857, xv, 57–59.—**Müller** (G.) Ueber die Wirkungen der verschiedenen Luftströmungen (Winde) auf die verschiedenen Organismen. Ztschr. d. deutsch. Chir.-Ver., Magdeb., 1850, iv, 361–366.—**Nieuwenhuis** (C. J.) Geneeskundige waarnemingen, vergeleken met weerkundige aanteekeningen gedurende het jaar 1812. Ἱπποκράτης, Rotterd., 1814, i, 103: 1816, ii, 14; 117; 340.— **Paroniants** (S.) Po voprosu meditsinskoĭ meteorologii. Med. Sbornik, Tiflis, 1867, iii, pt. 3, 1–9.—**Pendleton** (E. M.) Meteorology as a collateral science to the study of medicine. Atlanta M. & S. J., 1857-8, iii, 321–327. — **Pérez** (L.) Utilidad de las observaciones meteorológicas en la práctica de la medicina. Repert. Jalisc. de med. y cirug. práct., Guadalajara, 1874, i, 2-4.—**Pope** (J. H.) Climatology and epidemics. Tr. Texas M. Ass., Columbus, 1875, vii, 72–79.—**Prestel** (M. A. F.) Die Winde in ihrer Beziehung zur Salubrität und Morbilität. Ein Beitrag zur medizinischen Witterungs- und Klimakunde. Kl. Schrift. d. naturf. Gesellsch. zu Emden, 1872, xvi, 1–19. — **Ransome** (A.) & **Vernon** (G. V.) On the influence of atmospheric changes upon disease. Mem. Lit. & Phil. Soc. Manchester, Lond., 1862, 3. s., i, 164–185.— **Renauldin.** Météorologie et météores. Dict. d. sc. méd., Par., 1819, xxxiii, 122–228.—**Renou** & **Chereau** (A.) Météorologie. Dict. encycl. d. sc. méd., Par., 1873, 2. s., vii, 311–339.—**Reoch** (J.) Monthly prevalence of diseases. Lancet, Lond., 1873, ii, 225. — **Reuss.** Ueber den Einfluss einer herrschenden Luft- und Witterungsbeschaffenheit auf das Entstehen, Vorbereiten und Erlöschen der Volkskrankheiten, vorzüglich auf den allgemeinen Karakter der zu gleicher Zeit herrschenden Entzündungen und Fieber überhaupt und graduelle-entzündliche oder nervöse und pestartige Beschaffenheit der auf eine zufällige Art durch eine spezifische Anstekkung ausgekommenen exanthematischen Fieber insbe-

Meteorology (*Medical*).

sondere. J. d. pract. Heilk., Berl., 1817, xlv, 2. St., 3–105.—**Richardson** (B. W.) Lecture on meteorological readings in relation to surgical practice. Med. Times & Gaz., Lond., 1870, i, 115; 141; 174.—**Richter** (H. E.) Bericht über medicinische Meteorologie und Klimatologie. Schmidt's Jahrb., Leipz., 1874, clxiii, 65–118.—**Rossi** (F.) Osservazioni raccolte sopra tre costituzioni atmosferiche morbose durante il corso della carriera pratica. [3 cases.] Ann. univ. di med., Milano, 1867, cci, 53; 346.—**Roth.** Ueber den Einfluss der athmosphärischen Verhältnisse während der Jahre 1835–1839 (incl.), auf das Befinden der Menschen im Fürstenthum Lübeck und über die kritische Tendenz der durch den gen. epidemicus erzeugten Krankheiten. Mitth. a. d. Geb. d. Med., etc., Altona, 1840–41, viii, 5.–6. Hft., 1–14.—**Schneider.** Ueber meteorologische Beobachtungen und deren Anwendung in der Heilkunde. Allg. med. Ann., Altenb., 1811, pt. 2, 289; 481; 865: 1812, 97; 961; 1109: 1814, 793.—**Schreiber** (J.) Ueber die Stellung der Meteorologie in der Medicin. Oesterr. Ztschr. f. prakt. Heilk., Wien, 1871, xvii, 285; 301. ——. Meteorology in the service of medicine. An address delivered before the Austrian Meteorological Society. [*Transl. from:* Oesterr. Ztschr. f. Meteorol.] Richmond & Louisville M. J., Louisville, 1878, xxv, 126–135. *Also,* Reprint.—**Serrurier.** Remarques et faits relatifs à l'influence de la constitution atmosphérique sur le moral. J. de méd., chir., pharm., etc., Par., 1817, xl, 3–19.—**Société** de médecine de St.-Étienne et de la Loire. Ville de St.-Étienne. Tableau graphique indiquant les corrélations constatées entre le nombre des décès et les principales circonstances météorologiques de chaque jour pendant l'année 1882–3. Loire méd., St.-Étienne, 1883, ii, 1 tab. op. 56 : 1884, iii, 1 tab. op. 80.—**Sormani** (G.) L' età, la professione, il sesso, e la pressione barometrica nella mortalità per apoplessia, e per le altre affezioni endocraniche. Gior. di med. mil., Firenze, 1871, xix, 1–22.—**Tripe** (J. W.) An inaugural address on some of the relations of meteorological phenomena to man, delivered before the Society of Medical Officers of Health, October, 1882. Tr. Soc. M. Off. Health, Lond., 1882–3, 9–28. *Also:* San. Rec., Lond., 1882–3, n. s., iv, 197 ; 250. *Also :* Med. Times & Gaz., Lond., 1882, ii, 545–550. *Also,* Reprint.—**Weather** and mortality. [Edit.] Med. Times & Gaz., Lond., 1879, i, 93.—**Webster** (J.) The influence of weather on disease, and on the human frame. Lancet, Lond., 1859, i, 588.—**Weiglein.** Ueber Witterungs- und Jahreskrankheiten. Med. Jahrb. d. k. k. österr. Staates, Wien, 1845, i, 1 ; 139.—**Welcker** (F. G.) Einfluss der Luft und der Winde. Lit. Ann. d. ges. Heilk., Berl., 1832, xxiii, 146–154.—**Wiesing.** Die Witterungsverhältnisse des Jahres 1875. Cor.-Bl. d. allg. ärztl. Ver. v. Thüringen, Leipz., 1876, v, 289 : 1877, vi, 60 ; 116 ; 152. — **Witterungs-Kranckheiten** (Von), Ju. 1717–Ju. 1725. Samml. v. Nat.- u. Med.- . . . Gesch., Bresslau, Leipz., u. Budissin, 1718–26, i–xxxii, *passim.*—**Zimmermann** (K. G.) Ueber die Ursachen und den Zusammenhang der Witterungsphänomene, besonders rücksichtlich des Einflusses derselben auf das Häufigkeitsverhältniss der Krankheiten, und vorzüglich mit Bezug auf die Jahre 1844 und 1845. Ztschr. f. d. ges. Med., Hamb., 1846, xxxiii, 1–25, 1 tab.

Meteorology (*Observations and records of*).

See under names of countries and places.

Meteorology in relation to health. *See* **Royal** Meteorological Society.

Metford (Ellis Button). * De colica. 1 p. l., 34 pp. 8°. *Edinburgi, Balfour et Smellie,* 1777. [*Also, in :* P., v. 653.]

Metford (Gulielmus). * De febri puerperarum. 3 p. l., 50 pp. 8°. *Edinburgi, C. Stewart,* 1813. [P., v. 734; 863.]

Methæmoglobin.

See Hæmoglobin.

Methane.

Herter (E.) Ueber die physiologische Wirkung des Methan. Cong. périod. internat. d. sc. méd. Compt.-rend. 1884, Copenh., 1886, i, Sect. de physiol., 77–80.

Methe (Joh. Henr.) * De urinarum natura ac diversitate. 32 pp., 6 l. 4°. *Marburgi Cattorum, typ. P. C. Mülleri,* [1727].

de la Metherie (Jean-Claude) [1743–1817]. Vues physiologiques sur l'organisation animale et végétale. xxiv, 407 pp. 12°. *Amsterdam,* 1780.

Method.

See Graphic *method*; Hypodermic *injection, etc.*; Subcutaneous *surgery.*

Method of chymical nomenclature, proposed by Messrs. de Morveau, Lavoisier, Bertholet, and

Method of chymical nomenclature, [etc.]—cont. [Antoine François] de Fourcroy, to which is added, a new system of chymical characters, adapted to the nomenclature. By Messrs. Hassenfratz and Adet. Translated from the French, and the new chymical names adapted to the genius of the English language, by James St. John. xvi, 237 pp., 3 tab., 4 pl. 8°. *London, G. Kearsley,* 1788.

Method (On a) of cooling the air of rooms in tropical climates. 4 pp. 4° [*London,* 1849, *vel subseq.*]

Method (The) of practice in the small-pox. *See* **Williams** (Nathaniel).

Méthode agréable et facile, pour avoir des fruicts ès jardins, des herbages, racines, raisins, vins, chairs et bouïllons qui purgeront doucement et bénignement le corps, et par le moyen desquels on pourra donner remède à plusieurs maladies, sans peine et sans aucun dégoust. 78 pp. 16°. *Troyes, N. Oudot,* 1646.
Bound with : GUIBERT (Philbert). Le médecin charitable, etc. 16°. *Troyes,* 1645.

Méthode aisée pour conserver sa santé jusqu'à une extrême vieillesse, fondée sur les lois de l'œconomie animale, et les observations pratiques des meilleurs médecins, tant anciens que modernes. Trad. de l'anglois par M. L. de Préville. 3 p. l., viii, 509 pp., 2 l. 16°. *Paris, Prault jeune,* 1752.

Méthode asseurée et efficace pour guérir la maladie vénérienne sans salivation mercurielle. Composée en latin par un célèbre médecin d'Angleterre, et nouvellement mise en françois par le Sr. G. B. De S. Romain. 11 p. l., 128 pp. 16°. *Paris, L. d'Houry,* 1690.

Méthode (De la) en médecine, à propos du discours que M. Broussais a lu à l'Institut. [Par un interne des hôpitaux de Paris.] 8 pp. 8°. *Paris, H. Tilliard,* [*n. d.*] [*Also, in :* P., v. 1656.]

Méthode que l'on pratique à l'Hostel des Invalides pour guérir les soldats de la vérolle. 14 pp. 8°. *Paris, F. Muguet,* 1685.

Méthode à l'usage des malades pour l'emploi des différentes préparations des huiles pyrogénées animales. 4 pp. 8°. [*Paris*], *Baudouin & Cie.,* 1808. [P., v. 1746.]

Methodism.

SCHUBERT (J. S.) De laxitatis caussis disserit. 4°. *Lipsiæ,* [1772].
Dezeimeris (E.) Des principes du méthodisme, considérés comme source de la doctrine physiologique. J. compl. du dict. d. sc. méd., Par., 1824, xx, 3: 1825, xxi, 80.

Methodist Episcopal Hospital, Brooklyn, N. Y. General instructions for the guidance of architects in preparing designs for the . . . 7 pp. 8°. [*Brooklyn*], 1881.

Methodist General Hospital, Brooklyn, N. Y. Its origin, purposes, needs. 33 pp., 1 pl., 3 plans. roy. 8°. [*Brooklyn*], 1885.

Methodo de restituir a vida a's pessoas apparentemente mortas por affogamento ou suffocação; recommendado pela Sociedade humana de Londres; e descripção e figura do respirador de Mudge, cirurgião em Plymouth; com a maneira de usar delle, e hum summario dos seus effeitos nas tosses catarraes recentes, e noutros achaques do bofe; publicado tudo impresso por ordem do senhor Diogo Ignacio de Pina Manique. 31 pp., 1 pl. 12°. *Lisboa, typog. Nunesiana,* 1790. [P., v. 1258.]

Methodus curandorum morborum mathematica: qua morborum depellendorum ex astrorum concordanti influxu ratio certa et evidens ostenditur. Cui et locorum hylegialium, et thematum cœlestium structura adjecta. Nunc primum publici juris facta. 3 p. l., 54 pp. 8°. *Francofurti, excud. W. Richterus,* 1613.

Methomania.

See Dipsomania.

Methyl.

KLEEMANN (S.) * Ueber zwei Synthesen der Methyläthylalphaamidoessigsäure. 8°. München, 1883.

PANAJOTOW (G.) * Ueber Ortho-para-Dimethylchinaldin, dessen Umwandlungen, und über Ortho - para - Dimethylchinolin - a - Acrylsäure. [Erlangen.] 8°. München, 1886.

REGULATIONS for the preparation and sale of methylated spirit, issued by order of the commissioners of iuland revenue. 8°. London, 1855.

RICHARDSON (B. W.) Report on the physiological action of the methyl and allied series. 8°. London, [1869].

Cutting from: Rep. Brit. Ass. Adv. Sc., Lond., 1869, 405-421.

Also [Abstr.], in: Med. Times & Gaz., Lond., 1869, ii, 259

Debove (M.) De l'emploi du chlorure de méthyle. Bull. et mém. Soc. méd. d. hôp. de Par., 1887, 3. s., iv, 186-188. — Dubois (R.) & Roux (L.) Sur l'action anesthésique du méthylchloroforme. Compt. rend. Acad. d. sc., Par., 1887, civ, 1549-1551.—Hehner (O.) On the estimation of methylalcohol in presence of ethyalcohol. Analyst, Lond., 1887, xii, 25-29. — d'Ivors (C.) Chlorure de méthyle. N. dict. de méd. et chir. prat., Par., 1886, xl, 145-149.—Macfarlan (J. F.) On the methylated spirit, and some of its preparations. Pharm. J. & Tr., Lond., 1855-6, xv, 310-315. Also, Reprint. — Richardson (B. W.) Methylethyl ether. Asclepiad, Lond., 1886, iii. 361.—Shapiroff (B. M.) K izuchen. phiziol. deistvija tretich alkogol. na jivot. organ. [Physiological action of trimethylic alcohol in human organization.] Vrach, St. Petersb., 1887, viii, 388.—Traversa (G.) Sull' azione fisiologica e terapeutica del fenil-metil-carbonile. Gior. internaz. d. sc. med., Napoli, 1886, n. s., viii, 699; 799.

Methyl (Chloride of).

See, also, Neuralgia (Treatment of).

de Launay (H.) Deux observations relatives à l'emploi du chlorure de méthyle. Ann. méd.-chir. franç. et étrang., Par., 1885, i, 63-65. — Nussbaum. Methyl-Bichlorid mit Chloroform verglichen. Allg. Wien. med. Ztg., 1867, xii, 405.—Regnauld (J.) & Villejean. Études sur l'inhalation du formène et du formène monochloré (chlorure de méthyle). Compt. rend. Acad. d. sc., Par., 1885, c, 1024-1027. ———. Recherches sur les propriétés anesthésiques du formène et de ses dérivés chlorés. Bull. gén. de thérap., etc., Par., 1886, cx, 433; 490.—Tenneson & Bègue. Sur le chlorure de méthyle contre l'élément douleur dans des affections diverses. Bull. et mém. Soc. méd. d. hôp. de Par., 1885, 3. s., ii, 66-77. Also: Gaz. hebd. de méd., Par., 1885, 2. s., xxii, 155-157. — Vignard (E.) De l'emploi du chlorure de méthyle dans un certain nombre d'affections douloureuses. Gaz. méd. de Nantes, 1884-5, iii, 133; 137 [151].

Methyl (Iodide of).

KIRK (R.) On the vesicating properties of methyl iodide. Lancet, Lond., 1885, ii, 753-755.—Richardson (B. W.) Methyl iodide. Asclepiad, Lond., 1885, ii, 62.—Schwerin. Ueber Methylenjodid; ein Beitrag zur Kenntniss der Jodverbindungen. Centralbl. f. d. med. Wissensch., Berl., 1884, xxii, 130; 146. — Turnbull (J.) On iodide of methyle and therapeutical researches. Brit. M. J., Lond., 1869, i, 554.

Methyl (Salicylate of).

Rabuteau. Recherches sur les propriétés physiologiques et le mode d'élimination du salicylate de méthyle (essence de Gaultheria procumbens); action de cet éther sur la germination. Compt. rend. Soc. de biol., Par., 1885, 8. s., ii, pt. 2, 95-100.

Methylal.

Éloy (C.) Un nouvel hypnotique, le méthylal; ses propriétés physiologiques et ses usages thérapeutiques. Union méd., Par., 1887, 3. s., xliii, 100. — Lemoine (G.) Le méthylal, ses propriétés physiologiques et thérapeutiques. Gaz. méd. de Par., 1887, 7. s., iv, 205-208.—Mairet (A.) & Combemale. Recherches sur l'action physiologique et thérapeutique du méthylal. Montpel. méd., 1887, 2. s., viii, 495: ix, 67. Also: Progrès méd., Par., 1887, 2. s., vi, 3-8. Also [Abstr.]: Compt. rend. Acad. d. sc., Par., 1887, civ, 219; 1022. — Motrochin (M.) K vopr. o fiziol. deistvii metilala. [On physiological effect of methylal.] Sborn. rabot. proizved. lab. Anrepa, Charkoff, 1886-7, ii, 216-265. — Nicot (A.) Étude chimique et physiologique du méthylal. Nouv. remèdes, Par., 1886, ii, 458-461. — Personali (S.) Sull' azione fisiologica del metilal e sul suo potere ipnotico. Gior. d. r. Accad. di med. di Torino, 1886, 3. s., xxxiv, 293-310.

Methylamine.

See, also, Trimethylamine.

ROMENY (J.) * Over het methyleenmethylamine. [Leyden.] 8°. Amsterdam, 1878.

Behier. On acetate of methylamine. Practitioner, Lond., 1868, i, 207-210.—Œchsner de Coninck. De la recherche des alcaloïdes dans les méthylamines du commerce et dans les pétroles bruts. Compt. rend. Soc. de biol., Par., 1885, 8. s., ii, 359.

Methylaniline.

Jolyet (F.) & Cahours (A.) Sur l'action physiologique de la méthylaniline, de l'éthylaniline, de l'amylaniline comparée à celle de l'aniline. Compt. rend. Acad. d. sc., Par., 1868, lxvi, 1131.

Methylene, methyl-chloroform, etc.

MARSHALL (P.) Experiences with the bichloride of methylene. 8°. London, 1868.

MILLET (J.-E.) * Du bichlorure de méthylène comme agent anesthésique général. 4°. Strasbourg, 1868.

VILLEJEAN (E.-G.) * Recherches expérimentales sur les propriétés chimiques et physiologiques du chlorure de méthylène. 4°. Paris, 1886.

Brookhouse (J. O.) Methylene ether as an anæsthetic. Brit. M. J., Lond., i, 343.—Burroughs (J. E. B.) Note on the use of methyl-ethylic ether as an an æsthetic. Ibid., 1870, i, 515.—Dawson (B. F.) The use and comparative merits of the bichloride of methylene as an anæsthetic. Med. Rec., N. Y., 1874, ix, 252-255. — [Doctor Richardson's new anæsthetic, the methylic ether.] Tr. Odont. Soc. Gr. Brit., Lond., 1869-70, n. s., ii, 187-190.—Fayrer (J.) On the bichloride of methylene as an anæsthetic. Indian M. Gaz., Calcutta, 1868, iii, 275.—Hollaender (L.) Bichloride of methylene. Berl. klin. Wehnschr., 1867, iv, 519.—Jones (H. M.) Remarks on bichloride of methylene as an anæsthetic. Med. Press & Circ., Lond., 1873, xvi, 227.—Junker (F. E.) On a new apparatus for the administration of narcotic vapours, and some observations on the variations of pulse and respiration during the anæsthesia from bichloride of methylene (chloromethyl). St. Andrew's M. Grad. Ass. Tr. 1867, Lond., 1868, i, 213-220. ———. Bichloride of methylene before the Academy of Medicine of Paris. Brit. M. J., Lond., 1884, i, 430-452.—Kirk (R.) Remarks on bichloride of methylene. Ibid., 1883, ii, 1233.—Le Fort (L.) Sur le bichlorure de méthylène comme anesthésique. Bull. Acad. de méd., Par., 1856, 2. s., xv, 171-175.—McIntyre (J. H.) Bichloride of methylene used in a Junker's inhaler. St. Louis M. & S. J., 1883, xlv, 306-311. — Miall (P.) On bichloride of methylene; an account of one hundred cases of its use as an anæsthetic. Brit. M. J., Lond., 1870, i, 6.—Minkevich. Dvukhlorisuii methilen. [Bichloride of methylene.] Med. Sbornik, Tiflis, 1869, No. vi, pt. 2, 101-114.—Morisani (D.) & Bianchi (L.) Sull' anestesia per il bicloruro di metilene. Movimento, Napoli, 1878, x, 447; 465.—Moxey (D. A.) Inhalation of bichloride of methylene. Edinb. M. J., 1868, xiv. 323-325.—Nussbaum. Methyl-Bichlorid mit Chloroform verglichen. Aerztl. Int.-Bl., München, 1867, xiv, 690.—Panhoff (W.) Ueber die physiologischen Wirkungen des Methylenchlorids. Arch. f. Physiol., Leipz., 1881, 419-436.—Regnauld (J.) & Villejean. Études sur l'inhalation du formène bichloré (chlorure de méthylène) et du formène tétrachloré (perchlorure du carbon). Compt. rend. Acad. d. sc., Par., 1885, c, 1146-1148.—Rendle (R.) The bichloride of methylene. Brit. M. J., Lond., 1869, ii, 359. ———. On the use of protoxide of nitrogen gas; and on a new mode of producing rapid anæsthesia with bichloride of methylene. Ibid., 412.—Richardson (B. W.) On bichloride of methylene as a general anæsthetic. Med. Times & Gaz., Lond., 1867, ii, 423; 479. ———. On bichloride of methylene. Brit. M. J., Lond., 1869, ii, 487. ———. Methyl-ethylic ether: a new compound for the production of rapid general anæsthesia for short operations. Med. Press & Circ., Lond., 1870, n. s., ix, 245. ———. Methylene ether. Med. Times & Gaz., Lond., 1872, ii, 564. ———. On methylene ether or ethyl. Ibid., 1873, i, 164.—Rossi (P.) Risultamenti ottenuti nella scuola di chirurgia della R. Università di Padova col bicloruro di metilene, quale anestetico generale. Gazz. med. ital., prov. venete, Padova, 1871, xiv, 237-240.—Schmidt (C.) Das Methylenbichlorid als Anæstheticum. Aerztl. Mitth. a. Baden, Karlsruhe, 1873, xxvii, 179-181. — Tait (L.) Methylene ether as an anæsthetic. Brit. M. J., Lond., 1873, i, 254.—Tauber (E.) Ueber zwei neue Anæsthetica. I. Monochloræthylidenchlorid (Methylchloroform). Wien. med. Bl., 1880, iii, 1093-1095. Also: Centralbl. f. d. med. Wissensch., Berl., 1880, xviii, 775-778. Also: Allg. med. Centr.-Ztg., Berl., 1880, xlix, 1021-1023. ———. Ueber zwei neue Anæsthetica. II. Monochloræthylenchlorid, CH²Cl-CHCl². Wien. med. Bl., 1880, iii, 1095. Also: Centralbl. f. d. med. Wissensch., Berl., 1880, xviii, 778. Also: Allg.

Methylene, *methyl-chloroform, etc.*

med. Centr.-Ztg., Berl., 1880, xlix, 1023. — **Taylor** (B.) Case of apparent death from the inhalation of bichloride of methylene. and resuscitation. Lancet, Lond., 1876, ii, 462.—**Tourdes** (G.) & **Hepp.** Essai d'un nouvel anesthésique, le bichlorure de méthylène. Mém. Soc. de méd. de Strasb., 1867, vi, 216–231. *Also:* Gaz. méd. de Strasb., 1868, xxviii, 25–30. *Also:* Gaz. hebd. de méd., Par., 1868, 2. s., v, 115; 129.—**Wells** (T. S.) Bichloride of methylene (chloro-methyl) in general surgery. Lancet, Lond., 1871, i, 591.

Methylene (*Death from*).

Breisky. Rechtsseitige Parovarialcyste mit Achsendrehung des Stieles; Tod an Synkope während der Narkose mit sogenanntem Methylenbichlorid. Prag. med. Wchnschr., 1883, viii, 209–211.—**Burroughs** (J. E. B.) Death from bichloride of methylene. Brit. M. J., Lond., 1870, i, 460.—**Death** from bichloride of methylene. *Ibid.*, 1884, ii, 975 — **Death** from bichloride of methylene. Med. Press & Circ., Lond., 1872, n. s., xiv, 327.—**Junker** (F.) Remarks on death from methylene and on the use of other anæsthetics. Brit. M. J., Lond., 1883, ii, 104–107.— **Marshall** (P.) Death from bichloride of methylene. *Ibid.*, 1869, ii, 436. *Also:* Med. Times & Gaz., Lond., 1869, ii, 524. *Also:* Lancet, Lond., 1869, ii, 582.—**de Morgan** (C.) Death during the administration of bichloride of methylene. Brit. M. J., Lond., 1872, ii, 441.—**Richardson** (B. W.) Death from methylene. Asclepiad, Lond., 1885, ii, 58–61.—**Tait** (L.) Death under the administration of methylene ether. Med. Times & Gaz., Lond., 1873, ii, 3.— **Walser.** Ein Todesfall durch Methylenbichlorid. Mitth. d. Ver. d. Aerzte in Steiermark 1876–7, Graz, 1878, 62–66.

Methylkyanethine.

Walton (G. L.) The physiological action of methyl-kyanethine. J. Physiol., Lond., 1880–82, iii, 349–356. *Also:* Arch. f. exper. Path. u. Pharmakol., Leipz., 1881–2, xv, 419–426.

Methylstrychnine.

Faure (J.) *Pharmacologische Studien über schwefelsaures Methylstrychnin. 8°. *Dorpat*, 1880.

Schroff (C. D.) Vorläufige Mittheilung über die Einwirkung des salpetersauren Methylstrychnin auf den lebenden Organismus. Wchnbl. d. k. k. Gesellsch. d. Aerzte in Wien, 1866, xxii, 157–162.

Metidja.

Quesnoy. Topographie médicale de la plaine de la Métidja (Algérie). Rec. de mém. de méd. . . . . mil., Par., 1865, 3. s., xvi, 97; 216; 318.—**Villatte.** Topographie médicale de la Métidja. *Ibid.*, 1842, liii, 125–167.

Metis.

See **Hybridity.**

Metius (Gottlieb). *De construendo sceleto.

52 pp., 2 l. 4°. *Erfurti, lit. J. C. Heringi*, [1736].

Also, in: HALLER. Disp. anat. select. [etc.] 4°. *Gottingæ*, 1751, vi, 45–85.

Metivier (François-Alexis). * Sur la pleurésie.

32 pp. 8°. *Paris, an XI* [1803], v. 28.

Métivier (Louis-Auguste). *Aperçu sur la nature de la fièvre puerpérale. 30 pp. 4°. *Paris*, 1860, No. 114.

Métivier (Mathurin). * Sur l'hygiène des femmes enceintes. 37 pp. 4°. *Paris*, 1836, No. 214, v. 300.

Métivier (Théophile-Dieudonné). * Du croup.

66 pp. 4°. *Paris*, 1860, No. 82.

Metlinger (Bartholomæus). [Regiment der jungen Kinder.] [*Incipit:*] Wann nach Ansehung götlicher und menschlicher Ordenung unnd Gesaczt ein jeglich Vatter und Müter [etc.] [*In fine:*] Damit sich das vierd Capitel endet, und dardurch dises Büchlin. Dar von Got dem almechtigen Er würd und Lob gesagt sey, und seiner werden Müter der jungfrawen Marie. Geschehen, als man zalt nach Christi Geburt tauset vierhundert und in den lxxiii. Jar, an dem achten den Tag Sant Endris des zwölff Boten. 28 l. fol. [*Augsburg*, 1473.]

Metman (M. L.) Wetgeving op de krankzinnigen, bevattende: 1°. De Fransche wet van 30 Junij 1838, sur les aliénés, met de daarover bij de wetgevende Kamers gehouden discussiën;

Metman (M. L.)—continued.

benevens de Ordonnance du Roi, van 18 December 1839, relative aux établissemens publics et privés consacrés aux aliénés. 2°. De wet van Genève, d. d. 5. Februarij 1838, sur le placement et la surveillance des aliénés, en 3°. Gedachten over het ontwerp van wet, houdende bepalingen over de gestichten voor krankzinnigen en de wijze hunner opneming in en ontslag uit dezelve, den 28 December 1840 bij de Tweede Kamer der Staten-Generaal ingekomen, gevolgd door eene proeve van wet op de krankzinnigen, en eene memorie ter opheldering. 1 p. l., 112, 108*, 63** pp. 8°. *'s Gravenhage, J. Belinfante*, 1841. [P., v. 1223.]

Métoz (P.-F.-G.) *Sur le rhumatisme articulaire. 23 pp. 4°. *Paris*, 1835, No. 248, v. 289.

Métral (Albert). * De la résection sous-périostée du poignet, ses résultats définitifs. 104 pp. 4°. *Lyon*, 1882, No. 106.

Métral (Antoine) [1778–   ]. Description naturelle, morale et politique du choléra-morbus à Paris. vi, 162 pp. 12°. *Paris, Didot frères*, 1833.

Métras (Armand). *Rapports pathologiques de l'œil et des dents par action réflexe. 47 pp. 4°. *Paris*, 1873, No. 71.

Metrasse (G.) * Considérations sur l'usage et l'abus des purgatifs. vi, 7–19 pp. 4°. *Paris*, 1811, No. 83, v. 84.

de Metri (Nicolaus). Artzney Büch: von vilen herrlichen, treflichen, unnd bissher verborgenen Artzneyen, zü mancherley eusserlichen und innerlichen leybsgebrechen dienstlich. Von ihme erstlich vor vier unnd achtzig Jaren, ohngefehrlich, trewlich und mit höchstem fleiss, und grosser mühe und arbeyt zusamen getragen. Jetzundt aber durch Hieremiam Martium, von newem übersehen und in Truck verfertiget, allen Artzeten nicht allein lustig, sonder auch nothwendig zu lesen. 7 p. l., 332 pp., 12 l. 24°. [*Augspurg, M. Manger*], 1578.

Metric (The) Bulletin. Official journal of the American Metric Bureau. [Monthly.] Nos. 1–15, July, 1876, to Sept., 1877. 192 pp. 8°. *Boston*. Want no. 7, Jan., 1877.

Metric primer, a text-book for beginners. Prepared for the society by a practical teacher. 48 pp. 16°. *Boston*, 1878.

Metric system.

See **Weights,** *etc.*

Metric system of weights and measures. 9 pp. 8°. [*Boston*, 1876.]

Metritis.

See **Phlebitis** (*Uterine*); **Puerperal** *metritis;* **Uterus** (*Inflammation of*).

Metritis (*Puerperal*).

See **Puerperal** *metritis.*

Metroperitonitis.

See **Peritonitis; Peritonitis** (*Pelvic*); **Puerperal** *diseases;* **Puerperal** *metritis;* **Uterus** (*Inflammation, etc., of*).

Metrophlebitis.

See **Puerperal** *phlebitis.*

Metropolitan Association of Medical Officers of Health. The committee appointed by the association to enquire into the laws relating to slaughter-houses, the duties of medical officers under those laws, and the sanitary conditions under which slaughter-houses ought to be licensed. 3 pp. 8°. [*London*, 1856.] [P., v. 1620.]

———. Health and meteorology of the metropolis. Weekly returns. Communicated to the General Board of Health. v. 2, Nos. 1–42 and 44, Jan. 9 to Nov. 6, 1858. 180 pp. 8°. *London, G. E. Eyre & W. Spottiswoode*, 1858.

Metropolitan Association [etc.]—continued.
——. Health of the metropolis. Quarterly returns. Communicated to the General Board of Health. Nos. 1–3, Jan. to Sept., 1858. 8°. *London, G. E. Eyre & W. Spottiswoode*, 1858.
  Bound with the preceding.
——. The cattle plague. Return from the . . . of the number of cowsheds, of cows, and, so far as could be ascertained by inspection and inquiry, the number of cases of the cattle plague that have existed in each parish or district from 1st May to 13th Aug., 1865. 2 l. sm. 4°. [*London, B. Pardon*, 1865.]
——. Memorandum of a plan of united action in the case of an epidemic of cholera; to be communicated to vestries and district boards. 12 pp. 8°. *London*, [1866].
Metropolitan Asylums Board. Caterham Imbecile Asylum, Surrey. Annual reports of the committee of management and medical superintendent to the managers of the Metropolitan Asylums Board. 1.–11., 1870–71 to 1881; 15., 1885. 8°. *London*, 1871–86.
  9., for fifteen months ending Dec. 31, 1879.
——. Darenth Asylum and Schools for Imbeciles. Annual reports of the committee of management and the medical superintendent to the managers of the metropolitan asylum district. 1.–8., 1875–82; 11., 1885. 8°. *London*, 1876–86.
  Opened April 28, 1875.
——. Ambulance committee. Annual report of the committee of management and medical superintendent. 1., 1884–5. 28 pp., 1 map. 8°. *London, McCorquodale & Co.*, 1886.
  First report, Feb. 9, 1884, to Dec. 31, 1885.
——. Darenth Camps for Convalescing Small-pox Patients. Report of the medical superintendent on the working of the Darenth Camps for Convalescing Small-pox Patients. 1., 1884–5. 59 pp. 8°. *London, McCorquodale & Co.*, 1886.
  First report, for eighteen months, from opening, April, 1884, to Sept., 1885.
——. Eastern Hospitals (fever and small-pox). Annual reports of the medical superintendent to the committee of management for the year 1884. 68 pp. 8°. *London, McCorquodale & Co.*, 1886.
——. Léavesden Asylum (insane). Annual report of the medical superintendent to the committee of management for the year 1885. 41 pp. 8°. *London, McCorquodale & Co.*, 1886.
  Opened Oct. 9, 1870.
——. Hospital ships (Atlas and Castalia) for small-pox patients. Annual report of the medical superintendent to the committee of management for the year 1885. 26 pp. 8°. *London, McCorquodale & Co.*, 1886.
——. South-Eastern Hospital (fever and small-pox). Report of the medical superintendent to the committee of management for the year 1885. 34 pp. 8°. *London, McCorquodale & Co.*, 1886.
——. South-Western Fever Hospital. Annual report of the medical superintendent to the committee of management. 15., 1885. 39 pp. 8°. *London, McCorquodale & Co.*, 1886.
——. Metropolitan training ship "Exmouth" (for boys). Annual report of the committee of management to the managers of the metropolitan asylum district for the year 1885. 42 pp. 8°. *London, McCorquodale & Co.*, 1886.
——. Western Hospital (fever and small-pox). Annual report of the medical superintendent to the committee of management for the year 1885. 28 pp. 8°. *London, McCorquodale & Co.*, 1886.
Metropolitan Convalescent Institution, Piccadilly, W. Annual reports of the board of management to the governors and subscribers. 17., 1857; 19., 1859; 26., 1866; 27., 1867; 39., 1879;

Metropolitan Convalescent [etc.]—continued. 42., 1882. 8°. *London*, 1858–83. [26. & 27. *in:* P., v. 974.]
  Founded in 1840, being the first convalescent institution ever established. Provides an asylum in the country for the temporary residence of the convalescent and debilitated poor. Comprises three homes: one at Walton-on-Thames, for adults, 300 beds; one at Kingston Hill, for children, 170 beds; and one at Bexhill, near Hastings, for adults, 50 beds.
Metropolitan Ear and Throat Infirmary, London. Biennial report of the committee of management to the subscribers for the years 1882–3. 18 pp. 8°. *London, Hutchings & Crowsley*, 1884.
  Established 1838.
Metropolitan Female Reformatories. An exposure of the false statistics of the contagious diseases acts (women) contained in Parliamentary Paper No. 149, on the return of the assistant commissioner of metropolitan police. 16 pp. 8°. *London, W. Tweedie*, 1873.
——. A further answer by the . . . to police report for the year 1874 on the operation of the contagious diseases acts (Parliamentary Paper 97). 11 pp. 8°. [*London, Pardon & Son*, 1875?]
Metropolitan Free Hospital, London. Annual reports of the committee of management to the governors and subscribers. 25., 1860; 39.–46., 1874–81. 12°. *London*, 1861–82.
  1874–81 bound in 1 v. Instituted in 1836, for the gratuitous relief of the sick poor of every nation and creed, without the delay of a letter of recommendation.
——. History. 2 l. 4°. [*London*, 1884.]
——. Jubilee year of the . . . Special appeal. 2 l. 8°. [*London*, 1886.]
——. Diet scale. broadside fol. [*London, n. d.*]
——. Rules for the guidance of the resident medical officers. 1 sheet. fol. [*London, n. d.*]
  Bound with: Reports, 1874–81.
——. [Blank forms in use at the hospital.] various sizes. [*London, n. d.*]
  Bed cards. Diet list; daily requisitions by nurse. Obstetric patient. Out-patients. Casualty letter. Physician's letter. Surgeon's letter. Weekly return for publication.
  Bound with: Reports, 1874–81.
Metropolitan Health-of-Towns Association. *See* **Journal** of Public Health and Monthly Record of Sanitary Improvement. Published under the sanction of the . . .
Metropolitan Hospital-Sunday Fund, London, S. E. Annual reports of the council and the committee of distribution. 1.–5., 1873 to 1876–7; 7.–10., 1878–9 to 1881–2; 12.–14., 1883–5. sm. 4°. *London*, 1873–86.
——. [List of various churches, chapels, and congregations to appeal to in London and suburbs. Corrected to the 28. October, 1879.] 43 pp., interleaved. 4°. [*London*, 1879.]
  Reprinted every five years.
——. [Collection of blank forms, circulars, etc., used by the council.] v. s. [*London*, 1880–83.]
  A. Application from institutions desirous of participating in the funds.
  B. Circular letter to hospitals and dispensaries, requesting them to send in their applications for 1883.
  C. Circular letter transmitting forms.
  D. Analysis of accounts for dispensaries. Same for hospitals.
  E. Circular letter, relating to contributions received as the result of collections made on Hospital Sunday.
  F. Circular letter, transmitting blank receipts (to be filled up) for amount allowed.
  G. Abstracts of analysis. 12 sheets. 4°.
  No. I. Notice to clergymen of Hospital Sunday for 1882.
    II. Resolutions to be proposed at annual meeting, 1882.
    III. Secretary's acknowledgment of letter received.
      1. Circular letter, transmitting forms to clergymen.
      2. Return of amount collected.
      3. Circular letter soliciting donations.
      4. Secretary's acknowledgment of contributions received.
Metropolitan (The) Hospital Sunday Movement. Historical and helpful. The Lancet and

Metropolitan (The) Hospital [etc.]—cont'd. the fund. 47 pp. 8°. [*London*], *Lancet office,* [1885].

Metropolitan Imbecile Asylum, Caterham, Surrey. *See* **Caterham** Imbecile Asylum, Surrey.

Metropolitan Medical College. *See* **Journal** of Health of the . . .

Metropolitan medical relief. April, 1877. With appendices. 103 pp., 1 tab. 8°. *London, Spottiswoode & Co.,* 1877.
  1. Report on the social position of the out-patients of the Royal Free Hospital.
  2. Limits of unpaid service.
  3. First report of the medical committee of the Charity Organization Society, with rules for provident dispensaries.
  4. Report of a conference on out-patient relief in Dec., 1871.
  5. Correspondence relating to the memorial to the British Medical Association.
  6. Statement of metropolitan provident dispensaries in March, 1877.
  7. Metropolitan poor-law infirmaries and dispensaries.

Metropolitan Provident Medical Association, London. Annual report of the committee to the association for the year 1886. 11 pp. 8°. [*London,* 1887.]

Metropolitan Public Garden, Boulevard, and Playground Association, London. Annual report of the officers to the association. 2., 1883–4. 98 pp. 12°. *London,* [*Hutchings & Crowsley*], 1884.

Metropolitan Sanitary Association. The public health a public question. First report on the chief evils affecting the sanitary condition of the metropolis, with suggestions for their removal, and containing the proceedings of the public meeting held at Freemasons' Hall, Feb. 6, 1850, and of the deputations to the premier, the General Board of Health, and the chancellor of the exchequer. 102 pp. 8°. *London, by the association,* 1850.

Metropolitan Throat Hospital, N. Y. City. Constitution and by-laws. 16 pp. 16°. *New York, J. J. O'Brien,* 1874.
——. Annual reports of the trustees and medical superintendent to the subscribers. 1., 1874; 13., 1885. 12°. *New York,* 1875–86.
  Incorporated Jan. 3, 1874. No reports were printed from 1875 to 1884, inclusive.

Metropolitan training ship "Exmouth" (for boys). Annual report of the committee of management to the managers of the metropolitan asylums district. For the year 1885. 42 pp. 8°. *London, McCorquodale & Co.,* 1886.

Metropolitan Working Classes' Association for Improving the Public Health. [Miscellaneous papers.] 8°. *London, J. Churchill,* 1846–9. [P., v. 149.]
  1. On the ventilation of rooms, houses, workshops. 16 pp. 1846.
  2. Bathing and personal cleanliness. 16 pp. 1847.
  3. Drainage and sewerage. 16 pp. 1847.
  4. Exercise and recreation. 16 pp. 1847.
  5. The rearing and training of children. 16 pp. 1847.
  6. Water supply; especially for the working classes. 16 pp. 1847.
  7. On household cleanliness. 16 pp. 1849.

Metrorrhagia.
  See **Blood** (*Transfusion of*); **Hæmorrhage** (*Uterine*); **Menorrhagia.**

Metrorrhœa.
  See **Hydrorrhœa.**

Metrotome.
  See **Uterus-cervix** (*Incision of*).

Metsch (Joannes Christianus) [1796–]. *De blepharophthalmia blennorrhoica recens natorum. 61 pp. 8°. *Berolini, formis Brueschckianis,* 1821.

Metsch (Rudolphus Guilelmus) [1827–]. *De abortus origine. 32 pp. 8°. *Berolini, B. Schlesinger,* [1849].

Mettais (Hippolyte). *I. Des symptômes de l'encéphalite diffuse (méningo-encéphalite). II. [etc.] 18 pp. 4°. *Paris,* 1839, No. 101, v. 347.

Mettas (Barthélemy) [1854–]. *Des exostoses chez les adolescents. 83 pp. 4°. *Paris,* 1881, No. 281.

Mettauer (John P.) A memoir on stricture of the urethra. 45 pp., 2 pl. 8°. *Farmville, Va., Saunders & Cowan,* 1849.

Mette (Augustus Eduardus) [1802–]. *De metastasi lactea. 1 p. l., 28 pp. 8°. *Regiomonti, typ. Hartungianis,* [1827].

Mette (Carolus Gustavus). *De tabe dorsali. 31 pp. 8°. *Berolini, G. Schade,* [1864].

Mette (Célestin-Marie). *Quelques réflexions sur le traitement des malades affectés de lésions valvulaires du cœur. 46 pp. 4°. *Paris,* 1874, No. 453.

Mettegang (Ludovicus) [1812–]. *De diabete, præsertim mellito. 48 pp. 8°. *Berolini, typ. Friedlaenderianis,* [1838].

Mettenheimer (Carl Friedrich Christian) [1824–]. *Disquisitiones anatomico-comparativæ de membro piscium pectorali institutæ in Museo Regio Berolinensi. vi, 63 pp., 2 pl. 4°. *Berolini, A. Hirschwald,* 1847.
——. Nosologische und anatomische Beiträge zu der Lehre von den Greisenkrankheiten. Eine Sammlung von Krankengeschichten und Nekroskopien eigner Beobachtung. viii, 356 pp. 8°. *Leipzig, B. G. Teubner,* 1863.
——. Ueber die Verwachsung der Gefässhaut des Gehirns mit der Hirnrinde. Ein Beitrag zur pathologischen Anatomie des Gehirns und seiner häutigen Hüllen. 13 pp. 4°. *Schwerin, Stiller,* 1865.
——. Beobachtungen über die typhoiden Erkrankungen der französischen Kriegsgefangenen in Schwerin. 4 p. l., 87 pp. 8°. *Berlin, A. Hirschwald,* 1872.
——. Die Einführung einer ärztlichen Standesordnung. 32 pp. 8°. *Stuttgart, F. Enke,* 1878.
——. Leben und Wirken des weiland Geh. Med.-Raths Dr. F. W. Beneke, Professors der Medicin in Marburg, etc. Biographische Skizze. 1 p. l., 40 pp. 8°. *Oldenburg, Schulze,* [1883, *vel subseq.*].
——. Das Seebad Gross-Müritz an der Ostsee, und das Friedrich-Franz-Hospiz (Kinderasyl) daselbst. In Verbindung mit Oberforstmeister Garthe und Dr. med. Wagner beschrieben. 2 p. l., 60 pp., 1 map, 1 plan. 8°. *Rostock, W. Werther,* 1885.

Mettenius (Georg Heinrich) [1823–66].
  See **Reise** der österreichischen Fregatte Novara um die Erde. Botanischer Theil. 1. Bd. 4°. *Wien,* 1870.

Metternich (Antonius Franciscus) [–1827]. De urina, ut signo. 20 pp. 8°. *Moguntiæ, A. Crass,* 1784.
——. Dissertatio de tussi convulsiva infantum. *Moguntiæ,* 1777.
  In: FRANK (J. P.) Delect. opusc. med. 8°. *Ticini,* 1787, iii, 218–235.

Metting (Joh. Henricus). *De corde humano. 26 pp., 3 l. sm. 4°. *Lugd. Bat., J. Bos,* [1761].

Mettler (Arnold). *Ueber die wichtigsten Frakturen und Luxationen. 31 pp. 8°. *Würzburg, F. E. Thein,* 1846.

Mettler (Joh.) *Animadversiones in leges formationis sceleti, quibus annexæ sunt theses chirurgicæ. 29 pp. sm. 8°. *Tubingæ, typ. Reissianis,* [1816].

Mettmann.
  Mortalitäts-Statistik der Gemeinde Mettmann. Cor.-Bl. d. nied.-rhein. Ver. f. öff. Gsndhtspflg., Köln, 1873, ii, 189–193.

Metton (Alfred). *Étude sur le pityriasis rosé. 48 pp. 4°. *Paris,* 1877, No. 471.

Mettray.

See **Insane** (*Asylums for, etc.*), *by localities.*

de la Mettrie (Julien-Offray). *See* **La Mettrie** (Julien-Offray).

Mettrier (N.) * Sur la congestion cérébrale. 50 pp., 1 l. 4°. *Montpellier, Gras,* 1866, No. 58. c.

Metz (Ville de). Projet de distribution d'eau. Rapport fait au conseil municipal, dans sa séance du 29 janvier 1853, par M. Vander-Noot, ingénieur de la ville. 96 pp. 4°. *Metz, S. Lamort,* [1853].

——. Avis motivé et propositions de l'administration municipale sur les projets présentés par M. Vander-Noot, ingénieur de la ville, pour la distribution d'eau et la reconstruction des usines. Mémoire lu au conseil municipal dans les séances des 19 et 21 avril 1855, par M. Philippe-Félix Maréchal, maire de Metz. 4°. *Metz,* 1855.

Metz.

See, also, **Cholera** (*Asiatic, History, etc., of*), **Fever** (*Cerebro-spinal, History, etc., of*), **Fever** (*Malarial, History, etc., of*), **Fever** (*Typhoid, History, etc., of*), **Fever** (*Typhus, History, etc., of*), **Hospitals** (*Description, etc., of*), **Hospitals** (*Military*), *by localities;* **Measles** (*Epidemics of*); **Medicine** (*Military*).

MARÉCHAL (F.) Tableau historique, chronologique et médical des maladies endémiques, épidémiques et contagieuses qui ont régné à Metz et dans le pays messin depuis les temps les plus reculés jusqu'à nos jours. 8°. *Metz,* 1850.

—— & DIDION (J.) Tableau historique, chronologique et médical des maladies endémiques, épidémiques et contagieuses qui ont régné à Metz et dans le pays messin depuis les temps les plus reculés jusqu'à nos jours. 2 pts. in 1 v. 8°. *Metz,* 1850–61.

Didion aided in Pt. 2. Date on cover is 1863.

d'Arrest. Topographische Notizen über Metz. Deutsche mil.-ärztl. Ztschr., Berl., 1873, ii, 1; 65.—**Brault** (J.-C.) Topographie physique et médicale de Metz et de ses environs. Rec. de mém. de méd. . . . mil., Par., 1827, xxii, 1–245.—**Didion.** De l'assistance publique à Metz en 1867. Exposé d. trav. de la Soc. d. sc. méd. de la Moselle 1866, Metz, 1867, pp. i–lxxxvi.—**Études** statistiques sur la constitution médicale et la mortalité de la ville de Metz pendant les années 1850–60, 1862, 1864–9. *Ibid.* (1850), 1851, 61: (1851), 1852, 70: (1852), 1853, 93: (1853), 1854, 51: (1854), 1855, 37: (1855), 1856, 45: (1856), 1857, 61: (1857), 1858, 73: (1858), 1859, 69: (1859), 1860, 61: (1860), 1861, 111: (1862), 1863, 69: (1864), 1865, 117: (1865), 1866, 69: (1866), 1867, 83: (1867), 1868, 81: (1868), 1869, 9: (1869), 1870, 53.—**Géhin** (J.-B.) Rapport sur l'état de quelques fossés de la place de Metz au mois de juillet 1868. *Ibid.* (1868), 1869, 1–7.—**Langlois.** Analyse de l'eau ferrugineuse de la Bonne Fontaine, située à 3 kilomètres de Metz, sur la route de Lorry. *Ibid.* (1850), 1851, 125.—**Laveran.** Rapport fait à la Société des sciences médicales de la Moselle, sur les maladies qui ont régné à Metz depuis l'année 1838 jusqu'à l'année 1849. *Ibid.* (1848), 1849, 55–90.—**Maréchal** (F.) Recherches historiques, chronologiques et médicales sur les maladies endémiques, épidémiques et contagieuses qui ont régné à Metz et dans le pays messin, depuis les temps les plus reculés jusqu'à nos jours. *Ibid.* (1849). 1850, 109: (1851), 1852, 41: (1852), 1853, 63: (1856), 1857, 98: (1862), 1863, 99.—**Meinel.** Salubritätsverhältnisse und sanitäre Einrichtungen in Metz. Arch. f. öff. Gsndhtspflg., Strassb., 1880, v, 91–107.—**Renauld.** Observations sur la constitution physique, le caractère, les mœurs et les habitudes des Messins. Exposé d. trav. de la Soc. d. sc. méd. de la Moselle, Metz, 1838–41, 173.—**Schuster.** Résumé des observations météorologiques faites à Metz pendant l'année 1847. *Ibid.* (1847), 1848, 192–194.

Metz (*Siege of*).

See **Medicine** (*Military, History of*)—*Campaigns, etc.*

Metz (A.) The anatomy and histology of the human eye. xvi, 17–184 pp. 8°. *Philadelphia, office Med. & Surg. Reporter,* 1868.

——. An introductory address, before the students of the medical department of the Univer-

Metz (A.)—continued. sity of Wooster, delivered Oct. 4, 1871. 23 pp. 8°. *Cleveland, Spencer & Barker,* 1871.

Metz (August). * Ueber die Gewichtsveränderungen der Neugeborenen. 20 pp., 2 l., 1 tab. 8°. *Marburg, C. L. Pfeil,* 1873. c.

Metz (Carolus) [1824–]. * De gastro-enteromalacia. 26 pp., 2 l. 8°. *Berolini, typ. fratrum Schlesinger,* [1848].

Metz (E.) * De ulceribus ventriculi, præcipue de iis, quæ dicuntur hæmorrhagica. 22 pp., 1 l. 8°. *Bonnæ, formis F. Kruegeri,* [1864, *vel subseq.*]. c.

Metz (Franciscus Antonius). * Diss. sistens anginam parotidæam una cum thesibus ex universa medicina et chirurgia. iv, 32 pp. 4°. [*Wirceburg*], *F. E. Nitribitt,* [1801].

Metz (Georgius). * O temperaturie v peremejajoutsheisja lichoradkie, tifie, vospalenii legkich i legochnoi bugorchatkie. [Temperatures in intermittent and typhus fever, pneumonia, etc.] 22 pp, 1 l., 10 tab. 8°. *St. Petersburg,* 1862.

Metz (Hermann). * Ueber die Lösung des Oberschenkels aus dem Hüftgelenke. 44 pp. 8°. *Würzburg, F. E. Thein,* 1841.

Metz (Joh. Adamus). * De tactu regis Franciæ, quo strumis laborantes restituuntur. 7 l. sm. 4°. *Wittebergæ, lit. M. Henckelii,* [1675].

Metz (*Joh. Fridericus*) [1724–82].

Portrait in: **Collection**—van Kaathoven.

Metz (Joh. Philippus). * Diss. sistens diabetis observationem raram. 22 pp. sm. 4°. *Basileæ, J. H. Decker,* 1737.

Also, in: HALLER. Disp. ad morb. [etc.] 4°. *Lausannæ,* 1758, iv, 33–49.

Metz (Vitus Jacob) [1792–1866]. Ueber die Anwendung der Kälte nach gemachtem Kaiserschnitte. 19 pp. 8°. *Berlin, G. Reimer,* 1852.

Repr. from: Deutsche Klinik, Berl., 1852, iv.

——. The same. De l'emploi du froid après l'opération césarienne. 18 pp. 8°. *Aix-la-Chapelle,* 1856.

Metz (Vitus Nicolaus). * De teleangiektasia uteri. vii, 56 pp. 8°. *Groningæ, W. van Boekeren,* 1838.

Metzendorff (Joann. Mart.) [1805–]. * De asphyxia. 43 pp. 8°. *Berolini, typ. A. Petschii,* [1827]. [*Also, in:* P., v. 1548.]

Metzger.

See **von Pfeufer** (C.) Beobachtungen aus der Klinik, Dr. v. Pfeufer'schen Winter - Semester 1856–7. [etc.] 8°. [*Bamberg* (?), 1857.]—**Robert.** Recherches et considérations critiques sur le magnétisme animal, [etc.] 8°. *Paris,* 1824.

Metzger (A. D.) Ueber Irritabilität und Sensibilität als Lebensprincipien in der organisirten Natur. xiv, 118 pp. 12°. *Königsberg, Hartung,* 1794. [P., v. 1545.]

Metzger (Carl). Zusammenstellung sämmtlicher im Grossherzogthum Baden z. Z. giltigen Verordnungen über die Gebühren der Sanitätsdiener für amtliche Verrichtungen und Privatleistungen. Empfohlen durch Dr. Battlehner. viii, 68 pp. 12°. *Karlsruhe, G. Braun,* 1874.

Metzger (David). * De la lypémanie et plus particulièrement de la lypémanie anxieuse. 72 pp. 4°. *Paris,* 1884, No. 77.

Metzger (George A.) Plans for the proposed asylum for insane, to be located in northern New York. Plan A. 33 × 76 in. broadside. *Buffalo,* 1887.

Metzger (Joannes Ludovicus Fridericus). * De hactenus prætervisa nervorum lustratione in sectionibus hydrophoborum. 46 pp. 8°. *Tubingæ, typ. Schrammianis,* [1802].

Also, in: WEBER. Samml. med.-prakt. Diss. [etc.] 8°. *Tübingen,* 1824, iv, 1–69.

Metzger (Joh. Caspar). * De naturæ et artis effectu in medendo. 39 pp. sm. 4°. *Halæ Magdeb., lit. C. Henckelii,* [1708].

Metzger (Joh. Caspar)—continued.

——. Deutlich- und gründliche Beschreibung zweyer vortrefflichen Specificorum chymico-medicorum, davon das erste als ein metallisches Ant-Epilepticum, gegen die fallende Kranckheit und die Gichter, das zweyte aber als ein mineralisches Alexipharmacum, wider allerhand Arten, böser und gifftiger Kranckheiten, und in Specie, gegen die Kinder-Blattern, sich als souveraine Mittel erzeigen, wie solche, zum Nutzen vieler Krancken, mit allen nöthigen Umständen, die in und bey dem Gebrauch derselben zu beobachten sind, mit allem Fleiss und auf das deutlichste entworffen worden. 144 pp. 12°. *Strassburg, J. Beck,* 1724.

Metzger (Joh. Daniel) [1739–1805]. De argilla. 2 p. l., 44 pp., 1 l. 4°. *Argentorati, typ. J. H. Heitzii,* [1765].

——. *Nervorum primi paris historiam defendet. 1 p. l., 36 pp. 4°. *Argentinæ, Christmann et Levrault,* [1766].
    Also, in: SCRIPT. neurol. minores selecti. 4°. *Lipsiæ,* 1791, i, 108–126. *Also, in:* SANDIFORT. Thesaurus diss. [etc.] 4°. *Lugd. Bat.,* 1778, iii, 457–476.

——. Grundriss der Physiologie. 7 p. l., 133 pp. 16°. *Königsberg u. Leipzig, G. L. Hartung,* 1778.

——. Gerichtlich-medicinische Beobachtungen. 1. u. 2. Jahrgang. 2 v. in 1. 5 p. l., 153 pp.; 4 p. l., 192 pp. 16°. *Königsberg, J. J. Kauter,* 1778–80.

——. The same. 1. u. 2. Jahrg. 5 p. l., 154 pp.; 4 p. l., 192 pp. 12°. *Königsberg, F. D. Wagner u. K. G. Dengel,* 1781.

——. Beytrag zur Geschichte der Frühlings-Epidemie im Jahr 1782. 78 pp. 8°. *Königsberg u. Leipzig, G. L. Hartung,* 1782.
    Bound with: WITTWER (P. L.) Ueber den jüngsten epidemischen Katarrh. 8°. *Leipzig,* 1783.

——. [Pr.] de non negligendo linguæ latinæ et bonarum literarum studio ad commilitones admonitio. [Cum vita candidati Alexandri Magnus.] 8 pp. 4°. *Regiomonti, typ. G. L. Hartungii,* [1783].

——. [Pr.] de reue rupto observatio. [Cum vita candidati Christoph. Henr. Kruppa.] 8 pp. 4°. *Regiomonti, typ. G. L. Hartungii,* 1783.

——. Vermischte medicinische Schriften. 2. Aufl. 3 v. in 1. 284, 244, 432 pp. 12°. *Königsberg, K. G. Dengel,* 1784.

——. Opuscula anatomica et physiologica, retractata, aucta et revisa. viii, 208 pp., 4 l. 8°. *Gothæ, apud C. W. Ettingerum,* 1790.

——. Skizze einer pragmatischen Literärgeschichte der Medicin. 7 p. l., 448 pp., 1 l. 8°. *Königsberg, F. Nicolovius,* 1792.
    Another copy with which is bound the following.

——. Zusätze und Verbesserungen zu seiner Skizze einer pragmatischen Literärgeschichte der Medicin. 180 pp. 8°. *Königsberg, F. Nicolovius,* 1796.

——. Kurzgefasstes System der gerichtlichen Arzneiwissenschaft. xvi, 414 pp. 8°. *Königsberg u. Leipzig, Hartung,* 1793.

——. The same. Nach dem Tode des Verfassers revidirt, verbessert, mit den nöthigen Zusätzen . . . versehen von Christian Gottfried Gruner. 4. Ausg. xvi, 544 pp. 8°. *Königsberg u. Leipzig, A. W. Unzer,* 1814.

——. The same. Erweitert und berichtigt von Wilhelm Hermann Georg Remer. 5. Aufl. xv, 615 pp. 8°. *Königsberg u. Leipzig, A. W. Unzer,* 1820.

——. The same. Compendio di polizia medica del . . . recato dalla tedesca all' italiana favella con alcune viste del dottor Carlo Pietro Ferrari. 128 pp. 8°. *Venezia,* 1800. [P., v. 1122.]

Metzger (Joh. Daniel)--continued.

——. The same. Principes de médecine légale ou judiciaire, trad. de l'allemand, et augmentés de notes, par le Dr. J.-J. Ballard. xxiii, 504 pp. 8°. *Autun, Dejussieu,* 1812.

——. The same. xxiii, 504 pp. 8°. *Paris, Gabon,* 1813.

——. The same. Geregtelijke geneeskunde. Naar het Hoogdnitsch door Mr. J. van der Linden. xvi, 561 pp. 8°. *'s Gravenhage, J. Allart,* 1815.

——. Ueber Irritabilität und Sensibilität als Lebensprincipien in der organisirten Natur. xiv, 118 pp. 16°. *Königsberg, Hartung,* 1794. [*Also, in:* P., v. 1431.]

——. Ueber den menschlichen Kopf in anthropologischer Rücksicht; nebst einigen Bemerkungen über Dr. Galls Hirn- und Schädeltheorie. 133 pp. 12°. *Königsberg, Goebbels u. Unzer,* 1803.

——. Skizze einer medizinischen Enkyklopädie, für den Anfang des neunzehnten Jahrhunderts. Ein Leitfaden zu akademischen Vorlesungen. x, 139 pp. 12°. *Königsberg, Goebbels u. Unzer,* 1804.

——. Gerichtlich-medizinische Abhandlungen. Ein Supplement zu seinem: Kurzgefassten System der gerichtlichen Arzneywissenschaft. 2 v. in 1. 2 p. l., 136 pp.; 3 p. l., 128 pp. 12°. *Wien, A. Doll,* 1810.
    Also, Editor of: **Annalen** der Staatsarzneykunde, Züllichau, 1790–91.
    For Biography, see Krit. Jahrb. d. Staatsarznk., Berl., 1809, ii, 151–172. *Also:* Med. Briefwechsel, Halle, 1876, ii, 1–26.
    For Portrait, see Collection—van Kaathoven.—**Collection** of Portr. of Phys. & Men of Sc., 7.

——— & **Elsner** (Christoph Fried.) Medicinisch-gerichtliche Bibliothek. 4 St. in 1 v. viii, 476 pp., 5 l. 8°. *Königsberg, G. L. Hartung,* 1785[-6].

Metzger (Joh. Ulricus). *De vanitate medicamentorum pellentium in partu difficili. 3 p. l., 50 pp. 4°. *Argentorati, typ. M. Pauschingeri,* [1747].

Metzig (Joan. Heinrich Christian) [1804–69]. *De bubonibus syphiliticis. 22 pp., 1 l. 8°. *Berolini, lit. A. Petschii,* [1827].

——. Das Kleid des Soldaten vom ärztlichen Standpunkte aus betrachtet. Ein Beitrag zur Kriegs-Hygieine. xii, 158 pp., 1 l., 1 pl. 8°. *Lissa u. Leipzig, E. Günther,* 1837.

——. Gegen das Amputiren gleich nach schweren Verletzungen. 2 p. l., 81 pp., 1 l., 1 pl. 8°. *Lissa, E. Günther,* 1857. [P., v. 195.]

——. Der modificirte Sentin'sche Verband als vollkommenes Ersatzmittel der primairen Amputationen nach schweren Verletzungen. Ein Vortrag am 20. November 1859 in einer Versammlung von Aerzten und Freunden der Wissenschaft zu Lissa gehalten. Mit Anhang: Statuten des Sentin-Vereins. 64 pp. 8°. *Berlin, Nicolai,* 1860.

Metzinger (Joannes). *De singultu. 1781.
    In: LOUVAIN Diss. 8°. *Lovanii,* 1795, ii, 124–126.

Metzis (Davides). *De morbo hæmorrhoidali. 23 pp. 8°. *Jenæ, typ. Ratii,* 1858. c.

Metzke (Ernestus Augustus). *De morbis pulmonum ex mixtura formaque læsa explicandis. 32 pp. 4°. *Halæ, typ. Batheanis,* [1800].

Metzlar (A. G.) *Over radicaal operatie van breuken. 2 p. l., 61 pp. 8°. *Leiden, S. C. van Doesburgh,* 1880.

Metzler (Adamus). *De balsamis nativis. 29 pp., 1 l. 8°. *Vindobonæ, typ. Congregationis Mechitaristicæ,* 1836.

Metzler (Adolphus). *De medullæ spinalis avium textura. 57 pp. 8°. *Dorpat, typ. vid. J. C. Schünmanni et C. Mattieseni,* 1855.

Metzler (F. X.) *See* **Mezler** (F. X.)

Metzler (Johannes). *Zur Casuistik des Echinococcus hepatis. 33 pp., 1 l. 8°. *Berlin, G. Klemm*, [1886].

Metzner (Edmundus). *De carcinomate medullari. 13 pp. 8°. *Halis, typ. Orphanotrophei*, [1857].

Metzner (Jo. Christianus). *De somno meridiana. 13 l. sm. 4°. *Vitembergæ, prelo Gerdesiano*, [1706].

Metzner (Reinholdus Alexander). *De ætiologia scabiei. 30 pp. 8°. *Gryphiæ, typ. O. F. Zinckii*, [1849].

Metzquer (A.) *Sur les ulcères simples ou atoniques des extrémités. 25 pp. 4°. *Paris*, 1836, No. 358, v. 304.

Metzquer (Edmond). Étude clinique de la phthisie galopante. Preuves expérimentales de la non-spécificité et de la non-inoculabilité des phthisies. Ouvrage précédé d'une préface de M. le professeur Feltz. 219 pp. 8°. *Paris, A. Delahaye*, 1874.

Meuder (Carolus Henricus). *De urinæ se- et excretione ob multitudinem arteriarum renalium largiore casu quodam singulari illustrata. 1 p. l., 42 pp., 1 l., 1 pl. 4°. *Halæ ad Salam, ære Reyeriano*, [1763].
Also, in: SANDIFORT. Thesaurus diss. [etc.] 4°. *Lugd. Bat.*, 1778, iii, 123-144. Also [Abstr.], in: WEIZ (F. A.) Neue Ausz. [etc.] 12°. *Frankf. u. Leipz.*, 1774, i, 109-112.

Meuder (Ernestus Ludovicus). *Diss. sistens spicilegium de pedum ulceribus. 20 pp. 4°. *Wittenbergæ, lit. Tzschiedrichi*, [1802].
For Biography, see **Kreysig** (Frid. Ludovic.)

Meuder (Ernestus Petrus). *De febribus biliosis. 31 pp. 4°. *Halæ Magdeb., lit. C. Henckelii*, [1701].
———. The same. 32 pp. 4°. *Halæ Magdeb., recusa, typ. C. A. Zeitleri*, 1707.
———. The same. 32 pp. 4°. *Halæ Magdeb., lit. C. Henckelii*, 1726.

Meuder (Georg Christian). De contagiis idea nova et succincta seu malignitatis vere febrilis disquisitio physiologico-pathologica qua substantiarum macrocosmicarum in corpore animali maligne agentium ortus, indoles ac progressus in morbis omnibus acute malignis ex veris artis fundamentis, rationi et experimentiæ consentaneis, in usum publicæ utilitatis exhibetur, ubi simul causarum accidentalium effectus tumultuarii distinctius explanati, et rationibus a priori et posteriori perspicue evoluti sistuntur. 8 p. l., 78 pp. 12°. *Servestæ, G. W. Goeckingen*, 1725.

Meuder (Joannes Christianus Carolus). *De scirrho ejusque medela. 32 pp. 4°. *Vitembergæ, lit. A. C. Charisii*, [1800].

Meudon.

DE JUSSIEU (A. L.) *An clivi Meudonici situs, ut amœnus, sic salubris? Præses P. A. Pajon de Moncets. 4°. [*Paris*, 1771.]

Meugy (Jules). *Sur le diagnostic des tumeurs. 32 pp. 4°. *Paris*, 1859, No. 174, v. 634.

Meugy (P.-A.) *Sur la douleur physique. 31 pp. 4°. *Paris*, 1821, No. 115, v. 166.

ter Meulen (Gerard). *Over reflexprikkelbaarheid en peesreflexen aan de verlamde zijde bij cerebrale hemiplegiën. 2 p. l., 88 pp., 2 pl. 8°. *Amsterdam, J. H. & G. van Heteren*, 1879.

van der Meulen (Jacobus). *De inflammatione. 6 l. 4°. *Lugd. Bat., A. Elzevier*, 1682.

vander Meulen (Joh. Engberts). *Stereoscopie bij onvolkomen gezichtsvermogen. 2 p. l., 49 pp. 8°. *Utrecht, P. W. vande Weyer*, [1873].

Meulenbergh (Pet. Joh. Mathias). *De ruptura perinæi. 32 pp., 1 l. 8°. *Halis Sax., typ. Schmidtianis*, 1853. C.

Meuli (Joh.) *Die Veränderungen von Puls und Temperatur bei elevirten Gliedern. [Bern.] 2 p. l., 44 pp., 3 tab. 8°. *Leipzig, J. B. Hirschfeld*, 1882.

Meunier (Albin). *Étude parallèle des globules rouges et blancs du sang et des principaux éléments de l'urine dans quelques maladies aiguës. 66 pp., 3 pl. 4°. *Paris*, 1877, No. 264.

Meunier (Alcide-Félix). *De la contagion et de l'infection, spécialement étudiées dans le choléra. 42 pp. 4°. *Paris*, 1855, No. 205, v. 578.

Meunier (Alexius). *De aphthis. 1783.
In: LOUVAIN Diss. 8°. *Lovanii*, 1796, iii, 105-107.

Meunier (Antonin-Camille). *Contribution à l'étude des paraplégies par troubles de circulation de la moelle. 48 pp. 4°. *Paris*, 1885, No. 26.

Meunier (Augustin). *Doit-on employer l'acide hydrocyanique dans quelques affections de poitrine? 19 pp. 4°. *Paris*, 1823, No. 34, v. 178.

Meunier (Carl). *Zur Casuistik der Amputationen, insbesondere Amputatio femoris. 27 pp. 8°. *Greifswald, F. W. Kunike*, 1873. C.

Meunier (Édouard-Marie-Jules). *Étude sur la fièvre typhoïde à rechutes. 92 pp., 1 pl. 4°. *Paris*, 1883, No. 24.

Meunier (Ernst). *Statistik der chirurgischen Klinik zu Greifswald für das Sommersemester 1874, mit besonderer Berücksichtigung einzelner Fälle. 39 pp. 8°. *Greifswald, F. W. Kunike*, 1874.

Meunier (Félix)[1]. *Sur l'amputation du bras dans son articulation avec l'omoplate. 23 pp. 4°. *Paris*, 1815, No. 28, v. 108.

Meunier (Félix)[2]. *Considérations sur l'hépatite et les abcès du foie. 27 pp. 4°. *Paris*, 1850, No. 140, v. 499.

Meunier (Georges). *Du syphilome, ou gomme en nappe de la cavité buccale. 94 pp. 4°. *Paris*, 1882, No. 56.

Meunier (J.) *De la congestion pulmonaire dans les occlusions intestinales. 40 pp. 4°. *Paris*, 1878, No. 218.

Meunier (J.-A.-Alexandre). *Hémorrhagie produite par la lésion des intercostales; moyens proposés pour l'arrêter; ligature de ces artères. 34 pp. 4°. *Paris*, 1861, No. 111.

———. *Traitements chirurgicaux des collections de liquides qui se forment dans le thorax. 150 pp. 4°. *Paris*, 1861, No. 204.

Meunier (Jules). *Essai critique sur l'ictère des femmes enceintes à propos de l'épidémie de Paris, 1871-2. 64 pp. 4°. *Paris*, 1872, No. 213.

Meunier (Jules-Étienne-Ernest). *De l'atrophie des nerfs et des papilles optiques dans ses rapports avec les maladies du cerveau. 58 pp. 4°. *Paris*, 1864, No. 227.

Meunier (Léon). *Notes pour servir à l'histoire de la chorée vulgaire chez les vieillards. 38 pp. 4°. *Paris*, 1879, No. 299.

Meunier (Marie). *I. Tracer les caractères des ordres de la famille des rubiacées, désignées sous le nom d'aspérulées et de cinchonées. Faire l'histoire abrégée des médicaments fournis par ces deux ordres. II. [etc.] 36 pp. 4°. *Paris*, 1838, No. 332, v. 331.

Meunier (Théodore). *Étude sur l'affection vermineuse. 42 pp. 4°. *Paris*, 1867, No. 132.

Meunier (V.)
See **Coste** (Jean-Jacques-Marie-Cyprien-Victor). Embryogénie comparée [etc.] (Atlas.) fol. *Paris*, 1837.

Meunier (Valery). *Compte rendu d'une mission médicale au Guadarrama (Espagne). 54 pp. 4°. *Paris*, 1863, No. 21 & 24.

Meunier-Quéaux (Camille). *D'une anomalie rare dans la conformation de la matrice (uterus duplex semipartitus, globularis, bicollis). 54 pp., 1 pl., 1 l. 4°. *Paris*, 1879, No. 356.

Meurchin.

Mialhe. Rapport sur l'eau de Meurchin (Pas-de-Calais). Bull. Acad. de méd., Par., 1872, 2. s., i, 179.

Meurdefroy (Paul-Michel). * Sur les affections chroniques des reins. vi, 7–47 pp. 4°. *Paris*, 1823, No. 36, v. 178.

Meurein (Victor). Observations météorologiques faites à Lille, pendant les années 1855–6; 1858–9; 1866–7; 1878–9. 8°. *Lille, L. Danel*, 1857–80.
Repr. from: Rap. trav. Cons. centr. de salub. du dép. du Nord, Lille, 1855–66, 58; 166.

Meurer (Carl). * Ueber Krankheiten der Circulationsorgane bei Glaukom. 44 pp. 8°. *Würzburg, Becker*, 1884.

Meurer (Christophorus). Ein kurtz nützlich Haussregiment, darinnen gründtlichen vermeldet und angezeiget wird, wie ein Haussvater sich und sein Gesind vor der schrecklichen Seuche der Pestilentz hüten soll, oder, so jemandes von derselben angriffen, wie ihm zu Rettung seines Lebens vermittels Götlicher Gnaden zu helffen, und da auch letzlichen eines oder mehr aus einem Hause gestorben, das es nicht weiter einreisse, und ferner mehr schaden thun möge. Auff anordnung und väterliche Vorsorge eines Ehrnvesten Hochweisen Raths der stadt Leiptzig, gemeiner Bürgerschafft zu besondern nutz und frommen, mit allem trewen gebührenden fleisz gestellet. 3 p. l., 38 pp., 1 l. 4°. *Leiptzig, A. Lamberg*, 1598.
Bound with: SPREMBERG (J.) Kurtzer Bericht von zweyerley Geschlecht der pestilentischen Febern. 4°. *Bresslav*, 1568.

Meurer (Franciscus) [1808–   ]. * De vi atque potestate graviditatis in morbis. 32 pp. 8°. *Berolini, typ. Nietackianis*, [1835].

Meurer (Fridericus) Themata disputationis ordinariæ de vertigine, proposita a Francisco Kest. 10 l. sm. 4°. *Lipsiæ, J. Glück*, [1621].

Meurer (Fridericus) [1792–   ]. * De vitandis in præscribendo mercurio sublimato corrosivo vitiis. 31 pp. 4°. *Lipsiæ, lit. Staritzii*, [1826].
For Biography, see **Kuehn** (Carolus Gottlob.)

Meurer (Martin). * Beobachtungen über Febris recurrens. 30 pp. 8°. *Würzburg, Becker*, 1881.

Meurer (Paulus). * Quæstiones de contagiositate syphilidis secundariæ. 27 pp. 8°. *Gryphiæ, F. Hache*, 1859.

Meurer (Joannes Gottfridus Josephus). * De quadruplici hydrope in uno subjecto observato. 27 pp., 1 l. sm. 4°. *Erfordiæ, typ. J. C. Heringii*, [1745].

Meurer (Wolfgang) [1513–85]. De recta medendi ratione. Respondente Georgio Masbachio. Disputatio. 11 l. 4°. *Lipsiæ, J. Rhamba*, 1562.
For Portrait, see **Collection**—van Kaathoven.

von Meurers (Ludwig) [1849–   ]. * Die hämorrhagische Diathese und ihr Vorkommen bei Recurrens. 31 pp. 8°. *Berlin, M. Niethe*, [1873].

Meurers (Petrus Henricus). * De kyesteinio. 29 pp, 1 l. 8°. *Bonnæ, C. Krüger*, 1853.

Meurgey (Henri). * I. Des causes de la mort après la cystotomie périnéale. II. [etc.] 61 pp. 4°. *Paris*, 1845, No. 186, v. 435.

Meurin (Victor).
See **Nord** (*Département du*). Observations météorologiques. 8°. *Lille*, 1857–68.

Meuriot (André-Isidore). * De la méthode physiologique en thérapeutique et de ses applications à l'étude de la belladone. 164 pp. 4°. *Paris*, 1868, No. 68.

———. The same. Études de thérapeutique expérimentale. 159 pp. 8°. *Paris, P. Asselin*, 1868.

Meurisse (*Henricus Emmanuel.*) [– 1694].
Portrait in: **Collection**—van Kaathoven.

Meurissé (J.-L.-A.) * Quelques considérations générales sur les névroses et sur la méthode réfrigérante. 32 pp. 4°. *Paris*, 1836, No. 196, v. 299.

Meurisse (Martial - Xavier - Joseph). * Sur la tumeur et la fistule lacrymales. 24 pp. 4°. *Paris*, 1835, No. 180, v. 287.

Meurs.

See **Insane** (*Asylums for, etc.*), *by localities.*

Meurs (Alfred). * Des accidents qui peuvent suivre les opérations. 27 pp. 4°. *Paris*, 1850, No. 94, v. 499.

van Meurs (Lambertus Lucas). * Diss. inaug. sive systematis vasorum absorbentium succincta descriptio. 2 p. l., 52 pp., 3 l. 4°. *Harderovici, J. Mojen*, [1786]. [*Also, in :* P., v. 1477; 1578.]

van Meurs (Petrus). * De natura morbi a Thucydide descripti. 2 p. l., 107 pp. 8°. *Lugd. Bat., H. W. Hazenberg et soc.*, 1843.

Meurs (Rudolphus). * Remediorum quorundam externorum apparatum exhibens selectiorem. 1 p. l., 66 pp., 2 l. 4°. *Lugd. Bat., L. Herdingh*, 1793. [*Also, in :* P., v. 1479.]

Meursinge (Hendrik). * Verslag der verloskundige kliniek en polikliniek aan de Rijks-Universiteit te Leiden gedurende den cursus 1879–1880. 1 p. l., 83 pp. 8°. *Leiden, S. C. van Doesburgh*, 1881.

Meursinge (N.) Ontleedkundig onderzoek over eene aangeborene misvorming der beide handen. 23 pp., 4 pl. 4°. *Amsterdam, C. G. van der Post*, 1858.

Meursius (Joannes).
See **Antigonus** *Carystius*. Historiarum mirabilium collectanea [etc.] sm. 4°. *Lugd. Bat.*, 1619.—**Phlegontis** *Tralliani* quæ extant, opuscula [etc.] sm. 4°. *Lugd. Bat.*, 1620.

Meurthe (*Département de la*). Assistance publique. Rapports annuels sur le service départemental de l'assistance médicale et de la vaccine de Meurthe-et-Moselle. Lus au Comité central de l'assistance médicale et de vaccine. Par Edmond Simonin, directeur du service. 1., 1855; 6., 1860; 10.–12., 1864–66; 16., 1870; 25., 1879; 27., 1881. 8°. *Nancy*, 1856–82.
Reports for 1860, 1864–6, 1870, 1879, and 1881 contain 18., 22.–24., 28., 37., and 39., on vaccination.

———. Règlement relatif au service de l'assistance médicale et au service de la vaccine de la Meurthe. [20 mai 1869.] 28 pp. 8°. *Nancy, N. Collin*, 1869.

Meurthe (*Département de la*).

See **Cholera** (*Asiatic, History, etc., of*), *by localities.*

Meurthe - et - Moselle (*Département de*).

Assistance (L') médicale dans le département de Meurthe-et-Moselle, pendant l'année 1877. Rev. méd. de l'est, Nancy, 1878, x, 289–292.

Meurthe-et-Moselle (*Département de*). Rapports généraux sur les travaux des conseils d'hygiène publique et de salubrité du département de Meurthe-et-Moselle, pendant les années 1850–80. In 16 v. 8°. *Nancy*, 1852–81.
v. 1, by E. Simonin; 2 and 3, by L. Parisot; 4–11, by Demange; 12, by É. Claude; 13–16, by E. Delcominete.

Meuschen (F. C.)
See **Delius** (H. F.) Natuur- en geneeskundige verhandeling [etc.] 8°. *Amsterdam*, 1777.

Meuschen (Joh. Gerhardus). Disquisitio philologica de ritu salutandi sternutantes. Resp. Vito Henrico Hasenmüller. 24 pp. 4°. *Kiloni, lit. B. Reutheri*, [1704].

Meuse (*Département de la*). Rapports sur les travaux du Conseil d'hygiène publique et de salubrité du département de la Meuse, par Ach. Henriot, depuis le 1er août 1855 jusqu'au 1er août 1864. 2 v. in 1. 2 p. l., 140 pp., 5 tab. ; 2 l., 112 pp., 4 tab. 8°. *Bar-le-Duc, N. Rollin,* 1860–65.

Meusel (Christianus). De balneis veterum valetudinis caussa adhibitis. 32 pp. 4°. *Vitembergæ, ex off. Meyeriana,* [1611?]

Meusel (E.) * Osteopsathyrosis. 38 pp. 8°. *Würzburg, C. W. Becker,* 1840.

Meusel (Ernst). * Zur Lehre von den Folgen der Bronchectasie. 27 pp., 1 l. 8°. *Jena, J. Hermsdorf,* 1866. [P., v. 270.]

———. Die Krankheiten des Fusses.
In: HANDB. d. Kinderkr. (Gerhardt), Tübing., 1880, vi, 2. Abth., 553–618.

Meusell (Joannes Gottlob.) * Diss. sistens operationis hydrosarcoceles et hydro-hæmatoceles historiam. 18 pp. 4°. *Gottingæ, lit. Grapianis,* [1804].

Meusnier (Auguste). * De l'action de la digitale sur la fonction glycogénique. 44 pp. 4°. *Paris,* 1868, No. 269.

Meusnier (François). * Considérations générales sur l'hystérie. vi, 7–25 pp. 4°. *Paris,* 1817, No. 77, v. 131.

Meusnier (François-Paul-Émile). * De la dysenterie épidémique et de l'emploi des purgatifs salins dans le traitement de cette maladie. 25 pp. 4°. *Paris,* 1830, No. 99, v. 232.

Meusnier (Paul). * Étude sur la suette miliaire. 66 pp. 4°. *Paris,* 1872, No. 218.

Meuth (Camille). * Ueber das Fieber im Allgemeinen und dessen besondere Formen. 1 p. l., 82 pp. 8°. *Mainz, F. Kupferberg,* 1822.

———. Ueber die Wirkungen und den Gebrauch der Dampfbäder als Gesundheitserhaltungs- und Heilmittel. Nach eigenen und anderer Erfahrungen und mit besonderer Beziehung auf deren Anwendung gegen die ostindische Cholera. viii, 57 pp. 8°. *Zweibrücken, G. Ritter,* 1832.

Meuvret (Théophile-Victor). * Étude sur la pleurésie, particulièrement sur ses phénomènes physiques. 47 pp. 4°. *Paris,* 1863, No. 110.

Meverell.
See [**Pechey** (John)]. Some observations made upon the Blatta bizantina. sm. 4°. *London,* 1694.

Mewers (Jo. Frid. Aug.) * De hydrophobia. 32 pp., 2 l. 8°. *Halæ, formis F. Grunerti,* [1824].

Mewis (Christian). * Ueber puerperale Erkrankungen in der Strassburger Entbindungsanstalt. 63 pp., 19 ch. roy. 8°. *Strassburg, R. Schultz u. Comp.,* 1874.

Mexborough. Annual reports of the medical officer of health, for the urban sanitary district of Mexborough, for the years 1878 ; 1880. 12°. *Mexborough,* 1879–81.
1878; 1880, by Wm. Sykes.

———. *See, also:*
THORNE (T.) Report on the sanitary condition of Mexborough, with special reference to the prevalence of infectious diseases there. April, 1873. fol. *London,* 1873.

Mexia (L. M.) Tratado téorico-práctico de las enfermedades de los ojos, ó de las experiencias, observaciones y operaciones sobre las enfermedades que afligen este órgano. 2 v. ix, 235 pp., 1 tab., 2 l. ; 263 pp., 1 pl., 2 l. 12°. *Valladolid, H. Santander,* 1814.

Mexican *war.*
See **Medicine** (*Military, History of*) — *Campaigns, etc.*

Mexico. Instruccion formada para ministrar la vacuna, como único preservativo del contagio de las viruelas, y en defecto de su fluido inocular

Mexico—continued.
con el pus de esta ; del modo de conocer y distinguir las calidades de las naturales, y el método de curarlas. 25 pp. 12°. *México, M. Ontiveros,* 1814.

———. Army. Memoria del secretario de estado y del despacho de guerra y marina. 45 pp., 13 tab. 4°. *México, V. G. Torres,* 1845.

———. Reglamento del cuerpo médico - militar, espedido en virtud del decreto de 12 de Febrero de 1846. 23 pp., 10 l. roy. 8°. *México, establecimiento tipog. de Minerva,* 1846.

———. Cuerpo médico-militar. Detall del mismo. Parte que el que suscribe rinde al ciudadano subinspector del cuerpo como gefe del detall del expresado. México, Octubre 2 de 1871. pp. 391–396; 404–408. fol. [*México,* 1871?]
Cutting from: Revista militar.

———. Reports of the committee of investigation sent in 1873 by the Mexican government to the frontier of Texas. Transl. from the official edition made in Mexico. viii, 473 pp., 3 maps. 8°. *New York, Baker & Godwin,* 1875.

———. Memoria que el secretario de estado y del despacho de gobernacion presenta al Congreso de la Union, correspondiente al tiempo trascurrido desde el 15 de Diciembre de 1877 hasta de 31 de Diciembre de 1878. fol. *México,* 1879.
Contains 94 documents, each with separate pagination.

———. Secretaria de estado y del despacho de gobernacion. Resúmen general de la mortalidad habida en la ciudad de México durante el año de 1879 en los ocho cuarteles mayores que la componen, formado por el Consejo superior de salubridad del distrito federal. 1 sheet imp. broadside 4°. [*México,* 1880.]

———. Anales del ministerio de fomento de la República mexicana. Tomo 3. pp. 185–687. 8°. *México,* 1880.
Incomplete.

———. Boletin del Consejo superior de salubridad del distrito federal. 1.–3., Julio de 1880 á diciembre de 1883. fol. *México,* 1880–85.

———. República mexicana. Biblioteca de la secretaria de guerra y marina. Primera serie. Departamento del cuerpo médico. Reglamento para el servicio de hospitales militares, ambulancias y enfermerías en los cuarteles. 55 pp. fol. *México, I. Cumplido,* 1880.

———. República mexicana. Biblioteca de la secretaria de guerra y marina. Primera serie. Departamento del cuerpo médico. Reglamento general del cuerpo médico-militar. 50 pp. fol. *México, G. A. Esteva,* 1880.
Bound with preceding.

———. Medidas preservativas del cólera asiático que se han de poner en práctica en la República mexicana. 21 pp. 12°. [*México,* 1887.]

Mexico.
See, also, **Aguas** *calientes* ; **Anahuac** ; **Army** (*Mexican*) ; **Cholera** (*Asiatic, History, etc., of*), **Education** (*Medical*), etc., **Fever** (*Cerebro-spinal, History, etc., of*), **Fever** (*Malarial, History, etc., of*), **Fever** (*Typhoid, History, etc., of*), **Fever** (*Typhus, History, etc., of*), **Fever** (*Yellow, History, etc., of*), *by localities* ; **Guadalajara** ; **Hospitals** (*Descriptions, etc., of*), *by localities* ; **Irapuato** ; **Leprosy** (*History, etc., of*) ; **Medicine** (*History, etc., of*), *by nations, etc.* ; **Medicine** (*Military, History of*)—*Campaigns, etc.* ; **Merida** ; **Mexico** (*City of*) ; **Nervous** *system* (*Diseases of, Causes of*) ; **Orizaba** ; **Pharmacopœias** ; **Prostitution** (*History, etc., of*), *by localities* ; **Puebla** ; **Saltillo** ; **San Luis Potosi** ; **Vera Cruz.**

BONTE (A.) * Relation topographique et médicale d'une campagne sur les côtes occidentales du Mexique. 4°. *Montpellier,* 1866.

Mexico.

CUADRO que demuestra las diversas afecciones que causaron la mortalidad habida eu la ciudad de México durante el mes de setiembre de 1879, formado por el Consejo superior de salubridad del distrito federal. imp. fol. [*México*, 1879?]

DUGÈS (E.) *De l'influence du climat des altitudes mexicaines sur l'organisme humain. 4°. *Paris*, 1865.

GONZALEZ & AVENDAÑO (F.) Pachelion Marianum Mexici conspicuum suburbiis. 4°. *Mexici*, 1757.

GONZALEZ (E.) Cuadro gráfico comparativo por enfermedades, de las defunciones habidas en la municipalidad de México, el año de 1885. 1 chart, broadside. [*México*, 1886.]

JOURDANET (D.) Le Mexique et l'Amérique tropicale; climats, hygiène et maladies. 8°. *Paris*, 1864.

LARREY (F.-H.), *le baron*. Commission scientifique du Mexique. Programme d'instructions sommaires sur la médecine. 8°. *Paris*, 1864.

PEÑAFIEL (A.) Memoria sobre las aguas potables de la capital de México. 4°. *México*, 1884.

——. Nombres geográficos de México. Catálogo alfabético de los nombres de lugar pertenecientes al idioma "Nahuatl". Estudio jeroglífico de la matrícula de los tributos del Códice Mendocino. Dibujos de las "Antigüedades mexicanas" de Lord Kingsborough por el Sr. D. Carral y grabados por el Sr. A. H. Galaviz. fol. *México*, 1885.

POMMIER (C.-L.-F.) *Relation médicale d'une campagne dans le golfe du Mexique. 4°. *Montpellier*, 1868.

Beni (C.) Notizie sopra gli indigeni di México. Arch. per l' antrop., Firenze, 1882, xii, 1–17. *Also*, Reprint.—Buez (A.) Lettres médicales sur le Mexique. Gaz. hebd. de méd.. Par., 1862, ix, 737; 769; 785: 1863, x, 1; 17.—Charnay (D.) La civilisation toltèque. Rev. d'ethnog., Par., 1885, iv, 281–305.—Coindet (L.) Études statistiques sur le Mexique. Gaz. hebd. de méd., Par., 1864, 2. s., i, 129; 161; 234; 265; 371; 450; 545; 579; 674: 1865, 2. s., ii, 467. ——. De l'influence des altitudes sur les fièvres intermittentes, les diarrhées, les dyssenteries contractées dans les terres chaudes du Mexique. Rec. de mém. de méd.. mil., Par., 1866, 3. s., xvii, 273–303. ——. Climatologie ou climat des altitudes du Mexique. Phénomènes météorologiques. *Ibid.*, 1868. 3. s., xxi, 1–43. ——. Physiologie. De la respiration et de la circulation sur les altitudes du Mexique. *Ibid.*, 193; 290. ——. Hygiène des altitudes du Mexique. *Ibid.*, 1869, 3. s., xxii, 189; 273. ——. Le Mexique considéré au point de vue médico-chirurgical. Bull. Soc. méd. d'émulat. de Par., 1868–74, ii, 295; 372.—De la Torre (M.) La salubridad de México. An. Asoc. Larrey, México, 1876. ii, 172–181.—Didama (H. D.) Health resorts of Mexico. N. York M. J., 1886, xliv, 426. *Also:* Tr. Am Climat. Ass. 1886, N. Y., 1887, iii, 198–202.—Ehrmann. Géographie médicale; la route de Vera-Cruz à Mexico. Gac. méd. de México, 1864, i, 92–97.—G. (J.) Une expédition au Mexique de San-Luis dans les terres chaudes du Tamaulipas, ou journées de marche de la colonne Delloye dans cette contrée. Gaz. méd. de Par., 1868. 3. s., xxiii, 15; 159; 191; 703.—García (C.) Influencias meteorologicas en México, para el desarollo de ciertas enfermedades y en particular las intermitentes. Estudio, México, 1876, i, 256–263.—Guillard (A.) Mexique. Dict. encycl. d. sc. méd., Par., 1873, 2. s., vii, 464–498.—Hamy (E.-T.) Note sur une inscription chronographique de la fin de la période aztèque, appartenant au Musée du Trocadéro. Rev. d'ethnog., Par., 1883, ii, 193–202. ——. Commentaire sur un bas-relief aztèque de la collection Uhde. *Ibid.*, 438–451.—Heinemann (C.) Von der mexikanischen Expedition. Arch. f. path. Anat., etc., Berl. 1867, xxxix, 607–617.—Hester (A.) Medical and miscellaneous notes and observations in Mexico. N. Orl. M. & S. J., 1855-6, xii, 166–175.—Jourdanet. De la statistique du Mexique dans ses rapports avec l'acclimatement des différentes races humaines qui l'habitent. Gaz. méd. de Par., 1864, 3. s., xix, 438; 467; 484. ——. Études médicales sur le Mexique. Reponse à M. Coindet. Gaz. hebd. de méd.. Par., 1865, 2. s., ii, 145–151.—Lobato (J. G.) Meteorologia de México. Observador méd., México, 1874-6, iii, 42–48. ——. Consideraciones geográfico-higienicas sobre el territorio de México. *Ibid.*, 67–70. ——. De la alimentacion de las razas indigenas de México. comparada con la alimentacion adoptada por las razas criolla y extran-

Mexico.

jera. *Ibid.*, 170; 187; 205; 221. ——. Meteorología del valle de México. Desde el año de 1875. *Ibid.*, 1877, iv, 173–177.—McSherry (R.) Mexico and Mexican affairs. *In his:* Essays & Lect., 8°, Balt., 1869, 31–63.—Maler (T.) Notes sur la basse Mistèque. Rev. d'ethnog., Par., 1883, ii, 154–161, 1 pl. ——. Mémoire sur l'état de Chiapa (Mexique). *Ibid.*, 1884, iii, 295–342.—Mejía (D.) Estadística de mortalidad en México. Gac. méd. de México, 1879, xiv, 273–301, 3 tab. *Also*, Reprint.—Mendoza (G.) Agua sulfurosa potasso-sodica de la quinta Belendez. Gac. méd. de México, 1876, xi, 377.—Mendoza (G.) & Herrera (A.) Estudio sobre el origen del cloruro de sodio y el carbonato de sosa en el valle de México. *Ibid.*, 1866, ii, 85–91.—Noriega (T.) Apuntes sobre la beneficencia pública en México. Rev. méd.-quir. de México, 1883, i, no. 2, 4–7.—Olvera (J.) Corto ensayo sobre una constitucion médica especial de la primavera en México. Observador méd., México, 1873, i, 217–226.—Orvañanos (D.) Apuntes para el estudio del clima de México. Gac. méd. de México, 1879, xiv, 153; 198, 3 diag., 1 plan.—Schleiden (M. J.) Ueber Früchte, Gemüse und Droguen an der Westküste von Mexico. Jenaische Ann. f. Physiol. u. Med., Jena, 1850, i, 99–103.—Schmidt (H.) Briefe aus Mexico. Med. Cor.-Bl. d. württemb. ärztl. Ver., Stuttg., 1867, xxxvii, 253; 258; 285; 293; 301; 316; 333; 341; 349.—Soriano (M. S.) Itinerario de México á Morelia por Toluca. Gac. méd. de México, 1869, iv, 119–128.—Stricker (W.) Natur- und Heilkunde in Mexico. Ein Beitrag zur medicinischen Geographie. Ztschr. f. d. ges. Med., Hamb., 1847, xxxiv, 520–533.—Yule (A.) Medical topography of the coast of Mexico. Statist. Rep. Health Navy 1886, Lond., 1868, 174–176.

Mexico (*City of*).

See, also, Education (*Medical*), *etc.,* Fever (*Malarial, History, etc., of*), Hospitals (*Descriptions, etc., of*), Insane (*Asylums for, etc.*), *by localities.*

Lobato (J. G.) Meteorologia y constitucion médica de la capital, en los cuatro primeros meses del año. Observador méd., México, 1874-6, iii, 71.—Newton (R.) Medical topography of the city of Mexico. N. York J. M., 1848, i, 295–307.—Ortega (A.) Nota sobre el Hospicio de Pobres, considerado bajo el punto de vista de su salubridad. Gac. méd. de México, 1864-5, i, 499–509.—Pasalagua (M. A.) Algunas observaciones higiénicas sobre la ciudad de México, relativamente á los lagos que la rodean. *Ibid.*, 1873, viii, 45–55.—Peaslee (E. R.) Mexico as a residence for invalids. Med. Rec., N. Y., 1876, xi, 273; 290; 308; 835.—Reyes (J. M.) Estadística de mortalidad en la capital. Gac. méd. de México, 1864-5, i, 136.—Ruiz y Sandoval (G.) ¿Cual es la influencia patogénica que tienen los lagos sobre la ciudad de México? *Ibid.*, 1873, viii, 65–76.—Semeleder. Rapport sur les malades qui se sont présentés à la consultation gratuite donnée par les docteurs Schmidtlein et Semeleder, dans l'espace des derniers deux ans et trois mois. *Ibid.*, 1874, ix, 26; 46.—Strother (D. H.) Climate and health of the city of Mexico. Rep. Consuls U. S. on commerce, etc., Wash., 1881, No. iii, 16–21.

Mexico seeds.

PECHEY (J.) Some observations made upon the Mexico seeds, imported from the Indies, shewing their wonderful virtue against worms in the bodies of men, women, and children. Written by a countrey physitian to Dr. Burwell, president of the Colledge of Physitians in London. sm. 4°. *London*, 1695.

de Mey (Aloïse-François). *Recherches sur quelques affections chroniques de l'estomac. 32 pp. 4°. *Paris*, 1828, No. 50, v. 214.

Mey (Ernest). *Des rapports de la pleurésie et de la tuberculose. 43 pp., 3 tab. 4°. *Paris*, 1877, No. 421.

de Mey (Franciscus). *De mutatione sententiæ. 35 pp., 2 l. 4°. *Lugd. Bat., S. Luchtmans et fil.*, 1748. [P., v. 993.]

van der Mey (Gerrit Hendrik) jr. *De leer der ademhaling, historisch-kritisch toegelicht. [Utrecht.] 2 p. l., vi, 220 pp. 8°. *Amsterdam, Metzler & Basting*, 1876.

Mey (Joannes) [1619–78]. De admirando dextræ tubæ uterinæ hydrope. 5 l., 1 pl. 4°. *Ultrajecti, ex off. A. ab Eynden*, 1678.

For Biography, see Bayle (P.) Hist. & Crit. Dict. 2. ed. fol. *London*, 1737, iv, 179.

Mey (Léonard). *Sur le creux de l'aisselle. vi, 7–30 pp. 4°. *Paris*, 1817, No. 63, v. 131.

Mey (Max). Zur Aetiologie und Therapie der Lungenschwindsucht. 26 pp. 8°. *Leipzig, C. L. Hirschfeld*, 1875.

Mey (Philipp). *See* **May** (Philipp).

Meybachius (Joannes Godofred.) * Meditationes de inventione remediorum. 32 pp., 1 pl. sm. 4°. *Vitembergæ, ex off. Schlomachiana*, [1729].

Meyburg (Heinrich). * Ueber Milzbrand. 2 p. l., 31 pp. 8°. *Bonn, C. Georgi*, 1875.

Meye (Bruno). * Ueber Puerperal - Eclampsie. 29 pp., 1 l. 8°. *Halle, W. Plötz*, [1869].

Meye (Robertus Samuelis). * Abscessus pelvis subperitonæalis casus duo. 33 pp. 8°. *Halis Sax., formis Ploetzianis*, 1863. c.

Meyen (Franz Julius Ferdinand) [–1840]. * De primis vitæ phænomenis in fluidis formativis et de circulatione sanguinis in parenchymate. 27 pp. 4°. *Berolini, typ. Brueschckiänis*, 1826.

——. Untersuchungen über die Natur parasitischer Geschwülste im menschlichen Körper, insbesondere über den Mark- und Blutschwamm. 99 pp. 8°. *Berlin, Hirschwald*, 1828.

——. The same. An enquiry into the nature of parasitic tumors in general, and particularly those called medullary sarcoma and fungus hæmatodes. 52 pp. 16°. *Dublin, J. M. Leckie*, 1829.

——. A report on the progress of vegetable physiology during the year 1837. Transl. from the German, by William Francis. iv, 160 pp. 8°. *London, R. & J. E. Taylor*, 1839.

Meyen (Georg). * Ueber Icterus als Complication der croupösen Pneumonie. 46 pp. 8°. *Greifswald, C. Sell*, 1881.

Meyen (*Julius*).
Portrait in : **Collection**—van Kaathoven.

Meyenberg (Fridericus Conradus). * De spasmis eorumque quadruplici respectu. 53 pp., 1 l. 4°. *Halæ Magdeb., typ. J. C. Hilligeri*, [1754].

Meyenberg (Friederich Gabriel). * De hæmorrhoidibus hæreditariis. 36 pp., 2 l. sm. 4°. *Halæ Magdeb., lit. Hendelianis*, [1727]. [*Also, in :* P., v. 72.]

von Meyendorff (Fr.) * Einfluss des jugendlichen Alters auf die strafrechtliche Zurechnung. 47 pp. 8°. *Zürich, D. Bürkli*, 1862. c.

Meyer (A.)
Anatomische Charakteristik officineller Blätter und Kräuter. Abhandl. d. naturf. Gesellsch. zu Halle, 1882, xv, 445–497.

Meyer (Achille-Abraham). * Pseudo - paralysie générale d'origine saturnine. 42 pp. 4°. *Paris*, 1881, No. 325.

Meyer (Adamus Henricus). * Quædam de recto emeticorum usu. 18, 11 pp. 4°. *Lipsiæ, ex off. G. T. Hoehmii*, [1832].
For Biography, see **Kuehn** (Carolus Gottlob.)

Meyer (Adolf). * Ein Fall von Extrauterinschwangerschaft mit glücklichem Ausgang. 22 pp. 8°. *Erlangen, Junge u. Sohn*, 1874.

Meyer (Adolf Bernhard). * Beiträge zur Lehre von der elektrischen Nervenreizung. 35 pp. 8°. *Zürich, Zürcher u. Furrer*, 1867.

——. Das Hemmungsnervensystem des Herzens. Kritisches und Experimentelles. viii, 95 pp. 8°. *Berlin, A. Hirschwald*, 1869.

Meyer (Adolph Ludwig). * De causis quibusdam convulsionum imprimis vero animi affectibus immoderatis occasionalibus. 24 pp. 4°. *Gryphiswaldiæ, A. F. Röse*, 1773. [P., v. 59.]

Meyer (Adolphus)[1]. * De hepatis abscessibus. 30 pp. 8°. *Regiomonti Pr., typ. Dalkowskianis*, 1860. c.

Meyer (Adolphus)[2]. * Iridectomia quam vim habeat ad sanandas oculorum inflammationes, necnon ad tollenda mechanica visus impedimenta casibus nonnullis demonstratur. 24 pp. 4°. *Kiliæ, C. F. Mohr*, 1860.
In : SCHRIFT. d. Univ. zu Kiel, vii, 1860, vii, med. iii.

Meyer (Adolphus)[3] [1837–]. * De nephritide chronica post scarlatinam. 30 pp., 1 l. 8°. *Regimonti Pr., typ. Dalkowskianis*, 1863. c.

Meyer (Arminius). * De atrophia musculorum progressiva. 31 pp. 8°. *Regiomonti Pr., typ. Dalkowskianis*, 1858. c.

Meyer (August)[1]. Heil- und Pflege-Anstalt für Nerven-Kranke zu Eitorf a. d. Sieg. [Prospectus.] 2 l. 8°. [*Eitorf*, 1876.]

Meyer (August)[2] [1860–]. * Experimentelle Studien über den Einfluss des Ozons auf das Gehirn. 40 pp., 1 l. 8°. *Bonn, C. Georgi*, 1883.

Meyer (August Hermann). * Ueber die Gastrotomie. 38 pp., 1 l. 8°. *Leipzig, L. Schnauss*, [1862].

Meyer (Auguste). * Essai de quelques complications des plaies pénétrantes de poitrine. 1 p. l., 28 pp. 4°. *Strasbourg*, 1830, v. 61.

Meyer (Augustus). * De pachymeningitide cerebro-spinali interna. 56 pp. 8°. *Bonnæ, P. Neusser*, 1861. c.

Meyer (Augustus Bruno). * De tetano traumatico. 15 pp. 8°. *Jenæ, typ. A. Neuenhahni*, [1862].

Meyer (Augustus Eduardus). * De variolis modificatis. 47 pp. 8°. [*Dorpat*], *typ. Schünmanni*, 1827.

Meyer (Augustus Guilielmus). * Diss. sistens cogitata quædam de febre sic dicta puerperali, adnexa historia morbi punctione sanati. 36 pp. 4°. *Giessæ, typ. Braunii academicis*, 1804.

Meyer (Augustus Joannes Theodorus). * Symbolæ ad morbum Brightii. 46 pp., 1 l. 8°. *Halis Sax., typ. Colbatzkii*, [1846].

Meyer ([Augustus Robertus] Eduardus) [1818–]. * De morbosis urinæ alterationibus. 31 pp. 8°. *Berolini, typ. Nietackianis*, [1841].

Meyer (B. J.) Merkwaardige waarnemingen van behandeling en genezing door het dierlijk magnetismus en somnambulismus. Verrijkt met het portret van de somnambule Mejufvrouw Steffens. 1. deel. viii, 111, 135, 152 pp. 8°. *Rotterdam, J. Hendriksen*, 1826.

——. Een woord ter verdediging van het dierlijk magnetismus en somnambulismus tegen F. van der Breggen, Cornz. iv, 112 pp. 8°. *Rotterdam, T. J. Wynhoven & Hendriksen*, 1829.

Meyer (Benedict) [1807–]. * De entozoorum natura et indole. 35 pp., 2 l. 8°. *Berolini, typ. Nietackianis*, [1832].

——. Die Wurmkrankheiten des Menschen mit Versuchen an lebenden Thieren. 2. Aufl. v, 137 pp. 8°. *Leipzig, J. Wallerstein*, 1858.

Meyer (Benno). * Ueber Hysterie. 30 pp., 1 l. 8°. *Bonn, F. Krüger*, 1867.

Meyer (Bernhardus) [1767–1836]. De mercurialium in morbis venereis actione et usu commentatio. 109 pp. 8°. *Marburgi, in nova off. libraria academica*, 1790.
For Biography, see Med. Alm., Berl., 1838 (Nekrolog. Erinnerungen, etc.), 27–34.

Meyer (Bruno). Führer durch die Literatur der Gesundheitspflege, Naturheilkunde, Vegetarismus, Seelendiätetik für Freunde einer naturgemässen Lebensweise in Verbindung mit solchen herausgegeben von . . . 2. Aufl. 72 pp. 16°. *Rudolstadt i. Th., H. Hartung u. Sohn*, [1884].

Meyer (C. G. R.) [Twenty-five original drawings in water colors. Comparative myology.] Bound in 1 v. fol. [*n. p.*, 1840–47.]

Meyer (C.-R.) * I. Des causes des tubercules. II. [etc.] 27 pp. 4°. *Paris*, 1841, No. 274, v. 378.

Meyer (Caïus G.) * De episioraphia Frickiana. 16 pp. 8°. *Kiliæ, C. F. Mohr*, 1842. c.

Meyer (Carl)[1] [1848–]. * Ein Fall von Ulcus simplex in Verbindung mit Carcinom. 31 pp. 8°. *Berlin, G. Lange*, [1874].

Meyer (Carl)[2]. *Beiträge zur acuten Nephritis. 56 pp., 1 pl. 8°. *Strassburg, J. H. E. Heitz*, 1874.

Meyer (Carl)[3]. *I. Einwirkung von Bernstein-säurechlorid auf Acetanilid. II. Zur Kenntniss der Anhydrobasen. [Göttingen.] 30 pp. 8°. *Hannover, Gebr. Jänecke*, 1878.

Meyer (Carl)[4]. *Die Uterusfibroide in der Schwangerschaft, unter der Geburt und im Wochenbett. 82 pp. 8°. *Zürich, Zürcher u. Furrer*, 1887. C.

Meyer (Carl Joseph) [1798–]. Vollständiges Recept-Taschenbuch zur neuesten österr. Pharmakopöe. Für Aerzte und Wundärzte. Supplement zu dessen Handbuche der Pharmakologie als Erläuterung der österr. Pharmakopöe vom Jahre 1834. 1. Abth. x, 682 pp., 1 l. 16°. *Güns, Reichard*, 1836.

——. Pharmakologische Blätter zur Mittheilung und Besprechung des Neuesten und Wissenswerthesten aus dem Gebiete der Arzneimittellehre. Für praktische Aerzte und Wundärzte. vi, 386 pp. 8°. *Güns, C. Reichard*, 1840.

Meyer (Carolus) [1825–]. *Descriptio ossis frontis macrocephali. 29 pp., 2 pl. 8°. *Berolini, J. Plessner*, [1850].

Meyer (Carolus Albertus). *De pneumonia biliosa. 35 pp. 4°. *Lipsiæ, ex off. F. Andræi*, [1841].

For Biography, see **Clarus** (Jo. Christ. Aug.)

Meyer (Carolus Arnoldus). *De eximio ipecacuanhæ nec non aliorum quorundam emeticorum refracta dosi exhibitorum usu. 36 pp. 4°. *Gottingæ, F. A. Rosenbusch*, [1779].

For Biography, see **Murray** (Jo. Andreas).

Meyer (Carolus Fridericus)[1]. *De affectione cœliaca ex viscerum abdominalium infarctu oriunda. 32 pp. 4°. *Traj. ad Viadr., e typog. Apitziano*, [1794].

Meyer (Carolus Fridericus)[2]. *Diss. exhibens tineæ pathologiam. 2 p. l., 38 pp., 1 l. 4°. *Bonnæ, typ. H. Knirenschildi*, [1829].

For Biography, see Allg. Ztschr. f. Psychiat., etc., Berl., 1886, xliii, 331–333 (W. N.).

Meyer (Carolus Gottlieb). De discrimine motus elastici et vitalis fibrarum. 40 pp. 4°. *Altorfii, lit. vid. Meyeriæ*, [1735].

——. *De venæ sectione in hecticis sæpe noxia. 16 pp. 4°. *Altorfii Noricorum, typ. J. G. Meyeri*, [1738].

Meyer (Carolus Hermannus) [1823–]. *De talipede varo et nova correctione machinæ Stromeyerianæ. 31 pp., 1 pl. 8°. *Berolini, G. Schade*, [1846].

Meyer (Charles). *Essai sur les baraquements. 1 p. l., 22 pp. 4°. *Strasbourg, É. Huder*, 1870, 3. s., No. 302.

Meyer (Christian). *Ueber die Exarticulation des Unterschenkels im Kniegelenk. vi, 7–44 pp. 8°. *Würzburg, F. E. Thein*, 1847.

Meyer (Christianus David.) [1791–]. *De inflammationibus infantum internis generatim. 28 pp. 8°. *Berolini, T. Brüschcke*, [1819].

Meyer (Christianus Ludovicus). *De strumis earumque causis atque medela. [Jena.] 24 pp. 8°. *Hannoveræ, typ. L. Pöckwitzii*, [1817].

Meyer (Conradus). *De fissuris hominis mammaliumque congenitis; accedit fissuræ buccalis congenitæ cum fissura tubæ Eustachii et tympani complicatæ descriptio. 3 p. l., 44 pp., 2 l., 4 pl. fol. *Berolini, J. Sittenfeld*, [1835].

Meyer (D. L.) A method of making useful mineral collections. To which are added some experiments on a deliquescent calcareous earth, or native fixed sal ammoniac. 31 pp., 1 pl. 8°. *London, L. Davis*, 1775.

Meyer (Daniel). *De noxa potus frigidi. 22 pp. sm. 4°. *Halæ Magdeb., typ. C. Henckelii*, [1721].

Meyer (David). *De aurium cerumine. 40 pp. sm. 4°. *Argentorati, J. F. Spoor*, [1684].

Meyer (David) [–1835]. *De cerebri tumoribus. 24 pp., 1 pl. 4°. *Berolini, typ. Brüschckianis*, [1829].

Meyer (David) [1808–]. *De signis ex forma pupillæ. 26 pp., 3 l. 8°. *Berolini, F. Nietack*, [1831].

Meyer (Ed.) Direktorialbericht über die Verwaltung der Irren-Heil- und Pflege-Anstalt zu Brake, von der Eröffnung im Jahre 1811 bis Ende 1868. 32 pp. 4°. [*Brake*, 1869.]

——. Die Verwaltung der Heil- und Pflegeanstalt zu Brake. [27. Januar 1869.] pp. 181–187. 4°. [*Brake*, 1869.]

Beilage zu Nr. 13 des Regierungs- und Anzeigeblattes de 1869.

Meyer (Édouard)[1] [1838–]. *Du strabisme et spécialement des conditions de succès de la strabotomie. 112 pp., 2 pl. 4°. *Paris*, 1863, No. 122.

Meyer (Édouard)[2]. Maladies des yeux. Leçons sur la réfraction et l'accommodation professées à l'école pratique de la Faculté de médecine de Paris. Recueillies par le docteur A.-L. Roulet, revues et approuvées par le professeur . . . iv, 270 pp., 1 pl. 8°. *Paris, Chamerot & Lauwereyns*, 1869.

——. The same. Traité pratique des maladies des yeux. 2. éd. xx, 796 pp. 8°. *Paris, G. Masson*, 1880.

——. The same. 3. éd. xvi, 800 pp. 8°. *Paris, G. Masson*, 1887.

——. The same. Tratado práctico de las enfermedades de los ojos. Trad. por D. Pedro M. Brun. vii, 660 pp., 1 l. 8°. *Madrid, Moya y Plaza*, 1875.

——. The same. Handbuch der Augenheilkunde. Ins Deutsche übertragen und bearbeitet von W. Block. vi, 562 pp. 8°. *Berlin, H. Peters*, 1875.

——. The same. 2. Aufl. xvi, 587 pp. 8°. *Berlin, H. Peters*, 1879.

——. The same. 3. Aufl. xvi, 592 pp. 8°. *Berlin, H. Peters*, 1883.

——. The same. 4. Aufl. xviii, 602 pp. 8°. *Berlin, H. Peters*, 1886.

——. The same. A practical treatise on diseases of the eye. Transl., with the assistance of the author, from the 3. French ed., with additions as contained in the 4. German ed., by Freeland Fergus. xi, 637 pp., 1 pl. 8°. *London, C. Griffin & Co.*, 1887.

——. The same. xi (2 l.), 17–647 pp., 3 pl. 8°. *Philadelphia, P. Blakiston, Son & Co.*, 1887.

Also, Co-Editor of: **Revue** générale d'ophthalmologie, Paris, 1882.

—— & **de Montméja** (A.) Traité des opérations qui se pratiquent sur l'œil. viii, 275 pp., 22 phot. pl. 4°. *Paris, H. Lauwereyns*, 1871.

Meyer (Eduard)[1]. *Hepatitis suppurativa hervorgerufen durch Gallensteinbildung. 23 pp. 8°. *Göttingen, W. F. Kaestner*, 1868. C.

Meyer (Eduard)[2] [1859–]. *Ueber Infection durch todtfaule Früchte. 41 pp., 1 l. 8°. *Berlin, E. Müller*, [1883].

Meyer (Eduardus)[1] [1819–]. *De eclampsia parturientium. 27 pp., 2 l. 8°. *Berolini, typ. Nietackianis*, [1844].

Meyer (Eduardus)[2] [1823–]. *De tabe dorsuali. 31 pp. 8°. *Berolini, G. Schade*, [1847].

Meyer (Eduardus)[3]. *Disquisitiones de intoxicatione acuta phosphoro effecta. 47 pp. 8°. *Dorpati Livonorum, typ. E. J. Karowi*, 1861.

Meyer (Eduardus Simon.) *De perforatione fœtus sectione cæsarea. 32 pp. 8°. *Berolini, G. Lange*, [1860].

Meyer (Ernst)[1] [1845–]. *Ueber Fibromyome des Uterus. 32 pp. 8°. *Berlin, G. Lange*, 1871.

von Meyer (Ernst)[2]. * Ueber die in Steinkohlen eingeschlossenen Gase. 42 pp., 1 l. 8°. *Leipzig, Metzger u. Wittig, 1872.*

Meyer (Ernst)[3]. * Ueber rothe und blasse quergestreifte Muskeln. 19 pp. 8°. *Göttingen, W. F. Kaestner, 1875.*

Meyer (Ernst)[4]. * Klinischer Beitrag zur Lehre vom Wundstarrkrampf. 36 pp., 2 l. 8°. *Breslau, T. Schatsky,* [1887].

Meyer (Ernst Julius Jacob). Versuch einer medicinischen Topographie und Statistik der Haupt- und Residenz-Stadt Dresden. xx, 350 pp., 1 map, 3 pl. 4°. *Stolberg am Harz u. Leipzig, B. G. H. Schmidt,* 1840.

Meyer (Eugen). * Kritisch - historische Betrachtungen über Tabes dorsalis. 101 pp. 8°. *Strassburg, R. Schultz u. Comp.,* 1880.

Meyer (F.-E.-Gustave). * I. Des complications de la coqueluche. II. [etc.] 41 pp. 4°. *Paris,* 1841, No. 42, v. 378.

Meyer (F. H.) Aus der Havanna. Erfahrungen und Ansichten über die Fabrikation der ächten Cigarren ; nebst Mittheilungen über Tabackshandel, sowie nützlichen Winken für Fabrikanten zur Erzielung eines vorzüglichen und den Havanna-Cigarren gleichkommenden Frabrikats. 3. Ausg. 1 p. l., 53 pp. 12°. *Bremen, J. Kühtmann,* 1878.

Meyer (Felix) [1841–]. * De phosphoro veneno. 32 pp. sm. 8°. *Berolini, G. Lange,* [1866].

Meyer (Ferdinandus Augustus) [1807–]. * De morborum psychicorum curatione generatiora quædam. 42 pp., 3 l. 8°. *Berolini, F. Nietack,* [1830].

Meyer (Fernand). * De l'influence des émotions morales sur le développement des affections cutanées. 55 pp. 4°. *Paris,* 1876, No. 310.

Meyer (Franz)[1] [1858–]. * Zur Diagnose des Aneurysma arcus aortæ. 31 pp. 8°. *Berlin, L. Schumacher,* 1881.

Meyer (Franz)[2]. * Ein Fall von Echinococcus multilocularis. 36 pp., 1 l. 8°. *Göttingen, W. F. Kästner,* 1881.

Meyer (Frid. Aug.) De ozæna. Commentatio ad ... Matthæum Mederer. 39 pp., 1 pl. 8°. *Hamburgi, B. G. Hofmann,* 1785.
Also, in: Frank (J. P.) Delect. opusc. med. 8°. *Ticini,* 1792, xi, 249–273.

Meyer (Fridericus)[1]. * De operatione cataractæ. 31 pp. 8°. *Erlangæ, typ. Kunstmannianis,* [1810].
For Biography, see **Kühn** (Carolus Gottlob.)

Meyer (Fridericus)[2]. * De tussi convulsiva. 39 pp. sm. 4°. *Lipsiæ, lit. Staritii,* [1822].
For Biography, see **Kühn** (Carolus Gottlob.)

Meyer (Fridericus)[3] [1800–]. * De menstruatione ejusque anomaliis. 51 pp. 8°. *Berolini, formis Brüschckianis,* [1826].

Meyer (Fridericus Augustus). * Diss. sistens progressum digestionis. 98 pp. 8°. [*Dorpat*], *ex off. acad. J. C. Schünmanni,* 1823.

Meyer (Fridericus Guilelmus). * De hernia pulmonali. 31 pp. 8°. *Gryphiæ, F. G. Kunike,* [1843].

Meyer (Fridericus Gustavus) [1809–]. * De tumorum genu natura variisque speciebus. 38 pp., 1 l. 8°. *Berolini, typ. Nietackianis,* [1833].

——. Die Lehre von den Fracturen. xii, 322 pp. 8°. *Berlin, A. Förstner,* 1843.

Meyer (Fridericus Wilhelmus). * De abscessu ad coxam in febribus in lentam degenerantibus. 33 pp. sm. 4°. *Gottingæ, ex off. Schulziana,* [1759].

Meyer (Friedrich) [1852–]. * Ueber Schussverletzungen des Auges. 31 pp. 8°. *Berlin, G. Lange,* [1876].

Meyer (Friedrich Albert Anton) [1768–95]. * De cortice Angusturæ. 53 pp., 1 l. 8°. *Gottingæ, J. C. Dieterich,* [1790].

Meyer (G. M.)
See **Sammlung** auserlesener Recepte der neuesten Zeit. 11 v. 12°. *Erlangen,* 1833-9.

Meyer (Georg)[1]. * Ueber das Vorkommen des Leberzuckers in Krankheiten. [Zürich.] 39 pp. 8°. *Frankfurt a. M., A. Osterrieth,* 1858.

Meyer (Georg)[2]. * Ueber einige künstliche und natürliche Alkaloïde. 30 pp. 8°. *Kiel, P. Peters,* [1880].

Meyer (Georg)[3] [1860–]. * Ein Fall von Carcinoma hepatis idiopathicum. 36 pp. 8°. *Berlin, O. Francke,* [1882].

Meyer (Georg Hermann) [1815–]. * De musculis in ductibus efferentibus glandularum. 34 pp., 2 l. 8°. *Berolini, J. Sittenfeld,* [1837].

——. Untersuchungen über die Physiologie der Nervenfaser. vi, 316 pp. 8°. *Tübingen, H. Laupp,* 1843.

——. Die Phrenologie vom wissenschaftlichen Standpunkte aus beleuchtet. viii, 58 pp., 1 l. 8°. *Tübingen, H. Laupp,* 1844.

——. Lehrbuch der physiologischen Anatomie des Menschen. 2 pts. in 1 v. xviii, 396, 250 pp. 8°. *Leipzig, W. Engelmann,* 1856.

——. The same. 2. Aufl. xvi, 752 pp. 8°. *Leipzig, W. Engelmann,* 1861.

——. The same. 3. Aufl. xvi, 806 pp. 8°. *Leipzig, W. Engelmann,* 1873.

——. Die richtige Gestalt der Schuhe. Eine Abhandlung aus der angewandten Anatomie für Aerzte und Laien geschrieben. iv, 30 pp., 1 l. 8°. *Zürich, Meyer u. Zeller,* 1858.

——. The same. Procrustes ante portas. Why the shoe pinches; a contribution to applied anatomy. Transl. from the German, by John Stirling Craig. xiii, 15–55 pp. 16°. *Edinburgh, Edmonston & Douglas,* 1864.
Chiefly a reprint transl. from v. 2 of: Monatschr. d. Wissensch. Vereinschrift in Zürich, 1857.

——. The same. 24, 14, 4 pp., 4 l., 4 pl. 8°. *Boston, J. C. Plumer,* 1861. [*Also, in:* P., v. 227.]

——. The same. 29 pp., 1 pl. 18°. *New York, G. F. Nesbitt & Co.,* 1877.

——. Anleitung zu den Präparirübungen. Für den Gebrauch von Studirenden. 2. Aufl. viii, 216 pp. 8°. *Leipzig, W. Engelmann,* 1864.

——. The same. 3. Aufl. viii, 219 pp. 8°. *Leipzig, W. Engelmann,* 1873.

——. Die Entstehung unserer Bewegungen. 32 pp. 8°. *Berlin, C. G. Lüderitz,* 1868.

——. Stimm- und Sprachbildung. 32 pp. 8°. *Berlin, C. G. Lüderitz,* 1871.

——. Ueber Sinnestäuschungen. 2. Aufl. 36 pp. 8°. *Berlin, C. G. Lüderitz,* 1871.

——. Die Statik und Mechanik des menschlichen Knochengerüstes. viii, 402 pp. roy. 8°. *Leipzig, W. Engelmann,* 1873.

——. Die richtige Gestalt des menschlichen Körpers in ihrer Erhaltung und Ausbildung für das allgemeine Verständniss. vi (1 l.), 184 pp. 8°. *Stuttgart, Meyer u. Zeller,* 1874.

——. Ueber die Bedeutung des Nervensystems. Ein populärer Vortrag. 36 pp. 8°. *Stuttgart, Meyer u. Zeller,* 1874.

——. Der Mensch als lebendiger Organismus. Ein Hülfsbuch für Lehrer, Seminare und höhere Lehranstalten, sowie zum Selbstunterricht für Jedermann. viii, 330 pp. 8°. *Stuttgart, Meyer u. Zeller,* 1877.

——. Unsere Sprachwerkzeuge und ihre Verwendung zur Bildung der Sprachlaute. x, 367 pp. 12°. *Leipzig, F. A. Brockhaus,* 1880.

——. The same. The international scientific series. The organs of speech, and their application in the formation of articulate sounds. x, 349 pp. 8°. *New York, D. Appleton & Co.,* 1884.

Meyer (Georg Hermann)—continued.
———. William Harvey der Reformator der Physiologie. 32 pp. 8°. *Berlin SW., C. Habel,* 1880.

———. Zur genaueren Kenntniss der Substantia spongiosa der Knochen. 20 pp. 8°. *Stuttgart, J. G. Cotta,* 1882.
Repr. from: Beitr. zur Biologie. Jubiläumsschrift für Geheimerath v. Bischoff.

———. Ursache und Mechanismus der Entstehung des erworbenen Plattfusses, nebst Hinweisung auf die Indikationen zur Behandlung desselben. vi, 52 pp. 8°. *Jena, G. Fischer,* 1883.
1. Hft. of Studien über den Mechanismus.

———. Studien über den Mechanismus des Fusses in normalen und abnormen Verhältnissen. 1. Hft. Der Plattfuss. vi, 52 pp. 8°. *Jena, G. Fischer,* 1883.

———. Statik und Mechanik des menschlichen Fusses. Nach neuen Untersuchungen. vii, 119 pp. 8°. *Jena, G. Fischer,* 1886.
Second title-page of his: Studien über den Mechanismus [etc.] 2. Hft.

———. Studien über den Mechanismus des Fusses in normalen und abnormen Verhältnissen. 2. Hft. vii, 119 pp. 8°. *Jena, G. Fischer,* 1886.

Meyer (Georgius Justus Guilielmus). * De commercio inter hepar et cæterum organismum mutuo. 1 l. 4°. *Gottingæ, J. C. Baier,* [1806].

Meyer (Godofredus). * De fundamentis theoriæ medicæ. 48 pp. 8°. *Halæ Magdeb., lit. C. Henckelii,* [1704].

———. * De tertiana, febris genium universum manifestante. 56 pp. 4°. *Halæ Magdeb., lit. C. Henckelii,* [1706].

———. The same. 56 pp. 4°. *Recusæ Halæ Magdeb., lit. C. Henckelii,* 1715.
For Biography, see **Stahl** (Georgius Ernestus).

Meyer (Gottfried). * Zur Lehre von dem Mechanismus der Brucheinklemmung. 30 pp. 8°. *Bern, G. Michel,* 1878.

Meyer (Gotthelf Lotharius) [1841–82]. * De neonatorum tetano. 30 pp., 1 l. 8°. *Berolini, G. Schade,* 1864.

Meyer (Gustav)[1]. * Ueber Resection and Decapitation. vi, 7–64 pp. 8°. *Erlangen, Kunstmann,* 1829.

Meyer (Gustav)[2]. Handbuch der wundärztlichen Klinik, mit besonderer Rücksicht auf allgemeine Chirurgie und die chirurgischen Operationen. 2 v. x, 517 pp.; xii, 546 pp. 8°. *Berlin, F. A. Herbig,* 1840–41.

Meyer (Gustav)[3] [1841–]. * Ueber Aneurysma. 32 pp. 8°. *Berlin, G. Lange,* [1868].

Meyer (Gustav)[4]. * Ueber die antiseptische Wirksamkeit des Jodoforms. 19 pp. 8°. *Göttingen, E. A. Huth,* 1882.

Meyer (Gustavus) [1819–]. * De uteri inter partum spasmis. 37 pp., 1 l. 8°. *Berolini, typ. Schnitzerianis,* [1844].

Meyer (Gustavus Eduardus) [1801–]. * Quædam de morbo leproso inter rusticos Esthonos endemico. 71 pp. 8°. [*Dorpat*], *revaliæ ex off. C. Dullo,* 1824.

Meyer (H.) * Zur Behandlung des traumatischen Tetanus. 18 pp. 8°. *Würzburg, C. J. Becker,* 1862.

Meyer (Hans). * Beiträge zur Kenntniss des Stoffwechsels im Organismus der Hühner. 33 pp., 1 l. 8°. *Königsberg, E. J. Dalkowski,* 1877.

Meyer (Heinr.) * Knochenabscesse. 21 pp., 1 l. 8°. *Kiel, Schmidt u. Klaunig,* 1887.

Meyer (Heinr. Ferd.) * Die Indicationen zum Kaiserschnitt und zur Perforation, in ihrer Beziehung zur Frage: Hat die Mutter oder die Frucht bei einer Collision des Lebens mehr Recht auf Schonung von Seiten der Kunsthilfe? 57 pp. 8°. *Würzburg, C. Becker,* 1845.

Meyer (Heinricus).
See **Welsch** (Gottfried.) & **Meyer** (Heinricus). Anatome cerebri humani. 4°. *Lipsiæ,* [1639].

Meyer (Henricus). * De chlorosi virginum. 21 pp., 1 l. sm. 4°. *Lugd. Bat., J. et H. Verbeek,* 1728. [*Also, in:* P., v. 71.]

Meyer (Henricus Ernestus Ludovicus). * De opii usu in inflammationibus. 1 p. l., 18 pp., 1 l. 4°. *Gottingæ, in off. Barmeieriana,* [1800].

Meyer (Henricus Gottlob.) * De officio matris prolem lactandi. 32 pp. sm. 4°. *Wittenbergæ, prelo E. G. Eichsfeldi,* 1752.
For Biography, see **Langguth** (Geo. Aug.)

Meyer (Henricus Josephus). * De morbis glandularum salivalium capitis. 42 pp. 8°. *Bonnæ, typ. C. Georgii,* 1840.

Meyer (Henry).
See **Hôpital** (L') de Sct. Hans. oblong fol. *Copenhague,* 1884.

Meyer (Henry C.) Water-waste prevention; its importance and the evils due to its neglect. With an account of the methods adopted in various cities in Great Britain and the United States. With an appendix. 70 pp. 8°. *New York,* 1885.
Also, Editor of: **Sanitary** (The) Engineer, New York, 1880.

Meyer (Hermann). * Zur Toxicologie des Broms. 36 pp., 1 l. 8°. *Zürich, Zürcher u. Furrer,* 1870.

———. Ueber das Milchsäureferment und sein Verhalten gegen Antiseptica. 66 pp., 1 l., 1 tab. 8°. *Dorpat, H. Laakmann,* 1880.

Meyer (Hermann. Pet.) * De punctura vesicæ urinariæ in ischuria vesicali adhibenda. 1 p. l., 28 pp. 4°. *Marburgi Cattorum, typ. P. C. Mülleri,* 1727.

Meyer (Hermannus)[1] [1811–]. * De aëris in venas ingressu in operationibus chirurgicis. 28 pp., 2 l. 8°. *Berolini, typ. Nietackianis,* [1834].

Meyer (Hermannus)[2]. * De gastritide chronica. 38 pp. 8°. *Rostochii, lit. Adlerianis,* 1838. c.

Meyer (Hermannus Fridericus) [1807–]. * De balneis nonnulla. 32 pp. 8°. *Berolini, typ. Friedlaenderianis,* [1836].

Meyer (Hugo). * Ueber den Einfluss einiger flüchtigen Stoffe auf die Zahl der farblosen Zellen im Kreislauf. 1 p. l., 30 pp. 8°. *Bonn, P. Neusser,* 1874.

Meyer (Immanuel Ferd.) [–1813]. Versuch einer systematischen Enzyklopädie der gesammten Medizin. Nebst einer Abhandlung über das Studium der Medizin. viii, 374 pp. 8°. *Berlin, Schüppel,* 1807.
2. pt. wanting.

———. Repertorium der gesammten medizinischen Literatur. 2 v. in 1. 239 pp.; xvii, 532 pp., 1 l. 8°. *Berlin,* 1809.

———. Ueber die Natur der Entzündung; ein historisch-kritischer Versuch. 133 pp. 8°. *Berlin, J. E. Hitzig,* 1810.

———. Versuch einer kritischen Geschichte der Entzündungen. Erster Theil, oder Einleitung in die Geschichte der speciellen Pathologie und Therapie. xvi, 463 pp. 12°. *Berlin, F. Maurer,* 1812.

Meyer (Is.) [1847–]. * Die Lehre von der Entstehung der Herztöne. 30 pp. 8°. *Berlin, H. S. Hermann,* [1880].

Meyer (Isidorus). * De Joannis Christiani Reilii in physiologia dignitate. 2 p. l., 40 pp., 1 l. 8°. *Vratislaviæ, H. Lindner,* [1857].

Meyer (J. A.) Der Kurgast in Ober-Salzbrunn. 48 pp. 8°. *Berlin,* 1858.

Meyer (J. A. G.) Natur-Analogien, oder die vornehmsten Erscheinungen des animalischen Magnetismus in ihrem Zusammenhange mit den Ergebnissen der gesammten Naturwissenschaften, mit besonderer Hinsicht auf die Standpunkte und Bedürfnisse heutiger Theologie. lxiv, 412 pp. 8°. *Hamburg u. Gotha, F. u. A. Perthes,* 1839.

Meyer (J. Conradus). * De exstirpatione partium degeneratarum ossis maxillæ inferioris. [Göttingen.] 35 pp., 2 pl. 4°. *Berolini, typ. Feisterianis et Eisersdorffianis*, 1828.

Meyer (Jacobus) [1810–]. * De rarissimis duobus exemplis suppurationis cerebri, adnotationibus nonnullis adspersis necessariis. 18 pp., 2 pl., 1 l. 4°. *Halis, typ. Baentschianis*, [1832].

Meyer (James). How to prevent the spread of contagious diseases and epidemics. 24 pp. 8°. [*New York*, 1879.]
An advertisement of the Girondin disinfectant.

Meyer (Jep Heinrich) [1846–]. * Ein Beitrag zur Literatur der Fremdkörper in den Speisewegen aus eigner Praxis. 30 pp., 1 l. 8°. *Berlin, G. Schade*, [1881].

Meyer (Joachim). * De medici prudentia. 28 pp. 8°. *Landishuti, S. F. Storno*, 1820.

Meyer (Joann. Augustus). * De rubo idæo officinarum. 1 p. l., 26 pp., 1 l. 4°. *Halæ Magdeb., typ. J. C. Hilligeri*, [1744].

Meyer (Joannes). * De fistula ani. *Argentorati*, 1771.
In: WEIZ (F. A.) Neue Ausz. [etc.] 12°. *Frankfurt u. Leipzig*, 1780, xi, 115.

Meyer (Joannes Antonius) [1809–]. * De cholera asiatica. 35 pp. 8°. *Berolini, typ. Nietackianis*, 1838.

Meyer (Joannes Carolus)[1]. * De paracentesi vesicæ. ii, 3–65 pp., 1 l. 8°. *Erlangæ, typ. Hilpertianis*, 1798.

Meyer (Joannes Carolus)[2] [1780–1831]. * De fumi nicotianæ suctu. 35 pp. 4°. *Lipsiæ, J. Franz*, [1803].
For Biography, see **Platner** (Ernestus).

Meyer (Joannes Georgius) [1805–]. * De febre hectica. 32 pp. 8°. *Berolini, typ. A. Petschii*, [1830].

Meyer (Joannes Gottlob.) * De metaschematismo morborum. 40 pp. 4°. *Lipsiæ, ex off. Langenhemiana*, [1747].

Meyer (Joannes Michael.) * De difficili in observationes anatomicas epicrisi commentatio iii. 59 pp. 4°. *Erlangæ, ex off. Waltheriana*, [1773].

Meyer (Joh.)[1] * De fistula ani. 34 pp. 4°. *Argentorati, ex prelo J. Lorenzii*, [1771].

Meyer (Joh.)[2] * Einige Versuche über Strychnin-Vergiftung, als gerichtlich-toxicologischer Beitrag zu den Strychnin-Vergiftungen. 32 pp. 8°. *Bern, K. J. Wyss*, 1864. c.

Meyer (Joh.)[3] Berichte über die Idiotenanstalt in Kiel. 3.–6. (Juli 1864 bis Juli 1875). 8°. *Kiel*, 1866–75.

———. Prospectus über die Idiotenanstalt in Kiel. 2 l. 8°. *Kiel, C. F. Mohr*, 1868.

Meyer (Joh.)[4] [1855–]. * Ueber Placentarpolypen. 36 pp. 8°. *Berlin, G. Schade*, [1880].

Meyer (Joh.)[5] * Klinische Untersuchungen über das Verhalten der Ovarien während der Menstruation. 55 pp. 8°. *Dorpat, H. Laakmann*, 1883.

Meyer (Joh. Carol. Heinrich). * Delirii febrilis meletemata. 50 pp., 1 l. 8°. *Halæ, in off. Batheana*, [1797].

———. Grundriss der Physiologie des menschlichen Körpers zum Behuf seiner Vorlesungen entworfen. 4 p. l., 361 pp. 8°. *Berlin*, 1805.

Meyer (Joh. Casparus). * De morbis endemiis. 19 pp. 4°. *Lugd. Bat., A. Kallewier*, [1737].

Meyer (Joh. Conrad). * De clysmatibus. 27 pp. 4°. *Gottingæ, H. M. Grape*, [1786].
Also, in: FRANK (J. P.) Delect. opusc. med. 8°. *Ticini*, 1790, ix, 146–186.

Meyer (Joh. Conradus). * De phthisi. 6 l. sm. 4°. *Basileæ, typ. J. H. Meyeri*, [1678].

Meyer (Joh. Fridericus). * De spiritibus animalibus ex foro medico proscribendis. 36 pp. 4°. *Francof. cis Viadr., lit. J. C. Schwarzii*, [1723].

von Meyer (Joh. Friedrich) [1772–]. Wahrnehmungen einer Seherin. 1. Theil. x, 400 pp. 8°. *Hamburg, F. Perthes*, 1827.

Meyer (Joh. Jacobus). * De dysenteria. 48 pp. 8°. *Duisburgi, F. A. Benthon*, [1800].

von Meyer (Joh. Nep.) Einige neue Beobachtungen über das Wesen der Cholera morbus aus der Erfahrung geschöpft, in besonderer Beziehung auf die Haare als Leiter des Contagiums. 49 pp., 1 pl. 8°. *Wien, F. Tendler*, 1831. [P., v. 210.]

———. Ueber Sanitäts-Anstalten im Orient und über die Stellung der dortigen Aerzte. 26 pp. 8°. *Erlangen, Kunstmann*, 1840.

Meyer (Joh. Rudolphus). * De strangulationibus intestinorum in cavo abdominis. 37 pp. sm. 4°. *Argentorati, typ. J. H. Heitzii*, [1776].

Meyer (Jonas) [–1836].
See **Frank** (Joseph). Annalen des klinischen Instituts an der kaiserl. Universität zu Wilna. 8°. *Berlin*, 1810.

Meyer (Jorge Alberto). * Ueber einen Fall von multiplen Stenosen bei primärer Darmtuberkulose. 31 pp. 8°. *Heidelberg, C. Winter*, 1886.

Meyer (Joseph)[1]. Untersuchungen zur Therapie des Pleuritis. 335 pp. 8°. *Berlin, A. W. Schade*, 1863.
Repr. from: Ann. d. Char.-Krankenh. . . . zu Berl., 1863, xi.

Meyer (Joseph)[2]. * Ueber die Impfbarkeit der Tuberkulose. 31 pp. 8°. *Göttingen, G. Hofer*, 1873.

Meyer (Josephus). * Memoria Thomæ Sydenham. 30 pp., 1 l. 8°. *Halæ, typ. Gebaueriis*, [1833].

Meyer (Julius)[1] [1820–]. * De morbis false recteque dignoscendis. 32 pp. 8°. *Berolini, typ. Friedlaenderianis*, [1843].

Meyer (Julius)[2] [1844–]. * De natura morbi hypochondriaci. 31 pp. 8°. *Berolini, Nurnberg et Jeretyke*, 1867.

Meyer (Karl). * Die Behandlung der Blennorhöe des Thränenkanales. 60 pp., 1 l. 8°. *Zürich, F. Walder u. Sohn*, 1860.

Meyer (Karl Joseph). * Ein Wort über den Aderlass als Präservativ-Mittel. viii, 39 pp. 8°. *Würzburg, Kölisch*, [1798].

Meyer (L. C.) * Ueber das Kindbettfieber. 59 pp. 8°. *Würzburg, C. Becker*, 1844.

Meyer (L. N.) Sistemy kanalizatsii gorodov i sposoby ochistki grjaznoi kanalizatsionnoi vody. [Systems of canalization of cities, and means of purifying water by canalization.] iii, 62 pp., 15 pl. 8°. *Kieff, tipog. G. T. Korchak-Novitskago*, 1887.

Meyer (Leo). Festrede zur Jahresfeier der Stiftung der Universität Dorpat am 12. December 1871, nebst den Mittheilungen über die Preisaufgaben, sowie dem Universitäts-Jahresbericht für das Jahr 1871. 34 pp. 4°. *Dorpat, C. Mattiesen*, 1872.

Meyer (Leopold) [1852–]. * Uterinsygdomene som Sterilitetsårsag. 283 pp., 1 l. 8°. *Kjøbenhavn, Brødrene Salmonsen*, 1880.

Meyer (Levinus Bened.) * De ascitis origine et curatione. 51 pp. 8°. *Halæ, in off. Batheana*, [n. d.]

Meyer (Lothar) [1830–]. * Die Gase des Blutes. [Wurtzburg.] 61 pp., 1 l., 1 pl. 8°. *Göttingen, Dieterich*, 1857. [Also, in : P., v. 790.]

———. Ueber die Einwirkung des Kohlenoxydgases auf Blut. 11 pp. 8°. [n. p., 1857, vel subseq.] [P., v. 790.]

———. * De sanguine oxydo carbonico infesto. 12 pp., 1 l. 4°. *Wratislaviæ, typ. Grassii, Barthii et soc.*, 1858.

———. Chemische Analyse der Heilquellen zu Bad Landeck (Preussisch-Schlesien). Hrsg. von

Meyer (Lothar)—continued.
Dr. Langner. 26 pp. 8°. *Breslau, A. Gosohorsky*, 1863.

Meyer (Lucien). *Contribution à l'étude de la scarlatine hémorrhagique. 95 pp. 4°. *Paris, A. Davy*, 1887, No. 251.

Meyer (Ludovicus)[1]. *De cognoscenda et curanda chorea St. Viti. 24 pp. 8°. *Halæ, typ. Gebaueriis*, [1828].

Meyer (Ludovicus)[2] [1807-]. *De fuco crispo, seu lichene Carrageno. 29 pp., 1 l. 8°. *Berolini, typ. Nietackianis*, [1835].

Meyer (Ludovicus)[3] [1826-]. *Observationes quædam in tuberculosin. 31 pp. 8°. *Berolini, typ. fratrum Schlesinger*, [1852].

Meyer (Ludovicus Julius) [1810-]. *De cura cataractæ secundaria. 38 pp., 1 l. sm. 8°. *Berolini, typ. Nietackianis*, [1834].

Meyer (M. A.) Diätetische Verhaltungsregeln und erste Hülfe bei der asiatischen Cholera. 22 pp. 8°. *Hannover, Hahn*, 1848.

Meyer (Marie-Joseph-Édouard). *Recherches expérimentales sur la réfrigération des mammifères. 95 pp. 4°. *Lille*, 1886, 3. s., No. 24.

Meyer (Martinus). *Diss. sistens ideam de secretione in genere. 28 pp. 4°. *Argentorati, in off. Kürsneriana*, [1777].

Meyer (Mauritius)[1]. *De acologiæ chirurgicæ systemate. 38 pp., 1 pl. 4°. *Berolini, lit. A. Petschi*, [1827], v. 328.

Meyer (Mauritius)[2]. *De rupturis uteri et vaginæ una cum duobus casibus rupti in partu uteri et ruptæ vaginæ. 36 pp., 2 l. 8°. *Halis Sax., typ. Semmlerianis*, [1844].

Meyer (Max) [1845-]. *Klinische Beobachtungen über einige Formen von Rückwärtsbeugung der Gebärmutter. 43 pp. 8°. *Berlin, G. Schade*, [1869].

Meyer (Meyer Jacob) [1820-]. *De induratione telæ cellulosæ neonatorum. 32 pp., 2 l. 8°. *Berolini, typ. fratrum Schlesinger*, [1843].

Meyer (Moritz)[1]. Grundzüge der Militair-Chemie. 1 p. l., 246, xv pp. 8°. *Berlin, Schlesinger*, 1834.

Meyer (Moritz)[2] [1821-]. L'utilité de l'électricité et son emploi dans les maladies démontrés par des faits cliniques . . . Trad. de l'allemand par les soins de la société. 104 pp., 1 pl. 8°. *Gand, F. & E. Gyselynck*, 1852.
Repr. from: Ann. Soc. de méd. de Gand, 1852, xxx.

———. Die Elektricität in ihrer Anwendung auf praktische Medicin. 3. Aufl. xx, 423 pp. 8°. *Berlin, A. Hirschwald*, 1868.

———. The same. 4. Aufl. xx, 632 pp., 1 pl. 8°. *Berlin, A. Hirschwald*, 1883.

———. The same. Electricity in its relations to practical medicine. Transl. from the 3. German ed., with notes and additions, by W. A. Hammond. xxi, 497 pp. 8°. *New York, D. Appleton & Co.*, 1869.

Meyer (Moritz)[3]. *Zur Casuistik des geheilten Pneumothorax. 17 pp. 4°. *Kiel, C. F. Mohr*, 1878.
In: SCHRIFT. d. Univ. zu Kiel, xxv, 1878, vii, med. i.

Meyer (Moyses). *De tabe dorsuali. 35 pp. .8°. *Gottingæ, typ. Dieterichianis*, 1830.

Meyer (N.) *Ueber die physiologische Wirkung der Arsenik-Verbindungen. 32 pp. 8°. *Berlin, Thormann u. Goetsch*, [1873].

Meyer (Nicolaus) [1775-]. *Prodromus anatomiæ murium. 40 pp., 2 pl. sm. 4°. *Jenæ, typ. Prageri et soc.*, [1800].

———. Geschichte einer durch den Kaiserschnitt glücklich beendigten Entbindung. 74 pp., 1 pl. 12°. *Frankf. a. M., F. Varrentrapp*, 1821.

———. Ueber die Ursache des Erstickungstodes der Kinder in und gleich nach der Geburt.

Meyer (Nicolaus)—continued.
36 pp. 12°. *Frankf. a. M., F. Varrentrapp*, 1823.
For Biography, see **Loder** (Justus Christian.)
For Portrait, see **Collection**—van Kaathoven.

Meyer (Otto) [1860-]. *Ueber den Glycogengehalt embryonaler und jugendlicher Organe. 30 pp., 1 l. 8°. *Breslau*, 1884.

Meyer (Paul)[1] [1852-]. *Études histologiques sur le labyrinthe membraneux et plus spécialement sur le limaçon chez les reptiles et les oiseaux. 189 pp., 1 l. 8°. *Strasbourg, C.-G. Trübner*, 1876.

Meyer (Paul)[2]. *Beiträge zu den Functionen der Hirnteile des Frosches. 29 pp., 1 l. 8°. *Berlin, G. Schade*, [1881].

Meyer (Paul Oscar) [1856-]. *Zur Statistik über Affection der serösen Häute bei Nierenerkrankungen. 32 pp. 8°. *Berlin, M. Niethe*, [1881].

Meyer (Philippus) [1798-]. *Signa nonnulla ex naso atque olfactu. 43 pp. 8°. *Berolini, formis Brueschckianis*, [1820].

Meyer (Philippus Christianus). *De asthmate ejusque speciebus. 60 pp. sm. 4°. *Gottingæ, J. C. Dieterich*, [1779].
For Biography, see **Murray** (Jo. Andreas).

Meyer (Rudolf). *Zur Pathologie des Hirnabscesses. 99 pp., 1 l. 8°. *Zürich, Zürcher u. Furrer*, 1867. c.

———. Ueber die Endocarditis ulcerosa. Habilitationsschrift. 78 pp., 1 tab. 8°. *Zürich, Zürcher u. Furrer*, 1870.

Meyer (Rudolph). *Ueber die unglücklichen Ereignisse während und nach dem Aderlass. 39 pp. 8°. *Würzburg, F. Bauer*, 1833.

Meyer (S.) Report of one hundred joint resections treated at Professor Saxtorph's department, in Frederick's Hospital, Copenhagen. Statistics collected by S. Meyer. Transl. from the Danish, by Robert T. Morris. 41 pp. 8°. [*Newtown*, 1886.]
Repr. from: N. Eng. M. Month., Bridgeport, Conn., 1885-6, v.

Meyer (Salomon Leyser). *Virilis impotentiæ rationes. 40 pp. sm. 4°. *Traj. ad Viadr., typ. Winteriano*, [1782].

Meyer [**Meyr**] (Sebastian). Institutiones medicæ primæ. Omnes medicinæ locos solidaque totius artis fundamenta, distincte, breviter ordineque complectentes, quibusvis etiam literatis proficuæ, [etc.] 6 p. l., 226 pp. 18°. *Frib. Brisgoiæ, M. Böckler*, 1603.

———. Selectorum physicorum medicinalium, politicorum, aliorumque maxime memorabilium, exquisitorum, publicæ privatæque fælicitati servientium, sylloge prima. 188 pp. 18°. *Friburgi Brisgoiæ, ex typog. J. Strasseri*, 1617.

Meyer (Servatius). *De febri puerperali. 50 pp. 8°. *Gryphiæ, F. G. Kunike*, [1834].

Meyer (Siegismundus). *De situ viscerum abnormi. 1 p. l., 36 pp., 1 l. 8°. *Vratislaviæ, typ. R. Lucæ*. [1847].

Meyer (Theodor). *Untersuchungen über das Carcinom der Leber und einiger anderer pathologisch-anatomischer Abnormitäten desselben Organes. 60 pp., 1 l., 2 pl. 8°. *Basel, Schweighauser*, 1843.

Meyer (Theodorus B.) *Quæstiones de fontibus, ex quibus animalia et plantæ nitrogenium excipiant. 34 pp. 8°. *Dorpati Livonorum, typ. vid. J. C. Schünmanni et C. Mattieseni*, 1853.

Meyer (Valentin). *Observation sur un cas d'opération césarienne, pratiquée avec succès pour la mère et l'enfant, par M. le professeur Stoltz . . . suivie de réflexions sur l'ostéosarcôme du bassin, considéré comme cause de dystocie. 1 p. l., 45 pp. 4°. *Strasbourg*, 1847, No. 171, v. 13.

Meyer (Veit). Homöopatischer Führer für Deutschland und das Ausland. Enthaltend die Verzeichnisse der homöopathischen Aerzte und Anstalten Deutschlands, Englands, Frankreichs, Spaniens, Italiens, des übrigen Europa und Amerika's. vi–100 pp. 12°. *Leipzig, C. H. Reclam sen.*, 1856.
Also, Co-Editor of: **Homöopathische** Vierteljahrsschrift, Leipzig, 1851–61.—**Allgemeine** homöopathische Zeitung, Leipzig, 1853–72.

Meyer (Vincenzo).
Co-Editor of: **Archivio** di patologia infantile, Napoli, 1883.

Meyer (Vitus). * De hæmospasia seu de aëre expanso variis morbis adhibito. vi, 7–23 pp. 8°. *Lipsiæ, ex off. P. Reclami jun.*, [1842].

Meyer (W. H. Theodor). * Bestimmungen über die Intensität des freien Magnetismus in künstlichen Magneten, nebst Untersuchungen über Coërcitivkraft. [Marburg.] 31 pp., 2 pl. 8°. *Bonn, J. F. Carthaus*, 1857. c.

Meyer (Wilhelm)[1]. * Zwei Rückbildungsformen des Carcinoms. 30 pp., 1 l. 8°. *Zürich, E. Kiesling*, 1854. c.

Meyer (Wilhelm)[2] [1856–]. * Untersuchungen über den Bacillus des Abdominaltyphus. 37 pp., 1 l., 1 pl. 8°. *Berlin, G. Schade*, 1881.

Meyer (Wilhelm)[3]. * Ein Beitrag zur Behandlung der Rachitis mit Phosphor. 32 pp. 8°. *Kiel, Schmidt u. Klaunig*, 1885.

Meyer (Wilhelm Benedictus). * Ueber die künstliche Frühgeburt. 34 pp. 8°. *Jena, A. Neuenhahn*, 1869. [P., v. 304; 401.]

Meyer (Wilhelm H. A.) * Ueber systolische Einziehungen in der Gegend der Herzspitze. 31 pp. 8°. *Marburg, R. Friedrich*, 1881.

Meyer (Willy). * Die Behandlung der Skoliose nach Sayre'schem Princip mit Zuhülfenahme von Jacken aus plastischem Filz; nach Beobachtungen in der chirurgischen Klinik und Poliklinik zu Bonn. 37 pp., 1 l. 8°. *Bonn, C. Georgi*, 1880. c.

Meyer-Ahrens (Konrad) [1813–73]. Der Stich in den Jahren 1564 und 1565 im Zusammenhange mit den übrigen Epidemieen der Jahre 1562–1566. 1 p. l., 182 pp., 1 l. 8°. *Zürich, F. Schulthess*, 1848.

——. Die Bergkrankheit, oder der Einfluss des Ersteigens grosser Höhen auf den thierischen Organismus. xi, 130 pp. 8°. *Leipzig, F. A. Brockhaus*, 1854.

——. Die Heilquellen und Kurorte der Schweiz und einiger der Schweiz zunächst angrenzenden Gegenden der Nachbarstaaten. 2. Ausg. viii, 812 pp., 7 pl. roy. 8°. *Zürich, Orell, Füssli u. Comp.*, 1867.

—— & **Bruegger** (Chr. Gr.) Die Thermen von Bormio, in physikalisch-chemischer, therapeutischer, klimatologischer und geschichtlicher Beziehung. 135 pp. roy. 8°. *Zürich, Orell, Fuessli u. Comp.*, 1869.

—— & **Keiser-Muos.** Hotel, Kur- und Pensionshaus Schönfels auf dem Zugerberg, Ct. Zug (Schweiz). 41 pp. 8°. *Basel*, 1876.

—— & **Wiel** (Josef). Bonndorf und Steinamühle, zwei klimatische Curstationen auf dem Schwarzwalde. ii, 82 pp., 4 pl., 3 l., 2 maps. 8°. *Bonndorf u. Zürich, J. A. Binder*, 1873.

de Meyeren (Albertus). * De elephantiasi, nec non de casu quodam elephantiasis penis et scroti. 31 pp. 8°. *Halæ, typ. Ploetzianis*, 1865.

von Meyeren ([Carolus Augustus] Theophilus [Theodorus]) [1804–]. * De eclampsiæ diagnosi atque prognosi. 31 pp. sm. 8°. *Berolini, typ. J. F. Starckii*, [1825].

von Meyeren ([Joh.] Fridericus [Theophilus]) [1800–]. * De accuratiore phthisis nerveæ diagnosi. 26 pp. sm. 4°. *Berolini, typ. J. F. Starckii*, [1825].

Meyerheine (Ernestus) [1792–]. * De angina polyposa. 23 pp., 1 l. 8°. *Halæ, formis F. Grunerti*, [1823].
For Biography, see **Sprengel** (Curtius).

Meyerhoff (Jacobus) [1767–]. * De vestimentorum vi et efficacia deque optima ratione vestitus, præsertim virilis, apte instituendi; adjecta descriptione vestis virilis novæ, originis Germanicæ, quæ propositis conditionibus quam maxime respondeat, simulque subjuncto prodromo litterario de omni re vestiaria. vi, 29 pp., 1 pl. 4°. *Berolini, liberaria Maureri*, 1815.

Meyerhoff (Maximilianus Hugo Eduardus) [1843–]. * De rheumatismo articulorum acuto maximeque ejus therapia. 32 pp. 8°. *Berolini, G. Schade*, [1867].

Meyeringh (Ernst Friedrich). * Ueber die Behandlung von Oberschenkel-Fracturen durch permanente Extension mit Gewichten. 30 pp., 1 l. 8°. *Halle, Plötz*, [1872].

Meyerowitz (David) [1829–]. * De luxatione patellæ in partem superiorem congenita. 32 pp. 8°. *Berolini, Jacoby et Steinthal*, 1857.

Meyerowitz (Theodor). * Mikroskopische Untersuchungen über die normalen Hornhautzellen und deren Veränderungen bei der traumatischen Keratitis. 60 pp., 2 l. 8°. *Königsberg in Pr., J. Jacoby*, 1875.

Meyers (Arthur B. R.)
See **Seitz** (Joh.) Die Ueberanstrengung des Herzens [etc.] 8°. *Berlin*, 1875.

Meyers (J. Fred.)
See **United States.** *Treasury Department.* Letter from the Secretary . . . in compliance with a Senate resolution of March 11, 1873. 8°. [*Washington*, 1874.]

Meyers (Maurits). * Een geval van perichondritis laryngea laryngoskopisch onderzocht. viii, 47 pp. 8°. *Hoorn, Gebr. Vermande*, 1867.

Meyersohn (Bernhard). * Congenitale Defectbildungen an den Unterextremitäten eines Erwachsenen. 47 pp., 1 pl. 8°. *Greifswald, F. W. Kunike*, [1878].

Meyersohn (Moritz) [1849–]. * Zur Casuistik der Pulmonalklappenleiden. 32 pp. 8°. *Berlin, R. Boll*, [1872].

Meyerson (Albertus). * Sententiarum de inflammationis natura historia. 28 pp. 8°. *Jenæ, typ. Schlotteri*, 1846.

Meyerstein (Rudolph). * De pertussi. 43 pp. 8°. *Gottingæ, F. Baier*, 1831.

Meyfeld (Joannes Godofredus). * Diss. sistens historiam partus difficilis ex spastica strictura uteri circa placentam. 20 pp. 4°. *Altorfii, typ. J. G. Kohlesii*, [1732].

Meyhoeffer (Eduard). * Ueber die mechanische Behandlung der Hüftgelenksentzündung. 31 pp. 8°. *Greifswald, C. Sell*, 1884.

Meyhoeffer (Franciscus Fridericus). * De pneumatosi chronica intestinali. 31 pp. 8°. *Berolini, B. Schlesinger*, [1853].

Meyhoffer (Joh.) * Ueber acute Tuberculosis der Lungen. 81 pp., 1 l. 8°. *Zürich, E. Kiesling*, 1855.

Meyjes (Willem Christiaan Posthumus). Over traumatische beleedigingen van de wervelkolom. [Leiden.] 2 p. l., 92 pp., 2 l. 8°. *Amsterdam, ten Brink & de Vries*, 1859.

Meyjes (Willem Posthumus). * Kalomel als diureticum. 2 p. l., 80 pp., 2 l. 8°. *Amsterdam, ten Brink & de Vries*, 1887.

de Meyjounissas du Repaire (Guillaume-Puyjoli). * Du goître exophthalmique. 48 pp. 4°. *Paris*, 1867, No. 90.

Meyke (Wilhelm). * Beiträge zur Ermittelung einiger Hopfen-Surrogate im Biere. [Dorpat.] 44 pp., 1 tab. 8°. *Libau, V. Niemann*, 1878.

Meykow (Æmilius). * Comparatæ de radice rhei aliisque quibusdam substantiis investiga-

Meykow (Æmilius)—continued.
tiones. 36 pp. 8°. [*Dorpat*], *typ. H. Laak-manni*, 1858.

Meyl (Fr. Wilhelm). *Ein Beitrag zur Diagnostik der Neubildungen in der hintern Schädelgrube. 27 pp. 8°. *Jena, A. Neuenhahn*, 1869. [P., v. 270.]

Meyler (Antonius). *De melancholia. 24 pp. 8°. *Edinburgi, C. Stewart*, 1803. [P., v. 27.]

Meylert (Asa P.) Notes on the opium habit. 36 pp. 16°. *New York, G. P. Putnam's Sons*, 1884.

——. The same. 3. ed. iv pp., 1 p. l., 47 pp. 12°. *New York & London, G. P. Putnam's Sons*, 1885.

——. The same. 4. ed. vi (1 l.), 49 pp. 12°. *New York & London, G. P. Putnam's Sons*, 1885.

Meylett (Gulielmus Gough). *De calculosis. 1 p. l., 29 pp. 8°. *Edinburgi, A. Smellie*, 1798. [*Also, in:* P., v. 8.]

Meylor (J. J.)
See **Watson** (Thomas). Watson abridged; a synopsis of the lectures [etc.] 8°. *Philadelphia*, 1867.

de Meymar (Alexandre). *Contribution à l'étude du phlegmon diffus du membre supérieur. 33 pp., 1 l. 4°. *Paris*, 1882, No. 272.

Meyn (Andr. Ludw. Adolph). Die Asphyxie, in ihren staatsärztlichen und klinischen Beziehungen. 1 p. l., 172 pp. 8°. *Kiel, C. Bünsow*, 1843.

Meynard (J.) *I. Déterminer si des observations recueillies jusqu'à ce jour permettent d'établir que telle méthode de traitement de l'affection calculeuse est préférable à telle autre, suivant les pays, les âges, les habitudes, les professions. II. [etc.] 41 pp. 4°. *Paris*, 1840, No. 111, v. 363.

Meynard (J.-X.) *Étude sur l'oblitération de l'aorte abdominale par embolie ou par thrombose. 88 pp. 4°. *Paris*, 1883.

Meynard (Joseph). *Des indications et contre-indications opératoires. 31 pp. 4°. *Paris*, 1845, No. 175, v. 435.

Meynard (Louis-Gabriel). *Considérations sur les maladies nerveuses les plus communes aux filles à l'époque de la puberté. 24 pp. 4°. *Paris*, 1812, No. 23, v. 87.

Meynard (Pierre-Alphonse). *De la myélite. 26 pp. 4°. *Paris*, 1847, No. 169, v. 462.

Meyner (Ernst Albrecht). *Mittheilungen über Hautkrankheiten. 25 pp. 8°. *Jena, A. Neuenhahn*, 1868.

Meyners d'Estrey.
Editor of: **Revue** bibliographique universelle des sciences médicales, Paris, 1884.

Meynert (Theodor) [1833–]. Der Bau der Gross-Hirnrinde und seine örtlichen Verschiedenheiten, nebst einem pathologisch-anatomischen Corollarium. 68 pp., 4 pl. 8°. *Neuwied, J. H. Heuser*, 1872.
Repr. from: Vrtljschr. f. Phychiat., Neuwied, 1867–8, i.

——. Zur Mechanik des Gehirnbaues. 20 pp. 8°. *Wien, W. Braumüller*, 1874.

——. Skizzen über Umfang und wissenschaftliche Anordnung der klinischen Psychiatrie. 38 pp. 8°. *Wien, W. Braumüller*, 1876.
Repr. from: Psychiat. Centralbl., Wien, 1876, vi.

——. Die Windungen der convexen Oberfläche des Vorder-Hirnes bei Menschen, Affen und Raubthieren. 32 pp. 8°. *Berlin, A. Hirschwald*, 1877.
Repr. from: Arch. f. Psychiat., Berl., 1876–7, vii, 2. Hft.

——. Ueber Fortschritte im Verständniss der krankhaften psychischen Gehirnzustände. 54 pp. 8°. *Wien, W. Braumüller*, 1878.
Repr. from: Psychiat. Centralbl., Wien, 1877, vii.

——. Die acuten (hallucinatorischen) Formen des Wahnsinns und ihr Verlauf. 16 pp. 8° *Wien, Toeplitz u. Deuticke*, 1881.
Repr. from: Jahrb. f. Psychiat., Wien, 1881, ii.

Meynert (Theodor)—continued.
——. Psychiatrie. Klinik der Erkrankungen des Vorderhirns begründet auf dessen Bau, Leistungen und Ernährung. 1. Hälfte. x, 288 pp., 1 pl. 8°. *Wien, W. Braumüller*, 1884.

——. The same. Psychiatry; a clinical treatise on diseases of the fore-brain, based upon a study of its structure, functions, and nutrition. Transl. by B. Sachs. Pt. 1. The anatomy, physiology, and chemistry of the brain. ix pp., 1 l., 285 pp. 8°. *New York & London, G. P. Putnam's Sons*, 1885.

——. The same. Psichiatrija. Klinika zabolevanii peredniago mozga, osnovannaja na stroenii, otpravlenijach i pitanii. Perevod M. E. Liona, pod redaktsiei P. I. Kovalevskago. 323 pp. 8°. *Charkoff, M. F. Silberberg*, 1885.
Also, Co-Editor of: **Vierteljahrsschrift** für Psychiatrie, Neuwied und Leipzig, 1867–9.—**Psychiatrisches** Centralblatt, Wien, 1871–8.—**Jahrbücher** für Psychiatrie, Wien, 1879.

Meynet (C.-H.-Paul). *Épidémie d'érysipèle et d'ulcération de l'ombilic chez les nouveau-nés, observée à l'hospice de la Charité de Lyon. 54 pp. 4°. *Paris*, 1857, No. 156, v. 608.

Meynet (C.-Lucien). *Considérations sur quelques points de la physiologie et de la pathologie du cœur. 71 pp. 4°. *Paris*, 1858, No. 126, v. 621.

Meynet (G.) Assistance publique. Médecins municipaux. 15 pp. 8°. *Paris, A. Parent*, 1880.
Repr. from: J. d. conn. méd. prat., Par., 1880, xlvii.

Meynet (P.)
See **Vaccine** et vérole, etc. 8°. *Paris*, 1865.

Meynial (J.) *Quelques considérations sur la formation des hydropisies en général, leurs causes et leur traitement. 16 pp. 4°. *Paris*, 1831, No. 148, v. 242.

Meynier (Achille). *Essai sur l'amaurose, suivi de quelques propositions sur la médecine. 16 pp. 4°. *Strasbourg*, 1831, v. 62.

Meynier (J.) *Considérations sur l'emploi de la méthode inamovible dans le traitement des fractures des membres. 31 pp. 4°. *Strasbourg*, 1863, No. 714, 2. s., v. 37.

Meynier (J.-C.) *Étude des déviations de l'utérus gravide comme cause de dystocie. 68 pp. 4°. *Paris*, 1876, No. 132.

Meynier (J.-F.) *Considérations hygiéniques sur la femme pendant la gestation. vi, 7–29 pp. 4°. *Paris*, 1822, No. 22, v. 170.

Meynier (M.-L.-Gustave). *Recherches sur l'action toxique de quelques essences. 47 pp. 4°. *Paris*, 1859, No. 122, v. 634.

Meynier (Prosper). *Sur l'expectation. 32 pp. 4°. *Paris*, 1828, No. 177, v. 218.

Meynne (Amand). De la construction des casernes au point de vue de l'hygiène. 64 pp. 8°. *Bruxelles, J.-B. Tircher* 1847.

——. Hygiène militaire. Études sur la construction des casernes sur l'alimentation du soldat, et sur les fatigues de la vie militaire. 1 p. l., 79, 111, 63 pp. 8°. *Bruxelles, J.-B. Tircher*, 1856.

——. Éléments de statistique médicale militaire. 95 pp. 8°. *Bruxelles, Tircher*, 1859.

——. Topographie médicale de la Belgique. Études de géologie, de climatologie, de statistique et d'hygiène publique. xii, 582 pp., 1 map. 8°. *Bruxelles, H. Manceaux*, 1865.
Also, Editor of: **Archives** de médecine militaire, Bruxelles, 1848.

Meyr (Ignaz). Beiträge zur Augenheilkunde. 44 pp., 1 pl. 8°. *Wien, W. Braumüller*, 1850.

——. Compendium der Augenheilkunde. x, 333 pp., 1 pl. 8°. *Wien, W. Braumüller*, 1852.

——. The same. 2. gänzlich umgearbeitete und vermehrte Aufl. vi, 347 pp. 8°. *Wien, W. Braumüller*, 1866.

Meyr (Ignaz)—continued.

——. The same. 3. Aufl. vi, 358 pp. 8°. *Wien, W. Braumüller*, 1871.

——. The same. Beknopt handboek der oogheelkunde, uit het Hoogduitsch, door J. E. C. van Campen. viii, 298 pp. 8°. *Utrecht, van Heijningen & Post Uiterweer*, 1852.

——. Anleitung zur Wahl der Kurorte. Praktische Rathschläge für Aerzte und Kurbedürftige. x, 287 pp., 1 map. 8°. *Wien, W. Braumüller*, 1871.

Meyrac (F.-Eugène). * Des névralgies articulaires en rapport avec des fièvres intermittentes anciennes. 46 pp. 4°. *Paris*, 1841, No. 117, v. 378.

Meyrac (Joseph-Sylvain). * Essai séméiotique sur l'état de la langue dans les maladies aiguës. 34 pp. 8°. *Paris, an XI* [1803], v. 24.

Meyranx (Pierre-Stanislas) [1790–1832]. Observations sur la constitution médicale des mois de novembre, décembre et janvier des années 1819 et 1820, et sur les maladies qui se sont présentées pendant ce trimestre, à l'École clinique interne de Montpellier; et quelques réflexions sur le système de Broussais. 109 pp. 8°. *Montpellier, J.-G. Tournel*, 1821.

Meyrick (William). The new family herbal; or, domestic physician; enumerating, with accurate descriptions, all the known vegetables which are any way remarkable for medical efficacy; with an account of their virtues in the several diseases incident to the human frame. 469, 16 pp., 14 pl. 4°. *Birmingham, T. Pearson*, 1790.

de Meyrignac (Henri-Paul). * De l'empoisonnement par la strychnine. 40 pp. 4°. *Paris*, 1859, No. 225, v. 634.

de Meyserey. Méthode aisée et peu coûteuse, de traiter avec succès plusieurs maladies épidémiques, comme la suette, la fièvre miliaire, les fièvres pourprées, etc. 48 pp., 1 l. 12°. *Paris, Le Breton*, 1752. [P., v. 779.]

——. The same. 2. éd., revûe et augmentée. 58 pp. 8°. *Paris, Vve. Cavelier & fils*, 1753. [P., v. 1637.]

——. La médecine d'armée, contenant des moyens aisés de préserver de maladies, sur terre et sur mer, dans toutes sortes de païs et d'en guérir, sans beaucoup de remèdes ni de dépenses, les gens de guerre et autres de quelque condition qu'ils soient. 3 v. 12°. *Paris, Vve. Cavelier & fils*, 1754.

Meyssonerius (Hieremias). De peste libellus. In quo morbi essentia, causæ, signa et curatio, breviter pertractantur. 38 pp., 1 l. 16°. *Avenione, I. Bramereau*, 1607.

Meyssonnier (Lazare) [1602–72]. Théorie de la médecine d'une manière nouvelle et très-intelligible. 3 p. l., 7–53 pp., 7 l., 1 pl. 4°. [*Lyon, G. Barbier*, 1678.]

In: GUYON *Dolois* (L.) Le cours de médecine, etc. 4°. *Lyon*, 1678.

——. Traité des maladies vénéneuses, qui manquoit à ce cours. 7. éd. 12 pp. 4°. [*Lyon*, 1678.]

In: GUYON *Dolois* (L.) Le cours de médecine, etc. 4°. *Lyon*, 1678.

For Biography, see Ann. Soc. de méd. de Lyon, 1872, 2. s., xx, 67–72 (J.-G. Lavirotte). *Also:* Lyon méd., 1872, ix, 495–500 (J.-G. Lavirotte).

Mez (Joh. Fridericus). * Diss. sistens: Noli me tangere medicum, sive morbos quos tangere non licet. 29 pp., 3 l. sm. 4°. *Halæ Magdeb., typ. J. C. Hendelii*, [1751].

de Meza (Jacob Theophilus) [1756–1844]. Bemerkung eines durch kaltes Wasser geheilten Zahnschmerzes. Eine Streitschrift. 7 pp. 16°. *Kopenhagen, J. R. Thiele*, [1775].

16

de Meza (Jacob Theophilus)—continued.

——. Von dem Gebrauche der äusserlichen Artzneyen in der Artznéykunst. Erstes Capitel. 15 pp. sm. 8°. *Kopenhagen, J. R. Thiele*, [1776].

——. Tractatio de quibusdam notabilioribus objectis ad artem obstetricandi spectantibus tyronum usui destinata. 118 pp. 8°. *Hafniæ, C. G. Proft*, 1783.

de Meza (Justus Zadig).

See **Strack** (Carl). Medicinische Beobachtungen von der Petetschenkrankheit [etc.] 12°. *Copenhagen u. Leipzig*, 1777.

de Meza (Salomon Theophilus). Diatribæ medicæ tres. 176 pp. 8°. *Hafniæ, J. G. Rothe*, 1775.

CONTENTS.

I. De officio medico clinico.
II. De sanguinis missione.
III. De usu noxio et salubri vesicantium.

——. Fasciculus alter, inflammationes et dolores sistens. xxv pp., 1 l., 162 pp. 8°. *Hafniæ, C. G. Proft*, 1780.

——. Tentamen historiæ medicæ. viii, 248, 300 pp. 8°. *Hafniæ, C. G. Proft, fil. et soc.*, 1795.

Mezbourian (Nersès-Sahak). * Du diagnostic des bruits de souffle extracardiaques. 40 pp. 4°. *Paris*, 1874, No. 470.

Mezereum.

See **Daphne** *Mezereum.*

Mezger (Carl). * Beitrag zur anatomischen und chemischen Kenntniss des Holzes der Eperua falcata. [Erlangen.] 19 pp. 8°. *Halle a. S.*, 1884.

Mezger (Christophorus Daniel.) * De cuticula et cute. 52 pp. sm. 4°. [*Altdorfi*], *H. H. Meyer*, [1685].

——. * De lactatione. 40 pp. sm. 4°. *Altdorfi, H. Meyer*, [1685].

Mezger (Gottlob Immanuel Siegfried) & **Closs** (Joh. Fridericus). Disputatio de miraculorum indole, criterio et fine. 16 pp. 4°. *Tubingæ, typ. Loeffleriæ viduæ*, [1755].

Mezger (Joh. Georg). * De behandeling van distorsio pedis met fricties. [Leiden.] 2 p. l., 53 pp. 8°. *Amsterdam, C. van Helden*, 1868.

Mezger (Ludovicus). * De murorum recens illitorum exhalatione nociva. 31 pp. 8°. *Tubingæ, typ. Eifertianis*, [1832].

Mezger (*Martinus Christophorus*) [1625–90].

Portrait in: **Collection**—van Kaathoven.

Mezière (Victor). * De la puberté dans les deux sexes. 47 pp. 4°. *Paris*, 1846, No. 186, v. 448.

Mezler (Franz Xaver) [1756–1812]. Unfehlbares Wehrmittel gegen die Wuth- und Wasserscheue, welche auf Bisse wüthender Thiere folgen. 1 p. l., 80 pp. 12°. *Leipzig, Wagner u. Sohn*, 1781.

——. Von der Wassersucht. Eine gekrönte Preisschrift aus dem Lateinischen. Nebst einem Anhange über die Ansteckung. 3 l., 9–174 pp. 8°. *Ulm, J. K. Wohler*, 1787.

——. Von der schwarzgallichten Konstitution. Eine gekrönte Preisschrift. Aus dem Lateinischen. 198 pp. 8°. *Ulm, I. K. Wohler*, 1788.

——. Ueber die Vortheile des Fiebers in langwierigen Krankheiten. Eine Preissschrift. Aus dem Lateinischen. 218 pp. 12°. *Ulm, Wohler*, 1790.

——. Preisfrage. Welche Methode ist die beste, veraltete Geschwüre an den untern Gliedmassen zu heilen? Mit einem Anhange practischer Beobachtungen. 157 pp. 4°. *Wien, R. Graeffer u. Comp.*, 1792.

——. Versuch einer Geschichte des Aderlasses. 293 pp. 12°. *Ulm, Wohler*, 1793.

——. Ueber den Einfluss der Heilkunst auf die praktische Theologie. Ein Beytrag zur Pasto-

Mezler (Franz Xaver)—continued.
ralmedizin. 2. Aufl. 2 v. xxxii, 240 pp.; 242–568 pp. 12°. *Ulm, Wohler*, 1806.

——. Versuch eines Leitfadens zur Abfassung zweckmässiger medizinischer Topographien. xx, 189 pp., 2 tab., 1 pl., 1 l. 12°. *Freyburg u. Konstanz, Herder*, 1814.

——. Versuch einer medizinischen Topographie der Stadt Sigmaringen. xxviii, 381 pp., 1 l., 30 tab., 1 chart. 12°. *Freiburg, Herder*, 1822.
Also, Co-Editor of : **Medicinisch-chirurgische** Zeitung, Salzburg, 1790–93.

von Mezler von Andelberg (Franz Joseph) [1787–1858]. Sammlung auserlesener Abhandlungen über Kinder-Krankheiten. Aus den besten medicinisch-chirurgischen Zeitschriften und andern Werken der neuern Zeit zusammengestellt. 6 v. in 3. 8°. *Prag, G. Haase Söhne*, 1833–7.

——. Die Leistungen des kaiserl.-königl. Artilleriespitals zu Prag, nebst vorausgeschickten Betrachtungen über die Gesundheitspflege der Soldaten überhaupt und der Artilleristen insbesondere. viii pp., 1 l., 357 pp:, port., 3 l. 8°. *Prag, G. Haase Söhne*, 1839.

——. Der ärztliche Rathgeber für den Soldaten. Eine leichtfassliche Belehrung, wie sich der Krieger selbst kennen lernen soll, seine Gesundheit erhalten kann und sich bei Krankheiten und Unfällen zu benehmen hat, mit besonderer Rücksicht auf die Einrichtung und Verhältnisse der k. k. österreichischen Armee. xii, 592 pp. 12°. *Prag, F. Scheib*, 1846.

Mezler de Andelberg (Joannes Baptista). *De influxu anatomiæ pathologicæ in medicinam practicam. 80 pp., 2 l. 8°. *Pragæ, typ. filiorum T. Haase*, 1841.

Mezzabotta (E.) La verità sul cholera; la storia; i colpevoli, le rivelazioni; le conseguenze, i rimedii necessarii. 47 pp. 8°. *Roma, E. Perino*, 1883.

Mezzanotte (*Antonio*) [1786–   ].
DRAGOMANNI (F. G.) Biografia, [etc.] 8°. *Imola*, 1843.
Repr. from : Utile-Dulci, anno ii, nos. 4–5.

Mezzini (Augusto). Sulla emorragia cerebrale; considerazioni teorico-pratiche. 45 pp. 8°. *Bologna, Gamberini et Parmeggiani*, 1862.
Repr. from : Bull. d. sc. med. di Bologna, 1862, 4. s., xviii.

Mhichel (Adrien). *Réduction en masse des hernies étranglées. 68 pp. 4°. *Paris*, 1870, No. 70.

Mhow.
Weatherhead. [Observations made at Mhow.] Tr. M. & Phys. Soc. Bombay, 1840, iii, 204–206.

Miagliano. Regolamenti di pubblica igiene e polizia urbana. 32 pp. 8°. *Biella, G. Amosso*, 1886.

Mialaret (Gérard). *Contribution à l'étude des modifications de la sensibilité du membre supérieur consécutives aux sections nerveuses. 88 pp. 4°. *Paris*, 1881, No. 232.

Mialet (Antoine). *De la dysenterie. 26 pp. 4°. *Paris*, 1853, No. 292.

Mialhe (Louis)[1] [1807–86]. *Essai de propositions et d'observations pharmaceutiques. 44 pp. 4°. *Paris, Fain*, 1836.
For Biography, see France méd., Par., 1886, ii, 1536 (A. C.).

——. *Essai de propositions et d'observations chimiques et médicales. 40 pp. 4°. *Paris*, 1838, No. 26, v. 331.

——. *De la décomposition spontanée des êtres organisés, et des moyens de la prévenir. 52 pp. 4°. *Paris, Rignoux*, 1839.
Concours.

——. Considérations chimiques et thérapeutiques sur les différentes espèces de magnésie calcinée employées en médecine. 24 pp. 8°. *Paris, Lange, Lévy & Cie.*, 1844. [P., v. 1644.]
Repr. from : J. d. conn. méd. prat., Par., 1843–4, xi.

Mialhe (Louis)[1]—continued.
——. Mémoire sur les émanations du plomb et sur l'action physiologique des divers composés fournis par ce métal, lu à l'Académie royale de médecine, le 27 décembre 1842; suivi de quelques réflexions sur l'absorption des médicamens et des poisons. 24 pp. 8°. *Paris, Lange, Lévy & Cie.*, 1844. [P., v. 1666.]
Repr. from : J. d. conn. méd. prat., Par., 1843–4, xi.

——. Traité de l'art de formuler, ou notions de pharmacologie appliquée à la médecine. iv, cccvi, 220 pp. 8°. *Paris, Fortin, Masson & Cie.*, 1845.

——. Mémoire sur la digestion et l'assimilation des matières amyloïdes et sucrées. 26 pp. 8°. *Paris, V. Masson*, 1846. [P., v. 474; 1644.]

——. Mémoire sur la digestion et l'assimilation des matières albuminoïdes; lu à l'Académie des sciences le 3 août 1846. 1 p. l., 40 pp. 8°. *Paris, V. Masson*, 1847. [P., v. 474; 1203; 1644.]
Repr. from : Union méd., Par., 1847, i.

——. Recherches théoriques et pratiques sur les purgatifs. 36 pp., 1 l. 8°. *Paris, V. Masson*, 1848. [P., v. 803; 1644.]
Repr. from : Union méd., Par., 1848, ii.

——. Nouvelles recherches sur la cause et le traitement du diabète sucré ou glucosurie. 12 pp. 8°. [*Paris*, 1849.] [*Also, in :* P., v. 453; 1647.]
Repr. from : Bull. gén. de thérap., Par., 1849, xxxvi.

——. Nouvelles considérations chimiques et thérapeutiques sur le tartrate de potasse et de fer (tartrate ferrico-potassique). 7 pp. 8°. [*Paris, Hennuyer & Cie.*, 1850.]
Repr. from : Bull. gén. de thérap., etc., Par., 1850, xxxviii.

——. Die Receptirkunst, oder die Kenntniss der Pharmacologie in ihrer Anwendung auf die Medicin für Studirende und praktische Aerzte, ins Deutsche übertragen von Dr. R. Biefel. viii, 268 pp. 12°. *Breslau, Trewendt u. Granier*, 1852.

——. De l'albumine et de ses divers états dans l'économie animale. 48 pp. 8°. *Paris, F. Malteste & Cie.*, 1852. [P., v. 798; 1644.]
Repr. from : Union méd., Par., 1852, vi.

——. Du rôle chimique de l'acide carbonique dans l'économie animale. 15 pp. 8°. *Paris, F. Malteste & Cie.*, 1856.
Repr. from : Union méd., Par., 1856, x.

——. Chimie appliquée à la physiologie et à la thérapeutique. xxxii, 703 pp. 8°. *Paris, V. Masson*, 1856.

——. Considérations sur la destruction du sucre dans l'économie animale, présentées à la Société d'hydrologie médicale de Paris, en réponse à un travail de M. Fauconneau-Dufresne, le 6 avril 1857. 11 pp. 8°. *Paris, Germer-Baillière*, 1857. [*Also, in :* P., v. 1666.]
Repr. from : Ann. Soc. d'hydrol. méd. de Par. Compt.-rend., 1856–7, iii.

——. De la destruction des acides organiques dans l'économie animale envisagée au point de vue du régime à suivre à Vichy. 50 pp. 8°. *Paris, Germer-Baillière*, 1866.
Repr. from : Ann. Soc. d'hydrol. méd. de Par. Compt.-rend., 1866, xi.

——. Recherches sur la digestion, l'assimilation et l'oxydation organique cu vitale. 98 pp., 1 l. 8°. *Paris, E. Martinet*, 1879.

—— **& Pressat.** De la pepsine et de ses propriétés digestives. 32 pp. 8°. *Paris, V. Masson & fils*, 1860.

Mialhe (Louis)[2]. *De l'ictère grave essentiel. vi, 7–65 pp. 4°. *Montpeller, Boehm & fils*, 1864. [P., v. 47.]

Mialhes (J.-F.) *Sur la fièvre typhoïde, maladie plus généralement connue sous le nom de dothinentérite. 24 pp. 4°. *Paris*, 1831, No. 35, v. 238.

Miallet (Ernest-Daniel). *Du cancer de la langue et de son traitement. 38 pp. 4°. *Paris*, 1865, No. 274.

Miami Drake Medical Society. Constitution. 16 pp. 8°. *Dayton*, 1864.

Miami Medical College of Cincinnati. Annual announcements for the sessions of 1852–3 to 1882– 3 (1.–23.). 8°. *Cincinnati*, 1852–82.

List of students and graduates for the years 1852–3 to 1881–2 in announcement for subsequent years. Organized in 1852. In 1857 it coalesced with the Medical College of Ohio. In 1865 the connection was severed, and the school was reorganized under the old title.

——. Announcements of spring and summer sessions for 1853; 1867; 1872; 1873; 1876. 8°. [*Cincinnati*, 1853–76.]

——. History of the . . . and of its faculty and alumni. From the years 1852 to 1880, inclusive. 119 pp. 8°. *Cincinnati*, 1881.

Alumni Association, 1881.

Mianowski (*Joseph*) [1804–79].

[**Necrology.**] Gaz. lek., Warszawa, 1879, xxvi, 47.— **Nekrologia.** Medycyna, Warszawa, 1879, vii, 47.

Mianowski (Nicolaus) [–1844]. *Diss. therapiam febris nervosæ exhibens. 1 p. l., 40 pp. 8°. *Vilnæ, J. Zawadski*, [1807].

Miard (Antony). *Origine de la myopie, l'accommodation et les défauts de réfraction. 119 pp. 4°. *Paris*, 1870, No. 264.

——. Des troubles fonctionnels et organiques de l'amétropie et de la myopie en particulier, de l'accommodation binoculaire et ciliaire dans les vices de la réfraction. Recherches étiologiques des conditions d'existence des divers défauts réfractifs; nature et mécanisme des phénomènes physiologiques qu'ils comportent et des états pathologiques principaux qu'ils engendrent. Traitement de la myopie. viii, 460 pp. 8°. *Paris, J.-B. Baillière & fils*, 1872.

Mias (R.-N.) *Sur les passions considérées comme causes de maladies. 28 pp. 4°. *Paris*, 1836, No. 371, v. 305.

Miasm.

See, also, **Contagion**, *etc.*; **Effluvia**; **Fever** (*Malarial, Causes of*); **Gases** (*Irrespirable, etc.*); **Germ** *theory of disease, etc.*; **Malaria**, *etc.*; **Soil**.

BAERKEN (J. F.) Over contagium en miasma. 8°. *Tiel*, 1876.

BALESTRA (P.) Ricerche ed esperimenti sulla natura e genesi del miasma palustre. 2. ed. 8°. *Roma*, 1877.

BERTULUS (E.) Observations et réflexions sur l'intoxication miasmatique, considérée en général dans les différents états pathologiques qui en résultent, et plus spécialement dans la peste, le typhus, la fièvre jaune et le choléra-morbus épidémique. 8°. *Montpellier*, 1843.

BOISDON (A.) *Des effets produits sur l'organisme par les miasmes animaux non contagieux. 4°. *Paris*, 1861.

BRESLAUER (J.) *De miasmatibus et contagiis. 8°. *Vratislaviæ*, [1855].

BRESSY. Cours de miasmatique, traduit de la nature. 8°. *Paris*, 1832.

CHENAUD (L.) *De la réceptivité morbide de l'organisme à jeun. 4°. *Paris*, 1875.

DURAND-CLAYE (A.) Mémoire sur le desséchement du lac Fucino. 8°. *Paris*, 1878.

Repr. from: Ann. d. ponts et chaussées, 1878, xv, 1. sem.

FROEHLICH (J. B.) *De præcipuis miasmatum fontibus. 8°. *Landishuti*, 1812.

GERICKE (J. L.) *Diss. sistens miasmatologiam generalem. 4°. *Gottingæ*, [1775].

MALISCHEWSKI (H.) *Des principes miasmatiques. 4°. *Paris*, 1867.

PRADEAU (M.-E.-A.) *Parallèle des miasmes, des virus, des venins, des poisons et des médicaments. 4°. *Paris*, 1867.

Miasm.

ROMERSHAUSEN (E.) Das Miasma. Ueber wahrscheinliche Entstehung und Verbreitung desselben im Allgemeinen, und in besonderer Beziehung auf eine naturgemässe, richtige und schützende Construction der Abtrittsanlagen und Kloake. Eine physikalisch-technische Mittheilung an Sanitäts-Behörden, Aerzte, Ortsvorsteher, Bau-Unternehmer und Familienhäupter. 12°. *Marburg*, 1856.

SCHLEURHOLTS (L. T.) *De effluviorum paludosorum, in regione inprimis Groningana, origine, natura et efficacia noxia in corpus humanum. 8°. *Groningæ*, [1830].

ULFFERS (W. J.) *De miasmate contagioso. 4°. *Kiliæ Holsatorum*, 1773.

Bell (J.) On miasm as an alleged cause of fevers. Phila. J. M. & Phys. Sc., 1825, xi, 274–316. — **Bergman** (F. A. G.) Om miasmernas och contagiernas natur och verkningssätt. Upsala Läkaref. Förh., 1867–8, iii, 600–629. *Also,* Reprint.—**Bischof** (G.) Ueber die Natur der Miasmen, welche sich bei der Vermischung des Meerwassers mit süssem Wasser bilden. Org. f. d. ges. Heilk., Bonn, 1840–41, i, 479–493. — **Blue** (J. H.) Remarks on miasm. West. & South. M. Recorder, Lexington, Ky., 1843, ii, 67–71.—**Breyer** *et al.* Sur les miasmes. Bull. Soc. roy. d. sc. méd. et nat. de Brux., 1874, 2–12.—**Bryan** (J. M.) The origin of miasmatic disease. Brit. M. J., Lond., 1873, ii, 688.— **Burdel** (E.) Nouvelles recherches sur le miasme et l'impaludation. Bull. Acad. roy. de méd. de Belg., Brux., 1861, 2. s., iv, 98; 435: 1862, 2. s., v, 90. *Also,* Reprint.—**Carman** (B. R.) Remarks on the existence and mode of obviating the injurious effects of miasma, resulting from decomposition of vegetable matter. San Francisco M. Press, 1860, i, 5–8. — **Colin** (L.) Miasme. Dict. encycl. d. sc. méd., Par., 1873, 2. s., vii, 511–551. *Also,* Reprint.—**Correa de Serra** (E.-J.) Notice sur le miasme épidémique. Rev. de thérap. méd.-chir., Par., 1876, 320; 376; 430; 457. *Also, transl.* [Abstr.]: Salute, Genova, 1876, xi, 285; 297.—**Dalton** (N.) The analogy of miasmatic and electric changes in the production of disease. Tr. Ohio M. Soc., Columbus, 1861, 75–86.—**Diaz** (P.) El paludismo y el telurismo. Actas . . . Cong. region. de cien. méd. 1879, Cádiz, 1882, 722–728.—**Dyes** (A.) Ueber das Wesen und die Behandlung der miasmatischen Krankheiten. Deutsche Klinik, Berl., 1870, xxii, 227; 233. ——. Beitrag zur rationellen Behandlung der miasmatischen Krankheiten. *Ibid.*, 1873, xxv, 219; 231. — **Ferguson** (W.) On the nature and history of the marsh poison. Tr. Roy. Soc. Edinb., 1823, ix, 273–296. — **Friedmann.** Ueber die Quelle der Insalubrität der atmosphärischen Luft. Amtl. Ber. ü. d. Versamml. deutsch. Naturf. u. Aerzte 1864, Giessen, 1865, xxxix, 211–213. — **Gibbs** (O. C.) On miasmata. Med. & Surg. Reporter, Phila., 1862, vii, 6–9. — **Guérin** (J.) Des conséquences que peuvent avoir pour la santé publique les émanations cadavériques des armées. Gaz. méd. de Par., 1871, 3. s., xxvi, 83–86.—**Harvey** (W. F.) Miasmata. Cincin. Lancet & Obs., 1859, n. s., ii, 457: 1861, n. s., iv, 521.— **Hunt** (C. A.) Miasm and its effects on the human organism. West. Lancet, Cincin., 1853, xiv, 534–551. — **de Lassone.** Histoire de divers accidens graves, occasionnés par les miasmes d'animaux en putréfaction, et de la nouvelle méthode de traitement qui a été employée avec succès dans cette circonstance. Hist. Soc. roy. de méd. 1776, Par., 1779, i, pt. 2, 97–103.—**Lemaire** (J.) Recherches sur la nature des miasmes fournis par le corps de l'homme en santé. Gaz. méd. de Par., 1867, 3. s., xxii, 593; 657. *Also, transl.*: Chicago M. J., 1868, xxv, 97; 155.— **Miasmi** (I) ed i contagi, loro natura e modi di combatterne gli effetti; studii ed osservazioni. Imparziale, Firenze, 1879, xix, 144; 205; 283; 314; 372; 427. — **Mühry** (A.) Ueber die Natur der Miasmen, als vegetablische Organismen vorgestellt; aus geographischem Gesichtspunkte. (Malaria-Fieber, gelbes Fieber und indische Cholera.) Ztschr. f. rat. Med., Heidelb., 1854, n. F., v, 286–306.—**Nacquart.** Miasme. Dict. d. sc. méd., Par., 1819, xxxiii, 353–362.—**Natura** (Sulla) dei miasmi e dei contagi. [Rap. di Polli.] Atti . . . r. Ist. Lomb. di sc. e lett., Milano, 1867–71, v, pt. 1, pp. xxxix–l.—**Naumann.** Ueber das Wesen der Miasmen und der Contagien. Amtl. Ber. ü. d. Versamml. d. Gesellsch. deutsch. Naturf. u. Aerzte 1842, Mainz, 1843, xx, 268–274. — **Pantaleoni** (D.) Del miasma vegetale e delle malattie miasmatiche. Sperimentale, Firenze, 1870, xxvi, 218; 337; 446; 556. — **Paoli.** Einige Gedanken über die Miasmen. Allg. Ztg. f. Chir., Augsburg, 1843, iii, 325; 359.—**Pari** (A.) Sui miasmi, e sui contagi, non son le cognite che manchino per render scientifica la dottrina sui miasmi e sui contagi, è il gazzabuglio in cui furono gettate che impedisce vedervi chiaro. Gazz. med. pubb., Napoli, 1874, v, 161; 193; 225; 257; 289.— **Pech.** Ueber Miasmen und Contagien. Thierarzt, Wetzlar, 1877, xvi, 169; 193; 217; 241; 265. — **Poznanski.** L'air miasmatique et ses migrations. Bull. Acad. de méd., Par., 1868, xxxiii, 974–978. ——. La dynamique des mias-

Miasm.

mes. Bull. Soc. de méd. prat. de Par., 1868, 46–49.—**Roth** (T.) Ueber das Miasma. Vrtljschr. f. gerichtl. Med., Berl., 1878, n. F., xxix, 143 : 1879, n. F., xxx, 347.—**Satomi** (G.) [The nature of miasmata.] Ijishinbun, Tokio, 1880, no. 30, Sept. 15. — **Schleicher.** Teichmiasma. Med. Convers.-Bl., Hildburgh., 1831, ii, 263. — **Serrano** (N.) Sobre el concepto de virus ó de miasmas. Siglo méd., Madrid, 1865, xii, 161–165.— **Shurly** (E. L.) The poisons giving rise to the miasmatic order of zymotic diseases : their relationship. Detroit Rev. Med. & Pharm., 1876, xi, 410–419. — **Silvestrini** (G.) Sul miasma malarico ; studio sperimentale. Spallanzani, Modena, 1883, 2. s., xii, 135–147. *Also :* Gazz. med. ital., prov. venete, Padova, 1883, xxvi, 45–51.—**Smith** (B.) Miasm ; its probable origin and action. N. Orl. M. & S. J., 1873–4, n. s., i, 516–536.—**Tefft** (J. E.) On miasmata. Tr. M. Ass. Missouri. St. Louis, 1880, xxiii, 89–93.—**Torrellas** (L.) Miasmas y virus. Andalucía méd., Córdoba, 1881, vi, 153–160.—**Tuefferd** (H.) Des miasmes ; il n'y a pas de miasmes contagieux. Union méd., Par., 1865, 2. s., xxviii, 269.—**Verneuil** (A.) Du paludisme considéré au point de vue chirurgical. Rev. de chir., Par., 1881, i, 529 ; 881 : 1882, ii, 16 ; 279 ; 898. *Also* [Abstr.] : Rev. scient., Par., 1881, xxvii, 579–583.—**Wendrykowski.** Die Atmosphäre und die Miasmen. Org. f. d. ges. Heilk., Berl., 1857, vi, 341.—**Wildberg** (C. F. L.) Ueber das Miasma und Contagium überhaupt, und die Mephitis insbesondere. Jahrb. d. ges. Staatsarznk., Leipz., 1835, i, 4. Hft., 10–15.—**Winter.** Einige Bemerkungen über die Frage : Ob Miasmen, wenn sie auf lebende Organismen einwirken, primär die Solida oder die Fluida ergreifen? Med. Convers.-Bl., Hildburgh., 1831, ii, 369 – 376. — **Zambianchi.** Sui miasmi. Raccoglitore, Fano, 1844, xiv, 261–274.

Miaulet (J.) Nouveau système d'ablutions applicable aux établissements pénitentiaires, casernes, usines, etc. 15 pp., 1 pl. 8°. *Nîmes, C. Ballivet & Cie.*, 1880.

Mibelli (Vittorio).
See **Romiti** (Guglielmo). Sunto delle lezione di anatomia generale, etc. 8°. *Siena*, 1879.

Mican (D. Josephus Godefridus). * De lege revulsionis, ac derivationis virium systematis nervosi. 26 pp. 12°. *Pragæ, J. E. Diesbach*, [1784].

Micauld (Paul-Edmonde). * Influence du célibat sur la population. 42 pp. 4°. *Paris*, 1867, No. 280.

Micault (Paul). * Des tumeurs perlées aux doigts. 1 p. l., 44 pp., 1 l. 4°. *Nancy*, 1883, No. 183.

Mice (*Diseases of*).
See **Favus** in animals.

Micé (Léopold). De la rotation de la matière chez les êtres vivants. 76 pp. 4°. *Paris*, 1857, No. 80, v. 608.

———. Services mutuels que se rendent la médecine et les sciences dites accessoires. Leçon d'ouverture. 18 pp. 8°. *Bordeaux, A. Bellier*, 1872.
Repr. from : Gaz. méd. de Bordeaux, 1872, i.

———. De la fièvre charbonneuse et des moyens d'en préserver les animaux et, par suite, l'homme ; conférence faite à Bazas (Gironde), en février 1883, dans une séance publique solennelle du comice agricole de l'arrondissement. 40 pp. 8°. *Bordeaux, G. Gounouilhou*, 1883.
Repr. from : J. de méd. de Bordeaux, 1882–3, xii.

Michael (Bernhardus). * Quædam de partu arte præmaturo. 24 pp. 8°. *Jenæ, typ. Hochhausenii*, 1848.

Michael (Gustavus Theodorus). * De calore corporis humani in febri intermittente mutato. 28 pp., 1 l., 5 tab. 4°. *Lipsiæ, typ. J. S. Wassermanni*, [1855].

Michael (J.) Zur Physiologie und Pathologie des Gesanges. 18 pp. 8°. *Berlin, J. Sittenfeld*, [1876].
Repr. from : Berl. klin. Wchnschr., 1876, xiii.

———. Ueber Ohrensausen. 6 pp. 8°. *Berlin, E. Grosser*, 1884.
Repr. from : Deutsche Med.-Ztg., Berl., 1884, v.

Michael (J. Edwin). A critical historical and clinical study of Smith's anterior splint. 26 pp.

Michael (J. Edwin)—continued.
8°. *Brooklyn, N. Y., Annals of Anatomy & Surgery*, 1882.
Repr. from : Ann. Anat. & Surg., Brooklyn, 1882, v.

Michael (Jacobus). * De fontibus et fluminibus. Respondente Johanne Assingio. 7 l. 4°. [*Jenæ*], typ. *J. Weidneri*, 1613.

Michael (Johannes). Diss. pharmaceutico-therapeutica de natura tincturæ bezoardicæ, cum appendice collectanea ob naturam symbolicam et homogeneam, de mistura simplici ; his præfixæ sunt epistolæ honorariæ nonnullorum veteranorum medicorum. Opera et studio Godofredi Schultzii. 1 p. l., 197 pp., 1 l. 24°. *Halis Sax., sumpt. S. J. Hubneri*, 1678.

Michael (M.) * De syphiliticis affectionibus ductum aëriferorum. 3 p. l., 30 pp., 1 l. 8°. *Vratislaviæ, H. Lindner*, 1856. C.

Michael (Michel Isaacus). * De metrorrhagiis post partum insequentibus. 36 pp., 2 l. 8°. *Halis Sax., typ. Semlerianis*, [1844].

Michael (W. H.), **Corfield** (W. H.), & **Wanklyn** (J. A.) A manual of public health for the use of local authorities, medical officers of health, and others. Edited by Ernest Hart. viii, 374 pp. 12°. *London, Smith, Elder & Co.*, 1874.

Michaeli (Wilhelm) [1849–   ]. * Ueber Hysterie. 32 pp. 8°. *Berlin, G. Lange*, [1872].

Michaëlides (Jean). * Quelques considérations sur l'auscultation dans la grossesse. 35 pp. 4°. *Paris*, 1837, No. 205, v. 312.

Michælis. Die Krankheiten der Athmungsorgane. Begriff und Ziel der heutigen Schwindsuchtslehre in zwölf Vorträgen. 2 p. l., 104. 8°. *Elberfeld, E. Loss*, 1876.

———. Tisch für Lungenkranke, nebst einem Anhange: Schwindsuchtsprophylaxe im kindlichen Lebensalter. 141 pp., 3 l. 8°. *Elberfeld, E. Loll*, 1877.

———. Hals- und Lungen-Diätetik im Spiegel der pathologischen Entwicklungsprozesse. Diätetisch-praktischer Leitfaden für Behandlung und Verhütung der Hals- und Lungenleiden. 2. Aufl. 1 p. l., 224, vii pp. 8°. *Wüstegiersdorf bei Waldenburg i. Schl., M. Jacob*, [1882].

———. Die Pflege des Erkrankten Magens in sechzig Grundregeln nebst Tagesdiät. Diätetik und Hygieine gegen tiefergehende Erkrankungen des Magens. Für Aerzte und Laien. 64 pp. 8°. *Jena, H. Costenoble*, 1883.

———. Kampf und Schutz gegen beginnende Schwindsuchts-Krankheiten des Kehlkopfs und der Lungen in achtzig Lebensregeln, nebst Tagesdiät. Für Aerzte und Laien. 127 pp., 1 pl. 8°. *Jena, H. Costenoble*, 1884.

———. Die Pflege des erkrankten Magens. 2. Theil. Magen und Darm. Diätetik und Hygieine gegen die wechselseitigen und eigenartigen Erkrankungen des Magens und die damit zusammenhängenden Unterleibsstörungen in achtzig Aphorismen. Für Aerzte und Laien. 1 p. l., 79 pp. 8°. *Jena, H. Costenoble*, 1885.

———. Die Leberkrankheiten und Gallenstörungen in diätetischer, hygieinischer und prophylactischer Beziehung. Für Aerzte und Laien in sechzig Grundregeln nebst Tagesdiät. viii, 123 pp. 12°. *Jena, H. Costenoble*, 1886.

Michaelis (A.) * Ueber die Chloride und Oxychloride des Schwefels. [Carlsruhe.] 42 pp., 1 ch. 8°. *Giessen, W. Keller*, 1873.

Michaelis (Adolf). Zur Anwendung des Bromkalium gegen Epilepsie. 31 pp. 8°. *Göttingen, Hofer*, 1873.

Michaelis (Albert). * Ueber chronische Milztumoren im Kindesalter. 26 pp., 1 l. 8°. *Halle a. S., Plötz*, 1883.

Michaelis (Albert Carl Julius) [1826–86]. Compendium der Lehre von der Syphilis und der damit zusammenhängenden ähnlichen Krankheiten und Folgezustände für praktische Aerzte und Studirende. xv, 379 pp., 1 l. 8°. *Wien, W. Braumüller*, 1859.

——. The same. 2. Aufl. xvi, 367 pp. 8°. *Wien, W. Braumüller*, 1865.

Michaelis (Christ. Fridericus). * De hæmoptysi. 20 pp. 4°. *Vitenbergæ, lit. Hakianis,* [1732].

Michaelis (Christian. Frider.) [1754–1814]. De caussis commutatæ quarundam regionum fertilitatis. 26 pp. 4°. *Coburgi, ex off. Ahliana,* [1771].

——. Theses medicæ. 8 pp. sm. 4°. *Argentorati, typ. J. H. Heitzii,* 1776.

——. De angina polyposa sive membranacea. 7 p. l., 309 pp. 12°. *Gottingæ, typ. vid. A. Vandenhoeck,* 1778.

——. The same. Observations sur le croup, ou angine membraneuse. Trad. du latin par F. Ruette. 68 pp. 8°. *Paris, Allut,* 1810.

——. Etwas über den Blasensteinschnitt. 82 pp., 1 l., 2 pl. 4°. *Marburg, J. C. Krieger,* 1813.

*For Biography, see **Quelmalz** (Sam. Theo.)*
*See, also, **Nachrichten** von dem Leben und Schriften jeztlebender teutscher Aerzte, etc. 8°. Hildesheim, 1799, i, 379–385.*
*For Portrait, see **Collection**—van Kaathoven.*

Michaelis (Christianus Fridericus) [1727–   ]. * De orificii uteri cura clinica atque forensi. 34, xvi pp. sm. 4°. *Lipsiæ, ex off. Langenhemiana* [1756].

*See, also, **Adair** (Jacob Makkitrik). Physiologische und diätetische Schriften, [etc.] 8°. Zittau, 1788–91.—**Rowley** (William). Praktische Abhandlung über die Frauenzimmerkrankheiten, [etc.] 8°. Bresslau, 1790.—. Abhandlung über die vorzüglichsten Augenkrankheiten 8°. Bresslau, 1792.—**Rush** (Benjamin). Neue medicinische [etc.] 8°. Nürnberg, 1797.—**Stark** (William). Klinische und anatomische [etc.] 8°. Bresslau u. Hirschberg, 1789.*
*For Biography, see **Nachrichten** von dem Leben und Schriften jeztlebender teutscher Aerzte, etc. 8°. Hildesheim, 1799, i, 386–418.*

Michaelis (Curt). * Chirurgisch-humanistische Bemerkungen über die Schlachtfelder der neuesten Zeit. 25 pp. 8°. *Jena, Fischer u. Hermsdorf,* 1865.

Michaelis (E. O.) * De luxationis congenitæ patellæ duobus casibus. 28 pp. 8°. *Kiliæ, in libraria academica,* 1854.

Michaelis (Edgar) [1807–   ]. * Observationes quædam de catameniorum viis insolitis. 29 pp. 8°. *Berolini, typ. fratrum Unger,* [1830].

Michaelis (Eduard) [1824–   ]. * De scarlatina et morbis, qui eam sequuntur, adjecto insigni gangrænæ scarlatinosæ exemplo. 30 pp., 1 l. 8°. *Berolini, typ. Nietackianis,* [1847].

——. Albrecht von Graefe. Sein Leben und Wirken. viii, 196 pp., port. 8°. *Berlin, G. Reimer,* 1877.

——. Handwörterbuch der augenärztlichen Therapie zum Gebrauch für practische Aerzte. xi, 252 pp. 12°. *Leipzig, A. Abel,* 1883.

Michaelis (Ernst) [1860–   ]. * Zur Lehre von den Zwangsvorstellungen. 30 pp. 8°. *Berlin, M. Niethe,* [1882].

Michaelis (F. H.) Skizze von der Verbreitung des Cretinismus im Canton Aargau. fol. *Aarau, H. Böschlin,* 1843.

Michaelis (Ferdinandus) [1797–   ]. * De partibus constitutivis singularum partium sanguinis arteriosi et venosi. 31 pp. 8°. *Berolini, typ. Brüschckianis,* [1827]. [*Also, in:* P., v. 1535.]

Michaelis (Georgius Philip.) [1712–83]. * Diss. exhibens usum et abusum medicinæ in

Michaelis (Georgius Philip.)—continued. re publica. 2 p. l., 45 pp. 4°. *Marburgi, typ. P. C. Mulleri,* [1738].

——. De nexu scientiæ physicæ cum medicina. 12 pp. 4°. *Marburgi, ex off. Mülleriana,* [1764].

Michaelis (Germano). * Da injecção subcutanea em geral. 16 pp., 1 l. 4°. *Bahia, J. G. Tourinho,* 1870.

Michaelis (Godofr. Phil.) * Diss. sistens observationes circa placentæ ac funiculi umbilicalis vasa absorbentia. 16 pp. sm. 4°. *Gottingæ, J. G. Rosenbusch,* [1790].

——. Ueber die zweckmässigste Einrichtung der Feld-Hospitäler. xvi, 520 pp., 2 pl., 1 tab. 8°. *Göttingen, Dieterich,* 1801.

Michaelis (Gottlieb Augustus) [1712–   ]. * De anodynorum virtutibus venenorum. 50 pp. sm. 4°. *Vitembergæ, ex off. Eichsfeldiana,* [1735].
*For Biography, see **Stentzel** (Christian. Godofr.)*

Michaelis (Guilielmus). * De discrimine quod intercedit inter typhum abdominalem atque exanthematicum. 14 pp., 1 l. 8°. *Lipsiæ, P. Reclam jun.,* [1855].

Michaelis (Gustav Adolf) [1798–   ]. De induratione telæ cellulosæ recens natorum commentatio. 86 pp. 8°. *Kiliæ Holsatorum, in commissis bibliopolæ universitatis,* 1825.

——. Ueber die Retina, besonders über die Macula lutea und das Foramen centrale. 40 pp., 5 pl. 4°. [*n. p.,* 1838.]

——. Das enge Becken nach eigenen Beobachtungen und Untersuchungen. Hrsg. von Carl Conrad Theodor Litzmann. xiv pp., 1 l., 440 pp. 8°. *Leipzig, G. Wigand,* 1851.

——. The same. 2. Aufl. xii, 372 pp. sm. 8°. *Leipzig, G. Wigand,* 1865.

——. Unterricht für Hebammen. Neu bearbeitet und hrsg. von C. C. Th. Litzmann. 199 pp. 12°. *Kiel, C. F. Mohr,* 1862.

Michaelis (Gustavus). The gradual development of pharmacy. [Introductory address, Albany College of Pharmacy.] 17 pp. 8°. *Albany, N. Y., Burdick & Taylor,* 1886.

Michaelis (H. S.) C. F. v. Graefe in seinem 30jährigen Wirken für Staat und Wissenschaft. 98 pp. 8°. *Berlin, J. Petsch,* 1840.
Title-page wanting.
*See, also, **Vetch** (John). Geschichte der Ophthalmie, etc. 8°. Berlin, 1817.*

Michaelis (Joannes Fridericus). * De fallacia examinis chemici in exploranda intima thermarum natura. 35 pp. 4°. *Wittebergæ, lit. C. C. Dürrii,* [1767].
*For Biography, see **Langguth** (Geo. Aug.)*

Michaelis (Joannes Gottlieb.) Anevrysmatum cordis disq. anat.-med. vi, 50 pp. 8°. *Halæ, J. C. Hendel,* [1785].

Michaelis (Joh.)[1] [1607–67]. Opera medicochirurgica quotquot innotuerunt omnia. Ejus nempe I. Praxis clinica generalis ad Jonstoni ideam occupata circa affectus corporis humani universales, particulares et chirurgicos. II. Praxis clinica specialis casibus xxvi subitaneis monita praxeos generalia ad ægri lectum applicare docens. III. Apparatus formularum, seu annotationes in Morellum de præscriptione formularum. IV. Ordo visitandi officinas, libellus oppido rarus, cum annexis regulis pharmaceutico-chymicis. Accedit in fine: V. Clavis ad authoris polychresta, h. e. descriptio medicamentorum D. Michaelis quondam in secretis habitorum. frontispiece, 6 p. l., 747 pp., 13 l. 4°. *Norimbergæ, sumpt. J. Hofmanni,* 1688.
pp. 335–344 repeated; pp. 722–747 are erroneously marked 622–647. Title of § iv on p. 719 reads as follows: Ordo visitandi officinas. Ejusque regulæ pharmaceutico-chymicæ.

——. Opera quotquot haberi potuerunt omnia. I. Praxis clinica ad Jo. Jonstoni ideam comparata. II. Apparatus medicamentarius ad P. Mo-

Michaelis (Joh.)[1]—continued.
relli methodum præscribendi formulas remediorum. III. Animadversiones in Joh. Schroederi
pharmacopœiam. IV. Notationes ad Guerneri
Rolfincii chymiam. V. Officinas pharmaceu-
ticas visitandi ratio. VI. Medicamentorum familiar. syllabus. Editio altera ab innumeris
mendis repurgata et præclaris locupletata accessionibus. 11 p. l., 728 pp., 12 l., 103 pp., 2 l. 4°.
Norimbergæ, sumpt. hæred. J. Hoffmanni, 1698.
  See, also, **Drawitz** (Joh.) Bericht und Unterricht
von der Krankheit des schmerz-machenden Scharbocks
[etc.] 12°. *Leipzig*, 1658.—**Hartmann** (J.) Praxis
chymiatrica. 4°. *Lipsiæ*, 1633. ——. The same. 12°.
Francofurti, 1634.—**Lagus** (Daniel). Disputatio publica
de visu. 4°. *Regiomonti*, 1638.
  For Portrait, see **Collection**—van Kaathoven.—**Collection** of Portr. of Phys. & Men of Sc., 58.

Michaelis (Joh.)[2] * De apoplexia. 15 l. sm.
4°. *Hafniæ, lit. C. Weringii*, [1676].

Michaelis (Joh. Conrad). * De senum affectibus. 48 pp. 4°. *Halæ Magdeb., C. Henckel*,
[1710]. [P., v. 1391.]

Michaelis (Joh. Gottlob Daniel).
  See **Walter** (Joh. Gottlieb). Anatomische Beobachtungen. 4°. *Berlin u. Stralsund*, 1782.

Michaelis (Mauritius) [1811–   ]. * De ophthalmia syphilitica. 30 pp., 1 l. 8°. *Berolini*,
typ. Nietackianis, [1835].

Michaelis (Max) [1854–   ]. * Der Verwun-
deten-Transport im Gebirge. 30 pp., 1 l. 8°.
Berlin, G. Schade, [1877].

Michaelis (Philipp). Ueber die Durchkreuzung
der Sehenerven. Mit einigen Anmerkungen von
Soemmering. 55 pp. 16°. *Halle, J. C. Hendel*,
1790.

Michaelis (R.) & **Gordon** (J.) Die Canalisation der Stadt Dortmund. Gutachten im Auftrage der städtischen Behörden. 62 pp., 2 maps.
4°. *Dortmund, F. W. Ruhfus*, 1878.

Michaelis ([Rudolphus] Albertus) [1849–   ].
* De eclampsia gravidarum et pa[r]turientium.
32 pp. 8°. *Berolini, G. Lange*, [1864].

Michaëlis (Theodorus) [1815–   ]. * De diabete mellito. 28 pp., 2 l. 8°. *Berolini, typ.
Nietackianis*, [1838].

Michaelius Hornanus (Joh.) De oculo, seu de
natura visus, libellus. Accedunt dialogus de
æternitate et quædam poëmatia ejusdem auctoris. 7 p. l., 84 pp., 86 l. 16°. *Dordrechti, H.
Essæus*, 1645.

——. Oculi fabrica, actio, usus, seu de natura
visus libellus. 7 p. l., 84 pp., 11 l. 16°. *Lugd.
Bat., D. Lopez de Haro*, 1651.

——. The same. 7 p. l., 84 pp., 11 l. 16°.
Lugd. Bat., F. Moyaert, 1651.

——. De æternitate dialogus. 6 l. 16°. [*Lugd.
Bat., D. Lopez de Haro*, 1651.]
  Bound with his: Oculi fabrica, [etc.] 16°. *Lugd. Bat.*,
1651.

——. The same. 6 l. 16°. [*Lugd. Bat., D. F.
Moyaert*, 1651.]
  Bound with his: Oculi fabrica, [etc.] 16°. *Lugd. Bat.*,
1651.

——. Poëmatia quædam. 67 l. 16°. [*Lugd.
Bat., D. Lopez de Haro*, 1651.]
  Bound with his: Oculi fabrica, [etc.] 16°. *Lugd. Bat.*,
1651.

——. The same. 67 l. 16°. [*Lugd. Bat., F.
Moyaert*, 1651.]
  Bound with his: Oculi fabrica, [etc.] 16°. *Lugd. Bat.*,
1651.

Michaelsen (Hermann). * Ueber die Indication der Herniotomie und einige bei letzterer gefundene Anomalien. 23 pp. 4°. *Kiel, C. F.
Mohr*, 1877.
  In: SCHRIFT. d. Univ. zu Kiel. xxiv, 1877, vii, med. ix.

Michaelsen (Joh. Wilhelm) [1860–   ]. * Untersuchungen über Enchytraeus Möbii Mich. und
andere Enchytraeiden. 50 pp., 1 l., 3 pl. 8°.
Kiel, Lipsius u. Tischer, 1886.

Michahelles (G. C. C. W.) Das Malo di scar-
lievo in historischer und pathologischer Hinsicht
beschrieben. 64 pp. 8°. *Nürnberg, J. A. Stein*,
1833.

Michailescu. * Étude sur un fait de pleurésie
avec épanchement purulent d'emblée. 41 pp., 1 l.
4°. *Paris*, 1880, No. 437.

Michailoff (N. F.) Materialy k opredelenijou
fizicheskago razvitija i boliezennosti v selskich
schkolach Ruzskago uiezda Moskovskoi gubernii. [Material for statistics of physical development and morbidity in rural schools of
Ruzsk district, government of Moscow.] 42
pp., 4 diag. 8°. *Moskva, tipog. V. V. Isleneva*,
1887.

——. Obtshaja charakteristika dejatelnosti na-
shich vospitatelnych domov. [General features
of the foundling asylums.] 21 pp. 8°. *Moskva,
S. P Jakovleva*, 1887.

Michailoff (V. I.) Hipnotizm v sravnenii s
javlenijami jiznenno-magniticheshimi, v isklu-
chitelnom primenenii poslednich k lecheniu bolnich. [Hypnotism in comparison with the phenomena of bio-magnetism, excluding its application to treatment of diseases.] ii, 133 pp., 2 l.
8°. *Moskva, tip. A. I. Mamontova & Ko.*, 1886.

——. The same. ii, 137 pp., 1 l. 8°. *St. Petersburg*, 1886.

Michailovski (Jakov). * O vidielenii mocheju
rtuti pri terapevt. upotreb. eja v forme mazei.
[Presence of mercury in the urine after its application in the form of ointment.] 58 pp., 1
diag. 8°. *St. Petersburg*, 1886.

Michalevich (I.) * Obmien i usvoenie azot.
chastei pitshi pri tsinge. [Metamorphosis and
assimilation of nitrogenous matter of food in
scurvy. 34 pp., 6 tab. 8°. *St. Petersburg*, 1886.

Michalke (Carl). * Ueber die Verwachsung
des Herzbeutels mit dem Herzen. 38 pp. 8°.
Würzburg, 1880.

Michalke (Joh.) * Ein Beitrag zur Behandlung
des Bandwurmleidens. 20 pp. 8°. *Greifswald,
F. W. Kunike*, 1874.

Michallet (F.-Saint-Ange). * Coup-d'œil rapide
sur l'art de guérir. 19 pp. 4°. *Paris*, 1821, No.
150, v. 167.

Michaloff (Ivan H.) * Contribution à l'étude
de l'enchondrome avec métastases. 83 pp., 3 l.,
2 pl. 8°. *Genève, Taponnier & Studer*, 1882.

Michalon (Lucien). * Des insertions vicieuses
du placenta et des indications qui en découlent.
94 pp. 4°. *Paris*, 1869, No. 202.

Michalowicz (Edgard). * Dégénérescence
kystique des reins et du foie. 31 pp. 4°. *Paris*, 1876, No. 95.

Michalski (A.)
  See **Larrey** (Félix-Hippolyte), le baron. Observation
d'amputation [etc.] 8°. *Paris*, 1857.

Michalski (André). * I. Quelles sont les maladies de la peau qui consistent dans une coloration anormale? Établir les caractères de ces
maladies. II. [etc.] 47 pp. 4°. *Paris*, 1842,
No. 149, v. 393.

Michalski (Arthur). * De la méthode hypodermique, ou des injections sous-cutanées. 100
pp. 4°. *Paris*, 1862, No. 289.

Michalski (Franciscus). * De epilepsia. 31
pp. 8°. *Vratislaviæ, G. T. Korn*, [1830].

Michalski (L.) * Étude sur la première dentition. 1 p. l., 67 pp. 4°. *Paris*, 1872, No.
152.

——. Du sevrage. Conseils à ma fille, aux
jeunes mères et aux nourrices. 46 pp. 8°. *Paris, Delahaye & Cie.*, 1876.

Michalski (Ludwig). * Experimentelle Beiträge zur Frage über die Bedeutung der halbzir-
kelförmigen Kanäle des Ohrlabyrinths. 29 pp.
8°. *Greifswald, C. Sell*, 1876.

Michalsky (Carolus Oscarus). * Nonnulla de pneumothorace. 14 pp., 1 l. 8°. *Jenæ, typ. A. Neuenhahni*, 1863. C.

Michalsky (Joannes Joseph.) * De inflammatione tunicæ mucosæ tractus alimentarii folliculosa. 1 p. l., 39 pp. 8°. *Gryphiæ, F. G. Kunike*, [1839].

Michauck (Joh. Heinrich). * Ein Beitrag zur Pathologie des Uterus fibroides. 36 pp., 1 l. 8°. *Leipzig, Huethel u. Legler*, [1868]. [P., v. 304.]

Michaud (Antoine). * Sur l'inflammation de l'articulation coxo-fémorale, généralement connue sous le nom de luxation spontanée ou consécutive du fémur. 38 pp. 4°. *Paris*, 1836, No. 93, v. 296.

Michaud (C.) * I. Établir les caractères qui distinguent le lupus du visage des éruptions diverses qui peuvent se fixer dans cette région. II. [etc.] 47 pp. 4°. *Paris*, 1840, No. 309, v. 363.

Michaud (Claude-Florent). * Essai sur les tempéramens. 1 p. l., 15 pp. 4°. *Strasbourg*, 1808, v. 45.

Michaud (G.-L.)
See **Oettinger** (Édouard-Marie). Bibliographie biographique, etc. 8°. *Leipzig*, 1850.

Michaud (J.-D.-Albert). * De la mort subite dans l'état puerpéral par coagulums sanguins dans le cœur droit et l'artère pulmonaire. 1 p. l., 47 pp. 4°. *Strasbourg*, 1870, 3. s., No. 285.

Michaud (Jean-Clément). De l'assistance médicale dans les campag. es. 19 pp. 8°. *Chambéry, A. Pouchet & Cie.*, 1868.
Association des médecins de la Savoie.

Michaud (Jean-François-Marie-Antoine-Eugène). * Étude sur le traitement curatif des varices 80 pp. 4°. *Paris*, 1876, No. 255.

Michaud (Jules-Aimé). * Sur la méningite et la myélite dans le mal vertébral; recherches d'anatomie et de physiologie pathologiques. 100 pp., 3 pl. 4°. *Paris*, 1871, No. 163.
———. The same. 98 pp., 3 pl. 8°. *Paris, A. Delahaye*, 1871.

Michaud (P.) Avant-projet pour l'alimentation de Lyon en eaux de sources. 67 pp. roy. 8°. *Lyon, Pitrat aîné*, 1877.

Michaud (Pierre-Aimé). * I. Faire connaître les complications les plus fréquentes de la scarlatine; apprécier leur gravité, et indiquer le traitement qu'elles réclament. II. [etc.] 27 pp. 4°. *Paris*, 1840, No. 161, v. 363.

Michaut (Armand). * De la rétention d'urine causée par l'hypertrophie de la prostate et de son traitement. 44 pp., 1 l. 4°. *Paris*, 1878, No. 68.
———. * De l'angine de poitrine. 39 pp. 4°. *Paris*, 1878, No. 271.

Michaut (Paul). * Du collodion en thérapeutique. 56 pp. 4°. *Paris*, 1876, No. 382.

Michaux (*André*) [1746–1802].
Boott (F.) Memorial of the botanical labours of André Michaux. Edinb. J. M. Sc., 1826, i, 126–132.

Michaux (Benjamin). * De l'éveil d'un état constitutionnel (hystérie) à la suite de l'anesthésie par le chloroforme. 97 pp. 4°. *Paris*, 1886, No. 147.

Michaux (E.) [1856–]. * De la sidérose pulmonaire. 58 pp., 1 l. 4°. *Paris*, 1881, No. 373.

Michaux (Edwards). * La Guyane et ses établissements pénitentiaires. 70 pp. 4°. *Paris*, 1860, No. 8.

Michaux (Émile). * De l'influence menstruelle sur la production d'accidents rhumatismaux. 55 pp. 4°. *Paris*, 1876, No. 41.

Michaux (Flavien). * De la situation déclive du malade avec flexion du rachis et taxis dans la réduction des hernies. 44 pp. 4°. *Paris*, 1883, No. 195.

Michaux (François-André) [1770–1855]. Mémoire sur les causes de la fièvre jaune; le concours simultané de trois causes est nécessaire au développement de la fièvre jaune, ou résultat d'observations faites dans les ports de mer des États-Unis de l'Amérique du Nord. 22 pp. 8°. *Paris, Baillière*, 1852. [*Also, in:* P., v. 468; 1130.]
For Biography, see **Durand** (Élias). Biographical memoir of the late François-André Michaux. 4°. *Philadelphia*, 1856.
Repr. from: Tr. Am. Phil. Soc., Phila., 1856, xi.

Michaux (Maximilien) [1808–]. Rapport de la troisième section sur le mémoire de M. Didot, intitulé: Dépôts urineux et uréthrotomie, suivi des conclusions adoptées par l'Académie. 31 pp. 8°. *Bruxelles, J.-B. de Mortier*, 1847.
Repr. from: Bull. Acad. roy. de méd. de Belg., Brux., 1845–7, v–vi.
Bound with: DIDOT (A.) Mémoires, etc. 8°. *Dinant*, 1848.
———. Résection de la mâchoire supérieure. 107 pp., 1 l. 8°. *Bruxelles, J.-B. de Mortier*, 1853.
Repr. from: Bull. Acad. roy. de méd. de Belg., Brux., 1852–3, xii.
———. Nouvelles considérations sur les polypes naso-pharyngiens. iii, 105 pp., 5 pl. 8°. *Bruxelles, de Mortier fils*, 1863.
Repr. from: Bull. Acad. roy. de méd. de Belg., Brux., 1862, 2. s., v.
———. Quelques mots encore sur les polypes fibreux naso-pharyngiens volumineux à insertions larges et résistantes et à prolongements multiples. 56 pp. 8°. *Bruxelles, H. Manceaux*, 1867.
Repr. from: Bull. Acad. roy. de méd. de Belg., Brux., 1867, 3. s., i.

Michaux (Paul) [1854–]. * Contribution à l'étude du carcinôme de la parotide. xi, 92 pp. 4°. *Paris*, 1883.

Michaux (Victor). * De la méningite cérébro-spinale épidémique. 53 pp. 4°. *Paris*, 1852, No. 51, v. 529.

Michaux-Bellaire (Charles-Adolphe). * De l'amygdalite chronique. 23 pp. 4°. *Strasbourg*, 1854, No. 321, 2. s., v. 20.

Michéa (Claude-François) [1815–82]. * Des hallucinations. 21 pp. 4°. *Paris*, 1837, No. 159, v. 311.
———. Traité pratique, dogmatique et critique de l'hypochondrie. x, 486 pp. 8°. *Paris, Labé*, 1845.
———. Recherches chimiques sur le sang dans les névroses. 42 pp. 8°. [*Paris, Fain & Thunot*, 1848.] [*Also, in:* P., v. 804.]
Repr. from: Gaz. méd. de Par., 1848, 3. s., ii.
———. Du délire des sensations. Ouvrage couronné par l'Académie de médecine. xxii pp., 1 p. l., 343 pp. 8°. *Paris, Labé*, 1846.
———. The same. 2. éd. 111, 343 pp. 8°. *Paris, Labé*, 1851.
———. Du pronostic de l'épilepsie et du traitement de cette maladie par le valérianate d'atropine. Fragment d'un mémoire lu devant l'Académie impériale de médecine, précédé d'un extrait du rapport à l'Académie sur ce mémoire. 43 pp. 8°. *Paris, Labé*, 1858.
———. Recherches expérimentales sur l'emploi comparé des principaux agents de la médication stupéfiante dans le traitement de l'aliénation mentale. 112 pp. 8°. *Paris, E. Thunot*, [*n. d.*] [P., v. 478.]
———. The same. 2. éd. 112 pp. 8°. *Paris, Labé*, 1857.
Repr. from: Gaz. méd. de Par., 1852, 3. s., vii.

Michel[1].
See **Bertrand** (Jean-Baptiste) & **Michel**. Observations faites sur la peste, [etc.] 16°. *Lyon*, 1721.

Michel[2]. Nouvelles observations sur le pouls, par rapport aux crises. xxxiv, 118 pp., 1 l. 12°. *Paris, De Bure l'aîné*, 1757.

Michel[3]. Étude sur la nature et la cause présumée des accidents survenus parmi les ouvriers qui travaillent aux fondations à l'air comprimé du bassin de Missiessy à Toulon. 55 pp., 4 pl. 8°. *Paris, J.-B. Baillière & fils,* 1880.
Repr. from : Arch. de méd. nav., Par., 1880, xxxiii.

Michel (*Madame*). Les remèdes de bonnes femmes, ou moyens de prévenir, soigner et guérir toutes les maladies, [etc.] 104 pp., 1 pl. 32°. *Paris,* 1827.

Michel (A.-E.) * Quelques réflexions au sujet de la douleur en général et de sa pathogénie, avec indication sommaire de son traitement médical et chirurgical. vi, 7–106 pp., 1 l. 4°. *Montpellier,* 1878, No. 31.

Michel (Alph.) * Considérations sur la pneumonie, d'après les expériences de M. Magendie. 29 pp. 4°. *Paris,* 1838, No. 166, v. 331.

Michel (Alphonse-Armand) [1854–]. * Du pannus et spécialement de son traitement local par la poudre d'iodoforme. 36 pp. 4°. *Paris,* 1880, No. 471.

Michel (Augustus Ferdinandus). * De rachitide. 31 pp. 8°. *Berolini, G. Schade,* [1853].

Michel (Carl). Die Krankheiten der Nasenhöhle und des Nasenrachenraumes. Nach eigenen Beobachtungen. 1 p. l., 107 pp., 1 pl. 8°. *Berlin, A. Hirschwald,* 1876.

————. The same. Traité des maladies des fosses nasales et de la cavité nasopharyngienne d'après des observations personnelles. Trad. de l'allemand par le docteur A. Capart. 158 pp., 1 pl., 1 l. 8°. *Bruxelles, H. Manceaux,* 1879.

————. Du traitement des maladies de la gorge et du larynx. Études cliniques... Trad. de l'allemand par R. Calmettes. iv, 143 pp. 8°. *Bruxelles, A. Manceaux,* 1884.

Michel (Ch.-H.) * De la dysenterie. 35 pp. 4°. *Paris,* 1846, No. 40, v. 448.

Michel (Charles)[1]. * De la chlorose. 22 pp. 4°. *Paris,* 1836, No. 248, v. 301.

Michel (Charles)[2]. * Quelques considérations sur les plaies de la trachée et de l'emploi de la canule comme moyen hémostatique. 43 pp. 4°. *Paris,* 1877, No. 122.

Michel (Charles-Évariste). * Topographie médicale de l'île Maurice. 134 pp. 4°. *Paris,* 1842, No. 88, v. 393.

Michel (Denis). * De la grippe et de ses manifestations pulmonaires (pneumonie et bronchopneumonie). 91 pp., 8 ch. 4°. *Paris,* 1886, No. 172.

Michel (Denis-Frédéric). * Essai sur l'érysipèle. 15 pp. 4°. *Montpellier, J. Martel aîné,* 1824, No. 87. [P., v. 1331.]

Michel (E.-Adolphe). * De la variole anomale. 30 pp. 4°. *Paris,* 1867, No. 76.

Michel (Édouard - Isidore - Jules). * Considérations sur le rhumatisme cérébro-spinal. 45 pp., 1 l. 4°. *Strasbourg,* 1863, No. 713, 2. s., v. 37.

Michel (Évariste). * De l'ictère hémaphéique. 40 pp. 4°. *Paris,* 1868, No. 229.
See, also, **Langlebert** (Edmond). Traité théorique et pratique des maladies vénériennes, [etc.] 8°. *Paris,* 1864.
————. The same. Tratado teórico y práctico de las enfermedades venéreas. 8°. *Madrid,* 1877.

Michel (F.-J.-X.) * Sur l'emploi des eaux minérales de Plombières et de Luxeuil dans le traitement de quelques maladies chroniques. vi, 7–51 pp. 4°. *Paris,* 1823, No. 8, v. 177.

Michel (F.-M.-Eugène). * Des corps étrangers pénétrants de l'œil. 30 pp. 4°. *Paris,* 1859, No. 185, v. 634.

Michel (Félix). * Sur les fièvres intermittentes. 18 pp. 4°. *Paris,* 1831, No. 266, v. 245.

Michel (Francisque [François-Xavier]) [1809–]. Histoire des races maudites de la France et de

Michel (Francisque [François-Xavier])—cont'd. l'Espagne. 2 v. xii, 373; 341 pp. 8°. *Paris, A. Franck,* 1847.

Michel (François). * Études sur les accidents urémiques. 46 pp. 4°. *Strasbourg,* 1860, No. 527, 2. s., v. 29.

Michel (François-Jacques). * I. Du diagnostic des scrofules. II. [etc.] 34 pp. 4°. *Paris,* 1841, No. 275, v. 378.

Michel (François-Jules). * Observations pour servir à l'histoire de la névralgie du membre supérieur. 72 pp. 4°. *Paris,* 1858, No. 308, v. 621.

Michel (Friedericus). * Abhandlung über Geburtslagen, nebst Beschreibung und Abbildung eines neuen Gebärbettes. 2 p. l., 70 pp., 1 pl. 8°. *Prag, G. Haase,* 1824.
German text. Additional title is: De situ parturientium adnexa descriptione cubilis parturientibus dicati nuper inventi.

Michel (Gustave). * De l'érysipèle dans la convalescence à l'asile impérial du Vésinet. 44 pp. 4°. *Paris,* 1866, No. 131.

Michel (H.) De l'influence de l'eau potable sur la santé publique, ou recherches sur l'hygiène. viii, 92 pp. 12°. *Paris, Motteroz,* 1884.

————. Une épidémie de choléra dans les Basses-Alpes. 18 pp. 8°. *Annecy, J. Niérat & Cie.,* 1885.

Michel (Heinrich). * Ueber die Wirkung des Staphylococcus pyogenes albus auf die Milch. 24 pp. 8°. *Würzburg, P. Scheiner,* 1886.

Michel (Henri). * Contribution à l'étude de l'albuminurie transitoire dans quelques maladies du système nerveux. 94 pp. 4°. *Lyon,* 1885, No. 268.

————. The same. 94 pp. 8°. *Paris, J.-B. Baillière & fils,* 1885.

Michel (Hubert). * Des hydropisies en général, et spécialement de leur mécanisme ou de leurs divers modes de développement. 32 pp. 4°. *Paris,* 1845, No. 149, v. 435.

Michel (J.)[1] * Réflexions sur l'épidémie dysentérique qui régna en 1811 et 1812 à bord du vaisseau l'Auguste, dans l'escadre de l'Escaut. 22 pp. 4°. *Paris,* 1814, No. 105, v. 104.

Michel (J.)[2] Die histologische Structur des Iris-stroma. Programm zum Eintritt in die medicinische Facultät und in den Senat der königl. Friedrich-Alexanders-Universität zu Erlangen. 36 pp., 2 pl. 8°. *Erlangen, E. Besold,* 1875.

————. The same. Eine Monographie. 36 pp., 2 pl. 8°. *Erlangen, E. Besold,* 1875.

————. Die Prüfung des Sehvermögens und der Farbenblindheit beim Eisenbahnpersonal und bei den Truppen. 11 pp. 8°. *München, J. A. Finsterlin,* 1878.

Michel (J.-B.) * Des oreillons; études critiques sur leurs métastases. Orchite. 64 pp. 4°. *Paris,* 1868, No. 59.

Michel (J.-B.-Adrien). * Considérations physiologiques sur le corps thyroïde. 31 pp. 4°. *Paris,* 1850, No. 10, v. 499.

Michel (J.-B.-Edmond). * De l'endocardite dans l'état puerpéral physiologique, dans la fièvre puerpérale simple ou traumatique, et dans la fièvre puerpérale infectieuse. 83 pp. 4°. *Paris,* 1873, No. 145.

Michel (J.-M.-Aimé). * Des sympathies morbides, et des phénomènes secondaires dans les maladies. 31 pp. 4°. *Paris,* 1830, No. 158, v. 233.

Michel (J.-M.-J.) * Sur l'affection vermineuse. 23 pp. 4°. *Paris,* 1808, No. 96, v. 72.

Michel (*Jean*) [–1495].
CHEREAU (A.) Jean-Michel de Pierrevive, premier médecin de Charles VIII, roi de France, et le mystère de la passion. 8°. *Paris,* 1864.
Repr. from : Bull. de bibliopb.

Michel (Jean-Baptiste). * Sur la fièvre intermittente adynamique. 21 pp. 4°. *Paris*, 1812, No. 88, v. 89. [*Also, in* : P., v. 958.]

———. Statistique médicale de l'Hôpital militaire du Gros-Caillou, adressée au Conseil de santé des armées, suivie de recherches théoriques et pratiques sur les fièvres intermittentes et rémittentes, simples et pernicieuses, et sur les maladies typhoïdes. xxiv, 261 pp., 1 l. 8°. *Paris, Fortin, Masson & Cie.*, 1842.

Michel (Jean-Laurent-Auguste). * Sur le sarcocèle ou cancer du testicule. viii, 9–41 pp. 4°. *Paris*, 1817, No. 150, v. 134.

Michel (Jean-Simon-Eugène) [1819–83]. * I. Du traitement à mettre eñ usage contre les helminthes intestinaux. II. [etc.] 28 pp. 4°. *Paris*, 1841, No. 167, v. 378.

———. * Des muscles et des os au point de vue de la mécanique animale. 40 pp. 4°. *Strasbourg*, 1846, v. 12.
Concours.

———. * De la contractilité et des organes contractiles. 63 pp. 4°. *Strasbourg*, 1849, v. 15.
Concours.

———. Essai sur la chirurgie de Strasbourg ; lu dans la séance annuelle de la Société de médecine de Strasbourg le 6 juillet 1854. 92 pp., 1 pl. 8°. *Strasbourg, G. Silbermann*, 1855.
For Biography, see Rev. méd. de l'est, Nancy, 1883, xv, 289–298 (Gross *et al.*).

Michel ([Johannes Philippus] Carolus) [1843–]. * De favo. 26 pp. 8°. *Gryphiæ, F. Hache*, 1866.
c.

Michel (Joseph)[1]. * Sur la douleur et les anesthésiques en obstétrique. 34 pp. 4°. *Paris*, 1855, No. 127, v. 578.

Michel (Joseph)[2]. * Étude sur les arthropathies survenant dans le cours de l'ataxie locomotrice progressive. 95 pp. 4°. *Paris*, 1877, No. 93.

Michel (Joseph-Alfred). * Notes médicales récueillies à la Côte-d'Or (géographie et pathologie exotique). 43 pp. 4°. *Paris*, 1873, No. 183.

Michel (Jules). * Étude du jalap. 57 pp., 1 l. 4°. *Montpellier, Cristin, Serre & Ricome*, 1882, No. 313.
École supérieure de pharmacie.

Michel (Julius) [1843–]. * Ueber die Veränderungen des Sehnerven, der Netzhaut und Aderhaut bei der Epilepsie. 26 pp. 8°. *Würzburg, C. Becker*, 1867.
c.

———. Lehrbuch der Augenheilkunde. xvi, 674 pp., 2 pl. roy. 8°. *Wiesbaden, J. F. Bergmann*, 1884.
Also, Editor of : **Jahresbericht** über die Leistungen und Fortschritte im Gebiete der Ophthalmologie, Tübingen, 1877.

Michel (Léon-François). * Quelques considérations sur le crâne, surtout au point de vue des fractures. 42 pp. 4°. *Paris*, 1854, No. 93, v. 563.

Michel (Louis). * Sur l'ascite et la paracentèse. 23 pp. 4°. *Paris*, 1825, No. 77, v. 192.

Michel (Louis-Alfred). * Sur les rechutes de la fièvre typhoïde. 50 pp. 4°. *Paris*, 1864, No. 71.

Michel (Louis-Ernest). * De l'ictère des nouveau-nés. 28 pp. 4°. *Paris*, 1867, No. 61.

Michel (Ludovic). * Essai sur le diagnostic des tumeurs inguinales. 114 pp., 3 l., 1 tab. 4°. *Montpellier*, 1878, No. 51.

Michel (Marie-Ferdinand-Louis). * Étude clinique sur la fièvre typhoïde chez les vieillards. 56 pp., 1 l. 4°. *Montpellier*, 1884, No. 45.

Michel (Marx Friedrich). Einige Fälle aus der Entbindungs-Wissenschaft. 108 pp. 16°. *Frankfurt u. Leipzig*, 1781.

Michel (Middleton). * On organogeny. 21 pp. 8°. *Charleston, Burges & James*, 1846.

Michel (Middleton)—continued.

———. Poisoning by ergot in attempting criminal abortion ; with reflections upon some of the causes of sudden death. 30 pp. 8°. *Charleston, C. Canning*, 1850.
Repr. from: Charleston M. J. & Rev., 1850, v.

———. Introductory address, delivered before the class of the Medical College of South Carolina, Nov. 1, 1851. 31 pp. 8°. *Charleston, J. B. Nixon*, [1851].

———. Microscopic researches on the black vomit of yellow fever. 26 pp., 1 pl. 8°. *Charleston, Walker & James*, 1853.
Repr. from: Charleston M. J. & Rev., 1853, viii.

———. Monograph on the pathology of the pituitary body. 31 pp. 8°. *Charleston, S. C., James & Williams*, 1860.
Repr. from: Charleston M. J. & Rev., 1860, xv.

———. Cases of cataract extracted by the corneal-flap, with comments on Graefe's operation. 20 pp. 8°. *Charleston, Walker, Evans & Cogswell*, 1871.
Repr. from : Tr. South Car. M. Ass., 1871.

———. Anatomy of the bullet-track, and cicatrices of the wounds of entrance and exit. 14 pp. 8°. [*Charleston*, 1875.]
Repr. from: Charleston M. J. & Rev., 1875, n. s., ii.

———. Cancroid or epithelioma of the lower lip ; modified operation for its removal ; cure. 6 pp. 8°. [*Charleston*, 1875.]
Repr. from: Charleston M. J. & Rev., 1875, n. s., ii.

———. In memoriam. J. Lawrence Smith. 11 pp. 8°. *Charleston, S. C.*, 1884.
Repr. from: Year Book City of Charleston, S. C., 1883.

———. Effects consequent upon the section of the posterior muscles of the neck, with a short history of the cerebro-spinal fluid. 12 pp. 8°. [*n. p., n. d.*]

Michel (P.-J.-B.-E.) * Sur l'inflammation de la conjonctive. 40 pp. 4°. *Paris*, 1828, No. 48, v. 214.

Michel (R. Fraser). Monograph on hæmorrhagic malarial fever. 19 pp. 8°. *Montgomery, Ala.*, 1869.

———. Objections to the term "purpuræmia" being applied to the disease known as "hæmorrhagic malarial fever". 10 pp. 8°. *Montgomery, Ala.*, 1870.

———. Reflections on the anatomy and physiology of some parts of the eye. 11 pp. 8°. *Mobile*, 1871.

———. A history of break-bone-fever, as it prevailed in the city of Montgomery, Alabama, during the summer of 1866. 12 pp. 8°. *Charleston*, 1874.
Repr. from: Charleston M. J., 1874, i.

———. Epidemic yellow fever in Montgomery, Ala., during the summer of 1873. 17 pp. 8°. *Charleston*, 1874.

———. The same. 25 pp. 8°. *Montgomery, Barrett & Brown*, 1874.

Michel (Theodor). * Ueber Staubinhalationen. 24 pp., 1 l. 8°. *Bonn, J. F. Carthaus*, [1872].
c.

Michel (Vitus Paul). * Chemische Untersuchung eines Leberkonkrements. iv, 5–22 pp., 1 l. 8°. *Tübingen, G. Bähr*, 1832. [*Also, in* : P., v. 1516.]

Michel (William).
Co-Editor of : **Carolina** (The) Journal of Medicine, Science, and Agriculture, Charleston, 1825.

Michel Psellos. *See* Psellos [*or* Psellus] (Michel).

Michel de Trétaigne (Jean-Baptiste) baron [1780–1869].
See **Broussais** (Casimir-Anne-Marie). Lettre sur l'emploi du tartre stibié, etc. 8°. *Paris*, 1842.—**Mojon** (B.) Lois physiologiques. 8°. *Paris*, 1834.

Michelacci (Augusto). Saggi teorico-pratici di dermatologia. Anno primo. 2 p. l., 216 pp. 8°. *Firenze, Ricordi & Jouhaud*, 1865. [P., v. 1111.]

Repr. from: Sperimentale, Firenze, 1864–5, 4. s., xv.

———. Lezioni e cliniche di dermatologia. In compendio raccolte ed esposte dal Dott. Carlo Cassuto. 4 p. l., 277 pp.; 1 p. l., 189 pp., 1 l. 8°. *Firenze, N. Martini*, 1871.

Michelacci (Michele). I clisteri nutritivi e l' alimentazione per il retto. 15 pp. 8°. *Firenze, tipog. Cenniniana*, 1880.

Repr. from: Sperimentale, Firenze, 1880, 4. s., xlv.

Michelant (F.-J.-S.) * Sur la péritonite. 17 pp. 4°. *Paris*, 1820, No. 254, v. 160.

Michelena (Guillermo). * Des rétrécissements de l'urèthre. 43 pp., 1 pl. 4°. *Paris*, 1847, No. 29, v. 462.

———. Nueva teoria sobre el mecanismo del parto. 153 pp. 8°. *Nueva York, Hallet & Breen*, 1869.

Michelet (Charles) [1854–]. * Ueber Diphtherie. 28 pp., 2 l. 12°. *Berlin, G. Schade*, 1879.

Michelet (Honoratus).

See **Thomasseau** (Josephus). An ab ex lege inspirati aëris motu febres? 4°. [*Paris*, 1695.]

Michelet (Joseph-Théodore-Philippe). * Essai sur les rougeurs de la substance cérébrale, suivi de la description d'une disposition particulière de quelques artères du pli de l'aîne. 30 pp. 4°. *Paris*, 1827, No. 59, v. 205.

Michelet (Paulus Ludovicus) [1835–]. * De gonorrhœa. 32 pp. 8°. *Berolini, G. Lange*, 1859.

Micheli (*Pietro Antonio*) [1679–1736].

COCCHI (A.) Elogio di Pietro Antonio Micheli. 4°. *Firenze*, 1737.

Michelin (E.-F.-Maximilien). * Sur la gymnastique, et sur quelques-unes de ses applications en médecine. 56 pp. 4°. *Paris*, 1819, No. 264, v. 152.

Michelin (J.-B.-M.-E.) * I. De la dilatation avec amincissement du cœur. II. [etc.] 31 pp. 4°. *Paris*, 1844, No. 191, v. 421.

von Michelis (Alfred). * Einige Beobachtungen über den Geburtsverlauf bei engem Becken. 38 pp., 1 l. 8°. *Würzburg*, 1880.

de Michelis (Filippo). Trattato elementare di anatomia generale e descrittiva del corpo umano. 4 v. in 2. 8°. *Torino, G. Fodratti*, 1834–40.

Michelitz (Antonius) [1747–1818]. * Diss. exhibens systematicam salium divisionem. iv, 5–60 pp. 8°. *Viennæ, J. Thom*, [1776]. [*Also, in:* P., v. 429.]

Also, in: DE WASSERBERG. Op. min. med. et diss. 8°. *Vindobonæ*, 1776, iv, 345–391.

———. Scrutinium hypotheseos spirituum animalium. *Pragæ*, 1782.

In: SCRIPT. neurol. minores selecti. 4°. *Lipsiæ*, 1793, iii, 209–239. *Also, in:* KLINKOSCH (J. T.) Diss. med. select. Prag. 4°. *Pragæ et Dresdæ*, 1793, ii, 339–368.

———. Disquisitio physiologica caussarum respirationis. 72 pp. 8°. *Pragæ, W. Gerle*, 1783.

Also, in: KLINKOSCH (J. T.) Diss. med. select. Prag. 4°. *Pragæ et Dresdæ*, 1793, ii, 384–410.

———. Ueber den Nachtheil, den die heutige Frauentracht der Gesundheit bringt. viii, 9–45 pp. 8°. *Prag, C. Widtmann*, [1803].

Michelius (Jos.)

See **Libavius** (Andreas). *Novus de medicina veterum, [etc.] 12°. *Francof.*, 1599.

Michell (Charles L.) Fixed adhesive dressings in the treatment of skin diseases. 12 pp. 12°. *Philadelphia*, [1885].

Michell (Janus Petersen) [1760–95]. * De mirabili, quæ caput inter et partes generationi dicatas intercedit, sympathia. Præs. Bavius Voorda. 2

Michell (Janus Petersen)—continued.

p. l., 74 pp., 1 l. 4°. *Lugd. Bat., P. vander Eyk et D. Vygh*, [1781].

Also, in: SCHLEGEL (Jo. Christ. Traug.) Sylloge selectiorum opusculorum, etc. 8°. *Lipsiæ*, 1787, 1–152.

———. * Diss. acad. inquirens synchondrotomiæ pubis utilitatem in partu difficili. Præs. Gualtherus van Doeveren. 2 p. l., 58 pp., 1 l. 4°. *Lugd. Bat., P. vander Eyk et D. Vygh*, [1781].

———. Geneeskundige verhandeling over de oorzaken, onderscheiding en geneezing der febres catarrhales, welke zich sedert eenige jaaren meer dan voorheen in de Neederlanden vertoond hebben. 134 pp. 8°. *Eecloo, A. B. van Han*, 1795.

Michell (Joannes)[1]. *De intestinis crassis. 29 pp. 4°. *Lugd. Bat., S. et J. Luchtmans*, 1759.

Michell (Joannes)[2]. * Specimen exhibens aliquot animadversiones medicas. 1 p. l., 54 pp. 8°. *Lugd. Bat., apud vid. M. Cyfveer*, 1810.

Michell (W.) On difficult cases of parturition, and the use of ergot of rye. xv, 128 pp. 8°. *London, T. & G. Underwood*, 1828.

Michellet (Jules). * Considérations pathologiques sur la migraine. 22 pp. 4°. *Paris*, 1866, No. 227.

Michellet (L.-A.) * De l'usage extérieur de l'eau froide par affusions dans le traitement des fièvres essentielles et notamment des fièvres contagieuses des prisons, des hôpitaux. 22 pp. 4°. *Paris*, 1803, No. 68, v. C.

Michellier (Sigismondus). * I. De scapulæ fractura, etc. 12 pp. 4°. *Augustæ Taurinorum, Bianco*, [1818].

Michelon (Georges). * De l'iritomie. 80 pp. 4°. *Paris*, 1876, No. 471.

Michelot (A.) Analyse des recherches de MM. d'Arcet et de Puymaurin fils, sur les substances nutritives que renferment les os. 12 pp. 8°. *Paris*, [*Plassan & Cie.*], 1829. [P., v. 1633.]

Repr. from: Revue encyclopédique.

Michelot (Auguste-Marie-Léon). * Des luxations des quatre derniers doigts en arrière. 48 pp. 4°. *Paris*, 1883, No. 230.

Michelot (Jean-Baptiste-Marie). * Sur les hydropisies en général, et l'hydrothorax en particulier. 21 pp. 4°. *Paris*, 1815, No. 228, v. 115.

Michelotti (L.) Notizie sul cholera-morbus, ossia collezione delle principali memorie scritte intorno a questa malattia riportate nei varj giornali scientifici inglesi, francesi, tedeschi ed italiani dalla sua prima comparsa in Europa fino al presente; fatta e corredata delle opportune annotazioni e reflessioni e ridotta ad intelligenza comune da . . . 282 pp., 2 l. 8°. *Livorno, Signozzi*, 1831.

Also, Co-Editor of: **Mercurio** delle scienze mediche, Livorno, 1823–30.

Michelotti (Pietro Antonio) [1680–1740]. De separatione fluidorum in corpore animali. 2 p. l., 362 pp., 2 pl. 4°. *Venetiis, Pinellorum œre*, 1721.

For Biography, see Gior. di chir.-prat., Trento, 1823, v, pp. v–xxvii, port. (Abbate Maistrelli).

Michels (Adolf). * Ueber die Entstehung des ersten Herzkammertons. 31 pp. 8°. *Marburg, J. A. Koch*, [1870]. C.

Michels (Ambroise - François - Joseph). * Des fractures de l'olécrâne. 31 pp. 4°. *Strasbourg*, 1854, No. 318, 2. s., v. 20.

Michels (Ernst) [1863–]. * Zur Casuistik der Darm-Resectionen wegen maligner Tumoren. 30 pp., 1 l. 8°. *Berlin, G. Schade*, 1885.

Michels (Franc. Josephus) [1806–]. * De fracturis ossium pelvis et de eorum certo quodam casu. 23 pp. 8°. *Berolini, typ. A. Petschii*, [1829].

Michels (Hermann) [1847–]. * Ueber Carcinom der Niere. 34 pp. 8°. *Berlin, G. Lange*, [1872].

Michels (Josephus Ferdinandus). * De indagandæ historiæ morbi utilitate ad coguoscendos et curandos morbos. 1 p. l., 27 pp. 4°. *Argentorati, typ. J. H. Heitzii*, [1766].

Michels (Louis). Das Bad Kreuznach. Mittheilungen für Aerzte und Brunnengäste. 72 pp. 8°. *Berlin, A. Hirschwald*, 1859.

———. Die chronischen Frauenkrankheiten mit besonderer Berücksichtigung ihrer Behandlung im Bade Creuznach. 53 pp. 8°. *Berlin, Mitscher u. Röstell*, 1862.

———. The same. 2. Aufl. viii, 81 pp. 16°. *Berlin, Mitscher u. Röstell*, 1869.

———. The same. The chronic diseases of women, with special regard to their treatment in Creuznach. 2. ed. viii, 75 pp. 8°. *Berlin, Mitscher u. Röstell*, 1872.

———. Die Fibromyome des Uterus. 61 pp. 8°. *Stuttgart, F. Enke*, 1877.

———. The same. Contribution à l'étude des corps fibreux de la matrice. 36 pp. 8°. *Kreuznach, R. Schmithals*, [n. d.]

Michels (Wilhelm) [1834–   ]. * Ueber Diabetes. 32 pp. 8°. *Berlin, G. Lange*, [1868].

des Michels de Champorcin (Josephus Petrus). * Theoria convulsionis. 15 pp. 4°. *Monspelii, J. Martel*, 1759. [P., v. 1282.]

Michelsen (A.)
See **Hornemann** (Claud Jacob Emil). Vom Zustande des Menschen kurz vor dem Tode. 8°. *Gotha*, 1882.

Michelsen (Frederik Joh.) * Behandeling der scabies. [Utrecht.] 8°. *Amsterdam, C. G. van der Post*, 1877.

Michelsen (Julius). * De nervi quinti neuralgia, præmissa historia morbi. 31 pp. 4°. *Gryphiswaldiæ, F. G. Kunike*, 1863.   c.

Michelsen (Maximilianus). * De ulcere ventriculi chronico. 39 pp. 8°. *Gryphiswaldiæ, F. G. Kunike*, [1862].

Michelsen (Otto). * Ueber Puerperalpsychosen. 34 pp. 8°. *München, J. Schaumberg*, 1878.

Michelsen (Sigism. Henr.) * Impetiginum nova divisio. 24 pp. 8°. *Berolini, lit. A. Petschii*, [1826].

Michelson (Eduard). * Einige Versuche über die Todtenstarre des Muskels. 32 pp. 8°. *Dorpat, H. Laakmann*, 1872.

Michelson (Otto). * Ob amigdalinie v korie cheremuchie i siemenach vishni. [Amygdalin from the bark of the rock-cherry and cherrystones.] 12 pp. 8°. *St. Petersburg*, 1872.

Michelson (P.) Ueber Herpes tonsurans und Area Celsi.
In: SAMML. klin. Vortr., No. 120 (Chir., No. 36), Leipz, 1877, 977–1012, 2 pl.

Michelson (Paul Oscar). * Zur Histiologie der Vater-Pacini'schen Körperchen. 33 pp., 1 l. 8°. *Königsberg, E. J. Dalkowski*, 1868.

Michener (E.) [*et al.*]. Hand-book of eclampsia, or notes and cases of puerperal convulsions, comprising all the cases which have occurred during the present century within a radius of several miles around Avondale, Chester County, Pa., so far as can be ascertained. 68 pp. 16°. *Philadelphia, F. A. Davis*, 1883.

Michgorius (Willem Hendrik). * De lipomate, una cum duobus exemplis insignis hujus tumoris, in Nosocomio academico chirurgico observatis, et delineatis. 2 p. l., 27 pp., 2 pl., 1 l. 4°. *Groningæ, J. Römelingh*, 1824.

Michieli (Antonio). Della febbre, trattato medico-anatomico, teoretico, pratico, con in fine un discorso sopra la china-china del Dr. Gabriele Longobardi. xiii, 312 pp., 2 l., port. 4°. *Udine, A. del Pedro*, 1764.

Michiels (Ernest). * Étude sur la phlegmasia alba dolens. 36 pp., 2 l. 4°. *Montpellier, J. Martel aîné*, 1868, No. 11.   c.

Michiels (H.) * De la puberté chez la femme. 31 pp. 4°. *Paris*, 1846, No. 172, v. 448.

Michiels (Théophile). * Du traitement des fièvres intermittentes simples. 34 pp. 4°. *Paris*, 1852, No. 197, v. 529.

Michielsen (C. F.) Catalogus der bibliotheek van den militair-geneeskundigen dienst te Batavia; op last van den Chef over den geneeskundigen dienst opgemaakt; uitgegeven door de Vereeniging ter Bevordering van Geneeskundige Wetenschappen in Nederlandsch-Indië. 1 p. l., 226 pp., 1 l. 8°. *Batavia, Bruining & Wijt*, 1871.

Michigan. Report of joint committee on State prison to the senate and house of representatives of the State of Michigan. 15 pp. 8°. [*Lansing*, 1848?]

———. H. R. Report of the select committee appointed [by the legislature] to inquire concerning the character of a certain report alleged to have been made by the faculty of the university to the board of regents. House Doc. No. 24. 1850. 7 pp. 8°. [*Lansing*, 1850.]

———. H. R. Report of the select committee relative to establishing a homœopathic department in the University of Michigan. House Doc. No. 25. 1861. 16 pp. 8°. *Lansing*, 1861. [*Also, in:* P., v. 578.]

———. Annual reports of the adjutant-general of the State of Michigan. 1862–5. 6 v. 8°. *Lansing, State printer*, 1862–6.

———. Annual reports relating to the registry and return of births, marriages, and deaths in Michigan. By the secretary of state. 1.–15., 1867–81. 8°. *Lansing*, 1868–84.

———. Laws of Michigan concerning the solemnization of marriages, and the record and return of births, marriages, and deaths. 12 pp. 8°. [*Lansing*, 1871?]

———. Law of Michigan establishing a State board of health, providing for the appointment of a superintendent of vital statistics, and assigning certain duties to local boards of health. Approved April 12, 1873. 4 pp. 8°. [*Lansing*, 1873.]

———. Introduction, summary, and index to the statistics of Michigan, collected for the ninth census of the United States, June 1, 1870; compiled in the state department of Michigan, under the direction of the secretary of state, in accordance with an act of the legislature. Approved April 15, 1871. cxxiv, 700–711 pp. 8°. *Lansing, W. S. George & Co.*, 1873.

———. Census of the State of . . . 1874, collected by the supervisors and assessors, and compiled and published by the secretary of state, in accordance with an act of the legislature, approved Feb. 9, 1853, as amended by acts approved April 17, 1873, and April 1, 1875. c pp. 8°. *Lansing, W. S. George & Co.*, 1875.

———. Biennial report of the State librarian of the State of Michigan to the legislature, for the years 1875–6. vi, 50 pp. 8°. *Lansing, W. S. George & Co.*, 1876.

———. Laws of the State of Michigan relating to the public health. Compiled and published under the supervision of the secretary of state, in pursuance of joint resolution No. 18 of the session laws of 1875. 86 pp. 8°. *Lansing, W. S. George & Co.*, 1876.

———. Annual reports of the State inspector of illuminating oils of the State of Michigan, to the governor of the State. 1., 1877; 2., 1878. 8°. *Lansing*, 1878–9.

———. Saline statistics by the salt inspector of the State. Dec. 15, 1879. 1 sheet. fol. [*East Saginaw*, 1879.]

———. H. R. A bill to amend sections one and two of act number 138 of session laws of 1875,

Michigan—continued.

relative to subjects for dissection for the advancement of science. Approved April 27, 1875, the same being sections 2110 and 2111 of the compiled laws of 1871, as amended. File No. 213. H. of Rep. No. 30. Introd. by Mr. Sawyer. March 14, 1879. 2 pp. fol. [*Lansing,* 1879.]

——. H. R. A bill to amend sections 2, 4, 5, 6, 8, 9, 11, 12, 13, 18, and 19 of chapter 48 of the compiled laws of 1871, being compiler's sections 1779, 1781, 1782, 1783, 1785, 1786, 1788, 1789, 1790, 1795, and 1796, as amended by act number 140, of the session of 1875, approved April 28, 1875, also by act number 109, session of 1877, approved May 10, 1877, and act number 195, session of 1877, approved May 22, 1877, relative to the laying out, opening, locating, or constructing a water-course, ditch, or drain by township drain commissioners. State of Michigan. File No. 237. H. of Rep. No. 555. Originals introduced by Messrs. Pray, Chase, and Sharts. Substitute by committee on drainage for house bills number 64, 65, and 555. March 17, 1879. 10 pp. fol. [*Lansing,* 1879.]

——. H. R. Joint resolution for the prevention of adulteration of honey. State of Michigan. File No. 1. H. of Rep. No. 2. Introd. by Mr. Cheney. 1 sheet. fol. [*Lansing,* 1879.]

——. H. R. Joint resolution for the prevention of the adulteration of sugar. File No. 5. No. 5. Introd. by Mr. Blackman. Recommended by committee on public health. Jan. 23, 1879. 1 sheet. fol. [*Lansing,* 1879.]

——. H. R. A bill to authorize boards of health of cities, villages, and townships to furnish vaccination to the inhabitants thereof. File No. 6. No. 52. Introd. by Mr. Chase. Rep. by committee on public health. Jan. 18, 1879. 1 l. fol. [*Lansing,* 1879.]

——. H. R. A bill to amend section 1740 of the compiled laws of 1871, the same being section 49 of chapter 46, relative to boards of health in cities and villages. File No. 7. H. of Rep. No. 53. Jan. 18, 1879. Introd. by Mr. Chase. 1 l. fol. [*Lansing,* 1879.]

——. H. R. A bill to amend chapter 35 of the revised statutes of 1846, being chapter 46 of the compiled laws of 1871, by adding two new sections thereto, to stand as sections 51 and 52. File No. 98. No. 296. Introd. by Mr. Moe. Recommended by committee on public health. Feb. 19, 1879. 1 sheet. fol. [*Lansing,* 1879.]

——. H. R. A bill to prevent and punish the crime of criminal abortion. State of Michigan. File No. 100. H. of Rep. No. 355. Introd. by Mr. Kuhn. Recommended by committee on public health. Feb. 19, 1879. 1 l. fol. [*Lansing,* 1879.]

——. H. R. A bill to amend sections two (2) and six (6) of act number 181 of the session laws of 1875, as amended by act number 196 of the session laws of 1877, entitled "An act to provide for the inspection of illuminating oils, manufactured from petroleum or coal oils". File No. 53. Introd. by Mr. Willett. Jan. 30, 1879. 3 pp. fol. [*Lansing,* 1879.]

——. H. R. A bill relative to the duties of health officers of cities and villages. State of Michigan. File No. 110. H. of Rep. No. 259. Introd. by Mr. Chase. Recommended by committee on public health. Feb. 19, 1879. 1 l. fol. [*Lansing,* 1879.]

——. H. R. A bill to prohibit the sale of tobacco to minors. File No. 193. No. 574. Introd. by Mr. Blackman. Rep. without recommendation by committee on public health. March 14, 1879. 1 l. fol. [*Lansing,* 1879.]

Michigan—continued.

——. H. R. A bill to prevent the sale of unsound meat in the city of Detroit. State of Michigan. File No. 242. H. of Rep. No. 305. Introd. by Mr. Cottrell. Recommended by committee on public health. March 20, 1879. 2 pp. fol. [*Lansing,* 1879.]

——. H. R. A bill to prevent and to punish for the careless use of naphtha, gasoline, kerosene, or other products of petroleum. File No. 245. No. 678. Introd. by Mr. Hall. Recommended by committee on public health. March 20, 1879. 1 sheet. fol. [*Lansing,* 1879.]

——. H. R. A bill to provide for the compilation, printing, and distribution of the laws in regard to establishing water-courses and locating ditches and drains by drain commissioners. State of Michigan. File No. 250. H. of Rep. No. 124. Introd. by Mr. Pray. Recommended by committee on drainage. Lansing, March 20, 1879. 1 sheet. fol. [*Lansing,* 1879.]

——. H. R. A bill to establish an institution, under the name and style of "The Michigan Reformatory" for girls. File No. 346. Original No. 14, by Mr. Sawyer; original No. 493, by committee on State affairs; original No. 693, by Mr. Campbell. Substitute by house committee on education for house bills Nos. 14, 493, and 693. April 16, 1879. 7 pp. fol. [*Lansing,* 1879.]

——. H. R. A bill to prevent and punish the sending of any explosive substance to a person with intent to do grievous bodily harm. File No. 335. No. 385. Introd. by Mr. Henderson. April 16, 1879. 1 sheet. fol. [*Lansing,* 1879.]

——. H. R. A bill to provide for the holding of inquests upon the view of bodies of diseased persons, and to repeal sections 7970, 7971, 7972, 7973, 7974, 7975, 7976, 7977, 7978, 7979, 7980, 7981, 7982, and 7983, compiled laws of 1871, relative to inquests on the view of dead bodies. File No. 347. H. of Rep. No. 686. Introd. by Mr. Sawyer. Rep. without recommendation by committee on judiciary. Lansing, April 22, 1879. 5 pp. fol. *Lansing,* 1879.

——. H. R. A bill to authorize the board of control of State swamp lands to make an appropriation to drain and reclaim certain swamp and overflowed lands on section (16) sixteen, Yankee Springs township, Barry County. State of Michigan. File No. 372. H. of Rep. No. 431. Introd. by Mr. McAllister. Lansing, April 26, 1879. 1 sheet. fol. [*Lansing,* 1879.]

——. H. R. A bill to amend sections 1, 2, 3, 6, and 11, and to add a new section to stand as section 12 of act 181 of the session laws of 1875, as amended by act number 196 of the session laws of 1877, entitled "An act to provide for the inspection of illuminating oils manufactured from petroleum or coal oils. Reprint of file No. 53. No. 5. [Substitute reported by conference committee.] May 8, 1879. 5 pp. fol. [*Lansing,* 1879.]

——. H. R. A bill to authorize and empower the board of control of State swamp lands to make an appropriation of State swamp lands to drain and reclaim certain swamp and overflowed lands in town eight north, of range three east, being the town of Rush, Shiawassee County, State of Michigan. File No. 284. H. of Rep. No. 372. Introd. by Mr. Sharts. Lansing, March 28, 1879. 1 sheet. fol. [*Lansing,* 1879.]

——. H. R. A bill to appropriate 4,000 acres of any State swamp lands to drain Gun marsh, in the townships of Martin and Gun Plain, in Allegan County. State of Michigan. File No. 317. H. of Rep. No. 620. Introd. by Mr. Blackman. Lansing, April 2, 1879. 1 sheet. fol. [*Lansing,* 1879.]

Michigan—continued.

——. S. A bill to provide for the collection of the social statistics of Michigan, and to provide for the publication of said statistics, together with the statistics to be taken by the authority of the United States, in the year 1880. State of Michigan. No. 181. Senate. Introd. by Senator Moore. Feb. 19, 1879. Rep. favorably by committee on State affairs, and ordered printed March 31, 1879. 2 pp. fol. [*Lansing*, 1879.]

——. S. A bill to amend sections two, four, and six of act number 196 of the session laws of 1877, approved May 23, 1877, entitled "An act to amend act number one hundred and eighty-one of the session laws of 1875, entitled An act to provide for the inspection of illuminating oils manufactured from petroleum or coal oils". No. 41. Introd. by Senator Robbins, Jan. 8, 1879. . Rep. with amendments by committee on State affairs, Jan. 1879. 2 pp. fol. [*Lansing*, 1879.]

——. S. A bill to authorize the board of health of the township of Pentwater, Oceana County, State of Michigan, to remove and re-inter all the dead bodies and remains buried in cemetery on block 36 of the village of Pentwater, Oceana County . . . No. 134. Introd. by Senator Ambler, March 18, 1879. Rep. favorably by committee on public health and ordered printed, March 12(?), 1879. 1 l. fol. [*Lansing*, 1879.]

——. S. A bill to amend sections 2, 4, and 6 of act number 196 of the session laws of 1877, approved May 23, 1877, entitled "An act to amend act number 181 of the session laws of 1875, entitled An act to provide for the inspection of illuminating oils manufactured from petroleum or coal oils". No. 41. Introd. by Senator Robbins, Jan. 8, 1879. 2 pp. fol. [*Lansing*, 1879.]

——. S. A bill to protect the people of the State of Michigan from empiricism and quackery. State of Michigan. No. 27. Senate. Substitute reported by committee on public health for bill introduced by Senator Robbins, Jan. 10, 1879. 4 pp. fol. [*Lansing*, 1879.]

——. S. A bill to regulate the sale of medicines and poisons. No. 43. Introd. by Senator Benjamin, Jan. 24, 1879. Rep. by committee on public health, Jan. 31, 1879. 4 pp. fol. [*Lansing*, 1879.]

——. S. A bill to protect the people of the State of Michigan from empiricism and quackery. State of Michigan. No. 141. Senate. Reprint of Senate bill No. 27. Substitute reported by committee on public health for bill introduced by Senator Robbins, Jan. 10, 1879. Amended by committee on public health and ordered reprinted, March 14, 1879. 4 pp. fol. [*Lansing*, 1879.]

——. S. A bill to regulate the practice of dentistry. State of Michigan. No. 184. Senate. Substitute for senate bill number 129. Rep. by committee on public health and ordered printed, April 1, 1879. 2 pp. fol. [*Lansing*, 1879.]

——. S. A bill to authorize the board of control of State swamp lands to make an appropriation to drain and reclaim certain swamp lands in the townships of Ganges, Casco, and Clyde, in Allegan County. State of Michigan. No. 202. Senate. Introd. by Senator Lewis, Feb. 19, 1879. Rep. favorably by committee on public lands and ordered printed, April 11, 1879. 1 sheet. fol. [*Lansing*, 1879.]

——. S. A bill to provide for the safety of persons attending public assemblies. No. 206. Introd. by Senator McElroy, Feb. 17, 1879. Rep. favorably by committee on State affairs, and ordered printed, April 12, 1879. 2 pp. fol. [*Lansing*, 1879.]

Michigan—continued.

——. S. A bill making an appropriation to enable the State board of health to purchase meteorological instruments, and cause to be made and distributed reprints of articles published in the annual report of the secretary. State of Michigan. No. 240. Senate. Introd. by Senator Tyler, Feb. 19, 1879. Rep. favorably by committee on public health, and ordered printed May 24, 1879. 1 l. fol. [*Lansing*, 1879.]

——. Laws of Michigan concerning the manufacture, inspection, sale, and use of illuminating oils. 4 pp. 8°. [*Lansing*, 187-.]

——. H. R. A bill to amend section 2 of act No. 56 of the session laws of 1877, approved April 20, 1877, entitled "An act to amend sections 1692 and 1693, chapter 46, of the compiled laws of 1871, relative to boards of health and health officers in townships". State of Michigan. File No. 371. H. of Rep. No. 348. Introd. by Mr. Ballentine, April 8, 1881. 1 sheet. fol. [*Lansing*, 1881.]

——. H. R. A bill making an appropriation to enable the State board of health better to collect and disseminate information useful for the promotion of the public health. File No. 220. H. of Rep. No. 570. Introd. by Mr. Wilkins. March 14, 1881. 1 sheet. fol. [*Lansing*, 1881.]

——. H. R. A bill to regulate the manufacture and sale of adulterated foods and drugs. State of Michigan. File No. 299. H. of Rep. No. 644. Introd. by Mr. Root, March 23, 1881. 2 pp. fol. [*Lansing*, 1881.]

——. Michigan and its resources. Sketches of the growth of the State, its industries, agricultural productions, institutions, and means of transportation; descriptions of its soil, climate, timber, financial condition, and the situation of its unoccupied lands; and a review of its general characteristics as a home. [Compiled under authority of the State by Frederick Morley, commissioner of immigration.] 144 pp., 1 map. 8°. *Lansing, W. S. George & Co.*, 1881.

——. Michigan in the war. Compiled by John Robertson, adjutant-general. Rev. ed. 1039 pp., 3 port. 8°. *Lansing, W. S. George & Co.*, 1882.

Michigan.

See, also, **Blind**, **Deaf-mutes** (*Asylums for*); **Education** (*Medical*), etc., *by localities*; **Detroit**; **Fever** (*Cerebro-spinal, History, etc., of*), **Fever** (*Malarial, History, etc., of*), **Fever** (*Typhoid, History, etc., of*), *by localities*; **Grand Rapids**; **Greenville**; **Kalamazoo**; **Lansing**; **Mackinac**; **Medicine** (*History, etc., of*), *by nations, etc.*; **Monroe**; **Saginaw City**; **Saint Louis** *magnetic spring.*

KENNEDY (S.) The magnetic and mineral springs of Michigan, to which is prefixed an essay on the climate of Michigan. 8°. *Wilmington* (*Del.*), 1872.

McCRACKEN (S. B.) The State of Michigan; embracing sketches of its history, position, resources, and industries. Compiled under authority of the governor in the interests of emigration. 8°. *Lansing, Mich.*, 1876.

PIONEER Society of the State of Michigan. General circular [to the pioneers of Michigan, soliciting facts and materials towards the publication of a series of volumes to be entitled "Pioneer collections", in which the "Memories of other days" may be preserved in an authentic form. By the committee of historians. Feb. 28, 1876]. 8°. [*Lansing*, 1876.]

WINCHELL (A.) The Grand Traverse region. A report on the geological and industrial resources of the counties of Antrim, Grand Traverse, Benzie and Leelanaw in the lower peninsula of Michigan. 8°. *Ann Arbor*, 1866.

Michigan.

Baker (H. B.) A report on the death-rate of each sex in Michigan, and a comparison with Dr. Farr's life tables of healthy districts of England. Am. Pub. Health Ass. Rep. 1874-5, N. Y., 1876, ii, 125-138. *Also*, Reprint. —— The principal meteorological conditions in Michigan during the year 1881. Rep. Bd. Health Mich. 1881-2, Lansing, 1883, x, 444-512. ——. Principal meteorological conditions in Michigan in 1884. A compilation of reports by observers for the State board of health and for the United States Signal Service. *Ibid.*, 1884-5, Lansing, 1886, xiii, 1-86. ——. The time of greatest prevalence of each disease; contributions to the study of the causes of diseases. A statistical report based on weekly reports of diseases in Michigan during the year 1884, and preceding years. *Ibid.*, 87-151. ——. Climate and health in Michigan. [Revised from his paper in Descriptive America, 1884.] Detroit Lancet, 1885-6, n. s., ix, 145-150. *Also*, Reprint.— **Beech** (J. H.) On the topography and epidemic diseases of Michigan. Tr. Am. M. Ass., Phila., 1859, xii, 185-207. *Also*, Reprint.—**Corbin** (G. E.) Report to State Society on the diseases and topography of Livingston and Ingham Counties, Michigan. Penins. & Indep. M. J., Detroit, 1858-9, i, 12-15. *Also*, Reprint.—**Diseases** of Michigan in the years 1875-82. Rep. Bd. Health Mich., Lansing, 1875-6, iv, 141: (1876-7), 1878, v, 167: 1877-8, vi, 105: (1878-9), 1880, vii, 147: (1879-80), 1881, viii, 221: (1880-81), 1882, ix, 252: (1881-2), 1883, x, 282: (1882-3), 1884, xi, 1.—**Duffield** (S. P.) Report on the geological relation of the mineral waters of Michigan. Detroit Rev. Med. & Pharm., 1871, vi, 339-343.—**Goff** (W. W.) Medical topography of York Township, Washtenaw Co., Mich. Northwest. M. & S. J., Chicago & Indianap., 1850-51, vii, 415-418.—**Hazlewood** (A.) Water and the water supply in Michigan. Rep. Bd. Health Mich., Lansing, 1875-6, iv, 71-80.—**Kedzie** (R. C.) The meteorology of Central Michigan. *Ibid.* (1873-4), 1875, ii, 197 213. ——. Report on the water supply of Michigan. *Ibid.*, 1875-6, iv, 109-119. ——. Report on the resolutions, referred to the section on State medicine and public hygiene, on the use of alcoholic liquors, and the establishment of a national sanitary bureau, and the influence of drainage on public health in Michigan. Tr. Am. M. Ass., Phila., 1874, xxv, 401-424. ——. Report on the water supply of Michigan. *Ibid.*, 1876, xxvii, 357-370.—**Leach** (E.) Topography and diseases of Shiawassee County. Tr. M. Soc. Mich., Lansing, 1859, 43-52.— **Lyster** (H. F.) A study of the climate and topography of the lower peninsula of Michigan. Rep. Bd. Health Mich., Lansing, 1877-8, vi, 167-210. ——. Report on the work of the State board of health. Tr. Michigan M. Soc., Lansing, 1879, vii, pt. 3, 443-454.—**Principal** (The) meteorological conditions in Michigan during the years 1877-82. Rep. Bd. Health Mich., Lansing, 1877-8, vi, 211: (1878-9), 1880, vii, 335: (1879-80), 1881, viii, 303: (1880-81), 1882, ix, 403: (1881-2), 1883, x, 444: (1882-3), 1884, xi, 121.—**Report** of committee on the mineral springs and wells of Michigan. Tr. M. Soc. Mich., Lansing, 1871, 32-51.—**Report** on epidemics in Michigan. Tr. Am. M. Ass., Phila., 1852, v, 503-530.—**Sprague** (G.) Remarks on the topography of Michigan, and the diseases incident to its climate. West. Lancet, Cincin., 1845-6, iv, 289-301.—**Stockwell** (C. M.) Report to State Society on diseases and topography of north-eastern district of the State of Michigan. Penins. & Indep. M. J., Detroit, 1858-9, i, 136-142.—**Water-supply** (The) in its relations to health and disease, in some of the townships, cities, and villages of Michigan. Rep. Bd. Health Mich. 1874-5, Lansing, 1876, iii, 107: 1875-6, iv, 81: (1876-7), 1878, v, 143: (1878-9), 1880, vii, 279.— **Weekly** reports of diseases in Michigan, September, 1876, to December, 1882. *Ibid.*, 1875-6, iv, p. xlii: (1876-7), 1878, v, 237: 1877-8, vi, 253: (1878-9), 1880, vii, 395: (1879-80), 1881, viii, 365: (1880-81), 1882, ix, 305: (1881-2), 1883, x, 513: (1882-3), 1884, xi, 197.—**Willson** (G. B.) Report of the committee on vital statistics. Tr. M. Soc. Mich., Lansing, 1859, 75-81.

Michigan. *Eastern Michigan Asylum, at Pontiac.*

By-laws, rules and regulations of the . . . and by-laws of the joint boards of the Michigan and Eastern asylums. 48 pp. 8°. *Pontiac, Gazette Company's Printing House*, 1878.

——. Biennial reports of the trustees and medical superintendent to the legislature, for the years 1878-9 to 1883-4. 8°. *Lansing*, 1880-84.

——. Admission of private patients (conditions of). 1 sheet. 8°. [*Pontiac, n. d.*]

——. Visitors (rules for). 1 sheet. 8°. [*Pontiac, n. d.*]

——. [Blank forms in use in the hospital.] v. s. [*Pontiac*, 188-.]
Daily record.
Examination of urine.
History of patient.

Michigan. *Michigan Asylum for the Insane, at Kalamazoo.*

Annual reports of the board of trustees to the governor, for the years 1857, 1867, and 1871. 8°. *Lansing*, 1858-72.
Opened Aug. 29, 1859.

——. Biennial reports of the board of trustees to the legislature. 1.-13., 1859 to 1883-4. 8°. *Lansing*, 1861-84.
1. report dates from reorganization in 1859.

——. Report of the building commissioner. I. From the establishment of the asylum in 1848, under a joint board of trustees, until the dissolution of its connection with the asylum at Flint, in 1857. II. From its commitment to a distant board of trustees until its organization in 1859. III. From its organization to the present time. 66 pp. 8°. *Lansing, J. A. Kerr & Co.*, 1866.
Bound with: Biennial reports, 1-4.

——. By-laws, rules, and regulations of the Michigan Asylum for the Insane. Revised December, 1867. 31 pp. 8°. *Kalamazoo*, 1868.

——. Supplement to the report of the board of directors for the years 1867-8. Being observations on a form of nervous prostration (neurasthenia) culminating in insanity. By E. H. Van Deusen. 19 pp. 8°. *Lansing, W. S. George & Co.*, 1869.

——. By-laws, rules, and regulations of the . . . Revised Aug., 1879. 40 pp. 8°. *Kalamazoo*, 1879.

——. [Blank forms in use at the asylum.] fol. [*Kalamazoo*, 188-.]
History of patient.
Order for admission to insane asylum.
Order for pauper patients.
Present condition of patient.
Request for admission, bond, and physicians' certificate.

Michigan. *Michigan Institution for the Education of the Deaf and Dumb and the Blind, at Flint.*

Biennial reports of the board of trustees and officers to the governors of the State. 2., 1854-5 & 1855-6; 4.-7., 1858-9 to 1865-6; 9., 1868-9 & 1869-70; 10., 1870-71 & 1871-2. 8°. *Lansing*, 1856-72.
Reports for 1854-5 and 1855-6 are in: Reports Mich. Asyl. for Insane for same years.

Michigan. *Michigan School for the Blind, Lansing.*

Biennial report of the board of commissioners to the governor of the State. 2., 1882-3 & 1883-4. 58 pp., 1 tab. 8°. *Lansing, W. S. George*, 1885.

Michigan. *State Board of Health of Michigan.*

Circular No. 1. To the clerks of local boards, calling attention to the legal provisions relating to public health. Sept., 1873. 1 l. 4°. [*Lansing*, 1873.]
Established July 30, 1873.

——. Circular No. 2. To the physicians of Michigan, directing their attention to section 1735, compiled laws of 1871, which requires physicians to report cases of small-pox, or other dangerous diseases to the local board of health. Oct., 1873. 2 l. 4°. [*Lansing*, 1873.]

——. Circular No. 3. To the clerks of local boards, transmitting blank form for annual report for the year ending Sept. 30, 1873. Also, a form for record of a dangerous case. Sept., 1873. 2 l. 4°. [*Lansing*, 1873.]

——. Circular of the chairman of the committee on climate, etc., to physicians, requesting information on the climate, sewerage, and drainage in their vicinity. Nov. 10, 1873. 1 sheet. 4°. [*Detroit*, 1873.]

——. Annual reports of the secretary to the governor. 1.-12., 1873 to 1883-4. 8°. *Lansing*, 1874-85.
The 1. report for the 2 months ending Sept. 30. 1873.

——. Circular of the president to physicians, with a schedule of questions, requesting facts or

Michigan. *State Bd. of Health of Mich.*—cont'd.
statistics on the entailments of "alcoholism".
Jan. 1, 1874. 1 sheet. 4°. [*Kalamazoo*, 1874.]
——. The same. To officers in charge of public
institutions. 1 sheet. 4°. [*Kalamazoo*, 1874.]
——. Shadows from the walls of death; being
arsenical wall papers, gathered by R. C. Kedzie,
member of the board. 1, 86 specimen leaves.
4°. [*n. p.*], 1874.
——. Circular of the . . . The entailments of
alcohol; being the annual address of the president, H. O. Hitchcock. 32 pp. 8°. *Lansing,
W. S. George & Co.*, 1874.
——. Circular of the chairman of the committee
on epidemic, endemic, and contagious diseases,
to the presidents of local boards, calling attention to the law and their duties relative to dangerous diseases. April, 1874. 2 l. 4°. [*Grand
Rapids*, 1874.]
——. Circular No. 7. To correspondents relative to water-supply. Oct., 1875. 1 sheet. 4°.
[*Lansing*, 1875.]
——. Rules and regulations recommended for
adoption by local boards of health throughout
the State. Aug., 1875. 8 pp. 8°. [*Lansing*,
1875.]
——. Circular No. 19. To health officers of
townships [relating to their duties as sanitary
advisers of the local boards of health]. June,
1877. 1 l. 4°. [*Lansing*, 1877.]
——. [Blank forms used by.] 4°. [*Lansing*,
187-.]
A. Special report of the clerk of . . . on dangerous
diseases, to the State board.
B. Annual report of the clerk of . . . to the State board.
——. Restriction and prevention of scarlet fever.
April, 1877. 8 pp. 8°. [*Lansing*, 1877.]
——. The same. No. 72. Rev. ed. 8 pp. 8°.
[*Lansing*, 1884.]
——. Circular No. 25. Relative to notices of
diseases which endanger the public health;
duties of householders, physicians, and others.
Circular to supervisors and other officers of
townships. March, 1878. 8 pp. 8°. [*Lansing*,
1878.]
——. Circular No. 34. Being a modification of
circular No. 25, embodying one new law and one
amended law. Jan., 1880. 8 pp. 8°. [*Lansing*, 1880.]
——. No. 35. Circular to health officers, relative to the work of health officers and of local
boards of health in Michigan. Being a modification of circular No. 28. Jan., 1880. 3 pp. 8°.
[*Lansing*, 1880.]
——. List of books which will be found valuable to candidates for examination in sanitary
science, by the Michigan State board of health.
7 pp. 16°. *Lansing*, 1880.
Repr. from : Michigan M. News, Detroit, 1880, iii.
——. Proceedings and addresses at the sanitary
conventions, held under the direction of a committee of the State board of health and a committee of citizens. Jan. 7 & 8, 1880, at Detroit;
Jan. 31 & Feb. 1, 1883, at Pontiac; April 26 &
27, 1883, at Reed City; Dec. 13 & 14, 1883, at
Ionia; April 17 & 18, 1884, at Hillsdale; Jan. 1
& 2, 1886, at Kalamazoo. 6 Nos. 8°. *Lansing*,
1880-86.
Suppl. to : Rep. Bd. Health Mich. 1879-80, 1882-3, to
1884-5, Lansing, 1881, 1884-6, viii. xi-xiii.
——. Restriction and prevention of diphtheria.
8 pp. 8°. [*Lansing, n. d.*]
——. The same. Revised ed. of 1881. 8 pp.
8°. [*Lansing*, 1881.]
——. The same. 3. ed. Dec., 1881. 8 pp. 8°.
[*Lansing*, 1881.]
——. The same. No. 76. 4. ed. July, 1884.
6 pp. 8°. [*Lansing*, 1884.]

Michigan. *State Bd. of Health of Mich.*—cont'd.
——. Circular No. 46. Restriction and prevention of scarlet fever. Revised ed. 1881. 8 pp.
8°. [*Lansing*, 1881.]
——. Circular No. 47. Contagious diseases:
scarlet fever, diphtheria, small-pox, typhus
fever, etc. General rules for their prevention
and restriction. Dec., 1831. 1 l. 8°. [*Lansing*, 1881.]
——. No. 54. Prevention and restriction of
small-pox. 16 pp. 8°. [*Lansing*, 1882.]
Repr. from : Rep. Bd. Health Mich. 1880-81, Lansing,
1882, ix.
——. No. 55. The work of health officers and
of local boards of health in Michigan. April,
1882. 12 pp. 8°. [*Lansing*, 1882.]
——. No. 110. Report of the committee appointed by the Sanitary Convention at Ann Arbor, Michigan, March 1, 1882, on the sanitary
condition of the hospitals of the University of
Michigan, at Ann Arbor. pp. 124-135. 8°.
[*Lansing*, 1883?]
Cutting from : Rep. Bd. Health Mich. 1881-2, Lansing,
1883, x.
——. No. 75. Prevention and restriction of
cholera. Issued July, 1884. 4 pp. 8°. [*Lansing*, 1884.]
——. Health in Michigan. Monthly reports to
the State board. For Aug., 1884. 2 l. 8°. *Lansing*, 1884.
——. No. 211. Laws of Michigan relating to the
public health, in force Sept. 8, 1883. Compiled
by the secretary by direction of the board. 122
pp. 8°. *Lansing, W. S. George & Co.*, 1884.
Suppl. to : Rep. Bd. Health Mich. 1882-3, Lansing, 1884,
xi.
——. Report of proceedings of the Michigan
State board of health. Quarterly regular meeting, July 13, 1886. 13 pp. 8°. [*Lansing*, 1886.]
——. *See, also :*
SANITARY Convention. Health topics ably presented and discussed. Important papers and addresses by scientists and prominent citizens.
Held at Battle Creek under the auspices of the
State board of health. Report of the proceedings. [Supplement to Battle Creek Daily Jour-
nal, March, 1881.]

Michigan. *University of Michigan, Ann Arbor.*
Report of a special committee of the board of
regents of the University of Michigan, on the
organization of a medical department in the
university. [Jan. 9, 1849.] 8 pp. 8°. *Detroit,
Harsha & Wilcox*, 1849.
——. Annual catalogues of the officers and students [including the medical class] for the years
1853-4; 1854-5; 1856-7 to 1870-71. 8°. *Ann Arbor*, 1854-71.
1860-61 to 1870-71 bound in 1 v.
——. A general catalogue of the officers and
graduates from its organization, in 1837, to 1864.
[Including the graduates in medicine from 1851
to 1863.] 40 pp. 8°. *Ann Arbor, by the University*, 1864.
——. Annual reports of the president, made to
the board of regents, for the years 1866-7; 1872-3
to 1880-81. 8°. *Ann Arbor*, 1867-81.
1872-3 to 1880-81 bound in 1 v.
——. [Brief announcement to answer inquiries
for information prior to the publication of the
catalogue for 1868-9.] 20 pp. 8°. [*Ann Arbor*,
1868.]
Bound with : Catalogues, 1860-61 to 1870-71.
——. The Chemical Laboratory 8 pp. 8°.
[*Ann Arbor, Chase*, 1869.]
Repr. from : University Mag., April, 1869.
——. Report on a department of hygiene and
physical culture in the University of Michigan,
by a committee of the university senate. 18 pp.
8°. *Ann Arbor, by the University*, 1870.

Michigan. *Univ. of Mich., Ann Arbor—cont'd.*
——. Catalogue of the academic senate and of those who have received its regular and honorary degrees. A triennial catalogue. 88 pp. 8°. *Ann Arbor, by the University*, 1871.

——. Historical sketch of the University of Michigan. (Prepared in compliance with an invitation from the Commissioner of Education, representing the Department of the Interior in matters relating to the National Centennial of 1876.) By Charles Kendall Adams. 56 pp. 8°. *Ann Arbor, by the University*, 1876.

——. The Michigan University book, 1844–80. Compiled by Theodore R. Chase, class of "'49". 399 pp. 8°. *Detroit, Richmond, Backus & Co.*, 1881.

Michigan. *University of Michigan, Ann Arbor. College of Dental Surgery.* Annual announcements for the sessions of 1881–2 (7.); 1883–4 to 1885–6 (9.–11.). 8°. *Ann Arbor*, 1881–5.
Organized in 1875. List of graduates from 1875 to 1885 in: Announcement for 1885–6.

Michigan. *University of Michigan. Department of Medicine and Surgery, Ann Arbor.* Annual announcements for the sessions of 1851–2 to 1858–9 (2.–9.); 1860–61 (11.); 1864–5 (15.); 1868–9 (19.); 1870–71 (21.); 1871–2 (22.); 1876–7 to 1878–9 (27.–29.); 1880–81 (31.); 1881–2 (32.); 1885–6 (35.). 8°. *Detroit & Ann Arbor*, 1851–83.
List of students and graduates for the years 1851–2 to 1857–8; 1876–7 to 1880–81; 1882–3; 1884–5, in: Announcements for subsequent years.

——. A statement of the relations of the faculty of medicine and surgery in the University of Michigan to homœopathy. 12 pp. 8°. *Detroit, Tribune Printing Co.*, 1875.

——. Statement of the faculty of the department of medicine and surgery in the University of Michigan, regarding the action of the Michigan State Medical Society, and their relation to the introduction of homœopathy in the university. 9 pp. 8°. *Ann Arbor, Ann Arbor Pub. Co.*, 1876.

——. *See, also:*
MICHIGAN. *University of Michigan, Ann Arbor.* Report of a special committee of the board of regents of the University of Michigan on the organization of a medical department in the university. [Jan. 9, 1849.] 8°. *Detroit*, 1849.

Michigan. *University of Michigan. Homœopathic Medical College.* Annual announcement for the session of 1875 (1.). 8 pp. 8°. *Ann Arbor, Courier print*, 1875.

——. *See, also:*
MICHIGAN. H. R. Report of the select committee relative to establishing a homœopathic department in the University of Michigan. House Doc. No. 25, 1861. 8°. *Lansing*, 1861.

Michigan. *University of Michigan. School of Pharmacy.* Schedule of the course in pharmaceutical manipulation. 4 pp. 8°. *Ann Arbor*, [*n. d.*]

——. Schedule of course in qualitative analysis. Schedule of work in organic analysis for students in pharmaceutical chemistry. 2 galley sheets. [*Ann Arbor, n. d.*]

——. *See, also:*
Students' resolutions on the homœopathy complications. Penins. J. M., Detroit, 1876, n. s., i, 162–164. *Also*, Reprint.

Michigan College of Medicine, Detroit. Annual announcement for the session of 1880–81 to 1882–3 (1.–3.). 8°. *Detroit*, 1880–82.
List of students and graduates for the sessions of 1880–81; 1881–2 in: Announcements for subsequent years.

Michigan Dental Association. Transactions of 24.–26. annual meetings. 3 Nos. 8°. *Detroit*, 1879–81.

Michigan Free Eye and Ear Infirmary, Detroit. Biennial report of the . . . and eye and ear department of the Michigan College Hospital. 1., 1880–81 & 1881–2. 28 pp. 8°. *Detroit, G. S. Davis*, 1882.

Michigan Homœopathic College, Lansing. Annual announcement for the session of 1872–3 (2.). 7 pp. 8°. *Jackson, P. H. Van Dyne*, 1872.
List of students and graduates for the year 1871–2 in: Announcement for 1872–3.

Michigan Homœopathic Institute. Proceedings of annual meetings, 1855; 1860; 1865; 1867. 4 Nos. 8°. *Detroit*, 1855–67.

Michigan Homœopathic Journal.
Was title of nos. 8–9, v. 2, of: **Michigan** (The) Journal of Homœopathy, 1853–4.

Michigan (The) Journal of Homœopathy. Edited by John Ellis and S. B. Thayer. [Monthly.] [Commenced Nov., 1848.] Nos. 5, 7–9, v. 1; Nos. 6, 8–9, v. 2, March, 1849, to June, 1854. 8°. *Detroit*.
Title of nos. 8–9, v. 2, was: **Michigan** Homœopathic Journal. In v. 2 John I. Hewitt added as editor.

Michigan (The) Journal of Homœopathy; devoted to medical and surgical science. Published quarterly by the faculty of the Detroit Homœopathic College. Nos. 1–3, v. 1, July, 1872, to April, 1873. 8°. *Detroit*.
Nos. 2–3, E. R. Ellis, editor and publisher.

Michigan Medical Association. Journal of proceedings for the years 1849 and 1850. v. 1. 28 pp. 8°. *Jackson, R. S. Cheney*, 1850.

Michigan Medical News: a semi-monthly journal devoted to practical medicine. J. J. Mulheron, managing editor. v. 1–5, 1878–82. 8°. *Detroit.*
Ended. United with: **Detroit** (The) Clinic, forming: **Medical** (The) Age.

Michigan State Medical Society. Transactions, 1867–87. 4 v. 8°. [*r. p.*], 1867–87.

——. Action regarding homœopathy in the Michigan University, at its meeting in Ann Arbor, May 10, 11, and 12, 1876. 4 pp. 8°. [*n. p.*, 1876.]

——. State of Michigan. File No. 102. House of representatives. No. 258. [Introduced by Mr. Chase.] Ordered printed for the use of committee on public health, Feb. 19, 1879. A bill for the incorporation of the Michigan State Medical Society. 3 pp. fol. [*Lansing*, 1879.]

——. *See, also:*
Michigan State Medical Society. Transactions, 1855–8. Penins. J. M., Ann Arbor, Mich., 1854–5, ii, 481; 529: 1855–6, iii, 1; 481: 1856–7, iv, 575–581. *Continued in:* Penins. J. M., Detroit, 1858, v, 433–440.

Michigan State Pharmaceutical Association. Proceedings of the convention of druggists and the first annual meeting of . . . held at Lansing, Nov. 14 and 15, 1883. Also, constitution and by-laws, roll of members, etc. 67 pp. 8°. *Muskegon, Mich., J. Jesson*, 1883.

——. Proceedings, 1884–7. 4 Nos. 8°. [*v. p.*], 1885–7.

Michigan State Society of Rational Medicine. Transactions. 16 pp. 8°. *Detroit, McCormack & Co.*, 1881.

Michigan (The) University Medical Journal, conducted by the faculty of the medical department. [Monthly.] v. 1–3, March, 1870, to Feb., 1873. 8°. *Ann Arbor, R. A. Beale.*
Ended.

Michiner (Chas. B.)
See **Smith** (Horace J.) A plea for veterinary surgery. 8°. *Harrisburg*, 1879.

Michniewicz (Felician). * Die Quetschung als chirurgische Operation in ihrer neuesten Form. 67 pp. 8°. *Dorpat, Schünmanns Wittwe u. C. Mattiesen*, 1863.

Michniovski (S.) *Izsliedovanija zajivlenija otorvannich epiphizov. [Investigation of the separation of epiphyses.] 76 pp., 1 pl. 8°. *St. Petersburg*, 1864.

Michon (Henri) [1854–]. *Des moyens chirurgicaux employés comme traitement de la névralgie faciale rebelle. 94 pp. 4°. *Paris*, 1882, No. 115.

Michon (L.-A.-Joseph). *Étude d'histoire médicale. Documents inédits sur la grande peste de 1348. (Consultation de la Faculté de médecine de Paris; consultation d'un praticien de Montpellier; description de Guillaume de Machaut.) 68 pp. 4°. *Paris*, 1860, No. 127.

——. The same. 99 pp. 8°. *Paris, J.-B. Baillière & fils*, 1860.

Michon (Louis-Marie) [1803–66]. *Quelques propositions sur l'anatomie, la physiologie et la pathologie. 17 pp. 4°. *Paris*, 1832, No. 97, v. 251.

——. *De la carie et de la nécrose. 47 pp. 4°. *Paris*, 1832, No. 379. [*Also, in:* P., v. 494.]
Concours.

——. *Texture et développement de l'encéphale et de la moelle épinière. 47 pp. 4°. *Paris*, 1836. [P., v. 937.]
Concours.

——. *Des opérations que nécessitent les fistules vaginales. 245 pp. 4°. *Paris, Rignoux*, 1841. [*Also, in:* P., v. 935.]
Concours.

——. *Du cancer cutané. 151 pp., 2 pl. 4°. *Paris*, 1848. [*Also, in:* P., v. 479; 1660.]
Concours.

——. Mémoire et observations pour servir à l'histoire de l'application de la suture au traitement des plaies. 32 pp. 8°. *Paris, Hennuyer & Co.*, [n. d.]
Repr. from: Bull. gén. de thérap., etc., Par., 1850, xl.

——. *Des tumeurs synoviales de la partie inférieure de l'avant-bras, de la face palmaire du poignet, et de la main. 217 pp., 1 l., 2 pl. 8°. *Paris, J.-B. Gros*, 1851. [*Also, in:* P., v. 494.]
Concours.

——. The same. 220 pp., 2 pl. 8°. *Paris, Germer-Baillière*, 1851. [P., v. 754.]

——. Mémoire et observations sur quelques cas d'autoplastie de la face. 23 pp. 8°. *Paris, P. Dupont*, [1851, vel subseq.].
Repr. from: Rev. méd.-chir. de Par., 1851, ix.
For Biography, see Mém. Soc. de chir. de Par., 1874, vii, pp. xxxix-lvi (F. Guyon).

Michou (Casimir-Laurent). *De la congestion pulmonaire dans la fièvre typhoïde, principalement au point de vue du traitement. 50 pp. 4°. *Paris*, 1860, No. 68.

Michu (J.-L.) *De l'étude pratique des fièvres adéno-méningées (pituiteuses). vi, 7–31 pp. 4°. *Paris*, 1813, No. 39, v. 96.

——. Doctrine médicale expliquée d'après les théories enseignées depuis Hippocrate jusqu'à Broussais. 459 pp. 8°. *Paris, Compère jeune* [and others], 1824.

Mickaniewski (Witold). *Considérations sur la terminaison de l'orchite par suppuration. 52 pp. 4°. *Paris, A. Parent*, 1879, No. 159.

Mickel (Gustav). *Eine Diphtheritisepidemie im Jahre 1878–9. 51 pp. 8°. *Würzburg, Becker*, 1882.

Mickle (William Julius). General paralysis of the insane. vi pp., 1 p. l., 246 pp. 8°. *London, H. K. Lewis*, 1880.

——. The same. 2. ed. 1 p. l., 466 pp. 8°. *London, H. K. Lewis*, 1886.

Mickleham (R. S.)
See **Engineer** (An). The theory and practice of warming and ventilating public buildings. 8°. *London*, 1825.

17

Micksch (Henricus Julius). *De perforatione cranii. 27 pp. 4°. *Lipsiæ, lit. Staritzii*, 1828.
For Biography, see **Hanse** (Guil. And.)

Micksch (Josephus). *Diss. sistens historias atrophiæ ac emollitionis medullæ spinalis. 48 pp. 8°. *Pragæ, T. Thabor*, [1840].

de Mickwitz (Constantinus Eb.) *Nonnulla de tetani causa proxima et cura. 46 pp. 8°. *Dorpati Livonorum, typ. J. C. Schünmanni*, 1829.

Mickwitz (Eberhardus). *De usu belladonnæ in morsu canis rabidi. 23 pp. sm. 4°. *Jenæ, lit. Fiedlerianis*, [1795].
For Biography, see **Nicolai** (Ernestus Antonius).

Mickwitz (Henrik Joh.) *Om febris recurrens. 65 pp., 6 tab. 8°. *Helsingfors, J. C. Frenckell & Son*, 1866.

Mickwitz (Louis). *Vergleichende Untersuchungen über die physiologische Wirkung der Salze der Alcalien und alcalischen Erden. 104 pp., 1 l., 3 tab., 2 ch. 8°. *Dorpat, C. Mattiesen*, 1874.

Mickwitz (Theodorus). *De trunci anonymi ligatura. 40 pp. 12°. *Dorpati Livonorum, typ. J. C. Schuenmanni*, 1836.

Micolon de Blanval. Éloge de M. Duvernin . . . Lû dans l'assemblée publique de la Société royale des sciences, arts et belles-lettres de Clermont-Ferrand, le 27 août 1786. 32 pp. 8°. *Clermont-Ferrand, A. Delcros*, 1786. [P., v. 1388.]

Micrer. Tractatus suo discipulo Mirnefindo.
In: THEATRUM chemicum. 4°. Argentorati, 1660, v, 90–101.

Micridis (Pierre-Paul). *Étude sur le diagnostic des épanchements pleuraux. 46 pp. 4°. *Paris*, 1858, No. 196, v. 621.

Microbe.
See **Bacteria**; **Micro-organisms**.

Microcephalus.
See, also, **Cranium** (Abnormities, etc., of); **Dwarfs**, etc.; **Idiots**; **Idiots** (Pathology of).
VON BISCHOFF (T. L. W.) Anatomische Beschreibung eines mikrocephalen 8jährigen Mädchens, Helene Becker aus Offenbach. 4°. *München*, 1873.
Repr. from: Sitzungsb. d. math.-phys. Cl. d. k.-bayer. Akad. d. Wissensch. zu München, 1872, ii. [See, also, infra.]
DUCATTE (E.) *La microcéphalie au point de vue de l'atavisme. 4°. *Paris*, 1880.
Also [Abstr.], in: Rev. internat. d. sc. biol., Par., 1880, vi, 518–538.
GIACOMINI (C.) Una microcefala. 8°. *Torino*, 1876.
HOHL (A. F.) *De microcephalia. 8°. *Halæ*, [1827].
JANUSCH (A.) *Drei Fälle von Microcephalie. 8°. *Greifswald*, 1880.
KLÜPFEL (R.) *Beitrag zur Lehre von der Mikrokephalie. 8°. *Tübingen*, 1871.
MONTANÉ (L.) *Étude anatomique du crâne chez les microcéphales. 4°. *Paris*, 1874.
——. The same. 8°. *Paris*, 1874.
ONUFROWICZ (W.) *Das balkenlose Mikrocephalengehirn Hofmann. Ein Beitrag zur pathologischen und normalen Anatomie des menschlichen Grosshirnes. [Zürich.] 8°. *Berlin*, 1887.
Also, in: Arch. f. Psychiat., Berl., 1887, xviii, 305–328, 2 pl.
VAN SCHOUWEN (C.) *Over mikrocephalie. 8°. *Leiden*, 1876.
VOGT (C.) Mémoire sur les microcéphales ou hommes-singes. 4°. *Génève-Bâle*, 1867.
Repr. from: Mém. Inst. nat. Genévois, xi. [See, also, infra.] Also [Rev.], in: Bull. Soc. d'anthrop. de Par., 1867, 2. s., ii, 477–491 (Letourneau).
WOLFF (J.) *Morphologische Beschreibung eines Idioten- und eines Mikrocephalen-Gehirns. [Wurtzburg.] 4°. *Frankfurt a. M.*, 1885.

Microcephalus.

Adler (A.) A case of microcephalus. Pacific M. & S. J., San Fran., 1877, xx, 266–268.—**Adriani** (R.) Caso singolare di microcefalia. Sperimentale, Firenze, 1872, xxx, 413–433.—**Aeby** (C.) Beiträge zur Kenntniss der Mikrocephalie. Arch. f. Anthrop., Brnschwg., 1873–4, vi, 263 : 1874–5, vii, 1 ; 199. ———. Ueber das Verhältniss der Mikrocephalie zum Atavismus. Tagebl. d. Versamml. deutsch. Naturf. u. Aerzte, Cassel, 1878, li, 112–120. *Also*, Reprint. ———. Ein vierjähriger mikrocephaler Knabe mit theilweiser Verschmelzung der Grosshirnhemisphären. Arch. f. path. Anat., etc., Berl., 1879, lxxvii, 554–557.—**van Andel** (A. H.) Een microcephaal of zoogenaamd aapmensch. Nederl. Tijdschr. v. Geneesk., Amst., 1873, ix, 2. Afd., 89–102, 3 pl.—**Atlanta** (G.) I tre microcefali di Riola. Spallanzani, Modena, 1882, 2. s., xi, 546–553.—**Baillarger.** Ossification précoce du crâne chez les microcéphales. Bull. Acad. de méd., Par., 1855–6, xxi, 954–960. *Also:* Ann. méd.-psych., Par., 1856, 3. s., ii, 469–475. *Also:* Gaz. d. hôp., Par., 1856, xxix, 362. — **Baistrocchi** (E.) Sopra un idiota microcefalo ; reperto necroscopico e considerazioni. Riv. sper. di freniat., Reggio-Emilia, 1880, vi, 60, 2 pl. ; 273.—**Barlow** (T.) Brain of a microcephalous child. Tr. Path. Soc. Lond., 1876–7, xxviii, 8.—**Bastianelli** (G.) Sopra due casi di microcefalia. Bull. d. sc. med. di Bologna, 1859, 4. s., xi, 98 – 106. — **Beaunis.** Présentation d'un crâne et d'un cerveau d'idiot microcéphalie. Mém. Soc. de méd. de Nancy (1877–8), 1879, 99–108. — **Bertelsmann.** Ein Fall von Microcephalie. Berl. klin. Wchnschr., 1877, xiv, 266–268. — **Bischoff.** Ueber das Gehirn eines microcephalischen achtjährigen Mädchens, Helene Becker. [Abstr.] Sitzungsb. d. math.-phys. Cl. d. k.-bayer. Akad. d. Wissensch. zu München, 1872, ii, 163–171. [*See, also, supra.*]—**Bourneville** & **Wuillamié.** Note sur deux cas de microcéphalie. Bull. Soc. anat. de Par., 1881, lvi, 756–781. ———. Notes et observations sur la microcéphalie. Arch. de neurol., Par., 1882, iv, 52, 2 pl. : 1883, vi, 72, 2 pl.—**Brancaleone-Ribaudo** (P.) Un idiota microcefalo. Pisani, Palermo, 1881, 87–103, 1 pl.—**Broca** (P.) Sur un enfant microcéphale vivant. Bull. Soc. d'anthrop. de Par., 1875, 2. s., x, 541–543. ———. Sur un cas excessif de microcéphalie (encéphale de 104 grammes). *Ibid.*, 1876, 2. s., xi, 85–92. ———. Sur un microcéphale âgé de deux ans et demi ; anomalies viscérales régressives. *Ibid.*, 1880, 3. s., iii, 387–389.—**Brunati** (A.) Una microcefala. Arch. ital. per le mal. nerv., Milano, 1885, xxii, 148–159.—**Calderini** (G.) Una cretini ed una microcefala nell' Istituto ostetrico di Parma ; nota clinico-anatomica. Ann. di ostet., Milano, 1882, iv, 178–194.—**Calori** (L.) Di una bambina microcefalica e specialmente del suo cervello. Mem. Accad. d. sc. d. Ist. di Bologna, 1880, 4. s., i, 617–642, 4 pl.—**Cardona** (F.) D' una microcefalia. Arch. ital. per le mal. nerv., Milano, 1870, vii, 245–252.—**Chiari** (H.) Microcephalie bei einem 6jährigen Mädchen. Jahrb. f. Kinderh., Leipz., 1880, n. F., xv, 323–330, 2 pl.—**Chudzinski.** Sur le squelette d'un enfant microcéphale. Bull. Soc. d'anthrop. de Par., 1880, 3. s., iii, 563–568.—**Clarke** (C. K.) A case of microcephaly. Canad. J. M. Sc., Toronto, 1851, vi, 207.—**Davreux.** Un cas remarquable de microcéphalie. Ann. Soc. méd.-chir. de Liége, 1878, xvii, 329–331.—**Delisle** (F.) Observations d'une microcéphale de l'Asile des aliénées de Saint-Yon, près Rouen. Bull. Soc. d'anthrop. de Par., 1885, 3. s., viii, 526–529.—**Delorenzi** (G.) Intorno al cervello e al cranio di due microcefali. Gior. d. r. Accad. di med. di Torino, 1874, xxxvii, 567–588.—**Down** (L.) Cases of microcephalic skull. Tr. Path. Soc. Lond., 1868–9, xx, 284–286. —**Dursclen.** Cas remarquable de microcéphalie et asymétrie du cerveau. Ann. Soc. d'anat. path. de Brux. Bull., no. 30, 1880–81, 191–194, 1 pl.—**Eames** (J. A.) Case of microcephalic idiocy. Brit. M. J., Lond., 1875, ii, 523.—**Falkenheim** (A.) Ein 12jähriger Microcephale. Berl. klin. Wchnschr., 1882, xix, 284 – 287. — **Feijão** (O.) Caso de microcephalia. Correio med. de Lisb., 1880, ix, 217–219.—**Finci** (F.) Sur trois cas de microcéphalie observés en Italie. Cong. internat. d'anthrop. 1869, Copenhague, 1875, iv, 358–360.—**Flesch** (M.) Anatomische Untersuchung eines microcephalen Knaben. Festschr. z. 3. Saecularfeier . . . d. med. Fac. Würzb., Leipz., 1882, ii, 95–125, 3 pl. *Also* [Abstr.]: Verhandl. d. Berl. Gesellsch. f. Anthrop., 1882, 40–42. ———. Ueber Mikrocephalie. Cor.-Bl. d. deutsch. Gesellsch. f. Anthrop., etc., Brnschwg., 1882, xiii, 152–154.—**Flesch** (O.) Eine neue Microcephalen-Familie. Verhandl. d. Berl. Gesellsch. f. Anthrop., 1883, 72–77. ———. Ueber den anatomischen Befund am Rückenmarke zweier Mikrocephalen. Tagebl. d. Versamml. deutsch. Naturf. u. Aerzte, Magdeb., 1884, lvii, 365.—**Fraenkel.** Ueber einen Fall von Mikrokephalus. Wien. med. Presse, 1869, x, 43.—**Frickhöfer.** Ueber Mikrocephalus in Folge frühzeitiger Verknöcherung der Nähte und Fontanellen. Mitth. d. Ver. nassau. Aerzte, Weilburg, 1853, 68 – 73. — **Fridolin** (J.) Beschreibung eines Falles von Scaphocephalie bei einem microcephalen jungen Kinde, auf angeborener, theilweiser Verknöcherung der Pfeilnaht beruhend. Arch. f. Anthrop., Brnschwg., 1883–4, xv, 391–398, 2 pl. — **Frigerio** (L.) Caso di microcefalia con atrofia di molte circonvoluzioni. Arch. ital. per le mal. nerv., Milano, 1884, xxi, 353–361. ———. Caso di porencefalia posteriore destra da

causa traumatica. Ann. univ. di med. e chir., Milano, 1887, cclxxix, 46–52, 1 pl.—**Fürst** (C. M.) Tre fall af mikrocefali. Nord. med. Ark., Stockholm, 1881, xiii, no. 18, 1–22, 9 pl. *Also, transl.*: Arch. f. Anthrop., Brnschwg., 1882 – 3, xiv, 41 - 60.— **Gaucher** (E.) Microcéphalie et idiotie ; atrophie considérable des cornes frontales et sphénoïdales du cerveau ; arrêt de développement des os maxillaires : atrophie et contractures musculaires généralisées. Bull. Soc. anat. de Par., 1879, 4. s., iv, 31–34. *Also:* Progrès méd., Par., 1879, vii, 485.—**Giacomini** (C.) Presentazione di cranii e cervelli di microcefali. Atti Cong. gen. d. Ass. med. ital., Torino, 1876, vii, 150–152. ———. Una microcefala. Osservazioni anatomiche ed antropologiche. Gior. d. r. Accad. di med. di Torino, 1876, 3. s., xx, 774 ; 810 ; 873, 4 pl. ———. Contributo allo studio della microcefalia. Arch. di psichiat., etc., Torino, 1885, vi, 63–81, 2 pl.—**Gonzales** (E.) Altro caso di microcefalia. Arch. ital. per le mal. nerv., Milano, 1881, xviii, 13 – 15. — **Gore** (R. T.) Notice of a case of microcephaly. Anthrop. Rev., Lond., 1863, i, 168 ; 187.—**Gratiolet** (P.) Mémoire sur la microcéphalie considérée dans ses rapports avec la question des caractères du genre humain. Mém. Soc. d'anthrop. de Par., 1860–63, i, 61–67. *Also :* J. de la physiol. de l'homme, Par., 1860, iii, 110–116.—**Hamy** (E.-S.) Description d'un crâne de fœtus microcéphale avec déformation intra-utérine. Bull. Soc. d'anthrop. de Par., 1867, 2. s., ii, 507–511.—**Hill** (A.) The anatomy of a hydromicrocephalous brain. J. Anat. & Physiol., Lond., 1884–5, xix, 363–384, 2 pl.—**Hutchinson** (J.) Microcephalus (Aztec head), with indications of bilateral cerebral atrophy ; difficult birth, and severe convulsions during the first week of life. Brit. M. J., Lond., 1886, i, 1018.—**Jacobi** (A.) Premature ossification of the cranium ; microcephalic child. Tr. N. York Obst. Soc. (1876–8), 1879, i, 476. *Also :* Am. J. Obst ., N. Y., 1879, xii, 354. ———. Microcephalus. N. York M. J., 1880, xxxi, 396.—**Jacobi** (Mary P.) Case of microcephalus. Med. Rec., N. Y., 1881, xix, 645–650.—**Jensen** (J.) Schädel und Hirn einer Microcephalin. Arch. f. Psychiat., Berl., 1880, x. 735–759, 1 pl.—**Kormann** (E.) Fall von oxycephaler Microcephalie. Jahrb. f. Kinderh., Leipz., 1880–81, n. F., xvi, 174–177.—**Leidesdorf.** Vorstellung von Mikrocephalen. Anz. d. k. k. Gesellsch. d. Aerzte in Wien, 1884–5, 319–321. *Also :* Wien. med. Bl., 1885, viii, 715. *Also :* Wien. med. Wchnschr., 1885, xxxv, 771. — **Leopold** (J. H.) Microcephalus und Macrocephalus. N. Ztschr. f. Geburtsk., Berl., 1852, xxxiii, 349–351.—**Letourneau.** Un cas de microcéphalie. Bull. Soc. d'anthrop. de Par., 1885, 3. s., viii, 524.—**Lombroso** (C.) Lunghezza anormale dell' avambraccio ed altre anomalie in un maniaco microcefalo. R. 1st. Lomb. di sc. e lett. Rendic., Milano, 1870, 2. s., iii, 468. ———. Tre casi di microcefalia. *Ibid.*, 1871, 2. s., iv, 739–752. ———. Quarto caso di microcefalia. *Ibid.*, 1872, 2. s., v, 23–26. ———. Casi di microcefalia da influenza psichica nella gravidanza. Gior. d. r. Accad. di med. di Torino, 1885, 3. s., xxxiii, 720–728.—**Lukin** (M.) Sluchai plagio microcephaliæ. Vrach, St. Petersb., 1882, iii, 431.—**Maclaren** (J.) Clinical notes on a case of microcephaly. Edinb. M. J., 1874, xx, 296–300. *Also*, Reprint.—**Mantegazza** (P.) Di un caso di singolare microcefalia in una donna. R. 1st. Lomb. di sc. e lett. Rendic., Milano, 1870, 2. s., iii, 339–342.— **Merjeevski** (J.) Mikrotsefalizm. Arch. sudebnoi med., St. Petersb., 1871, vii, pt. 3, 1–22, 2 pl. *Also, transl*: Verhandl. d. Berl. Gesellsch. f. Anthrop., 1871 – 2, 100–122, 2 pl.—**Merjeevski** (J.) & **Bouchereau.** Note sur un cas de microcéphalie. Bull. Soc. anat. de Par., 1875, l, 381–386.—**Meynert** (T.) Fall von Mikrokephalie. Wchnbl. d. k. k. Gesellsch. d. Aerzte in Wien, 1868, viii, 293. *Also :* Wien. med. Wchnschr., 1868, xviii, 937.—**Microcephalism.** Brit. & For. M.-Chir. Rev., Lond., 1874, ii, 81–87.—**Mingazzini** (G.) & **Ferraresi** (O.) Sul cervello d' una ragazza microcefala. Arch. di psichiat., etc., Torino, 1886, vii, 575–581.—**Montané.** Un caso de microcefalia y escafocefalia. Crón. méd.-quir. de la Habana, 1877, iii, 442–447 —**Müller** (J.) Nachrichten über die beiden Microcephalen zu Kiwitsblott bei Bromberg. Med. Ztg., Berl., 1836, v, 7 ; 13.—**Neumann** & **Joseph** (G.) Eine 15jährige Mikrocephalin. Jahresb. d. schles. Gesellsch. f. vaterl. Cult., Bresl., 1878, lv, 235–243. — **Oldest** (The) living microcephalic. Med. Rec., N. Y., 1884, xxvi, 522.—**Pfluger** (E.) Microcephalie und Microphthalmie. Arch. f. Augenh., Wiesb., 1884–5, xiv, 1–11, 1 pl. *Also, transl.*: Arch. Ophth., N. Y., 1885, xiv, 91–97, 1 pl.—**Ponfick.** Demonstration einer Mikrocephalin, des Mädchens mit dem Vogelkopf. Jahresb. d. schles. Gesellsch. f. vaterl. Cult. 1884, Bresl., 1885, lxii, 154–157. *Also :* Breslau. aerztl. Ztschr., 1885, vii, 54.—**Pott** (R.) Ein microcephalisches Mädchen. Jahrb. f. Kinderh., Leipz., 1879, n. F., xiv, 273–276.—**von Rinecker.** Ein 10jähriges mikrocephales Mädchen. Verhandl. d. phys.-med. Gesellsch. in Würzb., 1881, n. F., xv, pt. 2, p. xi. ———. Vorstellung eines mikrocephalen Mädchens. Sitzungsb. d. phys. med. Gesellsch. zu Würzb., 1881, 86–90.—**Rüdinger** (N.) Ueber Hirne von neugeborenen und erwachsenen Microcephalen. Sitzungsb. d. math.-phys. Cl. d. k.-bayer. Akad. d. Wissensch. zu München, 1885, xv, 112 – 117. ———. Mittheilungen über einige mikrocephale Hirne.

Microcephalus.

München. med. Wchnschr., 1886, xxxiii, 161; 185; 205.—
Sander (J.) Beschreibung zweier Microcephalen-Ge-
hirne. Arch. f. Psychiat., Berl., 1868, i, 299–307, 2 pl.—
Sapolini. Caso di microcefalia parziale Ann. univ.
di med., Milano, 1870, ccxiii, 369–378.—**Scheiber** (S.-H.)
Sur l'enfant micro-céphale. Cong. internat. d'anthrop.
1876, Budapest, 1877, viii, 210–213. — **Scheuthauer** (G.)
Anthropologikus elöadások; microcephalia. Orvosi hetil.,
Budapest, 1881, xxv, 629–636.—**Schüle** (H.) Morpholo-
gische Erläuterung eines Microcephalen-Gehirns. Arch.
f. Anthrop., Brnschwg., 1872, v, 437–449, 1 pl.--**Shortt**
(J.) Description of a living microcephale. Mem. Anthrop. Soc. Lond., 1865–6, ii, 257–261. ———. A brief account of three microcephales. [Abstr.] J. Anthrop.
Inst., Lond., 1873–4, iii, 265, 2 pl.—**Shuttleworth** (E. G.)
Two cases of microcephalic idiocy. Brit. M. J., Lond.,
1875, ii, 454. ———. A case of microcephalic imbecility.
J. Ment. Sc., Lond., 1878, xxiv, 438–443, 1 pl. Also, Reprint.—**Spitzka** (E. C.) Concerning the case of microcephalus. Med. Rec., N. Y., 1881, xx, 48.—**Stark** (C.)
Mikrocephalie, fötale Encephalitis und amyloide Gehirn-
degeneration. Allg. Ztschr. f. Psychiat., etc., Berl., 1875,
xxxii, 260–332, 5 pl.—**Steinlechner-Gretschischni-
koff** (A.) Ueber den Bau des Rückenmarkes bei Microcephalen. Ein Beitrag zur Kenntniss des Einflusses des Vor-
derhirnes auf die Entwickelung anderer Theile des centralen Nervensystemes. Arch. f. Psychiat., Berl., 1886, xvii,
649–692, 1 pl.—**Steudel.** Margarethe Becker von Offenbach, ein microcephales Mädchen von 16 Jahren. Med.
Cor.-Bl. d. württemb. ärztl. Ver., Stuttg., 1886, lvi, 33–35.—
Tamburini (A.) Un caso di microcefalia. Arch. ital.
per le mal. nerv., Milano, 1881, xviii, 5–12. Also, Reprint.—
Theile (F. W.) Ueber Microcephalie. Ztschr. f. rat.
Med., Leipz. u. Heidelb., 1861, 3. R., xi, 210–249, 2 pl.
———. Beitrag zur Lehre von der Mikrocephalie. Schmidt's
Jahrb., Leipz., 1876, clxix, 95–104.—**Tirrizzi** (S. N.) Quattro microcefalia ed un clinocefalo in una famiglia. Atti d.
Accad. Gioenia di sc. nat. in Catania, 1881, 3. s., xv, 1–18, 1
pl.—**Topinard** (P.) Sur deux microcéphales. Bull. Soc.
d'anthrop. de Par., 1875, 2. s., x, 36–39. [Discussion], 54–
72.—**Venturi** (S.) Di un imbecille microcefala. Manicomio, Nocera, 1885, i, 5–31.—**Virchow** (R.) Zur Geschichte
der mikrocephalen Mähler. Arch. f. path. Anat, etc.,
Berl., 1867, xl, 295. ———. Eine Mikrocephale. Verhandl.
d. Berl. med. Gesellsch. (1877–8), 1879, ix, 2. Th., 12–16.
Also: Berl. klin. Wchnschr., 1877, xiv, 713. ———. Ueber
Microcephalie. Verhandl. d. Berl. Gesellsch. f. Anthrop.,
1877, 280–295. ———. Ueber Microcephalen. Ibid., 1878,
25–33. ———. Vorstellung der microcephalen Becker von
Offenbach. Verhandl. d. Berl. med. Gesellsch. (1883–4),
1885, xv, 272–275. Also: Berl. klin. Wchnschr., 1884, xxi,
691.—**Virgilio** (C.) Di un caso singolare di microcefalia.
Riv. sper. di freniat., Reggio-Emilia, 1875, i, 11–28.—**Vogt.**
(C.) Ueber die Mikrocephalen oder Affen-Menschen.
Arch. f. Anthrop., Brnschwg., 1867, ii, 129–284, 25 pl. [See,
also, supra.] ———. Ueber Mikrocephalie. Wien. med.
Wchnschr., 1869, xix, 1635; 1666. Also: Wien. med.
Presse, 1869, x, 1153; 1177. Also [Abstr.]: Allg. Wien.
med. Ztg., 1869, xix, 459–462.—**Voisin.** Cerveau micro-
céphale. Bull. Soc. d'anthrop. de Par., 1868, 2. s., iii, 651–
656.—**Wedl** (C.) Mikrokephalus bei einem Neugebore-
nen. Med. Jahrb., Wien, 1863, v, 149–152.—**Westbrook**
(B. F.) Microcephalus. Proc. M. Soc. County Kings,
Brooklyn, 1879–80, iv, 275.—**Wood** (H. C.) Microcepha-
lus; hydrocephalus. [Extr.] Arch. Pediat., Phila., 1884,
i, 748–752.—**Zaborowski.** Un cerveau de microcéphale.
Bull. Soc. d'anthrop. de Par., 1884, 3. s., vii, 101–104.—**Zoja**
(G.) Di un teschio boliviano microcefalo. Mem. r. Ist.
Lomb. di sc. e lett. Cl. di sc. matemat. e nat. 1873–6,
Milano, 1877, xiii, 53–60, 4 pl. Also: Arch. per l' antrop.,
Firenze, 1874, iv, 205–217, 4 pl. Also, Reprint.—**Zucker-
kandl** (E.) Ueber Mikrocephalie. Mitth. d. anthrop.
Gesellsch. in Wien, 1875, v, 138–148, 4 pl.

Micrococcus.

See, also, Bacteria; Eye (Inflammation of, Sym-
pathetic); Germ theory of disease, etc.; Gonorrhœa
(Causes of, etc.); Microorganisms; Pneumonia
(Causes of).

Cheyne (W. W.) Report on micrococci in relation to
wounds, abscesses, and septic processes. Brit. M. J.,
Lond., 1884, ii, 553; 599; 645.—**Duclaux** (E.) Influence
de la lumière du soleil sur la vitalité des micrococcus.
Compt. rend. Acad. d. sc., Par., 1885, ci, 395–398. Also:
Compt. rend. Soc. de biol., Par., 1885, 8. s., ii, 508–510.—
Finne (G.) Om Smaasoppene. [On micrococci.] Tidsskr. f. prakt. Med., Kristiania, 1886, vi, 145–153.—**Foà**
(P.) & **Bordoni-Uffreduzzi** (G.) Ulteriori ricerche
sul meningococco. Gior. d. r. Accad. di med. di Torino,
1886, 3. s., xxxiv, 53. Also, transl.: Deutsche med. Wchnschr., Berl., 1886, xii, 568.—**Gregg** (R. R.) The recognition of micrococci. Med. Rec., N. Y., 1882, xxii, 202–206.—
Hedenius (P.) Fall af spontan septichaemi med micrococcus septicus. Upsala Läkaref. Förh., 1873, viii,
529–533.—**von Jaksch** (R.) Ueber die Entwickelungs-
bedingungen des Micrococcus Ureæ, Pasteur. Centralbl.

f. d. med. Wissensch., Berl., 1880, xviii, 180.—**Manfredi**
(L.) Di un nuovo micrococco nella patogenesi di una
forma sperimentale di tumori da infezione; suoi rapporti
con la pneumonite. Gior. internaz. d. sc. med., Napoli,
1886, n. s., viii, 864–880, 3 pl. — **Micrococcus** (Der)
und seine Beziehung zu den Infections-Krankheiten.
Prakt. Arzt, Wetzlar, 1872, xiii, 145; 217; 241; 265.—**Perroncito** (E.) & **Ajroldi.** Sopra alcune particolarità relative alla tenacità di vita di speciali micrococchi. Gior. d.
r. Accad. di med. di Torino, 1885, 3. s., xxxiii, 809–812.—
Riess (L.) Ueber sogenannte Micrococcen. Centralbl.
f. d. med. Wissensch., Berl., 1873, xi, 530–533.—**Salmon**
(D. E.) On cultivation as a test for micrococci. Med.
Rec., N. Y., 1882, xxii, 454–457.—**Stein** (T.) Mikrokok-
ken und Bacterien. [From: Gartenlaube.] Ztscher. f.
mikr. Fleischschau, Berl., 1879–80, i, 97; 116.—**Sternberg**
(G. M.) The recognition of micrococci. Med. Rec., N.
Y., 1882, xxi, 368: xxii, 429. ———. Micrococcus Pasteuri.
Am. J. M. Sc., Phila., 1886, n. s., xcii, 123–131. Also: J.
Roy. Micr. Soc., Lond., 1886, 2. s., vi, 391–396.—**Vasil-
jeff** (N. P.) Ob uslovijach razvitija v krovenosnich so-
sudach kolonii mikrokokkov. [Conditions of development
of micrococci in blood-vessels.] Ejened. klin. gaz., St.
Petersb., 1882, ii, 374–376.—**Wernich** (A.) Untersuchun-
gen über Bacterien. VII. Versuche über die Infection
mit Micrococcus prodigiosus. Beitr. z. Biol. d. Pflanz.,
Bresl., 1879, iii, 105–118.

Microcosmo

(De) et macrocosmo dissert. ii.
20 pp. sm. 4°. Regiomonti Borussorum, typ.
Hartungianis, 1827.

Microcythemia.

Van Lair & **Masius.** De la microcythémie. Bull.
Acad. roy. de méd. de Belg., Brux., 1871, 3. s., v, 515–613,
1 pl. Also [Abstr.]: Rev. phot. d. hôp. de Par., 1872, iv,
17–22. Also [Abstr.]: Bull. Soc. de méd. de Gand, 1872,
xxxix, 272–289.

Microgale.

Dobson (G. E.) The anatomy of Microgale longi-
cauda, with remarks on the homologies of the long flexors
of the toes in mammalia. J. Anat. & Physiol., Lond.,
1881–2, xvi, 355–361.

Micrometer and micrometry.

Peuvion. Machines à faire les micromètres.
8°. Lille, [n. d.]

Repr. from: Mém. Soc. roy. d. sc., de l'agric. et d. arts de
Lille.

Weickert (C. F.) De micrometris duplicem
objecti imaginem proferentibus. 4°. Lipsiæ,
1811.

Harris (J.) Micrometer. In his: Lexicon techn., fol.,
Lond., 1708, 5 E²ᵇ.—**Hayden** (T.) A short notice of a ready
and simple mode of measuring microscopic objects. Dublin
Q. J. M. Sc., 1855, xix, 119–121, 1 pl.—**Malassez** (L.) Nouveaux procédés de micrométrie. Arch. de physiol. norm. et
path., Par., 1874, vi, 27–31.—**von Mohl** (H.) Ueber eine
neue Einrichtung des Schraubenmikrometers. Arch. f.
mikr. Anat., Bonn, 1865, i, 79–100.—**Robertson** (W.) On
micrometers applied to microscopes. Month. J. M. Sc.,
Lond. & Edinb., 1851, xii, 329–333.—**Welcker** (H.) Beschreibung eines genauen, leicht herstellbaren mikroskopischen Messapparates. Ztschr. f. rat. Med., Heidelb.,
1851, x, 1; 211, 2 pl.

Micronesia.

See Ethnology.

Microorganisms.

See, also, Air (Chemistry, etc., of); Bacteria;
Blood (Parasites in); Brownian motion; Fever
(Malarial, Causes of); Fever (Typhoid, Causes,
etc., of); Fever (Typhus, Causes, etc., of); Fungi
(Parasitic); Germ theory of disease, etc.; Germs
(Investigation of); Infusoria; Leprosy (Bacillus
of); Micrococcus; Microscopy (Manipulations,
etc., in); Milk (Abnormal, etc.); Photomicrographs, etc.; Phthisis (Causes, etc., of); Ptomaine; Saccharomyces; Tetanus (Causes of);
Tubercle (Bacillus of).

Baltus (E.) *Théorie du microzyma. Étude
théorique et pratique de la pyogénèse. 4°. Montpellier, 1874.

Béchamp (J.) *Des microzymas et de leurs
fonctions aux différents âges d'un même être.
4°. Montpellier, 1875.

Caizergues (L.) Les microzymas, ce qu'il
faut en penser. 8°. Paris, 1862.

Microorganisms.

EYFERTH (B.) Schizophyten und Flagellaten. Supplement-Heft zu der systematischen Naturgeschichte der mikroskopischen Süsswasserbewohner. 4°. *Braunschweig*, 1879.

DE FROMENTEL (E.) Études sur les microzoaires ou infusoires proprement dits, comprenant de nouvelles recherches sur leur organisation, leur classification et la description des espèces nouvelles ou peu connues. Planches et notes descriptives des espèces par Mme. J. Jobard-Muteau. 4°. *Paris*, 1874.

HARTING (P.) Redvoering bij gelegenheid van het 200-jarig feest, ter herdenking van Antony van Leeuwenhoek's ontdekking der mikroskopische wezens. 8°. [*n. p.*, 1875.]
Repr. from: Album der Natuur, 1875.

KINGZETT (C. T.) A precise investigation of some micro-organisms and soluble ferments, their chemical history and relation to disease, including also a practical study of the disinfecting value of "Sanitas" fluids. 8°. *London*, 1885.

MAGGI (L.) I piccoli benefattori dell' umanità. 8°. *Milano*, 1886.

TAXIS (A.) Recherches sur l'origine des microorganismes. 8°. *Marseille*, 1885.
Repr. from: Bull. d. Soc. d. horticul. et d. botan. de Marseille.

Barnard (W. S.) Micro-organisms and their effects in nature. Pop. Sc. Month., N. Y., 1879, xv, 764-772.—**Béchamp** (A.) Les microzymas, la pathologie et la thérapeutique. Montpel. méd., 1870, xxv, 141-153. ——. Microzyma et micrococcus. *Ibid.*, 1873, xxx, 44; 234. ——. Les microzymas dans leurs rapports avec les fermentations et la physiologie. Assoc. franç. pour l'avance. d. sc. Compt.-rend. 1875, Par., 1876, iv, 96-129. ——. Sur les microzymas géologiques; réponse à une récente communication de MM. Chamberland et Roux. Compt. rend. Acad. d. sc., Par., 1881, xcii, 1291. ——. Du rôle et de l'origine de certains microzymas. *Ibid.*, 1344-1347. ——. Sur les microzymas de la craie; réponse à la note de MM. Chamberland et Roux. *Ibid.*, 1467. ——. Les microzymas gastriques et la pepsine; remarques sur la note de M. A. Gautier du 6 mars dernier. *Ibid.*, 970-973. ——. Sur les microzymas comme cause de la décomposition de l'eau oxygénée par les tissus des animaux et des végétaux. *Ibid.*, 1882, xciv, 1653-1656. ——. Sur les propriétés et les fonctions des microzymas pancréatiques. Bull. Acad. de méd., Par., 1881, 2. s., x, 630-663. ——. Les microzymas des glandes stomacales et leur pouvoir digestif. *Ibid.*, 1882, 2. s., xi, 296-314. ——. Sur les microzymas gastriques. *Ibid.*, 347-357. ——. Les microzymas sont-ils des organismes vivants? Exposition d'une théorie expérimentale de l'antisepticité. *Ibid.*, 497-547. ——. Les microzymas et les zymases. Arch. de physiol. norm. et path., Par., 1882, 2. s., x, 28-62. ——. Les microzymas du foie et les microzymas du pancréas. *Ibid.*, 409-444. ——. Le choléra, les maladies contagieuses et les quarantaines, considérés dans leurs rapports avec la théorie du microzyma. Rev. méd. franç. et étrang., Par., 1883, ii, 721-731. ——. Sur l'origine des microzymas et des vibrioniens de l'air, des eaux et du sol, à propos d'une communication de M. Duclaux. Compt. rend. Acad. d. sc., Par., 1885, c, 181-184. ——. Sur la théorie du microzyma et le système microbien. Gaz. méd. de Par., 1886, 7. s., iii, 353; 365; 385; 409; 445; 509; 577; 601; 613.—**Béchamp** (A.) & **Estor** (A.) Des microzymas des organismes supérieurs. Montpel. méd., 1870, xxiv, 32-48.—**Béchamp** (J.) Des microzymas et de leurs fonctions aux différents âges d'un même être. Compt. rend. Acad. d. sc., Par., 1875, lxxxi, 226-229. ——. Sur un cas remarquable de réduction de l'acide nitrique et d'oxydation de l'acide acétique avec production d'alcool, sous l'influence de certains microzymas. Assoc. franç. pour l'avance. d. sc. Compt.-rend. 1876, Par., 1877, v, 314-317.—**Certes** (A.) Note relative à l'action des hautes pressions sur la vitalité des microorganismes d'eau douce et d'eau de mer. Compt. rend. Soc. de biol., Par., 1884, 8. s., i, pt. 2, 220-222. *Also:* Tribune méd., Par., 1884, xvi, 224.—**Chamberland** & **Roux.** Sur la non-existence du microzyma cretæ; réponse à une note de M. A. Béchamp. Compt. rend. Acad. d. sc., Par., 1881, xcii, 1347. ——. De la non-existence du microzyma cretæ. *Ibid.*, 1165.—**Christopher** (H.) The place in creation and the work in the economy of nature of micro-organisms. St. Louis M. & S. J., 1885, xlviii, 273; 361.—**Colin** (G.) De l'évolution des organismes microscopiques sur l'animal vivant, dans le cadavre et les produits morbides. [Extr.] Compt. rend. Acad. d. sc., Par., 1882, xcv, 1338.—**Dallinger** (W. H) The president's address. [Some septic organisms.] J. Roy. Micr. Soc., Lond., 1886, 2. s., vi, 193-207, 3 pl.—**Degagny**

Microorganisms.

(C.) Étude de divers micro-organismes à l'aide de solutions alcalines. Compt. rend. Soc. de biol., Par., 1884, 8. s., ii, pt. 2, 428-430.—**Estor** (A.) Contribution à l'étude des microzymas et des bactéries. Gaz. hebd. d. sc. méd. de Montpel., 1883, v, 301; 338; 377.—**Fiessinger** (C.) Note sur les organismes qui peuvent se développer dans les solutions phéniquées. Mém. Soc. de méd. de Nancy (1881-2), 1883, 76-81.—**Frankland** (E.) On chemical changes in their relation to micro-organisms. J. Chem. Soc., Lond., 1885, xlvii, 159-183.—**Frankland** (P. F.) On the multiplication of micro-organisms. Proc. Roy. Soc. Lond., 1886, xl, 526-544.—**Frenzel** (J.) Ueber die Mikrozymas in der Leber und im Pankreas. Biol. Centralbl.. Erlang., 1883, iii, 49-52.—**Gautier** (A.) Sur les modifications soluble et insoluble du ferment de la digestion gastrique. Compt. rend. Acad. d. sc., Par., 1882, xciv, 652-655.—**Künstler** (J.) Recherches sur les infusoires parasites; sur quinze protozoaires nouveaux. J. de microg., Par., 1883, vii, 583-585. ——. Sur la structure des flagellés. *Ibid.*, 1886, x, 17, 1 pl., 58.—**Marpmann** (G.) Ueber die Erreger der Milchsäure-Gährung. Ergnzngshft. z. Centralbl. f. allg. Gsndhtspflg., Bonn, 1885-6, ii, 117-132, 1 pl.—**Moniez** (R.) Note sur une nouvelle forme de sarcodine: le schizogenes parasiticus. J. de l'anat. et physiol., etc., Par., 1886, xx, 515-523, 1 pl.—**Sandri** (G.) Protorganismi, che appajono dopo morte, non provano ciò che avvenga durante la vita. Mem. r. Ist. Veneto di sc., lett. ed arti, Venezia, 1874-5, xviii, 239-252. *Also*, Reprint.—**Sherborn** (C. D.) & **Chapman** (F.) On some microzoa from the London clay exposed in the drainage-works, Piccadilly, London, 1885. J. Roy. Micr. Soc., Lond., 1886, 2. s., vi, 737-763, 3 pl.—**Sorokin** (N.) Eine neue Spirillum-Art. Centralbl. f. Bacteriol. u. Parasitenk., Jena, 1887, i, 465.—**Trélease** (W.) Observations on several zoogloeæ and related forms. Johns Hopkins Univ. Stud. biol. lab., Balt., 1884-7, iii, 193-216, 1 pl.—**Turró** (R.) Béchamp y Pasteur. Gac. méd. catal., Barcel., 1885, viii, 13; 45; 76; 109; 136; 269; 332; 429.

Microphone.

See, also, **Calculus** (*Urinary, Diagnosis of*).

BOEKMANN (O.) * Ueber den elektrischen Widerstand des Mikrophonkohlencontactes während der Bewegung. 8°. *Giessen*, 1884.

GIBOUX. Le microphone et ses applications en médecine. 8°. *Paris*, 1878.

Avezou (C.) Microphone de disposition spéciale applicable aux recherches physiologiques et en particulier à l'étude de la contraction musculaire. Progrès méd., Par., 1880, viii. 67; 88.—**Bianchi** (A.) Il telefono ed il microfono applicati alle scienze mediche; modalite di ascoltazione nella diagnosi medica. Ann. univ. di med. e chir., Milano, 1882, cclix, 193; 338; 402.—**Boudet.** Application du microphone à la clinique et aux recherches physiologiques. J. d. conn. méd. prat., Par., 1879, 3. s., i, 409. —**Brochin.** Des applications du téléphone et du microphone à la clinique. Gaz. d. hôp., Par., 1880, liii, 1025-1027.—**Eve** (E. J.) The microphone as a diagnosticator of the entire physical organism. Atlanta M. & S. J., 1885-6, n. s., ii, 229-231.—**Grassl** (W.) Das Microphon und seine diagnostische Verwerthung. Med.-chir. Centralbl., Wien, 1878, xiii, 555.—**Holland** (J. W.) A microphone for the heart. Louisville M. News, 1878, vi, 25.—**Ladendorf** (A.) Das Microphon als diagnostisches Hülfsmittel. Berl. klin. Wchnschr., 1878, xv, 565.—**Martius** (G.) Ueber die Einführung des Mikrophons in die praktische Medicin. Aerztl. Int.-Bl., München, 1882, xxix, 525-527.—**Mass** (H.) Ueber Anwendung des Microphons zu chirurgisch-diagnostischen Zwecken. Berl. klin. Wchnschr., 1878, xv, 535.—**Rijke** (P.-L.) Sur le microphone. Arch. néerl. d. sc. exactes, etc., Harlem, 1879, xiv, 76-96.—**Spillmann** (P.) & **Dumont** (P.) Des applications du microphone aux recherches cliniques. Arch. gén. de méd., Par., 1879, cxliii, 513-523.—**Trouvé** (G.) & **de Boyer** (H.) Microphone de disposition spéciale, applicable aux recherches physiologiques et en particulier à l'étude de la contraction musculaire. Progrès méd., Par., 1880, viii, 67.

Microphotography.

See Photomicrographs, *etc.*

Microphthalmus.

See **Eye** (*Abnormities, etc., of*); **Monsters** *from defect, etc., of brain, etc.*

Microphytes.

See Bacteria; Fungi; Microorganisms.

Micropia.

See Belladonna (*Effects of*) on the eye.

Micropyle.

André (J.) Sur la préparation du micropyle dans la coque des œufs de truite. J. de l'anat. et physiol., Par., 1875, xi, 197-202.—**Buchholtz** (R.) Ueber die Mikro-

Micropyle.

pyle von Osmerus eperlanus. Arch. f. Anat., Physiol. u. wissensch. Med., Leipz., 1863, 71 : 367, 1 pl.—**Reichert** (K. B.) Ueber die Micropyle der Fischeier und über einen bisher unbekannten, eigenthümlichen Bau des Nahrungsdottersreifer und befruchteter Fischeier (Hecht). *Ibid.*, 1856, 83–124, 1 pl.—**von Schlen** (D.) Beitrag zur Frage nach der Mikropyle des Säugethiereies. Gekrönte Preisschrift. Arch. f. Anat. u. Entwcklngsgesch., Leipz., 1882, 33–51, 1 pl.

Microscope (The).

Title, after 1883, of : **Microscope** (The) and its Relation to Medicine and Pharmacy.

Microscope *and microscopy.*

See, also, **Air** (*Chemistry, etc., of*); **Brownian** *motion* ; **Diatoms** ; **Histology** ; **Infusoria** ; **Instruments** (*Optical, etc.*); **Micrometer**, *etc.* ; **Microtomes**, *etc.* ; **Photomicrographs**, *etc.* ; **Toxicology** (*Use of microscope in*); **Urine**, **Water**, *Chemistry, etc., of.*

ABBE (E.) Beiträge zur Theorie des Mikroskops und der mikroskopischen Wahrnehmung. 8°. [*n. p.*, 1873.]

ADACHI KAN. Kenbikio Kensa Shishin. [Rules for microscopic examinations.] 12°. *Tokio*, 1882.
Japanese text.

ADAMS (G.) Micrographia illustrata, or the knowledge of the microscope explain'd ; together with an account of a new-invented universal, single or double microscope, either of which is capable of being applied to an improv'd solar apparatus. To which is added a translation of Mr. Joblott's observations on the animalcula . . . and a very particular account of that surprising phænomenon, the fresh-water polype, translated from the French treatise of St. Trembley. 4°. *London*, 1746.

———. The same. 2. ed. 4°. *London*, 1747.

———. The same. Likewise a natural history of aerial, terrestrial, and aquatic animals, etc., considered as microscopic objects. 4. ed. 8°. *London*, 1771.

———. Essays on the microscope ; containing a practical description of the most improved microscopes ; a general history of insects . . . an account of the various species and singular properties of the hydræ and vorticellæ ; a description of three hundred and seventy-nine animalcula . . . With atlas of 31 plates. 4°. *London*, 1787.

———. The same. 2. ed., with additions and improvements, by F. Kanmacher. 4°. *London*, 1798.

ADAN (H.-P.) Le microscope. Coup d'œil discret sur le monde invisible. 8°. *Bruxelles*, 1873.

———. Le monde invisible dévoilé. Révélations du microscope. 2. éd. 8°. *Bruxelles*, 1880.

ALESSANDRI (P. E.) Il microscopio e sua applicazione alla merceologia e bromatologia ; ad uso degli istituti e scuole tecniche, liceali, agrarie, industriali, commerciali, di farmacia, etc., commercianti, negozianti, farmacisti, etc. 8°. *Milano*, 1886.

AMICI (G.) De microscopj catadiottrici memoria. 4°. *Modena*, 1878.

ARNDT (A.) Das Mikroskop im Dienste des landwirthschaftlichen und gewerblichen Lebens sowie der Familie. Populäre Anweisung zur Behandlung und praktischen Verwendung desselben. 8°. *Berlin*, 1874.

BACHMANN (O.) Unsere modernen Mikroskope und deren sämtliche Hilfs- und Nebenapparate für wissenschaftliche Forschungen. Ein Handbuch für Histologen, Geologen, Mediziner, Pharmazeuten, Chemiker, Techniker und Studierende. 8°. *München u. Leipzig*, 1883.

BAILEY (J. W.) Microscopical observations made in South Carolina, Georgia, and Florida. 4°. *New York*, [*n. d.*]

BAILEY (L. W.) Notes on new species of microscopical organisms, chiefly from the Para River, South America. 8° *Cambridge*, 1861.
Repr. from : Boston J. Nat. Hist., vii.

BAKER (H.) The microscope made easy ; or, I. The nature, uses, and magnifying powers of the best kinds of microscopes described, calculated, and explained, for the instruction of such, particularly, as desire to search into the wonders of the minute creation, tho' they are not acquainted with optics. Together with full directions how to prepare, apply, examine, and preserve all sorts of objects, and proper cautions to be observed in viewing them. II. An account of what surprizing discoveries have been already made by the microscope, with useful reflections on them. And also a great variety of new experiments and observations, pointing out many uncommon subjects for the examination of the curious. 8°. *London*, 1742.

———. The same. 2. ed. 8°. *London*, 1743.

———. The same. 3. ed. 8°. *London*, 1744.

———. The same. Le microscope à la portée de tout le monde, ou description, calcul et explication de la nature, de l'usage et de la force des meilleurs microscopes, [etc.] Trad. de l'anglois . . . sur l'édition de 1743. 8°. *Paris*, 1754.

———. Employment for the microscope. (In two parts.) 8°. *London*, 1753.

———. The same. Beyträge zu nützlichem und vergnügendem Gebrauch und Verbesserung des Microscopii in zwey Theilen. Aus dem Englischen ins Deutsche übersetzt. sm. 8°. *Augsburg*, 1754.

———. Of microscopes and the discoveries made thereby. In 2 v. Vol. I. The microscope made easy. Vol. II. Employment for the microscope. A new ed. 8°. *London*, 1785.

BARKER (J.) On the illuminations of microscopic objects. 8°. [*n. p., n. d.*]
Read before the Royal Irish Academy, Jan. 10, 1870.

BAUSCH & LOMB Optical Company. Price list of microscopes, objectives, and accessories. 10. ed. 8°. *Rochester, N. Y.*, 1886.

———. The same. Illustrated catalogue of microscopes, objectives, and accessories. 11. ed. 8°. *Rochester, N. Y.*, 1887.

BEALE (L. S) How to work with the microscope. 8°. *London*, 1861.

———. The same. 3. ed. 8°. *London*, 1865.

———. The same. 4. ed. 8°. *London*, 1868.

———. Descriptive catalogue of microscopical specimens, illustrating the structure of certain tissues . . . exhibited at the president's soirée (British Med. Ass'n, 1868). 8°. *London*, 1868.

BECK (R.) A treatise on the construction, proper use, and capabilities of Smith, Beck, and Beck's achromatic microscopes. 8°. *London*, 1865.

——— & BECK (J.) A condensed list of a few of the most desirable microscopes, of moderate cost, and accessories, mounting implements, and materials, [etc.] 8°. [*Philadelphia*, 1883?]

BERLING (O.) Verzeichniss der wichtigsten Erscheinungen auf dem Gebiete der Mikroskopie. 8°. *Berlin*, 1886.

BERNARD (J.-G.) * Histoire des microscopes, ce que leur doit la médecine. 4°. *Paris*, 1886.

BION (N.) Traité de la construction et des principaux usages des instrumens de mathématique. Nouv. éd. 4°. *La Haye*, 1723.

BONANNI (P.) Observationes circa viventia, quæ in rebus non viventibus reperiuntur. Cum micrographia curiosa sive rerum minutissimarum observationibus, quæ ope microscopii recognitæ ad vivum exprimuntur. His accesserunt aliquot

Microscope *and microscopy.*

animalium testaceorum icones non antea in lucem editæ. Omnia curiosorum naturæ exploratorum utilitati et jucunditati expressa et oblata. sm. 4°. *Romæ,* 1691.

BONO (G. G.) Il microscopio e le sue applicazioni alle perizie di medicina forense, [etc.] 8°. *Genova,* 1863.

BORELLI (P.) De vero telescopii inventore, cum brevi omnium conspiciliorum historia, ubi de eorum confectione, ac usu, seu de effectibus agitur, novaque quædam circa ea proponuntur. Accessit etiam centuria observationum microcospicarum. 4°. *Hagæ-Comitum,* 1655.

BREWSTER (*Sir* D.) Description of a monochromatic lamp for microscopical purposes, etc., with remarks on the absorption of the prismatic rays by coloured media. 4°. *Edinburgh,* 1822.
Repr. from: Tr. Roy. Soc. Edinb.

BROCKLESBY (J.) The amateur microscopist; or, views of the microscopic world. A handbook of microscopic manipulation and microscopic objects. 8°. *New York,* 1871.

C. (E.) Bailey Microscopical Club; table showing the actual magnifying power of thirty-five microscopical objectives of various makers, as determined at a meeting of the Bailey Microscopical Club, held in New York, September 20, 1870. 8°. [*n. p., n. d.*]

CARPENTER (W. B.) The microscope and its revelations. 4. ed. 8°. *London,* 1868.

——. The same. 5. ed. Prepared with the assistance of H. J. Slack. 12°. *London,* 1875.

——. The same. 6. ed. 8°. *London,* 1881.

——. The same. 6. ed. 2 v. 8°. *New York,* 1883.

——. The same. With an appendix containing the applications of the microscope to clinical medicine, etc., by Francis Gurney Smith. 8°. *Philadelphia,* 1856.

CASTRACANE (F.) Cenni su l' esame microscopico di un fango estratto dal fondo del' Oceano Atlantico. 4°. [*Roma,* 1870.]
Repr. from: Atti Accad. pont. de' Nuovi Lincei, 1870, v.

——. Esame microscopico e note critiche su un campione di fango atlantico ottenuto nella spedizione del "Porcupine" nell' anno 1869. 4°. [*Roma,* 1871.]
Repr. from: Atti Accad. pont. de' Nuovi Lincei, 1871, i.

——. Su la illuminazione monocromatica del microscopio e la fotomicrografia e loro utilità. 4°. *Roma,* 1871.
Repr. from: Atti Accad. pont. de' Nuovi Lincei, 1871, iii.

——. Su la risoluzione delle linee di Nobert e su i progressi della micrografia. 4°. *Roma,* 1872.
Repr. from: Atti Accad. pont. de' Nuovi Lincei, 1872, vi.

——. La visione binoculaire in relazione alla micrografia. 4°. *Roma* 1874.

CATALOG mikroskopischer Injections - Präparate, welche durch Tausch oder Kauf zu beziehen sind von Prof. Hyrtl in Wien. 8°. *Wien,* 1873.

CATALOGUE of works on the microscope, and of those referring to microscopical subjects, in the library of Freeman C. S. Roper. 8°. [*London*], 1865.

CHEVALIER (A.) L'étudiant micrographe. Traité théorique et pratique du microscope et des préparations. 2. éd., augmentée... par Alph. de Brébisson, Henri van Heurck, G. Pouchet. 8°. *Paris,* 1865.

——. The same. 3. éd. 8°. *Paris,* 1882.

CHEVALIER (C.) Des microscopes et de leur usage. Description d'appareils et de procédés nouveaux, suivie d'expériences microscopiques ... et les notes de M. Le Baillif, et d'un mémoire sur les diatomées, etc., par M. de Brébisson. 8°. *Paris,* 1839.

Microscope *and microscopy.*

——. Rapports sur les instrumens inventés ou construits par... 8°. *Paris,* [*n. d.*]

CHUN (C.) Katechismus der Mikroskopie. 16°. *Leipzig,* 1885.

COLE (A. C.) Studies in microscopical science. 2 v. 8°. *London,* 1883–4.

COOKE (M. C.) One thousand objects for the microscope. 12°. *London & New York,* 1869.

CROSS (C. R.) On the focal length of microscopic objectives. Contributions from the physical laboratory of the Massachusetts Institute of Technology. 8°. [*Boston,* 1870.]

DAVIS (G. E.) Practical microscopy. 2. ed. 8°. *London,* 1882.

DECHALES (C. F. M.) Cursus seu mundus mathematicus. Editio altera ex manuscriptis authoris aucta et emendata, opera et studio... Amati Varcin... 4 v. fol. *Lugduni,* 1690.

DELLA TORRE (G. M.) Nuove osservazioni microscopiche. 4°. *Napoli,* 1776.

DESCRIPTION et usage du microscope. 16°. [*n. p., n. d.*]

DIDELOT (L.) *Du pouvoir amplifiant du microscope; détermination théorique et expérimentale. 4°. *Lyon,* 1886.

DIPPEL (L.) Das Mikroskop und seine Anwendung. 2 v. 8°. *Braunschweig,* 1867–9.

——. The same. 2. Aufl. 1. Theil, 1.–3. Abth. 8°. *Braunschweig,* 1882–3.

——. Handbuch der allgemeinen Mikroskopie. 2. Aufl. 1.–3. Abth. 8°. *Braunschweig,* 1882–3.
In his: Das Mikroskop und seine Anwendung. 8°. *Braunschweig,* 1882.

DRIELSMA (A.) Het mikroskoop in zijne toepassing bij de diagnose. Naar Bennett en Reinhard bewerkt, met aantekeningen en bijvoegsels vermeerderd, met eene voorrede van Prof. I. van Deen. 8°. *Tiel,* 1859.

EHRENBERG (C. G.) Mikrogeologische Studien über das kleinste Leben der Meeres-Tiefgründe aller Zonen und dessen geologischen Einfluss. 4°. *Berlin,* 1873.

ELSNER (F.) Mikroskopischer Atlas. Ein illustrirtes Sammelwerk zum Gebrauche für Gesundheitsbeamte, Apotheker, Drogisten, Kaufleute und gebildete Laien. 1.–5. Hft. fol. *Halle a. S.,* 1884–5.

FIDDIAN (T.) A paper on a new method of adjusting the focus of microscopes. 8°. [*Birmingham,* 1870.]

VON FLEISCHL (E.) Mikroskope. Medicin. 8°. *Wien,* 1877.
Repr. from: Bericht über die Weltausstellung in Philadelphia, 1876.

FLEMMING (W.) Ueber die heutigen Aufgaben des Mikroskops. Ein populärer Vortrag, gehalten in der Aula der Universität zu Rostock. 8°. *Rostock,* 1872.

FOSTER (M.) Report on modern microscopes and recent improvements in microscopical apparatus, with a special view to the requirements of medical students and practitioners. 8°. *London,* 1867.

FRANCOTTE (P.) Manuel de technologie microscopique applicable à l'histologie, l'anatomie comparée, l'embryologie et la botanique. 8°. *Paris,* [1886].

FREY (H.) Das Mikroskop und die mikroskopische Technik. Ein Handbuch für Aerzte und Studirende. 2. Aufl. 8°. *Leipzig,* 1865.

——. The same. 3. Aufl. 8°. *Leipzig,* 1868.

——. The same. 4. Aufl. 8°. *Leipzig,* 1871.

——. The same. 5. Aufl. 8°. *Leipzig,* 1873.

Microscope *and microscopy.*

──. The same. 6. Aufl. 8°. *Leipzig,* 1877.

──. The same. 7. Aufl. 8°. *Leipzig,* 1881.

──. The same. The microscope and microscopical technology. Transl. by George R. Cutler, M. D. From the 4. German ed. 8°. *New York,* 1872.

FRITSCH (G.) Ueber das stereoskopische Sehen im Mikroskop und die Herstellung stereoskopischer Mikrotypien auf photographischem Wege. 4°. *Berlin,* 1873.

FUSS (N.) Instruction détaillée pour porter les lunettes de toutes les différentes espèces au plus haut degré de perfection dont elles sont susceptibles, tirée de la théorie dioptrique de Mr. Euler le père et mise à la portée de tous les ouvriers en ce genre. Avec la description d'un microscope qui peut passer pour le plus parfait dans son espèce et qui est propre à produire tous les grossissemens qu'on voudra. 4°. *St.-Pétersbourg,* 1774.

──. The same. Umständliche Anweisung, wie alle Arten von Fernröhren in der grössten möglichen Vollkommenheit zu verfertigen sind. Aus des ältern Herrn Euler's Theorie der Dioptrik gezogen, und für alle Künstler in diesem Fache begreiflich gemacht. Aus dem Französischen übersetzt und mit einigen Zusätzten vermehrt, von Georg Simon Klügel. 4°. *Leipzig,* 1778.

GAGE (S. H.) Microscopical notes. 8°. [*Ann Arbor,* 1886.]
Repr. from: Microscope, Dec., 1886.

GARBINI (A.) Manuale per la tecnica moderna del microscopio nelle osservazioni zoologiche, istologiche ed anatomiche. 12°. *Verona,* 1885.

──. The same. 2. ed. 8°. *Verona,* 1887.

GÉRARD (R.) Traité pratique de micrographie appliquée à la botanique, à la zoologie, à l'hygiène et aux recherches cliniques. roy. 8°. *Paris,* 1887.

GIRARD (J.) Le monde microscopique des eaux. sm. 8°. *Paris,* 1872.

GLAISHER (J.) The president's address before the Royal Microscopical Society of London for the year 1867–8. 8°. [*n. p., n. d.*]

──. The president's address delivered before the Royal Microscopical Society, February 10, 1869. 8°. *London,* 1869.

GOECKEL (J. C.) *De microscopiis simplicibus et theoretice et practice consideratis. 4°. *Jenæ,* [1733].

GORING (C. R.) & PRICHARD (A.) Microscopic illustrations of a few new, popular, and diverting living objects . . . with accurate descriptions of the latest improvements in the new microscopes, [etc.] 8°. *London,* 1830.

──. Micrographia, containing practical essays on reflecting, solar, oxy-hydrogen gas microscopes, micrometers, eye-pieces, etc. Illustrated. 8°. *London,* 1837.

GOULD. Guide pour les recherches et observations microscopiques, contenant la description du microscope, la préparation des infusions végétales et des solutions salines. Trad. de la 7. éd. anglaise, avec figures et additions, par Julia de Fontenelle. 8°. *Paris,* 1836.

S' GRAVESANDE (W. J.) Mathematical elements of natural philosophy, confirm'd by experiments; or, an introduction to Sir Isaac Newton's philosophy. Written in Latin. Transl. into English by the late J. T. Desaguliers, and published by his son, J. T. Desaguliers. 6. ed. 2 v. 4°. *London,* 1747.

GRIENDELIUS (J. F.) Micrographia nova: sive nova et curiosa variorum minutorum cor-

Microscope *and microscopy.*

porum singularis cujusdam et noviter ab autore inventi microscopii ope adauctorum et miranda magnitudine repræsentatorum descriptio. 4°. *Norimbergæ,* 1687.

GRIFFITH (J. W.) & HENFREY (A.) The micrographic dictionary; a guide to the examination and investigation of the structure and nature of microscopic objects. 2. ed. 2 v. in 1. 8°. *London,* 1860.

──. The same. Edited by J. W. Griffith and Martin Duncan, assisted by the Rev. M. J. Berkeley and T. Rupert Jones. 3. ed. 2 v. 8°. *London,* 1871–4.

──. The same. 4. ed. 8°. *London,* 1883.

HAGER (H.) Das Mikroskop und seine Anwendung. 2. Aufl. 8°. *Berlin,* 1866.

──. The same. 4. Aufl. 8°. *Berlin,* 1874.

──. The same. 7. Aufl. 8°. *Berlin,* 1886.

──. The same. Kenbikio Yoho. [The use of the microscope. Transl. by Shibata Shokei.] 12°. *Tokio,* 1882.
Japanese text.

──. Le microscope; théorie; applications; traité pratique à l'usage des élèves des écoles du gouvernement, des chimistes, des pharmaciens, des agriculteurs, du commerce et de l'industrie, des laboratoires, des écoles d'arts et métiers, des établissements industriels et des gens du monde. Traduction et annotations sur la 4. éd. du Dr. . . . par L. Planchon et L. Hugounenq. Introd. par J.-E. Planchon. 12°. *Paris,* 1884.

HANNOVER (A.) On the construction and use of the microscope. Edited by John Goodsir. 8°. *Edinburgh,* 1853.

HARTING (P.) Das Mikroskop; Theorie, Gebrauch, Geschichte und gegenwärtiger Zustand desselben. Deutsch von F. W. Theile. 2. Aufl. 3 v. 8°. *Braunschweig,* 1866.

HARTNACK (E.) Preis-Courant der achromatischen Mikroskope. 8°. *Potsdam,* 1883.

HARTSOEKER (N.) Essay de dioptrique. 4°. *Paris,* 1694.

──. Principes de physique. 4°. *Paris,* 1696.

HAUSHOFER (K.) Mikroskopische Reactionen. Eine Anleitung zur Erkennung verschiedener Elemente und Verbindungen unter dem Mikroskop als Supplement zu den Methoden der qualitativen Analyse. 8°. *Braunschweig,* 1885.

HELLER (K. B.) Das dioptrische Mikroskop, dessen Einrichtung und Behandlung leichtfasslich dargestellt. 8°. *Wien,* 1856.

HEUMANN (G.) *Mikroskopische Untersuchungen an hungernden und verhungerten Tauben. 8°. *Giessen,* 1850.

VAN HEURCK (H.) Le microscope, sa construction, son maniement, et son application aux études d'anatomie végétale. 2. éd. 8°. *Anvers,* 1869.

──. The same. 3. éd. 12°. *Bruxelles,* 1878.

HOGG (J.) The microscope; its history, construction, and application; being a familiar introduction to the use of the instrument, and the study of microscopical science. 6. ed. 8°. *London,* 1867.

HOOKE (R.) Micrographia; or some physiological descriptions of minute bodies made by magnifying glasses; with observations and inquiries thereupon. fol. *London,* 1667.

──. Microscopic observations; or, wonderful discoveries by the microscope, illustrated by thirty-three copper-plates, curiously engraved; whereby the most valuable particulars in that celebrated author's Micrographia are brought together in a narrow compass, [etc.] fol. *London,* 1780.

Microscope *and microscopy.*

IMAYE MUSUTADA. Bioya Kenbikiyo. [A guide to chemical microscopy.] 12°. *Tokio,* 1876.

Japanese text.

INTERNATIONAL Exhibition of 1876. Hospital of the Medical Department, United States Army . . . No. 9. List of microscopical preparations from the Army Medical Museum. 8°. *Philadelphia,* 1876.

JOBLOT (L.) Descriptions et usages de plusieurs nouveaux microscopes, tant simples que composez; avec de nouvelles observations faites sur une multitude innombrable d'insectes, et d'autres animaux de diverses espèces, qui naissent dans les liqueurs préparées, et dans celles qui ne le sont point. 2 pts. 4°. *Paris,* 1718.

——. Observations d'histoire naturelle faites avec le microscope, sur un grand nombre d'insectes, et sur les animalcules qui se trouvent dans les liqueurs préparées et dans celles qui ne le sont pas, etc. Avec la description et les usages des différens microscopes, etc. 2 v. in 1. 4°. *Paris,* 1754.

KAMPF (C. L. F.) * Ueber die Untersuchung der Microscope und Theilungsfehler an den Kreisen des neuen Aequatoreals der Hamburger Sternwarte. [Göttingen.] 8°. *Altona,* 1868.

KING (J.) The microscopist's companion; a popular manual of practical microscopy. 8°. *Cincinnati,* 1859.

KLÜGEL (G. S.) Analytische Dioptrik in zwey Theilen. Der erste enthält die allgemeine Theorie der optischen Werkzeuge; der zweyte die besondere Theorie und vortheilhafteste Einrichtung aller Gattungen von Fernröhren, Spiegelteleskopen, und Mikroskopen. 4°. *Leipzig,* 1778.

KÖSTLIN (O.) Die mikroskopischen Forschungen im Gebiete der menschlichen Physiologie. Eine von der med. Facultät zu Tübingen gekrönte Preisschrift. 8°. *Stuttgart,* 1840.

KORISTKA (F.) Norme pratiche per l' uso del microscopio. 12°. [*Milano*], 1883.

LANKESTER (E.) Half-hours with the microscope, being a popular guide to the use of the microscope as a means of amusement and instruction. Illustrated from nature, by Tuffen West. 3. ed. 12°. *London,* 1860.

LARDNER (D.) The microscope. 8°. *London,* 1856.

LATTEUX (P.) Manuel de technique microscopique, ou guide pratique pour l'étude et le maniement du microscope. 2. éd. 12°. *Paris,* 1883.

——. The same. 3. éd. 8°. *Paris,* 1887.

LEDERMÜLLER (M. F.) Nachleese seiner mikroskopischen Gemüths- und Augen-Ergötzung. I. Sammlung, bestehend in zehen fein illuminirten Kupfertafeln, sammt deren Erklärung und einer getreuen Anweisung, wie man alle Arten Mikroskope geschickt, leicht und nüzlich gebrauchen solle. 4°. [*Nürnberg*], 1762.

——. Mikroskopische Gemüths- und Augen-Ergötzung: bestehend in ein hundert nach der Natur gezeichneten und mit Farben erleuchteten Kupfertafeln, sammt deren Erklärung. 4°. [*Nürnberg*], 1763.

——. Physikalisch-mikroskopische Zergliederung und Vorstellung einer sehr kleinen Winterknospe des Hippocastani seu Esculi, oder des wilden Rosskastanienbaums. fol. *Nürnberg,* 1764.

——. Phisicalisch mikroskopische Vorstellung und Zergliederung einer angeblichen Rokenpflanze, das Standten, Stek- oder Gerstenkorn insgemein genannt. Wobey die Embryonen der noch zarten und kaum 4. Wochen alten Aehre, mit ihrem Keim, dann Blüht und Befruchtungs-

Microscope *and microscopy.*

Theilen, ingleichen die Aehnlichkeit des Roken und Gerstengrases mit seiner Blüht und Frucht, sowohl natürlich als vergrössert sich abgebildet befinden; als der zugesicherte und verlangte Schluss des zergliederten Rokens. fol. *Nürnberg,* 1765.

LEE (A.-B.) & HENNEGUY (F.) Traité des méthodes techniques de l'anatomie microscopique; histologie, embryologie et zoologie. Avec une préface de M. Ranvier. 8°. *Paris,* 1887.

VAN LEEUWENHOEK (A.) Anatomia seu interiora rerum, cum animatarum tum inanimatarum, ope et beneficio exquisitissimorum microscopiorum detecta, variisque experimentis demonstrata, una cum discursu et ulteriore dilucidatione epistolis . . . datis comprehensa ab . . . 4°. *Lugd. Bat.,* 1687.

——. Arcana naturæ, ope et beneficio exquisitissimorum microscopiorum detecta, varisque experimentis demonstrata, una cum discursu et ulteriori dilucidatione; epistolis suis ad . . . quod . . . Londini floret, philosophorum collegium datis, comprehensa. Editio tertia. 4°. *Lugd. Bat.,* 1688.

——. The same. sm. 4°. *Delphis Batavorum,* 1695.

——. [Works.] 6 v. sm. 4°. *Leiden & Delft,* 1693–1718.

CONTENTS.

1. St. Ontledingen en ontdekkingen van levende dierkens in de teel-deelen van verscheide dieren, vogelen en visschen; van het hout met der selver meenigvuldige vaaten; van hair, vlees, en vis; alsmede van de groote meenigte der dierkens in de excrementen. 2. druk.
2. St. Vervolg, en tweede vervolg, der brieven.
3. St. Derde vervolg, en vierde vervolg der brieven.
4. St. Vijfde vervolg, en sesde vervolg der brieven.
5. St. Sevende vervolg.
6. St. Send-brieven . . . als aan andere aansienelijke en geleerde lieden, over verscheyde verborgentheden der natuure, namentlijk over het wonderlijk gestel van de veselen der spieren in veelderley gedierte; de pesen en deselver werking; verscheyde zuden, 't oog van een walvis, [etc.]

——. The select works of . . . containing his microscopical discoveries in many of the works of nature. Transl. from the Dutch and Latin editions published by the author, by Samuel Hoole. 2 v. in 1. 4°. *London,* 1798–1807.

LEREBOURS (N.-P.) Instruction pratique sur les microscopes, contenant la description des microscopes achromatiques simplifiés. 3. éd., précédé d'un aperçu sur les différents systèmes de microscopes. 8°. *Paris,* 1846.

LONG (R.) Instruktion über den zweckmässigen Gebrauch des zusammengesetzten Mikroskops. 8°. *Berlin,* [1886].

LUC-LÉO. L'industrie au xixe siècle. Les microscopes Chevalier, suivi d'une notice historique sur la plus ancienne maison de ce nom. 4°. *Paris,* 1878.

LYONS (R. [S.] D.) An apology for the microscope . . . introductory lecture. 8°. *Dublin,* 1851.

MCALLISTER (T. H.) Illustrated price list of microscopes, microscopic apparatus, lenses, etc. 3. ed. 8°. *New York,* 1877.

——. The same. 8°. *New York,* 1887.

MANDL (L.-L.) Traité pratique du microscope et de son emploi dans l'étude des corps organisés; suivi de recherches sur l'organisation des animaux infusoires par D.-C.-G. Ehrenberg. 8°. *Paris,* 1839.

MARTIN (B.) Optical essays, containing: I. A practical description of the several sorts of single, solar, and compound microscopes; with their apparatus, and latest improvements. II. The nature of vision in insects demonstrated by microscopic observations. III. A catalogue of all

Microscope *and microscopy.*

the principal microscopic objects. IV. The use of the reflecting telescope as an universal perspective for viewing every sort of object in the greatest perfection. V. The manner of computing the magnifying power in single and double microscopes. VI. A new method of applying a micrometer to take the dimensions of small objects. VII. An illustration of the whole in a great variety of figures on a large copper-plate. 8°. *London*, [*n. d.*]

———. A new and compendious system of optics, in three parts, viz: Part I. Catoptrics, or the doctrine of vision by rays reflected from mirrours or polished surfaces. Part. II. Dioptrics, or the theory of vision by rays refracted through lenses or transparent substances. Part III. A practical description of a great number of the most useful optical instruments and machines, and their construction shewn from the theory; viz, the eye, camera obscura, single and double microscopes, refracting and reflecting telescopes, perspective glasses, the magic lanthorn, etc. The manner of adapting micrometers to microscopes and telescopes of the reflecting sort. The whole explained, exemplified, and illustrated by a great variety of copper-plate figures as big as the life. 8°. *London*, 1740.

———. Micrographia nova; or a new treatise on the microscope, and microscopic objects. Containing: I. The description and use of two different reflecting microscopes, of a new form and structure, and furnish'd with a micrometer, viz, one design'd for the pocket, the other mounted on a ball and socket, which renders it of universal use. II. A large and particular account of all kinds of microscopic objects, to be found in the human body, in quadrupeds, in fowls, fishes, insects, reptiles, etc., in plants, and vegetables of every kind; in earths, minerals, and fossil substances; and various other miscellaneous subjects. With directions how to procure and prepare them for use; and divers occasional remarks interspersed thro' the whole. To which is added, an account of the camera obscura, and the solar microscope, or method of magnifying objects in a darken'd chamber, in every way by reflection and refraction. 4°. *Reading*, 1742.

———. New elements of optics, or the theory of the aberrations, dissipations, and colours of light; of the general and specific refractive powers and densities of mediums; the properties of single and compound lenses; and the nature, construction and use of refracting and reflecting telescopes and microscopes of every sort hitherto published. 8°. *London*, 1759.

———. Philosophia Britannica; or a new and comprehensive system of the Newtonian philosophy, astronomy, and geography, in a course of twelve lectures, with notes; containing the physical, mechanical, geometrical, and experimental proofs and illustrations of all the principal propositions in every branch of natural science; also a particular account of the invention, structure, improvement and uses of all the considerable instruments, engines, and machines; with new calculations relating to their nature, power, and operation. The whole collected and methodized from all the principal authors and public memoirs. 3. ed. 3 v. 8°. *London*, 1771.

MARTIN (J. H.) Microscopic objects figured and described. 8°. *London*, 1870.

MARTIUS (C.) Du microscope, et de son application à l'étude des êtres organisés et en particulier à celle de l'utricule végétale et des globules du sang. 4°. *Paris*, 1839.

MERKEL (F.) Das Mikroskop und seine Anwendung. 8°. *München*, 1875.

Microscope *and microscopy.*

MILLER (M. N.) Practical microscopy; a course of normal histology for students and practitioners of medicine. 8°. *New York*, 1887.

MÖLLER (J. D.) Institut für Mikroskopie. Preisverzeichniss mikroskopischer Präparate, Utensilien und Materialien zur Anfertigung derselben. 8°. *Berlin*, 1874.

———. The same. 8°. *Berlin*, 1883.

MOLYNEUX (W.) Dioptrica nova. A treatise of dioptricks, in two parts. Wherein the various effects and appearances of spherick glasses, both convex and concave, single and combined, in telescopes and microscopes, together with their usefulness in many concerns of human life, are explained. 4°. *London*, 1692.

MORIGGIA (A.) La microscopia. Prolusione al corso libero d' istologia normale umana nella R. Università di Torino per l' anno accademico 1864–5. 8°. *Torino*, 1865.

MOSER (A.) Anleitung zum Gebrauche des Mikroskops für Aerzte, Naturforscher und Freunde der Natur. 8°. *Berlin*, 1839.

VAN MUSSCHENBROEK (P.) Introductio ad philosophiam naturalem. 2 v. 4°. *Lugd. Bat.*, 1762.

NACHET (A.) Instruction sur l'application du microscope dans la production de la graine des vers à soie. 8°. *Paris*, 1872.

NÄGELI (C.) & SCHWENDENER (S.) Das Mikroskop; Theorie und Anwendung desselben. 8°. *Leipzig*, 1867.

N[EEDHAM ([J.] T.) An account of some new microscopic discoveries founded on an examination of the calamary and its wonderful milt-vessels . . . tending to prove, by an accurate description of their motion, action, etc., that the hitherto supposed animalcules in the semen of animals are nothing more than machines similar, tho' inconceivably less, to those discovered in this sea-production. Also, observations on the farina foecundans of plants; with a new discovery and description of the action of those minute bodies, analogous to that of the calamary's milt-vessels. And an examination of the pistil, uterus, and stamina of several flowers, with an attempt to shew how the seed is impregnated. Likewise observations on the supposed embryo sole-fish fixed to the bodies of shrimps; with a new discovery of a remarkable animalcule found single on the tail-part of each embryo. A description of the eels or worms in blighted wheat; and other curious particulars relating to the natural history of animals, plants, etc. 8°. *London*, 1745.

———. Nouvelles découvertes faites avec le microscope. Traduites de l'anglois avec un mémoire sur les polypes à bouquet et sur ceux à entonnoir par A. Trembley. 16°. *Leide*, 1747.

———. Nouvelles observations microscopiques, avec des découvertes intéressantes sur la composition et décomposition des corps organisés. 16°. *Paris*, 1750.

NIKIFOROV (M.) Kratkii uchebnik mikroskop. techniki. Posobie pri prakt. izuchen. patolog. gistologii. S predislov. J. F. Kleina. [Short manual of microscopical technics. Aid to the practical study of pathological histology. With a preface by J. F. Klein.] 8°. *Moskva*, 1885.

NOTCUTT (W. L.) A handbook of the microscope and microscopic objects; with descriptive lists of upwards of 1,780 objects, and full directions for obtaining, preparing, and viewing them. With twelve plates, including figures of sixty-one objects. 12°. *London*, 1859.

PACINI (F.) Sopra un nuovo meccanismo di microscopio specialmente destinato alle ricer-

Microscope *and microscopy.*

che anatomiche e fisiologiche. 8°. *Bologna*, 1845.

Repr. from: Nuovi ann. d. sc. nat. di Bologna, Novembre, 1845.

PAGET (J.) Report on the chief results obtained by the use of the microscope in the study of human anatomy and physiology. 8°. *London*, 1842.

See, also, infra.

PASCHIUS (G.) De novis inventis, quorum accuratiori cultui facem prætulit antiquitas, tractatus, secundum ductum disciplinarum, facultatum atque artium in gratiam curiosi lectoris concinnatus. Editio secunda. 4°. *Lipsiæ*, 1700.

PASSEMANT. Description et usage des télescopes, microscopes; ouvrages et inventions . . . 12°. *Paris*, [*n. d.*]

Bound with: SWEDENBORGIUS (Emanuel). *De infinito [etc.] 12°. Dresdæ et Lipsiæ*, 1734.

PEREIRA (J.) Lectures on polarized light, together with a lecture on the microscope . . . Edited by Baden Powell. 2. ed. 16°. *London*, 1854.

PORTA (J. B.) Magiæ naturalis, sive de miraculis rerum naturalium libri iiii. 24°. *Lugduni*, 1561.

———. Magiæ naturalis libri viginti, in quibus scientiarum naturalium divitiæ et deliciæ demonstrantur; jam de novo, ab omnibus mendis repurgati, in lucem prodierunt. 12°. *Francofurti*, 1597.

———. The same. Natural magic in twenty books. imp. 8°. *London*, 1669.

POWER (H.) Experimental philosophy in three books; containing new experiments, microscopical, mercurial, magnetical. With some deductions, and probable hypotheses, raised from them, in avouchment and illustration of the now famous atomical hypothesis. 4°. *London*, 1664.

PRITCHARD (A.) Microscopic illustrations of living objects, with researches concerning the methods of constructing microscopes and instructions for using them. Third edition. To which is added, a supplement on the verification of microscopic phenomena, and an exact method of testing microscopes. By C. R. Goring. 8°. *London*, 1845.

———. Microscopic objects, animal, vegetable, and mineral; with instructions for preparing and viewing them. 12°. *London*, 1847.

QUEKETT (J.) A practical treatise on the use of the microscope, including the different methods of preparing and examining animal, vegetable, and mineral structures. 8°. *London*, 1848.

———. The same. 2. ed. Library of illustrated standard scientific works. v. 6. 8°. *London*, 1852.

RALPH (T. S.) Observations and experiments with the microscope, on the chemical effects of chloral hydrate, chloroform, prussic acid, and other agents on the blood. 8°. [*n. p., n. d.*]

READE (J. B.) Address delivered before the Royal Microscopical Society at the anniversary meeting, February 9, 1870. 8°. *London*, 1870.

REINICKE (F.) Beiträge zur neuern Mikroskopie. 1.-3. Hft. 8°. *Dresden*, 1858-62.

REINSCH (P.) Das Mikroskop in seiner Bedeutung für die Erweiterung der Naturerkenntniss, für die Entwickelung der physikalischen, der beschreibenden und physiologischen Wissenschaften, wie auch für einige Zweige des bürgerlichen Lebens. Nebst einer übersichtlichen Darstellung seiner Einrichtung und seines Gebrauches. 8°. *Nürnberg*, 1867.

RIGOUT (A.) *De la recherche micro-chimique. 4°. *Paris*, 1865.

Microscope *and microscopy.*

ROBIN (C.) Du microscope et des injections dans leurs applications à l'anatomie et à la pathologie, suivi d'une classification des sciences fondamentales, de celle de la biologie et de l'anatomie en particulier. 8°. *Paris*, 1849.

———. Traité du microscope. Son mode d'emploi, ses applications à l'étude des injections, à l'anatomie humaine et comparée, à la pathologie médico-chirurgicale, à l'histoire naturelle animale et végétale, et à l'économie agricole. 8°. *Paris*, 1871.

SCHACHT (H.) Le microscope et son application spéciale à l'étude de l'anatomie végétale. Traduction française, publiée d'après la troisième édition allemande par M. Dalimier. 8°. *Paris*, 1865.

SCHLESINGER (R.) Mikroscopische Untersuchungen der Gespinnst-Fasern im rohen und gefärbten Zustande, nebst einem Versuche zur Erkennung der Shoddy-Wolle. Mit einem Vorwort von Emil Kopp. 8°. *Zürich*, 1873.

SCHOTT (G.) Magia universalis naturæ et artis, sive recondita naturalium et artificialium rerum scientia, cujus ope per variam applicationem activorum, cum passivis, admirandorum effectuum spectacula, abditarumque inventionum miracula, ad varios humanæ vitæ usus eruuntur. Opus quadripartitum. Pars I. Continet optica. II. Acoustica. III. Mathematica. IV. Physica. Singularum epitomen sequens præfatio obiter, accuratius vero uniuscujusque peculiare præloquium exponit. 4 v. in 2. 4°. *Herbipoli*, 1657-77.

———. De magia telescopica, sive de fabrica, usu et effectu prodigioso telescopii et microscopii.

In his: Magia universalis naturæ et artis. 4°. *Herbipoli*, 1657, 488-538.

SCHRADER (F.) De microscopiorum usu in naturali scientia et anatome. 16°. *Gottingæ*, 1681.

SCHRAUER (L.) Illustrated price-list of microscopes and microscopic apparatus. 8°. *New York*, [*n. d.*]

SLABBER (M.) Natuurkundige verlustigingen, behelzende microscopise waarneemingen van in- en uitlandse water- en land-dieren. 4°. *Haarlem*, 1778.

SLACK (H. J.) Marvels of pond-life; or, a year's microscopic recreations among the polyps, infusoria, etc. 8°. *London*, 1861.

SOMERVILLE (Mary). On molecular and microscopic science. 2 v. 8°. *London*, 1869.

STÖHR (P.) Lehrbuch der Histologie und der mikroskopischen Anatomie des Menschen mit Einschluss der mikroskopischen Technik. 8°. *Jena*, 1887.

STURMIUS (J. C.) Collegium experimentale, sive curiosum, in quo primaria hujus seculi inventa et experimenta physico-mathematica, speciatim campanæ urinatoriæ, cameræ obscuræ, tubi Torricelliani, seu baroscopii, antliæ pneumaticæ, thermometrorum, hygroscopiorum, telescopiorum, microscopiorum et cet., phænomena et effecta, partim ab aliis jam pridem exhibita partim noviter istis superaddita, per ultimum quadrimestre anni m.dc.lxxii. viginti naturæ scrutatoribus, ex parte illustri nobilique prosapia oriundis, et spectanda oculis subjecit, et ad causas suas naturales demonstrativa methodo reduxit, quodque nunc accessione multa, demonstrationum ac hypothesium veritatem porro illustrante, confirmante, et a nonnullorum cavillationibus vindicante, locupletatum amicorum quorundam suasu et consilio publicum adspicere voluit. 4°. *Norimbergæ*, 1676.

———. Tentaminum collegii curiosi quædam appendices sive auctaria quibus supplentur ea

Microscope *and microscopy.*

quæ partim in ipso collegio per discursum ad superiora phænomena et conclusiones oretenus annotata fuerunt, partim vero, istis nunc iterato lectis et sub incudem denuo revocatis, majoris evidentiæ ergo, addenda videbantur. 4°. *Norimbergæ*, 1676.

TECHNISCHES Institut für Anfertigung naturwissenschaftlicher Apparate und Utensilien. Dr. Robert Muencke. Utensilien zum mikroskopischen Gebrauche. Mit besonderer Berücksichtigung der Methoden nach Dr. Rob. Koch. 8°. *Berlin*, [1885].

VON THANHOFFER (L.) Das Mikroskop und seine Anwendung. Ein Leitfaden der allgemeinen mikroskopischen Technik für Aerzte und Studirende. 8°. *Stuttgart*, 1880.

TRABER (P. Z.) Nervus opticus sive tractatus theoricus, in tres libros, opticam, catoptricam, dioptricam distributus. In quibus radiorum a lumine, vel objecto per medium diaphanum processus, natura, proprietates et effectus, selectis, et rarioribus experientiis, figuris, demonstrationibusque exhibentur. fol. *Viennæ Austriæ*, 1690.

TRUTAT (E.) Traité élémentaire du microscope. Première partie. Le microscope et son emploi. 8°. *Paris*, 1883.

UNITED STATES. *War Department. Medical Department.* The World's Industrial and Cotton Centennial Exposition, New Orleans, La., 1884–5. Medical Department, United States Army. Exhibit class 4, No. 6. Description of the microscopes and microscopical preparations from the Army Medical Museum, Washington, D. C. 8°. *New Orleans*, 1884–5.

UNITED STATES. *War Department. Surgeon-General's Office.* Catalogue of the microscopical section of the United States Army Medical Museum. Prepared under the direction of the Surgeon-General, U. S. A., by Edward Curtis, assistant surgeon, U. S. A. 4°. *Washington*, 1867.

VERSUCH, bey angehende Frühlings-Zeit die Vergrösserungs-Werckzeüge zum nützlich u. angenehmen Zeitvertreib anzuwenden. Von dem Verfasser der mikroskopischen Gemüths- u. Augen Ergözung. fol. *Nürnberg*, 1764. Title page and text in German and French.

VOGEL (J.) Das Mikroskop und die Methoden der mikroskopischen Untersuchung in ihren verschiedenen Anwendungen. 3. Aufl. 8°. *Berlin*, 1879.

WELLS (S.), TREAT (Mary) & SARGENT (F. L.) Through a microscope; something of the science, together with many curious observations, indoor and out, and directions for a home-made microscope. 12°. *Chicago*, [1886].

WIESNER (J.) Einleitung in die technische Mikroskopie, nebst mikroskopisch-technischen Untersuchungen. 8°. *Wien*, 1867.

———. Mikroskopische Untersuchungen ausgeführt im Laboratorium für Mikroskopie und technische Waïrenkunde am k. k. polytechnischen Institute in Wien. 8°. *Stuttgart*, 1872.

WILLKOMM (M.) Die Wunder des Mikroskops, oder die Welt im kleinsten Raume. Für Freunde der Natur und mit Berücksichtigung der studirenden Jugend bearbeitet. 4. Aufl. 8°. *Leipzig*, 1878.

WINKLER (J. H.) Oratio qua quam mirabiles sint quamque necessariæ in animalibus parvitates exposuit. sm. 4°. *Lipsiæ*, [1739].

WONDERS (The) of the microscope; or, an explanation of the wisdom of the Creator in objects comparatively minute, adapted to the understanding of young persons. 12°. *London*, [*n. d.*]

[WOODWARD (H.)] The prize microscopes of the Society of Arts; with plain directions for working with them. 12°. *London*, 1859.

Microscope *and microscopy.*

WOODWARD (J. J.) Memorandum on Pleurosigma angulatum and Pleurosigma formosum. 4°. *Washington*, 1871.

———. Memorandum on the Surirella gemma. 4°. *Washington*, 1871.

———. Memorandum on the test podura. 4°. *Washington*, 1871.

———. Memorandum on the Amphipleura pellucida. 4°. *Washington*, 1871.

———. Memorandum on the nineteenth-band test-plate of Nobert. 4°. [*Washington*, 1872.]

WYTHES (J. H.) The microscopist; or, a complete manual on the use of the microscope. For physicians, students, and all lovers of natural science. 8°. *Philadelphia*, 1851.

———. The microscopist; a manual of microscopy and compendium of the microscopic sciences . . . 3. ed. 8°. *Philadelphia*, 1877.

YOUNG (T.) Remarks on the measurement of minute particles, especially those of the blood and of pus. *In his:* An introduction to medical literature, etc. 8°. *London*, 1823.

ZAHN (R. P. F. J.) Oculus artificialis teledioptricus sive telescopium, ex abditis rerum naturalium et artificialium principiis protractum nova methodo, eaque solida explicatum a comprimis e triplici fundamento physico seu naturali, mathematico, dioptrico et mechanico, seu practico stabilitum . . . nova plurima abstrusa curiosa technasmata recluduntur, ipsaque ars telescopiaria facillime addiscenda proponitur, adeoque telescopium ex tenebris in lucem asseritur. 3 pts. in 1 v. fol. *Herbipoli*, 1685–6.

ZEISS (C.) Illustrirter Katalog über Mikroskope und Nebenapparate. 8°. [*Jena*, 1879.]

ZENTMAYER (J.) Illustrated price list of microscopes, microscopic apparatus, and optical instruments. 7. ed. 8°. *Philadelphia*, [*n. d.*]

Abbe (E.) Ueber die Bestimmung der Lichtstärke optischer Instrumente; mit besonderer Berücksichtigung des Mikroskops und der Apparate zur Lichtconcentration. Jenaische Ztschr. f. Med. u. Naturw., Leipz., 1871, vi, 263–291. ——. Beiträge zur Theorie des Mikroskops und der mikroskopischen Wahrnehmung. Arch. f. mikr. Anat., Bonn, 1873, ix, 413–468. ——. Beiträge zur Theorie des Microscopes. Centralbl. f. d. med. Wissensch., Berl., 1874, xii, 197; 212. ——. Contribution à la théorie du microscope. J. de microg., Par., 1877, i, 23; 64; 107; 152; 245. ——. Ueber Stephenson's System der homogenen Immersion bei Mikroskop-Objektiven. Jenaische Ztschr. f. Naturw., Leipz., 1879, n. F., vi, 2. Supplhft., 3–16. *Also,* Reprint. ——. Ueber die Bestimmung der Brechungs-Verhältnisse fester Körper mittelst des Refractometers. Sitzungsb. d. Jenaisch. Gesellsch. f. Med. u. Naturw., 1879, 35–44. *Also,* Reprint. ——. Some remarks on the apertometer. J. Roy. Micr. Soc., Lond., 1880, iii, 20–31. ——. On the estimation of aperture in the microscope. *Ibid.*, 1881, 2. s., i, 388–423. ——. The relation of aperture and power in the microscope. *Ibid.*, 1882, 2. s., ii, 300; 460; 1883, 2. s., iii, 790–812. ——. Method of testing objectives. *Ibid.*, 1883, 2. s., iii, 120–126. *Also:* Micr. News, Lond., 1883, iii, 107–112. ——. Note on the proper definition of the amplifying power of a lens or lens-system. J. Roy. Micr. Soc., Lond., 1884, 2. s., iv, 348–351. ——. On the mode of vision with objectives of wide aperture. *Ibid.*, 20–26. ——. Ueber neue Mikroskope. Sitzungsb. d. Jenaisch. Gesellsch. f. Med. u. Naturw., 1886, 107–128. *Also, transl.:* J. Roy. Micr. Soc., Lond., 1887, 20–34.—**Abbott** (F.) Nobert's test plate, Moller's diatom type slide, and modern microscopes. Rep. Roy. Soc. Tasmania (1869), 1870, 35–41.—**Adolfo.** Teoria del microscopio. Ippocratico, Fano, 1872, 3. s., xxi, 5–46. — **Aievoli** (E.) Il fenolo nella tecnica microscopica. Riv. internaz. di med. e chir., Napoli, 1887, iv, 101–104. — **Albini** (G.) Guida elementare agli studii microscopici. Gior. veneto di sc. med., Venezia, 1859, 2. s., xiii, 234–243.—**Altmann** (R.) Ueber die Vorbemerkungen des Hrn. Prof. Abbe zu seinen Grenzen der geometrischen Optik. (Fortsetzung, das Mikroskop betreffend.) Arch. f. Anat. u. Entwcklngsgesch., Leipz., 1882, 52–59. ——. Ueber die Verbesserungsfähigkeit der Mikroskope. *Ibid.*, 1886, 64–68. — **d'Alton.** Ueber den Gebrauch des Mikroskops zur Anfertigung von Zeichnungen. Amtl. Ber. ü. d. Versamml. deutsch. Naturf. u. Aerzte, Aachen, 1849, xxv, 176–183.—**Anthony** (J.) On drawing prisms. J. Roy. Micr. Soc., Lond., 1884, 2. s., iv, 697–703.—**Application** (On the) of the microscope to

Microscope *and microscopy.*

scientific purposes. Lond. M. & Phys. J., 1843-4, i, 1-10.
Ayscough. A description of an universal microscope.
Universal Magazine, 1753, xii, 177, 1 pl.—**Bailey** (J. W.)
Some remarks on the Navicula Spencerii, and on a still
more difficult test object. Am. J. Sc. & Arts, N. Haven,
1849, 2. s., vii, 265-270. *Also,* Reprint. — **Barnard** (F.
A. P.) A new form of binocular for use with high powers
of the microscope. Am. Naturalist, Salem, 1871, iv, 696-
703. *Also,* Reprint.—**Beale** (L. S.) On a clinical microscope. Arch. Med., Lond., 1859, ii, 289-292. ———. The microscopic limit, and beyond. J. Roy. Micr. Soc., Lond.,
1881. 2. s., i, 181-202.—**Behrens** (W.) Winkel's Mikro-
meterocular mit vertical-beweglichem Mikrometer. Ztschr.
f. wissensch. Mikr., Brnschwg., 1885, ii, 41 - 43. ———.
Klönne und Müller's beweglicher Objecttisch. *Ibid.*, 502-
507.—**Bell** (T.) Observations on the use of the microscope, in investigations connected with anatomy, physiology, and pathology. Tr. M. Soc. Lond., 1846, n. s., i, 1-
24.—**Blackburn** (W.) The theory of aperture in the
microscope; a popular exposition. North. Microscopist,
Lond., 1882, ii, 325-334.—**Blackham** (G.-E.) Ouverture
angulaire des objectifs de microscope. J. de microg., Par.,
1878, ii, 463; 496, 1 pl. : 1879, iii, 23; 60, 2 pl. ———. The
evolution of the modern microscope. Proc. Am. Soc. Micr.,
Buffalo, 1882, v, 25-47.—**Bridgman** (W. K.) On the principles of illumination in connexion with polarization. J.
Quekett Micr. Club, Lond., 1874-7, iv, 171-176, 1 pl.—**Bruch**
(C.) Mikroskopische und mikrochemische Aufzeichnun-
gen. Ztschr. f. rat. Med., Heidelb., 1850, ix, 156-215, 1 pl.—
Brücke (E.) Die Elementarorganismen. (Aus den Si-
tzungsberichten der Wiener Akad. d. Wissensch.) Untersuch. z. Naturl. d. Mensch. u. d. Thiere, Giessen, 1862, viii,
495-522.—**Burch** (G. J.) On a perspective microscope.
[Abstr.] Proc. Roy. Soc. Lond., 1887, xlii, 49-52. — **Carpenter** (W. B.) Verslag van de, door het gebruik van het
microscoop, in de studie der anatomie en physiologie verkregene uitkomsten. *In:* Paget (J.) & Carpenter (W. B.)
Versl. over de verkregene, etc., 8°, Leiden, 1846, 96-157.—
Caruccio (A.) Sul nuovo microscopio solare e fotografico
del prof. F. Pacini. Imparziale, Firenze, 1868, viii, 442;
474.—**Chabry** (L.) Tube capillaire porte-objet et perforation des éléments cellulaires. Compt. rend. Soc. de biol.,
Par., 1886, 8. s., iii, 322.—**Chiusoli** (V.) Le grossissement
des appareils dioptriques. Rev. scient., Par., 1884, 3. s., vii,
62. *Also, transl.:* Ztschr. f. wissensch. Mikr., Brnschwg.,
1884, i, 558-560.—**Coulier.** Nouveau diaphragme gradué
pour les microscopes. Rec. de mém. de méd. . . . mil., Par.,
1868, 3. s., xx, 328-331.—**Cox** (J. D.) Telescopic field and
microscopic aperture. Am. Month. Micr. J., N. Y., 1882,
iii, 61-69. ———. A new form of microscope stand with
concentric movements. Proc. Am. Soc. Micr., Buffalo,
1883, vi, 147. ———. Robert B. Tolles and the angular
aperture question. *Ibid.*, vii, 5-39.—**Cramer** (C.) Ein
neuer beweglicher Objecttisch. Ztschr. f. wissensch.
Mikr., Brnschwg., 1886, iii, 5-14.—**Crisp** (F.) On some
recent forms of camera lucida. J. Roy. Micr. Soc., Lond.,
1879, ii, 21-24. ———. On the limits of resolution in the
microscope. *Ibid.*, 1885, 2. s., v, 968-973.—**Curtis** (L.)
The limits of the optical capacity of the microscope. Chicago M. J. & Exam., 1877, xxxv, 526-331.—**Dallinger**
(W. H.) On a new arrangement for illuminating and
centering with high powers. Month. Micr. J., Lond.,
1876, xvi, 165-169, 1 pl.—**Dalton** (J. C.) On the use of the
binocular microscope. Richmond M. J., 1867, iii, 30-34.—
De Vescovi (P.) Sul modo d' indicare e calcolare ra-
zionalmente l' ingrandimento degli oggetti microscopici
nelle immagini proiettate. Spallanzani, Roma, 1887, 2. s.,
xvi, 236 - 240. — **Dippel** (L.) Endomersions-Objective.
Ztschr. f. wissensch. Mikr., Brnschwg., 1884, i, 485-490.
———. Einige neue Mikroskopformen. *Ibid.*, 1885, ii, 309-319,
40. ———. Die apochromatischen Objective und Compen-
sationsoculare von Carl Zeiss. *Ibid.*, 1886, iii, 309-319.
———. A. Nachet's grosses Mikroskop No. 1. und dessen
Objectivform. *Ibid.*, 1886, iii, 457-460.—**Donders** (F. C.)
De aanwending van het mikroskoop bij het medisch-poli-
tisch onderzoek van voedingsmiddelen. Nederl. Lancet,
Gravenh., 1848-9, 2. s., iv, 559; 577.—**Edmunds** (J.)
Note on a new paraboloid illuminator for use beneath the
microscope stage. Month. Micr. J., Lond., 1877, xviii,
78-85. ———. Note on a revolver immersion prism for sub-
stage illumination. J. Roy. Micr. Soc., Lond., 1879, ii,
32-35.—**Engelmann** (T. W.) Beschreibung einer Gas-
kammer für mikroskopische Untersuchungen. Jenaische
Ztschr. f. Med. u. Naturw., Leipz., 1868, iv, 331-343.—
Éternod (A.) Des illusions d'optique dans les observations au microscope. Rev. méd. de la Suisse Rom., Genève,
1884, iv, 325-331. ———. Planche à dessin universelle pour
les laboratoires de microscopie. Internat. Monatschr. f.
Anat. u. Histol., Berl., 1885, ii, 269, 1 pl.—**Exner** (S.)
Ein Mikro-Refractometer. Arch. f. mikr. Anat., Bonn,
1885, xxv, 97-112, 1 pl.—**Fairfield** (F. G.) A new high-
power lens. Med. Rec., N. Y., 1878, xiii, 60.—**Fayel.** Le
microscope, avec son oculaire, employé comme chambre
claire et comme appareil à projections. Compt. rend. Soc.
de biol., Par., 1886, 8. s., iii, 405.—**von Fleisch** (E.) C.
Reichert's neuer beweglicher Objecttisch. Ztschr. f.
wi-sensch. Mikr., Brnschwg., 1885, ii, 289-295. ———.

Microscope *and microscopy.*

Ueber C. Reichert's vervollkommneten mechanischen Objecttisch. *Ibid.*, 1887, iv, 25-30.—**Flesch** (M.) Ueber
einige Verbesserungen an Seibert und Krafft's Mikroskop-
Stativ. Arch. f. mikr. Anat., Bonn, 1881-2, xx, 504.—
Focke (G. W.) Ueber die Anwendung des Mikroskopes.
Beitr. z. physiol. u. path. Chem. u. Mikr., Berl., 1843-4, i,
141-164.—**Francotte** (P.) Description du nouveau microscope à dissection de Zeiss. Bull. Soc. belge de micr.,
Brux., 1885-6, xii. 79-82, 1 pl.—**Frazer** (P.), jr. A mirror for illuminating opaque objects for the projecting microscope. Proc. Am. Phil. Soc., Phila., 1879 - 80, xviii,
503.—**Fripp** (H. E.) On the theory of illuminating apparatus employed with the microscope. J. Roy. Micr.
Soc., Lond., 1879, ii, 503 : 1880, iii, 742.—**Fritsch.** Ueber
Abbe's Beleuchtungsapparat. Arch. f. Physiol., Leipz.,
1878, 542-546.—**Gärtner** (G.) Ueber das elektrische Mikroskop. Med. Jahrb., Wien, 1884, 217-244, 1 pl.—**Gage**
(S. H.) Cataloguing, labeling, and storing microscopical
preparations. Proc. Am. Soc. Micr., Buffalo, 1883, vi, 169-
174. *Also,* Reprint.—**Gage** (S. H.) & **Smith** (T.) Section flattener for dry section cutting. Microscope, Detroit, 1884, iv, 25 - 27. *Also,* Reprint. — **Giacomini** (C.)
Nuovo microscopio per l' esame delle sezioni dell' intero
encefalo umano adulto. Gior. d. r. Accad. di med. di Torino, 1883, 3. s., xxxi, 412 - 420. — **Giltay** (E.) Ueber die
Lage des Brennpunktes resp. der Brennlinie der Doppel-
kugel oder des Hohlcylinders. Ztschr. f. wissensch. Mikr,
Brnschwg., 1884, i, 479-485. ———. Remarks on Prof. Abbe's 1850 on the proper definition of the amplifying power
of a lens or lens system. J. Roy. Micr. Soc., Lond., 1885,
2. s., v, 960-967.—**Giraud-Teulon.** Note sur la grandeur apparente des objets vus au moyen des instruments
d'optique. Base d'une appréciation exacte de leur pouvoir amplifiant. Bull. Acad. roy. de méd. de Belg., Brux.,
1862, 2. s., v, 427-432. [Rap. de Hairion], 588.—**Goldfuss**
(G. A.) Einige mikroskopische Beobachtungen über die
Metamorphose des vegetabilischen und animalischen Lebens. Abhandl. d. phys.-med. Soc. zu Erlang., 1810, i, 37-
46. 1 pl.—**Gruby** (D.) Description of a new microscope
for the use of medical practitioners at the bedside. Month.
J. M. Sc., Lond. & Edinb., 1846, vi (pt. 2), 418. — **Gund-
lach** (E.) An improvement in objectives. Proc. Am. Soc.
Micr., Buffalo, 1884, vii, 148-152.—**H.** (D. S.) Holman's
life slide for the microscope. J. Franklin Inst., Phila.,
1877, civ, 292. — **Hällstén** (K.) Ein Compressorium für
mikroskopische Zwecke. Ztschr. f. Biol., München, 1886,
n. F., iv, 404 - 407. — **Hagen** (H.) Ueber die Mikroskope Nordamerikas. Arch. f. mikr. Anat., Bonn, 1870,
vi, 205-224.—**Hall** (L. B.) An eye protector for use with
the monocular microscope. Med. & Surg. Reporter, Phila.,
1882, xlvi, 566. — **Harley.** Prof. Harley's compendiö-
ses Mikroskop. Arch. f. mikr. Anat., Bonn, 1865, i, 440-
442.—**Harris** (J.) Microscope. *In his:* Lexicon techn.,
fol., Lond., 1708, 5E²ᵇ⁻³ᵇ, 1 pl.—**Harting** (P.) Mikrometrische bepalingen en mikroskopische aanteekeningen.
Tijdschr. v. nat. Geschied. en Physiol., Leiden, 1840, vii,
165-209. ———. Beschrijving van eenen nieuwen verlich-
tingstoestel voor doorschijnende mikroskopische voor-
werpen. Nederl. Lancet, Gravenh., 1850-51, 2. s., vi,
457-472.—**Hayes** (B.) Histological anatomy and microscopical manipulation. Med. Times & Gaz., Lond., 1853, n.
n., vii, 132.—**Henning** (C.) "Augenschoner"; ein neuer
Hilfsapparat zum Mikroskop. Allg. Wien. med. Ztg.,
1881, xxvi, 175. — **Hénocque** (A.) Microscope. Dict.
encycl. d. sc. méd., Par., 1873, 2. s., vii, 560-607.—**Heschl.**
Zur Geschichte des zusammengesetzten Mikroskops.
Arch. f. mikr. Anat., Bonn, 1880, xviii, 391-402, 1 pl.—
Hewett (T. E.) An improved dissecting microscope.
J. & Proc. Roy. Soc. N. South Wales 1879. Sydney, 1880,
xiii, 185.—**Hildebrand** (H. E.) Ueber einen einfachen
und sehr gebrauchsfähigen Objectführer. Ztschr. f. wissensch. Mikr., Brnschwg., 1886, iii, 386-389.—**Hirst** (G.
D.) Notes on some recent objectives manufactured by
Carl Zeiss, of Jena. J. & Proc. Roy. Soc. N. South Wales
1879, Sydney, 1880, xiii, 175-179.—**Hitchcock** (R.) Aperture, angular and numerical. Am. Q. Micr. J., N. Y., 1878-9,
i, 284-287. ———. Recent studies on the theory of the microscope, and their practical results as regards the use of
the microscope in scientific investigations. N. York M.
J., 1884, xl, 337-340.—**Hockin** (C.), jr. On the estimation
of aperture in the microscope. J. Roy. Micr. Soc., Lond.,
1884. 2. s., iv, 337-347, 1 pl.—**Holman** (D. S.) Improved
glass slide for microscopes. Phila. M. Times, 1873, iii,
427.—**Holmes** (O. W.) New stand for the compound
microscope. Boston M. & S. J., 1858, lvii, 376 - 380. —
Holston (J. G. F.) Additional report on microscopes
and microscopy. Tr. Ohio M. Soc., Sandusky, 1857, xii
(app.), 103-108.—**Huizinga.** Ein Apparat zur microscopischen Anwendung der Gase. Centralbl. f. d. med. Wissensch., Berl., 1867, v, 675.—**Israel** (O.) Ueber eine Er-
wärmungsvorrichtung als Ersatz der heizbaren Object-
tische. Ztschr. f. wissensch. Mikr., Brnschwg., 1885, ii,
459-463.—**James** (F. L.) How to silver a mirror. Am.
J. Micr., N. Y., 1878, iii, 211-213.—**Kaiser** (E.) Ueber
die Entwicklung und gegenwärtige Stellung der Mikroskopie in Deutschland. Ztschr. f. Mikr., Berl., 1877, i, 1;
33; 97; 161: 1878, 225; 257. — **Lambl.** Ueber ein neues

Microscope *and microscopy.*

Taschen-Mikroskop von Amici. Wien. med. Wchnschr., 1858, viii, 413–415.—**von Lenhossék** (J.) Ein Poly-mikroskop. Arch. f. path. Anat., etc., Berl., 1877, lxx, 268–290, 2 pl. *Also, transl.:* Orvosi hetil., Budapest, 1877, 565; 590; 613.—**Lieberkühn** (J. N.) Description d'un microscope anatomique, ou d'un instrument, par le moyen duquel on peut affermir commodément et promptement des animaux en vie, les placer d'une manière convenable, et après avoir ouvert leur corps, examiner, à l'aide du mi-croscope, le contenu de quelques-unes de leurs parties. Trad. de l'allemand. Mém. de l'Acad. roy. de Prusse, Avignon, 1768, i, 101–110, 2 pl. ——. Description d'un microscope anatomique. *In his:* Diss. quatuor, 4°, Lon-dini, 1782. ——. Beschreibung eines Instrumentes zu den mikroscopischen Beobachtungen lebendiger Thiere. Phys. u. med. Abhandl. d. k. Acad. d. Wissensch. zu Berl., Gotha, 1783, iii, 39–42.—**List** (J. H.) Ueber einen Objecthalter mit Kugelgelenk. Ztschr. f. wissensch. Mikr., Brnschwg., 1885, ii, 341.—**Listing** (J. B.) Vorschlag zu feiner Ver-vollkommnung des Mikroskops auf einem abgeänderten di-optrischen Wege. Nachr. v. d. k. Gesellsch. d. Wissensch. u. d. Georg-Aug.-Univ., Götting., 1869, 1–7. ——. Nach-trag betreffend die neue Construction des Mikroskops. *Ibid.*, 108–116. ——. Notiz über ein neues Mikroskop von R. Winkel. *Ibid.*, 1870, 321.—**Löwit** (M.) Ein heizbarer Objecttisch für starke Vergrösserungen. Zt-schr. f. wissensch. Mikr., Brnschwg., 1885, ii, 43–46.—**Luys.** Instrument pour les coupes microscopiques. Bull. Soc. anat. de Par., 1868, xliii, 448.—**Malassez** (L.) Note sur la mesure des grossissements microscopiques. Arch. de physiol. norm. et path., Par., 1878, 2. s., v, 79–89. *Also:* Compt. rend. Soc. de biol. 1878, Par., 1880, 6. s., v, 19–21. *Also:* École prat. d. hautes études. Lab. d'histol. du Coll. de France. Trav., Par. (1877-8), 1879, iv, 114–124. ——. Correction des déformations produites par les chambres claires de Milne-Edwards et de Nachet. École prat. d. hautes études. Lab. d'histol. du Coll. de France. Trav., Par. (1877-8), 1879, iv, 188–196. ——. Chambre à air humide, graduée. Compt. rend. Soc. de biol. 1879, Par., 1880, 7. s., i, 323–326. ——. Sur les cham-bres claires en général et sur une chambre claire à 45°. Arch. de physiol. norm. et path., Par., 1884, 3. s., iv, 238–251. ——. Perfectionnement apporté à la chambre claire de Doyère et Milne-Edwards. Compt. rend. Soc. de biol., Par., 1884, 8. s., i. pt. 2, 510.—**Maravillas** del micro-scopio. Siglo. méd., Madrid, 1858, v, 41.—**Marshall** (J.) Description of the microscopic preparations sent by Dr. Straus, of Paris. Proc. Roy. M. & Chir. S. c. Lond., 1883-4, n. s., i, 203–208.—**Martinotti** (G.) Vecchi e nuovi strumenti della microscopia. Ztschr. f. wissensch. Mikr., Brnschwg., 1886, iii, 320–330. ——. Il timolo nella tecnica microscopica. *Ibid.*, 351–358.—**Mayall** (J.), jr. Immersion illuminators. J. Roy. Micr. Soc., Lond., 1879, ii, 27–31. ——. The microscope. J. Soc. Arts, Lond., 1886, xxxiv, 987; 1007; 1031; 1055; 1095.—**Merkel** (F.) Die Mikroskope von R. Winkel in Göttingen. Arch. f. mikr. Anat., Bonn, 1873, ix, 126–128.—**Meyer** (H.) Zwei neue Lupenträger. Untersuch. z. Naturl. d. Mensch. u. d. Thiere, Frankf. a. M., 1857, iii, 230–232.—**Michel.** Des théories furnies par le microscope. Gaz. méd. de Strasb., 1862, 2. s., ii, 81; 125.—**Michels** (J.) A home-made microscope. Pop. Sc. Month, N. Y., 1875, viii, 95–102.—**Microscope.** Dict. d. dict. de méd. (Suppl.), Par., 1851, 453–487.—**Microscope** (The). [*Transl. from:* "Aus der Natur, etc.", Leipz., 1858.] Rep. Smithson. Inst., Wash., 1860, 344–354. — **Microscopiques** (Les). Gaz. méd. de Par., 1866, xxi, 1; 19.—**Mitchell** (J.) De-scription of a new microscope suited for medical purposes, and of moderate price. Madras Q. J. M. Sc., 1863, vi, 435–438.—**Moeller** (J.) Reichert's Condensor. Ztschr. f. wissensch. Mikr., Brnschwg., 1885, ii, 339.—**Nachet.** Sur un nouveau microscope approprié au besoin des dé-monstrations anatomiques, et permettant à plusieurs per-sonnes l'observer ensemble. Gaz. méd. de Par., 1854, 3. s., ix; 61.—**Nägeli** (C.) Die Anwendung des Polarisa-tionsmicroscops auf die Untersuchung der organischen Elementartheile. *In his:* Beitr. z. wissensch. Botanik, 8°, Leipz., 1863, 3. Hft., 1–126, 7 pl.—**Nagura** (Osama). [The selection of a microscope.] Tokei M J., Tokio, 1886, no. 420. April 17.—**Nelson** (E. M.) Historic micro-scopy. J. Quekett Micr. Club, Lond., 1886, 2. s., ii, 222–229.—**Novaro** (B.) Técnica microscópica. An. Asoc. Circ. méd. argent., Buenos Aires, 1878-9, ii, 17; 109.—**Oppenheimer** (L. S.) Contributions from the micro-scopical laboratory of the University of Louisville. Louis-ville M. News, 1879, vii, 306, 1 pl.—**Ord** (W. M.) On some causes of Brownian movements. J. Roy. Micr. Soc., Lond., 1879, ii, 656–662.—**Ost** (J.) Ueber die Leistungs-fähigkeit der Mikrometerschraube. Ztschr. f. wissensch. Mikr., Brnschwg., 1885, ii, 295–300.—**Paget** (J.) Report on the results obtained by the use of the microscope in the study of human anatomy and physiology. Brit. & For. M. Rev., Lond., 1842, xiv, 259–296. *Also,* Reprint. *Also, transl. in:* Paget (J.) & Carpenter (W. B.) Versl. over de verkregene, etc., 8°, Leiden, 1846, 1–95. [*See, also, su-pra.*]—**Pelletan** (J.) Étude sur les microscopes étran-gers. J. de microg., Par., 1877, i, 186; 236; 285; 326: 1878,

Microscope *and microscopy.*

ii, 16; 114; 153. *Also, transl.:* Ztschr. f. Mikr., Berl., 1877-8, i, 65; 112; 129; 204; 275. ——. Promenades le long d'un ruisseau: le monde microscopique des eaux douces. J. de microg., Par., 1881, v, 124; 167.—**Piper** (R. U.) On the pictorial art in illustrating microscopic observations, with original drawings and descriptions. Chicago M. J., 1877, xxxiv, 193–200.—**Place** (F.) Ueber die Vergrösserung der Mikroskope, und über den optischen Einfluss der zwischen Object und Objectiv enthaltenen Substanzen. Arch. f. Anat., Physiol. u. wissensch. Med., Leipz., 1859, 184–196.—**Poulsen** (V. A.) Elektrisk Lys anvendt paa Mikrosko-pet samt en Beskrivelse af en af ... L. Nyrop konstrueret Lampe.] Hosp.-Tid., Kjøbenh., 1885, 3. R., iii, 81–87.—**Powell** (T.) A simple object finder for students' micro-scopes. Dublin Q. J. M. Sc., 1864, xxxviii, 286.—**Pur-kinje** (J.) Das Mikroskop, seine Anwendung und Ge-brauch bei physiologischen Untersuchungen. [Mit Anhang von R. Wagner.] Handwörterb. d. Physiol., Brnschwg., 1850, ii, 411; 441.—**Reeves** (H. A.) A circulation stage, a live-development slide, and an improved drawing reflector. J. Anat. & Physiol., Lond., 1877, xi, 403–405.—**Report** on modern microscopes and recent improvements in micro-scopical apparatus. Brit. M. J., Lond., 1867, ii, 321; 346; 371; 404.—**Richardson** (J. G.) Notes on the perform-ances of two one-fiftieth objectives. Phila. M. Times, 1874-5, v, 132. ——. Holman's siphon slide for the micro-scope. *Ibid.*, 1874, iv, 270.—**Riddell** (J. L.) Notes of mi-croscopic observations, by the aid of a superior achromatic objective combination, of the one twenty-first part of an inch focus. N. Orl. M. & S. J., 1849-50, vi, 791–794. ——. Selected items of observation, referring, chiefly, to the living microscopic organisms that abound in the waters of New Orleans and its vicinity. Embracing also some mat-ters pertaining to microscopic anatomy. *Ibid.*, 1851-2, viii, 530, 8 pl.; 667, 2 pl.: 1852-3, ix, 116, 4 pl.; 173. ——. Of the binocular microscope. *Ibid.*, 1853-4, x, 321–327.—**Robin** (C.) Sur un nouveau microscope approprié aux besoins des démonstrations anatomiques et permettant à plusieurs personnes d'observer ensemble. Compt. rend. Soc. de biol. 1853, Par., 1854, v, 141–145.—**Rochoux** (J.-A.) Principes de philosophie naturelle appuyés sur des observations microscopiques. Bull. Acad. roy. de méd., Par., 1842-3, viii, 193–224. *Also,* Reprint.—**Rogers** (W. A.) On Tolles' interior illuminator for opaque ob-jects; with note by R. B. Tolles. J. Roy. Micr. Soc., Lond., 1880, iii, 754–758.—**Royston-Pigott** (G. W.) On a searcher for aplanatic images applied to microscopes, and its effects in increasing power and improving defini-tion. Phil. Tr., Lond., 1870, clx, 591–603, 2 pl. *Also,* Re-print. ——. A further inquiry into the limits of micro-scopic vision, and the delusive application of Fraunhöfer's optical law of vision. J. Roy. Micr. Soc., Lond., 1879, ii, 9–20, 1 pl.—**Russell** (J. C.) Description of a new form of camera lucida. *Ibid.*, 25.—**Ryba.** Ueber die Prüfung des Brechungsvermögens durchsichtiger Körper durch das Mikroskop ohne directe Winkelmessungen. Vrtljschr. f. d. prakt. Heilk., Prag, 1852, ii, 95–119, 1 pl.—**Schäfer** (E. A.) Description of a new warm stage for the microscope. Physiol. Lab., Univ. Coll., Lond. Collected papers, 1874-5, Art. No. vii.—**Schiefferdecker** (P.) Ueber eine neue Construction der Mikrometerschraube bei Mikroskopen. Ztschr. f. wissensch. Mikr., Brnschwg., 1886, iii, 1–5.—**Schklarevsky** (A.) Ein heizbarer Objekttisch. Wien. med. Wchnschr., 1867, xvii, 1553–1555. *Also:* Arch. f. mikr. Anat., Bonn, 1868, iv, 342–344.—**Schmidt** (H. D.) The microscopic dissector. Am. J. M. Sc., Phila., 1859, n. s., xxxvii, 30–35.—**Schöbl** (J.) Ein neues Präparations-Mikroskop. Arch. f. mikr. Anat., Bonn, 1879, xvii, 165–167, 1 pl.—**Schröder** (H.) On a new camera lucida. J. Roy. Micr. Soc., Lond., 1883, 2. s., iii, 813–815.—**Schultze** (E. A.) Electrical illumination in microscopy; experiments and views of Drs. H. Van Heurck and T. Stein. J. N. York Micr. Soc., 1885, i, 1–6.—**Schultze** (M.) Die neuen Stein-heil'schen Loupen. Arch. f. mikr. Anat., Bonn, 1866, ii, 382–384.—**Schulze** (A.) On Abbe's apochromatic micro-objec-tives and compensating eye-pieces. J. Anat. & Physiol., Lond., 1886-7, xxi, 515–524.—**Selenka** (E.) Metallmodelle nach mikroskopischen Präparaten. Sitzungsb. d. phys.-med. Soc. zu Erlang., 1885-6, xviii, 26–28.—**Sharp** (H.) Notes upon Tolles's duplex front one-tenth immersion objec-tive, and of a comparative trial of the same with Zeiss's oil immersion one-eighth (No. 18), by both oblique and central light. J. & Proc. Roy. Soc. N. South Wales 1879, Sydney, 1880, xiii, 180–184.—**Smirnoff** (A.) Mikrostat; apparat dlja tochnago i sistemat. osmativ. mikroskop. preparat. i notirov. interesu. miest. [The microstat; an apparatus for exact and systematic examination of microscopic speci-mens.] Russk. Med., St. Petersb., 1886, iv, 455.—**Smith** (J. L.) The inverted microscope (a new form of micro-scope); with the description of a new eye-piece micrometer, and a new form of goniometer for measuring the angles of crystals under the microscope. Am. J. Sc. & Arts, N. Haven, 1852, n. s., xiv, 233–241. *Also,* Reprint.—**Sorby** (H. C.) The president's address, delivered before the Royal Microscopical Society, Feb. 2, 1876. Month. Micr. J., Lond., 1876, xv, 105–121. *Also,* Reprint. ——. The president's address. J. Roy. Micr. Soc., Lond., 1878, i, 1-

Microscope *and microscopy.*

18, 1 pl.—**Stearn** (C. H.) On the use of incandescence lamps as accessories to the microscope. *Ibid.*, 1883, 2. s., iii, 29–33.—**Stephenson** (J. W.) A catoptric immersion illuminator. *Ibid.*, 1879, ii, 36. ——. On a cata-dioptric immersion illuminator. *Ibid.*, 1885, 2. s., v, 207–211.—**Stodder** (C.) Nobert's test plate and modern microscopes. Am. Naturalist, Salem, 1869, ii, 93–101.—**Stricker** (S.) Ueber das elektrische Licht als Hilfsmittel für den mikroskopischen Unterricht. Med. Jahrb., Wien, 1883, 463–475.—**Sullivant** (W. S.) Notes on Mr. Chas. Stodder's paper entitled, "Norbert's test plate and modern microscopes". Am. J. Sc. & Arts, N. Haven, 1868, 2. s., xlvi, 347–351. *Also*, Reprint.—**Sullivant** (W. S.) & **Wormley** (F. G.) On the measurement of the striæ of diatoms. Am. J. Sc. & Arts, N. Haven, 1859, 2. s., xxvii, 249–252. *Also*, Reprint. ——. On Nobert's test plate and the striæ of diatoms. Am. J. Sc. & Arts, N. Haven, 1861, 2. s., xxxi, 12–17. *Also*, Reprint.—**Toison** (J.) Éclairage intensif en micrographie. J. d. sc. méd. de Lille, 1885, vii, 469–473.—**Valentin** (G.) Einige weitere Bemerkungen über Testobjecte für Mikroskope. Ztschr. f. rat. Med., Leipz. u. Heidelb., 1864, 3. R., xxi, 39–43. ——. Die Anwendung des binocularen Mikroskopes. *Ibid.*, 1869, xxxiv, 3. R., 214–239. ——. Beiträge zur Mikroskopie. Arch. f. mikr. Anat., Bonn, 1871, vii,140–156.—**Vanoye** (R.) Du microscope et de ses applications aux sciences d'observation. Arch. de la méd. belge, Brux., 1844, xiii, 92–102: xiv, 252–271: 1845, xvii, 61–73. — **Verbessertes** Mikroskop, insbesondere für Fleischbeschauer geeignet, von Franz Schmidt u. Haensch in Berlin. Hannov. Monatschr., 1879, ii, 145–147.—**Verweij** (L. H.) Een woord over de verdiensten van het microscopisch onderzoek. Boerhaave. Tijdschr., etc., Amst., 1846, n. s., v, 249–258.—**Vignal** (W.) Chambre chaude à régulateur direct pour le microscope. Arch. de physiol. norm. et path., Par., 1885, 3. s., vi, 1–10. *Also*: Compt. rend. Soc. de biol., Par., 1885, 8. s., ii, 255.—**Vogel** (J.) Mikroskope für Aerzte und Studirende. Arch. d. Ver. f. wissensch. Heilk. 1864, Leipz., 1865, n. F., i, 81–84. ——. Bezeichnungsweise sehr geringer mikroskopischer Grössen. *Ibid.*, 170.—**Wasserlein** (R.) Dr. Weber-Liel's Ohr-Mikroskop. Ztschr. f. Mikr., Berl.,1879–80, ii,175–179.—**Webb** (W.) The best, the most simple and unerring tests for objectives. J. Quekett Micr. Club, Lond., 1872, iii, 113–116. *Also*, Reprint. ——. On an improved finder. J. Roy. Micr. Soc., Lond., 1880, iii, 750–753.—**Wedl** (C.) Ueber eine Verbesserung des Objectträgers für Elektrisirung mikroskopischer Objecte. Arch. f. path. Anat., etc., Berl., 1878, lxxiv, 142.—**von Weinzierl.** Eine Lupe für Samenuntersuchungen. Ztschr. f. wissensch. Mikr., Brnschwg., 1887, iv, 42–44.—**Welcker** (H.) Unterscheidung von Erhöhungen und Vertiefungen unter dem Mikroskope. Ztschr. f. rat. Med., Leipz. u. Heidelb., 1859, 3. R., vii, 63–67. ——. Ueber die Ausmessung des senkrechten Durchmessers mikroskopischer Objecte und über die Ermittelung der chemischen Qualität aus dem Lichtbrechungsvermögen. Beitr. z. Anat. u. Physiol. (Eckhard), Giessen, 1860. ii, 45–58.—**Wollaston** (W. H.) Description of a microscopic doublet. Phil. Tr., Lond., 1829, 9–13, 1 pl.—**Woodward** (J. J.) Further remarks on the new-nineteen-band test-plate of Nobert, and on immersion lenses. Month. Micr. J., Lond., 1869, i, 289–294. ——. Note on the resolution of Amphipleura pellucida by certain objectives made by R. and J. Beck, and by William Wales. *Ibid.*, 1872, vii, 165. *Also*, Reprint. ——. Remarks on the resolution of the nineteenth band of Nobert's plate by certain objectives, especially by a new Tolles's immersion $\frac{1}{8}$th. Month. Micr. J., Lond., 1872, viii, 227–231. *Also*, Reprint. ——. Remarks on the nomenclature of achromatic objectives for the compound microscope. Am. J. Sc. & Arts, N. Haven, 1872, 3. s., iii, 406–414. *Also*, Reprint. ——. On the use of monochromatic sunlight as an aid to high power definition. Am. Naturalist, Salem, 1872, vi, 454–460. *Also*, Reprint. ——. A simple device for the illumination of balsam-mounted objects for examination with certain immersion objectives whose "balsam angle" is 90° or upwards. Month. Micr. J., Lond., 1877, xviii, 61–64. *Also*, Reprint. ——. Sur la lumière électrique, la lumière au magnésium [et la lumière oxycalcique] appliquées à la photo-micrographie. Bull. Soc. belge de micr., Brux., 1877–8, iv, pp. lxiv–lxxvi. [*See, also, supra.*] ——. The oblique illuminator; an apparatus for obtaining oblique illumination at definite angles. Am. Q. Micr. J., N. Y., 1878–9, i, 268–272. ——. Description of a new apertometer. *Ibid.*, 272–279. ——. Observations suggested by the study of Amphipleura pellucida, mounted in Canada balsam, by lamplight and sunlight, with various objectives. J. Roy. Micr. Soc., Lond., 1879, ii, 663–674. ——. Note on Abbe's experiment on Pleurosigma angulatum. *Ibid.*, 675. ——. Riddell's binocular microscopes; an historical notice. Am. Month. Micr. J., N. Y., 1880, i, 221–230.—**Wright** (L.) The lantern microscope. J. Roy. Micr. Soc., Lond., 1885, 2. s., v, 196–204.—**Zeiss** (C.) Ein neues Präparir-Mikroskop. Arch. f. mikr. Anat., Bonn, 1870, vi, 234–236. ——. Description of Professor Abbe's apertometer, with instructions for its use. J. Roy. Micr. Soc., Lond., 1878, i, 19–22, 1 pl.—**Zenger.** Ueber ein neues Universalmikroskop.

Microscope *and microscopy.*

Sitzungsb. d. k.-böhm. Gesellsch. d. Wissensch., Prag, 1874, 131–147.—**Zentmayer** (J.) Newly invented erecting prism for microscopes. Phila. M. Times, 1872, ii, 355.

Microscope (*Patents relating to*).

Allen (B. F.) Microscope. No. 352,639; Nov. 16, 1886.—**Bausch** (J. J.) Microscope. No. 230,688; Aug. 3, 1880. ——. Microscopic illuminator. No. 277,869; May 22, 1883. ——. Binocular microscope. No. 293,217; Feb. 12, 1884. ——. Microtome. No. 325,722; Sept. 8, 1885. ——. Microscope. No. 328,277; Oct. 13, 1885.—**Bulloch** (W. H.) Microscope. No. 215,878; May 27, 1879. ——. Turn-tables for microscopic slides. No. 226,648; April 20, 1880. ——. Objective attachments in microscopes. No. 287,904; Nov. 6, 1883.—**Deal** (H. J.) Microscope for examining flour and bolting cloths. No. 214,283; April 15, 1879.—**Fasoldt** (C.) Microscope. No. 334,009; Jan. 12, 1886.—**Gould** (F. B.) Microscopic photographic transparency. No. 271,838; Feb. 6, 1883.—**Griffith** (E. H.) Microscopist's turn-table. No. 354,130; Dec. 14, 1886.—**Kidder** (W. K.) Microscope. No. 295,770; March 25, 1884.—**Klippert** (C.) Microscopist's turn-table. No. 334,530; Jan. 19, 1886.—**McIntosh** (L. D.) Microscope. No. 273,752; March 13, 1883.—**Molera** (E. J.) & **Cebrian** (J. C.) Microscope. No. 230,320; July 20, 1880.—**Palmer** (C. W.) Glass slide for microscopes. No. 336,257; Feb. 16, 1886.—**Sidle** (J. W.) Turn-table for mounting microscopic objects. No. 235,030; Nov. 30, 1880.—**Tetlow** (D.) Microscope. No. 287,978; Nov. 6, 1883.

Microscope (The) and its relation to medicine and pharmacy. An illustrated bi-monthly journal. Edited and published by Charles H. Stowell and Louisa Reed Stowell. v. 1–7, April, 1881–7. 8°. *Ann Arbor, Mich.*
Current. v. 3 complete in 5 nos., April–Dec., 1883. In 1884 became monthly, title: **Microscope** (The).

Microscopic (The) Journal and Structural Record. Edited by Daniel Cooper. v. 1–2, 1841–2. 8°. *London, J. Van Voorst.*
In v. 2 George Busk added as editor.

Microscopical (The) Bulletin and Opticians' Circular. A bi-monthly magazine. Edited by Edward Pennock. v. 1–4, Dec., 1883, to Dec., 1887. 8°. *Philadelphia, J. W. Queen & Co.*
Current. v. 1 complete in 7 nos., Dec., 1883, to Dec., 1884: v. 2 commenced Jan., 1885. In June, 1885 (no. 3, v. 2), title became: **Microscopical** (The) Bulletin and Science News.

Microscopical (The) Bulletin and Science News.
Was title, after April, 1885, of: **Microscopical** (The) Bulletin and Opticians' Circular.

Microscopical (The) News and Northern Microscopist. An illustrated journal of practical microscopy. Edited by George E. Davis. [Monthly.] v. 3–4, 1883–4. 2 v. 8°. *London, D. Bogue.*
Ended. Title of v. 2 was: **Northern** (The) Microscopist and Microscopical News.

Microscopical Society of Liverpool. Annual reports. 13.-15., 1882–4. Abstract of proceedings; list of members; rules. 3 Nos. 8°. *Liverpool*, 1882–4.
——. Catalogue of the slides in the cabinets, and books in the library. 22 pp. 8°. *Liverpool, Turner, Rutledge & Co.,* 1884.

Microscopical Society of London. Catalogue of microscopic objects in the cabinet of . . . iv, 49 pp., 1 l. 8°. *London, E. Newman,* 1864.

Microscopy (*Journals and societies relating to*).

AMERICAN Journal of Microscopy. Devoted to the general dissemination of the knowledge of microscopic science. Published by George Mead & Co. [Monthly.] No. 1, v. 1. Nov. 1, 1870. 4°. *Chicago.*
No more published.

AMERICAN Journal of Microscopy. Devoted to the elucidation of scientific and popular microscopy. Edited by E. M. Hale. v. 1, April to July, 1871. 8°. *Chicago.*
No more published.

Microscopy (*Journals and societies re-relating to*).

AMERICAN (The) Journal of Microscopy and Popular Science. [Monthly.] v. 1–5; Nos. 1–8, v. 6, Dec., 1875, to August, 1881. 6 v. 8°. *New York.*

Said to be edited by John Phin.

AMERICAN (The) Monthly Microscopical Journal. Editor and publisher: Romyn Hitchcock. v. 1–8, 1880–87. 8°. *New York, 1880–82; Boston, 1883; Washington, D. C., 1884–7.*

Current.

AMERICAN Postal Micro-Cabinet Club, Troy, N. Y. Rules. 8°. [*n. p., n. d.*]

AMERICAN Postal Microscopical Club. Report [9., for 1883] and rules of the . . . 8°. *Troy, N. Y., 1884.*

———. Annual reports of the . . . for the years 1884–6 (10.–12.). 8°. *Troy, N. Y., 1885–7.*

AMERICAN (The) Quarterly Microscopical Journal; containing the transactions of the New York Microscopical Society. Edited by Romyn Hitchcock. v. 1, Oct., 1878, to July, 1879. 8°. *New York.*

Ended.

AMERICAN Society of Microscopists. Proceedings of the . . . 2.–8. Annual meetings, 1879–84. 8°. *Indianapolis, Columbus, Buffalo, 1880–85.*

ARCHIV für mikroskopische Anatomie, hrsg. von Max Schultze. v. 1–30, 1865–87. 8°. *Bonn.* Current. Also, index volume to v. 1–8 and to v. 1–20.

JOURNAL de micrographie. Réd.: J. Pelletan. [Monthly.] v. 1–11, May 15, 1877–87. 8°. *Paris.* Current.

JOURNAL (The) of Microscopy and Natural Science: the journal of the Postal Microscopical Society. Edited by A. Allen. [Quarterly.] v. 3–6, 1884–7. 8°. *London.* Current.

JOURNAL of the New York Microscopical Society. Edited by B. Braman. [Monthly.] v. 1–3, 1885–7. 8°. *New York.* Current.

JOURNAL (The) of the Postal Microscopical Society. Edited by A. Allen. [Quarterly.] v. 1–2, 1882–3. 8°. *London.*

JOURNAL (The) of the Quekett Microscopical Club. [Quarterly.] v. 1–6, 1868–81. 2. s., v. 1–3, March, 1882–7. 8°. *London.* Current.

JOURNAL of the Royal Microscopical Society. [Bi-monthly.] v. 1–3, March, 1878, to Dec., 1880. 2. s., v. 1–7, 1881–7. 8°. *London.* Current.

LENS (The). A quarterly journal of microscopy and the allied natural sciences; with the transactions of the State Microscopical Society of Illinois. Edited by S. A. Briggs. No. 1, v. 1, Oct., 1871. 56 pp., 1 pl. 8°. *Chicago, the State Microscopical Society of Illinois, 1871.*

No more published.

LENS (The). A quarterly journal of microscopy and the allied natural sciences; with the transactions of the State Microscopical Society of Illinois. Edited by S. A. Briggs. E. H. Sargent, C. Adams, O. S. Westcott, publishing committee. v. 1–2, Jan., 1872, to Dec., 1873. 8°. *Chicago, State Microscopical Society of Illinois.* Completed.

MALTWOOD's finder. 8°. [*London, 1859.*]

MICROSCOPE (The).

Title, after 1883, of: **Microscope** (The) and its Relation to Medicine and Pharmacy.

MICROSCOPE (The) and its Relation to Medicine and Pharmacy. Edited by Chas. H. Stowell and L. R. Stowell. [Bi-monthly.] v. 1–7, April, 1881–7. 8°. *Ann Arbor, Mich.*

Current. After 1883, title: **Microscope** (The).

Microscopy (*Journals and societies re-lating to*).

MICROSCOPIC (The) Journal and Structural Record. Edited by D. Cooper and George Busk. v. 1–2, 1841–2. 8°. *London.*

MICROSCOPIC (The) Miscellany; being selections from the Microscopic Journal. With illustrative diagrams, by J. Dinkel. Edited by D. Cooper. 8°. *London, 1847.*

Cuttings from: Micr. J., Lond., 1841-2—1847.

MICROSCOPICAL (The) Bulletin and Opticians' Circular. Edited by E. Pennock. [Bi-monthly.] v. 1–4, Dec., 1883–7. 8°. *Philadelphia, J. W. Queen & Co.* Current.

MICROSCOPICAL (The) News, and Northern Microscopist. Edited by G. E. Davis. [Monthly.] v. 3–4, 1883–4. 8°. *London.* Completed.

MICROSCOPICAL Society of Liverpool. Annual reports. 13.–15., 1882–4. Abstracts of proceedings, list of members, rules. 3 Nos. 8°. *Liverpool, 1882–4.*

———. Catalogue of the slides in the cabinets, and books in the library of the . . . 1884. 8°. *Liverpool, 1884.*

MICROSCOPICAL (The) Society of London. Catalogue of microscopic objects in the cabinet of . . . 8°. *London, 1864.*

MONTHLY (The) Microscopical Journal. Edited by H. Lawson. [2 v. annually.] v. 1–18, 1869–77. 8°. *London.* Completed.

NATIONAL Microscopical Congress. Proceedings of the National Microscopical Congress, held at Indianapolis, Aug. 14–19, 1878, and of the American Society of Microscopists, held at Buffalo, N. Y., Aug. 19–24, 1879. 8°. *Indianapolis, 1880.*

NORTHERN (The) Microscopist. Edited by G. E. Davis. [Monthly.] v. 1; Nos. 1–9, v. 2, Jan., 1881, to Sept., 1882. 8°. *London.*

NORTHERN (The) Microscopist and Microscopical News. Edited by G. E. Davis. [Monthly.] Nos. 9–12, v. 2, Oct. to Dec., 1882. 8°. *London.*

POSTAL (The) Microscopical Society. A classified list of objects shown from its commencement to the end of the 4th year, June, 1877. 4°. [*London*], 1878.

QUARTERLY Journal of Microscopical Science. Edited by E. Lankester and G. Busk. v. 1–8, 1853–60. N. s., v. 1–28, 1861–87. 8°. *London.* Current.

QUEKETT Microscopical Club. Catalogue of microscopical preparations in the cabinet of the . . . 8°. [*London, 1878.*]

SOCIÉTÉ belge de microscopie. Annales de la . . . v. 5–7, 1878–9 to 1880–81. 8°. *Bruxelles, 1879–83.*

———. Bulletins de la . . . v. 5–7, 1878–9 to 1880–81. 8°. *Bruxelles, 1879–83.*

———. Bulletins des séances. Procès-verbaux. Nos. 12–14, v. 3, 1876–7; Nos. 1–11, v. 9, 1882–3; Nos. 2, 4–6, 8, 9, v. 10, 1883–4. 8°. *Bruxelles, 1876–84.*

STATE Microscopical Society of Illinois. Charter, constitution, by-laws, and list of members. sm. 4°. *Chicago, 1870.*

ZEITSCHRIFT für Mikroskopie. Redigirt von E. Kaiser. [Monthly.] v. 1–2, Oct., 1877–80. 8°. *Berlin.* Ended.

ZEITSCHRIFT für Mikroskopie und Fleischschau. Hrsg. von H. C. J. Duncker. [Semimonthly.] v. 3–4, Jan., 1882, to April 20, 1885. 4°. *Berlin; Spandau.*

Microscopy (*Journals and societies relating to*).

ZEITSCHRIFT für mikroskopische Fleischschau und populäre Mikroskopie. Hrsg. von H. C. J. Duncker. [Semi-monthly.] v. 1–2, Dec., 1879, to Dec. 28, 1881. 4°. *Berlin u. Bernau.*

ZEITSCHRIFT für wissenschaftliche Mikroskopie und für mikroskopische Technik. Hrsg. von W. J. Behrens. [Quarterly.] v. 1–4, 1884–7. 8°. *Braunschweig.*
Current.

Société micrographique de Paris. J. de l'anat. et physiol., etc., Par., 1868, v, 326–334.

Microscopy (*Manipulations and preparations in*).

See, also, **Germs** (*Investigation of*); **Histology**; **Microtomes**, *etc.*; **Nervous** *system* (*Histology of*).

BACHMANN (O.) Leitfaden zur Anfertigung mikroskopischer Dauerpräparate. 8°. *München*, 1879.

BURG (J.) * Beitrag zur mikromechanischen Analyse. Veränderungen einiger Gewebe und Sekrete durch Magensaft. 8°. *Greifswald*, 1876.

COLE (A. C.) The methods of microscopical research; an introductory essay to studies in microscopical science. 8°. *London*, 1884.

DAVIES (T.) The preparation and mounting of microscopic objects. Edited by J. Matthews. 2. ed. 12°. *London*, [1873].
——. The same. 8°. *New York*, [*n. d.*]
——. The same. 2. ed. 8°. *New York*, 1874.

FRIEDLAENDER (C.) Microscopische Technik zum Gebrauch bei medicinischen und pathologisch-anatomischen Untersuchungen. 12°. *Kassel u. Berlin*, [1882].
——. The same. 2. Aufl. 8°. *Berlin*, 1884.
——. The same. A manual of microscopical technology for use in the investigations of medicine and pathological anatomy. Transl. by Stephen Yates Howell. 12°. *New York & London*, 1885.

GAGE (S. H.) Notes on microscopical methods for the use of laboratory students in the anatomical department of the Cornell University. 8°. *Ithaca*, 1886–7.

GROENLAND (J.), CORNU (M.), & RIVET (G.) Des préparations microscopiques tirées du règne végétal, et des différents procédés à employer pour en assurer la conservation. 8°. *Paris*, 1872.

GUY (W. A.) On the preservation and mounting of microscopic objects in minute tubes. 8°. [*London*, 1862.]

HEYDENREICH (L. L.) Metodi izsledov. ichich organizmov dlja vrachei, estestvoispitat., veterinarov, studentov i dr. [Method of examining lower organisms for physicians, naturalists, students, and others.] 8°. *St. Petersburg*, 1885.

MARTIN (J. H.) Microscopic objects figured and described. 8°. *London*, 1870.
——. A manual of microscopic mounting, with notes on the collection and examination of objects. 8°. *London*, 1872.

NORDMANN (O.) * Beiträge zur Kenntniss und namentlich zur Färbung der Mastzellen. 8°. *Helmstedt*, 1884.

PEYER (A.) Atlas der Mikroskopie am Krankenbette. 2. Aufl. 8°. *Stuttgart*, 1887.

ROBIN (C.) Mémoire sur les objets qui peuvent être conservés en préparations microscopiques transparentes et opaques, classés d'après les divisions naturelles des trois règnes de la nature. 8°. *Paris*, 1856.

SUFFOLK (W. T.) On microscopical manipulation. Being the subject-matter of a course of lectures. 12°. *London*, 1870.

Microscopy (*Manipulations and preparations in*).

——. The same. 12°. *Philadelphia*, 1870.

WOODWARD (J.-J.) Extrait de quelques travaux de . . . 8°. *Bruxelles*, 1878.
Repr. from : Bull. Soc. belge de micr., Brux., 1877–8, iv, pp. lxiv–lxxvi. [*See, also, infra.*]

Adler (H.) Vorläufige Mittheilung über eine mittelst Silber-Imbibition gemachte Beobachtung. Ztschr. f. rat. Med., Leipz. u. Heidelb., 1864, xxi, 3. R., 160–164, 1 pl.—**Afanassiew** (M.) Gram's method of staining applied to the examination of the micro-organisms in pneumonic and tuberculous sputum. Edinb. M. J., 1884–5, xxx, 717–726, 1 pl.—**Alferow** (S.) Nouveaux procédés pour les imprégnations de l'argent. Arch. de physiol. norm. et path., Par., 1874, 2. s., i, 694–697.—**Almén** (A.) Enkelt beredningssätt för lösligt berlinerblätt. [A simple way of preparing Berlin blue.] Upsala Läkaref. Förh., 1867–8, iii, 711–713.—**Arnold** (J.) Ueber das Verhalten des Indigcarmins in den lebenden Geweben. Centralbl. f. d. med. Wissensch., Berl., 1875, xiii, 865–867. — **Arnold** (J. W. S.) Hæmatoxylin as a staining material for animal tissue. Phila. M. Times, 1872, ii, 364. ——. The preparation of nervous tissue for histological examination. Am. Psych. J., N. Y., 1876, n. s., iii, 202–204. ——. Microscopical laboratories. Am. Month. Micr. J., N. Y., 1882, iii, 69–71.—**Aubert** (H.) Ueber die Anwendung des Glycerins zu mikroskopischen Untersuchungen. Wien. med. Wchnschr., 1855, v, 293.—**Babes** (V.) Ueber einige Färbungsmethoden, besonders für krankhafte Gewebe, mittelst Safranin und deren Resultate. Arch. f. mikr. Anat., Bonn, 1883, xxii, 356–365. — **Basslinger** (J.) Anwendung der Verdauungsversuche zur Microscopie, Unverdaulichkeit der lebenden Magenwand. Oesterr. Ztschr. f. prakt. Heilk., Wien, 1857, iii, 713–718.—**Beatty** (G. D.) Double staining of wood and other vegetable sections. Month. Micr. J., Lond., 1875, xiv, 57–59.—**Behrens** (W.) Bernsteinlack zum Verschliessen mikroskopischer Präparate. Ztschr. f. wissensch. Mikr., Brnschwg., 1885, ii, 54–57.—**Bergonzini** (C.) Sull' uso del collodio e del fenolo nella tecnica microscopica. Spallanzani, Modena, 1883, 2. s., xii, 196–200.—**Bermann** (I.) Some points on staining *in toto* and dry section cutting. Arch. Med., N. Y., 1881, v, 130–135. *Also*, Reprint.—**Beitman** (B.) Celloidin as an embedding mass. Chicago M. J. & Exam., 1884, xlix, 103. ——. Improved imbedding masses and a new sliding microtome. Chicago M. Rev., 1882, vi, 350.— **Bikfalvi** (K.) Beitrag zur Verwendung der Magenverdauung a's Isolationsmethode. Centralbl. f. d. med. Wissensch., Berl., 1883, xxi, 833–836.—**Birge** (E. A.) On a convenient method of imbedding. Am. Month. Micr. J., N. Y., 1882, iii, 73–75.—**Blochmann** (F.) Ueber Einbettungsmethoden. Ztschr. f. wissensch. Mikr., Brnschwg., 1884, i, 218–233.—**Borden** (W. C.) On electrical constant-temperature apparatus. Am. Month. Micr. J., Wash., 1887, viii, 131–133.—**Born** (C.) & **Wieger** (G.) Ueber einen neuen Unterguss. Ztschr. f. wissensch. Mikr., Brnschwg., 1885, ii, 346–348.—**Bozzolo.** Il regolatore del preparato al microscopio del Dr. C. Calliano. Gior. d. r. Accad. di med. di Torino, 1883, 3. s., xxxi, 210–214, 1 pl.—**Brandt** (O.) Das Tingiren mikroskopischer Präparate. Ztschr. f. Mikr., Berl., 1879–80, ii, 113–123.—**Brass** (A.) Die Anfertigung von zusammenhängenden Serienschnitten. Ztschr. f. wissensch. Mikr., Brnschwg., 1885, ii, 307. ——. Die Einbettungsmethode mit Benzol und das Schneiden leicht zerbrechlicher Objecte. *Ibid.*, 300–305.—**Broesicke** (G.) Die Ueberosmiumsäure in Verbindung mit der Oxalsäure als mikroskopisches Färbemittel. Centralbl. f. d. med. Wissensch., Berl., 1878, xvi, 833–836.—**Brücke** (E.) Erfahrungen über das lösliche Berlinerblau als Injectionsfarbe. Arch. f. mikr. Anat., Bonn, 1866, ii, 87–91.—**Bürkner** (K.) Ueber das Auer'sche Glasglühlicht als Lichtquelle für das Mikroskopiren. Ztschr. f. wissensch. Mikr., Brnschwg., 1887, iv, 35–38.—**Calberla** (E.) Eine Einbettungsmasse. Morphol. Jahrb., Leipz., 1876, ii, 445–448.—**Calliano** (C.) Un nuovo regolatore del preparato al microscopio. Arch. per le sc. med., Torino, 1883–4, vii, 167–170, 1 pl.—**Carpenter** (W. M.) Bayberry tallow as an embedding medium. Phila. M. Times, 1884–5, xv, 631.—**Certes** (A.) De l'emploi des matières colorantes dans l'étude physiologique et histologique des infusoires vivants. Compt. rend. Soc. de biol., Par., 1885, 8. s., ii, 197; 1886, 8. s., iii, 206–208.—**Clason** (E.) Histologisk technik. Upsala Läkaref. Förh., 1871, vi, 209–238.—**Coppinger** (C.) A new method of freezing tissues for the microscope. Lancet, Lond., 1876, i, 277.—**Cornil** (V.) Sur l'application du violet de méthylaniline dans la technique microscopique et sur les résultats obtenus par son emploi dans l'étude de la dégénérescence amyloïde des organes. Compt. rend. Soc. de biol., Par., 1875, 6. s., ii, 200–206. ——. Préparations au violet de méthylaniline. *Ibid.*, 215. ——. Sur la dissociation du violet de méthylaniline et sa séparation en deux couleurs sous l'influence de certains tissus normaux et pathologiques, en particulier par les tissus en dégénérescence amyloïde. Compt. rend. Acad. d. sc., Par., 1875, lxxx, 1288–1291. ——. Instruction sur le mode de

Microscopy (*Manipulations and preparations in*).

conservation des pièces anatomiques destinées à être examinées au microscope. Arch. de méd. nav., Par., 1884, xli, 495-504.—**Couch** (L. B.) Pieric acid, or a few comments on a bit of "master work". Homœop. Times, N. Y., 1878, vi, 94-101. *Also, Reprint.*—**Cuccati** (G.) Sopra una soluzione di carminio al carbonato di soda. Ztschr. f. wissensch. Mikr., Brnschwg., 1887, iv, 50.—**Curtis** (L.) On microscopical measurements. Rocky Mountain M. Rev., Denver, 1880-81, i, 271-276.—**Czokor** (J.) Die Cochenille-Carminlösung. Arch. f. mikr. Anat., Bonn, 1880, xviii, 412-414.—**Debes** (E.) Hilfsapparat zum Aussuchen und Legen von Diatomaceen. Ztschr. f. wissensch. Mikr., Brnschwg., 1886, iii, 330-336.—**Deecke** (T.) Preparations of tissues for microscopic examination; an account of the methods and apparatus employed. Am. J. Insan., Utica, 1876, xxxiii, 50-77.— **Donnadieu** (A.-L.) Des préparations entomologiques. J. de microg., Par., 1877, i, 147; 196.—**Dreschfeld** (J.) On a new staining-fluid. J. Anat. & Physiol., Lond., 1876, xi, 181.—**Duval** (M.) Procédé de coloration des coupes du système nerveux. J. de l'anat. et physiol., etc., Par., 1876, xii, 111. ———. Technique de l'emploi du collodion humide pour la pratique des coupes microscopiques. *Ibid.*, 1879, xv, 185-188.—**Ehrlich** (P.) Beiträge zur Kenntniss der Anilinfärbung und ihrer Verwendung in der mikroskopischen Technik. Arch. f. mikr. Anat., Bonn, 1876, xiii, 263-277. 1 pl. ———. Ueber das Methylenblau und seine klinisch-bakterioskopische Verwerthung. Ztschr. f. klin. Med., Berl., 1880-81, ii, 710-713. ———. Zur biologischen Verwerthung des Methylenblau. Centralbl. f. d. med. Wissensch., Berl., 1885, xxiii, 113-117.—**Errera** (L.) Sur l'emploi de l'encre de Chine en microscopie. Bull. Soc. belge de micr., Brux., 1884, x, 184-188.—**Eternod** (A.) Armoire à préparations microscopiques. Ztschr. f. wissensch. Mikr., Brnschwg., 1885, ii, 511-513. ———. Instruments destinés à la microscopie. *Ibid.*, 1887, iv, 39-42.—**Ewald** (C. A.) Die tinctorielle Methode Ehrlich's. Deutsche med. Wchnschr., Berl., 1881, vii, 20.—**Fafani** (A.) Nuovo metodo per colorire i preparati microscopici mediante una soluzione picro-anilinica. Sperimentale, Firenze, 1878, xli, 52-57.—**Fick.** Ueber eine Methode mikroskopische Objecte mathematisch genau zu zeichnen und insbesondere deren Flächenräume zu messen. Ztschr. f. rat. Med., Heidelb., 1853, n. s., iii, 273-278, 1 pl.—**Fischer** (E.) Eosin als Tinctionsmittel für mikroskopische Präparate. Arch. f. mikr. Anat., Bonn, 1875, xii, 349-352.—**Flemming** (W.) Eine Einbettungsmethode. *Ibid.*, 1873, ix, 123-125. ———. Ueber das E. Hermann'sche Kernfärbungsverfahren. *Ibid.*, 1880-81, xix, 317-330. ———. Mittheilungen zur Färbetechnik. Ztschr. f. wissensch. Mikr., Brnschwg., 1884, i, 349-361. ———. Notizen zur Färbetechnik. *Ibid.*, 517-519.— **Flesch** (M.) Bemerkungen zur Kritik der Tinctions Präparate. *Ibid.*, 464-477. ———. Einfache Vorrichtung zum Wiederauffinden wichtiger Stellen in mikroskopischen Präparaten. Arch. f. mikr. Anat., Bonn, 1881-2, xx, 502. ———. Zur Weigert'schen Hämatoxylinfärbung des centralen Nerven-Systems. Ztschr. f. wissensch. Mikr., Brnschwg., 1884, i, 564-566. ———. Zur Anwendung der Merkel'schen Doppelfärbung mit Indigo und Carmin. *Ibid.*, 1885, ii, 349-352. ———. Notiz zu Watney's Doppelfärbung mit Hämatoxylin. *Ibid.*, 353.—**Förster.** Ueber die Isolirbarkeit der Knochen-, Knorpel- und Bindegewebskörperchen. Arch. f. path. Anat., etc., Berl., 1860, xviii, 170.—**Francotte** (P.) Inclusion dans la paraffine. Bull. Soc. belge de micr., Brux., 1884-5, xi, 79-86, 2 pl.—**Friedländer** (C.) Notiz, die Färbung der Kapselmicrococcen betreffend. Fortschr. d. Med., Berl., 1885, iii, 757-760.—**Galli** (C.) Colorazione degli imbuti nelle fibre midollate periferiche col Bleu di China. Ztschr. f. wissensch. Mikr., Brnschwg., 1886, iii, 465-470 1 pl.—**Gelpke** (J.) Notiz zur Anwendung der Weigert'schen modificirten Hämatoxylin-Färbung auf das periphere Nervensystem. *Ibid.*, 1885, ii, 484-489.—**Gerlach** (J.) Ueber die Einwirkung von Farbstoff auf lebende Gewebe. Wissensch. Mitth. d. phys.-med. Soc. zu Erlang., 1858, i, 5-12. ———. Ueber die Einwirkung von Farbstoff auf lebende Gewebe. *Ibid.*, 1859, i, 1. Hft., 5-12.—**Giacomini.** Nuovo processo di conservazione delle sezioni microscopiche. Gazz. d. clin., Torino, 1885, xxii, 339; 355; 371. *Also:* Gior. d. r. Accad. di med. di Torino, 1885, 3. s., xxxiii, 762-789. *Also, Reprint.*—**Gibbes** (H.) On the double and treble staining of animal tissues for microscopical investigations; with a note on cleaning thin cover-glasses. J. Roy. Micr. Soc., Lond., 1880, iii, 390-393.—**Gierke** (H.) Färberei zu mikroskopischen Zwecken. Ztschr. f. wissensch. Mikr., Brnschwg., 1884, i, 62; 372; 497; 1885, ii, 13; 164. *Also, transl.:* Am. Month. Micr. J., Wash., 1886, vii, 13; 31; 52; 70; 97; 150.—**Goadby** (H.) A practical treatise on the art of making and preserving microscopical and other preparations. Med. Indep., Detroit, 1856, ii, 33; 91.—**Golgi** (C.) Un nuovo processo di tecnica microscopica. R. Ist. Lomb. di. sc. e lett. Rendic., Milano, 1879, 2. s., xii, 206-210.—**Goodale** (G. L.) A method for subjecting living protoplasm to the action of different liquids. Am. J. Sc., N. Haven, 1887, 3. s., xxxiii,

Microscopy (*Manipulations and preparations in*).

144.—**Gram** (C.) Ueber die Färbung der Schizomyceten in Schnittpräparaten. Cong. période. internat. d. sc. méd. Compt.-rend. 1884, Copenh., 1886, i (Sect. de path. gén., etc.), 116.—**Grancher** (J.) Des usages de la solution ammoniacale de carmin en histologie. Arch. de physiol. norm. et path., Par., 1871-2, iv, 770-776.—**Grenacher** (H.) Einige Notizen zur Tinctionstechnik, besonders zur Kernfärbung. Arch. f. mikr. Anat., Bonn, 1879, xvi, 463-471.—**Griesbach** (H.) Bemerkungen zur Injektionstechnik bei Wirbellosen. Arch. f. mikr. Anat., Bonn, 1882, xxi, 824-827. ———. Die Azofarbstoffe als Tinktionsmittel für menschliche und thierische Gewebe. *Ibid.*, 1883, xxii, 132-142.—**Groves** (J. W.) On stained sections of animal tissues, and how to prepare them. Am. J. Micr., N. Y., 1880, v, 25-34.—**Halford** (G. B.) On the use of "magenta" as an aid to investigation and diagnosis. Austral. M. J., Melbourne, 1864, ix, 196-198.—**Hamann** (O.) Eine neue Karminlösung. Internat. Monatschr. f. Anat. u. Histol., Berl., 1884, i, 346-348.—**Hamilton** (D. J.) On a method of combining Weigert's hæmatoxylene-copper stain for nerve-fibre with the use of the freezing microtome. J. Anat. & Physiol., Lond., 1886-7, xxi, 444-449.—**Hannover** (A.) Die Chromsäure, ein vorzügliches Mittel bei mikroskopischen Untersuchungen. Arch. f. Anat., Physiol. u. wissensch. Med., Berl., 1840, 549-558.—**Hansen** (A.) Eine bequeme Methode zum Einschliessen mikroskopischer Präparate. Ztschr. f. wissensch. Mikr., Brnschwg., 1886, iii, 482.—**Harris** (V.) On double staining nucleated blood-corpuscles with anilin dyes. Quart. J. Micr. Sc., Lond., 1883, n. s., xxiii, 292-301.—**Hayes** (B.) Histological anatomy and microscopical manipulation. Med. Times & Gaz., Lond., 1853, vi, 27; 83; 155; 263; 313; 391; 441; 547; 593; 645.—**Heidenhain** (R.) Eine neue Verwendung des Hämatoxylin. Arch. f. mikr. Anat., Bonn, 1884, xxiv, 468-470. ———. Eine Abänderung der Färbung mit Hämatoxylin und chromsauren Salzen. *Ibid.*, 1886, xxvii, 383.—**Heller.** Zur mikroskopischen Technik. Ztschr. f. wissensch. Mikr., Brnschwg., 1885, ii, 47.—**Henking** (H.) Technische Mittheilungen zur Entwicklungsgeschichte. *Ibid.*, 1886, iii, 470-479.—**Hensen** (V.) Ueber ein Instrument für mikroskopische Präparation. Arch. f. mikr. Anat., Bonn, 1866, ii, 46-55, 1 pl.—**Heschl.** Methylgrün als Tinktionsmittel für mikroskopische Präparate. Wien. med. Wchnschr., 1879, xxix, 25.—**Heydenreich** (L.) Ueber den besten Deckglaskitt. Ztschr. f. wissensch. Mikr., Brnschwg., 1885, ii, 333-338.—**His.** Ueber das Verhalten des salpetersauren Silberoxyds zu thierischen Gewebsbestandtheilen. Arch. f. path. Anat., etc., Berl., 1861 xx, 207-209, 1 pl.—**His** (W.) Ueber die Einwirkung des salpetersauren Silberoxydes auf die Hornhaut. Schweiz. Ztschr. f. Heilk., Bern, 1863, ii, 1-24. *Also, Reprint.*—**Hoeltge** (A.) Injection of microscopic preparations by means of compressed air. Clinic, Cincin., 1876, x, 169-172.—**Hoggan** (F. E.) On a new process of histological staining. J. Quekett Micr. Club, Lond., 1876, 180.—**Hunt** (J. G.) The preparation and preservation of tissues. Phila. M. Times, 1872, ii, 295. ———. Extract of hæmatoxylon in the preparation of staining of both vegetable and animal tissues. *Ibid.*, 1873, iii, 602.—**Jullien** (L.) Note sur une nouvelle méthode de coloration des éléments histologiques. Mém. Soc. d. sc. méd. de Lyon (1872), 1873, xii, pt. 1, 119-123. [Discussion], pt. 2, 138. *Also:* Lyon méd., 1872, x, 526-530.—**Kinne** (C. M.) A self-centering turntable. Am. J. Micr., N. Y., 1877, ii, 34.—**Klebs.** Die Einschmelzungs-Methode, ein Beitrag zur mikroskopischen Technik. Arch. f. mikr. Anat., Bonn, 1869, v, 164-166.—**Krönig.** Einschlusskitt für mikroskopische Präparate. *Ibid.*, 1886, xxvii, 657.—**Krukenberg** (A.) Ueber eine sehr vortheilhafte Methode der Zubereitung von Zahn- und Knochendurchschnitten für die mikroskopische Beobachtung. Arch. f. Anat., Physiol. u. wissensch. Med., Berl., 1849, 420-424.—**Krysiński** (S.) Photoxylin als Einbettungsmittel. Arch. f. path. Anat., etc., Berl., 1887, cviii, 217.—**Kultschitzky.** Carmintinction. Ztschr. f. wissensch. Mikr., Brnschwg., 1887, iv, 46-48. ———. Celloidin-Paraffin-Einbettung. *Ibid.*, 48.—**Lablovski** (M. D.) Iz zamietok po mikroskop. technike. [Microscopical technics.] Vrach, St. Petersb., 1885, vi, 655; 684.—**Landois** (L.) Die Imprägnation der Gewebe mit Schwefelmetallen. Centralbl. f. d. med. Wissensch., Berl., 1865, iii, 867.—[**Latteux.**] Nouveau appareil à injections histologiques. Mouvement méd., Par., 1875, xiii, 199.—**Lavdowsky** (M.) Myrtillus, ein neues Tinctionsmittel für thierische und pflanzliche Gewebe. Arch. f. mikr. Anat., Bonn, 1884, xxiii, 506-508.—**Leber** (T.) Zur Kenntniss der Imprägnationsmethoden der Hornhaut und ähnlicher Gewebe. Arch. f. Ophth., Berl., 1868, xiv, 3. Abth., 300-316.—**Libbey** (W.), jr. Celloidine as an embedding mass. [Abstr.] Am. Month. Micr. J., Wash., 1884, v, 183.—**Lieberkühn.** Von den Mitteln den Bau der Eingeweide kennen zu lernen. Phys. u. med. Ab handl. d. k. Acad. d. Wissensch. zu Berl., Gotha, 1783, iii, 310-314.—**Lindt** (O.) Ueber den Nachweis von Phloroglucin. Ztschr. f. wissensch. Mikr., Brnschwg., 1885, ii,

Microscopy (*Manipulations and preparations in*).

495–499.—**List** (J. H.) Zur Färbetechnik. *Ibid.*, 145–150. ——. Ueber Methoden, welche zum Studium der Structur von Drüsenzellen geeignet sind. *Ibid.*, 514–516. ——. Zur Verwendung des Anilingrüns. *Ibid.*, 222. ——. Notiz zur Färbetechnik. *Ibid.*, 1886, iii, 393. ——. Ueber eine kleine Abänderung am Reicherts'schen Objecthalter. *Ibid.*, 484.—**Loewe** (L.) Das Härten, Färben, und Schneiden anatomischer Präparate, sowie eine Modification des Ranvier'schen Microtoms. Ztschr. f. Mikr. Berl., 1879–80, ii, 123–139.—**Lovett** (E.) On an improved method of preparing embryological and other delicate organisms for microscopical examination. J. Roy. Micr. Soc., Lond., 1883, 2. s., iii, 785–789.—**Luchtmans** (G. J.) Iets over het vervaardigen van microscopische praeparaten, tot opheldering der structuur van sommige delen van het zenuwstelsel. Nederl. Tijdschr. v. Geneesk., Amst., 1863, vii, 564–567.—**Lustgarten** (S.) Victoriablau, ein neues Tinctionsmittel für elastische Fasern und für Kerne. Med. Jahrb., Wien, 1886, n. F., i, 285–289, 1 pl.—**Luys** (J.) Procédés pour décolorer les pièces et les coupes minces qui ont macéré dans la solution chromique et les rendre transparentes. J. de l'anat. et physiol., etc., Par., 1872, viii, 265–268.—**Malassez.** Coloration des bactéries par le violet de méthyle. Bull. Soc. anat. de Par., 1881, lvi, 670–674. *Also:* Progrès méd., Par., 1882, x, 523–525.—**Martinotti** (G.) Sulla colorazione doppia coll' ematossilina e coll' eosina. Osservatore, Torino, 1883, xix, 801–806. ——. Sull' uso dell' allume di cromo nella tecnica microscopica. Ztschr. f. wissensch. Mikr., Brnschwg., 1884, i, 361–366. ——. La picronigrosina nello studio delle alterazioni dei centri nervosi. *Ibid.*, 1885, ii, 478–484. ——. Un metodo semplice per la colorazione delle fibre elastiche. *Ibid.*, 1887, iv, 31–34.—**Marvin** (J. B.) Preservation of specimens for microscopical examination. Med. Herald, Louisville, 1879–80, i, 466.—**Mayer** (P.) Aus der Mikrotechnik. Internat. Monatschr. f. Anat. u. Physiol., Leipz., 1887, iv, 37–46.—**Meyer** (F.) Conservations-Flüssigkeit für mikroskopische Objecte. Arch. f. mikr. Anat., Bonn, 1877, xiii, 868.—**Meyer** (H.) Ueber farbige Kreiden für den anatomischen Unterricht. Arch. f. Anat., Physiol. u. wissensch. Med., Leipz., 1864, 678–681.—**Miller** (M. N.) Staining fluids for microscopic work. Med. Rec., N. Y., 1878, xiii, 97. ——. A new imbedding process for microscopic work. *Ibid.*, 1885, xxvii, 429.—**Mitchell** (C. L.) Staining with hæmatoxylon. Proc. Acad. Nat. Sc. Phila. (1883), 1884, 297–300.—**Mondino** (C.) Sull' uso del bicloruro di mercurio nello studio degli organi centrali del sistema nervoso. Ztschr. f. wissensch. Mikr., Brnschwg., 1885, ii, 157–163.—**Morland** (H.) On mounting media so far as they relate to diatoms. J. Quekett Micr. Club, Lond., 1887, 2. s., iii, 108–114.—**Morris** (W.) Notes on experiments in mounting the Amphipleura pellucida in media having a higher refractive index than Canada balsam. Australas. M. Gaz., Sydney, 1885–6, v, 124–130.—**Mounting** (On) and photographing microscopic objects. Nature, Lond., 1883–4, xxviii.—**Münster** (A.) Die Anfertigung der mikroskopischen Dauerpräparate. Ztschr. f. Mikr., Berl., 1878, i, 213; 289.—**Neumann** (E.) Die Picrocarminfärbung und ihre Anwendung auf die Entzündungslehre. Arch. f. mikr. Anat., Bonn, 1880, xxv, 130–150, 1 pl.—**Nörner** (C.) Beitrag zur Behandlung mikroskopischer Präparate. *Ibid.*, 1882, xxi, 351–356. ——. Zur Behandlung mikroskopischer Präparate. Ztschr. f. mikr. Anat., Brnschwg., 1886, iii, 19–23.—**Norris** (W. F.) & **Shakespeare** (E. O.) A new method of double staining. Am. J. M. Sc., Phila. 1877, n. s., lxxiii, 146–151.—**Oppenheimer** (L. S.) Letter from Vienna. Boston M. & S. J., 1877, xcvii, 204–206.—**Oschatz.** Ueber Herstellung und Aufbewahrung mikroskopischer Präparate. Beitr. z. physiol. u. path. Chem. u. Mikr., Berl., 1843–4, i, 128; 317.—**Pacini** (F.) Di alcuni metodi di preparazione e conservazione degli elementi microscopici dei tessuti animali e vegetali. Gior. internaz. d. sc. med., Napoli, 1880, ii, 337–350. *Also, transl.:* J. de microg., Par., 1880, iv, 136; 191; 235.—**Parker** (T. J.) On some applications of osmic acid to microscopic purposes. J. Roy. Micr. Soc., Lond., 1879, ii, 381–383.—**Passauer** (M.) Ueber das Erhärten des Canadabalsams auf den mikroskopischen Präparaten durch heisse Dämpfe. Ztschr. f. Mikr., Berl., 1879–80, ii, 194.—**Perls** (M.) Zur mikrotechnischen Verwerthung des Palladiumchlorids. Arch. f. path. Anat., etc., Berl., 1872, lvi, 463–467, 1 pl.—**Pommer** (G.) Ueber Methoden, welche zum Studium der Ablagerungsverhältnisse der Knochensalze und zum Nachweise kalkloser Knochenpartien brauchbar sind. Ztschr. f. wissensch. Mikr., Brnschwg., 1885, ii, 151–156.—**Quincy.** Hæmatoxyline as a coloring agent for microscopic specimens. Boston M. & S. J., 1873, lxxxviii, 252–254.—**Ralph** (T. S.) On the use of magenta and other dyes in the investigation of disease by the microscope. Austral. M. J., Melbourne, 1865, x, 310–314.—**Ranvier** (L.) Technique microscopique. Acide picrique (acide phénique trinitré; acide carbazotique; amer de Welter). Arch. de physiol. norm. et path., Par., 1868, i, 319–321. ——. Procédé pour faire apparaître les noyaux dans les tissus imprégnés d'abord par le nitrate d'argent.

Microscopy (*Manipulations and preparations in*).

Étude du carcinome à l'aide de l'imprégnation d'argent. *Ibid.*, 666–670. ——. Des applications de la purpurine à l'histologie. *Ibid.*, 1875, 2. s., i, 761–773. ——. De l'emploi de l'alcool dilué en histologie. *Ibid.*, 781–796.—**von Recklinghausen** (F.) Eine Methode, mikroskopische hohle und solide Gebilde von einander zu unterscheiden. Arch. f. path. Anat., etc., Berl., 1860, xix, 451. ——. Zur Geschichte der Versilberungsmethode. *Ibid.*, 1863, xxvii, 419–421.—**Reeves** (H. A.) How to fix aniline dyes. Brit. M. J., Lond., 1883, i, 450.—**Renaut** (J.) Sur l'éosine hématoxylique et sur son emploi en histologie. Compt. rend. Acad. d. sc., Par., 1879, lxxxviii, 1039–1042. ——. Sur le mode de préparation, et l'emploi de l'éosine et de la glycérine hématoxyliques en histologie. Arch. de physiol. norm. et path., Par., 1881, 2. s., viii, 640–648.—**Richardson** (B. W.) On a blue and scarlet double stain, suitable for nerve and many other animal tissues. J. Roy. Micr. Soc., Lond., 1881, 2. s., i, 573.—**Rindfleisch** (E.) Eine neue Injectionsmasse. Arch. f. path. Anat., etc., Berl., 1864, xxx, 602. ——. Blutuntersuchung. *Ibid.*, 603.—**Roberts** (W.) Note sur l'influence d'une solution de potasse et d'une température élevée sur l'origine et le développement des microphytes. [*Transl. from:* Proc. Roy. Soc. Lond., Dec. 21, 1876.] Monit. scient., Par., 1877, 3. s., vii, 590–592.—**Rossi** (A.) L' azione dell' acido osmico sulle cellule vegetali. Mem. Accad. d. sc. d. Ist. di Bologna, 1880, 4. s., i, 657–660, 1 pl.—**Rutherford** (W.) On some improvements in the mode of making sections of tissue for microscopic observation. J. Anat. & Physiol., Cambridge, 1871, v, 324–328.—**Schällibaum** (H.) Ueber ein Verfahren mikroskopische Schnitte auf dem Objectträger zu fixiren und daselbst zu färben. Arch. f. mikr. Anat., Bonn, 1883, xxii, 689.—**Schiefferdecker** (P.) Mittheilung, betreffend das von mir verwandte Anilingrün. Ztschr. f. wissensch. Mikr., Brnschwg., 1885, ii, 51–53; 1886, iii, 41–43. ——. Ueber einen Apparat zum Markiren. von Theilen mikroskopischer Präparate. *Ibid.*, 461–464. ——. Methode zur Isolirung von Epithelzellen. *Ibid.*, 483.—**Schmidt** (A.) Ueber das Aufbewahren mikroskopischer Präparate. Arch. d. Ver. f. wissensch. Heilk., Götting., 1858, iii, 269–278.—**Schultze** (M.) Essigsaures Kali zum Aufbewahren mikroskopischer Präparate. Arch. f. mikr. Anat., Bonn, 1871, vii, 180.—**Schulze** (F. E.) Eine neue Methode der Erhärtung und Färbung thierischer Gewebe. Centralbl. f. d. med. Wissensch., Berl., 1867, v, 193–195. ——. Ein Entwässerungsapparat. *Ibid.*, 1885–6, xxvi, 539–542.—**Sedgwick** (C.) Mounting chick embryos whole. Proc. Am. Ass. Adv. Sc. 1881, Salem, 1882, xxx, 115.—**Siredey** (A.) Instruction sur le mode de conservation des pièces anatomiques destinées à être examinées au microscope. Union méd. Par., 1884, 3. s., xxxvii, 1084–1087.—**Smirnow** (A.) Der Mikrostat; Apparat zur genauen und systematischen Untersuchung mikroskopischer Präparate und Notirung bemerkenswerther Stellen. Arch. f. mikr. Anat., Bonn, 1887, xxix, 384–388.—**Smith** (H. L.) A new mounting medium. Proc. Am. Soc. Micr., Buffalo, 1884, vii, 186–190. ——. Mounting media of high refractive index. *Ibid.*, 1885, viii, 86–90.—**Spee** (F.) Leichtes Verfahren zur Erhaltung linear geordneter, lückenloser Schnittserien mit Hülfe von Schnittbändern. Ztschr. f. wissensch. Mikr., Brnschwg., 1885, ii, 7–12.—**Squire** (P.) On a method of preserving the fresh-water medusa. J. Roy. Micr. Soc., Lond., 1883, 2. s., iii, 485.—**Standish** (M.) Celloidin, the new material for embedding specimens for microscopic section cutting; its method of use and its advantages. Am. J. Ophth. St. Louis, 1885, ii, 68–72. *Also, Reprint.*—**Stark.** Ueber die Bastian'sche Methode zur Aufhellung dünner Schnitte von Gehirn und Rückenmark. Deutsche Klinik, Berl., 1869, xxi, 94.—**von Stein** (S.) Einfache Vorrichtung für das Mikrotom zur Einbettung der Präparate. Centralbl. f. d. med. Wissensch., Berl., 1884, xxii, 100.—**Stein** (S. T.) Zur Technik der Injectionen. Arch. f. path. Anat., etc., Berl., 1867, xxxix, 180–183.—**Stevenson** (J.) A ready method of preparing sections of diseased tissues for the microscope. Edinb. M. J., 1875–6, xxi, 605–607.—**Stieda** (L.) Ueber die Anwendung des Kreosots bei Anfertigung mikroskopischer Präparate. Arch. f. mikr. Anat., Bonn, 1866, ii, 430–435.—**Stirling** (W.) On double and treble staining of microscopic specimens. J. Anat. & Physiol., Lond., 1880–81, xv, 349–354.—**Strasser** (H.) Ueber das Studium der Schnittserien und über die Hülfsmittel, welche die Reconstruction der zerlegten Form erleichtern. Ztschr. f. wissensch. Mikr., Brnschwg., 1886, iii, 179–195. ——. Ueber die Nachbehandlung von Serienschnitten bei Paraffineinbettung. *Ibid.*, 346–350. ——. Nachbehandlung der Schnitte bei Paraffineinbettung. *Ibid.*, 1887, iv, 44–46.—**Suffolk** (W. T.) On microscopical manipulation. Chem. News, Lond., 1869, xx, 145; 157; 169; 181; 193; 207; 219; 231; 243; 255; 265; 291; 301; 318.—**Tait** (L.) On the freezing process for section-cutting, and on various methods of staining and mounting sections. J. Anat. & Physiol., Lond., 1875, ix, 249–258.—**Thoma** (R.) Beitrag zur mikroskopischen Technik. Arch. f. path. Anat., etc., Berl., 1875, lxv, 36–47, 1 pl.—**Toldt** (C.) Ueber die neue-

Microscopy (*Manipulations and preparations in*).

ren Präparir-Methoden und die dadurch bedingten Fortschritte der Histologie. Wien. med. Wchnschr., 1871, xxi, 260–264.—**Tourneux** (F.) Technique microscopique; note sur l'emploi de la carthamine. Compt. rend. Soc. de biol. 1881, Par., 1882, 7. s., iii, 97.—**Tuke** (J. B.) On a handy method of examining morbid nervous tissues microscopically. Brit. M. J., Lond., 1874, ii, 304.—**Unna** (P. G.) Ueber weitere Versuche, Farben auf dem Gewebe zu erzeugen und die chemische Theorie der Färbung. Arch. f. mikr. Anat., Bonn, 1887, xxx, 38–48.—**Van Heurck** (H.) Nouvelle préparation du médium à haut indice (2. 4) et note sur le liquidambar. Bull. Soc. belge de micr., Brux., 1886-7, xiii, 20–24.—**Ville** (J.) Préparation de la masse neutre au carmin et à la gélatine. Gaz. hebd. d. sc. méd. de Montpel., 1882, iv, 87; 112.—**Vlacovich** (G.) Sopra l' uso dell' acido fenico nelle preparazioni microscopiche. Atti r. Ist. Veneto di sc.. lett. ed arti, Venezia, 1878, 5. s., iv, 851–868.—**Voinoff** (K. G.) Neskolko zamech. otnositel. nakleiki mikrosk. srezov na predmet. stekla. [On the different cements for mounting microscopic sections.] Ejened. klin. gaz., St. Petersb., 1887, vii, 411–416.—**W.** Double staining of vegetable tissues. Am. Month. Micr. J., N. Y., 1880, i, 81–83.—**Waddington** (H. J.) The action of tannin on the cilia of infusoria, with remarks on the use of solution of sulphurous oxide in alcohol. J. Roy. Micr. Soc., Lond., 1883, 2. s., iii, 185–188.—**Wedl** (C.) Ueber die Anwendung von Levulose zur Aufbewahrung mikroskopischer Präparate. Arch. f. path. Anat., etc., Berl., 1877, lxxi, 128–130.—**Weigert** (C.) Zur Technik der mikroskopischen Bakterienuntersuchungen; mit einem casuistischen Anhange. Ibid., 1881, lxxxiv, 275–315. ———. Ueber Schnittserien von Colloidinpräparaten des Centralnervensystems zum Zwecke der Markscheidenfärbung. Ztschr. f. wissensch. Mikr., Brnschwg., 1885, ii, 490–495. ———. Ueber Aufhellung von Schnittserien aus Celloidinpräparaten. Ibid., 1886, iii, 480.—**Whitman** (C. O.) Methods of microscopical research in the zoological station in Naples. Am. Naturalist, Phila., 1881, xv, 697; 772. Also, transl.: J. de microg., Par., 1882, vi, 558: 1883, vii, 18; 89; 188.—**Wickersheimer.** Conservirungsflüssigkeit. Ztschr. f. Mikr., Berl., 1879–80, ii, 192–194.—**Witt** (O. N.) Untersuchungen über einige zu mikroskopischen Zwecken verwandte Harze. Ztschr. f. wissensch. Mikr., Brnschwg., 1886, iii, 196–206.—**Woodward** (J. J.) On the use of aniline in histological researches, with a method of investigating the histology of the human intestine, and remarks on some of the points to be observed in the study of the diseased intestine in camp fevers and diarrhœas. Am. J. M. Sc., Phila., 1865, n. s., xlix, 106–113. ———. On the permanent preservation of histological preparations as practised at the Army Medical Museum, Washington, D. C. Ibid., 1869, n. s., lvii, 277–281. ———. Reply to Lionel S. Beale. [Controversy on the best material for the preservation of soft tissues.] Lens, Chicago, 1872, i, 208–210. Also, Reprint.—**Ziemacki** (J.) Zur Entfettung mikroskopischer Präparate von Eiter, Blut, Sputum, u. s. w., vor der Tinction in wässerigen Farbelösungen bei Untersuchung auf Mikroorganismen. St. Petersb. med. Wchnschr., 1885, n. F., ii, 130. **Zuppinger** (H.) Eine Methode Axencylinderfortsätze der Ganglienzellen des Rückenmarkes zu demonstriren. Arch. f. mikr. Anat., Berl., 1874, x, 255.

Microscopy (*Medical*).

See, also, **Diagnosis**; **Diagnosis** (*Chemical, etc.*); **Histology**; **Pathology**; **Toxicology**; **Urine** (*Chemistry, etc., of*).

BEALE (L. S.) The microscope and its application to clinical medicine. 8°. *London*, 1854.

———. The use of the microscope in clinical medicine. 8°. *London*, 1857.

———. The microscope in its application to practical medicine. 2. ed. 8°. *London*, 1858.

———. The same. 3. ed. 8°. *London*, 1867.

———. The same 3. ed. 8°. *Philadelphia*, 1867.

———. The microscope in medicine. 4. ed. 8°. *London & Philadelphia*, 1878.

BEAUREGARD (H.) & GALIPPE (V.) Guide de l'élève et du praticien pour les travaux pratiques de micrographie, comprenant la technique et les applications du microscope à l'histologie végétale, à la physiologie, à la clinique, à l'hygiène et à la médecine légale. 8°. *Paris*, 1880.

BENNETT (J. H.) On the employment of the microscope in medical studies. A lecture. 8°. *Edinburgh*, 1841.

Microscopy (*Medical*).

BIZZOZERO (G.) Manuale di microscopia clinica, con aggiunte risguardanti gli esami chimici più utili al pratico e l' uso del microscopio nella medicina legale. Seconda edizione completamente rifusa ed aumentata. 8°. *Milano*, 1882.

———. The same. Handbuch der klinischen Mikroskopie. Mit Berücksichtigung der wichtigsten chemischen Untersuchungen am Krankenbette und der Verwendung des Mikroskopes in der gerichtlichen Medicin. Autorisirte deutsche Original-Ausgabe besorgt von Alexander Lustig und Stefan Bernheimer. Mit einem Vorwort von Hermann Nothnagel. 8°. *Erlangen*, 1883.

———. The same. 2. Aufl. 8°. *Erlangen*, 1887.

———. The same. Manuel de microscopie clinique, avec des instructions sur l'emploi du microscope, en médecine légale, et sur les opérations d'analyse chimique les plus utiles au praticien. Trad. de l'italien par C. Firket. 8°. *Bruxelles*, 1883.

——— & FIRKET (C.) Manuel de microscopie clinique, microscopie légale, chimie clinique, technique bactérioscopique. 2. éd. française. 8°. *Paris & Bruxelles*, 1885.

COLLINGWOOD (C.) The influence of the microscope upon the progressive advance of medicine. An address. 8°. *Liverpool*, 1859.

COULIER (P.) Manuel pratique de microscopie appliquée à la médecine. 12°. *Paris*, 1859.

CUTTER (E.) Primer of the clinical microscope. Boston Optical Works. 8°. *Boston*, 1879.

DONNÉ (A.) Cours de microscopie complémentaire des études médicales; anatomie microscopique et physiologie des fluides de l'économie. 8°. *Paris*, 1844.

———. The same. Die Microscopie als Hilfswissenschaft der Medicin; microscopische Anatomie und Physiologie der thierischen Flüssigkeiten. Nach dem Französischen bearbeitet . . . von E. von Gorup-Besanez. 8°. *Erlangen*, 1846.

——— & FOUCAULT (L.) Cours de microscopie complémentaire des études médicales, anatomie microscopique et physiologie des fluides de l'économie. Atlas, fol. *Paris*, 1845.

DRIESEN (G. M.) * De microscopio, summo medici auxilio. 8°. *Berolini*, [1842].

VON DÜBEN (F. G. W. J.) * Öfversigt af de bidrag mikroskopet lemnat till den medicinska diagnostiken. 8°. *Stockholm*, 1855.

DUVAL (M.) & LEREBOULLET (L.) Manuel du microscope dans ses applications au diagnostic et à la clinique. 12°. *Paris*, 1873.

———. The same. 2. éd. 12°. *Paris*, 1877.

FRIEDLAENDER (C.) The use of the microscope in clinical and pathological examinations. 2. ed. Transl. . . . by Henry C. Coe. 8°. *New York*, 1885.

GIUDICI (V.) Il microscopio, e sue applicazioni agli studj medici. 8°. *Milano*, 1870.

HALTENBERGER (F.) * Mikroskopisch-pathologische Betrachtungen. [Munich.] 8°. *Würzburg*, 1867.

HARTING (P.) Over de belangrijkheid van mikroskopische onderzoekingen voor de geneeskunde. 8°. *Utrecht*, 1844.

HEINRICH (C. B.) Microscopische und chemische Beiträge zur practischen Medicin. 8°. *Bonn*, 1844.

HOEFLE (M. A.) De scheikunde en het mikroskoop aan het ziekbed. Eene bijdrage tot de geneeskundige herkennigsleer, vor den Nederduitschen lezer bewerkt door Dr. Henry Riehm. Met een woord tot inleiding van den hoogleeraar

Microscopy (*Medical*).

Dr. J. van Geuns. 8°. *Utrecht & Amsterdam*, 1852.

MERKEL (G. H.) Microscopy in medical practice; its necessity demonstrated in the investigation of disease. 8°. *New York*, 1881.

PEYER (A.) Die Microscopie am Krankenbette. sm. 4°. *Basel*, 1884.

———. The same. An atlas of clinical microscopy. Translated and edited by Alfred C. Girard. 1. Am. ed. 8°. *New York*, 1885.

———. The same. Atlas de microscopie clinique. Traduit sur la 2. éd. allemande par le Dr. Eugène De la Harpe. sm. 4°. *Paris*, 1887.

PORCHER (F. P.) Prize essay. Illustrations of disease with the microscope. Clinical investigations, aided by the microscope, and by chemical reagents; with microscopical observations of pathological specimens, medical and surgical, obtained in Charleston, S. C. A contribution intended to disclose the minute history of the diseases prevailing in this latitude, and to assist future students. With upwards of five hundred original drawings from nature, made at the time of the observations. Part first, with one hundred illustrations on wood. 8°. *Charleston, S. C.*, 1861.

REINHARD (H.) Das Mikroskop und sein Gebrauch für den Arzt. Mit Zugrundelegung des Werkes von Beale: "The microscope and its application to clinical medicine". 8°. *Leipzig u. Heidelberg*, 1857.

———. The same. 2. Aufl. 8°. *Leipzig*, 1864.

RICHARDSON (J. G.) A handbook of medical microscopy. 8°. *Philadelphia*, 1871.

ROSENBERG (D.) De microscopii usu in diagnostica. 4°. *Gottingæ*, [1847].

SAUREL (L.) * Du microscope au point de vue de ses applications à la connaissance et du traitement des maladies chirurgicales. 8°. *Paris*, 1857.
Concours.

SIMON (J. F.) Beiträge zur physiologischen und pathologischen Chemie und Mikroskopie in ihrer Anwendung auf die praktische Medizin. v. 1. 8°. *Berlin*, 1844.

STOEBER (V.) * De l'influence que l'analyse chimique et la micrographie ont exercée sur la pathologie et sur la thérapeutique. 4°. *Strasbourg*, 1845.
Concours.

STOWELL (C. H.) & STOWELL (L. R.) Microscopical diagnosis. 8°. *Detroit*, 1882.

VERDUC, le fils. Discours sur l'utilité du microscope, dans les découvertes d'anatomie, de physique et de médecine. 12°. [*n. p., n. d.*]

VOGEL (J.) Beiträge zur Kenntniss der Säfte und Excrete des menschlichen Körpers im gesunden und kranken Zustande. 1. Bd. Anleitung zum Gebrauch des Mikroskopes zur zoochemischen Analyse und zur mikroskopisch-chemischen Untersuchung überhaupt. 8°. *Leipzig*, 1841.

Allen (B. W.) Use and importance of the microscope to the medical profession. Tr. M. Soc. W. Virg., Wheeling, 1871, 242–249. — **Bennett** (J. H.) Histology and the use of the microscope. Lancet, Lond., 1845, i, 517–522.— **Burnett** (W. J.) Observations on the value of the microscope as a means for the diagnosis of disease. South. M. & S. J., Augusta, 1853, n. s., ix. 197–206. — **Cutter** (E.) The primer of the clinical microscope. Virginia M. Month., Richmond, 1879–80, vi, 376; 446.—**Danforth** (I. N.) The microscope in daily practice. Chicago M. J. & Exam., 1875, xxxii, 659; 737; 807; 1876, xxxiii, 116. — **De Hart** (J. N.) The microscope in its relation to medicine and cerebral pathology. *Ibid.*, 1879, xxxviii, 242–253. *Also*, Reprint.—**Edwards** (A. M.) The microscope in gynæcology. Tr. M. Soc. N. Jersey, Newark, 1875, 140–160.—**Falk** (F.) Bemerkungen über einige zweckdienliche Anwendungsweisen des Mikroskopes und des Spectralapparates

Microscopy (*Medical*).

für gerichtliche Zwecke. Vrtljschr. f. d. prakt. Heilk., Prag, 1869, ci, 40–58.— **Fischl** (J.) Zur praktischen Bedeutung der Mikroskopie bei Erkrankungen innerer Organe. Prag. med. Wchuschr., 1876, i, 853; 873.—**Forman** (D. M'L.) The microscope in medical jurisprudence. Tr. M. Soc. N. Jersey, Newark, 1876, 252–257.—**Gallard** (T.) Le microscope: ce qu'il a promis; ce qu'il a donné. Union méd., Par., 1859, 2. s., iii, 280–285. — **Heinrich** (C. B.) Ueber die Vortheile, welche der practische Arzt von der Anwendung des Mikroskopes bei Krankheiten der Respirationsorgane erwarten darf. Ztschr. f. rat. Med., Heidelb., 1846, iv, 71–90.—**Heitzmann** (C.) The aid which medical diagnosis receives from recent discoveries in microscopy. Richmond & Louisville M. J., Louisville, 1879, xxv, 255–275. — **Holmes** (O. W.) An address delivered at the annual meeting of the Boston Microscopical Society. Boston M. & S. J., 1877, xcvi, 601–612.—**Johnston** (C.), **McSherry** (R.) & **Wilkins** (J.) Report of the committee upon surgery. Proc. M. & Chir. Fac. Maryland 1854, Balt., 1855, 21–53.—**Michel.** Du microscope, de ses applications à l'anatomie pathologique, au diagnostic et au traitement des maladies. Mém. Acad. de méd., Par., 1857, xxi, 241–442, 5 pl. *Also*, Reprint.—**Mouncret.** De la microscopie dans ses rapports avec la médecine pratique. J. de méd., Par., 1844, ii, 177–182. — **Ollivier.** Nouvelle application de l'emploi du microscope dans les expertises médico-légales. Ann. d'hyg., Par., 1839, xxi, 219–223. — **Packard** (J. H.) The present state of microscopical science, medically considered. N. Am. M.-Chir. Rev., Phila., 1859, iii, 470; 658.—**Pfuhl.** Einiges über die Bedeutung der Mikroskopie des Auswurfs für den Militairarzt, sowie über deren Technik und wichtigsten Resultate. Deutsche mil.-ärztl. Ztschr., Berl., 1878, vii, 240–263. — **Prophetisches** über das Microscop. Von einem ungenannten franz. Arzte. Med. Alm., Berl., 1841, 73–85.—**Ramaer** (J. N.) Over de aanwending van het mikroskoop tot geneeskundig onderzoek. Arch. v. Geneesk., Amst., 1841, i, 305–368. *Also*, Reprint.—**Ritter** (B.) Ueber die Anwendbarkeit des Mikroskopes zu medizinisch-forensischen Zwecken. Ztschr. f. d. Staatsarznk., Erlang., 1853, lxv, 111–145.—**Schützenberger.** Les recherches microscopiques et la clinique médicale. [Discours.] Gaz. méd. de Strasb., 1860, xx, 49–54. — **Seiler** (C.) The judicious use of the microscope in medical practice. Proc. Phila. Co. M. Soc. 1880–81, Phila., 1881, iii, 23–25. *Also*: Phila. M. Times, 1880–81, xi, 193–195.—**Szokalski** (W.) O stanowisku mikroskopii i chemii w praktycznej medycynie. Pam. Towarz. Lek. Warszaw., 1855, xxxiv, 9–28. — **Virchow** (R.) Ueber die Reform der pathologischen und therapeutischen Anschauungen durch die mikroskopischen Untersuchungen. Arch. f. path. Anat., etc. Berl., 1847, i, 207–255.—**Ward** (R. H.) Medical microscopes. Tr. M. Soc. N. Y. 1872, Albany, 1873, 267–275. — **Wright** (J. W.) The microscope in its relation to disease. Proc. Connect. M. Soc., Hartford, 1886, n. s., iii, no. 3, 75–81.—**Wyss** (O.) Ueber die Bedeutung der Mikroskopie und Chemie in der ärztlichen Diagnostik. Wien. med. Presse, 1868, ix, 185; 209; 233. *Also*: Memorabilien, Heilbr., 1868, xiii, 85–92.

Microscopy (*Preparations of*).

See Microscopy (*Manipulations, etc., in*).

Microspectroscopy.

See Spectroscope, *etc.*

Microtomes *and microtomy.*

See, *also*, Microorganisms (*Manipulations, etc., in*).

HIS (W.) Beschreibung eines Mikrotoms. 4°. [*n. p., n. d.*]

LEE (A. B.) The microtomist's vade-mecum. A handbook of the methods of microscopic anatomy. 8°. *London*, 1885.

———. The same. 8°. *Philadelphia*, 1885.

MARSH (S.) Section-cutting. A practical guide to the preparation and mounting of sections for the microscope, special prominence being given to the subject of animal sections. 12°. *London*, 1878.

———. The same. 2. ed. 12°. *London*, 1882.

Barrett (J. W.) A new method of cutting sections for microscopical examination. J. Anat. & Physiol., Lond., 1884–5, xix, 94–96.—**Bickerstaff** (R.) A freezing microtome for use with ether spray. Dublin J. M. Sc., 1877, lxiv, 423.—**Brandt** (A.) Ueber ein Mikrotom. Arch. f. mikr. Anat., Bonn, 1871, vii, 175–179.—**Brass** (A.) Bemerkungen über die Mikrotommesser und ihre Behandlung. Ztschr. f. wissensch. Mikr., Brnschwg., 1885, ii, 305–307.—**Caldwell's** automatic microtome. Quart. J. Micr. Sc., Lond., 1884, n. s., xxiv, 648–654, 1 pl.—**Cathcart** (C. W.) New form of ether microtome. J. Anat. & Physiol., Lond., 1882–3, xvii, 401–403. *Also*: Edinb. Clin. & Path. J., 1883–4, i, 473–475. — **Curtis** (E.) An

Microtomes *and microtomy.*

apparatus for cutting microscopic sections of the eye. Tr. Am. Ophth. Soc., N. Y., 1871, viii, 60 - 68. — **Decker** (F.) Ein neuer Schnittstrecker. Arch. f. mikr. Anat., Bonn, 1884, xxiii, 537-543.—**von Dembowski** (T.) Ein neuer Apparat zur Controlle der Messerstellung im Mikrotom. Ztschr. f. wissensch. Mikr., Brnschwg., 1886, iii, 337-345.— **Duprat** (A.) Microtome de précision. Bull. Soc. anat. de l'ar. 1886, lxi. 355.—**Erdös** (J.) Eine Vorrichtung am Thoma'schen Mikrotom zum Schnellschneiden. Internat. Monatschr. f. Anat. u. Histol., Berl., 1885, ii, 343-346, 2 pl. *Also, transl :* Orvosi hetil., Budapest, 1885, xxix, 982-984. — **Fleming** (W. J.) A modification of Dr. Rutherford's freezing microtome. Month. Micr. J., Lond., 1875, xiv, 79-81. *Also:* Lancet, Lond., 1875, i, 855.—**Fletcher** (S. W.) A new microtome. Boston M. & S. J., 1879, c, 254-257.—**Francotte** (P.) Microtomes, méthodes d'inclusion et sériation des coupes. Bull. scient. dép. du nord, etc., Par., 1883, vi, 137-145. ——. Microtomes de Reichert. Bull. Soc. belge de micr., Brux., 1884-5, xi, 102-107, 4 pl.— **Fritsch** (G.) Ueber eine neue Modification des Rivet'schen Mikrotoms. Arch. f. Anat., Physiol. u. wissensch. Med., Leipz., 1874, 442-453. *Also,* Reprint.—**Gage** (S. H.) & **Smith** (T.) Serial microscopic sections. Med. Student, N. Y., 1883-4, i, 14-16.—**Golding-Bird** (C. H.) On a new microtome. J. Roy. Micr. Soc., Lond., 1884, 2. s., iv, 523.—**Gottschau** (M.) Mikrotomklammer für Keil- und planparallele Schnitte. Sitzungsb. d. phys.-med. Gesellsch. zu Würzb., 1881, 123-125. ——. Vorzüge und Nachtheile verschiedener Mikrotome und ihrer Hilfs-apparate. Ztschr. f. wissensch. Mikr., Brnschwg., 1884, i, 327-348.—**Grönland** (J.) Das Rivet'sche Mikrotom und seine Handhabung. Ztschr. f. Mikr., Berl., 1877, i, 8-15.—**Groves** (J. W.) A further improvement in the Groves-Williams ether freezing microtome. J. Roy. Micr. Soc., Lond., 1882, 2. s., ii, 755.—**von Gudden.** Ueber ein neues Microtom. Arch. f. Psychiat. u. Nervenkr., Berl., 1874, v, 229-234. ——. Katsch's Microtom. Arch. f. Psychiat., Berl., 1880, xi, 542.—**Hailes** (H. F.) On a new form of section-cutting machine. J. Quekett Micr. Club, Lond., 1874-7, iv, 243-245, 1 pl. ——. Sections and section cutting; with a description of a new poly-microtome for freezing. Am. J. Insan., Utica, N. Y., 1878-9, xxxv, 503-514. *Also,* Reprint. ——. An improved micro-tome; two hundred sections a minute, each $\frac{1}{2000}$ of an inch in thickness. Med. Rec., N. Y., 1880, xviii, 109. ——. An improved microtome. Science, N. Y., 1880, i, 187. ——. An improved freezing poly-microtome. Tr. M. Soc. N. Y., Syracuse, 1882, 279-281.—**Hatfield** (J. J. B.) Description of rotary section cutter. Proc. Am. Soc. Micr., Buffalo, 1884, vii, 171.—**Hawksley's** improved Valentin's knife. Lancet, Lond., 1870, i, 13.—**Henking** (H.) Neue Construction des Objecthalters am Schlitten-mikrotom, eine genaue Einstellung des Objectes bezweckend. Ztschr. f. wissensch. Mikr., Brnschwg., 1884, i, 491-496. ——. Ein einfaches Mikrotommesser. *Ibid.,* 1885, ii, 509-511.—**Henneguy.** Un microtome. Compt. rend. Soc. de biol., Par., 1882, 7. s., iv, 591.—**Henneguy & Vignal.** Sur quelques modifications apportées au microtome à bascule de la Société des instruments scientifiques de Cambridge. *Ibid.,* 1885, 8. s., ii, 647.—**Henschen** (S.) Tvenne mikrotomer. Upsala Läkaref. Förh., 1881, xvi, 311-321.—**Hildebrand** (H. E.) Improved microtome for cutting microscopic sections. Pharmacist, Chicago, 1885, xix, 105-107. *Also, transl.:* Ztschr. f. wissensch. Mikr., Brnschwg., 1885, ii, 343-345.— **His** (W.) Beschreibung eines Mikrotoms. Arch. f. mikr. Anat., Bonn, 1870, vi, 229-232.—**Holler** (A.) Ueber eine neue Schnittmethode für mikroskopische Präparate des Hirns und Rückenmarks. Mitth. d. Ver. d. Aerzte in Nied.-Oest., Wien, 1876, ii, 60-63.—**Hughes** (R.) An improved freezing microtome. J. Anat. & Physiol., Lond., 1876, ii, 615.—**Johnston-Lavis** (H. J.) & **Vosmaer** (G. C. J.) On cutting sections of sponges and other similar structures with soft and hard tissues. J. Roy. Micr. Soc., Lond., 1887, 200-204.—**Klebs** (E.) Eine Schneidemaschine zur Anfertigung mikroskopischer Präparate, nebst Bemerkungen über mikroskopisches Schneiden. Arch. f. exper. Path. u. Pharmakol., Leipz., 1876, vi, 205-215.—**Knives** for cutting sections. [Edit.] Am. J. Micr., N. Y., 1879, iv, 25-30.—**Körting.** Ein neues Mikrotom. Jenaische Ztschr. f. Naturw., Jena, 1880, n. F., vii, 193-195.—**Krause** (W.) Ueber Mikrotome. Arch. f. mikr. Anat., Bonn, 1876, xiii, 180.—**Lewis** (B.) On a new freezing microtome for the preparation of sections of the brain and spinal cord. J. Anat. & Physiol., Lond., 1877, xi, 537-539.—**Longstreth** (M.) Freezing microtome. Tr. Path. Soc. Phila., 1878, vii, 159. ——. The use of the freezing microtome. Boston M. & S. J., 1879, c, 632-636.—**Luys.** Instrument pour les coupes microscopiques. Bull. Soc. anat. de Par., 1868, xliii, 448.—**Malassez** (L.) Microtome de Roy perfectionné. Compt. rend. Soc. de biol., Par., 1883, 7. s., iv, 423-425. *Also:* Arch. de physiol. norm. et path., Par., 1884, 3. s., iv, 348-363.—**Martinotti** (G.) Un piccolo accessorio dei microtomi a slitta. Ztschr. f. wissensch. Mikr., Brnschwg., 1886, iii, 390-392.—**Nealey** (E. T.) A rapid method for making bone and teeth sections. Am. Month. Micr. J.,

Microtomes *and microtomy.*

N. Y., 1884, v, 142-144.—**Needham** (J.) On cutting sections of animal tissues for microscopical examination. Med. Press & Circ., Lond., 1873, xv, 491; 512.—**New** microtome of Dr. S. W. Fletcher. J. Roy. Micr. Soc., Lond., 1879, ii, 466-469.—**Pelletan** (J.) Microtome à levier (Hansen). J. de microg . Par., 1886, x, 507-512.—**Piana** (G. P.) Il microtomo del Prof. Ercolani. Arch. per le sc. med., Torino, 1876-7, i. 454-457.—**Pritchard** (U.) A simple form of freezing section machine. Lancet, Lond., 1875, ii, 833.—**Purkinje.** Der microtomische Quetscher, ein bei microscopischen Untersuchungen unentbehrliches Instrument. Arch. f. Anat., Physiol. u. wissensch. Med., Berl., 1834, 385-390, 1 pl. —**Revolving** automatic microtome. Johns Hopkins Univ. Stud. biol. lab., Balt., 1884-7, iii, 477-479.—**Rogers** (W. A.) On a new form of section-cutter. Proc. Am. Soc. Micr., Buffalo, 1884, vii, 191-193.—**Rohrbeck** (H.) Dr. R. Long's neues Mikrotom. Breslau. aerztl. Ztschr., 1886, viii, 284.—**Roy** (C. S.) A new microtome. J. Physiol., Lond., 1879-80, ii, 19-23. ——. Neues Schnellgefrier-Microtom. Arch. f. mikr. Anat., Bonn, 1880-81, xix, 137-143, 1 pl.—**Russell** (J. C.) Immersion microtome. Brit. M. J., Lond., 1880, i, 664.— **Rutherford** (W.) A new freezing microtome. Lancet, Lond., 1873, ii, 108. ——. On the freezing microtome; a reply to Mr. Lawson Tait. J. Anat. & Physiol., Lond., 1875, x, 178-185. ——. A combined ice and ether-spray freezing microtome. Lancet, Lond., 1885, i, 4-6.—**Ryder** (J. A.) On some points in microtomy. [Abstr.] Proc. Am. Ass. Adv. Sc. 1884, Salem, 1885, xxxiii, 565.—**Schiefferdecker** (P.) Ueber ein neues Mikrotom, nebst Bemerkungen über einige neuere Instrumente dieser Art. Arch. f. mikr. Anat., Bonn, 1875, xii, 91-102. ——. Kurze Mittheilung, mein Mikrotom betreffend. *Ibid.,* 1876, xii, 791. ——. Ueber ein neues Mikrotom. Ztschr. f. wissensch. Mikr., Brnschwg., 1886, iii, 151-164. —**Schmidt** (H. D.) Apparatus for making microscopic sections of tissue. Am. J. M. Sc., Phila., 1859, n. s., xxxvii, 35-40.—**Seiler** (C.) Immersion microtome. Phila. M. Times, 1879-80, x, 197. *Also:* Proc. Phila. Co. M. Soc., Phila., 1880, ii, 29. ——. Mechanical microtome. Tr. Path. Soc. Phila., 1880, ix, 184.—**Servel** (A.) Note sur un microtome. Arch. de physiol. norm. et path., Par., 1875, 2. s., i, 972-974.—**Smith** (R. S.) New method of section-cutting after freezing by means of ether spray. Lancet, Lond., 1878, i, 605.—**Sollas** (J.) An improvement in the method of using the freezing microtome. Quart. J. Micr. Sc., Lond., 1884, n. s., xxiv, 163.—**Spengel** (J. W.) August Becker's Schlittenmikrotom. Ztschr. f. wissensch. Mikr., Brnschwg., 1885, ii, 453-459.—**Sterling** (A. B.) Description of a section cutter for microscopical purposes. J. Anat. & Physiol., Lond., 1870, iv, 230-234.—**Taylor** (T.) Freezing microtome. Proc. Am. Ass. Adv. Sc. 1881, Salem, 1883, xxx, 119-121. *Also,* Reprint.—**von Thanhoffer** (L.) Ein Irrigationsmesser zur Anfertigung mikroskopischer Schnittpräparate. Arch. f. mikr. Anat., Bonn, 1880-81, xix, 315-317.—**Thoma** (R.) Ueber ein Mikrotom. Arch. f. path. Anat., etc., Berl., 1881, lxxxiv, 189-191. ——. Microtome à glissement et méthodes d'enrobage. J. de microg., Par., 1883, vii, 576 ; 939.—**Tricomi** (E.) Nuovo microtomo a mano. Riv. internaz. di med. e chir., Napoli, 1886, iv, 279-282.—**Vignal.** Sur le microtome congelant de Rutherford. J. de l'anat. et physiol., etc., Par., 1875, xi, 482-486. ——. Sur un microtome congelant par la vaporisation de l'ammoniaque. *Ibid.,* 1876, xii, 425-428.—**Waller** (B. C.) On a new form of section-knife especially adapted to the cutting of large sections. Edinb. M. J., 1878-9, xxiv, 893-895.—**Webster** (C. C.) A simple microtome. Chicago M. J. & Exam., 1885, l, 12.—**Weigert** (C.) Nowy mikrotom do dużych skrawków. [New microtome for large segments.] Gaz. lek., Warszawa, 1884. 2. s., iv, 1028 - 1032. *Also, transl.:* Ztschr. f. wissensch. Mikr., Brnschwg., 1885, ii, 326-333.— **Whitney** (J. E.) Rapid section cutting. Proc. Am. Soc. Micr., Buffalo, 1885, viii, 122.—**Williams** (R. P.) On cutting sections of the eyes of insects, and on a new instrument for that purpose. J. Quekett Micr. Club, Lond., 1874-7, iv, 4-10, 1 pl. ——. On a new method of cutting fresh frozen tissues. *Ibid.,* 154-156, 1 pl.

Microzymes.
See Microorganisms.

Micturition.
See Urination.

Miculci (Jo. Benjam.) *De scorbuto, ejusdemque tum genuinis, tum controversis causis, symptomatibus praecipuis, et cura. 20 pp. 4°. *Erfordiae, typ. J. H. Groschii,* 1717.

Mid-Cheshire Combined Sanitary District. Vital statistics and annual reports of the sanitary districts of Altrincham, Congleton, Nantwich, and Northwich, rural; Lymm, Middlewich, Nantwich, Northwich, Sandbach, and Winsford,

Mid-Cheshire Combined [etc.]—continued.
urban. By John Mapinson Fox, medical officer of health. 1.-4., 1878-81. fol. [*v. p.*],
1879-82.

1. and 2., London; 3., Manchester; 4., Warrington.

Middel (Klaas Kuiper). * Bijdrage tot de behandeling van het purulent pleuritisch exsudaat.
2 p. l., 56 pp. 8°. *Groningen, J. B. Huber*,
1879.

Middelbeek (Sebastianus). * De incremento
fœtus humani in utero. 32 pp., 3 l. sm. 4°.
Lugd. Bat., J. A. Langerak, 1719.

Middelburg.

Fokker (A. A.) & **de Man** (J. C.) Proeve eener geneesk. plaatsbeschrijving van de stad Middelburg, Prov.
Zeeland. Tijdschr. d. Nederl. Maatsch. t. Bevord. d. Geneesk., Arnhem, 1856, vi, 2. Afd., 41-136.—**de Man** (J. C.)
De afname der sterfte te Middelburg. Nederl. Tijdschr.
v. Geneesk., Amst., 1882, xviii, 901-907.

Middelburg (Henry Abraham). * De zitplaats
van het astigmatisme. 45 pp., 2 tab. 8°. *Utrecht,
P. W. van de Weijer*, 1863.

Middeldorpf (Albrecht Theodor) [1824-68].
* De glandulis Brunnianis. 1 p. l., 35 pp., 1 pl.
4°. *Vratislaviæ, typ. Grassii, Barthii et soc.*,
[1846].

——. Der Namen und das Wesen der Entzündung. 32 pp. 8°. *Breslau, E. Trewendt*, 1849.

——. Bemerkungen über Knochenbrüche. (Allgemeiner Theil.) 1 p. l., 46 pp., 1 l. 4°. *Breslau, R. Nischkowsky*, 1852.

——. Beiträge zur Lehre von den Knochenbrüchen. x, 150 pp., 5 pl. 4°. *Breslau, Trewendt
u. Granier*, 1853.

——. Die Galvanocaustik, ein Beitrag zur operativen Medicin. xvi, 272 pp., 4 pl. 8°. *Breslau, J. Max u. Comp.*, 1854. [*Also, in* : P., v.
1389.]

——. Ueberblick über die Akidopeirastik, eine
neue Untersuchungs-Methode mit Hilfe spitziger
Werkzeuge. 10 pp., 1 pl. 8°. [*Breslau, R.
Nischkowsky*, 1856.] [P., v. 876; 1389.]

Repr. from : Ztschr. f. klin. Med., Bresl., 1856, vii.

——. De polypis œsophagi, atque de tumore
ejus generis primo prospere exstirpato. iv, 24
pp., 1 pl. 4°. *Vratislaviæ, apud Max et soc.*,
1857.

——. Commentatio de fistulis ventriculi externis et chirurgica earum sanatione, accedente
historia fistulæ arte chirurgorum plastica prospere curatæ. 3 p. l., 33 pp., 2 pl. 4°. *Vratislaviæ, typ. Grassii, Barthii et soc.*, 1859.

——. Abrégé de la galvanocaustie. 14 pp. 8°.
Breslau, G.-T. Korn, 1864.

See, also, **von Pfolsprundt** (Heinrich). Buch der
Bündth-Ertznei . . . 1460 [etc.] 8°. Berlin, 1868.—**Ver-
ein** für physiologische Heilkunde. Der Namen und das
Wesen der Entzündung. 8°. Breslau, 1849.

For Biography, see Arch. f. klin. Chir., Berl., 1869, x,
397-420 (Klopsch). Also : Deutsche Klinik, Berl., 1868,
xx, 318. Also : Gazz. med. ital. lomb., Milano, 1868, 6. s.,
i, 399-401 (P. Schivardi). Also : Wien. med. Wchnschr.,
1868, xviii, 1023-1026.

Middeldorpf (Gustav). * Weitere Beiträge
zur Resection des Ellenbogengelenkes. [Wurtz-
burg.] 207 pp. 8°. *Berlin, L. Schumacher,
1886.

Middelschulte (Fritz). * Ein Beitrag zu den
primären desmoiden Geschwülsten der breiten
Gebärmutterbänder. 30 pp. 8°. *Greifswald,
J. Abel*, 1884.

Middendorf (Joannes Henricus) [1816-   ].
* De pulsus symptomatologia. 29 pp., 1 l. 8°.
Berolini, typ. Nietackianis, [1840].

von Middendorff (Al. Theodorus). * Quædam de bronchorum polypis, morbi casu observato illustrata. 83 pp. 8°. *Dorpati Livonorum,
typ. G. C. Schuenmanni*, 1837.

Middendorp (Albert Anton). * Verhandeling
over placenta prævia. [Utrecht.] 2 p. l., 57

Middendorp (Albert Anton)—continued.
pp., 2 l. 8°. *Amsterdam, Metzler & Basting*,
1870.

——. Het geneeskundig staatstoezicht en de
geneeskundige stand in Nederland. 38 pp. 8°.
Amsterdam, Scheltema & Holkema, 1878.

Middendorp (Harmen Anthonij). * Over de
doorborende chronische maagzeer. 3 p. l., 63
pp., 2 l. 8°. *Groningen, J. B. Wolters*, [1863].

Middendorp (Hendrik Willem). De aanwending der geneesmiddelen door de huid bij
cholera. 7 pp. 8°. *Groningen, R. J. Schierbeek*,
1866. [P., v. 185.]

——. Het vliezig slakkenhuis in zijne wording
en in den ontwikkelden toestand. 1 p. l., 111
pp., 3 pl. fol. *Groningen, J. Schierbeek*, [1867].

Middle (The) States Medical Reformer and Advocate of Innocuous Medication. J. S. Pretty-
man and Palemon John, editors and proprietors.
[Monthly.] Nos. 10-12, v. 1, Dec., 1854, to Feb.,
1855; Nos. 2, 4, 6, 8-12, v. 2, 1855-6; Nos. 1-3,
5-10, v. 3, 1856-7; No. 1, v. 4, May, 1857. 8°.
Millford, Del., 1854-5; *Millville, Pa.*, 1855-7;
Bloomsburg, Pa., 1857.

Title of v. 3-4 was: **Middle** (The) States Medical Reformer and Journal of Health. In 1858 continued as:
Eclectic (The) Medical Journal of Philadelphia.

Middle (The) States Medical Reformer and
Journal of Health.

Was title of v. 3-4 of: **Middle** (The) States Medical
Reformer and Advocate of Innocuous Medication.

Middleborough, *Massachusetts*.

Thompson (I.) Bill of mortality for Middleborough
in the years 1802 and 1803. Coll. Mass. Hist. Soc. 1804,
Bost., 1857, 235.

Middlebury.

See **Prostitution** (*History, etc., of*), by localities.

Middlebury College. Catalogus senatus academici et eorum qui munera et officia academica
gesserunt, quique aliquovis gradu exornati fuerunt, in Collegio Medioburiensi, Medioburiæ, in
Republica Viridimontana, anno 1871. 61 pp.
8°. *Medioburiæ, Knapp et sociis*, 1871.

Middlemore (Richard). Arrangement to be
adopted in the delivery of a course of lectures on
the diseases of the eye. 8 pp. 8°. *Birmingham,
J. C. Barlow*, 1832. [P., v. 515; 745.]

——. An address to the governors of the Birmingham General Hospital on the propriety of
appointing assistant surgeons to that institution.
15 pp. 8°. *Birmingham, J. Drake*, 1833. [P.,
v. 515.]

——. A treatise on the diseases of the eye and
its appendages. [Founded on a Jacksonian
prize essay for 1831.] 2 v. viii, 800 pp.; x, 844,
14 pp. 8°. *London, Longmans & Co.*, 1835.

——. An introductory lecture on the anatomy,
physiology, and diseases of the eye, delivered at
the Birmingham Royal School of Medicine and
Surgery, Oct. 4, 1839. 1 p. l., 30 pp. 8°. *London, Longman* [*and others*], 1839. [*Also, in* : P.,
v. 1442.]

Middlesborough.

Buchanan (G.) Report on the sanitary state of Mid-
dlesbrough-on-Tees, July 1, 1871. Collection of special reports, fol., Lond., i, no. 63.

Middlesex County, England. Annual report
of the coroner for the central district of Middlesex. 7., 1868-9. 38 pp. 8°. *London, R. Hardwicke*, 1871.

Repr. from : "Sessional Proc." Nat. Ass. Promot. Social Sc.

Middlesex County, England. *County Lunatic
Asylum at Colney Hatch.* The final report of
the committee appointed to provide an additional pauper lunatic asylum, and resolutions
of the court. Middlesex, Jan., general quarter

Middlesex County, England. *County Lunatic Asylum at Colney Hatch*—continued. sessions, 1852. 94 pp. 8°. *London, J. T. Norris,* 1852.

Corner-stone laid May 31, 1849; opened July 17, 1851.

———. Medical report of the female side of the Colney Hatch Lunatic Asylum. 1., 1851. 48 pp. 8°. *London, Walton & Mitchell,* 1852.

———. Annual reports of the committee of visitors and medical superintendent to her majesty's justices of the peace for the county of Middlesex. 1.-31., 1851-81. 8°. *London,* 1852-82.

1851-80 bound in 6 v. 1. report for 6 months, ending Dec., 31.

Middlesex County, England. *County Lunatic Asylum at Hanwell.* Annual reports of the resident physician to the visiting justices. 1.-14., 1831 to 1843-4. 8°. *London,* 1832-44.

1.-14. bound in 1 v.
The committee or visiting justices was appointed early in 1827, and made their first report in April of that year. Site purchased in 1828. Building completed in April, and opened May 16, 1831. From April, 1827, to Dec., 1845, the visiting justices made 77 reports. In 1846 the asylum was placed under control of a committee of visitors, who commenced a new series of annual reports, their 3. report being the 81. of the asylum.

———. The reports of the visiting justices to the quarter sessions, 1828–42. [Being the 1.–64. quarterly reports, 3. qr. 1827 to 3. qr. 1842.] 2 v. 208 pp., 4 l.; 244 pp. 8°. *London, M'Gowan & Co.,* 1842.

———. Quarterly reports of the visiting justices to her majesty's justices of the peace for the county of Middlesex. 1.-64., 4. qr. 1827 to 3. qr. 1842; 68., 3. qr. 1843; 72., 3. qr. 1844; 74., 75., and 77., 1., 2., and 4. qr. 1845. 8°. *London,* 1833-46.

1.-64. reprinted in 2 v., 1842. 23., 49.-59., 64., 68., 72., 74., 75., and 77. are in separate pamphlet form. For reports subsequent to 1845, see annual reports of the committee of visitors, who succeeded the visiting justices.

———. The special report of the committee of visitors, with appendices. [May general session, 1846.] 33, 8, 19, 4 pp., 1 pl., 1 plan. 8°. *London, J. T. Norris,* 1846.

———. An address from the visiting justices to the magistrates of the county of Middlesex. 19 pp. 8°. *London, J. T. Norris,* 1846.

Bound with: Special report. 8°. *London,* 1846.

———. Memorial of the guardians of Chelsea as to further accommodation for pauper lunatics of the county. Presented to the court at the May general session, 1846. 4 pp., 1 pl., 1 plan. 8°. *London, J. T. Norris,* 1846.

Bound with: Special report. 8°. *London,* 1846.

———. Additional accommodation for pauper lunatics. A return of reports made to the committee of visitors by the medical officers. Presented to the court May general session, 1846. 8 pp. 8°. *London, J. T. Norris,* 1846.

Bound with: Special report. 8°. *London,* 1846.

———. Annual reports of the committee of visitors and medical superintendent to her majesty's justices of the peace for the county of Middlesex. 3.-16., 1847-60; 19., 1863; 21., 1865. 8°. *London,* 1848-66.

For reports prior to 1847, see quarterly reports of the visiting justices. 10.-16. bound in 1 v.

Middlesex County Orphans' Home. Middletown. Annual report of the board of managers to the incorporators. 1., 1877-8. 19 pp. 8°. *Middletown, Pelton & King,* 1879.

Incorporated Feb. 28, 1877; opened June, 1878.

Middlesex East District Society. By-laws, with a list of officers and members. 13 pp. 8°. *Wakefield, W. H. Troombly,* 1876.

Middlesex Fells Association. Map of Middlesex Fells, showing the territory situated in various towns designed to be set apart as a public

Middlesex Fells Association—continued. domain for the preservation and production of forest trees and the water supply of many cities and towns. Compiled by Fuller and Whitney. Nov., 1882. 1 map. 4°. *Boston,* 1882.

———. Conditional obligation, public domain, and the new forestry law. (Chap. 255, acts of 1882.) An act authorizing towns and cities to provide for the preservation and reproduction of of forests. Approved May 25, 1882. 2 l. fol. [*Boston,* 1882.]

———. [Circular, on the importance of restoring the pines to the barren hills of Massachusetts. Jan 15, 1883.] 1 sheet. 8°. [*Boston,* 1883.]

Middlesex and Hertfordshire Combined Sanitary Districts. Annual reports on the sanitary condition of . . . for the years 1876; 1879. By C. E. Saunders, medical officer of health. 8°. *London,* 1877-80.

The combined district is composed of Barnet, Berkhamstead, Hemel Hempstead, Hendon, St. Albans, Watford, and Welwyn (rural districts); Barnet, East Barnet Valley, and Tring (urban districts).

Middlesex Hospital, London, W. The laws, orders, and regulations of the Middlesex Hospital, for the reception of sick and lame patients, and lying-in married women; revised and digested under proper heads, [etc.] ii, 64 pp. 8°. *London,* 1770.

Instituted in Aug., 1745. In 1747 a ward was opened for lying-in married women, but was given up in 1807. In 1792 a ward was fitted up, and endowed by Samuel Whitbread, for patients afflicted with cancer. Samaritan fund established in 1812. A medical school was established in connection with the hospital, May 7, 1835. Incorporated March 30, 1836.

———. List of the governors and subscribers of the Middlesex Hospital; with an abstract of the receipts and expenditure for the year 1816. 43 pp., 2 l. 12°. *London, J. Brettell,* 1817.

———. History of the . . . during the first century of its existence. Compiled from the hospital records, by Erasmus Wilson. xv, 296 pp. 8°. *London. J. Churchill,* 1845.

———. List of the governors and subscribers of the . . . with an abstract of the receipts and expenditures for the year 1851; and an account of the Samaritan fund of the hospital. 72 pp. 8°. *London, J. Truscott,* 1852.

———. Report on the cholera patients admitted into the [Middlesex] hospital during the year 1854. By S. W. Sibley, registrar. 28 pp., 8 tab. 8°. *London, J. Truscott,* 1855.

———. Report of the surgical staff of the Middlesex Hospital, to the weekly board and governors, upon the treatment of cancerous diseases in the hospital, on the plan introduced by Dr. Fell. vi, 114 pp. 12°. *London, J. Churchill,* 1857.

———. Reports of the medical and surgical registrars for the years 1869-76; 1878-83. 8°. *London,* 1870-85.

1869-75 bound in 2 v.

———. Historical account of the origin and progress of "The Middlesex Hospital", with a list of the governors and subscribers, and an account of the Samaritan fund of the hospital, for the year 1872, together with an abstract of the receipts and expenditure for the years 1871 and 1872. 87 pp., 4 l. 8°. *London, J. Smith & Co.,* 1873.

———. Annual reports of the weekly board to the governors and subscribers, for the years 1872; 1877. 8°. *London,* 1873-8.

Middlesex Hospital Medical School, London. Annual prospectuses for the sessions of 1876-7 (42.); 1878-9 to 1880-81 (44.-46.); 1884-5 (50.); 1887-8 (53.). 12° & 8°. *London,* 1876-87.

———. Prospectus for the summer session for 1886. 32 pp. 8°. [*London*], *Mitchell & Hughes,* [1886].

Middlesex Hospital Medical School—cont'd.

——. Regulations of the Middlesex Hospital College. 8 pp. 18°. [*London, Mitchell & Hughes*, 1887.]

Founded for the accommodation of the students in 1887.

Middlesex Institute, Malden. Annual report. 1., 1881–2. 12 pp. 8°. *Malden, G. A. Brown*, 1882.

Middlesex South District Medical Society. Constitution and by-laws, with a catalogue of the fellows of the Massachusetts Medical Society, residing in the Middlesex South Medical District. 12 pp. 12°. *Waltham, S. Hastings*, 1857.

——. The same. 16 pp. 12°. *Cambridge, Welch, Bigelow & Co.*, 1870.

Middleton (A. E.) All about mnemonics. 74 pp. 12°. *London, Simpkin, Marshall & Co.*, 1885.

Middleton (Amos). A chemical analysis of the Lemington waters, with a practical dissertation on their medical effects, and instructions for cold and warm bathing. 3. ed. xvii, 73 pp. 8°. *Warwick, H. Sharpe*, 1814.

Middleton (Conyers). De medicorum apud veteres Romanos degentium conditione dissertatio; qua contra viros celeberrimos Jac. Sponium et Rich. Meadium, servilem atque ignobilem eam fuisse ostenditur. 27 pp. 4°. *Cantabrigiæ, E. Jeffrey*, 1726. [*Also, in:* P., v. 1065.]

——. Oratio de novo physiologiæ explicandæ munere. 29 pp. 4°. *London, G. Thurlbourn*, 1732. [P., v. 753; 1065.]

Middleton (Edvardus). * De febris continuæ curatione. 46 pp. 8°. *Edinburgi, R. Allan*, 1802. [P., v. 20.]

Middleton (John). A short essay on the operation of lithotomy as it is performed by the new method above the os pubis . . . to which is added a letter relating to the same subject, from Mr. Macgill, of Edinburgh, to Dr. Douglas. 72 pp., 1 pl. 4°. *London, G. Strahan*, 1727. [*Also, in:* P., v. 1066.]

Middleton (Peter). A medical discourse, or an historical inquiry into the ancient and present state of medicine. The substance of which was delivered at opening the medical school, in the city of New-York. ii, 72 pp. [With portr. of Myles Cooper.] 8°. *New-York, H. Gaine*, 1769.

Middletown, *Connecticut.*

See, also, **Fever** (*Cerebro-spinal, History, etc., of*), **Hospitals** (*Descriptions, etc., of*), **Insane** (*Asylums for, etc.*), by localities.

CONNECTICUT Industrial School for Girls, Middletown. Annual reports of the board of directors to the legislature and to the benefactors and friends. 2.–16., 1870—84–5. 8°. *Hartford & Middletown*, 1872–86.

Middletown, *New York.*

See, also, **Insane** (*Asylums for, etc.*), by localities.

Report on the sewerage and drainage of Middletown. Rep. State Bd. Health N. Y., Albany, 1886, vi, 212–218.

Midland Institution for the Blind, Nottingham. Annual reports of the committee to the subscribers. 36., 1878–9; 38., 41., 1880–81 to 1884. 8°. *Nottingham*, 1879–84.

Midland (The) Medical Miscellany. A monthly magazine of medicine and materia medica. Published by Richardson & Co. v. 1–3; Nos. 37–42, v. 4, Jan., 1882, to June, 1885. 8°. *Leicester.*

In 1883, v. 2, title became: **Midland** (The) Medical Miscellany, and Provincial Medical Journal. In July, 1885, continued as: **Provincial** (The) Medical Journal.

Midland (The) Medical Miscellany, and Provincial Medical Journal. A monthly review of medical science, literature, and biography.

Was title of v. 2–3 of: **Midland** (The) Medical Miscellany, 1883–4.

Midland (The) Medical and Surgical Reporter and Topographical and Statistical Journal. [Quarterly.] v. 1–3, Aug., 1828, to May, 1832. 8°. *Worcester, Tymbs & Deighton.*

Ended.

Midland (The) Quarterly Journal of the Medical Sciences. v. 1; Nos. 1–3, v. 2, May, 1857, to July, 1858. 8°. *Birmingham, Cornish Brothers.*

Mid-Lothian.

Stevenson (W.) On the sanitary condition and general economy of the town of Musselburgh and parish of Inveresk, in the county of Mid-Lothian. San. Inquiry: Scotland, Lond., 1842, 130–152. *Also, Reprint.*

Mid-Lothian and Peebles District Lunatic Asylum, at Rosewell, by Edinburgh. Reports of the Mid-Lothian and Peebles district board of lunacy and the medical superintendent to the commissioners of supply of the counties of Mid-Lothian and Peebles. 1.–3., 1871–83. 8°. *Edinburgh*, 1878–83.

1. report, from July 1, 1871, to May 14, 1877; 2., May, 1877, to May, 1880; 3., May, 1880, to May, 1883. Opened in Nov., 1874.

——. Rules and regulations for the staff of the . . . 14 pp. 8°. [*Edinburgh, Lorimer & Gillies, n. d.*]

Midnight Mission, New York City. Annual report of the managers to the members and subscribers. 7., 1873–4. 33 pp. 16°. *New York, F. J. Huntington & Co.*, 1874.

Midol (G.-E.) * Sur l'hémoptysie. 1 p. l., 24 pp. 4°. *Strasbourg*, 1831, v. 62.

Midon (Charles) [1857–]. * Contribution à l'étude de la périostite externe chronique des membres. 53 pp., 1 l. 4°. *Paris*, 1881, No. 184.

Midrin (Pierre) * Essai sur la valeur physiologique et thérapeutique du phosphate de chaux dans les fractures. 31 pp. 4°. *Paris*, 1877, No. 96.

Midwifery.

See **Labor**; **Obstetrics**.

Midwives (*Education of, and laws relating to*).

See, also, **Hospitals** (*Maternity, etc.*); **Obstetrics**; **Obstetrics** (*Manuals on*); **Syphilis** (*Communication of*).

ABEGG (G. F. H.) Bericht über die königl. Hebammen-Lehr-Anstalt zu Danzig von 1819 bis 1868. 8°. *Danzig*, 1869.

AVELING (J. H.) English midwives; their history and prospects. 8°. *London*, 1872.

BADEN (Grand Duchy of). Dienstweisung für die Hebammen des Grossherzogthums Baden vom 22. November 1879. 12°. *Karlsruhe*, 1879.

BLUNT (J.) Man-midwifery dissected; or, the obstetric family instructors. For the use of married couples, and single adults of both sexes. Containing a display of the management of every class of labours by men and boy-midwives; also of their cunning, indecent, and cruel practices. Instructions to husbands how to counteract them. A plan for the complete instruction of women who possess promising talents, in order to supersede male practice. Various arguments and quotations proving that man-midwifery is a personal, a domestic, and a national evil. In fourteen letters. Addressed to Alexander Hamilton. Occasioned by certain doctrines contained in his letters to Dr. W. Osborn. 12°. *London*, [1793].

BRAUNSCHWEIG. Instruction für die Hebammen des Hergogthums Braunschweig. 8°. *Braunschweig*, 1867.

Midwives (*Education of, and laws relating to*).

BRENNECKE. Hebammen oder Diakonissinnen für Geburtshilfe? 8°. *Leipzig u. Neuwied*, 1884.

BRIEF van eenen vroedmeester ten platte lande, aan zijnen vriend en medebroeder te Amsteldam. Nopens het iets, betreffende de zogenaamde nieuwe wijze van vroedmeesters te maaken, door den stads vroedmeester Jan de Bree ter beoordeeling voorgedragen door David van Gesscher. 8°. *Amsterdam*, [1802].

CREDÉ (C. S. F.) Die preussischen Hebammen, ihre Stellung zum Staate und zur Geburtshülfe. Nach den Verordnungen der königlich preussischen Ministerien und Regierungen, der Landes-Gesetzbücher, sowie nach den Vorschriften des preussischen Hebammen-Lehrbuches. 8°. *Berlin*, 1855.

DELACOUX (A.) Biographie des sages-femmes célèbres, anciennes, modernes et contemporaines, avec 20 portraits. 4°. *Paris*, 1834.

DEUTSCH (C. F.) De necessitate obstetrices bene institutas publica auctoritate constituendi. 8°. *Erlangæ*, 1798.

DUNCAN (J. M.) On the advancement of midwifery education in Scotland. 8°. *Edinburgh*, 1856.

ESSICH [*or* ESSIG] (J. G.) Praktischer Unterricht für die Stadt- und Landhebammen. 12°. *Augsburg*, 1780.

——— F. Versuch einer Hebammenverbesserung zur Wohlfahrt und Bevölkerung des Staats und wie dieser Plan ohne grosse Schwierigkeiten zu bewerkstelligen. 16°. *Leipzig*, 1786.

FABBRI (G. B.) Brevi nozioni del corpo umano dettate per la scuola delle levatrici. 8°. *Bologna*, 1857.

GREGORY (G.) Medical morals, illustrated with plates and extracts from medical works, designed to show the pernicious social and moral influence of the present system of medical practice, and the importance of establishing female medical colleges and educating and employing female physicians for their own sex. 8°. *New York*, 1852.

[HAUCK (G.)] Tagebuchblätter. Zum Vortheil des Hebammen - Unterstützungs - Fonds. 18°. *Berlin*, 1852.

HEBAMMEN - LEHRANSTALT zu Breslau. Bericht über die Thätigkeit der . . . in den Jahren 1867–1877, von Dr. O. Dyhrenfurth. 8°. *Breslau*, 1878.

HECQUET (P.) De l'indécence aux hommes d'accoucher les femmes, et de l'obligation aux femmes de nourir leurs enfants. 12°. *Paris*, 1708.

———. The same. De l'indécence aux hommes d'accoucher les femmes. Ouvrage dans lequel on fait voir, par des raisons de physique, de morale et de médecine, que les mères n'exposeraient ni leurs vies, ni celles de leurs enfants en se passant ordinairement d'accoucheurs et de nourrices. 18°. *Bruxelles*, 1881.

HOCHEDLEN (Eines) und hochweisen Raths des heil. Rom. Reichs-Stadt Augsburg erneuerte Heb-Ammen-Ordnung. 4°. [*Augsburg*], 1750.

HOCHFÜRSTLICHE Wirtzburgische Hebammen-Ordnung vom Jahr 1739. fol. *Wirtzburg*, 1739.

ISTRUZIONI per le levatrici di Santa Corona nella r. città di Pavia, approvati dall' imp. r. governo coll' ossequiato decreto 1º marzo 1823. fol. *Pavia*, 1823.

JÄGERSCHMIDS (G. F.) Unterricht für die Hebammen in den badischen Landen. 2 v. in 1. 12°. *Carlsruhe*, 1775–6.

JAHN (G.) * De officio obstetricis, vom Amt der Heb-Amme. sm. 4°. *Erfordiæ*, [1723].

Midwives (*Education of, and laws relating to*).

JAHRESBERICHT über die Ereignisse königl. Landeshebammenschule zu Stuttgart im Jahr 1877. 4°. *Stuttgart*, 1878.

KATZENBERGER (J.) Hebammen-Catechismus, hauptsächlich zum Gebrauch für Wundärzte und Hebammen auf dem Lande. 12°. *Münster*, 1778.

KAUFMANN (G.) Leitfaden zum Hebammen-Unterrichte. 8°. *Hannover*, 1841.

———. The same. 8°. *Hannover*, 1850.

KURHESSISCHE Hebammen-Ordnung. (Auszug aus der Medizinal-Ordnung 10. Juli 1830, Abschnitt X, §§ 347–392.) 12°. *Cassel*, 1830.

LEIBLIN (P. J.) Ausführlicher Unterricht für die Hebammen in denen Hochfürstl. Brandenburg-Onolzbachischen Landen. 12°. *Anspach*, 1781.

LONICERUS (A.) Reformation, oder Ordnung für die Hebammen allen guten Policeyen dienstlich. Gestelt an einen erbarn Rath des heyligen Reichs-Statt Franckfurt am Meyn. 4°. [*Franckf. a. M.*], 1573.

MARTIN (C. A.) Geschichte und Lehr-Methode der k. Hebammen-Schule, dann Jahresbericht der Gebär-Anstalt zu München. 8°. *München*, 1848.

———. Betrachtungen über das Hebammenwesen in Bayern, dann Jahresbericht der Gebär-Anstalt zu München. 8°. *München*, 1850.

———. Sind Hebammen nothwendig? 8°. *München*, 1851.

———. Ueber die Privat-Gebär-Zimmer der Hebammen. 8°. *München*, 1855.

MARTIN (E. A.) Lehrbuch der Geburtshilfe für Hebammen. 8°. *Erlangen*, 1854.

———. The same. 2. Aufl. 8°. *Erlangen*, 1867.

———. The same. Leerboek der verloskunde voor vroedvrouwen. 2. ed. naar de laatste Duitsche uitgave bewerkt door Dr. H. W. Cramer. 8°. *Utrecht*, 1875.

———. Fragebuch zu dem Lehrbuch der Geburtshülfe für Hebammen. 8°. *Erlangen*, 1856.

MICHAELIS (G. A.) Unterricht für Hebammen. Neu bearbeitet und herausgegeben von C. C. Th. Litzmann. 12°. *Kiel*, 1862.

MORANT (G.) Winke für Ehemänner. Enthüllte Geheimnisse der männlichen Geburtshilfe. 2. Aufl. 8°. *Berlin*, 1870.

NAŘÍZENÉ, vydané od c. k. ministerium záležitostí vnitřních dne 4. června 1881, jímžto se vydává revidovaná instrukce bábám porodním. [Regulations . . . concerning instructions for midwives.] 12°. [*Prague?* 1881.]

NATH (R.) Die neue Stellung der preussischen Hebammen zum Staat und zur Geburtshülfe. Auf Grund der neueren Gesetzgebung und mit besonderer Berücksichtigung des neuen preussischen Hebeammen-Lehrbuches für Aerzte, besonders Medicinal-Beamte, zum Gebrauch bei den gesetzlichen Hebeammen-Nachprüfungen so wie für Hebeammen zum Selbstunterricht. 8°. *Stuttgart*, 1879.

NEUCHÂTEL (Canton of). Circulaire aux sages-femmes. Neuchâtel, le 2 août 1854. 8°. [*Neuchâtel*, 1854.]

NIHELL (Elizabeth). A treatise on the art of midwifery. Setting forth various abuses therein, especially as to the practice with instruments, [etc.] 8°. *London*, 1760.

———. The same. La cause de l'humanité, [etc.] 8°. *Paris*, 1771.

NOTHWENDIG- und nützlicher Unterricht, wornach sich die in des durchlauchtigsten Fürsten und Herrn, Herrn Bernhards, Herzogen zu Sach-

Midwives (*Education of, and laws relating to*).

sen . . . Landen, bestelte Hebammen oder Kind-Frauen, oder deren Stelle vertretende, und sonst männiglich, bey den schwangeren, kreysenden und gebährenden Weibern, vor-, in- und nach der Geburth, richten und halten sollen; nebst einer Anzeige etlicher Sprüche, Psalmen, Seufftzer und Gebethe, anstatt eines geistlichen Unterrichts bey dergleichen Zustande. 4°. *Meiningen*, 1682.

PRAKTISCHE Regeln für Hebammen. 12°. *Reval*, [1884].

PRAKTISCHER Unterricht der Hebammenkunst für die Hebammen. 16°. *Wirzburg*, 1779.

PROPRIETAS. An address to the public on the propriety of midwives instead of surgeons practising midwifery. 8°. *London*, 1825.

——. The same. 2. ed. 8°. *London*, 1825.

REGENSBURG. Regensburgische erneuerte und vermehrte Hebammenordnung. sm. 4°. [*Regensburg*], 1779.

REGLEMENTEN en ordonnantien aangaande de vroed-vrouwen en vroed-meesters. 4°. [*Amsterdam*], 1766.

RIECKE (V. H.) Kurtzer und deutlicher Unterricht für die Hebammen des löblichen Hertzogthums Würtenberg. Auf hoch-fürstl. gnädigsten Befehl verfertiget, mit Kupffern gezieret, und in Druck gegeben. 8°. *Stuttgart*, 1746.

SALZBURG (Duchy of). Hebammen-Ordnung im Kurfürstenthum Salzburg und in den Fürstenthümern Passau und Berchtolsgaden. fol. [*Salzburg*, 1805.]

SAXTORPH (D. M.) Umriss der Geburtshülfe für Wehmütter. Mit Genehmigung und vielen Vermehrungen des Verfassers aus dem Dänischen übersetzt von Karl Franz Schröder. 12°. *Koppenhagen u. Leipzig*, 1783.

SCHATZ (F.) Entwurf einer Hebammen-Ordnung für das Grossherzogthum Mecklenburg-Schwerin. 8°. *Rostock*, 1883.

VON SIEBOLD (A. E.) Geschichte der Hebammen-Schule zu Würzburg. 4°. *Würzburg*, 1810.

SOLINGEN (C.) Korte instructie wegens het ampt ende plicht der vroed-vrouwen. sm. 4°. [*Amsterdam*, 1691.]

——. Hand-Griffe der Wund-Artzney, nebst dem Ampt und Pflicht der Weh-Mutter wie auch sonderbare Anmerckungen von Frauen und Kindern denen ist beygefüget desselben Autoris Embryulcia oder Ausziehung einer todten Frucht aus dem Leibe der Mutter. Alles aus den Holländischen in das Hoch-Teutsche übersetzet und mit vielen Kupffern gezieret von einen Liebhaber der Wund-Artzney. Andere Aufflage. 4°. *Wittenberg*, 1712.

SOMMER (J. G.) Nohtwendiger Hebammen-Unterricht, wie eine Hebamme gegen Schwangere, Gebehrende und entbundene Weiber und deren Kinderlein, so wohl bey natürlichen als unnatürlichen Geburten sich zu erweisen; wie auch, wie sie bey solcher Weiber und Kinder Zufällen im Nohtfall einige diensame Mittel anzuwenden habe. Auff Hoch Gräfl. Schwartzburg. Herrschafft Verordnung und gnädigen Befehl aussgefertiget, und mit hierzu diensamen Kupffern erkläret. Welchem noch beygefügt ist ein Weiber und Kinder Pfleg-Büchlein, wie auch eine Anleitung zur Christlichen Kinderzucht. 18°. *Jena*, 1676.

STARK (J. C.) Hebammenunterricht in Gesprächen, nebst dem Verhalten und Vorschriften für Schwangere, Gebährende, Kindbetterinnen und neugebohrne Kinder. 12°. *Jena*, 1782.

STEIN (G. W.) Katechismus zum Gebrauche der Hebammen in den hochfürstlich hessischen

Midwives (*Education of, and laws relating to*).

Landen, nebst Hebammen-Ordnung und Anlagen. 16°. *Marburg*, 1801.

STEVENS (J.) Man-midwifery exposed; or, the danger and immorality of employing men in midwifery proved and the remedy for the evil found. Addressed to the Society for the Suppression of Vice. 8°. *London*, 1849.

——. The same. 3. ed. 8°. *London*, [1866?]

——. Extracts, etc., from: Man-midwifery exposed; or, the danger and immorality of employing men in midwifery proved, and the remedy for the evil found. Addressed to the Society for the Suppression of Vice; together with the celebrated letter of Sir Anthony Carlisle to the Times newspaper. 8°. [*London*, 1856?]

THEOPOLD. * Ueber das Hebammenwesen im Fürstenthum Lippe. Ein Beitrag zur Reform. [*Jena*.] 8°. *Detmold*, 1885.

THILENIUS (M. G.) Kurzer Unterricht für die Hebammen, Schwangeren und Wöchnerinnen auf dem Lande. 2. Aufl. 12°. *Cassel*, 1775.

TITSINGH (A.) Diana, ontdekkende het geheim der dwaazen, die zig vroedmeesters noemen. Ter eeren van chirurgia geschreeven. 4°. *Amsterdam*, 1750.

UNTERRICHT für Hebammen. Zum Gebrauch der Vorlesungen in der Ammenschule zu Mannheim. 16°. *Mannheim*, 1779.

Bound with: KATZENBERGER (L. J.) Katechetischer Unterricht, etc. 16°. *Frankfurt*, 1779.

UNTERRICHT für die pfälzischen Hebammen. Zum Gebrauch der Vorlesungen in der Ammenschule zu Mannheim. 2. Aufl. 12°. *Mannheim*, 1782.

VERORDNUNG des k. k. Ministeriums des Innern vom 4. Juni 1881, Z. 6183, mit welcher eine revidirte Hebammen-Instruction erlassen wird. 16°. *Wien*, 1881.

WACHS (O.) Die Organisation des preussischen Hebammenunterrichts nach den Anforderungen der Gegenwart. Ein Beitrag zur Vervollkommnung des Hebammenwesens. 8°. *Leipzig*, 1874.

WALTER (O.) Das Hebammenwesen im Grossherzogthum Mecklenburg-Schwerin. Seine Geschichte und sein gegenwärtiger Stand, nebst kurzen Vorschlägen zu einer Reform desselben. 8°. *Güstrow*, 1883.

WEIDMANN (J. P.) De officio artis obstetriciæ concedendo solis viris annotatio ulterior: Quomodo res ista intra virorum solas manus tradi possit? 4°. *Magontiaci*, [1807].

WIEDEMANN (C. R. W.) Unterricht für Hebammen. 12°. *Braunschweig*, 1802.

WÜRTTEMBERG. Dienstanweisung für die Hebamme des Königreichs Württemberg. 8°. *Stuttgart*, 1884.

Abhängigkeit (Ueber die) der Entbindungskunde und Entbindungskunst von dem Hebammen-Wesen. Beob. u. Bemerk. a. d. Geburtsh. u. gerichtl. Med., Götting., 1824, i, 53–104.—**Abstract** (An) of the laws and regulations with reference to midwives abroad. Med. Exam.. Lond., 1876, i, 108; 191. — **Adams** (J.) On midwives and accoucheurs. Med. & Phys. J., Lond., 1816, xxxv, 84–88.—**von Altenstein.** Circular-Verfügung wegen der künftigen Leitung des Hebammenwesens. Mag. f. d. ges. Heilk., Berl., 1824, xvi, 355–362. ——. Circular-Verfügung, betreffend die Zuziehung von Hebammen oder sogenannten Wickelfrauen bei Entbindungen. *Ibid.*, 1829, xxix, 205.—**Aperges** (D.) Ὀνοματοθεσία πρακτικωτέρα ἐπί τινων ἐν χρήσει τῆς Μαιευτικῆς ὁρῶν. Πρακτ. Συνόδου Ἑλλήνων ἰατρῶν, Ἀθήνησιν, 1883, 552–556.—**Arrêté** relatif à l'examen que devront subir les aspirantes au titre d'élève sage-femme. Union méd., Par., 1879, 3. s., xxviii, 431.— **Aveling** (J. H.) English midwives; their history and prospects. Lancet, Lond , 1872, i, 500; 533; 608; 749; 822. ——. On the instruction, examination. and registration of midwives. Brit. M. J., Lond., 1873, i, 308–310. — **Bachiller** (J. J. G.) Breves reflexiones sobre los grandes males que infieren á la sociedad las mal llamadas comadres ó parteras. Bol. de med., cirug. y farm., Madrid, 1851, época 2, 406.—**Barkmorske-**

Midwives (*Education of, and laws relating to*).

väsendet. [1851–59.] Sundh.-Coll. berät. om k. Med.-Verket i riket, Stockh.. 1853–61, i-ix, *passim.* — **Behm.** Nachrichten über das königl. Hebammen-Lehr-Institut zu Stettin. Prov.-San.-Ber. d. k. Med.-Coll. v. Pommern 1834, Stettin, 1835, 100–142. ———. Bericht über das königliche Hebammen-Lehr-Institut zu Stettin. *Ibid.*, 1837, Stettin, 1838, 153–159. ———. Bericht über die Leistungen des königlichen Hebammeninstituts zu Stettin während der Jahre 1834–59. Monatschr. f. Geburtsk. u. Frauenkr., Berl., 1861, xvii, 302 ; 366 : 452 : xviii, 60 ; 162.—**Beilby** (E.) Midwives in India. Med. Exam., Lond., 1877, ii, 536. — **Beitrag** zur Verbesserung des Hebammenwesens. Jahrb. d. ges. Staatsarznk., Leipz., 1837, iii, 49 – 57. — **Bennet** (H.) Women as practitioners of midwifery. Lancet, Lond., 1870, i, 887.—**van Berchem** (H.) Rapport fait à la Société de médecine pratique de la province d'Anvers établie à Willebroeck sur une lettre de la députation permanente du Conseil provincial d'Anvers, par laquelle celle-ci demande l'avis de la Société sur l'institution des sages-femmes dans les communes rurales. Ann. Soc. de méd. prat. de la prov. d'Anvers, Boom, 1848, 91–95.—**Bericht,** betreffend die Hebammen und Geburtshelfer in Amsterdam. Lucina, Marburg, 1811, vi, 93 ; 370.—**Beschikking** van den Minister van Binnenlandsche Zaken van 12 Junij, houdende kennisgeving aan de geneeskundigen en vroedvrouwen, gevestigd in Nederlandsche gemeenten, welke aan Belgie grenzen, van de in Belgie geldende wettelijke bepalingen op de uitoefening der geneeskunst. Versl. . . . v. h. geneesk. Staatstoez. 1868, Gravenh.. 1870, 584–591. — **Birnbaum** (F. H. G.) Bericht über die Leistungen der Hebammen Lehranstalt in Trier. Vom Jahre 1854–60. Monatschr. f. Geburtsk. u. Frauenkr., Berl., 1860, xvi, 353 ; 427. ———. Das Hebammenwesen in seiner Bedeutung für sich und für die allgemeine Gesundheitspflege. Centralbl. f. allg. Gsndhtspflg., Bonn, 1885, iv, 389 – 411.— **Bluff.** Ist es zweckmässig, den Hebammen die Operation der Wendung anzuvertrauen? J. f. Geburtsh., Frankf. a. M., 1832, 104–119.—**B[örner]** (P.) Der Hebammen-Unterricht und die Selbstverwaltung der Rheinprovinz. Deutsche med. Wchnschr., Berl., 1885, xi, 94. — **Brennecke.** Zur Reform des Hebammenwesens. Vrtljschr. f. gerichtl. Med., Berl., 1883, n. F., xxxix, 341–354.—**Broers** (H. J.) Naar aanleiding van de leer van het onderzoek voor verloskundigen- en vrouwen-artsen, bewerkt door A. E. Simon Thomas. Nederl. Tijdschr. v. Heel- en Verlosk., Utrecht, 1866–9, xvi, 515–527.—**Cambrelin.** Considérations relatives au degré d'instruction à exiger des sages-femmes. Bull. Acad. roy. de méd. de Belg., Brux., 1880, 3. s., xiv, 627–641.—**Chaudé** (E.) Les sages-femmes ont-elles le droit de traiter les maladies des femmes en général? Y a-t-il là, de leur part. exercice illégal dans la médecine? Les associations médicales peuvent-elles en poursuivre la répression? Ann. d'hyg., Par., 1883, 3. s., ix, 334–344.—**Cotti** (V.) I flebotomi surrogati dalle levatrici. Gior. d. r. Accad. di med. di Torino, 1870, 3. s., ix, 652–664.—**Daviller.** À propos de l'exercice illégal de la médecine par les sages-femmes. Bull. méd. d. Vosges, Rambervillers, 1887–8, ii, no. 5, 9–13.—**Deneke** (G. F. C.) Hebamme und Wochenbett. Centralbl. f. Gynäk., Leipz., 1883, vii, 622–626.—**Dieterich** (L.) Zur Frage der Reform des Hebammenwesens. Vrtljschr. f. gerichtl. Med., Berl., 1882, n. F., xxxvi, 91–98.—**Dohrn** (R.) Zustände des Hebammenwesens in Ostpreussen. Ztschr. f. Geburtsh. u. Gynäk., Stuttg., 1884, xi, 49–55.—**Dornblüth.** Das Hebammenwesen im Grossherzogthum Mecklenburg-Schwerin der Gesetzgebung und praktischen Ausführung nach kritisch erortert. Jahrb. d. ges. Staatsarznk., Leipz., 1840, vii, 16–39.—**Droits** et devoirs de la sage-femme: du viol et de l'attentat à la pudeur. J. d. sages-femmes, Par., 1875, iii, 52 ; 68 ; 76 ; 85 ; 123 ; 155 ; 162 : 1876, iv, 114 : 1877, v, 253 ; 260. — **Druhen.** De l'Institution des sages-femmes et de la réforme qu'elle réclame. Bull. méd. du nord, Lille, 1850, 89 ; 105 ; 137.—**Dyhrenfurth** (O.) Soll den Hebammen eine operative Hülfeleistung bei frischen Mittelfleischrissen gesetzlich gestattet sein? Antwort an Prof. Valenta. Arch. f. Gynaek., Berl., 1881, xviii, 50–52. ———. Ueber Reformen im Hebammenwesen. Jahresb. d. schles. Gesellsch. f. vaterl. Kult. 1881, Bresl., 1882, lix, 57–61. *Also :* Breslau. aerztl. Ztschr., 1881, iii, 97 ; 127.— **Education** (The) of midwives. Med. Times & Gaz., Lond., 1873, ii, 608.—**Erlass** königl. Oberpräsidiums der Provinz Schlesien vom 20. October 1884, betreffend Erfüllung der den Hebammen im sanitätspolizeilichen Interesse auferlegten Verpflichtungen in der Provinz Schlesien. Deutsche Vrtljschr. f. öff. Gsndhtspflg., Brnschwg., 1885, xvii, 523. — **Erlass** königlicher Regierung des Regierungsbezirks Königsberg vom 24. November 1884, betreffend Pflichten der Hebammen im Regierungsbezirk Königsberg. *Ibid.*, 524.—**Erlass** königl. Regierung des Regierungsbezirks Merseburg vom 3. October 1884, betreffend Verpflichtungen der Hebammen und nicht gewerbsmässige Ausübung der geburtshülflichen Thätigkeit im Regierungsbezirk Merseburg. *Ibid.*, 525.—**Erlass** königl. Regierung des Regierungsbezirks Minden vom 18. October 1884, betreffend Verpflichtungen der Hebammen

im Regierungsbezirk Minden. *Ibid.*, 526. — **F.** (C. P.) Einige Bemerkungen über Hebammen und ihre Bildung. Allg. med. Ann., Altenb., 1813, 169–180. — **Faure.** Rapport de la commission nommée pour étudier les moyens de remédier à la diminution croissante des sages-femmes dans le département. Bull. Soc. méd. de l'Yonne, Auxerre, 1877, xviii, pp. lviii–lxviii.—**Fehling** (H.) Ueber die Zahl und Thätigkeit der Hebammen im Königreich Württemberg. Med. Cor.-Bl. d. württemb. ärztl. Ver., Stuttg., 1882, lii, 9 ; 17 ; 25. ———. Soll die Wochenbettbesorgung der Hebamme verboten werden? Centralbl. f. Gynäk., Leipz., 1883, vii, 670.—**Finsen** (J.) Nogle Bemærkninger in Anledning af: "Et Spørgsmaal vedrørende Jordemodernes Kompetence ligeoverfor den private Læge" af Struckmann. [Remarks on Struckmann's article: A question concerning the competency of midwives as compared with private physicians.] Ugesk. f. Læger, Kjøbenh., 1885. 4. R., xii. 29–33.—**Floystrup** (A.) Om en Udvidelse af Lægens Virksomhed som Fødselshjælper. [Increase of demand for physicians as accoucheurs.] Hosp.-Tid., Kjøbenh., 1884, 3. R., ii, 319–324.— **Frage** (Zur) des Hebammenwesens. Wien. med. Bl., 1884, vii, 1524.—**Francis** (C. R.) Midwives in India. Med. Exam., Lond., 1877, ii, 496.—**Frari** (M.) Osservazioni sopra l' istituzione delle levatrici. Riv. veneta di sc. med., Venezia, 1886, v. 22–27.—**Fruitnight** (J. H.) The status of the midwife, legal and professional. Am. J. Neurol. & Psychiat., N. Y., 1884, iii, 518–537.—**Fuhrmann.** Zur Frage der beaufsichtigten Desinfektion der Hebammen. Centralbl. f. Gynäk., Leipz., 1883, vii, 459–461.—**Gebühren** für die Verrichtungen der Hebammen. Aerztl. Mitth. a. Baden, Karlsruhe, 1868, xxii, 177.—**Gesetz** vom 23. Februar 1837 für den Kanton Zürich wegen Erlernung und Ausübung des Hebammenberufs und wegen Anstellung von Hebammen. Jahrb. d. ges. Staatsarznk., Leipz., 1840, vi, 7-15.—**Graff.** Plan zur Errichtung eines Hebammeninstituts für Westpreussen. N. Mag. f. d. gerichtl. Arznk. u. med. Pol., Stendal, 1787, ii, 3. St., 25–38.—**Gumprecht.** Ueber das Examen der Hebammen. Mag. f. d. ges. Heilk., Berl., 1831, xxxv, 68–87.—**Härlin.** Ein Wort über Hebammenwahl und Hebammenvorprüfung. Med. Cor.-Bl. d. württemb. ärztl. Ver., Stuttg., 1845, xv, 89–94.— **Hart** (E.) [*et al.*]. Report of committee on the draft bill for the registration of midwives in England and Wales. Lancet, Lond., 1882, ii, 61–64.—**Hauff.** Ueber die von den Oberamtsärzten vorzunehmende Untersuchung der zu Hebammen gewählten Weibespersonen. Med. Cor.-Bl. d. württemb. ärztl. Ver., Stuttg., 1845, xv, 55 ; 113. — **Haussmann** (M.) Bemerkungen über die vaterländischen Unterrichtsanstalten für Geburtshülfe überhaupt und im besondern für Hebammen. Med. Cor.-Bl. d. württemb. ärztl. Ver., Stuttg., 1845, xv, 17–20.—**Hebammenfrage** (Zur). Cor.-Bl. d. ärztl. u. pharm. Kreis-Ver. im Königr. Sachsen, Leipz., 1867, iii, 19–22.— **Hebammen - Instruction** (Glossen zur) vom 4. Juni 1881. Oesterr. ärztl. Vereinsztg., Wien, 1882, vi, 57.—**Hebammen-Ordnung** (in Mailand). Samml. v. Nat.- u. Med.- . . . Gesch., Leipz. u. Budissin, 1724, xxiii, 352.—**Hebammenordnung** in Russland. Med.-chir. Ztg., Salzb., 1793, ii, 122–124.—**Hensgen.** Zur Reform des Hebammenwesens. Frauenarzt, Berl., 1886, i, 17 ; 76. *Also,* Reprint.—**Hervieux** (E.) Quelques mots de réponse à un article intitulé: La loi et les sages-femmes. J. d. sages-femmes, Par., 1877, v, 307.—**Hofmann.** Ueber die Unzulässigkeit zu gerichtlich-medizinischen Untersuchungen der weiblichen Geschlechtstheile Hebammen als sachkundige oder ehrbare Frauen als Zeuginnen beizuziehen. N. Ztschr. f. Geburtsk., Berl., 1850, xxvii, 157–160. ———. Ist zweckmässig und zulässig und ausführbar, in Universitätsstädten unehelich Gebärenden die Niederkunft nur in Gebärhäusern zu gestatten, in den Privatwohnungen der Hebammen aber zu verbieten? *Ibid.*, 1865, xxv, Supplhft., 209–225.—**Hohl.** Ueber das Hebammenwesen. Med. Argos, Leipz., 1839. i, 148–153.—**Holston** (J. G. F.) History of midwifery in Ohio. Tr. Ohio M. Soc., Sandusky, 1857, 38–64.—**Hugenberger** (T.) sen. Bericht aus dem Hebammen-Institute. Ihrer kaiserlichen Hoheit der Frau Grossfürstin Helene Pawlowna. zu St. Petersburg, für den xv-jährigen Cyclus von 1845 bis 1859 incl. St. Petersb. med. Ztschr. 1865, iv, 65 ; 129 ; 209. *Also,* Reprint.—**Ingerslev** (E.) Om en Udvidelse af Lægens Virksomhed som Fødselshjælper. Hosp.-Tid., Kjøbenh., 1884, 3. R., ii, 262 – 269. — **Institution** à la Faculté de médecine de Lyon d'un enseignement spécial pour les élèves sages-femmes. Lyon méd., 1882, xli, 32–34.— **Instrux** af 4de Novemb. 1881 for samtlige til Praxis berettigede Jordemødre paa Fær erne. Ugesk. f. Læger, Kjøbenh., 1881, 4. R., iv, 377–382.—**Justi** (H. E.) Etwas über die sehr nothwendige Verbesserung des Hebammenwesens in Sachsen, nebst einigen dahin gehörigen Beobachtungen. Arch. f. d. Geburtsh., Jena, 1787, i, 2. St., 35–53. — **Kirby** (T. W. B.) Midwives and midwifery. Lancet, Lond., 1842, i, 761.—**Kirsten** (T.) Ueber das Hebammenwesen in Sachsen. Monatschr. f. Geburtsk. u. Frauenkr., Berl., 1858, xii, 206–215.—**Klotz.** Die Neugestaltung des Hebammenwesens. Cor.-Bl. d. ärztl. u.

Midwives (Education of, and laws relating to).

pharm. Kreis-Ver. im Königr. Sachs., Leipz., 1867, iii, 14.—**Klusemann.** Wie weit gehen bei gewissen Fällen die Befugnisse der Hebammen? Mit Hinblick auf das Lehrbuch der Geburtskunde für die Hebammen in den k. preussischen Staaten. Vrtljschr. f. gerichtl. u. öff. Med., Berl., 1855, vii, 43-55. — **Koefoed** (P.) Om en Udvidelse af Lægêns Virksomhed som Fødselshjælper. [On the diffusion of the practice of accoucheurs.] Hosp.-Tid., Kjøbenh., 1884, 3. R., ii, 372-375. — **Köstlin** (O.) Ueber Veränderungen in der Tagebuchsführung der Geburtshelfer und Hebammen. Med. Cor.-Bl. d. württemb. ärztl. Ver., Stuttg., 1872, xlii, 154-158.—**Krieg.** Noch ein freimüthiges Wort über das Hebammenwesen. Wchnschr. f. d. ges. Heilk., Berl., 1839, 805-808.—**Kristeller.** Dass jede neugeprüfte Hebamme erst mehrere Jahre als Wickelfrau fungiren solle. Monatschr. f. Geburtsk. u. Frauenkr., Berl., 1860, xv, 11. — **Kuborn & Mascart.** L'Académie se permet d'attirer l'attention de M. le ministre sur la nécessité qu'il y aurait d'étendre le cercle des connaissances exigées des sages-femmes, afin de les mettre à même, en cas d'urgence et en l'absence du médecin, de faire des applications du forceps dans les cas simples. [Rap. de Kuborn.] Bull. Acad. roy. de méd. de Belg., Brux., 1876, 3. s., x, 272-336. [Discussion], 1875, 3. s., ix, 407; 1878, 3. s., xii, 25; 107; 206; 391; 514; 603; 844; 873; 1081; 1879, 3. s., xiii, 391; 460.—**Kurhessische** Verordnung vom 19. Juli 1838 über die Gründung einer allgemeinen Hebammenbehranstalt zu Marburg. Jahrb. d. ges. Staatsarznk., Leipz., 1839, v, 482-485.—**Kurze** Nachricht von den neuerrichteten Hebammen-Instituten in Schlesien. Repert. f. d. öff. u. gerichtl. Arzneyw., Berl., 1793, iii, 169-174.—**Lasser.** Verordnung des Ministeriums des Innern vom 25. März 1874 mit welcher eine Instruktion für Hebammen erlassen wird. Wien. med. Presse, 1874, xv. 441. ——. Instruction für Hebammen. Med.-chir. Centralbl., Wien, 1878, xiii, 448.—**Lettre** de la députation permanente du Conseil provincial d'Anvers, sur l'institution des sages-femmes dans les communes rurales. Ann. Soc. de méd. prat. de la prov. d'Anvers, Boom, 1848, 89.—**Levatrici** (Le) presso gli antichi romani. Osservatore, Torino, 1877, xiii, 33; 49; 65.—**Levy.** Landets Forsyning med Jordemødre. Kong. med. Selsk. Skr. 1846-7, Kjøbenh., 1848, 268-281.—**Levy** (F.) Om en Udvidelse af Lægens Virksomhed som Fødselshjælper. Hosp.-Tid., Kjøbenh., 1884, 3. R., ii, 224; 258.—**Liegeois** (C.) Un mot sur l'exercice illégal de la médecine par les sages-femmes. Concours méd., Par., 1882, iv, 453-455.—**Lindner.** Die Wendung im neuen und alten Hebammenlehrbuch. Vrtljschr. f. gerichtl. Med., Berl., 1880, n. F., xxxii, 169-175.—**Linkenheld** (J.) Der Hebammenunterricht und die Selbstverwaltung in der Rheinprovinz. Deutsche med. Wchnschr., Berl., 1885, xi, 246.—**Löffler** (A. F.) Praktische Lehren und Regeln für angehende Hebammen. Arch. f. d. Geburtsh., Jena, 1795, vi, 180-191. — **Löhlein** (H.) Zur Hebammenfrage. Deutsche med. Wchnschr., Berl., 1885, xi, 104; 121; 256.—**Louet** (E.) Notice historique sur les sages-femmes. Méd. contemp., Par., 1878, xx, 21; 33; 51.—**Lowndes** (F. W.) Women-midwives. Med. Times & Gaz., Lond., 1872, ii, 53. ——. On the registration of midwives. Brit. M. J., Lond., 1874, i, 159.—**Lutaud** (A.) Sages-femmes. Dict. encycl. d. sc. méd., Par., 1877, 3. s., vi, 110-130.—**Madsen** (E.) [et al.]. Jordemoderens Kompetence ligeoverfor den private Læge. Ugesk. f. Læger, Kjøbenh., 1885, 4. R., xii, 67; 92; 124; 172; 220.—**Manley** (T. H.) Women as midwives. Tr. N. York M. Ass. 1884, N. Y., 1885, i, 370-375.—**Martin** (E.) Ueber den naturgemässen Umfang des Hebammengeschäftes und die entsprechende Einrichtung des Hebammenunterrichts. Als Vorwort zu seinem Lehrbuch der Geburtshülfe für Hebammen. Monatschr. f. Geburtsk. u. Frauenkr., Berl., 1854, iv, 321-333.—**von Massenbach.** Die Verbreitung der Hebammen in preussischen Staate, mit besonderer Berücksichtigung des Regierungsbezirks Köslin. Ztschr. d. k. preuss. statist. Bureau's, Berl., 1881, xxi, 1-18.—**Mays** (W. H.) Midwives. West. Lancet, San Fran., 1879-80, viii, 447-449.—**Melioration** of midwives. Proceedings of the deputations of the Obstetrical Society of London to the Right Honorable James Stanfield, M. P. Obst. J. Gr. Brit., Lond., 1873, i, 617; 689.—**Mende** (L.) Unterrichts-Art der Hebammen in der Geburtshülfe in dem grossen Gebärhause zu Paris. Aus der Einleitung der Pratique des accouchemens der Madame Lachapelle, herausgegeben von Dugès, Paris, 1821. Mit Bemerkungen über die deutsche Geburtshülfe und über den Hebammen-Unterricht in der Entbindungs-Anstalt zu Göttingen. Beob. u. Bemerk. a. d. Geburtsh. u. gerichtl. Med., Götting., 1825, i, 3-26. ——. Von den Kunstfehlern der Hebammen, die ihnen rechtlich als Vergehungen zugerechnet werden können. Gem. deutsche Ztschr. f. Geburtsk., Weimar, 1830, v, 1-60.—**Mermann** (A.) Aphorismen über Hebammenwesen. Centralbl. f. Gynäk., Leipz., 1883, vii, 713-719. —— Erwiederung an Herrn Prof. Kehrer. Ibid., 1884, viii, 81-85.—**Meyer.** Die Hebammen-Lehranstalten im königlichen preuss. Regierungs-Bezirke Minden. J. f. Geburtsh., Frankf. a. M., 1827, vii,

Midwives (Education of, and laws relating to).

187-189.—**Meyer** (L.) Om en Udvidelse af Lægens Virksomhed som Fødselshjælper. Hosp.-Tid., Kjøbenh., 1884, 3. R., ii, 145-153.—**Meyer** (S.) I Anledning af L. Meyer's Artikel: Om en Udvidelse af Lægens Virksomhed som Fødselshjælper. Ibid., 205-210.—**Mitchell** (J. T.) On the necessity of adopting laws by which the wives of laboring classes and the poor shall have secured to them in their labours the attendance of qualified accoucheurs, female as well as male. Tr. Obst. Soc. Lond., 1873, xv, 3-9.—**Mombert** (M.) Hebammenunfug. Neuer Beitrag zur Quacksalberei. J. f. Geburtsh., Leipz., 1835, xiv, 135.—**Moppey.** Ueber die Stellung und Bildung der Hebammen. Deutsche Ztschr. f. d. Staatsarznk., Erlang., 1860, n. F., xvi, 3-20.—**Mourier.** Om Fødsler før Jordemoderens Ankomst til Barselkoner. Ugesk. f. Læger, Kjøbenh., 1875, xix, 3. R., 409-416. ——. Om Jordmoder-Instruxen i Henhold til Lov af 15de Maj 1875. Ibid., 1878, xxvi, 3. R., 161-173.—**Müller** (E. H.) Die die Hebammen betreffende Bestimmung der norddeutschen Gewerbe-Ordnung. Berl. klin. Wchnschr., 1870, vii, 138.—**Müller** (P.) Ueber Wiederholungscurse für Hebammen und über Ausbildungscurse für Wochenbettswärterinnen. Cor.-Bl. f. schweiz. Aerzte, Basel, 1885, xv, 594-597. — **Nath.** Mittheilungen über das Hebammenwesen im Regierungsbezirk Königsberg. Vrtljschr. f. gerichtl. Med., Berl., 1885, n. F., xlii, 393-403; xliii, 130-144.—**Necessità** (Della) di provvedere alla buona istituzione delle levatrici. Gior. Veneto di sc. med., Venezia, 1868, 3. s., viii, 861-872.—**Netolitzky** (A.) Hebammenwesen und Geburtstabellen. Wien. med. Presse, 1884, xxv, 1061; 1093; 1127; 1157; 1187; 1257.—**Neue** Ordnung und Instruction für die Hebammen in den hochfürstlichen Thurn und Taxischen Reichslanden, etc. Med.-chir. Ztg., Salzb., 1796, ii, 334-352.—**Neuschler.** Zur rechtlichen Stellung der Hebammen, besonders in Württemberg. Med. Cor.-Bl. d. württemb. ärztl. Ver., Stuttg., 1877, xlvii, 201; 209.—**Pauls.** Ueber Hebammen-Praxis. Med. Cor.-Bl. rhein. u. westfäl. Aerzte, Bonn, 1842, i, 307-311. — **Petermann** (A.) Von nicht verrichteter Amts-Verrichtung einer Weh-Mutter. In his: Casuum med.-leg., decas i, Leipz., 1708, 27-102. — **Peters.** Das Hebammenwesen im Regierungsbezirk Posen. Deutsche med. Wchnschr., Berl., 1878, iv, 167; 199; 213.— **Polizeiverordnung** vom 16. April 1884, betreffend die Hebammen in der Stadt Berlin. Deutsche Vrtljschr. f. öff. Gsndhtspflg., Brnschwg., 1885, xvii, 527.—**Praktische** Regeln für Hebammen, entworfen von der Gesellschaft praktischer Aerzte zu Riga. St. Petersb. med. Wchnschr., 1881, vi, 369.—**Preussen.** Bekanntmachung der königl. Regierung in Düsseldorf, betr. Hebammen, vom 7 Nov. 1879. Med.-Gesetzgeb., Berl., 1880, vi, 3.—**Pryor** (J. H.) The status of the midwife in Buffalo. N. York M. J., 1884, xl, 129-132.—**Puéjac** (Anna). Du progrès dans l'instruction des sages-femmes. Gaz. obst., Par., 1874, iii, 5-7. Also: Gaz. méd. de l'Algérie, Alger, 1874, 59. ——. Quelques notes biographiques sur les sages-femmes françaises. Gaz. obst., Par., 1879, viii, 145; 161; 177; 209.—**R.** Einige Worte über das Hebammenwesen. Allg. med. Ann., Altenb., 1807, 751-760. — **Rapport** de la Commission. Questions diverses—sages-femmes. Actes Cong. méd. de France 1845, Par., 1846, 238-267. — **Registration** (The) of midwives. Brit. M. J., Lond., 1874, i, 186. — **Registration** (The) of midwives. Ibid., 1873, i, 415.— **Registration** of midwives in England and Wales draft bill. Ibid., 1883, i, 222-224.—**Règlement** d'ordre intérieur de l'école d'enseignement pour les sages-femmes annexée à la Maternité de Liége. J. d'accouch., Liége, 1885, vi, 173-176.—**Rendu** (J.) Du degré d'instruction des élèves sages-femmes et des étudiants en médecine à l'étranger. Mém. et compt.-rend. Soc. d. sc. méd. de Lyon (1880), 1881, xx, 159-164.—**Richard** (T.) Ueber das Hebammenwesen, einige Ideen und Vorschläge. Allg. med. Ann., Leipz., 1820, 709; 855; 995. — **Ritter** (G.) Hebammen und Kindespflege. Prag. med. Wchnschr., 1878, iii, 332-334.—**Roche** (E.-H.) Projet d'organisation d'un cours d'accouchement à l'usage des élèves sages-femmes de campagne du département de l'Yonne. Bull. Soc. méd. de l'Yonne, Auxerre, 1868, 131-140.—**S.** Stück eines Hebammenunterrichts. Allg. med. Ann., Altenb., 1813, 451; 825; 1814, 445-485. — **S.** (J.) A midwifery diploma. Med. Times & Gaz., Lond., 1878, ii, 113.—**Sachsen:** Verordnung, Sorge für den Unterhalt der Hebammen betr., vom 24. August 1878. Med.-Gesetzgeb., Berl., 1879, v, 173. — **Sachsen-Weimar:** Dienstanweisung für die Hebammen und Beihebammen. Arch. d. deutsch. Med.-Gesetzgeb. u. öff. Gsndhtspflg., Erlang., 1858, ii, 402-404.—**Sandham** (W. H.) Midwives. Med. Press, Dubl., 1865, liii, 166. — **Schmid** (K.) Die Hebamme gegenüber dem Geburtshelfer. Med. Cor.-Bl. d. württemb. ärztl. Ver., Stuttg., 1846, xvi, 215.—**Schmidt** (J. H.) Bemerkungen über das Lehrbuch der Geburtskunde für die Hebammen in den königl. preussischen Staaten, von dem Verfasser dieses Lehrbuchs. N. Ztschr. f. Geburtsk., Berl., 1839, vii, 204-251.—**Schmidtmüller.** Welchen Wirkungskreis hat die Polizei den Hebammen anzuweisen? Ἀσκληπίειον, Berl., 1811, i, 65; 81.—**Schmitt** (J.)

Midwives (*Education of, and laws relating to*).

Antwort auf Prof. Valenta's in Laibach "Offene Frage: Soll den Hebammen eine operative Hülfeleistung bei frischen Mittelfleischrissen gesetzlich gestattet sein?" Aerztl. Int.-Bl., München, 1881, xxviii, 86.—**Schraube** (O.) Ein praktischer Fall zu Par. 201 des Straf-Gesetz-Buches. (Referring to fines imposed upon midwifes who neglect to call a physician in cases of emergency.) Vrtljschr. f. gerichtl. u. öff. Med., Berl., 1868, viii, 105–122.—**Schroeder.** Ueber die Reform des Hebammenwesens. Allg. deutsch. Hebam.-Ztg., Berl., 1887, ii, 1.—**Schwebes.** Wie weit gehn die Befugnisse der Hebammen? Mit besonderer Beziehung auf § 201, des neuen Strafgesetzbuches. Vrtljschr. f. gerichtl. u. öff. Med., Berl., 1856, x, 124–133.—**Second** vote des amendements adoptés dans la discussion de la proposition relative aux attributions des sages-femmes. Bull. Acad. roy. de méd. de Belg., Brux., 1879, 3. s., xiii, 718–726.—**von Siebold** (E.) Instruction für die Hebammen in Königreiche Baiern. J. f. Geburtsh., Frankf. a. M., 1817, ii, 221–258. ——. Die neue Organisation des Hebammenwesens im Königreiche Baiern. *Ibid.*, 175–258.—**Sir Patrick Dun's** Hospital: army midwives class. Brit. M. J., Lond., 1874, i, 595. — **Solingen** (C.) Ampt ende plicht der vroedvrouwen. *In his:* Alle de Med. e. Chir. Werk., 4°, Amst., 1698, 2. Deel, 122–199, 1 pl.— **Struckmann.** Et Spørgsmaal, vedrørende Jordemoderens Kompetence ligeoverfor den private Læge. Ugesk. f. Læger. Kjøbenh., 1885, 4. R., xi, 583–589; 4. R., xii, 34. [*See, also,* Finsen.]—**Theopold.** Ueber das Hebammenwesen im Fürstenthum Lippe. Deutsche med. Wchnschr., Berl., 1876, ii, 221.—**Thierfelder.** Platon über die Eigenschaften und Verrichtungen der Hebammen. Ztschr. f. Med., Chir. u. Geburtsh., Leipz., 1862, 399–404.—**Tott** (C. A.) Kurze Nachricht über das Hebammen-Wesen in Mecklenburg-Schwerin. N. Ztschr. f. Geburtsk., Berl., 1844, xvi, 386–409.—**Tribunal** civil de Toulon (Var): déclaration de naissance; secret professionnel; procès intenté à une sage-femme par la commission administrative. Union méd., Par., 1876, ii, 1–5.—**Valenta** (A.) Soll den Hebammen eine operative Hülfeleistung bei frischen Mittelfleischrissen gesetzlich gestattet sein? Arch. f. Gynaek., Berl., 1881, xvii, 45–49. *Also:* Oesterr. ärztl. Vereinsztg., Wien, 1881, v, 34.—**Verfügung**, betreffend die Tagebücher der Geburtshelfer und Hebammen. Med. Cor.-Bl. d. württemb. ärztl. Ver., Stuttg., 1872, xlii, 253–255.— **Verordnung**, die Dienst-Instruction für Hebammen betreffend. Jahrb. d. ges. Staatsarznk., Leipz., 1840, vii, 6.— **Voigtel.** Bericht über die Leistungen des königl. preussischen Hebammen-Instituts und der damit in Verbindung stehenden Gebäranstalt zu Magdeburg vom 1sten November 1826 bis Ende April 1827. J. f. Geburtsh., Frankf. a. M., 1828, viii, 830–834.—**Wachs.** Aphorismen zur Reform des preussischen Hebammenwesens, einschliesslich einer Kritik des von Herrn Prof. Dr. Litzmann in Kiel 1878 bearbeiteten officiellen Lehrbuchs. Vrtljschr. f. gerichtl. Med., Berl., 1882, n. F., xxxvii, 315–327: 1883, n. F., xxxviii, 123; 319.—**Walther** (A.) Zur Hebammenfrage. Centralbl. f. Gynäk., Leipz., 1884, viii, 305–310.—**Weatherill** (J.) Remarks on the employment of female midwives, and on the mode of executing the duties of the coronership at Liverpool. Lancet, Lond., 1831, ii, 207–209.— **Wildberg** (C. F. L.) Ueber die erforderliche Vorsicht bei der Untersuchung und Beurtheilung solcher medicinisch-gerichtlicher Fälle, in welchen eine Hebamme angeklagt, oder doch in den Verdacht gerathen ist, dass sie den während oder bald nach der Geburt erfolgten Tod einer Person verschuldet hat. Jahrb. d. ges. Staatsarznk., Leipz., 1838, iv, 214–222.—**Women** midwives. Med. Times & Gaz., Lond., 1872, i, 686.—**Wretlind** (E. W.) Böra läkare åtaga sig vården af normala förlossningar? [Should physicians attend natural labors?] Eira, Göteborg, 1884, viii, 283; 317. ——. Barnmorske-tillgången i Sveriges olika delar och betydelsen deraf. [The unequal distribution of midwives in Sweden and its consequences.] *Ibid.*, 1885, ix, 407–428.—**Young** (S. C.) Obstetrical reflections, suggested by passages in the first chapter of Exodus. N. Orl. M. & S. J., 1860, xvii, 834–838. — **Zittanische** erneuerte und vermehrte Hebammen-Ordnung. 1792. Arch. f. d. Geburtsh., Jena, 1792, iv, 592–614.—**Zulässigkeit** (Ueber die) der Hebammen als Sachverständige. Bl. f. gerichtl. Anthrop., Nürnb., 1855, 3. Hft., 20–30.

Midwives Home of Sir Patrick Dun's Hospital. *See* **Sir Patrick Dun's** Hospital Maternity. Midwives' Home.

Midy (Joannes). * An diluentia, in affectibus melancholicis, purgantibus præferenda? Præses: Joannes Franciscus Leaulté. 4 pp. 4°. [*Parisiis, Quillau*, 1737.]

——. * An quo major jactura virium, victus eo tenuior? Præses: Joannes Besse. 8 pp. 4°. [*Parisiis, Quillau*, 1737.]

Midy (L.) Essence of santal; its origin, preparation, and properties. 24 pp. 18°. *Paris*, 1882.

Midzu Ame.
Eldridge (Stuart). [On Midzu Ame (Japanese extract of malt).] Iji Shinshi, Tokei, 1884, no. 303, Jan. 19.

Mie (Amand-Isidore). * De la variole. 36 pp. 4°. *Paris*, 1848, No. 80, v. 474.

Mie (Ernestus). * De functionibus læsione nervorum alienatis. 40 pp. 8°. *Halæ, typ. Grunerti patris filiique*, [1818].

von Mieczkowski (Leo) [1846–]. * Fünfzig Fälle von Eclampsie. 39 pp. 8°. *Berlin, G. Lange*, [1869].

Miede (Bernardinus Gomesius). Ἀλογραφία sive diascepseon de sale libri quatuor, quorum 1 est de sale physico seu philosophico, 2 est de sale medico sive empirico, 3 est de sale geniali seu jocoso, 4 est de sale mystico . . . nunc vero denuo revisi . . . per Petrum Uffenbachium. 19 p. l., 679 pp., 8 l. 16°. *Ursellis, sumpt. J. Berneri*, 1605.

Mieg (Achilles) [1731–]. * De flatibus. 28 pp. 4°. [*Basil.*], *J. R. Im-Hof*, [1752].

Mieg (Joh. Rodolphus) [1694–1733]. * Plantarum nasturcinarum, quo vegetabilium horum structura naturalis, qualitates, vires atque usus in vita humana salubris breviter ac dilucide explicantur. 2 p. l., 92 pp., 1 l. sm. 4°. *Basileæ, typ. Thurnisiorum fratrum*, [1714].

Mieg (*Melchior*) [1759–1813].
CHAILLET. Oraison funèbre de Monsieur Melchior Mieg, docteur en médecine; prononcée à Colombier, le 15 août 1813. Précédée d'une notice sur la vie de M. Mieg. 8°. *Neuchâtel*, [1813].

Miege (Josephus). * De calomele. 44 pp., 1 l. 8°. *Pragæ, J. vid. Vetterl*, [1835].

Miehe (Adolph. Ferdin.) * Nonnulla de strychninii applicatione endermatica. [Göttingen.] 27 pp. sm. 8°. *Halæ, typ. H. Rufii jun.*, [n. d.]

Miehr (Wilhelm). Mittheilungen aus der Klinik für syphilitische und Haut-Krankheiten des Dr. Lindwurm. 1 p. l., 112 pp. 8°. *München, J. J. Lentner*, 1864.

Mielach (J. C.) Kleines Angedenken an Kreuth. Ein Handbüchlein des Wissenswürdigsten über die Verhältnisse dieser Molkenkur- und Badeanstalt. 135 pp., 3 pl. 12°. *München, G. Franz*, 1840.

von Mielęcki (Stanislaus) [1851–]. * Ueber Diabetes insipidus. 32 pp. 8°. *Berlin, G. Lange*, 1875.

Mielly (Louis). * Essai sur la périarthrite coxo-fémorale. 45 pp. 4°. *Paris, A. Derenne*, 1879, No. 93.

Miélot (Romain). * Sur les convulsions épileptiformes chez les femmes enceintes, ou éclampsie. 44 pp. 4°. *Paris*, 1836, No. 326, v. 303.

Miélot (Victor). * Sur la péritonite puerpérale aiguë. 20 pp. 4°. *Paris*, 1836, No. 303, v. 303.

Mierendorff (Otto). * De hydrope ovarii. 32 pp., 1 l. 8°. *Berolini, B. Schlesinger*, [1851].

Mierisch (Carolus Fridericus Guilielmus). * De incarceratione in annulo canalis inguinalis posteriore. 23 pp. 8°. *Lipsiæ, typ. Staritzii*, 1815.
C.

van Mierlo (Franciscus Gisbertus). * De potulentorum quorumdam virtute diætetica. 2 p. l., 46 pp. 8°. *Lugd. Bat., J. W. van Leeuwen*, 1846.

van Mierlo (Petrus Roverius). * Diss. continens aliquot observationes, e clinico viri clar. F. W. Krieger. 2 p. l, 36 pp. 8°. *Lugd. Bat., J. Hazenberg*, 1852.

Miers.
Chevallier. Rapport sur l'eau de Miers (Lot). Bull. Acad. de méd., Par., 1871, xxxvi, 765–767.—**Henry** (O.) Rapport sur une eau minérale découverte à Miers (Lot). *Ibid.*, 1855-6, xxi, 394.

Mierswa (Hieronymus). * De mechanismo valvularum semilunarium. 23 pp. 8°. *Gryphiæ, F. G. Kunike*, 1858.

Mierzejewski (M.) Études sur les lésions cérébrales dans la paralysie générale. 46 pp., 4 pl. 8°. *Paris, G. Masson*, 1875.

Mierziński (Stanislaus). Die Desinfections-mittel. 92 pp. 8°. *Berlin, J. Springer*, 1878 [1877].

———. Die Conservirung der Thier- und Pflanzenstoffe. 1 p. l., 166 pp. 8°. *Berlin, J. Springer*, 1878.

Miescher's *tube.*

Manz (W.) Beitrag zur Kenntniss der Miescher'schen Schläuche. Arch. f. mikr. Anat., Bonn, 1867, iii, 345–356, 1 pl.

Miescher [**Miescher-His**] ([Johann] Fridericus) [1811–]. * De ossium genesi, structura et vita. 4 p. l., 70 pp., 2 l., 2 pl. 4°. *Berolini, formis Nietackianis*, [1836].

———. De inflammatione ossium eorumque anatome generali; exercitatio anatomico-pathologica. xiv, 281 pp., 4 pl. 4°. *Berolini, G. Eichler*, 1836.

———. Die medizinische Facultät in Basel und ihr Aufschwung unter F. Plater und C. Bauhin mit dem Lebensbilde von Felix Plater. Zur vierten Säcularfeier der Universität Basel vi. September mdccclx, im Auftrage der medizinischen Facultät. 53 pp., 1 tab. 4°. *Basel, Schweighauser*, 1860.

Mieses (Samuel) [1841–]. * Perforatio vesicæ felleæ cum perihepatitide. 31 pp. 8°. *Berolini, G. Lange*, [1864].

Miessner (Gustav). *Zur Pathogenese der Knochencysten. [Erlangen.] 24 pp., 1 pl. 8°. *Berlin, E. Müller*, [1884].

Mieussens (Pierre-Joseph-Gustave). * De la dégénérescence graisseuse du cœur. 37 pp. 4°. *Paris*, 1882, No. 313.

Miéville (E.) * Nouvelle méthode de détermination quantitative du sens chromatique. Trad. de l'allemand par le Dr. Éperon. [Berne.] 27 pp. 8°. *Paris, A. Delahaye & E. Lecrosnier*, 1884.
Repr. from: Arch. d'ophth., Par., 1884, iv.

Miffre (Sylvain). * De la périnéorrhaphie. 43 pp. 4°. *Paris*, 1873, No. 60.

Migeod (Theodorus Georgius) [1823–]. * De ophthalmia nonnulla. 28 pp., 2 l. 8°. *Berolini, typ. Obstianis*, [1849].

Miglietta (Antonio) [1763–1826].
See Swediaur (F.) Trattato dei sintomi, degli effetti, della natura e del trattamento delle malattie sifilitiche. 8°. Napoli, 1830.
For Biography, see Esculapio napol., Napoli, 1839, xxv, 246–253.

Miglioranza (A.) Etiologia e terapia dell' antrace in genere. 3 l. roy. 8°. *Padova, L. Penada*, 1877.

———. La rabbia nell' uomo e negli animali domestici. 2. ed. 45 pp. 8°. *Milano*, 1885.

Migliori (U.) Igiene popolare. Dell' allatamento, ovvero il primo anno di vita dei bambini. Consigli pratici. 102 pp. 8°. *Firenze, A. Ciardelli*, 1886.

Mignard (Henri). * Étude sur les causes et le traitement de la paralysie. 46 pp. 4°. *Paris*, 1853, No. 43, v. 545.

Mignard (Jacques). Remarques sur les virus vénérien, scorbutique et goutteux, et la manière d'agir du mercure, avec les vrais remèdes pour guérir ces différentes maladies. 48 pp. 8°. *Paris, an IX* [1801].

Migne (Jacques-Paul) l'abbé [1800–].
See Poujol (F.-A.-A.) Dictionnaire de médecine-pratique [etc] fol. Paris, 1837.

Migneco (Giuseppe). Prolegomeni alla fisiologia igienica e patologica. 16 pp. 8°. *Catania, A. Pastore*, 1864. [P., v. 1459.]

———. Del chloroformio e di altri mezzi anestesiaci. Memoria inedita. 108 pp. 8°. *Augusta, D. Pattavina*, 1869. [P., v. 1459.]

Mignen (Gustave). * Essai sur les vertiges au point de vue du diagnostic. 66 pp., 1 l. 4°. *Paris*, 1873, No. 484.

Mignon (Alfred). * Du traitement des kystes de l'ovaire par la voie vaginale. 71 pp. 4°. *Paris*, 1878, No. 144.

Mignon (Camille). * Contribution à l'histoire des corps étrangers des voies digestives. 88 pp. 4°. *Paris*, 1874, No. 440.

Mignon (Jacques). * Du cowpox, ou vaccine primitive. 62 pp. 4°. *Paris*, 1848, No. 16, v. 474.

Mignon (Johan Diedrik). * Spec. sistens observationes quasdam patrium solum spectantes. 14 pp. 8°. *Groningæ, A. Groenewolt*, 1805.

Mignont (Sernin). * Sur les vomissements incoercibles pendant la grossesse. vi, 51 pp., 1 l. 4°. *Montpellier, Gras*, 1866, No. 6. c.

Mignot (Antoine-René). * Recherches sur les phénomènes normaux et morbides de la circulation, de la caloricité, et de la respiration chez les nouveau-nés. Des soins que réclame leur éducation. 60 pp. 4°. *Paris*, 1851, No. 30, v. 512.

———. Mémoire sur la contagion du muguet. 26 pp. 8°. *Paris, V. Masson*, 1857.

———. Traité d'hygiène élémentaire en six leçons. ii, 94 pp. 8°. *Paris, G. Masson*, 1872.

———. Des accidents, considérations sur leurs causes, leurs effets, et les moyens de les éviter. 11, 62 pp., 1 l. 8°. *Paris, V. Masson*, 1877.
See, also, Briquet (P.) & Mignot (Antoine-René). Traité pratique et analytique du choléra-morbus, [etc.] 8°. Paris, 1850.

Mignot (David). * Disputatio quædam de cynanche tracheali complectens. 2 p. l., 20 pp. 8°. *Edinburgi, C. Stewart*, 1813. [*Also, in:* P., v. 862.]

Mignot (Edmond). * Des corps étrangers organiques de l'articulation du genou. 39 pp. 4°. *Paris*, 1872, No. 180.

Mignot (Ernest). * De la chlorose. 68 pp. 4°. *Paris*, 1859, No. 59, v. 634.

Mignot (F.) * Sur quelques points de matière médicale et de thérapeutique. 21 pp. 4°. *Paris*, 1828, No. 55, v. 214.

Mignot (J.-Ch.) * Considérations générales sur l'hématurie. 19 pp. 4°. *Paris*, 1826, No. 72, v. 199.

Mignot (Jean-Louis). * Sur l'anémie, ses causes et son traitement. 15 pp. 4°. *Paris*, 1831, No. 207, v. 244.

Mignot (Laurent-Hippolyte). * Quelques considérations sur les affections cancéreuses. 32 pp. 4°. *Paris*, 1866, No. 266.

Mignot (Louis-Pascal). * De la chlorose. 35 pp. 4°. *Paris*, 1845, No. 108, v. 435.

Mignot (Maurice). * Des sueurs chez les phthisiques et de leur traitement par l'ergot de seigle. 64 pp. 4°. *Paris*, 1886, No. 139.

de Mignot (P.-Paul). * Sur les passions. 50 pp. 4°. *Paris*, 1836, No. 343, v. 304.

———. Notes et observations pratiques sur la dysenterie et la cholérine; formules; traitement de la cholérine par la quinine unie aux astringens. 34 pp. 8°. *Bordeaux, Balarac jeune*, 1847.

Mignot (Pierre-Victor). * Sur l'ophthalmie. 61 pp. 4°. *Paris*, 1807, No. 78, v. 131.

Mignot (Salvador). * De l'hépatite aiguë. 2 p. l., 20 pp. 4°. *Strasbourg*, 1837, v. 70.

Mignot (Victor-Adolphe). * Du catarrhe utéro-vaginal ou de leucorrhée. 35 pp. 4°. *Paris*, 1855, No. 243, v. 578.

Mignotte (J.-A.-Auguste). * Encore quelques pages sur la phthisie pulmonaire tuberculeuse. 52 pp. 4°. *Paris*, 1826, No. 173, v. 202.

Migon (Adolphe). * Histoire de l'éclampsie puerpérale. 38 pp. 4°. *Paris*, 1851, No. 201, v. 512.

Migraine.
See **Headache; Hemicrania.**

Miguel-Dalton (A.) * Les lésions des organes
génito-urinaires dans le diabète sucré. 31 pp.
4°. *Paris*, 1877, No. 83.

Miguet (E.) * Essai chimique et médical sur la
créosote. 50 pp. 4°. *Paris*, 1834, No. 151, v.
273.

——. The same. Recherches chimiques et médicales sur la créosote, sa préparation, ses propriétés, son emploi. 94 pp. 8°. *Paris, J. Rouvier & E. Le Bouvier*, 1834.

——. The same. Chemical and medical researches on kreosote, its preparation, properties,
and use. Transl. from the French, by William
Wetherill. vi, 7–49 pp. 8°. *Philadelphia, J.
Dobson*, 1835. [*Also, in* : P., v. 569; 571.]

Miguet (Frédéric). * Une ambulance pendant
le siége de Paris, 1870–71, au point de vue des
hôpitaux temporaires. 36 pp. 4°. *Paris*, 1872,
No. 222.

Miguet (Louis). * Du traitement de la phthisie
pulmonaire par le tartre stibié. 32 pp. 4°.
Paris, 1865, No. 159.

von Mihalkovics (Géza).
See **Hungary.** Das anatomische Institut der kön.
ung. Universität zu Budapest. 4°. *Budapest*, 1882.

von Mihalkovics (Victor). Entwicklungsgeschichte des Gehirns. Nach Untersuchungen
an höheren Wirbelthieren und dem Menschen.
viii, 195 pp., 7 pl. 4°. *Leipzig, W. Engelmann*,
1877.

Mihles (Samuel). Medical essays and observations relating to the practice of physic and surgery ; abridg'd from the Philosophical Transactions, from their first publication down to the
present time. v. 1. vii, 464, xv pp., 4 pl. 8°.
London, S. Birt, 1745.

——. The elements of surgery. In which are
contained all the essential and necessary principles of the art; with an account of the nature
and treatment of chirurgical disorders, and a
description of the operations, bandages, instruments, and dressings, according to the modern
and most approved practice. Adapted to the
use of the camp and navy, as well as of the domestic surgeon. 2 p. l., 324 pp., 6 l., 25 pl. 8°.
London, J. & P. Knapton, 1746.

——. The same. 2. ed., augmented by Alex.
Reid. 5 p. l., 368 pp., 7 l., 18 pl. 8°. *London,
R. Horsfield*, 1764.

Mijnlieff (Arie). * Cystotomia hypogastrica.
2 p. l., 92 pp. 8°. *Utrecht, Gebr. van der Post*,
1879.

Mik (Josephus). * De mania puerperarum. 29
pp. 8°. *Vindobonæ, A. de Haykul*, 1832.

Mikan (*Joh.*) [1769–].
Portrait in : **Portraiten-Galerie.** 4°. *Wien*, 1838,
No. 24.

Mikania.
See **Guaco.**

Mika-operation.
See **Genitals** (*Operations upon, Ceremonial, etc.*)

Miklis (Henricus) [1814–]. * De chorea St.
Viti. 18 pp., 3 l. 8°. *Berolini, typ. Neudorffia-
nis et soc.*, 1841.

von Miklucho-Maclay (N.) Beiträge zur
vergleichenden Neurologie der Wirbelthiere. I.
Das Gehirn der Selachier. II. Das Mittelhirn
der Ganoiden und Teleostier. 3 p. l., 74 pp., 7
pl. roy. 4°. *Leipzig, W. Engelmann*, 1870.

Miksche (Nicolaus). * Diss. sistens historiam
baryecoiæ cura Louvriana sanatæ, adnexa contemplatione baryecoiæ epicritica. 5 p. l., 51 pp.
8°. *Pragæ, J. Spurny*, 1830.

Mikulicz (Johann) [1850–]. Ueber die Beziehungen des Glycerins zu Coccobacteria septica

Mikulicz (Johann)—continued.
und zur septischen Infection. 75 pp. 8°. *Berlin*, 1878.
Repr. from : Arch. f. klin. Chir., Berl., 1878, xxii.

——. Eine neue osteoplastische Resections-
methode am Fusse. 8 pp., 1 pl. 8°. *Berlin,
L. Schumacher*, [1881].
Repr. from : Arch. f. klin. Chir., Berl., 1881, xxvi, Hft. 2.

——. Ueber Gastroskopie und Oesophagoskopie.
32 pp. 8°. *Wien, Urban u. Schwarzenberg*, 1881.
Repr. from : Wien. med. Presse, 1881, xxii.

——. Ueber Laparotomie bei Magen- und Darmperforation.
In : SAMML. klin. Vortr., Leipz., 1885, No. 262 (Chir., No.
83, 2307–2334).

Mikulinski (N. V.) Kratki kurs obtshei terapii
dlja vrachei i studentov. [Short course of general therapeutics for physicians and students.]
iv, 157 pp., 1 pl. 12°. *St. Petersburg*, 1883.

——. Povtoritel. kurs po dushevnim boliezniame.
[Repetition course on diseases of the mind.] 31
pp. 16°. *St. Petersburg, Med. Bibl.*, 1885.

——. Povtoritel. kurs po obtshei chirurg. patolog. i terapii. [Repetition course of general surgical pathology and therapeutics.] 379, viii pp.
12°. *St. Petersburg*, 1885.

——. Kratkii kurs uchenija o sifilise. [Study
of syphilis.] 429, 10, ix pp. 12°. *St. Petersburg*, 1885.

——. Kratkii kurs topograficheskoi anatomii
po Pirogovu, Richet i Tillaux. [Short course of
topographical anatomy, based upon Pirogoff,
Richet, and Tillaux.] 262, viii pp. 12°. *St.
Petersburg*, 1885.

Milan. Istruzioni per i medici-chirurghi comunali, 1858. 14 pp. fol. [*Milano*, 1859.]

——. Statuto pei medici-chirurghi comunali
nel regno L. V. 6 pp. fol. [*Milano*, 1859.]

——. Consiglio degli istituti ospitalieri di
Milano. Regolamento per servizio sanitario
nell' Ospitale maggiore e nell' annesso istituto
di Santa Corona. 48 pp. roy. 8°. *Milano, F.
Manini*, 1871.

——. Consiglio degli istituti ospitalieri di Milano. Regolamento amministrativo adottato dal
consiglio con deliberazione 3 gennajo 1872 e approvato dalla deputazione provinciale di Milano
con decreti 19 aprile 1872, N. 1704, e 24 maggio
1872, N. 2792. 38 pp. roy. 8°. *Milano, F. Manini*, 1872.

——. L' epidemia vajnolosa a Milano nel triennio 1870–71–72. Relazione dell' ufficio medico
municipale. 203 pp., 2 l. fol. *Milano, tipog. di
Luigi di G. Pirola*, 1872.

——. Ufficio statistico. Sezione sanitaria.
Bollettino necrologico mensile. Gennajo 1875
a dicembre 1884. fol. [*Milano*, 1875–85.]

——. Sul nuovo schema di regolamento igienico-
sanitario per l' Ospedale maggiore di Milano e
per l' annessoi istituto di S. Corona. Relazione
al Consiglio sanitario provinciale di Milano.
Dott. Gaetano Strambio, relatore. 28 pp. 8°.
Milano, tipog. del Riformatorio Patronato, 1884.

——. Regolamento igienico-sanitario degli istituti ospitalieri di Milano. Adottato dal Consiglio ospitaliero dapprima colla deliberazione 26
gennaio 1883, No. 2910, ed approvato dalla deputazione provinciale di Milano con sua deliberazione del 13 aprile, No. 2609, e successivamente,
nelle sedute consigliari 22, 23 e 24 dicembre
dello stesso anno cui fecero seguito i decreti di
definitiva approvazione 29 febbraio 1884, No.
1935 b (1323 div. 2ª), della prelodata rappresen-
tanza provinciale e 19 detto mese ed anno, No.
6029, del sig. prefetto di Milano. viii, 78 pp.
roy. 8°. *Milano, tipog. L. F. Cogliati*, 1884.

——. Regolamento igienico-sanitario dello spedale Ciceri, detto Fatebene-sorelle. Adottato

Milan—continued.

dal Consiglio ospitaliero colla deliberazione 25 febbraio 1883, No. 3006 del 1881, approvato dalla deputazione provinciale di Milano coll' ordinanza 4 maggio, detto anno, No. 2607, e reso esecutorio col decreto prefettizio 28 marzo 1884, No. 7620. 13 pp. roy. 8°. *Milano, tipog. L. F. Cogliati*, 1884.

——. Formulario farmaceutico degli istituti ospitalieri di Milano. 139 pp. 8°. *Milano, tipog. L. F. Cogliati*, 1885.

——. Sezione statistica. Bollettino demografico - sanitario - igienico - meteorico. [Monthly.] Anni 1–3, febbrajo 1885 a ottobre 1887. fol. [*Milano*, 1885-7.]
Want Jan., 1885.

——. Istruzione popolare sul colera dettati dalla commissione municipale straordinaria di sanità di Milano. 16 pp. 16°. *Milano, G. Pirola*, 1886.

——. Regolamento igienico-sanitario degli istituti ospitalieri di Milano. Adottato dal Consiglio ospitaliero colla deliberazione di seduta 6 novembre 1886, N. 2982. Ed approvato dalla deputazione provinciale di Milano con sua deliberazione del 23 dicembre 1886, N. 1249 B, communicata colla nota prefettizia 30 dic., detto anno, N. 24342. 72 pp. 8°. *Milano, tipog. L. F. Cogliati*, 1887.

Milan.

See, also, **Children** (*Hospitals, etc., for, Reports, etc., of*), **Cholera** (*Asiatic, History, etc., of*), **Education** (*Medical*), *etc.*, **Fever** (*Cerebro-spinal, History, etc., of*), **Fever** (*Typhoid, History, etc., of*), **Hospitals** (*Descriptions, etc., of*), **Hospitals** (*Management, etc., of*), **Hospitals** (*Maternity, etc.*), **Hospitals** (*Military*), **Hospitals** (*Ophthalmic, etc.*), *by localities*; **Measles** (*Epidemics of*); **Medicine** (*Clinical, Cases of*); **Pest** (*History, etc., of*), **Prostitution** (*History, etc., of*), *by localities.*

FERRARIO (G.) Statistica medica di Milano dal secolo xv, fino ai nostri giorni. 2 v. 8°. *Milano*, 1838–50.

PINI (G.) L' acqua potabile a Milano. Le acque del Brembo; il gozzo. 8°. *Milano*, 1881.

——. Pro aqua. sm. 8°. *Milano*, 1881.

SCHIZZI (F.) Dei lavori dell' Accademia fisiomedico-statistica di Milano nell' anno 1854–5. 8°. *Milano*, 1855.

Beretta (A.) La fognatura di Milano rispetto all' igiene. Gior. d. Soc. ital. d' ig., Milano, 1886, viii, 741–765, 1 plan.—**Bollettino** necrologico mensile della città di Milano, 1876-7. Ann. univ. di med. e chir., Milano, 1876, ccxxxv, 602: ccxxxvii, 573: 1877, ccxxxix, 569: ccxli, 586.—**Bono** (L.) L' ufficio medico municipale di Milano nell' anno amministrativo 1869–72 con proposta di varj provvedimenti igienici. Ann. univ. di med., Milano, 1872, ccxix, 449: ccxx, 47. *Also,* Reprint. *Continued in:* Gazz. med. ital. lomb. Milano, 1873, 6. s., vi, 153; 161; 169; 179. —Intorno all' ufficio sanitario del commune di Milano, nell' anno amministrativo 1870–71. Ann. univ. di med., Milano, 1873, ccxxiii, 3-59. *Also,* Reprint.—**Bonomi** (S.) Studii igienici intorno all' agro milanese. Ann. univ. di med., Milano, 1852, cxlii, 292. —Sul movimento della popolazione in Milano nel 1870. *Ibid.*, 1871, ccxvii, 297. — Intorno alla statistica mortuaria di Milano nel 1871. *Ibid.*, 1872, ccxxii, 493-544. *Also,* Reprint.—**Breganze** (N.) Rendiconto statistico-sanitario sui vajuolosi e petecchiosi ricoverati all' Ospitale succursale della Rotonda durante l' anno 1876. Gazz. med. ital. lomb., Milano, 1877, 7. s., iv, 71.—**Carrière** (E.) Lettre au docteur de Felippi, de la Gazette médicale de Milan, sur le climat du Milanais. Gaz. méd. de Par., 1845, 2. s., xiii, 465-470.—**Celoria** (G.) Variazioni periodiche e non periodiche della temperatura nel clima di Milano. R. Ist. Lomb. di sc. e lett. Rendic., Milano, 1874, 2. s., vii, 312–324.—**Chiara** (D.) L' anno clinico 1877. Osservatore, Torino, 1878, xiv, 536; 550; 582; 598; 615; 625; 661; 673; 689; 708; 725; 739. —**Costituzione** atmosferica, ossia malattie dominanti nella state del 1826. Gior. crit. di med. anal., Milano, 1826, iii, 266–279.—**Costituzione** medica, ossia malattie dominanti nella primavera del 1826. *Ibid.*, ii, 369–395. — **Donati** (P.) Un triennio in condotta a Casaleone. Ann. univ. di med., Milano, 1874, ccxxvii, 3–91.—**Ferrario** (G.) Statistica medica della città e dei corpi santi di Milano. Effem. d. sc. med., Milano, 1836, i, 1; 129; 257: 1837, iii,

Milan.

257. ——. Statistica dei matrimonj, dei nati-vivi, coll' epoca presumibile del loro concepimento, degli esposti e dei nati-morti per la sola città di Milano, dell' anno 1836. *Ibid.*, 1836. i, 32; 38; 142; 148; 270; 276: 1837, iii, 290.

——. Sull' istituzione di un ufficio sanitario di guardia notturna nella città di Milano. Atti Accad. fis.-med.-statist. di Milano, 1860-61, xvi, pp. xxxv–xxxix. —**Geromini** (F.) Del come formulare la nosostatistica delle infermerie per raggiungere il laudabile scopo. Ann. univ. di med., Milano, 1852, cxli, 225.—**Gherini** (A.) Relazione chirurgica dell' Ospedale militare provvisorio di S. Filippo. *Ibid.*, 1860, clxxiii, 411.—**de Giovanni** (A.) Rivista clinica sommaria degli ultimi quattro mesi dell' anno scolastico 1866-7. Gazz. med. ital. lomb., Milano, 1868, 6. s., i. 353; 375; 382; 390; 408; 413: 1869, 6. s., ii, 2.—**Osservazioni** meteorologiche della specola di Brera, 1864–6 e 1868–83. R. Ist. Lomb. di sc. e lett. Rendic. Cl. d. lett. e sc., mor. e polit., Milano, 1864–6, i–iii, *passim. Continued in:* R. Ist. Lomb. di sc. e lett. Rendic., Milano, 1868–83, 2. s., i–xvi, *passim.*—**Pavesi** (A.) Sulla condotta dell' acqua potabile per Milano. Atti Accad. fis.-med.-statist. di Milano, 1881, xxxvii, 78–87.—**Pavesi** (A.) & **Rotondi** (E.) Studj chimico-idrologici sulle acque potabili della città di Milano. Atti... r. Ist. Lomb. di sc. e lett., Milano, 1873–8, vi, pt. 2, 1–60, 4 pl. — **Pecorara** (A.) Sull' necessità di migliorare l' acqua potabile di Milano. Atti Accad. fis.-med.-statist. di Milano, 1875, xxxi, 16–25. — **Progetto** di regolamento edilizio per la città di Milano, approvato dal Collegio degli ingegneri ed architetti e dalla reale Società italiana d' igi·ne. Gior. d. Soc. ital. d' ig., Milano, 1884, vi, 559–590. — **Riassunto** statistico degli infermi curati nello Spedale maggiore di Milano, colla loro mortalità relativa annua per cento, e loro dimora media, distinti in maschi e femmine, dal 1848 al 1868 inclusivi. Atti Accad. fis.-med.-statist. di Milano, 1869, xxv, pp. xxxiii–xxxiv.—**Strambio** (G.) Delle malattie che hanno dominato in Milano durante il corrente anno 1829. Gior. anal. di med., Milano, 1829, xii, 267–279.—**Triberti** (A.) Rendiconto delle malattie curate nell' infermeria di S. Mauro e S. Vincenzo dello Spedale maggiore di Milano, nel mese di ottobre [1844], con alcune osservazioni e riflessioni sulla colica saturnina. Gazz. med. di Milano, 1844, iii, 445–449.—**Vigano** (F.) Acqua potabile; confutazioni e risposte. Atti Accad. fis.-med.-statist. di Milano, 1881, xxxvii, 62–69. ——. Relazione della Commissione academica sulle proposte del membro effettivo Ing.... intorno all' acqua potabile in Milano. *Ibid.*, 70-74.

Milan (Province of). Studii sui sordo-muti e rendiconto degli istituti per quelli poveri di campagna della provincia di Milano, annuario della commissione promotrice della loro educazione pel 1861–2. 190 pp., 1 l. 8°. *Milano, tipog. dell' Orfanotrofio dei maschi*, 1862. [P., v. 1426.]

——. Ospizio provinciale degli esposti e delle partorienti in Milano. Relazione generale per gli anni 1870, 1874–5, 1877, 1884, dei direttori R. Griffini e F. Gallarini. 8°. *Milano*, 1871–85.
1870, 1874–5, 1877, by Griffini; 1884, by Gallarini.

——. Rendiconto par gli anni dal 1876 al 1878 della commissione promotrice l' educazione dei sordo-muti poveri di campagna nella provincia di Milano. 92, 69 pp., 1 l. roy. 8°. *Milano, S. Giuseppe*, 1880.

——. Norme vigenti nella provincia di Milano per la cremazione dei cadaveri e per la conservazione delle ceneri. Approvate con decreti No. 6763, 1° ottobre 1878 e No. 4939, 2 aprile 1880 dal r. prefetto di Milano. 8 pp. sm. 4°. [*Milano*, 1884.]

——. Norme vigenti nella provincia di Milano per la cremazione dei cadaveri e per la conservazione delle ceneri. Approvate dal Consiglio superiore di sanità. 3 pp., 2 l. 8°. [*Milano, tipog. del Riformatorio Patronato*, 1885.]

——. Le condizioni sanitarie della ... Atti della commissione di inchesta nominata dal prefetto di Milano, comm. Achille Basile, per le indagini sulla pellagra. Pubblicazione fatta pei comuni in supplemento al foglio periodico della r. prefettura di Milano. 185 pp., 2 l., 5 tab. 8°. 5 diag. 4°. *Milano, tipog. del Riformatorio Patronato*, 1885.

——. Sulla reciprocità di trattamento gratuito dei malati poveri acuti negli ospitali Lombardo-Veneti. 16 pp. roy. 8°. *Mantova, F. Apollonia*, 1886.

Milan, *Tennessee.* Quarantine regulations [against all freight, baggage, and passengers coming from Memphis or any other infected point]. Mayor's office, July 20, 1879. broadside. [*Milan,* 1879.]

Milani (Giuseppe). Sulla scrofula. Memoria presentata al R. Istituto Lombardo di scienze, lettere ed arti, pel concorso di Fondazione Cagnola del 1860 ed onorata di premio d'incorragiamento. lxviii, 424 pp. 8°. *Milano, G. Bernardoni di Gio,* 1862.
Repr. from: Atti della Fondazione scientifica Cagnola, Milano, 1860-61, iii.

Milazzo. Regolamento di igiene pubblica del comune di Milazzo. 31 pp. 8°. *Messina,* 1877.

Milcent (Alphonse). *De la scrofule. 243 pp. 4°. *Paris,* 1846, No. 173, v. 448.

———. De l'intolérance et de la liberté scientifique dans les concours de médecine. 16 pp. 8°. *Paris, S. Raçon & Cie.,* 1854.

———. Jean-Paul Tessier; esquisse de sa vie, de son enseignement, de sa doctrine. 132 pp. 8°. *Paris, J.-B. Baillière & fils,* 1863.
Also, Co-Editor of: **Art** (L') médical, Paris, 1855-7.

Milchhoefer (Joannes Alexander) [1822-]. *De diagnosi morborum ventriculi. 32 pp. 8°. *Berolini, G. Schade,* [1848].

Milde (Carolus Augustus Joannes). *Nonnulla de tumoribus emphysematosis capitis. 16 pp. 8°. *Lipsiæ, typ. G. Kreysingi,* [1859].

Milde (Georgius Gottlob.) *De specificis eorumque operandi modo et usu. 26 pp., 3 l. 4°. *Halæ, J. C. Hilliger,* 1747.

Milde (Godofredus). *De fructuum horariorum et esculentorum usu et abusu. 28 pp. sm. 4°. *Erfordiæ, stanno Groschiano,* [1704].

Milde (J.)
See **Reise** der österreichischen Fregatte Novara um die Erde. Botanischer Theil. 1. Bd. 4°. *Wien,* 1870.

Milde (Julius).
See **Guenther** (Gustav Biedermann) & **Milde** (Julius). Die chirurgische Knochenlehre in Abbildungen, [etc.] 4°. *Hamburg,* 1850.

de Milde (Mattheus). *De peripneumonia utraque. 25 pp., 1 l. sm. 4°. *Lugd. Bat., apud H. Mulhovium,* [1722].

Mildenstein.
BAD Mildenstein. Reizender Sommerkurort verbunden mit einer klimatischen Kuranstalt. 12°. *Leipzig,* 1867.

———. Reizender von medicinischer Seite warm empfohlener Sommerkurort, [etc.] 12°. *Leisnig,* 1868.

Mildew.
See **Fungi.**

Mildmay Conference Hall, Mildmay Park, Middlesex. The cash accounts of the Mildmay institutions for the years 1877-83. obl. 24°. *London,* 1878-84.
The institutions under the management of Conference Hall are as follows: 1. Balls Pond Mission House. 2. Balls Pond Penny Bank. 3. Barnet Convalescent Home. 4. Bethnal Green Coffee and Lodging House. 5. Bethnal Green Hospital. 6. Brighton Convalescent Home. 7. Brighton Deaconess House. 8. Cabmen's Mission and Institute. 9. Conference Hall. 10. Cottage Hospital. 11. Deaconess House. 12. Deaf Mute Fund. 13. Female Workers' Association. 14. Home and Branch Mission. 15. Infirmary. 16. Invalid Home. 17. Invalid Kitchen. 18. Iron Room Mission. 19. Medical Mission Hospital. 20. Memorial Cottage Hospital. 21. Men's Night School. 22. Nursing House. 23. Open Air Mission. 24. Orphanage. 25. Probation House. 26. Servants' Home and Registry. 27. Shop Assistants' Home. 28. Training Home. 29. Workman's Hall.

———. Report of the Jaffa Medical Mission, under the superintendence of Miss Mangan. 6., 1883-4. 24 pp. 24°. *Moorfields, E. C.,* 1884.

Mildmay Deaconess Institution, Nursing Branch. [Circular relating to probationer

Mildmay Deaconess Institution, [etc.]—cont'd. nurses, with regulations, etc.] 2 l. 8°. [*London,* 1884?]
In connection with the Conference Hall, Mildmay Park, London, N.

Mildmay Memorial Hospital. *See* **Memorial** Cottage Hospital.

Mildmay Mission Hospital, Bethnal Green, London. Annual reports of the committee to the subscribers, for the years 1877-8 to 1886. 16° & 24°. *London,* 1878-87.

———. Statement of expenditures for nine years, ending 31 Dec., 1885. 1 broadside fol. *London, Bradbury, Wilkinson & Co.,* [1886].

———. Statistics of patients for nine years, ending 31st Dec., 1885. 1 broadside fol. [*London,* 1886.]

Mildner (Emanuel). *De galvanismi efficacia in cataractam destruendam. 24 pp. 8°. *Pragæ, typ. filiorum T. Haase,* 1843.

Mile End Old Town. *See* **London.** *Mile End Old Town.*

Mileham.
LEE (W.) Report to the General Board of Health, on a preliminary inquiry into the sewerage, drainage, and supply of water, and the sanitary condition of the inhabitants of the parish of Mileham. 8°. *London,* 1849.

Mileik (Andreas). *O vospalenii predstatelno jeliezi (prostatitis), v patol.-anat. otnoshenii. [Prostatitis from pathologico-anatomical point of view.] 26 pp. 8°. *St. Petersburg,* 1872.

Miles (Abijah J.) [1834-]. Report on smallpox, May 8, 1882. 15 pp. 8°. *Cincinnati, R. Clarke & Co.,* 1882.
Also, Co-Editor of: **Cincinnati** (The) Medical News, 1872-7.

Miles (F. T.) Peripheral paralysis. 16 pp. 8°. *New York, G. P. Putnam's Sons,* 1876.
No. 12, v. 2, Am. Clin. Lect., by Seguin, 325-340.

———. A contribution to regional diagnosis in brain lesion. 7 pp. 8°. *New York, G. P. Putnam's Sons,* 1877.
Repr. from: Tr. Am. Neurol. Ass., N. Y., 1877, ii.

———. Electricity in medicine. 17 pp. 8°. *Baltimore, J. H. Foster & Co.,* 1878.
Repr. from: Maryland M. J., Balt., 1878, ii.

Miles (Mason M.) & **Fogg** (David S.) Boston Vapor Bathing Institution, conducted by . . . 24 pp. 8°. *Boston, W. D. Ticknor & Co.,* 1850.

Miles (William J.) The horse's foot, and how to keep it sound. [From the 3. Lond. ed.] 70 pp. 12°. *New York, D. Appleton & Co.,* 1847.

———. Modern practical farriery; a complete guide to all that relates to the horse . . . With numerous illustrations and a series of anatomical plates, engraved from original drawings from nature, by Benjamin Herring. To which is added an essay on the diseases and management of cattle, sheep, and pigs, by J. I. Lupton. vii, iv, 536, 96 pp., 40 pl. 4°. *London, W. Mackenzie,* [1873, vel subseq.].

Milet (Eugène). *Des phlegmons et des abcès phlegmoneux de l'aisselle. 27 pp. 4°. *Paris,* 1855, No. 144, v. 578.

Milhau (François). *Essai sur l'enchatonnement du placenta. 51 pp. 4°. *Montpellier,* 1882, No. 17.

Milhau (Jean-Pierre). *Du mode de propagation du choléra épidémique. 38 pp. 4°. *Paris,* 1853, No. 14, v. 545.

Milhau (Joh. Ludovicus). *De carvi. 26 pp. sm. 4°. *Argentorati, typ. M. Pauschingeri,* [1740].

Milhauser (Joh. David.) *De atonia. 56 pp. sm. 4°. *Halæ Magdeb., typ. C. Henckelii,* [1716].

Milhet (J.-F.) *Sur l'érysipèle. 21 pp. 4°. *Paris,* 1812, No. 112, v. 91.

Milhet (Maurice). * Sur la fièvre ataxique continue simple. 20 pp. 4°. *Paris*, 1822, No. 137, v. 92.

Milianah.

Bruguière. Notice sur la topographie médicale de la ville de Milianah. Rec. de. mém. de méd. . . . mil., Par., 1844, lvi, 143–184.—**Pomel** (A.) Description et carte géologique du massif de Milianah. Bull. Soc. d. sc. . . . d'Alger, 1873, x, pp. i–iv; 9–184, 1 map.

Miliaria.

See, also, Fever (*Miliary*); Rheumatism (*Complications of, Cutaneous*); Sudamina; Sweating sickness.

ALLIONIUS (C.) Tractatio de miliarium origine, progressu, natura et curatione. 8°. *Augustæ Taurinorum*, 1758.

DE BORVILLE (H.-P.) * Sur la miliaire, considérée comme maladie symptomatique. 4°. *Paris*, 1822.

DEBIOL (A.) * Dissertation sur l'exanthème miliaire. 4°. *Paris*, 1811.

LOEBER (F.) * De exanthemate miliari et pemphigo. 4°. *Erfordiæ*, [1791].

PFLEIDERER (J. J.) * Quæstio medica an miliaria alba systematis nervosi soboles, occasione ictericæ miliis albissimis conspersæ noviter mota. 4°. *Tubingæ*, [1768].

SMIT (J.) * De miliaribus. 8°. *Groningæ*, [1817].

Balman (T.) Recurrent miliaria after scarlet fever. Brit. M. J., Lond., 1866, i, 36–38. — **Besnier** (E.) De la miliaire. Ann. de dermat. et syph., Par., 1873–4, v, 24–43.—**Bierbaum** (J.) Miliaria. J. f. Kinderkr., Erlang., 1865, xlv, 219–227.—**de Boret.** Considérations pratiques sur quelques maladies de la peau (miliaire). J. de méd. et chir. prat., Par., 1839, x, 15; 64; 116; 165; 223; 248; 303; 451.—**De la Vigne.** Miliaria. Gen.-Ber. d. k. rhein. Med.-Coll. 1841, Koblenz, 1844, 59.—**Hebra.** Miliaria. Allg. Wien. med. Ztg., 1864, ix, 204. — **Lyncker** (F.) Symptomatischer Wasserfriesel. Wchnschr. f. d. ges. Heilk., Berl., 1839, 520–523.—**Minich.** Sull' importanza da darsi alle eruzioni miliariformi, che si sviluppano nel decorso di alcune malattie. Gior. veneto di sc. med., Venezia, 1863, 2. s., xxi, 487–517. — **Müller** (F.) Ueber Miliarien. Vrtljschr. f. d. prakt. Heilk., Prag, 1845, ii, 82–88.—**Veiel.** Miliaria chronica. Deutsche Klinik, Berl., 1855, vii, 210.

Miliary *fever.*

See Fever (*Miliary*).

Milichius (*Jacobus*) [1501–59].

Portrait in: Collection—van Kaathoven.—Collection of Portr. of Phys. & Men of Sc., 197; 208.

Milieu.

See Environments.

Miling (Jo. Franc. Bernardus). * Mentis alienationum semiologia somatica. 1 p. l., 32 pp., 2 l. 4°. *Bonnæ, F. Baaden*, [1828].

Miliotti (Domenico). Della tabe dorsale (atassia locomotrice). ix (1 l.), 339 pp. 8°. *Milano, F. Vallardi*, [1886].

Militärärztliche Aphorismen. Populäre Abhandlungen aus dem Gebiete des Militär-Sanitätswesens. 1 p. l., 57 pp., 1 l. 8°. *München, J. A. Finsterlin*, 1878.

Militärärztliche Reformgedanken. Ein Project für das 20. Jahrhundert! 35 pp. 8°. *Wien*, 1886.

Repr. from: Wien. med. Bl., 1885, viii.

Militärärztliche Zeitung. Beilage zur Wiener Medizinal-Halle. 1862–4. 4°. *Wien, H. Engel u. Sohn.*

Militaerarzt (Der). (Beilage zur Wiener medizinischen Wochenschrift.) Redigirt von L. Wittelshöfer. v. 1–21, 1867–87. 4°. *Wien, L. W. Seidel u. Sohn.*

Current. Want no. 24, 1869; no. 12, 1873.

Militär-Arzt (Der) mit dem, was darum und daran ist, mikroskopisch und makroskopisch betrachtet. Militär- und Civil-Aerzten, Staats-

Militär-Arzt (Der)—continued.

männern wie auch dem geliebten Publicum zugeeignet. Nebst einem Traum über das Verhalten der Kleinstaaterei zum Menschen von einem Zweihänder. 2. Aufl. viii, 56 pp. 8°. *Essen, A. Silbermann*, 1883.

Militær - medicinske Selskab. Forhandlinger. 39 pp. 8°. *Kristiania*, 1886.

Suppl. to: Tidsskr. f. prakt. Med., Kristiania, 1886, vi, no. 22.

Militär - Sanität und freiwillige Hilfe im Kriege. [Dr. Wittelshöfer.] [Wiener Welt-Ausstellung 1873. Gruppe xvi, Section iii, Lit. E. Special-Katalog. Ausgegeben am 15. Juli 1873.] 51 pp., 2 l. 8°. *Wien, L. W. Seidel u. Sohn,* [*n. d.*]

Militär-statistisches Jahrbuch für die Jahre 1880, 1881 und 1882. Ueber Anordnung des k. k. Reichs-Kriegs-Ministeriums bearbeitet und hrsg. von der 3. Section des technischen und administrativen Militär-Comité. 1. Theil, 1885; 2. Theil, 1884. 4°. *Wien*, 1884-5.

Militairärztliche Bemerkungen aus dem Feldzuge 1866 gegen Oestreich und den deutschen Bund. 11 pp. MS. fol. [*n. p.*, 1867.]

Militair-Arzt (Der) im Felde und in Garnison, oder die Kunst, die Gesundheit des Kriegers zu erhalten, und wieder herzustellen, nebst Abhandlung über Aushebung der Recruten. Für Militair- und Commun-Behörden und Militair-Aerzte, so wie für Soldaten und Communal-Gardisten, hrsg. von einem Militair-Arzte. ix, 190 pp. 12°. *Meissen, F. W. Goedsche*, 1831.

Militaire-Artsenwet (De). Nos. 2–5. 8°. *Utrecht, J. G. van Terveen & Zoon*, 1880.

CONTENTS:

2. Proeve van een wetsontwerp tot regeling der van staatswege aan tot het leger behoorende personen te verstrekken genees- en heelkundige hulp en genees- en heelmiddelen, door Mavors medicator. 15 pp.

3. Proeve van een wetsontwerp regelende de samenstelling, benoeming en aanstelling, bezoldiging, bevordering, het pensioen en het ontslag van het personeel van den geneeskundigen dienst bij het leger, dor Mavors medicator. 32 pp.

4. Proeve van een wetsontwerp tot regeling der kleeding en uitrusting van het personeel en het materieel van den geneeskundigen dienst bij het leger, door Mavors medicator. 19 pp.

5. Aanteekeningen op de memoire van beantwoording van het voorloopig verslag omtrent het wetsontwerp tot regeling van de betrekkingen en rangen, de opleiding en de bevordering van het personeel der geneeskundige dienst bij de landmagt door Mavors medicator. 32 pp.

Militair-Wochenblatt. Hrsg. von A. Borbstaedt. [Semi-weekly.] v. 57–62, 1872-7. 6 v. 4°. *Berlin, E. S. Mittler u. Sohn.*

In 1873, von Witzleben became editor.

Military order of the Loyal Légion of the United States. Constitution and by-laws. 59 pp., 1 pl. 12°. *Philadelphia*, 1868. [P., v. 227.]

———. The same. 47, 45 pp. 8°. *Philadelphia*, 1877.

Military prison at Alcatraz Island, California. *See* United States. *War Department. Regulations for the government* [etc.] 8°. [*San Francisco*, 1873.]

Military Service Institution of the United States. Origin, progress, and condition of the . . . with a catalogue of the museum. 34 pp. 12°. [*New York*, 1880.]

Militchévitch (Demètre). * Considérations sur quelques troubles trophiques des ongles dans quelques maladies des centres nerveux. 64 pp. 4°. *Paris*, 1883, No. 234.

Militia.

See Army.

Militzer (Joannes Georgius). * De nonnullis moschi, muriatis oxyduli hydrargyri mitis et muriatis oxyduli ferri in organismo sano effectibus. 36 pp. 8°. *Erlangæ, typ. Jungeanis*, [*n. d.*]

Militzer (Rudolf). * Ueber das Malum Pottii. 23 pp. 8°. *Würzburg, Stahel, 1865.*

Milius (Abrahamus). De origine animalium et migratione populorum. Ubi inquiritur quomodo quaque via homines cæteraque animalia terrestria provenerint; et post deluvium in omnes orbis terrarum partes et regiones, Asiam, Europam, Africam, utramque Americam et terram Australem, sive Magellanicam, pervenerint. 68 pp. 24°. *Genevæ, apud P. Columesium, 1667.*

——. The same. Merckwürdiger Discurss von dem Ursprung der Thier, und Ausszug der Völcker . . . Auss dem Lateinischen in die teutsche Sprach versetzet, und mit vielen sinnreichen, seltenen Anmerkungen, denckwürdigen Begebenheiten, artigen wohlgefügten Fragen, auch einer medicinalischen Zugab, von der Fürtrefflichkeit dess Brod, und schädlichem Missbrauch dess Fleisch und Weine, etc., vermehret. Durch Joh. Christoph Bitterkraut. 6 p. l., 400 pp., 18 l. 18°. *Saltzburg, J. B. Mayr, 1670.*

Miljanitsch (Peter). * Zur Diagnose der Darmperforation im Typhus abdominalis. 18 8°. *Würzburg, P. Scheiner, 1884.*

Milk.

See, also, **Acid** (*Lactic*); **Breast**; **Butter**; **Dairies**; **Kefir**; **Koumiss**; **Lactation**; **Whey**.

ACOROMBONUS *Eugubius* (H.) Tractatus utilissimus de natura et usu lactis.
In: PLACITUS (S.) De medicamentis [etc.] 4°. *Norimbergæ*, 1538.

AKVILEFF (N.) * O vlijanii chloristago natrija na soderjanie kazeina, bielka i solei izvesti ve molokie. [Influence of chloride of sodium in increasing amount of casein, albumen, and phosphates in milk.] 8°. *St. Petersburg,* 1870.

ANDRÉ (E.) * Étude sur le lait. 4°. *Montpellier,* 1886.

BAINES (*Mrs.* M. A.) The comparative properties of human and animal milks. A new theory as to "essences", and a new interpretation of some physiological facts. 8°. *London,* 1860.

BIEDERT (P.) Untersuchungen über die chemischen Unterschiede der Menschen- und Kuhmilch. 8°. *Giessen,* 1869.

——. The same. 2. Ausg. 8°. *Stuttgart,* 1884.

BLANC (A.-H.) * Du lait et des matières émulsives analogues. 4°. *Paris,* 1832.

BOUCHARDAT (A.) & QUEVENNE (T.-A.) Du lait. 2 pts. in 1 v. 8°. *Paris,* 1857.

VAN BUEREN (R. L.) * Diss. sistens observationes microscopicas de lacte ejusque genesi. 8°. *Traj. ad Rhenum,* 1849.

CUHN (N. W.) * De lacte insonte. 4°. *Gottingæ,* [1737].

DAUTOUR (C.) * Du lait en pharmacie. 4°. *Montpellier,* 1885.

DOORSCHODT (H.) * De lacte. 4°. *Lugd. Bat.,* 1737.
Also, in: HALLER. Disp. anat. [etc.] 4°. *Gottingæ,* 1750, v, 739–776.

DUCLAUX (E.) Mémoire sur le lait. 8°. [*Paris,* 1882 ?]
Cutting from: Ann. de l'Inst. nat. agronomique, Par., 1882, vii, 23–138, 2 pl.

EGELING (J.) * De lacte. 4°. *Traj. ad Rhenum,* 1759.

FERRIS (S.) A dissertation on milk. 8°. *London,* [1785].

FJORD (N. J.) Tillæg til 18de Beretning. Forsøg paa Mejerivæsenets Omraade. Mælks Sammensætning og Benyttelse. Samt Bemærkn. af Red. af Tidsskr. for Landøkonomi og Dr. Panum. [Essay in the interest of dairies. Composition of milk, and its uses.] 8°. *Kjøbenhavn,* 1883.

Milk.

GABRILKO (A.) * K voprosu o vlijanii vodi na kolichestvo i kolichestv. sostave moloka. [Influence of water in increasing the quantity and quality of milk.] 8°. *St. Petersburg,* 1871.

GESNERUS (C.) Libellus de lacte, et operibus lactariis philologus pariter ac medicus. Cum epistola ad Jacobum Aujenum de montium admiratione. 16°. *Tiguri,* [1541].

GÖBEL (J. M.) * De lacte ejusque vitiis. 4°. *Lugd. Bat.,* 1684.

GOTTLIEB (R.) * De lacte. 8°. *Vindobonæ,* 1836.

DE GROOT (A. J.) * Verhandeling over de melk. 8°. *Groningen,* [1856].

GROS (G.) Recherches sur la vésiculation du lait. 8°. [*Moscou,* 1847.]

GÜNTHER (B. L.) * De lacte. sm. 4°. *Argentorati,* [1713].

HENRY (F. P.) Cartwright prize essay. Observations with the hæmacytometer upon the globular composition of the blood and milk. 8°. *Philadelphia,* 1881.

HIRD (W.) * De lactis natura et usu. 8°. *Edinburgi,* 1751.

HOFFMANN (M.) * Ueber die Verdaulichkeit des Caseïns aus erhitzter Milch. 8°. *Berlin,* [1881].

HUSSON (C.) Le lait, la crème et le beurre au point de vue de l'alimentation, de l'allaitement naturel, de l'allaitement artificiel et de l'analyse chimique. 12°. *Paris,* 1878.

IMPORTANT facts for the people, published by the officers of the Milk Dealers' Association, Chicago. 16°. *Chicago, Ill.,* 1879.

VAN DE KASTEELE (J. T.) * De analogia inter lac et sanguinem. 4°. *Lugd. Bat.,* 1780.
Also, in: JANSEN (W. H.) Collectio diss. select. 4°. *Dusseldorpii,* 1791, 59–108.

KINDLER (J. A.) * De lacte. 4°. *Halæ Magdeb.,* [1742].

KIRCHNER (W.) Beiträge zur Kenntniss der Kuhmilch und ihrer Bestandtheile nach dem gegenwärtigen Standpunkte wissenschaftlicher Forschung. 8°. *Dresden,* 1877.

LAINÉ (L.) * Du lait au point de vue physique, chimique et pharmaceutique. 4°. *Montpellier,* 1883.

LAURENTIUS (T. A.) * De lactis discussione. 4°. *Erfordiæ,* [1749].

LODIEU (J.) Die Milchkühe und der höchste Milchertrag. Vollständige und neue Darstellung der characteristischen Merkmale, nach denen man die Milchergiebigkeit einer Kuh leicht und genau beurtheilen kann, nebst Bemerkungen über die Mastung und das Mastvieh, sowie einer Kritik des Guénon'schen (Milchspiegel-) Systems und verschiedenen Abhandlungen über die Milch und ihre Bestandtheile, über Fütterung und Paarung, über Rindviehracen u. s. w. Ein von der landwirthschaftlichen Gesellschaft des Depart. Pas-de-Calais gekröntes Buch. Aus dem Französischen. 24°. *Stuttgart,* 1837.

MARTIN (B.) Traité de l'usage du lait. 24°. *Paris,* 1684.

MARTINY (B.) Die Milch, ihr Wesen und ihre Verwerthung. 2 v. in 1. 8°. *Danzig,* 1871.

MAUREL (J.-A.) * Du lait en général, sa digestion. De l'allaitement, du sevrage; hygiène des nouveau-nés. 4°. *Paris,* 1858.

NAUDIN (L.-S.-E.) * Des caractères microscopiques du lait. De la composition des globules de ce fluide. 4°. *Paris,* 1841.

NEUBECK (G.) * De lacte. 8°. *Berolini,* 1825.

NEUREITER (F. F.) * De dispositionibus lacteis. 8°. *Viennæ,* [1775].

NEW SOUTH WALES. An act establishing sanitary regulations in respect of the production

Milk.

and distribution of milk. No. xvii. [Assented to, 30th Sept., 1886.] fol. [*Sydney*, 1886.]

OTSERETSKOWSKY (N.) *De spiritu ardente ex lacte bubulo. 1778.

In: WITTWER. Delect. diss. med. 8°. *Norimbergæ*, 1781, iv, 152-175.

PARMENTIER (A.-A.) & DÉYEUX (N.) Précis d'expériences et observations sur les différentes espèces de lait, considérées dans leurs rapports avec la chimie, la médecine et l'économie rurale. 8°. *Strasbourg, an VII* [1799].

PETIT-RADEL (P.) Essai sur le lait, considéré médicinalement sous ses différens aspects, ou histoire de ce qui a rapport à ce fluide chez les femmes, les enfans et les adultes, soit qu'on le regarde comme cause de maladie, comme aliment, ou comme médicament. 8°. *Paris*, 1786.

PURE milk, and how to procure it. Tower dairy. 16°. *Cohasset, Mass.*, 1879.

RANDHAN (J. F.) De lactis origine brevis recensus. 4°. *Lipsiæ*, 1799.

ROERER (J. G. J.) *Diss. sistens monita quædam practica circa noxium et salutarem usum lactis, juxta Hippocratis Aphor. 64, sect. 5. 4°. *Erfordiæ*, [1739].

ROSNER (J. G. E.) *Nonnulla circa vires lactis notantur. 4°. *Lugd. Bat.*, 1756.

ROZANOFF (S.) *Moloko Peterburgskich korov i uslovija ego kontrolja na rynkach. [Milk of St. Petersburg cows, and means of control in the markets.] 8°. *St. Petersburg*, 1887.

RUSHMORE (J. H.) A treatise on aerated milk. 8°. *New York*, 1872.

SAILLET (J.) *Des laits fermentés et de leurs usages thérapeutiques. 4°. *Paris*, 1886.

SALACHAS (F.-J.) *Sur les usages du lait. 4°. *Paris*, 1873.

SARTORI (G.) Chimica agraria. Analisi del latte; guida pratica. 8°. *Napoli, Milano, Pisa*, 1887.

SCHLICHTINGIUS (J. D.) *De lacte. 4°. *Groningæ*, 1730.

SCHMIDT (A.) Ein Beitrag zur Kenntniss der Milch. 4°. *Dorpat*, 1874.

SIBOROTKIN (A.) *Ke voprosu o kolichestvie moloka i soderjanii ve neme jira i sachara pode vlijanieme vodi . . . [On the quantity of milk and influence of water on the fat and proportion of sugar.] 8°. *St. Petersburg*, 1871.

SLUIM (D.) *De lacte. 4°. *Lugd. Bat.*, [1716].

SOKOLOFF (P.) *O vlijanii chloristago natrija na kolichestvo moloka i na soderjanie ve neme jira i sachara. [Influence of choride of sodium in increasing fats and sugar in milk.] 8°. *St. Petersburg*, 1870.

STUKOVENKOFF (M.) *O vlijanii temperaturi jidkosti vvodimoi ve organizme ve formie pishi dli pitja na kolichestvo i kolichestvennii sostave moloka. [On the influence of temperature of liquids introduced into the organism upon the quantity and quality of milk.] 8°. *St. Petersburg*, 1871.

SZÁNTAY DE TASNÁD (J.) *De lacte. 8°. *Pestini*, [1834].

Hungarian text.

TREATISE (A) on milk, as an article of the first necessity to the health and comfort of the community. A review of the different methods of production, and suggestions respecting the best means of improving its quality, reducing its price, and increasing its consumption. 8°. *London*, 1825.

TROEGER (J. A.) *De lacte. 4°. *Erfordiæ*, [1724].

UNITED STATES. *Congress. Senate.* A bill to prevent the illegal sale of all imitations of dairy

Milk.

products, and for other purposes. 49. Cong., 1. sess., S., 1837, March 10, 1886. Introd. by Mr. Miller. 8°. [*Washington*, 1886.]

DE VISSCHER (A.) *Diss. sistens nosologiam lactis generalem. 4°. *Lugd. Bat.*, 1769.

VOGLER (V. H.) *De lacte. sm. 4°. *Helmestadi*, 1678.

DE WASSERBERG (F. X.) Examen chemicum lactis. 8°. *Vindobonæ*, 1775.

WESTPHAL (A.) *Candidati Alexander Bernh. Kölpin disp. indicit, insimulque de materia lactis disserit. sm. 4°. *Gryphiswaldiæ*, [1764].

WILL (J. G. F.) Ueber die Milchabsonderung. 4°. *Erlangen*, 1850.

YOUNG (T.) *De lacte. 8°. *Edinburgi*, 1761.

Also, in: SANDIFORT. Thesaurus diss. [etc.] 4°. *Roterodami*, 1769, ii, 525-557.

————. *De natura et usu lactis in diversis animalibus. 8°. *Edinburgi*, 1776.

ZAKRJEVSKI (C. F.) *O deistvii moloka na mocheotdelenie i kojno-legochnyja poteri. [On the effect of milk on urinary secretions and loss by excretion from skin and lungs.] 8°. *St. Petersburg*, 1887.

Also, in: Voyenno-med. J., St. Petersb., 1887, clviii, pt. 2, 79: clix, 1, 4 diag.

Ainda o leite. Correio med. de Lisb., 1874-5, iv, 111-114.—**Albrecht.** Du lait de vache comme succédané du lait de femme. Cong. internat. d'hyg. et de démog. Compt. rend. 1882, Genève, 1883, ii, 505-529.—**Allen** (A. H.) Note on the fat of porpoise milk. Analyst, Lond., 1886, xi, 190-194. ————. The preservation of milk samples for reference. *Ibid.*, 203-205.—**Allen** (A. H.) & **Chattaway** (W.) Suggestions for the more ready employment of Adams' method of determining fat in milk. *Ibid.*, 71-73.—**Andouard** (A.) & **Dézaunay** (V.) Influence de la pulpe de diffusion sur le lait de vache. Compt. rend. Acad. d. sc., Par., 1884, xcix, 443-445.—**Baginsky** (A.) Ueber die Verwendbarkeit der durch Einwirkung hoher Temperaturen (über 100° Cels.) dargestellten Milchconserven, als Kindernahrungsmittel. Arch. f. Kinderh., Stuttg., 1882-3, iv, 259; 397. ————. Ueber die Phosphorsäureverbindungen in der Milch. Ztschr. f. physiol. Chem., Strassb., 1882-3, vii, 354-361.—**Baron.** Influence de la nourriture des vaches sur la composition du lait; (second rapport de la Commission du lait). Rev. d'hyg., Par., 1884, vi, 590-594. [*See, also, infra*, Girard.] *Also:* Paris méd., 1884, ix, 519. *Also:* Ann. d'hyg., Par., 1884, 3. s., xii, 338-342. *Also:* J. d. conn. méd. prat., Par., 1884, 3. s., vi, 329-331.—**Basso-Arnoux** (G.) Rapidità colla quale gli olii essenziali ingeriti passano nel latte. Osservatore, Torino, 1884, xx, 424.—**Benzon.** Om Fattiges mangelfulde Mælkeforsyning paa Landet, dens Følger og mulige Afhjælpning. Ugesk. f. Læger, Kjøbenh., 1883, viii, 4. R., 57; 111.—**Berg** (W.) Zusätzliche Bemerkungen zu dem im vi. Hefte, vi. Jahrg. des Organs, S. 338, vom Collegen Hrn. Wendrykowski abgefassten, sehr geschätzten Aufsatze über die Eigenschaft und den Einfluss der Milch, etc. Org. f. d. ges. Heilk., Berl., 1858, vii, 96-100.—**Bernays** (A. J.) On milk, stale and fresh. St. Thomas's Hosp. Rep. 1883, Lond., 1884, n. s., xiii, 27-37.—**Biedert** (P.) Ueber die Eiweisskörper der Menschen- und Kuhmilch. Tagebl. d. Versamml. deutsch. Naturf. u. Aerzte, Berl., 1886, lix, 279-281. *Also:* Deutsche med. Wchnschr., Leipz., 1887, xiii, 105.—**Bischoff** (C.) Ueber polizeiliche Milchcontrole! Deutsche Vrtljschr. f. öff. Gsndhtspflg., Brnschwg., 1887, xix, 411-420.—**Bogomoloff** (T.) Ueber die Zusammensetzung der Milch. Centralbl. f. d. med. Wissensch., Berl., 1871, ix, 625-627.—**Bollinger** (O.) Ueber Kindermilch und über den Einfluss der Nahrung auf die Beschaffenheit der Kuhmilch. Deutsche Ztschr. f. Thiermed., Leipz., 1880, vi, 270-291.—**Borsarelli.** Nota intorno alla composizione delle ceneri di latte ed alla quantità di fosforo che possono contenere. Gior. d. r. Accad. di med. di Torino, 1865, 2. s., liv, 456-480.—**Bouchardat.** Expériences sur la décomposition du lait. Ann. d'hyg., Par., 1834, xi, 456-458.—**Braconnot** (H.) Mémoire sur le caséum et sur le lait; nouvelles resources qu'ils peuvent offrir à la société. Ann. de chim. et phys., Par., 1830, xliii, 337-351.—**Brame** (C.) Sur les globules du lait. Rec. d. trav. Soc. méd. d'Indre-et-Loire, Tours, 1857, 63-73.—**Branco** (A.) O leite. Correio med. de Lisb., 1874-5, iv, 85; 99.—**Brücke** (E.) Bemerkungen über die Bestimmung des specifischen Gewichtes der Milch. Arch. f. Anat., Physiol. u. wissensch. Med., Berl., 1847, 409-414.—**Bull** (E.) Steriliseret Melk. Tidsskr. f. prakt. Med., Kristiania, 1886, vi, 373-378.—**Camerer.** Versuche über den Stoffwechsel bei Ernährung mit Kuhmilch. Ztschr. f. Biol., München, 1880, xvi, 493-496.—**Centrifugemælken.** Ugesk. f. Læger, Kjøbenh., 1883, 4. R., viii, 465: 1884, 4. R., ix, 78.—**Chevalier** (A.) & **Henry** (O.) Mémoire sur le lait. J. de

Milk.

chim. méd., etc., Par., 1839, 2. s., v, 145; 193. *Also*, Reprint.—**Chichkoff** (L.) Note sur la composition chimique du lait. Bull. Soc. imp. d. nat. de Moscou (1880), 1881, lv, 141-144.—**Cold.** Om Centrifugemælk. Ugesk. f. Læger, Kjøbenh., 1883, 4. R., viii, 425-435.—**Coles** (W.) Milk and milk culture. St. Louis M. & S. J., 1883, xlv, 139-154.—**Davy** (J.) Miscellaneous observations on blood and milk. Tr. Roy. Soc. Edinb., 1845, xvi, 53-59.—**Delattre** (D.) Un côté de la question du lait. Gaz. d. hôp., Par., 1883, lvi, 227. *Also:* Marseille méd., 1883, xx, 261-264.—**Dogel** (A.) O svoistvach i perevariv. jenskago i korovjago moloka i tvorojini. [Degree of digestibility of woman's and cow's milk and curdled milk.] Vrach, St. Petersb., 1885, vi, 440; 461.—**Donders** (F. C.) Ontwikkeling van de vormbestanddeelen der melk. Onderzoek. ged. in h. physiol. Lab. d. Utrecht. Hoogesch., 1849-50, ii, 227-229, 1 pl.—**Doremus** (R. O.) Report of an address on milk, in its medico-legal aspects. Papers Med.-Leg. Soc. N. Y. (1875-8), 1886, 3. s., 222-228.—**Duclaux** (E.) Sur les matières albuminoïdes du lait. Compt. rend. Acad. d. sc., Par., 1884, xcviii, 373-375. ———. Sur la constitution du lait. *Ibid.*, 438-441. ———. Le lait et sa composition chimique. Rev. scient., Par., 1885, 3. s., ix, 685-690.—**Dumas.** Note sur la constitution du lait et du sang. Monit. scient., Par., 1871, 3. s., i, 778-783.—**Duquesnel** (H.) Lait. N. dict. de méd. et chir. prat., Par., 1875, xx, 58-86.—**Estudos** sobre o leite da mulher, da vacca, da jumenta e da cadella. J. Soc. d. sc. med. de Lisb., 1876, 2. s., xl, 225-229.—**Fazio** (E.) Il latte; sua importanza biologica. Gior. internaz. d. sc. med., Napoli, 1884, n. s., vi, 265-281.—**Finne** (G.) Steriliseret Melk. Tidsskr. f. prakt. Med., Kristiania, 1886, vi, 409-411.—**Firth** (R. H.) On the occurrence of a poisonous ptomaine in milk. Indian M. J., Calcutta, 1887, vi, 1-5.—**Fjord** (N. J.) Om Mælk, saaledes som den i sød og skummet Tilstand forekommer i de danske Meierier. Hyg. Medd., Kjøbenh., 1884, ii, 204-232.—**Fraas.** Zur Geschichte der Milchkugeln und Milchreactionen. Arch. f. path. Anat., etc., Berl., 1853, vii, 316-323.—**Girard** (C.) La nourriture des vaches laitières, et son influence sur la composition du lait. Rev. d'hyg., Par., 1884, vi, 361-405. [*See, also, supra*, Baron.] *Also:* Ann. d'hyg., Par., 1884, 3. s., xii, 228-257.—**Goppelsröder** (F.) Ueber praktische Milchuntersuchung. Centralbl. f. allg. Gsndhtspflg., Bonn, 1886, v, 278-288.—**Guérard.** Lait. Dict. de méd., 2. éd., Par., 1838, xvii, 438-470.—**Hammarsten** (O.) Om mjölkystningen och de dervid verksamma fermenterna i magslemhinnan. [On the curdling of milk and the persistent active fermentation in the mucous membranes of the stomach.] Upsala Läkaref. Förh., 1873, viii, 63-86.—**Hammerbacher** (F.) Ueber den Einfluss des Pilocarpin und Atropin auf die Milchbildung. Arch. f. d. ges. Physiol., Bonn, 1883-4, xxxiii, 228-239.—**Harrington** (C.) [*et al.*]. Reports of the analysts of milk. Rep. Bd. Health Mass. 1886, Bost., 1887, xviii, 115-154.—**Hermann** (L.) Ein Beitrag zur Kenntniss der Milch. Arch. f. d. ges. Physiol., Bonn, 1881-2, xxvi, 442-444.—**Hesse** (W.) Ein neuer Apparat zur Sterilisirung der Milch für den Hausgebrauch. Deutsche med. Wchnschr., Berl., 1886, xii, 323.—**Hoppe** (F.) Untersuchungen über die Bestandtheile der Milch und ihre nächsten Zersetzungen. Arch. f. path. Anat., etc., Berl., 1859, xvii, 417-451.—**Hueppe** (F.) Ueber die Zersetzungen der Milch und die biologischen Grundlagen der Gährungsphysiologie. Deutsche med. Wchnschr., Berl., 1884, x, 777; 796; 811.—**Ibañez** (J.) Estudio sobre la leche. Estudio, México, 1876, i, 308-310.—**Jimenez** (L. M.) Uso de la leche. Gac. méd. de México, 1869, iv, 140.—**Jolly.** Communication sur le lait. Bull. Soc. de méd. prat. de Par. (1880), 1881, 119-122.—**Joly** (N.) & **Filhol** (E.) Recherches sur le lait. Mém. d. concours . . . Acad. roy. de méd. de Belg., Brux., 1855, iii, 1-180, 2 pl. *Also*, Reprint.—**Kehrer** (F. A.) Zur Morphologie des Milchcaseïns. Arch. f. Gynaek., Berl., 1871, ii, 1-28. ———. Ueber die angeblichen Albuminathüllen der Milchkügelchen. *Ibid.*, 1871-2, iii, 495-502.—**Kemmerich** (E.) Untersuchungen über die Bildung der Milchfette. Centralbl. f. d. med. Wissensch., Berl., 1866, iv, 465-468. *Also*, Reprint.—**Kletzinsky** (V.) Ueber die Milch. Oesterr. Ztschr. f. prakt. Heilk., Wien, 1858, iv, 43; 139; 147.—**Lait** (Composition du). Ann. d'hyg., Par., 1849, xli, 221.—**L[amberges]** (A. K.) Περὶ τροφῶν; γάλα. Ἐφημ. ἑταιρ. ὑγιειν., Ἀθῆναι, 1883, 137-141.—**Lammerts van Bueren** (R.) Onderzoekingen over de melkbolletjes. Nederl. Lancet, Gravenh., 1848-9, 2. s., iv, 722-732. ———. De ontwikkeling van de vormbestanddeelen der melk. *Ibid.*, 1849-50, 2. s., v, 1-38, 1 pl.—**Lapchinski** (F. F.) K voprosu ob usvojaemosti moloka. [Assimilation of milk.] Vrach, St. Petersb., 1880, i, 479-481.—**Léger.** La caséine du lait pour l'émulsion des médicaments. Bull. et mém. Soc. de thérap., Par., 1887, 2. s., xiv, 96-98.—**Loeffler.** Ueber Bakterien in der Milch. Berl. klin. Wchnschr., 1887, xxiv, 607; 629. *Also:* Rundschau a. d. Geb. d. Thiermed. u. vergleich. Path., Osterwieck, 1887, iii, 269; 281; 289; 297.—**Mandl.** De la structure des globules du lait. [Rap. de de Lens.] Bull. Acad. de méd., Par., 1841-2, vii, 1157-1168.—**Marchand** (E.) Étude sur la fermentation lactique du lait, suivie de

Milk.

recherches sur la composition du lait sécrété par les vaches de différentes races. Assoc. franç. pour l'avance. d. sc. Compt.-rend. 1878, Par., 1879, vii, 411-433.—**Martens.** Rapport sur la question: Exposer l'état de nos connaissances sur le lait. Bull. Acad. roy. de méd. de Belg., Brux., 1854-5, xiv, 460-464. [Discussion], 501.—**Medin** (O.) Apparat för sterilisering af mjölk. Svens. Läk.-Sällsk. n. Handl., Stockholm, 1886, 197.—**Mittelstrass** (*Gebr.*). Ein neuer Milchprüfer. Ztschr. f. Untersuch. v. Lbnsmttln, Eichstätt u. Stuttg., 1880, iii, 159-161.—**Morabelli** (F.) Untersuchungen über die Natur einiger animalischen, und sonderlich einiger milchähnlichen Materien. Samml. auserl. Abhandl. z. Gebr. prakt. Aerzte, Leipz., 1807, xxiv, 461-476.—**Munk** (H.) Bewegung und Milchsecretion. Arch. f. Physiol., Leipz., 1883, Suppl.-Bd., 363-367.—**Musso** (G.) Chimica fisiologica; sugli stati del solfo nel latte, e sulla normale esistenza nel latte vaccino di solfati e solfocianati. R. Ist. Lomb. di sc. e lett. Rendic., Milano, 1877, 2. s., x, 396-410.—**Musso** (G.) & **Menozzi** (A.) Studj sull' albumina del latte e sulla genesi della ricotta. *Ibid.*, 1878, 2. s., xi, 399-416.—**Nasse.** Versuche über die Wärmefassungskräfte der Galle, der Milch und des Harns. Deutsches Arch. f. d. Physiol., Halle, 1815, i, 500-505. ———. Ueber die mikroskopischen Bestandtheile der Milch. Arch. f. Anat., Physiol. u. wissensch. Med., Berl., 1840, 259-266.—**Nencki** (L.) & **Fabian** (A.) O przetworach fermentowanych z mleka, a mianowicie o kumysie i kefirze. [On fermentative processes in milk, and especially in koumiss and kefir.] Gaz. lek., Warszawa, 1887, 2. s., vii, 53; 75; 167; 193.—**Newton** (W. K.) Reports of the milk inspector [1.-7.]. Rep. Bd. Health N. Jersey 1879-80, Camden, 1881, iv, 209: 1880-81, Mount Holly, 1881, v, 115: 1881-2, Woodbury, 1882, vi, 209: (1882-3), 1883, vii, 247: 1883-4, Trenton, 1884, viii, 219: 1884-5, ix, 263: (1885-6), 1887, x, 317. *Also*, Reprint of 6. report.—**Palm** (R.) Moloko, ego sostavnija chasti i preparati. [Milk, its component parts and preparations.] Voyenno-med. J., St. Petersb., 1886, clv, pt. 6, 95-134.—**Panum.** Bemærkninger om Mælks Næringsværdi. Hyg. Medd., Kjøbenh., 1884, ii, 232-242.—**Parmentier** & **Déyeux.** Mémoire sur la question suivante, proposée par la Société royale de médecine: Déterminer, par l'examen comparé des propriétés physiques et chymiques, la nature des laits de femme, de vache, de chèvre, d'ânesse, de brebis et de juments. Hist. Soc. roy. de méd. 1787-8, Par., 1790, ix, 415-524.—**Peddie** (A.) On the mammary secretion, and its pathological changes. Month. J. M. Sc., Lond. & Edinb., 1848-9, ix, 65-88, 1 pl. *Also*, Reprint.—**Pfeiffer** (E.) Ueber die Eiweisskörper der Milch und die Methoden ihrer quantitativen Bestimmung. Mitth. a. d. amtl. Lebensm.-Untersuch.-Anst. . . . zu Wiesb. 1883-4, Berl., 1885, 150-173.—**Piorry** (P.-A.) Lait artificiel ou lait-bouillon. *In his:* Clin. méd.-chir., 8°, Par., 1869, 70-78.—**Pirotta** (R.) & **Riboni** (G.) Studj sul latte. R. Ist. Lomb. di sc. e lett. Rendic., Milano, 1878, 2. s., xi, 866: 1879, 2. s., xii, 5; 69.—**Pooler** (H. A.) The milk supply of large cities and the improper mode in which it is conducted. Gaillard's M. J., N. Y., 1886, xlii, 587-602. *Also:* Med. News, Phila., 1886, xlix, 470-472.—**Possenti** (G. B.) Sul latte; studi chimici. Sperimentale, Firenze, 1859, 4. s., iv, 115-128.—**Quevenne** (T.-A.) Mémoire sur le lait. Ann. d'hyg., Par., 1841, xxvi, 5; 257.—**Rejchman** (I. M.) Badania nad trawieniem mleka w żołądku ludzkim, dokonane w celach klin. [Coagulation, digestion, and fermentation of milk.] Gaz. lek., Warszawa, 1884, 2. s., iv, 959; 1035.—**Rödén** (H.) Om blodserums inverkan på mjölkens koagulation med löpe. [Influence of blood serum in coagulation of milk by rennet.] Upsala Läkaref. Förh., 1886-7, xxii, 546-575.—**Rogers** (T. B.) Milk, from a medico-sanitary standpoint. J. Comp. M. & S., N. Y., 1885, vii, 101-139.—**Rohé** (G. H.) City feeding of milch-cows. Science, N. Y., 1887, ix, 440.—**Sartori** (G.) Sulla determinazione rapida della materia secca nel latte. Ann. di chim. e di farm., Milano, 1886, 4. s., iv, 98-105.—**Schaffer** (F.) Ueber den Einfluss der sexualen Erregung auf die Zusammensetzung der Kuhmilch. Mitth. d. naturf. Gesellsch. in Bern (1883), 1884, nos. 1064-1072, 63-66.—**Scherer.** Die Milch. Handwörterb. d. Physiol., Brnschwg., 1850, ii, 449-475.—**Schlossberger** (J.) Wird die Milch durch ihr Stagniren in der Milchdrüse sauer? Arch. d. Ver. f. gemeinsch. Arb. z. Förd. d. wissensch. Heilk., Götting., 1856, ii, 260-264.—**Schmidt** (F. A.) Ueber das Soxhlet'sche Milchkochverfahren. Centralbl. f. allg. Gsndhtspflg., Bonn, 1887, vi, 133-142.—**Schmidt-Mülheim.** Findet in der Milch eine Caseïnbildung auf Kosten des Albumins statt? Arch. f. d. ges. Physiol., Bonn, 1882, xxviii, 243-254. ———. Beiträge zur Kenntniss der Eiweiss-Körper der Kuhmilch. *Ibid.*, 287-312. ———. Beiträge zur Kenntniss der Milchsecretion. *Ibid.*, 1882-3, xxx, 602-620. ———. Ueber die Fortschritte auf dem Gebiete der Milchwirthschaft. Deutsche Ztschr. f. Thiermed., Leipz., 1883, ix, 146-159.—**Schreiner.** Ueber Kuhmilch: Veränderung derselben beim Kochen, Verhalten zu Säuren und Lab vor und nach dem Kochen, Quantitätsveränderung während der Lactationsperiode. Amtl. Ber. ü. d. Versamml. deutsch. Naturf. u. Aerzte, München, 1877, l, 218.—**Schübler.** Untersuchungen über die Milch und ihre

Milk.

nähern Bestandtheile. Deutsches Arch. f. d. Physiol., Halle, 1818, iv, 557–586, 2 pl. *Also, transl.: J.* compl. du dict. d. sc. méd., Par., 1819, iv, 311–327. — **Schwalbe** (C.) Ueber die Membran der Milchkügelchen. Arch. f. mikr. Anat., Bonn, 1872, viii, 269–273.—**Sebelien** (J.) Bidrag till Kundskaben om Mælkens Aeggehvidestoffer. [Albuminous bodies in milk.] Upsala Läkaref. Förh., 1885, xx, 334–351. *Also:* Overs. o. d. k. Danske Vidensk. Selsk. Forh., Kjøbenh., 1885. No. 1, 1–18. *Also, transl.:* Ztschr. f. physiol. Chem., Strassb., 1884-5, ix, 445–464.—**Short** (F. G.) Analysis of milk. Am. Chem. J., Balt., 1887-8, ix, 100–103.—**de Sinéty.** Recherches sur les globules du lait. Arch. de physiol. norm. et path., Par., 1874, 2. s., i, 479–488.—**Slack** (D. B.) Experiments on milk. Boston M. & S. J., 1843-4, xxix, 413–415.—**Something** about milk. Nature, Lond., 1879-80, xxi, 402–404.—**Strüve** (H.) Studien über Milch. J. f. prakt. Chem., Leipz., 1883, xxvii, 249 : 1884, n. F., xxix, 70; 110.—**Struve** (G. V.) O chimicheskom sostave moloka. [Chemical composition of milk.] Protok. zasiad. Kavkazsk. med. Obsh., Tiflis, 1882, xix, 309–318.—**Thierfelder** (H.) Zur Physiologie der Milchbildung. Arch. f. d. ges. Physiol , Bonn, 1883, xxxii, 619–625.—**Thomson** (W.) Note on the estimation of fat in milk. Analyst, Lond., 1886, xi, 73–75. — **Toussaint** (E.) Influence du lait des vaches nourries de drèches sur la santé et la mortalité des enfants du premier âge. Rev. d'hyg., Par., 1885. vii, 932. [Discussion]. 994 — **Van Stipriaan** (L. A.) & **Bond** (N.) Dissertatio qua respondetur ad quæstionem propositam a Societate regia medica, quæ exigit : "Ut determinetur, per examen comparatum proprietatum physicarum et chemicarum. natura lactis muliebris, vaccini, caprilli, asinini, ovilli et equini". Hist. Soc. roy. de méd. 1787–8, Par., 1799, ix, 525–628.— **Vernois** & **Becquerel** (A.) Recherches sur le lait. Ann. d'hyg., Par., 1853, xlix, 257 : l, 43.—**Vieth** (P.) On the composition of milk and milk products. Analyst, Lond., 1886, xi, 66–71 : 1887, xii, 39. ——. Notes on the complete analysis of milk. *Ibid.*, 1887, xii, 59–65.— **Volpe** (L.) Confronti fra il latte vaccino ottenuto durante continuo, eccessivo, prolungato lavoro, e quello avuto durante il riposo. Gior. d. Soc. ital. d' ig., Milano, 1884, vi, 530–535.—**Waage** (P.) Steriliseret Melk. Tidsskr. f. prakt. Med., Kristiania, 1887, vii, 5.—**Wawrinsky** (R.) Stockholms mjölkkommission. Hygiea, Stockholm, 1887, xlix, 269–273.—**Young** (P. A.) Milk in relation to public health. Edinb. Health Soc. Health Lect., 1885-6, 6. s., 55–78.—**Zahn** (F. W.) Untersuchungen über die Eiweisskörper der Milch. Arch. f. d. ges. Physiol., Bonn, 1869, ii, 598–611.

Milk (*Abnormal, poisonous*), *or as a cause of disease.*

See, also, **Cattle** (*Foot and mouth disease of*); **Cheese** (*Poisonous*); **Diphtheria** (*Causes, etc., of*); **Fever** (*Typhoid, Causes, etc., of*); **Ice-cream** (*Poisonous*); **Lactation** (*Abnormities of*); **Lactation** (*Pathology of*); **Milk** (*Metastases of*); **Milk** *and tuberculosis*; **Milk-sickness**; **Scarlatina** (*Causes, etc., of*); **Scrofula**; **Syphilis** (*Communication of*) *in lactation*; **Tyrotoxicon.**

BENZIN (J.) *Des altératious que le lait peut subir dans le sein de la mère, et de son influence sur la santé de l'enfant. 4°. *Paris*, 1838.

BEVERIDGE (R.) On a peculiar form of disease arising from milk contamination. 8°. *Aberdeen*, 1882.

Also [Abstr.], *in:* Brit. M. J., Lond., 1881, ii, 515.

CHEBERT (P.) & FROMAGE (C.-M.-F.) D'une altération du lait de vache, désignée sous le nom de lait bleu. 8°. *Paris, an XIII* [1805].

DAMOURETTE (F.-B.-E.) * Du lait, et de l'influence de ses altérations sur les maladies des enfants. 4°. *Paris*, 1854.

FINCKE (B. A. L.) * De lactis immutationibus et in specie de lacte cruento. 8°. *Halis Sax.*, 1849.

PELÉE DE VALONCOUR (A. B.) *An Parisiis a lacte valetudinum malarum Ilias? 4°. [*Paris*, 1765.]

ZORN (E.) Die Anomalien der Milch. 8°. *Jena*, 1880.

Ali-Cohen (C. H.) Typhus-infectie door melk ; een reeks van gevallen, te Groningen waargenomen. Nederl. Tijdschr. v. Geneesk., Amst., 1887, xxiii, 2. deel, 78–84.— **Axe** (J. W.) Milk in relation to public health. Veterinarian, Lond., 1885, lviii, 308; 384. —**Baldwin** (D. A.) Typhoid fever and milk. Med. Rec., N. Y., 1883, xxiv, 585.—**Becker** (A. R.) Milk as a vehicle of contagion. N. York M. J., 1878, xxviii, 507–509.—**Blyth** (A. W.)

Milk (*Abnormal, poisonous*), *or as a cause of disease.*

On the fatty metamorphosis of the albuminoids in milk and cheese. Analyst, Lond., 1878, iii, 230–235.—**Bond** (F. T.) On the dissemination of infectious disease by milk. San. Rec., Lond., 1880–81, n. s., ii, 299. — **Bourlier** (A.) Note sur des cas d'empoisonnements occasionnés par le lait de chèvre. Alger méd., 1885. xiii, 163–170. — **Bourquelot** (E.) Le microbe du lait bleu. Rev. scient., Par., 1884, 3. s., vii, 427–432.—**Britton** (T.) Milk supply. Is it desirable to take any, and what further, measures to prevent the spread of zymotic diseases through the milk supply of our towns? Tr. Nat. Ass. Promot. Social Sc. 1883, Lond., 1884, xxvii, 401–408. — **Brown** (W.) On an outbreak of typhoid fever in Carlisle, in which milk was the vehicle of infection, and where typhoid fever in the inmates of the dairy was associated with an infective fever among cows. San. Rec., Lond., 1887-8, n. s., ix, 10 – 15. — **Brush** (E. F.) Acute milk-poisoning. Med. Rec., N. Y., 1882, xxii, 424–426.—**Cameron** (C. A.) Illness caused by filth in milk. Dublin J. M. Sc., 1882, 3. s., lxxiii, 112–116.—**Cameron** (J.) Observations on a certain malady occurring among cows at a time when the milk produced by them disseminated scarlet fever. [Abstr.] Lancet, Lond., 1886, i, 927.—**Certain** (On) pathological conditions in milk as the cause of disease in infants. Lond. M. Gaz., 1845, n. s., i, 976–979.—**Chamberlain** (C. W.) Milk as a medium for the transmission of disease. Rep. Bd. Health Connect. 1882, Hartford, 1883, v, 233–255.—**Chambrelent.** De la présence des germes morbides dans le lait. Arch. de tocol., Par., 1884, xi, 498–506. — **Christie** (J.) On milk as a vehicle for the communication of disease. San. Jour. for Scotland, Glasg., 1876-8, i, 451-454.—**Clark** (J. S.) Disease in the milk-can. Boston M. & S. J.,1887, cxvii, 100.—**Colas.** Observations de lait bleu chez la vache, dans différents hameaux de la commune d'Ouanne. Bull. Soc. méd. de l'Yonne 1867, Auxerre, 1868, viii, 31–48. — **Collins** (J.) Notes on the precautions which have been taken against infection being conveyed by milk, and suggestions as to the necessity for further protection against the dangers of spreading disease. Tr. Nat. Ass. Promot. Social Sc. 1881, Lond., 1882, 622–625.—**Dufrénois.** Observations sur le danger d'allaiter les enfants après un accès de colère, ou l'abus des boissons alcooliques. J. de méd. et chir. prat , Par., 1833, iv, 401–404.—**Dugall** (J.) The dissemination of zymotic diseases by milk. Glasgow M. J., 1872-3, [4. s.], v, 312–331. — **Dupré** & **Lécuyer.** Transmission à l'espèce humaine de la péripneumonie contagieuse par le lait des vaches qui en sont atteintes. Ann. d'hyg., Par., 1885, 3. s., xiv, 87–99. *Also:* Union méd. et scient. du nord-est, Reims, 1885, ix. 195–208. — **Empoisonnement** par le lait provenant d'une vache soumise à un traitement mercuriel. Ann. d'hyg , Par., 1818, xxxix, 453.—**Ewart** (J. C.) On a new form of febrile disease associated with the presence of an organism distributed with milk from the Oldmill Reformatory School, Aberdeen. Proc. Roy. Soc. Lond., 1881, xxxii, 492–498.— **Fagan** (J.) Pseudo-membranous stomatitis produced by the milk of a cow with inflamed udder. Brit. M. J., Lond., 1869, ii, 489.—**Firmin.** Urticaire provoqué chez un enfant par le lait de sa nourrice. Bull. gén. de thérap., etc., Par., 1874, lxxxvi, 465.—**Firth** (R. H.) Report upon some obscure cases of poisoning by milk, apparently due to the presence of a ptomaine. Practitioner, Lond., 1887, xxxix, 75–80.—**Francis** (C. R.) Poison in milk. Indian M. Gaz., Calcutta, 1868, iii, 183.—**Gewisse** (Ueber) pathologische Zustände der Milch, als die Ursache von Krankheiten bei Säuglingen. J. f. Kinderkr., Berl., 1846, vi, 13–19. — **Girard.** Note sur l'influence de certaines altérations du lait comme cause de divers états pathologiques chez les nouveau-nés. Arch. de méd., Par., 1845, 4. s., viii. 192–200.—**Gooding** (J. C.) Disease of mouth and bowels from using the milk of cows affected with "foot and mouth disease". Med. Times & Gaz., Lond., 1872, i, 94. — **Graham** (A. R.) Cases of illness from drinking milk tainted with sewer-gases. Brit. M. J., Lond , 1874, ii, 742. — **Hagner** (C. E.) Cases of poisoning by milk. Tr. M. Soc. Dist. Columb., Wash., 1877, iv, 7.—**Hart** (E.) Milch und Wasser als Krankheitsursachen. Oesterr. ärztl. Vereinsztg., Wien, 1879, iii, 195; 205. ——. The influence of milk in spreading zymotic disease. Tr. Internat. M. Cong., 7. sess., Lond., 1881, iv, 491–544. *Also, transl.* [Abstr.]: Wien. med. Presse, 1881, xxii. 1139. ——. Milk supply. Is it desirable to take any, and what further, measures to prevent the spread of zymotic diseases through the milk supply of our towns? Tr. Nat. Ass. Promot. Social Sc. 1883, Lond., 1884, xxvii. 408–455.—**Haschek.** Muthmassliche Vergiftung durch Milch. Wien. med. Presse, 1866, vii, 42; 83.—**Heisch** (C.) On diseased milk. Analyst, Lond., 1878, iii, 249–251.—**Higginson** (F. J.) Poisoning by milk. Boston M. & S. J., 1829-30, ii, 305-308.—**Hill** (A.) Remarks on sewage-farm milk and butter. Analyst. Lond., 1885, x, 135–139. *Also* [Abstr.]: Polyclinic, Phila., 1885-6, iii, 20.—**Hüppe** (F.) Untersuchungen über die Zersetzung der Milch durch Mikroorganismen. Mitth. a. d. k. Gsndhtsamte, Berl., 1884, ii, 309.

Milk (*Abnormal, poisonous*), *or as a cause of disease.*

371. *Also* [Abstr.] : Breslau. aerztl. Ztschr., 1884, vi, 162.— **Infected** milk; the dangers of our milk supply. Med. Times & Gaz., Lond., 1878, i, 365.—**Jaillard.** Du lait des vaches atteintes de la maladie aphtheuse, dite cocotte. Rec. de mém. de méd. . . . mil., Par., 1876, xxxii, 191.— **Jameson.** Infected milk. Lancet, Lond., 1881, i, 27.— **Johnson** (M. M.) Milk; its nature, its contamination, and as a vehicle of contagion. Proc. Connect. M. Soc., Hartford, 1881, n. s., ii, no. 2, 180–188.—**Karsten** (H.) Notiz über blaue Flecken auf geronnener Milch. Deutsche Ztschr. f. Thiermed., Leipz., 1879, y, 326.—**Lécuyer** (H.) Le lait des vaches atteintes de péripneumonie contagieuse peut-il transmettre la maladie à l'espèce humaine? Rev. d'hyg., Par., 1887, ix, 221–229. *Also* [Abstr.]: Normandie méd., Rouen, 1887, iii, 118. — **Lécuyer** (H.) & **Dupré.** Mémoire sur la transmission à l'espèce humaine de la péripneumonie coutagieuse par le lait des vaches qui en sont atteintes. Ann. d'hyg., Par., 1885, 3. s., xiv, 87–97. [Discussion], 352–359. *Also:* Rev. d'hyg., Par., 1885, vii, 446; 551. — **Leffmann** (H.) Ropy or viscid milk. Agriculture of Pennsylv. Rep. State Bd. 1879, Harrisburg, 1880, 29–32. — **Mackay** (A. E.) Cases of poisoning by goat's milk. Edinb. M. J., 1861-2, vii, 825–827. — **Mackay** (G. A. D.) Milk and diseased cattle. San. Jour., Glasg., 1887-8, n. s., xi, 139–142. — **Mareschal.** Note sur un cas d'empoisonnement par des caillebottes. J. de la sect. de méd. Soc. acad. Loire-Inf., Nantes, 1839, xv. 244–248.—**Merkwürdiger** Fall einer zufälligen Vergiftung durch den Genuss saurer Milch, bei welchem auch die Priorität des Todes zur Sprache kam. Jahrb. d. ges. Staatsarznk., Leipz., 1835, i, 99–113.—**Milch** (Die) als Träger von Ansteckungsstoffen. Gesundheit, Elberfeld, 1877-8, iii, 212–215.—**Milch** und Wasser als Krankheitsursachen. Wien. med. Presse, 1879, xx, 1001; 1032.—**Milk** as a vehicle of infection. Practitioner, Lond., 1883, xxxi, 386 – 391. — **Moriggia.** Relazione delle sperienze fisio-tossicologiche sul latte di capre nutrite con erbe ed alcaloidi velenosi. Atti Accad. med. di Roma, 1877, iii, 16–19.—**Muter** (J.) Note on a curious case of dangerous milk. Analyst, Lond., 1878, iii, 357.—**Newton** (W. K.) & **Wallace** (S.) Cases of milk-poisoning, with remarks on tyrotoxicon. Med. News, Phila., 1886, xlix, 343–345. *Also:* Rep. Bd. Health N. Jersey 1885-6, Trenton, 1887, x, 318–325.—**Nichols** (A. H.) Report on the use of milk from cows affected with foot and mouth disease. Rep. Bd. Health Mass., Bost., 1871, ii, 426.—**Pattinson** (J.) On an abnormal sample of new milk. Analyst, Lond., 1876-7, i. 47–50.—**Pirrie** (J. M. G.) The milk fever epidemic in Aberdeen. Lancet, Lond., 1881, i, 657.—**Power** (W. H.) Milk-scarlatina in London in 1885; being a report on certain observed relations between scarlatina in various districts of London and milk supplied from a dairy farm at Hendon. San. Jour., Glasg., 1886-7, n. s., x, 140; 161.— **Propagation** (The) of milk through the medium of milk. *Ibid.*, 1887-8, n. s., xi, 142 – 145. — **Propagation** (The) of zymotic diseases through milk. Med. Times & Gaz., Lond., 1873, ii, 174. — **Reiset** (J.) Observations sur le lait bleu. Compt. rend. Acad. d. sc., Par., 1883, xcvi, 682; 745. — **Robinson** (M. K.) Outbreak of epidemic sore throat, following use of milk from cows suffering from aphthous fever. Practitioner, Lond., 1884, xxxii, 467–475.—**Schmidtmann** (H.) Geschichte einer tödtlichen Milchversetzung. J. d. pract. Heilk., Berl., 1832, lxxiv, 4. St., 63–71. — **Schmidt - Mülheim.** Untersuchungen über fadenziehende Milch. Arch. f. d. ges. Physiol., Bonn, 1881-2, xxvii, 490–510.—**Sergeant** (E) Symptoms of patients affected by drinking contaminated milk. Med. Times & Gaz., Lond., 1876, ii, 200. — **Simpson** (W. J.) On the spread of cholera through the medium of specifically polluted milk. Practitioner, Lond., 1887, xxxix. 144–156.—**Stadelmann.** Ueber die gesundheitsschädlichen Veränderungen der Milch der Kühe durch Krankheiten des Rindviehs. Vrtljschr. f. gerichtl. u. öff. Med, Berl., 1852, ii, 318–346.—**Sudakoff** (A.) Uslovija rasprostranenija bolieznei posredstvom moloka. [The propagation of diseases by infected milk.] Vestnik sudeb. med., etc., St. Petersb., 1883, ii, pt. 3, 63: iii, 103.— **Tait** (L.) The influence of milk in the propagation of contagious diseases. Brit. M. J., Lond., 1870, ii, 344.— **Thursfield** (W. N.) On the dissemination of infectious disease by milk; with suggestions for its more effectual prevention. Tr. Soc. M. Off. Health, Lond., 1880-81, 40–44. *Also:* San. Rec., Lond., 1880-81, n. s., ii, 243. — On cows' milk as a vehicle of infectious and epidemic disease to the community, with suggestions for the more effectua' prevention of such outbreaks. Internat. Health Exh. Confer., Lond., 1884, [no. 2], 152–197. *Also* [Abstr.]: Tr. Soc. M. Off. Health, Lond., 1883-4, 166–186. *Also* [Abstr.]: Med. Times & Gaz., Lond., 1884, i, 827–830.—**Toscani** (D.) Su di un caso di avvelenamento di molte persone mediante l' uso di latte caprino. Arch. di med., chir. ed ig., Roma, 1875, vii, 481–503.—**Tóthfalusi** (G.) A teheneknél előforduló betegségek befolynak a tej minőségére. [Hydrocephalus hydatidum (turnsick) in cows influencing the milk.] Államorvos, Budapest, 1878, iii, 153–157.—**Tur-**

ner (E.) The insanitary condition of milk-shops as bearing upon the dissemination of disease. San. Rec., Lond., 1877, vii, 49; 69; 85.—**Vacher** (F.) Milk supply. Is it desirable to take any, and what further, measures to prevent the spread of zymotic diseases through the milk supply of our towns? Tr. Nat. Ass. Promot. Social Sc. 1883, Lond., 1884, xxvii. 395–401.—**Valeri.** Rapporto sull' avvelenamento fortuito per latte di capra. Atti Accad. med. di Roma (1875-6), 1877, i, 70–73.—**Vallin** (E.) La souillure du lait par les germes morbides. Rev. d'hyg., Par., 1881, iii, 457–461.—**Vernois.** Note sur la diminution et la disparition des globules et par suite de la matière caséense dans le lait. Actes Soc. méd. d. hôp. de Par., 1852, 38–50.— **Vigir.** Lettre sur une couleur de rose éclatante, que prenoit, au bout de quelque tems, le lait d'une nouvelle accouchée. J. de méd., chir., pharm., etc., Par., 1770, xxxii, 222–225. ——. Lettre sur une couleur de rose que prenoit, au bout de quelque tems, le lait qui couloit de la mamelle d'une nouvelle accouchée. *Ibid.*, 1771, xxxv, 62–65.—**Warren** (J. H.) Poisonous milk. Boston M. & S. J., 1880, ciii, 505.—**Wigner** (G. W.) On some recent cases of diseased milk. Analyst, Lond., 1878, iii, 251–254. ——. Diseased milk. San. Rec., Lond., 1878, viii, 276–278.—**Willington** (H.) Affectable and infectable susceptibility of milk. Lancet, Lond., 1873, ii, 283.—**Zimmermann** (O. E. R.) Die blaue Milch. Ztschr. f. mikr. Fleischschau, Berl., 1881, ii, 76.

Milk (*Adulterations, analyses, and hygiene of*).

See, also, **Milk** (*Abnormal, etc.*); **Milk** (*Human*); **Milk** *and tuberculosis.*

ADAM (A.-F.) *Étude sur les principales méthodes d'essai et d'analyse du lait, suivie de la description d'un nouveau procédé pour l'analyse complète de ce liquide. 4°. *Paris*, 1879.

ANDREEVSKI (P. V.) * O sposobach izsledovanija prodajnago i razbavlennago vodojou moloka. [On method of investigation of salable and water-mixed milk.] 8°. *St. Petersburg*, 1883.

AUERBACH (L.) *Beitrag zur quantitativen Analyse der Milch. 4°. *Kiel*, 1868.

AXE (J. W.) Milk in relation to public health. 8°. *London*, 1885.

VON DER BECKE (W.) Die Milchprüfungs-Methoden; nach vergleichenden Untersuchungen bearbeitet und zusammengestellt von . . . mit einer Vorrede von J. König. 8°. *Bremen*, 1882.

BERGSMA (C. A.) Responsio ad quæstionem chemico-œconomicam a facultate disciplinarum mathematicarum et physicarum propositam: Instituatur lactis vaccini examen chemicum, ad hodiernam artis perfectionem accommodatum . . . 8°. [*n. p., n. d.*]

BOSTON. Annual reports of the milk inspector to the mayor and board of aldermen. 23., 1881-2; 26., 1884-5. 8°. [*Boston, 1882-5.*]

BUNGE (G.) * Der Kali-, Natron- und Chlorgehalt der Milch, verglichen mit dem anderer Nahrungsmittel und des Gesammtorganismus der Säugethiere. 8°. *Dorpat*, 1874.

CHRISTENN (G.) *Vergleichende Untersuchungen über die gegenwärtigen Methoden der Analyse der Milch, namentlich der Frauenmilch und Kuhmilch. 8°. *Erlangen*, 1876.

CITY of Charlestown [Mass.]. Extracts from acts in relation to the sale and inspection of milk, March 6, 1872. 1 sheet. [*Charlestown*, 1872.]

CONGREGAZIONE di carità di Arezzo. Regolamento per il servizio dei sussidi di latte. broadside. *Arezzo*, 1880.

CONSUMERS' Protective Association. To those who desire to have pure and good milk, the following facts are submitted. 8°. [*Boston, n. d.*]

COURT (In the) of general sessions, in and for the city and county of New York, at the December term, 1876. Hon. Josiah Sutherland presiding. The People *vs.* Daniel Schrumpf. Misdemeanor. Adulteration of milk. Argument of W. P. Prentice, counsel to the board of health, for the prosecution. 8°. *New York*, 1877.

Milk (*Adulterations, analyses, and hygiene of*).

CRAMER (G.) Die Mängel der Milchkontrole, mit besonderer Berücksichtigung vorgekommener Fehler; praktische Winke für Polizeibehörden und für Jedermann, welcher sich für gute Milchversorgung und zuverlässige Milchkontrole interessirt. 8°. *Biel*, 1882.

DIRR (F.-X.) Guide pratique pour constater les falsifications du lait. 8°. *Pontoise*, [1875].

FESER (J.) Der Werth der bestehenden Milchproben für die Milchpolizei, erläutert nach meist eigenen Untersuchungen und besonderer Berücksichtigung der neuen Vogel'schen Methode. 8°. *München*, 1866.

——. Die polizeiliche Controle der Markt-Milch. 8°. *Leipzig*, 1878.

FIESSINGER (C.-T.) * I. Comment reconnaître si le bi-oxyde de mercure est falsifié par le minium, par de la brique rouge, ou par des poudres végétales? II. Des caractères microscopiques du lait, de la composition des globules de ce fluide. III. [etc.] 4°. *Strasbourg*, 1840.

GOERLITZ (G.) * Die Milch in medicinisch-polizeilicher Hinsicht. 8°. *Würzburg*, 1837.

GOPPELSRÖDER (F.) Beitrag zur Prüfung der Kuhmilch, mit besonderer Berücksichtigung der Milchpolizei. 8°. *Basel*, 1866.

——. Ueber die Chemie und Prüfung der Kuhmilch. 4°. *Danzig*, [1872].
Repr. from: Milchzeitung, 1871–2.

How pure milk may be supplied to Boston at reasonable prices to consumer and fair returns to producer. A plan respectfully submitted to producers and consumers by a committee of the Worcester West Milk-Producers' Association. 8°. *Boston*, 1880.

KLUNK (O.) * Ueber die Coagulation der Milch durch Labflüssigkeit. 8°. *Giessen*, 1863.

LIEBE (H. A.) * De diversis lac probandi methodis. 8°. *Lipsiæ*, 1857.

LOCKE (J. M.) Report on the analysis of three specimens of milk, made at the request of the health officer of the city of Cincinnati. 8°. *Cincinnati*, 1870.

MAKRIS (C.) * Studien über die Eiweisskörper der Frauen- und Kuhmilch. 8°. *Strassburg*, 1876.

MASSACHUSETTS. *State Board of Health, Lunacy and Charity.* Results of inquiries conducted by the health department of the State board of health, lunacy, and charity, relative to the quality of milk as produced in Massachusetts. 8°. *Boston*, [1886].

MEIGS (A. V.) Milk analysis and infant feeding. A practical treatise on the examination of human and cows' milk, cream, condensed milk, etc., and directions as to the diet of young infants. 12°. *Philadelphia*, 1885.

MERCIER (E.) Le lait devant les tribunaux. Du galactomètre ou pèse-lait au point de vue des poursuites judiciaires et des pénalités édictées dans les règlements des fromageries. 12°. *Nantua*, 1882.

MÜLLER (C.) Anleitung zur Prüfung der Kuhmilch. 3. Aufl. 8°. *Bern*, 1872.

MÜLLER (G.) Milch and Milchcontrole. 8°. *Jena*, 1882.

NARDIUS (J.) Lactis physica analysis. 4°. *Florentiæ*, 1634.

NAVA (D.) & SELMI (G. F.) Sul caglio vitellino; memorie. 8°. *Milano*, 1857.

NEW ORLEANS Auxiliary Sanitary Association. Report on milk and dairies in the city of New Orleans, presented to the New Orleans Medical and Surgical Association, and unanimously adopted at their meeting held on Saturday, July 5, 1879. 8°. *New Orleans*, 1879.

Milk (*Adulterations, analyses, and hygiene of*).

NEWTON (W. K.) Some facts about the New Jersey milk adulteration act and the results of its enforcement. Notes on milk analyses, giving the results of 112 analyses and a brief account of methods. 8°. [*Paterson, N. J.*, 1884.]

NEW YORK City. Majority and minority reports of the select committee of the board of health appointed to investigate the character and condition of the sources from which cow's milk is derived for sale in the city of New York. Together with the testimony and the chemical and microscopical analyses of milks. Also, letters from distinguished physicians, etc. 8°. *New York*, 1858.

POGGIALE. Dosage du sucre de lait par la méthode des volumes ou à l'aide du saccharimètre de M. Soleil et détermination de la richesse du lait. 8°. *Paris*, 1856.

QUESNEVILLE (G.) * Nouvelles méthodes pour la détermination des éléments du lait et de ses falsifications. 4°. *Paris*, 1884.
Also, in: Monit. scient., Par., 1884, 3. s., xiv, 531–631.

——. The same. Neue Methoden zur Bestimmung der Bestandtheile der Milch und ihrer Verfälschungen. Deutsch von Victor Griessmayer. 8°. *Neuburg*, 1885.

RUGG (H. H.) Observations on London milk, showing its unhealthy character and poisonous adulterations; with remarks on the food of the cows, their pestilential places of confinement; with suggestions for remedying the evil. 8°. *London*, [*n. d.*]

SCHMIDT (F.) * Ueber Fettbestimmung in der Milch mittelst des Lactobutyrometers. 8°. *Göttingen*, 1878.

SEMBRITZKI (P.) * Beitrag zur Chemie der Milch. 8 . *Königsberg in Pr.*, 1885.
Also [Rev.], *in:* Arch. f. d. ges. Physiol., Bonn, 1885, xxxvii, 460–467.

SMOLENSKI (P. O.) Ob ispitanii dobrok. moloka v voyenno-vrach. zaveden. [Qualitative examination of milk in military medical establishments.] 8°. *St. Petersburg*, 1885.

STATE of New York. No. 213. In assembly, Jan. 7, 1880. [Introd. by Mr. Sheridan.] An act to amend an act entitled, "An act to amend chapter 467 of the laws of 1862, entitled, 'An act to prevent the adulteration of milk and prevent the traffic in impure and unwholesome milk'", passed May 2, 1864. fol. [*Albany*, 1880.]

TER KUILE (C. P.) * Verhandeling over de melk en hare vervalsching te Leyden. 8°. *Leyden*, 1857.

VIETH (P.) Die Milchprüfung-Methoden und die Controle der Milch in Städten und Sammelmolkereien. 8°. *Bremen*, 1879.

VOGEL (A.) Eine neue Milchprobe. 8°. *Erlangen*, 1862.

VULLYAMOZ (M. L.) * De sale lactis essentiali. 4°. *Lugd. Bat.*, 1756.

WANKLYN (J. A.) Milk-analysis, a practical treatise on the examination of milk and its derivatives, cream, butter, and cheese. 12°. *London*, 1874.

DE WASSERBERG (F. X.) Examen chemicum lactis.
In his: Op. min. med. et diss. 8°. *Vindobonæ*, 1775, ii, 85–158.

WIGNER (G. W.) Pure milk. 8°. *London*, 1884.
Also [Abstr.], *in:* Analyst, Lond., 1884, ix, 174–181.

ZABELIN (J.) * Podrobnii analize prodajnago moloka v S.-Peterburgie. [Analysis of milk sold in St. Petersburg.] 8°. *St. Petersburg*, 1873.

Milk (*Adulterations, analyses, and hygiene of*).

Abbott (L. F.) The milk supply of Boston, and the benefit to be derived from the spaying of cows. Boston M. & S. J., 1884, cx, 317–320. *Also:* J. Am. M. Ass., Chicago, 1884, ii, 402–404.—**Abraham** (A. C.) Note on the estimation of fixed oils and fats, with special reference to milk. Analyst, Lond., 1884, ix, 20–24.—**Act** (An) to regulate the sale and inspection of milk. Rep. Bd. Health N. Hampshire, Concord, 1883–4, iii, 305–308. **Adam** (A.) Nouveau procédé d'analyse du lait, donnant rapidement et directement les trois principes essentiels de ce liquide: beurre, lactose, caséine, sur un seul et même échantillon. J. de pharm. et chim., Par., 1878, xxviii, 4. s., 381–384. ——. Nouvelle méthode d'analyse du lait. Ann. d'hyg., Par., 1879, 3. s., i, 425–438. ——. Analyse du lait; améliorations et additions au procédé du Dr. . . . dosage volumétrique du beurre. J. de pharm. et chim., Par., 1880, 5. s., iii, 22–32.—**Adams** (M. A.) On a new method for the analysis of milk. Analyst, Lond., 1885, x. 46–54. [Discussion], 85–93. ——. On the treatment of sour milk intended for analysis. *Ibid.*, 99–103.—**Albenois.** Des altérations du lait; leur influence sur la santé. Marseille méd., 1881, xviii, 557–563.—**Allen** (A. H.) A critical examination of Dr. Voelcker's published statements on the composition of milk. Analyst, Lond., 1883, viii, 256–260.—**Ambühl** (G.) Die Milchkontrole im Kanton St. Gallen. Jahresb. ü. d. Verwalt. d. San.-Wes. d. Kanton's St. Gallen 1880, St. Gallen, 1881, 143–156.—**Amersfoordt.** De melkproever van Prof. Feser. Volksvlijt, Amst., 1878, 16–18.—**Analysing** sour milk; important evidence by Somerset House chemists. Analyst, Lond., 1883, viii, 128–132.—**Andouard** (A.) Variations de l'acide phosphorique dans le lait de vache. Compt. rend. Acad. d. sc., Par., 1887, civ, 1298–1300.—**Andrevski** (I. V.) O sposobach izsliedovanijach prodajnago i razbavlennago vodoiou moloka. [Method of testing milk in the market as to reduction by water.] Voyenno-med. J., St. Petersb., 1884, cxlix, pt. 7, 25; 115.—**d'Arcet & Petit.** Recherches et expériences sur les qualités chimiques du lait. Rev. méd. franç. et étrang., Par., 1839, i, 211–219.—**Arnold** (C.) Einige neue Reactionen der Milch. Repert. d. anal. Chem., Leipz., 1881, i, 226.—**Arnould** (J.) Législation sanitaire relative à la vente du lait. Bull. méd. du nord, Lille, 1879, xix, 12–29.—**Babcock** (J. F.) The average composition of milk, as reported by the leading authorities of the world. [*From:* Massachusetts Ploughman. Dec. 19, 1885.] Boston M. & S. J., 1886, cxiv, 7.—**Bacon** (C. S.) Results of an examination of the market milk of Chicago, and of the milk of cows fed on distillery refuse. J. Am. M. Ass., Chicago, 1884, ii, 365–368.—**Baertling** (F.) Ueber die neue Methode der Milchanalyse von Matthew A. Adams, nach vergleichenden Untersuchungen. Repert. d. anal. Chem., Leipz., 1886, vi, 411–415.—**Barruel.** Considérations hygiéniques sur le lait vendu à Paris comme substance alimentaire. Ann. d'hyg., Par., 1829, i, 404–419.—**Bartley** (E. H.) Rapid methods of testing milk. Proc. M. Soc. County Kings, Brooklyn, 1882–3, vii, 73–83.—**von Baumhauer** (E.-H.) Méthode d'analyse du lait. Arch. néerl. d. sc. exactes, etc., La Haye, 1869, iv, 239–265.—**Bell** (J.) [Processes used in the Somerset House laboratory in the analysis of milk, and especially the description of the process which is carried out there for the analysis of sour milk.] Analyst, Lond., 1883, viii, 141–144.—**Bell** (J. C.) On milk analysis. *Ibid.*, 1877–8, ii, 155–163. ——. On the difference in milk between the beginning and end of a delivery. *Ibid.*, 1879, iv, 163. ——. Samples of milk which have fallen below the society's standard. *Ibid.*, 1881, vi, 62–64.—**Berti** (G.) Relazione di un confronto fatto nello stabilimento esposti di Bologna fra bimbi a latte di donna ed a latte di bestia. Bull. d. sc. med. di Bologna, 1885, 6. s., xv, 366–377, 1 diag.—**Bestimmungen** zwischen der Control-Commission des Vereins für öffentliche Gesundheitspflege und dem Besitzer der Milchkur-Anstalt zu Hannover, Herrn Piltz. Wider d. Nahrungsfälscher, Hannov., 1881, iv, 17–19.—**Bichlmayr** (G.) Notiz über die Donné-Vogel'sche Milchprobe. Ztschr. f. Biol., München, 1865, i, 216–220, 1 pl.—**Biedert** (P.) Milch-Analyse und das Menschen- und Kuhcaseïn. Arch. f. path. Anat., etc., Berl., 1883, xci, 374–377.—**Bignamini** (A.) Sopra un metodo per dosare la saccarosa, lo zucchero invertito e la lattina, quando trovansi riuniti in un medesimo liquido, ed applicazione all' analisi del latte condensato con zuccaro di canna. Ann. di chim. applic. a med., Milano, 1884, 3. s., lxxviii, 5–10.—**Bird** (A.) Milk standards. Analyst, Lond., 1876–7, i, 80.—**Blanchard** (P.) Du lait. Santé, Brux., 1856–7, 2. s., viii, 150–156.—**Blyth** (A. W.) The composition of cows' milk in health and disease. J. Chem. Soc., Lond., 1879, xxxv, 530–539. ——. The composition of Devonshire cream. Analyst, Lond.. 1879, iv, 141.—**Blyth** (A. W.) & **Spencer** (A.) On the protection of milk from contamination, and the measures necessary for maintaining the purity of milk supplied to the metropolis and other towns. Tr. Soc. M. Off. Health, Lond., 1885–6, 73–91.—**Bond** (F. T.) Milk-testing. Brit. M. J., Lond., 1885, i, 622.—**Bonjean.** Le lait devant les tribunaux. Pharmacie de Lyon, 1876–7, ii, 291–293.—**Borch** (F. G.)

Milk (*Adulterations, analyses, and hygiene of*).

Om Undersøgelsen af Mælk ved Kjøbenhavns Mælkeforsyning. Ugesk. f. Læger, Kjøbenh., 1879, 3. R., xxviii, 71–74.—**Braconnat** (H.) Observations sur le lait bleu. J. de chim. méd., etc., Par., 1836, 2. s., ii, 625–628.—**Brasack.** Milch und Milchcontrole. Verhandl. u. Mitth. d. Ver. f. öff. Gsndhtspflg. in Magdeb. (1878) 1879, vii, 11–15.—**Brégi** (P.) Le lait à Paris. Mouvement méd., Par., 1879, xvii, 19.—**Brown** (W. T.) Milk and its adulterations. Cincin. Lancet & Obs., 1858, i, 577–587.—**Brush** (E. F.) Milk. Med. Rec., N. Y., 1881, xx, 149–151.—**Buchner** (E.) Anklage wegen Milchfälschung. Friedreich's Bl. f. gerichtl. Med., Nürnb., 1870, xxi, 53–57.—**Bukowski** (A.) Badanie mleka i mleko warszawskie. [Analysis of milk and of Warsaw milk.] Zdrowie, Warszawa, 1885, i, 21–27.—**Caldwell** (G. C.) & **Parr** (S. W.) Marchand de Fecamp's method for the determination of fat in milk. Am. Chem. J., Balt., 1885–6, vii, 238–246.—**Cameron** (C. A.) On the composition of the milk of a sow. Med. Press & Circ., Lond., 1869, vii, 390. ——. Amount of solids in milk. Analyst, Lond., 1879, iv, 11. ——. On the falsifications of milk. *Ibid.*, 49. ——. Results of analyses of the milk of forty-two cows. *Ibid.*, 1881, vi, 75–78.—**Canniff** (W.) Milk—the Toronto supply. San. Jour., Toronto, 1876, ii, 69–72.—**de Castro** (F. J.) La leche de perra. An. Soc. ginec. españ., Madrid, 1876, ii, 161; 193.—**Chambrelent & Moussous** (A.) Nouvelles expériences sur le passage des microbes dans le lait. Arch. de tocol., Par., 1884, xi, 305–309.—**Champouillon.** Du lait consommé dans la ville de Paris. Gaz. d. hôp., Par., 1853, xxvi, 291.—**Chandler** (C. F.) Report on the quality of the milk-supply during the year 1869. Rep. Metrop. Bd. Health 1869, N. Y., 1870, 426–436. *Also*, Reprint.—**Chevallier** (A.) fils. Le lait; comment peut-il être vendu pur? Quels moyens de reconnaître sa valeur? J. d. chim. méd., etc., Par., 1875, xlix, 81–86.—**Chevallier** (J.-B.-A.) Observations sur la vente du lait. Ann. d'hyg., Par., 1844, xxxi, 453–458. ——. De la nécessité de publier une instruction sur les moyens à mettre en pratique pour connaître si du lait est ou non allongé d'eau. *Ibid.*, 1855, 2. s., iii, 306–316. ——. Sur le commerce du lait pour l'alimentation de la population parisienne. J. de chim. méd., etc., Par., 1856, 4. s., ii, 633–646. *Also:* Ann. d'hyg., Par., 1856, 2. s., viii, 359–370. *Also*, Reprint.—**Chevallier** (J.-B.-A.) & **Henry** (O.) Mémoire sur le lait. J. de chim. méd., etc., Par., 1839, 2. s., v, 145; 193. *Also* [Abstr.]: Bull. Acad. de méd., Par, 1838–9, iii, 608.—**Chevallier** (J.-B.-A.) & **Reveil** (O.) Notice sur le lait; les falsifications qu'on lui fait subir; instruction sur les moyens à employer pour les reconnaître. J. de chim. méd., etc., Par., 1856, 4. s., ii, 342; 402.—**Cnyrim** (V.) Erfahrungen aus der Frankfurter Milchkuranstalt. Jahrb. f. Kinderh., Leipz., 1884, n. F., xxi, 225–275.—**Cohen** (L. A.) De jongste Engelsche wetgeving op het houden van melkkoeijen, den verkoop van melk, enz.; met eene aantekening over het verbreiden van besmettelijke ziekten. Nederl. Tijdschr. v. Geneesk., Amst., 1879, 2. R., xv, 513–518.—**Commaille** (A.) Analyse du lait de chatte. Rec. de mém. de méd. . . . mil., Par., 1867, 3. s., xviii, 69. ——. Mémoire sur le lait d'Alger. *Ibid.*, 1869, 3. s., xxii, 426–441. ——. Mémoire sur le lait de Marseille, et remarques sur le lait en général. *Ibid.*, xxiii, 64–74.—**Cook** (E. H.) On the analysis of milk, on its composition, and on the quality of the milk sold in Dublin and its suburbs. Med. Press & Circ., Lond., 1876, xxii, 211.—**Dancer** (J. B.) On the microscopical examination of milk under certain conditions. Chem. News, Lond., 1870, xxi, 5.—**Danckwortt.** Ueber polizeiliche Milchprüfungen. Monatschr. . . . d. San.-Pol., Berl., 1859, i, 193–201.—**Dean** (D. V.) The milk supply of St. Louis. Rep. Bd. Health St. Louis (1871) 1872, v, 59–69. *Also* [Abstr.]: St. Louis M. & S. J., 1872, n. s., ix, 21–27.—**Dechan** (M.) & **Maben** (T.) Notes on milk analysis. Analyst, Lond., 1884, ix, 186–189.—**Delarue.** Observations sur les moyens de reconnaître les falsifications du lait. Monit. scient., Par., 1859-60, ii, 425–429.—**Deutsch** (L.) Beitrag zur mikroscopischen Untersuchung der Milch. Jahrb. f. Kinderh., Leipz., 1875-6, ix, 309–318.—**Dietzsch** (O.) Ueber die neue Methode von F. Soxhlet zur Fettbestimmung der Milch, und das Lactobutyrometer von Marchand-Salleron. Repert. d. anal. Chem., Leipz., 1881, i, 33. ——. Ueber das specifische Gewicht der Kuhmilch. *Ibid.*, 129.—**Discussão** do relatorio ácerca da postura camararia destinada a evitar as falsificações do leite que so vende em Lisboa. Gaz. med. de Lisb., 1878, 4. s., v, 53; 63.—**Discussion** on milk analysis and standards. Analyst, Lond., 1886, xi, 1; 62.—**Divers.** London milk; second report, with analyses of the milk sold in different parts of London. Brit. M J., Lond., 1868, i, 356–358.—**Dormus** (R. O.) Milk in its medico-legal aspects. Sanitarian, N. Y., 1876, iv, 131–133.—**Dornblüth** (F.) Die Milchversorgung der Städte und ihre Reform. Deutsche Vrtljschr. f. öff. Gsndhtspflg., Brnschwg., 1880, xii, 413–424.—**Douaud** (C.-S.) Le lait et ses sophistications. Bordeaux méd., 1876, v. 289.—**Doubtful** milk adulteration. Local Gov. Chron., Lond., 1883, xvii, 527.—**Du Mesnil** (O.) La

Milk (*Adulterations, analyses, and hygiene of*).

surveillance du lait à Paris. Ann. d'hyg., Par., 1882, 3. s., viii, 305–308. — **Dumitreanu** (A.) A tejvizsgálatról, küönös tekintettel a fővárosi viszonyokra. [On the lactodensimeter.] Gyógyászat, Budapest, 1883, xxiii, 777–787. — **Duncan** (E.) Town milk; its uses and dangers. San. Rec., Lond., 1875, iii, 20–22. — **Dupre** (A.) On some points connected with milk analysis. Analyst, Lond., 1883, viii, 248–253. — **Durand.** Analyses de laits. Nice-méd., 1885–6, x, 49. — **Dutch** milk. San. Rec., Lond., 1879, x, 107. — **Duval** (J.) Sur un acide nouveau préexistant dans le lait frais de jument et nommé acide équinique. J. de l'anat. et physiol., Par., 1876, xii, 352–356. — **Dyer** (B.) Some analyses of milk. Analyst, Lond., 1881, vi, 59–62. — **Egger** (E.) Vergleichende Bestimmungen des Fettgehaltes der Milch durch Gewichtsanalyse, mittels des Lactobutyrometers und der neuen aräometrischen Methode von Soxhlet. Ztschr. f. Biol., München, 1881, xvii, 110–112. — **Einführung** (Ueber die) einer wissenschaftlichen Milchcontrole für die Zwecke des Lebensmittelmarktes. Med.-chir. Centralbl., Wien, 1886, xxi, 205; 217; 229; 241; 253; 289. — **Eklund** (F.) Sur le lait de Stockholm. J. d'hyg., Par., 1885, x, 45. — **Emmerich** (R.) Ueber die Bestimmung des Fettgehaltes der Milch. Ztschr. f. Biol., München, 1882, xviii, 1–16. — **Esbach** (G.) Analyse du lait; dosage du beurre et nouveau butyromètre. J. d. conn. méd. prat, Par., 1879, 3. s., i, 185; 192; 202; 210; 217; 226; 234; 242. *Also*, Reprint. —. Analyse du lait. *Ibid.*, 1880, xlvii, 19; 28; 36; 43; 53; 75; 100; 116; 124. — **Estcourt** (C.) Notes on the effect of low temperatures upon milk. Analyst, Lond., 1879, iv, 51. —. Valuation of milk solids instead of a limit or standard. *Ibid.*, 1883, viii, 245–248. —. Unreliability of analyses of samples of milk which have become partially decomposed by keeping. *Ibid.*, 1887, xiii, 168. — **Eyselein.** Ueber eine seltene Milchverunreinigung. Tagebl. d. Versamml. deutsch. Naturf. u. Aerzte, Eisenach, 1882, lv, 320. — **Faber** (H.) A new method of ascertaining the amount of fat in milk. Analyst, Lond., 1887, xii, 6–11. —. Some general results of milk analyses. *Ibid.*, 79–84. —. Testing skim-milk by the lactocrite. *Ibid.*, 130–132. — **Falsification** du lait. Rap. gén. Cons. d'hyg. pub. de la Seine 1849–58, Par., 1861, 198–210. — **Féry** (H.) Étude comparée sur le lait de la femme, de l'ânesse, de la vache et de la chèvre. J. d. conn. méd. prat., Par., 1883, l, 309; 317; 330; 353; 370; 402; 1884, li, 75; 83; 92. — **Fleury** (L.) D'une nouvelle méthode imaginée par M. Loyère pour déterminer la composition du lait. Gaz. d. hôp., Par., 1852, xxv, 421. — **Fodor** (J.) A tej Budapesten. [The milk in Budapest.] Közeg. és Törvény. Orvos., Budapest, 1883, 1–15. —. A tej piaczi vizsgálata. [The examination of market milk.] *Ibid.*, 99. *Also, transl.:* Arch. f. Hyg., München u. Leipz., 1884–5, ii, 365–367. — **Förslag** till anordningar för anskaffande af god komjölk i Stockholm. Hygiea, Stockholm, 1885, xlvii, 33–48. — **Frenzel** (J.) & **Weyl** (T.) Ueber die Bestimmung des Kuh-Caseïns durch Fällung mit Schwefelsäure. Ztschr. f. physiol. Chem., Strassb., 1884–5, ix, 246–252. — **Fuchs.** Ueber polizeiliche Untersuchung der Milch. Amtl. Ber. ü. d. Versamml. deutsch. Naturf. u. Aerzte 1858, Carlsruhe, 1859, xxxiv, 235–237. — **Fuchs** (D.) Ueber die unreine Milch in hygienischer Beziehung. Pest. med.-chir. Presse, Budapest, 1882, xvi, 574; 593; 614. —. Nachweis von Brunnenwasser in der gefälschten Milch. Deutsche Vrtljschr. f. öff. Gsndhtspflg., Brnschwg., 1881, xiii, 253–256. — **Fuchs** (D.) & **Péchy** (J.) A tiszta és a kereskedésbeli tej Budapesten. [Unadulterated articles and the market milk in Budapest.] Közeg. és Törvény. Orvos., Budapest, 1883, 41–49. *Also, transl.:* Pest. med.-chir. Presse, Budapest, 1883, xix, 752–755. — **Gædeken** (C. G.) Om Mælkens Beskaffenhed i større Byer. [Quality of milk in cities.] Hyg. Medd., Kjøbenh., 1879–80, n. R., iii, 54–69. — **Gamgee** (J.) Country versus town milk. Med. Times & Gaz., Lond., 1871, i, 38; 67. — **Gardner** (A. K.) Report of a committee appointed by the Academy of Medicine upon the comparative value of milk formed from the slop of distilleries and other food. Tr. N. York Acad. M., 1851–7, i, 31–49. *Also*, Reprint. — **Gaultier de Claubry** (H.) Sur la sophistication de lait au moyen de la matière cérébrale. Ann. d'hyg., Par., 1842, xxvii, 287–295. [Rap. de Henry.] Bull. Acad. de méd., Par., 1841–2, vii, 418–421. — **von Genser** (T. R.) Ueber die Verlässlichkeit der optischen Probe von A. Vogel bei der Untersuchung der Frauen- und Kuhmilch. Oesterr. Jahrb. f. Paediat, Wien, 1875, v, 149–164. — **Gerber** (N.) & **Radenhausen** (P.) Vorschläge zu einer einheitlichen Untersuchungsmethode der Milch. Schweiz. Wchnschr. f. Pharm., Schaffhausen, 1879, xvii, 327; 337; 346. — **Germany.** Technische Anhaltspunkte für die Handhabung der Milch-Kontrole; auf Grund stattgehabter Untersuchungen und Berathungen zusammengestellt im kaiserlichen Gesundheitsamte. Berlin, 1882. Arb. a. d. k. Gsndhtsamte, Berl., 1885, i, 24–45. — **Girard** (C.) Encore une falsification du lait. Gaz. hebd. d. sc. méd. de Bordeaux, 1882, iii, 397. —. Commerce du lait. Rev. d'hyg., Par., 1882, iv, 590–592. —. De la production et de la vente du lait à Paris.

Milk (*Adulterations, analyses, and hygiene of*).

Bull. Soc. de méd. pub. 1882, Par., 1883, v, 226–228. — **Girdwood** (G. P.) Analysis of milk. Canada M. & S. J., Montreal, 1874–5, iii, 385–388. — **Gomez** (J. M.) Sobre la adulteracion de la leche y otras sustancias. Siglo méd., Madrid, 1860, vii, 727. — **Gorup-Besanez** (E.) Untersuchungen über Milch. Arch. f. physiol. Heilk., Stuttg., 1849, viii, 717–719. — **Grangé** (J.) Le coupage du lait. J. d'hyg., Par., 1880, v, 81–83. *Also:* Gaz. obst., Par., 1880, ix, 68–73. — **Gray** (E. W.) Milk. Sanitarian, N. Y., 1875, iii, 64–71. — **Grenzzahlen** (Ueber) bei der Milchanalyse und über Schlempefütterung. Wider d. Nahrungsfälscher, Hannov., 1881, iv, 101–103. — **Grub** (F.) Zur Frage der besseren Milch-Versorgung grosser Städte. Cor.-Bl. d. nied.-rhein. Ver. f. öff. Gsndhtspflg., Köln, 1876, v, 142. — **Gruber** (M.) Ueber neuere Methoden der Milchuntersuchung. Mitth. d. Wien. med. Doct.-Coll., 1883, ix, 321; 332. *Also:* Mitth. d. Ver. d. Aerzte in Nied.-Oest., Wien, 1884, x, 6; 18. — **Gruner** (A.) Ueber Milchproben. Mitth. d. naturf. Gesellsch. in Bern, 1868, 74–84. — **Gscheidlen** (R.) Mittheilung zweier einfachen Methoden, den Zuckergehalt der Milch zu bestimmen. Arch. f. d. ges. Physiol., Bonn, 1877–8, xvi, 131–139. *Also* [Abstr.]: Amtl. Ber. ü. d. Versamml. deutsch. Naturf. u. Aerzte, München, 1877, l, 237. — **Guéneau de Mussy** (N.) La laiterie hygiénique d'Aylesbury à Londres. Rev. d'hyg., Par., 1881, iii, 834–849. — **Gustavson** (G.) O novich sposob. opred. jira v molokie, azota v organ. soedin., bielkov. veshestve i krachmala. [New method of analysis of fat in milk: nitrogenous combination, albumen and starch.] Vet. Vestnik, Charkoff, 1886, v, pt. 1, 1–19. — **Haines** (R.) Milk. J. Frankl. Inst., Phila., 1882, 3. s., lxxxiii, 269–281. *Also*, Reprint. — **Hamlet** (W. M.) On the estimation of fat in milk. Chem. News, Lond., 1881, xliii, 170. — **Hammarsten** (O.) Ueber den Gehalt des Caseïns an Schwefel und über die Bestimmung des Schwefels in Proteinsubstanzen. Ztschr. f. physiol. Chem., Strassb., 1884–5, ix, 273–309. — **Harker** (J.) Milk pathology. Brit. M. J., Lond., 1880, ii, 471. — **Hart** (E.) Milk and water. San. Rec., Lond., 1879, x, 305–309. — **Hearing** before the agricultural committee of the legislature on the adulteration of milk. Boston M. & S. J., 1863, lxviii, 81–88. — **Hehner** (O.) On some points in milk analysis. Analyst, Lond., 1882, vii, 60–64. —. On the relation between the specific gravity, the fat, and the solids not fat in milk. *Ibid.*, 129–135. —. Notes on milk analysis. *Ibid.*, 1883, viii, 253–256. — **Heisch** (C.) On the calculation of milk results. *Ibid.*, 1885, x, 22–26. — **Hennig** (C.) Ueber die Reaction der Kuhmilch. Jahrb. f. Kinderh., Leipz., 1875–6, n. F., ix, 357–361. — **Hessen.** Milchverkaufs-Ordnung für die Haupt- und Residenzstadt Darmstadt. Deutsche Med.-Ztg., Berl., 1881, ii, 49. — **Heusner.** Ueber Nutzen und Einrichtung der Milchcontrole in Städten. Deutscher Ver. f. öff. Gsndhtspflg. Ber. 1876, Brnschwg., 1877, iv, 43–63. — **Hill** (A.) Milk standards. Lancet, Lond., 1876, i, 759. *Also:* Analyst, Lond., 1876–7, i, 40–46. — **Hofmann.** Ueber polizeiliche Controle der Milch. Wider d. Nahrungsfälscher, Hannov., 1881, iv, 179–184. — **Hoppe-Seyler** (F.) Bestimmung des Milchzuckergehaltes der Milch mittelst des Soleil-Ventzke'schen Polarisationsapparates. Arch. f. path. Anat., etc., Berl., 1858, xiii, 276. —. Mittheilungen über die chemischen Verhältnisse der Kuhmilch. Verhandl. d. Gesellsch. f. Geburtsh. in Berl. (1858–9), 1860, xii, 89–92. *Also:* Monatschr. f. Geburtsk. u. Frauenkr., Berl., 1859, xiv, 185–188. —. Die Donné-Vogel'sche Milchprobe. Arch. f. path. Anat., etc., Berl., 1863, xxvii, 394–396. — **Hornemann** (E.) Nogle Bemærkninger om Melken og Melkesalget i Kjøbenhavn og om en mulig Control med samme. Hyg. Medd., Kjøbenh., 1858–9, ii, 152–179. — **Houzé de l'Aulnoit** (A.) Contribution à l'étude médico-légale de l'écrémage du lait au point de vue de l'allaitement artificiel. Bull. méd. du nord, Lille, 1878, xviii, 437–445. — **Howard** (C. C.) A preliminary report on the milk-supply of Columbus. Columbus M. J., 1883–4, ii, 502–506. — **Hueppe** (F.) Untersuchungen über die Zersetzungen der Milch durch Mikroorganismen. Mitth. a. d. k. Gsndhtsamte, Berl., 1884, ii, 309–371. — **Huppert.** Bericht über den Stand der Milchversorgungs-Frage in Prag. Prag. med. Wchnschr., 1879, iv, 234–236. — **Husson** (C.) Note sur les causes diverses qui peuvent rendre le lait plus aqueux. [*From:* L'Industrie laitière.] J. d'hyg., Par., 1883, viii, 16; 28; 41. — **Iliffe** (W.) Milk-poisoning. San. Rec., Lond., 1879–80, n. s., i, 340. — **Imlach** (F.) On the milk supply of Liverpool. [Abstr.] Liverpool M.-Chir. J., 1881, i, 102–107. — **Jacobi.** Ueber Production and Consumtion von Thiermilch in Breslau. Jahresb. d. schles. Gesellsch. f. vaterl. Kult. 1880, Bresl., 1881, lviii, 100–104. *Also:* Breslau. aerztl. Ztschr., 1880, ii, 184–186. — **Janke** (L.) Untersuchungen von Milch normal gefütterter Kühe. Hannov. Monatschr., 1880, iii, 41–45. —. Milchuntersuchungen. Repert. d. anal. Chem., Leipz., 1881, i, 84; 261. —. Beiträge zur Untersuchung der Milch. *Ibid.*, 1882, ii, 33–41. —. (Mittheilungen aus dem chemischen Laboratorium der Sanitätsbehörde zu Bremen.) A, Milchuntersuchungen. Veröffentl. d. k. deutsch. Gsndhtsam-

Milk (*Adulterations, analyses, and hygiene of*).

tes, Berl., 1882, vi, 21.—**Johnstone** (W.) Samples of milk which have fallen below the society's limit. Analyst, Lond., 1882, vii, 34–39. ———. An improved apparatus for milk analysis. *Ibid.*, 1885, x, 81–85. ———. Notes upon the use of acetic acid in milk analysis. *Ibid.*, 1886, xi, 22–32.—**Kemmerich** (E.) Beiträge zur Kenntniss der physiologischen Chemie der Milch. Centralbl. f. d. med. Wissensch., Berl., 1867, v, 417–419. ———. Beiträge zur physiologischen Chemie der Milch. Arch. f. d. ges. Physiol., Bonn, 1869, ii, 401–414.—**Kirchheim.** Ueber hygienische Einrichtung von Kuhställen, Molkereien und Milchläden. Deutsche Vrtljschr. f. öff. Gsndhtspflg., Brnschwg., 1879, xi, 468–474.—**Kletzinsky** (V.) Ueber die Fälschungen der Milch. Oesterr. Ztschr. f. prakt. Heilk., Wien, 1858, iv, 5–8. ———. Ueber Galactometer und Milcharäometer. *Ibid.*, 77; 97.—**Königs** (E.) Ueber die Controle der Milch seitens der Untersuchungsstation zu Crefeld, mit besonderer Rücksicht auf die Beurtheilung der mit Wasser gefälschten Marktmilch. Veröffentl. d. k. deutsch. Gsndhtsamtes, Berl., 1879, i i, 101. *Also*: Cor.-Bl. d. nied.-rhein. Ver. f. öff. Gsndhtspflg., Köln, 1879, viii, 83–85. *Also*: Hannov. Monatschr., 1879, ii, 55–60.—**Kotelnikoff** (V.) Opticheskii sposobe ispitaniia moloka. [Examination of milk.] Zdorovje, St. Petersb., 1879, v, 267–269 —**Kovalkovski** (K. P.) Prigod. apparata, nazv. " pioskop" dlja opredlen. jira v moloke. [Useful apparatus, called "pyoscope", to determine fat in milk.] Trudi Russ. Obsh. ochran. narod. zdravija (Protok.), St. Petersb., 1886. ii, no. 4, 110–114.—**Küchenmeister.** Was können wir praktische Aerzte aus den Versuchen des Prof. Wolff in Möckern über Milcherzeugung bei Kühen für das Ammenwesen lernen? Welche Versuche sind noch von uns anzustellen, um den rationellen Oekonomen gleichzukommen? Deutsche Klinik, Berl., 1854, vi, 72; 86.—**Labiche** (J.) Note à propos de la falsification du lait. J. de chim. méd., etc., Par., 1874, xlviii, 529–532.—**Lajoux** (H.) Remarques pratiques sur l'analyse du lait. Union méd. et scient. du nord-est, Reims, 1884, viii, 169–177.—**Lalieu.** Essai équioxalique du lait de vache. Ann. Soc. méd.-chir. de Liége, 1876, xv, 105–111.—**Leconte.** Note sur un nouveau procédé d'analyse du lait. Compt. rend. Soc de biol. 1854, Par., 1855, 2. s., i, 53–55.—**Lee** (A. E.) The way to get pure milk; how the matter is managed in Germany; the Milchkur-Anstalt at Frankfort-on-the-Main. Rep. Consuls U. S. on commerce, etc., Wash., 1881, no. 10, 264–268.—**Leeds** (A. R.), **Cornwall** (H. B.) & **Wallace** (S.) Specimen analyses of milk and methods. Rep. Bd. Health N. Jersey, Woodbury, 1883, vii, 232–235.—**Lehmann** (J.) Vorläufige Mittheilung über das Verhalten der Milch auf Thonplatten und über eine neue Methode der Casein- und Fettbestimmung in der Milch. Sitzungsb. d. math.-phys. Cl. d. k.-bayer. Akad. d. Wissensch. zu München, 1877, vii, 263–272.—**Liebermann** (L.) Volumetrische Methode zur Bestimmung des Fettgehaltes der Milch. Ztschr. f. anal. Chem., Wiesb., 1883, xxii, 383–390.—**Lies.** Mittheilungen aus der Kindermilchstation auf dem Kreuzkloster bei Braunschweig. Monatsbl. f. öff. Gsndhtspflg., Brnschwg., 1879, ii, 26–31.—**Löwit** (M.) Ueber die quantitative Bestimmung des Milchfettes. Arch. f. d. ges. Physiol., Bonn, 1874, ix, 65–71.—**Macdougald** (G. D.) Estimated cost of milk adulteration to the community of Dundee. San. Jour., Glasg., 1881–2, n. s., v, 148–150.—**Macnamara** (F. N.) Calcutta milk. Indian M. Gaz., Calcutta, 1873, viii, 171.—**Magnier** (L.) Altérations frauduleuses du lait. J. d. conn. méd prat., Par., 1876, 2. s., xliii, 227.—**Manchester.** Appeal against a conviction for selling milk adulterated with 4 per cent. water; reversal of judgment. Analyst, Lond., 1883, viii, 185–239. — **Marchand** (E.) Sur un nouveau procédé propre à déterminer la richesse du lait. [Rap. de Bussy.] Bull. Acad. de méd., Par., 1853–4, xix, 1101–1108. — Du lait considéré dans ses rapports avec la police judiciaire. J. de chim. méd., etc., Par., 1856, 4. s., ii, 561–572. ———. Analyse du lait. Assoc. franç. pour l'avance. d. sc. Compt.-rend. 1877, Par., 1878, vi, 394–401. — **Martin** (A.-J.) La laiterie lombarde de Milan. Bull. Soc. de méd. pub., Par., 1880, iii, 397–402. *Also*: Rev. d'hyg., Par., 1881, iii, 56–61. *Also* [Abstr.]: Ann. d'hyg., Par., 1881, 3. s., v, 165–167.—**Martin** (E. W.) Report on milk and its adulterations. Rep. State Bd. Health N. Y., Albany, 1884, iv, 429–442, 4 pl., 2 plans.—**Méhu** (C.) Sur la méthode de dosage du beurre du lait de M. E. Marchand. J. de pharm. et chim., Par., 1879, 4. s., xxix, 16–18. —**Meigs** (A. V.) Milk analysis. Proc. Phila. Co. M. Soc. 1881–2, Phila. 1882, iv, 146–152. *Also*: Phila. M. Times, 1881–2, xii, 660–664. *Also*, Reprint. ———. A criticism of Dr. Leeds's paper on "The composition and methods of analysis of human milk". Tr. Coll. Phys. Phila., 1884, 3. s., viii, 139–156.—**Meldon** (A.) Intravenous injection of milk. Brit. M. J., Lond., 1881, i, 228. — **Mendes de Leon** (M. A.) Het ijzergehalte van de melk. Onderzoekingen gedaan in het hyg. laboratorium te Amsterdam. Nederl. Tijdschr. v. Geneesk., Amst., 1886, xxii, 297–313.—**Milchuntersuchungen.** Veröffentl. d. k. deutsch. Gsndhtsamtes, Berl., 1882, vi, 43.—**Milchverkaufs-Ordnung** für die

Stadt Darmstadt. Deutsche Med.-Ztg., Berl., 1881, ii, 49. *Also*: Cor.-Bl. d. nied.-rhein. Ver. f. öff. Gsndhtspflg., Köln, 1881, x, 108.—**Milchverkaufs-Ordnung** von Weimar. (Stolps Ortsgesetze, Bd. xi.) Cor.-Bl. d. nied.-rhein. Ver. f. öff. Gsndhtspflg., Köln, 1880, ix, 72.—**Milk** adulteration in New Jersey. Analyst, Lond., 1883, viii, 123–125.—**Milk** analysis. [*From*: The Argus of March 27, 1876.] Austral. M. J., Melbourne, 1876, xxi, 89–94. — **Milk**, and its adulterations. Lancet, Lond., 1851, ii, 257; 279; 322. — **Millon** (E.) & **Commaille** (A.) Mémoire sur le lait. Monit. scient., Par., 1864, vi, 852–858.—**Miranda** (M. V.) Sucinta investigacion sobre los medios de reconocer la calidad de la leche así de las nodrizas, como de la vacas. Repert. méd.-habanero, Habana, 1842, 2. s., 33. — **Moleschott** (J.) Chemische und mikroskopische Notizen über die Milch. Arch. f. physiol. Heilk., Stuttg., 1852, xi, 696–708, 1 pl.—**Moncorvo** (C. A.) [Projecto de regulamento das amas de leite.] Gaz. med. da Bahia, 1876, 2. s., i, 496–504. *Also*, Reprint.—**Morales** (A.) Análisis de varias leches. Mem. Soc. méd.-farm. de Toluca, 1875, i, 39–44.—**Morgenstern** (J.) Ueber die Nothwendigkeit der Errichtung von Milchanstalten in Wien und seinen Vororten. Oesterr. ärztl. Vereinsztg., Wien, 1881, v, 51–53.—**Morris** (J.) Milk; its adulterations, analysis, etc. Maryland M. J., Balt., 1882–3, ix, 73–81. *Also*, Reprint.—**Morris** (J. C.) On the method of milk shipment in glass jars. J. Frankl. Inst., Phila., 1880, 3. s., lxxix, 49 - 52. ———. Milk supply in large cities. Sanitarian, N. Y., 1883, n. s., i, 737–740. ———. On milk supply in large cities. Boston M. & S J., 1884, cx, 315–317. [Discussion], 323–325. ———. The milk-supply of our large cities ; the extent of adulteration and its consequences ; methods of prevention. Am. Pub. Health. Ass. Rep. 1884, Concord, N. H., 1885, x, 246–252.—**Morse** (H. N.) & **Burton** (W. M.) A method for the determination of butter in milk. Am. Chem. J., Balt., 1887–8, ix, 222–331.—**Morse** (H. N.) & **Piggott** (C.) A method for the determination of butter in milk. *Ibid.*, 108–112.—**Mükisch.** Ueber die Gründung von Milchanstalten. Mitth. d. Ver. d. Aerzte in Nied.-Oest., Wien, 1882, viii, 1–10.—**Munita** (V.) De la leche ; sus adulteraciones y modo de reconocerlas. Gac. de sanid. mil., Madrid, 1883, ix, 590 ; 622.—**Munsell** (C. E.) Milk, fresh and condensed. Rep. State Bd. Health N. Y., Albany, 1884, iv, 269 - 311.—**Muter** (J.) On a rapid and accurate method of milk analysis ; with special reference to the examination of woman's milk. Lancet, Lond., 1871, i, 189. ———. Note on an ingenious adulteration of milk. Analyst, Lond., 1878, iii, 235. ———. Remarks on the estimation of milk sugar. *Ibid.*, 1880, v, 35–37. ———. A process for the estimation of the amount of cane sugar added to milk, together with the water thereby concealed. *Ibid.*, 37–40. ———. Notes on some old processes of milk analysis and on a rational view of milk standards. *Ibid.*, 1884, ix, 116–119.—**New** (A) and ingenious method of milk adulteration in Glasgow. San. Jour., Glasg., 1886–7, n. s., x, 307. — **Newton** (W. K.) Our milk supply. Rep. Bd. Health N. Jersey 1880. Camden, 1881, iv, 209 - 235. ———. Report of the milk inspector. *Ibid.*, Mount Holly, 1881, v, 115 - 121. ———. Report of the milk inspector. *Ibid.*, Woodbury, 1883, vii, 247–261.—**New York** Academy of Medicine. Report of the committee on city milk. Tr. N. York Acad. M., 1857–63, ii, 97–149, 7 pl.—**Nichols** (A. H.) & **Babcock** (J. F.) A report on the adulteration of milk. Rep. Bd. Health Mass., Bost., 1873–4, iv, 277–306.—**Notter** (J. L.) On the analysis of milk, etc. San. Rec., Lond., 1876, v, 67.—**Ogle** (J. W.) Milk and the microscope. Lancet, Lond., 1873, ii, 518.—**Opredielenii** (Ob) dostoinstva moloka. [Methods of defining the purity of milk.] Trudi Obsh. Russk. vrach. v. S.-Peterb., 1884, i, no. 1, 13–24.—**Ordem** da noite discussão do relatorio acerca de postura camararia destinada a evitar as falsificações do noite que se vende em Lisboa. J. Soc. d. sc. med. de Lisb., 1877, xli, 202–208.—**Otterson** (W. C.) & **Raymond** (J. H.) Milk ; its production and adulteration. Rep. Bd. Health Brooklyn, 1875–6, 109 - 120. — **Pabst** (J. A.) Les falsifications du lait à Paris. Rev. d'hyg., Par., 1881, iii, 502–514. *Also*: Bull. Soc. de méd. pub. 1881, Par., 1882, iv, 172 - 183. *Also* [Abstr.]: Ann. d'hyg., Par., 1881, 3. s., vi, 56–62.—**Pappenheim** (L.) Ueber polizeiliche Milchuntersuchungen. Arch. d. deutsch. Med.-Gesetzgeb. u. öff. Gsndhtspflg, Erlang., 1857, i, 5 ; 13 ; 21 ; 28 ; 38 ; 44.—**Parr** (S. W.) A test of certain methods for the estimation of the several albuminoids in cow's milk, and of the influence of the food on the relative proportions of these albuminoids. Am. Chem. J., Balt., 1885–6, vii. 246–249.—**Peltz.** Die Milch und ihre Fälschungen. Cor.-Bl. d. Naturf.-Ver. zu Riga, 1870, xviii, 44–46.—**Percy** (S. R.) Report of the committee on city milk, New York. Tr. M. Soc. N. Y., Albany, 1860, 31–66, 7 pl.—**Peters** (S.) Milk, good and bad. Med. & Surg. Reporter, Phila., 1884, 1, 257–259.—**Preusse.** Ueber technische Grundlagen für die polizeiliche Controle der Milch. Mitth. a. d. k. Gsndhtsamte, Berl., 1881, i, 1–17.—**Purdie.** Note on the chemical composition of the milk of the porpoise. Chem. News, Lond., 1885, lii, 170,—

Milk (*Adulterations, analyses, and hygiene of*).

Quevenne (T.-A.) Falsifications du lait. Ann. d'hyg., Par., 1842, xxvii, 241–286.—**Quinlan** (F. J. B.) Note upon a ready method of testing the purity of milk. Med. Press & Circ., Lond., 1883, n. s., xxxv, 552.—**Raimondi** (C.) & **de Pietra** (G.) Il latte considerato dal punto di vista della dietetica e dell' igiene, con speciale riguardo alle possibili adulterazioni ed ai modi più opportuni per riconoscerle. Gior. d. Soc. ital. d' ig.. Milano, 1882, iv, 375; 495. *Also*, Reprint.—**Renner.** Ueber Milch-Controle. Cor.-Bl. d. nied.-rhein. Ver. f. öff. Gsndhtspflg., Köln, 1876, v, 140–142.—**Report** on the present milk supply of London, with analyses of forty samples. Med. Times & Gaz., Lond., 1870, i, 69; 273.—**Report**, with analyses of the milk sold in various districts of London, shewing the degree and money-value of the adulterations practised. Brit. M. J., Lond., 1867, ii, 479.—**Richet** (C.) Note sur les réactions chimiques réductrices du lait et de l'urine. Compt. rend. Soc. de biol., Par., 1882, 7. s., iv, 233–235.—**Rossmann.** Mittheilungen aus der Kindermilchstation auf dem Kreuzkloster bei Braunschweig. Monatsbl. f. öff. Gsndhtspflg., Brnschwg., 1878, i. 13; 100.—**Rottier** (J. D.) Note sur la composition du lait vendu à Gand et sur les moyens de déterminer la pureté de ce produit. Ann. Soc. de méd. de Gand, 1881, lix, 207–216.—**Rueff.** Die Kontrole des Milchhandels. Arch. d. deutsch. Med.-Gesetzgeb. u. öff. Gsndhtspflg., Erlang., 1859, iii, 141; 148.—**Russell** (J. B.) On the existing sanitary regulation of the milk trade. San. Jour., Glasg., 1880–81, n. s., iv, 366: 1881–2, n. s., v, 1.—**Sambuc.** Procédé simple pour dévoiler la falsification du lait de vache par l'eau. Arch. de méd. nav., Par., 1879, xxxii, 81–95.—**Sapojnikoff** (N.) Kachestvennoe i kolichestvennoe izsledovanie prodajnago moloka v g. Kazani. [Qualitative and quantitative analysis of milk offered for sale in Kasan.] Zdorovje, St. Petersb., 1882, ix, 77–106.—**Sartori** (G.) Esperienze comparative per la rapida determinazione del burro nel latte con metodi diversi. Ann. di chim. e di farm., Milano, 1886, *4.* s., iii, 158–165.—**Schacht.** Ueber Milch-Analysen. Vrtljschr. f. gerichtl. Med., Berl., 1878, n. F., xxix, 401–406.—**Schacht** (J. E.) Amtlicher Bericht über die chemische Untersuchung einer dazu bestimmten Kuhmilch. Wehnschr. f. d. ges. Heilk., Berl., 1847, 749–752.—**Schlatter** (F.) Ueber Milchcontrole. Deutsche Vrtljschr. f. öff. Gsndhtspflg., Brnschwg., 1883, xv, 488–494.—**Schlossberger** (I.) Analyse der Milch eines Bocks. Arch. f. Anat., Physiol. u. wissensch. Med., Berl., 1844, 439–443.—**Schlossberger** (J.) Kritisches und Thatsächliches über die Reaktion der frischen Milch. Med. Cor.-Bl. d. württemb. ärztl. Ver., Stuttg., 1853, xxiii, 221–223.—**Schlotfeldt** (J.) Om Mælkeforsyning paa Landet. Ugesk. f. Læger, Kjøbenh., 1884, 4. R., ix. 145–148.—**Schmidt-Mülheim.** Ueber stickstoffhaltige Körper in der Kuhmilch. Arch. f. d. ges. Physiol., Bonn, 1882–3. xxx, 379–383. [*See, also, infra,* Schmoeger.] ———. Ueber das Vorkommen von Cholesterin in der Kuhmilch. *Ibid.*, 384. ———. Vergleichende Untersuchungen über die Bestimmung der Trockensubstanz in der Milch. *Ibid.*, 1883, xxxi, 1–11.—**Schmoeger** (M.) Einige Bemerkungen zu den von Dr. Schmidt-Mülheim jüngst veröffentlichten Arbeiten. *Ibid.*, 385–393.—**Schnutz.** Milch-, etc., Analysen (in Kiel, 1880–81). Veröffentl. d. k. deutsch. Gsndhtsamtes, Berl., 1882, vi, 9–12.—**Schröter** (R.) Untersuchungen über die Eiweisskörper der Menschenmilch und Kuhmilch. Jahrb. f. Kinderh., Leipz., 1887, n. F., xxvi, 362–371.—**Schultze** (H.) Mittheilungen der Controlestelle der Kindermilchstation auf der Domaine Krezzkloster zu Braunschweig. Monatsbl. f. öff. Gsndhtspflg., Brnschwg., 1879, ii, 119–125.—**Sellden** (H.) Om liquor ad serum lactis parandum. Upsala Läkaref. Förh., 1874, ix, 343–351.—**Shall** the sale of skim milk be permitted? San. Engin., N. Y., 1881–2, v, 540.—**Sharples** (S. P.) Specimens of milk from the vicinity of Boston. Proc. Am. Acad. Arts & Sc., Bost., 1876, n. s., iii, 149–156. ———. Milk analyses. *Ibid.*, 1877, n. s., iv, 98–112. ———. On the determination of fat in milk. Chem. News, Lond., 1881, xliii, 228.—**Shrady** (G. F.) Adulteration of milk. Med. Rec., N. Y., 1877, xii, 6; 1878, xiv, 371.—**Siddall** (J. D.) Contamination of milk. Lancet, Lond., 1884, i, 396.—**Simon** (J. F.) Ueber die Untersuchung der thierischen Milch. Ann. d. Staatsarznk., Freib., 1839, iv, 133–138.—**Simoni** (J. R.) Ensayo sobre la leche del estado de Yucatan. Emulacion, Mérida, 1873–4, i, 89–101.—**Skalweit** (I.) Ueber rationelle Verarbeitung der Milch und das Lefeldt'sche patentirte Centrifugal-Entrahmungs-Verfahren. Hannov. Monatschr., 1879, ii, 25–29.—**Smolenski** (P. O.) Ob ispitanii dobrokachest. moloka v voyenno-vrach. zavedenijach. [The military medical establishment for the supply of milk.] Voyenno-san. dielo, St. Petersb., 1885, v, 389; 401; 418.—**Soltmann** (O.) Zur Conservirung der Milch im Haushalt. Jahresb. d. schles. Gesellsch. f. vaterl. Kult. 1881, Bresl., 1882, lix, 129–134. *Also:* Breslau. aerztl. Ztschr., 1881, iii, 261–263.—**de Sousa Martins** (J. T.) Sobre os meios de fiscalisar a

Milk (*Adulterations, analyses, and hygiene of*).

pureza do leite exposto a venda em Lisboa. J. Soc. d. sc. med. de Lisb., 1877, xli, 141–155.—**Soxhlet** (F.) Aräometrische Methode zur Bestimmung des Fettgehaltes in der Milch. [*Extr. from a reprint from:* Ztschr. d. landwirthschaftl. Ver. in Bayern] Repert. d. anal. Chem., Leipz., 1881, i, 22–26. *Also, transl.:* Monit. scient., Par., 1881, 3. s., xi, 236–240. *Also, transl.:* Chem. News, Lond., 1881, xliii, 101; 111.—**Spiegelhalter** (J.) The local milk-supply [of St. Louis]; its sources and quality. Am. Pub. Health Ass. Rep. 1884, Concord, N. H., 1885, x, 320–326.—**Steiner** (S.) A piaczi tejről. [Market milk.] Közeg. és Törvény. Orvos., Budapest, 1884, 127–130.—**Stephens** (C. W.) Some analyses of milk and the determination of milk sugar. Analyst, Lond., 1885, x, 30–34.—**Stock** (W. F. K.) On a modification of Wynter-Blyth's apparatus for digestion in ether as applied to milk analysis. *Ibid.*, 1881, vi, 145.—**Storch** (C.) Die Untersuchung der Milch zum Zwecke der Marktcontrole. Oester. Vrtljschr. f. wissensch. Veterinärk., Wien, 1884, lxi, 195–216.—**Tables** de correction pour le lait avec sa crème, et pour le lait écrémé. J. de chim. méd., etc., Par., 1856, 4. s., ii, 14 tab. following p. 496.—**Thibaut.** Du lait à Lille et dans les hôpitaux. Bull. méd. du nord, Lille, 1879, xix, 62–71.—**Thomson** (W.) On the incongruity of the mode generally adopted in stating the results of milk analyses. Pub. Health, Lond., 1877, vii, 171. *Also:* Med. Press & Circ., Lond., 1877, xxiii, 213. *Also:* Analyst, Lond., 1877–8, ii, 94–96.—**Tisserand** (E.) De l'action du froid sur le lait et les produits qu'on en tire. Ann. de chim. et phys., Par., 1876, 5. s., vii, 554–569.—**Tolmatscheff.** Zur Analyse der Milch. Med.-chem. Untersuch. a. d. Lab. . . . . zu Tübing., Berl., 1867, 272–278.—**Toury** (W. P.) Report on cows' milk. Rep. Bd. Health 1873, Balt., 1874, 59, 2 tab.—**Torá y Ferrer** (B.) Estudios y aprovechamiento de la leche. Independ. méd., Barcel., 1877–8, ix. 435: 1878–9, x, 5; 27; 41.—**Tothfalusi** (G.) Egy szó fővárosunk tejkérdése érdekében. [An earnest word on adulteration of milk.] Közeg. és Törvény. Orvos., Budapest, 1879, 1–5.—**Trélat** (E.) La Société laitière d'Aylesbury. Bull. Soc. de méd. pub. 1881, Par., 1882, iv, 255–260.—**Uffelmann** (J.) Der Nachweis des Zusatzes kleiner Mengen Wassers zur Milch. Deutsche Vrtljschr. f. öff. Gsndhtspflg., Brnschwg., 1883, xv. 663–671.—**Untersuchung** der Kuhmilch. Wien. med. Wchnschr., 1853, iii, 311.—**Untersuchungen** von Milch normal gefütterter Kühe des Bremer Milchwirtschaftlichen Vereins. Veröffentl. d. k. deutsch. Gsndhtsamtes, Berl., 1878, ii, No. 24 (Beilage).—**Vacher** (F.) On the transmission of disease by milk. San. Rec., Lond., 1881–2, n. s., iii, 320–323.—**Van de Vyvere** (E.) Le lait de vache, sa composition et les moyens pratiques, considérés au point de vue légal. d'en reconnaître la falsification par l'eau. J. de pharm., Anvers, 1882, xxxviii, 261; 301; 357.—**Vandoni.** Dell' esame del latte. Gazz. med. di Torino, 1884, xxxv, 529–534.—**Vernois** (M.) & **Becquerel** (A.) Analyse du lait des principaux types de vache, chèvre, brebis, bufflesse. Ann. d'hyg., Par., 1857, 2. s., vii, 271–303. *Also*, Reprint.—**Vieth** (P.) On milk analysis. Analyst, Lond., 1882, vii, 53–60. ———. On the diminution of the solids in milk by decomposition. *Ibid.*, 213–215. ———. A point concerning milk control. *Ibid.*, 1883, viii, 2–4. ———. On an extensive series of milk analyses made during the year 1882. *Ibid.*, 33–37. ———. On condensed mare's milk. *Ibid.*, 81. ———. Milk analysis. *Ibid.*, 153. ———. Notes on milk, cream, skim milk, and buttermilk. *Ibid.*, 1884, ix, 56–64. ———. Notes on the examination and composition of milk and milk products. *Ibid.*, 1885, x, 67–71, 1 tab. ———. On the composition of mare's milk and koumiss. *Ibid.*, 218–221.—**Ville** (J.) Sur le mouillage du lait. Gaz. hebd. d. sc. méd. de Montpel., 1884, vi, 217–221.—**v. W.** (H.) & **S.** (E.) Ueber Milchkontrole in der Stadt Zürich. Bl. f. Gsndhtspflg., Zürich, 1878, vii, 209–212.—**Wall** (S.) Milk analysis at Manchester. Analyst, Lond., 1881, vi, 209.—**Watkins** (G. A.) Supply of milk in cities. Proc. . . . San. Convent. Detroit, Lansing, 1880, 82–86.—**Wein.** Ueber eine neue Methode der Casein- und Fettbestimmung in der Milch. Amtl. Ber. ü. d. Versamml. deutsch. Naturf. u. Aerzte, München, 1877, l, 220.—**Wigner** (G. W.) The milk supply of London. Analyst, Lond., 1883, viii, 243–245.—**Wiley** (H. W.) Determinations of lactose in milks by optical methods. Am. Chem. J., Balt., 1884–5, vi, 289–302.—**Willoughby** (E. F.) On the relation between the specific gravity, the fat, and the solids not fat in milk. San. Rec., Lond., 1882–3, n. s., iv, 92. *Also:* Analyst, Lond., 1882, vii, 176.—**Wilson** (A. C.) On a simple apparatus for the estimation of fat in milk. *Ibid.*, 1885, x, 55.—**Wittstein** (H. C.) Versuche zur Auffindung eines leichten, sichern und schnellen Verfahrens, die thierische Milch auf ihren Handelswerth zu prüfen. Beitr. d. San.-Pol., Berl., 1862, Hft. 4., 6–48.

Milk (*Analyses of*).

See **Milk** (*Adulterations, etc., of*); **Milk** (*Human*).

Milk (*Artificial, and substitutes for*).

See, also, **Infants** (*Food, etc., of*).

Clarke (D.) Artificial human milk. San. Rec., Lond., 1883-4, n. s., v, 420.—**Cumming** (W. H.) Artificial human milk. Atlanta M. Reg., 1882-3, n. s., ii, 385-434.—**Gubler.** Rapport sur les succédanés du lait en cas de disette de cet aliment. Bull. Acad. de méd., Par., 1870, xxxv, 753-765.—**Panum** (P.) Om kunstig Mælk og kunstige Celler. Biblioth. f. Læger, Kjøbenh., 1850, 3. R., viii, 1-12. *Also, transl.: Arch. f. path. Anat., etc., Berl., 1851, iv, 155-165.*

Milk (*Ass's*).

See, also, **Milk** *as a food, etc.*

Cyrnos (J.-M.) Le lait d'ânesse. J. d'hyg., Par., 1882, vii, 505; 519.—**Péligot** (E.) Mémoire sur la composition chimique du lait d'ânesse. J. de chim. méd., etc., Par., 1836, 2. s., ii, 571-577. *Also: J. d. conn. méd.-chir., Par., 1836-7, iv, pt. 1., 200-204.*—**Ralles** (C. G.) Tὸ ὄνειον γάλα, ὡς τροφὴ τῆς πρώτης ἡλικίας. Ἐφημ. ἑταιρ. ὑγιειν., Ἀθῆναι, 1883, i, 25-28.

Milk (*Chemistry of*).

See **Milk** (*Adulterations, etc., of*).

Milk (*Condensed*).

See **Milk** (*Preservation of*).

Milk (*Fungi in*).

von Hessling. Ueber den Pilz der Milch. Arch. f. path. Anat., etc., Berl., 1866, xxxv, 561-575, 1 pl.—**Müller** (G. A.) Ueber die Pilze der normalen Kuhmilch. Arch. f. wissensch. u. pract. Thierh., Berl, 1881, vii, 198-206, 1 pl.—**Rimmington** (F. M.) The conversion of lactine into oxalic acid by mucedinous fungi. Lancet. Lond., 1862, i, 499.—**Sigel.** Pilze in der Milch. Med. Cor.-Bl. d. württemb. ärztl. Ver., Stuttg., 1869, xxxix, 286.

Milk (*Human*).

See, also, **Colostrum**; **Lactation**; **Milk** (*Adulterations, etc., of*); **Milk** *as a food, etc.*

Bingel (G. A.) * Die Milch des Menschen und ihre Bedeutung für den Neugeborenen. 8°. *Würzburg*, 1861.

Denis (P.) * Du lait de femme à l'état physiologique. 4°. *Paris*, 1854.

Donné (A.) Du lait, et en particulier de celui des nourrices, considéré sous le rapport de ses bonnes et de ses mauvaises qualités nutritives et de ses altérations. 8°. *Paris*, 1837.

Guillot (L.-A.) * Étude générale des propriétés normales et des altérations pathologiques du lait de femme. 4°. *Paris*, 1867.

Knoche (A. G.) * De lacte mulierum. 8°. *Halis*, [1845].

Lachenal (G.) * De la quantité de caséine et d'azote contenue dans le lait de femme et dans le lait de vache. 8°. *Genève*, 1876.

Lebehot (L.) Étude sur le lait, suivie de considérations sur le choix d'une nourrice. 8°. *Caen*, 1858.

Makris (C.) * Studien über die Eiweisskörper der Frauen- und Kuhmilch. 8°. *Strassburg*, 1876.

Meggenhofen (C. A.) * Diss. sistens indagationem lactis muliebris chemicam. 8°. *Francof. a. M.*, 1826.

Mendes de Leon (M. A.) *Ueber die Zusammensetzung der Frauenmilch. 8°. *München*, 1881.

Also, in: Ztschr. f. Biol., München, 1881, xvii, 501-530.

Miller (J.) * De lacte humano. 8°. *Edinburgi*, 1805.

Müller (C. A.) * De vitiis lactis humani eorumque medela. 4°. *Jenæ*, 1746.

Ortlob (F.) De lacte humano. 4°. *Lipsiæ*, 1653.

Simon (J. F.) * De lactis muliebris ratione chemica et physiologica. 8°. *Berolini*, [1838].

———. The same. Die Frauenmilch nach ihren chemischen und physiologischen Verhalten dargestellt. 8°. *Berlin*, 1838.

von Stransky-Greiffenfels (H.) * Die Muttermilch. 8°. *München*, 1858.

Milk (*Human*).

Stricker (S.) Ueber contractile Körper in der Milch der Wöchnerin. 8°. [*Wien*, 1866.]

Repr. from: Sitzungsb. d. k. Akad. d. Wissensch., liii. [See, also, infra.]

Vasileff (A.) * K voprosu o vlijanii chaja na kolichestvo i kolichestv. sostave moloka. [Influence of tea on quantity and quality of milk.] 8°. *St. Petersburg*, 1871.

Vernois (M.) & **Becquerel** (A.) Du lait chez la femme dans l'état de santé et dans l'état de maladie. Mémoire suivi de nouvelles recherches sur la composition du lait chez la vache, la chèvre, la jument, la brebis et la chienne. 8°. *Paris*, 1853.

Voltelen (F. J.) * De lacte humano ejusque cum asinino et ovillo comparatione. 4°. *Traj. Batav.*, [1775].

d'Arcet & **Petit.** Recherches et expériences sur les qualités chimiques du lait, dans leurs rapports avec la santé des enfans et le choix des nourrices. Gaz. d. hôp., Par., 1839, 2. s., i, 113.—**B.** (A.) L'antagonisme du lait de femme et du lait de chienne. Abeille méd., Par., 1874, xxxi, 63.—**Béchamp** (A.) Sur la zymase du lait de femme. Bull. Acad. de méd., Par., 1883, 2. s., xii, 690-692. *Also:* Compt. rend. Acad. d. sc., Par., 1883, xcvi, 1508. — **Beigel** (H.) Vorläufige Mittheilung über die mikroskopische Zusammensetzung der Milch des Weibes. Arch. f. path. Anat., etc., Berl., 1868, xlii, 442-444, 1 pl.—**Biedert.** Ueber die Natur des Eiweisskörpers der Muttermilch. Berl. klin. Wchnschr., 1882, xix, 765.—**Boedeker** (C.) Die Zusammensetzung der Frauenmilch. Ztschr. f. rat. Med., Leipz. u. Heidelb., 1861, 3. R., x, 162-164.—**Bouchut.** De la numération des globules du lait pour l'analyse du lait de femme dans ses rapports avec le choix des nourrices et la direction de l'allaitement. Parisméd., 1883, 2. s., viii, 433-437.—**Brès** (Madeleine). Analyse du lait des femmes Galibis du Jardin d'acclimatation. Compt. rend. Acad. d. sc., Par., 1882, xcv, 567.—**Brunner** (T.) Ueber die Zusammensetzung der Frauenmilch. Arch. f. d. ges. Physiol., Bonn, 1873, vii, 440-458.—**Bunge** (G.) Der Kali-, Natron- und Chlorgehalt der Milch, verglichen mit dem anderer Nahrungsmittel und des Gesammtorganismus der Säugethiere. Ztschr. f. Biol., München, 1874, x, 295-335.—**Clarke** (J.) Observations on the properties commonly attributed by medical writers to human milk, on the changes it undergoes in digestion, and the diseases supposed to originate from this source in infancy. Lond. M. J., 1790, xi, 71-91.—**Coulier** (P.) & **Dechambre** (A.) Lait. Bibliographie. Dict. encycl. d. sc. méd., Par., 1868, 2. s., i, 129-171.—**Davis** (N. S.) On the changes in the composition and properties of the milk of the human female, produced by menstruation and pregnancy. Tr. Am. M. Ass., Phila., 1856, ix, 417-427. *Also,* Reprint. ——. On the changes in the composition and properties of the milk in the human female, produced by menstruation and pregnancy ; also, on the food most proper for infants when deprived of the milk of the mother. Tr. Illinois M. Soc., Chicago, 1860, x, 160-172. — **Devergie** (A.) Sur la valeur de l'examen microscopique du lait dans le choix d'une nourrice. Mém. Acad. de méd., Par., 1843, x, 206-222. *Also* [Rap. de M. Dubois]: Bull. Acad. de méd., Par., 1841-2, vii, 197-210.—**Dogel** (A. L.) Mikroskopicheskoe izsliedovanie formennîi elementov jeuskago moloka i vlijanie ich na kachestvo posliednjago. [Microscopical examination of milk of nurses, and its effect upon the child.] Vrach, St. Petersb., 1884, v, 271; 288; 306; 318.—**Dogiel** (A.) Einiges über die Eiweisskörper der Frauen- und der Kuhmilch. Ztschr. f. physiol. Chem., Strassb., 1884-5, ix, 591-615.—**Dolan** (T. M.) An experimental inquiry into human milk, and the effects of drugs during lactation on either nurse or nursling; with chemical analyses, by W. H. Wood. Practitioner, Lond., 1881, xxvi, 83; 165; 251; 331; xxvii, 120; 161.—**Donné.** Recherches sur le lait des nourrices. J. de chim. méd., etc., Par., 1837, 2. s., iii, 445-447.—**Escherich** (T.) Bakteriologische Untersuchungen über Frauenmilch. Fortschr. d. Med., Berl., 1885, iii, 231-236.—**Ewald.** Ueber den Uebergang von Arsenic in die Frauenmilch. Verhandl. d. Berl. med. Gesellsch. (1881-2) 1883, xiii, 143-145. — **Fernandez** (A. B.) Sobre la leche de muger. Siglo méd., Madrid, 1858, v, 108.—**Fleischmann** (L.) Ueber die Verlässlichkeit der mikroskopischen Frauenmilch-Untersuchung. Oesterr. Jahrb. f. Paediat., Wien, 1877, vii, 167-184. *Also,* Reprint.—**Guersent.** Lait. Dict. d. sc. méd., Par., 1818, xxvii, 126-170. — **Hélot.** Examen extemporané du lait de femme, procédé du compte-gouttes. Union méd. de la Seine-Inf., Rouen, 1884, xxiii, 101-107. — **Hoppe-Seyler** (F.) Ueber Trennung des Casein vom Albumin in der menschlichen Milch. Ztschr. f. physiol. Chem., Strassb., 1884-5, ix, 222: 533.—**Kehrer** (F. A.) Untersuchungen über den physiologischen Milchfluss der Stillenden. *In his:* Beitr. z. vergl. u. exp. Geburtsk., 4°, Giessen, 1875, 4. Hft., 39-62.—**Köl-**

Milk (*Human*).

pin (A. B.) & **Klix.** Obduktion eines plötzlich verstorbenen Kindes. Aufsätze u. Beob. a. d. gerichtl. Arzneyw., Berl., 1786, 4. Samml., 84–90. — **Lajoux.** Contributions à l'étude du lait de femme. Union méd. et scient. du nord-est, Reims, 1886, x, 220–229. *Also:* J. de pharm. et chim., Par., 1887, 5. s., xv, 407–411.—**Langgaard** (A.) Vergleichende Untersuchungen über Frauen-, Kuh- und Stutenmilch. Arch. f. path. Anat., etc., Berl., 1875, lxv, 1–9.— **Le Bon** (G.) Sur la composition comparée du lait de femme et de vache et sur une différence importante qui semble exister entre ces deux liquides. Bull. Soc. de méd. prat. de Par. (1878), 1879, 45–51. *Also:* France méd., Par., 1878, xxv, 338.—**Leeds** (A. R.) The composition and methods of analysis of human milk. Tr. Coll. Phys. Phila., 1883–4, 3. s., vii, 225–260, 1 diag. *Also:* Chem. News, Lond., 1884, 1, 263; 280; 289; 301. *Also:* J. Am. Chem. Soc., N. Y., 1884, vi, 252–279, 1 tab.—**Louis.** Du lait et en particulier de celui des nourrices, ses qualités nutritives, ses altérations, etc. Ann. d'hyg., Par., 1838, xx, 475–477.—**Marchand** (C.) De la composition anormale que peuvent présenter certains laits de femmes; de leur influence sur l'alimentation du nouveau-né et des moyens d'y remédier. Assoc. franç. pour l'avance. d. sc. Compt.-rend. 1877, Par., 1878, vi, 877–886.— **Meggenhofen** (C. A.) Chemische Untersuchungen über die Frauenmilch. Ztschr. f. Physiol., Darmstadt, 1829, iii, 274–282. *Also, transl.:* J. compl. du dict d. sc. méd., Par., 1829, xxxv, 322–329. — **Meigs** (A. V.) Proof that human milk contains only about one per cent. of casein; with remarks upon infant feeding. Proc. Phila. Co. M. Soc., Phila., 1883–4, vi, 92–112. *Also:* Arch. Pediat., Jersey City, 1884, i, 216–241. ——. A criticism of Dr. Leeds's paper on "The composition and methods of analysis of human milk". Chicago M. J. & Exam., 1885, 1, 534–551. *Also:* Tr. Coll. Phys. Phila., 1884–6, 3. s., viii, 139–156.— **Moner** (J.) Numeracion de los glóbulos de la leche de mujer bajo el punto de vista de la eleccion de nodriza y de la direccion de la lactancia. Independ. méd., Barcel., 1877–8, ix, 227–233.—**Moore** (W. D.) On the coagulability of human milk. Dublin Q. J. M. Sc., 1849, vii, 275; 492.— **Opitz.** Ueber die Begriffe "Milch" und "Colostrum". Centralbl. f. Gynäk., Leipz., 1884, viii, 513–517.—**P.** Von dem Vorzuge der Frauenmilch vor der Milch der Thiere, und von der Verbindlichkeit der Mütter, selbst zu stillen. Abhandl. u. Beob. v. einer Gesellsch. v. Aerzten in Hamb., 1776, 120–134.—**Payen.** Examen comparatif du lait de plusieurs femmes et du lait de chèvre. J. de chim. méd., etc., Par., 1828, iv, 118–126.—**Pellet** (H.) & **Biard** (L.) Composition du lait de vache et du lait de femme comparés aux divers laits sucrés et non sucrés. J. d'hyg., Par., 1883, viii, 165–168.—**Pfeiffer** (E.) Verschiedenes über Muttermilch. Berl. klin. Wchnschr., 1882, xix, 666; 684; 727: 1883, xx, 145; 158. ——. Kritische Untersuchungen über Muttermilch und Muttermilchanalysen. Jahrb. f. Kinderh., Leipz., 1882–3, n. F., xix, 463–482. ——. Zur quantitativen Analyse der Muttermilch, nebst einem Anhange über Kuhmilch. Ztschr. f. anal. Chem., Wiesb., 1882, xxii, 14–20. — **Przewoski** (E.) Nowy przykład większego wydzielania się mleka u mężczyzny. [New researches on the composition of milk in woman.] Gaz. lek., Warszawa, 1881, 2. s., i, 515–517.—**Radenhausen** (P.) Die Frauenmilch. Ztschr. f. phy-iol. Chem., Strassb, 1881, v, 13; 272.—**Rochrig** (A.) Experimentelle Untersuchungen über die Physiologie der Milchabsonderung. Arch. f. path. Anat., etc., Berl., 1876, lxvii, 119–146. *Also,* Reprint.—**Schlossberger** (J.) Menschliche Milch von höchst ungewöhnlichem Fettgehalt. Med. Cor.- Bl. d. württemb. ärztl. Ver., Stuttg., 1858, xxviii, 340.—**Schukowsky** (A.) Notiz über den Fettgehalt der Frauenmilch. Ztschr. f. Biol., München, 1873, ix, 432–434.— **Sourdat** (L.) Observation d'une inégale production et d'une différence de composition du lait pour les deux seins de la même femme. Compt. rend. Soc. de biol. 1870, Par., 1872, 5. s., ii, 106–109.—**Stenberg** (S.) Några iakttagelser och försök beträffande den kvantitativa bestämningen af ägghviteämnena uti kvinnomjölken. (C. r. Quelques observations et expériences pour déterminer la quantité de matières albuminoïdes que contient le lait de femme, no. 13.) Nord. med. Ark., Stockholm, 1877, ix, no. 7, 1–24. *Also,* Reprint.—**Stricker** (S.) Ueber contractile Körper in der Milch der Wöchnerin. [From: Sitzungsb. d. Wien. Akad. d. Wissensch.] Untersuch. z. Naturl. d. Mensch. u. d. Thiere, Giessen, 1870, x, 333–337.—**Tidy** (C. M.) On human milk. Clin. Lect. & Rep. Lond. Hosp., 1867–8, iv, 77–84. ——. On human milk. Lancet, Lond., 1871, i, 501.—**Tott** (C. A.) Ueber die Absonderung der Frauenmilch bei pathologischen Zuständen, nach Boisseau. N. Ztschr. f. Geburtsk., Berl., 1841, x, 28–32.—**Uffelmann** (J.) Ueber eine Frauenmilch, welche sich in der Verdauung wie Kuhmilch verhielt. Berl. klin. Wchnschr., 1882, xix, 683.— **Verrier** (E.) De l'analyse du lait de femme par l'accoucheur. Gaz. obst., Par., 1877, vi, 81–85.—**Vogel.** Infusorien in Frauenmilch Med. Cor.-Bl. d. württemb. ärztl. Ver., Stuttg., 1853, xxiii, 234–236.

Milk (*Hygiene of*).

See **Milk** (*Adulterations, etc., of*).

Milk (*Injections of*).

See **Milk** (*Transfusion of*).

Milk (*Medicated*).

See, also, **Lactation** (*Influence of food, etc., upon, and medication by*).

BERTHOLLET (C. L.) Diss. med. de lacte animalium medicamentoso. 4°. *Parisiis*, 1779.

Balestre. Note sur le lait phosphaté. Nice-méd., 1880–81, v, 203–205.—**Baréty** (A.) Contribution à l'étude des laits médicamenteux; le lait phosphaté: note sur son action thérapeutique dans diverses maladies. *Ibid.*, 1878–9, iii, 258–263.— **de Pietra Santa** (P.) Note sur la médication lacto-chlorurée dans les affections chroniques de la poitrine. Union méd., Par., 1860, 2. s., vi, 277: viii, 227–233.—**Suñé y Molist** (L.) Breves consideraciones sobre la eliminacion de los medicamentos por la secrecion lactea. Gac. méd. de Cataluña, Barcel., 1880, iii, 97–100.— **Taylor** (R. N.) Peptonized milk. Am. Pract. & News, Louisville, 1886, n. s., ii, 386–388. — **Therapeutische** (Ueber die) Anwendung arzneihaltiger Milch in verschiedenen Krankheiten, besonders bei Kindern. J. f. Kinderkr., Erlang., 1865, xlv, 229–238.

Milk (*Metastases of*).

See, also, **Lactation** (*Pathology of*); **Milk**-fever; **Phlegmasia** *dolens*; **Puerperal** *diseases*.

AIGNER (F.) *De metastasibus lacteis. 8°. *Vindobonæ*, 1826.

BALDINGER (E. G.) [Pr.] præmittuntur observationes de morbis ex metastasi lactis in puerperis 4°. *Jenæ*, [1772]. ·

Also, in: THESAURUS diss. med. [etc.] 4°. *Heidelb.*, 1784, 85–88.

BERENDT (N.) *De lactis metastasibus. 4°. *Gottingæ*, [1780].

Also, in: WEIZ (F. A.) Neue Ausz. [etc.] 12°. *Frankf. u. Leipz.*, 1781, xiv, 7–71. *Also, transl. in:* N. Samml. d. auserl. u. n. Abhandl. f. Wundärzte, Leipz., 1784, 6. St. 193–302.

BOSE (E. G.) [Pr.] de lacte aberrante, i–ii. 4°. *Lipsiæ*, [1772].

CLAEYS (C. E.) *De lactis metastasi. 4°. *Gandavi*, 1827.

CLEVE (J. D. M.) *Spec. sistens observationes medico-chirurgicas de aberratione lactis. 8°. *Lugd. Bat.*, 1796.

Also, transl. in: N. Samml. d. auserl. u. n. Abhandl. f. Wundärzte, Leipz., 1787, 17. St., 228–277.

EMBSER (J. J.) *De metastasi lactea. 4°. *Argentorati*, [1781].

GUTMANN (H. A. A.) *De metastasibus lactis. sm. 4°. *Vitebergæ*, 1797.

JOSEPH (I.) *De metastasi, inprimis lactea. 12°. *Halæ*, [1792].

METTE (A. E.) *De metastasi lactea. 8°. *Regiomonti*, [1827].

MONTAIN (G.-A.-C.) Du lait considéré comme cause des maladies des femmes en couche. 8°. *Paris*, 1808.

PELISSOT (F.) Observations sur les laits répandus. 8°. *Paris*, 1807.

PUZOS (N.) Mémoires sur les pertes de sang et le lait répandu, ou dépôts laiteux. 2. éd. 8°. *Paris, an IX* [1801].

Also, in his: Traité des accouchemens. 4°. *Paris*, 1759, 341–394.

RATZKY (J. L.) *De lactis metastasi causa febris puerperarum nuperrime rursus defensa. sm. 4°. *Jenæ*, [1789].

RÜST (J. C. F.) *De metastasibus lactis. 4°. *Gottingæ*, [1793].

SCHMIDT (D. C. G.) *De metastasibus lacteis. 4°. *Helmstadii*, [1796].

STURM (J. C.) *De metastasi lactea. 4°. *Argentorati*, [1773].

VOIGTEL (F. G.) *De metastasibus lacteis. 4°. *Halæ*, [1793].

WILLIARDTS (J. C.) *De metastasi lactis. 4°. *Tubingæ*, [1770].

WITSCHEL (C. G.) *De metastasibus inprimis lacteis. 4°. *Lipsiæ*, [1798].

Milk (*Metastases of*).

VAN WYNOXBERGEN (A.) *De metastasi lactis. 4°. *Lugd. Bat.*, 1781.

ZUCKER (L.) *De metastasi lactea. 8°. *Pestini*, 1836.

Bacchi (A.) Un caso di metastasi lattea con alquante considerazioni sulle metastasi umorali. Bull. d. sc. med. di Bologna, 1854, 4. s., i, 91–104.—**Balthazaar.** Von Versetzung der Milch. (Aus dem Holländischen.) N. Samml. d. auserl. u. n. Abhandl. f. Wundärzte, Leipz., 1785, 8. St., 210–213.—**Berncastel** jun. Milch-Metastase. Gen.-Ber. d. k. rhein. Med.-Coll. 1834, Koblenz, 1837, 107.—**Bluff.** Milchmetastase. Med. Convers.-Bl., Hildburgh, 1830, i, 67.—**Bonnet** (E.) Y a-t-il des maladies laiteuses? Courrier méd., Par., 1872, xxii, 250–252.—**Boyer.** Recherches et expériences sur les métastases laiteuses. Gaz. méd. de Par., 1834, 2. s., ii, 465–470. *Also:* Abeille. Brux., 1834, iii, 169–175.—**C.** Bemerkungen und Zweifel über die Milchversetzungen. Mag. v. Aerzte, Leipz., 1775–8, ii, 794–808.—**C.** Von der Metastasi lactis. Abhandl. u. Beob. v. einer Gesellsch. v. Aerzten in Hamb., 1776, 156–160.—**Coutenot** (F.) De l'action de l'huile de chènevis sur la sécrétion mammaire· observations de métastases laiteuses. Ann. méd. de la Flandre occid., Roulers, 1855, viii, 517–530.—**Dorfmüller.** Merkwürdige Erscheinungen nach einer sogenannten Milchmetastase. Hannov. Ann. f. d. ges. Heilk., 1839, iv, 537–540.—**Fleischmann** sen. Merkwürdiger Ausgang einer wahren Milchversetzung. J. d. pract. Heilk., Berl., 1836, lxxxii, 6. St., 7–10.—**Graefe** (E.) Merkwürdige Krankheitszufälle nach zurückgetretener Milch. *Ibid.*, 1826, lxiii, 2. St., 109–118.—**Hauser** (W.) Vicarisra: kidneys secreting milk. Oglethorpe M. & S. J., Savannah, 1859–60, ii, 408.—**Hirschel.** Noch ein Fall von wahrer Milchversetzung. J. d. pract. Heilk., Berl., 1831, lxxii, 2. St., 73–81.—**Marzuttini** (G. B.) Metastasi lattea, autossia. Mem. d. Soc. med.-chir. di Bologna, 1844, 2. s., iii, 338.—**de Meza** sen. De tumoribus chronicis a lactea metastasi observationes. Acta reg. Soc. med. Havn., 1791, ii, 142–154.—**Mitchell** (S. W.) A case of vicarious secretion of milk. Am. J. M. Sc., Phila., 1855, n. s., xxx, 83–85.—**Müller.** Notes of cases of unusual milk secretion. Customs Gaz. Med. Rep. 1875, Shanghai, 1876, x, 15–17.—**Planchon.** Observation sur une fièvre de lait, survenue à la suite d'un dépôt laiteux sur le bas-ventre, six semaines après la couche. J. de méd., chir., pharm., etc., Par., 1764, xxi, 112–119. ———. Observation sur un épanchement de lait sur le bas-ventre, accompagné de symptômes fâcheux, survenu les premiers jours des couches. *Ibid.*, 1766, xxiv, 408–443.—**Prässar.** Milchversetzung. Gen.-Ber. d. k. rhein. Med.-Coll. 1844, Koblenz, 1846, 78–80.—**Rasi** (D.) Racconto storico di una metastasi lattea. Bull. d. sc. med. di Bologna, 1842, 3. s., i, 303–310.—**Rehmann.** Fall von Milchmetastase. Med. Ann., Heidelb., 1841, vii, 487.—**Rommel** (P.) Von einer häufigen Ausführung der Milch durch den Nabel. Auserl. med.- chir.- . . . Abhandl. d. röm.-kais. Akad. d. Naturf., Nürnb., 1769, xviii, 371–375. *Also, transl.:* Misc. Acad. nat. curios. 1689, Norimb., 1690, decuria 2, viii, 451–455.—**Sachtleben** (D. W.) Ueber die Natur und Heilung der Milchversetzungen. Arch. f. d. Geburtsh., Jena, 1789, ii, 2. St., 1–57.—**Schmucker** (J. L.) Verschiedene Gattungen von Milchversetzungen, bei welchen die Operation angewandt werden musste. Verm. chir. Schrift., Berl. u. Stettin, 1779, ii, 27–48.—**Selle** (C. E.) Von Milchversetzungen. *In his:* N. Beitr. z. Nat.- u. Arzeneiw., 8°, Berl., 1783, pt. 2, 66–75.—**von Siebold** (A. E.) Beobachtung und Heilung einer merkwürdigen Milchversetzung oder eines Abscesses im Wochenbette. J. f. Geburtsh., Frankf. a. M., 1825–6, v, 274–304.—**Spiro.** Milcherbrechen bei einer stillenden Frau. Mitth. a. d. Geb. d. Heilk., Leipz., 1845, 213.—**Susewind.** Ein Fall von sogenannter Milchmetastase. Gen.-Ber. d. k. rhein. Med.-Coll. 1833, Koblenz, 1836, 80.—**Volz** (R.) Ueber Milchmetastase. Arch. f. d. ges. Med., Jena, 1842, ii, 525–535.—**Weber** (C. A.) Milchversatz auf's Gehirn und dessen Heilung. Ztschr. f. Med., Chir. u. Geburtsh., Magdeb., 1856, x, 409–414.—**Zimmermann.** Bemerkungen über die sogenannten Milchmetastasen. Arch. f. med. Erfahr., Berl., 1808, viii, 227–237.

Milk (*Poisonous*).

See Milk (*Abnormal, etc.*)

Milk (*Preservation of*).

CAZES (L.) *Du lait concentré en thérapeutique navale. 4°. *Paris*, 1877.

Albrecht. Le lait concentré sans sucre des usines de Vevey et Montreux. Bull. Soc. d. sc. nat. de Neuchât., 1882, xii, 3. cah., 468–472.—**Albrecht** (H.) Du lait de vache; procédés nouveaux pour le conserver. Rev. mens. d. mal. de l'enf., Par., 1884, ii, 49–55.—**Biedert** (P.) Ueber Milchconservirung. Berl. klin. Wchnschr., 1882, xix, 75.—**C.** Zur Aufbewahrung der Milch. Bl. f. Gsndhtspflg., Zürich, 1881, x, 111–114.—**Condensirte** (Die) Milch aus der Hernalser Condensations- Fabrik. Allg. Wien. med. Ztg., 1879, xxiv, 559.—**Conserves** de lait. Ann.

Milk (*Preservation of*).

d'hyg., Par., 1850, xliii, 197.—**Gaultier de Claubry.** De la conservation du lait. *Ibid.*, 1860, 2. s., xiii, 81–89.—**van Geuns** (J.) Gepasteuriseerde melk. Onderz., gedaan in het Hygien. Laboratorium te Amsterdam. Nederl.Tijdschr.v.Geneesk., Amst., 1885, 2. R., xxi, 1. Afd., 41–51. *Also, transl.:* Arch. f. Hyg., München u. Leipz., 1885–6, iii, 464–485.—**Guernsey** (J. C.) How condensed milk is prepared; its use as an article of diet for infants. Hahneman. Month., Phila., 1879, n. s., i, 203–211. ———. Reports from eminent authors on the use of condensed milk. St. Louis Clin. Rev., 1879–80, ii, 203–212.—**Hahn** (C.) Analyse de lait condensé. Schweiz. Wchnschr. f. Pharm., Schaffhausen, 1879, xvii, 45.—**de la Harpe** (P.) Considérations médicales sur le lait concentré sans sucre. Rev. méd. de la Suisse Rom., Genève, 1881, i, 712–718.—**Hehner** (O.) On condensed milk. Analyst. Lond., 1879, iv, 44–48.—**Hill** (A. B.) Condensed milk. Birmingh. M. Rev., 1884, xv, 7–12.—**Hoeber.** Ueber die veränderte Beschaffenheit der condensirten Milch. Prakt. Arzt, Wetzlar, 1877, xviii, 124–126.—**Hoffmann.** Kondensirte Milch als Nahrungsmittel kleiner Kinder. Aerztl. Mitth. a. Baden, Karlsruhe, 1872, xxvi, 103–107.—**Jacobi.** Ueber Conservirung der Milch. Jahresb. d. schles. Gesellsch. f. vaterl. Kult. 1882, Bresl., 1883, lx, 106–109.—**Jacquemin** (E.) Du lait au point de vue de sa conservation. Ann. d'hyg. Par., 1868, 2. s., xxix, 316–325.—**Klebs.** Ueber ein Verfahren zur Conservirung der Milch, vorzugsweise für die künstliche Ernährung kleiner Kinder. Prag. med. Wchnschr., 1878, iii, 221–223.—**Kraus** (B.) Die Wiener Milch-Condensations-Fabrik. Allg. Wien. med. Ztg., 1879, xxiv, 36.—**von Liebig** (H.) Condensirte Milch und ihre Anwendung. Aerztl. Int.-Bl., München, 1881, xxviii, 343.—**Manetti** (L.) & **Muso** (G.) L'acide salicylique dans l'industrie de la laiterie. Monit. scient., Par., 1876, 3. s., vi, 755–771.—**Pavesi** (A.) Chimica; sulla conservazione del latte, e su alcune qualità del presame. R. Ist. Lomb. di sc. e lett. Rendic., Milano, 1875, 2. s., viii, 716–722.—**Pouriau** (A.) Emploi de l'acide salicylique pour la conservation du lait. Monit. scient., Par., 1875, 3. s., v, 1016.—**Report** on solidified milk by the standing committee on public health and legal medicine. Read Dec. 6, 1854. Tr. N. York Acad. M., 1851–7, i. 179–189.—**Salkowski** (E.) Bericht über die Becker'sche Methode der Milchconservirung. Berl. klin. Wchnschr., 1882, xix, 77. *Also:* Verhandl. d. Berl. med. Gesellsch. (1881–2), 1883, xiii, 12–17.—**Scherff.** Ueber Milchconservirung. Arch. f. Kinderh., Stuttg., 1881–2, iii, 123.—**Soltmann.** Ueber Conservirung der Milch im Haushalt. Jahresb. d. schles. Gesellsch. f. vaterl. Kult. 1881, Bresl., 1882, lix, 129–134.—**Wigner** (G. W.) Milk preservatives. Analyst, Lond., 1879, iv, 88–90.

Milk (*Transfusion of*).

See, also, Cholera (*Asiatic, Treatment of*); Blood (*Transfusion of*).

BIEL (T.) *Einige Versuche über Milchinfusionen beim Hunde. 8°. *Greifswald*, 1879.

CULCER (D.) *Essai expérimental sur les injections intra-veineuses de lait. 4°. *Paris*, 1879.

Béchamp (J.) & **Baltus** (E.) Recherches expérimentales sur la valeur thérapeutique des injections intra-veineuses de lait. Compt. rend. Acad. d. sc., Par., 1879, lxxxviii, 1327–1329. *Also:* Ann. d. chim. et phys., Par., 1879, 5. s., xviii, 101–125.—**Bryson** (J.) Intravenous injections of milk in chronic Bright's disease. St. Louis Cour. Med., 1879, i, 523–528. — **Bullard** (W. E.) A successful case of intravenous injection of milk. N. York M. J., 1878, xxvii, 164–169, 1 pl. — **Castellano** (D.) Trasfusione di latte in anemia acuta. Riv. di chim. med. e farm., Torino, 1884, ii, 297–299.—**Coultcher** & **Laborde.** Essai expérimental sur les injections intra-veineuses de lait. Étude des effets immédiats et éloignés de l'introduction directe du lait dans la circulation. Tribune méd., Par., 1879, xi, 255; 291; 339; 403; 460; 484; 511. — **Helmuth** (W. T.) Intra-venous injection of milk. U. States M. Invest., Chicago, 1879, n. s., ix, 333–339. — **Howe** (J. W.) Transfusion of goat's-milk. N. York M. J., 1875, xxi, 507. ———. Transfusion of milk *versus* transfusion of blood. Med. Rec., N. Y., 1878, xiv, 443; 466: 1879, xv, 4. ———. Intra-venous injection of human milk. N. York M. J., 1880, xxxi, 383.—**Hunter** (C. T.) The intra-venous injection of milk: four cases with a description of the apparatus employed. Hosp. Gaz., N. Y., 1878, iv, 381–389. ———. The intravenous injection of milk in functional and organic anæmias. *In:* Notes Hosp. Pract. (Miller), 8°, Phila., 1879, pt. 1, 134.—**Laborde.** Des injections de lait dans les veines. Gaz. méd. de Par., 1879, 6. s., i, 100.—**Löffler.** Intravenöse Injection von Milch als Ersatz für die Bluttransfusion. Med.-chir. Centralbl., Wien, 1878, xiv, 399.—**Meldon** (A.) Intravenous injection of milk. Med. Press & Circ., Lond., 1879, n. s., xxviii, 345–348. ———. Intravenous injection of milk. Lancet, Lond., 1880, i, 76. ———. Case of intravenous injection of milk. *Ibid.*, 527. ———. Intravenous injection

Milk (*Transfusion of*).

of milk. Brit. M. J., Lond., 1880, ii, 349.—**Miglioranza** (D.) Injezioni intravenose di latte, sangue, urina, bile ed altre sostanze. Gazz. med. ital. lomb., Milano, 1883, 8. s., v, 207 ; 220 ; 237. *Also* [Abstr.] : Salute : Italia med., Genova, 1883, 2. s., xvii, 157.—**Moutard-Martin** (R.) & **Richet** (C.) Des causes de la mort par les injections intra-veineuses de lait et de sucre. Compt. rend. Acad. d. sc., Par., 1879, lxxxix, 107.—**Pepper** (W.) The intravenous injection of milk. Boston M. & S. J., 1878, xcix, 797–800. ———. Organic and functional anæmia, and milk-transfusion as a remedy. Phila. M. Times, 1878–9, ix, 54–58.—**Prout** (J. S.) Intra-venous injection of milk. Med. Rec., N. Y., 1878, xiii, 378.—**Roy** (G. C.) A case of intravenous injection of milk. Indian M. Gaz., Calcutta, 1879, xiv, 311.—**Thomas** (T. G.) Adeno-sarcoma of both ovaries; double ovariotomy; transfusion of milk; recovery. Am. J. Obst., N. Y., 1875–6, viii, 664–667. ———. The intra-venous injection of milk as a substitute for the transfusion of blood. Illustrated by seven operations. N. York M. J., 1878, xxvii, 449–465. *Also*, Reprint. *Also* [Abstr.] : Med. Rec., N. Y., 1878, xiii, 337.—**Vigezzi** (D.) Della infusione di latte e di quella di soluzione di cloruro sodico nelle vene, come cura dell' anemia acuta; studj sperimentali. Ann. univ. di med. e chir., Milano, 1883, cclxv, 143–173. — **Wulfsberg** (N.) Infusion af Melk. Norsk Mag. f. Lægevidensk., Christiania, 1877, 3. R., vii, 760–777.

Milk *as a cause of disease.*

See **Cattle** (*Tuberculosis in*); **Milk** (*Abnormal, etc.*)

Milk *as food or remedy.*

See, also, **Diabetes**, **Dropsy**, **Heart** (*Diseases of*), *Treatment of*; **Kefir**; **Koumiss**; **Phthisis** (*Treatment of*).

BARBOSA DA CUNHA (J.) *Acção physiologica e therapeutica do leite. 8°. *Rio de Janeiro*, 1883.

BAYLE (F.) De utilitate lactis ad tabidos reficiendos, et de immediato corporis alimento. *In his*: Dissertationes medicæ tres. 18°. *Hagæ-Comitis*, 1678, 75–98.

BERG (J.) Ueber Milch und Molken und ihre Bedeutung als Nähr- und Kurmittel. 8°. *Berlin*, 1870.

BORAK (J. B.) * De usu lactis medico. 8°. *Vindobonæ*, 1836.

BURGGRAFF (J. A. P.) * De mirabile lactis asinini in medendo usu. sm. 4°. *Halæ Maydeb.*, [1725].

CARRIÈRE (E.) Les cures de petit-lait et de raisin en Allemagne et en Suisse dans le traitement des maladies chroniques, et en particulier dans les névroses, les troubles fonctionnels des organes digestifs, les pléthores, la phthisie tuberculeuse et les affections chroniques des organes respiratoires, etc. 8°. *Paris*, 1860.

CORDIER (L.) * Des modifications imprimées aux hydropisies dyscrasiques par le lait. 4°. *Paris*, 1871.

DEBOVE. Du régime lacté dans les maladies. 8°. *Paris*, 1878.

DEJUST (É.) * Des applications thérapeutiques du lait. 4°. *Paris*, 1866.

DELSÉRIÈS (J.-A.-F.-N.-M.) * I. Du régime exclusivement lacté, et de ses effets sur l'économie animale. II. [etc.] 4°. *Paris*, 1839.

DESBOIS DE ROCHEFORT (L.) * An in dieta lactea tonicorum usus? 4°. [*Paris*, 1773.]

DURAND (L. - J. - A.) * Considérations sur l'usage du lait en thérapeutique. 4°. *Montpellier*, 1874.

FREYGANG (P.) * Die Milch und ihre Verwendung in der Diätetik. 8°. *Halle*, 1872.

GARLICHS (F. A. H.) * Ueber den medizinischen Gebrauch der Milch und der Molke. 8°. *Würzburg*, 1837.

GERVAIS (A.) * Du régime lacté dans quelques maladies de l'estomac, dans les hydropisies et les diarrhées. 4°. *Montpellier*, 1877.

GREISEL (J. G.) Tractatus medicus de cura lactis in arthritide, in quo indagata natura lactis

Milk *as food or remedy.*

et arthritidis tandem rationibus, et experientiis allatis diæta lactea optima arthritidem curandi methodus proponitur. 16°. *Viennæ Austriæ*, 1670.

HARTLEY (R. M.) An historical, scientific, and practical essay on milk as an article of human sustenance, with a consideration of the effects consequent upon the present unnatural methods of producing it for the supply of large cities. 8°. *New York*, 1842.

HEIM (J. H.) * Ueber den medicinischen Gebrauch der Molken. 8°. *St. Gallen*, 1824.

HENTSCHEL (G.) * De seri lactis virtute longe saluberrima. 4°. *Halæ Magdeb.*, [1725].

HOFFMAN (F.) A treatise of the extraordinary virtues and effects of asses' milk in the cure of various diseases, particularly the gout, scurvy, and nervous disorders; and of its peculiar nourishing and restorative qualities in all consumptive disorders, and even the decays of old age. 8°. *London*, 1754.

JAUFFRET (J. F.) * Acção physiologica e therapeutica do leite. 8°. *Rio de Janeiro*, 1883.

KARELL (P.) On the milk cure! Transl. from the author's manuscript, by E. L. Carrick. 8°. *Philadelphia*, 1870.
See, also, *infra*.

KUSSMANOFF (A.) * Die Ausscheidung der Harnsäure bei absoluter Milchdiät. 8°. *Dorpat*, 1885.

LAIT (Du) et de son emploi hygiénique. Conseils aux consommateurs et spécialement aux mères de famille. 8°. *Paris*, 1851.

LEBERT (H.) Ueber Milch- und Molkenkuren und über ländliche Kurorte für unbemittelte Brustkranke. sm. 8°. *Berlin*, 1869.
Also [Rev.], *in*: Wien. med. Presse, 1870, xi, 42–44.

LERSCH (B. M.) Die Kur mit Milch und den daraus gemachten Getränken (Molken, Kumys). Die Saisons-Kuren mit Milch und deren Präparaten, sowie mit Obst- und Kräutersäften. 2 v. 8°. *Bonn*, 1869.

MALLET (A.) Étude sur la médication lactée médicinale. Du lait phosphaté. 8°. *Nice*, 1881.

MANI (A.) On the use of milk-whey in the cure of disease, with an account of the establishment at Interlaken, in Switzerland, under the superintendence of . . . 8°. *London*, 1854.

NOLLAN (J. J.) * An senibus lac orillum? Præses C. F. Theroulde de Vallun. 4°. [*Paris*, 1769.]

REUSS (C. F.) * Novam methodum lacte caprillo viribus medicatis digestionis animalis et artis ope imprægnato morbis chronicis curabilibus cito, tuto, et jucunde medendi peritioribus medicis ulterius explorandam proponit. 4°. *Tubingæ*, [1769].

———. Neue praktische Versuche über die mit besondern Arzneykräften angeschwängerte Geiss- oder Ziegenmilch und deren vorzüglich schnelle, sichere und angenehme Wirkungen in manchen langwierigen Krankheiten. 16°. *Leipzig*, 1783.

RICHTER (M. F.) Der Milcharzt. Eine kurzgefasste Anweisung zum diätetischen und arzneilichen Gebrauche der süssen Milch, nebst einer nach den besten Quellen und Erfahrungen bearbeiteten Anleitung, viele der hartnäckigsten und gefährlichsten Krankheiten, als : Ausschläge, Auszehrung, Blutflüsse . . . durch den theils äusserlichen, theils innerlichen Gebrauch der süssen Milch leicht und sicher zu heilen. 4. Aufl. 16°. *Nordhausen*, 1844.

Milk *as food or remedy.*

——. The same. De melkarts. Eene beknopte handleiding voor het leefregelmatig en geneeskundig gebruik der zoete melk, benevens eene, naar de beste bronnen en waarnemingen zamengestelde handleiding om op eene gemakkelijke en zekere wijze, deels door uit-, deels door inwendig gebruik der zoete melk, onderscheidene der hardnekkigste en gevaarlijkste ziekten te genezen, [etc.] Naar de 5. uitgave, uit 't Hoogduitsch vertaald. 16°. *Nijmegen,* 1849.

RICHTER (G. G.) [Pr.] de insalubri lactis et vini miscela. 4°. *Gottingæ,* 1756.

ROSNER (G. E.) Disp. qua nonnulla circa vires lactis notantur.

In: HALLER. Disp. ad morb. [etc.] 4°. *Lausannæ,* 1760, vii, 226–248.

RUDENKO (T.) * K vopr. v molochnom lechenii. Ob usvoenii azot. veshestve korov. moloka i ob azot. metamorfoze pri absolut. molochnoi diete. [Milk cure. Assimilation of nitrogenous substances of milk, and on nitrogenous metamorphosis in absolute milk diet.] 8°. *St. Petersburg,* 1885.

RUPIN (É.) * De l'action du lait, comme contre-poison, sur quelques dissolutions métalliques. 4°. *Paris,* 1854.

SCHUBERT (C. F.) * De sero lactis recte præparando disserit. 4°. *Lipsiæ,* [1777].

SCHULZE (A.) Rathgeber für diejenigen, welche Milch- und Molkenkuren gebrauchen wollen. Eine Darstellung ihrer zweckmässigsten Anwendung und ihrer ausgezeichneten Heilwirkungen gegen hartnäckige und langwierige Krankheiten. Nebst Abhandlungen über die äusserliche Anwendung der Milch, die Heilkräfte der Buttermolken, sowie auch die Verbindung der Milch mit den verschiedenen Mineralbrunnen. 12°. *Quedlinburg u. Leipzig,* 1841.

SERVAES (B.) Ad Hipp. aphor. 64, sect. v. Lac dare capite dolentibus, malum. Malum etiam febricitantibus, et quibus præcordia elevata permurmurantia, et siticulosis. Malum et quibus biliosæ alvi egestiones in febribus acutis sunt, et quibus sanguinis multi egestio facta est. Convenit autem exhibere tabescentibus, non valde multum febrientibus, et in febribus longis, debilibus, nullo ex prædictis signis præsente, sed præter rationem consumptis.

In: LOUVAIN diss. 8°. *Lovanii,* 1796, iv, 136–144.

VIVANTE (C.) Della cura lattea. 8°. *Venezia,* 1874.

VOGEL (J. T.) * De connubio aquarum mineralium cum lacte longe saluberrimo. sm. 4°. *Halæ Magdeb.,* [1726].

WEBEL (C. G.) * De lactis cauto usu medico. sm. 4°. *Halæ Magdeb.,* [1730].

WEBER. Der Molkenkurort Streitberg in der fränkischen Schweiz. 8°. *Erlangen,* 1869.

WILL (G. P.) * De usu lactis antidoto. 4°. *Altorfii,* [1737].

ZELLER (F. J. B.) Die Molken-Kur in Verbindung der Mineral-Brunnenkur. Ein menschenfreundlicher Wink für Alle, denen daran gelegen ist, ihre Gesundheit zu erhalten und ihr Leben zu verlängern. 2. Aufl. 12°. *Würzburg,* 1828.

Aepli (J. M.) Fortsetzung der Untersuchung der Streitfrage: Ob die magern Molken ein Nahrungsmittel seyen? Gaz. de santé, Zürich, 1784. iii, 320–331.—**Aran** (F.-A.) De la cure du petit-lait. Bull. gén. de thérap., etc., Par., 1860, lix, 145–155.—**Ardoin.** De l'effet énervant du lait. J. d. conn. méd.-chir., Par., 1847–8, xv, pt. 1, 120–125. *Also* [Rap. de Collineau]: Bull. Acad. de méd., Par., 1853–4, xix, 1047–1052.—**Arnò** (F.) Nuovi casi comprovanti l'efficacia dell'uso terapeutico del latte. Spallanzani, Modena, 1882, 2. s., xi, 69–71.—**Asmus.** Ein Wort über die Milch als Heilmittel. Med. Ztg., Berl., 1838, vii, 183.—**Audhoui** (V.) De la diète lactée et de

20

Milk *as food or remedy.*

son rôle dans le traitement de la phthisie pulmonaire. Thérap. contemp., Par., 1881, i, 1; 17 — **Balestreri** (F. M.) Sulla dieta lattea nelle malattie giudicate incurabili. Ann. univ. di med., Milano, 1871, ccxv, 485–527.—**Banks** (J. T.) On the curative virtues of milk. Edinb. M. J., 1867–8, xiii, 416–421.—**Biedert** (P.) Neue Untersuchungen und klinische Beobachtungen über Menschen- und Kuhmilch als Kindernahrungsmittel. Arch. f. path. Anat., etc., Berl., 1874, lx, 352–379. *Also,* Reprint.—**Blaschko.** Ueber Milch- und Molkenkuren. Allg. med. Centr.-Ztg., Berl., 1858, xxvii, 329–332. — **Bokkenheuser** (V.) Om en paatænkt Mælkekuranstalt i Kjøbenhavn. Ugesk. f. Læger, Kjøbenh., 1884, 4. R., ix, 529–537.—**Brush** (E. F.) Observations on the digestion of milk. N. York M. J., 1879, xxx, 300–302. ——. Skimmed milk as an article of food. Med. Rec., N. Y., 1881, xx, 459–461. ——. One mode of improving cow's milk for human food. *Ibid.,* 539–541. — **Burghart** (G. H.) De curæ lactis et sanguinis antiquitatibus. Epistola ad C. de Helwich. Med. Siles. Sat., Wratisl. et Lips., 1737, v, 61–90.—**Burkart.** Die Stuttgarter Milchcuranstalt. Deutsche Vrtljschr. f. öff. Gsndhtspflg., Brnschwg., 1876, viii, 673–684. — **Carrière** (E.) Introduction à l'étude des cures de petit-lait et de raisin en Allemagne et en Suisse. Union méd., Par., 1860, 2. s., v, 241; 257. ——. Les cures de petit-lait et de raisin. Gaz. d. hôp., Par., 1862, xxxv, 250; 342. ——. Les cures de petit lait dans les maladies des femmes du monde et contre l'hypochondrie. *Ibid.,* 1864, xxxvii, 298.—**Carter** (W.) On the use of digested milk. Liverpool & Manchester M. & S. Rep., 1873, i, 42. — **Chapman** (E. N.) Milk with lime-water as food and medicine in the neuroses. Tr. M. Soc. N. Y., Syracuse, 1879, 354–365. *Also:* Sanitarian, N. Y., 1879, vii, 155–162. — **Chase** (W. B.) Note on peptonized milk diet. Tr. M. Soc. N. Y., Syracuse, 1885, 151–153.—**Chibret.** Sur l'action du régime lacté sur l'excrétion de l'urine. Compt. rend. Acad. d. sc., Par., 1887, civ, 1552.— **Cnyrim** (V.) Die Frankfurter "Milchcuranstalt". Deutsche Vrtljschr. f. öff. Gsndhtspflg., Brnschwg., 1877, ix, 820–825. ——. Ueber die Production von Kinder- und Kurmilch in städtischen Milchkuranstalten. *Ibid.,* 1879, xi, 239; 443. — **Dangers** (G) Die Milch als Nahrungsmittel für Kinder und Erwachsene. Deutsches Wchnbl. f. Gsndhtspflg. u. Rettungsw., Berl., 1885, ii, 105; 113.—**Debove.** Del régimen lácteo en las enfermedades. Version española de Federico Toledo. Génio méd.-quir., Madrid, 1878–9, xxiv–xxv, *passim.* — **De Simone** (A.) Tisichezza mesenterica incipiente venuta in seguito di cattivo metodo curativo, e compiutamente guerita per dieta di latte e rimedi antimoniali. Esculapio, Napoli, 1827, ii, 134–139.—**Donkin** (A. S.) On the curative influence of an exclusive milk diet. Lancet, Lond., 1876, ii, 921.— **Drescher.** Milch und Molken. Jahrb. f. Balneol., etc., Wien, 1879, viii, 30–50. — **Duckworth** (D.) On the insufficient use of milk as an article of diet in England. Practitioner, Lond., 1881, xxvi, 351–356. *Also:* Pop. Sc. Month., N. Y., 1881, xix, 491–494. — **Dujardin-Beaumetz.** Des aliments complets et du régime lacté. Bull. gén. de thérap., etc., Par., 1886, cxi, 1–19. *Also, transl.:* Boston M. & S. J., 1886, cv, 97–101.—**Dutt** (U. C.) The milk treatment in India. Indian M. Gaz., Calcutta, 1874, ix, 209.—**E.** Süsse Milch gegen Wassersucht. Med. Ztg. Russlands, St. Petersb., 1857, xiv, 388. — **Faber** (H.) Skizzen über einige Molken- und andere Kuranstalten der östlichen Schweiz. Med. Cor.-Bl. d. württemb. ärztl. Ver., Stuttg., 1861, xxxi, 38; 54; 61; 78; 87; 93; 100; 118; 124; 132; 141. ——. Skizzen über einige Molken- und andere Kurorte der mittlern Schweiz. *Ibid.,* 1862, xxxii, 92; 108; 116; 127; 134; 139. — **Faucus** (J.) Milk diet in disease. Indian M. Gaz., Calcutta, 1870, v, 10.—**Fazio** (E.) Sulla cura lattea. [*From his:* Climatologia ed igiene medica.] Riv. ital. di terap. ed ig., Piacenza, 1884, iv, 101–108. — **Fonssagrives.** Note sur le remplacement de l'huile de morue par la crème de lait dans le cas de répugnance invincible pour le premier de ces médicaments. Bull. gén. de thérap., etc., Par., 1861, lxi, 145.— **Forti** (F.) Cura degli spandimenti pleuritici con il latte. Ippocratico, Forlì, 1873, xxiii, 65–72. — **Foucart** (J.-B.) Observations et réflexions sur l'emploi de la diète lactée. Ann. de la méd. physiol., Par., 1826, x, 368–391. *Also,* Reprint.—**Friedländer.** Die Karpathen, ihre Molkencuren und Gesundbrunnen. Med. Jahrb. d. k. k. österr. Staates, Wien, 1839, xxviii, 576–587. — **Frühwald** (F.) Ueber die 1. Wiener Kindermilch-Anstalt. Ztschr. f. Therap. m. Einbezhng. d. Elect.- u. Hydrotherap., Wien, 1883, i, 217.—**Gallico** (E.) Effetti terapeutici della esclusiva dieta lattea in alcune affezioni morbose. Gazz. med. ital., prov. venete, Padova, 1878, xxi, 341; 349: 1879, xxii, 323. — **Grub** (F.) Prospect der Stuttgarter Milch-Cur-Anstalt. Cor.-Bl. d. nied.-rhein. Ver. f. öff. Gsudhtspflg., Köln, 1876, v, 88.—**Hacker.** Milchcuren. Summ. d. Neuest. u. Wissenswürd. a. d. ges. Med., Leipz., 1835, xi, 92–95.—**Heusner.** Ueber die Bedeutung der Milch als Nahrungsmittel. Cor.-Bl. nied.-rhein. Ver. f. öff. Gsndhtspflg., Köln, 1877, vi, 75–78.—**Heyfelder.** Notizen über die Molkenanstalten des Cantons Appenzell und über die Molkenkuren. J. d. pract. Heilk., Berl., 1836, lxxxii, 3. St., 86–95.—**Hoffmann** (F. A.) Betrachtungen über

Milk *as food or remedy.*

absolute Milchdiät. Ztschr. f. klin. Med., Berl., 1883–4, vii, Supplhft., 8–21. — **Horsley** (J.) The value of milk as an article of food. Chem. News, Lond., 1874, xxix, 224.—**Hubbard** (R.) The value of milk as an article of diet for the sick. Proc. Connect. M. Soc. 1864–7, N. Haven, 1867, 2. s., ii, 294–299.—**Hunter** (W.) Successful cure of a severe disorder of the stomach by milk taken in small quantities at once (with appendix). Med. Obs. Soc. Phys. Lond., 1784, vi, 310–330.—**Huss.** Några ord om så-kallade mjölkvassle-kuranstalter och om mjölkvasslans användande som therapeutiskt medel. Hygiea, Stockholm, 1853, xv, 737–744. — **Jobert.** De la médication lacto-alcoolique comme complément de la médication lactée. Gaz. d. hôp., Par , 1877, l, 501.—**Karell** (P.) Ueber die Milchkur. St. Petersb. med. Ztschr., 1865, viii, 193–220. *Also, transl.:* Arch. gén. de méd., Par., 1866, ii, 513 : 694. *Also, transl.:* Edinb. M. J., 1866–7, xii, 97–122.—**Labat.** La cure de petit-lait. Ann. Soc. d'hydrol. méd. de Par., 1873–4, xix, 39–63.—**La Carrière.** Les cures de petit lait. Le petit lait et les eaux sulfureuses. Gaz. d. hôp., Par., 1865, xxxviii, 282.—**Lammerts van Bueren** (R.) Vergelijkende digestie-proeven van verschillende melksoorten. Nederl. Lancet, Gravenh., 1848–9, 2. s., iv, 733–738.—**Laubender.** Einige Beobachtungen über Milchkuren. Allg. med. Ann., Altenb., 1801, 116–121. — **Leonhardt** (K.) Zur Frage der Einrichtung von Milchkur-Anstalten in den Städten. Cor.-Bl. d. nied.-rhein. Ver. f. öff. Gsndhtspflg., Köln, 1877, vi, 213. — **Leviseur.** Practische Bemerkungen über die Milch- und Molkenkuren. Wchnschr. f. d. ges. Heilk., Berl., 1837, 393 ; 411.—**Lill von Lilienbach** (A.) Milchcuranstalten. J. f. Gsndhtspflg., Wien, 1883, vii, 49 : 61. — **Lippe** (E.) Ueber Milch- und Molkenkuren. Wien. med. Presse, 1866, vii, 583–586.—**Loodiana.** Case of ascites ; with remarks on Karell's milk cure and thermometrics, by Dr. Johnston. Indian M. Gaz., Calcutta, 1867, ii, 77–79.—**Luzun** (P.) Essais de traitement par le lait de chienne. Bordeaux méd., 1875, iv, 341–343.—**Marius.** Einiges über Milch- und Molkenwein. Deutsche Klinik, Berl., 1873, xxv, 314 ; 321.—**Markiewicz** (S.) Wskazówki dotyczące sposobów użycia mleka krowiego dla niemowląt i dorosłych. [Manner of using cow's milk for infants and adults.] Medycyna, Warszawa, 1881, ix, 194 ; 211. — **Marsden** (W.) Limosis and parageusis. Canada M. J., Montreal, 1867, iii, 446–448. — **Martini.** Merkwürdige Wirkung der Kuhmilch auf eine chronische Kranke. Mag. f. d. ges. Heilk., Berl., 1831, xxxiv, 189–196.—**Méhu** (C.) Sur la présence de petites quantités de sucre dans les urines des personnes soumises à l'alimentation lactée. Ann. d. mal. d. org. génito-urin., Par., 1887, v, 340–345.—**Milk** diet ; sour milk, milk without sugar, koumis. Med. Times & Gaz., Lond., 1871, i, 70.—**Mitchell** (S. W.) On the use of skimmed milk as an exclusive diet in disease. Med. Times, Phila., 1870–71, i, 19 ; 213. — **Modry** (M.) Milch- und Molkencuren. Jahrb. f. Balneol., etc., Wien, 1876, vi, 54–69.—**Mojsisovics.** Ueber die Bereitung der Kuh- und Schafmolke und ihren medizinischen Gebrauch. Wien. med. Wchnschr., 1852, ii, 330.—**Morris** (J. C.) On cows' milk as food in health and for invalids. Proc. Phila. Co. M. Soc., 1879, i, 68–74. *Also :* Phila. M. Times, 1878–9, ix, 446–451.—**Niepce.** De la cure et des bains de petit lait dans les maladies nerveuses en général, et dans les maladies du cœur en particulier. Nice-méd., 1876–7, i, 234 ; 257 ; 294.— **Orzovensky** (K.) Die Molke. Wien. Med.-Halle, 1863, iv, 217 ; 226.—**Palmberg** (A.) Om Karellska mjölkkuren. Finska läk.-sällsk. handl , Helsingfors, 1873, xv, 81–100.--**Pécholier** (G.) Des indications de l'emploi de la diète lactée dans le traitement de diverses maladies et spécialement dans celui des maladies du cœur, de l'hydropisie et de la diarrhée. Montpel. méd., 1866, xvi, 289 : xvii, 1 ; 197. *Also* [Abstr.] Bull. gén. de thérap., etc., Par., 1866, lxxi. 443–449.—**Pletzer** (H.) Ueber Molkencuren und einige südliche Molkencurorte. Ztschr. f. prakt. Heilk. u. Med.-Wes., Hannov., 1866, iii, 201–215.— **Polansky.** Zur Charakteristik des Molkencurortes Roznau. Ztschr. d. k.-k. Gesellsch. d. Aerzte zu Wien, 1859, xv, 21–24.—**Rapin** (E) Journal d'un homme mis en nourrice à l'âge de 55 ans. Bull. Soc. méd. de la Suisse Rom., Lausanne, 1872. vi, 263–268.—**Reichmann** (M.) Experimentelle Untersuchungen über die Milchverdauung im menschlichen Magen, zu klinischen Zwecken vorgenommen. Ztschr. f. klin. Med., Berl., 1885, ix, 565–587.— *Also, transl.:* Gaz. lek., Warszawa, 1885, 2. s., v, 412–414. — **Richards** (V.) On the value of a purely milk diet in some forms of dropsy and general anasarca, and in elephantiasis arabum. Med. Times & Gaz., Lond., 1872, ii, 540. — **Richelot** (G.) Mémoire sur l'emploi thérapeutique des laits médicamenteux du Dr. Bouyer, de Saint-Pierre-de-Fursac. Union méd., Par., 1865, 2. s., xxvi, 35 ; 88 ; 137 ; 180 ; 233 ; 278. — **Richter** (H. E.) Ueber Milch- und Molken-Kuren. Schmidt's Jahrb., Leipz., 1870. cxlviii, 201 : 1875, clxviii, 281. *Also,* Reprint.— **Rosenthal.** Ueber Milchcuranstalten in grossen Städten. Verhandl. u. Mitth. d. Ver. f. öff. Gsndhtspflg. in Magdeb. (1879), 1881, vii, 64–72.—**Roubaud** (F.) Les cures de petit lait en Suisse, en Allemagne, dans le Tyrol et la Styrie. Gaz. d. hôp., Par., 1867, xl, 17 ; 29 ; 41 ; 53 ; 65 ;

Milk *as food or remedy.*

101 ; 109 ; 113 ; 149 ; 157 ; 169.—**Rudenko** (T. I.) K vopr. o molochnom lech. ; ob usvoenii azot. vetshestve korov. moloka i ob azot. metamorph. pri absolut. moloch. diete. [Milk diet. Assimilation of nitrogenous substances by cow's milk, and on nitrogenous metamorphosis in absolute milk diet.] Arch. klin. vnutren. boliez. Botkina, St. Petersb., 1886, x, 1–76.—**Schenck** (P. V.) Milk ; its uses and abuses. St. Louis Cour. Med., 1879, ii, 313–325. — **Spoof** (A. R.) Iakttagelser om Karell'ska mjölkkuren. Finska läk.-sällsk. handl., Helsingfors, 1876, xviii, 75–79.—**Straus** (I.) Lait, hygiène et diététique. N. dict. de méd. et chir. prat., Par., 1875, xx, 86–89.—**von Studzieniecki** (F) Die strenge Milch-Cur. Med.-chir. Centralbl., Wien. 1878, xiii, 290 ; 302 ; 314 ; 365 ; 374.—**Sweet** milk. Is it poisonous ? Buffalo M. J., 1858–9, xiv, 119–123.—**von Tott** (C. A.) Nutzen der Molken in einigen Fällen von hartnäckigen Abdominalleiden. J. d. pract. Heilk., Berl., 1838, lxxxvi, 3. St., 109–114.—**Trask** (J. D.) Practical suggestions in regard to milk as an article of diet. Med. Rec., N. Y., 1881, xix, 315.--**Tyson** (J.) Milk treatment of disease. J. Am. M. Ass., Chicago, 1884, ii, 626–630.—**Uffelmann** (J.) Studien über die Verdauung der Kuhmilch und über die Mittel, ihre Verdaulicheit zu erhöhen. Arch. f. d. ges. Physiol., Bonn, 1882, xxix, 339–386.—**Vanoye** (R.) De l'usage médicinal du lait. Ann. méd. de la Flandre occid., Roulers, 1852–3, vi, 353 ; 491.—**von Velsen.** Ueber die Milch und deren Anwendung in der Medizin. Arch. f. med. Erfahr., Berl., 1811, i, 14–24. —**Vives** (I.) De la leche considerada como elemento del régimen alimenticio de los enfermos militares. Gac. de sanid. mil., Madrid, 1882, viii, 231–242. — **Wiley** (H. W.) American milk. Science, Cambridge, 1885, v, 130. — **Winterniz** (W.) Ueber methodische Milch- und Diätenkuren. Wien. med. Presse, 1870. xi, 5 ; 49 ; 97 ; 140 ; 165 ; 193 ; 219 ; 245 ; 267 ; 289 ; 341 ; 382 ; 433.—**Zimermann** (G.) Bericht über die Bade-, Trink- und Molkenkur-Anstalt zu Luhatschowitz in Mähren. (Saison 1856.) Wien. med. Wchnschr., 1857, vii, 289 ; 313.

Milk (The) Journal.

Monthly review of the dairy, dairy produce, and poultry yard. v. 1–2, 1871–2. 4°. *London.*

v. 2, 1872, title: **Milk** (The) Journal and Farm Gazette.

Milk *and tuberculosis.*

See, also, **Cattle** (*Tuberculosis in*).

STEIN (G.) * Experimentelle Beiträge zur Infectiosität der Milch perlsüchtiger Kühe. 8°. *Berlin,* [1884].

Aufrecht. Eine Bemerkung zu Dr. May's Aufsatz : " Ueber die Infectiosität der Milch perlsüchtiger Kühe ". Arch. f. Hyg., München u. Leipz., 1883–4, i, 397–399.— **Bang** (B.) Om Tuberkulose i Koens Yver og om tuberkulös Mälk. Nord. med. Ark., Stockholm, 1884, xvi, no. 26, 1–22. *Also :* Tidsskr. f. Vet., Kjøbenh , 1884. 2. R., xiv, 290–316.—**Cressy** (N.) Transmission of bovine tuberculosis from infected milk. Proc. Connect. M. Soc., Hartford, 1881, n. s., ii, no. 2, 201–212.—**Macgillivray** (A. E.) Tuberculous milk. Vet. J. & Ann. Comp. Path., Lond., 1884, xix, 309–311.—**May** (F.) Ueber die Infectiosität der Milch perlsüchtiger Kühe. Arch. f. Hyg., München u. Leipz., 1883–4, i, 121–136, 1 pl.—**Olver** (H.) Tuberculosis in a cow, especially with reference to milk contamination ; [with notes by J. H. Steel]. Vet. J. & Ann. Comp. Path., Lond., 1881, xiii, 316–318. — **Richard** (E.) De la transmission de la tuberculose par le lait. [Rev. crit.] Rev. d'hyg., Par., 1884, vi, 35–38. — **Vallin** (E.) Danger du lait des vaches phthisiques. *Ibid.,* 1880, ii, 529–532.

Milk-cure.

See **Baden-Baden ; Badenweiler ; Bistritz ; Boll ; Boppard ; Gonten ; Kreuth ; Luhatschowitz ; Meran ; Milk** *as a food, etc.* ; **Salzbrunn ; Silvaplana ; Sinzig ; Würtemberg.**

Milk-fever.

See, also, **Breast** (*Inflammation, etc., of*) ; **Lactation** (*Pathology of*) ; **Milk** (*Metastasis of*) ; **Puerperal** *diseases* ; **Puerperal** *fever.*

BARCHEWITZ (A. G.) * De febris lacteæ diagnosi atque curatione. 8°. *Berolini,* [1825].

EICHINGER (J.) * Considérations sur la nature et les causes de la fièvre de lait. 4°. *Strasbourg,* 1865.

JOACHIMSOHN (S.) * De dirigendo febre lactea laborantium regimine. 4°. *Traj. ad Viadr.,* [1791].

MORY (P.-S.-A.) * De la prétendue fièvre de lait. 4°. *Paris,* 1863.

Milk-fever.

MOURETTE (I. - B.) *Quelques remarques critiques sur la fièvre de lait. 4°. *Paris*, 1859.

PARISI AB EICHENTHAL. *De galactopyra. 8°. *Vindobonæ*, [1835].

SCHAMBERGER (C. A.) *De caussis febris lacteæ hactenus dubiis. 8°. *Francof. ad Viadr.*, [1805].

THOMAS DES COLOMBIERS (C.) *Essai sur la fièvre dite de lait. 4°. *Paris*, 1863.

WAANDERS (H.) *Febris lactea puerperarum. 12°. *Herbipoli*, 1844.

WEISS (J. G. C.) *De febre lactea. 8°. *Erlangæ*, 1809.

ZILLES (J. - P.) *Dissertation sur la nature de la fièvre de lait. 8°. *Strasbourg, an VIII* [1800].

Bonté (M.) Observation sur la fièvre miliaire des femmes en couche. J. de méd., chir., pharm., etc., Par., 1757, vi, 29-45.—**Bouchut.** Bekommen Neugeborene auch ein Milchfieber? J. f. Kinderkr., Erlang., 1862, xxxix, 64-69.—**de Bourge.** Fièvre de lait avant l'accouchement. [Abstr.] Ann. Soc. de méd. prat. de la prov. d'Anvers, Boom, 1844-5, iii, 35-37. — **Buchheim** (C. F.) Das Milchfieber, Febris lactea. Allg. med. Ann., Leipz., 1823, 577 - 600. — [**Depaul.**] La fièvre de lait. Gaz. d. hôp., Par., 1875, xlviii, 353. — **Dumaz.** Fièvre de lait. Bull. Soc. méd. de Chambéry, 1875-7, v, 72-75, 1 tab.— **Esnoz.** Fiebre láctea que se hizo intermitente de tipo tercianario; malignidad de la misma; muerto á consequencia de metro-peritonitis consecutiva. Siglo méd., Madrid, 1869, xvi, 698.—**Gardien.** Lait (fièvre de). Dict. d. sc. méd., Par., 1818, xxvii, 170-177.—**Halbertsma** (T.) Zur Milchfieberfrage. Vorläufige Mittheilung. Centralbl. f. d. med. Wissensch., Berl., 1870, viii, 385-387.—**Howe** (S.) Milk fever; a treatise to show the relation which exists between the rise in temperature on the third to fifth day, and the beginning of the milk secretion. Am. J. Obst., N. Y., 1875-6, viii, 571-594, 4 pl. *Also*, Reprint.—**Löhlein** (H.) Ein typischer Milchfieberfall. Ztschr. f. Geburtsh. u. Gynäk., Stuttg., 1879, iv, 258-260. — **Macan** (A. V.) Milk fever. Obst. J. Gr. Brit., Lond., 1878-9, vi, 451-459. *Also*: Dublin J. M. Sc., 1878, lxv, 435-446.—**Mylius.** Etwas über das Milchfieber. Med.-chir. Ztg., Salzb., 1798, ii, 204-207.—**Neumann.** Das Milchfieber. N. Ztschr. f. Geburtsk., Berl., 1839, vii, 252-258.—**Planchon.** Observation sur un dépôt laiteux, accompagné d'une fièvre miliaire de même nature, survenu les premiers jours des couches. J. de méd., chir., pharm., etc., Par., 1771, xxxvi, 411-422. — ———. Observation sur une fièvre miliaire crystalline laiteuse, accompagnée d'aphtes, survenue à une femme nouvellement accouchée. *Ibid.*, 1772, xxxviii, 441-449. — ———. Sur la fièvre miliaire des femmes en couches, et sur leur traitement. *Ibid.*, 1780, liii, 340; 432.—**Razoux.** Dissertation en forme de lettre, contenant le détail d'une fièvre maligne laiteuse. *Ibid.*, 1772, xxxvii, 321-347.—**Reichard.** Eine heftige Raserey von zurückgetretener Milch, vorzüglich durch den Huxham'schen Spiessglas-Wein geheilt. Arch. f. d. Geburtsh., Jena, 1787, i, 2. St., 78-89.—**Richard.** Sur les fièvres laiteuses graves, improprement appelées fièvres puerpérales. Ann. clin., Montpel., 1813, xxx, 5; 105.—**Saint-Cyr** (F.) & **Chapelle** (F.) Le colostrum et la fièvre de lait chez les femelles de nos animaux domestiques, particulièrement chez la vache. J. de méd. vét. et zootech., Lyon, 1880, 3. s., v, 337; 393, 1 tab.: 1881, 3. s., vi, 5, 2 tab.—**Taylor** (B. D.) The so-called milk fever and antiseptic midwifery. Med. Rec., N. Y., 1877, xii, 343.—**Tott** (B.) Febris lactea. N. Ztschr. f. Geburtsk., Berl., 1851, xxx, 252.— **Viñas Cusí** (F.) Naturaleza de la fiebre láctea. Encicl. méd.-farm., Barcel., 1880, iv, 213; 229; 237; 239; 245.

Milk-leg.

See **Phlegmasia** *dolens*.

Milk-powder.

See **Nestlé's** *food*.

Milk-sickness.

See, *also*, **Cheese** (*Poisonous*).

BORLAND (S.) An essay on the milk sickness of the human subject, or the trembles of animals, embracing its history, cause, and treatment. 8°. *Little Rock, Ark.*, 1845.

HEERINGEN (E.) A discovery of the true cause of the disease called by the people trembles, or milk - sickness. 8°. *Louisville*, 1843.

Milk-sickness.

MCILHENNY. A treatise on the disease called the milk-sickness, or trembles. 8°. *Springfield*, 1843.

SEATON (J. S.) A treatise on the cause of the disease called by the people the milk-sickness, as it occurs in the Western and Southern States. 8°. *Louisville, Ky.*, 1841.

Also [Rev.], *in*: West. J. M. & S., Louisville, 1841, iv, 367-370.

Allen (Z.) Milk sickness. Illinois M. Recorder, Vandalia, 1878-9, i, 88-92.—**Anderson** (W.) Milk sickness and the Illinois legislature. Chicago M. J., 1867, xxiv, 163-165.—**Bailey** (F. K.) Milk-sickness. Tr. Illinois M. Soc., Chicago, 1858. 45-52.—**Barbee** (W. J.) Facts relative to the endemic disease called by the people of the West "milk-sickness". West. J. M. & S., Louisville, 1840, i, 178-190.—**Beach** (W. M.) Milk sickness. J. Am. M. Ass., Chicago, 1883, i, 71-75. *Also*: Tr. Ohio M. Soc. 1883, Columbus, 1884, xxxviii, 125-138.— **Beck** (J. C.) Milk-sickness. Northwest. M. & S. J., Chicago, 1857, xiv, 496. — **Beck** (L. C.) Facts relative to a disease generally known by the name of sick stomach, or milk sickness. N. York M. & Phys. J., 1822, i, 315 - 319. — **Bennett** (J.) Observations on the sick stomach, or milk sickness, as it appears in certain parts of Kentucky. West. Q. Reporter M., S. & Nat. Sc., Cincin., 1822, i, 353-357.—**Bowman** (J.) Milk sickness. Cincin. Lancet & Obs., 1870, xxii, 521. — **Boyles** (E. W.) Milk sickness. Chicago M. J., 1865, xxii, 139-141. — **Brewington** (W. J.) Milk sickness. Clinic, Cincin., 1876, x, 76. — **Bridgman** (W. S.) Milk sickness. *Ibid.*, 68.— **Buck** (J. B.) Remarks on the milk sickness, with cases. Med. Exam., Phila., 1840, iii, 792-795. — **Bürger.** Die Milchkrankheit der Nordamerikaner. Mag. f. d. ges. Heilk., Berl., 1825, xviii, 176 - 182. — **Byford** (W. H.) Milk sickness, poison, tires, etc. Nashville J. M. & S., 1855, ix, 460-473.—**Campbell** (J. L.) Milk-sick, or sick stomach. Physician & Surg., Ann Arbor, Mich., 1881, iii, 347-349.—**Carney.** Report on milk-sickness. Proc. M. Convent. Ohio, Columbus, 1847, 39-41.—**Chamberlin** (W. B.) Extracts from a dissertation on gastro-enteritis, commonly called sick stomach. Ohio M. Resposit., Cincin., 1826-7, i, 1.—**Chase** (S. C.) The cause of milk-sickness. Chicago M. J., 1861, xviii, 438-440. *Also*: Cincin. Lancet & Obs., 1861, iv, 347-349.—**Chesney** (J. P.) Milk sickness. St. Joseph M. & S. Reporter, 1880-81, i, 97-101.— **Coleman** (A.) Observations on the disease generally known by the name of sick stomach. West. Q. Reporter M., S. & Nat. Sc., Cincin., 1822, i, 133-141. *Also*: Phila. J. M. & Phys. Sc., 1822, iv, 322; 331.—**Compton** (J. W.) Milk-sickness. Indiana M. Reporter, Evansville, 1881, ii, 249-256.—**Converse** (J. N.) Remarks on milk-sickness and trembles. N. York J. M., 1853, [2.] s., xi, 358-363.— **Cosby** (A. D.) Pathology and treatment of milk-sickness. Atlanta M. & S. J., 1866-7, vii, B, 481.—**Crawford** (J.) Remarks on milk sickness. West. Lancet, Cincin., 1843-4, ii, 135. — **Crook** (J. W.) Twenty propositions on milk - sickness. Northwest. M. & S. J., Chicago, 1857, xiv, 489-492.—**Crooks** (C. V.) Milk-sickness, its causes and treatment. Med. & Surg. Reporter, Phila., 1873, xxix, 22-24.—**Crookshank** (N.) On the sick stomach of the Western country, or gastro-enteritis. Phila. J. M. & Phys. Sc., 1826, xii, 252-263. *Also*: Ohio M. Reposit., Cincin., 1826-7, i, 9-11.—**D.** Milk sickness. West. J. M. & S., Louisville, 1840, ii, 80.—**D.** Northern limits of milk-sickness. *Ibid.*, 1843, vii, 65.—**Davis** (C. W.) Treatment of milk sickness. Northwest. M. & S. J., Chicago, 1852-3, ix, 13.—**Davis** (K. H.) Milk-sickness. Atlanta M. Reg., 1881-2, i, 391-396.—**Dawson** (J.) Causes and treatment of milk-sickness. Proc. M. Convent. Ohio, Cincin., 1842, 45-51.—**De Bruler** (J. P.) Milk-sickness. Chicago M. J., 1858, xv, 206-209. — **Dewey** (J. S.) Milk sickness. Northwest. M. & S. J., Chicago, 1854-5, n. s., xi. 541-547.—**Dickey** (W.) An essay on milk sickness. West. Lancet, Cincin., 1852, xiii, 390-399.—**Disease** (A) in Ohio ascribed to some deleterious quality in the milk of cows. Med. Reposit., N. Y., 1812, xv, 92-94.—**Dixon** (M. L.) Milk sickness. Transylv. J. M., Lexington, Ky., 1833, vi, 157-163.—**Dorsey** (G. V.) Milk sickness. A question of priority. Clinic, Cincin., 1876, x, 100.— **Drake** (D.) The "sick stomach", or "milk sickness", of the Western States, ascribed to the Rhus radicans—by an unprofessional correspondent of the editor. West. J. M. & Phys. Sc., Cincin., 1836, ix, 243-247. ———. A memoir on the diseases called by the people "trembles", and the "sick-stomach" or "milk-sickness", as they have occurred in the counties of Fayette, Madison, Clark, and Green, in the State of Ohio. West. J. M. & S., Louisville, 1841, iii, 161-226. *Also*, Reprint.—**Drake** (D.) & **Yandell** (L. P.) Milk sickness, alias sick stomach; and its treatment. West. J. M. & S., Louisville, 1840, i, 84: ii, 80: 1841, iv, 75; 229: 1842, v, 235.—**Dumm** (S. C.) Epidemic gastritis, or milk-sickness, or malignant malarial fever. Cincin. Lancet & Clinic, 1878, n. s., i. 271. ———. Milk sickness treated with injections of brandy and milk.

Milk-sickness.

Ibid., 1879-80, n. s., iii, 209.— **Dunglison** (R.) Milk-sickness. Cycl. Pract. M. (Tweedie), Phila., 1845, iii, 314.— **Elder** (E. S.) Morbo lacteo. Tr. Indiana M. Soc., Indianap., 1874, xxiv, 113-129.— **Evans** (J. B.) Milk sickness—a mineral poison. Nashville J. M. & S., 1860, xviii, 110.— **Fisher** (G.) Milk sickness. Chicago M. Exam., 1861, ii, 538-542.— **Fulton** (A.) Milk sickness. Cincin. Lancet & Obs., 1873, xvi, 641-648. *Also:* Med. & Surg. Reporter, Phila., 1881, l, 449-453.— **Gardner** (J.) Milk-sickness; its microscopy. St. Louis M. & S. J., 1880, xxxviii, 288-294. *Also:* Indiana M. Reporter, Evansville, 1880, i, 145-151.— **Graff** (G. B.) On the milk sickness of the West. Am. J. M. Sc., Phila., 1841, n. s., i, 351-369.— **Gray** (S. S.) Milk-sickness. Tr. Ohio M. Soc., Cincin., 1877, xxxii, 81-90. ——. Milk-sickness. Ohio M. J., Columbus, 1881-2, i, 284-289.— **Haines.** [Facts relating to the disease generally known as the sick stomach.] West. Q. Reporter M., S. & Nat. Sc., Cincin., 1822, i, 141-144. *Also:* Phila. J. M. & Phys. Sc., 1822, iv, 331-333.— **Henry** (A. G.) Milk sickness. West. J. M. & S , Louisville, 1854, [4.] s., ii, 25.— **Hibberd** (J. F.) Observations on milk-sickness. West. Lancet, Cincin., 1844-5, iii, 445-461.— **Hogg** (S.) Fatal case of milksickness. West. J. M. & S., Louisville, 1842, vi, 253.— **Horne** (J.) Remarks on milk sickness. West. Lancet, Cincin., 1843-4, ii, 454 - 463. ——. Miasmata the exciting cause of the disease called milk sickness. *Ibid.*, Lexington, 1846-7, v, 397-410.— **Houser** (W. W.) Milk-sickness. Am. M. J., St. Louis, 1880, viii, 445-447.— **Howard** (E. J.) Mukosma. Syro, milk sickness, trembles, slows, tires, puking fevers, etc. Indiana J. M., Indianap., 1871-2, ii, 370-372. — **Hurd** (A.) Milk sickness. Clinic, Cincin., 1875, ix, 277 ; 290.— **Jackson** (J. M.) Milk-sickness. Louisville M. News, 1881, xii, 291-294.— **Jerry** (W.) The plant that causes milk-sickness. Med. & Surg. Reporter, Phila., 1867, xvi, 270.— **Johnson** (J. M) Milk-sickness; its pathology and treatment. Atlanta M. & S. J., 1866-7, vii, B, 289.— **Johnson** (L. B.) Thoughts on milk-sickness. Richmond & Louisville M. J., Louisville, 1874, xvii, 446-452.— **Jones** (G. W.) Upon the pathology of milk sickness. A thesis. Chicago M. Exam., 1862, iii, 267-283.— **Jones** (J. T.) A short essay on milk-sickness (colica trementia). E. Tennessee Rec. M. & S., Knoxville, 1852-3, i, 321-341.— **K.** (H. M.) Milk-sickness. Cincin. Lancet & Obs., 1862, v, 21-23.— **Kennedy** (J. F.) A reply to "Z. Allen on milk sickness". Illinois M. Recorder, Vandalia, 1878 - 9, i, 146.— **Landrum** (Z. C.) Rhus toxicodendron (the cause of milk sickness). A review of an article on this subject by S. C. Chase. Atlanta M. & S. J., 1861, vii, A, 1.— **Law** (J.) Milk-sickness. Vet. J. & Ann. Comp. Path., Lond., 1877, v. 161-174.— **Lea** (W. W.) Cursory remarks on a disease vulgarly called milk-sick. Phila. J. M. & Phys. Sc., 1821, ii, 50 - 55.— **Lescher** (J. J.) Milk sickness. Northwest. M. & S. J., Chicago & Indianap., 1850-51, vii, 124 - 132.— **Lewis** (J. T.) Cases of milk sickness, with some remarks on the treatment. Transylv. J. M., Lexington, Ky., 1829, ii, 241-245.— **Logan** (J. H.) The milk-sickness of upper Georgia and of other portions of the United States. Atlanta M. Reg., 1881-2, i, 458-469.— **Logan** (J. M.) Essay on trembles, alias animal poison. Northwest. M. & S. J., Chicago & Indianap., 1849-50, vi, 380 - 386.— **McAnelly** (C.) Observations on milk sickness. Transylv. J. M., Lexington, Ky., 1836, ix, 88-95.— **McCall** (A.) An account of the diseased state produced by taking into the stomach the milk or flesh of cows, which has acquired deleterious properties from a vegetable sometimes eaten by those animals. Phila. J. M. & Phys. Sc., 1822, iv, 318 - 321. ——. Observations on milk sickness. Am. M. Recorder, Phila., 1823, vi, 254-277. ——. Facts and observations on the mi k sickness, or sick stomach, of Tennessee. West. J. M. & Phys. Sc., Cincin., 1830, iii, 465-484. — **McClelland** (J. S.) Report on trembles, or milk sickness. Proc. Indiana M. Soc., New Albany, 1854, 43-50.— **McNutt** (J. H.) Observations on milk sickness. Illinois & Ind. M. & S. J., Chicago & Indianap., 1847-8, iv, 205-212.— **Maurel.** Swamp-sickness. Dict. encycl. d. sc. méd., Par., 1884, 3. s., xiii, 639-647.— **Mendenhall** (I.) Milk sickness. Cincin. Lancet & Obs., 1861, iv, 142 - 149. — **Milk** sickness. Maryland M. & S. J., Balt., 1839-40, i, 133.— **Milk** sickness. Chicago M. J., 1858, xv, 593 ; 645.— **Milk** sickness, or sick stomach. West. M. Gaz., Cincin., 1832 - 3, i, 101 ; 117.— **Milk** sickness, or trembles. Proc. Illinois M. Soc., Chicago, 1851, i, 33-37.— **Miller** (W. B.) Pathology and treatment of milk-sickness. Atlanta M. & S. J., 1867 - 8, viii, 57.— **Nagle** (I. E.) Milk sickness. Nashville J. M. & S., 1859, xvii, 289-295.— **Newman** (L. P.) Milk sickness. Chicago M. J., 1867, xxiv, 253. — **Nichols** (J. H.) Milk-sickness. Clinic, Cincin., 1876, x, 26. — **Patton** (J. C.) Milk sickness. Indiana J. M., Indianap., 1875, vi, 139-145.— **Philips** (W. H.) Pathology of milk sickness. Northwest. M. & S. J., Chicago, 1857, xiv, 7 - 12. ——. Milk sickness. Cincin. Lancet & Obs., 1877, xx, 130 - 150.— **Phillips** (N. F.) A case of milk sickness. Nashville J. M. & S., 1876, xvii, 61-63. — **Pickard** (J.) The pathology of milk sickness, in Parke County, Ind. Northwest. M. & S. J., Chicago, 1857, xiv, 260 - 262. — **Preston** (A. G.) Remarks on

Milk-sickness.

milk sickness. West. Lancet, Cincin., 1843-4, ii, 264.— **Pusey** (H. K.) Milk-sickness. Louisville M. News, 1880, ix, 16. ——. Notes on milk-sickness. *Ibid.*, 205.— **Rawlings** (J. W.) Trembles in stock, and milk-sickness in man. Tr. Drake Acad. M., Evansville, 1874, i, 50.— **Reagan** (J. A.) Milk sickness. Med. World, Phila., 1884, ii, 140. — **Reed** (N.) The milk sickness. Boston M. & S. J., 1856-7, lv, 273. — **Ruark** (S.) Milk sickness. Indiana M. Reporter, Evansville, 1880, i, 262 - 264. — **S.** Alleged causes of the milk sickness, or sick stomach. Transylv. J. M., Lexington, Ky., 1829, ii, 145.— **Sager** (J.) Milk-sickness and its etiology. Toledo M. & S. J., 1879, iii, 137-143.— **Sale** (F. H.) Milk sickness. Cincin. Lancet & Obs., 1871, n. s., xiv, 404-419.— **Sawyer** (A.) Milk-sickness; its cause and effects. Med. & Surg. Reporter, Phila., 1867, xvi, 249.— **Seaton** (J. S.) Remarks on a review of his essay on trembles, milk-sickness, etc. West. J. M. & S., Louisville, 1842, v, 64 - 69. [*See, also, supra.*]— **Schmidt** (C. H.) Milk sickness. Cincin. Lancet & Obs., 1877, xx, 411-413.— **Shelton** (A.) [*et al.*]. Observations on milk sickness, being extracts from inaugural dissertations submitted to the examination of the president, etc., of Transylvania University. 1836. Transylv. J. M., Lexington, Ky., 1836, ix, 85-95.— **Short** (C. W.) Alleged causes of milk-sickness. West. J. M. & S., Louisville, 1840, i, 231.— **Short** (H. S.) Milk sickness. Eclect. M. J., Cincin., 1875, xxxv, 211.— **Simpson** (D. L.) Extract from an inaugural thesis on milk sickness. Transylv. J. M., Lexington, Ky., 1839, xii, 146-150. — **Slack.** Ergodelateria. West. Lancet, Cincin., 1854, xv, 140-144.— **Smith** (C. H.) Milk sickness. Boston M. & S. J., 1867-8, lxxvii, 471. ——. Milk-sickness. Phila. M. Times, 1874-5, v, 186.— **Smith** (J. N.) On milk sickness. Inaugural dissertation. Transylv. J. M., Lexington, Ky., 1837, x, 236-246.— **Spalding** (J.) Milk sickness. West. M. Reporter, Chicago, 1881-2, iii, 266-274.— **Sutton** (G.) Preliminary report on milk sickness, as it prevails within the State of Indiana. Proc. Indiana M. Soc., Indianap., 1853, 176-178.— **Swan** (I. S.) Milk sickness. West. Lancet, Cincin., 1852, xiii, 671.— **Taylor** (G. B.) Facts and conjectures on the trembles and milksickness. West. J. M. & S., Louisville, 1842, vi, 181-185.— **Thompson** (S.) Milk sickness, or trembles. St. Louis M. & S. J., 1848-9, vi, 220-227. ——. Milksickness. Northwest. M. & S. J., Chicago, 1853, x, 225-234.— **Thompson** (S. W.) On milk-sickness; its etiology and treatment. West. J. M. & S., Louisville, Ky., 1853, 3. s., xi, 471-486. ——. An essay on milksickness. Northwest. M. & S. J., Chicago, 1854, xi, 385-401.— **Townshend** (N. S.) Milk-sickness. J. Comp. M. & S., N. Y., 1883, iv, 117-120.— **Travis** (J.) Observations on milk-sickness. West. J. M. & S., Louisville, 1840, ii, 101-104.— **Troy.** Case of milk sickness. Cincin. Lancet & Obs., 1861, iv, 283. — **Waggoner** (F. R.) Milk sickness; its etiology, pathology, diagnosis, and treatment. Penins. & Indep. M. J., Detroit, 1858-9, i, 658-662. ——. Milk sickness. *Ibid.*, 1859-60, ii, 5-10.— **Wagman** (J. V.) Morbid anatomy of milksickness. West. J. M. & S., Louisville, 1841, iv, 234.— **Walker** (J. W.) Milk-sickness. Science, N. Y., 1886, viii, 482.— **White** (C.) Observations on milk sickness. Transylv. J. M., Lexington, Ky., 1836, ix, 87.— **Wilkinson** (G. W.) Etiology of milksickness. Northwest. M. & S. J., Chicago, 1857, xiv, 151-159.— **Williams** (J. A.) Milk-sickness. Cincin. M. & S. News, 1863, iv, 165-171.— **Winans** (M.) Practical observations on the disease denominated milk-sickness, or sick-stomach. West. J. M. & S., Louisville, 1840, i, 190-193.— **Woodfin** (H. G.) Milk sickness. North Car. M. J., Wilmington, 1878, i, 13 ; 137.— **Wozencraft** (O. M.) Trembles and milksickness. Pacific M. & S. J., San Fran., 1873-4, xvi, 172 - 175.— **Wright** (G. W.) Observations on the atmosphere origin of the endemic sick stomach of particular situations in the Western States. West. M. & Phys. J., Cincin., 1827-8, i, 369-384.— **Wright** (G. W.) & **Bennett** (J.) Proposals for publishing by subscription a treatise on the endemic sick stomach of the Western States. *Ibid.*, 477.— **Yandell** (L. P.) An essay on milk-sickness. Transylv. J. M., Lexington, Ky., 1828, i, 309-321. ——. An inquiry into the nature of the disease called milk-sickness. West. J. M. & S., Louisville, 1852, 3. s., ix, 374-401. ——. Report on milk sickness. Proc. Kentucky M. Soc., Louisville, 1867-8, 88-96.

Milk-sugar.

See **Sugar** *of milk.*

Milk-tumors.

See **Breast** (*Tumors of, Cystic*).

Milkers' *cramp.*

See **Cramp** (*Dancers', etc.*)

Mill (John). The use of clairvoyance in medicine. 2. ed. vi, 7-40 pp. 8°. *London, W. Freeman,* 1858.

Mill (John Stuart) [1806-79]. The evidence of

... taken before the Royal Commission of 1870,

Mill (John Stuart)—continued.
on the administration and operation of the contagious diseases acts of 1866 and 1869. 24 pp. 8°. *London*, [1871?]
  Reprinted verbatim from the Blue-Book.
  For Biography, see Mind, Lond., 1879, iv, 211; 375; 520: 1880, v, 82–104 (A. Bain).

Millar (Alexander). *A probationary essay on lumbar abscess. 17 pp. 8°. *Edinburgh, Ballantyne & Co.*, 1831. [P., v. 1273.]

Millar (David). *De epilepsia. 36 pp. 8°. *Edinburgi, D. Paterson*, 1763. [P., v. 603.]

Millar (Jacobus). *De hepatitide. 2 p. l., 35 pp. 8°. *Edinburgi, A. Neill cum sociis*, 1795.

Millar (Joannes). *De renibus. 2 p. l., 58 pp. 8°. *Edinburgi, J. Pillans et fil.*, 1820.

Millar (John)[1]. *De fluxu lochiorum immodico. 2 p. l., 30 pp. 8°. *Edinburgi, Sands [and others]*, 1757. [*Also, in:* P., v. 645.]

———. Observations on the asthma and on the hooping cough. iii, iii, 207 pp. 8°. *London, T. Cadel*, 1769. [*Also, in:* P., v. 707; 1343.]

———. The same. Bemerkungen über die Engbrüstigkeit und das Hühnerweh. Nebst einem Anhange von der stinkenden Asa. Aus dem Englischen übersetzt. 7 p. l., 176 pp., 4 l. 8°. *Leipzig, C. Fritsch*, 1769.

———. Observations on anatomy, read before the Medical Society of London, and published at their request. viii, 101 pp., 1 l. 8°. *London, J. Johnson*, 1774.

———. Observations on the practice in the medical department of the Westminster General Infirmary; together with an arithmetical calculation of the comparative success of various establishments for the relief of the sick. By order of the governors. 3 p. l., 77 pp. 4°. *London*, 1777.

———. Observations on the management of the prevailing diseases in Great Britain, particularly in the army and navy, together with a review of that of other countries, and arithmetical calculations of the comparative success of different methods of cure. viii, 318 + pp. 4°. *London*, 1779.
  All after p. 318 wanting.

Millar (John)[2] [1839–72]. A plea in favour of the insane poor to the earl of Shaftesbury. 11 pp. 8°. *London, H. Renshaw*, 1859.

———. Hints on insanity. vi, 105 pp. 16°. *London, H. Renshaw*, 1861.

———. Notes on the recent epidemic in St. Petersburg. 9 pp. 8°. *Edinburgh, Oliver & Boyd*, 1865.
  See, also, **Manners** (Thomas). Cases of poisoning by susumber berries. 8°. *Edinburgh*, 1867.
  For Biography, see Brit. M. J., Lond., 1872, i, 171. *Also:* Lancet, Lond., 1872, i, 241.

Millar (Richard). Disquisitions in the history of medicine; part first, exhibiting a view of physic, as observed to flourish, during remote periods, in Europe and the East. 4, 338 pp., 1 l. 8°. *Edinburgh, W. Blackwood*, 1811.

———. Statements relative to the present prevalence of epidemic fever among the poorer classes of Glasgow; together with some suggestions, both for affording more adequate assistance to the sick and for checking the further progress of the contagion. In a letter addressed to the honorable the lord provost of Glasgow. 48 pp. 8°. *Glascow, J. Smith & Son*, 1818.

———. Clinical lectures on the contagious typhus, epidemic in Glasgow and the vicinity, during the years 1831 and 1832. 144 pp. 8°. *Glascow, J. Brash & Co.*, 1833.

Millar (William Barclay). *On dyspepsia, or indigestion. 2 p. l., 25 pp. 8°. *Edinburgh, J. Stark*, 1834.

Millard (Auguste). *De la trachéotomie dans le cas de croup; observations recueillies à l'Hôpital des enfants malades, années 1857 et 1858. 247 pp. 4°. *Paris, Rignoux*, 1858.

———. Rapport sur un cas d'anévrysme de l'aorte thoracique communiquant avec l'œsophage. 20 pp., 1 pl. 8°. *Paris, V. Masson & fils*, 1862. [P., v. 1667.]
  Repr. from: Bull. Soc. anat. de Par., 1861, xxxvi.

Millard (Charles) [–1836].
  See **Bloxam** (William). The cyclopædia of practical surgery [etc.] fol. *London*, 1836.

Millard (Henry B.) The climate and statistics of consumption. A paper read before the American Geographical and Statistical Society. With extensive additions by the author. 108, 4 pp. 8°. *New York, W. Radde*, 1861.

———. On diphtheria; illustrated by cases. 32 pp., 1 l. 8°. *New York, Boericke & Tafel*, 1879.
  Repr. from: N. Am. J. Homœop., N. Y., 1878–9, n. s., ix.

———. Researches in the minute anatomy of the epithelia of the kidney. 15 pp. 8°. [*New York*, 1882.]
  Repr. from: N. York M. J., 1882, xxxv.
  See, also, **Charcot** (Jean Martin). Lectures on Bright's disease, etc. 8°. *New York*, 1878. — **Reil** (W.) A monograph upon aconite, [etc.] 8°. *New York*, 1860.

Millard (William). A manual for the classification, training, and education of the feeble-minded, imbecile, and idiotic. xv, 191 pp. 8°. *London, Longmans [and others]*, 1866.

Millard De Montrion (J.-C.-C.-L.) *Sur l'érysipèle simple et phlegmoneux. 33 pp. 4°. *Paris*, 1837, No. 89, v. 308.

Millardet (A.) *Nouvelles recherches sur la périodicité de la tension. Étude sur les mouvements périodiques et paratoniques de la sensitive. 1 p. l., 79 pp., 6 ch. 4°. *Strasbourg*, 1869, 3. s., No. 191.

Millardet (P.-A.) *De l'hémorrhagie utérine avant, pendant et après l'accouchement. 36 pp. 4°. *Paris*, 1837, No. 235, v. 313.

Millars (Franciscus Xaverius)[1]. *De explorata kermes mineralis sive pulveris Carthusianorum in medendo efficacia. 3 p. l., 80 pp. sm. 4°. *Argentorati, typ. hœredum Pauschingerianorum*, [1752].

Millars (Franciscus Xaverius)[2]. *De medicamentis antepilepticis. 46 pp. 4°. *Argentorati, J. H. Heitz*, [1787].

Millar's *asthma.*
  See **Laryngismus** *stridulus.*

Millau.
  Gobley. Rapport sur l'eau minérale du Cambon, commune de Montjaux (Aveyron). Bull. Acad. de méd., Par., 1863–4, xxix, 277. — **Poggiale.** Rapport sur l'eau minérale du Cambon, commune de Montjaux (Aveyron). *Ibid.*, 1862–3, xxviii, 217.

Millault (Urban-Hippolyte). *De la chlorose. 60 pp. 4°. *Paris*, 1859, No. 182, v. 634.

Millbank.
  See **Prisons** (*Descriptions, etc., of*), by localities.

Millbrook.
  See **Fever** (*Typhoid, History, etc., of*), by localities.

Mille (A.) Rapport sur le mode d'assainissement des villes en Angleterre et en Écosse, présenté à M. le préfet de la Seine. 1 p. l., 33 pp., 1 map, 4 plans. 4°. *Paris, Vinchon*, 1854.

———. Assainissement des villes par l'eau, les égouts, les irrigations. iv pp., 2 l., 271 pp. 8°. *Paris, Vve. C. Dunod*, 1886.

Mille (Adolphe). *Considérations générales sur l'action et l'expectation en médecine. 19 pp. 4°. *Paris*, 1834, No. 81, v. 271.

Milledgeville.
  See **Insane** (*Asylums for, etc.*), by localities.

Millée (Ernest) [1856–   ]. *Étude sur la fièvre typhoïde à début grippal. 58 pp. 4°. *Paris*, 1884, No. 340.

Millefolium.

PETZSCHIUS (C. H.) * De millefolio, germ. Schaaf-Garben. 4°. *Halæ Magdeb.*, [1719].

Maumery. Lettre sur la vertu anti-spasmodique de l'infusion des sommités de mille-feuille (Millefolium vulgare album.) J. de méd., chir., pharm., etc., Par., 1770, xxxiv, 402–414. — **Mongin - Montrol.** Lettre sur une vertu spécifique et anti-spasmodique de la mille-feuille (Mille-folium vulgare album). *Ibid.*, 529–531. — **Normand de Sogny.** Lettre sur l'efficacité des sommités de mille-feuille dans plusieurs maladies. *Ibid.*, 1771, xxxv, 520–527.

Miller (A. G.) Organic stricture of the urethra, and its treatment by Holt's method. 9 pp., 1 pl. 8°. *Edinburgh, Oliver & Boyd*, 1868.
Repr. from: Edinb. M. J., 1868, xiii.

———. On polypus of the rectum. 7 pp. 8°. *Edinburgh, Oliver & Boyd*, 1870.
Repr. from: Edinb. M. J., 1870, xv.

———. The same. 10 pp. 8°. *Edinburgh, Colston & Son*, 1871.
Repr. from: Edinb. M. J., 1870, xv.

———. Remarks on the employment of bulbous bougies. 4 pp. 8°. *Edinburgh, Oliver & Boyd*, [1873].
Repr. from: Edinb. M. J., 1873, xix.
See, also, **Thomson** (Lawrence Ramsey). Case of tumour of the bones of the skull [etc.] 8°. *Edinburgh*, 1869.

Miller (A. W.)
Editor of: **Medical** Clippings and New Chemicals, Philadelphia, 1886.

Miller (*Aaron Wooley*) [1818–61].

Toner (J. M.) Obituary. Tr. Am. M. Ass., Phila., 1881, xxxii, 526.

Miller (Adam). Review of Dr. S. A. Latta's pamphlet, entitled "The cholera in Cincinnati, or a connected view of the controversy between the homœopathists and the Methodist Expositor; also, a review of the report read before the Homœopathic Association". 16 pp. 8°. *Cincinnati*, 1850.

Miller (Alexander). * A probationary essay on lumbar or psoas abscess. 16 pp. 8°. *Edinburgh, D. & W. Millar*, 1831. [*Also, in:* P., v. 1273.]

———. The same. 1 p. l., 16 pp. 8°. *Edinburgh, Ballantyne & Co.*, 1831.

———. An inquiry into the average mortality in lithotomic cases; with a few remarks on the operation of lithotrity. 44 pp. 8°. *Edinburgh, A. Shortreed*, 1831. [*Also, in:* P., v. 893.]

———. *See, also:*
TESTIMONIALS in favour of Alexander Miller, surgeon to the Royal Public Dispensary for the city and county of Edinburgh, etc., candidate for the situation of surgeon to the West Kirk Charity Workhouse. 8°. *Edinburgh*, [1834].

Miller (Antonius Engelbertus). * De respiratione et digestione. 16 pp. 8°. *Monachii, J. A. Giesser*, 1836.

Miller (August). * Ueber Delirium tremens. 15 pp. 8°. *Ingolstadt*, 1867.

Miller (Augustus Wolfgangus). Adagia quædam medicinalia doctrinæ promiscuæ discursibus illustrata. 1 p. l., 16 pp. 4°. [*Altdorf*], *lit. J. G. Kohlesii*, [1714].

———. * De febre maligna epidemica, quæ an. 1715 Lindaviæ in Lacu Acronio sitæ est grassata. 42 pp. sm. 4°. *Basileæ, typ. F. Lüdii*, 1716.

Miller (Ben. C.) The treatment of tank offal and the gases from rendering tanks. With a description of some of the processes in operation in Chicago. 7 pp., 2 pl. 8°. *Philadelphia, W. P. Kildare*, 1875.
Repr. from: J. Frankl. Inst., Phila., 1875.

Miller (Bloomfield J.) Mortuary experience of the Mutual Benefit Life Insurance Company, Newark, N. J., 1845–79. 16 pp., 15 l., 2 diag. 4°. [*Newark*, 1880?]

Miller (Charles). Case of hydrocephalus chronicus, with some unusual symptoms and appearances on dissection. 6 pp. 8°. [*n. p.*, 1826, *vel subseq.*]
Repr. from: Tr. Med.-Chir. Soc. Edinb., 1826, ii.

Miller (De Laskie) [1818–   ].
Co-Editor of: **Chicago** (The) Medical Journal, 1864–6.

Miller (Edmond). An account of the University of Cambridge, and the colleges there; being a plain relation of many of their oaths, statutes and charters; by which will appear the necessity the present members lie under of endeavouring to obtain such alterations as may render 'em practicable and more suitable to the present times; together with a few natural and easie methods, how the legislature may for the future fix that, and the other great nursery of learning, in the true interest of the nation and Protestant succession; most humbly propos'd to both houses of Parliament. 2. ed. 200 pp. 8°. *London, J. Baker*, 1717.

Miller (Edward) [1760–1812]. * De physconia splenica. 27 pp. 8°. *Philadelphia, G. Young*, 1789.

———. Report on the malignant disease which prevailed in the city of New York in the autumn of 1805. Addressed to the governor of the State of New York. 48 pp. 8°. *New York*, 1806.

———. The same. Histoire de la maladie maligne appelée fièvre jaune, avec ses effets pendant l'automne de 1805 à New-York, qui prouvent qu'elle n'est nullement contagieuse. Écrite en forme de lettre par le docteur E. Miller, médecin du gouvernement, et adressée par lui au gouverneur du dit état. Trad. de l'anglais par J.-D. Dupont. On a joint à cet intéressant ouvrage le rapport qui en a été fait à la Société de médecine par MM. Pinel et Moreau (de la Sarthe). 51 pp. 8°. *Paris, J. Charles*, 1806. [P., v. 476.]

———. The medical works of . . . collected, and accompanied with a biographical sketch of the author. By Samuel Miller. cxi, 392 pp. 8°. *New York, Collins & Co.*, 1814.
Also, Co-Editor of: **Medical** (The) Repository, New York, 1797–1814.
See, also, **Rush** (Benjamin). Facts intended to prove the yellow fever not to be contagious. 8°. *Philadelphia*, 1802.—**Thomas** (Robert). The modern practice of physic [etc.] 8°. *New York*, 1811. ———. The same. 8°. *New York*, 1813.
For Biography, see **Bush** (L. P.) Address before the Medical Society of Delaware, delivered at its annual meeting, held at Dover, June, 1855. [Life of Dr. Edward Miller.] 8°. *Wilmington, Del.*, 1856.—**Miller** (S.) A biographical sketch. *In:* MILLER (E.) Medical works of . . . 8°. *New York*, 1814, pp. xi–cxi.
See, also, Am. M. & Phil. Reg., N. Y., 1814, iii, 1–8, port. *For Portrait, see* **Collection** of Portr. (Libr.)

Miller (Eli P.) A treatise on the cause of exhausted vitality; or abuses of the sexual function. 131 pp. 8°. *New York, Gray & Green*, 1867.

———. The same. Vital force: how wasted and how preserved. 3. ed. vi, 131 pp. 12°. *New York, E. P. Miller*, 1874.

———. How to bathe; a family guide for the use of water in preserving health and treating disease. vi, 7–72 pp. 12°. *New York, American News Co.*, 1869.

———. The improved Turkish bath; what is it, who should take it, why, when, how, and where? 27 pp. 8°. *New York, Miller, Haynes & Co.*, 1871.

———. A father's advice; a book for every boy. 29 pp. 24°. *New York, E. P. Miller*, 1881.

———. A new treatment for piles or hemorrhoids, painful fissure, rectal ulcer, fistula, and other diseases of the rectum, without the use of the

Miller (Eli P.)—continued.
knife, ligature, clamp, écraseur, caustics, hot iron, etc., and by a process sure, safe, and painless. 32 pp. 8°. *New York, Miller, Haynes & Co.*, 1883.

Miller (*Erasmus Darwin*) [1813–81].
S. Biographical notice. Boston M. & S. J., 1881, cv, 584.—**Warner** (L. F.) Necrology. Tr. Am. M. Ass., Phila., 1882, xxxiii, 582–584.

Miller (Georg). *Beitrag zur Lehre von der multiloculären ulcerirenden Echinococcusgeschwulst in der Leber. 26 pp. 8°. *Tübingen, H. Laupp*, 1874.

Miller (Gerardus Andreas) [1718–62]. *Theses chymico-medicæ. 26 pp. 4°. *Argentorati, typ. S. Kürsneri*, [1740].

Miller (H. G.)
See **Snellen** (H.) & **Miller** (H. G.) Kan de cholera [etc.] 8°. [*Utrecht*, 1867.]

Miller (Henry) [1800–74]. *An inaugural thesis on the relation between the sanguiferous and nervous systems. 1 p. l., iv, 9–46 pp. 8°. *Lexington, W. G. Hunt*, 1822. [*Also, in:* P., v. 396; 762.]

——. An oration, pronounced on the anniversary of the K. A. Society of Hippocrates, in Lexington, Ky. 13 pp. 8°. *Lexington, T. T. Skillman*, 1822. [P., v. 396; 762.]

——. On the true value of experience in medicine; an introductory lecture. 21 pp. 8°. *Louisville, Ky., Prentice & Weissinger*, 1838.

——. Examination of the claims of homœopathy as a system of medical doctrine and practice; being a lecture delivered before the Medical Society of Louisville. 24 pp. 8°. *Louisville, Ky., G. H. Monsarrat & Co.*, [1847].

——. Report of the obstetric committee on anæsthesia in midwifery, and the speculum uteri. 29 pp. 8°. *Louisville, Webb & Levering*, 1853.
Repr. from: Tr. Kentucky M. Soc. 1852, Louisville, 1853.

——. Lectures in reply to the Croonian lectures for 1854, of Charles West, of London, on the pathological importance of ulceration of the os uteri. 71 pp. 8°. *Louisville, Ky., I. F. Brennan*, 1855.
Repr. from: West. J. M. & S., Louisville, 1855, 4. s., iii.

——. Lectures on inflammation and ulceration of the cervix uteri. 71 pp. 8°. [*Louisville?* 1855.]

——. The principles and practice of obstetrics, including the treatment of chronic inflammation of the uterus considered as a frequent cause of abortion. xix, 624 pp. 8°. *Philadelphia, Blanchard & Lea*, 1858.

——. Two cases of encysted tumour of the ovary successfully treated by excision; and an attempt to justify the operation of ovariotomy under certain circumstances. 26 pp. 8°. *Philadelphia*, 1859.
Repr. from: Am. J. M. Sc., Phila., 1859 n. s., xxxvii.

——. An address delivered before the American Medical Association at its thirteenth annual meeting. 28 pp. 8°. *Philadelphia, Collins*, 1860.

——. Brief notes of four additional cases of ovariotomy. 7 pp. 8°. [*Philadelphia*, 1869.]
Repr. from: Am. J. M. Sc., Phila., 1869, n. s., lxvii.

——. Thoughts on chronic inversion of the uterus; specially with reference to gastrotomy as a substitute for amputation of the uterus. 42 pp. 8°. *Louisville, Ky., Bell & Co.*, 1870.
Repr. from: Richmond & Louisville M. J., Louisville, 1870, ix.

——. Retrospect of uterine pathology and therapeutics in the United States; specially in regard to intra-uterine medication in chronic internal

Miller (Henry)—continued.
metritis. 37 pp. 8°. *New York, W. Baldwin & Co.*, 1871.
Repr. from: Am. J. Obst., N. Y., 1871, iv.
Also, Co-Editor of: **Louisville** (The) Journal of Medicine and Surgery, 1838.
For Biography, see Richmond & Louisville M. J., Louisville, 1872, xiii, 129–136, 1 pl. *Also:* Tr. Am. M. Ass., Phila., 1875, xxvi, 441–444 (S. D. Gross, E. S. Gaillard, J. M. Keller). *Also:* Tr. Kentucky M. Soc., Louisville, 1875, 38–43 (L. P. Yandell).

Miller (Henry J.)
See **Hogg** (Jabez). Sur les erreurs d'interprétation ayant rapport spécialement, etc. 8°. [*Bruxelles*, 1877.]

Miller (J.) Korerabio Ron. [A treatise on cholera; transl. by Yokoi Shinzo.] 2 (1 l.), 2, 61 pp. 12°. *Tokio*, 1878.
Japanese text.

Miller (J. F.) Synopsis of meteorological observations made at the observatory, Whitehaven, Cumberland, in the year 1853; including tables of the annual, monthly, and maximum daily fall of rain in the last nine years, at Seathwaite, Borrowdale, in the centre of the English lake district. 14 pp. 8°. *Edinburgh, Neill & Co.*, 1854.
Repr. from: Edinb. N. Phil. J., 1854.

Miller (J. P.) The hydatiform mole. The report of a case, together with a disquisition upon its history, pathology, etiology, diagnosis, prognosis, and treatment. 34 pp. 8°. *Wheeling*, 1879.
Repr. from: Tr. M. Soc. W. Virg., Wheeling, 1879.

Miller (Jacobus Vance). *De dyspepsia. 1 p. l., 32 pp. 8°. *Edinburgi*, 1808.

Miller (James)[1] [1812–1864]. A probationary essay on the dressing of wounds, as simplified and improved in modern surgery. 36 pp. 8°. *Edinburgh, A. Shortrede*, 1840. [P., v. 1200.]

——. An introductory lecture on surgery. 23 pp. 8°. *Edinburgh, W. Blackwood & Sons*, 1840.

——. Syllabus of lectures on the principles and practice of surgery. 15 pp. 8°. *Edinburgh, A. Shortrede*, 1841.

——. On the treatment of the hemorrhagic diathesis. 24 pp. 8°. [*Edinburgh, Balfour & Jack*, 1842.] [P., v. 1051; 1200.]
Repr. from: Lond. & Edinb. Month. J. M. Sc., 1842, ii.

——. An introductory lecture on pictorial anatomy. 32 pp. 8°. *Edinburgh, A. & C. Black*, 1842. [*Also, in:* P., v. 95.]

——. The principles of surgery. xii, 13–525 pp. 8°. *Philadelphia, Lea & Blanchard*, 1845.

——. The same. 3. ed. xvi, 760 pp. roy. 8°. *Edinburgh, A. & C. Black*, 1853.

——. The practice of surgery. xx, 14–496 pp. 8°. *Philadelphia, Lea & Blanchard*, 1846.

——. The same. Revised by the American editor. 4. Am. from the last Edinb. ed. xxxi, 34–682 pp. 8°. *Philadelphia, Blanchard & Lea*, 1857.

——. Surgical experience of chloroform. 60 pp. 8°. *Edinburgh, Sutherland & Knox*, 1848. [*Also, in:* P., v. 725; 1030; 1052; 1204.]

——. To the managers of the Royal Infirmary. 2 pp. 4°. [*Edinburgh*], 1852. [P., v. 919.]

——. Address to the Medico-Chirurgical Society of Edinburgh. 16 pp. 8°. *Edinburgh, Murray & Gibb*, 1857.

——. Prostitution considered in relation to its cause and cure. 38 pp. 8°. *Edinburgh, Sutherland & Knox*, 1859. [P., v. 1197.]
Repr. from: Edinb. M. J., 1858–9, iv, 1008–1033.

——. Alcohol: its place and power. (From the 19. Glasg. ed.) 179 pp. 12°. *Philadelphia, Lindsay & Blakiston*, 1859.

——. Neuenahr: a new spa on the Rhine. 35 pp. 8°. *Edinburgh, Oliver & Boyd*, 1861. [*Also, in:* P., v. 870; 1193.]

Miller (James)[1]—continued.

———. A system of surgery. [New ed.] xxv, 1387 pp. 8°. *Edinburgh, A. & C. Black*, 1864.
Being a 5. ed., in one volume, of the principles of surgery.
For Biography, see Edinb. M. J., 1864, x, 92–96. *Also:* Lancet, Lond., 1864, i, 735–736.

———. *See, also:*

LETTERS to the right honourable the lord provost, magistrates, and town council, against James Miller having the chair of surgery in the University of Edinburgh. 4°. [*Edinburgh,* 1842.]

TESTIMONIALS in favour of Mr. James Miller, candidate for the chair of surgery in the University of Edinburgh, 1842. 8°. [*Edinburgh,* 1842.]

——— & **Lizars** (John). Alcohol and tobacco. Alcohol: its place and power. The use and abuse of tobacco. 179, 138 pp. 8°. *Philadelphia, Lindsay & Blakiston*, 1870.

Miller (James)[2]. The pathology of the kidney in scarlatina; illustrated by cases. xiii, 177 pp. 8°. *London, T. & W. Boone*, 1850. [P., v. 1024.]

Miller (James H.) "Thomsonalgia." Report to the trustees of the Baltimore County Alms House, with contents; preceded by a few introductory remarks relating to the same. 19 pp. 8°. [*Baltimore,* 1836.]

Miller (Joannes)[1]. * De lacte humano. 1 p. l., 53 pp. 8°. *Edinburgi, A. Neill et socii*, 1805.

Miller (Joannes)[2]. * De rabie canina et hydrophobia contagiosa. [Landshut.] 30 pp. 8°. *Augustæ, J. Rösl*, 1823.

Miller (*John*)[1] [1774–1862].
Bradford (G. W.) Memoir of John Miller. Tr. M. Soc. N. Y., Albany, 1862, 449–460.

Miller (*John*)[2] [1800–38].
Biographical notice. Lancet, Lond., 1838, ii, 297–301; 1839, i, 744.

Miller (John Lindsay). On puerperal fever. 22 pp. 8°. *Glasgow,* 1878.
Repr. from: Glasgow M. J., 1878, xi.

Miller (John S.) A case of extensive recurrent sarcomatous disease. 3 pp. 8°. [*Philadelphia,* 1885.]
Repr. from: Proc. Phila. Co. M. Soc., Phila., 1885.

Miller (Joseph). Botanicum officinale, or a compendious herbal; giving an account of all such plants as are now used in the practice of physick, with their descriptions and virtues. 466 pp. 8°. *London, E. Bell*, 1722.

Miller (Josephus). * De ascite abdominali. 3 p. l., 58 pp. 8°. *Edinburgi, Balfour et Smellie*, 1792.

Miller (Josephus Ewing). * De gastritide. 1 p. l., 21 pp. 8°. *Edinburgi, R. Allan*, 1815. [P., v. 732.]

Miller (Ludovicus). * Disputatio physiologica de transpiratione insensibili. 28 pp. 4°. *Altdorffi*, 1680.

Miller (N. F.) Anatomicheskija i fiziologicheskija osobennosti dietskago organizma. [Peculiarities of the infantile organism.] xii, 263 pp. 8°. *Moskva*, 1885.

———. Dieti nedonoski i osobennosti ich bolieznei. Vtor. izd. [Prematurely born children, and their diseases.] 20 pp. 8°. *Moskva*, 1886.

———. Ospoprivivanie (vaktsinatsija). vii, 135 pp., 1 l. 8°. *Moskva, tip. A. A. Kartseva*, 1887.

Miller (Nathaniel) [1771–1850]. A dissertation, read before the Massachusetts Medical Society, on the importance and manner of detecting deep seated matter. 16 pp. 8°. *Boston, J. G. Scobie*, 1827.
For Biography, see Med. Communicat. Mass. M. Soc., Bost., 1854, viii, 171–174.

Miller (Patricius). * De scarlatina. 2 p. l., 31 pp. 8°. *Edinburgi, excud. A. Neill et socii*, 1804. [P., v. 30.]

Miller (Peter). *An essay on the means of lessening the pains of parturition. 38 pp. 8°. *Philadelphia, H. Maxwell*, 1804.
Also, in: CALDWELL (C.) Med. theses [etc.] 8°. *Philadelphia*, 1805, i.

Miller (Robert). * Upon the action of cold upon the human body, and its application to the cure of diseases. 28 pp. 8°. *Philadelphia, B. Graves*, 1807.

Miller (Samuel)[1]. * De dysenteria. 3 p. l., 49 pp. 8°. *Edinburgi, A. Smellie*, 1802. [P., v. 21.]

Miller (Samuel)[2]. A brief retrospect of the eighteenth century. Pt. 1 in 2 v. Containing a sketch of the revolutions and improvements in science, arts, and literature during that period. 2 v. xvi, 544 pp.; vi, 510 pp. 8°. *New York, F. & J. Swords*, 1803.

———. The guilt, folly, and sources of suicide; two discourses preached in the city of New York, Feb., 1805. 72 pp. 8°. *New York, F. & J. Swords*, 1805.
See, also, **Miller** (Edward). The medical works of . . . 8°. *New York*, 1814.—**Sergeant** (John). Observations and reflections on the design and effects of punishment, [etc.] 8°. *Philadelphia*, 1828.

Miller (Samuel M.) Notes of hospital practice. Pts. i–iv in 3 v. 8°. *Philadelphia*, 1879–82.

CONTENTS.
Pt. i. Philadelphia hospitals.
Pts. ii–iv. New York and Philadelphia hospitals.
Also, Editor of: **Clinical** (The) News, Philadelphia, 1880–81.

Miller (Stanislaus). * Materiali k patolog. gistol. bronchialnich jelezi pri razlichnich sostojanijach legkich. [Pathological histology of bronchial glands.] 49 pp., 1 pl. 8°. *St. Petersburg*, 1873.

Miller (T. Clarke). A contribution to the etiology, pathology, and therapeutics of cholera infantum. 18 pp. 8°. *New York, W. Wood & Co.*, 1879.
Repr. from: Am. J. Obst., N. Y., 1879, xii.

Miller (Thomas)[1]. * De pubertate. 1 p. l., 35 pp. 8°. *Edinburgi, Balfour et Smellie*, 1781.

Miller (Thomas)[2]. Introductory lecture on anatomy. 20 pp. 8°. *Washington, J. Gideon*, 1840.

———. An address to the graduates of the medical department of the Columbian College. 31 pp. 8°. *Washington, Blair & Rives*, 1842.

Miller (V.) * Iz nablondenii nad chachotochnini. (Vlijanie agaricina na poti chachotoch.) [Agaricine in the night-sweat of phthisis.] 114 pp., 1 l., 12 diag. 8°. *St. Petersburg*, 1885.

Miller (W. D.) Fermentation in the human mouth; its relation to caries of the teeth. The influence of antiseptics, filling materials, etc., upon the fungi of dental caries. The fungi of dental caries; their pure cultivation and effect upon lower animals. 41 pp. 8°. *New York*, 1884.
Repr. from: Independ. Pract., Balt., 1884, v.

———. Wörterbuch der Bacterienkunde bearbeitet von . . . Beilage zum "Jahrbuch der practischen Medicin, Jahrgang 1886". 3 p. l., 43 pp. 8°. *Stuttgart, F. Enke*, 1886.

Miller (Wesley). The germ-theory of Pasteur, and new discoveries of Dr. Wesley Miller to prevent diseases in domestic animals and mankind generally by vaccination. 21. 8°. [*n. p.,* 1881.]

———. Prevention of tubercular and other diseases, in man and domestic animals, by vaccination. 8 pp. 8°. [*New York,* 1882.]

———. New York Vaccine Co. Animal vaccine virus. New discoveries in the treatment of contagious or infectious diseases by vaccination or hypodermic injections. 2 l. 8°. [*New York,* 1882.]

Miller (William Allen) [–1870]. Elements of chemistry, theoretical and practical. 3 v. 8°. [*London*, 1862–4.]

CONTENTS.

Pt. 1. Chemical physics. 3. ed. *London, Parker, Son & Bourn*, 1863.
Pt. 2. Inorganic chemistry. 3. ed. *London, Longman & Co.*, 1864.
Pt. 3. Organic chemistry. 2. ed. *London, Parker, Son & Bourn*, 1862.
For Biography, *see* Lancet, Lond., 1870, ii, 523.

Miller (William H.)
Editor of: **San Francisco** (The) Medical Journal, 1856.

Milleradowics (Petrus Gabrielow). *De innocenti infectione venerea.
In: WEIZ (F. A.) Vollständ. Ausz. [etc.] 12°. *Leipzig u. Budissin*, 1774, vi, 121–124.

Millermann (L.) *De l'auto-inoculation traumatique. 63 pp. 4°. *Paris, A. Davy*, 1887, No. 118.

Millers.

SALDINI (C.) Modern corn-milling. Transl. by W. H. Thelwall. 8°. *London*, 1883.
Repr. from: Proc. Inst. Civil Engin., 1882–3, lxxi, pt. 1.
Chevallier (A.) Des accidents qui peuvent être observés dans les minoteries (moulins à farine); responsabilité des patrons envers leurs ouvriers. Ann. d'hyg., Par., 2. s., 1866, xxvi, 359–382.—**Duchesne** & **Michel** (E.) Les meuniers; étude d'hygiène professionelle. J. de méd. de Par., 1883, iv, 621–635. *Also:* Bull. Soc. de méd. prat. de Par. (1883), 1884, 18–23.—**Mercier** (T.) Voile préservateur pour les ouvriers fabricants et rhabilleurs de meules à moulins. Cong. internat. d'hyg. 1878, Par., 1880, ii, 444–447.—**Poincaré** (L.) Recherches expérimentales sur les effets des poussières de meunerie. Ann. d'hyg., Par., 1887, 3. s., xvii, 38–42.

Millet (A.) De l'emploi thérapeutique des préparations arsenicales. 2. éd. xxiii, 252 pp. 8°. *Paris, F. Savy*, 1865.
Prize essay.

Millet (A.-B.) *Sur la chlorose. 29 pp. 4°. *Paris*, 1833, No. 118, v. 260.

Millet (Alexandre-Auguste). *Coup-d'œil historique et médical sur Bicêtre (maison d'aliénés). 58 pp. 4°. *Paris*, 1842. No. 189, v. 393.

———. Du traitement de l'aliénation mentale. 50 pp. 8°. [*Paris, F. Malteste & Cie.*, 1842.]
Repr. from: Gaz. méd. de Par., 1842, 2. s., x.

———. Du choléra-morbus épidémique. xii, 440 pp. 8°. *Paris, Labé*, 1851.

———. Du seigle ergoté considéré sous les rapports physiologique, obstétrical et de l'hygiène publique. 163 pp. 4°. *Paris, J.-B. Baillière*, 1854.
Repr. from: Mém. Acad. de méd., Par., 1854, xviii.

———. Traité de la diphthérie du larynx. Croup. iv, 244 pp. 8°. *Paris, F. Savy*, 1863.

Millet (Charles)[1]. *Des luxations métatarso-phalangiennes du gros orteil. 1 p. l., 42 pp. 4°. *Strasbourg*, 1856, No. 363, v. 22.

Millet (Charles)[2]. *Quelques considérations sur la pneumonie latente. 86 pp., 1 l. 4°. *Montpellier*, 1875, No. 14.

Millet (Charles-Antoine). *De la fracture du col du fémur. 21 pp. 4°. *Paris*, 1825, No. 227, v. 196.

Millet (Cora), *née* **Robinet.** Conseils aux jeunes femmes sur l'éducation de la première enfance. 323 pp. 16°. *Paris, Dusacq*, [1855].

Millet (E.) L'angine arthritique. Traitement par les eaux d'Aix-les-Bains et de Marlioz. Obligation de l'examen laryngoscopique. 16 pp. 8°. *Paris, A. Delahaye & E. Lecrosnier*, 1885.

Millet (Eduardus). *Quædam de calculo, morbisque renum et vesicæ calculosis complectens. 3 p. l., 35 pp. 8°. *Edinburgi, G. Mudie et filii*, 1795.

Millet (Émile). *Étude statistique sur la maladie syphilitique, le chancre simple, et la blennorrhagie. 1 p. l., 76 pp. 4°. *Paris*, 1866, No. 82.

Millet (F.) *Sur les anus contre nature qui sont la suite des hernies gangrénées. 24 pp. 4°. *Paris*, 1822, No. 226.

Millet (Gonzague). *Recherches sur quelques points d'anatomie, de physiologie, et de pathologie placentaire. 103 pp. 4°. *Paris*, 1861, No. 97.

Millet (Jacobus Antonius). An mores parentum traducuntur ad sobolem? Præs. Claudius Antonius Renard. 4 pp. 4°. [*Parisiis, J. Quillau*, 1715.] [P., v. 1329.]

———. An in acutis, orgasmus a purgante? Præs. Franciscus Vernage. 4 pp. 4°. [*Parisiis, J. Quillau*, 1716.] [P., v. 1329.]

Millet (Joseph) [1851–86]. *De l'influence étiologique de l'alcoolisme sur la paralysie générale progressive. 51 pp. 4°. *Paris*, 1880, No. 440.
For Biography, *see* Encéphale, Par., 1886, vi, 511.

Millet (Jules-Émile). *Du bichlorure de méthylène comme agent anesthésique général. 1 p. l., 38 pp. 4°. *Strasbourg*, 1868, 3. s., No. 117.

Millet (L.-E.) *De la chlorose et de quelques maladies qu'on peut y rattacher. 44 pp. 4°. *Paris*, 1855, No. 187, v. 578.

Millet (Louis). *Essai sur la nature de l'éclampsie puerpérale. 1 p. l., 44 pp. 4°. *Strasbourg*, 1867, 3. s., No. 15.

Millet (Pierre). *Dyspepsie, ses rapports avec le rhumatisme. 40 pp. 4°. *Paris*, 1872, No. 273.

Millet (Pierre-Marie-Émile). *Des hémorrhagies utérines pendant la grossesse. 43 pp. 4°. *Paris*, 1871, No. 204.

Millet (V.) *Sur les fièvres intermittentes pernicieuses de Rome. vi, 7–38 pp. 4°. *Paris*, 1815, No. 54, v. 109.

Millet.

KURCHEMINOFF (K. P.) *Materialy k voprosu ob usvojaemosti azot-soderjatshich chastei pshena. [Assimilation of nitrogenous contents of millet.] 8°. *St. Petersburg*, 1887.

Milleter (Joh.) *De morbo Tsömör Hungaris endemio. 48 pp. 4°. *Lugd. Bat., C. Wishof*, 1717.
Also, in: HALLER. Disp. ad morb. [etc.] 4°. *Lausannæ*, 1760, vii, 639–676.

Millet-Lacombe (Georges). *De la vératrine dans la pneumonie. 35 pp. 4°. *Paris*, 1870, No. 276.

Millet-Lacombe (Pierre-C.) *Des hydropisies en général. 27 pp. 4°. *Paris*, 1845, No. 18.

Millett (Geo. Bown). Annual report of the medical officer of health for the port sanitary authority of Penzance for the years 1880; 1881. 12°. [*Penzance*, 1881–2.]

Millican (Kenneth W.) The evolution of morbid germs; a contribution to transcendental pathology. 6 p. l., 107 pp. 8°. *London, H. K. Lewis*, 1883.

Millie-Christina.

See **Monsters** (*Double*).

Millière (Jean-Pierre-Joseph). *Sur les exostoses. vi, 7–31 pp. 4°. *Paris*, 1814, No. 176, v. 106.

Millière (Victor). *Considérations sur l'agonie et son traitement. 1 p. l., 32 pp. 4°. *Strasbourg*, 1856, No. 367, v. 22.

Millies (Carolus Friderieus). *Collectanea de clysmatibus. 28 pp. 8°. *Lipsiæ, typ. Staritzii*, [1843].

Milliès-Lacroix (Adrien). *Essai sur l'emploi de l'extension continue dans le traitement de la coxalgie et des fractures du fémur. 58 pp. 4°. *Paris*, 1877, No. 499.

Milliet (André-Constant). *I. Quels sont les symptômes de la fièvre ataxique? II. [etc.] 33 pp. 4°. *Paris*, 1840, No. 297, v. 363.

Milliet (François-Simon). *De l'épistaxis. 24 pp. 4°. *Paris*, 1818, No. 7., v. 135.

Milliet (Joannis). Établissement médico-pneumatique de bains d'air. 22 pp. 8°. *Lyon, L. Perrin*, 1852, v. 460.

——. De l'air comprimé au point de vue physiologique. 40 pp. 8°. *Lyon, A. Vingtrinier*, 1856.

Milliez (Paul-Louis) [1858–]. *Contribution à l'étude du traitement de la syphilis par les injections sous-cutanées de peptône ammonique mercurique. 40 pp., 2 l. 4°. *Lille*, 1883, 2. s., No. 45.

Milligan (Gulielmus). *De cholera epidemica. 2 l., 3–20 pp. 8°. *Edinburgi, P. Neill*, 1822.

Millikin (Dan.) The extra-professional work of physicians. 20 pp. 8°. *Cincinnati*, 1884.

Millin de la Courveault (Joannes Nicolaus). *An conficiendæ bili a mesenterio oleum, a fæcibus liquor alkalinus? Præses: Honoratus Petiot. 8 pp. 4°. [*Parisiis, typ. vid. Quillau*, 1752.]

——. *Estne totus homo a natura morbus? Præses: Simon Antonius Bringaud. 8 pp. 4°. [*Parisiis, typ. vid. Quillau*, 1753.]

——. *An calvæ vehementius contusæ terebra? Præses: Claudius Josephus Gentil. 4 pp. 4°. [*Parisiis, typ. vid. Quillau*, 1754.]

See, also, **Nollan** (Joh. Jacobus.) *An impeditis lacrimarum viis parari debeat lacrimis artificiale iter, [etc.] 4°. [*Paris*, 1770.]

——— & **Morisot des Landes** (Petr. Jos.) Ergo Parisinis variolarum inoculatio. *Parisiis*, 1757.

In: HALLER. Disp. ad morb. [etc.] 4°. *Lausannæ*, 1758, v, 695–712.

Millingen (Edwin). *Ueber Insufficienz der Musculi recti interni und musculäre Asthenopie. 20 pp. 8°. *Würzburg, C. J. Becker*, 1871.

——. *Streitsätze. 4 l. 8°. *Würzburg, C. J. Becker*, 1871.

——. A tri-annual report of 5,703 cases of eye diseases seen and treated in private practice at Constantinople, in 1877, 1878, and 1879, and also a tabular analysis of 1,118 cases treated at the Imperial Naval Hospital. 6 p. l., 32 pp., 2 pl., 1 tab. 8°. *Constantinople*, [1881].

——. Augenheilanstalt in Constantinople. Bericht über die Jahre 1880 und 1881 (1. and 2.). 20 pp., 2 pl. 8°. *Salzburg, Zaunrith*, 1883.

Millingen (J. G.) The army medical officer's manual upon active service; or, precepts for his guidance in the various situations in which he may be placed. With observations on the preservation of the health of armies upon foreign service. x pp., 1 l., 267 pp., 1 pl. 8°. *London, Burgess & Hill*, 1819.

——. Observations sur la nature et le traitement du choléra morbus d'Europe et d'Asie. x, 54 pp. 8°. *Paris, Baillière*, 1831. [*Also, in :* P., v. 1042 ; 1262.]

——. Curiosities of medical experience. 2 v. 407, 411 pp. 8°. *London, R. Bentley*, 1837.

——. The same. 372 pp. 8°. *Philadelphia, Haswell, Barrington & Haswell*, 1838.

——. Aphorisms on the treatment and management of the insane; with considerations on public and private lunatic asylums, pointing out the errors in the present system. xii pp., 1 l., 202 pp. 24°. *London, J. Churchill*, 1840.

——. The same. 91 pp. 8°. *Philadelphia, Barrington & Haswell*, 1842. [*Also, in :* P., v. 199.]

——. Mind and matter, illustrated by considerations on hereditary insanity, and the influence of temperament in the development of the passions. vii, 464 pp. 8°. *London, H. Hurst*, 1847.

——. Recollections of republican France, from 1790 to 1801. 1 p. l., xvi, 378 pp. 8°. *London, H. Colburn*, 1848.

Millingen (James). Some observations on an antique bas-relief, on which the evil eye, or fasci-

Millingen (James)—continued. num, is represented. With further observations by S. Weston. 8 pp. 4°. *London*, 1818.
Royal Society of Antiquaries.

Millington (James). "Fining down" on natural principles without Banting. 54 pp. oblong 24°. *London, Field & Tuer*, [1884].

——. Are we to read sdrawkcab [backwards] or, what is the best print for the eyes? With an introduction by R. Brudenell Carter, F. R. C. S. xviii, 19–94 pp., 8 pl. 18°. *London, Field & Tuer*, [*n. d.*]

Millington (Thomas).
See **Cyprian** (Abraham). Epistola historiam, etc. 16°. *Lugd. Bat.*, 1700.

Million (Alexandre). *Sur l'accouchement laborieux terminé par le secours de la main. 43 pp. 4°. *Paris*, 1848, No. 53, v. 474.

Million (Prosper-Alexandre-Gabriel). *Sur les causes et le traitement de la phthisie pulmonaire. 82 pp. 4°. *Paris*, 1846, No. 207, v. 448.

Milliot (Benjamin). *Opite vozrojdenija normalnago chrustalika. [Experiments on regeneration of the lens.] 50 pp., 1 pl. 8°. *St. Petersburg*, 1868.

——. *De la régénération du crystallin chez quelques mammitères. 70 pp., 6 pl. 4°. *Paris*, 1871.

Milliot (Henri) [1860–]. *Recherches cliniques sur les rapports de la glycosurie et du paludisme. 48 pp. 4°. *Paris*, 1883, No. 283.

Milliot (Jean-Pierre). *Quelques considérations sur les abcès de la poitrine, leurs causes, etc. 24 pp. 4°. *Paris*, 1840, No. 363, v. 363.

Milliot (L.-Gustave). *Complications des tumeurs fibreuses de l'utérus. 68 pp. 4°. *Paris*, 1875, No. 28.

Milliot (Xavier). *Des fièvres pernicieuses. 25 pp. 4°. *Strasbourg*, 1851, No. 222, 2. s., v. 17.

Millioz (Humbert). *Sur le scorbut qui a régné à Alexandrie en Égypte, pendant le blocus de cette place, en l'an IX. 37 pp. 8°. *Paris, an XI* [1803], v. 22.

Milli (Guilio). Naturæ morbos decernentis arcanum opus, nova collustratum lucerna, ac duobus libris comprehensum. Quorum alter continet ea, quæ universim ad crises faciunt: alter Coacas Hippocratis et sigillatim morborum omnium enarrat eventa. 17 p. l., 610 pp. 4°. *Venetiis, typ. Ginammeis*, 1554.

Millon (Eugène) [1812–67]. *Du rapport philosophique des facultés de l'homme d'après le système phrénologique, et de quelques objections à ce système. 30 pp. 4°. *Paris*, 1836, No. 278, v. 302.

——. Éléments de chimie organique, comprenant les applications de cette science à la physiologie animale. v. 1 & 2. 636, 771 pp. 8°. *Paris, J.-B. Baillière*, 1845–8.

See, also, **Laveran & Millon** (Eugène). Mémoire sur le passage de quelques médicamens dans l'économie animale [etc.]. 8°. [*n. p., n. d.*]
For Biography, see Rec. de mém. de méd. . . . mil., Par., 1868, 3. s., xxi, 433–456 (Langlois).

Milloradovics (Petrus Gabrielow). De innocenti infectione venerea. 24 pp. 4°. *Halæ Magdeb., J. C. Hendel*, [1768].

——. *De surditate ex retropulsa crusta lactea orta. 16 pp. 4°. *Halæ Magdeb., J. C. Hendel*, [1769].

Millot (Auguste-Gabriel). *Du traitement des kystes de l'ovaire par le drainage. 43 pp. 4°. *Paris*, 1873, No. 66.

——. De l'hygiène publique et de la chirurgie en Italie. Compte-rendu à M. le ministre de l'instruction publique. 1. pt.: De l'hygiène publique en Italie. 1 p. l., iv, 182 pp. 8°. *Paris, J.-B. Baillière & fils*, 1876.

Millot (Auguste-Gabriel)—continued.

——. The same. 2. pt. : De la chirurgie en Italie. iii, 452 pp. 8°. *Paris, J.-B. Baillière & fils*, 1879.

——. De l'obstétrique en Italie. iv, 5–502 pp. 8°. *Paris, O. Doin*, 1882.

Millot (D.-B.-J.-L.) * Histoire pharmacologique du camphre. 1 p. l., 120 pp. 4°. *Strasbourg*, 1837, v. 70.

Millot (Gustave-Émile). * De quelques complications de la scarlatine observées dans une épidémie à l'Hôpital Saint-Éloi (service des militaires), dans le cours de l'année 1879–80. 64 pp., 2 l. 4°. *Montpellier*, 1880, No. 22.

Millot (J.) * Sur l'angine de poitrine. 29 pp. 4°. *Paris*, 1812, No. 90, v. 89.

Millot (J.-L.) * Du rhumatisme articulaire dans les affections des organes génitaux. 56 pp. 4°. *Paris*, 1873, No. 173.

Millot (Jacques-André) [1728–1811]. L'art de procréer les sexes à volonté, ou système complet de génération. 2. éd. xvi, 412 pp., 2 l., 2 pl. 8°. *Paris, Millot, an IX* [1801].

——. The same. 2. éd. xvi, 387 pp., 4 pl. 8°. *Paris, Millot, an IX* [1801].

Contains, in addition: Suppléments, pp. 385–412.

——. La gérocomie, ou code physiologique et phil·osophique, pour conduire les individus des deux sexes à une longue vie, en les dérobant à la douleur et aux infirmités ; par une société de médecins. 494 pp., port. 8°. *Paris, F. Buisson*, 1807.

——. Médecine perfective, ou code des bonnes mères. 2 v. vi, 602 pp. ; 622 pp. 8°. *Paris, L. Collin*, 1809.

——. Supplément à tous les traités, tant étrangers que nationaux, anciens et modernes, sur l'art des accouchements. 2. éd. 2 v. x, 11–506 pp., 2 pl. ; 1 l., 496 pp., 1 pl. 8°. *Paris, L. Collin*, 1809.

See, also, **Guilhermond.** Lettre au citoyen . . . sur son système de la génération. 8°. *Paris*, [1802].

For Portrait, see **Collection**—van Kaathoven.

Millot (Jules-Charles). * De la nature et des divers traitements de la fièvre typhoïde ou dothiénentérie. 34 pp. 4°. *Paris*, 1858, No. 65, v. 621.

Millot (Pierre-Raphael-Auguste). * De la constitution et des localités, sous le point de vue médical. 58 pp. 4°. *Paris*, 1849, No. 71, v. 487.

Millot-Carpentier (G.) Notes chirurgicales d'un médecin de campagne pour aider à la statistique (années 1876, 1877, 1878, 1879). 110 pp. fol. *Cambrai, J. Renaut*, 1880.

Millotianu (Michaelle). * Quelques considérations sur le pronostic des fractures par armes à feu étudié comparativement chez l'homme et chez la femme. 76 pp. 4°. *Paris*, 1871, No. 167.

Mills.

See **Flax** (*Manufacture, etc., of*).

Mills (Charles K.) [1845–]. Reflections on criminal lunacy, with remarks on the case of Guiteau. 26 pp. 8°. *Philadelphia*, 1882.

Repr. from : Tr. M. Soc. Penn., Phila., 1882, xiv.

——. Mental over-work and premature disease among public and professional men. iv, 34 pp. 8°. *Washington, Smithsonian Institution*, 1885.

Being No. 954, Smithson. Misc. Collect., and No. 9 of the "Toner Lectures".

——. Benjamin Rush and American psychiatry. 36 pp., port. 8°. [*New York*, 1886.]

Repr. from : Med.-Leg. J., N. Y., 1886–7, iv.

——. Practical lessons in nursing. The nursing and care of the nervous and the insane. 147 pp. 12°. *Philadelphia, J. B. Lippincott & Co.*, 1887.

See, also, **Kerlin** (Isaac N.) & **Mills** (Ch. K.) Three cases of progressive muscular degeneration. 8°. *Philadelphia*, 1880.

Mills (Daniel). * De ictero. 2 p. l., 31 pp. 8°. *Edinburgi, G. Creech*, 1793.

Mills (Edmund J.) On statistical and dynamical ideas in chemistry. (The atomic theory.) Pt. III. 18 pp. 8°. [*n. p.*, 1871.]

Repr. from : Lond., Edinb. & Dubl. Phil. Mag., Lond., 1871, 4. s., xlii.

Mills (George A.) How to keep teeth clean and healthful. 7 pp. 8°. [*Philadelphia*, 1879.]

Repr. from : Dental Cosmos, Phila., 1879, xxi : 1880, xxii.

——. Specialties and their advantages. 14 pp. 8°. *New York, Jenkins & Thomas*, [1882].

——. Pericementitis ; its manifestations in the oral cavity, and its serious effects upon the general health. 8 pp. 8°. *New York, Jenkins & Thomas*, [1882].

——. Riggs' disease (pericementitis, pyorrhea, alveolaris, diseased gums, loose teeth, etc.). 8 pp. 8°. *New York, Jenkins & McCowan*, [1885].

——. Dental specialists· of medicine and surgery, in the care and treatment of the disorders of the teeth and mouth. 10 pp. 8°. *St. Louis, J. H. Chambers & Co.*, 1886.

Repr. from : Arch. Dent., St. Louis, 1886, iii.

Mills (James). The horse-keeper's guide. 1. Am. ed. 86 pp., 1 pl. 16°. *New York, J. Mowatt & Co.*, 1834.

——. Horses ; the gentleman's guide· for the choice, treatment, and management of saddle, carriage, gig, and cart horses. 9. ed. 144 pp. 8°. *London, Dean & Son*, [1834, vel subseq.].

Mills (Lucius). Compendium of hygiene ; compiled for the use of the Winsted Hygiene Association. 190 pp. 8°. *West Winsted, Conn.*, 1855.

Mills (Rebecca). The influence of well-made stays on the health and beauty of woman, and the great injuries which ill-made ones inflict. vi, 88 pp., 10 pl. 8°. *London, Stewart & Murray*, 1841.

Mills (T. Wesley). Ueber die Ausscheidung der Oxalsäure durch den Harn. 9 pp. 8°. [*Berlin*, 1885.]

Repr. from : Arch. f. path. Anat., etc., Berl., 1885.

——. Outlines of lectures on physiology, with an introductory chapter on general biology, and an appendix containing laboratory exercises in practical physiology. 200 pp. 8°. *Montreal, W. Drysdale & Co.*, 1886.

See, also, **Hoppe-Seyler** (Felix). On the development of physiological chemistry, [etc.] 8°. [*New York*, 1884.]

Mills (Thomas). * De sonis et auditu complectens. 50 pp. 8°. *Edinburgi, R. Allan*, 1797. [P., v. 5.]

——. An essay on the utility of blood-letting in fever, illustrated by numerous cases ; with some inquiry into the seat and nature of this disorder. viii, 222 pp., 4 tab. 8°. *Dublin, Gilbert & Hodges*, 1813.

——. The same. 2. ed. With a supplement, containing cases and dissections which occurred in private practice. viii (1 l.), 327 pp., 4 tab. 8°. *Dublin, J. Cumming* [*and others*], 1816.

——. The morbid anatomy of the brain in typhous or brain-fever ; to which are added, cases of the present epidemic, with a few remarks on its nature and mode of treatment. 2. ed. 67 pp. 12°. *Dublin, Hodges & M'Arthur*, 1818. [P., v. 835.]

——. The same. Pathologische Anatomie des Gehirns bey'm Typhus, oder Gehirnfieber, mit beygefügten während der jetzigen Epidemie gesammelten Beobachtungen, und einigen Bemerkungen über die Natur und Behandlung desselben. Nach der zweyten englischen Ausgabe übersetzt von G. von dem Busch. ix, 79 pp., 1 l. 8°. *Bremen u. Leipzig, W. Kaiser*, 1820.

——. An account of the morbid appearances exhibited on dissection in various disorders of

Mills (Thomas)—continued.
the brain; with pathological observations, to which a comparison of the symptoms, with the morbid changes, has given rise. xvi, 239 pp. 8°. *Dublin, J. Cumming*, 1826.

——. The same. vii, 303 pp. 8°. *Dublin, J. Cumming* [*and others*], 1829.

Mill-stone *makers.*

    Peacock (T. B.) On French mill-stone makers' phthisis. Brit. & For. M.-Chir. Rev., Lond., 1860, xxv, 214-224. *Also*, Reprint. *Also* [Abstr.]: Med. Times & Gaz., Lond., 1860, ii, 263. *Also :* Tr. Path. Soc. Lond., 1860-61, xii, 36-40. ———. French mill-stone makers' phthisis. Brit. M. J., 1876, ii, 486-48². ———. Mill-stone makers' disease; siliceous matter found in the lung. Tr. Path. Soc. Lond., 1878, xxix, 31-34, 1 pl.

de Milly (Louis-Adolphe). * Sur les affections gastriques et leurs causes. 16 pp. 4°. *Paris*, 1828, No. 204, v. 219.

Milman (Francis). Animadversiones de natura hydropis ejusque curatione. xi, 172 pp. 8°. *Viennæ et Londini, R. Graeffer*, 1779.

——. The same. Animadversions on the nature and on the cure of the dropsy. Transl. from the Latin into English by F. Swediaur. 122 pp., 1 l. 8°. *London, J. Walter*, 1786.

    Bound with : WILKES (Richard). An historical essay on the dropsy. 8°. *London*, 1781.

——. An enquiry into the source from whence the symptoms of the scurvy and of putrid fevers arise, and into the seat which those affections occupy in the animal œconomy; with a view of ascertaining a more just idea of putrid diseases than has generally been formed of them. xx, 231 pp. 8°. *London, J. Dodsley*, 1782.

——. The same. Recherches sur l'origine et le siège du scorbut et des fièvres putrides; ouvrage trad. de l'anglois par M. Vigarous de Montagut. xxxii, 192 pp., 2 l. 8°. *Paris & Montpellier, P.-F. Didot jeune*, 1786.

    See, also, **Letter** (A) to Francis Milman, etc. 8°. *London*, 1813.—**Trotter** (Thomas). Observations on the scurvy [etc.] 8°. *Edinburgh*, 1786. ———. The same. 12°. *Philadelphia*, 1793.

Miln (Robertus). * De apoplexia sanguinea. xxix pp. 8°. *Edinburgi, G. Creech*, 1814.

Milne.
    See **Richard** (Louis Claude). A botanical dictionary [etc.] 12°. *New Haven*, 1817.

Milne (Alexander). Manual of materia medica and therapeutics, embracing all the medicines of the British Pharmacopœia, etc. 2. ed. 4 p. l., 256 pp. 12°. *Edinburgh, E. & S. Livingstone*, 1869.

——. The same. By William Craig. 4. ed. viii, 441 pp. 12°. *Edinburgh, E. & S. Livingstone*, 1879.

——. The principles and practice of midwifery, with some of the diseases of women. xxvii, 639 pp. 8°. *Edinburgh, E. & S. Livingstone*, 1871.

——. The same. 2. ed. 371 pp. 12°. *New York & London, Bermingham & Co.*, 1884.

——. How to nurse a child, or the management of children, and their diseases. xvi, 230 pp. 12°. *Edinburgh, E. & S. Livingstone*, 1880.

Milne (David). Observations on the probable cause of the failure of the potato crop, in the years 1845 and 1846. 53 pp., 1 pl. 8°. *Edinburgh & London, W. Blackwood & Sons*, 1847. [P., v. 1030.]

Milne (John). On construction in earthquake countries. With an abstract of the discussion upon the paper. Edited by James Forrest. 45 pp. 8°. *London*, 1885.
    Repr. from: Inst. Civ. Eng. Abstr. papers in for. trans. & period., Lond., 1885-6, lxxxiii, pt. 1.

Milne (Joshua).
    See **Lonsdale** (H.) The life of John Heysham, and his correspondence with Mr. Joshua Milne relative to the Carlisle bills of mortality. roy. 8°. *London*. 1870.

Milne (William). On some new infusoria. Read to the Glasgow Philosophical Society, 31st January, 1883. 5 pp., 1 pl. 8°. [*Glasgow*], 1883.

Milne-Edwards. *See* **Edwards**.

Milner (Ebenezer). On catalepsy, or trance. 20 pp. 8°. *Edinburgh, R. Inches*, 1850. [*Also, in :* P., v. 41; 446; 895; 919.]
    Repr. from: Edinb. M. & S. J., 1850, lxxiv.

Milner (Josephus D.) * De rheumatismo. 16 pp. 8°. *Edinburgi*, 1828.

Milner (Karl). * Ueber Krebs der Gekrösdrüsen. iv, 5-24 pp. 8°. *Tübingen, L. F. Fues*, 1856.

Milner (U. R.) Yellow fever not imported, nor contagious, but indigenous, and intrinsically identical with our paludal fevers. Preventable by well determined and wisely executed local sanitary measures. Quarantine a wide-spread calamity, and should not longer be tolerated. A lecture. 39 pp. 12°. *New Orleans, M. J. Scott*, 1880.

Milnes (Alfred).
    See **Is** vaccination desirable? 8°. *London*, 1885.

Milnor (*William H.*)
    Portrait in : **Collection** of Portr. (Libr.)

"**Milo**" [*pseudon.*]. Error of position; being a discussion of the ultra medical policy of the American Medical Association, as advocated by medical professors, Medicus and others; showing the policy to be adverse to the great interests and institutions of society, and the peace and prosperity of the nation. [In 4 numbers, No. 1.] 46 pp. 8°. *Nashville, W. F. Bang & Co.*, 1854.

——. "Catchings" for "catchings" to show what is caught; being a special undertaking in the way of "catchings", according to a proposition in the Nashville Medical Journal for May, 1855. 24 pp. 8°. *Nashville*, 1855.

Milon (Mathieu). * De l'action thérapeutique du chlorate de potasse. 34 pp. 4°. *Paris*, 1858, No. 267, v. 621.

Milon (Urbain-Eugène). * De la belladone et de son usage en thérapeutique. 32 pp. 4°. *Strasbourg*, 1859, No. 494, 2. s., v. 27.

Miloslavievitch (Étienne). * De l'endocardite rhumatismale. 44 pp. 4°. *Paris*, 1855, No. 26, v. 578.

Milroy (Gavin) [1805-86]. Quarantine and the plague; being a summary of the report on these subjects recently addressed to the Royal Academy of Medicine in France; with introductory observations, extracts from parliamentary correspondence and notes. 71 pp. 8°. *London, S. Highley*, 1846.

——. The cholera not to be arrested by quarantine; a brief historical sketch of the great epidemic of 1817, and its invasions of Europe in 1831-2 and 1847; with practical remarks on the treatment, preventive and curative, of the disease. 51 pp. 8°. *London, J. Churchill*, 1847.

——. Cholera (Jamaica). Return to an address of the House of Commons, dated 20 Feb., 1854, for a "copy of the report of . . . to the colonial office, on the cholera epidemic in Jamaica, 1850-51; and copies or extracts of despatches addressed to and received from the governor of Jamaica in relation to the said report". 147 pp., 3 maps. fol. [*London*, 1854.]

——. On the sickness and mortality in the French army during the campaign in Turkey and the Crimea in 1854-6. 23 pp. 8°. [*n. p.*, 1857, *vel subseq.*] [P., v. 324.]

——. Quarantine as it is and as it ought to be. Read before the public health section of the National Association of Social Science, 1858. 12 pp. 8°. *London, Savill & Edwards*, 1859.

——. Report on leprosy and yaws in the West Indies. Addressed to her majesty's secretary of state for the colonies. In continuation of paper

Milroy (Gavin)—continued.

presented to both houses of Parliament, May, 1871. 1 p. l., 104 pp. fol. *London, W. Clowes & Sons,* 1873.

For Biography, see Brit. M. J., Lond., 1886, i, 425. *Also:* Lancet, Lond., 1886, i, 425. *Also:* Tr. Epidemiol. Soc. Lond. (1885-6), 1887, n. s., v, 169.

Milschewsky (Guilielmus). * De gangræna nosocomiali. 42 pp. 8°. *Gryphiæ, F. G. Kunike,* [1850].

Milsonneau (Élie). * Contribution à l'étude de l'angine infectieuse simple primitive; manifestations ganglionnaires, adéno-phlegmon. 39 pp. 4°. *Paris, A. Parent,* 1885, No. 202.

Miltenberg.

See **Cholera** (*Asiatic, History, etc., of*), *by localities.*

Miltenberger (George W.) Oration before the Medical and Surgical Society of Baltimore, at their anniversary meeting, January 21, 1856. 17 pp. 8°. *Baltimore, J. W. Woods,* 1856.

——. Puerperal eclampsia. 29 pp. 8°. [*Baltimore, Guggenheimer, Weil & Co.,* 1886.]
Repr. from: Tr. M. & Chir. Fac. Maryland, Balt., 1886.

Miltenberger (Joseph-Théodore). * Du diagnostic différentiel des tumeurs développées dans l'hypochondre droit. 38 pp. 4°. *Paris,* 1850, No. 54, v. 499.

Miltner (Karl). * Statistisches und Experimentelles zur Pathogenese der Bauchfellentzündung. 34 pp. 8°. *Erlangen, E. T. Jacob,* 1887.

Milton (*District of*).

BUCHANAN (G.) Report on the sanitary state of Milton district, including the towns of Sittingbourne and Milton-next-Sittingbourne, July and August, 1870. fol. [*London,* 1870.]

Milton, *Indiana.*

See, also, **Fever** (*Malarial, History, etc., of*), *by localities.*

KERSEY (V.) Epidemics of Milton, Wayne County, Indiana. West. Lancet, Cincin., 1852, xiii, 672-676.

Milton, *Massachusetts.*

MILTON. A collection of papers relative to the transaction of the town of Milton, in the State of Massachusetts, to promote a general inoculation of the cow pox, or kine pock, as a never-failing preventive against small-pox infection. 48 pp. 8°. *Boston, J. Belcher,* 1809.

Milton (John Laws) [1820–]. On bubo and perinæal abscess. 32 pp. 8°. [*London, W. Tyler*], 1851. [P., v. 1188.]

——. On a new way of treating gonorrhœa. 3 p. l., 103 pp. 8°. *London, J. Churchill,* 1852.

——. Practical remarks on the treatment of spermatorrhœa and some forms of impotence. 2. ed. 30 pp. 8°. *London, S. Highley,* 1855.
Repr. from: Lancet, Lond., 1854, i.

——. The same. 3. ed. 30 pp., 1 l. 8°. *London, S. Highley,* 1855.

——. The same. 4. ed. 47 pp. 8°. *London, G. Philip,* 1856. [P., v. 1188.]

——. On the treatment of gonorrhœa without specifics. 2. ed. ix, 131 pp., 1 l. 8°. *London, J. W. Davies,* 1862.

——. The stream of life on our globe; its archives, traditions, and laws as revealed by modern discoveries in geology and palæontology. A sketch, in untechnical language, of the beginning and growth of life, and the physiological laws which govern its progress and operations. 2. ed. xxiv, 620 pp. 8°. *London, R. Hardwicke,* [1862, vel subseq.].

——. On the modern treatment of some diseases of the skin. vii, 117 pp. 8°. *London, R. Hardwicke,* 1865.

Milton (John Laws)—continued.

——. On the treatment of lupus. 27 pp. 8°. *London, R. Hardwicke,* 1866.

——. On the pathology and treatment of gonorrhœa. viii, 219 pp. 8°. *London, R. Hardwicke,* 1871.

——. The same. 5. ed. viii, 306 pp. 8°. *New York, W. Wood & Co.,* 1884.

——. The pathology and treatment of diseases of the skin. v, 358 pp., 4 pl. 8°. *London, R. Hardwicke,* 1872.

——. On the treatment of secondary syphilis. 16 pp. 8°. *Edinburgh, Oliver & Boyd,* 1875.
Repr. from: Edinb. M. J., 1875, xx.

——. The bath in diseases of the skin. x, 84 pp. 8°. *London, Chatto & Windus,* [1879, vel subseq.].

——. A history of syphilis. 2. ed. 84 pp. 8°. *London, Harrison & Sons,* 1880.

——. The laws of life, and their relation to the diseases of the skin. 154 pp. 12°. *London, Chatto & Windus,* 1882.

——. The hygiene of the skin. 2. ed. 104 pp. 8°. *London, Chatto & Windus,* 1883.

——. On dermatitis ferox. 8 pp. 8°. *Edinburgh, Oliver & Boyd,* 1886.
Repr. from: Edinb. M. J., 1886, xxxi.

——. The unity or duality of syphilis, historically considered. 12 pp. 8°. *Edinburgh, Oliver & Boyd,* 1886.

——. On the pathology and treatment of gonorrhœa and spermatorrhœa. x, 474 pp. 8°. *New York, W. Wood & Co.,* 1887.

——. The ligaments of the human body. 26 pp., 30 pl. 8°. *London, E. Lumley,* [n. d.]

Miltz (Arnoldus Petrus). * De febre et efflorescentia miliari. Von den sogenannten Friessel. 3 p. l., 30 pp., 8 l. sm. 4°. *Wirceburgi, J. J. C. Kleyer,* [1737].
See, also, **Orth** (Jo. M. A.) & **Miltz** (Arnoldus Petrus). Artium liberalium [etc.] 4°. *Wirceburgi,* 1737.

Milunovits (Alexander). * De rachitide. 3 p. l., 63 pp. 12°. *Viennæ, M. A. Schmidt,* 1816.

Milward (Eduardus).
See **Drake** (James). Orationes tres: de febre intermittente [etc.] 4°. *London,* 1742.

Milwaukee. *Health Department.* Annual reports to the mayor and common council of the city. 3.–7. (1869-70 to 1873); 9.–13. (1875-9). 8°. *Milwaukee,* 1870-80.

Seventh report changed from fiscal to calendar year. In 1878 the health department was reorganized by act of the legislature, approved Feb. 23, 1878. The powers vested in the board of health and health officer were conferred upon the commissioner of health. The 1. report of the commissioner is the 12. of the department.

——. Circular No. 1. To physicians, concerning their reports of contagious or infectious disease. 1 sheet. 4°. [*Milwaukee,* 1878.]

——. Circular No. 2. To officers in charge of cemeteries, directing their attention to chap. iii of the ordinance concerning the burial of the dead. Dec. 2, 1878. 1 sheet. 8°. [*Milwaukee,* 1878.]

——. Circular No. 3. To clergymen, undertakers, and others, forbidding communication with houses infected with any contagious disease, and ordering a private funeral in case of death. Dec. 2, 1878. 1 sheet. 8°. [*Milwaukee,* 1878.]

——. Circular No. 4. To physicians, requiring them to make daily reports of contagious cases under treatment, and the specific cause of any death. Dec. 2, 1878. 1 sheet. 8°. [*Milwaukee,* 1878.]

——. Circular No. 5. To families afflicted with diphtheria; and rules for their guidance. 2 l. 8°. [*Milwaukee, n. d.*]

——. Circular No. 6. Circular vom Gesundheits-Commissär an die durch Diphtherie heim-

Milwaukee. *Health Department*—continued.
gesuchten Familien. 2 l. 8°. [*Milwaukee, n. d.*]

——. Circular No. 7. To families affected with scarlet fever; and regulations condensed from circular issued by the State board of health of Massachusetts. 3 pp. 8°. [*Milwaukee, n. d.*]

——. Circular No. 8. Cirkular des Gesundheits-Kommissärs an die Familien, in denen Scharlachfieber herrscht. 3 pp. 8°. [*Milwaukee, n. d.*]

——. Circular No. 9. Rules for the collectors of garbage, offal, and dead animals. Also, rules for the people from existing ordinances. 1 sheet. 8°. [*Milwaukee, n. d.*]

——. Circular No. 10. Regeln, die vom Contractor für das Einsammeln von Küchenabfällen, Murath und todtem Vieh befolgt werden müssen. 1 sheet. 8°. [*Milwaukee, n. d.*]

——. Circular No. 11. Rules for night scavengers. 1 l. 8°. [*Milwaukee, 1879.*]

——. Circular No. 12. Rules for the regulation of the public baths on Canal street. May 14, 1879. 1 sheet. 8°. [*Milwaukee, 1879.*]

——. [Blank forms used by the health department.] v. s. [*Milwaukee, 1878–80.*]
No. 1. Report of sick cases.
No. 2. Transcript of report of sick cases.
No. 3. Report of cases recovered.
No. 4. Certificate of death.
No. 5. Burial permit.
No. 6. Monthly report of undertaker to health officer.
No. 7. Report of garbage contractor.
No. 8. Report of vaccination of children.
No. 9. Application for scavenger work.
No. 10. Permit to clean vault.
No. 11. Form of complaint.
No. 12. Notice served by police on parties complained of.
No. 13. Certificate admitting pupils to school after recovery from infectious disease.
No. 14. Order for abatement of minor nuisances.
No. 15. Order for abatement of graver nuisances, to make sewer connections, etc.
No. 16. Report of nuisance property to common council.
No. 17. Contract to remove offal and garbage.
No. 18. Notice to clean a vault, and the ordinance concerning scavengers.

——. Deaths caused by the Newhall House fire, Jan. 10, 1883. R. Martin, health commissioner. 1 sheet. 12°. [*Milwaukee, 1883.*]

——. Notice placed on the outside door of a house where diphtheria exists, and remains till after recovery and disinfection by an expert from the health office. 1 sheet. fol. [*Milwaukee, n. d.*]
In English and German.

——. Notice placed on the outside door of a house where scarlet fever exists, and remains till after recovery and disinfection by an expert from the health office. 1 sheet. fol. [*Milwaukee, n. d.*]
In English and German.

——. Notice placed on the outside door of a house where small-pox exists, and remains till after recovery and disinfection by an expert from the health office. 1 sheet. fol. [*Milwaukee, n. d.*]
In English and German.

——. *Health Department. Bureau of Vital Statistics.* Condensed statements of mortality. [Monthly.] Jan. to Dec., 1880; March to Dec., 1881; June, 1882, to Feb., 1886; April, 1886, to Dec., 1887. 4°. [*Milwaukee, 1880–88.*]

——. Reports of deaths in Milwaukee. [Weekly.] Dec. 8, 1883, to May 3, 1884; May 24 to Aug. 16; Aug. 30; Sept. 5, 19 to Oct. 25; Nov. 8, 15, 19; Dec. 13 to Jan. 3, 1885. 18°. [*Milwaukee, 1883–5.*]

Milwaukee Academy of Medicine. The progress of the Milwaukee test. Report of the standing committee on the test. 6 pp. 8°. [*Milwaukee, Wis.,* 1879.]

Milwaukee Academy of Medicine—continued.

——. Final report on the Milwaukee test of the thirtieth dilution. 4 pp. 8°. [*Milwaukee, Wis.,* 1880.]

Milwaukee City Medical Association. Constitution, by-laws, and code of medical ethics, adopted Dec. 9, 1847. 23 pp. 8°. *Milwaukee,* 1848.

Milwaukee Eye and Ear Infirmary. Annual report of the board of surgeons for the year 1873. 19 pp. 8°. *Milwaukee,* 1874.
Appendix contains a lecture on otology, by C. E. Houghman. Opened 1870.

Milwaukee Industrial School. *See* **Wisconsin** Industrial School for Girls, Milwaukee.

Milwaukee Orphan Asylum. Annual reports of the managers to their friends and subscribers. 19.–21., 1867–8 to 1869–70; 23., 1871–2; 24., 1872–3; 31., 1879–80; 33.–36., 1882–5. 8°. *Milwaukee,* 1868–86.
Established Jan. 4, 1850.

Milwaukee *test.*
See **Homœopathy** (*Attenuations, etc., of*).

Milz (Joannes Sigismundus). *De debilitate vera et spuria. 17 pp. 4°. *Jenæ, typ. Goepferdtii,* [1791].
For Biography, see **Loder** (Just. Ch.)

Milzbrand.
See **Anthrax; Charbon; Pustule** (*Malignant*).

Mimard (Frédéric). *De la chlorose, vulgairement pâles couleurs. 24 pp. 4°. *Paris,* 1837, No. 384, v. 317.

Mimerel (L.-A.) *Sur l'apoplexie sanguine. 15 pp. 4°. *Paris,* 1825, No. 55, v. 191.

Mimicry.
See **Imitation; Physiognomy.**

Mimis (Constantinus) [1806–]. *De catalepsi, adjecta catalepseos simulatæ historia. 32 pp. 8°. *Lipsiæ,* 1834.

Mimosa *pudica.*
Bert (P.) Sur les mouvements de la sensitive (Mimosa pudica). Compt. rend. Soc. de biol. 1867, Par., 1868, 4. s., iv, 99: (1869), 1870, 5. s., i, 248.—**Sigwart** (G. C. C.) Bemerkungen über die Bewegungen der Mimosa pudica, in welchen sich ein deutlicher Unterschied des äusseren und innern Eindruck zeigt, aus dem Institute für Cultur der Naturlehre der Organismen. Arch. f. d. Physiol., Halle, 1815, xii, 13–36.

Minadous (Aurelius). Tractatus de virulenta venerea. In quo omnium aliorum hac de re sententiæ considerantur; mali natura explicatur; caussæ et differentiæ aliaque, cum dogmatica curatione proponuntur. 8 p. l., 284 pp. 4°. *Venetiis, apud R. Meiettum,* 1596.

Minadous (Joh. Baptista). Tractatus de abusu non mittendi sanguinis in febribus malignis, etiamnum apparentibus exanthematibus, dictis petechis. Cui, tanquam appendix, additur ejusdemmet authoris disputatio, an exulceratio inter renes et jecur inhæreat. 3 p. l., 24 ff., 1 l. sm. 4°. *Venetiis, apud hæredes, M. Sessæ,* 1573.
Bound with: VIDIUS (Vidus). De febribus libri vii. sm. 4°. *Patavii,* 1595.

——. The same. De ratione mittendi sanguinis in febribus malignis, etiamnum apparentibus exanthematibus sive peticulis, doctissima disputatio. Cui accessit resolutio quæstionis an inter renes et jecur nob. Rhodigini inhæserit ulcus. 2 p. l., 24 ff., 1 l. 4°. *Venetiis, J. B. et J. B. Sessa,* 1597.

Minadous (Joh. Thomas) [–1615]. De arthritide. 82 ff. sm. 4°. *Patavii, apud F. Bolzettam,* 1602.

Mina' Morici (Giovanni). Su d' una aneurisma dell' arco dell' aorta. Memoria letta all' Accademia Peloritana li 14 marzo 1836. 13 pp. 8°. *Napoli,* 1836.
Repr. from: Filiatre-sebezio, Napoli, 1836.

Minarie (Eugène). * De l'hémorrhagie cérébrale. 22 pp. 4°. *Paris*, 1853, No. 192, v. 545.

das Minas.

DE ALMEIDA (F. J.) Exposição fiel da molestia da excellentissima Marqueza das Minas,
com hum discurso sobre a utilidade dos fructos.
16°. *Lisboa*, 1787.

Minas (Franciscus Xav.) * Diss. sistens sciagraphiam morborum cordis. xii, 72 pp. 12°.
Viennæ, typ. Congregationis Mechitaristicæ, 1817.

Minati (Carlo) [1824–]. Ostetricia minore.
Lezioni. xiv, 400 pp. 8°. *Milano, Napoli, Pisa,
U. Hoepli*, 1881.

——. Lo speculum delle partorienti inventato
per uso clinico. 20 pp., 1 pl. 8°. *Milano, frat.
Rechiedei*, 1885.

    Repr. from: Ann. univ. di med. e chir., Milano, 1885,
cclxxi.

——. Lo speculum delle partorienti. 8 pp. 8°.
Milano, F. Vallardi, 1885.

    Repr. from: Gazz. d. osp., Milano, 1885, vi.
    Also, Co-Editor of: **Gazzetta** medica italiana federa-
tiva toscana, Firenze, 1850–54. *Also:* **Tempo** (Il); giornale italiano di medicina, [etc.], Firenze, 1858.

Minch (G. N.) Prokaza (Lepra arabum) na juge
Rossii. [Leprosy in southern Russia.] xii; 344
pp., 14 pl. 8°. *Kieff, Univ. tipog.*, 1884–6.

    Repr. from: Univ. Izviestija, Kieff, 1884, xxiv: 1885,
xxv: 1886, xxvi.

Minchin (Humphrey). Contributions to craniology. 1 p. l., 26 pp. 8°. *Dublin, Hodges, Smith
& Co.*, 1856. [P., v. 1492.]

    Repr. from: Dublin Q. J. M. Sc., 1856, xxii.

Mind.

    See **Brain** *and mind*; **Emotions**; **Psychology**;
Psychology (*Physiological*).

Mind (*Condition of, Inquiry into*).

    See, also, **Criminals** (*Mental condition, etc., of*);
Criminals (*Mental condition, etc., of*)—*Special
cases*; **Dementia** (*Jurisprudence of*); **Epilepsy**
(*Jurisprudence of*); **Hallucinations**; **Insanity**
(*Diagnosis, etc., of*); **Insanity** (*Feigned*); **Insan-
ity** (*Homicidal*); **Insanity** (*Jurisprudence of,
Cases of*); **Kleptomania**; **Pyromania**; **Re-
sponsibility**; **Sexual** *instinct* (*Perversion of*);
Wills (*Jurisprudence of*).

BELL (C.) Speech of . . . to the jury, in the
. . . inquiry as to the sanity or insanity of Geo.
Francis Train. 8°. *New York*, 1873.

BIFFI (S.) Lettera al dottore A. Verga. [In-
vestigazione dello stato mentale di Giuseppe
Curti, che il 16 passato marzo uccideva la sposa
e il suocero.] 8°. *Milano*, 1858.

BURROWS (G. M.) A letter to Sir Henry Halford . . . touching some points of the evidence,
and observations of counsel, on a commission of
lunacy on Mr. Edward Davies. 8°. *London*,
1830.

CASES (The) of Gouldstone and Cole, and the
legal procedure in ascertaining the mental condition of prisoners. Ed. by D. H. Tuke and G.
H. Savage. 8°. *Lewes*, 1884.

    Repr. from: J. Ment. Sc., Lond., 1883–4, xxix.
    See, also, Savage and Tuke, *infra.*

DENNY (Lydia B.) Statement of . . . wife of
Reuben S. Denny, of Boston, in regard to her
alleged insanity. 12°. [*Boston*, 1862?]

[——. Letters and explanations relating to
and growing out of her proceedings to obtain a
divorce from her husband.] 8°. [*Boston*, 1864.]

GOUPIL (J.-M.-A.) Consultation médico-légale
pour le sergent-major P.-M.-H. Mendic, accusé
du crime de voies-de-fait envers ses supérieurs.
4°. [*Strasbourg*, 1825.]

GUALANDI (G.), BRUNELLI (C.) & SOLIVETTI
(A.) Il parere medico e i suoi 103 errori. roy.
8°. *Roma*, 1886.

Mind (*Condition of, Inquiry into*).

INQUIRY (An) into the state of mind of W. F.
Windham, esq., of Fellbrigg Hall, Norfolk, before
Samuel Warren, esq., Q. C., and a special jury,
upon the petition of General Windham, C. B.,
etc., the uncle of the alleged lunatic, and other
members of the family, at her majesty's court of
exchequer, Westminster, commencing Dec. 16,
1861. Illust. and unabridged ed. 8°. *London*,
1862.

JESSEN (W.) Ueber Zurechnungsfähigkeit.
Denkschrift zum Entwurfe eines Strafgesetzbuches für den Norddeutschen Bund. Abschnitt
iv, § 46 und 47. 8°. *Kiel*, 1870.

MOREL (B.-A.) Consultation médico-légale
sur l'état mental de Jeanson, accusé d'incendie
et de meurtre. Suivie du rapport présenté sur
ce travail à la Société de médecine légale par le
docteur J. Falret. 8°. *Paris*, 1869.

SOMBRE (D.) Refutation of the charge of
lunacy brought against him in the court of
chancery. 8°. *Paris*, 1849.

TAMASSIA (A.) Gli ultimi studi italiani sulla
imputabilità. Critica seconda. 8°. [*Roma*,
1877.]

TRIAL (The) and respite of George Victor
Townley, for wilful murder. With original doc-
uments and correspondence now first published;
Dr. [Forbes] Winslow's analysis of the convict's
mind, portraits, autographs, and plan. 12°.
Derby, [1864?]

    Alfaro (M.) & **Romero** (A.) Informe pericial sobre
el estado intelectual de la procesada Juana B. de P. Independ. méd., México, 1880, i, 153–155.—**Alvarado** (M.),
Carmona y Valle (M.) & **Rodriguez** (J. M.) Informe
pericial . . . acerca del estado mental del Sr. D. Agustin
Schulze . . . Observador méd., México, 1879–80, v, 55–
61.—**van Andel** (A. H.) & **Groskamp** (H. A.) Gerech-
telijkzielkundige verslag betreffende den van poging tot
moord verdachten J. M. Psychiat. Bl., Dordrecht, 1883, i,
161–173.—**Andreae** (A.) Zwei Gutachten über zweifelhafte Seelenzustände, nebst Bemerkungen. Mag. f. d. ges.
Heilk., Berl., 1837, xlix, 95; 179; 351.—**Arigo** (S.) &
Givogre (G. B.) Sulle condizioni psichiche di Giuseppe
Dossena, imputato di assassinio; studj, perizia e giudizio
medico-legale. *In:* Arigo (S.) Alcuni scrit. di med. e chir.,
8°, Lodi, 1885, 109–190.—**Arndt** (R.) Krankheit oder
Schamlosigkeit? Vrtljschr. f. gerichtl. u. öff. Med., Berl.,
1872, xvii, 49–70.—————. Freie Willensbestimmung oder
nicht? *Ibid.*, 232–247.—————. Blödsinnig oder wahnsinnig?
Gerichtsärztliches Gutachten. *Ibid.*, 1876, n. F., xxv, 52–
83.—**Aubanel.** Observations médico-légales sur l'état
mental d'un officier de l'armée d'Italie. Ann. méd.-psych.,
Par., 1851, iii, 443–465.—**von Autenrieth** (J. H. F.) &
Autenrieth (H. F.) Unzurechnungsfähigkeit aussspre-
chende Gutachten. In Betreff von Vermögensverwaltung.
In their: Gerichtl.-med. Aufs. u. Gutacht., 8°, Tübing.,
1846, 48–54.—————. Gutachten, welche unter grad-
weiser Annäherung bald zum einen, bald zum andern Zustand weder gänzliche Unzurechnungsfähigkeit, noch
volle Zurechnungsfähigkeit bestimmen. *Ibid.*, 118–252.—
Babé (J. M.) Informe sobre el estado mental de D.
B . . . C . . . Trab. Com. de med. leg. é hig. púb. de la r.
Acad. de cien. méd. . . . de la Habana, 1873, ii, 254–271.—
Bartsch. Gerichtsärztliches Erachten über den Gemüthszustand der Inquisitin Maria M. aus Rostock.
Ztschr. f. d. Staatsarznk., Erlang., 1845, xlix, 183–204.—
Baumes, Vigaroux & **Delpech.** Cas de médecine
légale, porté devant le tribunal de Strasbourg. Ann. clin.,
Montpel., 1815, xxxviii, 312–337.—**Begutachtungen**
über zweifelhafte psychische Zustände. Ztschr. f. d. Staatsarznk., Erlang., 1830, x, 95; 295.—**Béhier.** Rapport sur
une demande en annulation d'un acte de vente, fondée sur
l'état de santé de la venderesse pendant la passation de
son contrat. Soc. de méd. lég. de Par. Bull., 1871, ii, 32–
48.—**Behr.** Ober-Gutachten über den Geisteszustand
des wegen Majestäts-Beleidigung inhaftirten Arbeitsman-
nes Carl Eisfeld in Harzgerode. Allg. Ztschr. f. Psychiat., etc., Berl., 1861, xviii, 377–406.—**Benasach** (G.)
Informe sobre el estado mental de D. A . . . E . . . Trab.
Com. de med. leg. é hig. púb. de la r. Acad. de cien. méd.
. . . de la Habana, 1874, ii, 271–274.—**Bernay.** Ist die M.
P. als eine willenlose Person zu bezeichnen? Gutachten.
Vrtljschr. f. gerichtl. u. öff. Med., Berl., 1869, xi, 349–354.—
Bianchi (L.) Processo Conte. Arch. di psichiat., etc.,
Torino, 1887, viii, 65–80.—**Biermann.** Wie müssen,
vom ärztlichen Standpunkte aus, Fragen über psycholo-
gische Zurechnungsfähigkeit oder Zurechnungsunfä-
higkeit erörtert und entschieden werden? Ztschr. f. d.
Staatsarznk., Erlang., 1839, xxxviii, 1–24.—————. Gerichts-

Mind (*Condition of, Inquiry into*).

ärztliches Gutachten über einen in einen Zustand von Wahnsinn gerathenen Menschen, Behufs Anordnung polizeilicher Maassregeln. *Ibid.*, 1840, xxxix, 318–325. ——. Gutachten über einen anomalen Gemuthszustand, der zu einer officiellen gerichtsärztlichen Untersuchung Anlass gab. Hannov. Ann. f. d. ges. Heilk., 1842, n. F., ii, 525–536.—**Bietet** die Ehe bei Frauen Schutz gegen psychische Störung? Cor.-Bl. d. deutsch. Gesellsch. f. Psychiat., etc., Neuwied, 1857, ix, 97.—**Biffi** (S.) Psichiatria. A proposito d' una perizia medico-legale su un lipemaniaco condannato ai lavori forzati. R. Ist. Lomb. di sc. e lett. Rendic., Milano, 1876, 2. s., ix, 128–133.—**Bird** (F.) Nach welchen Principien bestimmen wir, ob ein Verrückter körperlich, geistig oder gar nicht arbeiten soll? Ztschr. f. d. Staatsarznk., Erlang., 1833, xiii (19. Suppl.),72–92.—**Blanche, Ball** & **Motet.** Rapport sur l'état mental de Sophie-Honorine, Sidonie et Camille Mercier. Tribune méd., Par., 1886, xviii, 445; 457; 469. ——. Rapport sur l'état mental d'Euphrasie Mercier. France méd., Par., 1886, ii, 1265–1269.—**Blumenstock** (L.) Barbara Ubryk, gerichtsärztlicher Bericht über deren Körper- und Geisteszustand. Wien. med. Wchnschr., 1870, xx, 333; 362; 394; 431; 465. ——. Sprawozdanie sądowo-lekarskie o stanie cielesnym i umysłowym Barbary Ubrykównéj. [Medico-legal opinion on the physical and mental condition of . . .] Przegl. lek., Krakow., 1870, ix, 91; 99; 123; 131; 139. ——. Zbrodnia czy obłąkanie. [Crime or aberration of mind?] Medycyna, Warszawa, 1885. xiii, 237 ; 257 ; 277; 302; 318; 525.—**Bodenmüller.** Gutachten über den angeblich gestörten Seelenzustand eines Inquisiten. Ztschr. f. d. Staatsarznk., Erlang., 1836, xxxi, 359–371.—**Boehr** (M.) Ein forensisch schwer zu beurtheilender Fall von Geistesstörung bei einem geschulten Verbrecher. Vrtljschr. f. gerichtl. Med., Berl., 1878, n. F., xxviii, 201–214.—**Bonnet** (H.) Rapport médico-légal sur le nommé Lejeune, atteint de folie raisonnante. Ann. méd.-psych., Par., 1865, 4. s., vi, 204–216. ——. Rapport médico-légal. *Ibid.*, 1866, 4. s., vii, 226–240.—**Bopp.** Nachträgliches in Bezug auf den (in Nro. vii des ersten Vierteljahrheftes dieser Zeitschrift, Jahrgang 1836) hinsichtlich seiner Geistescapacität, in Beziehung auf seinen Entschluss nach Amerika auswandern zu wollen, begutachteten Taubstummen. Ztschr. f. d. Staatsarznk., Erlang., 1837, 23. Ergnzngshft., 132–146.—**Bourneville** & **Teinturier** (E.) G. Townley. J. de méd. ment., Par., 1865, v, 100–114.—**Bouteille.** Rapport médico-légal sur l'état mental du nommé S . . . inculpé de concussion et d'abus de confiance. Gaz. méd.-chir. de Toulouse, 1883, xv, 49 ; 58.—**Brefeld** (F.) Gerichtsärztliches Gutachten nebst Superarbitrium und Rechtsspruch über den zweifelhaften Gemüthszustand eines bejahrten Juden, in Bezug auf Blödsinnigkeitserklärung und Versetzung in eine Irrenanstalt. Ztschr. f. d. Staatsarznk., Erlang., 1843, xlv, 132–207. ——. Excandescentia furibunda und Mania. Eine Parallele in Bezug auf Zurechnung und Blödsinnigkeits-Erklärung. *Ibid.*, 235–278.— **Brierre de Boismont** & **Boys de Loury.** Rapport médico-légal sur l'état mental de M. B. Ann. d'hyg., Par., 1850, xliv, 414–425. *Also:* Ann. méd.-psych., Par., 1850, ii, 636–644.—**Büchner** (E.) Gutachten über den Gemüthszustand eines Soldaten im Augenblick seines Vergehens im Dienste, durch thätliches Vergreifen am Vorgesetzten. Ztschr. f. d. Staatsarznk., Erlang., 1825, x, 39–72. ——. Aerztliches Gutachten über den zweifelhaften psychischen Zustand eines Inquisitin. *Ibid.*, 1839, 26. Ergnzngshft., 224–255. ——. Keine Tobsucht, aber erheblich geminderte Widerstandsfähigkeit gegen Gemüthsaffekte. Friedreich's Bl. f. gerichtl. Med., Nürnb., 1867, xviii, 337–347. ——. Ist die früher geistesgestörte A. B. nunmehr geistesgesund? *Ibid.*, 1869, xx, 387–392. ——. Selbstbestimmungsfähig oder nicht? (Untersuchung wegen Hausfriedensstörung.) *Ibid.*, 1870, xxi, 58–74.— **Bueno** (C.) Copia del proyecto de dictámen sobre el estado de Doña M. M. Corresp. méd., Madrid, 1884, xix, 197; 205; 249; 267; 294; 301.—**Buhl** (L.) & **Buchner** (L.) Gutachten über den Gesundheitszustand eines Verhafteten. Friedreich's Bl. f. gerichtl. Med., Nürnb., 1863, xiv, 112–116.—**Burckhardt** (G.) Gemeine Rachsucht, unerlaubte Selbsthülfe oder Wahnsinn? Ein psychiatrisches Gutachten. Vrtljschr. f. gerichtl. Med., Berl., 1879, n. F., xxxi, 235–251.—**de Cailleux** (G.) Rapport médico-légal sur l'état mental de Mme. Aglaé C . . . Fe H . . . Ann. méd.-psych., Par., 1860, 3. s., vi, 225–238.—**de la Calle** (L.) Consulta sobre el estado mental del negro Leoncio. Trab. Com. de med. leg. é hig. púb. de la r. Acad. de cien. méd. . . . de la Habana, 1873, i, 396–400.—**Caraza** (R.) Informe que el médico cirujano del hospital de San Hipólito que suscribe, rinde sobre el estado mental de Marcelino Domingo. Observador méd., México, 1879–80, v, 34–39.—**Carretaro** (J. F.) & **Carnicero** (P.) Declaraciones acerca de facultades intelectuales. España méd., Madrid, 1860, v, 149.—**Casper** (J. L.) Charlotte Luise Glaser. Ein seltener Fall von zweifelhaftem Wahnsinn. Vrtljschr. f. gerichtl. u. öff. Med., Berl., 1857, xii, 25–63.— **de Castro** (A.) Rapport médico-légal sur l'état mental de Hadji Abdullah, de Crimée, accusé d'un double meurtre et d'une tentative d'assassinat. Gaz. méd. d'Orient,

Mind (*Condition of, Inquiry into*).

Constantinople, 1883–4, xxvi, 167 ; 187 : 1884–5, xxvii, 5. ——. Rapport médico-légal sur l'état mental du nommé Moustapha, meurtrier de Hadji Panayoti. *Ibid.*, 1885–6, xxviii, 374 : 1886–7, xxix, 7.—**Chatelain.** Considérations médico-légales sur l'état mental de Marie Jenneret. Bull. Soc. méd. de la Suisse Rom., Lausanne, 1869, iii, 109–114.— **Chatelain** & **Langlois.** Rapport médico-légal sur l'état mental de la nommée G . . . (Adèle), inculpée d'infanticide. Rev. méd. de l'est, Nancy, 1887, xix, 353–361.— **Choulant** (L.) Gutachten der chirurgisch-medicinischen Academie zu Dresden über einen zweifelhaften Gemüthszustand. Ztschr. f. d. Staatsarznk., Erlang., 1842, xliv, 62–77.—**Clark** (D.) A psycho-medical history of Louis Riel. Am. J. Insan., Utica, 1887–8, xliv, 33–51.—**Collegii** Medici i Storfurstendömet Finland utlåtande i målet. (Sinnestillstånd.) [State of mind.] Finska läk.-sällsk. handl., Helsingfors, 1862, viii, 789 : 1871, xi, 989.—**Combes.** Double rapport sur l'état mental de Christine R . . . et de François M . . . inculpés l'une d'incendie volontaire, l'autre de parricide. J. de méd. ment., Par., 1863, iii, 293–297.— **Cram** (W. A.) Was he an idiot ? Pop. Sc. Month., N. Y., 1884, xxv, 110–113.—**Damerow.** Wiederaufnahmen in der Anstalt bei Halle, nebst gelegentlichen Bemerkungen über "zweifelhafte Gemüthszustände". Allg. Ztschr. f. Psych., etc., Berl., 1855, xii, 633–646.—**Delacour, Bruté** & **Lafitte.** Rapport sur l'état mental de L . . . (Pierre-Marie), inculpé de coups et blessures à son père ; alcoolisme chronique ; ordonnance de non-lieu. Ann. méd.-psych., Par., 1878, 5. s., xx, 55–60.—**Demleuthner.** Zur Theorie der Geisteskrankheiten ; veranlasst durch Nasse's Ansicht in Henke's Ztschr. f. d. Staatsarznk. 1831, 3. Hft., S. 1–45. Ztschr. f. d. Staatsarznk., Erlang., 1832, 17. Ergnzngshft., 284–288.—**Dictámen** de la comision de medicina legal sobre el "estado de la razon de un procesado". An. r. Acad. de med., Madrid, 1879, i, 209–218.—**Diez** (A.) Drei psychische Krankheitsfälle mit einigen gerichtlich-psychologischen Bemerkungen. Mag. f. phil., med. u. gerichtl. Seelenk., Würzb., 1831, 6. Hft., 215–239.—**Dioukoff.** Izsliedovanie sostojanija umstvennich sposobnoste M. i. zakliouchenie o tom vrache. [Examination into the state of mind of M.] Arch. sudebnoi med., St. Petersb., 1869, v, pt. 2, no. 1, 1–13.—**Droste** (A.) Medicina legalis in Sachen des Grafen Mortier. Ztschr. f. d. Staatsarznk., Erlang., 1848, lvi, 385–390.—**Dufour** (E.) Rapport médico-légal sur l'état mental du nommé Gay (Joseph-Étienne). Ann. méd.-psych., Par., 1880, 6. s., iv, 385–398. ——. Rapport médico-légal sur l'état mental du nommé Martin (Esprit). *Ibid.*, 399–410.—**Einfluss** (Ueber den) der Seelenstörung eines Angeklagten auf die Strafverhandlung. Bl. f. gerichtl. Anthrop., Nürnb., 1860, 3. Hft., 163–177.—**Erkenntniss** des Irrseins schliesst den Schwachsinn nicht aus. Cor.-Bl. d. deutsch. Gesellsch. f. Psychiat., etc., Neuwied, 1866, xiii, 290–293.—**Erpenbeck** (H.) Aerztliche Untersuchung und Begutachtung des Geisteszustandes des Kaufmanns Bernhard M. zu Z. Mag. f. d. ges. Heilk., Berl., 1838, li, 120–152.—**Eulenberg.** Gerichtsärztliche Untersuchung über einen zweifelhaften Geisteszustand. Cor.-Bl. d. deutsch. Gesellsch. f. Psychiat., etc., Neuwied, 1856, iii, 3–7.—**Falk** (F.) Gutachten über den Gemüthszustand des Dienstknechtes N. Deutsche med. Wchnschr., Berl., 1876, ii, 133–137. ——. Ueber den Gemüths-Zustand des der Blutschande angeklagten P. aus T. Vrtljschr. f. gerichtl. Med., Berl., 1877, n. F., xxvii, 19–29.—**Feroci** (A.) Parere intorno allo stato mentale di P. B. Raccoglitore med., Forlì, 1876, 4. s., vi, 335–353.—**Fisher** (T. W.) The Armstrong case. Alienist & Neurol., St. Louis, 1886, vii, 79–98. *Also,* Reprint.—**Flemming.** Ein Votum in Sachen der verminderten Zurechnungsfähigkeit. Allg. Ztschr. f. Psychiat., etc., Berl., 1865, xxii, 97–109. — **Fröhlich** (J. B.) Ueber Begriff und Eintheilung der psychischen Krankheitszustände ; Seelenkrankheiten ; Seelenstörungen, besonders zum medicinisch-gerichtlichen Behufe. Ztschr. f. d. Staatsarznk., Erlang., 1829, 10. Ergnzngshft., 120–162.—**Fuchs.** Gehirnerschütterung. Ein Beitrag zur Lehre von der Zurechnungsfähigkeit. *Ibid.*, 1838, xxxv, 47–53.—**Funaioli** (P.) Sullo stato intellettuale di G. M. di P., imputata di furto qualificato. Cron. d. manic. di Siena, 1882, viii, 90–97. ——. Sullo stato intellettuale di C. G. di S., imputato di ferimento. Perizia medico-legale. *Ibid.*, 1885, xi, 33–41. ——. Sullo stato intellettuale di M. E. di A. ; perizia medico-legale. *Ibid.*, 1886, xii, 58–66.—**Gambari** (G.) Relazione medico-legale sullo stato di mente di N. N. e sulle consequenze della malatia dalla quale è affetto. Arch. ital. per le mal. nerv., Milano, 1866, iii, 158–166.—**Gauster** (M.) Krank oder boshaft und zornmüthig? Allg. Ztschr. f. Psychiat., etc., Berl., 1877, xxxiii, 838–859.—**von Gellhorn.** Versuchter Todschlag im Zustande eines pathologischen Rausches. *Ibid.*, 1880, xxxvii, 44–54.—**Gellie.** Rapport médico-légal sur l'état mental de R . . . (Jean), inculpé d'homicide et de tentative de meurtre. Mém. et bull. Soc. de méd. et chir. de Bordeaux, 1879, 97–112.—**Gerichtsärztliche** Gutachten über zweifelhafte psychische Zustände. Ztschr. f. d. Staatsarznk., Erlang., 1822, ii, 399–418.—**Giacchi** (O.) Perizia medico legale. Raccoglitore med., Forlì, 1882, 4. s., xvii, 257–271.—**Gilson** (H.) Étude sur l'état mental de Louis Riel. Encéphale, Par.,

Mind (*Condition of, Inquiry into*).

1886, vi, 51-60.—**Giovanni** (A.) Considerazioni medico-legali sopra un accusato di borseggio trattenuto nelle carceri. Gior. d. r. Accad. di med. di Torino, 1878, xli, 257-266.—**Girard.** Monomanie d'ivresse par suite d'inconduite et d'une prédisposition nerveuse; rapport médico-légal pour obtenir l'interdiction. Gaz. méd. de Par., 1844, 2. s., xii, 746-748.—**Glaser** (G.) Ueber Zurechnungsfähigkeit. [From a work in press.] Jahrb. f. Psychiat., Leipz. u. Wien, 1887, vii, 322-336.—**Görck.** Zur Beleuchtung eines Falles von zweifelhafter Zurechnungsfähigkeit. Deutsche Ztschr. f. d. Staatsarznk., Erlang., 1865, n. F., xxiii, 137-146—**Górdon** (A.) Informe sobre el estado mental de D. R . . . Q . . . en causa por hurto. Trab. Com. de med. leg. é hig. púb. de la r. Acad. de cien. méd. . . . de la Habana, 1873, ii, 336-346. ——. Segundo informe sobre el estado mental de D. R . . . Q . . . en causa por hurto. Ibid., 346-355. ——. Informe relativo al estado mental de un procesado. Ibid., 1874, iii, 135-150.—**Graff.** A. Gutachten des grossherzogl. hess. Medicinal-Collegs zu Darmstadt über den angeblich geisteskranken Zustand des G. W. zu D. Ztschr. f. d. Staatsarznk., Erlang., 1830, x, 95-114. ——. Gutachten, eine Curatel-Verfügung betreffend. Ibid., 1833, xiii, 269-280. ——. Gutachten über den Gemüthszustand eines wegen Majestäts-Beleidigung öffentlicher Behörden Angeklagten. Ibid., 1838, xxxvi, 320-329.—**Graux** (P.-J.) [*et al.*]. Rapport médico-légal sur l'état mental d'Eugénie-Adélaïde Hayez. Ann. méd.-psych., Par., 1861, 3. s., vii, 569-587.—**Gray** (L. C.) The case of Maggie Keppel, the Brooklyn child-abductor. Am. J. Neurol. & Psychiat., N. Y., 1883, ii, 19-29.—**Griesinger.** Superarbitrium der königl. wissenschaftl. Deputation für das Medicinalwesen, betreffend eine Gemüthszustands-Untersuchung. Vrtljschr. f. gerichtl. u. öff. Med., Berl., 1867, vi, 269-294. ——. Gutachten der k. wissenschaftlichen Deputation für das Medicinalwesen über den Geisteszustand des P. Z. in A. Ibid., 1868, viii, 294-308.—**Guinier.** Rapport médico-légal sur un cas de sénilité ayant motivé la dation d'un conseil judiciaire. Rev. méd. de Toulouse, 1887, xxi, 309-317.—**Gutachten** über den Geisteszustand des, der Majestätsbeleidigung angeklagten B. G.; keine Geisteskrankheit. Samml. gerichtsärztl. Gutacht. d. Prag. med. Fak., Prag, 1858, 2. F., 313-317.—**Gutachten** über den Gemüthszustand einer nach Ehescheidung von ihrem Manne und durch eine anderweitige Heyrath nach Standeserhöhung strebenden jungen Frau. Ann. d. Staatsarznk., Züllichau, 1790-91, i, 2. St., 128-131.—**Gutachten** über den Gemüthszustand eines an krankhafter Zornmüthigkeit leidenden Menschen. Von Dr. X. Deutsche Ztschr. f. d. Staatsarznk., Erlang., 1855, n. F., vi, 105-123.—**Gutachten** (Das) der Landesgerichtsärzte im Prozesse Ulm-Windisch. Beurtheilt von einem Gerichtsarzte. Wien. med. Wchnschr., 1867, xvii, 104; 120; 136; 168; 182.—**Hardy** (W. L.) The Rhinelander case. Am. J. Neurol. & Psychiat., N. Y., 1884-5, iii, 664-690.—**Hecker** (E.) Dummheit oder krankhafter Schwachsinn? Irrenfreund, Heilbr., 1876, xviii, 153-166.—**Henke** (A.) Aerztlicher Bericht und Gutachten über den derzeitigen Geistes- und Gemüthszustand eines Frauenzimmers, in Bezug auf Fortbestand oder Aufhebung einer angeordneten Curatel. Ztschr. f. d. Staatsarznk., Erlang., 1836, xxxii, 225-243.—**Herzog.** Ueber die Vorsichtsmaassregeln, die bei Beurtheilung des Geisteszustandes von Personen in Betracht kommen, welche in dem Verdacht von Geisteszstörung stehen. Ztschr. f. d. ges. Med., Hamb., 1844, xxv, 433-449.—**Hitzig** (E.) Gutachten über den Gemüthszustand der unverehelichten A. P. Vrtljschr. f. gerichtl. Med., Berl., 1886, n. F., xlv, 254-271.—**Hoffmann.** Gutachten über den Gemüthszustand des Rechtspracticanten P. aus C. Jahrb. d. ges. Staatsarzn., Leipz., 1837, ii, 43-88.—**Hofmann** (J.) Ist der Student A. B., als er in überschwenglicher Liebe den Gegenstand derselben erschoss, vollkommen zurechnungsfähig oder beschränkt zurechnungsfähig gewesen? Ein Gutachten, als Beitrag zur Entscheidung der Kontroverse, was auf psychologischem Gebiete Zurechnungsfähigkeitsminderungsgrund und was Strafmilderungsgrund sei? Ztschr. f. d. Staatsarznk., Erlang., 1860, lxxix, 286-391. *Also, in his:* Aus dem Gerichtssaale, 8°, Erlang., 1860, 4. Hft., 1-106. ——. Eine Industrieritterin der höheren Stände. Anklage wegen Betruges und Wechselfälschung. Verhandelt vor dem k. Bezirksgerichte München links der Isar und dem k. Appellationsgerichte von Oberbayern. Ztschr. f. d. Staatsarznk., Erlang., 1863, lxxxv, 250-325. *Also, in his:* Aus dem Gerichtssaale, 8°, Erlang., 1864, 5. Hft., 1-76.—**Horn.** Gutachten über den Gemüthszustand eines Mädchens. Arch. f. med. Erfahr., Berl., 1817, i, 280-296.—**Hotzen.** Gutachten über den Geisteszustand des ehem. Districts-Schornsteinfegers H. in Bremen; Querulantenwahn. Friedreich's Bl. f. gerichtl. Med., Nürnb., 1874, xxv, 42-56.—**Huggard** (W. R.) The standard of sanity. Brit. M. J., Lond., 1885, ii, 1013.—**Informe** acerca del estado mental de D. S . . . M . . . Trab. Com. d. med. leg. é hig. púb. de la r. Acad. de cien. méd. . . . de la Habana, 1873, i, 158-168.—**Informe** con el fin de averiguar el estado mental de un individuo atacado de reblandecimiento cerebral. Ibid., 54-57.—**Informe** sobre el estado de las facultades intelectuales de Maria Garcia Casado. España

Mind (*Condition of, Inquiry into*).

méd., Madrid, 1861, vi, 602-605.—**Informe** sobre el estado mental de D. J . . . R . . . Trab. Com. d. med. leg. é hig. púb. de la r. Acad. de cien. méd. . . . de la Habana, 1873, i, 350-352.—**Jaumes** (A.) Le nommé T. doit il être considéré comme responsable? Montpel. méd., 1876, xxxvii, 289-298. ——. Détournements; rapport sur l'état mental de l'inculpé. Ibid., 1886, 2. s., vii, 453-500.—**Jendrássik** (J.) Orgyilkosság. s ennek beszámithatósága. [Assassination; mental condition of accused.] Közeg. és Törvény. Orvos., Budapest, 1877, 81-87.—**Jessen** (P.) Gutachten über einen zweifelhaften Gemüthszustand. Allg. Ztschr. f. Psychiat., etc., Berl., 1844, i, 262-321.—**Jurisprudence** médico-légale; aliéné; dommage résultant d'un crime commis par un aliéné; responsabilité des parents; responsabilité du maire de la commune: responsabilité civile de l'accusé. [*From:* Gaz. d. tribunaux, 1882.] Soc. de méd. lég. de France. Bull., Par., 1881-2, vii, 296.—**Kandinski** (V. C.) Sluchai somnitelnago dushevnago sostojanija pered sudom prisjajnich. [Doubtful state of mind in making oath before court.] Arch. psichiat., etc., Charkov, 1883, ii, no. 2, 1-70.—**Kelp.** Ueber die Zurechnungsfähigkeit des F. H. W—n aus B—e. Allg. Ztschr. f. Psychiat., etc., Berl., 1878, xxxv, 214-218. ——. Obergutachten, betreffend die Aufhebung der Curatel über den Arbeiter S. H. Ibid., 563-566. ——. Gutachten über den Geisteszustand des Füsiliers C. G. H . . . k. Ibid., 1879, xxxvi, 395-399.—**Kierski.** Willen- oder bewusstlos? Gutachten. Vrtljschr. f. gerichtl. u. öff. Med., Berl., 1869, xi. 345-348.—**Kirn** (L.) Verurtheilung einer Geistesgestörten; eine forensische Studie. Friedreich's Bl. f. gerichtl. Med., Nürnb., 1872, xxiii, 184-229.—**Klose** (C. S.) Bemerkungen über die gerichts-ärztlichen Untersuchungen gemüthskranker Zustände. Mag. f. d. ges. Heilk., Berl., 1833, xxxix, 404-517. ——. Zwei Begutachtungen eines Falles von zweifelhafter Narrheit. Ztschr. f. d. Staatsarznk., Erlang., 1841, xli, 350-365.—**König.** Bericht und Gutachten über einen angeblich an Stumpfsinn leidenden Landmann. Ztschr. f. d. Staatsarznk., Erlang., 1841, xli, 366-372.—**Kornfeld.** Motivirtes Gutachten über den geistigen Zustand des Dr. Phil. G . . . Arch. f. Psychiat., Berl., 1874, v, 262-270. ——. Motivirtes Gutachten in der Untersuchungs-Sache wider die unverehelichte P. H. aus A. Friedreich's Bl. f. gerichtl. Med., Nürnb., 1881, xxxii, 113-123.—**Koster.** Motivirtes Gutachten über den psychischen Zustand der Wittwe K. S. Irrenfreund, Heilbr., 1870, xii, 117-123. ——. Simulation und in Folge deren Geistesstörung; Gutachten über den Geisteszustand des Franz Joseph W. aus H. Ibid., 1883, xxv, 145-151. ——. Gutachten über den psychischen Zustand des Fabrikarbeiters B. A. L. aus B. zur Zeit Musketier eines Infanterie-Regiments. Ibid., 1884, xxvi, 33-37.—**von Krafft-Ebing** (R.) Gutachten über den Geisteszustand (Querulantenwahnsinn) des A. Lacroma. Ibid., 1863, xvii, 169-177. ——. Zweifelhafter Geisteszustand einer Frauensperson zur Zeit eines an ihr unternommenen Beischlafs. Ibid., 1878, xx, 177-188. ——. Zweifelhafter Geisteszustand (Geistesschwäche) eines wegen Cassadefects in Untersuchung stehenden Steuerbeamten. Friedreich's Bl. f. gerichtl. Med., Nürnb., 1878, xxix, 427-435. ——. Todschlag im Affect; zweifelhafter Geisteszustand (Epilepsie und dadurch bedingte krankhafte Gemüthsreizbarkeit) des Thäters. (Facultätsgutachten der Grazer med. Facultät.) Allg. Ztschr. f. Psychiat., etc., Berl., 1880, xxxvii, 40-43. ——. Gerichtsärztliche Gutachten über zweifelhafte Geisteszustände. Jahrb. f. Psychiat., Wien, 1882, iv, 39-51. ——. Drei Gutachten über zweifelhafte Geisteszustände. Friedreich's Bl. f. gerichtl. Med., Nürnb., 1882, xxxiii, 399-418. ——. Betrug; behauptete geistige Krankheit; blosse organische Belastung; gerichtsärztliches Gutachten. Ibid., 1885, xxxvi, 210-218.—**Krankengeschichte** (Eine) menschenfreundlichen praktischen Aerzten zur Beurtheilung vorgelegt. N. Mag. f. Aerzte, Leipz., 1792, xiv, 412-415.—**Krauss** (A.) War Anna Thormählen wirklich die Mörderin ihres Gatten, oder war ihre Selbstanklage eine falsche? Friedreich's Bl. f. gerichtl. Med., Nürnb., 1887, xxxviii, 153-185. ——. Der Criminalfall Marie Schneider nach Darstellung des Vertheidigers Dr. Friedmann im Tribunal, ii. Jahrg., p. 552, besprochen. Ibid., 258-275.—**Krügelstein.** Gutachten über zweifelhafte Gemüthszustände. Ann. d. Staatsarznk., Freib. i. Br., 1839, iv, 4. Hft., 59-97.—**Küttlinger.** Zur Lehre über die Beurtheilung versteckter Seelenkrankheiten und insbesondere über die Dauerhaftigkeit der Genesung früher an Geisteszerrüttung erkrankter Personen, in medicinisch-gerichtlicher Hinsicht. Ztschr. f. d. Staatsarznk., Erlang., 1829, xvii, 114-154.—**Kun** (T.) & **Lang** (B.) Elmeállapot megvizsgálása. [Examination of state of mind.] Államorvos, Budapest, 1883, 113; 121.—**Laehr.** Ueber die negativen Resultate bei gerichtlichen Gemüthszustandsuntersuchungen in Anstalten. [With discussion.] Allg. Ztschr. f. Psychiat., etc., Berl., 1878, xxxv, 255-260. ——. Ueber die Untersuchung zweifelhafter Geisteszustände in Anstalten. Ibid., 1883, xxxix, 601-605.—**Lafargue** & **Sisteray.** Rapport médico-légal sur l'état mental de D . . . (Bertrand), dit M . . . inculpé de tentative de viol. Mém. et bull. Soc. de méd. et chir. de Bordeaux, 1879, 112-

21

Mind (*Condition of, Inquiry into*).

122.—**Laffitte** (N.) Rapport médico-légal sur l'état mental de Marie G . . . Ann. méd.-psych., Par., 1865, 4. s., vi, 187–203. ——. Rapport sur l'état mental de M. K . . . séquestration d'office; demande de mise en liberté; expertises médico-légales; lypémanie avec idées de persécution, alcoolisme. Ann. méd.-psych., Par., 1879, 6. s., ii, 426–448.— **Landsberg.** Zwei dissentirende Gutachten und ein Superarbitrium des königl. Medicinal-Collegii über den Gemüthszustand des Stellenbesitzersohnes August H. zu B. bei M. Ztschr. f. d. Staatsarznk., Erlang., 1844, 33. Ergnzngshft., 140–208. — **Langvermisste** (Ueber eine) und bereits für todt gehaltene Person, nebst Untersuchung ihres jetzigen Gemüths- und Gesundheitszustandes. Aufsätze u. Beob. a. d. gerichtl. Arzeneyw., Berl., 1784, ii, 201– 208.—**Lauber** (J.) Gutachten, den Geisteszustand des Bauern A. B. von C. betr. Friedreich's Bl. f. gerichtl. Med., Nürnb., 1871, xxii, 58–64. ——. Gutachten die Curatel über A. B. von C., hier dessen Geisteszustand betreffend. *Ibid.*, 192–199.—**Lebredo** (J. G.) Consulta sobre el estado mental de D. P . . . H . . . Trab. Com. de med. leg. é hig. púb. de la r. Acad. de cien. méd. . . . de la Habana, 1873, i, 442–499. ——. Informe sobre el estado mental de D. J . . . M . . . C . . . *Ibid.*, ii, 138–153.—**Ledo** (J.) Consulta sobre documentos periciales y responsabilidad facultativa. *Ibid.*, i, 140–145. — **Legrand du Saulle.** De l'influence des congestions cérébrales et des attaques d'apoplexie sur la faculté de tester. Bull. Soc. de méd. prat. de Par., 1863, 65–68. ——. Sur l'état mental du sieur Lagarde. Ann. méd.-psych., Par., 1865, 4. s., vi, 369– 378. ——. Note médico-légale à l'occasion d'une donation entre-vifs à la période ultime d'une fièvre typhoïde ataxique. *Ibid.*, 1867, 4. s., ix, 439–443. ——. État mental des vieillards et des mourants. Concours méd., Par., 1880, ii, 247; 269. *Also* [Abstr.]: Praticien, Par., 1880, ii, 568. *Also, transl.*: Gac. méd. de Sevilla, 1880, ii, 224; 239. ——. Examen médico-légal de l'affaire T . . . opposition au mariage et instance en interdiction. Encéphale, Par., 1884, iv, 299–319. — **Lentz & Schrevens.** Rapport médico-légal sur l'état mental du nommé R . . . Bull. Soc. de méd. ment. de Belg., Gand et Leipz., 1875, no. 5, 19–48.— **Leuf** (A. H. P.) The Walsh case. Am. J. Neurol. & Psychiat., N. Y., 1882, i, 501–513. — **Leupoldt** (J. M.) Wahrheit oder wahnsinnige Einbildung? Ein ärztliches Gutachten über zweifelhaften psychischen Zustand. Auszugsweise mitgetheilt. Allg. Ztschr. f. Psychiat., etc., Berl., 1846, iii, 283–295.—**Lhomme.** Sur l'état mental du gendarme S . . . Ann. méd.-psych., Par., 1863, 4. s., ii, 338–348. — **Liman.** Bemerkungen zum forensischen Untersuchungs-Verfahren bei Geisteskranken, bei Gelegenheit eines Falles von streitiger Zurechnungsfähigkeit. Arch. f. Psychiat., Berl., 1868, i, 249–262. ——. Drei Gutachten über zweifelhafte Geisteszustände. Vrtljschr. f. gerichtl. Med., Berl., 1880, n. F., xxxii. 193–218: xxxiii, 1–34. ——. Verbrechen oder Wahnsinn? Prozess gegen den Rittergutsbesitzer Bötticher auf Zwecka wegen Meineides und Verleitung zum Meineide. *Ibid.*, 1885, n. F., xlii, 249–270. — **Litvinoff** (M.) Sluchai somnitelnago dushevnago sostojanija zavietshatelja. [Doubtful soundness of mind of a testator.] Sborn. sochin. po sudebnoi med., St. Petersb., 1881, i, pt. 1, 36–53. — **Locherer.** Zur Frage über die Zurechnungsfähigkeit von Taubstummen, zunächst behauptete Nothzüchtigung einer Taubstummen. Cor.-Bl. d. deutsch. Gesellsch. f. Psychiat., etc., Neuwied, 1855, ii, 139–141. ——. Gesuch des G. Z. in B. und dessen Ehefrau Chr. um Auflösung ihrer Ehe; ein Gutachten an Gr.-Herz. Landgericht G. über den Geisteszustand der Letzteren. *Ibid.*, 1856, iii, 17.— **Lombroso** (C.) Processo Peltzer. Arch. di psychiat., etc., Torino, 1883, iv, 130–134.—**von Ludwiger.** Eifersucht oder Geisteskrankheit? Motivirtes Gutachten. Vrtljschr. f. gerichtl. Med., Berl., 1883, n. F., xxxviii, 238–251.— **M.** Ist der Graf Chorinsky geistig gestört? Cor.-Bl. d. deutsch. Gesellsch. f. Psychiat., etc., Neuwied, 1868, xv, 194–196.—**Majno** (L.) Processo Barré e Lebiez. Arch. di psichiat., etc., Torino, 1883, iv, 232–238.—**Mallo** (P.) & **Wilde** (E.) Exámen fisiológico del estado mental de un individuo. Rev. méd.-quir., Buenos Aires, 1871–2, viii, 267–272.—**Mann** (E. C.) The psychological aspects of the trial of Edward Newton Rowell, at Batavia, New York. Am. Psychol. J., Phila., 1883–4, i, 381–411.—**Marzocchi** (S.) Lo stato della mente di un uxoricida. Gior. internaz. d. sc. med., Napoli, 1886, n. s., viii, 106–118.—**Maschka.** Majestätsbeleidigung, verübt von einem Epileptiker. Beantwortung der Frage über die Zurechnungsfähigkeit. Wien. med. Wchnschr., 1878, xxviii, 1221. ——. Gutachten über den Geisteszustand bei der Religionsstörung angeklagten J. P.; Verrücktheit. Vrtljschr. f. gerichtl. Med., Berl., 1879, n. F., xxxi, 218–224.—**Max-Simon** (P.) De l'expertise mentale. Lyon méd., 1885, i, 429–440.— **Meckel** (P. F.) Gutachten über den Gemüthszustand eines vermeinten Blöd- und Wahnsinnigen. N. Arch. d. prakt. Arznk. f. Aerzte, Leipz., 1790, 2. Th., 1–8.—**Medicina** legale; relazione di perizia sullo stato mentale di G. Pittarelli fu Felice. Indipendente, Torino, 1874, xxv, 99– 108.—**Mendel** (E.) Offene Antwort auf den offenen Brief des Herrn Dr. Wallichs. Vrtljschr. f. gerichtl. Med., Berl., 1886, n. F., xliv, 238; 444. — **Meuth.** Ueber ein einfaches

Mind (*Condition of, Inquiry into*).

Kriterium zur Beurtheilung zweifelhafter Geistes - Zustände. Verhandl. d. Ver. pfälz. Aerzte 1842–4, Kaiserslautern, 1845, 16–23. ——. Ein als Cause célèbre qualifizirter Assisenfall. *Ibid.*, 1847, 1–15.—**Meyer.** Gerichtlich-medicinisches Gutachten über einen zweifelhaften psychischen Zustand. Ztschr. f. d. Staatsarznk., Erlang., 1835, xxx, 152–197. — **Meynert** (T.) Superarbitrium bezüglich der Frage des Causalnexus zwischen eingetretenem Irrsinn und vorausgegangener Misshandlung. Psychiat. Centralbl., Wien, 1876, vi, 134–138.—**Miraglia** (B. G.) Sulla procedura neï giudizii criminali e civili per riconoscere l'alienazione mentale; osservazioni medico-psicologiche-legali. Boll. d. priv. manic. Fleurent, Napoli, 1880, vi, 7; 17.—**Möhsen.** Ueber die möglichst beste und gründlichste Bestimmung und Festsetzung der Begriffe in Ertheilung medizinischer Responsorum über zweifelhafte Gemüthszustände. Repert. f. d. öff. u. gerichtl. Arzneyw., Berl., 1791, ii, 28; 76.— **von Monakow.** Ein Fall von Selbstbeschuldigung bei Schwachsinn und Melancholie; motivirtes Obergutachten über den Geisteszustand der Anna Helena Br. von Biberach. Friedreich's Bl. f. gerichtl. Med., Nürnb., 1885, xxxvi, 24; 110.—**Mongeri** (L.) Consultation médico-légale sur l'état mental du sieur Oskan Arsénian. Gaz. méd. d'Orient, Constantinople, 1879–80, xxii, 35; 43; 51; 59.— **Mordret.** Rapport médico-légal sur l'état mental d'une jeune fille de douze ans et demi, prévenue d'un double assassinat. Ann. méd.-psych., Par., 1878, 5. s., xix, 103–106.— **Morel.** Rapport médical sur l'état mental de M. P . . . âgé de trente-sept ans, entré à Maréville le 21 décembre 1849. *Ibid.*, 1850, ii, 425–434.—**Morselli** (E.) & **Angelucci** (G.) Parere medico-forense sullo stato mentale di un uxoricida. Riv. sper. di freniat., Reggio-Emilia, 1880, vi, 101–139. — **Motet** (A.) [Rapport médico-légal; ordonnance de constater l'état mental de le nommé X . . . inculpé d'outrages à un ministre du culte, et de rébellion.] Ann. d'hyg., Par., 1883, 3. s., x, 243–250. ——. Médecine légale; examen de l'état mental de Delmet Gédéon, incendiaire. Encéphale, Par., 1883, iii, 474–481. ——. Examen de l'état mental du Sr. Chalenton, accusé de meurtre. *Ibid.*, 706–711. ——. État mental de B . . . inculpé de tentative de meurtre. Ann. d'hyg., Par., 1885, 3. s., xiii, 553–558. ——. Rapport sur l'état mental d'un individu inculpé d'assassinat et de tentative de meurtre. *Ibid.*, 1887, 3. s., xvii, 445–454. — **Nasse** (F.) Beiträge zur gerichtsärztlichen Begutachtung zweifelhaft psychischer Zustände. Ztschr. f. d. Staatsarznk., Erlang., 1831, xxii, 1–44.—**Neumann.** Zur Stellung der Sachverständigen in foro criminali. Allg. Ztschr. f. Psychiat., etc., Berl., 1883, xxxix, 521–532.—**Neumann** (A. C.) Verunstaltung des Körpers und Verwahrlosung des Geistes bei einem 20jährigen Manne als Anlass zur Anschuldigung seiner Geistesunfreiheit. Mag. f. d. ges. Heilk., Berl., 1834, xlii, 492–505. — **Niedermann** (G.) Orvosi észlelet és vélemény saját gyermekek meggyilkolásával vádolt N. N. elmeállapota felöl. [Mental condition of N. N., accused of murder.] Közeg. és Törvény. Orvos., Budapest, 1880, 81–85.—**Niess.** Gutachten über den zweifelhaften Gemüths-Zustand eines Mannes. Ann. d. Staatsarznk., Freib., 1845, x, 469–480. — **Obergutachten** des kgl. Medicinal-Collegiums der Provinz Schleswig-Holstein über den Geisteszustand des Maurers K. aus Gr.-B. Vrtljschr. f. gerichtl. Med., Berl., 1878, n. F., xxix, 209–220.— **Obergutachten** des königl. Medicinal-Collegiums der Provinz Brandenburg über den Geisteszustand des wegen betrüglichen Bankerotts, etc., angeklagten Banquiers Gustav J. *Ibid.*, 1886, n. F., xlv, 1; 201.—**Ordronaux** (J.) Case of Mrs. Jane C. Norton. (Value of testimony covering a period of past insanity). Am. J. Insan., Utica, N. Y., 1877, xxxiii, 352–390.—**Paganuzzi** (L.) Sullo stato di mente di Luigi Bozzato, imputato di parricidio; parere medico-legale. Riv. veneta di sc. med., Venezia, 1884, i, 89–103. ——. Sullo stato di mente di A. B., imputato di minaccie contro i parenti; parere medico-legale. *Ibid.*, 1885, ii, 321–337. — **Palmerini** (U.) In causa di reato di falsità. Riv. sper. di freniat., Reggio-Emilia, 1878, iii, 542–549. — **Parchappe.** Rapport médico-légal sur un cas d'interdiction. Ann. méd.-psych., Par., 1849, xiii, 339–350.—**Parchappe** [*et al.*] Sur Madame R . . . née B . . . pensionnaire à la maison impériale de Charenton. *Ibid.*, 1865, 4. s., vi, 338–368. — **Pavia** (A.) Processo Brusa. Arch. di psichiat., etc., Torino, 1887, viii, 289–293.—**Pécholier** [*et al.*]. Commentaire sur les articles 1974 et 1975 du code civil. Rente viagère constituée sur la tête d'une personne atteinte d'une affection cérébrale le jour de la passation du contrat, et qui a succombé moins de 20 jours après, par suite d'une attaque d'apoplexie; rapport médico-légal sur ce fait. Montpel. méd., 1873, xxx, 126–141.—**Peel** (A.) & **De Craene** (L.) Rapport médico-légal sur l'état mental du nommé T . . . Charles-Louis, prévenu d'incendie. Bull. Soc. de méd. ment. de Belg., Gand, 1885, no. 36, 32–38.— **Pelman** (C.) Ueber krankhafte Fragesucht (mit Furcht vor Berührung äusserer Gegenstände). Irrenfreund, Heilbr., 1876, xviii, 41; 57. ——. Einige gerichtlich medicinische Gutachten über zweifelhafte Gemüthszustände. Friedreich's Bl. f. gerichtel. Med., Nürnb., 1881, xxxii, 131; 161. ——. Gutachten, den Geisteszustand des Hermann G. betreffend. Brandstiftung von Seiten eines beschränkten und zu

Mind (*Condition of, Inquiry into*).

Geistesstörungen disponirten Menschen. *Ibid.*, 1885, xxxvi, 172-178.—**Perotti** (A.) Relazione di perizia sullo stato mentale del teolo_o sig. G. Battista P . . . Inuipendente, Torino, 1875, xxvi, 273-280. ———. Relazione di perizia sullo stato mentale di Cerione Luigi Gior. d. r. Accad. di med. di Torino, 1876, xxxix, 650-661.—**Pesta-lozza** (F.) Considerazioni dopo un processo per mancato omicidio. Guglielmo da Salic·to, Piacenza, 1882-3, iv, 235; 255.—**Pfeufer.** Tagebuch und Gutachten über die Geisteszerrüttung der Gräfin N. Arch. f. med. Erfahr., etc., Berl., 1825, i, 36-68. ———. Nachtrag zu meinem Tagebuche über die Geisterzerrüttung der Gräfin N. *Ibid.*, 1826, i, 397-410.—**Plasencia** (T.) Informe sobre el estado mental de D. D . . . G . . . Trab. Com. de med. leg. é hig. púb. de la r. Acad. de cien. méd. . . . de la Habana, 1873, ii, 73-78. — **Poutoppidan** (K.) Retsmedicinsk Kasuistik vedrørende den praktiske Afgjørelse af tvivlsomme Tilregnelighedstilfælde. [Responsibility of accused persons.] Ugesk. f. Læger, Kjøbenh., 1881, 4. R, iii, 81; 97.—**Ponza** (G. L.) Giudizio medico-legale per una tentata mutilazione Gior. d. r. Accad. di med. di Torino, 1864, 2. s., ii, 427; 1865, 2. s., lii, 99. *Also*, Reprint. — **Porta** *et al.* Rapporto su lo stato mentale di Giuseppe Curli, imputato di crimine per omicidio dello suocero e della propria moglie. Gazz. med. ital. iomb., Milano, 1859, 4. s, iv, 264; 340.— **Porto** (N.) O processo medico-legal Rego Pontes. Correio med. de Lisb., 1884, xiii, 53; 102.—**Prozess** (Der) Ulm - Windisch; Gutachten über den Geisteszustand des Baron Ulm; Kritik über dieses Gutachten von einem Anonymus und Gegenkritik von den k. k. Landesgerichtsärzten Dr. Haller und Prof. Dr. Schlager. Wien. med. Presse, 1867, viii, 512; 537; 560; 584; 610; 637; 667.—**Puch-stein.** Ueber den Gemüthszustand der unverehelichten Maria Krause zu Tonnin. Cor.-Bl. d. deutsch. Gesellsch. f. Psychiat., etc., Neuwied, 1874, xx, 101-103.—**Ramon Luis Miranda.** Informe para averiguar la fe cientifica que merecen las certificaciones facultativas ministradas a consecuencia del disparo de un tiro a D. I . . . V . . . Trab. Com. de med. leg. é hig. púb. de la r. Acad. de cien. méd. . . . de la Habana, 1873, i, 580-586.—**Ramon Zambrana.** Informe con el objeto de averiguar el estado de las facultades mentales del negro José Laffitte, antes, durante y despues del hecho, y cual de las cuatro declaraciones considera la Academia mas conforme con los principios de la ciencia. *Ibid.*, 1872, i, 64-79.— **Rehbein.** Aerztliches Gutachten über den Seelenzustand des inhaftirten Johann Tobias Bühning. Ztschr. f. d. Staatsarznk., Erlang., 1833, 18. Ergnzngshft., 229-254.—**Reiche.** H. Gerichtlich-medicinisches Gutachten über die Fähigkeit einer, an einer fixen Idee leidenden, Frau zur eigenen Verwaltung ihres Vermögens. *Ibid.*, 1830, x, 344-352.— **Renaudin** (E.) Rapport médico-légal sur l'état mental de la nommée D . . . veuve X . . . Ann. méd.-psych., Par., 1864, 4. s., iv, 200-212.—**Rodriguez** (F. F.) Consulta sobre el estado mental de D. J . . . R . . . Trab. Com. de med. leg. é hig. púb. de la r. Acad. de cien. méd. . . . de la Habana, 1873, i, 408-428. ———. Consulta para averiguar el estado mental del negro J. Martinez. *Ibid.*, 561-573.—**Responsabilité** (La) morale et la responsabilité sociale. [Discussion.] Ann. méd.-psych., Par., 1881, 6. s., v, 96; 270; 286; 484.—**Roggero** (G.) & **Ronconi** (L.) In causa di uxoricidio, parere medico-legale sullo stato di mente di Cattaneo Carlo. Boll. d. r. mauic. di Alessandria, 1882, iii, 18; 22; 27; 31; 35; 39; 43; 47.—**Rousselin** & **Lunier.** Étude médico-légale sur l'état mental de M. du P . . . Ann. méd.-psych., Par.,1870,5. s., iv, 56-89.—**Sander** (W.) Gutachten über den Gemüths-Zustand des Referendarius a. D. N. X. Arch. f. Psych., Berl., 1868. i, 655-675. ———. Gutachten über den Gemüthszustand der separirten Klara B. geb. F. Vrtljschr. f. gerichtl. u. öff. Med., Berl., 1872, xvii, 212-231. ———. Gutachten über den Gemüthszustand des Grafen B. von N. aus Z. Vrtljschr. f. gerichtl. Med., Berl., 1876, xxiv, 201-237. ———. Zwei Gutachten über zweifelhafte Gemüthszustände. *Ibid.*, 1878, n. F., xxviii. 40-61.—**Sane** or insane? Report of the medical commission on the case of John McGinnis. [Edit.] Med. News, Phila., 1884, xliv, 14.—**Savage** (G. H.) The case of Gouldstone. J. Ment. Sc., Lond., 1883-4, xxix, 534-539. [*See, also*, Cases, *supra.*]—**Schaeffer** (A. J.) Zwei gerichtliche Verhandlungen, enthaltend die ärztliche Untersuchung Geistesgestörter, in welchen das unzweifelhafte Ergebniss der Exploration, statt des nach dem Termine einzureichenden besonderen und motivirten Gutachtens sofort im Termin zu Protocoll gegeben wurde. (Ausgeführt nach Vorschrift der hohen Ministerial-Verfügung vom 14. November 1841.) *In his:* Samml. gerichtsärztl. Gutacht., 8°, Berl., 1848, 371-384.—**Schaitter** (J.) Watpliwy stan umysłowy mordercy. [Doubtful mental condition of a murderer.] Medycyna, Warszawa, 1883, xi, 50; 69; 85; 101.—**Schlager.** Die psychiatrische Begutachtung des Sultans Murad V. und dessen Thronentsetzung. Allg. Ztschr. f. Psychiat., Berl., 1877, xxxiv, 1-48.—**Schlager** & **Haller** (M.) Zum Process Ulm -Windisch. Wien. med. Wchnschr., 1867, xvi, 175.—**Schlangenhausen** (F.) Der Fall Hawranek. Allg. Ztschr. f. Psychiat., etc., Berl., 1884, xli, 390-394.—**Schlegel** (J. H. G.) Gutachten über den Gemüthszustand eines Menschen, über welchen

Mind (*Condition of, Inquiry into*).

die Streitfrage entstand: ob er fähig sey, sein Vermögen selbst zu verwalten. Mat. f. d. Staatsarzneiw. u. prakt. Heilk., Jena, 1800, i, 47-53. ———. Gutachten über den Gemüthszustand eines Mannes, welcher sich ins Wasser stürzte, aber gerettet wurde. *Ibid*, 1809, viii, 120-129. ———. Gutachten über den physischen und psychischen Zustand eines jungen Mannes. Jahrb. d. phil.-med. Gesellsch. zu Würzb., 1828, i, 3. Hft., 148-159. ———. Der geisteskranke E. B. zu R., den ihn betreffenden Acten zufolge beurtheilt. Ztschr. f. d. Staatsarznk., Erlang., 1829, ix, 446-452. ———. Ueber den zweifelhaften psychischen Gesundheitszustand eines Inquisiten. *Ibid.*, 1833, 19. Ergnzngshft., 127-149. ———. Gutachten über den psychischen Zustand eines früher an Manie und Melancholie leidenden Mannes, in Bezug auf eine angeordnete Curatel. *Ibid.*, 1836, 22. Ergnzngshft., 112-138. ———. Gutachten über den Geistes- und Gemüthszustand dës Fräuleins. Ann. d. Staatsarznk., Tübing., 1837, ii, 367-380.— **Schmelcher.** Gutachten über den Geisteszustand des Peter Kerz. Friedreich's Bl. f. gerichtl. Med., Nürnb., 1870, xxi, 198-204.—**Schneevoogt** (G. E. V.) & **van Hees** (C. C.) Geregtelijk-geneeskundig rapport omtrent den gemoedstoestand van Hendrik Aalders, beschuldigd van diefstal enz. Tijdschr. d. Nederl. Maatsch. t. Bevord. d. Geneesk., 's Gravenh., 1861, ii, 2. Afd., 195-217.— **Schneider** (P. J.) Obergerichtsärztliches Gutachten über zweifelhaften Seelenzustand. Deutsche Ztschr. f. d. Staatsarznk., Erlang., 1858, n. F., xi, 170-181.—**Scholz.** Zwangsvorstellungen; fälschliche Beschuldigung der Päderastie. Vrtljschr. f. gerichtl. Med., Berl., 1885, n. F., xliii, 222-230.—**Schreiber** (L.) Gutachten über einen zweifelhaften Gemüthszustand. Mag. f. d. ges. Heilk., Berl., 1836, xlvii, 307-338.—**Schumacher.** Ist Rupert L. geisteskrank? Friedreich's Bl. f. gerichtl. Med. Nürnb., 1871, xxii, 12-22. ———. Lebenscurrikel und Gutachten über den Geistes- und Gemüthszustand des Joseph R. *Ibid.*, 176-186. ———. Ist Jakob St. zurechnungsfähig, unzurechnungsfähig oder gemindert zurechnungsfähig? *Ibid.*, 1874, xxv, 457-465.—**Shteinberg** (S.) Analis psichicheskago sostojanija ph. [Medico-legal definition of mental condition.] Sborn. sochin. po sudebnoi med., St. Petersb., 1876, i, 30-61.—**Sicilia** (J.) Medicina forense; case práctico. España méd., Madrid, 1859, iv, 603; 619.—**da Silva Amado** (J. J.) Parecer sobra uma questão de medicina forense proposta â Sociedade das sciencias medicas de Lisboa. J. Soc. d. sc. med. de Lisb., 1879, xliv, 277-285.—**Skrzeczka** & **Virchow** (R.) Zurechnungsfähigkeit. (1869.) (Erörterung strafrechtlicher Fragen aus dem Gebiete der gerichtlichen Medicin. Eine Anlage zu den Motiven des Strafgesetz-Entwurfes f. d. Norddeutsch. Bund, p. 15.) *In:* Virchow (R.) Ges. Abhandl. a. d. Geb. d. öff. Med., 8°, Berl., 1879, ii, 505; 528.— **Snell.** Ein Gutachten über Zurechnungsfähigkeit. Allg. Ztschr. f. Psychiat., etc., Berl., 1879, xxxvi, 450-461.—**Solaville.** Rapport médico-légal sur l'état mental de Théodore X. Ann. méd.-psych., Par., 1878, 5. s., xx, 224-233.—**Speth.** Gerichtsärztliches Gutachten über den psychischen Zustand einer angeblich blödsinnigen Inquisitin. Ztschr. f. d. Staatsarznk., Erlang.. 1834, xxviii, 138-154.—**Sponholz.** Ueber Zurechnungsfähigkeit einer 79jährigen Wittwe, die sich eines Meineides bezüchtigt hatte. Cor.-Bl. d. deutsch. Gesellsch. f. Psychiat., etc., Neuwied, 1867, iv, 11-16.—**Steegmann.** Einige Bemerkungen zu der Abhandlung des . . . Dr. Mittermaier in Heidelberg "Ueber die zweckmässigste Art der gerichtlichen Fragestellung an Aerzte, bei Erforschung des geistigen Zustandes der Angeklagten und über das Verhältniss des Gerichts und der Medicinalbehörde in Bezug auf ärztliche Gutachten". [*From:* Hitzig's Ztschr. f. d. Criminalrechtspflege in den preussischen Staaten, Bd. ii, S. 235-261.] Ztschr. f. d. Staatsarznk., Erlang., 1831, 14. Ergnzngshft., 133-170.—**Sterne** (S.) Legal responsibility and accountability. Papers Med.-Leg. Soc. N. Y., 1882, 2. s., 277-287.—**Summing** (The) up in the Gilbert Scott case. [*From:* The Times.] Med. Times & Gaz., Lond., 1884, i, 536.—**Superarbitrium** der kgl. wissenschaftlichen Deputation für das Medicinalwesen in der Untersuchungssache wider den Invaliden L. aus W. Vrtljschr. f. gerichtl. Med., Berl., 1879, n. F., xxx, 209-231: xxxi, 1-19.—**Tarchini-Bonfanti** (A.) & **Tassani** (G.) Su lo stato mentale di G. Curti. Gazz. med. ital. lomb., Milano, 1859, 4. s., iv, 229; 237; 245; 436.—**Tebaldi** (A.) Voto medico-legale sopra lo stato mentale di Angelo B.; follia ereditaria con carattere impulsivo. Arch. ital. per le mal. nerv., Milano, 1873, x, 210-216.—**Teilleux.** Rapport médico-légal sur l'état mental d'Adèle-Hélène Brevard-Lacroix, femme Donnier-Blanc. Ann. méd.-psych., Par., 1865, 4. s, v, 419-454.—**Todtschlag** im Affect. Zweifelhafter Geisteszustand des Thäters. (Facultätsgutachten der Grazer med. Facultät.) Wien. med. Bl., 1880, iii, 1301-1303.—**Töl.** Beurtheilung eines zweifelhaften psychischen Zustandes bei einer Gebärenden. Ztschr. f. d. Staatsarznk., Erlang., 1826, xii, 48-72. — **Torino** (I.) Estado mental de A. Pagano; informe médico. An. d. Circ. méd. argent., Buenos Aires, 1883-4, vii, 852-878.— **Tott** (C. A.) Gutachten über den Seelenzustand mehrerer, ihm von der Oestbehörde zu D. vorgeführter Indivi-

Mind (*Condition of, Inquiry into*).

duen, zu gerichtlichen Zwecken. Mag. f. d. gerichtl. Arzneiw., Berl., 1832, ii, 23–35. ———. Gutachten über den Seelenzustand eines Landpredigers. Ztschr. f. d. Staatsarznk., Erlang., 1835, xxix, 467–470. ———. Zwei Gutachten über Irre. Jahrb. d. ges. Staatsarznk., Leipz., 1839, v, 181–183. — **Trélat.** Sur l'état mental de Victorine Despostes (dite Eugénie). Ann. méd.-psych., Par., 1861, 3. s., vii, 377–412. — **Tuke** (D. H.) The case of Cole, and the legal procedure in ascertaining the mental condition of prisoners. J. Ment. Sc., Lond., 1883–4, xxix, 539–543. [*See, also, supra,* Cases.] — **Unger.** Gutachten, die Untersuchung des Gemüthszustandes des zum Tode verurtheilten Bürgers Joh. Lampmann, etc., betreffend. Arch. f. med. Erfahr., etc., Berl., 1826, i, 459–484. — **Untersuchung** (Die) zweifelhafter Geisteszustände. Ztschr. f. d. Staatsarznk., Erlang., 1855, lxix, 27–207. — **Utlåtanden** i fråga om sinnesbeskaffenhet. [Twenty-three cases of inquiry into mental responsibility.] Vald saml. af k. Sundh.-Coll. utlåt. i jurisd. mål. Stockholm, 1857, 112–189. — **Vowinkel** (O.) Philipp Rückert alias Graf Thun; ein Beitrag zur Beurtheilung zweifelhafter Seelenstörungen. Deutsche Ztschr. f. d. Staatsarznk., Erlang., 1863, n. F., xxi, 389–441. — **Wallichs.** Sind Draak und Beckmann geisteskrank? Offener Brief an Dr. Mendel. Vrtljschr. f. gerichtl. Med., Berl., 1886, n. F., xliv, 327; 442. — **Warnung** (Zur) für Gerichtsärzte bei Schwurgerichten (zweifelhafte Zurechnungsfähigkeit); Gutachten, etc. Vrtljschr. f. gerichtl. u. öff. Med., Berl., 1853, iv, 256–275. — **Weiss** (A.) Kann Geisteszerrüttung die Folge von Misshandlungen ohne äussere Gewaltspuren sein? Liegt Geisteszerrüttung in Folge derartiger Misshandlungen oder Simulation vor? Arch. f. Psychiat., Berl., 1876, vi, 852–858. ———. Gutachten betreffend den Schulbesuch eines Schwachsinnigen. Vrtljschr. f. gerichtl. Med., Berl., 1878, n. F., xxix, 60–68. ———. Selbstmord, Selbsttödtung im Zustande geistiger Störung, oder Verunglückung im Wasser? Ein Beitrag zur Diagnose der Zurechnungsfähigkeit. Friedreich's Bl. f. gerichtl. Med., Nürnb., 1881, xxxii, 100; 200.— **Welter.** Zweifelhafte Seelenzustände. Cor.-Bl. d. deutsch. Gesellsch. f. Psychiat., etc., Neuwied, 1872, 1; 43; 79.— **Werres.** Untersuchung des Gemüthszustandes des Herrn v. X. auf N. T. in Bezug auf Aufhebung einer Curatel. Ztschr. f. d. Staatsarznk., Erlang., 1833, xiii, 281–331.— **Whitney** (J. O.) The Brown case. Boston M. & S. J., 1880, ciii. 261.— **Wilhelmi** (B.) Aufhebung einer wegen Geisteskrankheit instituirten Vormundschaft. Cor.-Bl. d. deutsch. Gesellsch. f. Psychiat., etc., Neuwied, 1873, 164–167.— **Wilks** (S.) Brief note of cases illustrating the importance of investigating the patient's environment in testing his sanity. J. Ment. Sc., Lond., 1882–3, n. s., xxviii, 549–552.— **Wille** (L.) Beitrag zur Lehre der zweifelhaften krankhaften Seelenzustände. Allg. Ztschr. f. Psychiat., Berl., 1864, xxi, 209–234. ———. Aerztliches Gutachten betreffend B. R. wegen sogenannter zweifelhafter Geistesstörung und der Frage seiner event. Versorgung. Vrtljschr. f. gerichtl. Med., Berl., 1879, n. F., xxx, 64–79. ———. Simulation oder Geistesstörung? Hirnkrankheit; Zurechnungsfähigkeit? Verhandlungsfähigkeit? Haftfähigkeit? Friedreich's Bl. f. gerichtl. Med., Nürnb., 1886, xxxvii, 81–110.— **Witlacil.** Der Prozess gegen die blödsinnige M. Kruger vom psychologischen, gerichtlichen und administrativen Standpunkte. Wien. med. Wchnschr., 1881, xxxi, 842; 865.— **Wittcke.** Gerichtsärztliches Gutachten über eine Blödsinnige. Ztschr. f. d. Staatsarznk., Erlang., 1838, xxxvi, 170–179. ———. Hat der alte A. F. aus Bosheit und überlegter Rache gehandelt oder ist er geisteskrank? *Ibid.*, 1858, lxxvi, 186–196.— **Wolfers** (P.) Medicinisch-gerichtliche Gutachten über den zweifelhaften Gemüthszustand der Regina K. zu Lemförde. *Ibid.*, 1831, 15. Ergnzngshft., 87–184.— **Wunderlich.** Gerichtsärztliches Gutachten über den körperlichen und geistigen Gesundheitszustand eines wegen unzulänglicher Geschäftsthätigkeit angeklagten Beamten. *Ibid.*, 1836, xxxi, 152–167.— **de Yebra** (G.) Dictámen médico-legal acerca de las facultades intelectuales de Dolores Tamis. Jurado méd.-farm., Madrid, 1884, v, 107–110.— **Zierl** (F.) Vergehen der Körperverletzung und drei Uebertretungen der Ruhestörung und des groben Unfugs; Schussverletzung am rechten Oberarme; Reflexpsychose (Aufregungszustände von epileptoidem Charakter). Friedreich's Bl. f. gerichtl. Med., Nürnb., 1883, xxxiv, 141–151.— **Ziino** (G.) In causa di ribellione con vie di fatto imputata ad un frenastenico; perizia frenologica. Morgagni, Napoli, 1883, xxv, 542–549.— **Ziliotto** (P.) & **Paganuzzi** (L.) Relazione sullo stato mentale di C. Pietro, imputato di detenzione d' arma vietata e di questua. Gior. veneto di sc. med., Venezia, 1878, 3. s., xxix, 525–542.— **Zimmermann.** Ein Richter erschiesst seine Gattin; ob in Folge psychischer Entartung? Friedreich's Bl. f. gerichtl. Med., Nürnb., 1879, xxx, 321; 452.— **Zweifelhafter** Ein) Gemüthszustand. Cor.-Bl. f. Aerzte u. Apoth. d. Grossherz. Oldenb., 1863, ii, 276–281.

Mind (*Diseases of*).

See **Insanity**; **Psychology** (*Medical, etc.*)

Mind (*Influence of, on the body*).

See, also, **Asthma**; **Attention**; **Bed-case**; **Belief**; **Body** and mind; **Brain** and mind; **Chorea** (*Epidemic*); **Civilization**; **Emotions**; **Ennui**; **Fear**; **Fœtus** (*Maternal influence on*); **Heart** (*Diseases of, Causes of*); **Homœopathy** (*Objections to, etc.*); **Hypnotism**; **Hysteria** (*Epidemic*); **Imagination**; **Imitation**; **Insanity** (*Treatment of, Mental, etc.*); **Jaundice** (*Causes, etc., of*); **Jealousy**; **Lactation** (*Pathology of*); **Magnetism** (*Animal*); **Metalloscopy**; **Mindcure**; **Miracles**; **Music**; **Nostalgia**; **Paralysis** (*Mental influence on*); **Presentiments**; **Psychology** (*Medical, etc.*); **Scrofula** (*Treatment of*) by king's touch; **Suggestion**.

ALBERTI (M.) [Pr.] de commercio animæ sive naturæ incorporeæ cum mediis et remediis corporeis. 4°. [*Halæ Magdeb.*, 1720.]

ANQUETIN (R.-A.-F.) *Considérations générales sur les effets des impressions morales vives considérées dans la production des maladies et la thérapeutique. 4°. *Paris*, 1835.

APOSTOLOVICS (J.) *Diss. exhibens modum quo affectus animi in corpus humanum agunt generatim. 4°. *Halæ*, 1757.

AUBRY (A.) *Étude sur les attractions et les répulsions de l'homme, leurs rapports avec la santé et la maladie. 4°. *Paris*, 1877.

AUCAIGNE (F.-S.) *De l'influence du moral sur le physique. 4°. *Paris*, 1835.

AZCARATE (H.) *Des passions, de leur influence comme cause de maladies et comme moyen thérapeutique. 4°. *Paris*, 1827.

BADELEY (J. C.) On the reciprocal agencies of mind and matter, and on insanity; being the Lumleian lectures, [etc.] 8°. *London*, 1851.

BAIN (A.) Mind and body. The theories of their relation. 8°. *New York*, 1873.

BANG (F. L.) *De ruina naturæ, vi ipsius naturæ in corpore humano seu de morte sine morbo quam moderato opponentium examini. Suppetias afferente Jano Buchave. sm. 4°. *Hafniæ*, [1767].

BARBIERUS (L.) De conjunctione animæ et corporis dissertatio. *In:* RAC. d' opusc. scient. e filol. 16°. *Venezia*, 1742, xxv, 183–235.

DE BEAUCHENE. De l'influence des affections de l'âme dans les maladies nerveuses des femmes, avec le traitement qui convient à ces maladies. Nouvelle édition, revue et augmentée du traitement des maux de nerfs des femmes enceintes. 8°. *Amsterdam*, 1783.

BÉDOR (H.) *Quelques considérations générales sur l'excitation subite des affections de l'âme. 4°. *Paris*, 1812.

BÉGIN (É.-A.) *De l'influence des travaux intellectuels sur le système physique de l'homme. 4°. *Strasbourg*, 1828.

BERTROU (G.-L.-B.) *De l'inquiétude et de son influence dans les maladies. 4°. *Paris*, 1817.

BOERHAAVE (A. K.) Impetum faciens dictum Hippocrati per corpus consentiens, philologice et physiologice, illustratum observationibus et experimentis passim firmatum. sm. 8°. *Lugd. Bat.*, 1745.

BRABANT (R. H.) *De valetudinis ex animo mutatione. 8°. *Edinburgi*, 1821.

BRECHT (C. J.) Trias exercitationum de mente et corpore examini . . . proponit. sm. 4°. *Francofurti cis Viadr.*, 1679.

BRIGHAM (A.) Remarks on the influence of mental cultivation and mental excitement upon health. 2. ed. 12°. *Boston*, 1833.

———. The same. 3. ed. 12°. *Philadelphia*, 1845.

BRILLANTOWSKI (S.) *De animi affectuum in motus musculares involuntarios efficacitate. 8°. *Berolini*, [1846].

Mind (*Influence of, on the body*).

BRODIE (B.) Mind and matter, or physiological inquiries. In a series of essays, intended to illustrate the mutual relations of the physical organization and the mental faculties. With additional notes by an American editor. 8°. *New York*, 1858.

BYSCHER (J. G.) * De perturbatione animi atque corporis. 4°. *Helmstadii*, [1738].

CABANIS (P.-J.-G.) Rapports du physique et du moral de l'homme. Précédés d'une table analytique par M. le comte Destutt de Tracy. Nouv. éd., augmentée d'une notice sur la vie de l'auteur. 3 v. 12°. *Paris*, 1824.

——. The same. Nouv. éd., contenant l'extrait raisonné de Destutt de Tracy, la table alphabétique et analytique de Sue, une notice biografique sur Cabanis, et un essai sur les principes et les limites de la science; des rapports du physique et du moral par le docteur Cerise. 12°. *Paris*, 1843.

CABBELL (J.) * De animi pathematibus quatenus morborum causis. 8°. *Edinburgi*, 1755.

CAHANIN (L.) * Des passions expansives, et de l'heureuse influence qu'elles exercent dans les maladies. 4°. *Paris*, 1818.

CAREL (V.-A.) * Quelques considérations sur l'influence morale, comme auxiliaire thérapeutique. 4°. *Paris*, 1835.

CHERUBIN (P.-J.-B.) * De l'influence du moral sur le physique de l'homme. 4°. *Paris*, 1840.

CHRISTOPH (A. B.) * De commotionum animi quarundum effectibus in corpus humanum. sm. 4°. *Vitebergæ*, [1794].

CLARK (G.) * De viribus animi pathematum in corpus humanum. 4°. *Lugd. Bat.*, 1727.

COMBEY (A.-A.) * De l'influence du moral sur l'organisme, soit à l'état de santé, soit à l'état de maladie. 4°. *Paris*, 1842.

COOKE (W.) Mind and the emotions considered in relation to health and disease. 8°. *London*, 1839.

——. A commentary of medical and moral life; or mind and the emotions, considered in relation to health, disease, and religion. 8°. *London*, 1852.

CORBIN (J.-L.) * Considérations générales sur l'influence du moral dans le développement et le traitement des maladies. 4°. *Paris*, 1833.

(ORP. An essay on the changes produced in the body by operations of the mind. 8°. *London*, 1791?

COTTE (P.-M.-J.-B.) * De quelques-unes des influences exercées par des émotions morales et des passions sur la production et la marche des maladies. 4°. *Strasbourg*, 1856.

COURBY (P.) * Des effets généraux des passions dans l'économie animale, et de leur influence chez les femmes grosses. 4°. *Paris*, 1807.

DOLEGA (E.) *Anima quid valeat ad corporis morbos et procreandos et debellandos. 8°. *Lipsiæ*, [1848].

DUHORDEL (V.) * Considérations médico-philosophiques sur l'influence du moral dans la production et le traitement des maladies. 4°. *Paris*, 1836.

DUNN (R.) Observations on the phenomena of life and mind. Read in the department of anatomy and physiology, at the meeting of the British Association at Dundee, Sept., 1867. 8°. *London*, 1868.

VAN ESSCHEN (P. J.) * De animi pathematum in corpus humanum agendi modo. 4°. *Gandavi*, [1828].

FLETCHER (R.) Sketches from the case book, to illustrate the influence of the mind on the body, with the treatment of some of the more important brain and nervous disturbances which arise from this influence. 8°. *London*, 1833.

Mind (*Influence of, on the body*).

FOISSAC. De l'influence du moral sur le physique. 8°. *Paris*, 1857.

Repr. from: Compt.-rend. Acad. d. sc. mor. et pol.

GAYE (B.) * De l'influence du moral sur le physique de l'homme. 4°. *Paris*, 1858.

VAN GEUNS (S. J.) * De corporum habitudine animæ hujusque virium indice ac moderatice. 4°. *Hardervici*, [1789].

GINSBERG (B.) * De consensu animi et corporis. 8°. [*Breslau*, 1825.]

GIRAUDON (F.) * Considérations générales sur le traitement moral des maladies. 4°. *Paris*, 1856.

DE GORTER (J.) Oratio de animi et corporis consensione mirabili, tam in secunda, quam adversa valetudine publice dicta die xii Junii 1730. 4°. *Lugd. Bat.*, 1731.

——. The same. sm. 4°. *Francofurti et Lipsiæ*, [1749].

GOULLARD (J.-C.-E.) * De l'influence des affections morales sur le résultat des opérations de la chirurgie. 4°. *Paris*, 1813.

GRUBER (A. J.) * De animi commotionum in corpus efficacia. 8°. [*Berlin*, 1843.]

GRUNOV (J. G.) * De noxa atque utilitate animi pathematum seu adfectuum in medicina. 4°. *Halæ Magdeb.*, [1745].

GUTERMANN (G. F.) * De efficacia animi pathematum in negotio sanitatis et morborum. 4°. *Tubingæ*, 1725.

HAASE (C. F.) * De parallelismo inter corpus et animam. 4°. *Lipsiæ*, [1812].

HAMAIDE (L.-A.) * De l'influence des causes morales dans les maladies. 4°. *Paris*, 1861.

HARDING (C. L.) Cogitationes posteriores de harmonia inter animam et corpus præstabilita. 4°. *Gottingæ*, [1738].

HÉLIE (J.) * Influence du moral dans les maladies. 4°. *Paris*, 1833.

HELT (F.) * De animi pathematum vi medica. sm. 4°. *Traj. ad Rhenum*, 1757.

VAN HENGHEL (D.) * De conjunctione mentis cum corpore humano. 4°. *Traj. ad Rhenum*, 1710.

HERRMANN (J. B.) * De viribus mentis in hominem. 8°. *Wirciburgi*, [1775].

HILSCHER (S. P.) [Pr.] I. de sensu corporis sanitatis conservandæ et redintegrandæ consiliario. 4°. *Jenæ*, [1729].

——. [Pr.] I. de remissione animorum magno sanitatis in litteratis præsidio. 4°. *Jenæ*, [1735].

——. [Pr.] de mutuo animæ cum corpore commercio et illius cogitatione alte defixa agoniam protrahente. 4°. [*Jena*, 1744.]

HIRZELIUS (J. C.) * De animi læti et erecti efficacia in corpore sano et ægro, speciatim grassantibus morbis epidemicis. 4°. *Lugd. Bat.*, 1746.

HOFFMANN (F.) [Pr.] de animæ ac corporis commercio. 4°. *Halæ Magdeb.*, [1695].

HOLLAND (P.) * Diss. pauca de mente, et ejus in corpus effectibus, exponens. 8°. *Edinburgi*, 1782.

JACKISCH (J. T.) * De vi animi affectuum noxia. sm. 8°. [*Berolini*, 1820.]

KNOTT (S.) * De animi in morbis et gignendis et sanandis potestate. 8°. *Edinburgi*, 1831.

KRAUSE (A. G. F.) & GROHMANN (J. F. R.) De damnis quæ ad corpus humanum ex imaginatione redundant. 4°. *Lipsia*, [1805].

KULM (J. A.) * De harmonia morum et morborum. sm. 4°. *Basileæ*, 1715.

LADEVI-ROCHE. Réponse au livre de Cabanis sur les rapports du physique et du moral. 8°. *Paris*, 1863.

LADMIRAULT (F.) * Aperçu de l'influence du moral sur les maladies. 4°. *Paris*, 1833.

Mind (*Influence of, on the body*).

LAGARRIGUE (J.) * Contribution à l'étude de l'influence du moral sur le physique, ou influence du système nerveux sur la nutrition. 4°. *Paris*, 1883.

LAMBERT (F. J.) * Diss. sistens perturbationum animi effectus medicinales in hominum morbos. 4°. *Argentorati*, 1811.

LARIVIÈRE (C.) * De l'influence des agents moraux, et de leur mode d'action sur l'organisme. 4°. *Paris*, 1855.

LEE (J.) * De viribus animi in corpus agentibus. 8°. *Edinburgi*, 1801.

LEIGHTON (J.) * De mente corporis imperatrice. 8°. *Edinburgi*, 1813.

LEROUX (F. N.) * De animi fortitudine in morbis. 4°. *Parisiis, an. XII* [1804].

LICETUS (F.) De rationalis animæ varia propensione ad corpus libri duo. 4°. *Patavii*, 1634.

VAN LUUNEN (T. J. M.) * De utili, quod animi cura in pluribus corporis humani morbis præstat. 8°. *Hagæ Comitum*, 1829.

MACKENZIE (P.) * De animi vi in morbis inducendis et curandis. 8°. *Edinburgi*, 1809.

MACLOUGHLIN (D.) * De animi auxilio ad morbos præcavendos aut sanandos. 8°. *Edinburgi*, 1810.

MANTHEY (J. G. L.) Gedanken von der gegenseitigen Wirkung des Körpers auf die Seele und der Seele auf den Körper. 12°. *Kopenhagen*, [1787].

MARAT (J.-P.) De l'homme, ou des principes et des loix de l'influence de l'âme sur le corps, et du corps sur l'âme. 3 v. 12°. *Amsterdam*, 1775-6.

DE MARÉES (C. G. H.) De animi perturbationum in corpus potentia. 4°. *Gottingæ*, [1775].

Also, in : SCRIPTORES neurol. minores selecti. 4°. *Lipsiæ*, 1795, iv, 344-378.

MARKS (E.) * Conjectural inquiry into the relative influence of the mind and stomach. 8°. *New York*, 1815.

MAROY (R. E.) * De animi pathematibus, eorumque in corpore effectibus. 4°. *Gandavi*, [1820].

MAUDSLEY (H.) Body and will; being an essay concerning will in its metaphysical, physiological, and pathological aspect. 8°. *New York*, 1884.

MEIER (H. L.) * De animi, ejusque affectuum quoad valetudinem, impressionibus in corpus. 4°. *Lugd. Bat.*, 1696.

MEYER (F.) * De l'influence des émotions morales sur le développement des affections cutanées. 4°. *Paris*, 1876.

MOORE (G.) The use of the body in relation to the mind. 12°. *New York*, 1847.

————. The power of the soul over the body, considered in relation to health and morals. 12°. *New York*, 1859.

————. The use of the body in relation to the mind. 8°. *New York*, 1859.

NAGY (M.) De potentia et impotentia animæ humanæ in corpus organicum sibi junctum, [etc.] sm. 4°. *Halæ Magdeb.*, 1729.

NEIKLER (J. F.) Diss. de medicina per incantationem. 4°. *Upsaliæ*, 1793.

NOBLE (D.) The human mind in its relations with the brain and nervous system. 8°. *London*, 1858.

NOËL (V.-A.) * De l'influence de l'imagination sur l'économie animale. 4°. *Strasbourg*, 1828.

OVERKAMP (T. C. G.) [Pr.] quo prælectiones suas indicit simulque de miranda admodum corporis mentisque tam in secunda quam adversa valetudine consentione pauca præfatur. 4°. *Gryphiswaldiæ*, [1752].

Mind (*Influence of, on the body*).

P. (D. G.) Dissertazione recitata nella sacra Accademia Fiorentina, nella quale si esamina se le forze della immaginazione possano alcuna volta nelle malattie nostre la perduta sanità restituirci.

In : DISSERTAZIONI e lett. [etc.] 8°. *Firenze*, 1750, ii, 131-156. *Also, transl. in :* PIÈCES intéressantes sur la médecine et la physiologie. 12°. *Paris*, 1782, 189-222.

PARRISH (J.) * An inaugural dissertation on the influence of the passions upon the body in the production and cure of diseases. 8°. *Philadelphia*, 1805.

PETIT (É.) * Essai sur l'influence de quelques affections morales dans les maladies chirurgicales des armées. 8°. *Paris, an XI* [1803].

PIETRI (J.-C.) * Sur l'influence du moral dans le développement et le traitement des maladies. 4°. *Paris*, 1836.

REICH (J. J.) * De passionibus animi corpus humanum varie alterantibus. 4°. *Halæ*, 1695.

RENZHAUSEN (C. L.) * De imperio animi in corpus. 4°. *Gottingæ*, [1808].

ROSE (H.) *An inaugural dissertation on the effects of the passions upon the body. 8°. *Philadelphia*, 1794.

SCHMID (Z. G.) * De mente sana in corpore sano. sm. 4°. *Halæ Magdeb.*, [1728].

SCHROEDER (J.) * Scrutinium commercii animæ et corporis, ac qui inde fluunt affectuum animi methodo mathematica, [etc.] sm. 4°. *Rostochii*, [1714].

SCHROEDER VAN DER KOLK (J. L. C.) Voorlezingen over het verband en de werking tusschen ligchaams- en zielskrachten bij mensch en dieren. 8°. *Utrecht*, 1843.

SEELMANN (J. G.) * De animæ ad restituendam sanitatem impotentia. 4°. *Helmstadii*, [1719].

SEGARD (C.-M.-J.) * De l'influence du moral sur le physique considérée au point de vue de la médecine. 4°. *Paris*, 1878.

SIEGLING (J. P.) *Animi vires in morborum curatione non esse negligendas. 4°. *Lipsiæ*, [1778].

STUTZER (J. A.) * Ideen über das Verhältniss der Seele zum Leib. 8°. *Landshut*, 1807.

THÉBERGE (P.-F.) * De l'influence qu'exerce le moral sur le physique de l'homme, étudiée dans ses rapports avec la pathologie et la thérapeutique et précédée d'un aperçu rapide sur la nature du moral. 4°. *Paris*, 1837.

THOROWGOOD (J. C.) The mind and its influence over the body. 12°. [*Barnet*, 1862.]

TITIUS (J. D.) & DE GERSDORFF (E. G. W.) De physico mentis in corpus regimine. 4°. *Wittebergæ*, [1780].

TUKE (D. H.) Illustrations of the influence of the mind upon the body in health and disease, designed to elucidate the action of the imagination. 2. ed. 2 v. 8°. *London*, 1884.

————. The same. 8°. *Philadelphia*, 1873.

————. The same. 2. Am. from 2. Eng. ed. 8°. *Philadelphia*, 1884.

Also [Abstr.]. *in :* J. Ment. Sc., Lond., 1870-71, xvi, 166; 351; 538: 1871-2, xvii, 153; 334: 1872-3, xviii, 8; 178; 369. *Also* [Rev.]. *in :* Edinb. M. J., 1873-4, xix, 341-350. *Also*, Reprint [of Rev.]. *Also* [Rev.]. *in :* Ann. méd.-psych., Par., 1874, 5. s., xii, 5-23 (Brierre de Boismont).

————. The same. Le corps et l'esprit. Action du moral et de l'imagination sur le physique. Traduit de l'anglais par V. Parant, précédé d'une introduction par A. Foville. 8°. *Paris*, 1886.

VERDRIES (J. M.) De æquilibrio mentis et corporis commentatio, qua harmonia, concordia et discordia utriusque hominis substantiæ, status hominis sani et morbosi, temperamenta et ex his provenientes animæ inclinationes, imaginationes,

Mind (*Influence of, on the body*).

nec non affectuum in corpus humanum vires, ex genuinis principiis declarantur, et ad experientiæ ac rationis leges expenduntur. Denuo recognita et maxima parte aucta. Accedit disquisitio de veneno canis et animalium rabidorum, et quem illud inferre solet morbo gravissimo, hydrophobia. sm. 4°. *Giessæ et Francofurti*, 1726.

VOETTINER (H.) * Ueber den Werth der Psychologie für die praktische Medicin im Allgemeinen und für die Psychiatrie ins Besondere. 8°. *Stuttgart*, 1839.

VOISIN (F.) * De l'utilité du courage et de la réaction morale dans les maladies. 4°. *Paris*, 1819.

VOSS (H. B. G.) * De animi commotionum in corpus efficacia præsertim ad procreandos et sanandos morbos. 8°. *Gottingæ*, 1819.

WELTZ (J. F.) * De medici officio circa animam in causa sanitatis: Ob die Medicin in Curen mit der Seele etwas zu schaffen habe? 4°. *Halæ Magdeb.*, [1745].

WICK (J. C.) * De animi affectuum in corpus efficacia. 4°. *Gottingæ*, [1796].

WINKLER (J. M.) * De nocivo animi affectuum et pathematum in hominum sanitatem imperio. 8°. [*n. p.*, 1822.]

WRIGHT (J. W.) A treatise on medical psychology; or, the influence of the mind over the health of the body, and sketch of practice; designed both for the use of practitioners of medicine and the people. sm. 8°. *Louisville*, 1866.

Allen (N. H.) The effects of mental emotions in producing asthma and dyspnœa in general. Boston M. & S. J., 1839, xxi, 42–46.—**Allier** (L.) Des influences morales en matière de thérapeutique. France méd., Par., 1863, x, 230–233.—**Amelung** (F.) Ueber die Seele des Menschen und ihre Verbindung mit dem Körper. Mag. f. phil., med. u. gerichtl. Seelenk., Würzb., 1829, 2. Hft., 1–46.—**Azam.** Le caractère dans les maladies. Ann. méd.-psych., Par., 1885, 7. s., ii, 386–406.—**Badeley** (J. C.) The Lumleian lectures for 1851. On the reciprocal agencies of mind and matter. Lond. M. Gaz., 1851, n. s., xii, 881; 952; 969; 1013; 1101.—**Beauchène.** Observation sur une leucophlegmatie produite par une affection de l'âme. J. gén. de méd., chir. et pharm., Par., 1808, xxxii, 371–375.—**Berry** (I. C.) Mental influence on the body in health and disease. Tr. M. Soc. W. Virg., Wheeling, 1874, 569–571.—**Bonnefoy.** Mémoire sur les passions de l'âme; année 1783. Mém. . . . pour les prix de l'Acad. roy. de chir., Par., 1819, v, 663–699. — **Borrichius** (O.) Alia imaginantium exempla. Acta med. et phil. 1677–9, Hafn., 1680, v, 137–140. *Also, transl.:* Collect. acad. d. mém., etc., Dijon, 1766, vii, 356.—**Braid** (J.) The power of the mind over the body; an experimental inquiry into the nature and cause of the phenomena attributed by Baron Reichenbach and others to a "new imponderable". Edinb. M. & S. J., 1846, lxvi, 286–312. *Also:* Med. Times, Lond., 1846, xiv, 214; 252; 273.—**Browne** (J. C.) Case of psychical intoxication. Med. Mirror, Lond., 1866, iii, 130–133.—**Buchner** (E.) Medicinalpfuscherei. Friedreich's Bl. f. gerichtl. Med., Nürnb., 1871, xxii, 338–359.—**Caldwell** (C.) Thoughts on moral medicine. Transylv. J. M., Lexington, Ky., 1836, ix, 401–430. *Also,* Reprint.—**Caldwell** (J. W.) Action of mental conditions upon the bodily organism. South. J. M. Sc., N. Orl., 1867, ii, 414–423. — **Cerise** (L.) Que sait-on de l'influence du moral sur les fonctions de sécrétion? Bull. Soc. méd.-prat. de Par., 1842, no. 36, 57; no. 37, 5. ———. Que faut-il entendre, en physiologie et en pathologie, par ces mots: Influence du moral sur le physique, influence du physique sur le moral? Ann. méd.-psych., Par., 1843, i, 1–21.—**Clifford** (W. K.) Body and mind. Fortnightly Rev., Lond., 1874, n. s., xvi, 714–736.—**Clough** (J.) The influence of the mind on physical organization. Boston M. & S. J., 1840, xxi, 410–415.—**Comins** (J. M.) Mental over the physical. Pub. Mass. Eclect. M. Soc., Bost., 1860–72, 120–125.—**Coriveaud** (A.) Études cliniques; du chagrin considéré comme cause indirecte de la mort; observation d'un cas de pleurésie compliquée de chagrin. J. de méd. de Bordeaux, 1879, i, 416; 428.—**Davis** (N. S.) The influence of mental anxiety on the development of tumors. Annalist, N. Y., 1848, iii, 25–28.—**Demangeon.** De l'imagination considérée dans ses effets directs sur l'homme et les animaux, et dans ses effets indirects sur les produits de la gestation. Hygie, Brux., 1829, vi, 567–572.—**Dendy** (W. C.) Psychotherapeia, or the remedial influence of mind. J. Psych. M., Lond., 1853, vi, 268–274.—**Denham** (J. F.) On the connection between morbid physical and moral phenomena. *Ibid.*, 1856, ix, 572–584. — **Droste** (A.) Practischer Beitrag zu der

Mind (*Influence of, on the body*).

Lehre von der Wechselbeziehung zwischen den psychischen und somatischen Krankheitsformen. Bl. f. Psychiat., Erlang., 1837, 2. Hft., 64–69.—**England** (W.) Case of fever caused by mental anxiety; conversion into the remittent type, with profuse hæmorrhage from the bowels. Med. Gaz., Lond., 1842, xxx, 462–465.—**Fauntleroy** (A. M.) Reciprocal action of morbid bodily and mental influences. Tr. M. & Chir. Fac. Maryland, Balt., 1882, 75–82.—**Faye** (F. C.) Nogle Bemærkninger om Forbindelsen mellem det mentale og det animalsk-organiske Livs Yttringer. Norsk Mag. f. Lægevidensk., Christiania, 1840, i, 205–246. — **Féré** (C.) La médecine d'imagination. Progrès méd., Par., 1884, xii, 309: 1886, 2. s., iv, 717; 741; 760. *Also,* Reprint.—**Fischer** (R.) Der feste Wille des Menschen als Heilmittel, und zwar als Präservativ-, als Vertilgungs- oder wenigstens Linderungsmittel in mannigfaltigen Krankheiten und krankhaften Gefühlen. Med. Jahrb. d. k. k. österr. Staates, Wien, 1841, xxxv, 292–301.—**Flint** (A.) On the agency of the mind in etiology, prophylaxis, and therapeutics. Am. Practitioner, Louisville, Ky., 1872, v, 1–15.—**Forwood** (W. S.) Practice of obeah or witchcraft by negroes; effects upon the mind and body. Med. & Surg. Reporter, Phila., 1871, xxv, 161–165.—**Foster** (T. A.) Effects of psychological influence upon disease. Tr. Maine M. Ass., Portland, 1871, iv, 63; 276.—**Fothergill** (J. M.) The mental aspects of ordinary disease. Pop. Sc. Month., N. Y., 1875, vi, 562–574. — **Gelpi** (J.) Fatales presentimientos de algunos infermos. Rev. de cien. méd., Barcel., 1877, iii, 340–342.—**Germe.** De l'influence morale dans les maladies, soit comme cause, soit comme traitement. France méd., Par., 1863, x, 146–149.—**Gibbons** (H.), sr. On some of the relations of body to mind. Pacific M. & S. J., San Fran., 1883–4, xxvi, 337–352. — **Gorton** (D. A.) Cure by faith. N. York M. Times, 1883–4, xi, 161–164. — **Haller** (C.) Ueber den Einfluss des Gemüthes als Krankheitsursache. Med. Jahrb. d. k. k. österr. Staates, Wien, 1839, n. F., xx, 387–398. — **Hauck.** Heftige Gemüthsbewegung als Ursache des Todes. Wchnschr. f. d. ges. Heilk., Berl., 1833, ii, 188. — **Hitchman** (J.) Effects of mental impressions on disease. Lond. M. Gaz., 1842, n. s., i, 406–408.—**Hofbauer.** Infectio psychica. Oesterr. med. Wchnschr., Wien, 1846, 1183–1188.—**Hohnbaum** (C.) Einige Worte über das Verhältniss von Leib und Seele, in Bezug auf des Hrn. Prof. Nasse's Abhandlung: Ueber die Abhängigkeit oder Unabhängigkeit des Irreseyns u. s. w. Ztschr. f. psych. Aerzte, Leipz., 1819, ii, 31–55. — **Hovell** (D. de B.) On neurosis from moral shock. Clin. Lect. & Rep. Lond. Hosp., 1867–8, iv, 404–414. — **Huber** (J. M.) Ein weiterer Beitrag über das Wechselverhältniss zwischen geistigem und physischem Leben. Oesterr. Ztschr. f. prakt. Heilk., Wien, 1857, iii, 593; 625.—**Jolly** (P.) De la volonté considérée comme puissance morale et comme moyen thérapeutique. Rev. méd. franç. et étrang., Par., 1837, i, 28–45. ———. L'imagination dans ses rapports avec la philosophie et la médecine. *Ibid.*, 1874, ii, 265; 297; 328. ———. La volonté considérée comme puissance morale et comme moyen thérapeutique. Gaz. méd. de Par., 1875, 4. s., iv, 497; 509; 533. *Also.* Gaz. d. hôp., Par., 1875, xlviii, 918; 925; 933; 942. *Also:* Abeille méd., Par., 1875, xxxii, 388; 397; 404. *Also:* Mouvement méd., Par., 1875, xiii, 647–652.—**Jones** (A. B.) The influence of the mental over man's physical forces. Tr. Ohio M. Soc., Cincin., 1872, 231–237.—**Kellogg** (A. O.) Considerations on the reciprocal influence of the physical organization and mental manifestations. Am. J. Insan., Utica, N. Y., 1854–5, xi, 217; 338: 1855–6, xii, 30; 111; 305: 1856–7, xiii, 1; 231: 1857–8, xiv, 145: 1858–9, xv, 366–376. — **Krebel** (R.) Umrisse zur Lehre über psychische Einflüsse in Bezug auf Krankheiten und deren Beseitigung. Med. Ztg. Russlands, St. Petersb., 1856, xiii, 65; 73; 81; 89.—**Laugier.** Observation sur les effets funestes des affections tristes de l'âme dans les maladies. J. de méd., chir., pharm., etc., Par., 1775, xliv, 117–133.—**Laura** (S.) Di un caso di cianosi da violenta emozione. Gazz. med. ital., prov. venete, Padova, 1863, vi, 109–111. — **Lebenheim.** Ueber die psychische Behandlung somatischer Krankheiten. Wchnschr. f. d. ges. Heilk., Berl., 1838, 489; 509. — **Le Grand** (J. N.) Mental excitement a remedy for disease; curious cases. N. Orl. M. News & Hosp. Gaz., 1858–9, v, 515–517. — **Leveillé.** Extrait des observations de M. A. Petit, D. M. et chirurgien en chef de l'Hôpital de Lyon, sur l'influence que peuvent avoir sur la santé les violentes et subites affections de l'âme. Rec. périod. Soc. de méd. de Par., 1798, iii, 426–441.—**Lorain.** Des émotions soudaines chez les femmes, développant instantanément des troubles nerveux persistants (hystérie, chlorose, chorée, paralysie agitante). Arch. gén. de méd., Par., 1875, i, 205–215.—**Luyckx.** Observation d'une profonde perturbation dans les systèmes nerveux de la vie organique et de celle de relation, produite sous l'influence de causes morales. Ann. Soc. de méd. d'Anvers, 1847, iv, 5–11. [Rap. de Berchem], 12.—**Maas** (C. A.) Fall einer rein psychischen Cur. Oesterr. med. Wchnschr., Wien, 1845, 1145–1152. — **Malden** (J.) Upon the reciprocal influence of the mind and body of man, in health and disease. Tr. Prov. M. & S. Ass., Lond., 1833, i, 109–122. — **Manley** (I.) Influence of mind upon the

Mind (*Influence of, on the body*).

body. Tr. M. Soc. Wisconsin, Milwaukee, 1881, xv, 64–75.—**Marquand.** De l'influence du moral sur le physique dans les maladies chirurgicales, et principalement dans les cas d'opération. J. de méd., chir., pharm., etc., Par., 1808, xvi, 101–106.—**Meier** (W.) Der Seele und des Leibes des Menschen Verhältniss, Wechselwirkung und Verbindung. Ann. f. d. ges. Heilk., Karlsruhe, 1827–8, iii, 1. Hft., 87–96.—**Mercier** (A.) On the influence of the mind on the origin, course, and termination of the diseases of the body. N. Orl. M. & S. J., 1857, xiv, 25–32.—**Michetti** (A.) Organicismo e mentalità. Arch. ital. per le mal. nerv., Milano, 1877, xiv, 39–52.—**Mind** and body. Med. Times & Gaz., Lond., 1872, ii, 462.—**Minichini** (D.) Discorso accademico su lo stato morale degli ammalati. Rendic. Accad. med.-chir. di Napoli, 1862, xvi, 56–62.—**Mitchell** (L. C.) The influence of mind in disease. N. Eng. M. Month., Bridgeport, Conn., 1885–6, v, 154–161. *Also:* Northwest. Lancet, St. Paul, 1885–6, v, 21–28.—**Moral** (On the) therapeutics of London. J. Psych. M., Lond., 1859, xii, 277–299.—**Moreau** (J.-L.) Observations sur un fait de médecine morale. Mém. Soc. méd. d'émulat. de Par., an v [1797], i, 40–43.—**Morselli** (E.) L' influenza del morale sul fisico, rassegna critica. Riv. sper. di freniat., Reggio-Emilia, 1886, xii, 120–130.—**Nasse.** Vereintseyn von Seele und Leib oder Einsseyn? Ztschr. f. psych. Aerzte, Leipz., 1820, iii, 1. Vrtljschr., 6–22.—**O'Neill** (H.) Psychological causes of disease. Pacific M. & S. J., San Fran., 1878, xxi, 159–164.—**Pamard.** Sur l'influence du moral sur le physique. Rev. méd. franç. et étrang., Par., 1836, iv, 47–55.—**Park** (J. R.) On the influence of mental impressions in producing change of function in the living body. J. Sc. & Arts 1817 [Am. rep.], N. Y., 1818, iv, 207–226.—**Petit** (M.-A.) Discours sur l'influence de la révolution française sur la santé publique. *In his:* Essai sur la médecine du cœur, 2. éd., 8°, Par., 1828, 177–213.—**Philips** (J.-P.) Coup d'œil sur la théorie des actions organoleptiques et sur l'influence réciproque de la pensée, de la sensation et des mouvements organiques. Ann. méd.-psych., Par., 1862, 3. s., viii, 270–281. *Also,* Reprint.—**Pistelli** (E. M.) Ricerche medico-legali sul momento in cui l' anima si divide dal corpo. Ann. univ. di med., Milano, 1826, xl, 127–138.—**Probst** (C. O.) The physical results of mental forces; or the action of mind on body. Columbus M. J., 1885–6, iv, 385–397.—**Reveillé-Parise.** Essai de thérapeutique morale. Bull. gén. de thérap., etc., Par., 1841, xxi, 5; 137.—**Ribes.** Des affections morales, et des passions considérées comme moyen thérapeutique. Rev. de thérap. du midi, Montpel., 1850, i, 289; 328.—**Richardson** (B. W.) Induced disease from the influence of the passions. Pop. Sc. Month., N. Y., 1875, viii, 60–66.—**Robert** (C.) Influence des émotions vives sur la production et sur la guérison de certaines maladies. J. d. conn. méd.-chir., Par., 1838–9, 109–111.—**Rouse** (W. H.) The influence of the mind on some of the organic functions of the body. Penins. J. M., Detroit, 1875, xi, 447–455.—**Russell** (J.) Illustrations of disease produced by mental influence. Brit. M. J., Lond., 1860, ii, 851; 874.—**Schuster.** Ueber die psychische Behandlung der Krankheiten als Hülfsmittel, die Wirkung der materiellen Heilmittel zu unterstützen. Mag. f. d. ges. Heilk., Berl., 1831, xxxiv, 489–526.—**Sealy** (J. H.) The imagination; its history and effects on the functions of the body in health and disease. *In his:* Medical essays, 12°, Lond., 1837, xiv, 1–91.—**Simpson** (H.) How the body may be influenced by the mind in sickness and health. Health Lect., Lond., 1878–9, ii, 35–56.—**Skvortsoff** (I. P.) O vlijanii duschevnago sostojanija chelovieka na proischojdenie, techenie i ischod bolieznei. [Influence of mental condition of man on the origin, course, etc., of disease.] Vrach. Vaidom., St. Petersb., 1880, v, 172.; 1752.—**Stearns** (J.) Address. Tr. M. Soc. N. Y., Albany, 1820, 13–29.—**Stinchfield** (A. W.) Psychological influences in health and disease. Tr. Minn. M. Soc., St. Paul, 1875, 30–40.—**Thibault.** Méloena déterminé par une affection vive de l'âme. Ann. clin. de Montpel., 1853, i, 207.—**Todd** (J. S.) Some thoughts and facts about the superstitions of medicine and mental influences as curative agents. Atlanta M. & S. J., 1885–6, n. s., ii, 709–718.—**Todd** (S. S.) Tranquilization as an elemen of cure. Tr. M. Ass. Missouri, St. Joseph, 1872, vi, 33–48.—**Van der Meersch** (D.-J.) Observation d'une maladie nerveuse rebelle, guérie subitement par un procédé moral, suivie de quelques rémarques sur ces espèces de cures. Ann. Soc. de méd. de Gand, 1865, xliii, 85–120. [Rap. de Ingels], 121–126.—**Van Vorhis** (F. J.) Psychical influence upon the organization of structures. Tr. Indiana M. Soc., Indianap., 1870, xx, 57–64. [Discussion], 64–66.—**Védie** (H.) De l'influence des causes morales sur l'économie et en particulier sur le système nerveux. Ann. méd.-psych., Par., 1874, xl, 5–35.—**Walker** (J. K.) On the influence of the depressing passions on the health and on disease. Tr. Prov. M. & S. Ass., Lond., 1841, ix, 471–480.—**Webber** (N. W.) Influence of the mind upon the body. Detroit Rev. Med. & Pharm., 1876, xi, 467–474.—**Williamson** (J.) Mental influence in physical disease. An inaugural thesis. Chicago M. J., 1869, xxvi, 65–84.—**Winslow** (F.) Influence of the mind on disease. Lond. M. Gaz., 1839, n. s., ii, 164–171.

Mind (*Overwork of*).

See, also, **Education** (*Hygiene of*); **Nervous system** (*Diseases of*).

WOOD (H. C.) Brain-work and over-work. 16°. *Philadelphia*, 1880.

Farquharson (R.) On overwork. Lancet, Lond., 1876. ii, 9.—**Fothergill** (J. M.) Mental strain; overwork and tension. San. Rec., Lond., 1874, i, 221–223.—**Franchi** (G.) L' abuso delle forze intellettuali. Medico di Casa, Milano, 1873, i, 4, 17.—**Johnson** (G.) Lectures on some nervous disorders that result from overwork and mental anxiety. Lancet, Lond., 1875, ii, 651: 1876, i, 233; 271.—**Josat.** De l'influence des travaux de l'esprit sur la santé. Investigateur. J. de l'Inst. hist., Par., 1847, 2. s., vii, 338–343.—**MacCabe** (F.) On mental strain and overwork. J. Ment. Sc., Lond., 1875, xxi, 388–402.—**Richardson** (B. W.) On physical diseases from mental strain. *Ibid.*, 1869–70, xv, 350–362. *Also:* Am. J. Insan., Utica, N. Y., 1869–70, xxvi, 449–469.—**Routh** (C. H. F.) Overwork and premature mental decay and their treatment. Proc. M. Soc. Lond., 1872–4, i, 19. *Also:* Med. Press & Circ., Lond., 1873, xv, 417; 439; 461. *Also,* Reprint.—**Wilks** (S.) On overwork. Lancet, Lond., 1875, i, 886. *Also:* San. Rec., Lond., 1875, iii, 54–56.—**Winslow** (F.) On softening of the brain arising from anxiety and undue mental exercise and resulting in impairment of mind. J. Psych. M., Lond., 1849, ii, 1–32.

Mind. A quarterly review of psychology and philosophy. Edited by George Croom Robertson. v. 1–12, 1876–87. 8°. *London, Williams & Norgate.*

Current. v. 10 contains general index to v. 1–10.

Mind (The), the breath, and speech; or practical remarks on stammering. viii, 9–48 pp. 12°. *London, J. Madden,* 1848.

Mind, life, and motion; with the law of their relations to matter. iv, 77 pp., 2 pl. 8°. *New York, J. F. Trow,* 1857.

With second title-page: Uncertainty of human testimony; conclusions not judgments. A letter to Hon. Wm. Kent.

Mind in animals.

See **Instinct.**

Mind in nature. A popular journal of psychical, medical, and scientific information. Published by the Cosmic Publishing Company. [Monthly.] v. 1–2, March, 1855, to Feb., 1887. 8°. *Chicago.* Ended.

Mind-cure.

See, also, **Magnetism** (*Animal*).

BARROWS (C. M.) Bread-pills; a study of mind-cure. What it is, and how to do it. 2. ed. 8°. *Boston,* 1885.

BARTOL (C. A.) Spiritual specifics. Mind in medicine. Embracing two sermons preached in the West Church, Boston, Mass., October 5 and 12, 1884. 12°. *New York,* 1884.

———. Spiritual specifics. Mind in medicine. No. 4. A sermon preached in the West Church, Boston. 8°. *Boston,* [1886.]

CHOATE (C. E.) True christianity; the basis of healing with mind. A lecture delivered in the Universalist Church, Chelsea, Mass., April 30, 1885. 12°. *Boston,* 1886.

———. The unfolding; or mind understood the healing power. 8°. *Boston,* 1886.

CHRISTIAN science and the Bible with reference to Mary Baker G. Eddy's Science and health. By Phare Pleigh. In review of a recent California essay. 12°. *Boston,* 1886.

DIAZ (Abby M.) Spirit as a power. 12°. [*Belmont,* 1886.]

———. The law of perfection. 24°. [*Belmont, Mass.,* 1886.]

DUTTON (G.) Ontology, or the science of being; a monograph, being an exposition of the mental cure, with a short chapter on hygiene. 8°. [*Boston, n. d.*]

EDDY (Mary B. G.) Defence of christian science against Rev. Joseph Cook and Dr. A. J. Gordon's religious ban. 12°. *Boston,* 1885.

Mind-cure.

——. Christian healing. A lecture delivered at Boston. 2. ed. 8°. *Cambridge*, 1886.

——. Science and health, with key to the Scriptures. 24. ed. 8°. *Boston*, 1886.

——. The people's idea of God; its effects on health and christianity. 2. ed. 8°. *Cambridge*, 1886.

EVANS (W. F.) The mental cure, illustrating the influence of the mind on the body, both in health and disease, and the psychological method of treatment. sm. 8°. *Glasgow*, 1870.

——. Mental medicine; a theoretical and practical treatise on medical psychology. 15. ed. 8°. *Boston*, 1872.

——. Soul and body, or the spiritual science of health and disease. 8°. *Boston*, 1876.

——. Healing by faith; or, primitive mindcure. Elementary lessons in Christian philosophy and transcendal medicine. 8°. *London*, 1885.

——. Esoteric christianity and mental therapeutics. 8°. *Boston*, 1886.

——. The primitive mind-cure. The nature and power of faith; or elementary lessons in christian philosophy and transcendental medicine. 5. ed. 8°. *Boston*, 1886.

HAZZARD (E. B.) The essence of mind-cure; what it is; what it is for; a primer of christian science. 12°. *New York*, 1886.

KIRCHGESSNER (E. M.) Preliminary lessons in metaphysics, or the science of christian healing. 12°. *Boston*, 1886.

MY physician, mind. Metaphysics in a nutshell. A concise treatise on mental and spiritual dynamics; their application as a therapeutic agent in the cure of all diseases, whether in acute or chronic form. In scope it covers the entire domain of man's relations to God, the neighbor, and the universe of things. 8°. *Topeka*, 1886.

NARRATIVE (A) of the late extraordinary cure wrought in an instant upon Mrs. Eliz. Savage (lame from her birth), without the using of any natural means. With the affidavits which were made before the right honorable the lord mayor, and the certificates of several credible persons, who knew her both before and since her cure. Enquired into with all its circumstances, by noted divines both of the Church of England and others; and by eminent physicians of the college; and many persons of quality, who have express'd their full satisfaction. With an appendix, attempting to prove that miracles are not ceas'd. 12°. *London*, 1694.

NICHOLLS (W. T.) Mind cure; its truths and fallacies from a common-sense standpoint. 12°. *Chicago*, 1886.

ROOT (Julia A.) Healing power of mind. A treatise on mind-cure, with original views on the subject and complete instructions for practice and self treatment. 2. ed. 12°. *Peoria*, 1886.

STUART (*Mrs.* E. G.) Healing power of thought. Lecture delivered in Hyde Park [Mass.], March 13, 1884. 12°. *Hyde Park, Mass.*, [1884].

WORD (The) of the Lord concerning sickness. Compiled by G. W. McCalla. 24°. *Philadelphia*, [n. d.]

Finley (Mary J.) The mind-cure. Med. Rec., N. Y., 1887, xxxii, 590–593.—Mitchell (L. C.) Mind or faith cure. Northwest. Lancet, St. Paul, 1885-6, v, 401–406.—Widney (J. P.) The faith cure fallacy. South. Calif. Pract., Los Angeles, 1886, i, 118–122. ——. Mind cure. *Ibid.*, 175–179.

Mind-Cure Journal. By Prof. A. J. Swarts.
[Monthly.] Nos. 1–3, v. 2, Oct. to Dec., 1885. 8°. *Chicago*.

A continuation of: **Mind-Cure** (The) and Science of Life. Continued in Jan., 1886, as: **Mental** Science Magazine and Mind-Cure Journal.

Mind-Cure (The) and Science of Life. Prof.
A. J. Swarts, editor and publisher. [Monthly.] Nos. 4, 6–8, 11, v. 1, Jan. to Aug., 1885. 8°. *Chicago*.

Continued in October, 1885, as: **Mind-Cure** Journal.

Minden. General - Verwaltungs - Bericht über
das Medicinal- und Sanitätswesen des Regierungs-Bezirks Minden für das Jahr 1880. Von Dr. Schulz-Hencke. 119 pp., 1 map, 1 tab. 8°. *Minden, J. C. C. Bruns*, 1882.

Minden.

SCHULTZ - HENCKE. Der Regierungs-Bezirk Minden. Eine medicinische Studie, nebst Verwaltungsbericht, über das Sanitäts- und Veterinär - Wesen für das Jahr 1875. 8°. *Minden*, 1877.

Mortalitäts-Statistik der Gemeinde Minden: 1. Januar bis 31. December 1874. Cor.-Bl. d. nied.-rhein. Ver. f. öff. Gsndhtspflg., Köln, 1876, v, 55–57.

Minder (Daniel). * De abortu, oder von der
unzeitigen Geburt. 27 pp., 2 l. sm. 4°. *Halæ Magdeb., typ. C. Hilligeri*, 1733.

Minder (Henry). * Des hémorrhagies utérines
qui si manifestent pendant la grossesse, pendant et après l'accouchement. 44 pp. 4°. *Paris*, 1864, No. 127.

Minderer (Joannes Martinus) [17 –1812]. * De
peste eique medendi methodo in ratione et experientia fundata. 52 pp. 4°. *Jenæ, typ. Goepferdtianis*, 1789.

——. The same. 52 pp. 4°. *Rigæ, J. F. Hartknoch*, 1789.

——. The same. Abermal ein Beytrag zur Kenntniss und Heilung der Pest. 161 pp. 16°. *Riga, J. F. Hartknoch*, 1790.

Minderer (Raymundus). De pestilentia liber
unus veterum et neotericorum observatione constans. 16 p. l., 386 pp. 12°. [*Vindobonæ*, 1608.]

——. Aloedarium marocostinum. 13 p. l., 235 pp., 3 l. 8°. *Augustæ Vindelicorum*, 1616.

——. Threnodia medica seu planctus medicinæ lugentis. 23 p. l., 597 pp., 9 l. 16°. [*Augustæ Vindelicorum, A. Aperger*], 1619.

——. Medicina militaris, seu libellus castrensis. Euporista ac facile parabilia medicamenta comprehendens. Id est: Gemaine Handstücklein zur Kriegs-Artzney gehörig. Mit wolgegründten Experimenten gezieret, und den gemainen Soldaten, Ritter und Knechten zum nutzen an Tag gegeben. 7 p. l., 232 pp., 4 l. 12°. *Augspurg, A. Aperger*, 1620.

Bound with: APOLLINARIS (Q.) Kurtz Handbuchlin [etc.] 12°. *Franckf. a. M.*, 1554.

——. The same. 4 p. l., 232 pp., 3 l. *Ingolstadt, W. Eder*, 1632.

——. The same. Medicina militaris. Das ist, gemeine Handstücklein zur Kriegs-Artzney gehörig. Mit wolgegründten Experimenten gezieret, und den gemeinen Soldaten, Ritter und Knechten zum Nutzen an Tag gegeben. Sampt angehengtem räthlichen Gutachten, die jetzt schwebende und unter den Soldaten mehrentheils grassirende Sucht betreffend. 383 pp., 4 l. 16°. *Nürnberg, J. Dümlern*, [1620].

——. The same. 319 pp., 26 l. 16°. *Augspurg, A. Aperger*, 1623.

——. The same. Medicina militaris; or, a body of military medicines experimented. Englished out of High-Dutch. 1 p. l., 30, 152 pp., 6 l. 8°. *London, W. Godbid*, 1674.

Bound with: BARBETTE (Paul). Thesaurus chirurgiæ [etc.] 8°. *London*, 1676.

——. Consilium, oder räthliches Gutachten, die jetzt schwebende und unter den Soldaten mehrertheils grassierende Sucht betreffend.

In his: Medicina militaris. 16°. *Augspurg*, 1623, 22 l.

See, also, **Barbette** (Paul). Thesaurus chirurgiæ [etc.] 3. ed. 8°. *London*, 1676.

Minderlein (Josephus). * De theoria genera-tionis. 32 pp. 8°. *Vindobonæ, F. Ludwig,* [1836].

Minderop (Gerardus Joannes Gustavus). *Twee ziektegevallen door den schrijver waargenomen. 2 p. l., 40 pp. 8°. *Leyden, P. Engels,* 1858.

Minding (Carolus Julius Augustus) [1808-   ]. * De vitæ functionum perturbationibus notiones generales. 29 pp., 1 l. sm. 8°. *Berolini, typ. Nietackianis,* [1833].

——. Nachtrag zu der Beleuchtung des literari-schen Treibens des Herrn Isaac Jacob Sachs, Redacteurs der medicinischen Central-Zeitung, ehedem der Gewerbszeitung, des Stadt- und Landboten und der Erinnerungsblätter, so wie alleinigen Inhabers der Buchhandlung Lieb-mann und Comp. in Berlin. iv, 43 pp. 12°. *Berlin, A. Hirschwald,* 1843.

——. Die vorzüglichsten Bäder und Heilquellen Mittel-Europa's. 70 pp. 16°. *Berlin, F. H. Morin,* 1846.

See, also, **von Behr** (Alfred) & **Minding** (Jul.) Taschen-Encyclopädie, etc. 12°. *Erlangen,* 1845-7.— **Sachs** (J. J.) Würdigung der zeitherigen [etc.] 8°. *Berlin,* 1843.

Also, Editor of : **Beiträge** zur physiologischen und pathologischen Chemie und Mikroscopie [etc.], Berlin, 1843-4.

Mindner (Daniel). * De abortu. 27 pp., 2 l. sm. 4°. *Halæ Magdeb., typ. J. C. Hilligeri,* [1733].

Mind-reading.

FRAZER (P.), jr. Mind reading. 8°. [*n. p., n. d.*]

Beard (G. M.) Muscle-reading versus "mind-read-ing". Detroit Rev. Med. & Pharm., 1875, xi, 520-527. ——. Physiology of mind-reading. Pop. Sc. Month., N. Y., 1876-7, x, 459-473. ——. Physiology of mind-reading. J. Sc., Lond., 1881, 3. s., iii. 407-419. ——. Some new experi-ments in muscle-reading (thought reading). Alienist & Neurol., St. Louis, 1883, iv, 175-182.— **Bishop** (W. I.) Muscle-reading. Science, N. Y., 1886, viii, 506. — **Cum-berland** (S. C.) A thought-reader's experiences. Nine-teenth Cent., Lond., 1886, xx, 867-885.— **Dessoir** (M.) Experiments in muscle-reading and thought-transference. [Transl.] Proc. Soc. Psych. Research, Lond., 1886-7, iv, 111-126.— **Gamale** (N. F) Otgadivanie muslei na razsto-janii. ("Suggestion mentale" Richet.) [Muscle-reading.] Vrach, St. Petersb., 1885, vi, 266 ; 304 — **Gley** (E.) Sur les mouvements musculaires inconscients en rapport avec les images ou représentations mentales. Tribune méd., Par., 1884, xvi, 354. — **Lyman** (H. M.) Notes of an interview with Brown, the "mind-reader". Chicago M. J., 1873, xxx, 505-570.— **McGraw** (T. A.) On mind-reading and allied morbid phenomena. Detroit Rev. Med. & Pharm., 1875, xi, 451-470. — **Mind-reading** and muscle-reading. [Edit.] Boston M. & S. J., 1886, cxv, 532.— **Prince** (M.) Thought-transference. *Ibid.,* 1887, cxvi, 107-112.— **Schmoll** (A.) Experiments in thought-transference. [Transl. from the German original.] Proc. Soc. Psych. Research, Lond., 1886-7, iv, 324-337.— **Sikorski** (I. A.) V chem sostoit t. naz. chtenie ili uznavanie mislei drugago ? [Is mind-read-ing. or the recognizing of thoughts by another, possible ?] Vrach, St. Petersb., 1884, iv, 853 ; 871.— **Symonds** (J. A.) On the relations between mind and muscle. *In his :* Misc., 8°, Lond., 1871, 265-292.

Minehead.

Clark (T.) Minehead as a winter residence for those suffering from chest diseases. Brit. M. J., Lond., 1877, i. 708.

Minel.

See **Indre** (Département de l'). Rapport général sur les travaux du Conseil central d'hygiène et de salubrité pour 1878. 8°. *Châteauroux,* 1879.

Minel (Charles-Camille). * De l'obésité 53 pp. 4°. *Strasbourg,* 1859, No. 472, 2. s., v. 26.

Miner (A. A.) Right and duty of prohibition. Argument before a joint special committee of the Massachusetts legislature, in the Hall of the House of Representatives. April 2, 1867. 122 pp. 8°. *Boston, Wright & Potter,* 1867.

Miner (Julius F.) [1823-86]. Ovariotomy by enucleation ; what it is and how to do it. 7 pp. 8°. *Buffalo, Baker, Jones & Co.,* 1875.

Repr. from : Buffalo M. & S. J., 1875, xiv.

Miner (Julius F.)—continued.

——. The same. 10 pp. 8°. *Philadelphia, Col-lins,* 1877.

Repr. from : Tr. Internat. M. Cong., Phila., 1876.

Also, Editor of : **Buffalo** (The) Medical and Surgical Journal, 1861-79.

For Biography, see Buffalo M. & S. J., 1886-7, xxvi, 233-237 [edit.]. *Also:* N. York M. J., 1886, xliv, 549. *Also:* Med. Press West. N. York, Buffalo, 1885-6, i, 690-693.

Miner (Thomas). Typhus syncopalis, sinking typhus, or the spotted-fever of New England, as it appeared in the epidemic of 1823, in Middle-town, Conn. iv, 5-48 pp. 8°. *Middletown, Conn.,* 1825. [*Also, in :* P., v. 248; 302.]

——. An address to the annual convention of the Medical Society of Connecticut, convened at Hartford May 10, 1837. 12 pp. 8°. *New Haven, B. L. Hamlen,* 1837.

Another copy bound with : Medical Society of Connecti-cut. Communications of the . . . 8°. *New Haven,* 1810.

——. The annual address to the candidates for degrees and licenses in the medical institution of Yale College, Feb. 26, 1839. 20 pp. 8°. *New Haven, B. L. Hamlen,* 1839. [*Also, in :* P., v. 257.]

—— & **Tully** (William). Essays on fevers and other medical subjects. x, 11-484 pp. 8°. *Middletown, E. & H. Clark,* 1823.

——. An examination of the strictures in the New England Journal for October, 1823, and in the North American Review for October, 1823, on Essays on fevers, etc. 32 pp. 8°. *Mid-dletown, Conn., E. & H. Clark,* 1823. [*Also, in :* P., v. 337 ; 761.]

Miner (W. W.)

Co-Editor of : **Buffalo** (The) Medical and Surgical Journal, 1877-9.

Mineral (The) spring waters of the world. Their chemical composition and therapeutic use. 30 l. 16°. *Boston, Rand, Avery & Co.,* [1876?]

Mineral Water Hospital, at Bath. *See* **Bath** General or Mineral Water Hospital.

Mineral *waters*.

See **Waters** (*Mineral*).

Mineralquelle (Die) und die Badenanstalt bei Wohenstein, historisch-topographisch, phy-sikalisch-chemisch und medicinisch-praktisch beleuchtet. vi, 7-83 pp., 1 pl., 1 diag. 16°. [*n. p.*], 1834.

Mineralquelle (Die) zu Niederselters, ihre Bestandtheile und Heilkräfte. 44 pp., 1 pl., 1 l. 8°. *Wiesbaden, L. Riedel,* [1838, *rel subseq.*].

Mineralquellen (Die) im Grossherzogthum Baden, deren Heilkräfte und Heilanstalten, in einer Sammlung medizinisch-theoretischer und praktischer Abhandlungen, zur Förderung für Wissenschaft und Kunst in diesem Theile der Heilkunde, und zum Leitfaden und Nutzen für Kranke, die an diesen Quellen Hülfe suchen. Hrsg. von W. L. Kölreuter. Erster bis dritter Jahrgang, 1820-22. 2 v. in 1. 1 p. l., xviii, 164 pp., 2 pl., 1 tab. ; xxiv, 268 pp., 1 l., 2 pl. 12°. *Carlsruhe u. Baden, D. R. Marr,* [1820-22].

Mineral-Quellen (Die) des Alexandrinen-Bades in Freienwalde a. O. [M. Wreschner, Be-sitzer.] 4 l. 8°. [*Freienwalde a. O.*], *A. Cohn,* [1873].

Mineralquellen (Die) und die Wasserheilan-stalt des Alexandrinen-Bades in Freienwalde a. Oder. [M. Wreschner, Besitzer.] 14 pp. 12°. *Berlin, M. Driesner,* [*n. d.*]

Minerals *in medicine*.

See, also, **Materia** *medica* ; **Metals.**

DUSART (L.-O.) De l'inanition minérale dans les maladies. Première partie. 12°. *Paris,* 1874. **Heckel** (E.) De quelques phénomènes de localisation minérale et organique dans les tissus animaux et de leur importance au point de vue biologique. J. de l'anat. et physiol., etc., Par., 1875, xi, 553-609, 2 pl. — **Polli** (J.)

Minerals *in medicine.*

De l'influence des matières minérales sur la nutrition de
l'organisme humain. J. de méd., chir. et pharmacol.,
Brux., 1871, liii, 224–235.—**Tuson** (R. V.) On the digestion of mineral substances. Lancet, Lond., 1871, ii, 812.—
Ullersperger (J. B.) Die mineralischen Elemente des
organischen Stoffwechsels im physiologisch-pathologisch-
therapeutischen Verhältnisse. Bl. f. Heilwissensch.,
München, 1871, ii, 89.

Mineralwasser (Das) von Geilnau, dessen Bestandtheile, Eigenschaften und Heilkräfte, nebst
einer kurzen Darstellung der örtlichen Verhältnisse der Heilquelle und den nähern Notizen
über die Füllung, Versendung und Behandlung
dieses Mineralwassers. 24 pp., 1 pl., 1 l. 8°.
Wiesbaden, A. Scholz, [*n. d.*]

Minerbi (Angelo). *De phlegmasia alba dolente. 31 pp. 8°. *Patavii, typ. V. Crescini*,
1834. [P., v. 946.]

Miners (*Diseases and hygiene of*).

See, also, **Anchylostoma** *duodenalis*; **Colic**
(*Lead*) *in relation to occupation*; **Heat** (*Effects
of*), *etc.*; **Hemeralopia**, *etc.*; **Lead-poisoning**
(*Causes of*); **Lungs** (*Carbon deposits in*); **Lungs**
(*Foreign deposits in*); **Nystagmus**; **Saint Go-
thard's** *tunnel epidemic.*

BALD (R.) A general view of the coal trade
of Scotland, chiefly that of the river Forth and
Mid-Lothian. To which is added an inquiry
into the condition of the women who carry coals
under ground in Scotland, known by the name
of bearers. With an appendix. 8°. *Edinburgh*,
1812.

BOËNS-BOISSAU (H.) Traité pratique des
maladies, des accidents et des difformités des
houilleurs. 8°. *Bruxelles*, 1862.

BONHOMME (T.-F.) *Étude sur l'anémie des
mineurs. 4°. *Montpellier*, 1865. c.

BOURGUET (É.) *Essai sur l'hygiène des
ouvriers houilleurs. 4°. *Montpellier*, 1864.

BRIZÉ-FRADIN. Secours à employer dans l'exploitation des mines de houille; préservatifs
contre les émanations métalliques, etc., suivi
d'un moyen nouveau pour enlever les asphyxiés.
8°. *Paris*, 1814.

BROCKMANN (C. H.) Die metallurgischen
Krankheiten des Oberharzes. 8°. *Osterode a.
H.*, [1851].

BUISSON (F.-J.-B.) *Étude médicale sur l'ouvrier houilleur. 4°. *Paris*, 1866.

CAUDRON (C.-A.-D.-F.) *Tableau historique,
et description générale de la maladie décrite
sous le nom d'anémie, et qui a attaqué tous les
ouvriers d'une galerie d'une mine de charbon de
terre en exploitation à Fresnes, département du
Nord. 4°. *Paris*, 1818.

COUCH (R. Q.) A statistical investigation into
the mortality of miners in the district of St. Ives,
and the agricultural population in the district
of St. Buryan. 8°. [*n. p.*, 1856?]

DAVY (*Sir* H.) On the safety lamp for coal
miners; with some researches on flame. 8°.
London, 1818.

FABRE (P.) Les mineurs et l'anémie. 8°.
Paris, 1834.

FABRE (S.-P.) De l'influence du travail sou-
terrain sur la santé des mineurs. 8°. *Paris*, 1878.

FRANCE. Instructions sur le caractère des
accidens auxquels les ouvriers mineurs sont exposés, et sur la nature des secours qui doivent
leur être administrés lorsque ces accidens ont
lieu. Rédigée par M. Salmade en exécution du
décret du 3 janvier 1813. 8°. *Paris*, 1813.

FRANTZ (A.) *Die Haftbarkeit und Entschä-
digungspflicht bei den Verunglückungen des
Bergbaus, besonders in Preussen, vom Standpunkte der Gesetzgebung und Volkswirthschaft
betrachtet. 8°. *Jena*, 1869.

Miners (*Diseases and hygiene of*).

FRYAR (M.) The sanitary condition of mines.
8°. [*n. p.*, *n. d.*]

GALLEZ (L.) Premiers secours aux ouvriers
houilleurs blessés. Manuel destiné aux employés et aux porions des charbonnages. 12°.
[*Bruxelles*, 1879.]

HAMMERSCHMIED (J.) Die sanitären Verhältnisse und die Berufskrankheiten der Arbeiter
bei den kais. königl. österreichischen Berg,-
Hütten- und Salinenwerken und Forsten. 8°.
Wien, 1873.

HANOT (G.) De la mortalité des ouvriers
mineurs. 8°. *Bruxelles*, 1846.

HUSTIN (J.-B.-F.-J.) *De la résistance du
houilleur aux grands traumatismes. 4°. *Paris*,
1880.

JOUANNET (A.) *Des troubles digestifs chez
les houilleurs et de leurs rapports avec l'anémie.
4°. *Paris*, 1880.

KUBORN (H.) Étude sur les maladies particulières aux ouvriers mineurs, employés aux exploitations houillères en Belgique. 8°. *Paris*,
1863.

MANOUVRIEZ (A.) Étude d'hygiène industrielle sur la houille et ses dérivés. De l'anémie
des mineurs dite d'Anzin. 8°. *Valenciennes*,
1878.

See, also, infra.

MOLL (E.) *Die Krankheiten der Bergarbeiter
im Allgemeinen und der Oberschlesiens insbesondere. sm. 8°. *Berlin*, [1869].

MOLLER (G.) *De aëre fodinarum metallicarum noxio. Von unterirrdischen bösen Wetter.
sm. 4°. *Halæ Magdeb.*, [1730].

PARACELSUS (A. T.) Von der Bergsucht oder
Bergkranckheiten drey Bücher. 4°. *Dilingen*,
1567.

POLECK (T.) Dr. Scheidemann und die wissenschaftliche Kritik. Eine Beleuchtung der
Scheidemann'schen Schrift: "Die Minenkrankheit, ihre wahre Ursache, Verhütung und Behandlung". 8°. *Berlin*, 1867.

RAYMOND (R. W.) The hygiene of mines. 8°.
[*New York*, 1879.]
Repr. from: Tr. Am. Inst. Mining Engineers.

REID (D. B.) Report on the sanatory condition of New Castle, Gateshead, North Shields,
Sunderland, Durham, and Carlisle, with remarks
on some points connected with the health of the
inhabitants in the adjacent mining district. fol.
[*London*, 1845.]

RICHE (C.) *Pathologie du houilleur. 4°.
Paris, 1874.

ROBERTON (J.) The insalubrity of the deep
Cornish mines, and, as a consequence, the physical degeneracy and early deaths of the mining
population. 8°. [*Manchester*], 1859.

SCHLOCKOW. Die Gesundheitspflege und medizinische Statistik beim preussischen Bergbau.
l. 8°. *Berlin*, 1881.

SCHNABEL (C.) *Geschichtliche Darlegung
und wissenschaftliche Begründung der metallurgischen Processe der Silber-Gewinnung aus sil-
berhaltigem Blei mit Hülfe von Zink unter besonderer Berücksichtigung dieser Processe auf
den Hüttenwerken des Oberharzes. 8°. *Jena*,
1879.

SCHOENFELD (M.) Recherches sur l'état sanitaire des houilleurs pendant la période de salubrité des mines en Belgique. 4°. *Bruxelles*, 1859.

TAYLER (W. W.) Practical observations on
the diseases of the Cornish miners. Part 1. Consumption. 8°. *London*, 1850.

Alison (S. S.) On the diseases, condition, and habits
of the collier population of East Lothian. Lancet, Lond.,
1841-2, i, 800; 854: ii, 90; 161.—**Anémie** (L') des mineurs, histoire, pathogénie, pathologie et thérapeutique.
[Rev.] Arch. gén. de méd., Par., 1878, 7. s., i, 606-620.—

Miners (*Diseases and hygiene of*).

Apuntes acerca de las enfermedades que padecen los mineros de Almadén. Bol. de méd., cirug. y farm., Madrid, 1843, 2. s., iv, 105; 113.—**Arnould** (J.) Note sur l'anémie des mineurs au sujet de deux ouvrages offerts à la Société centrale de médecine. Bull. méd. du nord, Lille, 1878, xvii, 405-410.—**Barham** (C.) The diseases of Cornish miners. Brit. M. J., Lond., 1871, ii, 253-255.—**Beaugrand** (E.) Mines; mineurs. (Hygiène publique et professionnelle.) Dict. encycl. d. sc. méd., Par., 1874, 2. s., viii, 216-252.—[**Bender.**] Zur Minenkrankheit: Aus dem Bericht über die in den Monaten August und September c. zu Coblenz stattgehabte Belagerungsübung. Deutsche mil.-ärztl. Ztschr., Berl., 1875, iv, 632-636.—**Bielczyk** (K.) Niektóre spostrzeżenia nad wpływem ropy (surowca nafty) i jéj gazów zdrowie górników. [Effect of crude naphtha and its gases on the health of miners.] Przegl. lek., Krakow., 1886, xxv, 273-275.—**Boens** (H.) Note sur la valeur des crachats noirs et sur les effets du poussier chez les houilleurs. Bull. Acad. roy. de méd. de Belg., Brux., 1862, 2. s., v, 645-667. [Discussion], 1863, vi, 429; 764: 1864, vii, 125; 228: 381.—**Bourguet.** De l'anémie chez les mineurs. Gaz. d. hôp., Par., 1877, l, 788; 812; 829; 836.—**Boyd** (J.) On mining exhalations. Edinb. M. J., 1871, xvii, 123-126. *Also*, Reprint. ———. On local hygienic influences. Edinb. M. J., 1875, xx, 137; 606.—**Burggraeve.** Rapport sur l'état physique et moral des enfants employés dans les manufactures, usines et mines de la Belgique. Bull. Acad. roy. de méd. de Belg., Brux., 1841-2, i, 675-717.—**Carpenter** (J. T.) Mining, considered with regard to its effects upon health and life. Tr. M. Soc. Penn., Phila., 1869, 5. s., ii, 487-491.—**Church** (J. A.) Accidents resulting from the heat of the Comstock mines. [*From:* Scientific American.] Month. J. Sc., Lond., 1879, 3. s., i, 796-800.—**Commissarischer** Bericht über die Erkrankungen durch Minengase bei der Graudenzer Mineurübung im Jahre 1873. Deutsche mil.-ärztl. Ztschr., Berl., 1875, iv, 379-503. *Also*, Reprint.—**Cox** (W. I.) Diseases of colliers in South Lancashire. Brit. M. J., Lond., 1857, 425; 491; 579. *Also:* J. Pub. Health & San. Rev., Lond., 1856-7, ii, 39; 374: 1857, iii, 48.—**Crocq.** Rapport sur la question mise au concours sur les maladies des houilleurs. Bull. Acad. roy. de méd. de Belg., Brux., 1865, 2. s., viii, 39.—**De Ferrari** (P. E.) Fiasca di salvamento per la respirazione nell' aria viziata delle solfare applicabile anche ai pompieri, alle fabbriche di prodotti chimici, allo spurgo dei pozzi neri, etc. Gior. d. Soc. ital. d' ig., Milano. 1884, vi, 218-228, 1 pl.—**De Lavacherie.** De l'hygiène des ouvriers mineurs et des premiers secours médicaux à leur donner en cas d'accidents. Bull. Acad. roy. de méd. de Belg., Brux., 1841-2, i, 111-161.—**Demarquette.** Essai sur les maladies des ouvriers des mines houillères de Courrières et de Dourges. Monit. d. hôp., Par., 1858, vi, 1164-1168. *Also* [Rap. de Devergie.]: Bull. Acad. de méd., Par., 1859-60, xxv, 214-218.—**Didot** (A.) Aperçu sur la condition des ouvriers et des enfants dans les manufactures, mines et usines de l'arrondissement de Dinant. Bull. Acad. roy. de méd. de Belg., Brux., 1847-8, vii, 126-202. [Rap. de Davreux], 98-102.—**Dransart.** De l'anémie chez les mineurs. Assoc. franç. pour l'avance. d. sc. Compt.-rend. 1882, Par., 1883, xi, 698-701.—**Effects** of the heat in the Nevada mines. Med. & Surg. Reporter, Phila., 1878, xxxiv, 153.—**Emploi** (Sur l') de la lampe de Davy. Ann. d'hyg., Par., 1846, xxxv, 58: xxxvi, 339.—**Erdmann.** Von den Krankheiten der Steinkohlenarbeiter in den Gebirgen des Plauenschen Grundes bei Dresden. J. d. pract. Heilk., Berl., 1831, lxxiii, 6. St., 3-21.—**Escolar** (S.) Notice sur les maladies qui affectent les ouvriers mineurs d'Almaden. Ann. Soc. de méd. prat. de la prov. d'Anvers, Malines, 1849, vii, 393-413.—**Ettmüller** (G.) Die Krankheiten der Silberhüttenarbeiter in den Freiberger Hüttenwerken. Arch. d. deutsch. Med.-Gesetzgeb. u. öff. Gsndhtspflg., Erlang., 1858, ii, 389; 396; 405.—**Evers.** Einige Fälle von Minenkrankheit. Deutsche mil.-ärztl. Ztschr., Berl., 1875, iv, 15-21.—**Fabre** (S.-P.) De l'anémie chez les mineurs. Ann. Soc. de méd. de St.-Étienne et de la Loire (1876), 1877, vi, 471-686. *Also*, Reprint. *Also* [Rap. de Lagout]: Soc. d. sc. méd. de Gannat. Compt.-rend., Par., 1879, xxxiii. 89-96. ———. De l'élévation de la température dans les houillères et des phénomènes qui s'y rattachent au point de vue hygiénique. Bull. Soc. de méd. pub., Par., 1877-9, i, 430-442. ———. Des conditions hygiéniques des houillères. Soc. d. sc. méd. de Gannat. Compt.-rend., Par., 1878. xxxii, 5-10. ———. De l'anoxhémie des houilleurs. *Ibid.*, 1879, xxxiii, 108-116. *Also* [Abstr.]: Progrès méd., Par., 1879, vii, 348. ———. De l'action d'un milieu humide sur l'organisme humain, étudiée spécialement chez les ouvriers mineurs. Rev. d'hyg., Par., 1880, ii, 313-317. ———. De l'état sanitaire des mineurs de nos jours. Gaz. méd. de Par., 1881, 6. s., iii, 6; 27. *Also*, Reprint. ———. La maladie des mineurs du Saint-Gothard et l'anchylostome duodénal. Gaz. méd. de Par., 1881, 6. s., iii, 181-191. ———. Règlementation des mines à grisou. *Ibid.*, 489-491. ———. Du rôle des poussières charbonneuses dans la pathologie du houilleur. France méd., Par., 1882, i, 569. ———. Nouvelles recherches sur l'hygiène des mineurs; des eaux dans les travaux de mine, au point de vue de l'hygiène professionnelle. Rev.

Miners (*Diseases and hygiene of*).

d'hyg., Par., 1883, v, 318-332. *Also*, Reprint. *Also:* Bull. Soc. de méd. pub. 1883, Par., 1884, vi, 123-137. ———. Les mineurs et l'anémie. Soc. d. sc. méd. de Gannat. Compt.-rend. 1883-4, Par., 1884, xxxviii, 143-150.—**Fanöe** (G.) De sanitare Forhold ved Ivigtut Kryolitbrud. 1866-76. Hosp.-Tid., Kjøbenh., 1877. iv, 2. R., 345-356.—**Förster.** Ueber eine Augenkrankheit der Bergwerk-arbeiter. Jahresb. d. schles. Gesellsch. f. vaterl. Kult., Bresl., 1876, 225-228.—**Fossion.** Rapport sur les maladies propres aux ouvriers employés aux travaux des exploitations houillères du royaume. Bull. Acad. roy. de méd. de Belg., Brux., 1857-8, 2. s., i, 601-614. ———. Rapport de la commission chargée d'examiner les mémoires envoyés au concours ouvert sur les maladies propres aux ouvriers employés aux travaux des exploitations houillères du royaume. *Ibid.*, 1861, 2. s., iv, 541-571.—**François.** Résumé et conclusions d'un mémoire sur l'anémie des mineurs en général. Bull. Acad. roy. de méd. de Belg., Brux., 1861, 2. s., iv, 464-469.—**Franz** (K.) Das Verhalten der Bergleute in den Steinkohlengruben zu Brustkrankheiten. Memorabilien, Heilbr., 1879, xxiv, 99-106.—**Gallez** (L.) L'ouvrier houilleur. Bull. Acad. roy. de méd. de Belg., Brux., 1869, 3. s., iii, 633-674. *Also*, Reprint. ———. Des secours immédiats à donner aux ouvriers houilleurs blessés. Bull. Acad. roy. de méd. de Belg., Brux., 1879, 3. s., xiii, 787-794.—**Gauchet** (A.) Maladies des mineurs. N. dict. de méd. et chir. prat., Par., 1876, xxii, 525-559. *Also, transl.* [Abstr.]: Andalucía méd., Córdoba, 1881, vi, 138-143.—**Giordano** (A.) Le disgrazie nelle miniere di zolfo e l' ordinanza della prefettura di Caltanissetta intorno a provvedimenti di pubblica sicurezza. Gior. d. Soc. ital. d' ig., Milano, 1883, v, 409-416.—**Goret** (G.) Lettre sur l'emploi des femmes dans les travaux souterrains. Bull. Acad. roy. de méd. de Belg., Brux., 1869, 3. s., iii, 5-11. [Discussion], 11; 99; 366; 483; 632; 730; 807; 927; 1044; 1239.—**Guinard** (A.) De l'anémie chez les mineurs. Ann. Soc. de méd. de St.-Étienne et de la Loire, 1876 (1877), vi, 353-470.—**Hallé.** Observations sommaires sur une maladie qu'on peut nommer anæmie, qui a attaqué tous les ouvriers d'une galerie dans une mine d'anthracite ou charbon de terre, en exploitation à Anzain, Frênes et Vieux-Condé, près Valenciennes. J. de méd., chir., pharm., etc., Par., 1805, ix, 3-17. ———. Observations additionnelles sur les quatre maladies dont il a été parlé dans la notice insérée dans le numéro de vendémiaire, an XIII. *Ibid.*, 138-144.—**Hanot** (G.) De la mortalité des ouvriers mineurs. Arch. méd. belge, Brux., 1845, xviii, 205-243: 1846, xix, 1; 121; 237.—**Health** (On the) of the mining population. Brit. & For. M.-Chir. Rev., Lond., 1865, xxxv, 363-373.—**Hesse** (W.) Das Vorkommen von primärem Lungenkrebs bei den Bergleuten der consortschaftlichen Gruben in Schneeberg. Arch. d. Heilk., Leipz., 1878, xix, 160-162. ———. Beitrag zur Grubenhygiene. Deutsche Vrtljschr. f. öff. Gsndhtspflg., Brnschwg., 1878, x, 279-284.—**Hinze.** Pathologische Fragmente über die Krankheiten der Berg- und Hüttenleute; aus einem grösseren, nächstens erscheinenden Werke mitgetheilt. Arch. f. med. Erfahr., Berl., 1825, ii, 202-211.—**Holland** (P. H.) In what way can the needless exposure of workmen to danger to life and health be best avoided, especially in collieries, mines, and manufactories? Tr. Nat. Ass. Promot. Social Sc. 1865, Lond., 1866, 377-382. [Discussion], 465-468.—**Jackson** (T. H.) Diseases of miners of Arkendale and Swaledale. Assoc. M. J., Lond., 1857, ii, 619.—**Josephson** (E.) Die Minenkrankheit. Preuss. mil.-ärztl. Ztg., Berl., 1861, ii, 9-16.—**Kauzler.** Die Minenkrankheit der Pioniere. Wehnschr. f. d. ges. Heilk., Berl., 1841, 476-478.—**Kuborn** (H.) Étude sur les maladies particulières aux ouvriers mineurs employés aux explorations houillères en Belgique. Mém. d. concours . . . Acad. roy. de méd. de Belg., Brux., 1860, v, 59-282. ———. Du rôle pathogénique des poussières charbonneuses des organes respiratoires des ouvriers mineurs. Bull. Acad. roy. de méd. de Belg., Brux., 1863, 2. s., vi, 204-274. [Rap. de Crocq], 27-38. [Discussion], 429; 764: 1864, vii, 125; 228; 381. ———. L'emploi des femmes dans les travaux souterrains des mines. *Ibid.*, 1868, 3. s., ii, 802-889. [Discussion], 1869, 3. s., iii, 11; 99; 366; 483; 632; 730; 927; 1044; 1058; 1239. ———. [Du travail des femmes et des enfants dans les mines de houille; réponse faite aux objections présentées à la Commission académique.] *Ibid.*, 1052-1212. *Also*, Reprint. — **Küpper** (F.) Krankheiten und Gefahren, welche den Bergmann in Steinkohlengruben bedrohen. Med. Cor.-Bl. rhein. u. westfäl. Aerzte, Bonn, 1845, iv, 268; 273; 292; 309; 323; 337.—**Langendorff.** Ueber die Gesundheitsrücksichten bei Anlage und Unterhaltung von Hüttenwerken. Ztschr. f. d. Staatsarznk., Erlang., 1857, lxxiii, 237-314, 1 pl.—**Lederle** (F.) Beobachtungen über die Krankheiten der Arbeiter der Silber- und Bleibergwerke und der Schmelzhütte im Münsterthal (Bez. Amt Staufen), nebst einigen Beiträgen zur Topographie und Statistik. Med. Ann., Heidelb., 1838, iv, 593-614. — **Lesage.** Note sur l'anémie des mineurs dite d'Anzin. Bull. méd. du nord, Lille, 1882, xxi, 56-59.—**Levy** (E.) Die Minenkrankheit. Allg. Wien. med. Ztg., 1877, xxii, 320; 331; 339.—**Life** (The), diseases, and death of the miner. Brit. & For. M.-Chir. Rev., Lond., 1860, xxvi, 39-67.—**Lobato**

Miners (*Diseases and hygiene of*).

(J. G.) Maduracion por las atmósferas deletéreas en las labores de las minas de metales argentiferos. Gac. méd. de México, 1875, x, 9; 28. — **Loewe.** Ueber die Schädlichkeiten, die in Steinkohlenbergwerken herrschen, und die dadurch veranlassten Krankheiten der Bergleute. J. d. pract. Heilk., Berl., 1838, lxxxvi, 6. St., 12–34. — **Logan** (T. M.) Accidents and explosives in mines. Rep. Bd. Health Calif. 1871–3, Sacramento, 1873, 141–150.— **Lorenzutti.** Antracosi. Resoc. san. d. osp. di Trieste, 1876, i, 80. — **Mallett** (G.) Remarks on accidents occurring to colliers. Assoc. M. J., Lond., 1855, ii, 929.— **Manouvriez** (A.) Mémoire sur les maladies et l'hygiène des ouvriers travaillant à la fabrication des agglomérés de houille et de brai. Cong. internat. d'hyg., Brux., 1876, i, 823–830. ———. De l'anémie chez les mineurs. Ann. Soc. de méd. de St.-Étienne et de la Loire (1876), 1877, vi, 123–352. [*See, also, supra.*] ———. État de l'anémie des houilleurs. Ann. Soc. de méd de St.-Étienne et de la Loire (1877–80), 1881, vii, 344–347. ———. De l'anémie des mineurs dite d'Anzin. Cong. périod. internat. d. sc. méd. Compt.-rend. 1877. Genève, 1878, v, 525–529. ———. État de l'endémie houillère d'Anzin; anémie des mineurs et maladies de brai. Ann. d'hyg., Par., 1885, 3. s., xiii, 164–166. — **Marten.** Die Schädlichkeiten und Krankheiten, denen die Kohlengruben-Arbeiter unterworfen sind. Vrtljschr. f. gerichtl. u. öff. Med., Berl., 1859, xvi, 264–277.— **Minenkrankheit** (Die). *Ibid.*, 1867, vii, 358–368.— **Note** sur l'éclairage des mines. Ann. d'hyg., Par., 1846, xxxv, 349.—**Observacion** de un calambrista con sudores y calentura, producidos por los trabajos de las minas de Almadén. Bol. de med., cirug. y farm.. Madrid, 1843, 2. s., iv, 241.—**Osler** (W.) Miners' phthisis. Canada M. & S. J., Montreal, 1879, vii, 452–454. *Also:* Montreal Gen. Hosp. Rep., 1880, i, 297–299.—**Panthel.** Ueber den Einfluss des Braunstein-Bergbaus auf die Gesundheit der Arbeiter. Med. Jahrb. f. Nassau, Wiesb., 1852, 652–662.— **Ploem** (J. C.) Eenige waarnemingen bij lood- en zinkmijn-arbeiders gedaan. Geneesk. Tijdschr. v. Nederl. Indië, Batav., 1854, iii, 202–212.—**Proust** (A.) Rapport sur les accidents auxquels sont exposés les ouvriers mineurs; instruction sur la nature des secours qui doivent leur être donnés. Bull. Acad. de méd., Par., 1881, 2. s., x, 336–356.— **Rawitz.** Zur Minenkrankheit. Preuss. militärärztl. Ztg., Berl., 1862, 121; 133. — **Remertz** (H.) Ueber die sanitätspolizeiliche Beaufsichtigung des Bergbaues. Vrtljschr. f. gerichtl. u. öff. Med., Berl., 1869, xi, 193–249.— **Riembault.** De l'anémie des mineurs. Ann. Soc. de méd. de St.-Étienne et de la Loire (1860), 1861, i, 748–755.— **Ripa** (L.) Le condizioni igieniche degli operai del Gottardo, e di altri congeneri lavori davanti alla Camera dei deputati. Atti Accad. fis.-med.-statist. di Milano, 1882, xxxviii, 143–148.—**Roberton** (J.) The insalubrity of the deep Cornish mines, and, as a consequence, the physical degeneracy and early deaths of the mining population. Tr. Manchester Statist. Soc., 1858–9, 43–66.—**Schaible.** Die Steinkohlengrube zu Berghaupten; ihr Einfluss auf die Gesundheit der Grubenarbeiter. Mitth. d. badisch. ärztl. Ver., Karlsruhe, 1857, xi, 33–40.— **Scheidemann** (T.) Die Minenkrankheit, ihre wahre Ursache, Verhütung und Behandlung. Vrtljschr. f. gerichtl. u. öff. Med., Berl., 1866, v, 177–253.—**Schirmer.** Die Krankheiten der Bergleute in den Grünberger Braunkohlengruben. Vrtljschr. f. gerichtl. u. öff. Med., Berl., 1856, x, 300–326. *Also, transl.* [Abstr.]: Ann. d'hyg., Par., 1859, 2. s., xi, 210–218. — **Schlockow.** Ueber die gesundheitsschädlichen Verhältnisse in den Bergwerken. Jahresb. d. schles. Gesellsch. f. vaterl. Kult. 1880, Bresl., 1881, lviii, 104–106. *Also:* Breslau. aerztl. Ztschr., 1881, iii, 115.—**Schoenfeld** (M.) Recherches sur l'état sanitaire des houilleurs pendant la période de salubrité des mines en Belgique. Mém. d. concours . . . Acad. roy. de méd. de Belg., Brux., 1855, iii, 261–424.—**Schwartz** (E.) Affections produites par les gaz résultant des mines de guerre. Ann. d'hyg., Par., 1877, 2. s., xlvii, 273–284.—**Seltmann.** Die Anthrakosis der Lungen bei den Kohlenbergarbeitern. Jahresb. d. Gesellsch. f. Nat.- u. Heilk. in Dresd., 1865, 108–129. — Die Lungenschwindsucht bei den Kohlenbergarbeitern. Sitzungsb. d. Gesellsch. f. Nat.- u. Heilk. zu Dresd., 1868–9, ii, 137–149.—**Senft** (H.) Der schlesische Steinkohlenbergbau in sanitätspolizeilicher Beziehung. Wien. med. Presse, 1879, xx, 1153; 1184; 1241; 1276. — **Sheafer** (H. C.) Hygiene of coal-mines. Cycl. Pract. M. (Ziemssen), N. Y.. 1879, xix, 27–264.—**Soviche** (J.) Nachricht von acht Leuten, die 136 Stunden lang in einer Steinkohlengrube abgesperrt waren. Gesundheit, Wien, 1837, n. F., i, 118–120.—**Sykes** (W.) Clinical notes and remarks on a disease of the eyes peculiar to colliers. Brit. M. J., Lond., 1881, ii, 77. — **Tanquerel des Planches** (L.) Note sur l'anémie d'Anzin. J. de méd., Par., 1843, i, 109–115. *Also:* Ann. de méd. belge, Brux., 1843, ii, 96–100. — **Thomson** (J. B.) The melanosis of miners. Edinb. M. J., 1858, iv, 226–235.—**Valat** (L.-J.-A.) Coup d'œil thérapeutique sur les caractères généraux des maladies des ouvriers des mines. Bull. gén de thérap., etc., Par., 1834, vii, 185–189. ———. Histoire médicale et statistique des ouvriers mineurs de la houillère de Decise (département de la Nièvre). Rev. méd. franç. et étrang., Par., 1835, i, 337–

Miners (*Diseases and hygiene of*).

366: ii, 30; 181.—**Virchow** (R.) The pathology of miners' lung. Edinb. M. J., 1858, iv, 204–243. *Also, Reprint.—* **Weickert** (H. E.) Ueber die Krankheiten der Hüttenarbeiter im Allgemeinen und über die im Jahre 1861 insbesondere. Ztschr. f. Med., Chir. u Geburtsh., Leipz., 1862, n. F., i, 414–429. ———. Ueber die Krankheiten der Arbeiter in den fiskalischen Hütten bei Freiberg vom J. 1862–75, mit Vorbemerkungen über die betr. Hüttenprocesse und die Arbeiter im Allgemeinen. Jahresb. d. Gesellsch. f. Nat.- u. Heilk. in Dresd., 1877, 14, 88.—**Wilson** (J.) An account of the disease called mill-reek by the miners at Leadhills. Essays & Obs. Soc. Edinb., 1754, i, 459–466. *Also:* 2. ed., Edinb., 1771, 517–526.—**Zuber** (C.) Mines (maladie des). Dict. encycl. d. sc. méd., Par., 1876, 2. s., xi, 353–357.

Minervini (Gabriele). Dell' epilessia. 214 pp. 8°. *Napoli, Tramater, 1847.*

———. Caso di ematuria grave comunicato all' Accademia medico-chirurgica di Napoli. 11 pp. 8°. *Napoli, F. Vitale, 1852.*

———. Monografia della clorosi. 2 p. l., 327 pp., 1 pl. 8°. *Napoli, Cataneo, 1853.*

———. Memorie fisiologiche riguardante la mestruazione. 126 pp., 1 l. 8°. *Napoli, Tramater, 1854.*

———. L' albuminuria in rapporto all' eclampsia. (Memoria letta a quell' Accademia medico-chirurgica di Napoli nella tornata del 28 luglio 1855.) 10 pp. 4°. [*Napoli*, 1855.]

———. Sulla scrofola messa a confronto colla tubercolosi e colla rachitide; ragionamenti due letti nelle tornate de' 17 giugno e 17 agosto 1855. 213–379 pp. 4°. [*Napoli*, 1855.]
Cutting from: Atti dell' Accademia pontaniana, Napoli, 1855, vii, pt. 2.

———. Trattato dell' eclampsie de' fanciulli extracerebrali, ossia provenienti da morbi che son posti fuori i centri nervosi, e della loro frequenza nella dentizione. (Lavoro approvato dall' Accademia medico-chirurgica di Napoli.) 278 pp., 1 l. 8°. *Napoli, Sebeto, 1857.*

Mines (*Ventilation of*).

See, *also*, **Ventilation**.

BLACKWELL (J. K.) Report on ventilation of mines. 25th March, 1850. fol. *London*, 1850.

BROWN (M. W.) A theory of mine ventilation. 8°. *Newcastle-on-Tyne*, 1884.

PHILLIPS (J.) Report on the ventilation of mines and collieries. fol. *London*, 1850.

Colquhoun (A.) The deterioration of the atmosphere in mines, caused by the explosion of nitro-glycerine preparations. Austral. M. J., Melbourne, 1881, n. s., iii, 252–256.—**Fairley** (W.) The theory and practice of ventilating coal mines. Van Nostrand's Engin. Mag., N. Y., 1882, xxvi, 186; 281.—**Murgue** (D.) Centrifugal ventilators for mines. [*From:* Proc. Inst. Civil Engin.] *Ibid.*, 1883, xxix, 222–228.

Mines (*Ventilation of*). [*Patents.*]

Beadle (J. L.) Mine ventilator. No. 47,694; May 16, 1865. — **Fisk & Westerman.** Mine ventilator. No. 45,918; Jan. 17, 1865. — **Greis** (W.) Apparatus for ventilating mines. No. 182,916; Oct. 3, 1876. — **Haupt** (H.) Ventilating mines. No. 48,065; June 6, 1865. — **Henry** (L. J.) Process for ventilating, purifying, and cooling the atmosphere of mines. No. 162,920; May 4, 1875.—**Jones** (J. B.) Mine ventilator. No. 102,681; May 3, 1870.— **Joseph** (T.) Cooling and ventilating mines, houses, etc. No. 181,945; Sept. 5, 1876. — **Kay** (J.) & **Rockefeller** (S) Ventilating apparatus for mines. No. 220,387; Oct. 7, 1879. — **McBroome** (J. R.) Furnace for ventilating mines. No. 239,816; April 5, 1881.—**Murphy** (F.) Mine-ventilating apparatus. No. 176,756; May 2, 1876. ———. Ventilating-apparatus for coal-mines. No. 163,098; May 11, 1875. ———. Ventilating apparatus for coal-mines. No. 176,757; May 2, 1876. — **Phillips** (W.) Means for ventilating mining shafts and tunnels. No. 294,805; March 4, 1884. — **Tessie du Motay** (C. M.) & **Beckwith** (L. F.) Method and means of ventilating mines, etc., and operating machinery therein. No. 219,037; Aug. 26, 1879.— **Weston** (M. L. D.) Apparatus for ventilating mines. No. 315,578; April 14, 1885.—**Williamson** (G. W.) Ventilating mines. No. 153,878; Aug. 4, 1874.—**Wilson** (T.), jr. Mine-ventilator. No. 325,034; Aug. 25, 1885.

Mingolsheim.

Speyer (A. F.) Die Schwefelquelle zu Mingolsheim im Grossherzogthum Baden. J. d. pract. Heilk., Berl., 1839, lxxxviii, 5. St., 48–61.

Mingoni (Josephus). Historia medica thermarum Patavinarum sive observationum medicopracticarum circa morbos iisdem thermis tractatos centuria prima. xxiv, cclxxxii pp. 4°. *Patavii, J. B. Penada,* 1775.

Minguet (Ferdinand-Timothée). * De la péritonite puerpérale aiguë. 20 pp. 4°. *Paris,* 1837, No. 270, v. 314.

Minguez (Perez M.)
    Editor of : **Diario** (El) médico-farmacéutico, Madrid, 1884.

Minich (Angelo) [1817–]. Degli apparecchi inamovibili e dell' estensione permanente nella cura delle malattie chirurgiche. 117 pp., 4 pl. 8°. *Venezia, G. Antonelli,* 1871.
    Repr. from : Atti r. Ist. Veneto di sc., lett. ed arti, 1870–71, 3. s., xvi.

――. Cura antisettica delle ferite e proposta di un nuovo metodo. 54 pp. 4°. *Venezia, G. Antonelli,* 1876.
    Repr. from : Mem. r. Ist. Veneto di sc., lett. ed arti, 1876, xix.

――. Sulla cura solvente di alcuni neoplasmi; memoria letta al r. Istituto Veneto di scienze, lettere ed arti nella seduta del 29 dicembre 1878. 17 pp. 8°. *Venezia, G. Antonelli,* 1879.

――. Commemorazione del professore Francesco Marzolo. 31 pp. 8°. *Venezia, G. Antonelli,* 1880.
    Repr. from : Atti r. Ist. Veneto di sc., lett. ed arti, 1880, vii.

――. Sulla lussazione divergente antero-posteriore del cubito. 34 pp. 8°. *Venezia, G. Antonelli,* 1880.
    Also, Co-Editor of : **Rivista** veneta di scienze mediche, Venezia, 1884.

Minier (Pierre-Joseph). * Il n'y a pas de phthisie sans inflammation préalable. vi, 7–24 pp. 4°. *Paris,* 1832, No. 198, v. 254.

Minière (Joseph-Xavier) [1859–]. * Emphysème traumatique considéré surtout comme complication des fractures de côtes. 47 pp. 4°. *Paris,* 1883.

Minière (Théodore). * Symptômes et diagnostic du testicule syphilitique. xii, 130 pp., 1 l. 4°. *Paris,* 1881, No. 229.

Minime (*Docteur*). La prostitution et la traite des blanches à Londres et à Paris. Études médicales et sociales sur la prostitution à Londres et à Paris; statistiques municipales; Saint-Lazare et Lourcine. Le tribut des vierges et la moderne Babylone. La prostitution et la police, [etc.] xci, 274 pp. 8°. *Paris, C. Marpon & Flammarion,* 1886.

――. Le Parnasse Hippocratique. Recueil de poésies fantaisistes tirées de différents auteurs plus ou moins drolatiques sur des sujets Hippocratiques de genres divers, hormis le genre ennuyeux. Nouv. éd. viii, 237 pp. 16°. *Paris, C. Marpon & E. Flammarion,* 1887.

Mining and Petroleum Standard and American Gas-Light Journal. Devoted to mining, petroleum, gas, water-supply, and scientific subjects generally. [Semi-monthly.] Bryant, Callender & Co., editors and proprietors. v. 8–9, July 2, 1866, to June 16, 1868. fol. *New York.*
    Want nos. 1–14, 20, v. 8; no. 12, v. 9. See **American** (The) Gas-Light Journal and Chemical Repertory for v. 10, *et seq.*

Ministers.
    See **Clergymen.**

Ministers' Seaside Home, Morthoe, North Devon. Report and statement of accounts for the year 1882. 4 pp. 4°. [*Bristol,* 1883.]

Minium.
    d'Astros (L.) L'industrie du minium à Marseille au point de vue de l'hygiène professionnelle. Marseille méd., 1885, xxii, 641–647. [Discussion], 682.—**Layet.** La fabrication du minium ; étude d'hygiène professionnelle et industrielle. Gaz. hebd. d. sc. méd. de Bordeaux, 1880, i, 183–188.

Minjak-Lagam.
    HAUSSNER (G.) * Ueber Minjak-Lagam. Ein Beitrag zur chemischen Kenntniss der Balsame aus der Familie der Dipterocarpeen. 8°. *Halle a. S.,* 1883.

Mink (Petrus Joh.) * Over het aneurysma cirsoïdeum van de hand. 72 pp., 1 l. 8°. [*Amsterdam, T. Horneer,* 1885.]

Minkowski (Oskar) [1858–]. * Ueber die Aenderungen der elektrischen Erregbarkeit des Gehirns nach Verschluss der Kopfarterien. 42 pp., 1 l. 8°. *Königsberg, Hartung,* [1881].

――. Ueber den Kohlensäuregehalt des arteriellen Blutes beim Fieber. 30 pp. 8°. *Leipzig, J. B. Hirschfeld,* 1885.
    Repr. from : Arch. f. exper. Path. u. Pharmacol., Leipz., 1885, xix.

Minkrevitch (Gabriel). * Razsujenie o nekotorych bolieznjach syvorotochno-suchojilnago sostava na konechnostjach loshadi. [Dissertation (veterinary) on some diseases affecting the tendinous insertions in horses.] 79 pp., 1 l. 8°. *St. Petersburg,* 1859.

Minks (Arthur). * Ueber Acidum carbolicum als neues Heilmittel. 36 pp. 8°. *Greifswald, F. W. Kunike,* 1869.   C.

Minneapolis. Statements of mortality of the city of Minneapolis. [Monthly.] By the health officer. Accompanied by an abstract of meteorological observations. April, 1882, to Nov., 1886. 8°. *Minneapolis,* 1882–6.

――. Annual report of the board of water commissioners of the city of Minneapolis, Minn. 2., 1882–3. 45 pp. 8°. *Minneapolis,* 1883.

――. Reports of deaths in Minneapolis. [Weekly.] Dec. 8 to 22, 1883; Jan. 5 to Nov. 1; Nov. 15, 1884, to Jan. 3, 1885. 18°. [*Minneapolis,* 1883–5.]

――. Annual report of the board of park commissioners of the city of Minneapolis to the legislature. 1., 1883–4. 16 pp., 3 plans. 8°. *Minneapolis, Johnson, Smith & Harrison,* 1884.
    Organized March 14, 1883.

――. Summary of mortality for the year 1883–4. 1 sheet. fol. *Minneapolis,* 1884.

Minneapolis.
    CLEVELAND (H. W. S.) Suggestions for a system of parks and parkways for the city of Minneapolis. Read at a meeting of the park commissioners, June 2, 1883. 8°. *Minneapolis,* 1883.
    UNIVERSITY of Minnesota, Minneapolis. Calendar for the year 1876–7. 8°. *Minneapolis,* 1877.
    Simpson (C.) Report of deaths in the city of Minneapolis from July 1, 1872, to May 20, 1873. Northwest. M. & S. J., St. Paul, Minn., 1872–3, iii, 79 ; 165 ; 242 ; 282 ; 325 ; 370 ; 402 ; 441 ; 488.

Minnequa.
    CRESSON (C. M.) & **HINKLE** (F.) Minnequa Springs, Bradford Co., Pa. Analysis of the water; therapeutical effects. 8°. *Philadelphia,* [1875].
    ―― ――. The same. 12°. *Williamsport, Pa.,* 1876.

Minner (Joh. Christophorus). * De pulmonum vomica. 10 l. sm. 4°. [*Vitembergæ*], *lit. Fingelianis,* [1700].

Minnesota. Minnesota; its progress and capabilities; being the second annual report of the commissioner of statistics for the years 1860 and 1861. 126 pp. 8°. *Saint Paul,* 1862.

――. Annual reports of the adjutant-general of the State of Minnesota for the years 1863–5. 3 v. 8°. *St. Paul,* 1864–6.

――. Annual report of the adjutant-general of the State of Minnesota for the year ending Dec.

Minnesota—continued.

1, 1866, and of the military forces of the State from 1861 to 1866. 805 pp. 8°. *Saint Paul, Pioneer Printing Company*, 1866.

——. Minnesota; its resources and progress; its beauty, healthfulness, and fertility: and its attractions and advantages as a home for immigrants. Compiled by the commissioner of statistics, and published by direction of the governor. 72 pp. 8°. *St. Paul, Press Printing Company*, 1870.

——. Statistics of the State of Minnesota. Being the annual reports of the commissioner of statistics to the governor of the State. N. s. 12., 1880; 13., 1881. 8°. *St. Peter & St. Paul*, 1881–2.

——. An act relating to infectious and epidemic diseases and the preservation of the public health. Approved March 3, 1883. 8 pp. 8°. [*St. Paul*, 1883.]

——. The geological and natural history survey of Minnesota. N. H. Winchel, State geologist. 1872–82. The geology of Minnesota. v. 1 of the final report. By N. H. Winchel, assisted by Warren Upham. Submitted March 10, 1882, and published under the direction of the Hon. Fred. von Baumbach. xii, 697 pp., 12 pl., 31 maps. fol. *Minneapolis, Johnson, Smith & Harrison*, 1884.

Minnesota.

See, also, **Deaf-mutes** (*Asylums, etc., for*); **Education** (*Medical*), *etc., by localities*; **Insane** (*Asylums for, etc.*), *by localities*; **Leprosy** (*History, etc., of*); **Minneapolis**; **Saint Paul**.

HEWITT (C. N.) Report on the climatology and epidemics of Minnesota. 8°. *Philadelphia*, 1831.

HISTORICAL Society of Minnesota. Annals for the years 1850 and 1851. 8°. *St. Paul*, 1851.

——. Annual reports of the Minnesota Historical Society for the years 1868, 1870, and 1876. 8°. *St. Paul*, 1869–77.

MATTOCKS (B.) Minnesota as a home for invalids. 12°. *Philadelphia*, 1871.

MINNESOTA. Minnesota, its resources and progress; its beauty, healthfulness, and fertility; and its attractions and advantages as a home for immigrants. Compiled by the commissioner of statistics, and published by direction of the governor. 8°. *St. Paul*, 1870.

Adams (B. F. D.) Minnesota as a resort in pulmonary affections. Boston M. & S. J., 1870, vi, 337–339.—**Carpenter** (F. D. Y.) Minnesota weather. Science, Cambridge, 1883, ii, 262–265.—**Climatology** and diseases of Minnesota; report of committee to annual meeting of State medical Society, February 7, 1871: published by request of the State Society. Northwest. M. & S. J., St. Paul, Minn., 1871, ii, 50–60.—**Finch** (J. E.) Report of the committee on epidemics, climatology, and hygiene. Minnesota M. Soc., St. Paul, 1874, 49–61.—**Finch** (W. W.) Physicians, the climate, and diseases in Minnesota Territory. Boston M. & S. J., 1854, xlix, 213.—**Hand** (D. W.) Diseases of Minnesota and the Northwest. Tr. Am. M. Ass., Phila., 1875, xxvi, 371–379.—**Hewitt** (C. N.) Report on the climatology and epidemics of Minnesota. *Ibid.*, 1871, xxii, 215–231: 1872, xxiii, 459–471. *Also, Reprint.*—**Jones** (T.) A plea for cold climates, in the treatment of pulmonary consumption; Minnesota as a health resort. N. York M. J., 1879, xxx, 269–300. *Also, Reprint.*—Midwinter treatment of phthisis in Minnesota; clinical study of thirteen cases, with results. Med. Rec., N. Y., 1880, xvii, 252–255.—**Leonard** (W. H.) Report on the meteorology of Minnesota, for the years 1875–6 and 1876–7. Rep. Bd. Health Minn. 1877, Minneap., 1878, vi, 43–53.—**Lewis** (G.) The climate of the State of Minnesota, and its adaptation to persons suffering from phthisis pulmonalis. Am. M. Times, N.Y., 1862, iv, 147: 162.—**Mattocks** (B.) The effects of climate upon the lungs, with special reference to Minnesota. Med. Rec., N. Y., 1869, iv, 121–123. ——. Has the climate of Minnesota changed within the past fifteen years? Northwest. M. & S. J., St. Paul, Minn., 1871, ii, 97–110.—**Record** of meteorological observations of Minnesota; taken under the direction of the State board of health. Rep. Bd. Health Minn. 1875, St. Paul, 1876, iv, 87–127.—**Report** of the committee on climatology and epidemics for 1871, Minnesota. Tr. Minn.

Minnesota.

M. Soc., Minneap., 1872, 60–76.—**Sanitary** (The) water survey of the State; chemical analyses of waters from lakes, rivers, springs, wells, cisterns, and from melted snow. Rep. Bd. Health Minn., St. Peter, 1881, viii, 127–141.—**Senkler** (A. E.) The peculiarities of the climate of Minnesota, with especial reference to its dryness, and the presence and operation of ozone (first report). *Ibid.*, St. Paul, 1876, 83–86.—**Staples** (F.) The influence of the climate of Minnesota upon diseases of the lungs and air passages. *Ibid.*, 55–67. ——. Report on the influence of climate on pulmonary diseases in Minnesota. Tr. Am. M. Ass., Phila., 1876, xxvii, 381–434. *Also, Reprint.*—**Sweeny** (W. W.) Endemic and epidemic diseases of Minnesota. Northwest. M. & S. J., St. Paul, 1870–71, i, 193–215.

Minnesota. *Minnesota Institution for the Education of the Deaf and Dumb, and the Blind, Faribault.* Annual reports of the directors and officers to the governor of Minnesota. 4.-6., 1865–6 to 1867–8; 8., 1869–70; 10., 1871–2; 12., 1873–4; 13., 1874–5. 8°. *St. Paul*, 1866–76.

Minnesota. *Second Minnesota Hospital for Insane, at Rochester.* Annual and biennial reports of the board of trustees and officers to the governor of the State. 1., 1877–8; 1.-3., bien., 1878–9 to 1883–4.

In: Rep. Minn. Hosp. Ins., St. Peter.

Minnesota. *State Board of Health of the State of Minnesota.* Annual reports to the governor of the State. 1.-10., 1872 to 1883–4. 8°. *Saint Paul & Minneapolis*, 1873–84.

——. The relations of scholastic methods to the health of pupils in the public schools. A preliminary inquiry into the subject. By the secretary of the State board of health. 41 pp. 8°. *Minneapolis, Johnson, Smith & Harrison*, 1878.

——. A plan for the completion of the organization of conference of State boards of health, proposed by the State board of Minnesota to the conference meeting in St. Louis, October 13, 1884. 2 l. 8°. [*n. p.*, 1884.]

——. Public Health, a monthly journal of State, municipal, family, and personal hygiene, and of veterinary sanitary science. The official publication of the State board of health of Minnesota. Edited by Chas. N. Hewitt, sec. of the board. v. 1–3. March, 1885, to Feb., 1888. 8°. *Red Wing*, 1885–8.

——. Minnesota from the standpoint of public health. Compiled by the secretary of the State board of health, as superintendent of Minnesota sanitary exhibit at the exposition in New Orleans in 1885. 17, 16 pp. 8°. *Saint Paul, W. T. Rich & Co.*, 1885.

——. Form 1. Sanitary inspection. Sanitary inspection of towns, villages, boroughs, and cities. 2 l. 8°. [*Red Wing*, 1885.]

——. Public health in Minnesota. The official publication of the State board of health. Published monthly, Red Wing, Minn. v. 1. Nos. 1–11. March, 1885, to Jan., 1886. 8°. [*Red Wing*, 1885–6.]

——. The organization, powers, and duties of local boards of health. An abstract of the laws of Minnesota relating thereto. Extra to "Public Health". 2 l. 8°. [*Red Wing*, 1886?]

Minnesota. *State Board of Medical Examiners.* Explanatory announcement. 3 pp. 8°. [*n. p.*, 1883.]

Minnesota; its advantages to settlers. Being a brief synopsis of its history and progress, climate, soil, agricultural and manufacturing facilities, commercial capacities, and social status; its lakes, rivers, and railroads; homestead and exemption laws; embracing a concise treatise on its climatology in a hygienic and sanitary point of view; its unparalleled salubrity, growth, and productiveness, as compared with the older States; and the elements of its future greatness and prosperity. 4. ed. 36 pp. 8°. *St. Paul*, 1867.

Minnesota Historical Society. Annual report for the year 1876. 26 pp. 8°. *St. Paul*, 1877.

Minnesota Hospital College, Minneapolis. Annual announcements of the collegiate department for the sessions of 1882–3 to 1886–7 (2.–6.). 8°. *Minneapolis*, 1882–6.

List of students and graduates for the sessions of 1881–2 to 1885–6, in announcements for subsequent years.

Minnesota Hospital for the Insane, at St. Peter. By-laws, rules, and regulations. 22 pp. 8°. *St. Paul, Pioneer Printing Co.*, 1867.

Bound with: Reports 1–9, 1866–7 to 1874–5.
Established March 2 and opened Dec. 6, 1866.

———. Annual and biennial reports of the board of trustees and officers to the governor of the state. 1.–12., 1866–7 to 1877–8; 1.–3., bien., 1878–9 to 1883–4. 8°. *St. Paul & Minneapolis*, 1868–84.

Reports for 1878–9 to 1883–4 are biennial, and include reports of both State hospitals for the insane, at St. Peter and Rochester.

———. [Blank forms in use at the hospital.] v. s. [*Minneapolis*, 188–.]

Abstract of personal and medical history. Notice to county clerk of discharge of patient. Questions to be answered by friends of patient.

———. Announcement for the spring session of 1886. 1 sheet. 8°. [*Minneapolis*, 1886.]

Minnesota (The) Medical Mirror. A monthly journal of the progress made in medicine, surgery, and pharmacy. Edited by N. M. Cook. v. 1–4, Dec., 1881, to March, 1885. 8°. *Cambridge City*.

No. 3, v. 4, last published.

Minnesota (The) Medical Monthly; a journal devoted to the interests of homœopathy and its practitioners in the Northwest. Editor: William E. Leonard. v. 1–2, May, 1886, to Oct., 1887. 8°. *Minneapolis*.

Current.

Minnesota (The) Medical and Surgical Journal. (Formerly the New York Medical and Surgical Journal.) Devoted to medicine, general science, and literature. Edited by Edward N. Fishblatt and W. Elmer Hubbard. [Monthly.] Nos. 4–11, v. 12, August, 1886, to March, 1887. 8°. *Minneapolis*.

Title of nos. 1–3, v. 12, and prior volumes, was: **New York** (The) Medical and Surgical Journal.

Minnesota State Homœopathic Institute. Transactions of 1867–82. vii, 223 pp. 8°. *Minneapolis, A. C. Bausman*, 1882.

Minnesota State Medical Society. Constitution and by-laws. 50 pp. 12°. *St. Paul, Goodrich & Somers*, 1856.

———. Transactions of 1869–85. 8°. *St. Paul & Minneapolis*, 1869–85.

Minnich (Joh. Alois). Baden in der Schweiz und seine warmen Heilquellen in medizinischer, naturhistorischer und geschichtlicher Hinsicht. xiii, 316 pp., 1 l., 6 pl., 1 map. 8°. *Baden, Höhr u. Langbein*, 1845.

———. The same. Les eaux thermales de Baden en Suisse, leur analyse chimique et leurs vertus thérapeutiques constatées par l'expérience, avec un aperçu descriptif et géognostique des environs de Baden, leur histoire naturelle, et des esquisses historiques concernant cette ville. viii, 365 pp., 5 pl., 1 ch. 8°. *Zurich, Meyer & Zeller*, 1846. [P., v. 1421.]

van Minninghen (Gerardus). * De jure codicillorum. 29 pp. 4°. *Lugd. Bat., S. Luchtman*, 1754. [P., v. 996.]

Minoliti (Felice). La ventilazione nei teatri in rapporto all' igiene. Conferenza letta il 17 aprile 1887 nel Circolo del Gabinetto di lettura. 30 pp. 8°. *Messina*, 1887.

Minonzio (Paolo). Il medico di collina, ossia quindici anni di servizio nella condotta medico-chirurgica di Carnage sui colli Varesini. Reso-

Minonzio (Paolo)—continued.
conto con osservazioni scientifico-pratiche intorno ai dettati più importanti della moderna scuola medica, e specialmente sull' uso ed in difesa del salasso. 600 pp., 1 tab. 8°. *Milano*, 1870.

Minoprio (Aloysius). * De tabe mesenterica infantili. 29 pp. 8°. *Ticini Regii, Fusi et socii*, [1842].

Minor (Carolus). * De typho. 2 p. l., 54 pp. 8°. *Edinburgi, A. Neill cum sociis*, 1793.

Minor (*Garry H.*) [1802–82].

Gilbert (C. H.) Obituary. Proc. Connect. M. Soc., Hartford, 1883, n. s., ii, no. 4, 178.

Minor (John C.) The relation of the law to medical education. 19 pp. 8°. *New York, W. R. Jenkens*, 1882.

———. Ethics and education. The annual address delivered November 14, 1883, before the New York Medico-Chirurgical Society. 36 pp. 8°. *New York*, 1884.

Repr. from: Tr. N. York M.-Chir. Soc., N. Y., 1884.
Also, Co-Editor of: **Medical** (The) Union, New York, 1873–4.

Minor (L. S.) K voprosu o pjanstve i ego lechenii v spetsialnych zavedenijach dlja pjanits. [The question of drunkenness and its treatment in special establishments for drunkards.] 99 pp. 8°. *St. Petersburg, tipog. M. M. Stasoulevitcha*, 1887.

Minor (Thomas C.) Erysipelas and child-bed fever. 131 pp., 2 tab. 8°. *Cincinnati, R. Clarke & Co.*, 1874.

———. Scarlatina statistics of the United States. 1 p. l., 55 pp. 8°. *Cincinnati, R. Clarke & Co.*, 1875.

———. Notes on the epidemiology of Ohio. 103 pp. 8°. [*Cincinnati*, 1877.]

Repr. from: Cincin. Lancet & Obs., 1877, xx.

———. Report on yellow fever in Ohio, as it appeared during the summer of 1878. 1 p. l., 122 pp. 8°. *Cincinnati*, 1878.

———. Athothis; a satire on modern medicine. viii, 194 pp. 12°. *Cincinnati, R. Clarke & Co.*, 1887.

See, also, **Study** on prostitution, [etc.] 8°. [*Cincinnati*, 1886.] — **Tardieu** (Ambroise). Feigned insanity. 8°. *Columbus*, 1882.

Minor (W. C.) Upon natural and artificial section in some chœtopod annelids. 43 pp. 8°. [*New Haven*, 1863.]

Repr. from: Am. J. Sc. & Arts, N. Haven, 1863, xxxv.

———. Post mortem examinations made at Knight U. S. A. Gen. Hospital. 20 l. 8°. *New Haven, Knight Hospital print*, 1864.

Minorca.

See, also, **Fever** (*Yellow, History, etc., of*), by localities.

Cleghorn (G.) Observations on the epidemical diseases in Minorca. From the year 1744 to 1749. To which is prefixed, a short account of the climate, productions, inhabitants, and endemial distempers of that island. 8°. *London*, 1751.

———. The same. 2. ed. 8°. *London*, 1762.
———. The same. 3. ed. 8°. *London*, 1768.
———. The same. 4. ed. 8°. *London*, 1797.
———. The same. With notes by Benjamin Rush. 8°. *Philadelphia*, 1809.

Foltz (J. M.) The endemic influence of evil government illustrated in a view of the climate, topography, and diseases of the island of Minorca, with an account of its medical faculty, etc. N. York J. M., 1843, i, 7–46. Also, Reprint.

Minot. De la nature et des causes de la fièvre, avec quelques expériences sur le quinquina, et des réflexions sur l'action de ce remède. 7 p. l., 176 pp. 18°. *Paris, R. Pepie*, 1684.

Minot—continued.

——. The same. De la nature et des causes de la fièvre; du légitime usage de la saignée et des purgatifs. Avec des expériences sur le quinquina, et des réflexions sur les effets de ce remède. 3. éd., reveuë et augmentée de quelques remarques sur l'opium. 5 p. l., 350 pp., 11 l. 12°. *Paris, L. d'Houry*, 1701.

——. The same. Nouv. éd. 5 p. l., 350 pp., 11 l. 16°. *Paris, L. d'Houry*, 1710.

——. The same. De la nature et des causes de la fièvre, des moyens d'en procurer la guérison; avec des réflexions sur le légitime usage de la saignée et des purgatifs, et sur les effets du quinquina, de l'opium, et des autres spécifiques. Nouv. éd., revue et augmentée d'un traité particulier sur les diverses préparations du quinquina, sur sa vertu et son action, et sur la manière de s'en servir dans toutes les différentes espèces de fièvres. 5 p. l., 350 pp., 11 l., 89 pp. 16°. *Paris, L. d'Houry*, 1722.

Minot (Charles Sedgwick).
See **Bowditch** (Henry P.) & **Minot** (C. S.) The influence of anæsthetics [etc.] 8°. *Boston*, 1874.

Minot (Francis). On hemorrhage from the umbilicus in new-born infants, with an analysis of forty-six cases. 11 pp. 8°. [*n. p.*, 1852.]
Repr. from: Am. J. M. Sc., Phila., 1822, n. s., xxiv.
For Portrait, see **Collection** of Portr. (Libr.)

Minot (J.) *Sur le mode d'action du calorique et du froid appliqué à l'économie animale. 26 pp. 4°. *Paris, an XIII* [1805], No. 446, v. 55. [*Also, in :* P., v. 1628.]

Minsch (Joh.) *Ein Fall von Cancroid der äusseren Genitalien des Weibes. 25 pp., 1 a. l. 8°. *Greifswald, C. Sell*, 1884.

Minsicht.
See **de Sgobbis** (Antonio). Universale theatro farmaceutico, etc. fol. *Venezia*, 1682.

Minssen (Heinrich). *Ueber gemischte Geschwülste der Parotis. 50 pp., 3 tab. 8°. *Göttingen, G. Hofer*, 1874.

Mint.
See **Mentha.**

de Minteguiaga (Fernando). *Sur la séméiologie des crachats considérée surtout au point de vue microscopique. 54 pp., 1 pl. 4°. *Paris*, 1868, No. 80.

Minter (Gustavus Guilielmus). *Diss. sistens prodromum zoologiæ generalis. 2 p. l., 31 pp., 1 l. 8°. [*n. p.*, 1836.]

Mintert (Franz). *Ueber Verletzungen und Schutz des Dammes in der Geburt. 44 pp., 1 l. 8°. *Halle a. S., R. Nietschmann*, 1881.

Minton (Henry). A practical homœopathic treatise on the diseases of women and children. Intended for intelligent heads of families and students in medicine. xxvi, 461 pp. 8°. *New York, W. Radde*, [1866].

——. Uterine therapeutics. 710 pp. 8°. *New York, A. L. Chatterton Publishing Co.*, 1884.
Also, Editor of : **Homœopathic** (The) Journal of Obstetrics and Diseases of Women and Children, New York, 1879–85.

Minutes of the proceedings of the committee, appointed on the 14 Sept., 1793, by the citizens of Philadelphia, the Northern Liberties and the District of Southwark, to attend to and alleviate the sufferings of the afflicted with the malignant fever prevalent in the city and its vicinity; with an appendix. 223 pp. 8°. *Philadelphia, R. Aitken & Son*, 1794.

——. The same. Printed by order of the select and common council of the city of Philadelphia. 243 pp., 1 tab. 8°. *Philadelphia, Crissy & Markley*, 1848.

Minutes of the proceedings of the Royal College of Physicians, relating to Dr. Isaac Schomberg,

22

Minutes of the proceedings [etc.]—continued. from Feb. 6, 1746, to Dec. 22, 1753. 52 pp. 8°. *London, J. Robinson*, 1754. [P., v. 1339.]

Minutilla (S.) Sulla etiologia, patogenesi e terapia del colera. 92 pp. 8°. *Palermo, frat. Vena*, 1884.

Minvielle (Eugène). *I. Décrire les divers genres de machines électriques, et donner leur théorie. II. [etc.] 31 pp. 4°. *Paris*, 1838, No. 185, v. 331.

Minvielle (Marie-François-Nic.) *De l'entérite, comme l'une des causes principales des coliques des enfants en bas âge. 1 p. l., 9 pp. 4°. *Strasbourg*, 1827, v. 56.

Minzior (Marie-Désiré-François-Edmond). *Quelques considérations sur l'étiologie et le traitement de la névralgie du trijumeau. 1 p. l., 32 pp. 4°. *Strasbourg*, 1865, 2. s., No. 887.

Mioche (Annet-Henri). *Quelques considérations sur la pratique de la médecine. 37 pp. 4°. *Paris*, 1864, No. 128.

Miocque (Edmond). *Propositions sur la phthisie pulmonaire. 23 pp. 4°. *Paris*, 1829, No. 77, v. 223.

Miomandre (J.) *Contribution à l'étude des surdités d'origine nerveuse. 40 pp. 4°. *Paris*, 1880, No. 365.

Mion (Louis-Joseph-Adolphe-Henri). *Des moyens externes de traitement dans la fièvre intermittente. 51 pp. 4°. *Paris*, 1873, No. 16.

Miorcec (Amand). *Étude sur la dengue d'après les travaux des médecins français et étrangers. 39 pp. 4°. *Paris*, 1876, No. 128.

Miot (Aristide). *Quelques remarques sur l'étude et la connaissance des maladies de l'oreille et sur les moyens physiques d'exploration du conduit auditif externe et de la membrane du tympan, à l'état normal adulte. 40 pp. 4°. *Paris*, 1871, No. 120.

Miot (C.) De la myringodectomie, ou perforation artificielle du tympan. 169 pp., 1 l. 8°. *Paris, A. Delahaye & Cie.*, 1877.

Miot (Camille). *De la cystalgie idiopathique. 58 pp. 4°. *Paris*, 1866, No. 155.

——. Traité pratique des maladies de l'oreille, ou leçons cliniques sur les affections de cet organe. 2 p. l., 464 pp., 4 pl. roy. 8°. *Paris, F. Savy*, 1871.

Miot (Léop.-G.-C.-F.) Recherches physiologiques sur l'innervation du cœur. 138 pp., 1 l. 8°. [*Bruxelles*, 1875.]

Miotat (Eugène). Suppression complète de la vidange. Assainissement des égouts et des habitations. 48 pp. 8°. *Paris, Ducher & Cie.*, 1881.

——. Assainissement de Paris. Suppression complète de la vidange. Le système diviseur appliqué à l'égout. 41 pp. 8°. *Paris, Ducher & Cie.*, 1882.

Miotti (Canciano). Breve ragguaglio delle vaccinazioni.
In : RAGGUAGLIO delle vaccina, etc. 8°. *Udine*, [1801], 251–254.

Miquel (*Alexis*) [1756–1838].
Portrait in : **Collection**—van Kaathoven.

Miquel (Alfred). *Du chloral et de son emploi après les opérations chirurgicales. 32 pp. 4°. *Paris*, 1874, No. 224.

Miquel (Antoine) [1796–1829]. Éloge de Xavier Bichat, suivi de notes historiques et critiques. 92 pp. 8°. *Paris*, 1823. [P., v. 581.]

——. Éloge de Parmentier. Discours qui a remporté le double prix proposé par l'Académie d'Amiens, pour l'année 1819. 60 pp. 8°. *Paris*, 1823. [*Also, in :* P., v. 581.]

——. Traité des convulsions chez les femmes enceintes, en travail et en couche. Mémoire qui a remporté le prix proposé par la Société de mé-

Miquel (Antoine)—continued.
decine de Paris pour l'année 1820. 164 pp. 8°. *Paris, Gabon & Cie.*, 1824. [*Also, in :* P., v. 581.]
——. The same. Abhandlung von den Konvulsionen der Schwangern, Gebärenden und Wöchnerinnen. Eine gekrönte Preisschrift. Aus dem Französischen. Hrsg. von Dr. Ludwig Cerutti. iv, 134 pp. 8°. *Leipzig*, 1824.
——. Lettres à un médecin de province, ou exposition critique de la doctrine médicale de M. Broussais. 2. éd., corrigée et augmentée d'une lettre sur les variations de la médecine physiologique. 2 p. l., 556 pp. 8°. *Paris*, 1826.
See, also, **Roche** (L.-C.) De la nouvelle doctrine médicale, etc. 8°. *Paris*, 1827.
Miquel (Charles). * I. Traitement de l'empoisonnement par les poisons narcotiques. II. [etc.] 25 pp. 4°. *Paris*, 1839, No. 217, v. 347.
Miquel (Dominique). * Sur la blennorrhagie. vi, 7–19 pp. 4°. *Paris*, 1818, No. 138, v. 139.
Miquel (F.-J.) * Du traitement des fractures du fémur, en combinant la demi-flexion et l'extension continue. vi, 7–34 pp., 1 pl. 4°. *Paris*, 1821, No. 146, v. 167.
Miquel (Fred. Anton. Guilielm.) [1811–71]. * Diss. exhibens veterum de jecore merita. viii, 89, iii pp., 1 l. 8°. *Groningæ, P. S. Barghoorn*, 1833.
Miquel (Jean-Édonard-Marcel-Marie) [1803–47]. *Editor of :* **Bulletin** général de thérapeutique médicale et chirurgicale, Paris, 1831–47.
For Biography, see Bull. gén. de thérap., etc., Par., 1847, xxxiii, 337–342.
Miquel (Jean-Félix). De la diphthérite. Lettre adressée à messieurs de la Société médicale d'Indre-et-Loire, pour éclairer quelques questions qui, malgré les travaux de M. Bretonneau et de ses élèves, sont encore restées litigieuses. 63 pp. 8°. *Tours*, 1848. [P., v. 453.]
——. Lettres d'un vétéran de l'école de Bretonneau. vii, 439 pp., 4 pl. 8°. *Tours, E. Mazereau & Cie.*, 1867.
——. Tribut à la chirurgie pratique du vétéran de l'école Bretonneau. xii, 6–347 pp., 13 pl. 8°. *Tours, E. Mazereau*, 1870.
——. Lettres du vétéran de l'école de Bretonneau à M. le professeur Bouillaud. 59 pp., 1 l. 8°. *Tours, E. Mazereau*, 1874.
Miquel (Joseph). * Étude clinique des blessures par l'obus et ses éclats. 47 pp. 4°. *Paris*, 1872, No. 344.
Miquel (M.-A.-N.) * Sur la néphrite. 12 pp. 4°. *Paris, an XIII* [1804], No. 370, v. 53.
Miquel (P.) Les organismes vivants de l'atmosphère. viii, 310 pp., 2 pl. 8°. *Paris, Gauthier-Villars*, 1883.
Miquel (R.) Der Landdrosteibezirk Osnabrück, seine klimatischen, Bevölkerungs- und gesundheitlichen Verhältnisse. Zugleich ein Bericht über Stand und Verwaltung der öffentlichen Gesundheitspflege mit besonderer Berücksichtigung der Jahre 1875–80. 1 p. l., 224 pp. 8°. *Osnabrück, G. Veith*, 1882.

Miquelon *Island.*
See, also, **Saint Pierre** *Island.*
GRAS (J.-G.-B.) * Quelques mots sur Miquelon. 4°. *Montpellier*, 1867.
Miquet (Frédéric). * Une ambulance pendant le siège de Paris 1870–71 au point de vue des hôpitaux temporaires. 36 pp. 4°. *Paris*, 1872, No. 222.
de Mirabeau (Honoré - Gabriel - Riquetti), Comte [1749–91]. Sur les actions de la Compagnie des eaux de Paris. 2. éd. xii, 36 pp. 8°. *Londres*, 1786.
——. Réponse ... à l'écrivain des administrateurs de la Compagnie des eaux de Paris. 2. éd. xii, 104 pp. 8°. *Bruxelles*, 1786.
Bound with preceding.

de Mirabeau (H.-G.-R.), Comte—continued.
——. *See also :*
Cabanis. Journal de la maladie et de la mort d'Honoré-Gabriel-Victor-Riquetti Mirabeau. *In his :* Œuvres complètes, 8°, Par., 1823, ii, 3–73. *Also, in :* Rev. de lit. méd., Par., 1877, ii, 86; 101; 117; 135; 168; 181; 203; 234; 265; 295; 363 : 1878, iii, 85; 144; 172; 225.
Mirabel (Alfred). * Des malformations des doigts et des orteils dans leurs rapports avec l'hérédité. 60 pp. 4°. *Paris*, 1873, No. 483.
Mirabel (Marc-Marmir). * De la parotidite dans la fièvre typhoïde. 54 pp., 1 l. 4°. *Paris*, 1883, No. 100.
Mirabello Monferrato. Regolamento di igiene pubblica approvato dal consiglio comunale in seduta delli 31 dicembre 1874. 30 pp. 8°. *Casale, P. Bertero*, 1882.

Miracles.
See, also, **Ecstasy**; **Imagination** *as a cause, etc., of disease ;* **Impostures.**
BELCHER (T. W.) Our Lord's miracles of healing considered in relation to some modern objections and to medical science. 8°. *London*, 1872.
MATTHEWS (W.) A collection of affidavits and certificates relative to the wonderful cure of Mrs. Ann Mattingly, which took place in the city of Washington, D. C., on the tenth of March, 1824. [Alleged miracle.] 8°. *Washington*, 1824.
MEZGER (G. I. S.) & CLOSS (J. F.) Disputatio de miraculorum indole, criterio et fine. 4°. *Tubingæ*, [1755].
MIRACLES. Philosophy of modern miracles; or, the relations of spiritual causes to physical effects, with especial reference to the mysterious developements at Bridgeport and elsewhere. By "a dweller in the temple". 8°. *New York*, 1850.
Belcher (T. W.) Reply to a criticism on "Our Lord's miracles of healing". Med. Times & Gaz., Lond., 1872, ii, 79 ; 106.—**Demoniacal** possession and miracles in the nineteenth century. *Ibid.*, 1869, ii, 8.—**Nagel** (L.) Die Heilwunder Jesu Christi, seiner Apostel und Einiger deren Vorfahren; medicinisch betrachtet und historisch zusammengestellt. Ztschr. d. deutsch. Chir.-Ver., Magdeb., 1850, iv, 290; 411: v, 91; 396.—**Pfeufer** (D. C.) Psychological and medical researches respecting the cures attributed to the prayers of Prince Hohenlohe (Alexander von). Edinb. M. & S. J., 1826, xxv, 63; 270.—**Ulrich.** Bemerkungen über die Wunderheilungen des Fürsten Hohenlohe und des Bauern Martin Michel, mit einem Rückblick auf die am Mittelrhein davon sichtbar gewordenen Wirkungen. Ztschr. f. d. Anthrop., Leipz., 1823, 397–412.

Mirage.
de Sesmaisons. Quelques observations sur les effets du mirage dans la région des Chott. Gaz. méd. de l'Algérie, Alger, 1868, xiii, 103–105.
Miraglia (Biagio G.) [1814–84]. Su le febbri periodiche; pensamenti patologico-pratici. 21 pp., 1 l. 8°. *Napoli*, 1842. [P., v. 1112.]
——. Della frenologia e della sua applicazione alla educazione ed alla giurisprudenza criminale, obbiezioni e risposte. 34 pp. 8°. *Napoli*, 1853. [P., v. 1141.]
——. Programma di un manicomio modello italiano seguito dall' applicazione dei precetti del programma alle riforme del R. Morotrofio di Aversa. vii, 140 pp., 5 pl. 12°. *Aversa, tip. del R. Morotrofio*, 1861.
——. Contro le vivisezioni degli animali, conferenze. 3. ed. 52 pp. 8°. *Napoli, L. Gargiulo*, 1884.
For Biography, see Arch. ital. per le mal. nerv., Milano, 1885, xxii, 211–218. *Also :* Manicomio, Nocera, 1885, i, 215–224.

Miral.
Henry (O.) Rapport sur l'eau minérale saline, chloroiodurée de Miral (Drôme). Bull. Acad. de méd., Par., 1860–61, xxvi, 101–103.

Miram (Joh. Ed.) * Zur Casuistik der spontanen Amputationen und ihrer Folgezustände. 51 pp., 1 pl. 8°. *Dorpat, Schnakenburg,* 1877.

Mirambeau (J.) [1793–1844]. * Dissertation sur le tétanos. 2 p. l., 32 pp. 4°. *Strasbourg, Levrault,* 1813.
  For Biography, see Bull. Soc. de méd. prat. de Par., 1844, no. 40, 123–134 (A. Lagasquie). *Also:* Gaz. d. hôp., Par., 1844, 193–195 (A. Lagasquie).

Miramond (Henri). * Sur la nature des fièvres continues, où l'on examine l'altération que les solides et les fluides subissent pendant ces maladies, et l'importance qu'on doit y attacher. 26 pp. 4°. *Paris,* 1825, No. 73, v. 192.

Miramond (Joseph-Benjamin). * De l'érysipèle spontané. 26 pp. 4°. *Paris,* 1852, No. 93, v. 529.

Miramond (P.-R.) * Sur l'affection épidémique qui s'est manifestée à la caserne de la rue de l'Oursine dans le mois de septembre 1828. 28 pp. 4°. *Paris,* 1829, No. 39, v. 222.

Miramont (P.-M.-L.-Artidore). * Du cancer en général. 31 pp. 4°. *Paris,* 1837, No. 111, v. 309.

Miran (Abel). * Essai sur l'éléphantiasis des Grecs. x, 11–40 pp., 1 l. 4°. *Montpellier,* 1870, No. 76.

Miranda. A book, divided into three parts, entitled: Souls, numbers, stars, on the neo-Christian religion. With confirmations of the old and new doctrines of Christ from wonders hitherto unheeded in the words and divisions of the Bible; in the facts and dates of history; and in the position and motions of the celestial bodies. v. 1, pts. 1–2. 394 pp., 2 l. 8°. *London, J. Morgan,* 1858–60.

Miranda (Manuel V.)
  Co-Editor of: **Repertorio** médico-habanero, Habana, 1842–3.—**Repertorio** médico-habanero y Boletin cientifico, Habana, 1843–4.

Miranda (Ramon-Luis). * De la paralysie du nerf moteur oculaire commun. 36 pp. 4°. *Paris,* 1861, No. 50.
  See, also, **Trabajos** de la Comision de medicina legal, etc. 3 v. 8°. *Habana,* 1872–4.

Mirande.
  See **Fever** (*Typhus, History, etc., of*), *by localities.*

Mirande (P.-Auguste). * Sur la colique de plomb. vi, 7–31 pp. 4°. *Paris,* 1825, No. 121, v. 193.

Mirandola.
  Marini (F.) Resoconto statistico-clinico dei malati osservati dal 1° settembre al 30 novembre 1863 nel' ospedale di S. Maria Bianca in Mirandola (sezione milit.). Gior di med. mil., Torino, 1864, xii, 665–691.

Mirandolle (Henricus). * De varia hydropis specie. [Leyden.] xvi, 121 pp., 3 l. 8°. *Hagæ Comitis, J. Roering,* 1839.

Mirano. Regolamento d' igiene del comune di Mirano. Approvato con deliberazione consigliare 16 febbraio 1886. 16 pp. roy. 8°. *Padova, tip. prov. Penada,* 1886.

Mirapeix (Jean). * Du mal perforant. 50 pp., 2 l. 4°. *Montpellier, Cristin, Serre & Ricome,* 1883, No. 35.

Mirassou (Alexandre). * De la dysenterie dans le fond de l'Afrique. 32 pp. 4°. *Paris,* 1854, No. 275, v. 563.

Mirault (Germanicus) [1796–1879]. * Sur l'anatomie et l'inflammation de la cornée transparente. 56 pp. 4°. *Paris,* 1823, No. 33, v. 178.

——. Sur une hydropisie particulière du globe de l'œil. 12 pp. 8°. [*Paris,* 1823.]
  Repr. from: Arch. gén. de méd., Par., 1823, ii.

——. Mémoire sur la ligature de la langue, et sur celle de l'artère linguale en particulier; précédé d'une observation de cancer de la langue

Mirault (Germanicus)—continued. guéri par la ligature de cet organe. 34 pp., 1 pl. 4°. [*Paris, n. d.*]
  Repr. from: Mém. Acad. de méd. 1833–4, Par., 1835, iv.

——. Du traitement de l'anévrisme externe par la compression indirecte et particulièrement par la compression exercée avec les doigts à l'occasion de deux nouveaux cas de guérison par l'emploi de ce procédé. Travail lu à la Société de médecine d'Angers dans sa séance de mars 1859. 16 pp. 8°. *Angers, imprimerie de Cosnier & Lachèse,* 1860.
  For Biography, see Bull. Soc. de méd. d'Angers (1879), 1880. n. s., vii, 78–84 (Farge).

Mirbach (Heribert). * Ueber einen Fall von Uterus duplex bicornis cum vagina duplici. 20 pp. 8°. *Würzburg, J. B. Fleischmann,* 1885.

Mirbane.
  See, also, **Nitrobenzole.**
  (**Vergiftungen** durch Mirbanöl.) Aerztl. Ber. d. k. k. allg. Krankenh. zu Prag (1875), 1877, 65.

de Mirbeck (Apollon). * Du tétanos chez l'adulte et en particulier du tétanos traumatique. 47 pp. 4°. *Strasbourg,* 1862, No. 610, 2. s., v. 32.

de Mirbeck (Louis). * Des fractures et des enfoncements du crâne du fœtus pendant l'accouchement. 1 p. l., 66 pp. 4°. *Strasbourg,* 1863, No. 684, v. 35.

Mire (Auguste). * Des procédés de névrotomie applicables au traitement de la névralgie sousorbitaire. 2 p. l., 41 pp. 4°. *Strasbourg,* 1863, No. 672, v. 35.

Mireau (Henri-Louis-Marie). * Sur les inconvéniens de l'amputation du moignon de la cuisse devenu conique. vi, 7–20 pp. 4°. *Paris,* 1815, No. 94, v. 110.

Mireur (Henri). * Sur les kystes hydatiques du foie. 50 pp. 4°. *Paris,* 1867, No. 10.

Mireur (Hippolyte). * Sur l'hérédité de la syphilis. 112 pp. 4°. *Paris,* 1867, No. 42.

——. La syphilis et la prostitution dans leurs rapports avec l'hygiène, la morale et la loi. 2 p. l., 475 pp. 8°. *Paris, G. Masson,* 1875.

——. La prostitution à Marseille. Histoire, administration et police hygiène. xiii, 15–404 pp. 8°. *Paris, E. Dentu,* 1882.

——. Étude historique et pratique sur la prophylaxie et le traitement du choléra, basée sur les observations fournies par l'épidémie de Marseille (1884). 2. éd. 193 pp. 8°. *Paris, G. Masson,* 1884.
  See, also, **Pornographe** (Le), etc. 8°. *Bruxelles,* 1879.

Mireur (Paul). * Des accès pernicieux à forme cérébro-spinale. Diagnostic et traitement. 70 pp., 1 l. 4°. *Montpellier,* 1882, No. 32.

Miriel (E.-C.-A.) * I. Décrire la période d'éruption de la variole; faire connaître les accidents qui peuvent la compliquer, et apprécier leur influence sur la marche et l'issue de la maladie. II. [etc.] 30 pp. 4°. *Paris,* 1848, No. 218.

Miriel [Jean-Joseph-Yves-Louis] [1779–1829]. * Réflexions sommaires sur l'importance du diagnostic, et sur les difficultés qu'il offre dans certain cas. 19 pp. 4°. *Paris,* 1810, No. 77, v. 80.

Miriel (P.-L.-M.-H.) * De quelques vices congéniaux de conformation de l'extrémité inférieure du tube digestif, et des moyens d'y remédier. 35 pp. 4°. *Paris,* 1835, No. 82, v. 284.

de Mirimonde (Léon-Pomme). L'art du dentiste en 1883. 11 l. 16°. *Paris, A.-P. de Mirimonde,* [1883].

Mirles. * Mikroorgan. broushnago tifa. [Microorganism in abdominal typhus.] 126 pp., 1 l. 8°. *St. Petersburg,* 1886.

Miron.
  Chereau (A.) Les quatre Miron. Union méd., Par., 1865, 2. s., xxv, 193; 209.

Miron (Valentineano Joan.) [1842–]. *Ueber den Bau der Milz. 29 pp., 1 l. sm. 4°. *Berlin, G. Schade*, [1869].

Miroudot (Henri). *Quelques considérations sur le ptérygion. 30 pp. 4°. *Paris*, 1862, No. 84.

Mirpied (Jean-Louis-Henri) [1844–]. *Des ulcères syphilitiques du membre inférieur et en particulier de "l'ulcus elevatum tertiaire". 34 pp. 4°. *Paris*, 1882, No. 222.

Mirrors.
See Looking-glass *makers (Diseases of)*.

Mirror-writing.
See Hand-writing.

Mirus (Adam Erdmann) & **Fischer** (Joh. Henricus). De monstris. 7 l. 4°. *Wittenbergæ, imp. M. Henckelius*, [1681].

Mirus (Albertus). *De pseudarthrosi. 24 pp., 1 l. 4°. *Jenæ, typ. Schlotterianis*, [1831].

Mirus (Christianus Fridericus Guilielmus). *Diss. sistens observationem dysenteriæ atque inflammationis arteriæ pulmonalis morbo syphilitico supervenientis una cum epicrisi. 2 p. l., 34 pp. 4°. *Lipsiæ, ex off. Richteri*, [1812].
For Biography, see **Kuehn** (Carolus Gottlob).

Mirus (Jo. Fridericus). De novo phosphoro æthereo. 11 pp. 4°. *Vitembergæ, ex off. C. Schroederi*, [1716].

Mirus (Samuel Gotth.) *De forma medicaminum pro curandis morbis apte et utiliter exhibenda. 40 pp. sm. 4°. *Lipsiæ, ex off. Stopffelia*, [1749].
For Biography, see **Quelmalz** (Samuel. Theodorus).

Miryachit.
See, also, Leaping *ague*.
Armangué y Tuset (J.) Mimicismo ó neurosis imitante (miryachit, jumping, latah). Rev. de cien. méd., Barcel., 1884, x, 547; 583; 613; 680; 715; 746; 777. *Also:* Rev. frenopát. barcel., 1884, iv, 290; 339; 368; 409; 443. *Also:* Clín. navarra, Pamplona, 1885, ii, nos. 8; 9; 10; 11; 13; 14; 15; 16; 17; 18; 19; 20; 21; 22; 23; 25. *Also,* Reprint.—**Beard** (G. M.) Experiments with the jumpers of Maine. [Read before the Am. Neurol. Ass., June, 1880.] Pop. Sc. Month., N. Y., 1880-81, xviii, 170–178.—**Gilles de la Tourette** (G.) Jumping, latah, myriachit. Arch. de neurol., Par., 1884, viii, 68–74. ——. Étude sur une affection nerveuse caractérisée par de l'incoordination motrice accompagnée d'écholalie et de coprolalie (jumping, latah, myriachit). Ibid., 1885, ix, 19; 158.—**Hammond** (W. A.) Miryachit, a newly described disease of the nervous system, and its analogues. N. York M. J., 1884, xxxix, 191. *Also:* Æsculapian, N. Y., 1884, i, 57–60. *Also:* Brit. M. J., Lond., 1884, i, 758. *Also, transl.:* Union méd., Par., 1884, 3. s., xxxvii, 706–708.—**Le Gendre** (P.) La maladie de Gilles de la Tourette (affection nerveuse caractérisée par de l'incoordination motrice, accompagnée d'écholalie et de coprolalie). Union méd., Par., 1885, 3. s., xl, 109–114. *Also, transl.:* St. Louis Cour. Med., 1885, xiv, 275–280.—**Neale** (R.) Miryachit, or lata. Brit. M. J., Lond., 1884, i, 884.—**Taylor** (H. M.) Nervous mimicry. Virginia M. Month., Richmond, 1886-7, xiii, 593–605.—**Vizioli** (F.) Sul miryachit e sul jumping, malattie del sistema nervoso. Gior. di neuropatol., Napoli, 1884, ii, 164–180.

Mirza-Ali. *Des hémorrhagies intestinales dans la fièvre typhoïde. 66 pp., 1 l. 4°. *Paris*, 1876, No. 445.

Mirza-Hussein-Khan. *De l'iodoforme donné à l'intérieur. 1 p. l., 63 pp. 4°. *Paris*, 1881, No. 318.

Miscarriage.
See Abortion.

Miscellanee medico-chirurgico-farmaceutiche; raccolte in Pisa nel 1844. Anno secondo. 108 pp. 8°. *Pisa, tipog. della Minerva*, [1844]. [P., v. 1419.]
Continuation of: **Giornale** toscano di scienze mediche, etc., and followed by: **Cimento** (Il) Pisa, 1844-6, etc.

Miscellaneous tracts relating to natural history, husbandry, and physick. To which is added the calendar of Flora. By Benj. Stilling-

Miscellaneous tracts [etc.]—continued.
fleet. 2. ed. xxxi, 391 pp., 11 pl. 8°. *London, R. & J. Dodsley*, 1762.

Miscellanies on homœopathy, edited by an association of homœopathic physicians. v. 1, Aug., 1838, to June, 1839. 216 pp. 8°. *Philadelphia, W. L. J. Kiderlen*, 1839.
Ended. Issued in bi-monthly numbers under title: **American** (The) Journal of Homœopathy.

Mischel (Aug. Christ. Gotthelf.) *Nonnulla de scarlatina. 22 pp. 8°. *Jenæ*, 1845.

Mischel (Franziscus Adolfus Gotthelf.) *De percussione et auscultatione chirurgiæ subsidiis. 16 pp. 8°. *Lipsiæ, typ. E. Stangii*, [1850].

Mischel (Joh. Alexander).
See **de Garengeot** (René-Jacques-Croissant). Splanchnologia sive anatomia viscerum, das ist: gründliche Abhandlung von allen Eingeweiden die in denen dreyen Cavitäten des menschlichen Cörpers enthalten, [etc.] 12°. Berlin, 1733.—**de Saint Yves** (Carl). Tractat von denen Krankheiten der Augen, etc. 12°. Berlin, 1730.

Mischel (Rudolf Oskar Gotthelf). *Ueber die in den Gelenken spontan sich bildenden fremden Körper (Gelenkmäuse). 26 pp. 8°. *Leipzig, C. E. Elbert*, 1865.
c.

Mischkovicsew (Maximus Nicolics). *De conio maculato. 54 pp., 1 l. 8°. *Budæ, typ. reg. scient. universitatis*, [1834]. [P., v. 1324.]

Mischner (Ferdinandus). *De morbo Brightii. 39 pp. 8°. *Gryphiswaldiæ, F. Hache*, [1861]. c.

Misco (Giovanni). Memoria anatomica sul numero e sulla disposizione dei fasci midollari componenti il midollo spinale umano. 22 pp., 1 pl. 8°. *Palermo, F. Lao*, 1842.

Misera (Franz). *Ueber die Masern. 23 pp. 8°. *Erlangen, C. H. Kunstmann*, 1837.

Miserere.
See Intestines *(Obstruction of)*.

Mises. Panegyrikus der jezigen Medicin und Naturgeschichte. 68 pp. sm. 8°. *Leipzig, C. H. F. Hartmann*, 1822.

——. Schutzmittel für die Cholera, nebst einem Anhange, enthaltend die vornehmsten Meinungen der Aerzte über den Sitz und das Wesen oder die nächste Ursache, die Contagiosität oder Nichtcontagiosität dieser Krankheit. iv, 164 pp. 8°. *Leipzig, L. Voss*, 1832. [P., v. 210; 1211.]

——. De cholera verdedigd. ·Naar het Hoogduitsch. iv, 106 pp. 8°. *Amsterdam, H. Frijlink*, 1833.

——. Lofrede op de hedendaagsche genees- en natuurkunde. 66 pp. 8°. *Amsterdam, H. Frijlink*, 1834.

von Mises (F.) Ueber die Nerven der menschlichen Augenlieder. 9 pp., 1 pl. 8°. *Wien*, 1882.
Repr. from: Sitzungsb. d. k. Akad. d. Wissensch. Math.-naturw. Cl., Wien, 1882, lxxxv, 3. Abth.

Misevitch (Anton). *K voprosu kolichestvennago opredelenija organicheskich veshestve v vode dlja pitja. [Quantitative analysis of organic substances in drinking-water.] 49 pp., 1 tab. 8°. *St. Petersburg*, 1874.

Miska (Christianus Guilielmus). *De damnis ex retardata abscessuum apertione. 1 p. l., 16 pp., 2 l. 4°. *Halæ ad Salam, stanno Curtiano*, [1765].
Also [Abstr.], in: WEIZ (F. A.) Vollständ. Ausz., [etc.] 12°. Budissin, 1769, i, 152–157.

Miskolcz.
Fodor (J.) Javaslat Miskolcz város köztisztaságaügyének rendezésére. [Proposition for the drainage of the city of Miskolcz.] Közeg. és Törvény. Orvos., Budapest, 1885, 21–28.

Mislerus (Joh. Jacobus). *De visus statu naturali et præternaturali. 1 p. l., 48 pp. 4°. *Gissæ, Karger*, 1680.

Misleus (Luca). *De marasmo senili. *Vindobonæ*, 1775.
In: DE WASSERBERG. Op. min. med. et diss. 8°. *Vindobonæ*, 1775, [ii], 427–445.

Misopædia.

See **Insanity** (*Anomalous, etc.*)

Missa (Henri). *Sur la toux convulsive. 44 pp. 4°. *Paris*, 1831, No. 230, v. 244.

Missa (Henricus Michaelis). Thesis in verba: Ergo herniosis ex scuto eburneo coriaceoque cingulo subligacula. [*Paris*, 1754.]

In: HALLER. Disp. chir. [etc.] 4°. *Lausannæ*, 1756, v, 623–652.

See, also, **Lafisse** (Claudius). *An lupiis caustica? 4°. [*Paris*, 1770.]

—— **& Despatureaux** (Guido D.) Thesis in ea verba: Ergo lui venereæ hydrargyrus camphoratus. *Paris*, 1756.

In: HALLER. Disp. ad morb. [etc.] 4°. *Lausannæ*, 1757, i, 525–532.

Missa (J.) *Sur les suites de couches. 20 pp. 4°. *Paris*, 1821, No. 101, v. 166.

Missa (M.-J.) *Sur les phénomèues chimiques de la respiration. viii, 9–46 pp. 8°. *Paris, an XI* [1803], v. 19.

Misset (Camille). *Étude sur la pathologie des glandes sébacées. 119 pp., 2 l., 2 pl. 4°. *Paris*, 1872, No. 179.

Misset (E.) *De l'inflammation du bord libre des paupières. 34 pp. 4°. *Paris*, 1859, No. 31, v. 634.

Missiaen (Ludovicus). *De emanatione et febre intermittenti paludosa. 35 pp. 4°. *Gandavi, typ. P. J. van Ryckegem*, [1828]. [P., v. 959; 1380.]

Missiles *and their extraction.*

See, also, **Bullet-extractors**, *etc.*; **Lead-poisoning** (*Causes of*); **Wounds** (*Foreign bodies in*).

VON BECK (B.) Ueber die Wirkung moderner Gewehrprojektile, insbesondere der Lorenz'schen verschmolzenen Panzer-Geschosse auf den thierischen Körper. imp. 4°. *Leipzig*, 1885.

CHESNEY (A.) *Étude sur l'enkystement des projectiles dans les plaies par armes à feu. 4°. *Paris*, 1874.

KLEFFEL (R.) *Ueber die Veränderungen und Wirkungen des Projectils beim Schiessen. 8°. *Berlin*, [1874].

KRÜGER (J. G.) *De nonnullis ad motum globuli e sclopeto explosi pertinentibus. 4°. *Halæ Magdeb.*, [1737].

KÜHN (C. G.) [Pr.] læsiones aëriæ expenduntur. 4°. *Lipsiæ*, 1814.

STENZEL (H.) *Ueber die Wirkung der modernen Handfeuerwaffen auf den menschlichen Organismus. 8°. *Berlin*, [1875].

STREICHER (P. E.) *Quædam de læsionibus ictu glandis sclopetariæ sic dicto aëreo exortis. 8°. *Berolini*, [1824].

ZEGERS (H. A.) *De hedendaagsche puntkogels, vooral die van het Beaumontgeweer en hunne werking. 8°. *Amsterdam*, 1876.

Allen (H.) Rib of an ox, showing the effects of pressure from an encysted connoidal rifle-ball. Phila. M. Times, 1870–71, i, 401.—**Bagnold.** On the wind of a commonball. Med. & Phys. J., Lond., 1817, xxxviii, 265–267.—**Bédoin.** Balle de chassepot simulant des effets d'une balle explosible. Cong. méd. de France 1872, Par., 1873, iv, 236. ——. Des balles explosibles; réflexions et faits relatifs à ce sujet. Union méd. de la Seine-Inf., Rouen, 1873, xii, 126–141. *Also,* Reprint. ——. Des balles explosibles. J. de méd. et pharm. de l'Algérie, Alger, 1879, iv, 4; 43; 75.—**Bell** (A. G.) Upon the electrical experiments to determine the location of the bullet in the body of the late President Garfield; and upon a successful form of induction balance for the painless detection of metallic masses in the human body. Am. J. Sc., N. Haven, 1883, 3. s., xxv, 22–61. *Also,* Reprint. ——. Sur un appareil permettant de déterminer, sans douleur pour le patient, la position d'un projectile de plomb ou d'autre métal dans le corps humain. Compt. rend. Acad. d. sc., Par., 1881, xc, 625–627. *Also:* France méd., Par., 1881, ii, 627–629. ——. Sur une méthode électrique servant à déterminer, par le moyen d'une aiguille, la position et la profondeur d'un projectile, ou autre substance métallique, dans le corps humain. Compt. rend. Acad. d. sc., Par., 1881, xciii, 717–719.—**Billroth** (T.) Die modernen Projektile und

ibre Wirkung auf die verschiedenen Theile des menschlichen Körpers; der erste Verband: freiwillige Hilfe in der ersten Linie. Militaerarzt, Wien, 1882, xvi, 33; 43.—**Bolton** (J.) Gunshot wound of the thigh; ball lodged in the condyle of the femur; detected by Nélaton's probe and canula forceps; successful removal. Confed. States M. & S. J., Richmond, 1864, i, 21.—**Bovet.** Einiges über Wirkung kleinkalibriger Handfeuerwaffen, insbesondere des Hebler-Gewehrs, Modell 1887. Cor.-Bl. f. schweiz. Aerzte, Basel, 1887, xvii, 746–751, 1 tab.—**Browne** (R. K.) Bullet-wound exploration. Am. M. Times, N. Y., 1862, v, 33.—**Bruce** (A.) The new bullets and the wounds produced by them. Med. Times & Gaz., Lond., 1867, ii, 455.—**Buck.** Noch einige Worte über die Luftstreifschüsse. J. d. Chir. u. Augenh., Berl., 1822, iv, 641–656. [*See, also, infra.* Ritter.]—**Busch.** Die Wirkung der sogenannten Luftstreifschüsse. Cor.-Bl. d. ärztl. Ver. d. Rhein-Prov., Bonn, 1868, iii, 10–12.—**Calhoun** (J. T.) A case of alleged contusion from the wind of a cannon ball. Med. & Surg. Reporter, Phila., 1862, vii, 573.—**Corlieu** (A.) Moyen facile de reconnaître la présence d'une balle dans les plaies par armes à feu. Gaz. d. hôp., Par., 1870, xliii, 398.—**Cortese** (F.) Degli effetti d'una palla spenta da fucile a retrocarica sopra un cranio doliocefalo allungato; cenni storici ed etnografici. Atti r. Ist. Veneto di sc., lett. ed arti, 1869–70, 3. s., xv, 2273–2298, 4 pl. ——. Sulle armi da fuoco attuali e sugli effetti dei loro projettili nell' organismo vivente. *Ibid.*, 1872–3, 4. s., ii, 291–331, 1 pl. *Also:* Gior. di med. mil., Firenze, 1873, xxi, 73–106.—**Davies** (R.) Extraction of bullets. Assoç. M. J., Lond., 1863, i, 538.—**Deneux.** Procédés pour reconnaître la présence et la nature des corps vulnérants métalliques engagés dans les plaies par armes de guerre. [Rap. de Legouest.] Bull. Acad. de méd., Par., 1872, 2. s., i, 876–886.—**Dupont** (L.) Sur les effets présumés du fluide électrique dans les coups des grosses armes à feu. Actes Soc. de méd. de Brux., 1808, ii, 285–304.—**Efecto** de los projectiles cónicos. Siglo méd., Madrid, 1860, vii, 29.—**Ellis** (D.) Observations on the nature and cause of certain accidents which sometimes occur in battle, and have been usually ascribed to the "wind of a ball". Edinb. M. & S. J., 1812, viii, 1–10.—**Emploi** du courant voltaïque pour la recherche des projectiles dans nos tissus. Gaz. d. hôp., Par., 1862, xxxv, 553.—**Ewich** (O.) Untersuchungen über die Unterschiede der Chassepot- und Zündnadelkugel-Verwundungen. Deutsche Klinik, Berl., 1870, xxii, 428–430.—**Forbes** (P.) Observations on the cause of death from what is called the wind of a ball. Edinb. M. & S. J., 1812, viii, 310–312.—**Garnett** (A. Y. P.) On the use of Nélaton's probe. Confed. States M. & S. J., Richmond, 1864, i, 22.—**Girdner** (J. H.) On the detecting and locating of metallic masses in the human body by means of the induction balance and the telephonic probe. N. York M. J., 1887, xlv, 393–396. *Also:* Med. News, Phila., 1887, i, 192.—**Goldsmith** (M.) The search for balls in old gun-shot wounds. N. York M. J., 1867–8, vi, 426–430.—**Gosselin.** Recherche au moyen de l'investigateur électrique et extraction d'une balle enkystée depuis 4 mois dans la première côte gauche. Bull. Acad. de méd., Par., 1870, xxxv, 730–733. *Also:* Bull. gén. de thérap., etc., Par., 1870, lxxix, 230–233.—**Harland** (H.) Extraction of a Waterloo bullet which had remained imbedded in the palm of the hand for upwards of fifty-nine years. Brit. M. J., Lond., 1874, ii, 275.—**van der Hegge Zijnen** (B. G.) Effect van den puntkogel, geschoten uit het achterlaadgeweer der Nederlandsche infanterie. Nederl. Tijdschr. v. Geneesk., Amst., 1869, 2. R., v, 1. Afd., 413–415.—**Heppner** & **Garfinkel.** Experimentelle Untersuchungen über die Wirkung der modernen Kleingewehrprojectile auf Lehmmassen und auf den menschlichen Körper. Centralbl. f. Chir., Leipz., 1874, i, 209; 225.—**Herrgott.** Lettre à propos de balles explosibles. Gaz. méd. de Par., 1871, xxvi, 242.—**Hirschfeld.** Ueber die Wirkungen des Chassepotgewehrs in sehr grosser Nähe, erläutert durch einen Fall von Schussverletzung des Oberschenkels aus einer Entfernung von einem Fuss. Deutsche mil.-ärztl. Ztschr., Berl., 1874, iii, 121–129.—**Ivanoff** (N. P.) K vopr. of deistvii sovremen. ognest. snarjadov. [On the effect of modern firearm projectiles.] Voyenno-med. J., St. Petersb., 1886, clvi, pt. 7, 319–336.—**Kemperdick.** Der electrische Kugelsucher. Deutsche Klinik, Berl., 1870, xxii, 375.—**Kocher** (T.) Ueber die Sprengwirkung der modernen Kleingewehr-Geschosse. Cor.-Bl. f. schweiz. Aerzte, Basel, 1875, v, 3; 29; 69. *Also,* Reprint. ——. Neue Beiträge zur Kenntniss der Wirkungsweise der modernen Kleingewehr Geschosse. Cor.-Bl. f. schweiz. Aerzte, Basel, 1879, ix, 65; 104; 133. *Also,* Reprint.—**Kolomnin** (S. P.) Sravnitel. ocherk deistvija na organ. razlich. pul: sphericheskoi svintsovoi i spherich. mednoi, cilindro-konich. i cilindro-oval. svintso i pantsir. cilindro-oval stalnoi. [Comparative researches into the effect on organism of spherical projectiles and spherical copper, cylindrico-conical and cylindrico-oval projectiles, and on cylindrico-oval steel breast-plates.] Ejeued. klin. gaz., St. Petersb., 1886, vi, 653; 673; 689; 713.—**Küster** (E.) Ueber die Wirkungen der neuern Geschosse auf den thierischen Körper. Verhandl. d. Berl. med. Ge-

Missiles *and their extraction.*

sellsch., 1873–4, v. pt. 2, 86–93. [Discussion], pt. 1, 81.—**Langenbeck** (B.) Ein neuer Kugelzieher. Deutsche Klinik, Berl., 1859, xi. 227. — **Larrey.** Sur l'extraction des corps étrangers qui compliquent les plaies d'armes à feu. Bull. Fac. de méd. de Par., 1809–11, ii (7. année), 135–141.—**Lecomte** (O.) De l'exploration des balles dans les plaies par armes à feu des os et des articulations. Rec. de mém. de méd. . . . mil., Par., 1863, 3. s., ix, 94–135. — **Le Courtois.** Note sur l'emploi des balles explosibles et les causes qui ont fait croire à leur usage; malléabilité, fragmentation, déformation des balles de plomb; étendue et gravité des plaies par armes à feu; de la fusion des balles de plomb dans les plaies. Bull. Soc. anat. de Par., 1871, xlvi, 398–406.—**Le Fort** (L.) Emploi de l'électricité pour découvrir la présence des corps étrangers métalliques enfoncés et perdus dans l'épaisseur des chairs. Bull. gén. de thérap., etc., Par., 1869, lxxvii, 92–95.—**Longmore** (T.) On the probable surgical effects in battle in case of the employment of projectiles of a more elongated form, such as the Whitworth projectiles. Army M. Dep. Rep. 1863, Lond., 1865, v, 500–504. *Also*, Reprint.—**Maisonneuve.** Extraction d'une balle enchatonnée depuis 5 ans dans l'os maxillaire supérieur. Monit. d. hôp., Par., 1853, i, 655.—**Maschek** (M.) Zwei Methoden, um mittels der Electricität metallene Projectile in Schusswunden mit Sicherheit zu diagnosticiren. Feldarzt, Wien, 1875, 5. — **Melicher** (L. J.) Kugelzieher, zur Entfernung der Kugeln aus Schusswunden. Oesterr. med. Wchnschr., Wien, 1848, 1189–1194.—**Melsens.** Balistique sur quelques effets de la pénétration des projectiles dans divers milieux et sur l'impossibilité de la fusion des balles de plomb dans les plaies produites par armes à feu. Arch. méd. belges, Brux., 1872, i, 348–353.—**Milliot** (B.) Nouveau moyen de diagnostic et d'extraction des projectiles en fonte et en plomb à noyaux de fer. France méd., Par., 1869, xvi, 765. ———. Du diagnostic et de l'extraction des projectiles, et particulièrement des projectiles en fonte de fer. Arch. gén. de méd., Par., 1872, 6. s., xix, 129–146.—**Mundy.** Ueber die Treffähigkeit, Geschwindigkeit und die Verschiedenartigkeit der Füllung der Projektile. Allg. mil.-ärztl. Ztg., Wien, 1872, xiii, 112–114. — **Neudörfer.** Die metallprüfende Sonde. Wien. Med.-Halle, 1863, iv, 86.—**Nicaise.** À propos des balles explosibles. Gaz. méd. de Par., 1871, 3. s., xxvi, 102–104.—**Nicolas.** De l'action explosive des projectiles d'infanterie, d'après les expériences de M. le Prof. Kocher. Bull. Soc. d. sc. nat. de Neuchâtel, 1883–4, xiv, 127–135.—**Observations** on the different hypotheses published to account for the effects ascribed to the wind of a ball. Edinb. M. & S. J., 1813, ix, 134–139. — **Pernet** (H.) Des balles explosibles. Gaz. d. hôp., Par., 1872, xlv, 123. — **Rapp.** Quelques mots sur l'échauffement subi par les balles pendant leur trajet à travers nos tissus. Rec. de mém. de méd. . . . mil., Par., 1872, 3. s., xxviii, 490–497.—**Reger.** Die Anforderungen der Humanität an die Kleingewehrprojectile. Deutsche mil.-ärztl. Ztschr., Berl., 1884, xiii, 575–592. *Also, transl.:* Voyenno-san. dielo, St. Petersb., 1885, v, 89; 97; 109. — **Reverdin** (J.-L.) Quelques expériences sur les effets du fusil Rubin. Rev. méd. de la Suisse Rom., Genève, 1884, iv, 704–716.—**Richter.** Ueber die sogenannten explosiven Wirkungen der Kleingewehrgeschosse. Tagebl. d. Versamml. deutsch. Naturf. u. Aerzte, Breslau, 1874, xlvii, 217–219.—**Ritter.** Refl·xionen über die Luftstreifschüsse. J. d. Chir. u. Augenh., Berl., 1822, iv, 120–133.—**Rodolfi** (R.) Specillo Nélaton, suoi vantaggi e inconvenienti, sonda elettrica. Gazz. med. ital. lomb., Milano, 1867, 5. s., vi, 127.—**Roscher.** Ueber die Flugbahn und die Wirkungen der Geschütz-Kugeln. Allg. Ztg. f. Mil.-Aerzte, Brnschwg., 1843, i. 305; 313.—**Roser** (W.) Ueber einige Verirrungen der Kriegschirurgie. Berl. klin. Wchnschr., 1867, iv, 145; 169; 181; 189; 213; 225. — **Roussin** (Z.) Assassinat par une arme à feu; intervention utile de l'analyse chimique. Ann. d'hyg., Par., 1875, 2. s., xliv, 100–106. — **Ruspini** (J. B.) A brief description of a newly invented instrument, for the extraction of balls from gunshot wounds. Med. & Phys. J., Lond., 1806, xv, 455–457, 2 pl.—**Sarazin.** Des effets produits par le projectile du fusil Chassepot sur le cadavre. Gaz. méd. de Strasb., 1867, xxvii, 223. — **Schoentjes** (H.) Note sur l'application de l'électricité à la recherche des projectiles dans le corps humain. Ann. Soc. de méd. de Gand, 1882, lx, 229–246, 1 pl. ———. Sur une application du téléphone à la recherche des projectiles dans le corps humain. *Ibid.*, 1885, lxiv, 207–210.—**Senftleben** (H.) Zur wundärztlichen Waffenkunde. Deutsche Klinik, Berl., 1870, xxii, 33; 41; 61. ———. On some effects of modern rifle projectiles. Lancet, Lond., 1875, ii, 524. — **Sonrier.** Des balles explosibles. Gaz. d. hôp., Par., 1872, xlv, 138.—**Spense** (J.) Observations on those accidents commonly ascribed to the wind of a ball. Edinb. M. & S. J., 1812, viii, 161–164.—**Surgeon** Tuson's bullet extractor. Med. Times & Gaz., Lond., 1870, ii, 464.—**Tardieu** (A.) Balles explosibles; balles fragmentées. Gaz. d. hôp., Par., 1872, xlv, 28; 34. — **Thierry.** Des balles explosibles. *Ibid.*, 1871, xliv, 610.—**Tolifree** (R.) Some remarks on the sudden death, without apparent injury or organic derangement, from the supposed wind of a cannon-ball. Balt. M. & S. J. & Rev., 1834, ii, 57–61.—**Trachez** (F.) Mémoire sur la manière des boulets et

Missiles *and their extraction.*

autres projectiles, lancés par la poudre à canon, lorsqu'ils nous frappent. J. de méd., chir. et pharm. mil., Par., 1816, ii, 227–237.—**Tuson** (J. E.) Description of a new bullet extractor. Med. Times & Gaz., Lond., 1870, ii, 152. ———. Dr. Tuson's bullet extractor. *Ibid.*, 489. ———. Description of a new bullet forceps. Indian M. Gaz., Calcutta, 1872, vii, 270.—**de V.** (J.) Heridas de arma de fuego causadas por haber reventado un cañon de escopeta. Gac. méd., Madrid, 1848, iv, 276.—**Vézien.** Sur un moyen simple de reconnaître avec certitude si un corps étranger caché au fond d'une plaie est une balle. Rec. de mém. de méd. . . . mil., Par., 1863, 3. s., ix, 308. — **Volkmann** (R.) Kugel zwischen Truncus anonymus und Trachea; Extraction. Deutsche Klinik, Berl., 1868, xx, 76.—**Wahl** (M.) Notiz über irisirende Farben an den Bleiprojectilen. Centralbl. f. Chir., Leipz., 1874, i, 577. — **Weitz** (M.) Die Ortsbestimmung einer Bleikugel oder irgend eines andern metallischen Gegenstandes im menschlichen Körper auf elektrischem Wege; (nach einer Zuschrift von M. A. Graham Bell an die Akademie der Wissenschaften in Paris). Deutsche med. Wchnschr., Berl., 1882, viii, 348.

Missing (The) Link Magazine. v. 14–19, 1878–83; n. s., v. 1, No. 10. 8°. *London*, 1878–84.

Contains notices of convalescent homes and institutions for nurses, cripples, and sick children.

Mission Hospital and Dispensary for Women and Children, Philadelphia. Mission Hospital and Relief Society for Women and Children, Philadelphia. [Announcement by the board of managers of its establishment, and appeal to the public for support.] 8 pp. 12°. *Philadelphia, Grant, Faires & Rodgers*, 1875.

Organized Jan., 1875; incorporated Jan. 15, 1876; closed Jan. 1, 1880.

———. Annual reports of the managers to the contributors and the public. 1.–5., 1875–9. 12° & 8°. *Philadelphia*, 1876–80.

Reports for 1877 and 1878 are printed abstracts; 1879, in MS. Full reports were not issued.

Mission Hospital and Relief Society for Women and Children, Philadelphia. *See* **Mission** Hospital and Dispensary for Women and Children.

Missionary Association of the University of Edinburgh. Report of the committee to the subscribers. 22., 1856–7. 12 pp. 8°. *Edinburgh, Paton & Ritchie*, 1857.

Missionary Hospital in the Western Suburbs of Canton. A report of the . . . under the care of Dr. [Benj.] Hobson, from Jan. 1, 1853, to June 30, 1854. 19 pp. 8°. [*Canton*, 1854.]

———. Report of the . . . for the year 1859–60. 13 pp. 8°. [*Canton*, 1860.]

First opened in April, 1848; closed in 1856, on account of hostilities; reopened in 1858.

Missions *and missionaries.*

See, also, **Negroes.**

EDINBURGH Association for Sending Medical Aid to Foreign Countries. Address to the students of medicine at the Scottish universities. 8°. *Edinburgh*, 1842.

EDINBURGH Medical Missionary Society. Quarterly paper. v. 3, Nos. 13 and 14, May and August, 1882; v. 4, No. 8. 8°. *Edinburgh*, [1882–5].

ILANGCHOW Medical Mission. Annual report of the . . . in connexion with the Church Missionary Society. 2., 1884. 8°. *Shanghai*, 1885.

KERR (J. G.) Medical missions at home and abroad. 8°. *San Francisco*, 1878.

LOWE (J.) Medical missions, their place and power. With introduction by Sir William Muir. 12°. *London*, 1886.

MEDICAL Missionary Society in China. Reports of the officers. 1.–3., 1838 to 1841–2; 6., 1844–5; 20.–43., 1858–81; 46., 1884. 8°. *Canton*, 1841–85.

MILDMAY Conference Hall. Report of the Jaffa Medical Mission, under the superintendence of Miss Mangan. 6., 1883–4. 24°. *Moorfields, E. C.*, 1884.

MILDMAY Mission Hospital, Medical Mission and General Mission Work, Bethnal Green, Lon-

Missions *and missionaries.*

don. Annual report of the committee to the subscribers, for the year 1886. 24°. *London*, 1887.

SCHWEIGGER. Ueber medicinische Missions-anstalten. 8°. [*n. p., n. d.*]
Repr. from: Sitzungsb. d. k. Akad. d. Wissensch. Math.-naturw. Cl., Wien, [1852].

WILLEY (N.) The mortality experience of American missionaries. Being a complete record of the mortality experience of the foreign missionaries of the A. B. C. F. M., from its organization to July 1, 1873, as compared with the American experience table of mortality. 8°. [*New York*, 1873.]
Repr. from: Insurance Monitor. Nov., 1873.

Barker (M. P.) Medical missions in heathen lands. Med. & Surg. Reporter, Phila., 1883, xlviii, 2-5.—**Keen** (W. W.) On medical-missionary work, with some notes on the condition of medicine in Japan. Tr. Coll. Phys. Phila., 1879. 3. s., iv, 13-25. — **Medical** Missionary Association of China. Constitution and by-laws of the . . . China M. Miss. J., Shanghai, 1887, i, 32-34.—**Medical** missions. Brit. & For. M.-Chir. Rev., Lond., 1875, lvi, 307-326.

Missirini (Melchiore). Pericolo di seppellire gli uomini vivi creduti morti. xxxix, 431 pp. 8°. *Milano, C. Branca*, 1837.

Missisquoi (The) Springs and their wonderful cures. 48 pp. 12°. *New York, A. Herrick & Sons*, [1868].

——. The same. 50 pp. 12°. [*Sheldon, Vermont, n. d.*]

Mississippi. Catalogue of the Mississippi State library, 1877. 194 pp. 8°. *Jackson, Power & Barksdale*, 1877.

——. Senate. A bill to be entitled "An act to amend the statutes in regard to boards of health". [Mississippi legislature, session of 1880.] S. B. No. 28. 9 pp. fol. [*Jackson*, 1880.]

——. An act to amend the statutes in regard to boards of health, approved March 4, 1880. 7 pp. 8°. *Jackson, Miss., J. L. Power*, 1880.

Mississippi.

See, also, **Blind** (*Asylums, etc., for*); **Brookhaven**; **Craven's** Creek (*Diseases of*); **Deafmutes** (*Asylums, etc., for*); **Fever** (*Cerebrospinal, History, etc., of*), **Fever** (*Malarial, History, etc., of*), **Fever** (*Typhoid, History, etc., of*), **Fever** (*Yellow, History, etc., of*), **Hospitals** (*Descriptions, etc., of*), *by localities*; **Jackson**; **Natchez**; **Pharmacy** (*Education in, etc.*)

HILGARD (E. W.) Report on the geology and agriculture of the State of Mississippi. 8°. *Jackson*, 1860.

UNITED STATES. *War Department. Engineer's Office.* Cypress Bayou. Letter from the Secretary of War, communicating a report of the Chief of Engineers, with an estimate of the cost for an improvement of Cypress Bayou, and the lakes between Jefferson and Shreveport. 48. Cong., 2. sess. H. R. Ex. Doc. 103. Jan. 21, 1885. 8°. [*Washington*, 1885.]

Evans (T. E.) On the medical history of the eastern part of Mississippi. [Pneumonia, pleuritis, intermittent, remittent, and inflammatory fevers.] N. Orl. M. & S. J., 1849-50, vi, 741-745.—**Hughes** (E. W.) Report on the topography and diseases of north Mississippi. Tr. Mississippi M. Ass., Jackson, 1876, ix, 94-101.—**Moore** (J. P.) Report on the epidemics and climatology of Mississippi. Tr. Am. M. Ass., Phila., 1871, xxii, 205-212.—**Phares** (D. L.) The spas of Mississippi. Tr. Mississippi M. Ass., Jackson, 1879, xii, 108-114.—**Pugh** (J. J.) On the medicinal waters of Mississippi; the artesian springs of Madison County. South. M. Rep. (Fenner), N. Orl., 1849, i, 379-381.

Mississippi. *Asylum for the Blind of the State of Mississippi, Jackson.* Annual and biennial reports of the trustees and superintendent to the governor of the State, for the years 1868-9; 1871-3; 1876-9. 8°. *Jackson*, 1869-80.

Mississippi. *Mississippi Institution for the Education of the Deaf and Dumb, at Jackson.* Annual and biennial reports of the trustees and superintendent to the governor of the State. 1.-3., 1871-3; 6., 1876; 7., 1877. Biennial: 3., 1882-3. 8°. *Jackson*, 1872-83.
This institution existed prior to 1861, but was broken up and the records lost during the war. Reorganized in 1871.

Mississippi. *Mississippi State Hospital, Vicksburg.* Annual report of the board of trustees and superintendent to the legislature, for the year 1870-71. 11 pp. 8°. *Jackson, Kimball, Raymond & Co.*, 1872.

Mississippi. *Natchez State Hospital.* Annual report of the board of trustees and superintendent to the legislature, for the year 1870-71. 8 pp. 8°. *Jackson, Kimball, Raymond & Co.*, 1872.

Mississippi. *State Board of Health of the State of Mississippi.* Annual reports to the legislature. 1. (1877); 2. (1878-9). 8°. *Jackson*, 1877-9.
Second report, from Jan., 1878, to Dec. 1, 1879.

——. Circular to the medical profession, soliciting information on the prevailing diseases in different parts of the State, Oct. 3, 1877. 1 sheet. 4°. [*Jackson*, 1877.]
Blank forms used by . . . 1877-9.
Form 3. Quarterly return of marriages.
Form 4. Quarterly return of births.
Form 5. Quarterly return of deaths.
Registration of a birth.
Registration of a death.
Receipt for books, blank forms, etc.

——. Trichina spiralis: [How to detect it in trichinous pork, and the means of destroying its vitality.] Jan. 7, 1878. 1 sheet. 4°. [*Jackson*, 1878.]

——. Circular suggesting the organization of local boards of health. Aug. 7, 1878. 1 sheet. 4°. [*Jackson*, 1878.]

——. Circular advising quarantines against yellow fever. Aug. 26, 1878. 1 sheet. 8°. [*Jackson*, 1878.]

——. Circular to the authorities of cities and towns where yellow fever has prevailed, on the importance of having houses disinfected before being reoccupied. With rules. Oct. 21, 1878. 1 sheet. 8°. [*Jackson*, 1878.]

——. Circular to circuit clerks on the registration of births, marriages, and deaths. Dec. 16, 1878. 1 sheet. 4°. [*Jackson*, 1878.]

——. To the medical profession of Mississippi. Circular soliciting co-operation in the registration of births, marriages, and deaths. Dec. 17, 1878. 1 sheet. 8°. [*Jackson*, 1878.]

——. Rules and regulations recommended for adoption by local boards of health throughout the State. 7 pp. 8°. [*Jackson, Power & Barksdale*, 1878?]

——. Circular to physicians, requesting full history of yellow fever. Feb. 10, 1879. 1 sheet. 4°. [*Jackson*, 1879.]

——. Opinion of attorney-general in reference to local quarantine. June 12, 1879. 1 sheet. 4°. [*Jackson*, 1879.]

——. Circular to president of county board of health, recommending a quarantine ordinance against yellow fever. June 16, 1879. 1 sheet. 4°. [*Jackson*, 1879.]

——. The same. To president of municipal board of health. June 20, 1879. 1 sheet. 4°. [*Jackson*, 1879.]

——. Circular to the county and municipal boards of health, requesting them to adopt the rules and regulations provided by the National Board of Health against infectious disease. July 16, 1879. 1 sheet. 4°. [*Vicksburg*, 1879.]

——. Small-pox. [A word of warning and advice to the people.] 1 sheet. 4°. [*Jackson*, 187-.]

Mississippi. *State Board of Health*—continued.

————. Sanitary rules and regulations. Suggestions in regard to general sanitation, disinfectants, and deodorants. Adopted April, 1880. 17 pp. 8°. *Jackson, Miss.*, 1880.

————. Quarantine rules and regulations. (Approved May 18, 1880.) 16 pp. 8°. *Jackson, J. L. Power*, 1880.

————. Disinfectants. 1 sheet. 4°. [*Jackson, n. d.*]

————. Memorandum for reporters on yellow fever. 1 sheet. 4°. [*Jackson, n. d.*]

Mississippi. *State Lunatic Asylum, at Jackson.* Annual and biennial reports of the trustees and superintendent to the legislature of Mississippi. 5., 1858–9; 16.–25., 1869–70 to 1879; 28., 1882; 29., 1883. 8°. *Jackson*, 1859–84.

Established March 4, 1848; opened Jan. 8, 1855. Reports for 1878 and 1879 and subsequent years are biennial.

Mississippi *River.*

See, also, **Inundations.**

EADS (J. B.) Report on the Mississippi jetties. Aug. 18, 1876. 8°. [*New York*, 1876.]

FOSTER (J. W.) The Mississippi valley; its physical geography, including sketches of the topography, botany, climate, geology, and mineral resources; and of the progress of development in population and material wealth. 8°. *Chicago*, 1869.

HUMPHREYS (A. A.) & ABBOT (H. L.) Report upon the physics and hydraulics of the Mississippi River [etc.] 4°. *Philadelphia*, 1861.

Professional papers of the Corps of Topographical Engineers, U. S. A., No. 4.

UNITED STATES. *War Department.* Letter from the Secretary of War, transmitting the annual report of the Mississippi River Commission. For the year 1884. 48. Cong., 2. sess. H. R. Ex. Doc. No. 64. Jan. 6, 1885. 8°. [*Washington*, 1885.]

Dowler (B.) Contributions to the hydrographical thermology and hygiene of the Mississippi River. N. Orl. M. & S. J., 1858, xv, 448–484.—**Forshay** (C. G.) A chapter of the hydrography of the Mississippi River. South. M. Rep. (Fenner), N. Orl., 1849, i. 63–76, 2 tab. ————. On the hydrography of the Mississippi River, for the year 1850. *Ibid.*, 1850, ii, 154–157, 1 tab.—**Mitchell** (R. W.) Mississippi River inspection service. Rep. Nat. Bd. Health 1880, Wash., 1882, ii, 617–635.—**Thornton** (G. B.) Sanitation of the Mississippi valley. Am. Pub. Health Ass. Rep. 1884, Concord, N. H., 1885, x, 214–223.

Mississippi State Dental Association. Constitution. 7 pp. 8°. *Vicksburg, Miss., Rogers & Groome*, 1875.

————. The constitution, by-laws, and code of ethics, adopted Jan. 17–18, 1882. 12 pp. 8°. *Jackson, Miss., C. Winkley*, 1882.

Mississippi State Pharmaceutical Association. Proceedings of the annual meeting, 1874. 8°. [*n. p.*], 1874.

Mississippi Valley Association of Dental Surgery. Proceedings of 1. annual meeting. 8°. *Cincinnati, E. Shepard*, 1845.

Mississippi Valley Medical Monthly. Editors and proprietors: J. J. Jones and Julius Wise. v. 1–7, 1881–7. 8°. *Memphis, Tenn.*

Current. Followed: **Arkansas** (The) Medical Monthly. In April, 1881, Dr. Wise became sole editor; in Oct., 1882, F. L. Sim became editor.

Mississippi Valley Sanitary Association. *See* **Sanitary** Council of the Mississippi Valley.

Missol (Léon). Notice historique sur l'ancien Hôpital de la Quarantaine, ou des pestiférés de Villefranche en Beaujolais et sur les épidémies de peste qui ont affligé la ville d'après les archives de la commune et de l'Hôtel-Dieu. 74 pp. 8°. *Lyon, A. Vingtrinier*, 1873.

Repr. from: Rev. du Lyonnais.

Missol (Noël-Léon). *De la compression, considérée comme cause d'accidents et comme moyen thérapeutique. 26 pp. 4°. *Paris*, 1854, No. 166, v. 563.

Missouri. Annual reports of the adjutant-general of the State of Missouri for the years 1864–5; 1871. 3 v. 8°. *Jefferson City*, 1865–72.

————. Annual reports of the commissioner of statistics to the general assembly of the State of Missouri. 1., 1866; 2., 1867. 8°. *Jefferson City*, 1867–8.

————. The registration law of the State of Missouri, passed at the adjourned session of the twenty-fourth general assembly; together with forms for notices and certificates, as contemplated by this act. 29 pp. 8°. *Jefferson City, Mo., E. Kirby*, 1868.

————. The acts establishing the State board of health, and regulating the practice of medicine and surgery in Missouri, with mode of procedure under the same. Compiled by Joseph C. Hearne, secretary. 32 pp. 8°. *St. Louis, Commercial Printing Co.*, 1883.

Missouri.

See, also, **Chariton**; **Cholera** (*Asiatic, History, etc., of*), **Education** (*Medical*), *etc.*, **Fever** (*Malarial, History, etc., of*), **Fever** (*Typhoid, History, etc., of*), *by localities*; **Kansas City**; **Saint Louis.**

AMMERMAN (C. R.) The medical and surgical directory of the State of Missouri for 1884 and 1885. Containing the names, post-office address, place and date of graduation, and school of practice of the physicians of the State; the names and residence of the officers and members of the various city, county, district, and State medical societies; of the Missouri members of the various national associations, regular, eclectic, and homœopathic; of the Missouri members of the various national societies of specialists; names and residence of the State board of health and of the State board of pharmacy; rosters of the U. S. examining surgeons for pensions for the State, and medical officers of the Missouri national guard. Also, medical colleges, State charitable institutions, hospitals, dispensaries, medical laws, mortality statistics, and census tables, showing how Missouri compares with her sister States in the number of her insane, idiotic, blind, deaf and dumb, and how the same are cared for; an article on fraudulent diplomas, and an index of the physicians of the State, alphabetically arranged, with reference page to register report. 8°. *Quincy*, 1885.

Blue (J. H.) Statistics of three hundred and thirty-three deaths in Chariton and the adjoining counties in Missouri, for the last ten years, with remarks. West. Lancet, Cincin., 1844–5, iii, 157–161.—**Reyburn** (T.) Report on the diseases of Missouri and Iowa. Tr. Am. M. Ass., Phila., 1855, viii, 83–323, 3 diag. *Also*, Reprint.—**Thompson** (J. E.) Topography and diseases of Bates County, Missouri. Boston M. & S. J., 1856, liv, 49; 269; 329; 489.—**Twyman** (L.) On the medical topography of Saint Charles County, Mo., with some account of the prevalent diseases from 1829 to 1841, inclusive. Missouri M. & S. J., St. Louis, 1845, i, 25–32.—**Wilcox** (J.) A report on the topography of the county of Boone, with some of the symptoms and treatment of dysentery and erysipelas, as they have prevailed in the Missouri River bottom, both in their endemic and epidemic forms. Tr. M. Ass. Missouri, St. Louis, 1852, ii, 97–100.

Missouri. *Missouri Institution for the Education of the Blind, St. Louis.* Annual and biennial reports of the trustees to the governor of the State. Annuals, 3., 1853–4; 5., 1855–6. Biennials, 6., 1866–7 & 1867–8; 9., 1872–3 & 1873–4. 8°. *Jefferson City & St. Louis*, 1854–74.

Missouri. *Missouri Institution for the Education of the Deaf and Dumb, Fulton.* Biennial reports of the commissioners and superintendent to the general assembly. 1.–15., 1853–84. 8°. *Jefferson City & Fulton*, 1859–85.

Opened Nov. 5, 1851. No report for 1861 and 1862; suspended for those years. 1.–5., reprinted by the pupils, 1882–3.

Missouri. *Missouri State Board of Health.* Proceedings of the . . . at its semi-annual meeting, held in the city of St. Louis, July 8–10, 1884, together with the report of the secretary. General rules for the restriction and prevention of small-pox, diphtheria, scarlet fever, Asiatic cholera, typhus fever, typhoid fever, etc., and a paper on hog cholera or swine plague, as read by Dr. W. B. Conery. 28 pp. 8°. *Hannibal,* [*Hannibal Print. Co.*. 1884].

———. Rules and regulations for the creation and establishing of boards of health in the several cities, towns, villages, and counties of the State, recommended by the board of health of the State of Missouri. 8 pp. 8°. [*St. Louis,* 1884.]

Missouri. *State Lunatic Asylum, at Fulton.* Annual and biennial reports of the board of managers and superintendent to the general assembly. 1.–3., 1851–2 to 1855–6; 5.–12., 1858–9 to 1875–6; 14.–16., 1878–9 to 1883–4. 8°. *Jefferson City,* 1853–85.
Opened Dec. 1, 1851. 1. report for one year.

———. A code of by-laws, rules, and regulations for the government of the board of managers, officers, and employés of the . . . with appendix. Revised, adopted, and ordered printed by authority of the board of managers. Nov. 24, A. D. 1873. 59 pp. 8°. *Columbia, Statesman office,* 1874.

Missouri. *State Lunatic Asylum, No. 2, St. Joseph.* Biennial reports of the board of managers and superintendent to the general assembly of the State. 2.–5., 1877–84. 8°. *Jefferson City, State Journal Co.,* 1879–85.

Missouri. *University of the State of Missouri, at Columbia.* Annual catalogues [including the medical department]. 1845–6 (4.); 1876–7 to 1884–5 (35.–43.). 8°. *Jefferson City,* 1846–85.
Founded 1820; organized 1840. For announcements and catalogues of the medical department from 1845–6 to 1854–5, see: Missouri Medical College, St. Louis. In the winter of 1845 Kemper Medical College was adopted as the medical department of the university. In 1855, by a change of charter, it became independent and assumed the title of Medical College of Missouri, St. Louis. In 1872, the curators determined to establish and maintain a permanent medical department, and a faculty was appointed Feb. 17, 1873.

———. Annual circular of the law school and of the medical school of the . . . for the session of 1877–8. pp. 114–129, 6 pl. 8°. [*Jefferson City,* 1877.]
Cutting from : Catalogue, 1876–7 (35.).

———. Report of the board of curators of the State University of the State of Missouri to the general assembly, for the years 1877 and 1878 (1.). 14 pp. 8°. *Jefferson City, Carter & Reagan,* 1879.

Missouri Clinical Record, a monthly journal of medicine and surgery. Editors: W. A. Hardaway and Alexander B. Shaw. v. 1, April, 1874, to March, 1875. 250 pp. 8°. *St. Louis.*
Established by the Missouri Medical College, Library Association, organized Feb. 12, 1874. Continued as **Saint Louis** Clinical Record.

Missouri Dental College, St. Louis. Annual announcements for the sessions of 1866–7 to 1872–3 (1.–7.); 1874–5 to 1885–6 (9.–20.). 8°. *St. Louis,* 1866–85.
List of students and graduates for the years 1866–7 to 1871–2; 1873–4 to 1876–7; 1878–9, in announcements for subsequent years. List of alumni from 1867 to 1879, in announcement for 1879–80.

Missouri (The) Dental Journal. A monthly record of medical science, devoted to the specialty of dentistry. Edited by Homer Judd. v. 1–15, 1869–83. 8°. *St. Louis,* 1869, *to March,* 1883; *Kansas City, April to Dec.,* 1883.
Ended. v. 5–8 edited by Henry S. Chase; v. 9 by H. Judd and W. H. Eames; v. 10–14 by C. W. Spalding; v. 15 by R. I. Pearson [*et al.*]. Followed in 1884 by : **Archives** (The) of Dentistry.

Missouri Eye and Ear Infirmary, St. Louis. Annual and biennial reports of the board of trustees to the public. 1.–2., 1876–7 to 1878–9. 8°. *St. Louis,* 1877–9.
Organized July 18, and incorporated Aug. 4, 1876. 2. report is for two years.

Missouri Medical College, Saint Louis. Annual announcements for the sessions of 1840–41 (1.); 1842–3 (3.); 1845–6 (6.); 1846–7 (7.); 1851–2 (12.); 1853–4 (14.); 1854–5 (15.); 1859–60 (20.); 1868–9 to 1873–4 (28.–33.); 1875–6 to 1883–4 (35.–43.). 8° & 4°. *Saint Louis,* 1840–83.
Organized in 1840, as the medical department of Kemper College. In 1845 it became the medical department of the University of the State of Missouri. In 1855, by a change of charter, it assumed above title. It was also formerly known as "McDowell's College" and Hospital. List of alumni from 1841 to 1883, in announcement for 1883–4. List of students and graduates for the years 1845–6; 1850–51; 1852–3; 1853–4; 1858–9; 1867–8 to 1872–3; 1874–5 to 1882–3, in announcements for subsequent years. 42. and 43. are 4°.

Missouri (The) Medical and Surgical Journal. Edited by R. F. Stevens. [Monthly.] v. 1–4, May, 1845, to July, 1848. 8°. *St. Louis.*
Nos. 7–12, v. 1, edited by J. N. McDowell and Thomas Barbour; in v. 2 Barbour sole editor; in v. 3–4 A. J. Coons added. No. 3, v. 4, last published; then merged in: **Saint Louis** (The) Medical and Surgical Journal.

Missouri State Dental Association. Minutes and proceedings of the Missouri State Dental Association (including the Missouri Dental College Association), from its organization, Oct. 31, 1865, to and including the eighteenth annual session, June 6, 1882. Compiled from the written records of the association, by W. H. Eames, recording secretary. 159 pp. 8°. *St. Louis,* 1883.

Missouri (The) Valley Medical Journal. A monthly journal of medicine, surgery, and the collateral sciences. Editors: W. C. Boteler, F. F. Hoyt [*et al.*]. v. 1, Jan. to Dec., 1882. 8°. *St. Joseph. Mo.*
Ended. Merged in: **Kansas** (The) Medical Index, forming: **Kansas** (The) and Missouri Valley Medical Index.

Missourium.

KOCH (A.) Description of the Missourium, or Missouri leviathan; together with its supposed habits, and Indian traditions concerning the location from whence it was exhumed. Also, comparisons of the whale, crocodile, and missourium with the leviathan, as described in 41st chapter of the book of Job. 8°. *Louisville,* 1841.

Missoux (T.-D.) * Quelques considérations sur les corps étrangers arrêtés dans les voies digestives, et un nouveau moyen d'extraction. vi, 7–28 pp. 4°. *Paris,* 1825, No. 76, v. 192.

Mistarlet (Léon). * Quelques cas de purpura chez les enfants. 34 pp. 4°. *Paris,* 1876, No. 252.

Mistler (J.-B.) * Considérations sur l'étranglement des hernies inguinales et crurales. 1 p. l., 72 pp. 4°. *Strasbourg,* 1830, v. 58 & 61.

Mistletoe.

COLBATCH (J.) A dissertation concerning mistletoe, a most wonderful specifick remedy for the cure of convulsive distempers. 2. ed., to which is added a second part. 8°. *London,* 1720.

———. The same. 3. ed. 12°. *London,* 1723.

———. The same. 6. ed. 12°. *London,* [*n. d.*]

Clos (J.-A.) Supplément aux observations de M. Duhamel, sur le guy, insérées dans les mémoires de l'Académie royale des sciences, année 1740. Hist. Soc. de méd.-prat. de Montpel., 1807, xvi, 1–11, 2 pl.—**Dixon** (J.) Case of poisoning by berries of the mistletoe; recovery. Brit. M.-J., Lond., 1874, i, 224.—**Hobbs** (A. G.) Mistletoe as an oxytoxic. Louisville M. News, 1878, v, 238.—**Kronfeld** (M.) Zur Biologie der Mistel (Viscum album). Biol. Centralbl., Erlang., 1887–8, vii, 449–464.—**Long** (W. H.) Viscum album (mistletoe) as an oxytocic. Louisville M. News, 1878, v, 132–134.—**Park** (R.) Note on the therapeutics of Viscum album. Practitioner, Lond., 1881, xxvii, 346.—**Payne**

Mistletoe.

(R. L.), jr. Mistletoe, its physiological action and some of its clinical applications. North Car. M. J., Wilmington, 1881, vii, 253–266. *Also* [Abstr.]: Med. & Surg. Reporter, Phila., 1887, lvii, 342–345.— **Turnipseed** (E. B.) Employment of the mistletoe (Viscum verticillatum Ell. Sk., non L.) to produce abortion. Charleston M. J. & Rev., 1851, vi, 448.

Mistral (Alexandre) [1852–]. * Essai clinique sur les troubles de la menstruation. 80 pp. 4°. *Paris*, 1881, No. 290.

Mitaine (Jules-Jean-Baptiste-Gabriel). * Considérations générales sur l'âge de l'adolescence. 33 pp. 4°. *Paris*, 1819, No. 118, v. 147.

Mitau.

See Cholera (*Asiatic, History, etc., of*), by localities.

Mitchel. De arte medendi apud priscos musices ope atque carminum epistola ad Antonium Relhan. 69 pp. 8°. *Londini, G. Johnston*, 1766.

Mitchel.

See **Robinson** (Henry). The new specialty for cancers and external tumors, [etc.] 2. ed. 8°. *London*, 1873.

Mitchel (Charles L.) Strictures of the urethra situated at or near the meatus; their causes, nature, and treatment. Together with a description of a new meatotome. 7 pp. 8°. [*n. p.*, 1882.]
Repr. from: Med. Times, Phila., 1882–3, xiii.

Mitchel (Joannes). * De febribus continuis, et præcipue de medelis in iis adhibendis. 4 p. l., 206 pp., 1 l. 8°. *Edinburgi, C. Stewart et socii*, 1802. [P., v. 22.]

Mitchell (Alfred).

See **Dana** (Israel Thorndike). History of the Portland School for Medical Instruction. 8°. *Portland*, 1874.

Mitchell (Andreas). * De dysenteria. 1 p. l., 35 pp. 8°. *Edinburgi, Balfour et Smellie*, 1789.

Mitchell (Arthur). Description of a new atmometer, or evaporometer. 4 pp. 8°. *London, W. Trounce*, [1856]. [P., v. 899.]
Repr. from: J. Soc. Arts, Lond., June 6, 1856.

———. On various superstitions in the northwest highlands and islands of Scotland, especially in relation to lunacy. 40 pp. 8°. *Edinburgh, Neill & Co.*, 1862.
Repr. from: Proc. Antiquarian Soc. Scotland, iv.

———. The insane in private dwellings. xii, 97 pp. 8°. *Edinburgh, Edmonston & Douglas*, 1864.

Mitchell (C. L.) A synoptical table of thoracic percussion and auscultation. Arranged from the works of Laennec, Hope, Louis, Piorry, Williams, and others, and the lectures of Barth, Roger, and Landouzy. 1 sheet. fol. *New York*, 1839.

———. Introductory lecture to the fall session of lectures in the Castleton Medical College. 16 pp. 8°. *Albany, C. Van Benthuysen & Co.*, 1844.

Mitchell (Charles Dundas). Essay on tic douloureux and other nervous affections. 19 pp. 8°. *Calcutta, Medical Journal press*, 1839. [P., v. 729.]

Mitchell (Charles L.) Fixed adhesive dressings in the treatment of skin diseases. 12 pp. 16°. *Philadelphia*, [1884].
Also, Editor of: **Clinical** Notes on the Local Treatment of Disease, Philadelphia, 1885.

Mitchell (Clifford). The practitioner's guide in urinalysis. 205 pp. 8°. *Chicago, Gross & Delbridge*, 1882.

Mitchell (Edward). A series of engravings representing the bones of the human skeleton; with the skeletons of the lower animals. The explanatory references by John Barclay. 7 pp., 45 l., 35 pl. 4°. *Edinburgh, E. Mitchell*, 1819–20.

———. Engravings of the ligaments, copied from the original works of the Caldanis, with descriptive letter-press. Revised and carefully com-

Mitchell (Edward)—continued.
pared with nature by Robert Knox. 13 l., 10 pl. 4°. *Edinburgh, Maclachlan & Stewart*, 1834.
See, also, **Scarpa** (Antonio). Engravings of the cardiac nerves, [etc.] 4°. *Edinburgh*, 1829. — **Scarpa** [*et al.*]. Engravings of the nerves, [etc.] 4°. *Edinburgh*, 1829.— **Sue** & **Albinus.** The anatomy of the bones, [etc.] 4°. *Edinburgh*, 1829.—**Tiedemann** (Frederic). Plates of the human body. 4°. *Edinburgh*, 1829.

Mitchell (*G. F.*) [1808–69].
Stevens (E. B.) Biographical sketch of G. F. Mitchell. Tr. Ohio M. Soc., Columbus, 1869, 177.

Mitchell (George E.) Puerperal state of fever. 30 pp. 8°. *Philadelphia, J. H. Oswald*, 1805. [*Also, in:* P., v. 388.]

Mitchell (*Gove*) [1781–1856].
Biographical notice. Tr. M. Soc. Penn., Phila., 1860, n. s., v, 133.

Mitchell (Gulielmus). * De scrofula. 1 p. l., 41 pp. 8°. *Edinburgi, R. et A. Foulis*, 1766. [P., v. 649.]

Mitchell (Gulielmus Somervell). * De animantium calore. 29 pp. 8°. *Edinburgi, E. Balfour*, 1800. [P., v. 15; 1553.]

Mitchell (*Henry*) [1784–1856].
Willard (A.) Biographical sketch of... Tr. M. Soc. N. Y., Albany, 1857, 85–90.

Mitchell (Howard E.) Bromide of ethyl, when and how to use it. 6 pp. 12°. *Troy, N. Y.*, [1883].

Mitchell (J. B.)
See **Koecker** (Leonard). An essay on the diseases of the jaws, [etc.] New ed. 8°. *London*, 1847.

Mitchell (J. H.) Introductory lecture delivered before the class of medical students at Willamette University for the session of 1867. 8 pp. 8°. *Salem, Oregon*, 1867.

Mitchell (J. W.) Hygienic hints to health seekers, while using the compound oxygen treatment. 15 pp. 12°. *Philadelphia, Collins*, 1872.

Mitchell (James). Account of a case in which hairs passed along the urine; with a short abstract of similar cases published by former authors. 4 pp. 8°. [*Edinburgh*, 1828.] [*Also, in:* P., v. 1523.]
Repr. from: Edinb. M. & S. J., 1828, xxx.

Mitchell (Joannes). * De phthisi pulmonali. 41 pp. 8°. *Edinburgi, Neill et soc.*, 1801. [P., v. 18.]

———. De scarlatina. 2 p. l., 23 pp. 8°. *Edinburgi, A. Neill et socii*, 1805.

Mitchell (John). Treatise on the falsifications of food, and the chemical means employed to detect them; containing water, flour, bread, milk, cream, beer, cider, wines, spirituous liquors, coffee, tea, chocolate, sugar, honey, lozenges, cheese, vinegar, pickles, anchovy sauce and paste, catsup, olive (salad) oil, pepper, mustard. xviii, 334 pp. 12°. *London, H. Baillière*, 1848.

———. A manual of practical assaying. 4. ed. Edited by William Crookes. xxxvi, 819, lv pp. 8°. *London, Longmans, Green & Co.*, 1873.

Mitchell (John Kearsley) [1793–1858]. An oration delivered before the Philadelphia Medical Society. 28 pp. 8°. *Philadelphia, I. Ashmead & Co.*, 1825. [P., v. 763.]

———. Observations on the treatment of curvatures of the spine. 19 pp. 8°. [*Philadelphia*, 1827.]
Repr. from: N. Am. M. & S. J., Phila., 1827, iv.

———. On the penetrativeness of fluids. 34 pp. 8°. *Philadelphia, J. R. A. Skerrett*, 1830.
Repr. from: Am. J. M. Sc., Phila., 1830–31, vii.

———. On a new practice in acute and chronic rheumatism. 12 pp. 8°. *Philadelphia, J. R. A. Skerrett*, 1831.
Repr. from: Am. J. M. Sc., Phila., 1831, viii.

Mitchell (John Kearsley)—continued.

——. Further cases and observations relative to rheumatism. 15 pp. 8°. *Philadelphia, J. R. A. Skerrett*, 1833.

Repr. from: Am. J. M. Sc., Phila., 1833, xii.

——. The wisdom of God, as displayed in the formation of water; an introductory lecture to a course of chemistry applied to the arts, during the winter session of 1833–34 of the Franklin Institute. 11 pp. 8°. *Philadelphia, T. K. Greenbank & Co.*, 1833.

——. The value of a great medical reputation, with suggestions for its attainment; a lecture introductory to the summer course of the Medical Institute. 20 pp. 8°. *Philadelphia, J. R. A. Skerrett*, 1834.

——. A lecture on some of the means of elevating the character of the working classes. 17 pp. 8°. *Philadelphia, J. Harding*, 1834.

Repr. from: J. Frankl. Inst., Phila., 1834, xiv.

——. The value of the practical interrogation of nature; a lecture. 22 pp. 8°. *Philadelphia, J. R. A. Skerrett*, 1834.

——. On the liquefaction and solidification of carbonic acid. 8 pp., 1 pl. 8°. [*Philadelphia*, 1838.]

Repr. from: J. Frankl. Inst., Phila., 1838, xxii.

——. On the usefulness of the medical profession, beyond the limits of the profession. A lecture, introductory to the course of practice of medicine in Jefferson Medical College. 30 pp. 8°. *Philadelphia, Merrihew & Thompson*, 1842.

——. Lecture introductory to the course on the practice of medicine in the Jefferson College. 24 pp. 8°. *Philadelphia, Merrihew & Thompson*, 1847.

——. On the cryptogamous origin of malarious and epidemic fevers. viii, 13–137 pp. 8°. *Philadelphia, Lea & Blanchard*, 1849. [P., v. 1017.]

——. Introductory lecture to the course of the practice of medicine, delivered in Jefferson Medical College. 24 pp. 8°. *Philadelphia, C. Sherman*, 1849.

——. Charge to the graduates of Jefferson Medical College. 24 pp. 8°. *Philadelphia, C. Sherman*, 1850.

——. Impediments to the study of medicine; a lecture, introductory to the course of practice of medicine. 28 pp. 8°. *Philadelphia, T. R. & P. G. Collins*, 1850.

——. On the progress of recent science. A lecture, introductory to the course of practice of medicine. 23 pp. 8°. *Philadelphia, T. K. & P. G. Collins*, 1851.

——. Charge to the graduates of Jefferson Medical College . . . With a list of the graduates. 16 pp. 8°. *Philadelphia, Collins*, 1857. [*Also, in:* P., v. 101.]

——. Five essays: [1. On the cryptogamous origin of malarious and epidemic fevers; 2. On animal magnetism; 3. On the penetrativeness of fluids; 4. On the penetration of gases; 5. On a new practice in acute and chronic rheumatism.] Edited by S. Weir Mitchell. xiv, 13–371 pp. 8°. *Philadelphia, J. B. Lippincott & Co.*, 1859.

For Biography, see Boston M. & S. J., 1850, xli, 38–41. *Also:* Charleston M. J., 1858, xiii, 122–127. *Also:* Med. & Surg. Reporter, Phila., 1858, xi, 307–311 (L. Turnbull). *Also:* N. Am. M. Chir. Rev., Phila., 1858, ii, 588–590. *Also:* Tr. M. Soc. Penn., Phila., 1859, n. s., iv, 93–98. *For Portrait, see* **Collection** of Portr. (Libr.)

——. *See, also:*

DICKSON (S. H.) The late Prof. J. K. Mitchell, M. D. Inaugural lecture. 8°. *Philadelphia*, 1858.

Mitchell (John S.) *An essay on the arbutus Uva ursi, and Pyrola umbellata and maculata

Mitchell (John S.)—continued.

of Linnæus. 35 pp. 8°. *Philadelphia, Eaken & Mecum*, 1803.

Mitchell (Joseph). *De hysteria. 1 p. l., 42 pp. 8°. *Edinburgi, Balfour et Smellie*, 1789.

Mitchell (Joseph). The conditions of health. A pamphlet for the people. 17 pp. 8°. *London, H. Michener*, 1871.

Mitchell (Joseph Thomas). Cholera; its physical phenomena, causes, and treatment; together with the sanitary arrangements and appliances for preserving health, necessary to be adopted at the time of the epidemic. 16 pp. 8°. *London, A. M. Pigott*, 1853.

Mitchell (Neal).

Co-Editor of: **Florida** (The) Medical and Surgical Journal, Jacksonville, 1885.

Mitchell (R.-D.) *Considérations sur la paralysie en général. 31 pp. 4°. *Paris*, 1835, No. 284, v. 290.

Mitchell (Robert). A general and historical treatise on cancer life; its causes, progress, and treatment. xii, 193 pp. 8°. *London, J. & A. Churchill*, 1879.

Mitchell (Robt. W.) Yellow fever in Memphis in 1873. 11 pp. 8°. *Louisville*, 1874.

Repr. from: Richmond & Louisville M. J., Louisville, 1874, xvii.

For Biography, see Mississippi Valley M. Month., Memphis, 1886, vi, 121.

Mitchell (S. L.)

Co-Editor of: **Western** (The) Medical Gazette, Cincinnati, 1832–5.

Mitchell (Samuel Weir) [1829–]. Researches upon the venom of the rattlesnake; with an investigation of the anatomy and physiology of the organs concerned. viii, 145 pp. 4°. [*n. p.*], 1860.

Smithson. Contrib. Knowl., Wash., 1860, xii.

——. On the treatment of rattlesnake bites, with experimental criticisms upon the various remedies now in use. 45 pp. 8°. *Philadelphia, J. B. Lippincott & Co.*, 1861.

Repr. from: N. Am. M.-Chir. Rev., Phila., 1861, v.

——. Experiments and observations upon the circulation in the snapping turtle, Chelonura serpentina, with especial reference to the pressure of the blood in the arteries and veins. 14 pp. 4°. *Philadelphia, C. Sherman & Son*, 1862.

——. Paralysis from peripheral irritation. 67 pp. 8°. *New York, J. Medole*, 1866. [*Also, in:* P., v. 105.]

Repr. from: N. York M. J., 1866, ii.

[——.] Case of George Dedlow. 8°. [*Boston*, 1866.]

Cutting from: Atlantic Month., Bost., 1866, xviii, 1–11.

——. On the retrogressive motions in birds produced by the application of cold to the cervical spine, with remarks on the use of that agent as an aid in physiological investigations. 15 pp. 8°. [*Philadelphia*], 1867. [P., v. 794.]

Repr. from: Am. J. M. Sc., Phila., 1867, n. s., liii.

——. Experimental contributions to the toxicology of rattle-snake venom. 34 pp. 8°. *New York, Moorhead, Simpson & Bond*, 1868.

Repr. from: N. York M. J., 1867–8, vi.

——. A list of the original memoirs of S. Weir Mitchell. 8 pp. 8°. *Philadelphia, J. B. Lippincott & Co.*, 1868.

——. Injuries of nerves, and their consequences. 377 pp. 8°. *Philadelphia, J. B. Lippincott & Co.*, 1872.

——. The same. Des lésions des nerfs et de leurs conséquences. Trad. et annoté avec l'autorisation de l'auteur par M. Dastre et précédé d'une préface par M. le professeur Vulpian. xlviii, 408 pp. 8°. *Paris, G. Masson*, 1874.

——. Wear and tear, or hints for the overworked. 4. ed. 59 pp. 16°. *Philadelphia, J. B. Lippincott & Co.*, 1874.

Mitchell (Samuel Weir)—continued.

——. The same. 5. ed. 76 pp. 12°. *Philadelphia, J. B. Lippincott & Co.*, 1887.

——. On some of the disorders of sleep. 13 pp. 8°. *Richmond*, 1875.

    Repr. from: Virginia M. Month., Richmond, 1875-6, ii.

——. On rest in the treatment of nervous disease. 20 pp. 8°. *New York, G. P. Putnam's Sons*, 1875.

    Is no. 4, v. 1, of: Am. Clin. Lect., by Seguin.

——. Neurotomy. With an examination of three [re]generated nerves, and notes upon neural repair, by R. M. Bertolet. 14 pp. 8°. [*Philadelphia*, 1876.]

    Repr. from: Am. J. M. Sc., Phila., 1876, n. s., lxxi.

——. The annual oration before the Medical and Chirurgical Faculty of Maryland, 1877. 18 pp. 8°. *Baltimore, Jones & Co.*, 1877.

    Repr. from: Tr. M. & Chir. Fac. Maryland, Balt., 1877.

——. Fat and blood, and how to make them. 101 pp. 12°. *Philadelphia, J. B. Lippincott & Co.*, 1877.

——. The same. 2. ed. 109 pp. 12°. *Philadelphia, J. B. Lippincott*, 1879.

——. The same. An essay on the treatment of certain forms of neurasthenia and hysteria. 4. ed. 166 pp. 8°. *Philadelphia, J. B. Lippincott Co.*, 1885.

——. The same. Du traitement méthodique de la neurasthénie et de quelques formes d'hystérie. Traduit par Oscar Jennings; avec une introduction par B. Ball. ix (1 l.), 169 pp. 8°. *Paris, O. Berthier*, 1883.

——. Nurse and patient, and camp cure. 73 pp. 24°. *Philadelphia, J. B. Lippincott & Co.*, 1877.

    Repr. from: Lippincott's Mag.

——. Address dedicatory of the new buildings erected by the University of Pennsylvania for its dental school and medical laboratories. 16 pp. 8°. *Philadelphia, J. B. Lippincott & Co.*, 1878.

——. Lectures on diseases of the nervous system, especially in women. xii, 13–238 pp., 5 pl. 8°. *Philadelphia, H. C. Lea's Son & Co.*, 1881.

——. The same. 2. ed. xii, 13–287 pp., 5 pl. 8°. *Philadelphia, Lea Bros. & Co.*, 1885.

——. A doctor's century. 4 l. sm. 4°. [*Philadelphia*, 1887.]

——. Celebration of the centennial anniversary of the institution of the College of Physicians of Philadelphia. Commemorative address. Delivered January 3, 1887. 40 pp. 8°. [*Philadelphia*, 1887.]

——. The rate of growth of the nails as a means of diagnosing certain forms of paralysis. 2 l. 12°. [*n. p., n. d.*]

    See, also, **Hammond** (William A.) & **Mitchell** (Samuel Weir) Experimental researches relative to corroval and vao, [etc.] 8°. [*Philadelphia*, 1859.]—**Reply** (A) to certain charges, [etc.] 8°. [n. p., 1885.]

—— & **Morehouse** (George R.) Researches upon the anatomy and physiology of respiration in the Chelonia. viii, 42 pp. 4°. *Washington*, 1864.

    Smithson. Contrib. Knowl., Wash., 1864, xiii.

——, **Morehouse** & **Keen** (W. W.), jr. Circular No. 6, Surgeon-General's Office, March 10, 1864. Reflex paralysis, the result of gunshot wounds, founded chiefly upon cases observed in the United States General Hospital, Christian street, Philadelphia. 17 pp. 12°. *Surgeon-General's Office, Washington*, 1864. [*Also, in:* P., v. 105.]

—— —— ——. Gunshot wounds and other injuries of nerves. vi, 9–164 pp. 12°. *Philadelphia, J. B. Lippincott & Co.*, 1864.

—— & **Reichert** (Edward T.) A partial study of the poison of Heloderma suspectum Cope, the Gila monster. 16 pp. 12°. *Philadelphia, Dorman*, 1883.

    Repr. from: Med. News, Phila., 1883, xlii.

Mitchell (S. W.) & **Reichert** (E. T.)—cont'd.

—— ——. Researches upon the venoms of poisonous serpents. ix, 186 pp., 5 pl. 4°. *Washington City*, 1886.

    Smithson. Contrib. Knowl., Wash., No. 647.

—— & **Wood** (H. C.) A report made to the College of Physicians of Philadelphia. 1 l. 4°. [*Philadelphia*, 1885.]

Mitchell (Thomas D.) Elements of chemical philosophy on the basis of Reid, comprising the rudiments of that science and the requisite experimental illustrations. xvi, 553 pp., 2 pl. 8°. *Cincinnati, Corey & Fairbank*, 1832.

——. Hints on the connexion of labor with study, as a preventive of diseases peculiar to students; and also as the best expedient for placing a good education within the reach of the poor. To which is appended the substance of an introductory lecture on medical education delivered in October, 1831. 85 pp. 12°. *Cincinnati, Corey, Fairbank & Co.*, 1832.

——. The annual oration of the Ohio Medical Lyceum. 32 pp. 8°. *Cincinnati, Truman, Smith & Co.*, 1834.

——. A cursory view of the history of chemical science, and some of its more important uses to the physician; being an introductory to the course of lectures for the session 1837–8. 22 pp. 8°. *Lexington, Finnell & Zimmermann*, 1837.

——. The pains and pleasures of a medical life, being an introductory to a course of lectures on materia medica and therapeutics. 23 pp. 8°. *Lexington, Ky., J. Virden*, 1839.

——. Annual address to the College of Physicians and Surgeons of Lexington; in which the principles and practice of medical ethics are illustrated and urged as essential to the welfare of the profession. 32 pp. 8°. *Lexington, Noble & Du lop*, 1839.

——. The good physician; being an introductory to the course of lectures on materia medica and therapeutics in the medical department of Transylvania University. 18 pp. 8°. *Lexington, Ky.*, 1842.

——. The reciprocal obligations of professors and pupils; an introductory lecture. 16 pp. 8°. *Lexington, N. L. Finnell*, 1845.

——. The character of Rush; an introductory to the course on the theory and practice of medicine, in the Philadelphia College of Medicine. 23 pp. 8°. *Philadelphia, J. H. Gihon*, 1848.

——. Lecture on epidemic cholera. 22 pp. 8°. *Philadelphia, Craig & Young*, 1849.

——. The study of medicine; an introductory lecture. 24 pp. 8°. *Philadelphia, Craig & Young*, 1849.

——. The past, the present, and the future of the medical profession in the United States of America; being a general introductory to the course of lectures in the third session of the Kentucky School of Medicine. 23 pp. 8°. *Louisville, Haldeman & Co.*, 1852. [*Also, in:* P., v. 544.]

——. Valedictory to the graduating class of the Philadelphia College of Medicine. 16 pp. 8°. *Philadelphia, T. K. & P. G. Collins*, 1852. c.

——. A lecture introductory to the course on materia medica and therapeutics in the Jefferson Medical College of Philadelphia. 31 pp. 8°. *Philadelphia, J. M. Wilson*, 1857.

——. Materia medica and therapeutics; with ample illustrations of practice in all the departments of medical science, and very copious notes of toxicology, suited to the wants of medical students, practioners, and teachers. 820 pp. 8°. *Philadelphia, J. B. Lippincott & Co.*, 1857.

——. Professor Mitchell's farewell to the graduating class of Jefferson Medical College. (With

Mitchell (Thomas D.)—continued.
a list of the graduates.) 12, 4 pp. 8°. *Philadelphia, Collins*, 1861.

———. The professor and the pupil; a general introductory lecture, delivered October 13th in Jefferson Medical College. 23 pp. 8°. *Philadelphia, H. B. Ashmead*, 1862.

Also, Editor of: **Transylvania** (The) Journal of Medicine and the Associate Sciences, Lexington, Ky., 1839.

For Biography, see Boston M. & S. J., 1852, xlv, 390-394 ("Cato").

Mitchell (Thomas R.) Practical remarks on the use of the speculum in the treatment of diseases of females. ix, 11-83 pp., 2 pl. 8°. *Dublin, Fannin & Co.*, 1849.

Mitchell (W. S.)
Co-Editor of: **Southern** (The) Journal of the Medical Sciences, New Orleans, 1866-7.—**New Orleans** (The) Journal of Medicine, 1868-70.

Mitchell (William). A family medical companion; a new medical work, devoted to the symptoms and remedies of one hundred and fifty diseases, embracing diseases of women and children. 191 pp. 8°. *Philadelphia, W. Brown*, 1835.

Mitchell Home, Torquay Institution for Trained Nurses. Annual report of the committee to the subscribers. 7., 1883. 8 pp. 8°. *Torquay, Directory office*, 1884.

———. Nurses for private families. Rules. 1 sheet. 4°. [*Torquay, n. d.*]

———. Rules for district nurses. 1 sheet. 4°. [*Torquay, n. d.*]

———. Rules for probationers and nurses. 1 sheet. 4°. [*Torquay, n. d.*]

Mitchill (Samuel Latham) [1764-1831]. *Circa novi genituram animalis. 3 p. l., 25 pp. 8°. *Edinburgi, Balfour et Smellie*, 1786.

———. Remarks on the gaseous oxyd of azote or of nitrogene, and on the effects it produces when generated in the stomach, inhaled into the lungs, and applied to the skin; being an attempt to ascertain the true nature of contagion, and to explain thereupon the phenomena of fever. 43 pp. 16°. *New York, T. & J. Swords*, 1795.

———. Explanation of the synopsis of chemical nomenclature and arrangement; containing several important alterations of the plan originally reported by the French academicians. 44 pp., 1 tab. 8°. *New York, T. & J. Swords*, 1801.

———. Observations on the Canada thistle. In a communication to David Hosack. 16 pp., 1 pl. 8°. [*New York*, 1810.]

Repr. from: Am. M. & Phil. Reg., N. Y., 1810, i.

———. A discourse pronounced by request of the Society for Instructing the Deaf and Dumb. 32 pp., 2 l. 8°. *New York, E. Conrad*, 1818.

———. Address to the officers composing the medical staff. 8 pp. 8°. *New York, E. Conrad*, 1820. [P., v. 747.]

———. Catalogue of the organic remains, which, with other geological and some mineral articles, were presented to the New York Lyceum of Natural History in August, 1826, by their associate. 40 pp. 8°. *New York, J. Seymour*, 1826. [P., v. 118.]

———. A discourse on the life and character of Thomas Addis Emmet. 26 pp. 8°. *New York, E. Conrad*, 1828.

Also, Co-Editor of: **Medical** (The) Repository, New York, 1797-1824.

For Biography, see **Francis** (J. W.) Reminiscences of Samuel Latham Mitchill, enlarged from Valentine's City Manual. 8°. *New York*, 1859.—**Gross** (S. D.) Lives of eminent American physicians. 8°. *Philadelphia*, 1861 (Francis), 267-288.—**Pascalis** (F.) Eulogy on the life and character of the Hon. Samuel Latham Mitchill, M. D., [etc.] 8°. *New York*, 1831.—**Some** of the memorable events and occurrences in the life of Samuel L. Mitchill, of New York. from the year 1786 to 1823 [with supplement to Feb., 1824]. 8°. [*n. p.*, 1824?]

For Portrait, see **Collection** of Portr. (Libr.)

Mites.
See **Acarus.**

Mitgau (L.) Bericht über die in Berlin, Amsterdam, Rochdale, Manchester, Croydon, Leamington und Abingdon eingeführten Systeme der Städtereinigung; unter Mitwirkung von Dr. R. Blasius, W. Clauss, H. Gebhard, W. Götte, J. Landauer, Dr. Rossmann, F. W. Schöttler. 58 pp., 1 plan. 8°. *Braunschweig, O. Haering u. Comp.*, 1880.

Mithobius (Burckhardus) [-1565]. Wie man sich für der hefftigen und tödtlichen seuche der Pestilentz bewaren sol, und so einer damit angegriffen, oder auch mit andern zufelligen kranckheiten behafft, mit was ertzney dem zuhelffen, Beyde reichen und armen, aus langer erfarung und den fürtrefflichsten Ertzten zusamen getragen. 61 l. 4°. *Erffurdt, S. Paul*, 1552.

Bound with: **Statmion** (Ch.) Ein kurtzer doch volkümlicher bericht [etc.] 4°. *Cobürgk*, 1551.

For Portrait, see **Collection**—van Kaathovon.—**Collection** of Portr. of Phys. & Men of Sc., 196.

Mithobius (Conradus). Disput. II. de curatione febris generatim, ejusdemque differentiis. 6 l. sm. 4°. *Jenæ, typ. T. Steinmanni*, [1598].

Mithobius (Georg. Ludovicus). *De abortu præcavendo. 34 pp., 3 l. 4°. *Halæ Magdeb., typ. J. C. Hilligeri*, [1739].

Mithobius de Mithofen (Joh. Christianus). *De fistula maxillari. 20 pp. 4°. *Halæ Magdeb., typ. J. C. Hilligeri*, [1735].

Mithoff (Aug. Ludov. Guilielmus). *Diss. sistens comparationem inter versionis negotium et operationem instrumentalem. 1 p. l., 62 pp. 8°. *Gottingæ, H. M. Grape*, [1788].

Mithoff (Hector Burchardus). *De sede irritamenti in epilepsia, adspersis practicis analectis. 22 pp. 4°. *Gottingæ, J. C. Dieterich*, [1788].

Mithridates.
See **Narcotics.**

Mitiffeu (A.-P.-H.-A.) *Sur les fistules à l'anus, et sur l'inutilité de l'opération pour la guérison des fistules incomplètes externes. 24 pp. 4°. *Paris*, 1812, No. 111, v. 91.

Mitiger (Joannes Henricus). *De nephritide vera ejusdemque curandi ratione legitima. 22 pp., 1 l. 4°. *Vitembergæ, lit. Kobersteinianis*, 1718.

Mitivié.
See **Sandon** (Léon). Plaidoyer contre les médecins, etc. 8°. *Bruxelles*, 1865.

Mitivié (Albert). *Quelques mots sur l'hérédité morbide. 62 pp. 4°. *Paris*, 1861, No. 95.

Mitivié [Jean-Étienne-Frumenthal] [1796-1871]. *Observations et réflexions pour servir à l'histoire de l'hydrocéphale aiguë chez les enfans. xii. 13-71 pp. 4°. *Paris*, 1820, No. 258, v. 162.

See, also, **Leuret** (François) & **Mitivié** (F.) De la fréquence du pouls, etc. 8°. *Paris*, 1832.

Mitjavila e Fisonel (Vicente).
See **Weikard** (Melchior Adam). Chave da prática medico-Browniana. 16°. *Lisboa*, 1800.

Mitkevich (Gregory). *K voprosu ob ostrotie tsentralnago zrienija i otnoshenii ego k granitsam polja zrienija v glazach razlichno refraktsii. [On acuteness of centralized sight and its relation to the limits of the field of vision in eyes of different refractive powers.] 28 pp. 8°. *St. Petersburg*, 1874.

Mitraud (Joseph-Antoine). *Quelques propositions sur les fractures de l'humérus. 13 pp. 4°. *Paris*, 1816, Nos. 49 & 91, v. 122.

———. Remarques sur les soins à donner à l'enfant pendant la première année de sa vie. viii, 9-25 pp. 4°. *Paris*, 1816, No. 49, v. 120.

Mitrofanoff (Demetrius). *O privivanii bugorchatki ve svjazi se sovremennime o nei uche-

Mitrofanoff (Demetrius)—continued.
nieme. [On inoculation of tubercle.] 30 pp.
8°. *St. Petersburg*, 1869.

Mitrophanow (Sila). * De spontaneo aëris
introitu in pulmonem. 33 pp. 4°. *Lugd. Bat.,
S. et J. Luchtmans*, 1765. [P., v. 1002.]

Mitry (Félix). * Études sur le ptosis congénital.
54 pp. 4°. *Paris*, 1885, No. 29.

Mitschein. Der Kinder-Arzt, oder fasslicher
Unterricht über die Erkennung, Verhütung und
Heilung der Kinderkrankheiten. Ein unent-
behrliches Hilfs- und Lesebuch für gebildete
Eltern. Nach Capuron, Feiler, Girtanner, Gorlis,
Henke, Hufeland, Jahn, Jörg, Meissner, Melin,
Rosenstein, Wendt, und Andern. vii, 285 pp.
18°. *Nordhausen, E. F. Fürst*, 1845.

Mitscherlich (Alfred). Der Cacao und die
Chocolade. vi, 129 pp., 3 pl. 8°. *Berlin, A.
Hirschwald*, 1859.

Mitscherlich (Carolus Gustavus) [1805–71].
Hydrargyri præparata usitatissima analytice
accuratius perscrutata. 32 pp. 8°. *Berolini,
typ. Brandesianis et Klewertianis*, [1829].

———. Bericht über Dr. Physick's Behandlung
der Coxarthrocace, im Auszuge mitgetheilt. 7
pp. 8°. [*Berlin*, 1831, *vel subseq.*]

———. Ueber die Wirkung des schwefelsauren
Kupferoxyds auf den thierischen Organismus.
29 pp. 8°. *Berlin, F. Sittenfeld*, 1837. [P., v. 698.]
Repr. from: Arch. f. Anat., Physiol. u. wissensch. Med.,
Berl., 1837.

———. De acidi acetici, oxalici, tartarici, citrici,
formici et boracici effectu in animalibus observato. 52 pp. 4°. *Berolini, formis Haynianis*, 1845.

———. Rede zur Feier des drei und fünfzigsten
Stiftungstages des königlichen medicinisch-
chirurgischen Friedrich-Wilhelms-Instituts am
2. August 1847. 18 pp. 8°. *Berlin, Gebr. Unger,*
[1847?]

———. Lehrbuch der Arzneimittellehre. 2. Aufl.
v. 1–3. 8°. *Berlin, G. Bethge*, 1847–61.

———. Rede zur Feier des ein und sechzigsten
Stiftungstages des königlichen medicinisch-
chirurgischen Friedrich-Wilhelms-Instituts am
2. August 1855. 26 pp. 8°. *Berlin, Gebr. Unger,*
[1855?]

———. Rede zur Feier des siebzigsten Stiftungstages des medicinisch-chirurgischen Friedrich-
Wilhelms-Instituts am 2. August 1864. 28 pp.
8°. *Berlin, Gebr. Unger*, [1864?]

Mitscherlich (Eilhard). Rede zur Feier des
ein und vierzigsten Stiftungstages des königli-
lichen medicinisch-chirurgischen Friedrich-Wilhelms-Instituts am 2. August 1835. 17 pp. 8°.
Berlin, Gebr. Unger, [1835?]

Mitscherlich (*Ernest*) [1794–   ].
Muspratt (S.) Biographical sketch of Ernest Mitscherlich. Lancet, Lond., 1850, n. s., ii, 660–663, port.

Mitsching (Car. Guil. Ferd.) * De articulatione
spuria et nova eam curandi methodo. 2 p. l.,
35 pp. 8°. *Hallæ, typ. Schimmelpfennigianis,*
[1822].

Mitsuma Kenzo.
See **Schultze.** Ikazensho Gank[w]ahen, etc. 12°.
Tokio, 1879.

Mittag (Albertus) [1820–   ]. * De urinæ sedi-
mentis. 28 pp., 2 l. 8°. *Berolini, typ. Nietackianis*, [1843].

Mittag (Fridericus Æmilius). * De pondere ac
pretio auscultationis et percussionis in morbis
organorum respirationis cognoscendis. 2 p. l.,
44 pp. 8°. *Gryphiæ, F. G. Kunike*, [1842].

Mittasch (Hans). * Die syphilitischen Erkrankungen der Augenlider, nebst zwei Beiträgen.
42 pp. 8°. *Würzburg, Becker*, 1883.

Mittelhaeusser (Joh. Daniel). * De incon-
tinentia urinæ ex partu globulis ligneis curanda,
occasione fœminæ eadem cum excretione fæcum

Mittelhaeusser (Joh. Daniel)—continued.
alvinarum per genitalia laborantis. 28 pp., 2 l.
sm. 4°. *Jenæ, lit. Nisianis*, [1716].
Also, in: HALLER. Disp. chir. [etc.] 4°. *Lausannæ,*
1755, iii, 597.

———. * Diss. fundamenta tractatus medici de
acquirenda et conservanda sobole brevi publico
dandi continens. 16 pp. 4°. *Jenæ, lit. Wertherianis*, [1720].
For Biography, see **Wedel** (Geo. Wolff.)

Mittelhaeuser (Lebr. Dan. Christoph). De
nodis articulorum et incurvatione ossium rachi-
tica. 4 l. 4°. *Jenæ, lit. Hellerianis*, [1747].

———. * Diss. sistens viam chyli ab intestinis ad
sanguinem. 20 pp. 4°. *Jenæ, lit. Tennemannianis*, [1752].
For Biography, see **Kaltschmied** (Carolus Fridericus).

Mittendorf (W. F.) Granular lids and contagious diseases of the eye. 2 p. l., 110 pp. 12°.
Detroit, G. S. Davis, 1886.

Mittendorffius (Bernhardus). Disputatio
physico-mathematica de ventis insolentibus et
inprimis eo, qui circa proxime præteritum ix de-
cemb. totam ferme Europam perflasse creditur,
cum appendice de recenti cometa. 22 l. 4°.
Wittebergæ, ex ergasterio Henckeliano, [1661].

Mittenwald.
See **Cholera** (*Asiatic, History, etc., of*), **Fever**
(*Typhus, History, etc., of*), *by localities.*

Mittenzweig (Bruno). * De carnis animalium
ægrotantium esu. 36 pp. 8°. *Berolini, G.
Schade*, [1853].

Mittenzweig (Hugo). * De eclampsia puerperali. 30 pp., 1 l. 8°. *Gryphiæ, F. Hache*, 1863. c.

———. Leitfaden für gerichtliche Obduktionen.
Ausgearbeitet auf Grund des Regulativs vom 13.
Februar 1875. viii, 112 pp. 8°. *Berlin, A.
Hirschwald*, 1878.

———. Die Bakterien-Aetiologie der Infections-
Krankheiten. viii, 135 pp. 8°. *Berlin, A. Hirschwald*, 1886.

———. The same. Bacteriën, de oorzaak van in-
fectieziekten. Naar het Duitsch door J. Schoondermark jr. ix, 111 pp. 8°. *Amsterdam, A. van
Klaveren*, [1886].

Mitterbacher (Bernard).
See **Damm** (Franz) & **Mitterbacher** (Bernard).
Untersuchung des Gisshübler-Sauerbrunns, [etc.] 8°.
Wien, 1798.

Mitterbacher (Carolus Rud.) * De organo
thymo. 35 pp. 8°. *Viennæ, typ. congregationis
Mechitaristicæ*, [1824].

Mitterbacher (Franciscus). De raro ventri-
culi casu cum vera morbi diagnosi. 47 pp. 8°.
Pragæ, typ. academicis, [1760].
Also, in: KLINKOSCH (J. T.) Diss. med. [etc.] 4°.
Pragæ et Dresdæ, 1775, i, 159–170.

———. De secretione urinæ fœminarum hysteri-
carum et de ea ut signo adfectionum earundem.
In: KLINKOSCH (J. T.) Diss. med. select. Prag. 4°.
Pragæ et Dresdæ, 1793, ii, 47–59.

Mittermaier (Carl J[oseph Anton]) [1787–
1867]. De principio imputationis alienationum
mentis in jure criminali recte constituendo. 62
pp. 4°. *Heidelbergæ, A. Osswald*, 1838.
See, also, **Gandolfi** (G.) Fondamenti di medicina
forensa analitica, etc. 8°. *Milano*, 1862–5.
For Biography, see J. de méd. ment., Par., 1868, viii,
279–286.

Mittermaier (Karl). Madeira und seine Be-
deutung als Heilungsort. Nach mehrjährigen
Beobachtungen für Aerzte geschildert. viii, 158
pp. 8°. *Heidelberg, J. C. B. Mohr*, 1855.
Bound with: SCHACHT (H.) Madeira und Tenerife. 8°.
Berlin, 1859.
Another copy bound with: RAMON PIÑA Y PEÑUELA (D.)
Topografía médica de la isla de Cuba. 8°. *Habana,*
1855.

———. Die Reinigung und Entwässerung der
Stadt Heidelberg, nebst einem Anhang über die

Mittermaier (Karl)—continued.

Wasserversorgung der Stadt. Denkschrift der von dem Heidelberger naturhistorisch-medicinischen Verein erwählten ärztlichen Commission: Prof. Dr. Friedreich, Knauff, Mittermaier, Moos. viii, 92 pp., 1 pl., 1 map. 4°. *Heidelberg, F. Bassermann,* 1870.

——. Die öffentliche Gesundheitspflege in Städten und Dörfern, mit besonderer Beziehung auf die Beseitigung der menschlichen Abfallstoffe. Im Auftrage der Centralstelle des landwirthschaftlichen Vereins in Baden. 1 p. l., 45 pp. 8°. *Karlsruhe, G. Braun,* 1875.

See, also, **Bahr** (Franciscus?) & **Mittermayer.** Einwirkung Madeira's auf Brustkranke. 8°. *Berlin,* 1861.

Mittermayer (Joannes). * De strumis ac scrophulis Bünsgensium. 24 pp., 1 pl. 4°. *Erfordiæ, typ. Groschianis,* [1723].

Mittermayr (Dominicus). * Ueber Rheumatismus acutus. 16 pp. 8°. *München, Kirschbaum u. Schuh,* 1872.

Mittheilungen des ärztlichen Vereines in Wien. Verantwortlicher Redacteur: J. Hock. [Fortnightly.] v. 3, Jan. 19, 1874, to Jan. 25, 1875. 1 v. 220 pp. 8°. *Wien, C. Finsterbeck.*
v. 3 complete in 15 nos.

Mittheilungen aus den amtlichen Berichten über die zum Ministerium des Innern gehörenden königlich preussischen Straf- und Gefängnissanstalten betreffend die Jahre 1858, 1859, resp. 1860. x, 402 pp., 1 l. 8°. *Berlin, W. Hertz,* 1861.

Mittheilungen des badischen ärztlichen Vereins. Besorgt durch Robert Volz. [Semimonthly.] v. 1-41, March 1, 1847-87. 8°. *Karlsruhe, G. Braun.*
Current. Want no. 10, v. 33, May 30, 1879. v. 1, 1847, complete in 17 nos ; v. 2 commenced Jan , 1848. In 1858, title became: **Aerztliche** Mittheilungen aus Baden. Dr. Volz died Jan. 22, 1882 ; Franz Neumann became editor.

Mittheilungen des Central-Vereins deutscher Zahnärzte, hrsg. von Dr. Moriz Heider. 1860. 2 p. l., 198 pp. 8°. *Wien, C. Gerold's Sohn.*

Mittheilungen über Cholera im engeren Verwaltungsbezirke Marktheidenfeld 1866. Speciell: Cholera-Epidemie zu Tiefenthal. Gedrucktes Manuscript. 131 pp., 1 ch. 8°. *Würzburg, F. E. Thein,* 1867.

Mittheilungen aus der dermatologischen Klinik des königlichen Charité-Krankenhauses zu Berlin, hrsg. von Ernst Schweninger. Hft. 1-3. 77 pp., 1 l., 2 pl.; 41 pp. 8°. *Berlin, Fischer,* 1887.

Mittheilungen aus einer am Johannistage 1832 in der Loge zu den drei Degen zu Halle gehaltenen Rede zum Besten der durch die Cholera Verwaiseten in Druck gegeben. 15 pp. 8°. *Halle, E. Anton,* 1832.

Mittheilungen aus dem Gebiete der gesammten Heilkunde. Hrsg. von einer medicinisch-chirurgischen Gesellschaft in Hamburg. v. 1-2, 1830-33. 8°. *Hamburg, Hoffmann u. Campe.*
Ended.

Mittheilungen aus dem Gebiete der Heilkunde. Im Vereine mit mehren practischen Aerzten Moskaus, hrsg. von H. Blumenthal, N. Anke und G. Levestamm. vii, 238 pp. 8°. *Leipzig, F. A. Brockhaus,* 1845.

Mittheilungen aus dem Gebiete der Medicin, Chirurgie und Pharmacie; in Verbindung mit einem Vereine von Aerzten und Pharmaceuten der Herzogthümer Schleswig und Holstein, hrsg. von C. H. Pfaff. v. 1-9, June 23, 1832, to May, 1843. 8°. *Kiel, Universitäts-Buchhandlung,* 1832-4; *Altona,* 1835-43.
v. 3-5, 1835-8. title also: **Practische** und kritische Mittheilungen [etc.], n. F., v. 1-3. v. 6-9, 1838-43, or v. 4-7, n. s., title also: **Practische** (C. H. Pfaff's) und kritische Mittheilungen, [etc.]; fortgesetzt von W. F. G. Behn, G. B. Günther, A. S. A. Meyn und G. A. Michaelis; redigirt von J. Samson.

Mittheilungen des heiligen Erzengels Raphael im Jahre 1855 durch den Mund der Crescentia Wolf, in Rapport mit den Mittheilungen seliger Geister, durch die Hand der Maria Kahlhammer. Hrsg. von Johann Schweykart. xi, 236 pp. 8°. *München, G. Franz,* 1856.

Mittheilungen aus dem Kölner Bürgerhospital. Hrsg. von Dr. Bardenheuer. 4. Hft. 8°. *Köln u. Leipzig,* 1886-7.
CONTENTS.
1. Hft. Osteoplastische Resection des Manubrium sterni. 79 pp., 10 pl.
2. Hft. Die Querexcision des Fusswurzelknochen, von Dr. J. Schmidt. 35 pp., 4 pl.
3. Hft. Die operative Behandlung der Hodentuberculose durch Resection der Nebenhoden, von Dr. Bardenheuer mit einer Einleitung von Dr. F. Bergkammer. xvi, 207 pp., 3 pl.
4. Hft. Interessante Kapitel aus dem Gebiete der Peritonealchirurgie. viii, 224 pp.

Mittheilungen aus dem magnetischen Schlafleben der Somnambüle Auguste K. in Dresden. 2. Ausg. xxii, 413 pp. 8°. *Dresden, R. Kuntze,* 1850.

Mittheilungen aus der medicinischen Klinik zu Würzburg. Hrsg. von C. Gerhardt und F. Müller. v. 1-2. xxix, 276 pp., 2 ch.; iv, 412 pp., 1 pl. 8°. *Wiesbaden, J. F. Bergmann,* 1885-6.

Mittheilungen an die Mitglieder des Centralvereins homöopathischer Aerzte. Nos. 1-16, May 20, 1872, to Sept. 20, 1877. 8°. *Württemberg u. Leipzig.*

Mittheilungen aus der ophthalmiatrischen Klinik in Tübingen. Hrsg. von Albrecht Nagel. Hft. 1-3, v. 1; Hft. 1-2, v. 2. 8°. *Tübingen, H. Laupp,* 1880-85.

Mittheilungen aus dem Osterlande. Gemeinschaftlich herausgegeben vom Gewerbe-Vereine, von der naturforschenden Gesellschaft und dem bienenwirthschaftlichen Vereine zu Altenburg. Nos. 1-2, v. 18, June, 1867. 8°. *Altenburg.*

Mittheilungen aus der thierärztlichen Praxis im preussischen Staate. C. Müller und F. Roloff. Neue Folge. v. 1-8, 1874-82. 8°. *Berlin, A. Hirschwald,* 1876-83.
Ended. A supplement to: **Archiv** für wissenschaftliche und praktische Thierheilkunde. v. 4-8 by Dr. Roloff and W. Schütz.

Mittheilungen des Vereines der Aerzte in Nieder-Oesterreich. Redacteur: Carl Kohn. [Semimonthly.] v. 1-13, April 15, 1875-87. 8°. *Wien, K. Czermak.*
Current. v. 1 complete in 17 nos., April to Dec., 1875; v. 2 commenced Jan., 1876. In 1881, v. 7, Dr. Kohn dropped.

Mittheilungen des Wiener medicinischen Doctoren-Collegiums, hrsg. vom Präsidium und redigirt vom Secretär des Collegiums, Dr. Leopold Hopfgartner. [Semi-monthly.] v. 1-13, Oct. 26, 1874-87. 8°. *Wien.*
Current. A continuation of: **Oesterreichische** Zeitschrift für practische Heilkunde. v. 2 commenced Jan., 1876.

Mittheilungen des württembergischen ärztlichen Vereins. Aus Auftrag desselben hrsg. von J. F. Blumhardt, G. Cless, G. Duvernoy, J. C. v. Frank [et al.]. v. 1, 1833-4. 596 pp. 8°. *Stuttgart, J. B. Metzler.*
Ended.

Mittié. Au comité de salut public. 12 pp. 12°. [*Paris*], an III [1795].

Mittié (Joannes Stanislaus) [1727-95]. * Utrum a gangliis nervi intercostalis partium omnium consensus? Præses: Joannes D'Arcet. 4 pp. 4°. *Parisiis, typ. F. A. Quillau,* 1764.

——. Questio medica: An quo uberior transpiratio, eo parcior fluxus menstruus? Præside Claudio Josepho Gentil. 4 pp. 4°. *Parisiis, typ. F. A. Quillau,* 1765.

Mittlacher (M. Zacharias). * De partu difficili. 12 l. 4°. [*Wittebergæ*], *lit. M. Henckelii,* 1675.

Mittlaender (Richard). * Das Verhältniss der Perforation zur Kephalothrypsie. 22 pp. 8°. *Leipzig, J. Klinkhardt.* [1870]. [P., v. 304.]

Mittler (Heinrich). Versuche über Transfusion des Blutes. 14 pp. 8°. [*Wien,* 1868.] [P., v. 802.]
Repr. from: Sitzungsb. d. k. Akad. d. Wissensch., 1868, lviii.

Mittmann (Eugenius) [1821–]. * De syphilidis historia notæ quædam. 36 pp. 8°. *Berolini, typ. Nietackianis,* [1844].

Mittmann (Josephus). * De luxatione patellæ, adjecta historia morbi. 44 pp. 8°. *Gryphiæ, F. G. Kunike,* 1850.

Mittre (Adolphe). * Notes sur le diagnostic et le traitement chirurgical des abcès du foie. 72 pp. 4°. *Lyon,* 1887, 1. s., No. 366.

Mittrich (Gustavus Adolphus). * De anomaliis systematis uropoëtici in scarlatina. 16 pp. 4°. *Lipsiæ, typ. Staritzii,* 1846.
c.

Mittweg (Aloysius Conradus). * De somno sano ac morboso. 1 p. l., 39 pp. 8°. *Halæ, formis J. C. Hendelii,* [1820].

Mittweg (Carl) [1843–]. Ueber Paralysis progressiva und die Erscheinung der Kleptomanie bei derselben. 34 pp. 8°. *Berlin, G. Schade,* [1869].

Mittweg (Carolus Henr. Aloys.) [1828–]. * De uteri polypis. 32 pp. 8°. *Berolini, G. Schade,* [1853].

Mitzkuner (Leon). * Zur Frage von der Entstehung der Divertikel der Harnblase. 21 pp. 8°. *Jena, M. Hermsdorf,* 1878.

Mitzky (Joannes Henricus). * De vario coffeæ potum parandi modo. 28 pp. sm. 4°. *Wittebergæ, lit. C. C. Dürrii,* [1782].
For Biography, see **Bochmer** (Geo. Rud.)

Miura (Igacushi Moritzi) [1857–]. * Beiträge zur Kenntniss der Gallencapillaren. 27 pp., 1 l., 1 col. pl. 8°. *Berlin, G. Schade,* [1884].

Mivart (St. George). On the genesis of species. xv, 296 pp. 8°. *London, Macmillan & Co.,* 1871.
——. The same. 314 pp. 8°. *New York, D. Appleton & Co.,* 1871.
——. Man and apes, an exposition of structural resemblances and differences bearing upon questions of affinity and origin. vi, 200 pp., 1 l., 41 pl. 8°. *London, R. Hardwicke,* 1873.
——. The same. vi, 1 p. l., 200 pp., 1 pl. 8°. *New York, D. Appleton & Co.,* 1874.
——. Lessons in elementary anatomy. xxviii, 535 pp. 16°. *London, Macmillan & Co.,* 1873.
——. The same. New ed. xxvi, 535 pp. 12°. *London, Macmillan & Co.,* 1879.
——. The common frog. vii, 158 pp. 12°. *London, Macmillan & Co.,* 1874.
——. The cat. An introduction to the study of backboned animals, especially mammals. xxiii, 557 pp. 8°. *London, J. Murray,* 1881.
See, also, **Wright** (C.) Darwinism. 8°. *London,* 1871.
——— & **Murie** (James). Observations on the anatomy of Nycticebus tardigradus. 18 pp. 8°. [*London,* 1865.] [P., v. 1488.]
Repr. from: Proc. Zool. Soc. Lond., Feb. 28, 1865.

Mivelle (Hippolyte-Joseph). * Des indications thérapeutiques fournies par l'appréciation des causes. II. [etc.] 53 pp. 4°. *Paris,* 1843, No. 173, v. 406.

Mixture ferro-manganique, préservateur des carènes de navires en fer. Vian & Cie. 19 pp. 8°. *Marseille, J. Clappier,* 1865.

Miyake Shiu. Biori Soron. [General pathology.] 3. ed. 3 p. l., 686 pp., 8 tab., 17 l. 12°. *Tokio,* 1882.
Japanese text.
——. Biori Kakuron. [Special pathology.] 2 v. 3 p. l., 912 pp., 8 tab., 10 l.; 6 p. l., 922 pp., 6 tab., 10 l. 12°. *Tokio,* 1882.
Japanese text.

Miyake Shiu—continued.
——. Biotai Boken Shiyo. [Pathological anatomy.] 4 p. l., 559 pp., 1 l. 12°. *Tokio,* 1882.
Japanese text.
——. Jirio Tsu-ron. [A treatise on general practice of medicine.] v. 1. 3 p. l., 151 pp., 2 l. 12°. *Tokio,* 1883.
Japanese text. Not completed.

Miye Genji.
See **Heath** (Christopher). Tikken Kaibo Gaku, etc. 3 v. 8°. *Osaka,* 1880.

Mizaldus [**Mizauld**] (Antonius) [1520–78]. Secretorum agri enchiridion primum, hortorum curam, auxilia, secreta, et medica præsidia inventu prompta, ac paratu facilia, libris tribus pulcherrimis complectens. 7 p. l., 180 ff. 16°. *Lutetiæ, apud F. Morellum,* 1560.
——. Alexikepus, seu auxiliaris hortus, extemporanea morborum remedia ex singulorum viridariis facile comparanda paucis proponens. Ad hæc, Dioclis Caristii epistola ad Antigonum, de tuenda valetudine per hortensia. 7 p. l., 267 pp., 6 l. 16°. *Lutetiæ, apud F. Morellum,* 1565.
——. The same. Alexikepus, seu auxiliaris et medicus hortus, rerum variarum, et secretorum remediorum accessione locupletatus. 11 p. l., 200 pp. 12°. *Coloniæ, apud J. Gymnicum,* 1576.
——. The same. 11 p. l., 107 ff., 5 l. 8°. *Parisiis, apud C. Morellum,* 1607.
Bound with his: Opusculorum pars prima. 8°. *Parisiis,* 1607.
——. The same. Artztgarten von Kreutern so in den Gärten gemeinlichen wachsen, und wie man durch dieselbigen allerhand Kranckheiten und Gebrechen eylendts heilen soll. Item ein Artztbüchlin, newe und wunderbare weiss begreiffend wie man allerley Frücht, Gartenkräuter, Wurtzel, Beer und Trauben artznen soll, dass man dieselb zum purgieren möge brauchen. Auch ein schöne weiss und kunstmancherley Wein zu machen, sampt einer Erzehlung etlicher geartzneten Wein, so für allerhand Kranckheiten nutzlich seind. Jetzund aber newlich verteutscht, durch Georgen Henisch von Bartfeld, vormals in teutscher Sprach nit gesehen worden. 4 p. l., 382 pp., 3 l.; 109 pp. 12°. *Basel, L. König,* 1616.
——. The same. Le jardin médicinal, enrichi de plusieurs et divers remèdes et secrets. Mis nouvellement en françois. 463 pp. 12°. [*Paris*], *J. Lertout,* 1578.
Bound with the following.
——. Le jardinage; contenant la manière d'embellir les jardins, les préserver de toute vermine, et en tirer remèdes propres aux maladies des hommes. Item, comme il faut enter les arbres, et les rendre médicinaux. Mis en françois [from the Latin]. 7 p. l., 399 pp. 12°. [*Paris*], *J. Lertout,* 1578.
——. Memorabilium aliquot naturæ arcanorum silvula, rerum variarum sympathias, et antipathias, seu naturales concordias et discordias, libellis duobus complectens. 88 pp. 32°. *Francofurti, apud J. Wechelum et P. Fischerum consortes,* 1592.
——. Harmonia superioris naturæ mundi et inferioris; una cum admirabili fœdere et sympatheia rerum utriusque. 7 p. l., 36 ff. 8°. *Parisiis, ex off. F. Morelli,* 1598.
Bound with his: Opusculorum pars prima. 8°. *Parisiis,* 1607.
——. Paradoxa rerum cœli ad Epiponum Philuranum et socios. 36 ff. 8°. *Parisiis, ex off. F. Morelli,* 1598.
Bound with his: Opusculorum pars prima. 8°. *Parisiis,* 1607.
——. Artificiosa methodus comparandorum hortensium fructuum, olerum, radicum, uvarum, vinorum, carnium et jusculorum, quæ corpus

Mizaldus [Mizauld] (Antonius)—continued.
elementer purgent, et variis morbis, absque ulla
noxa et nausea, blande succurrant. 7 p. l., 39 ff.
8°. *Parisiis, apud C. Morellum*, 1607.
 Bound with his: Opusculorum pars prima. 8°. *Parisiis*, 1607.

———. Dioclis Carystii medici, ab Hippocrate
fama et ætate secundi, aurea ad Antigonum
regem epistola, de morborum præsagiis, et
eorumdem extemporaneis remediis. Ad hæc,
Arnaldi a Villa-Nova medici præstantissimi consilium ad regem Aragonum, de salubri hortensium usu. De Syrmaismo, et ratione purgandi
vomitum, ex Ægyptiorum invento et formula.
Jos. Langio autore. 27 ff., 1 l. 8°. *Parisiis,
apud C. Morellum*, 1607.
 Bound with his: Opusculorum pars prima. 8°. *Parisiis*, 1607.

———. Opusculorum pars prima, in qua: Hortorum secreta, cultus et auxilia . . . illustrata.
De hortensium arborum insitione. Dendrana-
tome: seu exploratio et dissectio corporis arborei
in sua sigillatim membra et partes. De hominis
symmetria, proportione et commensuratione.
Alexikepus, seu auxiliaris et medicus hortus . . .
Artificiosa methodus comparandorum hortensium fructuum . . . 7 p. l., 132 ff. 8°. *Parisiis,
apud C. Morellum*, 1607.

———. Opusculorum pars secunda, in qua: Memorabilium utilium, ac jucundorum centuriæ
novem, in aphorismos arcanorum omnis generis
. . . digestæ. Harmonia superioris naturæ mundi
et inferioris . . . Paradoxa rerum cœli . . .
Opusculum de sena . . . Dioclis Carysti medici
. . . de morborum præsagiis . . . Joa. Langius
de Syrmaismo et ratione purgandi . . . Arnaldi
a Villa-Nova . . . de salubri hortensium usu.
Ejusdem Jo. Langii epistola, an caseus edendo
sit salubris . . . 14 p. l., 132 ff. 8°. *Parisiis,
apud C. Morellum*, 1607.
 Bound with preceding.

———. Opusculum de sena, planta inter omnes,
quotquot sunt, hominibus beneficentissima et
saluberrima. Accessit Proclus, De arcanis naturæ. 18 ff., 1 l. 8°. *Parisiis, apud C. Morellum*, 1607.
 Bound with his: Opusculorum pars prima. 8°. *Parisiis*, 1607.

———. Centuriæ ix memorabilium, utilium, ac
jucundorum in aphorismos arcanorum omnis
generis locupletes, perpulcre digestæ; accessit
his appendix nonnullorum secretorum, experimentorum, antidotorumque contra varios morbos, tam ex libris manuscriptis quam typis
excursis, collecta. Seorsum excusa, harmonia
cœlestium corporum et humanorum, dialogis
undecim astronomice et medice per Anton. Mizal-
dum elaborata et demonstrata. Item, memorabilium aliquot naturæ arcanorum sylvula, rerum
variarum sympathias et antipathias libellis ii
complectens. 15 p. l., 443 pp. 16°. *Francofurti, ex off. typog. N. Hoffmanni*, 1613.

Mizerski (Anastasius). *De chloroformii usu
inter partum. 28 pp. 8°. *Berolini, Rosenthal*,
[1861].

Mizonkuvich (Carol. Aloys.) *De sympathia
renum præcipue in statu morboso. 27 pp. 8°.
[*Dorpat*], *typ. J. C. Schünmanni*, 1816, v. 6.

Mladek (Henricus). *De bubone syphilitico.
25 pp. 8°. *Pragæ, J. H. Pospjsil*, [1838].

Mlinarich (Josephus). *De vermibus in corpore humano obviis. 40 pp. 8°. *Budæ, typ.
Reg. Univ. Hung.*, 1832. [P., v. 1321.]

Mlink (Isidor I.) [1850–]. *Ueber den Soor-
pilz. 31 pp. 8°. *Berlin, G. Schade*, [1877].

Mnichovski (A. K.) Jenstvennost. [Woman-
hood.] 74 pp. 16°. *Kieff, S. V. Kuljenko*, 1885.
———. Brak. [Marriage.] 106 pp., 1 l. 16°.
Kieff, E. T. Kerer, 1886.

Mnichovski (A. K.)—continued.
 ———. Tipi dushevnago razvitija. [Types of
development of mental disorders.] 1 p. l., 153
pp., 1 l. 16°. *Kieff, S. V. Kuljenko*, 1886.

Moacho (Mattheus Cesario Rodrigues). Relatorio geral do movimento vaccinico do reino de
Portugal e ilhas adjacentes durante os annos de
1850 a 1859 apresentado ao Conselho de saude
publica. (Appenso ao relatorio geral de serviço
da repartição de saude de 1862.) xiii, 298 pp.,
2 l. fol. *Lisboa, imp. nacional*, 1864.

Moale (William A.)
 See **Martin** (H. Newell) & **Moale** (William A.)
Handbook of vertebrate dissection. Pt. 2. How to dissect
a bird. 8°. *New York*, 1883. ———. The same. 8°.
New York, 1884.

Moat (C. W.) & **Greer** (J.) Rational arguments on the nature of true pathology, which, it
is presumed, prove the absurdity of dissection
and of the use of poisons, as necessary or useful
to the science of medicine. 2. ed. 8°. *Glasgow,
C. W. Moat*, [1832].
 In: Morison (J.) Morisoniana. 4. ed. 8°. *London*,
1834, ii, 339–378.

Moat (H. Shepheard). The mother's book of
hygeian midwifery; being a familiar treatise on
the security of health to females during that
most interesting period of their lives, the state
of pregnancy; with remarks on the management
of infants; founded on the doctrines of the
British College of Health. 108+ pp. 8°. *New
York, D. Mitchell*, 1837.

Moat (Thomas). The 1830 new year's gift to the
world, in a short treatise on the original cause
of the small-pox virus. Wherein it is proved to
be not only a necessary operation of nature, but
perfectly harmless and beneficial if judiciously
treated, etc. 8°. *Plymouth*, 1830.
 In: Morison (J.) Morisoniana. 3. ed. 8°. *London*,
1831, 373–392. *Also, in:* ———. The same. 4. ed. 8°.
London, 1834, i, 373–392. Also forms a part of the following
work.

———. The practical proofs of the soundness of
the hygeian system of physiology, selected from
the appendix of "Morisoniana", as incontrovertible testimonies to the afflicted of the inestimable value of Morison's vegetable universal
medicine, including "The origin of life and
cause of all diseases explained", [by James Mo-
rison], and an entirely new view of the origin
of the small-pox virus, etc. 168 pp. 8°. *Brooklyn, N. Y., H. S. Moat*, 1831.
 See, also, **Morison** (James). Morisoniana, etc. 3. ed.
8°. *London*, 1831.

Mobach (Elias).
 See **Hannemann** (J. L.) De anomalis et paradoxis
morborum curationibus. sm. 4°. *Kiliæ*, [1706].

Mobèche (Louis). * De la période prodromique
de la paralysie générale. 35 pp. 4°. *Paris*,
1874, No. 428.

Moberg (Wilhelm). * Om accommodationsbred-
den och refractionsanomalierna hos ögat. 62
pp. 8°. *Upsalæ, Edquist & Berglund*, 1862.

Mobile. Board of Health of the City of Mobile.
Annual reports to the mayor and city council.
1.–3. (1871–6) 8°. *Mobile*, 1872–7.

———. Monthly statements of mortality. July,
1875, to Dec., 1887. 4°. [*Mobile*, 1875–88.]
 The statements for Jan. to May, and for Nov. and Dec.,
1879, were not published. The port administration would
only authorize the publication during the existence of quarantine, viz, June to Oct.

Mobile.
 See, also, **Education** (*Medical*), *etc.*, **Fever**
(*Yellow, History, etc., of*), *by localities.*
 ANDERSON (W. H.) The city of Mobile and
the contiguous country about the Gulf coast, as
a winter resort for health and pleasure of invalids and others from the North and Northwest.
8°. *Mobile*, 1881.
 ———. The same. 8°. *Molile*, 1882.

Mobile.

SMITH (W. H.) History of the Mobile dumping ground. Sept. 17, 1872. fol. [*n. p.*, 1872.]

Anderson (W. H.) Report on the diseases of Mobile for the year 1850. Proc. M. Ass. Alabama 1850, Mobile, 1851, iv, 68–73. *Also:* South. M. Rep. (Fenner), N. Orl., 1850, ii, 307–314. ———. Report on the diseases of Mobile. Proc. M. Ass. Alabama, Mobile, 1854, vii, 39–50. — **Anderson** (W. H.) & **Ketchum** (G. A.) Report on the diseases of Mobile during the year 1852. *Ibid.* (1851), 1852, v, 24–30.— **Cochran** (J.) Endemic and epidemic diseases of Mobile, considered with special reference to their ætiology and prophylaxis. Tr. M. Ass. Alabama, Mobile, 1871, 225–268. *Also*, Reprint. ———. Mortuary and meteorological tables of the city of Mobile, for the year 1874. Tr. M. Ass. Alabama, Montgomery, 1875, 314–332.—**Fearn** (R. L.) On the diseases of Mobile, Alabama, from March 1 to the 1st of December, 1849. N. Orl. M. & S. J., 1849–50, vi, 745–751.—**Huestis** (J. W.) Topographical and medical sketches of Mobile for the year 1835. Am. J. M. Sc., Phila., 1836, xix, 65–85.—**Ketchum** (G. A.) Contributions to the vital statistics of Mobile. South. M. Rep. (Fenner), N. Orl., 1849, i, 281–286. ———. Notes on the topography, sanitary condition, and vital statistics of Mobile, Alabama. *Ibid.*, 1850, ii, 301–307. ———. Report on the diseases of Mobile for 1854. Proc. M. Ass. Alabama, Mobile, 1855, viii, 99–117. — **Lopez** (A.) Report on the diseases which prevailed in Mobile, for 1848; with an alphabetical list of the same appended. Read before the Alabama State Medical Association, March, 1849. N. Orl. M. & S. J., 1849–50, vi, 348–355.—**Moses** (G. A.) Report on the diseases of Mobile during the year 1871. Tr. M. Ass. Alabama, Mobile, 1872, 158–172, 2 pl.—**North** (S. B.) Meteorological table for Mobile. N. Orl. M. & S. J., 1850–51, vii, 121–123.—**Ross** (F. A.) Report of the diseases of Mobile, Alabama. Tr. M. Ass. Alabama, Mobile, 1870, 359–375.

Mobile medical profession. Rules of etiquette; rate of charges and fee-bill. 10 pp. 16°. *Mobile, J. F. Leavens*, 1838.

Mobile Medical Society. Constitution and by-laws, to which is annexed its charter, granted by the legislature December 21, 1841. 12 pp. 8°. *Mobile, Dade & Thompson*, 1843.

Mobitz (Friedrich). * Experimentelle Studien über die quantitativen Veränderungen des Hämoglobingehaltes im Blute bei septischem Fieber. 83 pp., 1 l., 3 pl. 8°. *Dorpat, H. Laakmann*, 1883.

Moch (Nathan). * Recherches sur l'étiologie, sur la nature et sur la prophylactique générale de la phthisie pulmonaire. 2 p. l., 84 pp. 4°. *Strasbourg*, 1846, No. 160, v. 12.

Mochinger (Jacobus). De catarrho. 11 l. 4°. *Jenæ, lit. G. Sengenwaldi*, 1651.

Mochner (Franciscus Joannes). * Conspectus partuum in Lechodochio Pragensi, a prima ejus origine usque ad finitum annum scholasticum, sive usque ad ultimam mensis Augusti 1825 celebratorum; necnon rerum memoratu dignarum in matribus et infantibus observatarum. 3 p. l., vi, 111 pp., 1 tab. 8°. *Pragæ, Kronberger et Weber*, 1826.

Mock (H.) Das Stahlbad Imnau in Hohenzollern. 67 pp., 1 l. sm. 8°. *Imnau, M. Frey*, 1873.

Mock (Hermann). * Ueber Eclampsie der Gebärenden. 30 pp., 1 l. 8°. *Halle, Sipke*, [*n. d.*] c.

Mockel (Henricus) [1815–]. * Quædam de congestione venosa et de morbis inde proficiscentibus. 31 pp. 8°. *Berolini, typ. Nietackianis*, [1842].

Mocquard (François). * Sur la docimasie pulmonaire et sur un caractère de respiration chez les nouveau-nés tiré des gaz contenus dans les poumons. 47 pp. 4°. *Paris*, 1873, No. 29.

Mocquin (Antoine) * D'un moyen nouveau de prévenir la péritonite consécutive à la kélotomie. 33 pp., 2 l. 4°. *Montpellier, J. Martel aîné*, 1866, No. 102. c.

Mocquin (L.) * Propositions sur divers points de chirurgie. 15 pp. 4°. *Paris*, 1830, No. 112, v. 232.

Mocquot (G.-P.) * Sur l'application du trépan au sternum, dans les cas de fracture, de carie, et

Mocquot (G.-P.)—continued. d'abcès au médiastin. 15 pp. 4°. *Paris, an XIII* [1805], No. 439, v. 55.

Mocquot (Gabriel). * Essai de pneumographie pour servir à l'étude des maladies des enfants. 2 p. l., 66 pp. 4°. *Paris*, 1875, No. 451.

Moczyński (Michael) [1825–]. * De atresia pudendi. 28 pp. 8°. *Berolini, B. Schlesinger*, [1850].

Modas (Jean-Baptiste). * Sur l'hydropisie du péricarde. 46 pp. 8°. *Paris, an X* [1802], v. 9.

Moddel (Marcus). Stromata materiæ medicæ sceptica. 20 pp. 4°. *Traj. ad Viadr.*, [1788].

Modderman (Rudolph Sicco Tjaden). * De leer der osmose. 4 p. l., vi, 174 pp., 2 l. 8°. *Leeuwarden, G. T. N. Suringar*, [1857].

Model (August). * Ein Fall von glandulärem Cystosarcom mit autogenem Atherom. 23 pp., 2 pl. 4°. *Erlangen, A. E. Junge*, 1858.

———. Zur Orientirung in der Trichinenfrage. Ein Wort für gebildete Laien. 28 pp. 8°. *Nordlingen, C. H. Beck*, 1866.

Model rules for provident dispensaries. By the medical committee of the Charity Organization Society. 16 pp. 8°. *London, Spottiswoode & Co.*, 1878.

Model (The) vaccine propagating establishment, etc. *See* **Wyeth** (John) & Bro. 8°. *Philadelphia*, 1885.

Modell (Joh. Georg) [1711–75]. * De borace nativa, a Persis Borech dicta. 36 pp. 4°. *Londini, C. Davis*, 1747.

———. The same. 40 pp. 4°. *Recusa Halæ Magdeb., typ. J. C. Hendelii*, 1749.

Modena. Regolamenti municipali di polizia urbania d' igiene pubblica e d' ornato. 48, 33, 8, 15 pp. 12°. *Modena, tipog. di A. E. A. Cappelli*, 1872.

Modena.

See, also, **Fever** (*Typhoid, History, etc., of*), **Hospitals** (*Descriptions, etc., of*), *by localities.*

RAMAZZINI (B.) De fontium Mutinensium admiranda scaturigine tractatus physico-hydrostaticus. 4°. *Mutinæ*, 1691.

Astegiano (G.) Saggio di meteorologia medica (delle malattie dominanti in Modena). Spallanzani, Modena, 1883, 2. s., xii, 225 ; 305.—**Machiavelli.** Sedici mesi allo spedale militare divisionale di Modena. Gior. di med. mil., Torino, 1864, xii, 473 ; 505.—**Ragona** (D.) Résumé des observations sur la météorologie faites à l'Observatoire royal de Modène, lat. 44° 38' 53", long. 0ʰ 34ᵐ 21ˢ E. de Paris; Hr. 63ᵐ 16 niv. mer ; année 1867. Mém. Soc. d. sc. nat. de Cherbourg, Par., 1868, xiv, 129–148.—**Ramazzini** (B.) De constitutione annorum 1690–91 ac de rurali epidemica, quæ Mutinensis agri, et vicinarum regionum colonos graviter afflixit. Misc. Acad. nat. curios. 1690, Norimb., 1691, 2. decuria, ix (app.), 15 : (1691), 1692, 2. decuria, x (app.), 79.—**Riccardi** (P.) Nuovo contribuzione all' antropologia del Modenese : note ed appunti intorno al peso, alla circonferenza toracica, alla capacità vitale, al diametro biacromiale, alla forza muscolare dei giovanetti e delle giovanette del comune di Modena. Gior. d. r. Accad. di med. di Torino, 1883, 3. s., xxxi, 383–412.

Modern (The) Cremastist. Devoted to the interests of funeral reform. M. L. Davis and W. U. Hensel, editors and publishers. [Monthly.] v. 1–2, 1886–7. 8°. *Lancaster, Pa.* Current.

Modern Life. Its moral, social, and physical health. A paper devoted to the health interests of the household. Edited by Jos. H. Warren and C. E. Warren. [Fortnightly.] Nos. 1–10, v. 1, Feb. 15, to June 21, 1887. 4°. *Boston.*

Modern (The) Physician and Family Adviser. A monthly journal of domestic medicine, hydropathy, and sanitary science. Edited by George Lade and E. B. Shuldham. v. 2, 1880. 1 v. 8°. *London.*

Modern (The) practice of the London hospitals, viz.: St. Bartholomew's, St. Thomas's, Guy's, St. George's, the Portuguese, and the Lock, at

Modern (The) practice [etc.]—continued.
Hyde-Park Corner. A new edition. v, 7–121 pp.
8°. *London, G. Lister,* [*n. d.*]
———. The same. 3. ed. xi, 229, xxii pp. 12°.
London, S. Crowder [*and others*], 1770.

Modern (The) quack, or medicinal impostor; in
three parts; with a supplement, displaying the
present set of pretenders to clap-curing, giving
judgment upon urine, etc., wherein their frauds
and abuses are laid open; rules, also, to know
and cautions against them; and, for the farther
security of the sick of any sort, a catalogue is
annexed of all the members of the Royal College
of Physicians, residing in town, with the places
of their several abodes or habitations. The second
edition, to which, as related to the same subject, are added by another hand, some remarks
upon Dr. Hancock's treatise, which he entitles:
Febrifugum magnum, or cold water the best cure
for fevers. 17 p. l., 206 pp. 8°. *London, T.
Warner,* 1724.

Modern (The) quacks detected. In three parts.
I. Exposing their qualifications and remedies.
II. Proving the insufficiency of the latter to
answer what is proposed by them. III. Unfolding the nature and ill consequences thereof.
Dedicated to the president of the Royal College
of Physicians in London; in which are exhibited
reasons why they ought to admit Dr. Schomberg
a member of their learned and honourable body.
By a London physician. 62 pp. 8°. *London,
M. Cooper,* 1752. [*Also, in :* P., v. 1338.]

Modern surgical instruments, chiefly of France
and Germany, illustrated. 16 pp., 8 pl. 8°.
London, H. Renshaw, 1844.

Moderna (La) medicina. Medicina; chirurgia;
medicina comparata; scienze affini, con particolare interesse sullo studio delle febbri, per cura
del dottore M. Gay. v. 1–6, April, 1878, to Dec.,
1886. 8°. *Torino.*

Moderne (Der) Laokoon, oder die Homöopathie
in Bayern. Ein offenes Wort an die Zunftmei-
ster. 83 pp. 8°. *Leipzig, O. Purfürst,* 1861.

Modificazioni ed aggiunte alla tariffa dei
medicinali per i servizi sanitari municipali di
Torino, approvate dalla giunta municipale il 16
dicembre 1886. 19 pp. 4°. *Torino, E. Botta,*
1887.

Modigliana.

See **Cholera** (*Asiatic, History, etc., of*), by localities.

Modin (Louis-Alfred). * Des eaux martiales de
Provins (Seine-et-Marne), et de leurs applications à la thérapeutique. 40 pp. 4°. *Paris,*
1852, No. 188, v. 529.

Modletyn.

LODGMAN VON AUEN (J. [R.]) Inventi neo
fontis aquas virtute salubris Sanct-Annæus ager
Modletinensis habet. Das ist : Neü erfundenes
Wasser Sanct Annæ genannt, welches viele
Krancke in der Noth schon erkannt, zu Modletyn
in dem Tschaslauer Creyss, dieses Königreichs
Böheimb. Von dessen Cräfften, Wirckung und
Gewalt wahrhaffter Bericht und kurtzer Inhalt.
12°. *Kuttenberg,* 1738.

Modlinski (Josephus). * Tentamen med. circa
rabiem. 19 pp. sm. 4°. *Monspelii, X. Jullien,*
1836.

Modo di preservarsi dal cholera-morbus. 8 pp.
8°. [*Roma, T. Ajani,* 1854.] [P., v. 872.]
Repr. from : Gior. di Roma, 1854.

Modo, et ordine ch' hà tenuto, e tiene Annibale
Patriarcha ; per la quale si sente haver sanato,
et sana tanti amalati di contaggio. Alla santità
di N. S. Papa Urbano VIII. 21 pp. sm. 4°. *Bologna, N. Tebaldini,* 1630.

Modo (Del) di prevenire e curare il cholera epidemico secondo i principii dell' omeopatia. 10
pp. 8°. [*Torino, Ceresole e Panizza,* 1854.]
[P., v. 1456.]

Modolea (V.) * Des positions inclinées de l'extrémité céphalique envisagées au point de vue
du diagnostic et du traitement. 38 pp. 4°.
Paris, 1873, No 423.

Modum.

See, also, **Fever** (*Typhoid, History, etc., of*), by
localities.
THAULOW (H. A.) Prospektus over Modums
Kuranstalt og Sanatorium i Norge ; vulgo, St.
Olafs Bad. 12°. [*n. p.,* 1882 ?]
Dedichen. Beretning fra Modums Bad, 1876-8. Norsk
Mag. f. Lægevidensk., Christiania, 1877, 3. R., vii, 229 :
1879, 3. R., ix, 382. — **Rasmussen** (V.) Om St. Olafs
Kildens Badeanstalt paa Modum. Hosp.-Tid., Kjøbenh.,
1869, xii, 57 ; 61.—**Thaulow** (H. A.) Om St. Olafs Kilden
paa Modum. Norsk Mag. f. Lægevidensk., Christiania,
1856, 2. R., x, 809 - 820. ———. Om St. Olafs Kildens Badeanstalt paa Modum og de Aarene 1857-61 her opnaaede
Curresultater. *Ibid.,* 1859, 2. R., xiii, 337 ; 467 : 1862, 2. R.,
xvi, 265.

Moe (Christophorus).
See **Gram** (Christophorus). De motu chyli [etc.] 4°.
Hafniæ, [1744].

Moebius (Christianus Gotthelf.) * De caussis
manifestis mortium repentinarum curiosius ca-
vendis. 24 pp. 4°. *Wittenbergæ, lit. C. C. Durrii,* [1772].
For Biography, see **Triller** (Daniel. Wilhelmus).

Moebius (Gothofred) [1611–64]. Anatomia cam-
phoreæ... 4 p. l., 104 pp. 4°. *Jenæ, J. L. Neuenhahn,* 1660.
Bound with his : Epitome [etc.] 4°. *Jenæ,* 1663.

———. Fundamenta medicinæ physiologica, in
quibus origo et natura medicinæ, doctrina de
animæ facultatibus, spiritibus ac temperamento,
necnon constitutio partium principaliorum naturalis, et præternaturalis, una cum earum usu
ex veterum et recentiorum sententiis ventil-
lantur, variisque observationibus illustrantur.
Publici Athenis Salanis proposita, nunc revisa,
et multis in locis correcta, et aucta. 2 p. l., 608
pp., port. 4°. *Jenæ, imp. J. Ludovici,* [1661].
Another copy bound with his : Epitome [etc.] 4°. *Jenæ,*
1663.

———. Synopses epitomes institutionum medicinæ in gratiam tironum concinnatæ. fol. *Jenæ,
typ. S. Krebsii,* 1662.
Printed on sheets lettered from A to Kk.

———. Epitome institutionum medicarum ...
7 p. l., 738 pp., 8 l. 4°. *Jenæ, S. Krebs,* 1663.
For Portrait, see **Collection**—van Kaathoven.—**Collection** of Portr. of Phys. & Men of Sc., 86.

Moebius (Jo. Gotthelff.) * De virgine ascitica
post paracenthesin purpura maligna exstincta.
1 p. l., 36 pp , 1 pl. 4°. *Lipsiæ, lit. J. Titii,*
[1725].
Also, in : HALLER. Disp. ad morb. [etc.] 4°. *Lausannæ,* 1758, iv, 329-352.
For Biography, see **Ettmüller** (Mich. Ern.)

Moebius (Joh.) De respiratione, cumprimis ut
in hominibus se habet. Disp. phys. 31 l. sm.
4°. *Jenæ, lit. J. J. Bauhoferi,* 1671.

Moebius (Joh. Fridericus). * Diss. sistens observationes medicas miscellaneas theoreticas et
practicas. 40 pp., 1 pl. sm. 4°. *Helmstadii, lit.
P. D. Schnorrii,* [1730].

Moebius (Mauritius Eduinus). * De chemica
chlorosis naturæ ejusque therapia. 16 pp. 8°.
Lipsiæ, typ. G. Staritzii, [1850].

Möbius (Otto). * Ueber die Foerster'sche Iri-
dektomia maturans zur künstlichen Reifung im-
maturer Katarakte. 13 pp., 1 l. 8°. *Kiel, Lipsius u. Fischer,* 1886.

Moebius (Paul) [1848-]. * Beiträge zur Physiologie und Pathologie der Varolsbrücke. 32
pp. 8°. *Berlin, G. Lange,* [1870].

Möbius (Paul Julius). Grundriss des deutschen Militair-Sanitätswesens. Ein Leitfaden für die in das Heer eintretenden Aerzte. xiii, 157 pp. 8°. *Leipzig, F. C. W. Vogel, 1878.*

———. Ueber die hereditären Nervenkrankheiten. *In:* SAMML. klin. Vortr., Leipz., 1879, No. 171 (Inn. Med., No. 57, 1505-1531).

———. Die Nervosität. xii, 191 pp. sm. 8°. *Leipzig, J. J. Weber, 1882.*

———. The same. 2. Aufl. xii, 195 pp. 12°. *Leipzig, J. J. Weber, 1885.*

———. Zur Pathologie des Halssympathikus. 37 pp. 8°. *Berlin, A. Hirschwald, 1884.* *Repr. from:* Berl. klin. Wchnschr., 1884, xxi.

———. Allgemeine Diagnostik der Nervenkrankheiten. iv, 338 pp. 8°. *Leipzig, F. C. W. Vogel, 1886.*

———. The same. Obshaja diagnostika nervnich boliezneï. Perev. s Niemetsk. S. Serebrennikoff i A. Feinberg. [General diagnosis of nervous diseases. From the German, by S. Serebrennikoff and A. Feinberg.] 360 pp. 8°. *St. Petersburg, 1886.* *In:* Ejem. jour. prakt. med., St. Petersb., 1886, ii. *Also, Co-Editor of :* **Schmidt's** Jahrbücher, Leipzig, 1886.

Moebius (Paulus Christoph.) *De catalepsi. 25 l. 4°. *Jenæ, typ. J. Nisi, 1671.*

Moebs (Alfred). *Beitrag zur Pathologie der Gehirnweichung. 33 pp., 1 l. 8°. *Breslau, R. Nischkowsky, 1887.*

Moebus (Joseph). *Beitrag zur Statistik der antiseptischen Behandlung complicirter Frakturen. 38 pp., 1 l. 8°. *Breslau, N. G. Korn, 1882.*

Moeckel (Augustus Fridericus). *De hydrorhachitide. 100 pp. 8°. *Lipsiæ, ex off. Glueckiana, [1822].* *For Biography, see* **Ludwig** (Christ. Frid.)

Moeckel (C. H. Aug.) *Quæ fuerit syphilidis forma ad seculi decimi quinti finem, quæritur. 52 pp. 8°. *Lipsiæ, typ. G. Voegelii filii, [1841].*

Moeckel (Henricus Augustus). *De diosma crenata, oleo crotonis tiglii, et carbone animali. 28 pp. sm. 4°. *Lipsiæ, typ. Staritzii, [1830].* *For Biography, see* **Haase** (Guil. And.)

Moeckel (Hermannus). *De periculis in operan 'a phimosi obviis. 23 pp. 8°. *Lipsiæ, typ. A. Edelmanni, [1861].*

Möder (Karl). Die Ventilation landwirthschaftlicher Gebäude; auf Veranlassung des landwirthschaftlichen Hauptvereins des Neustädter Kreises im Grossherzogthum Sachsen-Weimar. viii, 46 pp., 1 pl. 8°. *Weimar, B. F. Voigt, 1867.*

Mödling. Städtisches öffentliches Krankenhaus in Mödling. Aerztlicher Bericht des städtischen öffentlichen Krankenhauses in Mödling. 2., 1883. 27 pp., 2 pl. 4°. *Mödling, H. Büsing, 1848.*

Moeges (Anton). *Ueber embolische Verschleppung carcinomatöser Massen vom Magen zur Leber. 33 pp. 8°. *Erlangen, Junge u. Sohn, 1879.*

Moegling (Christianus Ludovicus). [1715-62]. *De peste. 28 pp. 4°. *Tubingæ, typ. J. Sigmundi, [1735].*

———. *Oratio de iis, quæ in curationis negotio contingunt, quandoque extra ordinem, et quam maxime de curationibus dictis vulgo et creditis miraculosis. 24 pp. sm. 4°. *Tubingæ, lit. et imp. Bauhofii ac Frankii, 1752.*

———. De tutissima methodo curandi morbos quam plurimos, eosque gravissimos. Disp. Respondente Ludovico Rudolpho Seubert. 14 pp. 4°. *Tubingæ, lit. Bauhofii atque Franckii, [1752].*

Moegling (Daniel) [1546-96]. *Portrait in:* **Collection**—van Kaathoven.—**Collection** of Portr. of Phys. & Men of Sc., 202.

Mögling (J.) *Ueber chirurgische Tuberculosen. 50 pp. 8°. *Tübingen, 1884.*

Mögling (Joh. Burckhardus). *De ictero. 16 pp. sm. 4°. *Tubingæ, J. H. Reis, [1679].*

Moegling (Joh. Theophilus). *De gemursa Pliniana, clavi pedis maligniori specie in Ephem. nat. curios. Cent. 11. obs. 92. notata, et casu peculiari medico-chirurgico aliisque quadantenus parallelis illustrata. 16 pp. 4°. *Tubingæ, lit. H. Franckii, 1722.*

Moegling (Joh. Ulricus). *See* **Krafft** (Georgius Wolffgang). Cogitationes in experimenta [etc.]. 4°. *Tubingæ, 1745.*

Möhl (Carl). *De morbis veneris. [Munich.] 24 pp. 8°. *Heilbronn, M. Schell, 1868.*

Möhl (Nicolai Christian) [1798-1830]. Ueber die Varioloiden und Varicellen. Aus dem Lateinischen übersetzt und mit Anmerkungen und Zusätzen herausgegeben von C. F. Th. Krause. 95 pp. 8°. *Hannover, Hahn, 1828.*

Möhling (A. Fr.) *Ueber die Femorocoxalgie oder das sogenannte freiwillige Hinken. 44 pp. 8°. *Würzburg, J. S. Richter, 1843.*

Möhlmann (Hermann). *Ueber das Carcinoma labii superioris. 30 pp. 8°. *Würzburg, A. Memminger, 1886.*

Moehring (Carol. Rodolph.) *De venenis et philtris propinatis aliisve modis applicatis. 15 l. sm. 4°. *Vitembergæ, prelo Hakiano, [1706].*

Moehring (Gotth.) [1802-]. *Anatomia normalis pathologica et physiologica glandulæ thyreoïdeæ. 30 pp. sm. 8°. *Berolini, typ. J. F. Starckii, [1825].*

Moehring (Gustavus Eduard.) [1819-]. *De hydrocephalo acuto. 31 pp. 8°. *Berolini, apud fratrum Schlesinger, [1846].* *See* **Voigt** (Gothofredus) & **Moehring** (Paulus Heinricus). Disputatio physica de amore ovis et lupi [etc.] 4°. *Wittebergæ, [1667].*

Moehring (Paull. Heur. Gerard.) [1710-92]. *De exostosi steatomatode claviculæ, ejusque felici sectione. 1 p. l., 19 pp., 2 l., 1 pl. 4°. *Gedani, ære Schreiberiano, [1732].* *Also, in:* HALLER. Disp. chir. [etc.] 4°. *Lausannæ, 1756, v, 653-666, 1 pl.

———. De quibusdam præjudiciis medicis. 16 pp. 4°. *[Gedani], ære Schreiberiano, [1732].*

———. *De inflammationis sanguineæ theoria mechanica. 38 pp. sm. 4°. *Vitembergæ, ære Hakiano, [1733].*

———. Mytulorum quorumdam venenum et ab eo natas papulas cuticulares epistola. 24 pp. sm. 4°. *Bremæ, G. G. Rump, 1742.* *Also, in:* HALLER. Disp. ad morb. [etc.] 4°. *Lausannæ, 1757, iii, 183-200.* *For Portrait, see* **Collection**—van Kaathoven.

Moehring (Rudolf) [1845-]. *Ueber die hygienische Bedeutung des Trinkwassers, im Besonderen für die Marine. 32 pp. 8°. *Berlin, G. Lange, [1872].*

Moehrlen (J. Paul). *Comparaison des médicaments et de leurs principes actifs. 1 p. l., 36 pp., 1 l. 4°. *Strasbourg, 1863, No. 697, v. 36.*

Moehsen (Joh. Carolus Wilhelmus) [1720?-95]. *De passionis illiacæ causis et curatione. 64 pp. sm. 4°. *Halæ Magdeb., lit. J. C. Hilligeri, [1742].*

———. Commentatio prima de medicis equestri dignitate ornatis. Præmissa est dissertatio de vera felicitate e studio et exercitio artis medicæ capienda, philosopho æque ac christiano digna. xxi, 164 pp. 4°. *Berolini, J. G. Bosse, [1767].*

———. Verzeichnis einer Samlung von Bildnissen, größtentheils berühmter Aerzte; sowohl in Kupferstichen, schwarzer Kunst und Holzschnitten, als auch in einigen Handzeichnungen: diesem sind verschiedene Nachrichten und Anmerkungen vorgesetzt, die so wohl zur Geschichte der Arzeneygelahrtheit, als vornehmlich zur Ge-

Moehsen (Joh. Carolus Wilhelmus)— continued. schichte der Künste gehören. 6 p. l., 243, 240 pp. 4°. *Berlin, F. W. Birnstiel*, 1771.

——. Geschichte der Wissenschaften in der Mark Brandenburg, besonders der Arzneiwissenschaft; von den ältesten Zeiten an bis zu Ende des sechszehnten Jahrhunderts, in welcher zugleich die Gedächtnismünzen berühmter Aerzte, welche in diesem Zeitraume in der Mark gelebt haben, beschrieben werden. 2 Theile. 3 p. l., 436 pp., 4 l.; 4 p. l., 576 pp., 3 l., 3 pl. 4°. *Berlin u. Leipzig, G. J. Decker,* 1773–81.
Second part has, also, title as follows: Beschreibung einer Berlinischen Medaillen-Sammlung, die vorzüglich aus Gedächtnismünzen berühmter Aerzte bestehet.

——. Beiträge zur Geschichte der Wissenschaften in der Mark Brandenburg von den ältesten Zeiten an bis zu Ende des sechszehnten Jahrhunderts. 7 p. l., 3–226, 1 pl. 4°. *Berlin u. Leipzig, G. J. Decker,* 1783.
See, also, **Schaarschmidt** (Samuel). Therapia generalis, [etc.] 16°. *Berlin,* 1755.
For Biography, see Med. Ephem. v. Berl., 1799, i, pt. 1, 118–130 (F.).
For Portrait, see **Collection**—van Kaathoven.—**Collection** of Portr. of Phys. & Men of Sc., 5.

à Möinichen (Henricus) [1631–1709].
See **Lyser** (Michael). Culter anatomicus. -2. ed. 12°. *Hafniæ,* 1665.

Moelaart (A. W.) *Tweetal ziektegevallen, waargenomen door den schrijver. 32 pp. 8°. *Leiden, D. J. Couvée,* 1861.

Mölle (Th.) *Ueber Behandlung der Epilepsie mit Osmiumsäure. 43 pp. 8°. *Strassburg, J. H. E. Heitz,* 1885.

Möllenbroccius (Valentinus Andreas) [— 1675]. De varis, seu arthritide vaga scorbutica tractatus. 7 p. l., 167 pp., 4 l. 16°. *Lipsiæ, hæred. G. Grossii,* 1663.

——. The same. Editione altera auctior et emendatior. 6 p. l., 284 pp., 33 l. 12°. *Lipsiæ, sumpt. J. Grossii et socii,* 1672.

——. Cochlearia curiosa. 5 p. l., 140 pp., 10 l. 12°. *Lipsiæ, sumpt. J. Grossii et socii,* 1674.
Bound with his : De varis, seu arthritide, [etc.] 12°. *Lipsiæ,* 1672.
See, also, **Dorncreilius** *ab Eberhertz* (Tobias). Medulla totius praxeos medicæ aphoristica, [etc.] sm. 4°. [*Erfurti*], 1656.

Moellendorff (Guilelmus). *Negotia comparata cum morbis, qui ex iis proveniunt. 31 pp. 8°. *Berolini, G. Schade,* [1852].

Mölleney (Wilhelm). *Zur Symptomatologie und Statistik der Trichinose, nebst einigen therapeutischen Versuchen. 63 pp. 8°. *Greifswald, C. Sell,* 1879.

Möllenhoff (Christianus). *Diss. sistens ægrum ictero calido laborantem. 28 pp. 4°. [*Jenæ*], *lit. Krebsianis,* [1716].
For Biography, see **Slevogt** (Jo. Had.)

Moellenthiel (Carol. Rudolph.) *De phthisi pulmonali. 54 pp. 4°. *Argentorati, J. H. Heitz,* [1785].

Mœller (A.) Du massage, son action physiologique, sa valeur thérapeutique, spécialement au point de vue du traitement de l'entorse. 27 pp. 8°. *Bruxelles, H. Manceaux,* 1877.

——. Du Daltonisme au point de vue théorique et pratique. Étude critique des méthodes d'exploration du sens chromatique, et rapport à M. le ministre des travaux publics sur la réforme des employés des chemins de fer affectés de Daltonisme en Suède, Norwège et Danemark. 146 pp. 8°. *Bruxelles, H. Manceaux,* 1879.

——. De la pneumothérapie. 29 pp. 8°. *Bruxelles, H. Manceaux,* 1880.

——. Les travaux à l'air comprimé. 51 pp. 8°. *Bruxelles, A. Vromant,* 1881.
Repr. from : Rev. d. questions scient., avril 1881.

Mœller (A.)—continued.
——. Thérapeutique locale des maladies de l'appareil respiratoire par les inhalations médicamenteuses et les pratiques aérothérapiques. vii, 325 pp., 2 pl. 8°. *Paris, J.-B. Baillière & fils,* 1882.

——. Le choléra d'après les découvertes modernes. 51 pp. 8°. *Bruxelles, A. Vromant,* 1885.
Repr. from : Rev. d. questions scient., octobre 1885.
See, also, **Warlomont.** Examen de la vision du personnel attaché aux chemins de fer. 8°. *Gand,* 1880.

Moeller (Augustus Julius) [1818–]. *De spasmodica pulmonum affectione. 48 pp. 8°. *Berolini, typ. Nietackianis.* [1840].

Möller (C. Ph.) Anthropologischer Beitrag zur Erfahrung der psychischen Krankheit oder der Standpunkt der psychischen Medizin, mit besonderer Rücksicht auf die nähere Bestimmung der Seele in ihrer Beziehung zum geistigen und leiblichen Leben. Ein Grundriss der Seelenheilkunde als wissenschaftlicher Versuch zur erfahrungsgemässeren systematischen Begründung und Vermittelung der Begriffe dieser Lehre. xxviii, 507 pp. 8°. *Mainz, F. Kupferberg,* 1837.

Moeller (Carl). *Ueber Scillipicrin, Scillitoxin und Scillin. 37 pp. 8°. *Göttingen, W. F. Kästner,* 1878.

Möller [Carl August Ferdinand]. Beiträge zur Psychologie aus den Schriften der Griechen und Römer. Nr. 1, enthaltend Aristoteles über das Gedächtniss und die Erinnerung. [Als Einladungsschrift zu der Prüfung der Schüler der Löbenicht'schen Stadtschule.] 16 pp. sm. 8°. *Königsberg, H. Degen,* [1817].

Möller (Carl Fingal). Bidrag till kännedomen af det religiösa vansinnet. Akad. Afh. 73 pp., 1 l. 8°. *Upsala, Edquist & K.,* 1860.

Möller (Carolus Guilielmus). *De metasyncrisi methodicorum in usum revocanda. 44 pp. 8°. *Halæ, typ. Batheanis,* [1795].

de Moeller (Carolus Lucian.) [1804–]. *De odorum effectibus. 55 pp. 8°. *Berolini, lit. A. Petschii,* [1826].

Möller (Detter). *Ueber Brüche des Tibiakopfes. 18 pp. 4°. *Kiel, C. F. Mohr,* 1875.
In: SCHRIFT. d. Univ. zu Kiel, xxii, 1875, vii, Med. xii,

Möller (F.) Die Heilkraft gewisser Bewegungen des Körpers bis in die spätern Lebensjahre zur gänzlichen Vertreibung hartnäckiger Hämorrhoiden, Gicht, Rheumatismus, Hypochondrie, Schwindel, Nervenschwäche, Brustbeschwerden und mehrerer anderer, durch sitzende oder unregelmässige Lebensweise entstandenen Krankheiten, nebst Angabe der bewährten einfachen und naturgemässen Mittel dagegen. Nach fünfzigjährigen Erfahrungen fasslich dargestellt von einem Nichtarzte. 10. Aufl. 88 pp. 8°. *Leipzig, C. Geibel,* 1870.

von Moeller (Fr. W.) Das königliche Soolbad bei Neusalzwerk ohnweit preussisch Minden in seinen medicinischen Wirkungen. Nebst einigen allgemeinen einleitenden Bemerkungen von C. von Oeynhausen. iv, 52 pp. 8°. *Berlin, Nicolai,* 1847.

——. The same. 2. Ausg. vi, 76 pp., 1 l. 8°. *Berlin, Nicolai,* 1849.

——. Bad Oeynhausen bei Rehme. Mit vorzüglicher Rücksicht auf die Methode, kurz dargestellt. vi pp., 1 l., 124 pp. 8°. *Berlin, A. Hirschwald,* 1850.

Möller (Friedrich). *Ueber Duplicität des Uterus und der Scheide. 33 pp., 1 l. 8°. *Bonn, J. F. Carthaus,* [1871].

Moeller (Georg H.) *Ueber das Hygroma patellare und seine Behandlung. 16 pp. 8°. *Leipzig, C. G. Naumann,* 1868. [P., v. 265.]

——. Internationales medizinisch - pharmazeutisches Wörterbuch in französischer, englischer und deutscher Sprache für den Gebrauch der

Moeller (Georg H.)—continued.
Aerzte und Apotheker im praktischen Verkehr mit fremdländischem Publicum. 2 p. l., 320 pp. sm. 4°. *München, J. Grubert, 1879.*
Also, French and English title-pages.

de Moeller (Guilielmus) [1801–]. *De musices et sonorum vi salutari. 40 pp. 8°. *Berolini, typ. J. F. Starckii,* [1824].

Moeller (H.) *Ueber die Intensität der Herztöne. 40 pp., 1 l. 8°. *Königsberg in Pr., Hartung,* 1879.

———. Grundzüge der Arzneimittelwirkung. 76 pp. 8°. *Jena, Dege u. Haenel,* 1881.
Vortr. f. Thieräzte, 4. St., 2. u. 3. Hft.

———. Klinische Diagnostik der äusseren Krankheiten der Hausthiere, mit besonderer Berücksichtigung der Lahmheiten des Pferdes. v pp., 1 p. l., 254 pp. 8°. *Stuttgart, F. Enke,* 1887.

Möller (Hans). *Ueber Darminfusionen von Thierblut. 43 pp. 8°. *Greifswald, J. Abel,* 1881.

Möller (J. D.) Institut für Mikroskopie. Preisverzeichniss mikroskopischer Präparate, Utensilien und Materialien zur Anfertigung derselben. 36 pp. 8°. *Berlin, G. F. O. Müller,* 1874.

———. The same. 40 pp. 8°. *Berlin, G. W. F. Müller,* 1883.

Möller (J. G.) Hydro-homöopathisches Taschenbuch der Thierheilkunde, oder die Krankheiten der Hausthiere und deren Heilung durch kaltes Wasser, vorzüglich aber durch homöopathische Mittel. Ein neues, alphabetisch bearbeitetes Noth- und Hülfsbuch für jeden Thierarzt und Viehbesitzer. Durchgesehen vom Mag. Lux. iv, 156 pp. 8°. *Leipzig, W. Lauffer,* 1839. [P., v. 1457.]

Moeller (Jac. Valentinus). *De medendi ratione per præsidia diætetica. 40 pp. sm. 4°. *Rostochii, typ. J. J. Adleri,* [1726].
For Biography, see **Burchard** (Christ. Mart.)

Möller (Jo. Georgius). *De affectibus animi. 20 pp., 2 l. 4°. *[Jenæ], lit. Nisianis,* 1695.

Moeller (Joann. Christophorus). *De ipecacuanha. 12 pp. 4°. *Erfordiæ, J. C. Goerling,* [1795].

Moeller (Joannes). *De viribus animæ humanæ ope medica firmandis. 79 pp. 8°. *Hafniæ, typ. J. R. Thiellii,* [1771].

Moeller (Joannes Franciscus Albertus). *De signo spasmi peripherici in febribus continentibus. 32 pp. sm. 4°. *Halæ ad Salam, stanno Curtiano,* [1765].

Moeller (Joannes Henricus). *Diss. exhibens nonnullas observationes circa tunicam retinam et nervum opticum. 2 p. l., 17 pp., 1 l., 1 pl. sm. 4°. *Halæ Magdeb., typ. J. C. Hilligeri,* [1749].
Also, in: HALLER. Disp. anat. [etc.] 4°. *Gottingæ,* 1751, vii, 136–205, 1 pl.

Moeller (Joannes Petrus). *Positiones chymicæ. 40 pp. 4°. *Kiliæ, lit. G. Bartschii,* [1752].

Moeller (Joannes Sigismundus). *Diss. in qua mortis subitaneæ non vulgaris causas et remedia exponit. 36 pp. 4°. *Wittenbergæ, lit. vid. Gerdesiæ,* [1723].

Moeller (Joh. Georg. Carol. Ludow.) *De fractura femoris. 40 pp. 8°. *Gryphiæ, F. Hache,* 1853.

Moeller (Joh. Wilhelmus). *Diss. exhibens criteria partus olim enixi diagnostica. 1 p. l., 23 pp. 4°. *Gottingæ, in off. acad. nova,* [1771].
See, also, **Sims** (Jakob). Bemerkungen über epidemische Krankheiten, [etc.] 8°. *Hamburg,* 1775.
For Biography, see **Vogel** (Rudolph August).

Moeller (Josef).
See **Real-Encyclopädie** der gesammten Pharmacie. 8°. *Wien u. Leipzig,* 1887.

Möller (Jul. Otto Ludov.) *Observata quædam anatomica de Auchenia lama. 40 pp. 8°. *Regimontii Pr., E. J. Dalkowski,* [1840].

Möller (Jul. Otto Ludov.)—continued.
———. De phænomenis acusticis, quæ in vasis sanguiferis observantur. 53 pp., 1 l. 8°. *Regimonti Pr., Samter et Rathke,* [1847].

Moeller (Julius)[1]. Symbolæ ad theoriam rheumatismi criticæ et experimentales. 39 pp. 8°. *Regiomonti Pr., typ. Dalkowskianis,* [1860]. c.

Moeller (Julius)[2]. *Ueber die käsigen Entartungen der Lymphdrüsen. 22 pp., 1 l. 8°. *Bonn, C. Georgi,* 1875.

Möller (Konrad). *Die Kohlensäureausscheidung des Menschen bei verkleinerter Lungenoberfläche. 23 pp. 8°. *München, R. Oldenburg,* 1878.

Moeller (Richard) [1846–]. *Ueber Beckentumoren als Complication von Geburten. 32 pp. 8°. *Berlin, G. Lange,* [1869]. c.

Moeller (Rudolf). *Quales secundinarum et fœtuum pondera inter se rationes habeant. 16 pp. 8°. *Rudolphopoli, G. Froebel,* 1858

Moeller (Rudolfus). *De versione cavo pelvis angusto facienda. 33 pp., 1 l. 8°. *Gryphiswaldiæ, F. G. Kunike,* 1867.

Moeller (Ulrich). *Ueber Endothel der Sehnenscheiden und Sehnen an den Muskeln der Extremitäten des Menschen. 29 pp. 8°. *Göttingen, G. Hofer,* 1873.

Moeller (Victor). *De colica saturnina. 2 p. l., 34 pp., 3 l. 8°. *Halæ, typ. H. Ruffii jun.,* [1831].

Möllers (Joh.)
See **Eichstadius** (Laurentius). "De osteologia humana," etc. 4°. *Dantisci,* 1648.

Moellmann (Guilelmus). *De alcoholica intoxicatione chronica. 31 pp. 8°. *Berolini, G. Schade,* [1862].

Moeltgen (Paulus Hubertus) [1813–]. *De morbis glandularum salivarium. 29 pp., 1 l. sm. 8°. *Berolini, typ. Nietackianis,* [1836].

Moench (Gustavus). *De vaginæ anatomia, physiologia et pathologia. 42 pp., 1 l. 8°. *Halæ, typ. Gebaueriis,* [1828].

Moenchs (Conrad). Arzneymittellehre der einfachen und zusammengesetzten gebräuchlichen Mittel. 4. Aufl. viii, 511 pp. 8°. *Marburg,* 1800.

Moenckeberg (Franciscus). *De nova catheteris forma, quam Amussat proposuit, quatenus cum structura anatomica urethræ conveniat. 26 pp. sm. 8°. *Gottingæ, C. E. Rosenbusch,* 1825.

Mœnig (Justus). Sterility and imbecility, in both sexes; their causes and their cure. With three introductory chapters on reproduction and generation, comparative and human. Condensed from the German, and adapted to the knowledge of the general reader by 'Ακεστής. iv, 5–100 pp. 12°. *London, T. Parton,* 1861.

Moennig (Balduinus) [1820–]. *De typo abdominali. 27 pp., 2 l. 8°. *Berolini, typ. Nietackianis,* [1843].

Moennikes (Franciscus Aloysius) [1838–]. *De pseudarthrosi. 32 pp. 8°. *Berolini, G. Lange,* [1864].

Moenninghoff (Otto). *Ueber frische Damnrisse. [Strasburg.] 19 pp. 8°. *Camen, W. Felting,* 1885.

Moens (Adriaan Isebree). Over de voortplantingssnelheid van den pols. viii, 76 pp. 8°. *Leiden, S. C. van Doesburgh,* 1877.

———. Die Pulscurve. 1 p. l., 145 pp. 8°. *Leiden, E. J. Brill,* 1878.

Moens (J. C. B.) De kinacultur in Azië 1854 t–m. 1882. Uitgegeven door de Vereeniging tot Bevordering der Geneeskundige Wetenschappen in Nederlandsch-Indië. 1 p. l., xii, 395 pp., 1 map, 33 pl. 4°. *Batavia, Ernst & Co.,* 1882.

Moens (M.-C.) *Sur le sarcocèle. 30 pp. 4°. *Paris,* 1807, No. 74, v. 67.

van de Moer (Joannes). * De gangræna sicca, in primis ratione habita gangrænæ spontaneæ siccæ. iv, 49 pp., 2 l. 8°. *Groningæ, C. M. van Bolhuis Hoitsema,* 1844. [P., v. 192.]

Mörgelin (J.) * Ueber angeborne Harnblasenspalte und deren Behandlung. 62 pp., 6 pl. 8°. *Bern, H. Blom,* 1855.

Moericke (Carolus Gottl.) * De aëre atmosphærico, ejusque vi quam in organismum animalem exserit. 38 pp. 4°. *Tubingæ, H. de L'Orme,* [1830].

Moericke (Joh. Gottlieb). * De febre tertiana intermittente soporosa utplurimum funesta, feliciter tamen curanda. 36 pp. 4°. *Tubingæ, lit. Cottaianis,* 1759.

Moerike (Carol. Fridericus). * De morbis acutis. 2 p. l., 96 pp., 1 l. 8°. *Stuttgardiæ,* [1793].

Mörike (Robert). * Ueber die Amputationen der Portio vaginalis. 30 pp., 1 l. 8°. *Berlin, G. Schade,* 1878.

Moehring (Fridericus). *See* **Moehring** (Georgius Fridericus).

Moering (Fridericus Gustavus). * Diss. sistens historiam choleræ, cum subsequente pleuroperipneumonia. 23 pp. 4°. *Lipsiæ, typ. Breitkopfii et Haertelii,* [1830].
For Biography, see **Weber** (Ernestus Henricus).

Moering (Georgius Fridericus). * Tentamen disquisitionis de linguæ integumentis. 32 pp. 8°. *Lipsiæ, typ. Staritzii,* [1845].

———. The same. 32 pp., 1 l. 8°. *Dorpat, typ. vid. J. C. Schünmanni et C. Mattieseni,* 1851.
This is a reprint of the preceding, with the addition of an "imprimatur" and a page of "theses". The author's name is given as "Fridericus".

Möring (Michel).
See **Paris.** Collection de documents pour servir à l'histoire des hôpitaux de Paris. 4°. *Paris,* 1881-2.

Moeringh (Cornelius Gerard.) * De visu. 76 pp., 2 l. 4°. *Lugd. Bat., J. et H. Verbeek,* 1729.

Moerire (Ludovicus Frieder. Leopoldus). * Diss. sistens expositionem physiologiæ et pathologiæ lienis. 38 pp. 8°. *Tubingæ, lit. Schoenhardtianis,* [1825].

de Moerisch (Joan. Wenc.) * Diss. sistens animal in sua elementa resolutum. 31 pp. 8°. *Viennæ, M. A. Schmidt,* [1782].

Moerlin (Jo. Christianus).
See **Carpzov** (Christian. Bened.) & **Moerlinus** (Jo. Christianus). De medicis ab ecclesia pro sanctis habitis. sm. 4°. *Lipsiæ,* [1709].

Moerlin (Julius Otto Carl) [1862–   ]. * Ueber indirecte Sternalfracturen. 30 pp. 8°. *Greifswald, J. Abel,* 1887.

Mörner (K. A. H.) * Bidrag till kännedomen om färgämnena i melanotiska svulster. 58 pp., 2 pl. 8°. *Stockholm, Kongl. Boktryckeriet,* 1886.

Moerner (Ludovicus). * De indicationibus et contraindicationibus amputationis. 27 pp. 4°. *Jenæ, typ. C. G. T. Jochii,* [1817].

Möers (Theodorus Ernestus Josephus Jacobus). * Diss. medicam variolarum præprimis malignarum rationem et curationem docentem exponit. 26 pp. 4°. *Wirceburgi, J. J. C. Kleyer,* [1746].

Moerschell (Mart. Jos.) * De apoplexia. [Munich.] 16 pp. 8°. *Amorbachii, typ. Volkhardtianis,* 1836.

Mœschlin (J.-L.) * Quelques considérations sur les maladies scrofuleuses et tuberculeuses chez l'ouvrier de fabriques au point de vue de l'hygiène et des moyens prophylactiques. 31 pp. 4°. [*Berne, Jenet & Reinert, n. d.*]

Moeser [Guilelmus Alexander Theodorus] [1839–   ]. * De cholelithiasi. 32 pp. 8°. *Berolini, G. Lange,* [1862].

Möser (Heinrich). * Die Diphtheritis im Juliushospitale in Würzburg vom Jahre 1878 bis Ende Mai 1882. 35 pp. 8°. *Kircheimbolanden, C. Thieme,* 1882.

Moeser (Hermann). * Zur Behandlung der Fehlgeburten. 35 pp. 8°. *Würzburg, A. Memminger,* 1887.

Moeser (Johannes Ludovicus). * De hæmorrhoidibus cæcis. 50 pp. 4°. *Halæ Magdeb., typ. C. Henckelii,* [1717].

Moesner (Theophilus Henricus). * De conformatione pupillæ artificialis. iv, 47 pp., 1 l. 8°. *Tubingæ, typ. Reissiansis,* [1823].

Möstner (Daniel. Fridericus). * De phlebotomia apud plethoricos catharsi præmittenda. 10 pp. 4°. *Francof. ad Viadr., J. C. Winter,* 1747.

Moethe, *dictus* **Baeumer** (Theodorus). * De delirio tremente. 24 pp. 8°. *Gryphiswaldiæ, F. G. Kunike,* 1863. C.

Moetig (Gottlieb. Fridericus). * De risus commodo et incommodo in œconomia vitali. Ob das Lachen zur Gesundheit nützlich oder schädlich sey. 26 pp., 1 l. 4°. *Halæ Magdeb., typ. J. C. Hendelii,* [1746].

Moffait (Louis). * Recherches sur la phlegmasie des membranes synoviales des articulations. 21 pp. 4°. *Paris,* 1810, No. 13, v. 78.

Moffat.

MACKAILE (M.) Moffet-well; or, a topographico-spagyricall description of the mineral wells at Moffet, in Annandale of Scotland. Translated, and much enlarged, by the author. As also the Oyly-well; or, a topographico-spagyricall description of the Oyly-well at St. Catharine's Chappel in the paroch of Libberton; to these is subjoyned, A character of Mr. Culpeper and his writing; by the same author. 16°. *Edinburgh,* 1664.

Garnett (T.) On the mineral waters of Moffat. Med. & Phys. J., Lond., 1799, ii, 354–360.—Horseburgh (W.) Experiments and observations upon the Hartfell Spaw, made at Moffat, 1750; and an account of its medicinal virtues so far as they have hitherto been discovered from experience. Essays & Obs. Phil. Soc. Edinb., 1754, i, 341–371.—Macadam (J.) Report on, and chemical analyses of. the Moffat mineral wells. Glasgow M. J., 1854–5, ii, 191; 295.

Moffat (John).
See **Hippocrates,** the prognostics and prorrhetics, from the original Greek, etc. 8°. *London,* 1788.

Moffat (Thomas). * De apoplexia hydrocephalica. 1 p. l., 37 pp. 8°. *Edinburgi, C. Stewart et socii,* 1800. [*Also, in:* P., v. 13.]

Moffatt (John). The French exhibition of horrors; a sermon on the sin of torturing animals, preached in the Middle Parish Church, Greenock, Scotland, Sept. 8, 1878; and in the Scotch kirks of Bayfield and Varna, Huron, Canada, July 6, 1879. 36 pp. 8°. *Toronto, Hunter, Rose & Co.,* 1879.

Moffet (Thomas). *See* **Mufettus** (Thomas).

Moffitt (Andrew) [–1882]. A manual of instruction for attendants on sick and wounded in the war. vii, 136 pp. 8°. *London, C. Griffin & Co.,* 1870.
For Biography, see Brit. M. J., Lond., 1882, i, 252.

Mog (Joh. Guilielmus). * De generibus et speciebus statuum præter naturalium qui in partibus fluidis contentisque corporis humani locum habent. 38 pp. sm. 4°. *Giessæ, ex off. Brauniana,* [1757].

Mogador.

OLLIVE (C.) Géographie médicale. Climat de Mogador et de son influence sur la phthisie. 8°. *Paris,* 1875.

Leared (A.) Mogador as a winter resort for invalids. Lancet, Lond., 1873, ii, 588–590.—Ollive. Du climat de Mogador et de son heureuse influence sur la phthisie pulmonaire et les affections de poitrine. Alger méd., 1875, iii, 91–93.—Seux père. Mogador et son climat. Marseille méd., 1869, vi, 829; 885.—Thevenin. Du climat de Mogador, sous le rapport des affections pulmonaires. Bull. Soc. d. sc. . . . . d'Alger, 1869, vi, 225–229. *Also:* Gaz. méd. de l'Algérie. Alger. 1869. xiv, 86.

Mogalla (Georg Philipp) [1766–1831]. Die Bäder bey Landeck. xii, 244 pp., 2 pl. 8°. *Breslau, Hirschberg,* 1799.

See, also, **von Krzowitz** (W. T.) Geschichte des schwarzen Staares [etc.] 8°. *Breslau,* 1790.

[**Mogaveri** (Giuseppe).] Ragguaglio intorno alla origine, prerogative, e privilegj della celebre Scuola Salernitana, e suo almo collegio di medici, et intorno a quanto è occorso per la osservanza di tutt' i suoi privilegj. 51 pp. 4°. [*Napoli,* 1737.]

Mogen (Joh. Wilhelm). Wahrhaffte, und von dem weltberühmten Medico Dr. Horsten approbirte Beschreibung des Nieder-Selterser Sauer-Brunnens, des vielen Nachfragens wegen, besonders auch, weilen von dessen führenden Mineralien ich die Proben selbst öffters genommen, wiederum zum Druck befördert worden A. 1692, durch D. Joh. Gregor Antoni, anjetzo aber wegen seither erlangter grossen Renommée und starcken Gebrauchs abermals zum Druck befördert von J. G. Hochheimer. 32 pp. 12°. *Leipzig,* 1724.

Mogen (Just. Conrad. Wilh.) * De aquis medicatis Fachingensibus. 36 pp. 4°. *Jenæ, lit. J. C. Tennemanni,* [1749].

Mogen (Philippus Wilhelmus). * De colica. 32 pp. 4°. [*Alldorffi*], *typ. H. Meyeri,* 1694.

Mogg (Matthias Ambrosius). * De crimine magica contra vulnera remedia adhibentium. 24 pp. sm. 4°. *Argentorati, typ. J. H. Heitzii,* [1763].

Mogigraphia.

See Cramp (*Writers'*).

Mogiljanski (J.) * Ke voprosu o dieistvii olova na jivotnii organizme. [Effect of tin on animal organism.] 66 pp. 8°. *St. Petersburg,* 1869.

Mogiljanski - Rusobtovski (I.) * O lechenii travmaticheskago stolubjaka. [Treatment of traumatic tetanus.] 46 pp. 8°. *St. Petersburg, tipog. E. Arnholda,* 1863.

Mogk (Carolus Fridericus Guilielmus). * De vi fluminis sanguinis in venarum cavarum systemate. 2 p. l., 43 pp., 2 l. 8°. *Marburgi Cattorum,* [*typ. Weigelii*], 1843.

Mogk (Julius). * Ueber die Lebercirrhose im Kindesalter, zugleich ein Beitrag zur Pathogenese der Lebercirrhose. 32 pp. 8°. *Giessen, C. von Münchow,* 1887.

Moglini (Blasius Stephanus Leopoldus). * I. De visu, etc. 20 pp. 4°. *Augustæ Taurinorum,* [1820]. [P., v. 945.]

Mohamed Ben-Si-El-Hadj-Benamar Nekkach. * Quelques mots sur les rétrécissements de l'œsophage et du cathétérisme de cet organe par la sonde Collin. 40 pp. 4°. *Paris,* 1880, No. 231.

———. The same. [Présentée le 16 juin 1880.] 38 pp. 4°. *Paris,* 1880, No. 257.

This is the same thèse as No. 231, presented June 2; names of professors on title-page, and the last two pages, containing "questions", being omitted.

Mohammed (Mirza) [1840–]. * De la valeur diagnostique du bruit de piaulement dans l'endocardite aiguë. 52 pp. 4°. *Paris,* 1879, No. 226.

Mohammed-Saïd. * De la chorée et de la douleur provoquée chez les choréiques. 86 pp. 4°. *Paris,* 1869, No. 39.

Mohamreh.

See Bassorah.

Mohaupt (Paulus). * Observationes de cholera asiatica in epidemia Sedinensi. 32 pp. 8°. *Gryphiswaldiæ, F. G. Kunike,* 1867.
C.

Mohawk *Valley.*

See New York (*State of*).

Mohen (Charles-Joseph). * De la phthisie pulmonaire. 37 pp. 4°. *Paris,* 1843, No. 246, v. 406.

von Mohl (Hugo) [–1872]. Principles of the anatomy and physiology of the vegetable cell. Transl. by Arthur Henfrey. 158 pp., 1 pl. 8°. *London, Van Voorst,* 1852.

Also, Co-Editor of: **Jahreshefte** des Vereins für vaterländische Naturkunde in Württemberg, Stuttgart, 1850-57. *Also, Editor of:* **Botanische** Zeitung, Berlin u. Leipzig, 1851-72.

Mohn (Carl Ehregott). * Die organische Schliessung des durchbrochenen harten Gaumens. 44 pp. 8°. *Leipzig, L. Schnauss,* [1862].

Mohn (H.) Havets Temperatur mellem Island, Skotland og Norge. 9 pp., 1 map. 8°. [*Kjøbenhavn,* 1869.]

Repr. from: Overs. o. d. k. Danske Vidensk. Selsk. Forh., Kjøbenh., 1869.

———. Om Tordenvejr i Norge i 1868. 55 pp., 6 ch. 8°. [*Kjøbenhavn,* 1869.]

Repr. from: Overs. o. d. k. Danske Vidensk. Selsk. Forh., Kjøbenh., 1869.

———. Norges Vind- og Stormstatistik. 48 pp. 8°. [*Kjøbenhavn,* 1869.]

Repr. from: Overs. o. d. k. Danske Vidensk. Selsk. Forh., Kjøbenh., 1869.

Mohnike (Gottl. Christ. Friedr.) Dr. Martin Luther und Philipp Melanchthon über den Arzt und seine Kunst. Der medicinischen Privatgesellschaft zu Stralsund an ihrem ein und fünfzigsten Stiftungstage. 32 pp. 8°. *Stralsund,* 1823.

Mohnike (Otto Theoph. Joan.) [1814–]. * De instinctu sexuali ejusque natura atque causis. 44 pp. 12°. *Berolini, typ. Feisterianis,* [1837].

———. The same. 1 p. l., 41 pp. 8°. *Berolini, Burmeister et Stange,* [1838].

———. Ueber geschwänzte Menschen. 112 pp., 1 l. 8°. *Münster, Aschendorff,* 1878.

Mohns (C.) * Ueber den Schornsteinfegerkrebs. 42 pp. 8°. *Jena, W. Ratz,* 1876.

Mohns (Joh.) * Beiträge zu den Resectionen der Knochen. 29 pp. 8°. *Jena, A. Neuenhahn,* 1866.

Mohr (A.) * Das Nervenfieber. 44 pp. 8°. *Würzburg, F. E. Thein,* 1841.

Mohr (Bernard). * Beiträge zur Kenntniss der organischen Hirnkrankheiten. 31 pp., 1 pl. 4°. *Würzburg, C. W. Becker,* 1833.

———. Beiträge zur pathologischen Anatomie, enthaltend die tödlich abgelaufenen Krankheitsfälle der medicinischen Abtheilung des Julins-Hospitals in Würzburg, vom 1. Mai bis 31. October 1837. vi pp., 1 l., 156 pp. 8°. *Stuttgart, P. Balz,* 1838.

———. Beiträge zu einer künftigen Monographie des Empyems. 151 pp. 8°. *Kitzingen, E. Koppling,* 1839.

———. Beiträge zur pathologischen Anatomie. Erste Folge, enthaltend die tödlich abgelaufenen Krankheitsfälle der medicinischen Abtheilung des Julius-Hospitals vom 1. November 1837 bis 31. October 1838. vi pp., 1 l., 527 pp. 8°. *Kitzingen, E. Köppling,* 1840.

Mohr (Carl Friedrich) [1806–79]. Commentar zur preussischen Pharmacopöe, nebst Uebersetzung des Textes. Nach der 6. Aufl. der Pharmacopœa Borussica. 2 v. xviii, 534 pp.; 487 pp., 1 tab. 8°. *Braunschweig, F. Vieweg u. Sohn,* 1847-9.

———. The same. 2. Aufl. 2 v. in 1. xx, 485, 459 pp., 1 tab. 8°. *Braunschweig F. Vieweg u. Sohn,* 1853-4.

———. The same. 3. Aufl. Nach der 7. Aufl. der Pharmacopœa Borussica. xxii, 702 pp., 1 tab. 8°. *Braunschweig, F. Vieweg u. Sohn,* 1865.

———. The same. Commentar zur Pharmacopœa Germanica, nebst Uebersetzung des Textes. xvii, 933 pp. 8°. *Braunschweig, F. Vieweg u. Sohn,* 1874.

Mohr (Carl Friedrich)—continued.
——. Lehrbuch der chemisch-analytischen Ti-
trirmethode. Nach eigenen Versuchen und systematisch dargestellt. 2. Aufl. xix, 588 pp.
8°. *Braunschweig, F. Vieweg u. Sohn*, 1862.
——. The same. 3. Aufl. xiv pp., 1 l., 707
pp. 8°. *Braunschweig, F. Vieweg u. Sohn*, 1870.
Also, Co-Editor of: **Annalen** der Pharmacie, Lemgo
u. Heidelberg. 1837.
See, also, **Blondlot** (Nicolas). Note sur une modification à la pipette graduée de Mohr. 8°. *Nancy*, [*n. d.*]
For Biography, see Pop. Sc. Month., N. Y., 1880, xvii,
402–404, port.

Mohr (Charles). The incompatible remedies of
the homœopathic materia medica. A paper read
before the Homœopathic Medical Society of the
County of Philadelphia. 9 pp. 8°. *New York,
& Philadelphia, Boericke & Tafel*, [1879].
——. Care of the mouth and teeth in infancy
and childhood. 10 pp. 8°. [*Philadelphia*, 1880.]
Repr. from : Hahneman. Month., Phila., 1880, n. s., ii.
——. Sanitary precautions in measles. 5 pp.
8°. [*Philadelphia*, 1880.]
Repr. from : Hahneman. Month., Phila., 1880, n. s., ii.

Mohr (Christianus). *De regionibus ad curam
phthiseos pulmonalis climaticam aptis. 12 pp.,
1 l. 4°. *Kiliæ, C. F. Mohr*, 1867.
In : SCHRIFT. d. Univ. zu Kiel, xiv, 1867; vii, Med. xi.

Mohr (Conradus). *Actio viscerum digestioni
famulantium physiologice et pathologice considerata. 90 pp. 8°. [*Herbipoli*], F. E. Nitri-
bitt, [1789].

Mohr (Francis) & **Redwood** (Theophilus).
Practical pharmacy; the arrangements, apparatus, and manipulations of the pharmaceutical
shop and laboratory. Edited, with extensive
additions, by William Procter, jr. xvi, 17–576
pp. 8°. *Philadelphia, Lea & Blanchard*, 1849.

Mohr (Franz). *Ueber Hepatitis suppurativa.
[Wurtzburg.] 23 pp. 8°. *Erlangen, A. E. Junge*,
1862.
——. Das Ophthalmophantom und der Augenspiegel als Optometer. 31 pp., 1 pl. 8°. *Würzburg, Stahel*, 1870.

Mohr (Georgius Fridericus). De machinæ humanæ vitiis eorumque causis dignoscendis atque
emendandis. Diss. prima. 24 pp. sm. 4°. *Tubingæ, lit. H. Franckii*, [1725].
——. Die gebährende Frau samt ihrer Leibesfrucht in Lebensgrösse sowol durch Kunst
abgebildet als auch von einem Todtengerippe
genommen, nach denjenigen Theilen des Leibes,
welche durch Unterweisung eines Hebammen-
meisters nicht nur allein die Wehemütter und
Wundärzte zu leichtern Begrif- und Verrichtung
deren nöthigsten Handgriffen in der Hebammenkunst, sondern auch die Eheweiber zu ihrem
Verhalt in Schwangerschaften und Geburten
kennen und verstehen sollen. 3. Aufl. 204 pp.,
2 l. 16°. *Hirschfeld, G. C. Mohr*, 1757.

Mohr (Gustav). *Ueber Benzylsulfonsäuren.
1 p. l., 38 pp. 8°. *Greifswald, J. Abel*, 1884.

Mohr (Joannes Michael.) *Diss. pertractans
miros nervorum morbos dæmoni subinde attri-
butus, quam una cum adnexis corollariis ex
omni parte medicinæ desumptis, [etc.] 3 p. l.,
38 pp. 4°. [*Herbipoli*], F. E. Nitribitt, [1768].

Mohr (Joh. Hubertus van der Meer). *See* **van
der Meer Mohr** (Joh. Hubertus).

Mohr (Michael Daniel). *Pathemata graviora
a flatuum caussa occulta oriunda. 1 p. l., xxiv
pp., 4 l. 4°. *Erlangæ, typ. M. J. D. Camerarii*,
[1759].

Mohr (Willy). *Zur Statistik der Spondylitis.
26 pp. 8°. *Würzburg, Thein*, 1886.

von Mohrenheim (Joseph Jacob) [–1799].
Abhandlung über die Entbindungskunst. Ver-
fasst auf höchstem Befehl Ihro Majestät der
Kayserinn aller Reussen, etc. Zum Nutzen ihres

von Mohrenheim (Joseph Jacob)—cont'd.
Reichs. v. 1. 6 p. l., 216 pp., 46 pl., 24 l. fol.
St. Petersburg, k. Akad. d. Wissenschaften, 1791.

Mohring (August. Francis. Ferdin.) *Diss.
sistens cogitata quædam de malo hypochondriaco
atque hysterico. 2 p. l., 19 pp. 4°. *Jenæ, typ.
Etzdorfii et soc.*, [1798].
For Biography, see **Nicolai** (Ernestus Antonius).

Mohrmann (Georgius Christianus Ludovicus).
*De gangræna et sphacelo, eorum causis et me-
dela. 33 pp. 8°. *Gottingæ, H. M. Grape*, [1798].

Mohs (Carolus Henricus). *De lupi forma et
structura nonnulla. 28 pp., 1 l., 1 pl. 8°. *Lipsiæ, typ. B. G. Teubneri*, [1855].

Mohs (Ernestus Joh. Rudolphus). *De monstris
et monstrositatibus corporis humani ac de vi
eorum ad vitam et valetudinem. 29 pp., 1 l. 8°.
Halæ, typ. Ploetzianis, 1864.   C.

Mohs (*Fried.*) [1774–   ].
Portrait in: **Portraiten-Gallerie.** 4°. *Wien*, 1838,
No. 18.

Mohs (Joann. Christoph.) *De ictero. 2 p. l.,
33 pp. 8°. *Berolini, typ. A. G. Schadii*, [1820].

Mohyus.
See **Deusingius** (Antonius). Sympathetici pulvis
examen. 16°. *Groningæ*, 1662.

Moigno [François-Napoléon-Marie] [1804–   ].
See **Tyndall** (John). Chaleur et froid [etc.] 8°. *Paris*, 1868. ——. Programme d'un cours [etc.] 8°. *Paris*,
1871. ——. La lumière [etc.] 8°. *Paris*, 1872.

Moilin (Tony). *De la pression du sang. 59
pp. 4°. *Paris*, 1858, No. 15, v. 621.
——. Leçons de médecine physiologique. xi,
296 pp. 8°. *Paris, A. Delahaye*, 1866.
——. Médecine physiologique. Maladies des
voies respiratoires, maladies des fosses nasales,
de la gorge, du larynx et de la poitrine. xi, 307
pp. 8°. *Paris, A. Parent*, 1867.

Moine (Charles). *Quelques recherches sur les
modifications de forme et de dimension du thorax
dans la pleurésie aiguë. 52 pp., 1 ch. 4°. *Paris*, 1872, No. 31.

Moineau (Jules) [1855–   ]. *De la marche des
plaies chez les scrofuleux. 40 pp. 4°. *Paris*,
1882, No. 76.

Moineau (P.-J.-Émile). *De la coqueluche.
46 pp. 4°. *Paris*, 1855, No. 318, v. 578.

Moinel (Paul-François). *Essai sur le lupus
scrofuleux des fosses nasales. 47 pp. 4°. *Paris*,
1877, No. 236.

Moinet (C.) Sur les eaux minérales. 12 pp.
8°. *Paris, A. Hennuyer*, 1878.
——. De l'action physiologique des eaux de Cauterets (Hautes-Pyrénées). 144 pp. 12°. *Paris, G. Masson*, 1878.

Moinet (Francis Walter) [–1886]. Hernia
simulating bubo. 1 l. 8°. *Edinburgh, Oliver &
Boyd*, [1871].
Repr. from : Edinb. M. J., 1870–71, xvi, pt. 2.
See, also, **Scoresby-Jackson** (R. E.) Note book of
materia medica, pharmacology, and therapeutics. 4. ed.
12°. *Edinburgh*, 1880.
For Biography, see Edinb. M. J., 1886–7, xxxii, 381.

Moinet (Jean-Charles). *De l'influence des climats chauds sur le traumatisme chez l'européen.
73 pp., 1 l. 4°. *Montpellier; Boehm & fils*, 1866,
No. 101.   C.
——. Des indications particulières de l'eau de
la Raillère. 136 pp. 8°. *Paris, G. Masson*,
1875.

Moingt.
Henry (O.) Rapport sur l'eau minérale découverte à
Moingt, arrondissement de Montbrison, département de la
Loire. Bull. Acad. de méd., Par., 1857–8, xxiii, 1053–1059.

Moir (D. M.) Outlines of the ancient history of
medicine; being a view of the progress of the
healing art among the Egyptians, Greeks, and
Arabians. v, 278 pp. 12°. *Edinburgh & London,
W. Blackwood & T. Cadell*, 1831.

Moir (D. M.)—continued.

——. Practical observations on malignant cholera, as that disease is now exhibiting itself in Scotland. vii, 52 pp. 8°. *Edinburgh, W. Blackwood,* 1832. [*Also, in :* P., v. 1040; 1061.]

——. The same. 2. ed. 71 pp. 8°. *Edinburgh & London, W. Blackwood & T. Cadell,* 1832.

Moir (James). Notes on Dr. Macintosh's treatise on the puerperal fever. 101 pp. 8°. *Edinburgh, Murray & Mitchell,* 1822.

——. Postscript to Mr. Moir's notes on Dr. Macintosh's treatise on puerperal fever. 23 pp. 8°. [*n. p., n. d.*] [P., v. 1617.]

Moir (Joannes Innes Allan). * De febre intermittente. 2 p. l., 18 pp. 8°. *Edinburgi,* 1828.

Moir (John). On retroflexion of the unimpregnated uterus; with cases illustrative of its causes and of a new mode of treatment. 12 pp. 8°. *Edinburgh, Murray & Gibb,* 1860.

Repr. from : Edinb. M. J., 1859-60, v, pt. 2.

——. Valedictory address on retiring from the president's chair of the Medico-Chirurgical Society of Edinburgh, 18th December, 1867. 11 pp. 8°. *Edinburgh, Oliver & Boyd,* 1868.

——. On croup; its nature and treatment. 41 pp. 8°. *Edinburgh, Oliver & Boyd,* 1878.

Repr. from : Edinb. M. J., 1878-9, xxiv.

Moireau (Charles-Symphor). * Du fer et de ses usages en médecine. 17 pp. 4°. *Paris,* 1834, No. 144, v. 273.

Moiroud (Anselme). * Recherches cliniques sur l'érysipèle médical deuthéropathique ou intercurrent. 70 pp., 1 l. 4°. *Paris,* 1881, No. 242.

Moiroud (Ernest). * Contribution à l'étude de l'épilepsie hémiplégique. 44 pp., 1 l. 4°. *Montpellier,* 1884, No. 50.

Moisan (Joseph-Marie). * Traitement général des plaies par armes à feu. 26 pp. 4°. *Paris,* 1849, No. 6, v. 487.

Moisè (Benvenisti). Legame degli esantemi completi e larvati colle lesioni del cuore sinistro e delle arterie. 45 pp. 8°. *Padova, G. R. Randi,* 1884.

Moise (Raphael). * De la laryngite diphthérique ou croup, et de son traitement. 48 pp. 4°. *Paris,* 1852, No. 272, v. 529.

Moisè *da Palermo.*

See **Hippocrates.** "Trattati di Mascalcia", etc. 8°. *Bologna,* 1865.

Moiseau (A.) * Sur les animaux vénéneux du département de la Vendée, et sur le traitement à employer contre leurs morsures et figures. 48 pp. 8°. *Paris, an XI* [1803], v. 30.

Moises (Hugh). Treatise on the blood, or general arrangement of many important facts relative to the vital fluid. With some cursory observations on the theory of animal heat. Interspersed with pathological and physiological remarks from the inductions of modern chemistry. iv, xx, 270 pp. 8°. *London, T. Evans & J. Stead,* [*n. d.*]

Moiset (Charles-Alphonse). * Sur la coqueluche. 20 pp. 4°. *Paris,* 1817, No. 13, v. 129.

Moissan (H.) Série du cyanogène. 323 pp. 8°. *Paris, G. Steinheil,* 1882.

Moissenet (J.) * De l'influence du solidisme sur la pratique médicale. 28 pp. 4°. *Paris, P. Dupont,* 1844.

Concours.

Moissenet (Joachim). * I. Histoire anatomique et physiologique des productions cartilagineuses. Des productions morbides libres dans les cavités séreuses. II. [etc.] 75 pp. 4°. *Paris,* 1840, No. 84, v. 363.

Moissinac (E.-M.-Ernest). * Quelques considérations sur les préparations arsenicales et sur l'emploi de l'acide arsénieux dans le traitement des fièvres intermittentes. 23 pp. 4°. *Paris,* 1863, No. 60.

Moisson (Fernand). * De l'anasarque sans albuminurie, spécialement considérée chez les enfants. 75 pp. 4°. *Paris,* 1867, No. 212.

Moisson (Louis). * Sur l'ulcère de Cochinchine. vi, 7-42 pp. 4°. *Montpellier,* 1864, v. 48.

Moisture.

See, also, **Air** (*Moisture of*); **Climate**; **Erysipelas** (*Causes of*); **Habitations**; **Hygiene** (*Naval*); **Hygrometer,** *etc.*; **Inundations**; **Irrigation**; **Meteorology** (*Medical*); **Miners** (*Diseases, etc., of*); **Phthisis** (*Causes, etc., of*); **Rice** *culture*; **Soil**; **Water** (*Subsoil*).

Beer (A.) * Ueber die Bestimmung der Feuchtigkeit der Wände und hygrometrische Bestimmungen zu hygienischen Zwecken im Allgemeinen. 8°. *Erlangen,* 1878.

Chanteux (M.-J.-M.) * De l'humidité et de son influence sur l'économie vivante. 4°. *Paris,* 1819.

Delaporte (J. J.) *An qui humidioribus vescantur diutius vivunt? 4°. [*Paris,* 1773.]

Fodéré (F.-E.) Traité du goitre et du crétinisme, précédé d'un discours sur l'influence de l'air humide sur l'entendement humain. 8°. *Paris, an VIII* [1800].

Haehnke (H.) * Ueber den schädlichen Einfluss feuchter Wohnungen. 8°. *Berlin,* [1873].

Kruse (M.-L.) Méthode pour le séchage des bâtiments. Présenté au Congrès d'hygiène et de sauvetage de Bruxelles par le comité danois. 4°. *Copenhague,* 1876.

Lamaury (G.-G.) * Influence de l'air humide sur l'économie animale. 4°. *Paris,* 1828.

Mezger (L.) * De murorum recens illitorum exhalatione nociva. 8°. *Tubingæ,* [1832].

Prosper (M.) Guerre à l'humidité, ou le secret de l'hydrofuge révélé à MM. les propriétaires. 2. éd. 16°. *Paris,* 1825.

Trossat (J.-E.) * De la chaleur humide envisagée comme agent modificateur de l'action nerveuse. 4°. *Montpellier,* 1879.

Beer (J.) Feuchte Wohnungen. Ztschr. f. gerichtl. Med., Wien, 1867, iii, 252; 265.—**Born** (C.F.) Ueber das frühe Bewohnen neuer Steinhäuser; eine Preisschrift. [*From:* Auswahl ökonomischer Abhandlungen, 8°, St. Petersb., 1793, iv.] Beitr. z. Arch. d. med. Poliz., Leipz., 1798, viii, 1. Samml., 84-126.—**Briggs** (R.) On the relation of moisture in air to health and comfort. J. Frankl. Inst., Phila., 1878, lxxv, 251-255. *Also.* Reprint.—**Chautard & Forthomme.** Sur une cause peu connue de l'humidité des appartements. Rev. méd. de l'est. Nancy, 1876, vi, 108-116.—**Dabney** (W. C.) The physiological and pathological effects of excessive soil moisture. Virginia M. Month., Richmond, 1875-6, ii, 781-789.—**Estelrich** (J. I.) Influencia de la humedad sobre el organismo. Abeja méd., Barcel., 1852, 2. s., vi, 293-301.—**Fleury.** Considérations sur l'influence qu'a exercée l'humidité à l'Hôtel-Dieu de Clermont pendant les mois d'avril et mai. Gaz. méd. de Par., 1857, 3. s., xii, 190-193.—**Fröbelius** (W.) Von der intermittirenden Trübung der wässerigen Feuchtigkeit. Med. Ztg. Russlands, St. Petersb., 1853, x, 115-119.—**Gaucher.** Influence de l'humidité sur les tissus vivants. Monit. d. sc. méd. et pharm., Par., 1860, 2. s., ii, 598.—**Glässgen** (J.) Ueber den Wassergehalt der Wände und dessen quantitative Bestimmung. Ztschr. f. Biol., München, 1874, x, 246-262, 1 pl.—**Heberden** (W.) In England few make any doubt of the great danger attending wet rooms, and damp cloaths, or beds. Is this opinion founded upon experience, or is it a prejudice, which has been suffered to grow up and get strength merely for want of being examined? Med. Tr. Roy. Coll. Phys. Lond., 1772. ii, 521-528.—**Hottinger-Goldschmid.** Die Bestimmung der Feuchtigkeit in den Neubauten. Bl. f. Gsndhtspflg., Zürich, 1880, ix, 201-205.—**von Jacquin.** Die Ursachen des schädlichen Einflusses der Feuchtigkeit neu erbauter Wohnungen auf die Gesundheit der Menschen. Med. Jahrb. d. k. k. österr. Staates, Wien, 1832, n. F., ii, 97-103.—**Krügelstein.** Von den Gefahren, welche für die Gesundheit durch das Bewohnen neuerbauter Häuser entstehen, und von den Mitteln, dieselben abzuwenden. Ann. d. Staatsarznk. Tübing., 1847, ii, 381-401.—**Lang** (C.) Ueber die Porosität einiger Baumaterialien. Ztschr. f. Biol., München, 1875, xi, 313-340, 2 pl., 2 tab. ——. Neuere Versuche über das hygroskopische Verhalten von Baumaterialien bei Temperaturen über und unter 0°. Ztschr. f. Biol., München, 1880, xvi, 443-454.—**Legler** (L.) Untersuchungen über den

Moisture.

Werth einzelner Methoden der Feuchtigkeitsbestimmung in der Atmosphäre und in Zimmerluft. Jahresb. d. chem. Centralstelle f. öff. Gsndhtspflg. in Dresd., 1882, x–xi, 43–49.—**Möller.** Ueber die Methoden zur Ermittelung der Feuchtigkeit in Gebäuden. Monatschr. . . . . d. San.-Pol., Berl., 1859, i, 337.—**Monoyer** (F.) Du rôle étiologique de la douche murale descendante dans le développement des psychronoses. Rev. méd. de l'est, Nancy, 1876, v, 219–222. [Discussion], 249; 251.—**Philippe** (G.) Damp; its causes, effects, prevention, and cure. [From: Les travaux publics, and The Builder.] Van Nostrand's Engin. Mag., N. Y., 1881, xxv, 476–478.—**Poincaré.** Sur l'hygroscopicité des matériaux de construction. Ann. d'hyg., Par., 1881, 3. s., vi, 36–39.—**Reinhard** (H.) Die relative Feuchtigkeit der Atmosphäre und ihre Wirkung auf den Menschen. Arch. f. Hyg., München u. Leipz., 1885–6, iii, 183–203.—**Woodbridge** (S. H.) Note on the relation of humidity to air-supply in ventilation. San. Engin., N. Y., 1885–6, xiii, 298.

Moisture in relation to heating and ventilation.

Allen (J. K.) Air-moistening. Rep. Bd. Health Mich. 1880, Lansing, 1881, viii, 146–148. Also, Reprint.—**Bouvet** (A.) Des variations du degré hygrométrique de l'air chauffé. Cong. internat. d'hyg. 1878, Par., 1880, ii, 323–333. Also: Rev. d'hyg., Par., 1880, ii, 92–107. — **Brackett** (C. F.) Hints with reference to the regulation of moisture in rooms. Rep. Bd. Health N. Jersey, Woodbury, 1882, vi, 123–126. — **Briggs** (R.) On the relation of moisture in air to health and comfort. J. Frankl. Inst., Phila., 1878, 3. s., lxxv, 10; 82; 168; 251. Also, Reprint.—**Curtis** (H.) [et al.]. The hygrodeik, and the proper means of hydrating our houses and halls of assembly. Boston M. & S. J., 1867–8. lxxvii, 49; 120; 146. Also, Reprint. — **Mantegazza** (P.) L'acqua sulle stufe. Medico di casa, Milano, 1879, vii, 33–35.

Moitessier (A.) * De l'urine. 83 pp. 4°. Paris, F. Thunot & Cie., 1856.
Concours.

——. * Recherches sur la dilatation du soufre. 31 pp., 1 pl. 4°. Montpellier, Boehm & fils, 1864. [P., v. 1704.]

——. * Recherches sur la salicine et les composés salicyliques. 78 pp. 4°. Montpellier, Boehm & fils, 1864. [P., v. 1704.]

——. * Thèses présentées à la Faculté des sciences de Montpellier. Thèse de chimie. Recherches sur la salicine et les composés salicyliques. Thèse de physique. Recherches sur la dilatation du soufre. 78, 31 pp., 1 pl. 4°. Montpellier, Boehm & fils, 1864, No. 26.

——. De l'emploi de la lumière polarisée dans l'examen microscopique des farines. 23 pp., 1 pl. roy. 8°. Paris, J.-B. Baillière & fils, 1866.
Repr. from: Mém. Acad. d. sc. et let., Montpellier, 1866.

——. La photographie appliquée aux recherches micrographiques. 333 pp., 3 pl. 8°. Paris, J.-B. Baillière & fils, 1866.

——. The same. Die Photographie als Hilfsmittel mikroskopischer Forschung. Nach dem Französischen, mit Autorisation des Verfassers deutsch bearbeitet, und durch zahlreiche Zusätze erweitert von Berthold Benecke. xiv, 265 pp., 3 l., 2 pl. 8°. Braunschweig, Vieweg u. Sohn, 1868.

——. Éléments de physique appliquée à la médecine et à la physiologie. vii, 601 pp. sm. 8°. Paris, G. Masson, 1879.

Moity (Charles-Casimir). * Des amygdales. 30 pp. 4°. Paris, 1858, No. 112, v. 621.

Moizard (Paul). * Étude sur les cas de diphthérie observés à l'Hôpital Sainte-Eugénie pendant l'année 1876. 72 pp. 4°. Paris, 1876, No. 493.

Moizard (Paulin). * Contribution à l'étude de la mammite chez l'homme. 83 pp. 4°. Paris, 1881, No. 414.

Moizin (Claude-Joseph) [1782–1849]. * Observations et réflections sur les effets du coup de pistolet, tiré dans la bouche. iv, 54 pp. 8°. Paris, an X [1802], v. 35.
For Biography, see Exposé d. trav. de la Soc. d. sc. méd. de la Moselle, Metz, 1849, 79–103 (P. Monard). Also: Gaz. méd. de Par., 1849, 3. s., iv. 155 (F. Jacquot). Also: Rec. de mém. de méd. . . . mil. Par., 1850, 2. s., 334–339 (Boudin).
For Portrait, see **Collection**—van Kaathoven.

Mojon (Benoît) [1784–1849]. Mémoire sur l'utilité de la musique, tant dans l'état de santé, que dans celui de maladie. Trad. de la 2. éd. italienne, avec notes, par C.-D. Muggetti. x, 11–48 pp. 8°. Paris, Fournier, 1803.
Bound with his: Mémoire sur les effets de la castration. 8°. Montpellier, an XII [1804].

——. Memoria sugli effetti della castratura nel corpo umano, trasmessa alla Società medica di emulazione di Genova li 28 giugno 1804. 19 pp. 8°. Genova, [1804].
Bound with his: Mémoire sur les effets de la castration. 8°. Montpellier, [1804].

——. The same. Mémoire sur les effets de la castration dans le corps humain. 35 pp. 8°. Montpellier, J.-G. Tournel, an XII [1804].

——. The same. 3. éd. vii, 9–35 pp. 4°. Gènes, J. Gravier, 1813. [P., v. 901.]

——. Leggi fisiologiche. 2. ed. xvii, 119, vi pp., 2 tab. 8°. Genova, I. Gravier, 1810.

——. The same. 3. ed. xxiv, 152 pp., 2 tab. 8°. Milano, G. Pirotta, 1821. [P., v. 1349.]

——. The same. Lois physiologiques. Trad. de l'italien, avec des additions et des notes, par le baron Michel. vii, xix, 287 pp. 8°. Paris, Béchet jeune, 1834.

——. Memoria sulla contrattilità della fibra animale, letta all' Accademia delle scienze ed arti di Genova. 18 pp. 12°. Genova, G. Gravier, 1814. [Also, in: P., v. 1349.]

——. Osservazioni notomico-fisiologiche sull' epidermide. 16 pp. 4°. Genova, G. Gravier, 1815. [P., v. 901.]

——. The same. 2. ed. 9–22 pp., 3 l. 4°. Genova, dalla fonderia Ponthenier, 1820. [P., v. 1578.]

——. Dissertazione sugli effetti della castratura nel corpo umano. 55 pp. 8°. Milano, G. Pirotta, 1822. [P., v. 1349.]

——. Conjectures sur la nature du miasme producteur du choléra asiatique. Trad. de l'italien par M. Julia de Fontenelle. 63 pp. 8°. Paris, J. Rouvier, 1833. [P., v. 491; 1354; 1657.]
See, also, **Poggi** (Junius). Aux rédacteurs des Annales de chimie, sur une nouvelle source de pétrole, [etc.] 8°. Paris, an XI [1803].
For Biography, see Union méd., Par., 1850, iv, 293–295 (P.-L.-B. Caffe). Also, Reprint.

Mojon (Giuseppe) [1777–1837]. Osservazioni sopra la tavola delle espressioni numeriche di affinità del cittadino Guyton Morveau. 6 pp. 8°. [n. p., 1802.]
Bound with: **Mojon** (B.) Mémoire sur les effets de la castration. 8°. Montpellier, [1804].

——. Memorie di chimica. 16 pp., 1 map. 8°. Genova, 1804.
Bound with: **Mojon** (B.) Mémoire sur les effets de la castration. 8°. Montpellier, [1804].

——. Descrizione mineralogica della Liguria. 26 pp. 12°. Genova, 1805.
See, also, **de Ferrari** (Luigi) & **Mojon** (Giuseppe). Analisi delle acque solforee e termali di Voltri. 8°. Genova, 1804.

Mojsisovics, Edler von Mojsvar (August). Leitfaden bei zoologisch-zootomischen Präpaririibungen. 2. Aufl. xii, 259 pp. 8°. Leipzig, W. Engelmann, 1885.

——. The same. Manuel de zootomie, guide pratique pour la dissection des animaux vertébrés et invertébrés, à l'usage des étudiants en médecine et des élèves qui préparent la licence ès sciences naturelles. Trad. de l'allemand et annoté, par J.-L. de Lanessan. 2 p. l., 368 pp. 8°. Paris, O. Doin, 1881.
A translation from the original edition.

Moj'sisovics, Edler von Mojsvár (Georg) [1799–1861]. * Diss. sistens actionem et usum therapeuticum balneorum simplicium tepidorum. 49 pp., 1 l. 8°. Vindobonæ, typ. Congregationis Mechitaristicæ, [1826].

Moj'sisovics, *Edler von Mojsvár* (Georg)—cont.
——. Darstellung der Aequilibrial-Methode der sicheren Heilung der Oberschenkelbrüche ohne Verkürzung. xii, 114 pp., 2 l., 4 pl. 8°. *Wien, Braumüller u. Seidel,* 1842.
——. The same. 2. Aufl. xii (1 l.), 114 pp., 2 l., 4 pl. 8°. *Wien, W. Braumüller,* 1851.
——. Darstellung einer sicheren und schnellen Heilmethode der Syphilis durch Jodpräparate. viii, 246 pp., 1 l. 8°. *Wien, Braumüller u. Seidel,* 1845.
For Biography, see Wien. med. Wchnschr., 1861, xi, 187–189 (Jos. Gruber).

Moke (Carolus Alexander). * De metastasi. 2 p. l., 14 pp., 2 l. 4°. *Lugd. Bat., apud Haak et soc.,* 1806. [*Also, in :* P., v. 1482.]

Mokmoko.
Schroff. Ueber Radix Mokmoko. Wien. Med.-Halle, 1864, v, 55.

Mokossinyi (Michaël). * De nutrice. 29 pp. 8°. *Pesthini, L. Landerer de Füskút,* [1822]. [*Also, in :* P., v. 1310.]

Mokrousoff (Iv.) * Materialy k voprosu o kolichestvennom opredelenii myshjaka v trupach jivotnych, im. otravlenych. [Instructions for quantitative analysis of arsenic in animal body in poisoning.] 46 pp., 1 l. 8°. *St. Petersburg, tipog. I. Habermana,* 1880.

Mol (Janus). * Diss. exhibens delineationem febris scarlatinæ anginosæ quæ exeunte potissimum a° 1780. Harderovici observata est. 56 pp., 1 l. 4°. *Harderovici, J. Moojen,* [1781].

de Mol (Joannes). * De hepatitide. 16 pp. 8°. *Marburgi, J. C. Krieger,* [1818].

Mol (Joannes Gerardus Jeremias Jacobus). *Spec. continens historiam eorum quæ proximo anno academico in clinico atque polyclinico chirurgico academiæ Rheno-Trajectinæ observata fuerunt. [Utrecht.] 3 p. l., 112 pp. 8°. *Amstelodami, typ. hered. H. van Munster et filius,* 1859.

Molander (J.) * Om Fosfornecros. [Upsala.] 36 pp. 8°. *Stockholm, N. Marcus,* 1855.

Molar.
Gonzalez y Crespo (M. J.) Memoria sobre las aguas hidro-sulfurosas de el Molar. Bol. de med., cirug. y farm., Madrid, 1837, iv, 218–222.—Memoria sobre las aguas minero-medicinales del Molar. España méd., Madrid, 1862, vii, 203 ; 219 ; 254 ; 283 ; 312.

Molard (Félix-Joseph). * I. Comment distinguer les taches de sperme des taches produites par la matière des écoulements blennorrhagiques, leucorrhagiques, etc.? II. [etc.] 26 pp. 4°. *Paris,* 1838, No. 180, v. 331.

Molard (J.-B.-M.-Paul). * Des plaies des articulations. 63 pp. 4°. *Paris,* 1848, No. 64, v. 474.

Molard (Jacques). * Du redressement dans les coxalgies, ses indications, moyens de l'obtenir. 40 pp. 4°. *Paris,* 1867, No. 183.

Molard (Victor). * Étude sur la pleurésie rhumatismale. 60 pp. 4°. *Paris,* 1870.

Molas (Louis). * Contribution à l'étude des hémorrhagies liées à l'éclampsie puerpérale. 48 pp., 1 l. 4°. *Paris,* 1877, No. 338.

Molasses.
Bauwens (C.) fils. · Note sur la présence de l'acétate de zinc dans la mélasse ou sirop commun. Bull. Soc. de méd. de Gand, 1853, xx, 104–108.—Cullimore (D. H.) On the preventive and remedial effects of molasses in scurvy and diseases connected with chronic starvation. Lancet, Lond., 1880, i, 186.—McCallum (A.), jr. Effect of molasses on the health. Med. & Surg. Reporter, Phila., 1879, xli, 351.

Molckenbour (Gerardus). * De ictero flavo. 7 l. 4°. *Harderovici, A. Sas,* 1685.

Mold.
See Fungi.

Mold Cottage Hospital. Annual reports of the committee to the subscribers. 4.-6., 1882-4. 8°. *Mold, Beresford & Co.,* [1883-5].

Moldau (Æmilius Adolarius). * De pulmonum tuberculosi. 29 pp., 1 l. 8°. *Jenæ, typ. A. Neuenhahni,* 1863.
C.

Moldavia.
See, also, Fever (*Malarial, History, etc., of*), Hospitals (*Description, etc., of*), by localities; Jassy; Sulina Island.
A Vernav (C.) * Rudimentum physiographiæ Moldaviæ. 8°. *Budæ,* 1836.
Dobronrawoff. Medico-topograficheskoe opisanie kniajestve Moldavii i Walachii. Voyenno-med. J., St. Petersb., 1834, xxiv, pt. 1, 189–214. Also, transl. : Wissensch. Ann. d. ges. Heilk., Berl., 1835, xxxi, 338–342.—Mitchtol (G.) Galatz i ego gospitali. [Hospitals in Galatz.] Med. pribav. k morsk. sborniku, St. Petersb., 1870, x, 377–396.—Vignard (V.) Notes pour servir à l'histoire médicale du delta du Danube. Gaz. méd. de Par., 1877, 4. s., v, 563.

Moldenhauer (Fritz). * Ueber die Reposition eingeklemmter Brüche mit Hülfe elastischer Binden. 64 pp. 8°. *Giessen, Brühl,* 1866. [P., v. 275.]
——. * Herr Professor Bock gegen die Heilkunst unserer Zeit. Eine kritische Analyse der jüngsten Ergüsse des Herrn Bock über die Aerzte und ihre Wissenschaft. 2. unveränderte Aufl. 54 pp. 12°. *Darmstadt u. Leipzig, E. Zurnin,* 1867.

Moldenhauer (Wilhelm). Die geburtshülflichen Operationen am Phantom. Ein Leitfaden für die Studirenden der Medicin. 27 pp. 8°. *Leipzig, O. Wigand,* 1875.
——. Die Krankheiten der Nasenhöhlen, ihrer Nebenhöhlen und des Nasen-Rachenraumes, mit Einschluss der Untersuchungstechnik. Zum Gebrauche für Aerzte und Studirende. viii, 198 pp. 8°. *Leipzig, F. C. W. Vogel,* 1886.

Moldenhawer (Car. Frid. Guil.) * De varia ustionem adhibendi ratione apud Hippocratem. 32 pp. 8°. *Berolini, ex off. A G. Schadii,* 1818.
Also, Co-Editor of : Neueste medizinisch-chirurgische Journalistik des Auslandes, Leipzig, 1831-3.

Moldenhawer (J.) Det Kongelige Blindeinstituts Historie tilligemed en Oversigt over Blindesagens Udvikling i Danmark fra 1811–83, udarbeitet i Anledning af Institutets 25-Aars-Jubilæum den 5. November 1883. 63 pp., 1 pl. 8°. *Kjøbenhavn, Hoffensberg Traps Etabl.,* 1883.

Moldt (Otto). * De angina membranacea ; accedit singularis casus laryngoscopia observatus. 27 pp. 8°. *Gryphiæ, F. Hache,* 1863.
C.

Mole.
Corthum (J.) De visu talparum. 4°. *Altenburgi,* 1671.
Freeman (R. A.) The anatomy of the shoulder and upper arm of the mole (Talpa europæa). J. Anat. & Physiol., Lond., 1885-6, xx, 201–219, 1 pl.—Ganser (S.) Vergleichend-anatomische Studien über das Gehirn des Maulwurfs. Morphol. Jahrb., Leipz., 1882, vii, 591–725, 5 pl.—Heape (W.) On the germinal layers and early development of the mole. Proc. Roy. Soc. Lond., 1881-2, xxxiii, 190–198.

Mole (*Pigmentary*).
See Nævus (*Pigmentary*).

Mole (*Uterine*).
See Dysmenorrhœa (*Membranous*); Pregnancy (*Molar*).

Mole (Léon). * Signes précis de début de la convalescence dans les maladies aiguës. 114 pp. 4°. *Paris,* 1870.

Moledo.
Ferreira (M. L.) [*et al.*]. As aguas mineraes de Moledo, sua composição chimica, acção physiologica e effeitos therapeuticos. 8°. *Coimbra,* 1871.

Molenaar (Andreas Jacobus). * Het ontstekingsproces en zijne uitgangen bij de weivliezen. 3 p. l., 37 pp., 1 l. 8°. *Groningen, R. J. Schierbeek,* 1868.

Molenaar (Comelis Anthonie). * Over het wezen der encephalopathia saturnina. 1 p. l., 80 pp. 8°. *Leiden, P. Somerwil*, 1883.

Molenaar (Dirk). * Bijdrage over pneumonie en hare behandeling. 1 p. l., 35 pp., 1 l., 2 tab. 8°. *Leyden, J. Hazenberg*, 1863.

Molenbroek (Matthys Herman). * Over tropische dysenterie. [Leyden.] 2 p. l., 45 pp. 8°. *Delft, J. H. Molenbroek*, 1856.

de Molènes (J.-J.-Marc). * De la migraine. 64 pp. 4°. *Paris*, 1853, No. 173, v. 545.

de Molènes (J.-J.-V.) * De l'aconitine cristalisée et de son azotate. 60 pp. 4°. *Paris*, 1874, No. 54.

de Molènes-Mahon (Paul) [1857–]. * Contribution à l'étude des maladies infectieuses. De l'érythème polymorphe. 215 pp. 4°. *Paris*, 1884, No. 61.

des Moles (Jacobus Verdelhan). An a globulosa sanguinis ad cutem adpellentis parte, Æthiopum color? [Præses: Urbannus de Vandenesse.] [1742.]
  In: SIGWART (G. F.) Quæst. med. Par. 4°. *Tubingæ*, 1789, ii, 293–300.

————. An senibus vinum parcius, dilutius? [Præses: Raymund de la Riviere.] [1743.]
  In: SIGWART (G. F.) Quæst. med. Par. 4°. *Tubingæ*, 1789, i, 207–211.

————. An quo præstantior in praxi medicus eo et vaticinii genio magis præditus? [Præses: Ludov. Hieron. Cosnier.] [1743.]
  In: SIGWART (G. F.) Quæst. med. Par. 4°. *Tubingæ*, 1789, i, 254–258.

Moleschott (Jacob) [1822–]. * De Malpighianis pulmonum vesiculis. 42 pp., 1 l., 1 pl. 8°. *Heidelbergæ, C. Groos*, 1845.

————. Physiologie des Stoffwechsels in Pflanzen und Thieren. xxii, 592 pp. roy. 8°. *Erlangen, F. Enke*, 1851.

————. Der Kreislauf des Lebens. Physiologische Antworten auf Liebig's chemische Briefe. vi, 485 pp. sm. 8°. *Mainz, V. von Zabern*, 1852.

————. The same. 4. Aufl. xviii, 556 pp. 12°. *Mainz, V. von Zabern*, 1863.

————. The same. 2 v. vi, 476 pp; 288 + pp. 8°. *Mainz, V. von Zabern*, 1877–8.
  Want all after p. 288 of v. 2.

————. The same. 5. Aufl. 2 v. vi, 476 pp., port.; 1 p. l., 771 pp. 8°. *Giessen, E. Roth*, 1887.

————. The same. La circulation de la vie. Lettres sur la physiologie en réponse aux lettres sur la chimie, de Liebig. Traduit de l'allemand, avec autorisation de l'auteur, par E. Cazelles. 2 v. in 1. xxviii, 201 pp., 1 l.; 233 pp., 1 l. 12°. *Paris, Germer-Baillière*, 1866.

————. Untersuchungen zur Naturlehre des Menschen und der Thiere. 10 v. 8°. *Frankf. a. M. u. Giessen, Meidinger Sohn u. Comp. u. E. Roth*, 1857–70.

————. Lehre der Nahrungsmittel. Für das Volk. 3. Aufl. xx, 239 pp. 8°. *Erlangen, F. Enke*, 1858.

————. Physiologie der Nahrungsmittel. Ein Handbuch der Diätetik. 2. Aufl. xxiv, 570, 254 pp., 355 tab. roy. 8°. *Giessen, Universitäts-buchhandlung*, 1859.

————. Untersuchungen über den Einfluss der Vagus-Reizung auf die Häufigkeit des Herzschlags. 32 pp., 1 pl. 8°. [*n. p.*, 1860.] [P., v. 790.]
  Repr. from: Untersuch. z. Naturl. d. Mensch. u. d. Thiere, Frankf. a. M., 1860, vii.

————. Physiologisches Skizzenbuch. ix (1 l.), 320 pp. 8°. *Giessen, Ferber*, 1861.

————. Zur Erforschung des Lebens. Rede beim Antritt der Professur für Physiologie an der Hochschule zu Turin. Gehalten am 16. December 1861. iv, 32 pp. 12°. *Giessen, Ferber*, 1862.

Moleschott (Jacob)—continued.
————. The same. Del metodo nella investigazione della vita; prima prolusione al corso di fisiologia sperimentale nella R. Università di Torino, letta il dì 16 dicembre 1861. 1 p. l., 28 pp. 8°. *Torino, E. Loescher*, 1862. [*Also, in:* P., v. 1429.]

————. Der bewegungvermittelnde Vorgang im Nerven kann auch von einer positiven Schwankung des Nervenstroms begleitet sein. 35 pp. 8°. [*n. p.*], 1862. [P., v. 790.]
  Repr. from: Untersuch. z. Naturl. d. Mensch. u. d. Thiere, Frankf. a. M., 1862, viii.

————. Die Grenzen des Menschen. Vortrag bei der Wiedereröffnung der Vorlesungen über Physiologie an der Turiner Hochschule. 56 pp. 16°. *Giessen, Ferber*, 1863.
  pp. 51–55 missing.

————. The same. Dei limiti della natura umana. Seconda prolusione al corso di fisiologia sperimentale nella R. Università di Torino, letta il dì 24 novembre 1862. 38 pp. 12°. *Torino, E. Loescher*, 1864.

————. L' unità della vita. Terza prolusione al corso di fisiologia sperimentale nella R. Università di Torino, letta il dì 23 novembre 1863. 52 pp. 12°. *Torino, E. Loescher*, 1864.

————. Eine physiologische Sendung. In der Turiner Gesellschaft für wissenschaftliche und litterarische Vorlesungen am 21. März 1864 vorgetragen von . . . 68 pp. 12°. *Giessen, E. Roth*, 1864.

————. The same. Eene physiologische zending; in de Vereeniging voor Wetenschappelijke en Letterkundige Voorlezingen te Turyn op den 21. Maart 1864 voorgedragen; uit het Hoogduitsch vertaald door Lupus. 67 pp. 8°. *Rotterdam, W. L. Stoeller*, 1864.

————. The same. Un ambasciata fisiologica esposta nella Società Torinese per letture scientifiche e letterarie, il dì 21 marzo 1864. 66 pp. 8°. *Torino & Firenze, E. Loescher*, 1866.

————. Natur- und Heilkunde. Vortrag bei der Wiedereröffnung der Vorlesungen über Physiologie an der Turiner Hochschule am 28. November 1864 gehalten. 52 pp., 1 l. 12°. *Giessen, E. Roth*, 1865.

————. Fisiologia e medicina. Quarta prolusione al corso di fisiologia sperimentale nella R. Università di Torino, letta il dì 28 novembre 1864. 44 pp. 12°. *Torino, E. Loescher*, 1865.

————. Patologia e fisiologia. Quinta prolusione al corso di fisiologia sperimentale nella R. Università di Torino, letta il dì 2 dicembre 1865. 39 pp. 12°. *Torino & Firenze, E. Loescher*, 1866.

————. The same. Pathologie und Physiologie. Vortrag bei der Wiedereröffnung der Vorlesungen über Physiologie an der Turiner Hochschule, am 2. December 1865 gehalten. 42 pp. 12°. *Giessen, E. Roth*, 1866.

————. Rath und Trost für Cholerazeiten. Insbesondere den Hausvätern gewidmet. 20 pp. 8°. *Giessen, E. Roth*, 1866.

————. The same. Consigli e conforti nei tempi di colera diretti alle singole persone ed in ispecie ai padri di famiglia. 16 pp. 8°. *Torino & Firenze, E. Loescher*, 1866.

————. The same. 3. ed. 15 pp. 12°. *Torino, E. Loescher*, 1884.

————. Sulla forma dell' arresto del cuore in seguito alla sovraeccitazione del nervo pneumogastrico. 10 pp. 8°. [*n. p., n. d.*] [P., v. 794.]
  Repr. from: Atti. d. r. Accad. d. sc. di Torino, 1866, 312.

————. Ursache und Wirkung in der Lehre vom Leben. Sechster Vortrag zur Wiedereröffnung der Vorlesungen über Physiologie an der Turiner Hochschule, gehalten am 8. Januar 1867. 39 pp., 1 l. sm. 8°. *Giessen, E. Roth*, 1867.

Moleschott (Jacob)—continued.

——. Sull' elettrotono primario e secondario dei nervi. 13 pp. 8°. *Torino*, 1870. [P., v. 802.]

Repr. from: Atti r. Accad. d. sc. di Torino, 1869, v.

——. Sugli effetti emodinamici della recisione dei nervi pneumogastrici. 23 pp. 8°. *Torino, Stamperia reale*, 1873. [P., v. 795.]

——. Dell' indole della fisiologia. Parole d' introduzione al corso di fisiologia sperimentale nell' Università di Torino, pronunziate il dì 12 dicembre 1875. 21 pp. 8°. *Roma, Torino & Firenze, E. Loescher*, 1876. [P., v. 1483.]

——. La fisiologia e le scienze sorelle. Prolusione al corso di fisiologia sperimentale nella Sapienza di Roma, pronunziata il dì 11 gennaio 1879. 25 pp., 1 l. 8°. *Roma, Torino & Firenze, E. Loescher*, 1879. [P., v. 1483.]

——. Ueber den Wassergehalt einiger Horngewebe des menschlichen Körpers. Ueber das Wachsthum der Horngebilde des menschlichen Körpers und die damit verbundene Stickstoffausgabe. 66 pp. 8°. *Giessen, E. Roth*, 1879.

Repr. from: Untersuch. z. Naturl. d. Mensch. u. d. Thiere, Giessen, xii.

——. Dei regolatori della vita umana. Discorso pronunciato nel solenne riaprimento della R. Università di Torino addì 16 novembre 1870. 3. ed. 28 pp. 8°. *Torino & Roma, E. Loescher*, 1880. [P., v. 1483.]

——. Veder nascere. Prolusione al corso di fisiologia sperimentale pronunziata il 5 novembre 1878 nell' Università di Torino. 23 pp. 8°. *Torino & Roma, E. Loescher*, 1880. [P., v. 1483.]

——. Sugli attributi generali dei nervi. Introduzione al corso di fisiologia sperimentale letta il 16 gennaio 1881. In occasione dell' inaugurazione del nuovo Istituto anatomico-fisiologico nell' Università di Roma. 23 pp. 8°. *Torino, E. Loescher*, 1881. [*Also, in:* P., v. 1483.]

——. Carlo Roberto Darwin. Commemorazione pronunziata a nome degli studenti dell' Università di Roma nel giorno 25 di giugno 1882. 45 pp. 8°. *Torino, E. Loescher*, 1882. [P., v. 1483.]

——. Ueber die allgemeinen Lebenseigenschaften der Nerven. Rede bei der Eröffnung des neuen anatomisch-physiologischen Instituts an der Universität zu Rom am 16. Januar 1881 gehalten. 26 pp. 12°. *Giessen, E. Roth*, 1882.

——. La conferenza sanitaria internazionale di Roma 20 maggio—13 giugno 1885. 37 pp. 8°. *Torino, E. Loescher*, 1885.

Also, Co-Editor of: **Holländische** Beiträge zu den anatomischen und physiologischen Wissenschaften, Düsseldorf u. Utrecht. 1846-8. *Also, Editor of:* **Untersuchungen** zur Naturlehre des Menschen und der Thiere, Frankfurt a. M., 1856-70. *See, also.* **Chapuis** (P.) & **Moleschott** (Jac.) Ueber einige Punkte, betreffend den Bau des Haarbalgs und der Haare der menschlichen Kopfhaut. 8°. [*Zürich*, 1860.]— **Hufschmid** (E.) & **Moleschott** (Jac.) Experimenteller Beweis der Theorie, nach welcher [etc.] 8°. [*Zürich*, 1861.]—**Mulder** (G. J.) Ueber den Werth und die Bedeutung der Naturwissenschaften für die Medicin. 8°. *Heidelberg*, 1844.—**Pagliani** (Luigi). Saggio sullo stato attuale, [etc.] 8°. *Torino*, 1872.—**Tiedemann** (Friedrich). Die Physiologie der Nahrungsmittel, etc. 8°. *Darmstadt*, 1850.

For Biography, see Pacific M. & S. J., San Fran., 1876, xviii, 345–350 (L. C. Lance).

——. *See, also:*

HARTING (P.) De Heer Jac. Moleschott, privaatdocent te Heidelberg, in zijne verhouding tegenover de geneeskundige faculteiten in Nederland. 8°. *Utrecht*, 1848.

—— & **Nauwerck** (Rob.) Untersuchungen über den Einfluss der Sympathicus-Reizung auf die Häufigkeit des Herzschlags. 16 pp. 8°. [*n. p.*, 1861.] [P., v. 790.]

Repr. from: Untersuch. z. Naturl. d. Mensch. u. d. Thiere, Frankf. a. M., 1862, viii.

Molesworth (*William*).

Portrait in: **Collection** of Portr. (Libr.)

Molet (Romain - Joseph). * I. Quelle est la valeur séméiologique des matières vomies ? II. [etc.] 44 pp. 4°. *Paris*, 1843, No. 142, v. 406.

Molewater (Janus Bastianus) [1813–64]. * De typho abdominali, sive febre typhoidea. 3 p. l., 118 pp. 8°. *Lugd. Bat., H. W. Hazenberg et socios*, 1840.

For Biography, see Nederl. Tijdschr. v. Geneesk., Amst., 1865, i, 65–72 (T. J. J. Schmidt).

Molgar.

Casares (A.) Aguas minerales de Molgar (Orense). Restaurador farm., Barcel., 1860, xvi, 43. *Also* [Abstr.]: Siglo méd., Madrid, 1860, vii, 394.

Molhant (Ernest-Henri-Augustin). * Étude sur la fistule borgne interne du rectum. 48 pp. 4°. *Lille*, 1886, 3. s., No. 22.

Molia (Jean-Louis-Léonce). * Des vomissements incoercibles pendant la grossesse. 40 pp. 4°. *Paris*, 1862, No. 166.

Molière (Gilbert). * Sur l'ophthalmie. 27 pp. 4°. *Paris*, 1817, No. 90.

Molière (*Jean-Baptiste-Poquelin*) [1622–73].

See, also, **Medicine** (*History, etc., of*), *by nations, etc.—France.*

NIVELET (F.) Molière et Gui Patin. (Molière et Gui Patin, satires médicales de Molière; Gui Patin et Théophraste Renaudot; la Faculté de Paris au xviie siècle; quelques critiques sur Gui Patin, son apologie.) 12°. *Paris*, 1880.

Molimbrochius (Andreas Valentinus). Cochlearia curiosa, or the curiosities of scurvygrass. Being an exact scrutiny and careful description of the nature and medicinal vertue of scurvygrass. In which is exhibited to publick use the most and best preparations of medicines, both Galenical and chymical, either for internal or external use, in which that plant, or any part thereof, is imployed. Englished by Tho. Sherley. 6 p. l., 195 pp., 14 l., 4 pl. 12°. *London, S. & B. Griffin*, 1676.

Molin. Notice sur Luxeuil et ses eaux minérales. 120 pp., 1 pl. 8°. *Paris, Mlle. Delaunay*, 1833. [*Also, in:* P., v. 915.]

Also, Editor of: **Journal** de la doctrine Hahnemannienne, Paris, 1840.

Molin (A.) * Sur la fièvre adynamique continue. 40 pp. 4°. *Paris*, 1820, No. 122, v. 157.

Molin (Auguste). * Sur l'angine scarlatineuse épidémique. 1 p. l., 16 pp. 4°. *Strasbourg*, 1833, v. 64.

Molin (Girolamo). Sopra la veterinaria di Pelagonio, pubblicata in Firenze nel 1826, qual opera originalmente latina. 54 pp. 8°. *Padova, tipog. del seminario*, 1828.

Molin (J.-Jacques). * Observations pratiques pouvant servir à éclairer l'étiologie de quelques fièvres intermittentes. 1 p. l., 9 pp. 4°. *Strasbourg*, 1829, v. 60.

Molin (Karl Fr.) *See* **Kwasser** (Israël). Läran om feber. Andra afdelningen. 16. delen. 8°. *Upsala*, 1839-44.

Molin (Louis-Just-Jean). * Des spécifiques en médecine. 64 pp. 4°. *Paris*, 1847, No. 139, v. 462.

Molina (Augusto). * Breves estudios sobre la infeccion purulenta. 34 pp. 8°. *México, I. Escalante*, 1873.

Molina (Rafael Martinez). *See* **Sabater** (Manuel Cárceles). Histero-ovariotomia, etc. 8°. *Madrid*, 1885.

Molinar de Carranza.

Rugama (H.) Baños minero-medicinales de Molinar de Carranza (encartaciones de Vizcaya). Bol. de med., cirug. y farm., Madrid, 1853, 2. s., iii, 277; 285.—**Tejada y España.** Los baños de Molinar de Carranza (Bilbao). Génio méd.-quir., Madrid, 1879, xxv, 274-276.

Molinard (Auguste). * De la fièvre typhoïde, nature, causes, traitement. 32 pp. 4°. *Paris,* 1848, No. 151, v. 475.

Molinari (Giambattista). Sull' allattamento dei bambini. Trattato teorico-pratico ad uso delle madri di famiglia. 74 pp. 8°. *Brescia,* 1872.

de Molinari (Philippe). Guide de l'homœopathiste, indiquant les moyens de se traiter soi-même dans les maladies les plus communes en attendant la visite du médecin. 2. éd. 256 pp., port. 8°. *Bruxelles, J.-B. Tircher,* 1861.
See, also, **de Bönninghausen** (C.) Les côtés du corps ainsi que les affinités, etc. Trad. de l'allemand par . . . 8°. *Bruxelles,* 1857.

Molinarius (Christ.) De miliarium exanthematum indole et tractatione disquisitio. 171 pp. 8°. *Vindobonæ, sumpt. H. J. Krüchten,* 1764.

Molinarus (Joh. Baptista). De apoplexia specimen. 3 p. l., 75 pp. 4°. *Viennæ,* 1753.

Molinella.
Calori (V.) Cenno storico e topografico de Molinella, e delle sue principali malattie dominanti. Bull. d. sc. med. di Bologna, 1860, 4. s., xiii, 5–32.

Molinerius (Cæsar Antonius). Brevis tractatus historico-medicus de pestilentiis quæ ad nostram, usque ætatem sevierunt. 42 pp. 4°. *Mediolani, typ. C. J. Quinti,* 1727.
Bound with: FIOCHETTO (Gianfrancesco). Trattato della peste [etc.] 4°. *Torino,* 1720.

Molinery (Victorius Franciscus). * I. Ex anatome. De mesenterio. II. [etc.] 12 pp. sm. 4°. *Augustæ Taurinorum, J. D. Verani,* 1748. [P., v. 979.]

Molines (L.) Contribution à l'étude de la colpohystérectomie totale dans les affections cancéreuses de l'utérus. 49 pp. 8°. *Montpellier, Boehm & fils,* 18-5.

Molinetti (Antonius). Dissertationes anatomicæ, et pathologicæ de sensibus et eorum organis. 2 p. l., 116 pp., 3 pl. sm. 4°. *Patavii, ex typog. M. Bolzetta de Cadorinis,* 1669
——. Dissertationes anatomico-pathologicæ quibus humani corporis partes accuratissime describuntur morbique singulas divexantes explicantur. 3 p. l., 338 pp., 1 tab., 2 pl. 4°. *Venetiis, apud P. Balleonium,* 1675.

Molinettus (Michael Angelus) [1645–1714]. Indicantur lectiones quas, Deo dante, in universam humani corporis fabricam professor publice habebit ad annum 1690. 4 pp. 4°. *Patavii, apud Cadorinum,* 1640. [P., v. 1234.]
For Portrait, see **Collection**—van Kaathoven.

Molineus (Richardus). * De peripneumonia notha. 35 pp. 8°. *Berolini, formis Brüschckianis,* [1825].

Molinié (Étienne-Adolphe). * I. Étudier la toux dans ses rapports avec les maladies de la plèvre. II. [etc.] 38 pp. 4°. *Paris,* 1841, No. 3, v. 378.

Molinié (Eugène). * Quelques notions générales sur l'empyème ou pyothorax. 42 pp. 4°. *Paris,* 1862, No. 144.

Molinié (J.) * De quelques indications dans le traitement de la fièvre typhoïde et des principaux moyens de les remplir. 116 pp., 1 l. 4°. *Montpellier, Boehm & fils,* 1883, No. 43.

Molinié (Jean). * Sur le zona. 45 pp. 8°. *Paris, an XI* [1803], v. 30.

Molinié (Jérôme). * Du traitement de l'érysipèle. 50 pp. 4°. *Paris,* 1856, No. 284, v. 593.

Molinié (P.-A.) * Sur la fièvre gastrique ou bilieuse. 19 pp. 4°. *Strasbourg, Levrault,* 1814.

Molinie (Raymond). * De l'écrasement linéaire. 40 pp. 4°. *Paris,* 1866, No. 151.

Molinier (A.)
See **Oribasius.** Œuvres, etc. 2 v. 8°. *Paris,* 1873-6.

Molinier (Auguste). * Sur la nature, les causes et le traitement de l'ictère. 1 p. l., 35 pp. 4°. *Strasbourg,* 1858, No. 447, v. 25.

Molinier (Mars). * Sur le fongus villeux, ou angiome villeux de la vessie. 72 pp. 4°. *Paris,* 1870, No. 219.

Molinius (Antonius). De diversa hominum natura, prout a veteribus philosophis ex corporum speciebus reperta est, cognoscenda liber. 107 pp. 12°. *Lugduni, J. Tornœsius,* 1549.

Molison (Thomas). * Essay on inguinal and femoral hernia. 24 pp. 8°. *Edinburgh, P. Neill,* 1822. [P., v. 1271.]
——. Remarks on the epidemic disease called cholera, as it occurred in Newcastle. 40 pp. 8°. *Edinburgh, M'Lachlan & Stewart,* 1832. [*Also, in:* P., v. 110; 893; 1061.]

Molitg.
CALMON (B.) * Des eaux de Molitg et de leur action thérapeutique. 4°. *Montpellier,* 1877.

Molitor. Notes sur la fièvre typhoïde qui a régné dans la garnison de Bruxelles pendant le premier semestre 1871. 61 pp. 8°. [*Bruxelles, H. Manceaux,* 1871.]
Repr. from: Arch. méd. belg., Brux., 1872, 3. s., i.

Molitor (Balthasar). * De crusta lactea. 1 p. l., 50 pp., 1 l. 12°. *Budæ, typ. C. Landerer viduæ,* [1783].

Molitor (Eduard). * Die Behandlung des Fiebers bei Typhus und Pneumonie. [Erlangen.] 33 pp. 8°. *München,* [*C. Wolf u. Sohn*], 1875.

von Molitor (F.) Der Durchfall der Kinder und seine Behandlung vom ärztlichen praktischen Standpunkte aus nach eigenen Beobachtungen und Erfahrungen. 32 pp. 8°. *Breslau, E. Morgenstern,* 1861.

Molitor (Francis. Joseph.) & **Mayr de Zinenau** (Henr. Joan. Andr.) De febre continua maligna et intermittente tertiana utraque ad Rhenum an. mdcxxxiv et mdcxxxv, epidemica et castrensi. *Heidelberg,* 1736.
In: HALLER. Disp. ad morb. [etc.] 4°. *Lausennæ,* 1758, v, 263–273.

Molitor (*Joh.*) [1631–64].
Portrait in: **Collection**—van Kaathoven.—**Collection** of Portr. of Phys. & Men of Sc., 171.

Molitor (Joh. Horatius). Tractatus de thermis artificialibus septem mineralium planetarum, in quo propositis aliorum authorum thermis, nostrarum thermarum ingredientia ac virtutes, una cum modo generationis mineralium in terræ visceribus exponuntur, quæstiones celebres thermas nostras attingentes solvuntur, ac quomodo corpus ante usum illarum præparandum explicatur. 10 p. l., 72 pp., 23 l. 16°. *Jenæ, S. Krebs,* 1676.
Bound with: WEDELIUS (G. W.) Theoremata medica, etc. 16°. *Jenæ,* 1677.

Molk (Alfred-Louis-Conrad). Des tumeurs congénitales de l'extrémité inférieure du tronc. 116 pp., 3 pl. 4°. *Strasbourg, F.-H. Le Roux,* 1868.

Molk (Jean-Conrad). * Considérations sur les causes et sur le traitement des courbures de la colonne vertébrale. 1 p. l., 36 pp. 4°. *Strasbourg,* 1828, v. 57.

Molkenboer (Julianus Henricus). * De colocynthide. 3 p. l., 67 pp. 8°. *Lugd. Bat., J. W. van Leeuwen,* 1840.

Molkenkur-Anstalt (Die) auf dem Schlosse Schöneck bei Boppard am Rhein von Baron von Ehrenkreutz. 68 pp., 1 pl. 12°. *Koblenz, W. Blum,* 1848.

Molkentin (Rudolf). Ein Beitrag zur Sicherstellung der Diagnose des occulten Rotzes. 69 pp., 1 pl. 8°. *Leipzig, Dege,* 1883.
Being Hft. 2-3, of: VORTR. f. Thierärzte, 1883, 6. s.

Molkow (Henricus). * De intestino cæco. 31 pp. 8°. *Berolini, typ. Nietackianis,* [1836].

Moll (Albert). Experimentelle Untersuchungen über den anatomischen Zustand der Gelenke bei andauernder Immobilisation derselben. 1 p. l., 122 pp., 3 pl. 8°. *Berlin, H. S. Hermann*, 1885.

Moll (Anthonie Theodoor). *Over het empyeem en zijne behandeling langs operatieven weg met opvolgende injectieën van tinctur jodii. viii, 87 pp., 1 l. 8°. *Leiden, J. Hazenberg*, 1864.

Moll (Antonius) [1786–1843]. *Generalia quædam circa theoriam, sic dictam, incitationis. 2 p. l., 56 pp., 4 l. 8°. *Lugd. Bat., M. Cyfveer, J. fil.*, 1806. [*Also, in :* P., v. 1482; 1606.]

———. Gemeenzame brieven over het Scheveninger-zeebad ten nut te van lijders, half-lijders en niet-lijders. viii, 215 pp., 5 pl. 8°. *Arnhem, D. K. Muller*, 1824.

———. Leerboek der geregtelijke geneeskunde voor genees- en regtskundigen. 3 v. 8°. *Arnhem, D. K. Muller u. Comp.*, 1825–6.

———. Beknopte beschrijving van den aziatischen braakloop (cholera asiatica), in deszelfs verschijnselen, kenteekenen, oorzaken, onderscheidene vormen, en geneeskundige behandeling; inzonderheid ten nutte der heelmeesters ten platten lande. 10 pp., 1 l., 73 pp. 8°. *Arnhem, D. K. Muller u. Comp.*, 1832. [P., v. 182.]

Also, Co-Editor of : **Practisch** Tijdschrift voor de Geneeskunde in al haren Omvang, Gorinchem, 1822–43.

For Biography, see Nederl. Lancet, Utrecht, 1843–4, vi, 64. *Also:* Pract Tijdschr. v. de Geneesk., Gorinchem, 1843, xxii, pp. xvii–xxiii (opposite p. 768) (C. von Eldik).

Moll (Arminius). *De chloroformii inhalationibus in arte obstetricia adhibendis. 32 pp. 8°. *Berolini, G. Lange*, [1861].

Moll (August Cornelis Henric). *Over het ontstaan en de operatieve behandeling van epispadie. [Utrecht.] 59 pp., 1 pl. 8°. *Rotterdam, Nijgh & van Ditmar*, 1875.

Moll (Christiaan Hendrik). *Over vreemde lichhamen in de luchtwegen. 72 pp. 8°. *Amsterdam, de Brakke Groud*, 1885.

Moll (Christophorus Jacobus). *De diathesi fibro-plastica. 26 pp., 2 l. 8°. *Bonnæ, formis F. Kruegeri*, [1860].

Moll (Eugen). *Die Krankheiten der Bergarbeiter im Allgemeinen und der Oberschlesiens insbesondere. 39 pp. 8°. *Berlin, G. Lange*, [1869].

van Moll (Franciscus Daniel Agatha Catharina). *Over de normale incongruentie der netvliezen. 59 pp., 2 pl. 8°. *Utrecht, J. G. Broese*, 1874.

Moll (Fridericus Guilelmus). *Brevis veterum de hepate doctrinæ explicatio. 42 pp., 3 l. 8°. *Berolini, typ. Nietackianis*, [1837].

Moll (Jacobus Antonius). *Diss. continens quædam de anatomia et physiologia palpebrarum. 1 p. l., 134 pp., 1 l., 3 pl. 8°. *Traj. ad Rhenum, P. W. van de Weijer*, 1857. [*Also, in :* P., v. 1098.]

With second title, text in Dutch: Bijdragen tot de anatomie en physiologie der oogleden.

Moll (Joannes Guilielmus). *De apoplexia biliosa. 40 pp. 4°. *Gottingæ, J. C. Dieterich*, [1780].

Also, in : FRANK (J. P.) Delect. opusc. med. 8°. *Ticini*, 1790, ix, 187–233.

For Biography, see **Richter** (Augustus Gottlieb.)

Moll (Joannes Petrus). *Diss. sistens sciagraphiam phthiseos nosologicam. 24 pp. 4°. *Tubingæ, typ. Reissianis*, [1789].

Moll (Joh. Christoph Albert). *Ueber den Sehnenschnitt. 42 pp. 12°. *Tübingen, L. F. Fues*, 1841.

Mollan (*John*) [1791–1877].

Obituary. Med. Press, Lond., 1877, n. s., xxiii, 269.

Molland. Catalogue de livres de médecine et de littérature composant la bibliothèque de M . . . 16 pp. 8°. *Paris, J.-B. Baillière & fils*, 1880.

Molland (J.-L.-Émile). *Epidémie typhoïde à l'hôpital Sainte-Eugénie (enfants malades pendant l'année 1857). 70 pp. 4°. *Paris*, 1859, No. 126, v. 634.

Mollard (Charles-Louis). *Sur l'hygiène des femmes enceintes. vi, 7–37 pp. 4°. *Paris*, 1815, No. 158, v. 112, 113.

Molle. *Sur l'inflammation essentielle de poitrine, ou péripneumonie. 21 pp. 4°. *Paris, an XII* [1804], No. 240, v. 49.

Møller (A. P.) Sundhedsvæsenets Ordning ved den danske Hær paa Garnisonsfod. Systematisk fremstillet efter de gjældende Forskrifter. xiii pp., 1 l., 287 pp. 8°. *Nyborg, V. Schønemann*, 1883.

Moller (Carolus Otto). *De divino in medicina. 32 pp. 4°. [*Altdorfii*], lit. H. Meyeri, [1695].

For Portrait, see **Collection**—van Kaathoven.—**Collection** of Portr. of Phys. & Men of Sc., 116.

Moller (Fridericus). *De colica. 7 l. sm. 4°. *Wittebergæ, C. Tham*, [1625].

Moller (Goddofredus). *De aëre fodinarum metallicarum noxio. Von unterirrdischen bösen Wetter. 52 pp. sm. 4°. *Halæ Magdeb., typ. J. C. Hendelii*, [1730]. [*Also, in :* P., v. 1386.]

Moller (Jacobus). Discursus de cornutis et hermaphroditis eorumque jure. 3. ed. 4 p. l., 211 pp., 2 l. 4°. *Berolini, J. G. Meyer*, 1708.

Moller (Joannes Fridericus). *De vera Peruviani corticis vi specifica. 34 pp. sm. 4°. *Goettingæ, lit. Barmeierianis*, [1768].

Møller (Joh. Eberhard). *Nogle anatomiske Jagttagelser. 7 pp. 12°. *Kjøbenhavn, J. R. Thiele*, [1776].

———. Beobachtungen vom Nutzen des Lein-Oels bey hartnäckigten Leibesverstopfungen. 7 pp. 8°. *Kopenhagen, J. R. Thiele*, [1778].

———. Bemerkung von Verletzung der vordern Schienbein-Pulsader. 7 pp. sm. 8°. *Kopenhagen, J. R. Thiele*, [1779].

Møller (Ove Ludvig). Gastrotomien. 1 p. l., 265 pp., 1 l. 8°. *Kjøbenhavn, Ursins Efterfølgers*, 1880.

Moller (Peter). Der Dorschleberthran und seine Zubereitung, nebst Angabe einer neuen Methode zur Gewinnung des reinen Medicinthrans. 24 pp. 8°. *Christiania, Brøgger u. Christie*, 1862.

Mollet (J.-M.) *Sur les signes diagnostiques des différentes tumeurs du scrotum. 58 pp. 8°. *Paris, an XI* [1803], v. 24. [*Also, in :* P., v. 769.]

Molleveaux (S.-V.) *Sur la coqueluche. 19 pp. 4°. *Paris*, 1831, No. 227, v. 244.

Mollheim (Ludovicus). *De noma seu stomatomalacia, adjecto morbi casu iterata applicatione ferri candentis sanato. 31 pp. 8°. *Berolini, typ. Nietackianis*, [1837].

Mollien (Auguste). *Accidents de l'uréthrotomie interne; indications et contre-indications de cette opération. 41 pp. 4°. *Paris*, 1867, No. 103.

Mollien (Charles). *De la pupille artificielle. 48 pp. 4°. *Paris*, 1862, No. 70.

Mollien (E.-L.-Z.) *Sur l'amaurose. 23 pp. 4°. *Paris*, 1827, No. 5, v. 204.

Mollière (Daniel). *Du nerf dentaire inférieur, anatomie et physiologie. Anatomie comparée. 86 pp. 4°. *Paris*, 1871, No. 132.

———. Recherches expérimentales et cliniques sur les fractures indirectes de la colonne vertébrale. 40 pp. 8°. *Lyon, A. Vingtrinier*, 1872.

Repr. from : Lyon méd., 1872, x.

———. Nuevos inconvenientes de la taxis forzada. Traducida por J. Casademunt. 15 pp. 8°. *Barcelona, J. Miret*, [1874, *vel subseq.*].

———. Note sur un cas de régénération osseuse. 8 pp. 8°. *Paris, J.-B. Baillière*, 1876.

———. Traité des maladies du rectum et de l'anus. xxiv, 758 pp. 8°. *Paris, G. Masson*, 1877.

Mollière (Humbert). Étude sur le vomissement dans les maladies chroniques du cerveau (paralysie générale et tumeurs). 16 pp. 8°. *Lyon, A. Vingtrinier,* 1874.

——. Recherches cliniques sur la nosographie du purpura hæmorrhagica et des affections pétéchiales. 32 pp. 8°. *Lyon, A. Vingtrinier,* 1874.
Repr. from: Lyon méd., 1873, xiv.

——. Études cliniques sur la physiologie pathologique de l'ictère grave. 24 pp. 8°. *Paris, A. Delahaye,* 1875.
Repr. from: Lyon méd., 1875, xviii.

——. Anévrysme de l'aorte pectorale traité par la galvano-puncture (mono-puncture positive); mort par déchirure interne du sac. Étude du mode de formation des caillots. 15 pp., 1 tab. 8°. *Lyon, T. Giraud,* 1882.

——. Sur un cas de phthisie consécutive à une hémoptysie (phthisis ab hemoptoe). Interprétation du phénomène. Communication faite à la Société des sciences médicales de Lyon. 14 pp., 1 tab. 8°. *Lyon, T. Giraud,* 1882.

——. Étude d'histoire médicale. Un précurseur Lyonnais des théories microbiennes. J.-B. Goiffon et la nature animée de la peste. 2 p. l., 152 pp., 1 pl. 8°. *Bâle, H. Georg,* [1886].

Molliet (Virgile) [1853–]. *De l'intoxication chronique par l'oxyde de carbone. 38 pp., 1 l. 4°. *Paris,* 1882, No. 1.

Mollin.
See Skin (*Diseases of, Treatment of*).

Mollina.
Perez (E. G.) Aguas minero-medicinales de la Capuchina. Anfiteatro anat., Madrid, 1873, i, 31.

Mollis.
See Fever (*Typhus, History, etc., of*), *by localities.*

Mollison (Patrick). A description of the pulmonic pulse. 2 pp. 8°. [*London,* 1837.]
Repr. from: Brit. Ann. Med., Pharm., etc., Lond., 1837, i.

Mollities *ossium.*
See Bones (*Softening of*).

Molloy (A.-C.-J.) *I. De la disposition des aponévroses de la main. II. [etc.] 49 pp. 4°. *Paris,* 1840, No. 226, v. 363.

Mollusca.
See, also, Fish (*Poisonous*); Liver (*Comparative anatomy of*); Mussels; Snails (*Poisonous*).

Adams (A.) & **Reeve** (L.) The zoology of the voyage of H. M. S. Samarang, under the command of Sir Edward Belcher, during the years 1843–46. Mollusca. Edited by Arthur Adams. 4°. *London,* 1848.

Albers (J. C.) Die Heliceen nach natürlicher Verwandtschaft systematisch geordnet. Zweite Ausgabe nach dem hinterlassenen Manuskript besorgt von Eduard von Martens. 8°. *Leipzig,* 1860.

Batelli (A.) Studio istologico degli organi sessuali complementari in alcuni molluschi terrestri. 8°. [*Pisa?* 1880.]
Cutting from: Atti Soc. tos. sc. nat., 1879, iv, 203–225, 1 pl.

Boll (F.) Beiträge zur vergleichenden Histologie des Molluskentypus. 8°. *Bonn,* 1869.

Cuvier (*Le baron*). Considérations sur les mollusques et en particulier sur les céphalopodes. 8°. [*Paris,* 1830.]
Repr. from: Ann. d. sc. nat., Par., 1830.

Dumortier (B.-C.) Mémoire sur les évolutions de l'embryon dans les mollusques gastéropodes. Lu à la séance du 8 mai 1835. · v. 10. 4°. [*n. p.,* 1835.]

Gill (T. N.) Arrangement of the families of mollusks. Prepared for the Smithsonian Institution. 8°. *Washington,* 1871.

24

Mollusca.
Grant (R. E.) On the existence and uses of ciliæ in the young of the gasteropodous mollusca, and on the causes of the spiral turn of univalve shells. 8°. [*Edinburgh,* 1827.]
Repr. from: Edinb. J. Sc., 1827, vii. *Also, transl. in:* Notiz. a. d. Geb. d. Nat.- u. Heilk., Weimar, 1827, xviii, 305–309. *Also, transl. in:* Ztschr. f. d. organ. Phys., Eisenach, 1827, i, 263–268.

Guiscardi (G.) Un genere di molluschi della famiglia delle neritide. . fol. [*Napoli,* 1856.]

Hogg (J.) The lingual membrane of mollusca, and its value in classification. 8°. [*London,* 1868.]

Keber (G. A. F.) *De nervis concharum. 8°. *Berolini,* [1837].

Köhler (H. J.) *Aristoteles de molluscis cephalopodibus (περὶ τῶν μαλακίων). 8°. *Dorpati,* 1820.

Kost (H.) *Ueber die Structur und chemische Zusammensetzung einiger Muschelschalen. 8°. *Hildburghausen,* 1853.

Lubbock (J.) On some Oceanic entomostraca collected by Captain Toynbee. 4°. [*n. p., n. d.*]
Repr. from: Tr. Linnean Soc. Lond., xxiii.

Ozenne (C.-M.-L.) *Essai sur les mollusques considérés comme aliments, médicaments et poisons. 4°. *Paris,* 1858.

Reincke (J.) Beiträge zur Bildungsgeschichte der Stacheln, etc., im Mantelrande der Chitonen. 8°. [*Leipzig,* 1868.]
Repr. from: Ztschr. f. wissensch. Zool., Leipz., 1868, xviii.

Roth (J. R.) *Molluscorum species, quas in itinere per Orientem facto, comites clarissimi Schuberti doctores M. Erdl et J. R. Roth collegerunt. Recensuit . . . sm. 4°. *Monachii,* 1839.

Schenk (A.) . * Diagnoses molluscorum terrestrium et fluviatilium circa Monachium indigenorum. 8°. *Monachii,* 1838.

Schlemm (T. F. G.) *De hepate ac bile crustaceorum et molluscorum quorundam. 4°. *Berolini,* [1844].

Todaro (F.) Sui primi fenomeni dello sviluppo delle salpe. 2ª comunicazione preliminare. 4°. *Roma,* 1882.
Repr. from: Atti d. r. Accad. d. Lincei. Cl. di sc. fis., matemat. e nat., Roma, 1882, 3. s., vi.

Treviranus (G. R.) Ueber die Zeugungstheile und die Fortpflanzung der Mollusken. 4°. [*n. p., n. d.*]
See, also, infra.

Woodward (S. P.) A manual of the mollusca. 2. ed. With an appendix of recent and fossil conchological discoveries to the present time, by R. Tate. With numerous illustrations by A. N. Waterhouse and T. W. Lowry. 12°. *London,* 1868.

Yarrow (H. C.) Report upon the collection of terrestrial and fluviatile mollusca made in portions of Colorado, Utah, New Mexico, and Arizona, during the years 1872, 1873, and 1874.
In: Rep. Exp. for Expl. west of 100. Meridian (Wheeler), v. Zoology. 4°. *Washington,* 1875.

Blanchard (R.) Note sur la présence des muscles striés chez les mollusques acéphales monomyaires. Compt. rend. Soc. de biol. 1880, Par., 1881, 7. s., ii, 133–135.—**Bonnet** (R.) Der Bau und die Circulationsverhältnisse der Acephalenkeime. Morphol. Jahrb., Leipz., 1877, iii, 283–327, 3 pl.—**Bourne** (A. G.) On the supposed communication of the vascular system with the exterior in pleurobranchus. Quart. J. Micr. Sc., Lond., 1885, n. s., xxv, 429–432, 1 pl.—**Bouvier** (E.-L.) La loi des connexions appliquée à la morphologie des organes des mollusques et particulièrement de l'ampullaire. Compt. rend. Acad. d. sc., Par., 1886, ciii, 162–165. ——. Sur le système nerveux typique des prosobranches dextres ou sénestres. *Ibid.*, 1274–1276.—**Brooks** (W. K.) Observations upon the early stages in the development of the fresh-water pulmonates. Johns Hopkins Univ. Stud. biol. lab. 1878-9, Balt., 1880, i, pt. 2, 73–104, 4 pl. ——. The anatomy and

Mollusca.

development of the Salpa-chain. *Ibid.*, 1884–6, Balt., 1887, iii, 451–475, 2 pl.—**Bütschli** (O.) Bemerkungen über die wahrscheinliche Herleitung der Asymmetrie der Gastropoden, spec. der Asymmetrie im Nervensystem der Prosobranchiaten. Morphol. Jahrb., Leipz., 1886–7, xii, 202–222, 2 pl.—**Carrière** (J.) Die Fussdrüsen der Prosobranchier und das Wassergefäss-System der Lamellibranchier und Gastropoden. Arch. f. mikr. Anat., Bonn, 1881–2, xx, 387–467, 3 pl.—**Clessin** (S.) Ueber Missbildungen der Mollusken und ihrer Gehäuse. Ber. d. naturh. Ver. in Augsburg, 1873, xxii, 21–107.—**Flemming** (W.) Untersuchungen über Sinnesepithelien der Mollusken. Arch. f. mikr. Anat., Bonn, 1870, vi, 439–471. ———. Ueber Organe vom Bau der Geschmacksknospen an den Tastern verschiedener Mollusken. *Ibid.*, 1884, xxiii, 141–148, 1 pl.—**Fournier** (E.) Mémoire sur la composition chimique des mollusques considérée dans ses rapports avec leur emploi médical. Monit. d. sc. méd. et pharm., Par., 1859, vii, 274; 283; 291.—**Fredericq** (L.) Sur l'organisation et la physiologie du poulpe. Bull. Acad. roy. d. sc. de Belg., Brux., 1878, 2. s., xlvi, 710–765. [Rap. de É. Van Beneden], 588–596. — **Garnault** (P.) Sur la glande à concrétions du Cyclostoma elegans. Compt. rend. Acad. d. sc., Par., 1887, civ, 708.—**Goodsir** (J.) On an undescribed form of gasteropod mollusk from the Firth of Forth. *In his:* Anat. Mem., 8°, Edinb., 1868, i, 420–424.—**Gray** (J. E.) A natural arrangement of mollusca, according to their internal structure. Lond. M. Reposit., 1821, xv, 229–239.—**Haller** (B.) Untersuchungen über marine Rhipidoglossen; erste Studie. Morphol. Jahrb., Leipz., 1883, ix, 1–98, 7 pl.—**von Ihering** (H.) Die Gehörwerkzeuge der Mollusken in ihrer Bedeutung für das natürliche System derselben. Sitzungsb. d. phys.-med. Soc. zu Erlang., 1876–7, 9. Hft., 35–65. *Also*, Reprint.—**Jobert.** Recherches sur le byssus des mollusques bivalves. Compt. rend. Soc. de biol. Par., 1882, 7. s., iv, 75–77.—**Jousset de Bellesme.** Recherches sur la digestion chez les mollusques céphalopodes. Compt. rend. Acad. d. sc., Par., 1879, lxxxviii, 428.—**Lankester** (E. R.) Contributions to the developmental history of the mollusca. Phil. Tr. 1875, Lond., 1876, clvi, 1–48, 12 pl.—**Livon** (C.) Recherches sur la structure des organes digestifs des poulpes. J. de l'anat. et physiol., etc., Par., 1881, xvii, 97–122, 3 pl.—**M'Intosh** (W. C.) On the nudibranchiate mollusca of St. Andrews, Edwardsia, and the polyps of Alcyonium digitatum. Proc. Roy. Soc. Edinb., 1862–6, v, 387–395. *Also*, Reprint.—**McMurrich** (J. P.) A contribution to the embryology of the prosobranch gasteropods. Johns Hopkins Univ. Stud. biol. lab., Balt., 1884–7, iii, 403–450, 4 pl.—**Owsjannikow** (P.) Histologische Studien über das Nervensystem der Mollusken; vorläufige Mittheilung. Mélanges biol. Acad. imp. d. sc. de St.-Pétersb., 1871, vii, 679–685.—**Rabl** (C.) Ueber die Entwicklung der Tellerschnecke. Morphol. Jahrb., Leipz., 1879, v, 562–660, 7 pl. ———. Beiträge zur Entwicklungsgeschichte der Prosobranchier. Sitzungsb. d. k. Akad. d. Wissensch. Math.-naturw. Cl., Wien, 1883, lxxxvii. 3. Abth., 45–60, 2 pl. — **Robin** (C.) Rapport à la Société de biologie, par la commission chargée d'examiner les communications de M. Souleyet, relatives à la question désignée sous le nom de phlébentérisme. Compt. rend. Soc. de biol. 1851, Par., 1852, iii, pt. 2, 5–132. *Also*, Reprint.— **Roule** (L.) Recherches histologiques sur les mollusques lamellibranches. J. de l'anat. et physiol., etc. Par., 1887, xxiii, 31–86, 5 pl.—**Schönn.** Untersuchung der Gewebe der Mollusken in polarisirtem Lichte. Jenaische Ztschr. f. Med. u. Naturw., Leipz., 1866, ii, 54–60.—**Steenstrup** (J.) Orientering i de Ommatostrephagtige Blæksprutters indbyrdes Forhold. Overs. o. d. k. Danske Vidensk. Selsk. Forh., Kjøbenh., 1880, 73–110, 1 pl.—**Treviranus** (G.-R.) Sur les organes génitaux et la génération des mollusques. J. compl. du dict. d. sc. méd., Par., 1825, xxi, 202; 307. [*See, also, supra.*]—**Triuchese** (S.) Véritable rein diffus chez quelques mollusques. [*Transl. from:* Rendic. r. Accad. d. sc. di Napoli.] Arch. ital. de biol., Turin, 1883, iv, 18–20.—**Vialleton** (L.) Sur l'innervation du manteau de quelques mollusques lamellibranches. Compt. rend. Acad. d. sc., Par., 1882, xcv, 461–463.—**Vignal** (W.) Structure de système nerveux des mollusques. *Ibid.*, 249–251.—**Warlomont** (R.) Étude de quelques points de la structure des firoles. J. de l'anat. et physiol., etc., Par., 1886, xxii, 331–350, 1 pl.—**Yung** (E.) De l'innervation du cœur et de l'action des poisons chez les mollusques lamellibranches. Compt. rend. Acad. d. sc., Par., 1881, xciii, 562–564.

Molluscoida.

Nitsche (H.) Beiträge zur Kenntniss der Bryozoen. Neue Folge. Habilitationsschrift. 8°. *Leipzig*, 1871.

Repr. from: Ztschr. f. wissensch. Zool, xxi.

Haddon (A. C.) On budding in polyzoa. Quart. J. Micr. Sc., Lond., 1883, n. s., xxiii, 516–555, 2 pl.—**Nitsche** (H.) On some interesting points concerning the mode of reproduction of the bryozoa. *Ibid.*, 1871, n. s., xi, 155–162.

Molluscum.

Babry (M.) * Étude clinique sur le molluscum pendulum. [Paris.] 4°. *Le Mans*, 1885.

Boudet (E.) Contribution à l'étude du fibroma molluscum. 4°. *Paris*, 1883.

Diaz de Bedoya (J.) * Du molluscum. 4°. *Paris*, 1856.

Faber (C. F.) * Die Hautkrankheit Molluscum. 8°. *Tübingen*, 1840.

Hürtile (K.) * Beiträge zur Kenntniss des Fibroma molluscum und der congenitalen Elephantiasis. [Tübingen.] 8°. *Jena*, 1886.

Jacobovics (M.-M.) Du molluscum; recherches critiques sur les formes, la nature et le traitement des affections cutanées de ce nom, suivies de la description détaillée d'une nouvelle variété. 8°. *Paris*, 1840.

Kittmann (R.) * Ueber das multiple Fibroma molluscum. 8°. *Würzburg*, 1884.

Lerefait (A.) * Contribution à l'étude des aberrations morphologiques des néoplasies et notamment du fibrome molluscum. 4°. *Paris*, 1885.

Morse (E. S.) Note on the extension of the coiled arms in rhynchonella. 8°. [*New Haven*, 1878.]

Also [Abstr.], *in:* Am. J. Sc. & Arts, N. Haven, 1879, 3. s., xvii, 257.

Müller (E.) * Ueber einen Fall von multiplen Fibromata mollusca und artificieller Elephantiasis arabum. 8°. *Würzburg*, [1882].

Philipp (H.) * Multiple sarcomatöse Geschwülste in der Haut (Sarcoma molluscum). 8°. *Berlin*, 1886.

Podlewski (O.) * Ein Beitrag zur Casuistik der Fibroma molluscum. 8°. *Berlin*, [1886].

Weissenborn (J. T.) * De exanthemate mollusco. 4°. *Lipsiæ*, [1829].

Allen (C. W.) Molluscum contagiosum; an analysis of fifty cases. J. Cutan. & Ven. Dis., N. Y., 1886, iv, 238–243. *Also*, Reprint *Also, transl.:* France méd., Par., 1886, ii, 1325–1330.—**Alvarenga** (P. F. C.) Molluscum. J. Soc. d. sc. med. de Lisb., 1853, 2. s., xiii, 48–50.—**Anderson** (I. W.) On molluscum simplex. J. Cutan. M., Lond., 1867–8, i, 60–63, 1 pl.—**Atkinson** (J. E.) Observations upon two cases of fibroma molluscum. N. York M. J., 1875, xxii, 601–610.—**Atlee** (W. L.) Case of molluscum, associated with fibro-cellular encysted tumour and encephaloid disease. Am. J. M. Sc., Phila., 1844, n. s., vii, 296–306.—**Barduzzi** (D.) Mollusco fibroso. Gior. ital. d. mal. ven., Milano, 1876, xi, 321–337.—**Beale** (L.) Molluscum. Tr. Path. Soc. Lond., 1854–5, vi, 313–316, 1 pl.—**Bergh** (R.) Tilfælde af Knudesot (Molluscosis fibrosa). Hosp.-Tid., Kjøbenh., 1876, 2. R., iii, 225; 241; 257.—**Bird** (W.) An instance of molluscum in a child of eight years, confined to the right side of the body. Lancet, Lond., 1863, ii, 248.—**Bourneville.** † Bull. Soc. anat. de Par., 1873, xlviii, 487.—**Bowman.** Molluscum tubercles removed by operation. Lancet, Lond., 1855, i, 289. ———. † Med. Chron., Montreal, 1857–8, v, 521–524.—**Brigham** (C. B.) A rare form of congenital cystic fibroma molluscum of the elbow; removal by operation; successful result. Tr. M. Soc. Calif., Sacramento, 1875, v, 67–69.—**Caillault** (C.) Recherches sur deux variétés assez rares d'acné décrites sous les noms de molluscum contagiosum et molluscum pendulum. Arch. gén. de méd., Par., 1851, 4. s., xxvii, 46; 316. *Also*, Reprint.—**Campana** (R.) Sui globi del mollusco contagioso. Gior. ital. d. mal. ven., Milano, 1886, xxi, 37–42. *Also*, Reprint.—**Candela** (P.) Molluscum péndulum generalizado. Rev. esp. de oftal., sif., etc., Madrid, 1879–80, iii, pt. 2, 116–1 8, 1 pl.—**Carrier** (A. E.) Clinical lecture. Fibroma, or molluscum fibrosum. Detroit Clinic, 1882, i, 42–45.—**Cuzenave** (A.) Du molluscum. [A propos de l'acné varioliforme de M. Bazin et d'une note communiquée par M. Caillault, sur une maladie analogue qui a été observée à l'hôpital des Enfants-Malades.] Ann. d. mal. de la peau, etc., Par., 1850–51, iii, 225–241.—**Cervera** (E.) Un caso notable de molluscum fibroso. Rev. esp. de oftal., sif., etc., Madrid, 1883–4, vii, pt. 1, 434–438.—**Challand.** Énumération des diverses affections décrites sous le nom générique de molluscum. [Rap. de Mallassez.] Bull. Soc. anat. de Par. (1871), 1873, xlvi, 151–157.—**Chassaignac.** Molluscum éléphantiasique. Bull. Soc. de chir. de Par. (1866), 1867, 2. s., vii, 194.—**Chausit.** Nature et traitement du molluscum. Monit. d. hôp., Par., 1855, iii, 417–419.—**Clark** (F. W.) A remarkable case of fibroma molluscum. Lancet, Lond., 1887, i, 1183.—**Córdova** (F.) Observacion de

Molluscum.

un caso de molluscum. Crón. méd.-quir. de la Habana, 1876, ii, 76–78.—**Corvisart** (L.) Tumeurs multiples de la peau (molluscum). Compt. rend. Soc. de biol. 1849, Par., 1850, i, pt. 2, 28.—**Craigie** (D.) Account of an instance of molluscum chronicum. Edinb. M. & S. J., 1851, lxxv, 105–120, 1 pl.—**Cruyl** (L.) Molluscum fibrosum congénital, observé à la clinique dermatologique de M. le Prof. E. Poirier. (Mémoire couronné au concours entre les élèves de la Faculté de médecine, 1881–2.) Ann. Soc. de méd. de Gand, 1883, lxi, 43–67.—**Decaisne** (G.) Molluscum adipeux. Bull. Soc. anat. de Par., 1876, li, 363. *Also:* Progrès méd., Par., 1876, iv, 661.—**Dick** (W.) A few remarks on molluscum, with two cases of molluscum non-contagiosum. Lond. M. Gaz., 1836–7, xix, 860–863.—**Dubois** (V.) Molluscum pendulum volumineux de la cuisse; ablation. Presse méd. belge, Brux., 1879, xxxi, 361.—**Dubois-Havenith.** Un cas de "molluscum contagiosum" communiqué par un nourrisson à sa mère. J. de méd., chir. et pharmacol., Brux., 1887, lxxxiv, 139–141.—**Dunglison** (R.) Molluscum. Cycl. Pract. M. (Tweedie), Phila., 1845, iii, 332.—**Engel** (J.) Anatomische Untersuchung eines Falles von Molluskum. Wien. med. Wchnschr., 1865, xv, 1485; 1501.—**Fagge** (C. H.) On the anatomy of a case of molluscum fibrosum. Med.-Chir. Tr., Lond., 1869–70, liii, 217–232, 1 pl. *Also* [Abstr.]: Proc. Roy. M. & Chir. Soc. Lond., 1871–4, vi, 298.—**Fourestié** (H.) Fibrômes molluscoïdes multiples. Union méd., Par., 1876, 3. s., xix, 226–228.—**Fowler** (C.) A case of molluscum. Tr. Prov. M. & S. Ass. 1838, Lond., 1839, vii, 364–371, 1 pl.—**Fremmert** (H.) Ueber Fibroma molluscum. St. Petersb. med. Ztschr., 1872–3, n. F., iii, 197–219, 1 pl.—**G.** (L.) Molluscum pendulum. Rev. phot. d. hôp. de Par., 1869, i, 61–64, 1 pl.—**Gamberini** (P.) Sul mollusco. Bull. d. sc. med. di Bologna, 1852, 3. s., xxi, 172–189. ———. Fibroma mollusco Virchow. Gior. ital. d. mal. ven., Milano, 1879, xiv, 103.—**García Duarte** (E.) Del molluscum; historia de un caso observado en la clínica . . . ¿ Podría aproximarse al grupo de las leproides? Prensa méd. de Granada, 1881, iii, 560; 577. *Also:* Rev. esp. de oftal., sif., etc., Madrid, 1881–2, v, pt. 2, 84–96.—**Geber** (E.) Az epithelioma molluscum (Virchow) universale esete különös tekintettel e bántalom lényegére. Orvosi hetil., Budapest, 1882, xxvi, 673; 701; 732, 1 pl. *Also, transl.:* Vrtljschr. f. Dermat., Wien, 1882, ix, 403–430, 1 pl. *Also, transl.:* Pest. med.-chir. Presse, Budapest, 1882, xviii, 685; 703.—**Gibert.** Quelques remarques sur la maladie tuberculeuse de la peau, désignée par Bateman sous le nom de molluscum, accompagnée d'une observation de molluscum sporadique. Rev. méd. franç. et étrang., Par., 1843, i, 5–13.—**Guéneau de Mussy.** Exposé des lésions anatomiques dans un cas de cette maladie rare de la peau décrite sous le nom de molluscum. Gaz. d. hôp., Par., 1831–2, v, 157.—**Hallin** (O. F.) †† Fall af Fibroma molluscum multiplex. Hygiea, Stockholm, 1871, xxxiii, 369–374.—**Hamlin** (A. C.) Case of molluscum fibrosum. Rep. Superv. Surg.-Gen. Mar. Hosp., Wash., 1882, 171, 1 pl. ———. A case of molluscum. *Ibid.,* 1883, 137.—**Hardy** (A.) Deux cas de molluscum; traitement par les onctions avec l'huile de cade. Gaz. d. hôp., Par., 1853, xxvi, 291. ———. Molluscum. N. dict. de méd. et chir. prat., Par., 1877, xxiii, 2–6.—**Hasse** (C. E.) † Deutsche Klinik, Berl., 1855, vii, 324.—**Hebra** (H.) Molluscum sebaceum. Aerztl. Ber. d. k. k. allg. Krankenh. zu Wien (1872), 1873, 298. ———. Molluscum fibrosum. *Ibid.* (1873), 1874, 206–208.—**Hopkins** (G. G.) Report of a case of molluscum fibrosum. Tr. M. Soc. N. Y., Syracuse, 1882, 328–331.—**Hyde** (J. N.) On a case of molluscum verrucosum, presenting certain unusual features. Edinb. M. J., 1879–80, xxv, 687–702, 2 pl. *Also,* Reprint.—**Jüngken** (J. C.) Molluscum simplex, durch Exstirpation geheilt. Deutsche Klinik, Berl., 1856, iii, 447–449.—**Juler** (C.) On molluscum fibrosum. Clinic, Cincin., 1873, v, 185–188.—**Kosiński.** Olbrzymiej wielkosci włókniak (fibroma molluscum); operacya; wyzdrowienie. [On nates; operation; recovery.] Pam. Towarz. Lek. Warszaw., 1873, lxix, 435–443.—**Lediard** (H. A.) Molluscum fibrosum and large pendulous fibroma; removal of growth; recovery. Lancet, Lond., 1887, ii, 62.—**Lehmann.** Fall der unter dem Namen Molluscum bekannten seltenen Hautkrankheit. Schweiz. Ztschr. f. Med., Chir. u. Geburtsh., Zürich, 1853, 334–336.—**McGarry** (J.) Molluscum; supposed cirrhosis. Med. Chron., Montreal, 1857–8, v, 238.—**M'Leod** (K.) Case of molluscum. Edinb. M. J., 1880–81, xxvi, 405–407, 1 pl.—**Malassez.** Observation d'un cas de molluscum pendulum; examen microscopique; réflexions sur le molluscum en général. Bull. Soc. anat. de Par. (1871), 1873, xlvi, 25–31, 1 pl.—**Marcacci** (G.) Di un raro esempio di fibroma-mollusco; storia e commenti. Gior. ital. d. mal. ven., Milano, 1879, xiv, 193–200. ———. Il fibroma mollusco e l' elefantiasi. Sperimentale, Firenze, 1879, xliv, 488–494.—**Michel.** Molluscum. Dict. encycl. d. sc. méd., Par., 1875, 2. s., ix, 87–102.—**Michel** (M.) Case of fibroma molluscum. Am. J. M. Sc., Phila., 1875, n. s., lxix, 124–131.—**Milner** (J. C.) Case of fibroma molluscum. J. Cutan. & Ven. Dis., N. Y., 1884, ii, 178.—**Mittendorf** (W. F.) Two epidemics of molluscum contagiosum. Tr. Am. Ophth. Soc., Bost., 1886, iv, pt. 2, 262–264.—**Modrzejewski** (E.) Wieloliczne, wrodzone włó-

Molluscum.

kniaki miękkie, tak zwane mięczaki nerwowłókniaki Recklinghausen 'a. [Case of multiform congenital fibroma molluscum.] Gaz. lek., Warszawa, 1882, 2. s., ii, 380; 406, 1 phot. *Also, transl.:* Berl. klin. Wchnschr., 1882, xix, 627–631. *Also, transl.:* Gaz. hebd. de méd., Par , 1882, 2. s., xix, 508–511.—**Mollusco** contagioso al dorso delle mani e alla faccia; estirpazione e cauterizzazione potenziale; guarigione. Clin. chir. (Mazzoni), Roma, 1884, viii–x, 275.—**Moore** (C. F.) Molluscum fibrosum seu simplex. Brit. M. J., Lond., 1885, ii, 739.—**Murchison** [C.] Specimen of skin affected with molluscum and the eruption of typhus. Tr. Path. Soc. Lond., 1862–3, xiv, 278.—**Murray** (J.) Three peculiar cases of molluscum fibrosum in children in which one or more of the following conditions were observed: Hypertrophy of the gums; enlargement of the ends of the fingers and toes; numerous connective-tissue tumours on the scalp and other parts of the surface of the body, with various superficial affections of the skin. Med.-Chir. Tr., Lond., 1872–3, lvi, 235–253, 1 pl. *Also* [Abstr.]: Proc. Roy. M. & Chir. Soc. Lond., 1871–5, vii, 146–148.—**Nagumowitsch** (L.) Ueber Molluscum simplex. Med. Ztg. Russlands, St. Petersb., 1844, i, 173.—**Nebel** (H.) Case of molluscum chronicum. Edinb. M. & S. J., 1852, lxxvii, 23–28.—**Nélaton.** Molluscum éléphantiasique; énorme tumeur, en forme de manteau, recouvrant les deux tiers du tronc; déformations du squelette; troubles dans les fonctions circulatoires, respiratoires et digestives; opération; autopsie; hypertrophie du derme et du tissu cellulaire sous-dermique; courbures anormales de la colonne vertébrale; lésions diverses des organes. Gaz. d. hôp., Par., 1865, xxxviii, 65; 70; 87; 98. *Also, transl.:* Wien. med. Wchnschr., 1865, xv, 354; 373; 389.—**Neret.** Observation sur le molluscum. Arch. gén. de méd., Par., 1845, 4. s., viii, 463–466.—**Octerlony** (J. A.) A case of molluscum simplex, with illustrations. Arch. Dermat., N. Y., 1874–5, i, 300–304. *Also,* Reprint.—**Ory** (E.) Molluscum pendulum généralisé. Bull. Soc. anat. de Par., 1875, l, 789.—**Parrish** (J.) Case of molluscum associated with encephaloid disease. N. Jersey M. Reporter, Burlington, 1852–3, vi, 417–421, 1 pl.—**Payne** (J. F.) Molluscum fibrosum and multiple fibro-neuromata. Brit. M. J., Lond., 1887, i, 1098.—**Philippson.** Molluscum fibrosum. Prakt. Arzt, Wetzlar, 1880, xxi, 244.—**Pick** (F. J.) Ueber das Molluscum. Wien. med. Wchnschr., 1865, xv, 900–905.—**Pollock** (G. D.) Report of a case of molluscum fibrosum, or fibroma; with observations. Med.-Chir. Tr., Lond., 1872–3, lvi, 255–266, 1 pl. *Also* [Abstr.]: Proc. Roy. M. & Chir. Soc. Lond., 1871–5, vii, 148–150. ———. Molluscum fibrosum. Tr. Path. Soc. Lond., 1874–5, xxvi, 219, 1 pl.—**Porcher** (F. P.) Case of molluscum fibrosum; tubercles of an unusual size. Am. J. M. Sc., Phila., 1878, n. s., lxxv, 145.—**Posadsky.** Fibroma molluscum multiplex congenitum. Arch. f. path. Anat., etc., Berl., lxxxvii, 380–382.—**Profeta** (G.) Mollusco fibroso. *In his:* Decennio di clin. dermo-sifil. di Palermo, 8°, 1878, 63–65, 1 pl.—**Purdon** (H. S.) On molluscum sebaceum. J. Cutan. M., Lond., 1867–8, i, 53.—**Purser.** Molluscum simplex. Dublin Q. J. M. Sc., 1871, lii, 221.—**Reclus** (P.) Molluscums fibreux et syphilomes de la région ano-rectale. Arch. gén. de méd., Par., 1885, 7. s., xvi, 271–282. ———. Du molluscum fibreux de la région ano-rectale. Gaz. d. hôp., Par., 1887, lx, 889.—**Remy** (C.) Molluscum; fibrômes multiples de la peau. Bull. Soc. anat. de Par., 1875, l, 786–789.—**Ritter** (H. P.) A description of two cases of non-contagious molluscum, or hypertrophy of the cellular tissue. Buffalo M. J., 1851–2, vii, 411.—**Sangster** (A.) A case of molluscum fibrosum, with some remarks on its histology. Tr. Clin. Soc. Lond., 1880, xiii, 166–172, 2 pl. *Also* [Abstr.]: Med. Press & Circ., Lond., 1880, n. s., xxix, 171.—**Schultze** (R.) Ein Fall von sehr grossem Fibroma molluscum an Kopf und Gesicht. Deutsche Ztschr. f. Chir., Leipz., 1880, xiii, 373–378, 2 pl.—**Smith** (H. H.) Case of molluscum developed by an injury and presenting, under the microscope, the characters of medullary cancer. Am. J. M. Sc., Phila., 1851, n. s., xxii, 396–404.—**Smith** (W. G.) Notes on molluscum sebaceum. Dublin J. M. Sc., 1878, lxvi, 371–377.—**Stokes.** Pachydermatocele, or fibro-molluscum. *Ibid.,* 1875, lix, 69–72.—**Taylor** (R. W.) On the mode of development and course of molluscum fibrosum and on the question of its relation to acrochordon and other cutaneous outshoots. J. Cutan. & Genito-Urin. Dis., N. Y., 1887, v, 41–51. *Also,* Reprint. ———. A further contribution to the study of molluscum fibrosum; etiology; fibromatous infiltration and its relation to keloid. *Ibid.,* 161–170.—**Thomson** (F. H.) Clinical lecture on molluscum. Lancet, Lond., 1840–41, ii, 256–260.—**Tillaux.** Molluscum pendulum du pied gauche. Rev. phot. d. hôp. de Par., 1872, iv, 385.—**Tompkins** (C.) Molluscum simplex. Virginia M. Month., Richmond, 1875–6, ii, 826.—**Trélat.** Transformation carcinomateuse d'un molluscum. France méd., Par., 1879, xxvi, 481–483.—**Venzetti.** Observation de fibrôme molluscum. Bull. Soc. de chir. de Par., 1867–8, 2. s., viii, 429–431.—**Verneuil.** Note sur la structure du molluscum, avec quelques remarques sur les productions homœomorphes. Compt. rend. Soc. de biol. 1854, Par., 1855, 2. s., i, pt. 2, 177–189.—**Viacent** (E.) Note pour servir à l'histoire du fibroma molluscum. Al-

Molluscum.

ger méd., 1886, xiv, 99-104.—**Virchow** (R.) Ueber Xanthelasma multiplex (Molluscum lipomatodes), nebst Notizen von Dr. Leber. Arch. f. path. Anat., etc., Berl., 1871, lii, 504-510, 1 pl.—**Wigglesworth** (E.), jr. Fibromata of the skin and subjacent tissues. Arch. Dermat., N. Y., 1875-6, ii, 193-202, 1 pl. *Also*, Reprint.—**Wood** (J.) Molluscum fibrosum. Tr. Path. Soc. Lond., 1878-9, xxx, 458-460.—**Worthington** (J. H.) Observations on molluscum, with a case. Am. J. M. Sc., Phila., 1845, n. s., x, 284-287.

Molluscum contagiosum.

RICHTER (C. L. J.) * De morbo cutaneo, qui dicitur molluscum contagiosum. sm. 8°. *Berolini*, [1865].

de Amicis (T.) Su di un caso della cosiddetta mycosis fungoide di Alibert. Movimento, Napoli, 1876, viii, 545-554.—**Angelucci** (A.) Sulla etiologia del mollusco contagioso; comunicazione preventiva. Gazz. med. di Roma, 1880, vi, 277. *Also, transl.*: Centralbl. f. d. med. Wissensch., Berl., 1881, xix, 49-51. — **Barraquer** (J.) Molluscum contagiosum, ó acné varioliforme de los párpados. Gac. méd. catal., Barcel., 1885, viii, 261-264.—**Bizzozero** (G.) Sulla struttura del mollusco contagioso. R. Ist. Lomb. di sc. e lett. Rendic., Milano, 1872, 2. s., v, 446-448. — **Bizzozero** (G.) & **Manfredi** (N.) Sullo sviluppo del mollusco contagioso. *Ibid*, 1870, 2. s., iii, 455-457. ———. Sul mollusco contagioso. Riv. clin. di Bologna, 1871, 2. s., i, 21-24, 1 pl. *Also*: Gior. ital. d. mal. ven., Milano, 1871, vi, pt. 1, 129-135. *Also*: Ann. di ottal., Milano, 1871-2, i, 33-39, 1 pl. ———. Sullo sviluppo del mollusco contagioso. R. Ist. Lomb. di sc. e lett. Rendic., Milano, 1874, 2. s., vii, 90-93. ———. Sul mollusco contagioso. Gior. ital. d. mal. ven., Milano, 1875, x, 409. ———. Sul mollusco contagioso. Arch. per le sc. med., Torino, 1876-7, i, 1-26, 1 pl. *Also, transl.* [Abstr.]: Centralbl. f. d. med. Wissensch., Berl., 1876, xiv, 114-116.—**Boeck** (C.) Et Tilfælde af Molluscum contagiosum. Norsk Mag. f. Lægevidensk., Christiania, 1872, ii, 386-389. ———. Ueber Molluscum contagiosum und die sogenannten "Molluscumkörper". Vrtljschr. f. Dermat., Wien, 1875, ii, 23-34, 1 pl.—**Bollinger.** Ueber die Ursache des Molluscum contagiosum. Tagebl. d. Versamml. deutsch. Naturf. u. Aerzte, Cassel, 1878, li, 159. *Also*: Med.-chir. Centralbl., Wien, 1879, xiv, 147. *Also*: Wien. med. Bl., 1878, i, 676. — **Campana.** Sui globi del mollu⸱co contagioso. Salute: Italia med., Genova, 1885, xix, 377. — **Caspary** (J.) Ueber Molluscum contagiosum. Vrtljschr. f. Dermat., Wien, 1882, ix, 205-212, 1 pl.—**Cotton** (R. B.) Report of some cases of molluscum contagiosum, with observations on its general history and pathology. Edinb. M. & S. J., 1848, lxix, 82-86.—**Crocker** (H. R.) The histology and pathology of molluscum contagiosum. Tr. Path. Soc. Lond., 1880-81, xxxii, 254-257.—**Duckworth** (D.) On the molluscum contagiosum of B⸱teman. St. Barth. Hosp. Rep., Lond., 1868, iv, 211: 1872, viii, 61. *Also*, Reprint (of pt. 2). ———. On four cases of molluscum contagiosum which occurred in one family. Tr. Clin. Soc. Lond., 1872, v, 205.—**Eames** (H.) On a case of molluscum contagiosum. Brit. M. J., Lond., 1872, ii, 680.—**Ebert.** Ueber Molluscum contagiosum. Allg. med. Centr.-Ztg., Berl., 1865, xxxiv, 62-66. ———. Ueber Molluscum contagiosum. Jahrb. f. Kinderh., Leipz., 1869-70, iii, 152-160, 1 pl.—**Fagge** (C. H.) Molluscum contagiosum. Guy's Hosp. Rep., Lond., 1870, 3. s., xv, 348-351.—**Ferrier** (D.) On molluscum contagiosum. Brit. M. J., Lond., 1872, ii, 682.—**Fox** (G. H.) Molluscum contagiosum. Tr. Am. Dermat. Ass. 1877, N. Y., 1878, i, 30. ———. A clinical study of molluscum contagiosum. Chicago M. J. & Exam., 1878, xxxvi, 466-475. *Also*, Reprint.—**Fox** (T.) & **Fox** (T. C.) The histology of molluscum contagiosum (Bateman). Tr. Path. Soc. Lond., 1879, xxx, 460-470, 1 pl. *Also*, Reprint.—**Henderson** (W.) Notice of the molluscum contagiosum. Edinb. M. & S. J., 1841, lvi, 213-218, 1 pl. *Also*, Reprint.—**Hutchinson** (J.) Molluscum contagiosum on the nipple of a mother and on the face of her child; an ulcerated molluscum looking like a chancre; history of contagion from another child. Med. Times & Gaz., Lond., 1867, ii, 649. ———. On some cases in which molluscum contagiosum occurred as a general eruption over the body and limbs of adults. Tr. Path. Soc. Lond., 1875-6, xxvii, 295-297. ———. Molluscum contagiosum. *In his*: Lect. Clin. Surg., Lond., 1878, i, 1-14.—**Kaposi.** Ueber das sogenannte Molluscum contagiosum. Mitth. d. Wien. med. Doct.-Coll., 1877, iii, 145-147. *Also*: Allg. Wien. med. Ztg., 1877, xxii, 159. *Also*: Vrtljschr. f. Dermat., Wien, 1877, iv, 333-362. — **Laache** (S.) Molluscum contagiosum giganteum. Nord. med. Ark., Stockholm, 1882, xiv, no. 21, 1-8.—**Lukomsky** (W.) Ueber Molluscum contagiosum. Arch. f. path. Anat., etc., Berl., 1875, lxv, 145-153, 1 pl.—**Mackenzie** (S.) Cases illustrating the communicability of, and some other points connected with, molluscum contagiosum. Tr. Clin. Soc. Lond., 1879, xii, 228-233. *Also*: Brit. M. J., Lond., 1879, i, 855. *Also*: Med. Times & Gaz., Lond., 1879, i, 633.—**Majocchi** (D.)

Molluscum contagiosum.

Sulla contagiosità del così detto mollusco contagioso; osservazioni cliniche e microscopiche. Gazz. med. di Roma, 1880, vi. 237 : 252; 289. ———. [Ricerche micologiche sul bacillo del mollusco contagioso.] Bull. d. r. Accad. med. di Roma, 1880, vi, no. 10, 67-71.—**Morison** (A.) & **Morison** (B. G.) Observations on the nature and affinities of molluscum contagiosum. Tr. Path. Soc. Lond., 1880-81, xxxii, 245-254. *Also* [Abstr.]: Brit. M. J., Lond., 1881, i, 768.—**Park** (R.) Three cases of molluscum contagiosum. Chicago M. J. & Exam., 1878, xxxvii, 593-595.—**Paterson** (R.) Cases and observations on the molluscum contagiosum of Bateman, with an account of the minute structure of the tumours. Edinb. M. & S. J., 1841, lvi, 279-288, 1 pl. *Also*, Reprint.—**Perroncito** (E.) Sur la nature parasitaire du mollusque contagieux de l'homme. Cong. périod. internat. d'ophth. Compt. rend. 1880, Milan, 1881, vi, pt. 2, 53-55, 1 pl.—**Renaut** (J.) Anatomie pathologique de l'acné varioliforme (molluscum contagiosum de Bateman). Ann. de. dermat. et syph., Par., 1880, 2. s., i, 397-407. *Also*: Lyon méd., 1880, xxxiv. 439-449.—**Retzius** (G.) Om molluscum contagiosum. Nord. med. Ark.. Stockholm, 1870, ii, no. 11, 1-26, 1 pl. *Also*, Reprint.—**Saugster** (A.) A contribution to the non-glandular theory of origin of molluscum contagiosum. Med.-Chir. Tr., Lond., 1880, 2. s, xlv, 149-159, 2 pl. *Also* [Abstr.]: Proc. Roy. M. & Chir. Soc. Lond., 1875-80, viii, 460-462. *Also* [Abstr.]: Brit. M. J., Lond., 1880, i, 327.—**Shah** (T. M.) Two cases of molluscum fibrosum with huge tumours. Indian M. Gaz., Calcutta, 1881, xvi, 169.—**Simon** (O.) Ueber Molluscum contagiosum. Vrtljschr. f. Dermat., Wien, 1876, iii, 400.—**Smith** (H. H.) Case of molluscum contagiosum; amputation. Med. Exam., Phila., 1851, n. s., vii, 96—**Smith** (W.) Molluscum contagiosum. Dublin Q. J. M. Sc., 1872, liii, 458.—**Squire** (B.) Molluscum contagiosum. Brit. M. J., Lond., 1872, i. 45.—**Startin** (J.) Case of molluscum contagiosum. Tr. Path. Soc. Lond., 1879-80, xxxi, 341. *Also*: Lancet, Lond., 1880, i, 564.—**Thin** (G.) The histology of molluscum contagiosum. J. Anat. & Physiol., Lond., 1881-2, xvi, 202-207, 1 pl. *Also* [Abstr.]: Tr. Path. Soc Lond., 1880-81, xxxii, 257.—**Turnbull** (W.) Notice of a case of molluscum contagiosum. Edinb. M. & S. J., 1841, lvi, 463.—**de Vincentiis** (C.) Mollusco contagioso multiplo delle palpebre. Movimento, Napoli, 1877, ix, 144-147.—**Virchow** (R.) Ueber Molluscum contagiosum. Arch. f. path. Anat. etc., Berl., 1865, xxxiii, 144-154, 1 pl.—**Virnicchi** (T.) Caso d'iperplasia cutanea molle multipla (molluscum multiplum) con singolare idrorachia. Movimento, Napoli, 1869, i, 9-14.

Mollweide (Car. Brand.) Demonstrationem novam propositionis, quæ theoriæ colorum Newtoni fundamenti loco est, exhibit. 15 pp., 1 pl. 4°. *Lipsiæ, ex off. Klaubarthia*, [1841].

Mollweide (Joannes Henricus). *De modo agendi metallorum in corpore humano. 36 pp. 4°. *Halæ Magdeb., typ. J. C. Hendelii*, [1752].

Mollweide (Julius Joannes). *De tremore artuum ejusque causis. 36 pp., 2 l. 4°. *Halæ Magdeb., typ. J. C. Hendelii*, [1752].

Molly (Guilelmus Henricus Fridericus) [1838-]. *De laryngitide crouposa. 31 pp. 12°. *Berolini, G. Lange*, 1861.

Molnar (Adamus). *Diss. sistens disquisitionem caussarum sterilitatis hominum utriusque sexus. 76 pp. 4°. *Halæ Magdeb., typ. J. C. Hendelii*, [1747].

Molnar (Joh.) Monographische Skizze über das Ofner Raitzerbad, vorgetragen in der Versammlung der Aerzte und Naturforscher in Pest im September 1863. 16 pp. 4°. *Pest, G. Enich*, 1863.

de Molo (Josephus). *Præcipue febrium intermittentium epidemiæ primis lineis adumbratæ. 16 pp. 8°. *Monachii, J. A. Giesser*, 1839.

von Molo (Th. J.) Ueber Epidemien im Allgemeinen und Wechselfieberepidemien insbesondere, nebst einer kurzen Darstellung der Schleimfieber-Epidemie in München im J. 1840. 295 pp. 8°. *Regensburg, G. J. Manz*, 1841.

Molokai.

See **Leprosy** (*Hospitals for*).

Molony (Michael Joseph). Rupture of the perinæum; its causes, prevention, and treatment. 63 pp. 12°. *Dublin, Fannin & Co.*, 1886.

Molsdorf (Alexandre). *Des hémorrhagies utérines pendant les derniers mois de la gros-

Molsdorf (Alexandre)—continued.
sesse et durant le travail. 50 pp. 4°. *Paris,*
1851, No. 51, v. 512.

Molter (August). *Ueber die Sensibilitätsver-
hältnisse der menschlichen Cornea. [Erlangen.]
34 pp. 8°. *Cassel, T. Fischer,* 1878.
Also forms: 2. Beilagehft. of : Klin. Monatsbl. f. Augenh.,
Cassel, 1878, xvi.

Molthan (J.) *Ueber Entzündung und Thrombose der Gehirnsinus. 48 pp., 2 l. 8°. *Giessen,*
W. Keller, 1862. C.

Moltherus (Georgius).
See **Petræus** (Henricus). De pleuritide. *In :* NOSOL.
harmonica dogmat. et hermet. 4°. *Marpurgi Cattorum,*
1615, i, 260–270. ———. De palpitatione cordis. *In :* NOSOL.
harmonica dogmat. et hermet. 4°. *Marpurgi Cattorum,*
1615, i, 362–373.

Moltherus (Joh.)
See **Petræus** (Henricus). De vitiis expulsionis ven-
triculi. *In :* NOSOL. harmonica dogmat. et hermet. 4°.
Marpurgi Cattorum, 1615, i, 400–413. ———. De peripneu-
monia. *In :* NOSOL. harmonica dogmat. et hermet. 4°.
Marpurgi Cattorum, 1615, i, 297–308.
For Portrait, see **Collection**—van Kaathoven.

Moltherus (Joh. Philippus). De sudore. 8°.
[*n. p., n. d.*]
In : AGONISMATA med. Marpurgensia. 4°. *Marpurgi*
Cattorum, 1618, 71–89.

Moltherus (Philippus Joh.)
See **Petræus** (Henricus). De ictero flavo et nigro. *In :*
NOSOL. harmonica dogmat. et hermet. 4°. *Marpurgi Cat-*
torum, 1616, ii, 263–278.

Moltrasio. Regolamento di pubblica igiene pel
comune di Moltrasio. 15 pp. roy. 8°. *Como,*
Bellasi & Bazzoro, 1886.

Moltrecht (Adolph). *Ueber Osteoaneurysma.
22 pp., 1 l. 8°. *Jena, A. Neuenhahn,* 1869. [P.,
v. 2-2.]

Molucca *nut.*
[PECHY (J.)] Some observations made upon
the Molucco nutts imported from the Indies ;
shewing their admirable virtues in curing the
collick, rupture, and all distempers proceeding
from the wind. Written by a doctor of physick
in the countrey to Dr. Castle, one of the Royal
Society in London. sm. 4°. [*London*], 1672.

Molweid (Christ. Henricus). *De sterilitate
sexus utriusque. 39 pp. sm. 4°. *Vitembergæ,*
lit. A. Kobersteinii, [1711].

Molwiz (Eberhard Friedrich) [1763–1812]. Nö-
thiger Unterricht für diejenigen, welche schlei-
chendes, verstektes und eingewurzeltes venerisches und Trippergift in ihrem Körper zu vermuthen Ursache haben. Mit Krankengeschichten
erläutert, wie die unentwikelten Keime sowohl
als auch die Ueberreste dieser Gifte, aus ihrem
verlarvten Zustande mit den gichtischen, rheumatischen, scrophulösen, herpetischen und andern hartnäckigen Krankheitsstoffen zu ent-
decken und zu heilen sind. 72 pp. 16°. *Leipzig, F. G. Jacobäer,* 1799.
———. The same. 3. Aufl. xvi, 110 pp. 8°.
Leipzig, F. G. Jacobäer, 1803.
———. The same. Instruction nécessaire pour les
personnes qui ont lieu de se croire infectées d'un
vice vénérien, assoupi, caché et invétéré ; dans
laquelle l'auteur explique, par le traitement de
beaucoup de malades, comment on peut découvrir et guérir le germe et les restes de ce funeste
poison, des rhumatismes, tantôt avec ceux des
écrouelles, des dartres et d'autres maladies opiniâtres. 63 pp. 12°. *Leipsic, F. G. Jacobäer,*
1800.
———. De natura impressionis venereæ. [Leip-
sic.] 26 pp. 4°. *Stutgardiæ,* 1801.

Moly.
Schwartz (W.) Ueber das μῶλυ des Homer. Ztschr.
f. Ethnol., Berl., 1882, xiv, 133–141.

Molyneux (William). Dioptrica nova. A treatise of dioptricks, in two parts. Wherein the

Molyneux (William) – continued.
various effects and appearances of spherick
glasses, both convex and concave, single and
combined, in telescopes and microscopes, together with their usefulness in many concerns of
humane life, are explained. 6 p. l., 301 pp., 43
pl. 4°. *London, B. Tooke,* 1692.

Molzahn (Georgius Andreas). *De ulcerum
externorum sanatione difficili ob illorum cum
morbis viscerum complicationem. 27 pp., 1 l.
sm. 4°. *Halæ ad Salam, stanno Schneideriano,*
[1762].
Also [Abstr.], *in :* WEIZ (F. A.) Vollständ. Ausz.,
[etc.] 12°. *Leipzig u. Budissin.* 1773, v, 19.

Momber (Antonius). *De kelotomiæ abusu tol-
lendo : vom Misbrauch des Bruchschneidens. 35
pp. sm. 4°. *Helmstadii, typ. P. D. Schnorri,*
[1728].
———. Tractat vom Nier- und Blasen-Stein, worin
selbiger eigentlich bestehe, dessen gründliche, innerliche als äuserliche Cur und Präservation,
nebst einem in Kupfer gestochenen curieusen Ab-
riss des von dem Herrn Hoff-Rath Heister aus
der Blase eines 40jährigen Bergmanns geschnit-
tenen wundersahm gebildeten Steins so zu Helmstädt 1735 glücklich vollentzogen. 6 p. l., 76 pp.,
1 pl. 8°. *Helmstädt. P. D. Schnorrn,* [1735].
Bound with : TOLET (F.) Tractätlein von der besten
Art und Weise den Blasen-Stein zu schneiden, etc. 8°.
Hannover u. Wolffenbüttel, 1694.

Momberger (Rudolph). *Beitrag zur Lehre
von der Hämophilie. 64 pp., 2 l. 8°. *Giessen,*
F. C. Pietsch, 1862. C.

Mombert (Philippus). *De imaginationis maternæ vi in fœtum. 49 pp., 1 l. 8°. *Marburgi,*
typ. Bayrhofferi, 1827.

de Momigny (J.-A.) *De la photophobie. 47
pp. 4°. *Paris,* 1846, No. 65, v. 442.

Momma (Joh. Wilhelmus). *De spiritibus chemicis. 1 p. l., 30 pp. sm. 4°. *Lugduni, Wishoff,*
[1725].

Momme (Julius Theodoricus) [1798–]. *De
calculis urinariis, corpore non inciso, e vesica
urinaria auferendis. 56 pp. 8°. *Halæ, typ. Gebaueriis,* [1833].
For Biography, see **Dzondi** (Car. Henr.)

Mommendey (G. C.) Rathgeber für Mütter
über das Verhalten der Schwangern und die Behandlung des neugeborenen Kindes und über die
Erkenntniss, Verhütung und Behandlung der
gewöhnlichen Kinderkrankheiten. vii, 79 pp.
16°. *Stuttgart, E. Müller,* 1873.

Mommer (Henricus). *De morborum generatione quædam. 32 pp. 8°. *Berolini, B. Schlesinger,* [1852].

de Mommerot (Claude). *Sur le croup. vi,
7–34 pp. 4°. *Paris,* 1807, No. 61, v. 67.

Mommeyer (Guil. Henr. J.) *De enteritide.
1786.
In : LOUVAIN Diss. 8°. *Lovanii,* 1796, iii, 404–427.

Mommsen [Jens Karl Friederich] [1852–].
Wider das "Post hoc ergo propter hoc". Ein
Beitrag zur Kenntniss einer in der speciellen
Therapie noch vielfach gebräuchlichen For-
schungsmethode, nebst Vorschlägen zur Verbesserung derselben. 28 pp. 8°. *Berlin, Fischer,*
1885.

Momon (Jules-Émile) [1852–]. *De la septicémie péritonéale à la suite de la kélotomie. 49
pp. 4°. *Paris,* 1822, No. 218.

Momordica.
Duprat (A.) Note sur l'action physiologique de la
Momordica Bucha. Compt. rend. Soc. de biol., Par., 1887,
8. s., iv, 133.—**Hancock** (J.) Observations and experiments upon the kusia, or koosia, of the Indians—the bitter
cucumber, Momordica operculata of Linnæus. Edinb. M.
& S. J., 1830, xxxiii, 93–100.—**Streubel** (C.) Von den
heilenden Kräfften der Momordicæ Ceylonicæ. Samml.
v. Nat.- u. Med.- . . . . Gesch., Leipz. u. Budissin, 1724, xxi,
216–218.

Momordica *elaterium.*
See **Elaterium,** *etc.*

Monachus *quidam Benedictinis ordinis.*
See **Sequitur** epistola [etc.]

Monaco.
See **Mentone.**

Monaco (Garibaldi). Manuale di medicina legale, redatto secondo le teorie dei più illustri autori moderni. iv, 534 pp. 8°. *Napoli, G. Jovene,* 1887.

Monaeus (*Joh. Conrad*). ·
Portrait in: **Collection** of Portr. of Phys. & Men of Sc., 194.

von Monakow (C.) Ueber die Grenzen der geistigen Gesundheit. Oeffentlicher Vortrag, [etc.] 24 pp. 8°. *Chur, Hitz u. Hail,* 1884.

Monantholius (Henricus). Ludus iatromathematicus, musis factus, ad averruncandum tres Academiæ perniciosissimos hostes, πολεμὸν, λιμν, λοδιμὸν. 3 p. l., 136 pp. 16°. *Parisiis, L. Delas,* 1597. [P., v. 1641.]

Monard (Charles)[1] [1795–1854]. * Considérations générales sur les scrophules. 24 pp. 4°. *Paris,* 1818, No. 209, v. 142.
For Biography, see Exposé d. trav. de la Soc. d. sc. méd. de la Moselle, Metz, 1853, 35–45.

Monard (Charles)[2]. * Considérations générales sur les concrétions sanguines qui se forment pendant la vie dans le cœur et les gros vaisseaux. 62 pp., 1 l. 4°. *Montpellier, Boehm & fils,* 1867, No. 57.

Monard (Jean). * Contribution à l'étude de la détermination du principe sulfuré des eaux minérales de Bagnères-de-Luchon; déductions pratiques. 64 pp. 4°. *Paris, A. Parent,* 1879, No. 498.

Monard (Pascal). * Considérations générales sur les fistules urinaires. 23 pp. 4°. *Paris,* 1818, No. 211, v. 142.

Monarda.
Atlee (E. A.) On the medicinal properties of the Monarda punctata. Am. M. Recorder, Phila., 1819, ii, 496–500, 2 pl.

Monardes (Nicolo) [1493–1588]. Sevillana medicina, que trata el modo conservativo y curativo de los qui abitan en la muy insigne ciudad de Sevilla; la qual sirve ya, puecha para qualquier otro lugar destos reynos. Obra antigua digna de ser leyda. 3 l., 135 ff. sm. 4°. *Sevilla, A. de Burgos,* 1545.

———. Dos libros. El uno trata de todas las cosas que traen nostras Indias occidentales, que sirven al uso de medicina, y como se ha de usar de la rayz del Mechoacan, purga excelentissima. El otro libro, trata de dos medicinas maravillosas que son contra todo veneno, la piedra bezaar, y la yerva escuerçonera. Con la cura de los venenados. Do veran muchos secretos de naturalesa y de medicina, con grandes experiencias. 132 l. 16°. *Serilla, S. Trugillo,* 1565.

———. Primera y segunda y tercera partes de la historia medicinal de las cosas que se traen de nuestras Indias occidentales, que sirven en medicina. Tratado de la piedra Bezaar, y de la yerva Escuerçonera. Dialogo de las grandezas del Hierro, y de sus virtudes medicinales. Tratado de la nieve y del bever frio. 6 l., 206 ff., 1 l. sm. 4°. *Sevilla, A. Escrivano,* 1574.
First Spanish edition of the collected works of Monardes. Comprises the preceding work with the addition of a third part. At the end a page of Italian MS., "Modo d' usar la triaca di smeraldi ", etc.

———. The same. Delle cose che vengono portate dall' Indie occidentali pertinenti all' uso della medicina, racolte e trattate dal Dottor . . . Parte prima, novamente recata dalla Spagnola nella nostra lingua Italiana, dove ancho si tratta

Monardes (Nicolo)—continued
de' veneni, e della lor cura, aggiuntivi dei indici; uno de' capi principali; l' altro delle cose più rilevanti, che si ritrovano in tutta '' opera. Parte seconda, con un libro appresso dell' istesso autore, che tratta della neve, e del bever fresco con lei. 7 p. l., 159 pp., 8 l.; 3 p. l., 140 pp. 16°. *Venetia, G. Ziletti,* 1575.

———. The same. Joyfull newes out of the new-found worlde. Wherein are declared, the rare and singuler vertues of divers herbs, trees, plantes, oyles and stones, with their applications as well to the use of physicke, as of chirurgery: which being well applyed, bring such present remedie for all diseases as may seeme altogether incredible; notwithstanding by practice found out to be true. Also the portraiture of the said hearbs very aptly described. Englished by John Frampton . . . Whereunto are added three other bookes treating of the bezaar stone, the herb escuerconera, the properties of iron and steele in medicine, and the benefit of snow. 3 p. l., 187 ff. 4°. *London, E. Allde,* 1596.
Gothic letter.

———. Modo et ordine come si ha da usare la radice Mechiocane, et delle sue excellentissime virtù et operationi, cavato da un trattato de alcuni simplici c' hora vengono dalle Indie occidentali. 7 l. 4°. *Milano,* 1570.

Monart (Henri). * Considérations sur l'adénite cervicale chez les soldats. 31 pp. 4°. *Paris,* 1875, No. 224.

Monassot (Jacques). * Étude sur la granulation des reins. 32 pp. 4°. *Paris,* 1835, No. 252, v. 289.

Monasterio y Correa (Raimundo).
See **Esquirol** (Jean-Étienne-Dominique). Tratado completo de las enagenaciones mentales. 8°. *Madrid,* 1856.

Monastirski (Nestor) [1847–]. * K patologii bugorchatoi prokazi (lepra tuberosa). 54 pp., 1 l., 4 pl. 8°. *St. Petersburg,* 1877.

———. O sovremennom lechenii ran. Lektsii, chitannija k Klinicheskom Institute Velikoi Knjagini Eleni Pavlovni vprodoljenie 1885-6 akademicheskago goda. [Modern treatment of wounds. Lectures delivered in the Clinical Institute, etc.] iv, viii, 248 pp. 8°. *St. Petersburg,* 1886.
Publications of: **Ejem.** journal prakt. med.

Monatliche Mittheilungen aus dem Gesammtgebiete der Naturwissenschaften. Organ des Regierungsbezirks Frankfurt, hrsg. von Ernst Huth. Jahrg. 4–5, April, 1886–7. 8°. *Frankf. a. O.*
Current.

Monatliche neu eröffnete Anmerkungen über alle Theile der Artzney-Kunst zusammen gebracht im Jahr 1679, durch Nicolaus de Blegny . . . aus dem Frantzösischen ins Teutsche übersetzet durch J. L. M. C. [Jan. to June, 1679.] 4 p. l., 163 pp. sm. 8°. *Hamburg, G. Schultze,* 1680.
A transl. of: **Nouvelles** (Les) découvertes, etc.; again transl. as: **Zodiacus** medico-gallicus.

Monatlicher Anzeiger über Novitäten und Antiquaria aus dem Gebiete der Medicin und Naturwissenschaft. Jahrg. 1874–87. 8°. *Berlin, Hirschwald.*
Current.

Monats-Ausgabe von Wolf's Vademecum für Medicin, Natur- und exacte Wissenschaften. Nos. 3–9, March to Sept., 1886. 8°. *Leipzig.*

Monatsblatt für medicinische Statistik und öffentliche Gesundheitspflege. Beilage zu: Göschen's Deutsche Klinik. 1856 to March 27, 1875. fol. *Berlin.*
Ended. Issued with: **Deutsche** Klinik.

Monatsblatt für öffentliche Gesundheitspflege. Hrsg. von dem Verein für öffentliche Gesundheitspflege im Herzogthum Braunschweig. Jahrg. 1–10, 1878–87. 8°. *Braunschweig, H. Bruhn.*
Current.

Monatshefte für praktische Dermatologie. Redigirt von H. von Hebra, O. Lassar und P. G. Unna. v. 1–6, March, 1882–7. 8°. *Hamburg u. Leipzig, L. Voss.*
Current. v. 2 commenced Jan., 1883. In 1886–7, contained supplements: "Dermatologische Studien".

Monatsschrift für Elektro-Homöopathie, redigirt von Dr. Med. Fewson. v. 1, March to Dec., 1887. 8°. *Danzig.*
Current.

Monatsschrift für exacte Forschung auf dem Gebiete der Sanitäts-Polizei. Hrsg. von Dr. Louis Pappenheim. Jahrg. 1–2, April, 1859, to July 11, 1862. 8°. *Berlin, J. Springer.*
Ended. v. 2 commenced Jan., 1860. Nos. 4–12, v. 2, appear also under title: **Beiträge** für exacte Forschung [etc.], Heft 1–4.

Monatsschrift für Geburtskunde und Frauenkrankheiten. Hrsg. von Busch, Credé, von Ritgen, von Siebold. [2 v. annually.] v. 1–34, 1853–69. 8°. *Berlin, A. Hirschwald.*
A continuation of: **Neue** Zeitschrift für Geburtskunde. Continued as: **Archiv** für Gynaekologie.

Monatsschrift für Medicin, Augenheilkunde und Chirurgie. Hrsg. von Dr. F. A. von Ammon. v. 1–3, 1838–40. 8°. *Leipzig, Weidmann.*
Ended. A continuation of: **Zeitschrift** für Ophthalmologie, 1831–37.

Monatsschrift für Ohrenheilkunde. Hrsg. von Josef Gruber, N. Rüdinger, F. E. Weber, Dr. Voltolini. Jahrg. 1–21, Oct., 1867–87. fol. & 8°. *Berlin.*
Current. v. 1 complete in 3 nos., Oct. to Dec., 1867; v. 2 commenced Jan., 1868. After 1875, v. 9, the words "sowie für Nasen-, Rachen-, Kehlkopf- und Luftröhren-Krankheiten" added to title.

Monatsschrift für Ohrenheilkunde sowie für Nasen-, Rachen-, Kehlkopf- und Luftröhren-Krankheiten.
Was title of: **Monatsschrift** für Ohrenheilkunde after 1875, v. 9.

Monatsschrift des Vereins deutscher Zahnkünstler. (Vereins-Organ.) Hrsg. vom Verein deutscher Zahnkünstler. Verantwortlicher Redakteur: Aug. Polscher. v. 3–7, April, 1883–8. 8°. *Dresden.*
Current. Title of v. 1–2 was: **Vierteljahresschrift** des Vereins deutscher Zahnkünstler.

Monavius (Fridericus) [1592–1659]. * Lanx satura rerum medicarum. 3 p. l., 154 pp., 1 l. 4°. *Tubingæ, typ. T. Werlini,* 1622.

——. Bronchotome nimirum gutturis artificiose aperiendi ἐγχείρησις cum appendice gemina tam elenchi affectuum ocularium hecatontadem ipsam excedentis, quam hypotyposeos febrium omnium. 3 p. l., 56 pp., 1 tab. 4°. *Montis Regii, typ. J. Reusneri,* 1644.
For Biography, see **Scheffelius** (C. S.) Vitæ professorum medicinæ in Acad. Gryphiswald. 4°. 1756, 153–176.

Monavius (Petrus) [1551–88].
See **Crato** à *Kraftheim* (Joannes). Consiliorum et epistolarum medicinalium liber [etc.] 8°. *Francofurti,* 1591–2.

Monay (Hyacinthe-Casimir). * Sur le goître. 18 pp. 4°. *Paris,* 1833, No. 72, v. 258.

Monbalon (François-Aristide). * Recherches sur la migraine. 38 pp. 4°. *Paris,* 1848, No. 63, v. 475.

Monbrun (J.-C.) * Considérations sur l'hygiène militaire. 33 pp. 4°. *Paris,* 1826, No. 15, v. 197.

Moncade (C.) * Étude sur l'étiologie de l'ascite. 78 pp. 4°. *Paris,* 1874, No. 209.

Moncamp (Evenor-Martin). * Sur les sympathies pathologiques. 69 pp. 4°. *Paris,* 1819, No. 152, v. 149.

Monceau (Henry). * Dissertation sur l'hémoptysie. 18 pp. 4°. *Paris,* 1803, No. 78, v. C.

Monceaux (C.-M.) * Sur quelques maladies des testicules qui exigent la castration. 21 pp. 4°. *Paris,* 1810, No. 42, v. 79.

Monceaux (P.-Victor). * Études cliniques sur le cancer de la matrice. 54 pp. 4°. *Paris,* 1855,– No. 14, v. 578.

Moncelon (Gabriel). * Sur l'allaitement étranger. 24 pp. 4°. *Paris,* 1825, No. 216, v. 196.

Moncetus (Joh. Benedictus).
See **Ægidius** (Romanus). Tractatus aureus . . . de formatione corporis humani in utero. 4°. *Parisiis,* 1515.

[du Monchaux (Pierre J.)] [1733–66]. Bibliographie médicinale raisonnée ; ou essai sur l'exposition des livres les plus utiles à ceux qui se destinent à l'étude de la médecine. Avec une lettre de du Monchaux, sur les commentaires de Vanswieten, et sur quelques autres ouvrages. xxxii, 468 pp., 39 pp., 2 l. 12°. *Paris, Ganeau,* 1756.

Monchique.

Ramos (D. T. de A.) Tentativa analytica sobre as aguas thermaes de Monchique. J. Soc. d. sc. med. de Lisb., 1839, x, 3 : 65.—**Soares** (A. A. de O.) Noticia das caldas de Monchique. *Ibid.,* 1837, vi, 73–88.

de Monchy (Franciscus Gulielmus). * De medico optimo naturæ et observatore et imitatore. 4 p. l., 136 pp., 1 l. 4°. *Lugd. Bat., typ. Bootianis,* [1774].

de Monchy (Hendrik Willem). * Vijf waarnemingen van gedeeltelijke verlamming der handen, met eenige opmerkingen aangaande dien ziektevorm. 2 p. l., 47 pp. 8°. *Leiden, J. Hazenberg, Corn. zoon,* 1855.

de Monchy (Solomon). * De opio. 52 pp., 4 l. 4°. *Lugd. Bat., J. Luzac,* 1739. [P., v. 53.]

——. An essay on the causes and cure of the usual diseases in voyages to the West Indies, together with the preservatives against them. In answer to the questions proposed by the Society of Sciences in Holland : What are the causes of the usual diseases among seamen in voyages to the West Indies ? and What are the means of preventing and of curing them ? To which essay the prize was adjudged. Transl. from the Dutch Philosophical Transactions. x, 175 pp. 8°. *London, T. Becket & P. A. De Hondt,* 1762. [*Also, in*: P., v. 547; 659.]

——. Remarks upon the mortality among the horned cattle ; containing directions for extirpating the infection, or, at least, for obstructing its progress. Transl. from the Low Dutch. 1 p. l., 43 pp. 8°. *London, T. Cadell,* 1770. [P., v. 661.]

Monciny (J.-P.) * Considérations sur la rage. 15 pp. 4°. *Paris, an XII* [1804], No. 273, v. 50.

van Monckhoven (D.) Photographic optics ; including the description of lenses and enlarging apparatus. Transl. from the French. 16, 259 pp., 5 pl. 8°. *London, R. Hardwicke,* 1867.

Monckton (Stephen) [1824–85]. The metaphysical aspect of natural history. 51 pp. sm. 4°. *London, H. K. Lewis,* 1885.
For Biography. see Lancet, Lond., 1885, ii, 695.

Monclair (Henri). * Du viburnum prunifolium, ses indications obstétricales. 52 pp. 4°. *Paris, A. Parent,* 1887, No. 256.

Moncoq (D.) * Procédé nouveau pour pratiquer la transfusion immédiate et instantanée du sang. 72 pp. 4°. *Paris,* 1864, No. 185.

——. Transfusion instantanée du sang. Solution théorique et pratique de la transfusion médiate et de la transfusion immédiate chez les ani-

Moncoq (D.)—continued.

maux et chez l'homme. 2. éd. 348 pp., 1 tab. 8°. *Paris, A. Delahaye*, 1874.

Moncorvo (Carlos Arthur). * Dyspepsias e seu tractamento. 2 p. l., 252 pp., 1 l. 4°. *Rio de Janeiro*, 1871.

——. Da acção abortiva do sulphato de quinina. 23 pp. 8°. *Rio de Janeiro*, 1874.

——. Da acção da genciana associada ao acido sulphurico. 29 pp. 8°. *Rio de Janeiro*, 1874.

——. De exercicio e ensino medico no Brazil. 203 pp. 12°. *Rio de Janeiro*, 1874.

——. Du diagnostic différentiel entre la dyspepsie essentielle et l'hypohémie intertropicale (oppilation); considérations cliniques. 16 pp. 8°. *Rio de Janeiro*, 1874.

——. Do emprego do chlorato de potassa na diarrhéa das crianças. 8 pp. 8°. *Rio de Janeiro, Brown & Evaristo*, 1875.

Repr. from: Rev. med., Rio de Jan., 1874-6, ii.

——. Do ainhum. Algumas considerações sobre esta molestia a proposito de um caso communicado á Academia imperial de medicina do Rio de Janeiro. 51 pp. 8°. *Rio de Janeiro, Brown & Evaristo*, 1876.

Repr. from: Rev. med., Rio de Jan., 1874-6, ii.

——. Projecto de regulamento das amas de leite. 11 pp. 8°. *Rio de Janeiro, J. G. Tourinho*, 1876.

Repr. from: Gaz. med. da Bahia, 1876, 2. s., i.

——. Do emprego do chlorato de potassa na diarrhéa das crianças. 40 pp. 8°. *Rio de Janeiro*, 1877.

Repr. from: Progresso med., Rio de Jan., 1876-7, i.

——. Do valor therapeutico das injecções hydricas subcutaneas. 38 pp., 1 l. 8°. *Rio de Janeiro*, 1877.

Repr. from: Progresso med., Rio de Jan., 1876-7, i-ii.

——. Da lienteria na infancia e do seu tractamento pelo acido chlorhydrico. 33 pp. 8°. *Rio de Janeiro*, 1879.

——. Estudo sobre o rheumatismo chronico nodoso na infancia e seu tractamento á proposito de um caso observado em uma menina de 2 annos e meio curado pelo emprego das correntes galvanicas. ii, 105 pp., 1 l. 8°. *Rio de Janeiro*, 1879.

——. Nota sobre a acção physiologica e therapeutica da Carica papaya (Mamoeiro). 25 pp. 8°. *Rio de Janeiro*, 1879.

——. Notas clinicas sobre duos casos de croup. 24 pp. 8°. *Rio de Janeiro*, 1879.

——. Da dilatação do estomago nas creanças e seu tratamento segundo as lições feitas na Policlinica do Rio de Janeiro. 79 pp. 8°. *Rio de Janeiro, G. Leuzinger & filhos*, 1883.

——. De la nature de la coqueluche et de son traitement par la résorcine. 96 pp., 1 l. 8°. *Rio de Janeiro, G. Leuzinger & fils; Paris, O. Berthier*, 1883.

——. The same. 87 pp. 8°. *Paris, O. Berthier*, 1885.

——. Contribution à l'étude de la sclérose multiloculaire chez les enfants. 85 pp. 8°. *Paris, O. Berthier*, 1884.

——. De l'emploi du chlorhydrate de cocaïne dans le traitement de la coqueluche. 11 pp. 8°. *Rio de Janeiro, Lombaerts & Cie.*, 1885.

Repr. from: União med., Rio de Jan., 1885, v.

Also, Co-Editor of: **Progresso** (O) medico, Rio de Janeiro, 1879-80. *Also, Co-Editor of:* **União** medico, Rio de Janeiro, 1881.

Moncouet (A.-A.-Léopold). * I. Du diagnostic et du pronostic de la chorée. II. [etc.] 24 pp. 4°. *Paris*, 1838, No. 245, v. 331.

Moncourrier (J.-F.) * Sur la phthisie pulmonaire. 28 pp. 4°. *Paris*, 1832, No. 37, v. 249.

Moncourrier (Léonard). * Sur le rachitis, ou l'ostéomalaxie. 58 pp. 8°. *Paris, an XI* [1803], v. 23.

Moncourrier (Léonard-Jean). * Sur les plaies d'armes à feu. 21 pp. 4°. *Paris*, 1834, No. 71, v. 271.

Moncreiff (Gulielmus). * De peste. 5 p. l., 73, 9 pp. 8°. *Edinburgi, C. Stewart*, 1814.

Moncreiff (John). An inquiry into the medicinal qualities and effects of the aerated alkaline water. Illustrated by experiments and cases. 1 p. l., 205 pp., 1 pl., 1 l. 8°. *Edinburgh, W. Creech*, 1794. [P., v. 121.]

——. The same. To which is prefixed a letter to the publisher, by a respectable physician of Baltimore. xii, 102 pp., 1 pl. 8°. *Baltimore, E. J. Coale*, 1810.

Moncrief [**Moncrieff**] (John). The poor man's physician, or the receipts of the famous John Moncrief, of Tippermalloch; being a choice collection of simple and easy remedies for most distempers, very useful for all persons, especially those of a poorer condition. 2. ed. To which is added the method of curing the smallpox and scurvy by the eminent Dr. Archbald Pitcairn. 1 p. l., 240 pp. 12°. *Edinburgh, J. Paton*, 1716.

——. The same. 3. ed. 1 p. l., 245 pp., 3 l. 12°. *Edinburgh, T. Heriot*, 1731.

——. The same. Tippermalluch's receipts. Being a collection of many useful and easy remedies for most distempers. 2. ed. viii, 128 pp. 16°. *Leith, W. Coke*, 1775.

Moncrieffe (Gulielmus). * De gonorrhœa virulenta. 1 p. l., 33 pp. 8°. *Edinburgi; Balfour, Auld et Smellie*, 1768. [*Also, in:* P., v. 133.]

Mondariz.

Andreu. Aguas minero-medicinales de Mondariz. Encicl. méd.-farm., Barcel., 1879, iii, 3.

Mondat (Vincent-Marie). * Essai physiologique et médical sur le diaphragme. 1 p. l., 21 pp. 4°. *Strasbourg*, 1810, v. 46.

——. Des hydropisies et de leur cure. 49 pp. 12°. *Paris, L. Colas*, 1817.

——. De la stérilité de l'homme et de la femme, et des moyens d'y remédier. viii, 172 pp., 1 l. 12°. *Paris, Migneret*, 1820.

——. The same. 4. éd. vi, 239, 1 tab., 2 pl. 8°. *Paris*, 1833.

——. The same. 5. éd. 270 pp., 1 l., 1 tab. 8°. *Montpellier, L. Castel*, 1840.

——. The same. On sterility in the male and female; its causes and treatment. Transl. from the 5. French ed. 248 pp. 8°. *New York, J. S. Redfield*, 1844.

——. Lettre à Monsieur Broussais (sur le choléra). 3 pp. 8°. [*Paris, 1832.*]

van der Monde (Hendrik Sebald). * Over het geneeskundig gebruik van het arsenigzuur; benevens eenige behandelingen met hetzelve, waargenomen in het Hospitaal der Kolonie: Ommerschans. xii, 100 pp. 8°. *Leyden, J. Hazenberg*, 1856.

Monde (Le) pharmaceutique. Journal des intérêts scientifiques et pratiques, moraux et professionnels du corps pharmaceutique. Publié sous la direction de Edmond Rousset. [Semimonthly.] Année 4-18, 1874-87. 15 v. 4°. *Paris.*

Current. Want nos. 6-24, v. 7 (1876). In Jan., 1877, v. 8, title became: **Monde** (Le) pharmaceutique et médical.

Monde (Le) pharmaceutique et médical.

Was title in 1877, *et seq.*, of: **Monde** (Le) pharmaceutique.

Monde (Le) thermal. Hydrologie, hydrothérapie, eaux minérales, bains de mer, résidences d'hiver. Directeur: A. Cazaux. [Weekly.] Année 23-28, 1880-85. 6 v. fol. *Paris.*

Mondelet (Frédéric). * Des différentes variétés d'orchites aiguës. 38 pp. 4°. *Paris*, 1857, No. 71, v. 608.

Mondelli (Francesco Saverio). Dissertazione medica sopra la podagra. 70 pp. 8°. [*Napoli*], 1794. [P., v. 1116.]

Mondellius (Franciscus). *De angina pectoris. 27 pp. 8°. *Ticini Regii, typ. Fusi et socii*, [1836].

Mondière (A.-T.) Monographie de la femme de la Cochinchine. Femmes annamite, chinoise, minh-huong, cambodgienne. Anthropométrie, physiologie, position sociale. Mémoire couronné par la Société d'anthropologie. (Prix Godard, 1881.) 40 pp. 8°. *Paris, G. Masson*, 1882.
Repr. from: Mém. Soc. d'anthrop. de Par., 1875–82, ii.

Mondière (Julien-Théophile). *Recherches sur l'inflammation de l'œsophage, et sur quelques points d'anatomie pathologique de cet organe. 44 pp. 4°. *Paris*, 1829, No. 118, v. 224.

Mondineu (Léon-Gaspard). *De quelques considérations sur la pathogénie et l'hygiène des Landes de l'arrondissement de Nérac. 30 pp. 4°. *Paris*, 1867, No. 168.

Mondini (Carolus). *De arteriarum tunicis. Dissertatio posthuma. 8 pp. 4°. *Bononiæ, ex typ. Annesii nobili*, 1817. [P., v. 1586.]

Mondini (Francesco). Osservazioni sul nero pigmento dell' occhio. 12 pp., 1 pl. 4°. *Bologna, stampe di Annesio Nobili*, 1818. [P., v. 1586.]

Mondino (Casimiro). Ricerche macro e microscopiche sui centri nervosi. 70 pp., 10 l., 9 pl. 8°. *Torino, unione tip.-editrice*, 1887.

Mondino de Foro [Mundinus Friulensis] (*Julio*) [–1340].
[**Biography.**] Janus, Gotha, 1853, ii, 391.

Mondino [or Mondini] da Luzzi [Mundinus de Lentiis] [1250–1325 (?)]. Anathomia Mundini emendata per doctorem Melerstat. 40 l. 4°. [*n. p., n. d.*]
Probably printed at Leipzig about 1493.

——. The same. Incipit anothomia Mundini. [*Ad finem:*] Explicit anothomia Mundini que emendata fuit per . . . Francischum Picium in florentissimo gymnasio Ticiensi impressa Papie per Jacob de Paucisdrapis de Burgofrancho 1507. 22 l. sm. 4°.

——. The same. Anatomia Mundini, ad vetustissimorum, e[o]rundemque aliquot manuscriptorum codicum fidem collata, justoque suo ordini restituta per Joannem Dryandrum. Adjectæ sunt quorumcunque partium corporis ad vivum expressæ figuræ. Adsunt et scholia non indocta, quæ prolixorum commentariorum vice esse possunt. 3 p. l., 67 pp. 4°. *Marpurgi, in off. C. Engeholphi*, [1541].

——. De omnibus humani corporis interioribus membris anothomia. [*Ad finem:*] Impressit Argentinæ, Martinus Flach, 1513.
See, also, **Berengarius** *Carpus* (Jacobus). Commentaria . . . super anatomia Mundini [etc.] 4°. [*Bononiæ*, 1521.]—**de Ketam** [*or* Ketham] (Joannes). Fasciculus medicinæ in quo continentur [etc.] fol. *Venetiis*, 1495. ——. Fasciculus medicinæ praxis [etc.] fol. [*Venetiis*, 1522.]—**Mesue** *Damascenus* (Joannes). Mesue cum expositione Mondini super canones [etc.] fol. *Venetiis*, 1495. ——. The same. fol. *Venetiis*, 1502. ——. The same. fol. *Lugduni*, 1510. ——. Opera. fol. *Venetiis*, 1581. ——. The same. fol. *Venetiis*, 1589. ——. The same. fol. *Venetiis*, 1602. ——. The same. fol. *Venetiis*, 1623. ——. De consolatione medicinarum simplicium [etc.] fol. *Lugduni*. 1525.
For Biography, see Ann. Anat. & Surg., Brooklyn, N. Y., 1882, xi, 35; 71 (G. J. Fisher). *Also:* Janus, Gotha, 1853, ii, 390 (A. W. E. T. Henschel).

Mondinus (Franciscus). Bicorporei humani monstri anatomica descriptio, una cum animadversionibus atque conjecturis nonnullis quæ ad illustrandam abnormium partium formationis rationem concurrunt. 96 pp., 1 l., 4 pl. 4°. *Bononiæ, ex off. Emygdii ab Ulmo et J. Tiocchi*, 1833.

Mondo (Il) termale. Guida pratica illustrata alle acque minerali, stabilimenti termali, bagni di mare, soggiorni estivi ed invernali. Tabella

Mondo (Il) termale—continued.
delle malattie, con indicazione della cura balneoclimatica. xcvi pp. 16°. *Milano*, [1887].

Mondon (L.-Clément). *Contribution à la chirurgie d'armée. 69 pp. 4°. *Paris, H. Jouve*, 1886, No. 252.

Mondon (Paul-Mathieu). *Températures locales et phthisie pulmonaire. [Paris.] 72 pp., 2 l. 4°. *Le Mans*, 1884, No. 312.

Mondorf.
MARCHAL (C.) Observations cliniques sur l'action des eaux de Mondorf employées isolément ou associées à l'hydrothérapie rationnelle. 8°. *Paris*, 1870.
Schmit. Étude sur les actions physiologique et thérapeutique de la source thermale de Mondorf. Bull. Soc. d. sc. méd. du gr.-duché de Luxemb., 1869, 113–135.

Mondot & Séguy (Georges). Le choléra en Espagne et les vaccinations anticholériques du docteur Ferrán. 14 pp. 8°. *Oran, A. Fouque & Cie.*, 1885.

Mondot (Émile). *Études sur le Sénégal. 34 pp. 4°. *Paris*, 1865, No. 270.

Mondot (Jean-Baptiste-Louis). *Étude sur la colique sèche, d'après des observations recueillies pendant une campagne de trois ans, dans les mers de Chine et de Cochinchine (du 22 février 1860 au 10 juillet 1863). vi, 7–70 pp. 4°. *Montpellier, Gras*, 1864. [P., v. 45.]

——. De la stérilité chez la femme. vii, 400 pp. 8°. *Paris, J.-B. Baillière & fils*, 1880.

Mondragon (Justiniano). *Valor semiotico de las alteraciones del dynamismo neumocardiaco. 22 pp. 8°. *México, J. Escalante*, 1874.

Mondragone.
Albini (G.) Nota su le acque termo-minerali di Monte Marsico, presso Mondragone. Rendic. Accad. med.-chir. di Napoli, 1868, xxii, 142–144.

Mondville (G.-E.-Auxence). *Sur la rage spontanée produite par des affections morales. 25 pp. 4°. *Paris*, 1821, No. 197, v. 168.

Mone (F. J.) Ueber Armen- und Krankenpflege früherer Zeit, mit Urkunden. 101 pp. 8°. *Karlsruhe, G. Braun*, 1861.

Mone (Franciscus Josephus). Historia statisticæ adumbrata. Præmissa est oratio de optimo genere tractandæ statisticæ deque hujus doctrinæ utilitate. viii, 200 pp. 4°. *Lovanii, F. Michel*, 1828.

Monégier-Sorbier (M.-P.) *Sur l'anasarque. 43 pp. 4°. *Paris*, 1814, No. 118, v. 104.

Moneglia (Gio. Andrea).
See **Ramazzini** (Gioseffo). Controversia medico-letteraria. 4°. *Modena*, 1758.

Monell (Gilbert C.) [1816–81]. Rheumatism, acute and chronic. A prize essay. 144 pp. 8°. *New York, H. G. Langley*, 1845.
For Biography, see Proc. Nebraska M. Soc., Omaha, 1883, 42–44.

Monera.
Häckel (E.) Monographie der Moneren. Jenaische Ztschr. f. Med. u. Naturw., Leipz., 1868, iv, 64, 2 pl. : 1870–71, vi, 23, 1 pl.

de Monès (Jean-Joseph-Éliacim). *Hygiène de la première année de la vie. 43 pp. 4°. *Paris*, 1840, No. 339, v. 363.

Monesia.
See, also, **Diarrhœa** (*Treatment of*).
BERNARD-DEROSNE. Notice sur le monésia. 8°. *Paris*, [1840].
See, also, infra.
Adrien. [Sur l'emploi du monésia.] J. d. conn. méd.-chir., Par., 1840–41, viii, pt. 1, 197–200. *Also:* Ann. de méd. belge, Brux., 1840, iv, 159–162. ——. Mémoire sur les effets thérapeutiques du monésia. J. d. conn. méd.-chir., Par., 1842–3, x, pt. 1, 133–137. — **Bernard-Derosne** [*et al.*]. Examen chimique et médical du monésia. *Ibid.*, 1840–41, viii, pt. 2, 3–20. [*See, also, supra.*]—**Bonetti** (E.) Esperienze terapentiche fatte colla monesia. Ann. univ. di med., Milano, 1841, xcvii, 646-648.—**Buchey** (E.) Du

Monesia.

monésia et des bons effets de son administration dans les affections scrofuleuses, etc. J. d. conn. méd.-chir., Par., 1839–40, vii, pt. 2, 157–159. *Also, transl.: Encicl. méd.-farm., Barcel., 1877, i, 52; 64.*—**Burnes** (R.) On the use of monesia. Med. Exam., Phila., 1840, iii, 517.—**Caminhoá** (J. M.) Parecer dos lentes da faculdade de medicina da côrte sobre o chicle do Canadá. Ann. Brasil. de med., Rio de Jan., 1876-7, xxviii, 136–140.—**Donovan** (M.) On the new medicine, monesia. Dublin M. Press, 1840, iii, 83.—**Forget.** Recherches chimiques et cliniques sur un nouveau médicament appelé monésia. Bull. gén. de thérap., etc., Par., 1839, xvi, 199–204. *Also:* Gaz. d. hôp., Par., 1839, 2. s., i, 193.—**Guibert.** Étude sur la monésia. Syn.: Cortex astringens brasiliensis; Cortex Buranhem. Rev. de thérap. méd.-chir., Par., 1867, 286–290.—**Halbout.** Nouvelles observations pratiques sur les effets thérapeutiques du monésia. J. d. conn. méd.-chir., Par., 1845-6, xiii, pt. 1, 20.—**Kappelhoff** (A.) Waarnemingen met het extractum monesiæ. [4 obs.] Boerhaave. Tijdschr., etc., Amst., 1842, n. s., i, 199–211.—**Lane** (A.) The extract of monesia. Lond. M. Gaz., 1843-4, xxxiii, 45.—**Laurand** (A.) Note sur le monésia. J. d. conn. méd.-chir., Par., 1846-7, xiv, pt. 1, 109–111.—**Martin-Saint-Ange** (G.-J.) De l'emploi du monésia en médecine. Gaz. méd. de Par., 1839, 2. s., vii, 661–664.—**Mascherpa** (G.) Esperienze cliniche fatte coll' estratto di monesia. Gazz. med. di Milano, 1843, ii, 401: 1846, v, 333.—**Nancrede** (J. G.) Remarks on the monesia. Med. Exam., Phila., 1840, iii, 215.

Monestier (Jules). * De la pustule maligne. 64 pp., 1 l. 4°. *Montpellier*, 1876, No. 52.

Monestier-de-Briançon.

Lacour (E.) Analyse des eaux minérales du Monestier de Briançon. Rec. de mém. de méd. . . . mil., Par., 1877, 3. s., xxxiii, 540–543.—**Poggiale.** Eau minérale du Monetier de Briançon (Hautes-Alpes). Bull. Acad. de méd., Par., 1879, 2. s., viii, 275.—**Tripier** (F.-M.) Analyse des eaux thermales du Monestier-de-Briançon. Rec. de mém. de méd. . . . mil., Par., 1835, xxxvii, 365–376.

de Monestrol (J.) La goutte. Mémoire sur les causes des maladies goutteuses et sur leur traitement par la méthode homœopathique. 95 pp. 8°. *Paris, J.-B. Baillière*, 1855.

——. De l'homœopathie en dehors des préjugés de ses adversaires et des exagérations de ses partisans. 71 pp. 12°. *Paris, J.-B. Baillière & fils*, 1861. [*Also, in:* P., v. 1455.]

See, also, **Perrussel** (C.) & **de Monestrol** [J.] De l'homœopathie, de sa doctrine, de ses prescriptions et du régime à suivre pendant le traitement des maladies aiguës ou chroniques. 3. éd. 12°. *Paris*, 1853.

de Monet, *Chevalier de Lamarck.* See **Lamarck** (Jean-Baptiste-Pierre-Antoine de Monet).

de Moneta (Christian Jakob) [–1792]. Abhandlung, dass die Kälte und das kalte Wasser in Catharrkrankheiten und Catharrhusten wahre Heilmittel sind. 3 p. l., 63 pp. 18°. *Warschau, M. Gröll*, 1779.

Monette (John W.) The epidemic yellow fevers of Natchez. An essay. 83 pp. 12°. *Natchez, Clarke, Newcomb & Crail*, 1838.

——. Observations on the epidemic yellow fever of Natchez and of the Southwest. 155 pp. 8°. *Louisville, Ky., Prentice & Weissinger*, 1842.

Money (Angel). Treatment of disease in children, including the outlines of diagnosis and the chief pathological differences between children and adults. xiii, 560 pp. 12°. *London, H. K. Lewis*, 1887.

——. The same. xiii, 560 pp. 8°. *Philadelphia, P. Blakiston, Son & Co.*, 1887.

Money (W.) A vade-mecum of morbid anatomy, medical and chirurgical, with pathological observations and symptoms. 2. ed. viii, 4, 51 pp., 1 l., 48 pl. 8°. *London, Burgess & Hill*, 1831.

Monfalcon (Jean-Baptiste) [1792–1874]. Mémoire sur l'état actuel de la chirurgie, ou précis des théories, procédés opératoires, bandages, cas rares, etc., publiés depuis la suppression de l'Académie royale de chirurgie. ix, 213 pp. 8°. *Paris, Lévèque*, 1816.

——. * De l'influence que l'âge exerce sur l'habilité du médecin. 9 pp. 4°. *Paris*, 1818, No. 164, v. 141.

Monfalcon (Jean-Baptiste)—continued.

——. Histoire médicale des marais, et traité des fièvres intermittentes causées par les émanations des eaux stagnantes. 2. éd. 528 pp. 8°. *Paris, Béchet jeune*, 1826.

——. Précis de bibliographie médicale. viii, 552 pp., 5 l. 16°. *Paris, Baillière*, 1827.

See, also, **Chervin** (Nicolas). Lettre à . . . sur la fièvre jaune [etc.] 8°. *Paris*, 1830.—**Terme** (J.-F.) & **Monfalcon** (J.-B.) Histoire statistique et morale des enfants trouvés [etc.] 8°. *Paris*, 1837. ——. Nouvelles considérations sur les enfants trouvés [etc.] 8°. *Paris*, 1838. ——. Histoire des enfants trouvés. 8°. *Paris*, 1840.

For Biography, see J. d. conn. méd. prat., Par., 1875, xlii, (A. Jeandet). *Also,* Reprint. *Also:* Lyon méd., 1874, xvii, 495–497 (A. Lacour).

—— & **de Polinière** (A.-P.-I) Hygiène de la ville de Lyon, ou opinions et rapports du conseil de salubrité du département du Rhône. xv, 377 pp. 8°. *Paris, J.-B. Baillière*, 1845.

——. Traité de la salubrité dans les grandes villes, suivi de l'hygiène de Lyon. viii, 10–551 pp. 8°. *Paris, J.-B. Baillière*, 1846.

Monfalcone.

Gorcy. Mémoire physique et médical sur la source thermale de Monte-Falcone, dans le Frioul. Rec. de mém. de méd. . . . mil., Par., 1817, iii, 221–255.—**Gruber** (I.) Authentische Notizen über die Bäder zu Monfalcone, aus dem italienischen Manuscripte übersetzt. Med. Jahrb. d. k. k. österr. Staates, Wien, 1839, n. F., xix, 393–396.—**von Hauer** (C.) Die warme Quelle von Monfalcone nächst Triest. Ztschr. d. k.-k. Gesellsch. d. Aerzte zu Wien, 1858, n. F., i, 690–694.

Monfange (Pierre-Désiré). * Sur le catarrhe des organes génitaux considéré chez la femme. 19 pp. 4°. *Paris*, 1816, No. 154, v. 124.

Monferrato (Jean-Fr.) * Du phlegmon des gaînes synoviales de la paume de la main. 48 pp., 1 l. 4°. *Paris*, 1879, No. 349.

Monfeuillard (Claude-Marie-Adolphe). * Sur la rage, considérée chez l'homme et les animaux. 32 pp. 4°. *Paris*, 1836, No. 33, v. 295.

Monfeuillard (Pierre-Ernest). * De l'emploi des iodures dans le traitement de l'albuminurie. 56 pp. 4°. *Paris*, 1869, No. 138.

Monfort (N.-G.) * Quelques propositions sur divers points de médecine. 16 pp. 4°. *Paris, an XII* [1804], No. 324, v. 51.

Monfrin (Benoît). * Considérations générales sur les maladies endémiques de la Basse-Bresse et de la Dombes, département de l'Ain. 1 p. l., 35 pp. 4°. *Strasbourg, F. G. Levrault*, 1817.

de Monfumat (Gabriel). * Études sur les polypes de l'utérus. 120 pp. 4°. *Paris*, 1867, No. 67.

——. The same. 115 pp., 2 l. 8°. *Paris, A. Asselin*, 1867.

Mongeal (Joseph). * De la syncope, considérée dans ses rapports avec la physiologie, la séméiologie et la thérapeutique. 35 pp. 4°. *Paris*, 1836, No. 89, v. 269.

Mongellaz (P.-J.) * Propositions sur les irritations intermittentes. vi, 7–31 pp. 4°. *Paris*, 1820, No. 214, v. 161.

——. Sur les irritations intermittentes, ou nouvelle théorie des maladies périodiques, fièvres larvées, fièvres pernicieuses, et des fièvres intermittentes en général. Exposé suivant la doctrine de M. Broussais, et appuyée d'un grand nombre d'observations. 2 v. xv, 464 pp.; 465–859 pp., 1 l. 8°. *Paris, Méquignon-Marvis*, 1821.

——. The same. Monographie des irritations intermittentes, ou traité théorique et pratique des maladies périodiques, des fièvres larvées, locales ou topiques, des fièvres pernicieuses, des fièvres rémittentes et intermittentes bénignes des auteurs et en général de tout ce qui offre de l'intermittence ou de la périodicité en pathologie. Nouv. éd. 2 v. 714 pp.; xv, 441 pp. 8°. *Bruxelles, Soc. enc. d. sci. méd.*, 1839.

Mongellaz (P.-J.)—continued.
——. Réflexions sur la théorie physiologique des fièvres intermittentes et des maladies périodiques. 178 pp. 8°. *Paris, Delaunay*, 1825.
——. L'art de conserver sa santé et de prévenir les maladies héréditaires, ou l'hygiène, appliquée à tous les âges, tous les sexes, tous les tempéramens, suivant les saisons et les professions diverses. xxiii, 624 pp. 8°. *Paris, Méquignon-Marvis*, 1828.

Mongenot (L.-A.) De la vaccine, considérée comme antidote de la petite vérole, avec un tableau de vaccinations, indiquant les noms, prénoms, âge, sexe et demeure des vaccinés; la date et la marche de leur vaccination; le nombre des piqûres faites à chaque bras; le nom des personnes qui ont fourni la matière, et les divers phénomènes qui ont eu lieu. xiv, 118 pp. 8°. *Paris, Méquignon l'aîné, an XI* 1802. [P., v. 1285; 1286.]

Mongeri (Louis). Études sur l'épidémie de choléra qui a régné à Constantinople en 1865, suivies d'un appendice sur la nature contagieuse du choléra et des devoirs des médecins sanitaires. 2 p. l., 102 pp., 1 map. 8°. *Constantinople, M. de Castro*, 1866. [P., v. 215.]
——. Notice statistique sur l'asile des aliénés "Solimanié" à Constantinople pour la période de dix ans comprise entre le 1er mars 1857, v. s., et le 28 février 1867, v. s. 58 pp. 8°. *Constantinople, M. de Castro*, 1867.

Monges (*John Armentaire*) [1858–1827].
Nancrede (J. G.) Obituary notice of John Armentaire Monges. Phila. J. M. & Phys. Sc., 1827, xiv, 338-343.

Mongibeaux (François). *De l'hémorrhagie cérébrale. 32 pp. 4°. *Paris*, 1848, No. 137, v. 475.

Mongie (Jules). *De l'aphasie. 54 pp., 2 l. 4°. *Paris*, 1866, No. 111.

Mongin (Jules-Laurent). *I. Symptômes du ramollissement sénile des centres nerveux. II. [etc.] 36 pp. 4°. *Paris*, 1838, No. 390, v. 331.

Mongin-Montrol (Charles). *Sur l'hypochondrie. 31 pp. 4°. *Paris*, 1823, No. 26, v. 177. [*Also, in*: P., v. 1640.]

[de Monginot (François).] De la guérison des fièvres par le quinquina. 146 pp., 1 l. 16°. *Paris, R. Guignard*, 1680.
——. The same. 4. éd. 1 p. l., 140 pp., 1 l. 16°. *Lyon, A. Briasson*, 1681.
——. The same. De febrium curatione per usum quinquinæ. *In*: FEBRIS china chinæ [etc.] 4°. *Ferrariæ*, 1687, 49-86.

Monginot (Louis-Eugène). *Des tumeurs syphilitiques des muscles et des tendons. 20 pp. 4°. *Paris*, 1851, No. 205, v. 512.

Mongird (Florentin). *Cancer du péritoine. 55 pp. 4°. *Paris*, 1884, No. 274.

Mongius (Joannes Paulus).
See **Avicenna.** Libri in re medica omnes [etc.] fol. *Venetiis*, 1564. ——. Arabum medicorum principis [etc.] fol. *Venetiis*, 1595.

Monglond (Henri). *De l'oignon, ou déviation du gros orteil. 37 pp., 1 l., 1 pl. 4°. *Paris*, 1876, No. 178.

Mongrand (E.) *Le bagne de Brest, considéré au point de vue hygiénique et médical. 66 pp. 4°. *Paris*, 1856, No. 55, v. 594.

Mongruel (L.-P.) Prodiges et merveilles de l'esprit humain sous l'influence magnétique. Verité du magnétisme, dégagée de toute exagération; son influence sur nos facultés, sur nos sens, sur nos organes matériels. Ce que c'est que le somnambulisme, [etc.] 92 pp. 18°. *Paris, chez l'auteur*, 1849. [*Also, in*: P.. v. 1255.]
Bound with: RICARD (J.-J.-A.) Lettres d'un magnétiseur. 16°. *Paris*, 1843.

Mongs (Peter). *Ueber Parotis-Tumoren. [Wurtzburg.] 31 pp. 8°. *M. Gladbach, E. Schnellmann*, [1886?]

Monguidi (Coriolano). Sulla ghiandola timo; ricerche di anatomia normale. 31 pp., 2 pl., 1 l. 8°. *Parma, L. Battei*, 1885.

Monguillem (Pierre). *De l'empoisonnement par les braises résultant de la combustion des bois peints. 72 pp. 4°. *Bordeaux*, 1884, 6. s., No. 21.

Monheim (Joh.-Peter-Joseph). Analyse des eaux thermales de Borcette, suivie de l'examen du gaz azote sulfuré dégagé des sources sulfureuses tant d'Aix-la-Chapelle que de Borcette. vii, 63 pp. 8°. *Aix-la-Chapelle, Schwartzenberg*, 1811.
——. Die Heilquellen von Aachen, Burtscheid, Spaa, Malmedy und Heilstein, in ihren historischen, geognostischen, physischen, chemischen und medizinischen Beziehungen. vii, 411 pp., 1 pl., 1 map. 8°. *Aachen u. Leipzig, J. A. Mayer*, 1829.
See, also, **von Sartorius** (G.) & **Monheim** (J. P. J.) Medicinisch-chemische Untersuchung einer an dreien Personen [etc.] 8°. *Cöln u. Aachen*, 1826.
For Portrait, see **Collection**—van Kaathoven.

Monier (Anne-François). *Aperçu physiologique sur les prédominances organiques relatives aux âges, considérées comme causes prédisposantes des maladies. 31 pp. 4°. *Paris*, 1825, No. 94, v. 192. [*Also, in*: P., v. 1576.]

Monier (Eugène)[1]. *Des résultats fournis par la médication salicylée en Angleterre dans le traitement du rhumatisme articulaire aigu. 60 pp. 4°. *Paris*, 1877, No. 87.

Monier (Eugène)[2] [1853–]. *Complications et conséquences de l'opération de l'empyème. 1 p. l., 97 pp. 4°. *Paris*, 1881, No. 288.

Monier (Gaston) [1850–]. *Influence des états constitutionnels et des altérations viscérales sur le traumatisme soit accidentel, soit chirurgical. [Paris.] 64 pp. 4°. *Havre*, 1885, No. 102.

Monier (Jules). *I. De l'influence du liquide spinal sur les fonctions de la moelle épinière. II. [etc.] 24 pp. 4°. *Paris*, 1841, No. 108, v. 378.

Monier (Louis-Ernest). *De la contusion des articulations. 39 pp. 4°. *Paris*, 1847, No. 183, v. 462.

Moniez (Romain-Louis). *Essai monographique sur les cysticerques. 190 pp., 1 l., 3 pl. 4°. *Lille, L. Danel*, 1880, No. 19.

Monin (Ernest). *Essai critique sur la pathogénie et l'étiologie des oreillons. 41 pp., 1 l. 4°. *Paris*, 1877, No. 540.
——. Obésité et maigreur. Essai d'hygiène pratique. 20 pp. 8°. *Paris*, 1882.
——. Publications de la Société française d'hygiène. La propreté de l'individu et de la maison. 44 pp., 1 l. 8°. *Paris*, 1884.
——. Un nouveau chapitre de séméiologie. Essai sur les odeurs du corps humain dans l'état de santé et dans l'état de maladie. Mémoire couronné par la Société de médecine pratique. [Prix biennal 1885.] 122 pp., 1 l. 12°. *Paris, G. Carré*, 1885.
——. Les propos du docteur, médecine sociale, hygiène générale à l'usage des gens du monde. ii, 324 pp. 8°. *Paris, E. Giraud & Cie.*, 1885.
——. L'hygiène de la beauté; formulaire cosmétique. Ouvrage précédé d'une lettre de Catulle Mendès. 1 p. l., xiv, 220 pp. 12°. *Paris, O. Doin*, 1886.
——. Les maladies épidémiques; hygiène et prévention. 175 pp. 18°. *Paris, Alcan*, 1887.
—— & **Maréchal** (Ph.) Stefano Merlatti; histoire d'un jeûne célèbre, précédée d'une étude anecdotique, physiologique et médicale sur le

Monin (Ernst) & **Maréchal** (Ph.)—cont'd.
jeûne et les jeûneurs. 2 p. l., 257 pp., 1 l. 12°.
Paris, C. Marpon & E. Flammarion, [1887].

Monin (Fréd.) Essai sur les eaux minérales de
Saint-Alban (Loire). 2. éd. 39 pp. 8°. *Lyon,
Mégret,* 1866.

——. Le bréviaire du médecin, précis de médecine rurale, d'économie et de philosophie médicales. Nouv. éd. xi, 386 pp., 1 l. 8°. *Paris,
J.-B. Baillière & fils,* 1869.

Monin (Marius-Eustache). * Des moyens de division des parties molles considérés au point de
vue de la douleur, de l'hémorrhagie et l'infection
purulente. 82 pp., 1 l. 4°. *Montpellier,* 1875,
No. 66.

Monin (Romain). * Considérations sur les
épanchemens dans l'intérieur du crâne par
causes externes. 25 pp. 4°. *Paris,* 1815, No.
200, v. 114.

Monique (Marc) [1859–]. * Des principales
applications de l'acide acétique, l'acide pyro-
ligneux rectifié, dans le traitement de la teigne
tondante et de quelques autres affections cutanées. 78 pp. 4°. *Paris,* 1883.

Moniteur (Le). Journal de médecine, de chi-
rurgie et de thérapeutique, paraissant les 1er, 8,
16 et 24 chaque mois sous la direction du docteur
P. Ménière (d'Angers). Année 1–2 (Nos. 1–45),
March 1, 1876, to June 1, 1877. 8°. *Paris, V.-
A. Delahaye & Cie.*
Issued semi-monthly in March to Oct., 1876. v. 1 ended
Dec. 24, 1876; v. 2 commenced Jan., 1877.

Moniteur (Le) des hôpitaux. Journal des progrès de la médecine et de la chirurgie pratiques,
rédigé par H. de Castelnau. Paraît 3 fois par
semaine. v. 1–9; Nos. 1–42, v. 10, Jan. 1, 1853,
to April 10, 1862. 4°. *Paris.*
Ended. In v. 4–10 subtitle, "Revue médico-chirurgicale de Paris". Suspended by decree of court, Aug. 11,
1859; continued, Aug. 23, 1859, as: **Moniteur** (Le) des
sciences médicales et pharmaceutiques, forming a 2. s. of
the periodical; v. 7 being composed, in part, of v. 1, 2. s.

Moniteur de l'hygiène publique.
Is subtitle of: **Médecin** (Le) in 1885 et seq.

Moniteur d'hygiène et de salubrité publique,
domestique, agricole, industrielle. Journal paraissant tous les mois sous la direction de A.
Chevallier fils. Année 1–4, Jan., 1866, to Nov.,
1869. 8°. *Paris.*
Want no. 2, v. 2; no. 10, v. 3; no. 12, v. 4.

Moniteur de la pharmacie belge. Organe des
intérêts professionnels. J. Fargeix, directeur.
[Monthly.] v. 1–8, July, 1880–87. 8°. *Bruxelles.*
Current. v. 1 complete in 6 nos., July to Dec., 1880; v.
2 commenced Jan., 1881.

Moniteur de la policlinique.
Is subtitle of: **Médecin** (Le), in 1878–85.

Moniteur (Le) de la santé; annales de l'hydrothérapie scientifique. [Semi-monthly.] Nos. 1–
2, année 1, March 12, 30, 1874. 32 pp. fol.
Paris.
Concurso.

Moniteur de la santé publique.
Is subtitle of: **Médecin** (Le), in 1875–8.

Moniteur (Le) des sciences médicales et phar-
maceutiques.
Was title of v. 7–10 of: **Moniteur** (Le) des hôpitaux,
Aug. 23, 1859, to April 10, 1862.

Moniteur (Le) scientifique. Journal des sciences
pures et appliquées. Compte-rendu des académies et sociétés savantes et revue des progrès
accomplis dans les sciences mathématiques, physiques et naturelles; travaux publiés à l'étranger;
revue des inventions nouvelles et industrie manu-
facturière des arts chimiques; journal mensuel
fondé et dirigé par le Dr. Quesneville. Première
série, v. 1–5, 1857–63 [7 années en 5 volumes];
2. s., v. 1–7, 1864–70; 3. s., v. 1–16, 1871–86; 4.
s., v. 1–3, 1888. 30 v. roy. 8°. *Paris.*
Current. In 1887, 2 v. annually.

Moniteur (Le) thérapeutique. Recueil mensuel des médications nouvelles. Directeur-gé-
rant: Édouard Pierre. Rédacteur en chef: Dr.
Duleau. Année 1–14, Oct., 1873–87. 8°. *Paris.*
Current. v. 5 complete in 15 nos., Oct., 1877, to Dec.,
1878; v. 6 commenced Jan., 1879.

Monitor (El) médico. Órgano de los intereses
científicos y profesionales del cuerpo médico.
Publicado bajo la proteccion de la Academia
libre de medicina de Lima. Redactor en jefe:
José Casimiro Ulloa. [Semi-monthly.] v. 1–3,
June 1, 1885, to Sept., 1887. sm. fol. *Lima.*
Current.

Monitor (El) médico-farmacéutico. Periódico
mensual de medicina, cirugía y farmacia. Director: E. Molina. No. 1, v. 1, April, 1883. 32
pp. 8°. *Nueva York.*
No more published.

Monitor (El) médico-farmacéutico ó industrial.
Periódico destinado á promover los intereses morales, científicos y materiales del Cuerpo médico-
farmacéutico ó industrial de Michoacan y los
particulares de la casa Atanasio Mier que lo pública. [Monthly.] v. 1, 1887. 4°. *Morelia,
México.*
Current. Each number paged separately.

Monitor (El) de la salud. Revista quincenal de
higiene pública, y de higiene y medicina domés-
ticas, [etc.] Publicada bajo la direccion del
Cárlos Ronquillo. Año 1–5, May 15, 1880, to
Dec. 30, 1884. 4°. *Barcelona.*
A supplement to: **Enciclopedia** médico-farmacéutica. v. 2 commenced Jan., 1881.

Monitor (El) de la salud de las familias y de la
salubridad de los pueblos. Revista de higiene
pública y privada; de medicina y economía do-
mésticas; de policía urbana y rural, etc. Publicada bajo la direccion del doctor Pedro Felípe
Monlau, con la colaboracion de varios profesores
y escritores distinguidos. [Semi-monthly.] v.
1–7, 1858–64. roy. 8°. *Madrid, C. Bailly-Bail-
lière.*

Monitore dei farmacisti. Si pubblica tutte le
domeniche. Antonio Corsi, responsabile. Nos.
1–25, anno 1, June 5 to Nov. 20, 1887. fol.
Roma.
Current. Each number paged separately.

Monitore (Il) medico-chirurgico. Giornale dei
medici comunali, diretto dal Dott. Norberto Perotti, [et al.]. [Semi-monthly.] Nos. 1–12, anno
1, Jan. 5 to June 20, 1884. 192 pp. 8°. *Ariccia.*

Monitore (Il) terapeutico. Raccolta mensile di
rimedi nuovi e ricette, diretto dal Dott. Nicola de
Dominicis. Anno 1–4, 1884–7. 8°. *Napoli.*
Current.

Moniz Sodré de Aragão (Egas Carlos).
* Funcções do grande sympathico. 53 pp. 4°.
Bahia, imp. na typog. do Diario, 1871.
Concurso.

——. * Diathese. 2 p. l., 105 pp. 4°. *Bahia,
typog. do Diario,* 1874.
Concurso.

Monjé (Joannes Jacobus). * De animi pathematibus, eorumque effectibus; necnon salutari
eorundem in morbis efficacia. 2 p. l., 33 pp., 1 l.
4°. *Lugd. Bat., A. et J. Honkoop et A. Koster,*
1785.

Monjou (Eugène). * Essai sur l'accouchement
prématuré artificiel considéré principalement au
point de vue des indications. 73 pp., 1 l. 4°.
Montpellier, 1873, No. 45.

Monk (Thomas H.) Outlines of a scheme for the
registration of the state of health, showing: 1.
The information which it is proposed to obtain; 2.
The method in which it is to be obtained; 3.
How it is to be utilized; 4. The benefits which
will be derived from it. 2 l. 4°. [*Toronto,*
1881.]

Monkewitz (Johann Heinrich). * Chemisch-medicinische Untersuchung über die Wandflechte (Lichen parietinus) und über die gebräuchlichsten Chinarinden. Eine akademische Streitschrift. 38 pp. 8°. *Dorpat, J. C. Schünmann,* 1817.

Monkeys.
See **Apes,** *etc.*

van Monkhoven (D.) Photography on collodion. 1 p. l., 54 pp. 8°. *New-York, H. H. Snelling,* 1856.

Monks.
BUXTORF (J. L.) Cura valetudinis religiosorum, ad normam naturæ, secundum rationis et experientiæ dictamen breviter delineata. 8°. *Basileæ,* 1768.
——. The same. 16°. *Basileæ,* 1770.

Monkur (*John C. S.*)
Portrait in : **Collection** of Portr. (Libr.)

Monlau (José). Nociones de fisiología é higiene con las nociones de anatomía humana correspondientes; obra escrita para uso de la juventud escolar, y estudio de la asignatura establecida en el plan vigente de estudios de segunda enseñanza, y revisada por Pedro Felípe Monlau. 3. ed. vi, 7–314 pp. 12°. *Madrid, M. Rivadeneyra,* 1872.

Monlau (Pedro Felípe) [1808–71]. Elementos de higiene pública. 2 v. xi, 468 pp. ; 471–894 pp. 8°. *Barcelona, D. P. Riera,* 1847.
——. The same. Arte de conservar la salud de los pueblos. 2. ed. revista, aumentada con un compendio de la legislacion sanitaria de España. 3 v. 12°. *Madrid, M. Rivadeneyra,* 1862.
——. The same. 3. ed. 2 v. viii, 368 pp.; 373–770 pp., 1 l. 8°. *Madrid, M. Rivadeneyra,* 1871.
——. Higiene de los baños de mar, ó instrucciones para su uso puramente higiénico, así como para el terapéutico ó curativo en las muchas enfermedades contra las cuales tienen probada eficacia, y manual práctico del bañista. xvi, 522 pp., 1 l. 12°. *Madrid, M. Rivadeneyra,* 1869.
——. Le mariage dans ses devoirs, ses rapports, et ses effets conjugaux au point de vue légal, hygiénique, physiologique et moral. Traduction libre refondue, corrigée et augmentée de: L'higiene del matrimonio, du docteur . . . par le Dr. P. Garnier. xxii pp., 1 l., 629 pp. 12°. *Paris, Garnier frères,* 1879.
Also, Editor of : **Monitor** (El) de la salud de las familias y de la salubridad de los pueblos, Madrid, 1858–64.
See, also, **Monlau** (José). Nociones de fisiología é higiene, etc. 12°. *Madrid,* 1872.—**Velpeau** (Alf. A. L. M.) Elementos de obstetricia. 8°. *Barcelona,* 1833.
For Biography, see Independ. méd., Barcel., 1870–71, ii, 116 ; 129 ; 141 (C. Ronquillo).

Monlaud (H.) * Propositions de médecine et de chirurgie. 16 pp. 8°. *Paris,* 1830, No. 179, v. 234.

Monlaud (Ph.-H.-Ch.) * Sur la puberté chez la femme. 23 pp. 4°. *Paris,* 1831, No. 165, v. 242.

Monlien (Adolphe-Frédéric). * Sur la métrite, ou inflammation de la matrice. 25 pp. 4°. *Paris,* 1819, No. 227, v. 151.

Monmouth.
PIRRIE [W.] Report on the sanitary condition of Monmouth. March 28, 1872. fol. *London,* 1872.

Monne (N.-B.) * Propositions de médecine et de chirurgie. 12 pp. 4°. *Paris,* 1823, No. 103, v. 180.

Monneins (François). * Sur la cystite chronique. 41 pp. 4°. *Paris,* 1833, No. 225, v. 262.

Monnereau [1847–]. * Recherches expérimentales sur le rôle de l'absorption cutanée dans l'intoxication et la paralysie saturnines. 60 pp. 4°. *Paris,* 1883, No. 320.

Monnereau (Pierre-Prosper). * De l'existence des maladies générales. 23 pp. 4°. *Paris,* 1837, No. 259, v. 314.

Monneret (A.) * Traitement de l'ophthalmie scrophuleuse. 60 pp., 1 l. 4°. *Montpellier, P. Grollier,* 1871, No. 66.

Monneret (Jules-Édouard-Auguste) [1810–68]. * Considérations générales sur les épidémies. 40 pp. 4°. *Paris,* 1833, No. 213, v. 262.
——. * Déterminer la part des causes occasionnelles dans la production des maladies. 63 pp. 4°. *Paris, Rignoux & Cie.,* 1838.
Concours.
——. Lettre sur le choléra-morbus en Orient et dans le nord de l'Europe. 29 pp. 8°. *Paris, E. Thunot & Cie.,* [1848]. [*Also, in :* P., v. 461.]
Repr. from : Gaz. méd. de Par., 1848, 3. s., iii.
——. Mémoire sur l'ondulation pectorale dans l'état physiologique et dans les maladies. 20 pp. 8°. *Paris, P. Dupont,* [1848?] [P., v. 465.]
Repr. from : Rev. méd.-chir. de Par., 1848, iv.
——. Note sur le choléra-morbus observé à Constantinople en 1847 et 1848. 16 pp. 8°. *Paris, J.-B. Baillière,* 1848.
——. * La goutte et le rhumatisme. 112 pp. 8°. *Paris, Rignoux,* 1851.
Concours.
——. De l'emploi du sous-azotate de bismuth à haute dose dans le traitement de diverses maladies. 32 pp. 8°. [*Paris, Hennuyer,* 1854.] [P., v. 1654.]
Repr. from : Bull. gén. de thérap., etc., Par., 1854, xlvii.
——. Du cancer du foie. 33 pp. 8°. *Paris, Rignoux,* 1855.
Repr. from : Arch. gén. de méd., Par., 1855, 6. s., v.
——. Traité de pathologie générale. 3 v. 8°. *Paris, B. Jeune,* 1857–61.
v. 3 in 2 pts.
——. De l'ictère hémorrhagique essentiel. 35 pp. 8°. *Paris, W. Remquet & Cie.,* 1859. [*Also, in :* P., v. 1666.]
Repr. from : Progrès, Par.
——. Des congestions dans les fièvres. 20 pp. 8°. *Paris, Rignoux,* [1860].
Repr. from : Arch. gén. de méd., Par., 1860, 6. s., xv.
——. Programme du cours de pathologie interne, fait à la Faculté de médecine de Paris pendant les années scolaires de 1861, 1862, 1863. Années 1–3. 170, 120 pp. 8°. *Paris, Béchet jeune,* 1861–3.
——. Traité élémentaire de pathologie interne. 3 v. 8°. *Paris, P. Asselin,* 1864–6.
CONTENTS.
v. 1. Maladies locales; du système nerveux; des organes de la circulation; de la respiration; de la digestion et du foie.
v. 2. Maladies du pancréas, des reins, de l'utérus, du péritoine, de la peau; des affections diathésiques; maladies virulentes; maladies syphilitiques; morve; rage; maladies venimeuses.
v. 3. Affections toxiques, ou empoisonnements; maladies du sang; maladies puerpérales; maladies paludéennes; fièvres essentielles; algidites.
——. Notice biographique sur les travaux scientifiques de Natalis Guillot. 3 pp. 8°. *Paris, F. Malteste & Cie.,* [1866].
Repr. from : Union méd., Par., 1866, 2. s., xxxvi.
See, also, **de Laberge** (Alexandre-Louis) & **Monneret** (J.-É.-A.) Compendium de médecine pratique [etc.] 8°. *Paris,* 1836–46.—**Pintado y Jordan** (Galo). Piretologia [etc.] 8°. *Madrid,* 1871.

Monnerot (Amynthe). * Considérations générales sur les maladies endémiques observées à l'hôpital du Gabon, pendant l'année 1864–5. 47 pp. 4°. *Montpellier, Boehm & fils,* 1868, No. 24.
c.

Monnet (Charles). Anatomie, ou la connoissance du corps humain détaillée dans chaque partie pour la facilité des personnes qui professent le dessin. Composée de 42 planches, d'après les

Monnet (Charles)—continued.
dessins originaux de . . . et la description générale des muscles, faite par Tanude. 42 pl. fol. *Paris, Jean, [n. d.]*

Monnet (L.-J.-F.) *Sur l'hystérie, appelée vulgairement vapeurs. 31 pp. 4°. *Paris,* 1808, No. 116, v. 72.

Monnet (Léon-Ernest). *De la kola (Sterculia acuminata); étude physiologique et thérapeutique. [Paris.] 106 pp., 1 l. 4°. *Lille,* 1884, No. 1.

Monnett (H.) The magic monitor and medical intelligencer; containing wonderful and elaborate revelations concerning the following subjects: Love, courtship, and marriage; how to prevent an increase of family; how to cure self-abuse and its results; the detection, prevention, and cure of all private diseases, etc. viii, 9–256 pp., 6 pl. 18°. *New York, H. Monnett & Co.,* 1857.

Monnier (A.) *Sur les calculs biliaires. 20 pp. 4°. *Paris,* 1834, No: 89, v. 271.

Monnier (Achille). *Contribution à l'étude des lésions de l'intestin à la suite de contusions abdominales. 35 pp. 4°. *Paris,* 1877, No. 292.

Monnier (Alexandre). Histoire de l'assistance dans les temps anciens et modernes. 1 p. l., 568 pp., 1 l. 8°. *Paris, Guillaumin & Cie.,* 1856.

Monnier (F.) *Des éruptions pemphigoïdes secondaires dans les fièvres éruptives. 64 pp. 4°. *Lyon,* 1880, No. 46.

Monnier (Henri). *Étude expérimentale et critique sur les luxations métacarpo-phalangiennes dorsales du pouce. [Berne.] 100 pp. 8°. *Lausanne, L. Corbaz & Cie.,* 1873.

Monnier (I.-L.) Le cabinet secret des grands préservatifs et spécifiques propres, contre la peste, fièvres pestilentielles, pourpres, petites vérolles et toutes sortes de maladies contagieuses. 4 p. l., 95 pp. 12°. *Paris, P. d'Arbisse,* 1666.

Monnier (Jean-Marie). *Sur la phthisie pulmonaire. 32 pp. 4°. *Paris,* 1821, No. 218, v. 169.

Monnier (Joseph-Honoré). *Sur quelques points de la luxation symptomatique du fémur; de l'anatomie pathologique, des causes et du mécanisme. 35 pp. 4°. *Paris,* 1850, No. 230, v. 499.

Monnier (L.) *Recherches sur les sources des œuvres d'Hippocrate. 35 pp., 2 l. 4°. *Montpellier,* 1875, No. 99.

Monnier (Léon-Pierre-Thomas). *Considérations physiologiques et thérapeutiques sur la transfusion du sang. 53 pp., 1 l. 4°. *Montpellier,* 1875, No. 6.

Monnier (Louis). *Sur quelques points de physiologie chirurgicale du membre inférieur comme introduction à l'étude de la coxalgie. 100 pp. 4°. *Paris,* 1886, No. 118.

———. The same. 100 pp. 8°. *Paris, G. Steinheil,* 1886.

le Monnier (Ludovicus Guillelmus).
See **Lalouette** (Joannes Franciscus Achilles). *An cereoli in plerisque urethræ fistulis sectione præstantiores? 4°. [Paris, 1774.]*

Monnier (Paul-Pierre-Marie). *Étude sur une variété de luxation du métatarse, luxation en dehors des métatarsiens. 50 pp. 4°. *Paris,* 1883, No. 179.

le Mönnier (René). *Observations sur quelques épidémies de Saint-Domingue, compliquées de symptômes de la fièvre dite jaune. 21 pp. 4°. *Paris,* 1810, No. 10, v. 78.

Monnik (Adriaan Johannes Willem). *Tonometers en tonometrie. 2 p. l., 59 pp., 2 pl. 8°. *Utrecht, Kemink & Zoon,* 1868.

———. Een nieuwe tonometer en zijn gebruik. 56 pp., 1 pl. 8°. [*Utrecht,* 1869.]
Repr. from: Versl. . . . Nederl. Gasth. v. Ooglijders 1868, Utrecht, 1869, x.

Monnikendam (Salomon). * Over splitsing van jodium- en bromiumverbindingen in het dierlijk lichaam. 2 p. l., 92 pp. 8°. *Amsterdam, Gebr. Schröder,* 1886.

Monnikhoff (I.)
See **Krauss** (Joannes Carolus). Nadere overweging van de aard [etc.] 8°. *Amsterdam,* 1819.

Monnot (Armand). *I. Décrire les éponges; discuter les opinions qu'on a émises sur leur nature; indiquer leur composition chimique et leur emploi médical et chirurgical. II. [etc.] 24 pp. 4°. *Paris,* 1840, No. 108, v. 363.

Monnot (Charles). * Contribution à l'étude du syphilome ano-rectal. 59 pp. 4°. *Paris,* 1882, No. 78.

Monnot (Étienne-Marie-Victor). * Sur la fièvre bilieuse et histoire d'une épidémie de cette nature. 1 p. l., 27 pp. 4°. *Strasbourg, Levrault,* 1813.

Monnot (Jean-Baptiste-Joseph). *Considérations générales sur les luxations et leur traitement. 1 p. l., 35 pp. 4°. *Strasbourg,* 1819, v. 49.

Monnot (Théodose-Dauphin). *Des abcès de la fosse iliaque interne. 56 pp. 4°. *Paris,* 1846, No. 90, v. 448.

Monnoye (Cyprien)[1]. * Des signes de la grossesse, de la fonction de l'accouchement, suivis du mécanisme de l'accouchement naturel dans la présentation de l'extrémité céphalique, première position. 41 pp. 4°. *Paris,* 1834, No. 333, v. 279.

Monnoye (Cyprien)[2]. *Des kystes muqueux du col de l'utérus et des polypes utéro-folliculaires. 36 pp. 4°. *Paris,* 1864, No. 195.

Monod (Charles). *De l'angiome simple souscutané circonscrit. (Nævus vasculaire souscutané. Angiome lipomateux. Angiome lobulé.) 86 pp., 2 pl. 4°. *Paris,* 1873, No. 95.

———. The same. . . . suivie de quelques remarques sur les angiomes circonscrits de l'orbite. 86 pp., 1 l., 2 pl. 8°. *Paris, J.-B. Baillière & fils,* 1873.

———. *Étude comparative des diverses méthodes de l'exérèse. 1 p. l., 115 pp. 8°. *Paris, J.-B. Baillière & fils,* 1875.
Concours.

———. Leçons de clinique chirurgicale faites à l'Hôpital Necker. 127 pp. 8°. *Paris, A. Delahaye & E. Lecrosnier,* 1884.

Monod (Eugène). *Étude clinique sur les indications de l'uréthrotomie externe. 3 p. l., 170 pp., 1 tab. 4°. *Paris,* 1880, No. 194.

Monod (Frédéric). *De la dilatation forcée du sphincter de l'anus considérée spécialement dans son application au traitement des hémorrhoïdes. 108 pp. 4°. *Paris,* 1877, No. 246.

Monod (Frédéric-Clément-Constant-Gustave) [1803–]. *Propositions sur l'anatomie pathologique des os. vi, 7–29 pp. 4°. *Paris,* 1831, No. 20. v. 238. [*Also, in:* P., v. 1607.]

———. * La section du col de l'utérus est-elle une opération rationnelle? et, dans le cas d'affirmative, indiquer les circonstances dans lesquelles il faut y avoir recours. 24 pp. 4°. *Paris,* 1832, No. 380.
Concours.

———. Conseils au sujet du choléra, suivi du: Choléra, sa nature et sa véritable cause, moyens de le prévenir et de le guérir, par Tissot. 32 pp. 18°. *Berne, B.-F. Haller & E. Mathey,* 1854.

———. The same. 2. éd. 34 pp., 1 l. 24°. *Paris, C. Meyrueis,* 1865.

Monod (Henri-Charles). De l'administration de l'hygiène publique à l'étranger et en France. Mémoire présenté au Conseil central d'hygiène et de salubrité publiques dans le Calvados, à l'occasion de l'exposition internationale d'hygiène de Londres. 104 pp., 1 l. fol. *Caen, F. Le Blanc-Hardel,* 1884.

Monod (Louis). *De l'encéphalopathie albuminurique aiguë et des caractères qu'elle présente en particulier chez les enfants. 172 pp. 4°. *Paris*, 1868, No. 144.

——. The same. 170 pp. 8°. *Paris, A. Delahaye*, 1868, v. 414.

Monods.
See **Infusoria.**

Monograph (A) on Erythroxylon coca. Its preparations and their medicinal applications. 31 pp. 12°. [*New York*, 1885, *vel subseq.*]

Monographia Syphilitica. A journal devoted to the treatment of diseases of the blood by "*succus alterans*". Edited by Geo. W. McDade. Nos. for Jan., 1884, to Jan., 1887. 8°. *Indianapolis, Ind., E. Lilly & Co.*
An advertisement.

Monographische Skizze über das Ofner Raitzenbad, vorgetragen von Johann Molnár, in der Versammlung der Aerzte und Naturforscher in Pest, im September 1863. 16 pp. 4°. *Pest, G. Emich*, 1863.

Monomania.
See **Insanity** (*Anomalous, etc.*); **Insanity** (*Partial*); **Kleptomania**; **Pyromania.**

Monopara.
Salensky (W.) Recherches sur le développement du Monopara vivipara (Borlasia vivipara Uljan). Arch. de biol., Gand, 1884, v, 517–571, 3 pl.

Monophthalmus.
See **Monsters** *from defect, etc., of brain, etc.*

Monorchis.
See **Testicle** (*Abnormities of*).

Monory (Léon). *Tumeurs solides des doigts (symptômes, diagnostic et traitement). 46 pp. 4°. *Paris*, 1873, No. 440.

Monot (C.) De l'industrie des nourrices et de la mortalité des petits enfants. 160 pp. 8°. *Paris, J.-B. Ballière & fils*, 1867.

——. De la mortalité excessive des enfants pendant la première année de leur existence, ses causes et des moyens de la restreindre. 64 pp. 8°. *Paris, J.-B. Baillière & fils*, 1872.

Monot (Charles). *Du chloroforme, considéré comme agent anesthésique dans la pratique chirurgicale. 43 pp. 4°. *Paris*, 1857, No. 142, v. 608.

Monoyer (Ferdinand). *Des fermentations. 158 pp. 4°. *Strasbourg*, 1862, No. 624, 2. s., v. 33.

——. *Applications des sciences physiques aux théories de la circulation. 86 pp. 4°. *Strasbourg*, 1863, v. 37.
Concours.

——. Une extraction de cataracte dans un cas de luxation spontanée et d'opacification du cristallin avec complications du côté du tractus uvéal et du corps vitré. 23 pp. 8°. *Strasbourg, G. Silbermann*, 1867.
Repr. from: Gaz. méd. de Strasb., 1867, xxvii.

——. De la cure radicale de certaines formes de tumeurs lacrymales, ou moyen de l'excision partielle du sac, du cathétérisme méthodique et des injections au sulfite de soude. 18 pp. 3°. *Paris, P. Asselin*, 1873.
Repr. from: Arch. gén. de méd., Par., 1873, 6. s., xxi.

Monphous (L.-N.-André). *De l'huile empyreumatique arabe de jaunes d'œuf dans le traitement des ulcères et plaies ulcéreuses. 54 pp., 1 l. 4°. *Bordeaux*, 1885, No. 8, 1885–6.

de Monquentin (Petrus Leonardus). Thermologia Badavino-Austriaca: das ist: kurtze jedoch warhaffte Beschreibung der Natur, Krafft, Eigenschafft und Gebrauch, des heylsamen Badwassers zu Baden alhie in Nider Oesterreich. Allen Badgästen in- und ausländischen zum besten in teutscher Sprach verfertigt und gestelt. 54 l. 32°. *Regenspurg, C. Fischer*, 1651.

Monrad (Laurentius) [–1836]. *De laude regiminis frigidi limitanda. 1 p. l., 67 pp. 12°. *Havniæ, typ. rid. Suare*, [1787].

Monraisse (P.-Adolphe). *Des palpitations. 30 pp. 4°. *Paris*, 1859, No. 251.

de Monravà (Antonio). Desterro critico das falsas anatomias, que hum anatomico novo deu a' luz, em Lisboa, neste presente anno de 1739. 23 p. l., 1 pl., 350 pp., 2 l. 4°. *Lisboa, A. I. da Fonseca*, 1739.

——. Operaçoens anatomicas, e cirurgicas, que tem feito no mez de janeiro deste prezente anno de 1739. 2 p. l., 21 pp. 4°. *Lisboa*, 1739.
Bound with the preceding.
For Portrait, see **Pradillo** (Joseph). Cirugia triunfante demonstrativa. 12°. *Madrid*, 1728-9, pt. ii.

Monribot (Pierre-Saint-Clair). *De la pellagre. 38 pp. 4°. *Paris*, 1865, No. 98.

Monro (Alexander)[1] [1697–1767]. The anatomy of the human bones. To which are added, an anatomical treatise of the nerves; an account of the reciprocal motions of the heart; and a description of the human lacteal sac and duct. 2. ed. 1. part: viii, 344 pp.; 2. part: iv, 41 pp. 12°. *Edinburgh, W. Monro*, 1732.

——. The same. 3. ed. ix, 324; 80 pp. 12°. *Edinburgh, W. Monro & W. Drummond*, 1741.

——. The same. 4. ed. ix, 395 pp. 16°. *Edinburgh, Hamilton & Balfour*, 1746.

——. The same. 7. ed. vii, 410 pp. 12°. *Edinburgh, E. Hamilton & J. Balfour*, 1763.

——. The same. A new ed. To which is added an essay on comparative anatomy. vii, 312, 12, 65 pp., port. 8°. *Edinburgh, W. Gordon & J. Dickson*, 1782.
The essay on comparative anatomy has a separate title-page and pagination, and is "third edition".

——. The same. Traité d'ostéologie. Trad. de l'anglois par M. Sue. 2 v. xxxii, 212 pp.; 213–316 pp., 31 pl. fol. *Paris, G. Cavelier*, 1759.

——. An anatomical treatise of the nerves; an account of the reciprocal motions of the heart; and a description of the human lacteal sac and duct. iv, 41 pp. 12°. *Edinburgh, W. Monro*, 1732.
Bound with his: The anatomy of the human bones. 2. ed. 12°. *Edinburgh*, 1732.

——. The same. [3. ed.] iv, 80 pp. 12°. *Edinburgh, W. Monro & W. Drummond*, [1741?]
Bound with his: The anatomy of the human bones [etc.] 3. ed. 12°. *Edinburgh*, 1741.

——. The same. Tractatus tres, de nervis eorumque distributione, de motu cordis et ductu thoracico, Latine redditi a G. Coopmans qui præter commentarium perpetuum adjecit librum de cerebri et nervorum administratione anatomica. Editio altera. 5 p. l., 251 pp. 8°. *Harlingæ, F. van der Plaats*, 1763.

——. The same. Bemerkungen über die Struktur und Verrichtungen des Nervensystems. Aus dem Englischen übersetzt, nebst einigen Anmerkungen und Zusätzen. 1 p. l., 96 pp., 13 pl. 4°. *Leipzig, Schwickert*, 1787.

——. Tentamina circa methodum partes animantium affabre injiciendi, easque injectas ac rite præparatas bene conservandi, ut usibus anatomicis et physiologicis inserviant. Anglico idiomate a . . . auctore scripta, nunc vero ob insignem usum latinitate donata, et notis quibusdam instructa a Joh. Christ. Fried. Bonegarde, qui et addidit figuram siphonis emendati, et methodum præparandi colorem cæruleum Berolinensem vulgo dictum. 83 pp., 1 pl. 16°. *Lugd. Bat., P. Bouk*, 1741.
Bound with: **Vieussens** (R.) Novum vasorum corporis humani systema. 16°. *Amstelodami*, 1705.

——. The same. 2. ed. 83 pp. 16°. *Lugd. Bat., J. Delbeek*, 1745.

Monro (Alexander)[1]—continued.

——. The history and progress of anatomy, from the earliest ages of the world down to this present time, to which is added an appendix on the uses of anatomy, and division of the parts of the body. Collected from the lectures of . . . 235, 16 pp. MS. 4°. *Edinburgh*, 1742.

——. An essay on comparative anatomy. 138 pp. 12°. *London, J. Nourse*, 1744.

——. A course of publick lectures in anatomy. Taken from him during the time of lecturing. By John Redman, student of physick and surgery in the same college. 2 v. MS. 131 l., 184 pp. 4°. [*Edinburgh*], 1746.

——. The physiology. Taken from him during his course of lectures, by John Redman. In proprium usum. MS. 144 pp. sm. 4°. [*Edinburgh*], 1746.

——. An account of the inoculation of small-pox in Scotland. vii, 53 pp. 8°. *Edinburgh, Drummond*, 1765. [*Also, in:* P., v. 660; 674; 1344.]

——. The works of . . . Published by his son, Alexander Monro, jr. To which is prefixed, the life of the author. xxiv, 791 pp., 7 pl., port. 4°. *Edinburgh, C. Elliot*, 1781.

See, also, **Schultze** [*or* **Schulze**] (Joh. Heinr.) Abhandlung von der Stein-Cur, etc. 16°. *Franckfurt u. Leipzig*, 1740.

For Biography, see **Duncan** (A.), sr. An account of the life and writings of the late Alex'r Mon-o, sen'r, M. D. . . . delivered as the Harveian oration at Edinburgh, for the year 1780. 8°. *Edinburgh & London*, 1780.

For Portrait, see **System** (A) of anatomy and physiology, etc. A new ed. 3 v. 8°. *Edinburgh*, 1801, v. 1.

Monro (Alexander)[2] [1733–1817]. * De testibus et de semine in variis animalibus. 1 p. l., 90 pp., 5 pl. 8°. *Edinburgi, G. Hamilton & J. Balfour*, 1755. [*Also, in:* P, v. 644.]

Also, in: SMELLIE. Thesaurus med. [etc.] 8°. *Edinburgi*, 1785, ii, 317–397, 5 pl.

——. De venis lymphaticis valvulosis et de earum in primis origine. 59 pp. 8°. *Berolini, imp. C. F. Henningius*, 1757.

——. The same. 62 pp. 8°. *Berolini, G. A. Lang*, 1761. [P., v. 909.]

——. The same. Editio altera, auctior et emendatior. 120 pp. 8°. *Edinburgi, Balfour, Auld et Smellie*, 1770. [P., v. 1540.]

——. Observations anatomical and physiological, wherein Dr. Hunter's claim to some discoveries is examined. 2 p. l., 80 pp., 2 pl. 8°. *Edinburgh, Hamilton, Balfour & Neill*, 1758. [*Also, in:* P., v. 715; 1540.]

——. Answer to the notes on the postscript to Observations anatomical and physiological. 16 pp. 8°. *Edinburgh*, 1758. [*Also, in:* P., v. 716.]

——. An expostulatory epistle to William Hunter. 30 pp. 8°. *Edinburgh, G. Hamilton & J. Balfour*, 1762.

——. A state of facts concerning the first proposal of performing the paracentesis of the thorax, on account of air effused from the lungs into the cavities of the pleuræ; and concerning the discovery of the lymphatic, valvular, absorbent system of vessels in oviparous animals. In answer to Mr. Hewson. 29 pp., 1 pl. 8°. *Edinburgh, Balfour, Auld & Co.*, 1770. [*Also, in:* P., v. 678; 1540.]

——. Surgery. [Lectures numbered 1 to 22.] MS. 2 v. 320, 322 pp. 8°. [*Edinburgh*, 1781?] No title-page.

——. Lectures upon surgery. [Numbered 96 to 123.] MS. 392 pp. 4°. [*Edinburgh*, 1781?] Same lectures as preceding, excepting that this copy has seven additional.

——. Observations on the structure and functions of the nervous system. x, 176 pp., 47 pl. fol. *Edinburgh, W. Creech*, 1783.

Monro (Alexander)[2]—continued.

——. The structure and physiology of fishes explained, and compared with those of man and other animals. 128 pp., 44 pl. fol. *Edinburgh, C. Elliot*, 1785.

Another copy bound with his: Observations on the structure [etc.] fol. *Edinburgh*, 1783.

——. A description of all the "bursæ mucosæ" of the human body; their structure explained, and compared with that of the capsular ligaments of the joints, and of those sacs which line the cavities of the thorax and abdomen; with remarks on the accidents and diseases which affect those several sacs, and on the operations necessary for their cure. 60 pp., 10 pl. fol. *Edinburgh, C. Elliot, T. Kay & Co.*, 1788.

——. The same. Abbildungen und Beschreibungen der Schleimsäcke des menschlichen Körpers. Umgearbeitet und vermehrt hrsg. von Johann Christian Rosenmüller. xii, 108 pp., 15 pl. fol. *Leipzig, Breitkopf u. Haertel*, 1799. Latin and German texts.

——. Description of a human male monster; illustrated by tables, with remarks. Read Nov. 6, 1792. 18 pp., 4 pl. 4°. [*Edinburgh*, 1792.] [P., v. 670.]

Repr. from: Tr. Roy. Soc. Edinb., 1789–93, iii.

Another copy bound with his: Experiments on the nervous system, [etc.] 4°. *Edinburgh & London*, 1793.

——. Experiments relating to animal electricity. (Read Dec. 3, 1792.) 11 pp. 4°. [*Edinburgh*, 1792.] [P., v. 670; 672.]

Repr. from: Tr. Roy. Soc. Edinb., 1789–93, iii.

——. Experiments on the nervous system, with opium and metalline substances; made chiefly with a view of determining the nature and effects of animal electricy. 43 pp. 4°. *Edinburgh & London, A. Neill & Co.*, 1793. [*Also, in:* P., v. 670.]

——. Observations of the muscles, and particularly of their oblique fibres; with an appendix, in which the pretention of Dr. Gilbert Blanc, that he first demonstrated the same effect to be produced by oblique muscles as by straight ones, with a less proportional decurtation of fibres, is proved to be unfounded. 78 pp., 4 pl. 4°. *Edinburgh, I. Dickson*, 1794. [P., v. 670.]

Another, but imperfect, copy bound with his: Experiments on the nervous system. 4°. *Edinburgh & London*, 1793.

——. Three treatises. On the brain, the eye, and the ear. viii, 9–263 pp., 20 pl. fol. *Edinburgh, Bell & Bradfute*, 1797.

——. Observations on hydrocephalus chronicus. 32 pp., 1 pl. 8°. *Edinburgh, A. Neill & Co.*, 1803. [P., v. 679.]

——. Observations on the causes which determine the form of the human skull. 34 pp., 6 pl. 4°. [*Edinburgh*, 1812, *vel subseq.*]

——. Essays and heads of lectures on anatomy, physiology, pathology, and surgery, with a memoir of his life, by his son [Alexander Monro[3]]. clix, 132 pp., 7 pl., port. 8°. *Edinburgh, Maclachlan, Stewart & Co.*, 1840.

See, also, **Anatomia** Britanica; a system of anatomy and physiology. 2. ed. 8°. *London*, 1808.—**Hunter** (William). Medical commentaries. Part I. [etc.] 4°. *London*, 1762.—**Innes** (John). A short description of the human muscles, chiefly as they appear on dissection. 12°. *Edinburgh*, 1784. ——. The same. New ed. 16°. *London*, 1791.—**Wood** (William). Copy of a correspondence between . . . and William Wood, 1807. 8°. [*Edinburgh*, 1807.]

For Biography, see **Duncan** (A.), sr. An account of the life, writings, and character of the late Dr. Alexander Monro *Secundus;* delivered as the Harveian oration at Edinburgh, for the year 1818. 8°. *Edinburgh*, 1818.

For Portrait, see **Collection** of Portr. (Libr.)

——. *See, also:*

NOTES on the postscript to a pamphlet entitled: Observations anatomical [etc.] 8°. *London*, 1758.

Monro (Alexander)[3] [1773–1859]. *De dyspha-gia. 2 p. l., 122 pp., 14 tab. 8°. *Edinburgi, A. Neill et socii*, 1797. [*Also, in:* P., v. 6; 698.]

——. Observations on crural hernia; to which is prefixed a general account of the other varie-ties of hernia. 4 p. l., 95, 16, 13 pp., 7 pl. 8°. *Edinburgh, W. Laing*, 1803.

——. The morbid anatomy of the human gul-let, stomach, and intestines. xxv, 567 pp., 1 l., 21 pl. 8°. *Edinburgh, A. Constable & Co.*, 1811.

——. The same. 2. ed. xxvii, 524 pp., 2 l., 6 pl. 8°. *Edinburgh, J. Carfrae & Son*, 1830.

——. Outlines of the anatomy of the human body in its sound and diseased state. 4 v. 8°. *Edinburgh, A. Constable & Co.*, 1813.

——. Engravings of the thoracic and abdom-inal viscera, and the canals connected with them; representing the natural appearance of those important parts immediately after death, and without being affected by previous disease. Drawn under the direction of, and with descript-ive letter-press by, Alexander Monro, jun. 1 p. l., 28, 3 pp., 5 pl. 4°. · *Edinburgh, T. Bryce & Co.*, 1814.

——. Observations on the different kinds of small-pox, and especially on that which some-times follows vaccination. Illustrated by a num-ber of cases. vi, 281 pp., 1 l., 2 pl. 8°. *Edin-burgh, A. Constable & Co.*, 1818.

——. Observations on the causes of the preval-ence of small-pox, and on the means of prevent-ing the dissemination of that disease. 8 pp. 8°. *Edinburgh*, [1825, *vel subseq.*]. [P., v. 698.]
Repr. from: Edinb. J. M. Sc., 1826, i.

——. Observations on spasm of the canals for the food, bile, and urine. 46 pp., 2 pl. 8°. *Edinburgh, P. Neill*, 1826. [P., v. 697.]

——. Illustrations of the anatomy of the pelvis. 2. ed. 25 pp., 9 pl. fol. *Edinburgh, Maclachlan & Stewart*, 1827.

——. The morbid anatomy of the brain. v. 1. Hydrocephalus. xix, 200 pp., 5 pl. 8°. *Edin-burgh, Maclachlan & Stewart*, 1827. [*Also, in:* P., v. 698.]

——. Observations on aneurism of the abdomi-nal aorta. 31 pp., 1 pl. 8°. *Edinburgh, P. Neill*, 1827. [P., v. 698; 1062.]

——. The anatomy of the urinary bladder and perinæum of the male. Illustrated by engrav-ings, with physiological, pathological, and sur-gical observations. ix, 90 pp, 5 pl. 8°. *Edin-burgh, Maclachlan, Stewart & Co.*, 1842. [P., v. 1200.]
See, also, **Monro** (Alexander)[2]. Essays and heads of lectures [etc.], with a memoir [etc.] 8°. *Edinburgh*, 1840.
For Biography, see Lancet, Lond., 1859, i, 331.

Monro (Donald) [1729–92]. *De hydrope. 1 p. l., 70 pp. 8°. *Edinburgi, Hamilton, Balfour et Neill*, 1753. [P., v. 737.]
Also, in: SMELLIE. Thesaurus med. [etc.] 8°. *Edin-burgi*, 1785, ii, 191–248.

——. The same. An essay on the dropsy, and its different species. 7 p. l., 172 pp. 12°. *Lon-don, D. Wilson & T. Durham*, 1755.

——. The same. 3. ed. xiv, 272 pp. 8°. *Lon-don, A. Millar [and others]*, 1765.

——. An account of the diseases which were most frequent in the British military hospitals in Germany from January, 1761, to the return of the troops to England in March, 1763. To which is added, an essay on the means of preserving the health of soldiers, and conducting military hospitals. xvi, 408 pp. 8°. *London, A. Millar [and others]*, 1764.

——. The same. Zusätze zu des . . . Beschrei-bung der Krankheiten, welche in den brittischen Feldlazarethen in Deutschland vom Januar 1761 bis zum März 1763 am häufigsten gewesen sind,

Monro (Donald)—continued.
von Begue de Presle. Aus dem Französischen übersetzt. 2 v. in 1. 6 p. l., 398 pp.; 5 p. l., 620 pp., 17 l. 8°. *Altenburg, Richter*, 1771.

——. An account of some neutral salts made with vegetable acids, and with the salt of amber. 40 pp., 1 pl. 4°. *London*, 1768. [P., v. 632.]

——. Médecine d'armée, ou traité des maladies les plus communes parmi les troupes, dans les camps et les garnisons. Trad. de l'anglois, avec des augmentations considérables par M. le Begue de Presle. 2 v. v. 1. Contenant le dis-cours préliminaire et l'introduction. v. 2. Con-tenant les symptômes, le traitement des mala-dies, etc. cclxiv, clix pp.; viii, 516 pp. 8°. *Paris, P.-F. Didot le jeune*, 1769.

CONTENTS.
1. Des recherches sur les progrès de la médecine d'ar-mée, et le catalogue des livres publiés sur ses diverses parties.
2. Les moyens de fortifier et conserver la santé des troupes dans les camps et les garnisons.
3. L'établissement et l'administration des hôpitaux mili-taires, soit fixes, soit ambulans, avec leurs règlemens.
4. Les symptômes, le traitement et les remèdes des maladies communes parmi les troupes dans les camps et les garnisons.

——. A treatise on mineral waters. 2 v. xxiv, 475 pp.; viii, 419 pp. 8°. *London, D. Wilson & G. Nichol*, 1770.

——. Prælectiones medicæ ex Cronii instituto, annis 1774, et 1775; et oratio anniversaria et Harveii instituto, die Octobris 18, anni 1775. 3 p. l., 199 pp. 8°. *London, G. Hay*, 1776. [*Also, in:* P., v. 1540.]

——. Observations on the means of preserving the health of soldiers, and of conducting mili-tary hospitals. And on the diseases incident to soldiers in the time of service, and on the same diseases as they have appeared in London. 2. ed. 2 v. xi (3 l.), 374, viii, 304 pp. 8°. *London, J. Murray*, 1780.

——. The same. Bemerkungen über die Mittel die Gesundheit der Soldaten zu erhalten und Feldlazarethe anzulegen, wie auch über die Krankheiten, welche die Soldaten im Lager be-fallen, und über die nämlichen Krankheiten, wie sie sich in London gezeigt haben. [2. Aufl.] 1 p. l., viii, 547 pp. 8°. *Altenburg, Richter*, 1784.

——. A treatise on medical and pharmaceutical chymistry, and the materia medica; to which is added, an English translation of the new edition of the pharmacopœia of the Royal College of Physicians of London, 1788. In 3 v. v. 3. 6 p. l., 464 pp. 8°. *London, T. Cadell*, 1788.
See, also, **Pringle** (John). Verhandeling over de le-gerziekten [etc.] 3 v. 8°. *Amsterdam*, 1785-8.

Monro (Georgius). *De suffocatione stridula. 3 p. l., 35 pp. 8°. *Edinburgi, Balfour et Smellie*, [1786].

Monro (Henry). On improving the condition of the insane. Public asylums for the middle classes. 23 pp. 8°. [*London*, 1851.]
Repr. from: J. Psych. M., Lond., 1851, iv.
Bound with the following.

——. Remarks on insanity. Its nature and treatment. xii pp., 2 l., 150 pp. 8°. *London, J. Churchill*, 1851. [*Also, in:* P., v. 41.]

——. Articles on reform in private asylums. viii, 87 pp. 8°. *London, J. Churchill*, 1852.
Another copy bound with his: Remarks on insanity. 8°. *London*, 1851.

Monro (John) [1715–91]. Remarks on Dr. Bat-tie's treatise on madness. 1 p. l., 60 pp. 8°. *London, J. Clarke*, 1758. [*Also, in:* P., v. 568.]

Monro (Thomas). Observations upon the evi-dence taken before the committee of the Hon. House of Commons for regulating mad-houses. [Also, observations of John Haslam.] 55 pp. 8°. *London, H. Bryer*, 1816.

Monro (William). Report to directors of the Dundee Royal Infirmary, with reasons for objecting to, and dissenting from, that part of the report of a majority of the medical officers of that institution, which recommends patients labouring under fever being treated in the same wards with those labouring under other diseases. 12 pp. 8°. *Dundee, Hill & Alexander*, 1849. [*Also, in :* P., v. 1017 ; 1023.]

Monroe, *Michigan.*
Douglass. Analysis of mineral water from a spring near Monroe, Mich. Penins. J. M., Ann Arbor, 1856–7, iv, 521.

Monroe (A. L.) Method of memorizing the materia medica. vii, 44, 6 pp. 16°. *Louisville, J. P. Morton & Co.*, 1882.

Monroe, *dit* **Roe** (Charles) [1852–]. *Étude sur le drainage capillaire par les crins. 67 pp., 5 tab. 4°. *Lyon, Vve. Chanoine*, 1879, No. 26.

Monroe *County, New York.*
See **New York** (*State of*).

Monroe *County, Virginia.*
See **Virginia** (*Mineral waters of*).

Monroe County Medical Society. Report of a committee on the subject of medical legislation to the Monroe County Medical Society, Rochester, Nov. 9, 1842. 15 pp. 8°. [*Rochester*, 1842.]
———. Report of a committee on Dr. Lovejoy's alleged new remedies. 15 pp. 8°. *Rochester, A. Strong & Co.*, 1858.
———. Constitution and by-laws, as amended at the annual meeting in June, 1871. 8 pp. 12°. *Rochester*, 1871.

Monroe County Penitentiary. Annual reports of the inspectors, superintendent, and other officers, to the board of supervisors of the county. 1., 1854–5 ; 7., 1860–61. 8°. *Rochester*, 1855–62.

Mons.
See, also, **Cholera** (*Asiatic, History, etc., of*), **Hospitals** (*Descriptions, etc., of*), *by localities;* **Medicine** (*Clinical, Cases of*).
Binard. Extrait du rapport médical de l'hôpital militaire de Mons. Arch. méd. belges, Brux., 1868, 2. s., vii, 81 : viii, 363.

van Mons (Charles Jacques) [1800–37]. * De infanticidio. 1 p. l., 60 pp. 4°. *Lovanii, C. J. De Mat*, 1822.
See, also, **Vleminckx** (J.-F.) Essai sur l'ophthalmie de l'armée des Pays-Bas. 8°. *Bruxelles*, 1825.
——— & **Marcq** (P.-A.) Rapport sur le choléra-morbus, adressé au Conseil supérieure de santé de la Belgique. 88 pp., 1 tab. 8°. *Bruxelles, J.-T. Tallois*, 1832.

van Mons (Jean-Baptiste) [1765–1842]. Censura commentarii a Wieglebo nuper editi, cui titulus : De vaporis aquei in aërem conversione. 40 pp. 4°. *Bruxellis, E. Flon*, [*n. d.*]
For Biography, see Arch. de la méd. belge, Brux., 1843, xi, 109–113 (A. Quételet). *Also :* Bull. Acad. roy. de méd. de Belg., Brux., 1842–3, ii, 851–881 (J.-S. Stas).

Mons (Laurent). * De la cystite dans la grossesse et dans l'accouchement. 66 pp., 1 l. 4°. *Paris*, 1877, No. 145.

Mons veneris.
Bethune (G. A.) Abscess of mons veneris. Extr. Rec. Bost. Soc. M. Improve., 1848–53, i, 156. — **Warren** (J. M.) Case of uncommon tumour of the mons veneris. Am. J. M. Sc., Phila., 1852, n. s., xxiii, 351. *Also, in his :* Surg. Obs., 8°, Bost., 1867, 269.

Monsão.
NOTICIA e ensaio sobre as aguas mineraes da villa de Monsão, contendo o melhoramento actual deste salutifero estabelecimento. 2. ed. sm. 8°. *Porto*, 1845.

Monsarrat (Jean-Bernard). * De la leucorrhée. 23 pp. 4°. *Paris*, 1855, No. 84, v. 578.

Monschen (Joannes Wolffgangus). * De epilepsia. 15 l. sm. 4°. *Francof. ad Viadr., lit. C. Zeitleri*, [1700].

Monscourt (G.-Joseph). * Du traitement de la fièvre typhoïde. 26 pp. 4°. *Paris*, 1852, No. 196, v. 529.

Monselise (Alessandro). La mano. Studj ed osservazioni di funzionalità anatomica. 2 p. l., 378, v pp., 1 l., 11 pl. 8°. *Verona, H. F. Münster*, 1877.
———. Le pieghe degli emisferi cerebrali ; memoria. 81 pp., 9 pl., 10 l. 8°. *Verona, Drucker & Tedeschi*, 1879.

Monserrat.
ARNÚS (M.) Historia topográfica, química y médica de la Puda de Monserrat, precedida de algunas generalidades de hidrología general y balnearia. 8°. *Barcelona*, 1863.

Monserrat y Riutort (*José*) [1814–81].
Aguilar y Lara. Necrología. Crón. méd., Valencia, 1880–81, iv, 737–741.

Monsey (*Messenger*) [1693–1788].
SKETCH (A) of the life and character of the late Dr. Monsey, physician to the Royal Hospital at Chelsea ; with anecdotes of persons of the first rank in church and state. 8°. *London*, 1789.
Portrait in : **Collection** of Portr. (Libr.)

Monsimier (J.-R.) * De l'hystérie. 22 pp. 4°. *Paris*, 1819, No. 169, v. 487.

Monski. Wahnsinn und Blödsinn pathologisch und pathogenetisch erörtert, mit einem Gutachten über einen Kranken, welcher in zweifelhafter Zurechnungsfähigkeit ein Mord-Attentat begangen. MS. 122 pp. fol. [*n. p.*], 1863.

Monski ([Carolus] Gustavus [Theodorus]). * De morbis tunicarum vaginalium testiculi et funiculi spermatici nonnulla. 31 pp. 8°. *Berolini, G. Schade*, [1848].

Monsnereau (Gustave). * Essai comparatif entre quelques-unes des principales ambulances sédentaires établies à Paris pendant le siége de 1870–71. 48 pp. 4°. *Paris*, 1871, No. 9.

Monson.
MASSACHUSETTS. *State Primary School at Monson.* Annual reports of the inspectors. 1.– 23., 1854 to 1875–6 ; 25., 1877–8. 8°. *Boston*, 1855–79.

Monson (Edward). The advantages of the separate system of drainage ; with a description of the works designed and carried out by the author at the town of Halstead, Essex. The evils and disadvantages of the metropolitan system of combined drainage. The cause of flooding from the low-level sewer, and how it might be prevented. A proposed method of sewage disposal for the metropolis, so as to prevent the present nuisance from the sewage and the silting up of the Thames. vi, 29 pp. 8°. *London, E. & F. N. Spon*, 1875.
———. Metropolitan sewage, and what to do with it ; a series of papers relating to the formation and expenditure of the Metropolitan Board of Works ; the separate system of drainage and the main drainage system ; the new stock brick-making process for utilizing sewage sludge ; a scheme of sewage disposal for the metropolis, and the author's scheme of drainage for the Lower Thames Valley, including an account of the competition and detailed estimates of cost ; the whole being a complete system of sewage clarification and purification. xx, 135 pp. 8°. *London, B. T. Batsford*, 1883.

Monsseau (Théodore-Antoine-François). * De l'ankylose. 32 pp. 4°. *Paris*, 1850, No. 166, v. 499.

Monsseaux (Charles - Joseph) * De l'emphysème du poumon. 26 pp. 4°. *Paris*, 1851, No. 222, v. 512.

Monsseaux (F. - Auguste). * Des rétrécissements de l'urèthre, et de leurs différents modes de traitement. 35 pp. 4°. *Paris*, 1854, No. 320, v. 563.

Monsseaux (Pierre-Joseph). * Sur les abcès ou tumeurs purulentes en général. 27 pp. 4°. *Paris*, 1821, No. 112, v. 166.

Monsters.

See, also, **Anatomy** (*Abnormities of*); **Anatomy** (*Essays, etc., on*); **Fœtus** (*Abnormities of*); **Fœtus** (*Maternal influence on*); **Labor** (*Complicated, etc.*), *from disproportion, etc., of the child*; **Nævus**; **Sacro-coccygeal** *region* (*Tumors of*); **Tumors** (*Congenital*); *and under names of organs and regions, e. g.*, **Breast**, **Extremities**, **Extremity** (*Upper*), **Eye**, **Genitals** (*Female*), **Hair**, **Placenta**, **Skin**, *Abnormities of.*

AHLFELD (F.) Die Missbildungen des Menschen. Eine systematische Darstellung der beim Menschen angeboren vorkommenden Missbildungen und Erklärung ihrer Entstehungsweise. 8°. Atlas, fol. *Leipzig*, 1880–82.

ALDROVANDUS (U.) Monstrorum historia. fol. *Bononiæ*, 1642.

In his: Opera. fol. *Bonon.*, 1646-8, xi.

BARDINET (M. - A.) Observations tératologiques. Hydrocéphales: I. Sirénomèle; II. Rhinencéphale; III. Cyclocéphale. 8°. *Paris*, 1839.

BATTIGLIANA (A. J.) * Contribucion al estudio de las monstruosidades fetales. 8°. *Buenos Aires*, 1884.

BAUHINUS (C.) De hermaphroditorum monstrosorumque partium natura ex theologorum, jureconsultorum, medicorum, philosophorum et rabbinorum sententia libri duo hactenus non editi. sm. 8°. *Oppenheim*, 1614.

BÉCHET (J.-F.) * Essai sur les monstruosités humaines, ou vices congéniaux de conformation. 4°. *Paris*, 1829.

BEER (F.) * Beiträge zu der Lehre von den Missgeburten. 8°. *Zürich*, 1850.

BENEKE (F. G.) De ortu et causis monstrorum disquisitio. 8°. *Gottingæ*, 1846.

BIERLING (C. T.) Monstra fœminina.

In his: Adversariorum curiosorum centuria prima. 4°. *Jenæ*, 1679, 40.

BISCHOFF (T. L. W.} Ueber Missbildungen, nebst einer Einleitung über die Literatur-Geschichte der Entwicklungs - Geschichte. 8°. *Braunschweig*, 1843.

Repr. from: WAGNER (R.) Handwörterbuch der Physiologie. v. 1. 8°. *Braunschweig*, 1842.

BOSCH (W. B.) * De monstris eorumque caussis. 4°. *Lugd. Bat.*, 1780.

BUSCH (J. D.) Beschreibung zweier merkwürdigen menschlichen Misgeburten, nebst einigen andern Beobachtungen aus der praktischen Entbindungskunst. 4°. *Marburg*, 1803.

BUSSON (J.) An ab origine monstra? Proponebat P. I. Poissonnier. [*n. p.*, 1743.]

In: SIGWART (G. F.) Quæst. med. Par. 4°. *Tubingæ*, 1789, i, 3-9.

CERUTTI (F. P. L.) [Pr.] rarioris monstri, in museo anatomico Lipsiensi adservati, descriptio anatomica. 4°. *Lipsiæ*, [1827].

CRAUSIUS (R. G.) [Pr.] de varietate lusuum naturalium, speciatim in animalibus, et cumprimis hominibus. i & iii. sm. 4°. *Jenæ*, [1705].

CURTIUS (C. W.) * De monstro humano cum infante gemello. 4°. *Lugd. Bat.*, 1762.

Also, in: WEIZ (F. A.) Neue Ausz., [etc.] 12°. *Frankfurt u. Leipzig*, 1775, iii, 57–82.

Monsters.

VAN DOEVEREN (G.) Specimen observationum academicarum ad monstrorum historiam, anatomen, pathologiam, et artem obstetriciam præcipue spectantium. 4°. *Groning. et Lugd. Bat.*, 1765.

DUMONT (F.-G.) * Sur l'agénésie, l'impuissance et la dysgénésie. 4°. *Paris*, 1830.

EHRMANN (C.-H.) Description de deux fœtus monstres, dont l'un acéphale et l'autre monopode. fol. *Strasbourg*, 1852.

ERPELS (J. P.) Nachricht von einer Frau, welche zugleich fünf Kinder, vier Missgeburthen und ein Mondkalb gebohren. 12°. *Halle im Magd.*, 1750.

FABER (G. F. C.) * Duorum monstrorum humanorum descriptio anatomica. 4°. *Berolini*, [1827].

FACICULI admirandorum naturæ accretio; of de speelende natuur kunstwerke, in verschyde misgeboorte voorgesteld, door een lievhebber die nog bloeyd door genade. [220 colored drawings of monstrosities, with MS. descriptions. By De Groot.] 1 v. 4°. 1736.

FERNAU (R. B.) * De causis monstrorum. 8°. *Berolini*, 1844.

FIGULUS (C. F. J.) * De monstrorum origine. 4°. *Vratislaviæ*, 1816.

FÖRSTER (A.) Die Missbildung des Menschen systematisch dargestellt. 2. Ausg. 4°. *Jena*, 1865.

FUCHS (R.) * De monstrorum genesi, exemplis duobus illustrata. 8°. *Berolini*, [1847].

GEOFFROY-SAINT-HILAIRE (I.) * Propositions sur la monstruosité, considérée chez l'homme et les animaux. 4°. *Paris*, 1829.

——. Histoire générale et particulière des anomalies de l'organisation. 3 v. & an atlas. 8°. *Bruxelles*, 1837.

GILBERT (M.) * Ueber einen durch amniotische Stränge verursachten Fall von Missbildung. 8°. *Berlin*, 1884.

GIULIO (G. C.) & ROSSI. Description d'un monstre, avec des recherches physiologiques sur les monstres, concernant particulièrement la question: s'il faut rapporter tous les monstres à des causes accidentelles. 4°. [*n. p., n. d.*]

Cutting from: Mém. de l'Acad. roy. d. sc. de Turin, 1802–3.

GRAETZ (H.) *Ueber zwei seltene Missbildungen. 8°. *Erlangen*, 1886.

'S GRAEUWEN (P.) Spec. med. inaug. cont. historiam trium fœtuum monstrosorum una cum adnexis animadversionibus. 4°. *Lugd. Bat.*, 1802.

GRUBER (W. L.) Missbildungen. Erste Sammlung. 4°. *St. Petersburg*, 1859.

Repr. from: Mém. Acad. imp. d. sc. de St.-Pétersb. Sc. math., phys. et nat., 7. s., ii, no. 2.

GUERIN (J.) Recherches sur les difformités congénitales chez les monstres, le fœtus et l'enfant. 8°. [Atlas, fol.] *Paris*, 1880[–82].

See, also, infra, de Quatrefages.

HALLER (A.) [Pr.] descriptio fœtus bicipitis, ad pectora connati, ubi in causas monstrorum ex principiis anatomicis inquiritur. 4°. *Hannoveræ*, 1739.

——. [Pr.] qua duorum monstrorum anatome continetur. 4°. *Gottingæ*, [1742].

——. [Pr.] suamque et Winslowi de monstris sententiam contra D. Lemery N. F. novis argumentis defendit. 4°. *Gottingæ*, [1745].

——. [Pr.] de monstrosis fabricis observationes profert. 4°. *Gottingæ*, 1753.

Also [Abstr.]. *in:* WEIZ (F. A.) Neue Ausz., [etc.] 12°. *Leipzig*, 1776, iv, 146.

HARTMANN (G. V.) Epistola, de bruto ex homine. 4°. *Erfordiæ*, 1733.

Monsters.

HEILAND (M.) Monstri hassiaci disquisitio medica. 4°. *Giessæ Hassorum*, [*n. d.*]

HERHOLDT (J. D.) Betragtninger over Misfostere i Almindelighed. 4°. *Kjöbenhavn*, 1828. *Repr. from:* Kongel. Danske Vidensk. Selskabs Skrifter.

——. Beschreibung sechs menschlicher Missgeburten mit 14 ausgemalten Kupfern. Nebst einem Anhange über den medicinischen Aberglauben, aus der Lehre von den Missgeburten entlehnt. 4°. *Kopenhagen*, 1830.

HERTWIG (J. G. F.) *De formatione epigenetica et monstrositate per defectum hujus formationis. 4°. *Landishuti*, [1821].

HOPPIUS (C. E.) *Anthropomorpha. 8°. *Upsaliæ*, 1760. *In:* LINNÆUS. Amœnitates acad. [etc.] 8°. *Lugd. Bat.*, 1764, vi, 63–76, 1 pl.

HUBER (J. J.) Observationes atque cogitationes nonnullæ de monstris. 4°. [With a letter from J. M. Gesner. 8°.] *Cassellis*, 1748.

INSFELDT (J. C.) *De lusibus naturæ. 4°. *Lugd. Bat.*, 1772.

IRENAEUS (M. C.) De monstris. Von seltzamen Wundergeburten. I. Was ein Monstrum oder Wundergeburt sey. II. Erzelung etlich hundert Wundergeburt nach Ordnung der Jarzal. III. Welches das aller grewlichste Monstrum sey. IV. Wer der Schoepfer der Wundergeburten sey. V. Woher sie sich hervorfachen und iren Offsprung haben. VI. Das sie Straffen der Stünden sein. VII. Was sie bedeuten und drauff erfolget. 1 v. 4°. [*Ad fin.:*] "*Getruckt zu Orsel, durch N. Henricum*", 1585.

JACKSON (J. B. S.) A descriptive catalogue of the monstrosities in the cabinet of the Boston Society for Medical Improvement. 8°. *Boston*, 1847.

JAEGER (G. F.) Vergleichung einiger durch Fettigkeit oder colossale Bildung ausgezeichneter Kinder und einiger Zwerge. 8°. *Stuttgart*, 1821.

JEROMIN (J. L.) *De morbis nisus formativi. 12°. *Dorpati*, 1815.

JOLY (N.) Mémoire sur un nouveau genre de monstres célosomiens, pour lequel l'auteur propose le nom de dracontisome. 8°. *Toulouse*, [1848?]

JOUARD (G.) Des monstruosités et bizarreries de la nature, principalement de celles qui ont rapport à la génération ... avec des réflexions philosophiques sur les monstrueux et dangereux empiétemens des sciences accessoires, telles que la chimie, la droguerie, etc., sur la vraie médecine, [etc.] 2 v. in 1. sm. 8°. *Paris*, 1806.

KALINKIUS (J.) *De monstris. 4°. *Wittebergæ*, 1657.

KELLER (E.) *Beiträge zur Casuistik und Theorie der Missbildungen. (Anencephalie mit Zwerchfellshernie und Acardie.) 8°. *Zürich*, 1886.

KLEIN (C. C.) Specimen inaugurale anatomicum sistens monstrorum quorundam descriptionem. 4°. *Stuttgardiæ*, 1793.

[KLINKENBERG (G. W.)] [A collection of sixty-five original drawings, in part colored, representing monstrosities in the museum of G. W. Klinkenberg at Leyden. With MS. notes.] 1 v. fol.

KOCH (H.) *De evolutionibus retardatis. 8°. *Jenæ*, [1835].

KOSTECKI (P.) *De monstrositatum origine. 8°. *Berolini*, [1819].

KURSNERUS (C.) Disput. physica de causa partus monstrosi, nuperrime nati, hujusque occasione de monstrorum humanorum in genere. sm. 4°. *Marburgi*, [1684].

Monsters.

LARCHER (O.-E.-F.) Mélanges de pathologie comparée et de tératologie. 8°. *Paris*, 1878.

LEMNIUS (L.) De miraculis occultis naturæ libri iiii. 18°. *Francofurti*, 1628.

LEUCKART (R.) De monstris eorumque caussis et ortu. 4°. *Gottingæ*, [1844].

LICETUS (F.) De monstrorum natura, caussis, et differentiis libri duo. 2. ed. 4°. *Patavii*, 1634.

——. The same. De monstris. Ex recensione Gerardi Blasii. Qui monstra quædam nova et rariora ex recentiorum scriptis addidit. Editio novissima. 4°. *Amstelodami*, 1665.

——. The same. Traité des monstres, de leur causes, de leur nature, et de leur différences. 4°. [*Leide*, 1708.]

LIETZAU (F. O.) *Historia trium monstrorum. Pars prior anatomica. 8°. *Regiomonti*, [1825].

LOWNE (B. T.) Descriptive catalogue of the teratological series in the museum of the Royal College of Surgeons of England. 8°. *London*, 1872.

LOMBARDIUS (C. P.) Exercitatio anatomica de monstro humano nupero. 4°. *Marburgi Cattorum*, 1684.

LYCOSTHENES [WOLFFHART] (C.) Prodigiorum ac ostentorum chronicon, quæ præter naturæ ordinem, motum, et operationem, et in superioribus et his inferioribus mundi regionibus, ab exordio mundi usque ad hæc nostra tempora, acciderunt, [etc.] roy. 8°. *Basileæ*, [1557].

——. The same. Wunderwerck. Oder Gottes unergründtliches vorbilden, [etc.] ... mit schönen Abbildungen gezierdt ... durch Johann Herold vertentscht. fol. [*Basle*, 1557?]

MADAI (C. A.) *Anatomen ovi humani fœcundati sed deformis, trimestri abortu elisi [etc.] 4°. *Halæ Magdeb.*, [1763]. *Also, in:* FASC. diss. anat.-med. 8°. *Amstelædami*, 1764, 1–62, 1 pl. *Also, in:* SCHLEGEL (J. C. T.) Sylloge oper. min. 8°. *Lipsiæ*, 1795, i, 389–420, 1 pl.

MAIERUS (M.) Tractatus de Voluci Arborea, absque patre et matre, insulis Orcadum, forma Anserculorum proveniente, seu de Ortu miraculoso potius, quam naturali vegetabilium, animalium, hominum et supranaturalium quorundam: Quo causæ illius et horum inquiruntur, et demonstrantur. 12°. *Francofurti*, 1619.

MECKEL (J. F.) Descriptio monstrorum nonnullorum cum corollariis anatomico-physiologicis. 4°. *Lipsiæ*, 1826.

MELONI-SATTA (P.) Teratologia in genere ed illustrazione di alcuni casi in specie. [Anno i.] 8°. *Sassàri*, 1885.

MIRUS (A. E.) & FISCHER (J. H.) De monstris. 4°. *Wittenbergæ*, 1681.

MOHS (E. J. R.) *De monstris et monstrositatibus corporis humani ac de vi eorum ad vitam et valetudinem. 8°. *Halæ*, 1864.

MÜLLER (E.) *Beitrag zur Casuistik der menschlichen Missgeburten. 8°. *Leipzig*, 1881. *Also, in:* Arch. f. Gynaek., Berl., 1881, xvii, 298–312, 1 pl.

MUSKKIN (M. M.) K uchen. o proischoj. vrojden. urodstve. Monstrum humanum kyphoscoliosi cum spina bif. consecutivisque ventroschysi seu abdom. hiatu compl. et genitalium extrem. inf. defectu depravatum. 8°. *St. Petersburg*, 1886.

NIGRISOLI (F. M.) Considerazioni intorno alla generazione de' viventi e particolarmente de' mostri fatte dal ... e da lui scritte al ... Dionisio Andrea Sancassani. 4°. *Ferrara*, 1712.

OTTENS (J.) *De lusibus naturæ naturam illustrantibus. 8°. *Hardervici*, 1799.

OTTO (A. W.) Seltene Beobachtungen zur Anatomie, Physiologie und Pathologie gehörig. 1. Hft. 8°. *Breslau*, 1816.

Monsters.

——. Monstrorum sexcentorum descriptio anatomica. fol. *Vratislaviæ*, 1841.

Also with the title: Museum anatomico-pathologicum Vratislaviæ.

PARÉ (A.) Deux livres de chirurgie. I. De la génération de l'homme [etc.] II. Des monstres tant terrestres que marins, avec leurs portraits, [etc.] 8°. *Paris*, 1573.

PIHRINGER (C.) * De monstro. Resp. Rudol. Gottfried Bürger. 4°. *Wittebergæ*, 1664.

POISSONNIER (P. I.) *An ab origine monstra? Præses J. Busson.

In: SIGWART (G. F.) Quæst. med. Par. 4°. *Tubingæ*, 1789, i, 3–9.

POSNER (C.) Curiöser Tractat von denen Miss-Geburthen, erster und ander Theil, aus dem Lateinischen ins Deutsche übersetzt von M. M. 16°. *Dressden u. Leipzig*, 1702.

PRINCETEAU. * Progrès de la tératologie depuis Isidore Geoffroy-Saint-Hilaire. 8°. *Paris*, 1886.

PROCHASKA (G.) Commentatio quædam in systema generationis et causas originis monstrorum.

In his: Adnot. acad. 8°. *Pragæ*, 1781, ii, 89–141.

PÜTTER (J. S.) * Historiæ naturalis fragmenta ex ostentis, prodigiis et monstris. 2 pts. fol. *Gottingæ*, 1784–5.

TEN RHYNE (W.) Dissertatio de monstris.

In his: Diss. de arthritide [etc.] 8°. *Londini*, 1683, 303–334.

ROLLIN (C. J.) * Duorum monstrorum anatomen et de causis monstrorum ulteriorem disquisitionem exhibens. sm. 4°. *Gottingæ*, [1742].

RUDOLPH (C. E.) *Monstrorum trium præter naturam cum secundinis coalitorum disquisitio. 4°. *Berolini*, 1829.

SCHENCKIUS (J. G.) Monstrorum historia memorabilis, monstrosa humanorum partuum miracula . . . Accessit analogicum argumentum de monstris brutis. sm. 4°. *Francofurti*, 1609.

SCHRÖDTER (A. D.) Lapsus naturæ in genere humano. 4°. *Jenæ*, [1689].

SCHUSTER (M. G.) Dissertatio physica de monstris. 4°. *Lipsiæ*, [1690].

SORBINUS (A.) Tractatus de monstris, quæ a temporibus Constantini hucusque ortum habuerint, ac iis quæ circa eorum tempore misere acciderunt. 16°. *Parisiis*, 1570.

STENGELIUS (G.) De monstris et monstrosis, quam mirabilis, bonus, et justus, in mundo administrando, sit Deus, monstrantibus. 16°. *Ingolstadii*, 1647.

STRICERIUS (J.) * De monstro. 4°. *Wittebergæ*, 1665.

SURINGAR (G. C.) * Dissertatio medica de nisu formativo ejusque erroribus. 4°. *Lugd. Bat.*, 1824.

TARENETSKI (A.) Anatomija i istorija razvitija tsiklopii u chelovieka s primiechanijami o razvitii prostvich urodov voobtshe. [Development of Cyclops-man, with remarks on the development of monsters in general.] 8°. *St. Petersburg*, 1882.

TARUFFI (C.) Storia della teratologia. 4 v. 8°. *Bologna*, 1881–6.

TILINGIUS (M.) De tuba uteri deque fœtu nuper in Gallia extra uteri cavitatem in tuba concepto; exercitatio anatomica, cui duorum monstrorum, unius Berolini, alterius vero in agro Marpurgensi nuper editorum, relatio est innexa. 18°. *Rinthelii*, 1670.

TRICESIMUS quartus thesauri picturarum tomus continens monstra relligionis horrenda et aliorum diversorum aliquot partuum animalium tam rationalium quam irrationalium congestus. Anno salutis restitutæ. MS. 4°. [*n. p.*], 1604.

Text in Latin and German.

Monsters.

VALENTINI (M. B.) De monstrorum Hassiacorum ortu atque causis, ad Joh. Dan. Dorstenium. 1684.

In his: Polychresta exotica [etc.] 4°. *Francof. a. M.*, 1700, 175–186. Also: Ibid., 1701, 175–186.

VORSTMAN (J. G.) * Beschrijving eener misvormde menschelijke vrucht. 8°. *Leiden*, 1857.

VROLIK (W.) Wenken over den oorsprong der misgeboorten en over de waarde van de leer der aangeboren misvormingen. 8°. *Amsterdam*, 1836.

Also, in: Tijdschr. v. nat. Geschied. en Physiol., Leiden, 1837–8, iv, 221–261.

——. Teratology. 8°. [*n. p., n. d.*]

Repr. from: Cycl. Anat. & Physiol.

WALLRICH (C.) De monstris. 4°. *Wittebergæ*, 1655.

WEINRICHIUS (M.) De ortu monstrorum commentarius. In quo essentia, differentiæ, causæ, et affectiones mirabilium animalium explicantur. 12°. [*Breslæ*], 1595.

WEKERLE (G.) * De monstris. 8°. *Pestini*, [1827].

WESTPHAL (J. C.) Natura peccans septenario problematum numero proposita. 4°. *Lipsiæ*, [1687].

Adam (A. M.) Contributions to teratology. Month. J. M. Sc., Lond. & Edinb., 1854, xviii, 241; 399: xix, 240; 515. Also, Reprint. — **Æquum** est, in fallor Domini, inchoavit Periander, ut memoratis productionibus enormibus, seu anomalis naturæ, regulares jam attingamus: nuper in examen adduximus sermonem habitum de generatione monstrorum: jam alius occurrit de animalibus perfectis: materia hæc priori non minus elegans, nec minus cognitu digna: cum porro in disquisitione hæc venire nequeat quin forma substantialis occurrat, de hac agendum erit, ob connexionem rerum harum mutuam; quo pacto utraque examini subjicientur: a Cleante expectamus deductionem hujus operis quandoquidem illam in se suscepit. Zodiacus med.-gall. 1682, Geneva, 1685, iv, 109–160.—**Ahlfeld** (F.) Ueber einen Monopus mit vollständigem Mangel der äusseren Genitalien und des Afters, nebst Bemerkungen, 1. zur Lehre von der Aetiologie der Sirenenbildung, und 2. zur Lehre von der Thätigkeit der fötalen Niere und Harnblase. Arch. f. Gynaek., Berl., 1879, xiv, 276–294. Also: Mitth. d. Gesellsch. f. Geburtsh. zu Leipz. (1879), 1880, pt. 2, 3–21. Also [Abstr.]: Deutsche med. Wchnschr., Berl., 1879, v, 376.—**Alischer.** Von Menschen, so von Pferden und Kühen gebohren worden. Samml. v. Nat.- u. Med.- . . . Gesch. 1722, Leipz. u. Budissin, 1724, xxi, 334–336.—**Amado** (J. J. da S.) Algumas reflexões a respeito da memoria do Sr. Professor T. Marques intitulada: Breve memoria sobre um exemplar de uma muito notavel monstruosidade, desconhecida até agora na especie humana e que se póde referir ao genero das pygomelias de J. G. Saint Hilaire. J. Soc. d. sc. med. de Lisb., 1864, 2. s., xxviii, 429–441.—**Animadversiones** de monstris humanis et in specie historia graviditatis quatuordecim annorum. Acta Acad. Cæs. reg. Joseph. med.-chir. Vindob., 1788, i, 196–208, 3 pl.—**Atthill.** Exhibition of a monster born in the Rotunda Lying-in Hospital. Obst. J. Gr. Brit., Lond., 1880, viii, 623.—**Bake** (H. A.) Twee waarneemingen van wanschepsels en daar uit afgeleide gevolgtrekkingen. Verhandel. en Waarn. t. Bevord. d. Genees-, Heel-, Verlos- en Scheik., Leyden, 1804, ii, 84–110.—**Barry** (M.) Further observations on the unity of structure in the animal kingdom, and on congenital anomalies, including "hermaphrodites"; with some remarks on embryology, as facilitating animal nomenclature, classification, and the study of comparative anatomy. Edinb. N. Phil. J., 1837, 345–364. Also, Reprint. — **Bartholinus** (T.) De naturæ abundantia et defectu. Acta med. et phil. Hafn. (1673), 1675, ii, 77. Also, transl.: Collect. acad. d. mém., etc., Dijon, 1766, vii, 211.—**Beach.** Ueber die Geburt einer Riesenfrucht. Vrtljschr. f. gerichtl. Med., Berl., 1879, n. F., xxxi, 191.—**Beale** (L. S.) Monstrosity and maternal impressions. Lancet, Lond., 1860, ii, 430.—**Beschriebenen** (Von dem) Leipzigischen Monstro, und einem andern in Schlesien und Polen, welches Letztere halb Mensch und halb Kalb soll gewesen seyn. Samml. v. Nat.- u. Med.- . . . Gesch. 1723, Leipz. u. Budissin, 1724, xxiv, 563–566.—**Born** (G.) Ueber Doppelbildungen beim Frosch und deren Entstehung. Jahresb. d. schles. Gesellsch. f. vaterl. Kult. 1882, Bresl., 1883, lx, 39–43. Also: Breslau. aerztl. Ztschr., 1882, iv, 162. —. Ueber die Furchung des Eies bei Doppelbildungen. Breslau. aerztl. Ztschr., 1887, ix, 169–174.—**Bryant.** Malformations and their causes. Lancet, Lond., 1838–9, i, 489. —**Burggraeve** (A.) Études sur les monstruosités considérées dans leurs rapports avec les lois de l'organogénie. Ann.

Monsters.

Soc. de méd. de Gand, 1837, iii, 37; 145, 2 pl.—**Calderini** (G.) Contributo alla diagnosi delle mostruosità del feto ed alla eziologia dell' idramnios. Ann. di ostet., Milano, 1882, iv, 101–107.—**Carli** (F.) Cenno su tre mostri venuti alla luce in altrettanti parti successivi. Bull. d. sc. med. di Bologna, 1863, 4. s., xix, 30–36.—**Carpenter** (J. G.) Report of a case of monstra deficientia. St. Louis M. & S. J., 1879, xxxvii, 281.—**Chabelard.** [Trois enfans monstrueux.] [*From:* Mém. Acad. roy. d. sc., 1746.] Collect. acad. d. mém., etc. Partie franç, Par. et Liége, 1785, x, 397.—**Chabry** (L.-M.) Processus tératologiques pendant la période de segmentation de l'œuf. Compt. rend. Soc. de biol., Par., 1887, 8. s., iv, 224.—**Chaussier & Adelon.** Monstruosités. Dict. d. sc. méd., Par., 1819, xxxiv, 154–263.—**Chevalier** (J.-M.) Observations pour servir à l'histoire des monstruosités humaines. J. de méd., chir., pharm., etc., Par., 1808, xvi, 369–373.—**Christian** (E. P.) Record of cases of fœtal abnormalities and monstrosities in my practice, with observations of embryonic nutrition. Tr. M. Soc. Mich., Lansing, 1876, 399–410.—**Clemens** (A.) Ueber Missgeburten und angeborene Missgestaltungen. J. f. Kinderkr., Erlang., 1863, xli, 74–78. — **Cnoeffelius** (A.) Infante monstroso cutem porcelli assati similem et duram ex parte gerente. Misc. Acad. nat. curios. 1673-4, Francof. et Lips., 1676, 51. *Also: Ibid.*, 1688, iv–v, 48. *Also, transl.:* Auserl. med.- chir-. . . . Abhandl. d. röm.-kais. Akad. d. Naturf. Nürnb., 1757, iv,72.—**Conant** (D. S.) The science, causes, and anatomical peculiarities of human monstrosities. Tr. N. York Acad. M., 1857-63, ii, 267–298. [Discussion], 362–373.—**Daley** (B.) A difficult labor and fœtal monstrosity. Peoria M. Month., 1882-3, iii, 424. — **Dareste** (C.) Mémoire sur la production de certaines formes de monstruosités simples. Compt. rend. Soc. de biol. 1863, Par., 1864, 3. s., v, 210–215. ——. Sur la production artificielle des monstruosités. Compt. rend. Acad. d. sc., Par., 1868, lxvi, 155–158. ——. Note sur le mode de formation des monstres syméliens. *Ibid.*, 185–187. ——. Nouvelles recherches sur la production des monstruosités dans l'œuf de la poule par une modification du germe antérieure à la mise en incubation. *Ibid.*, 1886, ciii, 355. — **Davaine** (C.) Monstres; monstruosité. Dict. encycl. d. sc. méd., Par., 1875, 2. s., ix, 201–264. — **Description** de deux monstres. [*From:* J. d. sçavans, 1672.] Collect. acad. d. mém., etc. Dijon, 1755, 269, 1 pl.—**Dickinson.** Monstrosities. Weekly M. Rev., Chicago, 1884, ix, 452–458.—**Dickson** (S. H.) Monstrosities. Richmond & Louisville M. J., Louisville, 1869, vii, 1–11. — **Dowler** (B.) Obstetrical cases and physiological remarks. N. Orl. M. & S. J., 1854-5, xi, 13–21.—**Düntzer.** Abgestorbenes Monstrum bei lebendem und wohlgebildetem Kinde. N. Ztschr. f. Geburtsk., Berl., 1842, xi, 364–366.—**Duméril.** Rapport fait sur un enfant monstrueux. Bull. Fac. de méd. de Par. (1809-11), 1812, ii, 23.—**Ectromélie.** Discussion. Bull. Soc. de chir. de Par. (1866), 1867, 2. s., vii, 383–385.— **Ehrmann** (C.-H.) Description de quelques monstruosités humaines. Répert. gén. d'anat. et physiol. path., Par., 1827, iv, 1–9, 1 pl.—**Engel.** Ueber Entstehung von Missgeburten durch äussere Bedingungen. Wien. med. Wchnschr., 1865, xv, 17; 33; 49.—**Engelmann** (G. J.) A teratological contribution. Illust. M. & S., N. Y., 1883, ii, 123–126, 1 pl.—**Falaschi** (E.) Descrizione di alcune mostruosità in un feto umano settimestre. Boll. d. Soc. tra i cult. d. sc. med. in Siena, 1884, ii, 54–56.—**Fisher** (G. J.) Does maternal mental influence have any constructive or destructive power in the production of malformations or monstrosities at any stage of embryonic development? Am. J. Insan., Utica, N. Y., 1869 - 70, xxvi, 241 – 295. *Also,* Reprint, under following title: Are malformations or monstrosities of the fœtus in utero ever produced by the power of maternal mental emotions?— **Formation** (Sur la) des monstres. [*From:* Mém. Acad. roy. d. sc., 1738-40.] Collect. Acad. d. mém., etc. Partie franç., Par. et Liége, 1785, viii, 325–334.—**Fox** (R.) Notices of monstrosities. Lancet, Lond., 1839, i, 471–473.—**Fuller** (A.) Monstrosities. Weekly M. Rev., Chicago, 1884, ix, 394 —**Gallez** (L.) Trois observations sur des enfants monstrueux. Bull. Acad. roy. de méd. de Belg., Brux., 1868, 3. s., ii, 1069–1080. [Rap. de M. de Roubaix], 992–996.—**Gammage** (W. L.) Case of twins, one being a monstrosity: uterine hæmorrhage. N. Orl. M. & S. J., 1856-7, xiii, 15–17.—**Gaston** (E.) Two cases of malformation. Med. Counsellor, Columbus, 1855, i, 561-563.—**Geoffroy-Saint-Hilaire** (E.) Philosophie anatomique des monstruosités humaines, etc. Rev. méd. franç. et étrang., Par., 1823, x, 243–256. ——. Considérations générales sur la monstruosité, et description d'un genre nouveau observé dans l'espèce humaine, et nommé Aspalasome. J. compl. du dict. d. sc. méd., Par., 1825, xxi, 236; 367. ——. Des adhérences de l'extérieur du fœtus, considérées comme le principal fait occasionnel de la monstruosité, et observations nouvelles à l'appui de cette théorie. Arch. gén. de méd., Par., 1827, xiv, 392–406. *Also,* Reprint. ——. Sur quelques dissentimens de théorie dans des questions de monstruosités. Rev. méd. franç. et étrang., Par., 1827, xxv, 277–283. *Also, transl.:* Arch. f. Anat. u. Physiol., Leipz., 1827, 328 - 334. — **Geoffroy-**

Monsters.

Saint-Hilaire (I.) Quelques remarques sur le traité de tératologie. Gaz. méd. de Par., 1837, 2. s., v, 431.— **Gerlach** (L.) Ueber die künstliche Erzeugung von Doppelbildungen beim Hühnchen. Sitzungsb. d. phys.-med. Soc. zu Erlang., 1880–81, 13. Hft., 5–18.—**Giraldès.** Monstruosités diverses chez un fœtus. Compt. rend. Soc. de biol. 1850, Par., 1851, ii, 152.—**Goldschmidt,** Fœtus monstrueux. Proc.-verb. . . . Soc. de méd. de Strasb., 1876 - 7, xii, 34 - 37. — **Gotaas.** Om tvende Misfostre. Norsk Mag. f. Lægevidensk., Christiania, 1853, 2. R., vii, 618–621.—**Guérin** (J.) Réponse à la lettre sur l'application de la méthode naturelle et la classification des monstres; par N. Jolly). Gaz. méd. de Par., 1866, 3. s., xxi, 470; 746: 1867, 3. s., xxii, 103; 477. ——. Nouvelle théorie des monstres. Tr. Internat. M. Cong., 7. sess., Lond., 1881, i, 425-427.—**Gurlt** (E. F.) Die neuere Literatur über menschliche und thierische Missgeburten. Arch. f. path. Anat., etc., Berl., 1878, lxxiv, 501 - 527. — **Gusserow.** Ueber zwei Missbildungen. Verhandl. d. Gesellsch. f. Geburtsh. in Berl. (1861-2), 1863, xv, 188–194. *Also:* Monatschr. f. Geburtsk. u. Frauenkr., Berl., 1863, xxi, 1–7, 1 pl.— **Hard** (A.) Six cases of monstrosities, or malformations, and one of puerperal convulsions. Tr. Illinois M. Soc., Chicago, 1859, 67–71.—**Hart** (S.) Five cases of congenital malformation, or monstrosity. Am. M. Month., N. Y., 1861, xvi, 175–214. *Also:* Tr. M. Soc. County Kings (1858-64), Brooklyn, 1865, i, 160–166.—**Hartmann** (P. J.) Anatome monstrosi crediti fœtus. Misc. Acad. nat. curios. 1686. Norimb., 1687, decuria 2, v, 176–179.—**Hénot.** Mémoire anatomique sur plusieurs fœtus humains monstrueux. Arch. gén. de méd., Par., 1830, xxiv, 313–334, 1 pl.—**Herrmann** (J. J.) Beschreibung zweyer Missgeburten. Med.-chir. Ztg., Innsbruck, 1822, iv, 93; 110.—**Hohl** (A.) Ein Beitrag zur Vervielfachung der Organe, ohne Erblichkeit in einer Familie. Arch. f. Anat. u. Physiol., Leipz., 1828, 177–180.—**Holub**(F.J.) Ueber Monstrositäten. Vrtljschr. f. d. prakt. Heilk., Prag, 1844, iv, 38–58.—**von Huyssen** (B.) Von einigen curieusen Monstris. Samml. v. Nat.- u. Med-. . . . Gesch. 1719, Bressl., 1720, vii, 70–76.—**Jackson.** Monstrosities. Boston M. & S. J., 1856, liv, 295.— **Jacobi.** A collection of anomalies in a monster. Med. Rec., N. Y., 1867-8, ii, 283.—**Jacquart** (H.) Anatomie comparée appliquée à la tératologie. Mémoire sur l'anatologie qui rapproche: 1° la disposition trouvée dans le système circulatoire des fœtus peracéphales de l'homme et des animaux; 2° le système lacunaire des animaux inférieurs; 3° enfin certaine portion du système lymphatique des ophidiens. Compt. rend. Soc. de biol. 1859, Par., 1860, 3. s., i, 235–243.—**Jacquet** (*Mme.*) Plusieurs cas de monstres dans des grossesses doubles et simples. J. d. sages- femmes, Par., 1875, iii, 114.—**Jaeckel** (J.) Beitrag zur Lehre über die ursprünglichen Missbildungen des Menschen. Org. f. d. ges. Heilk., Aachen, 1853, ii, 220–224.—**Jenisch.** Beschreibung einer Missgeburt. Med. Cor.-Bl. d. württemb. ärztl. Ver., Stuttg., 1837, vii, 129-131, 1 pl.—**Joly** (N.) Études sur un monstre humain, né à Toulouse, et affecté tout à la fois d'encéphalie, de pied-bot, de polydactylie, d'hermaphrodisme et d'inversion splanchnique générale. Gaz. méd. de Par., 1866, 3. s., xxi, 372. ——. Lettre sur l'application de la méthode naturelle et la classification des monstres. *Ibid.*, 1866, 3. s., xxi, 469: 1867, 3. s., xxii, 101; 473. [*See, also, supra,* Guérin (J.)]— **Kinnman** (S.) Beskrifning öfver tenne dubbelmissfoster jemte en kort framställning af några satser ur missbildningsbläran. [Description of three monsters, and a short sketch of theories of malformation.] Upsala Läkaref. Förh., 1871-2, vii, 264 - 288. — **Kneeland** (S.), jr. Four cases of malformed fœtus. Boston M. & S. J., 1857-8, lvii, 97–100.—**Koogler** (M. A.) A report of three human monstrosities. Am. J. M. Sc., Phila., 1882, lxxxiv, 129–132.—**Kottmeier.** Zur Casuistik der Missgeburten. Arch. f. path. Anat., etc., Berl., 1864, xxix, 610.—**Lammert** (G.) Ueber Missbildungen; Beiträge aus neuer und alter Zeit. *Ibid.*, 1861, xxii, 230-236, 1 pl.— **Lebedeff** (A.) Ueber die Entstehung der Anencephalie und Spina bifida bei Vögeln und Menschen. *Ibid.*, 1881, lxxxvi, 263–298, 3 pl.—**Lereboullet.** Tératologie. Proc.-verb. . . . Soc. de méd. de Strasb., 1858-63, i, 103–108.—**Leriche** (E.) Note sur quelques points de tératologie. Assoc. franç. pour l'avance. d. sc. Compt.-rend. 1873, Par., 1874, ii, 821–828.—**Lesauvage.** Quelques remarques sur le traité de tératologie de M. Isidore Geoffroy-Saint-Hilaire. Gaz. méd. de Par., 1837, 2. s., v, 431. *Also,* Reprint.—**Lippincott** (H.) & **Warrington** (J.) Cases of abnormal fœtuses; with remarks. Med. Exam., Phila., 1838, i, 269. —**Lombroso** (C.) Teratologia: caso singolare di macrosomia osservato all' Ospedale di Pavia. R. Ist. Lomb. di sc. e lett. Rendic., Milano, 1868, 2. s., i, 671-677.—**Lowne** (B.T.) Abstract of three lectures of teratology. Lancet, Lond., 1877, ii, 242; 392; 551.—**Lunel** (G.) Sur deux cas de polymélie (membres surnuméraires) observés chez la Rana viridis seu esculenta (Lin.). Mém. Soc. de phys. et d'hist. nat. de Genève, 1868, xix, 305-312, 1 pl.—**Lyford** (C.C.) Monstrosities. Am. Vet. Rev., N. Y., 1884-5, viii, 217-221.—**Macari** (F.) Mostro complesso. Salute: Italia med. Genova, 1883, 2. s., xvii, 73-75.—**Mitchell.** Arrested development of a fœtus. Canada Pract.,

Monsters.

Toronto, 1885, x, 121.—**Martin** (J.) Case of a succession of monstrous births occurring in the same female. Med. Exam., Phila., 1849, n. s., v, 23.—**Maughs** (G. M. B.) Remarkable monstrosities. Proc. St. Louis M. Soc. Missouri (1879), 1880, ii, 201.—**Mayer.** Beschreibung merkwürdiger Fälle aus zwei Klassen von Monstrositäten. J. d. Chir. u. Augenh., Berl., 1832, xviii, 521-547.—**Meckel.** Ueber die fehlerhafte erste Bildung der Wirbelsäule bei Monstrositäten. Verhandl. d. Gesellsch. f. Geburtsh. in Berl. (1852-3), 1853, vii, 95-101.—**Meckel** (J. F.) Beschreibung einer merkwürdigen Missgeburt. Deutsches Arch. f. d. Physiol., Halle, 1822, vii. 1-16, 1 pl. ——. Beschreibung einer merkwürdigen Missgeburt. Arch. f. Anat. u. Physiol., Leipz., 1826, i, 36-43.—**Mehrmann** (H. B.) Oakland's monstrosity; what is it? Calif. M. J., Oakland, 1886, vii, 52-55.—**Meissner** (F. L.) Ueber die angebornen Missbildungen des menschlichen Kindes. Monatschr. f. Geburtsk. u. Frauenkr., Berl., 1857, x, 415-435.—**Mekerttschiantz** (M.) Die Geburt und das Präparat einer Missbildung. Centralbl. f. Gynäk., Leipz., 1883, vii, 521-527.—**Mertins.** Ueber die nächste Ursache des Ansprungs (Crusta lactea, lactumen), nebst einigen Bemerkungen über die Entstehung widernatürlicher Lagen des Fötus und der Erzeugung von Aftergebilden (Molæ) krüpplicher und verkrüppelter Kinder. Jahrb. f. d. Lebens-Magnet., Leipz., 1819, ii, pt. 1, 147-159.— **Miles** (A. J.) Congenital malformations. Cincin. M. News, 1872, n. s., i, 201-207.—**Minkowski** (O.) Ueber Spaltungen im Thierkörper. Arch. f. exper. Path. u. Pharmakol., Leipz., 1883, xvii, 445-465.—**Monstres** (Sur les). [From: Mém. Acad. roy. d. sc., 1743.] Collect. Acad. d. mém., etc. Partie franç., Par. et Liége, 1785, ix, 202-211.— **Monstris** (De) Berolini ao. 1723 natis. Acta med. Berolin., 1726, decade 2, vi, 68-74, 1 pl.—**Monströsen** (Von einem) Kinde. Samml. v. Nat.- u. Med.- . . . Gesch. 1720, Leipz. u. Budissin, 1721, xi, 323.—**Montgomery** (E.) Cases of monstrosity. St. Louis M. & S. J., 1861, xix, 232-234.—**Mooney** (M. D.) Congenital malformations. Atlanta M. & S. J., 1874-5, xii, 354.—**Müller.** Beschreibung zweier Missgeburten. Oesterr. Vrtljschr. f. wissensch. Veterinärk., Wien, 1879, lii, 161-167.— **Müller** (A.) Beschreibung zweier Fälle von Missgeburten. Ztschr. f. Wundärzte u. Geburtsh., Stuttg., 1862, xv, 263-267, 1 pl.—**Müller** (A. D.) Et Tilfælde af Misdannelser hos et nyfødt Barn. [Case of malformation in new-born child.] Ugesk. f. Læger, Kjøbenh., 1868, 3. R., v, 329-335.—**Müller** (N.) & **Büchner** (J. G.) Von monströsen Gebuhrten. Samml. v. Nat.- u. Med.- . . . Gesch. 1722, Leipz. u. Budissin, 1724, xxii. 691.—**Murray** (J. J.) [Malformations due to arrested development may co-exist with malformations caused by intra-uterine disease of the fœtus.] Brit. & For. M.-Chir. Rev., Lond., 1860, xxvi, 509.—**Nachrichten** von sieben seltenen Monstrositäten. Mag. f. d. gerichtl. Arzneiw., Berl., 1832, ii, 212-214.—**Noeggerath** (E.) Monstrosity, probably composed of the human heart. N. York M. J., 1882, xxxv, 522. Also: Tr. N. York Obst. Soc. (1881-5), 1885, iii, 54.—**Norris.** Teratoma. N. York M. J., 1880, xxxii, 526.—**North** (J) On monstrosities. Lancet, Lond., 1840, i, 857; 913.—**Observations** sur les monstres humains, et en particulier sur l'histoire d'une grossesse de quatorze ans. Actes Acad. c. r. Joséphine méd.-chir. de Vienne, Montpel., 1792, i, 243-254.—**Olliver** (A.) Sur la pathogénie des vices de conformation. Bull. Soc. d'anthrop. de Par., 1878, 3. s., i, 150-155.—**Ollivier** & **Raige-Delorme.** Monstres; monstruosité. Dict. de méd., 2. éd., Par., 1839, xx, 169-213.—**Orth.** Drei menschliche Missgeburten. Arch. f. path. Anat., etc., Berl., 1872, liv, 492-500.—**Panum** (P. L.) Bidrag til Kundskabom Misdannelsernes Oprindelse. [Contributions to our knowledge of the origin of monsters.] Nord. med. Ark., Stockholm, 1869, i, no. 1, 1-25, pl. 1. ——. Beiträge zur Kenntniss der physiologischen Bedeutung der angebornen Missbildungen. Arch. f. path. Anat., etc., Berl., 1878, lxxii, 69; 165; 289, 2 pl.—**Pargamin.** Sluch. zamechat. urodstva. [Case of remarkable monster.] Russk. Med., St. Petersb., 1886, vi, 602.—**de Pedro** (M.) Tetratologia. Siglo méd., Madrid, 1868, xv, 147; 166; 554; 571; 598; 613.—**Pendleton** (J. M.) Observations on monstrosities. Phila. J. M. & Phys. Sc., 1826, n. s., iv, 289-297; 1827, n. s., v, 17-23.—**Penzig** (O.) Miscellanea teratologica. Mem. r. Ist. Lomb. di sc. e lett. Cl. di lett. e sc. matemat. e nat., Milano, 1883-5, 3. s., vi, 177-212, 4 pl.— **Percheron.** Difformités multiples chez un nouveau-né. Bull. Soc. méd. de Reims (1875), 1876, 70-72.—**Prioleau** (J. F.) Remarks on monstrosities. Tr. South Car. M. Ass., Charleston, 1882, 97-102.—**Prochaska.** Nachricht über zwey menschliche Missgeburten. Med. Jahrb. d k. k. österr. Staates, Wien, 1815-16, iii, 4. St., 104-116, 1 pl.— **Prochaska** (G.) Descriptiones quatuor monstrorum humanorum. In his: Adnot. acad., 8°. Pragæ, 1781, ii, 71-88, 3 pl.—**Purefoy** (R. D.) On a case of arrested development. Dublin J. M. Sc., 1881, lxxi, 260-262.— **de Quatrefages.** Observations à propos de la publication des "Œuvres du Dr. Guérin" (livraisons 1 à 3). Compt. rend. Acad. d. sc., Par., 1880, xci, 794.—**Rankin** (T. W.) Fœtal monstrosity. Cincin. Lancet & Clin., 1882, ix, 529.— **Rathke.** Beschreibung einiger Missbildungen des Men-

Monsters.

schen- und Thierkörpers. Deutsches Arch. f. d. Physiol., Halle, 1822, vii, 481-497.—**Rathke** (H.) Beschreibung zweier sehr seltenen Missgeburten. Arch. f. Anat. u. Physiol., Leipz., 1830, 368-395, 3 pl.—**Rauber** (A.) Die Theorien der excessiven Monstra. Arch. f. path. Anat., etc., Berl., 1878, lxxiii, 551-594, 2 pl.: lxxiv, 66-125.—**Reid** (J.) An account of some monstrosities. Ann. Anat. & Physiol., Edinb., 1850, i, 27-32.—**Relazione** di due parti mostruosi. In: Rac. d' opusc. scient. e filol., 16°, Venezia, 1748, xxxix, 519-532. — **Riecke.** Zur Lehre von den Bildungsfehlern des Menschen. J. d. Chir. u. Augenh., Berl., 1845, n. F., iv, 614-620. — **von Ritgen.** Ueber Entstehung von Missgeburten. Monatschr. f. Geburtsk. u. Frauenkr., Berl., 1855, vi, 1-21.— **Roché** (L.) Accouchement gémellaire; un des enfants cyclope; le deuxième hydrocéphale et bec de lièvie; difficulté de l'accouchement; description des deux enfants. Bull. Soc. méd. de l'Yonne 1870, Auxerre, 1872, xi, 42-50, 2 pl.— **Rodriguez y Palacios.** [Monstruosidades.] Gac. méd. de México, 1871, vi, 58-60.—**Roy** (V.-P.) Mémoire sur 1° un cas de cyclopie; 2° un cas de sycéphalie; 3° et un de polimélie. Ann. Soc. méd.-chir. de Bruges, 1841, ii, 189-209, 4 pl. Also: Arch. de la méd. belge, Brux., 1841, iv, 189-202.—**Sangalli** (G.) Teratologia; mole e mostri umani. R. Ist. Lomb. di sc. e lett. Rendic., Milano, 1875, 2. s., viii, 955.—**San Juan** (N.) Un caso de anomalia relativa á la ausencia de órganos únicos, segun la clasificacion de Geoffroy-Saint-Hilaire, ó ageneses de otros teratólogos. Escuela de med., México, 1879-80, i, no. 13, 8-10; no. 14, 6-8.—**Santlus.** Zur Lehre von den angeborenen Bildungsfehlern und dem Einflusse der Einbildungskraft auf die Entwickelung. J. f. Kinderkr., Erlang., 1856, xxvi, 194-203.—**von Scherer** (A.) Ritter. Zur vergleichenden Anatomie der Missgeburten, und einige Worte über ein sogenanntes Streben zur Hervorbringung eines möglichst unvollkommenen Organismus. Med. Jahrb. d. k. k. österr. Staates, Wien, 1824, n. F., ii, 263-273.—**Schultze** (B.) Ueber anomale Duplicität der Axenorgane. Arch. f. path. Anat., etc., Berl., 1853, vii, 479-531, 1 pl.—**Schwabe** (G.) Eine frühzeitige menschliche Frucht im bläschenförmigen Bildungszustande. Ztschr. f. Geburtsh. u. Gynäk., Stuttg., 1879, iv, 197-209.— **Sentex** (L.) Quelques mots sur deux cas de tératologie. J. de méd. de Bordeaux, 1886-7, xvi, 53-55. Also: Arch. de tocol., Par., 1886, xiii, 978-984. Also: Ann. d'hyg., Par., 1886, 3. s., xvi, 362-370.—**Silvester** (H. R.) Contribution to the science of teratology. Med.-Chir. Tr., Lond., 1858, xli, 73-110, 2 pl. Also [Abstr.]: Proc. Roy. M. & Chir. Soc. Lond. (1857-8). 1858, ii, 16-19. Also [Abstr.]: Lancet, Lond., 1857, ii. 628.—**Sinnett** (E.) Two cases of monstrosity. Tr. Ohio M. Soc., Cincin., 1872, 9-13. Also: Cincin. M. News, 1872, n. s., i, 357-360.—**Skrzeczka.** Leichnam; Lebensfähigkeit; Monstrum. Vrtljschr. f. gerichtl. u. öff. Med., Berl., 1865, n. F., iii, 263-286.— **Smellie** (W.) Of monsters. In his: A treatise on the theory and practice of midwifery; a new ed., 8°. Lond., 1779, i, 325-327: iii, 351-359.—**Sorbets** (L.) Fœtus hydrocéphale et fœtus n'ayant pas de cavité abdominale. Monit. d. sc. méd. et pharm., Par., 1860, ii, 662.—**Stalpart van der Wiel** (C.) Hondeken van een vrouw geboren. In his: Hond. seldz. aanmerk., 8°, Amst., 1682, 234-237.— **Steno** (N.) Embryo monstro affinis Parisiis dissectus. Acta med. et phil. Hafn. (1671-2), 1673, i, 200-203.—**de Superville** (D.) Some reflections on generation and on monsters; with a description of some particular monsters. Transl. from the French by P. H. Zollman. Phil. Tr., Lond., 1732-44, ix, 304-312.—**Tanner** (T. H.) A description of two fœtal monsters. Tr. Obst. Soc. Lond. (1860), 1861, ii, 247-250. Also, Reprint.—**Taxil St.-Vincent.** Observations sur quelques vices d'organisation. J. univ. d. sc. méd., Par., 1816, iii, 182-192.—**Terry** (C. C.) Remarks upon some recently reported cases of monstrosity. Am. J. Obst., N. Y., 1869-70, ii, 369-402. — **Thompson** (P. H.) Three monstrosities. Atlanta M. & S. J., 1885-6, n. s., ii, 592-595. —**Tiedemann** (F.) Observations sur l'état du cerveau et des nerfs dans les monstres. J. compl. du dict. d. sc. méd, Par., 1828, xxxi, 142; 208.— **Truchsess.** Beschreibung von zwei Missgeburten. Med. Cor.-Bl. d. württemb. ärztl. Ver., Stuttg., 1837, vii, 37-40.— **Tussau.** Observation d'un enfant monstre. Lyon méd., 1886, liii, 175.—**Valentini** (M. B.) De lusu et erroribus naturæ, ad Rudolphum Jac. Camerarium 1691. In his: Polychresta exotica etc., 4°, Francof. ad Mœnum, 1700, 166-175.—**Velasco.** Monstruosidades fetales. Anfiteatro anat., Madrid, 1873, i, 141.—**Verneau** (R.) Monstruosités. N. dict. de méd. et chir. prat., Par., 1877, xxiii, 8-35.—**Verrier.** Deux fœtus monstrueux. Gaz. méd. de Picardie, Amiens, 1885, iii, 167.—**Virey** (J.-J.) Monstre; considérations générales sur la formation des monstres parmi les animaux et les végétaux. Dict. d. sc. méd., Par., 1819, xxxiv, 131-154.—**Vrolik** (W.) Beschrijving eeniger merkwaardige misgeboorten. Verhandel. v. h. Genootsch. t. Bevord. d. Genees- en Heelk. te Amst., 1855, ii, 99-136, 9 pl. Also, Reprint.—**Warren** (J. M.) An account of two remarkable Indian dwarfs, exhibited in Boston under the name of Aztec children. Am. J. M. Sc., Phila., 1821, n. s., xxi, 285-293, 2 pl. Also, Reprint.—

Monsters.

Warynski (S.) & **Fol** (H.) Recherches expérimentales sur la cause de quelques monstruosités simples et de divers processus embryogéniques. Rev. méd. de la Suisse Rom., Genève, 1883, iii, 395–413, 3 pl.

Monsters (*Artificial production of*).

Dareste (C.) Recherches sur la production artificielle des monstruosités, ou essais de tératogénie expérimentale. 8°. *Paris*, 1877.

Boie (E. K.) K kasuistike urodstve u ptitse. [Production of monsters in birds.] Arch. vet. nauk, St. Petersb., 1885, xv, pt. 2, 9–13. — **Dareste** (C.) Nouvelles recherches sur la production artificielle des monstruosités dans l'espèce de la poule. Compt. rend. Soc. de biol. 1863, Par., 1864, 3. s., v, 158–160. —— Nouvelles recherches sur les conditions physiques de la production artificielle des monstruosités dans les embryons de poule soumis à l'incubation artificielle. Ibid., 1881, Par., 1882, 7. s., iii, 33. ——. Recherches sur la production des monstres, dans l'œuf de la poule, par l'effet de l'incubation tardive. Compt. rend. Acad. d. sc., Par., 1882, xcv, 254–256. ——. Recherches sur la production des monstruosités par les secousses imprimées aux œufs de poul. Ibid., 1883, xcvi, 511–513. ——. Nouvelles recherches sur la production des monstres, dans l'œuf de la poule, par l'effet de l'incubation tardive. Ibid., 444–446. — **Geoffroy-Saint-Hilaire.** Sur des déviations organiques provoquées et observées dans un établissement d'incubations artificielles. J. compl. du dict. d. sc. méd., Par., 1826, xxiv, 256–263. — **Vulpian** (A.) Expériences faites sur des embryons de grenouille et relative à l'influence des lésions des centres nerveux, pendant le développement embryonnaire, sur la production de certaines déformations. Arch. de physiol. norm. et path., Par., 1871–2, iv, 90–93.

Monsters (*Jurisprudence of*).

Jacobi (S.) Commentatio de monstris, quoad medicum forensem. 8°. *Halæ*, 1791.

Bierbaum (J.) Die Rechte der missgebildeten Neugebornen. Med. Ztg., Berl., 1850, xix, 147; 153. —— Das Rechtsverhältniss der missgebildeten Neugeborenen. Ztschr. f. d. Staatsarznk., Erlang., 1854, lxvii, 160–181. — **Geoffroy-Saint-Hilaire.** Des rapports de la tératologie avec la médecine légale. Ann. d'hyg., Par., 1837, xvii, 431–443. — **Géry** (L.-H.) Discussion tératologique et médico-légale sur un cas d'avortement ayant eu pour résultat l'expulsion d'un monstre prétendu acéphale. Rev. méd. franç. et étrang., Par., 1842, i, 20–54. — **Lonsdale** (H.) History of a monstrosity presenting remarkable peculiarities in the arrangement of the nervous system, with a brief inquiry into its teratological and medico-legal relations. Edinb. M. & S. J., 1843, lx, 324–340. — **Tardieu** (A.) & **Laugier** (M.) Contribution à l'histoire des monstruosités considérées au point de vue de la médecine légale à l'occasion de l'exhibition publique du monstre pygopage Millie-Christine. Ann. d'hyg., Par., 1874, 2. s., xli, 340–371. Also, Reprint.

Monsters (*Acardiac*).

See, also, **Blood** (*Circulation of, Fœtal*); **Monsters** (*Acephalous*).

Calori (L.) Di un mostro umano acardio e della ipotesi più probabile intorno alle cagioni della mancanza del cuore. 4°. *Bologna*, 1885. Repr. from: Mem. Accad. d. sc. d. Ist. di Bologna, 4. s., vi.

Claudius (M.) Die Entwicklung der herzlosen Missgeburten. 8°. *Kiel*, 1859.

Dickinson (W. H.) Description of a fœtus born without heart, brain, lungs, or liver. 8°. *London*, 1863.
Also, in: Proc. Roy. M. & Chir. Soc. Lond. (1861–4), 1864, iv, 237–239.

Elb (H.) *Ueber einen Fall von herzloser Missgeburt. 8°. *Leipzig*, [1869].

Eysell (C. G. A.) *Ueber einen menschlichen Acardiacus. 4°. *Marburg*, [1867].

Genth (C. P.) *Beitrag zur Kenntniss der herzlosen Missgeburten. 8°. *Berlin*, 1868.

Lehmann (O.) *Ein neuer Fall von Acardius amorphus (Amorphus Foerster). 8°. *Halle a. S.*, 1883.

Meïmaroglu (P. A.) *Ueber einen Acardiacus. 8°. *Halle a. S.*, 1879.

von Roques (C. P. H.) *Ueber einen menschlichen Acardiacus mit Nabelschnurbruch und Atresia ani. 4°. *Marburg*, 1864.

Monsters (*Acardiac*).

Schoenborn (C.) *De monstris acardiacis. 8°. *Berolini*, [1863].

Sippel (A.) *Ein menschlicher Acardiacus. 4°. *Marburg*, [1875].

Spliedt (O. J. F.) *Monstri acardiaci descriptio anatomica. 4°. *Kiliæ*, 1859.
Also, in: Arch. f. path. Anat., etc., Berl., 1860, xviii, 254–265.

van der Starp (A. T.) *Over het ontstaan der monstra acardiaca. 8°. *Utrecht*, [1875].

Adan (A. M.) Physiology of the circulation in the acardiac fœtus. Month. J. M. Sc., Lond. & Edinb., 1854, xix, 518–524. — **Ahlfeld** (F.) Die Entstehung der Acardiaci. Einldngsschr. z. Feier d. 25jähr. Besteh. d. Gesellsch. f. Geburtsh. zu Leipz., 1879, 20–59. — **Bompiani.** Illustrazione anatomica di un feto acardiaco, acormo. Bull. d. r. Accad. med. di Roma, 1885, xi, 146–156. — **Breus** (C.) Zur Lehre von den Acardiacis. Med. Jahrb., Wien, 1882, 57–72. 2 pl. ——. Erwiderung auf Ahlfeld's "Nachtäge zur Lehre von der Entstehung der Acardiaci". Arch. f. Gynaek., Berl., 1884, xxiii, 156. — **Brodie** (B. C.) Account of the dissection of a human fœtus, in which the circulation of the blood was carried on without a heart. Phil. Tr., Lond., 1809, xcix, 161–168. Also, transl.: Arch. f. d. Physiol., Halle, 1815, xii, 393–403. — **Calori** (L.) Sul sistema vascolare di un mostro umano acardio e anadenolinfemico. Mem. d. Accad. d. sc. d. Ist. di Bologna, 1869, 2. s., ix, 267–300, 3 pl. Also [Abstr.]: Rendic. Accad. d. sc. d. Ist. di Bologna, 1869–70, 9–13. — **Cederschjöld.** Fall af missfoster-acardiacus. Svens. Läk.-Sällsk. n. Handl., Stockholm, 1878, xl, 54. — **Combs** (R. C. F.) Acardiacus. Tr. N. York Obst. Soc. (1876–8), 1879. i. 19. — **Credé** (C. S. F.) Fall von Acardiacus. Monatschr. f. Geburtsk. u. Frauenkr., Berl., 1869, xxxiii, 296–302, 1 pl. — **Embleton.** Case of human monstrosity, with sketch; absence of the heart and lungs. Edinb. M. & S. J., 1841, lvi, 423–427. — **von Franque** (O.) Fall von Acardiacus. Beitr. z. Geburtsh. u. Gynaek., Würzb., 1869, vi, 136–138. — **Godin.** [Cœur remarquable par sa petitesse.] Bull. Soc. anat. de Par., 1836–7, xi, 108. — **Hall** (M.) On the circulation in the acardiac fœtus. Lond. & Edinb. Month. J. M. Sc., 1843, iii, 541–547. Continued in: Month. J. M. Sc., Lond. & Edinb., 1844, iv, 775. — **Hauptmann.** Monströse Ziegenfrucht; Acardiacus; Acephalus bipes. Arch. f. path. Anat., etc., Berl., 1870, l, 303. — **Hicks** (J. B.) & **Bankart** (J.) Dissections of acephalous monsters without head. heart, lungs, or liver. Guy's Hosp. Rep. 1866–7, Lond., 1868, 3. s., xiii, 456–461. 3 pl. — **Hildebrandt** (H.) Beschreibung einer herzlosen Missgeburt. Königsb. med. Jahrb., 1862, iii, 180–184. — **Holland** (G. C.) On the circulation in the acardiac fœtus. Edinb. M. & S. J., 1844, lxii, 156–178. — **Holst** (J. C.) Angeborener Herzfehler. J. f. Kinderkr., Erlang., 1865, xliv, 305–311. — **Houston** (J.) An account of a human fœtus without brain, heart, or lungs; with observations on the nature and cause of the circulation in such monsters. Dublin J. M. Sc., 1836, x, 204–220. ——. On the circulation of the blood in acardiac fœtuses. Ibid., 1843–4, xxiv, 337–354. — **Jackson** (J.) On the circulation in acardiac fœtuses. Lond. M. Gaz., 1843, xxxii, 467. — **Jackson** (J. S. B.) Case of monstrosity, in which the brain. heart, lungs, stomach, liver, spleen, pancreas, and right kidney were wanting. Am. J. M. Sc., Phila., 1837–8, xxi, 362–368. — **Koch** (G. W.) Ueber einen menschlichen Acardiacus. Arch. f. Gynaek., Berl., 1885, xxvi, 290–308, 1 pl. — **Kroner** (T.) & **Schuchardt** (K.) Ein Fall von Acardiacus amorphus. Arch. f. path. Anat., etc., Berl., 1882, xc, 443–455, 1 pl. — **Lahs.** Die Beschreibung eines Acardiacus. Sitzungsb. d. Gesellsch. z. Beförd. d. ges. Naturw. zu Marb. (1883), 1884, 39–44. — **Leboucq** (H.) Description anatomique d'un acardiaque humain paracéphalien (Geoffr.). Ann. Soc. de méd. de Gand, 1877, lv, 39–60, 2 pl. — **Le Cat** (C. N.) A monstrous human fœtus, having neither head, heart, lungs, stomach, spleen, pancreas, liver, nor kidnies; transl. from the French, by M. Underwood. Phil. Tr., Lond., 1767, lvii, 1–20, 2 pl. — **Lusk** (W. T.) Case of acardia. N. York M. J., 1874, xix, 176–179, 2 pl. — **Moldenhauer.** Anatomische Beschreibung eines Acardiacus. Arch. f. Gynaek, Berl., 1873, v, 337–342, 1 pl. Also: Mitth. d. Gesellsch. f. Geburtsh. zu Leipz. (1873), 1874, 1–6, 1 pl. — **Ogle** (J. W.) The circulation in the acardiac fœtus. Brit. M. J., Lond., 1871, ii, 490–492. — **Poppel** (J.) Ueber herzlose Missgeburten. Monatschr. f. Geburtsh. u. Frauenkr., Berl., 1862, xx, 249–271, 1 pl. Also, Reprint. ——. Beschreibung einer Acardiacus-Placenta. Monatschr. f. Geburtsk. u. Frauenkr., Berl., 1868, xxxii, 138–140, 1 pl. — **Report** of committee on case of acardiac monster. Am. J. Obst., N. Y., 1874–5, vi, 629–631. — **Simpson** (A. R.) Description of an acardiac fœtus. Tr. Edinb. Obst. Soc. (1874–7), 1878, iv, 384–389. Also: Edinb. M. J., 1877–8, xxiii, 46–50. Also: Obst. J. Gr. Brit., Lond., 1877–8, v, 681–685. — **Stalpart vander Wiel** (C.) Een kint sonder herssenen geboren. In his: Hond. seldz. aanmerk., 8°, Amst., 1682, 5–11.

Monsters (Acephalous).

See, also, Monsters (Acardiac).

BRERA (V. L.) Singulare mostruosità d' un feto umano, e congetture sul primitivo sviluppo dell' embrione. 4°. Verona, 1815.

Repr. from: Soc. ital. d. sc., xvii.

ELBEN (E.) De acephalis, sive monstris corde carentibus. 4°. Berolini, 1821.

GERGENS (P. J.) Anatomische Beschreibung eines merkwürdigen Acephalus. 4°. Giessen, 1830.

HEMPEL (C. F.) De monstris acephalis disquisitio anatomica. 4°. Hafniæ, 1850.

HERHOLDT (J. D.) Anatomisk Beskrivelse over fem menneskelige Misfostere. 4°. Kjøbenhavn, 1829.

Repr. from: Kongel. Danske Vidensk. Selskabs Skrifter.

KALEK (J. H.) Monstri acephali humani expositio anatomica. 4°. Berolini, [1825].

LAUFFER (J. J.) * Diss. med. qua infans sine cerebro natus consideratur. 4°. Halæ Magdeb., [1743].

LOCKE (J.) A strange and lamentable accident that happened lately at Mears-Ashby in Northamptonshire, 1642. Of one Mary Wilmore, wife to John Wilmore, rough mason, who was delivered of a childe without a head, and credibly reported to have a firme crosse on the brest, as this ensuing story shall relate. 8°. London, 1642.

Reprinted 1880.

MALHERBE. Observation d'acéphalie. 8°. [Nantes, n. d.]

MAPPUS (M.) Historia medica de acephalis. sm. 4°. Argentorati, 1687.

MONRO (A.) Description of a human male monster; illustrated by tables, with remarks. 4°. Edinburgh & London, 1793.

PFOTENHAUER (C. A.) * De monstro acephalo humano. 8°. Berolini, [1835].

RUDELT (J. P.) * Beschreibung einer kopflosen Missgeburt. 8°. Würzburg, 1829.

SAPOLINI (G.) Acefalia tetramerica. Lettera del . . . al Cristoforo Tommati. 8°. Milano, 1870.

SOWOIDNICH (E.) * De acephalo quodam humano. 8°. Vratislaviæ, 1847.

TIEDEMANN (F.) Anatomie der kopflosen Missgeburten. fol. Landshut, 1813.

TOEPPEN (H. A. M.) * De acephalo. 8°. Regimontii Pr., [1846].

VEENDAM (J. L.) * Over hoofdelooze misgeboorten. 8°. Leiden, 1869.

WULFSHEIN (S.) * Monstri acephali descriptio anatomica. 4°. Berolini, [1833].

Abortus septimestris monstrosus, sine cerebro et cranio, per 11 horas vivens. Acta med. Berolin., 1721, viii, 7-13.—Abraham (R.) Description of an acephalous fœtus. Lond. M. & Phys. J., 1827, n. s., ii, 135.—Adam (A. M.) The acephalous fœtus, and the physiology of its circulation. Month. J. M. Sc., Lond. & Edinb., 1854, xix, 515-524.—Allen. [A-typical acephale.] Austral. M. J., Melbourne, 1881, n. s., iii, 409.—Allison (J.) Acephalous fœtus. Prov. M. & S. J., Lond., 1842-3, v, 225.—Aymett (R. E.) An acephalous monster. South. Pract., Nashville, 1884, vi, 110.—Baxter (M.) Acephalous monstrosity. Nashville J. M. & S., 1881, n. s., xxvii, 15.—Beardsley (A.) Case of birth and dissection of an acrania. Brit. Rec. Obst. M. & S., Manchester, 1848, i, 168.—Beardsley (L. N.) An acephalous fœtus. Boston M. & S. J., 1858-9, lix, 39.—Beck. Case of acephalous fœtus. Dublin Hosp. Gaz., 1856, n. s., iii, 357.—Béclard. Mémoire sur les fœtus acéphales. Bull. Fac. de méd. de Par., 1814-15, iv, 447: 493: 1816-17, v, 488, 11 pl.—Bedengfield (J.) Monstrosity. Lancet, Lond., 1833, ii, 499.—Bevill (C.) A case of acephalus, with spina bifida. St. Louis Cour. Med., 1885, xiii, 280.—Beyer (G. W.) Ein Kind ohne Cranio und Haut. Samml. v. Nat.- u. Med.... Gesch. 1723, Leipz. u. Budissin, 1725, xxv, 311.—Bimar (A.) Sur un monstre acéphale; description et réflexions. Gaz. hebd. d. sc. méd. de Montpel., 1886, viii, 220-224.—Bonn (A.) Ontleedkundige beschrijving en aanmerkingen, over het maaksel en de voeding eener zeldzaame en wanstaltige

Monsters (Acephalous).

menschlijke vrucht, als van zes maanden dragts, ten zelfden tijde, nevens twee voldragene en welgemaakte kinderen geboren. Verhandel. d. Genootsch. t. Bevord. d. Heelk., Amst., 1794, iii, 123-192, 1 pl.—Bower (H. L.) Acephalous monsters. Med. Age, Detroit, 1883-4, ii. 64.—Boyce (L. R.) Acephalous monstrosity. Phila. M. Times, 1873-4, iv, 363. Also: Tr. M. Soc. County Albany, 1883, iii, 108.—Breschet (G.) Acéphalie. Dict. de méd., 2. éd., Par., 1832, i, 440-465.—Brewster (W. A.) Monster. Boston M. & S. J., 1830-31, iii, 176.—Brown (D.) A peculiar acephalous monster. Am. J. Obst., N. Y., 1884, xvii, 1021-1026. Also [Abstr.]: Med. News, Phila., 1884, xliv, 702.—Bryce (R.) Acephalous fœtus. Dublin Hosp. Gaz., 1856, n. s., iii, 357.—Burrows. Case of malformation of the head, constituting what is commonly called an acephalous fœtus. Med.-Chir. Tr., 3. ed., Lond., 1817, ii, 52-57.—Calderon y Martinez (J.) Un feto acéfalo. Anfiteatro anat., Madrid, 1876, iv, 243.—Calori (L.) Sopra un peracefalo umano. Mem. Soc. med.-chir. di Bologna, 1847, 2. s., iv, 345-383, 3 pl.—Chamberlain (W. M.) Acranial monster. N. York M. J., 1883, xxxvii, 93. Also: Tr. N. York Obst. Soc. (1881-5), 1885, iii, 147-149. - Chandelux. Rapport sur un cas de fœtus acéphale. Lyon méd., 1880, xxxv, 42-52. Also: Mém. et compt.-rend. Soc. d. sc. méd. de Lyon (1880), 1881, xx, 86-96.—Cintra (S.) Monstre unitaire de l'ordre des omphalosites, famille des acéphaliens, genre péracéphale. Ann. Soc. d'anat. path. de Brux., 1880, xxix, 93-96.—Cockell (F.), jr. Fœtal monstrosity [acephalic]. Tr. Obst. Soc. Lond. (1883), 1884, xxv, 110.—Cooper (W.) An account of an extraordinary acephalous birth. Phil. Tr., Lond., 1775, lxv, 311-321.—Courjon. Observation d'un monstre acéphalien, genre acéphale. Lyon méd., 1880, xxxv, 37-42. Also: Mém. et compt.-rend. Soc. d. sc. méd. de Lyon (1880), 1881, xx, 79-85.—Csap (J.) Ueber einen Acephalus. Ztschr. f. Nat.- u. Heilk. in Ungarn, Oedenburg, 1858, ix, 83. — Depaul. Note sur un fœtus acéphale. Compt. rend. Soc. de biol. 1857, Par., 1858, 2. s., iv, 132-137. Also [Abstr.]: Bull. Soc. anat. de Par., 1857, xxxii, 29. ———. Un fœtus acéphale. Bull. Acad. de méd., Par., 1874, 2. s., iii, 302-307. ———. Monstre acéphale. Ibid., 1875, 2. s., iv, 357-362. ———. Monstre appartenant à la famille des acéphaliens (genre péracéphale). Arch. de tocol., Par., 1875, ii, 234-241.—Depaul & Simonot. Description anatomique d'un monstre de la famille des acéphaliens. Bull. Acad. de méd., Par., 1856-7, xxii, 1152-1159.—van Deurs. Eine merkwürdige Missgeburt. [From: Arch. d. königl. dänischen Gesundheitscollegii ausgezogen von Otto.] Ztschr. f. d. ges. Med., Hamb., 1846, xxxiii, 99-101.—Doneaud. Observation sur un monstre acéphale. J. de méd., chir., pharm., etc., Par., 1772, xxxvii, 127.—Dubois. Monstre acéphale. Bull. Soc. de méd. et chir. de La Rochelle, 1878. no. 4, 52-54.—Du Castel. Deux cas d'acéphalie. Bull. Soc. anat. de Par., 1873, xlviii, 84.—Duckwell (F. A.) An acephalous monster. Med. Age, Detroit, 1884, ii, 30.—E. (A. J.) Acephalous fœtus; imperfect spinal column. Boston M. & S. J., 1841, xxiv, 123.—Elders (W. N.) Case of an acephalous monster. St. Louis M. & S. J., 1873, n. s., x, 316-318.—Ellis (B.) Description of a deformed fœtus. N. Am. M. & S. J., Phila., 1827, iii, 174, 1 pl.—Elmer (J.) Account of an imperfect fœtus. Phila. M. Museum, 1805-6, ii, 71. — Emmert. Ueber einen die hintere Gliedmasse eines Lamms vorstellenden Acephalus. Deutsches Arch. f. d. Physiol., Halle, 1820, vi, 1-9, 1 pl. — Enfant vivant sans tête. [Transl. from: Phil. Tr., Lond., 1667, by de Buffon.] Collect. acad. d. mém., etc., Dijon, 1755, ii, 88.—Erwin (R. W.) Acephalous monster. St. Louis M. & S. J., 1873, n. s., x, 520-522.—Felsenreich & Holl (M.) Acephalus monobrachius (Acardiacus). Med. Jahrb., Wien, 1880, 171-178, 1 pl.—Fenómeno. Siglo méd., Madrid, 1860, vii, 398.—Finaz. Observation sur un acéphale. J. univ. d. sc. méd., Par., 1821, xxiii, 120-128. — Flemming (R. N.) Acephalous fœtus. E. Tennessee Rec. M. & S., Knoxville, 1852-3, i, 130.—Fonssagrives & Gallerand. Description anatomique d'un monstre humain acéphalien paracéphale. Gaz. hebd. de méd., Par., 1865, 2. s., ii, 232-234.—Garland (G. W.) Acephalous monster. N. Hampshire J. M., Concord, 1850-51, i, 185.—Geddings (E.) Acephalous. Am. Cycl. Pract. M., Phila., 1834, i, 142-171.—Geoffroy-Saint-Hilaire (E.) Sur quelques conditions générales de l'acéphalie complète, lue à la Société philomatique, le 17 juin 1826. Rev. méd. franç. et étrang., Par., 1826, iii, 36-51. Also, Reprint.—Géry (L.-H.) Discussion tératologique et médico-légale sur un cas d'avortement qui a eu pour résultat l'expulsion d'un monstre prétendu acéphale. Rev. méd. franc. et étrang., Par., 1842, i, 20-51. Also, Reprint.—Getchell (F. H.) Monstrosity. Tr. Coll. Phys. Phila., 1863-74, n. s., iv, 189.—Gonzalez y Guerra (B.) Descripcion de un acéfalo, complicado con una transposicion de varias visceras torác cas y abdominales. Décadas de med. y cirug. práct., Madrid, 1822, v, 61-71.—Green (T.) Description of a monstrous child. Lond. M. Rev. & Mag., 1800, iii, 318.—Greene (W. T.) A case of acephalous monster. Brit. M. J., Lond., 1870, ii, 115.—Gripat (H) Monstre acéphale. Bull. Soc. anat. de Par. (1872), 1874, xlvii, 124-131. ———. Veau acéphale;

Monsters (*Acephalous*).

dissection. *Ibid.*, 601–606. ——. Notes sur un acéphale humain. Rev. phot. d. hôp. de Par., 1872, iv, 386–393, 1 pl.—**Hardey** (R.) Case of acephalo-cyclopean monstrosity. Tr. Obst. Soc. Lond. (1862), 1863, iv, 213–221.—**Harison** (B. D.) An acephalous monster. Canad. Pract., Toronto, 1883, viii, 41.—**Harker** (J.) Dissection of an abnormal four-toed fœtus without head or upper limbs. J. Anat.& Physiol., Lond., 1874–5, ix, 182–184.—**Harvey.** Acephalous monster born at the full period of pregnancy. Proc. Westminst. M. Soc., Lond., 1848–9, 21. *Also:* Lond. M. Gaz., 1848. n. s., vii, 1079. *Also:* Lancet, Lond., 1848, ii, 696.—**Heiberg** (J. F.) Beskrivelse over et menneskeligt Misfoster uden Hoved, Hals og Arme. Eyr, Christiania, 1831, vi, 281–291.—**Hélie** (P.) Observation d'acéphalie. J. de la sect. de méd. Soc. acad. Loire-Inf., Nantes, 1844, xx, 15–32.—**Hellwig** (J.) Infans acephalus. *In his:* Obs. phys.-med., 4°, Aug. Vindel., 1680, 1–6.—**Henckels** (J. F.) Anmerckungen von einer besondern Missgeburt, dergleichen meines Wissens noch nicht bekannt ist. *In his:* N. med. u. chir. Anmerck., 12°, Berl., 1769, i, 60–74.—**Hewitt** (G.) Acephalous monstrosity; absence of abdominal covering. Tr. Obst. Soc. Lond. (1866), 1867, viii, 316.—**Holt** (W.) Acephalous hermaphrodite monster. Lancet, Lond., 1861, i, 328.—**Hutchins** (E. R.) A case of monstrosity. Chicago M. J., 1869, xxvi, 704.—**Isaacs** (C. E) Dissection of an acephalous fœtus. N. York J. M., 1853, x, 205–207.—**Jackson** (J. B. S.) Monstrosity. N. Eng. Q. J. M. & S., Bost., 1842–3, i, 249–251. ——. A case of "acephalous fœtus", in which some of the abdominal organs were found in the posterior mediastinum, and a portion of intestine had passed through an opening in the bodies of the vertebræ so as to appear upon the back. Boston M. & S. J., 1858, lviii, 42–44. *Also:* Extr. Rec. Bost. Soc. M. Improve. (1856–8), 1859, iii, 191–194. ——. Case of an acephalous fœtus which lived about thirty-six hours. Boston M. & S J., 1859–60, lxi, 239. *Also:* Extr. Rec. Bost. Soc. M. Improve. (1859–61), 1862, iv, 63. ——. Acephalous fœtus, with dislocation of hip, and other complications. Boston M. & S. J., 1860, lxii, 127–129.—**Jänistus** (J.) Von einem neugebornen Kinde ohne Kopf. Auserl. med.- chir.- . . . Abhandl. d. röm.-kais. Akad. d. Naturf., Nürnb., 1756, iii, 418–420.—**Jeaffreson** (G. E.) An acephalous monster. Lancet, Lond., 1866, ii, 568.—**Kennedy** (E.) Acephalous fœtus, totally brainless, acutely sensitive. Brit. M. J., Lond., 1872, ii, 183. *Also:* Med. Press & Circ., Lond., 1872, n. s., xv, 209.—**Labbée** (E.) Un monstre acéphalien, genre acéphale. Réveil méd., Par., 1880–81, i, 216.—**Littré** (E.) De l'état du cœur et de quelques autres organes chez les acéphales. J. hebd. de méd., Par., 1830, vi, 481–487.—**Luzun.** Cas remarquable d'acéphalie; étude de cette monstruosité. Mém. Soc. d. sc. phys. et nat. de Bordeaux, 1868, vi, 145–162.—**M'Clintock.** Acephalous fetus. Dublin Q. J. M. Sc., 1867, xliv, 240.—**Malherbe.** Observation d'acéphalie. J. de la sect. de méd. Soc. acad. Loire-Inf., Nantes, 1855, xxxi, 195–199.—**Marcotte** (F. L.) Acephalus with spina bifida. St. Louis Cour. Med., 1883, ix, 430.—**Maurice** (E.-F.) Note sur un fœtus humain monstrueux de la famille des acéphaliens et du genre coccycéphale. Ann. Soc. de méd. de St.-Étienne et de la Loire (1867–71), 1872, iv, 22–32.—**Mayer** (C.) Geburt eines Acephalus. Verhandl. d. Gesellsch. f. Geburtsh. in Berl. (1844–5), 1846, i, 128; 180, 2 pl.—**Mercier.** [Acéphalie compliquée d'hydrocéphalie.] Bull. Soc. anat. de Par., 1836–7, xi, 108.— [**Méry.**] Sur un fœtus humain monstrueux. [*From:* Mém. Acad. roy. d. sc. de Par., 1720.] Collect. acad. d. mém., etc. Partie franç., Par., 1774, v, 275–277.—**Meulewaeter.** Description anatomique d'un monstre acéphale. Bull. Soc. de méd. de Gand, 1853, xx, 246–248.—**Miller** (E. D.) Acephalous fœtus carried much over the usual period of gestation. Boston M. & S.J., 1859–60, lxi, 501.—**Milward** (J.) Case of an acephalous monster. Tr. Obst. Soc. Lond. (1872), 1873, xiv, 140.—**Monro** (A.) Description of a human male monster. Tr. Roy. Soc. Edinb., 1794, iii, 215–230, 4 pl.—**Moreau.** Description d'un fœtus acéphale. Bull. Soc. anat. de Par., 1860, xxxv, 116–120.—**Mouser** (S. M.) The constant coincidence of excessive quantity of liquor amnii and acephalous children. Am. M. Bi-weekly, Louisville, 1878, viii, 241.—**Ollivier** (C.-P.) Description d'un acéphale monopède. Arch. gén. de méd., Par., 1825, vii, 414–418.—**O'Rielly** (W.), sr. Acephalous monsters. N. South Wales M. Gaz., Sydney, 1872–3, iii, 215.—**Phelan** (M.) Case of acephalous fœtus. Dublin M. Press, 1844, xii, 357–358.—**Pinson.** Un enfant monstrueux, qui n'avoit ni crâne, ni cervelle, ni cervelet, qui cependant vint au monde vivant, et vécut environ huit heures. [*From:* Mém. Acad. roy. d. sc. de Par., 1772.] Collect. acad. d. mém., etc. Partie franç., Par. et Liége, 1787, xv, 313. — **Pironet.** Description d'un fœtus humain monstrueux. Ann. Soc. de méd d'Anvers, Brux , 1840, 355–358. *Also:* Arch. de la méd. belge, Brux., 1840, iii, 87–90.—**Prochaska.** Nachricht über eine kopflose menschliche Missgeburt. Med. Jahrb. d. k. k. österr. Staates, Wien, 1819–20, v, 2. St., 64 – 68, 1 pl.—**Pulley** (J.) [Case of monstrosity.] Med. & Phys. J., Lond., 1800, iii, 138.—**Rendu** (H.) Description d'un fœtus humain monstrueux

Monsters (*Acephalous*).

de la famille des acéphaliens. Bull. Soc. anat. de Par., 1875, l, 352–360. 2 pl. *Also:* Progrès méd., Par., 1875, iii, 663; 668. — **Richard** (A.) Étude anatomique sur un fœtus acéphalien. Arch. gén. de méd., Par., 1852, 4. s., ii, 152 - 160. — **Rogers** (B.) Acephalous monster. Lancet, Lond., 1876, ii, 107.—**S.** (L. P.) Influence of maternal feelings; acephalous child. Boston M. & S. J., 1841, xxiv, 72. — **Sandifort** (G.) Ontleedkundige beschrijving en aanmerkingen over twee hoofdelooze misgeboorten. Genees-, heel-, . . . kundige Verhandel. v. h. k.-nederl. Inst. v. wetensch., etc., Amst., 1825, 1–40, 11 pl.—**Schelhammer** (G. C.) Von einer Misgeburt ohne Kopf. Auserl. med.- chir.- . . . Abhandl. d. röm.-kais. Akad. d. Naturf., Nürnb., 1770, xix, 235, 1 pl.—**Schmidt.** Potwor bezczaszkowy (acrania). Medycyna, Warszawa, 1875, iii, 774–776.—**Seeliger** (S.) Von einem menschlichen Monstro ohne Kopff, Brust und Armen. Samml. v. Nat.- u. Med.- . . . Gesch. 1722, Leipz. u. Budissin, 1723, xx, 626–634.—**Severance** (La G.) An acephalic monster. Fort Wayne J. M. Sc., 1882–3, ii, 14.—**Shirriff** (F. W.) Case of acephalous monster of seven months' fœtation, occurring in a primipara. Canada M. & S. J., Montreal, 1873–4, ii, 146–148. ——. Case of acephalous monster of seven months' fœtation. *Ibid.*, 385. — **Simonot.** Grossesse double; accouchement à sept mois; fœtus acéphale. Monit. d. hôp , Par., 1857, v, 157. *Also:* Bull. Soc. méd.-prat. de Par., 1859, 100–106.—**Smith** (T. H.) Case of acephalous monstrosity. Lancet, Lond., 1863, i, 373.—**Sommer** (F.) Merkwürdiger Acephalus bei einer Zwillingsgeburt, nebst dessen Abbildung. Med. Ann., Heidelb., 1844, x, 369–372.—**de Soyre.** Monstre acéphale. Bull. Soc. anat. de Par., 1873, xlviii, 224.—**Spaak.** Monstre acéphale dont s'est accouchée une femme atteinte d'hydropisie du péritoine compliquée d'hydramnios. Bull. Soc. roy. d. sc. méd. et nat. de Brux., 1873, 68.—**Strähler.** Beobachtung eines Acephalus. Med. Cor.-Bl. d. württemb. ärztl. Ver., Stuttg., 1834, iii, 249.—**Thomson** (W. S.) Short notes on a rare obstetric case, with specimen of acephalous fœtus. Glasgow M. J., 1881, [4. s.], xv, 21–23.—**Townsend** (W. E.) Acephalous female fœtus. Am. J. M. Sc., Phila., 1851, n. s., xxi, 339.—**Tuck** (H.) & **Jackson** (J. S. B.) Case of acephalus. Boston M. & S. J., 1876, xciv, 439–442. *Also:* Extr. Rec. Bost. Soc. M. Improve. (1874–9), 1880, vii (app.), pp. xxxii–xxxiv.—**Verco** (J. C.) Fœtal monster. Australas. M. Gaz., Sydney, 1886–7, vi, 160.—**Vernière** (A.) Mémoire sur les fétus acéphales. Répert. gén. d'anat. et physiol. path., Par., 1827, iii, 1–24.—**Virchow.** Eine Missgeburt (Acrania mit Spina bifida totalis). Verhandl. d. Gesellsch. f. Geburtsh. in Berl. (1856–7), 1858, x, 138–140, 1 pl.—**Wertheimer.** Observation de monstre peracéphale; considérations générales sur l'acéphalie. Bull. méd. du nord, Lille, 1880, 2. s., xx, 235–248, 1 pl.—**West** (J. W.) Acephalous fœtus. Prov. M. & S. J., Lond., 1842–3, v, 169.—**Westbrook** (B. F.) Acephalous monster. Proc. M. Soc. County Kings, Brooklyn, 1883–4, viii, 206.—**Willey** (J. M.) Birth of an acephalous infant. Calif. M. Gaz., San Fran., 1869–70, ii, 120.—**Wilson** (W. E.) Acephalic monsters. Colorado M. J., Denver, 1882, i, 14 - 19. *Also:* Rocky Mountain M. Times, Denver, 1882, i, 145–150.—**Winston** (C. K.) Acephalous monster. Nashville J. M. & S., 1868–9, n. s., iv, 411.—**Woodruff** (L.) Acephalous monsters. Columbus M. J., 1882, i, 252.

Monsters (*Double*).

See, also, **Eggs** (*Abnormal*); **Fœtus** *in fœtu*; **Monsters** *in animals, etc.*; **Siamese** *Twins*.

Alessandrini (A.) Annotazioni anatomiche risguardanti un mostro umano bicefalo e bispinale, Dicephalus bispinalis Gurlt. 4°. [*n. p.*, 1856.]

Cutting from: Mem. d. Soc. ital., 2. s., i, 37–51, 4 pl.

D'Alton (E.) *De monstrorum duplicium origine atque evolutione commentatio. 4°. Halis, 1848.

——. De monstris quibus extremitates superfluæ suspensæ sunt commentatio. Comment. de monstrorum duplicium origine atque evolutione altera pars. Accedit index monstrorum duplicium, quæ in collectione anatomica Halensi asservantur. 4°. *Halis Sax.*, 1853.

B. (T.) A trve and certaine relation of a strange-birth, which was borne at Stone-house in the parish of Plimmouth, the 20. of October, 1635. Together with the notes of a sermon . . . at the interring of the sayd birth. 8°. [*London*, 1635.] [Reprint], *London*, 1871.

von Baer (K. E.) Ueber doppelleibige Missgeburten, oder organische Verdoppelungen in Wirbelthieren. 4°. [*n. p.*, 1844.]

Monsters (*Double*).

———. The same. Als Anhang: Kleine Nachlese von Missgeburten, die an und in Hühner-Eiern beobachtet sind. 4°. *St. Petersburg*, 1845.
Repr. from: Mém. Acad. imp. d. sc. de St.-Pétersb. Sc. math., phys. et nat., iv.

BARDSLEY (J. L.) The retrospective address, delivered at the fifth anniversary meeting of the Provincial Medical and Surgical Association, held at Cheltenham, July 19 and 20, 1837. [With colored plate.] 8°. *Worcester*, [1837].

BARKOW (J. C. L.) * De monstris duplicibus verticibus inter se junctis. 4°. *Berolini*, 1821.

———. Monstra animalium duplicia per anatomen indagata, habito respectu ad physiologiam, medicinam forensem, et artem obstetriciam. Descripsit iconibusque illustravit . . . 2 v. 4°. *Lipsiæ*, 1828-36.

BARTELS (A. C.) * De janis inversis ac de duplicitate generatim. 4°. *Berolini*, [1830].

BECKER (A.) * Ueber einen Fall von Doppelmissbildung. 8°. *Würzburg*, 1863.

BECKER (E.) * Ein Fall von Bauchblasengenitalspalte mit Kloakenbildung und Dicephalus tripus dibrachius. 8°. *Göttingen*, 1881.

BERGHOLZ (S. T.) * De monstro duplici per implantationem ac de duplicitate. 8°. *Berolini*, [1840].

BESSE (H.) Diploteratology ; or a history of some of the most wonderful human beings that have ever lived in double form, and a scrutinizing view into the marvelously strange freaks of nature, and causes of same. 4°. *Delaware, Ohio*, 1874.

BEUTNER (F.) * Ein Fall von Doppelmissbildung (Thoracopagus tetrabrachius). 8°. *Erlangen*, 1880.

DE BILS (L.) Anatomische beschrijvinge van een wanschepsel, geboren op de elderschans buijten Aerdenburg ontleet. Briefs-gewijse gesonden door F. de Raet aen A. Parent. 4°. *Middelburgh*, 1659.

BRUNE (A. E.) Einiges über Doppelmissbildungen. 8°. *Berlin*, 1877.

BRUNNER (J. C.) * Fœtum monstrosum et bicipitem sistit. sm. 4°. *Argentorati*, [1672].

BUCH (J.) * De monstro humano distomo. 8°. *Halæ*, 1866.

BÜTTNER (C. G.) Anatomische Anmerckungen bey einem mit auswärtshänge dem Herzen lebendig gebornen Kinde, und dann bey Gelegenheit einer todt gebohrnen zwei-köpfigen Missgeburt, nebst Erörterung einiger curieusen Fragen. sm. 4°. *Königsberg u. Leipzig*, 1752.
Also, in his: Anat. Wahrnehm. 4°. *Königsberg*, 1769, 36-92, 3 pl.

BURDACH (K. F.) Berichte von der königlichen anatomischen Anstalt zu Königsberg. Sechster Bericht. Mit einer Uebersicht von parasitischen und gedoppelten Menschenkörpern. 8°. *Leipzig*, 1823.

———. Berichte von der königlichen anatomischen Anstalt zu Königsberg. Siebenter Bericht. Mit dem Beschlusse der Uebersicht von parasitischen und gedoppelten Menschenkörpern. 8°. *Leipzig*, 1824.

CALORI (L.) Intorno un peracefalo umano inserito col suo tralcio ombellicale in un tronco comune al tralcio di feto normale. fol. *Bologna*, 1855.
Repr. from: Mem. Accad. d. sc. d. Ist. di Bologna, v.

———. Descrizione di un mostro umano doppio opo-ectodimo, preceduta da un breve commentario sulle uova gemellifiche degli uccelli. 4°. *Bologna*, 1855.
Repr. from: Mem. Accad. d. sc. d. Ist. di Bologna, vi.

Monsters (*Double*).

CHRISTELL (G.) * De partu gemellorum coalitorum. sm. 4°. *Argentorati*, [1751].
Also, in: WEIZ (F. A.) Neue Ausz., [etc.] 12°. *Frankfurt. u. Leipzig*, 1780, xi, 174-201.

CURTIUS (C. W.) * De monstro humano cum infante gemello. 4°. *Lugd. Bat.*, 1762.

DANNENBERGER (J.) Tripes Haiterbacensis, cujus secundam considerationem dogmaticam sumsit. sm. 4°. *Tubingæ*, 1755.

DIETERICHS (L. M.) De fratribus Italis ad epigastrium connatis. 4°. *Ratisponæ*, 1749.

DISCOURS prodigieux de deux filles, nées à Paris le 17 janvier 1605. Lesquelles s'entretenoient par le ventre inférieur, ayant deux testes, quatre yeux, quatre bras, quatre jambes et deux natures. 12°. *Paris*, [n. d.]

DITTMER (L.) * Zur Lehre von den Doppelmissgeburten. 8°. *Berlin*, [1874].
Also, in: Arch. f. Anat., Physiol. u. wissensch. Med., Leipz., 1875, 356-401.

DUBÉ (P.) Histoire de deux enfans monstrueux, nées en la paroisse de Septfonds au duché de S. Fergeau, le 20 juillet 1649. 16°. *Paris*, 1650.

ENGELS (P.) * Ueber Xiphopagen. 8°. *Berlin*, [1873].

FANZAGO (F.) Storia del mostro di due corpi che nacque sul Bresciano in novembre 1802. 4°. *Padova*, 1803.

FATTORI (S.) De' feti che racchiudono feti, detti volgarmente gravidi . . . si aggiungono alcune considerazioni intorno alla generazione degli animali. fol. *Pavia*, 1815.

FAUST (B. C.) * Descriptionem anatomicam duorum vitulorum bicipitum et conjecturas de causis monstrorum exhibens. 4°. *Rintelii*, 1777.

FISHER (G. J.) Diploteratology; an essay on compound human monsters, comprising the history, literature, classification, description, and embryology of double and triple formation, including parasitic monsters, fœtus in fœtu, and supernumerary development. Pt. 1. 4°. *Albany*, 1868.
See, also, infra.

GERLACH (L.) Die Entstehungsweise der Doppelmissbildungen bei den höheren Wirbelthieren. roy. 8°. *Stuttgart*, 1882.

GERLING (C. L. H. T.) * Hypogastrodidymus in anatomia Marburgensi servatus tractatur. 4°. *Marburgi Cattorum*, 1845.

GERVAIS (H.-F.-P.) * Description anatomique d'un nouveau cas d'hétéradelphie, suivie d'un résumé des caractères propres à ce genre de monstruosités. 4°. *Paris*, 1877.

GRÆTZ (J. H.) De monstroso abortu Dessauiensi. 4°. *Servestæ*, [1694].

GRIMM (J. C.) Kurtze historische, physicalische und medicinische Relation einiger Mirabilium naturæ, oder Wunder-Dienge in der Natur, in specie von einem Monstro bicorporeo, oder von einer Wunder-Geburth, so in diesem 1700sten Jahr, den 16. Martii, von einer Frau in Pombseu, an das Tage-Licht gekommen. 4°. *Leipzig*, 1700.

GRONAU (L.) *Anatomische Bemerkungen über ein Diprosopus triopthalmus. 8°. *Rostock*, 1864.

GRUBER (W. L.) Anatomie eines Monstrum bicorporeum, eigenthümlicher (Thoraco-gastrodidymus). 4°. *Prag*, 1844.

HALL (R.) Description of a monstrous birth. fol. [n. p., n. d.]

HALLER (A.) Descriptio fœtus bicipitis, ad pectora connati, ubi in causas monstrorum ex principiis anatomicis inquiritur. 4°. *Hannoveræ*, 1739.

Monsters (*Double*).

——. [Pr.] disputationem inauguralem qua duorum monstrorum anatome continetur indicit. 4°. *Gottingæ*, 1742.

HELLMUTH (K.) * Zur Casuistik der Missbildungen. Ein Fall von congenitalem vollständigen Radiusdefect und von Dicephalus dibrachius tripus. 8°. *Erlangen*, 1881.

HENOP (W.) * Ein Fall von Dicephalus tribrachius. 4°. *Kiel*, 1877.

HESSE (E.) * Monstri bicipitis descriptio anatomica. 8°. *Berolini*, [1823].

HEUSER (C. V.) * Ueber ein Zwillingsei mit einem missbildeten Fötus. 8°. *Marburg*, 1864.

HIMLY (E. A. W.) Darstellung des Dualismus am normalen und abnormen menschlichen Körper, oder physiologische Erörterung seiner Zusammensetzung aus zwei Hälften und der auf mangelnder Vereinigung derselben beruhenden Missgeburten. 4°. *Hannover*, 1829.

HISTORY and medical description of the two-headed girl. Told in "her own peculiar way" by "one of them". 12°. *Buffalo, N. Y.*, 1869.

HOLME (E.) An account of a child with a double head. 4°. [*n. p.*, 1790.]

VON JAEGER (G. F.) Ueber zwey am Becken verwachsene männliche Kälber. 8°. [*Amsterdam*, 1858.]
Transl. from: Versl. . . . d. k. Akad. v. Wetensch., Letterk. [etc.], Amst., 1858, vii.

JEBE (L. F.) * De partubus monstrorum nonnullorum duplicium. 4°. *Kiliæ*, 1866.

KAESTNER (G.) * Monstri anatini bicorporei descriptio anatomica una cum disquisitione de ejus ortu. 4°. *Kiliæ*, 1860.

KLINKOSCH (J. T.) [Pr.] quo anatomicam monstri bicorporei monocephali descriptionem proponit. 4°. *Vetero Pragæ*, 1767.

KNATZ (K. H.) * Ueber Doppelmissbildungen. 8° & 4°. *Marburg*, 1856.

KORTÜM (E. G. A.) * Anatomische Beschreibung einer Doppelmissgeburt. 8°. *Greifswald*, 1875.
Also, in: Arch. f. path. Anat., etc., Berl., 1875, lxii, 441-463, 1 pl.

KRAUSE (H.) * Diss. exhibens descriptionem monstri humani bicorporei cum hemiacephalia. 8°. *Dorpati Livonorum*, 1826.

KREITNER (F.) * Descriptio monstri duplicati. 8°. *Nordlingæ*, 1826.

LAUTH (F.) * Essai et observations sur les diplogénésis, ou monstruosités doubles. 4°. *Paris*, 1834.

LENGELING (H.) * Ueber Duplicitas parasitica (Ischiopagus). 8°. *Bonn*, 1879.

LIEBENER (O.) * Ueber Sternopagen, mit besonderer Berücksichtigung der inneren Organisation. 8°. *Halle*, [1870].

LIESCHING (C. F.) * Tripes Heitersbacensis, cujus primam considerationem historico-dogmaticam defendendam sumsit. sm. 4°. *Tubingæ*, [1755].

LOCHER (J.) Carmen heroicum de partu monstrifero in oppido Rhain ad ripam Lyci adjacente ab egena femina edito anno Domini nonagesimo nono supra milesimum xv. kalendas decembris. 4°. [*Ad finem:*] Impressus hic libellus in Ingelstad[ie]nsi studio, [1489].

LÜRMAN (W.) * Ein Fall von Doppelmissbildung (Sternopagie). 4°. *Kiel*, 1874.

MECKEL (J. F.) De duplicate monstrosa commentarius. fol. *Halæ et Berolini*, 1815.

MONDINUS (F.) Bicorporei humani monstri anatomica descriptio. Una cum animadversionibus atque conjecturis nonnullis quæ ad illustrandam abnormium partium formationis rationem concurrunt. 4°. *Bononiæ*, 1833.

NEUBECK (A.) De dicephalo dibrachio. 4°. *Halis Sax.*, 1866.

Monsters (*Double*).

NÖLL (F.) * Ein Fall von Hemicephalie mit Epignathie. 8°. *Marburg*, 1882.

PALFYN (J.) Description anatomique, de la disposition surprenante de quelques parties externes et internes de deux enfans, nés dans la ville de Gand le 28 avril 1703, qui étoient joints par la partie inférieure des troncs de leurs corps. À laquelle on a ajoûté la description anatomique, de l'étrange disposition de quelques parties, d'un autre enfant gemeau, qui ne sont pas moins surprenantes, que dans les enfans précédens, né dans la même ville le 27 may 1703. Comme aussi un traité de la circulation du sang dans le fœtus, pendant qu'il est encore dans le sein de sa mère, avec une description très-exacte des conduits particuliers qui y concourent pour la confirmation de l'opinion des modernes contre le nouveau système de M. Mery, touchant l'usage du trou ovalaire. 12°. *Leide*, 1708.

——. The same. Anatomie, of ontleedkundige beschrijving, rakende de wonderbare gesteltenis van eenige uyt- en innerlijke deelen van twee kinderen, dewelke monstreuselijk aan malkander vereenigt zijn, onder met den tronk van 't lichaam, geboren binnen de stad van Gendt op den 28. April 1703. Waar bij gevoegd is de ontleedkundige beschrijving, aangaande de vreemde gesteltenis eeniger deelen van een ander kind, zijnde een tweeling, niet min wonderhaar, als in de bovengeseyde kinderen, geboren binnen deselve stad op den 27. Mey 1703. Als mede een zeer eurieuze verhandeling van de bijsondere wegen, die gevonden worden in de ongeboren kinderen, en waar door het bloed circuleert in dezelve, anders, als in de bejaarde personen. 8°. *Leyden*, 1733.

PETER (J. U.) * Monstri duplicis per implantationem expositio anatomica. 8°. *Turici*, 1844.

PRYTZ (L. J.) De monstro humano bicepite et bicorpore, trunces ad anteriora coalitis artusque duplicatis. Resp. C. Tengström. 4°. *Aboæ*, 1816.

RIOLANUS (J.) De monstro nato Lutetiæ anno Domini 1605. Disputatio philosophica. 8°. *Parisiis*, 1605.

RIPPMANN (T.) * Ueber einen bisher nicht beobachteten Fall multipler Intrafötation in- und ausserhalb der Schädelhöhle. 8°. *Zürich*, 1865.

ROLLIN (C. J.) * Dissertatio anatomico-medica duorum monstrorum anatomen et de causis monstrorum ulteriorem disquisitionem exhibens. sm. 4°. *Gottingæ*, 1742.

ROSENSTIEL (A.) * Monstri duplicis rarissimi descriptio anatomica. 4°. *Berolini*, [1824].

ROUGE (F.) * Beiträge zur Lehre des Geburtsmechanismus bei Doppelmissgeburten. 8°. *Giessen*, 1853.

SALM (A.) * De causis et origine monstrorum duplicium, adjecta descriptione anatomica monstri dicephali. 8°. *Gryphiæ*, 1858.

SANDIFORT (E.) [Twelve plates of double monsters from v. 2 of: Museum anatomicum Lugduno-Batavæ descriptum [etc.], Lugd. Bat., 1793.] fol. [*n. p., n. d.*]

SARNOW (H.) * Ueber die Formveränderungen der intermediären Schädelknochen beim Diprosopus. 8°. *Königsberg*, [1874].

SCHRAVEN (H.) * Ueber Sternopagen. sm. 8°. *Berlin*, [1869].

SERRES (E.-R.-A.) Recherches d'anatomie transcendante et pathologique. Théorie des formations et des déformations organiques, appliquées à l'anatomie de Ritta-Christine, et de la duplicité monstrueuse. 4°. *Paris*, 1832.

SKIBBE (G.) * Ein Thoracopagus. 8°. *Königsberg*, 1887.

Monsters (*Double*).

TACKE (R.) * De sternopago. 4°. *Halis Sax.*, [1864].

TARDIEU (A.) & LAUGIER (M.) Contribution à l'histoire des monstruosités considérées au point de vue de la médecine légale à l'occasion de l'exhibition publique du monstre pygopage Millie-Christine. 8°. *Paris*, 1874.

VERNOIS (M.) Loi universelle (attraction de soi pour soi), ou clef applicable à l'interprétation de tous les phénomènes de philosophie naturelle, par É. Geoffroy-Saint-Hilaire. Étude et analyse. 8°. *Paris*, 1839.

[VERO (Il) ritratto di un giovine con due teste.] roy. 8°. *Venetia*, 1695.

VILLENEUVE (A.-C.-L.) Description d'une monstruosité consistant en deux fœtus humains accolés en sens inverse par le sommet de la tête, suivie de remarques et d'observations à ce sujet. 4°. *Paris*, 1831.

VOTTEM (F.) Description de deux fœtus réunis par la tête. 8°. *Liége*, 1828.
Also [Abstr.], *in:* Compt. rend. Soc. d. sc. méd. et nat. de Brux , 1832, 5–8.

VROLIK (W.) Over dubbelde misgeboorten. 4°. *Amsterdam*, 1840.
Author's copy, interleaved and containing many manuscript notes and additions by Prof. Vrolik, MS. letters from Sandifort, etc.

WALTER (J. G.) Observationes anatomicæ. Historia monstri bicorporis duobus capitibus, tribus pedibus, pectore pelvique concreti. Curæ renovatæ de anastomosi tubulorum lactiferorum mammæ muliebris. Commenta terrestria. Venæ capitis et colli. fol. *Berolini*, 1775.

WALTHER (A. F.) [Pr.] partus monstrosi historiam et sectionem describit. 4°. [*Lipsiæ*, 1732.]

WEHRDE (F. G.) * De monstro rariore humano. 8°. *Halæ*, [1826].

WEINTRAUB (M. S.) * De duplicitate quadam monstrosa in capite vitulino animadversa. 8°. *Regimonti Pr.*, 1866.

WERTHER (G. C.) De monstro Hungarico. 4°. *Lipsiæ*, [1707].

WICHERT (C. E.) * Descriptio monstri duplicati. 8°. [*Dorpat*], 1824.

WILL (H.) *Anatomische Untersuchung einer Doppelmissbildung. 8°. *Würzburg*, 1863.

WIRTENSOHN (J.) * Duorum monstrorum duplicium humanorum descriptio anatomica. 4°. *Berolini*, [1825].

WOLFART (C. J.) * De fœtu monstroso duplici, hujusque occasione de pulmonum aquæ injectorum e- et submersione. 4°. *Marburgi Cattorum*, [1725].

ZAAIJER (A.) * Over monstra duplicia. 8°. *Leiden*, 1876.

ZIMMER (J. C.) Physiologische Untersuchungen über Missgeburten, nebst der Beschreibung und Abbildung einiger Zwillingsmissgeburten. 8°. *Rudolstadt*, 1806.

ZSCHOKKE (C. J. T.) * De janis. 4°. *Berolini*, 1827.

Aberle (M.) Geburtsgeschichte und anatomische Beschreibung einer zweyköpfigen menschlichen Missgeburt. Med.-chir. Ztg., Salzb., 1816, i, 225–240. — **Acton** (W.) Case of partial double monstrosity. (Ischiopage symélien of Geoffroy-Saint-Hilaire; heteradelphia of Vrolik.) Med.-Chir. Tr., Lond, 1845-6, xxix, 103–106, 1 pl. *Also*, Reprint. *Also* [Abstr.]: Lond. M. Gaz., 1846, n. s., ii, 521.—**Ahlfeld** (F.) Beiträge zur Lehre von den Zwillingen. Arch. f. Gynaek., Berl., 1874-5, vii, 210–286.—**Albrechtus** (J. S.) De monstroso gemellorum abortu salutari. Acta Acad. nat. curios., Norimb., 1737, iv, 411–416, 1 pl.—**Alischer** (S.) Zweyköpffiges Monstrum. Samml. v. Nat.- u. Med.- . . . Gesch. 1721, Leipz. u. Budissin, 1723, xvii, 89.—**Allen** (E.) Case of double monster, born at the full period of gestation. Prov. M. J., Lond., 1843, vi, 524.—**d'Alton.** Ueber das Entstehen von Doppelmissgeburten. Amtl. Ber. ü. d. Versamml. deutsch. Naturf. u. Aerzte 1847, Aachen, 1849, xxv, 168–175, 1 pl.—**Ancelet**

Monsters (*Double*).

(E.) Note sur un cas de pygomélie dans l'espèce humaine. Gaz. d. hôp., Par., 1869, xlii, 582 ; 590.—**Anger** (T.) Monstre double monocéphalien. Rev. phot. d. hôp. de Par., 1870, ii, 97, 2 pl.—**von Archenholz** (S.) Ein Monstrum. N. Mag. f. Aerzte, Leipz., 1793, xv, 492.—**Arnison** (G.) Remarkable fœtal malformation. Lancet, Lond., 1839-40, ii, 606–608.—**Ashburner** (J.) Duplex boys. Lond. M. Gaz., 1829-30, v, 135–137.—**Askham** (W. F.) Report of an extraordinary double-birth. Lancet, Lond., 1848, ii, 235.—**Badger** (G.) A rare case of monstrosity. Med. Rec., N. Y., 1869-70, iv, 166.—**Baker** (W.) A fœtus with two heads. Boston M. & S. J., 1839, xx, 237.—**Ball** (W. B.) A new edition of the Siamese twins. Virginia M. J., Richmond, 1858, x, 197–199, 1 pl.—**Bardescu.** Monstru dublu autositar, monomfalien, genul sternopag sex feminin. Progresul med. roman, Bucuresci, 1880, ii, 196.—**Barnsfather** (J.) A dicephalous hermaphrodite. Cincin. M. News, 1874, iii, 393–396. — **Battey.** [Case of a double monster.] Atlanta M. & S. J., 1874-5, xii, 154, 1 pl.—**Baur.** Ueber eine menschliche Doppelmissgeburt. Verh. d. phys.-med. Soc. zu Erlang., 1865-7, 1. Hft., 10–13.
——. Anatomie einer zweiköpfigen, dreiarmigen, dreibeinigen, weiblichen Doppelmissgeburt. Arch. f. Anat., Physiol. u. wissensch. Med., Leipz., 1867, 173; 311, 4 pl.—**Baynall** (G.) Duplex twins; some of the viscera common to both, and others distinct in each. Lond. M. Gaz., 1832, x, 348.—**Beaussier.** Sur deux enfans joints ensemble. J. de méd., chir., pharm., etc., Par., 1770, xxxiv, 90–92.—**Beer** (H.) † [Dicephalus.] Wien. med. Wchnschr., 1856, vi, 831.—**Beer** (J.) Ein fötales Zwillingsmonstrum. Deutsche Klinik, Berl., 1862, xiv, 453.—**Belgrave** (T. B.) Case of plural birth and monstrosity, the two fœtuses being joined at the vertices of the head. Tr. M. Soc. King's Coll., Lond., 1857-8, ii, 180–183. *Also:* Edinb. M. J., 1863-4, ix, 270–272.—**Benedini** (F.) Storia di un parto, e descrizione di un feto mostruoso bicorporeo dicefalo. Gazz. med. di Milano, 1844, ii, 25–28.—**Benito.** Parto dificil de dos gémelos adheridos por sus cavidades torácica y abdominal. Bol. de med., cirug. y farm., Madrid, 1844, 2. s., v, 109.—**Bentzien** (C.) Et Dobbeltmisfoster. Hosp.-Tid., Kjøbenh., 1877, iv, 409–413.—**Bérard.** Deux filles jumelles réunies par la poitrine et une grande partie du ventre jusqu'au dessous de l'ombilic (sternopages). Bull. Acad. de méd., Par., 1849-50, xv, 448–451.
——. Cas fort curieux de duplicité monstrueuse. *Ibid.*, 1851-2, xvii, 242.—**Berdot** (D. C. E.) Fetus biceps. Acta Helvet., Basileæ, 1767, vi, 179–185.—**Bérigny.** Des monstres diplogénèses. Bull. Acad. de méd., Par., 1843-4, ix, 1061.—**Bérigny & Dause** (P.) Observation d'un cas très rare de monstre humain. Monit. d. sc. méd. et pharm., Par., 1861, 2. s., iii, 409–412.—**Berjoan.** Un cas de monstre double autositaire. France méd., Par., 1876, xxiii, 712.—**Berry** (A.) Description of two children united together, and now living in the village of Arasoor, in the district of Bhavany. Tr. Med.-Chir. Soc. Edinb., 1826, ii, 35–38, 1 pl.—**Bert** (P.) Note sur un monstre double autositaire de la famille des monosomiens. Compt. rend. Soc. de biol. 1863, Par., 1864, 3. s., v, 132–137, 1 pl. *Also*, Reprint.——. Sur le monstre pygopage connu sous le nom de Millie-Christine. Bull. Soc. d'anthrop. de Par., 1873, 2. s., viii, 894–898. ——. Un monstre double. Médecin, Par., 1882, viii, no. 44, p. 1.—**Biaudet & Bugnion.** Histoire d'un monstre xiphopage. Rev. méd. de la Suisse Rom., Genève, 1882, ii, 121–144, 1 pl. *Also, transl.:* Med. Cor.-Bl. d. württemb. ärztl. Ver., Stuttg., 1882, lii, 233–238.—**Blackburn** (C. J.) Case of monstrosity. Transylv. J. M., Lexington, Ky., 1835, viii, 414.—**Blake** (J. E.) Analogue of the Siamese twins. N. York M. J., 1876, xxiii, 414.—**Blanks** (J. H.) A case of monstrosity. N. Orl. M. & S. J., 1881-2, n. s., ix, 424.—**Bleynie** (L.) Note sur un cas de tératologie. J. Soc. de méd. et de pharm. de la Haute-Vienne, Limoges, 1877, ii, 83–85.—**Blodgett** (A. W.) Description of a double monster; fœtus dicephalus, hydrocephalus, anencephalus, microcephalus. Boston M. & S J., 1881, cv, 194–197.—**Blot.** Sur deux monstres doubles autositaires et monomphaliens du genre sternopage. Bull. Acad. de méd., Par., 1877, 2. s., vi, 295–300.—**Blümlein.** Zwei Zwillingspaare mit seltener Missbildung. Vrtljschr. f. gerichtl. Med., Berl., 1874, n. F., xx, 70–80.—**Böhm.** Kurze Beschreibung des Verlaufes einer Geburt zweier, mit Brust und Unterleib verwachsener Kinder, nebst deren Behandlung bei der Entbindung. Mem. d. Heilk., Staatsarzneiw. u. Thierh., Züllichau, 1818, ii, 159–170. ——. Ein Fall verwachsener Zwillingsfrüchte (Xiphopagi) glücklich operativ getrennt. Arch. f. path. Anat., etc., Berl., 1866, xxxvi, 152–154.—**Boens.** À propos de Millie-Christine; du caractère propre et de la nature originelle des monstruosités de ce genre. Art méd., Brux., 1875, xi, 9–11.—**Bœrstler** (G. P.) Monstrosity. Ohio M. & S. J., Columbus, 1854-5, vii, 267–272. *Also:* Am. J. M. Sc., Phila., 1855, 2. s., xxx, 13–16, 2 pl.—**Boettcher** (A.) Zur Anatomie der xiphopagen Doppelbildungen. Dorpat. med. Ztschr., 1871, ii, 105–192, 1 pl. ——. Ueber einen Fall von Doppelmissbildung. *Ibid.*, 1873-4, v, 306–333, 2 pl.—**Boislinière** (L. C.) Case of double-headed monster. St. Louis M. & S. J., 1868, n. s., v, 412–414. *Also, transl.* [Abstr.]: Gaz. hebd. de méd., Par., 1869, 2. s., vi, 307.—**Boisot.** Sur un enfant

Monsters (*Double*).

monstrueux. [*From:* J. d. sçavans, 1682., Collect. acad. d. mém., etc., Dijon, 1755, i, 294.—**Bonini** (A.) Storia d' un feto mostruoso bicorporeo. Ann. univ. di med., Milano, 1834, lxxi, 257–260, 1 pl.—**Bordenave.** Description d'un enfant monstrueux né à terme. [*From:* Mém. Acad. roy. d. sc. de Par., 1776.] Collect. acad. d. mém., etc. Partie franç., Par. et Liége, 1787, xvi. 397–399, 2 pl.— **Borelli** (G. B.) Descrizione di due figlie gemelle riunite tra di loro nella regione epigastrica, e tuttora viventi al 55⁰ giorno; con riflessioni storico-teratologiche. Rac. di oss. clin.-patol., Torino, 1851–4, i, 4. fasc., 264–286. *Also, transl.:* Ann. clin. de Montpel., 1854–5, ii, 122; 151; 183.—**Borellus** (P.) Monstrum biceps, et testudineus tumor mirus. *In his:* Hist. et obs. med.-phys., 12⁰, Par., 1650, 153– 155.—**Borland** (J.) Account of a living duplex child. Lond. M. Gaz., 1829–30, v, 50–52.—**Bornemann.** Ein Fall von Doppelbildung. Arch. f. Gynaek., Berl., 1883, xxi, 205–210.—**van den Bosch.** Description d'un monstre double autositaire monomphalien ectopage. Bull. Acad. rôy. de méd. de Belg., Brux., 1879, 3. s., xiii, 268–282. *Also:* Ann. Soc. méd.-chir. de Liége, 1879, xviii, 193; 228, 1 pl. *Also, transl.:* Encicl. méd.-farm., Barcel., 1879, iii, 281; 289.—**Böttern.** Fødsel af et Misfoster med to fuldtudviklede Hoveder. Hosp.-Tid., Kjøbenh., 1876, 2. R., iii, 737–740.—**Boulant.** Monstre double monomphalien sternopage. Bull. Soc. anat. de Par., 1882, 4. s., vii, 130–133. *Also:* Progrès méd., Par., 1882, x, 950.—**Boulton** (T.) † Lancet, Lond., 1864, i, 517.—**Bourdel** (A.) Réflexions sur un fait de tératologie. Ann. clin. de Montpel., 1854–5, ii, 122; 151; 183; 205. *Also,* Reprint.—**Bourjot Saint-Hilaire.** Nouveau cas de monstruosité du genre hétéradelphe. Gaz. méd. de Par., 1832, iii, 701.—**Bouteiller** (J.) Monstre double parasitaire, famille des polyméliens, genre notomèle, variété nouvelle; un membre pelvien et un membre thoracique insérés sur la colonne vertébrale; spina bifida à l'endroit de cette insertion; kystes pileux entre les lames du spina bifida. Bull. Soc. anat. de Par., 1857, xxxii, 92–97. [Rap. de A. Goubaux], 97–110.—**Bouthier.** Fœtus monstrueux. [*From:* Mém. Acad. roy. d. sc. de Par., 1727.] Collect. acad. d. mém., etc., Par., 1781, vi, 417.—**Bozzetti** (C.) Ragguaglio di alcune notabili mostruosità umane. Ann. univ. di med., Milano, 1844, cxi, 5–30, 1 pl.—**Bradbury.** † Boston M. & S. J., 1858, lviii, 87.—**Braun** (C.) Ianiceps asymetros. Allg. Wien. med. Ztg., 1865, x, 313.—**Braun** (E.) Ein Fall von Doppelmissbildung. Wien. med. Presse, 1879, xx, 275–277.—**Bray** (A.) Observation sur un accouchement de deux jumeaux unis ensemble par la poitrine. Bull. Fac. de méd. de Par., 1814–15, iv (10. année), 184–188.—**Breschet** (G.) Des diplogénèses, ou déviations organiques par duplicité. Arch. gén. de méd., Par., 1823, iii, 523 : 1824, iv, 80.—**Brisebarre & Duvollier.** Description d'un fœtus monstrueux. J. de méd., chir., pharm., etc., Par., 1763, xviii, 66–69, 1 pl.— **Broca** (P.) Sur le monstre pygopage connu sous le nom de Millie-Christine. Bull. Soc. d'anthrop. de Par., 1873, 2. s., viii, 874–879. [Discussion], 880 : 1874, 2. s., ix, 14 : 147 ; 205. ——. Sur les doctrines de la diplogénèse. *Ibid.*, 156–180.—**Bromilow** (S.) Account of a male monster with two heads. Edinb. M. & S. J., 1841, lv, 435, 1 pl.— **Brown** (A.) Curious case of monstrosity. Med. Circ., Lond., 1854, iv, 193.—**Bruch** (C.) Ueber Missbildungen der Chorda dorsalis (Dichordus), nebst Bemerkungen über Doppelbildungen. Würzb. med. Ztschr., 1864, v, 1–35, 2 pl. ——. Ueber die Entstehung der Doppelbildungen. *Ibid.*, 1866, vii, 257–320, 2 pl.—**Brugisser.** Demonstration einer menschlichen Zwillingsmissbildung (Diprosopos). Verhandl. d. schweiz. naturf. Gesellsch., Aarau, 1880–81 lxiv, 59.—**Bry** (J.) Observation sur un accouchement de deux jumeaux unis ensemble par la poitrine. Bull. Fac. de méd. de Par., 1814–15, iv (10. année), 184–188. [Rap. de Desormeaux], 189–195.—**de Buchwald** (J. B.) Historia monstri gemelli coaliti et compositi, jam hac vice in pauciora redacta. Acta med. Hafn., n. ed., 1775, 18–29, 1 pl.—**Bucquoy.** Diplogénèse par juxtaposition; monstre homéadelphe à corps et à tête doubles. Bull. Soc. anat. de Par., 1852, xxvii, 495–498.—**Büchner** (A. E.) De fœtu masculino bicorporeo, circa abdomen concreto. Acta. Acad. nat. curios., Norimb., 1730, ii, 217–219, 1 pl.—**Bühring.** Zwei Köpfe bei einem Neugebornen; Abbinden des Einen. Wchnschr. f. d. ges. Heilk., Berl., 1844, 1–6.— **von Buhl.** Pathologisch-anatomische Demonstrationen. Aerztl. Int.-Bl., München, 1875, xxii, 83–85.—**Burke** (C. C.) Case of monstrosity. [Texarkana twins.] N. Orl. M. & S. J., 1880–81, n. s., viii, 1025. ——. The "Texas Siamese twins"; exhibited at the thirteenth annual session of the Texas Medical Association. Texas M. & S. Rec., Galveston, 1882, ii, 1–11.—**Buxtorf** (J.) Vir monstrosus. Acta Helvet., Basileæ, 1772, vii, 101–103, 1 pl.— **Calori** (L.) Di tre mostri doppi sicefali e particolarmente del giano. Mem. Accad. d. sc. d. Ist. di Bologna, 1882, 4. s., iv, 51–92, 5 pl. ——. Dell' iniope e del sinoto dei caratteri comuni e proprii de' varii sicefali e della loro genesi. *Ibid.*, 1883, 4. s., v, 143–184, 6 pl.—[**Capuron.**] Dystocie par monstruosité bicéphale du fœtus. Arch. gén. de méd., Par., 1846, 4. s., x, 352.—**Casanova** (J. N.) Description of a double fœtus. Tr. M. & Phys. Soc. Calcutta, 1831–3, vi, 490.—[**Cases.**] Monstri bicor-

Monsters (*Double*).

porei descriptio. Zodiacus med.-gall. 1683, Geneva, 1685, v, 250.—Zweyköpffigtes, doch einleibiges Monstrum. Samml. v. Nat.- u. Med.-.... Gesch. 1725, Leipz. u. Budissin, 1726, xxxii, 520.—[Deux filles qui se tenoient par l'estomach.] [*From:* Hist. Acad. roy. d. sc. de Par., 1702.] Rec. d. mém., Dijon, 1754, i, 747.—Un monstre. [*From:* J. d. sçavans, 1665.] Collect. acad. d. mém., etc., Dijon, 1755, i, 253.—Monstre double. [*From:* Mém. Acad. roy. d. sc. de Par., 1723.] Collect. acad. d. mém., etc. Partie franç., Par. et Liége, 1774, v, 305. — Sur un fœtus monstrueux. [*From:* Mém. Acad. roy. d. sc. de Par., 1724.] *Ibid.*, 306–308.—Kurze Beschreibung einer im vorigen Sommer hier gebornen zweileibigen Missgeburt. Ann. d. Staatsarznk., Züllichau, 1790–91, i, 2 St., 122–128.—Lusus naturæ. Phila. J. M. & Phys. Sc., 1824, viii, 469.—Autopsie cadavérique du corps de Ritta-Cristina. Bull. d. sc. méd., Par., 1829, xix, 169–172.—Notice sur Ritta-Christina. Clinique, Par., 1829, i, 200; 254.—Questions psyco-physiologiques et légales sur Ritta et Christina, enfant à deux têtes. Hygie, Brux., 1829, vi, 573.—Nouveaux détails sur l'autopsie de Ritta-Christina. Gaz. d. hôp., Par., 1829–30, ii, 306.—Diplogenesta. Facultad, Madrid, 1845–6, i, 463.— Nachricht über das junge, 14jährige, mit einer höchst interessanten Missgeburt verwachsene Mädchen, welches jetzt hier in Berlin zu sehen ist. J. f. Kinderkr., Berl., 1846, vi, 75–80, 1 pl.—The trisceles monster. Lond. M. Gaz., 1846, n. s., ii, 619.—Entwicklungsanomalien. (Kinder mit zwei Köpfen.) Oesterr. Ztschr. f. Kinderh., Wien, 1856–7, ii, 92–95.—Lusus naturæ. Med. Chron., Montreal, 1858–9, vi, 141.—Descrizione dei mostri conservati nel museo anatomo-patologico ticinese; opinioni sull' origine dei mostri doppi. Gior. di anat. e fisiol., Milano, 1867, iv, 284–305.—A human tripod. Lancet, Lond., 1868, ii, 397.— United twins. Med. Press & Circ., Lond., 1869, vii, 467.— Recherches anatomiques sur un monstre sternopage. [Concours du prix Portal.] [Rap. de Goubaux.] Bull. Acad. de méd., Par., 1875, 2. s., iv, 130–134.—Sluchai dvoinago urodstva (thoracodidymus). Sborn. sochin. po subdebnoi med., St. Petersb., 1879, iii, 108.—Monstrosity. Virginia M. Month., Richmond, 1879–80, vi, 252.—**del Castillo** (R.) Mónstruo compuesto sysomianos; derodymio. Andalucía méd., Córdoba, 1878, iii, 17–21, 1 pl. *Also* [Abstr.]: Génio méd.-quir., Madrid, 1878, xxiv, 284.— **Cauchois.** Monstre humain, né à Bolbec (Seine-Inférieure), envoyé au musée de l'École de médecine de Rouen par M. le Dr. C. Hélot; autopsie. Union méd. de la Seine-Inf., Rouen, 1875, xiii, 208–210.—**Cazeo.** Accouchement d'un enfant à terme ayant deux têtes, quatre bras, deux poitrines, un seul abdomen et trois extrémités inférieures. J. de méd. et chir. prat., Par., 1835, vi, 466–468.—**Chamejdes** (J.) Wiadomość o potworze urodzonym we wsi Radoszycach. [Living double monster.] Przegl. lek., Krakow., 1878, xvii, 553. *Also, transl.:* Wien. med. Presse, 1878, xix, 1576–1578. *Also, transl.:* Pacific M. & S. J., San Fran., 1878–9, xxi, 454–456.—**Chamousset.** Accouchement d'un fœtus monstrueux. Bull. Soc. méd. de Chambéry, 1875–7, No. v, 105–109.—**Chapman** (H. C.) Description of a monstrosity. Proc. Acad. Nat. Sc. Phila., 1876, pt. 1, 24–26.—**Chassanoil & Garnier** (P.) Observation de ziphopage, considérée au point de vue des manœuvres obstétricales. Union méd., Par., 1868, 3. s., v, 428.—**Chauveau** (A.) Remarques physiologiques à l'occasion d'un monstre double parasitaire hétéradelphe; circulation des monstres omphalosites; développement des nerfs et des muscles. J. de la physiol. de l'homme, Par., 1863, vi, 345–368. *Also* [Abstr.]: Mém. et compt.-rend. Soc. d. sc. méd. de Lyon, 1863–4, iii, pt. 2, 263–266.—**Chereau** (A.) Du monstre de la Châtre; rapport sur ce cas diplogénèse. Rev. méd. franç. et étrang., Par., 1845, iii, 184–195, 1 pl. *Also, transl.:* J. f. Kinderkr., Berl., 1846, vi, 161–167, 1 pl.—**Chilianus** (L. B.) Monstrous fœtus. Misc. Acad. nat. curios. 1682, Norimb., 1683, 2. decuria, i, 356, 1 pl. *Also, transl.:* Collect. acad. d. mém., etc., Dijon, 1755, iii, 516, 1 pl.—**Chrestien.** Sur un cas de dystocie; monstre à deux têtes. [Rap. de Capuron.] Bull. Acad. de méd., Par., 1845–6, xi, 461–472.—**Claudi.** Zusammengewachsene Zwillinge. Oesterr. med. Wchnschr., Wien, 1843, 197–200.—**Cleghorn** (J.) A case of monstrosity. Indian M. Gaz., Calcutta, 1871, vi, 178.—**Cleland.** On doublebodied monsters and the development of the tongue. J. Anat. & Physiol., Cambridge & Lond., 1874, viii, 250–260, 1 pl. ——. Remarkable double monstrosity of the head. *Ibid.*, 1878–9, xiii, 164–172, 1 pl.—**Clements** (H. J.) Case of triplets, with monstrosity. Lancet, Lond., 1887, ii, 755.— **Coirat** (P.) & **Rebatel** (F.) Baptiste et Jacques Tocci, un monstre double. Lyon méd., 1878, xxix, 274–280.— **Conquedo.** Monstri humani descriptio. Zodiacus med.-gall. 1681, Geneva, 1682, iii, 133–139.—**Cook** (A. B.) Joined twins; the obstetric and surgical management, with remarks. Richmond & Louisville M. J., Louisville, 1869, vii, 65–90, 1 pl. *Also,* Reprint.—**Corradi.** Fœtus with three legs. Lancet, Lond., 1865, i, 505.—**Coste.** Origine de la monstruosité double chez les poissons osseux; communication faite à l'Académie des sciences le 16 avril 1855. Gaz. méd. de Par., 1855, 3. s., x, 243 ; 257 ; 264.— **Court** (J.) Description of monster. Lancet, Lond., 1868, ii, 311.—**Cowan** (W.) Case of monstrosity. Penins. J. M.,

Monsters (*Double*).

Ann Arbor, Mich., 1854-5, ii, 49-52.—**Critchett.** Double monsters. Tr. Path. Soc. Lond., 1848-50, ii, 90-92.—**Crook** (W. E.) Notes of a case of monstrous birth. Austral. M. J., Melbourne, 1856, i, 204-206.—**Crosby** (A. B.) Case of Siamese twins; sloughing of the vesico-vaginal septum; operation for vesico-vaginal fistula; recovery. Michigan Univ. M. J., Ann Arbor, 1870-71, i, 577-582.—**Cuchet** (S.) [Un fœtus monstrueux, composé de deux corps réunis intérieurement et un peu latéralement par le ventre et par la poitrine.] [*From:* Mém. Acad. roy. d. sc., 1764.] Collect. acad. d. mém., etc. Partie franç., Par., 1786, xiii, 354.—**Czermak** (J.) Beschreibung eines doppelkörperigen Kalbes. Med. Jahrb. d. k. k. österr. Staates, Wien, 1834, n. F., vi, 480-486, 2 pl.—**D.** (B.) Eine seltene Zwillingsbildung (Bicephali tetrabrachii). Wien. med. Presse, 1881, xxii, 13.—**Damerow** (H.) Ueber Ritta-Christina und die Siamesen. Lit. Ann. d. ges. Heilk., Berl., 1830, xvi, 454-482.—**Danielebekoff** (A.) Opisanie Erivanskago uroda Saphar-Ali. [Description of the Ervan monster, Saphar-Ali.] Med. Sbornik, Tiflis, 1874, xx, pt. 4, 23-28.—**Dareste** (C.) Note sur un monstre appartenant à un nouveau type de la famille des polygnathiens. Compt. rend. Soc. de biol. 1859, Par., 1860, 3. s., i, 33. ———. Note sur un nouveau genre de monstruosités doubles appartenant à la famille des polygnathiens. *Ibid.,* 76. ———. De la duplicité monstrueuse. Bull. Soc. d'anthrop. de Par., 1875, 2. s., ix, 321-338. ———. Nouvelles recherches sur le mode de formation des monstres doubles. Compt. rend. Acad. d. sc., Par., 1887, civ, 715-717.—**Dauvé** (P.) Rapport sur un monstre double autositaire, né à Versailles le 21 mars 1861. Bull. Acad. de méd., Par., 1860-61, xxvi, 490; 581.—**Deakin** (S.) Case of posterior dichotomy. Brit. M. J., Lond., 1885, ii, 1104.—**Deane** (J.) The Leicestershire twins. Lond. M. Gaz., 1838, xxii, 109-111.—**De Camp** (S. G. J.) Connected sisters. Boston M. & S. J., 1829-30, ii, 518.—**Decerfz.** Note sur un enfant monstre, né dans l'arrondissement de la Châtre. Compt. rend. Acad. d. sc., Par., 1845, xxi, 486-489.—**Degner** (J. H.) Von einem zweyleibichten Fœtu. Samml. v. Nat.- u. Med.- ... Gesch. 1724, Leipz. u. Budissin, 1725, xxvii, 101-104. ———. Von monströsen Geburten. *Ibid.* (1724), 1726, xxix, 195.—**De Jumné.** Note sur un monstre double sycéphalien. Bull. Soc. de méd. de Gand, 1854, xxi, 179-181.—**Dekigallas** (I.) Περὶ δίδύμου τινὸς τέρατος. Ἰατρικὴ Μέλισσα, Ἀθῆναι, 1854-5, ii, 277.—**Delacroix.** Fœtus à deux têtes. Bull. Soc. méd. de Reims, 1872, No. xi, 24-26.—**Delafield** (E.) † Am. M. Recorder, Phila., 1822, v, 286-290.—**Delmas.** Observation d'un enfant à deux têtes. Hist. Soc. de méd.-prat. de Montpel., 1808, xvii, 227-230. ———. Observation d'hétéradelphie. J. Soc. de méd.-prat. de Montpel., 1841, iii, 210-222, 1 pl.—**De Marco** (V.) † Osservatore med., Palermo, 1882, 3. s., xii, 114.—**Demichelis** (F.) Relazione sull' esterna disposizione di un mostro umano singolare e vivente. nato in Sassari. Ann. univ. di med., Milano, 1829, l, 381-385, 1 pl.—**Depaul.** [Fœtus à deux têtes.] Bull. Soc. anat. de Par., 1852, xxvii, 45. ———. [Monstre à deux faces.] *Ibid.,* 1855, xxx, 243-247. ———. [Deux jumeaux du sexe masculin, soudés par l'abdomen.] *Ibid.,* 1857, xxxii, 283-285. *Also, transl.* [Abstr.]: Siglo méd., Madrid, 1857, iv, 368.—**Derien** (G.) Accouchement laborieux d'un fœtus à terme à deux corps très bien conformés et développés, unis depuis le haut du thorax jusqu'à l'ombilic commun, terminé avec succès pour la mère sans opération sanglante. [Rap. de Capuron.] Bull. Acad. roy. de méd., Par., 1847-8, xiii, 1048-1060. *Also:* Union méd., Par., 1848, ii, 305; 310.—**Deslongchamps** (E.) Mémoire sur un monstre double monomphalien de provenance humaine, constituant un genre nouveau désigné sous le nom de rachipage. Compt. rend. Soc de biol. 1851, Par., 1852, iii, pt. 2, 221-225.—**Detharding** (G. G.) Historia partus monstri bicorporei monocephali hujusque descriptio; accedit disputatio de monstro sine cerebro. Nova acta phys.-med. Acad. nat. curios., Bonnæ, 1821, x, pt. 2, 693-710. *Also,* Reprint.—**Deutsch** (M.) Seltener Fall von Doppelmissbildung. Wien. med. Presse, 1875, xvi, 437-439.—**Dönitz** (W.) Beschreibung und Erläuterung von Doppelmissgeburten. Arch. f. Anat., Physiol. u. wissensch. Med., Leipz., 1865, 113; 129, 2 pl.; 512; 610, 2 pl.: 1866, 518; 529, 2 pl. *Also,* Reprint.—**D'Orsonnens** (T.-E. d'O.) Cas d'ischiopagie. Abeille méd., Montréal, 1879, i, 38-44.—**Dubrueil.** Description de deux doubles monstres humains, et création du genre ischiadelphe. Éphém. méd. de Montpel., 1827, vi, 293-297.—**Dumont.** Note sur un fœtus bicéphale. Ann. Soc. de méd. de Gand, 1839, v, 465-467.—**Dungan** (J. B.) Double-headed monster. N. Orl. M. News & Hosp. Gaz., 1857-8, iv, 129.—**Dunster** (E. S.) Remarks on double monsters. Penins. J. M., Detroit, 1874, x, 241-253. *Also,* Reprint.—**Dureau** (A.) Les monstres composés. Gaz. méd. de Par., 1873, 4. s., ii, 665-674. ———. Sur un monstre double du genre xiphopage. Gaz. obst. de Par., 1874, iii, 65.—**Durston** (W.) Twins fastened together at the breast. Phil. Tr. 1698-1700, 4. ed., Lond., 1731, iii, 301. *Also, transl.:* Collect. acad. d. mém., etc., Dijon, 1755, ii, 288, 1 pl.—**Eastman** (J.) Report of a case of double-headed monstrosity. J. Am. M. Ass., Chicago, 1884, ii, 88.—**Eban** (J.) Przypadek konczyn dolnych nadliczbowych potwornych. [Mon-

ster with three legs.] Gaz. lek., Warszawa, 1883, 2. s., iii, 9; 32.—**Ebermaier.** Kurze Nachricht von einem ohne besondere Kunsthülfe gebornen zweiköpfigen Kinde. N. Jahrb. d. teutsch. Med. u. Chir., Elberfeld, 1822, vi, 1. St., 24-31, 1 pl.—**Ebsworth** (A.) A child with two heads. Med. Times, Lond , 1843-4, ix, 266.—**Ehrmann.** Fœtus monstrueux (dérodelphe). Gaz. méd. de Strasb., 1858, xviii, 77.—**Ellis** (C.) Autopsy of the double monster (ischiopagus tripus) born in Ohio, and lately exhibited in Boston. Boston M. & S. J., 1871, lxxxv, 218-223. *Also:* Extr. Rec. Bost. Soc. M. Improve. (1866-74), 1876, vi (app.), 141-151.—**Ellis** (R.) & **Embleton** (D.) On a rare form of twin monstrosity. Tr. Obst. Soc. Lond. (1865), 1866, vii, 160-164.—**Elwood** (D. M.) A remarkable double monstrosity. Med. & Surg. Reporter, Phila., 1874, xxx, 257-259.—**von Embden.** History and description of a remarkable monstrosity at Cadiz. Lond. M. & Phys. J., 1819, xlii, 104-109.—**Engström.** Zwillings-Monstruosität. J. f. Kinderkr., Erlang., 1868, li, 137.—**Eschricht.** Gesichtsverdoppelung mit Mangel an Gehirn und Rückenmark. Arch. f. Anat., Physiol. u. wissensch. Med., Berl., 1834, 268-272, 1 pl.—**Eve** (F. S.) Description of a double-headed human female monster, born at the full term of gestation. Tr. Obst. Soc. Lond. (1880), 1881, xxii, 74-78.—**Eve** (J. A.) A case of adherent fœtuses. South M. & S. J., Augusta, 1852, n. s., viii, 76-81.—**Facsebeck** (F.) Ueber Doppelbildung. Arch. f. Anat., Physiol. u. wissensch. Med., Berl., 1842, 61-72, 3 pl.—**Farge.** Segment supérieur (tête et cou) d'un monstre double polynathien. Bull. Soc. de méd. d'Angers (1867), 1868, n. s., lxx, 50-52.—**Fauchien.** Observation d'un fétus double. [Rap. de Gilbert.] J. gén. de méd., chir. et pharm., Par., 1803, xvi, 172-176.—**Fedoroff** (I. I.) K uchen. ob urodstvach. Dvoinoe urodstvo u cheloveka. Monstrum congenitum humanum; dicephalus tetrabrachius tripus. Zamiech. o razvitii dvoin. urodstva. Russk. Med., St. Petersb., 1886, iv, 361-364.—**Ferrand.** Description d'un monstre parasitaire de la famille des polyméliens. Monit. d. sc. méd. et pharm., Par., 1861, 2. s., iii, 993-996.—**Fevry.** A monstrous double birth in Lorrain. Phil. Tr. 1719-33, Lond., 1734, vii, pt. 3, 688, 1 pl.—**Fiedler** (W.) Ein Naturspiel seltener Art. Wien. med. Presse, 1872, xiii, 946.—**Finkelstein** (W.) Ein Fall von Doppelmissgeburt; Thoraco-Gastropagus. Berl. klin. Wchnschr., 1883, xx, 81.—**Fisher** (G. J.) Double monstrosity. Am. M. Month., N. Y., 1857, viii, 229. ———. Diploteratology; an essay on compound human monsters, comprising the history, literature, classification, description, and embryology of double and triple formation, including the so-called parasitic monsters, fœtus in fœtu, and supernumerary formation of parts or organs in man. Tr. M. Soc. N. Y., Albany, 1865, 232, 2 pl.: 1866, 207, 19 pl.: 1867, 396, 6 pl.: 1868, 276, 6 pl. *Also,* Reprint. ———. Double monsters. Phila. M. Times, 1870-71, i, 376. ———. Case of a rare variety of human diprosopic monster, with observations on the genus diprosopus. Ann. Anat. & Surg. Soc. Brooklyn, N. Y., 1880, ii, 193-197.—**Fitzhugh** (T.) A monstrosity; a second Rita-Christina. Texas Cour.-Rec. Med., Fort Worth, 1883-4, i, no. 5, 6-8.—**Flügel.** Beiträge zur Geschichte verwachsener Zwillinge. Med. Cor.- Bl. bayer. Aerzte, Erlang., 1848, ix, 91-108, 1 pl.—**Fonssagrives.** Description anatomique d'un monstre humain sycéphalien synote. Arch. gén. de méd., Par., 1859, 5. s., xiii, 677-684.—[**Force** (J. F.)] A bicephalic monster. Med. & Surg. Reporter, Phila., 1875, xxxiii, 318.—**Formento** (F.) fils. Relation d'un cas de monstruosité fort remarquable. J. Soc. méd. de la N.-Orléans, 1860-61, ii, 196-198.—**Foston** (W. H.) Case of bicephalous monster (a twin child). Madras Q. J. M. Sc., 1867-8, xii, 226, 1 pl.—**Fourdrignier.** Monstre double sternopage vivant. Bull. Soc. d'anthrop. de Par., 1884, 3. s., vii, 500-502.—**Fränkel** (E.) Ueber den Mechanismus, die Diagnose und die Leitung der Geburt bei Thoracopagen. Breslau. aerztl. Ztschr., 1884, vi, 1-4.—**Fränkel** (M.) Ein Bicephalus. Arch. f. path. Anat., etc., Berl., 1870, xlix, 143.—**Francis** (R. S.) On a curious instance of double fœtal malformation. Lancet, Lond., 1846, ii, 560.—**Fribe** (M.) Von einer zweyköpfichten Missgeburt. Auserl. med.- chir- ... Abhandl. d. röm.-kais. Akad. d. Naturf., Nürnb., 1756, iii, 253, 1 pl.—**Frühauf.** Ein Fall von pathologischer Zwillingsbildung. Berl. klin. Wchnschr., 1870, vii, 506.—**Fubini** (S.) & **Mosso** (A.) Gemelle xiphoide juncti. Gior. d. r. Accad. di med. di Torino, 1878, xli, 13-26, 1 pl. *Also, transl.:* Mouvement méd., Par., 1878, xvi, 168; 181.—**Garden** (A.) Note of a case of heteradelphic monstrosity. Indian M. Gaz., Calcutta, 1881, xvi, 95.—**Gardiner** (J. H.) Monstrosity. [Double headed.] Canad. Pract., Toronto, 1884, ix, 136.—**Gayraud** (E.) Accouchement prématuré artificiel dans un cas de grossesse gémellaire compliqué d'hydroamnios; fœtus monstrueux (acéphalien péracéphalien). Montpel. méd., 1870, xxiv, 16-32.—**Genersich** (A.) Missgeburt mit zwei Gesichten (Heteroprosopus). Allg. Wien. med. Ztg., 1882, xxvii, 19. *Also:* Pest. med.-chir. Presse, Budapest, 1882, xviii, 62.—**Geoffroy-Saint-Hilaire** (E.) Mémoire sur un enfant quadrupède, né et vivant à Paris; monstruosité déterminée sous le nom générique d'iléa-

Monsters (*Double*).

delphe. Gaz. méd. de Par., 1830, i, 340. *Also*, Reprint.
——. Rapport sur un enfant double, du genre ischiadelphe, suivi de considérations et de réflexions sur la monstruosité double. J. compl. du dict. d. sc. méd., Par., 1830, xxxvii, 133–145.—**Gerlach** (L.) Zur Bildungsgeschichte der vorderen Verdoppelung. Sitzungsb. d. phys.-med. Soc. zu Erlang., 1885–6, xviii, 92–94. — **Gerold.** Monströse Duplicität. Klin. Ztschr. f. Chir. u. Augenh., Halle, 1836–7, i, 467–469.—**Gholson** (S. C.) Singular case of monstrosity. Cincin. Lancet & Obs., 1859, n. s., ii, 34–40.—**Gibson** (B.) Description of an extraordinary human fœtus. Phil. Tr., Lond., 1810, 123–135, 2 pl. *Also*, Reprint. — **Gichrl.** Ueber Doppelmissbildungen. J. d. Chir. u. Augenh., Berl., 1843, n. F., ii, 484–501.—**Gil y Fernandez** (A.) Observacion de una monstruosidad. Facultad, Madrid, 1845–6, i, 230.—**Giné.** Union de las dos cabezas por los huesos occipitales ausiliada por el lado derecho por un hueso supernumerario comun á los dos y que llamo tercer parietal del mismo lado. Independ. méd., Barcel., 1870–71, ii, 282–285. *Also:* Pabellon méd., Madrid, 1871, xi, 460–462. *Also, transl.:* Med. Press & Circ., Lond., 1872, xiv, 76–78.—**Gintrac** (E.) Recherches anatomiques des deux monstres doubles monocéphales. *In his:* Mém. et obs. de méd. clin , 8°. Bordeaux, 1830, 309–324, 1 pl.—**Girard & Berlioz.** Jacques et Baptiste Tocci, monstre double sysomien, à variété xyphoïdienne. J. Soc. de méd. et pharm. de l'Isère, Grenoble, 1878, ii, 243–250.—**Girard de Cailleuse.** Note sur un monstre xyphodime. Gaz. méd. de Par., 1859, 3. s., xiv, 105.—**Gockel** (E.) Partus gemellorum monstrosus. *In his:* Gallicinium med.-pract., 4°, Ulmæ, 1700, 148–153.—**Godson** (C.) Double monster. Tr. Obst. Soc. Lond. (1878), 1879, xx, 171–(1879), 1880, xxi, 88. ——. Monster; "double syncéphalien"; dissection by D'A. Power. *Ibid.* (1886), 1887, xxviii, 68–70.—**Golay.** Monstre janiceps. Bull. Soc. anat. de Par., 1876, li, 525–532. [Rap. de Raymond], 1877, lii, 608. *Also:* Progrès méd., Par., 1876, iv, 8c5; 1877, v, 91.—**Gomez Torres** (A.) Noticia de un monstruo compuesto, autositario, sysomiano, xiphodymo, segun la clasificacion de G. de Saint-Hilaire. Crón. méd.-quir. de la Habana, 1876, ii, 116–121.—**Goodell** (W.) Clinical lecture on monstrosities; illustrated by a remarkable living double monster. Phila. M. Times, 1870–71, i, 333. ——. Double monsters. *Ibid.*, 440.—**Goodeve** (H. H.) Account of a human monstrosity in the museum of the Medical College. [Union of twins.] Tr. M. & Phys. Soc. Calcutta, 1835–42, viii, pp. xxxi–xxxiv.—**Gosselin** (L.) Observation de monstruosité double (sternopagie) qui a rendu l'accouchement difficile et nécessité l'embryotomie. Arch. gén. de méd., Par., 1847, 4. s., xiv, 72–81.—**Goubaux** (A.) [Crâne d'un monstre qui avait deux bouches.] Compt. rend. Soc. de biol. 1868, Par., 1869, 4. s., v, 25. ——. Mémoire sur un monstre de l'espèce bovine de la classe des monstres doubles autositaires de la famille des monosomiens et du genre opodyme, suivi de quelques remarques sur les monstres de la famille des monosomiens et de la création d'un genre nouveau, genre synopodyme. *Ibid.*, 127–145. ——. Mémoire sur un monstre double, autositaire, monomphalien que l'on propose de nommer dérodymo-thoradelphe; observation recueillie sur un individu de l'espèce bovine. *Ibid.* (1869), 1870, 5. s., i, pt. 2, 81–97.—**Goujon.** Cas de monstruosité. Compt. rend. Soc. de biol. 1866, Par., 1867, 4. s., iii, 47. — **Grabowski** (L.) O potworze dwulicowym. [Double monster.] Gaz. lek., Warszawa, 1873, xiv, 147.—**Greiner** (A.) Vereinigte Zwillinge mit zwei Köpfen, einem einzich vollkommen ausgebildeten Rumpfe und nicht vollzähligen Gliedmassen. Oesterr. med. Wchnschr., Wien, 1846, 321–324.—**Greisel** (J. G.) Anatome monstri gemellorum humanorum. Misc. Acad. nat. curios., Lips., 1670, i, 152, 1 pl. *Also, transl.:* Auserl. med.- chir.- . . Abhandl. d. röm.-kais. Akad. d. Naturf., Nürnb., 1755, i, 113, 1 pl.—**Gross.** Les monstres doubles parasitaires hétérotypiens ou épigastriques et la séparation des monstres doubles en général; rapport sur une observation de Lardier. Mém. Soc. de méd. de Nancy (1876–7), 1878, 1–26, 1 pl. *Also:* Rev. méd. de l'est, Nancy, 1877, vii, 166; 236; 270, 1 pl. *Also:* Arch. de tocol., Par., 1877, iv, 282; 340. *Also*, Reprint.—**Grosse** (T.) Künstliche Geburt eines zusammengewachsenen Zwillingspaares. St. Petersb. med. Wchnschr., 1885, n. F., ii, 79.—**Grünwald.** Eine neue lebende menschliche Doppelmissbildung. Arch. f. path. Anat., etc., Berl., 1879, lxxv, 561.—**Grützbach.** Beschreibung einer monströsen Doppelgeburt. Allg. med. Ann., Altenb., 1803, pt. 2, 95.—**Guerdan** (A.) Beschreibung einer synotischen Missgeburt. Monatschr. f. Geburtsk. u. Frauenkr., Berl., 1857, x, 176–206.—**Habershon** (S. O.) Anatomical description of a double fœtus. Guy's Hosp. Rep., Lond., 1857, 3. s., iii, 116–122, 2 pl.—**Hackedorn** (M. R.) A bicephalic monstrosity. Med. & Surg. Reporter, Phila., 1870, xxiii, 417.—**Hadley** (G. P.) United twin monstrosity. Brit. M. J., Lond., 1875, i, 508.—**Halberg.** Zwillingsgeburt; das zweite Kind eine Doppelmissbildung mit drei Füssen; Extraction desselben am Steiss. Berl. klin. Wchnschr., 1875, xii, 534.—**Handyside** (P. D.) Observations on the arrested twin development of Jean Battista dos Santos, born at Faro, in Portugal, in 1846. Edinb. M. J., 1865–6, xi, 833–842. *Also*, Reprint. ——. Further observations

Monsters (*Double*).

on arrested twin development. Edinb. M. J., 1868–9, xiv, 772–774. *Also*, Reprint.—**Hanks** (H.) On a case of united children, or double monstrosity. Tr. Obst. Soc. Lond. (1861), 1862, iii, 414–417.—**Hard** (N.) Bi-cephalous fœtus; use of forceps, etc. West. M.-Chir. J., Keokuk, 1850–51, i, 225–227.—**Harris** (M.) Two fœtuses completely joined at the thorax and abdomen. Liverpool & Manchester M. & S. Rep., 1876, iv, 273. — **Harris** (W. P.) Rare case of "monster". Indian M. Gaz., Calcutta, 1867, ii, 73 — **Hart** (E.) Jean Battista dos Santos; two developed penes, and a large central third leg. Lancet, Lond., 1865. ii, 124. *Also, transl.:* Compilador méd., Barcel., 1868–9, iv, 189–193.—**Hartmannus** (P. J.) De sceleto gemellorum coalitorum janiformi. Misc. Acad. nat. curios. 1701–5, Norimb., 1706, 3. decuria, ix–x, 341–344. —**Harvey** (P.) Case of united twins. Am. J. M. Sc., Phila., 1866, n. s., lii, 403–405.—**Hatté.** Observation sur un enfant à trois jambes. J. de méd., chir., pharm., etc., 2. éd., Par., 1783, ii, 227–231, 1 pl. — **Hawkins** (W. H.) A case of monstrosity. N. Orl. M. & S. J., 1861, xviii, 1–6. — **Heaton** (J. D.) United twins. [The "Biddenden Maids"; lived A. D. 1100.] Brit. M. J., Lond., 1869, i, 363.—**Hecker** (C.) Ueber einen Epignathus. Monatschr. f. Geburtsk. u. Frauenkr., Berl., 1865, xxv, 1–9, 1 pl.—**Hein** (R.) Beschreibung einer seltenen Missgeburt und Bemerkungen über ihr Entstehen. Ztschr. f. Geburtsh. u. Gynäk., Stuttg., 1881, vi, 352–357, 1 pl —**Hellwig** (J.) Infantes bicorporei. *In his:* Obs. phys.-med., 4°, Aug. Vindel., 1680, 25–27. ——. Infans monstrosus ac veluti biceps. *Ibid.*, 27–29. ——. Gemellæ corporibus concretæ. *Ibid.*, 35–40. ——. Itali fratres in pectore connati. *Ibid.*, 44–49.—[**Helsen.**] Accouchement d'un monstre double monomphalien; ectopage. Rev. méd., Louvain, 1886, v, 352.—**Hennig.** Doppelmissbildung mit verschmolzenen Köpfen. Arch. f. Gynaek., Berl., 1874, vii, 389.—**Hervieux** (E.) [Sur les monstres doubles polyméliens.] Bull. Acad. de méd., Par., 1874, 2. s., iii, 20–32. ——. L'enfant à quatre jambes, et la femme à deux têtes. Arch. de tocol., Par., 1874, i, 39–52.—**Heschl.** Malformation by duplication of the lower half of the body. Brit. M. J., Lond., 1877, ii, 934. — **Hewitt** (G.) Case of united children, or double monstrosity. Lancet, Lond., 1861, ii, 570.—**Hildreth** (S. P.) A case of twins united along the course of the sternum to the insertion of the umbilical cord. Med. Reposit., N. Y., 1822, vii, 361–363.—**Hill** (A.) Dissection of a double monster (epignathus). J. Anat. & Physiol., Lond., 1884–5. xix, 190–197. *Also* [Abstr.]: Brit. M. J., Lond., 1884, ii, 965.—**Hilliard.** One-headed twin monster. Obst. J. Gr. Brit., Lond., 1880. viii, 91.—**Himly** (E. A. W.) G. Vrolik's Abhandlung über zerstreute Theile eines zweiten Kindes in einer Geschwulst an der linken Wange einer siebenmonatlichen menschlichen Frucht. Arch. f. Anat. u. Physiol., Leipz., 1832, vi, 397–410, 3 pl.—**Hobart** (H. S.) Case of double monster. Dublin Q. J. M. Sc., 1860, xxix, 328–337, 2 pl.—**Hochstetter** (C. F.) Geburt zweier mit einander verwachsener Kinder. Med. Cor.-Bl. d. württemb. ärztl. Ver , Stuttg., 1834–5, iv, 31.—**Höhne.** Anastomose der Blutgefässe einer zusammengewachsenen Zwillingsnachgeburt. Ztschr. f. Chir. v. Chir., Osterode u. Gos'ar, 1845, ii, 89.—**Hoffmann** (J. M.) De monstro gemello. Misc. Acad. nat. curios. 1685, Norimb., 1705, 2. decuria, iv, 288–290, 3 pl. *Also, transl.:* Collect. acad. d. mém., etc., Dijon, 1755, iii, 664–666, 1 pl. *Also, transl.:* Auserl. med.- chir.- . . . Abhandl. d. röm.- kais. Akad. d. Naturf., Nürnb., 1765, xiv, 245–248, 2 pl. ——. Fœtu monstroso. Misc. Acad. nat. curios. 1687, Norimb., 1707, 2. decuria, vi, 333–336. *Also, transl :* Collect. acad. d. mém., etc., Dijon, 1766, vii, 467.—**Home** (E.) An account of a child with a double head. Phil. Tr., Lond., 1790, lxxx, 296–305, 2 pl. *Also:* Med. Facts & Obs., Lond., 1791, i, 164–175, 1 pl. ——. Some additions to a paper, read in 1790, on the subject of a child with a double head. Phil. Tr., Lond., 1799, 28–30, 2 pl.—**Horner** (W. E.) Account of a double female fœtus. Am. J. M. Sc., Phila., 1831, viii, 349–352, 1 pl.—**Horrocks** (P.) Dicephalous fœtus. Tr. Obst. Soc. Lond. (1884), 1885, xxvi, 326–328.—**Houel.** Description de trois monstres sycéphaliens. Compt. rend. Soc. de biol. 1857, Par., 1859, 2. s., iv, pt. 2, 297–305. ——. Mémoire sur les monstres ischiopages, premier genre de la famille des monomphaliens (I. Geoffroy-Saint-Hilaire). Bull. Soc. anat. de Par., 1873, xlviii, 263–273.—**Hubbard** (L.) Case of a deformed fœtus. Cases & Obs. M. Soc. N.-Haven County, 1788, 38 - 42. —**Hubbard** (S.) Cause of the blending of twins, and their being of the same sex. Buffalo M. J., 1851–2, vii, 546.—**Hubert** (E.) Note sur un monomphalien - xipho - ischio - page. Bull. Acad. roy. de méd. de Belg., Brux., 1861, 2. s., iv, 857–867, 2 pl. [Rap. de Poelman], 60–67. [Discussion]. 682; 808. *Also* [Abstr.]: Gaz. obst., Par., 1874, iii, 89–94, 1 pl. — **Hünerwolffius** (J. A.) De fœmellis duabus monstrosis. Misc. Acad. nat. curios. 1690, Norimb., 1691, 2. decuria, ix, 170, 1 pl.—**Hugenberger** (T.) Die Geburtsgeschichte einer Doppelmissgeburt. St. Petersb. med. Ztschr., 1868, xv, 371–374.—**Hurford** (C.) Twin female monster. Tr. Obst. Soc. Lond. (1883), 1884, xxv, 111.—**Hott** (H. J.) Peculiar case of triplets. [A double monster.]

Monsters (*Double*).

Brit. M. J., Lond., 1887, ii, 880.—**Incoronato** (A.) Di un caso d' ischiopagia umana. Arch. di med., chir. ed ig., Roma, 1875, vii, 790-828, 4 pl. ——. Di un caso vivente di pygomelia umana. Resoc. Accad. med.-chir. di Napoli, 1876, xxx, 91-99, 1 pl.—**Irion.** Durch grosse Missbildung der Frucht sehr schwer gewordene Wendungsoperation. Ztschr. f. Wundärzte u. Geburtsh., Stuttg., 1851, iv, 319-326, 1 pl.—**Jackson** (I.) Descriptive account of a bicephalous fœtus. Med. & Phys. J., Lond., 1821, xlv, 128-133.—**Jackson** (J. B. S.) Two fœtuses united, face to face, from the umbilicus to the upper third of the sternum. Boston M. & S. J., 1858, lviii, 274-277. *Also*: Extr. Rec. Bost. Soc. M. Improve. (1856-8), 1859, iii (suppl.), 147-150. ——. An imperfect head upon the top of the head of a child otherwise well formed. Boston M. & S. J., 1858, lviii, 159-161. ——. The Carolina sisters. *Ibid.*, 1869, lxxx, 414-416.—**Jacobs** (J.) Beschrijving van het dubbel-kind Srie Sedono en Srie Gati. Geneesk. Tijdschr. v. Nederl.-Indië, Batav., 1880, n. s., ix, 187-193, 1 pl.—**Jacquemin.** Notice sur deux jumelles nées à Langenneufnach (Bavière) et dont le sequelette a été présenté au Congrès des naturalistes et des médecins d'Allemagne. Expérience, Par., 1839, iii, 104-106.—**Jagor** (F.) Triplicitas monstrosa inferior. Arch. f. path. Anat., etc., Berl., 1870, l, 296, 1 pl.—**Jakin** (J.) Case of duplex monster. Med. Times, Lond., 1848-9, xix, 7.—**Jay** (F. F.) Double monstrosity. Tr. Obst. Soc. Lond. (1864), 1865, vi, 222.—**Johnson** (T. D.) Monstrosity; hepatotomy children. Pacific M. & S. J., San Fran., 1868-9, n. s., ii, 166-170.—**Johnston** (B. R.) Twin-monstrosity; alleged maternal impression. Brit. M. J., Lond., 1885, i, 653.—**Johnston** (W. J.) Singular case of monstrosity. Boston M. & S. J., 1847-8, xxxvii, 77.—**Joly** (N.) Une lacune dans la série tératologique, remplie par la découverte du genre iléadelphe. Compt. rend. Acad. d. sc., Par., 1875, lxxxi, 207-211. —**Joly** (N.) & **Peyrat.** Études sur un monstre humain bifemelle du genre pygopage, né à Mazères (Ariège). Bull. Acad. de méd., Par., 1874, xxxviii, 52-56, 1 pl. *Also*: Gaz. méd.-chir. de Toulouse, 1874, vi, 41-43.—**Jones** (L.) Female twin monster. Tr. Obst. Soc. Lond. (1885), 1886, xxvii, 305.—**Jouon.** Description d'un monstre double sycéphalien iniope. J. de la sect. de méd. Soc. acad. Loire-Inf., Nantes, 1864, xl, 13-22, 2 pl.—**Julia de Fontenelle** (J.-S.-E.) Sur la monstruosité à deux têtes, dont chacune a été baptisée séparément sous les noms de Ritta et Cristina. Rev. méd. franç. et étrang., Par., 1829, iv, 237-244.—**Jung.** Doppel-Kind. Gen.-Ber. d. k. rhein. Med.-Coll. 1836, Koblenz, 1839, 200-203.—**Kennard** (D.) Account of the birth of a fœtus with two heads. Assoc. M. J., Lond., 1854, i, 459.—**Kerambrun.** Monstruosité; deux fœtus réunis par le thorax. J. d. conn. méd.-chir., Par., 1847-8, xv, pt. 2, 231-234.—**Kidgell** (S. W.) Birth of a double fœtus. Lond. M. Gaz., 1834-5, xv, 371.—**Kieter** (A.) Anatomische Beschreibung von mit den Köpfen zusammengewachsenen Zwillingen. Med. Ztg. Russlands, St. Petersb., 1856, xiii, 257; 265.—**King** (J. K.) An unusual case of monstrosity. Edinb. M. J., 1887-8, xxxiii, 125, 1 pl.—**Klapp** (J.) A description of the birth and form of a human monster. Phila. M. Museum, 1809, vi, 248-257, 1 pl.—**Klauber** (T.) Künstliche Entbindung einer Frau von einem Doppelkinde. Med. Ann., Heidelb., 1846, xii, 319.—**Kleber** (J. C.) Berigt, aangaande de verlossing van twee aan elkanderen vastzittende wanschapen kinderen. Handel. v. h. genoot. Genootsch., Amst., 1778, iii, 478-480.—**Kleemann.** Zwillingspaar, dem siamesischen ähnlich. Med. Ztg., Berl., 1838, vii, 11.—**Klein** (A.) Eine Zwillingsmissgeburt (Hypogastrodydimus), lebend zur Welt gekommen. Wien. med. Presse, 1871, xii, 1329-1332. *Also, transl.:* Am. J. Obst., N. Y., 1872-3, v, 253-257.—**Klein** (K. C.) Beschreibung zweier mit den Wirbeln verwachsener Kinder. Jahrb. d. teutsch. Med. u. Chir., Nürnb., 1813, iii, 17-22, 1 pl. ——. Beschreibung eines zweiköpfigen Mädchens. Deutsches Arch. f. d. Physiol., Halle, 1817, iii, 374-384. ——. Janusmissgeburten. *Ibid.*, 1818, iv, 551-557, 2 pl.—**Klinkosch** (J. T.) Programma, quo anatomicam monstri bicorporei monocephali descriptionem proponit. *In his:* Diss. med. select. Pragenses, 4°, Pragæ et Dresdæ, 1775, i, 219-234, 6 pl.—**Knapp** (M. L.) Bicephalous fœtus. N. York J. M., 1851, vii, 202.—**Knox.** A curious case of lusus naturæ. Med. Comment. 1791, Lond., 1792, 2. decade, vi, 291-297. — **Kœhler** (A.) Anatomical characters of a bicipital monster. Med. Rec., N. Y., 1871-2, vi, 402.—**von Kölliker.** Zwei Fälle von Doppelmissbildung beim Menschen. Sitzungsb. d. phys.-med. Gesellsch. zu Würzb., 1885, 19.—**Köllinger.** Janusmissbildung. Verhandl. d. phys.-med. Gesellsch. in Würzb., 1850, i, 280.—**König** (E.) Gemelli sibi invicem adnati feliciter separati. [Cartilaginous band from ensiform cartilage to umbilicus.] Misc. Acad. nat. curios. 1689, Norimb., 1690, 2. decuria, viii, 305-307, 1 pl. *Also, transl.:* Auserl. med.-chir.-... Abhandl. d. röm.-kais. Acad. d. Naturf., Nürnb., 1769, xviii, 273-276, 1 pl.—**Koller** (G.) Eine seltene Missgeburt. Wien. med. Wchnschr., 1856, vi, 670. — **Krause** (E.) An den Brustkörben verwachsene, ausgetragene Zwillinge weiblichen Geschlechts. Allg. med. Centr.-Ztg., Berl., 1875, xliv, 133. — **Krauss** (F.) Ein Fall von Sternothoracopa-

Monsters (*Double*).

gus tetrabrachius. Jahresb. d. schles. Gesellsch. f. vaterl. Kult. 1883, Bresl., 1884, lxi, 67. — **Kulmus** (J. A.) Von zwey zusammengewachsenen Kindern, nebst deren anatomischen Section. Samml. v. Nat.- u. Med.-.... Gesch. 1724, Leipz. u. Budissin, 1725, xxvii, 207-210.— **Labbée** (E.) Un nouveau monstre (hétéradelphe). Mouvement méd., Par., 1877, xv, 17. — **Labbée** (H.) Des monstres doubles. *Ibid.*, 1875, xiii, 193-196.— **Laforgue.** Mémoire sur un enfant à deux têtes, né à Bagnères-de-Luchon, le 16 septembre 1855. J. de méd., chir. et pharm. de Toulouse, 1856, 3. s., i, 65-73, 1 pl.— **Lamprey** (R. O.) Plural monstrosities. Brit. Gynæc. J., Lond., 1885, i, 128-130.— **Langer** (C.) Zur Anatomie des Gehörorganes doppelleibiger Missgeburten. Oesterr. med. Wchnschr., Wien, 1846, 609-620. — **Lanzonus** (J.) De monstro mentulato et bicorpori. Misc. Acad. nat. curios., Lips. et Francof., 1694, 3. decuria, i, 185, 1 pl. — **Lardier** (P.) Observation d'un cas de monstre composé double parasitaire hétéradelphe; portion parasitaire séparée de l'autosite par l'écraseur linéaire; guérison. Union méd., Par., 1877, 3. s., xxiii, 535; 561. *Also*: Rev. méd. de l'est, Nancy, 1877, vii, 166-172, 1 pl. *Also*: Arch. de tocol., Par., 1877, iv, 282-287. [*See, also,* Gross, *supra*.]—**Larkins** (J. M.) A child with two heads. Nashville J. M. & S., 1883, xxxii, 135-137.— **Larrey** (F.-H.) Anomalie des membres pelviens. Bull. Acad. de méd., Par., 1860-61, xxvi, 261-265. ——. Cas de monstruosité autositaire. *Ibid.*, 581-583. *Also*, Reprint. ——. [Sur un cas de monstruosité, mélomélie.] Bull. Acad. de méd., Par., 1874, 2. s., iii, 29-32. *Also*, Reprint. ——. [Observation de monstruosité dite pygopage, recueillie par N. Joly et Peyrat et communiquée à l'Académie de médecine le 20 janvier 1874.] Bull. Acad. de méd., Par., 1874, 2. s., iii, 51-56. *Also*, Reprint.—**Launay-Hanet.** Description d'un enfant monstrueux. J. de méd., chir., pharm., etc., Par., 1764, xxi, 44-48.—**Lavialle.** Sur un fœtus monstrueux. [Rap. de Baudeloque et Dupuytren.] Bull. Fac. de méd. de Par., 1804-8, i (2. année), 201-207.— **Leclerc.** Deux jumeaux réunis par la face antérieure du tronc. Mém. et compt.-rend. Soc. d. sc. méd. de Lyon (1885), 1886, xxv, pt. 2, 67. — **Legge** (F.) Embrione duplice in un blastoderma unico. Riv. clin. di Bologna, 1886, 3. s., vi, 206. — **Leisching.** Description d'un enfant né avec trois jambes. Rec. périod. d'obs. de méd., de chir. et pharm., Par., 1757, vi, 45-47.—**Lemon** (E.) Rare case of monstrosity. Ohio M. & S. J., Columbus, 1852-3, v, 537.— **von Lenhossék.** Nachricht von einigen menschlichen Doppelmissgeburten, nebst kurzen physiologischen Bemerkungen über ähnliche Monstrositäten. Med. Jahrb. d. k. k. österr. Staates, Wien, 1820, vi, 2 St., 125; 3. St., 125, 3 pl. — **Lenoel.** Accouchement de deux jumeaux unis par le ventre. Soc. méd. d'Amiens. Bull. (1863), 1864, iii, 35-43.—**Leopold.** Geburt von zwei zusammengewachsenen Kindern. Ztschr. f. Wundärzteu. Geburtsh., Stuttg., 1853, iv, 96-100, 1 pl. — **Leray** (C.) Observation sur une naissance monstrueuse de deux filles jumelles unies ensemble, avec des remarques sur la section de la symphysis. J. de méd., chir., pharm., etc., Par., 1778, l, 436-460, 1 pl.—**Lereboullet.** [Un fœtus humain à deux têtes.] Proc.-verb. .... Soc. de méd. de Strasb. (1858-63), 1864, i, 59-61. — **Leroux.** Monstre double, bifemelle, de la famille des monomphaliens, à unions sous et sus ombilicale, appartenant en même temps aux deux genres ischiopage et xyphopage de Geoffroy-Saint-Hilaire. Compt. rend. Soc. de biol. 1863, Par., 1864, 3. s., v, 45-47.—**Lesauvage.** Observation nouvelle d'accouchement d'un fœtus double monstrueux, avec quelques remarques sur le mécanisme de l'accouchement dans le cas de diplogénèse monstrueuse. Arch. gén. de méd., Par., 1848, 4. s., xviii, 444-454.—**Levison** (F.) Om dobbeltmisfostrenes genese med särligt hensyn på sternopagerne. Nord. med. Ark., Stockholm, 1878, x, 1-30, 1 pl. — **Liebman** (C.) Di un caso di ischiopagia e del parto di mostri doppi in genere. Morgagni, Napoli, 1874, xvi, 264; 340. — **Lindemann** (M.) Geburt einer Doppelbildung, beendigt durch Abtrennung eines Kopfes mittels des Braun'schen Schlüsselhackens, mit günstigem Ausgange für die Mutter. Monatschr. f. Geburtsk. u. Frauenkr., Berl., 1869, xxxiii, 457-461.— **Little** (G. W.) A case of twins united at the umbilicus, in which the connection was cut and the perfect child survived. West. J. M. & Phys. Sc., Cincin., 1836, ix, 38-41.— **Livingstone** (J.) An account of a lusus naturæ. Phila. J. M. & Phys. Sc., 1821, ii, 148-153.—**Loescher** (H.) Beschreibung eines Doppelkindes. Med. Ztg., Berl, 1854, xxiii, 229. ——. Ein zweiköpfiges Monstrum. Monatschr. f. Geburtsk. u. Frauenkr., Berl., 1858, xi, 432-438, 1 pl.—**Look** (E. S.) [Remarkable case of two children united.] Month. M. News, Louisville, 1860, ii, 71.—**Lopez** (M.) Monstruo notable y relativamente perfecto. Génio méd.-quir., Madrid, 1880, xxvi, 446-448.—**Louvois.** [Enfant monstrueux.] [*From:* Hist. Acad. roy. d. sc. de Par., 1706.] Rec. d. mém., Dijon, 1754, ii, 330.—**Lowe** (W.) Case of double monster. Med. Times & Gaz., Lond., 1862, i, 121.—**Lunadei** (G.) Lettera intorno una bambina nata con due teste, e risposta del Giovanni Bianchi intorno questo mostro. *In:* Rac. d' opusc. scient. e filol., 16°, Venezia, 1740, xxii, 85-92.—**Lyell.** Birth of a double monster. Mouth. J. M. Sc., Lond. & Edinb., 1848-9, ix,

26

Monsters (*Double*).

133, 1 pl.—**McCallum** (D. C.) A description of the conjoined twins, Marie-Rosa Drouin. Tr. Obst. Soc. Lond. (1878), 1879, xx, 120–122, 2 pl. *Also:* Canada M. Rec., Montreal, 1878–9, vii, 43, 1 pl. *Also:* Canada M. & S. J., Montreal, 1878–9, vii, 97–99, 1 pl. *Also* [Abstr.]: Obst. J. Gr. Brit., Lond., 1878–9, vi, 235. *Also, transl.:* Abeille méd., Montréal, 1879, i, 47–50, 1 pl.—**McCaskey** (G. W.) Lusus naturæ (double monster). [*From:* Fort Wayne Gazette.] Fort Wayne J. M. Sc., 1822–3, ii, 23.—**M'Clintock.** A case of double monstrosity. Dublin Q. J. M. Sc., 1866, xlii, 192–194.—**Macdonald** (A.) On a diprosopus triophthalmus monster. Tr. Edinb. Obst. Soc. (1874–7), 1878, iv, 1–10. *Also:* Edinb. M. J., 1874–5, xx, 702–708, 1 pl. *Also:* Obst. J. Gr. Brit., Lond., 1875–6, iii, 48–54.—**de Macédo** (A.) Cas de tératologie. Rev. phot. d. hôp. de Par., 1869, i, 103, 1 pl.—[**McFarlane** (S.)] Case of difficult labor with a bicephalous fœtus. Am. J. Obst., N. Y., 1876, ix, 83.—**Mackay** (E.) A description of a double monocephalic human monster, which was transmitted to this country from South America, by Robert Mackay, British consul at Maracaylis, Venezuela. Edinb. M. & S. J., 1841, lv, 76–81.—**McKenzie.** Double monstrosity. St. Louis M. & S. J., 1884, xlvi, 522–526.—**Mackinder** (D.) Malformation of twins. Lancet, Lond., 1842–3, i, 173.—**M'Laurin** (H. N.) Twin monster. Tr. Obst. Soc. Lond. (1880), 1881, xxii, 155. *Also:* Obst. J. Gr. Brit., Lond., 1880, viii, 415.—**McMaster** (H. S.) A monstrous birth; two heads and two necks on one body. Tr. Nat. Eclect. M. Ass. 1877–8, N. Y., 1879, vi, 465–469. —**Macquelyn** (M. J.) Beschrijving van eene wanstaltige menschelijke vrucht van zeven maanden dragts, veroorzaakt door eene gedeeltelijke samergroeijing van twee vruchten. Geneesk. Mag., Delft, 1801, i, 2. st., 1–27, 4 pl.—**Manlove** (J. E.) Remarkable case of monstrosity. Nashville Month. Rec. M. & Phys. Sc., 1858–9, i, 656–658. *Also:* Nashville J. M. & S., 1859, xvi, 481–484.—**Manson.** Amputation of a child's head. Edinb. M. J., 1859–60, v, 692.—**Marchal.** Veau monstrueux, bicéphale, avec spina bifida. J. d. conn. méd.-chir., Par., 1843–4, xi, pt. 1, 87.—**Marchand.** Die böhmischen Schwestern Rosalia und Josepha. Breslau. aerztl. Ztschr., 1881, iii, 237–240.—**Marchand** & **Boulland** (H.) Monstre sternopage; étude obstétricale et anatomique. Arch. de tocol., Par., 1882, ix, 641–647.—**Marcy** (H. O.) & **Fitz** (R. H.) A case of double monstrosity; union upon the anterior median line from clavicle to umbilicus. Boston M. & S. J., 1871, lxxxv, 17–20.—**de la Mare.** Observation sur un accouchement d'un enfant mal conformé, et d'une espèce de tête attachée au même placenta. J. de méd., chir., pharm., etc., Par., 1770, xxxiii, 515–517.—**Marin** (R.) Parto de una niña monstruosa con dos cabezas. Bol. de med., cirug. y farm., Madrid, 1845, 2. s., vi, 105–108.—**Marisy.** Description d'un enfant monstrueux. J. de méd. chir., pharm., etc., Par., 1771, xxxvi, 312–314.—**Marjolin.** Enfant à trois membres inférieurs; trois cuisses, trois jambes, trois pieds. Bull. Soc. de chir. de Par. (1861), 1862, 2. s., ii, 55.—**Marnitz** (C.) Fall einer Geburt von zusammengewachsenen Zwillingen. Org. f. d. ges. Heilk., Berl., 1857, vi, 197–200.—**Marques** (T.) Mémoire sur un cas remarquable de monstruosité, inconnue jusqu'à présent dans l'espèce humaine, appartenant à la classe des monstres doubles hétérotypiens de M. I. Geoffroy de St.-Hilaire, et que l'on pourrait avec beaucoup de probabilité ranger dans l'ordre des polyméliens, genre pygomèle du même auteur. [*Transl. from:* Rev. med. portugueza.] J. de méd., chir. et pharmacol., Brux., 1865, xl, 411–427.—**Marsden** (W.) The united African twins. Med. Chron., Montreal, 1856, iii, 81–87. — **Marshall** (E.) Double monstrosity. Lancet, Lond., 1865, ii, 548.—**Martin** (J.) A case of twins united by the umbilicus. West. J. M. & Phys. Sc., Cincin., 1830, iii, 290.—**Martinez y Molina** (R.) Description de un monstruo bicéfalo del órden de los ruminantes; consideraciones sobre el dualismo orgánico. Siglo méd., Madrid, 1857, iv, 67.—**Marvin** (L. I.) Case of monstrosity. Med. & Surg. Reporter, Phila., 1867, xvi, 82.—**Mather** (A.) A case of monstrous birth. Med. Facts & Obs., Lond., 1793, iv, 107–111.—**Mato Montero** (D.) Parto doble distócico; monstruosidad por union; mecanismo del parto; resultado satisfactorio. Jurado méd.-farm., Madrid, 1880, i, 146–148.—**Matteucci** (A.) Un caso di riunione di due feti umani, ossia di mostro sinadelfo, del genere Dipygus tetrabrachius (Forster) o deraldelfo (G. S. Hylaire). Ippocratico, Fano, 1869, 3. s., xv, 119–122.—**Maunoir.** Particulars concerning the structure of a monstrous fœtus. Med.-Chir. Tr., Lond., 1816, vii, 257–263.—**de Maurans.** Un monstre double. Semaine méd., Par., 1882, ii, 173.—**Maurice** (E.-F.) Note sur un monstre humain femelle, à trois membres pelviens; d'un genre et d'une famille tératologiques encore incertains. Ann. Soc. de méd. de St.-Étienne et de la Loire (1872–5), 1876, v, 583–610, 1 pl. *Also, Reprint.*—**Mayer** (C.) Eine Missgeburt mit einem Parasiten auf der Brust. J. d. Chir. u. Augenh., Berl., 1827, x, 44–60, 1 pl. ——. Ueber Doppelmissbildungen und deren Eintheilung durch zwei eigne Fälle erläutert. *Ibid.*, 61–76, 1 pl. *Also, transl.:* J. compl. du dict. d. sc. méd., Par., 1828, xxx, 59–66. ——. Drei merkwürdige Doppel-Missgeburten, untersucht und beschrieben. Zt

Monsters (*Double*).

schr. f. Physiol., Darmstadt, 1829, iii, 240–248.—**Mayor** (A.) Note sur un monstre du genre janiceps. Bull. Soc. anat. de Par., 1881, lvi, 496–535. *Also:* Progrès méd., Par., 1882, x, 169; 224; 244. ——. Contribution à l'étude des monstres doubles; des monstres du genre janiceps. Arch. de physiol. norm. et path., Par., 1882, 2. s., ix, 127–161, 1 pl.—**Mays** (C. E.) Case of embryotomy. [Double-faced monster.] Med. Brief, St. Louis, 1886, xiv, 154–156.—**Meadows** (A.) Case of plural birth and monstrosity. Tr. M. Soc. King's Coll., Lond., 1856–7, i, 236.—**Meigs** (C. D.) Case of double fœtus. Am. J. M. Sc., Phila., 1857, n. s., xxxiii, 45–47, 1 pl.—**Meloni-Satta** (P.) & **Pintor-Pasella** (G.) Derodimo rarissimo. Spallanzani, Modena, 1882, 2. s., xi, 231–243, 1 pl.—**Ménage.** Observation d'un fœtus bi-céphale. J. de la sect. de méd. Soc. acad. Loire-Inf., Nantes, 1839, xv, 199–204.—**Merindolus** (A.) Quid monstra, quæ ex plurium coagmentatione coivisse apparent: unum, aut plura esse, discernat. *In his:* Ars medica, fol., Aquis-Sextiis, 1633, 375–379.—**Mikimara Kakizaku.** [A double monstrosity.] Iji Shinshi, Tokei, 1883, no. 300, Dec. 29.—**Miller** (H. V. M.) Account of a case of double monstrosity. South. M. & S. J., Augusta, 1854, n. s., x, 79–84.—**Mitchell** (J. K.) An account of a monster. Phila. J. M. & Phys. Sc., 1821, iii, 78–86, 1 pl. *Also:* Lond. M. Reposit., 1821, xvi, 441–447.—**Mitchell** (T. D.) Newport twins, analogous to the celebrated Siamese twins. West. M. Gaz., Cincin., 1832–4, i, 295.—**Mitchell** (W. J.) A child having two perfectly formed and fully developed heads and necks. Richmond & Louisville M. J., Louisville, 1868, v, 186.—**Montané** (L.) Descripcion de un monstruo doble heterotipico perteneciente al genero heterodimo. An. r. Acad. de cien. méd. . . . de la Habana, 1878–9, xv, 416–427. *Also, transl.* [Abstr.]: Lancet, Lond., 1885, ii, 1205.—**Montgomery** (E. E.) A case of double monster. Phila. M. Times, 1875, v, 485.—**Montgomery** (W. F.) Account of a very remarkable case of double monster; with some observations on the subject of double monstrosity. Dublin Q. J. M. Sc., 1853, xv, 257–280, 4 pl.—**Monti** (L.) Descrizione anatomica di un mostro umano doppio del genere derodimo. Mem. Acad. d. sc. d. Ist. di Bologna, 1880, 4. s., i, 713–725, 6 pl.—**Moore** (J. W.) Notice of two children whose bodies were united anteriorly, and lived some time after birth. Am. J. M. Sc., Phila., 1829, v, 252, 1 pl.—**Moore** (M.) A case of two-headed monstrosity. Lancet, Lond., 1882, i, 986.—**Moreno** (F.-F.) Description de deux fœtus adhérens l'un à l'autre, nés à Cadix en 1818. J. univ. d. sc. méd., Par., 1820, xviii, 125–127, 1 pl. *Also, transl.* [Abstr.]: Med. Reposit., N. Y., 1820, n. s., v, 425.—**Morgan** (W.) A duplex child. Lond. M. Gaz., 1830, vi, 117.—**Morin.** Sur un fétus monstrueux. [*From:* Hist. d. mém. Acad. roy. d. sc. de Par., 1715.] Collect. acad. d. mém., etc , Par., 1770, iv, 440.—**Morlanne** & **Charneil.** Observation d'un fétus né avec deux têtes. Rec. période. Soc. de méd. de Par., 1801, xi, 19–24.—**Mowat** (J.) The description of a monstrous fœtus. Essays & Obs. Phil. Soc. Edinb., 1756, ii, 266–272.—**Müller** (N.) Monstrum von zusammen-gewachsenen Zwillingen, und deren Section. Samml. v. Nat.- u. Med.-. . . Gesch. 1721, Leipz. u. Budissin, 1723, xvii, 178.—**Muggeridge** (H. H.) An extraordinary birth. Lancet, Lond., 1872, i, 538.—**Mullin** (J.) Duplicitas monstrosa. Canada M. Rec., Montreal, 1874–5, iii, 365.—**Murphy** (J.) Double monster. Tr. Obst. Soc. Lond. (1880), 1881, xxii, 109. *Also* [Abstr.]: Obst. J. Gr. Brit., Lond., 1880, viii, 288. *Also:* Extr. Rec. Bost. Soc. M. Improve. (1874–9), 1880, vii, 64.—**Naef.** Entbindung einer Frau von einem monströsen zeitigen Kinde mit zwey nebeneinander stehenden Köpfen. N. Denkwrdgktn. f. Aerzte u. Geburtsh., Götting., 1797, i, 188–204.—**Nannizzi** (D.) Relazione anatomica d' un doppio feto. *In:* Rac. d' opusc. scient. e filol., 16°, Venezia, 1748, xxxix, 505–532.—**Nesterus** (J. M.) De fœtu monstroso. Misc. Acad. nat. curios. 1675–6, Francof. et Lips., 1688, vi–vii, 59, 1 pl. *Also, transl.:* Auserl. med.-chir.-. . . Abhandl. d. röm.-kais. Akad. d. Naturf., Nürnb., 1759, vi, 56. — **Neugebauer** (L. A.) Kilka słów o potworach podwójnych czyli bliźniętach zrosłych (monstra duplicia sive gemini coaliti). Gaz. lek., Warszawa, 1873, xv, 17; 33; 49; 68; 81; 105; 116.—**Neullier** (J.) Cas rare et curieux d'un enfant montrueux comparable à Ritta-Christina. Bull. gén. de thérap., etc., Par., 1835, ix, 290–293. *Also:* Ann. de méd. belge, Brux., 1836, i, 179–181. *Also:* Gaz. d. hôp., Par., 1836, x, 13.—**Niess.** Fall eines mit zwei Köpfen geborenen Kindes, nebst einer Beschreibung und Abbildung desselben. Monatschr. f. Geburtsk. u. Frauenkr., Berl., 1853, i, 433–437, 1 pl.—**Nockher.** Entbindung einer Missgeburt mit zwei Köpfen. Gen.-Ber. d. k. rhein. Med.-Coll. 1836, Koblenz, 1839, 138; 203. *Also:* Wchnschr. f. d. ges. Heilk., Berl., 1839, 542–554.—**Normand.** Observation sur deux jumeaux accolés dos à dos. Bull. Fac. de méd. de Par., 1818–19, vi (13. année), 1–5.—**O'Donovan** (R. W.) Case of double monster. Dublin Q. J. M. Sc., 1851, xii, 482.—**Oliphant** (J.) Account of an uncommon case in midwifery, where a preternatural adhesion of twins had taken place. Med. Comment. 1785, Lond., 1786, x, 249–255.—**Ollivier.** Diplogénèse. Dict. de méd., 2. éd., Par.,

Monsters (*Double*).

1835, x, 396-420.—**de Oria** (A.) Extraccion de un feto de dos cabezas. Siglo méd., Madrid, 1872, xix, 262. *Also, transl.:* Rec. d. trav. Soc. méd. d'Indre-et-Loire 1872, Tours, 1873, lxx, 40-44.—**Orye** (A.) Notice sur un enfant monstrueux né le 30 août 1826, dans la commune de Benais. Précis de la const. méd. d'Indre-et-Loire, Tours, 1827, 76-79.—**Otto** (R.) Ueber einen Epignathus. Arch. f. Gynaek., Berl., 1878, xiii, 167-181, 1 pl.—**de Padua** (J. M.) Historia de hum parto difficultoso por causa de monstruosidade dobrada, cuja peça foi offerecida para o museu da Sociedade das sciencias medicas de Lisboa. J. Soc. d. sc. med. de Lisb., 1840, xi, 134-141, 1 pl.—**Palfrey** (J.) [Monster with two heads.] Tr. Obst. Soc. Lond. (1877), 1878, xix, 40; 97, 1 pl.—**Pancoast** (W. H.) Strange case of monstrosity; heteradelphia; operation by the écraseur. Med. & Surg. Reporter, Phila., 1859, i, 405-407. ———. The Carolina twins. Phot. Rev. M. & S., Phila., 1870-71, i, 43-57, i, 1 pl. *Also* [Abstr.]: Tr. M. Soc. Penn., Phila., 1873, ix, pt. 2, 115-117.—**Pappenheim** (S.) Ueber eine dreifüssige Missgeburt. Arch f. Anat., Physiol. u. wissensch. Med., Berl., 1840, 534.—**Parsons** (J.) An account of a preternatural conjunction of two female children. Phil. Tr. 1743-50, Lond., 1756, xi, 1209-1215, 1 pl.—**Parsons** (S. N.) Case of monstrosity. Prov. M. & S. J., Lond., 1840-41, i, 294.—**Pasi** (C. A.) Storia di un monosomio dicefalo. Bull. d. sc. med. di Bologna, 1837, 2. s., iii, 90-95, 1 pl.—**Pasquet-Labroue.** Observation sur un cas de monstre double autositaire. Union méd., Par., 1875, 3. s., xx, 642-644.—**Patinus** (C.) Monstrum biceps masculinum. Misc. Acad. nat. curios. 1691, Norimb., 1692, 2. decuria, x, 72, 1 pl. *Also, transl.:* Auserl. med.-chir.- . . . Abhandl. d. röm.-kais. Akad. d. Naturf., Nürnb., 1771, xx, 60, 1 pl.—**Patterson** (A.) The Siamese twins. Glasgow M. J., 1887, [4.] s., xxvii, 19-21.—**Paulleus.** Historia monstruosi infantis, nati in Castro de Loire. Zodiacus med.-gall. 1679, Geneva, 1680, i, 152-155, 1 pl.—**Percival** (T.) An account of a double child. Phil. Tr. 1751-2, Lond., 1753, xlvii, 360-362.—**Pereira** (J. A.) Notice of a bicephalous and bisomatous child, born at Galle, in the island of Ceylon. Edinb. M. & S. J., 1844, lxi, 58.—**Pertsch.** Ein Fall von Xiphopagie aus dem 10. Jahrhunderte. Arch. f. path. Anat., etc., Berl., 1871, liii, 138.—**Petit.** Description d'un fétus difforme. [*From:* Hist. d. mém. Acad. roy. d. sc. de Par., 1716.] Collect. acad. d. mém., etc., Par., 1770, iv, 441-444.—**Peyerus** (J. C.) De gemellis monstrosis, coalitis partibus obscœnis. Misc. Acad. nat. curios. 1683, Norimb., 1698, 2. decuria, ii, 267.—**Pfeifer** (M. D. G.) Case of double-headed monster; delivery without mutilation. Am. J. M. Sc., Phila., 1846, n. s., xii, 80-87.—**Phillips** (J.) Case of dicephalous monstrosity. Tr. Obst. Soc. Lond. (1886), 1887, xxviii, 278.—**Phillips** (J. J.) & **Dalton** (B. C. N.) A short account of the delivery of a two-headed monster. Guy's Hosp. Rep., Lond., 1871, 3. s., xvi, 455-461, 2 pl.—**Pichartus.** Monstrum bicorporeum. Zodiacus med.-gall. 1679, Geneva, 1680, i, 129.—**Pigeolet.** Monstruosité (janiceps). Bull. Soc. roy. d. sc. méd. et nat. de Brux., 1875, 54.—**Pigné.** [Un fœtus simple supérieurement, double inférieurement et postérieurement.] Bull. Soc. anat. de Par., 1846, xxi, 12. ———. [La duplicature des germes.] *Ibid.*, 144. ———. †† *Ibid.*, 205. ———. [Fœtus simple à l'extérieur, sauf que l'un des membres supérieurs est terminé par deux avant-bras; duplicatures de plusieurs des organes thoraciques et abdominaux.] *Ibid.*, 206-208. ———. [Un monstre double, monocéphale, bimane seulement, mais ayant quatre membres abdominaux.] *Ibid.*, 1847, xxii, 169.—**Pilat.** Hydropisie de l'amnios; grossesse gémellaire; monstre pigopage; mort d'un des fœtus avec dégénérescence graisseuse; accouchement à six mois et demi. Ann. de gynéc., Par., 1879, xii, 133-138. *Also:* Bull. méd. du nord, Lille, 1879, xviii, 187-192.—**Pilcher** (L. S.) Double monsters; description of the specimens in the museum of the Brooklyn Anatomical and Surgical Society. Ann. Anat. & Surg. Soc, N. Y., 1880, ii, 19-33.—**Pincott** (R.) Notes on twin monsters, exhibited at the meeting of the Medical Society of Victoria, July 3, 1867. Austral. M. J., Melbourne, 1867, xii, 272.—**Pippingsköld.** Dubbel-missbildning. Finska läk.-sällsk. handl., Helsingfors, 1879, xxi, 298.—**Playfair** (W. S.) On the mechanism and management of delivery in cases of double monstrosity. Tr. Obs. Soc. Lond. (1866), 1867, viii, 300-312. ———. Conjoined twins. *Ibid.* (1880), 1881, xxii, 265. *Also:* Lancet, Lond., 1881, i, 15.—**Poelman** (C.) Description de deux monstres doubles monomphaliens, sternopages et ischiopages. Ann. Soc. de méd. de Gand, 1849, xxiv, 149-157, 2 pl. ———. Note sur une monstruosité double iléadelphe. Bull. Soc. de méd. de Gand, 1857, xxiv, 292-294, 1 pl.—**Poland** (A.) Contribution to the anatomy of double monsters. Guy's Hosp. Rep., Lond., 1848, 2. s., vi, 248-262, 3 pl.—**Poletti** (L.) † Mostro diplogenetico. Rendic. Accad. med.-chir. di Ferrara 1841, Bologna, 1843, 56-60: (1846-49), 1850, 177-179.—**Portal.** Relazione di un mostro umano. Mercurio d. sc. med., Livorno, 1825, iii, 15.—**Préfet.** Description d'un fœtus monstrueux. Hist. Soc. de méd.-prat. de Montpel., 1805, xiv, 5-7.—**Preuss.** Seltener Fall von Doppelbildung; Kind mit Sacralgeschwulst, in welcher Theile eines Fœtus gefühlt und leb-

Monsters (*Double*).

hafte Bewegungen wahrgenommen werden. Arch. f. Anat., Physiol. u. wissensch. Med., Leipz., 1869, 267-272, 1 pl.—**Prieger** (H.) Entbindungsgeschichte zusammengewachsener, ausgetragener Zwillingsmädchen. N. Ztschr. f. Geburtsk., Berl., 1851, xxix, 112-117.—**Prochaska** (G.) Descriptio anatomica fœtus humani bicipitis monocorporei. *In his:* Adnot. acad., 8°, Pragæ, 1780, i, 49-81, 1 pl.—**Proschko** (J.) Zwillinge mit zusammengewachsener Bauchhaut; Steisslage; Entwicklung derselben. Med.-chir. Centralbl., Wien, 1878, xiii, 4.—**Prus.** Observation de monstruosité double. Rev. méd. franç. et étrang., Par., 1848, ii, 449-458.—**Puech** (A.) Étude sur un monstre double, compliqué de deux autres monstruosités. Ann. clin. de Montpel., 1856-7, iv, 28; 56; 88, 1 pl.—**Ragotzky.** Duplicitas monstrosa superior neben ausgebildeten Zwillingen. Arch. f. path. Anat., etc., Berl., 1870, l, 297.—**Ramsbotham** (F. H.) A description of the united African twins, now being exhibited at the Egyptian Hall, Piccadilly. Med. Times & Gaz., Lond., 1855, n. s., xi, 313.—**Ranking** (S. A.) Case of united twins three months old. Indian M. Gaz., Calcutta, 1877, xii, 158.—**Ratel.** Cas d'accouchement rendu impossible par la conformation monstrueuse d'un fœtus dont les parties supérieures étaient doubles. Bull. Fac. de méd. de Par., 1818-19, vi (13. année), 32-35.—**Rauber** (A.) Die Theorien der excessiven Monstra. Arch. f. path. Anat., etc., Berl., 1877, lxxi, 133-206, 3 pl. ———. Zur Beurtheilung der pluralen Monstra; ein Nachtrag zur Radiationstheorie derselben. *Ibid.*, 1883, xci, 564-567.—**Raygerus** (C.) Anatomia monstri bicipitis. Misc. Acad. nat. curios., Lips., 1670, i, 25-27. *Also, transl.:* Collect. acad. d. mém., etc., Dijon, 1755, iii, 6. *Also, transl.:* Auserl. med.-chir.- . . . Abhandl. d. röm.-kais. Akad. d. Naturf., Nürnb., 1755, i, 19-21.—**Rear** (W.) [Twins firmly attached to each other from the junction of the upper with the middle third of the sternum above to two inches above the pubes below.] Canada Lancet, Toronto, 1877-8, x, 301.—**Reddy** (J.) A case of sterno-omphalopage. Med. Chron., Montreal, 1858-9, vi, 289-292.—**Regnoli** (G.) Sulla estrazione di un feto mostruoso. Ann. univ. di med., Milano, 1826, xxxviii, 218-231, 1 pl.—**Reichert** (C. B.) Anatomische Beschreibung zweier sehr frühzeitiger Doppel-Embryonen von Vögeln, zur Erläuterung der Entstehung von Doppel-Missgeburten. Arch. f. Anat., Physiol. u. wissensch. Med., Leipz., 1864, 744-766, 2 pl.—**Reiner** (M.) Glücklich vorgenommene unblutige Trennung zweier zwischen Sitzknorren und Steisse miteinander verwachsener Kinder. Wien. med. Wchnschr., 1858, viii, 560; 575; 593; 887.—**Retzius** (A.) Monstrum duplex monomphalicum. J. f. Kinderkr., Erlang., 1855, xxiv, 317.—**Richard.** Description de deux enfans unis ensemble, ne formant qu'un seul tronc depuis le cou jusqu'audessus du nombril, ayant deux têtes, trois bras et quatre jambes. J. de méd., chir., pharm., etc., Par., 1773, xxxix, 405-409.—**Ricoigne.** Cas remarquable de monstruosité (monstres homœadelphes ectopages). Monit. d. hôp., Par., 1854, ii, 619-621.—**Rintel** jun. & **Krieger.** Geburt zweier mit einander verwachsenen Kinder. Verhandl. d. Gesellsch. f. Geburtsh. in Berl. (1844-5), 1846, i, 140; 181, 1 pl.—**von Ritgen.** Ueber die Entstehung von Doppelmissgeburten auf gemeinsamem Dotter. Monatschr. f. Geburtsk. u. Frauenkr., Berl., 1856, viii, 193-213, 1 pl.—**Robinson** (C. C.) [Case of monstrosity, or united twins.] Buffalo M. & S. J., 1862-3, ii, 97-108.—**Robinson** (H.) A case of two-headed monstrosity. Brit. M. J., Lond., 1876, ii, 44.—**Rodriguez** (J. M.) Descripcion de un monstruo humano diplogenésico, monocéfalo, autositario, oníxsido, noviable. Gac. méd. de México, 1869, iv, 145; 161, 1 pl. ———. Parto de una monstruosidad synota. *Ibid.*, 1872, vii, 253-260.—**Rogers** (J. F.) Case of double monstrosity. Tr. Obst. Soc. Lond. (1869), 1870, xi, 128-131.—**Rogowicz** (J.) Pygopagi (monstrum duplicia). Medycyna, Warszawa, 1879, vii, 542.—**Rohde.** Geburt eines Sternopagus. Centralbl. f. Gynäk., Leipz., 1878, ii, 289.—**Rohrer.** Ueber ein zweiköpfiges Kind, welches am 13. Oct. 1836 im Dorfe Targanice geboren wurde. Med. Jahrb. d. k. k. österr. Staates, Wien, 1838, n. F., xv, 91-96.—**Rolland.** Observation sur un accouchement dans lequel l'enfant avait deux têtes. J. de méd., chir., pharm., etc., Par., 1815, xxxii, 244-246.—**von Rościszewski** (S.) Zur Kenntniss der Dignathie. Arch. f. path. Anat., etc., Berl., 1875, lxiv, 540-556, 2 pl.—**Rothe** (H.) Die Geburt einer verwachsenen Doppelfrucht. Arch. f. Gynaek., Berl., 1870, i, 340-346.—**Ruggles.** A double-headed fœtus. N. York M. & S. Reporter, 1845-6, i, 340.—**Ruhl** (W. D.) A monstrosity. Weekly M. Rev., Chicago, 1884, x, 108.—**Rul-Ogez.** Cas de monstruosité. Ann. Soc. de méd. d'Anvers, 1851, viii, 526-528.—**Rzadkowski** (M.) Potwór bliźniaczy, czyli zroślak jednogłowy i jednopępkowy (monstrum duplicium s. geminus coalitus monocephalus et monomphalus). Medycyna, Warszawa, 1879, vii, 743-747.—**S.** (J. G.) Von einem menschlichen Monstro. Samml. v. Nat.- u. Med. . . . Gesch. 1717-18, Bresl., 1718-20, 1992-1994.—**Saint-Ange** (M.) Note sur quelques circonstances de la naissance, de la vie et de la mort de la fille bicéphale (Rita-Christina). J. hebd. de méd., Par., 1830, vi, 42-49.—**Salcher.** Fall von einer Doppelmissgeburt. Oesterr. med. Wchnschr., Wien,

Monsters (*Double*).

1847, 225-231.—**Salmon** (G. H.) On a singular freak of ature. Nashville J. M. & S., 1857, xiii, 236-238.—**Saltzmann** (J.) De fœtu monstroso bicorporeo, manu obstetricia extracto. Acta Acad. nat. curios., Norimb., 1737, iv, 232-245, 2 pl.—**Sangalli** (G.) I mostri doppi. Mem. r. Ist. Lomb. di sc. e lett. Cl. di sc. matemat. e nat. 1870-72, Milano, 1873, 3. s., xii, 301-328. *Also*, Reprint.———. Breve relazione delle due gemelle della Carolina del Nord. R. Ist. Lomb. di sc. e lett. Rendic., Milano, 1873, 2. s., vi, 379-382.—**Sarkies** (J. C.) Lusus naturæ. Indian J. M. & Phys. Sc., Calcutta, 1839, n. s., iv, 346, 1 pl.—**Sarluis** (J.) Waarneming van eene door de kunst ten einde gebragte, zur moeijelijke verlossing, veroorzaakt door eenen gedeeltelijk ineengesmolten tweeling (heteradelphos). Boerhaave. Tijdschr., etc., Amst., 1842, n. s., i, 425, 2 pl.: 1844, n. s., iii, 319.—**Sauve** (C.) Monstre xiphodyme ou dicephalus tetrabrachius. Rev. méd.-phot. d. hôp. de Par., 1875, vii, 137, 2 pl.—**Schaffler.** Beschreibung einer Geburt von zusammengewachsenen Zwillingen. J. f. d. Chir., Geburtsh. u. gerichtl. Arznk., Jena, 1806, iv, 541-547.—**Scharfius** (B.) Monstrum a constrictione. Misc. Acad. nat. curios. 1683, Norimb., 1698, 2. decuria, ii, 254-256, 1 pl.—**Scheiber** (S. H.) Die Anatomie eines Doppelmonstrums. Med. Jahrb., Wien, 1874, 187-216, 1 pl.—**Scheuthauer** (G.) Gastrodidymus exomphalus. Allg. Wien. med. Ztg., 1865, x, 325.—**Schmidtmüller.** Beschreibung und Abbildung missgebildeter Zwillinge und ihrer Placenta. Lucina, Leipz., 1808, iv, 252-265.—**Schœllhammer.** Dystocie et tératologie Bull. Soc. méd. du Haut-Rhin, Strasb., 1864, ii, 296-298.—**Schönfeld** (F.) Eine Doppelgeburt. Monatschr. f. Geburtsk. u. Frauenkr., Berl., 1859, xiv, 378-380.—**Schroeckius** (L.) De gravidæ symptomatibus singularibus et partu gemellorum monstroso. Misc. Acad. nat. curios. 1678-9, Norimb., 1693, ix-x, 354, 1 pl. *Also, transl.:* Auserl. med.- chir.- . . . . Abhandl. d. rom.-kais. Akad. d. Naturf., Nürnb., 1761, ix, 216.—**Schultze** (B.) Ueber die Entstehung der Doppelmonstra. Verhandl. d. Gesellsch. f. Geburtsh. in Berl. (1855-6), 1857, ix, 65-106, 2 pl. *Also:* Monatschr. f. Geburtsk. u. Frauenkr., Berl., 1856, vii, 247-285, 1 pl.———. Erwiderung auf die in Betreff meiner Arbeiten über Entstehung der Doppelmonstra vom Herrn von Ritgen gemachten Bemerkungen. Monatschr. f. Geburtsk. u. Frauenkr., Berl., 1857, ix, 459-464.—**Schwarz.** Beschreibung und Abbildung einer merkwürdigen menschlichen Missgeburt, in Gemeinschaft mit Dr. Wankel in Hünfeld. Gem. deutsche Ztschr. f. Geburtsk., Weimar, 1827, i, 521-540.—**Scultetus** (J.) De duobus monstris. Misc. Acad. nat. curios. 1672, Lips. et Francof., 1681, iii, 346-351, 1 pl. *Also, transl.:* Auserl. med.- chir-. . . Abhandl. d. rom.-kais. Akad. d. Naturf., Nürnb., 1756, iii, 337, 1 pl.—**Sextex** (L.) Note sur un cas de mélomélie. Mém. et bull. Soc. de méd. et chir. de Bordeaux, 1875, 59-64. *Also:* Bordeaux méd., 1875, iv, 129-131.—**Serres.** Mémoire sur l'organisation anatomique des monstres hétéradelphes; appliquée à la pathologie. Arch. gén. de méd., Par., 1828, xvi, 321-352.———. Observations sur la duplicité monstrueuse, faites à l'occasion de la communication de M. de Quatrefages. Monit. d. hôp., Par., 1855, iii, 281.—**Sevelle.** Description anatomique d'un enfant double. J. de méd., chir., pharm., etc., Par., 1786, lxviii, 468-475.—**Sherman & Furry.** Monstrosity, double. Am. M. J., St. Louis, 1882, x, 433.—**Shiland** (A. W.) Case of united twins (xyphopages). Am. J. Obst., N. Y., 1875-6, viii, 156-158. *Also:* Med. Ann., Albany, 1881, ii (Tr. M. Soc. County Albany), 181.—**Shultz** (H. N.) Case of a double-headed monster. Med. & Surg. Reporter, Phila., 1864, n. s., xi, 279.—**Siegenbeek van Heukelom.** Een dubbelmonster. Nederl. Tijdschr. v. Geneesk., Amst., 1887, xxiii, 225-241, 5 pl.—**Siegwart** (A. J. D.) Historia gemellorum coalitorum monstrosa pulchritudine spectabilium. *In:* Weiz (F. A.) Neue Ausz., (ed.) 12°, Leipz., 1776, iv, 147: v, 136.—[**da Silva Cardeira** (L.)] Raros vicios de conformação, caracterisados exteriormente por tres pernas e dois membros viris. Escholiaste med., Lisb., 1864, xv, 186.—**Simmonds** (M.) Ein parasitischer Steisszwilling. Arch. f. path. Anat., etc., Berl., 1880, lxxxii, 374-376, 1 pl.—**Simmons** (W.) A case of monstrosity. Med. Facts & Obs., Lond, 1800, viii, 1-18, 1 pl.—**Simpson** (A.) Double monstrosity. Edinb. M. J., 1862-3, viii, 475.—**Sims** (J. T.) & **Farrar** (G. W.) A double monster. Med. & Surg. Reporter, Phila., 1881, xlv, 446.—**Skipton** (H. S.) Case of twins; with union of the bodies of the children. Dublin M. Press, 1842, vii, 328.—**Soeneus.** Cas de monstruosité double. Ann. Soc. méd.-chir. de Bruges, 1801, 2. s., ix, 144-150, 2 pl. [Rap. de Van Biervliet], 151-156.—**Sorel** (E.) Adjonction fatale. Soc. méd. d'Amiens. Bull. (1873-4), 1875, 201-204.—**Spessa** (A. A.) Parto bicorporeo. Bull. d. sc. med. di Bologna, 1840, 2. s., ix, 113-118.—**Spruijt** (J.) Waarneming eener verlossing van aaneengegroeide tweelingen. Pract Tijdschr. v. de Geneesk., Gorinchem, 1829, viii, 374-376.—**Staub.** Die Geburt und die Beschreibung einer gedoppelten Missgeburt. Med. Ztg., Berl., 1857, xxvi, 5.—**Stedman** (J.) A case of united children, or double monstrosity. Boston M. & S. J., 1881, cv, 583-586.—**Steele.** A case of a double-headed human monstrosity. Med. Arch. St. Louis, 1869,

Monsters (*Double*).

iii, 148-154.—**Stein** (G. W.) jun. Zwillingsmissgeburt. Ann. d. Geburtsh., etc., Leipz., 1808, 1. St., 57-66.—**Stokes** (J. G.) Description of a double monster. Med. Exam., Chicago, 1874, xv, 433-435.—**Stuart** (C.) Case of difficult labour, in consequence of twins joined by the breast. Month. J. M. Sc., Lond. & Edinb., 1851, xii, 5.—**Swayne** (J. G.) Case of double monstrosity. Tr. Obst. Soc. Lond. (1860), 1861, ii, 320-323.———. Case of double monstrosity. *Ibid.* (1866), 1867, viii, 1-3.—**Tadlock** (A. B.) The Cardwell twins. Nashville J. M. & S., 1873, n. s., xi, 65-71.—**Talko** (J.) Materyjał do teratologii; potwory podwójne (monstra duplicia). Pam. Towarz. Lek. Warszaw., 1875, lxxi, 198-207.—**Tanner** (T. H.) Description of two fœtal monstrosities. Lancet, Lond., 1860, i, 598.—**Tardieu.** L'examen du monstre connu sous le nom de Millie-Christine. Bull. Acad. de méd., Par., 1874, 2. s., iii, 36-45. *Also:* Abeille méd., Par., 1874, xxxi, 17. *Also:* Gaz. obst., Par., 1874, iii, 14-16. *Also:* France méd., Par., 1874, xxi, 50.—**Tarenetski** (A.) Dvoinie urodi s razdieleniem nijnei polovini tiela. [Double monster classified as Dipygus tetrabrachius.] Voyenno-med. J., St. Pctersb., 1880, cxxxvii, pt. 2, 219-254, 1 pl.—**Taruffi** (C.) Dottrine sulla formazione dei mostri doppi. Bull. d. sc. med. di Bologna, 1878, 6. s., ii, 5; 81; 241.———. Intorno ad un nuovo gruppo di mostri appartenente al genere Dicephalus dibrachius (Förster). Mem. Accad. d. sc. d. Ist. di Bologna, 1880, 4. s., ii, 665-673, 1 pl.———. Sui gemelli monocorii; studi critici. Bull. d. sc. med. di Bologna, 1881, 6. s., vii, 313-347.———. Intorno al genere ileopago (ileadelphus di St. Geoffroy Saint-Hilaire). *Ibid.*, 1881, 6. s., viii, 385-417.———. Nota intorno ai derodimi (Dicephalus dibrachius Förster). Spallanzani, Modena, 1882, 2. s., xi, 281-287.—**Tatum** (W. B.) [A case of a double monster.] Nashville J. M. & S., 1858, xv, 296.—**Taylor** (R.) An account of a monstrous birth. Phil. Tr., Lond., 1700-20, v, 304.—**Teissier.** Monstre bicéphale, cause de dystocie. Rev. de thérap. méd.-chir., Par., 1868, 564-567.—**Telfair** (D. A.) Case of malformation [double monster]. N. Eng. J. M. & S., Bost., 1816, v, 250-252.—**Teljer** (G. J.) Beschrijving der verlossing eener voldragende vrucht, met twee gelijkvormige ligchamen, door burst en buik onderling vereenigd. Nederl. Lancet, Gravenh., 1849-50, 2. s., v, 39-54.—**Thiernesse.** Description d'un monstre double monocéphalien. Bull. Acad. roy. de méd. de Belg., Brux., 1847-8, vii, 804-809. *Also:* Gaz. méd. de Par., 1849, 3. s., iv, 145.—**Thomas.** Case of difficult labor with a bicephalous fœtus. Am. J. Obst., N. Y., 1876, ix, 82.—**Thomas** (S. J.) Report of a case of double monster. Austral. M. J., Melbourne, 1856, i, 202-204.—**Thomason** (T. J.) [Twin male fœtuses, connected anteriorly in median line from clavicle to umbilicus; have a common cord inserted at umbilical juncture.] Tr. M. Soc. N. Jersey, Newark, 1864, 116. *Also* [Abstr.]: Med. & Surg. Reporter, Phila., 1864, xi, 161.—**Thompson** (C. S.) A monstrosity of the Siamese twins type. Brit. M. J., Lond., 1880, i, 897.—**Thompson** (W. E.) A monster presenting the union of two fœtuses. West. M. & Phys. J., Cincin., 1827-8, i, 598.—**Thomson** (A.) Remarks upon the early condition and probable origin of double monsters. Lond. & Edinb. Month. J. M. Sc., 1844, iv, 479; 568; 639.—**Tinelli** (G.) Storia di un mostro bicorporeo monocefalo. Ann. univ. di med., Milano, 1830, liii, 256-316, 1 pl.—**Toms** (W.) Case of male twins united from the axilla to the spine of the ileum. Lond. M. & Phys. J., 1824, li, 292-295.—**Torkos** (J. J.) Observationes anatomico-medicæ de monstro bicorporeo virgineo a. 1701, die 26 Oct. in Pannonia . . . in lucem edito, atque a. 1723, die 23 Febr. Posonii in Cænobio Monialum S. Ursulæ morte functo ibidemque sepulto. [Helena-Judith.] Phil. Tr. 1757-8, Lond., 1758-9, l, 311-322, 2 pl. *Also, transl.* [Abstr.]: Anfiteatro anat. españ., Madrid, 1874, ii, 78. *Also, transl.* [Abstr.]: France méd., Par., 1874, xxi, 49-51.—**Torlese** (J.) Account of a monstrous birth. Phil. Tr., Lond., 1782, lxxii, 44, 1 pl.—**Torres** (A. G.) Noticia de un mónstruo compuesto, autositario, sysomiano, xiphodymo, segun la clasificacion de G. de Saint-Hilaire. Siglo méd., Madrid, 1876, xxiii. 232-235. *Also:* An. Soc. ginec. españ., Madrid, 1876, ii, 80-88. *Also:* Anfiteatro anat., Madrid, 1876, iv, 68; 83; 102.—**Townsend** (R. M.) Bicephalic monstrosity, ischiopagus tripus. Phot. Rev. M. & S., Phila., 1870-71, i, 58-60, 1 pl.———. Pygopagus symmetros. Med. & Surg. Reporter, Phila., 1871, xxiv, 264-267.—**Trout** (M.) Singular freak of nature in malformation. Med. Counselor, Columbus, 1855, i, 74. **Tweedie** (A. C.) Singular double monster. Lancet, Lond., 1876, ii, 313.—**Tymowski.** Baptysta i Jakób Focci. Gaz. lek., Warszawa, 1879, xxvi, 77.—**Valenta** (A.) Geburt eines Dicephalus tribrachius dipus. Memorabilien, Heilbr., 1879, xxiv, 241-246.—**Valentin** (G.) Ein Beitrag zur Entwickelungsgeschichte der Doppelmissgeburten. Arch. f. physiol. Heilk., Stuttg., 1851, x, 1-39, 1 pl.—**Valentin** (L.) Détails ultérieurs sur un enfant à deux têtes superposés. J. gén. de méd., chir. et pharm., Par., 1807, xxx, 408-414.—**Valentin & Hisselsheim.** Recherches sur le développement des monstres doubles. Compt. rend. Soc. de biol. 1852, Par., 1853, iv, 99-102.—

Monsters (*Double*).

Valentini (C. M.) Anatomia fœtus monstrosi Gelnhusæ die iv Apr. a. 1728 editi. Acta Acad. nat. curios., Norimb., 1730, ii, 283.—**Valentini** (M. B.) De monstris Hassiacis recens natis. Misc. Acad. nat. curios. 1684, Norimb., 1685, 2. decuria, iii, 190–192, 2 pl. *Also, transl. :* Auserl. med.-chir.- . . . Abhandl. d. röm.-kais. Akad. d. Naturf., Nürnb., 1764, xiii, 157–159, 1 pl. ——. De monstrorum Hassiacorum ortu atque causis epistola ad J. D. Dorstenium. Misc. Acad. nat. curios. 1684, Norimb., 1685, 2. decuria, iii, 473–486. *Also,* Reprint. *Also, transl. :* Auserl. med.- chir.- . . . Abhandl. d. röm.-kais. Akad. d. Naturf., Nürnb., 1764, xiii, 372–378.—**Valtorta** (G.) Parto confeto mostruoso. Gior. veneto d. sc. med., Venezia, 1875, 3. s., xxiii, 167–174.—**Van Bambeke.** Note sur une monstruosité iléadelphe observée chez l'homme. Bull. Soc. de méd. de Gand, 1866, xxxiii, 199–204, 1 pl. [Rap. de Poelman], 207.—**Veit** (G.) Ueber die Leitung der Geburt bei Doppelmissgeburten. Samml. klin. Vortr., No. 164–165, Leipz., 1879 (Gynäk., No. 48), 1273–1326.—**Velasco.** Duplogenesia génito-urinaria y de miembros abdominales. Siglo méd., Madrid, 1864, xi. 796.—**de la Vergne.** Observation sur un enfant à deux têtes. J. de méd., chir., pharm., etc., Par., 1788. lxxv, 483–489.—**Verhaeghe.** Notice sur deux enfants unis ensemble à la façon des jumeaux siamois, dits jumelles flamandes. Gaz. d. hôp., Par., 1849, xxii, 378. *Also, transl. :* Med. Times, Lond., 1849, xx, 26.—**du Verney.** Observation sur deux enfans joints ensemble. [*From :* Mém. Acad. roy. d. sc. de Par., 1706.] Rec. de mém., Dijon, 1754, ii, 395–403, 1 pl.—**Villeneuve.** Description d'une monstruosité consistant en deux fœtus humains accolés en sens inverse par le sommet de la tête ; suivie de remarques et d'observations à ce sujet. Gaz. d. hôp., Par., 1730–31, iv, 305. ——. Observation sur un cas de monstruosité, consistant en deux enfans du sexe féminin, qui ont vécu un mois accolés directement et dans le même sens par la partie inférieure du tronc. Bull. Acad. de méd., Par., 1838–9, iii, 210.—**Villette.** Monstre de Vieux-Moulin. J. d. progr. d. sc. méd., Par., 1828, viii, 157–187, 4 pl.—**Virchow** (R.) Ueber die sogenannte "zweiköpfige Nachtigall". Verhandl. d. Berl. med. Gesellsch. (1871–3), 1874, iv, 252–263. *Also* [Abstr.] : Berl. klin. Wchnschr., 1873, x, 97. ——. Die xiphodymen Brüder Tocci. Verhandl. d. Berl. Gesellsch. f. Anthrop., 1886, 47–50. ——. Photographien eines indischen Heteradelphus. *Ibid.,* 373.—**Virdung ab Hartung** (O. P.) De monstroso gemello. Acta Acad. nat. curios., Norimb., 1737, iv, 297.—**Vollgnad** (H.) De monstroso fœtu. Misc. Acad. nat. curios. 1672, Lips. et Francof., 1681, iii, 446. *Also, transl. :* Auserl. med.- chir.- . . . Abhandl. d. röm.-kais. Akad. d. Naturf., Nürnb., 1756, iii, 445, 1 pl.—**Wagner.** Geburtsfall bei Thoracopagus tripus. Aerztl. Mitth. a. Baden, Karlsruhe, 1882, xxxvi, 123–126.—**Wahrendorffius** (J. P.) Fœtus bicorporeus. Acta Acad. nat. curios., Norimb., 1737, iv, 574–576, 1 pl —**Walsh** (R. J.) Short notes of a midwifery case, with fœtal monster. Dublin M. Press, 1863, l, 207.—**Walter** (J. G.) De monstro bicorpori, duobus capitibus, quatuor brachiis, tribus pedibus, pectore, pelvique concreto. *In his :* Observat. anat., fol., Berl., 1775, 1–32, 6 pl.—**Wands** (J. A.) A case of Siamese twins. Brit. M. J., Lond., 1887, i, 1273.—**Warrington.** Skeleton of double-bodied monster. Tr. Coll. Phys. Phila., 1850–53, n. s., i, 90–94.—**Watson** (W.) Double monster ; post-mortem examination. Med. Times & Gaz., Lond., 1872, ii, 90 ; 100.—**Webb** (H. G.) A monster. Lancet, Lond., 1879, i, 143. — **Weddeburn** (A. J.) Description of a double monster. N. Orl. M. & S. J., 1845–6, ii, 161–168, 1 pl.— **Werner** (O.) Eine Doppelmissgeburt. Berl. klin. Wchnschr., 1876, xiii, 467.—**de Wersier.** Accouchement naturel de jumeaux unis latéralement. Ann. Soc. de méd. d'Anvers, 1844, i, 452–454, 1 pl. [Rap. de Matthyssens], 454–456.—**West** (J. W.) Bicephalous child, born at the full period of gestation. Lond. M. Gaz., 1845, n. s., i, 140.—**West** (R. U.) Account of a case in which two fœtuses were united at the sternum, with only one liver and one common heart. Edinb. M. & S. J., 1847, lxviii, 385–394, 1 pl. *Also,* Reprint.—**Wettengel** (E.) Interesting case of monstrosity. Am. J. Obst., N. Y., 1871–2, iv, 451–454, 1 pl. [Report of A. Koehler], 545.—**Wetzel.** Ein seltener Fall von Doppelmissgeburt. München. med. Wchnschr., 1887, xxxiv, 80.—**Weyher.** Ein Fall von Zwillingsmissgeburt (Dicephalus nach Barkow). Cor.- Bl. d. Ver. nassau. Aerzte, Weilburg, 1857, 36.—**Wheeler** (C. A.) A case of a remarkable monstrosity. Boston M. & S. J., 1859–60, lxi, 487. *Also :* N. Orl. M. & S. J., 1860, xvii, 290.—**White** (M. E.) [An account of a double-headed fœtus.] Dublin M. Press, 1839, i, 212.—**Wilcke.** Geburt monströser Zwillinge. Prov. San.-Ber. d. k. Med.-Coll. v. Pommern 1837, Stettin, 1838, 142.—**Wilder** (B. G.) Lateral asymmetry in the brains of a double human monster. Proc. Am. Ass. Adv. Sc. 1873, Salem, 1874, xxii, pt. 2, 250, 1 pl. ——. The papillary representative of two arms of a double human monster, with a note on a mummied double monster from Peru. *Ibid.,* 251–256.—**Wilkins** (R.) Description of a lusus naturæ. Madras Q. J. M. Sc., 1861, ii, 347, 1 pl.—**Willige** (F.) Wahrnehmung einer zweiköpfigen Miss-

Monsters (*Double*).

geburt und Verwachsung der Placenta. Ztschr. f. Chir. v. Chir., Osterode u. Goslar, 1845, ii, 307–313.—**Willis** (R. W.) Account of the birth of a double monster, with description. Atlanta M. & S. J., 1874–5, xii, 154, 1 pl.—**Wills** (W.) Double monstrosity, with account of the delivery. Tr. Obst. Soc. Lond. (1865), 1866, vii, 6–8.—**Winslow.** Remarques sur les monstres, à l'occasion d'une fille de douze ans, au corps de laquelle étoit attachée la moitié inférieure d'un autre corps ; et à l'occasion d'un faon à deux têtes, disséqué par ordre du roi ; avec des observations sur les marques de naissance. [*From :* Mém. Acad. roy. d. sc. de Par., 1733.] Collect. acad. d. mém., etc. Partie franç., Par. et Liége, 1784, vii, 164–204, 8 pl.—**Witt** (O. M.) Dubbelt missfoster. Hygiea, Stockholm, 1856, xviii, 338–342.—**Wolf.** Anatomische Beschreibung einer zweiköpfigen Missgeburt. Med. Jahrb. f. d. Herzogth. Nassau, Wiesb., 1859, 5.–6. Hft., 714–725.—**Wooden** (J. L.) Pair of twins à la Siamese. Cincin. Lancet & Obs., 1860, n. s., iii, 669.—**Woodworth** (B. S.) & **Ruhl** (W. D.) A two-headed monster. Obst. Gaz., Cincin., 1882, v, 343–345.—**Wyman** (J.) Description of a double fœtus. Boston M. & S. J., 1866, lxxiv, 169–176. *Also :* Extr. Rec. Bost. Soc. M. Improve. (1862–6), 1867, v (app.), 261–270.—**Yarrow** (E. G.) Double monster. Obst. J. Gr. Brit., Lond., 1880, viii, 220.—**Yeisuke Tuzai.** [A case of twins united throughout thorax and abdomen.] Iji Shinshi, Tokei, 1883, no. 293, Nov. 10.—**Zwicke** (F.) Ein Monstrum. Med.-chir. Centralbl., Wien, 1876, xi, 568.

Monsters (*Quadruple*).

Rodriguez (J. M.) Descripcion de un monstruo humano cuádruple, nacido en Durango el año de 1868. Gac. méd. de México, 1870, v, 17 ; 33, 3 pl. *Also,* Reprint.

Monsters (*Shapeless*). [*Anidian, etc.*]

See, also, **Monsters** (*Acardiac*).

Glasor (J.) * Ein Amorphus globosus. 4°. *Giessen,* 1852.

Grambs (J. J.) Anatomische Beschreibung eines monströsen Gewächses, welches in dem Leibe einer Frauen, von drey und fünfftsig Jahr, an ein gewisses Stück des Mesenterie angewachsen, und achtzehen Pfund schwer ausgewachsen gefunden worden. 4°. *Franckfurt a. M.,* 1730.

Blanchard (R.) Ein Fall vom abortiven Bluthofe (Panum) beim Menschen. Mitth. a. d. embryol. Inst. d. k. k. Univ. in Wien, 1877–80, i, 193–197, 1 pl.—**Boulton** (T.) Account of a monstrous fœtus without head, chest, and arms. Lancet, Lond., 1838–9, i, 611–613.—**Calori** (L.) Di un anideo umano trilobato. Rendic. Accad. d. sc. d. Ist. di Bologna, 1868–9, 86–90.—**Cornil** & **Causit.** Un cas de monstre anidien chez l'homme. Compt. rend. Soc. de biol. 1865, Par., 1866, 4. s., ii, 222–225.—**Gamgee** (J.) Anidian monsters. Veterinarian, Lond., 1855, xxviii, 320–327, 1 pl. *Also,* Reprint.—**Hannäus** (G.) De abortu bulliformi. Misc. Acad. nat. curios. 1685, Norimb., 1705, 2. decuria, iv, 221–223. *Also, transl. :* Auserl. med.- chir.- . . . Abhandl. d. röm.-kais. Akad. d. Naturf., Nürnb., 1765, xiv, 190.—**Hartmann** (P. J.) De duobus abortibus humanis oviformibus. Misc. Acad. nat. curios. 1701–5, Norimb., 1706, 3. decuria, ix–x, 350–359.—**Kleinwächter** (L.) Ueber die zweite Frucht einer Zwillingsgeburt, ein Amorphus. Vrtljschr. f. d. prakt. Heilk., Prag, 1872, cxiv, 104–111. — **Lanzoni** (J.) Partus mirabilis Scandiani editus 26 Maji a. 1690. Misc. Acad. nat. curios. 1690, Norimb., 1691, 2. decuria, ix, 73–76. *Also, transl. :* Auserl. med.- chir.- . . . Abhandl. d. röm.-kais. Akad. d. Naturf., Nürnb., 1770, xix, 66–69.—**Martou.** [Monstre dont la conformation bizarre avait quelque analogie avec celle d'un ours.] Bull. Soc. de méd. de Gand, 1839, v, 128–131.—**Morisani** (D.) [Anatomia patologica di un mostro amorfo.] Ann. clin. d. osp. incur., Napoli, 1879, iv, 293–321, 1 pl.—**Noeggerath.** Monstrosity, probably composed of the human heart. N. York M. J., 1882, xxxv, 522.—**Novi** (R.) Un caso di teratologia. Ann. clin. d. osp. incur., Napoli, 1880, v; 117.

Monsters (*Triple*).

Blasius (G.) Observationes medicæ rariores. Accedit monstri triplicis historia. 16°. *Amstelodami,* 1677.

Martin de Pedro (E.) Estudios de teratología con motivo de un extraordinario caso de monstruo triple. 8°. *Madrid,* 1879.

Geoffroy-Saint-Hilaire. Note sur le triencéphale. Arch. gén. de méd., Par., 1823, ii, 101–104.—**Philipeaux** (J.-M.) Monstre humain triple par inclusion. Compt. rend. Soc. de biol. 1873, Par., 1875, 5. s., v, pt. 2, 87–90. *Also :* Gaz. méd. de Par., 1873, 4. s., ii, 546.

Monsters (*Vegetable*).

Crausius (R. W.) [Pr.] de naturæ in regno vegetabili lusibus. sm. 4°. *Jenæ,* [1706].

Monsters (*Vegetable*).

KIRSCHLEGER (F.) * Essai historique sur la tératologie végétale. 4°. *Strasbourg,* 1845.

MOQUIN-TANDON (A.) Éléments de tératologie végétale, ou histoire abrégée des anomalies de l'organisation dans les végétaux. 8°. *Paris,* 1841.

RATZEBURG (J. T. C.) * Animadversiones quædam ad peloriarum indolem definiendam spectantes. 4°. *Berolini,* [1825].

Godron (D.-A.) Des races végétales qui doivent leur origine à une monstruosité. Mém. Acad. de Stanislas 1873, Nancy, 1874, 4. s., vi, 77–95. ———. Nouveaux mélanges de tératologie végétale. Mém. Soc. d. sc. nat. de Cherbourg, 1874, xviii, 318–352.—**Heckel** (É.) Introduction à l'étude de la tératologie végétale; tératologie et tératogénie générales. Rev. scient., Par., 1880, 2. s., xviii, 820–828.—**Kickx** (J.-J.) Notice sur les ascidies tératologiques. Bull. Acad. roy. d. sc. de Belg., Brux., 1863, 729–738, 1 pl. *Also,* Reprint.—**Strasburger** (E.) O wiel ozarodkowości. [Monstrosities in plants.] Rozpr. . . . wydz. matemat.-przyr. Akad. Umiej. w Krakow., 1878, v, 9–32, 4 tab.

Monsters *in animals, birds, fish, etc.*

See, also, **Monsters** (*Artificial production of*); **Penis** (*Abnormities, etc., of*).

ALESSANDRINI (A.) Descrizione di un vitello mostruoso mancante di porzione del midollo spinale. 8°. *Bologna,* 1829.

———. Descrizione di un vitello mostruoso. 8°: *Bologna,* 1830.

BLUMENTHAL (M. E.) * De monstroso vituli sceleto. 8°. *Regimonti,* [*n. d.*]

CANESTRINI (G.) Intorno a due uccelli mostruosi. 8°. *Modena,* 1870.

Repr. from: Ann. d. Soc. d. nat., Modena, ann. v.

CAVANNA (G.) Ancora sulla polimelia nei batraci anuri. Sopra alcuni visceri del gallo cedrone (Tetrao urogallus Linn.). roy. 8°. *Firenze,* 1879.

DARESTE (C.) Recherches sur les conditions de la vie et de la mort chez les monstres ectroméliens, célosomiens et exencéphaliens, produits artificiellement dans l'espèce de la poule. 8°. *Lille,* 1863.

VAN DEEN (I.) Anatomische Beschreibung eines monströsen, sechsfüssigen Wasser-Frosches (Rana esculenta). 4°. *Leiden,* 1838.

DELPLANIQUE (P.) Études tératologiques. 1. Des difformités congénitales produites sur le fœtus par la contraction musculaire. Les veaux à tête de chien, ou niatas. 4°. *Paris,* 1885.

GURLT (E. F.) Ueber thierische Missgeburten. Ein Beitrag zur pathologischen Anatomie und Entwickelungs-Geschichte. 4°. *Berlin,* 1877.

HAMBERGER (G. E.) [Pr.] de cyprino monstroso rostrato. i et iii. sm. 4°. *Jenæ,* [1748].

HERZBERG (J.) * Monstri vitulini descriptio anatomica. 4°. *Berolini,* [1825].

VON JAEGER (G. F.) Beobachtung eines Stierkalbs mit einem Nebenkopfe. 8°. [*Amsterdam,* 1858.]

Transl. from: Versl. . . . d. k. Akad. v. Wetensch. Afd. Natuurk., Amst., 1858, vii.

JOLY (N.) Études anatomiques sur un agneau bimale du genre synotus. 8°. *Toulouse,* 1843.

Repr. from: J. de méd. et chir. de Toulouse, 1843.

———. Mémoire sur un agneau monstrueux constituant un nouveau genre (Déromèle) dans la famille des monstres doubles polyméliens. 8°. *Toulouse,* [1868].

Repr. from: Mém. de l'Acad. imp. d. sc. de Toulouse, 1868, 6. s., vi.

———. Sur deux cas très-rares de mélomélie observés chez le mouton. 8°. *Toulouse,* [1869].

Repr. from: Mém. Acad. imp. d. sc., inscrip. et belles-lettres de Toulouse, 1869, 7. s., i.

KERSTEN (H.) * Capitis trichechi rosmari descriptio osteologica. 8°. *Berolini,* [1821].

Monsters *in animals, birds, fish, etc.*

KOCH (H.) * Ueber die künstliche Herstellung von Zwergbildungen im Hühnerei. 4°. *Stuttgart,* 1884.

LARCHER (O.-E.-F.) Mélanges de pathologie comparée et de tératologie. 8°. *Paris,* 1878.

LE BLOND (C.) Recherches d'anatomie et de physiologie sur un embryon monstrueux de la poule domestique circonscrit dans l'existence solitaire d'un cœur. 8°. *Paris,* 1834.

MENSINGA (W. P. J.) * Monstri gallinacei bicorporei bicephali descriptio anatomica, una cum disquisitione de ejus ortu. 4°. *Kiliæ,* 1861.

MULLER (H. F.) * Descriptio anatomica pulli gallinacei extremitatibus superfluis præditi, simul cum disquisitione physiologica de ortu monstrorum duplicium parasiticorum. 4°. *Kiliæ,* 1859.

PANCK (J. E.) * De bicipiti monstro agnino. 12°. *Dorpati Livonorum,* 1831.

PAPI (C.) Una osservazione di mostruosità del rachide e del torace in un asinello. 8°. *Parma,* 1885.

PLANCUS (J.) De monstris ac monstrosis quibusdam, ad Josephum Puteum . . . epistola. fol. *Venetiis,* 1749.

SCHMIDT (A.) * Ovis bicorporis descriptio, adjunctis notationibus de monstrorum duplicium ortu in genere. 8°. [*Dorpat*], 1858.

THEMEL (J. C.) Commentatio medica qua nutritionem fœtus in utero per vasa umbilicalia solum fieri occasione monstri ovilli sine ore et faucibus nato ostenditur. 4°. *Lipsiæ,* 1751.

Also, in: FASC. diss. anat.-med. 8°. *Amstelædami,* 1764, 121–173, 1 pl.

VOGELGESANG (J. A.) * De perocephalo aprosopo fœtus ovini. 8°. *Regiomonti Pr.,* [1837].

VORBILDUNG deren Missgeburten dieses 1620. Jahrs, welcher hie bevor gedacht worden. 4°. [*n. p.,* 1620.]

WIESE (J. E. P.) * De monstris animalium. 4°. *Berolini,* 1812.

Agneau (Sur un) fœtus monstrueux. [*From:* Hist. Acad. roy. d. sc. de Par., 1703.] Rec. de mém., Dijon et Auxerre, 1754, ii, 15–17.—**Amat** (C.) Œuf de poule complet inclus dans un autre. Compt. rend. Soc. de biol., Par., 1885, 8. s., ii, 256. — **Atkinson** (J. C.) Feline monstrosity. Lond. M. Gaz., 1833, xii, 294.—**Auber.** Description d'un monstre. [Two-headed calf.] J. de méd., chir., pharm., etc., Par., 1761, xv, 45–52. — **Aucante.** Lettre sur une production monstrueuse. *Ibid.,* 1770, xxxii, 13–16.—**B.** Monstrosity in a calf. Boston M. & S. J., 1862, lxvi, 26.— **Baer.** Ueber einen Doppel-Embryo vom Huhne, aus dem Anfange des dritten Tages der Brütung. Arch. f. Anat. u. Physiol., Leipz., 1827, 576–586. — **Barkow.** Ueber eine lebende (3 Tage alte) Missgeburt vom Kalbe mit doppeltem Gesichte, einfachem Hinterkopfe und Leibe, welche er kurz als Diprosopus tetrophthalmus oculis intermediis septo membranaceo separatis definirte. Ausz. a. d. Uebers. d. Arb. u. Veränd. d. schles. Gesellsch. f. vaterl. Kult. Jahresb. d. med. Sect., Bresl., 1841, 10; 17.— **Barrier.** Tératologie vétérinaire; monstre de la famille des otocéphaliens (crotaphocéphale). Compt. rend. Soc. de biol. 1876, Par., 1877, 6. s., iii, 271–279. ———. Sur les veaux cynocéphales. *Ibid.,* 1885, 8. s., ii, 213–215.—**Bartholinus** (T.) Monstrum agninum duplex. Acta med. et phil. Hafn. (1674–5), 1677, iii, 53, 1 pl. — **Beach.** A remarkable monstrosity. Boston M. & S. J., 1875, xcii, 595. *Also:* Extr. Rec. Bost. Soc. M. Improve. (1874–9), 1880, vii, 20–22. — **Bert.** Note sur deux poulets déradelphes. Compt. rend. Soc. de biol. 1863, Par., 1864, 3. s., v, 23–26. — **Bochefontaine.** Monstruosité unithoracique chez une chienne; atrophie de l'omoplate et de la moelle cervicale du côté correspondant. Arch. de physiol. norm. et path., Par., 1881, 2. s., viii, 286–297. — **Boeck** (C. B.) Et Kalvemisfoster paa Røraas. Eyr, Christiania, 1836–7, xi, 151–154. — **Bourgeois.** Observation sur un agneau monstrueux. J. de méd., chir., pharm., etc., Par., 1764, xx, 264–266. — **Brand.** Dicephalus bispinalis von einer Kuh. Wchnschr. f. Thierh. u. Viehzucht, Augsburg, 1883, xxvii, 329. — **Bricon** (P.) Poulet pygomèle (quatre membres postérieurs, deux anus, etc.). Bull. Soc. anat. de Par., 1884, lix, 483. *Also:* Progrès méd., Par., 1885, 2. s., i, 148. — **Bruch** (C.) Ueber Dreifachbildungen. Jenaische Ztschr. f. Med. u. Naturw., Leipz., 1871–3, vii, 142–175, 1 pl. — **Bugnion** (É.) Description de quelques alevins de truite monstrueux. Bull. Soc.

Monsters *in animals, birds, fish, etc.*

vaudoise d. sc. nat., Lausanne, 1879, 2. s., xvi, 463–466.—
Caldani (F.) Memoria sopra un agnello mostruoso,
con alcune osservazioni sopra la midolla spinale. Ann.
univ. di med., Milano, 1824. xxix, 92–94.—**Calori** (L.) Di
un mostro eteropago suino anatomia. Mem. Accad. d. sc.
d. Ist. di Bologna, 1876, 3. s., vii, 395–411, 2 pl. — **Carlet**
(G.) Sur une truite mopse. J. de l'anat. et physiol., etc.,
Par., 1879, xv, 154–160. — **Cathcart** (C. W.) Dissection
of a lamb with fissure of the sternum and transposition
of the origin of the right subclavian artery. J. Anat. &
Physiol., Lond., 1873–4, viii, 321–326. — **Cattie** (J. T.)
Notice sur deux monstrûosités observées chez le gallus
domesticus, L. Bull. Acad. roy. d. sc. de Belg., Brux.,
1883, 3. s., v, 119–126, 1 pl.—**Chabry** (L.) Monstres nouveaux chez les ascidies. Compt. rend. Soc. de biol., Par.,
1885, 8. s., ii, 42–44. ———. Contribution à l'embryologie
normale et tératologique des ascidies simples. J. de l'anat.
et physiol., etc., Par., 1887, xxiii, 167–319, 5 pl.— **Cist** (J.)
Account of a singular lusus naturæ in the fœtus of a sheep.
Phila. J. M. & Phys. Sc., 1824, viii, 470, 1 pl. — **Colin.**
[Un veau monstrueux.] Bull. Soc. anat. de Par., 1848, xxiii,
136.—**Contamine** (J. M.) Cas remarquable de dystocie
fœtale, déterminé par un monstre autosite, célosomien,
schistosome réfléchi, agénosome, aproctéisen. [In a cow.]
Ann. de méd. vét., Brux., 1886, xxxv, 477–486.—**Dareste.**
Déviation chez un agneau, résultant d'une compression
exercée par l'amnios. Bull. Soc. d'anthrop. de Par., 1881, 3.
s., iv, 816. ———. Sur la viabilité des embryons monstrueux
de l'espèce de la poule. Compt. rend. Acad. d. sc., Par.,
1883, xcvi, 1672–1674. ———. Mémoire sur un cas de cébocéphalie observé chez un poulain. J. de l'anat. et physiol.,
etc., Par., 1885, xxi, 346–355, 2 pl. — **Dareste** (C.) Mémoire sur la production artificielle des monstruosités de
l'espèce de la poule. Compt. rend. Soc. de biol. 1861, Par.,
1862, 3. s., iii, pt. 2, 157–187.— **Davaine.** Duplicité de la
face chez les oiseaux. Gaz. méd. de Par., 1850, 3. s., v,
875.—**Dobrosmisloff** (A.) Urodliv. ploda korovi; schis-
tosoma reflexu.n. [Birth of a monster in a cow.] Uchen.
zapiski Kazan. Vet. Inst , 1886, iii, 140–142.—**Dugès** (A.)
Description d'un cas de monstruosité. Rev. méd. franç.
et étrang., Par., 1835, i, 197–204.—**Duplay.** Note sur
un coq monstrueux polymélien, genre ischiomèle. Bull.
Soc. anat. de Par., 1865, xl, 355 – 359. — **Duval** (M.) &
Hervé (G.) Sur un monstre otocéphalien. Compt.
rend. Soc. de biol., Par., 1883, 7. s., iv, 76 – 78. — **Ercolani** (G. B.) Osservazioni teratologiche sopra un pseu-
dacormo bovino pseudacormus aprosopus Erc. Mem.
Accad. d. sc. d. Ist. di Bologna, 1876, 3. s., vii, 63–100, 2
pl.—**Fahnestock** (S.) An account of a singular malfor-
ma tion of the heart, liver, and spleen in a hog. Am. M.
Recorder, Phila., 1823, vi, 282–284.—**Feldmann.** Schis-
tosoma reflexum. Arch. vet. nauk, St Petersb., 1884, iii,
pt. 3, 119.—**Fingerhuth.** Beschreibung eines seltenen
missgebildeten Kalbsfötus mit mangelnden Bauchdecken,
Becken und hintern Extremitäten. Arch. f. Anat. u. Physiol., Leipz., 1826, i, 109–111, 1 pl.—**Fougeroux.** [Un
monstre formé de deux lapins réunis depuis la tête
jusqu'au bas du sternum] [*From*: Mém. Acad. roy. sc.,
1759.] Collect. acad. d. mém., etc. Partie franç., Par. et
Liége, 1769, xii, 381.—**Gadeau de Kerville** (H.) Note
sur un canard monstrueux appartenant au genre pygomèle. J. de l'anat. et physiol., etc., Par., 1884, xx, 462–464,
1 pl. ———. Description de quatre monstres doubles (2
chats et 2 poussins), appartenant aux genres synote, iniodyme, opodyme et ischiomèle. *Ibid.*, 1885, xxi, 304–308, 1
pl.—**Galindo** (J.) Vicio de conformacion en un borrego.
Observador méd., México, 1872–4, ii, 14.—**Galvez** (D. F.)
Anomalia notada en un chivo. An. r. Acad. de cien. méd.
. . . de la Habana, 1865–6, ii, 190–196.—**Gay** (M.) Sopra
un mostro ovino (Ciclope perostomo arnico). Medico vet.,
Torino, 1878, 5. s., i, 193–195, 1 pl.—**Geoffroy.** Observation sur l'excès et le défaut du nombre des parties d'un
poulet et de deux chiens. J. de méd., chir. et pharm.,
etc., 2. éd., Par., 1755, iii, 266–273.—**Gluge & Deron-
baix.** Observation d'un chien cyclope. Arch. de la méd.
belge, Brux., 1840, iii, 115–117.—[**Goadby** (H.)] A lusus
naturæ. Med. Indep., Detroit, 1856, i, 102–104.—**Goddard** (Q. J.) Beschrijving eener kalfs-misgeboorte, met
epicrisis. Nederl. Tijdschr. v. Geneesk., Amst., 1860, iv,
469.—**Goubaux** (A.) Description d'un monstre du genre
célosome, de l'espèce bovine. Compt. rend. Soc. de biol.
1868, Par., 1869, 4. s., v, 161–164 ———. Mémoire sur un
monstre de l'espèce bovine, classe des parasitaires, famille
des polyméliens, genre notomèle (I. Geoffroy-Saint-Hilaire).
Ibid., pt. 2, 45 – 61. ———. Mémoire sur les fissures mé-
dianes, ou les ectrogénies symétriques chez les animaux
domestiques. *Ibid.*, 1872, Par., 1874, 5. s., iv, pt. 2, 121–144.
———. Tératologie vétérinaire; genre agnathe; des monstres doubles polygnathes. Arch. de tocol., Par., 1877,
iv, 193–207. ———. Mémoire sur un veau monstrueux du
genre dérodyme. *Ibid.*, 1878, v, 641–650. ———. Tératologie vétérinaire; mémoire sur l'ectromélie quadruple.
Ibid., 1879, vi, 129–146. ———. Tératologie vétérinaire;
classe des monstres doubles autositaires, famille des monosomiens; mémoire sur un monstre du genre atlodyme.
Ibid., 1882, ix, 214; 278 —**Guichard** (A.) Deux monstruosités semblables chez un fœtus humain et chez un

Monsters *in animals, birds, fish, etc.*

poulet. Bull. Soc. de méd. d'Angers (1879), 1880, n. s., vii,
104–106, 2 pl.—**Guillebeau** (A.) Un cas d'épignathie
chez le veau. Arch. de physiol. norm. et path., Par., 1881,
2. s., viii, 205–223, 1 pl.—**Hable** (F.) Missgeburt beim
Rind mit grossen Cysten um den Kopf. Oesterr. Vrtljschr. f. wissensch. Veterinärk., Wien, 1884, lxi, 217–221.—
Hammericus (F.) Monstra varia animalium. Acta
med. et phil. Hafn. (1671-2), 1673, i, 53, 1 pl.—**Heckel** (É.)
Note sur un cas de monstruosité observé dans les pattes du
poulet. J. de l'anat. et physiol., etc., Par., 1887, xxiii, 320–
323 —**Hoffmann** (M.) De agno monstroso. Misc.
Acad. nat. curios. 1678–9, Norimb., 1693, ix-x, 32–37, 1 pl.
Also, transl.: Collect. acad. d. mém., etc., Dijon, 1755, iii,
363–366, 1 pl. *Also, transl.:* Auserl. med.- chir.- . . . Abhandl. d. röm.-kais. Akad. d. Naturf., Nürnb., 1761, ix, 22–
26, 1 pl.—**Jaeger** (G.) Missbildung des Kopfes eines
Kalbes und eines Lammes mit rüsselartigem Fortsatze an
der Stirn und Annäherung dazu bei einem neugeborenen
Rinde, als Nachtrag zu den (Jahrg. 1829, iii. Hft., p. 202
des Arch.) beschriebenen missgebildeten Schädeln eines
Lammes und einer Ziege. Arch. f. Anat. u. Physiol.,
Leipz., 1830, 105–119.—**Joly** (N.) Description anatomique
d'un agneau du genre dérodymé, suivie de réflexions sur
les phénomènes physiologiques que ce monstre eut présentés s'il eut vécu. J. de méd. et chir. de Toulouse, 1844-
5, viii, 222 – 232. — **Krushinski** (L.) Sluchai rojdenija
korovoju tudovishnago uroda. [Birth of a monster calf.]
Arch. vet. nauk, St. Petersb., 1885, xv, pt. 3, 49–55.—**Larcher** (O.) Note pour servir à l'histoire de la pygomélie
chez les oiseaux. J. de l'anat. et physiol., etc., Par., 1872,
viii, 408 – 416. — **Lavocat.** Considérations sur un veau
anide. [Abstr.] Compt. rend. Acad. d. sc., Par., 1866,
lxiii, 972–974.—**Leblond** (C.) Embryon monstrueux de
la poule ordinaire. [Rap. de Pascal.] Exposé d. trav. de
la Soc. d. sc. méd. de la Moselle 1831-8, Metz, 1840, 68–72.—
Lereboullet. Formation des monstres doubles chez les
poissons. Gaz. méd. de Par., 1855, 3. s., x, 315.—**Loiset.**
Note concernant un veau atteint d'ectrodactylie. Bull.
méd. du nord, Lille, 1846-8, i, 106–108. ———. Veau gastro-
mèle. *Ibid.*, 181.—**Longo** (T.) Due casi di nanosomo ca-
niforme. Medico vet., Torino, 1882, xxix, 49–51.—**Lvoff**
(K.) K kazust. vrojden. urodstve. [Congenital monstrosity.] Uchen. zapiski Kazan. Vet. Inst., 1885, ii, 219–221.—
Macalister (A.) Notes on an instance of cranial deformity in a domestic cat, with remarks on its probable
origin. Med. Press & Circ., Dubl., 1867, n. s., iv, 290–292.—
McIntosh (W. C.) Notes on the structure of a monstrous kitten. J. Anat. & Physiol., Lond., 1868, 366–373.—
Magendie (F.) Anatomie d'un chien cyclope et astome.
Rev. méd. hist. et phil., Par., 1821, vi, 323–328.—**Maggi**
(L.) Mostruosità d' un gambero d' acqua dolce (Astacus
fluviatilis). R. Ist. Lomb. di sc. e lett. Rendic., Milano,
1881, 2. s., xiv, 333–342.—**Magniaux.** Canard à trois
pattes. Bull. Soc. anat. de Par., 1868, xliii, 399. — **Martin** (J.-G.) Sur l'existence d'un cloaque observé chez un
chien sans prolongement caudal. *Ibid* , 1827, 2. éd., 1844,
ii, 49 – 54.— **Martinet** (L.) Sur les poulets pentadac-
tyles. Bull. Soc. d'anthrop. de Par., 1878, 3. s., i, 147–
149.—**Martini** (E.) Considérations sur les monstruosités animales. Arch. gén. de méd., Par., 1824, iv, 568–579.—
von Martius (H.) Beschreibung eines äusserst merkwürdigen Huhns mit menschenähnlichem Profil. J. d.
Chir. u. Augenh., Berl., 1829, xii, 305–316.—**Merindol.**
Sur un chevreau monstrueux. [*From:* J. d. sçavans, 1683.]
Collect. acad. d. mém., etc., Dijon, 1755, i, 297, 1 pl.—
Meyer (O.) Ein Fall von Verdopplung der Allantois
und der äusseren Genitalien. Schrift. d. naturf. Gesellsch.
in Danzig, 1882, n. F., v, 15–17.—**Michels** (J.) A fowl
monstrosity. [*From:* Scientific American.] Am. M. Bi-
Weekly, Louisville, 1878, viii, 160. — **Missbildungen.**
Deutsche Ztschr. f. Thiermed., Leipz., 1878, [1. Supplhft.],
41–43.—**Moncil** (G. C.) Case of a deformed calf. N.
York J. M., 1846, vii, 43–48.—**Monströsen** (Von einem)
doppeltgeschwänzten Hühner-Ey. Samml. v. Nat.- u.
Med.- . . . Gesch. 1719, Bressl., 1720, viii, 587–589.—**Morot** (C.) Anomalie congénitale du membre postérieur
gauche d'un jeune veau; absence des deux onglous, des
deux phalanges ungéales et des deux petits sésamoïdes;
développement incomplet des deux phalangines. Bull. et
mém. Soc. centr. de méd. vét., Par., 1886, n. s., iv, 681–
683. — **Oggioni** (P.) Mostro peccorino per difetto dal
quale si rileva chiaramente che il feto nell' utero materno
non si nutre che per la via ombellicale. Verhandl. d.
schweiz. naturf. Gesellsch. 1844, Chur, 1845, xxix, 126–
133.—**Ostapenko** (A. P.) Teratologicheskie materiali.
Arch. vet. nauk, St. Petersb., 1882, i, pt. 2, 1–14.—**P.** (P.)
Two calves brought forth of different cows, but of the
same bull, without any fore legs, but otherwise well
formed and healthy. Belmont M. J., Bridgeport, Ohio,
1859, 64.—**Paterson** (A. M.) On some monstrosities in
a Dorking fowl. J. Anat. & Physiol., Lond., 1886-7, xxi,
180–184, 1 pl. — **Paulicki.** Thoracopagus beim Kalb.
Deutsche Ztschr. f. Thiermed., Leipz., 1883, ix, 253–257.—
Pavesi (P.) Toradelfia di uno scorpione. R. Ist. Lomb.
di sc. e lett. Rendic., Milano, 1881, 2. s., xiv, 329–332.—
Piana (G. P.) Osservazioni anatomo-istologiche intorno
a cinque mostri bovini del gen. amorphus di Gurlt, con

Monsters *in animals, birds, fish, etc.*

alcune considerazioni sulla loro teratogenia. Mem. Accad. d. sc. d. Ist. di Bologna, 1882, 4. s., iv, 795-819, 2 pl.— **Pigné.** D'un chevreau cyclocéphale. Bull. Soc. anat. de Par., 1841, xvi, 138.—**Pouchet.** Note sur quelques cas tératologiques chez le poulet. Compt. rend. Soc. de biol. 1877, Par., 1879, 6. s., iv, 211-213. — **Pouchet** (G.) Sur des cyprins monstrueux (C. auratus) venant de Chine. J. de l'anat. et physiol., etc., Par., 1870-71, vii, 561-569, 1 pl. *Also,* Reprint.— **Pouchet** (G.) & **Beauregard.** Veau monstrueux iniodyme. Compt. rend. Soc. de biol., Par., 1882, 7. s., iv, 521-523.—**Quatrefages.** Formation des monstres doubles chez les poissons. Gaz. méd. de Par., 1855, 3. s., x, 183. ——. De la monstruosité double chez les poissons. *Ibid.*, 300-302. ——. Mémoire sur un pigeon monstrueux du genre déradelphe, Déradelphe synanencéphale. Assoc. franç. pour l'avance. d. sc. Coumpt.-rend. 1877, Par., 1878, vi, 627-640.—**Rauber** (A.) Ueber Doppelbildung bei Wirbelthieren. Arch. f. path. Anat., etc., Berl., 1878, lxxii, 443. ——. Gastrodidymus des Lachses. *Ibid.*, 1879, lxxv, 553. ——. Gibt es Stockbildungen (Cormi) bei den Vertebraten? Morphol. Jahrb., Leipz., 1879, v, 167-190, 2 pl. — **Rayer.** Sur plusieurs monstres de lièvre et de perdreau. Compt. rend. Soc. de biol. 1862, Par., 1863, 3. s., iv, 111.—**Reutzius** (S. A.) De monstro agnino Norwegico. Acta med. et phil. Hafn. (1674-5), 1677, iii, 99.—**Rieck** (M.) Perocephalus aotus (Gurlt) vom Schwein. Rev. f. Thierh., Wien, 1887, x, 1-3.—**Roloff** (F.) Missgeburten. Arch. f. wissensch. u. prakt. Thierh., Berl., 1876, ii, 401-404.—**Rose** (D. D.) A monstrosity. Weekly M. Rev., Chicago, 1884, x, 401.— **Samelsohn.** Fall von Diprosopus triophthalmus bei einem neugeborenen Kätzchen. Sitzungsb. d. nied.-rhein. Gesellsch. f. Nat.- u. Heilk. zu Bonn, 1880, 206.—**Schaaffhausen.** Ueber die thierischen Missbildungen. *Ibid.*, 1870, 18-20.—**Schläpfer.** Skizze eines natürlichen Systems der angebornen Monstrositäten der Thiere. Ann. d. allg. schweiz. Gesellsch. f. d. ges. Naturw., Bern, 1824-5, ii, 1-32.— **Schmidt-Rimpler.** Eine ungewöhnliche Miss- und Hemmungsbildung an einem Kalbsauge. Amtl. Ber. ü. d. Versamml. deutsch. Naturf. u. Aerzte, München, 1877, l, 334.—**Schütz.** Zur Kenntniss der Dignathie. Arch. f. wissensch. u. prakt. Thierh., Berl., 1879, v, 1-21, 1 pl.—**Serres** (A.) Essai sur une théorie anatomique des monstruosités animales. Rev. méd. hist. et phil., Par., 1821, vi, 180-199.—**Storch** (C.) Beiträge zur Anatomie der thierischen Missgeburten. Oesterr. Vrtljschr. f. wissensch. Veterinärk., Wien, 1883, lix, 141-155. ——. Ein Fall von Cyclopie bei einem Kalbe. *Ibid.*, 1884, lxii, 112-115.—**Strahl** (C.) Eine Missbildung am Flusskrebs. Arch. f. Anat., Physiol. u. wissensch. Med., Leipz., 1859, 333-336.—**Studiati** (C.) Di un caso raro di mostruosità in un feto vitellino (Schistozomus reflexus). Gior. di anat., fisiol. e patol. d. animali, Pisa, 1874, vi, 81-92.—**Szymkiewicz.** Beitrag zur Lehre von den künstlichen Missbildungen am Hühnereie. Sitzungsb. d. k. Akad. d. Wissensch. Math.-naturw. Cl. 1875, Wien, 1876, lxxii, 139-147, 1 pl.—**Taruffi** (C.) Mostruosità delle uova d' uccelli. Gior. di anat., fisiol. e patol. d. animali, Pisa, 1886, xviii, 254; 326: 1887, xix, 16-44.—**Thiernesse.** Rapport sur un monstre double monomphalien de l'espèce porcine, compliqué de rhinocéphalie chez l'un des sujets composants; formation d'un nouveau genre appelé gastropage. Bull. Acad. roy. de méd. de Belg., Brux., 1850-51, x, 240-250, 2 pl.—**Tiedemann** (F.) Beschreibung einiger seltenen Thier-Monstra. Ztschr. f. Physiol., Heidelb., 1831, iv, 121-124, 1 pl.—**Van Bambeke** (C.) Description anatomique d'un amorphe globuleux (amorphus globosus, Gurlt) appartenant à l'espèce bovine, suivie de quelques considérations sur ce genre de monstruosité. Ann. Soc. de méd. de Gand, 1866, xliv, 75-110, 3 pl. [Rap. de Poelman], 111. ——. Note sur une inclusion rencontrée dans un œuf de poule. Livre jubil. publié p. la Soc. de méd. de Gand, etc., 1884, 395-410, 1 pl.— **Van Steenkiste** (C.) Description anatomico-tératologique d'un chevreau diplocéphale à corps simple (2me genre de la diplogénèse). Ann. Soc. méd.-chir. de Bruges, 1845, vi, 85-98, 1 pl.— **de Ville.** Histoire anatomique d'un chat monstrueux. [*From:* J. d. scavans, 1680.] Collect. acad. d. mém., etc., Dijon, 1755, i, 286, 1 pl.—**Vulpian.** Note sur un chat monstrueux (groupe des monstres doubles monosomiens, genre opodyme, I. Geoffroy-Saint-Hilaire). Gaz. méd. de Par., 1855, 3. s., x, 18.—**Walley.** On a congenital cranial tumour in a calf. Tr. Edinb. Obst. Soc. (1871-4), 1875, iii, 68-70. ——. Deformed fœtus of a cow (ectopia). *Ibid.*, 334.—**Ward** (T. O.) Absence of the left foot in a cat. Tr. Path. Soc. Lond., 1857-8, ix, 460.— **Weyenbergh** (H.) Remarques sur un monstre hydrocéphalique, extrait mort d'une vache. Bol. Acad. nac. de cien. exact., Córdoba, 1875-8, ii, pt. 1, 58-65.—**Wilckens** (M.) Bemerkungen über einen doppelten linken Vorderfuss vom Kalbe. Oesterr. Monatschr. f. Thierh., Wien, 1879, iv, 25-27.—**Wilson** (J.) A fœtal monstrosity. Vet. J. & Ann. Comp. Path., Lond., 1880, x, 156-158.—**Wyman** (J.) Cyclopism in a pig. Boston M. & S. J., 1858-9, lix, 121.—**Wyman** (J.) Double pig. *Ibid.*, 1861, lxiv, 535.— **Yates** (C. C) Account of a monster. Phila. M. Musuem, 1807-8, iv, 254-256.

Monsters *from defect or malformation of abdomen and thorax.*

See, also, **Bladder** (*Exstrophy of*); **Hermaphrodites**; **Hypospadias**; **Monsters** (*Acardiac*); **Monsters** *in animals, etc.;* *and under names of regions and viscera, e. g.,* **Abdomen, Genitals, Heart,** *Abnormities of.*

Barkow (H. C. L.) Ueber Pseudacormus, oder den scheinbar rumpflosen Kopf. fol. *Breslau,* 1854.

Bassini (E.) Vizio di conformazione dell' ano, dell' intestino retto e dell' apparato urogenitale (cloaco uro-genitale). *In his:* De clin. operat. 8°. *Genova,* 1878, 97-99.

Bellard (E.-M.-G.) * Contribution à l'étude des monstres célosomiens. 4°. *Lille,* 1882. *Also* [Abstr.], *in:* Ann. de gynéc., Par., 1882, xviii, 212-225.

Brandau (J. V.) * Ueber eine menschliche Missgeburt mit zwei abnormen Nabelvenen. 4°. *Marburg,* [1862].

Büttner (C. G.) Anatomische Anmerkung und Beweiss aus der Natur des Cörpers, dass ein Kind, mit dem aus der Brust gewachsenen und heraushängenden Hertzen und fehlenden Hertzbeutel, so wohl im Mutterleibe wachsen, zunehmen und vollkommen, als auch lebendig gebohren werden, und nach der Geburt noch einige Zeit leben könne. sm. 4°. *Königsberg,* 1747.

——. The same. Anatomische Anmerckungen bey einem mit auswärtshängendem Herzen lebendig gebornem Kinde, und dann bey Gelegenheit einer todt gebohrnen zwey - köpfigen Missgeburt, nebst Erörterung einiger curieusen Fragen. [2. Aufl.] 4°. *Königsberg u. Leipzig,* 1752.

Calori (L.) Di tre celosomi umani (Celosomiens Isid. Geoffroy-Saint-Hilaire) notabili per rispetto alla tocologia ed alla distribuzione teratologica di cotale famiglia di mostri. 4°. *Bologna,* 1863. *Repr. from:* Mem. Accad. d. sc. d. Ist. di Bologna, 2. s., ii. *See, also, infra.*

Coen (E.) Descrizione anatomica di un feto senza reni e senza utero, con altre anomalie. 8°. *Milano,* 1884.

Dehn (M.) * Descriptio anatomica monstri cum eventratione. 8°. *Berolini,* [1864].

Eisenach (H. P.) * Ein weiblicher Fötus ohne Harn-, Darm- und Geschlechtsöffnungen, daneben Meropus. 8°. *Rotenburg,* [1873].

Eschenbach (C. E.) Partus monstrosi. *In his:* Obs. quædam anat.-chir.-med. rariora. 4°. *Rostochii,* 1753-5, 8-14. *Also: Ibid.* Editio altera. 12°. *Rostochii,* 1769, 5-18.

Fleischmann (G.) * De vitiis congenitis circa thoracem et abdomen. 4°. *Erlangæ,* [1810].

Fried (G. A.) * Fœtus intestinis plane nudis extra abdomen propendentibus natus. sm. 4°. *Argentorati,* 1760. *Also, in:* Sandifort. Thesaurus diss. [etc.] 4°. *Roterodami,* 1768, i, 311-324.

Jensen (J.) * Descriptio monstri cum ligamentis amnioticis. 4°. *Kiliæ,* 1866. *In:* Schrift. d. Univ. zu Kiel, xiii, 1866, vii, Med. ii.

Koch (E. A.) * Diss. inaug. . . . exhibens monstri humani rarioris descriptionem. 12°. *Dorpati Livonorum,* 1836.

Krüger (G.) * Ueber eine Missbildung mit Perinealbruch und offener Blase. 8°. *Rostock,* [1872].

Leucke (A. G.) * De monstro quodam humano. 4°. *Halis Sax.,* 1854.

de Lucretis. Descrizione di un mostro notomizzato in San Severo, e pensieri sulla formazione de' medesimi. MS. 4°. [*San Severo,* 1807.]

Manniske (G. A.) * Diss. monstri humani rarioris descriptionem continens. 4°. *Jenæ,* [1831].

Monsters *from defect or malformation of abdomen and thorax.*

NICHOLSON (G.) * De monstro humano sine trunco nato. 4°. *Berolini*, 1837.

NIEMEYER (C. E.) * Singularis in fœtu puellari recens edito abnormitatis exemplum descriptum et illustratum. 4°. [*Halæ*, 1814.]

PACINI (L.) Di un fanciullo mostruoso per difetto di organizzazione; lettera chirurgico-anatomica diretta all' Tommaso Biancini. 8°. *Pisa*, 1834.

SACHS (W.) * Ueber einen Fall von Eventration. 8°. *Marburg*, 1877.

SCHAEFER (P.) * Descriptio anatomico-pathologica monstri cum eventratione. 4°. *Bonnæ*, [1837].

SCHEPLER (T.) Adspirante numine sapientissimo! monstrum humanum ventribus sine proportione et mutilis artubus, Wittebergæ d. xxx Augusti, natum, animo lustrandum sistit in publico. 4°. *Wittebergæ*, [1674].

ULRICH (G. L.) * Diss. inaug. med. deformationem fœtus humani rariorem describens. 4°. *Marburgi Cattorum*, 1833.

WEDEL (E. E. L.) * Dissertatio medica monstri humani rarioris descriptionem continens. 4°. *Jenæ*, 1830.

Adler (S.) Ein fötaler Bildungsfehler. Med.-chir. Centralb., Wien, 1876, xi, 195.—**Adradas** (C. L.) Un caso teratológico. An. de cien. méd., Madrid, 1876, ii, 385-390.—**Anatomische** Beschreibung einer überaus fehlerhaften Bildung der Brust- und Baucheingeweide eines neugebornen Kindes, welches 58 Stunden gelebt hat. J. d. pract. Heilk., Berl., 1805, xxii, 2. St., 110-121.—**d'Arcy** (H.) Inversion splanchnique. Monstruosité par inclusion? Abeille méd., Par., 1875, xxxii, 310.—**Arnold** (J.) Ein Fall von Cor triloculare biatriatum, Communication der Lungenvenen mit der Pfortader und Mangel der Milz. Arch. f. path. Anat., etc., Berl., 1868, xlii, 449-472, 1 pl.—**Atthill.** Exhibition of a monster born in the Rotunda Lying in Hospital. Dublin J. M. Sc., 1880, lxix, 533.—**B.** Exomphale du foie par arrêt de développement. Gaz. d. hôp., Par., 1873, xlvi, 1098.—**Baena** (A.) Monstruosidad notable. España méd., Madrid, 1861, vi, 483.—**Baistrocchi** (E.) Osservazioni sopra un feto avente anomalie di sviluppo degli organi genito-urinari. Riv. clin. di Bologna, 1882, 3. s., ii, 216-222.—**Barrett** (T. B.) Malformation of a fœtus. Lancet, Lond., 1834-5, i, 349.—**Barrier** (G.) Description d'un monstre du genre célosome. Compt. rend. Soc. de biol. 1875, Par., 1876, 6. s., ii (Mém.), 29-45.—**Baster** (J.) Description of a monstrous fœtus, without any distinction of sex. Phil. Tr., Lond., 1744-50, x-xi, 1208.—**Batalla** (J. L.) Observacion de un feto de todo tiempo, que al nacer carecia de la pared anterior del abdómen, y que murió á los cuatro dias de su nacimiento. Siglo méd., Madrid, 1874, xxi, 823.—**Bauchêne** fils. Description du squelette d'un enfant hydrocéphale offrant une conformation singulière de la partie inférieure du tronc. Bull. Fac. de méd. de Par. 1809-11, ii (6. année), 27-29.—**Beale** (J. S.) On a case of deficiency of development of the superior, posterior, and anterior aspect of the fœtus. Lancet, Lond., 1858, ii, 280.—**Becker** (A.) Eine seltene Missbildung des Menschen. Berl. klin. Wchnschr., 1887, xxiv, 675-677.—**Béclard.** Notice descriptive d'un fœtus né avec des vices très-singuliers de conformation, et en particulier avec une adhérence du cœur à la voûte palatine. Bull. Fac. de méd. de Par. (1812-13), 1814, iii, 293-296.—**Behrendt** (S.) Spaltbildung des Cœcum, der Blase und Genitalien; Spina bifida; Defect der Bauchmuskeln um den Nabel. Arch. f. path. Anat., etc., Berl., 1874, lx, 298-300.—**Bellmunt** (O.) Observacion de un feto monstruoso. Anfiteatro anat., Madrid, 1876, iv, 148.—**Berti** (A.) Rara mostruosità in un fanciullo. Gazz. med. ital., prov. venete, Padova, 1858, i, 100.—**Beschrijving** van een wanschepsel. Boerhaave. Tijdschr., etc., Amst., 1843, n. s., ii, 477-480, 1 pl.—**Bevern.** Beschreibung eines zweijährigen durch eine zu frühzeitige Entwickelung monströsen Kindes; nebst Sectionsbericht. J. d. pract. Heilk., Berl., 1802, xiv, 3. St., 141-149.—**Blagden** (R.) Letter. Account of a monstrous birth. Med. Times & Gaz., Lond., 1861, ii, 336.—**Bousquet.** Observation sur un fœtus mal conformé. Rec. périod. d'obs. de méd., chir. et pharm., Par., 1757, vi, 128-130.—**Borellus** (P.) Infans monstrosa cum duplici vesica urinaria, recto intestino, atque utero extra locum naturalem suis. *In his:* Obs. med. communicatæ, 12°, Parisiis, 1657, 76.—**Bourneville** & **Bricon.** Ectromélie unilatérale; rein unique; inclusion de la verge; cloaque vésico-rectal; tumeur mixte (fibro-sarcome) du périnée, etc. Bull. Soc. anat. de Par., 1886, lxi, 238-247.

Monsters *from defect or malformation of abdomen and thorax.*

Also: Progrès méd., Par., 1886, 2. s., iv, 651; 672.—**Bouteillier** (J.) Description d'un fœtus monstrueux d'une espèce nouvelle. Monit. d. hôp., Par., 1853, i, 777; 801; 945. *Also:* Bull. Soc. anat. de Par., 1853. xxviii, 299-317.—**Boylston** (W. H.) Case of monstrosity. Boston M. & S. J., 1837, xvi, 382.—**Brandon** (W. C.) A case of monstrosity. South. M. & S. J., Augusta, 1851, n. s., vii, 591-594.—**Braun.** Beschreibung einer angeborenen auffallenden Missbildung. Ann. d. Staatsarznk., Freiburg, 1844, ix, 164-168.—**Breschet** (G.) Account of a congenital monstrosity. Med.-Chir. Tr., Lond., 1817-18, ix, 433-442.—**Brosillon.** Observation sur une monstruosité. J. de méd., chir., pharm., etc., 2. éd., Par., 1755, iii, 35-39.—**Brown** (E. T.) Fœtal monster. Ohio M. & S. J., Columbus, 1851-2, iv, 229.—**Browning.** Notes of a case of monstrosity. Indian M. Gaz., Calcutta, 1886, xxi, 219-221, 1 pl.—**Bruchet.** Sur un enfant monstrueux. [*From:* J. d. sçavans, 1683.] Collect. acad. d. mém., etc., Dijon, 1755, i, 297, 1 pl. — **Büttner** (C. G.) Anatomische Anmerkung von einem mit auswärts hangenden Herzen den 27. Sept. 1745 allhie lebendig gebornen, getauften und den andern Tag gestorbenen wohlgebildeten Kinde, weiblichen Geschlechts, mit Erklärung unterschiedener Fragen. *In his:* Anat. Wahrnehm, 4°, Königsb., 1769, 36-58, 2 pl. —, Wahrnehmung einer mit offenen Brust und Unterleibe, nebst den herausgehängenen Eingeweiden, allzu todt gebornen unreifen oder unzeitigen Frucht, männlichen Geschlechts. *Ibid.*, 121-131.—**Bunde.** Eine merkwürdige Missgeburt. [*From:* Arch. d. k. dänischen Gesundheitscollegii ausgezogen von Otto.] Ztschr. f. d. ges. Med., Hamb., 1844, xxv, 254.—**Burggraeve.** Cas remarquable de monstruosité. Ann. Soc. de méd. de Gand, 1844, xiv, 208.—**Byford.** A remarkable case of malposition and deficiency of the thoracic and abdominal viscera in a fœtus. Am. J. M. Sc., Phila., 1853, n. s., xxvi, 271.—**Calderini** (G.) Illustrazione di un feto umano abortivo mostruoso. Gior. d. r. Accad. di med. di Torino, 1874, 3. s., xvi, 229-243.—**Calori** (L.) Sopra un voluminoso tumore congenito esteso dalla pelvi ai piedi con apparente complicazione di ernia, o sventramento. Bull. d. sc. med. di Bologna, 1858, 4. s., x, 368. ———. Di tre mostri celosomi umani notabili per rispetto alla tocologia ed alla distribuzione teratologica di cotale famiglia di mostri. *Ibid.*, 1863, 4. s., xix, 36-39. [*See, also, supra.*]—**Canton** (E.) Description of a fœtal monster, with eventration. Lancet, Lond., 1849, ii. 266. *Also.* Reprint.—**Carolina** (L.) Raro caso di ettopia. Spallanzani, Modena, 1878, vii, 68-70.—**Chambon** (E.) Description d'un monstre célosomien, suivie de quelques considérations sur la parturition. Compt. rend. Soc. de biol. 1869, Par., 1870, 5. s., i, pt. 2, 211-232.—**Chamorro** (B.) Eventracion umbilical congénita curada á pesar de haber quedado al exterior un trozo cólon transverso. Anfiteatro anat., Madrid, 1874, ii, 27.—**Chance** (E. J.) Arrest of development in the fœtus. Lancet, Lond., 1863, i, 110.—**Clay.** Delivery of a deformed fœtus; accidental postpartum hæmorrhage. Lancet, Lond., 1871, ii, 261.—**Coales** (J.) Absence of the pleuræ; absence of a portion of the intestines. *Ibid.*, 1840, ii, 937.—**Coffin** (M.) Fœtal monstrosity. Tr. Obst. Soc. Lond. (1882), 1883, xxiv, 98-100.—**Colomiatti** (V. F.) Sopra un caso di arresto di sviluppo dell' intestino posteriore. Arch. per le sc. med., Torino, 1878-9, iii, no. 2, 1-15, 1 pl. *Also* [Abstr.]: Osservatore, Torino, 1878, xiv, 737-739.—**Conover** (S. B.) [Specimen belonging to the family of fœtal monsters.] Cincin. Lancet & Obs., 1867, x, 245-247.—**Corey** (L.) A singular case of malformation. [Reversed pelvis.] West. J. M., Indianap., 1868, iii, 282. *Also:* Med. & Surg. Reporter, Phila., 1868, xviii, 316.—**Coutagne** (E.) Note sur un fœtus monstrueux présentant des vices de conformation aussi nombreux que remarquables. Gaz. méd. de Lyon, 1859, xi, 94.—**Czermak** (J. J.) Eine seltene menschliche Missbildung. Med. Jahrb. d. k. k. österr. Staates, Wien, 1834, xv, 142-149.—**Darling** (J. A.) Birth of a monster. Boston M. & S. J., 1852, xlvi, 403.—**Darling** (W.) Case monstrosity. N. York J. M., 1844, ii, 377. *Also,* Reprint.—**Debouie.** [Imperforation congénitale du vagin; inversion de l'estomac et de la rate.] Bull. Soc. anat. de Par., 1857, xxxii, 59.—**De Camin** (F.) Storia d' una singolare deformità congenita, e riflessioni sopra di un fatto analogo. Ann. univ. di med., Milano, 1825, xxxvi, 127-132. — **De Crespigny** (E.) Case of monstrosity; congenital malformation. Tr. M. & Phys. Soc. Bombay (1852-3), 1855, n. s., ii, 322.—**De la Vigne.** Missbildung durch Vorfall sämmtlicher Eingeweide des Unterleibs. Gen.-Ber. d. k. rhein. Med.-Coll. 1839, Koblenz, 1842, 190.—**Delbovier.** Développement énorme de la vessie et des parois abdominales chez un fœtus d'environ huit mois. Ann. Soc. d. sc. méd. et nat. de Brux., 1842, 36-40. *Also:* Arch. de la méd. belge, Brux., 1842, viii, 10-13, 1 pl.—**Delore** (X.) Description d'un monstre célosomien aspalasome, avec réflexions. Montpel. méd., 1860, v, 444-455.—**De Moulon** (A.) Scherzi di natura altremodo singolari osservati nella sezione cadaverica di una giovinetta d' anni 14. Ann. univ. di med., Milano, 1827, xliv, 44-48.—**Dentan** (P.) Description d'un fœtus atteint de fissure abdominale avec hernie

Monsters *from defect or malformation of abdomen and thorax.*

funiculaire. Bull. Soc. méd. de la Suisse Rom., Lausanne, 1879. xiii, 158-161, 1 pl.—**Depaul.** [Extroversion de la vessie; absence du pénis; spina bifida.] Bull. Soc. anat. de Par., 1842, xvii, 213.—**Depaul.** Éventration fœtale par arrêt de développement; présentation de l'épaule. Gaz. d. hôp., Par., 1873, xlvi, 1073.—**Dickson.** Case of monstrosity. Med. Times, Lond., 1850, n. s., i, 81.—**Dickson.** Case of fœtal monstrosity, in which the placenta was affixed to the region of the abdominal walls, etc. Month. J. M. Sc., Lond. & Edinb., 1851, xiii, 82-84.—**Dickson** (S. H.) Case of monstrosity. South. J. M. & Pharm., Charleston, 1846, i, 496.—**Dinmore** (R.) A case of monstrous birth. Lond. M. J., 1790, xi, 339-342.—**Doran** (A.) Dissection of the genito-urinary organs in a case of fissure of the abdominal walls. J. Anat. & Physiol., Lond., 1880-81, xv, 226-234, 1 pl.—**Drew** (J.) Curious birth, and lusus naturæ; [abdominal parietes wanting.] Med. Times & Gaz., Lond., 1855, n. s., xi, 236 —**Dubois** (P.) Rapport sur deux cas de monstruosité. Mém. Acad. de méd., Par., 1835, iv, 475-488.—**Dubreuil.** Fœtus monstrueux célosomien; spina-bifida de la région dorsale; absence complète des ertèbres lombaires; inversion des membres inférieurs. Gaz. méd. de Par., 1849, 3. s., iv, 944-946.—**Duchateau** (A.-R.-P.) Observation d'un fœtus monstrueux. J. compl. du dict. d. sc. méd., Par., 1821, viii, 377.—**Duhamel.** Exomphale congénitale volumineuse. Mém. Soc. de méd. de Strasb. (1872-3), 1874, x, 100-104. — **Duvernoy** (J. G.) Von einer Missgeburt ohne Arme. Phys. u. med. Abhandl. d. k. Akad. d. Wissensch. in Petersb., Riga, 1783, ii, 311-332. — **Duvigneau.** Accouchement d'un enfant monstrueux. J. de méd., chir., pharm., etc., Par., 1790, lxxxv, 61-66. —**Elsholtius** (J. S.) De puella monstrosa, Berolini nuper nata. Misc. Acad. nat. curios. 1673-4, Francof. et Lips., 1676, iv-v (app.), 80, 1 pl. *Also: Ibid.* (1673-4), 1688, iv-v (app.), 67, 1 pl.— **Emanuel** (M.) Case of malformation in a child. Med. Exam., Phila., 1851, n. s., vii, 429.—**Eppinger.** Anatomischer Beitrag zu der Mittheilung Prof. v. Ritter's, "Ein-Fall von angeborener Lücke des Brustkorbes". Oester. Jahrb. f. Pädiat., Wien, 1876, vii, 201-214. —**Estéban** (R. M.) Un caso notable de obstetricia. Génio méd.-quir., Madrid, 1875, xxi, 188. — **Estep** (W.) A case of lusus naturæ. Med. Counsellor, Columbus, 1885, i, 147.—**Eves** (A.) Eventration and other deviations from the natural state of the fœtus. Lancet, Lond., 1844, i, 469.—**F[eigneau]x.** Monstruosité spéciale. Art méd., Brux., 1875-6, xi, 40.—**Feto** monstruo. Anfiteatro anat., Madrid, 1873. i, 262.—**Fleury** & **Duchamp.** Fœtus monstrueux; éventration; adhérence des membranes; absence des organes génitaux externes et de l'anus; persistance d'un cloaque; rein unique; bassin fendu; scoliose; spina bifida latéral; pied bot. Ann. Soc. de méd. de St.-Étienne et de la Loire, 1883, viii, 312-315. — **Fracys.** Vice de conformation du genre diastématiscs chez un nouveau-né. Bull. Soc. de méd. de Gand, 1849, xvi, 306-309.— **Fredet** fils. Note sur un monstre humain. Ann. Soc. de méd. de St.-Étienne et de la Loire (1867-71), 1872, iv, 139-147. *Also:* Rev. méd. franç. et étrang., Par., 1869, ii, 289-295. — **Friese.** Merkwürdige Missgeburt. Wchnschr. f. d. ges. Heilk., Berl., 1841, 848. — **Fuller** (A. P.) Case of malformation. Boston M. & S. J., 1835, xii, 348-350.— **Garbiglietti** (A.) & **Moriggia** (A.) Descrizione di celosomo dirino con exencefalia idrocefalica. Gior. r. Accad. di med. di Torino, 1870, 3. s., ix, 65-74, 1 pl.—**Gastelier.** Observation sur un fœtus monstrueux. J. de méd., chir., pharm., etc., Par., 1773, xxxix, 27-42.—**Gayton** (W.) Case of monstrosity. Tr. Obst. Soc. Lond. (1865), 1866, vii, 56. *Also:* Am. J. M. Sc., Phila., 1867, n. s., liii, 418.—**Goldschmidt.** Accouchement d'un fœtus monstrueux. Gaz. méd. de Strasb., 1875, xxxiv, 40.— **Griffith** (G. de G.) Curious monstrosity. Tr. Obst. Soc. Lond. (1869), 1870, xi, 5-7.—**Günsburg** (F.) Missbildungen im Verhältniss zu consecutiven pathologischen Entwicklungsvorgängen. Arch. f. d. ges. Med., Jena, 1846, viii, 293-305: 1849, x, 158-173.—**Hall** (A.) A case of monstrosity. Tr. Obst. Soc. Lond. (1867) 1868, ix, 271-275.— **Hallett** (C. H.) Observations illustrating the anatomical structure and physiological history of monsters with eventration. Edinb. M. & S. J., 1847, lxviii, 303-342, 3 pl.— **Hamy** (E.-T.) Description d'un fœtus monstrueux, présentant une atrésie des voies urinaires et de l'intestin transformés en cloaque, et l'absence d'organes génitaux. J. de l'anat. et physiol., etc., Par., 1884, xx, 193-200, 1 pl.— **Harrison** (J. B.) Case of monstrosity. Dublin Q. J. M. Sc., 1852, xiii, 229-231. *Also* [Abstr.]: Lond. J. M., 1850, ii, 79. — **Hartmannus** (P. J.) Anatome monstri. Misc. Acad. nat. curios. 1691, Norimb., 1692, decuria 2, x, 258-262, 1 pl. *Also, transl.:* Auserl. med.- chir.- . . . Abhandl. d. röm.-kais. Akad. d. Naturf., Nürnb., 1771, xx, 223-226, 1 pl.—**Harvey** (A.) Case of presentation of the bladder in labour. Edinb. M. & S. J., 1855, lxxxii, [case book, 29-31].— **Harvey** (R. S.) Case of mal-nutrition during fetal life. Cincin. Lancet & Obs., 1874, xvii, 264.— **Heath** (C.) Fœtus presenting several remarkable deformities and malformations. Tr. Path. Soc. Lond., 1858-

Monsters *from defect or malformation of abdomen and thorax.*

9, x, 304. *Also:* Lancet, Lond., 1859. i, 391. — **Hein** (R.) Beschreibung einer Missgeburt. [Fehlen der vorderen Bauchwand mit Ektopia viscerum und mangelhafter Entwickelung der Extremitäten.] Arch. f. path. Anat., etc., Berl., 1873, lviii, 326-328, 1 pl.—**Helbing** (H.) Partieller Rippenmangel und pleuritisches Exsudat als angeborene Bildungsanomalie. Aerztl. Mitth. a. Baden, Karlsruhe, 1860, xiv, 21. — **Heroldt** (C.) Widernatürliche Geburt eines monströsen Kindes. Arch. f. d. Geburtsh., Jena, 1787-8, i, 1. St., 37-47, 2 pl.—**Hetzell** (D. G.) Monstrosity; possibly from maternal impression. Med. & Surg. Reporter, Phila., 1876, xxxv, 442.—**Hill** (J. W.) Case of monstrosity. Med. & Phys. J., Lond., 1810, xxiv, 61-63.— **Hirigoyen** (L.) Monstre célosomien, agénosome, spina-bifida. J. de méd. de Bordeaux, 1884-5, xiv, 275.—**Hodge** (H. L.) Fœtal monstrosity presenting protrusion of the abdominal contents. Med. Times, Phila., 1870-71, i, 324.— **Hodges** (R. M.) Monstrosity; anterior parietes of the abdomen deficient, peculiar form of spina bifida. Am. J. M. Sc., Phila., 1854, n. s., xxviii, 394. *Also:* Extr. Rec. Bost. Soc. M. Improve. (1854-5), 1856, ii, 123. — **Hoefnagels** (J.-J.) Observation d'un cas de monstruosité. Ann. Soc. de méd. d'Anvers, Brux., 1840, 65-68, 1 pl. *Also:* Arch. de la méd. belge, Brux., 1840, i, 109-114, 1 pl.— **Höring.** Beschreibung einer menschlichen Missgeburt. Med. Cor.-Bl. d. württemb. ärztl. Ver., Stuttg., 1837, vii, 126-128.—**Holmes** (T. M.) A monstrosity. Atlanta M. & S. J., 1885-6, n. s., ii, 474.—**Houel.** Monstre célosomien du genre agénosome. Gaz. méd. de Par., 1851, 3. s., vi, 50-52. *Also:* Compt. rend. Soc. de biol. 1850, Par., 1851, ii, 107-117. ——. Anatomie d'un monstre humain célosomien. *Ibid.* 1851, Par., 1852, iii, 51. ——. [Éventration; spina bifida; torsion ainsi que les fesses et les jarrets sont dirigés en avant.] Bull. Soc. anat. de Par., 1850, xxv, 184-190. ——. [Vices de conformation sous-ombilicales; vessie exstrophiée; absence des organes génitaux externes, de pubis et de symphyse pubienne; spina bifida et pied-bot.] *Ibid.*, 1862, xxxvii, 156-159.—**Housley** (J.) Arrest of development in the fœtus. Lancet, Lond., 1864, i, 195.— **Hubbauer.** Geburtshergang bei einer Missgeburt und Beschreibung der Letzteren. Ztschr. f. Wundärzte u. Geburtsh., Stuttg., 1871, xxiv, 262.—**Hunter** (J. H.) Case of monstrosity. Am. J. M. Sc., Phila., 1858, n. s., xxxv, 294.—**Hupier.** Sur un fœtus monstrueux qui a donné lieu à un accouchement laborieux. Bull. Fac. de méd. de Par. (1809-11), 1812, ii, 102-104.—**Imlach** (F.) Dissection of a malformed fœtus having deficiency of anterior abdominal wall. Edinb. M. J., 1872-3, xviii, 415-418. ——. Case of cloaca in a child. Tr. Edinb. Obst. Soc. (1871-4) 1875, iii, 66-68.—**Istad** (H. L.) Et Misfoster med en særegen Dannelse af Urinveiene og Fødselsdelene. Eyr, Christiania, 1832, vii, 12.—**Jackson** (J. S. B.) Monstrosity. [Case.] Boston M. & S J., 1865-6, lxxiii, 101. *Also:* Extr. Rec. Bost. Soc. M. Improve. (1862-6), 1867, v, 177.—**Jakins** (W. V.) Rare form of fœtal deformity. Austral. M. J., Melbourne, 1878, xxiii, 189.—**Jung.** Seltsame Misgestaltung eines ausgetragenen Kindes. N. Jahrb. d. teutsch. Med. u. Chir., Hamm, 1824, viii, 2. St., 15-17.—**Johnson** (J. G.) Fœtal malformation. N. York J. M., 1859, 3. s., vi, 392.—**Johnston** (W.) A case of false conception. West. Lancet, Cincin., 1846-7, v, 31.—**Léautaud.** Description d'un enfant monstrueux. J. de méd., chir., pharm., etc., Par., 1781, lv, 76-79.—**Lemoigne** (A.) Cenni intorno ad un mostro celosomo. Gazz. med. ital. lomb., Milano, 1869, 6. s., ii, 297-300, 1 pl.—**von Lenhossék.** Nachricht von einem menschlichen Fötus, der mit einem Bauchbruche, in welchem das Herz, die Leber, und der grössere Theil des Dünndarmes enthalten waren, geboren wurde. Med. Jahrb. d. k. k. österr. Staates, Wien, 1820-21, vi, 2. St., 68-78.—**Leopold.** Fall von Spaltung der Harnblase, Cloakenbildung und Hydrorrhachis. Monatschr. f. Geburtsk. u. Frauenkr., Berl., 1861, xvii, 357-363, 1 pl.—**Lippincott** (H.) & **Warrington** (J.) Case of abnormal fœtuses. Med. Exam., Phila., 1838, i, 269. —**van Lissa** (V.) Waarneming eener monstrositas per excessum, gesproten uit eene weelderige vormingskracht, zonder eenige ziekelijke afwijking der vrucht. Nederl. Lancet, Utrecht, 1839-40, ii, 310-312, 1 pl.—**Litchfield** (T.) An account of a delivery of a monstrosity after a painful labor; with an engraving and examination of the fœtus. Lancet, Lond., 1850, i, 50.— **Littré** (A.) Observations sur un fœtus humain monstrueux. [*From:* Hist. Acad. roy. d. sc. de Par., 1701.] Rec. de mém., Dijon, 1754, i, 672-677. ——. Sur un fœtus humain monstrueux. [*From:* Mém. Acad. roy. d. sc. de Par., 1709.] *Ibid.*, ii, 702-706.—**Long** (R. W.) A case of monstrosity. Chicago M. J., 868, xxv, 568-570.—**Losada** (F.) Ectromelia abdominal derecha. An. r. Acad. de med., Madrid, 1880, ii, 43-50.—**de Macedo e Valle** (L. A.) Un nouveau cas de tératologie. [Trad. du portugais.] Ann. Soc. de méd. d'Anvers, 1865, xxvi, 49-55, 1 pl. [Rap. de Kums]. 55-58.—**Mackay** (E.) Account of a child born within eight months, presenting important anomalies in its development. Lond. & Edinb. Month. J. M. Sc., 1841, i, 403-405.—**Martin.** Vorlegung eines Präparates von Eventration mit beiderseitiger Hydronephrose und Uterus didel-

Monsters *from defect or malformation of abdomen and thorax.*

phys, nebst offener Harnblase und Dickdarm mit deutlicher Oeffnung des Dündarmes und ausgebildetem Mastdarme bei einem acht Monate alten Neugeborenen. Monatschr. f. Geburtsk. u. Frauenkr., Berl., 1864, xxiv, 161-165. *Also:* Verhandl. d. Gesellsch. f. Geburtsh. in Berl. (1864), 1865, xvii, 77-81.—**Martin** (E.) Mémoire sur un cas de persistance des canaux de Muller; oblitération des voies urinaires; neutralité sexuelle. J. de l'anat. et physiol., etc., Par., 1878, xiv, 20-33, 1 pl.—**Martin** (E.) & **Letulle.** Étude d'un monstre pleuro-célosomien. *Ibid.*, 1876, xii, 561-574, 2 pl.—**Martinez y Molina** (R.) Ectopia de las visceras contenidas en las dos grandes cavidades esplánicas. Siglo méd., Madrid, 1855, ii, 58.—**Maury.** Description d'un fœtus monstrueux. Bull. Soc. de méd. de Poitiers, 1849, No. xv, 34-39, 2 pl.—**Mayer.** Beschreibung einer Missgeburt mit völligem Mangel der Organe des Urinsystems, so wie auch sehr mangelhafter Entwickelung der Geschlechtstheile und der Cauda equina des Rückenmarks. Ztschr. f. Physiol., Darmstadt, 1827, ii, 36-46. ——. Ueber eine Missbildung; Verkehrung sämmtlicher Eingeweide. Arch. f. path. Anat., etc., Berl., 1864, xxix, 389-394, 1 pl.—**Meadows** (A.) Case of monstrosity. Tr. Obst. Soc. Lond. (1862), 1863, iv, 255-259. ——. Case of monstrosity, with remarks on the influence of maternal impressions on the fœtus in utero. *Ibid.* (1865), 1866, vii, 84-94, 2 pl.—**Meckel von Hemsbach** (H.) Anatomische Geschichte frühgeborner Drillinge, unter denen einer monströs ist; gemeinschaftliche Eihäute; Anastomose der Nabelgefässe in der Plazenta; Nabelbruch; Atrophie des Herzens; Mangel der Leber; medianer Wolfsrachen; Umschlingung des Nabelstrangs. Illust. med. Ztg., München, 1852, i, 99-102, 1 pl.—**Meissner** (F. L.) Kurze Beschreibung einer sehr merkwürdigen Missgeburt. J. f. Geburtsh., Frankf. a. M., 1826, vi, 333-336.—**Méry.** Sur un autre monstrueux. [*From:* Hist. d. mém. Acad. roy. d. sc. de Par., 1716.] Collect. acad. d. mém., etc. Partie franç., Par., 1770, iv, 445-447.—**Metcalf** (J. G.) Case of monstrosity. Boston M. & S. J., 1839, xx, 341-343.—**Miles** (M.) Case of monstrosity. Northwest. M. & S. J., Chicago, 1852-3, ix, 111.—**Milford** (F.) Case of an infant monster. N. South Wales M. Gaz., Sydney, 1870-71, i, 48; 122, 2 pl.—**Mills** (T. W.) Case of congenital ectopia of abdominal organs. Canad. J. M. Sc., Toronto, 1880, v, 35.—**Milner** (U. R.) [A deformed fœtus.] N. Orl. J. M., 1869, xxii, 789-792.—**Möller.** Notiz über eine ungewöhnliche Missbildung. Arch. f. path. Anat., etc., Berl., 1864, xxix, 205-207, 1 pl.—**de Moerloose** (*Mlle.*) Un cas intéressant de tératologie (célosomien plenrosome). [Rap. de P. Albrecht.] Presse méd. belge, Brux., 1884, xxxvi, 385-387. —**Montault.** Exposition raisonnée d'un cas d'accouchement et de monstruosité humaine; présentation d'un bras et des intestins par un fœtus affecté d'éventration; version de l'enfant qui offrait plusieurs vices de conformation remarquables; prompt rétablissement de la mère. Expérience, Par., 1837-8, i, 145-150. — **Montgomery** (J. E.) A case of monstrosity. Memphis M. Recorder, 1856-7, v, 420-422.—**Montgomery** (W. F.) Description of a very remarkable malformation in a fœtus, in which nearly all the abdominal viscera and the intestinal canal were external to the body. Dublin M. Tr, 1830, n. s., i, 375-383, 3 pl.—**Morean** (A.) Rapport sur un fœtus monstrueux du genre célosomien présenté par le docteur Pruneau. Bull. Soc. anat. de Par., 1858, xxxiii, 473-476 —**Morel.** Fœtus monstrueux. Rev. méd. de l'est, Nancy, 1874, ii, 458.—**Müller** (A.) Beschreibung einer Missgeburt. Ztschr.f.Wundärzte u. Geburtsh., Stuttg., 1865, xviii, 258.—**Mulot.** On the particular conformation of a fœtus, which led to some difficulty to determine its position in utero. Med. & Phys J., Lond., 1803, ix. 461.—**Murdoch** (J.) Dissection of a human monster Edinb. M. & S J., 1821, xvii, 315-317.—**Myschkin** (M. M.) Monstrum humanum kyphoscolioticum cum spina bifida deque univocivisque abdominis hiatu completo et genitalium extremitatumque inferiorum defectu. Arch. f. path. Anat., etc., Berl., 1887, cviii, 146-164, 1 pl.—**Naudin.** Notice sur un fœtus portant une monstruosité singulière. J. gén. de méd., chir. et pharm, Par., 1816, lv, 342-350.—**Neugebauer** (L.) Ueber das Auftreten der Leber im Nabel, als Fehler der ersten Bildung; eine pathologisch-anatomische Untersuchung. N. Ztschr. f. Geburtsk., Berl., 1850, xxvii, 64-78, 1 pl.—**Novi** (J.) Breve descrizione di un feto mostro. Ann. clin. d. osp. incur., Napoli, 1882, n. s., vii, 87-94, 3 pl. — **Oberrit.** Eine seltene Missgeburt. Wien. med. Presse, 1872, xiii, 1215.— **Observacion** de un feto monstruoso. An. Soc. ginec. españ., Madrid, 1876, ii, 295-298.—[**O'Connor.**] Case of monstrosity; deficiency of the abdominal walls, of the cartilages of the ribs, and a part of the diaphragm; hernia of the heart. Dublin Q. J. M. Sc., 1861, xxxi, 454.—**Oswald** (J. W. J.) Fœtal monstrosity. Tr. Obst. Soc. Lond. (1882), 1883, xxiv, 75.— **Owen** (A. P.) Arrest of development in the fœtus. Lancet, Lond., 1863. i, 25.— **Pachstein.** Seltene Monstrosität. Preuss. Med.-Ztg., Berl., 1861, n. F., iv, 134.— **Pacini** (L.) Ragguaglio anatomico-fisiologico intorno

Monsters *from defect or malformation of abdomen and thorax.*

ad un mostro umano. Ann. univ. di med., Milano, 1843, cvi, 457-472, 1 pl. — **Packard.** Monstrosity [malformed fœtus]. Proc. Path. Soc. Phila. (1860-66), 1867, ii, 89.— **Patoun.** Extract of letter from Dr. . . . of Aberdeen, containing an account of a singular case of monstrosity. Edinb. M. & S. J., 1807, iii, 374-376. — **Pelvet.** Note sur un fœtus célosomien, voisin du genre aspalasome. Compt. rend. Soc. de biol. 1865, Par., 1866, 4. s., ii, 75-87.—**Petit.** Monstro pleurosome. Bull. méd. du nord, Lille, 1874, xiv, 177-181.—**Patrick** (S.) [Case of monstrosity.] Calif. State M. J., Sacramento, 1856-7, i, 273.— **Philipeaux** (J.-M.) Note sur un fœtus monstrueux à éventration complète, du sexe féminin. Compt. rend. Soc. de biol. 1873, Par., 1874, 5. s., v, 93-97.— **Pinnock** (R. D.) † Obst. J. Gr. Brit., Lond., 1878-9, vi, 430-432. *Also:* Australas. M. Gaz., Sydney, 1883-4, iii, 101. — **Pithie** (A. D.) A rare monstrosity. Brit. M. J., Lond., 1879, ii, 641. — **Poli** (B.) [Uomo mostruoso di Macao.] Ann. univ. di med., Milano, 1839, xci, 19, 1 pl.—**Puech** (A.) Note sur divers vices de conformation observés chez une fille. Gaz. d. hôp., Par., 1857, xxx, 586.—**Rankin** (D. N.) Deficiency of the integuments of the abdomen and spina bifida in the same child. Am. J. M. Sc., Phila., 1867, n. s., liii, 273 — **Ranvier.** Scissure du sternum; ectopie du cœur; absence du canal artériel; deux veines caves supérieures chez un fœtus de 8 mois. Compt. rend. Soc. de biol. 1863, Par., 1864, 3. s., v, 93.—**Raphael** (B. I.) Unique malformation of an infant. West. J. M. & S., Louisville, 1849, 3. s., iv. 110.—**von Recklinghausen.** [Zwei Präparate von Missbildungen, welche als Unica betrachtet werden müssen.] Verhandl. d. phys.-med. Gesellsch. in Würzb. (1866-8), 1869, n. F., i, p. xv.—**Reil.** Merkwürdige Missbildung. Illust. med. Ztg., München, 1853, iii, 83-92.—**Renault** (P.) Tumeur sacro-coxcygienne congénitale. Bull. Soc. anat. de Par., 1884, lix, 647-649.— **Reuss.** Beschreibung einer Missgeburt mit "Kloakbildung". Arch. f. physiol. Heilk., Stuttg., 1856, xv, 523-529.—**Revolat.** Observation sur la conformation singulière d'un enfant. J. gén. de méd., chir. et pharm., Par., 1806, xxvii, 370-382.—**Rich.** Monstrosity. Liverpool M.-Chir. J., 1885, v, 194.—**del Riego** (A.) Observacion rara de un feto monstruo sin cordon ombilical. Bol. de med., cirug. y farm., Madrid, 1843, 2. s., iv, 108-110.— **Ritter** (G.) Ein Fall von angeborener Lücke des Brustkorbes. Oesterr. Jahrb. f. Pädiat., Wien, 1876, vii, 101-107. [*See, also, supra,* Eppinger.]—**Rolfe** (W. D.) Case of lusus naturæ. Lond. M. & Phys. J., 1827, n. s., iii, 50, 1 pl.—**Sacré** (J.) Description d'un monstre agénosome. Ann. Soc. d'anat. path. de Brux., 1861, 28-31. *Also:* J. de méd., chir. et pharmacol., Brux., 1861, xxxii, 41-44. ——. Description d'un monstre cyllosome. Ann. Soc. d'anat. path. de Brux., 1863, 27-30, 1 pl.—**Sampson** (H.) De fœtu monstrosissimo. Misc. Acad. nat curios. 1672, Francof. et Lips., 1681, iii, 279. *Also, transl.:* Collect. acad. d. mém., etc., Dijon, 1755, iii, 158.—**Sandifort** (E.) Observatio de fœtu monstroso, cujus viscera abdominalia omnia una cum corde extra corpus propendebant. Acta Helvet., Basileæ, 1772, vii, 56-61, 1 pl.—**Sanfrutos** (R.) Fénomeno curioso. Siglo méd., Madrid, 1860, vii, 287.— **Sappey** (C.) Monstre célosomien du genre agénosome. Compt. rend. Soc. de biol. 1859, Par., 1860, 3. s., i, 250.— **Sauri** (J. R.) Teratologia; extroversion de la vejiga; deformidad de los riñones y uréteres; duplicacion del aparato genital. Emulacion. Mérida, 1877-9, iii, 191-194.— **Saxtorph** (M.) Observatio de fœtu aperto abdomine, visceribusque abdominalibus solo peritonæo tectis nato. Acta reg. Soc. med. Havn., 1783, i, 191-195. *Also, transl. in his:* Ges. Schrift. geburtsh., 8°, Kopenh., 1804, 281-285. ——. Beschreibung zweyer Kinder, denen die Bedeckungen des Unterleibes fehlten. *In his:* Ges. Schrift. geburtsh., 8°, Kopenh., 1804, 312-329.—**Schatz** (F.) Geburt eines Monstrums; drei Fälle von einhörnigem Uterus. Arch. f. Gynaek., Berl., 1870, i, 153-155, 1 pl.— **Scheiber** (S. H.) Einige angeborene Anomalien beobachtet im pathologisch-anatomischen Institut zu Bukarest. Med. Jahrb., Wien, 1875, 257-264, 1 pl.—**Schmidt** (J.) De monstro fœminini sexus. Misc. Acad. nat. curiós. 1673-4, Francof. et Lips., 1688, iv-v, 26.—**Schmidt** (J. A.) Sonderbare angeborne Missbildung eines Kindes weiblichen Geschlechts. J. d. pract. Heilk., Berl., 1806, xxiv, 3. St., 147-162.—**Schuller** (M.) Ein Fall von seltener Missbildung. Ztschr. d. k.-k. Gesellsch. d. Aerzte zu Wien, 1853, ii, 503-506.—**Schultze** (B. S.) Ein Fall von Heterotaxie der Bauch- und Brusteingeweide und wahrscheinlichen Offenstehen des Foramen ovale, nebst allgemeinen Bemerkungen über die Genese dieser beiden Bildungsfehler. Arch. f. path. Anat., etc., Berl., 1881, xxii, 209-230.—**Schupmann** (A.) Hemmungs-Bildung in den Bauchdecken; Vorfall der Eingeweide des Unterleibes bei einem neugeboren völlig ausgetragenen und sonst gut gebildeten Mädchen. J. f. Geburtsh., Leipz., 1837, xvi, 111-120. — **Scotti** (G.) Mostruosità. Gazz. med. ital. lomb., Milano, 1850, 3. s., i, 353-355. — [**Semple.**] [Monstra deficientia.] N. Orl. J. M., 1868. xxi, 734-736.—**Sewall** (J. G.) A case of congenital malformation. N. York J.

Monsters *from defect or malformation of abdomen and thorax.*

M., 1854, [2.] s., xii, 194–197.—**Simon-Cheffe.** Monstruosité; ectopie intestinale; spina-bifida; pieds bots. Gaz. d. hôp., Par., 1856, xxix, 262.—**Sinclair** (E. B.) Case of malformation in a foetus, with fissure of the pubic and hypogastric regions. Dublin Q. J. M. Sc., 1851, xii, 481.—**Snively** (J. N.) Remarkable case of monstrosity. Med. & Surg. Reporter, Phila., 1871, xxiv, 383.—**Soper** (J.) Singular case of monstrosity. Lancet, Lond., 1829-30, ii, 56.—**Spessa** (A. A.) Ipotiposi di un mostro straordinario, ed osservazioni intorno al medesimo. Mem. Soc. med.-chir. di Bologna, 1838, 2. s., i, 117–127. — **Steger** (F. E. H.) Congenital malformation. Nashville M. Rec. M. & Phys. Sc., 1858-9, i, 208–213.—**Teissier.** Description d'un foetus monstrueux célosomien, offrant des particularités sans analogues dans la science. Mém. Soc. méd. d'émulat. de Lyon, Par. et Lyon, 1842, i, 1–8.—**Teratologia.** Siglo méd., Madrid, 1867, xiv, 822–824.— **Terrill** (J. E. G.) † Atlanta M. & S. J., 1857-8, iii, 651. — **Thorner** (E.) Ueber eine Hemmungs-Bildung des Amnion bei einem menschlichen Fötus, verbunden mit anderweitigen Missbildungen. Arch. f. Anat., Physiol. u. wissensch. Med., Leipz., 1869, 200–206, 1 pl.—**Tonelli** (G.) Rapporto di mostruosa trasposizione dei visceri addominali in un feto umano, osservata in Paliano presso Roma. Ann. univ. di med., Milano, 1837, lxxxii, 441–452.—**Tourneux** (F.) & **Wertheimer** (E.) Description d'un monstre célosomien avec spina bifida (hydrorachis interna). J. de l'anat. et physiol., etc., Par., 1882, xviii, 578–587.—**Tucker** (J.) Account of a foetal monster. Lond. M. Reposit., 1827, [3.] s., v, 401. — **Vejas** (P.) Eine seltene Missbildung. Arch. f. path. Anat., etc., Berl., 1886, civ, 72–80, 1 pl.— **Velpeau.** Dissertation sur un foetus monstrueux. J. hebd. d. progr. d. sc. et inst. méd., Par., 1834, i, 277–291.— **Verger** (D.) Observacion de una criatura monstruosa por defecto. Arch. de la med. españ., Madrid, 1846, i, 334–337.—**Virchow** (R.) Ein Fall von Transposition der Eingeweide und ausgedehnten Localerkrankungen beim Neugebornen. Arch. f. path. Anat., etc., Berl., 1861, xxii, 426–433. ——. Ueber eine Missgeburt, Exocardie, Hydrocephalie, Verwachsung der Eihäute mit dem Fötus. Monatschr. f. Geburtsk. u. Frauenkr., Berl., 1862, xx, 16–18. *Also:* Verhandl. d. Gesellsch. f. Geburtsh. in Berl. (1861-2), 1863, xv, 88. — **Vosselmann** (C.) Sur un cas de singulière disposition des viscères chez un enfant nouveau-né. Gaz. méd. de Strasb., 1876, xxxv, 16.—**Vrolik** (G.) Mémoire sur un foetus monstrueux né au bout du 8me mois de la grossesse en même temps qu'un enfant bien conformé. *In his:* Mém. sur . . . anat. et de physiol., 4°, Amst., 1822, 25–64, 5 pl. ——. Mémoire sur un vice de conformation, accompagné de la dénudation de la moitié antérieure de la vessie, et de la division partielle du pénis. *Ibid.*, 95–101, 2 pl.—**Walton** (E.) Cas d'éventration. Rev. méd.-phot. d. hôp. de Par., 1874, vi, 131, 1 pl. — **Wasseige** (A.) fils. Observation d'un cas de monstruosité remarquable. Bull. Acad. roy. de méd. de Belg., Brux., 1861, 2. s., iv, 221–232, 1 pl. [Rap. de Spring], 185–190. — **Watt** (J.) Case of monstrosity. Glasgow M. J., 1831, iv, 130–132. — **Wedl** (C.) Rauchspalte eines sechsmonatlichen menschlichen Fötus. Med. Jahrb., Wien, 1863, v, 143–148, 2 pl.—**Williams** (S. W.) Case of monstrosity, with some remarks on moles, marks, etc. Am. J. M. Sc., Phila., 1835, xvi, 88–91. —**Wilson** (H. S.) Malformed foetus. Obst. J. Gr. Brit., Lond., 1879-80, vii, 29.—**Winkler** (F. N.) Ist Ektopia viscerum vielleicht nur eine Folge abnormer Muskelinsertionen an der Rückseite des Rumpfes? Arch. f. Gynaek., Berl., 1877, xi, 564–567.—**Wolfart.** † Ἀσκληπίειον, Berl., 1811, i, 745–752, 1 pl. — **Xarrié** (A. C.) Una monstruosidad. Anfiteatro anat., Madrid, 1879, vii, 60. *Also:* Rev. de cien. méd., Barcel., 1879, v, 36–40. — **Yeatman** (J. C.) A remarkable instance of fatal malformation. Lond. M. & Phys. J., 1824, lii, 367–369, 1 pl.

Monsters *from defect or malformation of brain, cranium, or face.*

See, also, **Brain, Cranium,** *Abnormities of*; **Encephalocele; Eye, Face,** *Abnormities, etc., of*; **Hydrencephalocele; Hydrocephalus** (*Congenital*); **Monsters** (*Acardiac*); **Monsters** (*Acephalous*; **Monsters** *in animals, etc.*; **Nose** (*Abnormities of*).

DE ASSIZ E SOUZA VAZ (F.) Descripção de hum feto monstruozo exposto na caza da Roda da cidade do Porto. 8°. *Porto*, 1837.

BAART DE LA FAILLE (J.) Jets over den epignathus. Eene teratologische bijdrage. 4°. *Groningen*, 1874.

[BELHOMME.] Observation d'ectrogénie assymétrique. 8°. [*n. p., n. d.*]

BENTKOWSKI (L.-H.) * Étude sur un monstre exencéphalien. 4°. *Montpellier*, 1885.

Monsters *from defect or malformation of brain, cranium, or face.*

BIANCINI (T.) Di una anencefalia; osservazione anatomica. 8°. *Pisa*, 1829.

BOUTIN (E.) * Diss. sistens descriptionem monstri humani. 4°. *Berolini*, [1817].

BUCH (J.) * De monstro humano distomo. 8°. *Halæ*, 1866.

BUSCH (F.) * De raro quodam exemplo monstrositatis humanæ. 8°. *Berolini*, 1866.

CALORI (L.) Sopra una nuova specie di mostro umano exencefalico vissuto trent' ore. 8°. *Bologna*, 1860.
Repr. from: Mem. Accad. d. sc. d. Ist. di Bologna, x.

CARUS (C. G.) Entwickelung der Form eines Angesichts auf einem cyclopischen Auge; sehr merkwürdiger Fall einer Missgeburt. 4°. [*n. p.*, 1839.]
Repr. from: Nova acta phys.-med. Acad. nat. curios., xix.

CERTAINE (A) relation of the hog-faced gentlewoman called Mistris Tannakin Skinker, who was borne at Wirkham, a neuter towne betweene the emperour and the Hollander, scituate on the river Rhyne, who was bewitched in her mother's wombe in the yeare 1618 and hath lived ever since unknowne in this kind to any but her parents and a few other neighbours, and can never recover her true shape, tell she be married, etc. Also, relating the cause, as it is since conceived, how her mother came so bewitched. 4°. *London*, 1640.

CERUTTI (F. P. L.) Inest rarioris monstri, in museo anatomico Lipsiensi adservati, descriptio anatomica. 4°. *Lipsiæ*, 1827.

CHARVET (A.) Cébocéphalie avec adhérence du placenta au crâne et à la face sur un foetus humain. 8°. *Grenoble*, 1874.

DELLE CHIAIE (S.) Istoria anatomico-teratologica intorno ad una bambina rinocefalo-monocola. fol. *Napoli*, 1840.

CROSNIER (É.) * Étude sur quelques cas de monstruosités foetales pseudencéphales-encéphalocèles, avec anomalies du côté de la face, de l'appareil oculaire et des membres. 4°. *Paris*, 1875.

DESORMEAUX (A.-J.) & GERVAIS (P.) Description d'un foetus humain monstrueux devant former un genre à part sous le nom de pseudacéphale. 4°. *Paris*, 1860.
Repr. from: Acad. d. sc. de Montpel. Mém. de la sect. d. sc.

ELSÆSSER (H.) * Ueber eine widernatürliche Verdünnung des Hinterhauptbeins bei einem Kinde. sm. 8°. *Tübingen*, 1837.

FRIDERICUS (G.). Monstrum humanum rarissimum recens in lucem editum in tabula exhibet, simulque observationibus pathologicis aliisque illuc pertinentibus breviter illustrat. 4°. *Lipsiæ*, 1737.

——. The same. sm. 4°. *Lipsiæ*, 1737.

GEBAUER (J.) * De monstro cyclopeo. 8°. [*Dorpat*], 1833.

GERET (A.) & HÜTTLINGER (P.) * Infans monstrosus Wittebergæ, d. 30. Augusti anno 1674 natus. 4°. *Wittebergæ*, [1674].

GRILLENZONI (C. E.) Sopra un caso di emicefalia nella specie umana. Osservazioni presentate all' Accademia medico-chirurgica di Ferrara il 5 marzo 1841. 8°. [*Bologna*, 1841·]
Repr. from: Nuovi Ann. d. sc. nat. di Bologna, vi. *See, also, infra.*

HALLER (A.) Indicit anatomen fetus cranii parte et cerebro destituti, centesimum nempe cadaver quod in hoc theatro secuit. Ad D. xxvi. Mart. mdccxliii. fol. *Gottingæ*, 1743.

——. [Pr.] de fetu humano septimestri sine cerebro edito agit. sm. 4°. *Gottingæ*, [1745].

Monsters *from defect or malformation of brain, cranium, or face.*

HANNOVER (A.) Den menneskelige Hjerneskals Bygning ved Anencephalia og Misdannelsens Forhold til Hjerneskallens Primordialbruck. 4°. *Kjøbenhavn,* 1882.

Cutting from: Vidensk. Selsk. Skr., 6. R., Naturvidenskabelign og Mathematisk, Afd. 1. 8., 369-395, 2 pl. *See, also, infra.*

HENSCHE (C. A.) * Quædam de anencephalia. 8°. *Halis Sax.,* 1854.

JADELOT (J.-F.-N.) Description anatomique d'une tête humaine extraordinaire, suivie d'un essai sur l'origine des nerfs. 8°. *Paris,* 1799.

JAHN (C. A. B.) * De cyclopia. 8°. *Berolini,* [1860].

JOLY (N.) & GUITARD (I.) Mémoire sur un enfant nosencéphale adhérent à son placenta, et né vivant à Toulouse le 26 juillet 1850. 8°. *Toulouse,* [1850].

Repr. from: Mém. Acad. nat. d. sc. de Toulouse.

JOURDAN (C.) * Description anatomique d'un cas de cyclopie. 4°. *Paris,* 1833.

JUNGBLUTH (B.) * De anencephalis. 8°. *Berolini,* [1843].

KLINKOSCH (J. T.) [Pr.] quo sectiones et demonstrationes suas anatomicas, publicas, hyemales, anni academici 1766 indicit, et anatomen partus capite monstroso proponit.

In his: Diss. med. [etc.] 4°. *Pragæ et Dresdæ,* 1775, i, 199-208, 1 pl.

———. [Pr.] quo anatomen partus capite monstroso proponit.

In: WEIZ (F. A.) Neue Ausz., [etc.] 12°. *Leipzig,* 1777, vi, 11-18.

KNACKSTEDT (C. E. H.) Anatomische Beschreibung einer Missgeburt, welche ohne Gehirn und Hirnschädel lebendig geboren wurde, als eine Einladungsschrift abgefasset. 4°. *St. Petersburg,* 1791.

KNAPE (G. A. E. T.) * Monstri humani maxime notabilis descriptio anatomica. 4°. [*Berlin,* 1823.]

KOEPPEL (P. K. E. E.) * Ueber die Verschmelzung der Augen bei einfachen und Doppel-Missgeburten. sm. 8°. *Berlin,* [1867].

KROMBHOLZ (J. V.) Anatomische Beschreibung eines sehr merkwürdigen Anencephalus. 8°. *Prag,* 1830.

Repr. from: Abhandl. d. k. böhm. Gesellsch. d. Wissensch., Prag, 1830.

LAROCHE (V.) * Essai d'anatomie pathologique sur les monstruosités ou vices de conformation primitifs de la face. 4°. *Paris,* 1823.

LAULAIGNE (J.) * Contribution à l'étude de l'anencéphalie. Diagnostic pendant la grossesse et l'accouchement. 4°. *Paris,* 1883.

Also, in: Ann. de gynéc., Par., 1883, xix, 401-431, 3 pl.

LINDFORSS (P. P.) * Diss. descriptionem monstri anatomicam proponens. 4°. *Helsingforsiæ,* [1822].

LÖFDAHL (C. J.) * De fetu monstroso, judicio medici submisso. 8°. *Lundæ,* 1837.

LOMBARDINI (L.) Intorno ad un mostro appartenente al genere rhinocephalus di I. Geoffroy-Saint-Hilaire. 4°. [*n. p., n. d.*]

Cutting from: Scienze cosmolog., vii, 1-25, 1 pl.

LOSCHGE (F. H.) * De commodis quibusdam ex singulari infantum calvariæ structura oriundis. 4°. *Erlangæ,* 1785.

LUECKE (A. G.) * De monstro quodam humano. 4°. *Halis Sax.,* 1854.

MATTERSDORF (H.) * De anencephalia cum novissimi casus anencephali post partum vivi expositione. 4°. *Berolini,* [1836].

MYLIUS (L. H.) * De puella monstrosa. sm. 4°. *Lipsiæ,* 1717.

Monsters *from defect or malformation of brain, cranium, or face.*

NAGEL (E.) * De anencephalia quædam cum descriptione monstri unis. 8°. *Gryphiæ,* [1865].

NIEDER (F. X.) * De anencephalo casus singularis. 8°. *Monachii,* 1834.

NOODT (G. W.) De monstro quodam humano. 8°. *Schoonhoviæ,* 1839.

OBSERVATION d'ectrogénie asymétrique. 8°. [*Paris,* 1848.]

PEGASUS (J. B. R.) Monstrum apud orbem natum. Nonis Martiis natum, 1513. 12°. [*n. p., n. d.*]

A poem.

PIERQUIN, *de Gembloux.* Histoire naturelle du Berri et réflexions philosophiques sur un adamide ailé. 8°. *Châteauroux,* [*n. d.*]

PRUNEAU (E.) * Dissertation sur l'anencéphalie. 4°. *Paris,* 1837.

RADDATZ (E. J.) * De cyclopia. 4°. *Berolini,* 1829.

ROSENBERG (A.) * Ueber einen Fall von Missbildung. 8°. *Berlin,* [1886].

RUDOLPH (C. E.) * Monstrorum trium præter naturam cum secundinis coalitorum disquisitio. 4°. *Berolini,* [1829].

RUPPERSBERG (J.) * Ein Fall von Hirnbruch mit Spaltbildungen des Gesichts und Truncus. (Mit Abbildung.) 8°. *Marburg,* [1872].

RUSCHE (E.) * Ein Fall von Hydrocephalus congenitus mit Spina bifida. 8°. *Marburg,* 1880.

SANDIFORT (E.) Anatome infantis cerebro destituti. 4°. *Lugd. Bat.,* 1784.

SAPOLINI. Caso di microcefalia parziale. 8°. *Milano,* 1870.

SCHÖN (W.) * Ueber Verkümmerung des Zwischenkiefers mit gleichzeitiger Missbildung des Gehirns. 8°. *Berlin,* [1870].

SPEER (C. G.) * De cyclopia, sive unione partium capitis in statu normali disunclarum. 8°. *Halæ,* [1819].

STEIN (C. E.) * Ein Fall von Hämicephalie mit Verwachsung zwischen Kopf und Placenta. 8°. *Marburg,* 1879.

TESDORPF (P. H.) * Beschreibung und Erklärungsversuch einer mit amniotischen Bändern behafteten menschlichen Missbildung. 8°. *München,* 1883.

TORRALBAS (J. I.) Estudio teratológico de un caso de exencefalia. 8°. *Carácas,* 1876.

ULLERSPERGER. * Pathologisch-anatomische Beschreibung zweyer Missgeburten. 8°. *Würzburg,* 1822.

VORSTMAN (J. G.) * Beschrijving eener misvormde menschelijke vrucht. 8°. *Leiden,* 1857.

VROLIK (W.) Over den aard en oorsprong der cyclopie. 4°. *Amsterdam,* 1834.

WEBER (M. I.) Specimen malæ conformationis encephali capitis et pelvis viri rarissimum et memoratu dignissimum. 8°. *Bonnæ ad Rhenum,* 1828.

WEDEKIND (J. G.) * De cyclopia. 4°. *Groningæ,* 1830.

Adam (M.) A case of a malformed male fœtus, born at the full time. Month. J. M. Sc., Lond. & Edinb., 1853, xvii, 191.—**Adams** (W. W.) Fœtal malformation. Northwest. M. & S. J., Chicago 1856-7, xiii, 215-217.—**Adamson** (T. J.) A singular case of infant monstrosity. Med. Counsellor, Columbus, 1856, ii, 313-315.—**Ahlfeld.** Ueber Schmauzengeburten beim Menschen. Arch. f. Gynaek., Berl., 1877, xii, 159-162, 1 pl.—**Albrecht** (J. S.) De fœtu abortivo, scroti virilis nævum in nucha gæstante. Acta Acad. nat. curios., Norimb., 1733, iii, 290-292.—**Allan** (R.) Dissection of a human astomatous cyclops. Lancet, Lond., 1848, i, 227.—**Allen** (Z.) A case from practice. Illinois M. Recorder, Vandalia, 1878-9, i, 251.—**Allouneau** (A.) Observation sur une anencéphalie compliquée d'amyélée suivie de réflexions sur cette monstruosité. J. compl. du dict. d. sc. méd , Par., 1829, xxxiii, 169-181.—**de Alquen.** Fall eines vollständigen Anencephalus. N. Jahrb. d. teutsch. Med. u. Chir., Hamm, 1825, x, 1. St., 77-79.—**An-**

Monsters *from defect or malformation of brain, cranium, or face.*

drew (W.) Monstrous female fœtus. Lancet, Lond., 1838-9, i, 332.—**Anselin.** Observation sur un enfant dont la tête étoit monstrueuse. J. de méd., chir., pharm., etc., Par., 1771, xxxv, 336-341.—**Arellano** (A.) Una niña monstruosa. Periód. Acad. de med. de Mégico, 1839-40, iv, 389-392, 1 pl.—**Arloing.** Monstruosités de la famille des cyclocéphaliens et des genres ethnocéphale et rhinocéphale. Mém. et compt.-rend. Soc. d. sc. méd. de Lyon (1867), 1868, vii, 338.—**Arnold.** Beschreibung einer merkwürdigen Missgeburt. Med. Cor.-Bl. d. württemb. ärztl. Ver., Stuttg., 1834, iii, 165.—**Arnold** (J.) Beschreibung einer Missbildung mit Agnathie und Hydropsie der gemeinsamen Schlundtrommelhöhle. Arch. f. path. Anat., etc., Berl., 1867, xxxviii, 145-172, 2 pl.—**Arnott** (J.) Case of supposed prolonged gestation and monstrosity. Tr. M. & Phys. Soc. Bombay (1882), 1883, [3.] s., ii, 91-93.—**Atkin** (J. M.) Case of an encephalic monstrosity. Dublin M. Press, 1857, xxxvii, 101.—**Atlee** (W. F.) Account of a monster of the genus peracephalus. Am. J. M. Sc., Phila., 1858, n. s., xxxv, 370-373.—**Bacqué** (J.) Observation d'une fille née au terme de neuf mois, portant un vice de conformation du crâne, privée de cerveau, de cervelet et de moelle allongée. Ann. Soc. de méd.-prat. de Montpel., 1806, viii, 64-69.—**Bailey** (F. A.) Case of a monstrosity. [Acrania.] Proc. Oregon M. Soc., Portland, 1881, viii, 81.—**Bailly** [*et al.*]. Rapport de la commission chargée d'examiner le monstre envoyé par M. le docteur Cambray. Bull. méd. du nord, Lille, 1846-8, i, 164-166.—**Baker** (L. W.) Case of monstrosity. Am. J. M. Sc., Phila., 1862, n. s., xliv, 278.—**Bambaren.** Descripcion de un monstruo ciclocefaliano, del género de etnocéfalos. Gac. med. de Lima, 1860-61, v-vi, 125-128, 1 pl.—**Bang** (J.) De monstro Hafniæ 1767 nato. Soc. med. Havn. collect., 1774, i, 92-94, 1 pl.—**Bardinet** (A.) Observations tératologiques. Bull. Soc. anat. de Par., 1838, xiii, 196-264.—**Baudry.** Fœtus monstrueux. *Ibid.*, 1874, xliv, 312.—**Bayle.** Lettre contenant la description d'un fœtus venu au monde vivant, dans lequel on n'a point trouvé de cerveau. J. de méd., chir., pharm., etc., Par., 1766, xxv, 518-522.—**Beadle.** Anencephalous fœtus. N. York J. M., 1846, vi, 22.—**Beardsley** (A.) Birth of an acranial fœtus; with an account of the dissection. Med. Times & Gaz., Lond., 1856, n. s., xii, 200.—**Beauchamp** (J. F.) Fœtus with absence of cranial bones. Am. J. M. Sc., Phila., 1870, n. s., lix, 571.—**Beauchêne** fils. Description du squelette d'un enfant hydrocéphale offrant une conformation singulière de la partie inférieure du tronc. Bull. Fac. de méd. de Par. (1809-11), 1812, ii, 27-29.—**Béclard.** Rapport sur un cas de monstruosité. *Ibid.*, 1812-13, iii, 229-232.—**Belhomme.** Observation d'ectrogénie asymétrique. Bull. Soc. méd.-prat. de Par., 1847, 22-31. *Also,* Reprint.—**Bellouard** (V.) Fœtus anencéphale. Bull. Soc. anat. de Par., 1877, lii, 114. *Also:* Progrès méd., Par., 1877, v, 353.—**Beltran** (J. A.) Teratologia y parto prematuro, producido por una contusion abdominal, con expulsion de un feto que contiene un ojo en la parte media é inferior de la cara, y los pabellones del oido en la parte superior de la region cervical anterior. Génio méd.-quir., Madrid, 1880, xxvi, 258.—**Benda.** Demonstration eines Falles von Hyperrhinencephalie. Berl. klin. Wchnschr., 1886, xxiii, 889.—**Bernier.** Lusus naturæ. Union méd. du Canada, Montréal, 1876, v, 249.—**Bertrand** (P.) & **Fricant** (A.) Observation sur une conception extraordinaire. Précis d. trav. Soc. méd. de Boulogne-sur-Mer, 1836-9, 167-169.—**Beschreibung** eines monströsen Fötus. Museum d. Heilk., Zürich, 1794, ii, 204-211, 2 pl.—**Beuttenmüller.** Monstrositäten an Neugebornen beobachtet. Med. Cor.-Bl. d. württemb. ärztl. Ver., Stuttg., 1832-3, i, 188.—**Billaudeau.** Monstre rhinocéphale. Rev. phot. d. hôp. de Par., 1873, v, 143, 2 pl.—**Bimar.** Note sur un monstre pseudencéphalien. Gaz. hebd. d. sc. méd. de Montpel., 1886, viii, 349; 385.—**Blackshear** (J. E.) A monstrosity. Atlanta M. & S. J., 1887, n. s., iv, 203.—**Blandin** (F.) Description d'un anencéphale, suivie de quelques réflexions sur les causes de l'anencéphalie. J. hebd. de méd., Par., 1828, i, 107-114.—**Blot** (H.) Note sur un exemple remarquable de notencéphale compliqué de spina bifida. Union méd., Par., 1849, iii, 441.—**Borrichius** (O.) Monstrum Liundbyense. Acta med. et phil. Hafn. (1673), 1675, ii, 158-160.—**Bouchardus** (F.) De infante monstroso Lugduni in viam publicam, die v Martii a. 1671 exposito. Misc. Acad. nat. curios. 1672, Lips. et Francof., 1681, iii, 14-16. *Also, transl.:* Auserl. med.-chir. . . . Abhandl. d. röm.-kais. Akad. d. Naturf., Nürnb., 1756, iii, 21-23, 1 pl.—**Bouillé.** Note sur un fœtus anencéphale. Bull. Acad. de méd., Par., 1843-4, ix, 115-118.—**Bouillet.** Observation d'un cas d'anencéphalie. Expérience, Par., 1843, xii, 273.—**Bourneville.** Anencéphalie. Rev. phot. d. hôp. de Par., 1870, ii, 31-33.—**Bouteillier** (J.) Monstre humain pseudencéphalien, genre nosencéphale; arrêt de développement de la face; déplacement herniaire des viscères thoraciques et abdominaux. Union méd., Par., 1868. 3. s., v, 570.—**Boyce** (L. R.) Anencephalic monster. Tr. M. Soc. County Albany (1870-80), 1883, iii, 108.—**Bradley.** Arrest of develop-

ment; the facial bones entirely absent, and the thigh bones and bones of the fore arm rudimentary. Brit. M. J., Lond., 1871, i, 508.—**Brainard** (D.) Account of an anencephalous fœtus, with an unusual malformation of the heart. Illinois M. & S. J., Chicago, 1844-5, i, 22-24.—**Bramwell** (B.) Photographs of a case of cyclopean monstrosity. Edinb. M. J., 1880-81, xxvi, 550, 1 pl.—**Brechtfeld** (J. H.) Sur un monstre né à Systoft dans un canton de Danemark. Collect. acad. d. mém., etc., Dijon, 1766, vii, 384.—**Breed** (J. E.) Case of monstrosity; deficiency of posterior parts of cranium and spinal column; deformity of genital organs, etc. Am. J. M. Sc., Phila., 1849, n. s., xviii, 408-410.—**Brenzinger.** Eine Missgeburt. Aerztl. Mitth. a. Baden, Karlsruhe, 1877, xxxi, 43-46.—**Breschet** (G.) Notice sur deux enfans nouveau-nés hydrocéphales et manquant de cerveau. J. compl. du dict. d. sc. méd., Par., 1822, xiii, 202-206. *Also:* J. de physiol. expér., Par., 1822, ii, 269-276.—**Breus** (C.) Geburt einer Missbildung: Hernia funiculi umbilicalis, Hydrocephalus. Wien. med. Wchnschr., 1881, xxxi, 300-302.—**Broca** (P.-P.) Rapport sur quelques monstruosités. Bull. Soc. anat. de Par., 1849, xxiv, 292-306. ———. Sur un fœtus exencéphale. Bull. Soc. d'anthrop. de Par., 1879, 3. s., ii, 467.—**Browning** (W. G.) Case of premature labor; fœtal malformation. Cincin. Lancet & Obs., 1859, ii, 213-218. — **Brück** (A. T.) Psychische Bildungs-Rückschritte in Verbindung mit Skeletabnormitäten. Wchnschr. f. d. ges. Heilk., Berl., 1834, 49-56.—**Bruneel.** Trois monstres anencéphales mis au monde par la même mère. Ann. Soc. méd.-chir. de Bruges, 1854, 2. s., ii, 73-84.—**Büttner** (C. G.) Wahrnemung von der besondern Beschaffenheit eines den 19. Oct. 1752, allhie todtgebornen Kindes, weiblichen Geschlechts, welches, nebst einem vorhero lebendig gebornen Knäblein, in Mutterleibe zwar seine vollkommene Reife am Körper und andern Gliedmassen erhalten, aber am Kopf keine Hirnschaal, auch kein grosses noch kleines Gehirn gehabt. *In his:* Anat. Wahrnehm., 4°, Königsb., 1769, 92-109. ———. Beweiss, dass ein Kind ohne Hirnschaal, grossem und kleinem Gehirn, lebendig geboren werden, und einige Stunden leben könne. *Ibid.*, 109-121. ———. Anatomische Wahrnehmungen von einer ohne Kopf, Arme und innern Eingeweiden gebornen Missgeburt. *Ibid.*, 188-202, 1 pl.—**Buffiere.** A child born without a brain. Phil. Tr., Lond., 1700, iii, 26.—**Burns** (W.) Cyclopean monstrosity. Boston M. & S. J., 1863, lxviii, 153.—**Burt** (W. J.) Case of ectrogenesis. Daniel's Texas M. J., Austin, 1885, i, 73.—**Busey** (S. C.) Congenital hydrocephalus, hernia cerebri, spina bifida, cranio-tabes. Tr. M. Soc. Dist. Columb., Wash., 1876, iii, 40.—**Cairns.** Anencephalous fœtus. Obst. J. Gr. Brit., Lond., 1875-6, iii, 55.—**Calori** (L.) Storia di un mostro umano anencefalo con imperforazione del naso e con labbro leporino mediano complicato. Mem. d. Soc. med.-chir. di Bologna, 1838, 2. s., i, 193-223, 1 pl. ———. Descrizione anatomica di un mostro umano exencefalo. *Ibid.*, 297-317, 3 pl. ———. Descrizione anatomica di un iperencefalo umano. *Ibid.*, 417-438, 4 pl. ———. Sopra un mostro umano rinocefalico e pseudencefalico ad un tempo (rhinopseudencephalus). *Ibid.*, 531-557, 3 pl. ———. Di un porencefalo umano singolare per alcune parti soprannumerarie simbianti a dermocimache. Mem. Accad. d. sc. d. Ist. di Bologna, 1880, 4. s., ii, 27-36, 1 pl.—**Campá.** Una monstruosidad obstetricia. Independ. méd., Barcel., 1871-2, iii, 54. ———. Monstruo exencefálico-celosomiano. Crón. méd., Valencia, 1883-4, vii, 449-460. ———. Cuatro palabras más sobre el monstruo exencefálico-celosomiano. *Ibid.*, 481-486. *Also:* Med. contemp., Madrid, 1884, i, 291-295.—**Campbell** (W.) An account of malformation of the head, cervical spine, diaphragm, etc. Edinb. M. & S. J., 1830, xxxiv, 109.—**Candela.** Un caso de celosoma exencefálico. Progreso ginec., Valencia, 1884, i, 49-61.—**Caradec.** Relation d'un cas de monstruosité; monstre cyclocéphale anopse. Compt. rend. Soc. de biol. 1866, Par., 1867, 4. s., iii, pt. 2, 117-126. *Also:* Gaz. méd. de Par., 1867, 3. s., xxii, 42-45. *Also* [Abstr.]: Compt. rend. Acad. d. sc., Par., 1866, lxiii, 806-808.—**Carafi** (J.-M.) Monstre anencéphale présentant plusieurs vices de conformation; bec de lièvre commissural génial à gauche; bec de lièvre latéral; coloboma de la paupière inférieure et de l'iris à droite. Bull. Soc. anat. de Par., 1881, lvi, 733-736. *Also:* Progrès méd., Par., 1882, x, 618.—**Carlyle.** Casts of the head of an anencephalous fœtus, with description of the labour. Tr. Obst. Soc. Lond. (1869), 1870, xi, 35-37.—**Castelin.** Observation d'un monstre exencéphalien. Bull. méd. du nord, Lille, 1846-8, i, 60-62.—**Cazeaux** (P.) Description d'un monstre peracéphale, suivie de quelques réflexions sur le mécanisme de la circulation dans cette espèce de monstruosité. Compt. rend. Soc. de biol. 1851, Par., 1852, iii, pt., 211-220. *Also:* Gaz. méd. de Par., 1853, 3. s., viii, 422-424.—**Cerutti** (L.) Beschreibung einer seltenen Missgeburt, welche sich in der Sammlung des anatomischen Theaters zu Leipzig befindet. Arch. f. Anat. u. Physiol., Leipz., 1828, 192-208, 2 pl. — **Chailly-Honoré.** Fœtus anencéphale monstrueux, extrait par la section du col, d'une épaule, et

Monsters *from defect or malformation of brain, cranium, or face.*

l'aplatissement de la poitrine à l'aide du céphalotribe, chez une fille primipare de 43 ans, dont le bassin est rétréci. Bull. Acad. de méd., Par., 1842-3, viii, 879-883. *Also,* Reprint.—**Chamberlain** (W. M.) An anencephalic monster. N. York M. J., 1883, xxxvii, 93.—**Chantreuil.** Monstre anencéphale. Bull. Soc. anat. de Par., 1868, xliii, 111-115. — **Charlier** (E.) Observation d'un monstre humain pseudencéphale. Ann. Soc. méd. chir. de Liége, 1865, iv, 241-263. ———. Observation d'un monstre humain notencéphale. *Ibid.*, 287-301, 1 pl.—**Charrin.** Fœtus anencéphale. Lyon méd., 1873, xiii, 223-226. *Also:* Mém. Soc. d. sc. méd. de Lyon (1873), 1874, xiii, pt. 2, 60-63. — **Chilianus** (L. B.) Monstrosus fœtus. Misc. Acad. nat. curios. 1682, Norimb., 1683, decuria 2, i, 356, 1 pl. — **Clark** (R. O.) Anencephaloid fœtus. Med. Times & Gaz., Lond., 1866, ii, 408.—**Clark** (W. E. C.) Case of monstrosity. Glasgow M. Exam., 1831-2, i, 210. — **Claus** (E.) Anencephalie (Hemicephalie) eines künstlich entwickelten Kindes. Ztschr. d. nordd. Chir.- Ver., Magdeb., 1847, i, 591-597. — **Clauzure.** Note sur un monstre à tête de cyclope. Rev. méd. franç. et étrang., Par., 1830, ii, 59.—**Cleland.** On the brain in cyclopians. J. Anat. & Physiol., Lond., 1877-8, xii, 518-525, 1 pl.— **Clericus.** Puella sine cerebro nata. [Cum dissertatione in præcedentem historiam Des-Noves.] Zodiacus med.-gall. 1681, Geneva, 1682, iii, 54-57. — **Clermont.** Observation de fœtus notencéphale. Mém. et compt.-rend. Soc. d. sc. méd. de Lyon, 1866-7, vi, 17-25. *Also:* Gaz. méd. de Lyon, 1866, xviii, 332-335.—**Clippinger** (H. G.) An anencephalus monster. Med. & Surg. Reporter, Phila., 1879, xl, 152.—**Close** (T.) Singular monstrosity; with a single eye-ball! Boston M. Intellig., 1825-6, iii, 71. — **Cohen & Durr.** Case of monstrosity. Charleston M. J. & Rev., 1852, vii, 67.—**Colleville** (G.) Fœtus de 6 mois ½; monstre exancéphalien. Bull. Soc. anat. de Par., 1883, lviii, 213-215. *Also:* Progrès méd., Par., 1883, xi, 974. — **Collomb** (B.) Observation sur un enfant monstrueux. *In his:* Œuvres méd.-chir., 8°, Lyon, 1798, 458-463. *Also, transl.:* Arch. f. d. Physiol., Halle, 1800, iv, 213-219.— **Comucci** (E.) Di un mostro emicefalo nato nella clinica ostetrica di S. Maria Nuova di Firenze. Gazz. med. ital. feder. tosc., Firenze, 1852, 2. s., ii, 282-285. -- **Cone & Mott.** Case of monstrosity. Buffalo M. J., 1851-2, vii, 476-478. — **Conspectus** historiarum notabiliorum sine cerebro et calvaria natorum. Acta med. Berolin. 1721, viii, 13-21.—**Coote** (H.) Upon the cranial bones of the anencephalous fœtus. Med. Times & Gaz., Lond., 1852, n. s., iv, 488-490.— **Corson** (E. R.) Note on a curious malformation in an infant. Homœop. Times, N. Y., 1880-81, viii, 177—**Cotting.** Malformation. Boston M. & S. J., 1855, lii, 300.—**Craig** (W.) & **Symington** (J.) Case of a full-grown male fœtus, exhibiting the rare malformation of a cyclops. Tr. Med.-Chir. Soc. Edinb., 1885-6, n. s., v, 178-182, 1 pl. *Also:* Edinb. M. J., 1886-7, xxxii, 193-197, 1 pl.— **Credé** (S. C. F.) Eine Missbildung durch amniotische Fäden und Bänder. Monatschr. f. Geburtsk. u. Frauenkr., Berl., 1869, xxxiii, 441-457, 1 pl. — **Cremer.** Monophthalmos. Gen.-Ber. d. k. rhein. Med.-Coll. 1834, Koblenz, 1837, 217.—**Culver** (E. V.) On a case of monstrosity. South. M. & S. J., Augusta, 1852, n. s., viii, 604-606.—**Curran** (J. W.) Case of monstrosity dependent on mental shock. Brit. M. J., Lond., 1867, ii, 468.— **Dalton** (J. C.) Case of malformation of the cranium, encephalon, and spinal cord. Am. J. M. Sc., Phila., 1850, n. s., xix, 340-350. — **Dantscher.** Beschreibung eines menschlichen Cyclops. Oesterr. med. Wchnschr., Wien, 1847, 801-808. — **Danyau.** Anencéphalie avec tumeur sur la région fronto-pariétale; bride membraneuse partant de cette tumeur et allant s'enrouler autour de la jambe gauche; section incomplète de ce membre; insertion de cette bride sur la face fœtale du placenta; autopsie. Bull. Soc. de chir. de Par. (1861), 1862, 2. s., ii, 423-429. *Also:* Gaz. d. hôp., Par., 1861, xxxiv, 345.—**Dareste** (C.) Sur le mode de formation des monstres anencéphales. Compt. rend. Acad. d. sc., Par., 1866, lxiii, 448-451. ———. Mémoire sur le mode de formation des monstres anencéphales. Compt. rend. Soc. de biol. 1866, Par., 1867, 4. s., iii, 109-112. ———. Recherches sur le mode de formation de la cyclopie. Compt. rend. Acad. d. sc., Par., 1877, lxxxiv, 1038-1041. ———. Sur un nouveau type de la monstruosité simple, l'omphalocéphalie, ou hernie ombilicale de la tête. *Ibid.*, 1075-1077. ———. Recherches sur le mode de formation des monstres otocéphaliens. *Ibid.*, 1880, xc, 191-193.— **Davaine** & **Robin** (U.-M.) Observations pour servir à l'histoire de quelques monstruosités de la face. Compt. rend. Soc. de biol. 1849, Par., 1850, i, 43-51. *Also:* Gaz. méd. de Par., 1849, 3. s., iv, 903-906. — **Debierre** (C.) Sur un monstre cyclocéphalien du genre rhinencéphale. Compt. rend. Soc. de biol., Par., 1886, 8. s., iii, 184-186. — **Defilippi.** Fœtus humain dépourvu d'encéphale et de moelle-épinière ou fœtus amil-acéphale. Gaz. hebd. de méd., Par., 1855, ii, 552.— **De-Kegulas.** Περί τέρατος τινος. Ἰατρικὴ Μέλισσα, Ἀθῆναι, 1858-9, vi, 130.—**Delacour** (C.) Note sur un cas de monstruosité du genre paracéphale (classe des acépha-

liens). Gaz. d. hôp., Par., 1858, xxxi, 483.— **Delore** (X.) Note sur un fœtus notencéphale. Mém. et compt.-rend. Soc. d. sc. méd. de Lyon, 1866-7, vi, 241. *Also:* Gaz. méd. de Lyon, 1867, xix, 110. —. Monstre paracéphalien omocéphale. Mém. et compt.-rend. Soc. d. sc. méd. de Lyon (1867), 1868, vii, 248-252. ———. Monstre pseudo-encéphalien. *Ibid.*, 306.—**Delorenzi** (G.) Osservazioni intorno al cervello e al cranio di due microcefali. Gior. d. r. Accad. di med. di Torino, 1874, 3. s., xv, 567; 612, 1 pl.— **Deluen** (L.) Observation d'un enfant monstrueux. J. de la sect. de méd. Soc. acad. Loire-Inf., Nantes, 1845, xxi, 107-119. — **Del-Vesco** (P.) Otto parti di bambini anencefali. Gazz. med. ital., prov. venete, Padova, 1859, ii, 149.—**Dendy.** Cat-head monster. Med. Times & Gaz., Lond., 1853, n. s., vi, 483.— **Deroubaix.** Observations sur un monstre anencéphale, présentant une incurvation remarquable du rachis, une soudure de plusieurs côtes, et un pied-bot. Ann. de méd. belge, Brux., 1840, iii, 93-98.— **Destrés.** Description d'un anencéphale, avec disposition anormale des viscères principaux. Tr. méd., Par., 1833, xii, 359-367. — **Deydier.** Histoire d'une fausse-couche singulière, suivie peu de tems après d'une grossesse extraordinaire. Rec. périod. d'obs. de méd., de chir. et pharm., Par., 1757, vi, 410-421. — **Dick** (W.) Case of hyperencephalous monstrosity, conjoined with other monstrous formations. Lond. M. Gaz., 1836-7, xix, 897-899.— **Dickinson** (W. H.) Description of a fœtus born without heart, brain, lungs, or liver. Med.-Chir. Tr., Lond., 1863, xlvi, 141-148, 2 pl. — **Dolignon.** Observation sur un enfant monstrueux auquel manquoient le cerveau et le crâne. J. de méd., chir., pharm., etc., Par., 1786, lxvi, 91-94.—**Duane** (W. N.) Description of a human monster. Am. J. M. Sc., Phila., 1829-30, v, 377-379.—**Dubois** (E.) [Un cas d'anencéphale.] Bull. Soc. anat. de Par., 1847, xxii, 441-445.—**Dufour.** Mémoire concernant un fœtus qui a été tiré du sein de sa mère, au terme de huit mois et demi, et qui a été trouvé sans cerveau, cervelet, moëlle allongée, et même sans celle de l'épine. J. de méd., chir., pharm., etc., Par., 1771, xxxv, 325-336.—**Dugès** (A.) Mémoire sur les altérations intra-utérines de l'encéphale et de ses enveloppes. Éphém. méd. de Montpel., 1826, i, 292: ii, 132; 275, 1 pl. ———. Observations de monopsie et d'aprosopie. Rev. méd. franç. et étrang., Par., 1827, iv, 407-447.—**Dulles** (C. W.) Note on a case of anencephalous monster. Maryland M. J., Balt., 1886-7, xvi, 135.—**Duméril.** Rapport fait sur une demande de son excellence le ministre de l'intérieur, relatif à un enfant monstrueux. Bull. Fac. de méd. de Par., 1809-11, ii (6. année), 23.—**Dumont-Pallier.** Fœtus anencéphale. Bull. Soc. anat. de Par., 1856, xxxi, 245. ———. Observation d'un monstre de la famille des pseudencéphaliens, genre nosencéphale de M. Geoffroy-Saint-Hilaire. Compt. rend. Soc. de biol. 1856, Par., 1857, 2. s., iii, 167-170.— **Duncan** (J. M.) A dissection of a monstrous fœtus with distended abdomen. Edinb. M. J., 1870, xvi, 163-167. ———. Some points ascertained in the dissection of an anencephalous fœtus; with preparation. Tr. Edinb. Obst. Soc. (1871-4), 1875, iii, 72-74.—**Dupré** (L.) Monstre anencéphale. Montpel. méd., 1878, lx, 429-434, 2 pl.—**Duval** (M.) Sur un monstre otocéphale. Compt. rend. Soc. de biol. 1881, Par., 1882, 7. s., iii, 145-147. *Also:* Gaz. méd. de Par., 1881, 6. s., iii, 255. — Nouvelle communication sur un monstre otocéphale. Compt. rend. Soc. de biol., Par., 1883, 7. s., iv, 253.—**Duvernoy** (J. G.) Beschreibung einer Missgeburt in Casan. Phys. u. med. Abhandl. d. k. Akad. d. Wissensch. in Petersb., Riga, 1782, i, 410-422.—**Egelston** (J. Q.) Labor complicated with monstrosity. Iowa M. J., Keokuk, 1854-5, ii, 12-14.—**Einem** (Von) monströsen Fœtu. Samml. v. Nat.- u. Med.. . . . Gesch. 1720, Leipz. u. Budissin, 1722, xiii, 328-330.—**Eller.** Description d'un monstre cyclope mis au monde à Berlin le 19 de février de l'année 1755. Rec. périod. d'obs. de méd., de chir. et pharm., Par., 1757, vi, 347-360. *Also:* Mém. Acad. roy. de Prusse, Avignon, 1768, iv, 167-189, 8 pl. *Also:* Collect. acad. d. mém., etc., Par., 1770, ix, 24-32, 8 pl.— **Elsässer.** Angeborener Wasserkopf (Acranios). Med. Cor.-Bl. d. württemb. ärztl. Ver., Stuttg., 1850, xx, 65.—**English** (F. E.) Case of monstrosity. Chicago M. J., 1874, xxxi, 213-215.—**Eustache** (G.) Études tératologiques; mémoire sur un fœtus dérencéphale (de la famille des anencéphaliens). J. d. sc. méd. de Lille, 1878-9, i, 166-190, 1 pl. *Also.* Reprint. *Also:* Arch. de tocol., Par., 1879, vi, 84-107, 1 pl. ———. Études de tératologie humaine, fœtus cyclope et fœtus acéphale. Arch. de tocol., Par., 1884, xi, 309-326. *Also:* J. d. sc. méd. de Lille, 1884, vi, 473; 568.—**Facen** (J.) Osservazione teratologica. Gior. veneto di sc. med., Venezia, 1859, 2. s., xiii, 765.—**Faréon.** Un monstre. Union méd. de la Louisiane, N.-Orl., 1852, i, 83.—**Fede & Armanni.** Di un nuovo mostro per raro caso di idromeningocele cefalo-rachidiano. Ann. clin. d. osp. incur., Napoli, 1877, n. s., ii, 214-232, 2 pl.—**Fenton.** Case of anencephalous monster. Month. J. M. Sc., Lond. & Edinb., 1852, xv, 170.—**Fernet.** [Un fœtus monstrueux mort né, qui présente des vices de conformation multiples.] Bull. Soc. anat. de Par., 1864, xxxix,

Monsters *from defect or malformation of brain, cranium, or face.*

130.— **Ferrandi** (A.) Feto mostruoso ottimestre, di sesso femineo, mancante della volta del cranio, del braccio destro, di parte del costato e delle pareti abdominali. Gazz. med. ital. lomb., Milano, 1857, 4. s., ii, 27.—[**Finn** (W. H.)] Anencephalic fœtus born at full term. Proc. Path. Soc. Phila. (1866-70), 1871, iii, 137.—**Firor**·(S. V.) Case of anencephalous monster. Am. Pract., Louisville, 1872, vi, 354-356.—**Fitzpatrick** (J.) Account of a case of monstrosity. N. York M. & Phys. J., 1826, v, 317-319.—**Folet** (H.) Sur le vice de conformation d'un monstre anencéphalien. Bull. méd. du nord, Lille, 1869, x, 129-135.—**Foot** (A. W.) Remarks upon a fœtus with hernia cerebri; complete fissure of the spinal column, and absence of the spinal cord (amyelia). Med. Press, Dubl., 1865, 2. s., xi, 435 - 438. ——. Report of the dissection of a monster. Dublin Q. J. M. Sc., 1867, xliv, 251-253.— **Foucher** (A.) Cas de notencéphalie. Abeille méd., Montréal, 1879, i, 30-33.—**Fouilloux.** Monstre acéphale pseudencéphalien. Bull. Soc. anat. de Par., 1869, xliv, 180.—**Francis** (D. J. T.) A short account of a one-eyed human monster. Lond. M. Gaz., 1844, xxxiv, 580-582.— **Frantz** (J. G.) Beschrijving eener vrouwelijke misgeboorte. Nederl. Tijdschr. v. Geneesk., Amst., 1860, iv, 273 - 275.— **Gacon.** Description d'un enfant monstrueux. J. de méd., chir., pharm., etc., Par., 1773, xxxix, 42 - 45.— **Gadaud.** Crâne de fœtus thlipsencéphale. Bull. Soc. d'anthrop. de Par., 1868, 2. s., iii, 153-156.—**Gaddi** (P.) Mostruosità. Gazz. med. ital. lomb , Milano, 1855, 3. s., vi, 180.— **Galloupe** (I. F.) Combination of cyclopia and anterior hydrencephalocele. Boston M. & S. J., 1880, cii, 135. ——. Cyclops, with anterior hydrencephalocele *Ibid.*, 495.—**Gandy.** Observation sur un enfant né, au terme de neuf mois, sans cerveau, ni cervelet, ni moëlle allongée. Hist. Soc. de méd.·prat. de Montpel., 1806, xv, 330-333.—**Garbiglietti** (A.) & **Moriggia** (A.) Descrizione di celosomo dirino con exencefalia idrocefalica. Gior. d. r. Accad. di med. di Torino, 1870, 3. s., ix, 65 - 74, 1 pl. *Also,* Reprint.— **Garmann** (C. F.) De mentula ex capite. Misc. Acad. nat. curios. 1672, Lips. et Francof., 1681, iii, 61-63. *Also, transl.:* Auserl. med - chir.· · · . Abhandl. d. röm.·kais. Akad. d. Naturf., Nürnb., 1756, iii, 53-56, 1 pl.—**Garnett** (A. Y. P.) Cyclops monstrosity. Tr. M. Soc. Dist. Colomb., Wash., 1876, ii,83-90.—**Garrett** (J. W. B) Singular case of monstrosity. West. J. M. & S., Louisville, 1850, 3. s., vi, 1-6.— **Gauche**(P.) Note sur un cas d'anencéphalie. Ann. Soc. de méd. de St.-Étienne et de la Loire (1877-80), 1881, vii, 331-343.—**Geoffroy-Saint-Hilaire.** D'un nouvel anencéphale humain, sous le nom d'anencéphale de Patare, confirmant par l'autorité de ses faits la nouvelle théorie sur la formation des monstres, et fournissant de nouveaux élémens aux caractères de genre anencéphale. J. univ. d. sc. méd., Par., 1824, xxxvi, 129 - 151, 1 pl. ——. Sur l'anencéphale de Patare. *Ibid.*, 1825, xxxix, 257-267. ——. Sur des monstruosités humaines caractérisées par le défaut de moelle cérébro-spinale, et nommées anencéphales. Extrait d'un mémoire qui a paru dans les troisième et quatrième cahiers des Mémoires du Mus. d'hist. nat., tome 12, comprenant les pages 233-293. Arch. gén. de méd., Par., 1825, ix, 41-55. ——. Sur une monstruosité humaine d'un caractère encore inconnu. Rev. méd. franç. et étrang., Par., 1825, i, 372-377. *Also, transl.:* Arch. f. Anat. u. Physiol., Leipz., 1827, 323-328. ——. Rapport sur plusieurs monstruosités humaines anencéphaliques. Rev. méd. franç. et étrang., Par., 1827, i, 269-283.—**Geoffroy-Saint-Hilaire** (I.) Remarques générales sur les monstres anencéphaliens. Gaz. obst. et gynéc. de Par., 1875, iv, 211-215.—**Gintrac** (E.) Note sur un monstre exencéphalien (pleurencéphale). J. de méd. de Bordeaux, 1856, 2. s., i, 445-454. ——. Considérations sur la cyclocéphalie. *Ibid.*, 1860, 2. s., v, 153-167. *Also,* Reprint.—**Girolamo** (C.) Istoria di un mostro raniforme. *In:* Rac. d'opusc. scient. e filol., 16°, Venezia, 1729, ii, 469-490.— **Göller** (G. C.) Abortus humani monstrosi hist. anatom. Misc. Acad. nat. curios. 1683, Norimb., 1698, decuria 2, ii, 311-318, 1 pl. *Also, transl.:* Auserl. med.- chir.· · · . Abhandl. d. röm.·kais. Akad. d. Naturf., Nürnb., 1763, xii, 268-273, 1 pl.— **Goffart** (L.) Description de deux monstruosités humaines. Ann. Soc. méd.·chir. de Liége, 1862, i, 5-13.— **Golay** (E.) Fœtus hydrocéphale avec vices de conformation des quatre membres. Progrès méd., Par., 1876, iv, 512.—**Goode** (B. P.) Anencephalic fœtus. Cincin. Lancet & Clinic, 1881, n. s., vi, 566.—**Gosselin.** Examen d'un fœtus monstrueux anencéphale manquant de nez et d'yeux. Compt. rend. Soc. de biol. 1850, Par., 1851, ii, 177-180. ——. Description d'un fœtus cyclope. *Ibid.*, 1852, Par., 1853, iv, 28.—**Graham** (A.) A case of malformation. Brit. M. J., Lond., 1883, ii, 1125.—**Grammar** (R. B.) A wonderful monstrosity. Texas Cour.·Rec. Med., Fort Worth, 1884-5, ii, 153.—**Gramshaw** (F. S.) A veritable monster. Lancet, Lond., 1879, i, 467.—**Grattan** (E.) An anencephalous fœtus. Liverpool M. & S. Rep., 1871, v, 173.—**de Grazia y Alvarez** (A.) Exposicion abreviada de un hecho curioso para la historia de los vicios de conformacion. Siglo méd., Madrid, 1858, v, 370.—

Monsters *from defect or malformation of brain, cranium, or face.*

Greene (W. W.) Case of monstrosity. Penins. J. M., Ann Arbor, Mich., 1855-6, iii, 369.—**Greenhalgh.** Case of monstrosity. Lancet, Lond., 1844, ii, 411. -- **Gregory** (D. G.) A remarkable deformity in a human fœtus. West. J. M. & S., Louisville, 1845, 2. s., iv, 271.—**Gregory** (W.) An account of a monstrous fœtus, resembling a hooded monkey. Phil. Tr., Lond., 1732 - 44, viii - ix, 314-316.— **Griffith** (T.) Case of lusus naturæ. Phila. M. Museum (1807), 1808, iv, 252-254.—**Grillenzoni** (C. E.) Alcune osservazioni sopra un caso di emiaccefalia nella specie umana. Rendic. Accad. med.-chir. di Ferrara 1811, Bologna, 1843, 6 ; 65, 2 pl. [*See, also, supra.*]— **Gros.** [Monstre exencéphalien.] Mém. et compt -rend. Soc. d. sc. méd. de Lyon (1877), 1878, xvii, pt. 2, 151.— **Grosz** (L.) Cyclopie. Ztschr. f. Nat.- u. Heilk. in Ungarn, Oedenburg, 1857, viii, 34.—**Grüber** (J.) Mangel des Gehirns und Schädelgewölbes in einem erst nach vollendetem zehnten Schwangerschaftsmonate (Sonnenmonat) gebornen Kinde. Oesterr. med. Wchnschr., Wien, 1845, 864-866,—**Guelliot** (O.) Monstre nosencéphale. Union méd. et scient. du nord-est, Reims, 1883, vii, 185-189.— **Guillaumet.** Monstre pseudoanencéphale mort-né à neuf mois de grossesse, avec rupture spontanée de la poche sanguine avant la naissance. Bull. Soc. anat. de Par., 1874, xlix, 751-754.—**Guillot** (N.) Addition à l'histoire de la notencéphalie. Expérience, Par., 1838, ii, 497-506.— **Guthrie** (J.) Case of a newborn child, in which the brain and the greater part of the cranium were wanting. Edinb. M. & S. J., 1826, xxvi, 28.—**von Haartman** (C.) Ett missfoster, i flere afseenden märkvärdigt. Finska läk.-sällsk. handl., Helsingfors, 1841-3, i, 193-196, 1 pl.— **Habgood** (H.) Anencephalous monster ; curious family history. Brit. M. J., Lond., 1876, i, 505.—**Hadaway** (J.) Two cases of encephalon monsters. Lancet, Lond., 1862, ii, 646. — **Hall** (A. B.) Case of cyclopic malformation. Boston M. & S. J., 1861-2, lxv, 263. ——. Cases of cyclopic malformation. Brit.-Am. J., Montreal, 1861, ii, 485-488.—**Hallez.** Monstre pseudo-anencéphale. Bull. Soc. anat. de Par., 1868, xliii, 65.—**Hamilton** (J. A.) An anencephalous child. Louisville M. News, 1884, xviii, 410.—**Hamilton** (J. K.) Case of monstrosity. Atlanta M. & S. J., 1866-7, vii[b], 478-480.—**Hamilton** (P. J.) Monster with a head resembling a dog's. Northwest. M. & S. J., Chicago & Indianap., 1848-9, v, 455-457.—**Hamy** (E. T.) Monstre anencéphalien pseudencéphale, développement imparfait de la face. Bull. Soc. anat. de Par., 1869, xliv, 75. ——. Note sur un nouveau type de monstre exencéphalien. Compt. rend. Soc. de biol. 1874, Par., 1875, i, 6. s., 146-148. ——. Le nosencéphale pleurosome de Pondichéry. J. de l'anat. et physiol., etc., Par., 1874, x, 294-310, 1 pl.—**Hannover** (A.) Anencephaly. [Abstr. of original memoir, by J. F. Knott.] Dublin J. M. Sc., 1883,-lxxv, 396-401. [*See, also, supra.*] ——. Sur la structure du crâne humain dans l'anencéphalie, la cyclopie et la synotie et sur les rapports de ces monstruosités avec le cartilage primordial du crâne. [Abstr., transl] Cong. périod. internat. d. sc. méd. Compt.-rend. 1884, Copenh., 1886, i, Sect. de path. gén., etc., 71-87.—**Hard** (J.) A case of monstrosity ; a child with a dog's head. Chicago M. J. & Exam., 1884, xlviii, 246.—**Hargadine** (R. W.) Fœtal monstrosity. Am. J. M. Sc., Phila., 1870, n. s , lix, 135. *Also:* Proc. Path. Soc. Phila. (1866-70), 1871, iii, 135.— **Harrison** (E. B.) Case of monstrosity connected with dropsy of the amnion. West. Lancet, Cincin., 1855, xvi, 216-218.—**Hartshorne** (F. H.) Two cases of hemicephalous monsters. Assoc. M. J., Lond., 1856, 422. — **van Hasselt.** Fœtus pseudoanencéphale. Presse méd. belge, Brux., 1876-7, xxix, 251.—**Hathwell** (C. A.) Singular case of malformation. Northwest. M. & S. J., Chicago & Indianap., 1850 - 51, vii, 50-53.—**Hayem** (G.) & **Clado.** Un cas de monstruosité. Bull. Soc. anat. de Par., 1881, lvi, 742-744. *Also:* Progrès méd., Par., 1882, x, 632.— **Hecker** (C.) & **Buhl** (L.) Unvollkommene Cyklopie. Monatschr. f. Geburtsk. u. Frauenkr., Berl., 1868, xxxi, 430-433, 1 pl.—**Helie** (T.) Observation d'anencéphale. Rev. méd. franç. et étrang., Par., 1832, ii, 427-442.—**Henderson** (W. W.) A monstrosity. Obst. Gaz., Cincin., 1879-80, ii, 540-545.—**Hershey** (D. W.) A case of monstrosity. Kansas City M. J., 1874, iv, 137.—**Heyfelder.** Hémicéphalie compliquée avec l'absence de la voûte palatine et l'adhésion de l'arrière-faix à la tête de l'enfant (hyperencephalus ex conjunctione placentæ abnormi cum fœtus corpore, d'après Geoffroy). Rev. méd. franç. et étrang., Par., 1839, ii, 228-230.—**Heyman.** Vollkommener Monoculus (Cyclops). Deutsches Arch. f. d. Physiol., Halle, 1820, vi, 527-534, 1 pl.—**Highet** (J.) Curious monstrosity, accompanied by spontaneous expulsion of the placenta, without hæmorrhage. Lancet, Lond., 1878, i, 456.—**Hildreth** (C. T.) Case of notencephale. Med. Mag., Bost., 1834-5, iii, 3-16, 2 pl. *Also,* Reprint.—**Hinton** (J.) Case of monstrous birth. Assoc. M. J., Lond., 1863, 191.—**Hintz** (F. E. B.) Obstetrical anomaly. Balt. Month. J. M. & S., 1830-31, i, 493.—**Hird.** Anencephalous monstrosity. Med. Times, Lond., 1851, n. s., ii, 21.— **Hirigoyen** (L.) Observation d'un fœtus cynocéphalien.

Monsters *from defect or malformation of brain, cranium, or face.*

Mém. et bull. Soc. de méd. et chir. de Bordeaux, 1878, 225–238. *Also:* Gaz. méd. de Bordeaux, 1877, vii, 293; 306.—**Historia** eines Monstri. Samml. v. Nat.- u. Med.- . . . Gesch. 1717-18, Bresl., 1718-20, 85-87. — **Hittner** (H. M.) Description of a remarkable case of defective development; the subject, a child eight years of age; with a woodcut. Cincin. Lancet & Obs., 1865, viii, 592-594.—**Hodge** (H. L.) Pseudencephalous fœtus. Proc. Path. Soc. Phila. (1860-66), 1867, ii, 80. ———. Monstrosity. Tr. Path. Soc. Phila. (1871-3), 1874, iv, 233.—**Hofer** (J.) fils. Observatio monstri humani. Acta Helvet., Basileæ, 1758, iii, 366-369, 3 pl.—**Hoffman** (D. B.) A case of deformity in utero. Pacific M. & S. J., San Fran., 1867-8, x, 501-503. — **Hoffmann** (J. M.) De fœtu monstrosi. Misc. Acad. nat. curios. 1687, Norimb., 1707, decuria 2, vi, 333-336. *Also, transl.:* Auserl. med.- chir.- . . . Abhandl. d. röm.-kais. Akad. d. Naturf., Nürnb., 1767, xvi, 307-310, 1 pl.—**Hoffmann** (M.) Anatome partus cerebro carentis. Misc. Acad. nat. curios. 1671, Francof. et Lips., 1688, ii, 60-64. *Also, transl.:* Auserl. med.- chir.- . . . Abhandl. d. röm.-kais. Akad. d. Naturf., Nürnb., 1756, ii, 70-75, 1 pl.—**Hohl** (A.) Geschichte eines Microcephalen; seine Geburt, äussere Beschaffenheit und Erhaltung am Leben durch 70½ Stunde, nebst Zusätzen. Ztschr. f. Geburtsh. u. prakt. Med., Halle, 1828, i, 173-188. 2 pl.—**Holub** (F. J.) Merkwürdige Missgeburt. Vrtljschr. f. d. prakt. Heilk., Prag, 1846, i, 156 —**Hou** (J.) A case of anencephalia. Tr. Indiana M. Soc., Indianap., 1877, xxvii, 101.—**Houel.** [Un fœtus de huit mois qui présente plusieurs anomalies, savoir: Une hernie du cerveau et du cervelet; un développement incomplet de l'œil gauche; une éventration latérale, etc.] Bull. Soc. anat. de Par., 1849, xxiv, 217-220. ———. Description d'un nouveau genre de la famille des monstres paracéphaliens. *Ibid.*, 1850, xxv, 268-298. ———. Observation d'un monstre de la famille des pseudencéphaliens. Compt. rend. Soc. de biol. 1865, Par., 1866, 4. s., ii, pt. 2, 29-40. *Also:* Gaz. méd. de Par., 1866, 3. s., xxi, 90-94.—**Houel & Arnault.** Fœtus pseudencéphalien (genre nosencéphale). Bull. Acad. de méd., Par., 1857-8, xxiii, 298-302. — **Hubbard** (T. W.) Anencephalous fœtus. Brit. M. J., Lond., 1878, i, 752.— **Hubbauer** (O.) Beschreibung einer mittelst Perforation zur Welt beförderten Missgeburt. Ztschr. f. Wundärzte u. Geburtsh., Stuttg., 1858, xi, 115.— **Huber.** Ein Fall von Partus serotinus, nebst Notizen über Geburten hemicephalischer Früchte. Aerztl. Int.-Bl., München, 1874, xxi, 105.—**Hulme** (J. D.) Another monster. Lancet, Lond., 1864, ii, 481.—**Humes** (M. D.) Beiträge zur Lehre über die Entstehung der Exencephalie. Oesterr. Jahrb. f. Paediat. 1876, Wien, 1877, vii, 114-118, 1 pl. — **Hunt** (E. B.) An account of experiments and a post-mortem examination; illustrating the physiology of the excito-motor system of nerves. Buffalo M. J., 1853-4, ix, 183-185.—**Hunton** (A.) A case of monstrosity. North. Lancet, Plattsburgh, N. Y., 1851, iii, 92-94.—**Isaacs** (C. E.) Anencephalous fœtus. N. York J. M., 1850, [2.] s., iv, 330. — **Izquierdo** (G.) Abortos repetidos; feto monstruoso. Siglo méd., Madrid, 1861, viii, 116.—**Jackson** (J. B. S.) Monstrosity. Boston M. & S. J., 1859-60, lxi, 237. *Also:* Extr. Rec. Bost. Soc. M. Improve. (1859-61), 1862, iv, 61. ———. † Boston M. & S. J., 1865, lxxii, 82. *Also:* Extr. Rec. Bost. Soc. M. Improve. (1862-6), 1867, v, 164. ———. Anencephalous fœtus. Boston M. & S. J., 1865-6, lxxiii, 359. ———. Notencephalus. *Ibid.*, 1875, xcii, 599. ———. Rhinencephalus and some allied forms of monstrosity. *Ibid.*, 1878, xcviii, 66-73. *Also:* Extr. Rec. Bost. Soc. M. Improve. (1874-9), 1880, vii (app.), pp. xlii-xlix.—**Jacobæus** (M.) De monstro Norwegico. Acta med. et phil. Hafn. (1673), 1675, ii, 80, 3 pl.—**Jacobi.** Case of monopus. Am. J. Obst., N. Y., 1873-4, vi, 633. ———. Fœtal monstrosity. N. York M. J., 1875, xxi, 622.—**Jaeger** (G.) Beschreibung eines durch Vereinigung der Augenhöhlen, Mangel der Nase, Verkürzung des Oberkiefers und Aufwärtskrümmung des Unterkiefers missgebildeten Kopfes eines Lammes und einer Ziege. Arch. f. Anat. u. Physiol., Leipz., 1829, iv, 202-208. — **James** (C.) An anencephaloid monster. Tr. Obst. Soc. Lond. (1880), 1881, xxii, 241.—**Johnston** (C.) Description of a pseudencephalic monster. Am. J. M. Sc., Phila., 1862, n. s., xliv, 96-99.—**Joly** (N.) Études sur un monstre humain né à Toulouse, et affecté tout à la fois d'exencéphalie, de pied-bot, de polydactylie, d'hermaphrodisme et d'inversion splanchnique générale. France méd., Par., 1866, xiii, 343.—**Jones** (C. H.) Account of the dissection of a pseudencephalic fœtus. Lond. M. Gaz., 1846, n. s., xxxvii, 897-901, 1 pl.—**Jones** (E.) Anencephalous fœtus with spina bifida; history of a case. Tr. Obst. Soc. Lond. (1869), 1870, xi, 209. — **Josias.** Fœtus anencéphale. Bull. Soc. de méd. prat. de Par., 1859, 67-70.—**Joy** (J. H.) Case of twin pregnancy; birth of an anencephalous monster without arms, shoulders, or thorax. Lancet, Lond., 1872, i, 465.—**Juvet.** Observation sur un enfant monstrueux. J. de méd., chir., pharm., etc., Par., 1761, xiv, 244-248.—**Keen** (W. W.) Anencephalic fœtus born at full time. Proc. Path. Soc. Phila. (1866-70), 1871, iii, 137. *Also:* Am. J. M. Sc., Phila., 1870, n. s., lix, 408.—**Kennedy.** Small anen-

cephalic fœtus. Canada M. & S. J., Montreal, 1883-4, xii, 602-604.—**Kidd** (G. H.) Description of a monster by excess of development. Dublin Hosp. Gaz., 1856, n. s., iii, 82-84.—**Kildal** (S. N.) Beretning om den mærkelige Vanskabning eller Misfosteret Brede Norman Tanoen. Eyr, Christiania, 1835, x, 293-299.—**Kilian** (L. B.) Von einer Missgeburt. Auserl. med.- chir.- . . . Abhandl. d. röm.-kais. Akad. d. Naturf., Nürnb., 1762, xi, 196-198.—**Kilseil** (J.) Fœtal monstrosity. Prov. M. & S. J., Lond., 1850, 540.—**Költsch.** Ein Acranius mit Spina bifida und Exophthalmos. Monatschr. f. Geburtsk. u. Frauenkr., Berl., 1857, x, 19-22.—**Kraus** (J.) Ein Fall von Anencephalus. Allg. Wien. med. Ztg., 1866, xi, 272.—**Kretschmar** (O.) Hemicephalus. N. Ztschr. f. Geburtsk., Berl., 1848, xxv, 110-112.—**Krieg.** Geburt eines Hemicephalus. Wchnschr. f. d. ges. Heilk., Berl., 1843, 543-546.—**Krimer** (W.) Merkwürdige Missbildung bei einem Neugeborenen. J. f. Chir. u. Augenh., Berl., 1829, xiii, 609-611, 1 pl.—**Kundrat** (H.) Arhinencephalie als typische Art von Missbildung. Graz, 1882. Wien. med. Bl., 1882, v, 1395-1397.—**L.** (N.) Account of a male child born without a brain. Med. & Phys. J., Lond., 1815, xxxiv, 104-106.—**Labuze.** Fœtus mal conformés; absence de la voûte du crâne; exomphale. Bull. Soc. anat. de Par., 1870, xlv, 385.—**Lacroix** (E.) Observation d'un fœtus cyclope, suivie de considérations sur le nisus formativus. Tr. méd., Par., 1833, xiii, 141-156.—**Laforgue** (H.) Mémoire sur un cyclope rhinocéphale humain, né à Toulouse. J. de méd., chir. et pharm. de Toulouse, 1860, 3. s., v, 273-279.—**Lambert** (A.-P.) Observation sur un cas d'anencéphalie, causée probablement par une hydropisie des ventricules cérébraux. J. Soc. méd. de la N.-Orléans, 1839, i, 49; 99. — **Langlet.** Anencéphalie; sa production par l'hydrocéphalie. Bull. Soc. méd. de Reims (1876), 1877, xv, 180-184.—**Langston** (T.) Case of monstrosity; with specimen. Tr. Obst. Soc. Lond. (1868), 1869, x, 37.—**Lannelongue.** Bec-de-lièvre rare chez un monstre exencéphalien; à gauche, le bec-de-lièvre est latéral et étendu jusqu'à la paupière inférieure; à droite, il est commissural. Bull. et mém. Soc. de chir. de Par., 1881, n. s., vii, 483-488.—**Larcher** (O.) Cyclope, cyclopie. Dict. encycl. d. sc. méd., Par., 1880, xxiv, 538-545. — **Lardier** (E.) Naissance d'un monstre nosencéphalien (Geoffroy-Saint-Hilaire). Mém. Soc. de méd. de Nancy (1885-6), 1887, pp. xlviii-liv.— **Larsh** (N. B.) Akephaloid monster. Chicago M. J., 1870, xxvii, 205.—**Laurent.** Monstre anencéphalien. Bull. Soc. anat. de Par., 1881, lvi, 620. *Also:* Progrès méd., Par., 1882, x, 463.—**Lauwers** (E.) Un cas d'anencéphalie; remarques sur la genèse de l'hydramnios. Rev. méd., Louvain, 1885, iv, 241-247.—**de Lavergne.** Observation d'un enfant né sans cerveau. J. gén. de méd., chir. et pharm., Par., 1816, lvi, 175-177.—**Lavialle.** Sur un fœtus monstrueux. [Rap. de Baudelocque et Duportren.] Bull. Fac. de méd. de Par. (1804-8). 1812, i, 2. année, 201-207.—**Lawrence** (W.) Account of a child born without a brain, which lived four days. Med.-Chir. Tr., Lond., 1814, v, 165-224, 1 pl.—**Lebedeff** (A.) Ueber Entstehung der Anencephalie und Spina bifida bei Vögeln und Menschen. Tr. Internat. M. Cong., 7. sess., Lond., 1881, i, 178-181. — **Lecadre.** Remarques sur un cas d'anencéphalie. Rev. méd. franç. et étrang., Par., 1830, i, 433-440.— **Leclerc.** Monstre anencéphale. Mém. et compt.-rend. Soc. d. sc. méd. de Lyon (1885), 1886, xxv, pt. 2, 66.—**Ledel** (S.) De fœtu monstroso. Misc. Acad. nat. curios. 1687, Norimb., 1707, vi, 152.—**Lee** (C. A.) Monstrosity; fœtus born at the full period; lived but a few minutes. Am. J. M. Sc., Phila., 1835-6, xvii, 65.—**Lee** (R.) Account of a fœtus of 7 months, with its placenta partially adherent to a nævus occupying the scalp and dura mater. Med.-Chir. Tr., Lond., 1839, xxii, 300-309.— **von Lenhossék.** Beschreibung einer menschlichen Missgeburt mit einem Auge und andern merkwürdigen Deformitäten des Kopfs. N. Jahrb. d. teutsch. Med. u. Chir., Bonn, 1621, iii. 1-17, 1 pl.—**Levy** (C. E.) Beschreibung einer Missgeburt mit vollständiger Wirbelspalte und einem Darmbruche in der Rückgrathshöhle. Arch. f. Anat., Physiol. u. wissensch. Med., Berl., 1845, 22-33, 2 pl.—**Lichliter** (D. C.) An anencephalic monster. Cincin. Lancet & Clinic, 1881, vi, 493-495.—**Linck** (J. H.) Fœtus humanus monstrosus similitudinem leonis habere, sed perperam, putatus. Acta Acad. nat. curios., Norimb., 1727, i, 128-133, 1 pl.—**Littré.** Sur un fétus monstrueux qui n'avoit qu'un œil. [*From:* Hist. d. mém. Acad. roy. d. sc. de Par., 1717.] Collect. acad. d. mém., etc. Partie franç., Par. et Liége, 1770, iv, 468.—**Llave** (A.) Niño monstruo. Anfiteatro anat., Madrid, 1874, ii, 62.—**Löw** (A.) Fœtus, qua caput. monstrosus. Misc. Acad. nat. curios. 1690, Norimb., 1691, decuria 2, ix, 200-202, 1 pl.—**Lombardini** (L.) Illustrazione di un monstro con faccia bipartita. Gior. di anat., fisiol. e patol. d. animali, Pisa, 1869, i, 65-80. ———. Intorno ad un caso d' idrencefalocele congenito. *Ibid.*, 1873, v, 193-206, 1 pl.—**Lonsdale** (H.) History of a monstrosity presenting remarkable peculiarities in the arrangement of the nervous system; with a brief inquiry into its teratological and med-

Monsters *from defect or malformation of brain, cranium, or face.*

ico-legal relations. Edinb. M. & S. J., 1843, lx, 324–340. *Also*, Reprint —**Lorain** (P.) [Une monstruosité remarquable.] Bull. Soc. de chir. de Par. (1861), 1862, 2. s., ii, 394.—**Lowther** (G.) Case of extraordinary abnormal deviations in the development of a fœtus (seven months) as demonstrated in an autopsical examination. Obst. J. Gr. Brit., Lond., 1880, viii, 335–337.—**Lucia** (C.) Niña pseudencefaliana que vivio 34 horas. Siglo méd., Madrid, 1856, iii, 187.—**Lussana** (P.) Due casi di completa anencefalia. Gazz. med. ital. lomb., Milano, 1861, 4. s., vi, 329.—**Luton** (A.) Description d'un fœtus monstrueux paracéphalien omphalosite unitaire. Compt. rend. Soc. de biol. 1854, Par., 1855, 2. s., i, pt. 2, 315–329.—**Macari** (F.) Mostro rarissimo presentato, descritto e commentato, e discussione relativa. Gior. d. r. Accad. di med. di Torino, 1865, 2. s., liii, 501.—**McCollough** (J. R.) A monstrosity. Physician & Surg. Ann Arbor, Mich., 1884, vi, 105.—**M'Junkin** (D. W.) † South. M. & S. J., Augusta, 1836–7, i, 294–296.—**Mackall.** Case of anencephalous monster. Tr. M. Soc. Dist. Colomb., Wash., 1876, ii, 90–94.—**Maggi** (L.) Sulle emiterie aritmetiche. R. Ist. Lomb. di sc. e lett. Rendic., Milano, 1879, 2. s., xii, 298–306.—**Mahot.** Rapport sur un fœtus hyperencéphale. J. de la sect. de méd. Soc. acad. Loire-Inf., Nantes, 1845, xxi, 81–90. —**Malherbe.** Observation de notencéphalie. Ibid., 1840, xvi, 11–21, 2 pl. *Also*, Reprint.—**Malherbe** (A.) Description d'un monstre cyclopien rhinocéphale. Bull. Soc. anat. de Par., 1879, liv. 115–117. *Also:* Bull. Soc. anat. de Nantes 1878-9, Par., 1879, ii, 68–70. *Also:* J. de méd. de l'ouest, Nantes, 1879, 2. s., iii, 154–156. *Also:* Progrès méd., Par., 1879, vii, 664.—**de Man** (J. C.) Waarneming over monstrositeit door vergroeijing van de huid voor de geboorte. Nederl. Tijdschr. v. Geneesk., Amst., 1874, 2. R., x, 433–440.—**Manlove** (J. E.) Remarks on a case of an acephalous monster. West. J. M. & S., Louisville, 1845, 3. s., iv, 401–405.—**Manz** (W.) Ueber das Auge hirnloser Missgeburten und über Erscheinungen des Gehirndrucks im Auge. Ber. ü. d. Verhandl. d. naturf. Gesellsch. zu Freib. i. Br., 1868–9, v, 2 Hft., 109–111. ———. Das Auge der hirnlosen Missgeburten. Arch. f. path. Anat., etc., Berl., 1870, li, 313–349, 1 pl.—**Marcot.** Mémoire sur un enfant monstrueux. [*From:* Hist. d. mém. Acad. roy. d. sc. de Par., 1716.] Hist. Soc. roy. d. sc. à Montpel., 1778, ii, pt. 2, 461–480. *Also* [Abstr.]: Collect. acad. d. mém., etc. Partie franç., Par., 1770, iv, 447–452.—**de la Mardière.** Monstre cyclope. Bull. Soc. de méd. de Poitiers, 1858, xxvii, 48–50, 1 pl.—**de la Mare.** Observation sur un enfant à face monstrueuse, et sans crâne. J. de méd., chir., pharm., etc., Par., 1770, xxxiii, 517.—**Marye.** Observation d'une nouvelle monstruosité, suivie de quelques remarques sur l'anencéphalie. Arch. gén. de méd., Par., 1827, xiv, 379–385.—**Masse** (E.) Monstre anencéphale à langue trifide; observation de M. le Dr. Septours. Assoc. franç. pour l'avance. d. sc. Compt.-rend. 1875, Par., 1876, iv, 1106–1111.—**Maurice** (E.-F.) Note sur un fœtus monstrueux pseudencéphale. Ann. Soc. de méd. de St.-Étienne et de la Loire (1865-6), 1867, iii, 565–577. ———. Note sur un monstre humain de la famille des pseudencéphaliens et du genre nosencéphale. *Ibid.* (1881), 1882, viii, pt. 2, 154–159. *Also:* Loire méd., St.-Étienne, 1882, i, 36–40.—**Mauricet** (A.) Observation d'un fœtus anencéphale. Compt. rend. Soc. de biol. 1862, Par., 1863, 3. s., iv, 18–20.—**Mayer.** Beschreibung eines Monoculus. Mag. f. d. ges. Heilk., Berl., 1824, xvii, 329–332. —**Mayer** (E.) Acrania monsters, with report of a case. Am. J. M. Sc., Phila., 1882, n. s., lxxxiii, 118–122.—**Mazirel** (P.) Waarneming eener monstrositas per defectum en hydrocephalus, met eenen doodelijken afloop voor moeder en vrucht. Nederl. Lancet, Utrecht, 1843–4, vi, 379–382. —**Meckel** (A.) Monströse Larve eines Fötus. Arch. f. Anat. u. Physiol., Leipz., 1828, 149–155, 2 pl. ———. Theilweiser Hirn- und Schädelmangel. *Ibid.*, 156–159. ———. Bemerkungen über einen Kalbscyklopen. *Ibid.*, 159–166.—**Meckel** (J.-F.) Description d'une monstruosité remarquable. J. compl. du dict. d. sc. méd., Par., 1822, xiii, 335–344.—**Mendenhall** (E.) A monstrous birth. Cincin. Lancet & Obs., 1869, xii, 212–215. —**Méry** (J.) Remarques sur un fœtus monstrueux. [*From:* Mém. Acad. roy. d. sc. de Par., 1709.] Rec. de mém., Dijon, 1754, ii, 707–709. —**Mezeray.** Un enfant monstrueux, cyclope. [*From:* Mém. Acad. roy. d. sc., 1761.] Collect. acad. d. mém., etc. Partie franç., Par., 1786, xiii, 313.—**Michaal.** Anencephalus und zugleich Spätgeburt. Ztschr. d. nordd. Chir.-Ver., Magdeb., 1848, ii, 470–476. —**Mikertchjants** (M. G.) Demonstrirnja preparate uroda cheilo-gnatho-palato schisis. Protok. zasaid. Kavkazsk. med. Obsh., Tiflis, 1883–4, xx, 46–53.—**Mollière** (D.) Un fœtus anencéphale. Gaz. méd. de Lyon, 1868, xx, 254. *Also:* Mém. et compt.-rend. Soc. d. sc. méd. de Lyon (1868), 1869, viii, 55–59.—**Monro** (A.) Description of a human male monster. Tr. Roy. Soc. Edinb., 1794, iii, pt. 2, 215–230, 4 pl. *Also*, Reprint.—**Monstrum** ohne Augen und sonst ungestalt. Samml. v. Nat.- u. Med.- . . . Gesch. 1725, Leipz. u. Budissin, 1726, xxxii, 520.—**Montrose** (S. L.) Case of large congenital cranial tumour. Tr. Edinb.

Monsters *from defect or malformation of brain, cranium, or face.*

Obst. Soc. (1871-4), 1875, iii, 22–25.—**Moore** (A. A.) Anencephalic monster. Am. J. M. Sc., Phila., 1867, n. s., liii, 281.—**Morel.** Étude anatomique d'un monstre anencéphale (pseudencéphalien de Geoffroy-Saint-Hilaire), avec division complète de la colonne vertébrale, absence de la moelle épinière, exstrophie de l'estomac, exstrophie de la vessie, utérus et vagin bifides, aorte double, anomalies multiples. Rev. méd. de l'est, Nancy, 1878, x, 33–42, 1 pl.—**Morisani** (D.) Di un nuovo mostro per raro caso di idro-meningocele cefalo-rachidiano. Movimento, Napoli, 1877, ix, 225; 246, 1 pl. — **Morland.** Anencephalous fœtus. Boston M. & S. J., 1860, lxii, 160.—**Morris** (O. W.) Case of monster. E. Tennessee Rec. M. & S., 1852–3, i, 247. — **Moussu.** Note relative à deux cas de cyclocéphalie. Bull. et mém. Soc. centr. de méd. vét., Par., 1886, n. s., iv, 63–66.—**Mulvany** (J.) Remarkable monstrosity. Brit. M. J., Lond., 1883, i, 1063.—**Munro** (H.) Malformation in a new-born child. Lancet, Lond., 1864, ii, 462. — **Nagel.** Todtgeborenes Kind mit sehr grossem Wasserkopfe und verunstalteten Extremitäten. Oestdr. med. Wchnschr., Wien, 1843, 1345–1350. — **Negri** (P.) Osservazione di una singolare lesione riscontrata in un feto estratto col cranioclaste. Ann. di ostet., Milano, 1880, ii, 98–107. — **Nicholls** (J.) Malformation; maternal influences (cyclopia). St. George's Hosp. Rep., Lond., 1869, iv, 215.—**Nicod.** Description d'un fœtus anencéphale, avec hernie du foie, et de presque tout le tube intestinal par l'ombilic. J. gén. de méd., chir. et pharm., Par., 1819, lxviii, 321–332.—**Nicoll** (A. Y.) & **Arnold** (R. D.) Account of an anencephalus, or human monstrosity without a brain and spinal marrow. South. M. & S. J., Augusta, 1837–8, ii, 10–18. *Also:* Am. J. M. Sc., Phila., 1838, xxii, 253–257. *Also:* Lancet, Lond., 1837–8, i, 202–204. —**Nitot** (E.) Description d'un fœtus humain monstrueux du genre paracéphale. Ann. de gynéc., Par., 1876, vi, 99–106. *Also:* Bull. Soc. anat. de Par., 1876, li, 356–362. *Also:* Progrès méd., Par., 1876, iv, 671.—**Nolleson** fils. Observation sur un fœtus monstrueux de sept mois. J. de méd., chir., pharm., etc., Par., 1768, xxix, 514–518. — **Norris-Cane** (J. B.) Remarkable monstrosity. Med. Press & Circ., Lond., 1872, n. s., xiv, 268. — **Okel** sen. Merkwürdige Missgeburten. Verm. Abhandl. . . . v. einer Gesellsch. pract. Aerzte zu St. Petersb., 1854, viii, 185–188, 1 pl.—**Olier.** Observation d'un fœtus anencéphale. Compt. rend. Soc. de biol. 1850, Par., 1851, ii, 106–110. — **Ollivier** (*d'Angers*). Enfant monstrueux. [Case.] Bull. Acad. de méd., Par., 1837–8, ii, 95; 99. *Also* [Abstr.]: Arch. gén. de méd., Par., 1837, 2. s., xv, 244; 352.—**Packard.** Anencephalous monster, with spina bifida, and failure of development of the anterior abdominal walls. Proc. Path. Soc. Phila. (1860–66), 1867, ii, 83. — **Paddock** (L. S.) A case of monstrosity. Proc. Connect. M. Soc., Hartford, 1876, 75. — **Palmer.** Anencephalous fetus, with eventration. Am. J. Obst., N. Y., 1878, xi, 632.—**Parada y Santin** (J.) Monstruo autosito ectro-parameliano. An. de obst., ginecopat. y pediat., Madrid, 1881, 2. ép., i, 329–331. — **Paterson** (A.) Notes of a case of anencephalous fœtus born co-twin with a healthy child. Tr. Edinb. Obst. Soc. (1874–7), 1878, iv, 376. — **Paterson** (J.) Case of monstrosity. Glasgow M. Exam., 1831–2, i, 159. — **Pearse** (J. S.) † Med. Times & Gaz., Lond., 1853, vii, 412.—**Pearson** (J. C.) A monster. Louisville M. News, 1885, xix, 355.— **Peschier.** Beschreibung einer merkwürdigen Missgeburt. Aus dem französischen Manuscripte übersetzt von Locher-Balber. Lit. Ann. d. ges. Heilk., Berl., 1826, v, 406–409.—**Petit.** Description d'un monstre pseudencéphalien (genre thlipsencéphale). Bull. méd. du nord, Lille, 1866–8, 2. s., vii-ix, 329–334. ———. Monstre cébocéphale. *Ibid.*, 1875, xv, 473–478.—**Pézérat** (P.) Observation sur un fœtus monstrueux. J. compl. du dict. d. sc. méd., Par., 1827, xxix, 252–262.—**Philippart** (A.) Observation sur un monstre anencéphale. Bull. Soc. de méd. de Gand, 1836, ii, 175–177. *Also:* Ann. Soc. de méd. de Gand, 1836, ii, 275–281. *Also:* Ann. de méd. belge, Brux., 1837, i, 174.—**Picco** (A. F.) Caso di mostruosità diplencefalica od iniodiploencefalo. Gior. d. r. Accad. di med. di Torino, 1869, 3. s., viii, 14–19.—**Pinard.** Pseudencéphale, bec de lièvre double, mains et pieds bots, ectrodactylie de la main gauche et polydactylie du pied droit, absence d'organes génitaux externes et internes et d'orifice anal, pharynx imperforé, fistule trachéo-œsophagienne. Bull. Soc. anat. de Par., 1873, xlviii, 685–688.—**Pittman** (W. H.) A monstrosity. South. Pract., Nashville, 1884, vi, 319.—**Planchon.** Monstre pseudencéphale, cyclocéphale. Bull. Soc. anat. de Par., 1868, xliii, 541–543.—**Plazanet.** Description d'un fœtus monstrueux. J. de méd., chir., pharm., etc., Par., 1772, xxxvii, 498–505.—**Poelman** (C.) Description d'un monstre paracyclocéphale. Ann. Soc. de méd. de Gand, 1850, xxv, 229–242, 2 pl. ———. Note sur une monstruosité cyclocéphalienne. Bull. Soc. de méd. de Gand, 1856, xxiii, 223–225. ———. Description d'un cyclope iniencéphale. *Ibid.*, 1862, xxix, 320–323, 2 pl.—**Polaillon.** Présentation d'un fœtus anencéphale né à terme, dans le service d'accouchements de la Maternité de Cochin. Bull. Soc. de chir. de

Monsters *from defect or malformation of brain, cranium, or face.*

Par., 1874, 3. s., iii, 435.—**Poland** (A.) Exencephalous monster. Tr. Path. Soc. Lond., 1846–8, i, 177. ———. An account of the dissection of two anencephalous monstrosities. Guy's Hosp. Rep., Lond., 1847, 2. s., v, 77–92, 2 pl.—**Pole** (T.) [Deformed fœtus.] Med. & Phys. J., Lond., 1800, iii, 397; 497.—**Polis** (G. S.) Von einem Mädgen, welches mit einem seltsamen Wasserkopf gebohren wurde. Auserl. med.- chir.-.... Abhandl. d. röm.-kais. Akad. d. Naturf., Nürnb., 1766, xv, 339–341, 1 pl.—**Pooley** (J. H.) Case of congenital deformity. Med. Gaz., N. Y., 1870, iv, 257.—**Pope** (H. C.) Anencephaloid fœtus. Tr. Obst. Soc. Lond. (1881), 1882, xxiii, 178.—**Popham** (J.) Hemicephalic infant; protrusion of the membranes of the brain through a fissure of the occipital bone; supernumerary fingers and toes. Tr. Cork M. & S. Soc., Dubl., 1866–7, 70–72.—**Popham** (W. H.) Curious case of monstrosity. Lancet, Lond., 1832, i, 356.—**Port & de Méric** (H.) Deformed fœtus. Med. Press & Circ., Lond., 1874, n. s., xvii, 111.—**Prestat.** Description d'un fœtus monstrueux présenté à la Société anatomique. Bull. Soc. anat. de Par., 1837, xii, 167–175.—**Püllen.** Beschreibung eines Anencephalus. Gen.-Ber. d. k. rhein. Med.- Coll. 1834, Koblenz, 1837, 218.—**Purple** (S. S.) A literary, historical, and practical sketch of acrania, "brainless", or pseudencephalous monsters; with the report of a case. N. York J. M., 1850, [2.] s., v, 40–57, 1 pl. *Also,* Reprint.—**Putnam** (Mary C.) Note on a case of human nosencephalian monster who lived 29 hours. Arch. Scient. & Pract. M. & S., N. Y., 1873, i, 342; 446.—**Quail** (C. E.) Case of monstrosity. Tr. M. Soc. Penn., Phila., 1870, 6. s., pt. 1, 163.—**Rarísimo** fenómeno. An. Soc. ginec. españ., Madrid, 1876, ii, 270–272.—**Rayer.** Sur un monstre anencéphalien dont une partie du cuir chevelu adhère à l'amnios dans un point correspondant au placenta. Gaz. méd. de Par., 1855, 3. s., x, 701. *Also:* Compt. rend. Soc. de biol. 1855, Par., 1856, 2. s., ii, 103.—**Raygerus** (C.) De capite monstroso sine cranio et cerebro. Misc. Acad. nat. curios. 1672, Lips. et Francof., 1681, iii, 427.— **Rebsamen.** Cyclopen-Missbildung mit schweinrüsselförmigem Rudimente der Nase bei einem menschlichen Fötus männlichen Geschlechtes. Schweiz. Ztschr. f. Nat.- u. Heilk., Heilbronn, 1837, ii, 38–40.—**Rechnitz** (G.) Ungewöhnlicher Fall angeborner Missbildung. Ztschr. f. Nat.- u. Heilk. in Ungarn, Oedenburg, 1857, viii, 259.—**Redmond** (L.) A child without calvaria or brain. Chicago M. J., 1869, xxvi, 15.—**Reid** (T.) [Case of anophthalmos binocularis.] Glasgow M. J., 1878, [4. s.], x. 281.—**Reiset** (S.) Von einem Gehirn, so ausserhalb der Hirnschale lag, und welches durch einen Schreken gekommen, den eine schwangere Frau von einer Kaze hatte. Auserl. med.- chir.-.... Abhandl. d. röm.- kais. Akad. d. Naturf., Nürnb., 1763, xii, 231–234.—**Renard.** Description d'un fœtus monstrueux. J. de méd., chir., pharm., etc., Par., 1765, xxiii, 118–128.—**Report** of a committee appointed by the Pathological Society of Philadelphia to examine the specimen of imperfect-cyclops monster presented by Dr. F. H. Gross. Phila. M. Times, 1874–5, v, 481–483.—**Rern.** Kurze Beschreibung eines monströs geborenen Kindes. Med. Cor.-Bl. d. württemb. ärztl. Ver., Stuttg., 1838, viii, 392.—**Retsin.** Description d'un fœtus monstrueux péracéphalien. Ann. Soc. méd.-chir. de Bruges, 1855, 2. s., iii, 321–326, 2 pl.— **Reynier** (L.) Un notencéphale. Écho méd., Neuchât., 1859, iii, 512.—**Ribbert** (H.) Beitrag zur Entstehung der Anencephalie. Arch. f. path. Anat., etc., Berl., 1883, xciii, 396–400.—**Richard** (A.) Sur la composition de la tumeur des monstres pseudencéphaliens. Compt. rend. Soc. de biol. 1851, Par., 1852, iii, 68–71.—**Richardson** (W. L.) Case of anencephalic monster, with spina bifida and umbilical hernia. Boston M. & S. J., 1877, xcvii, 174.—**Ridgeway** (N. B.) An anencephalous monster, with spina bifida. Ohio M. Recorder, Columbus, 1880–81, v, 406.—**Rieken** (H. C.) Beschreibung einer merkwürdigen Bildungshemmung. J. d. Chir. u. Augenh., Berl., 1831–2, xvii, 471–477.—**Riez** (J.) Hydrocéphalie; spina bifida; fractures spontanées; pieds-bots. Presse méd. belge, Brux., 1875–6, xxviii, 3.—**Rindfleisch.** Ein Fall von Anencephalie und Spina bifida. Arch. f. path. Anat., etc., Berl., 1860, xix, 546–548.—**Ritter** (C.) Das Auge eines Acranius histologisch untersucht. Arch. f. Augenh., Wiesb., 1881–2, xi, 215–218.—**Ritter** (J.) Singular case of malformation of the mouth, nose, and palate of an infant at birth. Med. & Surg. Reporter, Phila., 1866, xv, 506.— **Roberts** (D. L.) Two cases of monstrosity. Tr. Obst. Soc. Lond. (1868), 1869, x, 269–273, 1 pl.—**Robin de Kyavalle.** Observation sur un monstre sans cerveau, ayant la tête figurée comme celle d'un crapaud, né entre le cinquième et sixième mois de conception. J. de méd., chir., pharm., etc., Par., 1770, xxxii, 151–157.—**Rodgers** (J. W.) A monstrosity. Med. Arch., St. Louis, 1871–2, vii, 551.— **Rodriguez** (J. M.) Descripcion de un monstruo humano derencéfalo. Porvenir, México, 1870–71, iii, 47–70, 1 pl. ———. Descripcion de un feto hidrocéfalo, ectrodáctyle. Gac. méd. de México, 1871, vi, 129–136.—**Roe** (W.) A case of cyclopian monster. Dublin Q. J. M. Sc., 1871, li,

Monsters *from defect or malformation of brain, cranium, or face.*

146–149.—**Römer** (A.) Anatomische Bemerkungen über einen Cyclopen-Kindeskopf. Med. Jahrb. d. k. k. österr. Staates, Wien, 1837, xxiii, 453–459.—**Roloff.** Courte description d'un monstre humain. (Traduit du latin.) [*From:* Mém. Acad. roy. d. sc. de Berl.] Collect. acad. d. mém., etc. Partie franç., Par., 1774, xii, 17–22, 2 pl. *Also:* Mém. Acad. roy. de Prusse, Avignon, 1774, viii, 46–58.—**Rosenfeld** (J.) Egy iméntszülött, kiviselt hemikephalus leirata. [Recent birth, which proved to be a hemicephalus.] Orvosi Tár, Pest, 1845, 49–53.—**Ross** (W.) A curious monster, which lived for some time after birth. Tr. Obst. Soc. Lond. (1867), 1868, ix, 31, 1 pl.—**Rotureau.** Absence des os de la partie supérieure du crâne, de la région cervicale, spina-bifida, traces de cuir chevelu entourant les lobes cérébraux et l'écartement de la colonne vertébrale jusqu'à la région lombaire. Bull. Acad. de méd., Par., 1850–51, xvi, 176.—**Roux** (G.) Monstre nosencéphale. Lyon méd., 1874, xv, 496–498.—**Roy** (V.-P.) Mémoire sur trois cas de monstruosité, savoir: un cas de cyclocéphalie et un de polymélie. Rev. méd. franç. et étrang., Par., 1841, iii, 36–69.—**de la Rue.** Observation sur un monstre cyclope. Rec. périod. d'obs. de méd., de chir. et pharm.. Par., 1757, vii, 278–281.—**Sanderson** (W. B.) Case of monstrosity. Prov. M. & S. J., Lond., 1842, iv, 269.—**Sandifort** (G.) Ontleedkundige beschrijving van twee herselnooze misgeboorten. Genees-, heel-, ... kundige Verhandel. v. h. k.-nederl. Inst. v. Wetensch., etc., Amst., 1824, 23, 4 pl.—**Sangalli** (G.) Teratologia; casi speciali di anencefalia, con appunti sulla loro etiologia. R. Ist. Lomb. di sc. e lett. Rendic., Milano, 1877, 2. s., x, 24.—**Sapolini** (G.) Circa un feto trimestre pseudoncefalo. Lettera al Prof. Tommati. Ann. univ. di med., Milano, 1868, cciii, 138.——. Descrizione di tre mostrini della famiglia dei ciclocefalici, ossia di due rinocefali e di un ciclocefalo propriamente detto. *I bid.*, cciv, 321.———. Teratologia; succinta descrizione di due mostri, l'uno umano, l'altro vitellino, appartenenti alla famiglia degli otocefalici, e precisamente al genere triocefalo. R. Ist. Lomb. di sc. e lett. Rend'c., Milano, 1869, 2. s., ii, 415–422. *Also,* Reprint. *Also:* Ann. univ. di med., Milano, 1869, ccviii, 134.—**Sappey.** Cas de cyclopie. Compt. rend. Soc. de biol. 1859, Par., 1860, 3. s., i. 46.—**Saussol.** Un monstre cyclocéphalien rhinocéphale. Gaz. hebd. d. sc. méd. de Montpel., 1886, viii, 458.—**Schaack.** Présentation d'un fœtus pseudencéphale. Mém. et compt.- rend. Soc. d. sc. méd. de Lyon, 1866–7, vi, 69. *Also:* Gaz. méd. de Lyon, 1866, xviii, 389.— **Schelhase** (E. F.) Von einem monströsen Mädgen. Auserl. med.- chir.-.... Abhandl. d. röm.-kais. Akad. d. Naturf., Nürnb., 1764, xiii, 257, 1 pl.———. Von einem monströsen Knaben ohne Gehirn. *Ibid.*, 259.—**Schermerhorn** (B.) Case of monstrosity (malformation of face, etc.). Am. J. M. Sc., Phila., 1872, n. s., lxiii, 570.— **Schleifer.** Zur Geschichte des menschlichen Anencephalus. Oesterr. med. Wchnschr., Wien, 1844, 197–199.— **Schmidt** (F. J. I.) Ontleedkundig onderzoek van eene misvormde menschelijke vrucht (cébocéphalie G. St. Hilaire). Verhandel. v. h. Genootsch. t. Bevord. d. Geneesen Heelk. te Amst., 1857, ii, 1. St., 181–193, 1 pl.— **Schmidt** (J.) Die Zergliederung einer Missgeburt weiblichen Geschlechtes. Auserl. med.- chir.-... Abhandl. d. röm.-kais. Akad. d. Naturf., Nürnb., 1757, iv, 42.— **Schneider** (J.) Geburtsgeschichte und Beschreibung eines durch die Zange entbundenen Kindes ohne Gehirn- und Rückenmark. Lucina, Leipz., 1807–8, iv, 270–281.— **Schofield.** The delivery of a monster. Tr. Obst. Soc. Lond. (1879), 1880, xxi, 71–73.—**Schultze** (B.) Fall von angebornem Wasserkopf, Spina bifida lumbo-dorsalis u. Klumpfüssen. Verhandl. d. Gesellsch. f. Geburtsh. in Berl. (1856–7), 1858, x, 142–148, 1 pl. *Also:* Monatschr. f. Geburtsk. u. Frauenkr., Berl., 1857, x, 5-12, 1 pl.—**Schwarz.** Deformitäten am Kopfe einer menschlichen Missgeburt, nebst einigen Bemerkungen über den psychischen Einfluss der Mutter auf die Bildung der Leibesfrucht. Gem. deutsche Ztschr. f. Geburtsk., Weimar, 1829, iv, 182–222.— **Scott** (J.) A monoculous male fœtus. Lancet, Lond., 1862, i, 633.—**Seguin.** Brainless child. N. York M. J., 1878, xxvii, 535.—**Septours** (A.) Observation sur un cas de monstre anencéphale; langue trifide; bec-de-lièvre; spina bifida considérable, avec rupture spontanée de la poche dans le sein de la mère. Union méd., Par., 1876, 3. s., xxi, 209–214. *Also:* Mouvement méd., Par., 1876, xiv, 153–155.—**Sequira.** Brief account of face monstrosity. Tr. Obst. Soc. Lond., 1863–4, v, 195.—**Shepherd** (F. J.) The musculus sternalis and its occurrence in (human) anencephalous monsters. J. Anat. & Physiol., Lond., 1884–5, xix, 311–319, 1 pl.———. On the musculus sternalis occurring in anencephalous monsters. Tr. Acad. M. Ireland, Dubl., 1885, iii, 439–446, 1 pl.—**von Siebold** (E.) Entbindungsgeschichte und Beschreibung eines monströsen Kindes, nebst Abbildung des sehr merkwürdigen abnormen Kopfgebildes. Lucina, Leipz., 1802–4, i, 394–400.—**Simons.** [Sketch of the head of a monstrosity, in which the right orbit and right side of the face was occupied by a soft, pulpy tumor.] Prov. M. J., Lond.,

Monsters from defect or malformation of brain, cranium, or face.

1844, vii, 193.— **Simpson** (T. P.) A monstrosity. Tr. M. Soc. Penn., Phila., 1883, xv, 335.— **Smith** (C. H.) A child born without calvaria or encephalon. West. J. M., Indianap., 1869, iv, 209.— **Smith** (R. M.) & **Parker** (A. J.) Dissection of a human otocephalic cyclops monstrosity. Am. J. M. Sc., Phila., 1882, lxxxiv, 132–140.— **de Soemmerring** (S. T.) Specimen malæ conformationis encephali capitis et pelvis viri rarissimum et memoratu dignissimum. Nova acta phys.-med. Acad. nat. curios., Bonnæ, 1828, xiv, pt. 1, 109–126, 5 pl.— **Spalding** (S. C.) † Tr. M. Soc. Penn., Phila., 1877, xi, pt. 2, 728.— **Spessa** (A.-A.) Mémoire sur un enfant complétement privé de cerveau, de cervelet et de moelle allongée, et qui a vécu onze heures. Gaz. méd. de Par., 1833, 2. s., i, 46. Also, transl.: [Abstr.]: Lancet, Lond., 1832–3, i, 570. Also, transl.: [Abstr.]: Lond. M. Gaz., 1832-3, xi, 559.— **Stapfer.** Pseudencéphalie. Ann. de gynéc. Par., 1885, xxiii, 127–131.— **Stevens** (R. P.) Instrumental delivery; singular deformity of the fœtus. Boston M. & S. J., 1844, xxx, 52–54.— **Stevenson** (J. M.) Case of monstrosity. Med. & Surg. Reporter, Phila., 1864-5, xii, 223.— **Stienon.** Fœtus exencéphale avec complication de spina bifida; description de cette monstruosité. Ann. Soc. d'anat. path. de Brux., 1873, xxii, 96–101.— **Stout** (S. H.) A case of abnormal reproduction. Texas Cour.-Rec. Med., Fort Worth, 1885-6, iii, 133–135.— **Stratford** (S. I.) Fœtal monstrosity; deficiency of the cranial bones. Midland M. & S. Reporter, Worcester, 1828-9, i, 197, 1 pl.— **Stryker** (P. J.) Case of monstrous birth. Phila. M. Museum, 1809, vi, 144–146.— **Stuart** (F. H.) Microcranial monster, with cleft palate, colon terminating in the bladder, talipes varus in a marked degree. Ann. Anat. & Surg. Soc. Brooklyn, N. Y., 1880, ii, 230–234.— **Suchier.** Geburt eines Hemicephalus. J. f. Geburtsh., Frankf. a. M., 1830-31, x, 555–560.— **Suckling** (C. B.) A rare case of monstrosity; hydrencephalocele. Med. Times & Gaz., Lond., 1873, i, 85.— **Svitzer.** Nachricht von einem weiblichen Hemicephalus, bei welchem ein Theil der Unterleibseingeweide auf dem Rücken in einem Sacke zwischen dem Kopf und dem Rückgrat lag. Arch. f. Anat., Physiol. u. wissensch. Med., Berl., 1839, 35–38, 1 pl.— **Talko** (J.) Ein Fall von Gehirnhernie, bedingt durch unregelmässige und frühzeitige Synostosen der Schädelknochen. Arch. f. path. Anat., etc., Berl., 1871, lii, 563–566. ———. Przypadek malooocznosci (mikrophthalmos) z wrodzona torbiela surowicza pod powiekami dolnemi. [Microphthalmos; congenital ectropion.] Medycyna, Warszawa, 1876, iv, 590–592.— **Tanchis** (B.) Breve cenno descrittivo sopra un caso di anencefalia in un feto a maturità. Spallanzani, Modena, 1873, ii, 381–383.— **Taylor** (J. S.) Case of monstrosity. West. Lancet, Cincin., 1854, xv, 470–472.— **Taylor** (W. T.) † Am. J. M. Sc., Phila., 1871, n. s., lxii, 574.— **Terlaak** (G. C.) Exencephalus. Boerhaave. Tijdschr., etc., Amst., 1842, n. s., i, 526–528, 2 pl.— [**Ternisien.**] Rapport sur un monstre peracéphale. Bull. Acad. de méd., Par., 1874, 2. s., iii, 1096–1101.— **Thibault.** Observation sur un enfant monstrueux. J. de méd., chir., pharm., etc., Par., 1761, xv, 434.— **Thiebault.** Description d'un monstre humain. Méd. éclairée, Par., 1791, ii, 36–38.— **Thomas** (J. H.) Monstrosity. Brit. M. J., Lond., 1881, i, 594.— **Thompson** (J. A.) Description of a cyclopean monster. Tr. Obst. Soc. Lond. (1873), 1874, xv, 35–38.— **Thys.** Anencéphale; présentation de la face; vagissement utérin. [Avec rapport.] Ann. Soc. de méd. d'Anvers, 1846, 694; 699.— **Tiedemann.** Beobachtungen über die Beschaffenheit des Gehirns und der Nerven in Missgeburten. Ztschr. f. Physiol., Darmstadt, 1829, iii, 1–44. ———. Beschreibung des Hirns und Rückenmarks einer Missgeburt mit Uebermass in der Bildung. Ibid., 235–239, 2 pl.— **Tilgen.** Merkwürdige Missgeburt. Gen.-Ber. d. k. rhein. Med.-Coll. 1840, Koblenz, 1841, 170.— **Tinley** (T.) Malformed fœtus. Brit. M. J., Lond., 1876, ii, 8.— **Touzeau** (N.) Description d'un monstre humain du genre podencéphale. J. de la sect. de méd. Soc. acad. Loire-Inf., Nantes, 1831, vii, 12–19.— **Troussel-Delvincourt.** Observation d'enfant anencéphale. N. Jour. de méd., chir., pharm., etc., Par., 1821, x, 162–172.— **Tyson** (E.) An infant with the brain depressed into the hollow of the vertebræ. Phil. Tr., Lond., 1700, iii, 26.— **Ullersperger** (J. B.) Monstruosidades fetales. Anfiteatro anat., Madrid, 1873, i, 191.— **Ulrich.** Ueber einige im Herzogthum Niederrhein vorgekommene interessante Missgeburten. Deutsches Arch. f. d. Physiol., Halle, 1820, vi, 522–526, 1 pl.— **Underhill.** Agnathous and hydrocephalic fœtus. Tr. Edinb. Obst. Soc., 1885-6, xi, 79.— **Valtorta** (G.) Parto ottimestre di feto mostruoso. Gior. veneto di sc. med., Venezia, 1875, 3. s., xxii, 657.— **Verga** (A.) Sugli anencefali umani. R. Ist. Lomb. di sc. e lett. Rendic., Milano, 1876, 2. s., ix, 303–310, 1 pl.— **Verrier.** Sur un fœtus anencéphale. Gaz. obst. et gynéc. de Par., 1875, iv, 193–198. Also [Abstr.]: Bull. acad. de méd., Par., 1875, 2. s., iv, 721.— **Vicq d'Azyr.** Observation sur un fœtus monstrueux. Hist. Soc. roy. de méd. 1776, Par., 1779, 315.— **Vigla.** De l'aprosopie, ou absence congéniale de la face. Arch. gén. de méd., Par., 1849, ii, 25–35.— **Vir-**

Monsters from defect or malformation of brain, cranium, or face.

chow. Beschreibung einer Missgeburt (Acrania mit Spina bifida). Verhandl. d. Gesellsch f. Geburtsh. in Berl. (1856-7), 1858, x, 138–141. Also: Monatschr. f. Geburtsk. u. Frauenkr., Berl., 1857, x, 2–4.— **Wannamaker** (W. C.) A case of anencephalus, Tr. South Car. M. Ass., Charleston, 1886, 37. Also: Am. J. Obst., N. Y., 1886, xix, 794.— **Watkins** (J. M.) Delivery of an anencephalic fœtus. N. Orl. M. & S J., 1880-81, n. s., viii, 25.— **Weber** (E.) Geburt eines Hemicephalus männlichen Geschlechtes, welcher noch 38 Stunden nach der Geburt lebte. Monatschr. f. Geburtsk. u. Frauenkr., Berl., 1857, ix, 366–370.— **Wepfer** (J. J.) De puella sine cerebro nata, historia. Misc. Acad. nat. curios. 1672, Lips. et Francof., 1681, iii, 175–203. Collect. acad. d. mém., etc, Dijon, 1755, iii, 137–152. Also, transl. [Abstr.]: Auserl. med.-chir.-... Abhandl. d. röm.-kais. Akad. d. Naturf., Nürnb., 1756, iii, 193–198.— **Wertheimer.** Description d'un monstre péracéphale: considérations générales sur l'acéphalie. Bull. scient. dép. du nord, etc., Par., 1880, iii, 321–332.— **West** (R. U.) Description of an anencephalian monster. Tr. Obst. Soc. Lond. (1859), 1860, i, 105–107. Also: Lancet, Lond., 1859, i, 511.— **Westbrook** (B. F.) Acranial monster. Ann. Anat. & Surg. Soc., Brooklyn, 1879, i, 96. ———. Acranial monster. Proc. M. Soc. County Kings, Brooklyn, 1879–80, iv, 274.— **White.** [An interesting specimen of monstrosity.] Buffalo M. J., 1858-9, xiv, 537.— **Wieber** (G.) Anencephalic monster. Proc. M. Soc. County Kings, Brooklyn, 1879-80, iv, 94.— **Wiedemeister.** Den macerirten Schädel eines Kindes. Allg. Ztschr. f. Psychiat., etc., Berl., 1877, xxxiv, 685.— **Williams** (N. W.) A monstrosity. Calif. M. J., Oakland, 1886, vii, 537.— **Windrif.** Présentation à la Société d'un fœtus monstrueux paracéphale, etc. Bull. méd. du nord, Lille, 1865, vi, 179; 217.— **Withers** (O.) Case of abnormal development of a fœtus. Brit. M. J., Lond., 1884, ii, 807.— **Wittmann.** Description d'un fœtus pseudencéphale. [Soc. d. sc. méd. et nat. de Malines.] Arch. de la méd. belge, Brux., 1841, vi, 177, 1 pl.— **Witzel** (O.) Hemicephalus mit grossen Lebercysten, Cystennieren und einer Reihe anderer Missbildungen. Centralbl. f. Gynäk., Leipz., 1880, iv, 561–564.— **Worbe** (J.-F.-S.) Description d'un fœtus monstrueux. Bull. Fac. de méd. de Par. (1804–8), 1812, i, 46–50.— **Wrangell.** Monströser Anhang am Hinterkopf eines Neugeborenen. Ztschr. f. d. ges. Med., Hamb., 1839, xi, 95.— **Wyman.** Spina bifida in an anencephalous fœtus. Boston M. & S. J., 1862, lxvi, 452. ———. Fœtus with protrusion of the membranes of the brain; transposition of viscera; malformation of throat; and encysted disease of the kidneys. Ibid., 1863, lxviii, 385. ———. Description of an anencephalous fœtus with unusual malformation. Ibid., 1864-5, lxxi, 49–52. Also: Extr. Rec. Bost. M. Improve. (1862–6), 1867, v (app.), 101–103, 1 pl. ———. Malformed fœtus, with numerous fractures of the bones. Boston M. & S. J., 1866-7, lxxv, 19.— **Ygonin.** Observation sur un cas de monstruosité. J. de méd. de Lyon, 1845, viii, 426–430.— **Zartmann.** Missgeburt. Gen.-Ber. d. k. rhein. Med.-Coll. 1840, Koblenz, 1841, 169.— **Zchender** (W.) Case of a monster with the eyes covered with skin, kryptophthalmia. Rep. Internat. Ophth. Cong. 1872, Lond., 1873, iv, 86–94, 1 pl. Also, Report.— **von Ziemssen.** Fall von Agenesia cerebralis unilateralis. Sitzungsb. d. phys.-med. Soc. zu Erlang., 1871–2, iv, 59–62.— **Zwinger** (J. R.) Hydrocephalus cum defectu calvariae. Acta Helvet., Basileæ, 1751, i, 1–12.— **Zwinger** (T.) Puellus sine cerebro natus, ad momentum vivens. Misc. Acad. nat. curios. 1691, Norimb., 1692, decuria 2, x, 386–388, 1 pl.

Monsters from defect or malformation of limbs.

See, also, **Amputation** (Intra-uterine); **Extremities** (Lower), **Extremities** (Upper), Abnormities of.

BEHN (H. J.) *De monopodibus. 4°. Berolini, [1827].

BOERHAAVE (A. K.) Historia anatomica infantis cujus pars corporis inferior monstrosa. 4°. Petropoli, 1754.

CALORI (L.) Sopra un sirenomelo. 4°. Bologna, 1860.

Repr. from: Mem. Accad. d. sc. d. Ist. di Bologna, x.

Monsters *from defect or malformation of limbs.*

VAN CAMPEN (M. J.) * Puellæ monstrosæ delineatio. 4°. *Lugd. Bat.*, 1793.

CHAILLY-HONORÉ (N.-C.) Cas de monstruosité. 8°. [*Paris*, 1842.]

DALKOWSKI (E. J.) * De monopodia. 8°. *Regimonti Pr.*, 1855.

DANIEL (C. F.) Anhang zu der D. Christ. Friedr. Daniels medicinischen Gutachten beygefügten Abhandlung von einer siebenmonatlichen Misgeburt, etc., welcher die Beantwortung der Göttingischen Recension enthält. 8°. *Leipzig*, 1777.

DIECKERHOFF (F. H. C.) * De monopodia. 8°. *Halæ*, 1819.

DREIBHOLZ (E.) * Beschreibung einer sogenannten Phokomele. 8°. *Berlin*, [1873].

FRIEDLIEB (T.) Monstrosi fœtus descriptio atque delineatio. 4°. *Altonæ*, 1803.

HELLWIG (G.) * Beschreibung eines männlichen Amelus von 66 Jahren. 8°. *Halle*, 1867.

HEMPEL (A.) * Ueber Sirenenmissbildung. sm. 8°. *Berlin*, [1869].

HÜESKER (B. W.) * De vitiis syngeneticis, adjecta monstri sireniformis descriptione. 8°. *Gryphiæ*, [1841].

HUMMEL (J. C.) * Spec. continens observationem de monstro cui nomen phocomelus. 8°. *Lugd. Bat.*, 1819.

KLEIN (A. A. H. H.) * Zur Anatomie des Amelus. 8°. *Cassel*, 1872.

KOEHLER (E.) * Diss. sistens descriptionem monstri humani monopodis, adjectis nonnullis de monopodia animadversionibus. sm. 4°. *Jenæ*, [1831].

LANGSDORFF (C. G.) * De sympodia. Diss. sistens descriptionem anatomicam infantis parte inferiore monstrosi. fol. *Heidelbergæ*, 1846.

LEVY (M. M.) * De sympodia seu monstrositate sireniformi, cum anatomica ejusmodi monstri descriptione. 8°. *Havniæ*, 1833.

MAJER (F. T.) * De fœto humano monopodio. 4°. *Tubingæ*, [1827].

MEYERSOHN (B.) * Congenitale Defectbildungen an den Unterextremitäten eines Erwachsenen. 8°. *Greifswald*, [1878].

Also, in: Arch. f. path. Anat., etc, Berl., 1879, lxxvi, 330-353, 1 pl.

MÜLLER (C.) * Diss. inaug. anatomico-pathologica sistens monstri humani rarissimi descriptionem. 8°. *Halis Sax.*, [1831].

NYGREEN (C. J.) * De fetu monstroso, judicio medici submisso. 8°. *Lundæ*, 1840.

ORSOLATO (G.) Storia e descrizione anatomica di un mostro umano appartenente alle Sirene; alcune considerazioni relative. 8°. *Padova*, 1855.

ROSENBAUM (A. S.) * De singulari cujusdam fœtus humani monstrositate. 8°. *Regimontii*, [1828].

ROSSI (F. J. A.) * Diss. sistens fœtus monstrosi Holmiæ nati descriptionem et delineationem. 4°. *Jenæ*, [1800].

SACHSSE (C. D.) * Descriptio infantis monstrosæ. 4°. *Lipsiæ*, 1803.

SÄNGER (W. M. H.) * Beschrijving van eene misvormde menschelijke vrucht, benevens eenige opmerkingen omtrent de zoogenaamde aangeboren Engelsche ziekte (rachitis congenita). 8°. *Leyden*, 1857.

SCHÜSSLER (P. J. F.) * Ueber die Bildungsfehler der Extremitäten, nebst anatomischer Beschreibung einer missbildeten Oberextremität. 4°. *Marburg*, [1861].

SERLO (M. L.) * Monstrorum extremitatibus carentium exempla tria. 8°. *Berolini*, [1826].

WAGNER (E.) * Anatomische Untersuchung eines Monstrum perobrachium. 8°. *Würzburg*, 1862.

Also, in: Würzb. med. Ztschr., 1862, iii, 44-57, 2 pl.

Monsters *from defect or malformation of limbs.*

WIESING (H. T.) * De humana quadam inferiorum extremitatum monstrositate. 8°. *Halæ*, 1836.

WOLFF (F.) * De sympodia. 8°. [*Dorpat*], 1856.

WOLFF (G. P. J.) * Specimen anatomico-pathologicum de monstris sireniformibus. 8°. *Amstelodami*, 1839.

Adams (W.) Fœtus with arrested development. [Phocomelus.] Tr. Path. Soc. Lond., 1872-3, xxiv, 263.—**Ahlfeld** (F.) Ueber einen Monopus mit vollständigem Mangel der äusseren Genitalien und des Afters, nebst Bemerkungen 1) zur Lehre von der Aetiologie der Sirenenbildung und 2) zur Lehre von der Thätigkeit der fötalen Niere und Harnblase. Arch. f. Gynaek., Berl., 1879, xiv, 276-294.—**Arango y Lamar** (F.) Descripcion de un feto ectromélico. An. r. Acad. de cien. méd. . . . de la Habana, 1875-6, xii, 107-112. *Also:* Crón. méd.-quir. de la Habana, 1875, i, 125-128.—**Arentz** (L. H.) † Eyr, Christiania, 1832, vii, 9-12.—**Arnold.** † [Amelus.] Med. Cor.-Bl. d. württemb. ärztl. Ver., Stuttg., 1834-5, iv, 129.—**Austin** (T. M.) † Austral. M. J., Melbourne, 1878, xxiii, 105.—**Ball.** Sur un cas d'ectromélie chez l'homme. Bull. Soc. d'anthrop. de Par., 1878, 3. s., i, 136-139.—**Barzellotti** (G.) † Ann. univ. di med., Milano, 1828, xlv, 574-582, 1 pl.—**Bassett.** † [Monopus.] Prov. M. & S. J., Lond., 1852, 45.—**Behr** (G. H.) De viro, brachiis ac manibus penitus destituto, varia tamen pedibus suis peragente. Acta Acad. nat. curios., Norimb., 1740, v, 177-181, 1 pl.—**Behr** (S.) Eine Missgeburt mit fehlenden Unterschenkeln. Aerztl. Int.-Bl., München, 1855, ii, 363.—**Benito** (F.) Peromelia; mónstruo sin miembros inferiores y el brazo derecho bastante defectuoso; cabeza y tronco regulares; fenómeno particular de una niña viable. Crón. de l. hosp., Madrid, 1854, ii, 54.—**Bennett** (J. C.) An account of a singular case of fœtal monstrosity. West. J. M. & Phys. Sc., Cincin., 1830, iii, 213-215.—**Bernays** (A. C.) Aborted ovum and fœtal monstrosity. St. Louis M. & S. J., 1878, xxxv, 115.—**Blanckmeister** (L.) Bericht über eine interessante Missgeburt (Phocomele, oder Robben-Glieder-Bildung). Ztschr. f. Med., Chir. u. Geburtsh., Leipz., 1868, n. F., vii, 251-254.—**Blin** (L.) Conformation vicieuse des quatre membres; observation . . . suivie d'un rapport sur l'interprétation de ce fait et sur les causes des difformités congéniales par P. Broca. Bull. Soc. anat. de Par., 1852, xxvii, 376-406. *Also,* Reprint.—**Bondet.** Nouvel exemple de phocomélie. Mém. et compt.-rend. Soc. d. sc. méd. de Lyon, 1864-5, iv, pt. 2, 37-39. *Also:* Gaz. méd. de Lyon, 1864, xvi, 390.—**Bougard.** Enfant affectée de divers vices de conformation tant aux extrémités supérieures qu'aux inférieures. J. de méd., chir. et pharmacol., Brux., 1847, v, 853-856.—**Boulland** (C.) Observation d'un monstre symélien affecté d'arrêt de développement des membres supérieurs et de plusieurs autres organes. Bull. Soc. de méd. et pharm. de la Haute-Vienne, Limoges, 1868, 314-320.—**Brandt.** Ein Fall von angebornem Defect der Extremitäten. Arch. f. path. Anat., etc., Berl., 1882, lxxxvii, 195, 1 pl.—**Braun.** Monstrum Menhemii ab uxore judaica Dreifuss dicta enixum. Ann. d. Staatsarznk., Freib. i. Br., 1840, v, 149, 1 pl.—**Breschet.** Description d'un vice de conformation congénial. Bull. Fac. de méd. de Par., 1814-15, iv (11. année), 325-331. ———. Description d'un vice congénial de conformation de tous les membres. *Ibid.*, 1820, vii (15. année), 33-39, 1 pl.—**Broca** (P.) Anomalie des quatre membres par défaut, amputations congéniales des auteurs. Bull. Soc. anat. de Par., 1852, xxvii, 275; 294. ———. Localisations cérébrales sur le cerveau d'un ectromélien. Bull. Soc. d'anthrop. de Par., 1878, 3. s., ii, 669-673. ———. Note sur les monstres ectroméliens. Rev. d'anthrop., Par., 1882, 2. s., v, 193-200.—**Burke** (G. W.) A case of arrest of development in the human fœtus. Proc. Connect. M. Soc., Hartford, 1877, 101-104.—**Cam** (T. C.) † Med. & Phys. J., Lond., 1802, vii, 385, 1 pl.—**Camelli.** † Morgagni, Napoli, 1873, xv, 431-434.—[**Cases.**] Account of a living child aged two months and ten days, which had been born without limbs. Med. & Phys. J., Lond., 1803, ix, 63.—[Only one perfect limb, the left arm.] Boston M. & S. J., 1847, xxxvi, 92-96.—Lancet, Lond., 1857, i, 431.—Feto monopodo. Anfiteatro anat., Madrid, 1873, i, 251.—**du Cauroy.** Un monstre par excès. [*From:* J. d. sçavans, 1696.] Collect. acad. d. mém., etc., Dijon, 1766, vii, 26.—**Cederschiöld.** Foster med förvridna lemmar. [Monster with deformed lower limbs.] Förh. v. Svens. Läk.-Sällsk. Sammank., Stockholm, 1869, 31.—**Chancerel.** Hémimèle congénitale. Année méd., Caen, 1876, i, 6.—**Chantreuil.** Note sur un monstre phocomélien. Bull. Soc. anat. de Par. (1868), 1874, xliii, 191-195.—**Charon** (E.) [Monstre hémimèle et hectromèle.] Ann. Soc. d'anat. path. de Brux., 1876-7, xxvi, 85-87. ———. [Un monstre ectromélien, se rapprochant du phocomèle.] *Ibid.*, 1879-80, xxix, 187-191, 1 pl. *Also:* Presse méd. belge, Brux., 1880, xxxii, 201. *Also:* J. de méd., chir. et pharmacol., Brux., 1880, lxxi, 15-18.—**Choate** (D.) Mon-

Monsters *from defect or malformation of limbs.*

strosity. Extr. Rec. Bost. Soc. M. Improve. (1874–9), 1880, vii, 64.—**Claudot** (M.) Note sur un cas de monstruosité par absence d'un des membres supérieurs et difformité de l'autre. J. de l'anat. et physiol., etc., Par., 1874, x, 207–217. *Also* [Abstr.]: Compt. rend. Acad. d. sc., Par., 1874, lxxviii, 427.—**Collignon** (R.) Note sur un cas tératologique rare ; arrêt de développement en longueur des humérus. Bull. Soc. d'anthrop. de Par., 1886, 3. s., ix, 28.—**Collineau.** Sur un cas de phocomélie thoracique unilatérale. *Ibid.*, 1878, 3. s., i, 167–173.—**Coni.** Mónstruo unitario de la familia de los ectromelianos. Rev. méd.-quir., Buenos Aires, 1882–3, xix, 301–304, 1 pl.—**Creighton.** † Dublin M. Press, 1847, xviii, 387.—**Cruveilhier.** Note sur un cas de monopodie. Bull. Soc. anat. de Par. 1827, 2. éd., 1844, ii, 205–208. — **Cullen** (T. F.) A male monstrosity. Tr. M. Soc. N. Jersey, Newark, 1875, 125–128.—**Cunningham** (S. B.) † South. M. & S. J., Augusta, 1845, i, 120.—**Davis** (E. W.) A child born without arms. Med. Herald, Louisville, 1885–6, vii, 338.—**Davis** (J. T.) Congenital malformations. Med. & Surg. Reporter, Phila., 1871, xxiv, 112.—**Debout.** Nouveaux faits de phocomélie. Bull. Soc. de chir. de Par. (1863), 1864, 2. s., iv, 103–107.—**Delore.** Plusieurs cas d'ectromélie. Mém. et compt.-rend. Soc. d. sc. méd. de Lyon, 1863–4, pit, pt. 2, 146–149. ———. Ectromélie syndactyle. *Ibid.*, 1864–5, iv, pt. 2, 42–44. *Also* [Abstr.]: Ann. Soc. de méd. de Lyon, 1864, 2. s., xii, pt. 2, 55–57.—**Depaul.** Monstre uromèle. Bull. Soc. de chir. de Par., 1871–2, 2. s., xii, 141.—**Dreyfous** (F.) Arrêt de développement des membres supérieurs ; ectrodactylie ; altération des méninges localisée à la région des centres moteurs. Bull. Soc. anat. de Par., 1878, liii, 197–199.—**Dubreuil.** [Un fœtus phocomèle.] *Ibid.*, 1862, xxxvii, 404.—**Dumont** (H.) [Une monstruosité affectant les deux membres thoraciques. Rap. de Tillaux.] Bull. Soc. de chir. de Par. (1866), 1867, 2. s., vii, 380–382.—**Dunn.** Case of syreniform monster. Med. Times, Lond., 1844, x, 19.—**Dziecku** (O) bez czlonków. [Child without limbs.] Pam. Towarz. Lek. Warszaw., 1851, xxvi, pt. 2, 57–67.—**Edmundson** (J.) † Dublin M. Press, 1860, xliii, 483.—**Eschricht.** Ueber die Fötalkrümmungen, namentlich in Bezug auf die Bedeutung der angeborenen Verdrehungen der Bauchglieder. Deutsche Klinik, Berl., 1851, iii, 467–470.—**Eve** (P. F.) A short account of Master S. K. G. Nellis, born without arms, and of his performances with his toes. South. M. & S. J., Augusta, 1836–7, i, 522–524.—**F.** (P.) Vicios de conformacion. Anfiteatro anat., Madrid, 1873, i, 215.—**Fages** (J.) Anatomie d'un monstre ectromélien (phocomélie pelvienne double, hémimélie thoracique gauche). Gaz. hebd. d. sc. méd. de Montpel., 1885, vii, 517 ; 529. — **Feijão** (F. A. O.) Monstro ectromeliano. J. Soc. d. sc. med. de Lisb., 1877, xli, 132–141.—**Field** (N.) A remarkable case of deformity. Louisville J. M. & S., 1838, i, 67–71.—**Fischer** (A. R.) K kazuistikie urodstve utrobnago ploda ; micromelus. Vrach, St. Petersb., 1884, v, 331.—**Förster.** † Ann. f. d. ges. Heilk., Karlsruhe, 1832, iv, 2. Hft., 147, 1 pl. — **Freudenberg.** Ein Perobrachius. Allg. med. Centr.-Ztg., Berl., 1886, lv, 349.—**Frost** (H. C.) A marked case of non-development. Physicians' & Surgeons' Invest., Buffalo, 1887, viii, 1.—**Garden** (A.) Case of malformation of the lower half of the body. Indian M. Gaz., Calcutta, 1873, viii, 179.—**Gelauff** (S. P. G.) Waarneming eener verlossing van eene eigenaardige wanvormige vrucht. Boerhaave. Tijdschr., etc., Amst., 1843, n. s., ii, 335, 1 pl.—**Gerrard** (J.) Unusual fœtal deformity ; retention of placenta. Month. J. M. Sc., Lond. & Edinb., 1855, xx, 348. — **Giraud** (F.) † Marseille méd., 1881, xviii, 545–548.—**Goodman.** † Atlanta M. & S. J., 1867–8, viii, 420. — **Goubaux** (A.) De l'ectromélie et de l'amputation spontanée des membres chez les animaux domestiques. Compt. rend. Soc. de biol. 1864, Par., 1865, 4. s., i, pt. 2, 119–140. *Also:* Gaz. méd. de Par., 1865, 3. s., xx, 207 ; 223.—**Gouriet.** Exemple curieux d'anomalie multiple. Gaz. d. hôp., Par., 1857, xxx, 15. — **Goyraud** (G.) Fœtus monstrueux ; réunion des deux membres abdominaux par une masse charnue ; absence de l'appareil urinaire et des organes sexuels extérieurs ; imperforation du rectum. *Ibid.*, 1829–30, ii, 381.—**Greb** (J.) Beschreibung einer Missbildung. (Mangel der Diaphyse und oberen Epiphyse des linken Oberschenkelknochens, Verkürzung der Extremität). Würzb. med. Ztschr., 1864, v, 120–123, 1 pl.—**Greene** (W. T.) Congenital malformations. Brit. M. J., Lond., 1867, ii, 547.—**Gruber** (W.) Zergliederung oberer Extremitäten mit angeborenen Defecten an der Hand. Arch. f. Anat., Physiol. u. wissensch. Med., Leipz., 1863, 319–338, 1 pl.—**Grushetski.** † [Case of monstrosity.] Russk. Med., St. Petersb., 1885, iii, 775. — **Guérin** (E.) Vices de conformation nombreux et graves observés chez un nouveau-né. Rev. phot. d. hôp. de Par., 1869, i, 93.—**Gunning** (A. F.) A case of congenital malformation. Austral. M. J., Melbourne, 1880, n. s., ii, 485. — **Haskler** (W.) Peromelus, oder eine besondere Art von Bildungshemmung. Ztschr. f. Nat.- u. Heilk. in Ungarn, Oedenburg, 1859, x, 58.— **Hastings** (C.) Description of a monster, in whom the upper and inferior extremities were entirely wanting. Tr

Monsters *from defect or malformation of limbs.*

Med.-Chir. Soc. Edinb., 1826, ii, 39–41, 1 pl. *Also:* Edinb. J. M. Sc., 1826–7, ii, 100.—**Hauck.** [Geburt eines Monopoden.] Wchnschr. f. d. ges. Heilk., Berl., 1833, i, 556.—**Heath** (W. L.) Notes on the dissection of a malformed child. Tr. Obst. Soc. Lond. (1881), 1882, xxiii, 195–202.—**Hellwig** (J.) Infans cum capite naturali, sed corpore plano, sine manibus et pedibus, instar pupæ infantilis. *In his:* Obs. phys.-med., 4°, Aug. Vindel., 1680, 18–20.—**Hernando** (I.) Feto con defecto de partes ó agenesia. Siglo méd., Madrid, 1858, v, 172. — **Hervás y Casado** (J.) † [Ectromele.] Anfiteatro anat., Madrid, 1876, iv, 172.—**Hervé** (G.) Sur un cas d'hémimélie. Bull. Soc. d'anthrop. de Par., 1886, 3. s., ix, 752. — **Heusinger** (C. F.) Beobachtung einer Missgeburt mit Verwachsung der Haut und des Amnions, Mangel der rechten unteren Extremität u. s. w. Ztschr. f. d. organ. Phys., Eisenach, 1828, ii, 208–213. — **Hewett** (W.) Singular case of fœtal non-development. Med. Times, Lond., 1851, n. s., iii, 434.—**Hitzig.** Hæmatorrhachis, Syringomyelie, abnorme Structur des spinalen Markmantels. Tagebl. d. Versamml. deutsch. Naturf. u. Aerzte, Magdeb., 1884, lvii, 134–137.—**van der Hoeven** (L.) Over phocomele. Nederl. Tijdschr. v. Geneesk., Amst., 1884, 2. R., xx, 13–19 — **Holst** (J.) Beschreibung des Beckens und der Geschlechtstheile eines 40 Jahre alten weiblichen Amelus. *In his:* Beitr. z. Gynäk. u. Geburtsk., 8°, Tübing., 1867, ii, 145–148. — **Hottinger** (J. H.) De monstruo humano absque sexu, pedibus, etc., in excrescentiam caudiformem definente. Misc. Acad. nat. curios. 1704–5, Norimb., 1706, decuria 2, ix–x, 413–416, 1 pl.—**Houel.** [Fœtus monstrueux ; la peau tellement en excès qu'elle forme partout de larges plis qui sont, pour ainsi dire, flottant.] Bull. Soc. anat. de Par., 1850, xxv, 149. ———. Observations de monstres ectroméliens. Compt. rend. Soc. de biol. 1853, Par., 1854, v, pt. 2, 211–221. *Also* [Abstr.]: Bull. Soc. anat. de Par., 1854, xxix, 13–15. ———. Monstre symélien. Bull. Soc. anat. de Par. (1871) 1873, lxvi, 258. ———. Sur un cas de monstruosité. Bull. et mém. Soc. de chir. de Par., 1878, n. s., iv, 382–386.—**Hulke** (J. W.) A case of complete absence of both the upper limbs and of faulty development of the right lower limb. Med.-Chir. Tr., Lond., 1876–7, lx, 65–69, 1 pl.—**Isaacs** (C. E.) An account of a case of monstrosity. N. York M. & S. Reporter, 1847, ii, 89–95.—**Jackson** (J. B. S.) † (Siren.) Boston M. & S. J., 1869, lxxx, 33–35. *Also:* Extr. Rec. Bost. Soc. M. Improve. (1866–74), 1876, vi (app.), 74–78. ———. Deficiency of the extremities. Extr. Rec. Bost. Soc. M. Improve. (1874–9), 1880, vii, 35.—**Jacobæus** (O.) Monstra cruribus intortis, et capreæ figura. Acta med. et phil. Hafn. (1674–5), 1677, iii, 97–99.—**Jacobi.** Congenital deficiency of the right thigh. Am. J. Obst., N. Y., 1871, iv, 548. ———. A phocomelus with insufficient development of osseous tissue. Tr. N. York Obst. Soc. (1876–8), 1879, i, 308. *Also:* Am. J. Obst., N. Y., 1878, xi, 143. — **Jäger** (C. G.) Fall einer Missbildung per defectum. Ztschr. d. deutsch. Chir.-Ver., Magdeb., 1850, iv, 377. — **Jean** (A.) Cas d'hémimélie (avant-bras gauche). Bull. Soc. anat. de Par., 1877, lii, 144–146.—**Johnson** (S. P.) † [Monopodus.] Virginia M. J., Richmond, 1858, xi, 351.—**Julliard** (G.) Mémoire sur un monstre appartenant à la famille des syméliens et sur les causes de la symélie. Compt. rend. Soc. de biol. 1868, [Par., 1869, 4. s., v, pt. 2, 63–76. *Also:* Gaz. méd. de Par., 1869, 3. s., xxiv, 199 ; 212.—**Krahe** (C.) A monstrous child. Phil. Tr. 1698-1700, 4. ed., Lond., 1731, iii, 304, 1 pl. *Also, transl.:* Collect. acad. d. mém., etc, Dijon, 1766, vii, 71, 1 pl. — **Krauss** (E.) Ueber einen Fall von Syringomyelie. Arch. f. path. Anat., etc, Berl., 1885, ci, 304–315, 1 pl.—**Larcher** (O.) Syméliens. Dict. encycl. d. sc. méd., Par., 1884, 3. s., xiii, 663–669.—**Laroche** (V.) [*et al.*]. Rapport sur un fœtus monstrueux monobrache. Arch. gén. de méd., Par., 1830, xxiii, 506–518.—**Larrey.** Phocomélie thoracique unilatérale gauche. Bull. Soc. de chir. de Par. (1870), 1871, 2. s., xi, 258–260.—**Laval** (V.) Un enfant né sans jambes et avec un seul bras. Union méd., Par., 1878, 3. s., xxvi, 41–43. — **Lecadre.** Monstruosité par défaut, ou privation des extrémités abdominales et de l'avant-bras gauche. Compt. rend. Soc. de biol. 1852, Par., 1853, iv, 8.—**Lenhossék.** Beschreibung einer menschlichen Missgeburt, bey welcher das ganze Muskel-System mangelt, nebst einigen physiologischen Bemerkungen. Med. Jahrb. d. k. k. österr. Staates, Wien, 1819–20, v, 4. St., 109–132, 1 pl.—**Lissauer.** Eine Missgeburt mit Mangel der Extremitäten. Allg. med. Centr.-Ztg., Berl., 1871, xl, 805.—**Little.** Casts of a peculiar fœtal malformation. Tr. Path. Soc. Lond., 1846–8, i, 331–334. — **Losada** (C. F.) Ectromelia abdominal del lado derecho. Gac. de sanid. mil., Madrid, 1880, vi, 120–124, 1 pl.—**Lutz** (F. J.) A living boy, with congenital absence of the limbs. St. Louis M. & S. J., 1877, xiv, 578–581. — **McClintock.** Skeleton of a monstrous fœtus. Dublin Q. J. M. Sc., 1857, xxiii, 218–220.—**Macdougall** (J.) † (Phocomelos.) Tr. Edinb. Obst. Soc. (1876-7), 1878, iv, 50–52. *Also:* Edinb. M. J., 1874–5, xx, 940. *Also:* Obst. J. Gr. Brit., Lond., 1875–6, iii, 126.—**M'Ghie** (J.) Case of congenital malformation

Monsters *from defect or malformation of limbs.*

and abnormal presentation. Glasgow M. J., 1858–9, vi, 47, 1 pl.—**Maclaren** (W.) Case of siren-like malformed fœtus at full time, with a well-formed penis on the posterior aspect of the body. Edinb. M. J., 1873-4, xix, 590–592.—**Macloughlin.** Case of a child born without limbs. Med. Times & Gaz., Lond., 1853, n. s., vii, 604.—**Marduel.** Un monstre symélien uromèle. Ann. Soc. de méd. de Lyon, 1868, 2. s., xvi, pt. 2, 27–29.—**Martin** (E.) & **Le-tulle** (M.) Contribution à la tératologie; monstre unitaire; hémimélie. J. de l'anat et physiol., etc , Par., 1877, xiii, 371–390, 1 pl.—**Martinez y Molina** (R.) Cuatro palabras sobre el mónstruo sin estremidades que actualmente llama la atencion en esta córte. Siglo méd., Madrid, 1856, iii, 114.—**de Martino** (G.) & **Renzone** (R.) Ricerche anatomiche e considerazioni su di un feto umano con osso intermascellare e con altre rare e rilevanti anomalie. Rendic. Accad. med.-chir. di Napoli, 1871, xxv, 5–14.—**Maurice** (E.-F.) Note sur un monstre humain hémimèle. Ann. Soc. de méd. de St.-Étienne et de la Loire (1877–80), 1881, vii, 48–52.—**Mayet.** Cas d'ectromélie. Mém. et compt.-rend. Soc. d. sc. méd. de Lyon, 1866-7, vi, 288–291. *Also:* Gaz. méd. de Lyon, 1867, xix, 161.—**Meadows** (A.) & **Bannister** (A. J.) [Monstrosity, with caudal appendage in place of the lower extremities.] Tr. Obst. Soc. Lond. (1867), 1868, ix, 112–116.—**Meckel** (J. F.) Ueber die Verschmelzungsbildungen. Arch. f. Anat. u. Physiol., Leipz., 1826, i, 238–310.—**de Mesquita** (A. J.) † J. Soc. d. sc. med. de Lisb., 1856, 2. s., xviii, 58–67.—**Mestre** (A.) Caso de ectromelia. An. r. Acad. de cien. méd. . . . de la Habana, 1866-7, iii, 316–318.—**Michalski.** Angeborne Anomalien der organischen Entwicklung (Monstra per defectum). Preuss. Med.-Ztg., Berl., 1862, n. F., v, 355.—**Miller** (N. F.) Urodstva konechnostei. [Monsters as to extremities.] Trudi Obsh. Russk. vrach. v. Mosk., Moskva, 1885, 121–135, 1 pl.—**Milroy** (D.) † [Siren] Edinb. M. J., 1858–9, iv, 1098–1101.—**Milward** (J.) † Tr. Obst. Soc. Lond. (1872), 1873, xiv, 141.—**Mitchell** (S.) † Boston M. & S. J., 1859, lx, 178.—**Moores** (W. L.) † Cincin. M. Repert., 1868, i, 202.—**Moré.** † Gaz. méd. de Par., 1847, 3. s., ii, 991.—**Moreau.** [Enfants offrant plusieurs exemples d'amputations spontanées] Bull. Soc. anat. de Par., 1847, xxii, 395.—**Morgan** (J. H.) Siren monster. Tr. Path. Soc. Lond., 1886, xxxvii, 555.—**Nagel.** Beschreibung einer männlichen Missgeburt, welche in der Sternalgegend zwei obere Extremitäten, dann ein Becken mit den untern Extremitäten und den Sexual-Organen überzählig besass. Oesterr. med. Wchnschr., Wien, 1845, 257–261—**Neale** (L. E.) Fœtal monstrosity. Maryland M. J., Balt., 1886-7, xvi, 337.—**O'Farrell** (G.) A case in which both legs were amputated in utero. Phila. M. Times, 1873-4, iv, 277.—**Osiander** (J. F.) Monstrum horrendum. J. f. Geburtsh., Frankf. a. M., 1829, ix, 277.—**Paget.** Monstrosity in a child, following a fright to the mother in the third month of pregnancy. Med. Times & Gaz., Lond., 1865, ii, 333. *Also:* Canada M. J., Montreal, 1865-6, ii, 165–167.—**Palmer** (E.), jr. Extraordinary case of monstrosity. Med. Mag., Bost., 1834, iii, 327–330.—**Parada y Santin** (J) Sobre un mónstruo ameliano. Rev. de med. y cirug. práct , Madrid, 1881, viii, 109–119.—**Petermann** (B. B.) & **Rudorff.** Von dem beschriebenen Leipzigischen Monstro, und einem andern in Schlesien und Polen, welches letztere halb Mensch und halb Kalb soll gewesen seyn. Samml. v. Nat.- u. Med.- . . . Gesch. 1723, Leipz., 1724, xxiv, 563–566, 1 pl.—**Petit.** Description et dissection d'un monstre uromèle. Bull. méd. du nord, Lille, 1869, x, 337–360.—**Plant** (W. T.) An anomalous monstrosity. Obst. Gaz., Cincin., 1878-9, i, 398.—**Prochaska.** Beschreibung einer menschlichen Missgeburt mit umgekehrten untern Gliedmassen. Med. Jahrb. d. k. k. österr. Staates, Wien, 1811–12, i, 4. St., 155–164, 1 pl.—**Ranke** (H.) Bemerkungen über ein fünf Monate altes Kind mit angebornem Mangel aller Gliedmassen. Arch. f. path. Anat., etc., Berl., 1880, lxxxii, 360–374, 1 pl.—**Rasori.** Peromelia e micromelia. Gazz. d. osp., Milano, 1882, iii, 403–405.—**Raverty** (G. A.) A case of monstrosity. Brit. M. J., Lond., 1883, i, 1116.—**Reisel** (S.) Infans truncus sine artubus. Misc. Acad. nat. curios. 1689, Norimb., 1690, decuria 2, viii, 136, 1 pl. *Also, transl.:* Auserl. med.- chir. . . . Abhandl. d. röm.-kais. Akad. d. Naturf., Nürnb., 1769, xviii, 122, 1 pl.—**Renaut.** Sur deux cas d'ectrodactylie et un cas d'hémimèle. Bull. Soc. anat. de Par. (1870), 1874, xlv, 224.—**Retzius** (A.) Tvenne fall af missbildning med bålens förkortning genom benens sammansmältning (Nanocormus *Gurlt*). Förh. v. de skandin. Naturf. 1844, Christiania, 1847, 326–330.—**Richter.** Eine Missgeburt. Med. Cor.-Bl. d. württemb. ärztl. Ver., Stuttg., 1872, xlii, 133.—**Rieding.** Geburt eines monströsen Fötus. Prov.-San.-Ber. d. k. Med.-Coll. v. Pommern 1837, Stettin, 1838, 141.—**Ringhoffer.** Beschreibung einer menschlichen Missgeburt. Arch. f. path. Anat., etc., Berl., 1860, xix, 28–42, 1 pl.—**Rivetius.** Monstrosus infans. Zodiacus med.-gall. 1680, Geneva, 1682, ii, 79, 1 pl.—**Robin** (C.) Cas de tératologie. Rev. phot. d. hôp. de Par., 1869, i, 113, 2 pl.—**Roderique** (A.) Case of monstrosity. Am. J. M. Sc., Phila., 1835, xvi, 249. — **Rodriguez** (J.

Monsters *from defect or malformation of limbs.*

M.) Teratología; estudio sobre varias monstruosidades ectromelianas y mas particularmente sobre Pedro Salinas. Gac. méd. de México, 1872, vii, 381; 397. *Also,* Reprint.—**Roger** (H.) Note sur un exemple de double main-bot congéniale, avec absence du radius, observé sur un enfant à terme. Union méd., Par., 1851, v, 562. *Also:* Bull. Soc. méd. d. hôp. de Par. (1849–52), 1861, i, 249–253.—**Sachero** (G.) Descrizione d' un neonato mostruoso. Ann. univ. di med., Milano, 1830, lv, 95–103, 1 pl.—**Scellier.** Description anatomico-pathologique d'un fœtus monobrache, monopode et agame, parvenu à peu près au terme de la naissance, mais cependant mort avant l'accouchement. Arch. gén. de méd., Par., 1823, iii, 415–418. — **Schabel.** † Med. Cor.-Bl. d. württemb. ärztl. Ver., Stuttg., 1854, xxiv, 103.—**Sentex** (L.) Note sur un cas de mélomélie. Gaz. d. hôp., Par., 1882, lv, 99. *Also, transl.:* Arch. f. Kinderh., Stuttg., 1882-3, iv, 232. ——. Phocomélie accompagnée d'ectrodactylie. J. de méd. de Bordeaux, 1886-7, xvi, 53. — **Sewall.** † [Apodia.] N. York M. Times, 1854, iii, 128.—**Sim** (F. L.) Fœtal monstrosity. Mississippi Valley M. Month., Memphis, 1883, iii, 13–15.—**Simmons** (W.) A case of malformation. Med. & Phys. J., Lond., 1800, iv, 189–191, 1 pl.—**Skinner** (N. C.) Singular fœtal malformation. Med. Exam., Phila., 1854, n. s., x, 461–465.—**Smiley** (G. P.) Remarkable monstrosity. St. Louis Cour. Med., 1882, vii, 271–273. — **Smith.** Doubtful case; infant born without legs. Lancet, Lond., 1837-8, i, 409.—**Snow** (G. W.) Case of arrest of development of both upper extremities. Tr. N. York Obst. Soc. (1876-8), 1879, i, 20.—**Solger** (B.) Fall von Monobrachius. Jahresb. d. schles. Gesellsch. f. vaterl. Kult. 1876, Bresl., 1877, liv, 225. — **de Souza Fontes** (J. R.) Ein lebender Knabe mit angebornem Mangel der Glieder. Arch. f. path. Anat., etc.. Berl., 1877, lxxi, 107–111, 1 pl.—**Spencer** (R. H.) A curious monster. Med. Rec., N. Y., 1885, xxviii, 258.—**Stadthagen.** Angeborener hochgradiger Defect sämmtlicher vier Extremitäten, fehlendes Schwanzbein und zurückgebliebene Schwanzverlängerung bei einem lebenden Neugeborenen. Monatschr. f. Geburtsk. u. Frauenkr., Berl., 1860, xvi, 321–331.—**Stein.** Eine sirenenartige Missgeburt von chinesischen Eltern; beschrieben und für die Lehre von der Diagnose der vorliegenden Theile bei der Geburt benutzt. N. Ztschr. f. Geburtsk., Berl., 1841, x, 338–344. — **Stricker** (G.) Doppelseitiger angeborner Defect des Radius und des Daumens. Arch. f. path. Anat., etc.. Berl., 1864, xxxi, 529. ——. Grossartiger Defect an beiden Vorderarmen und Händen eines Neugebornen. *Ibid.*, 1878, lxxii, 144.—**Tassani** (A. F.) Mostro monopodo. Gazz. med. ital. lomb., Milano, 1848, 2. s., i, 274.—**Tassin** père. Observation d'hémimélie thoracique droite. Bull. Soc. méd. de l'Yonne, Auxerre, 1870, xi, 10–12, 2 pl.—**Taylor** (S. F.) A case of monstrosity. N. York M. J., 1883, xxxvii, 260.—**Thompson** (B.) † Phila. M. Museum, 1806, ii, 17–20, 1 pl. — **Troisier.** Hémimélie thoracique du côté droit; examen de la moelle épinière. Bull. Soc. anat. de Par. (1870), 1873, xlvi, 140–142. *Also:* Arch. de physiol. norm. et path., Par., 1871-2, iv, 72–82, 1 pl.—**Verrier** (E.) Note concernant un fœtus ectromélien. Gaz. obst., Par., 1879, viii, 193–196. *Also* [Abstr.]: Ann. de gynéc., Par., 1879, xii, 65. ——. Dystocie tératologique; note sur un cas d'éventration fœtale avec un seul membre inférieur, considéré au point de vue de la dystocie. Médecin prat., Par., 1882, iii, 589–593. *Also* [Abstr.]: Bull. Acad. de méd., Par., 1882, 2. s., xi, 1434. — **Vianna** (C.) (Monstruosidade sem braços nem pernas.) Gaz. med. de Lisb., 1856, iv, 84–87, 1 pl. — **Villard** (F.) Arrêts de développement multiples; hémi-phocomélie. Rev. phot. d. hôp. de Par., 1871, iii, 164–167. — **Vincent** (A. F.) Remarkable monstrosity, consequent upon maternal impressions. Nashville J. M. & S., 1883, xxxii, 68. — **Wall** (O. A.) † [Monopodus.] Med. Arch., St. Louis, 1872, viii, 330.—**Wedemeyer.** Mangelhafte Ausbildung der Extremitäten. J. d. Chir. u. Augenh., Berl., 1826, ix, 113 — **Willis** (E. C.) Hereditary formations. Lancet, Lond., 1857, ii, 258.

Monsters *from defect or malformation of spine.*

See, also, Sacro-coccygeal *region* (*Tumors of*); Spina *bifida*; Spine (*Abnormities of*).

NICHOLSON (G.) * De monstro humano sine trunco nato. 4°. *Berolini*, [1837].

Also, transl. [Abstr.]: Arch. f. Anat., Physiol. u. wissensch. Med., Berl., 1837, 328–334, 4 pl.

REMBE (J.) * Beitrag zur Lehre von der Wirbelspalte, nebst einigen anderen Entwicklungsanomalieen. 8°. *Erlangen*, 1877.

RUMPHOLZ (C.) * De monstro trunco carente. 4°. *Halis Sax.*, [1848].

SÄNGER (W. M. H.) * Beschrijving van eene misvormde menschelijke vrucht, benevens eenige

Monsters *from defect or malformation of spine.*

opmerkingen omtrent de zoogenaamde aangeboren Engelsche ziekte (rachitis congenita). 8°. *Leyden*, 1857.

Bax. Accouchement prématuré: présentation de la plaie; malformation congénitale; double pied-bot et spina-bifida cranio-cervical; autopsie. Soc. méd. d'Amiens. Bull. (1873-4), 1875, 179-193. [Rap. de Peulevé], 194-200.—**Blanchot** (E. F.) De monstro singulari, sine collo et spina dorsi a meretrici prognato. Acta Acad. nat. curios. 1748-50, Norimb., 1752, ix, 350-356, 1 pl.—**Cabot.** Sacral teratoma. Boston M. & S. J., 1878, xcviii, 112-114.—**Folet** (H.) [Anatomie tératologique; anomalies des vertèbres et des côtes] Bull. méd. du nord, Lille, 1870-71, xi, 319-328. *Also*, Reprint.—**Giraud** (J. T.) † Med. & Phys. J., Lond., 1803, x, 171-173, 1 pl.—**Green** (W. A.) Remarkable case of malformation. South. M. & S. J., Augusta, 1858, n. s. xiv, 451.—**Löffler** (A. F.) Ein pathologisches Naturspiel eines monströsen Kindes mit einer kopfähnlichen Geschwulst am Heiligbein hängend. N. Arch. f. d. Geburtsh., etc., Jena, 1798-1800, i, 2.-3. St., 145-151, 1 pl.—**Mayer.** Ueber eine Missgeburt; Kopf ohne Rumpf (Acormus). Arch. f. path. Anat., etc., Berl., 1864, xxix, 380-389, 1 pl.—**Millar** (W. S.) Description of a fœtus presenting remarkable deviations from normal structure. Lancet, Lond., 1858, i, 60-62.—**Porro** (E.) Sopra un caso di straordinario atteggiamento di feto mal conformato, ed osservazioni sopra alcuni difficoltà accompagnanti la nascita di feti mostruosi o malati. Gazz. med. ital. lomb., Milano, 1873, xxxiii, 393; 404; 409, 1 pl.: 1874, xxxiv, 1. ———. Distocia grave per gravissima e strana mostruosità. *Ibid.*, 185-187, 1 pl.—**Sänger.** Monstrum mit eigenthümlichen Dys- und Aplasien der Wirbelsäule und des Beckens. Arch. f. Gynaek., Berl., 1879, xiv, 306-308.—**Soriano** (M.) Feto monstruo; lordosis. Gac. méd. de México, 1867-8, iii, 78-80.—**Whitfield** (G.) Case of fœtal monstrosity; labor retarded thereby. N. Orl. J. M., 1870, xxiii, 479-481.—**Vanverts.** Cas rare de monstruosité. Bull. méd. du nord, Lille, 1860, 2. s., i, 147-150.

Monsters *by inclusion.*

See **Fœtus** *in fœtu.*

Monstruosité autositaire. (Enfants jumeaux réunis par le crâne.) Communiquée à l'Académie impériale de médecine le 16 avril 1861. 3 pp. 8°. *Paris, L. Martinet*, [1861].

Repr. from: Bull. Acad. de méd., Par., 1861, xxvi.

Monsummano.

GRANDEAU (L.) Notice sur la grotte thermale de Monsummano (Toscane). 8°. *Paris*, 1864.

Turchetti (O.) Guida pei bagni a vapore naturale della Grotta di Monsummano, con osservazione pratiche. Ann. univ. di med., Milano, 1869, ccix, 457: cex, 3.—**W.** Die Dampfgrotte von Monsummano. Prag. med. Wchnschr., 1883, viii, 152; 164.

Monsummano e Monte-Vettolini. Regolamento comunale di igiene pubblica. 33 pp. 8°. *Pescia, Vannini*, 1873.

du Mont (Nicolaus). Exercitatio medica de chyli secretione et distributione. 5 l. 4°. *Basileæ, typ. J. Bertschius*, [1690].

Montag (Joh. Ernst). * Ueber die Harnruhr. 43 pp. 8°. *Würzburg, Becker*, 1850.

Montagard (Émile). * De la vaginite aiguë et chronique. 72 pp. 4°. *Paris*, 1877, No. 263.

Montagk (Car. Anton. August.) * In philosophiam medicam introductio. 34 pp., 1 l. 8°. [*Berolini*], *formis Brueschckianis*, [1823].

Montagna (Giuseppe). Sopra alcune malattie del corpo umano; cenni teorico-pratici. Si aggiunge un discorso anatomico dello stesso autore. 98 pp. 8°. *Verona, V. Crescini*, 1831.

———. Sul perfezionamento della litotomia nel Veneto; cenni storici. 22 pp. 8°. *Parma, Carmignani*, 1844. [P., v. 1108.]

Montagnac (Barthélemy). * Étude clinique sur la dilatation des bronches. 68 pp., 2 l. 4°. *Montpellier*, 1874, No. 39.

Montagnac (Léonard). * Sur la pleurésie. 22 pp. 4°. *Paris*, 1834, No. 162, v. 273.

Montagnan (J.) * Quelques considérations sur l'utilité de l'anatomie pathologique pour la thérapentique. 32 pp. 4°. *Paris*, 1836, No. 138, v. 298.

Montagnana.

See **Cholera** (*Asiatic, History, etc , of*), *by localities.*

Montagnana (*Angelus*) [–1678].

Portrait in: **Collection**—van Kaathoven.

Montagnana (Bartholomæus) [–circa 1460]. Consilia... Tractatus tres de balneis patavinis; de compositione et dosi medicinarum; antidotarium ejusdem. 7 p. l., 387 ff., 1 l. fol. [*Venetiis*], *sumpt. B. Locatellus*, 1497.

———. The same. Consilia... cum tribus tractatibus de balneis Patavinis, et de compositione et dosi medicinarum ac antidotario. Consilia domini Antonii Cermisoni Patavini. Tractatus de animali theria domini Francisci Caballi. 6 p. l., 413 ff. fol. [*n. p., n. d.*]

Folio 406 is blank. The treatises of Montagnana end with fol. 354. The treatise of Cermisonus ends with: Venetiis per Simonem de Luere, 9 Septembris, 1514.

———. De balneis, et utilitatibus juvamentisque eorum, ac regulæ et modus quem observare debent.

In: GATENARIA (Marcus). Omnes, quos scripsit, libri, [etc.] fol. *Basileæ*, 1537, 274-291.

———. Selectiorum operum in quibus ejusdem consilia variique tractatus alii, tum proprii tum adscititii, continentur liber unus et alter... revisi, relecti, locupletati a Petro Uffeubachio. 3 p. l., 1309 pp., 7 l. fol. *E paltheniano musarum Francofurtensium collegio*, 1604.

See, also, **Illustrium** in re medica. 16°. *Patavini*, 1556.

Montagnana (Bartholomæus)[2] [–1525]. De morbo gallico consilium.

In: LUISINUS (A.) Aphrodisiacus, [etc.] Ed. emend. fol. *Lugd. Bat.*, 1728, 957-966.

Montagnana (Marcus Antonius). De herpete, phagedæna, gangræna, sphacelo, et cancro, tum cognoscendis, tum curandis, tractatio accuratissima. 7 p. l., 107 ff. 4°. *Venetiis, apud P. Meiettum*, 1589.

Montagne (Angel). * Contribution à l'étude de l'alimentation, envisagée au point de vue physiologique (en particulier à l'hôpital et dans l s établissements de bienfaisance de la ville du Havre). [*Paris.*] 93 pp. 4°. *Havre*, 1885, No. 268.

———. The same. 93 pp., 1 tab. 8°. *Paris, G. Steinheil*, 1885.

Montagne (Édouard). Histoire de la prostitution dans l'antiquité. 96 pp. roy. 8°. *Paris, A. Fayard*, [1872].

Montagne (J.-L.) * Étude clinique sur le salol. 68 pp. 4°. *Lyon, imprimerie nouvelle*, 1887, 1. s., No. 353.

Montagne (Jean-François-Camille) [1784-1866]. Sylloge generum specierumque cryptogamarum. 498 pp. 8°. *Parisiis, J.-B. Baillière*, 1856.

For Biography, see Gaz. méd. de Par., 1866, xxi, 757-763. *Also:* Rec. de mém. de méd.... mil., Par., 1866, 3. s., xvi, 81-96 (Larrey). *Also*, Reprint.

Montagnon (Félix). De la fréquence des localisations et des reliquats prostatiques dans la blennorrhagie et de leur rôle dans la blennorrhée. 16 pp. 8°. *Lyon*, 1885.

———. * Contribution à l'étude des abcès de la cornée. Du prognostic et du traitement des grands abcès de la cornée. 1 p. l., 82 pp. 4°. *Lyon*, 1887, 1. s., No 376.

Montagu (George). An essay on sponges, with descriptions of all the species that have been discovered on the coast of Great Britain. (Read 7th March, 1812.) 56 pp., 14 pl. 8°. [*n. p.*, 1812.] [P., v. 726.]

Montagut (J.-George). * Propositions sur quelques maladies des voies urinaires, et sur l'opération du cathétérisme. 11 pp. 4°. *Paris*, 1810, No. 60, v. 79.

Montaignac (Albert). * De l'ulcère artério-athéromateux du pied (autrement dit mal perforant). 94 pp. 4°. *Paris*, 1868, No. 274.

Montaigu-lez-Combrailles.

See **Fever** (*Typhus, History, etc., of*), *by localities.*

Montain jeune. Mémoire sur plusieurs points d'anatomie, de chirurgie et de l'art des accouchemens. 35 pp. 8°. [*Paris, Migneret,* 1817.] [P., v. 1524.]

Repr. from : J. de méd., chir., pharm., etc., Par., 1817, xxxviii.

Montain (F.-P.) * I. Établir le diagnostic et le traitement du rupia. II. [etc.] 43 pp. 4°. *Paris,* 1841, No. 224, v. 378.

Montain (Gilbert-Alphonse-Claude) [1780-1853]. * Quelques propositions sur les maladies laiteuses. 8 pp. 4°. *Paris,* 1808, No. 77, v. 71.

———. Du lait considéré comme cause des maladies des femmes en couche. x, 11–67 pp. 8°. *Paris, Brunot-Labbé,* 1808. [P., v. 131.]

———. Discours sur quelques parties de l'hygiène publique et privée, prononcé pour l'ouverture des cours de l'École secondaire de médecine de Lyon, à Hôtel-Dieu. 16 pp. 8°. *Lyon, L. Perrin,* 1832. [P., v. 132.]

———. Mémoires de thérapeutique médico-chirurgicale ; médication pneumatique ; sangsues artificielles ; section du fillet et de la luette ; agrafe labiale ; staphyloraphie ; périnoraphie ; accouchements secs ; rétention d'urine ; soudes à dilater ; alcoolé sécalique ; extrait cynarique ; sulfure de chaux, etc. iv, 88 pp., 1 l., 1 pl. 8°. *Paris, J.-B. Baillière,* 1836.

For Biography, see Ann. Soc. de méd. de Lyon, 1855, 2. s., iii, 148–170 (Brachet). *Also,* Reprint. *Also :* Gaz. méd. de Lyon, 1855, vii, 109–121.

Montajone.

See **Cholera** (*Asiatic, History, etc., of*), *by localities.*

Montalban (*Ovidius*) [1601–1672].

Portrait in : **Collection**—van Kaathoven.

Montalcino. Statuto organico dello Spedale di Montalcino. 23 pp. 8°. *Montalcino, Donnoli,* 1883.

Montaldo (Giambattista). Il controstimolo dedotto dall' analisi fisio patologica dell' infiammazione. Commentario di . . . xii, 13–117 pp. 8°. *Genova, F. Pagano,* [1828]. [P., v. 1350.]

Montalègre (Audibert-Sylvain). * Sur l'étiologie de la mort du fœtus dans le sein de sa mère. 38 pp. 4°. *Paris,* 1852, No. 287, v. 529.

Montalembert (J.-F.-Charles). * Sur la stomatite en général, ou inflammation de la bouche. 17 pp. 4°. *Paris,* 1826, No. 38, v. 198.

Montalier (Charles-Louis-René). * De la myotomie pour le redressement immédiat dans la coxalgie et en particulier des sections du couturier et du fascia lata. 44 pp. 4°. *Paris, A. Parent,* 1879, No. 188.

Montalier (Pierre-Charles). * De l'angine couenneuse. 39 pp. 4°. *Paris,* 1848, No. 205, v. 475.

de Montallegry. Hypochondrie-spleen, ou névroses trisplanchniques. Observations relatives à ces maladies, et leur traitement radical. xvi, 144 pp. 8°. *Paris, Fortin, Masson & Cie.,* 1841.

Montalti (Ciro). Lo Spedale civile di Ravenna nell' anno 1879. Con annotazioni su la cura delle febbri intermittenti, la toracentesi, e la miliare. 80 pp. 8°. *Ravenna, E. Lavagna,* 1880.

Montaltus (Hieronymus). De homine sano libri iii, in quorum primo agitur de natura et substantia hominis ; in altero de his quæ ad ipsam

Montaltus (Hieronymus)—continued. substantiam labefactandam ejusque functiones violandas valent ; in tertio denique de facultate qua hæc propulsare, et proinde illam tueri valemus. 7 p. l., 506 pp., 7 l. 12°. *Francofurti, apud J. Wechelum et P. Fischerum consortes* 1591.

Montan.

See **Cholera** (*Asiatic, History, etc., of*), *by localities.*

Montaña de Monserrate (Bernardino) [1483–]. Libro de la anothomia del hombre . . . En el qual libro se trata de la fabrica y compostura del hombre, y de la manera como se engendra y nasce, y de las causas por que necessariamente muere. Juntamente con una declaraciõ de un sueño que soño el illustrissimo señor Don Luys Hurtado de Mendoça, Marques de Mondejar . . . El qual sueño debaxo de una figura muy graciosa, trata brevemente la dicha fabrica del hombre, con todo lo de mas que en este libro se contiene. 8 p. l., 136 ff. fol. *Valladolid, S. Martinez,* 1551.

Title-page in red and black. The "Sueño del marques de Mondejar" has a separate title-page, commencing "Sigue se un coloquio del Illustrissimo señor Don Luys Hurtado de Mendoça", [etc.]

Montana *Territory.*

See, also, **Dakota** *Territory.*

STRAHORN (R. E.) The resources of Montana Territory, and attractions of Yellowstone National Park ; facts and experiences on the farming, stock-raising, mining, lumbering, and other industries of Montana, and notes on the climate, scenery, game, fish, and mineral springs. 8°. *Helena,* 1879.

Montañana (Pedro). Examen de un practicante boticario, substituto de el maestro en el despacho de las medicinas. Recopilado por . . . 7 p. l., 304 pp. 16°. *Zaragoza, J. de Casas,* [1728].

Montanari (L.) Cenno sull' organismo umano ed importanza dell' acqua su di esso specie in rapporto alla salute. Conferenza di presidio. 26 pp. 8°. *Roma, Z. C. Voghera,* 1886.

Repr. from : Riv. mil. ital., 1886.

Montanceix (J.-Delage). * Propositions et observations sur le traitement de quelques maladies. 27 pp. 4°. *Paris,* 1829, No. 138, v. 225.

Montané (Louis). * Étude anatomique du crâne chez les microcéphales. 74 pp., 3 l., 6 pl. 4°. *Paris,* 1874, No. 79.

———. The same. 76 pp., 2 tab., 1 l., 6 pl. 8°. *Paris, J.-B. Baillière & fils,* 1874.

Montané (Louis-Justin-Marie-Cyprien). * Du traitement curatif de la varicocèle et en particulier de son traitement par l'isolement des veines 1 p. l., 43 pp. 4°. *Strasbourg,* 1868, 3. s., No. 63.

Montaner (Pietro).

See **Masdevall** (Joseph). Relazione dell' epidemie sofferte nel principato di Catalogna. 12°. *Venezia,* 1790.

Montanier (Joseph-Henri) [1824–72]. * De la maladie de Bright. 43 pp. 4°. *Paris,* 1849, No. 8, v. 487.

———. Quelques considérations sur le traitement de la syphilis à propos de la discussion à la Société de chirurgie. 56 pp. 8°. *Paris, P. Asselin,* 1867.

Repr. from : Gaz. d. hôp., Par., 1867, xl.

———. Les facultés de médecine de province avant la révolution. 43 pp. 8°. *Saint-Germain, L. Toinon & Cie.,* 1868.

Repr. from : Rev. de Par , 1868.

———. * Des conditions pathogéniques et de la valeur séméiologique de l'albuminurie. 55 pp. 4°. *Paris, Maulde & Renou,* 1857.

Concours.

Montanier (Joseph Henri)—continued.

——. Du traitement par les bougies de la blennorrhée, ou goutte militaire. 15 pp. 8°. *Paris, P. Asselin,* 1863.

Repr. from: Gaz. d. hôp., Par., 1863, xxxvi.

See, also, **Maisonneuve** (Jacques-Giles) & **Montanier** (Joseph-Henry). Traité pratique des maladies vénériennes, [etc.] 8°. *Paris,* 1853.

Montano (Joseph). *Note sur une opération de polype naso-pharyngien par la galvano-caustic physique. 44 pp. 4°. *Paris,* 1872, No. 434.

Montanus (Joannes Augustus). *De curatione ulcerum per puris resorptionem. 20 pp. 4°. [*Erfordiæ*], *ex off. Nonnii,* [1769].

Montanus (Joannes Baptista) [1498–1552]. Metaphrasis summaria eorum quæ ad medicamentorum doctrinam attinent, excerpta ab accuratis auditoribus ex quotidianis prælectionibus in Patavino gymnasio publice explicatis. 64 pp. 16°. *Patavii, excud. J. Fabrianus,* 1550.

——. De differentiis medicamentorum et causis diversarum virium ac facultatum in medicamentis, tractatus pulcherrimus exceptus ex ore enarrantis quartam partem primi libri Avicennæ. 46 pp. 32°. *Wittebergæ,* 1551.

——. Summaria declaratio eorum quæ ad urinarum cognitionem maxime faciunt. 1 p. l., 52 pp. 4°. *Viennæ, E. Aquila,* 1552.

——. In tertiam primi epidemiorum sectionem explanationes. A Valentino Lublino Polono collectæ. 7 p. l., 260 pp. 16°. *Venetiis, apud B. Constantinum,* 1554.

——. Consultationum medicinalium centuria prima, a Valentino Lublino Polono quam accurate collecta. 7 p. l., 628 pp. 12°. *Venetiis, apud V. Valgrisium,* 1554.

——. De excrementis lib. ii, a Valentino Lublino Polono in studiosorum communem utilitatem dati. Alter de fecibus, alter de urinis, quibus accessit quæstio ejusdem quomodo medicamentum æquale vel inæquale dicatur. Tractatus etiam utilissimus, de morbo gallico. 39, 52, 20, 29 ff. 12°. *Venetiis, apud B. Constantinum,* 1554.

Another copy bound with his: In nonum librum [etc.] 12°. *Venetiis,* 1554.

——. Opuscula. I. De characterismis febrium. II. Quæstio de febre sanguinis. III. De uterinis affectibus. A Valentino Lublino Polono collecta. 3 p. l., 110 pp., 1 l. 12°. *Venetiis, apud B. Constantinum,* 1554.

——. De morbo gallico tractatus. 20 ff. 12°. *Venetiis, apud B. Constantinum,* 1554.

Another copy bound with his: In nonum librum [etc.] 12°. *Venetiis,* 1554.

——. The same. Ejusdemque de eodem epistolæ quædam ex consultationibus centuriarum medicinalium ipsius excerptæ.

In: LUISINUS (A.) Aphrodisiacus, [etc.] Ed. emend. fol. *Lugd. Bat.,* 1728, 553–584.

——. In libros Galeni de arte curandi ad Glauconem explanationes. 3 p. l., 562 ff. 16°. *Venetiis, apud B. Constantinum,* 1554.

——. Quæstio in qua examinatur quomodo medicamentum dicatur æquale aut inæquale, videlicet, calidum, frigidum, humidum, aut siccum. 29 ff. 12°. *Venetiis, apud B. Constantinum,* 1554.

Another copy bound with his: In nonum librum [etc.] 12°. *Venetiis,* 1554.

——. In nonum librum Rhasis ad Mansorem regem Arabum expositio. A Valentino Lublino Polono, medicis posteritatique eorum fideliter communicata. 11 p. l., 344 ff. 12°. *Venetiis, apud B. Constantinum,* 1554.

——. Explicatio eorum quæ pertinent, tum ad qualitates simplicium medicamentorum, tum ad eorundem compositionem. 3 p. l., 61 pp. 16°. *Venetiis, apud B. Constantinum,* 1555.

Bound with preceding.

Montanus (Joannes Baptista)—continued.

——. De coctione et præparatione humorum.

In: CRATO (Joannes). Methodus θεραπευτική, etc. 12°. *Basileæ,* [1555], 171–179.

——. De succo melancholico et atra bile sententia.

In: CRATO (Joannes). Methodus θεραπευτική, etc. 12°. *Basileæ,* [1555], 142–160.

——. Idea et characterismus doctrinæ Hippocraticæ, propositus studiosis in prælectione aphorismorum Hippocratis.

In: CRATO (Joannes). Methodus θεραπευτική, etc. 12°. *Basileæ,* [1555], 76–141.

——. Sententia de generatione pituitæ: contra eos qui affirmant, pituitam in ventriculo generari.

In: CRATO (Joannes). Methodus θεραπευτική, etc. 12°. *Basileæ,* [1555], 163–170.

——. Sententia excellentissimi Montani διαιτητικὴν demonstrans, sive de alimentis et victus ratione, a Joanne Cratone exposita.

In: CRATO (Joannes). Methodus θεραπευτική, etc. 12°. *Basileæ,* [1555], 180–190.

——. In quartam fen primi canonis Avicennæ lectiones, a Valentinus Lublino Polono collectæ. 4 p. l., 283 ff. 12°. *Venetiis, apud B. Constantinum,* 1556.

——. In primi lib. canonis Avicennæ primam fen profundissima commentaria. Adjecto nuper secundo, quod ·nunquam antea fuerat typis excusum: De membris capite. Censore Jano Matthæo Durastante. 14 p. l., 651 pp. 16°. *Venetiis, typ. V. Valgrisii et B. Constantini,* 1557.

——. In secundam fen primi canonis Avicennæ in qua agitur de causis, ægritudinibus, accidentibus, pulsibus, et urinis. 20 p. l., 832 pp. 8°. *Venetiis, ex off. V. Valgrisii et B. Constantini,* 1557.

——. Opuscula varia ac præclara: in quibus tota fere medicina methodice explicatur, quorum nomina sequens pagina declarat. Omnia, post alios eruditos viros qui in eis corrigendis desudarunt, nunc tandem Hieronymi Donzellini opera ab infinitis propé mendis vindicata. 27 p. l., 349 pp., 1 tab., 9 l. 12°. *Basileæ, apud P. Pernam,* 1558.

——. In nonum librum Rhasis ad r. Almansorem lectiones primi anni publicæ professionis in academia Patavina summa fide, atque diligente cura emendatæ, et integritati restitutæ a Joanne Cratone . . . cum ejusdem luculenta præfatione. 12 p. l., 686 pp. 8°. *Basileæ,* 1562.

——. Consultationum medicarum opus absolutissimum. In quo ad consilia omnia prius edita . . . accesserunt centum fere nunquam antea typis expressa . . . studio . . . Jo. Cratonis. 9 p. l., 1024 col. fol. [*Basileæ, H. P. et P. Perna,* 1565.]

Title-page mutilated.

——. Consultationes medicæ, olim quidem Joannis Cratonis opera atque studio correctæ, ampliatæque, nunc vero post secundæ editionis appendicem et additiones, insigni novorum consiliorum auctario ex Ludovici Demoulini Rochefortii codicibus exornatæ. 9 p. l., 1120 col., 15 l. fol. [*Viennæ*], 1583.

——. Defensio librorum suorum de morbis, adversus Thomam Erastum. 3 p. l., 164 ff., 1 l. 4°. *Venetiis, apud F. Zilettum,* 1584.

Another copy bound with: FRACASTORIUS (H.) Opera omnia, etc. 3. ed. 4°. *Venetiis,* 1584.

——. De uterinis affectibus.

In: GYNÆCIORUM, etc. 4°. *Basileæ,* 1586, ii, 197–251.

——. The same. De affectibus uterinis libellus, cum ejusdem x. consiliis muliebribus.

In: SPACHIUS (I.) Gynæciorum, [etc.] fol. *Witebergæ,* 1597, 303–330.

——. Problematum partim physicorum, partim medicorum, ex . . . scriptis accurate selectorum liber unus. Nunc primum editus studio et opera

Montanus (Joannes Baptista)—continued.
Martini Weindrichii Vratislaviensis. 23 p. l.,
521 pp., 20 l. 12°. *Witebergæ, ex off. Cratoniana,*
1590.

See, also, **Rucius** *Carmignolius* (Dominicus). Quæsita
iv. medicinalia. 12°. [*Turini*], 1551. — **Cervetto** (Giuseppe). Di Giambattista da Monte e della medicina italiana nel secolo xvi. 8°. *Verona,* 1839.—**Crato** (Joannes).
Ad artem medicam isagoge [etc.] 12°. *Venetiis,* 1560.—
Erastus (Thomas). Varia opuscula. [No. 7.] fol.
Francof. a. M., 1590.—**Solenander** (Reinerus). Consilium medicinalium sectiones quinque [etc.] fol. *Francofurti,* 1596. ——. The same. fol. *Francofurti,* 1609.
For Portrait, see **Collection**—van Kaathoven.—**Collection** of Portr. of Phys. & Men. of Sc., 120.

Montanus (Joannes Sigismundus). * De lethalitate vulnerum. 8 pp. 4°. *Harderovici, J.
Moojen,* 1750.

Montargis.

See **Cholera** (*Asiatic, History, etc., of*), *by localities.*

Montargis (Gustave). * I. Déterminer l'influence de l'inflammation du péricarde sur le
développement de l'hypertrophie du cœur. II.
[etc.] 68 pp. 4°. *Paris,* 1844, No. 177, v. 421.

Montauban.

Guiraud. Des mouvements de population à Mon-
tauban depuis le commencement du siècle et particulièrement dans les vingt dernières années. Ann. de démog.
internat., Par., 1881, v, 278-320.

Montaudon (Charles). * Sur les rétrécissemens organiques de l'urètre, et sur les accidens
qui en sont la suite. 7-25 pp. 4°. *Paris,* 1821,
No. 136, v. 167.

Montaudon (Martial-Victor). * Sur le tempérament lymphatique. 30 pp. 4°. *Paris,* 1822, No.
78, v. 172.

Montaudon-Bousseresse (Léonard). * I.
Des caractères anatomiques de l'inflammation
des tissus fibreux, fibro-cartilagineux et cartila-
gineux. II. [etc.] 31 pp. 4°. *Paris,* 1844, No.
166, v. 421.

Montauit (J.-J.-H.) Observations médicales,
recueillies à l'Hôpital Saint-Louis, dans le service
de M. le docteur Manry. 26 pp. 8°. [*Paris,
Crapelet,* 1829.] [P., v. 912.]
——. * Sur l'hémiplégie faciale, ou perte du
mouvement et de l'expression de l'un des côtés
du visage, par lésion de la septième paire des
nerfs (portion dure), nerf respiratoire de la face
de M. Ch. Bell. 28 pp. 4°. *Paris,* 1831, No.
300, v. 246.
——. Des fièvres typhoïdes et du typhus, histoire
et description de ces affections; analogies et
différences qui existent entre elles; mémoire honoré d'une médaille de 500 francs par l'Académie
royale de médecine dans la séance publique de
1837. 230 pp. 4°. *Paris, J.-B. Baillière,* 1838.
——. * Des moyens à l'aide desquels on peut distinguer les névroses des lésions dites organiques.
46 pp. 8°. *Paris,* 1838.
Concours.

Montaut (F.) * De la fièvre éruptive hémorrhagique observée à Bordeaux en 1847 et 1848.
40 pp. 4°. *Paris,* 1849, No. 73, v. 487.

de Montaux (Chambon). *See* **Chambon de
Montaux** (Nicolas).

Montaz (Léon-Genevey). * Recherches sur la
trace indélébile du chancre syphilitique; ses
caractères. 91 pp. 4°. *Lyon,* 1880, No. 43.

Montazeau (M.-P.-Hippolyte). * Sur l'apoplexie. 21 pp. 4°. *Paris,* 1820, No. 51, v. 155.

de Montbel (Guillaume-Isidore), le baron [1787-
1845]. Lettre sur le choléra de Vienne en Autriche. Avec des notes par M. Guyon. 23 pp.
8°. *Paris,* 1832. [P., v. 491.]

Montbéliard.

See **Fever** (*Cerebro-spinal, History, etc., of*), *by
localities.*

Montbrehain.

See **Cholera** (*Asiatic, History, etc., of*), *by localities.*

Montbrison.

Lefort (J.) Eau de Fontfort (commune de Montbrison, Loire). Bull. Acad. de méd., Par., 1878, 2. s., vii,
1109.—**Royère** (J.-T.-E.) Topographie physique et médicale de la ville de Montbrison, chef-lieu du département
de la Loire. Rec. de mém. de méd. . . . mil., Par., 1831,
xxx, 1-59.

Montbrun.

Lazare (H.) * Étude sur les eaux minérales
de Montbrun (Drôme). 4°. *Paris,* 1876.

Henry (O.) Rapport au sujet des sources sulfureuses
de Montbrun (département de la Drôme). Bull. Acad. de
méd., Par., 1857-8, xxiii, 219-222.

Mont-Cassel.

Windrif. Essai sur les eaux ferrugineuses du Mont-
Cassel. Bull. méd. du nord, Lille, 1863, iv, 65-83.

Montceau.

See **Fever** (*Typhus, History, etc., of*), *by localities.*

Mont-Cenis.

Desgaultière (P.) Essai sur la topographie médicale
du Mont-Cénis. Rec. de mém. de méd. . . . mil., Par.,
1817, iii, 81-139.

Mont-Dauphin.

Charmeil. Mémoire sur la topographie médicale de
la ville de Montdauphin et de ses environs. J. de méd.
mil., Par., 1784, iii, 397-443.—**Tripier** (F.-M.) Analyse
des eaux thermales du Plan-de-Phazi, près de Mont-Dau-
phin. Rec. de mém. de méd. . . . mil., Par., 1836, xxxix,
332-351.

Mont Dore.

See, also, **Bourboule** (*La*).

D'**Ambert de Serilhag** (J.) * Les eaux du
Mont-Dore; leurs effets physiologiques, leur
action thérapeutique sur les affections chroniques des voies digestives. 4°. *Montpellier,*
1877.

Bertrand (M.) Recherches sur les propriétés
physiques, chimiques et médicinales des eaux du
Mont-d'Or, département du Puy-de-Dôme. 8°.
Paris, 1810.
——. The same. 2. éd. 8°. *Clermont-
Ferrand,* 1823.
——. Mémoire sur l'établissement thermal
du Mont-d'Or, et les antiquités que l'on vient
d'y découvrir. 8°. *Clermont-Ferrand,* 1819.

Brosson (E.) Notice sur les eaux minérales
et sur l'établissement thermal du Mont-Dore
(Puy-de-Dôme). 8°. *Clermont-Ferrand,* 1856.
——. The same. 8°. *Moulins,* 1858.

Chabory-Bertrand (E.) Études médicales
sur les eaux minérales du Mont-Dore. Première
partie. 8°. *Paris,* 1859.

Geay (E.) Le Mont-Dore et ses indications
thérapeutiques. Lettres adressées au Dr. Le-
cuyer. 12°. *Paris,* 1885.

Goupil des Pallières. Notice sur les eaux
du Mont-Dore, présentée à l'Académie de médecine. 8°. *Paris,* 1859.

Joal (J.) * Essais médicaux sur les eaux du
Mont-Dore. 4°. *Paris,* 1875.

Leymerie (A.) Notice familière sur la géologie du Mont-d'Or Lyonnais. 8°. *Lyon,* 1838.

Mascarel (J.) Nouvelles recherches sur
l'action curative des eaux du Mont-Dore dans la
phthisie pulmonaire. 8°. *Paris,* 1865.

Bertrand. Note sur la température des eaux thermales, et plus particulièrement sur celle des eaux du Mont-
d'Or. Bull. Acad. de méd., Par., 1836-7, i, 604-606. ——.
Temperatur der Thermen und besonders derer von Mont-
Dore. J. d. pract. Heilk., Berl., 1838, lxxxvi, 4. St., 118-
124.—**Boudant.** Du traitement aux eaux du Mont-Dore,
du coryza chronique et de l'ozène. Lyon méd., 1870, v,
166-171.—**Cazalis** (J.) Étude sur les sueurs qui se produisent sous l'influence du traitement par les eaux du
Mont-Dore. Ann. Soc. d'hydrol. méd. de Par. Compt.-
rend., 1876-7, xxii, 248-270.—**Chateau.** Le Mont-Dore
et La Bourboule; parallèle de ces deux stations. Gaz. méd.

Mont Dore.

de Bordeaux, 1877, vi, 198–200.—**Delpit.** De l'Auvergne, de ses eaux minérales, et particulièrement de celles du Mont-d'Or. J. univ. d. sc. méd., Par., 1818, x, 137–164.—**Dufresne** (F.) Excursion aux stations thermales de Royat, du Mont-Dore, de Saint-Hectaire et de Vichy. Union méd., Par., 1871, 3. s., xii, 601; 625; 637.—**Labat.** Étude sur le pays et sur les eaux du Mont-Dore (Auvergne). Ann. Soc. d'hydrol. méd. de Par., 1883-4, xxix, 425–456.—**Laronde** (C.) De la médication thermale du Mont Dore, dirigée contre certaines manifestations internes de nature rhumatismale et goutteuse; communication verbale. Soc. d. sc. méd. de Gannat. Compt. rend., 1861-2, xvi, 77–84. *Also :* Union méd., Par., 1862, 2. s., xv, 263–266.—**Lefort.** Étude chimique des eaux minérales du Mont-Dore. Ann. Soc. d'hydrol. méd. de Par. Compt.-rend., 1862, viii, 461–522. *Also* [Abstr.]: Union méd., Par., 1862, 2. s., xv, 89–92.—**Mascarel** (J.) Des effets des eaux thermales du Mont-Dore dans le traitement du coryza et de l'aphonie. Gaz. hebd. de méd., Par., 1862, ix, 324–329. ———. Des effets thérapeutiques généraux et spéciaux des eaux du Mont-Dore. Bull. gén. de thérap., etc., Par., 1881, c, 413–416.—**Richelot** (G.) Études médicales sur le Mont-Dore. Union méd., Par., 1859, 2. s., ii, 267; 280; 297; 315; 1860, 2. s., vi, 421; 434; 1861, 2. s., x, 193; 227; 275; 324; 377. ———. De la cure thermale du Mont-Dore dans le traitement des affections rhumatismales. *Ibid.*, 1866, 2. s., xxx, 410; 432; 449. ———. Du climat du Mont-Dore pendant la saison des bains. *Ibid.*, 1867, 3. s., ii, 49–57. ———. De la cure thermale du Mont-Dore dans le traitement des affections chroniques du larynx et en particulier de l'aphonie. *Ibid.*, 1869, 3. s., vii, 315; 356; 401; 439. ———. Observation de tuberculose pulmonaire commençante, avec altération grave de la santé générale, heureusement enrayée par la cure thermale du Mont-Dore. *Ibid.*, 1872, 3. s., xiii, 734; 749. ———. Étude sur la nature et les propriétés thérapeutiques de l'eau minéro-thermale du Mont-Dore; parallèle sommaire de l'eau du Mont-Dore et de La Bourboule. *Ibid.*, 1874, 3. s., xvii, 669; 690; 709. ———. Discussion sur la nature arsenicale des eaux du Mont-Dore. Ann. Soc. d'hydrol. méd. de Par., 1875-6, xxi, 491–536. *Also :* Union méd., Par., 1876, 3. s., xxi, 646; 657; 707; 736; 749. ———. Note sur les indications thérapeutiques des sources du Mont-Dore. Union méd., Par., 1880, 3. s., xxix, 653; 689. ———. Sources thermales du Mont-Dore (Puy-de-Dôme); considérations pratiques sur quelques effets du traitement Montdorien. *Ibid.*, 1881, 3. s., xxxi, 821–825.—**Scoutetten.** Procès-verbal des expériences sur l'état électrique des eaux du Mont-Dore. Gaz. d. hôp., Par., 1865, xxxviii, 353.—**Seney.** Étude clinique des eaux du Mont-Dore (souvenirs d'un baigneur). J. de thérap., Par., 1880, vii, 321; 375.—**Terrier** (F.) Note sur l'emploi de la pulvérisation de l'eau du Mont-Dore en inhalations. Gaz. hebd. de méd., Par., 1884, 2. s., xxi, 640–642.—**Thomson** (W.) A holiday at Mont-Dore. Dublin J. M. Sc., 1887, 3. s., lxxxiv, 265–274.—**Vacher** (L.) Mont-Dore als Luftcurort. Jahrb. f. Balneol., etc., Wien, 1879, viii, 160.

"**Mont Dore**" (The) of Bournemouth. [Abridged prospectus of the directors.] 6 pp., 1 plan. 8°. [*London, J. & A. Churchill*, 1881.]

———. Residential and bath establishment. 20 pp. 16°. [*n. p.*, 1885.]

———. Hotel and Bath Establishment, Bournemouth. [Circular of the manager, Oct. 18, 1886.] 2 l. 4°. [*London*, 1886.]

do Monte (João Pedro Xavier). O homem medico de si mesmo, ou sciencia, e arte nova de conservar cada hum a si proprio a saude, e destruir a sua doença, dirigida ao bem commum. 1 p. l., 179 pp., 2 l. 12°. *Lisboa, A. V. da Silva*, 1760. [*Also, in :* P., v. 1256.]

Monteagudo.

Maza (M. A.) La mortandad habida en Monteagudo en 1885 no fué debida al pantano y si á otras causas. Génio méd.-quir., Madrid, 1886, xxxii, 594–596.

Monte-Alfeo.

Brugnatelli (T.) & **Pelloggio** (P.) Analisi dell' acqua minerale di Monte Alfeo; e nota intorno all' azione del solfo sull' acqua e sui carbonati terrosi. R. Ist. Lomb. di sc. e lett. Rendic., Milano, 1874, 2. s., vii, 333–338.—**Lupi** (P.) Cenni sopra l'acqua minerale di Monte Alfeo. Gior. di r. Accad. di med. di Torino, 1876, xxxix, 247; 268.—**Schivardi** (P.) L'acqua minerale solforosa di Monte Alfeo. Idrologia, Firenze, 1886, viii, 141–146.

Monte Argentario. Regolamento sulla pubblica igiene. 25 pp. 8°. *Siena, L. Lazzeri*, 1882.

Monteath (George Cunningham) [1788–1828]. *See* **Weller** (C. H.) A manual of the diseases of the human eye, etc. 8°. *Glasgow*, 1821.

Montebello Sulphur and Iron Springs, Newbury, Vt. 8 pp. 24°. [*Newbury*, 1874.]

Montecalvus (*Jacob*).

Portrait in : **Collection**—van Kaathoven.

Monte Castellaccio.

Gioachino (C.) Sulle acque minerali Imolesi dette del Monte Castellaccio; osservazioni pratiche e regole da tenersi nell' uso loro. Seconda edizione con aggiunte e correzioni. 8°. *Imola*, 1839.

Monte-Catini.

See, also, **Poretta.**

Barzellotti (G.) Bagni termali e minerali di Monte Catini nella Val di Nievole illustrati con nuova analisi chimica e nuove osservazione pratiche. 4°. *Pisa*, 1823.

Bicchierai (A.) Dei bagni di Montecatini. [With atlas.] 2 v. 4° & fol. *Firenze*, 1788.

Maluccelli (S.) Dell' attività e dell' uso de' bagni minerali di Montecatini. 8°. *Pisa*, 1810.

Maunoir (R.) * La Porrette et Monte-Catini. 8°. *Florence*, 1848.

Barzellotti (G.) Sopra i miglioramenti fatti in quest' anno 1829 ai Bagni di Montecatini in Val di Nievole a vantaggio della salute umana. N. Mercurio d. sc. med., Livorno, 1829, iii. 242–255.—**Dupuis.** Analyse des eaux minérales de Monte-Catini. Rec. de mém. de méd. . . . mil., Par., 1860, 3. s., iv, 164–168.—**Giulj** (G.) Dell' influenza, che sembrano avere le correnti eletriche per ristabilire la salute in alcune malattie dietro l'uso dei bagni d'acqua salina ed in ispecie di quelli di Monte Catini in Toscana. Bull. d. sc. med. di Bologna, 1840, 2. s., ix, 199–229.—**Labat.** Étude. La station et les eaux de Montecatini, Italie (Toscane). Ann. Soc. d'hydrol. méd. de Par. Compt.-rend., 1875-6, xxi, 56–79.—**Perier** (J.-A.-N.) Notice sur les eaux minérales de Monte-Catini, suivie d'une note sur les étuves de Monsummano (Toscane). Rec. de mém. de méd. . . . mil., Par., 1860, 3. s., iv, 149–164.—**S.** (A.) Azione fisiologica ed efficacia terapeutica delle acque di Montecatini in alcune malattie del cavallo. Gior. d. anat., fisiol. e patol. d. animali, Pisa, 1872, iv, 165–167.

Montée (Joseph-Augustin). * Sur la gastrite aiguë. 16 pp. 4°. *Paris*, 1837, No. 412, v. 318.

Montefeltro.

Badaloni (G.) Il Montefeltro e le sue acque minerali. Idrologia, Firenze, 1885, vii, 197; 260.

Monteferrante (R.) Manuale pratico di ricerche tossicologiche. vii, 122 pp., 10 tab. 12°. *Napoli, stabilimento tipog. dell' Unione*, 1872.

Montefusco (Alfonso). Consigli pratici contro il cholera. 20 pp. 8°. *Napoli, C. La Cava*, 1885.

———. Diagnosi delle malattie di cuore; studio semiotico-clinico. 164 pp. 8°. *Napoli, E. Detken*, 1887.

Monteggia (Giovanni Battista) [1762–1815]. Fasciculi pathologici. 3 p. l., 142 pp. 12°. *Mediolani, typ. J. Marelli*, 1789.

———. Annotazioni pratiche sopra i mali venerei. 1 p. l., viii, 255 pp. 8°. *Milano, G. Galeazzi*, 1794.

———. Istituzioni chirurgiche. 2. ed. 8 v. in 4. 8°. *Milano, G. Maspero*, 1813–15.

———. The same. 3. ed. 4 v. in 2. 8°. *Firenze, G. Piatti*, 1820.

———. The same. Aumentado di numerose aggiunte per cura di G. B. Caimi. 7 v. in 3. 8°. *Milano, G. Truffi*, 1829–30.

For Biography and Portrait, see **Acerbi** (F. E.) Della vita di Giambatista Monteggia. 8°. *Milano*, 1816. *See, also*, Gaz. med. ital. lomb., Milano, 1864, 5. s., iii, 381–384 (C. Bazzoni). *Also :* Ann. univ. di med., Milano, 1867, ccii, 561–564 (C. Fumagalli). *See, also*, **Fritze** (Joannes Fridericus). Compendio sopra le malattie veneree. 8°. *Pavia*, 1795.—**Stein** (G. G.) Arto ostetricia, [etc.] 8°. *Venezia*, 1816. *For Portrait, see* **Collection**—van Kaathoven.

de Montègre (Antoine-François-Jenin) [1779–1818]. * Quelques vues sur les tempéraments et leurs principales différences dans les deux sexes. 11 pp. 4°. *Paris, an XII* [1804], No. 184, v. 47.

de Montègre (Antoine-François-Jenin)—cont.
——. Du magnétisme animal et de ses partisans, ou recueil de pièces importantes sur cet objet. Précédé des observations récemment publiées. 139 pp. 8°. *Paris, D. Colas*, 1812.
——. Expériences sur la digestion dans l'homme, présentées à la première classe de l'Institut de France, le 8 septembre 1812. Suivies du rapport des commissaires nommés par l'Institut. 55 pp. 8°. *Paris, Le Normant & Colas fils*, 1814.
——. Des hémorroïdes, ou traité analytique de toutes les affections hémorroïdales. vi, 232 pp. 8°. *Paris, l'auteur*, 1817. [P.; v. 1684.]
——. The same. 2. éd. xlvii, 360 pp. 8°. *Paris, Mlle. Delaunay*, 1830.
——. The same. Die Hämorrhoiden, ihre Erkenntniss, alle ihre Zufäll und Folgen und ihre Heilung. x, 374 pp. 8°. *Leipzig, W. Engelmann*, 1821.
——. The same. Ueber die Erkenntniss und Behandlung der Hämorrhoiden. Nach dem Französischen für praktische Aerzte und Hämorrhoidal-Patienten deutsch bearbeitet, und mit Anmerkungen versehen, von Dr. F. J. Wittemann. 186 pp., 9 l. 16°. *Pesth, C. A. Hartleben*, 1843.
For Biography. see J. univ. d. sc. méd., Par., 1819, xiii, 359-364 (Broussais).

de Montegre (Horace) [1806–64]. * Sur les plaies pénétrantes de la poitrine et les lésions du cœur. 38 pp. 4°. *Paris*, 1836, No. 6, v. 294.
——. Notice historique sur la vie, les travaux, les opinions médicales et philosophiques de F.-J.-V. Broussais, précédée de sa profession de foi, et suivie des discours prononcés sur sa tombe. 156 pp., 1 pl. 8°. *Paris, J.-B. Baillière*, 1839.

Montegut (L.) * Étude sur le rhumatisme articulaire aigu. 46 pp., 1 l. 4°. *Montpellier, Boehm & fils*, 1867, No. 53. C.

Montégut-Ségla.
Henry (O.) Analyse chimique de l'eau minérale naturelle de Montégut-Ségla (Haute-Garonne). Bull. Acad. de méd , Par., 1849-50, xv, 911-914.

Monteil (A.-Alexis). Histoire agricole de la France. L'agriculture, les cultivateurs et la vie rurale depuis l'époque gauloise jusqu'à nos jours, avec introduction, supplément et notes par Charles Louandre. 387 pp., 7 pl. 12°. *Paris, P. Daffis*, 1872.
——. Histoire financière de la France, depuis les premiers temps de la monarchie jusqu'à nos jours. Avec introduction, supplément et notes par Charles Louandre. 360 pp., 12 pl. 12°. *Paris, P. Daffis*, 1872.
——. Histoire de l'industrie française et des gens de métiers. Introduction, supplément et notes par Charles Louandre. 2 v. 320 pp., 6 pl. ; 320 pp., 4 pl. 12°. *Paris, P. Daffis*, 1872.
——. La magistrature française, les lois et les gens de loi, depuis les premiers temps de la monarchie jusqu'à nos jours, avec introduction, notes et supplément par Charles Louandre. Parlement, présidiaux, justices royales, cours seigneuriales, cours d'exception, basoches gens de roi, avocats, procureurs, notaires, greffiers, huissiers, etc. iv, 364 pp., 2 pl. 12°. *Paris, P. Daffis*, 1873.
——. La médecine en France, hommes et doctrines depuis l'antiquité jusqu'à nos jours, avec introduction, notes et supplément par A. Le Pileur. Ouvrage publié sur la dernière édition de l'histoire des Français des divers états, couronnée deux fois par l'Académie française. 438 pp. 12°. *Paris, Bibliothèque Nouvelle, P. Dupont*, [1874].

Monteils (E.) Histoire de la vaccination. Recherches historiques et critiques sur les divers moyens de prophylaxie thérapeutique employés contre la variole depuis l'origine de celle-ci

Monteils (E.)—continued.
jusqu'à nos jours. xlii, 422 pp. 8°. *Paris, A. Delahaye*, 1874.

Monteils (J.-B.-M.-Amédée). * Des flux diarrhéiques chez les enfants. Des ulcérations et granulations simples du col de l'utérus. 62 pp. 4°. *Paris*, 1849, No. 232, v. 487.

Monteiro (Antonio-Peregrino-Maciel) [1804–'68]. * Sur la nature, les symptômes de l'inflammation de l'arachnoïde, et son rapport avec l'encéphalite. 53 pp. 4°. *Paris*, 1829, No. 76, v. 223.
For Biography, see Brazil. Biogr. Ann. [Macedo], Rio de Jan., 1876, iii, 101–104.

Monteiro (J. C.)
Co-Editor of : **Centro** (O) pharmaceutico portuguez, Porto, 1876.

Monteiro (João Franco). Mais factos para a vida moral, da Eschola medico-cirurgica de Lisboa. 29 pp. 8°. *Lisboa, J. B. de A. Gouveia*, [1842, vel subseq.]. [P., v. 1264.]
——. Ueber das gelbe Fieber. 50 pp., 1 l. 8°. *Leipzig, A. Edelmann*, 1883.

Monteiro (Jone-Vaz). * Du rhumatisme en général. 46 pp. 4°. *Paris*, 1845, No. 116, v. 435.

Monteiro (Ramiro Affonso). * Funcções do grande sympathico. 45 pp. 4°. *Bahia, J. G. Tourinho*, 1871.
Concurso.
——. * Pathologia geral do elemento pernicioso nas molestias. 136 pp. 8°. *Bahia, J. G. Tourinho*, 1874.
Concurso.

Monteiro (W. A.)
Co-Editor of : **University** (The) Literary Magazine, Charlottesville, Va., 1856.

Monteiro da Silva (Joaquim Antonio). *Amputação utero-ovarica. 5 p. l., 69 pp., 1 l. 8°. *Rio de Janeiro, E. R. da Costa*, 1883.

Monteiro de Carvalho (Antonio Junio). * Hemorrhagia uterina durante o delivramento e suas indicações. 26 pp., 1 l. 4°. *Bahia, J. G. Tourinho*, 1874.

Monteith (Joannes). * De dolore. 8°. *Edinburgi*, 1726.
In : SMELLIE. Thesaurus med. [etc.] 8°. *Edinburgi*, 1778, i, 1–16.

Montel (Michel). * De l'épilepsie infantile. 86 pp. 4°. *Lyon*, 1887, 1. s., No. 356.

Monteloy (M.) * Sur la carie du corps des vertèbres. 15 pp. 4°. *Paris*, 1813, No. 123, v. 98.

Monte di Misericordia.
Palermi (P.) Le terme del Monte di Misericordia in Casamicciola (Ischia) dopo il terremoto del 4 marzo 1881 ; sommarie osservazioni e analisi chimiche. Morgagni, Napoli, 1881, xxiii, 286–291.

Montén (Andreas Ulr.) [1805–84]. Observationes circa exanthema scarlatinosum. 8 pp. 4°. *Londoni Gothorum, ex off. Berlingiana*, [1832].
For Biography, see Eira, Göteborg, 1884, viii, 413–416.

Montenegro.
See, also, **Medicine** (*History, etc., of*), *by nations, etc.* ; **Medicine** (*Military, History of*)— *Campaigns, etc.*
Boulongne (A.) Le Monténégro, le pays et ses habitants. Rec. de mém. de méd. . . . mil , Par., 1868, 3. s., xxi, 465–518. *Also*, Reprint. — **Hickl.** Erlebnisse in Montenegro (von Oktober 1875 bis März 1876). Wien. med. Wchnschr., 1876, xxvi, 727 ; 751 ; 823 ; 1159 ; 1231 ; 1877, xxvii, 639 ; 807 ; 903 ; 1099. — **Tedeschi.** Notice médicale sur le Monténégro. Rec. de mém. de méd. . . . mil., Par., 1860, 3. s., iii, 273–294. — **Weiser** (M. E.) Sanitäts-Verhältnisse und Volksheilmittel in Montenegro. Allg. Wien. med. Ztg., 1875, xx, 245 ; 255.

Montenegro (M. V.) Estudio abreviado de las fiebres miasmáticas mas frecuentes i efectos de la malaria, en los climas calidos, despues de quince años de práctica en países intertropicales. 53 pp. 8°. *Cartagena, A. Araujo*, 1883.

Montenegro (M. V.)—continued.

——. Estudio fisiolójico de los sentidos. 17 pp. 8°. *Cartajena, A. Araujo,* 1883.

Montennis (Albert). *Étude clinique de la fièvre et des antipyrétiques nouveaux dans les maladies des enfants. 150 pp. 4°. *Paris,* 1886, No. 275.

——. Nouvel appareil à extension continue pour le traitement des fractures de cuisse et de la coxalgie. 72 pp. 8°. *Paris, G. Steinheil,* 1887.

Monte-Ortone.

Berti (A.) Considerazioni mediche sulle acque solforate fredde di Montortone, S. Daniele e della Costa D'Arquà. Atti r. Ist. Veneto di sc., lett. ed arti, Venezia, 1876–7, 5. s., iii. 241–246.—**Bizio** (G.) Analisi chimica delle acque solforate fredde di Monte Ortone, S. Daniele e della Costa di Arquà. Gior. veneto di sc. med., Venezia, 1871, 3. s., xv, 203–218.

de Montépin.

See **Chervin** (Nicolas). Pétition adressée à la Chambre des députés à l'effet d'obtenir [etc.] 8°. *Paris,* 1853.
——. Pétition adressée à la Chambre des députés sur la nécessité d'une prompte réforme [etc.] 8°. *Paris,* 1833.

Monterey.

King (W. S.) Medical topography, climate, diseases, etc., of Monterey, Cal. Am. J. M. Sc., Phila., 1853, n. s., xxv, 386–392.

Montero (L. M.)

Co-Editor of: **Escuela** médica, Carácas, 1874–6.

Monte Romboli.

Franchini (E.) L'acqua minerale di Monte Romboli in Casale di Val di Cecina (provincia di Pisa). Idrologia, Firenze, 1882, iv, 141; 169; 202.

Monteros (José-E.) *Du traitement des fistules urinaires chez la femme [et tableaux synoptiques des observations des fistules vésico-vaginales opérées par les divers procédés]. 218; 39 pp., 1 l., 17 pl. 4°. *Paris,* 1864, No. 139.

Monterossi (Pasquale). Manuale di chirurgia minore. 3. ed. 188 pp. 8°. Atlas, 12 pl., 4°. *Napoli, V. Puzziello,* 1854.

Montesano.

See **Rheumatism** (*Epidemics, etc., of*).

Montesano (Giuseppe Antonio Maria) [1779–1839]. Articolo estratto dalla Gazzetta privilegiata di Venezia 29 settembre 1831, N. 219. Al . . . Dott. Stëer. [On cholera morbus.] 2 l. 8°. [*Padova,* 1831.] [P., v. 941.]

See, also, **Stëer** (M.) Epistola, etc. 8°. [*n. p.,* 1831.] For Biography, *see* **Zannini** (P.) Biografia di Giuseppe Montesanto. Ediz. seconda. 8°. *Venezia,* 1841. Repr. from: Biog. degl' Italiani illustri del sec. xviii, pubb. dal E. de Tipaldo (v. viii fasc. ii)

See, also, Ann. univ. di med., Milano, 1841, xcviii, 648.

Montesaurus (N.) De dispositionibus quas vulgares mal franzozo appellant, tractatus.

In: **Luisinus** (A.) Aphrodisiacus, [etc.] Ed. emend. fol. *Lugd. Bat.,* 1728, 113–124.

Montes de Oca (Francisco). *Amputacion en la mano. Modificacion en la desarticulacion del hombro. Operacion de la fimosis. Extirpacion del testículo. 26 pp., 6 pl. roy. 8°. *México, Leon & White,* 1874.

For Portrait, see **Escuela** de med., México, 1883–4, v, no. 4.

Montes de Oca (*Juan José*) [1806–76].

Necrologia. Rev. méd.-quir., Buenos Aires, 1875–6, xii, 434–442.

Montesquiu.

Garrigou (F.) La source gazeuse bicarbonatée de Montesquiù (Pyrénées-Orientales). Rev. méd. et scient. d'hydrol., Toulouse, 1887, iv, 225–233.

de Montessus (Ferdinand de Bernard). *Notice sur l'épilepsie saturnine, ou occasionnée par le plomb. 78 pp. 4°. *Paris,* 1845, No. 92, v. 430.

Montet (Adrien). *De la kérato-conjonctivite phlycténulaire. 40 pp. 4°. *Paris,* 1866, No. 192.

de Montet (Charles). *Dissertation sur un cas d'hydropisie de matrice, simulant une grossesse. 30 pp. 8°. *Berne, C. Rœtzer,* 1843.

Montet (Jean-Jacques). *Quelques considérations sur les hémorrhagies utérines qui peuvent avoir lieu avant, pendant et après l'accouchement. 25 pp. 4°. *Paris,* 1829, No. 17, v. 221.

Montet (Michel). *Sur la convalescence. 23 pp. 4°. *Paris,* 1816, No. 110, v. 122.

Montet-Lalainguette (P.) *Sur les écrouelles. vi, 7–21 pp. 4°. *Paris,* 1824, No. 69, v. 185.

de Montéty (J.-Lucien). *De la ration alimentaire en général; application au soldat. 80 pp., 1 l. 4°. *Paris, A. Parent,* 1886, No. 71.

Montevarchi. Servizio medico-chirurgico nei due anni 1883, 1884 nello Spedale della Misericordia in Montevarchi. Resoconto statistico della sezione di chirurgia, pel Dott. Giuseppe Pacinotti, direttore sanitario. xiv, 48 pp. fol. *Firenze, tipog. Cenniniana,* 1885.

Monteveglio.

Vanni (L.) Osservazioni fisico-chimiche intorno all' acqua marziale carbonato magnesiana di Monteveglio. 8°. *Bologna,* 1827.

Monteverde (Dionysio). *Du choléra-morbus. 16 pp. 4°. *Paris,* 1833, No. 356, v. 266.

Monteverdi (Angelo). Sull' epidemia cholerosa dell' anno 1867 nei comuni del Due Miglia e del Corpi Santi. Relazione. 100 pp. 8°. *Cremona, Ronzi & Signori,* 1868.

——. Dimostrazione di una nuova importantissima virtù medicamentosa della china e dei snoi preparati. 279 pp. 8°. *Cremona, Ronzi & Signori,* 1870.

——. Contributo alla constatazione della virtù medicamentosa del solfato di chinina di eccitare l'azione fisiologica delle fibre muscolari dell' utero, vescica, intestino, vasi sanguigni, ecc. 14, 41, 59 pp. 8°. *Milano, frat. Rechiedei,* [1873].

Consists of extracts from various journals, etc. Repr. from: Ann. univ. di med., Milano, 1872, ccxxi: 1873, ccxxii.

——. Studi sopra l'azione del miasma palustre e del solfato di chinina. 184 pp. 8°. *Milano, frat. Rechiedei,* 1874.

Repr. from: Ann. univ. di med., Milano, 1874, ccxxix.

——. Note sur un moyen simple, facile, prompt et certain de distinguer la mort vraie de la mort apparente de l'homme. 20 pp., 6 pl. roy. 8°. *Crémone, Ronzi & Signori,* 1874.

Also, Editor of: **Bullettino** del Comitato medico Cremonese, Cremona, 1885.

Monte-Vettolini.

See **Monsummano** e Monte-Vettolini. Regolamento comunale di igiene pubblica. 8°. *Pescia,* 1873.

Montevideo.

See, also, **Fever** (*Yellow, History, etc., of*), *by localities.*

Saurel (L.-J.) Essai d'une climatologie médicale de Monte-Video et de la république orientale de l'Uruguay (Amérique du Sud). 8°. *Montpellier,* 1851.

Féris. Contributions à la géographie médicale. Montévidéo; topographie médicale, météorologie, pathologie. Arch. de méd. nav., Par., 1879, xxxii, 241–257.—**Martin de Moussy.** Ojeada sobre la constitucion médica de Montevideo durante los últimos quince años 1840 à 1854. Rev. méd.-quir., Buenos Aires, 1870, vii, 47; 82; 99.—**Melcior** (C.) Noticias médicas sobre la estacion naval del sur de América en el puerto de Montevideo. Bol. de med. nav., San Fernando, 1880, iii, 5; 30; 54; 73.

Monteville (Frédéric). La vérité de l'homœopathie prouvée par le simple exposé de sa véritable doctrine, fortifiée par les tristes aveux des médecins allopathes, jugés par eux-mêmes, suivie d'un coup d'œil sur son utilité, ses progrès, ses obstacles, son avenir et de quelques conseils pour la pratique homœopathique. ix, xxvii, 79 pp. 12°. *Namur, Woitrin-Bourdillon,* 1871.

Montfaucon.

MOURET (L.-A.) *Aperçu de la statistique médicale du canton de Montfaucon, département de la Haute-Loire, suivi de quelques propositions de médecine et de thérapeutique. 4°. *Paris*, 1835.

Montfort(C.) * De peritonitide puerperali simplici et complicata. 24 pp. 4°. *Parisiis*, 1809, No. 42, v. 75.

Montfort (Franciscus). *Tentamen medico-practicum circa hanc quæstionem quid in peri-pneumonicis morbis conferat anni diathesis, quid in illis ex vesicantibus sperandum. 43 pp. 8°. *Monspelii, J. F. Picot*, 1789. [P., v. 1091.]

Montfort (Léon). *Des eaux potables et de leur purification. 2 p. l., 56 pp. 4°. *Paris*, 1874, No. 385.

Montfort (Léon-Constantin). *Étude sur les déchirures de la vulve et du périnée pendant l'accouchement. 106 pp. 4°. *Paris*, 1869, No. 17.
———. The same. 103 pp. 8°. *Paris, A. Delahaye*, 1869.
Title-page wanting.

Montforte.
See **Fever** (*Cerebro-spinal, History, etc., of*), *by localities.*

Montfort-l'Amaury.
Will. Topographie de la ville et de l'Hôtel-Dieu de Montfort-l'Amaury. J. de méd., chir., pharm., etc., Par., 1785, lxv, 361–375.

de Montgarny (Jean-Baptiste-Tite Harmand) [1790–1823].
See **Dictionnaire** des termes de médecine, [etc.] 8°. *Paris*, 1823.

de Montgeron (Louis-Basile-Carré) [1686–1754].
See **Mathieu** (P.-F.) Histoire des [etc.] 12°. *Paris*, 1864.—**Préservatif** contre les faux principes et les maximes dangereuses établies par . . . [etc.] 16°. [n. p.], 1750.

Montgolfier (*Jacques-Étienne*) [1745–99] & **Montgolfier** (*Joseph-Michel*) [1740–1810].
Portraits in: **Collection** of Portr. of Phys. & Men of Sc., 87.

de Montgolfier (René). *Contribution à l'étude des convulsions de l'enfance étudiées spécialement au point de vue de l'hérédité. 100 pp. 4°. *Lyon, A. Waltener & Cie.*, 1883, 1. s., No. 191.

Montgomery, *Alabama.*
See, also, **Fever** (*Cerebro-spinal, History, etc., of*), *by localities* ; **Fever** (*Yellow, History, etc., of*), *by localities—United States.*
Ames (S.) & **Boling** (W. M.) Report of the committee appointed at the annual meeting of the Alabama Medical Association, held at Selma, the 8th and 9th of March, 1848, to take an account of the diseases which occurred in the city of Montgomery, and vicinity, in 1848. N. Orl. M. & S. J., 1849-50, vi, 1 tab., foll. p. 360.—**Weatherly** (J. S.) Report upon the diseases of the city and county of Montgomery. Tr. M. Ass. Alabama, Mobile, 1870, 415–417.

Montgomery (*David*).
See **Homicide**, *etc.—Cases, etc.*

Montgomery (E. E.) Is craniotomy justifiable? 8 pp. 8°. [*Philadelphia*, 1883.]
Repr. from: Med. Times, Phila., 1882-3, xiii.
———. Abdominal surgery; seven cases. 14 pp. 8°. *Philadelphia, F. A. Davis*, 1885.
———. The bromide of ethyl as an anesthetic in labor. 12 pp. 8°. *New York, W. Wood & Co.*, 1885.
Repr. from: Am. J. Obst., N. Y., 1885, xviii.

Montgomery (Edmund). On the formation of so-called cells in animal bodies. vi, 56 pp. 8°. *London, J. Churchill & Sons*, 1867.
See, also, **Esmarch** (Fr.) On the use of cold in surgery [etc.] 8°. *London*, 1861.

Montgomery (Edward) [1816–83]. A plea for the antiphlogistic treatment of disease. 20 pp. 8°. *St. Louis*, 1872.
Repr. from: Med. Arch., St. Louis, 1872, viii.
Also, Co-Editor of: **Humboldt** (The) Medical Archives, St. Louis, 1870–73.
For Biography, see J. Am. M. Ass., Chicago, 1883, i, 548 (J. M. Toner). Also: St. Louis M. & S. J., 1883, xlv, 559–562 (G. M. B. Maughs).

Montgomery (Howard B.) [–1869]. Report on the sanatory condition of Honore, with reference to the non-appearance of cholera in an epidemic form. 24 pp. 8°. *Madras, S. C. Graves*, 1856. [P., v. 922.]
Repr. from: BALFOUR (Edward). The localities in India exempt from cholera. 8°. Madras, 1856.
Also, Co-Editor of: **Madras** (The) Quarterly Journal of Medical Science, 1860–69.

Montgomery (James). * De phthisi pulmonali. 26 pp. 8°. *Edinburgi, A. Smellie*, 1817.
———. An essay on the phrenology of the Hindoos and negroes; together with strictures thereon, by Corden Thompson. v, 6–62 pp. 8°. *London, E. Lloyd & Co.*, 1829. [P., v. 1050.]

Montgomery (Joseph Fauntleroy) [1812–83]. The ethics of the medical profession. [Read before the Sacramento Society for Medical Improvement.] 14 pp. 8°. *San Francisco, J. H. Carmany & Co.*, 1871.
———. Burns and scalds; their treatment, with cases. 24 pp. 8°. *San Francisco, J. F. Brown*, 1872.
———. The treatment of typhoid fever. 28 pp. 8°. *Sacramento, F. A. Springer*, 1873.
Repr. from: Tr. M. Soc. Calif. 1872-3, Sacramento, 1873.
———. Fracture of the inferior maxillary bone. 17 pp. 8°. *Sacramento, Cal., H. S. Crocker & Co.*, 1875.
Repr. from: Tr. M. Soc. Calif. 1874-5, Sacramento, 1875.
———. Annual address delivered before the Sacramento Society for Medical Improvement. March 23, 1875. 8 pp. 8°. *San Francisco, Woman's Publishing Co.*, 1875.
Repr. from: Pacific M. & S. J., San Fran., 1874-5, viii.
———. Report of the committee on medical education, made by the Medical Society of the State of California. 20 pp. 8°. *Sacramento, Sacramento Leader Printing Office*, 1876.
Repr. from: Tr. M. Soc. Calif. 1875-6, Sacramento, 1876.
For Biography, see J. Am. M. Ass., Chicago, 1883, i, 716 (J. M. Toner). Also: Pacific M. & S. J., San Fran., 1883-4, xxvi, 363–366 (F. W. Hatch).

Montgomery (Robert). * De variola. 2 p. l., 22 pp. 8°. *Edinburgi, A. Neill cum sociis*, 1792.

Montgomery (*Thomas Johnson*) [1812–77].
Steele (A. J.) Necrology. Tr. Am. M. Ass., Phila., 1878, xxix, 718. Also: Tr. M. Ass. Missouri, St. Louis, 1878, 154.

Montgomery (William Fetherston [H.]) [1797–1859]. Catalogue of the preparations in the museum of . . . 32 pp. 8°. *Dublin, T. & S. Courtney*, 1830.
———. Catalogue of the preparations in the museum of . . . Oct. 31, 1834. 31 pp. 8°. *Dublin, G. Folds*, 1834. [P., v. 744.]
———. An exposition of the signs and symptoms of pregnancy, the period of human gestation, and the signs of delivery. xxiv, 344 pp., 11 pl. 8°. *London, Sherwood, Gilbert & Piper*, 1837.
———. The same. With some other papers on subjects connected with midwifery. 2. ed. xx, 706 pp., 7 pl., port. 8°. *London, Longman [and others*], 1856.
———. The same. v (1 l.), 220 pp. 8°. *Philadelphia, A. Waldie*, 1839.
———. The same. v (1 l.), 220 pp. 8°. *Philadelphia, Carey & Hart*, 1841.

Montgomery (W. F. [H.])—continued.

——. The same. From 2. Lond. ed. xxiii, 568 pp., 2 col. pl. 8°. *Philadelphia, Blanchard & Lea*, 1857.

——. Observations on the incipient stage of cancerous affections of the womb. 20 pp. 8°. [*Dublin*, 1842.]

Repr. from: Dublin J. M. Sc., 1841-2, xx.
For Biography, see Dublin Q. J. M. Sc., 1862, xxxiii, 250-253. *Also*: Lancet, Lond., 1860, n. s., i, 24. *Also*: Med. Times & Gaz., Lond., 1859, xl, 664.
See, also, **Barker** (F.) & **Montgomery** (Wm. F.) Observations . . . on the Dublin Pharmacopœia [etc.] 8°. *Dublin*, 1830.

Montgomery County, England. *See* **Lunatic** Asylum for the counties of Salop and Montgomery and for the boroughs of Much Wenlock, Shrewsbury, and Oswestry.

Montgomery County Medical Society. Constitution and by-laws. 24 pp. 8°. *Dayton*, 1857.

——. The same. 24 pp. 8°. *Dayton*, 1868.

Monthesaurus (Dominicus).
See **Sethus** (Simeon). Syntagma per elementorum ordinem, etc. 12°. *Basileæ*, 1561.

Monthiers (J.-H.) * Des cyanures doubles. 44 pp. 4°. *Paris, Poussielgue*, 1847. [P., v. 1699.]

Monthly (The) Abstract of Medical Science. A digest of the progress of medicine and the collateral sciences; being a supplement to the "Medical News and Library". v. 1–6, July, 1874, to Dec., 1879. 8°. *Philadelphia, H. C. Lea.*

A continuation of the American reprint of: **Ranking's** Abstract. v. 1 complete in 6 nos., July to Dec., 1874; v. 2 commenced Jan., 1875. After 1879, united with: **Medical** (The) News and Library, forming: **Medical** (The) News and Abstract.

Monthly (The) American Journal of Geology and Natural Science. By G. W. Featherstonhaugh. No. 4, v. 1, October, 1831. pp. 145–192. 8°. *Philadelphia, H. H. Porter.*

Monthly (The) Archives of the Medical Sciences. Edited by [James] Hunter Lane. v. 1, January to May, 1834. 484 pp. 8°. *London, J. Churchill; Liverpool, T. Kaye.*
Ended.

Monthly Bulletin of the Operations of the Cincinnati Branch United States Sanitary Commission. Feb., 1863, to April, 1865. 8°. *Cincinnati, Ohio.*

Monthly (The) Gazette of Health, or general and periodical collection of all new discoveries relative to the means of preserving health, curing diseases, promoting domestic economy, etc. Edited by Richard Reece. v. 1–16, 1816–31. 8°. *London, Sherwood & Co.*

v. 2–5, sub-title: "or Popular Medical, Dietetic and General Philosophical Journal". v. 6–16, sub-title: "or Medical, Dietetic, Anti-empirical" [etc.] v. 2–7 are 3. and 4. ed. v. for 1831 [v. 16] is v. 1, new series, with running title: **Monthly** Gazette of Practical Medicine. Dr. Reece died in 1831.

Monthly Gazette of Practical Medicine.
Was running title of v. 16 of: **Monthly** (The) Gazette of Health, 1831.

Monthly (The) Homœopathic Independent.
Was title, after Nov., 1868, of: **Homœopathic** (The) Independent, St. Louis.

Monthly (The) Homœopathic Observer.
Was title on covers, in 1864, of: **American** (The) Homœopathic Observer.

Monthly (The) Homœopathic Review. Edited by John Ozanne. v. 1–32, July, 1856, to 1888. 8°. *London, W. Headland; H. Turner & Co.*
Current. v. 2 complete in 18 nos., July, 1857, to Dec., 1858; v. 3 commenced Jan., 1859. v. 2–8 edited by John Ryan; in v. 9, W. Bayes and A. C. Pope added; in v. 11, H. R. Madden added; in v. 14, Dr. Madden dropped; v. 20 et seq., by Dr. Pope and D. Dyce Brown.

Monthly (The) Index to Current Periodical Literature. Proceedings of learned societies and government publications. A complete, classi-

Monthly (The) Index [etc.]—continued.
fied record of the English periodical literature of the world, except fiction. v. 1–3, July, 1880, to Dec., 1881. 8°. *New York, published at the office of the "American Bookseller".*

Monthly International Journal of Anatomy and Histology.
Was title, on cover, of reprint of no. 1, v. 1, of: **Internationale** Monatsschrift für Anatomie und Histologie, Berlin, 1884.

Monthly (The) Journal of Foreign Medicine. Edited by Squire Littell, jr. [2 v. annually.] v. 1–3, Jan., 1828, to June, 1829. 8°. *Philadelphia, E Littell.*
Also under title: "**Spirit** of the European Medical Journals".

Monthly (The) Journal of Medical Literature, and American Medical Students' Gazette. Edited by E. Bartlett. Nos. 1–3, v. 1, January to March, 1832. 96 pp. 8°. *Boston, Carter & Hendee.*
Nos. 2–3 published at Lowell, Mass.; title: **Monthly** (The) Journal of Medical Literature and the Literature of Science.

Monthly (The) Journal of Medical Science.
Was title of v. 5–19 of: **London** (The) and Edinburgh Monthly Journal of Medical Science, 1845–54.

Monthly (The) Journal of Medicine.
Was title of v. 20 of: **London** (The) and Edinburgh Monthly Journal of Medical Science, 1855.

Monthly (The) Journal of Medicine, containing selections from European journals, the transactions of learned societies, etc., and embracing a concise analysis of the medical journals of the United States. Conducted by an association of physicians. [2 v. annually.] v. 1–6, Jan., 1823, to Dec., 1825. 8°. *Hartford, Conn., Huntington & Hopkins.*
No. 12, v. 6, last published.

Monthly (The) Journal of Medico-Chirurgical Knowledge. Edited by A. Trousseau [et al.]. Transl. [from the French] by H. B. Lefèvre. Nos. 1–3, v. 1, Oct. to Dec., 1833. 8°. *London, Smith, Elder & Co.*
A transl. of: **Journal** des connaissances médico-chirurgicales, Paris, 1833 [et seq.].

Monthly (A) Journal of Popular Medicine; explaining the nature, causes and prevention of diseases, the immediate management of accidents, and the means of preserving health. Conducted by Charles Thomas Haden. [2 v. annually.] v. 1–2, March, 1821, to Feb., 1822. 8°. *London, Simkin & Marshall.*

Monthly (The) Journal of Science, [etc.]
Was running title of v. 2–12, v. 1, 3. s., of: **Journal** (The) of Science, [etc.], London, 1879.

Monthly Journal of the Southern Illinois Medical Association. Edited by C. W. Dunning and Horace Wardner, committee on publication. v. 1–2, Aug., 1877, to Dec., 1878. 8°. *Cairo, Ill.*
Want no. 10, v. 2, Nov., 1878. v. 1 complete in 6 nos., Aug., 1877, to Jan., 1878; v. 2 commenced Feb., 1878.

Monthly (The) Magazine of Pharmacy, Chemistry, Medicine, etc. Published by Burgoyne, Burbidges, Cyriax, and Farries. Nos. 114, 126, Sept., 1885, Sept., 1886. 4°. *London.*

Monthly Medical Monitor. An outspoken expositor of social and sanitary reform. Sara B. Chase, editor and proprietor. No. 1, v. 1, May 1881. 4 pp. 4°. *New York.*

Monthly (The) Medical News. Edited by S. M. Bemiss and J. W. Benson. [2 v. annually.] v. 2–3, Jan. to Dec., 1860. 2 v. 8°. *Louisville, Ky.*
Title of v. 1, 1859, was: **Semi-Monthly** Medical News. In v. 3 Dr. Benson sole editor.

Monthly (The) Medical Reprint. A reproduction of the most valuable articles published in eight leading British medical journals. Nos. 1–5, v. 1, July to Nov., 1868. 320 pp. roy. 8°. *New York, J. Hillyer.*
Ended.

Monthly (The) Microscopical Journal. Transactions of the Royal Microscopical Society, and record of histological research at home and abroad. Edited by Henry Lawson. [2 v. annually.] v. 1–18, Jan., 1869, to Dec., 1877. 8°. *London, R. Hardwicke.*
Ended. Dr. Lawson died Oct. 4, 1877. Followed, in 1878, by: **Journal** of the Royal Microscopical Society.

Monthly (The) Mirror. Devoted to free thought in medicine, science, and general literature. Edited by Robert A. Gunn. v. 1, June, 1873, to May, 1874. 576 pp. 8°. *New York, B. J. Stow.*
Continued, in July, 1874, as: **Medical** (The) Mirror.

Monthly (The) Miscellany, and Journal of Health.
Was title of no. 1, v. 1, Jan., 1846, of: **Journal** (The) of Health and Monthly Miscellany, Boston.

Monthly (The) Monitor and People's Health Journal. Conducted by Calvin M. Fitch and John W. Sykes. No. 1, v. 1, Sept., 1858. 8°. *Pittsburgh, Pa.*

Monthly (The) Record of the Five Points House of Industry, New York City. No. 7, v. 1; No. 12, v. 18, 1874–5; Nos. 8, 9, 12, v. 26, 1882–3; Nos. Nos. 11, 12, v. 27, 1883–4. 8°. *New York,* 1854–84.

Monthly (The) Register of the Philadelphia Society for Organizing Charity. v. 1–9, Nov. 15, 1879, to 1888. 4°. *Philadelphia.*
Current.

Monthly Retrospect of the Medical Sciences. Edited by A. Fleming and W. T. Gairdner. v. 1–2, Feb., 1848, to Dec., 1849. 8°. *Edinburgh, Sutherland & Knox.*
In v. 2 George E. Day added as editor.

Monthly (The) Review of Dental Surgery. v. 1–8, June, 1872, to Dec., 1879; also, Nos. 1–3, v. 9, Jan. to March, 1880. 8°. *London, Smith, Elder & Co.*
In v. 1–2 no editors named; v. 3–5 edited by Oakley Coles; v. 6–9 by Thomas Gaddes. v. 6 complete in 7 nos., June to Dec., 1877; v. 7 commenced Jan., 1878.

Monthly (The) Review of Dental Surgery; being the journal of the British Dental Association. Edited by Alfred Coleman and Joseph Walker. [N. s.] v. 1, Jan. to Dec., 1880. 8°. *London, Smith, Elder & Co.*
Continued as: **Journal** (The) of the British Dental Association.

Monthly (The) Review of Medicine and Pharmacy. Edited by Richard V. Mattison. v. 2–5, 1879–82. 4 v. roy. 8°. *Philadelphia, Keasbey & Mattison.*
Title of v. 1, 1878, was: **Philadelphia** (The) Druggist and Chemist. In 1883 continued as: **Quinologist** (The).

Monthly (The) Sanitary Record. The official organ of the Ohio State board of health. Dr. C. O. Probst, editor. No. 1, v. 1, January, 1888. 16 pp. 8°. *Columbus, O.*
Current.

Monthly (The) Stethoscope and Medical Reporter. G. A. Wilson and R. A. Lewis, editors and proprietors. v. 1–2, Jan., 1856, to May, 1857. 8°. *Richmond, Va.*
Ended. 5 nos. in v. 2.

Monthly (The) Supplement to the American Journal of Obstetrics. Edited by Paul F. Mundé. v. 1, 1882. 8°. *New York, W. Wood & Co.*

Monthus (J.-B.) *I. Quelle est la valeur des signes fournis par le sang avant sa coagulation? II. [etc.] 34 pp. 4°. *Paris,* 1838, No. 269, v. 331.

Monthus (Théodore-Adolphe). *Sur la pneumonie double. 1 p. l., 287 pp., 5 tab. 4°. *Paris,* 1868, No. 243.

[**Monti** (Alfonso).] Stranezze ed assurdità della omiopatia! Un morto nel 1852 rispondeva nel 1841 ad un opuscolo del 1856. 107 pp. 8°. *Firenze, tipog. Tofani,* 1856. [P., v. 1451.]

28

Monti (Alois) [1839–]. Epidemische Cholera.
In: HANDB. d. Kinderkr. (Gerhardt), Tübing., 1877, ii, 587–646.
——. Krankheiten der Nieren.
In: HANDB. d. Kinderkr. (Gerhardt), Tübing., 1878, iv, 3. Abth., 357–494.
——. Krankheiten der Nebennieren.
In: HANDB. d. Kinderkr. (Gerhardt), Tübing., 1878, iv, 3. Abth., 495–504.
——. Hyperämie und Blutung des Rückenmarkes und seiner Häute.
In: HANDB. d. Kinderkr. (Gerhardt), Tübing., 1879, v, 1. Abth., 361–372.
——. Ueber Croup und Diphtheritis im Kindesalter. viii, 384 pp. 8°. *Wien, Urban u. Schwarzenburg,* 1884.
——. *See, also:*
Quellen zu den Publicationen des Dr. Alois Monti auf dem Gebiete der Kinderheilkunde. Wien. med. Bl., 1880, iii, Beilage, 16.

Monti (Benedetto) [1799–1869]. Dell' uomo come soggetto ed oggetto della pubblica igiene e della polizia medica. 26 pp. 8°. *Milano, De-Cristoforis,* 1859. [P., v. 1144.]
——. Della igiene pubblica, della polizia medica, della medicina legale e della loro coordinazione sintetica e del principio unitivo nel quale si congiungono. Prolusione letta nella R. Università di Bologna. 22 pp. 8°. *Bologna, regia tipografia,* 1860.
——. Dei concetti fondamentali della fisiologia, igiene, patologia e terapia e della redintegrazione di essi in un concetto supremo. Lettera all' eccelmo. Sig. Dott. Rignon. 30 pp. 8°. *Fano, G. Lana,* 1862. [P., v. 1132.]
Repr. from: Ippocratico, Fano, 1862, 3. s., i.
For Biography, see **Zani** (I.) Cenni necrologici del Prof. Benedetto Monti. Letti alla Società medico-chirurgica di Bologna nella tornata del dì settembre 1869. 8°. Bologna, 1869.

Monti (Giambattista). Istruzioni contro il colera. 56 pp. 12°. [*Fermo,* 1884.]

Monti (Giuseppe). Rendiconto economico-amministrativo sui cronici di Milano nell' Ospedale Maggiore pel biennio 1875–6, con studii pratici per la ricostituzione dei tre grandi istituti sanitario-caritativi giusta la mente del R. ministero. 74 pp., 1 l. 8°. *Milano, tipog. fratelli Rechiedei,* 1877.
Repr. from: Ann. univ. di med., Milano, 1877, ccxli.

Monti (Ignaz). Medicinische Dictata. Aus dem Italiänischen übersetzt. 270 pp. 12°. *Stutgart, J. B. Mezler,* 1781.

Monti (*Lorenzo*) [1841–81].
Necrologia. Pisani, Palermo, 1881, 224. *Also, transl.:* Alien. & Neurol., St. Louis, 1881, ii, 703.

Monti (Luigi). La diagnostica delle malattie dedotta in modo facile dalla chimica ed esposta per uso dei medici pratici. 383 pp. 8°. *Venezia, P. Naratovich,* 1866.
——. Studio antropologico sui crani dei delinquenti. 24 pp. 4°. *Bologna, Gamberini & Parmeggiani,* 1884.

Monticelli (Teodoro). Sulla economia delle acque da ristabilirsi nel regno di Napoli; memoria. 3. ed. vii, 90 pp. 8°. *Napoli,* 1820.

Montier (Constant). *Sur l'hydrocèle de la tunique vaginale. 33 pp. 4°. *Paris,* 1827, No. 21, v. 204.

Montier (Émile). *Parallèle entre l'opération césarienne et l'embryotomie. 52 pp. 4°. *Paris,* 1855, No. 97, v. 578.

Montieri.
Cozzi (A.) Ricerche geologiche e mineralogiche sopra Montieri e sue adiacenze. 8°. *Firenze,* 1842.

de Montigny (*Etienne-Mignot*) [1714–82].
Éloge de . . . Hist. de la Soc. roy. de méd. 1780–81, Par., 1785, 85–100.

de Montigny (Hippolyte). *Sur un cas d'oblitération artificielle du vagin (méthode indirecte du traitement des fistules vésico-vaginales). 44 pp. 4°. *Paris*, 1873, No. 88.

Montilla.

See, also, **Cholera** (*Asiatic, History, etc., of*), **Fever** (*Malarial, History, etc., of*), *by localities.*

de Aguayo y Trillo (J. M.) Enfermedades reinantes en Montilla en el otoño de 1857. Siglo méd., Madrid, 1857, iv, 403: 1858, v, 2. ———. Noticia de las enfermedades que han reinado en la ciudad de Montilla, provincia de Córdoba, 1860. *Ibid.*, 1861, viii, 168; 199; 259; 371.

Montillot (G.) *De la rétention d'urine envisagée comme symptôme. 34 pp. 4°. *Paris*, 1862, No. 122.

Montin (Abrahamus).

See **Lindforss** (Martinus Joannes) & **Montin** (Abrahamus). De abscessu lymphatico [etc.] 4°. *Helsingforsiæ*, [1833].

Montin (Laur.) *Splachnum. *Upsaliæ*, 1750. *In:* LINNÆUS. Amœnitates acad. [etc.] 8°. *Lugd. Bat.*, 1764, ii, 2. ed., 242–260, 1 pl.

Montinho (A. F.) Duas palavras a respeito da obra do Snr. Duque de Saldanha intitulada: Estado da medicina em 1858. 14 pp. 8°. *Porto*, 1858. [P., v. 1255.]

Montini (Lodovico). *Sull' anatomia patologica. 24 pp. 8°. *Pavia, eredi Bizzoni*, [1855]. [P., v. 1416.]

Montisianus (Marcus Antonius).

See **Bucius** (Dominicus). Quæsita medicinalia iv juxta Hippocratis, [etc.] 12°. [*Montis Regali*], 1551.

Montius (Pamphilus). Methodus medendi. clxiii pp. 16°. *Augustæ Vindel., excud. H. Steynerus*, 1540.

Montlovier (Denis-Laurent). *Sur la péritonite aiguë. 25 pp. 4°. *Paris*, 1817, No. 170, v. 134.

Mont-Luc (A.-F.-M.-Falvard). *Considérations générales sur les phénomènes des maladies. 32 pp. 4°. *Paris*, 1808, No. 138, v. 73.

de Montmahoux (Étienne) [1793–]. *Considérations médicales sur les moyens employés pour conserver la beauté. 32 pp. 4°. *Paris*, 1815, No. 299, v. 117.

———. Manuel médico-légal des poisons, précédé de considérations sur l'empoisonnement; des moyens de le constater; du résultat d'expériences faites sur l'acétate de morphine et les autres alcalis végétaux; suivi d'une méthode de traiter les morsures des animaux enragés et de la vipère; d'un précis sur la pustule maligne; des secours à donner aux personnes empoisonnées, noyées ou asphyxiées, etc.; rédigé sous les yeux de M. le professeur Chaussier. xv, 375 pp., 19 pl. 18°. *Paris, Compère jeune*, 1824.

Montmajou.

Moitessier (A.) Les eaux minérales de Montmajou. Gaz. hebd. d. sc. méd. de Montpel., 1880, ii, 421–423.

Montmasson (Auguste). *De la gangrène du poumon. 46 pp. 4°. *Paris*, 1856, No. 233, v. 594.

de Montméja (A.) Pathologie iconographique du fond de l'œil. Traité d'ophthalmoscopie, comprenant la théorie, la description et le maniement des divers ophthalmoscopes, l'étude du fond de l'œil normal et pathologique, un atlas de 40 sujets dessinés et coloriés d'après nature. 2 p. l., 48 pp., 10 pl., 10 l. roy. 4°. *Paris, H. Lauwereyns*, 1870.

———. *Diagnostic des cataractes et parallèle des opérations qui sont applicables à leur traitement. 74 pp. 4°. *Paris*, 1871, No. 14.

Also, Co-Editor of: **Revue** photographique des hôpitaux de Paris, 1869–76.

See, also, **Hardy** (Alfred) & **de Montméja** (A.) Clinique photographique de l'Hôpital Saint-Louis. 8°. *Paris*, 1868.—**Meyer** (Édouard) & **de Montméja** (A.) Traité des opérations qui se pratiquent sur l'œil. 4°. *Paris*, 1871.

Montméja (Pierre-Romain). *Quelques considérations sur l'état aigu de l'inflammation du poumon. vi, 7–38 pp. 4°. *Paris*, 1823, No. 5, v. 177.

de Montmollin (Henri). *De la fistule vésico-vaginale. [Zurich.] 32 pp., 1 pl. 8°. *Neuchâtel, J. Attinger*, 1864.

Montmorency.

See, also, **Fever** (*Typhus, History, etc., of*), *by localities.*

Beauchêne [*et al.*]. Analyse chimique de l'eau minérale de la source de Montlignon, près Montmorency. J. gén. de méd., chir., et pharm., Par., 1803, xviii, 52–60.—**Cotte** (L.) Observations météorologiques, faites à Montmorency pendant les ans IV–V. Rec. périod. Soc. de santé de Par., 2. éd., an v [1797], i, 48; 138; 223; 303; 398; 484: ii, 54; 112; 185; 303; 356; 450: an vi [1797–8], iii, 58; 132:—**Cotte** (R.-P.) Mémoire sur la topographie médicale de Montmorency et de ses environs. Hist. Soc. roy. de méd. 1779, Par., 1782, iii, pt. 2, 61–83.

Montoya (Eugène). *De la dilatation de l'estomac consécutive à la fièvre typhoïde. 48 pp. 4°. *Paris*, 1884, No. 321.

Montozon (A.-L.-Henri). *De l'heureux emploi de la teinture d'iode dans le traitement de la dysenterie chronique. 32 pp. 4°. *Paris*, 1856, No. 11, v. 594.

de Montozon (Joseph-Jean-Arnaud). *Considérations générales sur l'hystérie. viii, 9–28 pp. 4°. *Paris*, 1832, No. 228, v. 255.

Montpellier (Auguste). *Sur le traitement du croup. 120 pp., 1 l. 4°. *Montpellier, J. Martel*, 1864. [P., v. 45.]

Montpellier.

See, also, **Cholera** (*Asiatic, History, etc., of*), **Education** (*Medical*), *etc.*, **Fever** (*Malarial, History, etc., of*), **Fever** (*Typhoid, History, etc., of*), **Hospitals** (*Descriptions, etc., of*), **Insane** (*Asylums for, etc.*), *by localities;* **Medicine** (*Clinical, Cases of*).

GUINIER (H.) Des conditions sanitaires de la ville de Montpellier. 8°. *Montpellier*, 1863.

MEYRANX (P.-S.) Observations sur la constitution médicale des mois de novembre, décembre et janvier des années 1819 et 1820, et sur les maladies qui se sont présentées pendant ce trimestre à l'École clinique interne de Montpellier, et quelques réflexions sur le système de Broussais. 8°. *Montpellier*, 1821.

POITEVIN (J.) Essai sur le climat de Montpellier, contenant des vues générales sur la nature et la formation des météores, et les principaux résultats des observations faites à Montpellier depuis l'établissement de la ci-devant Académie des sciences de cette ville; ouvrage qui peut servir de suite aux mémoires publiés par cette compagnie 4°. *Montpellier*, 1803.

Bourrely (J.) Quelques mots sur les maladies observées pendant les mois d'août et septembre à Hôtel-Dieu St.-Éloi de Montpellier. Gaz. méd. de Montpel., 1842–3, iii, nos. 23; 26; 30.—**Castan** (A.) De l'influence de la température sur la mortalité de la ville de Montpellier. Montpel. méd., 1870, xxiv, 1; 97.—**Crova** (A.) Observations météorologiques faites à la citadelle de Montpellier pendant l'année 1875. Acad. d. sc. de Montpel. Mém. de la sect. d. sc., 1872–5, viii, 641–648.—**Garimond** (E.) Statistique des hôpitaux de Montpellier au point de vue de l'influence du climat sur le développement et la marche de la phthisie pulmonaire. Gaz. méd. de Par., 1860, 3. s., xv, 8; 18.—**Girbal** (A.) Constitution médicale de Montpellier pendant les mois d'avril, mai, juin, juillet et décembre 1849, et janvier, février et mars 1850. Rev. de thérap. du midi. Montpel., 1850, i, 609; 637; 669: 1851, ii, 7; 45; 71; 116; 138; 207; 244; 400; 471; 485; 526; 717; 753. ——. Études cliniques sur les principales maladies observées à l'Hôtel-Dieu Saint-Éloi du 22 août au 1er novembre 1857. Montpel. méd., 1859, ii, 493: iii, 1; 481: 1860, iv, 393.—**Mejan** (T.) Éphémérides météorologico-médicales, 1803–15. Ann. Soc. de méd.-prat. de Montpel., 1803, i: 1806, x, *passim. Continued in:* Hist. Soc. de méd.-prat. de Montpel., 1805, xiv: 1815, xxxviii, *passim.*—**Mourgue de Montredon.** Observations sur les naissances, les mariages et les morts à Montpellier pendant dix années consécutives, de 1772 à 1781 inclusivement. Hist. Soc. roy. de méd. 1780–81, Par., 1785, iv, pt. 1, 378–392, 3 tab.—**Roche** (E.) Ré-

Montpellier.

sumé des observations météorologiques faites à la Faculté des sciences de Montpellier pendant les années 1864–7. Acad. d. sc. de Montpel. Mém. de la sect. d. sc., 1864–5, vi, 209; 3ᵒ9; 1867–71, vii, 1; 127. ———. Le climat actuel de Montpellier, comparé aux observations du siècle dernier. Ibid. (1881), 1882, x, 329–384, 6 diag.—**Saintpierre** (C.) Introduction à l'étude médicale du climat de Montpellier. Montpel. méd., 1868, xx, 524–544.

Montpellier mineral waters.

Bertin (E.) Nouvelle notice sur les eaux minérales thermales acidules de Foncaude. J. Soc. de méd.-prat. de Montpel., 1846, xiii, 182–203. ———. Des eaux minérales acidules thermales de Foncaude, de leurs effets et de leur usage dans le traitement des maladies qu'elles peuvent guérir. Acad. d. sc. de Montpel. Mém. de la sect. de méd., 1849–53, i, 305–407. Also, Reprint.—**Moitessier** (A.) Analyse d'une eau minérale récemment découverte aux environs de Montpellier. Montpel. méd., 1860, v, 466–471.

Montpellier médical.

Journal mensuel de médecine, rédigé par MM. Bérard, Lordat [et al.]. [Monthly; 2 v. annually.] v. 1–50, June, 1858, to June, 1883; 2. s., v. 1–9, July, 1883, to Dec., 1887. 59 v. 8ᵒ. Montpellier.

Current. In 1860, **Revue** thérapeutique du midi merged in this journal. In July, 1887, became semi-monthly.

Mont-de-Piété de Paris.

Notice sur le . . . et compte général des recettes et dépenses de cet établissement pendant l'année 1828. 10 pp., 4 l., 3 tab. 4ᵒ. [Paris, Éverat, 1829.]

Montreal.

Report on the proposed enlargement of the Montreal water-works, together with an historical sketch of the works up to present date. In accordance with instructions from the water committee by Louis Lesage, superintendent. 23 pp., 3 pl., 2 plans, 1 tab. 8ᵒ. Montreal, J. Starke & Co., 1873.

———. Rapport annuel du surintendant de l'aqueduc de Montréal, pour l'année 1873. 43 pp. 8ᵒ. Montréal, L. Perrault & Cie., 1874.

———. Annual reports on the sanitary state of the city of Montreal. By the health officer to the board of health, for the years 1877–83. [By A. B. La Rocque.] 8ᵒ. Montreal, 1878–84.

1877–81 bound in 1 v.; 1879, 1880 are also bound with: Rep. on the accounts of the corporation. 8ᵒ. Montreal, 1880–81. 1882, 1883 bound with: Rep. of the corporation. 8ᵒ. Montreal, 1884–5.

———. Mortality of Montreal. Statement of deaths in the city during the month of Nov., 1879. 2 l. sm. 4ᵒ. [Montreal, 1879.]

———. Reports on the accounts of the corporation of the city of Montreal, and reports of the city officials for the years 1879–84. 6 v. 8ᵒ. Montreal, L. Perrault & Son, 1880–85.

———. Annual reports of the superintendent of the Montreal water-works, for the years 1879–84. 8ᵒ. Montreal, 1880–85.

1879–84 bound with: Rep. on the accounts of the corporation. 8ᵒ. Montreal, 1880–85.

———. Annual reports of the chief of police, for the years 1879–85. 8ᵒ. Montreal, the Perrault Printing Co., 1880–86.

1879–84 bound with: Rep. on the accounts of the corporation. 8ᵒ. Montreal, 1880–85.

———. Annual report of the harbour commissioners of Montreal, for the year 1885. 67 pp. 8ᵒ. Montreal, 1886.

———. Mortalité de la cité de Montréal. [Monthly.] Jan., 1887. 8ᵒ. Montréal, la compagnie d'imprimerie Perrault, 1887.

Montreal.

See, also, **Cholera** (Asiatic, History, etc., of), by localities; **Deaf-mutes** (Asylums, etc., for); **Education** (Medical), etc., **Fever** (Cerebro-spinal, History, etc., of), **Fever** (Typhus, History, etc., of), **Hospitals** (Descriptions, etc., of), **Hospitals** (Maternity, etc.), by localities.

Carpenter (P. P.) On the vital statistics of Montreal. (Supplement to the Montreal Gazette.) 8ᵒ. [Montreal, 1867.]

Montreal.

Hovey & **Dawson**. Health map of Montreal, showing the annual death-rate per thousand for the average of the years 1876, '77, and '78, resulting from small-pox, typhoid fever, and diphtheria. 4ᵒ. [Montreal, 1879.]

Watt (A. A.) Notes on the principles of population. Montreal compared with London, Glasgow, and Manchester, with an examination of the vital statistics, by P. P. Carpenter. 8ᵒ. Montreal, 1869.

Repr. from: "Witness", and "Daily News". Also, in: Canada M. J., Montreal, 1869–70, vi, 248; 307.

Arnoldi (A. F. C. T.) [et al.]. Report of the Montreal Self-Supporting Dispensary. Montreal M. Gaz., 1844, i, 120.—**Bill** of mortality for the city of Montreal, from 31st Dec., 1845, to 29th Feb., 1848. Brit.-Am. J. M. & Phys. Sc., Montreal, 1845–6, i: 1847–8, iii, passim.—**Bowie** (J.) Sick report of the immigrants arrived at the Montreal immigrant sheds, for the years 1843 and 1844. Brit.-Am. J. M. & Phys. Sc., Montreal, 1845–6, i, 146–148.—**Edwards** (J. B.) On the filtration of the public water supply. Pub. Health Mag., Montreal, 1875–6, i, 1–3. ———. Montreal water supply. Ibid., 36–40.—**Fenwick** (G. E.) Medical statistics of the city of Montreal. Brit.-Am. J., Montreal, 1861, ii, 383; 390; 431; 439; 479; 489; 527; 1862, iii, 33. Also, Reprint. ———. Mortality of the city of Montreal in March and April, May, June, July, Aug., Sept., Oct., Nov., and Dec., 1864. Canada M. J., Montreal, 1865, i, 101; 153; 205; 303; 349.—**Girdwood** (G. P.) On the water supply and drainage of Montreal. Canada M. J., Montreal, 1870–71, vii, 18–40.—**Grenier** (G.) Tableau des maladies traitées au dispensaire de l'Asile de la Providence, depuis le 15 février 1872, jusqu'au 15 avril de la même année. Union méd. du Canada, Montréal, 1872, i, 221.—**Hall** (A.) Observations on the mortality of the city of Montreal, for the year 1846. Brit.-Am. J. M. & Phys. Sc., Montreal, 1847–8, iii, 141–144. ———. Mortality of the city of Montreal during the year 1860. Brit.-Am. J., Montreal, 1861, ii, 79–81. ———. Mortality of Montreal. Ibid., 130–132.—**Health** (The) of Montreal. San. Engin., Lond., 1880, i, 69.—**King** (T. D.) Register of thermometer and barometer, Montreal, Feb. and March, April and May, 1872. Canada M. J., Montreal, 1871–2, viii, 480; 576. ———. Monthly summary of meteorological observations taken at No. 26 Beaver Hall, Montreal, June, July, Aug., Sept., 1872. Canada M. & S. J., Montreal, 1872–3, i, 144; 240.—**Larocque** (A. B.) Sanitary matters in Montreal. Ibid., 1874–5, iii, 499–502. ———. Rapport de l'état sanitaire de la cité de Montréal pour l'année 1878. Abeille méd., Montréal, 1879, i, 357–360.—**Mondelet** (W. H.) Principal causes of the mortality of Montreal, and modes of prevention. Canada M. J., Montreal, 1868–9, v, 12; 53; 157.—**Monthly** meteorological register at Montreal, March, 1845, to Feb., 1851. Brit.-Am. J. M. & Phys. Sc., Montreal, 1845–6, i: 1849–50, v, passim. Continued in: Brit.-Am. M. & Phys. J., Montreal, 1850–51, n. s., vi, passim.—**Mortality** of the city and suburbs of Montreal, for 1875–7. Pub. Health Mag., Montreal, 1875–6–1876–7, passim.—**Salubrité** de la cité de Montréal comparée à d'autres villes et prouvée par les tableaux suivants. Abeille méd., Montréal, 1880, ii, 390–392.—**Smallwood** (C.) Abstract of meteorological observations taken at the Montreal Observatory, latitude 45ᵒ 31' N., longitude 4ʰ 54ᵐ 11ˢ W. of Greenwich; height above level of the sea, 182 feet. For the months of March, April, May, June, July, Aug., Sept., Oct., Nov., and Dec., 1864. Canada M. J., Montreal, 1864–5, i, 103; 155; 207; 256; 302; 351.

Montreal College of Pharmacy.

Annual announcements of the lecture department. Syllabus of lectures, regulations, and terms, for the session of 1878–9 (11.); 1881–2 (14.). 8ᵒ. Montreal, 1879–81.

Montreal Dispensary.

Dispensaires de l'Asile des Sœurs de la Providence et des Dames de l'Hôpital-Général de Montréal. Union méd. du Canada, Montréal, 1873, ii, 567–571.—**Montreal** Dispensary. Semi-annual report, from 1st May, 1853, to 1st May, 1858. Med. Chron., Montreal, 1853–4, i, 245; [255]: 1854–5, ii, 82: 1855–6, iii, 37: 1856–7, iv, 39: 1857–8, v, 95: 1858–9, vi, 46.

Montreal General Hospital.

Annual reports of the governors to the corporation at the annual meetings. 36.–63., 1857–8 to 1884–5. 8ᵒ. Montreal, 1858–85.

36.–61. bound in 1 v.

———. The by-laws of the . . . as amended and finally passed by the governors, and approved by the corporation of the Society of the Montreal General Hospital, on the 16th of May, 1876, to

Montreal General Hospital—continued.
which is prefixed a copy of the original and of the amended charter. 22 pp. 8°. *Montreal, Lovell Printing and Publishing Co.*, 1876.
Bound with: Reports 36.; 61., 1857–8 to 1882–3.

———. Pathological reports, by William Osler. 1., 1876–7; 2., 1877–9. 8°. *Montreal*, 1878–80.
2. *repr. from:* Montreal Gen. Hosp. Rep. Clin. & Path., 1880, i.

———. By-laws of the . . . as amended and finally passed by the governors, and approved by the corporation of the Society of the Montreal General Hospital, on the 17th May, 1881. 24 pp. 8°. *Montreal, J. Lovell & Son*, 1881.
Bound with: Reports 36.-61., 1857–8 to 1882–3.

———. Letter to the governors, relating to the plans for the new pavilions. To be considered at the quarterly meeting in May, 1884. By Andrew Robertson. 14 pp. 8°. [*Montreal*, 1884.]

———. By-laws of the . . . as amended and finally passed by the governors and approved by the corporation of the Society of the Montreal General Hospital, on the 19th day of May, 1885. 23 pp. 8°. *Montreal, J. Lovell & Son*, [1885].

Montreal (The) Medical Gazette; being a monthly journal of medicine and the collateral sciences. Edited by Francis Badgley and Wm. Sunderland. v. 1, 1844–5. 8°. *Montreal, Lovell & Gibson.*

Montreal Veterinary College. Annual announcement for the session of 1883–4 (17.). 16 pp. 8°. *Montreal, Canada Printing Company*, 1883.

Montreuil-sur-Mer.
See **Fever** (*Typhus, History, etc., of*), by localities.

Montreul (Henri). * Physiologie et pathologie de la sueur. 38 pp. 4°. *Paris*, 1866, No. 314.

Montreux.
STEIGER. Montreux am Genfer See als klimatischer Winteraufenthalt und Traubenkurort. 12°. *Stuttgart*, 1876.

de Montrœil. Sommaire des bandes et bandages. 23 pp. 12°. [*Rouen*, 1680.]
Bound with: DE MARQUE (J.) Méthodique introduction à la chirurgie. 12°. *Rouen*, 1680.

Montrond.
Chavanis. Les eaux minérales de Montrond. Loire méd., St.-Étienne, 1883, ii, 185–199.

Montrond-Geyser.
Dulac (P.) Étude sur les eaux de Montrond-Geyser. Loire méd., St.-Étienne, 1885, iv, 29–39.

Montrose. Annual reports on the health of Montrose. By the medical officer of health to the local authority, for the years 1880–83. 12°. *Montrose*, 1881–4.
1880–82, by Sam. Lawrence

Montrose.
See **Hospitals** (*Descriptions, etc., of*), **Insane** (*Asylums for, etc.*), by localities.

Montrose Royal Infirmary and Dispensary. *See* **Royal** Infirmary and Dispensary of Montrose.

Montrose Royal Lunatic Asylum. *See* **Royal** Lunatic Asylum of Montrose.

Montrose Station.
Andrews (H.), jr. Report upon a nuisance occasioned by swamp lands at Montrose Station, Westchester county. Rep. State Bd. Health N. Y., Albany, 1886, vi, 200, 1 map.

Mont-Saint-Aubert.
See **Fever** (*Malarial, History, etc., of*), by localities.

Mont-Saint-Bernard.
Cloquet (H.) Aperçu sur la topographie médicale de l'Hospice du Mont-Saint-Bernard. Rédigé en partie d'après des notes du R. P. Bisela. N. Jour. de méd., chir., pharm., etc., Par., 1820, vii, 29–37.

Mont-Saint-Michel.
Ledain (H.) Extrait d'un essai sur la topographie médicale du Mont-Saint-Michel. Arch. gén. de méd., Par., 1833, 2. s., ii, 346; 457.

Montségur (Jean-Baptiste-Amédée). * Du diagnostic de la grossesse utérine. 31 pp. 4°. *Paris*, 1844, No. 236, v. 421.

Montserrat.
Badham (J.) Some account of the diseases usually treated in Montserrat. Lond. M. Gaz., 1833, xii, 238; 460.

Montuus (Hieronimus). Compendiolum curatricis scientiæ longe utilissimum. Adjecta insuper est ejusdem: Sylloge de purgationibus. 254 pp., 3 l. 12°. *Lugduni, apud J. Tornæsium et G. Gazeium*, 1556.

———. De medica theoresi liber primus. 122 pp., 8 l. 24°. *Lugduni, apud J. Tornæsium et G. Gazeium*, 1556.
Bound with preceding.

———. Selecta aliquot in aphorismos redacta, quorum sectiones tres sunt. 56 pp. 24°. *Lugduni, apud J. Tornæsium et G. Gazeium*, 1556.
Bound with preceding.

———. De his quæ ad rationalis medici disciplinam, munus, laudes, consilia, et præmia pertinent, libellus cum appendice. 38 pp. 24°. *Lugduni, apud J. Tornæsium et G. Gazeium*, 1556.
Bound with preceding.
See, also, **Montuus** (Sebastianus). Dialexeon [etc.]

———. De admirandis facultatibus, quarum causæ latentes cæcæque ac plerisque omnibus ignotæ sunt, centuriæ duæ cum aliquot decuriis. 56 pp. 24°. *Lugduni, apud J. Tornæsium et G. Gazeium*, 1556.
Bound with preceding.

———. Opuscula juvenilia. 32 pp. 24°. *Lugduni, apud J. Tornæsium et G. Gazeium*, 1556.
Bound with preceding

———. De activa medicinæ scientia commentarii duo. Quorum primus de salubritate non modo tuendæ sanitatis, verumetiam producendæ ad multos annos vitæ rationem modumque docet. Alter vero universales, qui ad morborum curationes pertinent, canones explanat. 7 p. l., 323 pp., 6 l. 12°. *Lugduni, apud J. Tornæsium et G. Gazeium*, 1557.

———. Halosis febrium. Quæ omnium morborum gravissimæ sunt, libri ix. Chirurgica auxilia ad aliquot affectus . . . Morbi item venerei . . . De infantium febribus . . . In 1 v. 8 p. l., 166 pp.; 3 p. l., 78 pp.; 3 p. l., 25 pp., 1 l. 8°. *Lugduni, apud J. Tornæsium et G. Gazeium*, 1558.

———. Anasceues morborum. Tomus primus [–quartus]. 4 v. in 1. 559 pp., 5 l. sm. 4°. *Lugduni, apud J. Tornæsium*, 1560.

Montuus (Sebastianus) [1480–]. Annotatiunculæ . . . in errata recentiorum medicorum per Leonardum Fuchsium collecta: Apologetica epistola pro defensione Arabum a domino Bernardo Unger composita: Epistola responsiva pro Græcorum defensione in Arabum errata, a domino Symphoriano Campegio composita. 1v ff., 1 l. 12°. *Lugduni*, 1533.

———. Dialexeon medicinalium libri duo, nunc recens in lucem prolati. Adjectus est de his quæ ad rationalis medici disciplinam, munus, laudes, consilia et præmia pertinent, libellus. 3 p. l., 184 pp., 12 l. 4°. *Lugduni, apud M. Parmanterium*, 1537.
The treatise Adjectus est de his [etc.] is by Hieronymus Montuus.
See, also, **Fuchs** (Leonhard). Paradoxorum medicinæ libri tres. fol. *Basileæ*, 1535. ———. The same. 12°. *Parisiis*, 1555.

Montvale Spring.
Mitchell (J. B.) Analysis of Montvale Spring; efficacy and properties of mineral waters. E. Tennessee Rec. M. & S., Knoxville, 1852–3, i, 357–363.

du Montvert (Raoul). Les fleurs et secretz de médecine, lequel traictans de plusieurs remèdes, receptes, et conservatoires pour le corps humain contre toutes maladies comme de peste, fiebvres, pleurésies, enfleures, caterres, gravelles, et plusieurs aultres. Compilé par . . . puis traduict de latin en françois; lequel livre Ypocras envoya à Jalius, lequel estoit malade de plusieurs maladies tant extérieures qu'intérieures. Nouvellement imprimé. 8 p. l., 79 ff., 1 l. 24°. *Paris*, [1500?]
———. The same. 8 p. l., 68 ff. 24°. *Poictiers, Bouchet*, [1544].

Monument to Jenner. Considerations and suggestions in its favor. [With the report of committee, appointed by the Suffolk District Medical Society, to receive subscriptions. Boston, Sept. 1, 1851.] 3 pp. 4°. [*Boston*, 1851.]

Monument to Joseph Lovell, late Surgeon-General of the Army of the United States. [Signed by T. G. Mower, C. S. Tripler, and Benjamin King, committee on behalf of the medical staff. April, 1844.] 2 l. fol. [*n. p.*, 1844.]

Monvenoux (A.-J.) *I. De la nature de la coqueluche et de ses causes. II. [etc.] 31 pp. 4° *Paris*, 1840, No. 281. [P., v. 363.]

Monvenoux (Frédéric) [1857–]. * Documents relatifs à la présence des matières grasses dans l'urine. Première série suivie d'une nomenclature raisonnée des travaux qui ont paru jusqu'à ce jour sur les entozoaires de la chylurie et de l'hémato-chylurie. [Paris.] vii, 1106 pp., 11 pl., 10 l. 4°. *Lyon, Pitrat aîné*, 1884, No. 362.

Monvenoux (Joseph). *Considérations sur les méthodes récentes employées dans le traitement de la rage. 60 pp. 4°. *Paris*, 1876, No. 91.

Mony (Adolphe-S.-P.-D.) *Considérations sur l'étranglement de l'intestin par les brides péritonéales. 64 pp., 2 pl. 4°. *Paris*, 1860, No. 171.

Monza. Regolamento di polizia urbana per la città di Monza. 25 pp. roy. 4°. [*Milano*, 1866.]

Monza.
See **Hospitals** (*Descriptions, etc., of*), by localities.

Monzel (Matthias). * De secretione cutanea. 40 pp. 8°. *Berolini, typ. Brüschckianis*, [1829]. [*Also, in:* P., v. 1548.]

Moodie (John). A medical treatise, with principles and observations to preserve chastity and morality, with four plates of an apparatus for the same purpose; and principles and observations to preserve the beauty, expression and youth of the face, so much destroyed by stuffing, sea bathing and the evils of tight lacing, [etc.] iv, 91, 8 pp. 8°. *Edinburgh, Stevenson & Co.*, 1848.

———. New and original opinions as to the sounds of the heart and circulation, and abscesses, their physiology and treatment; and contagion and puerperal fever, their causes; and the cause of contagion in various diseases. vi, 96 pp. 12°. *Edinburgh*, 1850.

———. A new strict entail of £1,500 a year or less, for one hundred years, and the evils of national loans, benefits of private endowments, many important legal changes, and change in the Scotch appeal judicature of Scotland. 69 pp. sm. 8°. *Edinburgh*, 1850.

Moody (*Anson*) [1792–1855].
Catlin (B. H.) Biographical sketch of Anson Moody, M. D., of New Haven. Proc. Connect. M. Soc. 1860–63, N. Haven, 1863, 2. s., i, 125–128.

Moody (G. W.) Veratrum viride. 8 pp. 8°. *Nashville, Harslock & Ambrose*, [1887].
Repr. from: Tr. M. Soc. Tennessee, Nashville, 1887.

Moody (*George*) [–1887].
Barr (G. W.) [*et al.*]. Obituary. Med. & Surg. Reporter, Phila., 1887, lvi, 256.

Moody (*George Anson*) [1821–77].
Lyon (E. B.) Obituary. Proc. Connect. M. Soc., Hartford, 1878, 201.

Moody (*Horace P.*) [1835–69].
Necrological notice. Tr. M. Soc. Penn., Phila., 1870, 6. s., i, 92.

Moody (Jacobus). * De causis et formis febrium epidemicarum communium. 1 p. l., 40 pp. 8°. *Edinburgi, Balfour et Smellie*, 1772.

Moody (Loring). The higher demands of humanity. 2 l. 8°. [*Boston*, 1880.]

Mooers (*Benjamin J.*) [1787–1869].
de Forris (T.) Biographical sketch of Benjamin J. Mooers. Tr. M. Soc. N. Y., Albany, 1870, 309–312.

Mook (Friedrich).
See [Ferguson (John)]. Bibliographia Paracelsica. 8°. *Glasgow*, 1877.

Mook (Kurt). * Ueber den Grund des Eintrittes der Geburt. 35 pp. 8°. *Würzburg, C. J. Becker*, 1872.

Mook (M.-C.) * Contribution à l'étude de l'anatomie pathologique et du traitement de l'eczéma. 64 pp., 1 l. 4°. [*Paris*], 1880, No. 61.

Mookerjee (Gunga Persaud). The principles and practice of medicine in Bengali. v. 1. lv, 712 pp. 8°. *Calcutta, C. B. Lewis*, 1869.
Hindostanee text. Only one volume published.

Moolenaar (Joh.) * De asthmate. 6 l. sm. 4°. *Traj. ad Rhenum, F. Halma*, 1689.

Moolenburgh (Joh.) * De dilatatione bronchiorum. 2 p. l., 45 pp. 8°. *Lugd. Bat., apud L. Herdingh et filium*, 1840.

Mooltan.
Hogg (F. R.) Change of air, with special reference to Mooltan. Indian M. Gaz., Calcutta, 1878, xiii, 141–143.— Lyons (R. T.) The station of Mooltan [a famous town in India; its history and description]. Indian Ann. M. Sc., Calcutta, 1864–5, ix, no. 18, 145–186.

Moon (*Influence of*).
See, also, **Asthma** (*Causes of*); **Astrology**; **Fever** (*Malarial, Causes of*); **Fevers** (*Causes of*); **Solar** *and lunar influence.*

BALFOUR (F.) A treatise on the influence of the moon in fevers. 8°. *Calcutta*, 1784.

———. The same. 8°. *Edinburgh*, [*reprinted*], 1785.

———. A treatise on putrid intestinal remitting fevers, in which the laws of the febrile state and sol-lunar influence being investigated and defined, are applied to explain the nature of the various forms, crises, and other phænomena of these fevers; and thence is deduced an improved method of curing them. 8°. *Edinburgh*, 1790.

———. A treatise on the action of sol-lunar influence, in which it is inferred, from observations on the urine, etc., that it occasions the daily and lunar revolutions observable in the state of fevers of other diseases, and of health, by producing coincident changes in the condition of the constrictive power and balance of the vascular system; and that there is reason to believe that sol-lunar influence exerts its dominion over every production, and in every operation and revolution in nature. 8°. *Edinburgh*, 1791.

———. A treatise on sol-lunar influence in fevers, etc. 8°. *Calcutta*, 1794.

———. A collection of treatises on the effects of sol-lunar influence in fevers and other diseases. 8°. *Calcutta*, 1805.

———. Observations respecting the remarkable effects of sol-lunar influence in the fevers of India; with the scheme of an astronomical ephemeris, for the purposes of medicine and meteorology. This treatise was read before the Asiatic Society, at their meeting, on the 7th July, 1802, and was printed as the first paper in the viiith vol. of their transactions early in 1803. 8°. [*n. p., n. d.*]

Moon (*Influence of*).

GERIKE (P.) * De influxu lunæ in corpus humanum. 4°. *Halæ Magdeb.*, [1724].

GUITARD (J.) * Sur l'influence des corps célestes sur l'économie animale, considérée comme cause déterminante et procatarctique des maladies. 4°. *Montpellier, an VI* [1798].

HAGEN (F. C.) De lunæ viribus in hæc inferiora et inprimis oceanum. 4°. [*n. p.*], 1700.

MEADE (R.) De imperio solis ac lunæ in corpora humana, et morbis inde oriundis. *In his:* Opera medica. 12°. *Gottingæ*, 1748, i. *Also, in his:* Opera ad editiones anglicas, [etc.] 12°. *Parisiis*, 1751, 411-483.

——. The same. Mechanica expositio venenorum; accedit tractatus de imperio solis ac lunæ in corpora humana et morbis unde oriundis. 16°. *Francof. ad Mœnum*, 1763.

——. The same. A treatise concerning the influence of the sun and moon upon human bodies, and the diseases thereby produced. Transl. from the Latin by T. Stack. 8°. *London*, 1758. *Also, in his:* Med. works. 4°. *London*, 1762, pp. cxlix-clxii, 163-206.

NUMAN (A.) Over den invloed der maan in hare verschillende standen op het voorstellingsvermogen der dieren. 8°. [*n. p., n. d.*]

RASCHIG (C. E.) * De lunæ imperio in valetudinem corporis humani nullo. 4°. *Vitebergæ*, [1787].

Behr. Ueber die Mondblindheit. Ztschr. f. d. Ophth., Dresd., 1830-31, i, 238; 277.—**Berncastle** (J.) Influence of the moon's rays. Lond. M. Gaz., 1843, xxxii, 22.—**Berthier.** De l'influence de la lune sur l'organisme en général, et l'épilepsie en particulier. J. de méd. ment., Par., 1865, v, 345-352.—**Chatterjee** (S. C.) The effect of lunar influence on disease. Indian M. Gaz., Calcutta, 1880, xv, 154-156.—**Creniceanu** (G.) A somnambulismus erős holdfény mellet. [Somnambulism in bright moonshine.] Szemészet, Bud.pest, 1886, 83.—**Foissac** (P.) The influence of the lunar phases on the physical and moral man. St. Louis M. & S. J., 1855, xiii, 502-517.—**Giraud** (H.) A commentary upon a tabular statement of the number of paroxysms of malarious intermittent fever that occurred in 146 medical charges in the Bombay Presidency in the year 1861, arranged as data for determining the question of the moon's influence upon these fevers. Tr. M. & Phys. Soc. Bombay (1862), 1863, n. s., viii, 235-245.—**Jackson** (R.) Some observations on the connexion of the new and full moon with the invasion and relapse of fevers. Lond. M. J., 1787, viii, 25; 300.—**Johnson** (J.) The alleged connection between the phases of the moon and the quantity of rain. Charleston M. J., 1854, ix, 452-456.—**Lartigue** (G. B.) Lunar influence. *Ibid.*, 731-743.—**Laycock** (T.) On lunar influence; being a fourth contribution to proleptics. Lancet, Lond., 1842-3, ii, 438-444.—**Lind** (J.) Some remarks on the supposed influence of the moon on fevers. Lond. M. J., 1787, viii, 145-147.—**Mädler** (J. H.) Hat der Mond einen Einfluss auf Krankheiten? Med. Alm., Berl., 1838, 48-55.—**Moore** (W. J.) On lunar influence over malarious fevers. Indian M. Gaz., Calcutta, 1869, iv, 112; 139. *Also*, Reprint. ——. On maladies attributed to lunar influence — rheumatism, paralysis, ocular, etc. Indian M. Gaz., Calcutta, 1869, iv, 180-182.—**Murray** (J.) Cases illustrative of the influence of lunar agency as an occasional cause of periodical exacerbations in various chronic diseases. Tr. M. & Phys. Soc. Bombay, 1837-9, ii, 171-180.—**Peet** (J.) An enquiry into the evidence which is recorded in relation to the influence of the lunar changes upon certain forms of disease. *Ibid.*, 1843, vi, 210-230.—**Py.** Cas de médecine-pratique, venant à l'appui des observations transmises concernant l'influence de la lune sur le retour périodique de certaines maladies. Ann. clin., Montpel., 1809, xx, 31-56.—**Schiaparelli** (G. V.) Dell' influenza della luna sulle vicende atmosferiche. Mem. r. Ist. Lomb. di sc. e lett. Cl. di lett. e sc. matemat. e nat., Milano, 1867, x, 1-26.—**Schimmel** (W. C.) Maanblindheid. Tijdschr. v. veeartsenijk. en veeteelt, Amst., 1886, xiii, 274-287.—**Thompson** (G.) On the supposed influence of the moon's rays as a cause of disease in tropical climates. Lond. M. Gaz., 1842-3, xxxi. 780.— **Tranzieri** (A.) Memoir on a periodical difficulty of breathing, tending to prove the influence of the moon on the human body. Med. & Phys. J., Lond., 1802, viii, 401-411.—**Winslow** (F.) On lunar influence in the production of bodily disease. Lancet, Lond., 1856, i, 254-257.

Moon (Robert C.)

See **Laurence** (John Zachariah) & **Moon** (Robt. C.) A handy-book of ophthalmic surgery [etc.] 8°. *Philadelphia*, 1866.

Moon (W.) Mathew, chapter 5, in type for the blind. 26 pp. oblong 8°. [*London*], *Moon's*, [*n. d.*]

Moonblindness.

See **Hemeralopia**, *etc.*

Moons (P.-J.) Lettre sur l'emploi d'un caustique particulier dans le traitement du cancer externe. 16 pp. 8°. *Bruxelles*, 1841. *Repr. from:* Bull. méd. belge, Brux., 1841, viii.

de Moor (Bartholomæus) [1649-1724]. Cogitationum de instauratione medicinæ, ad sanitatis tutelam, morbos profligandos, nec non vitam prorogandam, libri tres. 14 p. l., 440 pp., 3 pl., 1 l. 12°. *Amstelædami, excud. G. Borstius*, 1695.

——. Veris œconomiæ animalis, seu potius humanæ, principiis innixæ pathologiæ cerebri delineatio practica: in qua, morborum soporosorum, per notas characteristicas, distinctio: nec non spasmorum accuratior distributio traditur. 7 p. l., 593 pp., 10 l. 4°. *Amstelædami, excud. G. Borstius*, 1704.

——. Oratio de hypothesibus medices. [Groningen.] 35 pp. 4°. *Amstelædami, apud R. et G. Wetstenios*, 1706.

de Moor (Bartholomæus Hermannus). * Diss. in aphorismum Hippocraticum xxviii, sectionis vi. Εὐνοῦχοι οὐ ποδαγριῶσιν, οὐδὲ φαλακροὶ γίγνονται. 1 p. l., 3 l., 38 pp. sm. 4°. *Lugd. Bat., S. Luchtmans*, 1736. [*Also, in:* P., v. 989.]

Moor (Edward). Hindu infanticide. An account of the measures adopted for suppressing the practice of the systematic murder by their parents of female infants; with incidental remarks on other customs peculiar to the natives of India. xxvii, 306 pp. 4°. *London, J. Johnson & Co.*, 1811.

Moor (Gideon E.) Analysis report on the Granger water-gas, together with a brief description of the process and apparatus. vii, 8-65 pp., 1 pl. sm. 4°. *Philadelphia, A. O. Granger & Co.*, 1885.

Moor (Joh.) Das in Zürich befindliche kyphotisch-querverengte Becken, nebst einem Vorwort von Prof. Dr. Breslau. 76 pp., 5 pl. 8°. *Zürich, Orell, Füssli u. Comp.*, 1865.

Moor (Thomas).

See **Lindley** (J.) The treasury of botany, [etc.] 8°. *London*, 1870.

Mooradabad.

See **Hospitals** (*Descriptions, etc., of*), by localities.

Moore (Alexander). * Diss. quædam de dyspepsia et melancholia dyspeptica complectens. 2 p. l., 50 pp. 8°. *Edinburgi, J. Moir*, 1820.

Moore (Ann).

See **Statement** (A) of facts [etc.] 8°. *Burton-on-Trent*, 1813.

Moore (Benjamin Thomas). An epitome of the chromo-thermal system of medicine, in a metrical letter addressed to J.W. Cox. 8 pp. 8°. *London*, 1856.

Moore (Carolus). * De usu vesicantium, quæ cantharides recipiunt in febribus. 1 p. l., 17 pp. sm. 4°. *Edinburgi, Hamilton, Balfour et Neill*, 1752.

Moore (Charles). A full inquiry into the subject of suicide, to which are added (as being closely connected with the subject) two treatises on duelling and gaming. 2 v. in 1. 17 p. l., 388 pp., 2 l.; 7 p. l., 405 pp., 12 l. 4°. *London, J. F. & C. Rivington*, 1790.

Moore (Charles Frederick). Suggestions for improvements in the sewerage of cities and towns. 12 pp. 8°. *Dublin, Hodges & Smith*, 1854.

——. Sanitary improvement; the best safeguard against puerperal fever, and many other diseases. 9 pp. 8°. *Dublin, Fannin & Co.*, 1869.

Moore (Charles Hewitt) [1821-70]. An account of some unusual occurrences during the cure of a popliteal aneurism. 8 pp. 8°. [*London*, 1864.]

——. The antecedents of cancer. 53 pp. 8°. *London, T. Richards*, 1865

——. The same. 1 p. l., ix, 53 pp. 8°. *London, T. Richards*, 1865. [P., v. 1197.]
  Repr. [with additions] *from :* Brit. M. J., Lond., 1865, xviii.

——. Rodent cancer; with photographic and other illustrations of its nature and treatment. xiii, 128 pp., 2 pl. 8°. *London, Longmans* [*and others*], 1867.
  See, also, **Rokitansky** (Carl). A manual of pathological anatomy 8°. *London*, 1849-54.
  For Biography, see Brit. M. J., Lond., 1870, i, 641.

——— & **Murchison** (Charles). On a method of procuring the consolidation of fibrin in certain incurable aneurisms. With the report of a case in which an aneurism of the ascending aorta was treated by the insertion of wire. 21 pp. 8°. [*London*, 1864.]

Moore (Chas. W.) A review of the most important advances in surgery, medicine, and pharmacy in the last forty years. 16 pp. 12°. *San Francisco*, 1887.
  Repr. from : Pacific Rec. M. & Pharm., San Fran., 1886-7, i.

Moore (Daniel M.) * On pulmonary consumption. 19 pp. 8°. *Baltimore, S. Hall*, 1813. [P., v. 380.]

Moore (David). * On ophthalmia. 3 p. l., 30 pp. 8°. *Philadelphia, B. Graves*, 1807.

Moore (E. M.) Treatment of the clavicle when fractured or dislocated. 2 pp., 1 pl. 8°. [*Rochester, N. Y.*, 1870.]
  Revised repr. from : Tr. M. Soc. N. Y., Albany, 1870.

——. A luxation of the ulna not hitherto described, with a plan of reduction and mode of after-treatment; including the management of Colles' fracture. 12 pp., 4 pl. 8°. *Albany, Weed, Parsons & Co.*, 1872.
  Repr. from : Tr. M. Soc. N. Y., Albany, 1870.
  See, also, **Pennock** (Caspar Wistar) & **Moore** (E. M.) Report of experiments on the action of the heart [etc.] 8°. *Philadelphia*, 1839.

Moore (*Edward Bucknam*) [1801-78].
  Toner (J. M.) Necrology. Tr. Am. M. Ass., Phila., 1878, xxix, 719-722.

Moore (*Eli Hurdman*) [1814-78].
  Hazlett (R. W.) Necrology. Tr. Am. M. Ass., Phila., 1878, xxix, 722.

Moore (Frederick F.) Old-school and new-school therapeutics; read before the Cambridge Society for Medical Improvement, December 22, 1879. Revised and enlarged. 59 pp. 8°. *Boston, A. Mudge & Son*, 1880.

Moore (George). An enquiry into the pathology, causes, and treatment of puerperal fever; being an essay for which the Fothergillian gold medal was conferred on the author, by the Medical Society of London, in March, 1835. xii, 247 pp. 8°. *London, S. Highley*, 1836.

——. The use of the body in relation to the mind. x, 431 pp. 8°. *London, Longman* [*and others*], 1846.

——. The same. x, 356 pp. 12°. *New York, Harper & Bros.*, 1847.

——. The same. vii, 356 pp. 8°. *New York, Harper & Bros.*, 1859.

——. Health, disease, and remedy familiarly and practically considered in a few of their relations to the blood. xi, 372 pp. 8°. *London, Longman* [*and others*], 1850.

——. The same. xii, 13-320 pp. 8°. *New York, Harper & Bros.*, 1850.

——. The same. xii, 13-320 pp. 8°. *New York, Harper & Bros.*, 1854.

Moore (George)—continued.

——. Man and his motives. vii, 348 pp. 12°. *London, Longman* [*and others*], 1852.

——. The power of the soul over the body, considered in relation to health and morals. vi, 7-270 pp. 12°. *New York, Harper & Bros.*, 1859.

——. The desire for intoxicating liquors a disease; its causes, its effects, and its cure, with the danger of a relapse, together with illustrative sketches: The good salesman: The would-be politician, etc. 216 pp. 12°. *Baltimore, Sherwood & Co.*, 1864.

——. On some diseases of the nose, throat, air-tubes, and lungs, and their local treatment. 103 pp., 1 l. 8°. *London, Simkin, Marshall & Co.*, 1867.

——. Scarlatina; its prevention by belladonna and carbolic acid; their success and mode of use. American revised ed., by Edwin A. Lodge. 23 pp. 8°. *Detroit,* [*E. A.*] *Lodge,* [1870, *vel subseq.*].

——. Summer catarrh, or hay fever; its causes, symptoms, and treatment. 54 pp. 12°. *London, J. Epps & Co.*, [1870].

Moore (James)[1]. A method of preventing or diminishing pain in several operations of surgery. 1 p. l., 50 pp., 1 pl. 8°. *London, T. Cadell*, 1784. [*Also, in :* P., v. 702; 1155.]

——. A dissertation on the process of nature in the filling up of cavities, healing of wounds, and restoring parts which have been destroyed in the human body; which obtained the prize-medal, given by the Lyceum Medicum Londinense, for the year 1789. 76 pp. 4°. *London, J. Richardson*, 1789.

——. An essay on the materia medica. In which the theories of the late Dr. Cullen are considered; together with some opinions of Mr. Hunter and other celebrated writers. xiii (1 l.), 330 pp. 8°. *London, T. Cadell*, 1792.

——. A reply to anti-vaccinists. 70 pp. 8°. *London, J. Murray*, 1806. [P., v. 432.]

——. The history of the small-pox. viii, 312 pp. 8°. *London, Longman* [*and others*], 1815.

——. The history and practice of vaccination. iv, 300 pp. 8°. *London, J. Callow*, 1817.
  See, also, **Adams** (Joseph). Observations on morbid poisons [etc.] 8°. *London*, 1795.

Moore (James)[2]. A practical reply to Sir B. Brodie's letter on homœopathy; with cases, showing the efficacy of homœopathic treatment in the disease of animals. 49 pp. 8°. *Edinburgh, Oliver & Boyd*, 1861.

——. La maladie pulmonaire du bétail, ou pleuro-pneumonie, guérissable par l'homœopathie; avec des avis par . . . Trad. de l'anglais sur la septième édition. 16 pp. 8°. *Bruxelles, Tircher & Manceaux*, 1863.

——. Outlines of veterinary homœopathy; comprising horse, cow, dog, sheep, and dog diseases, and their homœopathic treatment. 7. ed. xxiii, 295 pp. 12°. *London, H. Turner & Co.*, 1874.

——. The same. 9. ed. xxiii, 295 pp. 12°. *London & Leamington, Leath & Ross*, 1882.

——. Dog diseases treated by homœopathy. 4. ed. 180 pp. 18°. *London, J. Epps & Co.*, [*n. d.*]

Moore (Joannes). * De febribus intermittentibus. 17 pp. 8°. *Edinburgi, Abernethy et Walker*, 1808.

Moore (John)[1] [1730-1809]. Medical sketches. In 2 pts. xii, 537 pp. 8°. *London, A. Strahan & T. Cadell*, 1786.

——. The same. 1. Am. ed. vi, 271 pp. 8°. *Providence, Carter & Wilkinson*, 1794.
  For Portrait, see **Collection**—van Kaathoven.—**Collection** of Portr. (Libr.)

Moore (John)[2]. * On digitalis purpurea, or foxglove, and its use in some diseases. 36 pp., 2 pl. 8°. *Philadelphia, Way & Groff*, 1800.
  Also, in : CALDWELL (C.) Med. theses [etc.] 8°. *Philadelphia*, 1805, i, 195-214.

Moore (John)[3]. The structure of the lungs anatomically and physiologically considered, with a view to exemplify or set forth, by instance or example, the wisdom, power, and goodness of God, as revealed and declared in holy writ. The Warneford prize essay for the year 1844. 3 p. l., 106 pp., 1 l., 5 pl. 8°. *London, Longman & Co.*, 1845. [*Also, in:* P., v. 90.]

——. Annual reports on the sanitary condition of Leicester, to the local board of health. 3.–5., 1855–57; 7.–14., 1859–66. 8°. *Leicester,* 1856–67.

——. A full report of [his] speech delivered at the Medical Institution, Jan. 28, 1859, on the occasion of passing the law for the exclusion of future homœopathists from that institution. 8 pp. 12°. *Liverpool, Benson & Mallet,* 1859.

Moore (John S.)
Co-Editor of: **Saint Louis** (The) Medical and Surgical Journal, 1848–56. Also, Co-Editor of: **Humboldt** (The) Medical Archives, St. Louis, 1870-73.

Moore (John William). Notes on "Mean temperature in its relation to disease and mortality", with special reference to the city of Dublin. 107–122 pp. 8°. [*Dublin,* 1869.]
Repr. from: Dublin Q. J. M. Sc., 1869, xlviii.

——. On an aspirator for use in thoracentesis, invented by Dr. Vald. Rasmussen, of Copenhagen. 5 pp., 1 pl. 8°. *Dublin, J. Falconer,* 1871.
Repr. from: Dublin Q. J. M. Sc., 1871, lii.

——. Crystallization of nitrate of urea from urine. 10 pp. 8°. [*Dublin,* 1873.]
Repr. from: Dublin J. M. Sc., 1873, lvi.

——. Meteorology in its bearing on health and disease. 32 pp., 5 diag. 8°. *Dublin, A. Thorn,* 1873.

——. The medical history of the Meath Hospital; an address introductory to the session 1875–76. 20 pp. 8°. *Dublin, J. Falconer,* 1875.

——. A case of pyæmia attended by sudden destruction of the eye. 10 pp. 8°. [*Dublin,* 1876.]
Repr. from: Dublin J. M. Sc., 1877, lxiv.

——. Two cases illustrative of the clinical history of secondary pleuritis in phthisis. 7 pp. 8°. [*Dublin,* 1877.]
Repr. from: Dublin J. M. Sc., 1877, lxiv.

——. A case of typhus with hyperpyrexia. 6 pp. 8°. [*Dublin,* 1878.]
Repr. from: Dublin J. M. Sc., 1878, lxv.

——. In memoriam. William Stokes, M. D., D. C. L., F. R. S., etc. 16 pp. 8°. [*Dublin,* 1878.]
Repr. from: Dublin J. M. Sc., 1878, lxv.

——. A case of phlegmonous erysipelas, followed by pyæmic hemiplegia. 6 pp. 8°. *Dublin,* 1879.
Repr. from: Dublin J. M. Sc., 1879, lxvii.

——. Homes for convalescents from acute infective diseases. 10 pp., 2 pl. 8°. *Dublin,* 1879.
Repr. from: Dublin J. M. Sc., 1879, lxviii.

——. The microcosm of disease; an address introductory to the session 1879–80. 24 pp. 8°. *Dublin,* 1879.

——. Medical reports of the Fever Hospital and House of Recovery, Dublin. 75., 1878–9; 77., 1880–81; 78., 1881–2; 80., 1883–4. 8°. *Dublin,* 1879–84.
In: FEVER Hosp., etc. Reports of com. of management.

——. A case of exanthematic fever resembling epidemic cerebro-spinal meningitis. 7 pp. 8°. [*Dublin,* 1880.]
Repr. from: Dublin J. M. Sc., 1880, lxx.

——. On the compulsory notification and registration of infectious diseases. 9 pp. 8°. [*Dublin,* 1880.]
Repr. from: Dublin J. M. Sc., 1880, lxix.

——. A case of stenosis of the pulmonary valves. 4 pp. 8°. [*n. p.,* 1881.]
Repr. from: Dublin J. M. Sc., 1881, lxxii.

Moore (John William)—continued.
——. Is it (*a*) desirable that there should be a system of compulsory notification of infectious diseases; and, if so (*b*), what is the best method of carrying such a system into effect? and (*c*) what is the best mode of enforcing the isolation of cases of infectious disease? 11 pp. 8°. [*Dublin,* 1881.]
Repr. from: Dublin J. M. Sc., 1881, lxxii.

——. Medical report of the Fever Hospital and House of Recovery, Cork-street, Dublin, for the year ending 31st March, 1881. 25 pp. 8°. [*Dublin,* 1881.]
Repr. from: Dublin J. M. Sc., 1881, lxxii.

——. Clinical note on enteric fever. 8 pp. 8°. [*Dublin,* 1883.]
Repr. from: Dublin J. M. Sc., 1883, lxxvi.

——. Discussion on the present epidemic of scarlet fever in Dublin. 9 pp. 8°. [*Dublin,* 1884.]
Repr. from: Dublin J. M. Sc., 1884, lxxvii.

——. Large gall stones passed per anum. 6 pp. 8°. *Dublin,* 1885.
Repr. from: Dublin J. M. Sc., 1885, lxxix.

——. Sanitary organization in Ireland in its medical aspect. 18 pp. 8°. *Dublin,* 1885.
Repr. from: Dublin J. M. Sc., 1885, lxxix.

——. In memoriam. Benjamin George Mac-Dowell, M. D. 4 pp. 8°. [*Dublin,* 1885.]
Repr. from: Dublin J. M. Sc., 1885, lxxx.

——. A retrospect of clinical teaching in Dublin; being an introductory address delivered on the occasion of the opening of the first session of the Carmichael College Medical Science Association, Tuesday, February 16, 1886. 12 pp. 8°. *Dublin, J. Falconer,* 1886.

——. Remarks on the climate of Dublin, based upon twenty years' observations. 19 pp. 8°. *Dublin, J. Falconer,* 1886.
Repr. from: Dublin J. M. Sc., 1886, lxxxii.

——. The present and the future of state medicine. 20 pp. 8°. *Dublin, J. Falconer,* 1887.
Repr. from: Dublin J. M. Sc., 1887, 3. s., lxxxiii.

——. A case of calculous pyelitis, followed by albuminoid disease. 7 pp. 8°. *Dublin, J. Falconer,* 1887.
Repr. from: Dublin J. M. Sc., 1887, 3. s., lxxxiii.
See, also, **Manual** of public health for Ireland. 8°. *Dublin,* 1875. — **Stokes** (William). Lectures on fever. 8°. *London,* 1874. ——. The same. 8°. *Philadelphia,* 1876.

Moore (Josephus). * De dysenteria. 2 p. l., 64 pp., 2 l. 8°. *Glasgoviæ, R. Chapman,* 1814.

Moore (Levi) [1827–80]. Address delivered before the Medical Society of the County of Albany, November 13, 1866. 11 pp. 8°. *Albany, Van Benthuysen & Sons,* 1867.
For Biography, see Med. Ann., Albany, 1882, iii [Tr. M. Soc. County Albany, 366] (J. M. Bigelow). *Also:* Tr. M. Soc. N. Y., Syracuse, 1883, 279–281 (J. M. Bigelow).

Moore (Matthæus Scott). * De podagra. 3 p. l., 30 pp. 8°. *Edinburgi, G. Mudie et filii,* 1798.

Moore (Norman). * Observations on the shape of the chest in cases of hypertrophy of the heart. 32 pp., 2 pl. 8°. *London, Bradbury, Agnew & Co.,* 1873.

——. * The cause and treatment of rickets. 35 pp. 8°. *London, Bradbury, Agnew & Co.,* 1876.

——. On two Roman tombs discovered in digging the foundations of the new buildings of the medical school at St. Bartholomew's Hospital. 9 pp. 8°. [*London,* 1878.]
Repr. from: Proc. Lond. & Middlesex Archæol. Soc., 1878, v.

——. The illness and death of Henry, Prince of Wales, in 1612. A historical case of typhoid fever. 18 pp. 8°. *London, J. E. Adlard,* 1882.

Moore (Robert). On the sewerage of Kansas City, being a review of a paper on the same sub-

Moore (Robert)—continued.
ject by O. Chanute. Read March 12, 1884. 8 pp.
8°. [St. Louis], 1884.
*Repr. from : J. Ass. Engineering Soc., [St. Louis], 1884.
See, also, Leete (James M.) & Moore (Robert). The
sanitary condition of St. Louis, etc. 8°. St. Louis, 1885.*

Moore (S. W.) Notes of demonstrations on physiological chemistry. viii (1 l.), 58 pp. 12°.
London, Smith, Elder & Co., 1874.

Moore (Samuel). * De rachitide. 35 pp. 8°.
Edinburgi, Balfour et Smellie, 1778.

Moore (Samuel W.) [1786-1854]. * On the medical virtues of the white oxide of bismuth; with some preliminary observations on the chemical properties of that metal. 39 pp. 8°. *New York, T. & J. Swords*, 1810. [P., v. 826.]

———. A memoir of the life and character of John Watts. With an address to the gentlemen who were graduated doctors of medicine at the annual commencement of the College of Physicians and Surgeons, held April 5, 1831. 28 pp. 8°. *New York, G. & C. & H. Carvill*, 1831.
For Biography, see N. York M. Times, 1855, iv, 5-8 (C. R. Gilman). Also, Reprint.

Moore (Sanford). Notes with a Prussian Sanitäts detachment in the Loire ca npaign, 1870. 35 pp., 1 pl. sm. 8°. *London, Pardon & Son*, 1872.
See, also, Prussia. Prussian War Office. Instructions for military surgeons in training sick-bearers. 12°. London, 1876.

Moore (Thomas)[1]. * De dysenteria. 2 p. l., 31 pp. 8°. *Edinburgi, C. Stewart*, 1815. [P., v.734.]

Moore (Thomas)[2]. Valedictory address to the graduating class of the Homœopathic Medical College of Pennsylvania. 16 pp. 8°. *Philadelphia, King & Baird*, 1861.

———. Homœopathy, the science of therapeutics; its natural law and the essential conditions of that law. Annual address before the Homœopathic Medical Society of the State of Pennsylvania. 42 pp. 8°. *Germantown, W. H. Bonsall*, 1873.

———. Dietetics in relation to infants and young children. 14 pp. 8°. *Philadelphia, Sherman & Co.*, 1877.
Repr. from : Hahneman. Month., Phila., 1877-8, xiii.

Moore (W. J.) A manual of the diseases of India. xix, 220 pp. 12°. *London, J. Churchill*, 1861.

———. The same. 2. ed. vi, 638 pp. 8°. *London, J. & A. Churchill*, 1886.

———. Health in the tropics; or, sanitary art applied to Europeans in India. xvi, 318 pp. 8°.
London, J. Churchill, 1862.

———. On lunar influence over malarious fevers. 12 pp. 8°. [*Calcutta*, 1869.]
Repr. from : Indian M. Gaz., Calcutta, 1869, iv.

———. The value of quinine. 10 pp. 8°. [n. p., 1870, vel subseq.]
Repr. from : Indian M. Gaz., Calcutta, 1870, v.

———. A manual of family medicine for India. xvi, 519 pp. 8°. *London, J. & A. Churchill*, 1874.

———. Malarious fevers and rainfall in Rajpootana. 10 pp. 8°. [n. p., 1876, vel subseq.]
Repr. from : Indian M. Gaz., Calcutta, 1876, xi.

———. The other side of the opium question. 95 pp. 8°. *London, J. & A. Churchill*, 1882.

Moore (William)[1]. Elements of midwifery, or the arcana of nature, in the formation and production of the human species elucidated; comprehending an anatomical description of the female organs of generation, with physiological observations on their destined offices. To which are added, instructions to the accoucheur how to proceed in every case that is possible for the fœtus to present in utero; together with a full investigation of the causes of those disorders to which women and children are liable during the first month, with the most rational method of

Moore (William)[1]—continued.
obviating them. 234 pp. 8°. *London, J. Johnson*, 1777. [P., v. 514.]

Moore (William)[2] [1754-1824]. * De bile, morbisque nonnullis qui ab ea oriuntur. 42 pp. 8°.
Edinburgi, Balfour et Smellie, 1780.
For Biography, see Med. Repository, N. Y., 1824, n. s., viii, 460-462.

Moore (William)[3] [1826–]. On infantile mortality, and the establishment of hospitals for sick children; read before the Dublin Obstetrical Society, January 8, 1859. 27 pp. 8°. *Dublin, Fannin & Co.*, 1859.

———. On some of the more prominent causes of excessive mortality in early life. 21 pp. 8°.
Dublin, Fannin & Co., 1861.

———. Some remarks on the nature and treatment of pulsating thyroid gland, with exophthalmos (Graves' disease). 12 pp. 8°. *Dublin, Fannin & Co.*, 1865.

———. A case of bronzed skin (melasma) without disease of the supra-renal capsules. 1 p. l., 7 pp. 8°. *Dublin, J. Falconer*, 1871.
Repr. from : Dublin Q. J. M. Sc., 1871, lii.

Moore (William Daniel) [1813-71]. An outline of the history of pharmacy in Ireland. 55 pp. 8°. *Dublin, Hodges & Smith*, 1848.
Repr. from : Dublin Q. J. M. Sc., 1848, xi.

———. Experiments as to the existence of sugar in the urine of the fœtus. 8 pp. 8°. [n. p., 1855, vel subseq.] [P., v. 590.]
*See, also, Dahl (Ludwig). Heller's pathological chemistry of the urine [etc.] 8°. Dublin, 1855.—Rassmussen (Vald.) On hæmoptysis [etc.] 8°. Edinburgi, 1868.— Continued observations on hæmoptysis [etc.] 8°. Edinburgi, 1869. ———. A contribution to the normal and pathological histology of the kidneys. 8°. [n. p., n. d.]— Salomon (Ernst). On the pathological elements of general paresis [etc.] 8°. London, 1862.
For Biography, see Brit. M.J., Lond., 1871, ii, 571. Also: Med. Times & Gaz., Lond., 1871, ii, 604.*

Moore (William Oliver). Diseases of the eye occurring in affections of the kidney. 16 pp. 12°. [*New York*, 1886.]
Repr. from : N. York M. J., 1886, xliii.

———. A clinical lecture on herpes zoster. 12 pp. 8°. [*New York*, 1886.]
Repr. from : Quart. Bull. Clin. Soc. N. Y. Post. Grad. M. School & Hosp., N. Y., 1886, ii.

———. The ophthalmoscope in general medicine. 13 pp. 8°. *Montpelier, Vt., Argus & Patriot Printing House*, 1887.
Repr. from : Tr. Vermont M. Soc., Montpelier, 1886.

Moore & Gardiner's imperishable raw hide artificial limbs. 19 pp. 12°. *New York, H. Croker*, 1866.

Moore Street Home for Crippled and Orphan Boys, London, W. Annual reports of the committee to the subscribers, for the years 1876–81; 1883. 16°. *London*, 1877–84.

Moorehead (Joh.) * De theoriarum physiologicarum certitudine observationes quasdam complectens. 2 p. l., 28 pp. 8°. *Edinburgi, Abernethy et Walker*, 1813.

Mooren (Albert) [1828–]. Die verminderten Gefahren einer Hornhautvereiterung bei der Staarextraction. 43 pp. 8°. *Berlin, A. Hirschwald*, 1862.

———. Ophthalmiatrische Beobachtungen. 1 p. l., 345 pp. 8°. *Berlin, A. Hirschwald*, 1867.

———. Ueber sympathische Gesichtsstörungen. 2 p. l., 169 pp. 8°. *Berlin, A. Hirschwald*, 1869.

———. Ophthalmologische Mittheilungen aus dem Jahre 1873. 122 pp. 8°. *Berlin, A. Hirschwald*, 1874.

———. Fünf Lustren ophthalmologischer Wirksamkeit. vi, 311 pp. 8°. *Wiesbaden, J. F. Bergmann*, 1882.

———. Hauteinflüsse und Gesichtsstörungen. 55 pp. 8°. *Wiesbaden, J. F. Bergmann*, 1884.

Moores (Daniel). * De febre remittente Marilandica. 1 p. l., 30 pp. 8°. *Edinburgi, Balfour et Smellie*, 1787.

Moorhead (J.)
Co-Editor of: **Western** (The) Quarterly Journal of Practical Medicine, Cincinnati, 1837.

Moorhead (Joannes N.) * De phthisi pulmonali tuberculosa. 1 p. l., 20 pp. 8°. *Edinburgi, P. Neill*, 1821. [*Also, in:* P., v. 1071.]

Moorhead (Robertus). * De pneumonia. 1 p. l., 18 pp. 8°. *Edinburgi, O. Neill*, 1821. [*Also, in:* P., v. 1071.]

Moorhouse (Henricus). * De ascite. 2 p. l., 50 pp. 8°. *Edinburgi, Balfour et Smellie*, 1785.

Moorman (John J.) Water from the White Sulphur Springs, Greenbrier County, Va. With practical remarks on its medical properties, and applicability to particular diseases. 8 pp. 8°. [*n. p.*, 1840, *rel subseq.*]

————. A brief notice of a portion of a work by Wm. Burke, entitled "The mineral springs of Western Virginia". With preliminary remarks on the relative virtues of the saline and gaseous contents of the White Sulphur water. 52 pp. 8°. *Philadelphia, Merrihew & Thompson*, 1843.

————. The Virginia springs, with their analysis; and some remarks on their character, together with a directory for the use of the White Sulphur water, and an account of the diseases to which it is applicable; to which is added, a review of a portion of Wm. Burke's book on the mineral springs of Western Virginia, etc., and an account of the different routes to the springs. xii, 219 pp., 1 l., 1 map. 12°. *Philadelphia, Lindsay & Blakiston*, 1847.

————. The Ohio White Sulphur Springs, with observations at the Ohio White Sulphur, in 1858, by W. W. Dawson. 72 pp., 1 pl., 1 map. 8°. *Cincinnati, Moore, Wilstach, Key & Co.*, 1859.

————. The mineral waters of the United States and Canada. With a map and [4] plates, and general directions for reaching mineral springs. 507 pp. 12°. *Baltimore, Kelly & Piet*, 1867.

————. Virginia White Sulphur Springs, with the analysis of its waters, the diseases to which they are applicable, etc. 27 pp., 1 map. 12°. *Baltimore, Kelly, Piet & Co.*, 1869.

————. The same. 31 pp., 1 plan. 12°. *Baltimore, The Sun Printing Office*, 1876.

————. The same. And some account of society and its amusements at the springs. 30 pp., 1 map. 12°. *Baltimore*, 1879.

————. The same. 31 pp., 1 pl. 8°. *Baltimore*, 1880.

————. Mineral springs of North America; how to reach and how to use them. 1 p. l., 294 pp., 1 l. 12°. *Philadelphia, J. B. Lippincott & Co.*, 1873.

Moormann (Alexander). * De morbo hæmorrhagico Werlhofii. 43 pp. 8°. *Berolini, typ. Brüschckianis*, [1829].
For Portrait, see **Collection**—van Kaathoven.

Moorrees (*Conrad Frans Anne*) [1835–78].
Dumontier. Necrologie. Nederl. mil. geneesk. Arch., etc., Utrecht, 1878, ii, 612–614.

van Moorsel (Amandus Hubertus). * De hepatitide. 1 p. l., 23 pp. 4°. *Lugd. Bat., P. Pont*, 1829.

van Moorsel (Franciscus). * De pleuritide vera. 23 pp. 4°. *Lugd. Bat., A. Koster*, 1772.

Moorss (Henricus). * De perfrigerio. 19 pp. 4°. *Berolini, B. Schlesinger*, [1853].

van de Moortele (Felix). * Specimen med.-phil. de natura syphilidis. 40 pp. 4°. *Leodii, typ. fratrum Jeunehomme*, [1829]. [P., v. 959.]

Moortgat (Émile).
See **Loreta** (P.) Description d'un nouvel [etc.] 8°. *Bruxelles*, 1882.

Moos (Joseph M.) Ueber das Verfahren und die ersten Hülfleistungen in der Cholera. 2 l. fol. *Freiburg, Herder*, [*n. d.*]

Moos (Salomon) [1831–]. * Ueber den Harnstoff- und Kochsalz-Gehalt des Urins in verschiedenen Krankheiten, insbesondere im Typhus und im Intestinalcatarrh. 53 pp. 8°. *Göttingen, Dieterich*, 1856.

————. Untersuchungen und Beobachtungen über den Einfluss der Pfortaderentzündung auf die Bildung der Galle und des Zuckers in der Leber. Habilitationsschrift zur Erlangung der "Venia docendi" an der Universität Heidelberg. 30 pp. 8°. *Leipzig u. Heidelberg, C. F. Winter*, 1859.

————. Klinik der Ohrenkrankheiten. ix, 348 pp. 8°. *Wien, W. Braumüller*, 1866.

————. 1. Pathologische Beobachtungen über die physiologische Bedeutung der höheren musikalischen Töne. 2. Kleinere Mittheilungen. 25 pp. 8°. *Carlsruhe*, 1872.
Repr. from: Arch. f. Augen- u. Ohrenh., Carlsruhe, 1872, ii, 2. Abth.

————. Beiträge zur normalen und pathologischen Anatomie und zur Physiologie der Eustachischen Röhre. 58 pp., 1 l., 7 pl. 8°. *Wiesbaden, C. W. Kriedel*, 1874.
Also, Co-Editor of: **Archiv** für Augen- und Ohrenheilkunde, Carlsruhe u. Wiesbaden, 1869–78.—**Archives** (The) of Ophthalmology and Otology, New York, 1869–79.—**Archives** of Otology, New York, 1879.—**Zeitschrift** für Ohrenheilkunde, Wiesbaden, 1879.
See, also, **Mittermaier** (Karl). Die Reinigung und Entwässerung der Stadt Heidelberg [etc.] 4°. *Heidelberg*, 1870.

Moosbrugger (Paul). * Ueber Aktinomykose des Menschen. 57 pp., 1 pl. 8°. *Tübingen, H. Laupp*, 1886.

Moosherr (Herrmann). * Ueber das pathologische Verhalten der kleineren Hirngefässe. 42 pp., 1 l. 8°. *Würzburg, E. Thein*, 1854.

Moosmair (Moriz). * Ueber den Abdominal-Typhus. 23 pp. 8°. *München, E. Mühlthaler*, 1874.

Mootz (Franciscus). * Diss. sistens catarrhum ventriculi et intestinorum. 28 pp. 8°. *Pragæ, typ. filiorum T. Haase*, 1846.

de Mooy (C.) *See* **De Mooy**.

Mopillier le jeune. Dissertation contre l'usage des sétons, des cautères, et des vésicatoires, et par occasion contre celui des ventouses, des scarifications, des épispastiques ou attractifs, et même des sangsues, dans le traitement des maladies internes; suivie de quelques remarques contre le choix des différentes saignées. 54 pp. 16°. *Paris, Chaubert*, 1744. [P., v. 1392.]

Mopinot (Pierre-Jules-Adolphe). * I. Du diagnostic de scrofules. II. [etc.] 36 pp. 4°. *Paris*, 1839, No. 8, v. 347.

Moquette (J. B.), jr.
See **van Wijk** (J.) Vrijmoedige gedachten. 8°. *Rotterdam & Leyden*, 1833.

Moquette (Janus Samuel Theodorus). De conio maculato. 3 p. l., 39 pp. 8°. *Lugd. Bat., A. van Benten*, 1845.

Moquin-Tandon [Chrétien-Horace-Bénédicte-Alfred] [1804–36]. Éléments de tératologie végétale, ou histoire abrégée des anomalies de l'organisation dans les végétaux. xii, 403 pp. 8°. *Paris, P.-J. Loss*, 1841.

————. Monographie de la famille des hirudinées. Nouv. éd., revue et augmentée. 2 v. 8°. *Paris*, 1846.

————. Observations sur les spermatophores des gastéropodes terrestres androgynes. 10 pp. 4°. *Paris, Mallet-Bachelier*, 1855.

————. Éléments de zoologie médicale, contenant la description détaillée des animaux utiles à la médecine et des espèces nuisibles à l'homme, particulièrement des venimeuses et des parasites, précédée de considérations générales sur l'organi-

Moquin-Tandon [C.-H.-B.-A.]—continued. sation et sur la classification des animaux et d'un résumé sur l'histoire naturelle de l'homme. xvi, 428 pp. 12°. *Paris, J.-B. Baillière & fils, 1860.*

——. The same. Elements of medical zoology. Transl. and edited by Robert T. Hulme. xiv, 423 pp. 8°. *London, H. Baillière, 1861.*

——. Éléments de botanique médicale, contenant la description des végétaux utiles à la médecine et des espèces nuisibles à l'homme, vénéneuses ou parasites, précédée de considérations sur l'organisation et la classification des végétaux. 2. éd. xx, 543 pp. 8°. *Paris, J.-B. Baillière & fils, 1866.*

——. The same. 3. éd. xx, 543 pp. 8°. *Paris, Londres, Madrid, etc., J.-B. Baillière & fils, 1875.*

For Biography, see Gaz. d. hôp., Par., 1864, xxxvii, 513–515 (H. Baillon). *Also:* Union méd., Par., 1864, 2. s., xxiv, 244; 250 (H. Baillon).

Mora (A.) *Étude clinique sur quelques complications de la pleurésie. 80 pp. 4°. *Paris, 1874, No. 290.*

Mora (Eugène). *Contribution à l'histoire des plaies des os. 32 pp. 4°. *Paris, 1870, No. 24.*

Mora (Henri-Pierre-Claude) [1854–]. *De la dyspnée et des troubles cardiaques d'origine réflexe chez les tuberculeux. 36 pp., 1 l. 4°. *Paris, 1881, No. 408.*

Mora (J.-L.) *Des localisations spinales du rhumatisme. 76 pp. 4°. *Paris, 1876, No. 141.*

Mora (Jean). *Considérations générales sur l'inflammation aiguë du foie, suivies des sentences et observations d'Hippocrate, sur la dysenterie. 26 pp. 4°. *Paris, an XIII [1805], No. 475, v. 56.*

Mora (Pietro).
See **Ratier** (M. F.) Formulario pratico degli ospedali [etc.] 16°. *Padova, 1824.*

Mora (Virgile). *Des hémorrhagies dans l'hystérie. 75 pp. 4°. *Paris, 1880, No. 200.*

de Moraaz (Samuel. Antonius). *De herniis, et præsertim de femorali incarcerata, citra kelotomiam reposita. 1 p. l., 31 pp., 2 l. 4°. *Hardervici, J. Moojen, 1770.* [P., v. 56.]

Morache (Georges-Auguste) [1837–]. *Essai sur l'anémie globulaire et ses rapports avec la dyspepsie. 63 pp. 4°. *Strasbourg, 1859, No. 479, 2. s., v. 27.*

——. Pékin et ses habitants. 164 pp. 8°. *Paris, J.-B. Baillière & fils, 1869.*

——. Des trains sanitaires. Étude sur l'emploi des chemins de fer pour l'évacuation des blessés et malades en arrière des armées. 55 pp., 1 pl. 8°. *Paris, J. Dumaine, 1872.*
Repr. from: J. d. sc. militaires.

——. Traité d'hygiène militaire. x, 1040 pp. 8°. *Paris, J.-B. Baillière & fils, 1874.*

——. The same. 2. éd. viii, 926 pp. 8°. *Paris, J.-B. Baillière & fils, 1886.*

——. La médecine légale, son exercice et son enseignement. 30 pp. 8°. *Paris, J.-B. Baillière & fils, 1880.*

Morachevski (M.) *K voprosu o vydelenii vodjanych parov i uglekisloty kojejou lichoradjashich bolnych. [On insensible exhalation of water and carbonic acid by the skin in fever.] 33 pp., 1 l. 8°. *St. Petersburg, tipog. J. Treja, 1884.*

Morachi (Marino). *Ueber die Pathologie der Dysenterie. 20 pp. 8°. *Würzburg, C. J. Becker, 1860.* C.

Morael (F.-J.) *Sur l'ascite. 21 pp. 4°. *Paris, 1816, No. 206, v. 125.*

de Moraes Sarmento (Joze-Joaquim). *De l'emploi du nitrate d'argent dans le traitement de l'amygdalite simple. 26 pp. 4°. *Paris, 1837, No. 278, v. 314.*

Moraeus (Franciscus). De maligna febre paroxisante; opus consultationes et super unam quamque medici, per totum morbi decursum operation·m, utilissimas novellas, practicas observationes continens. 7 p. l., 412 pp. 16°. *Francofurti, J. B. Zubrodt, 1670.*

Moraht (Otto). *De lingua. 2 p. l., 35 pp. 8°. *Halæ, typ. Rufit jun., 1829.*

Moral (The) Reformer and Teacher on the Human Constitution. Wm. A. Alcott, editor. [Monthly.] v. 1–2, Jan., 1835, to Dec., 1836. 8°. *Boston, Light & Horton.*
See **Library** (The) of Health, etc., for continuation.

Moral *responsibility.*
See **Responsibility.**

de Morales (Sebastian Alfredo). Anuario de la seccion de ciencias físicas y naturales del Liceo de Matanzas. Año 1, tomo 1, xxx, 274 pp., 3 tab. 8°. *Matanzas, J. Curbelo y hermano, 1866.*

Moralès Alpaca (José-A.) Note sur un nouveau portelacs et sur un forceps à trois courbures. 8 pp. 8°. *Bruxelles, H. Manceaux, 1868.*
Repr. from: Bull. Acad. roy. de méd. de Belg., Brux., 1868. 3. s., ii.

Morales Perez (Antonio). Tratado de operatoria quirúrgica. Con un prólogo por Juan Creus y Manso. 2 v. xxxii, 749, 735 pp. 8°. *Barcelona, sucesores de Ramirez y Ca., 1882.*

Moralis (Georgius). Enchiridium medicum, ethicum, et theologicum; sive magni Hippocratis Coi aphorismorum sect. vii. in quibus, facta sacrarum sententiarum ad aphorismos collatione, brevissima elicitur methodus, dignoscendarum, præsagiendarum, et curandarum animi simul, atque corporis ægritudinum. 29 p. l., 546 pp., 8 l. 12°. *Venetiis, apud Juntas, 1655.*

Morality.
See **Ethics** (*Medical*); **Medicine** *and religion.*

Morals.
See **Psychology.**

Morand.
See **Traité** de la taille au haut appareil [etc.] 16°. *Paris, 1728.*

Morand (Albert). *De la rupture centrale du périnée. 87 pp. 4°. *Paris, 1869. No. 113.*

Morand (*Anto. Joannes*).
Portrait in: **Collection**—van Kaathoven.

Morand (Auguste). *Recherches sur la cataracte congénitale. 44 pp. 4°. *Paris, 1858, No. 151, v. 621.*

Morand (J.) *Sur l'acupuncture, et ses effets thérapeutiques. 57 pp. 4°. *Paris, 1825, No. 25, v. 190.*

Morand (Jean-Sylvaire-Louis). *Note sur quelques cas de guérison de l'infection purulente. 68 pp. 4°. *Paris, 1880, No. 143.*

Morand [Joannes Franciscus Clemens] [1726–84]. Lettre traduite du latin sur feu M. [Sauveur-François] Morand, adressée aux différentes académies des pays étrangers, dont il étoit. 16 pp. 12°. *Paris, 1774.*
See, also. **Bertin** (Exupère-Joseph). *An specificum viperæ morsus antidotum alkali volatile? 4°. [*Parisiis,* 1749.]—**Bertin** (Exupère-Joseph) & **Morand** (J.-F.-C.) Thesis in hæc verba, ergo specificum, etc. 4°. *Parisiis,* 1749.—**Chomel** (Jean-Baptiste-Louis) & **Morand** (J.-F.-C.) Thesis in hæc verba, ergo tumidis hæmorrhoidibus hirudines. 4°. *Parisiis,* 1750. *In:* HALLER. Disb. ad morb. 4°. *Lausannæ,* 1758, iv, 117–124.—**Le Roy** (Paulus). *Utrum in corpore humano fluidarum duntaxat partium deperditio et reparatio? 4°. [*Parisiis,* 1751.]—**Macquart** (Ludovicus Carolus Henricus). An prægnantibus crebro periculosa catharsis, etc. 4°. [*Parisiis,* 1771.]—**Sallin** (Carolus). *An in partu difficili sola manus instrumentum? 4°. [*Parisiis,* 1762.]
For Portrait, see **Collection**—van Kaathoven.

Morand (Louis). *De l'érysipèle phlegmoneux, de sa terminaison par gangrène, et des injections

Morand (Louis)—continued.
toniques comme moyen thérapeutique propre à en arrêter les progrès. 25 pp. 4°. *Paris*, 1836, No. 50, v. 295.

——. Mémoires et observations cliniques de médecine et de chirurgie. xii, 262 pp., 1 l., 2 pl. 8°. *Tours, R. Pornin & Cie.*, 1844. [*Also, in:* P., v. 466; 1678.]

Morand (Paul). * De la septicémie gangréneuse aiguë. viii, 9–60 pp. 4°. *Montpellier*, 1877, No. 5.

Morand (Philibertus) [–1787]. * De febre multos sanante morbos. 1 p. l., 20 pp. 4°. *Traj. ad Rhenum, I. Broedelet*, 1761.

——. Verhandeling over het kolijck van Poitou, mitsgaders een naauwkenrig onderzoek van deszelvs oorzaaken, kenteekenen, toevallen, en wijze om dezelve te verhoeden; en gemakkelijk, vijlig, en spoedig door gepaste hulpmiddelen te geneezen. Beneevens verscheiden geneeskundige waarneemingen, over deeze ziekte, en inzonderheid over die lammigheid, die gemeenlijk op deeze ziekte komt te volgen alles door eigen ondervinding van een reeks van gevallen, beschreeven. 100 pp. 16°. *Amsterdam, F. Sundorff*, 1763.

Morand (S.) Memoir on acupuncturation, embracing a series of cases drawn up under the inspection of M. Julius Cloquet, Paris, 1825. Transl. from the French by Franklin Bache. 1 p. l., 87 pp. 12°. *Philadelphia, R. Desilver*, 1825.

Morand (Sauveur-François) [1697–1773]. A dissertation on the high operation for the stone. Transl. from the French by John Douglas, to which is added an appendix containing an account of 60 odd patients cut after this method by various hands; with some general inferences from the whole. As also a short syllabus of the chirurgical operations, and of the anatomia chirurgis scitu summe necessaria. 165 pp., 1 l. 8°. *London, E. Symon*, 1729.

——. Description d'un hermaphrodite, que l'on voyoit à Paris en 1749. 4 pp., 3 pl. 4°. [*Paris*, 1749, *vel subseq.*] [P., v. 630.]

——. Histoire de la maladie singulière, et de l'examen du cadavre d'une femme, devenue, en peu de tems, toute contrefaite par un ramollissement général des os. Communiquée à la Faculté de médecine de Paris, dans plusieurs assemblées du prima mensis. 112 pp., 1 pl. 12°. *Paris, Vve. Quillau*, 1752.

——. Recueil pour servir d'éclaircissement détaillé sur la maladie de la fille d'un tireur de pierres du village de S. Geomes, près Langres, laquelle depuis plusieurs années jettoit des pierres, tantôt par la voie des urines, et à qui on en a tiré de la vessie à douze reprises différentes. 150 pp., 2 l. 16°. *Paris, Delaguette*, 1754.

——. Opuscules de chirurgie. 2 pts. in 1 v. 2 p. l., 253 pp.; viii, 306 pp. 4°. *Paris, G. Desprez & P.-A. Le Prieur*, 1768–72.
See, also, **Gem** (Richard). An account of the remedy for the stone. 8°. *London*, 1741.
For Biography, see **Morand** (J.-F.-C.) Lettre traduite du latin sur feu M. [Sauveur-François] Morand, adressée aux différentes académies des pays étrangers, dont il étoit. 12°. *Paris*, 1774.
For Portrait, see **Collection**—van Kaathoven.

Morandi (Antonio). Trattato universale teorico e pratico dei parti, necessario alle mammane, ai chirurghi, ed ai medici. Nel quale si descrivono tutte le malattie che succedono dopo il concepimento, durante la gravidanza, nel parto e nel puerperio, col metodo curativo di ciascheduna. 399 pp. 8°. *Graziosi, Venezia*, 1788.

Morandi (Joannes Baptista). Historia botanica practica, seu plantarum, quæ ad usum medicinæ pertinent, nomenclatura, descriptio, et virtutes, cum ab antiquis, tum a recentibus celebrium

Morandi (Joannes Baptista)—continued.
auctorum scriptis desumptæ, ac aëneis tabulis delineata, atque ad vivum ex prototypo expressæ, nec non in classes xxxv distributæ, ut facilius cujusque simplicis genus, ac species dignoscantur. 4 p. l., 32, 164 pp., 67 pl. fol. *Mediolani, apud J. Galeatium*, 1761.

Morando (Felice). Riflessioni dirette all' anonimo, che sotto il nome di Paolo Francesco Giaccheri ha preteso difendere questo medico, accusato d' aver avvelenato Gio. Batista Bobbio. 18 pp. 4°. *Genova, G. Caffarelli*, 1788. [P., v. 901.]

Morange (André-Numa). * I. Quelle est la valeur séméiologique du carus? II. [etc.] 26 pp. 4°. *Paris*, 1840, No. 302, v. 363.

Morani (Antoine-François). * Des formes de la fièvre intermittente pernicieuse observées en Cochinchine. 73 pp., 3 l. 4°. *Montpellier, L. Cristin & Cie.*, 1868, No. 26. c.

Morano (Francesco). Contribuzione alla terapia delle vie lagrimali. 11 pp., 1 pl. 8°. *Napoli, V. Morano*, 1886.

Morano sul Po. Regolamento di pubblica igiene del comune di Morano sul Po. 12 pp. roy. 8°. *Casale, tipog. P. Bertero*, 1880.

Morant (Georg). Winke für Ehemänner. Enthüllte Geheimnisse der männlichen Geburtshilfe. 2. Aufl. 60 pp. 8°. *Berlin, T. Grieben*, 1870.
Gesundh., Wohlst. u. Glück, iii, 15. Lfg.

Morar.
See **Cholera** (*Asiatic, History, etc., of*), *by localites*).

Morasch (Joannes Adamus) [1682–1734]. Nucleus physiologicus seu institutionum medicarum liber 1. Brevi et singulari methodo juxta veterum et neotericorum mentem, ad discentium commodum expositus, chymico-mechanice decisus. Defendentibus . . . Joanne Baptista Nerf, et Georgio Henrico Freisinger. 8 p. l., 369 pp. 16°. *Eustadii, F. Strauss*, 1711.

——. Ignavum caput ferulis academicis submissum, i. e., tractatus medico-practicus de affectibus cataphoricis, seu soporosis; defendente Wolfgango Pergbaur. [1723.] 2 p. l., pp. 505–560, 2 l. sm. 4°. *Ingolstadii, T. Grass*, [*n. d.*]
Repr. [cutting] *from his:* Prælectiones acad. [etc.] 4°. *Ingolstadii*, 1725, 505–560.

——. Insanum caput Anticyris academicis submissum, i. e., tractatus medico-practicus de affectibus paraphoricis seu deliriis; defendente Joanne Georgio Vogel. [1723.] 3 p. l., pp. 361–488, 3 l. sm. 4°. *Ingolstadii, T. Grass*, [*n. d.*]
Repr. [cutting] *from his:* Prælectiones acad. [etc.] 4°. *Ingolstadii*, 1725, 361–488.

——. Prælectiones academicæ ex medicina practica de febribus et capitis morbis, habitæ in . . . Universitate Ingolstadiana, et . . . per partes publicis disputationibus subjectæ, nunc in unum digestæ volumen a . . . 3 p. l., 806 pp., 9 l.; 110 pp., 1 l. 4°. *Ingolstadii, typ. vid. Graffianæ*, 1725.

Morasch (Josephus Ignatius). Dissertatio de oleis. 16 pp. sm. 4°. *Ingolstadii, M. A. Schleigin*, [1760].

Morat (J.-P.) * Contribution à l'étude de la moelle des os. 40 pp. 4°. *Paris*, 1873, No. 370.
See, also, **Duplay** (Simon) & **Morat** (J.-P.) Recherches sur la nature et la pathogénie de l'ulcère perforant du pied [etc.] 8°. *Paris*, 1873.

Morattus (Petrus). Racconto de gli ordini e provisioni fatte ne' lazaretti in Bologna, e suo contado in tempo del contagio dell' anno 1630. 3 p. l., 124 pp. 4°. *Bologna, C. Ferroni*, 1631.

Moravia.
See, also, **Brünn**; **Cholera** (*Asiatic, History, etc., of*), *by localities*; **Datschitz**; **Koritschau**; **Luhatschowitz**; **Physician's** *aid societies, etc.*
MELION. Ueber die balneographische Literatur Mährens. 8°. [*n. p.*, 1856?]

Moravia.

SANITÄTS-BERICHT des k. k. Landes-Sanitäts-rathes für Mähren für die Jahre 1880–81. 4°. *Brünn,* 1-82-3.

Entwurf des Gesetzes betreffend die Organisation des Sanitätsdienstes in den Gemeinden giltig für die Markgrafschaft Mähren. Oesterr. ärztl. Vereinsztg., Wien, 1879, iii. 125 - 127. — **Gesetz,** giltig für die Markgrafschaft Mähren, betreffend die Organisirung des Sanitätsdienstes in den Gemeinden. Med.-chir. Centralbl., Wien. 1883, xviii, 506 - 516. — **Gesundheitsverhältnisse** Mährens im Jahre 1876. Oesterr. ärztl. Vereinsztg., Wien, 1878, ii, 175; 181; 191. — **Mährische** (Der) Landes-Sanitäts-Gesetzentwurf. *Ibid.,* 1879, iii, 127-132. — **Pluskal** (F. S.) Zur Kunde der sämmtlichen, bisher bekannt gewordenen Mineralwässer Mährens, mit Rücksicht auf ihre geognostischen Verhältnisse. Med. Jahrb. d. k. k. österr. Staates, Wien, 1847, lxi. 311: lxii, 67; 323: 1848, lxiii, 79; 198: lxiv, 59; 191; 331. — **Steiner** (J.) Ueber den Gesundheitsstand in Mähren im Jahre 1814. Eine pathographische Skizze. Beob. u. Abhandl. . . . v. österr. Aerzten, Wien, 1819, i, 88–112.

Moravitz (Ferdinandus). * Quædam ad anatomiam blattæ Germanicæ pertinentia. 54 pp., 1 pl. 8°. *Dorpati, typ. H. Laakmanni,* 1853.

Morawa (Josephus). * Nonnulla quæ in generatione notatu digna sunt. 1 p. l., 18 pp., 1 l. 4°. *Vratislaviæ, typ. Kreuzero-Scholzianis,* [1820].

Morawek (Adolphus) [1818–55]. * De anasarcæ speciebus, adnexis casibus in nosocomio generali Prægeno observatis. 63 pp. 8°. *Pragæ, typ. fil. T. Haase,* 1842.

For Biography, see Aerztl. Int.-Bl., München, 1855, ii, 609.

Morawitzky (S.) O narkoticheskich i nekotorych drugich jadovitych veshestvach, upotrebljaemych naselemiem Ferganskoi oblasti. [Narcotics and other poisons used in Ferghana.] ii, 27 pp. 8°. *Kazan, tipog. imp. Univ.,* 1886.

Repr. from: Trudi Obsh. Estestvois. pri Imp. Kazan. Univ., xv, pt. 2.

Morax (Jean). * Recherches sur la nature, le diagnostic et le traitement des affections couenneuses du larynx. 157 pp. 4°. *Paris,* 1864, No. 137.

Morbi Gallici curandi ratio exquisitissima, a variis iisdemque peritissimis medicis conscripta: nempe Petro Andrea Mattheolo Senensi. Joanne Almenar, Hispano, Nicolao Massa . . . Nicolao Poll, Veneto, Benedicto de Victoriis . . . his accessit Angeli Bolognini de ulcerum exteriorum medela opusculum perquam utile. Ejusdem de unguentis . . . ad maligna ulcera conficiendis lucubratio. 299 pp., 4 l. 4°. *Basileæ, J. Beb,* 1536.

Last leaf of index wanting.

———. The same. 279 pp., 8 l. 8°. *Lugduni, S. de Gabiano et frat.,* 1536.

Morbieu (Alfred). * Quelques considérations sur la nécrose. 51 pp. 4°. *Paris,* 1857, No. 64, v. 608.

Morbihan (Département du). Comptes rendus des épidémies, des épizooties et des travaux des conseils d'hygiène du Morbihan en 1867–74; 1876–9; 1881; 1885. Par Alfred Fouquet et Alph. Mauricet. 8° & 4°. *Vannes,* 1868–86.

1867-73 by Fouquet; 1874-9, 1881, and 1885 by Mauricet. 1878-9, 4°.

———. *See, also :*

Atgier. Étude d'ethnographie et de géographie médicale dans le département du Morbihan. Arch. de méd. et pharm. mil., Par., 1886, vii, 376-384.

Morbility.

See **Disease** (*Registration of*); **Meteorology** (*Medical*); **Statistics** (*Medical, etc.*)

Morbo (De) democratico antiquissimo insaniæ genere. Diss. inaug. medico-historica prima quam sine consensu et auctoritate [etc.] . . . ipsis calendis Græcis privatim defendet auctor. Sociis: A. Corn. Celso, M. Tull. Cicerone, T. Livio. [Friedrich Wilhelm's Univ.] 16 pp. 8°. *Gedani, typ. E. Groningii,* 1850.

Morbus anglicanus sanatus; or a remarkable cure of an inveterate scurvy, made public for the benefit of those who labour under the same troublesome disorder; in a letter from a country clergyman to his son in London. Concluding with a contrivance or two for saving the lives of those who shall happen to be in the upper rooms of a house when the lower are on fire. 31 pp. 8°. *London, J. & T. Curtis,* 1766.

Morbus *Hungaricus.*

See **Fever** (*Typhus*) *in armies, etc.*

Morbus *maculosus.*

See **Purpura.**

Morbus *niger.*

See **Melæna.**

Morbus *Scythicus.*

BOSE (E. G.) [Pr.] de Scytharum νόσῳ θηλείᾳ ad illustrandum locum Herodoti. 4°. [*Lipsiæ,* 1778.]

GRAFF (C.) * Θήλεια νοῦσος seu morbus fœmineus Scytharum. 8°. *Wirceburgi,* [*n. d.*]

NEBEL (E. L. W.) De morbis veterum obscuris. Sectio i. 12°. *Giessæ,* 1794.

STARK (C. G.) De νόσῳ θηλείᾳ apud Herodotum prolusio. 4°. *Jenæ,* 1827.

Beaugrand (E.) Maladie des Scythes, maladie féminine (θηλεία νοῦσος). Dict. encycl. d. sc. méd , Par., 1876, 2. s., iv, 283–286. — **Broca** (P.) Sur la maladie des Scythes. Bull. Soc. d'anthrop. de Par., 1877, 2. s., xii, 537–541. — **Friedreich** (J. B.) Θηλεια νοῦσος. Mag. f. d. phil., med. u. gerichtl. Seelenk., Würzb., 1829, i, 71–77. — **Hammond** (W. A.) The disease of the Scythians (morbus feminarum) and certain analogous conditions. Am. J. Neurol. & Psychiat., N. Y., 1882, i, 339–355. — **Lereboullet** (L.) Contribution à l'étude des atrophies testiculaires et des hypertrophies mammaires observées à la suite de certaines orchites (féminisme). Gaz. hebd. de méd., Par., 1877, 2. s., xiv, 533; 549. — **Liégeois** (C.) Atrophie testiculaire. féminisme. *Ibid.,* 605. — **Maladie** des Scythes. Dict. de méd. (Nysten), 12. éd., 8°. Par., 1865, 893. — **Marandon de Montyel.** De la maladie des Scythes. Ann. méd.-psych., Par., 1877, 5. s., xvii, 161–174. — **Martin** (E.) Réflexions à propos de la mutilation génitale et de ses conséquences morales. Gaz. hebd. de méd., Par., 1877, 2. s., xiv, 591. — **Rosenbaum** (J.) Νοῦσος θήλεια. *In his:* Geschichte der Lustseuche im Alterthume, 8°, Halle, 1845, 2. Aufl., 141-219. *Also:* 8°, Halle, 1888, 4. Aufl., 145-227. *Also, transl.:* Arch. de la méd. belge, Brux., 1846, xix, 376: xx, 129.— **Sprengel** (K.) Médecine des Scythes. *In his:* Histoire de la méd. Trad. de l'allemand sur la 2. éd., par A.-J.-L. Jourdan, 8°, Par., 1815, i, 206–210.

Morcillo y Olalla (Juan). Breves consideraciones acerca de la hipofagia, principalmente aplicables á las necesidades, usos y costumbres de los Españoles. 50 pp., 1 l. 8°. *Madrid, L. Maroto y Roldan,* 1877.

Morcrette (Auguste - Ernest). * Essai sur les abcès d'origine dentaire et les accidents qui les accompagnent. 43 pp. 4°. *Paris,* 1873, No. 364.

Mordagne (Henri). * Relation de deux épidémies de choléra observées en 1885 à La Cassaigne et à Courtauly (Aude). 48 pp. 4°. *Paris,* 1885, No. 20.

Mordecai (*Edward Randolph*) [1825–66].

[**Obituary** notice.] South. J. M. Sc., N. Orl., 1867, ii, 189.

Mordey (W.)

See **Haslewood** (W.) & **Mordey** (W.) History and medical treatment of cholera [etc.] 8°. *London,* 1832.

Mordhorst (Carl). * Einige Fälle von spontaner Linsenluxation. 10 pp., 1 l. 4°. *Kiel, C. F. Mohr,* 1868.

In: SCHRIFT. d. Univ. zu Kiel, xv, 1868, vii, Med. vi.

———. Ursache, Vorbeugung und Behandlung der Lungenschwindsucht. Nebst einem Anhang: "Weshalb erkranken die Bewohner des Hochlandes nie an der Lungenschwindsucht?" viii, 80 pp. 8°. *Berlin, T. C. F. Enslin,* 1874.

———. Zur Entstehung der Scrophulose und der Lungenschwindsucht.

In: SAMML. klin. Vortr., Leipz., 1879, No. 175 (Inn. Med., No. 59, 1569–1584).

Mordhorst (Carl)—continued.

——. Antwort auf Herrn Dr. Ziemssen's "Offene Erwiderung auf Herrn Dr. Mordhorst's Wiesbaden gegen chronischen Rheumatismus, Gicht, etc." 14 pp. 8°. *Wiesbaden, L. Schellenberg,* 1885.

——. Wiesbaden gegen chronischen Rheumatismus, Gicht, Ischias, etc., und als Winter-Aufenthalt. 48 pp. 8°. *Wiesbaden, J. F. Bergmann,* 1885.

——. Wiesbaden als Terrain-Curort zur Behandlung von Herz- und Lungenkrankheiten, Bleichsucht, Fettsucht, etc. Im Auftrage des Wiesbadener Curvereins veröffentlicht. 19 pp., 1 map. 8°. *Wiesbaden, H. Isselbaecher,* 1886.

Mordicus (Gulideolus).

See **Hippocrates.** De significatione mortis, etc. *In :* GANIVETUS (Joannes). Amicus medicorum. 24°. *Lugduni,* 1550, 551-585.

Mordret (A.-F.) * Sur l'extension continuelle dans les fractures compliquées et obliques de la jambe, avec la description d'un appareil pour opérer cette extension sans secousses, sans beaucoup de douleur, et à l'aide duquel on peut réduire et panser seul toutes ces fractures, et transporter sûrement les blessés. vi, 7-25 pp., 1 pl. 4°. *Paris,* 1815, No. 143, v. 112.

——. Souvenirs médico-philosophiques d'un médecin de province, suivies d'observations. x, 345 pp. 8°. *Paris, J.-B. Baillière,* 1845.

Mordret (Ambroise-Eusèbe). * Des hémorrhagies des fosses nasales. 47 pp. 4°. *Paris,* 1847, No. 161, v. 462.

——. Traité pratique des affections nerveuses et chloro-anémiques considérées dans leurs rapports qu'elles ont entre elles. viii, 488 pp. 8°. *Paris, A. Delahaye,* 1861.

——. Rapport sur le service militaire de santé dans la ville du Mans du 19 août 1870 au 20 avril 1871. Adressé à M. le ministre de la guerre le 11 juin 1871. (Guerre de 1870-71.) 51 pp. 8°. *Le Mans, E. Monnoyer,* 1871.

——. Considérations sur la sensibilité dans ses rapports généraux avec les phénomènes psychiques. (Fragment d'une étude sur la folie.) 64 pp. roy. 8°. *Paris, J.-B. Baillière & fils,* 1879. *Repr. from :* Bull. Soc. d'agric., sc. et arts de la Sarthe.

——. De la folie à double forme. Circulaire-alterne. Mémoire récompensé par l'Académie de médecine. 255 pp. 8°. *Paris, J.-B. Baillière & fils,* 1883. *Repr. from :* Bull. Soc. d'agric., sc. et arts de la Sarthe.

Mordtmann (A. D.) * Einige Beobachtungen über Morbus Brightii. 30 pp. 8°. *Würzburg, C. J. Becker,* 1861. C.

von Mordwinoff. Ein Wort über Homöopathie, nebst einem Briefe und Verzeichniss über die im Gouvernement Saratoff in Russland bei Cholerakranken mit dem glücklichsten Erfolge angewandten homöopathischen Heilmittel. Ins Deutsche übersetzt von J. Ekkenstein. 17 pp. 8°. *Dresden, Arnold,* 1832.

Moré (Otto). * De voce et lingua humana. 40 pp. 8°. *Gryphiswaldiæ, F. G. Kunike,* 1862. C.

Moré (Philippe-Eutrope). * Essai sur la topographie médicale du département de La Charente-Inférieure. 26 pp. 4°. *Paris,* 1835, No. 80, v. 284.

More extracts from the critical review, etc. *See* [Dancer (Thomas)].

More "hints", and more to the purpose, on the tendency of the projected changes in the requisite qualifications of candidates for a medical degree in the University of Edinburgh, and in the ceremony of conferring it. By a new 'un. 27 pp. 8°. *Edinburgh, A. Black,* 1824.

More Light. Devoted to the advancement of general knowledge and to useful information

More Light—continued. pertaining to health. O. P. Rice, M. D., editor. No. 1, v. 1, May, 1874. 2 l. fol. *Boston.*

More public parks! How New York compares with other cities. Lungs for the metropolis. The financial and sanitary aspects of the question. 23 pp., 5 pl. 8°. *New York,* 1882.

Morea.

GITTARD (P.-É.) * Sur la constitution physique du Péloponèse, et son influence sur le caractère et les maladies de ses habitans. 4°. *Paris,* 1834.

Morea (Vitangelo). Storia della peste di Noja. xxxii, 488 pp., 3 tab. 8°. *Napoli, A. Trani,* 1817.

Moreali (Giam-Battista). Delle febbri maligne e contagiose. Nuovo sistema teorico-pratico. Scoperta fatta nella medicina da . . . 9 p. l., 229 pp., 1 l. sm. 4°. *Modena, F. Torri,* 1739.

——. The same. In questa nuova edizione aggiuntovi una ritrattazione dell' autore, e molte altre cose. Nuova ed. 3 p. l., 360 pp. 8°. *Venezia, G. Corona,* 1746.

Moreau.

See **Villain** (L.) & **Bascou** (V.) Manuel de l'inspecteur des viandes [etc.] 8°. *Paris,* 1886.

Moreau. * Réflexions sur la législation des blessures. 28 pp. 4°. *Paris,* 1831, No. 172, v. 243.

Moreau (Alexis). * Recherches sur la fièvre puerpérale épidémique observée à la Maternité de Paris en 1843 et 1844. 46 pp. 4°. *Paris,* 1844, No. 205, v. 421.

——. * Thèse sur cette question : Jusqu'à quel point l'anatomie pathologique a-t-elle éclairé le diagnostic et le traitement des affections chirurgicales? 31 pp. 8°. *Paris, L. Martinet,* 1847. [P., v. 454.] Concours.

——. * Des grossesses extra-utérines. 142 pp. 4°. *Paris, W. Remquet & Cie.,* 1853. Concours.

——. The same. 142 pp., 1 l. 8°. *Paris, Germer-Baillière,* 1853. [*Also, in :* P., v. 1680.]

Moreau (Armand). Expériences sur l'intestin. 7 pp. 8°. [*Paris, Cusset & Cie.,* 1870.] [P., v. 802.] *Repr. from :* Gaz. méd. de Par., 1870, n. s., xxiv.

Moreau (Camille). Recherches sur la structure de la corde dorsale de l'amphioxus. 22 pp., 1 pl. 8°. *Bruxelles, F. Hayez,* 1875. *Repr. from :* Bull. Acad. roy. de méd. de Belg., Brux., 1875, xxxix. *In:* UNIVERSITÉ de Liége. Recher. lab. d'embryog. [etc.] 8°. *Bruxelles,* 1876, i.

Moreau (Edme-Charles-Léonard). * De l'entérite folliculeuse. 26 pp. 4°. *Paris,* 1836, No. 209, v. 300.

Moreau (Edmundus Thomas). Quæstio medica : An præter genitalia sexus inter se discrepent? 8 pp. 4°. *Parisiis, Quillau,* 1750.

——. * An in vulneribus sclopetorum ictu factis ad præcavendam gangrænam, incisiones et aqua maris? Præses: Antonius Pepin. 4 pp. 4°. [*Parisiis, Quillau,* 1752.] *See, also,* **Solier** (Joannes Ludovicus Maria). *An sclopetorum vulnera venenata? 4°. *Parisiis,* 1754.

Moreau (Élie-Auguste-Marie). * Des diverses modalités cliniques de la grippe. 84 pp. 4°. *Paris,* 1885, No. 21.

Moreau (Émile). * De l'albuminurie. 46 pp. 4°. *Paris,* 1850, No. 223, v. 499.

Moreau (F.) * I. Des complications de la phthisie pulmonaire tuberculeuse. II. [etc.] 87 pp. 4°. *Paris,* 1842, No. 244, v. 393.

Moreau (F.-Armand). * Propositions sur quelques formes d'affections puerpérales, et sur une éruption particulière de la période d'invasion de la variole. 34 pp. 4°. *Paris,* 1854, No. 1.

Moreau (François-Joseph) [1789–1862]. * Sur la disposition de la membrane caduque, sa formation et ses usages. 34 pp. 4°. *Paris*, 1814, No. 186, v. 107.

——. Considérations sur les perforations du périnée et sur le passage de l'enfant à travers cette partie. 19 pp. 8°. *Paris, Cosson*, [1830]. [P., v. 908.]

——. Traité pratique des accouchemens. Atlas de planches exécutées d'après nature par Émile Beau, sur les préparations anatomiques de M. Jacquemier. 30 l., 60 pl. fol. *Paris, Germer-Baillière*, 1837.

——. The same. 30 l., 60 col. pl. fol. *Paris, Germer-Baillière*, 1837.

——. The same. Icones obstetricæ; a series of 60 plates illustrative of the art and science of midwifery, in all its branches. Edited, with practical observations and tables, by J. S. Streeter. 5 pp., 30 l., 3 pp., 60 pl. fol. *London, H. Baillière*, 1842.
Title-page of this edition gives author's name as A. L. Moreau.

——. The same. Atlas de 60 planches sur l'art des accouchemens. Nouveau tirage. 30 l., 60 pl. fol. *Paris, Germer-Baillière*, 1845.

——. Traité pratique des accouchemens. 2 v. in 1. xiv, 564 pp.; 1 p. l., 500 pp. 8°. *Paris, Germer-Baillière*, 1838.
The first edition of the atlas accompanied this work.

——. The same. 2 v. xiv, 564 pp.; 1 p. l., 500 pp. 8°. *Paris, Germer-Baillière*, 1841.

——. The same. 2 v. in 1. xiv, 564 pp.; 500 pp. 8°. *Paris*, 1858.

——. The same. A practical treatise on midwifery; exhibiting the present advanced state of the science. Transl. from the French by Thos. Forrest Betton, and edited by Paul B. Goddard. 235 pp., 80 pl. 4°. *Philadelphia, Carey & Hart*, 1844.
For Biography, see Union méd., Par., 1862, 2. s., xvi, 324–332 (Gosselin).
For Portrait, see **Collection**—van Kaathoven.— **Collection** of Portr. (Libr.) — **Portraits** of Celebrated French Surg. & Phys., no. 43.

Moreau (Georges). * De la diphthérie cutanée. 37 pp., 1 l. 4°. *Paris, P. Dupont*, 1879, No. 205.

Moreau (Gustave). * De la congestion pulmonaire dans le rhumatisme articulaire sub-aigu. 1 p. l., 108 pp., 1 l. 4°. *Nancy*, 1876, 1. s., No. 34.

Moreau (Henri). * De l'hémorrhagie cérébrale. 27 pp. 4°. *Paris*, 1853, No. 162, v. 545.

Moreau (J.-F.) * Sur la péripneumonie simple. 14 pp. 4°. *Paris, an XIII* [1805], No. 466, v. 56.

Moreau (J.-I.) * Analyse physiologique et siége des phénomènes caractéristiques de l'hystérie. viii, 9–32 pp. 4°. *Paris*, 1822, No. 12, v. 170.

Moreau (Jacques-Joseph) [1804–84]. * De l'influence du physique relativement au désordre des facultés intellectuelles, et en particulier dans cette variété du délire désignée par M. Esquirol sous le nom de monomanie. 25 pp. 4°. *Paris*, 1830, No. 127, v. 232.

——. Études psychiques sur la folie. 17 pp. 8°. *Paris, Lacour et Cie.*, 1840. [P., v. 1399.]

——. Mémoire sur le traitement des hallucinations par le Datura stramonium. 43 pp. 8°. *Paris, J. Rouvier & E. Le Rouvier*, 1841.

——. Lettres médicales sur la colonie d'aliénés de Ghéel (Belgique). 39 pp. 8°. *Paris, Bourgogne & Martinet*, [1843.]
Bound with: Ann. méd.-psych., Par., 1849, xiii.

——. Du hachisch et de l'aliénation mentale. Études psychologiques. viii, 431 pp. 8°. *Paris, Fortin, Masson & Cie.*, 1845.

——. Un chapitre oublié de la pathologie mentale. 77 pp. 8°. *Paris, V. Masson*, 1850. [P., v. 37.]
Repr. from: Union méd., Par., 1850, iv.

Moreau (Jacques-Joseph)—continued.

——. Mémoire sur les causes prédisposantes héréditaires de l'idiotie et de l'imbécilité. 32 pp. 8°. *Paris, F. Malteste & Cie.*, 1853. [P., v. 1645.]
Repr. from: Union méd., Par., 1853, vii.

——. De l'étiologie de l'épilepsie et des indications que l'étude des causes peut fournir. 175 pp. 4°. *Paris, J.-B. Baillière & fils*, 1854.
Repr. from: Mém. Acad. de méd., Par., 1854, xviii.

——. De l'identité de l'état de rêve et de la folie. 48 pp. 8°. *Paris, L. Martinet*, [1855.]
Repr. from: Ann. méd.-psych., Par., 1855, 3. s., i.

——. Traité pratique de la folie névropathique (vulgo, histérique). xxiv, 206 pp., 1 l. 8°. *Paris, Germer-Baillière*, 1869.
Also, Co-Editor of: **Annales** médico-psychologiques, Paris, 1855–62.
For Biography, see Bull. et mém. Soc. méd. d. hôp. de Par., 1885, 3. s., i, 412–415 (Desnos).
See, also, **Ritti**. Éloge de J. Moreau (*de Tours*). Ann. méd.-psych., Par., 1887, 7. s., vi, 112–145.

Moreau (Jacques-Louis) [1771–1826]. Éloge de Félix Vicq-d'Azyr, suivi d'un précis des travaux anatomiques et physiologiques de ce célèbre médecin. 56 pp. 8°. *Paris, Laurens, an VI* [1798]. [*Also, in:* P., v. 1388.]

——. Esquisse d'un cours d'hygiène, ou de médecine appliquée à l'art d'user de la vie et de conserver la santé; extrait d'une partie des leçons d'hygiène faites pour la première fois au Lycée républicain, en l'an VIII. Ouvrage, ou mieux, dessein et fragments d'un ouvrage, ayant pour objet de montrer l'hygiène comme l'ensemble des données et des résultats que l'histoire naturelle de l'homme et la médecine doivent fournir pour concourir à perfectionner le physique de l'espèce humaine, et pour asseoir sur des bases communes l'art de conserver la santé, la morale et le bonheur, accompagné de notes, de deux tableaux analytiques, et d'un précis d'histoire naturelle de l'homme et de physiologie, présenté comme introduction. xxiv, 97 pp., 1 l. 8°. *Paris, Tiger* [*and others*], [1801]. [P., v. 1643.]

——. Traité historique et pratique de la vaccine, qui contient le précis et les résultats des observations et des expériences sur la vaccine, avec un examen impartial de ses avantages et des objections qui leur sont opposées, et tout ce qui concerne la pratique du nouveau mode d'inoculation. xvi, 346 pp. 8°. *Paris, Bernard, an IX* [1801].

——. The same. Tratado histórico y práctico de la vacuna. Trad. por D. F. X. De Balmis. xl, 368 pp., 1 pl., port. 8°. *Madrid, imprenta real*, 1803.

——. * Sur la gangrène humide des hôpitaux. 19 pp. 8°. *Paris, an XI* [1803], v. 26.

——. Mélanges de littérature et de philosophie médicales. 25 pp. 8°. *Paris, an XIII* [1805].

——. Rêve. 56 pp., 1 tab. 8°. [*Paris*, 1821.]
Repr. from: Dict. d. sc. méd., Par., [1821.]

——. Discours prononcé dans la séance publique annuelle de l'Académie royale de médecine. 24 pp. 12°. *Paris, Migneret*, 1826. [*Also, in:* P., v. 470.]
See **Vicq-d'Azyr** (Félix). Planches pour les œuvres de . . . [etc.] 4°. *Paris*, [1805.]

Moreau (Jean-Baptiste).
Portrait in: **Collection**—van Kaathoven.

Moreau (Jean-Chéri). * Propositions sur les hydropisies du tissu cellulaire et des membranes séreuses, considérées d'une manière générale. 8 pp. 4°. *Paris*, 1828, No. 96, v. 216.

Moreau (Jean-Philippe). * De la nature du goître exophthalmique. 40 pp. 4°. *Paris*, 1867, No. 158.

Moreau (Jean-Raphael-Jules). * Considérations générales sur les hémorrhagies spontanées. 23 pp. 4°. *Paris*, 1830, No. 16, v. 229.

Moreau (Joseph-A.-E.) * De l'ictère chez les nouveau-nés. 38 pp. 4°. *Paris*, 1858, No. 163, v. 621.

Moreau (Joseph-Frédéric). * De la température dans quelques états pathologiques de l'enfance. 46 pp. 4°. *Paris*, 1858, No. 23, v. 621.

Moreau (Jules). * Du traitement médical de la diphthérie et en particulier de son traitement par le cubèbe. 64 pp. 4°. *Paris*, 1870, No. 118.

Moreau (Jules-Albert). * Influence des diathèses (scrofule et syphilis) en chirurgie. 36 pp. 4°. *Paris*, 1872, No. 303.

Moreau (Jules - Henri). * Recherches sur la trachéotomie. 135 pp. 4°. *Paris*, 1877, No. 473.

Moreau (Jules-M.-É.-B.) * Considérations sur la nostalgie. 29 pp. 4°. *Paris*, 1848, No. 138, v. 475.

Moreau (Jules-Michel-Ferdinand). * De l'emploi topique de l'huile de croton tiglium dans l'anasarque. 41 pp. 4°. *Paris*, 1864, No. 198.

Moreau (L.) * Considérations sur l'effet et l'abus des alimens. 16 pp. 4°. *Paris*, 1807, No. 72, v. 67.

Moreau (L.-E.) Eaux thermales de Hammam-Meskhoutine, Algérie. 125 pp., 1 pl., 1 map. 8°. *Bone, Dagand*, 1858.

Moreau (Louis). * Des affections syphilitiques tertiaires des bourses séreuses. 32 pp. 4°. *Paris*, 1873, No. 360.

Moreau (Louis - Auguste). * Contribution à l'étiologie des varices. 43 pp. 4°. *Paris*, 1877, No. 368.

Moreau (Louis-Augustin). * Sur la péripneumonie compliquée d'affection bilieuse. 15 pp. 4°. *Paris*, 1823, No. 11, v. 177.

Moreau (Louis-Léo). * Nouveau procédé d'auscultation pour le diagnostic des pierres de la vessie, suivi de quelques propositions. 36 pp. 4°. *Paris*, 1837, No. 247, v. 314.

Moreau (M.-J.) * Considérations générales sur les dyspepsies, des formes flatulente et acide en particulier. 46 pp. 4°. *Paris*, 1864, No. 6.

Moreau (Marc-François). * Des maladies des femmes en couche, observées à l'Hôpital Saint-Louis pendant l'année 1820. x, 11–52 pp. 4°. *Paris*, 1821, No. 45, v. 164.

——. Réflexions et observations sur les anévrismes de l'aorte ascendante, ouverts dans le péricarde. 16 pp. 8°. [*Paris, Vve. Thuau*, 1830.]

Repr. from: J. hebd. de méd., Par., 1830, vi.

——. Mémoire sur l'épidémie miliaire (suette miliaire, suette des Picards, fièvre miliaire) qui a régné en 1821 dans la commune du Mesnil-Saint-Denis, et autres lieux du département de l'Oise. 36 pp. 8°. *Paris, J.-B. Baillière*, 1832. [P., v. 488.]

——. Histoire statistique du choléra-morbus dans le quartier du Faubourg Saint-Denis (5me arrondissement) pendant les mois d'avril, mai, juin, juillet, août et septembre [1832]. 3 p. l., 68 pp. 8°. *Paris*, 1833.

——. Histoire statistique du choléra asiatique de 1849 dans le 5e arrondissement municipal de Paris. 60 pp., 1 l. 8°. *Paris, Labé*, 1859. [*Also, in:* P., v. 461.]

Moreau (Matheus-Victor). * Quædam de læsionibus et symptomatibus affectionis typhodis. 43 pp. 4°. *Leonii, ex typ. fratrum Jeunehomme*, [1830].

Moreau (Nicolas). * De l'insolation comme cause de mort subite au Sénégal. 42 pp., 1 l. 4°. *Montpellier, Boehm & fils*, 1866, No. 91.   c.

Moreau (P.-F.) * Observations pratiques relatives à la résection des articulations affectées de carie. 87 pp., 2 pl. 4°. *Paris, Farge, an XI* [1803].

Moreau (P.-F.)—continued.
——. The same. Versuch über die Resection der Knochenextremitäten cariöser Gelenke. Aus dem Französischen übersetzt von Carl Krause. Mit einer Vorrede beg'eitet von Dr. Georg Wedemeyer. xvi, 127 pp. 8°. *Hannover, Helwing*, 1821.

See, also, **Park** (H.) & **Moreau** (P. F.) Cases of excision of carious joints, [etc.] 12°. *Glasgow*, 1866.

Moreau (P.-J.) Lettre à monsieur le ministre de l'intérieur sur l'assainissement des villes et la conservation des engrais. 21 pp. 12°. *Bruxelles, Decq*, 1848.

Moreau (Paul). * De la contagion du suicide à propos de l'épidémie actuelle. 80 pp. 4°. *Paris*, 1875, No. 129.

——. Des troubles intellectuels dus à l'intoxication lente par le gaz oxyde de carbone. 70 pp., 1 l. 8°. *Paris, P. Asselin*, 1876.

——. De la folie jalouse. 109 pp, 1 l. 8°. *Paris, P. Asselin*, 1877.

——. De la démence dans ses rapports avec l'état normal des facultés intellectuelles et affectives. 59 pp., 1 l. 8°. *Paris, Asselin*, 1878.

——. Des aberrations du sens génésique. 304 pp. 8°. *Paris, Asselin & Cie.*, 1880.

——. The same. 3. éd. 320 pp. 8°. *Paris, Asselin & Cie.*, 1883

——. De l'homicide commis par les enfants. 196 pp. 8°. *Paris, Asselin & Cie.*, 1882.

——. Fous et bouffons; étude physiologique, psychologique et historique. vii, 283 pp. 12°. *Paris, J.-B. Baillière & fils*, 1885.

Moreau (Pierre-Alphonse). * Du délire dans la pneumonie. 36 pp. 4°. *Paris*, 1864, No. 68.

Moreau (R.-M.-Charles). * Des hémorrhagies de l'utérus. 62 pp. 4°. *Paris*, 1859, No. 62, v. 634.

Moreau (Raoul). * Essai sur les fractures transversales simples de la rotule. 44 pp. 4°. *Paris*, 1874, No. 207.

Moreau (Renatus) [1587–1656]. De missione sanguinis in pleuritide, ubi demonstratur ex qua corporis parte detractus ille fuerit a duobus annorum millibus, ex omnium pene medicorum græcorum, latinorum, arabum, barbarorum exacta enumeratione, juxta temporum quibus floruere seriem instituta. Adjuncta est Pet. Brissoti . . . vita. 3 p. l., 118 pp., 3 l. 12°. *Parisiis, A. Pacard*, 1622.

Bound with: BRISSOTUS (Petrus). Apologetica discepatio [etc.] 12°. *Parisiis*, 1622.

——. The same. 3 p. l., 146 pp., 3 l. 12°. *Halæ, C. H. Hemmerde*, 1742.

Bound with: SCHULZE. Compendium historiæ, etc. 12°. *Halæ Magdeb.*, 1742.

See, also, **Brissotus** (Petrus). Apologetica disceptatio [etc.] 12°. *Parisiis*, 1622.—**Martinus** (Joannes). Prælectiones in librum Hippocratis. 8°. *Parisiis*, 1637.—**Salernum** (School of). Schola Salernitana [etc.] 8°. *Parisiis*, 1625.—**Schulze** (Jo. Henricus). Compendium historiæ medicinæ [etc.] 16°. *Halæ Magdeb.*, 1742.—**Sylvius** *Ambianus* (Jacobus). Opera medica [etc.] fol. *Genevæ*, 1635.

For Portrait, see **Collection**—van Kaathoven.

Moreau (René)[1]. * I. Faire connaître les causes et le pronostic de l'érysipèle en général; de l'emploi des topiques dans le traitement de l'érysipèle. II. [etc.] 29 pp. 4°. *Paris*, 1838, No. 200, v. 331.

Moreau (René)[2]. * Recherches cliniques et expérimentales sur l'empoisonnement aigu par le plomb et ses composés. 112 pp. 4°. *Paris*, 1875, No. 432.

——. The same. 109 pp. 8°. *Paris, Vve. A. Delahaye & Cie.*, 1876.

Moreau (Simon-René). * Sur l'hygiène des enfans dans le premier âge. vii, 7–26 pp. 4°. *Paris*, 1817, No. 194, v. 128.

Moreau (Sylvain). * Considérations sur le choix d'une nourrice. 19 pp. 4°. *Paris*, 1828, No. 171, v. 218.

Moreau (T.) *Sur un point d'hygiène militaire. 20 pp. 4°. *Paris*, 1810, No. 11, v. 78.

Moreau (Urbain). *Hydronéphrose. 52 pp. 4°. *Paris*, 1868, No. 120.

Moreau[-Boutard] (Louis-M.-A.) De deux autres modes de suture intestinale. 14 pp. 4°. *Paris*, 1837, No. 200, v. 312.

——. Précis de chirurgie élémentaire; leçons professées à l'Hôpital militaire de perfectionnement du Val-de-Grâce, en 1843 et 1844. iv, 5–184 pp. 12°. *Paris, Fortin, Masson & Cie.*, 1845.

Moreau - Christophe (Louis - Mathurin) [1799–]. De la mortalité et de la folie dans le régime pénitentiaire, et spécialement dans les pénitentiers de Philadelphie, d'Auburn, de Genève et de Lausanne. 100 pp., 1 l. 8°. *Paris, Baillière*, 1839.

——. Raison des faits communiqués par Ch. Lucas, à l'Académie des sciences morales, sur quelques détenus cellulés. 35 pp. 8°. *Paris, J.-B. Baillière*, 1839.

Moreau de Jonnès (A.-C.) Ethnogénie caucasienne. Recherches sur la formation et le lieu d'origine des peuples éthiopien, chaldéens syriens, hindous, perses, hébreux, grecs, celtes, arabes, etc. xxiii, 468 pp., 1 l., 2 maps. 8°. *Paris, J. Cherbuliez*, 1861.

Moreau de Jonnès (Alexandre) [1778–]. Monographie du trigonocéphale des Antilles, ou grande vipère fer-de-lance de la Martinique. 42 pp. 8°. [*Paris*], *Migneret*, [1816].

——. Essai sur l'hygiène militaire des Antilles; envoyé aux administrateurs et aux chefs du service de santé des colonies, des ports et des hôpitaux de terre et de mer, par ordre de LL. EEx. les ministres de la guerre et de la marine. 83 pp. 8°. *Paris, imp. Migneret*, 1817.

——. Tableau du climat des Antilles, et des phénomènes de son influence sur les plantes, les animaux et l'espèce humaine. 83 pp. 8°. *Paris, Migneret*, 1817.
Bound with preceding.

——. Monographie historique et médicale de la fièvre jaune des Antilles; et recherches physiologiques sur les lois du développement et de la propagation de cette maladie pestilentielle. 384 pp. 8°. *Paris, Migneret*, 1820.

——. Notice sur la maladie pestilentielle, importée aux îles de France et de Bourbon, et désignée sous le nom de choléra-morbus de l'Inde. Lue à l'Académie royale des sciences dans sa séance du 16 avril 1821. 20 pp. 8°. *Paris, imp. de Migneret*, 1821.

——. Rapport au Conseil supérieur de santé sur la maladie pestilentielle désignée sous le nom de choléra-morbus de l'Inde et de Syrie. 52 pp., 1 map. 4°. *Paris, imp. royale*, 1824.

——. Notice sur les enquêtes officielles constatant la contagion de la fièvre jaune et de la peste. 27 pp. 8°. *Paris, Rignoux*, [1825].

——. Rapport au Conseil supérieur de santé sur l'irruption du choléra pestilentiel en Russie, pendant l'été et l'automne de 1830. 12 pp. 12°. *Paris*, 1830. [P., v. 1410.]
Repr. from: Rev. encyclopédique (Dec., 1830).

——. Rapport au Conseil supérieur de santé sur le choléra-morbus pestilentiel, les caractères et phénomènes pathologiques de cette maladie, les moyens curatifs et hygiéniques qu'on lui oppose, sa mortalité, son mode de propagation et ses irruptions dans l'Indoustan, l'Asie orientale, l'archipel Indien, l'Arabie, la Syrie, la Perse, l'empire Russe et la Pologne. 356 pp., 1 l., 1 map. 8°. *Paris, de Cosson*, 1831. [P., v. 1042.]
Another copy bound with: DELPECH (J.) Étude du choléra-morbus. 8°. *Paris*, 1832.

——. The same. Intorno al cholera-morbus pestilenziale, ai carratteri e fenomeni patologici,

Moreau de Jonnès (Alexandre)—continued. [etc.] Trad. con note del Girolamo Novati. 3 p. l., 278 pp., 1 l., 1 map. 8°. *Milano, G. Silvestri*, 1831.

[**Moreau de Saint-Élier** (*L'abbé*).] Traité de la communication des maladies et des passions; avec un essai pour servir à l'histoire naturelle de l'homme. 1 p. l., 224 pp. 12°. *La Haye, J. van Duren*, 1738.
Bound with: KIRKPATRICK (J.) Naaukeurig verhaal van het succes.[etc.] 12°. *Amsterdam*, 1739.

Moreaud (Angel). *Considérations sur quelques cas de rhumatisme articulaire accompagnés de lésions cardiaques observés chez des vieillards. 68 pp. 4°. *Paris*, 1874, No. 65.

Moreaud (Ernest). *Contribution à l'étude des concrétions fibrineuses de l'aorte. 74 pp. 4°. *Paris*, 1864, No. 156.

Moreaud (P.) *Considérations sur la nostalgie. 24 pp. 4°. *Paris*, 1829, No. 176, v. 226.

Moreau-Lajarige (Jean-Baptiste-Adolphe). *Sur la variole. 27 pp. 4°. *Paris*, 1833, No. 245, v. 263.

Moreau-Marmont (J.) Mémoire sur la thérapeutique des anomalies de l'appareil dentaire. 30 pp., 1 l. 8°. *Paris, P. Asselin*, 1878.
Repr. from: Arch. gén. de méd., Par., 1878, 7. s., ii.

Moreau-Wolf (F.) Des rétrécissements de l'urèthre et de leur guérison radicale et instantanée par un procédé nouveau, la divulsion rétrograde. 100 pp. 8°. *Paris, A. Delahaye*, 1870.
See, also, **Chéron** (Jules) & **Moreau-Wolf.** Des services que peuvent rendre les courants continus [etc.] 8°. *Paris*, 1870.

Moreaux (Eugène) [1852–]. *Marche de la paralysie générale chez les alcooliques. 91 pp. 4°. *Paris*, 1881, No. 127.

Morehead (Charles) [1807–82]. Notes on Bright's disease of the kidney, as observed chiefly in the clinical wards of the Jamsetjee Jejeebhoy Hospital, at Bombay. 47 pp. 8°. [*Bombay*, 1850.] [P., v. 1023.]
Repr. from: Tr. M. & Phys. Soc. Bombay, 1849–50, x.

——. An introductory lecture delivered in the Grant Medical College on June 15, 1850. 36 pp. 12°. *Bombay, Y. Graham*, 1850.

——. An introductory lecture delivered in the Grant Medical College at Bombay on June 15, 1853. v, 45 pp. 8°. *Bombay, Bombay Education Society's Press*, 1853. [P., v. 923.]

——. An account of the system of clinical instruction and examination followed in the Grant Medical College at Bombay, with remarks on medical education. 34 pp., 1 pl. 8°. [*Bombay*, 1853.] [P., v. 923.]
Repr. from: Grant Med. College Reports. 7., 1852–3. 8°. *Bombay*, 1853.

——. A clinical report on the cases of pneumonia treated in the clinical ward of the Jamsetjee Jejeebhoy Hospital during the six years from 1848 to 1853. 44 pp. 8°. [*n. p.*, 1854, *vel subseq.*]
Repr. from: Tr. M. & Phys. Soc. Bombay, 1854, No. ii, n. s.

——. Clinical researches on disease in India. 2. ed. xx, 774 pp. 8°. *London, Longman* [*and others*], 1860.
For Biography, see **Memorial** of the life and work of Charles Morehead, edited by Hermann A. Haines. 12°. *London*, 1884.
See, also, Brit. M. J., Lond., 1885, i, 236. *Also:* Lancet, Lond., 1882, ii, 468. *Also:* Med.-Chir. Tr., Lond., 1883, lxvi, 3 (J. Marshall). *Also:* Med. Times & Gaz., Lond., 1882, ii, 286.

Morehead (D. C.)
See **Hawthorne** (George Stuart). Cholera; its cure and prevention. The true pathological nature of cholera, [etc.] 8°. *New York*, 1849.

Moreheid (J. N.) Lives, adventures, anecdotes, amusements, and domestic habits of the Siamese twins, one of the greatest wonders of the present time; being two perfectly formed persons,

Moreheid (J. N.)—continued.
whose bodies, by a singular caprice of nature, are united together as one. 24 pp., port. 8°. *Raleigh, N. C.*, 1850.

Morehouse (George Read) [1829–].
See **Mitchell** (S. Weir) & **Morehouse** (George R.) Researches upon the anatomy and physiology of respiration in the Chelonians. 4°. *Washington*, 1863-4. ——. —— & **Keen** (W. W.) Circular No. 6, 1864. 12°. [*Washington*, 1864.]

Moreira (Manoel Carlos Cleto). *Rachitismo. 2 p. l., 53 pp., 1 l. 4°. *Rio de Janeiro, E. et H. Laemmert*, 1875.

Moreira de Almeida (Americo Vespucio). *Tratamento da angina diphtherica. 2 p. l., 38 pp., 1 l. 4°. *Bahia, J. G. Tourinho*, 1869.

Morejon (Antonio Hernandez) [1773–1836]. Ensayo de ideológia clínica, ó de los fundamentos filosóficos para la enseñanza de la medicina y cirujía. 3 p. l., 334 pp. 18°. *Madrid, D. C. Martinez*, 1821.

——. Bellezas de medicina práctica descubiertas en el ingenioso caballero Don Quijote de la Mancha, compuesto por Miguel Cervantes Saavedra. 25 pp. 12°. *Madrid, T. Jordan*, 1836.

——. The same. Étude médico-psychologique sur l'histoire de Don Quichotte. Trad. et annotée par J. M. Guardia. 28 pp. 8°. *Paris, J.-B. Baillière & fils*, 1858.

——. Historia bibliográfica de la medicina española; opera póstuma. 7 v. 8°. *Madrid*, 1842–52.

For Biography, see Bibliot. méd.-castr. españ., Madrid, 1852, vii, 35–39 (J. J. Piernas). *Also:* Bol. de med., cirug. y farm., Madrid, 1836, iii, 333–336. *Also:* Gaz. méd., Par., 1863, 3. s., xxxiv, 479–483 (J.-M. Guardia).

Morel[1]. Mémoire et observations sur l'application du feu au traitement des maladies; guérison d'une maladie du foie opérée par le moxa; suivis de vues générales sur la médecine, et de quelques préceptes en forme d'aphorismes. xi, 13–315 pp. 8°. *Paris, Le Normant*, 1813.

Morel[2]. *Étude sur le traitement des fractures simples et compliquées du corps de l'humérus. 53 pp., 1 l. 4°. *Paris*, 1878, No. 177.

Morel (A.-Armand). *De la phthisie laryngée. 30 pp. 4°. *Paris*, 1854, No. 186, v. 563.

Morel (Antoine). *Quelques généralités sur les maladies du cœur. 32 pp. 4°. *Montpellier*, 1837, No. 134. [P., v. 1081.]

Morel (Auguste). *Considérations sur le varus, gutta-rosea (groupe des dermatoses dartreuses). 26 pp. 4°. *Paris*, 1834, No. 329, v. 279.

Morel (Bénédict-Augustin) [1809–73]. *I. Comparer les avantages et les inconvénients des tailles périnéales et hypogastriques dans les cas de grosse pierre chez l'adulte et le vieillard. II. [etc.] 34 pp. 4°. *Paris*, 1839, No. 279, v. 347.

——. Mémoire sur la manie des femmes en couches, précédé de quelques réflexions sur la direction à suivre dans l'étude des maladies mentales. 72 pp. 8°. *Paris, Cosse & Gaultier-Laguionie*, 1842. [P., v. 1399.]

——. Pathologie mentale en Belgique, en Hollande et en Allemagne. Des journaux de psychiatrie en Allemagne. 8 pp. 8°. [*Paris, Bourgogne & Martinet*, 1845.]
Repr. from: Ann. méd.-psych., Par., 1845, vi.

——. Considérations sur les causes du goître et du crétinisme endémiques à Rosières-aux-Salines (Meurthe). 32 pp., 1 pl. 8°. *Nancy, Vagner*, 1851.

——. Études cliniques. Traité théorique et pratique des maladies mentales considérées dans leur nature, leur traitement, et dans leur rapport avec la médecine légale des aliénés. 2 v. xviii, 471 pp., 1 l., 14 pl.; 600 pp., 3 tab., 10 pl. 8°. *Nancy & Paris, V. Masson*, 1853.

——. Y a-t-il plus d'aliénés aujourd'hui qu'autrefois? ou de l'influence de la civilisation sur le

Morel (Bénédict-Augustin)—continued.
développement de la folie. Discours de réception lu en séance publique de l'Académie impériale des sciences, belles-lettres et arts de Rouen, le 7 août 1857. 47 pp. 8°. *Rouen, A. Péron*, 1857.

——. Traité des dégénérescences physiques, intellectuelles et morales de l'espèce humaine, et des causes qui produisent ces variétés maladives. Accompagné d'un atlas. xix, 700 pp., 8°; atlas, 23 pp., 12 pl., fol. *Paris, J.-B. Baillière*, 1857.

——. Mélanges d'anthropologie pathologique et de médecine mentale. Swedenborg; sa vie, ses écrits, leur influence sur son siècle, ou coup d'œil sur le délire religieux. 64 pp. 8°. *Rouen, A. Péron*, 1859. [*Also, in:* P., v. 787.]
Repr. from: Précis Acad. imp. d. sc., etc., de Rouen.

——. Souvenirs scientifiques d'un voyage dans le midi de la France et dans la Savoie, en octobre 1859. 27 pp. 8°. *Rouen*, [1860].
Repr. from: Précis Acad. imp. d. sc., etc., de Rouen, 1859-60.

——. Traité des maladies mentales. xvi, 866 pp. 8°. *Paris, V. Masson*, 1860.

——. D'une forme de délire suite d'une surexcitation nerveuse se rattachant à une variété non encore décrite d'épilepsie, épilepsie larvée. 28 pp. 8°. *Paris, V. Masson & fils*, 1860.
Repr. from: Gaz. hebd. de méd., Par., 1860, vii.

——. Le non-restraint ou l'abolition des moyens coercitifs dans le traitement de la folie, suivi de considérations sur les causes de la progression dans le nombre des aliénés admis dans les asiles. 107 pp. 8°. *Paris, V. Masson & fils*, 1860.

——. De la folie héréditaire; rapport médico-légal sur un individu qui comptait des aliénés dans son ascendance paternelle et maternelle et qui a été condamné pour outrages aux mœurs; précédé de considérations sur les actes immoraux des aliénés. xi, 29 pp. 8°. *Paris, V. Masson & fils*, 1862.

——. De la formation du type dans les variétés dégénérées, ou nouveaux éléments d'anthropologie morbide, pour faire suite à la théorie des dégénérescences dans l'espèce humaine. 40 pp., 5 pl. 4°. *Paris, J.-B. Baillière & fils*, 1864.

——. Du goître et du crétinisme, étiologie, prophylaxie, traitement, programme médico-administratif, précédé d'une lettre de Mgr. Billiet, cardinal-archevêque de Chambéry. xvi, 79 pp., 2 l. 8°. *Paris, P. Asselin*, 1864.

——. Traité de la médecine légale des aliénés dans ses rapports avec la capacité civile et la responsabilité juridique des individus atteints de diverses affections aiguës ou chroniques du système nerveux, d'infirmités congénitales (surdi-mutité, cécité), d'arrêts de développement cérébral (idiotie, imbécillité), etc. 1er fascicule. Considérations préliminaires. Historique. vii, 160 pp. 8°. *Paris, V. Masson & fils*, 1866.

——. Le procès Chorinski. Étude médicolégale. 32 pp. 8°. *Rouen, C.-F. Lapierre & Cie.*, 1868.
Repr. from: Nouvelliste de Rouen, 28 juillet 1868.

——. Consultation médico-légale sur l'état mental de Jeanson, accusé d'incendie et de meurtre. Suivie du rapport présenté sur ce travail à la Société de médecine légale par le docteur J. Falret. 109 pp., 1 l. 8°. *Paris, J.-B. Baillière & fils*, 1869.
For Biography, see Ann. méd.-psych., Par., 1874, 5. s., xii, 85–108 (A. Motet). *Also,* Reprint. *Also:* Arch. gén. de méd., Par., 1873, i, 589–600 (Ch. Lasègue). *Also:* Union méd., Par., 1873, 3. s., xv, 757–761. *Also:* Union méd. de la Seine-Inf., Rouen, 1873, xii.

——. *See, also:*
Lévy (A.) Rapport sur les travaux anthropologiques de M. le Dr. Morel. *In:* Morel (B.-A.) Mélanges d'anthrop. path. 8°. *Rouen*, 1859, 21–26.

Morel (C.-L.) *Essai sur quelques-unes des hémorrhagies utérines qui ont lieu pendant la

Morel (C.-L.)—continued.
grosse, avant et après la parturition. 1 p. l., 16 pp. 4°. *Strasbourg*, 1808, v. 45.

Morel (Ch.) * Sur l'apoplexie. 22 pp. 4°. *Paris*, 1806, No. 78, v. 62.

Morel (Charles). * Recherches sur le point de départ et l'évolution de l'athérome artériel. 22 pp., 1 pl. 4°. *Paris*, 1855, No. 118, v. 578.

Morel (Charles-Basile) [1823–84]. * Développement et structure du système musculaire. 30 pp. 4°. *Paris, Lacour*, 1856.
Concours.

——. Traité élémentaire d'histologie humaine normale et pathologique, précédé d'un exposé des moyens d'observer au microscope; accompagné d'un atlas de 34 planches dessinées d'après nature par J.-A. Villemin. iv, 278 pp.; atlas, 31 pp., 34 pl. 8°. *Paris, J.-B. Baillière & fils*, 1864.

——. The same. 3. éd. viii, 418, 76 pp., 36 pl. 8°. *Paris, J.-B. Baillière & fils*, 1879.

——. The same. Compendium of human histology. Transl. and edited by W. H. Van Buren. 207 pp., 28 pl. 8°. *New York, Baillière Bros.*, 1861.

——. Le cerveau, sa topographie anatomique. v, 48 pp., xvii pl. 4°. *Paris, J.-B. Ballière & fils*, 1880.

——**& Duval** (Matthias). Manuel de l'anatomiste. (Anatomie descriptive et dissection.) xiv, 1152 pp. 8°. *Paris, Asselin & Cie.*, 1882.

Morel (Charles-Ernest). * Des affections rhumatismales. 64 pp. 4°. *Paris*, 1834, No. 271, v. 277.

Morel (Charles - Narcisse). * Réflexions sommaires sur l'inflammation. 21 pp. 4°. *Paris*, 1836, No. 204, v. 300.

Morel (Daniel) [1809–]. * De signis morborum, quæ ex faciei habitu petuntur. 44 pp., 2 l. 8°. *Berolini, typ. Nietackianis*, [1836].

Morel (E.-E.-Henri). * Quelques considérations sur les phlegmasies et les abcès du foie en Algérie. 50 pp. 4°. *Paris*, 1852, No. 257, v. 529.

Morel (Émile). * Des complications cardiaques de la blennorrhagie. 45 pp., 1 l. 4°. *Paris*, 1878, No. 269.

Morel (Eugène). * Contribution à l'étude des épithéliomas du maxillaire supérieur et en particulier de l'épithélioma térébrant. 40 pp. 4°. *Paris*, 1879, No. 334.

Morel (Florent). * Considérations sur la phthisie pulmonaire. 27 pp. 4°. *Paris*, 1821, No. 111, v. 166.

Morel (G.-C.-Louis). * Essai sur le croup. 23 pp. 4°. *Strasbourg*, 1833, v. 64.

Morel (Gustave). * De la hernie étranglée. 55 pp. 4°. *Paris*, 1859, No. 222, v. 634.

Morel (Henri). * De l'emphysème vésiculaire des poumons. 27 pp. 4°. *Paris*, 1852, No. 309, v. 529.

Morel (J.-B.) * I. Des influences qui agissent plus particulièrement sur le système circulaire, de manière à y déterminer un état pathologique. II. [etc.] 36 pp. 4°. *Paris*, 1841, No. 291, v. 378.

Morel (J.-C.-N.) * Sur la suette miliaire observée à Saint-Valery-en-Caux en 1832 et en 1833. 24 pp. 4°. *Paris*, 1834, No. 205, v. 275.

Morel (J. S.)
See **Bernard** (Claude). Lecture on the physiology of the heart [etc.] 8°. *Savannah*, 1867.

Morel (J.-T.) * Sur le melæna, ou la maladie noire. 25 pp. 4°. *Paris, an XIII* [1805], No. 456, v. 55.

Morel (Jacques). * De l'anesthésie appliquée à la lithotritie. 20 pp. 4°. *Paris*, 1853, No. 219, v. 545.

Morel (Jacques-Charles-Aimé). * Essai sur les épanchemens dans les plèvres. 1 p. l., 26 pp. 4°. *Strasbourg*, 1830, v. 61.

Morel (Jacques-Philibert). Discours anatomiques prononcés dans l'amphithéâtre de chirurgie. 4 p. l., 506 pp., 21. 18°. *Chalon-sur-Saône, J. Nanty*, 1716.

Morel (Jacques-Pierre-Louis). * Sur les causes qui contribuent le plus à rendre cachectique et rachitique la constitution d'un grand nombre d'enfans de la ville de Lille. 12 pp. 4°. *Paris*, 1812, No. 140, v. 92.

Morel (Jean-Louis). * Sur la cataracte. vi, 7–29 pp. 4°. *Paris*, 1824, No. 93, v. 185.

Morel (Joseph). * Propositions de physiologie et de pathologie. 12 pp. 4°. *Paris*, 1824, No. 47, v. 184.

Morel (Jules). * Étude sur un point de traitement des anévrysmes cirsoïdes. 48 pp. 4°. *Paris*, 1873, No. 439.

Morel (Jules-Albert). * Sur la scarlatine. 23 pp. 4°. *Paris*, 1829, No. 242, v. 228.

Morel (L.-H.-Ernest). * Diagnostic de la cataracte. 50 pp., 1 pl. 4°. *Paris*, 1862, No. 134.

Morel (Léon) [1853–]. * Essai sur la persistance du trou de Botal chez l'adulte. 58 pp., 1 l. 4°. *Paris*, 1881, No. 68.

Morel (Léon-Pierre-Hyacinthe). * De l'action dès alcalins dans le traitement des maladies. 34 pp. 4°. *Paris*, 1866, No. 70.

Morel (Louis-Anselme). * De la désarticulation tibio-tarsienne (procédé nouveau). 42 pp. 4°. *Paris*, 1847, No. 250, v. 462.

Morel (Louis-Camille). * Recherches à propos de la transfusion du sang. 27 pp. 4°. *Paris*, 1856, No. 91, v. 594.

Morel (Louis-Gabriel).
See **Richter** (August-Gottlieb). Traité des plaies de tête. 8°. *Colmar*, [n. d.].

Morel (Nestor). * Contribution à l'étude de la méningite tuberculeuse de l'adulte. Quelques observations de formes anormales. 84 pp. 4°. *Paris*, 1887, No. 239.

Morel (Pierre-François-Siméon). * Essai sur la topographie physique et médicale de la ville de Dieppe, suivi de quelques propositions sur les bains de mer, sur les conditions les plus favorables à leur emploi, et les maladies auxquelles ils ont paru le mieux convenir jusqu'à présent. vi, 7–68 pp. 4°. *Paris*, 1824, No. 34, v. 184.

Morel (V.) Nouveau traitement des affections des voies respiratoires et des intoxications du sang par les injections rectales gazeuses d'après la méthode du Dr. L. Bergeon. 45 pp., 1 l. 8°. *Paris, G. Masson*, 1885.

——. The same. New treatment of the affections of the respiratory organs and of blood poison by rectal injections of gases after the method of Dr. Bergeon. Transl. from the French by L. E. Holman. 21 pp. 8°. *Philadelphia, J. W. Queen & Co.*, [1887].

Morel (Vital-Ambroise). * Sur l'encéphalite. 15 pp. 4°. *Paris*, 1829, No. 235, v. 227.

Morel (*William Richard*).
Brief memoir on the professional character of William Richard Morel. Tr. Ass. Apoth., etc., Lond., 1823, i, 387–391.

Morel d'Arleux (Jules-Paul). * Considérations sur la résection du coude et particulièrement sur la pratique de cette résection en Angleterre. 78 pp., 1 l. 4°. *Paris*, 1874, No. 230.

Morel de Rubempré (M.-J.) Les secrets de la génération, ou l'art de procréer à volonté des filles ou des garçons, de faire des enfants d'esprit, de les orner du don de la beauté, de les avoir sains et robustes; précédé de la description des parties naturelles de l'homme et de la femme, avec l'indication de l'usage particulier de chacune d'elles; terminé par l'exposition des moyens propres à se conserver une grande puissance en amour jusqu'à l'âge le plus avancé;

Morel de Rubempré (M.-J.)—continued.
suivi de l'art d'être mère sans le concours des
hommes. 11. éd. 294 pp., 1 pl. 16°. *Bruxelles,
Hauman, Cattoir & Cie.*, 1837.

——. Codice preservativo della sifilide o malattie veneree. Preceduto dalla sposizione de'
segni esterni ed interni da' quali si conosceranno
le persone che ne sono infetti. Dal francese voltato in italiano da Giuseppe Raffaele Perrelli.
155 pp., 2 l. 8°. *Napoli, Partenope,* 1843. [P.,
v. 1112.]

Morel-Deville (Achille). * Érysipèle traumatique. 37 pp. 4°. *Paris,* 1844, No. 146, v. 421.

Morell (C. F.) Chemische Untersuchung einiger
der bekanntern und besuchtern Gesundbrunnen
und Bäder der Schweiz, insbesonders des Cantons
Bern. Nebst einer Beschreibung der neuesten
Untersuchungs-Methoden; durch eigene Erfahrungen vermehrt und bestätiget. 9 p. l., 385
pp., 1 pl. 12°. *Bern, E. Haller,* 1788.

Morell (Cornelius Gualtherus De Prill). * De
inflammatione diaphragmatis. iv, 47 pp. 8°.
Lugd. Bat., C. C. van der Hoek, 1840.

Morell (Joannes). * De regione inguinali. 20
pp. 4°. *Monachii, I. Rösl,* 1837.

Morel-Lavallée (A.) * Contribution à l'étude
de la symphyse cardiaque. 162 pp. 4°. *Paris,*
1886, No. 102.

——. The same. 162 pp. 8°. *Paris, G. Steinheil,* 1886.

Morel - Lavallée (Victor-Auguste-François)
[1811–65]. * Des luxations de la clavicule. 53
pp. 4°. *Paris,* 1842, No. 90, v. 393.

——. Essai sur les luxations de la clavicule,
présenté à l'Académie de médecine le 14 février
1843. 151 pp. 8°. *Paris, J.-B. Baillière,* 1844.

——. * Sur les rétractions accidentelles des
membres. 77 pp. 4°. *Paris, Hauguelin & Bautruche,* 1844.
Concours.

——. * Sur l'ostéite et ses suites. 54 pp. 4°.
Paris, D.-E. Bautruche, 1847.
Concours.

——. * Sur les luxations compliquées. 68 pp.
4°. *Paris, Hennuyer & Co.*, 1851.
Concours.

——. * Sur les corps étrangers articulaires. 11
pp., 4 pl. 4°. *Paris,* 1853.
Concours.
For Biography, see Mém. Soc. de chir. de Par., 1869, vii,
pp. vii–xiv (Legouest). *Also :* Rev. de lit. méd., Par., 1876,
i, 207 (D.-F.-B.).

Morelle (Émile). * I. Exposer les symptômes
et le diagnostic de la syphilide vésiculeuse. II.
[etc.] 19 pp. 4°. *Paris,* 1840, No. 85, v. 363.

Morelle (Émile-François-Joseph) [1834–].
* Recherches des leucomaïnes dans la rate. 31
pp. 4°. *Lille,* 1886, 3. s., No. 19.

——. * L'air atmosphérique. 126 pp. 8°. *Paris, A. Parent,* 1886.
Concours.

Morellet (Félix). * Le caoutchouc; origines
botaniques, procédés de récolte. 70 pp., 2 pl.
4°. *Paris, Vert aîné,* 1884.
École supérieure de pharmacie de Paris, no. 3.

Morelli (Carlo) [1816–79]. La pellagra nei
suoi rapporti medici e sociali. 279 pp. 8°.
Firenze, Murate, 1856.

——. Guida pratica e razionale alla cura dei
morbi cronici della pelle. 2 p. l., 1064, 8 pp.,
11 pl. roy. 8°. *Firenze, Murate,* 1857.

——. The same. 1064, 8 pp., 11 pl. 8°. *Firenze, G. Ferroni,* 1872.

——. Le carceri penitenziali della Toscana.
Studi igienici. 123 pp., 2 tab. 8°. *Firenze, N.
Fabbrini,* [1860]. [P., v. 1134.]

——. Il riordinamento degli studj medici e della
medicina pubblica nel regno d'Italia. 96 pp.

Morelli (Carlo)—continued.
8°. *Milano, Soc. d. Ann. univ. d. sc. e indust.*,
1862. [P., v. 1145.]
Repr. from: Ann. univ. di med., Milano, 1862, clxxix.
Also, Co-Editor of: **Tempo** (Il); giornale italiano di
medicina, [etc.], Firenze, 1858.
For Biography, see Ann. univ. di med. e chir., Milano,
1879, ccil, 525–528.

——— **& Nesti** (Leopoldo). Istoria clinica della
difterite osservata nella città di Firenze e suoi
dintorni dal 1862 al 1872. 1 p. l., 160 pp., 1 pl.,
1 l. 8°. *Firenze, typ. Cenniniana,* 1873.

Morelli (Gio. Batt.) Rendiconto clinico della
sezione chirurgica maschile diretta dal dottor
Giovanni Mori, medico-chirurgo, direttore dell'
ospedale in Brescia. 109 pp. 8°. *Brescia, F.
Apollonio,* 1884.

Morelli (Joannes Silvester). * I. De sanguinis
circuitu, etc. 19 pp. 4°. *Augustæ Taurinorum,
Bianco,* [1818]. [P., v. 944.]

Morelli (Luigi). Istruzioni al popolo sul modo
di vivere e diportarsi in caso d'invasione colerica; sperimenti e studi. 9 pp. 8°. *Caltanissetta, tipog. Giacopino,* 1884.

——. Relazione sulle proposte delle opere da
farsi, come più necessarie al miglioramento
igienico della città di Brescia. 10 pp., 1 map.
roy. 8°. [*Brescia, Apollonio,* 1886.]

Morelli (Pasquale). Studio critico sulla cura
dei tumori emorroidarii interni. 206 pp., 1 l.,
1 pl. 8°. *Napoli,* 1873.
Repr. from: Morgagni, Napoli, 1873, xv.

Morello (Franciscus). Medicinale patrocinium
in sanguinis circulationem. 72 pp. 4°. *Neapoli,
ex off. Bulifoniana,* 1678.

[**Morello** (Paolo).] Note sull' omeopatia in
occasione del colèra. 20 pp. 12°. [*Firenze,*
1854.] [P., v. 1456.]

——. Prolegomeni della storia della medicina
nelle sue attinenze colla civiltà, corso del 1861
nell' Università di Palermo. viii, 252 pp. 8°.
Palermo, B. Virzi, 1861. [P., v. 1430.]

——. Orazione inaugurale per l' apertura degli
studi nell' anno scolastico 1863, letta nell' aula
della Università di Palermo il 16 novembre 1862,
coll' intervento del commissario regio commendatore A. De Monale. 39 pp. 8°. *Palermo,
Morvillo,* 1862. [P., v. 1426.]

Morellus *Cabilonensis* (Joannes). De febre purpurata, epidemia et pestilente, quæ ab aliquot
annis in Burgundia et omnes fere Galliæ provincias misere debacchatur, medica dissertatio :
in qua de pestilentium febrium natura, causis,
signis, et curatione breviter disseritur. 5 p. l.,
132 pp. 12°. *Lugduni, J. A. Huguetan,* 1641.

Morellus (Petrus). Formulæ remediorum studio
et opera Jo. Jacob à Brunn. Cujus accedit systema materiæ medicæ. 10 p. l., 296, 187 pp.
18°. *Patavii, P. Frambott,* 1647.

——. The same. Methodus præscribendi formulas remediorum. Cum adjuncto materiæ
medicæ systemate. Aucta, variisque modis illustrata, nunc pro 2. ed. recensita a Gerardo
Blasio. 16 p. l., 578 pp., 3 l. 18°. *Amstelodami,
apud C. Commelinium,* 1665.

——. The same. Recensita, aucta, illustrata a
Gerardo Blasio. 3. ed. 8 p. l., 578 pp., 1 pl.
24°. *Amsterodami, H. et T. Boom,* 1680.
See, also, **Michaelis** (Joh) Opera medico-chirurgica
[etc.] 4°. *Norimbergæ,* 1688. ——. Opera quotquot haberi potuerunt omnia [etc.] 4°. *Norimbergæ,* 1698.

Morelot (Léon). * De la valeur pronostique des
éruptions miliaires dans le rhumatisme articulaire aigu. 52 pp. 4°. *Paris,* 1870, No. 230.

Morelot (Simon). Cours élémentaire théorique
et pratique de pharmacie-chimique, ou manuel
du pharmacien-chimiste, contenant la description de tous les médicaments usités en médecine ;
la définition des diverses opérations pharma-

Morelot (Simon)—continued.
ceuto-chimiques; l'indication de tous les procédés connus . . . l'exposition des vertus, de l'usage, et des doses des médicaments, tant magistraux qu'officinaux. 2. éd., augmentée . . . par F.-V. Mérat. 3 v. 8°. *Paris, Méquignon-Marris*, 1814.

Morély (Jacques-Henri-Julien). * Sur l'hygiène de quelques communes des arrondissemens de Tulle et de Brives, et sur quelques moyens d'y perfectionner la médecine rurale. 25 pp. 4°. *Paris*, 1834, No. 245, v. 276.

Morély (Jean-Paul). * Nouvelles considérations sur la transfusion du sang. 50 pp. 4°. *Paris*, 1864, No. 73.

Moreno (Eduardo). Algas termales. Descripcion micrográfica de algunas especies presentadas en la exposicion de minería, aguas minerales, etc. 44 pp. 8°. *Madrid, M. Minnesa*, 1883.

Moreno de la Tejera (Vicente). Campaña sanitaria en el año 1884. 86 pp. 8°. *Madrid, W. Montegrifo*, 1885.

Moreno y Fernandez (José). Del cólera, sus caracteres, orígen y desenvolvimiento, causas, naturaleza y curacion; historia de esta enfermedad durante la invasion que ha sufrido Sevilla en 1854, con algunas consideraciones generales sobre el mismo padecimiento, tomadas de su estudio en los diferentes pueblos que ha recorrido. 219 pp., 2 l. 8°. *Sevilla*, 1855.

——. El espíritu de Cláudio Bernard como fisiólogo y como médico. Leccion pronunciada el primer dia de clase en la de fisiología humana. 52 pp. 8°. *Sevilla, C. M. Santigosa*, 1880.

Moréno y Maïz (Thomas). * Recherches chimiques et physiologiques sur l'érythoxylum coca du Pérou et la cocaïne. 92 pp. 4°. *Paris*, 1868, No. 6.

——. The same. 1 p. l., 90 pp., 1 l., 1 pl. 8°. *Paris, L. Leclerc*, 1868.

de Morentin (Manuel Martinez). Tratado de la higiene, ó sea, salud y enfermedad. Con un pequeño apendice. xvi (1 l.), 454 pp. 12°. *London, Trübner & Co.*, 1864.

Morer (Eugène). * Du suicide en France; étude statistique. 39 pp. 4°. *Paris*, 1878, No. 122.

Morer (Sauveur). Du délire dans les maladies aiguës; fréquence, pathogénie et valeur pronostique de ce symptôme dans quelques maladies aiguës du poumon. 2 p. l., 56 pp. 4°. *Paris*, 1872, No. 473.

Morère (H.-A.) * Sur les fistules stercorales. 28 pp. 4°. *Paris*, 1831, No. 37, v. 238.

Moreschi. Trattamento delle fratture dell' estremità inferiore del radio. 8 pp. 8°. *Recanati, Pupilli*, 1886.

Moreschi (Alessandro). Avviso al pubblico sull' antidoto, ossia preservativo del vajuolo. viii, 70 pp. 8°. *Venezia, F. Andreola*, 1801. [*Also, in:* P., v. 1423.]

——. Del vero e primario uso della milza nell' uomo e in tutti gli animali vertebrati. xxx, 256 pp. 8°. *Milano, G. G. Destefanis*, 1803.

——. Commentarium de urethræ corporis glandisque structura, vi. idus Decembris ann. m.dccc.x. detecta ab. i. r. scientiarum, literarum artiumque instituto approbatum. Accedunt de vasorum splenicorum in animalibus constitutione, nec non de utero gravido epitomæ. xii, 59 pp., 4 pl. fol. *Mediolani, typ. J. Pirottæ*, 1817.

Morescotti (Alfonso). Compendium totius medicinæ; in quo de complexionum arcanis indiciis, morborum præcipuorum causis, prognosticis et signis, deque fabrica receptorum breviter tractatur. Additis formulis remediorum Petri Gorræi. 448 pp., 3 l. 16°. *Herbornæ, typ. C. Corvini*, 1588.

Morescotti (Alfonso)—continued.
——. The same. In utilitatem filii sui Ornedi Morescotti collectum. Additis formulis remediorum Petri Gorræi. 399 pp., 4 l. 16°. *Herbornæ Nassoriorum*, 1604.

Morescotti (Ornedi).
See **Morescotti** (Alfonso). Compendium medicinæ totius. 16°. *Herbornæ Nassoviorum*, 1604.

Morestin (Charles-Amédée). * Sur les tumeurs sanguines des os. 59 pp. 4°. *Paris*, 1862, No. 101.

Moret (A.) * De l'exhalation cutanée et de la sécrétion de la sueur, au point de vue de la pathologie et de la thérapeutique. 34 pp. 4°. *Paris*, 1856, No. 79, v. 594.

Moret (Bernard). * Sur l'érysipèle. 19 pp. 4°. *Strasbourg, F.-G. Levrault*, 1817.

Moret (Joseph-Étienne-Hippolyte). * Considérations médicales sur les frictions. 18 pp., 1 l. 4°. *Montpellier, Concourdan, an XII* [1804].

Moret (Jules). * Des manifestations syphilitiques chez la femme enceinte et les nouvelles accouchées. 104 pp. 4°. *Paris*, 1875, No. 238.

Moret (Louis). * Contribution à l'étude du traitement des fièvres intermittentes par les injections hypodermiques de sulfovinate de quinine. 38 pp., 1 l. 4°. *Montpellier*, 1876, No. 82.

Moret (Paul). * Des complications péri-utérines de la blennorrhagie. 52 pp. 4°. *Paris*, 1878, No. 305.

Moret (Richard). * Des rétrécissements organiques du canal de l'urèthre. 54 pp. 8°. *Strasbourg*, 1867, 2. s., No. 975.

Morétin (Claude-Marie-Joseph). * Dissertation sur l'abus des médicamens dans le traitement des maladies. 38 pp. 8°. *Strasbourg, P.-J. Dannbach, an VIII* [1800].

Morétin (L.-F.-C.-M.) * De l'étiologie du goître endémique, et de ses indications prophylactiques et curatives. 104 pp., 1 map. 4°. *Paris*, 1854, No. 142, v. 563.

Moreton (Corbet). *See* **Wem Union.**

Moretti (Ange-Benoît). * Sur l'hygiène de la digestion. 50 pp. 4°. *Paris*, 1851, No. 131, v. 512.

Moretti (F.) Traité pratique des écoulements des organes génitaux des femmes et des ulcérations de la matrice, suivi d'observations et d'un formulaire des médicaments les plus usités pour ces maladies, terminé par le mode d'exploration des organes et par l'indication des caustiques à employer pour la cautérisation. vii, 96 pp. 8°. *Paris, Germer-Baillière*, 1845.

Moretti (Gian Pietro). L' afta epizootica. Studiata nella sua forma clinica e nelle sue conseguenze sui bovini con figure di preparati microscopici dimostranti la probabile natura parassitaria del suo agente infettivo. 85 pp., 1 l. 12°. *Milano, fratelli Dumolard*, 1886.

Morettini (Ugolino). Il chirurgo sul campo di battaglia. Compendio di chirurgia militare. vii, 238 pp. 8°. *Todi, Z. Foglietti*, 1883.

Moreuw (Édouard). * De l'alimentation forcée des aliénés. 59 pp. 4°. *Paris*, 1880, No. 203.

Morf (Heinrich). Gratulationsschrifft der Universität Bern an die Universität Zürich zu deren fünfzigjährigen Stiftungsfeier, vom 2. und 3. August 1883. El poema de José nach der Handschrift der Madrider Nationalbibliothek. xv, 65 pp. 4°. *Leipzig, W. Drugulin*, 1883.
Arabic text.

Morgagni (Il). Opera periodica di medicina e chirurgia; diretta dal Dott. Pietro Cavallo [*et al.*]. [Monthly.] Anno 1–29, 1857–87. 8°. *Napoli.*
Current. Nothing published in 1859 or in 1861. In 1862, v. 4, Prof. Salvatore Tommasi became editor. In 1884-7, has a supplement, Bolletino delle cliniche. In 1885-7, has a 2. part, published weekly, title: **Riviste.**

Morgagni (Joannes Baptista) [1682–1771]. Adversaria anatomica prima ab eo nuper in eadem academia publice lecta, multis deinde accessionibus, novisque icouismis adaucta, et viris præstantissimis, ejusdem academiæ principi, ac sodalibus d. d. d. ·3 p. l., 48 pp., 4 pl. 4°. *Bononiæ, F. Pisarri*, 1706.

——. Nova institutionum medicarum idea. xxiii pp. 4°. *Patavii, apud J. Coronam*, 1712.
Bound with his: Adversaria anatomica omnia [etc.] 4°. *Patavii*, 1719.

——. The same. Nova institutionum medicarum idea medicum perfectissimum adumbrans. 21 pp. 4°. *Lugd. Bat., J. A. Langerak*, 1740.
Bound with his: Adversaria anatomica omnia. 4°. *Lugd. Bat.*, 1740–41.

——. Adversaria anatomica omnia [i–vi] (quorum tria posteriora nunc primum prodeunt). 4°. *Patavii, J. Cominus*, 1719.
In six parts, each with separate title-page and pagination.

——. The same. Adversaria anatomica omnia (i–vi). 4°. *Lugd. Bat., J. A. Langerak*, 1723.
——. The same. Adversaria anatomica omnia. [i–vi.] 4°. *Lugd. Bat., J. A. Langerak*, 1740–41.
——. The same. Adversaria anatomica omnia. [i–vi.] xvi, 244 pp., 11 pl., port. fol. *Venetiis, typ. Remondini*, 1762.
Paged consecutively, each part having a separate title-page.

——. In Aur. Corn. Celsum et Q. Ser. Samonicum epistolæ. In quibus de utriusque auctoris variis editionibus, libris quoque manuscriptis, et commentatoribus disseritur. 117 pp. 4°. *Hagæ-Comitum, R. Alberts*, 1724.
——. The same. 117 pp. 4°. *Lugd. Bat., J. van Kerckhem*, 1735. [P., v. 1268.]

——. Epistolæ anatomicæ duæ novas observationes et animadversiones complectentes, quibus anatome augetur, anatomicorum inventorum historia evolvitur, utraque ab erroribus vindicatur. 9 p. l., 308 pp., 1 l. 4°. *Lugd. Bat., J. a Kerkhem*, 1728.
——. The same. Epistolæ anatomicæ duæ, novas [etc.] viii, 96 pp. fol. *Venetiis, ex typog. Remondiniana*, 1762.
Another copy bound with his: Epistolæ anat. duodeviginti, etc. fol. *Patavii*, 1764. *And, also, one bound with his:* Adversaria anat. omnia. fol. *Venetiis*, 1762.

——. De sedibus et causis morborum per anatomen indagatis libri quinque. Dissectiones, et animadversiones, nunc primum editas complectuntur propemodum innumeras, medicis, chirurgis, anatomicis profuturas. 2 v. xcvi, 298 pp.; 450 pp., port. fol. *Venetiis, ex typog. Remondiniana*, 1761.
——. The same. 2. ed. 2 v. lxxxiv, 256 pp.; 388 pp., port. fol. *Patavii, sumpt. Remondini*, 1765.
——. The same. 4 v. in 2. 4°. *Lovanii, e typog. academica*, 1766–7.
——. The same. Præfatus est S. A. D. Tissot. 3 v. 4°. *Ebroduni in Helvetia*, 1779.
——. The same. 9. ed., auctoris vita et triplici rerum nominumque indice illustrata; curantibus F. Chaussier, et N. P. Adelon. 8 v. 8°. *Lutetiæ, M. C. Compère jun.*, 1820–23.
——. The same. Editionem reliquis emendatiorem et vita auctoris auctam curavit Justus Radius. 6 v. 12°. *Lipsiæ, sumpt. L. Vossii*, 1827–9.
——. The same. Recherches anatomiques sur le siége et les causes des maladies. Trad. du latin par A. Desormeaux et J.-P. Destouet. 10 v. 8°. *Paris, Caille & Ravier*, 1820–24.
Also, in: Encycl. des sc. méd., 41 v., 8°, Par., 1834–46, 7. div. [v. 5–6].
——. The same. Pathologisch-anatomische Untersuchungen über den Sitz und die Ursachen der Krankheiten. Nach der lateinischen Urschrift

Morgagni (Joannes Baptista)—continued.
bearbeitet von M. S. Krüger. 1. Lfg. 192 pp. 8°. *Berlin, W. Schüppel*, 1836.
——. The same. Delle sedi e cause delle malattie anatomicamente investigate. Libri cinque recati nella lingua italiana, con note di F. Chaussier e N. P. Adelon. 3 v. 8°. *Firenze, S. Coen*, 1839–40.
——. The same. The seats and causes of diseases investigated by anatomy. In five books, containing a great variety of dissections, with remarks. Transl. from the Latin by Benjamin Alexander. 3 v. 4°. *London, A. Millar & T. Cadell*, 1769.
——. The same. Abridged and elucidated, with copious notes, by William Cooke. 2 v. xxiv, 577 pp.; 693 pp. 8°. *London, Longman [and others]*, 1822.
——. The same. 2 v. xvii, 519 pp.; 616 pp. 8°. *Boston, Wells & Lilley; Philadelphia, H. C. Carey & I. Lea*, 1824.
——. Opera omnia. 5 v. in 2. fol. *Patavii, sumpt. J. Remondini (Venet.)*, 1762–5.
CONTENTS.
Tom. 1. Continens adversaria anatomica omnia. xxxvi, 214 pp., 10 pl., port.
Tom. 2, pars 1. ... epistolas anatomicas duas. viii, 96 pp.
Tom. 2, par. 2 et 3. ... epistolas anatomicas duodeviginti Ant. M. Valsalvæ. xii, 427 pp.
Tom. 3. ... libros priores duos de sedibus, et causis morborum per anatomen indagatis. lxxxiv, 256 pp.
Tom. 4. ... tres reliquos libros de sedibus, et causis morborum per anatomen indagatis. 388 pp.
Tom. 5. ... opuscula miscellanea tres in partes divisa. vi, 120, 75, 84 pp.
——. Opuscula miscellanea. 3 pts. vi, 120, 75, 84 pp. fol. *Venetiis, typ. Remondini*, 1763.
Bound with his: Adversaria anatomica omnia. fol. *Venetiis*, 1762.
——. Epistolæ anatomicæ duodeviginti ad scripta pertinentes celeberrimi viri Antonii Mariæ Valsalvæ. xxi, 427 pp. fol. *Pativii, sumpt. Remondinianis*, 1764.
See, also, **Celsus** (Aurelius Cornelius). De medicina libri octo [etc.] 2. ed. 8°. *Basileæ*, 1748. ——. The same. 8°. *Lipsiæ*, 1766.—**Cocchius** (Antonius Cælestinus). Epistolæ physico-medicæ. 8°. *Parisiis*, 1732.— **Valsalva** (Antonius Maria). Opera [etc.] 4°. *Venetiis*, 1740.
For Biography, see Ann. d. mal. de l'oreille, du larynx, etc., Par., 1883, ix, 149; 213 (J.-A.-A. Rattel). *Also:* Bull. d. sc. med. di Bologna, 1868, 5. s., v, 241–299: 1869, 5. s., vii, 241–276 (C. Versari). *Also:* Gaz. méd. de Par., 1875, 4. s., iv, 265; 349 (R. Lepine). *Also:* Gior. di anat. e fisiol., Pavia, 1864–5, i, 148–163.
For Portrait, see **Collection**—van Kaathoven.—**Collection** of Portr. of Phys. & Men of Sc., 125.—**Raccoglitore**, Fano, 1839, iv.

——. See, also:
Corradi (A.) Dei consulti e d' altri scritti inediti del Morgagni. R. Ist. Lomb. di sc. e lett. Rendic., Milano, 1874, 2. s., vii, 198–206. — **Desgenettes** (R.) Notice sur quelques manuscrits de Morgagni restés inédits. J. compl. du dict. d. sc. méd., Par., 1825, xxiii, 50–52.—**Robolotti** (F.) Dei manoscritti autografi e dei consulti medici e chirurgici di G. B. Morgagni. Gazz. med. ital., prov. venete, Padova, 1872, xv, 17–19.—**Versari** (C.) Quarto opuscolo intorno G. B. Morgagni e alla sua medicina. Bull. d. sc. med. di Bologna, 1870, 5. s., ix, 268–315. —— . Quinto opuscolo intorno a G. B. Morgagni. *Ibid.*, 1871, 5. s., xii, 5–39. ——. Sesto, ed ultimo opuscolo intorno a G. B. Morgagni sulle sue sentenze filosofiche, mediche, e sopra varii ammonimenti di lui. *Ibid.*, 1872, 5. s., xiii, 5–40.

Morgan (C. Lloyd). Animal biology; an elementary text-book. xxii (1 l.), 370 pp. 12°. *London, Rivingtons*, 1887.
Morgan (Carolus). *De podagra. 42 pp. 8°. *Edinburgi, R. Allan*, 1796. [*Also, in:* P., v. 4.]
Morgan (Charles E.) [1833–67]. Electro-physiology and therapeutics; being a study of the electrical and other physical phenomena of the muscular and other systems during health and disease, including the phenomena of the electrical fishes. xvi, 714 pp. 8°. *New York, W. Wood & Co.*, 1868.
For Biography, see Med. Rec., N. Y., 1867, ii, 311.

Morgan (Ethelbert Carroll). A contribution to the study of laryngeal syphilis. 17 pp. 8°. [*Richmond*, 1879.]
Repr. from: Virginia M. Month., Richmond, 1879, v.

———. Diphthonia paralytica. 6 pp. 8°. *Washington*, 1879.
Repr. from: Nat. M. Rev., Wash., 1879, i.

———. Cystic tumor of the epiglottis. 4 pp. 8°. [*New York*, 1882.]
Repr. from: Arch. Laryngol., N. Y., 1882, iii.

———. Diphthonia, or double voice. 10 pp. 8°. *New York*, 1882.
Repr. from: Arch. Laryngol., N. Y., 1882, iii.

———. Clinical lecture. [Laryngeal fibroma; relaxed pharynx.] 11 pp. 12°. [*Baltimore*, 1883.]
Repr. from: Maryland M. J., Balt., 1883–4, x.

———. Aphonia due to chronic alcoholism. Paralysis of the lateral crico-arytenoids. 8 pp. 8°. *Chicago*, 1884.
Repr. from: J. Am. M. Ass., Chicago, 1884, iii.

———. Extraction of a glosso-epiglottic myxosarcoma by means of the fingers; to which are added two cases of palato-pharyngeal tumor and a bibliography of pharyngeal growths. 15 pp. 8°. *New York, G. P. Putnam's Sons*, 1884.
Repr. from: Tr. Am. Laryngol. Ass., N. Y., 1883, iv.

———. Submucous laryngeal hemorrhage. 3 pp. 12°. *New York*, 1885.
Repr. from: Med. Rec., N. Y., 1885, xxvii.

———. The value of the snare in performing uvulotomy. 3 pp. 12°. [*Baltimore*, 1885.]
Repr. from: Maryland M. J., Balt., 1885–6, xiv.

———. The question of hæmorrhage following uvulotomy. Report of twenty-three cases of obstinate uvular hæmorrhage; description of a uvular clamp; bibliography. 27 pp. 8°. *New York, D. Appleton & Co.*, 1886.
Repr. from: N. York M. J., 1886, xliv. *Also, in:* Tr. Am. Laryngol. Ass. 1886, N. Y., 1887, viii.

———. The bursa pharyngea and its relation to naso-pharyngeal diseases. 16 pp. 12°. *Baltimore*, 1887.
Repr. from: Maryland M. J., Balt., 1887, xvi.

Morgan (Frances Elizabeth). * Ueber progressive Muskelatrophie. 2 p. l., 58 pp., 1 l. 8°. *Zürich, J. Schabelitz*, 1870.

Morgan (*Frederick*) [1791–1877].
Woodward (A.) Obituary. Proc. Connect. M. Soc., Hartford, 1878, 211–213.

Morgan (George T.) First principles of surgery, being an outline of inflammation and its effects. xiv, 210 pp. 8°. *London, S. Highley*, 1837.

———. The same. An outline of inflammation and its effects; being the first principles of surgery. viii, 134 pp. 8°. *Philadelphia, A. Waldie*, 1838. [P., v. 392.]
American Medical Library.

———. The same. viii, 134 pp. 8°. *Philadelphia, Carey & Hart*, 1841.

———. The same. First principles of surgery; being an outline of inflammation and its effects. xiv, 780 pp. 8°. *London, S. Highley*, 1840.
Same as preceding in the first seven sections, but has seven additional sections.

Morgan (Hill). * De dyspepsia. 4 p. l., 19 pp. 8°. *Edinburgi, R. Allan*, 1797.

Morgan (J.) The dangers of chloroform, and the safety and efficiency of ether as an agent in securing the avoidance of pain in surgical operations. With a description of an ether-inhaler and its mode of administration. vi, 7–45 pp. 8°. *London, Baillière, Tindall & Cox*, 1872.

Morgan (*James*) [1802–59].
Paddock (L. S.) Biographical sketch of James Morgan. Proc. Connect. M. Soc., N. Haven, 1860–63, n. s., i, 65.

Morgan (James Ethelbert) [1822–]. Introductory to the course of medical lectures, delivered in the medical department of Georgetown College, session 1856–57. 14 pp. 8°. *Washington, T. McGill*, 1857.

———. Valedictory delivered at the commencement of the medical department of Georgetown College, March 19, 1863. 11 pp. 8°. *Washington, D. C., Gibson Bros.*, 1863.
See, also, **Science** lectures for the people. 1. s. Elementary physiology. 8°. Manchester, 1871.

——— & **Cowan** (Frank). Addresses delivered at the annual commencement of the medical department of Georgetown College, March 2, 1869, with a catalogue of the faculty and students. 15 pp. 8°. *Washington*, 1869.

Morgan (Joannes). * De dysenteria. 3 p. l., 43 pp. 8°. *Edinburgi, A. Neill et socii*, 1798.

Morgan (John)[1] [1735–89]. Πύοποίησις, sive tentamen medicum de puris confectione. viii, 55 pp., 1 tab. 8°. *Edinburgi, typ. Academicis*, 1763. [P., v. 645.]

———. A discourse upon the institution of medical schools in America . . . with a preface containing, amongst other things, the author's apology for attempting to introduce the regular mode of practicing physic in Philadelphia. vii, xxvi pp., 1 l., 63 pp. 12°. *Philadelphia, W. Bradford*, 1765.

———. A recommendation of inoculation according to Baron Dimsdale's method. 18 pp. 8°. *Boston, J. Gill*, 1776.

———. A vindication of his public character in the station of director-general of the military hospitals and physician-in-chief to the American Army, anno 1776. xliii, 158 pp. 8°. *Boston, Powers & Willis*. 1777.
For Biography, see N. Am. M. & S. J., Phila., 1827, iv, 362–386. Also: Phila. J. M. & Phys. Sc., 1820, i, 439–442 (B. Rush).
For Portrait, see **Collection** of Portr. (Libr.)

Morgan (John)[2] [1797–1847]. A lecture on tetanus, delivered in Guy's Hospital. Published at request of his pupils. iv, 38 pp. 8°. *London, S. Highley*, 1833. [*Also, in:* P., v. 114.]

———. Lectures on diseases of the eye. x, 221 pp., 18 col. pl. 8°. *London, S. Highley*, 1839.
For Biography, see Lond. M. Gaz., 1847, n. s., v, 778–780. Also: Med. Times & Gaz., Lond., 1871, i, 50.

——— & **Addison** (Thomas). An essay on the operation of poisonous agents upon the living body. viii, 91 pp. 8°. *London, Longman [and others]*, 1829. [P., v. 114.]
Another copy, in which the name of Addison appears first.

Morgan (John)[3] [1829–76]. Nouveau procédé pour la conservation des viandes alimentaires, breveté s. g. d. g. Trad. de l'anglais. 32 pp. 8°. *Paris, Malé*, 1865.

———. Practical lessons in the nature and treatment of the affections produced by the contagious diseases; with an account of the primary syphilitic poison and its communicability, etc. With an appendix on the recent report of the royal commission on the contagious diseases act, and its application to the voluntary hospital system. viii, 335 pp., 3 col. pl. 8°. *Philadelphia & London, Baillière, Tindall & Cox*, 1872.
For Biography, see Med. Times & Gaz., Lond., 1876, i, 295.

Morgan (John)[4]. A warning against quackery, with a brief narrative of the sufferings of the author. 32 pp. 16°. *Boston, G. B. Rand*, 1851.

Morgan (John C.) Valedictory address delivered at the nineteenth annual commencement of the Homœopathic Medical College of Pennsylvania, March 2, 1867. With catalogue of matricu-

Morgan (John C.)—continued.

lants and graduates, session of 1866-7. 23 pp. 8°. *Philadelphia, A. J. Tafel,* [1867].

———. Introductory lecture, delivered at the Hahnemann Medical College, Philadelphia. 8°. *Wilmington, Del., H. & E. F. James,* 1867.

———. The action and classification of medicines, in connection with the anatomy of temperaments. 44 pp. 8°. *Albany, C. Van Benthuysen,* 1868.

Repr. from: Tr. Homœop. M. Soc., N. Y., 1868, vi.

———. Introductory address delivered at the opening of the course of lectures for 1870-71 at the Hahnemann Medical College, October 10, 1870. iv, 35 pp. 8°. *Philadelphia, W. P. Kildare,* 1870.

———. Diet of infants and young children. 22 pp. 8°. *Philadelphia, W. P. Kildare,* 1873.

———. The same. 2. ed. 50 pp. 24°. *Philadelphia, J. Hogan,* 1882.

———. Address delivered by the president of the Homœopathic Medical Society of Pennsylvania, at the eighteenth annual session. 13 pp. 8°. *Pittsburgh, Stevenson & Foster,* 1882.

Repr. from: Tr. Homœop. M. Soc. Penn., Altoona, 1882.

Morgan (John Edward). Manchester and Salford Sanitary Association. Reports of the health of Manchester and Salford. Compiled from the weekly returns of the Sanitary Association and presented to the committee. 3. qr. of 1863 to 4. qr. of 1866. 8°. *Manchester,* 1863-7.

Bound with: Manchester and Salford San Assoc. Rep. (1863-6), 1864-7, xi-xiv.

———. The danger of deterioration of race from the too rapid increase of great cities. [With an appendix.] 64 pp. 8°. *London, Longmans* [and others], 1866.

———. Town life among the poorest; the air they breathe and the houses they inhabit. 47 pp. 12°. *London, Longmans* [and others], 1869.

———. University oars; being a critical enquiry into the after health of the men who rowed in the Oxford and Cambridge boat race, from the year 1829 to 1869. Based on the personal experience of the rowers themselves. xvi, 397 pp. 8°. *London, Macmillan & Co.,* 1873.

———. The Victoria University; why are there no medical degrees? An address. 28 pp. 8°. *Manchester, J. E. Cornish,* 1881.

See, also, **Science** lectures for the people. 1. s. 8°. Manchester, 1871.

Morgan (Lewis Henry) [1818–]. Circular in reference to the degrees of relationship among different nations. 33 pp. 8°. [*Washington,* 1860.]

Smithson. Misc. Collect., Wash., 1860, ii.

———. Systems of consanguinity and affinity of the human family. xii, 590 pp., 14 pl. 4°. *Washington, D. C.,* 1869.

Smithson. Contrib. Knowl., Wash., 1869, xvii. For Biography, see Pop. Sc. Month., N. Y., 1880-81, xviii, 114-121, port. (J. W. Powell).

Morgan (M.) Biographical memoir of Dr. John Davis, late of Chester County, Pennsylvania. 15 pp. 8°. *Philadelphia,* 1828. [P., v. 761.]

Morgan (Samuel). The text-book for domestic practice; being plain and concise directions for the administration of homœopathic medicines in simple ailments. 191 pp. 24°. *New York,* [n. d.]

Morgan (Th. Ch.) Sketches of the philosophy of life. x (1 l.), 466 pp. 8°. *London, H. Colburn,* 1819.

———. Essai philosophique sur les phénomènes de la vie. Trad. de l'anglais, sous les yeux de l'auteur, avec des corrections et des additions. 475 pp., 1 l. 8°. *Paris, P. Dufart,* 1819.

Morgan (Thomas)[1]. Philosophical principles of medicine, in three parts. lviii, 440 pp., 1 pl. 8°. *London, J. Osborne,* 1725.

CONTENTS.

1. A demonstration of the general laws of gravity, with their effects upon animal bodys.

2. The more particular laws, which obtain in the motion and secretion of the vital fluids, applied to the principal diseases and irregularities of the animal machine.

3. The primary and chief intentions of medicine in the cure of diseases, problematically propos'd and mechanically resolv'd.

———. The same. lxxii, 440 pp., 1 pl. 8°. *London, J. Osborn & T. Longman,* 1730.

———. The mechanical practice of physick, in which the specifick method is examin'd and exploded; and the Bellinian hypothesis of animal secretion and muscular motion considered and refuted. With some occasional remarks and scholia on Dr. Lobb's treatise of the small-pox, Dr. Robinson on the animal œconomy, and Professor Boerhaave's account of the animal spirits and muscular motion. xvi, 362 pp., 3 l. 8°. *London, T. Woodward,* 1735.

Morgan (Thomas)[2]. *De dolore capitis. 1 p. l., 36 pp. 8°. *Edinburgi, Balfour, Auld et Smellie,* 1769. [*Also, in:* P., v. 652.]

Morgan (William). The homœopathic treatment of indigestion, constipation, and hæmorrhoids. Edited, with notes and annotations, by A. E. Small. 166 pp., 1 pl. 8°. *Philadelphia, Rademacher & Sheek,* 1854.

———. Tic douloureux; its causes, symptoms, and treatment. 41 pp. 8°. *London, H. Baillière,* 1856. [P., v. 1187.]

———. Diphtheria; its pathology and treatment, with cases. 31 pp. 8°. *London, H. Turner & Co.,* 1861. [P., v. 1187.]

Repr. from: Month. Homœop. Rev., Lond., 1861, v.

———. Contagious diseases, their history, anatomy, pathology, and treatment; with comments on the contagious diseases acts. xix, 194 pp. 8°. *London, Homœopathic Publishing Company,* 1877.

———. The liver and its diseases, both functional and organic; their history, anatomy, chemistry, pathology, physiology, and treatment. xx, 244 pp. 12°. *London, Homœopathic Publishing Company,* 1877.

———. The signs and concomitant derangements of pregnancy, their pathology and treatment, to which is added a chapter on delivery; the selection of a nurse; and the management of the lying-in chamber. 1. ed. xix, 136 pp. 18°. *London, Homœopathic Publishing Company,* 1877.

Morgante (Luigi). Osservazioni intorno l' articolo del poligrapho Veronese del dicembre 1831, intitolato. Pietro Maggi sulla difficoltà della diagnosi delle malattie chirurgiche. 30 pp. 8°. *Padova, tipi del Seminario,* 1832.

Morganti (Giuseppe). Sopra lo sviluppo dei ciprini dopo essere usciti dell' uovo e norme sulla fecondazione artificiale dei pesci di Mauro Rusconi; dissertazione inedita letta dall' autore nell' adunanza del giorno 14 dicembre 1843 all' I. R. Istituto lombardo-veneto di scienze, lettere ed arti. 20 pp., 7 pl. fol. *Pavia, frat. Fusi,* 1854.

Morgen (Fridericus Julius). *Observationes quædam de utriusque sexus præter sexualia differentia e physiologia et pathologia peritæ. 69 pp. 8°. *Regimonti Borussorum, C. Paschke,* [1832].

Morgen (Joh. Fridericus). *Diss. exhibens observationum anatomico-pathologicarum bigam cum epicrisi. 1 p. l., 26 pp. 4°. *Regiomonti, typ. G. L. Hartungii,* [1792].

Morgen (Julius Robertus Eduardus) [1812–]. *De noma infantum. 29 pp. 8°. *Berolini, typ. Natorffianis,* 1837.

Morgenbesser (Henricus). * De amauroseos ætiologia. 26 pp. 8°. *Halis, typ. Ploetzianis,* [1845].

Morgenbesser (Joh. Gottfried). * De fœtus non vitalis partu dirigendo. 54 pp., 1 pl. 4°. *Francof. ad Viadr., lit. J. C. Winteri,* [1767].

——. Abhandlung von der Nothwendigkeit des Zufühlens. 1. St. Nebst einer Anzeige seiner Vorlesungen. 8 pp. 4°. *Breslau, Grassi,* [1773].

——. Lehrbuch für Hebammen. xliv, 284 pp. 8°. *Breslau u. Leipzig, W. G. Korn,* 1805.

Morgenbesser (Michael). * De vomito. 3 p. l., 75 pp. 4°. *Lipsiæ, ex off. Langenhemiana,* [1738].

Also, *in :* HALLER. Disp. anat. [etc.] 4°. *Gottingæ,* 1750, i, 249–311.

For *Biography, see* **Walther** (Aug. Fred.)

Morgenroth (Theodorus). * De pneumonitide biliosa. 35 pp. 8°. *Barutha, F. C. Birner,* 1830.

Morgenstern (Emil). * Ueber das Vorkommen von Microorganismen bei Puerperalfieber. 43 pp. 8°. *Würzburg, P. Scheiner,* 1886.

Morgenstern (Fridericus Simon) [1737–82]. * De antimonii crudi usu interno. 51 pp., 1 l. sm. 4°. *Halæ, J. F. Grunert,* [1750].

See, *also,* **Tissot** (S. A. D.) Practische Vertheidigung des Einpropfens der Pocken [etc.] 8°. *Halle,* 1756.

Morgenstern (Gottlob). * Diss. proponens catarrhum suffocativum. 10 l. sm. 4°. [*Erfurt,* 1713.]

Morgenstern (Joh. Bened.) * De exanthematibus, speciatim de purpura 32 pp., 1 pl., 7 l. 4°. *Jenæ, typ. Ritterianis,* [1749].

For *Biography, see* **Kaltschmied** (Carolus Fridericus).

Morgenstern (Jul. Ott.) * De rara herniæ cruralis specie in muliere observata. 44 pp., 2 l., 1 pl. 8°. *Halis, typ. Ruffianis,* [1843].

Morgenstern (Julius) [1814–]. * De dothienenteritide. 32 pp. 8°. *Berolini, typ. Hachtmannianis,* [1839].

Morgenstern (Michael). Untersuchungen über den Ursprung der bleibenden Zähne. Ausgeführt in dem Institute der normalen Histologie zu Genf. vi (1 l.), 114 pp., 4 pl. 8°. *Leipzig, A. Felix,* 1885.

Repr. from : Deutsche Monatschr. f. Zahnh., Leipz., 1884, ii : 1885, iii.

Morgenstern (Rudolf). * Das chirurgische Nähmaterial. [Strasburg.] 46 pp. 8°. *Berlin, L. Schumacher,* 1880.

Morgon (T.-A.) * Considérations sur l'éducation physique des enfans nouveau-nés. 18 pp. 4°. *Paris,* 1828, No. 207, v. 219.

Morgue.

See **Cadaver** (*Care, etc., of*); **Death** (*Apparent*), etc.

Morgue (Claude). * De l'uréthrite, considérée à l'état aigu et à l'état chronique, et de son traitement. 1 p. l., 27 pp. 4°. *Strasbourg,* 1827, v. 56.

Morhardt (Georgius). * De hydrocephalo interno acuto. 50 pp., 1 l. 8°. *Pestini, J. T. Trattner de Petróza,* 1823. [*Also, in :* P., v. 1311.]

Morhardus (Joannes). De sede atque differentiis febrium, disputatio. 15 l. 4°. *Tubingæ, per A. Hockium,* 1585.

Morhéry. Avis aux femmes et aux médecins, suivi d'un exposé à l'Académie impériale de médecine sur l'emploi du fixateur utéro-vaginal. Nouvel appareil destiné à guérir radicalement la stérilité par déviation, les descentes et autres affections des organes génitaux de la femme. 19 pp., 1 pl. 8°. *Paris, Baillière & fils,* [1864].

Morhéry (A.-Robin). * Réflexions sur les passions et leur influence sur l'organisme. 1 p. l., 31 pp. 4°. *Strasbourg,* 1831, v. 62.

Morhofius (Danielis Georgins). Oratio de intemperantia in studiis, et eruditorum qui ex ea oriuntur morbis. 11 l. sm. 4°. *Kiloni, typ. J. Reumanni,* 1672.

——. Dissertationes academicæ et epistolicæ, quibus rariora quædam argumenta erudite tractantur, omnes in unum volumen collatæ et consensu filiorum editæ. Accessit auctoris vita, quæ tum lectiones ejus academicas, tum scripta edita et edenda, elogia item ac judicia clarorum virorum exhibet ; et præfatio Johannis Burchardi Maji, qua institutum hujus operis declaratur. 3 p. l., 143 pp., 3 l. ; 616 pp., 22 l., 1 pl. 4°. *Hamburgi, G. Liebernickel,* 1699.

Mori (Giovanni). Osservazioni anatomiche sulla patologia dell' orecchio. 107 pp., 1 l., 3 pl. 4°. *Pavia,* 1876.

See, *also,* **Morelli** (Gio. Batt.) Rendiconto clinico della sezione chirurgica maschile, etc. 8°. *Brescia,* 1884.

Mori (Robusto). Relazione sullo stato sanitario e sulla mortalità del comune di Cesena nell' anno 1879. 33 pp. 8°. *Cesena, Collini,* 1880.

——. Buffalini (Maurizio). Discorso. 208 pp., 1 l., 1 port. phot. roy. 8°. *Cesena, G. Vignuzzi,* 1883.

Morian (Richard). * Zur Casuistik der Kopfverletzungen. [Wurtzburg.] 16 pp. 8°. *Berlin, L. Schumacher,* 1883.

Moriancour (J.-G.-V.-Ernest). * De l'hémorrhagie utérine consécutive à l'accouchement. 30 pp. 4°. *Paris,* 1856, No. 173, v. 594.

Moriarty. * A description of the mercurial lepra. 64 pp. 12°. *Dublin, Gilbert & Hodges,* 1804.

Moriarty (Merion M.) * De febre continua, ut sese habuit in nosocomii regii Edinensis cubiculis clinicis æstate anni 1820, curante Jacobo Home. 2 p. l., 36 pp. 8°. *Edinburgi, Abernethy et Walker,* 1821, v. 3. [*Also, in :* P., v. 1071.]

Moriarty (Morteus) * De colica pictonum. 33 pp. 4°. *Edinburgi, R. Allan,* 1804. [P., v. 30.]

Moribana Soji. Hikachiusha Yoriaku. [On hypodermic medication.] 2 p. l., 15 ff. 8°. *Osaka,* 1873.

Japanese text.

——. Naika Zensho. [Practice of medicine.] 3 v. 8°. *Osaka,* 1877.

Japanese text.

——. Gekk(w)a Shindan Gaku. [On surgical diagnosis.] 2, 3, 413, 23, 3, 9 pp. 8°. *Osaka,* 1881.

Japanese text.

Moricand (Alexandre). * De quelques causes de l'amaurose. 43 pp. 4°. *Paris,* 1856, No. 74, v. 594.

Morice (Albert) [1848–77]. * De la dengue (fièvre éruptive des pays chauds) et de sa distribution géographique. 59 pp. 4°. *Paris,* 1875, No. 227.

For *Biography, see* Lyon méd., 1877, xxvi, 321–325 (L. Jullien).

Morice (Gaston) [1856–]. * Ce qu'il faut entendre par appareils hyponarthéciques, leur histoire, leurs avantages, leurs indications. 60 pp. 4°. *Paris,* 1880, No. 450.

Morice (J.) Mémorial de médecine dosimétrique vétérinaire, comprenant: 1° les lois fondamentales de la méthode dosimétrique; 2° ses avantages pour la médecine vétérinaire; 3° la thérapeutique des principales maladies internes de nos animaux domestiques ; 4° un aperçu sur les médicaments dosimétriques. xi, 204 pp. 12°. *Paris, C. Chanteaud & Cie.,* 1879.

Also, *Co-Editor of :* **Medical** (The) Review according to the dosimetric method of Dr. Burggraeve, New Orleans, 1882–4.

Morice (Paul). * De la fièvre intermittente simple ou bénigne. 47 pp. 4°. *Paris,* 1849, No. 4, v. 487.

Morice (René-Nicolas-Marin). * Sur l'hydro-thorax. 17 pp. 4°. *Paris*, 1813, No. 162, v. 100.

Moriceau (Charles-Gustave). * Considérations étiologiques relatives aux habitans des campagnes dans le département de la Loire-Inférieure. 33 pp. 4°. *Paris*, 1828, No. 179, v. 217.

Moriceau (P.-Louis). * De l'érythème noueux. 41 pp. 4°. *Paris*, 1861, No. 44.

Moricheau - Beauchamp (René-Pierre) [1776-1832]. De la nuit et de son influence sur les malades. Mémoire couronné par la Société de médecine de Bruxelles, dans sa séance publique du 2 vendémiaire, an 14. 1 p. l., 68 pp. 8°. *Paris, Capelle & Renaud; Poitiers, Catineau*, 1808. [*Also, in :* P., v. 1643.]

Moricheau-Beaupré. *See* **Beaupré** (Moricheau).

Morici (Giovanni Mina). Sulle febbri periodiche de' dintorni, e della città di Messina. Memoria letta nella seduta del 9 febbraro 1835 alla classe delle scienze fisiche della R. Accademia Peloritana di Messina. 2. ed. 37 pp. 8°. *Messina, G. Fiumara*, 1837. [P., v. 1130.]

Moricourt (Jules). * De la nature des affections considérées cliniquement cancéreuses. 82 pp. 4°. *Paris*, 1864, No. 44.

Moride (Édouard). * Études physiologiques de la plante, sous les rapports chimiques et physiques. 28 pp. 4°. *Paris,* [*Lacour & Maistrasse fils*], 1843. [P., v. 1698.]

Morienvalle (D.) * Contribution à l'étude de l'érysipèle du pharynx. 50 pp. 4°. *Paris, A. Parent*, 1879, No. 97.

Morier (Gabriel). * De l'uréthrite blennorrhagique. 28 pp. 4°. *Paris*, 1850, No. 49, v. 499.

Morieu (Antoine). * Dissertation contenant en abrégé un traité mécanique et raisonné sur l'art de l'accouchement. 26 pp., 2 l. 4°. *Gripswalde, A. F. Röse*, 1769.

Moriez (Robert). * La chlorose. 160 pp., 5 diag. 4°. *Paris*, 1880.
Concours.

Moriez (Robert-Joseph). * De l'impaludisme dans ses rapports avec les lésions traumatiques. xiii, 14-72 pp. 4°. *Paris*, 1876, No. 202.

Moriggia (Aliprando) [1830-   ]. La microscopia. Prolusione al corso libero d' istologia normale umana nella R. Università di Torino per l'anno accademico 1864-5. 26 pp. 8°. *Torino, R. Iona*, 1865. [P., v. 1144.]

——. Sperienze fisio-tossicologiche sulla delfina. 8 pp. 4°. [*Roma*, 1878.]
Repr. from : Atti d. r. Accad. d. Lincei. Cl. di sc. fis., matemat. e nat., Roma, 1877-8, 3. s., ii.
See, also, **Garbiglietti** (Antonio) & **Moriggia** (A.) Descrizione di celosomo dirino [etc.] 8°. *Torino*, 1870.

Morigi (*Nicola*) [1746-1836].
Speranza. Tributo alla memoria. Effem. d. sc. med., Milano, 1839, xii, 5-33.

Morillion (Hippolyte). * Sur l'hypertrophie du cœur. 35 pp. 4°. *Paris*, 1828, No. 153, v. 217.

Morillon (Auguste). * Recherches pour servir à l'histoire jusqu'ici incomplète du spina bifida. 44 pp., 2 pl. 4°. *Paris*, 1865, No. 22.

Morillon (Ernest). * Identité en général et signes professionnels en particulier. 48 pp. 4°. *Paris*, 1865, No. 28.

Morillon (Hippolyte). * Diagnostic différentiel des tumeurs du testicule. 26 pp. 4°. *Paris*, 1848, No. 95, v. 475.

Morillon (J.-C.-J.) * Sur la petite vérole. 28 pp. 8°. *Paris, an X* [1802], v. 5.

Morin (A.) Hôpital Sainte-Eugénie. Rapport de la Commission des arts insalubres, sur l'hôpital construit à Lille par M. Mourcou, architecte des hospices, année 1873. 4 pp. 4°. *Lille, Lefebvre-Ducrocq*, 1875.

Morin (A.-S.) Du magnétisme et des sciences occultes. ix, 532 pp. 8°. *Paris, Germer-Baillière*, 1860.

Morin (Alphonse). * Considérations générales sur l'emploi des médicaments à haute dose dans le traitement du rhumatisme. 1 p. l., 20 pp. 4°. *Strasbourg*, 1843, No. 121, v. 9.

Morin (Antoine). * Des perforations intestinales dans le cours de la fièvre typhoïde. 80 pp. 4°. *Paris*, 1869, No. 135.

Morin (Arsène). * Sur la péritonite, considérée dans son état aigu. 25 pp. 4°. *Paris*, 1824, No. 36, v. 184.

Morin (Arthur). Mécanique pratique. Études sur la ventilation. 2 v. iii, 610, 407 pp., 16 pl. 8°. *Paris, L. Hachette & Cie.*, 1863.

——. Manuel pratique du chauffage et de la ventilation. viii, 148 pp., 2 pl. 8°. *Paris, L. Hachette & Cie.*, 1868.
See, also, **Degen** (Ludwig). Practisches Handbuch für Einrichtungen der Ventilation und Heizung. 2. ed. 8°. *München*, 1878.

Morin (Auguste). * Sur la gale. 1 p. l., 14 pp. 4°. *Strasbourg*, 1830, v. 61.

Morin (C.)[1] * Sur la péripneumonie aiguë. vi, 7-25 pp. 4°. *Paris*, 1818, No. 86, v. 137.

Morin (C.)[2] Le camp de Châlons en 1858 au point de vue hygiénique et médical. Hygiène des camps en général. 2 l., 136 pp. 8°. *Paris, J. Masson*, 1858.

Morin (E.) Om renlighet personlig och inomhus. 51 pp. 12°. *Stockholm, U. Fredrikson*, 1885.

Morin (Edme-Auguste). * Analyse physiologique des aberrations de l'intelligence. 1 p. l., 15 pp. 4°. *Strasbourg*, 1825, v. 54.

Morin (Edmond)[1]. * De l'action du courant électrique sur les matières albuminoïdes du sang. 35 pp. 4°. *Paris*, 1861, No. 143.

Morin (Edmond)[2]. * De la glucosurie passagère dans l'anthrax. 43 pp. 4°. *Paris*, 1872, No. 157.

Morin (Eugène)[1] [1847-   ]. * Des maladies, et en particulier des affections pulmonaires, résultant de la suppression brusque des menstrues. 50 pp. 4°. *Paris*, 1878, No. 356.

Morin (Eugène)[2] [1858-   ]. * Contribution à l'étude de la tuberculose péritonéo-pleurale subaiguë. 59 pp. 4°. *Paris*, 1885, No. 173.

Morin (F.-R.) * Propositions sur les voies d'excrétion des principes qui entrent dans la composition du sang, et des substances qui sont accidentellement introduites dans ce fluide. 10 pp. 4°. *Paris*, 1824, No. 45, v. 184.

Morin (F.-Victor). * De la monomanie homicide. 31 pp. 4°. *Paris*, 1830, No. 162, v. 233.

Morin (François). * Considérations sur les fièvres paludéennes des possessions françaises de Madagascar. 42 pp., 1 l. 4°. *Montpellier, Boehm & fils*, 1866, No. 3.   c.

Morin (François-Amable-Frédéric). * À propos du traitement de la pneumonie. 71 pp., 6 tab. 4°. *Strasbourg*, 1867, 3. s., No. 57.

Morin (G.)
See **Gouguenheim** (Achille). Des névroses du larynx, etc. 8°. *Paris*, 1883.

Morin (Gabriel-Hyacinthe). * De l'hypochondrie. 32 pp. 4°. *Paris*, 1831, No. 34, v. 238.

Morin (Georges - Herbland). * D'une variété d'exanthème observée dans l'embarras gastrique aigu fébrile (fièvre gastrique, fièvre synoque). 40 pp. 4°. *Paris*, 1885, No. 90.

——. The same. 44 pp. 8°. *Paris, J. Steinheil*, 1886.

Morin (Henri). * De l'influence des privations et des excès sur la tuberculisation. 46 pp. 4°. *Paris*, 1856, No. 159, v. 594.

Morin (J.) Manuel théorique et pratique d'hygiène, ou l'art de conserver sa santé. 2. éd. 1 p. l., 372 pp. 18°. *Paris, Roret*, 1835.

Morin (J.-C.) *Sur les accidens qui suivent et reconnaissent pour cause la taille dite latéralisée. vi, 7–17 pp. 4°. *Paris*, 1813, No. 14, v. 95.

Morin (Jacques). * I. Des fièvres intermittentes larvées. II. [etc.] 29 pp. 4°. *Paris*, 1840, No. 244, v. 363.

Morin (Jean) [1858–]. *Traitement chirurgical de l'éléphantiasis du scrotum ; deux observations d'oschéotomie. 73 pp., 4 pl. 4°. *Paris*, 1885, No. 92.

Morin (*Joannes Baptista*) [1583–1656].
Portrait in: **Collection**—van Kaathoven.—**Collection** of Portr. of Phys. & Men of Sc., 47.

Morin (Joseph)[1]. * Considérations générales sur l'érosion, suivies de l'exposition chalcographique de quelques cas d'érosion de l'estomac. 20 pp., 3 pl. 4°. *Paris*, 1806, No. 108, v. 63.

Morin (Joseph)[2]. * Propositions de médecine et de chirurgie. 20 pp. 4°. *Paris*, 1833, No. 293, v. 264.

Morin (Jules). * Considérations thérapeutiques sur les ferrugineux, suivies de quelques réflexions de philosophie médicale, et d'un nouveau traitement de la blennorrhagie vénérienne. 29 pp. 4°. *Paris*, 1837, No. 414, v. 318.

Morin (Laurent-Michel). * Sur le catarrhe pulmonaire aigu. 24 pp. 4°. *Paris*, 1824, No. 223, v. 189.

Morin (Léonce). * I. Énumérer les maladies propres à l'âge adulte. Déterminer si la physiologie est assez avancée pour que l'on puisse expliquer d'une manière satisfaisante la prédominance de certains accidents morbides chez les adultes. II. [etc.] 25 pp. 4°. *Paris*, 1840, No. 354, v. 363.

Morin (Marcel). * Essai sur le traitement local de l'acné et de la couperose. 58 pp. 4°. *Paris*, 1883, No. 169.

Morin (Paul-Alexandre). * De l'éclampsie puerpérale. 1 p. l., 56 pp. 4°. *Strasbourg*, 1864, No. 803, v. 41.

Morin (Paul-Raoul). * Pensées et réflexions philosophiques sur le génie médical, suivies d'un essai sur la sensibilité. 67 pp. 4°. *Paris*, 1846, No. 82, v. 448.

Morin (Z.-Th.) * Sur l'hystérie. vi, 7–41 pp. 4°. *Paris*, 1831, No. 126, v. 241.

Morinda.
Féris (B.) Doundaké. Dict. encycl. d. sc. méd., Par., 1884, xxx, 512.

Moringa.
Holmes (E. M.) Note on Murungai or Murungah. Lancet, Lond., 1883, i, 947.

Moringlane (Joseph-Wrimouth). * Essai sur l'hépatite chronique, précédé de quelques considérations physiologiques sur le foie. 27 pp. 4°. *Paris*, 1837, No. 123, v. 309.

Morini (D.) Sopra un caso di avvelenamento acuto di fosfora. Studio clinico e anatomo-patologico. 27 pp. 8°. *Bologna, Fava & Garagnani*, 1884.

Morinière (Prudent). * Sur la péritonite des nouvelles accouchées, et son traitement par les frictions mercurielles. 23 pp. 4°. *Paris*, 1824, No. 178, v. 187.

Moris (Paul-Eugène). * Sur l'emploi thérapeutique du phosphore. 32 pp. 4°. *Paris*, 1868, No. 169.

Morisani (Ottavio) [1835–]. Manuale delle operazioni ostetriche. 2. ed., interamente rifata ed accresciuta. vi, 208 pp., 1 pl. 8°. *Napoli, libreria Detken & Rocholl*, 1878.
Title on cover gives date 1881.

——. La ostetricia in quadri sinottici da servire come guida ai pratici ed agli studenti. 3. ed. 18 ch. roy. 8°. *Napoli, G. Jovene*, 1885.

Morisani (Ottavio)—continued.
——. Manuale di ostetricia ad uso degli studenti e de' medici pratici. 2. ed., ampliata e riveduta dall' autore sulla precedente redatta per cura del Dott. Vincenzo Vivenzio. iv, 448 pp. 12°. *Napoli, G. Jovene*, 1887.
See, also, **Verrier** (Eugène). Manuale pratico di ostetricia. 2. ed. 8°. *Napoli*, 1875.

Morison (Alexander)[1] [1779–1866]. * De hydrocephalo phrenitico. 77 pp. 8°. *Edinburgi, A. Smellie*, 1799. [*Also, in :* P., v. 12.]

——. Heads of a course of lectures on mental diseases. 72 pp. 8°. *Edinburgh, P. Neill*, 1824.

——. The same. Outlines of lectures on mental diseases. 2. ed. viii, 150 pp., 13 pl. 8°. *London, Rees [and others]*, 1826.

——. The physiognomy of mental diseases. 290 pp., 106 pl. 8°. *London, G. Odell*, 1838–40.
Published in separate numbers, paged consecutively. No. 12 (pp. 155–169) missing.

——. The same. 2. ed. 2 p. l., 271 pp., 100 pl. 8°. *London, Longman & Co.*, 1843.

——. A paper, suggesting the propriety of the study of the nature, causes, and treatment of mental diseases, as forming part of the curriculum of medical education. Read before the Society for Improving the Condition of the Insane, 1st July, 1844. 8 pp. 8°. *London, G. Odell*, 1844.

——. Outlines of lectures on the nature, causes, and treatment of insanity. Edited by his son, Thomas Coutts Morison. 4. ed., much enlarged. xiv, 481 pp., 22 pl., port. 8°. *London, Longman [and others]*, 1848.

——. The same. Lectures on insanity, for the use of students. Edited by his son. 5. ed., with notes by the editor, etc. xiv, 488 pp., 25 pl. 8°. *Edinburgh, Maclachlan & Stewart*, 1856.
See, also, **Tuke** (Daniel H.) Rules and list of members, etc. 8°. *London*, 1854.
For Biography, see Lancet, Lond., 1866, i, 331.
For Portrait, see **Collection**—van Kaathoven.

Morison (Alexander)[2]. On bone absorption by means of giant cells. 7 pp. 8°. *Edinburgh, Oliver & Boyd*, [1873].
Repr. from: Edinb. M. J., 1873, xix.

Morison (Carolus). * De dysenteria. 40 pp. 8°. *Edinburgi, A. Neill et socii*, 1800. [*Also, in :* P., v. 14.]

Morison (Franciscus). * De dyspepsia. 43 pp. 8°. *Edinburgi, Balfour et Smellie*, 1787.

Morison (James)[1] [1768–1840]. Morisoniana ; or, family adviser of the British College of Health. Being a collection of the works of . . . comprising : Origin of life, and true cause of diseases explained. Important advice to the world. Letter on cholera morbus of India. Anti-Lancet, in six numbers. More new truths. Forming a complete manual for individuals and families . . . With an appendix containing a short treatise on the origin and eradicability of the small-pox [by T. Moat], numerous well-authenticated cures, and other interesting matter. 3. ed. xvi (4 l.), 604 pp., 34 l., 3 pl., port. 8°. *London, College of Health*, 1831.

——. The same. 4. ed., with additional articles. 2 v. xxi (6 l.), 629, lxvii pp., 3 pl., port. ; xvi, 793, lx pp., port. 8°. *London*, 1833–4.
v. 1 same as 3. ed. v. 2 comprises : Valuable extracts from the first six monthly numbers of the Hygeian Journal ; also, extracts from other London periodicals, etc. Also : Rational arguments on the nature of true pathology, etc., by C. W. Moat and J. Greer.

——. The same. La causa verdadera de las enfermedades y modo de curarlas, [etc.] [Trad. del ingles por A. Eusberg.] 198 pp. 12°. *Barcelona, D. J. Oliveres*, 1844.

——. Practical proofs of the soundness of the hygeian system of physiology, giving incontrovertible testimony to the afflicted of the inestimable value of . . . vegetable universal medicines ;

Morison (James)[1]—continued.
including, with other matter, "The origin of life,
and cause of all disease explained"; an entirely
new view of the origin of the small-pox virus,
and of its being most certainly eradicable, or rendered harmless, and sundry cases of cure; with
most important information connected with the
successful promulgation of the hygeian system
in the United States of America. xi, 202 pp., 2
pl. 3. ed. 12°. *New York, H. S. Moat,* 1832.
———. An essay, or tract, on the vitality of the
warm blood and air. Am. ed., by Elisha North.
29 pp. 8°. *New York, the author,* 1835.
For Biography, see **Biographical** (A) sketch of James
Morison, the hygeist. 12°. *London,* 1873.
For Portrait, see **Collection**—van Kaathoven.

Morison (*James*)[2] [1818–82].
Obituary. Boston M. & S. J., 1882, cvi, 621.

Morison (Joannes). *De mania. 24 pp. 8°.
Edinburgi, Abernethy et Walker, 1808.

Morison (John)[1].
See **Complete** (A) report of the trial of Miss Madeline
Smith, [etc.] 2. ed. 8°. *Edinburgh,* 1857.

Morison (John)[2]. The anti-vaccination or conscience play. 16 pp. 12°. *London,* 1873.

Morison (*Robert*) [1620–83].
[**Biography.**] *In:* BAYLE (P.) Hist. & Crit. Dict.
(transl. Des Maizeaux). 2. ed. fol. *London,* 1737, iv, 270.
Portrait in: **Collection**—van Kaathoven.

Morison (Robert B.) Bacteria and their pres-
ence in syphilitic secretions. 4 pp., 1 pl. 8°.
[*Baltimore,* 1883.]
Repr. from: Maryland M. J., Balt., 1882-3, ix.

———. Ergebnisse der Behandlung von Hautkrankheiten mit Unna'schen Präparaten. (Aus
dem engl. Manuscript übersetzt.) 6 pp. 8°.
Berlin, 1885.
Repr. from: Deutsche med. Wchnschr., Berl., 1885, xi.

Morison (Thomas Coutts). On the distinction
between crime and insanity. An essay to which
the Society for Improving the Condition of the
Insane awarded the premium of twenty guineas.
33 pp. 8°. *London, G. Odell,* 1844.
See, also, **Johnston** (David). Statements, etc., respecting the cases of Christina and David Hutcheon. 8°.
[*Montrose?* 1852.] — **Morison** (Alexander). Outlines of
lectures on the nature, causes, and treatment of insanity.
4. ed. 8°. *London,* 1848.

Morisot des Landes (Petr. Jos.)
See **Millin de la Courveault** (Joan. Nicol.) &
Morisot des Landes (Petr. Jos.) Ergo Parisinis
variolarum inoculatio. *Parisiis,* 1757. *In:* HALLER.
Disp. ad morb. [etc.] 4°. *Lausannæ,* 1758, v, 695-712.

Morisse (Anthime-Onézime). * I. Quels sont les
avantages et les inconvénients des résections?
II. [etc.] 27 pp. 4°. *Paris,* 1838, No. 377, v.
331.

Morisse (J.) *Du polype fibreux de la cavité
utérine. 13 pp. 4°. *Paris,* 1833, No. 86, v. 259.

Morisse (Lucien). * De la médication intestinale antiseptique par l'eau sulfo-carbonée. 80
pp., 1 l. 4°. *Paris,* 1886, No. 223.
———. The same. 80 pp., 1 l., 4 tab. 8°. *Paris,*
G. Steinheil, 1886.

Morisseau (L.-F.) *Coup-d'œil physiologique
sur certains résultats de l'organisation. 26 pp.
4°. *Paris,* 1832, No. 122, v. 251.

Morisset (J.-Paul). * De l'influence des marais
sur la santé des hommes. 31 pp. 4°. *Montpellier,* 1837, No. 175. [P., v. 1081.]

Morisset (J.-S.) *Sur le scorbut. 18 pp. 4°.
Paris, 1809, No. 41, v. 75.

Morisset (Martial). *Étude sur la pression
intra-labyrinthique. 98 pp. 4°. *Paris,* 1878,
No. 319.

Morisson (François-Firmin). *Sur les pieds-
bots. 30 pp. 4°. *Paris,* 1847, No. 17, v. 462.

Morisson (François-Marie). *Sur l'hématurie,
ou pissement de sang. 14 pp. 4°. *Paris,* 1827,
No. 30, v. 204.

Morisson (Georges). * Quelques considérations
sur l'œdème et en particulier sur l'œdème des
membres inférieurs. 53 pp. 4°. *Paris,* 1878,
No. 193.

Morisson (Louis-Paulin-Auguste). * Quelques
mots sur les causes et la nature de la fièvre puerpérale. 40 pp. 4°. *Strasbourg,* 1861, No. 590,
2. s., v. 31.

Morisson (Raoul). *D'une forme de céphalalgie rhumatismale algie du péricrâne. 64 pp.
4°. *Paris,* 1872, No. 336.

Moritz (Carolus Ludovicus). *Specimen topo-
graphiæ medicæ Dorpatensis. 80 pp. 8°. *Dorpati Livonorum, ex off. J. C. Schünmanni,* 1823.

Moritz (Emanuel) [1836–] *Untersuchun-
gen über die Entwickelung der quergestreiften
Muskelfaser; eine Abhandlung. 41 pp., 1 pl.
8°. *Dorpat, C. Schulz,* 1860.
———. Ueber Asthma bronchiale. 27 pp. 8°.
St. Petersburg, 1884.

Moritz (Ernestus). *Observationes nonnullæ
de febribus intermittentibus larvatis. 36 pp.
8°. *Regimontii Pr., C. Paschke,* [1836].

Moritz (Ferdinandus Constantinus). *De convulsionum therapia. 38 pp. 8°. *Francof. ad
Viadr., typog. Apitziano,* [1792].

Moritz (Frider. Augustus) [1804–]. *Observationes quædam in uteri morbos organicos.
30 pp., 1 l. 8°. *Berolini, typ. A. Petschii,* [1830].

Moritz ([Friedrich Ernst] M[ax]). *Ueber
einige Präparate des Gelsemium sempervirens.
30 pp., 1 l. 8°. *Greifswald, C. Sell,* 1879.

Moritz (Guilielmus)[1]. *De lini cathartici vi purgante observationes. 32 pp. 8°. *Dorpati Livonorum, typ. J. C. Schuenmanni,* 1835.

Moritz (Guilelmus)[2] [1838–]. *De epilepsia.
32 pp. 8°. *Berolini, G. Lange,* 1860.

Moritz (Ludovicus) [1810–54]. *De pathologia
ac diagnosi aneurysmatum internorum. 1 p. l.,
40 pp., 1 pl., 2 l. 4°. *Vratislaviæ, typ. Grassii,
Barthii et soc.,* [1835].

Moritz (Siegmund). *Unterbrochener Wintrich'-
scher Schallwechsel. Ein Beitrag zur Cavernen-
Diagnostik. 19 pp. 8°. *Würzburg, Stahel,* 1877.

Morival (Jules). *Traitement des vomissements incoercibles de la grossesse. 58 pp., 1 l.
4°. *Paris,* 1884, No. 165.

Moriz (Eduard). *Die Wendung auf den Kopf.
33 pp. 8°. *Königsberg, E. J. Dalkowski,* 1873.

Moriz (Guil. Theod. Eduard.) *De mutationibus pathologicis tractus intestinorum et ventriculi quoad anatomen nonnulla. 32 pp. 8°. *Regimontii Pr., typ. Hartungianis,* [1838].

Morizot (Marie-Gabriel-Hyacinthe). *La chlorose. 68 pp. 4°. *Paris,* 1841, No. 56, v. 378.

Morland (Joseph). Disquisitions concerning the
force of the heart, the dimensions of the coats
of the arteries, and the circulation of the blood.
2 p. l., 88 pp. 8°. *London, J. Lawrence,* 1713.

Morland (Pierre). *Propositions sur divers
objets de médecine. 34 pp. 4°. *Paris, an XIII*
[1805], No. 508, v. 57.

Morland (William Wallace). Diseases of the
urinary organs. A compendium of their diagnosis, pathology, and treatment. 579 pp. 8°.
Philadelphia, Blanchard & Lea, 1858.
———. The morbid effects of the retention in the
blood of the elements of the urinary secretion.
(Fiske fund prize essay.) 83 pp. 8°. *Philadelphia, Blanchard & Lea,* 1861.
———. Florida and South Carolina as health resorts. 20 pp. 8°. *Boston, J. Campbell,* 1873.

Morlanne (Étienne-Pierre) [1772–]. Mémoire et observations sur plusieurs cas importants de l'art des accouchements, recueillis en
1835 et 1837 à la clinique de l'École pratique du
département de la Moselle. 34 pp., 2 pl. 4°.
Metz, Dosquet, 1838.

Morlard (Victor).
See **Hornemann** (Claude Jacob Emil). De l'inhumation, de la crémation [etc.] 8°. *Copenhague*, 1876.

Morlet (C.-F.) * De la levée du premier appareil dans les plaies simples qui doivent suppurer. 29 pp. 4°. *Paris*, 1838, No: 195, v. 331.

Morlet (E.) * I. Établir les différences qui existent entre les inflammations des membranes séreuses et les inflammations des membranes muqueuses, sous le point de vue de l'anatomie pathologique et de la séméiologie. II. [etc.] 42 pp. 4°. *Paris*, 1838, No. 372, v. 331.

Morley (Charles). Elements of animal magnetism; or process and application for relieving human suffering. 27 pp. 12°. *New York, Fowler & Wells*, 1847.

———. The same. 24 pp. 8°. *New York, Fowlers & Wells*, [1847].

Morley (Frederick).
See **Michigan** and its resources. 8°. *Lansing*, 1881.

Morley (Henry). A tract upon interrupted health and sick-room duties. 23 pp. 8°. *London, C. Edmonds*, 1847. [P., v. 149; 754.]

———. Jerome Cardan. The life of Girolamo Cardano, of Milan, physician. 2 v. xii, 304 pp.; iv, 328 pp. 8°. *London, Chapman & Hall*, 1854.

———. The life of Henry Cornelius Agrippa von Nettesheim, doctor and knight, commonly known as a magician. 2 v. xii, 304, 332 pp. 8°. *London, Chapman & Hall*, 1856.

Morley (John). An essay on the nature and cure of the king's evil; deduced from observation and practice. With additions, and a great variety of cases and their remedies, with a plate of the herb "Vervain"; published for the good of mankind, particularly the common people. 4. ed. vii, 9-48 pp., 1 pl. 8°. *London, J. Buckland*, 1768.

———. The same. 10. ed. iv, 5-60 pp., 1 pl. 8°. *London, J. Buckland*, 1773. [P., v. 661.]

———. The same. With additions, and above sixty cases (some never before publish'd). 12. ed. 80 pp. 8°. *London, J. Buckland*, 1774.
Half of last leaf is missing; plate wanting.

———. The same. 14. ed. iv, 5-80+ pp., 1 pl. 8°. *London, J. Buckland*, 1775.

———. The same. 17. ed. iv, 5-89 pp., 1 pl. 8°. *London, J. Buckland*, 1777. [P., v. 605.]

———. The same. 89 pp., 1 pl. 8°. *London, J. Buckland*, 1782. [P., v. 432.]

———. The same. 27. ed. iv, 5-89 pp., 1 pl. 8°. *London, J. Buckland*, 1790.

———. The same. iii, 4-89 pp., 1 col. pl. 8°. *London, G. & T. Wilkie*, 1791. [P., v. 636.]

———. The same. 31. ed., revised. viii, 7-51 pp., 1 pl. 8°. *New York*, 1861.
From the London ed. of 1797.

Morlière (L.-F.-A.) Quelques idées sur la cause prochaine des fièvres et sur la nature de la contagion. 64 pp. 8°. *Compiègne, J. Escuyer*, 1845. [P., v. 1357.]

Morlok (G.) Die Heizung durch Zimmeröfen . . . Bericht erstattet im Auftrag des königl. württ. Ministeriums für die Verkehrsanstalten. viii, 97 pp., 44 pl. roy. 8°. *Stuttgart, J. B. Metzler*, 1870.

Morlot (Édouard). * Sur une forme grave de l'épilepsie. 1 p. l., 44 pp., 2 l. 4°. *Paris*, 1881, No. 314.

Morlot (Ferdinand) [1853–]. * Contribution à l'étude de l'atrophie du testicule. 63 pp. 4°. *Paris*, 1881, No. 361.

Morlot (J.-B.) * De la méningite aux différents âges. 43 pp. 4°. *Paris*, 1846, No. 98, v. 448.

Mormiche (M.) * Contribution à l'étude de l'adénome palatin. 46 pp. 4°. *Paris*, 1883, No. 51.

Mormonism.
Furley (C. C.) The physiology of Mormonism. San Francisco M. Press, 1863, iv, 1-4.

Mormyeus.
See **Fish** (*Electrical*).

Mornac. Naika Suyo. [The treatment of internal disease. Transl. by Takamatsu Riöoun.] 10 v. 12°. *Tokio*, 1883.
Japanese text.

Mornac (Antoine-Émile). * De la fièvre en elle-même. 34 pp. 4°. *Paris*, 1856, No. 279, v. 594.

Mornac (Jean-Baptiste-Gabriel). * Sur quelques plaies d'armes à feu. 23 pp. 4°. *Paris*, 1821, No. 177, v. 168. [*Also, in:* P., v. 50.]

Mornac (Jean-Joseph). * Sur la phthisie tuberculeuse, avec des propositions sur cette maladie. vi, 7-20 pp. 4°. *Paris*, 1809, No. 106, v. 77.

Mornand (Félix). La vie des eaux, avec des notes sur la vertu curative des eaux par le docteur Rouraud. 2. éd. 386 pp. 12°. *Paris, L. Hachette & Cie.*, 1856.

Mornard (Henri). * Sémiologie des éruptions cutanées dans la fièvre typhoïde. 36 pp. 4°. *Paris*, 1875, No. 159.

Mornay (C.-M.-B.-Frédéric). * Sur la gangrène des extrémités supérieures et inférieures. 23 pp. 4°. *Strasbourg, Levrault*, 1816.

Mornese. Regolamento di polizia mortuaria del comune di Mornese. 11 pp. 12°. *Novi, tip. Camusso*, 1884.

Morning.
Regius (J.) * Diss. inaug. qua expenditur cur aurora musis sit amica; warum die Morgenstunde Gold im Munde habe. 4°. *Halæ*, [1745].

Morning, Noon, and Night. A medical and miscellaneous annual for the years 1870-72 (2.-4.). 8°. *New York, Crump*, [1869-71].

Moro (Giacopo). Anatomia ridotta all' uso de' pittori e scultori. 23, 25 pp., 19 pl., 1 l. fol. *Vinegia, presso G. F. Valvasense*, 1679.
Another copy bound with: **Cesio** (Carlo). Eine herrliche Anweisung . . . von der Anatomie [etc.] fol. *Augspurg*, 1708.

Morocco.
See, also, **Cholera** (*Asiatic, History, etc., of*), by localities; **Medicine** (*Military, History, of*), **Campaigns, etc.**—*Spain*; **Mogador**; **Tangiers**.
Notes on the sanitary state of Moorish towns, and on the climate and diseases of Morocco. Med. Times & Gaz., Lond., 1877, ii, 96.—**Quedenfeldt.** Anthropologische Aufnahmen von Marokkanern. Verhandl. d. Berl. Gesellsch. f. Anthrop., 1887, 32-37.—**Rohlfs** (G.) Beiträge zur Geschichte der Medicin und medicinischen Geographie Marokko's. Deutsches Arch. f. Gesch. d. Med. u. med. Geog., Leipz., 1878, i, 183-193.—**Schousboe** (P.-K.-A.) Observations sur le règne végétal au Maroc. Bull. Soc. d. sc. . . . . d'Alger, 1874, 1-202, 8 pl.—**Stirling** (J.) The races of Morocco. J. Anthrop. Soc. Lond., 1870-71, viii, pp. clxix-clxxiii.

Moroche (Edme-Jean). * I. Des symptômes de la métrite chronique dans ses différentes formes. II. [etc.] 27 pp. 4°. *Paris*, 1842, No. 146, v. 393.

Morochovets (Leon). * Zakony pitshevarenija. [Function of digestion.] 54 pp., 1 l. 8°. *St. Petersburg, tipog. B. G. Janpolskago*, 1881.

Morocomio centrale maschile in San Servolo di Venezia. See **Manicomio** centrale maschile in S. Servolo di Venezia.

Morong (Thomas). The beneficence of pain. An essay read before the Young Ladies' Institute in Iowa City, 23d June, 1858. 7 pp. 8°. *Iowa City, J. Duncan & Crouse*, 1858.

Moroni (Ercole). Storia del curaro; studii critici ed esperimentali. 463 pp., 1 l. 8°. *Milano, F. Gareffi*, 1867.

Moronus (Matthias). Directorium medico-practicum, sive indices duo præternaturalium affectuum, cum distinctorum tum implicatorum, de

Moronus (Matthias)—continued.
quibus extant gravissimorum virorum consultationes, epistolæ, quæstiones, responsiones, observationes, historiæ, etc. Medicis, præsertim ty-
ronibus, quæ consimilibus in casibus imitentur
exempla, præmonstrantes. Jam primum in Germania editi, variisque auctorum exemplis aucti,
opera et studio Sebastiani Schefferi. 11 p. l., 494
pp., 8 l. sm. 4°. *Francof. a. M., sumpt. vid. J. G.
Schönwetteri*, 1663.

Morosinus (R. D. Franciscus). Tractatus de
scorezzis primo in unum collectus, deinde divisus
in plures propositiones, in fine positas, pro opportunitate loci, temporis, personarum, propug-
nandas. 1. ed. 60 pp. 12°. *Laudæ, typog. A.
Pallavicinis*, 1783. [P., v. 1074.]

Morot (Pierre). * Sur l'ulcère simple du duodénum. 44 pp. 4°. *Paris*, 1865, No. 276.

Morotrofia (R.)
See **Miraglia** (B. G.) Programma di un manicomio,
modello italiano. 12°. *Aversa*, 1861.

Moroux [1855–]. * Des rapports de la cirrhose du foie avec la péritonite tuberculeuse.
64 pp. 4°. *Paris*, 1883, No. 367.

Morovaja boliezne cholora i kak uberech. neja.
Nastavlenie dlja prostago narodo. [Cholera and
how to prevent it; advice for common people.]
24 pp. 8°. *Kazan, typ. Gubernsk. pravlen.*, 1885.

Morozoff (Dimitrius). * Anatomija pitshevoda
i k ucheniou o rakovom sujenii etogo organa i
ego lecheniou kateterizatsiei, elektrolizom i gas-
trostomiei. [Anatomy of œsophagus, and study
on cancerous diseases of this organ and their
treatment by catheterization, electrolysis, and
gastrotomy.] 216 pp., 1 l., 2 pl. 8°. *St. Petersburg, tipog. J. N. Skorochodova*, 1887.

Morpain (Alphonse) [1826–70]. * Études anatomiques et pathologiques des grandes lèvres.
54 pp. 4°. *Paris*, 1852, No. 278, v. 529.

——. Sarcocèle encéphaloïde; ablation au moyen de la galvano-caustique thermique; cicatrisation. 7 pp. 8°. *Paris, E. Martinet*, [1871].
See, also, **Amussat** (Alphonse) fils & **Morpain** (Alphonse). Galvano-caustique thermique [etc.] 8°. *Paris*,
1865. — **Remak** (Robert). Galvanothérapie [etc.] 8°.
Paris, 1860.
For Biography, see Bull. Soc. méd.-prat. de Par. (1868–
72), 1873, no. 65–69, 12 (Collineau).

Morpeth. Speech of Viscount de Morpeth in
the House of Commons, on Tuesday, 10th February, 1848, on moving for leave to bring in a
bill for promoting the public health. 37 pp. 8°.
London, J. Ridgway, 1848. [P., v. 162.]

Morphine *and its salts.*
See, also, **Anæsthetics**; **Atropine** (*Physiological, etc., effects of*); **Endermic** *method*; **Fœtus** (*Effects of medicines on*); **Heart** (*Diseases of,
Treatment of*); **Insanity** (*Treatment of*); **Opium**
habit.

CZVAINA (J.) * De morphio. 8°. *Pestini*,
[1835].
GAILLARD (B.) * Propositions sur les effets
des sels de morphine. 4°. *Paris*, 1832.
HENNELLE (C.) * Nouvelles recherches sur le
mode d'action du principe de Derosne et de la
morphine. 4°. *Paris*, 1825.
HOPPE (J. G.) * De morphio et acido meco-
nico. 4°. *Lipsiæ*, [1820].
KANZMANN (T.) Beiträge für den gerichtlich-
chemischen Nachweis des Morphins und Narco-
tins in thierischen Flüssigkeiten und Geweben.
8°. [*Dorpat*], 1868.
KINDSCHER (F. L. E.) * De morphio. sm. 8°.
Berolini, [1828].
VON KOSTIN (E.) * Ueber das essigsaure Morphium, dessen Wirkung und Anwendung am
Krankenbette, und seine Bereitungsart. 8°.
München, 1838.

Morphine *and its salts.*
KRAGE (W.) * Ueber Albuminurie und Glycosurie nach Morphium. 8°. *Anklam*, 1878.
LEVACHER-DE-BOISVILLE (F.-S.) * De la morphine, ou principe-actif de l'opium. 4°. *Paris*,
1817.
NIELAND (J. J.) * De opii et morphini effectuum comparatione. 8°. *Berolini*, [1825].
PETIT (E.-A.) * Sur la morphine et les préparations d'opium. 4°. *Paris*, 1862.
TROUSSEAU (A.) & BONNET. Essai thérapeutique et médico-légal sur les effets des sels de
morphine. 8°. *Paris*, 1831.
See, also, infra.
VALENCIENNES (A. -A.) * Recherches cliniques sur l'oxydation de la morphine et sur l'extraction de la castorine. 4°. *Paris*, 1861.
WOLTERS (A.) * Contributions à l'étude de la
morphine et du morphinisme. 4°. *Montpellier*,
1883.
Anrep (V. K.) & **Kushnerenko** (D.) K vopr.
o sudbe morfija v organizme. [What becomes of morphia in the organism?] Sborn. rabot. proizved. lab.
Anrepa, Charkoff, 1886–7, ii, 193–215. — **Audhoui** (V.)
Recherches expérimentales sur l'action toxique et médicale du chlorhydrate de morphine. Thérap. contemp.,
Par., 1881, i, 49–56. — **Bally** (V.) Observations sur les
effets thérapeutiques de la morphine ou narcéine. Mém.
Acad. de méd., Par., 1828, i, 99–180. — **Bell** (J. C.) Iodic
acid test for morphia. Analyst, Lond., 1879, iv, 181. —
Beraudi. Sugli effetti della morfina e del suo acetato sul
corpo umano. Ann. univ. di med., Milano, 1828, xlviii, 551–
564. — **Bernard** (C.) Des effets physiologiques de la morphine et de leur combinaison avec ceux du chloroforme.
Bull. gén. de thérap., etc., Par., 1869, lxxvii, 241–256. —
Bernatzik (W.) Ueber die Wirksamkeit chloroform-
haltiger Lösungen von Morphin und Caffeïn. Wien. med.
Presse, 1867, viii, 659; 689. — **Bertini** (B.) Osservazioni
pratiche sull' utilità dell' acetata di morfina. Gior. d. Soc.
med.-chir. di Torino, 1845, xxii, 309–319. — **Bricheteau.**
D'un moyen simple et facile pour éviter aux malades la douleur du vésicatoire. Bull. gén. de thérap., etc., Par., 1868,
lxxv, 481. — **Bruneau** (L.) Recherche de la morphine
dans l'urine. [Extrait d'un mémoire intitulé : Du passage
de quelques médicaments dans les urines. Paris, 1880.]
Bull. scient. dép. du nord, etc., Par., 1880, iii, 238–240. —
Brunton (T. L.) & **Cash** (J. T.) Temperaturerniedri-
gende Wirkung des Morphins auf Tauben. Centralbl. f.
d. med. Wissensch., Berl., 1886, xxiv, 241. — **Burr** (H. N.)
A case of morphine idiosyncrasy. Med. & Surg. Reporter, Phila., 1887, lvii, 206. — **Byrd** (H. L.) Parturient effects of the sulphate of morphia. Oglethorpe M. & S. J.,
Savannah, 1858–9, i, 73–75. Also: Med. & Surg. Reporter,
Phila., 1869, xxi, 111–113. — **Cabadé** (E.) Note sur un effet insolite du chlorhydrate de morphine. Gaz. hebd. de
méd., Par., 1887, 2. s., xxiv, 522–524. — **Calvet** & **Laborde.** Recherches expérimentales sur l'action physiologique et toxique de la morphine, à l'état aigu et chronique. Tribune méd., Par., 1876, viii, 530; 552: 1877, ix, 2;
29; 40; 64; 113; 135; 161. — **Cervello** (V.) & **Valenti**
(S.) Sopra gli effetti combinati della morfina e della
paraldeide. Ann. di chim. med.-farm., Milano, 1885, 4. s.,
i, 65–78. — **Chastaing.** Sur la fonction complexe de la
morphine et sa transformation en acide picrique; de sa
solubilité. Compt. rend. Acad. d. sc., Par., 1882, xciv,
44. — **Chouppe** (H.) Note sur un accident qui peut se
produire à la suite des injections sous-cutanées de chlorhydrate de morphine; des précautions à prendre pour l'éviter.
Compt. rend. Soc. de biol. 1876, Par ., 1877, 6. s., iii, 78–80. —
Coe (H. C.) Peculiar phenomena following an injection
of morphine. N. York M. J., 1887, xlvi, 267. — **van den
Corput** (E.) Du cyanhydrate de morphine et de ses
usages thérapeutiques. Presse méd. belge, Brux., 1854–5,
vii. 149; 157; 165. — **Curci** (A.) Azione della morfina
sulla circolazione del sangue. Sperimentale, Firenze, 1883,
li, 449–467. — **Davey** (N. F.) Taraxacum a source of fallacy in testing for morphine. Med. Times & Gaz., Lond.,
1857, xv, 229. — **Demarquay.** Conférences sur l'association de la morphine et du chloroform, et sur un nouveau
mode d'administration de cet agent. Gaz. d. hôp., Par.,
1872, xlv, 770; 786; 795; 809; 817. — **Donáth** (G.) A morphin sorsa a szervezetben. [The disposal of morphine in
the organism.] Orvosi hetil., Budapest, 1866, xxx, 713;
745. Also, transl. · Arch. f. d. ges. Physiol., Bonn, 1885–6,
xxxviii, 528–548. — **Dublanc** jeune. Sur un réactif propre à indiquer la présence des sels de morphine dissous
dans un liquide, dans le rapport d'un à dix mille en poids,
suivi d'un procédé pour analyser, à l'aide de ce réactif, les
liqueurs animales qui contiennent la morphine. J. de
pharm., Par., 1824, x, 425–431. Also, transl. [Abstr.] :
Arch. f. d. ges. Naturl., Nürnb., 1824, iii, 101–108. — **Dupré** (A.) Some observations on the iodic acid test for
morphia. Guy's Hosp. Rep., Lond., 1863, 3. s., ix, 323–

Morphine *and its salts.*

327. *Also :* Chem. News, Lond., 1863, viii, 267.—**Dupuy** [*et al.*]. Expériences sur l'action de l'acétate de morphine dans les animaux, et sur les moyens de reconnaître l'empoisonnement par cette substance. J. gén. de méd., chir. et pharm., Par., 1824, lxxxvi, 13-30.—**Ebrard.** Mémoire sur un mode nouveau d'employer l'hydrochlorate de morphine dans les odontalgies, les névralgies frontales et dans quelques névralgies trifaciales. J. de méd. de Lyon, 1845, ix, 5-20.—**Fantonetti** (G.) Ulteriori osservazioni sull' uso terapeutico della morfina data internamente. Gior. per serv. ai progr. d. patol., Venezia, 1836, iv, 203-213.—**Fate** (On the) of morphia in the living organism. Ann. Chem. Med., Lond., 1881, ii, 109-111.—**Fazio** (E.) Sulla tollerabilità degli oppiati ed in ispecie della morfina. Movimento, Napoli, 1880, 2. s., ii, 70-78.—**Filehne** (W.) Ueber die Einwirkung des Morphins auf die Athmung. Arch. f. exper. Path. u. Pharmakol., Leipz., 1878-9, x, 442, 2 pl.: 1879, xi, 45. ———. Zur Morphinwirkung. Sitzungsb. d. phys.-med. Soc. zu Erlang., 1879, 'ii, 47.—**Florio** (F.) Solubilità della morfina e preparazione di alcuni suoi sali. Riv. di chim. med. e farm., Torino, 1883, i, 214-220.—**Fort.** Leccion sobre la morfina. [Transl.] Rev. méd. de Chile, Sant. de Chile, 1885-6, xiv. 50-54.—**Frickenhaus.** Ueber eine unerwünschte Nebenwirkung des Morphium muriaticum (per os oder subcutan) und deren untrügliche Vermeidung. Allg. med. Centr.-Ztg., Berl., 1875, xliv, 1061.—**Friedberger.** Uvangenehme Folgen der Morphiuminjection bei einem Pferde. Wchnschr. f. Thierh. u. Viehzucht, Augsburg, 1877, xxi, 121; 129.—**Fristedt** (R. F.) Om den farmakologiska gruppen morfin, efter W. v. Schroeder. Upsala Lâkaref. Förh., 1884, xix, 182-189.—**Galvani di Domenico** (A.) Nuovo processo per estrarre la morfina dall' oppio direttamente spoglia di narcotina. Ann. univ. di med., Milano, 1831, lviii, 311-314.—**Gil y Municio** (P.) Procedimientos por la estraccion de la morfina. Siglo méd., Madrid, 1864, xi, 597; 614; 660; 681.—**Grasset & Amblard.** Note sur les propriétés convulsivantes de la morphine. Gaz. hebd. de méd., Par., 1882, 2. s., xix, 123. *Also* [Abstr.]: Compt. rend. Acad. d. sc., Par., 1881, xciii, 973-975.—**Gregory** (W.) On a process for preparing economically the muriate of morphia. Edinb. M. & S. J., 1831, xxxv, 331-338.—**Grimaux** (E.) Sur quelques réactions de la morphine et de ses congénères. Compt. rend. Acad. d. sc., Par., 1881, xciii, 217-219. ———. Sur une nouvelle série de bases dérivées de la morphine. *Ibid.*, 591-593. ———. Sur la transformation de la morphine en codéine et en bases homologues. J. de l'anat. et physiol., etc., Par., 1881, xvii, 329.—**Gscheidlen** (R.) Ueber die physiologischen Wirkungen des essigsauren Morphiums. Untersuch. a. d. physiol. Lab. in Würzb., Leipz., 1869, ii, 3-66.—**Hartwig** (M.) Eine Erfahrung mit Morphium. Med.-chir. Cor.-Bl. f. deutsch-am. Aerzte, Buffalo, 1883, i. No. 5, 13-15.—**Hünefeld.** Beiträge zur Chemie des Morphiums, zur Beförderung der gerichtlichen Chemie und in Bezug auf den Castaingschen Prozess. Arch. f. med. Erfahr., Berl., 1826, i, 411-458.—**Johnson** (W.) Endermic application of sulphate of morphia. Med. & Surg. Reporter, Phila., 1860, n. s., iv, 155-157.—**Jolly.** Ueber örtliche Morphiumwirkung. Arch. f. Psychiat., Berl., 1877, viii, 215.—**Kennedy** (T. J.) Parturient effects of the sulphate of morphia. Med. & Surg. Reporter, Phila., 1869, xxi, 191.—**Kersch.** Das Morphium und seine physiologische Wirkung auf den thierischen Organismus nach eigens angestellten Versuchen und nach Beobachtungen am Krankenbette. Memorabilien, Heilbr., 1871, xvi, 1; 25.—**Labbé** (L.) & **Goujon** (E.) Sur l'action combinée de la morphine et du chloroforme. Gaz. d. hôp., Par., 1872, xlv, 251.—**Landrieux.** Bromhydrate de morphine. J. de thérap., Par., 1879, vi, 121; 201.—**Landsberg** (E.) Untersuchungen über das Schicksal des Morphins im lebenden Organismus. Arch. f. d. ges. Physiol., Bonn, 1880-81, xxiii, 413-433.—**Laurence** (J. Z.) The antiphlogistic powers of morphia illustrated by its use in the treatment of acute inflammations of the sclerotic and iris. Med. Times & Gaz., Lond., 1859, n. s., xix, 651.—**Lefort** (J.) Études chimiques et toxicologiques sur la morphine, suivies d'observations sur son passage dans l'économie animale. Bull. Acad. de méd., Par., 1860-61, xxvi, 817.—**Lenhartz.** Ueber den Antagonismus von Morphin und Atropin vom klinischen und experimentellen Standpunkte. Tagebl. d. Versamml. deutsch. Naturf. u. Aerzte, Berl., 1886, lix, 205-207. *Also* [Abstr.]: Deutsche Med.-Ztg., Berl., 1886, vii, 932.—**Leoni** (B.) Intorno agli effetti prodotti dall' uso esterno dell' acetato di morfina impiegato nella sciatica, ed alcuni riflessi su 'l modo d' agire di questo medicamento. Gazz. med. ital. lomb., Milano, 1852, 3. s., i, 11-13.—**Lindo** (D.) Morphia reactions. Chem. News, Lond., 1878, xxxviii, 65.—**Little** (J. L.) A remarkable case of morphine tolerance by an infant. Am. J. Obst., N. Y., 1878, xi, 374-377. *Also,* Reprint.—**Luppi** (G.) Sur les propriétés thérapeutiques du sulfate double de morphine et de strychnine; lettre à M. le docteur G. Grimelli. Gaz. méd. de Par., 1857, 3. s., xii, 438; 458; 475. ———. Deuxième lettre sur l'action et les usages thérapeutiques du sulfate double de morphine et strychnine, adressée à M. le docteur G. Grimelli. *Ibid.*,

Morphine *and its salts.*

1858, 3. s., xiii, 804; 829.—**Lutz & Fonssagrives.** Morphine. Dict. encycl. d. sc. méd., Par., 1875, 2. s., ix, 487-516.—**Magendie.** Note sur l'emploi de quelques sels de morphine comme médicamens. N. Jour. de méd., chir., pharm., etc.. Par., 1818, i, 23-28.—**Marc.** Anwendung ausserordentlicher Gaben von Morphium. Med. Cor.-Bl. bayer. Aerzte, Erlang., 1850, xi, 303.—**Marmé.** Az oxydimorphin kimutatása. Gyógyszerészi hetil., Budapest, 1885, xxiv, 50; 65; 82.—**Mayer** (E.-L.) & **Wright** (G.-R.-A.) Recherches sur les polymères de la morphine et leurs dérivés. Monit. scient.. Par., 1873, 3. s., xv, 659-672.—**Mazzola** (G.) Lettera al Dott. A. Quadri (sugli effetti dell' acetato di morfina). Ann. univ. di med., Milano, 1826, xl, 156-165.—**Melion** (J.) Wirkungen des essigsauren Morphiums; beobachtet am Krankenbette. Med. Cor.-Bl. d. württemb. ärztl. Ver., Stuttg., 1844, xiv, 137-143.—**Michiels** (J.) Note sur quelques modifications au procédé de Gregory pour la préparation du chlorhydrate de morphine, d'après une nouvelle propriété reconnue à ce sel alcaloïde. [Rap. de Vandevelde.] Ann. Soc. de méd. d'Anvers, 1842, 196; 206. ———. Notice sur un procédé pour obtenir la morphine cristallisée sans intermédiaire de l'alcool. *Ibid.*, 376-378.—**Nothnagel.** Ueber die Wirkungen des Morphin auf den Darm. Verhandl. d. Cong. f. innere Med., Wiesb., 1882, i, 132-137. *Also :* Arch. f. path. Anat., etc., Berl., 1882, lxxxix, 1-8.—**Orfila** (P.) Mémoire sur la morphine, ou sur le principe actif de l'opium. N. Jour. de méd., chir., pharm., etc., Par., 1818, i, 3-22.—**Ott** (I.) Morphia and gelsemium. Arch. Med., N. Y., 1884, xi, 79-81.—**Petit** (A.) Sur un procédé de dosage rapide de la morphine dans l'opium. J. de pharm. et de chim., Par., 1879, xxix, 159-162. *Also:* Monde pharm., Par., 1879, x, 157.—**Picard** (P.) Sur l'action de la morphine chez les chiens. Compt. rend. Acad. d. sc., Par., 1878, lxxxvi, 1144-1147. ———. Sur les phénomènes qui suivent les injections de chlorhydrate de morphine. Compt. rend. Soc. de biol. 1878, Par., 1880, 6. s., v, 13-15, pt. 2.—**Picard** (P.) & **Rebatel.** Action des sels de morphine sur le cœur. *Ibid.*, 145.—**Pierce** (F. M.) On the physiological action of some new morphine and codeine derivatives. Practitioner, Lond., 1875, xiii, 437-442.—**Pontoppidan** (K.) & **Christensen** (O. T.) En ny Reaktion paa Morfin-Urin. Hosp.-Tid., Kjøbenh., 1884, 3. R., ii, 625-627.—**Quadri** (A.) La morfina in pratica, o cenni sulla medesima. Ann. univ. di med., Milano, 1824, xxxi, 169: 1825, xxxiv, 100.—**Reale** (N.) Nuovo processo di dosamento della morfina e nuova reazione chimica di essa. Resoc. Accad. med.-chir. di Napoli, 1882, xxxvi, 85-90.—**Révay** (J.) Kisérletek a sósavas apomorphinnak gyógygyakerlatba hozatala körül. [Therapeutic effects of hydrochlorate of morphia.] Magy. orv. és term.-vizsg., Budapest, 1875, 174-179.—**Ricotti** (M.) Sull' uso esterno dell' acetato di morfina. Ann. univ. di med., Milano, 1829, li, 36-45.—**Robertson** (M.) On the medicinal effects of the salts of morphia, especially the muriate, with a new mode of preparing it. Edinb. M. & S. J., 1832, xxxvii, 278-295. *Also,* Reprint.—**Ruiz del Cerro** (A.) Esposicion sucinta de las propiedades físicas, químicas y medicinales de la morfina. Bibliot. méd.-castr. españ., Madrid, 1852, vii, 337-348.—**Sancho del Rio** (J.) Morfina y separacion de los demas alcaloides que le acompañan en el opio. Union de l. cien. méd., Cartagena, 1883-4, i, 108; 123; 140; 157; 172. *Also:* Encicl. méd.-farm., Barcel., 1883, vii, 751; 768.—**Sandras** (S.) Recherches sur les propriétés thérapeutiques de la morphine. Gaz. méd. de Par., 1830, i, 66-68.—**Santoliquido** (R.) Sul meccanismo del vomito da morfina. Terap. mod., Napoli, 1887, i, 5-13.—**Schmitt.** Sur le dosage de la morphine dans l'opium. Bull. Soc. de pharm. de Bordeaux, 1880, xx, 74-83. *Also:* J. d. sc. méd. de Lille, 1880, ii, 598-605.—**von Schroeder** (W.) Untersuchungen über die pharmakologische Gruppe des Morphins. Arch. f. exper. Path. u. Pharmakol., Leipz., 1883, xvii, 96-144.—**Schuld** (J. F.) Langdurig gebruik van groote giften acetas morphii. N. pract. Tijdschr. v. de Geneesk., Gorinchem, 1856, n. s., ii, 79-81.—**Selmi** (F.) Dell' uso dell' acido iodidrico iodurato per riconoscere gli alcaloidi dell' oppio. Mem. Accad. d. sc. d. Ist. di Bologna, 1875, 3. s., vi, 217-221.—**Serres.** Observation sur un effet remarquable de l'application extérieure de l'acétate de morphine dans une affection particulière de l'estomac et des intestins; recueillie par J. Dubourg. Arch. gén. de méd., Par., 1826, x, 431-437.—**Smith** (E.) On the efficacy of small doses of morphia in hooping cough, chronic bronchitis, and phthisis. Edinb. M. J., 1855-6, ii, 1001-1010.—**Sorokin** (I.) O daiistvii morphiya na organizm zhivotnikh. [Action of morphia on the animal organism.] Med. Vestnik, St. Petersb., 1863, viii, 79.—**Sprott** (J.) Effects of morphine not mentioned by medical writers. N. Orl. J. M., 1869, xxii, 506.—**Squire** (P.) [*et al.*]. Bi-meconate of morphia. Lond. M. Gaz., 1838-9, xxiii, 861-863.—**Staples** (E.) Practical observations on the preparation of morphia, etc. N. Am. M. & S. J., Phila., 1829, vii, 433.—**Strambio** (G.) Su 'l azione dell' acetato e solfato di morfina. Gior. crit. di med. anal., Milano, 1827, vi, 186: vii, 221.—**Trousseau** (A.) & **Bonnet.** Considérations sur les effets produits par les sels de morphine. Bull. gén. de thérap., etc., 2. éd., Par., 1832, ii,

Morphine *and its salts.*

72-101. [*See, also, supra.*]—**Tully** (W.) Results of experiments with, and observations upon, sulphate of morphine. Boston M. & S. J., 1832-3, vii, 28-33.—**Vögen.** Endermatische Anwendung des Morphiums. Gen.-Ber. d. k. rhein. Med.-Coll. 1840, Koblenz, 1841, 55 —**Wiglesworth** (A.) On morphia as a parturifacient. Obst. J. Gr. Brit., Lond., 1877-8, v, 368-382. — **Witkowski** (L.) Ueber die Morphiumwirkung. Arch. f. exper. Path. u. Pharmakol., Leipz., 1877, vii, 247-270. ———. Zur Wirkung des Morphiums und des Chloralhydrats. Deutsche med. Wchnschr., Berl., 1879, v, 513-515. ———. Zur Morphiumwirkung. *Ibid.*, 667. — **Wormley** (T. G.) Notes on some of the chemical reactions of morphia. Ohio M. & S. J., Columbus, 1859-60, xii, 260-264. *Also:* Chem. News, Lond., 1860, ii, 137-139.— **Wyman** (M.) & **Horsford** (E. N.) On valerianate of morphia. Proc. Am. Ass. Adv. Sc. 1849, Bost., 1850, ii, 92.—**Zanetti** (G.) Uso dell' acetato di morfina nelle malattie di petto. Gazz. med. di Milano, 1845, iv, 339-341.

Morphine (*Antagonisms of*).

BAKKER NIEMEIJER (J. H.) * Over antagonisme tusschen morphine en atropine. 8°. *Gouda*, 1883.

KNAPSTEIN (A.) * Ueber die gleichzeitige Wirkung von Atropin und Morphium. 8°. *Bonn*, [1878].

———. Sind Atropin und Morphin Antidote? Neue Versuche nebst einer Abfertigung der Angriffe des Herrn Dr. Hans Heubach. 8°. *Bonn*, 1879.

KONING (I. J.) * Over de antagonistische werking van het morphium en de atropine. 8°. *Arnhem*, 1870.

Alexander (W.) Prolonged suspension of vitality through the subcutaneous injection of morphia and atropine. Med. Times & Gaz., Lond., 1883, i, 582.—**Beatty** (T. C.) Morphia an antidote to strychnine. Lancet, Lond., 1871, ii. 907.— **Bennett** (J. H.) Antagonism between tea, coffee, cocaine, theine, caffeine, and guaranine, on the one hand, and morphia on the other. Brit. M. J., Lond., 1874, ii, 615; 697; 771. — **Brouardel** (P.) & **Boutmy** (E.) De l'antagonisme de la morphine et de l'atropine. Ann. d'hyg., Par., 1881, 3. s., v, 497-505. *Also, Reprint.*—**Brown-Séquard.** Sur l'importance de l'emploi simultané de la morphine et de l'atropine dans la plupart des cas où l'on doit faire usage de l'une de ces substances. Compt. rend. Soc. de biol., Par., 1883, 7. s., iv, 289.—**Clarke** (J. M.) A case showing the antidotal effect of atropia over morphia. Med. Rec., N. Y., 1885, xxvii, 514.— **Coomes** (M. F.) Physiological research in regard to the action of morphia and atropia. Med. Herald, Louisville, 1885-6, vii, 452-455.— **Couzier.** Empoisonnement par l'atropine; traitement par la morphine en injections sous-cutanées, par le café et les révulsifs; guérison. Bull. et mém Soc. de thérap. 1875, Par., 1876, 2. s., ii, 17-20.—**Discussion** sur l'antagonisme de l'atropine et de la morphine. Ann. d'hyg., Par., 1881, 3. s., v, 172-195.— **Farnsworth** (P. J.) A case of poisoning by morphia and atropia. Iowa State M. Reporter, Des Moines, 1884-5, ii, 99.—**Haldeman** (J. S.) Report of a case showing the antidotal virtues of the Veratrum viride in morphia poisoning. Cincin. Lancet & Clinic, 1879, n. s., iii, 458.—**Hetherington** (S. M.) Case of morphia poisoning treated with atropine; recovery. Med. Press & Circ., Lond., 1878, n. s., xxvi, 22.— **Heubach** (H.) Antagonismus zwischen Morphin und Atropin. Berl. klin. Wchnschr., 1878, xv, 767-771. *Also, Reprint.*—**Joy** (D. A.) Atropia as an antidote for morphia. Physician & Surg., Ann Arbor, Mich , 1881, iii, 65.— **King** (C. F.) A case of poisoning by sulphate of morphia treated by atropia. Med. News, Phila., 1882, xl, 68.— **King** (E. W.) Attempted suicide by taking morphine and strychnine; their antagonistic action well shown. Louisville M. News, 1880, x, 160.—**Lenhartz.** Ueber den Antagonismus zwischen Morphin und Atropin vom klinischen und experimentellen Standpunkte. Deutsche med. Wchnschr., Berl., 1886, xii, 712.—**Lockridge** (J. E.) Atropia versus morphia. Indiana M. J., Indianap., 1883-4, ii, 157-160.—**Oglesby** (R. T.) On the relative effects of morphia and atropia on the temperature of the body. Practitioner, Lond., 1870, iv, 27-33.—**Reese** (J. J.) Antagonism of morphia and hydrocyanic acid. Am. J. M. Sc., Phila., 1871, n. s., lxi, 133-139.— **Shipman** (N. N.) A case of morphia poisoning treated with atropia hypodermically. Cincin. Lancet & Clinic, 1878, n. s., i, 110.—**Sircar** (J. K.) A case of morphia poisoning successfully treated with hypodermic injection of sulphate of atropia. Indian M. Gaz., Calcutta, 1879, xiv, 259. — **Smith** (J. H.) A case of morphia poisoning treated successfully by large doses of atropia. Med. News, Phila., 1882, xl, 318.— **Stuver** (E.) Poisoning by ten grains sulphate of morphia treated by sulphate of atropia; recovery. *Ibid.*, xli, 592.

Morphine (*Hypodermic use of*).

See, also, **Morphine** *habit.*

ALTVATER (P.) Die Morphium-Einspritzungen (subcutane Injectionen). Deren Wesen und Wirkung, unschädliche und schädliche Anwendung, Abminderung und Abgewöhnung; nach eigenen, in vieljährigem Selbstgebrauch gewonnenen Erfahrungen, für Jedermann fasslich dargestellt als sicherer Führer für Aerzte und Laien. 2. Aufl. 8°. *Auerbach a. B.*, 1879.

CROMBIE (J. M.) A new and easy method for the subcutaneous application of morphia, without the pain, risk, and expense of the hypodermic syringe. 8°. *London*, 1873.

HILSMANN (F. E. T.) * Ein Beitrag zur hypodermatischen Injection des Morphium. 8°. *Arnsberg*, [1874].

KANE (H. H.) The hypodermic injection of morphia; its history, advantages, and dangers. Based on the experience of 360 physicians. 12°. *New York*, 1880.

OBERPRIELER (J.) * Ueber die subcutane Anwendung des Morphium bei Anomalien der Wehenthätigkeit. 8°. *München*, 1874.

Allbutt (C.) On the abuse of hypodermic injections of morphia. Practitioner, Lond., 1870, v, 327-331.—**Anstie** (F. E.) On the effects of the prolonged use of morphia by subcutaneous injection. *Ibid.*, 1871, vi, 148-157.— **Audhoui** (V.) Note sur les injections hypodermiques de chlorhydrate de morphine. Thérap. contemp., Par., 1881, i. 534.—**Babcock** (L. F.) Cases illustrating the use of morphia hypodermically. N. York M. J., 1870, xii, 181.—**Barclay** (J.) Some cases in which the hypodermic injection of morphia was employed with good results Med. Press & Circ., Lond., 1869, n. s., viii, 433; 509.—**Barr** (D. M.) The hypodermic use of morphia. Med. & Surg. Reporter, Phila., 1879, xli, 423-426.—**Bassetti** (A.) Le iniezioni di solfato di morfina nelle malattie nervose. Gazz. med. ital. lomb., Milano, 1877, 7. s., iv, 281.—**Blackwell** (E. T.) Illustrations of the use of large hypodermics of morphine, and the dangers attending them. Phila. M. Times, 1880-81, xi, 776-778.—**Cecil** (J. G.) Acetate of morphia for hypodermic injection. Med. Herald, Louisville, 1879-80, i, 493.—**Chamberlin** (J.) Death from hypodermic injection of morphia. Canada M. J., Montreal, 1872, viii, 251-253.—**Chouppe** (H.) Note sur un accident possible à la suite des injections sous-cutanées de chlorhydrate de morphine; précautions à prendre pour l'éviter. Rev. méd. franç. et étrang., Par., 1876, i, 423-425. *Also:* Rev. méd. du midi, Montpel., 1876, ii, 27. — **Ciramelli.** Le iniezioni ipodermiche di idroclorato di morfina. Gior. internaz. d. sc. med., Napoli, 1879, n. s., i, 984-987.— **Claus.** Ueber die Verbindung der Morphiumeinspritzungen mit Atropin. Allg. Ztschr. f. Psychiat., etc., Berl., 1877, xxxiii, 529-554.—**Coggeshall** (W. H.) The hypodermic use of sulphate of morphia. Virginia M. Month., Richmond, 1883 4, x, 151-170. — **Discussion** on the effects of the hypodermic application of morphine. Bull. N. York Acad. M. (1862-6), 1866, ii, 318-321.—**Dumas** (A.) Moyen de rendre inoffensives les injections de morphine; action antiémétique de l'atropine. Bull. gén. de thérap., etc., Par., 1881, c, 534-539.—**Estlander** (I. A.) Om subkutana insprutningar af morfin vid sårros. Nord. med. Ark., Stockholm, 1871, iii, no. 4, 1-5.—**Evans** (H. Y.) The hypodermic employment of the sulphate of morphia in fifty distinct cases. Med. Times, Phila., 1870-71, i, 264.— **Evershed** (A.) On the hypodermic injection of morphia. Med. Times & Gaz., Lond., 1869, i, 463.—**Fiedler** (A.) Ueber den Missbrauch subcutaner Morphiuminjectionen. Deutsche Ztschr. f. prakt. Med., Leipz., 1874, i, 231; 239.—**Freeman** (H. W.) On the hypodermic injection of morphia. Brit. M. J., Lond., 1865, i, 639-641.— **Gibbons** (H.), sr. Hints on the hypodermic use of morphia. Pacific M. & S. J., San Fran., 1878-9, xxi, 6-8.— **Greenley** (B.) The hypodermic use of morphia as a supporter of the heart's action. South. M. Rec., Atlanta, 1879, ix, 325.—**Griffith** (G. de G.) On the hypodermic administration of morphia as a means of cure in cases of pain. Med. Press, Dubl., 1865, iv, 241.—**Hendrick** (O.) On the value of hypodermic injections of morphia in obstetric practice. Richmond & Louisville M. J , Louisville, 1869, viii, 397-399.—**Hergt.** Ueber subcutane Morphiuminjectionen. Allg. Ztschr. f. Psychiat., etc., Berl., 1876, xxxiii, 261-275.—**Jennings** (C. E.) The subcutaneous injection of morphia. Lancet, Lond., 1884, i, 562.—**Jones** (C. H.) On circumstances influencing the safety of subcutaneous injection of morphia. Tr. Clin. Soc. Lond., 1871, iv, 72-74.—**Jones** (G. E.) Some observations on the deep injections of morphia. Cincin. Lancet & Clinic, 1878, n. s., i, 85. — **Jones** (W. H.) The reckless injection of morphine hypodermically. Cincin. Lancet-Clinic, 1887, n. s., xviii, 195.—**Kormann** (E.) Die Anwendung sub-

Morphine (*Hypodermic use of*).

cutaner Morphium-Injectionen unter der Geburt und in den ersten Tagen des Wochenbettes. Monatschr. f. Geburtsk. u. Frauenkr., Berl., 1868, xxxii, 114-127.—**Kühn** (J.) Ueber subcutane Morphiuminjectionen. Ztschr. f. Med., Chir. u. Geburtsh., Leipz., 1867, n. F., vi, 453-465.—**Lafargue** (G.-V.) Lettres sur l'inoculation de la morphine avec la lancette. [Rap. de Martin-Solon.] Bull. Acad. de méd., Par., 1836, i, 13; 40: 249. ———. Dei vantaggi terapeutici dell' inoculazione della morfina e di altri medicamenti energici. Bull. d. sc. med. di Bologna, 1847, 3. s., xii, 261; 379.—**Lawson** (H.) Subcutaneous injection of morphia in the treatment of sciatica, lumbago, and brachialgia. Med. Times & Gaz., Lond., 1876, ii, 671-673.—**Lebert.** Ueber die subcutane Anwendung des Morphium's als Mittel, um die Schmerzen der Geburt und die Krampfwehen zu mildern. Berl. klin. Wchnschr., 1866, iii, 109-111.—**Levick.** [Prolonged hypodermic injections of morphia without bad effects.] Tr. Coll. Phys. Phila. (1856-62), 1863, n s., iii, 471-474.—**Levier** (E.) Osservazioni pratiche sulle iniezioni sottocutanee di morfina. Imparziale, Firenze, 1870, x, 133; 161.—**Martin** (C.) Quelques notes sur les solutions des sels de morphine pour injection hypodermique. Rec. d. trav. Soc. méd. d'Indre-et-Loire, Tours, 1874-5, lxxii, 53.—**Mengus** (J.) Quelques mots sur les injections hypodermiques de morphine et résultats inespérés obtenus dans deux cas de rhumatismes musculaires, grace à cette méthode de traitement. Abeille méd., Par., 1874, xxxi, 111.—**Moutard-Martin** & **Richet** (C.) Contribution à l'étude des injections intra-veineuses de lait et de sucre. Compt. rend. Soc. de biol. 1879, Par., 1880, 7. s., i, pt. 2, 65-80. *Also:* Gaz. méd. de Par., 1879, 6. s., i, 588; 600; 624.—**Müller.** Ueber subcutane oder hypodermatische Injection von schwefelsaurem Morphium. Cor.- Bl. f. d. Aerzte u. Apoth. d. Grossherz. Oldenburg. 1860-61, i, 249-253.—**Ogle** (W.) Injection of acetate of morphia into the cellular tissue of the arm in delirium tremens. Med. Times & Gaz., Lond., 1860, ii, 54.—**Oliver** (G.) On hypodermic injection of morphia. Practitioner, Lond., 1871, vi, 75-80. *Also:* Canada M. J., Montreal, 1872, viii, 91-96.—**Ortille.** Des bons effets obtenus par les injections hypodermiques de morphine associée à l'atropine. Bull. gén. de thérap., etc., Par., 1876, xc, 547.—**Parker** (W. W.) Subcutaneous injection of morphia in facial neuralgia and subacute rheumatism. Richmond & Louisville M. J., Louisville, 1868, v, 41-45.—**Picard** (P.) Sur les phénomènes qui suivent les injections du chlorhydrate de morphine. Gaz. méd. de Par., 1878, 4. s., vii, 143.—**Ross** (J.) The hypodermic administration of morphia. Canada M. J., Montreal, 1866, ii, 433-439.—**Santoliquido** (R.) Se le iniezioni ipodermiche di morfina hanno azione locale. Gior. internaz. d. sc. med., Napoli, 1882. n. s., iv, 1279-1300.—**Schütz.** Ueber subcutane Morphiuminjectionen. Vrtljschr. f. d. prakt. Heilk., Prag, 1874, cxxii, 103-114.—**Seguin** (E. C.) Subcutaneous use of sulphate of morphia in cases of malarial neuralgia. N. York M. J., 1867, v, 402-409.—**Sellman** (W. A. B.) The hypodermic injection of morphia. Maryland M. J., Balt.. 1881-2, viii, 79-87.—**Sleightholme** (J. P.) Hypodermic morphia in a general hospital. Practitioner, Lond., 1871, vii, 25-28.—**Sommerbrodt** (J.) Ueber hypodermatische Morphium-Injektionen. Wien. med. Presse, 1865, vi, 1113; 1142; 1165; 1187.—**Speer** (J. R.) Death from the hypodermic use of morphia. Atlanta M. & S. J., 1871-2, ix[b], 546.—**Spender** (J. K.) The hypodermic action of morphia. Brit. M. J., Lond., 1860, i, 436.—**Stuart** (J. A. E.) Tartrate of morphia as an agent for hypodermic injection. Edinb. M. J., 1878-9, xxiv, 809.—**Terson.** Des injections sous-cutanées de morphine dans les affections douloureuses des yeux. Rev. méd. de Toulouse, 1868, ii, 257-265.—**Vibert** (E.) Études pratiques sur les injections sous-cutanées de morphine. J. de thérap., Par., 1875, ii, 129; 214: 453; 577; 625; 752; 787: 1876, iii, 8.—**Warren** (E.) A lecture on the subcutaneous injection of morphia. Med. & Surg. Reporter, Phila., 1867, xvi, 101; 161.—**Weinlechner** (J.) Morphium aus Gewohnheit und in steigender Dosis bis zu 40 Gran täglich injicirt; zahllose Hautabscesse; Heilung. Ber. d. k. k. Krankenanst. Rudolph-Stiftung in Wien (1874), 1875, 524.—**Wiener** (S.) Ein Beitrag zum Missbrauche der Morphin-Injektionen. Wien. med. Presse, 1880, xxi, 432.—**Wilson** (E. T.) Notes on the subcutaneous injection of morphia. St. George's Hosp. Rep., Lond., 1869, iv, 19-30.

Morphine (*Toxicology of*).

See, also, **Morphine** (*Antagonisms of*); **Morphine** *habit*.

DALBANNE (N.) *Essai sur quelques accidents produits par la morphine. 4°. *Paris*, 1877.

KREYSSIG (C. B.) *Casus intoxicationis per morphium aceticum. 8°. *Lipsiæ*, 1855.

SAISSINEL (A.-P.) *De quelques accidents de l'emploi de la morphine. 4°. *Paris*, 1883.

Alexander (S.) Ein Fall von Morphium-Vergiftung. Wien. med. Presse, 1865, vi, 754.—**Alleged** poisoning by

30

Morphine (*Toxicology of*).

morphine. Superior court of Buffalo. Frances C. Dustin, administratrix of James E. Dustin, deceased, against Merrell Eugene Shaw, M. D. Buffalo M. & S. J., 1867-8, vii 121-129.—**Almagro** [*et al.*]. [Suspected poisoning by morphia.] Bol. de med., cirug. y farm., Madrid, 1847, 3. s., ii, 244.—**Anderson** (L. B.) Case in which unusual phenomena followed the administration of "sulphate of morphia". Am. J. M. Sc., Phila., 1848, n. s., xvi, 347.—**Anstie.** Poisoning with morphia. Med. Times & Gaz., Lond., 1863, i, 134.—**Barry** (W. M.) Poisoning by morphine; successfully treated with strychnia. Daniell's Texas M. J., Austin, 1886-7, ii, 274.—**Bayles** (G. A.) Case of poisoning by sulphate of morphia. Virginia M. Month., Richmond, 1875-6, ii, 188-194.—**Bergeron** (G.) & **L'Hote** (L.) Sur les inconvénients que présente, au point de vue des réactions physiologiques. dans les cas d'empoisonnement par la morphine, la substitution de l'alcool amylique à l'éther dans le procédé de Stas. Compt. rend. Acad. d. sc., Par., 1880, xci, 390-393.—**Binz** (C.) Ueber den arteriellen Druck bei Morphium-Vergiftung. Deutsche med. Wchnschr., Berl., 1879, v, 615; 627: 1880, vi, 149.—**Blanton** (W. H.) Was it morphia? Louisville M. News, 1883, xv, 203.—**Bonjean** (J.) Empoisonnement par une forte dose d'acétate de morphine; (guérison). J. de chim. méd., etc., Par., 1844, 2. s., x, 692-699. *Also:* Ann. d'hyg., Par., 1845, xxxiii, 150-157.—**Bossart.** Cas d'empoisonnement par le chloral et la morphine. Rev. méd. de la Suisse Rom., Genève, 1885, v, 679.—**Bourchardat.** Thérapeutique de l'empoisonnement par la morphine, et les médicaments qui en contiennent, suivie de quelques réflexions sur la recherche de la morphine dans les urines. Bull. gén. de thérap., etc., Par., 1861, lxi, 360-362.—**Cabell** (J. L.) Case of coma following the hypodermic injection of morphia in a moderate dose, and exhibiting certain peculiar characters which served to obscure the diagnosis. Richmond & Louisville M. J., Richmond, 1871, xi, 255-260.—**Caillé** (A.) Ein Fall von Morphium-Vergiftung bei einem Kinde. N. Yorker med. Presse, 1886, ii, 192.—**Carpenter** (J. G.) Three cases of morphine narcosis; recovery. St. Louis M. & S. J., 1882, xliii, 219.—**Cartaz** (A.) Un cas d'intoxication par la morphine. France méd., Par., 1878, xxv, 593. *Also:* Bull. Soc. clin. de Par. (1878), 1879, ii, 192.—**Castara** (J.-S.) Empoisonnement par l'acétate de morphine. J. de chim. méd., etc., Par., 1831, vii, 135-139.—**Chafee** (W. C.) Sixteen grains of sulphate of morphia taken at one time; recovery. Med. & Surg. Reporter, Phila., 1882, xlvii, 697.—**Comanos** (A.) Ueber eine merkwürdige, toxische Nebenwirkung des Morphium muriaticum. Berl. klin. Wchnschr., 1882, xix, 631.—**Courtenay** (J. H.) Peculiar effects produced by the administration of hydrochlorate of morphia. Brit. M. J., Lond., 1879, ii, 615.—**Davis** (J. D. S.) A case of morphia poisoning. Weekly M. Rev., Chicago, 1883, viii, 93.—**Davy** (R. B.) Case of morphia poisoning. Cincin. Lancet & Clinic, 1880, n. s., iv, 101-105.—**Dawson** (J.) Case of poisoning from the taking of nearly a drachm of morphine. Ohio M. & S. J., Columbus, 1850-51, iii, 525.—**Desportes** (E.) Recherches expérimentales sur l'empoisonnement lent par l'acétate de morphine. Rev. méd. franç. et étrang., Par., 1824, iv, 70-82.—**Dow** (T. C.) Morphia-poisoning; patient, aged four years, relieved by belladonna and electricity. Virginia M. Month., Richmond, 1877-8, iv, 670-672.—**Dragendorff** (G.) Beiträge zur gerichtlichen Chemie. IV. Ueber das Morphin. Pharm. Ztschr. f. Russland, St. Petersb., 1884, xxiii, 713-721.—**Dubay** (M.) Meghiusult önmérgezés esete 0.75 grm. morph. mur. bevétele után. [Unsuccessful attempt at suicide by taking 0.75 grm. of muriate of morphia.] Gyógyászat, Budapest, 1886, xxvi, 97-99. *Also, transl.:* Pest. med.-chir. Presse, Budapest, 1886, xxii, 277.—**Duke** (J. M.) Morphia poisoning treated by atropia. Clinic, Cincin., 1872, iii, 229.—**Egan** (C. J.) Poisoning by morphia. Med. Times & Gaz., Lond., 1876, i, 248.—**Eliot** (L.) A case of poisoning by sulphate of morphia; recovery. Med. Rec., N. Y., 1886, xxix, 555.—**Empoisonnement** d'une fille de 5 ans par le sulfate de morphine. Clin. d. hôp., Par., 1829, iv, 108.—**Everitt** (R. A.) Notes on a case of poisoning with sulphate morphia. Detroit Rev. Med. & Pharm., 1875, x, 659-661.—**Fénykövy** (A.) Zwei Fälle von Morphin-Vergiftung. Wien. med. Presse, 1883, xxiv, 208.—**Ferris** (J. S.) Anomalous symptoms in a case of morphia-poisoning. Brit. M J., Lond., 1871, ii, 555.—**Fick.** Ueber die Blutdruckschwankungen im Herzventrikel bei Morphium-Narcose. Verhandl. d. Cong. f. innere Med., Wiesb., 1886, v, 92-103.—**Fielitz.** Fahrlässige Tödtung eines Kindes durch Verwechslung von Morphium mit Calomel. Vrtljschr. f. gerichtl. Med., Berl., 1883, n. F., xxxviii, 82-87.—**Fisson.** Sur l'empoisonnement par l'acétate de morphine. Bull. Soc. de méd. de la Sarthe 1851, Le Mans, 1852. 42-44.—**Fontenelle** (J.) Empoisonnement par l'acétate de morphine. J. de chim. méd., etc., Par., 1829, v, 410-412.—**Foulke** (C.) Case of overdose of morphia during labour; unconscious delivery; recovery. Am. J. M. Sc., Phila., 1848, n. s., xv, 568.—**Fox** (T. C.) Eruption produced by morphia. Brit. M. J., Lond., 1879, i, 969.—**Frua** (C.) Un caso di avvelenamento dall' acetato di morfina guarito

Morphine (*Toxicology of*).

coll' uso di una ingente dose di infuso di caffè. Gazz. med. di Milano, 1846, v, 185.—**Haldemann** (J. S.) Morphia and its antidotes. Cincin. Lancet & Clinic, 1879, n. s., iii, 141-14:.—**Halla**. Morphium-Vergiftung. Med.-chir. Centralbl., Wien, 1878, xiii, 567.—**Harnan** (W.) A case of morphine narcosis. N. Orl. M. & S. J., 1885-6, n. s., xiii, 701.—**Heymanns**. Vergiftungszufälle durch Morphium. Wchnschr. f. d. ges. Heilk., Berl., 1837, 402.— **Hill**. Symptoms of morphine poisoning. St. Louis M. & S. J., 1881, xli, 626.—**Hill** (P. E.) A case of morphia poisoning by hypodermic injection; recovery. Lancet, Lond., 1882, ii, 527.—**Holst** (V.) Eine acute Morphium-Vergiftung. St. Petersb. med. Wchnschr., 1882, vii, 421. — **Houston** (M. H.) Speedy death from a large dose of sulphate of morphia. Am. J. M. Sc., Phila., 1843, n. s., vi, 372. — **Hudson** (A. S.) The undefined poisonous quantity of morphine. Med. & Surg. Reporter, Phila., 1881. xliv, 591-593.—**Hughes** (C. H.) [et al.]. Report of committee on the case of H. W. Hagemann, whose death had been attributed to hypodermic injection of morphia, administered by Dr. C. F. V. Ludwig. Proc. St. Louis M. Soc. Missouri, 1878, i, 156-160.— **Hull** (A. P.) Poisoning by morphia. Phila. M. Times, 1875-6, vi, 581.—**Husemann** (T.) Beiträge zur Diagnostie der acuten Vergiftung mit Morphin. Deutsche Klinik, Berl., 1874, xxvi, 5; 19; 41; 59; 73.—**Jakovski** (I. L.) Sluchai tjajelago otravl. morfiem izliech. atropin. [Serious case of poisoning by morphia cured by atropine.] Vrach, St. Petersb., 1885, vi, 733. — **Jenkins** (A. R.) Ten grains of sulphate of morphine without vomiting; recovery. Indiana M. Reporter, Evansville, 1881, ii, 201-203.—**Jones** (H. E.) A phenomenon of partial morphianarcotism. Med. Rec., N. Y., 1881, xx, 734.—**Judkins** (W.) A case of morphia poisoning in a child aged fifty hours. *Ibid.*, 1885, xxviii, 151. — **Kapff**. Chronische Morphium-Vergiftung am eigenen Leib beobachtet. Med. Cor.-Bl. d. württemb. ärztl. Ver., Stuttg., 1876, xlvi, 174-176. — **Kern** (H.) Ueber Morphium-Erythem. Wien. med. Presse, 1883, xxiv, 568.—**Kimmel** (J. A.) Recovery after taking fourteen grains of morphia. Cincin. Lancet & Clinic, 1881, n. s., vii, 308. ———. What constitutes a poisonous dose of morphine? Med. & Surg. Reporter, Phila., 1881, xliv, 611.—**Klob** (J.) Zur pathologischen Anatomie der Vergiftungen; Morphium-Vergiftung . . . Wien. med. Presse, 18..8, ix, 521; 545. — **Kobert** (E. R.) Ein Fall von Morphiumvergiftung. Allg. med. Centr.-Ztg., Berl., 1880, ii, 86.—**Kratter** (J.) Ueber einen Fall von Vergiftung durch Morphin. Mitth. d. Ver. d. Aerzte in Steiermark 1878, Graz, 1879, xv, 85.—**Krauss** (A.) Eine Morphiumvergiftung. Friedreich's Bl. f. gerichtl. Med., Nürnb., 1883, xxxix, 370-382. — **Kussmaul** (A.) Ein Fall wahrscheinlicher Morphinvergiftung. Deut-che Ztschr. f. d. Staatsarznk., Erlang., 1857, n. F. ix, 398-434.— **von Langsdorff** (T.) Fahrlässige Tödtung durch Morphium-Vergiftung. Vrtljschr. f. gerichtl. Med., Berl., 1885, n. F., xliii, 212-221.—**Lassaigne** (J.-L.) Mémoire sur la possibilité de reconnaître, par les moyens chimiques, la présence de l'acétate de morphine chez les animaux empoisonnés par cette substance vénéneuse. Rev. méd. franç. et étrang., Par., 1824, i, 96-107.—**Lemen** (L. E.) Case of attempted suicide from the ingestion of thirty-six grains of morphia, which remained in the stomach five hours; recovery. Boston M. & S. J., 1887, cxvi, 443.— **Lenhartz** (H.) Experimentelle Beiträge zur Kenntniss der acuten Morphinvergiftung und des Antagonismus zwischen Morphin und Atropin. Arch. f. exper. Path. u. Pharmakol. Leipz., 1886-7, xxii, 337-366.—**Levin** (P. A.) Morfinmissbruket och morfinförgiftning. Eira, Göteborg, 1882, vi, 712-724. — **Löwenstein** (M. G.) Elixir acidum Halleri gegen Narcosis durch Morphium. Med. Ztg. Russlands, St. Petersb., 1846, iii, 59.—**Lyon** (T.) [Eight grains of sulphate of morphine taken; recovery.] Tr. M. Soc. Penn., Phila., 1878, xii, pt. 1, 326.— **Marmé** (W.) Untersuchungen zur acuten und chronischen Morphin-Vergiftung. Deutsche med. Wchnschr., Berl., 1883, ix, 197.—**Maschka** (J.) Angebliche Vergiftung eines Kindes mit Morphium in Folge unzweckmässiger ärztlicher Ordination. Oesterr. Ztschr. f. prakt. Heilk., Wien, 1860, vi, 244-247. ——. Beitrag zur Lehre von den Vergiftungen. Vrtljschr. f. d. prakt. Heilk., Prag, 1867, xcvi, 23-25.—**Merkwürdige** Criminaluntersuchung zu Paris wegen Vergiftung mit essigsaurem Morphium. Ztschr. f. d. Staatsarznk., Erlang., 1823, vi, 473-486.—**van Minden** (J. J.) Een geval van morphinevergiftiging. Nederl. mil. geneesk. Arch., etc., Utrecht, 1879, iii, 379-382.—**Miner** (J. F.) A case of morphine poisoning apparently relieved by a'ropine. Buffalo M. & S. J., 1869-70, ix, 134-136.—**Model** (A.) Eine Morphiumvergiftung. Aerztl. Int.-Bl., München, 1871, xviii, 572.— **Morse** (G. M.) Attempted suicide from the ingestion of fifty-one grains of morphine, the greater part of which remained in the stomach thirteen hours; recovery. Boston M. & S. J., 1887, cxvi. 603.—**Nutt** (C. M.) Alarming narcosis from a small dose of morphia. Louisville M. News, 1881, xi, 267. — **Oppenheimer** (Z.) Ueber einen Fall von angeblicher Morphiumvergiftung. Deutsche Ztschr. f. d. Staatsarznk., Erlang., 1867, n. F., xxv, 341-373.—**Orfila**

Morphine (*Toxicology of*).

Observation d'empoisonnement par l'acétate de morphine. Arch. gén. de méd., Par., 1829, xx, 211-220. ———. Empoisonnement par la morphine. Ann. d'hyg., Par., 1852, xlviii, 359-369.—**Park** (R.) Some cases in which morphia has been administered in large doses hypodermically. Practitioner, Lond., 1880, xxiv, 424-433.—**Parsons** (J.) Case of fatal poisoning in an infant by sulphate of morphia, with the results of six experiments upon dogs Leavenworth M. Herald, 1867-8, i, 13-16.—**Pellacani** (P.) Singolare decorso di un avvelenamento per morfina; ricerca medico - forense. Riv. sper. di freniat., Reggio - Emilia, 1885, xi, pt. 2, 83-89.—**Pfister** (J. H.) Krankheitserscheinungen und Leichenerfund nach einer zufälligen Selbstvergiftung durch morphium-haltigen Alkohol. Schweiz. Ztschr. f. Nat.- u. Heilk., Heilbr., 1837, ii, 283 - 288. — **Picard** (P.) Sur les causes secondes des phénomènes morbides de l'empoisonnement par la morphine. Gaz. d. hôp., Par., 1880, liii, 60-62.—**Pollock** (C.) Morphia poisoning. Med. & Surg. Reporter, Phila., 1882, xlvi, 615.— **Praeger** (H.) An extraordinary case of morphia poisoning. *Ibid.*, 430.—**Prentiss** (D. W.) Case of poisoning by morphia: death. Am. J. M. Sc., Phila., 1867, n. s., liii, 562.— **Prentiss** (J. L.) Poisoning with morphine. Chicago M. J., 1866, xxiii, 559.—**Radcliffe** (S. I.) Case of poisoning by acetate of morphia, in a child aged seven months. Am. M. Month., N. Y., 1861, xvi. 410-412.—**Reamy** (T. A.) Case of fatal narcosis in an adult from one-fourth grain of morphia hypodermically. Cincin. Lancet & Clinic, 1885, n. s., xiv, 1-14. *Also:* Med. News, Phila., 1885, xlvi, 18-24.—[**Report** upon the communication of Dr. Chas. F. V. Ludwig, with accompanying affidavits respecting the death of Mr. W. H. Hageman.] St. Louis M. & S. J., 1878, xxxv, 156-160.—**Reyher** (G.) Ungewöhnliche Erscheinungen bei einem Falle von Vergiftung durch Morphin. Deutsches Arch. f. klin. Med., Leipz., 1868, iv, 602-609.—**Ribbing**. (Morfinförgiftning, idiosynkrasi.) Hygiea Stockholm, 1877, xxxix, 519-522.—**Rodzevich** (G. B. I.) Vizdorovlenie poslie otravlenija 8 granami soljanokislago morfija. [Recovery after a dose of 8 grains of acetate of morphia.] Vrach. Vaidom., St. Petersb., 1883, viii, 4162-4164. — **Salviat** (T.) Observation d'un cas d'empoisonnement par l'acétate de morphine. Union méd. de la Gironde, Bordeaux, 1859, iv. 314-316. *Also:* J. de chim. méd., etc., Par., 1859, 4. s., v, 587-591.—**Saunders** (W. H.) The Ruth-Medlicott poisoning case. Michigan Univ. M. J., Ann Arbor, 1871-2, ii, 641-652. *Also:* Chicago M. Times, 1872, iv, 19-27.—**Scheibe** (E.) Zur Reingewinnung des Morphiums bei gerichtlichen Untersuchungen. Pharm. Ztschr. f. Russland, St. Petersb., 1883, xxii, 49-51.—**Schwarz** (J.) Beitrag zur Geschichte der Morphium-Vergiftungen. Wien. med. Presse, 1865, vi, 1193.— **Schweig** (G. M.) An extraordinary case of poisoning by morphia; recovery. N. York M. J., 1874, xix, 278-281.— **Schweninger** (E.) Bemerkungen über den Morphiumtod. Deutsché med. Wchnschr., Berl., 1879, v, 436-439. *Also, in his:* Ges. Arb., 8°, Berl., 1886, i, 143-151.—**Sears** (M. H.) Morphine poisoning; the intravenous injection of milk as a treatment for acute poisoning by sulphate of morphia, with operation and notes of two cases so treated. Tr. Colorado M. Soc., Denver, 1884, 107-111.—**Selmi** (F.) Sul modo di estrarre e riconoscere la morfina nei casi di avvelenamento. Mem. Accad. d. sc. d. Ist. di Bologna, 1877, 3. s., viii, 527-556, 1 pl. *Also, transl.* [Abstr.]: Monit. scient., Par., 1878, 3. s., viii, 877-891.—**Severi** (A.) Breve osservazione sopra un caso d' avvelenamento acuto per morfina. Boll. d. Soc. tra i cult. d. sc. med. in Siena, 1884, ii, 41-43.—**Shearer** (T. W.) A case of poisoning by morphine. Iowa State M. Reporter, Des Moines, 1885-6, iii, 236.—**Shearman** (C. J.) Poisoning by morphia; a case with symptoms simulating strychnine poisoning. Med. Times & Gaz., Lond., 1857, xiv, 235.—**Shepard** (C. U.) jr. A case of morphine poisoning; suicide; discovery of the drug in the stomach and its contents; analysis by H. D. Geddings Tr. South Car. M. Ass., Charleston, 1880, xxx, 25-27.—**von Siebold** (E.) Fahrlässige Vergiftung eines neugeborenen Kindes durch Morphium. Monatschr. f. Geburtsk. u. Frauenkr., Berl., 1860, xvi, 60-64.—**Silberstein**. Ein absonderlicher Fall einer Morfiumintoxication im Verlaufe einer acuten Miliartuberkulose. Med.-chir. Centralbl, Wien, 1882, xvii, 184.—**Souchon** (E.) On relapses following recoveries from overdoses of injections of morphine. N. Orl. M. & S. J., 1886-7, n. s., xiv, 437-439.—[**Soujcou.**] Empoisonnement par quatre grammes d'acétate de morphine, suivi de guérison. Gaz. méd. de Par., 1844. 2. s., xii, 599.—**Taylor** (W. H.) A case of morphia-atropia poisoning, with an inquiry as to the antagonism of the two substances in toxic doses. Cincin. Lancet & Obs., 1875, xviii, 9-16. — **Theegarten**. Zur Casuistik der Morphiumvergiftung. Pharm. Ztschr. f. Russland, St. Petersb., 1887, xxvi, 273; 289.—**Tomlinson** (S. C.) Morphia sulph. grs. jss., swallowed by mistake by a little girl four years old; recovery. Indiana J. M., Indianap., 1871-2, ii, 121. — **Townsend** (W. E.) Large dose of morphia taken as a stimulant. Boston M. & S. J., 1860-61, lxiii, 262.—**Trask** (J. D.) Morphine-poisoning successfully treated by atropia and electricity. N. York M. J., 1874, xx, 165-175. *Also*, Reprint.—**Tup-**

Morphine (*Toxicology of*).

per (A. M.) Unusual effect of a hypodermic injection of morphia. Boston M. & S. J., 1879, ci, 619.—**Uhle** (F.) Ein Fall von akuter Morphiumvergiftung. Wien. med. Wchnschr., 1886, xxxvi, 1114-1116.—**Watkins** (C.) Case of poisoning by morphia. Richmond & Louisville M. J., Louisville, 1870, x, 453-455.—**Weickert.** Vergiftung eines 5 Tage alten Kindes durch Morphium (gr. ¼. 0,015). Jahrb. f. Kinderh., Leipz., 1868-9, n. F , ii, 445-447.—**Weist** (J. R.) A case of poisoning, by sulphate of morphia, treated by belladonna. Cincin. J. M., Indianap., 1867, ii, 265-274.—**Wertheimber** (A.) Morphiumvergiftung eines 14 Tage alten Kindes mit günstigem Ausgange. Deutsches Arch. f. klin. Med., Leipz., 1879, xxiv, 350-352.—**Wimmer.** Medicinal-Vergiftung durch essigsaures Morphium. Vrtljschr. f. gerichtl. u. öff. Med., Berl., 1868, n. F., ix, 284-298.—**Winterbotham** (L.) Case of poisoning, by a grain of acetate of morphia, in a child. Lancet, Lond., 1883, i, 8 —**Würth.** Ueber einen Fall von Morphiumvergiftung bei einem 10 Wochen alten Kinde. Deutsche Ztschr. f. d. Staatsarznk., Erlang., 1868, n. F., xxvi, 100-124. — **Zepuder** (F.) Fall von akuter Morphin-Vergiftung eines eilfwöchentlichen Kindes; Heilung. Wien. Med.-Halle, 1861, ii, 135.

Morphine *habit.*

See, also, **Opium** *habit.*

BALL (B.) The morphine habit (morphino-mania). With four lectures on the borderland of insanity; cerebral dualism; prolonged dreams; insanity in twins. Transl. from the French for the Humboldt Library. 8°. *New York*, 1887.

BROERS (J.) * Alcoholisme, morphinisme, chloralisme, op zich zelf en in verband met el-kaar beschouwd. [Leiden.] 8°. *Beverwijk*, [1886].

BURKART (R.) Die chronische Morphiumver-giftung in Folge subkutaner Morphiuminjek-tionen und deren Behandlung. 8°. *Bonn*, 1877.

Also [Rev.], *in:* Irrenfreund, Heilbr., 1877, xix, 108-112.

————. Weitere Mittheilungen über die chro-nische Morphiumvergiftung in Folge subkutaner Morphiuminjectionen und deren Behandlung. 8°. *Bonn*, 1878.

————. Die chronische Morphiumvergiftung und deren Behandlung durch allmähliche Entzie-hung des Morphium. 8°. *Bonn*, 1880.

ERLENMEYER (A.) Die Morphiumsucht und ihre Behandlung. Auf Grund eigener Beobach-tung und Erfahrung. 2. Aufl. 8°. *Leipzig u. Neuwied*, 1883.

————. The same. 3. Aufl. roy. 8°. *Berlin, Leipzig u. Neuwied*, 1887.

GAUDRY (C.) * Contribution à l'étude du mor-phinisme chronique et de la responsabilité pé-nale chez les morphinomanes. 4°. *Paris*, 1886.

JACQUET (A.-J.-B.) * De quelques accidents produits par l'abus de la morphine. 4°. *Paris*, 1882.

JOUET (D.) * Étude sur le morphinisme chro-nique. 4°. *Paris*, 1883.

LEVINSTEIN (E.) Weitere Beiträge zur Patho-logie der Morphiumsucht und der Morphiumver-giftung. Vortrag gehalten in der Berliner Ge-sellschaft am 22. November 1876. 8°. *Berlin*, 1876.

————. Die Morphiumsucht. Eine Monogra-phie nach eignen Beobachtungen. 8°. *Berlin*, 1877.

————. The same. 3. Aufl. 8°. *Berlin*, 1883.

————. The same. La morphiomanie. Mo-nographie basée sur des observations person-nelles. 8°. *Paris*, 1878.

————. The same. Morbid craving for mor-phia. Transl. by Charles Harrer. 8°. *London*, 1878.

Also [Rev.], *in:* Ugesk. f. Læger, Kjøbenh., 1877, xxiv, 1; 17.

LEVINSTEIN (W.) * Sehstörungen in Folge chronischen Gebrauchs von Chloral, Morphium und Nicotin. 8°. *Berlin*, [1883].

PONTOPPIDAN (K.) Den kroniske Morfinisme. 8°. *Kjøbenhavn*, 1883.

Morphine *habit.*

SCHMIDT (C.) Die Heilung der durch Mör-phiumgenuss verursachten Nervenzerrüttung und Willensschwäche. Eine psychologisch-me-dizinische Aufgabe. 8°. *Berlin u. Neuwied*, 1887.

STAMMLER (D.) Die Morfiumsucht und der Morfiummarasmus. 12°. *München*, 1885.

WACH (C. H. J.) * Ein Beitrag zur Patholo-gie und Therapie der chronischen Morphium-Vergiftung. 8°. *Jena*, 1880.

ZEPPENFELDT (A.) * Ueber Morphinismus. 8°. *Würzburg*, 1879.

Andrews (J. B.) Case of excessive hypodermic use of morphia; three hundred needles removed from the body of an insane woman. Am. J. Insan., Utica, N. Y., 1872-3, xxix, 13-20. *Also*, Reprint. ————. Report of two cases of morphia and cocaine habit. Tr. N. York M. Ass. 1886, Concord, N. H., 1887, iii, 68-77. — **Arima Taro.** ┼ Tokei Zasshi, Osaka, Dec. 15, 1881.—**Averbeck** (H.) Die Morphiumsucht; die akute Neurasthenie bei der plötzli-chen Entziehung des Morphium und deren allgemeine Be-deutung für die Beurteilung der Wirkung von Reiz- und Genussmitteln. Deutsche Med.-Ztg., Berl., 1887, viii, 421; 433; 443; 453; 463.—**Ball** (B.) La morphinomanie. Rev. scient., Par., 1884, xxxiii, 449: xxxiv, 1. ————. Des lésions de la morphinomanie et de la présence de la morphine dans les viscères. Bull. Acad. de méd., Par., 1887, 2. s., xviii, 525-530. — **Ball** (B.) & **Jennings** (O.) Sur certains ca-ractères du pouls chez les morphinomanes. Compt. rend. Acad. d. sc., Par., 1887, civ, 864. ————. Considéra-tions sur le traitement de la morphinomanie. Bull. Acad. de méd., Par., 1887, 3. s., xvii, 373-377. *Also:* Tribune méd., Par., 1887, xix, 159-162. *Also:* France méd., Par., 1887, i, 466-470. *Also:* Encéphale, Par., 1887, vii, 295-301.— **Boulton** (P.) An extraordinary morphia case. Lancet, Lond., 1882, i, 343.—**Braithwaite** (J.) A case in which the hypodermic injection of morphia was suddenly discon-tinued after its use daily in large doses for seven years. Ibid., 1878, ii, 874.—**Bulova.** Ein Fall von acutem Mor-phinismus. Prag. med. Wchnschr., 1879, iv, 165. — **Bur-kart** (R.) Ueber die Behandlungsmethode der chroni-schen Morphiumvergiftung. Deutsche med. Wchnschr., Berl., 1879, v, 499-501. ————. Die Behandlung der chroni-schen Morphium-Vergiftung. Wien. med. Presse, 1880, xxi, 704; 736; 803. ————. Zur Pathologie der chronischen Morphiumvergiftung; Statistik. Deutsche med. Wchn-schr., Berl., 1883, ix, 33-36. ————. Ueber Wesen und Be-handlung der chronischen Morphiumvergiftung. Samml. klin. Vortr., Leipz., 1884, No. 237 (Inn. Med., No. 83), 2159-2200. — [**Ca.**] Et Tilfælde af kronisk Morfinisme. Ugesk. f. Læger, Kj benh., 1886, 4. R., xiii, 413-421.— **Clarke** (J. St. T.) The sudden discontinuance of hypo-dermic injections of morphia after protracted use. Lancet, Lond., 1879, i, 70. ————. Treatment of the habit of in-jecting morphia by suddenly discontinuing the drug. Ibid., 1884, ii, 491.—**Cramer** (G.) Rasche Heilung von Mor-phiumsucht. Memorabilien, Heilbr., 1887, n. F., vii, 147.— **Dana** (S. W.) Delirium closely resembling mania à potu, following the free use of morphine. Med. Rec., N. Y., 1884, xxvi, 64.—**Després.** Des abcès gommeux du mor phinisme. Gaz. d. hôp., Par., 1882, lv, 1066-1069.—**Dun-can** (H. S.) The morphia habit; how is it most usually contracted, and what is the best means to diminish it? Nashville J. M. & S., 1885, n. s., xxxv, 246-248.—**Engel** (H.) Ein Beitrag zur Kenntniss der Morphiumsucht und deren Behandlung; Wirkung der Tinctura avenæ sativæ. Med.-chir. Cor.-Bl f. deutsch.-am. Aerzte, Buffalo, 1883, i, No. 8, 1-5.—**Erlenmeyer** (A.) Die Recidive der Mor-phiumsucht. Centralbl. f. Nervenh., Coblenz, 1879, ii, 505-509. ————. Ueber die Wirkung des Cocaïn bei der Morphiumentziehung. Ibid., Leipz., 1885, viii, 289-299. ————. Considérations sur la morphinomanie et son traite-ment. Encéphale, Par., 1886, vi, 677-708.—**Fischer** (A.) Ein Fall von Morphiumsucht. Wien. med. Wochnschr., 1878, xxviii, 1346.—**Folet** (H.) Morphinisme et morphio-manie. [With discussion.] Bull.-méd. du nord, Lille, 1878, xviii, 197-223.—**Gans** (E.) Ein Fall von Morphinismus chronicus geheilt durch langsame Entziehung des Mor-phin. Centralbl. f. d. ges. Therap., Wien, 1883, i, 219-224.—**Garnier** (P.) Morphinisme avec attaques hystéro-épileptiques causées par l'abstinence de la dose habituelle du poison; vol à l'étalage. Rapport médico-légal. Ann. d'hyg., Par., 1886, 3. s., xv, 302-316. ————. De l'état mental et de la responsabilité pénale dans le morphinisme chro-nique. Ann. méd.-psych., Par., 1886, 7. s., iii, 351-378.— [**Georgantes** (A.)] Μορφινομανία. Γαληνός, Ἀθῆναι, 1885, II′, 25; 42; 54; 81; 205; 236.—**Gerne** (P.) Des usages et de l'abus de la morphine. Concours méd., Par, 1882, iv, 450; 482.—**Gibbons** (H.) Letheomania; the result of the hypodermic injection of morphia. Pacific M. & S. J., San Fran., 1869-70, xii, 481-495. *Also:* Oregon M. & S. Reporter, Salem, 1869-70, i, 207-214. *Also*, Reprint.— **Gossmann** (J.) Ueber chronischen Morphiummiss-brauch. Deutsche med. Wchnschr., Berl., 1879, v, 431;

Morphine habit.

450; 463.—**Grasset** (J.) Traitement du morphinisme chronique et de la morphinomanie. Semaine méd., Par., 1885, v, 75.—**Grilli.** Il morfinismo. Imparziale, Firenze, 1881, xxi, 166-173.—**Güntz** (J. E.) Ueber Morphinismus. Memorabilien, Heilbr., 1879, xxiv, 534-544.—**H.** (J. T.) The abuse of morphia. Guy's Hosp. Gaz., Lond., 1878, n. s., iii, 130: 1879, n. s., iv, 8.—**Harrington** (Harriet L.) Case of enteritis complicated with the morphia habit. Physician & Surg., Ann Arbor, Mich., 1884, vi, 20-23.—**Hinkley** (L. S.) A remarkable case of the excessive use of morphine. N. York M. J., 1884, xxxix, 354.—**Jablonowski** (W.) Morfinizm. Przegl. lek., Krakow., 1883, xxii, 465-467.—**Jaeckel.** Zur Behandlung der Morphiumsucht mittelst Cocain. Deutsche Med.-Ztg., Berl., 1885, ii, 913-915.—**Jammes** (L.) Quelques cas de morphinomanie chez les animaux. Compt. rend. Acad. d. sc., Par., 1887, civ, 1195.—**Jennings** (O.) Sur un nouveau mode de traitement de la morphinomanie. Encéphale, Par., 1887. vii, 198-221. Also, Reprint. ———. Sur l'arrêt (inhibition) du besoin de la morphine par la nitro-glycérine associée à la spartéine. Tribune méd., Par., 1887, xix, 303-308. Also, transl.: Lancet, Lond., 1887, i, 1278-1280.—**Johansen** (J. P. G.) Et Tilfælde af kronisk Morfinisme, behandlet med Hypnotisme. Ugesk. f. Læger, Kjøbenh., 1887, 4. R., xvi, 1-6.—**Josselyn** (E. E.) An analysis of twelve cases of the morphia habit. Med. Reg., Phila, 1887, i, 195-198.—**Kaczorowski.** Pryczynek do leczenia morfinizmu. [Contribution to treatment of morphinism.] Medycyna, Warszawa, 1887, xv, 453; 474.—**Kane** (H. H.) Rapid and easy cure of a case of morphine habit of twelve years' standing; amount used, sixteen grains per day. Med. & Surg. Reporter, Phila., 1881, xliv, 649-652. Also: N. Orl. M. & S. J., 1881, n. s., ix, 103-108. ———. Some medico-legal aspects of morphia-taking; with special reference to "the Lamson case". Alienist & Neurol., St. Louis, 1882, iii, 419-433.—**Krage** (W.) Zum chronischen Morphium-Missbrauch. Deutsche med. Wchnschr., Berl., 1879, v, 487.—**Kunz.** Die Morphiumsucht vor Gericht. Aerztl. Int.-Bl., München, 1880, xxvii, 25.—**Lancereaux.** Du morphinisme chronique. Semaine méd., Par., 1884, 2. s., iv, 233. ———. Du morphinisme chronique. Union méd., Par., 1887, 3. s., xliii, 61; 74.—**Landowski** (P.) Le morphinisme et son traitement. J. de thérap., Par., 1882, ix, 164-178.—**Langer** (L.) Morphinismus. Med. Jahrb., Wien, 1881, xi, 480.—**Levinstein** (E.) Die Morphiumsucht. Tagebl. d. Versamml. deutsch. Naturf. u. Aerzte, Graz, 1875, xlviii, 66-68. ———. Die Morphiumsucht. Berl. klin. Wchnschr., 1875, xii, 646-649. Also: Verhandl. d. Berl. med. Gesellsch. 1875-6, vii, pt. 2, 14-23. Also, transl.: Bull. gén. de thérap., etc., Par., 1876, xc, 348-356. Also, transl.: Lond. M. Rec., 1876, iv, 55. ———. Zur Pathologie, Therapie, Statistik, Prognose und gerichtsärztlichen Bedeutung der Morphiumsucht. Berl. klin. Wchnschr., 1880, xvii, 73-77. Also: Verhandl. d. Berl. med Gesellsch. (1879-80), 1881, xi, pt. 2. 72-85. Also: Allg. med. Centr.-Ztg., Berl., 1880, xlix, 318. Also: Med.-chir. Centralbl., Wien, 1880, xv, 295; 309; 332; 344. Also, transl.: St. Louis Cour. Med., 1880, iii, 452-462.—**Levinstein** (W.) Frühzeitige Atrophie des gesammten Genitalapparates in einem Fall von Morphiummissbrauch. Centralbl. f. Gynäk., Leipz., 1887, xi, 633-639.—**Loose** (A.) The rapid spread of the morphia habit (by subcutaneous injection) in Germany; a village of morphia takers. [Transl. by H. H. Kane.] Maryland M. J., Balt., 1881-2, viii, 337-341.—**Loveland** (J. A.) Morphia habit. Boston M. & S. J., 1881, civ, 301.—**Lussana** (F.) Un caso di morfinismo cronico e relative questioni proposte. Riv. di chim. med. e farm., Torino, 1884, ii, 446-448.—**Lutaud.** Des troubles fonctionnels de l'utérus dans la morphinomanie; indications thérapeutiques. Union méd., Par., 1887, 3. s., xliii, 984-988. Also: Arch. de tocol., Par., 1887, xiv, 644-650.—**Lyman.** Morphia habit. Extr. Rec. Bost. Soc. M. Improve. (1874-9), 1880, vii, 106-108.—**Marandon de Montyel.** Contribution à l'étude de la morphinomanie. Ann. méd.-psych., Par., 1885, 7. s., i, 45-64.—**Marmé** (W.) Ueber die sog. Abstinenzerscheinungen bei Morphinisten. Centralbl. f. klin. Med., Leipz., 1883, iv, 241.—**Meine** Heilung vom Morphinismus. Berl. klin. Wchnschr., 1887, xxiv, 102.—**Møller** (O. S.) Anledning af "Et Tilfælde af kronisk Morfinisme". Hosp.-Tid., Kjøbenh., 1886, 3. R., iv, 1206-1210. [See, also, infra, Petræus.]—**Morphiumsucht** (Die) Gesundheit, Frankf. a. M., 1880, v, 202-206.—**Motet.** Morphinomanie. Ann. d'hyg., Par., 1883, 3. s., x, 22-36. ———. Rapport médico-légal sur Annette G . . . (hystérie et morphiomanie). Arch. de neurol., Par., 1886, xi, 398-405.—**Müller** (F.) Ueber Morphinismus. Wien. med. Presse, 1880, xxi, 297; 332; 361.—**Nankivell** (J. H.) Case of a morphia habitué said to have taken daily forty grains of morphia hypodermically; temporary abstention; relapse; death. Lancet, Lond., 1884, ii, 913.—**Nothnagel** (H.) Morphinismus. Allg. Wien. med. Ztg., 1884, xxix. 368.—**Notta** (M.) La morphine et la morphiomanie. Arch. gén. de méd., Par., 1884, ii, 385; 561. ———. De la recherche de la morphine dans l'urine des morphiomanes. Union méd., Par., 1884, 3. s., xxxviii, 409-413.—**Obersteiner** (H.) Chronic morphinism. Brain, Lond., 1879-80, ii, 449-465.

Morphine habit.

———. Further observations on chronic morphinism. Ibid., 1882-3, v, 324-331. ———. Der chronische Morphinismus. Wien. Klinik, 1883, ix, 61-84. ———. Die Morphiumsucht und ihre Behandlung. Cong. périod. internat. d. sc. méd. Compt.-rend. 1884. Copenh., 1886. Sect. de psychiat. et névrol., iii, 10-14. ———. Olvera (J.) ¿Los morfomaniáticos son aptos para ciertas acciones civiles? ¿Son responsables de sus actos? Gac. méd., Méjico, 1886, xxi, 205-210.—**Otis** (R. M.) Prolonged use of hypodermic injections of morphine. Boston M. & S. J., 1872, lxxxvi, 231.—**Papin** (T. L.) Morphia and the morphia habit. St. Louis Cour. Med., 1883, ix, 18-23.—**Peeters** (J.-A.) Du morphinisme. Bull. Soc. de méd. ment. de Belg., Gand, 1883, no. 31, 54: 1884, no. 32, 19.—**Petit** (L.-H.) Des accidents qui peuvent survenir chez les morphiomanes; morphinisme et traumatisme. Bull. gén. de thérap., etc., Par., 1879, xcvi, 119: 171; 212; 262: 318; 362; 412; 453.—**Petræus.** Et Tilfælde af kronisk Morfinisme. Hosp.-Tid., Kjøbenh., 1886, 3. R., iv, 1141-1147. [See, also, supra, Møller.]—**Pichon** (G.) Considérations sur la morphinomanie et sur son traitement. Encéphale, Par., 1886, vi, 307-335.—**Pilliet.** Note sur les lésions histologiques de l'intoxication morphinique subaigüe. Compt. rend. Soc. de biol., Par., 1887, 8. s., iv, 586-588.—**Rambaud** (L.) Morphine et morphiomanes. [Résumé.] Par., 1884, no. 42, 3; no. 43, 5; no. 46, 4; no. 49, 3; no. 51, 2; no. 52, 2.—**Rank** (C.) Ueber die Bedeutung des Cocains bei der Morphiumentziehung. Med. Cor.-Bl. d. württemb. ärztl. Ver., Stuttg., 1885, lv, 169-173.—**Read** (A. N.) Morphinism and alcoholism treated with cocaine. Gaillard's M. J., N. Y., 1886, xli, 369.—**Regnard** (P.) Deux poisons à la mode: la morphine et l'éther. Rev. scient., Par., 1885, xxxv, 545-556.—**Richardson** (B. W.) Morphia habitués and their treatment. Asclepiad, Lond., 1884, i, 1-31. Also [Abstr.]: Lancet, Lond., 1883, ii, 1046. ———. Discovery of morphine in the urine of a morphine habitué. Asclepiad, Lond., 1884, i, 356-358.—**Ricklin** (E.) Le morphinisme. Gaz. méd. de Par., 1880, 6. s., ii, 387; 403.—**Rizat** (A.) Morphinomanie; rétrécissement spasmodique du canal de l'urèthre. Encéphale, Par., 1883, iii, 344-352.—**Rochard.** Rapport sur un mémoire du docteur Combes, concernant les altérations dentaires chez les morphinomanes. Bull. Acad. de méd., Par., 1885, 2. s., xiv, 585-588.—**Sanchez** (F. I.) Apuntes sobre la morfiomania. Tésis inaugural. [Résumé.] Rev. méd.-quir. de México, 1883, i, 39.—**Schmidbauer** (J.) Ueber den Einfluss des Morphinismus auf die civil- und strafrechtliche Zurechnungsfähigkeit. Friedreich's Bl. f. gerichtl. Med., Nürnb., 1886, xxxvii, 377-397.—**Sharkey** (S. J.) The treatment of morphia habitués by suddenly discontinuing the drug. Lancet, Lond, 1883, ii, 1120.—**da Silva Lima** (J. F.) Morphinomania por abuso das injecções hypodermicas. Gaz. med. de Bahia. 1879, 2. s., iv, 297-310.—**Smidt** (H.) Zur Kenntniss der Morphinismuspsychosen. Arch. f. Psychiat., Berl., 1886, xvii, 257-273.—**Smidt** (H.) & **Rank** (C.) Ueber die Bedeutung des Cocain bei der Morphiumentziehung. Berl. klin. Wchnschr., 1885, xxii. 592-596.—**Stécoulis** (C.) Deux cas de morphiomanie. Gaz. méd. d'Orient, Constantinople, 1881-2, xxiv, 115-120.—**Strahan** (S. A. K.) Treatment of morphia habitués by suddenly discontinuing the drug. Lancet, Lond., 1884, i, 561.—**Thaon.** Abus des injections de morphine; leur efficacité dans la phthisie avancée. Nice-méd., 1876, i, 24-27.—**Thomsen** (R.) Zur Casuistik combinirten Morphium-Cocain-Psychosen. Charité-Ann. 1885-6, Berl., 1887, xii, 405-420.—**Voisin** (A.) Traitement et guérison d'une morphinomane par la suggestion hypnotique. Rev. de l'hypnot. expér. et thérap., Par., 1886, i, 161-163. Also. Reprint.—**Wallé.** Die Morphiumsucht und die Physiologie der Heilungsvorgänge; auf Grund neuester Beobachtungen dargestellt. Deutsche Med.-Ztg., Berl., 1885, i, 469; 481; 493. Also, Reprint.—**Zampakos** (D.) Περὶ μορφινισμοῦ, ἢ τῆς διὰ μορφίνης χρονίας δηλητηριάσεως. Πρακτ. Συνόδου Ἑλλήνων ἰατρῶν, Ἀθήνησιν, 1882, 46-60. Also, transl.: Encéphale, Par., 1882, ii, 413; 603. Also, Reprint. ———. Contribution à l'étude de la morphéomanie. Encéphale, Par., 1884, iv, 658-683.

Morphinism.

See **Morphine** habit.

Morphiomania.

See **Morphine** habit.

Morphœa.

See, also, **Keloid**; **Vitiligo**.

PAUTRY (H.) *Essai sur la morphœa alba (variété de lésion trophique de la peau). [Paris] 4°. Châteauroux, 1883.

Abbe (R.) Case of morphœa. Arch. Dermat., Phila., 1880, vi, 143.—**Baker** (W. M.) Morphœa, or circumscribed scleroderma, affecting the left side of the face and scalp. Tr. Path. Soc. Lond., 1876-7, xxviii, 245.—**Baptista** (J.) Extracto de huma memoria inedita, existente no Arch. da Soc. das sc. med. de Lisb., sobre a morfea de Lafões. J. Soc. d. sc. med. de Lisb., 1838, vii, 260-264.—

Morphœa.

Bronco (J. M. A.) jr. Ensalos com assucú no tratamento da morphea no Hospital de S. Lazaro. *Ibid.*, 1851, 2. s., ix, 228–236. — **Bulkley** (L. D.) Two cases of morphœa, with remarks on the disease and its differential diagnosis. Arch. Dermat., N. Y., 1876–7, iii, 100–105. *Also*, Reprint. ——. Case of morphœa. Arch. Dermat., Phila., 1880, vi, 144. — **Cattaneo** (A.) Fitopatologia; sui microfiti che producono la malattia delle piante, volgarmente conosciuta col nome di nero, fumago o morfea. R. Ist. Lomb. di sc. e lett. Rendic., Milano, 1877, 2. s., x, 513–520. — **Crocker** (H. R.) The histology and pathology of morphœa and its relation to scleroderma adultorum. Tr. Path. Soc. Lond., 1879–80, xxxi, 315–322. *Also* [Abstr.]: Lancet, Lond., 1879, ii, 692. *Also* [Abstr.]: Brit. M. J., Lond., 1879, ii, 736. *Also* [Abstr.]: Med. Times & Gaz., Lond., 1879, ii, 570. *Also* [Abstr.]: Arch. Dermat., Phila., 1880, vi, 54–56. ——. A case of morphœa with raised patches arranged in the course of nerves. Tr. Clin. Soc. Lond., 1880, xiii, 116. — **Duckworth** (D.) A case of morphœa. *Ibid.*, 1876, ix, 78–80. — **Foster.** Morphœa, or scleroderma. Arch. Dermat., Phila., 1879, v, 54–56. — **Fox** (T.) Morphœa alba, and its treatment. Lancet, Lond., 1874, ii, 510. ——. Clinical lecture on morphœa ("Addison's keloid"). Lancet, Lond., 1876, i, 843–845. — **Fox** (T.) & **Farquhar** (T.) On morphœa. *In their*: On certain endemic skin and other diseases of India [etc.], 8°, Lond., 1876, 1 (app.); 3; 37. — **Gaskoin** (G.) On morphœa alba or leuce, with cases. Brit. M. J., Lond., 1877, i, 425. *Also*: Proc. Roy. M. & Chir. Soc. Lond. (1875–80). 1880, viii, 221. ——. A case of morphœa. Med.-Chir. Tr., Lond., 1879, lxii, 169–175. — **Graham** (J. E.) Case of morphœa. Arch. Dermat., Phila., 1880, vi, 140. — **Hutchinson** (J.) Morphœa, taking the arrangement of zoster on chest and arm, twenty years' duration; recent single patch on back. Brit. M. J., Lond., 1886, ii, 149. — **Jamieson** (W. A.) Morphœa affecting large areas of trunk and limbs; cure. Edinb. M. J., 1879–80, xxv, 648. ——. Case of morphœa associated with alopecia areata. Arch. Dermat., N. Y., 1881, vii, 141–143. — **Lallemand.** Einiges über die Morpheia in Rio de Janeiro. Schmidt's Jahrb., Leipz., 1849, lxiv, 90–105. — **Mackenzie** (S.) A case of symmetrical morphœa, associated with alopecia areata. Tr. Clin. Soc. Lond., 1886, xix, 308–310. — **de Magalhães** (J. L.) A morphéa no Brazil, especialmente na provincia de S. Paulo. Rio de Jan., 1882. [Rev.] Gaz. med. da Bahia, 1883–4, 3. s., i, 12; 122; 280; 358; 497; 557. — **Molinari** (G. B.) Di un caso clinico di morfea alba. Gazz. med. ital. lomb., Milano, 1877, 7. s., iv, 301. — **Morrow** (P. A.) Case of morphœa. Arch. Dermat., Phila., 1879, v, 158. [Discussion], 266. *Also, in*: Gibney (V. P.) A case of scleroderma, vel morphœa, 8°, [N. Y., 1879], 5. — **Nettleship** (E.) & **Higgens** (C.) A case of morphœa in the region of the first and second divisions of the fifth nerve, with paralysis of the intra-ocular branches of the third nerve. Tr. Clin. Soc. Lond., 1882–3, xvi, 199–202. *Also*: Lancet, Lond., 1883, i, 867. *Also*: Brit. M. J., Lond., 1883, i, 961. — **Ramos** filho. Do tratamento da morphéa. Rev. med., Rio de Jan., 1874–6, ii, 54–58. — **Robinson** (A. R.) Case of morphœa. Arch. Dermat., Phila., 1880, vi, 142. — **Sangster** (A.) Notes on a case of morphœa. Med. Times & Gaz., Lond., 1879, ii, 340. — **Startin** (J.) Morphœa alba. Tr. Path. Soc. Lond., 1881–2, xxxiii, 384. — **Stowers** (J. H.) Case of morphœa alba. Brit. M. J., Lond., 1874, ii, 517. — **Streatfeild** (J. F.) & **Hutchinson.** A case of unilateral morphœa, with exostoses and corneal opacity; with remarks. Tr. Clin. Soc. Lond., 1880, xiii, 362–365. *Also*: Med. Press & Circ., Lond., 1880, n. s., xxix, 456. *Also*: Med. Times & Gaz., Lond., 1880, i, 703.

Morphologisches Jahrbuch. Eine Zeitschrift für Anatomie und Entwickelungsgeschichte. Hrsg. von Carl Gegenbaur. [Quarterly.] v. 1–13, 1875–87. 8°. *Leipzig, W. Engelmann*. Current.

Morphology.

See, also, Anatomy; Biology; Extremities; Function; Histology.

BEITRÄGE zur Morphologie und Morphogenie. Untersuchungen aus dem anatomischen Institut zu Erlangen. Hrsg. von Leo Gerlach. 1., 1883. 4°. *Stuttgart*, 1884.

BONDESEN (V.) Hvilken er den almindelige Plan for Bygningen af Ledene i det menneskelige Legeme; og i hvilke Hovedretninger forekommer denne Plan modificeret i det Enkelte. [What is the general plan in structure of limbs in the human body, and in which of them is this plan modified individually?] 12°. *Kjøbenhavn*, 1846.

CARUS (J. V.) System der thierischen Morphologie. 8°. *Leipzig*, 1853.

CLINE (H.) On the form of animals. 12°. *Northampton, [n. d.]*

CORNAY (J.-E.) Éléments de morphologie humaine. Première partie, physionomie de relation. Localisation physionomique des plis faciaux représentatifs des différents actes de relation. Seconde partie, physionomie naturelle, genèse des formes et loi d'ordre universel. Troisième partie, physionomie anormale, appréciation des lois, des théories, des faits, pour servir à l'étude des races. 8°. *Paris*, 1847–50.

FREITAG (J.) Disputatio medico-philosophica de formarum origine, quam adversus venerandæ antiquitati repugnantem neotericorum doctrinam auditoribus suis exhibet . . . defendente eam Henrico Welman. 12°. *Groningæ*, 1633.

GOODSIR. Detailed abstracts of papers on: 1. The morphological relations of the nervous systems in the annulose and vertebrate types of organization. 2. The morphological constitution of the skeleton of the vertebrate head. 3. The morphological constitution of limbs. Communicated to the Cheltenham meeting of the British Association, August, 1856. 8°. [*Edinburgh*, 1857.] *Repr. from:* Edinb. N. Phil. J., 1857, n. s., v.

HASSE (C.) Die Beziehungen der Morphologie zur Heilkunde. 8°. *Leipzig*, 1879.

HENLE (J.) Allgemeine Anatomie. Lehre von den Mischungs- und Formbestandtheilen des menschlichen Körpers. 8°. *Leipzig*, 1841.

VON KÖLLIKER (A.) Der jetzige Stand der morphologischen Disciplinen mit Bezug auf allgemeine Fragen. Rede des Vorsitzenden der anatomischen Gesellschaft, gehalten bei Eröffnung der ersten Versammlung in Leipzig am 14. April 1887. 8°. *Jena*, 1887.

NOVAG (L.) Grundsätze der physischen Erziehung des Menschen. 2. Aufl. 8°. *Wien*, 1842.

OGER (L.) *Considérations physiologiques sur la forme naturelle et la forme apparente de quelques organes et en particulier sur la forme naturelle et la form apparente des artères. 4°. *Strasbourg*, 1870.

REEVES (H. A.) Human morphology; a treatise on practical and applied anatomy. v. 1. The limbs and the perinæum. 8°. *London*, 1882.

REINKE (J.) Morphologische Abhandlungen. 8°. *Leipzig*, 1873.

SCHMIDT (J. H.) Zwölf Bücher über Morphologie überhaupt und vergleichende Noso-Morphologie insbesondere. 2 v. in 1, 8°; atlas, fol. *Berlin*, 1831.

SUCCOW (G.) *De morphologiæ legibus cum stœchiologiæ principiis accurate comparandis. 8°. *Jervæ*, [1829].

WIEDERSHEIM (R.) Morphologische Studien. Heft 1. 8°. *Jena*, 1880.

Addison (W.) The law of morphology, or metamorphosis of the textures of the human body. Prov. M. & S. J., Lond., 1847, 33; 60; 90; 116; 169; 199; 229; 259; 313; 340; 505. — **Collingwood** (C.) On homomorphism; or, organic representative form. Proc. Lit. & Phil. Soc. Liverp., 1860, xiv, 181–216. — **García** (S. M.) Estudio morfológico del hombre comparado con los monos. Mem. Soc. anat. españ., Madrid, 1875, iii, 141–164. — **Geddes** (P.) Entwickelung und Aufgabe der Morphologie. Jenaische Ztschr. f. Naturw., Jena, 1884, n. F., xi. 1–39. — **Gegenbaur** (C.) Die Stellung und Bedeutung der Morphologie. Morphol. Jahrb., Leipz., 1875, i, 1–19. — **de Giovanni** (A.) Studi morfologici sul corpo umano, a contribuzione della clinica. Gazz. med. ital, prov. venete, Padova, 1884, xxvii, 37; 81; 100; 138. *Also* [Abstr.]: Arch. clin. ital., Roma, 1884, xiv, 154–157. — **Hinton** (J.) On physical morphology, or the laws of organic form. Brit. & For. M.-Chir. Rev., Lond., 1858, xxii, 482–495. — **Langer** (C.) Ueber Form- und Maassverhältnisse des Körpers. Wien. med. Wchnschr., 1880, xxx, 1357; 1392; 1881, xxxi, 673; 703. — **Maggi** (L.) Applicazione di alcuni concetti morfologici dell' organizzazione animale alla medicina.

Morphology.

Gazz. med. ital. lomb., Milano, 1883, 8. s., v, 277–281.—**Parker** (W. K.) What is morphology? Nature, Lond. & N. Y., 1878, xviii, 255–257. *Also*: Pop. Sc. Month. Suppl., N. Y., 1878, 357–360. *Also, transl.*: Rev. internat. d. sc, Par., 1879, iii, 24–32.—**Recent** morphological speculations. I. On alternation of generations. II. The origin of vertebrates. III. Non-segmented animals. Nature, Lond., 1884, xxx, 67; 225; 308.—**Roux** (W.) Beiträge zur Morphologie der functionellen Anpassung. 2. Ueber die Selbstregulation der morphologischen Länge der Skeletmuskeln. Jenaische Ztschr. f. Naturw , Jena, 1883. n. F., ix. 358–427. ——. Beiträge zur Morphologie der functionellen Anpassung. Arch. f. Anat. u. Entwcklngsgesch., Leipz., 1883, 76, 1 pl.: 1885, 120.—**Sedgwick** (A.) On the origin of metameric segmentation and some other morphological questions. Quart. J. Micr. Sc., Lond., 1884, n. s., xxiv, 43–82, 2 pl.

Morpurgo (Victor) [–1856].
See **Clairat** & **Morpurgo** (Victor). Cas d'abcès par congestion avec carie, etc. 8°. *Paris*, 1839.

Morra (Joseph). * I. De fluxu lochiali, etc. 15 pp. 4°. *Augustæ Taurinorum, V. Bianco*, [1818]. [P., v. 944.]

Morra (Vincent). Du croup laryngien et de son identité avec la diphtérite. 29 pp. 8°. *Naples, Rinaldi & Sellitto*, 1880.

Morrell (G. Herbert). Supplement to the anatomy of the mammalia, containing dissections of sheep's heart and brain, rat, sheep's head, and ox's eye. pp. 153–269, 1 tab. 8°. *London, Longman & Co.*, 1872.

Morrell (J. Conyers). The sanitary question and treatment of town's refuse. 24 pp. 8°. *Manchester, J. Heywood*, 1868. [*Also, in*: P., v. 1432.]

——. The high death rate. An answer to the question "What is to be done?" Being the substance of a paper read before the Manchester and Salford Sanitary Association, March 19, 1869. 19 pp., 2 pl. 12°. *Manchester, Powlson & Sons*, 1869.

Morrell (Robert). * On animal heat. 30 pp. 8°. *New York, T. & J. Swords*, 1810.

Morren (Carolus Franciscus Antonius). Specimen academicum exhibens tentamen biozoogeniæ generalis, quo continentur leges primitivæ apparitionis entium organicorum ad superficiem telluris, eorumque speciei propagationis per generationem, novæ inquisitiones de modo quo producuntur entozoa intestinalia et spadspermoes, quo vero propagantur infusoria, vegetabiliaque microscopica. 1 p. l., 35 pp., 1 l. 4°. *Bruxellis, H. Remy*, 1829.

Morren (Petrus Jacobus). * De pertussi. 26 pp. 4°. *Heidelbergæ, J. M. Gutmann*, 1823.

Morrhua.

DYCE (R.) On the identity of Morrhua punctata and Morrhua vulgaris. 8°. [*London*, 1860.]
Repr. from: Ann. & Mag. Nat. Hist., Lond., 1860, 3. s., v, 366–369, 2 pl.

Morrhuol.

CHAZEAUD (E.) * Études cliniques sur le morrhuol (extrait de l'huile de foie de morue brune). 4°. *Paris*, 1887.
Lafage (J.) Du morrhuol, ou principe actif de l'huile de foie de morue. Bull. gén. de thérap., etc., Par., 1885, cix. 417–419.

Morries (John Davie). Observations on the chemical and physiological properties of the empyreumatic oils of foxglove, henbane and tobacco. 7 pp. 8°. *Edinburgh, J. Stark*, [*n. d.*]
Repr. from: Edinb. M. & S. J., 1833, xl.

Morrill (F. Gordon). A case of typhlitis, with some statistics of the disease. 5 pp. 8°. *Cambridge, Riverside Press*, 1875.
Repr. from: Boston M. & S. J., 1875, xciii.

Morrill (Frederic). The gentleman's medical adviser, and sure guide to health and long life. Designed to illustrate the author's new system of botanical practice in the cure of all diseases

Morrill (Frederic)—continued.
incident to exposure, early indiscretions, etc. 80 pp. 24°. *Boston, Mass.*, 1869.

Morrill (G. H.)
Co-Editor of: **Western** (The) Homœopathic Observer, St. Louis, 1868–70.

Morrill (S. E.) A treatise of practical instructions in the medical and surgical uses of electricity, including instructions in electrical diagnosing and a new method of general and local electrization. Also clinical experiences of fifteen years. x, 11–249 pp., 2 l. 8°. *Kalamazoo*, 1882
Also, Editor of: **World's** Electropathic Journal, Three Rivers, Mich., 1885.

Morris, *Illinois*.

Armstrong (P. A.) Sanitary survey of Morris. Rep Bd. Health Illinois 1885, Springfield, 1886, viii, 199–208.

Morris (Albert J. T.) A treatise on meteorology; the barometer, thermometer, hygrometer rain-gauge, and ozonometer; with rules and regulations to be observed for their correct use To which are appended some of the latest discoveries and theories of scientific men respecting various solar and terrestrial phenomena. viii, 98 pp. 12°. *Edinburgh, R. Grant & Son*, 1866.

Morris (Beverly R.) Observations on the construction of hospitals for the insane. 18 pp. 8° *London, H. Renshaw*, 1844.
Repr. from: Yorkshire Gazette.

Morris (Caspar) [1806–84]. Appeal on behalf of the sick. 48 pp. 8°. *Philadelphia, Lindsay & Blakiston*, 1851.

——. Lectures on scarlet fever. 2 p. l., 104 pp. 8°. *Philadelphia, Lindsay & Blakiston*, 1851.

——. An essay on the pathology and therapeutics of scarlet fever. 192 pp. 8°. *Philadelphia Lindsay & Blakiston*, 1858.

——. Hospital construction and organization. *In*: HOSPITAL plans. Johns Hopkins Hospital, Baltmore. 8°. New York, 1875, 172–268, 3 pl.
For Biography, see Med. & Surg. Reporter, Phila., 1884 l, 416.

Morris (Charles). * On the Prunus virginiana commonly known in the United States by the name of wild cherry-tree. 45 pp. 8°. *Philadelphia, J. Geyer*, 1802.

Morris (Corbyn).
See **Collection** (A) of the yearly bills of mortality from 1657 to 1758 inclusive. 4°. London, 1759.

Morris (Edward). Water-lords tyranny, espionage, and imposition on the city, and the doing of the magistrates court, exposed. 30 pp. 12° [*York*, 1854?]

Morris (Edwin). Fibro-cellular tumour of the right labium pudendum successfully removed 4 pp. 8°. [*n. p.*, 1858.] [P., v. 725.]

——. A practical treatise on shock after surgical operations and injuries; with especial reference to shock caused by railway accidents. vi 88 pp. 8°. *London, R. Hardwicke*, 1867.

Morris (Henricus Sutherland). * Diss. exhibens casum singularem morbi medullæ spinalis et gangliorum nervorum spinalium, cum adnotationibus. 35 pp. 4°. *Bonnæ, typog. Thormanniana* [1827].

Morris (Henry) [1844–]. Surgical disease of the kidney. viii, 548 pp., 6 pl. 16°. *London Cassell & Co.*, 1885.

Morris (J. Cheston).
See **Lehmann** (C. G.) Manual of chemical physiolog [etc.] 8°. *Philadelphia*, 1856.

Morris (Jacobus Maury). * De cynanche maligna. 1 p. l., 26 pp. 8°. *Edinburgi, J. Ballantyne*, 1805.

Morris (James). Germinal matter and the contact theory. 23 pp. 8°. *London, J. Churchill & Sons*, 1867.

——. The same. An essay on the morbid poisons, their nature, sources, effects, migration

Morris (James)—continued.
and the means of limiting their noxious agency.
2. ed. viii, 111 pp. 8°. *London, J. Churchill,*
1867.

———. Irritability; popular and practical sketches
of common morbid states, and conditions bordering on disease, with hints for management, alleviation, and cure. xi, 114 pp. 8°. *London,*
J. Churchill & Sons, 1868.

Morris (John). Local causes of insanitation in
Baltimore. 22 pp. 8°. *Baltimore,* 1878.
Repr. from: Rep. Bd. Health Maryland, Annapolis, 1878,
ii.

———. Milk; its adulterations, analysis, etc. 9
pp. 8°. [*Baltimore,* 1882.]
Repr. from: Maryland M. J., Balt., 1882-3, ix.

———. Hydrops chorii. (Presentation of two
bags of waters.) 8 pp. 8°. *Baltimore,* 1883.
Repr. from: Med. Chron., Balt., 1883, i.

Morris (Malcolm) [1849–]. Skin diseases,
including their definition, symptoms, diagnosis,
prognosis, morbid anatomy, and treatment. A
manual for students and practitioners. x, 288
pp. 8°. *London, Smith, Elder & Co.,* 1879.

———. The same. 320 pp. 8°. *Philadelphia,*
H. C. Lea, 1880.
Also, Co-Editor of: **American** (The) Journal of the
Medical Sciences, Philadelphia, 1886.
For Biography, see Midland M. Misc., Leicester, 1885,
iv, 201, port.

———. The book of health. xi, 1079 pp. 8°.
London, Paris & New York, Cassell & Co., 1883.

———. Ethics of the skin. 22 pp. 8°. *London,*
W. Clowes & Sons, 1884.
Internat. Health Exh. Lect., No. 1 [7?].

———. The management of the skin and hair.
vi, 7-109 pp. 8°. *London, Cassell & Co.,* [1886?]

Morris (Max) [1859–]. *Ueber die Behandlung der Febris intermittens mit Salicylsäure.
29 pp., 1 l. 8°. *Berlin, M. Cohn,* [1883].

Morris (Moreau). Epidemic cerebro-spinal meningitis. 26 pp., 1 map. 8°. *New York, Tower,*
Gildersleeve & Co., 1873.

———. Medical supervision in distinction from
medical selection in life insurance. Quarterly
report. Appendix. Confirmatory evidence of
the value of medical supervision by T. S. Lambert. Remarks upon biometry incidental to Dr.
Morris's report by W. H. Dwinelle. 17, 15 pp.
8°. *New York,* [1874].

———. Biometry; its relation to the practice of
medicine. 16 pp. 8°. *New York, J. F. Trow &*
Son, 1875.

———. The same. 30 pp. 8°. [*n. p.,* 1875.]

———. The same. New ed. 30 pp. 8°. [*n. p.,*
1875.]
Repr. from: Med. Rec., N. Y., 1875, x.
See, also, **New York** (State of). Metropolitan Board
of Health of the City of New York. Special report upon
the operations of the New York Rendering Company. 8°.
New York, 1868.

Morris (Richard L.) Memoir of the late Francis
U. Johnston, read . . . before the New York
Academy of Medicine . . . with an extract from
the funeral sermon in his memory, preached by
Rev. Henry Anthon. 20 pp., 1 pl. 8°. [*New*
York, 1858.]

Morris (Robert).
See **Edinburgh** (The) Medical and Physical Dictionary [etc.] 4°. *Edinburgh,* 1807.

Morris (Robert T.) How we treat wounds to-
day. A treatise on the subject of antiseptic
surgery which can be understood by beginners.
vi, 161 pp. 12°. *New York & London, G. P.*
Putnam's Sons, 1886.
See, also, **Meyer** (S) Report of one hundred joint resections, etc. 8°. [*Newtown,* 1886.]

Morris (Trevor). *De variis sententiis quod ad
contagii vires in morbis pestilentibus. 2 p. l.,
27 pp. 8°. *Edinburgi,* 1820.

Morris (W. A.), **McLaughlin** (J. W.) &
Swearingen (R. M.) A review of Dr.
Wooten's review of the causes that led to the
death of the late Adjt. Gen. John B. Jones. 44
pp. 12°. *Austin, Texas, E. von Boeckmann,*
1882.

Morris (William). Covered service-reservoirs,
with an abstract of the discussion upon the
paper. Edited by James Forrest. 64 pp., 4 pl.
8°. *London, pub. by the Institution,* 1883.
Repr. from: Proc. Inst. Civil Engineers, Lond., 1882-3,
lxxiii, pt. 3.

———. Textile fabrics. A lecture delivered in
the lecture room of the Exhibition, July 11, 1884.
29 pp. 8°. *London, W. Clowes & Sons,* 1884.
Internat. Health Exh., Lect. no. 23.

Morris (*William Winder*) [1784–1857].
Bush (L. P.) Necrology. Tr. Am. M. Ass., Phila.,
1878, xxix, 723.

Morrison (John). Medicine no mystery; being
a brief outline of the principles of medical
science; designed as an introduction to their
general study as a branch of a liberal education.
xxxii, 165 pp. 8°. *London, Hurst, Chance & Co.,*
1829.

Morrison (*John M*) [1836–80].
Bailey (F. H.) Obituary. Tr. Am. M. Ass., Phila.,
1880, xxxi, 1079.

Morrison (R. T.) Die Anwendung einer Knochen - Resections - Maschine, insbesondere für
zahnärztliche Zwecke. 4 pp. 8°. [*Berlin,*
1873.]
Repr. from: Allg. med. Centr.-Ztg., Berl., 1873, xlii.
Also, Editor of: **Dental** (The) Headlight, Nashville,
Tenn., 1883-4.

Morrison's *pills.*
See **Medicines** (*Patent, etc.*); **Toxicology**
(*Cases, etc., of*).

Morrisson (Félix). *Sur la métrite aiguë, ou
inflammation aiguë du tissu de l'utérus. 31 pp.
4°. *Paris,* 1827, No. 8, v. 204.

Morristown.
See **Insane** (*Asylums for, etc.*), *by localities.*

Morrovalle. Statuto organico dell' Ospedale
civico di Morrovalle. Approvato con decreto
regio in data maggio 1884. 6 pp. 8°. *Civita-*
nova-Marche, Natalucci, 1884.

Morrow.
See **Fever** (*Cerebro-spinal, History, etc., of*),
by localities.

Morrow (Prince Albert). Case of morphœa.
In: GIBNEY (V. P.) A case of scleroderma vel morphœa. 8°. [*New York,* 1879.] *Repr. from:* Arch. Dermat., N. Y., 1879, v, 5.
Also, Co-Editor of: **American** (The) Eclectic Medical
Review, New York, 1868-72.—**Journal** of Cutaneous
and Venereal Diseases, New York, 1882.

Morrow (T. V.) A few thoughts on the necessity of medical reformation, in a lecture delivered
before the class of the Reformed Medical School
of Cincinnati, Ohio, Nov. 6, 1843. 16 pp. 8°.
Cincinnati, A. Derrough, 1844.

———. Introductory address, delivered before the
class of the Eclectic Medical Institute, Cincinnati, Ohio, at the commencement of the session,
November, 1847. 20 pp. 8°. *Cincinnati,* 1847.
[P., v. 424.]
Also, Co-Editor of: **Western** (The) Medical Reformer
and Eclectic Journal, Cincinnati, 1847-8.—**Eclectic** (The)
Medical Journal, Cincinnati, 1849.
See, also, **Jones** (I. G.) The American eclectic practice
of medicine. To which are appended the posthumous
writings of T. V. Morrow. 2 v. 8°. *Cincinnati,* 1853-4.

Morsbach (Engelbert). *Das papilläre Kystom
in seiner klinischen Bedeutung. [Halle.] 60
pp., 1 l. 8°. *Dortmund, K. Wörle,* 1881.

Morsbach (Franciscus Adolphus) [1823–].
*De cantharidibus. 28 pp., 2 l. 8°. *Berolini,*
B. Schlesinger, [1850].

Morsch (Fridericus Otto) [1814–]. * De signis vitiorum cordis organicorum generalibus, adjecta morbi historia. 32 pp. 8°. *Berolini, typ. Friedlænderianis*, [1837].

Morse (David Appleton) [1840–]. Report on dipsomania and drunkenness. 52 pp. 8°. [*Dayton, Ohio*, 1873.]
Repr. from : Tr. Ohio M. Soc., Dayton, 1873.

———. Report on monomania. 46 pp. 8°. [*n. p.*, 1874.]
Repr. from : Tr. Ohio M. Soc., Piqua, 1874.

———. Report on general paralysis. 120 pp. 8°. [*n. p.*, 1874.]
Repr. from : Tr. Ohio M. Soc., Piqua, 1874.

———. The mind; an introductory lecture. 28 pp. 8°. *Cincinnati*, 1875.

———. Mental and nervous disorders. Review of nervous disorders, insanity, and medical jurisprudence. 8 pp. 8°. [*n. p.*, 1876.]

———. A review of the literature of nervous disorders and insanity for the year 1878. 4 pp. 8°. [*Cincinnati*, 1878.]
Repr. from : Cincin. Lancet & Clinic, 1879, n. s., ii.

———. Cerebral circulation. The duties of the medical witness and his privileges. The mind; lectures delivered. 72 pp. 8°. *Dayton*, 1879.

———. The doctrines of the human will as interpreted by the courts. 7 pp. 8°. [*Toledo*, 1880.]
Repr. from : Toledo M. & S. J., 1880, iv.

Morse (E. Malcolm). A treatise on the hot sulphate springs of El Paso de Robles . . . With a description of its natural beauties and improvements, and how to get there. Edited by W. W. Messer, jr. 38 pp., 1 l. 8°. *San Francisco, H. S. Crocker & Co.*, 1875.

Morse (Edward S.) On the oviducts and embryology of terebratulina. 2 pp., 1 l., 1 pl. 8°. [*New Haven*, 1872.]
Repr. from : Am. J. Sc. & Arts, N. Haven, 1872, iv.

———. On the systematic position of the brachiopoda. 60 pp., 1 pl. 8°. *Boston, A. A. Kingman*, 1873.
Repr. from : Proc. Bost. Soc. Nat. Hist., 1873, xv.

———. Note on the extension of the coiled arms in Rhychonella. 1 l. 8°. [*n. p.*, 1878.]
Repr. from : Am. J. Sc. & Arts, N. Haven, 1869, xvii. *Also, Co-Editor of:* **American** (The) Naturalist, Salem, Mass., 1867–71.
For Portrait, see **Science**, N. Y., 1886, viii, no. 185.

———. Man in the tertiaries. An address before the section of anthropology of the American Association for the Advancement of Science. 15 pp. 8°. *Salem, Mass., Salem Press*, 1884.
Repr. from : Proc. Am. Assoc. Adv. Sc., Salem, Mass., 1884 xxxiii.

Morse (Jedidiah). A sermon preached before the Humane Society of the Commonweath of Massachusetts, at their semi-annual meeting, June 9, 1801. 53 pp. 8°. *Boston, J. & T. Fleet*, 1801.

———. A report to the Secretary of War of the United States, on Indian affairs, comprising a narrative of a tour performed in the summer of 1820, under a commission from the President of the United States, for the purpose of ascertaining, for the use of the Government, the actual state of the Indian tribes in our country. 400 pp., 1 map, port. 8°. *New Haven, Howe & Spalding*, 1822.

Morse (John Frederick) [1856–]. * Eingangspforten der Infectionsorganismen. 31 pp. 8°. *Berlin, P. Lange*, [1881].

Morse (John Frederick) [1815–74].
Editor of: **California** (The) State Medical Journal, Sacramento, 1856–7. *Also, Co-Editor of:* **Pacific** (The) Medical and Surgical Journal, San Francisco, 1864.
For Biography, see Tr. M. Soc. Calif. 1875–6, Sacramento, 1876, 158–160.

Morse (Lucius D.) Popular exposition of homœopathy. 6. ed. 24 pp. 12°. *St. Louis, H. C. G. Luyties*, 1878.

Morse (Samuel Finley Breese) [1791–1872].
See **Taylor** (W. B.) An historical sketch of Henry's contribution to the electro-magnetic telegraph [etc.] 8°. *Washington*, 1879.

Morse (Verranus). The renewal of prescriptions. Proceedings of the East River and other medical societies, and a paper, with an appendix. 16 pp. 8°. *New York, East River M. Ass.*, 1869.

Morse (Willard H.) New therapeutical agents. 208 pp. 8°. *Detroit, G. S. Davis*, 1882.

Morse Dispensary of Cooper Medical College, San Francisco. Annual reports by the officers for the years 1885; 1886. 8°. *San Francisco, W. A. Woodward & Co.*, 1886-7.
Report for 10 months, ending Nov. 14, 1885.

Morselli (Enrico Agostino) [1852–]. La transfusione del sangue. 2 p. l., 603 pp. 8°. *Roma, Torino, Firenze, E. Loescher*, 1876.

———. L' uccisore dei bambini, Carlino Grandi. Relazione del processo e degli studii medico-legali dei perite Prof. Livi, Prof. Bini et Dott. Morselli. 2 p. l., 183 pp., 4 tab., 1 pl. 8°. *Reggio-Emilia, S. Calderini & figlio*, 1879.

———. Critica e riforma del metodo in antropologia fondate sulle leggi statistiche e biologiche dei valori seriali e sull' esperimento. 1 p. l., 178 pp. 8°. *Roma, eredi Botta*, 1880.

———. Introduzione alle lezioni di psicologia patologica e di clinica psichiatrica. 75 pp. 8°. *Torino, E. Loescher*, 1881.

———. Il metodo clinico nella diagnosi generale della pazzia. II. Esame fisico degli alienati. 55 pp. 8°. *Milano, F. Vallardi*, 1882.
Coll. ital. di lett. s. med., Milano, 1882, ii, no. 12.

———. Un carattere atavico dell' evoluzione umana. 14 pp. 8°. *Milano, Torino, frat. Dumolard*, [1882].
Repr. from : Riv. di filos. scient., 1882, i.

———. Suicide; an essay on comparative moral statistics. ix, 388 pp., 4 tab. 12°. *New York, D. Appleton & Co.*, 1882.
Internat. scient. series.

———. Manuale di semejotica delle malattie mentali. Guida alla diagnosi della pazzia per i medici, i medico-legiste e gli studenti. v. 1. xii, 438 pp. 8°. *Milano, F. Vallardi*, 1885.

———. Il magnetismo animale, la fascinazione e gli stati ipnotici. 2. ed. viii, 427 pp. 12°. *Torino, Roux & Farale*, 1886.
Also, Co-Editor of: **Rivista** sperimentale di freniatria e di medicina legale, Reggio-Emilia, 1875.—**Archivio** di psichiatria, antropologia criminale e scienze penali, Torino e Roma, 1885.

——— & **Buccola** (Gabriele). L' Istituto psichiatrico di Torino. Contributo clinico alla dottrina della pazzia sistematizzata primitiva. 94 pp. 8°. *Torino, Celanza & Comp.*, 1883.

Morshead (E. A.) Tables of the physiological action of drugs. 16 pp. 12°. *London, H. K. Lewis*, 1880.

Morson (Gualterus S.) * De canalis alimenti scirrho. 3 p. l., 31 pp. 8°. *Edinburgi, J. Moir*, 1821.

Morstatt (Joh. Henricus). Exostosis singulari exemplo illustrata. 24 pp., 1 l., 1 pl. 4°. *Tubingæ, typ. Fuesianis*, [1781].

Morsus (Joachimus).
See **Liddel** (Duncan). Ars medica [etc.] Ed. ultima. 8°. *Hamburgi*, 1610.—**Medici** Londinensis eximii epistola de Isaaci Casauboni [etc.] 4°. *Lugd. Bat.*, 1619.

Mortagne (Richard - Parfait - Modeste - Désiré). * Sur les âges. 33 pp. 4°. *Paris*, 1830, No. 150, v. 233.

Mortal *wounds.*
See **Wounds** (*Jurisprudence of*).

Mortality.
See **Armies** (*Diseases, etc., of*); **Infants** (*Mortality of*); **Statistics** (*Medical, etc.*); **Temperature** (*Effects of*), etc.

Mortality *in children.*
See **Labor** (*Statistics of*).

Mortality *tables.*
See **Life-tables.**

Mortara.
See **Cholera** (*Asiatic, History, etc., of*), *by localities.*

Mortegiani (Franciscus). Novæ observationes de oculo humano. 24 pp. 8°. *Neapoli, C. Eboli,* 1814. [P., v. 1112.]

Mortehan (Henricus Josephus). * Tractatus de pleuritide. 51 pp. 4°. *Parisiis, an. XIII* [1805], No. 405, v. 54.

Mortet (Toussaint). * Sur l'extraction des dents à l'aide d'un instrument nouvellement inventé. 35 pp., 1 tab. 8°. *Paris, an XI* [1802], v. 16.

Morthereux (J.) * Réflexions sur les causes et la nature de la colique dite de Madrid. 35 pp. 4°. *Paris,* 1816, No. 62, v. 121.

Morthier & Cornaz. Le libre exercice de la médecine dans le canton de Neuchâtel. 66 pp. 8°. *Neuchâtel, J. Attinger,* 1869.

Morthier (Paul. Carol. Freder.) * De eczemate. 17 pp. 8°. *Turici, ex off. Zürcheri et Furreri,* 1846. [*Also, in :* P., v. 586.] c.

Mortier. Discours prononcé à son entrée en exercice comme chirurgien en chef de l'Hôtel-Dieu de Lyon, le 30 décembre 1823. Imprimé par ordre de l'administration. 54 pp. 8°. *Lyon, Durand & Perrin,* 1824.

Mortier (Denis). * Sur l'ophthalmie. 13 pp. 4°. *Paris,* 1814, No. 30, v. 101.

Mortification.
See **Gangrene.**

de Mortillet (Gabriel).
Editor of : **Matériaux** pour l'histoire positive et philosophique de l'homme, 1864–9.—**L'Homme,** Paris, 1884.
For Portrait, see **L'Homme,** Par., 1884. i, 298–300 (de Bulhouse).

Mortimer (Cromwell). An address to the public, containing narratives of the effects of certain chemical remedies in most diseases ; particularly exemplified in the histories of various cases, both medical and chirurgical, attested by the patients themselves or by their friends ; whereby it appears that these medicines have cured many distempers with single doses, and given great relief in the gout, and some disorders usually pronounced incurable. To which is prefixed a preface, giving an account of the uses and operations of these particular remedies, with practical remarks on some diseases ; and a few hints relating to virtues, not commonly known, of some medicines already in use. 1 p. l., xviii pp., 1 l. ; 104 pp., 2 l. 8°. *London, C. Davis,* 1714. [P., v. 1336.]

———. The same. xviii, 104 pp., 3 l. 8°. *London, C. Davis,* 1745.

———. * De ingressu humorum in corpus humanum. 30 pp. 4°. *Lugd. Bat.,* 1724.
In : HALLER. Disp. anat. [etc.] 4°. *Gottingæ,* 1748, iii, 620–654. Also, in : DE OBERKAMP (F. J.) Collect. diss. 4°. *Francof. a M.,* 1767, i, 313–342.

Morton (A. Stanford). Refraction of the eye ; its diagnosis and the correction of its errors, with chapter on keratoscopy. viii, 57 pp. 8°. *London, H. K. Lewis,* 1881.

———. The same. 3. ed. viii, 67 pp., 2 pl. 8°. *Philadelphia, P. Blakiston, Son & Co.,* 1886.

Morton (Bowditch). Handbook of first aid to the injured ; prepared at the request of the Society for Instruction in First Aid to the Injured. 2. ed. Frontispiece, 90 pp. 12°. *New York, M. B. Brown,* [1884].

Morton (Carolus)[1]. * De corde. 6 l. 4°. *Lugd. Bat., A. Elzevier,* 1683.

Morton (Carolus)[2]. * De tussi convulsiva dissertatio et theses medicæ. [Leyden.] 2. ed. 29 pp., 1 l. 4°. *Londini,* 1748.

Morton (Edward). Remarks on the subject of lactation ; containing observations on the healthy and diseased conditions of the breast-milk ; the disorders frequently produced in mothers by suckling ; and numerous illustrative cases, proving that, when protracted, it is a common cause, in children, of hydrencephalus, or water in the brain, and other serious complaints. ix pp., 1 l., 63 pp. 8°. *London, Longmann [and others],* 1831. [P., v. 395.]

Morton (Geo. W.)
See **New York** (City of). Laws and ordinances relative to the preservation of the public health. 8°. *New York,* 1860.

Morton (Henry). Carbonic oxide ; is it a harmless anæsthetic or a virulent poison ? 12 pp. 8°. *New York,* 1878.
Repr. from : Am. Gas-Light J., N. Y., March 2 and 16, 1878.
Also, Editor of : **Journal** of the Franklin Institute of the State of Pennsylvania, Philadelphia, 1867–70.

Morton (J. Chalmers). An agricultural experience of 300,000 tons of north London sewage, 1867. 31 pp., 2 ch. 8°. *London, F. Warne & Co.,* 1868.

———. Report on the disposal of the sewage of West Derby. 12 pp. 12°. *Liverpool, E. Smith & Co.,* 1869.

———. Our water supply ; a local study. 48 pp. 8°. *London, Bradbury, Agnew & Co.,* 1884.

Morton (Jacob). * De phthisi pulmonali. 25 pp. 8°. *Edinburgi, E. Balfour,* 1800. [*Also, in :* P., v. 13.]

Morton (James). Case of lithotomy by the lateral operation in a female. Extraction of three stones and a bone ; sequelæ of an extra uterine conception. 12 pp. 8°. [*Glasgow, W. Mackenzie,* 1855.] [P., v. 1558.]
Repr. from : Glasgow M. J., 1854–5, 2. s., ii.

———. History of a case of fracture of the femur, bearing chiefly on the diagnosis of such lesions. 8 pp. 8°. *Edinburgh, Oliver & Boyd,* 1870.
Repr. from : Edinb. M. J., 1870–71, xvi.

———. The treatment of spina bifida by a new method. viii, 120 pp., 6 pl. 8°. *Glasgow, J. Maclehose,* 1877.

———. The same. With a paper on the pathology of spina bifida, by John Cleland. 228 pp., 4 l., 4 pl. 8°. *London, J. & A. Churchill,* 1887.

Morton (John). A novel view of the causes producing typhoid fever, etc., and plan of treatment. vi, 7–14 pp. 8°. *Sydney, J. Sands,* 1875.

———. Annual report of the medical officer of health to the Guilford urban sanitary authority for the year 1881. 8 pp., 1 tab. 8°. *Guilford, West Surry Times,* 1882.

Morton (John W.)
See **Menees** (Thomas) & **Morton** (John W.) Addresses delivered at the public commencement [etc.] 8°. *Nashville,* 1867.

Morton (Richard) [1635–98]. Phthisiologia, seu exercitationes de phthisi tribus libris comprehensæ. Totumque opus variis historiis illustratum. 11 p. l., 411 pp., 1 l. 8°. *London, S. Smith,* 1689.

———. The same. Phthisiologia, seu exercitationum de phthisi libri iii. 11 p. l., 455 pp. 18°. *Ulmæ, apud D. Bartholomæ,* 1714.

———. The same. Phthisiologie, oder Abhandlung von der Schwindsucht. Aus dem Lateinischen übersetzt. xvi, 292 pp. 8°. *Helmstedt, J. H. Kühnlin,* 1780.

Morton (Richard)—continued.
——. Πυρετολογία: seu exercitationes de morbis universalibus acutis. 40 p. l., 430 pp., 9 l., 1 tab. 8°. *Londini, S. Smith,* 1692.

——. The same. Πυρετολογία. Pars altera: sive exercitatio de febribus inflammatoriis universalibus. 23 p. l., 511 pp., 8 l. *Londini, S. Smith et B. Walford,* 1694.

——. Opera medica. In tres tomos distributa. 8°. *Amstelodami, D. Donati,* 1696.

CONTENTS.

1. De phthisi.
2. De morbis universalibus acutis.
3. De febribus inflammatoriis.

——. The same. Opera medica, quibus additi fuere tractatus sequentes . . . 4°. *Genevæ, Cramer et Perachon,* 1696.

CONTENTS.

1. Morton (R.) Phthisiologia, sive tractatus de phthisi in iii libros comprehensus totumque opus variis historiis illustratum. 5 p. l., 155 pp., port.
2. Morton (R.) Pyretologia, sive tractatus de morbis acutis universalibus variis historiis illustrata. 13 p. l., 163 pp., 2 l., 1 tab.
3. Morton (R.) Pyretologia, sive tractus de febribus inflammatoriis universalibus variis historiis illustrata. 14 p. l., 207 pp., 4 l.
4. Harris (Gualt.) Tractatus de morbis acutis infantum. 3 p. l., 44 pp.
5. Cole (Guliel.) Novæ hypotheseos, ad typos excogitatæ hypotyposis, etc. 5 p. l., 95 pp., 2 l.
6. Cole (Guliel.) Tractatus de secretione animali. 3 p. l., 72 pp.
7. Lister (Martin.) Tractatus de quibusdam morbis chronicis. 3 p. l., 100 pp.
8. Lister (M.) Tractatus de variolis, etc. 40 pp.
9. Sydenham (Thomæ.) Processus integri in morbis fere omnibus curandis. 3 p. l., 44 pp.

——. The same. Opera medica, in quatuor tomos distributa, quibus additi tractatus sequentes . . . Editio ultima. 4 v. in 2. 12°. *Amstelodami, apud D. Donati,* 1699.

CONTENTS.

1. Morton (R.) Phthisiologiæ. 6 p. l., 206 pp., 2 tab., port.
2. Morton (R.) Exercitationes de morbis universalibus acutis. 23 p. l., 242 pp., 6 l.
3. Morton (R.) Πυρετολογία, [etc.] 19 p. l., 318 pp., 9 l.
4. Harris (G.) De morbis acutis infantum. 1698. 3 p. l., 51 pp., 2 l.
5. Cole (G.) Novæ hypotheseos, [etc.] 1698. 15 p. l., 143 pp.
6. Cole (G.) De secretione animali. 1698. 7 p. l., 93 pp.
7. Lister (M.) Octo exercitationes medicinales de quibusdam morbis chronicis. 1698. 3 p. l., 196 pp., 2 l.

——. The same. Opera medica. Editio novissima, in qua præter tractatus varios, prioribus subjunctos, alii rursus ad majorem illustrationem, et utilius augmentum adjiciuntur. 4°. *Genevæ, sumpt. Perachon et Cramer,* 1727.

CONTENTS.

1. Morton (R.) Phthisiologia . . . de phthisi, in iii libros comprehensus totumque opus variis historiis illustratum. 7 p. l., 155 pp.
2. Leigh (Carol.) Phthisiologia lancastriensis, cui accessit tentamen philosophicum de mineralibus aquis in eodem comitatu observatis. 47 pp.
3. Morton (R.) Pyretologia . . . de morbis acutis universalibus, etc. 13 p. l., 163 pp., 1 tab., 2 l.
4. Morton (R.) Pyretologia . . . de febribus inflammatoriis universalibus, variis historiis illustrata. 14 p. l., 207 pp., 4 l.
5. Dissertationes in novam, tutam ac utilem methodum inoculationis, seu transplantationis variolarum . . . cum criticis notis in varios autores de hoc morbo scribentes a Jacobo a Castro. Altera methodus prælecta a Gualtero Harris. Tertia byzantina dicta . . . publice ventilata ab Antonio le Duc. 5-36 pp.

——. The same. Opera medica, quibus præter tractatus varios prioribus subjunctos, alii rursus ad majorem illustrationem et utilius augmentum adjiciuntur, quorum enumeratio ac explicatio in subsequenti pagina continentur. Editio novissima, omnibus hucusque editis auctior et emendatior. Cum elenchis rerum et in-

Morton (Richard)—continued.
dicibus necessariis. 2 v. sm. 4°. *Lugduni, apud P. Bruyset et socios,* 1737.

CONTENTS.

1. Morton (R.) Phthisiologia, [etc.] 5 p. l., 155 pp.
2. Morton (R.) Pyretologia . . . de morbis acutis universalibus, etc. 13 p. l., 163 pp., 2 tab., 2 l.
3. Morton (R.) Pyretologia . . . de febribus inflammatoriis, etc. 14 p. l., 207 pp., 4 l.
5. Cole (G.) Novæ hypoteseos, [etc.] 4 p. l., 103 pp., 4 l.
6. Cole (G.) De secretione animali. 3 p. l., 72 pp.
7. Lister (M.) De quibusdam morbis chronicis. 16, 100 pp.
8. Lister (M.) De variolis, etc. 40 pp.
9. Sydenham (T.) Processus integri in morbis fere omnibus curandis, [etc.] 3 p. l., 44 pp.
10. Leigh (C.) Phthisiologia, [etc.] 46 pp.
11. Dissertationes in novam, [etc.] pp. 47-80.
12. Ketelaer (Vincent). Commentarius medicus de aphthis nostratibus seu Belgarum sprouw. pp. 81-102.
13. Sidobre (Anton.) De variolis et morbillis. pp. 103-160.
14. Harris (G.) De morbis acutis infantum, etc. 84 pp., 3 l.

For Portrait, see **Collection**—van Kaathoven.—**Collection** of Portr. (Libr.)

Morton (Samuel George) [1799–1851]. * De corporis dolore. 4 p. l., 37 pp. 8°. *Edinburgi, P. Neill,* 1823. [*Also, in :* P., v. 577.]

——. Introductory lecture to a course of demonstrative anatomy, delivered Dec. 11, 1830. 16 pp. 8°. *Philadelphia, Mifflin & Parry,* 1831.

——. Illustrations of pulmonary consumption, its anatomical characters, causes, symptoms, and treatment. xiii, 7–183 pp., 12 pl. 8°. *Philadelphia, Key & Biddle,* 1834.

——. The same. To which are added, some remarks on the climate of the United States, the West Indies, etc. 2. ed. xiv, 15–349 pp., 13 pl. 8°. *Philadelphia, E. C. Biddle,* 1837.

——. Crania Americana; or, a comparative view of the skulls of various aboriginal nations of North and South America. To which is prefixed an essay on the varieties of the human species. v, 296 pp., 78 pl., 1 map. fol. *Philadelphia, J. Dobson,* 1839.

——. Catalogue of skulls of man, and the inferior animals, in the collection of . . . 48 pp. 8°. *Philadelphia, Turner & Fisher,* 1840.

——. The same. 3. ed. x pp., 37 l. 8°. *Philadelphia, Merrihew & Thompson,* 1849. [*Also, in :* P., v. 845.]

——. A memoir of William Maclure, esq., late president of the Academy of Natural Sciences of Philadelphia. 37 pp., 1 l., 1 pl. 8°. *Philadelphia, T. K. & P. G. Collins,* 1841.

——. The same. 2. ed. 33 pp., port. 8°. *Philadelphia,* 1844.

——. Brief remarks on the diversities of the human species, and on some kindred subjects; being an introductory lecture delivered before the class of Pennsylvania Medical College. 24 pp. 8°. *Philadelphia, Merrihew & Thompson,* 1842.

——. An inquiry into the distinctive characteristics of the aboriginal race of America. 2. ed. 48 pp. 8°. *Philadelphia, J. Penington,* 1844.

——. Crania Ægyptica; or, observations on Egyptian ethnography, derived from anatomy, history, and monuments. 67 pp., 14 pl. 4°. *Philadelphia, J. Penington,* 1844.

Repr. from : Tr. Am. Phil. Soc., Phila., 1844, ix.

——. Some observations on the ethnography and archæology of the American aborigines. 19 pp. 8°. *New Haven, B. L. Hamlen,* 1846.

Repr. from : Am. J. Sc. & Arts, N. Haven, 1846, 2. s., ii.

——. Hybridity in animals and plants, considered in reference to the question of the unity of the human species. 23 pp. 8°. *New Haven, B. L. Halem,* 1847.

Repr. from : Am. J. Sc. & Arts, N. Haven, 1817, 2. s., iii.

Morton (Samuel George)—continued.
———. An illustrated system of human anatomy, special, general, and microscopic. xix, 17–642 pp. 8°. *Philadelphia, Grigg, Elliot & Co.*, 1849.

———. Biographical notice of the late George McClellan, M. D. 10 pp. 8°. *Philadelphia*, 1849. [*Also, in:* P., v. 161.]

———. Observations on the size of the brain in various races and families of man. 4 pp. 8°. [*n. p.*, 1849.]
Repr. from: Proc. Acad. Nat. Sc. Phila., 1849.

———. Additional observations on hybridity in animals and on some collateral subjects; being a reply to the objections of the Rev. John Bachman, D. D. 53 pp. 8°. *Charleston, Walker & James*, 1850.
Repr. from: Charleston M. J. & Rev., 1850, v.

———. Letter to the Rev. John Bachman, D. D., on the question of hybridity in animals, considered in reference to the unity of the human species. 18 pp. 8°. *Charleston*, 1850.

———. Notes on hybridity, designed as a further supplement to a memoir on that subject in a former number of this journal. Being a second letter to the editors of the Charleston Medical Journal and Review. 8 pp. 8°. *Charleston*, 1851.
Repr. from: Charleston M. J. & Rev., 1851, vi.
See, also, **Mackintosh** (John). Principles of pathology, and practice of physic. 2. Am. ed. 8°. *Philadelphia*, 1837. ———. The same. 4. Am. ed. 8°. *Philadelphia*, 1844.
For Biography, see **Gross** (S. D.) Lives of eminent American physicians. 8°. *Philadelphia*, 1861, 582–604 (S. B. Hunt).—**Meigs** (C. D.) A memoir of Samuel George Morton, [etc.] 8°. *Philadelphia*, 1851.—**Patterson** (H. S.) Memoir of the life and scientific labors of Samuel George Morton. *In:* NOTT (J. C.) & GLIDDON (G. R.) Types of mankind. 8°. *Philadelphia*, 1854, pp. xvii–lvii.—**Wood** (G. B.) A biographical memoir of Samuel George Morton. 8°. *Philadelphia*, 1853. *Also, in his:* Introductory lect., Univ. of Pa. 8°. *Philadelphia*, 1859, 435–455.
See, also, Boston M. & S. J., 1850, xlii, 56–58. *Also:* Med. Exam., Phila., 1851, n. s., vii, 382–385. *Also:* Tr. Coll. Phys. Phila., 1850, n. s., i, 372–388 (G. B. Wood).
For Portrait, see **Collection** of Portr. (Libr.)

Morton (Thomas). The surgical anatomy of the perinæum. 1 p. l., 80 pp., 4 pl. 8°. *London, Taylor & Walton*, 1838.
Also, in: MORTON (T.) & CADGE (W.) The surgical anatomy [etc.] 8°. *London*, 1850, 1–80, 4 pl

———. The surgical anatomy of the groin, the femoral, and popliteal regions. 81–207 pp., 8 pl. 8°. *London, Taylor & Walton*, 1839.
Also, in: MORTON (T.) & CADGE (W.) The surgical anatomy [etc.] 8°. *London*, 1850, 81–207, 8 pl.

———. The surgical anatomy of inguinal herniæ, the testis and its coverings. 210–330 pp., 5 pl. 8°. *London, Taylor & Walton*, 1841.
Also, in: MORTON (T.) & CADGE (W.) The surgical anatomy [etc.] 8°. *London*, 1850, 210–330, 5 pl.

———. Engravings illustrating the surgical anatomy of the head and neck, axilla, bend of the elbow, and wrist, with descriptions. 24 pp., 8 pl. 8°. *London, Taylor & Walton*, 1845.
Also, in: MORTON (T.) & CADGE (W.) The surgical anatomy [etc.], [with the addition of a commentary by Wm. Cadge]. 8°. *London*, 1850, 331–371, 5–24 pp., 8 pl.

———— & **Cadge** (William). The surgical anatomy of the principal regions of the human body. 4 p. l., 371, 5–24 pp., 25 pl. 8°. *London, Taylor, Walton & Marberly*, 1850.
This entire work is by Morton, with the exception of the commentary on the head and neck and upper limb, by Wm. Cadge. 1 pl. missing.

Morton (Thomas George) [1835–]. Transfusion of blood and its practical application. 35 pp. 8°. *New York, G. P. Putnam*, 1877.
No. 1, v. 3, Am. Clin. Lect., by Seguin, 1–35.

———. The effects of heat.
In: INTERNAT. Encycl. Surg. [Ashhurst], N. Y., 1882, ii, 217–250. *Also, transl. in:* ENCYCL. internat. de chir. [Ashhurst], Par., 1883, ii, 707–746.

Morton (Thomas George)—continued.
———. On the antiseptic treatment of wounds. Clinical lectures. 35 pp. 12°. [*Philadelphia*, 1886.]
Repr. from: Phila. M. Times, 1886-7, xvii.

———. On asymmetry of the lower limbs as a cause of lateral spinal curvature, with a description of a new method for readily and accurately determining any variation in the lengths of the lower extremities. 28 pp. 8°. [*Philadelphia*, 1886.]
Repr. from: Phila. M. Times, 1886-7, xvii.

———. Clinical lecture on cases of painful affection of the foot. 22 pp. 12°. [*Philadelphia*, 1886.]
Repr. from: Phila. M. Times, 1886-7, xvii.

———. The duty of the State and the obligations of directors of the poor, with the policy of the State committee on lunacy, with regard to the management and care of the insane in the State of Pennsylvania. Read at the annual meeting of the association of directors of the poor at Gettysburg, Oct. 18, 1887. 27 pp. 8°. *Harrisburg, E. K. Meyers*, 1887.

———— & **Hunt** (William). Surgery in the Pennsylvania Hospital, being an epitome of the practice of the hospital since 1756; including collations from the surgical notes, and an account of the more interesting cases from 1873 to 1878; with some statistical tables; with papers by John B. Roberts and Frank Woodbury. x, 9–348 pp., 2 pl. 8°. *Philadelphia, J. B. Lippincott & Co.*, 1880.

Morton (W. J. T.) On calculous concretions in the horse, ox, sheep, and dog; being the substance of two essays read before the Veterinary Medical Association. 83 pp., 4 pl. 8°. *London, Longman* [*and others*], 1844.

———. A manual of pharmacy for the student of veterinary medicine; containing the substances employed at the Royal Veterinary College, with an attempt at their classification, and the pharmacopœia of that institution. 7. ed. xv, 568 pp. 12°. *London, Longmans* [*and others*], 1868.

Morton (William J.) Mount Desert and typhoid fever during the summer of 1873. 8 pp. 8°. [*Boston*, 1873.]
Repr. from: Boston M. & S. J., 1873, lxxxix.

———. South African diamond fields and the journey to the mines. 28 pp. 8°. *New York*, 1877.

———. Anæsthetic inhalation. Rival claimants to the discovery. Dr. Long's claim criticised; the priority of Dr. Morton's announcement maintained. 3 l. 8°. [*New York*, 1879.]
Repr. from: N. York Times, Sept. 9, 1879.

———. The invention of anæsthetic inhalation; or, discovery of anæsthesia. 48 pp. 8°. *New York, D. Appleton & Co.*, 1880.
Repr. from: Virginia M. Month., Richmond, 1880, vi.

———. A contribution to the subject of nerve-stretching. In 1. Lateral sclerosis; 2. Paralysis agitans; 3. Athetosis; 4. Chronic transverse myelitis; 5. Sciatica; 6. Reflex epilepsy. 31 pp. 8°. *New York*, 1882.
Repr. from: J. Nerv. & Ment. Dis., N. Y., 1882, ix.

———. Neurological specialism. Presidential address delivered at the annual meeting of the New York Neurological Society, May 1, 1883. 12 pp. 8°. [*n. p.*, 1883.]
Repr. from: J. Nerv. & Ment. Dis., N. Y., 1883, vii.
Also, Editor of: **Neurological** Contributions, New York, 1879-81.—**Journal** (The) of Nervous and Mental Disease, New York, 1882-5.

[**Morton** (William T. G.)] Circular. Morton's letheon. [Cautioning those who attempt to infringe upon his legal rights.] 14 pp. 8°. *Boston, Dutton & Wentworth*, [1846].

———. Remarks on the proper mode of administering sulphuric ether by inhalation. 44 pp. 12°. *Boston, Dutton & Wentworth*, 1847.

[**Morton** (William T. G.)]—continued:

——. Mémoire sur la découverte du nouvel emploi de l'éther sulfurique, suivi des pièces justificatives. 60 pp. 8°. *Paris, E. Bautruche,* 1847.

——. On the loss of the teeth, and the modern way of restoring them, as practiced by . . . 2. ed. 32 pp. 24°. *Boston, W. A. Hall,* 1848.

——. On the physiological effects of sulphuric ether, and its superiority to chloroform. 24 pp. 8°. *Boston, D. Clapp,* 1850.

See, also, **Anæsthetics** (*History of.*)

——— & **Whitman** (Francis). On the loss of the teeth and the modern way of restoring them, as practised by . . . 23 pp., 1 pl. 24°. *Boston, Damrell & Moore,* 1847.

Morton Testimonial Association. A representation to Congress by the . . . covering a portion of the new and recently received petitions, memorials, resolutions, and letters from a large number of the American Medical Association, scientific societies, professors, and surgeons of the principal colleges and hospitals, surgeons, officers, and wounded soldiers of the Federal Army, etc., urging compensation for the use of anæsthetics in the Army and Navy. Submitted to the Thirty-eighth Congress and printed for the use of its members. 67 pp. 8°. [*Washington*, 1864 ?]

Mortreuil (Alfred) [1856–]. * Contribution à l'étude des pseudo-étranglements de l'intestin, iléus traumatique. 55 pp. 4°. *Paris,* 1883, No. 306.

Morus (Horatius). Tabulæ universam chirurgiam miro ordine complectentes, ex eruditioribus medicis collectæ. 39 pp. fol. *Venetiis, apud G. Zilettum et soc.,* 1622.

Morvan.

GAGNIARD (E.) * Topographie médicale du Morvan Avallonnais. 4°. *Paris,* 1859.

Morvan (Augustin-Marie). * De l'anévrysme variqueux. 75 pp. 4°. *Paris,* 1847, No. 41, v. 462.

Morvan (Charles-Étienne-Alfred). * De l'ictère, et de ses rapports avec les diverses maladies du foie et de l'appareil excréteur de la bile. 30 pp. 4°. *Paris,* 1848, No. 156, v. 475.

Morvan (Stephanus Yvo). * De medici obstetricantis officio in partubus fortuito præternaturalibus. viii, 9–32 pp. 4°. *Parisiis,* 1817, No. 183, v. 128.

Morvan (Yves). * Quelques considérations sur les fièvres paludéennes du Gabon. 46 pp., 2 l. 4°. *Montpellier, L. Cristin & Cie.,* 1865, No. 20. c.

Morwitz (E.) Geschichte der Medicin. [Zweiter Band, enthaltend: Chronologisch - systematische Zusammenstellung der medicinischen Literatur.] 2 v. xxvi, 472, x, 342 pp. 12°. *Leipzig, F. A. Brockhaus,* 1848–9.

Forms Abth. 4 of: Encyklopaedie d. med. Wissensch. 12°. *Leipzig,* 1844–9.

Morwitz (Eduardus). * De scotomatibus. 27 pp. 8°. *Berolini, typ. fratrum Schlesinger,* 1841.

Morwyng (Peter).

See **Gesner** (Conrad). The treasure of Euonymus. Transl. by . . . [etc] 4°. *London,* 1559.

Mory (Emil). * Einige neue toxicologische Versuche über die Wirkungen des Wismuths. 32 pp. 8°. *Bern, B. F. Haller,* 1883.

Mory (François) [1861–]. * De la mort apparente des nouveau-nés. 53 pp. 4°. *Paris,* 18~7, No. 285.

Mory (P.-S.-A.) * De la prétendue fièvre de lait. 31 pp. 4°. *Paris,* 1863, No. 107.

Mosan (Jacob).

See **Wirtzung** [*or* **Wirsung**] (Christopher). Praxis medicinæ universalis, or a generall practise of physicke, [etc.] sm. fol. *London,* 1599. ——. The general practice of physicke. fol. *London,* 1617.

Mosander (Carl Gustaf) [1797–].

Co-Editor of: **Tidskrift** for Läkare och Pharmaceuter, Stockholm, 1835–8.

Mosbach.

Schürmayer (J. H.) Bericht über die Verhandlungen des Vereins Badischer Medicinal-Beamter zur Förderung der Staatsarzneikunde in der am 14. August 1843 zu Mosbach abgehaltenen General-Versammlung, die gesetzliche Einführung der Revaccination betr. Ann. d. Staats arznk., Freiburg, 1844, ix, 89–117. *Also,* Reprint.

Mosberg (Paul). * Syphilis hereditaria tarda. 72 pp. 8°. *Würzburg, P. Scheiner,* 1883.

Moscatelli (Carlo). Sul colera indiano; riflessioni pratiche. 38 pp., 1 l. 8°. *Napoli, G. Palma,* 1837. [P., v. 1131; 1137.]

Moscatelli (Regulus). * Untersuchungen über das Vorkommen von Zucker und Gallenfarbstoff im normalen menschlichen Harn. 14 pp. 8°. *Erlangen, Junge u. Sohn,* 1880. s. D.

Moscati (Pietro) Conte [1739–1824]. Von dem körperlichen wesentlichen Unterschiede zwischen der Structur der Thiere und der Menschen. Eine akademische Rede gehalten auf dem anatomischen Theater zu Pavia. Aus dem Italienischen übersetzt von Johann Beckmann. 3 p. l., 100 pp. 16°. *Göttingen, Wittwe Vandenhoeck,* 1771.

——. Neue Beobachtungen und Versuche über das Blut und über den Ursprung der thierischen Wärme. Aus dem Italiänischen übersetzt von Carl Heinrich Köstlin. 4 p. l., 3–56 pp. 16°. *Stutgart, J. B. Mezler,* 1780.

——. Osservazioni ed esperienze sul sangue fluido, e rappreso; sopra l' azione dell' arterie; e sui liquori che bollono poco riscaldati nella macchina pneumatica. 84 pp. 8°. *Napoli, G. M. Porcelli,* 1788. [P., v. 429.]

See, also, **Rasori** (G.) Analisi del preteso genio d' Ippocrate. 8°. *Milano,* 1799.

Mosch (Carl Friedrich) [1785–]. Die Bäder und Heilbrunnen Deutschlands und der Schweiz. Ein Taschenbuch für Brunnen- und Bade-Reisende bearbeitet. 2 v. :96, 167 l., 28 pl., 1 map. 12°. *Leipzig, F. A. Brockhaus,* 1819.

——. The same. 2 v. in 1. 214, 186 l., 1 map. 12°. *Leipzig, F. A. Brockhaus,* 1820.

Moschard (A.-S.-C.-H.) * Sur la fièvre adynamique ou putride. 34 pp. 4°. *Paris,* 1808, No. 84, v. 71.

Moschard (George).

See **Villbourg** (Charles-Ant.) Médecine vétérinaire, [etc.] 12°. *Berne,* 1785.

Mosche (Hermann). * Ueber Hydrophthalmie. 33 pp. 8°. *Würzburg, C. W. Becker,* 1834.

Moscherosch (J. D.) * De lege naturæ quod in corpore animali spasmum excipiat atonia spasmo proportionata. 32 pp. sm. 4°. *Helmstadii, P. D. Schnorr,* [1754].

Moschion. Περὶ γυναικείων παθῶν, id est, Moschionis . . . de morbis muliebribus liber unus: cum Conradi Gesneri scholiis et emendationibus, nunc primum editus opera ac studio Caspari Wolphij. Continentur hoc libro quæ ad gravidarum et puerperarum, itemque infantium curam pertinent clxii distincta capitibus; multa quædam etiam nova atqne a veteribus antehac nunquam tradita: preterea medica nonnulla alia autoris incerti. 3 p. l., 63 pp. 4°. *Basileæ, per T. Guarinum,* 1566.

Greek text.

Also, in: SPACHIUS (I.) Gynæciorum, etc. fol. *Argentinæ,* 1597, 1–28.

——. The same. Περὶ τῶν γυναικείων παθῶν. Moschionis de mulierum passionibus liber, quem ad mentem manuscripti græci in bibliotheca Cæsareo-regia Vindobonensi asservati, tum propriis correctionibus emendavit, additaque versione latina edidit F. O. Dewez. x (6 l.), 240 pp. 12°. *Viennæ, R. Gräffer et soc.,* 1793.

See, also, **Wolphius** (Caspar). Harmonia gynæciorum, etc. *In:* GYNÆCIORUM . . . commentarii, etc. 8°. *Basileæ,* 1586, i.

Moschkau (Alfred).
Editor of: **Gesundheitswacht**, Leipzig, 1876–8.

Moschkowitsch (S.) * Ueber Pemphigus syphiliticus. 1 p. l., 19 pp. 8°. *Würzburg, J. M. Richter,* 1882.

Moschkowsky (Joseph). * Ueber congenitale Stenose der Pulmonalis. 25 pp., 1 l. 8°. *Königsberg, Hartung,* 1872.

Moschner (Paul [Carl Albert]) [1859–   ]. * Beiträge zur Histologie der Magenschleimhaut. 31 pp. 8°. *Breslau, Genossenschafts-Buchdruckerei,* 1885.

Moscho (Stavrus Poliso). * De mensium vitiis. 40 pp. 8°. *Halæ, in off. Batheana,* 1800.

Moschus.
See, also, **Musk.**
EDWARDS (A.-M.) * Recherches anatomiques, zoologiques et paléontologiques sur la famille des chevrotains. 4°. *Paris,* 1864.

von Moschzisker (Franz Adolph). A guide to the diseases of the eye, and their treatment. For the use of students and young practitioners. xi, 13–174 pp. 8°. *Baltimore, Cushings & Bailey,* 1856.

———. On the use of the artificial membrana tympani in cases of deafness depending upon perforation or destruction of the natural organ. 40 pp. 8°. *Philadelphia, Town,* 1857.

———. Medical and surgical science in the United States, specialities, empiricism, etc. ; enlarged from an article published in the New Orleans Picayune of Feb. 14, 1860. 28 pp. 18°. *New Orleans,* 1860.

———. The ear, its diseases and their treatment. xix, 13–319 pp., port. 8°. *Philadelphia, Martin & Randall,* 1864.

———. Medici nugæ. 2. ed. 28 pp. 8°. *Philadelphia, S. P. Town,* 1879.

Moscow (Government of). Sbornik statisticheskich sviedienii po Moskovskoi gubernii. Otdiel sanitarnoi statistiki. Izdanie Moskovskago gubern. zemstva. Tom iii. Pt 8 & 9. 2 v. iii, 370, 55 pp., 15 tab. ; iv, 292, 85 pp., 23 plans. roy. 8°. *Moskva, tipog. A. Kartser,* 1883.

CONTENTS.

Moscow.
See, also, **Children** (*Hospitals, etc., for, Reports, etc., of*); **Cholera** (*Asiatic, History, etc., of*), *by localities*; **Education** (*Medical*), *etc.—Russia*; **Fever** (*Cerebro-spinal, History, etc., of*), **Fever** (*Relapsing, History, etc., of*), **Foundlings**, *etc.*, **Hospitals** (*Descriptions, etc., of*), **Hospitals** (*Military*), **Hospitals** (*Ophthalmic, etc.*), **Insane** (*Asylums for, etc.*), **Medicine** (*Clinical, etc.*), **Prostitution** (*History, etc., of*), *by localities.*

KRATKII med. otchet Moskovsk. gorodskoi bolnitsi za 1879 g. [Diseases in Moscow in 1879.] 8°. *Mosk.,* 1880.

MURATOFF (A.) * Materiali dlja akucherskoi statistiki goroda Moskvi. [Births in the city of Moscow.] 8°. *Moskva,* 1879.

SOCIÉTÉ impériale des naturalistes de Moscou. Bulletins. Meteorologische Beobachtungen ausgeführt am meteorologischen Observatorium der landwirthschaftlichen Academie zu Moskau. 1882; 1. Hlfte. 1883. obl. 4°. *Moskau,* 1883.

Bonnafont. Notice sur quelques établissements scientifiques et de bienfaisance de la ville de Moscou. Union méd., Par., 1874, n. s., xviii, 941 ; 957.—**Bubnoff** (S. F.) Niekotor. dannija dlja san. otsenki Moskov. pochvi. [On the sanitary state of the Moscow soil.] Sborn.

Moscow.
rabot. hyg. lab. Moskov. Univ., Mosk., 1886, i, 178–195.—**Levestamm** (G.) Die Krankheitenconstitution in Moskau während der Jahre 1841 und 184?. Mitrh. a. d. Geb. d. Heilk.. Leipz., 1845, i, 1–11. — [**Ostroglasow.**] Die Sterblichkeitsverhältnisse der Stadt Moskau im Jahre 1878. Veröffentl. d. k. deutsch. Gsndhtsamtes, Berl., 1879, iii, 151. ———. Sterblichkeitsverhältnisse der Stadt Moskau im Jahre 1879. *Ibid.,* 1880, v, 16.—**Sterblichkeitsverhältnisse** in Moskau im Jahre 1881. *Ibid.,* 1882, vi, 12.—**Peskoff** (P. A.) O stemni rasprostraneniya zemskoi vrachebnoi pomoshihi i o bolaiznosti selskago nascleniya v' 3-kh meditsinskikh uchastkakh Moskovskago uaizda. [Sickness in the three medical subdistricts of the district of Moscow, and the means for affording medical aid to the rural population.] Sborn. sochin. po sudebnoi med., St. Petersb., 1877, sec. 2, 63–124.—**Vivoz** nechistot iz Moskvi. [Removal of dirt from Moscow.] Zdorovje. St. Petersb., 1876, ii, 74.—**Vodostokakh** (O) G. Moskvi. [On the sewers of Moscow.] *Ibid.,* 192.—**Weinberg** (J.) Observations météorologiques faites à l'Institut des arpenteurs (dit Constantin) de Moscou. Bull. Soc. imp. d. nat. de Moscou, 1867, xl, no. 4, suppl., 1–15: 1868, xli, no. 4, suppl., 1–9: 1869, xlii, no. 4, suppl., 1–21: 1870, xliii. nos. 3 and 4, suppl., 11–37 ; 2. suppl., 1–13: 1871, xliv. nos. 3 and 4, suppl., 1–15: 1872, xlv, no. 4, suppl., 1–24: 1873, xlvi, no. 4, suppl., 1–24: xlviii, no 4, suppl., 1–24: 1878, lii, no. 4, 27: 1881, lvi, no. 1, 1–27: 1882, lvi, 1–27.

Mosdorffius (Johannes Godofredus). * De febre intermittente in genere. 32 pp. sm. 4°. *Jenæ, lit. Krebsianis,* [1690].

Mose (Franz) [1862–   ]. * Ueber Exenteratio bulbi. 20 pp. 8°. *Kiel, A. F. Jensen,* 1887.

Moseder (Joh. Fridericus)[1]. * Theses medicas varii argumenti subjiciet. 16 pp. sm. 4°. *Argentorati, M. Pauschinger,* [1741].

Moseder (Joh. Fridericus)[2]. * Examen de compositione et usu argillæ. 50 pp. 4°. *Argentorati, typ. J. H. Heitzii,* [1773].

———. * De dysenteria quam excepit aphonia cum epicrisi. 28 pp., 1 l. 4°. *Argentorati, typ. J. H. Heitzii,* [1775].

Moseley (Benjamin) [–1819]. Observations on the dysentery of the West Indies, with a new and successful method of treating it. iv, 24 pp. 8°. *Jamaica, printed ; London, reprinted from the 2. ed. by T. Becket,* 1781. [P., v. 557 ; 604.]

———. A treatise on tropical diseases, and on the climate of the West Indies. xix, 544 pp. 8°. *London, T. Cadell,* 1787.

———. The same. A treatise on tropical diseases, on military operations, and on the climate of the West Indies. 2. ed. xv, 556 pp. 8°. *London, T. Cadell,* 1789.
Another copy bound with his: A treatise on tropical diseases, etc. 8°. *London,* 1787.

———. The same. 3. ed. xv, 568 pp. 8°. *London, T. Cadell,* 1792.

———. The same. 3. ed. xiii, 568 pp. 8°. *London, G. G. & J. Robinson,* 1795.

———. The same. 4. ed. xvi, 670 pp. 8°. *London, Cadell & Davies,* 1803.

———. The same. Abhandlung von den Krankheiten zwischen den Wendezirkeln und von dem Klima in Westindien. Aus dem Englischen übersetzt. 7 p. l., 462 pp., 1 l. 12°. *Nürnberg u. Altdorf, Monath u. Kussler,* 1790.

———. A treatise concerning the properties and effects of coffee. 5. ed. xxvii, 80 pp. 8°. *London, J. Sewell,* 1792.

———. Medical tracts. 1. On sugar. 2. On the cow-pox. 3. On the yaws. 4. On obi, or African witchcraft. 5. On the plague, and yellow fever of America. 6. On hospitals. 7. On bronchocele. 8. On prisons. 2. ed., with considerable additions. iv, 3–276 pp. 8°. *London, J. Nichols,* 1800.

———. The same. 2. ed., with considerable additions. iv, 3–276 pp. 8°. *London, F. N. Longman & O. Rees,* 1804.

———. A treatise on the lues bovilla, or cow pox. xxiii, 142 pp. 8°. *London, Longman [and others],* 1805.

Moseley (Benjamin)—continued.

———. Commentaries on the lues bovilla, or cow pox. xv, 184 pp., 1 l. 8°. *London, Longman [and others]*, 1806.

———. On hydrophobia, its prevention and cure. With a dissertation on canine madness; illustrated with cases. 5. ed. 74 pp. 8°. *London, Longman & Co.*, 1809.

See, also, **Vaccine** (La) combattue dans le pays où elle a pris naissance. 8°. *Paris,* 1807.

Moseley (Francis Xavier). On the causes of epidemic fever in great cities. 30 pp., 1 l. 8°. *London, Whittaker & Co.*, 1838.

Moseley (George). Insanity curable. Mental disorders and nervous affections of recent origin or long standing; their cause are now successfully treated by a new especial method. 63 pp. 8°. *London, J. & A. Churchill*, 1886.

Moseley (William E.) The influence, from a clinical standpoint, of cicatricial tissue in the angles of the lacerated cervix. 12 pp. sm. 8°. [*New York*, 1886.]

Repr. from: N. York M. J., 1886, xliv.

Moseley (William Willis). Eleven chapters on nervous or mental complaints, and on two great discoveries, by which hundreds have been, and all may be, cured with as much certainty as water quenches thirst or bark cures ague. 2. ed. xiv, 15–151 pp., 1 pl. 8°. *London, Simpkin, Marshall & Co.*, 1838.

Moselle (*Département de la*).

See, also, **Alsace-Lorraine**; **Cholera** (*Asiatic, History, etc., of*), *by localities;* **France.**

Guyot (P.) Les sources minérales du département de la Moselle. Gaz. d. eaux, Par., 1879, xxii, 355; 363; 369; 379: 1880, xxiii, 52; 76.

Mosely (Ephraim). Teeth; their natural history; with the physiology of the human mouth, in regard to artificial teeth. vii, 56 pp. 16°. *London, R. Hardwicke*, 1862.

Mosén (Frans Gerhard.)

See **Hwasser** (Israël). Om colik. 2. delen. 8°. *Upsala,* 1837-9. *See, also,* **Liedbeck** (Petrus Jacobus) & **Mosén** (Frans Gerhard). * Morbi scarlatinæ expositio. sm. 4°. *Upsaliæ,* [1835].

von Mosengeil (Karl) [1840–]. * Beitrag zur Geschichte der osteoplastischen Resectionen. 32 pp. 8°. *Berlin, G. Lange,* [1868].

Mosengel (Heinricus Josua) * De longævitate ex aëris temperie. 32 pp. sm. 4°. *Halæ Magdeb., typ. Hendelianis,* [1728].

Mosenthal (Moritz). * Geburtshilfliche Operationslehre bei Eucharius Roesslin, Walther Reiff und Jacob Rueff. 26 pp. 8°. *Würzburg, Becker,* 1887.

Moser (Adolphus) [1810–]. * De cultus nexu et discrimine scientiarum naturalium et medicarum. 40 pp., 2 l. 8°. *Berolini, typ. Nietackianis,* [1833].

———. Anleitung zum Gebrauche des Mikroskops für Aerzte, Naturforscher und Freunde der Natur. 3 p. l., 163 pp., 1 pl. 8°. *Berlin, Liebmann u. Comp.,* 1839.

———. Lehrbuch der Geschlechtskrankheiten des Weibes, nebst einem Anhang enthaltend die Regeln für die Untersuchung der weiblichen Geschlechtstheile. xviii, 684 pp., 1 l. 8°. *Berlin, A. Hirschwald,* 1843.

———. Die medicinische Diagnostik und Semiotik, oder die Lehre von der Erforschung und der Bedeutung der Krankheitserscheinungen bei den innern Krankheiten des Menschen. xii, 520 pp. 12°. *Leipzig, F. A. Brockhaus,* 1845.

Also forms Abth. 3 of: Encyklopädie d. med. Wissensch. 12°. *Leipzig,* 1844-9.

Also, Co-Editor of: **Analekten** der Chirurgie, Berlin, 1837-9.

See, also, **Busch** (Dietrich Wilhelm Heinrich) & **Moser** (A.) Handbuch der Geburtskunde [etc.] 8°. *Berlin,* 1840-43.

Moser (Albert). Verzeichniss des medicinischen Bücherlagers von . . . in Tübingen. Nos. 34, 38, 41, 50, 52, 56, 58, 59, 60, 61, 63. 8°. *Tübingen, H. Laupp,* 1875-85.

Moser (Edmundus) [1819–]. De compressionis vi physiologica et therapeutica. 29 pp. 8°. *Berolini, typ. Friedlaenderianis,* [1843].

Moser (Ernst). * Ueber die organischen Substanzen des Mainwassers, bei Würzburg. Ein Beitrag zur Frage der Flussverunreinigung. 15 pp. 8°. *Würzburg, Stahel,* 1887.

Moser (Fr. Xaverio). * De miliaria. 17 pp. 8°. *Monachii, J. Deschler,* 1842.

Moser (Franciscus Ludovicus). * De theoria et therapia famis caninæ. 1 p. l., 19 pp. 4°. *Herbipoli, typ. hær. Zinck,* [1694].

Moser (Franz Ser.) * Einige Beobachtungen über die Wirkung des neutralen salicylsauren Natrons. [Munich.] 30 pp. 8°. *Leipzig, J. B. Hirschfeld,* 1877.

Moser (Friedrich). * Ueber die Ruhr. 21 pp. 8°. *Würzburg, C. J. Becker,* 1856.

Moser (Gottlob Friedrich). * Das Gaumensegel des Menschen verglichen mit dem der Säugethiere. 30 pp. 8°. *Tübingen, H. Laupp,* 1868.

Moser (Isaacus) [1819–]. * De morbo hydrocephaloide. 28 pp., 2 l. 8°. *Berolini, typ. Nietackianis,* [1843].

Moser (J. P.) Homöopathische Lebensregeln für Gesunde und Kranke. Ein Wort der Belehrung für Jedermann. 2. Aufl. 80 pp., 4 pl. 16°. *Hagen i. W., H. Risel u. Comp.,* 1886.

Homöopathischer Hausschatz, Hft. 1.

———. Die Diphtheritis (brandige Halsbräune, Rachencroup) und ihre sicherste homöopathische Heilung. Ein Wort der Belehrung für alle Eltern. 2. Aufl. 48 pp. 12°. *Hagen i. W., H. Risel u. Comp.,* 1886.

Homöopathischer Hausschatz, Hft. 2.

———. Homöopathische Heilerfolge. Beiträge zur homöopathischen Krankenbehandlung (mit Angabe der Heilmittel). 4. Aufl. 1 p. l., xvi, 350 pp. 8°. *Hagen i. W., H. Risel u. Comp.,* 1886.

Moser (Joh.) Das Alter des Menschen und die Wissenschaft. 39 pp. 8°. *Frankf. a. M. u. Luzern,* 1885.

Forms Hft. 2, v. 6, of: Frankfurter zeitgemässe Broschüren, neue Folge, 377–415.

Moser (Louis-Auguste). * Quelques considérations sur le dicrotisme du pouls dans diverses pyrexies et phlegmasies, et en particulier dans la fièvre typhoïde. 31 pp., 2 pl. 4°. *Paris,* 1872, No. 158.

Moser (Ludwig) [1805–]. * De vitæ atque morbi notionibus. 42 pp., 1 l. 8°. *Berolini, typ. Brüschckianis,* [1828].

———. Die Gesetze der Lebensdauer, nebst Untersuchungen über Dauer, Fruchtbarkeit der Ehen, über Tödtlichkeit der Krankheiten, Verhältniss der Geschlechter bei der Geburt, über Einfluss der Witterung u. s. w. und einem Anhang, enthaltend die Berechnung der Leibrenten, Lebensversicherungen, Wittwenpensionen und Tontinen. xxviii, 399 pp., 2 diag. 8°. *Berlin, Veit u. Comp.,* 1839.

———. Das Wesen der Cholera. Der wahre Schutz vor derselben. Ihre sicherste und schnellste Heilung. 16 pp. 8°. *Ulm, Gebr. Nübling,* 1854.

Moser (Wenc. Leop.) * Diss. sistens historias synopticas ophthalmiarum duarum, phænomenis et decursu singularium, in clinico ophthalmiatrico Pragensi tractatarum. 18 pp., 1 l. 8°. *Pragæ, J. H. Pospjsil,* [1838].

Moser (Wolfgangus Henricus). * De ortu dentium, et symptomatibus quæ circa dentitionem

Moser (Wolfgangus Henricus)—continued.
infantum occurrunt. 36 pp. sm. 4°. *Tubingæ, typ. Fuesianis*, 1770.

Moses *Maimonides* (Abu Amrân Musa Ben Meimun) [1139–1208]. Tractatus rabi Moysi quem domino et magnifico soldano Babilonii transmisit [de regimine sanitatis]. 40 l. 4°. *Florentie, apud Sanctum Jacobum de Ripolis*, [*circa* 1478].

———. Incipiunt aphorismi excellentissimi Raby Moyses secundum doctrinam Galieni medicorum principis. 133 l. sm. 4°. *Bononie, B. Hector*, 1489.
Following the foregoing, in like type and paper, but beginning with sig. A 1, is: **Janus** *Damascenus.* Aphorismi [et liber Rhasis de secretis in medicina].

———. Tractatus de regimine sanitatis ad Soldanum regem. 16 l. sm. 4°. *Augustæ Vindel.*, 1518.
Also, in: DE GRADI (Joan. Matth.) Consiliorum. fol. *Venetiis*, 1514, ff. 105–110.

———. [De regimine vitæ quinque tractatus.]
In: DE GRADI (Jo. Matth.) Consilia secundum viam Avicennæ ordinata. 2. ed. fol. *Lugduni*, 1535, ff. 89–93.

———. Aphorismi, ex Galeno medicorum principe collecti; nunc vero ad usum studiosorum medicinæ ab interitu vindicati, et jam primum in lucem editi. Item locorum quorundam apud Gaienum sibi ipsis contradicentium castigatio et notatio. Denique, Joannis Damasceni aphorismi utilissimi ad filium. 39 p. l., 542 pp. 18°. *Basileæ, ex off. Henricpetrina*, 1579.
For Biography, see Ann. Soc. de méd. d'Anvers, 1846, 149–159 (L. Ali-Cohen). *Also:* Deutsches Arch. f. Gesch. d. Med. u. med. Geog., Leipz., 1879, ii, 463–478 (Oppler).

Moses (G. A.) Hysterectomy, in malignant disease. 7 pp. 8°. [*St. Louis*, 1882.]
Repr. from: St. Louis Cour. Med., 1882, viii.

Moses (I.) Surgical notes of cases of gun-shot injuries occurring during the advance of the Army of the Cumberland, 1863. 20 pp. 8°. [*n. p., n. d.*] [P., v. 194.]
Repr. from: Am. J. M. Sc., Phila., 1864, n. s., xlvii.

Moses (Julius). *Ein und sechzig Fälle von Abort aus der geburtshilflichen Universitäts-Poliklinik zu Breslau (mit Bemerkungen über Aetiologie, Symptomatologie und Therapie). 2 p. l., 37 pp. 8°. *Breslau*, [1884].

Moses (Levy) [1811–]. * De exanthemate miliari. 32 pp. 8°. *Berolini, typ. Friedlaenderianis*, [1837].

Moses (Moses P.) *Experimentelle Untersuchungen über die Wirkung der Canthaniden-tinctur und die dadurch hervorgebrachten örtlichen Hautveränderungen, nebst Schlussbetrachtungen, Bemerkungen über die Wundheilung, etc. 143 pp. 8°. *Würzburg, Becker*, 1885.

Moses (Simon) [1841–]. * De pneumothorace nonnulla. 32 pp. 8°. *Berolini, G. Schade*, [1863].

Moses Ben Maimon. *See* **Moses** *Maimonides.*

Mosesinno (Jacobus) [1803–]. * De methodo diuretica. 35 pp. 8°. *Berolini, lit. A. Petschii*, [1827].

Mosetig (Albert). Ueber die Anomalien bei der Herniotomie der Leisten- und Schenkelbrüche 55 pp. 8°. *Wien, Tendler u. Comp.*, 1867.

von Mosetig-Moorhof (Albert) Ritter. Der Jodoform-Verband.
In: SAMML. klin. Vortr., Leipz., 1882, No. 211 (Chir., No. 68), 1811–1864.

———. Sechs gemeinverständliche Vorträge über die erste Hilfe bei plötzlichen Unglücksfällen. 62 pp. roy. 8°. *Wien*, 1884.

———. Handbuch der chirurgischen Technik bei Operationen und Verbänden. vi, 883 pp. 8°. *Wien, Toeplitz u. Denticke*, 188[5]–6.

von Mosetig-Moorhof (A.) Ritter—cont'd.
———. The same. Rukovodstvo k chirurgicheskoi technike pri operatsijach i povjazkach. Perevod s vtor. Nemetskago izdanija E. Salitsheva. 725 pp., 1 l. 8°. *St. Petersburg*, 1887.
In: Ejem. jour. prakt. med., St. Petersb., 1887, iii.

———. Vorlesungen über Kriegschirurgie. viii, 332 pp. 8°. *Wien u. Leipzig, Urban u. Schwarzenberg*, 1887.

Mosgrove (Frederick J.) A practical treatise on congestion and inactivity of the liver; showing some of the effects produced by these disorders on the most important organs of the body. Illustrated by cases. vi, 120 pp. 12°. *London, Simpkin, Marshall & Co.*, 1843.

———. Practical remarks on the predisposing causes and treatment of the Asiatic cholera. 43 pp. 12°. *Bombay, T. Graham*, 1849.

Mosheim (Henricus). De icteri origine probabilia. 30 pp., 1 l. 8°. *Halæ, formis F. Gruneti filii*, [1816].

von Mosheim (Johann Lorenz). Neue Nachrichten von dem berühmten spanischen Arzte Michael Serveto, der zu Geneve ist verbrannt worden. 108 pp. 4°. *Helmstaedt, C. F. Weygand*, 1750.

Mosher (Alanson). Learned quackery exposed, or the difference shown between poisons and medicines. 37 pp. 16°. *Schoharie, Gallup & Lawyer*, 1846.

Mosher (Jacob Simmons) [1834–83]. Catalogue of a portion of the carefully selected library of the late J. S. Mosher, comprising miscellaneous literature and a large and curious collection of criminal trials. 44 pp. 12°. *Albany, J. McDonough*, 1884.

———. Catalogue of the medical and scientific portion of the library of the late J. S. Mosher, comprising many scarce books on insanity, yellow fever, sanitation, medical journals, reports, etc. 21 l. obl. 18°. [*Albany*, 1884.]
For Biography, see Med. Ann., Albany, 1883, iv, 184–188. *Also:* Med. Rec., N. Y., 1884, xxiv, 188. *Also:* Tr. M. Soc. N. Y., Syracuse, 1885 (W. G. Tucker). *Also*, Reprint.

Mosimann (Lucien) [1860–]. *Contribution à l'étude du traitement de la péritonite aiguë. 32 pp. 4°. *Paris*, 1881, No. 333.

Mosino (Philipp). Das Russische rothe Kreuz, 1877–78 in Rumänien; nach dem amtlichen russischen Berichte des ehem. General-Delegirten Wirkl. Staatsrathes P. A. von Richter frei bearbeitet und erläutert. viii, 288 pp., 1 map, 7 plans, 6 tab. 8°. *Berlin, Stuhr*, 1880.

Moskovskaya gazeta, izdavaemaya obshtshestvom russkich vratchei. [Moscow Medical Gazette. Issued by the Society of Russian Physicians.] [Weekly.] v. for 1866–8; v. 19–21, 1876–8. 6 v. 4°. *Moskva*.
Commenced about 1858. Want no. 28 in 1878 (v. 21).

Moskovskii gubernija. Sbornik statisticheskich svedenii po Moskovski gubernii. Otdel sanitar. statistiki. T. iii. pt. 9. Sanitar. izsledov. fabrichnich zavedenii Mosk. uezda. Chart iii. F. F. Erismann. [Examinations of manufacturing establishments of the Moscow district.] ii, 292, 85 pp., 23 diag. 8°. *Moskva*, 1883

Moskovskii vratchebnii Journal; izdavremii A. Poluninim. [Moscow Medical Journal.] v. for 1854–9. 5 v. 8°. *Moskra*.

Moskovskii vratchebnii Vestnik; izdawaiemii sostriashtchim pri Imperatorskom Moskovskom Universitete, fiziko-meditsinskim obshtshestvom. [Moscow Medical Courier. Issued by the Physico-Medical Association of the Imperial Moscow University.] [Fortnightly.] v. 1–3, Sept. 10, 1873, to Dec. 29, 1876. 4°. *Moskva*.

Mosler (Carol.) * De scarlatinæ epidemia Gryphiæ annis hujus sæculi lv et lvi observata. 31 pp. 8°. *Gryphiæ, F. G. Kunike,* 1856.

Mosler (Friedrich). * Beiträge zur Kenntniss der Urinabsonderung bei gesunden, schwangeren und kranken Personen, insbesondere quantitative Bestimmung der phosphorsauren Verbindungen. 20 pp., 2 l. 8°. *Giessen, J. Ricker,* 1853. C.

——. Untersuchungen über den Einfluss des innerlichen Gebrauches verschiedener Quantitäten von gewöhnlichem Trinkwasser auf den Stoffwechsel des menschlichen Körpers unter verschiedenen Verhältnissen. Erste vom Verein f. g. A. gekrönte Preisschrift. 1 p. l., 73 pp. 8°. *Göttingen, Vandenhoeck u. Ruprecht,* 1857.
Repr. from: Arch. d. Ver. f. wissensch. Heilk., Leipz., 1857, iii, Hft. 3.

——. * Untersuchungen über den Uebergang von Stoffen aus dem Blute in die Galle. 19 pp. 4°. *Giessen, W. Keller,* 1857.

——. Helminthologische Studien und Beobachtungen. vi, 89 pp., 2 pl. 8°. *Berlin, A. Hirschwald,* 1864.

——. Zur Casuistik des Hautskleremes bei Erwachsenen. 9 pp. 8°. [*Berlin, G. Reimer,* 1865.]
Repr. from: Arch. f. path. Anat., etc., Berl., 1865, xxxiii.

——. Ueber Transfusion defibrinirten Blutes bei Leukämie und Anämie. 23 pp., 1 pl. 8°. *Berlin, A. Hirschwald,* 1867.

——. Erfahrungen über die Behandlung des Typhus exanthematicus mit Berücksichtigung dabei erforderlicher prophylaktischer Maassregeln. vii, 126 pp., 1 l., 1 pl. 8°. *Greifswald,* 1868.

——. Die Pathologie und Therapie der Leukämie. vi, 283 pp. 8°. *Berlin, A. Hirschwald,* 1872.

——. Ueber den Nutzen der Einführung grösserer Mengen von Flüssigkeit in den Darmkanal bei Behandlung interner Krankheiten. Ein Vortrag, gehalten im Greifswalder medicinischen Vereine. 10 pp. 8°. *Berlin, J. Sittenfeld,* 1873.
Repr. from: Berl. klin. Wchnschr., 1873, x.

——. Klinische Symptome und Therapie der medullaren Leukämie. 37 pp. 8°. *Berlin, A. Hirschwald,* 1877.
Repr. from: Berl. klin. Wchnschr., 1876, xiv.

——. Ueber Lungen-Chirurgie. Vortrag gehalten beim zweiten Congiesse für innere Medicin zu Wiesbaden am 20. April 1883. Erweitert durch eine Uebersicht der gesammten Literatur des Gegenstandes. 1 p. l., 72 pp. 8°. *Wiesbaden, J. F. Bergmann,* 1883.

——. Ueber Milz-Echinococcus und seine Behandlung. Eine Monographie. 75 pp. 8°. *Wiesbaden, J. F. Bergmann,* 1884.

——. Ueber die medicinische Bedeutung des Medinawurmes (Filaria medinensis). 25 pp. 8°. *Wien u. Leipzig, Urban u. Schwarzenberg,* 1884.

——. Bericht über die Benutzung unserer transportablen Baracke während der Wintermonate 1886-7. 7 pp. 8°. *Berlin u. Leipzig, G. Thieme,* 1887.
Repr. from: Deutsche med. Wchnschr., Berl., 1887, xiii.

——. Exacte Versuche über die Wirkungen des Friedrichshaller Bitterwassers auf den Stoffwechsel und klinische Beobachtungen über die Heilwirkung des Friedrichshaller Bitterwasssers gegen verschiedene Krankheiten. Ein Auszug aus der im Archiv für gemeinschaftliche Arbeiten veröffentlichten Abhandlung. 15 pp. 8°. *Würzburg, M. Walz,* [n. d.]
See, also, **Handbuch** d. spec. Path. (Ziemssen), Leipz., 1875, viii, 2. Hlfte. *Also:* **Cyclopedia** Pract. M. (Ziemssen), N. Y., 1878, viii.

Mosler (Leo). * Die Tuberculose der weiblichen Genitalien. [Breslau.] 42 pp., 1 l. 8°. *Berlin, J. Sittenfeld,* 1883.

Mosmant (Charles-Antoine). * Influence des alimens sur les sécrétions. vi, 7–29 pp. 4°. *Paris,* 1830, No 121, v. 232.

Mosmant (Eugène-Gustave). * Sur la congestion cérébrale. 38 pp. 4°. *Paris,* 1858, No. 153, v. 622.

Mosnier (Antoine). * Sur l'ophthalmie. vi, 7–41 pp. 4°. *Paris,* 1825, No. 120, v. 193.

Mosnier (Ernest). * Contribution à l'étude de quelques symptômes de la chlorose. 75 pp. 4°. *Paris,* 1883, No. 99.

Mosnier (Louis-Théodore). * De l'emploi du seigle ergoté à faibles doses, dans les cas d'inertie de matrice et les hémorrhagies après la délivrance. 55 pp. 4°. *Paris,* 1837, No. 93, v. 308.

Mosny (Ernest). * De l'influence des moyens abortifs dans les accidens réputés primitifs de la syphilis, relativement aux accidents secondaires. 63 pp. 4°. *Paris,* 1848, No. 203, v. 475.

Mosovius (Mauritius Adolphus). * De calculorum animalium eorumque inprimis biliariorum origine et natura. 44 pp., 1 pl. 8°. *Berolini, typ. A. G. Schadii,* [1812].

Mosquera (José-Antonio). * Quelques réflexions à propos d'un cas de rétrécissement de l'orifice auriculo-ventriculaire gauche. (Autopsie: triple bruit; bruit anormal au second temps.) 35 pp. 4°. *Paris,* 1860, No. 189.

Mosqueron (A.) * Des accidents développés chez les ouvriers teinturiers par l'emploi du bichromate de potasse. 49 pp. 4°. *Paris,* 1880, No. 233.

Mosquinot (M.-J.-J.-R.) * Considérations sur le traitement de névralgies. 67 pp. 4°. *Paris,* 1854, No. 40, v. 563.

Mosquito.

See, also, **Filaria.**

Dowler (B.) Researches into the natural history of the mosquito. N. Orl. M. & S. J., 1855–6, xii, 63; 176.—**Finlay** & **Delgado.** Colonias de tetrágenos sembradas por mosquitos. An. r. Acad. de cien. méd. . . . de la Habana, 1887–8, xxiv, 205–210, 1 pl.—**Johnston** (C.) Auditory apparatus of the culex musquito. Quart. J. Micr. Soc., Lond., 1855, iii, 95–102, 1 pl. *Also,* Reprint.—**King** (A. F. A.) Insects and disease; mosquitoes and malaria. Pop. Sc. Month., N. Y., 1883, xxiii, 644–658.—**Stevenson** (J.) Mosquito-bite. Edinb. M. J., 1881–2, xxvii, 692.—**Thin** (G.) Mosquito bites. Lancet, Lond., 1881, ii, 398.

Moss.

Lediard (H. A.) Experience with moss as a surgical dressing. Brit. M. J., Lond., 1887, ii, 829.

Moss (Albertus Parry). * De apoplexia. 41 pp. 8°. *Edinburgi, A. Neill et soc,* 1807.

Moss (Lemuel). Annals of the United States Christian Commission. 752 pp., 7 pl., port. 8°. *Philadelphia, J. B. Lippincott & Co.,* 1868.

Moss (W.) A familiar medical survey of Liverpool; addressed to the inhabitants at large. Containing observations on the situation of the town, the qualities and influence of the air, the employments and manner of living of the inhabitants, the water, and other natural and occasional circumstances whereby the health of the inhabitants is liable to be particularly affected. With an account of the diseases most peculiar to the town, and the rules to be observed for their prevention and cure, including observations on the cure of consumptions. The whole rendered perfectly plain and familiar. vii, 130 pp. 12°. *Liverpool, J. & W. Lowndes,* 1784.

——. The same. The Liverpool guide; including a sketch of the environs, with a map of the town, and directions for sea bathing. 4. ed., en-

Moss (W.)—continued.
larged. 1 p. l., 192 pp. 12°. *Liverpool, W. Jones*, 1801.
One map missing.

Moss (William). An essay on the management and nursing of children in the earlier periods of infancy; and on the treatment and rule of conduct requisite for the mother during pregnancy, and in lying-in. Including the diseases to which the mother and child are liable; with the methods of curing, and particularly of preventing, many of those diseases. The whole addressed as well to the medical faculty as to the public at large, and purposely adapted to a female comprehension, in a manner perfectly consistent with the delicacy of the sex. xxxi, 32–372 pp. 8°. *London, J. Johnson*, 1781.

——. The same. An essay on the management, nursing, and diseases of children from the birth; and on the treatment and diseases of pregnant and lying-in women, with remarks on the domestic practice of medicine. 2. ed. To which is now added, the treatment and diseases of children at more advanced periods of childhood. xii, 472 pp., 1 l. 8°. *Egham, C. Boult*, 1794.

——. An essay on the management and feeding of infants. 104 pp. 8°. *Philadelphia, B. Johnson*, 1808.
Repr. [Abstr.] *from his:* An essay on the management and nursing [etc.] 8°. *London*, 1781.

Mossakowski (Paul). Statistischer Bericht über 1145 französische Invaliden des deutsch-französischen Krieges 1870–71. [Basel.] 36 pp. 8°. *Leipzig, J. B. Hirschfeld*, 1872.

Mossdorf (Ferdinand). * Ueber die Methode durch gewaltsame Streckung die Contracturen des Kniegelenkes zu heilen. 22 pp. 8°. *Leipzig, Huethel u. Legler*, [1867].

Mossdorf (Godofredus Christophorus). * De lilio convallium. 28 pp., 2 l. 4°. *Halæ Magdeb., lit. J. C. Hilligeri*, [1742].

Mossdorff (Joh. Fridericus). * De valetudinariis imaginariis, von Menschen die aus Einbildung kranck werden. 32 pp. sm. 4°. *Halæ Magdeb., typ. J. C. Hendelii*, [1721].

——. The same. 32 pp. sm. 4°. *Halæ Magdeb., typ. J. C. Hendelii, recusa* 1723.

Mossdorff (Theodorus). * Synopsis calculorum urinariorum. 40 pp. sm. 4°. *Jenæ, typ. Schreiberi et soc.*, [1820].

Mossé (A.) * Étude sur l'ictère grave. 178 pp., 1 l., 2 tab. 4°. *Paris, A. Parent*, 1879, No. 495.

——. *Accidents de la lithiase biliaire. 158 pp. 4°. *Paris*, 1880.
Concours.

——. Observation de grande hystérie chez l'homme; crises convulsives arrêtées par la compression du testicule gauche; état léthargique. 15 pp. 8°. [*Montpellier*, 1887.]

Mosse (*Bartholomew*) [1712–59].
Biographical notice. Dublin Q. J. M. Sc., 1846, ii, 565, port.

Mosse (Marcus) [1808–]. * De transpirationis et sudoris dignitate. 38 pp., 1 l. 8°. *Berolini, typ. Nietackianis*, [1832].

Mossel (Émile). * Des kystes séreux du cou. 36 pp. 4°. *Paris*, 1868, No. 194.

Mossel (Jules-Marc-André). * Sur la vératrine. 1 p. l., 96 pp. 4°. *Paris*, 1868, No. 78.

Mosselage (Fridericus Christianus). * De hydrope ex spiritus vini abusu. 24 pp. 4°. *Harderovici, J. Moojen*, 1749.

van Mossevelde (Josephus). * De usu balneorum in morbis. 30 pp. 4°. *Gandavi, Vanderhaeghe-Maya*, [1830]. [P., v. 1384.]

Mossier (François). * Des luxations traumatiques des cinq dernières vertèbres cervicales.

Mossier (François)—continued.
41 pp. 4°. *Strasbourg, E.-P. Le Roux*, 1869, 3. s., No. 158.

Mossier (Joannes Baptista Amabilis). * De digestione. 16 pp. 8°. *Monspelii, J. F. Picot*, 1789. [P., v. 1091.]

Mossier (Joseph). * Considérations sur les fièvres intermittentes en général. 17 pp. 4°. *Paris*, 1825, No. 171, v. 195.

Mossin (Christian. Ludovic.) * Præsidia sanitatis et vitæ longæ e decalogo. 1 p. l., 32 pp. sm. 4°. *Hafniæ, typ. J. G. Hopffneri*, [1741].

Mossin (Joh.) filius. * Demonstratur continuatio connubii theoriæ et praxeos in studio medico. 20 pp. sm. 4°. *Harniæ, ex off. Rotmeriana*, [1734].

Mossin (Joh. R.) *Ueber die Anilocra mediterranea. 31 pp., 1 pl. 8°. *St. Petersburg*, 1870.

Mossmann (Paul). * Sur un cas d'hystéro-épilepsie chez l'homme. Relation entre les attaques et une lésion périphérique. 1 p. l., 45 pp., 3 pl. 4°. *Nancy*, 1883, No. 162.

Mosso (Angelo). Sul polso negativo e sui rapporti della respirazione addominale e toracica nell' uomo. 68 pp. 8°. *Torino, V. Bona*, 1878.
Repr. from: Arch. per le sc. med., Torino, 1878, iii.

——. Sulle variazioni locali del polso nell' antibraccio dell' uomo. 93 pp., 11 tab. 8°. *Torino*, 1878.
Repr. from: Atti d. r. Accad. d. sc. di Torino, 1877, xiii.

——. Sulla circolazione del sangue nel cervello dell' uomo. Memoria del . . . letta nella seduta del 7 dicembre 1879.
Cutting from: Atti d. r. Accad. d. Lincei. Cl. di sc. fis., matemat. e nat., Roma, 3. s., v, 237–358, 9 pl.

——. Die Diagnostik des Pulses in Bezug auf die localen Veränderungen desselben. vii, 65 pp., 7 pl. 8°. *Leipzig, Veit u. Comp.*, 1879.

——. Applicazione della bilancia allo studio della circolazione sanguigna nell' uomo. 15 pp., 1 ch. roy. 8°. *Roma, Salviucci*, 1884.
Repr. from: Atti r. Accad. d. Lincei, 1883-4.

——. La paura. 309 pp. 12°. *Milano, fratelli Treves*, 1884.

——. The same. La peur; étude psycho-physiologique, trad. de l'italien sur la 3. éd., avec autorisation de l'auteur par Félix Hément. (Bibliothèque de philosophie contemporaine.) viii, 179 pp. 12°. *Paris, F. Alcan*, 1886.

——. Le precauzioni contro il colera e le quarantene. 31 pp. 8°. [*Roma, E. Botta*, 1884.]
Repr. from: Nuova antologia, Roma, 1884, 2. s., xlvii.

——. Le università italiane e lo stato. 35 pp. 8°. *Roma, E. Botta*, 1884.
Repr. from: Nuova antologia, Roma, 1884, 2. s., xlviii, fasc. 21.

——. La respirazione periodica e la respirazione superflua o di lusso. 62 pp., 8 pl. imp. 8°. *Roma, V. Salviucci*, 1885.
Repr. from: Mem. d. Cl. d. sc. fis., matemat. e nat., 4. s., i.

——. L' istruzione superiore in Italia. 19 pp. 8°. *Roma, tipog. d. Camera d. deputati*, 1886.
Repr. from: Nuova antologia, fasc. 20.

——. L' istruzione superiore in Italia. 23 pp. 8°. *Roma, tipog. d. Camera d. deputati*, 1886.
Repr. from: Nuova antologia, vi, fasc. 23.

—— & **Pellacani** (P.) Sulle funzioni della vescica. Memoria letta nella seduta del 1 maggio 1881. 64 pp., 7 pl. 8°. [*Roma*, 1881.]
Repr. from: Atti d. r. Accad. d. Lincei. Cl. di sc. fis., matemat. e nat., Roma, 1881, 3. s., xii.

Mosso (Ugolino). Sulla azione delle sostanze che per mezzo del sistema nervoso aumentano o diminuiscono la temperatura animale. 17 pp. 8°. *Torino, E. Loescher*, 1886.

Most. Moshi Yakuron. [Most's materia medica, transl. by Yema Ringen.] 3 v. 8°. *Kioto*, 1867.
Japanese text.

Most (Chr. Geor. Bern.) * De cirsocele seu hernia varicosa. 48 pp. 8°. *Halæ, typ. Trampianis*, [1796].

Most (Georg. Frieder.) [1794–]. * Diss. sistens brevem phthiseos pulmonalis exulceratæ descriptionem. 69 pp. 12°. *Gottingæ, J. C. Baier*, [1817].

——. Influenza Europæa, oder die grösseste Krankheits - Epidemie der neuern Zeit. Ein Versuch zur Beantwortung der Fragen: Was ist die Influenz? Wie war sie früher beschaffen? Woher entstand dieselbe? Aus welchen Gründen können wir ihre Wiedererscheinung im Jahre 1822 mit Wahrscheinlichkeit in Europa vermuthen? Wie wird sie dann beschaffen seyn? Durch welche Mittel kann man ihr Grenzen setzen? Für Aerzte und Nichtärzte. xlviii, 254 pp., 2 l. 8°. *Hamburg, Perthes u. Besser*, 1820.

——. La guérison de l'épilepsie, par un nouveau procédé, puissant, efficace, et peu conteux; appuyée par de nombreux exemples, rapportés par . . . avec des notes de l'auteur, ajoutées en 1824. Trad. de l'allemand, par Ch. de G . . . iii, 124 pp., 1 l. 8°. *Paris, Rey & Gravier*, 1825.

——. Versuch einer kritischen Bearbeitung der Geschichte des Scharlachfiebers und seiner Epidemien von den ältesten bis auf unsere Zeiten. 2 v. xii, 300 pp.; vi, 367 pp. 8°. *Leipzig, F. A. Brockhaus*, 1826.

——. Encyklopädie der gesammten medicinischen und chirurgischen Praxis, mit Einschluss der Geburtshülfe, der Augenheilkunde und der Operativchirurgie. Im Verein mit mehreren praktischen Aerzten und Wundärzten bearbeitet und hrsg. von . . . 2. Aufl. 2 v. viii, v–xxxii, 1048 pp.; 1138 pp. 8°. *Leipzig, F. A. Brockhaus*, 1836-7.
   v. 1. A—Humectantia.
   v. 2. Hyalitis—Zymosis.

——. Ueber Liebe und Ehe in sittlicher, naturgeschichtlicher und diätetisch - medicinischer Hinsicht; nebst einer Anleitung zur richtigen physischen und moralischen Erziehung der Kinder. 3. Aufl. 414 pp., 1 l. 8°. *Leipzig, F. A. Brockhaus*, 1837.

——. Ausführliche Encyklopädie der gesammten Staatsarzneikunde. Im Vereine mit mehreren Doctoren der Rechtsgelahrtheit, der Philosophie, der Medicin und Chirurgie, mit praktischen Civil-, Militair- und Gerichtsärzten und Chemikern bearbeitet und hrsg. von . . . Für Gesetzgeber, Rechtsgelehrte, Policeibeamte, Militairärzte, gerichtliche Aerzte, Wundärzte, Apotheker und Veterinärärzte. 2 v. xviii, 1132 pp., 1 l.; 1190 pp.; 1 l., 336 pp. 8°. *Leipzig, F. A. Brockhaus*, 1838-40.
   v. 1. A—K.
   v. 2. L—Z.
   Supplement, A—Z.

——. Ueber alte und neue medicinische Lehrsysteme im Allgemeinen und über Dr. J. L. Schönlein's neuestes natürliches System der Medicin insbesondere. Ein historisch-kritischer Versuch. 1 p. l., 413 pp. 8°. *Leipzig, F. A. Brockhaus*, 1841.

——. Denkwürdigkeiten aus der medicinischen und chirurgischen Praxis: v. 1. xx, 378 pp., 1 l. 8°. *Leipzig, F. A. Brockhaus*, 1842.
   No more published.

——. Die sympathetischen Mittel und Curmethoden. Diss. xvi, 175 pp. 8°. *Rostock, Eberstein u. Otto*, 1842.
                      c.

——. Encyclopedisch woordenboek der praktische geneesmiddelleer, naar de beste bronnen en eigene veeljarige ondervinding bewerkt door . . . Naar het Hoogduitsch. 2 v. 1 p. l., 503

Most (Georg. Frieder.)—continued.
pp.; 1 p. l., 560 pp., 1 l. 8°. *Amsterdam, H. Frijlink*, 1843.

Most important errors ·in chemistry, electricity, and magnetism pointed out and refuted; and the polarity of the magnetic needle accounted for and explained. By a fellow of the Royal Society. iv, 5–47 pp. 8°. *London, J. Ridgway*, 1846.

Mostafa el Soubky. * Dissertation historique et médicale sur la peste. 61 pp. 4°. *Paris*, 1837, No. 401, v. 318.

Mostaganem.

   See **Cholera** (*Asiatic, History, etc., of*), *by localities.*

Mosterts (Henricus Guilelmus). * De myocarditide, addita historia morbi. 35 pp. 8°. *Gryphiæ, F. G. Kunike*, 1858.
                      c.

Mosthaff (Antonius). * Diss. sistens disquisitionem an in morborum curatione ad formam respiciendum. 22 pp., 1 l. 4°. *Gottingæ, H. Dieterich*, [1802].

Mosthaff (Fr.) Die Homöopathie in ihrer Bedeutung für die Entwicklung der Medizin als Kunst und Wissenschaft. 1. u. 2. Theil. iv, 155 pp. 8°. *Heidelberg, K. Groos*, 1843.

Motais (Ernest). * Symptomatologie de la congestion chronique du foie. 36 pp. 4°. *Paris*, 1870, No. 119.

——. Notions générales sur le strabisme. Résultats de 26 opérations de strabisme. 94 pp., pl., 3 phot. pl., 1 l. 8°. *Angers, P. Lachèse & Dolbeau*, 1881.

——. Hygiène professionnelle. Hygiène de la vue chez les typographes. 45 pp., 1 l. 8°. *Paris, J.-B. Baillière & fils*, 1883.

——. Anatomie de l'appareil moteur de l'œil de l'homme et des vertébrés. Déductions physiologiques et chirurgicales (strabisme). [2 pts.] 303 pp., 14 pl. 8°. *Paris, A. Delahaye & E. Lecrosnier*, 1887.
   1. pt. is repr. from: Arch. d'opht., Par., 1884-6, iv-vi.

Motard (Louis-Claude-Adolphe). * De l'arsenic, considéré comme médicament et comme poison. 28 pp. 4°. *Paris*, 1835, No. 276, v. 290.

——. * Du sang considéré sous les rapports anatomique, physiologique et chimique. 40 pp. 4°. *Paris*, 1835, No. 415, v. 290.
   Concours.

——. * Des eaux stagnantes, et en particulier des marais et des desséchemens. 68 pp. 4°. *Paris*, 1838. [P., v. 1695.]
   Concours.

——. Essai d'hygiène générale. 2 v. 496 pp., 1 l.; 592 pp., 1 l. 8°. *Paris, I. Pesron & J.-B. Baillière*, 1841.

——. Traité d'hygiène générale. 2 v. iv, 876, 824 pp. 8°. *Paris, J.-B. Baillière & fils*, 1868-9.

Motel (Jules) [1858–]. * Sur un cas de mort subite par embolie pulmonaire. 34 pp., 1 l. 4°. *Paris*, 1884, No. 252.

Motet (Auguste). De la possibilité et de la convenance de faire sortir certaines catégories d'aliénés des asiles spéciaux et de les placer, soit dans des exploitations agricoles, soit dans leurs propres familles. 22 pp. 8°. *Lyon, A. Vingtrinier*, 1865.

——. Les aliénés devant la loi. 48 pp. 8°. *Paris, J.-B. Baillière & fils*, 1866.

——. Atrophie musculaire progressive. 8°. *Paris, E. Martinet*, 1866.
   Cutting from: Guide du méd. praticien, Valleix, 5. éd., Par., 1866, i, 997–1028.

——. Névroses. 8°. *Paris, E. Martinet*, 1866.
   Cutting from: Guide du méd. praticien, Valleix, 5. éd., Par., 1866, i, 641–686.

Motet (Auguste)—continued.

——. Éloge de Félix Voisin. 28 pp. 12°. *Paris, J.-B. Baillière & fils*, 1873.
Repr. from: Ann. méd.-psych., Par., 1873, 5. s., x.

——. Éloge de Morel. 36 pp. 12°. *Paris, J.-B. Baillière & fils*, 1874.
Repr. from: Ann. méd.-psych., Par., 1874, 5. s, xii.

——. Éloge de G. Ferrus; lu à la séance publique annuelle de la Société médico-psychologique du 27 mai 1878. 31 pp. 8°. *Paris, E. Donnaud*, 1878.
Repr. from: Ann. méd.-psych., Par., 1878, xx.

——. Broadmoor Criminal Lunatic Asylum. 48 pp. 8°. *Paris, Boudet*, 1881.
Repr. from: Ann. méd.-psych., Par., 1881, 6. s., vi.

——. Accès de somnambulisme spontané et provoqué. Prévention d'outrage public à la pudeur; condamnation; irresponsabilité; appel, infirmation et acquittement; relation médico-légale. 16 pp. 8°. *Paris, J.-B. Baillière & fils*, 1881.

——. Les faux témoignages des enfants devant la justice. 20 pp. 8°. *Paris, J.-B. Baillière & fils*, 1887.
See, also, **Miraglia** (B.) Relazione sui lavori e titoli del Augusto Motet. Resoc. Accad. med.-chir. di Napoli, 1877, xxxi, 170-174.—**Statistique** (la) générale des aliénés de 1854 à 1860. 8°. *Paris*, 1867.

Mothe. Mélanges de médecine et chirurgie, ou mémoires sur les pansemens, luxations, opérations chirurgicales, maladies syphilitiques, paralysie, etc. 2 v. xix, 23-445 pp., 1 pl.; xii, 426 pp., 1 pl. 8°. *Paris, Baillière*, 1812-27.

Mothe (Adrien-Ambroise-Antoine). * De l'acupuncture dans la mort apparente des asphyxiés. xviii, 19-50 pp., 1 l. 4°. *Montpellier*, 1878, No. 35.

Mothe (B.) * Sur le cathétérisme. 21 pp. 4°. *Paris*, 1830, No. 280, v. 237.

Mothe (J.-M.) * Sur la variole. 18 pp. 4°. *Paris*, 1826, No. 141, v. 201.

Mothe (Joseph-Hilarion). * De la tumeur et de la fistule lacrymale. 34 pp. 4°. *Paris*, 1857, No. 262, v. 608.

Motheau (René). * Traitement de la tuberculose pulmonaire par les injections intestinales de gaz carbonique chargé de vapeurs médicamenteuses. 40 pp. 4°. *Paris*, 1887, No. 134.

Motherby (G.) [A new] medical dictionary or general repository of physic. Containing an explanation of the terms and a description of the various particulars relating to anatomy, physiology, physic, surgery, materia medica, chemistry, [etc.] 2. ed. vi pp., 359 l., 24 pl. fol. *London, J. Johnson*, 1785.

——. The same. 5. ed., revised and corrected, with considerable additions, by George Wallis. 811 pp., 34 pl. fol. *London, S. Hamilton*, 1801.

Motherby (Gulielmus). * De epilepsia. 46 pp. 8°. *Edinburgi, C. Stewart et socii*, 1799. [*Also, in:* P., v. 11.]

Motherby (Robertus) [1808-]. * De atresia punctorum lacrymalium. 31 pp. 8°. *Berolini, typ. A. Petschii*, [1831].

Motheré (A.-Maximilien). * De la fièvre intermittente simple. 30 pp. 4°. *Paris*, 1854, No. 131, v. 563.

Mother-of-pearl (*Workers in*).
Duchesne (L.) & **Michel** (E.) Les nacriers; étude d'hygiène professionnelle. Rev. d'hyg., Par., 1882, iv, 656-665.—**Layet** (A.) Nacriers (hygiène professionnelle). Dict. encycl. d. sc. méd., Par., 1876, 2. s., xi, 361-367.—**Mahier** & **Chevallier**. Mémoire sur les ouvriers qui travaillent les coquilles de nacre de perle. Ann. d'hyg., Par., 1852, xlviii, 241-251.

Mothers.
See **Women** (*Diseases, etc., of, Popular treatises on*).

Mothers (*Duties of*).
See **Children** (*Hygiene, etc., of*); **Infants** (*Hygiene, etc., of*).

Mothers' (The) book, containing the management of children, by Amie M. Hale. What every mother should know, by Edward Ellis. The mental culture and training of children, by Pye Henry Chavasse. 3 v. in 1. 12°. *Philadelphia, P. Blakiston, Son & Co.*, [1880].

Mother's-marks.
See **Fœtus** (*Maternal influence on*); **Nævus**.

Motherwell (*James Bridgeham*) [1815-86].
Obituary. Austral. M. J., Melbourne, 1886, viii, 224.

Motion.
See **Force**.

Motion (*Animal and vital*).
See **Cilia**, *etc.*; **Locomotion**; **Mechanics** (*Animal*); **Movement**, *etc.* (*Organic*); **Muscles**.

Motion (*Organic*).
See **Movement**, *etc.* (*Organic*).

Motion (*Sense of*).
See **Movement** (*Sense of*).

Motion as a remedy.
See **Exercise** *as a remedy*; **Nervous** *system* (*Diseases of, Treatment of*); **Orthopædia**.

Motref (Jean-Pierre-François). * Sur le catarrhe aigu de la vessie. 25 pp. 4°. *Paris*, 1818, No. 144, v. 139; 140.

Motreuil (Jean - Armand). * Conseils hygiéniques à une jeune mère et aux personnes qui l'entourent. 17 pp. 4°. *Paris*, 1832, No. 237, v. 255.

Motschenbacher (J. Chr.) * Wie werden Kranke, unbeschadet der Sicherheit der Kur, wohlfeil behandelt? 32 pp. 8°. *Erlangen, Hilpert*, 1840.

Mott (*Mrs.*) The ladies' medical oracle; or, Mrs. Mott's advice to young females, wives, and mothers; being a non-medical commentary on the cause, prevention, and cure of the diseases of the female frame; together with an explanation of her system of European vegetable medicine for the cure of diseases, and the patent medicated champoo baths; to which is added, an explanation of the gift, and an exposition of the numerous fabricated reports "a weak invention of the enemy". Printed and published for the authoress. 213 pp., 1 pl. 12°. *Boston*, 1834.

Mott (Albert J.) Alcohol and total abstinence. 22 pp. 8°. *London, W. H. Allen & Co.*, 1884.
Repr. from: Nat. Rev., May, 1884.

Mott (Alexander Brown) [1826-]. Surgical operations. Series No. 1. 26 pp., 3 pl. 8°. [*New York*], 1856-7.

CONTENTS.

I. Remarks on deformities from burns; with a successful operation on a formidable case.
II. Case of wound of the internal jugular vein, successfully treated by ligature.
III. Case of exostosis occupying the orbit and nasal cavity, successfully removed, and vision restored.

——. Advantages of clinical teaching. An address introductory to the regular course of lectures at the Bellevue Hospital Medical College, N. Y. 30 pp. 8°. *New York, C. A. Alvord*, 1868.
See, also, **Mott** (Valentine). Catalogue of the surgical and pathological museum of . . . and of his son . . . 8°. *New York*, 1858.
For Biography, see Med. & Surg. Reporter, Phila., 1864-5, xii, 409-411.
For Portrait, see **Collection** of Portr. (Libr.)

Mott (Henry A.) Complete history and process of manufacture of artificial butter. 2. ed. 27 pp. 12°. *New York, J. F. Trow & Son*, 1876.

Mott (Henry A.)—continued.

——. A brief history of the Mége discovery. Oleomargarine butter, or butterine. "The microscope and chemical analysis in the hands of the most skilful and distinguished scientists demonstrating its purity." 30 pp. 8°. *New York, Trow,* 1880.

——. Heveenoid; the rubber of the future. 13 pp. 8°. *New York, Trow,* 1880.

——. The practical determination of the value of the sugars of commerce. 19 pp. 8°. *New York,* 1880.

——. The air we breathe and ventilation. Mott series. No. 2. 81 pp., 25 pl. 16°. *New York, J. Wiley & Sons,* 1883.

——. Essay on electricity and description of apparatus for sale by the New York Electric Novelty Co., designed for colleges, high schools, and other institutions of learning. 26 pp. 8°. *New York,* [1886].

Mott (Hugo). * Der Gebärmutterkrebs. 30 pp. 8°. *Würzburg, Becker,* 1879. C.

Mott (J. Varnum). A paper on medicated ice. 7 pp. 8°. *New York, Mucklow & Simon,* 1877.

Mott (Lucretia). A sermon to the medical students, delivered at Cherry street meeting, Philadelphia. 21 pp. 8°. *Philadelphia, W. B. Zeiber,* 1849.

Mott (Valentine) [1785–1835]. *An experimental inquiry into the chemical and medical properties of the Statice limonium of Linnæus. 58 pp., 1 pl. 8°. *New York, T. & J. Swords,* 1806.

——. Reflections on securing in a ligature the arteria innominata, to which is added a case in which this artery was tied by a surgical operation. 46 pp., 2 pl. 8°. [*New York,* 1819.] [P., v. 746; 817.]

——. A biographical memoir of Wright Post, M. D. Delivered as an introductory lecture. 32 pp. 8°. *New York, E. Conrad,* 1829. [*Also, in:* P., v. 833.]

——. Travels in Europe and the East. 452 pp. 8°. *New York, Harper & Bros.,* 1842.

——. A biographical memoir of John Revere, M. D. 40 pp. 8°. *New York, J. H. Jennings,* 1847. [*Also, in:* P., v. 235.]

——. An inaugural address, delivered before the New-York Academy of Medicine, February 7, 1849. To which is prefixed, an address by Dr. J. W. Francis to the president elect. 24 pp. 8°. *New-York, H. Ludwig & Co.,* 1849.

——. An introductory discourse, delivered in the University of New York, session 1849–50. 32 pp. 8°. *New York, Jennings & Harrison,* 1850.

——. Reminiscences of medical teaching and teachers in New York. An address introductory to a course of lectures at the College of Physicians and Surgeons, New York, session of 1850–51. 32 pp. 8°. *New York, J. H. Jennings,* 1850.

——. Catalogue of the surgical and pathological museum of Valentine Mott, and of his son, Alexander B. Mott. iv, 78 pp., 1 l. 8°. *New York, W. M. Taylor,* 1858.

——. Address before the graduates of 1860 of the University Medical College of New York. 25 pp. 8°. *New York, Miller, Mathews & Clasback,* 1860.

——. Eulogy on the late John W. Francis, being a discourse on his life and character, delivered before the New York Academy of Medicine, May 29, 1861. 33 pp. 8°. *New York, S. S. & W. Wood,* 1861.

——. Pain and anæsthetics; an essay, introductory to a series of surgical and medical monographs. (Prepared by request of the Sanitary Commission.) 16 pp. 8°. *Washington, Government Printing Office,* 1862.

Mott (Valentine)—continued.

——. The same. 2. ed. 16 pp. 8°. *Washington, McGill & Witherow,* 1863.

——. On hæmorrhage from wounds, and the best means of arresting it. 16 pp., 4 pl. 8°. *New York, A. D. F. Randolph,* 1863. [*Also, in:* P., v. 194.]

See UNITED STATES Sanitary Commission. R.

Also, Co-Editor of: **New York** (The) Medical Magazine, 1814–15.—**Medical** (The) and Surgical Register, New York, 1818–20.

See, also, **Vanderbergh** (F.) Letter to . . . in reply to his valedictory [etc.] 8°. *New York,* 1850.—**Velpeau** (A. A. L. M.) New elements of operative surgery [etc.] 8°. *New York,* 1847.

For Biography, see **Gross** (S. D.) Memoir of Valentine Mott. 8°. *Philadelphia,* 1868.—**Post** (A. C.) Eulogy on the late Valentine Mott. 8°. *New York,* 1866.

See, also, Ann. univ. di med., Milano, 1868, cciii, 360–362 (C. Fumagalli). *Also:* Boston M. & S. J., 1851, xliii, 370–374. *Also:* Frank Leslie's Illust. Newspaper, N. Y., 1856, i, no. 20, 318–320, port. *Also:* Lancet, Lond., 1865, i, 553. *Also:* Med. & Surg. Reporter, Phila., 1864, ii, 311 ; 329 (S. W. Francis). *Also:* Pacific M. & S. J., San Fran., 1865–6, viii, 163–174 (H. H. Toland). *Also:* Richmond & Louisville M. J., Louisville, 1869, vii, 110–113, port. *Also:* Tr. M. Soc. N. Y., Albany, 1866, 304–316 (S. B. Gunning).

For Portrait, see **Collection** of Portr. (Libr.)

——. *See, also:*

FAIR play is a jewel. 8°. *New York,* 1819.

FRANCIS (J. W.) Address to the president elect, Valentine Mott, [etc.] 8°. *New York,* 1849.

——. Report of Prof. Valentine Mott's surgical cliniques, [etc.] 8°. *New York,* 1860.

——. Memoir of the life of Valentine Mott, [etc.] 8°. *New York,* 1865.

PUBLIC dinner to Valentine Mott. 8°. [*New York,* 1835.]

WOOD (I.) An inaugural address delivered before the New York Academy of Medicine, etc. 8°. *New York,* 1850.

WOOD (J. R.) Early history of the operation of ligature of the primitive carotid artery, [etc.] 8°. *New York,* 1857.

Remarks on a pamphlet entitled : "Reflections on securing in a ligature the arteria innominata, to which is added a case in which this artery was tied by a surgical operation". By Valentine Mott, [etc.] Am. M. Recorder, Phila., 1819, ii, 73–81. *Also, repr. under title:* Fair play is a jewel. 8°. *New York,* 1819.

Mott (J. L.) **Iron Works.** Illustrated catalogue of the plumbing and sanitary department of the J. L. Mott Iron Works. 176 pp. 8°. *New York, E. D. Slater,* [1878].

——. 1884. Catalogue D. The bath room illustrated ; also, fixtures for laundry, kitchen, and butler's pantry. 82 pp. 4°. *New York,* 1884.

——. 1885. Price list of catalogue D. The bath room illustrated. 31 pp. 8°. *New York,* 1885.

Motta (Eduardo Augusto). Da anemia do cerebro em geral e particularmente da ischemia cerebral e amollecimento consecutivo; memoria apresentada à Academia real das sciencias de Lisboa. 117 pp., 6 l. 4°. *Lisboa, typ. Acad. real d. sc.,* 1874.

Motta (L.)

See **Bertani** (Agostino). Su 'l colera, [etc.] 8°. *Milano,* 1854.

da Motta Andrade (Mathias Arthur). * Dissertação do diagnostico e tratamento das paralysias periphericas. 6 p. l., 79 pp., 1 l. 8°. *Rio de Janeiro, Laemmert & Co.,* 1886.

Motta Baluffi.

See **Cholera** (*Asiatic, History, etc., of*), by localities.

Motta Maia. Estudo sobre o ensino medico na Austria e na Allemanha. Terceiro relatorio semestral apresentado á Faculdade de medicina do Rio de Janeiro. 316 pp., 2 tab. 8°. *Paris, A. Parent,* 1877.

da Motta Silva (Joaquim). * Rheumatismo articular agudo. 2 p. l., 30 pp., 1 l. 4°. *Bahia, J. G. Tourinho,* 1871.

Motte. Chirurgie infantile. 25 pp. 8°. [*Bruxelles,* 1875, *vel subseq.*]
Repr. from: Bull. Acad. roy. de méd. de Belg., Brux., 1876, 3. s., x.

Motte (Charles-Adolphe). * Sur les luxations spontanées ou consécutives du fémur. 27 pp. 4°. *Paris,* 1817, No. 177, v. 128.

de la Motte (Guillaume-Mauquest). *See* **La Motte** (Guillaume-Mauquest).

Mottet (P.) * Réflexions sur quelques substances médicinales indigènes. 15 pp. 4°. *Paris,* 1833, No. 19, v. 257.

————. De la brûlure et de la congélation; appréciations cliniques fournies par la colonne expéditionnaire du 22 février au 24 avril 1852. 15 pp. 8°. *Paris, J.-B. Baillière,* 1852.

————. Nouvel essai d'une thérapeutique indigène, ou études analytiques et comparatives de phytologie médicale exotique. xvi, 17–812 pp. 8°. *Paris, J.-B. Baillière,* 1852.

Mottini (Pietro). Della pellagra e principalmente dell' opera del Dott. Teofilo Roussel di Parigi sulla stessa pubblicata nello scorso 1845. 18 pp. 8°. *Milano, G. Ghius*i, 1846.
Repr. from: Gazz. med. ital. lomb., Milano, 1846, v.

Mottley (Edward). The vital statistics of the town of Margate for the twelve years ending June, 1849, compiled from the records at the register office for the purpose of ascertaining the sanitary condition of the town. Revised ed. 24 pp. 8°. *Margate, T. H. Keble,* 1850.

————. A report on the sanitary condition of the town of Margate from the year 1837 to 1862; being a statistical account of the numbers dying and the cause of death of the inhabitants, visitors, and inmates of the infirmaries. By order of the council of the borough. 2. ed. 31 pp., 1 diag. 8°. *London, Simpkin, Marshall & Co.,* [1862?]

————. Statistical examination of the Margate death-rate, for the five years 1863–67. By order of the council of the borough of Margate. 15 pp. 8°. *Margate, T. H. Keble,* 1868.

Motton-Richard (Louis-Antoine). * I. Établir les caractères qui distinguent le prurigo de la gale. II. [etc.] 20 pp. 4°. *Paris,* 1839, No. 130, v. 347.

Moty (Fernand). * Sur une épidémie de pourriture d'hôpital. 64 pp., 1 tab. 4°. *Paris,* 1871, No. 179.

Moty (Jules). * Des anévrysmes de l'aorte thoracique. 68 pp. 4°. *Paris,* 1877, No. 553.

Motz (G. D.) * De structura, usu et morbis ovariorum. 40 pp., 2 l. 4°. *Jenæ, typ. Gæpferdtii,* 1789. [P., v. 59.]

Mouat (Frederic John) [1816–]. Observations on the nosological arrangement of the Bengal medical returns, with a few cursory remarks on medical topography and military hygiene. 1 p. l., 64 pp. 8°. *Calcutta, Sanders & Cones,* 1845.

————. An atlas of anatomical plates of the human body, with descriptive letter press in English and Hindustani. Published by order of government. 50 col. pl. and text. fol. *Calcutta, Bishop's College Press,* 1849.

————. Reports on jails visited and inspected in Bengal, Behar, and Arracan. iv, 338, lxxvi pp., 2 plans. 8°. *Calcutta, F. Carbery,* 1856.

————. The Andaman Islands; with notes on Barren Island. [Report of the committee appointed Nov. 20, 1857, to select a site for the establishment of a penal settlement.] xvii, 131 pp., 6 pl., 1 plan. 8°. *Calcutta, C. B. Lewis,* 1859.
Selections from the records of the government of India (home department), No. xxv.

Mouat (Frederic John)—continued.

————. On prison statistics and discipline in lower Bengal. 44 pp. 8°. [*n. p.,* 1860, *vel subseq.*] [P., v. 952.]

————. Report on the diet of prisoners in the jails of the lower provinces of the Bengal Presidency. [With Appendix No. II, shewing in detail the strength, admissions, deaths, dietary, and cubical space of the three quinquennial periods of 1839 to 1843, 1844 to 1848, and 1852 to 1856, in the jails of the lower provinces, with abstracts of the same.] 6, 7, [1 l.], 52, 122, xcvii pp. 4°. *Calcutta, Alipore Jail press,* 1860.

————. Report on the classified dietary of 1862 for prisoners in the jails of the lower provinces of the Bengal Presidency. [With appendix showing the results of the new dietary, as exhibited by the weights of the prisoners subjected to it, on admission and discharge; the sickness and mortality that prevailed among them; and the cost of the measure during the continuance of the experiment, viz, from the 1st of May to the 31st of October, 1862.] 12, 123, xxiii pp., 17 tab. 4°. *Calcutta, Alipore Jail press,* 1863.
Bound with preceding.

————. The New Zealand war of 1863–5. Special report on wounds and injuries received in battle. 56 pp. 8°. [*n p.,* 1865, *vel subseq.*] [P., v. 421.]
Repr. from: Med. & Surg. Hist. of the New Zealand war.

————. Memorandum on the duties, etc., of inspectors of sanitary arrangements. 7 pp. fol. [*n. p.*], 1858.

————. A visit to some of the battle-fields and ambulances of the north of France. 18 pp. 8°. [*London,* 1871.]

————. The death tribute of England to India; being an examination of the deaths and invaliding of officers of H. M. British forces serving in India, from 1861 to 1870, inclusive, considered with special reference to the question of the present value of European life in India. 73 pp., 1 tab. 8°. *London, C. & E. Layton,* 1875.

————. Repression of crime; address delivered before the Social Science Congress at Dublin, Oct. 4, 1881. 22 pp. 8°. *London, Spottiswoode & Co.,* 1881.

————. Memorial of . . . to the right honourable the secretary of state for India, in council. 8°. [*n. p., n. d.*]
See, also, **Hickey** (W. R. Gilbert). The carbonization or dry distillation system, etc. 8°. *Darjeeling,* 1869.

————. *See, also:*
ADDRESSES, etc., presented to Dr. F. J. Mouat on his retirement from her majesty's Indian service. Calcutta, November, 1870. 8°. *London,* 1871.
RECORD of the public services in India of F. J. Mouat. fol. [*n. p., n. d.*]
————. The same. Record of public services in India. 8°. [*Bengal, n. d.*]
UNIVERSITIES in India. 8°. [*n. p., n. d.*]

———— **& Snell** (H. Saxon). Hospital construction and management. xiv, 78, 280, 60 pp., 1 l., 52 pl., 1 map. 4°. *London, J. & A. Churchill & Co.,* 1883[–84].

Mouat (James). * Disp. quædam de inflammatione complectens. 2 p. l., iv, 36 pp. 8°. *Edinburgi, Abernethy et Walker,* 1812. [P., v. 861.]

———— **& Wyatt** (John). Report of Drs. . . . [in reference to the medical concerns of the Russian army]. Sept., 1856. 11 pp. fol. [*London, War Department,* 1856.] [P., v. 1080.]

Moubis (J. B. H.)
Co-Editor of: **Tijdschrift** voor Veeartsenijkunde en Veeteelt, Amsterdam, 1879.

Moucelot (Philippe). * Sur la grenouillette. 1 p. l., 18 pp. 4°. *Strasbourg,* 1805, v. 43.

Mouchard (M.)
See de St. Ives. A new treatise of the diseases of the eyes. 8°. *London*, 1741.

Mouche (Aimé). *Quelques mots sur le régime alimentaire des femmes enceintes et de son influence sur le volume et le poids du fœtus. 50 pp., 3 l. 4°. *Montpellier, L. Cristin & Cie.*, 1866, No. 42. c.

Mouchet (Alphonse). *Des affections secondaires du choléra, observées dans l'épidémie de 1866. 76 pp. 4°. *Paris*, 1867, No. 131.
———. The same. 74 pp., 1 l. 8°. *Paris, A. Delahaye*, 1867.

Mouchet (Henri). *I. Quels sont les divers modes de préparation de l'extrait d'opium? Comparer la composition chimique des extraits obtenus par des procédés différents; étudier les préparations dont l'extrait d'opium fait la base. II. [etc.] 21 pp. 4°. *Paris*, 1842, No. 127, v. 393.

Mouchon (Émile). Monographie des principaux fébrifuges indigènes, considérés comme succédanés du quinquina. 151 pp. 8°. *Lyon, A. Vingtrinier*, 1856.

Mouchot (Alphonse). *Quelques considérations sur la scille dans les hydropisies. 36 pp. 4°. *Paris*, 1871, No. 70.

Mouchot (Jean-Marie-Émile). *Essai sur la rétinite dite pigmentaire, suivi de six observations sur cette maladie. 70 pp., 3 pl. 4°. *Strasbourg*, 1868, 3. s., No. 103.
———. The same. 1 p. l., 69 pp., 2 pl. sm. 4°. *Paris, J.-B. Baillière*, 1868.

Mouchot (Justin-Martial). *De la rage, ou hydrophobie rabique. 40 pp. 4°. *Paris*, 1848, No. 107, v. 475.

Mouchotte (C.-I.-H.) *Des blessures de l'œil par les corps étrangers. 36 pp. 4°. *Paris*, 1873, No. 280.

Moudan (Pierre-Louis-Gabriel) [1856–]. *Recherches expérimentales et cliniques sur les atrophies des membres dans les affections chirurgicales. (Système musculaire et système osseux.) 255 pp. [Lyon.] 4°. *Valence*, 1882, No. 149.

Mouette (Thomas). *Sur la pleurésie chronique. 29 pp. 4°. *Paris*, 1818, No. 16, v. 135. [*Also, in:* P., v. 1640.]

Mouffet [or **Moufit**]. *See* Mufettus (Thomas).

Mougenc de Saint-Avid (F.-E.) *Étude sur le chancre non infectant de l'utérus et ses rapports avec le chancre mou du vagin. 50 pp., 1 l. 4°. *Paris*, 1856, No. 167.

Mougeot (de l'Aube). Nouvelles instructions pour se préserver du choléra. 16 pp. 12°. *Paris, J. Michelet*, 1883.

Mougeot (Albert). *Contribution à l'étude des ruptures variqueuses vulvaires pendant la grossesse. 48 pp. 4°. *Paris*, 1883, No. 180.

Mougeot (J.-B.) *Essai zoologique et médical sur les hydatides. 75 pp. 8°. *Paris, an XI* [1803], v. 26.

Mougeot (J.-B.-A.) *Recherches sur quelques troubles de nutrition consécutifs aux affections des nerfs. 1 p. l., 154 pp. 4°. *Paris*, 1867, No. 43.

Mougeot (Jean-Baptiste-Félix). *I. Du sang à l'état normal et chez les individus atteints de pneumonie. II. [etc.] 43 pp. 4°. *Paris*, 1843, No. 60, v. 406.

Mougeot (Jean-Baptiste-Paul). *Pseudo-étranglement causé par des adhérences de l'intestin hernié. 35 pp. 4°. *Paris*, 1874, No. 351.

Mougeot (Joseph-Antoine). *Quelques considérations générales sur les hernies du bas-ventre. 30 pp. 4°. *Paris*, 1837, No. 173, v. 311.

Mougeot (Pierre-Bonaventure-Alfred). *I. Des causes de l'hypertrophie du cœur. II. [etc.] 38 pp. 4°. *Paris*, 1844, No. 120, v. 421.

Mougin (Ch.-Léon). *De l'épididymite caséeuse. 86 pp. 4°. *Paris*, 1873, No. 216.
———. The same. 83 pp. 8°. *Paris, A. Delahaye*, 1873.

Mougin (L.) Les épidémies dans la ville de Vitry-le-François, et dans son arrondissement. ii, 76 pp. 8°. *Vitry-le-François, Vve. Tavernier & fils*, 1886.

Mouginez (Jean-Bapt.-Benj.) *Essai sur l'autocratie de la nature, envisagée spécialement sous le rapport des crises dans les maladies aiguës. 1 p. l., 19 pp. 4°. *Strasbourg*, 1822, v. 50.

Mouillard. *Du traitement des tumeurs érectiles en particulier par les injections de chloral. 1 p. l., 40 pp. 4°. *Paris*, 1876, No. 374.

Mouillard (Eugène-Auguste). *I. Des passions, sous le point de vue séméiologique. II. [etc.] 30 pp. 4°. *Paris*, 1841, No. 255, v. 378.

Mouilleron (Louis). *Contribution à l'étude des corps étrangers de la cavité oculaire. 78 pp., 1 l. 4°. *Paris*, 1878, No. 77.

[**Mouilleseaux**] [1739–1811]. Appel au public sur le magnétisme animal, ou projet d'un journal pour le seul avantage du public et dont il serait le coopérateur. 100 pp. 8°. [*n. p.*], 1787.

Mouilleseaux (P.-F.) *I. Du mouvement vibratoire dans les corps solides; balance de torsion, ses usages. II. [etc.] 23 pp. 4°. *Strasbourg*, 1839, No. 37, v. 4.

Mouillet (F.) *Sur la hernie ombilicale des enfans. 32 pp. 8°. *Paris, an XI* [1803], v. 38.

Mouisset (Alphonse). *Quelques considérations sur la suette miliaire. 86 pp., 3 l. 4°. *Montpellier, L. Cristin & Cie.*, 1866, No. 98. c.

Mouktar (M.) *Du diagnostic différentiel de l'adénopathie trachéo-bronchique, avec la tuberculose au début. 135 pp. 4°. *Paris*, 1886, No. 235.

Moula (Paul). *De l'atrésie de la membrane hymen. ix, 11–86 pp., 2 l. 4°. *Montpellier*, 1878, No. 70.

Moulard. *Des fractures transversales de la rotule et de leur traitement. 43 pp. 4°. *Paris*, 1877, No. 198.

Moulard (Irénée-Marc). *Contribution à l'étude de l'ictère dans les phénomènes secondaires de la syphilis. 52 pp. 4°. *Paris*, 1879, No. 561.

Mould (G. W.)
See Six introductory lectures, etc. 12°. *Manchester*, 1884.

Moulds.
See Fungi.

Moule (Henry). National health and wealth, instead of the disease, nuisance, expense, and waste caused by cess-pools and water-drainage. 15 pp. 8°. *London, Bradbury & Evans*, 1859.
———. The same. 2. ed. 26 pp. 8°. *London, Bradbury & Evans*, 1861. [P., v. 880.]
———. The same. 3. ed., revised. 17 pp. 8°. *London, Bradbury & Evans*, 1864.
———. Manure for the million. To the cottage gardeners of England. 6 pp. 16°. [*Whitefriars, Bradbury & Evans*, 1862.] [P., v. 1487.]
———. The dry earth system. The advantages of the dry earth system in the disposal of sewage and excreta. 8 pp. 8°. *London, W. Macintosh*, [*n. d.*]

Moulenq (F.-P.) *De la fièvre typhoïde. 28 pp. 4°. *Paris*, 1848, No. 145, v. 475.

Moulié (P.) *Sur la fièvre jaune observée au Cap-Français, île Saint-Domingue, pendant les années 10 et 11. vi, 7–26 pp. 4°. *Paris*, 1812, No. 155, v. 92.

Moulin (Aart. Jurriaan). *Over het bepalen der temperatuur, en het gebruik der chinine bij typhus. 1 p. l., 48 pp., 1 tab. 8°. *Leiden, S. C. van Doesburgh*, 1864.

Moulin (Charles). * Considérations sur quelques points de la médecine et de la chirurgie. 38 pp. 4°. *Paris*, 1848, No. 123, v. 475.

Moulin (Charles-François-Constant). * Introduction à la pathologie de la race nègre dans les pays chauds. 36 pp. 4°. *Paris*, 1866, No. 211.

Moulin (Étienne) [1795–1871]. * Sur l'apoplexie, ou hémorrhagie cérébrale; considérations nouvelles sur les hydrocéphales; description d'une hydropisie cérébrale particulière aux vieillards. x, 11–115 pp. 4°. *Paris*, 1819, No. 269, v. 153.

——. Traité de l'apoplexie. 224 pp. 8°. *Paris, J.-B. Baillière*, 1819.

Another copy bound with: LECIEUX [*et al.*]. Médecine légale [etc.] 8°. *Paris*, 1819.

——. Mémoire sur les inflammations de poitrine, leur nature, leurs symptômes et leur traitement. 33 pp. 8°. *Paris, C.-L.-F. Panckoucke*, 1827. [P., v. 929.]

Repr. from: J. compl. du dict. d. sc. méd., Par., 1827, xxviii.

——. Cathétérisme rectiligne, ou nouvelle manière de pratiquer cette opération chez l'homme. (Sondes droites et positions particulières du chirurgien et du malade.) Méthode ayant, dans beaucoup de cas de rétention d'urine, sur toutes celles employées jusqu'ici, les avantages d'une exécution plus facile et d'un succès plus certain; avec un procédé opératoire propre à l'auteur pour guérir les rétrécissemens de l'urètre, suivi d'un nouveau moyen de réunir et cicatriser les déchirures de la vulve et du périnée produites par l'accouchement. ii, 184 pp., 10 pl. 8°. *Paris, F.-M. Maurice*, 1834.

——. The same. Nouveau traitement des rétentions d'urine et des rétrécissemens de l'urètre par le cathétérisme rectiligne, suivi d'un mémoire sur les déchirures de la vulve et du périnée, produites par l'accouchement. xiv, 184 pp., 10 pl. 8°. *Paris, J.-B. Baillière*, 1834.

Same as the preceding, except title-page and preface.

——. Hygiène et traitement du choléra-morbus. Coup-d'œil historique sur l'épidémie de Paris de 1832. 38 pp. 8°. *Paris, J.-B. Baillière*, 1832.

——. Un mot sur le Congrès médical. 14 pp. 8°. *Paris, J.-B. Baillière*, 1845. [P., v. 467.]

Moulin (Eugène-J.) * Considérations pratiques sur le choléra-morbus des Indes. 76 pp. 4°. *Paris*, 1833, No. 22, v. 257.

Moulin (Félix). * Du phénol, ou acide phénique. 41 pp., 1 l. 4°. *Montpellier*, 1886, No. 390.

Ecole de pharmacie.

Moulin (J.-A.-M.) * Des ulcères de la matrice, et de leur traitement. 35 pp. 4°. *Paris*, 1840, No. 237, v. 363.

Moulin (Léopold). * De la médication antithermique dans le traitement de la fièvre typhoïde. 59 pp., 2 l. 4°. *Montpellier*, 1883, No. 8.

Moulin (Victor). * Sur la maladie endémique des climats chauds, vulgairement appelée fièvre jaune. 31 pp. 4°. *Paris, an XIII* [1805], No. 454, v. 55.

Moulinet (Charles). * Sur l'hygiène des vieillards. 3 pp. 4°. *Paris*, 1818, No. 121, v. 139.

Moulinet (Léonce). * De l'influence de la grossesse sur l'innervation. 64 pp. 4°. *Paris*, 1860, No. 50.

Moulinet (Paul) [1855–]. * Des rapports entre la vaccine et certaines maladies de peau. Influence réciproque. 65 pp. 4°. *Paris*, 1884, No. 235.

Moulinié (Jean) [1787–1842]. * Brûlures. 24 pp. 4°. *Paris*, 1812, No. 87, v. 89.

——. Notice sur les bains, suivie du prospectus des nouveaux bains de Bordeaux. vii, 116 pp. 8°. *Bordeaux, Brossier*, 1826.

Moulinié (Jean)—continued.

——. Question médico-légale sur la viabilité. Extraits de certificats, rapports et consultations, suivis de réflexions qui leur sont relatives. 44 pp. 12°. *Bordeaux, Castillon*, [1826].

——. Maladies des organes génitaux et urinaires, exposées d'après la clinique chirurgicale de l'Hôpital de Bordeaux. 2 v. 4 p. l., 336 pp., 4 l., 1 pl.; 416 pp., 4 l., 1 pl. 8°. *Paris, Germer-Baillière*, 1839.

——. Considérations cliniques sur les engorgemens. 152 pp., 3 l. 8°. *Paris, Germer-Baillière*, 1840.

——. Le médecin de mer. xv, 550 pp. 8°. *Paris, Germer-Baillière*, 1841.

——. Du bonheur en chirurgie. Recueil de faits cliniques. ccxxiii pp., 2 l. 8°. *Paris, Germer-Baillière; Bordeaux, Lawalle*, 1842.

——. The same. Vom Glücke in der Chirurgie. Eine Sammlung klinischer Fälle. Aus dem Französischen übersetzt, mit Vorwort und einigen Notizen begleitet von R. Berend. x, 171 pp. 8°. *Hannover, C. F. Kins*, 1844.

Moulinier (Achille-Adolphe). * De l'endocardite dans les fièvres éruptives, nature et fréquence. 84 pp. 4°. *Paris*, 1879, No. 431.

Moulinier (Pierre-Paul-Émile). * I. Des symptômes du cancer de la matrice. II. [etc.] 30 pp. 4°. *Paris*, 1844, No. 109, v. 421.

Moulins.

Jemois. Histoire des constitutions météorologiques et maladies qui ont régné depuis le mois de nivôse de l'an onze, jusqu'à celui de brumaire inclusivement. Ann. Soc. de méd.-prat. de Montpel., 1804, iv, 5–36.—**Michel & Simard.** Topographie médicale de la ville et des hôpitaux de Moulins. J. de méd., chir., pharm., etc., Par., 1788, lxxvi, 361–388.

des Moulins (Scipio). * De febribus. 16 pp. 4°. *Lugd. Bat., A. Elzevier*, 1701.

Moulins (Tiburce). * Du croup; son traitement médical. 114 pp., 3 l. 4°. *Montpellier, J. Martel aîné*, 1867, No. 64. C.

Moulins-la-Marche.

See **Fever** (*Typhoid, History, etc., of*), by localities.

Moulion (André-Marie). * Quelques réflexions sur la colique métallique et son traitement. 21 pp. 4°. *Paris*, 1830, No. 180, v. 234.

Moullin (Joh.) Quæstio medica: An perturbationes motum cordis sanguinisque augeant minuant? Præses: Jacobus Fourneau. *Paris*, 1721.

In: HALLER. Disp. anat. [etc.] 4°. *Gottingæ*, 1749, iv, 413–424.

Moullin de Marguery. Traité des eaux minérales nouvellement découvertes au village de Passy, près Paris. Dans lequel sont expliquées leur nature minérale, la différence des sources, leurs qualités, leurs vertus et leurs effets sur le corps humain. 7 p. l., 415 pp., 5 l. 12°. *Paris, F. Barois*, 1723.

de Moulon (Amédée-Mathieu). Il cholera asiatico in Trieste, negli anni 1835 e 1836. 112 pp. 8°. *Marsiglia, eredi Feissat aîné & Demonchy*, 1839.

——. Du typhus tétanique, vulgairement connu sous le nom de méningite cérébro-spinale qui a régné à Trieste en 1868. 21 pp. 8°. *Trieste, F. H. Schimpff*, 1868.

de Moulon (Amedeus). De positivæ electricitatis vel per excessum a negativa, vel per defectum necessitate instituendi discriminis, in therapeutico usu ejusdem fluidi. 31 pp. 8°. *Patavii, typ. Seminarii*, 1826.

Moulson (Richardus). * De chorea. 3 p. l., 40 pp. 8°. *Edinburgi, Abernethy et Walker*, 1816. [P., v. 558.]

Moulton (Ferdinand).

See **Mayo** (Robert) & **Moulton** (Ferdinand). Army and Navy pension laws [etc.] 8°. *Washington*, 1852.

——. The same. 4. ed. 8°. *Washington*, 1861.

Moulton (G.-C.)   Des aliénés, et de l'établissement projeté pour l'amélioration de leur sort dans
le canton de Genève. 27 pp. 8°. *Genève, Lador,*
1830. [P., v. 809.]

Moultrie (James) [1793-1869]. On the organic
function of animals. 2 p. l., 20 pp. 8°. *Charleston, Burges & James,* 1844.

———. Introductory lecture to the course of phy-
siology in the Medical College of the State of
South Carolina. 15 pp. 8°. *Charleston, Walker,
Evans & Co.,* 1856.

  For Biography, see **Wragg** (William T.) Memoir of
Dr. James Moultrie [etc.] 8°. *Charleston,* 1869. *See,
also,* Charleston M. J., 1857, xii, 827–833. *Also:* Tr. Am.
M. Ass., Phila., 1878, xxix, 724 (J. M. Toner).
  For Portrait, see **Collection** of Portr. (Libr.)

Moultrie (Joannes) [1793–]. * De febre maligna biliosa Americæ. 24 pp., 4 l. sm. 4°.
Edinburgi, ex off. E. Flaminii, 1749.

———. The same. De febre maligna biliosa
Americæ, anglice, the yellow fever, edidit iterum et præfatus est E. G. Baldinger. 2 p. l.,
26 pp., 4 l. 4°. *Longosalissæ, imp. J. C. Martini,* 1768.

———. The same. Traité de la fièvre jaune.
Trad. par M. Aulagnier. Auquel il a joint des
notes de l'ouvrage du docteur Makithrik sur
cette maladie. viii, 65 pp. 8°. *Paris, Méquignon, an XIII* [1805].
  The name of author is printed on title-page as L. Moultrie.

———. The same. Ueber das gelbe Fieber. Mit
Zusätzen und Anmerkungen von Karl Paulus.
xvi, 89 pp. 12°. *Bamberg u. Würzburg, J. A.
Göbhardt,* 1805. [*Also, in:* P., v. 1393.]
  For Biography, see N. Jersey M. Reporter, Burlington,
1855, viii, 73–80, port.

Mouly (A.) * Contribution à l'étude de l'aï, de
son étiologie en particulier. 42 pp. 4°. *Paris,*
1876, No. 253.

Mouly (Auguste). * Essai sur la pneumonie
rhumatismale. 51 pp., 2 tab., 2 l. 4°. *Montpellier,* 1878, No. 26.

Mouly (Jean-Placide) [1857–]. * Étude sur
le champ visuel et ses anomalies dans quelques
affections oculaires. 62 pp., 1 l. 4°. *Paris,*
1881, No. 168.

Mouly (P.) [1849–]. * Contribution à l'étude
de l'héméralopie dans les affections hépatiques.
43 pp. 4°. *Paris,* 1881, No. 217.

Moumiet (Auguste). * I. De la syncope. II.
[etc.] 25 pp. 4°. *Paris,* 1842, No. 100, v.
393.

Moumiet (J.-H.) * Recueil de quelques observations de médecine et de chirurgie pratique.
31 pp. 4°. *Paris,* 1817, No. 79, v. 131.

Mounaud (Jean-Baptiste). * Sur le typhus
contagieux. vi, 7–35 pp. 4°. *Paris,* 1817, No.
107, v. 132.

Mounds *and mound-builders.*

  See, also, **Craniology**; **Ethnology**; **Indians**
(*North American*); **Man** (*Primitive, etc.*)

  Wyman (J.) Fresh-water shell mounds of
the St. John's River, Florida. 4°. *Salem, Mass.,*
1875.

  Derby (O. A.) The artificial mounds of the island of
Marajó, Brazil. Am. Naturalist, Phila., 1879, xiii, 224–
229.—**Farquharson** (R. J.) Recent explorations of
mounds near Davenport, Iowa. Proc. Am. Ass. Adv. Sc.
1875, Salem, 1876, xxiv, pt. 2, 297–315, 6 pl.

Mounet (Jean-Paul). * De la congestion pulmonaire alcoolique. 40 pp. 4°. *Paris,* 1880, No.
404.

Mounier (G. J. D.) De zoogenaamde prosti-
tutie-regeling te Utrecht, in hare onhoudbaar-
heid voorgesteld, naar aanleiding van de jongste
zittingen van den gemeenteraad. 46 pp., 1 l.
8°. *Utrecht, J. Bijleveld,* 1884.

Mounier (G. J. D.)—continued.
———. Het beginsel van politietoezicht op de
prostitutie, getoetst aan moraal, recht en hy-
giëne. Beschouwingen naar aanleiding van het
strafproces in de zaak van Neeltje F . . . voor den
Hoogen Raad der Nederlanden. Bevattende een
groot aantal officieele stukken. xii, 286 pp. 8°.
[*Utrecht*], *W. A. Beschoor,* 1885.

Mounier (Gustave-Antoine). * Du permanganate de potasse et de ses propriétés désinfec-
tantes. 44 pp. 4°. *Paris,* 1878, No. 357.

Mounier (Henri). * Esquisses d'anatomie topographique. Régions ilio-costale, dorso-lombaire,
périnéale. 2 p. l., 55 pp., 1 pl. 4°. *Strasbourg,*
1865, 2. s., No. 856.

Mounier (J.-C.) * Sur les fractures en général.
23 pp. 4°. *Paris,* 1833, No. 331, v. 266.

Mounier (Jacques-Alfred). * De la fièvre intermittente à l'île de Nossi-Bé de Madagascar. 47
pp. 4°. *Paris,* 1849, No. 56, v. 487.

Mounier (Léopold). De la culture de la bet-
terave et de son utilisation pratique en vue de
remplacer momentanément la culture de la
vigne dans le département de la Charente. 37
pp., 1 l. 8°. *Angoulême, Lugeol & Cie.,* 1881.

Mounier (Martin-Émile). * Quelques considérations sur la fièvre. 52 pp. 4°. *Paris,* 1868,
No. 253.

Mounier (Rodolphe). * De la commotion cérébrale. 45 pp. 4°. *Paris,* 1834, No. 119, v. 272.

Mounstein (A.) * Ueber die spontane Gangrän und Infarcte. 43 pp., 1 pl. 8°. *Strassburg, K. J. Trübner,* 1884.

Mount Aboo.

  Lownds (T. M.) Remarks on Mount Aboo. Tr. M.
& Phys. Soc. Bombay (1855–6), 1857, n. s., iii, 163–189.—
Moore. The sanitary condition of hill stations. with
especial reference to Mount Aboo; with statistical tables,
compiled from the Aboo Sanitarium Hospital records, and
other sources. *Ibid.* (1862), 1863, n. s., iii, 146–200.—
Ogilvy (J.) General topographical and medical account of Mount Aboo. *Ibid.* (1860), 1861, n. s., vi, 192–
216.—**Roe** (W. C.) Annual report of the Sanatarium,
Mount Aboo, for the year ending March 31, 1859. *Ibid.*
(1859), 1860, n. s., v, 222–229.

Mount Auburn Cemetery. Annual report of
the trustees, together with the reports of the
treasurer and superintendent [for the year] 1872.
10 pp. 8°. *Boston, Barker, Cotter & Co.,* 1873.

Mount Clemens.

  Shotwell (A. N.) Mineral waters of Mt. Clemens,
Mich., in leucorrhœa. St. Louis M. J., 1886, xiii, 339–344.
Also: Therap. Gaz., Detroit, 1886, 3. s., ii, 534–536.

Mount Holly Springs, Cumberland Co., Pennsylvania. 7 pp. 16°. *Washington, Judd & Detweiler,* [1887].

Mount Hope Cemetery of the city of Boston.
See **Boston.**

Mount Hope Retreat, near Baltimore. Annual
reports of the physician to the guardians. 1.–11.,
1842–3 to 1853; 13., 1855; 14., 1856; 16.–43., 1858–
85. 8°. *Baltimore,* 1843–86.

  Opened by the Sisters of Charity in Oct., 1840. Soon
after removed to the present site. Dr. Wm. H. Stokes
became connected with the institution in Sept., 1842, from
which period the first report commences. Changes in
title: Original title, "Mount St. Vincent's Hospital in the
city of Baltimore". In 1844, called "Mount Hope Hospital". In 1845, "Mount Hope Institution, near Baltimore". In 1865, a new building was erected, and called
"Mount Hope Retreat", making two institutions under
one management, the title being "Mount Hope Institution
and Retreat". In 1871 the title reads "Mount Hope Retreat and Mount Hope Institution". The new building,
Mount Hope Retreat, being used for the insane, and the
old one, Mount Hope Institution, for inebriates. In 1875
Mount Hope Institution was converted into a general hospital, under title of "Mount Hope Hospital". From 1876
to date, reports are for Mount Hope Retreat only.

Mount Pleasant.

  See **Education** (*Medical*), *etc.*; **Insane** (*Asylums for, etc.*), *by localities.*

Mount Sinai Hospital, N. Y. City. Act of incorporation and by-laws of the Jews' Hospital in New York, 5618, corresponding with the year 1857. 16 pp. 16°. *New York, C. A. Alvord*, 1857.
Bound with : Reports.
Incorporated Jan. 5, 1852. Opened June, 1855, as "Jews' Hospital in New York". Changed title in 1866. 18. report for 11 months, Jan. to Nov., 1872.

———. Annual reports of the directors and the medical and surgical staff to the members and patrons. 2., 1856; 6., 1860; 10.–25., 1864 to 1878–9; 27.–31., 1880–81 to 1884–5. 8°. *New York*, 1857–86.

———. Rules and regulations for officers and superintendent. March, 1869. Adar 5627. 12 pp. 16°. *New York, Bunce & Co.*, 1869.
Bound with : Reports.

———. Ceremonies attending the laying the corner-stone of the new building, May 25, 1870. 24 pp. 8°. *New York, D. Taylor*, 1870.
Bound with : Reports.

———. Proceedings attending the ceremonies of laying the corner-stone of the new building, May 25, 1870. 22 pp. 8°. [*New York*, 1870.]
Bound with : Reports.

———. Act of incorporation and by-laws. 21 pp. 12°. *New York, Hebrew Orphan Asylum Printing Establishment*, 1872.
Bound with : Reports.

Mount Tátra.
Szontagh (A.) Tátravidéki gyógyító és nyaraló helyek. [Mount Tátra as a health resort.] Államorvos, Budapest, 1884, ix, 57–72.

Mount Vernon, *Indiana.*
See Cholera (*Asiatic, History, etc., of*), Fever (*Typhoid, History, etc., of*), *by localities.*

Mount Vernon. Sanitary code of the board
of health of the village of Mount Vernon, N. Y. Unanimously adopted Feb. 14, 1882. [*n. p., n. d.*] Newspaper cutting.

Mount Vernon, *New York.*
See, also, Children (*Hospitals, etc., for, Reports, etc., of*).
Andrews (H.), jr. Report on the sewerage of Mount Vernon, Westchester County. Rep. Bd. Health N. Y. 1884, Albany, 1885, v, 419–433, 2 pl. *Also,* Reprint.—
Gardiner [*et al.*] A report on the sewerage of Mt. Vernon. Rep. State Bd. Health N. Y. 1884, Albany, 1885, v, 419–433, 2 plans.—**Report** of the sewerage of Mt. Vernon. *Ibid.*, 1886, vi, 235–264.

Mount Vernon Ladies' Association of the
Union. Report of the meeting of 1872. 8°. [*n. p.*], 1872.

Mountain Sanitarium for Pulmonary Diseases,
Asheville, N. C. [Circular letter announcing the establishment of, by Wm. Gleitsmann.] 2 l. 4°. [*n. p.*; 1875.]
Opened June 1, 1877.

———. Biennial report of the proprietor and physician in charge to the public. By Wm. Gleitsmann. 1., 1875–6 to 1876–7. 8 pp. 8°. *Baltimore, Sherwood & Co.*, 1877.
Opened June 1, 1875.

Mountains.
See, also, Alps (*The*); Altitude; Andes; Fever (*Mountain*); Goitre, *by localities*; Health resorts; Himalayas.
Adolphus (C. M.) De incolatus montani salubritate. Resp. Christ. Gott. Grünwaldus. 4°. *Lipsiæ*, 1721.
Assmann (C. G.) De vi singulari quam natura et conditio regionum montanarum exserat in metallicorum aliorumque hominum natura indoleque formanda. sm. 4°. *Vitembergæ*, [1789].
Delachaux (L.) * Physiologische Wirkung der Bergluft auf Gesunde und auf Kranke. [Wurtzburg.] 8°. *Berne*, 1871.
Deserin (J.-P.-A.) * Quelques considérations sur les pays de montagnes. 4°. *Paris*, 1830.

Mountains.
Ennemoser (J.) * De montium influxu in valetudinem hominum, vitæ genus, et morbos. sm. 8°. *Berolini*, 1816.
———. The same. 12°. *Berolini*, 1816.
Georgeon (J.-B.) * Quelques considérations générales sur l'hygiène dans les campagnes de la partie montagneuse des Vosges. 4°. *Strasbourg*, 1863.
Meyer-Ahrens (C.) Die Bergkrankheit, oder der Einfluss des Ersteigens grosser Höhen auf den thierischen Organismus. 8°. *Leipzig*, 1854.
Payot (A.) * Du mal des montagnes considéré au point de vue de ses effets, de sa cause, et de son traitement. 4°. *Paris*, 1881.
Le Tenneur (T.) * An magis amœna quam salubris in montium clivis habitatio? Præses F. Bernard. 4°. [*Paris*, 1773.]
Billings (J. S.) Abstract of special reports by army medical officers on the effect of mountain climates upon health. Am. Pub. Health Ass. Rep. 1875, N. Y., 1876, ii, 148–150.—**Brachet** (J.-L.) Note sur les causes de la lassitude et de l'anhélation dans les ascensions sur les montagnes les plus élevées. J. de méd. de Lyon, 1843, iv, 402–414. *Also:* Rev. méd. franç. et étrang., Par., 1844, iii, 356–368. *Also,* Reprint.—**Branchat y Prada** (R.) El mal de montañas. Prensa méd. de Granada, 1881, iii. 1–8.—**Brodowski** (W.) Ieszcye słów kilka o dzialaniu ścisnionego powietrza na organizm ludzki w stanie zdrowia i choroby. [On the influence of climate of high altitudes on health and disease.] Gaz. lek., Warszawa, 1869, vi, 816 ; 845 ; 865. — **Cunningham** (P.) The pathological effects produced by localities (particularly mountain elevations). Lond. M. Gaz., 1834, xiv, 207; 520.—**Edmondson** (W.) Report on altitude; its influence on health. Rep. Bd. Health Colorado 1876, Denver, 1877, i, 21: (1877), 1878, ii, 39.—**Escherich.** Die quantitativen Verhältnisse des Sauerstoffes der Luft, verschieden nach Höhenlage und Temperatur der Beobachtungsorte. Aerztl. Int.-Bl., München, 1877, xxiv, 339–344. — **Flechner** (A. E.) Betrachtung der Gebirgsluft und der Lebensweise der Gebirgsbewohner in Bezug ihres Einflusses auf Blutbereitung und auf das Vorkommen gewisser Krankheitsformen. Med. Jahrb. d. k. k. österr. Staates, Wien, 1840, xxxii, 1–10. — **Forel.** Untersuchungen über die Körperwärme des Menschen bei Bergbesteigungen. Verhandl. d. schweiz. naturf. Gesellsch. 1871, Frauenfeld, 1872, liv, 79.—**Fryer** (B. E.) The influence of the high altitudes and climate of the table-land country of the Rocky Mountain region upon health and disease. Am. Pub. Health Ass. Rep. 1875, N. Y., 1876, ii, 141–148.—**Gardner** (W. H.) Some remarks on diseases peculiar to mountainous regions. Am. J. M. Sc., Phila., 1876, n. s., lxxii, 56–63.—**Jourdanet** (D.) Nature du mal de montagnes. *In his:* Le Mexique et l'Amérique tropicale, sm. 8°, Par., 1864, 85–110. — Invloed van hooggelegen plaatsen op de gezondheid der bewoners. Schat d. Gezondh., Gorinchem, 1865, viii, 129–137.—**Koch** (C. A. L.) Ueber den Einfluss der Gebirge und der Gebirgsformationen auf die Krankheiten der Menschen. Monatschr. f. med. Augenh. u. Chir., Leipz ,1838, i, 351–368.—**von Liebig** (G.) Ueber die Bergkrankheit und Indicationen für Höhenkurorte bei Lungenleiden. Deutsche med. Wchnschr., Berl., 1880, vi, 205 ; 222. — **Loewe.** Ueber das Alpenklima. Verhandl. d. Berl. med. Gesellsch. (1865–6), 1867, i, 3. Hft., 280–293.—**Lortet** (L.) Deux ascensions au Mont-Blanc en 1869; recherches physiologiques sur le mal des montagnes. Lyon méd., 1869, iii, 79–103.—**Marcet** (W.) Summary of an experimental inquiry into the function of respiration at various altitudes. Proc. Roy. Soc. Lond., 1878, xxvii, 293–304.—**Martin** (J. R.) Suggestions for the investigation of mountain climates in the East Indies. Lancet, Lond., 1858, i, 161.—**Mermod** (A.) Nouvelles recherches physiologiques sur l'influence de la dépression atmosphérique sur l'habitant des montagnes. Bull. Soc. vaudoise d. sc. nat. 1877–8, Lausanne, 1879, xv, 65–104, 3 tab.—**Parat** & **Martin.** Observations médicinales sur les principaux effets du froid et du chaud sur le sommet des hautes montagnes. Rec. d. actes Soc. de santé de Lyon, an vi [179?], i, 273–301.—**Perroncito** (E.) Der Dochmius und verwandte Helminthen in ihren Beziehungen zu der sogenannten Bergkachexie. Centralbl. f. d. med. Wissensch., Berl., 1881, xix, 435.—**de Pietra-Santa.** Les climats de montagne. J. d'hyg., Par., 1878, iii, 564 ; 574.—**Pöppig** (E.) Ueber die Puna auf den Peruanischen Anden. Beitr. z. prakt. Heilk., Leipz., 1836, ii, 305–311.—**Rey.** Influence sur le corps humain des ascensions sur les hautes montagnes. Rev. méd. franç. et étrang., Par., 1842, iv, 320–344.—**Schillinger** (F.) A bányász-as-zályról (cachexia montana). Gyógyászat, Budapest, 1881, xxi, 49–51.—**Speer** (S. T.) On the nature and causes of the physiological phenomena comprised in the term "mountain sickness", more especially as experienced among the

Mountains.

higher Alps. Assoc. M. J., Lond., 1853, i, 49; 80.—**Tóth** (I.) Bányászaszály (cachexia montana), s ennek oktana. Orvosi hetil.. Budapest, 1883, xxvii, 323; 349; 380; 470; 525; 559; 672; 787; 907; 1032; 1056; 1296. *Also, transl.*: Pest. med.-chir. Presse, Budapest, 1884, xx, 135; 161; 181; 203.—**de Ujfalvy** (C.) Quelques observations sur le mal de montagne éprouvé par des voyageurs en Asie centrale. Bull. Soc. d'anthrop. de Par., 1880, 3. s., iii, 397–400.

Mountain-sickness.

See Mountains.

Mouphe.

Babaeff (A. N.) Nieskalko slov o Mouphe. [Some remarks on Mouphe.] Med. Sbornik, Tiflis, 1886, no. 41, 68–77.

de Moura (Adolpho Marcondes). * Estudo clinico da reunião immediata. 4 p. l., 74 pp., 1 l. 8°. *Rio de Janeiro, J. D. de Oliveira, 1883.*

de Moura (Fiel-Antonio). * Du choléra épidémique. 38 pp. 4°. *Paris, 1850*, No. 24, v. 499.

de Moura (José Affonso). Apreciação dos meios empregados na cura dos estreitamentos organicos da urethra. 43 pp. 4°. *Bahia, J. G. Tourinho,* 1871.
Concurso.

Moura-Bourouillou. Cours complet de laryngoscopie, suivi des applications du laryngoscope à l'étude des phénomènes de la phonation et de la déglutition. 100 pp. 8°. *Paris, A. Delahaye,* 1861.

——. Traité pratique de laryngoscopie et de rhinoscopie, suivi d'observations. 2. tirage. 198 pp. 8°. *Paris, A. Delahaye,* 1865.

——. L'acte de la déglutition, son mécanisme. 63 pp., 3 pl. 8°. *Paris, A. Delahaye,* 1867.

——. Angines aiguës ou graves, origine, nature, traitement. 68 pp. 8°. *Paris, A. Delahaye,* 1870.

——. Revue clinique. Laryngopathies. Classification, statistique. viii, 109 pp., 1 l. 8°. *Paris, A. Delahaye,* 1874.

Mourain (Pierre-Alexandre). * Sur la dysenterie aiguë. 15 pp. 4°. *Paris, 1830*, No. 106, v. 232.

Mourao-Pitta (C.-A.) * Du climat de Madère et de son influence thérapeutique dans le traitement des maladies chroniques en général et en particulier de la phthisie pulmonaire. xxx, 31–263 pp. 4°. *Montpellier, 1859*, No. 68.

Mourcet (Jean-Étienne). * Sur le cancer externe et son traitement. 21 pp. 4°. *Paris,* 1831, No. 33, v. 238.

Mourcou.
See **Morin** (A.) Hôpital Sainte-Eugénie. Rapport de la Commission des arts insalubres. 4°. *Lille, 1875.*

Moure (E.-J.) Manuel pratique des maladies des fosses nasales et de la cavité naso-pharyngienne. iii, 304 pp., 4 pl. 12°. *Paris, O. Doin,* 1886.
Also, Editor of: **Revue** mensuelle de laryngologie, d'otologie et de rhinologie, Bordeaux, Paris, 1880.
See, also, **Mackenzie** (Morell). Traité pratique des maladies du larynx [etc.] 8°. *Paris, 1882.*

Moure (J.-G.-Amédée-Pisani). * Considérations générales médico-hygiéniques et philosophiques sur les âges. 34 pp. 4°. *Paris, 1834*, No 241, v. 275; 276.

—— & **Martin** (J.-Henri). Précis de thérapeutique spéciale, de pharmaceutique et de pharmacologie. viii, 628 pp. 12°. *Paris, Fortin, Masson & Cie.,* 1845.

Moure (J.-Gabriel). * Des rapports de certaines névroses, et en particulier de l'asthme, avec les polypes muqueux du nez et avec les sténoses nasales en général. 52 pp., 1 l. 4°. *Bordeaux,* 1883, 6. s., No. 1.

Moure (R.) * Des accidents de la paracentèse abdominale dans l'ascite. 46 pp. 4°. *Paris,* 1873, No. 391.

Mouremans (Josephus). * Diss. summariam expositionem complectens de legibus formationis necnon actionis systematis nervosi centralis. 40 pp. 4°. *Gandavi, P. J. Van Ryckegem,* [1829]. [*Also, in*: P., v. 959.]
Also, Editor of: **Journal** du dispensaire Hahnemann de Bruxelles, 1862-7.
See, also, **Hippocrates.** Les aphorismes [etc.] 2 v. 8°. *Paris, 1864.*

Mouret (Adolphe) [1860–   ]. * De la néphrite infectieuse consécutive à l'ostéo-périostite. 53 pp., 1 l. 4°. *Paris, 1883,* No. 349.

Mouret (Amand). * De la coïncidence de l'hépatite ou des abcès du foie avec la dysenterie, dans les pays chauds. 30 pp. 4°. *Paris, 1853,* No. 52, v. 545.

Mouret (J.-N.) * Sympathies morbides entre les poumons et les intestins. viii, 9–33 pp. 4°. *Paris, 1828,* No. 226, v. 219.

Mouret (Louis-Auguste). * Aperçu de la statistique médicale du canton de Montfaucon, département de la Haute-Loire, suivi de quelques propositions de médecine et de thérapeutique. 36 pp. 4°. *Paris,* 1835, No. 194, v. 287.

Moureton (Louis). * Étude sur la tuberculisation des vieillards. 66 pp. 4°. *Paris, 1863,* No. 123.

Mourette (J.-B.) * Quelques remarques critiques sur la fièvre de lait. 36 pp. 4°. *Paris,* 1859, No. 192, v. 634.

Mourey (Jean-François-Gabriel-Jules). * Étude sur la trépanation. 42 pp. 4°. *Paris, 1877,* No. 307.

Mourey (S.) [1848–   ]. * Des kystes de la grande lèvre et de leur traitement par la ligature élastique. 80 pp. 4°. *Paris, 1882,* No. 15.

Mourgué (Ch.-L.) Journal des bains de mer de Dieppe, ou recherches et observations sur l'usage hygiénique et thérapeutique de l'eau de mer. Première livraison. 2 p. l., 127 pp., 1 pl. 8°. *Paris, Seignot; Dieppe, Corsange,* 1823. [P., v. 582.]

——. Considérations générales sur l'utilité des bains de mer dans le traitement des difformités du tronc et des membres. 81 pp., 1 l. 8°. *Paris, J.-P. Roret,* 1828.

Mourgue (Jacques-Augustin) [1734–1818]. Plan d'une caisse de prévoyance et de secours présenté au conseil général de l'administration des hospices et secours à domicile de Paris. 63 pp., 1 l., 7 tab. 12°. *Paris, imp. des Hospices civils,* 1809.

Mourgue (Paul). * Quelques mots sur la pourriture d'hôpital et un nouveau mode de pansement des plaies. 60 pp., 2 l. 4°. *Montpellier, L. Cristen & Cie.,* 1873, No. 67.

Mourgues (Jean-Léon). * Sur les granulations intra-utérines et sur leur traitement par l'abrasion suivie de la cautérisation. 44 pp. 4°. *Paris,* 1861, No. 207.

Mourier (Auguste). * Des effets physiologiques et thérapeutiques des préparations d'argent. 42 pp. 4°. *Paris, 1871,* No. 197.

Mourier (Fredericus Ferdinandus) [1804–   ]. Dissertationis de inflammatione corneæ transparentis scrofulosa pars prior. 92 pp. 8°. *Havniæ, A. Seidelin,* [1832].

Mourier (Henri-L.) Des causes de la stérilité chez l'homme et chez la femme et de leur traitement. 130 pp. 8°. *Paris, A. Delahaye,* [1866].

Mourier (P. P. F.) Om Prostitutionslovgivningen. 40 pp. 8°. *Kjøbenhavn, V. Thaning & Appel,* 1884.

Mourlet (Claude-Pierre-Étienne). * De la néphrite dite albumineuse. 31 pp. 4°. *Paris,* 1846, No. 168, v. 448.

Mourlhon (P.-M.-Lucien). * Propositions de médecine et de chirurgie. 20 pp. 4°. *Paris,* 1835, No. 87, v. 284.

Mourlion (Henri). * Essai sur la pathogénie de la fièvre traumatique et de l'infection purulente. 32 pp. 4°. *Paris*, 1880, No. 125.

Mourlon (François-Aug.-Léandre). * Considérations sur l'emploi du chloroforme dans le traitement de certaines affections chirurgicales. 29 pp. 4°. *Strasbourg*, 1853, No. 287, 2. s., v. 19.

Mouronval (J.-F.-J.) * Recherches sur les causes de la gale, faites à l'Hôpital Saint-Louis pendant les années 1819, 1820 et 1821. viii, 9–25 pp. 4°. *Paris*, 1821, No. 130, v. 167.

——. Recherches et observations sur le prurigo. vii, 40 pp., 1 tab. 4°. *Paris, Croullebois,* 1823.

——. The same. Faites à l'Hôpital Saint-Louis et dans les départemens du Pas-de-Calais et de la Somme. 2. éd. x, 97 pp., 1 tab. 8°. *Paris, Baillière,* 1836.

Mouronval (Saint-Ange). * Considérations sur les lésions traumatiques cavitaires. 23 pp. 4°. *Paris*, 1872, No. 161.

Mouroux (Charles-Félicité). * Sur l'estomac, et en particulier sur les gastralgies ou maladies nerveuses de cet organe. 36 pp. 4°. *Paris*, 1829, No. 11, v. 221.

Mourraille (J.-J.-Gustave). * De la fièvre typhoïde. 54 pp. 4°. *Paris*, 1854, No. 300, v. 563.

Mourret (François). * De la première dentition, et des accidents qui la compliquent. 38 pp. 4°. *Paris*, 1847, No. 106, v. 462.

Mourruau (Émile). * Du traitement du trachome conjonctival par la cautérisation. 41 pp. 4°. *Paris*, 1887, No. 163.

Mourson (Joseph). * De la médication antiseptique dans la fièvre typhoïde, avec quelques considérations sur la nature de cette fièvre et sur celle de la forme putride. 92 pp. 4°. *Paris*, 1869, No. 284.

Moursou (J.) Étude clinique sur l'asphyxie locale des extrémités et sur quelques autres troubles vasomoteurs dans leurs rapports avec la fièvre intermittente. 43 pp. 8°. *Paris, J.-B. Baillière & fils,* 1880.

Repr. from: Arch. de méd. nav., Par., 1880, xxxiii.

——. De la fièvre typhoïde dans la marine et dans les pays chauds. Prix de médecine navale (1884). 311 pp. 8°. *Paris, O. Doin,* 1885.

Mouse.

See **Muridæ.**

Mousnier (E.)

See **Papillaud** (L.) & **Mousnier** (E.) Arséniate d'antimoine [etc.] 8°. *Marennes,* 1872.

Mousnier-Lompré. * Quelques considérations sur l'hygiène des campagnes d'une partie du Limousin. vi, 7–16 pp. 4°. *Paris,* 1832, No. 31, v. 248.

Mousnier-Lompré (Antoine). * De la goutte dans ses rapports avec les lésions traumatiques. 35 pp. 4°. *Paris,* 1876, No. 44.

Moussaud (A.) * De la périostite phlegmoneuse. 44 pp. 4°. *Paris,* 1872, No. 300.

Moussaud (Alexis-Augustin). * Des inclusions fœtales. 68 pp. 4°. *Paris,* 1861, No. 179.

Moussaud (François-Joseph). * Quelques considérations sur l'influence morale dans les maladies. 20 pp. 4°. *Paris,* 1835, No. 309, v. 291.

Moussaux (L.) * Sur la fièvre scarlatine. 33 pp. 8°. *Paris, an X* [1802], v. 6.

Mousse (Arthur). * Causes de la mort subite. 64 pp. 4°. *Paris,* 1877, No. 364.

Mousseaux-Laurent [1776–1851].

Degott. Notice nécrologique sur Laurent Mousseaux. Exposé d. trav. de la Soc. d. sc. méd. de la Moselle, Metz, 1852, 28–36.

Moussel (Modeste). * Traitement curatif de la diathèse scrophuleuse par l'usage des bois sudorifiques, des préparations mercurielles et des eaux minérales de la province de Naples. 32 pp. 4°. *Paris,* 1835, No. 78, v. 284.

Moussette (Paul-Gustave). * De l'albuminurrhée, considérée dans ses relations avec les maladies. 38 pp. 4°. *Paris,* 1855, No. 316, v. 578.

Moussier (Auguste). * De la taille périnéale chez l'homme. 42 pp. 4°. *Paris,* 1866, No. 71.

Moussillac (J.-Félix). * Fragmens cliniques sur quelques maladies de l'utérus. 37 pp. 4°. *Paris,* 1835, No. 155, v. 286.

Moussous. Étude historique et pratique sur le traitement de la syphilis. 30 pp. 8°. *Bordeaux, G. Gounouilhou,* 1867.

Moussous (André-Charles). * Contribution à l'étude des atrophies musculaires succédant aux affections articulaires. Recherches anatomo-pathologiques. 70 pp. 4°. *Bordeaux,* 1885, 7. s., No. 26.

——. The same. 66 pp., 1 l. 8°. *Bordeaux, O.-L. Farraud frères,* 1885.

——. De la mort chez les phtisiques. 164 pp. 8°. *Paris, G. Steinheil,* 1886.

Moussous (Louis-Dominique). * Des principales altérations physiques et chimiques du sang. 46 pp. 4°. *Paris,* 1846, No. 23, v. 448.

Moussu (Amédée-Charles-Eugène). * De la résection de l'articulation tarso-métatarsienne. Nouveau procédé opératoire. 18 pp., 1 l. 4°. *Strasbourg,* 1863, No. 718, 2. s., v. 37.

de Moussy [1810–70].

Nécrologie. Rev. d'anthrop., Par., 1872, i, 165.

Moustapha (Mahmoud). *See* **Mahmoud-Moustapha.**

Moustardier (Louis). * I. Faire l'histoire de l'anasarque symptomatique, d'une modification dans le tissu de la peau, d'un obstacle à la perspiration cutanée. II. [etc.] 41 pp. 4°. *Paris,* 1843, No 154, v. 406.

Moustelon (Émile). * Considérations sur les hémorrhagies de la délivrance. viii, 9–74 pp., 1 l. 4°. *Montpellier,* 1875, No. 17.

Mousteu (Urbain-Camille). * Considérations cliniques sur la lithotritie et la taille. 51 pp. 4°. *Paris,* 1862, No. 35.

Moutard-Martin. * Propositions sur les différentes espèces d'angine. 39 pp. 4°. *Paris,* 1806, No. 55, v. 61.

Moutard-Martin (Eugène). * Des accidents qui accompagnent l'établissement de la menstruation. De la chlorose en particulier. 67 pp. 4°. *Paris,* 1846, No. 198, v. 448.

——. Mémoire sur la valeur du sulfate de cinchonine dans le traitement des intermittentes, adressé au directeur de l'administration générale de l'assistance publique à Paris. 44 pp. 4°. *Paris, J.-B. Baillière & fils,* 1860.

Repr. from: Mém. Acad. de méd., Par., 1860, xxiv.

——. La pleurésie purulente et son traitement. 203 pp. 8°. *Paris, Delahaye,* 1872.

Moutard-Martin (Robert). * Étude sur les pleurésies hémorrhagiques, néomembraneuse, tuberculeuse et cancéreuse. 162 pp., 1 l. 4°. *Paris,* 1878, No. 23.

——. The same. 162 pp., 1 l. 8°. *Paris, A. Delahaye & Cie.,* 1878.

—— & **Richet** (Charles). Recherches expérimentales sur la polyurie. 48 pp. 8°. *Paris, G. Masson,* [1881.]

Repr. from: Arch. de physiol. norm. et path., Par., 1881, 2. s., xiii.

Moutet (Abel-Jérémie). * De l'ongle incarné. 29 pp. 4°. *Strasbourg,* 1863, No. 661, 2. s., v. 34.

——. Mémoires de médecine et de chirurgie. 2. s. vii, 411 pp. 8°. *Paris, P. Asselin,* 1864.

Repr. from: Montpel. méd., 1859–64, iii–xii, *passim.*

Moutet (Jean-Frédéric) [1824–75]. * De l'influence des travaux et de l'enseignement du pro-

Moutet (Jean-Frédéric)—continued.
fesseur Delpech sur le développement de la chirurgie. 142 pp., 1 l. 8°. *Montpellier, J. Martel aîné*, 1855.
Concours.

———. Examen des principales contre-indications de la lithotritie. 82 pp., 1 l. 8°. *Montpellier, Boehm*, 1859.

———. The same. 3. s. 455 pp., 5 pl. 8°. *Paris, P. Asselin*, 1872.
Also, Co-Editor of: **Année** médicale et scientifique, Montpellier, Paris, 1863–6.
For Biography, see Montpel. méd., 1875, xxxiv 289–296.

Moutet (Louis). * Recherches sur l'existence d'un signe caractéristique dans chaque fracture des membres. 54 pp., 2 l. 4°. *Montpellier*, 1879. No. 16.

Moutet (Louis-Xavier). * Recherches et considérations physiologiques et médicales sur la chlorose. 24 pp. 4°. *Paris*, 1837, No. 239, v. 313.

Mouth.

See, also, **Gums**; **Jaws**; **Lips**; **Palate**; **Pharynx**; **Tongue**; **Tonsils**.

DENNIS (J. M.) The mouth and teeth in health and disease. 8°. *London*, 1884.

FEUERSTEIN (W.) * Die Muskulatur der Mundspalte beim Menschen. 8°. *Bern*, 1878.

GREEN (S. F.) The mouth. 16°. *Manippay*, 1877.
Tamil text.

KARMEL (J.) * Ueber die Resorption in der Mundhöhle. 8°. *Dorpat*, 1873.
Also [Abstr.], in: Deutsches Arch. f. klin. Med., Leipz., 1873–4, xii, 466–480.

LECLUSE. Nouveaux élémens d'odontologie, contenant l'anatomie de la bouche, ou la description de toutes les parties qui la composent, et de leur usage, et la pratique abrégée du dentiste, avec plusieurs observations. 12°. *Paris*, 1754.

LÖWE (L.) Beiträge zur Anatomie der Nase und Mundhöhle. 2. Aufl. 4°. *Leipzig*, 1883.

SCHMIDT (F. T.) Det follikulære kjertelvæv i Mundhulens og Svælgets Slimhinde hos Mennesket og Pattedyrene. 8°. *Kjøbenhavn*, 1862.

SEVERIN (F.) * Untersuchungen über das Mundepithel bei Säugethieren, mit Bezug auf Verhornung, Regeneration und Art der Nervenendigung. 8°. *Kiel*, 1885.
Also [Abstr.], in: Arch. f. mikr. Anat., Bonn, 1885–6, xxvi, 81–88, 1 pl.

WATT (J. J.) Anatomico-chirurgical views of the nose, mouth, larynx, and fauces. fol. *London*, 1809.

Aeby (C.) Die Muskulatur der menschlichen Mundspalte. Arch. f. mikr. Anat., Bonn, 1879, xvi, 651–664, 1 pl.—**Beauregard** (H.) Appareil buccal des insectes de la tribu des vésicants. Compt. rend. Soc. de biol., Par., 1883, 7. s., iv, 204–206.—**Dwight** (T.) A new demonstration of the cavities of the mouth. nose, and pharynx. Boston M. & S. J., 1883, cix, 244.—**Epstein** (A.) Zur Hygiene der Mundhöhle neugeborener Kinder. Arch. f. Kinderh., Stuttg., 1883–4, v, 292–304.—**Gubler** [et al.]. Bouche. Dict. encycl. d. sc. méd., Par., 1869, i, 177–267.—**Hamann** (O.) Die Mundarme der Rhizostomen und ihre Anhangsorgane. Jenaische Ztschr. f. Naturw., Jena, 1881, n. F., viii, 243–285, 3 pl.—**His** (W.) Vogelschnabel und Säugethier-Lippe. Fortschr. d. Med., Berl., 1885, iii, 492–494.—**Kölliger.** Beiträge zur Anatomie der Mundhöhle. Verhandl. d. phys.-med. Gesellsch. in Würzb., 1851, ii, 169.—**Langer** (C.) Ueber den Musculus orbicularis oris. Med. Jahrb., Wien, 1861, i, 87–91.—**Magitot** (E.) Étude d'anatomie topographique et chirurgicale sur la bouche. Dict. encycl. d. sc. méd., Par., 1876, x, 178–211.—**Naylor** (J.) Resonance of the mouth cavity. Nature, Lond., 1881, xxiv, 100; 126.—**Petit.** De quelques-unes des fonctions de la bouche. [*From:* Hist. d. mém. Acad. roy. d. sc. de Par., 1715] Collect. acad. d. mém., etc., Par., 1770, iv, 430–439.—**Rappin.** Micro-organismes de la cavité buccale des animaux. Gaz. méd. de Nantes, 1886-7, v, 139.—**Reichel** (P.) Beitrag zur Morphologie der Mundhöhlendrüsen der Wirbelthiere. Morphol. Jahrb., Leipz.,

Mouth.

1882, viii, 1–72, 1 pl.—**Rex** (H.) Ein Beitrag zur Kenntniss der Muskulatur der Mundspalte der Affen. *Ibid.*, 1886-7, xii, 275–286, 1 pl.—**Stricker** (S.) Untersuchungen über die Papillen in der Mundhöhle der Froschlarven. [*Extr. from:* Sitzungsb. d. math.-naturw. Cl. d. k. Akad. d. Wissensch., 1857, Oct.] Untersuch. z. Naturl. d. Mensch. u. d. Thiere, Frankf. a. M., 1858, iv, 241–245, 1 pl.

Mouth (*Abnormities and deformities of*).

See, also, **Cheek** (*Fissure of*); **Face** (*Surgery of*); **Idiots** (*Pathology of*); **Jaws** (*Abnormities of*); **Mouth** (*Surgery, etc., of*).

COLES (J. O.) On deformities of the mouth, congenital and acquired, with their mechanical treatment. 2. ed. 8°. *London*, 1870.

JAHN (A. T. F. A.) * Pauca de operatione synechiarum oris internarum. 8°. *Lipsiæ*, 1856.

KINGSLEY (N. W.) A treatise on oral deformities as a branch of mechanical surgery. 8°. *New York*, 1880.

MEYER (C.) * De fissuris hominis mammaliumque congenitis; accedit fissuræ buccalis congenitæ cum fissura tubæ Eustachii et tympani complicatæ descriptio. fol. *Berolini*, [1835].

RAMSAY (R.) & COLES (J. O.) The mechanical treatment of deformities of the mouth, congenital and accidental. 8°. *London*, 1868.
Also [Abstr.], in: Lancet, Lond., 1868, i, 404; 435, 1 pl.

REMACLY (E.) * De fissura genæ congenita. 8°. *Bonnæ*, 1864.

Albers. Ueber die Abnormitäten des Mundes und der Sprache der blödsinnigen Kinder. Verhandl. d. naturh. Ver. d. preuss. Rheinl. u. Westphal., 1862, 107.—**Atresia** oris. [Case.] Indian Ann. M. Sc., Calcutta, 1864, no. 17, 191.—**Atrésie** de la bouche, consécutive au scorbut; accidents gastralgiques; opérations suivies de succès. Gaz. d. hôp., Par., 1860, xxxiii, 422.—**Bentley.** Great contraction of the mouth following cancrum oris. Tr. Path. Soc. Lond., 1846–8, i, 88.—**Blanckmeister.** Fehler der ersten Bildung in der Mundhöhle an einem Neugeborenen. Ztschr. f. Med., Chir. u. Geburtsh., Leipz., 1868, n. F., vii, 519–521.—**Bondi.** Eigenthümliche Neigung zur Verwachsung des Mundes. J. d. Chir. u. Augenh, Berl., 1825, vii, 473–477.—**Büchnerus** (A. E.) Infans ore clauso et concreto natus. Acta Acad. nat. curios., Norimb., 1730, ii, 210–217.—**Cayley** (H.) Case of atresia oris. Indian M. Gaz., Calcutta, 1872, vii, 184.—**Harlan** (G C.) A case of congenital deformity of the mouth. Med. Times, Phila., 1870–71, i, 401.—**Hart** (C. A.) Excessive contraction of the mouth following scarlet fever; relieved by a new operation. N. York M. J., 1867, v, 499–503.—**Heyfelder.** Verengerung des Mundes in Folge von Ptyalismus mercurialis. Arch. f. physiol. Heilk., Stuttg., 1845, iv, 600–602.—**M.** Método operatorio del doctor Creus para corregir la oclusion bucal, debida á cicatrices de la mucosa gingival. Anfiteatro anat., Madrid, 1878, vi, 28.—**Morgan** (J. H.) Case of contracted mouth operated upon successfully. Med. Press & Circ., Lond., 1869, viii, 159. ———. Two cases of congenital macrostoma, accompanied by malformation of the auricles and by the presence of auricular appendages. Med. Times & Gaz., Lond., 1881, ii, 613. Also: Proc. Roy. M. & Chir. Soc. Lond. (1881), 1882, ix, 94–96.—**Mutter** (T. D.) Case of deformity of the mouth, from a burn, successfully treated by Dieffenbach's method. Am. J. M. Sc., Phila., 1837, xx, 341–346, 1 pl.—**Pitet.** Arrêt de développement de la voûte palatine. Bull. Soc. anat. de Par., 1848. xxiii, 182–184.—**Schmitt** (J.) Heilung einer Mundhöhlenverwachsung. Verhandl. d. k. k. Gesellsch. d. Aerzte zu Wien, 1843 ii, 299–308. — **Smith** (T.) A very unusual congenital deformity. Lancet, Lond, 1876, i, 13.—**Sourrouille** (A.) Vices de conformation de la bouche chez un nouveau-né. Gaz. d. hôp., Par., 1883, lvi, 707.—**Stankiewicz** (W.) Zwężenie otworu ustnego (atresia oris): przywrócenie tegoz za pomocą operacyi (stomatopoesis). Pam. Towarz. Lek. Warszaw., 1877, lxxiii, 149–151.—**Van Duyse.** Macrostomes congénitaux avec tumeurs préauriculaires et dermoïde de l'œil. Ann. Soc. de méd. de Gand, 1882, lx, 141–169, 1 pl.

Mouth (*Abscess of*).

See **Abscess** (*Sublingual, etc.*)

Mouth (*Cancer of*).

See, also, **Noma**; **Tongue** (*Cancer of*).

ESCHER (T.) * Ueber die Exstirpation des Mundbodencarcinoms. 8°. *Zürich*, 1874.

FEUILLETAUD (G.) * Contribution à l'étude du traitement chirurgical des cancers du plancher de la bouche. 4°. *Paris*, 1886.

Mouth (*Cancer of*).

GUILLOT (F.-M.-S.) Complications pulmonaires de l'épithélioma buccal. 4°. *Paris*, 1881.

HOMOLLE (S.-G.) Des scrofulides graves de la muqueuse bucco-pharyngienne (angines scrofuleuses graves; lupus de la gorge). 4°. *Paris*, 1875.

―――. The same. 8°. *Paris*, 1875.

JESSETT (F. B.) On cancer of the mouth, tongue, and alimentary tract, their pathology, symptoms, diagnosis, and treatment. 8°. *London*, 1885.

OSTROM (H. I.) Epithelioma of the mouth. 12°. *New York*, 1885.

Alberti (V.) Estirpazione di un epitelioma della cavità della bocca. Spallanzani, Modena, 1881, 2. s., x, 72-77.—**Baker** (M.) Three cases of epithelioma of the tongue and floor of the mouth. Lancet, Lond., 1884, ii, 732.—**Bassini** (E.) Al pavimento della bocca e parte anteriore della lingua; 1 caso (cancro). *In his:* Clin. operat., 8°, Genova, 1878, 53-60.—**Berti** (A.) Asportazione di un epitelioma al pavimento della bocca. Spallanzani, Modena, 1880, 2. s., ix, 186-189.—**Birkett.** Case of epithelioma of the mucous membrane of the mouth. Lancet, Lond., 1863, i, 579.—**Blache** (R.) Épithélioma de la langue et du plancher de la bouche; résection du maxillaire inférieur. Bull. Soc. anat. de Par., 1865, xl, 175-177.—**Bouisson.** Du cancer buccal chez les fumeurs. Montpel. méd., 1859, ii, 539: iii, 19. *Also* [Abstr.]: J. de chim. méd., etc., Par., 1860, 4. s., vi, 565-569.—**Cancer** of tongue and mouth; résumé of 76 cases for the 4 years 1882, 1883, 1884, and 1885. Middlesex Hosp. Rep. 1885, Lond., 1887, 161-170.—**Cancer** of the tongue and mouth. [23 cases.] *Ibid.*, 171-184.—**Carcinom** des Mundbodens. [Case.] Jahresb. ü. d. chir. Abth. d. Spit. zu Basel (1883), 1884, 24.—**Carcinom** des Mundbodens und des Unterkiefers. [Case.] *Ibid.*, 25-27.—**Castex** (A.) Des tumeurs malignes de l'arrière-bouche (clinique et intervention chirurgicale). Rev. de chir., Par., 1886, vi, 44; 130.—**Chenantais.** Épithéliome pavimenteux lobulé de la commissure buccale. Bull. Soc. anat. de Nantes 1879, Par., 1880, iii, 66.—**Clarke** (W. F.) Tubercular lupus of tongue, palate, and gums. Tr. Path. Soc. Lond., 1875-6, xxvii, 148.—**Douglass** (T.) Cases of disease of the mucous membrane. South. M. & S. J., Augusta, 1858, n. s., xiv, 744-747.—**Eder** (A.) Carcinoma buccæ sinistræ. *In his:* Aerztl. Ber. 1882, 8°, Wien, 1883, 17-20.—**Graverre** (E.) Épithélioma de la bouche; opération; pneumonie; mort. Bull. Soc. anat. de Par., 1886, lxi, 321-323. *Also:* Progrès méd., Par., 1886, 2. s., iv, 762.—**d'Héran.** Du cancer de la cavité buccale. J. d. conn. méd. prat, Par., 1858-9, xxvi, 351; 365.—**Heyfelder** (O.) [Eine härtliche, unebene Geschwulst in der Wangenschleimhaut.] Deutsche Klinik, Berl., 1849, i, 21.—**Lange.** Carcinoma of the floor of the mouth. Med. Rec., N. Y., 1881, xix, 106.—**Leidenfrost** (J. G.) De cancro scorbutico ejusque differentiis a cancro carcinomatoso. *In his:* Opusc. phys.-chem. et med., 12°, Duisburgi ad Rhenum, 1797, ii, 1-85.—**Malherbe.** Cancroïde de la bouche (épithéliome lobulé). Bull. Soc. anat. de Nantes 1880, Par., 1881, iv, 78-80.—**Moore.** Cancer in the floor of the mouth and in the subjacent lymphatic glands; treatment by the ligature of the lingual artery and division of the gustatory nerve, and by injections of acetic acid. Med. Times & Gaz., Lond., 1866, ii, 444.—**Parmentier.** [Tumeur épithéliale du plancher de la bouche.] Bull. Soc. anat. de Par., 1854, xxix, 204-207.—**Paul** (J.) Removal of a cancerous tumor from below the tongue. Edinb. M. J., 1858-9, iv, 200-204.—**Polaillon.** Épithélioma de l'amygdale, du voile du palais et de la base de la langue; ligatures primitives de la linguale gauche et de la carotide primitive droite; ablation de la masse morbide avec l'anse galvanique et le thermocautère; hémiplégie consécutive à gauche; récidive du cancer; mort par hémorrhagie foudroyante un mois et demi après l'opération. Gaz. méd. de Par., 1885, 7. s., ii, 3-6. ―――. Quelques réflexions sur les larges ablations de cancers de la bouche, de l'isthme du gosier et du pharynx. Bull. et mém. Soc. de chir. de Par., 1886, n. s., xii, 576-583. *Also:* Gaz. méd. de Par., 1886, 7. s., iii, 337; 349; 361.—**Prewitt.** Epithelioma of the mouth. St. Louis Cour. Med., 1882, vii, 459.—**Richard.** Sur quelques cas de cancer de la cavité buccale. Bull. Soc. de chir. de Par., 1857-8, viii, 213-215.—**Richet.** Cancer du plancher buccal. *Ibid.* (1860), 1861, 2. s., i, 430-436.—**Roux** fils. Du cancer sublingual. Gaz. d. hôp., Par., 1858, xxxi, 154.—**Seppilli** (G.) Cancro della retro-bocca con diffusione alla fossa media sinistra del cranio ed atrofia delle cellule del ganglio cervicale superiore sinistro del simpatico. Arch. ital. per le mal. nerv., Milano, 1886, xxiii, 183-192.—**Spence.** Sublingual cancroid ulcer; operation; recovery. Lancet, Lond., 1875, i, 858.—**Verneuil.** Diverses formes de cancroïdes de la bouche; gommes péri-articulaires; gommes de la parotide. J. de méd. et chir. prat., Par., 1876, xlvii, 396-400. ―――. Épi-

Mouth (*Cancer of*).

thélioma buccal; glycosurie reconnue à l'avance et rapidement dissipée par le traitement; opération; point d'accidents traumatiques locaux ni généraux; mort 75 heures après, par la pneumonie et coma diabétique. Bull. et mém. Soc. de chir. de Par., 1884, n. s., x, 379-390.—**Weiss** (T.) Cancer du plancher buccal et de la langue; section du maxillaire par le procédé de Sédillot; guérison. *In his:* Mém. sur quelques cas de chir., 8°, Nancy, 1883, 80-90.

Mouth (*Diseases of*).

See, also, Aphthæ; Dentistry; Glass-blowing, *etc.*; Gums (*Diseases of*); Jaws (*Diseases of*); Mercury (*Toxicology of, etc.*); Mouth (*Gangrene of*); Mouth (*Inflammation, etc., of*); Palate (*Diseases of*); Psoriasis (*Buccal*); Ranula; Salivation; Teeth, Tongue, Uvula, *Diseases of.*

ALBRECHT (E.) Klinik der Mundkrankheiten. Erster Bericht, 1855-60. 8°. *Berlin*, 1862.

BLACHE (M.-J.-G.) * Recherches sur une production particulière de la membrane muqueuse de la bouche qui se manifeste dans les derniers temps des maladies chroniques. 4°. *Paris*, 1824.

BOHN (H.) Die Mundkrankheiten der Kinder. 8°. *Leipzig*, 1866.

BRANDT (J. T.) * De lepræ in membrana faucium, narium, nec non oris mucosa obviæ diagnosi. [Dorpat.] 8°. *Rigæ*, 1825.

BRESSLER (H.) Die Krankheiten der Nasen- und Mundhöhle, der Zähne und des Gesichts, nach Deschamps, Cloquet, Weinhold, [etc.] 8°. *Berlin*, 1840.

CALI (G.) Sulla patologia, terapia ed igiene del vestibolo della bocca e dei denti. 8°. *Napoli*, 1884.

CHRUTSHOFF (I. I.) Polnii zubo-vrachebnii kurs. Chast pervaja: Gistologija, anatomija i fiziologija zubov i polosti rta. [Complete medico-dental course. Part I. Histology, anatomy, and physiology of the teeth and cavity of mouth.] 8°. *St. Petersburg*, 1885.

COLES (J. O.) Deformities of the mouth, congenital and acquired, with their mechanical treatment 2. ed. 8°. *London*, 1870.

―――. The same. 3. ed. 8°. *London*, 1881.

DALIBON. Hygiène des dents et des gencives et conseils pour guérir soi-même toutes les maladies de la bouche. 8°. [*Paris, n. d.*]

DUBINSKI (T.) * Bismutnii difterite polosti rta. [Effects of bismuth on mouth.] 8°. *St. Petersburg*, 1839.

FORESTUS *Alcmarianus* (P.) De ægritudinibus labiorum, gingivarum, dentium, oris ac linguæ. *In his:* Obs. et curat. med. 8°. *Lugd. Bat.*, 1591, xiv, 367-504.

GARIOT (J.-B.) Traité des maladies de la bouche, d'après l'état actuel des connaissances en médecine et en chirurgie, qui comprend la structure et les fonctions de la bouche, l'histoire de ses maladies, les moyens d'en conserver la santé et la beauté, et les opérations particulières à l'art du dentiste. 8°. *Paris*, 1805.

―――. The same. Treatise on the diseases of the mouth, [etc.] Transl. by J. B. Savier. 8°. *Baltimore*, 1843.

HELMKAMPFF (H.) Diagnose und Therapie der Erkrankungen des Mundes und Rachens sowie der Krankheiten der Zähne. 8°. *Stuttgart*, 1886.

HEURNIUS (J.) De morbis oculorum, aurium, nasi, dentium et oris, liber. Editus post mortem auctoris ab ejus filio Othone Heurnio. 4°. [*Lugd. Bat.*], 1608.

―――. The same. 4°. *Lugd. Bat.*, 1608.

JOURDAIN-BERCHILLET (A.-L.-B.) A treatise on the diseases and surgical operations of the mouth, and parts adjacent; with notes of inter-

Mouth (*Diseases of*).

esting cases, ancient and modern. Transl. from the French. 8°. *Baltimore*, 1849.

———. The same. Transl. from the last French ed. 8°. *Philadelphia*, 1851.

MALTERRE (P.-L.) * Études sur le diagnostic différentiel de quelques maladies de la peau qui peuvent affecter la muqueuse buccale. (Eczéma, impétigo, pemphigus, psoriasis.) 4°. *Paris*, 1857.

MAYNARD (P.-F.) * Des maladies de la muqueuse buccale chez les enfants à la mamelle. 4°. *Strasbourg*, 1845.

MEIBOM (H. J.) Gegründetes Bedencken über einen Gestanck aus dem Munde, benebst der Untersuchung und Wiederlegung des darin befindlichen Visi reperti. Mit Anmerckungen von Paul Gottlieb Werlhof. 4°. *Franckfurt u. Leipzig*, 1743.

VON OPPOLZER. Vorlesungen über die Krankheiten der Mundhöhle, der Speicheldrüsen, des Rachens und der Speiseröhre, bearbeitet von E. Ritter von Stoffella. 8°. *Erlangen*, 1872.

PATRICK (J. J. R.) Oral electricity and the new departure. 8°. *Belleville*, 1881.

PELAEZ (F. A.) Tratado de las enfermedades de la boca sobre todas las partes del arte del dentista. 16°. *Madrid*, 1795.

PUCCI (F.) Studj teorico-pratici per la cura e conversazione dei denti e malattie della bocca. 8°. *Venezia*, 1871.

SCHECH (P.) Die Krankheiten der Mundhöhle, des Rachens und der Nase. Mit Einschluss der Rhinoskopie und der local therapeutischen Technik. roy. 8°. *Wien*, 1885.

———. The same. Diseases of the mouth, throat, and nose. Including rhinoscopy and methods of local treatment. Transl. by R. H. Blaikie. 8°. *Edinburgh*, 1886.

SCHMITT (A.) Die Krankheiten des Mundes und der Zähne, ihre Behandlung und Heilung. 8°. *Wien*, 1850.

SOCIETY for the Advancement of Oral Science. [Constitution and by-laws.] 16°. [*n. p.*, *n. d.*]

Albrethsen (V.) Lidt om Mundsygen og dens Overførelse paa Mennesker. [Diseases of the mouth and their treatment.] Hosp.-Tid., Kjøbenh., 1870, xiii. 37. — **Arkövy** (J.) Das Papillom in der Mundhöhle. Pest. med.-chir. Presse, Budapest, 1878, xiv. 926–930. — **Bénard** (P.) Le psoriasis buccal (de Bazin) observé et traité aux eaux minérales de Saint-Christan. Mém. et bull. Soc. de méd. et chir. de Bordeaux (1885), 1886, 258–312. — **Bierbaum** (J.) Krankheiten des Mundes und Schlundes. J. f. Kinderkr., Erlang., 1857, xxviii, 297–309. — **Bohn** (H.) Zur Geschichte der Mundkrankheiten. Deutsche Klinik, Berl., 1867, xix, 136–138. ——— Die Mundkrankheiten. Handb. d. Kinderkr. (Gerhardt), Tübing., 1879, iv, 2. Abth., 3–128. — **Bordenave.** Maladies de l'intérieur de la bouche: I. Excroissance fongueuse des gencives. [6 obs.] II. Sur la gangrène scorbutique des gencives dans les enfans. [Par feu M. Berthe.] III. Sur les effets rapides de la pourriture aux gencives. [Par M. Capdeville.] IV. Sur des tumeurs sublinguales. V. De la rescission des amygdales tuméfiées. [16 obs.] Mém. Acad. roy. de chir., Par., 1774, v. 272–485, 2 pl. — **Boyer & Roux.** Prolapsus de la membrane muqueuse labiale; considérationes générales. Gaz. d. hôp., Par., 1828-9, i, 31. — **Broers** (H. J.) Over enkele aandoeningen van mond en keelholte. Nederl. Tijdschr. v. Heel en Verlosk., Utrecht, 1864, xiv, 278; 327, 1 pl. *Also, Reprint.* — **Busch.** Die Poliklinik für Zahn- und Mundkrankheiten in dem neu begründeten zahnärztlichen Institut an der Universität Berlin. Deutsche med. Wchnschr., Berl., 1885, xi, 407; 423. — **Caponotto** (A.) Malattie della faccia, naso, bocca, fauci; casi 32. Osservatore, Torino, 1883, xix, 241; 257.— **Cohen** (J. S.) Diseases of the mouth and tongue. Syst. Pract. M. (Pepper), Phila., 1885, ii, 321–378. — **Cormack** (E. A.) The mucous membrane of the mouth, with special reference to its physiology and pathology, and the part played by its secretions in the production of dental caries. Brit. J. Dent. Sc., Lond., 1886, xxix, 486; 535; 577.— **Diseases** of the mouth. St. Louis Cour. Med., 1879, ii, 503.— **Epstein** (A.) Zur Aetiologie einiger Mundkrankheiten und zur Hygiene der Mundhöhle bei neugeborenen Kindern. Prag. med. Wchnschr., 1884, ix, 121; 155.— **Fischl** (R.) Statistischer Beitrag zur Frage der Prophylaxis der Mundkrankheiten des Säuglings. *Ibid.*, 1886,

Mouth (*Diseases of*).

xi, 389–392. — **Frédericq** (A.) Du chlorate de potasse dans les affections malignes de la bouche. Ann. Soc. méd. d'émulat. de la Flandre occid., Roulers, 1848, ii, 244–247.— **Fremmert** (H.) Zur Casuistik der Leukoplakie. St. Petersb. med. Wchnschr., 1885, n. F., ii, 4. — **Glasgow** (W. C.) A case of leucoplakia buccalis; recovery. N. York M. J., 1887, xlvi, 461.— **Grigorow.** Erythema exsudativum papulatum der Mundschleimhaut. St. Petersb. med. Wchnschr., 1879, iv, 469.— **Hamonic** (P.) De la leucoplasie buccale dans ses rapports avec la syphilis. Ann. méd.-chir. franç. et étrang., Par., 1886, ii, 193–204.— **Harvey** (P. F.) Chronic hyperplasia of the oral mucosa, with cornification of its epithelium. Am. J. M. Sc., Phila., 1886, n. s., xcii, 110–120.— **Hauner.** Mundkrankheiten der Kinder. Deutsche Klinik, Berl., 1852, iv, 272–275. — **Heath** (C.) Injuries and diseases of the mouth, fauces, tongue, palate, and jaws. Internat. Encycl. Surg. (Ashhurst), N. Y., 1885, v, 493–549. *Also, transl.:* Encycl. internat. de chir. (Ashhurst), Par., 1886, v, 507–554.— **Henoch.** Fall von acuter Anschwellung des Bodens der Mundhöhle. Charité-Ann. 1879, Berl., 1881, vi. 509–511.— **Hohl** (R.) Zur Casuistik der Mundkrankheiten. Deutsche Vrtljschr. f. Zahnh., Nürnb., 1870, xi, 178–183. *Also, Reprint.*—**Joseph.** Beitrag zur Therapie der Leucoplakia. Deutsche med. Wchnschr., Berl., 1885, xi, 738.— **Leloir** (H.) Note sur l'anatomie pathologique et la nature du psoriasis lingual. Bull. Soc. anat. de Par., 1883, lviii, 485–488. ——— Recherches sur la nature et l'anatomie pathologique de la leucoplasie buccale (psoriasis buccal). Compt. rend. Acad. d. sc., Par., 1887, civ, 1747-1749. *Also:* J. d. conn. méd. prat., Par., 1887, 3. s., ix, 234. ——— Recherches sur l'anatomie pathologique et la nature de la leucoplasie buccale (psoriasis buccal). Arch. de physiol. norm. et path., Par., 1887, 3. s., x, 86–106, 2 pl.— **Luther** (H.) Ueber eine eigenthümliche Krankheit der Mundhöhle. J. d. pract. Heilk., Berl., 1840, xc, St. 1, 110.— **Macgregor** (A. D.) On the value of boric acid in various conditions of the mouth. Brit. M. J., Lond., 1886, ii, 63.— **Miller.** Die Anwendbarkeit einiger Antiseptika bei der Behandlung der Krankheiten der Mundhöhle und der Zähne. Deutsche med. Wchnschr., Berl., 1885, xi, 552–554.— **Mitchell** (J. K.) Encephaloid disease of the mouth. Tr. Path. Soc. Phila. (1883–5), 1886, xii, 63–66.— **Morrow** (P. A.) Keratosis follicularis, associated with fissuring of the tongue and leukoplakia buccalis. J. Cutan. & Ven. Dis., N. Y., 1886, iv, 257–265. *Also* [Abstr.]: Med. Rec., N. Y., 1886, xxx, 304. *Also* [Abstr.]: Med. News, Phila.,1886, xlix, 295. *Also* [Abstr.]: Am. M. Ass., Chicago, 1886; vii, 302.— **Münlig.** Zur Pathologie der Mundschleimhaut. Ztschr. d. k.-k. Gesellsch. d. Aerzte zu Wien, 1852, i, 28-48.— **Pensa** (G.) Sulle malattie delia bocca dei bambini. Imparziale, Firenze, 1864, iv, 262; 308; 346; 397; 434; 469; 504. — **Pollock** (G.) Diseases of the mouth. Syst. Surg. (Holmes), Lond., 1864, iv, 76–138. *Also: Ibid.*, 2. ed., N. Y., 1870, iv, 398-495.— **Pospelow.** Ein Fall von Erythema nodosum auf der Schleimhaut der Mundhöhle. St. Petersb. med. Wchnschr., 1876, No. 40. — **Reclus** (P.) Cancroïdes et leucoplasie des muqueuses buccale et vaginale. Gaz. hebd. de méd., Par., 1887, 2. s., xxiv, 420–424. — **Reid** (J. G.) Oral chemistry. Tr. Illinois Dent. Soc., Chicago. 1886, xxii, 139–149.— **Rhein** (M. L.) Oral hygiene. N. Eng. J. Dent., Springfield, Mass., 1884, iii, 356–361. *Also, Reprint.* — **Ritter.** Dauerndes Aufhören epileptischer Krampfanfälle nach der Behandlung eines kranken Mundes. Deutsche Monatschr. f. Zahnh., Leipz., 1886, iv, 247. — **Ruppius.** Beobachtungen über eine eigne Krankheit des Mundes. Allg. med. Ann., Leipz., 1820, 1565–1574. — **Russell** (J. W.) Treatment of diseases of the mouth. Independ. Pract., N. Y., 1884, v, 408–414. — **Schrakamp.** Zur Differentialdiagnose der Erkrankungen der Mundhöhle. Deutsche med. Wchnschr., Leipz., 1887, xiii, 892–894.— **Servaes.** Ueber eine (in 4 Fällen beobachtete) neuralgische Affection des Zahnfleisches der Zunge und des harten Gaumens. Allg. Ztschr. f. Psychiat., etc., Berl., 1871-2, xxvii, 335-337. — **Smith** (J. S.) Oral disease and caseous phthisis. Med. & Surg. Reporter, Phila., 1886, lv, 422.— **Somma** (L.) Su alcune malattie della bocca poco note nella prima infanzia. Gior. internat. d. sc. med., Napoli, 1882, n. s., iv, 1197–1214.— **Squarey** (C. E.) Diseases of the mouth. Syst. Med. (Reynolds), Lond., 1871, iii, 3–26.— **Starbuck** (W. C.) The possibilities of hereditary transmissions of oral lesions. Independ. Pract., N. Y., 1884, v, 483–487. — **Thomas** (L.) Traitement des varices de la bouche, du pharynx et du larynx. Cong. internat. de laryngol. 1880, Milan, 1882, i, 235–237.— **Trautmann** sen. Ueber die Heilkraft der Herba Agrimoniæ in Krankheiten der Mund- und Schlundhöhle. Summ. d. Neuest. u. Wissenswürd. a. d. ges. Med., Leipz., 1837, v, 19–21 — **Vogel** (A.) Krankheiten der Lippen und der Mundhöhle. Handb. d. spec. Path. (Ziemssen), Leipz., 1874, vii, 1. St., 1–116. *Also, transl.:* Cycl. Pract. M. (Ziemssen), N. Y., 1876, vi, 733–860.— **Wertheim.** Ueber die häufige Verwechselung von Chlorkalium und chlorsaurem Kali, in Lösungen als Mundwasser verwendet. Ber. d. k. k. Krankenanst. Rudolph-Stiftung in Wien (1881), 1882, 261. *Also:* Med. Jahrb., Wien, 1882, 7.

Mouth (*Diseases of*) *in pregnancy*.

See **Mouth** (*Inflammation of*) *in pregnancy*.

Mouth (*Exploration and semeiology of*).

See, *also*, **Auscultation** *of mouth*; **Tongue** (*Semeiology of*).

BRUCK (J.) jun. Das Stomatoscop zur Durchleuchtung der Zähne und ihrer Nachbartheile durch galvanisches Glühlicht. Nebst einem Anhang, das Stomatoscop zur Erleuchtung des Rachenraumes zu benutzen. 8°. *Breslau*, 1865.

DIMEY (N.-A.) * Séméiologie de la cavité buccale. 4°. *Paris*, 1848.

HARTMANN (A. J.) De stomatoscopia medica. 4°. *Vitembergæ*, [1786].

LAFFIN (J.) * Contribution à l'histoire de la séméiologie buccale. Étude des arcades alvéolo-dentaires. 4°. *Paris*, 1876.

ZIMMERMANN (J. C. P.) * De ore ut signo. sm. 4°. *Halæ Magdeb.*, [1752].

Adelmann (G. F. B.) Adelmanns Mundspiegel. Beitr. z. Heilk., Riga, 1853, ii, 1 pl. opposite p. 42.—[**Chassaignac**.] Nouveau spéculum oris. Gaz. d. hôp., Par., 1853, xxvi, 491.—**Fleming** (A.) Note on the mouth speculum. Month. J. M. Sc., Lond. & Edinb., 1848-9, ix, 171.—**Galippe.** Note sur l'examen de la bouche et de l'appareil dentaire dans les établissements consacrés à l'instruction publique. Rev. d'hyg., Par., 1883, v, 889-907.—**Goodwillie** (D. H.) Oral speculum. Med. Rec., N. Y., 1884, xxv, 278.—**Gubler** (A.) [Bouche.] Séméiologie. Dict. encycl. d. sc. méd., Par., 1869, x, 211-249.—**Klopsch.** Ueber das Stomatoskop von Julius Bruck jun., und die Verwendung des galvanischen Glühlicht's zu diagnostischen Zwecken. Wien. med. Wchnschr., 1866, xvi, 108-110.—**Magitot.** Instructions relatives à l'examen de la bouche et des dents dans les écoles. Ann. d'hyg., Par., 1885, 3. s., xiv, 360-377. *Also*: Rev. d'hyg., Par., 1885, vii, 558-571.—**Mathieu.** Spéculum de la bouche. [Rap. de Ricord.] Bull. Acad. de méd., Par., 1850-51, xvi, 434-436.—**Price** (P. C.) On a convenient instrument for examining the base of the tongue and epiglottis. Lancet, Lond., 1859, ii, 643.—**Rhodes** (W. A.) The mouth in the insane. J. Brit. Dent. Ass., Lond., 1884, v, 413-415.—**Roser.** Ueber die Anwendung eines zweiklappigen Mundspiegels bei Kindern. Arch. f. physiol. Heilk., Stuttg., 1846, v, 87.—**Seemann.** Ein neues Mundspeculum. Deutsche med. Wchnschr., Berl., 1881, vii, 387.—**Smith** (J.) On a speculum adapted for employment during operations on the mouth, under chloroform. Month. J. M. Sc., Lond. & Edinb., 1854, xviii, 333-335.—**Spengler.** Zur Untersuchung der Mund- und Rachenhöhle. Arch. f. path. Anat., etc., Berl., 1860, xviii, 556-558.—**Vollmar** (E.) Ein Mundspiegel. Ztschr. f. Wundärzte u. Geburtsh., Stuttg., 1851, iv, 314-318, figs. 1-9.—**Yates** (H.) Speculum oris. Med.-Chir. Rev., Lond., 1843, xxxix, 570.

Mouth (*Gangrene of*).

See, *also*, **Measles** (*Complications, etc., of*); **Mercury** (*Toxicology of, etc.*); **Noma**.

BLONDEAUX (E.-J.) * De la stomatite ulcéreuse des enfants et de la nécrose du maxillaire dans cette affection. 4°. *Paris*, 1851.

VAN BUUREN (B.) * De stomacace. 8°. *Groningæ*, 1850.

CORDOËN (H.-F.) * Essai sur la gangrène de la bouche des enfans. 4°. *Paris*, 1830.

DAVONNEAU (É.) * De la gangrène de la bouche chez les enfans. 4°. *Paris*, 1855.

DUBOIS (N.) * Dissertation sur une gangrène de la bouche, particulière aux eufans, précédée de la définition et de la division de la gangrène en général. 4°. *Paris*, 1823.

MAHIEUX (S.-C.) * De la gangrène de la bouche chez les enfans. 4°. *Paris*, 1855.

TOURDES (J.) * Du noma, ou du sphacèle de la bouche chez les enfants. 4°. *Strasbourg*, 1848.

Adams (A. L.) A case of idiopathic gangrenous stomatitis. Edinb. M. J., 1862-3, viii, 154.—**Anderson** (H. M.) Report of two cases of gangrena oris. Memphis M. Recorder, 1855, iii, 169-171.—**Anderson** (R. S.) Two cases of cancrum oris. Med. Arch., St. Louis, 1869, iii, 483-486. ———. Gangrenous stomatitis. History of two cases. *Ibid.*, 591-595.—**Bainbridge** (W.) Idiopathic gangrene of the mouth; disease of the mouth from unfit or deficient food. Lancet, Lond., 1839-40, i, 509-511.—**Barker** (T. H.) Case of cancrum oris, with necrosis of a large portion of the inferior maxillary bone, followed by recov-

ery. Prov. M. & S. J., Lond., 1852, 611.—**Barlow** (W. F.) Cancrum oris, not a result of mercury. Lancet, Lond., 1842-3, ii, 120.—**Baron.** Mémoire sur une affection gangréneuse de la bouche, particulière aux enfans. Bull. Fac. de méd. de Par., 1816-17, v, 145; 151.—**Barth** fils. Gangrène spontanée de la gencive; extension rapide de l'eschare; état général grave, intoxication putride; autopsie. Bull. Soc. clin. de Par. (1878), 1879, ii, 183-187.—**Baudelocque.** Gangrène de la bouche; cautérisation avec le nitrate acide de mercure; guérison. Gaz. méd. de Par., 1834, 2. s., ii, 102. *Also*: Abeille, Brux., 1834, i, 208.—**Behrend** (F. J.) Einige Bemerkungen über die entzündlichen, geschwürigen und brandigen Affektionen des Mundes bei Kindern und über deren Unterscheidung. J. f. Kinderkr., Erlang., 1853, xx, 344-355.—**Berkley** (H. J.) Notes on a case of gangrena oris (?) in a man of twenty-five. Maryland M. J., Balt., 1883-4, x, 226.—**Birkett** (J.) Necrosis of the symphysis and portions of the horizontal rami of the lower jaw, consequent upon cancrum oris; reparation of the loss thus sustained by the development of new bone. Tr. Path. Soc. Lond., 1855-6, vii, 284.—**Bouchut.** Ueber die Stomatitis ulcero-membranosa und über deren Einfluss auf die Kiefernekrose. J. f. Kinderkr., Erlang., 1863, xli, 253-257.—**Bouchut** (E.) De la gangrène de la bouche chez les enfants. Paris méd., 1881, vi, 25.—**Bouillaury.** Stomatite terminée par gangrène. Rev. de thérap. du midi, Montpel., 1857, xi, 223-228.—**Bouneau.** Gangrène de la bouche survenue pendant le cours d'une pneumonie avec tubercules pulmonaires; mort. Gaz. d. hôp., Par., 1833, vii, 49.—**Brackett** (C.) Cases of cancrum oris. Northwest. M. & S. J., Chicago, 1852-3, ix, 11. ———. Cancrum oris. Chicago M. J., 1860, n. s., iii, 638-640.—**Brown** (J. B.) Gangrenous erosion of the face. Boston M. & S. J., 1829-30, ii, pt. 2, 679-682.—**Browne** (R. K.) Report on gangrene of the mouth and fauces, observed at the U. S. General Marine Hospital, New Orleans, La. Tr. M. Soc. N. Y., Albany, 1863, 289-307. ———. Gangrene of the mouth and fauces. Am. M. Times, N. Y., 1863, vi, 50-52.—**Brydon** (W.) Case of cancrum oris in the adult. Brit. M. J., Lond., 1882, ii, 838.—**Burrows.** Cancrum oris. Lancet, Lond., 1851, i, 621.—**Bystroff** (N.) Zamietka otak nazvaiemoy stomacace u dietey. [Observation on so-called stomacace (cancer aquaticus) in children] Med. Vestnik, St. Petersb., 1867, 456-458.—**C.** De la gangrène de la bouche chez les enfans, et de son traitement. Bull. gén. de thérap., etc., Par., 1834, vii, 318-323.—**Carroll** (T.) Observations on cancrum oris as it appeared in the Cincinnati Orphan Asylum from Feb., 1842, to May, 1847. West. J. M. & S. Louisville, 1847, 3. s., viii, 93-127.—**Cases** of cancrum oris. Lancet, Lond., 1857, ii, 325. *Ibid.*, 1868, ii, 601.—**Chaloin.** Cas de gangrène de la muqueuse buccale produite par le froid. Rap. gén. trav. Soc. d. sc. méd. de Gannat, 1855-6, x, 19.—**Chipault** (A.) [Une gangrène de la bouche qui a provoqué une necrose du maxillaire supérieur, et consécutivement une infection purulente.] Bull. Soc. anat. de. Par., 1862, xxxvii, 444.—**Clendinning** (J.) Gangrene of the mouth. Lancet, Lond., 1841-2, i, 811.—**Cleveland** (W. F.) Case of ulcerative stomatitis in an adult, terminating fatally in sloughing phagedena (cancrum oris). Med. Times & Gaz., Lond., 1860, i, 288.—**Coates** (B. H.) Description of the gangrenous ulcer of the mouths of children. N. Am. M. & S. J., Phila., 1826, ii, 1-24.—**Collin** (J. G.) Anmärkningar om stomacace hos barn. Hygiea, Stockholm, 1843, v, 414-424.—**Cook** (W. C.) Cancrum oris; two rare cases. Nashville M. News, 1887, i, 162-164. *Also*: Nashville J. M. & S., 1887, n. s., xl, 341-344.—**Corse.** Gangrena oris. Am. J. M. Sc., Phila., 1858, n. s., xxxvi, 493. *Also*: Tr. Coll. Phys. Phila. (1856-62), 1863, n. s., iii, 191.—**Cory** (E. A.) Fatal cancrum oris; inquest. Lancet, Lond., 1840, ii, 872-874. —**Courbon-Pérusel.** Observation d'un ulcère à la bouche, du genre de ceux que Van-Swieten a appelés chancres aquatiques. Bull. Fac. de méd. de Par., 1820-21, vii, 376-379.—**Crandell** (R. O.) Cancrum oris. Tr. M. Ass. South. Central N. Y., Auburn, 1852, 55.—**Crane.** † Med. Rec., N. Y., 1866-7, i, 18.—**Cripps** (W. H.) Diseased jaw-bone from case of cancrum oris. Tr. Path. Soc. Lond., 1879-80, xxxi, 242.—**Croly.** Cancrum oris. Dublin M. Press, 1863, xlix, 391-394.—**Cuming** (T.) Observations on an affection of the mouth in children. Dublin Hosp. Rep., 1827, iv, 330-348.—**Daugherty** (W. H.) Phagedenia oris in adults. Cincin Lancet & Obs., 1865, viii, 531-533.—**Dawson** (J.) Cancrum oris. Ohio M. & S. J., Columbus, 1854-5, vii, 182.—**Descamps.** Observations sur la gangrène humide et scorbutique des gencives. J. de méd., chir., pharm., etc., Par., 1803, vi, 114-121.—**Destrées.** Observation d'une gangrène de la bouche, suite d'une entérite. J. gén. de méd., chir. et pharm., Par., 1821, lxxv, 303-311.—**Dowse** (T. S.) Clinical and pathological notes on ulcerative stomatitis (noma), gangrenous stomatitis (cancrum oris), and the clinical resemblance of the latter to malignant pustule, or charbon. Med. Exam., Lond., 1877, ii, 45-48.—**Drew** (J.) A report of two cases of sloughing phagedæna. Lancet, Lond., 1850, i, 206-208.—**Dudart** (G.) Observation de stomatite gangréneuse avec nécrose de toute la branche horizontale gauche du maxillaire inférieur. Ann. Soc. de méd. d'An-

Mouth (*Gangrene of*).

vers, 1850, xi, 123-128.—**Duke** (B. F.) Cancrum oris. South. M. Rec., Atlanta, 1881, xi, 451.—**Duncan** (J. F.) On the administration of mercury in cases of cancrum oris. Dublin Q. J. M. Sc., 1852, xiv. 265-273.—**Dunn** (R.) † Inquest. Lancet, Lond., 1843, i, 60-62. *Also:* Lond. M. Gaz., 1843, i, 57. *Also:* Prov. M. J., Lond., 1843-4, vii, 38-40.—**Edgar** (W. S.) Cancrum oris. St. Louis M. & S. J., 1870, n. s., vii, 398-403.—**Espina** (A.) Un caso de gangrena de la boca. Rev. de med. y cirug. práct., Madrid, 1878, ii, 200-205.—**Estevez y Fernandez** (A.) Un caso de gangrena de la boca (úlcera corrosiva de Hipócrates). *Génio* méd.-quir., Madrid, 1882, xxviii, 19. *Also, transl.:* Courrier méd., Par., 1882, xxxii, 63.—**Eve** (E. A.) An essay on gangrenopsis. South. M. & S. J., Augusta, 1837, i, 731-737.—**Farre.** Gangrenous stomatitis. Lancet, Lond., 1859, ii, 534. — **Féraud** (L.) Observation de gangrène de la bouche. [Rap. de Blache.] Bull. Acad. de méd., Par., 1859-60, xxv, 120-125.—**Fleming** (C.) Cancrum oris. Dublin Hosp. Gaz., 1856, n. s., iii, 100-102.—**Forbes** (S. S.) [Four cases of cancrum oris.] Tr. M. Ass. Alabama, Mobile, 1871, 135-137.—**Forster** (J. C.) † Death. Guy's Hosp. Rep., Lond., 1875, 3. s., xx, 22.—**Fuller** (A. P.) Case of gangrenopsis. Boston M. & S. J., 1835, xiii, 319.—**Glauner.** Der feuchte Mundkrebs der Kinder. Ztschr. f. rat. Med., Heidelb., 1854, n. F., v, 180-211, 1 pl.—**Glynn.** A paper on cancrum oris. Brit. M. J., Lond., 1869, i, 248.—**Godelier.** Gangrène de la bouche localisée au niveau de la 2ᵐᵉ grosse molaire inférieure gauche; invasion rapide d'un état adynamique, très-grave; mort; septicémie. Gaz. d. hôp., Par., 1861, xxxiv, 437.—**Gray** (J.) Cancrum oris. Glasgow M. J., 1856-7, [2. s.], iv, 16-21.—**Guersent.** Stomatites couenneuses; terminaison par gangrène; autopsie. Clinique, Par., 1830, ii, 123-125.—**Guibert** (T.) Mémoire sur la gangrène de la bouche chez les enfans. J. compl. du dict. d. sc. méd., Par., 1829, xxxiv, 331-340. — **Hall** (M.) On a peculiar species of gangrenous ulcer, which affects the face in children. Edinb. M. & S. J., 1819, xv, 547-553. ———. Case of phagedena oris on which an inquest was held. Lancet, Lond., 1839-40, i, 409.—**Hallopeau** (H., & **Tuffier.** Note sur un cas d'herpès phlycténoïde de la face avec gangrène des muqueuses buccale et pharyngée. Union méd., Par., 1882, 3. s., xxxiii, 965-971.—**Harris** (C. A.) Ulceration of the gums and exfoliation of the alveolar processes of children resulting from general debility or defective nutrition. Maryland M. & S. J., Balt., 1840, i, 424-429.—**Heath** (C.) Cancrum oris; spread of the disease; absence of microorganisms in the blood; autopsy. Med. Times & Gaz., Lond., 1884, i, 661-663.—**Hempstead** (G. S. B.) Erosion of the face. Boston M. & S. J., 1830-31, iii, pt. 1, 30-33.—**Hengst** (D. A.) A case of gangrena oris. Med. & Surg. Reporter, Phila., 1883, xlviii, 33.—**Herme.** Fall einer gelungenen Heilung des Wasserkrebses der Kinder. Arch. f. med. Erfahr.. Berl., 1810, ii, 567-577.—**Hervez.** De la gangrène de la bouche chez les enfants. J. de méd., Par., 1846. iv, 44-46.—**Holmes.** Portion of the jaw-bones, which exfoliated in a case of cancrum oris, perforating the cheek. Tr. Path. Soc. Lond., 1862-3, xiv, 225-227.—**Honert.** Eine Gangræna oris, anscheinend abgewendet durch die Darreichung grösserer Mengen eines feurigen Weines. Deutsche Klinik, Berl., 1867, xix, 326.—**Howard** (G. C.) On calomel in gangrenopsis. Boston M. & S. J., 1835, xii, 411-413.—**Howe** (J. J.) Remarks on an ulceration of the mouth, of a peculiar character, as it occurs in the New York Alms-House. Med. Repository, N. Y., 1821, n. s., vi, 304-311.—**Hubbard** (C.) Erosion of the face. Boston M. & S. J., 1830-31, iii, pt. 1, 12-14.—**Huber.** Ueber den mikroskopischen Befund bei Stomacace. Aerztl. Int.-Bl., München, 1884, xxxi, 67.—**Hunt** (H.) Remarks on cancrum oris, and the gangrenous erosion of the cheek of Mr. Dease and Dr. Underwood, and more particularly on the efficacy of the chlorate of potash in the treatment of those diseases. Med.-Chir. Tr., Lond., 1843, xxvi, 142-153. ———. Remarques sur l'ulcère gangréneux de la bouche chez les enfants (cancrum oris), et sur l'efficacité du chlorate de potasse dans le traitement de cette maladie. Rev. méd.-chir. de Par., 1847, i, 4-9.—**Ingals** (E. F.) † Med. Exam., Chicago, 1872, xiii, 133.—**Jackson** (S.) On the gangrenopsis or gangrenous erosion of the cheek. Am. M. Recorder, Phila., 1827, xii, 66-96.—**Jobert.** Perforation complète de la joue à la suite d'une gangrène; génioplastie; guérison. Gaz. d. hôp., Par., 1853, xxvi, 275.—**Juvera** (R.) Breves reflexiones sobre la gangrena de la boca. Observador méd., México, 1874-6, iii, 311.—**Keiller** (A.) Communication on cancrum oris, or noma; cases in which recovery had taken place after exfoliation and sloughing of considerable portions of the jaw and cheek. Month. J. M. Sc., Lond. & Edinb., 1848, viii, 888. ———. On cancrum oris. Edinb. M. J., 1861-2, vii, 919-934. *Also, transl.:* J. f. Kinderkr., Erlang, 1862, xxxix, 22-38.—**Kittredge** (C. S.) Paper on cancrum oris. West. Lancet, San Fran., 1872-3, i, 141-149.—**Krasin.** K vopr. ob etiologii gangren tsheki (noma). Vrach. Vaidom., St. Petersb., 1880, v, 1945-1947. *Also, transl.:* France méd., Par., 1881, xxxiii, 657-661.—**Kühn** (E.) Fall von Mundfäule und schnelle Heilung derselben nach Anwendung der Iodine. Summ.

Mouth (*Gangrene of*).

d. Neuest. u. Wissenswürd. a. d. ges. Med., Leipz., 1835, iii, 97-99.—**Lanyon** (R.) On phagedæna oris. Lancet, Lond., 1839-40, i, 793.—**Lavacherie.** De la gangrène de la bouche avec nécrose des os maxillaires. J. de méd., chir. et pharmacol., Brux., 1844, ii, 53-59.—**Lavit.** Gangrène de la bouche: traitement par la créosote camphrée; guérison. Bull. gén. de thérap., etc., Par., 1867, lxxiii, 412-414. — **Léveillé.** Observation sur une gangrène de la face développée chez un adulte, et semblable à celle qu'on dit être particulière aux enfans. Bull. Fac. de méd. de Par., 1819, vi, 443-446.—**Macguire** (C. J.) Bismuth as a specific for cancrum oris. Med. Rec., N. Y., 1883, xxiii, 113-117.—**Malécot & Huet.** Gangrène de la bouche; autopsie; estomac bilobé avec ulcère rond de sa face postérieure; lame de verre enkystée dans le péricarde. Bull. Soc. anat. de Par., 1881, lvi, 196-201.—**Malle** (P.) Gangrène à la partie interne de la bouche; autopsie. Rec. de mém. de méd. . . . mil., Par., 1837, xliii, 258-271.—**Menger** (R.) [Gangrene of the mouth.] Texas M. & S. Rec., Galveston, 1881, i, 98-100.—**Merriman** (R. A.) Some account of affections of the face, considered in relation to the appearance of a new disease of this part, designated, by Dr. Jackson, gangrænopsis. Boston M. & S. J., 1829-30, ii, pt. 2, 758-761.—**de Meza** sen. De cancro aquoso. Acta reg. Soc. med. Havn. (1782-8), 1791, ii, 102-105.—**Miller** (J. G.) Three cases of cancrum oris successfully treated with a saturated solution of iodine. Kansas City M. J., 1879, iii, 211-214.—**Montgomery** (J. E.) Cancrum oris. Nashville J. M. & S., 1858, xv, 453-459.—**Moore** (S. W.) A case of mortification of the cheek, in which pyrolignous acid was employed with advantage. Med. Reposit., N. Y., 1822, n. s., vii, 237 - 240. — **Obre** (H.) Gangrene of the mouth successfully treated by the actual cautery. Lancet, Lond., 1840, ii, 649. ———. Remarks on gangrene of the face, and its treatment. Edinb. M. & S. J., 1814, lxi, 103-107.—**Odin.** Gangrène aiguë de la bouche chez un adulte; mort. Mém. Soc. d. sc. méd. de Lyon (1876), 1877, xvi, 160-162.—**O'Gorman** (P. W.) Caucrum oris in an European soldier; enlarged spleen; pancreatic disease; post mortem results. Indian M. Gaz., Calcutta, 1882, xvii, 14.—**Owsley** (W. T.) Case of cancrum oris, following typhoid pneumonia, in a boy thirteen years old. Virginia M. & S. J., Richmond, 1856, vii, 383-385.—**Packard** (G.) Case of gangrenous erosion of the face. Boston M. & S. J., 1830-31, iii, pt. 1, 337-339.—**Paget.** Cancrum oris, consequent on fever: death. Med. Times & Gaz., Lond., 1862, ii, 253. — **Parham** (F. W.) A case of gangrenous stomatitis (cancrum oris); successfully treated by the thermocautery. N. Orl. M. & S. J., 1886-7, n. s., xiv, 211-213.—**Pétaver** (J.) Gangrène des tonsiles, de la luette et de la partie interne de la joue droite. Bull. Soc. méd. de la Suisse Rom., Lausanne, 1871, v, 367.—**Poland** (A.) Phagedæna of tongue, gums, and lips; rapid recovery. Guy's Hosp. Rep., Lond., 1850-51, 2. s., vii, 331. — **Priestley** (W. O.) Abstract of a clinical lecture on a case of cancrum oris. Brit. M. J., Lond., 1871, ii, 577.—**Putegnat.** De la stomatite gangréneuse. Gaz. hebd. de méd., Par., 1865, 2. s., ii, 118-124. *Also,* Reprint.—**Reese** (W. P.) A case of gangrenous stomatitis. N. Orl. M. & S. J., 1850-51, vii, 40.—**Rendu.** Stomatite ulcéro-membraneuse terminée par gangrène; nécrose des os maxillaires supérieur et inférieur (incomplète); néphrite catarrhale; autopsie. Bull. Soc. anat. de Par., 1872, 2. s., xvii, 440-443.—**Rey.** Observation sur une affection gangréneuse de la joue, chez un enfant de trente mois, traitée avec le chlorure de soude. Rev. méd. franç. et étrang., Par., 1823, xi, 184-196.—**Ritchie** (R. P.) Observations on the inflammations of the mouth in children, with an illustrative case of cancrum oris. Tr. Edinb. Obst. Soc. (1869-71), 1872, iii, 428-434, 1 pl.—**S.** (J.) Mortification of the lower lip. Bost n M. & S. J., 1835-6, xiii, 93.—**Santopadre** (T.) Stomatite gangrenosa, edema della glottide; morte per asfissia. Riv. clin. di Bologna, 1869, viii, 75-79.—**Seguy** (F.) Affection gangréneuse de la joue. Gaz. méd. de Montpel., 1842-3, iii, no. 4.—**Shearer** (G.) Four cases of cancrum oris. Customs Gaz. Med. Rep. 1872, Shanghai, 1873, iv, 45.—**Siebert.** Der Wasserkrebs der Lippen (Cancer aquaticus; Waterkanker). J. d. pract. Heilk., Berl., 1811, xxxiii, 6. St., 74-91, 1 pl.—**Smith** (G. S.) Cancrum oris, or gangrenous stomatatis; two fatal cases. Med. Press & Circ., Dubl., 1866, ii, 61-63.—**Smith** (L.) Gangrene of the mouth; clinical notes. Med. Rec., N. Y., 1872, vii, 452.—**Sprague** (S. L.) Cancrum oris. Boston M. & S. J., 1863, lxix, 357.—**Stokes.** Cancrum oris. Dublin Q. J. M. Sc., 1863, xxxvi, 453-455.—[**Symonds** (J. A.)] Gangræna oris. Syst. Pract. M. (Tweedie), Phila., 1841, iv, 66-69.—**Taupin** (C.) Stomatite gangréneuse; sa nature, ses causes, son traitement. J. d. conn. méd.-chir., Par., 1838-9, vi, pt. 2, 134-145. *Also:* Ann. de méd. belge, Brux., 1839, ii, 112-123.—**Trelles** (P.) Terapéutica de la gangrena de la boca en los niños. Gac. méd., Madrid, 1848, iv, 2; 9—**Tweed** (T. M.) Observations on cancrum oris. West. Lancet, Cincin., 1847, vi, 12-17.—**Tyson.** Case of cancrum oris. Guy's Hosp. Gaz., Lond., 1874, iii, 132.—**Vogel.** Stomacace gangrænosa. Med. Cor.-Bl. d. württemb. ärztl. Ver., Stuttg., 1836, vi, 383.—**Volcan** (H.) Memoria sobre el cáncer, particularmente de la boca, y la causa de su fre-

Mouth (*Gangrene of*).

cuente ocurrencia en este pais. Union méd., Carácas, 1883, iii, 161 ; 182.—**Waldhauer.** Ein Fall von Verwachsung der Wange nach Stomatitis mercurialis. Beitr. z. Heilk., Riga, 1857, iv, pt. 2, 103–109.—**Walker** (E. F.) A fatal case of gangrene of the mouth. N. York M. J., 1878, xxvii, 159–162.—**Waring** (T. S.) A case of gangrenous erosion of the cheeks. Charleston M. J., 1856, xi, 298–300.—**Webb** (W. T.) Observations on cancrum oris, or sloughing sore mouth of children. Med. Exam., Phila., 1839, ii, 549–551.—**Webber** (S.) On gangrenous erosion of the cheek. Am. J. M. Sc., Phila., 1829, vi, 41–45.—**White** (J.) Cases of gangrene of the mouth. West. J. M. & S., Louisville, 1840, ii, 422–433.—**Wilks** (S.) Cancrum oris, etc., in children. Guy's Hosp. Rep., Lond., 1860, 3. s., vi, 142–145.—**Wood.** Necrosis of superior maxilla following cancrum oris. Med. Times & Gaz., Lond., 1872, ii, 145.—**Worthington** (T.) Case of gangrænopsis. Am. M. Recorder, Phila. 1828, xiii, 293–296.—**Young** (J.) Observations on the gangrenous sore mouth of children. Am. J. M. Sc., Phila., 1831, viii, 106–108.

Mouth (*Hæmorrhage from*).

See, also, Artery (*Carotid, Ligature of*) ; Hæmatemesis ; Hæmoptysis ; Menstruation (*Abnormal, etc.*)

DUBOIS-DELAMOTTE (L.) * Du diagnostic différentiel des hémorrhagies qui ont lieu par la bouche. 4°. *Paris*, 1851.

LEHARDELAY (C.-F.-A.) * Diagnostic différentiel des hémorrhagies qui se font par la bouche. 4°. *Paris*, 1845.

LE MARQUAND (J.) * De la stomatorrhagie. 4°. *Paris*, 1815.

LOTTE (L.-P.) * Diagnostic différentiel des hémorrhagies qui se font par la bouche. 4°. *Paris*, 1844.

RENARD (N.-L.) * Diagnostic différentiel des hémorrhagies qui se font par la bouche. 4°. *Paris*, 1847.

ROI (É.-É.) * Du diagnostic différentiel des hémorrhagies qui se font par la bouche. 4°. *Paris*, 1845.

Berg. Blutung aus der Schleimhaut der Mundhöhle. Med. Cor.-Bl. d. württemb. ärztl. Ver., Stuttg., 1852, xxii, 38.—**Droste** (A.) Fall von Stomatorrhagie. Wchnschr. f. d. ges. Heilk., Berl., 1833, 689–691.—**Salomon.** Freiwillige Blutung aus dem Munde mit tödtlichem Ausgang. Ibid., 1845, 732–736.—**Zarlenga** (R.) Stomatorragia ricorrente per flebonosi. Filiatre-sebezio, Napoli, 1845, xxix, 164–168.

Mouth (*Inflammation and ulceration of*).

See, also, Aphthæ ; Mercury (*Toxicology of, etc.*) ; Mouth (*Gangrene of*) ; Salivation.

ARGUELLO (J.) * Des stomatites fétides dans les intoxications par le plomb, l'arsenic et le phosphore. 4°. *Paris*, 1878.

BENJAMIN (J.) * De variis stomatitidis speciebus nonnulla. 8°. *Berolini*, [1841].

BORBERG (A.) * De stomatitidis variis generibus. 8°. *Berolini*, [1854].

BRUNEAU (J.) * Des ulcérations tuberculeuses de la bouche. 4°. *Paris*, 1887.

CAMERARIUS (A.) & LINSENMANN (C. L.) Exercitatio academica, sistens ægram purpura alba majori laborantem. 4°. *Tubingæ*, [1723].

CHAUVIN (G.) * Des ulcérations de la bouche et de leur diagnostic. 4°. *Paris*, 1874.

COUTEMOINE (E.) * Contribution à l'étude de la stomatite ulcéro-membraneuse chez les personnes âgées (depuis 40 ans). 4°. *Paris*, 1881.

DEVAUX-BIDON (M.-P.) * Dissertation sur la stomatite en général, et spécialement sur la stomatite pseudo-membraneuse. 4°. *Paris*, 1831.

EVENS (B. J.) * De cavi oris catarrho. 8°. *Halis Sax.*, 1862.

FROELICH (C.-C.-E.) * Du chlorate de potasse et de l'emploi de ce médicament dans les stomatites gangréneuses, ulcéreuses et mercurielles. 4°. *Strasbourg*, 1856.

LANSORNE (C.-H.-N.) * Sur la stomatite pseudo-membraneuse. 4°. *Paris*, 1830.

32

Mouth (*Inflammation and ulceration of*).

MESSIER (L.) * De la stomatite ulcéro-membraneuse. 4°. *Paris*, 1855.

MONTALEMBERT (J.-F.-C.) * Dissertation sur la stomatite en général, ou inflammation de la bouche. 4°. *Paris*, 1826.

RAVET (G.) * Séméiologie des ulcérations de la cavité buccale chez le nouveau-né. 4°. *Paris*, 1877.

SANLAVILLE (C.) * De la stomatite et de ses variétés. 4°. *Paris*, 1848.

TUJAGUE (J.) * Du phlegmon diffus sous-muqueux de la bouche. 4°. *Paris*, 1874.

Abbot. Use of chlorate of potash in stomatitis. Boston M. & S. J., 1858, lviii, 280–282.—**Acebes** (A.) Gengivitis simple ; estomatitis ; gengivitis ulcerosa ; ulceracion cancerosa ; caquexia consecutiva ; muerte. Rev. méd., Guadalajara, 1876, iii, 103–106. — **Aguilhon de Sarran.** Sur la pathogénie de la stomatite ulcéro-membraneuse. Rev. mens. d. mal. de la bouche. Par., 1881-2, i, 9–11.—**Angelot.** Observations sur l'emploi du chlorure de chaux dans le traitement des ulcérations de la bouche. Rev. méd. franç. et étrang., Par., 1827, ii, 49–57.—**Archambault.** De la stomatite ulcéro-membraneuse avec traitement par le chlorate de potasse. Ibid., 1882, ii, 78–81.—**Barth.** Ulcérations de la bouche de nature spéciale. Union méd., Par., 1847, i, 531 ; 539. ———. Stomatite et glossite idiopathiques; émissions sanguines ; guérison rapide. Ibid., 1870, 3. s., ix, 937–939.—**Beitz.** Stomatite ulcéro-membraneuse chez un adulte. Gaz. d. hôp., Par., 1868, xli, 34.—**Bergeron** (J.) Note sur l'emploi du chlorate de potasse dans le traitement de la stomatite ulcéreuse (ulcéro-membraneuse couenneuse). Rec. de mém. de méd. . . . mil., Par., 1855, 2. s., xvi, 1–46. ———. Stomatites. Dict. encycl. d. sc. méd., Par., 1883, 3. s., xii, 146–216.—**Boissier.** Stomatite ulcéro-membraneuse ; adynamie profonde ; cachexie ; mort. Bull. Soc. anat. de Par., 1875, l, 219.—**Bouchut.** De la stomatite ulcéro-membraneuse et de son influence sur la nécrose des maxillaires. Union méd., Par., 1863, n. s., xvii, 243–248. — **Brissaud** (E.) Stomatite et endocardite infectieuses. Progrès méd., Par., 1885, 2. s., i, 311–313.—**Brunzlow.** Einige Worte über die Ursachen der sogenannten Mundfäule und über die Uebertragbarkeit der Maulseuche der Thiere auf Menschen in Form jeder Krankheit. Wchnschr. f. d. ges. Heilk., Berl., 1840, 409 ; 433.—**Caffort** (J.-P.) Recherches et observations sur la stomatite. Arch. gén. de méd., Par., 1832, xxviii, 56–75.—**Catelan** (J.-A.) De la stomatite ulcéreuse épidémique. Arch. de méd. nav., Par., 1877, xxviii, 122 ; 161 ; 241, 1 map. Also, Reprint. ———. De la stomatite ulcéreuse épidémique à bord des navires. Bull. Soc. de méd. pub. 1877-9, Par., 1879, i, 88–102.—**Chauffard** (A.) Stomatites. N. dict. de méd. et chir. prat., Par., 1882, xxxiii, 681–698.—**Corson** (H.) The Rhus glabrum, a remedy for stomatitis. Med. & Surg. Reporter, Phila., 1887, lvi, 325–328. Also, Reprint.—**Delvaux** (P.) À propos des considérations de M. le Dr. Isidore Henriette sur la gengivite ulcéreuse des enfants. J. de méd., chir. et pharmacol., Brux., 1858, xxvi, 341–344.—**Dolbeau.** Leçons sur le diagnostic général des ulcères de la bouche ; cours de pathologie chirurgicale de . . . École de méd., Par., 1876-7, 1–6.—**Drée.** Mémoire sur la stomatite. Rec. de mém. de méd. . . . mil., Par., 1833, xxxv, 169–189.—**Drey** (J.) Abscesse in der Mundhöhle. Med. Ztg. Russlands, St. Petersb., 1853, x, 132.—**Dumont.** Considérations sur la stomatite ulcéreuse des enfants. Ann. Soc. de méd. de Gand, 1846, xvii, 245–252.—**Dunglison** (R.) Stomatitis. Cycl. Pract. M. (Tweedie), Phila., 1845, iv, 275. — **Eggeling & Ellenberger.** Stomatitis pustulosa contagiosa der Pferde. Arch. f. wissensch. u. prakt. Thierh., Berl., 1878, iv, 334–358.—**Eigenthümliche** (Ueber eine) Form von Stomatitis, genannt Stomatitis nodosa. J. f. Kinderkr., Erlang., 1862, xxxix, 202–205.—**Eraud** (J.) Stomatite aphteuse, entretenue par des cautérisations au nitrate d'argent ; grenouillette parotidienne aiguë. Province méd., Lyon, 1887, ii, 661–663.—**Fischl.** Entzündung der Mundschleimhaut, Oedem des submucösen Bindegewebes, Erstickungszufälle. Allg. Wien. med. Ztg., 1863, viii, 62.—**Gilbert.** Du mode d'action du chlorate de potasse dans la stomatite ulcéro-membraneuse. Gaz. méd. de méd., Par., 1856, iii, 395–398.—**Gradowicz** (E.) Stomatitis diphtheritica adultorum. Med. Ztg. Russlands, St. Petersb., 1850, vii, 129–131.—**Guersant & Blache.** Stomatite. Dict. de méd., 2. éd., Par., 1844, xxviii, 577–603.—**Hall** (G. W.) Ulcerative stomatitis. Missouri Clin. Rec., St. Louis, 1874-5, i, 188.—**Hardy.** Notice sur une stomatite épizootique observée sur les chevaux du 3e régiment de lanciers. Arch. méd. belges, Brux., 1865, 2. s., ii, 322–324.—**Henriette** (I.) De la gengivite ulcéreuse chez les enfants et de son traitement. J. de méd., chir. et pharmacol., Brux., 1858, xxvi, 221–230.—**Holt** (H. D.) [Sore mouth treated with iodide of potash.] N. York J. M., 1848, x, 372.—**Hutchinson** (J.) On a form of inflammation of the lips and mouth which sometimes ends fatally, and is usually attended by some disease of the skin. Proc.

Mouth (*Inflammation and ulceration of*).
Roy. M. & Chir. Soc. Lond., 1885–7, n. s., ii, 284–287. *Also:* Brit. M. J., Lond., 1887, i, 1333. — **Ingels.** Les différentes stomatites, leurs caractères et leur traitement. [Rap.] Ann. Soc. de méd. de Gand, 1865, xliii, 159–161. — **Jadelot.** Stomatite pseudo-membraneuse; quelques réflexions sur cette maladie chez l'enfant. Gaz. d. hôp., Par., 1844, 2. s., vi, 385. — **Jardin.** Sur les différentes stomatites, leurs caractères differentiels et sur leur traitement. Ann. Soc. de méd. de Gand, 1868, xlvi, 181–334. — **Krackau** (C.) Stomatitis gangraenosa. Deutsche Monatschr. f. Zahnh., Leipz., 1885, iii, 519–526. — **Kussmaul** (A.) Stomatitis septica bei einem kräftigen jungen Manne mit sehr raschem tödtlichem Ausgange. Mitth. d. badisch. ärztl. Ver., Karlsruhe, 1853, vii, 57–64. — **Laborde** (J.-V.) De la valeur du chlorate de potasse dans le traitement des gingivites chroniques, avec ou sans pyorrhée alvéolo-dentaire. Bull. gén. de thérap., etc., Par., 1858, liv, 289–301. — **Laboulbène** (A.) Note sur la stomatite ulcéro-membraneuse; examen histologique de la membrane mortifiée ou nécrohymène. Gaz. hebd. de méd., Par., 1878, xxv, 536. — ——. De la stomatite ulcéro-membraneuse. Gaz. d. hôp., Par., 1879, lii, 113–115. — **Livingston** (B.) The value of bismuth in the treatment of ulcerative stomatitis and noma. Am. J. Obst., N. Y., 1883, xvi, 441; 545. — **Löwenstamm.** Zur Stomatitis exsudativa. Med.-chir. Centralbl., Wien, 1876, xi, 531. — **Longtin** (S.-A.) Diagnostic général des ulcères chirurgicaux de la bouche. Union méd. du Canada, Montréal, 1877, vi, 145–151. — **Maréchal.** Stomatite ulcéreuse. Arch. belges de méd. mil., Brux., 1862, xxx, 174–177. — **Mayr.** Stomatitis diphtheritica. Jahrb. f. Kinderh., Wien, 1859–60, iii, 273. — **Mende** (D. L.) Ueber die Mundfäule, in den Jahren 1806–1809. J. d. pract. Heilk., Berl., 1809, xxix, 10. St., 24–48. — **Menger** (R.) Hemorrhage of the mouth in a child aged 9 days, affected with stomatitis parasitica; autopsy and microscopic examination. Daniel's Texas M. J., Austin, 1887–8, iii, 35–40. — **Müller.** Bemerkungen über Mundgeschwüre. Med. Cor.-Bl. d. württemb. ärztl. Ver., Stuttg., 1832–3, i, 67. — **Neuhof.** Beobachtung einer besondern Art von Mundfäule. J. d. pract. Heilk., Berl., 1810, xxxi, 11. St., 85–103. — **Nielsen** (L.) Gangraenøs Mundbetændelse hos Kvæget. [Stomatitis gangraenosa in cattle.] Tidsskr. f. Vet., Kjøbenh., 1885, xv, 12–19. — **Parrot.** Des ulcérations buccales chez les nouveau-nés. Gaz. d. hôp., Par., 1879, lii, 883–886. — **Paulet.** De la stomatite érythémateuse idiopathique et de son traitement. Congrès méd. de France 1865, Par., 1866, iii, 238–244. — **Pavloff** (E.) Sluchai sibirsko jazvi i vijiganie eja pomoshiou apparata Pakelona. [Ulcer of mouth, involving cheek, treated by Paquelin's cautery.] Med. Vestnik, St. Petersb., 1880, xx, 81; 89. — **Payne** (J. F.) Stomatitis and coryza combined with impetigo. St. Thomas's Hosp. Rep. 1883, Lond., 1884, n. s., xiii, 305–309. — **Pereiro Pull** (F.) Concepto general de las estomatitis. Rev. de enferm. de niños, Madrid, 1883, i, 321–326. — **Pfeufer** (C.) Der Mundböhlenkatarrh. Ztschr. f. rat. Med., Heidelb., 1849, vii, 180–183. — **Pinilla** (A.) El clorato de potasa contra la estomatitis mercurial. Siglo méd., Madrid, 1857, iv, 395. — **Quaife** (F. H.) A case of stomatitis with jaundice. Australas. M. Gaz., Sydney, 1886–7, vi, 224. — **Ribes** (F.) Sur la stomatite pseudo-membraneuse. Rev. méd. franç. et étrang., Par., 1831, iv, 368–409. *Also,* Reprint. — **Richardson** (H.) Case of fatal aphthous ulceration of the mouth. Lancet, Lond., 1846, ii, 608. — **Rossi.** Note sur la stomatite folliculaire hétérométrique de la ligne médiane de la voûte palatine, appelée vulgairement, en Égypte, bouton de l'enfance. Gaz. méd. de Par., 1862, 3. s., xvii, 29–31. — **Routier** (A.) Stomatite ulcéromembraneuse ou nécrohyménique. France méd., Par., 1878, xxv, 797; 805. — **da Silva** (J. A.) Estomatites; 16 casos. Escholiaste med., Lisb., 1861, xii, 264–267. — **da Silva Cardeira** (L.) Historia da estomatite ulcerosa em Portugal; bibliographia. *Ibid.*, 10; 23; 36; 54; 68; 85; 103; 120. — **Simas.** Sobre o emprego do chlorato de potassa, principalmente na stomatite ulcerosa. *Ibid.*, 1887, viii, 460–463. — **Skoloff** (N.) Laichenie katarralnago vospaleniya zaiva i gortani rastvorom aidkikh shchelochei. [Treatment of catarrhal inflammation of the mouth and throat with a solution of caustic alkali.] Med. Vestnik, St. Petersb., 1869, ix, 431. — **Sourrouille** (J.) Ulcérations multiples de la cavité buccale et du tube digestif par la morphine à haute dose. Gaz. d. hôp., Par., 1885, lviii, 541. — **Souza da Silveira.** Observação de um caso de stomatite erythematosa com caracter intermittente. Ann. Brasil. de med., Rio de Jan., 1879–80, xxix, 325–327. — **Stomatite** (De la) par pincement des gencives ou de la muqueuse buccale entre les dents molaires, et de son traitement par l'alun. Bull. gén. de thérap., etc., Par., 1835, viii, 174–178. — [**Symonds** (J. A.)] Stomatitis; or inflammation of the mouth. Syst. Pract. M. (Tweedie) Phila., 1841, iv, 60–66. — **Talma** (A.) Observations sur l'emploi du chlorure d'oxide de sodium dans les maladies de la bouche. [With remarks by J. F. Vleminckx.] Biblioth. méd., Brux., 1828, v, 113–131. — **Troschel.** Beitrag zur Lehre von der Stomatocace. Med. Ztg, Berl., 1838, vii, 175–177. — **Wharton** (H. R.) Seven cases of gangrenous stomatitis. Med. & Surg. Reporter, Phila., 1887,

Mouth (*Inflammation and ulceration of*).
lvii, 373–376. — **Wigglesworth** (E.) & **Cushing** (E. W.) Buccal ulcerations of constitutional origin. Arch. Dermat., N. Y., 1882, viii, 1–18. *Also,* Reprint. — **Wilcox** (R.) The smart-weed as a remedy for mercurial salivation and aphthous stomatitis. Am. J. M. Sc., Phila., 1848, n. s., xvi, 247. — **Wilson** (J.) Cases of ulcerative stomatitis with yellow palms. Glasgow M. J., 1871–2, [4. s.], iv, 377. — **Wolff** (J.) Cases of hæmorrhage from the mouth. Lancet, Lond., 1835–6, i, 863–865. — **Wright** (E.) Case of pseudo-membranous stomatitis. Med. Times & Gaz., Lond., 1853, vi, 198.

Mouth (*Inflammation of*) in pregnancy and lactation.

Didsbury (H.) * De l'état des gencives chez les femmes enceintes, et de son traitement. 4°. *Paris*, 1883.

Ludlam (R.) Stomatitis materna. 8°. [*Chicago, n. d.*]

Backus (F. F.) On the form of sore mouth peculiar to nursing women. Am. J. M. Sc., Phila., 1841, n. s., i, 114–116 — **Bennet** (J. C.) An account of some sporadic cases of apthous sore mouth, occurring in pregnant females, and attended with some unusual symptoms. West. J. M. & Phys. Sc., Cincin., 1831, iv, 346. — **Brandon** (D. S.) Stomatitis materna; what is its pathology? Treatment with turpentine. South. M. & S. J., Augusta, 1860, n. s., xvi, 1–5. — **Byford** (W. H.) On stomatitis materna. Am. J. M. Sc., Phila., 1853, n. s., xxv, 392–398. — **Castleman** (A. S.) Stomatitis materna. Northwest. M. & S. J., Chicago, 1853, x, 88–90. — **Chambers** (W. M.) Stomatitis materna. Tr. Illinois M. Soc., Chicago, 1857, vii, 106–122. — **Coventry** (C. B.) "Stomatitis materna"; the sore mouth of nursing women. Buffalo M. J., 1847–8, iii, 513–525. — **Eiselt** (J. N.) Zahnfleisch-Hypertrophie während der Schwangerschaft. Med. Jahrb. d. k. k. österr. Staates, Wien, 1840, xxxi, 560. — **Ellis** (L. S.) Stomatitis materna. Chicago M. J., 1860, xvii, 200–208. — **Ely** (W. W.) On the treatment of nursing sore mouth. Boston M. & S. J., 1848–9, xxxix, 41–43. — **Evans** (J.) On the use of cod-liver oil in nursing sore mouth. Northwest. M. & S. J., Chicago & Indianap., 1854–2, viii, 199–201. — **Faulkner** (L.) Chlorate of potash in stomatitis materna. Virginia M. J., Richmond, 1857, ix, 465–467. — **Fountain** (E. J.) Treatment of stomatitis materna by the syrup of the phosphates. N. Am. M.-Chir. Rev., Phila., 1860, iv, 89–91. — **Green** (J. N.) Stomatitis materna. Chicago M. J., 1859, n. s., ii, 137–139. — **Hale** (E.), jr. Remarks on the sore mouth of nursing women. Med. Communicat. Mass. M. Soc., Bost., 1836, v, 34–45 — **Hall** (J. W.) Stomatitis materna. Cincin. Lancet & Obs., 1858, i, 193–196. — **Harris** (J. O.) Stomatitis materna. Chicago M. J., 1858, n. s., i, 650–660. — **Hollister** (J. H.) Report on the sore mouth of nursing women. Tr. Il inois M. Soc. 1858, Chicago, 1859, viii, 35–49. — **Hubbard** (J. C.) Anatomical lesions in stomatitis materna and their treatment. Am. J. M. Sc., Phila., 1853, n. s., xxv, 269. — **Hurd** (E. P.) Treatment of stomatitis materna. Med. Rec., N. Y., 1878, xiii, 449. — **Hutchinson** (D.) Stomatitis of pregnant, and nursing women. Northwest. M. & S. J., Chicago, 1852–3, ix, 529–535. ——. Stomatitis materna. West. Lancet, San Fran., 1855, xvi, 193–216. ——. What are the causes and nature of that disease incident to pregnancy and lactation, characterized by inflammation and ulceration of the mouth and fauces, usually accompanied by anorexia, emaciation, and diarrhœa, and what is the best mode of treatment? Fiske fund prize essay. Am. J. M. Sc., Phila., 1857, n. s., xxxiv, 369–386. — **Kilburn** (J.) Aphtha in women during lactation, and its cure by nitrate of silver gargle. Lancet, Lond., 1838–9, i, 521. — **Knapp** (M. L) An inquiry into the nature of the anomalous affection known in the United States by the appellation of the nursing sore-mouth, or puerperal anæmia. N. York J. M., 1855, n. s., xiv, 345–381. — **McClelland** (J. S.) Report on stomatitis materna. Tr. Indiana M. Soc., Indianap., 1856, 48–52. — **M'Gugin** (D. L.) On stomatitis materna. Tr. Am. M. Ass., Phila., 1858, xi, 749–776. — **McKee** (W. H.) Stomatitis materna. Tr. M. Soc. N. Car., Wilmington, 1857, viii, 22–26. — **Maris** (G. W.) Sore mouths of nursing women. Ohio M. & S. J., Columbus, 1854–5, vii, 359–367. — **Pallen** (M. M.) Observations on stomatitis materna, or nursing sore-mouth. St. Louis M. & S. J., 1859, xvii, 116–118. ——. Stomatitis materna. *Ibid.*, 1869, n. s., vi, 305–308. — **Pinard** (A.) & **Pinard** (D.) De la gingivite des femmes enceintes et de son traitement. Bull. gén. de thérap., etc., Par., 1877, xcii, 157–162. *Also,* Reprint. — **Pitcairn** (J.) A case of disease of the gums which occurred during pregnancy. Dublin Hosp. Rep. 1818, ii, 309–311 — **Pray** (T. J. W.) Nursing sore mouth; its nature, causes, and treatment. Tr. N. Hampshire Med. Soc., Concord, 1857, iv, 35–62. — **Prince** (D.) Stomatitis materna. Chicago M. J., 1859, n. s., ii, 400–402. — **Reeve** (J. C.) Stomatitis materna cured by the syrup of the phosphates. N. Am. M.-Chir Rev., Phila., 1858, iii, 1053–1055. — **Richardson** (J.) Reflex lesions of the oral cavity associated with pregnancy.

Mouth (*Inflammation of*) *in pregnancy and lactation.*

[*From:* Tr. Am. Dent. Ass., 1882.] Missouri Dent. J., St. Louis, 1883, xv, 97-103.—**Shanks** (L.) On endemic sore mouth and diarrhœa, peculiar to nursing women. Am. J. M. Sc., Phila., 1842, n. s., iv, 300-304.—**Shields** (P. S.) An essay on the sore-mouth peculiar to nursing females. West. J. M. & S., Louisville, 1852, 3. s., ix, 21-28.—**Taylor** (B. W.) Remarks on a species of sore mouth peculiar to nursing women. Am. J. M. Sc., Phila., 1843, n. s., v, 119-122.—**Wilson** (I. P.) Stomatitis materna. St. Louis M. & S. J., 1869, n. s., vi, 408.—**Wright** (C O.) Stomatitis materna. Am. J. Obst., N. Y., 1877, x, 511-513.

Mouth (*Inflammation of*) *in soldiers.*

BERGERON (R.-L.) * De la stomatite en général, et en particulier de la stomatite ulcéreuse chez les soldats. 4°. *Paris*, 1851.

FEUVRIER (J.-B.) Stomatite ulcéreuse des soldats. Relation d'une épidémie. 8°. *Paris*, 1875.

See, also, infra.

MAGET (L.-G.) * Étude sur l'étiologie de la stomatite ulcéreuse des soldats et des marins. 4°. *Paris*, 1879.

PÉCHAUD (J.-J.) * De la stomatite ulcéreuse spécifique chez les soldats en particulier. 4°. *Strasbourg*, 1863.

Alard. Note sur une maladie nouvellement décrite et très-fréquente parmi les soldats de l'armée d'Espagne (fégarite, fégrite ou figar). J. de méd., chir., pharm., etc., Par., 1812, xxiv, 354-364. — **Bergeron** (E.-J.) De la stomatite ulcéreuse des soldats et de son identité avec la stomatite des enfants, dite couenneuse, diphthéritique, ulcéro-membraneuse. Rec. de mém. de méd. . . . mil., Par., 1858, 2. s., xxi, 51-232. *Also,* Reprint. *Also* [Abstr.]: Arch. gén. de méd., Par., 1859, ii, 446-459. *Also* [Rap. de Roger]: Union méd., Par., 1859, 2. s., ii, 249-255. *Also:* Bull. Soc. méd. d. hôp. de Par. (1858-61) 1861, iv, 264-273.— **Catelan** (J.-A.) De la stomatite ulcéreuse épidémique à bord des navires. Ann. d'hyg., Par., 1877, xlviii, 319-332. *Also* [Abstr.]: Tribune méd., Par., 1877, ix, 375-378. — **Delpech.** Lettre sur l'efficacité du chlorure de chaux dans une affection ulcéreuse de la bouche, propre aux jeunes soldats en garnison. Mém. d. hôp. du midi, Par., 1829, i, 422-426.—**Feuvrier.** Relation d'une épidémie de stomatite ulcéreuse observée au dépôt du 59e de ligne à Auxerre (Yonne). Rec. de mém. de méd. . . . mil., Par., 1873, 3. s., xxix, 449-465.—**Hunter** (G. Y.) Report on a peculiar mouth affection prevalent among the men of the Indian expeditionary force. Lancet, Lond., 1878, ii, 249.—**Léonard.** Notice sur une stomatite épidémique; sur son mode de propagation et sur l'emploi du sulfate d'alumine pour la combattre. Rec. de mém. de méd. . . . mil., Par., 1835, xxxviii, 296-303. — **Malapert** (A.-F.) Considérations hygiéniques sur quelques maladies, et particulièrement sur les stomatites occasionnées par l'encombrement des troupes dans les bâtimens où elles sont casernées. Ibid., 1838, xlv, 280-302. — **Note** sur l'inflammation ulcéreuse de la bouche et des gencives parmi les troupes. Ibid., 1830, xxviii, 129-140.—**Payen** & **Gourdon.** Mémoire sur les stomatites et les gingivites affectant un caractère épidémique et contagieux, qui se sont montrées dans l'Hôpital militaire de Toulon, pendant l'année 1829. Ibid., 1841, 141-169.—**Pereira e Horta** (P.) Considerações sobre a estomatite dos soldados, denominada especifica pelo Sr. Dr. Bergeron, medico civil do hospital civil de Santa Eugenia em Paris, na sua monographia de la stomatite ulcéreuse des soldats. Escholiaste med. Lisb., 1861, xii, 168-173.—**Raddock** (C. E.) Report on an outbreak of stomatitis in the 31st regiment native infantry. Indian M. Gaz., Calcutta, 1878, xiii. 240. — **Rica y Ravassa.** De la stomatitis de los soldados. Rev. de sanid. mil. españ., Madrid, 1864, i, 141; 213; 317.

Mouth (*Injuries of*).

See Teeth (*Fractures, etc., of*).

Mouth (*Nerves of*).

de Carvalho (J. P.) Prova experimental de que os nervos vaso-dilatadores da região bucco-facial existem no cordão cervical do grande sympathico. Rev. d. cursos prat. e theor. da Fac. de med. do Rio de Jan., 1885-6, ii, 1s9-202.—**Dastre** & **Morat.** Sur les nerfs vaso-dilatateurs des parois de la bouche. Compt. rend. Acad. d. sc., Par., 1880, xci, 441-443. ———. Réflexe vaso-dilatateur des parois buccales. Compt. rend. Soc. de biol. 1881, Par., 1882, 7. s., iii, 112. ———. Des nerfs sympathiques dilatateurs des vaisseaux de la bouche et des lèvres. Compt. rend. Acad. d. sc., Par., 1882, xcv, 161-163. ———. De l'influence exercée par le nerf dépresseur de Ludwig et Cyon sur la circulation bucco-labiale.

Mouth (*Nerves of*).

Compt. rend. Soc. de biol., Par., 1882, 7. s., iv, 462-466. *Also* [Abstr.]: Gaz. d. hôp., Par., 1882, lv, 265.—**Elin** (E.) Zur Kenntniss der feineren Nerven der Mundhöhlenschleimhaut. Arch. f. mikr. Anat., Bonn, 1871, vii, 382-388, 1 pl. *Also* [Abstr.]: Centralbl. f. d. med. Wissensch., Berl., 1871, ix, 225.—**Laffont.** De l'origine des nerfs vaso-dilatateurs de la région bucco-labiale. Compt. rend. Soc. de biol. 1880, Par., 18s1, 7. s., ii, 297-300.—**Myers** (W.) The influence of the nervous system on the health of the mouth. Cincin. Lancet & Clinic, 1878, n. s., i, 467.—**Zlobikowski** (T.) Nowe poszukiwania nad nerwem zebojezykowym prof. Sappey'a. [Nerves of teeth and tongue.] Gaz. lek., Warszawa, 1870, viii, 625-630.

Mouth (*Organisms in*).

See, also, Perlèche; Saliva; Teeth (*Caries of*).

McQUILLEN (J. H.) Oral organisms. 8°. [*n. p.*, 1875.]

RAPPIN (G.) *Contribution à l'étude des bactéries de la bouche à l'état normal et dans la fièvre typhoïde. 4°. *Paris*, 1881.

Bechamp [*et al.*]. Du rôle des organismes microscopiques de la bouche (ou de Leuewenhoeck) dans la digestion en général, et particulièrement dans la formation de la diastase salivaire. Montpel. méd., 1867, xix, 456-460. *Also,* Reprint.—**Black** (G. V.) Micro-organisms of the oral cavity. Tr. Illinois Dent. Soc., Chicago, 1886, xxii, 180-208.—**Miller** (W. D.) Biological studies on the fungi of the human mouth. Independ. Pract., N. Y., 1885, vi, 227; 283. ———. The comma-bacilli of the human mouth. Brit. M. J., Lond., 1885, i, 935. ———. Fermentation in the human mouth; its relation to caries of the teeth; the influence of antiseptics, filling materials, [etc.], upon the fungi of dental caries; the fungi of dental caries; their pure cultivation and effect upon the lower animals; biological studies on the fungi of the human mouth. *In:* The American system of dentistry, roy. 8°, Phila., 1886, 791-828.—**Sternberg** (G. M.) Der Micrococcus der Sputumsepticämie (M. Pasteuri, Sternberg). Deutsche med. Wchnschr., Leipz., 1887, xiii, 44.—**Vignal** (W.) Sur l'action des micro-organismes de la bouche et des matières fécales sur quelques substances alimentaires. Compt. rend. Soc. de biol., Par., 1887, 8. s., iv, 547. ———. Sur l'action des micro-organismes de la bouche et des matières fécales, sur quelques substances alimentaires. Compt. rend. Acad. d. sc., Par., 1887, cv, 311-313. ———. Recherches sur les micro-organismes de la bouche. Arch. de physiol. norm. et path., Par., 1886, 3. s., viii, 325-391, 8 pl.

Mouth (*Semeiology of*).

See Mouth (*Exploration, etc., of*).

Mouth (*Surgery and wounds of*).

See, also, Artery (*Carotid, Ligature of*); Dentistry; Lips (*Plastic surgery of*); Mouth (*Abnormities, etc., of*); Mouth (*Cancer of*); Palate (*Plastic surgery of*); Tongue (*Excision of*); Tongue (*Wounds of*).

ANDRIEU (E.) Traité de prothèse buccale et de mécanique dentaire. 8°. *Paris*, 1887.

BAUMANN (F.) Quelques considérations anatomiques, avec observations des affections buccales les plus fréquentes et de la prothèse dentaire. 8°. [*Paris*], 1872.

BUSOLT (O.) * Ueber die Lagerung der Kranken bei Operationen in und an der Mundhöhle. 8°. *Jena*, 1875.

DÖBBELIN (C. B.) * De uniendis vulnerum oris. 8°. *Halæ*, [1817].

GARRETSON (J. E.) A treatise on the diseases and surgery of the mouth, jaws, and associate parts. 8°. *Philadelphia*, 1869.

———. The same. A system of oral surgery; being a consideration of the diseases and surgery of the mouth, jaws, and associate parts. 2. ed. 8°. *Philadelphia*, 1873.

WEDGWOOD (J. J.) Progress of dentistry and oral surgery. 4. ed. 16°. *London*, 1885.

WITZEL (A.) Ueber Cocain-Anästhesie bei Operationen in der Mundhöhle. 8°. *Hagen i. W.*, 1886.

Allen (D. P.) Partial narcosis in operations on the mouth; chlorate of potash poisoning cases. Med. Rec., N. Y., 1881, xix, 330.—**Andrews** (E.) Restraint of hæmorrhage during operations in the mouth. Med. Exam., Chicago, 1874, xv, 169.—**Annandale** (T.) On the

Mouth (*Surgery and wounds of*).

value of the dependent position of the head in operations on the mouth and throat. Lancet, Lond., 1879, ii, 685.—**de la Barre** fils. De l'emploi du caoutchouc dans différents cas de stomatonomie. Compt. rend. Acad. d. sc., Par., 1844, xviii, 377.—**Bottini.** Fibro-encondroma della tonsilla destra invadente il cavo faringeo, e la coana e proteso nella regione sovrajoidea, esportato dal cavo orale. Gazz. d. osp., Milano, 1885, vi, 98–100.—**Briddon.** Excision of tongue and floor of the mouth, ligation of both lingual arteries. Med. News, Phila., 1883, xlii, 628.—**Bryant** (T.) Case of deformity of the mouth, after sloughing of the cheek from fever; operation and recovery. Guy's Hosp. Rep., Lond., 1862, 3. s., viii, 289, 3 pl. ——. The surgery of the mouth, pharynx, abdomen, and rectum, including hernia. *In his:* Clin. Surg. 8°, Lond., 1860–64, pt. iii, 153–253.—**Busch.** Eine Stomatopoësis. Sitzungsb. d. nied.-rhein. Gesellsch. f. Nat.- u. Heilk. zu Bonn, 1879, 415.—**Caselli** (A.) Delle emorragie della bocca da lesioni violente e da operazioni chirurgiche; nuovo instrumento per frenarle. Bull. d. sc. med. di Bologna, 1878, 6. s., ii, 299–308.—**Coleman** (A.) An instrument for keeping the mouth open in operations under chloroform. Med. Times & Gaz., Lond., 1861, i, 105.—**Collier** (M.) Removal of the tongue and floor of the mouth for extensive epithelioma. Lancet, Lond., 1885, ii, 340.—**Colombier.** Observation sur un coup de pistolet tiré dans la bouche. J. de méd. mil., Par., 1782, i, 222–239.—**Demarquay.** Instrument dilatateur, de la mâchoire. Bull. Soc. de chir. de Par., 1851, ii, 17–19.—**Deswatines.** Quelques considérations sur un cas d'occlusion de la bouche, suite de sphacèle scorbutique, et sur le procédé employé pour en empêcher le récollement. Cong. méd. de France, Par., 1863, i, 334–341.—**Dulles** (C. W.) An interesting gunshot wound. Phila. M. Times, 1876-7, vii, 79.—**Elliott** (W. St. G.) Gunshot wounds of the mouth. N. York M. J., 1879, xxix, 267–281.—**Goodwillie** (D. H.) Extirpation of the bones of the nose and mouth by the use of the surgical engine. Med. Rec., N. Y., 1879, xvi, 28–31. *Also,* Reprint. ——. An address on oral surgery, delivered before the American Medical Association. Tr. Am. M. Ass., Phila., 1882, xxxiii, 469–484. *Also,* Reprint.—**Grant** (H. McG.) Paper on oral surgery, with cases, treatment, and results. South. Dent. J., Atlanta, 1882, i, 363–367.—**Gussenbauer** (C.) Ueber das Schlussresultat der im verflossenen Jahre referirten Stomatoplastik. Verhandl. d. deutsch. Gesellsch. f. Chir., Berl., 1878, vii, pt. 2, 77, 1 pl. ——. Ueber Stomatoplastik. Wien. med. Presse, 1885, xxvi, 406. *Also:* Prag. med. Wchnschr., 1885, x, 117–119.—**Hernu** (J. J.) Observation sur un coup de pistolet dans la bouche. J. de chir. (Desault), Par., 1792, iii, 236–240.—**Hublé** (M.) Examen d'un cas de suicide par coup de feu dans la bouche; alcoolisme et pachyméningite chronique; irresponsabilité. Ann. d'hyg., Par., 1887, 3. s., xvii, 285–291.—**Keith.** Ingenious mechanism. St. Louis M. & S. J., 1879, xxxvi, 259.—**Kent** (J. T.) Fatal hemorrhage; blunder of a dentist. Am. M. J., St. Louis, 1879, vii, 314–316.—**Kraus** (E.) Ein durch 7 Wochen im Munde zurückgehaltener fremder Körper; Extraction desselben. Allg. Wien. med. Ztg., 1866, xi, 200.—**Lecerf.** Atrésie accidentelle de l'orifice buccal; chéiloplastie. Bull. méd. du nord, Lille, 1886, xxv, 524–526 — [**Legouest.**] Large fistule du plancher buccal guérie par une opération anaplastique. Bull. gén de thérap., etc, Par., 1863, lxiv, 319–323.—**Ludwig.** Heilungsgeschichte einer merkwürdigen, durch einen Schuss in den Mund bewirkten Verwundung. Mag. f. d. ges. Heilk., Berl., 1832, xxxviii, 191–204, 1 pl.—**Luer.** Appareil désigné sous le nom d'écarteur des joues. Bull. Acad. de méd., Par., 1861-2, xxvii, 76.—**McQuillen** (J. H.) A case of oral surgery. Dental Cosmos, Phila., 1875, xvii, 397–401. *Also,* Reprint.—**Manoury.** Plaie d'arme à feu dans la bouche, avec fracture à la mâchoire inférieure; trou à la voûte et au voile du palais; balles perdues dans les fosses nasales; déglutition impossible; introduction par le nez dans l'œsophage d'une sonde, portée pendant un mois. J. de chir. (Desault), Par., 1791, i, 8–18. *Also* [Abstr.]: J. de méd.- chir., pharm., etc., Par., 1791, lxxxxi, 214–225.—**de Marchettis** (P.) Lingua, ex vulnere sclopeti curato, partibus subjectis arcte coalescens, cum impedita locutione, perita sectione separata ac restituta. *In his:* Obs. med.-chir. [etc.], 8°, Lond., 1729, 46. *Also, transl. in his:* Rec. d'obs. rares, [etc.], 8°, Par., 1858, 89.—**Marjolin.** Plaie d'arme à feu intéressant la face et l'intérieur de la cavité buccale. Bull. Soc. de chir. de Par., 1852, iii, 61–66. — **Marquez.** Note sur une opération de stomatoplastie. Gaz. méd. de Strasb., 1864, xxiv, 75.—**Mason's** gag. Lan et, Lond., 1886, i, 260.—**May** (B.) On a case of excision of the tongue with a large portion of lower jaw and floor of mouth for epithelioma; recovery. *Ibid.,* 1882, i, 947–949.—**de Medici** (T.) Di un nuovo divaricatore orale. Raccoglitore med., Forlì, 1877, 4. s., viii, 171–173, 1 pl.—**Minkewitsch** (J.) Fehlen der Nase; Bildung eines künstlichen Mundes. Arch. f. path. Anat., etc., Berl., 1867, xli, 433–437. ——. Spostrzezenia chirurg.; narzady trawienia [mouth. lips, and palate]; warge zajęczą. Gaz. lek., Warszawa, 1881. 2. s., i, 389; 568. — **Monod** (C.) Trachéotomie préventive dans une ablation d'un cancer du

Mouth (*Surgery and wounds of*).

plancher de la bouche. Bull. et mém. Soc. de chir. de Par., 1886, n. s., xii, 126–129. ——. De la trachéotomie préventive dans les opérations faites sur la bouche. *Ibid.,* 140–146.—**Mussey** (W. H.) An instrument for keeping the jaws apart during operations in the mouth or throat. Cincin. Lancet & Obs., 1868, n. s., xi, 517.—**Napier** (W. D.) [A desirable process of operating on the mouth without causing pain to the patient.] Proc. M. Soc. Lond., 1874-5, ii, 23.—**Nichet.** Coup de feu à la face; perforation du plancher de la bouche; autoplastie; guérison. Gaz. méd. de Par., 1836, 2. s., iv, 454.—**Parker** (W. T.) A new mouth gag. Med. Rec., N. Y., 1883, xxiv, 250.—**Parmele** (G. L.) Some points in oral surgery of interest to the general practitioner. Proc. Connect. M. Soc., Hartford, 1883, n. s., ii, no. 4, 111–121. *Also,* Reprint.—**Pollosson.** De l'incision commissurale coudée; moyen d'agrandir l'orifice buccal dans la chéiloplastie. Mém. et compt.-rend. Soc. d. sc. méd. de Lyon (1885), 1886, xxv, pt. 2, 3–41. — **Power** (W.) The "lingual depressor", a new surgical instrument. Dublin M. Press, 1840, iv, 228.—**Préterre.** De la prothèse buccale. J. de méd., chir. et pharmacol., Brux., 1862, xxxiv, 217; 325. ——. Des restaurations buccales (divisions palatines syphilitiques, congénitales ou acquises de la voûte et du voile); restaurations des maxillaires après leur ablation totale ou partielle. Cong. méd. de France 1863, Par., 1863, i, 222–235.—**Privat.** Restaurations buccales; appareils prothétiques exécutés dans les hôpitaux, notamment à l'Hôpital de la Pitié. *In his:* À propos de la "greffe prothésique dentaire?" 8°, Par., 1886, 17–19.—**Redier** (J.) Appareils prothétiques de la bouche; description générale; indications; accidents. J. d. sc. méd. de Lille, 1880, ii, 365; 522; 605. *Also,* Reprint.—**Rivet.** Note sur une lésion de la bouche produite par une nouvelle arme à feu, la sarbacane-fusil. Rec. de mém. de méd. . . . mil., Par., 1876, xxxii, 467–473.—**Roe** (J. O.) Combined mouth-gag and cheek retractor. Med. Rec., N. Y., 1880, xviii, 193.—**Rose** (E.) Ueber die anhaltend tiefe Narkose bei blutigen Mundoperationen. Arch. f. klin. Chir., Berl., 1879, xxiv, 429–437.—**Roux.** Coup de pistolet tiré dans la bouche; hémorrhagie mortelle au bout de sept jours. Gaz. d. hôp., Par., 1845, 2. s., vii, 189. — **Sachs.** Ueber ein Mittel, bei widerspenstigen Kranken das Oeffnen des Mundes zu erzwingen. Berl. klin. Wchnschr., 1871, viii, 603 —**Sauve** (L.) Wystrzat z pistoleta w gebe. [Pistol-shot in the mouth.] Pam. Towarz. Lek. Warszaw., 1841, vi, 444–447. — **Schmidt** (H.) Beiträge über die Anwendung des Cocaïn. 2. Serie. Cocaïnanästhesie bei Operationen im Munde. Wien. med. Wchnschr., 1887, xxxvii, 1263–1265.—**Simon** (G.) Plastik der Defecte in den Wandungen der zugängigen Körperhöhlen: des Mundes, der Scheide und des Mastdarmes. Vrtljschr. f. d. prakt. Heilk., Prag, 1867, xciii, 1–61.—**Smith** (H.) Foreign body in the pterygoid region. Lancet, Lond., 1883, i, 821.—**Stimson** (L. A.) A pharyngeal obtunder for use during operations on the mouth and nasal passages. Ann. Anat. & Surg., Brooklyn, N. Y., 1883, vii, 268–270.—**Textor** (K.) Ueber künstliche Mundbildung. J. d. Chir. u. Augenh, Berl., 1847, n. F., vi, 385–395. — **Toscano.** Seltener Verwundungs-Fall. [Eine Kugel, in der obern Zungenbeingegend, in den Kopf geschossen, durchschoss die Zunge, den Gaumen und das linke Nasendach, wo sie ihren Ausweg nahm; eine zweite Kugel, nachher applizirt, hatte denselben Eingang wie die erste, sie durchschoss die Zunge, den linken Oberkiefer, das vordere halbe Siebbein, die innere Wand und die obere vordere Parthie der rechten Augenhöhle, welches permanente Schliessung der rechten Augenlider bewirkte, ferner das mittlere Stirnbein in der Form eines Baumblattes, durch welches die Kugel ihren Ausweg nahm; Tod nach 54 Tagen.] Wien. med. Wchnschr., 1865, xv, 1256.—**Türck** (L.) Ueber eine neue Zungenspatel. Allg. Wien. med. Ztg., 1861, vi, 100.—**Velpeau.** Oblitération de la bouche; anaplastie des lèvres; modification du procédé de M. Dieffenbach; succès complet. Gaz. d. hôp., Par., 1840, 2. s., ii, 378.—**Vidéky** (F.) A szájüreg deformitásairól és az itt előforduló hiányok müleges pótlásáról. [Deformities of mouth, and treatment.] Orvosi hetil., Budapest, 1882, xxvi, 1293–1296.—**Wawra.** Ueber einen in dem Winkel, welchen der Boden der Mundhöhle mit dem Kiefer bildet, vorgefundenen fremden Körper. Wien. med. Presse, 1873, xiv, 247. — **Weinlechner.** Lupus an der Oberlippe, am Zahnfleische und harten Gaumen, mit scrophulöser Hauterkrankung im Gesichte, durch Auskratzung geheilt. Aerztl. Ber. d. k. k. allg. Krankenh. zu Wien (1882), 1883, 252.—**Weiss** (W.) Macrostoma. Aerztl. Ber. d. k. k. allg. Krankenh. zu Prag (1881), 1883, 186–188.—**Westmoreland** (W. F.) [Plastic operation for mouth contracted by cicatrices.] Atlanta M. & S. J., 1884-5, n. s., i, 212–217.—**Wilms.** Heilung einer Verwachsung der innern Oberfläche der Wange mit dem Zahnfleische und dem Kieferknochen. Allg. med. Centr.-Ztg., Berl, 1858, xxvii, 417.—**Windle** (B. C. A.) An instrument for the administration of anæsthetics through the nose in operations about the mouth and face. Brit. M. J., Lond., 1884, i, 18.—**Wölfler** (A.) Zur Wundbehandlung im Munde. Arch. f. klin. Chir., Berl., 1881-2, xxvii, 419–456, 1 pl.

Mouth (*Syphilis of*).

See, also, **Chancre** (*Abnormities of*); **Tongue** (*Syphilitic disease of*).

EYTING (G.) * De methodo, ulcera venerea oris et palati curandi, casibus quibusdam illustrata. 8°. *Jenæ*, [1801].

HÉRAUD (A.) * Étude diagnostique sur deux cas de syphilome bucco-lingual. 4°. *Paris*, 1880.

Audouard. Buccite syphilitique, guérie par un traitement fondé sur la sympathie de la gorge avec les organes de la génération, ou sympathie génito-buccale. Rev. méd. franç. et étrang., Par., 1837, ii, 27–36.—**Belousoff** (P. P.) O form. projav. perv. sifilit. poraj. na slizis. oboloch. polosti rta. [Forms of hereditary syphilitic affections of mucous membranes in cavities of mouth.] Trudi Obsh. Russk. vrach. v. Moskve, 1887, ii (Venereal), 20–32.—**Borrichius** (O.) Ex faucibus aqua mercuriali inconsulte tactis cœcitas. Acta med. et phil. Hafn. (1671–2), 1673, i, 147. *Also, transl.*: Collect. acad. d. mém.. etc., Dijon, 1766, vii, 164.—**Epithelial** (The) discolorations of the oral mucous membranes in syphilitic subjects. Arch. d. Heilk., Leipz., 1875, xvi, 433.—**Fischer** (G.) Gummigeschwülste an der Innenfläche der Wange und im sublingualen Raum der Mundhöhle. Deutsche Ztschr. f. Chir., Leipz., 1883, xix, 127–129.—**Fournier.** Des syphilides muqueuses buccogutturales. Gaz. d. hôp., Par., 1881, liv, 523.—**Galet** (J.) Inflammation syphilitique de l'arrière-bouche. Éphém. méd. de Montpel., 1828, ix, 277–280.—**Gross** (F.) À propos du chancre buccal. Rev. méd. de l'est, Nancy, 1879, xi, 145.—**Kinsman** (D. N.) Chancre of the gum. Cleveland M. Gaz., 1885–6, i, 494.—**Lydston** (G. F.) Syphilis in its relations to dental and oral urgery. J. Am. M. Ass., Chicago, 1886, vi, 652–657.—**de Méric.** Syphilitic gangrene of the mouth, with impending suffocation. Lancet, Lond., 1859, i, 213.—**Mulhall** (J. C.) Some phases of buccal syphilis. St. Louis Cour. Med., 1887, xviii, 97–107.—**Pedley** (F. N.) Syphilis about the mouth. Brit. J. Dent. Sc., Lond., 1881, xxiv, 49–54. *Also*: Dental Adv., Buffalo, 1881, xii, 65–70. *Also*: Am. J. Dent. Sc., Balt., 1881–2, 3. s., xv, 6–13.—**Reignier.** [Destruction partielle de la voûte palatine.] Bull. Soc. anat. de Par., 1834, ix, 92.—**Rollet** (J.) [Bouche]; maladies vénériennes et syphilitiques. Dict. encycl. d. sc. méd., Par., 1869, x, 249–267.—**Schuster.** Die Epitheltrübungen der Mundschleimhaut bei Syphilitischen. Arch. d. Heilk., Leipz., 1875, xvi, 433–440.—**Sigmund.** Ueber Syphilis an der Mundschleimhaut. Wien. med. Wchnschr., 1863, xiii, 273; 289; 321; 465; 513; 593. ———. Ueber die Zunahme syphilitischer Erkrankungen der Mundschleimhaut. *Ibid.*, 1865, xv, 917–920.—**Spillmann** (P.) Contribution à l'étude du chancre buccal. Rev. méd. de l'est, Nancy, 1878, x, 292–295.—**Stirling** (R. A.) The local treatment of syphilitic affections of the mouth. Austral. M. J., Melbourne, 1885, n. s., vii, 158–161.

Mouth (*Tuberculosis of*).

See, also, **Pharynx**, **Tongue**, *Tuberculosis of*.

DESPLOUS (J.) * De la tuberculose de l'arrière-bouche. 4°. *Paris*, 1879.

DUCROT (L.) * Étude sur la tuberculose de la bouche, et en particulier sur sa forme curable. 4°. *Paris*, 1879.

GELADE (E.) * De la tuberculose bucco-pharyngée (phthisie buccale). 4°. *Paris*, 1878.

Abercrombie (J.) On three cases of acute tubercular ulceration of the fauces. Brit. M. J., Lond., 1886, ii, 923.—**Babès.** Bacilles de la tuberculose dans une ulcération périnéale, dans la tuberculose du vagin et dans une ulcération de la lèvre inférieure. Bull. Soc. anat. de Par., 1883, lviii, 341–344. *Also, transl.*: Orvosi hetil., Budapest, 1883, xxvii, 860–862.—**Boeckel** (E.) Ulcères tuberculeux de la bouche. Gaz. méd. de Strasb., 1872–3, xxxii, 8.—**Browne** (L.) Tuberculose buccale, linguale et pharyngée. Cong. internat. de laryngol. 1880, Milan, 1882, i, 104–112.—**Chamberlain** (C. W.) Tuberculosis of the mouth and pharynx. Proc. Connect. M. Soc., Hartford, 1881, 78–81.—**De Blois** (T. A.) Cases of buccal tuberculosis. Tr. Am. Laryngol. Ass., N. Y., 1884, vi, 99–105. *Also*: N. York M. J., 1884, xl, 505–507.—**Delavan** (D. B.) Seven cases of buccal tuberculosis; with remarks upon tubercular ulceration of the tongue. Tr. Am. Laryngol. Ass., 1886, N. Y., 1887, viii, 197–210. *Also*: N. York M. J., 1887, xlv, 536–541. *Also*, Reprint.—**Eichhoff** (J.) Ein Fall von ausgebreiteter Tuberculose der Mundschleimhaut. Deutsche med. Wchnschr., Berl., 1881, vii, 413.—**Finger** (E.) Beitrag zur Kenntniss des Miliartuberkels. (Miliartuberculose der Mundspeicheldrüsen, Zungen- und Mundschleimhaut und äusseren Haut.) Med. Jahrb., Wien, 1883, 99–122, 1 pl. *Also*: Med.-chir. Centralbl., Wien, 1885, xx, 447; 459; 470. *Also*: Allg. Wien. med. Ztg., 1883, xxviii, 33; 46. *Also*: Aerztl. Ber. d. k. k. allg. Krankenh. zu Wien (1882) 1883, 155–162.—**Hansemann** (D.) Ueber die Tuberculose der

Mouth (*Tuberculosis of*).

Mundschleimhaut. Arch. f. path. Anat., etc., Berl., 1886, ciii, 264–275. —**Julliard** fils. Note sur l'ulcère tuberculeux de la bouche. Bull. Soc. méd. de la Suisse Rom., Lausanne, 1870, iv, 104–112. *Also*, Reprint. *Also*: Gaz. méd.-chir. de Toulouse, 1875, vii, 34–38.—**Le Dentu** (A.) Note sur un cas d'ulcère tuberculeux des gencives, de la joue, du voile du palais et des deux lèvres. Assoc. franç. pour l'avance. d. sc. Compt.-rend. 1876, Par., 1877, v, 884–886.—**Peter.** Sur la tuberculisation buccale. Gaz. méd. de Par., 1880, 6. s., ii, 6; 18; 102; 114; 142.—**Quenu.** Ulcération tuberculeuse de la muqueuse palatine; perforation de la voûte palatine. Bull. Soc. clin. de Par. (1878), 1879, ii, 194–198.—**Reclus** (P.) Tuberculose buccale. Gaz. hebd. de méd., Par., 1887, 2. s., xxiv, 691–695.—**Reverdin** (A.) Ulcères tuberculeux de la bouche. Mém. Soc. de méd. de Strasb., 1872, ix, 173–176.—**Richet.** Des ulcérations tuberculeuses de la bouche, en général, à propos d'un cas d'ulcération tuberculeuse des lèvres. France méd., Par., 1877, xxiv, 25; 33.—**Routier** (A.) Tuberculose bucco-pharyngée; phthisie buccale. *Ibid.*, 1879, xxvi, 113; 122. —**Schliferowitsch** (P.) Ueber Tuberculose der Mundhöhle. Deutsche Ztschr. f. Chir., Leipz., 1887, xxvi, 527–593.—**Testi** (A.) Contribuzione allo studio della tubercolosi boccale e faringea. Boll. d. osp. . . . di Fermo, 1880, i, 25–33.—**Trélat** (U.) Note sur l'ulcère tuberculeux de la bouche et en particulier de la langue. Arch. gén. de méd., Par., 1870, i, 35–47.

Mouth (*Tumors of*).

See, also, **Calculus** (*Salivary*); **Epulis**; **Gums**, **Jaws**, **Palate**, *Tumors of*; **Ranula**; **Submaxillary** *region*, **Tongue**, *Tumors of.*

BARBÈS (É.) * Contribution à l'étude des kystes dermoïdes du plancher de la bouche. 4°. *Paris*, 1879.

BERTHERAND (E.-L.) * Recherches sur les tumeurs sublinguales. 4°. *Strasbourg*, 1845.

Also, in: J. de méd., chir. et pharmacol., Brux., 1849, viii, 3; 123.

BOIS (A.) * Étude sur quelques tumeurs de la bouche et de l'arrière-bouche. 4°. *Paris*, 1858.

FAURE (P.) * De l'épithélioma du plancher de la bouche. 4°. *Paris*, 1884.

LABAT (E.) * Les lipomes buccaux. 4°. *Paris*, 1874.

LARRIEU (L.) * Contribution à l'étude de l'épithélioma du plancher de la bouche. 4°. *Paris*, 1879.

Ammerman (G. K.) Removal of tumor from the mouth; successful. Chicago M. Exam., 1864, v, 458–460.—**Ansiaux** (O.) Kyste congénital du plancher de la bouche. Ann. Soc. méd.-chir. de Liége, 1862, i, 204–207.—**Arkovy.** On papilloma of the oral cavity; [discussion]. Tr. Odont. Soc. Gr. Brit., Lond., 1881, n. s., xiii, 16–28.—**Bacot** (J.) Case of a steatomatous tumor under the tongue. Lond. M. & Phys. J., 1826, lv, 375–377.—**Baistrocchi** (E.) Contribuzione allo studio dei neoplasmi dell' organo dello smalto. Gazz. d. osp., Milano, 1883, iv, 76; 91.—**Bakó** (S.) A paquelin-féle thermo-cauter, höetetö, alkalmazása álképletek kiirtására. [Removal of fungoid tumor of mouth by thermo-cautery.] Gyógyászat, Budapest, 1880, xx, 489–494. — **Bertherand.** Tumeurs sublinguales. [Rap. de Larrey.] Bull. Soc. de chir. de Par., 1848–50, i, 374–378.—**Bickersteth** (E. R.) Removal of pterygo-maxillary tumors by the mouth. Lancet, Lond., 1871, ii, 156; 186. —**Bouilly.** Tumeur généralisée chez un enfant. Bull. Soc. anat. de Par., 1871, xlvi, 297–303.—**Bowman.** Large sebaceous cyst under the tongue; excision; recovery. Med. Times & Gaz., Lond., 1853, n. s., vii, 678.—**Brady** (G. S.) On a case of sublingual tumour partially removed by operation. *Ibid.*, 1867, i, 3 6.—**Broca.** [Liquide extrait d'une tumeur de la bouche.] Bull. Soc. anat. de Par., 1853, xxviii, 49.—**Buck** (G.) [Tumor under the tongue.] N. York M. Times, 1856, v, 208.—**Cabot.** Tumor from the roof of the mouth. Boston M. & S. J., 1863–4, lxix, 322. *Also*: Extr. Rec. Bost. Soc. M. Improve., 1867, v, 245–249.—**Cameron** (W. L.) Removal of a large tumor from the mouth. Tr. M. & Phys. Soc. Bombay (1847–8), 1849, ix, 217–219. — **Cardone** (F.) Mixoma papillare della cavità orale di un bambino. Arch. ital. di laringol., Napoli, 1887, vii, 132–134.—**Castex** (A.) Des tumeurs malignes de l'arrière-bouche (clinique et intervention chirurgicale). Rev. de chir., Par., 1886, vi, 44; 130; 304. — **Chassaignac.** Hydrocèle sublinguale. Bull. Soc. de chir. de Par., 1853–4, iv, 23. ———. [Kyste de la région sus-hyoïdienne.] Bull. Soc. anat. de Par., 1858, xxxiii, 274.—**Churchill** (F.) Fatty tumour simulating ranula. Tr. Path. Soc. Lond., 1871–2, xxiii, 234–237. *Also*: Med. Times & Gaz., Lond., 1872, i, 160.—**Combalat.** Sur une observation de kyste dermoïde du

Mouth (*Tumors of*).

plancher de la bouche. Bull. et mém. Soc. de chir. de Par., 1881, n. s., vii, 505–511.—**Cruveilhier.** [Tumeur sublinguale.] Bull. Soc. anat. de Par., 1862, xxxvii, 44.—**Dardignac** (J.) Observation de tumeur dermoïde du plancher buccal. [Rap. de Chauvel.] Bull. et mém. Soc. de chir. de Par., 1883, u. s., ix, 710–712. *Also:* Rev. de chir., Par., 1884, iv, 655–660. — **Dehler.** Atheromatöse Cyste unter der Zunge. Oesterr. Ztschr. f. prakt. Heilk., Wien, 1857, iii, 41–44.—**Denis.** Observation sur une tumeur fongueuse dans la bouche, extirpée et guérie par M. Denis. J. de méd., chir., pharm., etc., Par., 1763, xix, 365.—**Després.** Lipôme sous-lingual. Bull. Soc. de chir. de Par., 1873, 3. s., ii, 208–213. ——. Tumeur veineuse du plancher de la bouche; anévrysme artério-veineux; ligature des deux artères linguales. Bull. et mém. Soc. de chir. de Par., 1879, n. s., v, 794–800. ——. Kyste dermoïde du plancher de la bouche. Gaz. d. hôp., Par., 1881, liv, 298.—**von Dumreicher.** Exstirpation eines Sarcom's aus der Mundhöhle. Allg. Wien. med. Ztg., 1856, i, 50.—**Ferguson** (W.) Removal of a fibrous tumor from the roof of the mouth. Lancet, Lond., 1871, ii, 676. — **Fergusson.** Vascular tumours of the mouth. *Ibid.*, 1857, i, 62. — **Ferron.** Observation de kyste dermoïde du plancher de la bouche. Gaz. hebd. de méd., Par., 1887, 2. s., xxiv, 150–152.—[**Gaillet.**] Kystes muqueux du plancher de la bouche et de la région thyrohyoïdienne. Gaz. d. hôp., Par., 1851, 3. s., iii, 171.—**Godoy y Rico** (J.) Epitelioma de la boca; operacion; muerte por pneumonia. Gac. méd. de Granada, 1884, ii, 104–110.—**Gruget.** Tumeur du plancher buccal; hypertrophie glandulaire; épithéliome au début? Bull Soc. anat. de Nantes 1881, Par., 1882, v, 35. *Also:* J. de méd. de l'ouest, Nantes, 1882, xvi, 250. — **Güterbock** (P.) Ueber eine Dermoidcyste am Boden der Mundhöhle (Kiemengangcyste). Arch. f. klin. Chir., Berl., 1878, xxii, 985–989.—**Guyon** (F.) & **Thierry** (É.) Note sur l'existence temporaire de kystes épidermiques dans la cavité buccale chez le fœtus et les nouveau-nés. Arch. de physiol. norm. et path., Par., 1869, ii, 368; 530.—**Halke.** Case of a large sebaceous cyst beneath the tongue. Med. Times & Gaz., Lond., 1862, ii, 628.—**Heyfelder** (J. F.) Exstirpation eines umfangreichen Pseudoplasma in der Mundhöhle, nebst Resection der rechten Unterkieferhälfte. [Case.] Deutsche Klinik, Berl., 1860, xii, 111.—**Hoefle** (M. A.) Balggeschwulst unter der Zunge. Jenaische Ann. f. Physiol. u. Med., Jena, 1851, ii, 273.—**Hofmokl.** Lipoma in regione sublinguali; Exstirpatio; Jodoformbehandlung; Heilung in 10 Tagen. Ber. d. k. k. Krankenanst. Rudolph-Stiftung in Wien (1883), 1884, 284. *Also:* Med.-chir. Centralbl., Wien, 1885, xx, 172.—**Jackson** (R. J.) Fibrous tumor of 35 years' standing, occupying the whole of the buccal cavity; removal; fatal result. Indian M. Gaz., Calcutta, 1870, v, 227–229.—**Jamieson** (H. G.) Case of tumour of the superior jaw. Am. M. Recorder, Phila., 1821, iv, 222–230, 1 pl. *Also, transl.* [Abstr.]: Arch. f. med. Erfahr., Berl , 1821, i, 542–546.—**Johnston** (D.) Removal of a large cancerous sub-lingual tumor along with part of the lower jaw. Edinb. M. J., 1867–8, xiii, 436–439.—**Kühn** (F. A.) Iets over een mond-uitwas. ʼΙπποκράτης, Rotterd., 1828, vii, 45–51.—**Leoni** (P.) Istoria clinica di una ciste del pavimento della bocca. Gior. med di Roma, 1867, iii, 321–347, 1 pl.—**Linhart.** Dermoid-Cyste unter der Zunge. Oesterr. Ztschr. f. prakt. Heilk., Wien, 1858, iv, 257–260.—**Liston** (R.) Tumour of the mouth; operation. Lancet, Lond., 1842–3, i, 745.—**Lundquist** (G.) Polyp i munhålan; operation. *In:* Bergstrand (C. H.) Chir. iakttagelser, 8°, Upsala [1842], 1848, 201–213.—**March** (C. J.) Multiple papillary tumors of the labial, buccal, and glossal mucous membrane. St. Louis Cour. Med., 1880, iv, 236. — **Marchant** (G.) Note sur les kystes dermoïdes du plancher buccal. Bull. Soc. anat. de Par., 1886, lxi, 653–676. *Also:* Progrès méd., Par., 1887, 2. s., v, 462; 481; 504.—**de Marchettis** (P.) Tumor meliceris, a parte sub lingua, ubi raninæ, sensim per partem dextram colli, juxta jugulares venas, et carotides arterias, ad fauces exporrectus, respiratione intercipiens, sectione perfecte sanatus. *In his:* Obs. med.-chir. [etc.], 8°, Lond., 1729, 44–46. *Also, transl. in his:* Rec. d'obs. rares [etc.], 8°, Par., 1858, 86–89.—**Monod** (C.) Grenouillette hydatique. Bull. Soc. anat. de Par., 1869, xliv, 209–211. ——. Lipome du plancher de la bouche. Bull. et mém. Soc. de chir. de Par., 1881, n. s., vii, 365–367.—**Montfumat.** Kyste buccal. Bull. Soc. anat. de Par., 1865, xl, 301–303.—**Morris** (H.) Dermoid cyst in floor of mouth treated by excision of part of cyst-wall, and plugging with lint soaked in iodine liniment; subsequently, death from cancer of the œsophagus. Med. Times & Gaz., Lond., 1884, i, 43. ——. Dermoid cyst containing hair in the floor of the mouth; removal through an incision below the jaw. *Ibid.*, 44.—**Nicaise.** Kyste dermoïde canaliculé de la bouche. Bull. et mém. Soc. de chir. de Par., 1881, n. s., vii, 498.—**Niedzwiecki** (P.) Wyrosłe brodawkowate mnogie błowy śluzowej, warg, jamy ustnej, języka i. t. d. [Growths in mucous membrane of lips, mouth, etc.] Gaz. lek. Warszawa, 1882, 2. s., ii, 896–899.—**Padieu** (A.) Kyste dermoïde de la partie latérale droite du plancher de la bouche. Soc. méd. d'Amiens. Bull. (1873-4), 1875, xiii–xiv, 173–178. ——

Mouth (*Tumors of*).

Tumeur fibro-kystique volumineuse de la cavité buccale, à la face interne de la lèvre supérieure, chez une femme de 76 ans; opération; guérison. Gaz. méd. de Picardie, Amiens, 1885, iii, 165.—**Palumbo** (A.) [Un tumore follicolare della grundezza di una noce nell' interno della sua bocca, che impedivale la masticazione dei cibi.] Filiatresebezio, Napoli, 1845, xxix, 22.—**Pandolfi** (O.) Descrizione di una speciale neoplasia osservata sotto la lingua dei bambini. Resoc. Accad. med.-chir. di Napoli, 1875, xxix, 62–64.—**Patterson.** Tumour of the mouth; operation; death. Glasgow M. J., 1880, [4. s.], xiii, 242.—**Poelman** (C.) Description d'une tumeur cystique pédiculée, observée chez un fœtus. Bull. Soc. de méd. de Gand, 1855, xxii, 10–13, 1 pl.—**Poland** (S.) Three cases of cystiform tumour under the tongue. Guy's Hosp. Rep., Lond., 1850–51, 2. s., vii, 338–340.—**Poulain.** Sçavoir, si, dans le cas d'une tumeur abscédée aux environs de la bouche, on ne pourroit pas donner issue à la matière par une ouverture pratiquée dans l'intérieur de cette cavité. J. de méd., chir., pharm., etc., Par., 1768, xxviii, 79–83.—**Reclus** (P.) Des kystes dermoïdes du plancher buccal. Gaz. hebd. de méd., Par., 1887, 2. s., xxiv, 75–79. *Also:* Gaz. d. hôp., Par., 1887, lx, 1105–1107.—**Reinvillier.** Tumeur obturant complètement la bouche d'un enfant nouveau-né. Gaz. d. hôp., Par., 1850, 3. s., ii, 63.—**Remarques** sur certaines tumeurs de la bouche formées par l'hypertrophie des glandules salivaires de la muqueuse buccale; procédé très-simple pour leur ablation. Bull. gén. de thérap., etc., Par., 1852, xlii, 58–64.—**Riberi** (A.) Énorme tumore cistico sottolinguale. *In his:* Raccolti d. opere minori, etc., 8°, Torino, 1851, ii, 451–453.—**Richelot** (L.-G.) Ablation d'un épithéliome intra-buccal chez un diabétique. Union méd., Par.. 1883, 3. s., xxxv, 781–784.—**Rothman** (A.) Ein Papillom im Munde. Oesterr.-ungar. Vrtljschr. f. Zahnh., Wien, 1887, iii, 203–209. *Also, transl.:* Orvosi hetil.. Budapest, 1887, xxxi, 1461–1464.—**Rushworth** (J.) The case of Dr. James Keil. *In:* Beckett (W.) A collection of chirurgical tracts, 8°, Lond., 1740, 61-77.—**Sarazin.** Quelques tumeurs de la cavité buccale et des fosses nasales. Rev. méd. de l'est, Nancy, 1880, xii, 139; 180.—**Schmalz.** Entfernung einer zungenförmigen Geschwulst aus dem Innern des Mundes. Summ. d. Neuest. u. Wissenswürd. a. d. ges. Med., Leipz., 1835, ii, 307.—**Schulzen** (S.) Von einem Stein unter der Zunge, der durch den Schnitt glüklich ware herausgenommen worden. Auserl. med - chir- . . . . Abhandl. d. röm. kais. Akad. d. Naturf., Nürnb., 1756, iii, 1–4.—**Sewell.** Fatty tumour in the situation of ranula beneath the tongue, successfully removed from an old man 86 years of age. Med. Times & Gaz., Lond , 1872, i, 160. — **Smith** (H.) Removal of an enormous polypoid tumor from behind the palate. Lancet, Lond , 1867, ii. 515.—**Smith** (W. J.) Large sublingual-cyst, treated by puncture and drainage. *Ibid.*, 1872, i, 468.—**Suque** (J.) Kyste pileux du plancher de la cavité buccale. France méd , Par., 1854, i, 214.—**Syme** (J.) Removal of a large encysted tumor of the mouth. Lond. & Edinb. Month. J. M. Sc., 1843, iii, 497.—**Tumoren** im Boden der Mundhöhle; 3 Fälle; 1 Tod. Jahresb. ü d. chir. Abth. d. Spit. zu Basel (1880), 1881, 23–26.—**Vanzetti** (T.) Atheroma ingentis molis basi linguæ adhærens, et in regione inframaxilari propendes; punctio quinquies reiterata, denique incisio tumoris. *In his:* Ann. scholæ clin. chir., etc , 8°, Charcoviæ, 1846, 72–75, 1 pl.—**Velpeau.** Tumeur au-dessous de la langue, qui communique avec une autre tumeur située sous l'angle de la mâchoire du côté droit; diagnostic différentiel; nature; traitement; de la conjonctivite papuleuse. Gaz. d. hôp , Par., 1849, 3. s., i, 62.—**Verneuil.** Kyste de la base de la langue. Bull. Soc. anat. de Par., 1853, xxviii, 8. ——. Kyste dermoïde du plancher de la bouche. *Ibid.*, 1872, 2. s., xvii, 110–112.—**Vittadini** (A.) Voluminoso tumore steatomatoso sottolinguale. Gazz. med. ital. lomb., Milano, 1865, 5. s., iv, 61. — **Wagner** (C.) Case of sub-lingual fallicular cyst, with sebaceoid contents. Arch. Clin. Surg., N. Y., 1877, i, 261.—**Wardrop.** On a mode of removing tumors growing within the mouth, attached to the bones. Lancet, Lond., 1834, ii, 829.—**Warren** (J. M.) Encysted tumor under the tongue, resembling ranula. *In his:* Surg. Obs., 8°, Bost., 1867, 92. ——. Venous erectile tumor of mouth, lip, and tongue. *Ibid.*, 462–464.—**Watson** (P. H.) Case of tumor originating in the pterygoid fossa, and developing towards the buccal cavity, successfully removed. Lancet, Lond.. 1869, i, 744. *Also, Reprint.*—**Weinlechner.** Epithelialcarcinom am Boden der Mundhöhle und an der unteren Fläche der Zungenspitze; Exstirpation. Aerztl. Ber. d. k. k. allg. Krankenh. zu Wien (1882), 1883, 241.—**Wright** (J. W.) Rare congenital, composite, non-encysted, hairy lipoma of the mouth. Bull. N. York Path. Soc., 1881, 2. s., i, 11-14.

Mouth (*Ulceration of*).

See **Mouth** (*Inflammation, etc., of*).

Mouth (*Wounds of*).

See **Face** (*Wounds, etc., of*); **Mouth** (*Surgery, etc., of*).

Mouth-breathing.

CATLIN (G.) The breath of life, or mal-respiration and its effects upon the enjoyments and life of man. 8°. *New York*, 1861.

———. The same. 8°. *New York*, 1864.

———. The same. 8°. *London*, 1862.

PINCKARD (F.) The sanitary brace, a simple mechanical invention intended to force the closure of the mouth during sleep, and thereby absolutely compel the nose to perform all that nature designed in the act of breathing. 8°. *New Orleans*, 1869.

WAGNER (C.) Habitual mouth-breathing. Its causes, effects, and treatment. 12°. *New York*, 1881.

Moutier (Alexandre). *Étude sur le fongus bénin du testicule. 76 pp. 4°. *Paris*, 1875, No. 178.

Moutier (Edmond-Augustin). *De la perforation intestinale dans la fièvre typhoïde. 32 pp. 4°. *Paris*, 1855, No. 66, v. 578.

Moutier (Louis-Alexandre) [1857–]. *Contribution à l'histoire de la protection de l'enfance à Rome. 43 pp. 4°. *Paris*, 1884, No. 365.

Moutier (U.) *Propositions sur le catarrhe utérin, ou la leucorrhée. vi, 7–22 pp. 4°. *Paris*, 1808, No. 75, v. 71.

Moûtiers, *France*.

Gobley. Rapport sur les eaux de Salins et les eaux mères de Moûtiers (Savoie). Bull. Acad. de méd., Par., 1863-4, xxix, 278. — **Laissus** (C.) Sulle acque termali clorurate di Salins (Moûtiers, Savoia). Gior. Accad. di med. di Torino, 1869, 3. s., viii, 287-295.

Moutillard (Victor). *I. De l'œdème des centres nerveux. II. [etc.] 68 pp. 4°. *Paris*, 1841, No. 211, v. 379.

Moutin (J.) *Sur la fistule à l'anus. 4°. *Paris*, 1818, No. 67, v. 137.

Moutin (L.) Le nouvel hypnotisme. 220 pp., 1 pl. 12°. *Paris, Perrin & Cie.*, 1887.

Moutinho (A. F.) Breves reflexões ao autor do opusculo: A homœopathia; o que é, e o que vale. 32 pp. sm. 8°. *Porto, Braz Tisana*, 1852. [P., v. 1249.]

Mouton (Alexandre)[1]. *Essai sur le choléra-morbus. 1 p. l., 30 pp. 4°. *Strasbourg*, 1826, v. 55.

———. *Sur les maladies qui peuvent simuler les hernies inguinales et crurales. 23 pp. 4°. *Strasbourg*, 1826, v. 51; 55.

Mouton (Alexandre)[2]. *Sur l'imagination, considérée dans ses rapports avec les maladies. 35 pp. 4°. *Paris*, 1835, No. 135, v. 286.

Mouton (Alphonse-Marie). *Du traitement des fractures par le pansement ouaté. 39 pp. 4°. *Paris*, 1877, No. 22.

Mouton (Auguste). *Influence de l'utérus sur le système physique et moral de la femme. 37 pp. 4°. *Paris*, 1834, No. 140, v. 273.

Mouton (Célestin). *De la scarlatine. 38 pp. 4°. *Paris*, 1854, No. 180, v. 563.

Mouton (Émile-Garnier). *Des tumeurs hypertrophiques et vasculaires de l'urèthre chez la femme. 46 pp. 4°. *Paris*, 1876, No. 209.

Mouton (Eugène). La physionomie comparée; traité de l'expression dans l'homme, dans la nature et dans l'art. 3 p. l., 595 pp., port. 8°. *Paris, P. Ollendorff*, 1885.

See, also, **Sergi** (G.) La psychologie physiologique, [etc.] 8°. *Paris*, 1880.

Mouton (Gustave). *Des convulsions de l'enfance. 30 pp. 4°. *Paris*, 1856, No. 228, v. 594.

Mouton (Henri) [1858–]. *Du traitement de l'empyème chronique par des résections de côtes (procédé d'Estlander). [Paris.] 86 pp., 1 l. 4°. *Le Mans*, 1883.

Mouton (Leonardus Petrus). *De oculorum in morbis habitu. vi, 68 pp. 8°. *Lugd. Bat., C. C. van der Hoek*, 1833.

Mouton (Louis-Charles-Ernest). *Du calibre de l'œsophage et du cathétérisme œsophagien. 118 pp. 4°. *Paris*, 1874, No. 47.

———. The same. 118 pp. 8°. *Paris, A. Delahaye*, 1874.

Mouton (Marie-Luglien-Charles). *Quelques considérations sur l'hémorrhagie rachidienne. 26 pp. 4°. *Strasbourg, G. Silbermann*, 1867, 3. s., No. 35.

Mouton (Philibert). *Sur la hernie ombilicale, ou exomphale. 27 pp. 8°. *Paris, an X* (1802), v. 11.

Moutte (H.) *Étude sur le rôle pathogénique de l'eau. 44 pp., 1 l. 4°. *Montpellier*, 1874, No. 36.

Moutton (C.-Olivier). *Des hémorrhagies utérines avant, pendant et après l'accouchement. 44 pp. 4°. *Paris*, 1852, No. 267, v. 530.

Mouva.

Garrigou (F.) La source bicarbonatée ferrugineuse du Mouva, près Queyrac (Médoc-Gironde). Rev. méd. et scient. d'hydrol., Toulouse, 1887, iv, 249-252.

Mouvement (Le) hygiénique. Revue d'hygiène publique et privée. Comité de rédaction: H. Barella [*et al.*]. [Monthly.] v. 1–3, Dec., 1884-7. 8°. *Bruxelles*.

Current. v. 1 complete in 13 nos., Dec., 1884, to Dec., 1885 ; v. 2 commenced Jan., 1886.

Mouvement (Le) médical. Annales de l'hydrothérapie scientifique. (La santé publique et l'association médicale.) Rédacteur en chef: N. Pascal. [Weekly.] Années 4–17; Nos. 1–13, v. 18, Jan. 7, 1866, to March 27, 1880. 15 v. 8° & 4°. *Paris*.

In July, 1872, sub-title became : **Journal** international de médecine, de chirurgie et de pharmacie. Rédacteurs : N. Pascal, Bourneville, Kraus (de Vienne). In 1873 E. Labbée added as editor ; after 1873 Labbée sole editor. No. 13, v. 18, probably last published. Continued as : **Réveil** (Le) médical.

Mouveroux (François). *Compression des nerfs récurrents; trachéotomie. 42 pp., 1 l. 4°. *Paris*, 1880, No. 151.

Mouyane (P.) *Sur la pleurésie simple. 18 pp. 4°. *Paris, an XIII* (1804), No. 329, v. 52.

du Mouza (Charles-Auguste) [1852–]. *Quelques cas de chirurgie conservatrice à l'Hôpital maritime de Clermont-Tonnerre (Brest) pendant les années 1880, 1881, 1882. 85 pp., 1 l. 4°. *Paris*, 1883, No. 352.

Mouzaïa-les-Mines.

Bertherand (A.) Notice sur les eaux alcalines gazeuses de Mouzaïa-les-Mines (province d'Alger), précédée de considérations sur la genèse des eaux minérales et thermales, d'après la tradition arabe. Ann. Soc. d'hydrol. méd. de Par., 1857-8, iv, 455-473.

Mouzard (Adolphe-Ambroise). *Sur les avantages de l'allaitement maternel. 22 pp. 4°. *Paris*, 1836, No. 201, v. 299.

Mouzat (Achille). *Sur la scarlatine. 17 pp. 4°. *Paris*, 1833, No. 351, v. 266.

Mouzin (Alexis).

See **Pamard** (Alfred) & **Mouzin** (Alexis). Compterendu des travaux du Conseil d'hygiène publique et de salubrité du département de Vaucluse. 8°. *Avignon*, 1876.

Mouzon (Charles). *Étude sur la valeur séméiologique des hémoptysies, principalement dans certaines formes de maladies du cœur. 72 pp. 4°. *Paris*, 1885, No. 333.

Movement (*Sense of*).

MACH (E.) Grundlinien der Lehre von den Bewegungsempfindungen. 8°. *Leipzig*, 1875.

Vierordt (K.) Die Bewegungsempfindung. Ztschr. f. Biol., München, 1876, xii, 226-240.

Movement *and motion* (*Organic*).

See, also, **Cilia**, *etc.* ; **Leaping** ; **Life** ; **Locomotion** ; **Muscles**.

BORELLI (G. A.) Philosophia de motu animalium ex unico principio mechanico-statico deducta. fol. *Amstelodami*, [1704].

Movement *and motion* (*Organic*).

———. De motu animalium. Editio nova ... dissertationibus physico-mechanicis de motu musculorum, et de effervescentia et fermentatione, Joh. Bernoullii aucta et ornata. 4°. *Neapoli,* 1734.

———. The same. 4°. *Hagæ Comitum,* 1743.

DEHOUX (J.-B.) * Du mouvement organique et de la synthèse animale. 4°. *Paris,* 1861.

ENDTZ (J.-A.) * De motu corporis animalis, sive conscientia voluntaria. 8°. *Groningæ,* 1825.

GENDRIN (A.-N.) Recherches physiologiques sur la motilité. [Mémoire lu au Cercle médical, le 24 décembre 1821, et inséré dans les annales de cette société.] 8°. *Paris,* 1822.

DE GORTER (D.) * De motu vitali. 4°. *Harderovici,* 1736.

JANUS (J. F. C.) * Systema motuum microcosmicum, secundum principia psychologismi medici. 4°. *Halæ Magdeb.,* [1748].

MÜHLPFORT (J. A.) * Diss. phys. quinta qua motus animalis e fundamentis genuinis erutus. sm. 4°. *Wittenbergæ,* [1694].

MÜLLER (F. H.) * De motu corporis ejusque influxu in sanitatem et morbos. 8°. *Vindobonæ,* 1840.

MULLER (J.) De natura motus animalis et voluntarii exercitatio singularis, ex principiis physicis, medicis, geometricis et architectonicis deducta. sm. 4°. *Giessæ,* 1617.

PAULI (J, G.) [Pr. de fibra motrice.] 4°. [*Lipsiæ,* 1717.]

RADCLIFFE (C. B.) The philosophy of vital motion. 8°. *London,* 1851.

———. Vital motion as a mode of physical motion. 8°. *London,* 1876.

STRICKER (S.) Studien über die Bewegungsvorstellungen. 8°. *Wien,* 1882.

WHYTT (R.) An essay on the vital and other involuntary motions of animals. 2. ed. 8°. *Edinburgh,* 1763.

WLOKKA (W. M.) * De ratione motus medica. 8°. *Jenæ,* [1802].

ZURNER (N.) * De viventibus mobilibus a seipsis secundum sententiam Aristotelis aliorumque veterum et contra modernam scholam Cartesianam. 4°. *Jenæ,* 1697.

Arloing (S.) Dissociation ou association nouvelle des mouvements instinctifs sous l'influence de la volonté; contribution à la dénomination de la nature des actes instinctifs. Compt. rend. Soc. de biol., Par., 1885, 8. s., ii, 648–652. — Bechtereff (V. M.) Eksperiment. izsliedovanija nad krugovimi dvijenijami u jivotnich. [Experiments on circular motions in animals] Ejened. klin. gaz., St. Petersb., 1881, i, 585. — Budde (E.) Ueber metakinetische Scheinbewegungen und über die Wahruehmung der Bewegung. Arch. f. Physiol., Leipz., 1884, 127–152.—Cornish (K. H.) Remarks on the laws of animal motion; with a new theory thereon. Lancet, Lond., 1857, ii, 518.—Couty. Sur la distinction physiologique de deux classes de mouvements. Compt. rend. Acad. d. sc., Par., 1884, xcviii, 687–689.—Delaunay (G.) Les mouvements centripètes et centrifuges. Rev. scient., Par., 1880, 2. s., xix, 608–610. *Also*: Assoc. franç. pour l'avance. d. sc. Compt.-rend. 1880, Par., 1881, ix, 880–882. — Dupuy (P.) Du rôle du mouvement dans l'ordre vital. Gaz. méd. de Par., 1864, 3. s., xix, 649; 679. — Féré (C.) Le mouvement considéré comme dynamogène; influence de sa direction; expression des émotions. Compt. rend. Soc. de biol., Par., 1885, 8. s., ii, 629–632.—von Fleischl (E) Ueber willkürliche Bewegungen. Wien. med. Bl., 1878, i, 932; 968.—Heidenhain (R.) Notizen über die Bewegungserscheinungen, welche das Protoplasma in Pflanzenzellen zeigt. Stud. d. physiol. Inst. zu Bresl., 1863, ii, 52–68.—Inman. On voluntary and involuntary motions, with an account of the organs by which they are produced. Proc. Lit. & Phil. Soc. Liverp., 1847, iii, 34–39.—Jürgensen (T.) Ueber die in den Zellen der Vallisneria spiralis stattfindenden Bewegungserscheinungen. Stud. d. physiol. Inst. zu Bresl, 1861, i, 87–109.—Lereboullet (A.) Note sur les mouvements rhythmés dans l'organisme animal. Gaz. méd. de Par., 1857, 3. s., xii, 538. — Purkinje (J. E.) & Valentin (G.) De motu vibratorio animalium vertebratorum. Nova acta phys.-med. Acad. nat. curios., Vratislaviæ et

Movement *and motion* (*Organic*).

Bonnæ, 1835, xvii, 843–854, 2 pl. — Rojas (F. de P.) Determinacion de los movimientos voluntarios en nuestro organismo. Gac. méd. catal., Barcel., 1881, i, 729–738.—Sanderson (J. B.) On the discoveries of the past half century relating to animal motion. Med. Times & Gaz., Lond., 1881, ii, 354–359. — Savory (W. S.) On motion in plants and animals. Lancet, Lond., 1862, ii, 79; 107. — Spence (P.) Voluntary motion. Pop. Sc. Month., N. Y., 1878, xiii, 444–455. — Stricker (S.) Bemerkungen über die Bewegungs-Vorstellungen. Wien. med. Bl., 1882, v, 5; 36.

Movement-cure.

See, also, Exercise *as a remedy;* Gymnastics.

FAESBECK. Die Methode der Bettgymnastik in Verbindung mit Massage. 12°. *Braunschweig,* 1887.

GEORGII (A.) Kinésithérapie, ou traitement des maladies par le mouvement, selon la méthode de Ling. Suivi d'un abrégé des applications de la théorie de Ling à l'éducation physique. 8°. *Paris,* 1847.

LING (P. H.) The gymnastic free exercises. Arranged by H. Rothstein; translated, with additions, by M. Roth. A systematized course of gymnastics without apparatus, [etc.] 16°. *Boston,* 1853.

ROTH (M.) A short sketch of the movement-cure, or rational medical gymnastics, and of the Russian bath, and the use of these hygienic means for the treatment of many chronic diseases. 8°. *London,* 1860.

ROTHSTEIN (H.) Die gymnastischen Freiübungen nach dem System P. H. Ling's reglementarisch dargestellt. 4. Aufl. 12°. *Berlin,* 1861.

SCHEUSTRÖM (R.) Gymnastique médicale suédoise, ou l'art de guérir les maladies au moyen de mouvements bien co-ordonnés, et exécutés par le médecin-gymnaste sur le corps du malade, ou par le malade lui-même. 8°. *Paris,* 1876.

TAYLOR (G. H.) An exposition of the Swedish movement-cure, embracing the history and philosophy of this system of medical treatment, with examples of single movements and directions for their use in various forms of chronic disease, forming a complete manual of exercises, together with a summary of the principles of general hygiene. 8°. *New York,* [1860].

———. Paralysis and other affections of the nerves; their cure by vibratory and special movements. 16°. *New York,* 1871.

Broberg (B. H.) Treatment of chronic disorders by Swedish movements and massage. Canada Lancet, Toronto, 1887-8, xx, 101–104.—Henschen (S. E.) Några ord om sjukgymnastiken såsom undervisningsämne för läkare och dess förhållande till kliniken. [Gymnastics for the sick, with directions.] Upsala Läkaref. Förh., 1884-5, xx, 134–145. *Also* [Rev.]: *Ibid.,* xii.—Karlsjoc (W. J.) Facts in regard to the Swedish movement-cure. Proc. Phila. Co. M. Soc. 1880–81, Phila., 1881, iii, 38–46. *Also*: Phila. M. Times, 1880–81, xi, 257–264.—Macgowan (D. J.) On the movement cure in China. China. Imp. Customs. Med. Rep., Shanghai, 1885, no. 29, 42–52. *Also,* Reprint.—Nebel (H.) Briefe aus Schweden. Deutsche med Wchnschr., Berl., 1887, xiii, 869; 914; 940; 959. *Also,* Reprint.

Movements (*Abnormal*).

See, also, Chorea; Convulsions; Miryachit; Spasm.

Bechterew (W.) Thierversuche über zwangsweise Rollbewegungen um die Längsaxe. St. Petersb. med. Wchnschr., 1882. vii, 45–47. — Paget (G. E.) Cases of morbid rhythmical movements, with observations. Edinb. M. & S. J., 1847, lxvii, 60–80.—Pendleton (L. W.) Involuntary action. Tr. Maine M. Ass., Portland, 1876, 312–331.

Movements (*Co-ordination of*).

See Co-ordination *of movements.*

Movimento (Il). Giornale di medicina e chirurgia. Diretto dal Prof. Dr. Michele del Monte. (Con appendice: Ricordi pel medico-pratico.)

Movimento (Il)—continued.
[Monthly.] Anno 15–16, July, 1883, to June, 1885. 2 v. 8°. *Napoli.*
Title of v. 1–14 was: **Movimento** (Il) medico-chirurgico. v. 15 complete in 6 nos., July to Dec., 1883; v. 16 complete in 12 nos., Jan., 1884, to June, 1885.

Movimento (Il) medico-chirurgico. Compilato dal Dott. A. D' Ambrosio [*et al.*], e sotto la speciale direzione del Prof. Michele del Monte. [3 times a month.] v. 1–14, 1869–82. 4° & 8°. *Napoli.*
Want pp 16–33, v. 6 (in Feb., 1874). v. 11–14, 1879–82, are also called v. 1–4, 2. s. v. 10, 1878, contains general index to v. 1–10. v. 11–12, 1879–80, contain a supplement: **Rivista** clinica e terapeutica. 1879 is semi-monthly: in 1880, became monthly. In July, 1883, continued as: **Movimento** (Il).

Mowbray (G. M.) Nitro glycerine, as used in the construction of the Hoosac Tunnel. [Read before the Albany Institute, Oct. 17, 1871.] 17 pp. 8°. [*n. p.*, 1871.]

Mowbray (John). Midwifery brought to perfection by manual operation, illustrated in a lecture, containing: I. The reasons and motives for instituting and undertaking the performance of a compleat course of midwifery. II. An enquiry into the merit of such a new and laborious enterprise. III. A disquisition upon the excellency of the art of midwifery, in its own nature. IV. The regular method and different steps to be taken in order to qualify and accomplish pupils, both in the theory and practice of this most useful science. xviii, 46 pp. 8°. *London, J. Holland,* 1725.

———. The female physician, containing all the diseases incident to that sex in virgins, wives and widows; together with their causes and symptoms, their degrees of danger, and respective methods of prevention and cure. To which is added the whole art of new improved midwifery, comprehending the necessary qualifications of a midwife, and particular directions for laying women in all cases of difficult and preternatural births, together with the diet and regimen of both the mother and child. xxiv, 420 pp., 2 l. 8°. *London, S. Austen,* 1730.

Mowris (J. A.) Reform; medicine and morals. No. 3. An address delivered before the Onondaga Medical Society, at Syracuse, N. Y., June 14, 1870. 2 l. 8°. [*n. p., Durston's Book Store,* 1870.]

Moxa.

See, also, **Epilepsy** (*Treatment of*); **Joints** (*Diseases of, Treatment of*); **Phthisis** (*Treatment of*).

AVERY (J. F.) *De usu moxæ. 8°. *Edinburgi,* 1821.

COTHENET (C.-J.-B) *Dissertation médico-chirurgicale sur le moxa ou cautère actuel. 4°. *Paris,* 1808.

CRETIN (J.) *Propositions sur l'application et les effets du moxa. 4°. *Paris,* 1809.

DUCHEK (J.) *De moxibustione; adnexa historia synoptica pareseos rheumaticæ faciei. 8°. *Pragæ,* [1836].

FELDMANN (A. C.) *De moxa. 8°. *Festini,* [1831].

VON GEHEMA (J. A.) Eroberte Gicht durch die Chinesche Waffen der Moxa. Worin aus gnugsamer Erfahrung angewiesen wird, dass die beste, geschwindeste, kürtzeste, sicherste und bequemste Genesung, so bisshero noch erfunden worden, bestehe, in dem alhier angeführten Methodo oder Curirungs-Kunst. 16°. *Hamburg,* 1683.

GIRGENSOHN (J.) *De moxa. 8°. [*Dorpat*], 1833.

HALLMAN (J. G.) *De moxæ atque ignis in medicina rationali usu. 4°. *Upsaliæ,* [1788].

Moxa.

HEYMANN (C. F.) *De moxa. 8°. *Berolini,* 1826.

HONGO (M.) Shin Kiu Choho Jikki Komoku. [Handbook of moxa and acupuncture.] obl. 12°. *Osaka,* 1718.

IDELER (K. W.) *De moxæ efficacia in animi morborum medela. 8°. *Berolini,* [1831].

LAPIERRE, *dit* DUPERRON (P.-C.-A.) *Du moxa. 4°. *Paris,* 1851.

LARREY (D. J.) On the use of the moxa as a therapeutical agent. Transl. from the French, with notes, and an introduction containing a history of the substance by Robley Dunglison. 8°. *London,* 1822.
See, also, infra.

LINDNER (C. G.) *De moxis ex remediis domesticis incongrue applicatis. 4°. *Halæ,* [1729].

MARCON (L.-I.) *Dissertation sur l'action du moxa. 4°. *Paris,* 1826.

MOREL. Mémoire et observations sur l'application du feu au traitement des maladies; guérison d'une maladie du foie opérée par le moxa, [etc.] 8°. *Paris,* 1813.

OEHME (C. G.) *Moxæ historiam adumbrandi specimen. 8°. *Halis,* [1845].

ORTIGUIER (B.) *Essai médico-chirurgical sur le moxa, et sur l'ustion en général, et ses différens modes d'application. 4°. *Paris,* 1821.

PIOLLET (P.) *Du moxa, et de son application au traitement de la carie qui attaque les os du tronc; carie ordinairement accompagnée de dépôt par congestion, et généralement regardée alors comme incurable. 4°. *Paris,* 1817.

VILDIEU (É.-G.) *Dissertation sur le moxa, et de son emploi dans le rhumatisme chronique. 4°. *Paris,* 1823.

WALLACE (W.) A physiological enquiry respecting the action of moxa and its utility in inveterate cases of sciatica, lumbago, paraplegia, epilepsy, and some other painful paralytic and spasmodic diseases of the nerves and muscles. 8°. *Dublin,* 1827.

WITTHOFF (S. A.) *De usu moxæ. 4°. *Lundæ,* 1799.

Barde. Cinq observations sur l'emploi du moxa dans diverses maladies. Rev. méd. hist. et phil., Par., 1820, i, 4. livr., 139–149.—**Bartholinus** (T.) De moxa. Acta med. et phil. Hafn.•(1677–9), 1680, v, 7–11.—**Boyle** (J.) Cases and observations illustrating the application of moxa to the treatment of chronic affections of the limbs. Lond. M. & Phys. J., 1827, n. s., iii, 309–314.—**Cooper** (B. B.) An indolent sore, resisting ordinary treatment, but speedily cured by the electric moxa. Med. Times, Lond., 1851, n. s., ii, 553–555.—**Cramer** (J. G.) Modification apportée à la confection des moxas. Écho méd., Neuchât., 1857, i, 762.—**Frank** (L.) Ueber Moxa. Med.-chir. Ztg., Salzburg, 1795, ii, 183–188.—**von Graefe** (C. F.) Ueber leicht anwendbare Moxen. J. d. Chir. u. Augenh., Berl., 1837, xxvi, 526–535.—**Hara, Sei.** [On the old Japanese practice with the moxa.] Iji Shinbun, Tokio, 1885, no. 165, Aug. 5.—**Kæmpfer** (E.) Moxa, præstantissima cauteriorum materia, Sinensibus Japonibusque multum usitata. *In his:* Amœnitatum exoticarum [etc.], 4°, Lemgoviæ, 1712, 589–599.—**Larrey** (D.-J.) Notice d'un mémoire ayant pour titre: Observations sur les bons effets du moxa, secondé par l'application de l'ammoniaque. Mém. Soc. méd. d'émulat. de Par. (an v), an vi [1798], i, 199. ———. Moxa. Dict. d. sc. méd., Par., 1819, xxxiv, 459–474. ———. De l'usage du moxa. *In his:* Rec. de mém. de chir., 8°, Par., 1821, 1–160. 2 pl. [*See, also, supra.*]—**Leney** (J.) Use of moxa in rheumatism. Lond. M. Gaz., 1842, xxx, 608–610.—**Pascal.** Observations sur l'usage du moxa des Chinois, ou du cylindre de coton, employé selon la méthode de feu M. Ponteau. J. de méd., chir., pharm., etc., Par., 1784, lxi, 268; 595: 1786, lxvi, 280–288: 1788, lxxvii, 74–85. ———. Observations sur l'usage du moxa, pour la guérison des ulcères, avec des moyens d'en perfectionner l'application. Méd. éclairée, Par., 1792, iv, 336–346.—**Perez** (J. L.) Observacion en confirmacion de la eficacia de las moxas en las flemasias crónicas de los órganos pulmonales. Décadas méd.-quir. y farm., Madrid, 1821, ii, 275–280.—**Perula** (J. B.) Eficacia del moxa contra las flegmasias rebeldes de pecho. Bol. de med., cirug. y farm., Madrid, 1836, iii, 233–235.—**Potet.** Du moxa. Ann. de la méd. physiol., Par., 1830, xviii, 288–291.—**von**

Moxa.

Reichert (K. W. G.) Ein Beitrag zur Geschichte der Moxa. Deutsches Arch. f. Gesch. d. Med. u. med. Geog., Leipz., 1879, ii, 45; 145.—**Richter.** Kautelen zum Gebrauch der Moxae. J. d. Chir. u. Augenh., Berl., 1845, xxxiv, 146.—**Rivera** (J. A.) Observaciones prácticas sobre la eficacia de la moxá en las flemasias crónicas de pecho. Décadas de med. y cirug. práct., Madrid, 1822, v, 329–357.—**Saddler.** Ueber die Anzeige zur Anwendung der Moxa; nebst dahin gehörigen Krankengeschichten. Ztschr. f. d. ges. Med., Hamb., 1836, iii, 234–247.—**Souville.** Observation sur l'application du moxa, dans une douleur de sciatique. J. de méd. mil., Par., 1783, ii, 470–479.—**Stockwell** (W. H.) On moxa. Transylv. J. M., Lexington, Ky., 1835, viii, 151–169.—**Use** (The) of the moxa in Japan in the xviii. century. [From: Kæmpfer's Japan.] Sei-i-Kwai M. J., Tôkyô, 1887, vi, 180–182. — **Vaidy** (J.-V.-F.) Observation sur les bons effets du moxa dans le traitement des inflammations chroniques des organes de la respiration. J. compl. du dict. d. sc. méd., Par., 1820, vi, 9–16. ———. Faits constatant l'efficacité du moxa dans le traitement des phlegmasies chroniques des organes de la respiration. J. gén. de méd., chir. et pharm., Par., 1820, lxxii, 55–68. Also: Bull. Fac. de méd. de Par., 1820–21, vii, 148–159.—**Valentin** (L.) Sobre los buenos efectos de la adustion en el esternon en un caso de expectoracion purulenta. Décadas méd.-quir. y farm., Madrid, 1821, ii, 24–32.—**Valentini** (M. B.) De moxa atque podagra. In his: Polych. exot., 4°, Francof. ad M., 1701, 197–203, 1 pl.—**Wade** (R.) Cases in which moxa was successfully applied. Lond. M. & Phys. J., 1828, n. s., iv, 473–478.—**Wedel** (G. W.) De moxa germanica. Misc. Acad. nat. curios. 1682, Norimb., 1683, decuria 2, i. 14–19. Also, transl.: Collect. acad. d. mém., etc., Dijon, 1755, iii, 456–458. Also, transl.: Auserl. med.- chir.- . . . Abhandl. d. röm.-kais. Akad. d. Naturf., Nürnb., 1762, xi, 10–13.

Moxey (Georgius Todd). * De puerperarum hysteritide. 3 p. l., 26 pp. 8°. Edinburgi, P. Neill, 1821.

Moxhay (W. Watkinson) [–1885].
Obituary. Brit. M. J., Lond., 1885, i, 1131.

Moxly (J. H. Sutton). An account of a West Indian sanatorium and a guide to Barbados. xii, 209 pp. 12°. London, S. Low [and others], 1886.

Moxon (Walter) [1836–86]. How should we study medicine? The lecture introductory to session 1868-9 at Guy's Hospital. 36 pp. 8°. London, F. Bentley & Co., [1868, vel subseq.].

———. A case of inflammation of the aorta, causing contraction of its ascending part and fatal ischæmia. 4 pp., 1 l., 1 pl. 8°. [n. p., 1871, vel subseq.]

———. On the pathological nature of tumours. 77 pp. 8°. [n. p., 1872, vel subseq.]

———. Pilocereus senilis and other papers. 3 p. l., 262 pp. 12°. London, S. Low [and others], 1887.

See, also, **Wilks** (Samuel) & **Moxon** (Walter). Lectures on pathological anatomy. 2. ed. 8°. London, 1875. For Biography, see Brit. M. J., Lond., 1886, ii, 234–236. Also: Lancet, Lond., 1886, ii, 273–276. Also: Med.-Chir. Tr., Lond., 1887, lxx, 20–23 (G. D. Pollock).

Moxter (Heinrich). * Ueber einen Fall von Granularatrophie der Niere. 40 pp. 8°. Würzburg, Becker, 1881.

Moxter (Philipp) [1858–   ]. * Therapie des Nabelschnurfalls bei Schädellage. 38 pp., 1 l. 8°. Berlin, A. Haack, [1882].

Moy (Adrien). * Du tampon en obstétrique. 38 pp. 4°. Paris, 1875, No. 198.

Moye (Eugène). * Considérations sur l'influence exercée par le système sanguin sur le système nerveux, et sur les applications qui en résultent pour la pathologie. 105 pp. 4°. Strasbourg, 1853, No. 270, 2. s., v. 19.

Moye (Georges). * Contributions à l'étude du retour des battements dans les anévrysmes poplités et de l'extrémité inférieure de la fémorale après la ligature de cette artère. 120 pp. 4°. Paris, 1874, No. 492.

Moye (Léon). * De l'affection généralement connue sous le nom d'engorgement tuberculeux du testicule. 36 pp. 4°. Strasbourg, 1855, No. 348, 2. s., v. 21.

Moyen de guérir du choléra morbus, et de s'en préserver. [Communiqué par un médecin hongrois.] 2 pp. 8°. [Paris, L.-E. Herhan, n. d.]

Moyle (John). Chirurgus marinus; or, the sea chirurgion. Being instructions to junior chirurgic practitioners, who design to serve at sea in this imploy. In two general parts. The first part contains necessary directions, how the chirurgion should furnish himself with medicines, instruments, and necessaries, fit for that office; together with a medicinal catalogue, and an exemplary invoyce. The second part contains the surgions practice at sea; which practical part serves as well at land as at sea. 4. ed. 11 p. l., 326 pp.. 5 l. 12°. London, E. Tracy, 1702.

———. The experienced chirurgion; deliver'd under the following heads: I. Preternatural tumors and ulcers. II. Affects thereupon. III. Wounds and contusions. IV. Fractures of the skull. V. Luxations and sprains. VI. Fractures of the limbs and other bones. Wherein are occasionally handled the chirurgical part in the stone, the gout, the rhumatism, the dropsie, the scurvey, the king's evil, the confirmed itch, the leprosie, and the French pox. With an anatomical description of the parts treated of; besides the chirurgical part in the vermis Africanus, never treated of before, the concussio cerebri, etc. To which are added the best approv'd remedies now in use for most distempers incident to humane bodies, by sea or land. Collected from Dr. Bates, and Dr. Fuller's pharmacopeia, and others of the best modern authors. By a Dr. of physick. Very necessary for all chirurgions and other persons that have not the conveniency of a physician's advice. 3 p. l., 320 pp., 4 l. sm. 8°. London, W. Davis, 1703.

———. Chyrurgic memoirs, being an account of many extraordinary cures which occurred in the series of the author's practice, especially at sea [etc.] 3 p. l., 128 pp., port. 12°. London, D. Brown [and others], 1708.

———. The present ill state of the practice of physick in this nation truly represented, and some remedies thereof humbly proposed to the two Houses of Parliament. By a member of the College of Physicians. 34 pp. 8°. [n. p., 1702.]

Moynac (Léon). * Du traitement des hernies par le caoutchouc. 3 pp., 1 l. 4°. Paris, 1875, No. 13.

———. The same. 33 pp. 8°. Paris, A. Delahaye, 1875.

———. Manuel de pathologie générale et de diagnostic. xii, 759 pp. 12°. Paris, H. Lauwereyns, 1877.

———. The same. 3. éd. xii, 726 pp. 12°. Paris, H. Lauwereyns, 1883.

———. The same. Manual de patología general y de diagnóstico, traducido al castellano por el doctor Don Estéban Sanchez Ocaña. vii, 687 pp. 8°. Madrid, Moya y Plaza, 1878.

———. The same. Manuel de pathologie et de clinique médicales. 3. éd. 1 p. l., 715 pp. 18°. Paris, Lauwereyns, [1880].

———. Manuel d'anatomie descriptive. 2 v. 814, 581 pp. 12°. Paris, H. Lauwereyns, 1880–81.

CONTENTS.

I. Manuel de l'amphithéâtre.
II. Splanchnologie; organes des sens; embryologie.

———. Éléments de pathologie et de clinique chirurgicales. 3. éd. 2 v. viii, 766 pp ; 738 pp. 12°. Paris, H. Lauwereyns, 1881.

———. Conseils aux personnes qui souffrent des voies génito-urinaires. 392 pp. 12°. Paris, G. Steinheil, 1886.

Moyne (F.-Numa). * I. Des indications dans la convalescence. II. [etc.] 70 pp. 4°. Paris, 1841, No. 261, v. 379.

Moyne (Giuseppe). Il servizio oculistico nelle già ferrovie romane. Lettera al Sig. Comm. L. T. Kossuth, direttore dell' esercizio delle strade ferrate del Mediterraneo. xx pp. 8°. *Firenze, tipog. cooperativa,* 1885.

Suppl. to: Boll. d' ocul., Firenze, 1885-6, viii, no. 1.

Moyne (J.-P.) * Sur le crétinisme et l'idiotisme. 28 pp. 4°. *Paris,* 1814, No. 80, v. 103.

Moynier (Eugène). * De la chorée. 142 pp. 4°. *Paris,* 1855, No. 48, v. 578.

——. Des morts subites chez les femmes enceintes ou récemment accouchées. iv, 5–167 pp. 8°. *Paris, V. Masson,* 1858.

——. Des accidents graves qui surviennent dans le cours de la rougeole et de la scarlatine. 290 pp. 8°. *Metz, J. Verronnais,* 1860.

Repr. from: Exposé d. trav. de la Soc. d. sc. méd. de la Moselle, Metz, 1860.

Moynier (Gustave). Note sur les travaux du comité international, fondateur de l'œuvre des secours aux militaires blessés, lue à la conférence internationale de Berlin le 27 avril 1869. 8 pp. 8°. *Berlin, J. F. Starcke,* 1869.

——. Droit des gens. Étude sur la convention de Genève pour l'amélioration du sort des militaires blessés dans les armées en campagne (1864 et 1868). 376 pp. 8°. *Paris, J. Cherbuliez,* 1870.

——. Note sur la création d'une institution judiciaire internationale propre à prévenir et à réprimer les infractions à la convention de Genève. Lue au Comité international de secours aux militaires blessés, dans sa séance du 3 janvier 1872. 1 l., 12 pp. 8°. *Genève, Soullier & Wirth,* 1872.

——. The red cross, its past and its future. Transl. by John Furley. viii, 9–188 pp. 12°. *London, Cassell, Petter, Galpin & Co.,* 1883.

—— & **Appia** (L.) La guerre et la charité. Traité théorique et pratique de philanthropie appliquée aux armées en campagne. ix, 10–401 pp. 8°. *Genève, Cherbuliez,* 1867.

—— ——. The same. Help for sick and wounded. Transl. by John Furley. Together with other writings on the subject by officers of her majesty's service. xix, 467 pp. 8°. *London, J. C. Hotten,* 1870.

Moynier (Jean-Baptiste). * Sur l'ophthalmie, ou l'inflammation de la membrane externe de l'œil. vi, 7–19 pp. 4°. *Paris,* 1815, No. 80, v. 110.

Moynier (Joseph). *Sur la péritonite. vi, 7–25 pp. 4°. *Paris,* 1817, No. 200, v. 128.

Moyret (P.-J.-A.) * Essai sur la brûlure, suivi de quelques propositions de médecine et de chirurgie. 27 pp. 4°. *Paris,* 1831, No. 77, v. 240.

M[oysant].

See le V[acher de la Feutrie], M[oysant] & la M[acellerie]. Dictionnaire de chirurgie. 2 v. sm. 8°. *Paris,* 1767.

Moysant (Léon). * Du prurigo. 42 pp. 4°. *Paris,* 1858, No. 99, v. 622.

See, also, **Hardy** (Alfred). Leçons sur les maladies de la peau, [etc.] 8°. *Paris,* 1859-60. ——. Leçons sur les maladies dartreuses, etc. 8°. *Paris,* 1868.

Moyse (D.) * Étude historique et critique sur les fonctions et les maladies du pancréas. 60 pp., 1 pl. 4°. *Paris,* 1852, No. 170, v. 530.

Moysen (Marie-Bernard). * Des âges, et de leur influence sur les maladies. vi, 7–30 pp. 4°. *Paris,* 1824, No. 172, v. 187.

Moyses (Raby). *See* **Moses Maimonides.**

Mozac (M. S.) * Recherches sur le furoncle. 28 pp. 4°. *Paris,* 1837, No. 117, v. 309.

Mozambique.

de Almeida (A. N. C. P.) Excerptos de um relatorio sobre o serviço de saude na estação naval de Moçambique nos annos 1867, 1868 e 1869. J. Soc. d. sc. med. de Lisb., 1876, 2. s., xl, 28; 58; 89. — **Cabral** (F. J.) Relatorio

Mozambique.

sobre as doenças observadas na cidade de Moçambique desde 1866 a 1869. *Ibid.,* 147; 183; 211; 248; 265. — **Roquete** (A.-P.) Note sur la topographie médicale de Mozambique. Arch. de méd. nav., Par., 1868, ix, 161–168. — **de Salis** (J. N.) Esboço ácerca das molestias de Moçambique. J. Soc. d. sc. med. de Lisb., 1876, 2. s., xl, 271; 317; 338.

Mozambique (*Ulcer of*).

See **Ulcers** (*Endemic*).

de Moze (Henri-Brunel). * De la paralysie du nerf moteur oculaire commun. 87 pp. 4°. *Montpellier, L. Cristin & Cie.,* 1-64, v. 46.

Mozer (Alexander). * Ein Beitrag zur Geschichte der Ligatur der Arteria lingualis bei Operationen an der Zunge. 29 pp. 8°. *Rostock, C. Boldt,* 1868.

C.

Mozian (Krikor-Nersèh). * De la maladie de Bright. 54 pp. 4°. *Paris,* 1854, No. 289, v. 563.

Moziman (Louis). * Relation d'une épidémie d'accidents intermittents observés dans les environs de Lacaune pendant l'hiver de 1864. De leur cause, des moyens de les prévenir et de les combattre. xii, 13–78 pp., 2 l. 4°. *Montpellier, J. Martel aîné,* 1864. [P., v. 45.]

Mozzio. Regolamento di polizia urbana e rurale per il comune di Mozzio. 18 pp. 8°. *Domodossola, Porta,* 1878.

Mozzoni (Giuseppe). Che sieno il coléra e le febbri tifoidee. Saggio di fisica sintetica applicata alle malattie ora dominanti e digressione sulla diffusione de' veri. Memoria . . . letta ad alcuni amici. Con note dell' autore. 92 pp. 8°. *Milano, G. Chiusi,* 1855.

Mraovich (Alexander). * Diss. sistens quædam de hydrargyrosi. vi, 21 pp. 8°. *Viennæ, J. P. Sollinger,* 1825.

Mrs. Day (The) fund. 2 l. 8°. *St. Andrews,* [*n. d.*] [P., v. 1294.]

Mseno.

Reuss (F. A.) Physisch-chemische Beschreibung des Gesundbrunnens und Bades zu Msseno auf der hochfürstlich Kinskyschen Herrschaft Slonitz im Rakonitzer Kreise. 8°. *Dresden,* 1799.

Staněk (W. S.) * Die Mineralwässer und die Bäder zu Mseno (Mscheno) in Böhmen rakonitzer Kreise. 8°. *Prag,* 1832.

Mucci (Domenico) [–1885]. Varici guarite coll' elettrolisi. 7 pp. 8°. *Firenze, tipog. Cenniniana,* 1881.

Repr. from: Sperimentale, Firenze, 1881, xlviii.

——. Manuale di elettroterapia-galvanica, informato alle più recenti innovazioni scientifico-pratiche. 438 pp. 16°. *Piacenza, G. Tedeschi,* 1883.

For Biography, see Gazz. clin. di elettroter., Palermo, 1885, iii, 182 (edit.).

Mucci (Gregorio). Collezione di memorie medicofisiche. 70 pp. 8°. *Napoli,* 1804. [P., v. 1116; 1125.]

Much Wenlock. *See* **Lunatic** Asylum for the Counties of Salop and Montgomery and for the Boroughs of Much Wenlock, Shrewsbury, and Oswestry.

Much Woolton.

Rawlinson (R.) Report to the General Board of Health, on a preliminary inquiry into the sewerage, drainage, and supply of water, and the sanitary condition of the inhabitants of the township of Much Woolton, in the county palatine of Lancaster. 8°. *London,* 1852.

Mucha (Eduardus). * Diss. exhibens remediorum hæmostaseos in artuum amputatione perficiendæ disquisitionem. 1 p. l., 51 pp. 8°. *Vratislaviæ, A. Brehmer et Minuth,* [1835].

Mucha (J. Wolfgangus). * De morbo puerperali. 22 pp., 1 l. 8°. *Viennœ, ex typog. vid. A.
Pichler,* [1838].

Mucilage.

QUENTIN (L.) * Du principe mucilagineux,
et de ses usages en thérapeutique. 4°. *Paris,*
1854.

  Langlebert (A.) Propriétés des graines mucilagi-
neuses; du lin; du sésame. Bull. gén. de thérap., etc.,
Par., 1882, ciii, 549–551.

Mucin.

LANDWEHR (H. A.) * Untersuchungen über
das Mucin der Galle und das der Submaxillardrüse. 8° *Strassburg,* 1881.

  Also, in: Ztschr. f. physiol. Chem., Strassb., 1881, v, 371–
383.

WAELCHLI (G.) * Ueber die Fäulniss des
Elastin und Mucin. 8°. *Leipzig,* 1878.

  Hammarsten (O.) Bidrag till kännedomen om mu-
cinet och de mucinliknande ämnena. Upsala Läkaref.
Förh., 1883–4, xix, 381–406. *Also, transl.:* Arch. f. d. ges.
Physiol., Bonn, 1885, xxxvi, 373–456. ———. Ueber die
mucinartigen Substanzen und ihr Verhältniss zu den Eiweissstoffen. Cong. périod. internat. d. sc. méd. Compt.-
rend. 1884, Copenh., 1886. i, sect. de physiol., 3–10.—**Jern-
ström** (E. A.) Några bidrag till kännedomen om muci-
net. [On mucins.] Upsala Läkaref. Förh., 1879–80, xv,
434–439.—**Landwehr** (H. A.) Untersuchungen über das
Mucin von Helix pomatia und ein neues Kohlenhydrat
(Achrooglycogen) in der Weinbergschnecke. *Ibid.*, 1881–
2, vi, 74–77. ———. Ueber Mucin, Metalbumin und Paralbumin. *Ibid.*, 1883–4, viii, 114–121.—**Reissner** (F.) Ueber
gelösten Schleimstoff (Mucin) im menschlichen Harn.
Arch. f. path. Anat., etc., Berl., 1862, xxiv, 191–197.

Muck (Ferdinandus). * De ganglio ophthalmico
et nervis ciliaribus animalium a medicorum ordine præmio ornata. vi, 7–94 pp., 2 pl. 4°.
Landishuti, J. Thomann, 1815. [*Also, in:* P., v.
814.]

Muck (Gulielmus). * De semiologia oculi. 15
pp. 8°. *Monachii, J. Deschler,* 1838.

Muck (Rudolph). * Ueber Gut- und Bösartig-
keit des Carcinoms. 38 pp. 8°. *Würzburg, J.
Kayser,* 1850.
                                 C.

Muckermann (Clemens) [1838–   ]. * De
scarlatina. 30 pp., 1 l. 8°. *Berolini, G. Schade,*
[1862].

Muckley (William J.) The student's manual of
artistic anatomy, with plates of the bones and
surface muscles of the human figure, together
with a description of the origin, insertion, and
use of the muscles. 26 l., 25 pp. 8°. *London,
Baillière, Tindall & Cox,* 1878.

Mucous *membranes.*

  See **Membranes** (*Mucous*).

Mucous *tubercules.*

  See **Condyloma**.

Mucus.

  See, also, **Asphyxia** *from bronchial mucus;*
Mucin; Pus: Saliva.

BENTZIUS (A. C.) * De pituita vitrea insipida.
4°. *Altdorffi,* [1690].

BUCHHEIM (R.) * Meletemata quædam de al-
bumino, pepsino et muco. 4°. *Lipsiæ,* [1845].

DARWIN (C.) Experiments establishing a criterion between mucaginous and purulent matter.
8°. [*Edinburgh,* 1778?]

  ———. The same. Experiments establishing
a criterion between mucaginous and purulent
matter. And an account of the retrograde motions of the absorbent vessels of animal bodies in
some diseases. [With a preface by E. Darwin.]
8°. *London,* 1780.

GAUBIUS (J.) * De pituita. 4°. *Harderovici,*
1698.

GORN (C. A.) * De pituita. 4°. *Lipsiæ,* 1718.

  Also, in: HALLER. Disp. anat. [etc.] 4°. *Gottingæ,*
1751, vii, 373–419.

VON GRUITHUISEN (F. P.) Naturhistorische
Untersuchungen über den Unterschied zwischen

Mucus.

Eiter und Schleim durch das Mikroskop. 4°.
München, 1809.

HEBOLD (O.) * Ein Beitrag zur Lehre von der
Sekretion und Regeneration der Schleimzellen.
8°. *Bonn,* [1879].

HEULE (B.) * De muco et morbis a muco
oriundis. 4°. *Lugd. Bat.,* 1790.

HOFFBAUER (C. H.) * De ignobili muco in-
grato multorum nobilium hospite. 4°. *Halœ
Magdeb.,* [1734].

LORLEBERG (J. C. C.) * Physiologia muci
primarum viarum. 4°. *Wittenbergæ,* [1789].

MAERKL (G. B.) * De polyblennia. 8°. *Straubingæ,* 1835.

MONTANUS (J. B.) Sententia de generatione
pituitæ: contra eos qui affirmant, pituitam in
ventriculo generari.

  In: CRATO (J.) Methodus θεραπευτική, etc. 12°.
Basileæ, [1555], 163–170.

PATERSON (A.) * Soderjanie jirov v mokrotie.
[Fat in mucus.] 8°. *St. Petersburg,* 1871.

SCHLEIM (Der) vorzüglich der Kinder und
alten Leute, oder Entstehung, Ursachen, Kennzeichen, Natur und Heilung der in jedem Alter
sich bildenden, sehr gefährlichen Verschleimung
des Bluts, der Brust, des Magens und der Eingeweide, mit beigefügten, durch eigene Erfahrung
bestätigten, vorzüglichen Mitteln und Recepten.
2. Aufl. 8°. *Frankf. a. M.,* 1821.

SCOTT (D.) * De genere mucoso in corpore
animali præsertim humano. 8°. *Edinburgi,*
1812.

STARKOFF (I.) * Soderjanie vielkovich tiele
ve mokrotie. [Albuminous bodies in mucus.]
8°. *St. Petersburg,* 1871.

TILANUS (J. G. R.) * De saliva et muco.
8°. *Amstelodami,* 1849.

DE WISINGER (R.) * De pituita. 12°. *Monachii,* 1836.

  Beale (L. S.) On the vital changes occurring in the
mucus-corpuscle. Assoc. M. J., Lond., 1863, i, 262; 315.—
Biedermann (W.) Zur Histologie und Physiologie der
Schleimsecretion. Sitzungsb. d. k. Akad. d. Wissensch.
Math.-naturw. Cl., Wien, 1887, xciv, 3. Abth., 250–272, 2
pl.—**Chambers** (T. K.) On the formation of mucus and
pus. Lancet, Lond., 1863, ii, 153; 182; 212.—**De Giovanni** (A.) Alcune osservazioni microscopiche sopra il
sangue, il muco ed il pus. Gazz. med. ital. lomb., Milano,
1870, 6. s., iii, 313–316.—**Duncan** (J. M.) Clinical lecture on retention of mucus. Med. Times & Gaz., Lond.,
1879, ii, 629–631.—**Eberth** (C. J.) Zur Entstehung der
Schleimkörper. Arch. f. path. Anat., etc., Berl., 1861, xxi,
106–115, 1 pl.—**Gruby.** Mucus. Verhandl. d. k. k. Gesellsch. d. Aerzte zu Wien, 1842, i, 188–194.—**Heule.** Ueber
Schleim- und Eiterbildung und ihr Verhältniss zur Oberhaut. J. d. pract. Heilk., Berl., 1838, lxxxvi, 5. St., 3–62, 1 pl.
Also, transl.: Lancet, Lond., 1839, ii, 286–294.—**Kelsch** &
Kiener. Sur la sécrétion muqueuse et la formation des
moules dans les tubuli du rein, à l'état normal et à l'état
pathologique. Compt. rend. Soc. de biol. 1880, Par., 1881,
7. s., ii, 348–350. *Also:* Gaz. méd. de Par., 1880, 6. s., ii,
647.—**Kemp** (G.) On the composition of mucus. Lond.
M. Gaz., 1841-2, xxx, 672–674.—**Mandl** (L.) Mémoire sur
les rapports qui existent entre le sang, le pus, le mucus et
l'épiderme. Gaz. méd. de Par., 1840, 2. s., viii, 417–422.—
Ranvier (L.) Des vacuoles des cellules caliciformes, des
mouvements de ces vacuoles et des phénomènes intimes de
la sécrétion du mucus. Compt. rend. Acad. d. sc., Par.,
1887, civ, 819–822.—**Rossbach** (M. J.) & **Aschenbrandt** (T.) Beiträge zur Physiologie und Pathologie
der Schleimsecretion in den Luftwegen; vorläufige Mittheilungen. Monatschr. f. Ohrenh., Berl., 1881, xv, 41;
113.—**Simon** (F.) Ueber Schleim und Eiter. J. d. pract.
Heilk., Berl., 1841, xciii, 5. St., 3–14.—**Tigri** (A.) Sulla
composizione istologica primativa del mucco. Bull. d. sc.
med. di Bologna, 1859, 4. s., xi, 380–386.

Mud *baths.*

  See **Baths** (*Mud*).

Mudar.

PIEROT (J.) * De mudar sive Calotropi gigan-
tea R. Br. 8°. *Lugd. Bat.,* 1839.

  Cumin (W.) Remarks on the medicinal properties of
madar, and on the effects of bichromate of potass on the
human body. Edinb. M. & S. J., 1827, xxviii, 295–302.

Mudar.

Also: Am. M. Recorder, Phila., 1828, xiii, 315–322.—**Duncan** (A.) Observations on the bark of the root of the Calotropis mudarii. Edinb. M. & S. J., 1829, xxxii, 60–74. ———. On mudarine, the active principle of the bark of the root of the Calotropis mudarii, Buch., and the singular influence of temperature upon its solubility in water. Lancet, Lond., 1830–31, ii, 641–643.—**Playfair** (G.) On the madar and its medical uses. Tr. M. & Phys. Soc. Calcutta, 1823–5, i, 77–102, 1 pl.

Muddock (J. E.) The "J. E. M." guide to Davos-Platz, with analytical notes on the food, air, water, and climate, by Philip Holland. 2. ed. viii, 132 pp. 12°. *London, Simpkin, Marshall & Co.*, 1882.

Mudge (Henry). Physiology, health, and disease, demanding abstinence from alcoholic drinks, and prohibition of their common sale; being a course of five lectures. With illustrations and appendix; to which is added The Distracted Village. A tale. viii, 124 pp. 8°. *London, W. Tweedie*, 1859. [P., v. 1432.]

Mudge (John) [1720–93]. A dissertation on the inoculated small-pox; or, an attempt towards an investigation of the real causes which render the small-pox by inoculation so much more mild and safe than the same disease when produced by the ordinary means of infection. vii (1 l.), 152 pp., 1 pl. 16°. *London, E. Allen*, 1777. [P., v. 1435.]

———. A radical and expeditious cure for a recent catarrhous cough. Preceded by some observations on respiration; with occasional and practical remarks on some other diseases of the lungs. To which is added a chapter on the vis vitæ, so far as it is concerned in preserving and reinstating the health of an animal. Accompanied with some strictures on the treatment of compound fractures. xvi, 252 pp. 16°. *London, E. Allen*, 1778. [P., v. 1435.]

———. The same. 5. ed. xx, 231 pp., 1 pl. 16°. *London, J. G. Kaven*, 1783.

———. The same. Abhandlung von dem catarrhalischen Husten, in welcher zugleich eine gründliche und geschwinde Heilungsart desselben mitgetheilet wird. Nebst einigen Bemerkungen über die Lebenskraft des menschlichen Körpers, und über die Behandlung complicirter Beinbrüche. Aus dem Englischen übersetzt. 5 p. l., 126 pp., 1 pl. 12°. *Leipzig, Weidmanns Erben u. Reich*, 1780.

For Portrait, see **Collection**—van Kaathoven.—**Collection** of Portr. (Libr.)

Mücke (Die). Ein volksthümliches Correspondenz-Organ für alle Freunde der Natur und Warheit. Hrsg. und redigirt von Carl Baunscheidt. [28 Nos. annually.] Jahrg. 1–2, 1861–2; 16–28, 1876–88. 14 v. 8°. *Bonn.*
Current.

Muecke (Benjamin Gottfried). * Historia tetani nuper observati cum epicrisi caussarum hujus morbi. 24 pp. sm. 4°. *Jenæ, lit. Kirchnerianis*, [1770].
Also [Abstr.], in: WEIZ (F. A.) Vollständ. Ausz. [etc.] 12°. Leipzig u. Budissin, 1774, vi, 125–129.

Muecke (Carl) [1845–]. * Ueber Vaccination und Revaccination. 32 pp. 8°. *Berlin, G. Lange*, [1872].

Muecke (Franciscus). * De ossium fungo medullari aneurysma simulante. 27 pp. 8°. *Gryphiæ, F. G. Kunike*, [1856].

Muecke (Georgius A.) [1823–]. *Analecta ad medicinam scholæ methodicæ. 26 pp., 1 l. 8°. *Vratislaviæ, E. Klein*, 1847.

Muecke (Joannes Henricus). * De persicaria acida Jungermanni. 26 pp. sm. 4°. *Halæ Magdeb., typ. J. C. Hilligeri*, [1735].

Mueckl (Gustav Adolph). *Ueber die Placenta prævia. 16 pp. 8°. *München, J. Deschler*, 1845.

Müehr (Ferdinandus Josephus). * De achoribus. 1 p. l., 32 pp., 2 l. 12°. *Budæ, typ. C. Landerer, viduæ*, [1783].

Muegel (Fridericus) [1818–]. * De diabete pathologia. 30 pp., 1 l. 8°. *Berolini, typ. Nietackianis*, [1840].

Mügge (Friedrich). * Ein Fall von Dermoidcyste des Ovarium. 41 pp. 8°. *Göttingen, Dieterich*, 1876.

Muehl (Gustave-Adolphe). * Sur le rachitisme. 1 p. l., 90 pp. 4°. *Strasbourg*, 1847, No. 174, v. 13.

Mühlbach (*Mart.*)
Portrait in: **Collection** of Portr. of Phys. & Men of Sc., 136.

Mühlbauer (Franz Xaver). * Ueber Transplantation der Cornea. 85 pp., 1 l. 8°. *München, Wild*, 1840.

———. Beitrag zur Lehre von den Blutcrasen vom pathologisch-anatomischen Standpunkte aus betrachtet. iv, 48 pp. 8°. *Erlangen, F. Enke*, 1845.

———. Die Lehre von der Percussion und Auscultation mit Berücksichtigung der pathologischen Anatomie der Brustorgane für den praktischen Arzt. viii, 90 pp. 8°. *Erlangen, F. Enke*, 1847.

———. The same. De leer der percussie en auscultatie met betrekking tot de pathologische anatomie der borstorganen, ten behoeve van practische artsen zamengesteld. Uit het Hoogduitsch vertaald en het aanteekeningen voorzien door Dr. C. Gobée. 1 p. l., 96 pp. 8°. *Leiden, J. H. Gebhard & Comp.*, 1847.

Mühlbauer (Josephus). * De ulceribus tractus intestinalis. 16 pp. 8°. *Monachii, J. Deschler*, 1839.

Mühlbaur (Francisco). * De hæmoptysi. 15 pp. 8°. *Augustæ Vindel., G. Geiger jun.*, 1839.

Mühlbaur (Maximilianus). * De statu morborum nosocomii Augustani sectionis chirurgicæ anno 1836–7. 19 pp. 8°. *Augustæ Vindel., G. Geiger*, 1837.

Mühle (F.) * Ein Fall von Anus præternaturalis und dessen Behandlung. 24 pp. 8°. *Erlangen, E. T. Jacob*, 1880.

Mühlebach (Friedrich). Beschreibung einer Dysenterie-Epidemie von 19 Fällen in der Gemeinde Mühlheim a. Bach. 26 pp., 1 pl. 8°. *Freiburg in Baden, H. M. Poppen u. Sohn*, 1877.

Mühlenbach ([Friedrich Wilhelm] Georg) [1854–]. * Zur Aetiologie und Statistik der phlyctänulären Augenentzündungen. 31 pp. 8°. *Greifswald, J. Abel*, 1878.

Mühlenbeck (H. Gustave). * Sur la docimasie pulmonaire. 1 p. l., 21 pp. 4°. *Strasbourg*, 1822, v. 50.

———. The same. 1 p. l., 21 pp. 4°. *Strasbourg, F.-G. Levrault*, 1822.

Mühlenbein (Carolus Georgius Fridericus). * De staphylomate scleroticæ. 44 pp., 1 pl. 8°. *Gottingæ, J. H. Meyer*, 1834.

Mühlenbein (*G. A. H.*) [1764–].
Portrait in: **Collection**—van Kaathoven.—**Collection** of Portr. (Libr.)

Mühlenthor (Joh.) Das Leben und Streben Samuel Hahnemanns, des Erfinders und Begründers der homöopathischen Irrlehre. Nach den besten Quellen geschildert. 35 pp. 8°. *Potsdam, H. Vogler*, 1834.

von Mühler.
See **Preussische** Pharmakopöe. 7. Ausg. 8°. *Berlin*, 1862.

Mühlfeld (*Eugen.*)
Portrait in: **Collection**—van Kaathoven.

Mühlhäuser (Friedr. Aug.) Ueber Epidemieen und Cholera, insbesondere über Cholera in Speier 1873. 2 p. l., 104 pp., 2 ch. 8°. *Mannheim, J. Schneider*, 1875.

Mühlhäuser (H.)
  See **Schaarschmidt** (U.) & **Mühlhäuser** (H.)
  S chulsanatorium Fridericianum zu Davos (Schweiz). 8°.
  [*Davos-Platz,* 1886.]

Mühlhaus (Albert). * Ueber Probepunktionen
und Punktionen bei Pleuritis exsudativa; Statistik der seit 1872 bis jetzt im Julius-Hospitale
zu Würzburg bei Pleuritis exsudativa zur Ausführung gekommenen Probepunktionen und
Punktionen. 49 pp. 8°. *Würzburg, Becker,*
1882.

Mühlhausen (Friderich). Iagttagelse om
Tobaksrøgens Nytte hos Druknede. 7 pp. 12°.
Kiøbenhavn, J. R. Thiele, [1776].

——. Pandebenet. En Prøve af et Forsøg paa en
fuldstændig og paa Chirurgien anvendt dansk
Beenlære. 8 pp. 12°. *Kiøbenhavn, J. R. Thiele,*
1778.

Mühlhausen (Godeschalcus). * De cruditate,
coctione et crisi. 47 pp. 4°. *Lugd. Bat., J.
Heyligert,* [1740].

Mühlhausen (Joseph). * Ueber die Behandlung des Lympho-Sarcom. 28 pp., 1 l. 8°.
Bonn, I. F. Carthaus, [1873].

Mühlhausen (Josephus Joh.) * De asthmate
thymico infantum. vi, 7–37 pp. 8°. *Lipsiæ,
typ. Breitkopfio-Haertelianis,* 1837.
  For Biography, see **Weber** (Ernestus Henricus).

Mühlibach (Nicolaus Theodorus). Inquisitio
optico-physiologica de visus sensu ; in qua, viso-
rum imaginem objectorum, perceptioni, situ haud
inverso, uti hucusque docuerunt, repræsentari,
plane evincitur. xiv, 15–80 pp. 8°. *Vindobonæ,
in bibliopolio Camesinano,* 1816.

Mühlig. Conférence sanitaire internationale.
Appendice au rapport de la commission des mesures hygiéniques. La désinfection appliquée
au choléra. Travail revu et approuvé par la
commission. 18 pp. fol. [*n. p* , 1866, *vel subseq.*]

Muehlmann (Carolus) [1821–   ]. * De partu
præmaturo artificiali. 29 pp., 1 l. 8°. *Berolini,
G. Schade,* 1845.

Muehlmann ([Carolus Gustavus] Adolphus).
[1800–   ]. * De graviditatis diagnosi sæpe
dubia. 43 pp. 8°. *Berolini, lit. A. Petschii,*
[1826].

Mühlpauer (Joannes Maximil. Josephus). * De
febre catarrhali passim hactenus epidemia. 16
pp. 4°. *Altorfii Noric., typ. J. G. Kohlesii,* [1730].

Mühlpfort (Joh. Adolphus). * Diss. phys.
quinta qua motus animalis e fundamentis genuinis erutus. 16 l. sm. 4°. *Wittenbergæ, typ. M.
Schultzii,* [1694].

Muehmler ([Joh. Ferdinand] Wilhelm) [1845–
    ]. * Beobachtungen über Typhus exanthema-
ticus. 24 pp. 8°. *Greifswald, F. W. Kunike,*
1868.
                                                C.

Mühry (Adalbertus Adolphus) [1811–   ]. Ad
parasitorum malignorum imprimis ad fungi medullaris oculi historiam symbolæ aliquot. viii,
48 pp., 4 pl. 4°. *Gottingæ, sumpt. Dieterichianis,*
1833.

——. Darstellung und Ansichten zur Vergleichung der Medicin in Frankreich, England und
Deutschland. Nach einer Reise in diesen Ländern im Jahre 1835. x, 283 pp., 2 pl. 12°. *Hannover, Hahn,* 1836.

——. The same. Observations on the compar-
ative state of medicine in France, England, and
Germany. Transl. from the German by Edward
G. Davis, M. D. 126 pp. 8°. *Philadelphia, A.
Waldie,* 1838.

——. Ueber die historische Unwandelbarkeit
der Natur und der Krankheiten. 50 pp. 16°.
Hannover, Hahn, 1844.

——. Die geographischen Verhältnisse der
Krankheiten, oder Grundzüge der Noso-Geogra-
phie, in ihrer Gesammtheit und Ordnung und mit

Mühry (Adalbertus Adolphus)—continued.
einer Sammlung der Thatsachen dargelegt. 1.
Thl. Allgemeine Gesetze und Lehren der Noso-
Geographie. 2. Thl. Thesaurus noso-geographi-
cus, oder geordnete Sammlung noso-geographi-
scher Berichte, mit hinzugefügten Commenta-
tionen. 2 v. in 1. xiv, 224 pp. ; x, 284 pp., 1 map.
8°. *Leipzig u. Heidelberg, C. F. Winter,* 1856.

——. Klimatologische Untersuchungen, oder
Grundzüge der Klimatologie in ihrer Beziehung
auf die Gesundheits-Verhältnisse der Bevölke-
rungen. Mit einer geographisch geordneten, die
gesammte Erde umfassenden Sammlung klima-
tographischer Schilderungen. 2 Abth. xviii (2
l.), 816 pp., 2 pl. 8°. *Leipzig u. Heidelberg, C.
F. Winter,* 1858.

——. Klimatographische Uebersicht der Erde,
in einer Sammlung authentischer Berichte, mit
hinzugefügten Anmerkungen, zu wissenschaftli-
chem und zu praktischem Gebrauch. Mit einem
Appendix. xvi, 744 pp. 8°. *Leipzig u. Heidelberg, G. F. Winter,* 1862.

——. Untersuchungen über die Theorie und das
allgemeine geographische System der Winde.
Ein Beitrag zur Begründung einer rationellen
Lehre von den Luftströmen, für den Gebrauch
der Klimatologie und der Nautik. xvi, 253 pp.,
1 map. 8°. *Göttingen, Vandenhoeck u. Ruprecht,*
1869.
  See, also, **Mühry** (Carl). Medicinische Fragmente.
  8°. *Hannover,* 1841.—**Petermann** (A.), **von Freeden**
  (W.) & **Mühry** (A.) Papers on the eastern and northern extensions of the Gulf stream [etc.] 4°. *Washington,*
  1871.

Mühry (Carl) [1806–40]. Medicinische Fragmente betreffend eine allgemeine Lehre des See-
bodens und der Seebäder und die Identitätsfrage
der Kuhpocken und Menschenpocken. Hrsg. mit
einigen Zusätzen von Adolph Mühry. xvi, 168
pp., 2 tab. 8°. *Hannover, Hahn,* 1841.

Muehry (Ed. Ch. A.)
  Co-Editor of: **Hannoversche** Annalen für die gesammte Heilkunde, 1844–6.

Muehry (Georg. Carol.) De spinæ dorsi distor-
sionibus et pede equino. Disquisitio patholo-
gico-therapeutica. 60 pp., 3 tab. 4°. *Gottingæ,
typ. Dieterichianis,* 1829.

Mühry (Georgius Fridericus). * De aëris fixi
inspirati usu in phthisi pulmonali. 3 p. l., 68 pp.
4°. *Gottingæ, J. C. Dieterich,* [1796].

——. Rathschläge und Vorsichtsregeln, seinen
Mitbürgern gegen die bevorstehende Cholera zur
Beachtung empfohlen. 16 pp. 12°. *Hannover,
Gebr. Jänecke,* 1831.
  See, also, **Niemeyer** (Ludwig Heinrich Christian).
  Materialien zur Erregungstheorie. 8°. *Göttingen,* 1800.—
  Portal (Anton). Beobachtungen über die Natur und
  Behandlung der Lungenschwindsucht. 2 v. in 1. 8°.
  Hannover, 1799–1802.

Muehsam (Eduardus) [1840–   ]. * De effectu
acidi sulphurici in organismum, imprimis in renes. 32 pp. 8°. *Berolini, H. S. Hermann,*
[1862].

Mühsam (Josef) [1852–   ]. * Fünf Fälle von
Meningitis tuberculosa. 32 pp. 8°. *Berlin, M.
Niethe,* [1874].

Mühsam (Siegfried). Apotheken-Manual. Anleitung zur Herstellung von in den Apotheken
gebräuchlichen Präparaten, welche in der Pharmacopœa Germanica, Editio altera, keine Aufnahme gefunden haben. 2. Aufl. 157 pp. 8°.
Leipzig, Denicke, 1885.

——— & **Baginsky** (A.) Die Hausapotheke,
enthaltend die unentbehrlichen Hausmittel. 28
pp., 2 l. 8°. *Berlin, Denicke,* [1875, *vel subseq.*].

Mükisch (S. A.) Beyträge zur Kenntniss des
kindlichen Organismus. viii, 316 pp. 8°. *Wien,
C. Gerold,* 1825.

Muel (Jean-François-Octave). * Sur la dysenterie. 17 pp. 4°. *Paris,* 1836, No. 105, v. 297.

Mülberger (Arthur). * Ueber Geschwülste im Becken und ihren Einfluss auf den Verlauf der Geburt. [Tübingen.] 40 pp. 8°. *Stuttgart, C. F. Cotta's Erben, 1872.*

Mülberger (Friederich). * Ueber die Bedeutung der Irrenanstalten zur Verhütung des Selbstmordes der Geisteskranken. 32 pp. 8°. *Würzburg, Becker, 1886.*

Mülberger (Georgius Fridericus). Schediasma physicum de montibus. 20 pp. 4°. *Argentorati, typ. J. H. Heitzii,* [1736].

Müldner (Josephus). * De meteorismo intestinali. 32 pp. 8°. *Pragæ, T. Thabor,* 1838.

Mülenfeld (J.) * O peptonach voloknini. 27 pp. 8°. *St. Petersburg,* 1872.

Mülerius (*Nicolaus*) [1564-1630].
Portrait in: **Collection** of Portr. of Phys. & Men of Sc., 195.

Mülerius (*Petrus*) [1590-1647].
Portrait in: **Collection** of Portr. of Phys. & Men of Sc., 195.

Mülhäuser (Heinrich).
See **Schaarschmidt** (Ulrich) & **Mülhäuser** (Heinrich). Schulsanitorium für Knaben Fridericianum zu Davos-Platz (Schweiz). 8°. [*Berlin,* 1887.]

Mülhausen. Erneuert und verbesserte Medicinal, Apothecker, Chirurgorum, und andere dahin gehörige Ordnungen, etc., samt beygefügt-revidirter Taxa, derer in hiesigen privilegirten Apothecken befindlicher Waaren und Artzeneyen, auch selbigen ertheiltes Privilegium, etc. Eines hochedlen und hochweisen Raths der käyserlichen Freyen- und des Heiligen Reichs-Stadt Mühlhausen in Thüringen R. R. Zu jedermanns Wissenschaft und Nachricht von neuem in den Druck gegeben. 14 l. sm. 4°. *Mühlhausen, M. Käyser,* 1715. [P., v. 1411.]

———. Revidirte und erneuerte Apotheker-Taxa aller Medicamenten, Materialen, Specereien und Waaren, welche man bey denen privilegirten und geschwornen Apothekern in der käyserlichen Reichs-Stadt Mühlhausen zu Kauffe findet. 3 p. l., 95 pp., 14 l. sm. 4°. *Mühlhausen, M. Käyser,* 1715. [P., v. 1411.]
German and Latin text.

Mülhausen.
See, also, **Diphtheria** (*History of*).
Hack (C.) Statistische Mittheilungen über die Stadt Mülhausen 1873-5. 8°. *Mülhausen i. E.,* 1877.
Kestner (G.) Die Wasserversorgung der Stadt Mülhausen. Arch. f. öff. Gsndhtspflg., Strassb., 1887, xii, 70-98.—Kochlin (J.) & Kestner. Witterung und Sterblichkeit in Mülhausen während der Jahre 1875, 1876 u. 1877. *Ibid.,* 1876, i, 129: 1877, ii, 151: 1878, iii, 82.

Mülheim-am-Rhein, *Prussia.*
d'Alquen. Beiträge zu einer näheren Darstellung der Krankheits-Constitution des verflossenen Jahres 1825, zunächst in der Stadt und Umgegend von Mülheim am Rhein, mit vorzugsweiser Berücksichtigung der letzteren Jahres-Hälfte. N. Jahrb. d. teutsch. Med. u. Chir., Hamm, 1826, xii, 117–139.

Mülich (Joannes Fridericus). * De variolarum insitione modesta epicrisis. 16 pp. sm. 4°. *Altorfii Noricorum, typ. M. D. Meyeri,* [1723].

Müller.
See **Établissement** hydrothérapique de Bretiège près d'Anet, canton de Berne. [Circular.] 4°. *Berne,* 1843.

Mueller.
Co-Editor of: **Correspondenzblatt** für die Aerzte und Apotheker des Grossherzogthums Oldenburg, Oldenburg, 1860-65.

Müller (A.) * Drei Fälle von Hydrops ovarii. 30 pp. 8°. *Rostock, C. Boldt,* 1857.

Müller (Achatius). * De astrobolismo. 73 pp. 4°. *Francof. ad Viadr., J. Coepfelius,* [1690].

Mueller (Adam). * Ueber Alkoholismus im Allgemeinen und sein Vorkommen und seine Behandlung in der Greifswalder medicinischen

Mueller (Adam)—continued.
Klinik im Besonderen. 50 pp. 8°. *Greifswald, F. Hache,* 1868. c.

Mueller (Adam-P.) * Sur le traitement des tumeurs blanches. 59 pp. 4°. *Strasbourg,* 1853, No. 300, 2. s., v, 19.

Mueller (Adamus) [1835-]. * De struma. 29 pp., 1 l. 8°. *Halis Sax., typ. orphanotrophei,* 1862. c.

Mueller (Adolf). * Ueber 176 Fälle von Tyfuserkrankungen im Augsburger Krankenhaus während des Jahres 1869. 27 pp. 8°. *Erlangen, E. T. Jacob,* 1870.

Müller (Adolphus) [1813-]. * De chorea S. Viti. 24 pp., 2 l. 8°. *Berolini, typ. fratrum Schlesinger,* [1837].

Müller (Adolphus Adalbertus) [1806-]. * De dentitione prima. 29 pp. 8°. *Berolini, lit. A. Petschii,* [1828].

Müller (Adolphus Ferdinand) [1804-]. * De ratione, quæ morbos inter et ætates diversas intercedat. 31 pp. 8°. *Berolini, lit. A. Petschii,* [1828].

Müller (Alb.) Nachtrag zur Kenntniss der Wirkungen der Weissenburg-Therme im Simmenthal, Kanton Bern. 22 pp. 8°. *Bern, Stämpf,* 1872.

———. Weissenburg in Brustkrankheiten und speziell bei Lungenphthise. 22 pp. 8°. *Bern, Stämpf,* 1875.

———. * Statistische Beiträge zur Beleuchtung der Hereditätsverhältnisse bei der Lungenschwindsucht. 37 pp. 8°. *Bern, H. Körber,* 1876.

———. * Beitrag zur Lehre von der traumatischen Cataract. [Basel.] 55 pp. 8°. *Solothurn, J. Gassmann Sohn,* 1883.

Mueller (Albert W.) * Ueber Pulver-Verbrennung mit letalem Ausgang. 20 pp. 8°. *Leipzig, J. Klinkhardt,* 1870.

Mueller (Albertus) [1805-]. * De usu vesicantium. 28 pp. 4°. *Lipsiæ, typ. Staritzii,* [1830].
For Biography, see **Haase** (Guilielmus Andreas).

Müller (Alexander)[1]. Das Complementär-Colorimeter. Ausführlicheres über Construction und Anwendung desselben für Chemiker, Hüttenprobirer, Metallurgen, Pharmaceuten, Coloristen, Physiker, Meteorologen u. s. w. 32 pp., 1 pl. 8°. *Chemnitz, G. Ernesti,* 1854. [P., v. 1501.]

Mueller (Alexander)[2]. Die Ziele und Mittel einer gesundheitlichen und wirthschaftlichen Reinhaltung der Wohnungen, besonders der städtischen. 89 pp. 8°. *Dresden, C. A. Werner,* 1869.

Mueller (Alfredus [Georgius Carolus]) [1842-]. * De peritonitide acuta, præcipue ex perforatione orta. 31 pp. 8°. *Berolini, G. Schade,* [1866].

Mueller (Alwin). * Der Mittelohrkatarrh und dessen Behandlungsweisen. 15 pp. 8°. *Leipzig, C. G. Naumann,* [1870]. [P., v. 361.]

Müller (Andreas Christoph). Paralysin. 16 l. 4°. [*Wittebergæ*], *lit. Meyerianis,* [1670].

Mueller (Andreas Hadrianus Valentinus Fridericus) [1798-]. * De perforatione calli præternaturalis ossis femoris atque de curatione articuli spurii et spinæ ventosæ per setaceum cuneiforme. 20 pp., 2 l. 8°. *Halæ, formis Schimmelpfennigianis,* [1826]. [*Also, in:* P., v. 139.]

Müller (Anton) [-1827]. Die Irren-Anstalt in dem königlichen Julius-Hospitale zu Würzburg und die sechs und zwanzigjährigen ärztlichen Dienstverrichtungen an derselben. Mit einem Anhange von Krankengeschichten und Sektions-Berichten. Ein Wort zu seiner Zeit. xiv, 280 pp., 1 l. 8°. *Würzburg, Stahel,* 1824.

Müller (Anton Benjamin). * De locis in ischuria adfectis. 36 pp. 8°. *Halæ, typ. Trampianis,* [1791, *vel subseq.*].

Mueller (Antonius)[1]. *Diss. experimenta circa chylum sistens. 64 pp. 8°. *Heidelbergæ, J. Engelmanni,* 1819.

Müller (Antonius)[2]. *Diss. sistens adnotationes ætiologicas de phthisi pulmonali apud sexum sequiorem. 30 pp., 2 l. 8°. *Halis Sax., typ. Grunerti patris filiique,* [1820].

Mueller (Arminius)[1]. *De insania puerperarum. 2 p. l., 54 pp. 8°. *Gryphiæ, F. G. Kunike,* 1834.

Mueller (Arminius)[2]. *De valgi pedis ætiologia quædam. 24 pp., 2 l. 8°. *Wolgastiæ, F. Elsner,* 1846.

Müller (August)[1] [1810–75]. Verzeichniss der naturhistorischen und medicinischen Bücher aus dem Nachlasse August Müller's, Professors der Anatomie zu Königsberg in Pr. vi, 264 pp. 8°. *Glogau, E. Mosche,* 1876.

Müller (August)[2]. *Die Ornis der Insel Salanga, sowie Beiträge zur Ornithologie der Halbinsel Malakka. Eine zoogeographische Studie. [Erlangen.] 96 pp., 2 tab. 8°. *Naumburg a. S., G. Pätz,* 1882.

Müller (August)[3].
See **Ibn Abi Usaibi'a.** Hrsg. von August Müller. roy. 8°. *Königsberg i. Pr,* 1884.

Müller (August F.) Supplement to the Catalogue raisonné of the medical library of the Pennsylvania Hospital. pp. 713–810. 8°. *Philadelphia, Collins,* 1867.

Mueller (Augustus) [1818–]. *De ossificatione retinæ aliarumque oculi partium. 32 pp., 2 l. 8°. *Halis, formis expr. Ploetzianis,* 1843.

Mueller (Augustus [Henricus]) [1840–]. *De scarlatina. 31 pp. 8°. *Berolini, G. Schade,* [1865].

Müller (Barwardus Joh.) *De vita longa. 20 pp. 4°. *Rintelii, J. G. Enax,* [1721].

Mueller ([Benjamin Carolus] Leopoldus) [1824–]. *De liquido cerebro-spinali. 31 pp. 8°. *Berolini, G. Schade,* [1847].

Müller (Benjaminus). *Diss. qua uterus gravidus physiologice et pathologice consideratus exposita simul ejusdem structura sinuosa ac orificiorum menses et lochia fundentium fabrica. 32 pp., 1 pl. 4°. *Witebergæ, lit. viduæ Gerdesiæ,* [1725].

Mueller (Bernhardus Josephus). *De lithiasi et lithotomia. 29 pp. 8°. *Vratislaviæ, H. Lindner,* [1856]. [Also, in: P., v. 295.]

Müller (Bonaventura). *De inflammatione. 9 l. sm. 4°. *Lipsiæ, lit. Wittigavianis,* [1686].

Mueller (C.)[1] Einige Bemerkungen über die asiatische Cholera für Aerzte nach eigener Erfahrung gesammelt auf einer zur Beobachtung des Uebels unternommenen Reise. 47 pp. 8°. *Hannover, Lamminger,* 1848.
See, also, **Ophthalmologische** (Der) Congress zu Brüssel 1857. 8°. *Hannover,* 1858.

Mueller (C.)[2]
Co-Editor of : **Mittheilungen** aus der thierärztlichen Praxis im preussischen Staate, Berlin, 1874–6.
See, also, **Gurlt** (Ernestus Fridericus). Handbuch der vergleichenden Anatomie [etc.] roy. 8°. *Berlin,* 1873.

Mueller (C. F.)
Co-Editor of : **Archiv** für wissenschaftliche und practische Thierheilkunde, Berlin, 1875.

Müller (C. W.) Zur Einleitung in die Elektrotherapie. xii, 187 pp. 8°. *Wiesbaden, J. F. Bergmann,* 1885.

CONTENTS.
I. Nothwendigkeit, Möglichkeit und Bedingungen einer sicheren Strommessung. Das absolute astatische Vertical-Galvanometer.
II. Präcisere Bestimmung der Stromstärke für die elektrotherapeutische Praxis in Form der Stromdichte.

Müller (Carl). *Ueber die künstliche Frühgeburt. 78 pp. 8°. *Würzburg, C. W. Becker,* 1837.

Mueller (Carl Albert). *Ueber Wesen und Behandlung des Tetanus. 1 p. l., 16 pp. 8°. *Leipzig, C. G. Naumann,* [1866].

Müller (Carl Friedr. Otto). *Ueber tuberculöse Sehnenscheidenentzündung. 22 pp. 8°. *Würzburg, C. W. Becker,* 1887.

Mueller (Carl Friedrich)[1]. *Versuche über den Verlauf der Netzhautermüdung. 32 pp., 1 pl. 8°. *Zürich, Zürcher u. Furrer,* 1866.

Müller (Carl Friedrich)[2]. *Ueber das Vorkommen von Eisen im Harn bei verschiedenen Krankheiten und nach der Zufuhr von Eisenpräparaten. 15 pp. 8°. *Erlangen, Junge u. Sohn,* 1882.

Müller (Carl Hermann Alfred) [1844–]. *Ueber Luftathmen der Frucht während des Geburtsacts, nebst Mittheilung eines dahin einschlagenden Falles. 29 pp., 1 l. 8°. *Marburg, C. L. Pfeil,* 1869.

Mueller (Carl Wilhelm). *Die vitale Lungencapacität und ihre diagnostische Verwerthung. 52 pp. 8°. *Leipzig, E. Polz,* 1868.
Repr. from : Ztschr. f. rat. Med., Leipz., 1868, xxiii.

Mueller (Carolus)[1] [1806–]. *Diss. sistens monstri humani rarissimi descriptionem. 1 p. l., 26 pp., 1 pl. 8°. *Halis Sax., typ. Schimmelpfinnigianis,* [1831].

Müller (Carolus)[2]. *Tractatus de aqua Püllnaensi. 3 p. l., 36 pp., 2 l. 8°. *Pragæ, typ. filiorum T. Haase,* 1834.

——. Das Pullnaer Bitterwasser in kurzer Uebersicht. 30 pp., 1 l. 12°. *Wien, J. P. Sollinger,* 1844.

——. The same. Les eaux minérales de Püllna. 35 pp. 12°. *Vienne, J.-P. Sollinger,* [1843].

Müller (Carolus)[3]. *De placenta prævia. 33 pp. 12°. *Dorpati, typ. J. C. Schünmanni,* 1835.

Mueller (Carolus)[4] [1829–]. *De pulmonum hæmorrhagia. 28 pp., 2 l. 8°. *Berolini, F. Schlesinger,* [1855].

Mueller (Carolus Antonius) [1836–]. *De cornibus cutaneis. 31 pp., 1 pl. 8°. *Gryphiæ, F. Hache,* 1861.
C.

Müller (Carolus Augustus)[1]. *De vitiis lactis humani eorumque medela. 1 p. l., 39 pp. 4°. *Jenæ, lit. J. C. Croekeri,* 1746.

Müller (Carolus Augustus)[2]. *De notione et pretio cognitionis medico-empiricæ specimen. 22 pp. 4°. *Lipsiæ, ex off. Klaubarthia,* [1802].
For Biography, see **Platner** (Ernestus).

Mueller (Carolus Frid.) *Diss. sistens delineationem morborum intestini recti et præsertim carcinomatis intestini recti. 32 pp. 4°. *Tubingæ, typ. Schoenhardtianis,* [1827].

Mueller (Carolus Frider. Guil.) *De chorea Sancti Viti. 27 pp., 1 l. 8°. *Jenæ, typ. Schlotteri,* 1839.

Mueller (Carolus Fridericus Gustavus). *De diagnosi coxariorum morborum graviorum. 27 pp. 8°. *Lipsiæ, ex off. O. Leiner,* 1846.
C.

Mueller (Carolus Guilelmus) [1816–]. *De sympathia contagiosa. 40 pp., 1 l. 8°. *Berolini, typ. Nietackianis,* [1839].

Mueller (Carolus Hermannus). *De singulari in puerperarum pudendis exulceratione. 24 pp. 4°. *Lipsiæ, ex off. Breitkopfio-Haerteliana,* [1828].
For Biography, see **Kuehn** (Carolus Gottlob).

Müller (Carolus Joannes Georgius). *Analecta in pathologiam et therapiam bubonum venereorum. 63 pp. 8°. *Dorpati, ex off. J. C. Schünmanni,* 1820.

Müller (Carolus Josephus). *De prognosi apoplexiæ. 40 pp. 8°. *Halæ, typ. J. C. Hendelii,* 1792.

Mueller (Carolus Julius Maximilianus) [1834–]. *De curatione vulnerum sclopetariorum artuum ossibus illatorum. 35 pp. 8°. *Berolini, G. Schade,* [1859].

Mueller (Carolus Mauritius). * De pneumonia infantium. 24 pp. 4°. *Lipsiæ, typ. G. Staritzii,* [1843].

For Biography, see **Clarus** (Jo. Christ. Aug.)

Müller (Casparus). * De tussi. 30 pp., 2 l. 12°. *Moguntiæ, apud J. J. A. hæred. Hæffner,* [1784].

Müller (Christian). Analyse de la source sulfureuse de Heustrich dans l'Oberland bernois, avec des notices sur d'autres eaux sulfureuses de la Suisse. 30 pp. 8°. *Aarau, E. Albrecht,* 1867.

——. Anleitung zur Prüfung der Kuhmilch. 3. Aufl. 1 p. l., 86 pp., 2 tab. 8°. *Bern, Haller,* 1872.

Mueller (Christian F.) * Ein Beitrag zur chirurgischen Pathologie der Vena femoralis. 38 pp., 1 l. 8°. *Leipzig, O. Wigand,* 1868. [P., v. 298.]

Müller (Christian Gottlieb). * Dysenteriam ex principiis chemiæ sublimioris perlustratam . . . proponit. 36 pp. 4°. *Halæ Magdeb., apud J. C. Hendelii vid.,* [1764].

Müller ([Christian Gustav] Wilhelm) [1857–]. * Beitrag zur Kenntniss der Fortpflanzung und der Geschlechtsverhältnisse der Ostracoden, nebst Beschreibung einer neuen Species der Gattung Cypris. 26 pp., 1 l., 2 pl. 8°. *Greifswald, C. Sell,* 1880.

Mueller (Christianus Fridericus) [1799–]. * Diss. de hydrargyro muriatico corrosivo. 36 pp., 1 l. 8°. *Halæ, typ. F. A. Grunerti patris fil.,* [1825].

Müller (Christianus Godofredus). * De angina polyposa seu membranacea. 24 pp. 4°. *Vitebergæ, lit. hæred. C. H. Graesleri,* [1814].

Müller (Christoph). * Versuche über die physiologischen Wirkungen des Toluchinoxalins und des Chinolins. 23 pp. 8°. *Erlangen, Junge u. Sohn,* 1885.

Müller (Clotar). * De febre inflammatoria, quæstionum ante hos viginti quinque annos a patre Mauricio Guilielmo Müllero propositarum pars altera. 23 pp. 8°. *Lipsiæ, typ. F. Ruckmanni,* [1835].

Müller (Clotar Moriz) [–1877]. * De juglandis regiæ viribus. 31 pp. 8°. *Lipsiæ, typ. F. A. Brockhausii,* [1843].

——. Systematisch-alphabetisches Repertorium der gesammten homöopathischen Arzneimittellehre nach den sämmtlichen Aeltern und bis auf die neuste Zeit herab genau zusammengestellten Quellen der Pharmakodynamik. viii, 944 pp. 8°. *Leipzig, T. O. Weigel,* 1848.

——. Die Homöopathie, oder die Reform der Heilkunde. Eine Darstellung der Grundsätze und Lehren der Homöopathie mit ausführlicher Angabe ihres Verfahrens zur Heilung der Krankheiten. xiv, 186 pp. 8°. *Leipzig, O. Wigand,* 1854.

——. Die Quellen der Arzneimittellehre. Eine kritische Beleuchtung der herrschenden Ansichten. Zur Beherzigung für Aerzte jeder Richtung. viii, 117 pp. 8°. *Leipzig, C. F. Fleischer,* 1860. [Also, in : P., v. 1458.]

——. Der homöopathische Haus- und Familienarzt. Eine Darstellung der Grundsätze und Lehren der Homöopathie zur Heilung der Krankheiten. 6. Aufl. xvi, 220 pp. 8°. *Leipzig, O. Wigand,* 1867.

——. Die Homöopathie in Amerika und der Welt-Congress in Philadelphia. 53 pp. 8°. *Leipzig, W. Schwabe,* 1876.

Repr. from : Internat. homöop. Presse, Leipz., 1875–6, vi–vii.

Also, Co-Editor of : **Homöopathische** Vierteljahresschrift, Leipzig, 1850–61. Also, Editor of : **Internationale** homöopathische Presse, Leipzig, 1872–7.

Müller (Conradus Guilielmus Augustus). * Diss. observationes medicas et chirurgicas conti-

Müller (Conradus Guilielmus Augustus)—cont. nens. xx pp. 4°. *Helmstadii, C. G. Fleckeisen,* [1798].

Müller (Daniel). Ausführlicher und warhaffter Bericht von den Rathmanusdorffischen nahe bey Stassfurth gelegenen Wunder-Heil und Gesund-Brunen, in welchen zu finden: I. Desselben Ursprung und Anfang. II. Die Natur und Würckung, welche sowohl aus einem gelehrten Judicio Medico, als grosser Anzahl glückl. curirter desperater Patienten erwiesen wird. III. Eine dienliche Art und Methode denselben nützlich zu gebrauchen. IV. Ein Entwurff des Gottesdiensts, nebst dem besondern Brunnen-Gebet. Auff wiederholtes Verlangen zur fernern Ausbreitung, göttlicher Ehre und seinen Neben-Christen zum Nutz entworffen. 30 pp. sm. 4°. *Leipzig, C. Hendler,* 1701.

Müller (Daniel). * De caussis quare ingens Europæorum multitudo præmatura morte Bataviæ pereat ; et de mali hujus remediis. 37 pp., 1 l. 12°. *Gottingæ, H. M. Grape,* [1798].

Müller (Daniel Traugott). Pietatem primum esse officiorum a doctore scholastico observandorum comprobat. 16 pp. 4°. *Dresdæ, typ. Harpeterianæ viduæ,* [1765].

Müller (Daniele). * De therapeutis sententiæ nuper defensæ maxime opposita. 39 pp. 4°. *Lipsiæ, lit. Schedianis,* [1724].

Müller (Detlef). * Ueber Echinococcus. [Wurtzburg.] 25 pp. 8°. *Glogau, E. Mosche,* 1885.

Mueller (E. H. Th.) * Der einfache chronische Katarrh des Mittelohres. 31 pp. 4°. *Kiel, C. F. Mohr,* 1868.

In : SCHRIFT. d. Univ. zu Kiel, xv, 1868, vii, Med. xi.

Mueller (Eberhard). * Ein Beitrag zur Lehre von der sogenannten Pseudoleukämie. [Tübingen.] 1 p. l., 33 pp. 8°. *Berlin, J. Sittenfeld,* 1867.

Müller (Eduard)[1]. * Ueber primäres Blasencarcinom. 23 pp. 4°. *Kiel, C. F. Mohr,* 1878.

In : SCHRIFT. d. Univ. zu Kiel, xxv, 1878, vii, Med. xvii.

Müller (Eduard)[2] [1857–]. * Ein Uterusfibroid mit Verkalkungen. 16 pp., 1 l., 1 pl. 8°. *Marburg, C. L. Pfeil,* 1882.

Müller (Eduard)[3]. Die Hochschule Bern in den Jahren 1834–84. Festschrift zur fünfzigsten Jahresfeier ihrer Stiftung. v, 227 pp. 8°. *Bern, K. J. Wyss,* 1884.

Mueller (Eduard Heinrich) [1809–75]. * De ustionibus. 55 pp. 8°. *Berolini, typ. frat. Unger,* [1831].

——. Entwurf einer medicinisch-topographischen Skizze der Stadt Stettin. vi, 145 pp., 1 tab. 8°. *Berlin,* 1843.

——. Mittheilungen über die Choleraepidemie zu Berlin im Jahre 1850, in statistischer und sanitätspolizeilicher Beziehung. 58 pp. 8°. [*Berlin,* 1851.]

——. Die Quarantaine gegen das gelbe Fieber. 42 pp. 8°. [*Berlin,* 1853, vel subseq.]

——. Die Cholera-Epidemie in Berlin im Jahre 1855. 86 pp. 8°. *Berlin,* 1856.

Repr. from : Ann. d. Char.-Krankenh. . . . zu Berl., 1856, vii, 1–86.

——. Die Cholera-Epidemie zu Berlin im Jahre 1866. Amtlicher Bericht erstattet im Auftrage der kön. Sanitäts-Commission. vi, 160 pp., 1 map. 4°. *Berlin, T. C. F. Enslin,* 1867.

——. Ueber Pockenimpfung und über die Bedeutung der Glycerinlymphe für die öffentliche Gesundheitspflege. 26 pp. 8°. *Berlin, J. Sittenfeld,* 1869.

Repr. from : Vrtljschr. f. gerichtl. u. öff. Med., Berl , 1869, n. F., xi.

——. Berlin's Sanitätswesen. Ein Führer für Fremde und Einheimische. viii, 141 pp. 12°. *Berlin, T. C. F. Enslin,* 1870.

Mueller (Eduard Heinrich)—continued.

———. Die Cholera-Epidemie zu Berlin im Jahre 1873. Amtlicher Bericht. 1 p. l., 58 pp. fol. *Berlin, T. C. F. Enslin,* 1874.

Also, Co-Editor of : **Archiv** der deutschen Medicinal-gesetzgebung und öffentlichen Gesundheitspflege, Erlangen, 1857–9. *Also, Editor of :* **Preussische** Medicinal-Zeitung, Berlin, 1861-4.

Mueller (Eduardus Albert) [1815–   ]. * De colica saturnina. 33 pp., 1 l. 8°. *Berolini, typ. fratrum Schlesinger,* [1839].

Mueller (Eduardus Theodorus). * De resectione ossium carpi et metacarpi. [Leipsic.] 22 pp., 1 l. 8°. *Misniæ, C. Cato,* 1852.   c.

Müller (Emil). * Zur Casuistik der Hirntumoren. 51 pp. 8°. [*Dorpat*], *H. Laakmann,* 1869.

Müller (Émile). * De la grossesse utérine prolongée indéfiniment, ou rétention illimitée de l'œuf dans la matrice (missed labour des Anglais). 1 p. l., 171 pp. 4°. *Nancy,* 1877, 1. s., No. 51.

———. The same. Ouvrage couronné par la Faculté de médecine de Nancy. 176 pp. 4°. *Paris, J.-B. Baillière,* 1878.

Mueller (Enno Rudolph). * De vexis artis medicæ præcipuis. 4 p. l., 52 pp., 1 l. 4°. *Halæ Magdeb., typ. J. C. Hilligeri,* [1740].

Müller (Erich). * Ueber einen Fall von multiplen Fibromata mollusca und artificieller Elephantiasis Arabum. 36 pp. 8°. *Würzburg, Bonitas-Bauer,* [1882].

Mueller (Ernestus). * De angina membranacea, asthmate Millari et tussi convulsiva. 48 pp. 8°. [*Dorpat*], *typ. J. C. Schuenmanni,* 1833.

Mueller (Ernestus [Carolus Bernardus]) [1819–   ]. * De diabete. 30 pp., 1 l. 8°. *Berolini, typ. Nietackianis,* [1845].

Müller (Ernestus Guilelmus Ludovicus) [1792–   ]. * De scarificatione et cucurbitulis. 3 p. l., 35 pp. 8°. *Berolini, ex off. Starckiana,* [1817].

Müller (Ernst)[1]. * Ueber das Auftreten der constitutionellen Syphilis im Darmkanale. 22 pp. 8°. *Erlangen, A. E. Junge,* 1858.

Müller (Ernst)[2]. * Untersuchungen über die Ausscheidung des Quecksilbers durch den Harn während der Inunctionscur. [Erlangen.] 23 pp. 8°. *Hameln, G. F. Becker,* 1879.

Müller (Ernst)[3]. * Beitrag zur Casuistik der menschlichen Missgeburten. [Tübingen.] 16 pp., 1 pl. 8°. *Leipzig, A. T. Engelhardt,* 1881.

———. Die Hasenscharten der Tübinger chirurgischen Klinik in den Jahren 1843–1885. 1 p. l., 89 pp., 2 pl. 8°. *Tübingen, H. Laupp,* 1886.

Repr. from : BRUNS (P.) Beiträge zur klinischen Chirurgie. 8°. *Tübingen,* 1886, ii.

Müller (Eugen). * Ueber die intracapsuläre Exstirpation der Kropfcysten. 24 pp., 1 l. 8°. *Tübingen, H. Laupp jun.,* 1885.

von Mueller (Ferdinand) Baron. *See* **Von Mueller** (Ferdinand).

Mueller (Ferdinand). * Ueber Typhus exanthematicus. 38 pp., 1 l., 3 tab. 8°. *Jena, A. Neuenhahn,* 1868.

Mueller (Ferdinand Adolph Heinrich Joseph). Ueber das Gesichts-Aeussere nach seiner Fülle, Farbe und Temperatur im krankhaften Zustande des menschlichen Organismus. 45 pp. 8°. *Tübingen,* 1833.

———. Einige worte über die Heilsysteme von Broussais, Rasori und Hahnemann. Eine Vorlesung. 12 pp. 8°. *Zürich, O. Füssli u. Comp.,* 1834.

Mueller (Ferdinandus Augustus) [1816–   ]. * De delirio tremente. 35 pp. 8°. *Gryphiæ, F. G. Kunike,* [1841].

Müller (Franciscus)[1]. * De caussis perturbati catameniorum profluvii, et huic pedisequa chlorosi addita sparsim therapia. vii, 9–51 pp. 12°. *Pragæ,* [*F. Gerzabek*], 1817.

Müller (Franciscus)[1]—continued.

———. Vitæ vivendæ ratio in gratiam Caroli quarti a magistro gallo medico et mathematico conscripta. Cui adnexa est lucubraciuncula sistens præstantiam et utilitatem scientiæ artis medicæ, indolemque medicorum. 62 pp., 1 l. 8°. *Pragæ, typ. Schollensis,* [1819].

Mueller (Franciscus)[2] [1811–   ]. * De ictero. 40 pp. 8°. *Berolini, typ. Nietackianis,* 1837.

Müller (Franciscus)[3]. * Diss. sistens tractatum de carcinomate. 30 pp., 1 l. 8°. *Pragæ, A. Spinka,* 1842.

Mueller (Franciscus Henricus) [1812–   ]. * De variis pulmonum hæmorrhagiis. 32 pp. 8°. *Berolini, G. Lange,* [1865].

Mueller (Franz)[1]. Lehrbuch der Anatomie der Haussäugethiere, mit besonderer Berücksichtigung des Pferdes, und physiologischen Bemerkungen. 2. Aufl. xiii, 551 pp. roy. 8°. *Wien, W. Braumüller,* 1871.

Also, Co-Editor of: **Vierteljahresschrift** für wissenschaftliche Veterinärkunde, Wien, 1851–62. — **Oesterreichische** Vierteljahrsschrift für wissenschaftliche Veterinärkunde, Wien, 1863.

Müller (Franz)[2]. Exploration des cavités naturelles du corps humain par la lumière électrique. 16 pp. 8°. *Paris, Yves. Renou, Maulde & Cock,* 1879.

Imperfect; wants pp. 8–9.

Repr. from : J. Union méd. autrichienne, Vienne, 1er juillet 1879.

———. Die acute atrophische Spinallähmung der Erwachsenen (Poliomyelitis anterior acuta). Eine klinische Studie. 2 p. l., 105 pp., 1 pl. 8°. *Stuttgart, F. Enke,* 1880.

Müller (Franz Carl)[1]. * Ueber psychische Erkrankungen bei acuten fieberhaften Krankheiten. [Strasburg.] 82 pp. 8°. *Kiel, C. F. Mohr,* 1881.

Müller (Franz Carl)[2]. * Railway-spine. 34 pp. 8°. *Würzburg, Kohl u. Hecker,* 1884.

Müller (Franz Rudolph). * Die beschwerliche und schmerzhafte Menstruation, ihre Ursachen und Heilung. 37 pp. 8°. *München, J. A. Giesser,* 1838.

Müller (Franz Xaver). * Untersuchungen über die Vertheilung der Farben und Geruchsverhältnisse in der Familie der Rubiaceen. 38 pp., 1 pl. 12°. *Tübingen, C. H. Reifs jun.,* 1831. [P., v. 1507.]

Müller (Fridericus) [1824–   ]. * De graviditate extrauterina. 2 p. l., 59 pp. 8°. *Gryphiæ, F. G. Kunike,* [1848].

Mueller (Fridericus) [1839–   ]. * De resectionibus, præcipue de resectione articulationis cubiti. 42 pp. 8°. *Berolini, G. Lange,* [1864].

Mueller (Fridericus Augustus) [1772–   ]. * De hysterotomia. viii, 36 pp. 4°. *Lipsiæ, lit. Klaubarthiis,* [1800].

———. Einige Worte über die Methode der Bildung angehender Geburtshelfer, nebst einer Anzeige des seit 1803 in Leipzig bestehenden Privat-Entbindungs-Instituts. 24 pp. 4°. *Leipzig, F. Richter,* [1808].

For Biography, see **Haase** (J. G.)

Mueller (Fridericus Gottlieb). * De venæsectionis etiam reiteratæ usu in febribus inflammatoriis imo exanthematicis. 62 pp. 4°. *Argentinæ, ex off. Pauschingeriana,* 1743.

Mueller ([Fridericus] Guilelmus) [1822–   ] * De cyanosi et tuberculosi. 64 pp., 1 l. 8°. *Berolini, G. Schade,* [1845].

Mueller ([Fridericus Guilelmus] Carolus) [1837–   ]. * De stenosi œsophagi. 32 pp. 8°. *Berolini, G. Lange,* [1863].

Müller (Fridericus Heliod.) * De motu corporis ejusque influxu in sanitatem et morbos. 27 pp. 8°. *Vindobonæ, C. Ueberreuter,* 1840.

Mueller (Fridericus Justus). * Analecta che-
mica de vitro antimonii exhibens. 1 p. l., 28 pp.,
4 l. sm. 4°. *Gottingæ, typ. J. C. L. Schulzii,* [1757].
Also, in: VOGEL (R. A.) Opusc. med. selecta, etc. 4°.
Gottingæ, 1768, 147–174.
For Biography, see **Brendel** (Jo. God.)

Müller (Friedrich)[1]. * Diss. sistens oculi humani anatomico-physiologicam descriptionem.
viii, 154 pp. 8°. *Viennæ, typ. hæred. van Ghelen,*
1819.

——. Die Cholera und die Anwendung der
Kälte als einfachstes Schutz- und Haupttheilmit-
tel derselben mit Berücksichtigung der durch die
Untersuchung mit dem Horchrohre erhaltenen
Resultate. iv, 162 pp., 1 l. 8°. *Wien, F. Beck,*
1832.

Müller (Friedrich)[2]. Erfahrungen über den Ge-
brauch und die Wirksamkeit der Heilquellen zu
Homburg vor der Höhe. 44 pp. 8°. *Frankf. a.
M., F. Wilmans,* 1838.

——. The same. Kurze Abhandlung über den
Gebrauch und die Wirksamkeit der Heil-Quellen
zu Homburg vor der Höhe mit Belegen nach
eignen Beobachtungen. Neue Aufl. 68 pp. 8°.
Homburg vor der Höhe, L. Schick, 1845.

——. The same. 7. Aufl. iv, 77 pp., 1 l. 8°.
Homburg vor der Höhe, L. Schick, 1857.

——. Compendium der Staatsarzneikunde für
Aerzte, Juristen, Studirende, Pharmaceuten und
Geschworene. Nebst einem Anhange, enthaltend die gerichtliche Chemie von Friedrich Mann.
8 p. l., 286 pp. 12° *München, J. Palm,* 1855.

Müller (Friedrich)[3].
See **Reise** der österreichischen Fregatte Novara um
die Erde. Linguistischer Theil. 4°. *Wien,* 1867. An-
thropol. Theil. 3. Abth. 4°. *Wien,* 1868.

Müller (Friedrich)[4] [1848–]. * Beitrag zur
Kenntniss der Wirkung des Chlornatriums. 21
pp., 1 l. 8°. *Marburg, C. L. Pfeil,* [1872]. c.

Müller (Friedrich)[5]. Ueber die diagnostische
Bedeutung der Tuberkelbacillen. 8 pp. 8°.
Würzburg, Stahel, 1883.
Being No. 1 of: Verhandl. d. phys.-med. Gesellsch. zu
Würzb., 1883. n. F., xviii.

Müller (Friedrich), **Schmidt** (Constantin
August) & **König.** Preisschriften über die
Schaafpockenimpfung, deren zweckmässigste
Anwendung und Verrichtung. Bekannt gemacht und mit Zusätzen von der königlichen
märkisch-ökonomischen Gesellschaft zu Potsdam. viii (1 l.), 150 pp. 8°. *Potsdam, Hor-
vath,* 1837.

Mueller (Friedrich Conrad). Medicinisch-klini-
sches Taschenbuch der rationellen Heilkunde
mit Anführung der Rademacher'schen Erfah-
rungsheillehre, nebst einem Anhange, enthaltend die Grundzüge der Percussion und Auskul-
tation und einen Auszug der Hydropathie und
Pharmacodynamik, einschliesslich der Analyse
der Mineralwässer, für Studirende und Aerzte.
vi, 684 pp. 12°. *Erlangen, F. Enke,* 1854.

Mueller (Friedrich Ernst). * Ueber die Hæmatocele retrouterina. 27 pp. 8°. *Leipzig, L.
Schnauss,* 1862. c.

Mueller (Friedrich Wilhelm)[1]. Ueber einige
Schönheiten von Carlsbad nach Gesner bear-
beitet, nebst einigen Gedichten. 15 l. 12°.
Prag, 1792.

Müller (Friedrich Wilhelm)[2]. * Das Thebaïn.
37 pp. 8°. *Marburg, C. L. Pfeil,* [1868].

——. Die Prostitution in socialer, legaler und
sanitärer Beziehung, die Nothwendigkeit und
der Modus ihrer Regelung. 35 pp. 8°. *Erlangen, F. Enke,* 1868.

——. Compendium der Geschichte, Pathologie
und Therapie der venerischen Krankheiten. xv,
336 pp. 8°. *Erlangen, F. Enke,* 1869.

——. Die venerischen Krankheiten im Alterthum. Quellenmässige Erörterungen zur Ge-

Müller (Friedrich Wilhelm)[2]—continued.
schichte der Syphilis. xvi, 148 pp. 8°. *Erlangen, F. Enke,* 1873.

——. Klinische Pharmacopöe. Die gebräuchlichen Arzneimittel der deutschen Medicin, ihre
Wirkung und Anwendung, nebst 400 beliebten
Receptformeln für innere und äussere Krankheiten. vi, 128 pp. 12°. *Stuttgart, F. Enke,*
1875.

——. Pathologie und Therapie des Harnröhren-
trippers. xii, 186 pp. roy. 8°. *Stuttgart, F.
Enke,* 1875.

——. Der Arzneischatz des praktischen Arztes.
Charakteristik, Dosirung, Anwendungsweise und
Anwendungsfall aller wichtigen Arzneimittel,
unter Berücksichtigung der einschlägigen Indi-
cationen und Methoden. 1 p. l., 140 pp. 8°.
Stuttgart, F. Enke, 1877.

——. Grundriss der Pathologie und Therapie
der venerischen Krankheiten für praktische
Aerzte und Studirende. viii, 172 pp. 8°. *Leipzig, Veit u. Comp.,* 1884.

——. Ueber die dermaligen Behandlungs-Me-
thoden der venerischen Krankheiten. 64 pp.
8°. *München, M. Ernst,* 1886.

Müller (Fritz). Systematische Zusammenstellung der Medizinal-Gesetze des Kantons Bern.
viii, 175 pp. 8°. *Bern, G. Hünerwadel,* 1867.

——. Facts and arguments for Darwin. Transl.
from the German by W. S. Dallas. iv, 144 pp.,
2 l. 8°. *London, J. Murray,* 1869.

Müller (G. A. Alfred). Zur Therapie der syphilitischen Krankheiten, mit besonderer Berücksichtigung der im äussern Krankenhause bei
Bern üblichen und eingeführten Heilmethoden.
148 pp. 16°. *Bern, J. A. Weingart,* 1852.

Müller (G. D. Richard). * Angeborener Zwerch-
fellbruch. 29 pp. 8°. *Marburg, Bayrhoff,* [1856].

Müller (G. E.) * Zur Theorie der sinnlichen
Aufmerksamkeit. [Göttingen.] 1 p. l., 136 pp.
8°. *Leipzig, A. Edelmann,* [1874, *vel subseq.*].

Mueller (Gaeander Guil. Ferd.) * De lithoto-
miæ administratione. 39 pp. 8°. *Halæ, typ.
Batheanis,* 1797.

Müller (Georg)[1]. * Ueber Augina. 16 pp. 8°.
München, C. Wolf, 1839.

Müller (Georg)[2]. Milch und Milchcontrole.
Vortrag, gehalten in dem thierärztlichen Verein
für den Regierungsbezirk Leipzig. 47 pp. 8°.
Jena, Dege u. Hænel, 1882.
Vorträge für Thierärzte, 4. s., Hft. 11–12.

Müller (George)[3]. * Seltene Folgen der Endocarditis. 16 pp., 1 l. 8°. *Jena, Frommann,* 1887.

Müller (Georg Adam). * Von dem Einflusse der
atmosphärischen Luft auf den menschlichen Organismus. 84 pp. 12°. *Würzburg, F. Bauer,* 1832.

Müller (Georg Alfred)[1]. Veterinär-Receptir-
und Dispensirkunde. Auf Grundlage der Pharmacopœa Germanica, ed. altera. viii, 196 pp.
12°. *Berlin, P. Parey,* 1885.

Müller (Georg Alfred)[2]. * Beitrag zur Kenntniss des Oxyhämoglobins im Blute der Haus-
säugethiere und des Hausgeflügels. [Erlangen.]
40 pp. 8°. *Leipzig, G. Wolf,* 1886.

Müller (George). New orphan houses (for
2,050 children) on Ashley Down, Bristol. Brief
narrative of facts relative to the . . . and the
other objects of the Scriptural Knowledge Institution for Home and Abroad. (Being the reports
of the institution.) 23., 1861–2 to 1862–3; 36.–
45., 1874–5 to 1882–3. 8°. *London,* 1862–83.

Mueller (Georgius Henricus). Series experimentorum in musculis et nervis animalium
quorundam institutorum horumque organorum
functionem s. effectus naturales illustrantium.
Stuttgardiæ, 1793.
In: SCRIPT. neurol. minores selecti. 4°. *Lipsiæ,* 1795,
iv, 170–180.

Müller (Georgius Ludovicus). * De diabete præsertim mellito. 1 p. l., 5–74 pp. 8°. *Gottingæ, F. E. Huth*, 1822.

Mueller (Gerhard) [1845–]. * Ueber Ileus. 27 pp. 8°. *Greifswald, F. Hache*, 1869. c.

Müller (Gerhard Andreas) [1718–62]. Betrachtungen über die Art und Weise der Mitwürckung derer Nerven zu denen musskulösen Zusammenziehungen. 7 p. l., 119 pp. 16°. *Franckf. a. M., J. G. Garbe*, 1753.

See, also, **Mead** (Richard). Medizinische Erinnerungen, [etc.] 16°. *Frankf. a. M.,* 1759.

Müller (Godofredus). * De rheumatismo. 54 pp. sm. 4°. *Halæ Magdeb., lit. C. Henckelii,* [1707]. [*Also, in :* P., v. 1391.]

Müller (Godofredus Guilielmus) [1709–99]. * De situ uteri obliquo in gravidis et ex hoc sequente partu difficili. 24 pp. sm. 4°. *Argentorati, typ. G. A. Piesckeri,* [1731].

For Portrait, see **Collection**—van Kaathoven.

Müller (Gottfridus Polycarpus). De temperamentorum propensionumque humanarum connexione. Resp. Joh. Godofredo Am Enden. 39 pp. 4°. *Lipsiæ, typ. hæredum Brandenburgerianorum,* [1708].

——. Meditationes in œconomiam generationis animalium . . . Resp. Joh. Zacharia Platnero. 48 pp. 4°. *Lipsiæ, lit. I. Titii,* [1715].

——. De signatura corporum naturalium physica. Respondens Johannes Casparus Troeger. 31 pp. 4°. *Lipsiæ, lit. Schedianis,* [1716].

Müller (Gottfried Wilhelm). * De mechanica operandi ratione medicamentorum sic dictorum alterantium. 24 pp. 4°. *Halæ, typ. C. A. Zeitleri,* [1698].

——. XXIV Kupfer-Tafeln, welche die Knochen des ganzen menschlichen Körpers vorstellen. 22 l., 24 pl. 4°. *Frankf. a. M., F. Varrentrapp,* 1749.

——. XII Kupfertafeln, welche die meisten kleinern und zarten Mäuslein an dem menschlichen Körper vorstellen. 9 l., 12 pl. 4°. *Frankfurt u. Leipzig, J. B. Eichenberg, dem Aeltern,* 1755.

——. The same. Mit drey Figuren vermehrt. 11 l., 15 pl. 4. *Frankfut u. Leipzig, J. C. F. Diehl,* 1769.

Müller (Gottlieb Samuel). * De stimulo naturæ parcius addendo. 30 pp. 4°. *Wittenbergæ, lit. C. C. Dürrii,* [1776].

For Biography, see **Boehmer** (Geo. Rudolphus).

Müller (Gottlob). * Physiologiæ et pathologiæ pilorum quædam fragmenta. 2 p. l., 24 pp. 8°. *Wratislaviæ, typ. Kreuzero-Scholzianis,* 1816.

Mueller (Guilielmus Erdmannus Ludovicus). * Diss. sistens phthisis purulentæ pulmonum ejusque in corpus humanum effectuum examen. 17 pp. 4°. *Jenæ, lit. Goepferdtii,* [1795].

For Biography, see **Gruner** (Christ. Gottfr.)

Mueller (Guilielmus Theophilus Carolus Fridericus). * De evolutione organismi nec non de evolutionum morbis. 54 pp. 8°. *Wirceburgi, F. E Nitribitt,* 1818.

Mueller (Gustav). * Die Prosopalgie und ihre Heilung durch die Neurectomie. 27 pp. 4°. *Kiel, C. F. Mohr,* 1875.

In : SCHRIFT. d. Univ. zu Kiel, xxii, 1875, vii, Med. vi.

Mueller (Gustavus) [1840–]. * De sputorum dignitate diagnostica. 32 pp. 8°. *Berolini, G. Schade,* [1865].

Müller (Gustavus Eduardus). * De ulcere ventriculi perforante. 12 pp. 4°. *Kiliæ, C. F. Mohr,* 1865.

In : SCHRIFT. d. Univ. zu Kiel, xii, 1865, vii, Med. vi.

Mueller (Gustavus Eduardus Rudolphus) [1826–]. * De epilepsia ejusque connexu cum traumate et rheumate. 32 pp. 8°. *Berolini, Rosenthal et soc.,* 1861.

Mueller (H. A. Eduardus) [1835–]. * De cataractæ ætiologia experimenta. 26 pp., 1 l., 1 tab. 8°. *Bonnæ, typ. Carthausianis,* [1858]. c.

Müller (H. F. J.) * Nonnulla de lithotritia. vi, 7–19 pp. sm. 4°. *Kiliæ, ex offic. C. F. Mohr,* 1840.

Müller (Heinrich)[1]. * Ueber den Nabelbruch, mit einem neuen Vorschlage zu seiner Behandlung. vi, 67 pp., 5 pl. 4°. *Erlangen, Kunstmann,* 1841.

Müller (Heinrich)[2] [1820–64]. * Beiträge zur Morphologie des Chylus und Eiters. 79 pp. 8°. *Würzburg,* 1845.

——. Abhandlung über den Bau der Molen. 87 pp. 8°. *Würzburg, Bonitas-Bauer,* 1847.

——. Ueber die entoptische Warnehmung der Netzhautgefässe, insbesondere als Beweismittel für die Lichtperception durch die nach hinten gelegenen Netzhautelemente. 39 pp., 1 pl. 8°. *Würzburg, Stahel,* 1855. [P., v. 1561.]

——. Anatomisch-physiologische Untersuchungen über die Retina des Menschen und der Wirbelthiere. 1 p. l., 122 pp., 2 pl. 8°. *Leipzig, W. Engelmann,* 1856.

Repr. from: Ztschr. f. wissensch. Zool., Leipz., 1856, viii, 1–122.

——. Ueber die Entwickelung der Knochensubstanz, nebst Bemerkungen über den Bau rachitischer Knochen. 147–233 pp., 2 pl. 8°. *Leipzig, W. Engelmann,* 1858.

Cutting from: Ztschr. f. wissensch. Zool., Leipz., 1858, ix, 147–233.

——. Gesammelte und hinterlassene Schriften zur Anatomie und Physiologie des Auges. I. Band, gedruckt, zusammengestellt und hrsg. von Otto Becker. xxviii, 400 pp., 5 pl. 8°. *Leipzig, W. Engelmann,* 1872.

——. Ueber das Vorkommen von Resten der Chorda dorsalis bei Menschen nach der Geburt und über die Verhältnisse zu den Gallerigeschwülsten am Clivus. 28 pp., 1 pl. 12°. [*Leipzig, E. Polz, n. d.*] [P., v. 1505.]

See, also, **von Kölliker** (Albert) & **Müller** (H.) Bericht über die während der Sommersemester 1853 und 1854 [etc.] 8°. [*n. p.,* 1854.] ——. Zweiter Bericht über die im Jahr [etc.] 8°. *Würzburg,* 1856.

For Biography, see Wien. med. Wchnschr., 1864, xiv, 331.

——. *See, also :*

Verzeichniss der schriftstellerischen Arbeiten von Heinrich Müller. Würzb. med. Ztschr., 1865, vi, pp. xxxii-xxxxvi.

Mueller (Heinrich)[3]. * Symptome des Alkoholismus, nebst Mittheilung einiger Fälle von chronischer Alkohol-Vergiftung. 20 pp. 8°. *Würzburg, C. J. Becker,* 1868.

Mueller (Heinrich)[4] [1845–]. * Ueber die Syphilis der Circulationsorgane. 32 pp. 8°. *Berlin, G. Lange,* [1868].

Müller (Heinrich)[5]. * Ueber Ostitis cranii traumatica purulenta. 1 p. l., 26 pp., 1 l. 8°. *Breslau, C. H. Storch u. Comp.,* [1871].

Müller (Heinrich)[6] [1851–]. * Ueber den Einfluss wiederholter Schwangerschaft auf die Prognose der Geburt bei engem Becken. 18 pp., 1 l. 8°. *Marburg, J. A. Koch,* 1874.

Müller (Heinrich)[7] [1858–]. * Zur Entstehungsgeschichte der Bronchialerweiterungen. [Halle.] 36 pp., 2 l. 8°. *Ermsleben a. H., A. Busch,* 1882.

Müller (Heinrich)[8]. * Ein Fall von Hirnsyphilis mit Erweichungs-Herd in Hirnschenkel und Veränderungen au den Kernen der Medulla oblongata unter dem Bilde einer apoplektiformen Bulbärparalyse, verbunden mit hochgradiger Ataxie. [Göttingen.] 36 pp. 8°. *Helmstedt, J. C. Schmidt,* 1886.

Müller (Henricus). * De gastricismo et methodo gastrica. 34 pp. 8°. *Halis Sax., typ. Grunerti vatris filiique,* [1820].

Mueller (Henricus Adolphus) [1796 – 1829]. * Signa præcipua ex colore cutis in morbis. 42 pp. 8°. [*Berolini*], *formis Brueschckianis,* [1820].

Müller (Henricus Conradus). * De phlegmasia alba dolente. 34 pp. 4°. *Gottingæ, J. H. Meyer,* [1833].

Mueller (Henricus Rudolphus). * De eorum, quæ vel e leviori vulnera ratione inter dissecanda cadavera accepta proveniunt, differentia et natura. 1 p. l., 36 pp. 4°. *Lipsiæ, ex off. Hirschfeldii,* [1831].

For Biography, see **Haase** (Guilielmus Andreas).

Müller (Hermann)[1]. * Ueber Typhus abdominalis. x, 86 pp. 8°. *Freiberg i. Br., F. Wagner,* 1845.

Müller (Hermann)[2]. * Das Brechmittel. 16 pp. 8°. *München, C. R. Schurich,* 1853.

Mueller (Hermann)[3]. Das Arznei-Dispensir-Recht der homöopathischen Aerzte. iv, 64 pp. 8°. *Berlin, R. Gaertner,* 1862.

Also, Co-Editor of : **Pharmaceutische** Zeitung, Bunzlau und Berlin, 1876.

Müller (Hermann)[4]. * Die Sporenvorkeime und Zweigvorkeime der Laubmoose. [Wurtzburg] 25 pp. 8°. *Leipzig, W. Engelmann,* 1874.

Repr. from : Arb. d. botan. Inst. in Würzb., iv. Hft.

Müller (Hermann)[5]. Die progressive perniciöse Anämie nach Beobachtungen auf der medicinischen Klinik in Zürich. 2 p. l., xiv, 250 pp. 8°. *Zürich, C. Schmidt,* 1877.

Müller (Hermann)[6] [1861–]. * Beitrag zur Casuistik und Lehre der Carbolsäurevergiftung durch Verschlucken derselben. 37 pp., 1 l. 8°. *Halle a. S., C. A Kaemmerer u. Comp.,* 1885.

Müller (Hermann)[7]. * Einige seltenere congenitale Neubildungen an Kopf und Gesicht. 37 pp., 1 pl. 8°. *Jena, A. Neuenhahn,* 1885.

Mueller (Hermann [Eugen August Albert]) [1859–]. * Zur Aetiologie der Parotitis. 30 pp., 1 l. 8°. *Halle, E. Karras,* 1883.

Mueller (Hermann Reinhold) [1846–]. * Ueber Aphasie. 32 pp. 8°. *Berlin, G. Lange,* [1871].

Mueller (Hermannus)[1]. * De histologicis pulmonum desorganisationibus. 30 pp. 8°. *Marburgi, typ. Bayrhofferi Acad.,* 1837.

Mueller (Hermannus)[2]. * De ectropio ejusque curatione chirurgica exemplo illustrata. 23 pp., 1 pl. 4°. *Jenæ, typ. Schreiberi,* [1840].

Mueller (Hermannus Fridericus Vollrath) [1816–]. * De abscessu lumbali. 34 pp. 8°. *Berolini, Nietackianis,* [1839].

Müller ([Hermannus] Ludovicus) [1827–]. * De iridis motu. 28 pp., 1 l. 8°. *Bonnæ, Krüger,* 1851.

Müller (Hieronymus). De clepsydrarum tum vulgatioribus tum rarioribus quibusdam, itemque, nonnullis aliis horum similibus phænomenis et effectibus. horumque omnium genuinis causis. 13 l. 4°. *Alldorffi, typ. H. Meyeri,* [1674].

Mueller (Hugo)[1]. * Ueber Luftröhrengeschwülste. 37 pp. 8°. *Jena, W. Ratz,* 1865.

Müller (Hugo)[2] [1846–]. * Zur Casuistik der Cyklitis. 52 pp. 8°. *Greifswald, F. W. Kunike,* 1873. C.

Müller (Iwan).

See **Galen** (Claudius). Libellum qui inscribitur Ὅτι ἄριστος ἰατρὸς καὶ φιλόσοφος recensuit et explanavit. 4°. *Erlangæ,* 1873.

Mueller (J.) * De hæmoptysi. 14 pp. 4°. *Parisiis,* 1809, No. 28, v. 75.

Müller (J. B.) Die neuesten Resultate über das Vorkommen, die Form und Behandlung einer ansteckenden Augenliederkrankheit unter den Bewohnern des Niederrheins durch Thatsachen belegt. 2 p. l., 192 pp., 2 pl. 8°. *Leipzig, C. H. F. Hartmann,* 1823.

Müller (J. D. Heinr.) * Ueber das Wesen der Rhachitis. vi, 7 – 28 pp. 8°. *Würzburg, F. E. Thein,* 1840.

Müller (J. H.) * Ueber die Krankheiten des Magens. 22 pp. 4°. *Zürich,* 1822.

Müller (J.-Jacques). * Sur le tétanos traumatique. 34 pp. 4°. *Strasbourg,* 1802, v. 43.

Müller (J. M.) Die Gicht, ihre Ursache und ihr Wesen so wie deren Heilbarkeit; mit einem Anhange von Krankengeschichten. 13. Aufl. v, 6–23 pp. 8°. *Coburg, G. Sendelbach,* 1865.

――――. Die Hämorrhoiden, ihre Entstehung, ihre Folgen und deren Heilbarkeit. 16 pp. 8°. *Coburg, G. Sendelbach,* 1865.

――――. The same. 4. Aufl. 16 pp. 12°. *Leipzig, W. Baensch,* 1867.

Mueller (J. O.)

Editor of : **Zeitschrift** des Vereins der homöopathischen Aerzte Oesterreichs, Wien, 1857.

Mueller (Jacob). * Der Harn als diagnostisches und kritisches Moment am Krankenbett. 40 pp. 8°. *Würzburg, F. E. Thein,* 1850.

Mueller (Jacobus)[1]. * Natura choleræ indicæ. 2 p. l., 33 pp. 8°. *Pestini, J. Beimel,* [1832]. [*Also, in :* P., v. 1320.]

Müller (Jacobus)[2]. * De angina parotidea. 16 pp. 8°. *Monachii, J. Deschler,* 1840.

Müller (Jo. Gottlieb). * De eo quod in cognoscendis et curandis morbis est præcipuum. 1 p. l., 24 pp. 4°. *Erfordiæ, lit. J. H. Groschii,* [1717].

Müller (Jo. Ludolfus Arnoldus). * Lithonthrypticorum examen. 1 p. l., 36 pp. 8°. *Halæ, typ. Trampianis,* [1797].

Müller (Joachimus Ludovicus) * De ossis femoris luxatione. 26 pp., 1 l. 4°. *Halæ Magdeb., lit. J. C. Hilligeri,* [1738].

Müller (Joan. Godof.) * De vase dorsali insectorum. 22 pp. 8°. *Berolini, typ. J. F. Starckii,* [1816].

Mueller (Joannes) [1835–]. * De cavi narium carcinomatibus, scirrho atque fungo medullari. Addita est historia morbi mollis sarcomatis in hac regione observati. 35 pp., 1 l. 8°. *Gryphiæ, F. Hache,* 1861. c.

Mueller (Joannes. Abraham Theodor.) * De clematide vitalba Linn. ejusque usu medico. 28 pp. 4°. *Erlangæ, typ. Kunstmannianis,* [1736].

Mueller ([Joannes Adolphus] Oscarus [Honoratus]) [1820–]. * De decapitatione crurotalana propter cariem. 31 pp. 8°. *Berolini, G. Schade,* [1845].

Mueller (Joannes Albertus). * De vulneribus ductuum excretoriorum decolorum. 30 pp. 8°. *Tubingæ, typ. Reissianis,* 1819.

Müller (Joannes Carol. Sam.) * De optima lympham vaccinam asservandi ratione. 30 pp. 8°. [*Halæ*], *typ. Orphanotrophii,* [1811].

Müller (Joannes Carolus Andreas). Rudimenta doctrinæ Hippocraticæ veræ. 2 p. l., 64 pp. 8°. *Halæ, formis Grunerti patris filiique,* 1815.

Müller (Joannes Christianus)[1]. * De dolorum ad partum genuinorum anomalia. 32 pp., 1 l. 8°. *Vindobonæ, A. Pichler,* 1826.

Mueller (Joannes Christianus)[2] [1726–70]. * De vulnere per se lethali homicidam non excusante. 28 pp. sm. 4°. *Lipsia, ex off. Langenhemia,* [1758].

For Biography, see **Ludwig** (Christ. Gottlieb). De medicinæ studio non præcipitando. [In memoriam Joh. Christ. Müller.] 4°. *Lipsiæ,* 1772.

Mueller (Joannes Christianus Guilielmus). * De viribus ac usu mercurialium. 27 pp. sm. 4°. *Jenæ, lit. Fickelscherrii.* [1775].

For Biography, see **Neubauer** (Joannes Ernestus).

Müller (Joannes Conradus)[1] [1789–1869]. Meditationes nonnullæ de cephalotomia seu perforatione cranii. Resp. Samuele Jacobo Ballin. 1

Müller (Joannes Conradus)[1]—continued.
p. l., 151 pp. 8°. *Havniæ, ex off. typ. Trieri,*
1835.
For Biography, see Biblioth. f. Læger, Kjøbenh., 1869,
5. R., xviii, 484–489.

Müller (Joannes Conradus)[2]. * De adenophy-
mate inguinali. 23 pp. 8°. *Turici, typ. Meyeri,*
1838. [*Also, in :* P., v. 586.]

Müller (Joannes Ehrenfried. Mauritius). * Diss.
sistens methodorum atque instrumentorum ad
pupillam artificialem formandam inventorum
historiam. vi, 7–27 pp., 1 pl. 4° *Jenæ, typ.
Schreiberi et soc.*, [1825].

Müller (Joannes Franciscus). * De marasmo
senili. 30 pp., 1 l. 8°. *Halæ, typ. F. D. Frankii,*
[1800].

Müller (Joannes Franciscus Conradus). * Sistit
fasciculum observationum circa arnicam quas
una cum selectioribus quibusdam ex universa
medicina positionibus submittit. 3 p. l., 39 pp.
4°. [*Bamberg*], *typ. J. G. Klietsch,* [1776].

Mueller (Joannes Fridericus)[1]. * De statu mixto
somni et vigiliæ quo dormientes multa vigilan-
tium munera obeunt. 34 pp., 2 l. sm. 4°. *Gottingæ, E. Luzac,* [1756].
For Biography, see **Richter** (Georgius Gottlob).

Mueller (Joannes Fridericus)[2]. * De ortu morborum contagiosorum ex fermento et acrimonia
specifica deducto. 26 pp. 4°. *Jenæ, ex off.
Stranckmanniana,* [1793].

Mueller (Joannes Fridericus)[3]. * Diss. sistens
vitandam vegetabilium venenatorum Germaniæ
permutationem cum oleribus. 46 pp. 4°. *Erfordiæ,* 1806.

Mueller (Joannes Fridericus Arnoldus). * De
viribus vitri antimonii cerati ad rationes suas
revocatis. 32 pp. sm. 4°. *Halæ Magdeb., typ.
J. C. Hilligeri,* [1757].

Müller ([Joannes] Fridericus [Christophorus])
[1800–]. * Diss. sistens nonnulla de variis arthritidis formis earumque decursu et curatione.
24 pp., 1 l. 8°. *Halis, typ. Baentschianis,* [1835].

Müller (Joannes Georgius). * De pellentium remediorum usu, abusu ac damno in parturientibus. 24 pp., 6 l. 4°. *Halæ Magdeb., typ. J.
C. Hendelii,* [1746].
For Biography, see **Gmelin** (Jo. Frid.)

Mueller (Joannes Godofredus)[1]. * Diss. sistens
theoriam inflammationis. 27 pp. 4°. *Jenæ, ex
off. Fickelscherrio-Stranckmanniana,* [1789].
For Biography, see **Loder** (Just. Christ.)

Mueller (Joannes Godofredus)[2] [1802–]. * De
syphilidis primariæ curatione sine mercurio. 30
pp., 2 l. 8°. *Berolini, typ. G. C. Nauckii,* 1832.

Mueller (Joannes Gottgetreu). * De medicamentorum congruo delectu in curandis morbis
perquam necessario. 36 pp. sm. 4°. [*Halæ
Magdeb.*], *ex off. Hendeliana,* [1758].

Müller (Joannes Guilielmus). * De morbis infantum. 32 pp. 4°. *Halæ Magdeb., typ. J. C.
Hilligeri,* [1746].

Müller (Joannes Henricus). * Vitia quædam
circa infantum educationem physicam commissa.
28 pp. 4°. *Erlangæ, typ. Ellrodtianis,* [1786].

Müller (Joannes Ludovicus)[1]. * De aëre sive
tentamen novæ methodi medicinam per principia physica scientifice tractandi in aëris exemplo exhibitum. 60 pp. 4°. *Erfordiæ, typ. J.
H. Groschii,* [1713].

Müller (Joannes Ludovicus)[2]. * De fungo articu-
lari, cum annexa ejusdem argumenti observatione. 1 p. l., 44 pp. 4°. *Gottingæ, lit. J. H.
Schulzii,* [1780].
For Biography, see **Richter** (Augustus Gottlieb).

Müller (Joannes Philippus). * De palpebrarum
affectibus.
In : WEIZ (F. A.) Vollständ. Ausz. [etc] 12°. *Leipzig u. Budissin,* 1773, v, 110.

Müller (Joannes Sigismund). * Raram de calculo vesicæ observationem atque epicrisin proponit.
In : WEIZ (F. A.) Vollständ. Ausz. [etc.] 12°. *Leipzig u. Budissin,* 1774, vi, 82–89.

Mueller (Joannes Theodorus Ludovicus) [1814–
]. * De induratione medullæ spinalis. 2 p. l.,
36 pp., 2 l. 8°. *Bonnæ, C. et F. Krüger,* [1842].

Mueller (Joh.)[1] * Diss. medicamentorum anti-
monialium conspectum sistens. 85 pp. 8°. *Havniæ, F. W. Thiele,* [1787].

Müller (Joh.)[2] [1801–58]. * Diss. sistens com-
mentarios de phoronomia animalium. 44 pp.,
1 l., 2 tab. sm. 4°. *Bonnæ, typ. C. F. Thormanni,*
[1822].

——. De respiratione fœtus; commentatio physiologica, in Academia Borussica Rhenana præmio ornata. xiv, 225 pp., 1 pl. 8°. *Lipsiæ, apud
C. Cnoblochium,* 1823. [*Also, in :* P., v. 1515.]

——. Ueber die Entwickelung der Eier im Eier-
stock bei den Gespenstheuschrecken und eine
neuentdeckte Verbindung des Rückengefässes
mit den Eierstöcken bei den Insecten. 118 pp.,
6 pl. 4°. [*Bonn,* 1825.]
Repr. from : Nova acta Acad. nat. curios., Bonnæ, 18.5,
xii, pt. 2, 555–672, 6 pl.

——. Ueber die phantastischen Gesichtserscheinungen. Eine physiologische Untersuchung mit
einer physiologischen Urkunde des Aristoteles
über den Traum. x, 117 pp. 8°. *Coblenz, J.
Holscher,* 1826.

——. Zur vergleichenden Physiologie des Ge-
sichtssinnes des Menschen und der Thiere, nebst
einem Versuch über die Bewegungen der Augen
und über den menschlichen Blick. xxxii, 462
pp., 8 pl. 8°. *Leipzig, C. Cnobloch,* 1826.

——. Grundriss der Vorlesung über die Physiologie. xiv, 102 pp., 1 l. 8°. *Bonn, T. Habicht,*
1827. [P., v. 1519.]

——. Grundriss der Vorlesungen über allgemeine Pathologie. 44 pp., 1 l. 8°. *Bonn, T.
Habicht,* 1829.

——. Bildungsgeschichte der Genitalien, aus
anatomischen Untersuchungen an Embryonen
des Menschen und der Thiere, nebst einem Anhang über die chirurgische Behandlung der Hy-
pospadia. xviii, 152 pp., 4 pl. 4°. *Düsseldorf,
Arnz,* 1830.

——. De glandularum secernentium structura
penitiori earumque prima formatione in homine
atque animalibus. Commentatio anatomica.
131 pp., 17 pl. fol. *Lipsiæ, sumpt. L. Vossii,* 1830.

——. Handbuch der Physiologie des Menschen
für Vorlesungen. 2 v. viii, vi–xvi, 852 pp. ; vi,
780 pp., 2 l., 1 pl. 8°. *Coblenz, J. Hölscher,*
1834–40.

——. The same. 2 v. 1 p. l., 741 pp. ; vi, 780
pp., 1 l. 8°. *Coblenz, J. Hölscher,* 1840–44.
1. Bd. is 4. Aufl.

——. The same. Elements of physiology.
Transl. from the German, with notes, by William
Baly. xxvi (2 l.), 1058, 22 pp., 1 pl. 8°. *Lon-
don, Taylor & Walton,* 1837[–8].

——. The same. 2. ed. 2 v. xxxviii, 1671 pp.,
2 l., 4 pl. 8°. *London, Taylor & Walton,* 1840–43.

——. The same. Arranged from the 2. Lond.
ed., by John Bell. xix, 13–886 pp. 8°. *Philadelphia, Lea & Blanchard,* 1843.

——. The same. Manuel de physiologie. Trad.
de l'allemand sur la dernière édition, avec des
additions, par A.-J.-L. Jourdan. 2. éd., revue et
annotée par É. Littré. 2 v. xxiv, 800 pp. ; 842
pp., 4 pl. 8°. *Paris, J.-B. Baillière,* 1851.

——. Rede zur Feier des zwei und vierzigsten
Stiftungstages des königlichen medicinisch-
chirurgischen Friedrich-Wilhelms-Instituts, am
2ten August 1836. 27 pp. 8°. *Berlin, Gebr.
Unger,* [1836].

Müller (Joh.)[2]—continued.

——. Ueber die organischen Nerven der erectilen männlichen Geschlechtsorgane des Menschen und der Säugethiere. 50 pp., 4 pl. 4°. *Berlin, F. Dümmler,* 1836.

——. Gedächtnissrede auf Carl Asmund Rudolphi. In der öffentlichen Sitzung der Akademie der Wissenschaften zu Berlin vom 6ten August 1835 gelesen. 24 pp. 4°. *Berlin, F. Duemmler,* 1837.

——. Ueber den feinern Bau und die Formen der krankhaften Geschwülste. 1. Lfg. 60 pp., 1 l., 4 pl. fol. *Berlin, G. Reimer,* 1838.

——. The intimate structure of secreting glands. With the subsequent discoveries of other authors, by Samuel Solly. xv, 166 pp., 4 pl. 8°. *London, J. Butler,* 1839.

——. Ueber die Compensation der physischen Kräfte am menschlichen Stimmorgan, mit Bemerkungen über die Stimme der Säugethiere, Vögel und Amphibien. Fortsetzung und Supplement der Untersuchungen über die Physiologie der Stimme. 54 pp., 4 pl. 8°. *Berlin, A. Hirschwald,* 1839.

——. The same. ii, 52 pp., 4 pl. 8°. *Berlin,* [*Gebr. Unger*], 1839. [*Also, in:* P., v. 1555.]

——. On the nature and structural characteristics of cancer, and of those morbid growths which may be confounded with it. Transl. from the German, with notes, by Charles West. 5 p. l., 182 pp., 8 pl. 8°. *London, Sherwood, Gilbert & Piper,* 1840. [*Also, in:* P., v. 891; 1560.]

——. Ueber die Lymphherzen der Schildkröten. Vorgetragen in der königlichen Akademie der Wissenschaften zu Berlin am 14. October 1839. 7 pp., 1 pl. 4°. *Berlin, Druckerei der k. Akad.,* 1840.

——. Gerichtlich - chemische Untersuchungen ausgeführt unter Professor G. J. Mulder's Leitung im Laboratorium zu Utrecht. Aus dem Holländischen für deutsche Juristen, Aerzte und diejenigen bearbeitet, welche sich mit diesem Zweige der Chemie beschäftigen müssen. iv, 121 pp. 18°. *Berlin, E. H. Schroeder,* 1848.

——. The physiology of the senses, voice, and muscular motion, with the mental faculties. Transl. from the German. With notes by William Baly. (From Müller's Elements of Physiology and supplement.) xvii, 849–1419, 32, 22 pp. 8°. *London, Taylor, Walton & Maberly,* 1848.

——. Beleuchtung der Dr. Casper'schen Abhandlung über Vergiftung durch Colchicum, Reagens auf Colchicin, vom medizinisch-chemischen und gerichtlich - medizinischen Standpunkte. 35 pp. 8°. *Berlin, W. Logier,* 1855.

Also, Editor of: **Archiv** für Anatomie, Physiologie und wissenschaftliche Medicin, Berlin und Leipzig, 1834–58.
See, also, **Wagner** (Rudolph). Zur vergleichenden Physiologie des Blutes. 8°. *Leipzig,* 1833.
For Biography, see **Dubois-Reymond** (E.) Gedächtnissrede auf Johannes Müller. 4°. *Berlin,* 1860. *Repr. from:* Abhandl. d. k. Akad. d. Wissensch. zu Berl., 1859.—
Virchow (R.) Johannes Müller. Eine Gedächtnissrede. 8°. *Berlin,* 1858. *Also, transl. in:* Edinb. M. J., 1858, iv, 452; 527. *Also,* Reprint.
See, also, Aerztl. Int.-Bl., München, 1858, v, 278. *Also:* Ibid., 1859, vi, 235 (Emil Harless). *Also:* Allg. med. Centr.-Ztg., Berl., 1858, xxvii, 286. *Also:* Arch. gén. de méd., Par., 1858, ii, 240–244. *Also:* Brit. & For. M.-Chir. Rev., Lond., 1858, xxvii, 285–303. *Also:* Deutsche Klinik, Berl., 1858, x, 306–308 (A. Göschen). *Also:* Med. Times & Gaz., Lond., 1858, xvii, 66–68. *Also:* Nederl. Tijdschr. v. Geneesk., Amst., 1858, ii, 301–303 (W. Berlin). *Also:* Wien. med. Wchnschr., 1858, viii, 419–423 (E. Brücke).
For Portrait, see **Collection**—van Kaathoven.

Mueller (Joh.)[3] Grundriss der Physik und Meteorologie. Für Lyceen, Gymnasien, Gewerbe- und Realschulen, sowie zum Selbstunterrichte. 5. Aufl. xviii, 538 pp. 8°. *Braunschweig, F. Vieweg u. Sohn,* 1856.

Mueller (Joh.)[3]—continued.

——. The same. Principles of physics and meteorology. 1. Am. ed. xii, 25–635 pp., 2 col. pl. 8°. *Philadelphia, Lea & Blanchard,* 1848.

——. Lehrbuch der kosmischen Physik. Zugleich als dritter Band zu sämmtlichen Auflagen von Mueller-Pouillet's Lehrbuch der Physik. 3. Aufl. 791 pp., 25 pl., 8°; atlas, 40 pl., 4°. *Braunschweig, F. Vieweg u. Sohn,* 1872.
See, also, **Raspail.** Neues Heilverfahren [etc.] Hrsg. von Dr. J. Müller. 8°. *Bern,* [1885].

Mueller (Joh.)[4] Ueber epidemische Krankheiten, insbesondere die asiatische Cholera. 32 pp. 8°. *Würzburg, Bonitas-Bauer,* 1855.

Mueller (Joh.)[5] [1844–]. * Ueber knorpelige Exostosen an den Epiphysen der langen Röhrenknochen. 20 pp. 4°. *Kiel, C. F. Mohr,* 1869.
Also, in: SCHRIFT. d. Univ. zu Kiel, xvi, 1869, vii, Med. ii.

Müller (Joh.)[6] * Pneumonie nach Nephritis. 29 pp. 8°. [*Würzburg*], *Becker,* 1882.

Müller (Joh.)[7] * Untersuchungen über das Verhalten des Convolvulins und Jalapins im Thierkörper. 29 pp., 1 l. 8°. *Dorpat, Schnakenburg,* 1885.

Müller (Joh.)[8] * Beiträge zur Tracheotomie. Bericht über 349 derartige im Hamburger allgemeinen Krankenhause ausgeführte Operationen. [Wurtzburg.] 16 pp., 1 tab. 8°. *Altona, H. W. Kobner u. Comp.,* 1886.

Müller (*Joh. Caspar*).
Portrait in: **Collection**—van Kaathoven.

Müller (Joh. Casparus Antonius). * De sede et indole pleuritidis. 44 pp. sm. 4°. *Gissæ, ex off. Brauniana,* [1754].

Müller (Joh. Christianus)[1] * Novorum pharmacorum technicorum pharmacopœæ Danicæ vires, usus et doses. 1 p. l., 58 pp. 8°. *Kilonii, lit. M. F. Bartschii,* [1779].

Mueller (Joh. Christianus)[2] * De diarrhœa. 16 pp. 12°. *Havniæ, typ. vid. L. N. Svare,* [1786].

Mueller (Joh. Christianus Friedr.) [1799–]. * De concretione morbosa cordis cum pericardio, casibus aliquot illustrata. 1 p. l., 43 pp. 8°. *Bonnæ, typ. Thormannianis,* [1825].

Müller (Joh. Christoph). * De mictione cruenta. 16 pp. sm. 4°. *Erfordiæ, charactere Groschiano,* [1636].

——. * De pulvere sympathetico. 19 pp. sm. 4°. *Erfurti, typ. J. H. Groschii,* [1687].

Müller (Joh. Fridericus)[1] De corpore raro et denso. 7 l. 4°. *Servestæ, excud. J. E. Bezelius,* [1687].

Müller (Joh. Fridericus)[2] [1761–]. * Genitalium sexus sequioris, ovi, nutritionis fetus atque nexus inter placentam et uterum brevis historia. 37 pp. 4°. *Jenæ, lit. Fickelscherrianis,* [1780].
Also, in: SCHLEGEL (J. C. T.) Sylloge op. min. [etc.] 8°. *Lipsiæ,* 1795, i, 187–216. *Also* [Abstr.], *in:* WEIZ (F. A.) Neue Ausz. [etc.] 12°. *Frankfurt u. Leipzig,* 1781, xiv, 188–194.

Mueller (Joh. Friedrich)[1] * Ueber die arzeneiliche Wirkung und Anwendung der Iodine. 55 pp. 8°. *Würzburg, F. E. Thein,* 1832.

Müller (Joh. Friedrich)[2] * Das allgemein gleichmässig verengte Becken, und dessen Einfluss auf die Geburt. [Munich.] 64 pp. 8°. *Kircheimbolanden, C. Thieme,* 1880.

Müller (Joh. Georg). * De dispositione ad morbos hæreditaria. 28 pp. 4°. *Gottingæ, H. M. Grape,* [1794].

Mueller (Joh. Georgius). De partu hominis post mortem matris moderante. 29 pp., 1 l. 4°. *Vitembergæ, formis S. Kreusigii,* [1714].

Mueller (Joh. Godofredus). * De attentione medico-practica. 40 pp. sm. 4°. *Halæ Magdeb., typ. C. Henckelii,* [1711].

Müller (Joh. Gottwerth).

   See **Lange** (Joh. Henricus). Dubia cicutæ vexata. sm. 4°. *Helmstadii,* [1764].

Müller (Joh. Guilielmus). * De morbis infantum. 32 pp. sm. 4°. *Halæ Magdeb., typ. J. C. Hilligeri,* 1746.

Müller (Joh. Heinricus).

   See **Walther** (Joh.) De lapidibus in genere. 4°. *Lipsiæ,* 1648.

Müller (Joh. Jakob). * Untersuchungen über den Drehpunct des menschlichen Auges. 22 pp, 1 l., 2 pl. 4°. *Zürich, Zürcher u. Furrer,* 1868.

Müller (Joh. Ludovicus). * De morbis tartareis. 32 pp. 4°. *Jenæ, lit. Krebsianii,* [1695].

   For Biography, see **Wedelius** (Geo. Wolff.)

Müller (Joh. Matthias). * De inflammatione vesicæ urinariæ. 16 pp. 4°. [*Altdorffi*], *lit. J. G. Kohlesii,* 1703.

   ——. Casus medico-chirurgicus, effractura cranii et subsecutis gravissimis symptomatibus divina gratia ex voto curatis, cum notis de capite ejusque affectibus, in quibus extracta plurimorum auctorum anatomica atque practica, [etc.] 2 p. l, 131 pp. 16°. [*Francof. a. M.*], *lit. G. M. Mayeri,* 1712.

   ——. Casuum medico-chirurgicorum de capitis præcipue passionibus rariorum, Deo benedicente feliciter curatorum, decas, una cum promissis auctorum, horumque allegatorum librorum, nec non rerum et verborum indicibus. 1 p. l., 40 pp. 16°. [*n. p.,* 1712.]

   ——. Observationum et curationum medico-chirurgicarum rariorum decades II. I. De præcipuarum corporis humani partium affectibus, cum scholiis, in quibus exempla ab auctore ultra centum, longeque numerosiora a multis aliis notata parallela continentur. II. De capitis præcipue passionibus historiarum resolutionibus. Una cum annexo tractatulo de effractura cranii, nec non insecutis gravissimis symptomatibus, divina gratia ex voto curatis. Cum notis de capite ejusque affectibus anatomicis physiologico practicis, pathologicis atque therapeuticis ex quamplurimis auctoribus extractis ut et rerum et auctorum, horumque allegatorum librorum indicibus. 4 p. l., 24 pp. 16°. *Norimbergæ, apud W. Michahellem,* 1714.

Müller (Joh. Michael). * De gangræna et sphacelo, vom heissen und kalten Brand. 9 l. 4°. [*Erfurt*], *typ. J. H. Groschii,* [1712].

Müller (Joh. Nicolaus).

   See **Valentinus** (Michael. Bernhardus). Prodromus historiæ naturalis Hassiæ [etc.] 4°. *Gissiæ Hassorum,* [1707].

Müller ([Joh. Oswald] Oscar) [1860–]. * Ueber das serös-purulente Oedem. 32 pp. 8°. *Berlin, G. Lange,* [1883].

Mueller (Joh. Paul) [1838–]. * Untersuchung über einige Derivate des Camphers. vi, 40 pp. 8°. *Greifswald, F. W. Kunike,* 1864.
                                  C.

Mueller (Joh. Ulricus). * De mania seu insania. 23 pp. sm. 4°. *Argentorati, typ. E. Welperi,* 1654.

Müller (Joh. Valentin) [1756–1813]. * Diss. sistens nævorum origines. 2 p. l., 87 pp., 1 l. 4°. *Jenæ, lit. Fickelscherrianis,* [1778].

   ——. De scirrho speciatim mammarum. 80 pp. 4°. *Jenæ, lit. Fickelscherrianis,* [1779].

   ——. Abhandlung von der Drüsenverhärtung, besonders der Brüste, und ihrer Behandlungsart mit äussern und innern Heilmitteln. 160 pp. 12°. *Leipzig, Weygand,* 1784.

   ——. Praktisches Handbuch der medicinischen Galanteriekrankheiten. Zum Gebrauch für Aerzte und Wundärzte mit den nöthigen Recepten. viii, 296 pp. 8°. *Marburg,* 1788.

   ——. The same. 2. Aufl. ix, 416 pp., 5 l. 8°. *Marburg,* 1802.

Müller (Joh. Valentin)—continued.

   ——. Medizinisches praktisches Handbuch der Frauenzimmer-Krankheiten, zum Gebrauch der Aerzte und des schönen Geschlechts. 4 Th. in 2 v. 16°. *Frankfurt u. Leipzig, Jäger,* 1788–95.

   ——. Entwurf der gerichtlichen Arzneywissenschaft nach juristischen und medicinischen Grundsätzen für Geistliche, Rechtsgelehrte und Aerzte. 4 v. 8°. *Frankf. a. M., Andrea,* 1796–1801.

   ——. Beweiss, dass die Kuhpocken mit den natürlichen Kinderblattern in keiner Verbindung stehen, und also ihre Einimpfung kein untrügliches Verwahrungsmittel gegen die natürlichen Blattern seyn könne. vi, 72 pp., 1 l. 16°. *Frankf. a. M., Jäger,* 1801.

   ——. Praktische Bemerkungen über die Kur des halbseitigen Kopfwehes oder sogenannten Migraine, mit beigefügten diätetischen Vorschriften und bewährten Arzneimitteln für Nervenkranke und Hypochondristen. viii, 167 pp. 12°. *Frankf. a. M., H. L. Brönner,* 1813.

   Also, Co-Editor of: **Frankfurter** medicinische Annalen für Aerzte, Wundärzte, Apotheker und denkende Leser aus allen Ständen, 1789.

   See, also, **K.** (J. A.) Erinnerungen gegen den Beweis des . . . 16°. *Frankf. a. M.,* 1801.

   For Biography, see **Gruner** (Christ. Goth.)

Müller (Joh. [Wilh. Hub.]) [1846–]. * Zur Casuistik der Gehirntumoren. 22 pp. 8°. *Greifswald, F. Hache,* [1874].

Mueller (Joh. Wilhelm). Vita humana ex fune pendens. 18 pp., 1 pl. sm. 4°. *Tubingæ, J. C. Reisl,* [1692].

Müller (Josephus). * De affectione carcinomatosa pylori. 16 pp. 8°. *Monachii, C. Wolf,* 1837.

   ——. Systematische Darstellung des Medicinal-Wesens in den deutsch-illyrischen, böhmisch-galizischen und italienischen Provinzen des österreichischen Kaiserstaates, nach authentischen Quellen bearbeitet. Abth. 1–4. ix, 86 pp., 1 l.; 172 pp., 2 tab.; vi (1 l.), 382 pp.; 167 pp., 1 l. 8°. *Wien, Braumüller u. Seidel,* 1843–4.

CONTENTS.

   Abth. 1. Oeffentlicher Medizinal-Dienst.
   Abth. 2. Oeffentliche Hygiene.
   Abth. 3. Oeffentliche Krankenpflege.
   Abth. 4. Oeffentliche Hygiene.

   ——. Das Apotheker-Wesen in den k. k. österreichischen, k. preussischen, k. baierischen, k. würtembergischen, k. sächsischen, k. hannoveranischen, churfürstlich und grossherzoglich hessischen, grossherzoglich badischen und mecklenburgischen, herzoglich nassau'schen und braunschweig'schen, fürstl. hohenzollern'schen, etc., Staaten, mit besonderer Rücksicht auf die Bildung, das Pflichtverhältniss und die Gewerbsrechte des pharmaceutischen Personals, die deutschen Landes-Pharmakopöen und die landesüblichen Arzneitaxen. 3 p. l., 258 pp., 1 l. 8°. *Wien, Braumüller u. Seidel,* 1844.

Müller (Josephus Ferdinandus). * De balneorum particularium usu. 53 pp., 1 l. 12°. *Viennæ, M. A. Schmidt,* 1781. [P., v. 1074.]

   Also, in: EYEREL. Diss. med. [etc.] 8°. *Viennæ,* 1792, iv, 136.

Mueller (Julius)[1] [1817–79]. * Ueber Resektion des Unterkiefers ohne Verletzung der äussern Haut, oder mit möglichster Schonung derselben. 24 pp. 8°. *Erlangen, J. P. A. Junge,* 1847. [*Also, in :* P., v. 224.]

   See, also, **Fischer** (H.) & **Mueller** (Julius). Angebliche Phosphorvergiftung. "Wie lange lässt," etc. 8°. *Berlin,* [1876].

   For Biography, see Aerztl. Int.-Bl., München, 1879, xxvi, 382.

Müller (Julius)[2]. * Beitrag zur Statistik und Casuistik der Geschwülste der weiblichen Brust. 28 pp. 8°. *Greifswald, F. Hache,* [1873].

Müller (Julius)[3]. *Ein Beitrag zur Lehre von der medullaren Leukämie. 36 pp. 8°. *Erlangen, Junge u. Sohn,* 1879.

Müller (Julius)[4]. *Die jährliche Periode des atmosphärischen Niederschlages in der Schweiz. [Bern.] 16 pp., 1 pl. 4°. *Zürich, Zürcher u. Furrer,* 1883.

Müller (Julius)[5]. *Ueber die Diagnose der Extrauterinschwangerschaft. 120 pp. 8°. *Strassburg, E. Hubert u. E. Haberer,* 1884.

Mueller (Julius Augustus) [1806–]. *De adjumentis quibus natura utitur ad evolutionem hominis perficiendam physicam et psychicam. 54 pp., 1 l. 8°. *Berolini, typ. Brüschckianis,* [1829].

Mueller (Julius Carolus) [1821–]. *De tumoribus. 61 pp. 8°. *Gryphiæ, F. G. Kunike,* [1844].

Müller (Julius [Friedrich Melchior]) [1850–]. *Beitrag zur Statistik und Casuistik der Geschwülste der weiblichen Brust. 28 pp. 8°. *Greifswald, F. Hache,* [1873].

Müller (Karl)[1]. *Statistik der menschlichen Entozoën. 31 pp. 8°. *Erlangen, E. T. Jacob,* 1874.

Müller (Karl)[2] [1859–]. *Ueber Azo- und Hydrazosulfobenzolamid. 28 pp. 8°. *Greifswald, J. Abel,* 1881.

Müller (Karl Ernst) [1855–]. *Neue Helminthocecidien und deren Erzeuger. 50 pp., 1 a. l. 8°. *Berlin,* [*Mesch u. Lichtenfield*]. 1883.

Müller (Konrad) [1857–]. *Vergleichende Untersuchung der anatomischen Verhältnisse der Clusiaceen, Hypericaceen, Dipterocarpaceen und Ternstroemiaceen. [Kiel.] 38 pp., 1 l., 1 pl. 8°. *Leipzig, W. Engelmann,* 1882.
Repr. from: Botan. Jahrb., ii, 5. Hft.

Müller (L.-A.-C.-F.) *Dissertation sur le spasme en général, et l'affection vaporeuse en particulier. 100 pp. 4°. *Strasbourg, Levrault,* 1813.

Müller (Leopold). Die Typhus-Epidemie des Jahres 1868 im Kreise Lötzen (Regierungs-Bezirk Gumbinnen), besonders vom ätiologischen und sanitäts-polizeilichen Standpunkte aus dargestellt. v, 101 pp., 1 map. 8°. *Berlin, A. Hirschwald,* 1869.

Mueller (Louis-Armand). *Considérations générales sur la maladie dite fièvre typhoïde. 38 pp. 4°. *Paris,* 1857, No. 6, v. 608.

Müller (Louis-Auguste). *Sur le baromètre et ses usages. 44 pp. 4°. [*Lausanne*], *Hignou & Cie.,* [*n. d.*]
Concours.

Mueller (Ludovicus)[1]. *De ophthalmia gonorrhoica. 22 pp. 8°. *Monachii, typ. G. Jaquet,* 1832.

Mueller (Ludovicus)[2] [1836–]. *De myelitide. 31 pp., 1 l. 8°. *Berolini, G. Schade,* 1864.
c.

Müller (Ludwig)[1]. Ueber den wechselseitigen Einfluss des menschlichen Körpers und der menschlichen Seele aufeinander. Ein anthropologisch-medizinischer Versuch. 16 pp. 4°. *Zweibrücken, G. Ritter,* 1830.

———. *Ueber Augenwassersucht, nebst Beschreibung und Abbildung eines unter der Form des Staphyloma corneæ pellucidum auftretenden Falles. 36 pp., 1 pl. 8°. *Würzburg, C. W. Becker,* 1833.

Müller (Ludwig)[2]. *Experimentelle Studien über eine Krankheits- und Todesursache in faulenden Stoffen, das sogenannte "putride Gift". 35 pp. 8°. *München, J. Deschler,* 1867.

Mueller (Ludwig)[3]. Das corrosive Geschwür im Magen und Darmkanal (Ulcus ventriculi perforans s. chronicum rotundum), und dessen Behandlung. x, 274 pp., 1 l., 3 pl. 8°. *Erlangen, F. Enke,* 1860.

Müller (Ludwig)[4] [1852–]. *Ueber Querbrüche der Kniescheibe. 30 pp., 1 l. 8°. *Berlin, G. Schade,* [1876].

Mueller (Ludwig)[5] [1857–]. *Ueber das Verhältniss der acuten Miliartuberculose zu käsigen Heerden. 8°. *Berlin, A. Haack,* 1879.

Müller (M.)
See **Mededeelingen** over de echte [etc.] 12°. *Utrecht,* [1875].

Mueller (Martin Gustav Adolph). *De iodii in organismum humanum effectu. 20 pp. 4°. *Lipsiæ, typ. G. Staritzii,* [1843].
For Biography, see **Joerg** (Jo. Christ. God.)

Müller (Mathias) [1848–]. *Ueber Hæmoglobin und Chinin. 29 pp., 1 l. 8°. *Bonn, C. Georgi,* 1872. [*Also, in:* P., v. 1367.]

Müller (Max). *Behandlung der Pleuritis exsudativa mit Chlornatrium. 48 pp. 8°. *Greifswald, J. Abel,* 1884.

Mueller (Maximilianus)[1]. *Observationes anatomicæ de vermibus quibusdam maritimis. 1 p. l., 30 pp., 1 l., 3 pl. 4°. *Berolini, G. Schade,* [1852]. [P., v. 796.]

Mueller (Maximilianus)[2]. *De parametritide acuta. 3 p. l., 39 pp., 1 l. 8°. *Vratislaviæ, typ. A. Neumanni,* 1865.
c.

Müller (Maximilianus Augustus). *De mercurio præcipitato rubro. 34 pp. 4°. *Monachii, C. Wolf,* [1835].

Müller (Moritz). *Ueber tonische und klonische Krämpfe des Nervus facialis. 24 pp. 8°. *Würzburg, Becker,* 1882.

Müller (Moritz Wilhelm) [1784–]. *De febre inflammatoria quæstiones. 1 p. l., 74 pp. 8°. *Lipsiæ, G. Bruder,* [1810].

———. Zur Geschichte der Homöopathie. iv, 100 pp. 8°. *Leipzig, C. H. Reclam,* 1837.
Also, Co-Editor of: **Jahrbücher** der homöopathischen Heil- und Lehranstalt zu Leipzig, 1833-4.
See, also, **Gehler** (Joannes Carolus) & **Mueller** (Mauritius Guilelmus). *De adsuetudine. 4°. *Lipsiæ,* [1807].
For Biography, see **Ludwig** (Christ. Frid.)
For Portrait, see **Collection** –van Kaathoven.—**Collection** of Portr. (Libr.)

——— & **Beck** (Christianus Fridricus Henricus). De schola Lipsiensium clinica. Commentatio historica. 37 pp. 8°. *Lipsiæ, G. Bruder,* [1809].

Müller (Nicolaus)[1]. *De nephritide spuria. 9 l. sm. 4°. [*Erfordiæ*], typ. J. H. Groschii, [1712].

Mueller (Nicolaus)[2]. *De actione virium alterna. 60 pp. 8°. *Jenæ, typ. Fiedleri,* [1794].
For Biography, see **Nicolai** (Ernestus Antonius).

Mueller (Nicolaus Wolfgangus). *De callo ossium. 32 pp. sm. 4°. [*n. p.*], lit. H. Meyeri, [1707].

Mueller (Otto)[1] [1831–]. *De variis hydrocelen curandi methodis. 1 p. l., 30 pp., 1 l. 8°. *Bonnæ, formis C. Georgii,* 1857.

Müller (Otto)[2]. Der Selbstmord. Eine psychiatrische Skizze. viii, 96 pp. 8°. *Harburg, G. Elkan,* 1859.

Müller (Otto)[3] [1837–]. *De apoplexia ischæmica. 32 pp. 8°. *Berolini, G. Lange,* [1861].

———. Berichte über die Heilanstalt für Nervenkranke bei Blankenburg am Harz, von den Jahren 1866–72 (1.–3.). 8°. *Braunschweig, F. Vieweg u. Sohn,* 1867–72.

———. Prospectus der Curanstalt für Nervenkranke in Blankenburg am Harz. [Mai 1875.] 2 l. 4°. [*Braunschweig, J. Krampe,* 1875.]

Mueller (Otto)[4] [1841–]. *Ueber acute Phosphorvergiftung. 33 pp. 8°. *Berlin, G. Schade,* [1867].

Mueller (Otto)[5] [1845–]. *Ueber die granulöse Augenkrankheit in den europäischen Armeen. 34 pp. 8°. *Berlin, G. Lange,* [1869].

———. The same. 2. Aufl. 33 pp. 12°. *Preuss. Stargardt, F. Kienitz,* 1870.

Müller (Otto [Friedrich]) [1844–]. * Ueber Kehlkopfpolypen und ihre Behandlung mit specieller Berücksichtigung der Galvanocaustic. 28 pp., 1 l. 8°. *Halle, Plötz*, [1872]. c.

Müller (Paul). * Ueber das Verhältniss der specifischen Wärme bei Gasen und Dämpfen. 46 pp., 1 pl. 8°. [*Breslau*, 1882.]

Müller (Paul [Friedrich Theodor Ehrenfried]) [1859–]. * Ueber zwei Fälle von Ektopia vesicæ, nebst Beiträgen zur operativen Behandlung derselben. 30 pp., 1 l. 12°. *Greifswald, C. Sell*, 1883.

Mueller ([Paul. Lud.] Guilelmus) [1819–]. * De hydrophobia. 28 pp., 2 l. sm. 8°. *Berolini, typ. fratrum Schlesinger*, 1843.

Mueller (Paul Samuel). *Convulsionum et epilepsiæ infantum ex leviori dolore prodeuntium rationes medicas proponit. 29 pp., 1 l. sm. 4°. *Halæ Magdeb., lit. Curtianis*, [1757].

——. Leges naturæ tensionem et laxitatem fibrarum totius corporis humani inter se semper esse proportionales stabiliet. 23 pp. sm. 4°. *Halæ, ex off. Fürstenia*, 1757.

Mueller (Peter) [1836–]. * Ueber utero-vaginale Atresien und Stenosen. 18 pp. 8°. *Würzburg, Stahel*, 1868. c.
Repr. from: Beitr. z. Geburtsk. u. Gynaek., Würzb., 1868, v, 1. Hft.

——. Das Esmarch'sche Verfahren zur Herstellung künstlicher Blutleere und seine Anwendung in der Geburtshilfe. 3 pp. 8°. *Wien*, 1874.
Repr. from: Wien. med. Presse, 1874, xv.

——. Ueber die Wendung auf den Kopf und deren Werth für die geburtshilfliche Praxis.
In: SAMML. klin. Vortr., Leipz., 1874, No. 77 (Gynäk., No. 25), 579–598.

——. Ein eigenthümlicher Bildungsfehler des Cervix uteri. 7 pp. 8°. *Stuttgart, F. Enke*, [1878].
Repr. from: Ztschr. f. Geburtsh. u. Gynäk., Stuttg., 1878, iii, 1. Hft.

——. Eine Vierlingsgeburt. 7 pp., 1 pl. 8°. *Stuttgart, F. Enke*, [1878].
Repr. from: Ztschr. f. Geburtsh. u. Gynäk., Stuttg., 1878, iii, 1. Hft.

——. Anatomischer Beitrag zur Frage vom Verhalten des Cervix während der Schwangerschaft. 5 pp., 1 l. 8°. *Berlin*, 1878.
Repr. from: Arch. f. Gynaek., Berl., 1878, xiii, 1. Hft.

——. Ein Kaiserschnitt mit Exstirpation des Uterus. Mit Bemerkungen über das einschlägige Verfahren. 8 pp. 8°. *Leipzig*, 1878.
Repr. from: Centralbl. f. Gynäk., Leipz., 1878, ii.

——. Der moderne Kaiserschnitt, seine Berechtigung und seine Stellung unter den geburtshülflichen Operationen. vi, 75 pp. 8°. *Berlin, A. Hirschwald*, 1882.

——. Des Berner Stadtarztes Wilhelm Fabricius Hildanus, Leben und Wirken. Rede zur Feier des 48. Stiftungstages der Universität Bern am 18. November 1882. 26 pp., 1 l., port. 8°. *Leipzig, J. B. Hirschfeld*, 1883.

——. Die Sterilität der Ehe. Entwicklungsfehler des Uterus. xxii, 300 pp. 8°. *Stuttgart, F. Enke*, 1885.
55. Lfg. of: Deutsche Chirurgie.

——. Die Unfruchtbarkeit der Ehe. xv, 193 pp. 8°. *Stuttgart, F. Enke*, 1885.

——. Ueber das Einpressen des Kopfes in den Beckenkanal zu diagnostischen Zwecken.
In: SAMML. klin. Vortr., Leipz., 1885, No. 264 (Gynäk., No. 73), 1887–1906.

Müller (Petrus)[1]. De annulo pronubo, vulgo vom Jaworts- oder Trau-Ring hypomnema, cui accessit de modo ac usu computationis graduum dissertatio. 3. ed. 108 pp. 4°. *Jenæ, typ. et sumpt. J. J. Bauhoferi*, 1680.

Müller (Petrus)[2]. * Spec. sistens meletemata circa morbos quosdam incurabiles. 30 pp. sm. 8°. *Havniæ, N. Möller*, [1778]. .
For Biography, see **de Obelitz** (Balthasar Gebhardus).

Mueller (Petrus Jeremia). Diss. phys. de somno . . . una cum defendente Herlovio Flensborg. 16 pp. sm. 4°. *Havniæ, lit. N. Mölleri*, [1765].

——. Diss. phys. de pinguedine corporis . . . cum defendente Jano Bükhave. 12 pp. sm. 4°. *Hafniæ, typ. A. H. Godiche*, [1766].

Mueller (Petrus Josephus) [1834–]. * De carcinomate uteri. 32 pp. 8°. *Berolini, G. Lange*, [1859].

Mueller (Philippus)[1]. *See* **Muller** (Philippus).

Müller (Philippus)[2]. * De necrosi ossium. 35 pp., 1 pl. 4°. [*Fuldæ*], *A. Neu*, [1832].

Müller (Philippus Jacobus). [Medicina biblica.] 4 l. fol. *Argentorati, typ. J. H. Heitzii*, [1785].

Müller (Richard). Akiurgische Vorträge. Repetitorium für die medicinische Staats-Prüfung bearbeitet. iv, 248 pp. 8°. *Berlin, Gutmann*, 1875.

Mueller (Richard Hermann). Ueber Peripachymeningitis. 30 pp., 1 l. 8°. *Königsberg, Gruber u. Longrien*, 1868. c

Müller (Rudolf)[1] [1859–]. * Beitrag zur Statistik der Schieloperation. 36 pp. 8°. *Berlin, E. Müller*, [1884].

Müller (Rudolf)[2]. *Ueber Urämie. 16 pp. 8°. *Erlangen, Junge u. Sohn*, 1885.

Müller (Rudolph). Schädigen die Kirchhöfe die Gesundheit der Lebenden? 32 pp. 8°. *Dresden, E. L. Knecht*, 1885.

Mueller (Rudolph L.) *Ueber Masernepidemien. 15 pp. 8°. *Leipzig, H. Springer*, 1870. [P., 294.]

Mueller (Samuel. Fridericus). * Observationes de morbis mulierum ex scabie repulsa propullulantibus. 32 pp. 8°. *Tubingæ, Schramm*, [1813].

Müller (Theodor) [1851–]. * Statistik der Amputationen der königlichen chirurgischen Klinik zu Breslau, vom Jahre 1877 bis März 1884. 65 pp., 1 l. 8°. *Breslau, F. W. Jungfer*, 1884.

Müller (Theophilus). * De medicis balneis artificialibus. 11 l. 4°. *Lipsiæ, typ. vid. J. Wittigau*, [1672].

——. The same. 24 pp. 4°. *Lipsiæ, imp. N. Scipionis*, [1672].
Also, in: ETTMÜLLER (M.) Diss. xiix med. 4°. Francof. et Lips., 1685.

Müller (Vincent. Henr.)
See **Engelhart** (Joh. Henr.) De dysenteria. Resp. Vincent. Henr. Müller. 4°. *Lundæ*, [1780].

Müller (Vincenz). Specielle Beschreibung der Heilquellen, Mineralbäder und Molkencur-Anstalten des Königreichs Bayern. 2. vermehrte und verbesserte Aufl. viii, 544 pp., 10 pl. 8°. *Augsburg, M. Rieger*, 1847.

Mueller (Wernerus Guilielmus). * De differentiis naturarum respectu climatum. 57 pp., 5 l. 4°. *Halæ Magdeb., typ. J. C. Hendelii*, [1746].

Müller (Wilhelm)[1]. *Ueber Struktur und Entwicklung des Tuberkels in den Nieren. 26 pp. 8°. *Erlangen, A. E. Junge*, 1857.

——. Ueber die chemischen Bestandtheile des Gehirns. 48 pp. 8°. *Erlangen, A. E Junge*, 1857.

——. Beiträge zur Theorie der Respiration. 40 pp. 8°. *Wien, K. Gerold's Sohn*, 1858.
Repr. from: Sitzungsb. d. k. Akad. d. Wissensch. Math.-naturw. Cl., Wien, 1858, xxxiii, 99.

——. Ueber den feineren Bau der Milz. vi, 115 pp., 6 pl. 4°. *Leipzig u. Heidelberg, C. F. Winter*, 1865.

——. Beiträge zur pathologischen Anatomie und Physiologie des menschlichen Rückenmarks. 41 pp., 2 pl. 4°. *Leipzig, L. Voss*, 1871.

Müller (Wilhelm)[2]. * De febri typhosa. 39 pp. 8°. *München, J. Gotteswinter et Mössl*, 1866.

Müller (Wilhelm)[3]. * Die Lebergranulation als Causalmoment des Magengeschwürs. 23 pp. 8°. *Würzburg, Becker, 1878.*

Müller (Wilhelm)[4]. *Untersuchungen über das Verhalten der Lymphdrüsen bei der Resorption von Blutextravasaten. 38 pp. 8°. *Göttingen, W. F. Kaestner, 1879.*

Müller (Wilhelm)[5]. * Ueber das Auftreten von Sepsis bei Diabetes. 19 pp. 8°. *München, J. A. Finsterlin, 1882.*

Müller (Wilhelm)[6]. Die Massenverhältnisse des menschlichen Herzens. 1 p. l., 220 pp. 8°. *Hamburg u. Leipzig, L. Voss, 1883.*

Mueller (Wilhelmus). * De pernionibus. 28 pp. sm. 4°. *Jenæ, lit. S. A. Mülleri,* [1680].

——. * De convulsione. 20 pp. sm. 4°. *Jenæ, typ. vid. S. Krebsii,* 1684.

Mueller (Xaverius). * De usu argenti nitrici in morbis ventriculi. 53 pp., 1 l. 8°. *Tubingæ, typ. Elfertianis,* [1829].

Mueller de Berneck (Franciscus). * Nonnulla de causis phthiseos pulmonalis. 28 pp. 4°. *Lipsiæ, lit. Staritzii,* [1830].
For Biography, see **Haase** (Guilielmus Andreas).

Mueller von Löwenstein (Fridericus). Lexicon medico-Galeno-chymico-pharmaceuticum, oder: gründliche Erklärung achtzehen tausend medicinischer Nahmen . . . 4 p. l., 312 pp. fol. *Franckf. a. M., M. Endters,* 1661.

Müllerklein (Clemens). * Ueber die venerischen Krankheiten. [Wurtzburg.] 63 pp. 12°. *Karlstadt, T. B. Dürr,* 1853.

Mueller-Pouillet.
See **Fick** (Adolf). Die medizinische Physik, [etc.] 8°. *Braunschweig,* 1856.

Müller's *canal.*
RELIQUET. Persistance du canal de Müller. Hydronéphrose du rein et de l'uretère droits. Pyélo-néphrite calculeuse du rein gauche très hypertrophié. 8°. *Paris,* 1887.
Boogaard (J. A.) Persistentie der Müllersche gangen bij een volwassen man. Versl. . . . d. k. Akad. v. Wetensch. Afd. Natuurk., Amst., 1876. 2. s., ix, 266–270, 1 pl.—**Dohrn** (F. A. R.) Zur Kenntnis der Müller'schen Gänge und ihrer Verschmelzung. Schrift. d. Gesellsch. z. Beförd. d. ges. Naturw. zu Marb., 1872, ix, 251–259, 3 pl.—**Frank** (L.) Rudimente des vorderen Endes der Müller'schen Gänge beim frisch geborenen Hengstfohlen. Deutsche Ztschr. f. Thiermed., Leipz., 1883, ix, 289.—**Ord** (W. M.) Malformation of the genital organs of a man, with persistence of one of the ducts of Müller. Med. Times & Gaz., Lond., 1879, ii. 542.—**Remy** (C.) Sur l'utricule prostatique et le canal de Müller chez l'homme. J. de l'anat. et physiol., Par., 1879, xv, 175–184, 2 pl.

Muelmann (Paulus). * De insomniis. 7 l. sm. 4°. *Lipsiæ, typ. hæredum Lambergianorum,* [1630].

Mümler (J. L. C.)
See **Königliche** Academie der Wissenschaften zu Berlin. Physikalische und medicinische Abhandlungen, [etc.] 8°. *Gotha,* 1781–6.

Münch (A.) Das Armen-Soolbad in Rheinfelden (Canton Aargau); Mittheilungen über Gründung, Haushalt und Erfolge der Anstalt. 15 pp. 8°. *Zürich, J. Herzog,* 1868.
Repr. from: Schweiz. Ztschr. f. Gemeinnützigk., Jahrg., 1868.

Münch (Alfred Rud. Wilh.) *Ueber cariöse Erkrankungen des Fussskeletes. [Basel.] 1 p. l., 38 pp. 8°. *Leipzig, J. B. Hirschfeld,* 1879.

Münch (Aloys). *Abhandlung über die Wirkungen des Weins. 14 pp. 4°. *Giessen,* 1815.

Münch (Burchard Friedrich) [1759–1830]. De belladonna efficaci in rabie canina remedio. 47 pp. 4°. *Gottingæ, F. A. Rosenbusch,* [1781].
Also, in: FRANK (J. P.) Delect. opusc. med. 8°. *Ticini,* 1785, i, 248–328.

——. Practische Abhandlung von der Belladonna und ihrer Anwendung, besonders zur Vorbauung und Heilung der Wuth nach dem Bisse von tollen Hunden. xvi, 408 pp., 2 pl. 12°. *Göttingen, J. C. Dieterich,* 1785.

Muench (Eduard). * Ueber Embolie der Arteria centralis retinæ. 28 pp. 8°. *Giessen, W. Keller,* 1866, v. 293.

Münch (Eugen). * Ueber die Bauchnaht. [Wurtzburg.] 18 pp. 8°. *Bamberg, Humann,* 1884.

Münch (Franciscus) [1802–]. * De cupri viribus in corpus humanum. 37 pp. 8°. *Berolini, formis Brüschckianis,* [1833].

Münch (Georgius). * De febre nervosa versatili ac stupida. 24 pp. 8°. [*Landshut*], 1811.

Münch (Gustav). * Beitrag zur Lehre von dem osteomalakischen Frauenbecken. 24 pp., 4 pl. 8°. *Giessen, W. Keller,* 1851.

Münch (Joannes Georgius) [1793–]. * De cardialgia. 1 p. l., 41 pp., 1 l. 8°. *Berolini, Plateni,* [1818].

Muench (Joannes Godofredus) [1832–]. * De carcinomate testiculorum. 22 pp., 1 l. 8°. *Gryphiæ, F. Hache,* 1858. c.

Münch (Joannes Henricus). * Diss. sistens observationes practicas circa usum belladonnæ, in melancholia, mania, et epilepsia. 2 p. l., 32 pp., 1 l. sm. 4°. *Gottingæ, J. C. Dieterich,* [1783].

München.
See **Munich.**

München in naturwissenschaftlicher und medicinischer Beziehung. Führer für die Theilnehmer der 50. Versammlung deutscher Naturforscher und Aerzte. vi, 278 pp., 1 l., 1 map. 8°. *Leipzig u. München, G. Hirth,* 1877.

Muenchenberg (Augustus). * Fungus medullaris duræ matris et pericranii. 2 p. l., 34 pp., 1 pl. 8°. *Regimontii Pr., E. J. Dalkowski,* [1842].

Münchener (Zur). Canalisationsfrage. Vorträge, gehalten im ärztlichen Bezirks-Vereine München. Zwei Vorträge von H. Ranke. Entgegnung von v. Pettenkofer. Vortrag von Kerschensteiner. Vortrag von Rudolf Emmerich. Schlusswort von H. Ranke. 128 pp. 8°. *München, J. A. Finsterlin,* 1879.
Repr. from: Aerztl. Int.-Bl., München, 1879, xxvi.

Münchener medicinische Wochenschrift. (Früher Aerztliches Intelligenz-Blatt.) Organ für amtliche und praktische Aerzte. Hrsg. von Dr. Bollinger [*et al.*]. Redacteur: B. Spatz. Jahrjang 33–35, 1886–8. fol. *München, J. A. Finsterlin.*
Current. Title of v. 1–32 was: Aerztliches Intelligenz-Blatt.

Münchenrod (Georgius).
See **Naboth** (Martinus). De organo auditus. Respondente G. Münchenrod. sm. 4°. *Lipsiæ,* [1703].

von Münchhausen (Otto).
Portrait in: **Collection** of Portr. of Phys. & Men of Sc., 166.

Muenchheimer (Mauritius) [1807–]. * De catarrho vesicæ urinariæ. 29 pp., 1 l. 8°. *Berolini, typ. Nietackianis,* [1832].

Münchmeyer (Carol. Aug. Adalb.) Commentatio de differentia quæ intercedit inter epilepsiam et eclampsiam. iv, 63 pp. 4°. *Gottingæ, typ. Dieterichianis,* [1830].

Münchmeyer (E. E.) * Ueber das Alter des Varioloid. 40 pp. 8°. *Würzburg, C. A. Zürn,* 1835.

Münchmeyer (Emil). Die Cardialgie nach den neuesten Quellen und eigenen Beobachtungen pathologisch und therapeutisch dargestellt. 1 p. l., 144 pp. 8°. *Lüneburg, Herold u. Wahlstab,* 1843.

Münchmeyer (Ernest. Henric. Guilielmus). Commentatio de viribus oxygenii in procreandis et sanandis morbis. 64 pp. 4°. *Gottingæ, H. Dieterich,* [1801].

Münchmeyer (Friedrich Adelbert). * Ein Fall von Tuberkulose des Herzbeutels. 31 pp., 1 pl. 8°. *Würzburg, P. Scheiner,* 1883.

von Münchow (L. D.)
See **Werneburg** (J. F. Ch.) Die richtige Katoptrik. 4°. [*n. p., n. d.*]

Münck (Sebastianus). *De febre quotidiana intermittente. 12 pp. 4°. *Argentorati, J. F. Le Roux*, [1754].

Muencke (Robert).
See **Technisches** Institut für Anfertigung naturwissenschaftlicher Apparate, etc. 8°. *Berlin*, [1885].

Münden.
See **Insane** (*Asylums for, Reports, etc., of*), by *localities—Königshof.*

Muennich (August). *Welches ist das beste Mittel zur Verhütung der Placentarretention? 2 p. l., 24 pp., 1 l. 8°. *Breslau, O. Raabe*, 1876.

Muennich (Ernestus) [1836–]. *De pneumothorace. 31 pp. 8°. *Berolini, G. Schade*, [1859].

Muennich (Frid. Guil. Alex. Franc.) [1814–]. * De gravidarum parturientium et puerperarum eclampsia. 32 pp., 2 l. 8°. *Halæ, C. Grunert*, [1838].

Münnich (Henricus Fridericus) [1806–]. *Glossomantia, sive de signis a lingua depromendis. 32 pp. 8°. *Berolini, typ. A. Petschii*, [1830].

Münnich (Joannes Fridericus). *De peripneumonia. 1 p. l., 20 pp. 4°. *Halæ ad Salam, ære Hendeliano*, [1772].

Münnich (Joh. Andreas). *De diarrhœa biliosa. 20 pp., 2 l. 4°. *Halæ Magdeb., typ. J. C. Hilligeri*, [1729].

————. Relatio physico-medica, oder kurzer doch gründlicher Bericht von zweyen, durch einen Donner-Schlag im vergangenen Sept. 1731 zu Osterwieck gerührten Personen, davon die Eine gleich todt geblieben, die Andere aber noch gerettet worden ist . . . Zuerst als ein pflicht-mässiges Attestat dem wohl-löblichen Judicio daselbst schrifftlich übergeben, nachgehends aber, auf Ersuchen, etwas vermehrter, in gegenwärtiger Form zum Druck be. 3 p. l., 19 pp. 4°. *Halberstadt, Schoppen*, 1732.

Münnich (Joh. Friedricus). *De diarrhœa serosa. 21 pp., 1 l. 4°. *Halæ Magdeb., typ. J. C. Hilligeri*, [1729].

Münnich (Joh. Gust. Ad.) Beschreibung der Brause-Badeanstalt in der Kaserne des Kaiser Franz Garde-Grenadier-Regiments No. 2. 10 pp., 1 pl. 8°. [*Berlin*], *W. Greve*, 1880.
Repr. from: Deutsche mil.-ärztl. Ztschr., Berl., 1880, vi.

Münnich (Paulus Joannes Wilhelmus). *De caussis determinantibus ancipitem eventum morborum in nosocomiis occurrentium. 24 pp. 4°. *Halæ Magdeb., ex off. Hendeliana*, [1762].

Münninghoff. Das eigentliche Wesen der Krankheiten. Enthaltend zugleich die Physiologie des thierischen Magnetismus und des Hellsehens. Auch für Nicht-Aerzte verständlich dargestellt. ix (1 l.), 155 pp. 8°. *Leipzig, W. Besser*, 1881.

Münscher (Otto). *Ein Fall von Trismus neonatorum mit einigen Bemerkungen über die Aetiologie dieser Krankheit. 24 pp., 2 l. 8°. *Marburg, N. G. Elwert*, 1876.

Münster. General-Bericht über das Medizinal- und Sanitäts-Wesen im Regierungs-Bezirk Münster im Jahre 1882. Vom Regierungs- und Medizinal-Rath Dr. Hoogeweg. Durch Erlass Sr. Excellenz des Herrn Cultus-Ministers zum Druck bestimmt. 95 pp. 8°. *Münster, Coppenrath*, 1883.

Münster, *Westphalia.*
See, also, **Fever** (*Cerebro-spinal, History, etc., of*), *by localities;* **Medicine** (*Clinical, Cases of*).
Sendschreiben eines rheinischen Arztes an Herrn P . . . zu C . . . über einige, in dem Un-

Münster, *Westphalia.*
terricht von dem Collegium der Aerzte zu Münster angenommene Grundsätze. 16°. [*Rheine*], 1778.

Münster (Carl Julius) [1847–]. *Die unblutige forcirte Erweiterung des Afters in ihrer diagnostischen und therapeutischen Verwerthung. 32 pp. 8°. *Greifswald, F. W. Kunike*, 1873.

Münster (Fridrich Gottlieb). *Diss. exhibens monita quædam discrimen spectantia quod inter morbos universales et topicos vulgo assumitur. 45 pp., 2 l. 8°. *Gottingæ, typ. Barmeierianis*, [1801].

Muenster (Hermann). *Wendung, Zange und künstliche Frühgeburt bei verengtem Becken mit Rücksicht auf die exspectative Behandlung. 39 pp. 8°. *Königsberg, H. Hartung*, 1870.

Muenster (Joannes Elias) [1797–]. * De balneo animali. 98 pp. 8°. [*n. p.*], *formis Brueschckianis*, [1832].

von Münster (Walter Alfons) [1848–]. *Casuistische Beiträge zur Kenntniss der präcornealen und conjunctivalen melanotischen Neubildungen. 30 pp., 1 l., 1 pl. 8°. *Halle, J. G. Lipke*, 1872. C.

Münsterlingen.
See **Hospitals** (*Descriptions, etc., of*), **Insane** (*Asylums, etc., for*), *by localities.*

Muenter (Fridericus [Adolphus]) [1843–]. *Ad symptomatologiam morborum cerebri. De apoplexia duplici et tumore, glioma, in ponte Varolii. 30 pp., 1 l. 8°. *Halis Sax., formis Plœtzianis*, [1866]. C.

Münter (Gustav Wilhelm). Versuch einer neuen Theorie der Verrichtungen des Gehirns und Nervensystems, enthaltend eine physiologische Beweisführung, dass das centrale und peripherische Nervensystem für den Organismus das ist, was die Genitalien für die Erhaltung der Gattung sind. viii, 63 pp. 8°. *Leipzig, A. Reimann*, 1838.

————. Anatomische Grundlagen zur Seelenlehre des Menschen und der Thiere. viii, 190 pp., 1 pl. 8°. *Halle, R. Mühlmann*, 1846.

————. Geschichtliche Grundlagen zur Geisteslehre des Menschen, oder die Lebensäusserungen des menschlichen Geistes im gesunden und krankhaften Zustande. Für Gebildete aller Stände. viii, 208 pp. 8°. *Halle, C. E. M. Pfeffer*, 1850.

Münter (M.) Der Untergrund der Stadt Halle an der Saale, beschrieben und auf einer Karte dargestellt. 32 pp., 1 ch. 8°. *Halle, G. E. Barthel*, 1869.
No. 1 of the: Publicationen d. Ver. f. öffentl. Gesundh. in Halle.

Münz (Martinus) [1785–1848] **& Raab** (Ferdinandus). Dissertatio de cortice peruviano et radice ipecacuanhæ, eorumque surrogatis. 1 p. l., 233 pp. 8°. *Landishuti, J. Thomann*, [1810].

Münzberger (Leopold [Wilhelm]) [1858–]. *Ueber das pathologisch-anatomische Substrat der Erosionen an der Portio vaginalis uteri. 35 pp., 1 l. 8°. *Halle, E. Karras*, 1881.

Muenzel (Arminius). *De necrosi ossium. 32 pp. 8°. *Jenæ, typ. A. Neuenhahni*, 1853.

Muenzel (Eduard). *Ueber amyloide Degeneration der Niere. 17 pp. 8°. *Jena, A. Neuenhahn*, 1865.

Münzenthaler (Augustus Josephus). *Diss. sistens observationes et annotationes quasdam de anenrysmatibus et præcipue veris. vi, 7–20 pp., 2 pl. sm. 4°. *Landishuti, J. Thomann*, 1820.

————. Versuch über die Amputationen in den Gelenken. 44 pp. 8°. *Leipzig, P. G. Kumi*, 1822.

Münzinger (Wilhelm). *Das Tübinger Herz. Ein Beitrag zur Lehre von der Ueberanstrengung des Herzens. [Tübingen.] 23 pp. 8°. *Leipzig, J. B. Hirschfeld*, 1877.

Mürcke (Andreas). *De viribus sanguinis et solidorum motum facientibus curatius definiendis. 28 pp. 4°. *Lipsiæ, ex off. Langenhemia*, [1772].

For Biography, see **Bose** (Ernestus Gottlob).

Mürdel (Matthæus). *Diss. sistens annotationes de velamentis fœtus. 32 pp. 12°. *Tubingæ, typ. Reissianis*, 1821.

Mürer (T. C.) *De causis cophoseos surdomutorum indagatu difficilibus. Commentatio brevis sectionibus cadaverum ut plurimum illustrata. 25 pp., 1 pl. 12°. *Hafniæ, B. Schlesinger*, [1825].

Müri (Hans). *Das Recht an der Wasserquelle. 1 p. l., 86 pp. 8°. *Bern, R. F. Haller-Goldschach*, 1886.

Mürling (Josephus Martinus). Prima corporis physici principia. 16 pp. 4°. *Wittebergæ, lit. Tschidiichianis*, [1754].

Muermann (Georgius) [1813–]. *De ossium decapitatione. 36 pp., 2 l. 8°. *Berolini, typ. Natorffianis*, [1837].

Mürset (Alfred). *Untersuchungen über Intoxications-Nephritis (Aloin, Oxalsäure). [Bern.] 1 p. l., 30 pp., 1 pl. 8°. *Leipzig, J. B. Hirschfeld*, 1885.

Mueser (Frid. Guil.) [1812–]. *De hernia diaphragmatis. 32 pp., 2 l. 8°. *Berolini, typ. Nietackianis*, [1835].

Muesmann (J.) *Der Darmcatarrh der Kinder. [Wurtzburg.] 16 pp. 8°. *Augsburg, J. M. Kleinle*, 1861

Müthler (Gustav). *Ein Fall von Bronchostenose durch ein Sarcom bedingt. 32 pp. 8°. *Berlin, G. Lange*, [1873].

Mütter (Thomas Dent) [1811–59]. A lecture on loxarthrus, or club-foot. 104 pp. 8°. *Philadelphia, Hooker & Claxton*, 1839.

———. The salt sulphur springs, Monroe County, Va. 32 pp. 8°. *Philadelphia, T. K. & P. G. Collins*, 1840.

———. On recent improvements in surgery. An introductory lecture to the course on the principles and practice of surgery in Jefferson Medical College. 52 pp. 8°. *Philadelphia, Merrihew & Thompson*, 1842. [*Also, in:* P., v. 847.]

———. Cases of deformity from burns, successfully treated by plastic operations. 23 pp. 8°. *Philadelphia, Merrihew & Thompson*, 1843.

———. A report on the operations for fissures of the palatine vault. 28 pp. 8°. *Philadelphia, Merrihew & Thompson*, 1843.

———. Syllabus of the course of lectures on the principles and practice of surgery, delivered in the Jefferson Medical College, Philadelphia. Pts. 1–3. pp. 11–206. 8°. *Philadelphia, Merrihew & Thompson*, 1843.

Pt. 1 incomplete; wants pp. 1-10.

———. The same. 206 pp. 8°. *Philadelphia, Barrett & Jones*, 1846.

———. The same. 212 pp. 8°. *Philadelphia, J. H. Jones*, 1848.

———. The same. 212 pp. 8°. *Philadelphia, J. H. Jones & Co.*, 1855.

———. Cases of deformity of various kinds successfully treated by plastic operations. 38 pp., 2 pl. 8°. *Philadelphia, Merrihew & Thompson*, 1844. [P., v. 114.]

———. Introductory for 1844-5, on the present position of some of the most important of the modern operations of surgery. 34 pp. 8°. *Philadelphia, Merrihew & Thompson*, 1844. [*Also, in:* P., v. 408.]

———. Lecture introductory to a course on the principles and practice of surgery in the Jeffer-

Mütter (Thomas Dent)—continued.
son Medical College. 26 pp. 8°. *Philadelphia, Merrihew & Thompson*, 1847.

———. Charge to the graduates of Jefferson Medical College of Philadelphia. Delivered March 8, 1851. With a list of the graduates. 28 pp. 8°. *Philadelphia, T. K. & P. G. Collins*, 1851.

———. Catalogue of the pathological museum of Prof. T. D. Mütter. 60 pp., 1 l. 8°. *Philadelphia*, 1856.

For Biography, see **Pancoast** (J.) A discourse commemorative of the late Professor T. D. Mütter. 8°. *Philadelphia*, 1859.

See, also, Med. & Surg. Reporter, Phila., 1859, n. s., ii, 113–118 (R. J. Lewis). Also: N. Am. M.-Chir. Rev., Phila., 1858, iii, 571–574. Also: Tr. M. Soc. Penn., Phila., 1860, n. s., v, 148–154 (J. Pancoast).

Muettrich (Æmilius). *De rationibus quibus constituatur, num domus quædam imprimis nova satis exsiccata sit, ut sine damno valetudinis habitari possit. 31 pp. 8°. *Regimonti Pr., typ. Dalkowskianis*, 1857.

Muettrich (T. A.) *Quid valeat temperatura ad variandos constantes opticos tartari natrionati. 32 pp., 1 pl. 8°. *Regimonti Pr., typ. Dalkowskianis*, 1863.
C.

Mützenberg (Ernst). *Ueber das Vorkommen der vasculären Welle in der Carotiscurve. 54 pp., 2 diag. 8°. *Bern, P. Haller*, 1885.

Mufettus [**Muffet, Moffet, Moufet,** etc.] (Thomas) [–1600?]. De jure et præstantia chymicorum medicamentorum dialogus apologeticus. Accesserunt etiam epistolæ quædam medicinales ad medicos aliquot conscriptæ. 111 pp. 12°. *Francofurti, apud hæred. A. Wecheli*, 1584.

———. Health's improvement; or, rules comprizing and discovering the nature, method, and manner of preparing all sorts of food used in this nation, corrected and enlarged by Christopher Bennet. 2 p. l., 296 pp. sm. 4°. *London, S. Thomson*, 1655.

———. The same. To which is now prefix'd a short view of the author's life and writings, by Mr. Oldys, and an introduction by R. James. xxxii, 398 pp. 12°. *London, T. Osborne*, 1746.

Also, in: THEATRUM chemicum. 4°. *Argentorati*, 1659, i, 64-108.
For Biography, see **Aikin** (J.) Biog. mem. 8°. *London*, 1780, 168–175.

Mugdan (Otto). *Untersuchung der Fäces von Nierenkranken auf Harnstoff und kohlensaures Ammoniak. 16 pp. 8°. *Erlangen, E. T. Jacob*, 1884.

Muggetti (C. D.)
See **Mojon** (Benoît). Mémoire sur l'utilité de la musique [etc.] 8°. *Paris*, 1803.

Mugino (Gioseppo). Trattato breve sopra la preservatione et cura della peste. Con le vere cagioni di cognoscere se l'infermità, che regna di presente in Milano, et luoghi circonvicini, sia vera pestilenza, et da quali cagioni sia dependuta. 5 p. l., 70 pp. sm. 8°. *Milano, J. M. Meda*, 1577.

Mugna (Gio. Batt.)
See **Giacomini** (Giacomandrea). La clinica medica pei chirurghi [etc.] 8°. *Padova*, 1836. ———. Opera . . . publicate per cura di G. B. Mugna e F. Coletti. 8°. *Padova*, 1852.

Mugnier (Eugène). *De la folie consécutive aux maladies aiguës. 100 pp. 4°. *Paris*, 1865, No. 38.

Mugnier (Lucien). *Des lésions tardives de l'intestin consécutives au traumatisme de l'abdomen sans trace apparente de contusion sur les parois abdominales. 70 pp. 4°. *Paris*, 1883, No. 176.

Mugnier-Motta (A.) *Contribution à l'étude des sutures tendineuses. 55 pp., 2 l. 4°. *Montpellier*, 1885, No. 35.

Muguet.
See **Aphthæ**; **Mouth** (*Inflammation of*).

Muguet (Félix). * Des fils métalliques capillaires pour la réunion des plaies, et de leur emploi comme sétons dans les petits abcès ganglionnaires du cou. 50 pp. 4°. *Paris*, 1862, No. 30.

Muhammad Ben Zakhariah Alrazi (Abu Bekr). *See* **Rhazes** [Abu Bekr Muhammad Ben Zakhariah Alrazi].

Muhammad 'Ulwi *Khân*. Khulâsat Attajârib. [The result of experiments. A comprehensive compendium of medicine, composed in Persian by . . .] 724 pp. sm. fol. *Lukhnow, A. H.* 1283 [1866].

Muhammed (Mir) Hussein ul Khurâsâni Shîrazî. Makhzan al-Adwiya. [Dictionary of medicaments.] 582, 70 pp. fol. *Bombay*, [1866].
A medical dictionary in Persian text.

Muhlenberg (Henry). Catalogus plantarum Americæ septentrionalis, huc usque cognitarum indigenarum et cicurum; or, a catalogue of the hitherto known native and naturalized plants of North America, arranged according to the sexual system of Linnæus. iv, 112 pp. 8°. *Lancaster, W. Hamilton*, 1813.

——. Descriptio uberior graminum et plantarum calamariarum, Americæ septentrionalis indigenarum et cicurum. ii, 295 pp. 8°. *Philadelphia, S. W. Conrad*, 1817.
See, also, **Smith** (*Sir* James Edward). A grammar of botany. 8°. *New York*, 1822.

Muhlenberg (W. A.) A plea for a church hospital in the city of New York. In two lectures . . . With an appendix, containing the constitution, etc., of St. Luke's Hospital. 55 pp. 8°. *New York, Stanford & Swords*, 1850.

Muhlenbruck (Simon. Henricus). * De usu venæsectionis in febribus acutis. 24 pp. 4°. *Halæ Magdeb., apud J. C. Hendelii viduam*, [1766].

Muhlert (Wilhelm). * Beiträge zur Kenntniss über das Vorkommen der Tuberkelbacillen in tuberkulösen Organen. 36 pp. 8°. *Göttingen, L. Hofer*, 1885.

Muhlius (Benedictus) [1693–]. * De febrium intermittentium theoria et therapia. 3 p. l., 53 pp. sm. 4°. *Helmstadii, typ. H. D. Hammii*, [1721].

——. Vernunftmässige und durch Erfahrung bestätigte Präservir-Cur, welche in einer Anweisung, wie man durch wenige und sichere Mittel die Gesundheit erhalten, und die sonst gewöhnlichen Zufälle entweder gar abwenden oder doch wenigstens erträglich machen könne; denen, die ihre Gesundheit lieb haben und solche zu conserviren bemühet sind, eröfnet, und auf Verlangen einiger Freunde entworfen. x, 258 pp., 9 l. 12°. *Lemgo, J. H. Meyer*, 1743.
For Biography, see **Spies** (Joh. Car.)

Muhr (Adolphus Æm. Guil.) [1788–1836]. * De partibus ossium excidendis. 29 pp., 1 pl. 12°. *Berolini, formis Brüschckianis*, 1823.

Muhrbeck (K.) * De hæmoptysi. 28 pp., 1 l. sm. 4°. *Londini Gothorum, C. G. Berling*, [1768].

de Muiller (Carolus Guilielmus). Physiologia systematis vasorum absorbentium. 62 pp. 4°. *Lipsiæ, ex off. Klaubarthia*, [1793].
For Biography, see **Haase** (J. G.)

Muiller (Joh. Fridericus). De luxu gravissimorum morborum fonte. 3 p. l., 48 pp. 4°. *Lipsiæ, ex off. Sommeria*, [1787].
For Biography, see **Gehler** (Joannes Carolus).

Muilman (Gisbertus Verzyl). *An ex celebrata hactenus opinione de plethora universali vel particulari vera fluxus menstrui causa explicari possit? 1 p. l., 59 pp. 4°. *Leidæ, H. Mostert*, 1772. [*Also, in:* P., v. 1473.]

Muir (G. W.) Sanitary condition of Glasgow and the failure of the improvement act in improving the health of the community. Exposed

Muir (G. W.)—continued.
in letters to the Marquis of Salisbury and Dr. Alfred Carpenter, of Croydon, Surrey. 24 pp. 8°. *Glasgow, W. Portrus & Co.*, 1884.

Muir (M. M. Pattison). Practical chemistry for medical students; specially arranged for the first M. B. course. 64 pp. 16°. *London, Macmillan & Co.*, 1878.

Muir (William).
See **Lowe** (John). Medical missions [etc.] 12°. *London*, 1886.

Muir (*Sir William Mure*) [1818–85].
Obituary. Brit. M. J., Lond., 1885, i, 1271. *Also:* Lancet, Lond., 1885, i, 1107.

Muirhead (Claud). Relapsing fever in Edinburgh during the first five months of the year 1870. 24 pp., 6 tab. 8°. *Edinburgh, Oliver & Boyd*, 1870.
Repr. from: Edinb. M. J., 1870–71, xvi.

Muis (Joan). Redelijke heelkonstoeffening, of heelkonstige aenmerkingen na de vaste gronden der waerachtige, filozofie opgelost . . . en vertaelt door David van Hoogstraten. Vyfde tiental. 9 p. l., 62 pp.; 2 l., 33 pp.; 8 l., 32 pp.; 3 l., 26 pp.; 5 l., 72 pp.; 1 l., 20 pp. 12°. *Rotterdam, F. van Hoogstraten*, 1684–5.
See, also, **Barbette** (Paul). Chirurgia, notis ac observationibus rarioribus illustrata [etc.] 12°. *Amstelædami*, 1693.

Mujarrabât-Akbarî [Great Experiences]. 64 l. 4°. [*n. p., n. d.*]
Work written in Persian, in the so-called "ta' alik" method of writing. The main title, in the center of the title-page, is: "Mujarrabât-Akbari", and a secondary title, printed on top, is as follows: "Aun shibâ-naksh abdân saqimân, we feiz eser berâï'ilâj hakîmân . . ." "Health spending help for sick nobles, and abundance of records on the treatment by physicians . . ."

Mul (Joh.) * De fluore albo. 11 l. 4°. *Lugd. Bat., A. Elzevier*, 1694.

de Mulder (Benedictus). * De erysipelate. 19 pp. 4°. *Gandavi, J. Begyn*, [1822]. [P., v. 958; 961.]

Mulder (Dedericus). * De rabie hydrophobica. 12 pp. sm. 4°. *Lugd. Bat., A. Elzevier*, 1707.

Mulder (Didericus H.) * De ischuria vera ac spuria. 48 pp., 3 l. 4°. *Lugd. Bat., C. de Pecker*, 1766. [P., v. 56.]

Mulder (Gerardus Joh.) [1802–80]. Commentatio de entozoïs. 108 pp. 8°. *Traj. ad Rhenum, O. J. van Paddenburg*, 1823.

——. Commentatio de aquis Rheno-Trajectinis, earumque adhibitione. 158 pp., 1 l. 8°. *Traj. ad Rhenum, O. J. van Paddenburg*, 1824.

——. * De opio ejusque principiis, actione inter se comparatis. 122 pp. 8°. *Traj. ad Rhenum, ex off. J. Altheer*, 1825. [*Also, in:* P., v. 1027.]

——. Verslag wegens den staat der genees-, heel-, verlas- en artsenijbereidkundige school te Rotterdam, uitgebragt ter gelegenheid van het derde algemeene examen der kweekelingen aan dezelve, op den 17. September 1830. 34 pp. 8°. *Rotterdam, M. Wijt*, 1830.

——. Over de waarde der natuurkundige wetenschappen voor de geneeskunde. 35 pp. 8°. *Rotterdam, H. A. Kramers*, 1842.

——. Het streven der stof naar harmonie; eene voorlezing. 40 pp. 8°. *Rotterdam, H. A. Kramers*, 1844.

——. Ueber den Werth und die Bedeutung der Naturwissenschaften für die Medicin. Eine Rede, gehalten bei der Eröffnung seiner chemischen Vorlesung an der Universität zu Utrecht. Aus dem Holländischen übersetzt von Jac. Moleschott. 36 pp. 8°. *Heidelberg, C. F. Winter*, 1844.

——. Versuch einer allgemeinen physiologischen Chemie; mit eigenen Zusätzen des Verfassers für diese deutsche Ausgabe seines Werkes. Nach

Mulder (Gerardus Joh.)—continued.
dem Holländischen von H. Kolbe. 2 v. (paged consecutively). xii, 1289, 15 pp., 20 pl. 8°. *Braunschweig, F. Vieweg u. Sohn,* 1844–51.

——. Gebangan's water, eene iodium houdende watersoort van Neêrlandsch Indië. 18 pp. 8°. *Rotterdam, H. A. Kramers,* 1845.

——. The chemistry of vegetable and animal physiology. Transl. from the Dutch, by Dr. Fromberg. With an introduction and notes by James F. W. Johnston. Pts. 1–4. iv, 28, 827 pp., 20 pl. 8°. [*Edinburgh,* 1845–9.]
Half-title and advertisement to pt. 3 inserted between pp. 346–347, and to pt. 4 between pp. 614–615.

——. The same. 1. Am. ed., with notes by B. Silliman. 176 pp. 8°. *New York, Wiley & Putnam,* 1845.

——. Liebig's questions to Mulder tested by morality and science. Transl. by P. F. H. Fromberg. vii, 122 pp. 8°. *London, W. Blackwood & Sons,* 1846.

——. De voeding in Nederland, in verband tot den volksgeest. 1 p. l., 77 pp. 8°. *Rotterdam, H. A. Kramers,* 1847.

——. De voeding van den neger in Suriname. 36 pp. 8°. *Rotterdam, H. A. Kramers,* 1847.

——. Untersuchungen über die Galle und ein Wort über Protein. Unter des Verfassers Mitwirkung übersetzt von Dr. A. Völcker. xv, 172 pp. 8°. *Frankf. a. M., S. Schmerder,* 1847.

——. Chemische Untersuchungen, unter des Verfassers Mitwirkung übersetzt von Dr. A. Völcker. Drittes Hft. 1 p. l., 293–384 pp. 8°. *Frankf. a. M., S. Schmerder,* 1849.

——. De voeding van Nederlanders. 84 pp. 8°. *Rotterdam, H. A. Kramers,* 1854.

——. Redevoeringen, den 27en en 28en Maart 1854, bij gelegenheid der overdragt van het rectoraat aan de Hoogeschool te Utrecht. 70 pp. 8°. *Utrecht, Gieben u. Dumont,* 1854.

——. Die Chemie des Weines. Aus dem Holländischen von Karl Arenz. xii, 405 pp. 16°. *Leipzig, J. J. Weber,* 1856.

——. The same. The chemistry of wine. Edited by H. Bence Jones. xii, 390 pp. 12°. *London, J. Churchill,* 1857.

——. Die Chemie des Bieres. Aus dem Holländischen übersetzt von Chr. Grimm. x, 472 pp. 16°. *Leipzig, J. J. Weber,* 1858.

——. Water van Goenong Saharie. 8 pp. 8°. *Utrecht,* 1860.

——. Het geneeskundig hooger onderwijs in Nederland in 1865. 24 pp. 8°. *Rotterdam, H. A. Kramers,* 1865.

——. Adres aan zijne excellentie den minister van binnenlandsche zaken, betreffende het nieuwe geneeskundige staats-bestuur. 24 pp. 8°. *Rotterdam, H. A. Kramers,* 1866.

——. De scheikundige middelen der Nederlandsche regering tegen de verspreiding der cholera. 47 pp. 8°. *Rotterdam, H. A. Kramers,* 1866. [P., v. 213.]

——. De natuurkundige methode en de verspreiding der cholera. 348 pp., 2 l. 8°. *Rotterdam, H. A. Kramers,* 1866.

——. Ontleding van Deventer ijzer. 32 pp. 8°. [*n. d., n. p.*]
See, also, **Müller** (Joh.) Gerichtlich-chemische Untersuchungen. 18°. *Berlin,* 1848.—**Sasse** (Augustus). De cholera [etc.] 8°. *Amsterdam,* 1867.—**Vosmaer** (Jacobus). Institutiones semeioticæ [etc.] 8°. *Lugd. Bat.,* 1878.

——. See, also :
Giltay (K. M.) Beschouwing van de levenschets van G. J. Mulder, door hem zelven geschreven. Nederl. Tijdschr. v. Geneesk., Amst., 1882, 2. Afd., 195–201.—**Snellen** (H.) Openingsrede. (Wie was Mulder en wat was hij?) Handel. d. Nederl. Maatsch. t. Bevord. d. Geneesk., Amst., 1880, 66–78.

Mulder (Gerardus Joh.) & **van der Pant** (D. F.) De cholera in Rotterdam. 172 pp. 8°. *Rotterdam, M. Wijt & Zonen,* 1832. [P., v. 204.]

—— & **Roelants** (J. M. A.) Bijdrage tot de geschiedenis der thans in ons vaderland heerschende ziekte. vii, 24 pp. 8°. *Rotterdam, Mensing & van Westreenen,* 1826.

Mulder (Jan Andries) [1807–47]. Tabulæ vasorum corporis humani. 4 tab. imp. fol. *Lugd. Bat., S. et J. Luchtmans,* 1839.

——. Verhandeling over het scheelzien en deszelfs behandeling, voornamelijk door de oogspiersnede (myotomia ocularis), met waarnemingen gestaafd. Uit het Latijn vertaald door J. P. T. van der Lith. viii, 98, vii pp., 3 pl. 8°. *Utrecht, R. Natan,* 1841.
Pl. 2 missing.

——. Aanteekeningen omtrent eene splijting van den voorwand der piswerktuigen. 28 pp., 2 pl. 8°. [*n. p., n. d.*]
Repr. from : Nederl. Lancet, Gravenh., 1845–6, 2. s., i.
See, also, **Kramer** (W.) Raad en waarschuwing omtrent doofheid. Ter behartiging van oorlijders en derzelver artsen. Mit een voorbericht van J. A. Mulder. 8°. *Utrecht,* 1843.

Mulder (Jan). *Bijdrage tot de leukaemie. vii, 64 pp. 8°. *Leyden, P. Engens,* 1856.

Mulder (Jan Sonius). *Eenige belangrijke uitkomsten van de laatste jaren ter beantwoording van de vraag, in hoe ver de aziatische cholera voor eene besmettelijke ziekte moet worden gehouden. 39 pp., 3 l. 8°. *Groningen, J. B. Wolters,* 1860. [*Also, in:* P., v. 185.]

Mulder (Joannes Cornelius). *Diss. sistens observationem fracturæ vertebrarum colli cum adnexa epicrisi. 1 p. l., 31 pp. 8°. *Traj. ad Rhenum, J. Altheer,* [1832].

Mulder (Joannis). Oratio de meritis Petri Camperi in anatomiam comparatam. 112 pp. 4°. *Groningæ, T. Spoormaker,* 1808. [P.,v. 1576.]

Mulder (Joh.) [1769–1810]. *Spec. phys. generalia quædam de calore, et modo quo specifice corporibus inest. 2 p. l., 46 pp., 3 l. 4°. *Franequeræ, G. Coulon,* 1790.

——. *Historia litteraria et critica forcipum et vectium obstetriciorum. [Leyden.] viii, 210 pp., 1 l., xi pl., 4 tab., 4 l. 8°. *Franequeræ,* [1793].

——. The same. viii, 210 pp., 2 l., 11 pl., 4 tab. 8°. *Lugd. Bat., A. et J. Honkoop,* 1794.

——. Redevoering over de redenen, waarom de Nederlanders in het algemeen zeer weinig tot verbetering en uitbreiding van de heel- en verloskunde hebben toegebragt. 59 pp. 4°. *Leeuwarden, D. van der Sluis,* [1797].

——. Oratio de meritis Petri Camperi in anatomiam comparatam, habita die xv. Junii, ciɔiɔcccviii, cum in Academia Groningana physiologiæ, anatomes, chirurgiæ et artis obstetriciæ docendæ munus auspicaretur. Accedunt annotationes biographicæ et literariæ, atque descriptio musei Camperiani. 1 p. l., 112 pp. 4°. *Groningæ, T. Spoormaker,* 1808.

Mulder (Joh. Andreas). *De strabismo, ejusque curandi ratione imprimis per myotomiam ocularem, observationibus probatam. viii, 90, iv pp. 8°. *Traj. ad Rhenum, C. van der Post,* 1840.

Mulder (Marten Edsge). *Over parallelle rolbewegingen der oogen. [Utrecht.] 2 p. l., 74 pp., 1 pl. 8°. *Amsterdam, J. H. De Bussy,* 1874.

Mulder (Nicolaus). *De functione hepatis in disquisitione zoötomica illius visceris nixa. 1 p. l., 146 pp. 8°. *Lugd. Bat., apud viduam M. Cyfreer,* 1818.

Mulders (Aart). *De respiratione. 36 pp. sm. 4°. *Lugd. Bat., Q. Visser,* 1744.

Mule.

See **Horse**; **Hybridity.**

Mulé (Jules). * Quelques considérations sur le traitement des bubons inguinaux. 44 pp. 4°. *Paris*, 1879, No. 401.

Mulert(Carolus). * Diss. enchondromatis casum rariorem sistens. 21 pp. 8°. *Lipsiœ, typ. B. G. Teubneri*, [1852].

Mulert ([Ernst] Otto [Joh.]) [1858–]. * Ein Beitrag zu den fibrösen Neubildungen der Haut. 30 pp. 8°. *Berlin, M. Niethe*, 1881.

Mulert (Guilielmus Fridericus). * Meletemata quædam de hernia ovarii. [Dorpat.] 52 pp. 8°. *Mitaviœ, typ. J. F. Steffenhagen et fil.*, 1848.

Mulert (Henricus) [1824–]. * De usu vaporum chloroformi obstetricio. 39 pp. 8°. *Berolini, G. Schade*, [1848].

Mulette (Charles). * Contribution à l'étude de la pneumonie typhoïde. 106 pp., 1 l. 4°. *Paris*, 1886, No. 276.

Muleur (Georges). * Essai historique sur l'affection calculeuse du foie depuis Hippocrate jusqu'à Fourcroy et Pujol (1801–1802). 258 pp. 4°. *Paris*, 1884, No. 320.

Mulford (*Isaac B.*) [1843–82].
    Obituary. Med. & Surg. Reporter, Phila., 1882, xlvii, 644.

Mulh. Essai sur l'art de faire vivre l'homme sous l'eau et sur les divers travaux qu'il peut faire, même pour le service des bâtimens sousmarins et flottans. xvii (2 l.), 20–256 pp., 2 pl. 8 . *Pau, E. Vignancour*, 1836.

Mulhall (Michael G.) Dictionary of statistics. 2 p. l., 504 pp., 16 pl. 8°. *London, G. Routledge & Sons*, 1884.

Mulheron (John J.) The collective investigation of diphtheria, as conducted by the Therapeutic Gazette, Detroit, Michigan; with editorial summary. 1 p. l., 120 pp. 8°. *Detroit, Mich., G. S. Davis*, 1883.
    Also, Co-Editor of: **Peninsular** (The) Journal of Medicine, Detroit, 1875–6. Also, Editor of: **Michigan** Medical News, Detroit, 1878–82.—**Medical** (The) Age, Detroit, 1883.

Mulle (Louis-Prosper). * Sur la hernie inguinale. 29 pp. 4°. *Paris*, 1834, No. 287, v. 278.

Muller. * Des hydropisies en général, et spécialement de leur mécanisme et de leurs divers modes de développement. 35 pp. 4°. *Paris*, 1847, No. 78, v. 462.

Muller (Abraham). * Theses medicæ inaugurales. 19 pp. 4°. *Lugd. Bat., G. Wishoff*, 1764. [P., v. 55.]

——. Historische beschrijving, van den loop der ziekte een's agtjaarigen lijders, wiens beide voeten door de koude volkomen verstorven waren: nevens de opgaave der adviesen van eenige voornaame mannen, en het voorgevallene in onderscheidene consultatien. 3 l , 66 pp. 8°. *Rotterdam, P. Holsteyn*, 1776.

Muller (Anatole). * Considérations sur un cas de gangrène foudroyante par cause d'endartérite. 2 p. l., 34 pp., 1 l., 1 pl. 4°. *Nancy*, 1881, 1. s., No. 128.

Muller (Antonius Statius). Adversariorum argumenti physico medici collectio. lxiii pp. 4°. *Erlangœ, lit. Waltherianis*, 1775.
    In: DELIUS (H. F.) Adversaria. Fasc. I. 4°. Erlangœ, 1778.

Muller (Auguste)[1]. * De l'emploi de l'eau froide et de la glace en chirurgie. 36 pp. 4°. *Paris*, 1849, No. 162, v. 487.

Muller (Auguste)[2]. * Des appareils plâtrés. 75 pp. 4°. *Strasbourg*, 1867, 2. s., No. 997.

Muller (Auguste)[3]. * Des signes de la mort fournis par l'appareil de la vision. 1 p. l., 43 pp. 4°. *Strasbourg, E. P. Le Roux*, 1870, 3. s., No. 301.

Muller (Auguste)[4]. * De l'atrophie du nerf optique dans les affections cérébrales. 28 pp. 4°. *Paris*, 1871.

Muller (Christianus). Exercitatio anthropologica de cute. Resp. Christophoro Heinrico Kauderbach. 13 l. 4°. *Lipsiœ, lit. J.-E. Hahnii*, [1661].

Muller (Christianus Carolus). De perversa pathologiam discendi, docendi atque exercendi methodo rectæ ad medicinam viæ opposita. 48 pp., 1 l. 4°. *Vitembergœ, typ. E. G. Eichsfeldii*, [1733].

——. * De cephalæa cum immoderato hæmorrhoidum fluxu sæpius repetente. 36 pp. sm. 4°. *Halœ Magdeb., typ. J. C. Hilligeri*, [1735].

Muller (Daniel Gottfried). * De vi consuetudinis rationaliter explicanda. 1 p. l., 39 pp. 4°. *Halœ Magdeb., typ. J. C. Hilligeri*, [1734].

Muller (Eugène). * De l'opération de la pupille artificielle. 40 pp. 4°. *Strasbourg*, 1859, No. 477, 2. s., v. 26.

Muller (Frederik). Catalogus van de bibliotheek der Vereeniging ter Bevordering van de Belangen des Boekhandels. xiv, 144 pp. 8°. *Amsterdam*, 1855.

——. Supplement op den Catalogus [etc.] 91 pp. 8°. *Amsterdam*, 1868.
    Bound with preceding.

——. Catalogue de la bibliothèque d'histoire naturelle de médecine et d'autres sciences de feu M. G. Vrolik. xvi, 154 pp. 8°. *Amsterdam, F. Muller*, 1860. [P., v. 1519.]

——. Curiosa medica. Auteurs anciens sur les sciences médicales, spécialement sur la peste, l'obstétrie, [etc.] 30 pp. 8°. *Amsterdam*, 1884.

——. The same. Spécialement sur la chirurgie, la peste, l'hygiène, la pharmacie, etc. Portraits de centenaires, nains, etc. Figures de monstres. 34 pp. 8°. *Amsterdam*, 1887.

——. Portraits de médecins, naturalistes, astronomes, mathématiciens et physiciens néerlandais et flamands. 104 pp. 8°. *Amsterdam*, [n. d.]
    Bound with: VAN DER WILLIGEN. Portraits. 8°. Amsterdam, [n. d.]

——. Portraits de médecins, naturalistes, astronomes, mathématiciens et physiciens de l'Allemagne, de l'Autriche, de la Suisse, du Danemarc et de la Suède. 152 pp. 8°. *Amsterdam*, [n. d.]
    Bound with: VAN DER WILLIGEN. Portraits. 8°. Amsterdam, [n. d.]

——. Portraits de médecins, naturalistes, mathématiciens, physiciens, philosophes, astronomes, voyageurs, etc., de France et de Suisse.
    In: MULLER (F.) & Co. Portraits de médecins, etc. 8°. Amsterdam, [n. d.], 130–152.

Muller (Frederik Joh.) * Over den invloed van eenige zuren en alcaliën op de spieren van de maag. 2 p. l., 72 pp., 1 l. 8°. *Utrecht, J. van Druten*, 1884.

Muller (Georg. Guilielm. Carol.) * De febre biliosa subjuncta observatione exostoseos rarioris in cranio repertæ. 34 pp. 4°. *Argentorati, lit. J. H. Heitzii*, [1782].

Muller (Georges). * I. Quels sont les changements et les altérations anatomiques immédiats qu'on observe dans l'affection scrofuleuse de la colonne vertébrale, ou mal de Pott, considérée aux différentes époques de son développement. II. [etc.] 36 pp. 4°. *Paris*, 1842, No. 35, v. 393.

Muller (Georgius Ferdinandus). * De damnis et diarrhœa intempestive suppressa oriundis. 48 pp. sm. 4°. *Altorfii, lit. J. G. Meyeri*, [1742].

——. De diarrhœa puerperarum. 30 pp., 1 l. sm. 4°. *Altorfii, typ. J. G. Meyeri*, [1745].

Muller (Georgius Henricus). * De acido hydrocyanico. [Leyden.] 4 p. l., 91 pp. 8°. *Hagæ Comitum, A. van Hoogstraten*, 1835.

Muller (Gerardus). * De atresia felici operatione curata. 27 pp. 4°. *Groningœ, H. Spandaw*, 1763.

Muller (Godefried Theodoor Adolf Wolterbeek). * Over de hooge steensnijding. 1 p. l., 80 pp. 8°. *Leiden, J. Hazenberg, Corns. zoon*, 1862.

Muller (Gottlob David). * De bezoardicorum emolumento et detrimento. 48 pp. sm. 4°. *Vitembergæ, lit. vid. Gerdesiæ*, [1735].

Muller (Henricus Fredericus) * Descriptio anatomica pulli gallinacei extremitatibus superfluis præditi simul cum disquisitione physiologica de ortu monstrorum duplicium parasiticorum. 12 pp., 1 l., 2 pl. 4°. *Kiliæ, C. F. Mohr*, 1859. *In:* SCHRIFT. d. Univ. zu Kiel, vi, 1859, vii, Med. x.

Muller (J. M. F.)
See à **Bergen** (Carol. Augustus) & **Muller** (J. M. F.) De morbo epidemico spasmodico convulsivo [etc.] 4°. *Francof. ad Viadr.*, 1742. *In:* HALLER. Disp. ad morb. [etc.] 4°. *Lausannæ*, 1757, i, 75-96.

Muller (J. T. V.) Guia teórico-práctica para combatir las enfermedades de la vid. Traducido por M. P. O. y adicionado con apéndices que contienen entre otros trabajos una memoria de Mr. Millardet sobre las cepas americanos que resisten á la filoxera y otra de Mr. Dumas sobre los medios de combatir la filoxera. viii, 183 pp. 8°. *Madrid, Gaspar*, 1882.
Biblioteca agrícola ilustrada.

——. Tratado de la falsificacion de los vinos, sus carácteres, efectos en la economía y procedimientos prácticos para reconocer su presencia, obra util é indispensable á los comerciantes de vinos, cosecheros y peritos, traducido y adicionado notabilmente por R. M. O. 94 pp. 8°. *Madrid, Gaspar*, 1882.
Biblioteca agrícola ilustrada.

de Muller (J. W.) baron. Des causes de la coloration de la peau et des différences dans les formes du crâne au point de vue de l'unité du genre humain. 74 pp. 4°. *Stuttgart, imp. roy.*, 1853.

Muller (Jacobus). De natura motus animalis et voluntarii exercitatio singularis, ex principiis physicis, medicis, geometricis et architectonicis deducta. 13 l. sm. 4°. *Giessæ, typ. C. Chemlini*, 1617.

Muller (Jean-Baptiste). * Remarques sur le traitement du croup. 34 pp. 4°. *Strasbourg*, 1842, No. 101, 2. s., v. 8.

Muller (Jeremias). * De usu et abusu potus thee in genere, præcipue vero in hydrope. 24 pp. 4°. *Kiliæ*, [1692].

Muller (Jo. J.) De rupto in partu utero. *Basileæ*, 1745.
In: HALLER. Disp. chir. [etc.] 4°. *Lausannæ*, 1755, iii, 489-524.

Muller (Joannes Andreas Petrus). * De phimosi et paraphimosi eorumque curatione. 27 pp. 4°. *Erfordiæ, J. C. Goerling*, [1797].

Muller (Joannes Antonius). * De habitu phthisico. viii, 80 pp., 1 l. 8°. *Traj. ad Rhenum, ex off. van Paddenburg et soc.*, 1838.

Muller (Joannes Bernhardus). * De melancholia. 40 pp. sm. 4°. *Jenæ, lit. Marggrafianis*, [1727].
For Biography, see **Hilscher** (Sim. Paul.)

Muller (Joannes Caspar.) * Polypos capitis exponit. 28 pp., 4 l. sm. 4°. *Jenæ, typ. P. Ehrichi*, [1699].
See, also, **Wedelius** (Ern. Hen.) & **Muller** (J. C.) De peritonæo. 4°. *Jenæ*, [1696].
For Biography, see **Slevogt** (Jo. Had.)

Muller (Joannes Christianus Gottlob). * De angina maligna. 22 pp. 4°. *Erfordiæ, S. H. R. Nonne*, [1773].

Muller (Joannes Godofredus). * De venenis acutis. 82 pp. 4°. *Vitebergæ, lit. E. G. Eichsfeldii*, [1732].

——. The same. * De venenis acutis (von schnellem Gifft). 82 pp. 4°. *Vitebergæ, E. G. Eichsfeldii*, [1732].

34

Muller (Joannes Paulus). * De phrenitide. 13 l. 4°. *Helmæstadi, typ. H. Mulleri*, 1643.

Muller (Joh.) De ephialte seu incubo. 19 l. 4°. *Lipsiæ, typ. C. Fleischeri*, [1688].

——. * Spec. med. de febre amatoria. 28 pp., 4 l. sm. 4°. *Jenæ, lit. Krebsianis*, [1689].
For Biography, see **Faschius** (Aug. Hen.)

Muller (Joh. Christianus). * Disp. exhibens morbum regium. 7 l. 4°. *Erffordiæ, typ. Groschianis*, [1707].

Muller (Joh. Ernestus). * De cornu cervi ejusque vi bezoardica. 11 l. 4°. *Erfordiæ, lit. D. Sumphi*, [1704].

Muller (Joh. Fridericus). * Diss. sistens casum peculiarem de morbo motuum habituali ex imaginatione sub ructuum schemate enato. 32 pp. sm. 4°. *Halæ Magdeb., typ. J. C. Hendelii*, [1732]. [*Also, in :* P., v. 69; 73.]

Muller (Joh. Jacobus). * De melancholia attonita raro litteratorum affectu. 28 pp. 4°. *Jenæ, lit J. F. Ritteri*, [1741].
For Biography, see **Teichmeyer** (Hermannus Fridericus).

Muller (Joh. Leonardus). * Verhandeling over eenige der oorzaken van plotselingen dood in het kraambed. 34 pp., 2 l. 8°. *Groningen, H. R. Roelfsema*, [1856].

Muller (Joh. Sigismundus). * Raram de calculo vesicæ observationem atque epicrisin proponit. 1 p. l., 35 pp., 1 pl. sm. 4°. *Argentorati, typ. J. H. Heitzii*, [1768].

Muller (Joseph-Robert) [1850–   ]. * Contribution à l'étude de l'intervention chirurgicale chez les calculeux. 127 pp., 2 l. 4°. *Lille*, 1883, 2. s., No. 52.

Muller (Lambertus Fredericus Antonius). * De motibus quos dicunt reflexos. [Utrecht.] xxvi, 158 pp., 1 l. 8°. *Amstelodami, C. L. van Langenhuysen*, 1855.

Muller (Lambertus Reinier). * De febre intermittente. 1 p. l., 92 pp., 3 l. 8°. *Groningæ, H. Eekhoff, H. fil.*, 1809.

Muller (Louis-Antoine). * La fièvre puerpérale existe-t-elle ? 1 p. l., 64 pp. 4°. *Strasbourg*, 1846, No. 158, v. 12.

Muller (M. J. E.)
Co-Editor of : **Natuur-** en geneeskundig Archief voor Neêrlandsch Indië, Batavia, 1844-6.

Muller (Matth. Christianus). De laterna magica. 36 pp., 1 pl. 4°. *Jenæ, H. Beyer*, [1704].

Muller (P.) * Des extraits de viande au point de vue physiologique. 48 pp. 4°. *Paris*, 1871, No. 77.

Muller (Paul) [1862–   ]. * Essai sur la dyspepsie cardiaque. 73 pp. 4°. *Paris, A. Parent*, 1886, No. 277.

Muller (Paul) [1858–   ]. * De la toux utérine. 83 pp. 4°. *Paris*, 1887, No. 274.

Muller (Paulus Christianus). * Diss. ægrum hæmoptysi laborantem sistens. 2 p. l., 24 pp. 4°. *Lipsiæ, lit. Schniebesianis*, [1728].
For Biography, see **Schacher** (Polyc. Gottlieb).

Muller (Petrus Joh.) * Spec. med. inaug. exhibens observationes quasdam therapeuticas de fibra adstringenda. 1 p. l., 34 pp., 3 l. 8°. *Groningæ, B. van der Kamp*, [1822].

Muller (Philippus) [1585-1659]. Miracula et mysteria chymico-medica libris quinque enucleata. 3. ed. Accesserunt his : 1. Tyrocinium chymicum. 2. Novum lumen chymicum; summa horum juxta seriem capitum et tractatuum ad calcem invenienda est. 12 p. l., 493 pp. 24°. [*Friborgi*], imp. C. Bergeri, 1616.

——. The same. 4. ed. 10 p. l., 493 pp., 2 l. 16°. *Wittebergæ, sumpt. C. Bergeri*, 1623.

——. The same. Miracula chymica et mysteria medica. 10 p. l., 191 pp. 32°. *Parisiis, M. Mondiers*, 1644.

Muller (Philippus)—continued.
——. The same. 9 p. l., 379 pp., 1 l. 32°.
Amstelodami, A. J. Valckenier, 1656.
For *Portrait, see* **Collection**—van Kaathoven.

Muller (Rudolphus Joh. Petrus). * Spec. med.
inaug. continens casum spondylarthrocacis. 1
p. l., 20, iii, 7 pp. 8°. *Groningæ, H. Roelfsema*,
[1851].

Muller (Sigismundus). * De motu sanguinis
naturali, nonnaturali et mixto. 20 pp. 4°.
Erfordiæ, typ. J. H. Groschii, 1719.

Muller (Theodorus Andreas). * De conscientia
medica. 48 pp. sm. 4°. [*Halle*], *J. C. Hendel*,
[1724].

Muller (Theodorus Leopoldus Guillielmus).
* Diss. med. inaug. continens historiæ dyna-
micæ organicæ ætatem Stahlianam. 37 pp. 8°.
Lugd. Bat., P. H. van den Heuvell, 1844.

Muller (Wilhelm Henr.) * De thymo. 24 pp.
4°. *Lovanii*, 1706.
In: HALLER. Disp. anat. [etc.] 4°. *Gottingæ*, 1747,
ii, 455–479.

——. * De ἀνκύλωσι. 14 pp., 1 l., 1 pl. 4°.
Lugd. Bat., A. Elzevier, 1707.
Also, in: HALLER. Disp. chir. [etc.] 4°. *Lausannæ*,
1755, iv, 539–547, 1 pl.

Muller (Wolffgang Sigismundus). * De erube-
scentibus et venarum capitis subitaneo tumore.
32 pp. sm. 4°. *Lipsiæ, ex off. Langenhemiana*,
[1739]. [*Also, in :* P., v. 58.]
For *Biography, see* **Platner** (Jo. Zach.)

Muller, *dictus* **Wohlheimer** (Fridericus
Christianus). * Diss. opii correctionem genui-
nam et usum . . . proponit. 31 pp., 2 l. 4°.
Halæ Magdeb., lit. C. Henckelii, [1702].
——. The same. 31 pp. 4°. *Recusa, Halæ
Magdeb., typ. J. C. Hilligeri*, 1730.

Mullois (Georges) [1854–]. * Contribution à
l'étude de la congestion pulmonaire et rénale
dans l'étranglement herniaire avec algidité. 73
pp., 1 l. 4°. *Paris*, 1881, No. 331.

Mullon (Henri). * Causes et pronostic des hémorrhagies intestinales survenant dans la fièvre
typhoïde. 62 pp., 1 l. 4°. *Paris*, 1876, No. 102.

Mullot (Albert). * Du vertige auriculaire consécutif aux injections de liquide dans le conduit
auditif externe. 44 pp. 4°. *Paris*, 1885, No.
48.

Mullot (L.-N.-P.) * Sur le bubonocèle. 30 pp.
8°. *Paris, an XI* [1803], v. 30.

Mullot (Laurent) fils. * Sur la péritonite des
femmes en couches. 15 pp. 4°. *Paris*, 1816,
No. 195, v. 125.

Mullye.
Tytler (J.) Remarks on the climate of Mullye. Tr.
M. & Phys. Soc. Calcutta, 1827-9, iv, 359–376.

Mulnier (Richard) [1844–]. * Ueber Basedow'sche Krankheit. 39 pp. 8°. *Berlin, G.
Lange*, [1869].

Mulnier (Sam. Ferd. Amad. Paulus) [1837–].
* De calculis biliaris. 32 pp. 8°. *Berolini, G.
Lange*, [1863].

Mulock (Thomas). British lunatic asylums,
public and private ; with an appendix containing the case of Doctor Peithman, and special
references to the cases of Lady Lytton Bulwer
and Mrs. Turner. 50 pp. 12°. *London, Hill &
Halden*, 1858.

Mulot (Albert). * D'une complication des fractures. 35 pp. 4°. *Strasbourg, Christoph*, 1869,
3. s., No. 207.

Mulot (Henry-Michel-Jean). * Quelques considérations sur une épidémie de dysenterie. 30 pp.
4°. *Paris*, 1853, No. 303, v. 546.

Mulsant (E.) Notice sur le docteur Jules
Sichel. 30 pp. 8°. *Lyon, Associat. typog. Regard*,
1869.
Repr. from : Ann. Soc. Linnéenne de Lyon, n s., xvii.

Mulzer (Josef). * Ueber Thoraxmessungen. 47
pp. 8°. *Würzburg, Becker*, 1879.
c.

Mumia *nativa persica.*

Kæmpfer (E.) Muminahi, seu mumia nativa persica.
In his : Amœnitatum exoticarum [etc.], 4°, Lemgoviæ,
1712, 516–524.—**Schoberus** (G.) De mumia persica : i. e.
remedio in Asia celeberrimo. Acta Acad. nat. curios.,
Norimb., 1727, i (app.), 150–157.

Mumm (Ernst). * Ueber Verschliessung der
Scheide bei Blasen-Scheidenfisteln. 32 pp. 8°.
Marburg, C. L. Pfeil, [1858].

Mumm (Franz Anton). * Ueber die Unempfindlichkeit des Rückenmarks insbesondere der vordern Stränge desselben gegen Reize. 17 pp., 1 l.
8°. *Greifswald, F. Hache*, [1869].
c.

Mummery (John R.) On the relations which
dental caries (as discovered amongst the ancient
inhabitants of Britain, and amongst existing aboriginal races) may be supposed to hold to their
food and social conditions. 74 pp., 2 tab. 8°.
London, Wyman & Sons, 1870.
Repr. from : Tr. Odont. Soc. Gr. Brit., Lond., 1869-70,
n. s., ii.

Mummies *and mummy.*

See, also, **Embalming.**

BELLONIUS (P.) De admirabili operum antiquorum et rerum suspiciendarum præstantia
liber primus. De medicato funere, seu cadavere condito, et lugubri defunctorum ejulatione
liber secundus. De medicamentis nonnullis,
servandi cadaveris vim obtinentibus liber tertius. 8°. *Parisiis*, 1553.

CONSTANTIN (M.) * De methodis balsamandi
cadavera humana, juxta antiquos et recentiores.
8°. *Pestini*, [1834].
Hungarian text.

CORNALIA (E.) Illustrazione della mummia
peruviana esistente nel Civico Museo di Milano.
fol. *Milano*, 1860.
Repr. from : Atti . . . r. Ist. Lomb. d. sc. e lett., Milano,
1860, ii.

CZERMAK (J. N.) Beschreibung und mikroskopische Untersuchung zweier ägyptischer Mumien. 8°. [*Prag*, 1852.]
Repr. from : Sitzungsb. d. k. Akad. d. Wissensch.
Math.-naturw. Cl., Wien, 1852, ix.

HENDEWERCK (G. B.) * De mumia. 4°.
Halæ Magdeb., [1737].

VON ISENFLAMM (H. F.) Ueber Mumien.
In his : Anat. Untersuchungen. 8°. *Erlangen*, 1822,
301–320.

JOLY (N.) Notice sur une momie américaine,
du temps des Incas, trouvée dans la Nouvelle-
Grenade. 8°. *Toulouse*, [n. d.]
Repr. from : Mém. Acad. nat. d. sc. de Toulouse.

KETTNER (F. G.) Μουμία τῶν Αἰγυπτίων, sive
historicum schediasma de mumiis Ægyptiacis
deque egregia Lipsiensi in bibliotheca instructis-
sima magnifici senatus quondam visa. 2. ed.
12°. *Lipsiæ*, 1703.

—— & SUSCHKY (J. S.) De mumiis Ægyptiacis. 4°. *Lipsiæ*, [1694].

LANGGUTH (C. A.) De bestiis Ægyptiorum studio conversis in mumias. 4°. *Vitebergæ*, [1808].

LANZONI (J.) Tractatus de balsamatione cadaverum, in quo non tantum de pollinctura apud
veteres, sed etiam de variis balsamandi cadavera modis apud recentes multa curiosa breviter
exponuntur. 18°. *Genevæ*, [1693].

LECHE (J.) * De mumia Ægyptiaca. sm. 4°.
Londini Gothorum, [1739].

NEICHEL (C.) * De pollinctura cadaverum
humanorum juxta antiquos et recentes. 8°.
Pestini, [1-21].

PANCERI (P.) La mummia peruviana del
Museo nazionale di Napoli. Nota letta nella
tornata del dì 26 gennaio 1868 della Accademia
Pontaniana. 4°. *Napoli*, 1868.
Repr. from : Atti Accad. Pontaniana, ix.

Mummies *and mummy.*

PARÉ (A.) Discours. À sçavoir: de la mumie, des vénins, de la licorne et de la peste. sm. 4°. *Paris*, 1582.

PETTIGREW (T. J.) A history of Egyptian mummies and an account of the worship and embalming of the sacred animals by the Egyptians, with remarks on the funeral ceremonies of different nations, and observations on the mummies of the Canary Islands, of the ancient Peruvians, Burman priests, etc. 4°. *London*, 1834.

PICKERING (C.) The Gliddon mummy case in the museum of the Smithsonian Institution. 4°. *Washington*, 1870.

REINHARDT (J.) Quinque mumias bestiarum Ægyptiacas describendo prolusit. sm. 4°. *Havniæ*, 1824.

TENTZELIUS (A.) Medicina diastatica, hoc est singularis illa et admirabilis ad distans, et beneficio mumialis transplantationis operationem et efficaciam habens, quæ ipsa loco commentarii in tractatum tertium de tempore seu philosop. D. Theoph. Paracelsi, multa, eaque selectissima abstrusioris philosophiæ et medicinæ arcana continet, [etc.] 32°. *Erfurti*, [1661].

UNCOVERING the mummy of Rameses II., king of Egypt, the oppressor of the Jews in the time of Moses.. The mummy of the Egyptian king, Rameses II., of the nineteenth dynasty (about 1400 to 1250 B. C.), stripped of its coverings. From photographs. 2 l. fol. *Boston*, 1886.

Boudet [*et al.*]. Rapport sur plusieures substances provenant d'une momie d'Égypte. Mém. Acad. de méd., Par., 1833, iii, pt. 2, 46-62.—**Brébant.** Notes sur un curieux procédé d'embaumement et de momification constaté sur deux cadavres trouvés à Reims dans des cercueils de plomb. Union méd. et scient. du nord-est, Reims, 1886, x, 290-305.—**Brouardel.** Sur un cas de momification d'un cadavre; applications médico-légales. Bull. Acad. de méd., Par., 1886, 2. s., xv, 793-811.—**Brownlie** (J. R.) On certain mummy teeth. J. Brit. Dent. Ass., Lond., 1886, vii, 401-403.—**Cailliaud** (F.) Rapport de M. Mareschal sur la momie donnée à la Société académique. J. de la sect. de méd Soc. acad. Loire-Inf., Nantes, 1826, ii, 180-196.—**Dalrymple** (J.) An account of the examination of two bodies, found in the vaults of the ruins of Wymondham Abbey, in Norfolk. Med. Q. Rev., Lond., 1835, iii, 169-171, 1 pl.—**Fouquet.** Observations relevées sur quelques momies royales d'Égypte. Bull. Soc. d'anthrop. de Par., 1886, 3. s., ix, 578-590.—**Granville** (A. B.) An account of the opening of an Egyptian mummy. Med. & Phys. J., Lond., 1821, xlvi, 377-379.—**Maddox** (R. L.) On the different tissues found in the muscle of a mummy. J. Roy. Micr. Soc., Lond., 1887, pt. 4, 537-544, 1 pl.—**Mareschal de Rougeres.** Lettre contenant quelques observations sur les effets de la momie. J. de méd., chir., pharm., etc., Par., 1767, xxvi, 466-469.—**Maspero** (G.) Unbandaging of Egyptian mummies. [Transl.] San. World, Lond., 1886, vi, 5.—**Mummification** der Leichen amerikanischer Indianer. Allg. Ztschr. f Epidemiol., Erlang., 1874, i, 157.—**Senéze** (V.) & **Noctzli** (J.) Sur les momies découvertes dans le haut Pérou. Bull. Soc. d'anthrop. de Par., 1877, 2. s., xii, 640.—**de Sevelinges.** Observation sur les effets de la momie d'Égypte. J. de méd., chir., pharm., etc, Par., 1759, xi, 224-227.—**Warren** (J. C.) Description of an Egyptian mummy presented to the Massachusetts General Hospital, with an account of the operation of embalming in ancient and modern times. Boston J. Phil. & Arts, 1823-4, i, 164; 269, 2 pl. *Also*, Reprint.

Mummification.

See Cadaver (*Jurisprudence of*); Mummies, etc.

Mumps.

See, also, Parotid *gland* (*Inflammation of*).

BAUER (A. C.) * De parotitide. 8°. *Lugd. Bat.*, 1840.

BRUN (P.) * Considérations sur les oreillons. 4°. *Montpellier*, 1873.

CARPENTIER (L.) * De l'oreillon considéré comme maladie générale et éruptive. 4°. *Paris*, 1869.

COMBEAU (E.) * Des oreillons, considérés comme maladie générale, et de l'atrophie consécutive à l'orchite épidémique. 4°. *Paris*, 1867.

Mumps.

CORDES (C. E.) * De angina parotidea. 8°. *Gottingæ*, [1829].

DE CREVOISIER D'HURBACHE (M.-J.-C.-H.) * Des oreillons idiopathiques. 4°. *Strasbourg*, 1847.

ELSNER (C. F.) [Pr.] in proœmio spicilegium ad anginam maxillarem præmittitur. sm. 4°. *Regiomonti*, [1787].

GAILHARD (J.) * Étude sur la maladie appelée oreillons, sa nature, ses expressions, ses rapports, etc. 4°. *Montpellier*, 1877.

GASTET (M.) * Sur les oreillons. 4°. *Montpellier*, 1876.

HAILLOT (J.-C.) * De l'oreillon et de ses complications. 4°. *Paris*, 1876.

HOPFF (J. G.) * De angina parotidea. 8°. *Gottingæ*, [1799].

KARTH (A.) * Étude sur une forme grave d'oreillons. 4°. *Paris*, 1883.

LAMOTTE (D.) * Étude sur les oreillons. 4°. *Montpellier*, 1876.

LEMARCHAND (A.) * Des oreillons chez le soldat. 4°. *Paris*, 1876.

MACHADO (V. - C.) * Essai sur les oreillons sous-maxillaires. 4°. *Paris*, 1880.

MALABOUCHE (É.) * Étude sur la maladie désignée généralement sous le nom d'oreillons. 4°. *Montpellier*, 1867.

METZ (F. A.) * Diss. sistens anginam parotidæam una cum thesibus ex universa medicina et chirurgica. 4°. [*Wirceburg*, 1801.]

MÜLLER (J.) * De angina parotidea. 8°. *Monachii*, 1840.

PHILIPP (C.) * De parotitide. 8°. *Berolini*, [1846].

PINET (C.) * De l'état de nos connaissances sur l'affection ourlienne, ou oreillons. 4°. *Paris*, 1878.

ROPAS (T.) * Essai sur les oreillons. 4°. *Paris*, 1869.

SALLAUD (É.-A.) * Des oreillons, de leur nature, de leurs soi-disant métastases. 4°. *Montpellier*, 1868.

SETA (F.-M.) * Des oreillons. 4°. *Paris*, 1869.

TOURTELLE (J. F.) * Dissertation sur les oreillons. 4°. *Paris*, 1828.

VIDAL (A.) * Des oreillons. 4°. *Paris*, 1871.

VIÉLA (L.) * Considérations sur les oreillons examinés principalement au point de vue de la fièvre. 4°. *Paris*, 1886.

Albers. Angina submaxillaris. Med. Cor.-Bl. rhein. u. westfäl. Aerzte, Bonn, 1844, iii, 222-224.—**Atkinson** (T. P.) Liability of young children to mumps. Stethoscope, Richmond, 1855, v, 1-3.—**Béhier.** Les oreillons. Courrier méd., Par., 1874. xxiv, 347-350. *Also:* École de méd., Par., 1876-7, 1-8.—**Billroth.** Fall von Angina parotidea. Mag. f. d. ges. Heilk., Berl., 1831, xxxv, 27-30.—**Bosc.** Réflexions et observations sur l'oreillon et la parotide. Bull. Soc. anat. de Par. 1829, 2. éd., 1846, iv, 61.—**Bougard.** De l'oreillon. J. de méd., chir. et pharmacol., Brux., 1866, xlii, 22-31.—**Brush** (E. C.) Parotitis. Columbus M. J., 1884-5, iii, 435-444.—**Chenery** (F.) Mumps; a reply to Dr. F. M. Wilson's inquiry. Boston M. & S. J., 1875, xciii, 87.—**Chomel & Louis.** Observations sur les oreillons. Gaz. d. hôp., Par, 1830-31, iv, 335.—**Chrétien** (H.) Parotide. Dict. encycl. d. sc. méd., Par., 1885, 2. s., xxi, 378-474.—**Davezac.** Parotide suppurée; broncho-pneumonie; mort. Mém. et bull. Soc. de méd. et chir. de Bordeaux (1885), 1886, 12-14.—**Debout** (*d'Estrées*) (A. E.) On gouty parotitis and gouty orchitis. Brit. M. J., Lond., 1887, i, 569.—**d'Heilly** (E.) Oreillons. N. dict. de méd. et chir. prat., Par., 1878, xxv, 93-109.—**van Dommelen.** Angina parotidea (bauerwetzel, mumps, oreillons). N. pract. Tijdschr. v. de Geneesk., Gorinchem, 1856, n. s., ii, 261-265.— **Dumarest** (A.) Note sur quelques particularités des oreillons. Lyon méd., 1876, xxii, 109-111.— **Fehr** (M.) Ueber das Wesen des Mumps. Arch. f. klin. Chir., Berl., 1876-7, xx, 600-621.— **Fournié** (H.) Contribution à l'histoire épidémiologique et clinique des oreillons. Rec. de mém. de méd. . . . mil., Par., 1881, xxxvii, 509-536.— **Fremmert** (H.) Die Parotitis: nach Beobachtungen im Hospital. Deutsches Arch. f. klin. Med., Leipz., 1885-6, xxxviii, 389-432.— **Gabbi** (U.)

Mumps.

Ritardo del polso in un caso di parotite epidemica. Raccoglitore med., Forlì, 1886, 5. s., i, 547–560. — **Gallozzi** (C.) Storia ed osservazione clinica d' una rara forma morbosa della parotide. Gior. internaz. d. sc. med., Napoli, 1881, n. s., iii, 27–30.—**Groffier.** Remarques sur les affectious catarrhales, connues sous le nom de parotides simples, et vulgairement appelées ourles; sur les formes particulières sous lesquelles elles se reproduisent quelquefois; et sur le traitement qui leur convient. Ann. Soc. de méd.-prat. de Montpel., 1806, viii, 311–327.—**Groner** (F. J.) Specific for parotitis. Physician & Surg., Ann Arbor, Mich., 1881, iii, 307.—**Habran.** Parotide à répétition. Union méd. et scient. du nord-est, Reims, 1880, iv, 137.—**Hamilton** (R.) An account of a distemper, by the common people in England vulgarly called the mumps. Tr. Roy. Soc. Edinb., 1790, ii, pt. 2, 59–72. Also: Lond. M. J., 1790, xi, 190–211.—**Holmes** (T. M.) A case of metastatic parotiditis terminating in suppuration; recovery. Atlanta M. & S. J., 1887, n. s., iv, 205–209.—**Holt** (L.) Parotitis; being a summary of all the cases found in the records of the Bellevue Hospital. Med. Gaz., N. Y., 1881, viii, 351.—**Isham** (A. B.) Parotiditis, or mumps; a theory of its etiology, and the rationale of the secondary manifestations, or so-called metastases. Am. J. M. Sc., Phila., 1878, n. s., lxxvi, 369–378. Also, transl.: Med.-chir. Centralbl., Wien, 1879, xiv, 86; 97; 134; 158. — **Jaccoud** (S.) Sur un cas d'oreillons. In his: Leçons de clin. méd. . . . (1883–4), 8°, Par., 1885, 497–516. Also [Abstr.]: J. de méd. et chir. prat., Par., 1884, lv, 56–58. — **Jacob.** Les oreillons au point de vue épidémiologique et clinique. Rec. de mém. de méd. . . . mil., Par., 1875, 3. s., xxxi, 529–568. — **Keith** (S.) A case of suppuration of the parotid following ovariotomy. Edinb. M. J. 1886-7, xxxii, 306.—**Laveran** (A.) Du pronostic et de la prophylaxie des oreillons chez l'adulte, et en particulier de l'orchite ourlienne. Union méd., Par., 1878, 3. s., xxvi, 159; 169; 184. Also: Bull. et mém. Soc. méd. d. hôp de Par. (1878), 1879, 2. s., xv. 61–72. Also: Gaz. d. hôp., Par., 1878, li, 444–446. ——. Oreillons. Dict. encycl. d. sc. méd , Par., 1882, 2. s., xvii, 310–363.—[**Liégey.**] Un mot sur les adénites en général et l'oreillon en particulier. J. de méd., chir. et pharmacol., Brux., 1866, xliii, 133–136.—**Little** (J. P.) Very young children not liable to the mumps. Stethoscope, Richmond, 1854, iv, 576. [See, also, supra, Atkinson (T. P.)]—**Manby** (A. R.) Note on the incubation of mumps. Brit. M. J., Lond., 1878, i, 642.—**Margianti** (E.) Studio analitico sui così detti orecchioni. Gior. med. d. r. esercito, etc., Roma, 1886, xxxiv, 780; 902. — **Mercklen.** Deux observations de parotidite. France méd., Par., 1878, xxv, 313–315.—**Murat.** Oreillon. Dict. d. sc. méd., Par., 1819, xxxviii, 129–137.— **Parsons** (H.) Observations on cynanche parotidea, or mumps. Lond. M. Reposit., 1817, vii, 205–207.—**Peirson** (A. L.) Observations upon parotitis, or mumps. N. Eng. J. M. & S., Bost., 1824, xiii, 116–119.—**Prager** (P.) Ueber Parotitis catarrhalis s. epidemica. Wien. med. Bl., 1887, x, 302.—**Recent** observations on mumps. Brit. M. J., Lond., 1879, ii, 311.—**Records** (B. F.) Parotitis. Cincin. Lancet & Obs., 1872, xv, 394–397.— **Reig Gascó** (J.) Importancia de las parotiditis idiopáticas ó paperas. Gac. de sanid. mil., Madrid, 1884, x, 390–395.—**Renard** (E.) Note sur l'albuminurie et les oreillons. Arch. de méd. et pharm. mil., Par., 1885, vi, 185–189.—**Rinaldi.** Quelques mots sur les oreillons. J. de méd. et pharm. de l'Algérie, Alger, 1876–7, i, 38.—**Ringer** (S.) Parotitis. Syst. Med. (Reynolds), Lond., 1866, i, 227–233.—**Rizet.** Note sur les oreillons. Bull. méd. du nord, Lille, 1865, 2. s., vi, 418–423.—**Roskoten** (R.) Idiopathic parotitis, or mumps. Peoria M. Month., 1884-5, v, 677–679.—**Schwerin.** Fall von Mumps. Deutsche med. Wchnschr., Berl., 1883, ix, 146.—**Siedamgrotzky &** **Hofmeister.** Chemische Zusammensetzung des Speichels der Parotis vom Rinde. Ber. ü. d. Veterinärw. im Königr. Sachs., Dresd., 1878, xxiii, 123.—**Smolinski** (P.) Ueber Parotitis. St. Petersb. med. Wchnschr., 1878, iii, 339.—**Sorel** (F.) Note sur quelques particularités observées dans le développement des oreillons. Rev. mens. de méd. et chir., Par., 1878, ii, 266–273.—**Strambio** (G.) Pratiche osservazioni intorno agli orecchioni. Gior. anal. di med., Milano, 1828, ix, 241–244.—**Testa** (B.) Intorno la virtù terapeutica del jaborandi contro gli orecchioni. Morgagni, Napoli, 1878, xx, 544–547.—**Vallejo Lobon** (M.) Parotitis afectando la forma epidémica. Rev. de med. y cirug. práct., Madrid, 1886, xviii, 225–238.—**Von** **Iffland** (A.) Cynanche parotidæa. Montreal M. Gaz., 1844, i, 233. — **Wagner** (B.) Zur Incubationszeit der Parotitis. Jahrb. f. Kinderh., Leipz , 1868–9, n. F., ii, 335.—**Ward** (B. S.) Parotitis in the aged. N. Orl. M. & S. J., 1858-9 xv, 169–173.—**Wendt** (E. C.) A contribution to the pathological histology of acute parotitis. N. York M. J., 1880, xxxii, 248–261.

Mumps (Causes and contagion of).

BERTH (P.) * Ueber Parotitis nach gynäcologischen Operationen. 8°. Greifswald, 1886.

MONIN (E.) * Essai critique sur la pathogénie et l'étiologie des oreillons. 4°. Paris, 1877.

Mumps (Causes and contagion of).

MUELLER (H.) * Zur Aetiologie der Parotitis. 8°. Halle, 1883.

SCHMALLE (R.) * Ein Fall von Parotitis nach einer Hämorrhoiden-Operation. 8°. Greifswald, 1886.

Boinet. Note sur le microbe des oreillons. Lyon méd., 1885, xlviii, 285–289. Also: Mém. et compt.-rend. Soc. d. sc. méd. de Lyon (1884), 1885, xxiv, pt. 2, 210–215.— **Capitan & Charrin.** Étiologie des oreillons. Compt. rend. Soc. de biol. 1881, Par., 18-2, 7. s., iii, 192. ——. Microbes dans les oreillons. Ibid., 358.—**Colin** (L.) Rapport des oreillons avec les fièvres éruptives. Bull. et mém. Soc. méd. d. hôp. de Par. (1876), 1877. 2 s., xiii, 56–70. Also: Union méd., Par., 1876, 3. s., xxi, 437; 462; 499. — **Cousin** (A.) Que les oreillons doivent être mis au rang des éruptives frustes. Union méd., Par., 1869, vii, 679–681.—**Curtis** (B. F.) Parotitis complicating gonorrhœa. N. York M. J., 1887, xlv, 346.—**Jaccoud.** Du caractère infectieux de l'affection ourlienne. Gaz. d. hôp., Par., 1885, lviii, 547. — **Ollivier.** Étiologie et pathogénie des oreillons. Praticien, Par., 1885, vii, 306–308.— **Ollivier** (A.) De la contagiosité et du contage des oreillons. Rev. mens. d. mal. de l'enf., Par., 1885, iii. 297–307, 1 pl.—**Paget** (S.) Parotitis after injury or disease of the abdomen or pelvis. Lancet, Lond., 1887, i, 314. Also: Brit. M. J., Lond., 1887, i, 613–616. Also. transl.: Wien. med. Bl., 1887, x, 684; 720.—**Trousseau.** Des oreillons; leur nature contagieuse. Gaz. d. hôp., Par., 1843, 2. s., v, 405.

Mumps (Complications and sequelæ of).

BICH (O.) * De l'atrophie testiculaire consécutive aux oreillons; de ses conséquences et de son traitement. 4°. Paris, 1883.

BOUTEILLIER (G.-L.-F.) * Des oreillons et de leur métastase chez la femme. 4°. Paris, 1866.

DEBIZE (F.) * De l'état typhoïde dans les oreillons. 4°. Paris, 1869.

DÜHRSSEN (A.) * Ueber chronische Parotitis mit consecutiver Speichelgeschwulst, nebst einer Zusammenstellung der bisher veröffentlichten Fälle ven Sialodochitis Stenoniana und Whartoniana. 8°. Berlin, [1884].

MICHEL (J.-B.) * Des oreillons; études critiques sur leurs métastases. Orchite. 4°. Paris, 1868.

SPIRE (F.-J.-P.) * De l'orchite métastatique des oreillons. 4°. Paris, 1851.

Aitken (C.) Mumps, orchitis, rheumatic fever, chorea. Brit. M. J., Lond., 1887, i, 155.—**Appleyard** (A.) Case of mumps, with endocardial murmurs, high temperature and metastasis to testes. Lancet, Lond., 1882, i, 101.— **Armstrong** (S. T.) Parotitis accompanied with orchitis; eventual suppuration and atrophy of testicle. N. Orl. M. & S. J., 1882-3, n. s., x, 678.—**Beale.** Case of cyanche parotidea, with metastasis. Med. Times & Gaz., Lond., 1875 i, 416.—**Benoit** (E.) Observation de métastase des oreillons sur le testicule. Gaz. d. hôp., Par., 1854, xxvii, 74.—**Bethune.** Deafness following mumps. Boston M. & S. J., 1861, lxiv, 390.—**Bienfait.** Albuminurie consécutive à des oreillons. Bull. Soc. méd. de Reims, 1873, xii, 79.—**Billoir.** De l'oreillon survenant dans l'orchite blennorrhagique. Gaz. hebd. de méd., Par., 1859, vi, 617.— **Boinet** (E.) De quelques complications rares des oreillons. Mém. et compt.-rend. Soc. d. sc. méd. de Lyon (1884), 1885, xxiv, 297–303. Also: Lyon méd., 1885, xlviii, 141–146.—[**Bourru.**] Complications des oreillons chez l'adulte. Paris méd., 1885, x, 409; 421. — **Boutelle** (J. T.) Cases of mumps complicated with epididymitis. Boston M. & S. J., 1876, xciv, 384–386. — **Brunner** (G.) Ein Fall von completer einseitiger Taubheit nach Mumps. Ztschr. f. Ohrenh., Wiesb., 1882, xi, 229–232. Also, transl.: Arch. Otol., N. Y., 1882, xi, 102–105.—**Bürkner** (K.) Ein Fall von plötzlichem Verlust des Hörvermögens auf einem Ohre im Verlaufe von Mumps. Berl. klin. Wchnschr., 1883, xx. 193.—**Burne** (J.) Case of epidemic mumps, complicated with parotitis, orchitis, nephritis, albuminuria, convulsions; recovery. Prov. M. & S. J., Lond., 1851, 623–625.—**Burnett** (S. M.) Absolute loss of hearing-power in both ears accompanying an attack of mumps. Arch. Otol., N. Y., 1885, xiv, 19. ——. Affections of the eye accompanying mumps. Am. J. M. Sc., Phila., 1886, n. s., xci, 86–89.—**Buxton** (A. St. C.) Complete suppression of saliva after mumps. Lancet, Lond., 1883, i, 1087. — **Calmettes.** Sur une conséquence peu connue des oreillons. France méd., Par., 1882, ii, 85–89.— **Carbajal** (A. J.) Un caso de parotiditis catarral doble, complicada de estrechamiento del canal de Stenon, y cálculo salivar consecutivo. Gac. méd., Méjico, 1886, xxi, 94–104.—**Cardozo Teixeira** (J. J.) Papeiras terminando por orchites. Escholiaste med., Lisb., 1862, xiii, 343–345 —

Mumps (*Complications and sequelæ of*).

Carlier. Observations de métastase des oreillons sur les testicules. Gaz. d. hôp., Par., 1854, xxvii, 113.—**Chambers** (T. R.) Annular disease of the ear; a sequel of mumps. Tr. M. Soc. N. Jersey, Newark, 1884, 230.—**Chaumier** (E.) Note sur les manifestations articulaires des oreillons. Concours méd., Par., 1883, v, 650.—**Cheatham** (W.) Parotitis followed by total deafness of one ear. Am. Pract. & News, Louisville, 1886, n. s., i, 133.—**Connor** (L.) Mumps as a cause of sudden deafness. Am. J. M. Sc., Phila., 1884. n. s., lxxxviii, 401–409.—**Desprès.** Vaginalité métastatique des oreillons avec phlébite d'une varicocèle. France méd., Par., 1877, xxiv, 209. ——. Orchite des oreillons. Gaz. d. hôp., Par., 1879, lii, 1059. ——. Orchite des oreillons, orchite ourlienne. *Ibid.*, 1883, lvi, 393.— **Discussion** sur une épidémie d'oreillons et sur les orchites et les atrophies des testicules. Tr. méd., Par., 1831, iii, 26–32.— **Éloy** (C.) Les déterminations de la fièvre ourlienne sur l'appareil auditif. Union méd., Par., 1885, 3. s., xl, 145–149.—**Emond** (E.) Observation d'oreillons suppurés. Gaz. d. hôp., Par., 1867, xl, 448.—**Fischer** (A. F.) Parotiden-Metastase auf das linke Ovarium und merkwürdige Heilung derselben. Mag. f. d. ges. Heilk, Berl., 1823, xv, 509–512.—**Flögl** (J.) Epidemisches Auftreten von Orchitis als Complication einer idiopatischen Parotitis. Aerztl. Cor.-Bl. f. Böhmen, Prag, 1874, ii, 18.—**Fournié.** Complications du côté des organes des sens dans le cours des oreillons. [From a prize memoir.] Arch. de méd. et pharm. mil, Par., 1885, v, 205–227.—**Gautier** (V.) Oreillon épidémique chez une femme en couches et chez son nouveau-né. Rev. méd. de la Suisse Rom., Genève, 1883, iii, 81–85.—**Gérard.** Deux épidémies d'oreillons au 10e dragons; contribution à l'étude de l'atrophie testiculaire consécutive à l'orchite oreillarde. Rec. de mém. de méd. . . . mil, Par., 1878, 3. s., xxxiv, 561–566.—**Gillet.** Mort subite dans un cas d'oreillons. Gaz. d. hôp., Par., 1873, xlvi, 1122.—**Glénereau.** Sur une épidémie d'oreillons compliqués d'accidents cérébraux. Bull. gén. de thérap., etc., Par., 1884, cvi, 464–468.—**Granier.** Des oreillons, des orchites métastatiques et des atrophies testiculaires consécutives. Lyon méd., 1879, xxxi, 285–296. [Discussion], 301–304. *Also:* Mém. et compt.-rend. Soc. d. sc. méd. de Lyon (1879), 1880, xix, 132–144, pt. 2. [Discussion], 78–81.—**Grisolle.** De l'atrophie des testicules consécutive aux oreillons. Gaz. d. hôp., Par., 1866, xxxix, 221.—**Grisolle & Fournier** (A.) Oreillons avec manifestation vulvaire. J. de méd. et chir. prat., Par., 1867, xxxviii, 198.—**Haldeman** (F. D.) Unusual metastasis in mumps, with report of three fatal cases. J. Am. M. Ass., Chicago, 1887, viii, 543–545.—**Hall** (W.), jr. Mumps and orchitis. Brit. M. J., Lond., 1881, i, 966.—**Harlan** (G. C.) Case of sudden deafness from mumps. Med. News, Phila, 1883, xlii, 326.—**Harlow** (E. A. W.) Case of cynanche parotidæa, with metastasis. Boston M. & S J., 1861–2, lxv, 151.—**Hatry.** Considérations sur des troubles visuels observés avec l'altération de la papille et de la zone péripapillaire, chez les malades atteints d'oreillons pendant l'hiver de 1875–6. Rec. de mém. de méd. . . . mil., Par., 1876, 3. s., xxxi, 305–316, 1 pl.—**Hitchcock** (A.) Case of retrocedent mumps, with hemiplegia and coma; recovery. Boston M. & S J., 1842, xxvi, 301.—**Hixson** (C.) Absorption of the testes from metastasis of mumps. Med. Exam., Phila., 1850, n. s., vi, 582.—**Homans** (C. D.) sr. Mumps in a pregnant woman; premature labour, followed by the appearance of the same disease in the infant, twenty-four hours after its birth. Am. J. M. Sc., Phila., 1855, n. s, xxix, 56. *Also:* Extr. Rec. Bost. Soc. M. Improve. (1854–5), 1856, ii, 138.—**Irwin.** Instance of metastatic action between an inflamed parotid gland and the meninges of the brain. Tr. Wisconsin M. Soc., Milwaukee, 1874, viii, 13.—**Jacob.** Les oreillons au point de vue épidémiologique et clinique; un cas de mort par oreillon. Rec. de mém. de méd. . . . mil., Par., 1875, xxxi, 529–568.—**Jahn.** Merkwürdige Metastase. Med. Convers -Bl., Hildburgh., 1832, iii, 174.—**Janson-Zuède.** Note sur les manifestations cérébrales des oreillons. Ann. Soc. méd.-chir. de Liége, 1884, xxiii, 181–183.—**Joffroy** (A.) De la paralysie ourlienne. [Extr.] Progrès méd., Par., 1886, 2. s., iv, 1009.—**Juloux** (A.) Contribution à l'étude des oreillons et de l'orchite métastatique. Rec. de mém. de méd. . . . mil., Par., 1882, xxxii, 478–483.—**Knapp** (H.) A case of bilateral deafness from mumps. Arch. Otol., N. Y., 1882, xi, 385–387. *Also, transl.:* Ztschr. f. Ohrenh., Wiesb., 1883, xii, 121–123.—**Lannois.** Surdité complète survenue chez un soldat pendant l'évolution des oreillons huit mois auparavant. Mém. et compt.-rend. Soc. d. sc. méd. de Lyon (1883), 1884, xxiii, pt. 2, 119.—**Lannois** (M.) & **Lemoine** (G.) Pseudo-rhumatisme des oreillons. Rev. de méd., Par, 1885, v, 192–202. —— ——. Des manifestations méningitiques et cérébrales des oreillons. (Contribution à l'étude des troubles nerveux consécutifs aux maladies aiguës.) Arch. de neurol., Par., 1886, xi, 1–15.—**Leale** (C. A.) Pyæmic parotitis. Tr. N. York Acad. M., 1883, 2. s., iii, 33–57.—**Lees.** A case of parotiditis with metastasis to the brain and testicles in a gentleman aged forty-five years. Dublin Q. J. M. Sc., 1854, xviii, 457.—**Léger.** Observation d'oreillons à répétition. Gaz. méd. de Picardie, Amiens, 1886, iv, 54.—**Le-**

Mumps (*Complications and sequelæ of*).

moine (G.) & **Lannois** (M.) De la surdité complète unilatérale ou bilatérale consécutive aux oreillons. Rev. de méd., Par., 1883, iii, 713–725. *Also* [Abstr.]: J. de méd. et chir. prat., Par., 1884, lv, 22.—**Lindsley** (H.) Two cases of mumps, with metastasis to the brain, both terminating fatally. Stethoscope & Virg. M. Gaz., Richmond, 1851, i, 15.—**Logan** (H. V.) Metastasis in parotitis. Med. News, Phila., 1882, xl, 569. —**Longuet** (R.) Des lésions des divers organes et appareils dans les oreillons. Union méd., Par., 1885, 3. s., xxxix, 673; 725: xl, 121.—**McSherry** (R.) Mumps; with an unusual sequel. J. Am. M. Ass., Chicago, 1885, iv, 627.—**Maximowitsch** (J.) Ein Fall von Parotitis mit nachfolgender Meningitis. St. Petersb. med. Wchnschr., 1880, v, 185.—**Meynet** (P.) Observation d'oreillons suivis de métastase sur les ovaires, recueillie chez une jeune fille de 16 ans. Mém. et compt.-rend. Soc. d. sc. méd. de Lyon, 1866–7, vi, 33–38. *Also:* Gaz. méd. de Lyon, 1866, xviii, 357–359.—**Michalski** (L.) Oreillons; convulsions; mort. Union méd., Par., 1885, 3. s., xl, 316–318.—**Minot** (F.) Case of cynanche parotidæa, with metastasis to the testicle, and cerebral complication; convalescence in ten days. Am. J. M. Sc., Phila., 1850, n. s., xx, 377–380.—**Monro.** Case of parotitis followed by orchitis and meningitis; high temperature; recovery. Lancet, Lond., 1883, ii, 280.—**Moos** (S.) Erworbene Taubstummheit nach Mumps. Ztschr. f. Ohrenh., Wiesb., 1882-3, xii, 112. ——. Ein Fall von partieller Labyrinthaffection nach Mumps. Berl. klin. Wchnschr., 1884, xxi, 36. — **Moure** (E. J.) Sur un cas de perte complète de l'ouïe à la suite des oreillons. Rev. mens. de laryngol., etc., Bordeaux, 1882, iii, 297–303.—**Newmarch** (B. J.) Parotitis, double orchitis, hydrocele of tunica vaginalis. Australas. M Gaz., Sydney, 1884–5, iv, 160.—**Nimier** (H.) De la récidive des oreillons. Arch. gén. de méd., Par., 1883, ii, 93–95.—**Osborn** (S.) Parotitis and acute orchitis. Brit. M. J., Lond., 1879, ii, 476.—**Page** (R. C. M.) Orchitis dependent on mumps. Virginia M. Month., Richmond, 1877–8, iv, 121.—**Phares** (D. L.) Mumps; metastasis. Tr. Mississippi M. Ass., Jackson, 1883, xvi, 114.—**Pierce** (F. M.) Mumps (parotitis) as a cause of ear disease. Med. Chron., Manchester, 1884–5, i, 505–510.—**Pollard** (T.) Mumps terminating fatally; occurring in "Bellevue Hospital", Richmond, Va. Atlanta M. & S. J., 1860–61, v, 462.—**Pontoppidan** (K.) Deliria post parotit. epidemic. Hosp.-Tid., Kjøbenh., 1883, 3. R., i, 1057–1059. — **Radcliffe** (S. J.) Parotitis, translation to testis and brain, with threatened acute mania; recovery. Phila. M. Times, 1873-4, iv, 721.—**Reamy** (T. A.) Metastasis of mumps to the testicles, treated by the application of cold. Med. Counsellor, Columbus, 1855, i, 313.—**Rindzun** (I.) Sluchai ischeznov. parotita vslied. prisoedinenija roji. [Disappearance of parotitis soon after the appearance of erysipelas.] Med. Obozr., Mosk., 1886, xxv, 893.—**Robbins** (C. W.) Metastasis of mumps. Chicago M. J. & Exam., 1881, xlii, 279.—**Roosa** (D. B. St. J.) Disease of the ear occurring during the course of parotitis. Arch. Otol., N. Y., 1883, xii. 1–13. *Also, transl.:* Ztschr. f. Ohrenh., Wiesb., 1883, xii, 240–251.—**Roubaud.** Note sur les orchites partielles selon la classification de M. Vidal (de Cassis); orchite parenchymateuse métastatique des oreillons. Union méd., Par., 1847, i, 237.—**Salter** (T.) Abortion produced by metastasis in cynanche parotidæa. Lond. M. Gaz., 1849, n. s., ix, 106.—**Seitz** (J.) Taubheit nach Mumps. Cor.-Bl. f. schweiz. Aerzte, Basel, 1882, xii, 641–643.—**Seligsohn** (M.) Ueber Taubheit nach Mumps. Berl. klin. Wchnschr., 1883, xx, 267; 283. *Also:* Verhandl. d. Berl. med. Gesellsch. (1882–3), 1884, xiv, pt. 2. 86–101.—**Shapard** (J. C.) Mumps; meningitis. Nashville J. M. & S., 1887, n. s., xxxix, 116–118.—**Shreve** (O. B.) A case of metastasis of mumps to the testes and the brain. Boston M. & S. J., 1875, xcii. 739.—**Skelly** (J. I.) Orchitis following parotiditis. Med. Rec., N. Y., 1881, xix, 357.—**Snead** (A.) Metastasis of mumps to the brain and uterus. Stethoscope & Virg. M. Gaz., Richmond, 1851, i, 322–324.—**Sorel.** De l'orchite dite métastatique dans les oreillons. Rec. de mém. de méd. . . . mil., Par., 1877, 3. s., xxxiii, 225–245. ——. Contribution à la thermométrie clinique de la fièvre dans l'orchite symptomatique des oreillons. Rev. mens. de méd. et chir., Par., 1877, i, 280–288. — **Talon.** Observation d'atrophie du nerf optique consécutive à des oreillons. Arch. de. méd. et pharm. mil., Par., 1883, i, 103–108.—**Todd** (C. A.) Deafness after mumps. Tr. M. Ass. Missouri, St. Louis, 1884, 22–25. *Also:* St. Louis Cour. Med., 1884, xii, 97–100.—**Tott** (C. A.) Fall von Mumps-Metastase und anomalem Verlaufe dieser Krankheit. Ztschr. f. d. ges. Med., Hamb., 1841, xvii, 477. — **Trousseau** (A.) Notes sur quelques accidents dans la maladie connue sous le nom d'oreillons, ourles, etc. Arch. gén. de méd., Par., 1854, i, 69–72. — **Tuckey** (T. P.) On some peculiar symptoms following parotitis. Med. Press & Circ., Lond., 1875, n. s., xx, 167.—**Van Bibber** (J.) Three cases of metastatic insanity, following parotiditis. Med. News, Phila, 1885, xlvii, 678.—**Védrènes** (A.) Orchite ourlienne observée, en 1881, à l'École polytechnique, dans le cours d'une épidémie d'oreillons. Rec. de mém. de méd. . . . mil. Par., 1882, xxxviii, 167–180. — **Velpeau.** Oreillons; orchite métastatique,

Mumps (*Complications and sequelæ of*).

France méd., Par., 1866, xiii, 95-97 — **Venturini** (E.) Caso di meningite in un' epidemia di orecchioni. Bull. d. sc. med. di Bologna, 1866, 5. s., ii, 169-180. — **Wamsley** (F. H.) Mumps; metastasis to brain. Lancet, Lond., 1878, ii, 312. — **Williamson** (J. M.) On a fatal case of acute delirious mania complicated with parotitis. *Ibid.*, 1886, i, 487.

Mumps (*Epidemics of*).

Buhl (B.) * Beiträge zur Kenntniss der Parotitis epidemica und ihres Fieberverlaufs. 8°. *Würzburg*, 1882.

Glubrecht (C. F. H.) * De parotitide epidemica. 8°. *Gryphiæ*, [1839].

Guasco (P.) *Étude sur une épidémie d'oreillons ayant sévi dans la garnison de Toulouse en 1881. 4°. *Paris*, 1883.

Jobard (V.-E.) * Relation de deux épidémies d'oreillons observées sur des émigrants hindous. 4°. *Paris*, 1875.

Plagneux (E.) *Quelques considérations sur une épidémie d'oreillons observée à Rochefort (1885). 4°. *Paris*, 1885.

Allexich (G.) Sulla parotite epidemica. Gazz. med. ital., prov. venete, Padova, 1883, xxvi. 105. — **Andrä.** Eine Mumps-Epidemie. Mag. f. d. ges. Heilk., Berl, 1823, xv, 138 – 140. — **Burtseff** (N. A.) Epidem. periparotite. Vrach, St. Petersb., 1885, vi, 767; 786; 856. — **Calmette** (E.) Oreillons et fièvres éruptives; affinités et analogues. Arch. gén. de méd, Par., 1883, ii, 455 – 467. — **Chauvin.** Relation d'une épidémie d'oreillons survenue au 111e de ligne. Rec. de mém. de méd. . . . mil., Par., 1876, xxxii, 473 – 478. — **Delmas.** Rapport sur une épidémie mixte d'oreillons et de pneumonies. Arch. de méd. et pharm. mil., Par., 1883, ii, 349-354. — **Dogny.** Oreillons ou parotidites qui ont régné épidémiquement sur le 1er régiment d'infanterie légère, pendant son séjour à Mont-Louis, Pyrénées orientales, en 1828. Précis de la const. méd. d'Indre-et-Loire, Tours, 1820, 52 – 57. ——. Oreillons ou parotidites qui ont régné épidémiquement dans le 1er régiment d'infanterie légère en 1827, à Mont-Louis. Rec. de mém. de méd. . . . mil., Par., 1831, xxxi, 319 – 328. — **Eisenmann.** Epidemie von Parotitis polymorpha in Passau. Arch. f. d. ges. Med., Jena, 1842, iii, 275 – 277. — **Eklund** (F.) Några ord om den epidemiska parotitis och dennas vegetabiliska miasma. Eira, Göteborg, 1880, iv, 584-597. — **Gola** (D.) Della parotitide epidemica osservata in Milano nei mesi di maggio e giugno. Gazz. med. ital. lomb., Milano, 1849, 2. s., ii, 261-263. — **Graves** (R. J.) Epidemic of mumps. Dublin Q. J. M. Sc., 1851, ix, 9 – 11. — **Gripouilleau.** Note sur une épidémie d'oreillons qui a régné à Montlouis pendant l'année 1865. Rec. d. trav. Soc. méd. d'Indre-et-Loire, Tours, 1865, 7 – 9. — **Hamersley** (A.) Observations on cynanche parotidæa, as it occurred in the New York State prison during the winters of 1821-2. Med. Reposit., N. Y., 1822, n. s., vii, 413-422. — **Hamilton** (R.) Account of some circumstances respecting the cynanche parotidea, as it lately appeared in the neighbourhood of Ipswich. Med. Comment., Edinb., 1787, decade 2, i, 390. — **Helmkampff** (H.) Parotitis epidemica s. polymorpha. Deutsche Med.-Ztg., Berl., 1886, vii, 519-522. — **Horst.** Beobachtung einer epidemischen Parotitis in Cöln und der Umgegend während der Jahre 1840-41. Ztschr. f. d. ges. Med., Hamb., 1848, xxxix, 1 – 10. — **Jarnuszkiewicz** (W.) Epidemiczne zapalenie ślinianek przyusznych i jąder (parotitis et orchitis idiopatica epidem.). Medycyna, Warszawa, 1881, ix, 421-424. — **Jimeno** (E. M.) Una epidemia rara. Encicl. méd. farm., Barcel., 1882, vi, 180. — **Joseph** (G.) Bemerkungen über die vom Januar bis März 1864 epidemischen genuinen Ohrspeicheldrüsenerkrankungen. Berl. klin. Wchnschr., 1864, i, 297 – 299. — **Jourdan.** Relation d'une épidémie d'oreillons au 28e bataillon de chasseurs à Dax. Rec. de mém. de méd. . . . mil, Par., 1878, 3. s., xxxiv, 537-552. — **Laurens.** Note sur une épidémie d'oreillons au 83e régiment de ligne à Albi. *Ibid.*, 1876, 3. s., xxxii, 603 – 605. — **Leichenstern** (O.) Parotitis epidemica. Handb. d. Kinderkr. (Gerhardt), Tübing., 1877, ii, 647-674. — **Leitzen** (E) Angina parotidea, im Sommer 1837 zu Halle, und namentlich in der Franke'schen Stiftung daselbst, epidemisch beobachtet. J. d. pract. Heilk., Berl., 1838, lxxxvi, 4. St., 101–110. — **Lucchetti** (F.) Osservazioni sulla cinanche parotidea che domino epidemicamente in Monticelli di Rocaguglielma. Raccoglitore med. di Fano, 1856, xiv, 320 – 325. — **Lühe.** Eine Parotitis-Epidemie. Berl. klin. Wchnschr., 1879, xvi, 600-602. — **Madamet.** Épidémie d'oreillons observée au 1er hussards en 1877. Rec. de mém. de méd. . . . mil., Par., 1878, 3. s., xxxiv, 552 – 561. — **Mahéo** (S.) Note sur une épidémie d'oreillons survenue à bord du trois-mats Latona, de Londres, conduisant de Pondichéry et Karikal à la Guadeloupe un convoi d'émigrants indiens, an 1880 – 81. Arch. de méd. nav., Par., 1884, xli, 147 – 151. — **Mangor**

Mumps (*Epidemics of*).

(C. E.) Historia cynanches parotideæ, Viburgi 1772 epidemicæ. Acta reg. Soc. med. Havn., 1791, ii, 165-175. — **Miller** (C. H.) Epidemic metastatic parotiditis. Med. & Surg. Reporter, Phila., 1881, xliv. 529. *Also*: South. Pract., Nashville, 1881, iii, 241. — **Miquel.** Beschreibung einer Bauerwetzel-Epidemie. Arch. f. med. Erfahr., Berl., 1822, ii, 120 - 131. — **Nikolski** (D. P.) K statistike epidem. periparotita. Med. Obozr., Mosk., 1887, xxvii, 661 – 672. — **Noble** (A.) History of an endemic cynanche parotidea, on board his majesty's ship Ardent, on its passage to Monte Video. Edinb. M. & S. J., 1808, iv, 304-306. — **Nogueira** (R. Z.) Historia da epidemia de bexigas e sarampo, que tem grassado na Ilha Terceira desde os principios do mez de Nov. de 1844. J. Soc. d. sc. med. de Lisb., 1845, xxii, 201-210. — **von Nymann** (J.) Parotitis epidemica. Arch. f. Kinderh., Stuttg., 1880, i, 73 – 80. — **Olivi** (D.) Breve cenno sulla parotite epidemica, osservata nel 1839, nel circondario esterno di Senigallia. Raccoglitore, Fano, 1839, iv, 89-91. — **Pampoukes** (P. S.) Ἐπιδημικὴ ὑπογενίτις. Γαληνὸς, Ἀθῆναι, 1884, IΑ΄, 392-394. — **Pellengahr** (A.) Einige Bemerkungen über die im Sommer und Spätjahre 1827 zu Münster in Westfalen beobachtete Parotitis epidemica. Abhandl. u. Beob. d. aerztl. Gesellsch. zu Münster, 1829, i. 177-189. — **Penzoldt** (F.) Ueber eine Varietät der Parotitis epidemica. Deutsche med. Wchnschr., Berl., 1878, iv, 523. — **Pollak** (S.) Ueber das epidemische Vorkommen der Parotitis. Wien. med. Presse, 1875, xvi, 264. — **Ressiguier** (C.) Histoire d'une épidémie d'oreillons qui a régné à Montpellier en 1848. Rev. méd.-chir. de Par., 1850, vii, 204; 329. — **Riget.** Note sur une épidémie d'oreillons. Arch. gén. de méd., Par., 1866, i, 355-358. — **Rilliet.** Mémoire sur une épidémie d'oreillons qui a régné à Genève pendant les années 1848 et 1849. Gaz. méd. de Par., 1850, 3. s., v, 22; 42. — **Roth** (F.) Ueber die Incubation und Uebertragbarkeit der Parotitis epidemica. München. med. Wchnschr., 1886, xxxiii, 345. — **Schiede.** Memoria sobre la epidemia que esta reinando en Mégico desde abril de 1836. Periód. Acad. de med. de Mégico, 1836-7, i, 47-52. — **Servier.** De l'épidémie d'oreillons qui a régné dans la garnison de Bayonne, pendant les mois de février et mars 1878. Rec. de mém. de méd. . . . mil., Par., 1878, 3. s., xxxiv, 529-537. — **Settekorn.** Das Auftreten der Parotitis epidemica unter dem Militär zu Stettin im Winter 1879–80 und im Frühjahr 1880. Deutsches Arch. f. klin. Med., Leipz., 1880-81, xxviii, 308-316. — **Soltmann** (O.) Zur Mumps-Epidemie in Breslau 1877-8. Jahrb. f. Kinderh., Leipz., 1878, n. F., xii, 409-414. — **Spengler.** Die Mumps-Epidemie zu Herborn im Winter 1851 auf 1852. Med. Ztg., Berl., 1852, xxi, 183-185. — **Troitski** (I. V.) Epidem. periparot. istorija odnoi schkolnoi epidemii. Vrach, St. Petersb., 1886, vii, 595; 615. — **Tsantes** (R.) Ἐπιδημικὴ ὑπογενίτις. Γαληνὸς, Ἀθῆναι, 1884, IΒ΄, 5-8. — **Woollen** (L. J.) History of an epidemic of parotitis in Switzerland County. Tr. Indiana M. Soc., Indianap., 1872, 25-29.

Mumssen (Dietericus). Leutarum obstructionum theoriam delineat. xvi pp. 4°. *Lipsiæ, ex off. Salbachiana*, [1763].

——. * De corde rupto. 42 pp., 1 l. sm. 4°. *Lipsiæ, ex off. Langenhemia*, [1764].

Also [Abstr.], *in:* Weiz (F. A.) Neue Ausz. [etc.] 12°. *Frankfurt u. Leipzig*, 1774, i, 65-80.

For Biography, see **Ludwig** (Christ. Gott.)

Mumssen (Jacobus). * De plethoræ differentiis. 36 pp. 4°. *Lipsiæ, ex off. Langenhemia*, [1766].

For Biography, see **Plaz** (Ant. Guil.)

For Portrait, see **Collection**—van Kaathoven.

Munaret (Jean-Marie-Placide) [1805–]. Du médecin de campagne et de ses malades, mœurs et science. v. 1. xvi, 427 pp., 1 l. 8°. *Paris, Baillet*, 1837.

——. The same. 2. éd. xvi, 554 pp., 1 l. 8°. *Paris, Germer-Baillière*, 1840.

——. Dispensaire spécial pour le traitement des vénériens indigents de la ville de Lyon, son but et ses moyens. 32 pp. 8°. *Lyon, L. Boitel*, 1841.

——. Lettre à messieurs les médecins, membres du Congrès scientifique de France à Lyon, qui s'intéressent à la réorganisation médicale. 15 pp., 1 l. 8°. [*Lyon, Mougin-Rusand*, 1841.]

——. Notice sur Mathias Mayor, sa vie et ses travaux. 2 p. l., 104 pp., port. 8°. *Paris, Germer-Baillière*, 1847.

——. Causeries du mois. 14 pp. 8°. *Lyon, Rodanet*, 1850.

Repr. from: Gaz. méd. de Lyon, 1850, ii.

Munaret (Jean-Marie-Placide)—continued.

——. Supplique au président de la république en faveur de la création d'une maison et d'une caisse de retraite pour les médecins vieux et infirmes. 8 pp. 8°. [*Lyon, Mougin-Rusand*, 1852.]
Repr. from: Union méd., Par., 1852, vi.

——. Lettre à M. le docteur Diday sur les eaux de Saint-Galmier. 8 pp. 8°. *Lyon, Mougin-Rusand*, 1852.

——. Éloge historique de Charles Pravaz; lu à l'Association des médecins du Rhône dans la séance générale annuelle du 18 mai 1854. 52 pp. 8°. *Lyon, A. Vingtrinier*, 1854.

——. Iconautographie de Jenner. 69 pp., 1 l. 8°. *Paris, Germer-Baillière & F. Savy*, 1860. [P., v. 1669.]

——. Le médecin des villes et des campagnes. 3. éd. xxiv, 600 pp. 12°. *Paris, Germer-Baillière*, 1862.

——. Le bréviaire du médecin. Précis de médecine rurale, d'économie et de philosophie médicales. 15 pp. 8°. *Lyon, A. Vingtrinier*, 1868.
Repr. from: J. de méd. de Lyon.

——. Notice sur T.-C.-É.-Édouard Auber; sa vie et ses travaux. 1 p. l., 32 pp. 12°. *Lyon, A. Vingtrinier*, 1874.

——. Travaux et titres scientifiques, 1826–76. 16 pp. 8°. *Lyon, A. Vingtrinier*, 1876.
See, also, **Loreau.** De l'exercice illégal de la médecine, etc. 12°. *Lyon,* 1857.
For Biography, see [**F.** (Ed.)] Notice sur M. Munaret, docteur en médecine. 8°. *Meaux*, [1844, *vel subseq.*]. *Repr. from:* Biogr. des gens de lettres.

Munch (Ernest). * De l'accouchement artificiel après la mort. 1 p. l., 59 pp. 4°. *Strasbourg*, 1864, No. 757, v. 39.

Munck af Rosenschöld (Eberhard Zacharias) [1775–1837]. De rheumatismo acuto. 1 p. l., 42 pp. 4°. *Lundæ, typ. Berlingianis*, 1790.

——. * De hæmorrhagiis. 18 pp. 4°. *Lundæ, typ. Berlingianis*, [1794].

Muncke (Georg. Guil.) [Pr.] disquisitiones de relatione mutua inter tellurem et atmosphæram quoad calorem et fluidum electricum. 42 pp., 2 l., 2 pl. 4°. *Heidelbergæ, typ. J. M. Gutmanni*, [1819].

Mund (H.) Einführung in die naturgemässe Gesundheitspflege und arzneilose Heilkunde. 32 pp. 8°. *Hannover, Schmorl u. von Seefeld*, 1887.

Mundanus (Theodorus).
See **Dickinson** (E.) Epistola . . . De quintessentia philosophorum, [etc.] 8°. *Oxoniæ*, 1686.

Munday (George).
See **London.** City of London sewers. Report of James Walker, etc. 4°. [*London*, 1848.]

Munde (Carl). Genaue Beschreibung der Gräfenberger Wasserheilanstalt und der Priessnitzischen Curmethode. Nebst einer Anweisung über siebenzig der am häufigsten vorkommenden Krankheiten, als: Gicht, Rheumatismus, Syphilis, Hämorrhoiden, Hypochondrie, Fieber, Entzündungen, Cholera, Influenza und eine Menge anderer chronischer und acuter Uebel, durch Anwendung des kalten Wassers mit Schwitzen, nach der Gräfenberger Curmethode gründlich zu heilen. 3. Aufl. xx, 223 pp. 8°. *Leipzig, A. Frohberger*, 1839.

——. The same. Die Gräfenberger Wasserheilanstalt und die Priessnitzische Curmethode. 6. Aufl. viii, 256 pp. 8°. *Leipzig, Hartleben*, 1845.

——. Hydrothérapeutique, ou l'art de prévenir et de guérir les maladies sans le secours des médicamens, par l'eau, la sueur, le bon air, l'exercice, le régime et le genre de vie. viii, 424 pp. 12°. *Paris, J.-B. Baillière*, 1842.

——. Memorien eines Wasserarztes. 2. Ausg. 2 v. in 1. xxxvi, 286 pp.; x, 371 pp. 8°. *Dresden u. Leipzig, Arnold*, 1847.

Munde (Carl)—continued.

——. Zimmerluft, Ventilation und Heizung Ein Beitrag zur wohlfeilen Verbesserung der verdorbenen Luft, welche wir während der kalten Jahreszeit in unseren Wohnungen athmen, und welche eine der Hauptursachen der Vermehrung und Verschlimmerung von Krankheiten ist. 2. Aufl. iv, 40 pp. 8°. *Leipzig, Arnold*, 1877.
Repr. from 12. *Aufl. of his:* Hydrotherapie, oder Wasserheillehre.

Mundé (Paul Fortunatus) [1846–]. The indications for hystero-trachelorrhaphy, or the operation for laceration of the cervix uteri. 20 pp., 2 col. pl. 8°. *New York, W. Wood & Co.*, 1879.
Repr. from: Am. J. Obst., N. Y., 1879, xii.

——. Minor surgical gynecology. A manual of uterine diagnosis and the lesser technicalities of gynecological practice for the use of the advanced student and general practitioner. xi, 381 pp. 8°. *New York, W. Wood & Co.*, 1880.

——. The same. Including general rules for gynecological operations and the operations for lacerated cervix and perineum, and prolapsus of uterus and vagina, for the use of the advanced student and general practitioner. 2. ed. xxii, 552 pp. 8°. *New York, W. Wood & Co.*, 1885.

——. The diagnosis and treatment of obstetric cases by external (abdominal) examination and manipulation. 114 pp. 8°. *New York, W. Wood & Co.*, 1880.
Repr. from: Am. J. Obst., N. Y., 1879–80, xii–xiii.

——. Clinical observations on reflex genital neuroses in the female. 11 pp. 8°. [*Chicago*, 1886.]
Repr. from: J. Nerv. & Ment. Dis., Chicago, 1886, xi.

——. The value of antipyrine in puerperal fever. 6 pp. 8°. [*New York*, 1886.]
Repr. from: N. York M. J., 1886, xliv.

——. A plea for intra-uterine medication. 13 pp. 8°. [*New York*, 1887.]
Repr. from: N. York M. J., 1887, xlv.

——. A sketch of the management of pregnancy, parturition and the puerperal state, normal and abnormal. 2 p. l., 110 pp. 12°. *Detroit, G. S. Davis*, 1887.

——. Three cases of pregnancy complicated by ovarian tumors. Ovariotomy; recovery. 11 pp. 12°. [*New York*, 1887.]
Repr. from: N. York M. J., 1887, xlvi.

——. De l'électricité comme agent thérapeutique en gynécologie. Traduit avec l'autorisation de l'auteur et annoté par P. Ménière. 2 p. l., 72 pp. roy. 8°. *Paris, O. Doin*, 1888.
Also, Editor of: **American** (The) Journal of Obstetrics and Diseases of Women and Children, New York, 1873.
See, also, **Discussion** on the influence of medicine, etc. 8°. *New York*, 1877.

Mundella (Aloisius). Epistolæ medicinales, nunc ab ipso autore auctæ et recognitæ, in quibus variæ et difficiles quæstiones utiliter tractantur; Galeni atque aliorum medicorum loci obscuri et implicati illustrantur et explicantur. Ejusdem annotationes in Antonii Musæ Brasavolæ simplicium medicamentorum examen. 15 p. l., 655 pp. 12°. *Basileæ, M. Ising*, [1538].

——. Dialogi medicinales decem, nunc primum in lucem editi: in quibus multa et varia tum artis theoremata, tum historiæ et experimenta doctissime explicantur. 7 p. l., 117 ff., 15 l. 8°. *Tiguri, apud Froschoverum*, 1551.

——. Theatrum Galeni, hoc est: universæ medicinæ a medicorum principe Galeno diffuse sparsimque traditæ promptuarium, quo vel indicis loco in omnes Galeni libros, vel locorum communium instar in re medica, lector eruditus

Mundella (Aloisius)—continued.
magna commoditate nec minori facilitate ute-
tur. 685 l. fol. *Basileæ, per Eusebium Episco-
pium et Nicolai frateris hæredes,* 1568.

———. The same. Epistolæ medicinales variorum quæstionum et locorum insuper Galeni difficilium expositionem continentes [etc.] 7 p. l.,
263 pp. 4°. *Basileæ, apud M. Isingrinium,* 1543.
See, also, **Epistolæ** medicinales [etc.] fol. *Lugd.
Bat.,* 1556.

Mundigl (J[oseph]). Comparativ-physiologisch
und nosologische Ansichten von den Krankheiten des Menschen und der vorzüglichsten
Hausthiere, insbesondere von dem Fieber als
sporadisch- und epidemischer Krankheitsform.
xlii, 146 pp., 1 l. 8°. *München, Lentner,* 1818.

———. Klinische Beyträge, herausgegeben bey
Gelegenheit der den 30. August statt findenden
öffentlichen Preise-Vertheilung. xvi, 104 pp.,
2 l. 8°. *München, Lentner,* 1820.

Mundinus Friulensis (Julius). *See* **Mondino de Foro** (Julio).

Mundinus de Lentiis. *See* **Mondino** [*or*
Mondini] **da Luzzi.**

Mundium.

See **Cholera** (*Asiatic, History, etc., of*), *by
localities.*

Mundius (Henr.) Opera omnia medico physica,
tractatibus tribus comprehensa : de aëre vitali ;
de esculentis ; de potulentis. Una cum appendice
de parergis in victu ut chocolata, coffe, thea,
tabaco, etc. 10 p. l., 362 pp. 8°. *Lugd. Bat.,
P. Vander Aa,* 1685.

Mundorff (Fridericus Carolus). * De cataractæ
morbis secundariis. 23 pp. 8°. *Wirceburgi, C.
G. Becker,* 1831.

Mundt (Ernestus Edmundus) [1804–]. * De
thoracum abusu noxio. 31 pp. 8°. *Berolini,
lit. A. Petschii,* [1828].

von Mundy (Jaromir) [1822–]. De l'institution des colonies d'aliénés. Gheel et ses adversaires. 16 pp. 8°. *Bruxelles, Tircher,* 1860.

———. Gheel est un asile patronal et nullement
une colonie, moins encore un établissement d'aliénés. 5 pp. 8°. *Bruxelles, Tircher,* 1860.

———. Fünf Kardinal-Fragen der administrativen Psychiatrie. 36 pp. 8°. *Osnabrück, Rack-
horst,* 1862.
Repr. from: Med. Aehrenlese, Osnabrück, 1860–63,
v–viii.

———. Sur les divers modes de l'assistance publique appliquée aux aliénés. Discours prononcé
dans les séances de la Société médico-psychologique à Paris le 26 décembre 1864 et le 16 janvier 1865. 60 pp. 4°. *Paris, A. Marc,* 1865.

———. Beiträge zur Reform des Sanitätswesens
in Oesterreich. 1 p. l., 205 pp., 1 l. 8°. *Wien,
C. Gerold's Sohn,* 1868.

———. Die Militärsanität der Zukunft. 30 pp.
8°. *Wien, L. W. Seidel u. Sohn,* 1882.
Repr. from : Militärarzt, Wien, 1881, xv.

———. Der Transport von Kranken und Verle-
tzten in grossen Städten. 73 pp., 2 l., 12 pl.
12°. *Wien, C. Reisser u. M. Werthner,* 1883.

———. Ueber das freiwillige Rettungswesen in
Europa.
In : VORTR. ü. Gsndhtspflg. u. Rettungsw. 8°. *Berlin,*
1883, i, 17–27.
See, also, **Billroth** (Th.) & **von Mundy** (J.) Ueber
den Transport der im Felde Verwundeten und Kranken.
8°. *Wien,* 1874.—**Rapport** sur l'ambulance de l'ambas-
sade d'Autriche-Hongrie à Paris. 8°. *Versailles,* 1871.—
Souveräner Malteser Ritter-Orden Grossprioriat von
Böhmen. Studien über den Umbau und die Einrichtung
von Güterwaggons. 8°. *Wien,* 1875.—**Wiener** freiwillige Rettungs-Gesellschaft. Das elektrische Licht, etc.
8°. *Wien,* 1884.

Munford (S. E.) A question in state medicine.
16 pp. 8°. *Indianapolis, W. B. Burford,* 1884.

Munich. Das neue öffentliche Krankenhaus zu
München. Die Bedingungen zur Aufnahme der
Kranken in dasselbe, die Eröffnung einer Ver-
sicherungs-Anstalt für Nichtarme, und die Festsetzung der Verpflegungsgebühren für bezah-
lende Gäste. Auf allerhöchsten Befehl bekannt
gemacht, durch die kön. besondere Administration der Wohlthätigkeits-Stiftungen der Haupt-
und Residenzstadt München. 30 pp. 12°.
München, F. S. Storno, 1813.

———. Tags-Rapport über den Stand der Brech-
ruhr-Kranken in der königl. Haupt- und Residenz-Stadt München und deren Vorstädten.
Vom 25sten October 1836 bis 21sten Januar 1837.
89 l. fol. *München,* [1837].

———. Städtisches allgemeines Krankenhaus in
München. Instruction für den Direktor. 22 pp.
12°. *München, J. G. Weiss,* 1850.

———. Berichte über die Verhandlungen und
Arbeiten der vom Stadtmagistrate München nie-
dergesetzten Commission für Wasserversorgung,
Canalisation und Abfuhr. 1., 1874 u. 1875 ; 2.,
1876 u. Anfang 1877 ; 3., 1877 ; 4., 1878 u. 1879. 9
v. 4°. *München, A. Ackermann,* 1876–80.
Four reports and 5 appendices.

CONTENTS OF THE APPENDICES.

Anhang IV. Zum 1. Ber. Die Canalisation der kgl.
Haupt- und Residenzstadt München. Bericht im Auftrage
des Magistrates erstattet von J. Gordon. iv, 57 pp., 10
plans. 4°. *München,* 1876
Anhang I. Zum 2. Ber. Die Wasserversorgung der Stadt
München. Vorprojekt im Auftrage der beiden Gemeinde-
Collegien bearbeitet von A. Thiem. 1 p. l., 85 pp , 15 plans.
4°. *München,* 1877 ?
Anhang II. Project im Auftrage der beiden Gemeinde-
collegien verfasst von P. Schmick. 1 p. l., 21 pp., 8 plans.
4°. *München,* 1877.
Anhang III. 3. Nachtrag zu dem im Auftrage beider
Gemeindecollegien erstatteten Berichte von B. Salbach.
47 pp., 3 plans. 4°. *München,* 1877.
Beilage VII. Zum 3. Ber. Bericht der Münchener Com-
mission über die Besichtigung der Canalisations- und Be-
rieselungs-Anlagen in Frankfurt a. M., Berlin, Danzig
und Breslau sowie der Liernur-Anlagen in Amsterdam,
Leiden, und Dordrecht. iv, 122 pp , 1 map, 4 plans. 4°.
München, 1879.

———. Uebersicht der Geburten und Sterbefälle
in München, während des 1. Vierteljahres 1877.
(Einzelnabdruck aus den Mittheilungen des
städtischen statistischen Bureaus.) 13 pp. 4°.
München, J. Bolster, 1877.

———. Annalen der städtischen allgemeinen
Krankenhäuser zu München. Im Verein mit den
Aerzten dieser Anstalten hrsg. von Prof. Dr.
v. Ziemssen. v. 1–3, 1874–9. 8°. *München,*
1878–86.

———. Berichte über die Geburten und Sterbefälle in München während die Jahre 1880, 1–82,
1884, mit Rückblicken über die Vorjahre. Veröffentlicht vom statistischen Bureau der Stadt
München. 54 pp., 4 diag. 4°. *München, J.
Lindauer,* 1881–5.

Munich.

See, also, **Children** (*Hospitals, etc., for, Reports,
etc., of*), **Cholera** (*Asiatic, History, etc., of*),
Education (*Medical*), *etc.,* **Fever** (*Malarial,
History, etc., of*), **Fever** (*Typhoid, History, etc.,
of*), **Fever** (*Typhus, History, etc., of*), **Hospitals**
(*Descriptions, etc., of*), **Hospitals** (*Maternity,
etc.*), **Hospitals** (*Ophthalmic, etc.*), **Hospitals**
(*Orthopædic*), **Insane** (*Asylums for, Reports, etc.,
of*), *by localities ;* **Measles** (*Epidemics of*) ; **Medicine** (*Clinical, etc.*), *by localities.*

ALLIOLI (J. F.) Ueber den Genius der Krank-
heitskonstitution zu München im Allgemeinen,
und den Genius der Krankheiten des Jahres 1821
im Besondern. 4°. *München,* 1822.

BAYR (E.) * De charactere morborum Monachii anno 1831–2 observato. 8°. *Monachii,*
1832.

Munich.

BEETZ (F.) Die Gesundheitsverhältnisse der k b. Haupt- und Residenzstadt München. Ein hygienischer Führer für Einheimische und Fremde. 8°. *München*, 1882.

BRUNNER (F.) & EMMERICH (R.) Die chemischen Veränderungen des Isarwassers während seines Laufes durch München nach Analysen. Nach den beiden von der medicinischen Facultät der kgl. Maximilians - Universität gekrönten Preisschriften zusammengestellt von Dr. Rudolf Emmerich. 8°. *München*, 1878.

GORDON (J.) Die Canalisation der kgl. Haupt- und Residenzstadt München. Bericht im Auftrage des Magistrates erstattet. 4°. *München*, 1876.

HEMMER (M.) Münchens Sanitätskarten, bearbeitet nach 1. der allgemeinen Sterblichkeit, 2. der Sterblichkeit der Kinder im 1. Lebensjahre, 3. der Sterblichkeit der Personen über dem 1. Lebensjahre, 4. der Sterblichkeit an zymotischen Krankheiten. roy. 8°. *München*, 1877.

HOEFLER (G.) * De charactere morborum Monachii anno 1832–3 observato. 8°. *Monachii*, 1833.

JAHRBÜCHER des ärztlichen Vereins zu München. Jahrgänge 1–4, 1835–42. 8°. *München*, *A. Weber.*

MARTIN (A.) Topographie und Statistik des kgl. bayer. Landgerichtes Au bei München, mit Berücksichtigung der medizinischen Verhältnisse desselben. 8°. *München*, 1837.

VON PETTENKOFER (M.) Das Kanal- oder Siel-System in München. 8°. *München*, 1869.

SATZUNGEN für die Studirenden der Ludwigs-Maximilians Universität in München. 4°. [*München*, 1827.]

WIBMER (C.) Medizinische Topographie und Ethnographie der k. Haupt- u. Residenzstadt München. Hrsg. von einer Commission des ärztlichen Vereins in München. 3 v. in 1. 8°. *München*, 1862–3.

WINTERHALTER (L.) Zur Kanalisation von München. I. Dr. Varrentrapp's Brief an Bürgermeister Dr. Erhardt. II. Dr. Varrentrapp als Hygieniker im Frankfurter Collegium. III. Auszug aus : Les systèmes d'évacuation des eaux et immondices d'une ville par M. le Dr. van Overbeek de Meijer. 8°. *München*, 1880.

Dieterich (L.) Witterungs- und Krankheitsconstitution zu München [April 1833 bis Dec. 1836]; mit besonderer Berücksichtigung der Influenza. Wchntl. Beitr. z. med. u. chir. Klin., Leipz., 1833–4, iii, 245–256. *Continued in:* Beitr. z. prakt. Heilk., Leipz., 1834, i, 196; 338; 699: 1836, ii, 357–361: iii, 177–182: 1837, iv, 197–205.— **Emmerich** (R.) Zur Münchener Canalisationsfrage. Aerztl. Int.-Bl., München, 1879, xxvi, 334; 346.—**Fch.** Hygieinisches aus München. Deutsche med. Wchnschr., Berl., 1876, ii, 353–356.—**Geigel.** Ueber die Einrichtung von Gesundheitsräthen nach dem Gutachten des Obermedicinalausschusses zu München. Deutsche Vrtljschr. f. öff. Gsndhtspflg., Brnschwg., 1875, vii, 312–321.—**Graf** (L.) Bericht der kön. Univ. Poliklinik zu München. 1864–7. Deutsche Klinik, Berl., 1868, xx, 437; 448; 456; 470.—**Hofmann.** Jahresbericht der geburtshülflichen Poliklinik, München, 1850–51. *Ibid.*, 1853, v, 40; 52; 81; 103; 150; 165; 201; 246; 256.—**Kerchensteiner.** Zur Münchener Canalisationsfrage. Aerztl. Int.-Bl, München, 1879, xxvi, 324 – 326. — **Liernur.** The Munich sewers as illustrating how the subsoil and subsoil water of towns are polluted by sewage. Pub. Health, Lond., 1876, iv, 428. — **Majer** (C.) Die Sterblichkeit in München. Nürnberg und Augsburg während der Jahre 1871 und 1872. Aerztl. Int.-Bl., München, 1873, xx, 677; 702.— **Plank.** Bemerkungen über die Abfassung medicinischer Länder-, Bezirks- und Ortsbeschreibungen überhaupt, und Versuch eines medicinisch-topographischen Entwurfes von der königl. bayerischen Haupt- und Residenzstadt München insbesondere. Ztschr. f. d. Staatsarznk., Erlang., 1828, 9. Ergnzngshft., 215–307.—**Ranke** (H.) [*et al.*]. Zur Münchener Canalisationsfrage. [With discussion] Aerztl. Int-Bl., München, 1879, xxvi, 243; 258; 270; 281; ·293; 303; 314; 324; 334; 346; 358; 370.—

Munich.

Renk. Ueber Ventilation, Beheizung und Beleuchtung des grossen Odeonsaales zu München. Gesundh.-Ingenieur, München, 1887, x, 224; 289.—**Richard.** L'hygiène à Munich. [Rev. crit.] Rev. d'hyg., Par., 1885, vii, 982: 1886, viii, 32; 398.—**Sailer.** Ueber das Mortalitäts-Verhältniss in München. Jahrb. d. ärztl. Ver. zu München, 1835, i, 226: 1836, ii, 391.—**Seitz** (F.) Die Krankheitsconstitution zu München vom Mai 1841 bis zum Juli 1843; [also] 4. Quartal 1845. Med. Cor.-Bl. bayer. Aerzte, Erlang., 1844, v, 97; 113; 129; 145; 161; 177: 1846, vii, 266; 273. ——. Die Krankheiten zu München in den Jahren 1875, 1876, 1877, 1878, 1879, 1880, 1881, 1882 und 1883, und ihre Verhütung. Aerztl. Int.-Bl., München, 1877, xxv, 533–536; 1878, xxv, 25; 35; 54; 64; 547: 1879, xxvi, 21; 34; 44; 53; 67: 1880, xxvii, 569: 1881, xxviii, 27; 49; 64; 73: 1882, xxix, 571 · 1883, xxx, 16; 35; 47; 77; 89; 110: 1885, xxxii, 65; 75; 88; 107; 131; 143. ——. Rückblick auf die im Jahre 1884 u. 1885 zu München herrschenden Krankheiten. München. med. Wchnschr., 1887, xxxiv, 5; 22; 40; 57; 77.—**Stand** (Der) der Kanalisationsfrage in München. Gesundheit, Frankf. a. M., 1881, vi. 115–117.—**Uebersicht** der Sterbefälle in München 1875–6. Aerztl. Int.-Bl., München, 1875–7, xxii-xxiv, *passim.*—**Uebersicht** der Geburts- und Sterblichkeitsverhältnisse der Stadt München in den Jahren 1876–82: 1884. Veröffentl. d. k. deutsch. Gsndhtsamtes, Berl., 1877, i, No. 4: 1878, ii, No. 4: 1879, iii, 34: 1880, iv, 74: 1881, v, 35: 1882, vi. 69: 1883, vii, 155: 1885, ix. 49.—**V.** (E.) L'Institut hygiénique de Munich. Rev. d'hyg., Par., 1879, i, 194–197.—**Varrentrapp** (G.) Offener Brief an Herrn Dr. Erhardt, ersten rechtskundigen Bürgermeister von München betreffend Dr. L. Winterhalter's Schrift: "Zur Kanalisation von München". Deutsche Vrtljschr. f. öff. Gsndhtspflg., Brnschwg.. 1880, xii, 545–566. *Also*, Reprint.—**von Weckbecker-Sternfeld** (F.) Zur Thätigkeit der Ortsgesundheits-Commissionen. Aerztl. Int.-Bl., München, 1879, xxvi, 209–211.—**Wibmer** (C.) Études sur la statistique médicale de la ville de Munich. [Trad. par le docteur E.-L. Berthrand.] J. de méd., chir. et pharmacol., Brux.. 1871, liii, 493–510. ——. Beitrag zur medicinischen Statistik der Stadt München. Aerztl. Int.-Bl., München, 1878, xxv, 190; 203.—**Wolffhügel** (G.) München eine "Peststadt"? Deutsche Vrtljschr. f. öff. Gsndhtspflg., Brnschwg., 1876, viii, 523–541.

Municipal Hospital, Philadelphia. *See* Philadelphia. Report of the Municipal Hospital.

Municipal *hygiene.*

See **Hygiene** (*Municipal*).

Munier (Alfred). * Des indications dans le traitement de la pleuro-pneumonie primitive chez l'adulte. 117 pp. 4°. *Montpellier, Boehm & fils*, 1865, No. 50.
c.

Munier (Henry). * Considérations sur les maladies de l'œil consécutives à la fièvre typhoïde et particulièrement sur un cas de névro-rétinite. 27 pp. 4°. *Paris*, 1874, No. 84.

Munier (Honoré). * Considérations sur le palper abdominal en obstétrique. 42 pp., 1 l. 4°. *Pari*, 1879, No. 61.

Munier (Joannes Baptista).
See **Saillant** (Carolus Jacobus). *An in vulneribus unicum linteum carptum? 4°. [*Paris*, 1772.]

——. *An omni sexui, omni ætati, omni temperamento, salubris caffé potus? Præses: Ludovicus Hieronymus Cosnier. [1743.]
In: SIGWART (G. F.) Quæst. med. Par. 4°. *Tubingæ*, 1789, i, 192–206.

Munier (Joh. Claudius). *An venæ spermaticæ structura secretioni seminis favet? [1743.] Præses: Joh. Franciscus Gez.
In: SIGWART (G. F.) Quæst. med. Par. 4°. *Tubingæ*, 1789, i, 44–47.

——. *An suppresso et immoderato catameniorum fluxui aperientia? Præses: A. J. Seron.
In: HALLER. Disp. anat. [etc.] 4°. *Gottingæ*, 1750, v, 197–232. *Also, in:* SIGWART (G. F.) Quæst. med. Par. 4°. *Tubingæ*, 1789, i, 289–326.
See, also, **Mauduyt de la Varenne** (Petrus Joannes Claudius). *An tumoris cancrosi radicitus ablati regeneratio rursus chirurgiæ tradenda? 4°. *Parisiis*, 1760.—**Paris** (Joannes Franciscus). *An variolis balneum? 4°. *Parisiis*, 1745. ——. *An post gravem, ab ictu vel casu violento, [etc.] 4°. *Parisiis*, 1746.

Munier (Joseph). * Ueber die Spaltung des Acetessigesters und einiger seiner Derivate durch Schwefelsäure. 26 pp. 8°. *Würzburg, Becker*, 1880.
c.

Munier (M.) De l'alcool en thérapeutique. 43 pp. 8°. *Troyes, imp. Dufour-Bouquot,* 1867.
Repr. from: Bull. Soc. méd. de l'Aube, 1867.

Munier (Maria Zorobabel). *An dysentericis anodyna? Præses: Joannes Baptista Jumelin. 4 pp. 4°. [*Paris, Quillau,* 1775.]

——. *Utrum in ascite paracentesim tardare, malum? Præses: Claudius Antonius Caille. 4 pp. 4°. [*Paris, Quillau,* 1776.]

Munière (Paul). *De l'ictère consécutif à la septicémie puerpérale. 1 p. l., 40 pp., 2 l. 4°. *Nancy,* 1876, 1. s., No. 40.

Munk (Emanuel) [1809–   ]. *Nonnulla de corde sano et morboso. 36 pp., 2 l. 8°. *Berolini, typ. Nietackianis,* [1835].

Munk (Hermann) [1839–   ]. Untersuchungen über das Wesen der Nerven-Erregung. v. 1. xviii, 482 pp. roy. 8°. *Leipzig, W. Engelmann,* 1868.

——. Ueber die Functionen der Grosshirnrinde; gesammelte Mittheilungen aus den Jahren 1877–80; mit Einleitung und Anmerkungen. x, 133 pp., 1 pl. 8°. *Berlin, A. Hirschwald,* 1881.

Munk (Immanuel) [1852–   ]. *Versuche über die Wirkung des Cryptopin. 32 pp. 8°. *Berlin, Thormann u. Goetsch,* [1873].

——. Physiologie des Menschen und der Säugethiere. Ein Lehrbuch für Studirende. viii, 546 pp. 8°. *Berlin, A. Hirschwald,* 1881.

——. The same. 2. Aufl. viii, 592 pp. roy. 8°. *Berlin, A. Hirschwald,* 1888.

Munk (Joh.) Sieben neue Fälle von Uterus-Ruptur mit Rücksicht auf vaterländische Literatur. iv, 5–40 pp. 8°. *Tübingen, F. Fues,* 1874.

Munk (Michael) [1812–   ]. *De hæmorrhoidibus ac tumorum hæmorrhoidalium anatomia et causis. 34 pp., 3 l. 8°. *Berolini, J. Sittenfeld,* [1842].

Munk (Nicolaas). *Ueber den Einfluss der Witterung auf die Croupsterblichkeit in den Niederlanden. [Heidelberg.] 77 pp. 8°. *Leyden, P. W. M. Trap,* 1885.

Munk (Philippus) [1832–71]. *De cupro in organica rerum natura obvio. 28 pp., 2 l. 8°. *Berolini, G. Nietack,* [1856].

——. Ueber das Wesen der Homöopathie. 1 p. l., 44 pp. 8°. *Bern, J. Dalp,* 1868.
For Biography, see Cor.-Bl. f. schweiz. Aerzte, Bern, 1871, i, 33–37 (E. Klebs).

—— & **Leyden** (E.) [1832–71]. Die acute Phosphor-Vergiftung. Mit besonderer Rücksicht auf Pathologie und Physiologie experimentell bearbeitet. 1 l., 188 pp. 8°. *Berlin, A. Hirschwald,* 1865. [*Also, in:* P., v. 1457.]

Munk (Reinhold). *Ein Beitrag zu den Dermoidcysten des Ovarium. 19 pp. 8°. *Tübingen, Fues u. Kostenbader,* 1885.

Munk (S.) *De vomitu. 16 pp., 1 l. 8°. *Pragæ, J. Spurny,* [1837].

Munk (William). A memoir of the life and writings of John Ayrton Paris. 30 pp. 8°. *London, Bell & Daldy,* 1857.

——. The roll of the Royal College of Physicians of London; compiled from the annals of the college and from other authentic sources. 2 v. v. 1, 1518 to 1700; v. 2, 1701 to 1800. xvi, 472 pp.; ix, 429 pp. 8°. *London, Longman [and others],* 1861.

——. The same. Comprising biographical sketches of all the eminent physicians whose names are recorded in the annals from the foundation of the college in 1518 to its removal in 1825 from Warwick Lane to Pall Mall East. 2. ed. 3 v. 8°. *London,* 1878.

——. Euthanasia; or medical treatment in aid of an easy death. vi (1 l.), 105 pp. 16°. *London & New York, Longmans, Green & Co.,* 1887.

Munkátsy (Nicolaus). *De coordinatione nosocomiorum. 44 pp., 2 l. 8°. *Budæ, typ. reg. univ. Hungaricæ,* [1834]. [P., v. 1324.]
Hungarian text.

Munn (*Jephtha B.*) [1780–1863].
Munn (J. L.) Obituary. Tr. M. Soc. N. Jersey, N. Y., 1864, 72.

Munnich (Adrianus Joh.) *Onderzoekingen over de bloedkleurstof. 60 pp. 8°. *Leiden, S. C. van Doesburgh,* 1868.

Munnicks (Joannes) [1652–1711]. De re anatomica liber. 10 p. l., 239 pp., 7 l. 8°. *Traj. ad Rhenum, A. Schouten,* 1697.

——. Anatomia nova qua juxta neotericorum inventa tota res anatomica breviter et dilucide explicatur; editio novissima. Frontispiece, 6 p. l., 229 pp., 5 l., 19 pl. 8°. *Lugduni, sumpt. J. Tenet,* 1699.

——. Praxis chirurgica. 507 pp., 2 l. 4°. *Amsterdam,* 1715.
Title-page wanting.

——. The same. Cheirurgia ad praxin hodiernam adornata, in qua veterum pariter ac neotericorum dogmata dilucide exponuntur. 3 p. l., 557 pp., 2 l. 8°. *Amstelodami, apud L. Malcomesium,* 1721.

Munniks (Jacobus). *De atropa belladona, præcipue exhibens ejus vires venenatas ac medendi rationes, septem observationibus confirmatas. 1 p. l., 58 pp., 3 l. 4°. *Groningæ, T. Spoormaker,* [1803].

——. *Observationes variæ. 3 p. l., 78 pp., 7 pp. 4°. *Groningæ, W. Kamerling,* 1805.

Munniks (Wynoldus) [1744–1806]. *De lue venerea, ejusque præcipuis auxiliis, inter quæ illustrissimi Zwietenii et clarissimi Plenkii remedia potissimum examinantur. 50 pp., 1 l. 4°. *Lugd. Bat., E. Luzac,* 1769. [P., v. 54.]

——. *De summis quas anatome habet, deliciis. 1 p. l., 50 pp., 1 l. 4°. *Groningæ, H. Spandaw,* 1771.
Also [Abstr.], *in:* WEIZ (F. A.) Neue Ausz. [etc.] 12°. *Leipzig,* 1777, vi, 5–7.

Munot (J.-Victor). *Contribution à l'étude de l'élimination de l'urée dans la phthisie pulmonaire. 43 pp. 4°. *Paris,* 1881, No. 255.

Muñoz (A.) Memoria descriptiva de una epidemia de viruela ocurrida en Olias del Rey (Toledo) en los años de 1882–3. 45 pp. 8°. *Madrid, J. J. Menendez,* 1885.

——. Las inyecciones hipodérmicas. 395 pp. 8°. *Madrid, J. J. Menendez,* 1886.

Munoz (José-Joaquin). *Du traitement de l'hydrocèle. 30 pp. 4°. *Paris,* 1852, No. 79, v. 530.
Also, Co-Editor of: **Anales** de la real Academia de ciencias médicas, físicas y naturales de la Habana, 1864–6.

Muñoz (Juan Fourquet).
See **Sanchez** (Julian Calleja). Tratado de anatomia humana. 3 v. 8°. *Valladolid,* 1869–72.

Muñoz (Luis). Observaciones sobre las cuestiones mas importantes que se refieren á la vacuna. 76 pp. 8°. *México, Lara,* 1869.

Muñoz y Miguel (*Francisco*) [18 –84].
Espina (A.) [Obituary.] Rev. de med. y cirug. práct., Madrid, 1884, xiv, 147–149, port.—**Huertas** (F.) [Obituary.] Rev. esp. de oftal., sif., etc., Madrid, 1884, viii, 41, port.

Muñoz y Sanchez (*Justo*) [1783–1857].
Guijarro (L.) Noticia biográfica. Siglo méd , Madrid, 1858, v, 33.

Munro (A. Campbell). Annual reports on the health and sanitary condition of the borough of South Shields. 10., 1884; 1885. 8°. *South Shields,* 1885–6.

——. Annual reports on the health and sanitary condition of the borough of Jarrow, by the medical officer of health, for the year 1885. 17 pp., 1 tab. *Jarrow-on-Tyne,* 1886.

Munro (Æneas). The science and art of nursing the sick. 2 p. l., 231 pp. 12°. *Glasgow, J. Maclehose,* 1873.

——. Deaths in childbed and our lying-in hospitals; together with a proposal for establishing a model maternity institution for affording clinical instruction and for training nurses. xv, 222 pp., 2 pl. 8°. *London, Smith, Elder & Co.,* 1879.

——. Dissertation on the use of the stethoscope in obstetrics. 34 pp. 8°. *Glasgow, J. Maclehose,* [*n. d.*]

Munro (Andreas). * De phthisi pulmonali. 30 pp. 8°. *Edinburgi, typ. G. Mudie et filii,* 1797. [P., v. 5.]

Munro (Donald). An account of the diseases which were most frequent in the British military hospitals in Germany, from January, 1761, to the return of the troops to England in March, 1763. To which is added an essay on the means of preserving the health of soldiers, and conducting military hospitals. 408 pp. 8°. *London, A. Millar & Co.,* 1764.

Munro (Gulielmus). ** De tetano. 1 p. l., 66 pp. 8°. *Edinburgi, Balfour et Smellie,* 1783.
Also, in: SMELLIE. Thesaurus med. [etc.] 8°. *Edinburgi,* 1785, iv, 325–357.

Munro (Hugh). A compendious system of the theory and practice of modern surgery, arranged in a new nosological and systematic method, different from any yet attempted in surgery; in the form of a dialogue. 352 pp., 10 l., 1 tab. 8°. *London, A. Guthrie,* 1792.

——. The same. 288 pp. 12°. *London, F. Hodson,* 1800.

Munro (*Pierre Antoine Conefroy*) [1811–82].
Obituary. Canada M. Rec., Montreal, 1881–2, x, 215.

Munro (W.) Notes on cases of yellow fever in St. Kitts, W. I., during 1868–69–70. 23 pp., 1 map. 8°. *Edinburgh, Oliver & Boyd,* 1871.
Repr. from: Edinb. M. J., 1871–2, xvii.

Munroe (Henry) [1818–87]. The physiological action of alcohol. 24 pp. 8°. *New York,* [1865, *vel subseq.*].

——. Alcohol not food. 2 pp. 8°. [*n. p., n. d.*]
——. Is alcohol a necessary of life? 22 pp. 8°. [*n. p., n. d.*]
For Biography, see Lancet, Lond., 1887, i, 245.

Munroe County Board of Health, Mississippi. Quarantine notice! [In consequence of the prevalence of yellow fever in Memphis, Tenn.] July 21, 1879. broadside 4°. [*Aberdeen,* 1879.]

Munsch (Julius) [1838–]. * De trichiniasi. 35 pp. 8°. *Gryphiswaldiæ, F. G. Kunike,* 1863. c.

Munschina (Édouard). *Contribution à l'étude des accidents laryngés chez les ataxiques. 59 pp. 4°. *Paris,* 1885, No. 1.

Munsell (Henry). The Dublin practice of midwifery. With notes and additions by Chandler R. Gilman. x, 11–292 pp. 8°. *New York, W. E. Dean,* 1845.

Munsell (Joel). A catalogue of the books and pamphlets issued from the press of . . . from the year 1828 to 1870. 191 pp. 8°. *Albany,* 1872.

Munson (*Æneas*).
Portrait in: **Collection** of Portr. (Libr.)

Munson (Franklin Avery) [1852–78]. The errors of refraction demonstrated by a new and original model. 11 pp. 8°. *Albany, N. Y., G. C. Riggs,* 1877.
Repr. from: N. York M. J., 1877, xxv.
For Biography, see Med. Ann., Albany, 1882, iii [Tr. M. Soc. County Albany, 366] (J. B. Stonehouse).

Munson (George S.) A case of chronic suppurative otitis, with exostosis of the auditory

Munson (George S.)—continued.
canal, abscess of the brain; autopsy. 17 pp. 8°. *Albany, Burdick & Taylor,* 1882.
Repr. from: Med. Ann., Albany, 1882, iij.

Munster (Godofredus Sigism.) * De macie et atrophia infantum. 39 pp. sm. 4°. *Kilonii, lit. G. Bartschii,* 1754.

van Munster (Jacobus). * De hydrope, ascite et paracentesi. 38 pp., 3 l. sm. 4°. *Lugd. Bat., C. Wishoff,* 1723. [P., v. 78.]

Munster (Joannes). Discussio eorum quæ ab Abrahamo Schopffio, in generalis suæ, omnium præsidiorum medicorum, universalium et topicorum disquisitionis, libri tertii sectione quarta, cum de aliis quibusdam ad purgandi negotium spectantibus theorematis, tum vero maxime de purgatione principio morborum instituenda, contra magnum illud magni Hippocratis i. aphot. 22. oraculum scripta sunt; quibus duæ accesserunt ejusdem argumenti appendices: una, contra Hieronymum Capovacceum; altera, contra Hieronymum Mercurialem. 3 p. l., 325 pp. 12°. *Francofurti, typ. J. Bratheringii,* 1603.
Bound with: HAFENREFFER (S.) Raphael artem medicam, [etc.] 12°. *Francofurti,* 1629.

van Munster (Joh.) Een zestal verloskundige operatien en waarneemingen, zo omtrent het verlossen van vrouwen door de sectio sijmphisis ossis pubis, of doorsnijding der schaambeensvereeniging, als wegens het openen eener toegegroeide baarmoder. Met een' aanprijzenden brief van Petrus Camper; benevens een' anderen onlangs bekomen brief van G. J. van Wy. iv, 5–61 pp. 8°. *Amsterdam, J. W. Yntema & Co.,* 1804.

Munster (Joh. Christianus). De diversis obstructionum caussis et remediis. 16 pp. 4°. *Francof. ad Viadr., ex off. J. C. Winteri,* [1750].

Muntaner (Lorenzo).
Editor of: **Revista** balear de medicina, farmacia y veterinaria, Palma de Mallorca, 1885.

Muntendam (Didericus Joannes). * Diss. sistens quædam de sanguinis detractione. 1 p. l., 51 pp, 1 l. 8°. *Amstelædami, C. G. van der Post,* 1848.

Muntendam (Stephanus). * De atelectasi pulmonum. [Leyden.] 1 p. l., 56 pp., 2 l. 8°. *Amstelodami,* 1848.

Munthé (A.) *Prophylaxie et traitement des hémorrhagies post partum. 71 pp. 4°. *Paris,* 1880, No. 330.

Munting (Abrahamus). Aloidarium, sive aloës mucronato folio Americanæ majoris, aliarumque ejusdem speciei historia. In quâ floridi illius temporis, loci, naturæ, culturæ, nec non qualitatum ratio paucis enarratur. 33 pp., 9 l. 4°. [*Amstelodami*], 1680.
Bound with his: De vera antiquorum herba Britannica, etc. 4°. *Amstelodami,* 1681.

——. De vera antiquorum herba britannica ejusdemque efficacia contra stomacaccen, seu scelotyrben, Friscis et Batavis de scheurbuijck. Dissertatio historico-medica. 12 p. l., 231 pp., 32 pl., port. 4°. *Amstelodami, apud H. Sweerts,* 1681.

Muntingh (Fredericus Gulielmus). *Annotationes de nonnullis diureticis. 3 p. l., 12 pp. 8°. *Lugd. Bat., J. W. van Leeuwen,* 1834.

Muntinghe (Hermannus). * Spec. med. inaug. exhibens nonnulla de necessitudine inter febres intermittentes et morbos nervosos. 1 p. l., 27 pp., 2 l. 8°. *Groningæ, H. R. Roelfsema,* [1852].

Muntok.
Lindgreen (J. J.) Geneeskundige topographie van Muntok. Tijdschr. d. Vereen. t. Bevord. d. geneesk. Wetensch. in Nederl. Indië, Batav., 1857, v, 839–889.

Munzer (Carl) [1864–]. * Zur Kenntniss der Vergiftungen durch Oxalsäure. 28 pp., 2 l. 8°. *Berlin, O. Francke,* [1887].

Munzert (Fridericus Christianus). * De metrorrhagia gravidarum. 32 pp. 8°. *Erlangæ, Kunstmann*, [1834].

Munzert (H. Ch. A.) * De hydrocele. vi, 7–23 pp. 8°. *Erlangæ, Kunstmann*, [1842].

Muquardt (C.) Catalogue d'une collection d'ouvrages de médecine et d'entomologie. 26 pp. 8°. *Bruxelles*, 1885.

Murad V.

Schlager. Ueber die psychiatrische Begutachtung des Geisteszustandes Sultans Murad V. Allg. Wien. med. Ztg., 1876, xxi, 315.

Muræna.

CLARK (A.) Observations on the anatomy of the skin of a species of muræna. 8°. [*London, n. d.*]

Repr. from : Tr. Micr. Soc. Lond.

Robin (C.) Sur la structure des corps rouges du congre (Muræna conger L.). J. de l'anat. et physiol., etc., Par., 1883, xix, 528–537, 1 pl.

Muraire.

See **Robert** (L.-M.-J.) Observations sur la fièvre jaune, etc. 8°. *Marseille*, 1822.

Murakami (Toki). Bai So Hi Roku Hiyo Ki. [A treatise on syphilis.] 2 v. 2, 3, 4, 2, 41 pp. ; 53 pp. 8°. *Kioto*, 1808.

von Muralt (Carl). * Die Staarextraction der ophthalmologischen Klinik in Zürich 1870 – 80. 2 p. l., 70 pp. 8°. *Zürich, O. Füssli u. Comp.*, 1881.

von Muralt (Joh.) [1645–1733]. Vade mecum anatomicum, sive clavis medicinæ, pandens experimenta de humoribus, partibus et spiritibus. 11 p. l., 593 pp., 8 l., 1 pl. 24°. *Tiguri, typ. D. Gessneri*, 1677.

———. Anatomisches Collegium in welchem alle und jede Theile dess menschlichen Leibes zusamt denen Kranckheiten und Zufällen welchen sie unterworffen, nach ihren aus den neuesten Lehr-Sätzen untersuchten Ursachen und bewährt darwider befundenen Artzney-Mitteln beschrieben worden. Mit einer Erklärung der fürnehmsten in der Artzney gebräuchlichen Kräuter, vorgetragen zu Zürch, auf einer löblichen Gesellschäfft zum schwartzen Garten. 9 p. l., 775 pp., 43 l. 16°. *Nürnberg, W. M. Endters*, 1687.

———. Hippocrates Helveticus: oder der getreu-sichere, und wohl-bewährte Eydgnössische Stadt-, Land- und Hauss-Artzt in welchem eine klare und wahrhaffte Beschreibung innerlicher Gebrechen und Kranckheiten des menschlichen Leibs und aller dessen Gliederen, nach den besten Grund-Sätzen der Heilkunst enthalten ; sammt Entdeckung der gewissesten, kräfftigsten, wohl-befundenen und bewährtesten Artzney-Mitteln, welche wider dieselbigen heilsamlich können gebraucht werden. Zu Nutz und Frommen der Eydgnössischen Einwohneren und anderen der Preiss-würdigen Artzneykunst Liebhabern, an das Tagliecht gegeben, und zu unaussprechlicher Bequemlichkeit dem Alphabet nach vorgestellet. Frontispiece, 15 p. l., 1046 pp., 12 l. 8°. *Basel, E. & J. G. Königen*, 1692.

———. Aretæi, Neu-Eröffneter Balsamischer Gesundheit-Schatz, wieder die ansteckende Seuche an Menschen und Viehe. 102 pp. 12°. *Zürich*, 1714.

For Portrait, see **Collection** of Portr. of Phys. & Men of Sc., 189.

———. *See, also :*

Meyer-Ahrens (C.) Die Arztfamilie von Muralt [etc.] Arzt in Zürich. Schweiz. Ztschr. f. Heilk., Bern, 1862, i, 268 ; 423 : 1863, ii, 25–47.

de Muralto (Joh. Conradus). * De iliaca passione. 23 pp. 4°. *Basileæ, typ. E et J. Georgius*, [1693].

See, also, **Welsch** (Christianus Ludovicus) & **de Muralto** (Joh. Conradus). Compendiosam naturalis [etc.] 4°. *Basileæ*, [1692].

de Muralto (Leonardus). * De parorchidio. [Gottingæ.] 28 pp., 1 tab. 4°. *Berolini, typ. Feisterianis et Eisersdorffianis*, 1828.

Muramatsu Sekizo. Yojo Kunmo. [Hygiene in time of cholera.] 2 p. l., 34 pp., 1 l. 12°. *Tokio*, 1880.

Japanese text.

Muranges (Barthélemy). * I. Du cancer du pharynx. II. [etc.] 28 pp. 4°. *Paris*, 1839, No. 56, v. 346.

Muraour (P.-A.) * Sur la fistule lachrymale. 24 pp. 4°. *Paris*, 1818, No. 44, v. 136.

Murat (A.-L.) [–1837]. * La glande parotide considérée sous ses rapports anatomiques, physiologiques et pathologiques. iv, 5–84 pp. 8°. *Paris, an XI* [1803]. [*Also, in :* P., v. 1078.]

Murat (J.-A.) * De l'empoisonnement par les substances végétales. 1 p. l., 23 pp. 4°. *Strasbourg*, 1811, v. 47.

Murat (Jean-Baptiste-Arnaud) [1793–]. Mémoire sur la question proposée par la Société de médecine de Bruxelles: La nuit exerce-t-elle une influence sur les maladies ? Y a-t-il des maladies où cette influence est plus ou moins manifeste ? Quelle est la raison physique de cette influence ?

In : Actes Soc. de méd. de Brux., 1806, i, 91–266.

———. Mémoire qui a remporté le premier prix au jugement de la Société de médecine de Toulouse, dans la séance du 10 novembre 1806, sous la question proposée en ces termes : Déterminer quels sont les avantages ou les inconvéniens de la multiplicité des nomenclatures, relativement aux travaux des anatomistes, des physiologistes et des nosographes vi, 7–182 pp. 8°. *Montpellier, A. Seguin*, 1807.

See, also, **Influence** (De l') de la nuit sur les maladies. 8°. *Bruxelles*, 1806.

Murat (Jn.-Louis). * Sur le tétanos traumatique. viii, 9–49 pp. 4°. *Paris*, 1816, No. 232, v. 126.

Murat (Joseph-François-Victor). * La méthode de l'analyse, appliquée à l'étude des maladies chroniques. 37 pp. 4°. *Paris*, 1818, No. 248, v. 143.

Muratet (A.) * D'un cas d'anévrysme de la carotide interne. Diagnostic différentiel d'avec les tumeurs du voile du palais. viii, 9–40 pp., 1 l. 4°. *Montpellier, Firmin et Cabirou frères*, 1883, No. 40.

Muratoff (Alexander). * Materiali dlja akucherskoi statistiki goroda Moskvi. 77 pp., 1 l. 8°. *Moskva*, 1879.

Muratoff (I.) * Materiali k izsledov. zdorovja fabrichnich rabochich i mjasinkov posred. opredelenija rosta, viesa, okrujnosti grudi i jiznennoi emkosti legkich. [Sanitary condition of factory workers and butchers, comparing size, weight, circumference of chest, and vital capacity.] 74 pp., 1 diag. 8°. *St. Petersburg*, 1885.

Muratori (Lodovico Antonio) [1672–1750]. Del governo della peste e delle maniere di guardarsene, trattato diviso in politico, medico et ecclesiastico, da conservarsi et aversi pronto per le occasioni, che Dio tenga sempre lontane. xxxii, 437 pp. 12°. *Modena, B. Soliani*, 1714.

———. The same. Ed in questa seconda edizione accresciuto dall' autore con nuove aggiunte poste in fine del lontane. 2. ed. xxviii, 383 pp., 1 l. 4°. *Torino, P. G. Zappata*, 1721.

Another copy bound with : FIOCHETTO (Gianfrancesco). Trattato della peste, [etc.] 4°. *Torino*, 1720.

———. Li tre governi politico, medico, ed ecclesiastico utilissimi, anzi necessari in tempo di peste, autenticati da quanto è accaduto in moltissime città, e provincie secondo l' opportunità usata nelle precauzioni, e rimedj. Aggiuntovi il dettaglio della peste, che ultimamente ha desolata Marsiglia, pubblicato dai medici che hanno

Muratori (Lodovico Antonio)—continued.
operato in essa, e con alcune osservazioni dell' autore. 4. ed. xxiii, 366 pp. 12°. *Lucca, D. Ciuffetti & F. M. Benedini*, 1743.

——. Delle forze dell' intendimento umano, osia il pirronismo confutato. Opposto al libro del preteso M. Huet intorno alla debolezza dell' umano intendimento. 2. ed. 1 p. l., xxxviii, 348 pp., 2 l. 12°. *Venezia, presso G. Pasquali*, 1748.

——. Della forza della fantasia umana. 2. ed. xii, 212 pp. 12°. *Venezia, presso G. Pasquali*, 1753.
Bound with the preceding.

——. Reflexiones sobre el buen gusto en las ciencias y en las artes. Traduccion libre de las que escribio en italiano . . . con un discurso sobre el gusto actual de los Españoles en la literatura, por Juan Sempere y Guarinos. 2 p. l., 296 pp. 8°. *Madrid, en la imp. de A. de Sancha*, 1782.
See, also, **Tortus** (Franciscus). Therapeutice specialis ad febres. [etc.] 4°. *Venetiis*, 1755. ——. The same. 4°. *Francofurti et Lipsiæ*, 1756.

Murché (Vincent T.) Animal physiology. A specific subject of instruction in public elementary schools. Blackie's elementary text-books. 144 pp. *London, Blackie & Son*, [1884].

Murchison (Charles) [1830-79]. On the experiments of Dr. Casimiro Sperino, of Turin, on the subject of syphilization. 4 pp. 8°. *Edinburgh, Sutherland & Knox*, [1851, *vel subseq.*].
Repr. from: Rep. Phys. Soc. Edinb.

——. Contributions to the pathology of morbid growths. 24 pp. 8°. *Edinburgh, Sutherland & Knox; London, Simpkin, Marshall & Co.*, 1852. [P., v. 894; 1558.]
Repr. from: Month. J. M. Sc., Lond. & Edinb., 1852, xiv.

——. Medical notes on the climate of Burmah, and on the diseases which have there prevailed among European troops. 70 pp. 8°. *Edinburgh, Neill & Co.*, 1855. [*Also, in :* P., v. 1188.]
Repr. from: Edinb. M. & S. J., 1855, i.

——. On gastro-colic fistula. A collection of cases and observations on its pathology, diagnosis, etc. 35 pp. 8°. [*Edinburgh, Murray & Gibb*, 1857.] [*Also, in :* P., v. 1188.]
Repr. from: Edinb. M. J., 1857, iii.

——. Contributions to the etiology of continued fever, or an investigation of various causes which influence the prevalence and mortality of its different forms. 88 pp., 4 tab. 8°. *London, J. E. Adlard*, 1858. [P., v. 1025.]
Repr. from: Med.-Chir. Tr., Lond., 1858, xli.

——. Remarks on the changes which are supposed to have taken place in the type of continued fever. 6 pp. 8°. [*Edinburgh, Murray & Gibb*, 1858.] [P., v. 1197.]
Repr. from: Edinb. M. J., 1858-9, iv.

——. Remarks on the classification and nomenclature of continued fevers. 12 pp. 8°. *Edinburgh, Murray & Gibb*, 1858. [*Also, in :* P., v. 1197.]
Repr. from: Edinb. M. J., 1858-9, iv.

——. A treatise on the continued fevers of Great Britain. xiv, 638 pp., 5 pl., 10 diag. 8°. *London, Parker, Son & Bourn*, 1862.

——. The same. 2. ed. xix, 729 pp., 5 col. pl., 19 diag. roy. 8°. *London, Longmans, Green & Co.*, 1873.

——. The same. Die typhoiden Krankheiten, Flecktyphus, recurrirender Typhus, Ileotyphus und Febricula. Deutsch herausgegeben mit einem Anhange: Die Epidemie des recurrirenden Typhus in St. Petersburg 1864-5, von Dr. W. Zuelzer. xviii, 729 pp., 6 pl. 8°. *Braunschweig, F. Vieweg u. Sohn*, 1867.

Murchison (Charles)—continued.
——. The same. La fièvre typhoïde, traduit par le Dr. Lutaud, accompagné de notes et précédé d'une introduction par M. Henry Guéneau de Mussy. lvi (lvi bis—lvi quinque), 409 pp., 3 pl., 4 tab. 8°. *Paris, Germer-Baillière & Cie.*, 1878.

——. Hydatid tumors of the liver; their dangers, their diagnosis, and their treatment. 26 pp. 8°. *Edinburgh, Oliver & Boyd*, 1865.

——. On a peculiar disease of the cranium, hyoid bone, and fibula, with a report by a committee of the Pathological Society. 8 pp., 1 l., 3 pl. 4°. *London*, 1866.
Repr. from: Tr. Path. Soc. Lond., 1865-6, xvii.

——. Clinical lectures on diseases of the liver, jaundice, and abdominal dropsy. xxi, 556 pp. 8°. *New York, W. Wood & Co.*, 1868.

——. The same. Klinische voordragten over ziekten van de lever, geelzucht en buikwaterzucht. Uit het Engelsch door Dr. J. C. ten Noever de Brauw. ix, 327 pp. 8°. *Tiel, H. C. A. Campagne*, 1870.

——. The same. Leçons cliniques sur les maladies du foie, suivies des leçons s r les troubles fonctionnels du foie. Traduites sur la seconde édition avec l'autorisation de l'auteur et annotées par le Dr. Jules Cyr. xii, 660 pp. 8°. *Paris, A. Delahaye & Cie.*, 1878.

——. Clinical lectures on diseases of the liver, jaundice, and abdominal dropsy, including the Croonian lectures on functional derangements of the liver, delivered at the Royal College of Physicians in 1874. Edited by T. Lauder Brunton; the section on tropical diseases by Joseph Fayrer. 3. ed. xviii (1 l.), 702 pp. 8°. *London, Longmans, Green & Co.*, 1885.

——. On the period of incubation of typhus, relapsing fever, and enteric fever. 20 pp. 8°. [*London*, 1871, *vel subseq.*]
Repr. from: St. Thomas's Hosp. Rep., Lond., 1871, n. s., ii.

——. On functional derangements of the liver, being the Croonian lectures delivered at the Royal College of Physicians in March, 1874. xvi, 182 pp. 8°. *London, Smith, Elder & Co.*, 1874.

——. The same. xvi, 182 pp. 8°. *New York, W. Wood & Co.*, 1875.
See, also, **Frerichs** (Fred. Theod.) A clinical treatise on diseases of the liver. [etc.] 8°. *New York*, 1860-61. ——. The same. 8°. *New York*, 1879. — **Lackersteen** (M. H.) The physiology of digestion, [etc.] 8°. *Chicago*, 1884. — **Moore** (Charles H.) & **Murchison** (Charles). On a method of procuring the consolidation of fibrin in certain incurable aneurisms, [etc.] 8°. [*n. p., n. d.*] — **Van Derveer** (Albert). Report of ten cases of gastric ulcer, etc. 8°. *Albany*, 1880.
For Biography, see Brit. M. J., Lond., 1879. i, 648-650. *Also :* Lancet, Lond., 1879, i, 645. *Also :* Med. Rec., N. Y., 1879, xv, 478. *Also :* Med. Times & Gaz., Lond., 1879, i, 522.

——. *See, also :*
Watson (*Sir* Th.) Presentation of address and testimonial to Dr. Murchison. Med. Times & Gaz., Lond., 1874, i, 455-457.

Murcia.
See **Cholera** (*Asiatic, History, etc., of*), by localities.

Murder.
See **Asphyxia, Cadaver,** *Jurisprudence of*; **Contusions; Criminals** (*Mental condition, etc., of*)**; Homicide,** *etc.*; **Insanity** (*Homicidal*).

"**Murder** will out." The Ashland tragedy. The crow bar and ax, the silent witnesses. A history of the killing of Fanny Gibbons, Emma Carico, and Robbie Gibbons. 1 p. l., 52 pp. 8°. *Ashland, Ky., J. M. Huff*, [1882].

Murdfield (Franz) [1851-]. * Ein Beitrag zur Kenntniss des Lichen exsudativus ruber. 23 pp. 8°. *Greifswald, F. W. Kunike*, 1875.

Murdoch (Donald). A few remarks on the necessity for further suppression of infectious disorders (fevers). 31 pp. 8°. *London, E. Stanford,* 1880.

Murdoch (Gilbert). Special report of the commissioners of sewerage and water supply, for the city of Saint John and town of Portland, on the formation of anchor ice. 30 pp., 5 plans. 8°. *Saint John, N. B., Daily News,* 1881.

——. Special report on the water supply of Saint John (East) and town of Portland. To the commissioners of sewerage and water supply. 59 pp., 1 map, 2 diag. 8°. *Saint John, N. B., J. & A. McMillan,* 1883.

——. Review of the report of Hurd Peters, on the water supply of the cities of St. John and Portland. 59 pp., 2 tab. 8°. *Saint John, N. B., J. & A. McMillan,* 1884.

Murdoch (James). Practical observations on the extraction of the placenta. iv, 48 pp. 8°. *Edinburgh, Caw & Elder,* 1818.

Murdoch (Robertus). * De gonorrhœa. 2 p. l., 16 pp. 8°. *Edinburgi, G. Hamilton & J. Balfour,* 1754.

Murdoch (William). * Quelques propositions et considérations sur les maladies des enfans et les maladies mentales. 20 pp. 4°. *Paris,* 1832, No. 199, v. 254.

[**Mure** (B.)] Publication de l'Institut homéopathique du Brésil. Doctrine de l'école de Rio Janeiro et pathogénésie brésilienne, contenant une exposition méthodique de l'homéopathie, la loi fondamentale du dynamisme vital, la théorie des doses et des maladies chroniques, les machines pharmaceutiques, l'algèbre symptomatologique, la classification philosophique des esprits médicinales, et trente-six expériences pures. lx, 367 pp. 8°. *Paris, Institut homéopathique,* 1849.

——. Materia medica or provings of the principal animal and vegetable poisons of the Brazilian Empire; and their application in the treatment of disease. Transl. from the French, and arranged according to Hahnemann's method, by Charles I. Hempel. 218 pp. 8°. *New York, W. Radde,* 1854.

——. Le médecin du peuple; enseignement mettant à la portée des hommes de conscience et de bon vouloir les procédés les plus parfaits et les récentes découvertes de l'art de guérir, indiquant les moyens pratiques de traiter toutes les maladies de l'homme et des animaux selon les principes de l'homœopathie. Revu, augmenté et mis en meilleur ordre par Sophie Liet. 504 pp. 12°. *Paris, J.-B. Baillière & fils,* 1883.

——. L'homœopathie pure; exposé complet des connaissances nécessaires au traitement des malades, contenant la solution scientifique de tous les points encore douteux du nouvel art, la physiologie et la pathologie nouvelles. l'algèbre médicale et ses applications, les tables logarithmiques pour le choix instantané du médicament, etc., suivi de nombreux documents inédits, et orné de gravures, revu, augmenté et mis en ordre par Sophie Liet. vii, 208 pp., 1 pl. 8°. *Paris, J.-B. Baillière & fils,* 1883.

—— & **Gatti** (P.) Il cholera-morbus vinto colla scienza. 2. ed., con appendice. 52 pp. 8°. *Genova, A. Moretti,* [1854]. [P., v. 1456.]

Mure (Georgius). * De dyspepsia. 1 p. l., 27 pp. 8°. *Edinburgi, A. Smellie,* 1798. [*Also, in*: P., v. 7.]

Murelle (Lucien-Sénateur). * De l'anesthésie locale par réfrigération, au point de vue chirurgicale. 42 pp. 4°. *Paris,* 1855, No. 257, v. 578

Muret (C.) * De la suture des os faite avec des fils; ses indications. 56 pp. 4°. *Paris,* 1873, No. 122.

Muret (D.-J.-P.) * Sur les épanchemens du péricarde. 1 p. l., 27 pp. 4°. *Strasbourg,* 1833, v. 64.

Muret (Henri) [1804–86]. * Sur le traitement des principaux dérangemens des menstrues, considérées dans les différens âges de la femme. 31 pp. 4°. *Paris,* 1826, No. 39, v. 198.

For Biography, see Rev. méd. de la Suisse Rom., Genève, 1886, vi, 776.

Muret (J.-V.-Charles). * Des écrasements des doigts. Dangers de l'amputation. 27 pp. 4°. *Paris,* 1853, No. 196, v. 546.

Muret (Maurice). * Ueber die therapeutische Verwerthung des Naphthalins, besonders bei Typhus abdominalis. [Strasburg.] 74 pp., 1 l. 8°. *Basel, M. Werner-Riehm,* 1886.

Muret (Rodolphe). * Essai sur l'opération de la cataracte; suivi du parallèle des deux méthodes (l'abaissement et l'extraction), et de quelques réflexions sur les accidens qui peuvent les suivre. [Paris.] 2 p. l., 57 pp. 4°. *Strasbourg, Levrault,* 1813.

Murga (D. Leopoldo). La verdad de la inoculación anticolérica del Dr. Ferrán en relación con la epidemia colérica en Valencia. Memoria presentada á la excma. diputación provincial de Sevilla. 119 pp., 9 pl. 8°. *Sevilla, J. M. Ariza,* 1885.

Murgulovié (Ljubomir). * Drei Fälle von Unterbindung der Arteria femoralis. 22 pp., 1 l. 8°. *Jena, H. Pohle,* 1884.

Muriated *tincture of iron.*
    See Iron (*Chloride of*).

Muridæ.
    NICATI (C.) Commentatio de mure domestico, silvatico atque arvali. 8°. *Traj. ad Rhenum,* 1822.

    Dobson (G. E.) Note on the mandibular dentition of the shrews. J. Anat. & Physiol., Lond., 1885–6, xx, 359.—**Shufeldt** (R. W.) Description of Hesperomys Truei, a new species belonging to the subfamily Murinæ. Proc. U. S. Nat. Mus., Wash., 1885, viii, 403–408, 1 pl.

Murie (James). Observations upon Presbytes albigena, Gray, and Colobus guereza, Rüppel. 6 pp. 8°. [*London,* 1865.] [P., v. 1488.]
    Repr. from: Proc. Zool. Soc. Lond., 1865.

——. On the anatomy of a fin-whale (Physalus antiquorum, Gray) captured near Gravesend. 23 pp. 8°. [*London,* 1865.] [*Also, in*: P., v. 1488.]
    Repr. from: Proc. Zool. Soc. Lond., 1865.

——. On the myology of Hyrax capensis. 24 pp. 8°. [*London,* 1865.] [*Also, in*: P., v. 1488.]
    Repr. from: Proc. Zool. Soc. Lond., 1865.

——. On deformity of the lower jaw in the cachalot (Physeter macrocephalus, Linn.). 8 pp. 8°. [*London,* 1865.] [*Also, in*: P., v. 1488.]
    Repr. from: Proc. Zool. Soc. Lond., 1865.

——. On the identity of the hairy-nosed wombat (Phascolomys lasiorhinus, Gould), with the broad-fronted wombat (P. latifrons, Owen), with further observations on the several species of the genus. 18 pp., 1 pl. 8°. [*London,* 1865.] [P., v. 1488.]
    Repr. from: Proc. Zool. Soc. Lond., 1865.

——. Note upon the abnormality of a tailfeather in a male Sœmmering's pheasant. 1 l. 8°. [*London,* 1865.] [P., v. 1488.]
    Repr. from: Proc. Zool. Soc. Lond., 1865.

——. On the movement of the symphysis of the lower jaw in the kangaroos. 7 pp. 8°. [*London,* 1866.] [P., v. 1488.]
    Repr. from: Proc. Zool. Soc. Lond., 1866.
    See, also, **Mivart** (St. George) & **Murie** (James). Observations on the anatomy, etc. 8°. *London,* 1865.

Murie (Raoul-Enghéraud) [1859–]. * De la résection du pylore dans les lésions organiques de l'estomac. 86 pp. 4°. *Paris,* 1883.

Murie (Victor). * Sur le croup. 25 pp. 4°. *Paris,* 1824, No. 16, v. 183.

Murillo (A.) Vacunacion obligatoria. Discurso pronunciado en la Camara de diputados. (Session del 6 de julio de 1883.) 27 pp. 8°. *Santiago de Chile, J. Nuñez,* 1883.

Murillo (Thomas). Novissima, verifica, et particularis hypochondriacæ melancholiæ curatio, et medela. 35 p. l., 320 pp., 13 l. 16°. *Lugduni, C. Bourgeat,* 1672.

Murino (Alessio). Manuale di medicina teorico-pratica compilato sugli autori più recenti. 301 pp. 8°. *Roma, tipog. Editrice Romana,* 1873.

———. Lezioni di medicina popolare e preventiva. 1 p. l., x, 241 pp., 1 l. 12°. *Roma, Barbèra,* 1875.

———. Il colèra asiatico e la sua cura; lezione popolare. 14 pp. 12°. [*n. p., n. d.*] [P., v. 854.]

Muriset (Eloi). *Der Schmerz. 60 pp. 8°. *Würzburg, C. J. Becker,* 1866.   c.

Murisier (John). *Ueber die Formveränderungen, welche der lebende Knochen unter dem Einflusse mechanischer Kräfte erleidet. [Wurtzburg.] 29 pp., 1 pl. 8°. *Leipzig, J. B. Hirschfeld,* 1875.

Murmurs.

See, also, **Auscultation;** **Auscultation** (*Sounds, etc., in*); **Auscultation** *of heart, etc.*; **Blood-vessels** (*Murmurs in*); **Heart** (*Murmurs, etc., of*).

Bailly. Recherches sur le souffle utérin après l'accouchement. Arch. de tocol., Par., 1874, i, 449–471.—**Hohl.** Klinische Mittheilungen über das Uterin-Placentarstellengeräusch. Deutsche Klinik, Berl., 1849, i, 61.—**Jenner** (W.) Clinical lecture on the influence of pressure in the production and modification of palpable vibrations, and murmurs, perceptible over the heart and great vessels, larynx and lungs. Med. Times & Gaz., Lond., 1856, n. s., xii, 203–205.—**Physical** (On the) theory of murmurs, vascular, cardiac, and respiratory. Brit. & For. M.-Chir. Rev., Lond., 1873, lii, 13–32.—**Seidel** (M.) Ueber Reibegeräusche am Peritoneum. Deutsche Klinik, Berl., 1865, xvii, 465; 485.

Muro (Vincenzo). Sulla epidemia cholerica napoletana del 1884. 44 pp. 8°. *Napoli, A. Tocco & Comp.,* 1885.

Muron (Antoine) [–1874]. *Pathogénie de l'infiltration de l'urine. 76 pp. 4°. *Paris,* 1872, No. 44.

———. The same. 72 pp. 8°. *Paris, A. Delahaye,* 1872.

For Biography, see Compt. rend. Soc. de biol., Par., 1875, pp. xiii–xvi (Laborde).

Murphy.

See **Portal** (Antoine). Observations sur la nature et le traitement de la phthisie pulmonaire [etc.] 8°. *Paris,* 1809.

Murphy (Carolus). *De cynanche maligna. 2 p. l., 26 pp. 8°. *Edinburgi, A. Neill et socii,* 1805.

Murphy (Charles).

Co-Editor of: **University** (The) Medical and Surgical Journal of Philadelphia, 1864.

Murphy (Edward A.) Notes on electro-surgery, with cases and operations. 15 pp. 8°. *Chicago, Lakeside Press,* 1874.

Repr. from: Med. Invest., Chicago, 1874, xi.

———. Yellow fever; its treatment and prevention. [Homœopathic.] 25 pp. 8°. [*n. p.,* 1876, *vel subseq.*]

Murphy (Edward William) [1802–77]. Advantages of medical association; an address read to the Harveian Society at the opening of its 14th session. 15 pp. 8°. *London, Taylor & Walton,* 1844. [*Also, in:* P., v. 895.]

———. A report of the obstetric practice of the University College Hospital, London. 53 pp., 1 l., 1 pl. 8°. *Dublin, Hodges & Smith,* 1844. [P., v. 888.]

———. Lectures on natural and difficult parturition. xii, 263 pp. 8°. *London, Taylor & Walton,* 1845.

Murphy (Edward William)—continued.

———. The same. 281 pp. 8°. *New York, S. S. & W. Wood,* 1846.

———. Introductory lecture delivered at University College, London. 12 pp. 8°. *London, Wilson & Ogilvy,* 1846.

Repr. from: Lond. M. Gaz., 1846, n. s., iii.

———. Chloroform in the practice of midwifery. [Read at the Harveian Society, February 5, 1848.] 28 pp. 8°. *London, Taylor & Walton,* 1848. [*Also, in:* P., v. 1204.]

———. Further observations on chloroform in the practice of midwifery. 43 pp. 8°. *London, Taylor, Walton & Maberly,* 1850. [*Also, in:* P., v. 39; 725.]

Repr. from: Month. J. M. Sc., Lond. & Edinb., 1848-9, ix.

———. Lectures on the principles and practice of midwifery. xviii, 616 pp., 7 pl. 8°. *London, Taylor, Walton & Maberly,* 1852.

———. The same. 2. ed., enlarged and revised. xx, 735 pp. 8°. *London, Walton & Maberly,* 1862.

———. Lectures on preternatural and complex parturition and lactation. 2 p. l., 259–616 pp., 7 pl. 8°. *London, Taylor, Walton & Maberly,* 1852.

Second part of his: Lectures on the principles and practice of midwifery. 8°. *London,* 1852.

———. What is puerperal fever? A question proposed to the Epidemiological Society, London. 31 pp. 8°. *Dublin, McGlashan & Gill,* 1857.

Repr. from: Dublin Q. J. M. Sc., 1857, xxiv.

———. The same. De la fièvre puerpérale. Traduit de l'anglais par M. le docteur Gentil. 31 pp. 8°. *Paris, Germer-Baillière,* 1858. [P., v. 1345.]

Repr. from: Rev. étrang. méd. chir.

———. The Cæsarean section. 31 pp. 8°. *Dublin, McGlashan & Gill,* 1859. [P., v. 89.]

Repr. from: Dublin Q. J. M. Sc., 1859, xxvii.

———. Introductory lecture on the history of midwifery. Delivered at University College, May 1, 1864. 24 pp. 8°. *London, Saunders, Otley & Co.,* 1864. [P., v. 89.]

———. On the comparative claims of craniotomy and the Cæsarean section in a certain class of labors, and on the use of a new pelvimeter. 8 pp. 8°. *Dublin, J. Falconer,* 1864. [P., v. 89.]

Repr. from: Dublin Q. J. M. Sc., 1864, xxvii.

For Biography, see Brit. M. J., Lond., 1877, i, 122. *Also:* Med. Times & Gaz., Lond., 1877, i, 217.

Murphy (Joh.) *De hydrocephalo acuto. 3 p. l., 18 pp. 8°. *Edinburgi,* 1824.

Murphy (John A.) [1825-   ]. An introductory address, delivered to the students of the Miami Medical College, of Cincinnati, Oct. 30, 1854. 24 pp. 8°. *Cincinnati, T. Wrightson & Co.,* 1855.

Also, Co-Editor of: **Cincinnati** (The) Medical Observer, 1856-7.—**Cincinnati** (The) Lancet and Observer, 1858-73.—**Cleveland** (The) Medical Gazette, 1860-61.

For Biography, see Tr. Ohio M. Soc., Columbus, 1880, xxxv, 25.

Murphy (Joseph). A natural history of the human teeth, with a treatise on their diseases from infancy to old age, adapted for general information; to which are added, observations on the physiognomy of the teeth, and of the projecting chin. iv (1 l.), 160 pp. 8°. *London, J. Callow,* 1811.

Murphy (P. J.) Practical observations, showing that mercury is the sole cause of what are termed secondary symptoms. xiii, 14–107 pp. 8°. *London, J. Churchill,* 1839.

Also, Co-Editor of: **Chemist** (The), London, 1847.

Murphy (Patricius). *De rheumatismo. 1 p. l., 29 pp. 8°. *Edinburgi, P. Neill,* 1821, v. 3. [*Also, in:* P., v. 1071.]

Murphy (Patrick J.) Observations regarding the effects of trachelorrhaphy on fertility and parturition. 6 pp. 8°. [*n. p.*], 1883.
Repr. from: Am. J. Obst., N. Y., 1883, xvi.

Murphy (Shirley Foster). Annual reports of the medical officer of health, on the sanitary condition of St. Pancras, Middlesex, to the vestry. 23.–26., 1878–81 ; 29., 1884. 8°. *London*, 1879–85.

——. Vestry of St. Pancras to the sanitary committee. [Letter of the medical officer of health, on the importance of the local sanitary authority having power to inspect and regulate bakehouses. July 5, 1882.] 3 pp. fol. [*London*, 1882.]

——. Report on the recent outbreak of enteric fever in Saint Pancras. 24 pp. 8°. *London, Mutchener*, 1883.

——. Monthly reports of the medical officer of health, on the sanitary condition of Saint Pancras, Middlesex, to the sanitary committee. Nos. 1–4, Jan. to April, 1883. 8°. *London*, 1883.

——. Report to the Local Government Board, on an outbreak of enteric fever in St. Albans, Oct. 17, 1884. 8 pp. fol. *London, Her Majesty's Stationery Office*, 1884.
Official copy.

——. The same. 8 pp. fol. *London, Eyre & Spottiswoode*, 1884.

——. Infectious disease and its prevention. 2 p. l., 69 pp. 8°. *London, W. Clowes & Sons*, 1884.
International Health Exhibition. Handbooks [No. 20].

——. Report to the Local Government Board, on the sanitary condition of Gravesend. Aug. 22, 1885. 5 pp. fol. *London, Her Majesty's Stationery Office*, 1885.
Official copy.

——. The same. 5 pp. fol. *London, ptd. for Her Majesty's Stationery Office*, 1885.

——. Memorandum on diphtheria. Collective investigation committee. 4 pp. 8°. [*London, n. d.*]
See, also, **Our** homes, etc. 8°. *London*, 1883.

de Murr (Christophor. Theophil.) Adnotationes ad bibliothecas Hallerianas, botanicam, anatomicam, chirurgicam et medicinæ practicæ, cum variis ad scripta Michaelis Serveti pertinentibus. 1 p. l., 67 pp. 4°. *Erlangæ, I. I. Palm*, 1805.

Murrain.
See **Epizootic** *diseases*.

Murraté (Édouard). * Des troubles mentaux dans l'asystolie. 38 pp. 4°. *Paris*, 1880, No. 44.

Murray. Surgeon . . .'s paper, on the patent aperient solution of magnesia. 22 pp., 1 l. 8°. *Newry, A. Wilkinson*, 1817. [P., v. 1063.]

Murray (Adolphus) [1751–1803]. Fundamenta testaceologiæ. 1 p. l., 43 pp., 2 pl. 4°. *Upsaliæ, ex off. Edmanniana*, [1771]. [P., v. 623.]
Also, in: LINNÆUS. Amœnitates acad. [etc.] 8°. *Erlangæ*, 1785, viii, 1o7–150, 3 pl.

——. * Observationes anatomicæ, circa infundibulum cerebri, ossium capitis in fœtu structuram alienam, partemque nervi intercostalis cervicalem. 1 p. l., 31 pp., 1 pl. sm. 4°. *Upsaliæ, ex prelo Edmanniano*, [1772].
Also, in: SCRIPTORES neurol. minores selecti. 4°. *Lipsiæ*, 1792, ii, 242–250.

——. * Descriptio arteriarum corporis humani in tabulas redacta, cujus partem primam publice ventilandam exhibet Johannes Theophilus Nathhorst. 23 pp. sm. 4°. *Upsaliæ, J. Edman*, [1780].

——. The same. . . . cujus partem secundam publice ventilandam exhibet Ericus Odhelius. 30 pp., 1 l. sm. 4°. *Upsaliæ, J. Edman*, [1781].

——. The same. . . . cujus partem tertiam publice ventilandam exhibet Andreas Hesselius. 30 pp., 1 l. sm. 4°. *Upsaliæ, J. Edman*, [1782].

Murray (Adolphus)—continued.

——. The same. . . . cujus partem quartam et ultimam publice ventilandam exhibet Johannes Gustavus Hallman. 32 pp., 1 l. sm. 4°. *Upsaliæ, J. Edman*, [1783].

——. The same. [Parts i–iv.] vi, 7–120 pp. 4°. *Upsaliæ, J. F. Edman*, 1798.

——. The same. A description of the arteries of the human body. Reduced to tables. Transl. from the original by Arch. Scott. xx, 172 pp. 8°. *Edinburgh, C. G. & J. Robinson*, 1801. [*Also, in:* P., v. 685.]
Incomplete; wants 18 pp. of index.

——. The same. Transl. from the Latin, under the inspection of James Macartney. iv, 106 pp. 8°. *London, J. Debrett*, 1801.

——. The same. Transl. from the original, by Archibald Scott. xix, 172 pp. 8°. *Philadelphia, T. Dobson*, 1810.

——. The same. xix, 172 pp. 8°. *Philadelphia, J. Webster*, 1816.

——. Diss. academica de sensibilitate ossium morbosa. *Upsaliæ*, 1780.
In: SCRIPTORES neurol. minores selecti. 4°. *Lipsiæ*, 1795, iv, 252–263. *Also, in:* FRANK (J. P.) Delect. opusc. med. 8°. *Ticini*, 1793, xii, 267–302.

——. In gangrænam scroti observatio, animadversionibus nonnullis illustrata. *Upsaliæ*, 1783.
In: FRANK (J. P.) Delect. opusc. med. 8°. *Ticini*, 1791, x, 260–301.

——. Diss. anatomico-chirurgica de cirsocele. *Upsaliæ*, 1784.
In: FRANK (J. P.) Delect. opusc. med. 8°. *Ticini*, 1791, x, 302–360.

——. [Afhandling om anatomiens framsteg i nyare tider.] 101 pp. 8°. [*Stockholm, J. P. Linde*, 1795.]
See, also, **Lauth** (Thomas). Scriptorum latinorum de aneurysmatibus collectio, [etc.] 4°. *Argentorati*, 1785.

Murray (Alex.) Treatment of ulcers by electricity. 8 pp. 8°. [*New York*, 1873.]

——. Electricity, as used in parturition, postpartum hemorrhage, and resuscitation of new-born infants. 16 pp. 8°. *New York, E. O. Jenks*, [1875].
Repr. from: Psych. & Med.-Leg. J., N. Y., 1875, ii.

Murray (Andreas). * De hepatitide maxime Indiæ Orientalis. 1 p. l., 56 pp., 2 l. 8°. *Gottingæ, J. C. Dieterich*, [1779].
For Biography, see **Murray** (Jo. Andreas).

Murray (Carlos). Avisos interessantes á humanidade, ou collecçaõ de alguns artigos concernentes á restauração da vida dos affogados, e outros casos de morte apparente, ou animação suspensa; extrahidos dos escriptos publicados em Inglaterra por ordem da Sociedade humana, instituida na corte, e cidade de Londres em 1774. Trad. do original inglez por Francisco Manoel de Oliveira. Medallion title-plate, 144 pp. 16°. *Lisboa, F. L. Ameno*, 1788.

Murray (David). First commencement exercises of the Albany College of Pharmacy, department of pharmacy of Union University, with the address delivered to the graduating class. 8 pp. 8°. [*Albany*, 1882.]

Murray (George). Aërial locomotion; a descriptive treatise of a practical method of traversing the atmosphere. 36 pp., 8 pl. 12°. *Liverpool, C. Tinling & Co.*, [*n. d.*]

Murray (Henricus Nanton). * Quædam de dysenteria complectens. 2 p. l., 28 pp. 8° *Edinburgi*, 1825.

Murray (J.) An author's conduct to the public, stated in the behaviour of Dr. William Cullen. ii, 41 pp. 8°. *London, J. Murray*, 1784.

Murray (J. Clark). A handbook of psychology. x, 422 pp. 8°. *London, A. Gardner*, 1885.

Murray (J. Jardine). Case of extraction from the pharynx of a needle which had penetrated

Murray (J. Jardine)—continued.
the neck; with remarks. 12 pp. 8°. *Edinburgh, A. Jack*, 1859.
——. The danger of ill-constructed and neglected cisterns. 8 pp. 8°. *Brighton, G. Wakeling*, 1872.
Repr. from: Lancet, Lond., 1871, ii.

Murray (J. Monro). The physiological action of napellina and aconitia. 28 pp. 12°. [*n. p.*, 1876, *vel subseq.*]
Repr. from: Phila. M. Times, 1875-6, vi.

Murray (Jacobus). *De phthisi pulmonali. 1 p. l., 34 pp. 8°. *Edinburgi, Balfour et Smellie*, 1777.

Murray (Jacobus Thomson). *De cynanche maligna. 2 p. l., 20 pp. 8°. *Edinburgi, G. Creech*, 1793.

Murray (James). A dissertation on the influence of heat and humidity; with practical observations on the inhalation of iodine, and various vapours, in consumption, catarrh, croup, asthma, and other diseases. xiii, 305, xviii pp., 1 tab. 8°. *London, Longman & Co.*, 1829.
——. Observations on the medical and surgical agency of the air pump. Read before the British Association in 1835. 63 pp. 8°. *Dublin, Hodges & Smith*, 1836.
——. Observations on fluid magnesia, with papers read before the British and other associations. 16 pp. 8°. *London, Simpkin, Marshall & Co.*, 1840.
——. Electricity as a cause of cholera or other epidemics, and the relation of galvanism to the action of remedies. 1 p. l., 160 pp. 8°. *Dublin, J. McGlashan*, 1849.

Murray (Joannes Andreas) [1740-97]. *Fata variolarum insitionis in Suecia. 3 p. l., 36 pp. 4°. *Gottingæ, typ. Pockwitzii et Barmeieri*, [1763]. [*Also, in:* P., v. 620; 1472.]
——. Commentatio de arbuto uva ursi exhibens descriptionem ejus botanicam, analysin chemicam, ejusque in medicina et œconomia varium usum. 65 pp. sm. 4°. *Gottingæ, apud Pockwitzium et Barmeierum*, 1765. [*Also, in:* P., v. 632.]
——. De vermibus in lepra obviis, juncta leprosi historia et de lumbricorum setis observationes reg. societati scientiarum Gotting. prælectæ. xvi, 76 pp., 2 l., 2 pl. 8°. *Gottingæ, C. Dieterich*, 1769.
——. Enumeratio librorum præcipuorum medici argumenti. xxviii, 100 pp. 8°. *Lipsiæ, Weygand*, 1773.
——. Medicinisch-practische Bibliothek. 3 v. sm. 8°. *Göttingen, J. C. Dieterich*, 1774-8.
——. Apparatus medicaminum tam simplicium quam præparatorum et compositorum in praxeos adjumentum consideratus. 6 v. 8°. *Gottingæ, J. C. Dieterich*, 1776-92.
v. 4. Post mortem auctoris edidit Ludov. Christoph. Althof. Want pt. 2 of v. 1 and 2.
——. The same. 6 v. 8°. *Gottingæ*, 1784-94.
v. 1 and 2, "edito altera curante Ludovico Christoph. Althof". v. 6, "post mortem auctoris edidit Ludov. Christoph. Althof".
——. The same. 6 v. in 3. 8°. *Venetiis, S. Valle*, 1795.
——. [Pr.] de tempore corticis peruviani in tussi convulsiva exhibendi. [Cum vita candidati Josephi Gerson.] 11 l. 4°. *Gottingæ, J. C. Dieterich*, [1776].
——. De limitanda laude librorum medicorum practicorum usu populari destinatorum. 32 pp. sm. 4°. *Gottingæ, J. C. Dieterich*, [1779].
——. [Pr.] observationum et animadversionum super variolarum insitione satura, sectio prima. [Cum vitis candidatorum C. H. Haeseler, A. C. Waitz, P. C. Meyer, et D. C. Rauh.] 20 pp. 4°. *Gottingæ, J. C. Dieterich*, [1779].

35

Murray (Joannes Andreas)—continued.
——. The same. Sectio secunda. [Cum vitis candidatorum M. a Paecken, C. G. Berg, A. Roesslein, et T. G. Schroeder.] 20 pp. 4°. *Gottingæ, J. C. Dieterich*, 1779.
Bound with preceding.
——. The same. Sectio tertia et novissima. [Cum vitis candidatorum G. P. Lehr, T. F. Trendelenburg, C. H. Westmüller, et J. F. A. Becker.] 18 pp. 4°. *Gottingæ, J. C. Dieterich*, 1779.
Bound with preceding.
——. [Pr.] spinæ bifidæ ex mala ossium conformatione initia persequutus. [Cum vitis candidatorum H. I. Ruer, A. Murray, J. F. Behrens, et C. A. Meyer.] 26 pp. sm. 4°. *Gottingæ, J. C. Dieterich*, 1779.
——. [Pr.] de febribus epidemicis Romæ falso in pestium censum relatis. [Cum vita candidati J. C. Gatterer.] viii pp. fol. *Gottingæ, J. C. Dieterich*, [1782.]
——. [Pr.] de medendi tineæ capitis ratione paralipomena. [Cum vitis candidatorum L. Krüger, M. Matthias, J. Victor, et H. Siegel.] 26 pp. 4°. *Gottingæ, J. C. Dieterich*, 1782.
——. [Pr.] vindiciæ nominum trivialium stirpibus a Linneo impertitorum. [Cum vita candidati J. G. Carelson.] 23 pp. 4°. *Gottingæ, J. C. Dieterich*, 1782.
——. [Pr.] de materia arthritica ad verenda aberrante disquisitio. Sectio prior. [Cum vitis candidatorum S. C. Philites, L. G. Haselberg, C. G. T. Kortum, et J. H. A. Niemeyer.] 22 pp. sm. 4°. *Gottingæ, J. C. Dieterich*, 1785.
——. The same. Sectio posterior. [Cum vitis candidatorum F. G. Büttner, J. F. E. Heine, R. H. Stender, et D. A. F. J. Kosegarten.] 19 pp. sm. 4°. *Gottingæ, J. C. Dieterich*, 1785.
——. The same. Sectio prior et posterior.
In: FRANK (J. P.) Delect. opusc. med. 8°. *Ticini*, 1786, ii, 1-61.
——. Opuscula in quibus commentationes varias tam medicas quam ad rem naturalem spectantes retractavit, emendavit, auxit. 2 v. xxii, 392 pp.; vi, 500 pp., 5 pl. 8°. *Gottingæ, J. C. Dieterich*, 1785-6.
——. De laude magnetismi sic dicti animalis ambigua. 24 pp. 4°. *Gottingæ, J. C. Dieterich*, [1789].
——. Vorrath von einfachen, zubereiteten und gemischten Heilmitteln zum Gebrauche practischer Aerzte bearbeitet. 2. Aufl. herausgegeben und übersetzt von Ludwig Christoph Althof. 1280 pp., 6 l. 8°. *Göttingen, J. C. Dieterich*, 1793.
See, also, **Rosén von Rosenstein** (Nils). Anweisung zur Kenntniss der Kinderkrankheiten. 12°. *Göttingen u. Gotha*, 1768. ——. The same. 12°. *Wien*, 1787. ——. The same. 6. Aufl. 8°. *Göttingen*, 1798.

Murray (Joannes Rogerus). *De abortu. 1 p. l., 38 pp. 8°. *Edinburgi, Balfour et Smellie*, 1787.

Murray (John)[l] [–1820]. Elements of materia medica and pharmacy. 2 v. xv, 394 pp.; viii, 351 pp. 8°. *Edinburgh, W. Creech* [*and others*], 1804.
——. The same. 2 v. in 1. xii, 13-447 pp. 8°. *Philadelphia, B. & T. Kite*, 1808.
——. The same. System of materia medica and pharmacy. With notes by N. Chapman. 2 v. vi, 399 pp.; iv, 384 pp. 8°. *Philadelphia, T. Dobson*, 1815.
——. The same. 2 v. vi, 399 pp.; iv, 384 pp. 8°. *New York, S. Wood & Sons*, 1821.
——. The same. Including translations of the Edinburgh, London, and Dublin pharmacopœias. With notes and additions by John B. Beck, M. D. From the 4. and last Edinb. ed. viii, 560 pp. 8°. *New York, E. Duyckinck* [*and others*], 1824.

Murray (John)[1]—continued.

——. The same. 6. ed. With notes and additions by John B. Beck, M. D. 584 pp. 8°. *New York, W, E. Dean,* 1834.

——. A supplement to the first edition of a system of chemistry, containing a view of the recent discoveries in the science. 150 pp. 8°. *Edinburgh, Brown & Crombie & W. Creech,* 1809. [P., v. 682; 1176.]

——. Supplement to the 3. ed. of: Elements of chemistry. 39 pp. 8°. [*n. p., n. d.*] [P., v. 664.]

——. Elements of chemistry. 6. ed. 2 v. xvi, 716 pp.; vii, 752 pp., 6 pl. 8°. *Edinburgh, A. Black,* 1828.

——. Syllabus of the course of lectures on mineralogy and geology ... with a classification of minerals in the order followed in the course, and an explanation of the chief mineralogical terms. 30 pp. 8°. *Edinburgh, J. Walker,* [*n. d.*]

Murray (John)[2]. *A probationary essay on the formation and solution of urinary calculi. 35 pp. 8°. *Edinburgh, P. Neill,* 1826.

——. A treatise on pulmonary consumption; its prevention and remedy. x, 156 pp. 8°. *London, Whittaker, Treacher & Arnot,* 1830.

——. The same. 2. ed. xxiv, 186 pp. 8°. *London, Longman* [*and others*], 1831.

——. Remarks on the disease called hydrophobia; prophylactic and curative. ix (1 l.), 86 pp. 8°. *London, Longmans* [*and others*], 1830.

——. On the topography of Meerutt, and the principal diseases which prevailed in the 1st brigade of horse artillery at that place. Printed by order of government. 59 pp., 1 plan. 8°. *Calcutta, G. H. Huttmann,* 1839.

——. The plague and quarantine. Remarks on some epidemic and endemic diseases (including the plague of the Levant), and the means of disinfection; with a description of the preservative phial. Also a postscript on Dr. Bowring's pamphlet. viii, 54 pp., 1 pl. 8°. *London, Relfe & Fletcher,* 1839. [P., v. 640.]

——. Practical observations and researches on ventilation and disinfection, inclusive of other essential provisions connected with sanitary regulations, and the health of towns. 34 pp. 8°. *London, Whittaker & Co.,* 1850. [P., v. 149.]

——. Topography and diseases of Futtehpore Seekree. Reprinted from the selections from public correspondence. 8 pp., 1 map. 8°. [*Agra,* 1852.] [P., v. 952.]

——. Report on the attack of cholera in the central prison at Agra in 1856. 23 pp., 1 tab. 8°. *Agra, Secundra Orphan press,* 1856. [*Also, in:* P., v. 859.]

——. Report on the attack of epidemic cholera in Agra and Central India during the year 1861. [With appendix.] 11 pp., 1 l. 8°. [*Agra, R. Miller,* 1861.] [P., v. 1025.]

——. Report on the attack of epidemic cholera in the Agra and Gwalior circle during the year 1862. [With appendix.] 5, iv pp., 6 tab. 8°. [*Agra?* 1863.]

——. The second siege of Paris. The ambulances and hospitals of Paris under the Commune. 1 p. l., 24 pp. 8°. *London, T. Richards,* 1871.

——. Observations on the pathology and treatment of cholera, the result of forty years' experience. vi, 58 pp. 12°. *London, Smith, Elder & Co.,* 1874.

——. The same. 2. ed. 1 p. l., 58 pp. 12°. *London, Smith, Elder & Co.,* 1884.

Murray (John)[3] [1835–75].
Obituary. Glasgow M. J., 1875, n. s., vii, 129–134.

Murray (*John*)[4] [1843–73].
Obituary. Brit. M. J., Lond., 1873, ii, 478.—**Obituary.** Lancet, Lond., 1873, ii, 577.—**Obituary.** Med. Times & Gaz., Lond., 1873, ii, 452.

Murray (John C.) Snuff taking; its utility in preventing bronchitis, consumption, etc. (With prescriptions.) 64 pp. 12°. *London, J. Churchill & Sons,* 1870.

——. The same. 2. thousand. viii, 66 pp. 8°. *London, J. Churchill & Sons,* 1870.

Murray (*John L.*) [1784–1859].
Biographical notice of the late John L. Murray. Month. M. News, Louisville, 1860, ii, 44–46.

Murray (John W. B.) *On neuralgia. 71 pp. 8°. *New York, J. Seymour,* 1816. [*Also, in:* P., v. 746.]

Murray (Joseph). *De l'apoplexie pulmonaire. 38 pp. 4°. *Paris,* 1865, No. 25.

Murray (Patricius) *De asthmate. 1 p. l., 32 pp. 8°. *Edinburgi, Balfour, Auld et Smellie,* 1769.

Murray (Petrus). *De aëribus. 51 pp. 8°. *Edinburgi, A. Neill et socii,* 1802. [P., v. 21; 634.]

Murray (Robertus)[1]. *De lue venerea. 1 p. l., 24 pp. 8°. *Edinburgi, Neill et socii,* 1813. [*Also, in:* P., v. 865.]

Murray (Robertus)[2]. *De circulatione sanguinis in foetu. 1 p. l., 23 pp. 8°. *Edinburgi, Schaw et filium,* 1815. [P., v. 735.]

Murray (T.) The Murray specific for gout and rheumatism; with prefatory observations on gout, and notices of patients and testimonials. 16 pp. 12°. *London, T. Murray,* [*n. d.*]

Murray (Thomas Archibald) [–1802]. * De phænomenis et natura morbi ex submersione oriundi. 1 p. l., 44 pp. 8°. *Edinburgi, A. Neill cum sociis,* 1796. [*Also, in:* P., v. 4.]

——. Remarks on the situation of the poor in the metropolis, as contributing to the progress of contagious diseases; with a plan for the institution of houses of recovery for persons infected by fever. vii, 47 pp. 8°. *London, J. Hatchard,* 1801.

Murray (William). The rapid cure of aneurism by pressure; illustrated by the case of Mark Wilson, who was cured of aneurism of the abdominal aorta in the year 1864. 43 pp. 8°. *London, J. & A. Churchill,* 1871.

Murray (William H. H.) The perfect horse. How to know him. How to breed him. How to drive him. How to shoe him. With an introduction by Henry Ward Beecher, and a treatise on agriculture and the horse by George B. Loring. Containing illustrations of the best trotting stock-horses in the United States, done from life, with their pedigrees, records, and full descriptions. xi, 480 pp., 14 pl. roy. 8°. *Boston, I. R. Osgood & Co.,* 1873.

Murray Royal Asylum, Perth. (Copy.) Warrant for charter of incorporation in favour of James Murray's Royal Asylum for Lunatics. (Dated March 5, 1827.) 14 pp. 8°. [*Perth,* 1827?]

Founded by James Murray, who, in the years 1813–14, left a portion of his fortune to build, in the city of Perth, an asylum for the reception of lunatic persons. Plans were approved in 1822 and completed in 1826. Chartered March 5, and opened July 1, 1827.

——. Annual reports of the physician superintendent to the directors. 1.–41., 1827–8 to 1867–8; 53., 1880–81; 54., 1881–2. 8°. *Perth,* 1828–82.

1.–41. bound in 2 v. 39.–41. is a triennial report.

——. James Murray's Royal Asylum for Lunatics, near Perth. [Circular of the directors, announcing the purchase of the Mansion House of Pitcullen, for the reception of private patients of the first class.] 2 l. 4°. [*Edinburgh, W. E. Lizars,* 1850]. [P., v. 1291.]

Murray Royal Asylum, Perth—continued.

———. Regulations and by-laws of James Murray's Royal Asylum for Lunatics, at Perth. Published by order of the directors. 24 pp. 8°. *Perth, J. Dewar, jr.*, 1858. [P., v. 223.]

———. General regulations. [Including the petition, statement, medical certificates, sheriff's order, and obligation required for admission.] 4 pp., 2 l. fol. [*Perth, n. d.*]

———. Regulations for bath rooms. 1 sheet. fol. [*Perth, n. d.*]

———. [Blank forms in use at the asylum.] v. s. [*Perth, n. d.*]

CONTENTS.

Attendants' leave list.
Form for application for situation.
Lists of patients, weekly.
Notice that patient needs clothing.
Obligation to be signed by attendants and servants.
Requisition for removal of a non-recovered patient.

Murray's fluid magnesia To the president and members of the London Medical Society. 16 pp. 8°. [*Wolverhampton, J. Bridgen*], 1839. [P., v. 1202.]

Murree.

Ince (J.) The Murree Sanitarium. Indian M. Gaz., Calcutta, 1871, vi, 31; 44.—**Murree**; its topography and medical history. Indian Ann. M. Sc., Calcutta, 1854-5, ii, 111-142, 1 tab.

Murrell (William) [1851-]. What to do in cases of poisoning. 2. ed. 1 p. l., 96 pp. 24°. *Detroit, Mich., G. S. Davis*, 1882.

———. The same. 4. ed. 1 p. l., 212 pp. 18°. *London, H. K. Lewis*, 1884.

———. The same. 5. ed. vi, 220 pp. 18°. *London, H. K. Lewis*, 1887.

———. Nitro-glycerine as a remedy for angina pectoris. 3 p. l., 78 pp. 12°. *Detroit, G. S. Davis*, 1882.

———. Massage as a therapeutic agent. 3 pp. 8°. *London*, 1886.

Repr. from: Brit. M. J., Lond., 1886, i.

———. Massage as a mode of treatment. vi (1 l.), 78 pp. 12°. *London, H. K. Lewis*, 1886.

———. The same. 3. ed. vi (1 l.), 143 pp. 12°. *London, H. K. Lewis*, 1887.

———. The same. vi (1 l.), 78 pp. 8°. *Philadelphia, P. Blakiston, Son & Co.*, 1886.

———. The same. 2. ed. vi (1 l.), 100 pp. 8°. *Philadelphia, P. Blakiston, Son & Co.*, 1887.

Murri (Augusto) [1841-]. Del potere regolatore della temperatura animale. Studio critico-sperimentale. 79 pp. 8°. *Firenze, tipog. Cenniniana*, 1873.

Repr. from: Sperimentale, Firenze, 1873, xxxi.

———. Sulla teoria della febbre indagini. 132 pp. 8°. *Fermo, Bacher*, 1874.

———. La diagnosi delle lesioni sifilitiche del cervello. 74 pp. 8°. *Bologna, Gamberini & Parmeggiani*, 1876.

———. Della emoglobinuria da freddo. 242 pp. 8°. *Bologna, Fava & Garagnani*, 1880.

See, also, **Traube** (L.) Lezioni cliniche sui sintomi delle malattie degli apparati, etc. 8°. *Napoli*, 1868.

[**de**] **Murrieta** (Juan Luciano). Tratado de las enfermedades de la piel, seguido del formulario del célebre dermatólogo Biett, y de la esplicacion de las láminas de Thibert, del gabinete dermatológico de la Facultad de medicina de la Universidad de Madrid. xlvii, 354 pp., 1 l. 8°. *Madrid, Compañía de imp. y libreros del Reino*, 1848.

Murry (Bartholomæus). An fœtui sanguis maternus alimento? Præses Josephus de Jussieu. 4 pp. 4°. *Paris, Quillau*, 1735. [P., v. 701.]

Murry (John). Descriptive account of a new shower bath, constructed on a principle not hitherto applied to that machine; also, an apparatus for restoring suspended animation. 2.

Murry (John)—continued.

ed. 41 pp., 1 pl. 8°. *London, Whittaker & Co.*, 1831.

Mursick (Geo. A.) A case of complete intestinal occlusion by pressure of an ovarian tumor; ovariotomy; death. 4 pp. 8°. [*New York*, 1882]

Repr. from: Am. J. Obst., N. Y., 1882, xv. no. 2.

Mursinna (Christian Ludewig) [1744-1823]. Medicinisch-chirurgische Beobachtungen, nebst einigen Anmerkungen darüber. 2 v. xvii, 221 pp., 1 l.; vi (1 l.), 184 pp. 16°. *Berlin, C. F. Himburg*, 1782-3.

———. Abhandlung von den Krankheiten der Schwangern, Gebärenden und Wöchnerinnen. 2 v. xxii (1 l.), 317 pp., 1 l.; 1 p. l., 344 pp. 12°. *Berlin, C. F. Himburg*, 1784-6.

———. The same. 2. Aufl. 2 v. in 1. xiii, 278 pp.; 1 p. l., 319 pp. 8°. *Berlin, C. F. Himburg*, 1792.

———. Beobachtungen über die Ruhr und die Faulfieber. xvi, 256 pp. 8°. *Berlin, C. F. Himburg*, 1787.

———. Berichtigung des Sendschreibens des Herrn Hofrath Hagen in Berlin an den Herrn Hofrath Stark in Jena über zwey schwere Geburtsfälle. 56 pp. 8°. *Berlin, C. F. Himburg*, 1791.

———. Medicinisch-chirurgische Beobachtungen, nebst einigen Anmerkungen darüber. 2. Aufl. vi, 406 pp. 8°. *Berlin, C. F. Himburg*, 1796.

———. Neue medicinisch-chirurgische Beobachtungen. xvi, 549 pp. 8°. *Berlin, C. F. Himburg*, 1796.

———. Rede über die Vereinigung der Medizin mit der Chirurgie, gehalten am fünfzehnten Stiftungstage der königlichen medizinisch-chirurgischen Pepiniere. Berlin, den zweiten August 1809. 15 pp. 8°. *Berlin, C. S. Spener*, [1809].

———. Rede über die alte und neue Chirurgie, gehalten am siebenzehnten Stiftungstage der medicinisch-chirurgischen Pepiniere, am 2ten August 1811. 30 pp. 8°. *Berlin, C. S. Spener*, 1812.

See, also, **Lämmerhirt** (Ludewig). Taschenbuch über Beinbrüche. 12°. *Berlin*, 1805.—**Rheineck** (Joh.) Medizinische und chirurgische Beobachtungen [etc.] 8°. *Berlin*, 1815.

For Biography, see 'Ασκληπίειον, Berl., 1811, i, 385-394. *Also:* Med.-chir. Ztg., Salzb., 1811, iii, 189-192.

For Portrait, see **Collection**—van Kaathoven.

Murtough (Peter). Condensed history of the great yellow fever epidemic of 1878. Personal sketches and incidents, full particulars of the Father Mathew Camp, list of cities and towns visited by the scourge, and names of the victims of the fever in Memphis. 103 pp. 8°. *Memphis, S. C. Toof & Co.*, 1879.

Murville (François-Joseph) [1801-61]. *Considérations sur le sommeil. viii, 9-35 pp. 4°. *Paris*, 1824, No. 114, v. 186.

For Biography, see Rec. de mém. de méd. . . . mil., Par., 1861, 3. s., v, 253-256 (M. Ladureau).

Mury (Narcisse-Désiré). *Du cancer de l'utérus, et de sa thérapeutique. 27 pp. 4°. *Paris*, 1826, No. 41, v. 198.

Mus (Leonardus). *Spec. sistens rationalem methodum curandi et præcavendi quosdam mammarum muliebrium læsam lactationem concernentes morbos. 26 pp. 4°. *Duisburgi ad Rhenum, F. A. Benthon*, [1770].

Musa (Antonius). Libellus utilissimus de botanica.

In: MEDICI antiqui omnes qui latinis [etc.] fol. *Venetiis*, 1547, ff. 223.

See, also, **Ackermann** (Joannes Christianus Gottlieb.) De Antonio Musa, Octaviani Augusti medico, [etc.] 4°. *Altorfii*, 1786.—**Crell** (Joh. Fridericus). Antonium Musam Augusti medicum observationibus varii generis illustratum sistit. 4°. *Lipsiæ*, [1725].—**Salernum** (School of). De conservanda bona valetudine. 8°. *Francofurti*, 1545.

Musa ben Maimon.   *See* **Moses** *Maimonides.*

Musa *paradisiaca.*

Kestner. Der Platanenstaub und sein Einfluss auf die Gesundheit. Arch. f. öff. Gsndhtspflg., Strassb., 1879, iv, 162–167.

Musæum Franc. Calceolari jun. veronensis a Benedicto Ceruto medico incæptum, et ab Andrea Chiocco . . . luculenter descriptum et perfectum, in quo multa ad naturalem moralemque philosophiam spectantia, non pauca ad rem medicam pertinentia erudite proponuntur et explicantur. 23 p. l., 746 pp., 1 pl. fol. *Veronæ, apud A. Tamum,* 1622.

Musæus (Carolus). * De unguibus monstrosis, et cornuum productione in puella cornigera Lalandiæ. 26 pp., 1 pl. sm. 4°. *Hafniæ, typ. J. S. Martini,* [1716].

Musaeus (Joannes Theodorus). * De paracentesi thoracis et abdominis. 15 pp. sm. 4°. *Jenæ, typ. Gollnerianis,* [1697].

For Biography, see **Slevogt** (Jo. Had.)

Musatti (Cesare). Cremazione e medicina forense. Lettura tenuta all' Ateneo veneto il 20 luglio 1876. 44 pp., 1 l. 8°. *Padova, P. Prosperini,* 1876.

————. Il solfito di soda nell' allattamento artificiale e nei catarri intestinali dei bambini. 4 pp. 8°. *Padova,* 1880.

Repr. from: Gazz. med. ital., prov. venete, Padova, 1880, xxiii.

————. Storia di un' ipertrofia prostatica vinta colla cauterizzazione termo-galvanica. 8 pp. 8°. *Milano,* 1885.

Repr. from: Gazz. d. osp., Milano, 1885, vi.

Muscæ *volitantes.*

See, also, **Vitreous** *humor (Diseases, etc., of).*

ANDREAS (C. G.) * De maculis oculorum volaticis. 4°. *Lugd. Bat.,* 1725.

BRENNER (J.), *Ritter von Felsach.* * De myodesopsia respectu diagnostico et ætiologico. 8°. *Vindobonæ,* 1833.

DANION (J.-M.) * Étude sur la myodésopsie. 4°. *Paris,* 1866.

FEUILLERADE (L.-C.) * De la myiodopsie, ou des mouches volantes et fixes. 4°. *Paris,* 1864.

GÖDEKENN (J. H.) * De maculis punctulis scintillis aliisque corpusculis visui obversantibus. 4°. *Francof. ad Viadr.,* 1747.

NEUBER (A. W.) Ueber schwebende Flecke im Auge, oder den sogenannten Mückentanz, nach Beobachtungen an sich selber. 8°. *Hamburg,* 1830.

Also [Abstr.], *in:* Pfaff's prakt. u. krit. Mitth. a. d. Geb. d. Med., Altona, 1839–40, vii, Hft. 11–12, 1–45.

ROTHKEPPEL (C. W.) * Phantasmata ante oculos volitantia, oculorum adfectus singularis. 4°. *Erlangæ,* 1751.

SCHOLZ (C. F.) * De muscis volitantibus. 8°. *Berolini,* [1853].

VOGLER (J. H. C.) * De maculis ante oculos volitantibus. sm. 4°. *Helmstadii,* [1795].

WELLER (E. C. A.) * Nonnulla de muscis volitantibus. 8°. *Lipsiæ,* 1857.

ZILLIOX (I.) * Essai sur la pseudoblepsie, ou imaginations perpétuelles de Maître Jean. 4°. *Strasbourg,* 1837.

Andreæ (A.) Ueber das Flockensehen. J. d. Chir. u. Augenh., Berl., 1825, viii, 16; 214. — **Andrieux.** Quelques réflexions pratiques sur la myodepsie et sur son traitement. Bull. gén. de thérap., etc., Par., 1840, xix, 274–278. — **Appia.** De l'œil vu par lui-même. Arch. d'opth., Par., 1853, i, 49–65. — **Brewster** (D.) On the optical phenomena, nature, and locality of muscæ volitantes; with observations on the structure of the vitreous humour, and on the vision of objects placed within the eye. Tr. Roy. Soc. Edinb., 1842–3, xv, 377–385. — **Demours.** Extrait d'un mémoire sur des filamens, taches mobiles, globules, et toiles d'araignées très-déliées qui paroissent voltiger devant les yeux. J. de méd., chir., pharm., etc., Par., 1788, lxxiv, 274–289. — **Fano.** Essai sur la myodésopsie, ou sur les mouches volantes et fixes. Union méd.,

Muscæ *volitantes.*

Par., 1864, 2. s., xxiii, 84; 131; 180: 215.—**Fenner** (C. S.) Muscæ volitantes. Am. Pract., Louisville, 1876, xiii, 19–22.—**Galezowski** (X.) Études sur les flocons du corps vitré, synchysis (floconeux). Ann. d'ocul., Brux., 1864, li, 61–76. — **Giraud-Teulon.** Myiodopsie. Dict. encycl. d. sc. méd., Par., 1876, 2. s., xi, 219–223.—**Griffith** (*Mrs.*) Air bubbles in the fluids of the eye (muscæ volitantes). N. York Lancet, 1842, ii, 209; 225.—**Hay** (G.) Apparent movement of muscæ. Tr. Am. Ophth. Soc., N. Y., 1869, 6. sess., 71.—**Iago** (J.) Opthalmoscopic muscæ volitantes in a very myopic eye. Med. Times & Gaz., Lond., 1861, i, 465–467. — **Jouon.** Note sur la myodésopsie. J. de la sect. de méd. Soc. acad. Loire-Inf., Nantes, 1862, xxxviii, 47–61.—**Panas.** Les mouches volantes. Progrès méd., Par., 1887, 2. s., v, 435–437. — **Parfait-Landrau.** Cas de pathologie oculaire, relatif à des corpuscules voltigeant dans la chambre postérieure de l'œil, et donnant lieu à des images fantastiques. Rev. méd. franç. et étrang., Par., 1828, iv, 203–207.—**Riley**(T. C.) The significance of specks or opacities before the eyes. Med. & Surg. Reporter, Phila., 1886, liv, 450–452.—**Ruete** (T.) Ueber die Gesichtserscheinungen, welche von Körperchen abhängen, die sich in, oder auf dem Auge selbst befinden. Hannov. Ann. f. d. ges. Heilk., 1844, n. F., iv, 443–457. *Also* [Abstr.]: Amtl. Ber. ü. d. Versamml. deutsch. Naturf. u. Aerzte 1843, Gratz, 1844, xxi, 296–298. — **Sichel.** De la myiodopsie et des scotomes. Monit. d. hôp., Par., 1859, vii, 643–647. — **Sotteau.** Recherches sur les apparences visuelles sans objet extérieur, connues sous le nom vulgaire de mouches volantes. [Rap. de Stacquez.] Ann. Soc. de méd. de Gand, 1842, xi, 49; 98. — **Stark** (J.) On the nature, locality, and optical phenomena of muscæ volitantes. Edinb. M. & S. J., 1843, lx, 399–410. *Also,* Reprint. — **Steifensand.** Ueber die im Auge selbst befindlichen Gesichtsobjecte, besonders das Mückensehen. Monatschr. f. Med., Augenh. u. Chir., Leipz., 1838, i, 203–211.— **Tavignot.** Pseudo mouches volantes simulant une amaurose. Union méd., Par., 1851, v, 14. — **Wallace** (W. C.) Cases of muscæ volitantes; with remarks on their proximate cause. Lond. M. Gaz., 1838–9, xxiii, 109–114. — **Ware** (J.) On the muscæ volitantes of nervous persons. [4 cases.] Med.-Chir. Tr., Lond., 1814, v, 255–277.

Muscale *button.*

Briggs (J. R.) "Muscale buttons;" physiological effects; personal experience. Med. Reg., Phila., 1887, i, 276.

Muscardine.

See **Silk-worms** (*Diseases of*).

Muscarine.

See, also, **Amanita** *muscaria;* **Atropine** (*Physiological, etc., effects of*); **Fungi** (*Toxicology of*).

JORDAN (S. N.) * Beiträge zur Kenntniss der pharmakologischen Gruppe des Muscarins. 8°. *Leipzig,* 1877.

Also, in: Arch. f. exper. Path. u. Pharmakol., Leipz., 1877, viii, 15–30.

Boehm (R.) Ueber das Vorkommen und die Wirkungen des Cholins und die Wirkungen der künstlichen Muscarine. Arch. f. exper. Path. u. Pharmakol., Leipz., 1885, xix, 87–100.—**Chouppe** (H.) La muscarine. Gaz. hebd. de méd., Par., 1876, 2. s., xiii, 259; 291.—**Gaskell** (W. H.) On the action of atropia and muscarin upon the heart of the frog. Tr. Internat. M. Cong., 7. sess., Lond., 1881, i, 508–511.—**Harnack** (E.) Untersuchungen über Fliegenpilz-Alkaloïde. Arch. f. exper. Path. u. Pharmakol., Leipz., 1875, iv, 168–190.—**Högyes** (F.) Die Wirkung des Muscarins auf die Circulationsorgane. Arch. f. Physiol., Leipz., 1882, 37–45. — **Kobert** (R.) Ueber die Deutung der Muscarinwirkung am Herzen. Arch. f. exper. Path. u. Pharmakol., Leipz., 1885-6, xx, 92–115, 1 pl.— **Krenchel** (V.) Over de werking van muscarine op de accommodatie en de pupil. Onderzoek. ged. in h. physiol. Lab. d. Utrecht. Hoogesch., 1874-5, 3. R., iii, 22–38. *Also:* Versl. . . . Nederl. Gasth. v. Ooglijders, Utrecht, 1874, xv, 36–52. *Also, transl.:* Hosp.-Tid., Kjøbenh., 1874, 2. R., i, 145–155. *Also, transl.:* Arch. f. Ophth., Berl., 1874, xx, 1. Abth., 135–150.—**Merunowicz** (J.) Die Strömung der Bauchlymphe nach der Vergiftung mit Muscarin, Nicotin und Veratrin. Arb. a. d. physiol. Anst. zu Leipz. (1876), 1877, xi, 117–142. — **Morshead** (E. A.) The action of muscarin on the human body. Lancet, Lond., 1877, ii, 198–200.—**Nawrocki** (F.) Przyczynek do działania muskarynu. [Effects of muscarin.] Przegl. lek., Krakow, 1880, xix, 221–223. *Also, transl.:* Vrach. Vaidom., St. Petersb., 1880, v, 1953–1956.—**Prevost** (J.-L.) Note relative à l'antagonisme mutuel de l'atropine et de la muscarine. Compt. rend. Acad.d. sc., Par., 1877, lxxxv, 630.—**Prevost** (J.-L.) & **Monnier** (D.) Note relative à l'action physiologique de la muscarine, principe toxique de l'Agaricus muscarius. Compt. rend. Soc. de biol. 1874, Par., 1875, 6. s, i, 183–188 — **Schliephake** (H.) Ueber die Einwirkung des Muscarins auf das menschliche Auge. Mitth. a. d. ophth. Klin. in Tübing., 1880, 51–57.—**Schmiedeberg** (O.) Bemerkungen über die Muscarinwirkung. Arch. f. exper. Path.

Muscarine.

u. Pharmakol., Leipz., 1881, xiv, 376–378.—**Schmiede-berg** (O.) & **Harnack** (E.) Ueber die Constitution und Darstellung des Muscarins. Centralbl. f. d. med. Wissensch., Berl., 1875, xiii, 598. ————. Ueber die Synthese des Muscarins und über muscarinartig wirkende Ammoniumbasen. Arch. f. exper. Path. u. Pharmakol., Leipz., 1876, vi, 101–112.—**Sondén** (C. M.) Om muscarin, den giftiga alkaloiden i flugswampen. Upsala Läkaref. Förh., 1869–70, v, 245–253.—**Trümpy** (D.) & **Luch-singer** (B.) Die Wirkung von Muscarin und Atropin auf die Schweissdrüsen der Katze. Arch. f. d. ges. Physiol., Bonn, 1878, xviii, 501–503.—**Weinzweig** (E.) Ueber das Verhalten des mit Muscarin vergifteten Herzens gegen seine Nerven. Arch. f. Physiol., Leipz., 1882, 527–539, 2 pl.

Muscat.

See, also, **Bassadore.**

Peters (C. T.) Medico-topographical report of Muscat. Tr. M. & Phys. Soc. Bombay, 1876, n. s., xii, 152–174.

Muscat (Ernestus Ludovicus) [1797–1832]. *De metamorphosi gelatinosa ventriculi et ceterarum tubi intestinalis partium infantum. 45 pp. 8°. *Berolini, formis Brüschckianis*, [1825].

Muschaweckh (Joanne Baptista). *De morbis ægris et medicamentis aphorismi medici. 14 pp. 8°. *Monachii, F. Wild*, 1839.

Muscle (Chemistry and histology of).

See, also, **Electro-physiology**; **Fibre** (*Animal*); **Meats**; **Muscles**; **Muscular** *sense*; **Musculine**; **Urea.**

Arnold (J.) Das Gewebe der organischen Muskeln, mit einer Tafel. 8°. *Leipzig*, 1869.

Brecht (H.) *De musculi agentis chemismo nonnulla. 8°. *Berolini*, [1864].

da Costa Simões (A. A.) Histologia e physiologia geral dos musculos. Secção I. Histologia dos musculos. Tomo i. 8°. *Coimbra*, 1878.

Cramer (F.) *Ueber das Verhalten der quergestreiften Muskelfaser bei traumatischer Entzündung. 8°. *Frankfurt*, 1870.

Dobie (W. M.) Observations on the minute structure and mode of contraction of voluntary muscular fibre. 8°. [*London*, 1849.]
Repr. from: Ann. & Mag. Nat. Hist., Lond., 1849, iii.

Du Bois-Reymond (E.) De fibræ muscularis reactione, ut chemicis visa est, acida. 4°. *Berolini*, 1859.

Dwight (T.), jr. The structure and action of striated muscular fibre. 8°. [*Boston*, 1873.]
Repr. from: Proc. Bost. Soc. Nat. Hist., 1873, xvi.

Ficinus (H. R.) *De fibræ muscularis forma et structura. 4°. *Lipsiæ*, [1836].

Grunmach (E.) *Ueber die Structur der quergestreiften Muskelfaser bei den Insecten. 8°. *Berlin*, [1872].

Gubler (J.) *Ueber die Längenverhältnisse der Fleischfasern einiger Muskeln. 8°. *Zürich*, 1860.

ab Holst (J.) *De structura musculorum in genere et annulatorum musculis in specie observationes microscopicæ. 8°. *Dorpati Livonorum*, 1846.

Klein (T.) *Ueber Entwicklungs- und Kreislaufverhältnisse kleinzelliger Rundzellensarkome der Muskeln. 8°. *Burg*, 1886.

Kölliker (A.) Ueber die Cohnheim'schen Felder der Muskelquerschnitte. 8°. *Würzburg*, 1866.

Meyer (E.) *Ueber rothe und blasse quergestreifte Muskeln. 8°. *Göttingen*, 1875.
Also, in: Arch. f. Anat., Physiol. u. wissensch. Med., Leipz., 1875, 217–232.

Muys (W. G.) Investigatio fabricæ, quæ in partibus musculos componentibus extat. Dissertatio prima de carnis musculosæ fibrarumque carnearum structura, quatenus sine vasis sanguiferis, nervis, nervosisque villis, atque membranis spectantur. 4°. *Lugd. Bat.*, 1741.

————. Musculorum artificiosa fabrica, observationibus copiosissimis et experimentis physicis

Muscle (Chemistry and histology of).

demonstrata atque iconibus manu autoris delineatis illustrata. 4°. *Lugd. Bat.*, 1751.

Nasse (O.) Zur Anatomie und Physiologie der quergestreiften Muskelsubstanz. 8°. *Leipzig*, 1882.

Piotrovski (A.) *O mishechnome fermentie. [On muscular ferments.] 8°. *St. Petersburg*, 1867.

Povarin (M.) *K voprosu o vlijanii sna na myshetchnujou silu cheloveka. [Influence of sleep on muscular strength of man.] 4°. *St. Petersburg*, 1883.

Ritter (E.) *Des propriétés physiques du tissu musculaire. 4°. *Strasbourg*, 1863.

Rollett (A.) Ueber freie Enden quergestreifter Muskelfäden im inneren der Muskeln. 8°. *Wien*, 1856.

————. Untersuchungen über den Bau der quergestreiften Muskelfasern. 1. Theil. 4°. *Wien*, 1885.
Repr. from: Denkschr. d. math.-naturw. Cl. d. k. Akad. d. Wissensch., xlix.

Solger (E.) *De musculi calore. 8°. *Vratislaviæ*, [1862].

Steffan (P.) *Die kernähnlichen Gebilde des Muskelprimitivbündels. 8°. *Erlangen*, 1860.
Also, in: Ztschr. f. rat. Med., Leipz. u. Heidelb., 1861, 3. R., x, 204–237, 2 pl.

Sundevall (C. J.) Om muskelbyggnaden i foglarnas extremiteter. 8°. *Stockholm*, 1855.
Repr. from: Nat.- forsk.- Sällsk. forhandl., 1851.

Wagner (H.) *Beiträge zur vergleichend chemischen Physiologie der Muskelsubstanz. 8°. *Würzburg*, 1885.

Warren (J.) *Beiträge zur physiologischen Chemie des Muskels. 8°. *Bonn*, 1880.

Wydler (F.) *Ueber die Bestandtheile des menschlichen Muskelextracts. 8°. *Würzburg*, 1848.

Aducco (V.) La reazione dell' orina in rapporto con il lavoro muscolare. Gior. d. r. Accad. di med. di Torino, 1887, 3. s., xxxv, 42–56.—**Aeby** (C.) Ueber die Beziehungen der Faserzahl zum Alter des Muskels. Ztschr. f. rat. Med., Leipz. u. Heidelb., 1862, 3. R., xiv, 182–199, 1 pl.—**Apelson** (O.) Bidrag till kännedomen om extremiteternas bygnad hos den tvåtåige sengångaren, Cholœpus didactylus. [Structure of terminal fibres of muscles.] Upsala Läkaref. Förh., 1880–81, xvi, 122–144. — **Arnold** (J.) Ueber die Abscheidung des indigschwefelsauren Natrons im Muskelgewebe. Arch. f. path. Anat., etc., Berl., 1877, lxxi, 1–16, 1 pl.—**Astaschewsky.** Ueber die Säurebildung und den Milchsäuregehalt der Muskeln. Ztschr. f. physiol. Chem., Strassb., 1880, iv, 397–406. — **Balser** (H.) Entwicklung quergestreifter Muskelfasern in Pseudomembranen. Ztschr. f. rat. Med., Heidelb., 1846, iv, 17–20.—**Barry** (M.) Note regarding the structure of muscle. Lancet, Lond., 1842–3, i, 167. ————. Neue Untersuchungen über die schraubenförmige Beschaffenheit der Elementarfasern der Muskeln, nebst Beobachtungen über die muskulöse Natur der Flimmerhärchen. Arch. f. Anat., Physiol. u. wissensch. Med., Berl., 1850, 529–596, 2 pl. ————. Renewed inquiries concerning the minute structure of muscle, with observations on the muscularity of cilia. Lond., Edinb. & Dubl. Phil. Mag., Lond., 1852, iv, 81; 177, 2 pl. *Also,* Reprint. *Also:* Edinb. M. & S. J., 1853, lxxix, 54–81. — **Berlin** (W.) Ueber die quergestreiften Muskelfaser. Arch. f. d. holländ. Beitr. z. Nat.- u. Heilk., Utrecht, 1857–8, i, 417–470.—**von Bibra** (E.) Ueber das Muskelfleisch des Menschen und der Wirbelthiere. Arch. f. physiol. Heilk., Stuttg., 1845, iv, 536–581.—**Bierdermann** (W.) Zur Lehre vom Bau der quergestreiften Muskelfaser. Sitzungsb. d. k. Akad. d. Wissensch. Math.-naturw. Cl. 1876, Wien, 1877, lxxiv, 49–62, 1 pl.—**von Biesiadecki** (A.) & **Herzig** (A.) Die verschiedenen Formen der quergestreiften Muskelfasern. [*From:* Sitzungsb. d. k. Akad. d. Wissensch. Math.-naturw. Cl., Wien, xxx, No. 13.] Untersuch. z. Naturl. d. Mensch. u. d. Thiere. Giessen, 1860, vi, 105–109. — **Bremer** (L.) Ueber die Muskelspindeln, nebst Bemerkungen über Structur, Neubildung und Innervation der quergestreiften Muskelfaser. Arch. f. mikr. Anat., Bonn, 1883, xxii, 318–356, 2 pl. — **Brücke** (E.) Ueber den Bau der Muskelfasern. Resultate von Untersuchungen, die mit Hülfe des polarisirten Lichtes angestellt wurden. [*From:* Sitzungsb. d. k. Akad. d. Wissensch. Math.-naturw. Cl., Wien, 1857, Juli.] Untersuch. z. Naturl. d. Mensch. u. d. Thiere, Frankf. a. M., 1858, iv, 89. — **Budge** (J.)

Muscle (*Chemistry and histology of*).

Ueber einige chemische Mittel, welche zur Unterscheidung zwischen der Muskelfaser und der mittleren Arterienhaut dienen. Arch. f. Anat.. Physiol. u. wissensch. Med., Berl., 1842, 367-371. ———. Bemerkungen über Structur und Wachsthum der quergestreiften Muskelfasern Arch. f. physiol. Heilk., Stuttg., 1858, n. F., ii, 71-79. 1 pl. ———. Ueber die Genauigkeit meiner Methode der Muskelfaserzählung. Arch. f. path. Anat., etc., Berl., 1859, xvii. 196-199. — **Bunge** (G.) Analyse der anorganischen Bestandtheile des Muskels. Ztschr. f. physiol. Chem., Strassb., 1884-5, ix, 60-62. — **Campbell** (H. F.) Observations on the law governing muscular fibre. South. M. & S. J., Augusta, 1851, n. s., vii, 139-142.— **Capezzuoli** (S.) Sulla composizione della carne muscolare di diversi vertebrati; studi chimici comparativi. Gazz. med. ital. feder. tosc., Firenze 1854, iv, 65; 73.— **Chandelon** (T.) Ueber die Einwirkung der Arterienunterbindung und der Nervendurchschneidung auf den Glycogengehalt der Muskeln. Arch. f. d. ges. Physiol., Bonn, 1876, xiii, 626-630. — **Cohnheim** (J.) Ueber den feineren Bau der quergestreiften Muskelfaser. Arch. f. path. Anat., etc.. Berl., 1865, xxxiv, 606-622, 1 pl. *Also, in his:* Ges. Abhandl., 8°, Berl., 1885, 35-50. — **Deiters** (O.) Beitrag zur Histologie der quergestreiften Muskeln. Arch. f. Anat. Physiol. u. wissensch. Med., Leipz., 1861, 393-424. 1 pl.—**Demant** (B.) Beitrag zur Lehre über die Zersetzung des Glycogens in den Muskeln. Ztschr. f. physiol. Chem., Strassb., 1879 iii. 200-204. ———. Beitrag zur Chemie der Muskeln. *Ibid.,* 241-249. ———. Zur Kenntniss der Extractivstoffe der Muskeln. *Ibid.,* 381-390. ———. Ueber das Serumalbumin in den Muskeln. *Ibid.,* 1880, iv, 384-386. ———. Zur Frage nach dem Harnstoffgehalt der Muskeln. *Ibid.,* 419-422. — **Discussion** on the microscopical appearances of striped muscle during rest and contraction. Tr. Internat M. Cong., 7. sess., Lond., 1881, i, 270-272. — **Duval** (M.) Muscle; anatomie et physiologie. N. dict. de méd. et chir. prat., Par., 1877, xxiii. 209-262.—**Eberth** (C. J.) Die Elemente der quergestreiften Muskeln. Arch f. path. Anat., etc., Berl., 1866, xxxvii, 100-124, 1 pl. — **Emery** (C.) Sur la structure des fibres musculaires striées de quelques vertébrés; résumé. [*Transl. from:* Mem. Accad. d. sc. d. Ist. di Bologna, 1882. 4. s., iii.] Arch. ital. de biol., Turin, 1882, ii, 133.— **Engelmann** (T. W.) Mikroskopische onderzoekingen omtrent den bouw en de beweging der dwarsgestreepte spierzelstandigheid. Onderzoek. ged. in h. physiol. Lab. d. Utrecht. Hoogesch., 1873, 3. R., ii, 151-241, 2 pl. *Also, transl.:* Arch. f. d. ges. Physiol., Bonn, 1873, vii, 33; 155, 2 pl. ———. Ueber Bau, Contraction und Innervation der quergestreiften Muskelfasern. Cong. périod. internat. d. sc. méd. Compt. rend. 1879, Amst., 1880, vi, 562-583. ———. Ueber den Bau der quergestreiften Substanz an den Enden der Muskelfasern. Onderzoek. ged. in h. physiol. Lab. d. Utrecht. Hoogesch., 1882, 3. R., vii, 141-148.—**Fano** (G.) & **Baldi** (D.) Gli albuminoidi della linfa e del sangue nel lavoro muscolare. Sperimentale, Firenze, 1883, iii, 3-12.—**Fick** (A.) Ueber die Anheftung der Muskelfasern an die Sehnen. Arch. f Anat., Physiol. u. wissensch. Med., Berl., 1856, 425-432, 1 pl.— **Flemming** (W.) Ueber Bindesubstanz und Gefässwandung im Schwellgewebe der Muscheln. Arch. f. mikr. Anat., Bonn, 1877, xiii, 818-867, 3 pl.—**Folwarczny** (C.) Ueber die Reaction des frischen Muskelfleisches. Wchnbl. d. k. k. Gesellsch. d. Aerzte in Wien, 1862, xviii, 25-28.— **Froriep** (A.) Ueber das Sarcolemm und die Muskelkerne. Arch. f. Anat. u. Physiol., Leipz., 1878, 416-428.— **Giuliani** (M.) Sopra i rapporti dei muscoli coi tendini. Atti Accad. med. di Roma, 1883-6, 2. s., ii, 75-86, 2 pl.— **Gleiss** (W.) Ein Beitrag zur Muskelchemie. Arch. f. d. ges Physiol., Bonn, 1887, xli, 69-75.—**Golgi** (C) Contribuzione all' istologia dei muscoli volontarj. Ann. univ. di med. e chir., Milano, 1880, ccli, 250-261. *Also:* R. Ist. lomb. di sc. e lett. Rendic., Milano, 1880, 2. s., xiii, 25-31. ———. Annotazioni intorno all' istologia normale e patologica dei muscoli volontari. Arch. per le sc. med., Torino, 1881, v, 194-236, 2 pl.—**Goodfellow** (S. J.) Some remarks on the internal structure of voluntary muscle. Lond. Phys. J., 1843-4, i, 97-103.—**Grützner** (P.) Ueber einige chemische Reactionen des thätigen und unthätigen Muskels. Arch. f. d. ges. Physiol., Bonn, 1873, vii, 254-263.—**Gubler.** Ueber die Längenverhältnisse der Skeletmuskelfasern. Aus der Inauguralabhandlung des . . . mitgetheilt von A. Fick. Untersuch. z. Naturl. d. Mensch. u. d. Thiere, Giessen, 1860, vii, 251-264. — **Haeser** (H.) Ueber Amici's Untersuchungen, betreffend den Bau der

Muscle (*Chemistry and histology of*).

Primitivfasern der Muskeln. Deutsche Klinik, Berl., 1859, xi, 206.—**Halliburton** (W. D.) On muscle plasma. J. Physiol., Lond. & Cambridge, 1887, viii, 133-202. *Also* [Abstr.]: Brit. M. J., Lond., 1887, ii, 227. *Also* [Abstr.]: Proc. Roy. Soc. Lond., 1887, xlii, 400. — **Harless** (E.) Ueber die chemische Veränderung des Muskel-Saftes durch Wärme und Bewegung. Aerztl. Int. Bl., München, 1860, vii, 154.—**Haycraft** (J. B.) Upon the cause of the striation of voluntary muscular tissue. Proc. Roy. Soc. Lond., 1880-81, xxxi, 360-379, 1 pl. *Also:* Quart. J. Micr. Sc., Lond., 1881, n. s., xxi, 307-329. — **Hensen** (V.) Ueber ein neues Structurverhältniss der quergestreiften Muskelfaser. Arb. a. d. Kieler physiol. Inst. (1868), 1869, i, 1-26, 2 tab. ———. Nachträgliche Bemerkungen über die Structur der quergestreiften Muskeln. *Ibid.,* 172-176.— **Heppner** (C. L.) Ueber ein eigenthümliches optisches Verhalten der quergestreiften Muskelfaser. Arch. f. mikr. Anat., Bonn, 1869, v, 137-144, 1 pl. — **Hermann** (L.) Ueber den Längs- und Querwiderstand der Muskeln. Arch. f. d. ges. Physiol., Bonn, 1886, xxxix, 490-498. — **Home** (E.) The Croonian lecture. On the structure of a muscular fibre from which is derived its elongation and contraction. Phil. Tr., Lond., 1826, cxvi, pt 1, 64-68, 1 pl.— **Jahn** (A.) & **Welcker** (H.) Die kernähnlichen Gebilde der quergestreiften Muskelfaser und die Frage nach der Existenz eines plasmatischen Gefässsystems der Muskeln. Ztschr. f. rat. Med., Leipz. u. Heidelb., 1861, 3. R., x, 238-262, 1 pl.—**Jolly** (L.) Du mode de distribution des phosphates dans les muscles et les tendons. Compt. rend. Acad. d. sc., Par., 1879, lxxxix, 958.—**Jousset de Bellesme.** Sur les anastomoses des fibres musculaires striées chez les invertébrés. *Ibid.,* 1882, xcv, 1003.—**Klemensiewicz** (R.) Ueber lacunäre Usur der quergestreiften Muskelfasern. Sitzungsb. d. k. Akad. d. Wissensch. Math.-naturw. Cl., Wien, 1879, lxxix, 3. Abth., 162-176, 1 pl. *Also* [Abstr.]: Oesterr. ärztl. Vereinsztg., Wien, 1879, iii, 138. — **Kœhler** (R.) Sur la morphologie des fibres musculaires chez les échinorhynques. Compt. rend. Acad. d. sc., Par., 1887, civ, 1634-1636. ———. Recherches sur les fibres musculaires de l'Echinorhynchus gigas et de l'E. heruca. *Ibid.,* 1192-1194. — **Krause** (W.) Ueber den Bau der quergestreiften Muskelfaser. Ztschr. f. rat. Med., Leipz. u. Heidelb., 1868, 3. R., xxxiii, 265: 1869, 3. R., xxxiv, 110. ———. Die Querlinien der Muskelfasern in physiologischer Hinsicht. Ztschr. f. Biol., München, 1869, v, 411, 2 pl.: 1870, vi, 453. — **Krukenberg** (C. F. W.) Vergleichend-physiologische Beiträge zur Chemie der contractilen Gewebe. Untersuch. a. d. physiol. Inst. d. Univ. Heidelb., 1879-80, iii, 198-220. ———. Weitere Untersuchungen zur vergleichenden Muskelchemie. *In his:* Vergleich.-physiol. Stud., 8°, Heidelb., 1882, 2. R., 143-147.—**Kühne** (W.) Die Muskelspindeln. [Ein Beitrag zur Lehre von der Entwickelung der Muskeln und Nervenfasern] Arch. f. path. Anat., etc., Berl., 1863, xxviii, 528-538, 1 pl. ———. Ueber den Farbstoff der Muskeln. *Ibid.,* 1865, xxxiii, 79-94.—**Latham** (P. W.) On the origin and formation of lactic acid, creatine, and urea in muscular tissue. [Abstr.] Lancet, Lond., 1885, i, 493. *Also:* Med. Times & Gaz., Lond., 1885, i, 674.—**Lebert.** Résumé d'un mémoire sur la structure de la fibre musculaire du mouvement volontaire et du cœur dans les diverses classes d'animaux. Gaz. méd. de Par., 1849, 3. s., iv, 938-941. *Also:* Compt. rend. Soc. de biol. 1849. Par., 1850, i, 53-61. — **Leydig** (F.) Ueber Tastkörperchen und Muskelstruktur. Arch. f. Anat., Physiol. u. wissensch. Med., Leipz., 1856, 150-159, 1 pl.—**von Limbeck** (R.) Ueber morphologische Verschiedenheiten quergestreifter Muskelfasern. Prag. med. Wchnschr., 1885, x, 437-439.—**Lister** (J.) On the minute structure of involuntary muscular fibre. Tr. Roy. Soc. Edinb., 1856-7, xxi, 549-557, 1 pl.—**McDonnell** (R.) On the recent researches concerning the sugar of muscle. J. Anat. & Physiol., Lond., 1866-7, i, 275-280.— **Macnamara** (C.) On the minute anatomy of muscle. Indian M. Gaz., Calcutta, 1866, i, 237. ———. Striped muscle. Med. Times & Gaz., Lond., 1866, ii, 526.—**Marcet** (W.) Remarks on the brine of salt meat, and on the distribution of albumen through muscular tissue. J. Chem. Soc. Lond., 1864, xvii, 405-415. *Also,* Reprint.—**Marey.** Recherches expérimentales sur la morphologie des muscles. Compt. rend. Acad. d. sc., Par., 1887, cv, 446-451. *Also:* France méd., Par., 1887. ii, 1355-1358. — **Margo** (T.) Neue Untersuchungen über die Entwicklung, das Wachsthum, die Neubildung und den feineren Bau der Muskelfasern. [*From:* Sitzungsb. d. k. Akad. d. wissensch. Math.-naturw. Cl., Wien, xxxvi.] Untersuch. z. Naturl. d. Mensch. u. d. Thiere, Giessen, 1860, vi, 327-349. ———. Ueber die Muskelfasern der Mollusken. Ein Beitrag zur vergleichenden Structur und Entwicklungs-Lehre des Muskelgewebes. [*From:* Sitzungsb. d. k. Akad. d. wissensch. Math.-naturw. Cl., Wien.] *Ibid.,* vii, 165-189, 1 pl.—**Marshall** (C. F.) Observations on the structure and distribution of striped and unstriped muscle in the animal kingdom, and a theory of muscular contraction. Quart. J. Micr. Sc., Lond., 1887-8, n. s., xxviii, 75-107, 1 pl.—**Martin** (H.) Recherches sur la structure de la fibre musculaire striée et sur les analogies de structure et de fonction entre le tissu musculaire et les cellules à baton-

Muscle (*Chemistry and histology of*).

nets (protoplasma strié). École prat. d. hautes études. Lab. d'histol. du Coll. de France. Trav., Par., 1882, 173–218, 1 pl. *Also:* Arch. de physiol. norm. et path., Par., 1882, 2. s. x, 465–510, 1 pl.—**Martyn** (S.) On the anatomy of muscular fibre. Arch. Med., Lond., 1861-2, iii, 227–234 — **Mayer** (S.) Zur Histologie des quergestreiften Muskels. Weitere Beitrag zur Lehre von den Transformationsprozessen in unversehrten Geweben. Biol. Centralbl., Erlang., 1884-5, iv, 129–137. ———. Die sogenannten Sarkoplasten. Anat. Anz., Jena, 1886, i, 231–235.—**Melland** (B.) A simplified view of the histology of the striped muscle-fibre. Quart. J. Micr. Sc., Lond., 1885, n. s., xxv, 371–390, 1 pl.—**Merkel** (F.) Der quergestreifte Muskel. II. Der Contractionsvorgang im polarisirten Licht. Arch. f. mikr. Anat., Bonn, 1873, ix. 293–307, 1 pl.—**Mettenheimer** (C.) Ueber eine eigenthümliche Art von Querstreifung an den Muskeln der Anneliden. Arch. f. Anat., Physiol. u. wissensch. Med., Leipz., 1860, 361–363, 1 pl.—**Moleschott** (J.) & **Battistini** (A.) Sur la réaction chimique des muscles striés et des diverses parties du système nerveux à l'état de repos et après le travail. Arch. ital. de biol., Turin, 1887, viii, 90–124.—**Munk** (H.) Entgegnung. [Kommentar zur neuesten Literatur der quergestreiften Muskelfaser.] Wien. med. Wchnschr., 1858, viii, 216–218. [*See, also, infra,* Rollet.]—**Muys.** Observations on the texture of the muscles. Phil. Tr. 1700-20, Lond., 1731, v, 392–394. — **Nasse** (O.) Zur mikroskopischen Untersuchung des quergestreiften Muskels. Arch. f. d. ges. Physiol., Bonn, 1878, xvii, 282–290. — **Nikolaides** (R.) Ueber di mikroskopischen Erscheinungen bei der Contraction des quergestreiften Muskels. Arch. f. Physiol., Leipz., 1885, 150–156. — **Paneth** (J.) Zur Frage nach der Natur der Sarkoplasten. Anat. Anz., Jena, 1887, ii, 136–138. — **Petersen** (P.) Ueber die Schwankungen im Wasser-, Fett- und Stickstoffgehalt des Fleisches. Ztschr. f. Biol., München, 1871, vii, 166–178.—**Picard.** Sur l'albumine des muscles du chien. Compt. rend. Soc. de biol. 1880, Par., 1881, 7. s., ii, 145–147.—**Pisano** (G.) Studi istologici sul fascio muscolare primitivo striato. Gior. di med., farm. e vet. mil., Firenze, 1870, xviii, 901 – 922.—**Plósz.** Ueber die Beschaffenheit der doppelbrechenden Substanzen der quergestreiften Muskelfasern. Med.-chem Untersuch. a. d. Lab. . . . zu Tübing., Berl., 1871, 510–516.—**Prochaska** (G.) De carne musculari tractatus anatomico-physiologicus. Oper. minor. pars i, 1800, 159–272, 6 pl.—**Ranke** (J.) Untersuchung über die chemischen Bedingungen der Ermüdung des Muskels. Arch. f. Anat., Physiol. u. wissensch. Med., Leipz., 1863, 422: 1864, 320.—**Ranvier** (L.) Du spectre musculaire. Compt. rend. Acad. d. sc., Par., 1874, lxxviii, 1572-1575. *Also:* Arch. de physiol. norm. et path., Par., 1875, 2. s., i, 774–780.—**Remak** (R.) Ueber die Zusammenziehung der Muskelprimitivbündel. Arch. f. Anat., Physiol. u. wissensch. Med., Berl., 1843, 182–189.—**Renaut** (J.) Note sur les disques accessoires des disques minces dans les muscles striés, présentée par M. Cl. Bernard. Compt. rend. Acad. d. sc., Par., 1877, lxxxv, 964–967.—**Retzius** (G.) Zur Kenntniss der quergestreiften Muskelfaser. Biol. Untersuch., Stockholm, 1881, i, 1–26, 2 pl.—**Richet** (C.) Sensibilité, nutrition, physiologie pathologique des muscles. Rev. de méd., Par., 1881, 1024–1043. — **Rippmann** (T.) Ueber das Vorkommen von Theilungen der Muskelfasern in der Zunge der Wirbelthiere und des Menschen. Ztschr. f. rat. Med., Leipz. u. Heidelb., 1862, 3. R., xiv, 200–202. — **Robin** (C.) Musculaire (tissu). § 1. Anatomie. Dict. encycl. d. sc. méd., Par., 1876, 2. s., x, 501-651, 4 pl.—**Rollett** (A.) Untersuchungen zur näheren Kenntniss des Baues der quergestreiften Muskelfasern. [*From:* Sitzungsb. d. k. österr. Akad. d. Wissensch. Math.-naturw. Cl., Wien, 1856, xxi, 176.] Untersuch. z. Natul. d. Mensch. u. d. Thiere, Frankf. a. M., 1857, iii, 345–370, 1 pl. *Also,* Reprint. ———. Commentar zur neuesten Literatur der quergestreiften Muskelfaser. Wien. med. Wchnschr., 1858, viii, 165. [*See, also, supra,* Munk (H.)]—**Ronjon** (A.) Note sur les derniers éléments auxquels on puisse parvenir par l'analyse histologique des muscles striés. Compt. rend. Acad. d. sc., Par., 1875, lxxxi, 375.—**Rouget** (C.) Sur les phénomènes de polarisation qui s'observent dans quelques tissus des végétaux et des animaux et en particulier dans le tissu musculaire. J. de la physiol de l'homme, Par., 1862, v, 247–271, 1 pl.—**Ruppert** (H.) Ueber den Stickstoffgehalt des Fleisches. Ztschr. f. Biol., München, 1871, vii, 354–360.—**Sachs** (C.) Die quergestreifte Muskelfaser. Arch. f. Anat., Physiol. u. wissensch. Med., Leipz., 1872, 607–648, 2 pl.—**Sarokow.** Beitrag zur Physiologie des Muskelstoffwechsels. Arch. f. path. Anat., etc., Berl., 1864, xxviii, 544–551.—**Schäfer** (E. A.) On the structure of striped muscular fibre. Proc. Roy. Soc. Lond., 1872-3, xxi, 242–245.—**Schipiloff** (Catherine) & **Danilevsky** (A.) Ueber die Natur der anisotropen Substanzen des quergestreiften Muskels und ihre räumliche Vertheilung im Muskelbündel. Ztschr. f. physiol. Chem., Strassb., 1881, v, 349–365.—**Schultze** (M.) Ueber Muskelkörperchen und das was man eine Zelle zu nennen habe. Arch. f. Anat., Physiol. u. wissensch. Med., Leipz., 1861, 1–27.—**Schwalbe** (G.) Ueber den feineren Bau der Muskelfasern wirbelloser

Muscle (*Chemistry and histology of*).

Thiere. Arch. f. mikr. Anat., Bonn, 1869, v, 205–247, 2 pl.— **Sczelkow.** Zur Histologie der quergestreiften Muskeln. Arch. f. path. Anat., etc., Berl., 1860, xix, 215–220, 1 pl.— **Stintzing** (R.) Fortgesetzte Untersuchungen über die Kohlensäure der Muskeln. Arch. f. d. ges. Physiol., Bonn, 1879-80, xx, 189–200.—**von Thanhoffer** (L.) Beiträge zur Histologie des quergestreiften Muskels und der Nervenendigung in demselben. Biol. Centralbl., Erlang., 1881, i, 349–351 ———. Beiträge zur Histologie und Nervenendigung der quergestreiften Muskelfasern. Arch. f. mikr. Anat., Bonn, 1882-3, xxi, 26–44, 2 pl.—**Thin** (G.) On the minute anatomy of muscle and tendon, and some notes regarding the stricture of the cornea. Edinb. M. J., 1874-5, xx, 238–251, 3 pl. ———. On the structure of muscular fibre. Quart. J. Micr. Sc., Lond., 1876, n. s., xvi, 251–259, 1 pl.—**Unger** (L.) Untersuchungen über die quergestreiften Muskelfasern des lebenden Thieres. Med. Jahrb., Wien, 1879, 1. Hft., 61–66.—**Wagener** (G. R.) Ueber die Muskelfaser der Evertebraten. Arch. f. Anat., Physiol. u. wissensch. Med., Leipz., 1863, 211–233, 2 pl. ———. Ueber die Entwicklung und den Bau der quergestreiften und glatten Muskelfasern. Sitzungsb. d. Gesellsch. z. Beförd. d. ges. Naturw. in Marb., 1867, 82–88. ———. Ueber die Querstreifen der Muskeln. *Ibid.*, 1872, 25–33. ———. Ueber die quergestreiften Muskelfasern des Herzens. *Ibid.*, 1872, 141–154. ———. Ueber die quergestreifte Muskelfibrille. Arch. f. mikr. Anat., Bonn, 1873, ix, 712–725, 1 pl. ———. Ueber einige Erscheinungen an den Muskeln lebendiger Corethra plumicornis; Larven. *Ibid.*, 1874, x, 293–310, 2 pl. ———. Ueber die Entstehung der Querstreifen auf den Muskeln und den davon abhängigen Erscheinungen. Arch. f. Anat. u. Entwcklngsgesch., Leipz., 1880, 253–279, 2 pl. *Continued in:* Arch. f. d. ges. Physiol., Bonn, 1882-3, xxx, 511–535, 1 pl.—**Weber** (E.) Note sur les noyaux des muscles striés chez la grenouille adulte. Arch. de physiol. norm. et path., Par., 1874, vi, 489–495.—**Weber** (O.) Ueber die Betheiligung der Muskelkörperchen und der quergestreiften Muskeln an den Neubildungen, nebst Bemerkungen über die Lehre von der Specificität der Gewebselemente. Arch. f. path. Anat., etc., Berl., 1867, xxxix, 254–269, 1 pl.—**Weismann** (A.) Ueber die Verbindung der Muskelfasern mit ihren Ansatzpunkten. Ztschr. f. rat. Med., Leipz. u. Heidelb., 1861, 3. R., xii, 126–144, 2 pl. ———. Zur Histologie der Muskeln. *Ibid.*, 1865, 3. R., xxiii, 26–45.—**Weyl** (T.) Histoische Notiz zur Muskelchemie. Ztschr. f. physiol. Chem., Strassb., 1882-3, vii, 185.—**Windle** (B. C. A.) On the myology of Erethizon epixanthus. J. Anat. & Physiol., Lond., 1887-8, xxii, 126–132.—**von Wittich.** Beiträge zur Histologie der quergestreiften Muskeln. Königsb. med. Jahrb., Königsb., 1861-2, iii, 46-51.—**Zaleski** (S. S.) Das Eisen und das Hämoglobin im blutfreien Muskel. Centralbl. f. d. med. Wissensch., Berl., 1887, xxv, 66; 98. *Also, transl.:* Arch. slaves de biol., Par., 1887, iii, 435–441.

Muscle (*Development and growth of*).

DEITERS (O. F. C.) * De incremento musculorum observationes anatomico-physiologicæ. 8°. *Bonnæ,* 1856.

FOREL (F. A.) * Einige Beobachtungen über die Entwicklung des zelligen Muskelgewebes. Beiträge zur Entwicklungsgeschichte der Najaden. 8°. *Würzburg,* 1866.

KRASKE (P.) Experimentelle Untersuchungen über die Regeneration der quergestreiften Muskeln. 4°. *Halle,* 1878.

LUEDEKING (R.) * Untersuchungen über die Regeneration der quergestreiften Muskelfasern. 8°. *Strassburg,* 1876.

MORITZ (E.) * Untersuchungen über die Entwickelung der quergestreiften Muskelfaser. 8°. [*Dorpat*], 1860.

SCHMITZ (G.) * De incremento musculorum observationes physiologicæ. 8°. *Gryphiæ,* 1858.

VON VILLERS (A.) * Ueber Muskelwachsthum. [Jena.] 8°. *Leipzig,* 1881.

WESTHOLT (J.) * Ueber Muskelregeneration. 8°. *Würzburg,* 1874.

ZABIELIN (A.) * O vozrojdenii mishtse pri traumatizmie. [Regeneration of muscles in wounds.] 8°. *St. Petersburg,* 1870.

ZEUKER (F. A.) Ueber die Regeneration des quergestreiften Muskelgewebes; eine historisch-kritische Untersuchung zur theoretischen Pathologie. 4°. *Leipzig,* 1864.

Billroth (T.) Ueber die Neubildung quergestreifter Muskelfasern in einer Hodengeschwulst. Deutsche Klinik, Berl., 1855, vii, 73.—**Braidwood** (P. M.) On the development of striped muscular fibre in the vertebrata.

Muscle (*Development and growth of*).

Brit. & For. M.-Chir. Rev., Lond., 1866, xxxvii, 447–458, 1 pl.—**Budge** (J.) Ueber das Wachsthum der Muskeln. Ztschr. f. rat. Med., Leipz. u. Heidelb., 1861, 3. R., xi, 305–313.—**Calberla** (E.) Studien über die Entwicklung der quergestreiften Muskeln und Nerven der Amphibien und Reptilien. Arch. f. mikr. Anat., Bonn, 1875, xi, 442–458, 2 pl.—**Chappuis.** Die morphologische Stellung der kleinen hintern Kopfmuskeln. Ztschr. f. Anat. u. Entwcklngsgesch., Leipz., 1876–7, ii, 287–297, 1 pl.—**Dutrochet** (R.-J.-H.) Recherches sur la formation de la fibre musculaire. Gaz. méd. de Par., 1831, ii, 411–415. *Also*, Reprint.—**Eberth** (C. J.) Zur Entwicklungsgeschichte der Muskeln. Arch. f. mikr. Anat., Bonn, 1866, ii, 504–506, 1 pl.—**Fox** (W.) On the development of striated muscular fibre. Phil. Tr., Lond., 1866, clvi, 101–112, 2 pl.—**Hermann** (L.) Untersuchungen über die Entwicklung des Muskelstroms. Arch. f. d. ges. Physiol., Bonn, 1877, xv, 191–232, 1 pl.—**Heschl.** Ueber die Neubildung quergestreifter Muskeln und cavernöse Tumoren. Arch. f. path. Anat., etc., Berl., 1854, viii, 126.—**Hoffmann** (C. E. E.) Ueber die Neubildung quergestreifter ǀ Muskelfasern, insbesondere beim Typhus abdominalis. *Ibid.*, 1867, xl, 505–518, 1 pl.—**Kaczander** (J.) Beiträge zur Entwicklungsgeschichte der Kaumuskulatur. Mitth. a. d. embryol. Inst. d. k. k. Univ. in Wien, 1885, n. F., i, 17–23, 1 pl.—**Macalister** (A.) On the embryogeny of the muscular system. Dublin J. M. Sc., 1877, lxiii, 317–328.—**Peremeschko** (P.) Die Entwickelung der quergestreiften Muskelfasern aus Muskelkernen. [Eine an Froschmuskeln angestellte Untersuchung mit Berücksichtigung der Arbeit von Kühne: Ueber die peripherischen Endorgane der motorischen Nerven, 1862.] Arch. f. path. Anat., etc., Berl., 1863, xxvii, 116–126, 2 pl.—**Petrowsky.** Zur Frage über das Wachsthum der Muskelfasern und der Muskeln beim Frosch. Centralbl. f. d. med. Wissensch., Berl., 1873, xi, 769–772.—**Robin** (C.) Mémoire sur la naissance et le développement des éléments musculaires de la vie animale et du cœur. Compt. rend. Soc. de biol. 1854, Par., 1855, 2. s., i, 201–207. *Also*: Gaz. méd. de Par., 1855, 3. s., x, 387–389.—**Rouget** (C.) Mémoire sur le développement embryonnaire des fibres musculaires de la vie animale et du cœur. J. de la physiol. de l'homme, Par., 1863, vi, 459–465.—**Schulze** (F. E.) Beitrag zur Entwickelungsgeschichte der quergestreiften Muskelfaser. Arch. f. Anat., Physiol. u. wissensch. Med., Leipz., 1862, 385–392, 1 pl.—**Salvia** (E.) Sul trapiantamento dei muscoli e sulla rigenerazione delle fibre muscolari. Gazz. d. osp., Milano 1885, vi, 156; 172; 179. *Also* [Abstr.]: Riv. clin. e terap., Napoli, 1884, vi, 507–510.—**Stilling** (H.) & **Pfitzner** (W.) Ueber die Regeneration der glatten Muskeln. Arch. f. mikr. Anat., Bonn, 1886, xxviii, 396–412, 1 pl.—**Surbled** (G.) Sur la genèse de la fibrille musculaire. Bull. Soc. philomat., Par., 1878, 7. s., ii, 150.—**Trinchese** (S.) Comment les fibres musculaires en voie de développement s'unissent aux fibres nerveuses. [*Transl. from*: Atti d. r. Accad. d. Lincei. Cl. di sc. fis., matemat. e nat., Roma, 1886, ii, Rendic.] Arch. ital. de biol., Turin, 1886, vii, 376–378.—**Weismann** (A.) Ueber das Wachsen der quergestreiften Muskeln nach Beobachtungen am Frosch. Ztschr. f. rat. Med., Leipz. u. Heidelb., 1861, 3. R., x, 263–284, 2 pl. ——. Ueber die Neubildung quergestreifter Muskelfasern. Eine Erwiderung an Herrn Prof. Budge. *Ibid.*, xii, 354–359.—**Will** (F.) Einige Worte über die Entstehung der Querstreifen der Muskel. Arch. f. Anat., Physiol. u. wissensch. Med., Berl., 1843, 353–364.—**Wutzer.** Ueber die Möglichkeit der Bildung von Muskelfasern durch pathologische Processe. *Ibid.*, 1834, 451–456.

Muscle (*Fistula of*).

See **Fistula** (*Muscular*).

Muscle (*Growth of*).

See **Muscle** (*Development, etc., of*).

Muscle (*Histology of*).

See **Muscle** (*Chemistry, etc., of*).

Muscle (*Influence of drugs on*).

See, *also*, **Curare**; **Guanidine**; **Nux** *vomica*.

BRACKMANN (H.) * Ueber die Wirkung verschiedener Gifte auf die Form der quergestreiften Muskelfaser. 8°. [*Würzburg*], 1886..

CLOSTERMEYER (T.) * Beeinflussung des lebenden Warmblütermuskels durch Curare, Guanidin, Veratrin. 8°. *Würzburg*, 1877.

FLIESCHER (J. H.) * Tetanisirende Gifte und ihr Antidot. [Göttingen.] 8°. *Heiligenstadt*, 1877.

FLÖEL (O.) * Die Wirkung der Kalium- und Natrium-Salze auf die glatte Muskulatur verschiedener Thiere. [Jena.] 8°. *Bonn*, 1884.

Also, in: Arch. f. d. ges. Physiol., Bonn, 1884-5, 157–173.

Muscle (*Influence of drugs on*).

KIESSLING (A.) * Beiträge zur Kenntniss der spezifischen Wirkungen der Kaliumsalze auf die Muskelsubstanz. 8°. *Würzburg*, 1886.

KLEMPTNER (I.) * Ueber die Wirkung des destillirten Wassers und des Coffeins auf die Muskeln und über die Ursache der Muskelstarre. 8°. *Dorpat*, 1883.

NEUMANN (W.) * Ueber toxicologische Verschiedenheiten functionell verschiedener Muskelgruppen. Ein Beitrag zu der Lehre von den Muskelgiften. 8°. *Bern*, 1883.

REISER (K.) * Die Einwirkung verschiedener Reagentien auf den quergestreiften Muskelfaden. 8°. *Zürich*, 1860.

Brunn (E.) Ueber die Wirkung einiger Gifte auf gereizte Muskeln. St. Petersb. med. Ztschr., 1862, ii, 206–208.—**Brunton** (T. L.) & **Cash** (J. T.) Influence of heat and cold upon muscles poisoned by veratria. J. Physiol., Lond., 1883–4, iv, 1–17.—**Buchheim** & **Eisenmenger.** Ueber den Einfluss einiger Gifte auf die Zuckungscurve des Froschmuskels. Beitr. z. Anat. u. Physiol. (Eckhard), Giessen, 1874, v, 73–145.—**Bufalini** (G.) & **Tassi** (F.) Dell' influenza di alcuni alcaloidi sulla eccitabilità muscolare. Boll. d. Soc. tra i cult. d. sc. med. in Siena, 1883, i, 89–91.—**Kobert** (E. R.) Ueber den Einfluss verschiedener pharmakologischer Agentien auf die Muskelsubstanz. Arch. f. exper. Path. u. Pharmakol., Leipz., 1881–2, xv, 22–80. [*See, also, infra*, Rossbach (J. M.)]—**Kunkel** (A. J.) Ueber eine Grundwirkung von Giften auf die quergestreifte Muskelsubstanz. Arch. f. d. ges. Physiol., Bonn, 1885, xxxvi, 353–372. ——. Ueber die Beeinflussung der Muskeln durch Gifte und andere Ernährungsstörungen. Sitzungsb. d. phys.-med. Gesellsch. zu Würzb., 1887, 53.—**Laborde** (J.-V.) Les poisons dits musculaires et le sulfo-cyanure de potassium; étude de critique expérimentale. Compt. rend. Soc. de biol. 1879, Par., 1880, 7. s., i, pt. 2, 107–149; *see, also*, pt. 1, 255. *Also*: Gaz. méd. de Par., 1880, 6. s., ii, 116; 143; 189; 283; 295; 347; 462.—**Lewin** (H. L.) Ueber den Einfluss des Tannins auf die Elasticität des Muskels. Arch. f. Physiol., Leipz., 1880, 277–280.—**Panormoff** (A.) Wpływ soli potasowych na tkankę mięśniową. [Effect of salts of potassium on muscular fibres.] Gaz. lek., Warszawa, 1882, 2. s., ii, 1027; 1041.—**Paschkis** (H.) & **Pal** (J.) Ueber die Muskelwirkung des Coffeins, Theobromins und Xanthins. Med. Jahrb., Wien, 1886, n. F., i, 611–617.—**Quinquaud** (C.E.) Action, mesurée au dynamomètre, des poisons dits musculaires sur les muscles de la vie de relation. Compt. rend. Soc. de biol., Par., 1884, 8. s., i, pt. 2, 739–743. *Also* [Abstr.]: Gaz. d. hôp., Par., 1885, lviii, 29.—**Rabuteau.** Sur divers poisons curarisants de l'ordre des ammoniums quaternaires. Compt. rend. Soc. de biol., Par., 1885, 8. s., ii, 138–143. ——. Sur les poisons curarisants; alun de phényldiméthylallylammonium. *Ibid.*, 152–156. ——. Sur les poisons curarisants de l'ordre des ammoniums quaternaires, iodures et oxydes de phényldiméthylpropylammonium et de phényldiméthylisobutylammonium. *Ibid.*, pt. 2, 61–64.—**Ringer** (S.) Report on the influence of rhombic sodium-phosphate and sodium-bicarbonate on muscular contraction. Brit. M. J., Lond., 1884, ii, 114–118. ——. Further experiments regarding the influence of small quantities of lime potassium and other salts on muscular tissue. J. Physiol., Lond., 1886, vii, 291–308, 1 diag. ——. Regarding the action of lime, potassium, and sodium salts on skeletal muscle. *Ibid.*, 20–24.—**Ringer** (S.) & **Buxton** (D. W.) Concerning the action of calcium, potassium, and sodium salts upon the eel's heart and upon the skeletal muscles of the frog. *Ibid.*, 15–19. ——. Upon the similarity and dissimilarity of the behaviour of cardiac and skeletal muscle when brought into relation with solutions containing sodium, calcium and potassium salts. *Ibid.*, 288–295.—**Ringer** (S.) & **Morshead** (E. A.) Concerning the action of common salt, sulphate of atropia, bromide of conia and sulphate of nicotine on muscular irritability. *Ibid.*, 1879–80, ii, 252–260. — **Rossbach** (M. J.) Beeinflussung des lebenden Warmblütermuskels durch Curare, Guanidin, Veratrin. Arch. f. d. ges. Physiol., Bonn, 1876, xiii, 607–626, 1 pl. ——. Bemerkungen zu Kobert's Arbeit über den Einfluss verschiedener pharmakologischer Agentien auf die Muskelsubstanz. *Ibid.*, 1881-2, xxvii, 372–382.—**Rossbach** (M. J.) & **von Anrep** (B.) Einfluss von Giften und Arzneimitteln auf die Länge und Dehnbarkeit des quergestreiften Muskels. *Ibid.*, 1879–80, xxi, 240–247, 3 pl.—**Rossbach** (M. J.) & **Clostermeyer** (T.) Einwirkung des Curare, Guanidin und Veratrin auf den lebenden Warmblütermuskel. Verhandl. d. phys.-med. Gesellsch. in Würzb., 1877, n. F., xi, 153–172.—**Szpilman** (J.) & **Luchsinger** (B.) Atropin und glatte Muskelfaser. Arch. f. d. ges. Physiol., Bonn, 1881, xxvi, 459–463.

Muscle (*Physiology of*).

See, also, **Cadaver** (*Attitudes of*); **Cadaver** (*Experiments on*); **Dynamometer**; **Electrophysiology**; **Exercise**; **Irritability**; **Movements** *and motion* (*Organic*); **Muscle** (*Chemistry, etc., of*); **Myograph**; **Nerves**; **Nervous** *system* (*Electrophysiology of*); **Rigor** *mortis*; **Tetanus**; **Urea**.

BARTHOLOMAEUS (J.) & BARTHOLOMAEUS (M.) * De pandiculatione. 4°. [*Lipsiæ*, 1648.]

BELL (C.) On the nervous circle which connects the voluntary muscles with the brain. 4°. *London*, 1826.

BÉRARD. Application de la galvanisation localisée à l'étude des fonctions musculaires par . . . Dr. Duchenne (de Boulogne). 8°. *Paris*, 1851.

BERGONIÉ (J.) Contribution à l'étude des phénomènes physiques du muscle. 8°. *Bordeaux*, 1883.

BERNARD (F.-A.) * De l'élasticité du tissu musculaire et des phénomènes physiques de l'activité des muscles. 4°. *Strasbourg*, 1853.

BERNOULLI (J.) Meditationes mathematicæ de motu musculorum. 4°. [*Lugd. Bat.*, 1710.]

——. The same. . . . Editio secunda. Accedunt Petri Antonii Michelotti Tridentini animadversiones x. Ad ea, quæ cl. vir Jacobus Keill M. D. protulit in tentamine v. quod est de motu musculari. 4°. *Venetiis*, 1721.

VON BEZOLD (A.) Ueber den Beginn der negativen Stromesschwankung im gereizten Muskel. (Jena, 18. November 1861.) 8°. [*n. p., n. d.*]
Repr. from: Monatsber. d. k. Akad. d. Wissensch. zu Berl.

BILLING (J. J.) De motu musculorum. 4°. *Lipsiæ*, [1780].

BLANE (G.) A lecture on muscular motion; read at the Royal Society. 4°. *London*, [1788].

——. The same. The Croonian lecture on muscular motion; read at the Royal Society, November 13th and 20th, 1788. Corrected and enlarged. 4°. *London*, 1790.
Also, in his: Select dissertations. 8°. *London*, 1822, 229–283.

BORUTTAU (C.) Contractiones musculorum illæ, quæ post aquæ injectionem observantur, num nervorum irritatione efficiantur an musculorum ipsorum? 8°. *Regimonti Pr.*, 1862.

BOUDET DE PARIS. * De l'élasticité musculaire. 4°. *Paris*, 1880.

BOULTON (R.) A treatise of the reason of muscular motion; or the efficient causes of the contraction of a muscle, wherein most of the phænomena about muscular motion are explained. 16°. *London*, 1697.

BOUR (J. P.) * Ueber die verschiedene Erregbarkeit functionell verschiedener Nerv-Muskelapparate. 4°. *Würzburg*, 1875.
Also, in: Arb. a. d. physiol. Lab. d. Würzb. Hochsch., 1876, iii, 253–269.

BRANDT (G.-H.) * Des phénomènes de contraction musculaire observée chez des individus qui ont succombé à la suite du choléra ou de la fièvre jaune. 4°. *Paris*, 1855.

BRONDGEEST (P. Q.) * De tono musculorum voluntati subditorum. 8°. *Traj. ad Rhenum*, 1860.
Dutch text.
Also, transl. [Abstr.] *in:* Arch. f. d. holländ. Beitr. z. Nat.- u. Heilk., Utrecht, 1859–60, ii, 329–357, 1 pl.

BRÜCKE (E.) Ueber das Verhalten lebender Muskeln gegen Borsäurelösungen. 8°. [*Wien*, 1867.]
Repr. from: Sitzungsb. d. k. Akad. d. Wissensch. Math.-naturw. Cl., Wien, lv.

——. Ueber den Einfluss der Stromesdauer auf die elektrische Erregung der Muskeln. 8°. [*Wien*, 1867.]
Repr. from: Sitzungsb. d. k. Akad. d. Wissensch. Math.-naturw. Cl., Wien, lvi.

Muscle (*Physiology of*).

——. Ueber das Verhalten entnervter Muskeln gegen discontinuirliche elektrische Ströme. 8°. [*Wien*, 1868.]
Repr from: Sitzungsb. d. k. Akad. d. Wissensch. Math.-naturw. Cl., Wien, lviii.

VAN BRUGGE (F. R.) * De actione musculorum. 4°. *Lugd. Bat.*, 1777.

BRUN (J.) * Otia phisiologica, quorum primum, de circulatione; secundum, de pulsu arteriarum; tertium, de motu musculari. 4°. *Avenione*, 1753.

BULFFINGER (J. W.) * Fibra motrix animata, sive diss. academ. de medio motus animalis. 4°. *Tubingæ*, 1716.

CADET (S.) Considerazioni intorno l' ipotesi di nervi che avebbero per ufficio d' infrenare la contrattilità o la tonicità muscolare e ricordo di alcune sperienze cimentate nel laboratorio fisiologico della r. Università di Roma. 4°. *Roma*, 1876.
Repr. from: Atti d. r. Accad. d. Lincei, 2. s., iii.

CHAILLY (J.-N.) * Sur le mouvement musculaire; si le fluide galvanique peut en être considéré comme la cause. 8°. *Paris, an XI*, [1803].

[CROONE (W.)] De ratione motus musculorum. 4°. *Londini*, 1664.

——. The same. 2. ed. 24°. *Amstelodami*, 1667.

DEIDIER (A.) * De motu musculari. *Monspelii*, 1699.
In: HALLER. Disp. anat. [etc.] 4°. *Gottingæ*, 1748, iii, 411–419.

DEUSINGIUS (A.) Exercitatio de motu musculorum.
In his: Exercitationes de motu animalium, etc. 16°. *Groningæ*, 1661, 1–66.

DISSERTATION qui a remporté le prix proposé par l'Académie royale des sciences et belles-lettres de Pruss, sur le principe de l'action des muscles, avec des pièces qui ont concouru. 4°. *Berlin*, 1753.
German text.

DU BOIS-REYMOND (E.) Gesammelte Abhandlungen zur allgemeinen Muskel- und Nervenphysik. 2 v. 8°. *Leipzig*, 1875–7.

DUFOUR (M.) * La constance de la force et les mouvements musculaires. 8°. *Lausanne*, 1865.

ENGELHARDT (E.) * De vita musculorum observationes et experimenta. 8°. *Bonnæ*, [1841].

ENGELMANN (T. W.) Ueber Reizung der Muskelfaser durch den constanten Strom. 4°. [*n. p., n. d.*]

ENGELS (A.) * De tono musculorum animalium. 8°. *Bonnæ*, 1861.

ETTINGER (F. J.) Relationen zwischen Blut und Erregbarkeit der Muskeln. 8°. *Nürnberg*, 1860.

EULENBURG (A.) * De argumentis irritabilitatis muscularis recentioribus. 8°. *Berolini*, [1861].

FLINT (A.), jr. On the source of muscular power. Arguments and conclusions drawn from observations upon the human subject, under conditions of rest and of muscular exercise. 12°. *New York*, 1878.

FONTANA (F.) Réflexions sur le mouvement des muscles.
In his: Traité sur le venin de la vipère. 4°. *Florence*, 1781, iii, 239–266. *Also, transl.:* 8°. *Napoli*, 1787, iii, 210–242. *Also, transl.:* 8°. *London*, 1787, ii, 277–310.

FREYLACH (E. G.) * De fibrarum matricium indole. 8°. *Halæ*, [1809].

FUNKE (O.) [Pr.] über den Einfluss der Ermüdung auf den zeitlichen Verlauf der Muskelthätigkeit. 4°. *Freiburg*, 1873.
Also, in: Arch. f. d. ges. Physiol., Bonn, 1873–4, viii, 213–252, 1 pl.

Muscle (*Physiology of*).

GOLDHAGEN (J. F. G.) * Dubitationes de quadam caussæ motus muscularis explicatione. 4°. *Halæ ad Salam*, [1765].

GOTTSCHED (J.) De motu musculorum. 4°. *Regiomonti*, 1694.

Also, in: HALLER. Disp. anat. [etc.] 4°. *Gottingæ*, 1748, iii, 359–410, 2 pl.

GOUPIL (J.-M.-A.) * La contractilité musculaire étant donnée, considérer les muscles en action, particulièrement dans la station, dans la progression, dans le saut, dans l'action de saisir et de grimper. 4°. *Strasbourg*, 1833.

GROTH (E.) * De musculorum qui appellantur organici tono. 8°. *Berolini*, [1863].

GRUBERT (E.) * Ein Beitrag zur Physiologie des Muskels. 8°. *Dorpat*, 1883.

HAASE (J. G.) De adminiculis motus muscularis. 4°. *Lipsiæ*, 1785.

HANDBUCH der Physiologie, bearb. von H. Aubert [*et al.*]. 1. Bd., 1. Th. Physiologie der Bewegungsapparate. 8°. *Leipzig*, 1879.

HANKO (F.) * De fibris motricem facultatem exercentibus. 8°. *Traj. ad Viadr.*, [1797].

HANRIOT (M.) * De l'électricité musculaire. 4°. *Paris*, 1880.

HEIM (P. A.) * De motu musculari ejusdemque morbis. 4°. *Gottingæ*, [1806].

HERINGA (A.) * De motu musculorum. 4°. *Lugd. Bat.*, 1741.

HERMANN (L.) * De tono ac motu musculorum nonnulla. 8°. *Berolini*, 1859.

———. Untersuchungen über den Stoffwechsel der Muskeln, ausgehend vom Gaswechsel derselben. 8°. *Berlin*, 1867.

———. Weitere Untersuchungen zur Physiologie der Muskeln und Nerven. 8°. *Berlin*, 1867.

———. Untersuchungen zur Physiologie der Muskeln und Nerven. 3. Hft. 8°. *Berlin*, 1868.

HOLMGREN (F.) Om den elektriska strömfluktuationen hos den arbetande muskeln. 8°. *Upsala*, 1873.

VON HUMBOLDT (F. H. A.) Versuche über die gereizte Muskel- und Nervenfaser, nebst Vermuthungen über den chemischen Process des Lebens in der Thier- und Pflanzenwelt. 2 v. 8°. *Posen*, 1797.

———. The same. Expériences sur le galvanisme, et en général sur l'irritation des fibres musculaires et nerveuses. Trad. de l'allemand, avec des additions, par J.-Fr.-N. Jadelot. 8°. *Paris*, 1799.

HUNTER (J.) Croonian lecture on muscular motion, No. 1.

In his: Observations on certain parts of the animal œconomy, [etc.] 8°. *London*, 1837, 195–276.

DE JAGER (P.) * Iets over spier-irritabiliteit. 8°. *Groningen*, [1861].

JONES (R.) * De motus muscularis causa. 4°. *Lugd. Bat.*, 1735.

Also, in: HALLER. Disp. anat. [etc.] 4°. *Gottingæ*, 1751, vii, 533–559, 1 pl. *Also, in:* DE OBERKAMP (F. J.) Collect. diss. 4°. *Francof. a. M.*, 1767, i, 459–480.

KAUFMANN (K.) * Ueber Contraction der Muskelfaser. 8°. *Göttingen*, 1873.

Also, in: Arch. f. Anat., Physiol. u. wissensch. Med., Leipz., 1874, 273–285, 1 pl.

KAY (J. P.) * De motu musculorum. 8°. *Edinburgi*, 1827.

KEILL (J.) An account of animal secretion, the quantity of blood in the humane body, and muscular motion. 8°. *London*, 1708.

KLUENDER (T. H. W.) * Voruntersuchung über den zeitlichen Verlauf der Muskelzuckung. 4°. *Kiel*, 1869.

Also, in: Arb. a. d. Kieler physiol. Inst. (1868), 1869, 107–130.

KNORZ (F.) * Ein Beitrag zur Bestimmung der absoluten Muskelkraft. 8°. *Marburg*, 1865.

Muscle (*Physiology of*).

KOEHLER (J. F.) * De vi musculorum absque cerebro et medulla spinali. 8°. *Halæ*, [1818].

KRIMER (J. F. W.) * De vi musculorum in partibus a reliquo corpore sejunctis. 8°. *Halæ*, [1818].

KRONECKER (H.) * De ratione qua musculorum defatigatio ex labore eorum pendeat. 8°. *Berolini*, [1863].

KÜGLER (E.) * Ueber die Starre des Säugethiermuskels. 8°. *Dorpat*, 1883.

KÜHN (J. F.) * Diss. qua nonnulla muscularis motus momenta perlustrantur. 4°. *Gottingæ*, 1755.

Also [Abstr.], *in:* WEIZ (F. A.) Neue Ausz. [etc.] 12°. *Frankfurt u. Leipzig*, 1782, xv, 14–17.

LALLEMANT (J.) An actio muscularis a solis spiritibus? *Paris*, 1745.

Also, in: HALLER. Disp. anat. [etc.] 4°. *Gottingæ*, 1748, iii, 421–428.

LANGRISH (B.) A new essay on muscular motion, founded on experiments, observations, and the Newtonian philosophy. 4°. *London*, 1733.

———. The Croonian lectures on muscular motion, read before the Royal Society in the year 1747, being a supplement to the Philosophical Transactions for that year. 4°. *London*, 1748.

Also [Abstr.], *in:* Phil. Tr., Lond., 1743–50, xi, 1181–1205.

LAVES (M.) * Ueber das Verhalten des Muskelglycogens nach der Leberexstirpation. 8°. *Königsberg i. Pr.*, 1886.

LEROI (F. J.) * De irritabilitate musculorum. [Leiden.] 8°. *Rotterodami*, 1846.

LESSHAFT (P.) Des divers types musculaires et de la façon différente dont s'exprime la force active des muscles. (Matériaux d'une anatomie générale du système musculaire.) 4°. *St.-Pétersbourg*, 1884.

Repr. from: Mém. Acad. imp. d. sc. de St.-Pétersb., 7. s., xxxii, no. 12.

LEVY (M.) * Ueber den Einfluss der Dehnung auf die Muskelkraft. 8°. *Berlin*, 1886.

LONGET (F.-A.) Recherches expérimentales sur les conditions nécessaires à l'entretien et à la manifestation de l'irritabilité musculaire avec applications à la pathologie. 8°. *Paris*, 1841.

LOSTALOT-BACHOUÉ (J.-P.) * Quelques considérations sur les actes automatiques des muscles en général, suivies de quelques propositions physiologiques et pathologiques sur quelquesuns de ces actes en particulier. 4°. *Paris*, 1827.

MACKALL (L.) An essay on the law of muscular action. 8°. *Washington*, 1859.

———. The same. 2. ed. 8°. *Washington*, 1865.

———. Essays on muscular action, written in 1843 and 1844. 8°. *Washington*, 1860.

MACKINTOSH (J.) * De actione musculari. 8°. *Edinburgi*, 1787.

MANDELBAUM (A.) * Beiträge zur Lehre über die physiologische Bedeutung des Muskelglycogens, seine Verwerthung bei der Contraction. 8°. *Königsberg*, 1881.

VAN MANSVELT (A. P.) * Over de elasticiteit der spieren. 8°. *Utrecht*, 1863.

MARHERR (P.) Quæ sint causæ musculorum motrices, actiones horum, actionum effectus cordis, auricularum, arteriarum, diaphragmatis, musculorum abdominalium, vesicæ? 4°. *Viennæ*, [1761].

MOJON (B.) Memoria sulla contrattilità della fibra animale. Letta all' Accademia delle scienze ed arti di Genova. 8°. *Genova*, 1814.

MOLESCHOTT (J.) Sull' elettrotono primario e secundario dei nervi. 8°. *Torino*, 1870.

Repr. from: Atti d. r. Accad. d. sc. di Torino, 1869, v.

NÄGELI (W.) * Beiträge zur Lehre der elektrischen Muskelreizung. 8°. *Zürich*, 1861.

Muscle (*Physiology of*).

OOSTERDYK (H. G.) *De motu musculorum. 4°. *Traj. ad Rhenum*, 1754.

PAPILLON (S.) *Propositions sur l'élasticité des muscles. 4°. *Paris*, 1824.

PARSONS (J.) The Crounian lectures on muscular motion, for the years 1744 and 1745. 4°. *London*, 1745.
  Also [Abstr.], *in:* Phil. Tr., Lond., 1743-50, xi, 1114-1181, 8 pl.

PFEFFINGER (J.) *De vi musculari. sm. 4°. *Argentorati*, 1754.

PFLÜGER (E.) Untersuchungen über die Physiologie des Electrotonus. 8°. *Berlin*, 1859.

PLACE (T.) *De contractie-golf der willekeurige spieren. 8°. *Utrecht*, 1867.
  Also, in: Onderzoek. ged. in h. physiol. Lab. d. Utrecht. Hoogesch., 1867-8, 2. s., i, 73-138, 2 pl.

POHL (E.) *Diss. . . . pertractans motum organismi humani. 8°. *Pragæ*, 1843.

PREYER (W.) Das myophysische Gesetz. 8°. *Jena*, 1874.

PROCHASKA (G.) De carne musculari tractatus anatomico-physiologicus. 8°. *Viennæ*, 1778.
  Also, in his: Op. minor. anat., etc. 8°. *Viennæ*, 1800, 161-272, 6 pl.

PUGH (J.) A treatise on the science of muscular action. 8°. *London*, 1794.

RADCLIFFE (C. B.) Dynamics of nerve and muscle. 8°. *London*, 1871.

RANKE (G. J.) Der galvanische Leitungs-Widerstand des lebenden Muskels. 8°. *Ausbach*, 1862.

RANKE (J.) Tetanus. Eine physiologische Studie. 8°. *Leipzig*, 1865.

VON RAUM (J.) *Die wirkliche Dauer der einfachen Muskelzusammenziehung. 8°. *Berlin*, 1878.

REGNIER (J.-B.) *Considérations sur la force musculaire, suivies de la description et de l'exposition chalcographique d'un nouvel instrument pour mesurer cette force. 4°. *Paris*, 1807.

RICHET (C.) Physiologie des muscles et des nerfs. Leçons professées à la Faculté de médecine en 1881. 8°. *Paris*, 1882.

ROCHA (M.) *Física médica, el calor en sus relaciones con la contraccion muscular. 8°. *México*, 1873.

ROSENTHAL (I.) Allgemeine Physiologie der Muskeln und Nerven. 12°. *Leipzig*, 1877.

ROSENTHAL (L.) *De tono cum musculorum tum eo imprimis qui sphincterum tonus vocatur. 8°. *Regimonti Pr.*, [1857].

ROTTBÖLL (C. F.) De motus muscularis causis præsertim occasionalibus. sm. 4°. *Hafniæ*, [1752].

SAMT (P.) *Der Electrotonus am Menschen. sm. 8°. *Berlin*, [1868].

SCHIFF (J. M.) Lehrbuch der Physiologie des Menschen. I. Muskel- und Nervenphysiologie. 8°. *Lahr*, 1858-9.

SCHMULEVITCH (J.) *O vlijanii sogrevanija myshts na ich mechanicheskujou rabotu. 8°. *St. Petersburg*, 1869.
  Also, in: Voyenno-med. J., St. Petersb , 1869, ii, pt. 1, 115.

SCHÖNHEYDER (J. H.) *De resolutione et impotentia motus muscularis. 8°. *Hafniæ*, [1768].

SCHOEPSS (C. G.) *Diss. sistens musculorum, quibus volandi motus perficitur, in omnium atque familiarum avibus comparationem et descriptionem. 8°. *Halæ*, [1829].

SMITH (T.) *De actione musculari. 8°. *Edinburgi*, 1767.

———. The same. [With appendix.] 8°. *Edinburgi et Londini*, 1767.
  Also, in: SMELLIE. Thesaurus med. 8°. *Edinburgi*, 1785, 78-115.

Muscle (*Physiology of*).

SÖNNERBERG (J.) & AGARDH (C. A.) Quæstio physiologica, quæ et qualis est musculorum vis formam ossium mutandi. 4°. *Lundæ*, [1801].

SOLGER (E.) *De musculi calore. 8°. *Vratislaviæ*, [1862].

STEINMANN (F.) Ueber den Tonus der willkürlichen Muskeln. 8°. *St. Petersburg*, 1871.
  Cutting from: Bull. Acad. imp. d. sc. de St.-Pétersb., 1870-71, vii, 787-807.

STROSCHEIN (E.) *Ueber passive Bewegungen des menschlichen Körpers während der Muskelruhe. 8°. *Jena*, 1885.

STUART (A.) Dissertatio de structura et motu musculari. 4°. *Londini*, 1738.

———. Three lectures on muscular motion, read before the Royal Society in the year 1738; as appointed by the will of Lady Sadleir, pursuant to the design of her first husband, William Croone . . . Wherein the elasticity of fluids and the immediate cause of the cohesion and elasticity of solids are proved by experiments, etc, and shewn to arise from the same principle as gravity; with a general scheme of muscular motion, founded on anatomy, experiments, etc 4°. *London*, 1739.
  Also [Abstr.], *in:* Phil. Tr., Lond., 1732-44, ix, 277-304, 1 pl.

TAPIE (J.) Travail et chaleur musculaires. 8°. *Paris*, 1886.

DE VARIGNY (H.-C.) Thèses présentées à la Faculté des sciences de Paris pour obtenir le grade de docteur és sciences naturelles. 1re Thèse. Recherches expérimentales sur la contraction musculaire chez les invertébrés. 2e thèse. Propositions données par la Faculté. 8°. *Poitiers*, 1886.

VOLKMANN (A. G.) Commentatio de elasticitate musculorum. 4°. *Halis*, 1866.

VULPIAN (A.) Recherches expérimentales sur la contractilité des vaisseaux du foie et des reins, des uretères, et sur la durée de la contractilité du cœur après la mort chez les mammifères. 8°. *Paris*, [n. d.]

WALLIS (G.) *De motu musculorum. 8°. *Edinburgi*, 1812.

WATTERS (J. H.) An essay on muscular action and its condition. The 9th of a series of articles published in the St. Louis Medical Journal "On Life". 8°. *St. Louis*, 1857.

WATZEL (C. T.) *Diss. sistens semiologiam motuum musculorum voluntariorum. 8°. *Pragæ*, 1839.

WILLIS (T.) De motu musculari.
  In his: Affectionum quæ dicuntur hystericæ, etc. 16°. Lugd. Bat., 1671, 104-162, 2 pl.

———. De ratione motus musculorum.
  In his: Cerebri anatome [etc.] 4°. *Genevæ*, 1676.

WINTER (F.) *De moto musculorum. 4°. *Lugd. Bat.*, [1736].
  Also, in: HALLER. Disp. anat. [etc.] 4°. *Gottingæ*, 1748, iii, 431-472. *Also, in:* DE OBERKAMP (F. J.) Collect. diss. 4°. *Francof. a. M.*, 1767, i, 481-522, 1 pl.

DE WITTICH (G.) Experimenta quædam ad Halleri doctrinam de musculorum irritabilitate probandam instituta. 4°. *Regiomonti*, [1857].

WUNDT (W.) Die Lehre von der Muskelbewegung. Nach eigenen Untersuchungen bearbeitet von . . . 8°. *Braunschweig*, 1858.

YPEUS (A.) Observationes physiologicæ de motu musculorum voluntario et vitali. 8°. *Leovardiæ et Franequeræ*, 1775.

Abildgaard (P. C.) Aliquid ad physiologiam musculorum pertinens. Acta reg. Soc. med. Havn., 1783, i, 470-476.—**Adamkiewicz** (A.) Die normale Muskelfunction betrachtet als das Resultat eines Gleichgewichts zweier antagonistischer Innervationen und die atonische Ataxie und die spastische Parese der Muskeln als die beiden Endaffecte einer Störung dieses Gleichgewichts. Ztschr. f. klin. Med., Berl., 1881, iii, 450-464.—**Aeby** (C.) Die Reizung der quergestreiften Muskelfaser durch Ketten-

Muscle (*Physiology of*).

ströme. Arch. f. Anat., Physiol. u. wissensch. Med., Leipz., 1867, 688–712. ———. Die Fortpflanzungsgeschwindigkeit der Reizung in der quergestreiften Muskelfaser. Arch. f. d. ges. Physiol., Bonn, 1875, x, 465–467. — **Albrecht** (J.), **Meyer** (A.) & **Giuffrè** (L.) Untersuchungen über die Erregbarkeit der Nerven und Muskeln bei Längs- und Querdurchströmung. *Ibid.*, 1879–80, xxi, 462–478.—**von Anrep** (B.) Studien über Tonus und Elasticität der Muskeln. *Ibid.*, xxi, 226–240, 2 pl.— **Armsby** (H. P.) The source of muscular power. Pop. Sc. Month., N. Y., 1879, xv, 812–825.—**Arnold** (J. W. S.) On muscular phenomena. Med. Rec., N. Y., 1875, x, 289; 337.—**Auerbach** (L.) Ueber den Muskeltonus. Ausz. a. d. Uebers. d. Arb. u. Veränd. d. schles. Gesellsch. f. vaterl. Kult. Jahresb. d. med. Sect., Bresl., 1856, 7–10. ———. Ueber Muskelkontraktionen durch mechanische Reizung am menschlichen Körper. Verhandl. d. Breslau. med. Sekt. (Sekt. d. schles. Gesellsch. f. vaterl. Kult.), Bresl., 1859–60, 32–38. ———. Ueber die Wirkungen topischer Muskelreizung. Abhandl. d. schles. Gesellsch. f. vaterl. Kult. Abth f. Naturw. u. Med., Bresl., 1861, 3. Hft., 291–326.—**Baierlacher** (E.) Physiologische Studien im Gebiete der elektrischen Muskelerregung vom Nerven aus. Ztschr. f. rat. Med., Leipz. u. Heidelb., 1859, 3. R., v, 233–267. ———. Ueber Muskelbewegungen beim Menschen. *Ibid.*, 1860, 3. R., viii, 263–266.—**Barlow** (W. F.) A supplement to some observations on the muscular contractions which occasionally happen after death from cholera. Lond. M. Gaz., 1850, n. s., xi, 654; 739.—**Barzelotti** (J.) Prüfung einiger neuern Theorien über die nächste Ursache der Muskelzusammenziehung. Arch. f. d. Physiol., Halle, 1805, vi, 168–221.—**Beaunis** (H.) Note sur la forme de la contraction musculaire réflexe. Gaz. méd. de Par., 1883, 6. s., v, 598; 610; 626. *Also* [Abstr.]: Compt. rend. Soc. de biol., Par., 1883, 7. s., v, 528–532. *Also* [Abstr.]: Compt. rend. Acad. d. sc., Par., 1883, xcvii, 841. *Also* [Abstr.]: Gaz. d. hôp., Par., 1883, lvi, 981.—**Béclard** (J.) De la contraction musculaire, dans ses rapports avec la température animale. Arch. gén. de méd., Par., 1861, i, 24; 157; 257. *Also*, Reprint.—**Benedikt** (M.) Untersuchungen über das Zuckungsgesetz der motor. Nerven. Wien. med. Presse, 1870, xi, 529; 553; 582; 612; 629.—**Bernoulli** (D.) Versuch einer neuen Theorie der Bewegung der Muskeln. Phys. u. med. Abhandl. d. k. Akad. d. Wissensch. in Petersb., Riga, 1782, i, 3–28.—**Bernstein** (J.) Gegenbemerkung über die Anfangszuckung. Arch. f. d. ges. Physiol., Bonn, 1871–2, v, 318–320. ———. Ueber das myophysische Gesetz des Herrn Preyer. *Ibid.*, 1872, vi, 403–412. ———. Ueber die myophysischen Untersuchungen von Preyer. Zweite Kritik. *Ibid.*, 1873, vii, 90–100. ———. Ueber den Electrotonus und die innere Mechanik des Nerven. *Ibid.*, 1873–4, viii, 40–60, 1 pl. ———. Ueber Electrotonus. Antikritik. *Ibid.*, 498–505. ———. Ueber die Höhe des Muskeltones bei elektrischer und chemischer Reizung. *Ibid.*, 1875, xi, 191–196. ———. Ueber den Einfluss der Reizfrequenz auf die Entwickelung der Muskelkraft. Arch. f. Physiol., Leipz., 1883, Suppl.-Bd., 88–104, 1 pl.—**Bernstein** (J.) & **Steiner** (J.) Ueber die Fortpflanzung der Contraction und der negativen Schwankung im Säugethiermuskel. Arch. f. Anat., Physiol. u. wissensch. Med., Leipz., 1875, 526–551.—**Berry** (G. A.) & **Rutherford.** Note on Pflüger's law of contraction. J. Anat. & Physiol., Lond., 1876, x, 604–608.—**Bertacchini** (P.) Contribuzione allo studio delle correnti elettriche nei muscoli. Rassegna di sc. med., Modena, 1887, ii, 270; 316.— **von Bezold** (A.) Zur Physiologie des Electrotonus. Allg. med. Centr.-Ztg., Berl., 1859, xxviii, 193–195. ———. Ueber einige Zeitverhältnisse, welche bei der directen elektrischen Erregung des Muskels in's Spiel kommen. [*From*: Monatsber. d. k. preuss. Akad. d. Wiss. zu Berl., 5. Dec. 1860.] Untersuch. z. Naturl. d. Mensch. u. d. Thiere, Giessen, 1860, vii, 590–594.—**Biedermann** (W) Ueber die polaren Wirkungen des elektrischen Stromes im entnervten Muskel. Sitzungsb. d. k. Akad. d. Wissensch. Math.-naturw. Cl., Wien, 1879, lxxix, 3. Abth., 289–320, 1 pl. ———. Ueber die durch chemische Veränderung der Muskelsubstanz bewirkten Veränderungen der polaren Erregung durch den elektrischen Strom. *Ibid.*, 1879, Wien, 1880, lxxx, 3. Abth., 367–410, 1 tab. ———. Ueber die Abhängigkeit des Muskelstromes von localen chemischen Veränderungen der Muskelsubstanz. *Ibid.*, 1880, lxxxi, 3. Abth., 74–114. ———. Ueber rhythmische, durch chemische Reizung bedingte Contractionen quergestreifter Muskeln. *Ibid.*, 1880, Wien, 1881, lxxxii, 3. Abth., 257–275. ———. Ueber scheinbare Oeffnungszuckung verletzter Muskeln. *Ibid.*, 1882, lxxxv, 3. Abth., 144–171. *Also*, Reprint. ———. Ueber das Herz von Helix pomatia. (Ein Beitrag zur vergleichenden Physiologie der Muskeln.) *Ibid.*, 1884, lxxxix, 3. Abth., 19–55.—**Bilharz** (A.) & **Nasse** (O.) Elektrotonus im modificirten Nerven. Arch. f. Anat., Physiol. u. wissensch. Med., Leipz., 1862, 66–89.—**Billroth** (T.) Ueber eine Art der Bindegewebs-Metamorphose der Muskel- und Nervensubstanz. Arch. f. path. Anat., etc., Berl., 1855, viii, 260–268. *Also*, Reprint.—**Bizzozero** (G.) Fisiologia; sulla vitalità degli elementi contrattili. R. Ist. Lomb. di sc. e lett.

Muscle (*Physiology of*).

Rendic., Milano, 1868, 2. s., i, 679–681.—**Blasius** (E.) Ueber den Tonus. Arch. f. path. Anat., etc., Berl., 1863, xxviii, 83–157.—**Bleuler** (E.) & **Lehmann** (K.) Hat Abkühlung eines Nervenstückes oberhalb der Reizstelle Einfluss auf die zeitlichen Verhältnisse der Zuckung? Arch. f. d. ges. Physiol., Bonn, 1879–80, xx, 362–364. ———. Ueber den Einfluss der Länge des Nervenstückes auf die Absterbezeit der Muskeln. *Ibid.*, 364.—**Blix** (M. G.) Bidrag till läran om muskelelasticiteten. Upsala Läkaref. Förh., 1874, ix, 555–577. ———. Ett bidrag till kännedomen om muskelus spänning och det mekaniska arbetet vid kontraktionen. *Ibid.*, 1885, xx, 161–174. ———. Till belysning af frågan: Huruvida värme omsättes till mekaniskt arbete vid muskelkontraktionen. [Mechanical action of heat in producing contraction of muscles.] *Ibid.*, 1881, xvi, 569–619.—**Bloch** (A.-M.) Expériences sur les sensations de contraction musculaire. Compt. rend. Soc. de biol., Par., 1884, 8. s., i, 31–33. ———. Expériences sur la contraction musculaire provoquée par une percussion du muscle chez l'homme. J. de l'anat. et physiol., etc., Par., 1885, xxi, 19–27. *Also* [Abstr.]: Compt. rend. Soc. de biol., Par., 1884, 8. s., i, pt. 2, 576.—**Bochefontaine** & **Couty.** Influence de l'oxyde de carbone sur la durée de la contractilité musculaire. Gaz. méd. de Par., 1875, 4. s., iv. 617–620.— **Böttcher** (A.) Ueber Ernährung und Zerfall der Muskelfasern. Arch. f. path. Anat., etc., Berl., 1858, xiii, 227, 1 pl.; 392.—**Bohr** (C.) Om Loven for den tetaniske Sammentræknings Højde, betragtet som Funktion af de tetaniserende Irritationers Antal i Tidsenheden og af den enkelte Irritations Styrke. Overs. o. d. k. Danske Vidensk. Selsk. Forh., Kjøbenh., 1881, No. 3, 171–191. — **Bordoni** (L.) Osservazioni sul decorso della contrattilità elettromuscolare nei muscoli gemelli della rana. Boll. d. Soc. tra i cult. d. sc. med. in Siena, 1886, iv, 13–16.—**Boudet de Pâris.** Effets du curare, de la chaleur et de la section des nerfs moteurs sur l'excitabilité et l'élasticité musculaires. *In*: Marey (E.-J.) Physiol. exp., 8°, Par., 1880, 155–174.—**Bouvier.** Sur la contraction et la rétraction musculaires. Bull. Acad. de méd., Par., 1842–3, viii, 1195.— **Bowman** (W.) On the minute structure and movements of voluntary muscle. Phil. Tr., Lond., 1840, cxxx, 457–501. ———. Additional note on the contraction of voluntary muscle in the living body. *Ibid.*, 1841, cxxxi, 69–72.—**Brodhurst** (B. E.) The etiology of muscular retraction. Med. Times & Gaz., Lond., 1854, n. s., viii, 105; 483.—**Brown-Séquard** (C.-E.) Mouvements rhythmiques de muscles respirateurs et locomoteurs après la mort. Compt. rend. Soc. de biol. 1849, Par., 1850, i. 158–160. ———. Des rapports qui existent entre l'irritabilité musculaire, la rigidité cadavérique et la putréfaction. *Ibid.*, 173–175. ———. De l'influence du système nerveux, du galvanisme, du repos et de l'action sur la nutrition des muscles. *Ibid.*, 195–197. ———. Preuve nouvelle à l'appui de la doctrine de Haller relative à l'indépendance de l'irritabilité musculaire. *Ibid.*, 1850, Par., 1851, iii, 101–103. ———. Recherches sur le rétablissement de l'irritabilité musculaire chez un second supplicié, plus de quatorze heures après la mort. *Ibid.*, 103. ———. Récherches sur le rétablissement de l'irritabilité musculaire chez un supplicié treize heures après la mort. *Ibid.*, pt. 2, 147–153. *Also*: Gaz. méd. de Par., 1851, 3. s., vi, 421–423. *Also*, Reprint. ———. On the nutrition of muscles during their contraction. Med. Exam., Phila., 1852, n. s., viii. 428–430. ———. Recherches sur l'irritabilité musculaire. J. de la physiol. de l'homme, Par., 1859, ii, 75–83. ———. Du rhythme dans le diaphragme et dans les muscles de la vie animale, après leur séparation des centres nerveux. *Ibid.*, 115–119. ———. Leçon Croonienne sur les relations entre l'irritabilité musculaire, la rigidité cadavérique et la putréfaction. *Ibid.*, 1861, iv, 266–278. ———. Recherches sur l'augmentation de la tonicité musculaire et sur l'inhibition de la propriété essentielle des tissus contractiles. Compt. rend. Soc. de biol., Par., 1885, 8. s., ii, 206–208.—**Brücke** (E.) Ueber das Verhalten der entnervten Muskeln gegen den constanten Strom. Sitzungsb. d. k. Akad. d. Wissensch. Math.-naturw. Cl., Wien, 1874, lxx, 144–150. ———. Ueber die Wirkungen des Muskelstromes auf einen secundären Stromkreis und über eine Eigenthümlichkeit von Inductionsströmen, die durch einen sehr schwachen primären Strom inducirt worden sind. *Ibid.*, 1875, lxxi, 13–26. *Also*. Reprint. ———. Ueber willkürliche und krampfhafte Bewegungen. Sitzungsb. d. k. Akad. d. Wissensch. Math.-naturw. Cl. 1877, Wien, 1878, lxxvi, 237–279, 4 pl.—**Brückner** (A.) Ueber das Ausbleiben der Zuckung gelähmter Nervenmuskel bei momentaner Unterbrechung des constanten electrischen Stromes. Deutsche Klinik, Berl., 1865. xvii, 291.— **Buch** (M.) O kolebanijach mushechnoi sili cheloviéka v techenii dnija. [Muscular force displayed in the course of a day.] Vrach, St. Petersb., 1883, iv, 690; 709. *Also*, *transl.*: Berl. klin. Wchnschr., 1884, xxi, 436–439.—**Budge** (J.) Ueber die Ursache der willkührlichen und unwillkührlichen Bewegungen. Org. f. d. ges. Heilk., Bonn, 1842–3, ii, 311–332. ———. Beweis, dass das Dubois'sche Gesetz vom Muskelstrom unhaltbar ist. Deutsche Klinik, Berl., 1861, xiii, 207–210. ———. Ueber das Dubois'sche Gesetz des Muskelstromes. *Ibid.*, 1862, xiv, 415–417.— **Bufalini** (G.) Dell' azione dei sali ammoniacali e

Muscle (*Physiology of*).

d' idrossilammina sulla eccitabilità muscolare. Boll. d. Soc. tra i cult. d. sc. med. in Siena, 1885, iii, 207–209.— ——. Sul decorso dell' eccitabilità muscolare in alcuni avvelenamenti acutissimi. *Ibid.*, 229–239, 1 pl.—**Bufalini** (G.) & **Tasi** (F.) Dell' influenza di alcuni alcaloidi sulla eccitabilità muscolare. *Ibid.* (1883), 1885, i, 89–91. *Also*: Riv. di chim. med. e farm., Torino, 1884, ii, 303–306.—**Burdon-Sanderson** (J.) On the electro-motive properties of muscle. Med. Press & Circ., Lond., 1877, xxiii, 37; 119. ——. A report on Prof. L. Hermann's recent researches on the electro-motive properties of muscle. Jour. Physiol., Lond., 1878–9, i, 196–212.—**Carlet** (G.) Sur le retour de la contractilité dans un muscle où cette propriété a disparu sous l'influence de courants d'induction énergiques. Compt. rend. Acad. d. sc., Par., 1877, lxxxiv, 193. ——. Expériences sur la tonicité musculaire. *Ibid*, 562–564. — **Carlisle** (A.) The Croonian lecture on muscular motion. Phil. Tr., Lond., 1805, xcv, 1–30. *Also*, Reprint.—**Carre.** De la contractilité idio-musculaire. Gaz. hebd. de méd., Par., 1868, 2. s., v, 161–165.—**Carson** (J.) On muscular motion. Liverpool M. Gaz., 1833, i, 113–116.—**Cash** (J. T.) Der Zuckungsverlauf als Merkmal der Muskelart. Arch. f. Physiol., Leipz., 1880, Suppl.-Bd., 147–160. *Also*, Reprint. *Also*, *transl.*: J. Anat. & Physiol., Lond., 1880–81 xv, 431–445.—**Chauveau** (A.) De la contraction produite par la rupture du courant de la pile, dans le cas d'excitation unipolaire des nerfs. Compt. rend. Acad. d. sc., Par., 1875, lxxxi, 1038–1041.—**Chauveau** (A.) & **Kaufmann.** Conséquences physiologiques de la détermination de l'activité spécifique des échanges ou du coefficient de l'activité nutritive et respiratoire dans les muscles en repos et en travail. *Ibid.*, 1887, civ, 1352–1359. ——. Expériences pour la détermination du coefficient d'activité nutritive et respiratoire des muscles en repos et en travail. *Ibid.*, 1126–1132. ——. Nouveaux documents sur les relations qui existent entre le travail chimique et le travail mécanique du tissu musculaire ; de l'activité nutritive et respiratoire des muscles qui fonctionnent physiologiquement sans produire de travail mécanique. *Ibid.*, 1763–1771. *Also*: France méd., Par., 1887, ii, 1165–1169.—**Chirone** (V.) La doppia attività muscolare e l' azione della chinina ; risporta ai Dott. A. Mosso e L. Pagliani. Riv. clin. di Bologna, 1876, 2. s., vi, 203; 225; 291.—**Chmoulevitch** (J.) *See* Schmulevitch, *infra*.—**Chvostek** (F.) Einige Bemerkungen über die knollenförmigen und wellenförmigen Muskelcontractionen. Allg. Wien. med. Ztg., 1883, xxviii, 26; 34; 151; 163.—**Cohnstein** (J.) Beitrag zur Lehre vom Muskeltonus. Allg. med. Centr.-Ztg., Berl., 1861, xxx, 801. ——. Kurze Uebersicht der Lehre des Muskeltonus. Arch. f. Anat., Physiol. u. wissensch. Med., Leipz., 1863, 165–172.—**Couty** (L.) Étude relative à l'influence de l'encéphale sur les muscles de la vie organique, et spécialement sur les organes cardio-vasculaires. Arch. de physiol. norm. et path., Par., 1876, 2. s., iii, 665–756.—**Cyon** (E.) Ueber den Tonus der willkürlichen Muskeln. Mélanges biol. Acad. imp. d. sc. de St-Pétersb., 1871, vii, 787–807. — **Czermak** (J.) Ueber secundäre Zuckung vom theilwiese gereizten Muskel aus. [*From*: Sitzungsb. d. k. Akad. d. Wissensch. Math.-naturw. Cl., 1857, Mai.] Untersuch. z. Naturl. d. Mensch. u. d. Thiere, Frankf. a. M., 1858, v, 141–144. ——. Vorläufige Mittheilung über das Myochronoskop und über das electromotorische Verhalten des Muskels während der sogenannten idiomuskulären Zuckung. Allg. med. Centr.-Ztg., Berl., 1861, xxx, 353.—**Danilevski** (V. J.) Termofiziologicheskija muskulov. [Thermophysiology of muscles.] Med. Vestnik, St. Petersb., 1879, xix, 251; 259. — **Danilevsky** (A.) Ueber die Abhängigkeit der Contractionsart der Muskeln von den Mengenverhältnissen einiger ihrer Bestandtheile ; Beitrag für eine zukünftige Theorie der Contraction. Ztschr. f. physiol. Chem., Strassb., 1882–3, vii, 124–160, 1 tab.—**Danilewsky** (B.) Ein Beitrag zur Physiologie der Muskelathmung. Centralbl. f. d. med. Wissensch., Berl., 1874, xii, 721–725. ——. Thermodynamische Untersuchungen der Muskel. Arch. f. d. ges. Physiol., Bonn, 1879–80, xxi, 109–152. *Also* [Abstr.] : Centralbl. f. d. med. Wissensch., Berl., 1879, xvii, 97–99. *Also*, *transl.* [Abstr.]: Med. Vestnik, St. Petersb., 1879, xix, 251; 259.—**Debrou** (T.) Mémoire sur les mouvements involontaires qui sont exécutés par des muscles de la vie animale. Arch. gén. de méd., Par., 1847, xv, 72; 222.—**Dionisio** (I.) Ricerche sulla influenza che diversi agenti esercitano sulla eccitabilità galvanica dei muscoli nell' uomo sano. Osservatore, Torino, 1887, xxxviii, 481.—**Donders.** Over de wetten van den electrotonus, getoetst aan den invloed van den constanten stroom op den n. vagus. Proc.-verb. v. de Vergad. d. k. Akad. v. Wetensch., Afd. Natuurk., Amst., 1869–70, no. 2, 2–6. — **Dowler** (B.) Experimental researches on the post-mortem contractibility of the muscles, with observations on the reflex theory. N. York J. M., 1846, vi, 305–339. *Also*, Reprint. — **Draper** (J. C.) The production of muscular force. Med. Rec., N. Y., 1867, ii, 247–249.—**Du Bois-Reymond** (E.) Note sur la loi du courant musculaire, et sur la modification qu'éprouve cette loi par l'effet de la contraction. Ann. de chim. et phys., Par., 1850, 3. s., xxx, 119–128. ——. Ueber

Muscle (*Physioloyy of*).

das angebliche Fehlen der unipolaren Zuckung bei dem Schliessungsinductionsschlage. Arch. f. Anat., Physiol. u. wissensch. Med., Leipz., 1860, 857. *Also*, Reprint. ——. Ueber das Gesetz des Muskelstromes, mit besonderer Berücksichtigung der M. gastroknemius des Frosches. Arch. f. Anat., Physiol. u. wissensch. Med., Leipz., 1863, 521; 649, 2 pl. *Also*, Reprint. ——. Ueber die Erscheinungsweise des Muskel- und Nervenstromes bei Anwendung der neuen Methoden zu deren Ableitung. Arch. f. Anat., Physiol. u. wissensch. Med., Leipz., 1867, 257–310. ——. Ueber die elektromotorische Kraft der Nerven und Muskeln. *Ibid.*, 1867, 417–497, 1 pl. ——. Neue Versuche über den Einfluss gewaltsamer Formveränderungen der Muskeln auf deren elektromotorische Kraft. Monatsb. d. k. Akad. d. Wissensch. zu Berl., 1867, 572–597. ——. Experimentalkritik der Entladungshypothese über die Wirkung von Nerv auf Muskel. *Ibid.*, 1874, 520–560. ——. Ueber den Einfluss körperlicher Nebenleitungen auf den Strom des M. gastroknemius des Frosches. Arch. f. Anat., Physiol. u. wissensch. Med., Leipz., 1871, 561–607. ——. Ueber die negative Schwankung des Muskelstromes bei der Zusammenziehung. *Ibid.*, 1873, 517: 1875, 610: 1876, 123; 342. — **Dupuy** (P.) De la contraction musculaire dans ses rapports avec la chaleur animale. Cong. méd. de France (Bordeaux, 1865), Par., 1866, iii, 859–874. ——. De la contraction musculaire dans ses rapports avec la circulation sanguine. Gaz. méd. de Par., 1866, 3. s., xxi, 623; 641. ——. De la chaleur et du mouvement musculaire. *Ibid.*, 1867, 3. s., xxii, 493; 524; 567; 580; 641; 673. ——. Considérations sur le mouvement musculaire. *Ibid.*, 1869, 3. s., xxiv, 4; 83; 99; 129. *Also*, Reprint. ——. De la fatigue musculaire. Gaz. méd. de Par., 1869, 3. s., xxiv, 435; 475; 542. ——. De certains phénomènes relatifs à la contraction musculaire. *Ibid.*, 1871, 3. s., xxvi, 155; 165.—**Edinger** (L.) Untersuchungen über die Zuckungscurve des menschlichen Muskels im gesunden und kranken Zustande. Ztschr. f. klin. Med., Berl., 1883, vi, 139–160.—**Engel** (J.) Ueber Muskelreizbarkeit. Ztschr. d. k.-k. Gesellsch. d. Aerzte zu Wien, 1849, v, 205; 252.—**Engelmann** (T. W.) Ueber den Ort der Reizung in the Muskelfaser bei Schliessung und Oeffnung eines constanten elektrischen Stromes. Jenaische Ztschr. f. Med. u. Naturw., Leipz., 1867, iii, 445–447. *Also*, *transl.*: Onderzoek. ged. in h. physiol. Lab. d. Utrecht. Hoogesch., 1867–8, 2. s., i, 267–270. ——. Ueber Reizung der Muskelfaser durch den constanten Strom. Jenaische Ztschr. f. Med. u. Naturw., Leipz., 1868, iv, 295–306. *Also*, *transl.*: Onderzoek. ged. in h. physiol. Lab. d. Utrecht. Hoogesch., 1868–9, 2. s., ii, 128–145. ——. Beiträge zur allgemeinen Muskel- und Nerven-Physiologie. Arch. f. d. ges. Physiol., Bonn, 1870, iii, 247; 403. ——. Ueber Reizung der Muskeln und Nerven mit discontinuirlichen electrischen Strömen. *Ibid.*, 1871, iv, 3–33, 2 pl. *Also*, *transl.*: Onderzoek. ged. in h. physiol. Lab. d. Utrecht. Hoogesch., 1872, 3. s., i, 103–145, 2 pl. ——. Bemerkungen zur Theorie der Sehnen- und Muskelverkürzung. Arch. f. d. ges. Physiol., Bonn, 1873–4, viii, 95–97. ——. Ueber den Einfluss des Blutes und den Nerven auf das elektromotorische Verhalten künstlicher Muskelquerschnitte. *Ibid.*, 1877, xv, 328–334. *Also*: Onderzoek. ged. in h. physiol. Lab. d. Utrecht. Hoogesch., 1878, 3. s., v, 13–22. *Also*, *transl.*: Arch. néerl. d. sc. exactes, Harlem, 1878, xiii, 428–436. ——. Vergleichende Untersuchungen zur Lehre von der Muskel- und Nervenelektricität. Onderzoek. ged. in h. physiol. Lab. d. Utrecht. Hoogesch., 1877, 3. s., iv, 281–324. *Also*, *transl.*: Arch. néerl. d. sc. exactes, etc., Harlem, 1878, xiii, 305–343. ——. Neue Untersuchungen über die mikroskopischen Vorgänge bei der Muskelcontraktion. Arch. f. d. ges. Physiol., Bonn, 1878, xviii, 1–25, 1 pl. *Also*: Onderzoek. ged. in h. physiol. Lab. d. Utrecht. Hoogesch., 1878–80, 3. s., v, 128–160, 1 pl. [pl. wanting]. *Also*, *transl.*: Arch. néerl. d. sc. exactes, etc., Harlem, 1878, xiii, 437–465, 1 pl. ——. Mikrometrische Untersuchungen an contrahirten Muskelfasern. Arch. f. d. ges. Physiol., Bonn, 1880, xxiii, 571–590. *Also*: Onderzoek. ged. in h. physiol. Lab. d. Utrecht. Hoogesch., 1881, 3. s., vi, 43–67. *Also*, *transl.*: Arch. néerl. d. sc. exactes, etc., Harlem, 1881, xvi, 279–302. ——. Ueber den faserigen Bau der contractilen Substanzen, mit besonderer Berücksichtigung der glatten und doppelt schräggestreiften Muskelfasern. Onderzoek. ged. in h. physiol. Lab. d. Utrecht. Hoogesch., 1881, 3. s., vi, 325–361, 1 pl. *Also*: Arch. f. d. ges. Physiol., Bonn, 1881, xxv, 538–565, 1 pl. ——. Ueber den Einfluss örtlicher Verletzungen auf die electrische Reizbarkeit der Muskeln. Nach Versuchen von J. W. van Loon van Iterson. Arch. f. d. ges. Physiol., Bonn, 1881-2. xxvi, 97–136.—**Enko** (P.) Beitrag zur Lehre von der Muskelcontraction. Arch. f. Physiol., Leipz., 1880, 95–111.—**Erb** (W.) Ueber electrotonische Erscheinungen am lebenden Menschen. Deutsches Arch. f. klin. Med., Leipz., 1867-8, iii, 513–528.—**Erlenmeyer** (A.) Ueber die "paradoxe Muskelcontraction". Centralbl. f. Nervenh., Coblenz, 1880, iii, 345–350.—**Essai** sur le mouvement musculaire. Rec. périod. d'obs. de méd., de chir. et pharm., Par., 1756, v, 436–443.—**Ewald** (J. R.) Aendert sich das Volumen eines Muskels bei der Contraction? Arch. f. d. ges. Physiol., Bonn, 1887, xli, 215–239.—**Exner** (S.) Ein

Muscle (*Physiology of*).

Schulversuch aus der Muskelphysiologie. Sitzungsb. d. k. Akad. d. Wissensch. Math.-naturw. Cl., Wien, 1874, lxx, 155. ——. Ueber optische Eigenschaften lebender Muskelfasern. Arch. f. d. ges. Physiol., Bonn, 1886-7, xl, 360-393, 2 pl. — **Féré** (C.) Contribution à la physiologie des mouvements volontaires. Compt. rend. Soc. de biol., Par., 1885, 8. s., ii, 223-227. — **Fick** (A.) Ueber theilweise Reizung der Muskelfaser. Untersuch. z. Naturl. d. Mensch. u. d. Thiere, Frankf. a. M., 1857, ii, 62-70. ——. Experimenteller Beitrag zur Lehre von der Erhaltung der Kraft bei der Muskelzusammenziehung. Untersuch. a. d. physiol. Lab. d. Züricher Hochschule, Wien, 1869, 1. Hft., 1-16. ——. Ueber das Abklingen des Elektrotonus. *Ibid.*, 129-137. ——. Die "Uebermaximalen" Zuckungen betreffend. Centralbl. f. d. med. Wissensch., Berl., 1869, vii, 611. ——. Ueber die Aenderung der Elasticität des Muskels während der Zuckung. Arch. f. d. ges. Physiol., Bonn, 1871, iv, 301-315, 1 pl. ——. Einige Demonstrationen zur Erläuterung der Muskelarbeit. Verhandl. d. phys.-med. Gesellsch. in Würzb., 1872, n. F., iii, 254-259, 1 pl. *Also:* Untersuch. a. d. physiol. Lab. in Würzb., 1873, 175-180, 1 pl. ——. Ueber die Wärmeentwickelung bei der Muskelzuckung. Arch. f. d. ges. Physiol., Bonn, 1877-8, xvi, 59-90. ——. Zur verschiedenen Erregbarkeit funktionell verschiedener Nervenmuskelpräparate. *Ibid.*, 1882-3, xxx, 596. ——. Myothermische Fragen und Versuche. Verhandl. d. phys.-med. Gesellsch. in Würzb., 1884, n. F., xviii, 299-321, 1 pl. ——. Versuche über Wärmeentwicklung im Muskel bei verschiedenen Temperaturen. *Ibid.*, 1885, n. F., xix, 61-72. ——. Myographische Versuche am lebenden Menschen. Arch. f. d. ges. Physiol., Bonn, 1887, xli, 176-189. — **Fieber** (F.) Ueber die elektro-muskuläre Kontraktilität und Sensibilität in verschiedenen Affektionen des Nervensystems und die Modifikationen ihrer Erregung. Wien. med. Wchnschr., 1868, xviii, 853; 869; 885. — **Fisher** (W. R.) The effects of tension and relaxation of muscle upon electro-muscular contractility. N. York M. J., 1873, xvii, 495-498. — **Fitzgerald** (G. F.) On the superficial tension of fluids and its possible relation to muscular contractions. Scient. Tr. Roy. Dubl. Soc., 1878, n. s., i, 95-99. — **von Fleischl** (E.) Ueber das Verhalten von Käfermuskeln gegen Reize. Centralbl. f. d. med. Wissensch., Berl., 1875, xiii, 469. ——. Ein mikrostroboskopischer Reizversuch. Arch. f. Physiol., Leipz., 1886, 67-71. — **Fordyce** (G.) The Croonian lecture on muscular motion. Phil. Tr., Lond., 1788, lxxviii, 23-36. — **Foster** (M.), jr. The elements of muscular strength. Fortnightly Rev., Lond., 1866, vi, 189-199. — **Frankland** (E.) Sur la source de la force musculaire. [Extrait de son ouvrage intitulé: Experimental researches in pure, applied and physical chemistry, London, 1878.] Monit. scient., Par., 1879, 3. s., ix, 467-493. — **Fraser** (W.) Description of a piece of mechanism on the supposed principle of muscular action. Lond. M. Gaz., 1848, n. s., vii, 366-370. — **Fredericq** (L.) Chaleur et travail musculaire. Rev. scient., Par., 1887, xxxix, 466. — **Freusberg.** Zur elektrischen Erregbarkeit gelähmter Muskeln. (Eine Theorie der Molecularbewegung im gesunden und gelähmten Muskel.) Arch. f. Psychiat., Berl., 1878-9, ix, 244; 434. — **von Frey** (M.) Versuche über den Stoffwechsel des Muskels. Arch. f. Physiol., Leipz., 1885, 533-562. ——. Reizungsversuche am unbelasteten Muskel. *Ibid.*, 1887, 195-203. — **Friedrich** (J. J.) Untersuchung des physiologischen Tetanus mit Hilfe des strompürfenden Nervmuskelpräparates. Sitzungsb. d. k. Akad. d. Wissensch. Math.-naturw. Cl. 1875, Wien, 1876, lxxii, 413-426. — **Fuchs** (F.) Ueber die Regel der Muskelzuckungen in der offenen galvanischen Kette. Ztschr. f. Biol., München, 1872, viii, 100-123. ——. Ueber die Gleichgewichtsbedingungen für den erregten und den unerregten Muskel. Arch. f. d. ges. Physiol., Bonn, 1873, vii, 421-440, 1 pl. ——. Ueber die Anwendung der mechanischen Wärmetheorie auf den Muskel. *Ibid.*, 1877, xv, 536-553. ——. Ueber die Gleichgewichtsbedingung für den Muskel. *Ibid.*, 553-572. ——. Ueber die Gleichungen der Muskelstatik mit Zugrundelegung der Förderung des kleinsten Stoffumsatzes. *Ibid.*, 1878-9, xix, 67-78. — **Gad** (J.) Ueber Zeichenwechsel der Stromesschwankung innerhalb des Latenzstadiums bei der Einzelzuckung des Froschgastroknemius. Arch. f. Physiol., Leipz., 1877, 37-65. ——. Ueber das Latenzstadium des Muskelelementes und des Gesammtmuskels. *Ibid.*, 1879, 250-268. — **Garreau** (P.) De l'action de la volonté sur les muscles. Rev. méd. franç. et étrang., Par., 1865, i, 321-327. — **Gaskell** (W. H.) Ueber die Aenderungen des Blutstroms in den Muskeln durch die Reizung ihrer Nerven. Arb. a. d. physiol. Anst. zu Leipz. (1876), 1877, xi, 45-88, 2 pl. — **von Gendre** (A.) Ueber das Verhalten eines dem Muskel zugeleiteten Stromes während des Tetanus. Arch. f. d. ges. Physiol., Bonn, 1884-5, xxxv, 49-54. — **Gluge.** Note sur la transformation de la contraction musculaire tonique en contraction rhythmique. Bull. Acad. roy. d. sc. de Belg., Brux., 1874, 2. s., xxxvii, 830. — **Godman** (J. D.) Notes on the actions of the muscular system. Phila. J. M. & Phys. Sc., 1825. x, 270-279. — **Goldzieher** (W.) Zur Kenntniss des Elektrotonus. Arch. f. d. ges. Physiol., Bonn, 1870, iii, 240-246. — **Gruenhagen** (A.) Ue-

Muscle (*Physiology of*).

ber die unipolare Zuckung. Ztschr. f. rat. Med., Leipz. u. Heidelb., 1865, 3. R., xxiv, 153-168. ——. Notiz über das Verhalten der negativen Stromesschwankung zur sogenannten parelectronomischen Schichte des natürlichen Muskelquerschnitts. *Ibid.*, 1867, 3. R., xxix, 285-287. ——. Ueber das Wesen und die Bedeutung der elektromotorischen Eigenschaften der Muskeln und der Nerven. *Ibid.*, 1868, 3. R., xxxi, 46: 1869, 3. R., xxxvi, 132. ——. Zur Theorie des physikalischen Electrotonus. *Ibid.*, 1868, 3. R., xxxiii, 256. ——. Ueber das zeitliche Verhalten von An- und Kat-Electrotonus während und nach der Einwirkung des polarisirenden Stromes. Arch. f. d. ges. Physiol., Bonn, 1871, iv, 547-550. ——. Versuche die secundäre Muskelzuckung betreffend. *Ibid.*, 1871-2, v, 119-122. — **Grützner** (P.) Zur Physiologie und Histologie der Skelettmuskeln. Breslau. aerztl. Ztschr., 1883, v, 257. ——. Zur Muskelphysiologie. *Ibid.*, 1887, ix, 1-3. — **Gruithuisen.** Resultate der Versuche über die Volumsverminderung, welche die Muskeln bey ihrer Contraction erleiden. Med.-chir. Ztg., Salzb., 1811, iv, 91-95. — **Gscheidlen** (R.) Ueber das Reductionsvermögen des thätigen Muskels. Arch. f. d. ges. Physiol., Bonn, 1873-4, viii, 506-519. — **Gulliver** (G.) On the state of the blood and muscles in animals killed by hunting and by fighting. Edinb. M. & S. J., 1848, lxx, 367-370. — **Hall** (M.) Ueber den Zustand der Irritabilität in den Muskeln gelähmter Glieder. Arch. f. Anat., Physiol. u. wissensch. Med., Berl., 1839, 200-219, 1 pl. ——. On the irritability of the muscular fibre. Lond. J. M., 1849, i, 710-714. — **Harless** (E.) Experimente zur Lehre von der Muskelirritabilität. Arch. f. Anat., Physiol. u. wissensch. Med., Berl., 1847, 228-231. ——. Die Muskelkrämpfe bei der Nervenvertrocknung. Ztschr. f. rat. Med., Leipz. u. Heidelb., 1859, 3. R., vii, 219-257. ——. Untersuchungen an der Muskelsubstanz. Sitzungsb. d. k.-bayer. Akad. d. Wissensch. zu München, 1860, 93. ——. Ueber physikalische und chemische Vorgänge in der Muskelsubstanz. Deutsche Klinik, Berl., 1860, xii, 160-163. — **Heidenhain** (R.) Die Wiederherstellung der erloschenen Muskelerregbarkeit durch constante galvanische Ströme. Allg. med. Centr.-Ztg., Berl., 1856, xxv, 545-547. ——. Noch ein Wort, die Wiederherstellung der erloschenen Muskelerregbarkeit betreffend. *Ibid.*, 585-587. ——. Historisches und Experimentelles über Muskeltonus. Arch. f. Anat., Physiol. u. wissensch. Med., Berl., 1856, 200-229, 1 pl. ——. Beitrag zur Kenntniss des Zuckungsgesetzes. Arch. f. physiol. Heilk., Stuttg., 1857, n. F., i, 442-481. ——. Vorläufige Mittheilung einiger Resultate, betreffend die Wärme-Entwicklung in den Muskeln bei ihrer Thätigkeit. Centralbl. f. d. med. Wissensch., Berl., 1863, i, 545-547. ——. Ueber Ad. Fick's experimentellen Beweis für die Gültigkeit des Gesetzes von der Erhaltung der Kraft bei der Muskelzusammenziehung. Nach Versuchen der Herren Studirenden Leopold Landau und Carl Pacully mitgetheilt von . . . Arch. f. d. ges. Physiol., Bonn, 1869, ii, 423-432. — **Heidenhain** (R.) & **Colberg** (A.) Versuche über den Tonus des Blasenschliessmuskels. Arch. f. Anat., Physiol. u. wissensch. Med., Berl., 1858, 437-452, 1 pl. — **Heidenreich.** Die Muskelcontraction scheint uns dennoch ein imponderables Agens zu entwickeln. N. med.-chir. Ztg., München, 1846, i, 97-103. — **Heinike.** Versuche über die Irritabilität der Muskeln und deren Zusammenhang mit der Todtenstarre. Deutsche Klinik, Berl., 1858, x, 420-422. — **Heinrich** (J.) Zur Funktionsfähigkeit der Muskel und Sehnen. Wien. med. Presse, 1872, xiii, 1212-1214. — **Heitzmann** (C.) Muscle- and nerve-action. J. Nerv. & Ment. Dis., N. Y., 1884, n. s., ix, 232-241. — **Helmholtz** (H.) Ueber den Stoffverbrauch bei der Muskelaktion. Arch. f. Anat., Physiol. u. wissensch. Med., Berl., 1845, 72-83. ——. Messungen über den zeitlichen Verlauf der Zuckung animalischer Muskeln und die Fortpflanzungsgeschwindigkeit der Reizung in den Nerven. *Ibid.*, 1850, 276-364, 1 pl. — **Henke** (W.) Die absolute Muskelkraft; Antikritik. Ztschr. f. rat. Med., Leipz. u. Heidelb., 1868, 3. R., xxxiii, 148-152. — **Henry** (W. C.) A critical and experimental inquiry into the relations subsisting between nerve and muscle. Edinb. M. & S. J., 1832, xxxvii, 11-20. *Also,* Reprint. — **Hering** (E.) Ueber die Methoden zur Untersuchung der polaren Wirkungen des elektrischen Stromes im quergestreiften Muskel. Sitzungsb. d. k. Akad. d. Wissensch. Math.-naturw. Cl., Wien, 1879, lxxix, 3. Abth., 237-262. ——. Ueber Veränderungen des elektromotorischen Verhaltens der Muskeln in Folge elektrischer Reizung; nach Untersuchungen von E. Hering und W. Biedermann. *Ibid.*, 1884, lxxxviii, 3. Abth., 415-437. *Also,* Reprint. ——. Ueber Du Bois-Reymond's Untersuchung der secundär-elektromotorischen Erscheinungen am Muskel. Sitzungsb d. k. Akad. d. Wissensch. Math.-naturw. Cl., Wien, 1884, lxxxviii, 3. Abth., 445-471. *Also,* Reprint. — **Hermann** (L.) Beitrag zur Erledigung der Tonusfrage. Arch. f. Anat., Physiol. u. wissensch. Med., Leipz., 1861, 350-360. ——. Ueber das Verhältniss der Muskelleistungen zu der Stärke der Reize. *Ibid.*, 369-393. ——. Weitere Untersuchungen über die Ursache der electromotorischen Erscheinungen an Muskeln und Nerven. Arch. f. d. ges. Physiol., Bonn, 1870, iii, 15-46: 1871, iv, 149-182.

Muscle (*Physiology of*).

——. Kleinere Beiträge zur Lehre von der Muskelstarre. *Ibid.*, 182–195. ——. Ueber die Abnahme der Muskelkraft während der Contraction. *Ibid.*, 195–201. ——. Weitere Untersuchungen über den Electrotonus, insbesondere über die Erstreckung desselben auf die intramusculären Nervenenden. *Ibid.*, 1873, vii, 301–322, 1 pl. ——. Experimentelles und Kritisches über Electrotonus. *Ibid.*, 1873-4, viii, 258–275. ——. Entgegnung an Herrn T. W. Engelmann. *Ibid.*, 275–277. ——. Zur Aufklärung und Abwehr. *Ibid.*, 1874, ix, 28–34. ——. Braucht der bei der Anlegung eines künstlichen Querschnitts auftretende Muskelstrom zu seiner Entwickelung Zeit? Centralbl. f. d. med. Wissensch., Berl., 1875, xiii, 705–708. ——. Neue Messungen über die Fortpflanzungsgeschwindigkeit der Erregung im Muskel. Arch. f. d. ges. Physiol., Bonn, 1875, x, 48–55. ——. Bemerkung zur Fortpflanzungsgeschwindigkeit der Erregung im Muskel. *Ibid.*, 639. ——. Ueber den Verkürzungsrückstand der Muskeln. *Ibid.*, 1875-6, xiii, 370–372. ——. Versuche mit dem Fall-Rheotom über die Erregungsschwankung des Muskels. *Ibid.*, 1877, xv, 233–245, 1 pl. ——. Untersuchungen über die Actionsströme des Muskels. *Ibid.*, 1877-8, xvi, 191–262. ——. Ueber den Actionsstrom der Muskeln im lebenden Menschen. *Ibid.*, 410-420. ——. Ueber die Abhängigkeit des Absterbens der Muskeln von der Länge ihrer Nerven. *Ibid.*, 1880, xxii, 37-40. ——. Ueber das Verhalten der optischen Constanten des Muskels bei der Erregung, der Dehnung und der Contraction. *Ibid.*, 240–251. ——. Untersuchungen zur Lehre von der electrischen Muskel- und Nervenreizung. *Ibid.*, 1882-3, xxx, 1: 1883, xxxi, 99. ——. Ueber das galvanische Wogen des Muskels. *Ibid.*, 1886, xxxix, 597–623.—**Herroun** (E. F.) & **Yeo** (G. F.) Note on the sound accompanying the single contraction of skeletal muscle. J. Physiol., Lond., 1885, vi, 287–292.—**Hingston** (W. H.) Muscular fatigue. Brit.-Am. J., Montreal, 1861, ii, 4–7.—**Hohnbaum.** Unwillkührliche Muskelbewegung in sonst gelähmten Theilen. Med. Convers.-Bl., Hildburgh., 1831, ii, 364–366.—**Holmgren** (F.) Ueber die negative Schwankung des Muskelstromes im nervenfreien Muskelgewebe Centralbl. f. d. med Wissensch., Berl., 1864, ii, 180 ——. Ueber die elektrische Stromschwankung am thätigen Muskel. *Ibid.*, 291–293. ——. Om den verkliga naturen af den "positiva strömfluctuationen" id en enkel muskelryckning. Upsala Läkaref. Förh., 1866-7, ii, 3. Hft., 160–173. *Also, transl.*: Arch. f. Anat., Physiol. u. wissensch. Med., Leipz., 1871, 237–251. ——. Ur muskelphysiologiens senaste utvecklingshistoria. Upsala Läkaref. Förh., 1868-9, iv, 657–691.—**Home** (E.) The Croonian lecture on muscular motion. Phil. Tr., Lond., 1795, lxxxv, 1, 1 pl. ; 202 : 1796, lxxxvi, 1, 1 pl. *Also, transl. of* pp. 202–220: Arch. f. d. Physiol., Halle, 1797, ii, 87–108.—**Horsley** (V.) & **Schäfer** (E. A.) Experiments on the character of the muscular contractions which are evoked by excitation of the various parts of the motor tract. J. Physiol., Lond., 1886, vii, 96–110, 1 pl.—**Houghton** (S.) Observations on the rate at which muscular action takes place, and the quantity of work stored up in muscle deducible from that rate. Brit. & For. M.-Chir. Rev., Lond., 1863, xxxi, 276–279. ——. Source of muscular power. Med. Times & Gaz., Lond., 1867, ii, 269.—**Humilewski** (G.) Ueber den Einfluss der Muskelcontractionen der Hinterextremität auf ihre Blutcirculation. Arch. f. Physiol., Leipz., 1886, 126–148, 1 pl. —**Jacks** (T. M.) Muscular contraction; its rationale. South. J. M. & Phys. Sc., Nashville, 1854, ii, 237–244.—**Jendrássik** (A. E.) Erster Beitrag zur Analyse der Zuckungswelle der quergestreiften Muskelfaser. Arch. f. Anat., Physiol. u. wissensch. Med., Leipz., 1874, v, 513–597. ——. Ueber die Ursachen der in den quergestreiften Muskeln unter der Einwirkung constanter Ströme auftretenden Strömungserscheinungen. Arch. f. Physiol., Leipz., 1879, 300–341.—**Jones** (T. W.) Muscle a neuro-magnetic apparatus. Lond. M. Gaz., 1843-4, xxxiii, 77.—**Jürgensen** (T.)-Ueber den Tonus der willkürlichen Muskeln. Stud. d. physiol. Inst. zu Bresl., Leipz., 1861, i, 139–162.—**Kilner** (W. J.) Some experiments upon, and explanatory of, the physical properties of muscle. St. Thomas's Hosp. Rep. 1884, Lond., 1886, n. s., xiv, 43–59.—**Knorz** (F.) Die Grösse der absoluten Muskelkraft aus Versuchen neu berechnet. Ztschr. f. rat. Med., Leipz. u. Heidelb., 1865, 3. R., xxiv, 247–260, 2 pl. —**Krause** (W.) Die Contraction der Muskelfaser. Arch. f. d. ges. Physiol., Bonn, 1873, vii, 508–514.—**Krauss.** Die Extensoren in ihrem Verhältniss zum normalen psychischen Impulse und zur krankhaften Affection des Sensoriums. Allg. Ztschr. f. Psychiat., etc., Berl., 1853, x, 89–96.—**von Kries** (J.) Zur Kenntniss der willkürlichen Muskelthätigkeit. Arch. f. Physiol., Leipz., 1886, Suppl.-Bd., 1–16.—**Kronecker** (H.) Ueber die Form des minimalen Tetanus. *Ibid.*, 1877, 571–573.—**Kronecker** (H.) & **Hall** (G. S.) Die willkürliche Muskelaction. *Ibid.*, 1879, Suppl.-Bd., 11–47.—**Kronecker** (H.) & **Stirling** (W.) Ueber die sogenannte Anfangszuckung. *Ibid.*, 1878, 394–400.—**Kühne** (W.) Recherches expérimentales sur l'excitabilité des muscles et des nerfs. Compt. rend. Soc. de biol. 1858, Par., 1859, 3. s., i, 81. ——. Ueber di-

Muscle (*Physiology of*).

recte und indirecte Muskelreizung mittelst chemischer Agentien. Ein Beitrag zur Lehre von der selbständigen Reizbarkeit der Muskelfaser. Arch. f. Anat., Physiol. u. wissensch. Med., Leipz., 1859, 213–253. ——. Ueber Muskelzuckungen ohne Betheiligung der Nerven. *Ibid.*, 314–333. ——. Ueber die chemische Reizung der Muskeln und Nerven und ihre Bedeutung für die Irritabilitätsfrage. *Ibid.*, 1860, 315–354. ——. Ueber das Verhalten des Muskels zum Nerven. Untersuch. a. d. physiol. Inst. d. Univ. Heidelb., 1879, iii, 1–148, 1 pl.—**Kupffer** (C.) Ueber das Hemmungsvermögen der Muskeln gegenüber lokaler Erregung, nach Prof. Dr. Fick. Ztschr. f. rat. Med., Leipz. u. Heidelb., 1858, 3. R., ii, 160–162, 1 pl.—**Laborde** (J.-V.) Température des muscles pendant la contraction. Progrès méd., Par., 1880, viii, 50. ——. Modifications de la température liées au travail musculaire ; l'échauffement primitif du muscle en travail est indépendant de la circulation. Compt. rend. Soc. de biol., Par., 1887, 8. s., iv, 304–307.—**Lamansky** (S.) Neue Versuche, die übermaximalen Zuckungen betreffend. Centralbl. f. d. med. Wissensch., Berl., 1869, vii, 17; 804. ——. Ueber die negative Stromesschwankung des arbeitenden Muskels. Arch f. d. ges. Physiol., Bonn, 1870, iii, 193–204.—**Latham.** On the death-struggle of a muscular fibre. Med. Times & Gaz., Lond., 1880, ii, 709.—**Laulanié** (F.) Note sur les phénomènes histologiques de la secousse et de l'onde musculaires et leur signification physiologique. Gaz. méd.-chir. de Toulouse, 1884, xvi, 279–281.—**Lautenbach** (B. F.) The idio-muscular contraction. Phila. M. Times, 1879-80, x, 641–643.—**Lavdowsky** (M.) Ueber die Contractilität des Muskelprotoplasma. Centralbl. f. d. med. Wissensch., Berl., 1871, ix, 769–772.—**Leber** (T.) Ueber den Einfluss der Leistung mechanischer Arbeit auf die Ermüdung der Muskeln. Ztschr. f. rat. Med., Leipz. u. Heidelb., 1863, 3. s., xviii, 262–288, 2 pl.—**Lee** (F. S.) Ueber die elektrischen Erscheinungen, welche die Muskelzuckung begleiten. Arch. f. Physiol., Leipz., 1887, 204–223.—**Legros & Onimus.** De la contraction des muscles de la vie végétative. J. de l'anat. et physiol., etc., Par., 1869, vi, 413–436. ——. Musculaire (tissu) ; physiologie. Dict. encycl. d. sc. méd., Par., 1876, 2. s., x, 1–696.—**Lesshaft** (P.) De l'influence sur le système nerveux, des conditions mécaniques qui sont faites à l'exercice musculaire. Internat. Monatschr. f. Anat. u. Histol., Leipz., 1886, iii, 81–102.—**Letheby** (H.) Remarks on Mr. Wharton Jones' opinion of muscle being a neuro-magnetic apparatus. Lond. Physiol. J., 1843-4, i, 77-79.—**Liebig** (G.) Ueber die Respiration der Muskeln. Arch. f. Anat., Physiol. u. wissensch. Med., Berl., 1850, 393–416.—**von Liebig** (J.) Ueber die Gährung und die Quelle der Muskelkraft. Sitzungsb. d. k.-bayer. Akad. d. Wissensch. zu München, 1869, ii, 323; 393. *Also, transl.*: Monit. scient., Par., 1871, xiii, 894: 1872, xiv. 7.—**Loeb** (J.) Muskelthätigkeit als Maass psychischer Thätigkeit. Arch. f. d. ges. Physiol., Bonn, 1886, xxxix, 592–597.—**Longet** (A.) & **Matteucci** (C.) Sur la relation qui existe entre le sens du courant électrique et les contractions musculaires dues à ce courant. Ann. méd.-psych., Par., 1844, iv, 317–327.—**Lovén** (C.) Om naturen af de normala muskelkontraktionerna. (C. r. Sur la nature des contractions musculaires volontaires.) Nord. med. Ark., Stockholm, 1881, xiii, no. 5, 1–8. ——. Ueber den Muskelton bei elektrischer Reizung sowie über einige in Zusammenhang damit stehende elektrisch-akustische Erscheinungen. Arch. f. Physiol., Leipz., 1881, 363–381.—**Luchsinger** (B.) Ueber W. Preyer's: "Myophysische Untersuchungen". Arch. f. d. ges. Physiol., Bonn, 1872, vi, 395–403. ——. Antwort auf W. Preyer's Rechtfertigung seiner "Myophysischen Untersuchungen". *Ibid.*, 642–646. ——. Kritisches und Experimentelles zu Herrn W. Preyer's myophysischem Gesetz. *Ibid.*, 1873-4, viii, 538–550. ——. Zur verschiedenen Erregbarkeit functionell verschiedener Nervmuskelapparate. *Ibid.*, 1882, xxviii, 60. — **Lukjanow** (S. M.) Wärmelieferung und Arbeitskraft des blutleeren Säugethiermuskels. *Ibid.*, 1886, Suppl.-Bd., 117–183, 1 pl.—**McGiffert** (W. C.) On the relations of nerve and muscle. Med. Rec., N. Y., 1880, xviii, 275.—**Mackall** (L.) The action of the voluntary muscles. Buffalo M. & S. J., 1861-2, i, 307; 335.—**McLaurin** (H. N.) A view of the present state of our knowledge of the question of muscular irritability. Edinb. M. J., 1863-4, ix, 22–36.—**Marey.** Nature de la contraction dans les muscles de la vie animale. Compt. rend. Acad. d. sc., Par., 1860, lxii, 1171–1175. ——. Études graphiques sur la nature de la contraction musculaire. J. de l'anat. et physiol., etc., Par., 1866, iii, 225; 403. ——. De la contractilité et de la secousse musculaire. Gaz. hebd. de méd., Par., 1867, 2. s., iv, 754 : 1868, 2. s., v, 21; 101; 131. ——. Phénomènes intimes de la contraction musculaire. Compt. rend. Acad. d. sc., Par., 1868, lxvi, 202-205. ——. Rôle de l'élasticité dans la contraction musculaire. *Ibid.*, 293. ——. Des variations électriques des muscles et du cœur en particulier, étudiées au moyen de l'électromètre de M. Lippmann. *Ibid.*, 1876, lxxxii, 975–977. ——. La décharge électrique de la torpille comparée à la contraction musculaire. Cong. périod. internat. d. sc. méd. Compt.-rend., Genève, 1878, 92–102.—**Martini.** Nota sul meccanismo della contra-

Muscle (*Physiology of*).

zione muscolare. Rendic. Accad. med.-chir. di Napoli, 1853, vii, 31–34.—**Matteucci** (C.) Electro-physiological researches; physical and chemical phenomena of muscular contraction. Phil. Tr., Lond., 1857, cxlvii, 129–143.—**Mayer.** Ueber die spontane Bewegung der Muskelfibrillen der niedern Thiere. Arch. f. Anat., Physiol. u. wissensch. Med., Berl., 1854, 214–219. ———. Ueber spontane Bewegung der Muskelfibrille. *Ibid.*, 1856, 321.—**Meissner** (G.) Ueber das Verhalten der muskulösen Faserzellen im contrahirten Zustande. Ztschr. f. rat. Med., Leipz. u. Heidelb., 1858, 3 R., ii, 316–320, 1 pl. ———. Zur Kenntniss des elektrischen Verhaltens des Muskels. *Ibid.*, 1861, 3. R., xii, 344–353.—**Meissner** (G.) & **Cohn** (F.) Ueber das elektrische Verhalten des thätigen Muskels. *Ibid.*, 1862, 3. R., xv, 27–59, 2 pl.—**Mendelssohn** (M.) Étude sur l'excitation latente du muscle chez la grenouille et chez l'homme, à l'état sain et à l'état pathologique. *In:* Marey (E.-J.) Physiol. exp., 8°, Par., 1880, 99–153. *Also* [Abstr.]: Compt. rend. Acad. d. sc., Par., 1879, lxxxix, 367–370. *Also* [Abstr.]: Compt. rend. Soc. de biol. 1879, Par., 1880, 7. s., i, 279–282. *Also* [Abstr.]: Gaz. méd. de Par., 1879, 6. s., i, 460; 544. ———. Ueber die paradoxe Muskelcontraction. St. Petersb. med. Wchnschr., 1881, vi, 81–83. ———. Quelques recherches relatives à la mécanique du muscle. Gaz. méd. de Par., 1881, 6. s., iii, 657. *Also:* Compt. rend. Soc. de biol. 1881, Par., 1882, 7. s., iii, 303–307. ———. Sur le tonus des muscles striés. Gaz. méd. de Par., 1881, 6. s., iii, 619. *Also:* Compt. rend. Soc. de biol 1881, Par., 1882, 7. s., iii, 281–284. ———. Influence de l'excitabilité du muscle sur son travail mécanique. Compt. rend Acad. d. sc., Par., 1882, xcv, 1234–1237.—**Merkel** (F.) Ueber die Contraction der gestreiften Muskelfaser. Arch. f. mikr. Anat., Bonn, 1880–81, xix. 649–702, 1 pl.—**Meyer** (A. B.) Die übermaximale Zuckung. Centralbl. f. d. med. Wissensch., Berl., 1868, vi, 721–725. ———. Kritik der "neuen Versuche" des Herrn S. Lamansky, die übermaximale Zuckung betreffend. *Ibid.*, 1869, vii, 161–164. ———. Die Muskelzuckung in ihrer Abhängigkeit von der Stärke elektrischer Nervenreizung. Untersuch. a. d. physiol. Lab. d. zürich. Hochsch., Wien, 1869, 36–40.—**Milrad** (K.) Ueber den Einfluss veränderter Muskelerregbarkeit auf die Folgen der mechanischen Muskelreizung. Arch. f. exper. Path. u. Pharmakol., Leipz., 1885–6, xx, 217–242.—**Minot** (C. S.) Die Bildung der Kohlensäure innerhalb des ruhenden und erregten Muskels. Arb. a. d. physiol. Anst. zu Leipz. (1876), 1877, xi, 1–24. — **Moilin.** Expérience servant à établir les lois fondamentales de la contraction musculaire. Compt. rend. Soc. de biol. 1858, Par , 1859, 3. s., i, 181–183.—**Mommsen** (J.) Beitrag zur Kenntniss des Muskeltonus. Arch. f. path. Anat., etc., Berl., 1885, ci, 22–36.—**Montgomery** (E.) Zur Lehre von der Muskelcontraktion. Arch. f. d. ges. Physiol., Bonn, 1881, xxv, 497–537, 1 pl.—**Morat & Toussaint.** Variations de l'état électrique des muscles dans la contraction volontaire et le tétanos artificiel, étudiées à l'aide de la patte galvanoscopique. Compt. rend. Acad. d. sc., Par., 1876, lxxxii, 1269–1272. ———. Influence de la fatigue sur les variations de l'état électrique des muscles pendant le tétanos artificiel. *Ibid.*, lxxxiii, 155–159. ———. Variations de l'état électrique des muscles dans le tétanos produit par le passage du courant continu, étudiées à l'aide de la contraction induite. *Ibid.*, 834–836. ———. Variations de l'état électrique des muscles dans les différents modes de contraction. Arch. de physiol. norm. et path., Par., 1877, 2. s., iv, 156–182.—**Müller** (J. W.) Ueber die Präexistenz des Muskelstromes und über die Veränderungen der Stromverhältnisse nach der Entblössung. Arch. f. Anat., Physiol. u. wissensch. Med., Leipz., 1870, 208–226.—**Munk** (H.) Forsøg til en Beregning af Muskelkraften. Eyr, Christiania, 1827, ii, 31–45.—**Munk** (H.) Nachweis des Muskelstromes am unenthäuteten Frosche ohne Aetzung der Haut. Arch. f. Anat., Physiol. u. wissensch. Med., Leipz., 1869, 649–653. ———. Ueber die Abhängigkeit des Absterbens der Muskeln von der Länge ihrer Nerven. Arch. f. Physiol., Leipz., 1880, 169–175.—**Murray** (R. M.) The physiological effect of thermal stimuli on non-striped muscular tissue. Tr. Edinb. Obst. Soc., 1885–6, xi, 55–68, 3 diag.—**Nasse.** Ueber eine besondere Einwirkung des Wassers auf die Muskelreizbarkeit. Deutsches Arch. f. d. Physiol., Halle, 1816, ii, 78–85.—**Navalichin** (J.-G.) Genèse et mort des fibres musculaires chez l'animal supérieur adulte à l'état normal. Arch. slaves de biol., Par., 1886, i, 134–138. ———. Myothermische Untersuchungen. Arch. f d. ges. Physiol., Bonn, 1876–7, xiv, 293–329, 1 pl. —**Nawrocki** (F.) Beiträge zum Stoffwechsel im Muskel. Centralbl. f. d. med. Wissensch., Berl., 1865. iii, 417: 1866, iv, 385. *Also,* Reprint. — **Neumann.** Zur Muskelwirkungs-Frage. Med. Ztg., Berl., 1858, n. F., i, 210. — **Neumann** (E.) Ueber das verschiedene Verhalten gelähmter Muskeln gegen den constanten und inducirten Strom und die Erklärung desselben. Deutsche Klinik, Berl., 1864, xvi, 65–69. ———. Eine Versuchsreihe, betreffend das Absterben der Erregbarkeit in Muskeln und Nerven. Arch. f. Anat., Physiol. u. wissensch. Med., Leipz., 1864, 554–567.—**Nigetiet** (F.) & **Hepner** (S.) Versuche über die Abhängig-

Muscle (*Physiology of*).

keit des Stoffumsatzes in den thätigen Muskeln von ihrer Spannung. Arch. f. d. ges. Physiol., Bonn, 1870, iii, 574–578.—**Nikolaides** (R.) Ueber die Curve, nach welcher die Erregbarkeit des Muskels abfällt. Arch. f. Physiol., Leipz., 1886, Suppl.-Bd., 27–30.—**Nipher** (F. E.) On the mechanical work done by a muscle before exhaustion. Am. J. Sc. & Arts, N. Haven, 1875, 3. s., ix, 130–137.—**Norris** (R.) Researches on muscular irritability and the relations which exist between muscle, nerve, and blood. J. Anat. & Physiol., Lond., 1866–7, i, 217–236.—**Onimus**, Expériences sur un supplicié. Gaz. hebd. de méd., Par., 1875, 2. s., xii, 246.—**Orschansky** (S.) Ueber die Reactionszeit eines willkürlichen Impulses und einer willkürlichen Hemmung. Neurol. Centralbl., Leipz., 1887, vi, 265–267.—**Orshanski** (I. G.) O vlijanii raboti i ustalosti na suchojilnie refleksi i elektricheskuju vozbudimost mushts i nervov u chelovieka. [Influence of labor and rest on tendons, and electrical excitability of muscles and nerves.] Vrach, St. Petersb., 1884, v, 523.— **Oughton** (T.) Composition, resolution, and abeyance of secondary perceptions. Lancet, Lond., 1882, ii, 1068.—**Park** (J. R.) On the laws of muscular motion. J. Sc. & Arts, 1816 [Am. ed.], N. Y., 1817, ii, [223–]246. ———. An inquiry into the varieties of muscular motion, and their connection with peculiarity of texture in the moving organ. *Ibid.*, 1817 [Am. ed.], N. Y., 1818, iii, 296–315.—**Pasternatzky** (J.) Recherches expérimentales sur l'origine du tremblement qui accompagne les mouvements volontaires, ou tremblement intentionnel. Arch. de physiol. norm. et path., Par., 1881, 2. s., viii, 328–342.—**Pawlow** (J.) Wie die Muschel ihre Schaale öffnet; Versuche und Fragen zur allgemeinen Muskel- und Nervenphysiologie. Arch. f. d. ges. Physiol., Bonn, 1885, xxxvii, 6–31, 4 diag.—**Peckham** (G.) Rhythmical myoclonus. Arch. Med., N. Y., 1883, ix, 97–117.—**Pflüger** (E.) Vorläufige Mittheilung über die Ursache des Ritterschen (Oeffnungs-) Tetanus. Allg. med. Centr.-Ztg., Berl., 1859, xxviii, 17–19. ———. Ueber die Ursache des Oeffnungstetanus. (Ein Beitrag zur Lehre vom Gesetze der Zuckung.) Arch. f. Anat., Physiol. u. wissensch. Med., Leipz., 1859, 133–149.—**Pfündel.** Ueber krankhafte Irritabilität oder unwillkührliche Muskelbewegung und ihre Behandlung. J. d. pract. Arznk. u. Wundarznk., Jena, 1796, ii, 2. St., 243–270.—**Pick** (A.) Zur Lehre von der Wirkungen der mechanischen Muskelreizung. Prag. med. Wchnschr., 1884, ix, 123; 126; 136; 145.—**Plateau** (F.) Recherches sur la force absolue des muscles des invertébrés. 1re partie: Force absolue des muscles adducteurs des mollusques lamellibranches. Bull. Acad. roy. d. sc. de Belg., Brux., 1883, 3. s., vi, 226–259, 1 pl. ———. Recherches sur la force absolue des muscles des invertébrés (deuxième partie). Force absolue des muscles fléchisseurs de la pince chez les crustacés décapodes. *Ibid.*, 1884, 3. s., vii, 450–474, 1 pl.—**Poole** (T. W.) On the necessity for a modification of certain physiological doctrines regarding the inter-relations of nerve and muscle. N. Eng. M. Month., Bridgeport, Conn., 1887–8, viii, 74; 109.—**Poore** (G. V.) On the influence of the continuous galvanic current over voluntary muscular action. Practitioner, Lond., 1873, x, 37–43.—**Powell** (T.) New theories concerning the construction and action of the muscular and nervous elements. Med. Advocate, N. Y., 1886, iii, 89–93.—**Prévost & Dumas.** Mémoire sur les phénomènes qui accompagnent la contraction de la fibre musculaire. J. de physiol. expér., Par., 1823, iii, 301–344.—**Preyer** (W.) Rétablissement de l'irritabilité des muscles roides. Rec. d. trav. Soc. méd. allem. de Par., 1864–5, 37–53. *Also* [Abstr.]: Gaz. méd. de Par., 1864, 3. s., xix, 812. *Also, transl.* [Abstr.]: Centralbl. f. d. med. Wissensch., Berl., 1864, ii, 769–773. ———. Myophysische Untersuchungen. Arch. f. d. ges. Physiol., Bonn, 1871–2, v, 294; 483, 1 pl. : 1872, vi, 237; 567. ———. Erklärung. Arch. f. d. ges. Physiol., Bonn, 1873, vii, 200. [*See, also, supra,* Bernstein (J.)] ———. Ueber elektrische Muskelreizung. Jenaische Ztschr. f. Naturw., Leipz., 1874, viii, 281–292. ———. Ueber Muskelruhe und Gedankenlesen. Sitzungsb. d. Jenaisch. Gesellsch. f. Med. u. Naturw., 1885, 1–19.—**Quetelet** (A.) Considérations sur la théorie de la population, et expériences sur la force musculaire de l'homme aux différens âges. Ann. d'hyg., Par., 1834, xii, 294–311.—**Quinquaud** (C.-E.) De la force motrice, mesurée au dynamomètre lorsqu'on excite directement le nerf ou le muscle. Compt. rend. Soc. de biol., Par., 1885, 8. s., ii, 14–17. ———. Expériences sur la contraction musculaire et la chaleur animale. *Ibid.*, 1886, 8. s., iii, 410.—**Radcliffe** (C. B.) The physical theory of muscular contraction (a sketch of the argument with alterations and additions). Med. Times & Gaz., Lond., 1855, n. s., x, 591; 615; 639. *Also,* Reprint.—**Ranke** (J.) Untersuchung über die chemischen Bedingungen der Ermüdung des Muskels. No. 1 u. 2. Arch. f. Anat., Physiol. u. wissensch. Med., Leipz., 1863, 422: 1864, 320. ———. Das Gesetz des Electrotonus. Centralbl. f. d. med. Wissensch., Berl., 1867, v, 257–259.—**Ranvier.** Note sur les vaisseaux sanguins et la circulation dans les muscles rouges. Compt. rend. Soc. de biol. 1874, Par., 1875, 6. s., i, 28–31. — **Redding** (J.) Muscular contractility. Proc. Am. Soc. Micr., Buffalo, 1881, iv, 17–27, 1 pl. *Also:* Cincin. M. News, 1882, n.

Muscle (*Physiology of*).

s., xi, 436-446. — **Regnard** (P.) Sur la cause de la rigidité des muscles soumis aux très hautes pressions. Compt. rend. Soc. de biol., Par., 1884, 8. s., i, pt. 2, 310. ————. Les phénomènes de la vie sous les hautes pressions ; la contraction musculaire. Compt. rend. Soc. de biol., Par., 1887, 8. s., iv, 265-269.—**Regnauld** (J.) Recherches sur les courants musculaires. Compt. rend. Acad. d. sc., Par., 1854, xxxviii, 890-894. *Also*, Reprint.— **Reinbold** (T.) Einige Bemerkungen über die bei der Bewegung des Muskels in Betracht kommende Kraft, u. die Anwendung des Begriffs "activ u. passiv" auf die Bewegung des Muskels. Schmidt's Jahrb., Leipz., 1846, l, .82-86.— **Remak** (R.) Ueber die Verdickung der Muskeln durch constante galvanische Ströme. Deutsche Klinik, Berl., 1857, ix, 435.—**Renaut** (J.) Nouvelle méthode de dissociation des muscles des animaux supérieurs, sur un nouveau procédé de dissociation du faisceau musculaire primitif des muscles volontaires, en fibrilles. Compt. rend. Soc. de biol. 1876, Par., 1877, 6. s., iii, 189. — **Rendu** (A.) Des divers modes de contractilité musculaire ; influence de cette contractilité dans la production et dans les phénomènes consécutifs des luxations et des fractures. Rev. méd. franç. et étrang., Par., 1843, i, 374-393.—**Reydellet.** Muscle. Dict. d. sc. méd., Par., 1819, xxxiv, 560-624. — **Richardson** (B. W.) The Croonian lecture ; on muscular irritability after systemic death. Proc. Roy. Soc. Lond., 1872-3, xxi, 339-348. *Also* [Abstr.]: Med. Times & Gaz., Lond., 1873, ii, 262-265.—**Richet** (C.) De la forme de la contraction musculaire des muscles de l'écrevisse. Compt. rend. Acad. d. sc., Par., 1879, lxxxviii, 868-870. ————. De l'excitabilité du muscle pendant les différentes périodes de sa contraction. *Ibid.*, lxxxix, 242-244. ————. De l'excitabilité rythmique des muscles et de leur comparaison avec le cœur. *Ibid.*, 792-794. *Also* [Abstr.]: Gaz. méd. de Par., 1879, 6. s., i, 614. ————. Recherches sur la contraction musculaire de l'écrevisse. Cong. périod. internat. d. sc. méd. Compt. rend. 1879, Amst., 1880, vi, 554-560. ————. De l'ondre secondaire du muscle. Compt. rend. Acad. d. sc., Par., 1880, xci, 828. *Also:* Gaz. méd. de Par., 1880, 6. s., ii, 631. ————. Phénomènes chimiques de la contraction musculaire. Rev. scient., Par., 1881, 3. s., i, 206-215. ————. Notes sur quelques faits relatifs à l'excitabilité musculaire. Compt. rend. Soc. de biol., Par., 1882, 7. s., iv, 21-23. ————. De diversorum musculorum diversa irritabilitate. Arch. f. d. ges. Physiol., Bonn, 1883, xxxi, 146.—**Roeber** (H.) Beitrag zur Kenntniss des Elektrotonus. Arch. f. Anat., Physiol. u. wissensch. Med., Leipz., 1869, 623-631, 1 pl. ————. Ueber die Natur der negativen Nachwirkung des Tetanus auf die elektromotorische Kraft der Muskeln. *Ibid.*, 1870, 615-641. — **Röhmann.** Ueber Bildung und Ausscheidung von Milchsäure und Zucker bei der Muskelthätigkeit (nach Versuchen von W. Marcuse). Jahresb. d. schles. Gesellsch. f. vaterl. Kult., Bresl., 1887, lxiv, 39-42. — **Rollett** (A.) Ueber die verschiedene Erregbarkeit functionnell verschiedener Nervmuskel-Apparate. Sitzungsb. d. k. Akad. d. Wissensch. Math.-naturw. Cl., Wien, 1874, lxx, 7, 3 pl.; 1875, lxxi, 33, 1 pl.; 1876, lxxii, 349, 3 pl. ————. Ueber die verschiedene Erregbarkeit functionell verschiedener Muskelapparate. [Rev.] Centralbl. f. d. med. Wissensch., Berl., 1875, xiii, 337-339.—**Rosenbach** (P.) & **Schtscherbak** (A.) Graphische Untersuchung der Muskelzuckung bei Entartungsreaction. Neurol. Centralbl., Leipz., 1886, v, 337-344.—**Rosenthal** (J.) Ueber der relative Stärke der directen und indirecten Muskelreizung. Untersuch. z. Naturl. d. Mensch. u. d. Thiere, Frankf. a. M., 1857, iii, 185-194. ————. Ueber die Arbeitsleistung der Muskeln. Sitzungsb. d. phys.-med. Soc. zu Erlang., 1879-80, xii, 15-26. *Also:* Arch. f. Physiol., Leipz., 1880, 187-196. — **Rosenthal** (M.) Untersuchungen und Beobachtungen über das Absterben der Muskeln und den Scheintod. Med. Jahrb., Wien, 1872, 389-413.—**Rossbach** (M. J.) & **Hartenck** (K.) Muskelversuche an Warmblütern. Arch. f. d. ges. Physiol., Bonn, 1877, xv, 1-11, 1 pl.—**Roth** (O.) Experimentelle Studien über die durch Ermüdung hervorgerufenen Veränderungen des Muskelgewebes. Arch. f. path. Anat., etc., Berl., 1881, lxxxv, 95-109.—**Roth** (W.) Ueber neuromusculäre Stämmchen in den willkürlichen Muskeln. Centralbl. f. d. med. Wissensch., Berl., 1887, xxv, 129-131.—**Rouget** (C.) Phénomènes microscopiques de la cont. action musculaire ; striation transversale des fibres lisses. [Extr.] Compt. rend. Acad. d. sc., Par., 1881, xcii, 1446-1449. ————. Note sur des photographies microscopiques relatives à la structure des muscles et aux phénomènes de la contraction musculaire. *Ibid.*, 1866, lxii, 1314-1317. —**Roux** (W.) Beiträge zur Morphologie der functionellen Anpassung. 2. Ueber die Selbstregulation der morphologischen Länge der Skeletmuskeln. Jenaische Ztschr. f. Naturw., 1882-3, n. F., ix, 358-427. *Also*, Reprint. — **Rozanoff** (I.) K voprosu o kolebanijach muschechnoi sili u cheloveka. [On the variations of muscular force in man.] Vrach, St. Petersb., 1885, vi, 8-10. — **Rubner** (M.) Versuche über den Einfluss der Temperatur auf die Respiration des ruhenden Muskels. Arch. f. Physiol., Leipz., 1885, 38-66. — **Runge.** Der Elektrotonus am Lebenden. Deutsches Arch. f. klin. Med., Leipz., 1870, vii, 356-384.—**Rutherford** (W.) Electrotonus. J.

Anat. & Physiol., Lond., 1867-8, ii, 87-103.—**Sadler** (W.) Ueber den Blutstrom in den ruhenden, verkürzten und ermüdeten Muskeln des lebenden Thieres. Arb. a. d. physiol. Anst. zu Leipz., 1870, iv, 77-100, 1 pl. — **Samkowy.** Ueber den Einfluss der Temperatur auf den Dehnungszustand quergestreifter und glatter Muskulatur verschiedener Thierklassen. Arch. f. d. ges. Physiol., Bonn, 1874, ix, 399-402, 1 pl. — **Sansom** (A.) Mémoire sur la source du travail musculaire et sur les prétendues combustions respiratoires. J. de l'anat. et physiol., etc., Par., 1880, xvi, 473-534. *Also* [Abstr.]: Compt. rend. Acad. d. sc., Par., 1880, xci, 336-338. — **Sarlandière** (J.) Des différences de l'action musculaire considérée physiologiquement. Ann. de la méd. physiol., Par., 1830, xviii, 41-80.—**Schäfer** (E. A.) An improved method of directly determining the velocity of the contraction-wave in curarised muscle. Rep. Brit. Ass. Adv. Sc. 1882, Lond., 1883, lii, 575.—**Schäfer** (E. A.) [*et al*.] On the rhythm of muscular response to volitional impulses in man. J. Physiol., Lond., 1886, vii, 111-117, 1 pl.—**Schiff** (M.) Ueber die peristaltische Bewegung quergestreifter Muskeln. Untersuch. z. Naturl. d. Mensch. u. d. Thiere, Frankf. a. M., 1857, i, 84-89. ————. Ueber directe Reizung der Muskeln mit besonderer Beziehung auf die von Dr. W. Wundt vertheidigten theoretischen Ansichten. *Ibid.*, 1858, v, 181-191.—**Schiffer** (J.) Ueber Wärmebildung im erstarrenden Muskel. Centralbl. f. d. med. Wissensch., Berl., 1867, v, 849. ————. Ueber die Wärmebildung erstarrender Muskeln. Arch. f. Anat., Physiol. u. wissensch. Med., Leipz., 1868. 442-464. — **Schipiloff** (Catherine). Ueber die Entstehungsweise der Muskelstarre. Centralbl. f. d. med. Wissensch., Berl., 1882, xx, 291-294.—**Schmulewitsch** (J.) Zur Muskelphysiologie und Physik. Med. Jahrb., Wien, 1868, xv, 3-36, 1 pl. *Also*, Reprint. *Also* [Abstr.]: Centralbl. f. d. med. Wissensch., Berl., 1867, v, 81-83. ————. Études sur la physiologie et la physique des muscles. J. de l'anat. et physiol., etc., Par., 1868, v, 27-47, 1 pl. ————. Zur Frage über das Wesen der Muskelcontraction. Centralbl. f. d. med. Wissensch., Berl., 1870, viii, 609-611. ————. Ueber den Einfluss des Blutgehaltes der Muskeln auf deren Reizbarkeit. Arch. f. Physiol., Leipz., 1879, 479-512.—**Schoenlein** (K.) Zur Frage nach der Natur der Anfangszuckung. *Ibid.*, 1882, 356-368. ————. Ueber rhythmische Contractionen quergestreifter Muskeln auf tetanische Reizung. *Ibid.*, 369-386. ————. Ueber das Verhalten des secundären Tetanus bei verschiedener Reizfrequenz. *Ibid.*, 347-356.—**Schultz-Schultzenstein.** Ueber Selbstbewegung der Muskelfaser. Arch. f. Anat., Physiol. u. wissensch. Med., Berl., 1855, 265-268.— **Segura** (A.) Fenómenos que por el método gráfico se observan en la contraccion muscular. Porvenir, México, 1870-71, iii, 424-454.—**Sewall** (H.) On the effect of two succeeding stimuli upon muscular contraction. J. Physiol., Lond., 1879-80, ii, 164-190, 1 pl. *Also:* Johns Hopkins Univ. Stud. biol. lab. 1878-9, Balt., 1880, i, pt. 2, 29-56, 1 pl.—**Sikorski.** Sur la tension des muscles comme substratum de l'attention. Arch. de neurol., Par., 1885, x, 145-157.—**da Silva Jones** (G.-M.) Du mécanisme de la contraction musculaire et de ses rapports avec l'innervation du cœur et des vaisseaux. [Résumé of his Diss. inaug.: O mecanismo da contracção muscular, Lisboa, 1880.] J. Soc. d. sc. med. de Lisb., 1883, xlvii, 88 ; 97.— **Smith** (R. M.) Die Temperatur des gereizten Säugethiermuskels. Arch. f. Physiol., Leipz., 1881, 105-152. *Also, transl.*: Arch. Med., N. Y., 1884, xi, 279 : xii, 1.—**Sokollovski.** Izsledovanie mishetchnoy systemy. [Investigation of the muscular system.] Moskov. med. Gaz., 1866, no. 42, 347.—**von Solbrig.** Die Beziehungen des Muskeltonus zur psychischen Erkrankung. Allg. Ztschr. f. Psychiat., etc., Berl., 1871-2, xxviii, 369-389.— **Stannius.** Untersuchungen über Muskelreizbarkeit. Arch. f. Anat., Physiol. u. wissensch. Med., Berl., 1847, 443-462. ————. Fortgesetzte Untersuchungen über Muskelreizbarkeit. *Ibid.*, 1849, 588-592. ————. Untersuchungen über Leistungsfähigkeit der Muskeln und Todtenstarre. Arch. f. physiol. Heilk., Stuttg., 1852, xi, 1-25.— **Stillman** (J. M.) The source of muscular energy. Pop. Sc. Month., N. Y., 1883-4, xxiv, 377-387.—**Stintzing** (R.) Fortgesetzte Untersuchung über die Kohlensäure der Muskeln ii. Arch. f. d. ges. Physiol., Bonn, 1880, xxiii, 151-161.—**Straub**(M.) De spier beschouwd als samentrekbare band. Nederl. mil. geneesk. Arch., etc., Utrecht, 1886, x, 1-11.—**Stricker** (S.) Das Zuckungs-Gesetz : eine Anklageschrift gegen Herrn Prof. v. Fleischl in Wien im Betreff seines im Archiv von Dubois Reymond (Heft i, 1882) unter dem Titel : "Das Zuckungsgesetz" publicirten Aufsatzes. Wien. med. Bl., 1882, v, 236 ; 266, 299 ; 330 ; 393.—**Sustschinsky** (P.) Ueber den Muskeltonus in den hinteren Extremitäten des Frosches und über den Einfluss einiger Gifte auf denselben. Centralbl. f. d. med. Wissensch., Berl., 1871, ix, 529-531.—**Tarkhanoff** (I.) Pribavlenie k' phiziologii mishechnago okochenainiya. [Contribution to the physiology of muscular numbness.] Med. Vestnik, St. Petersb., 1869, ix, 67.—**Tiegel** (E.) Die Zuckungshöhe des Muskels als Function der Lastung. Arch. f. d. ges. Physiol., Bonn, 1875-6, xii, 133-140. ————. Ueber Tetanisiren durch Influenz. *Ibid.*, 141. ————.

Muscle (*Physiology of*).

Ueber Muskelcontractur im Gegensatz zu Contraction. *Ibid.*, 1876, xiii, 71–83, 1 pl. ——. Weitere Untersuchungen über die Wirkung einzelner Inductionsschläge auf den Sceletmuskel und seinen Nerven. *Ibid.*, 272–284. ——. Vom Einfluss der Reizortes am Nerven auf die Zuckungshöhe des Muskels. *Ibid.*, 598–606. ——. Ueber den Einfluss einiger willkürlich Veränderlichen auf die Zuckungshöhe des untermaximal gereizten Muskels. Arb. a. d. physiol. Anst. zu Leipz. (1875), 1876, x, 1–50. ——. Ueber den Gebrauch eines Condensators zum Reizen mit Inductionsapparaten. Arch. f. d. ges. Physiol., Bonn, 1876-7, xiv, 330–340, 1 pl. — **Tigerstedt** (R.) Untersuchung über die Latenzdauer der Muskelzuckung in ihrer Abhängigkeit von verschiedenen Variabeln. Arch. f. Physiol., Leipz., 1885, Suppl., 111–265, 6 pl. *Also, transl.* [Abstr.] : Nord. med. Ark., Stockholm, 1885, xvii, no. 12, 1–30.—**Tschirjew** (S.) Ueber die Erregbarkeit des Nerven und des Muskels in Quer- und Längsrichtung. Centralbl. f. d. med. Wissensch., Berl., 1877, xv, 369. ——. Tonus quergestreifter Muskeln. Arch. f. Physiol., Leipz., 1879, 78–89, 1 pl. ——. Zur Lehre vom Elektrotonus. *Ibid.*, 1883, Suppl.-Bd., 280–301.—**Valentin** (G.) Ueber die Wechselwirkung der Muskeln und der sie umgebenden Atmosphäre. Arch. f. physiol. Heilk., Stuttg., 1855, xiii, 431–478. ——. Die Wirkung der zusammengezogenen Muskeln auf die sie umgebenden Luftmassen. *Ibid.*, n. F., i, 285–366, 1 pl. ——. Eudiometrische Studien über Muskeln und Nerven. *Ibid.*, 1859, n. F., iii, 441–485. ——. Note sur la partie respective des solides et des liquides sur l'action des nerfs et des muscles. Bull. Acad. roy. de méd. de Belg., Brux., 1862, 2. s., v, 799–802. ——. Einige Erfahrungen über den Einfluss der Dehnung der Muskelfasern auf die Zusammenziehungsgrösse derselben. Ztschr. f. Biol., München, 1878, xiv, 305–334. ——. Die Leistung des nur gespannten und nicht vorher gedehnten Muskels. *Ibid.*, 1879, xv, 349–363. ——. Die Untersuchung der Verkürzungserscheinungen der Muskelfasern in polarisirtem Lichte. Arch. f. d. ges. Physiol., Bonn, 1879-80, xxi, 307–327. ——. Die Abhängigkeit der Gestalt der Muskelcurve von dem Verkürzungsgange. Ztschr. f. Biol., München, 1880, xvi, 129–178. ——. Einige Bemerkungen über Beschleunigungswerthe des Verkürzungsganges der Muskeln. *Ibid.*, 1881, xvii, 157–164.— **de Varigny** (H.) Sur la période d'excitation latente des muscles des invertébrés. Compt. rend. Acad. d. sc., Par., 1884, xcix, 334–337. ——. Sur le tétanos rythmique dans les muscles d'invertébrés marins. Compt. rend. Soc. de biol., Par., 1885, 8. s., ii, 751–753. ——. Sur la contraction idiomusculaire chez les invertébrés marins. *Ibid.*, 1886, 8. s., iii, 139. ——. Sur le tétanos rythmique chez les muscles d'invertébrés. Arch. de physiol. norm. et path., Par., 1886, 3. s., vii, 151–171.—**de Vauréal.** Recherches sur l'irritabilité musculaire et la rigidité cadavérique. Union méd. Par., 1866, xxxii, 2. s., 403.—**Virchow** (R.) Tonus und Atonie. Arch. f. path. Anat., etc., Berl., 1853, vi, 139.— **Vizioli** (F.) Fatti e teoria delle contratture muscolari che cessano durante il sonno. Morgagni, Napoli, 1870, xii, 835–842.—**Voelkers** (C.) Ueber combinirte Bewegungen und Mitbewegungen. Arch. f. Anat., Physiol. u. wissensch. Med., Berl., 1838, 469–481.—**Voichvil** (I.) Materiali k ucheniou ob otnoshenii kalibra nervov k koje i mushtsam chelovieka. [Calibre of nerve fibres in the muscular system.] Voyenno-med. J., St. Petersb., 1883, cxlviii, pt. 2, 247–298.—**Voit** (C.) Ueber die Entwicklung der Lehre von der Quelle der Muskel-Kraft und einiger Theile der Ernährung seit 25 Jahren. Ztschr. f. Biol., München, 1870, vi, 305–401.—**Volkmann** (A. W.) Versuche über Muskelreizbarkeit. Arch. f. Anat., Physiol. u. wissensch. Med., Berl., 1857, 27–45. ——. Versuch und Betrachtungen über Muskelcontractilität. *Ibid.*, 1858, 215–288, 1 pl. ——. Erwiederung auf die im Schlusshefte des Müller'schen Archivs gegen mich gerichtete Abhandlung E. Weber's über Muskelreizbarkeit. Arch. f. Anat., Physiol. u. wissensch. Med., Leipz., 1860, 145–161. ——. Controle der Ermüdungseinflüsse in Muskelversuchen. *Ibid.*, 705–768. ——. Die Ermüdungsverhältnisse der Muskeln. Arch. f. d. ges. Physiol., Bonn, 1870, iii, 372–403. ——. Von den Beziehungen der Elasticität zur Muskelthätigkeit. *Ibid.*, 1873, vii, 1–18, 1 pl.—**Voorhoeve** (N. A. J.) Ueber das Entstehen der sogenannten Fibrincylinder. Arch. f. path. Anat., etc., Berl., 1880, lxxx, 247–268.—**Weber** (E.) Expériences sur la contraction de la fibre musculaire. Arch. gén. de méd., Par., 1846, Suppl., 9–12. ——. Die Muskelbewegung. Handwörterb. d. Physiol., Brnschwg., 1846-50, iii, 2. Abth., 1–122. ——. Ueber die Elasticität der Muskeln. Arch. f. Anat., Physiol. u. wissensch. Med., Berl., 1858, 506–557. ——. Dritte Erwiederung auf Volkmann's dritte Abhandlung über Muskelirritabilität. *Ibid.*, Leipz., 1861, 248; 530, 1 pl. ——. Ueber Eduard Weber's Entdeckungen in der Lehre von der Muskelcontraction. *Ibid.*, Berl., 1846, 483–527.—**Wedenskij** (N.) Zur Methodik der telephonischen Beobachtungen über die galvanischen Muskelwirkungen während des willkürlichen Tetanus. Mélanges biol. Acad. imp. d. sc. de St.-Pétersb., 1880-83, xi, 519–521. ——. Ueber die telephonischen Erscheinungen im Muskel bei künstlichem und natürlichem Teta-

Muscle (*Physiology of*).

nus. Arch. f. Physiol., Leipz., 1883, 313–325. *Also, in:* Arb. a. d. spec. physiol. Abth. d. physiol. Inst. d. Univ. Berl., 1883, [No. 19]. ——. Ueber die Ursachen des Ritter-Rollet'schen Phänomens am Fusse des Frosches. Centralbl. f. Physiol., Leipz. u. Wien, 1887-8, i, 256; 269.— **Werner.** Untersuchungen über den Zustand der Muskeln in der Zeit ihrer Ruhe, zur Begründung einer wissenschaftlichen Therapie der Skoliosen leitend. Med. Ztg., Berl , 1849, xviii, 199; 205; 209. ——. Untersuchungen über den Zustand der willkürlichen Muskeln zur Zeit ihrer Thätigkeit, zur Begründung einer wissenschaftlichen Therapie der Skoliosen leitend. *Ibid.*, 1850, xix, 51; 55. — **Westphal** (C.) Eine Art paradoxer Muskelcontraction. Tagebl. d. Versamml. deutsch. Naturf. u. Aerzte, Baden-Baden, 1879, lii, 316. *Also:* Centralbl. f. Nervenh., Coblenz, 1880, iii, 417.—**Weyl** (T.) & **Zeitler** (H.) Ueber die Reaction des thätigen Muskels und über die Rolle der Phosphorsäure beim Muskeltetanus. Sitzungsb. d. phys.-med. Soc. zu Erlang., 1881-2, xiv, 119–12⁶. *Also:* Ztschr. f. physiol. Chem., Strassb., 1882, vi. 557–565.—**von Wittich.** Ueber eigenthümliche Muskelcontractionen, welche das Durchströmen von destillirtem Wasser hervorruft. Arch. f. path. Anat., etc., Berl., 1858, xiii, 421–436.— **Wolf** (C.) Du courant galvanique opposé à la contraction musculaire. Gaz. méd. de Strasb., 1853, xiii, 1–6.— **Wundt** (W.) Ueber das Gesetz der Zuckungen und die Modification der Erregbarkeit durch geschlossene Ketten. Arch. f. physiol. Heilk., Stuttg., 1858, n. F., ii, 354–400. [*See, also, supra,* Schiff.] ——. Ueber den Verlauf idiomuskulärer Zusammenziehungen. Amtl. Ber. ü. d. Versamml. deutsch. Naturf. u. Aerzte 1858, Carlsruhe, 1859, xxxiv, 200–202. ——. Ueber den Verlauf der Muskelzusammenziehung bei directer Muskelreizung. Arch. f. Anat., Physiol. u. wissensch. Med., Leipz., 1859, 549–552, 1 pl. ——. Ueber die Erregbarkeitsveränderungen im Electrotonus und die Fortpflanzungsgeschwindigkeit der Nervenerregung. Arch. f. d. ges. Physiol., Bonn, 1870, iii, 437–440.—**Yeo** (G. F.) The minimal interval at which the summation of two maximal stimuli occurs in striated muscle. J. Physiol., Lond., 1885, vi, 122–132.—**Yeo** (G. F.) & **Cash** (T.) On the relation between the active phases of contraction and the latent period of skeletal muscle. *Ibid.*, 1883-4, iv, 198–221.—**Zasietski** (N. A.) O vlijanii mushechnich dvijenii na obmien azot. vetshest. [Muscular motion in the promotion of metamorphosis of nitrogen.] Vrach, St. Petersb., 1885, vi, 868; 885.—**Zelenski** (A.) Zur Frage von der Muskelirritabilität. Arch. f. path. Anat., etc., Berl., 1862. xxiv, 362–428.—**Zuradelli** (C.) Sulla tonicità muscolare; osservazioni fisiologiche e patologiche. Gazz. med. ital. lomb., Milano, 1861, 4. s., vi, 429; 437: 1862, 5. s., i, 7; 18; 25. ——. Studii sulla contrattilità elettrica e volontaria. Ann. univ. di med., Milano, 1866, cxcvii, 241; 453. *Also:* Gazz. med. ital. lomb., Milano, 1866, 5. s., v, 39; 103; 265: 1867, 5. s., vi, 190; 278; 364.

Muscle (*Regeneration of*).

See **Muscle** (*Development, etc., of*).

Muscle (*Smooth*).

See, also, **Intestines** (*Movements of*).

BENEKE (R.) * Zur Lehre von der hyalinen (wachsartigen) Degeneration der glatten Muskelfasern. [Strasburg.] 8°. *Berlin*, 1885.

EYLANDT (A.) * Observationes microscopicæ de musculis organicis in hominis cute obviis. 4°. *Dorpati*, 1850.

HELLWIG (G.) * De musculis lævibus. 8°. *Vratislaviæ*, [1861].

LARGER (R.) * Essai critique et expérimental sur les muscles lisses en général et sur quelques-uns en particulier; leur anatomie, leur physiologie normale et pathologique. 4°. *Strasbourg*, 1870.

PLEWKIEWICZ (M.) * Mikrometrische Beobachtungen über glatte Muskelfasern. 8°. *Greifswald*, 1868.

VAN RHYN (C. G.) * De motu peristaltico in genere. 4°. *Lugd. Bat.*, 1765.

SCHWARZENBERG (J. C. G. E.) * De structura et functione musculorum lævium. 8°. *Marburgi Cattorum*, 1847.

WALTHER (C. R.) * Nonnulla de musculis lævibus. 8°. *Lipsiæ*, [1851].

Arnold (J.) Ueber die Neubildung von glatten Muskelfasern in pleuritischen Schwarten. Arch. f. path. Anat., etc., Berl., 1867, xxxix, 270–289, 1 pl.—**Busachi** (T.) Sulla scissione indiretta delle fibre muscolari liscie in seguito ad irritazione. Gior. d. r. Accad. di med. di Torino, 1886, 3. s., xxxiv, 55. *Also:* Gazz. d. clin., Torino, 1886, xxiii, 209. ——. Ueber die Regeneration der glatten Muskeln. Centralbl. f. d. med. Wissensch., Berl., 1887,

Muscle (*Smooth*).

xxv, 113.—**Capparelli** (A.) Sulla fisiologia dei muscoli lisci. Gior. d. r. Accad. di med. di Torino, 1883, 3. s., xxxi, 303–317. *Also, transl.* [Abstr.]: Arch. ital. de biol., Turin, 1882–3, ii, 291–302.—**Fick** (A.) Vorläufige Ankündigung einer Untersuchung über die Physiologie der glatten Muskelfaser. Wien. med. Wchnschr., 1860, x, 577–580.—**Fischel** (W.) Eine neue Reaction zur Erkennung glatter Muskelfasern. Prag. med. Wchnschr., 1879, iv, 39. — **Grünhagen** (A.) & **Samkowy.** Ueber das Verhalten isolirter glatter Muskeln bei electrischer Reizung. Arch. f. d. ges. Physiol., Bonn, 1875, x, 165–173.—**Gscheidlen** (R.) Beiträge zur Lehre von der Nervendigung in den glatten Muskelfasern. Arch. f. mikr. Anat., Bonn, 1877, xiv, 321–332, 1 pl. — **Jakimovitsch.** Ueber die Regeneration der glatten Muskelfasern. Centralbl. f. d. med. Wissensch., Berl., 1879, xvii, 897.—**Kölliker** (A.) Beiträge zur Kenntniss der glatten Muskeln. *Cutting from:* Ztschr. f. wissen-ch. Zoologie, 1. Bd., 1. Hft., Leipz., 48–87, 4 pl.—**Lister** (J.) On the minute structure of involuntary muscular fibre. Tr. Roy. Soc. Edinb., 1853–7, xxi, pt. iv, 549–557. *Also,* Reprint. *Also* [Abstr.]: Proc. Roy. Soc. Edinb., 1850–57, iii, 413–416.—**Lukjanow** (S. M.) Ueber die Kerne der glatten Muskelzellen bei Salamandra macul. 2. Abh. Arch. f. mikr. Anat., Bonn, 1887, xxx, 545–558, 2 pl.—**Mazoon** (I. F.) Untersuchungen über die Gewebselemente der glatten Muskeln und über die Existenz dieser Muskeln in der menschlichen Milz. Arch. f. path. Anat., etc., Berl., 1854, viii, 25–40, 1 pl.—**Moleschott** (J.) Bequemes mikrochemisches Verfahren zur Untersuchung der glatten Muskeln. Wien. med. Wchnschr., 1859, ix, 785–788. ——. Ein Beitrag zur Kenntniss der glatten Muskeln. Untersuch. z. Naturl. d. Mensch. u. d. Thiere, Giessen, 1860, vi, 380–402.—**Moleschott** (J.) & **Piso-Borme** (G.) Ueber das Vorkommen gabelförmiger Theilungen an glatten Muskelfasern. *Ibid.*, 1865, ix, 1–6, 1 pl.—**Ranvier.** Propriétés physiologiques des fibres musculaires lisses. Progrès méd., Par., 1880, viii, 287–289.—**Salvioli** (G.) Contribuzione alla istologia patologica delle fibre muscolari liscie; nota preventiva. Osservatore, Torino, 1879, xv, 609–612.—**Schwalbe** (G.) Beiträge zur Kenntniss der glatten Muskelfasern. Arch. f. mikr. Anat., Bonn, 1868, iv, 392–406, 1 pl.—**Sertoli** (E.) Contribuzioni alla fisiologia generale dei muscoli lisci. R. Ist. Lomb. di sc. e lett. Rendic., Milano, 1882, 2. s., xv, 567–582. *Also, transl.:* Arch. ital. de biol., Turin, 1883, iii, 78–94.—**Tolotschinoff.** Ueber das Verhalten der Nerven zu den glatten Muskelfasern der Froschharnblase. Arch. f. mikr. Anat., Bonn, 1869, v, 509–511.—**de Varigny** (H.) Sur quelques points de la physiologie des muscles lisses chez les invertébrés. Compt. rend. Acad. d. sc., Par., 1885, c, 656–658.

Muscle (*Sounds of*).

Blake (C. J.) Summary of results of experiments on the perception of high muscular tones. Tr. Am. Otol. Soc., Bost., 1872, 74–79.—**Boudet de Paris.** Recherches sur le bruit musculaire. Gaz. méd. de Par., 1880, 6. s., ii, 121–123. *Also:* Compt. rend. Soc. de biol. 1880, Par., 1881, 7. s., ii, 40–44. *Also* [Abstr.]: Progrès méd., Par., 1880, viii, 108. *Also* [Abstr.]: J. d. conn. méd. prat., Par., 1880, xlvii, 66. ——. Appareil microphonique pour la constatation des bruits musculaires. Rev. méd. franç. et étrang., Par., 1880, i, 323–328. — **Boudet de Paris** & **Brissaud** (E.) Recherches microphoniques sur le bruit musculaire des membres contracturés. Progrès méd., Par., 1879, vii, 981.— **Heitler** (M.) Ein Fall von Muskeltönen. Med. Jahrb., Wien, 1875. 265–268.—**Helmholtz** (H.) Ueber das Muskelgeräusch. [*From:* Monatsb. d. k. Akad. d. Wissensch., Berl., 1864, 307.] Arch. f. Anat., Physiol. u. wissensch. Med., Leipz., 1864, 766–768. ——. Ueber den Muskelton. Verhandl. d. naturh.-med. Ver. zu Heidelb., 1865–8, iv, 88–90.—**Hueter** (C.) Zur Dermatophonie. Berl. klin. Wchnschr., 1879, xvi, 461; 481.—**MacWilliam.** Ueber das Muskelgeräusch. Centralbl. f. d. med. Wissensch., Berl., 1887, xxv, 657.—**Natanson.** Ueber Muskelton. Amtl. Ber. ü. d. Versamml. deutsch. Naturf. u. Aerzte 1860, Königsb., 1861, xxxv, 126–129. — **Plessen** (L.) Ueber Haut-, Muskel- und Sehnengeräusche; einige historische Bemerkungen zu Prof. C. Hueter's Untersuchungen über Dermatophonie, Myophonie und Tendophonie. Wien. med. Bl., 1879, ii, 135–137.—**Stein** (T.) Trouvé's Controlversuche über Töne und Geräusche der Muskeln. Centralbl. f. d. med. Wissensch., Berl., 1880, xviii, 177–180.—**Trouvé** (G.) & **de Boyer** (H.) Microphone de disposition spéciale applicable aux recherches physiologiques et en particulier à l'étude de la contraction musculaire. Compt. rend. Soc. de biol. 1880, Par., 1881, 7. s., ii, 30–36.

Muscle (*Striated*).

See, also, Muscle (*Chemistry, etc., of*); Muscle (*Development, etc., of*); Muscles (*Nerves of*).

VON BIESIADECKI (A.) & HERZIG (A.) Die verschiedenen Formen der quergestreiften Muskelfasern. 8°. *Wien,* 1858. *Repr. from:* Sitzungsb. d. k. Akad. d. Wissensch. Math.-naturw. Cl., Wien, 1858, xxxiii.

Muscle (*Striated*).

BORN (G.) *Beiträge zur Entwicklungsgeschichte der quergestreiften willkürlichen Muskeln der Säugethiere. 8°. *Berlin,* [1873].

BRAIDWOOD (P. M.) On the development of striped muscular fibre in the vertebrata; being part of a graduation thesis for which a gold medal was awarded by the Senatus academicus of the Edinburgh University, August, 1863. 8°. [*n. p., n. d.*]

HARTENECK (K.) *Untersuchungen über Ermüdung und Erholung des quergestreiften Muskels der Warm- und Kaltblüter. 8°. *Würzburg,* 1877. *Also, in:* Verhandl. d. phys.-med. Gesellsch. in Würzb., 1877, n. F., xi, 175–201.

HERZIG (A.) Spindelförmige Elemente quergestreifter Muskeln. 8°. *Wien,* 1858. *Repr. from:* Sitzungsb. d. k. Akad. d. Wissensch. Math.-naturw. Cl., Wien, 1858, xxx.

LEVEN (L.) *Experimentelle Untersuchungen über die Regeneration der quergestreiften Muskelfasern unter besonderer Berücksichtigung der Karyokinese. 8°. *Halle a. S.,* 1887.

PLACE (T.) *De contractie-golf der willekeurige spieren. 8°. *Utrecht,* 1867.

RACHMANINOFF (I.) *K voprosu o regeneratsii poperechno-polosatych myshechnych volokon. [On regeneration of transversally striated muscular fibres.] 8°. *St. Petersburg,* 1881.

ROLLETT (A.) Untersuchungen zur näheren Kenntniss des Baues der quergestreiften Muskelfaser. 8°. *München,* [1857]. *Cutting from:* Sitzungsb. d. math.-phys. Cl. d. k.-bayer. Akad. d. Wissensch. zu München, 1857, xxiv, 291–313, 1 pl.

STEUDEL (E.) *Zur Kenntniss der Regeneration der quergestreiften Muskulatur. [Tübingen.] 8°. *Stuttgart,* 1887.

Babinski (J.) Sur la présence dans les muscles striés de l'homme d'un système spécial constitué par des groupes de petites fibres musculaires entourées d'une gaine lamelleuse. Compt. rend. Soc. de biol., Par., 1886, 8. s., iii, 629–631.—**Biedermann** (W.) Ueber rhytmische Contractionen quergestreifter Muskeln unter dem Einflusse des constanten Stromes. Sitzungsb. d. k. Akad. d. Wissensch. Math.-naturw. Cl., Wien, 1883, lxxxvii, 3. Abth., 115–136, 2 diag.—**von Ebner** (V.) Die Histologie des quergestreiften Muskels. Cong. périod. internat. d. sc. méd. Compt. Rend. 1884, Copenh., 1886, i, Sect. d'anat., 23–29.—**Engelmann** (T. W.) Bemerkungen zu einem Aufsatz von F. Merkel: "Ueber die Contraktion der gestreiften Muskelfaser". Arch. f. d. ges. Physiol., Bonn, 1881, xxvi, 501–515. *Also:* Onderzoek. ged. in b. physiol. Lab. d. Utrecht. Hoogesch., 1882, 3. R., vii, 122–140. ——. Ueber den Bau der quergestreiften Substanz an den Enden der Muskelfasern. Arch. f. d. ges. Physiol., Bonn, 1881, xxvi, 531–536, 1 pl.—**Erbkam** (R.) Beiträge zur Kenntniss der Degeneration und Regeneration von quergestreifter Muscular nach Quetschung. Arch. f. path. Anat., etc., Berl. (1880), 1882, lxxix, 49–75, 1 pl.—**Flögel** (J. H. L.) Ueber die quergestreiften Muskeln der Milben. Arch. f. mikr. Anat., Bonn, 1872, viii. 69–80. — **Fraenkel** (E.) Ueber Veränderungen quergestreifter Muskeln bei Phthisikern. Arch. f. path. Anat., etc., Berl., 1878, lxxiii, 380–398, 1 pl.—**Hällstén** (K.) Directe Reizung der quergestreiften Muskeln mittels des constanten Stromes. Ztschr. f. Biol., München u. Leipz., 1886, xxiii, 486–508, 1 pl.—**Heidelberg** (M.) Zur Pathologie der quergestreiften Muskeln. Arch. f. exper. Path. u. Pharmakol., Leipz., 1878, viii, 335–354.—**Hensen** (V.) Nachträgliche Bemerkungen über die Structur der quergestreiften Muskeln. Arb. a. d. Kieler physiol. Inst. (1868), 1869, 172–176.—**Hoggan** (G.) & **Hoggan** (Frances Elizabeth). Lymphatiques des muscles striés. Cong. périod. internat. d. sc. méd. Compt.-rend. 1877, Genève, 1878, v, 704–709. *Also:* Compt. rend. Soc. de biol. 1879, Par., 1880, 7. s., i, 197–199.— **von Kries** (J.) Untersuchungen zur Mechanik des quergestreiften Muskels. Arch. f. Physiol., Leipz., 1880, 348, 1 pl. : 1885, 67.—**Kronecker** (H.) Ueber die Ermüdung und Erholung der quergestreiften Muskeln. Arb. a. d. physiol. Anst. zu Leipz., 1872, vi, 177–266, 6 pl.—**Kunckel** (J.) Sur le développement des fibres musculaires striées chez les insectes. Compt. rend. Acad. d. sc., Par., 1872, lxxv, 359–362.—**Laulanié** (F.) Sur les phénomènes intimes de la contraction musculaire, dans les faisceaux primitifs striés. *Ibid.*, 1885, ci, 705–707. *Also* [Abstr.]: Gaz. méd.-chir. de Toulouse, 1885, xvii, 249.—**Macallum**

Muscle (*Striated*).

(A. B.) On the nuclei of the striated muscle-fibre in Necturus (menobranchus) lateralis. Quart. J. Micr. Sc., Lond., 1886–7, n. s., xxvii, 461–466, 1 pl.—**Mayer** (S.) Ueber einige Bewegungserscheinungen an quergestreiften Muskeln. Prag. med. Wchnschr., 1881, vi, 4, 14; 26. ———. Einige Bemerkungen zur Lehre von der Rückbildung quergestreifter Muskelfasern. Ztschr. f. Heilk., Prag, 1887, viii, 177–190.—**Melland** (B.) A simplified view of the histology of the striped muscle fibre. Stud. Biol. Lab. Owens Coll., Manchester, 1886, i, 225–241, 1 pl.—**Merkel** (F.) Der quergestreifte Muskel. Arch. f. mikr. Anat., Bonn, 1872, viii, 244–268. ———. Ueber die Contraction der gestreiften Muskelfaser. *Ibid.*, 1880–81, xix, 649–702, 1 pl. — **von Millbacher** (H.) Beitrag zur Pathologie des quergestreiften Muskels. Deutsches Arch. f. klin. Med., Leipz., 1881–2, xxx, 304–331, 2 pl.—**Montgomery** (E.) Zur Frage über die Structur und Contraction quergestreifter Muskelfasern. Centralbl. f. d. med. Wissensch., Berl., 1870, viii, 163.—**Newman** (D.) New theory of contraction of striated muscle, and demonstration of the composition of the broad, dark bands. J. Anat. & Physiol., Lond., 1878–9, xiii, 549–576, 2 pl.—**Nicolaides** (R.) Ueber die karyokinetischen Erscheinungen der Muskelkörper während des Wachsthums der quergestreiften Muskeln. Arch. f. Physiol., Leipz., 1883, 441–444, 1 pl.—**Oehl** (E.) Sullo sviluppo de' muscoli striati e sulle loro differenze di struttura, di composizione chimica e di pigmentazione. Morgagni, Napoli, 1864, vi, 114–149, 1 pl. *Also*, Reprint.—**Popoff** (L.) Zur Pathologie der quergestreiften Muskelfasern. Centralbl. f. d. med. Wissensch., Berl., 1873, xi, 690–693. — **Ranvier** (L.) De quelques faits relatifs à l'histologie et à la physiologie des muscles striés. Arch. de physiol. norm. et path., Par., 1874, 2. s., i, 1–15, 1 pl.—**Rollett** (A.) Zur Kenntniss des Zuckungsverlaufes quergestreifter Muskeln. Sitzungsb. d. k. Acad. d. Wissensch. Math.-naturw. Cl., Wien, 1884, lxxxix, 3. Abth., 346–353, 1 diag.—**Rossbach** (J. M.) & **Hartenck** (K.) Ueber Ermüdung und Erholung des quergestreiften Muskels der Warm- und Kaltblüter. Verhandl. d. phys.-med. Gesellsch in Würzb., 1877, n. F., xi, 172–201. — **Tizzoni** (G.) Sulla fisio-patologia del tessuto muscolare striato. Gazz. d. osp., Milano, 1885, vi, 243.—**Valentin** (G.) Einiges über Ermüdungscurven quergestreifter Muskelfasern. Arch. f. d. ges. Physiol., Bonn, 1882, xxix, 506–508, 1 diag.—**Virchow.** Pathol. Neubildung von quergestreiften Muskelfasern. Verhandl. d. phys.-med. Gesellsch. in Würzb., 1850, i, 189.

Muscle (*Transplantation of*).

Budge (J.) Ueber die Fortpflanzung der Muskeln. Untersuch. z. Naturl. d. Mensch. u. d. Thiere, Giessen, 1860, vi, 40–50, 1 pl.—**Gluck** (T.) Ueber Muskel- und Sehnenplastik. Arch. f. klin. Chir., Berl., 1881, xxvi, 61–66, 1 pl.—**Helferich** (H.) Ueber Muskeltransplantation beim Menschen. Verhandl. d. deutsch. Gesellsch. f. Chir., Berl., 1882, xi, pt. 2, 212–218, 1 pl. *Also* : Arch. f. klin. Chir., Berl., 1882–3, xxviii, 562–568. — **Howard** (B.) Muscle-grafting : its elucidation of the physiological action in the cicatrization induced by skin-grafting. N. York M. J., 1871, xiv, 275–280.

Muscle-reading.

See **Mind-reading**.

Muscles.

See, *also*, **Anæsthesia** (*Muscular*) ; **Anatomy** (*Artistic*) ; **Arm** ; **Body** (*Human, Attitude of*) ; **Contractility** ; **Co-ordination** *of movements* ; **Creatin**, *etc.* ; **Dynamoscopy** ; **Effort** ; **Electrophysiology** ; **Fascia** ; **Glycogen** ; **Heat** (*Animal*) ; **Latissimus** *dorsi* ; **Leaping** ; **Locomotion** ; **Muscle** (*Chemistry, etc., of*) ; **Neck** ; **Nervous** *system* (*Electrophysiology of*) ; **Nervous** *system* (*Reflex action of*) ; **Position** ; **Shoulder** ; **Tendons**.

ABRÉGÉ de myologie. 12°. [*Paris*, 1747.]

ADAMY (J. V.) * Cogitata quædam de adipis origine, de musculorum motu, et de perspirationis cutaneæ processu. 8°. *Herbipoli*, 1815.

ALBINUS (B. S.) Historia musculorum hominis. 4°. *Leidæ Batav.*, 1734.

———. The same. Ed. altera, Notis aucta. 4°. *Francofurti et Lipsiæ*, 1784.

———. The same. 4°. *Bambergæ et Wirceburgi*, 1796.

———. The same. Ed. notisque illustravit D. Joannes Jacobus Hartenkeil. 4°. *Bambergæ et Wirceburgi*, 1796.

ANFANGSGRÜNDE der Muskellehre. fol. *Wien*, 1786.

Muscles.

BAJARD (J.-F.) * Remarques sur l'anatomie chirurgicale du système musculaire. 4°. *Paris*, 1819.

BARCLAY (J.) The muscular motions of the human body. 8°. *Edinburgh*, 1808.

BARTH (J.) Muskellehre nach den zwey Hauptverhältnissen, ihrer Lage und Verbindung untereinander, wie auch nach ihren allgemeinen und besondern Verrichtungen. fol. *Wien*, 1819.

BERNSTEIN (J.) * De animalium evertebratorum musculis nonnulla. 8°. *Berolini*, [1862].

BLUNDELL (J. W. F.) The muscles and their story from the earliest times ; including the whole text of Mercurialis and the opinions of other writers, ancient and modern, on mental and bodily development. 12°. *London*, 1864.

BOCK (L.) * Ueber Analogien der Knochen und Muskeln. 8°. *Nürnberg*, 1832.

BOESSEL (G. D.) * De usu myologiæ medico. 4°. *Halæ Magdeb.*, [1730].

BRÖSIKE (G.) Cursus der normalen Anatomie des menschlichen Köpers. 1. Hälfte : Knochen-, Bänder- und Muskel-Lehre. 8°. *Berlin*, 1887.

BROWNE (J.) A compleat treatise of the muscles, as they appear in humane body, and arise in dissection ; with diverse anatomical observations not yet discover'd. fol. *In the Savoy* [*London*], 1681.

———. Myographia nova sive musculorum omnium (in corpore humano hactenus repertorum) accuratissima descriptio, in sex prælectiones distributa [etc.] fol. *Londini*, 1684.

———. The same. fol. *Lugd. Bat.*, 1687.

———. The same. Myographia nova ; or, a graphical description of all the muscles in humane body, as they arise in dissection. Together with an accurate and concise discourse of the heart, and its use ; as also of the circulation of the blood, and the parts of which the sanguinary mass is made and framed. Written by the late learned Dr. Lower. fol. *London*, 1697.

———. The same. Verteutschte neue Beschreibung derer in dem menschlichen Körper befindlichen Musculen, darinnen eines jeden Nahmen und natürliches Lager in Kupffer-Stichen vorgestellet auch derselben Ursprüng, Einpflantzungen und Gebrauch, deutlich beschrieben wird, nebst dem, was so wohl der Autor als andere auffs neueste hierinn entdecket, mit einigen neuen Kupffer-Blatten, samt einer Vorrede von den Fundamentis Myologiæ, und durchgehends nöthigen Anmerckungen vermehret von Christian Maximilian Spencer. fol. *Berlin*, 1704.

BUDDEUS (A.) * De musculorum actione et antagonismo. 4°. *Lugd. Bat.*, 1721.

B[ULWER] (J.) Pathomyotomia, or a dissection of the significative muscles of the affections of the minde. Being an essay to a new method of observing the most important movings of the muscles of the head, as they are the neerest and immediate organs of the voluntarie or impetuous motions of the mind, with the proposall of a new nomenclature of the muscles. 16°. *London*, 1649.

CARPENTER (W. B.) On the influence of suggestion in modifying and directing muscular movement, independently of volition. 8°. [*n. p.*, 1852.]

CASSEBOHM (J. F.) Methodus secandi et contemplandi corporis humani musculos, in usum medicinæ et chirurgiæ studiosorum. 12°. *Halæ Magdeb.*, 1740.

CHAPPIUS (H.) * Die morphologische Stellung der kleinen hintern Kopfmuskeln. [*Bern.*] 8°. *Leipzig*, 1876.

Muscles.

CHAUSSIER. Exposition sommaire des muscles du corps humain, suivant la classification et la nomenclature méthodiques adoptées au cours public d'anatomie de Dijon. 12°. *Dijon*, 1789.

CLOQUET (J.) Engravings of the muscles, carefully copied from the folio plates of . . . by Edward Mitchell. 4°. *Edinburgh*, 1832.

DA COSTA SIMÕES (A. A.) Histologia e physiologia geral dos musculos. Secção I. Histologia dos musculos. Tomo I. 8°. *Coimbra*, 1878.

COUES (E.) & SHUTE (D. K.) Neuro-myology; classification of the muscles of the human body with reference to their innervation and new nomenclature of the muscles. 12°. *New York*, 1887.

DE COURCELLES (D. C.) Icones musculorum capitis . . . cum expositione papillarum cutanearum icone singulari. Met eene Nederduitsche verklaring over deselve. 4°. *Lugd. Bat.*, [1743].

COWPER (W.) Myotomia reformata; or, a new administration of the muscles of the humane bodies; wherein the true uses of the muscles are explained, the errors of former anatomists concerning them confuted, and several muscles not hitherto taken notice of described; to which are subjoined a graphical description of the bones and other anatomical observations. 8°. *London*, 1694.

——. Myotomia reformata; or, an anatomical treatise on the muscles of the human body. To which is prefix'd an introduction concerning muscular motion. fol. *London*, 1724.

DENONVILLIERS (C.-P.) *Comparaison des deux systèmes musculaires. 4°. *Paris*, 1846. Concours.

DOUGLAS (J.) Myographiæ comparatæ specimen; or, a comparative description of all the muscles in a man and in a quadruped, shewing their discoverer, origin, [etc.]; to which is added an account of the muscles peculiar to a woman. [With an appendix.] 16°. *London*, 1707.

——. The same. With an etymological table and several useful indexes. 16°. *Edinburgh*, 1750.

——. The same. New ed. 8°. *Dublin*, 1755.

——. The same. 8°. *London & Edinburgh*, 1763.

——. The same. New ed. To which is now added an account of the blood-vessels and nerves. 8°. *Edinburgh*, 1775.

——. The same. New ed., with additions. 12°. *Dublin*, 1777.

——. The same. Descriptio comparata musculorum corporis humani et quadrupedis. 8°. *Lugd. Bat.*, 1729.

——. The same. 8°. *Lugduni*, 1734.

DURSY (E.) Die Muskellehre in Abbildungen zum Gebrauche bei Präparirübungen und Vorlesungen. 5 Lfg. in 3. 4°. *Tübingen*, 1856.

——. Anatomischer Atlas; nach Originalzeichnungen entworfen. 1. Abth.: Muskeln und Blutgefässe. 4°. *Lahr*, 1861.

GALIEN. Du mouvement des muscles, livre deux, nouvellement traduict de latin en françoys par monsieur maistre Jehan Canappe, docteur en médecine. 16°. *Lyon*, [1541].

GANTZER (C. F. L.) *De musculorum varietate. 8°. *Berolini*, [1813].

DE GARENGEOT (R.-J.-C.) Miotomie humaine et canine, dans laquelle on instruit les élèves en chirurgie, de la manière de disséquer les muscles de l'homme et des chiens. 16°. *Paris*, 1724.

——. The same. Miotomie humaine et canine, ou la manière de disséquer les muscles de l'homme et des chiens; suivie d'une miologie, ou histoire abrégée des muscles. 2. éd. 12°. *Paris*, 1728.

——. The same. 3. éd. 2 v. 12°. *Paris*, 1750.

Muscles.

GAUTIER [D'AGOTY (J.)] Essai d'anatomie en tableaux imprimés, qui représentent au naturel tous les muscles de la face, du col, de la tête, de la langue et du larinx, d'après les parties disséquées et préparées par Duverney. Comprenant huit grandes planches dessinées, peintes, gravées et imprimées en couleur et grandeur naturelles. elephant fol. *Paris*, 1745.

GAVARD (H.) Traité de miologie, suivant la méthode de Desault. 8°. *Paris*, 1802.

GERVAIS (P.) Planches murales d'histoire naturelle. [Muscles.] fol. *Paris*, [1885].

GLEIS (J. G.) *Diss. med. exhibens myologiam, sive musculorum tam in genere, quam in specie doctrinam ad usum practicum accommodatam. 4°. [*Würzburg*, 1738.]

GUENTHER (G. B.) & MILDE (J.) Die chirurgische Muskellehre iu Abbildungen. Neue Ausg. 4°. *Hamburg*, 1850.

HAFIZ (M.) *Sur la circulation dans les muscles de la vie de relation. 4°. *Paris*, 1871.

HAINDL (A. F.) *Anleitung zur Darstellung der Muskeln des menschlichen Körpers. 8°. *Prag*, 1829.

HALLER (A.) [Pr.] observationes quasdam myologicas addit. 4°. *Gottingœ*, [1742].

HAUGHTON (S.) On the muscular mechanism of the hip-joint in man; on the muscular mechanism of the leg of the ostrich; on the muscular anatomy of the lion; on the muscular anatomy of the crocodile; and other scientific papers read before the Royal Irish Academy. 8°. *Dublin*, 1866.
Cutting from: Proc. Roy. Irish Acad., i.

DE HEIDE [*or* HEYDE] (A.) Ontledinge des mossels, en ontleed-, genees- en heelkundige waarnemingen. Uit het Latijn vertaalt door Theod. Jansson van Almeloveen. 16°. *Amsteldam*, 1684.

HEILENBECK (J.) *De musculis dorsi et cervicis comparatis. 8°. *Berolini*, [1836].

HOOPER (R.) Anatomical plates of the bones and muscles, diminished from Albinus, for the use of students in anatomy and artists, accompanied by explanatory maps. 3. ed. 12°. *London*, 1807.

——. The same. 12°. *London*, 1818.

HUGHES (R.) The motor nerves of the muscles; being a tabular view of the muscles of the body, with the nerves which supply them. 16°. *London*, 1858.

HUMPHRY (G. M.) Observations in myology, including the myology of cryptobranch, lepidosiren, dog-fish, ceratodus, and pseudopus pallasii, with the nerves of cryptobranch and lepidosiren and the disposition of muscles in vertebrate animals. 8°. *Cambridge & London*, 1872.

INNES (J.) A short description of the human muscles, chiefly as they appear on dissection. Together with their several uses, and the synonyma of the best authors. A new ed., greatly improved by Alex. Monro. 12°. *Edinburgh*, 1784.

——. The same. A new ed., improved by Alex. Monro. 16°. *London*, 1791.

——. The same. New ed., with notes, practical and explanatory, by R. Hunter. 12°. *London*, 1822.

JEFFREYS (J.) An inquiry into the comparative forces of the extensor and flexor muscles, connected with the joints of the human body. 8°. *London*, 1822.

VON JÜNGLING (N. F. L.) *Diss. . . . sistens prodromum myographiæ infantis. 8°. *Dorpati*, 1803.

KÜHNE (W.) Myologische Untersuchungen. 8°. *Leipzig*, 1860.

Muscles.

LANNEGRACE (P.-J.-J.) * Myologie comparée des membres. 4°. *Montpellier*, 1878.

LAUTH (T.) Élémens de myologie et de syndesmologie. 2 v. in 1. 8°. *Bâle*, 1798.

LEWIS (G.) Plates of the muscles of the human body; drawn from nature and engraved by... Accompanied by explanatory references. 4°. *London*, 1834.

LODER (J. C.) [Pr.] prima myologiæ elementa. Pt. i–v. 4°. *Jenæ*, 1802–[3].

LUYTEN (A.) * De musculorum rubore. 8°. *Traj. ad Rhenum*, 1840.

MARTIN (R.) * Ueber Gelenkmuskeln beim Menschen. 8°. *Erlangen*, 1874.

MERCER (J.) Anatomical observations on the analogous structure and uses of the lingualis and panniculus carnosus muscles. 8°. *Edinburgh*, 1841.

MEYER (C. G. R.) [Twenty-five original drawings in water-colors. Comparative myology.] Bd. in 1 v. fol.

MONRO (A.) Observations of the muscles, and particularly of their oblique fibres; with an appendix, in which the pretention of Dr. Gilbert Blane, that he first demonstrated the same effect to be produced by oblique muscles as by straight ones, with a less proportional decurtation of fibres, is proved to be unfounded. 4°. *Edinburgh*, 1794.

MOREL (C.) * Développement et structure du système musculaire. 4°. *Paris*, 1856.

MÜLLER (G. W.) XII Kupfertafeln, welche die meisten kleinern und zarten Mäuslein an dem menschlichen Körper vorstellen. 4°. *Frankfurt. u. Leipzig*, 1755.

MURIE (J.) On the myology of Hyrax capensis. 8°. *London*, 1865.
Repr. from: Proc. Zool. Soc. Lond., April 11, 1865.

NEBEL (F.) Die Muskeln, Knochen und Bänder des menschlichen Körpers. Vorwort, Revision und Neuordnung des Textes von Dr. J. Herm. Baas. imp. fol. *Tübingen*, 1885.

NIPHER (F. E.) On the variation in the strength of a muscle. 8°. *St. Louis, Mo.*, 1875.

POHL (J. C.) [Pr.] de apta musculorum disquisitione et divisione disserit. 4°. *Lipsiæ*, [1772].

QUAIN (J.) The muscles of the human body in a series of plates. 2 v. fol. *London*, 1839.

RAMEUX (J.-F.) * Considérations sur les muscles. 4°. *Paris*, 1834.

READ (A.) A treatise of all the muscles of the whole body. sm. 4°. *London*, 1650.

RICHTER (C. H.) * Ex mechanicis, de vesica tanquam potentia mechanica considerata, ejusdemque usu in explicando animalium membrorum per musculos motu . . . disputabit. 4°. *Coburgi*, 1698.

ROBERT (A.) * Quelques considérations physiologiques et pathologiques sur certains appareils musculaires faisant fonction de sphincters. 4°. *Strasbourg*, 1865.

ROEDERER (J. G.) [Pr.] et animadversiones de arcubus tendineis musculorum originibus continuat. 4°. *Gottingæ*, [1760].

ROMANSON (H. W.) * Myologiska dissectioner, eller afhandling om musklerne i menniskokroppen. Pts. i–xviii. 8°. *Upsala*, 1820–38. Imperfect.

SAMBACH (C.) Myologia, oder die Wissenschaft und Lehre von denen äusserlichen Fleischteilen oder Muskeln des menschlichen Leibes, vor Mahler, Bildhauer und Zeichner, wie auch für alle diejenigen, so dass Bild des Menschen es seye in was vor Materia oder Handlung es immer wolle, wahrhaft vor zu stellen willens sind, aus welcher Erlernung man fähig wird, einer jeden Figur ihre richtige Bezeichnung, Caracter,

Muscles.

und die Grossheit oder wahrhaftes Wesen in Umriss zu geben, wie auch die Muskeln an gehörigen Ort zu setzen. MS. fol. [*n. p., n. d.*]

SANDIFORT (E.) Descriptio musculorum hominis. 4°. *Lugd. Bat.*, 1781.

SCHAARSCHMIDT (A.) Myologische Tabellen. 3. Aufl. 8°. *Berlin*, 1765.

SCHNEIDEMÜHL (G.) Repetitorium der Muskellehre bei den Haussäugethieren, gleichzeitig ein Leitfaden für die Präparirübungen für Studirende und Thierärzte. 12°. *Hannover*, 1884.

SCHOENER (T.) * Ueber das Verhältniss der Musculatur zum Knochengerüste. 8°. *Würzburg*, 1865.

SCHUH (F.-C.) * Quelques considérations médicales sur les muscles. 4°. *Strasbourg*, 1853.

SCHUMACHER (C. F.) * Einige myologische Bemerkungen bei Zerlegung verschiedener Leichname. 8°. *Kopenhagen*, [1779].

VON SÖMMERRING (S. T.) Lehre von den Muskeln und Gefässen des menschlichen Körpers. Umgearbeitet von Friedrich Wilhelm Theile. 2 Abth. bd. in 1 v. 8°. *Leipzig*, 1841.

STENO (N.) De musculis et glandulis observationum specimen. Cum epistolis duabus anatomicis. 24°. *Amstelodami*, 1664.

———. The same. 12°. *Hafniæ*, 1664.

———. Elementorum myologiæ specimen; seu musculi descriptio geometrica. Cui accedunt canis carchariæ dissectum caput, et dissectus piscis ex canum genere. sm. 8°. *Amstelodami*, 1669.

STOCK (J. C. F.) * Diss. varias de musculis meditationes sistentem. sm. 4°. *Jenæ*, [1758].

STROSCHEIN (E.) * Ueber passive Bewegungen des menschlichen Körpers während der Muskelruhe. 8°. *Jena*, 1885.

TARIN. Myographie, ou description des muscles du corps humain. 4°. *Paris*, 1753.

TEISSLER (C.) * Diss. sistens anatomico-physiologicam musculorum voluntariorum descriptionem. 8°. *Pragæ*, 1835.

THAETZ (J.) * De musculorum regeneratione experimentis illustrata. 8°. *Berolini*, [1843].

THEILE (F. W.) Gewichtsbestimmungen zur Entwickelung des Muskelsystems und des Skelettes beim Menschen. Durch eine biographische Notiz eingeleitet von W. His. 4°. *Halle*, [1884].
Cutting from: Nova Acta der Ksl. Leop.-Carol.-Deutschen Akademie der Naturforscher, Band xlvi, Nr. 3, 135–471.

TUSON (E. W.) Myology. 2. ed. fol. *London*, 1828.

VALENTIN (G.) * Historiæ evolutionis systematis muscularis prolusio. 4°. *Vratislaviæ*, [1832].

VETTER (A. R.) Neueingerichtete Muskellehre für Schüler der Arzneikunde. 16°. *Wien*, 1790.

WALTER (J. G.) Myologisches Handbuch zum Gebrauch derjenigen, die sich in der Zergliederungskunst üben auf dem anatomischen Theater in Berlin. 3. Aufl. 16°. *Berlin*, 1795.

WALTHER (A. F.) Teneriorum musculorum humani corporis anatome repetita, qua observationes anatomicorum cum suis contulit, tabulam faciei internæ adjecit, omnia ad idonei exempli novissimæ sectionis fidem exegit, et in usum auditorum convertit. 4°. *Lipsiæ*, 1731.
Also in: HALLER. Disp. anat. [etc.] 4°. *Gottingæ*, 1751, vi, 605–634, 1 pl.

———. Observationes novas de musculis. 4°. *Lipsiæ*, [1733].

WIGHT (J. S.) The principles of myodynamics. 8°. *New York*, 1881.

WOLFF (W.) * Ueber den Zusammenhang des Muskels mit der Sehne. 8°. *Berlin*, 1877.

Muscles.

Abbate (V.) Ricerche sulle ramificazioni ed anastomosi di alcune fibre nei muscoli sfinterici, nei muscoli a ventaglio, e in quelli a movimento rapido in alcuni mammiferi. Osservatore med., Palermo, 1876, 3. s., vi, 36–39, 1 pl.—**Bardeleben** (K.) Muskel und Fascie. Jenaische Ztschr. f. Naturw., Leipz., 1881, n. F.; viii, 390–417. — **Beaunis** (H.) Recherches sur la contraction simultanée des muscles antagonistes. Gaz. méd. de Par., 1885, 7. s., ii, 325; 339. *Also* [Abstr.]: Compt. rend. Soc. de biol., Par., 1885, 8. s., ii, 345–347.—**Bonora** (C.) Un po' di miologia applicata e derivata dalla clinica. Raccoglitore med., Forlì, 1875, 4. s., iv, 433–447.—**Cash** (T.) & **Yeo** (G. F.) On the variations of latency in certain skeletal muscles of some different animals. Proc. Roy. Soc. Lond., 1883, xxxv, 281–292.—**Chassaignac** (E.) Note sur le système musculaire. Bull. Soc. anat. de Par., 1834, ix, 19–22. *Also, in his:* Extr. d'un mém. [etc.], 8°, Par., [n. d.], 8–11.—**Chatin** (J.) Structure des éléments musculaires chez les distomiens. Bull. Soc. philomat. de Par., 1881–2, 7. s., vi, 200–202.—**Cleland** (J.) On the actions of muscles passing over more than one joint. J. Anat. & Physiol., Lond., 1866–7, i, 85–93.—**Cunningham** (D. J.) The relation of nerve-supply to muscle-homology. Tr. Internat. M. Cong., 7. sess., Lond., 1881, iv, 166.—**Dobson** (G. E.) On the comparative variability of bones and muscles, with remarks on unity of type in variations of the origin and insertion of certain muscles in species unconnected by unity of descent. J. Anat. & Physiol., Lond., 1884–5, xix, 16–23.— **Dugniolle** (J.-F.) Considérations sur les muscles et leurs fonctions. Arch. de la méd. belge, Brux., 1853, l, 133: li, 10—**Eldridge** (S.) On an apparatus for teaching the action of the muscles. Nat. M. J., Wash., 1870–71, i, 410.—**Exner** (S.) Ueber Lumen-erweiternde Muskeln. Sitzungsb. d. k. Akad. d. Wissensch. Math.-naturw. Cl., Wien, 1877, lxxv, 6–14.—**Fick** (A.) Statische Betrachtung der Muskulatur des Oberschenkels; mit einer einleitenden Bemerkung von C. Ludwig. Ztschr. f. rat. Med., Heidelb., 1850, ix, 94–106.—**Fick** (A. E.) Ueber zweigelenkige Muskeln. Arch. f. Anat. u. Entwcklngsgesch., Leipz., 1879, 201–239, 1 pl.—**Flint** (A.) The source of muscular power, as deduced from observations upon the human subject under conditions of rest and of muscular exercise. J. Anat. & Physiol., Lond., 1877–8, xii, 91–141.— **Fredericq** (L.) Note sur la contraction des muscles striés de l'hydrophile. Bull. Acad. roy. d. sc. de Belg., Brux., 1876, 2. s., xli, 583–594, 2 pl.—**Führer** (F.) Beiträge zur chirurgischen Myologie. Arch. f. path. Anat., etc., Berl., 1851, iii, 313–398. *Also,* Reprint.—**Gadow** (H.) Observations in comparative myology. J. Anat. & Physiol., Lond., 1881–2, xvi, 493–514 —**Giraudi** (H.) Observations myologiques. J. gén. de méd., chir. et pharm., Par., 1813, xlvi, 353–370.—**Goodsir** (J.) Notes on the general morphology of the muscles. *In his:* Anat. Mem., 8°, Edinb., 1868, i, 451. ——. Notes on the morphology of the muscles of the limbs. *Ibid.*, 452–455.—**Gruber** (W.) Ueber den normalen Musculus peroneo-tibialis bei den Hunden (Homologon des gleichnamigen, aber anomalen Musculus bei dem Menschen), nebst Vorbemerkungen über die gekannte Unterschenkelmusculatur dieser Thiere. Arch. f. Anat. u. Entwcklngsgesch., Leipz., 1878, 438, 1 pl., 481. *Also, in his:* Beob. a. d. menschl. u. vergl. Anat., 4°, Berl., 1879, Hft. 1, 59–75, 2 pl.—**Grützner** (P.) Ueber physiologische Verschiedenheiten der Skeletmuskeln. Breslau. aerztl. Ztschr., 1883, v, 189–191.—**Halbertsma** (H. J.) Ueber eine Verbindung zwischen dem M. lattissimus dorsi und dem M. triceps brachii des Menschen; ein Analogon des M. anconæus quintus der Thiere. Arch. f. d. holländ. Beitr. z. Nat.- u. Heilk., Utrecht, 1858, i, 54–59.—**Haswell** (W. A.) Some points in the myology of the common pigeon. J. Anat. & Physiol., Lond., 1882–3, xvii, 218; 404.—**Haughton** (S.) Three lectures on the principle of least action in nature illustrated by animal mechanics. Brit. M. J., Lond., 1871, i, 549; 577; 603; 631; 659. *Also,* Reprint.—**Herrick** (C. L.) Certain homologous muscles. Science, N. Y., 1886, vii, 396.—**von Hoffmann** (G.) Morphologische Untersuchungen über die Muskulatur. Ztschr. f. Geburtsh. u. Frauenkr., Stuttg., 1875–6, i, 448–473, 1 pl.—**Hoggan** (G.) & **Hoggan** (Frances Elisabeth). Études sur les lymphatiques des muscles striés. J. de l'anat. et de la physiol., etc., Par., 1879, xv, 584–611, 2 pl.—**Hulin** (A.) Note préliminaire sur l'action réciproque des muscles antagonistes: étude clinique et expérimentale. Tribune méd., Par., 1884, xvi, 403.—**Humphry** (G. M.) On the disposition and homologies of the extensor and flexor muscles of the leg and forearm. J. Anat. & Physiol., Lond., 1868–9, iii, 320–334. ——. The myology of the limbs of the unau, the aï, the two-toed anteater, and the pancolin. *Ibid.*, 1869–70, iv, 17–78. ——. On the disposition of muscles in vertebrate animals. *Ibid.*, 1871–2, vi, 293–376. ——. Lectures on human myology. Brit. M. J., Lond., 1872, i, 657; 685; ii, 4: 33; 57; 85. *Also* [Abstr.]: Med. Times & Gaz., Lond., 1872, ii, 49; 131.—**Hyrtl** (J.) Entdeckung zweier neuer Muskel. Ztschr. d. k.k. Gesellsch. d. Aerzte zu Wien, 1844, i, 115–117, 1 pl.—**Imbert** (A.) Contribution à la mécanique des muscles du membre supérieur chez l'homme. J. de l'anat. et physiol., etc., Par., 1884, xx, 85–

Muscles.

105.—**Isenflamm** (H. F.) Ueber die Muskeln des Kindes. *In his:* Anat. Untersuchungen, 8°, Erlang., 1822, 45–66.—**Johnson** (G.) The Lumleian lectures on the muscular arterioles; their structure and function in health and in certain morbid states. Brit. M. J., Lond., 1877, i, 443; 473; 539; 577.—**Kennedy** (H.) On the strength of muscle. Med. Press & Circ., Lond., 1875, n. s., xix, 246–248.—**Koster** (W.) Sur quelques points de la mécanique du corps humain. Arch. néerl. d. sc. exactes, etc., La Haye, 1867, ii, 88–114.—**Lebert.** Sur quelques points de l'anatomie comparée des muscles et de la formation des os. Compt. rend. Soc. de biol. 1849, Par., 1850, i, 76. *Also* [Abstr.]: Tribune méd., Par., 1881-2, xiii, 440.—**Lombard** (W. P.) Die räumliche und zeitliche Aufeinanderfolge reflectorisch contrahirter Muskeln. Arch. f. Pysiol., Leipz., 1885, 408–489.—**Macalister** (A.) On the homologies of the flexor muscles of the vertebrate limb. J. Anat. & Physiol., Lond., 1867-8, ii, 283–289. ——. The myology of the cheiroptera. Phil. Tr. 1872, Lond., 1873, clxi, 125–171, 4 pl.—**Mercer** (J.) Anatomical observations on the analogous structure and uses of the lingualis and panniculus carnosus muscles. Lond. M. Gaz., 1841, xxviii, 346–349. *Also,* Reprint.—**Monro** (A.) Observations on the muscles, and particularly on the effects of their oblique fibres. Tr. Roy. Soc. Edinb., 1794, iii, 250–265. — **Müller** (E.) Ueber Associationsgruppen und Mitbewegungen willkührlicher Muskeln. Verhandl. d. schweiz. naturf. Gesellsch., Glarus, 1851, xxxvi. 118–126.— **Mussey** (R. D.) A short notice of an improved method of teaching myology. Ohio M. Reposit., Cincin., 1826-7, i, 50.—**Ollivier** & **Raige-Delorme.** Muscles. Dict. de méd., 2. éd., Par., 1839, xx, 333–371.—**Ramsay** (A.) Observations on the vis insita musculorum, the laws of which seem to have been overlooked, in some measure, by natural philosophers, in explaining muscular attachments and their phenomena. Med. & Phys. J., Lond., 1814, xxxi, 288–295. — **Ranvier** (L.) Note sur les vaisseaux sanguins et la circulation dans les muscles rouges. Arch. de physiol. norm. et path., Par., 1874, 2. s., i, 446–449, 1 pl. *Also:* Gaz. méd. de Par., 1874, 4. s., iii, 43. ——. Des muscles rouges et des muscles blancs chez les rongeurs. Compt. rend. Acad. d. sc., Par., 1887, civ. 79.— **Renaut** (J.) & **Debove.** Nouvelle méthode de dissociation des muscles des animaux supérieurs, sur un nouveau procédé de dissociation du faisceau musculaire primitif des muscles volontaires en fibrilles. Compt. rend. Soc. de biol. 1876, Par., 1877, 6. s., iii, 189.—**Rossi** (A.) Sul modo di terminare dei nervi nei tendini e nei muscoli degli uccelli. Mem. Accad. d. sc. d. Ist. di Bologna, 1882, 4. s., iv, 783–788, 1 pl. —**Schlagdenhauffen.** Considérations mécaniques sur les muscles. J. de l'anat. et physiol., etc., Par., 1872, viii, 550 : 1873, iv, 271. — **Schönn.** Anatomische Untersuchungen im Bereiche des Muskel- und Nervengewebes. Jenaische Ztschr. f. Med. u. Naturw., Leipz., 1866, ii, 26–60.—**Sebastian** (A. A.) Bijdragen tot de anatomie der spieren van de bovenste en onderste ledematen van den mensch. Nederl. Laucet, Gravenh., 1846-7, 2. s., ii, 165–212.—**Shufeldt** (R. W.) A review of the muscles used in the classification of birds. J. Comp. M. & S., N. Y. & Phila., 1887, viii, 321–344.—**Source** (The) of muscular power. Pop. Sc. Month., N. Y., 1878, xii, 729–736.—**Testut** (L.) Note sur la solidarité des groupes musculaires homologues. Gaz. méd. de Bordeaux, 1876, v, 273 ; 293. — **Voprosu** (K) ob ischislenii mekhanicheskoi raboti chelovaika. [On determination of the mechanical power of man.] Med. pribav. k morsk. sborniku, St. Petersb., 1878, xviii, 492–500.— **Weber** (C. O.) Bindegewebskörper der Muskulatur. Arch. f. path. Anat., etc., Berl., 1859, xvi, 411.—**Weitbrecht** (J.) Von der Wirkung der Muskeln, die von ihrer Direktion abhängt. Phys. u. med. Abhandl. d. k. Akad. d. Wissensch. in Petersb., Riga, 1783, 501–524 —**Welcker** (H.) Beiträge zur Myologie. Ztschr. f Anat. u. Entwcklngsgesch., Leipz., 1875, i, 173–204. — **Werner.** Untersuchungen über den Antagonismus der Muskeln und das Gleichgewicht, welches sie einander halten sollen, zur Begründung einer wissenschaftlichen Therapie der Skoliosen leitend. Med. Ztg., Berl., 1850, xix, 71.—**Winslow.** De l'action des muscles en général et de l'usage de plusieurs en particulier. [*From:* Hist. d. mém. Acad. roy. d. sc. de Par., 1719.] Collect. acad. d. mém., etc. Partie franç., Par., 1770, iv, 499–504. — **Wood** (J.) On a group of varieties of the muscles of the human neck, shoulder, and chest, with their transitional forms and homologies in the mammalia. Phil. Tr., Lond., 1870, clx, pt. 1, 83–116, 3 pl.

Muscles (*Abnormities of*).

See, also, **Extremity** (*Lower*), **Extremity** (*Upper*), *Abnormities of.*

BJÖRKSTÉN (G. R.) * Anatomisk beskrifning öfver några hos menniskan observerade anomalier. 8°. *Helsingfors,* 1862.

CIVININI (F.) Sul nuovo anomalo muscolo minino gluteo. 4°. *Pisa,* [1836].

Muscles (*Abnormities of*).

DULLE (J.) *Diss. anat. nonnullas musculorum varietates exhibens. 8°. *Landishuti*, [1813].

FICK (A.) Untersuchungen über Muskel-Arbeit. 4°. [*Basel*, 1867.]

FRÖHLICH (F.) *Der Mangel der Muskeln, insbesondere der Seitenbauchmuskeln. 8°. *Würzburg*, 1839.

GRUBER (W. L.) Die supernumerären Brustmuskeln des Menschen. 4°. *St. Petersburg*, 1860.

Repr. from: Mém. Acad. imp. d. sc. de St.-Pétersb. Sc. math., phys. et nat., 7. s., iii, no. 2.

HOFFMANN (C. J.) *De aliquibus musculorum differentiis. 4°. *Altorfii*, [1772].

ROSENMÜLLER (J. C.) De nonnullis musculorum corporis humani varietatibus. 4°. *Lipsiæ*, [1804].

SELS (H. J.) *Diss. anatomica musculorum varietates sistens. 8°. *Berolini*, [1815].

TESTUT (L.) Les anomalies musculaires chez l'homme expliquées par l'anatomie comparée; leur importance en anthropologie. Précédé d'une préface par Mathias Duval. 8°. *Paris*, 1884.

Also [Abstr.], *in:* Rev. scient., Par., 1884, xxxiii, 369–372. *Also* [Rev.], *in:* Gaz. méd. de Par., 1885, 7. s., ii, 41–44.

WOOD (J.) Additional varieties in human myology. 8°. [*London*], 1865.

Repr. from: Proc. Roy. Soc. Lond., 1865, xiv.

Abraham (P. S.) Notes on the occurrence of the musculus sternalis in human anencephalous fœtus. Tr. Acad. M. Ireland, Dubl., 1883, i. 301–304, 1 pl.—**Alezais.** Anomalie musculaire. [Biceps.] Tribune méd., Par., 1881-2, xiii, 604. ———. Anomalies musculaires; de l'arc axillaire. Marseille méd., 1886, xxiii, 86–89.—**Anderson** (R. J.) A variety of the mylopharyngeus and other unusual muscular abnormalities. J. Anat. & Physiol., Lond., 1879-80, xiv, 357-359, 1 pl. ——— Vorkommen eines Musculus tibio-tarsalis sive tensor fasciæ plantaris. Arch. f. path. Anat., etc., Berl., 1880, lxxxi, 574.—**Andzelevich** (F.) Sluchai anomalii deltovidnoi mishtsi. Voyenno-med. J., St. Petersb., 1876, cxxvi, 239.—**Antonelli** (G.) Su di un muscolo presternale, con altre anomalie. Resoc. Accad. med.-chir. di Napoli, 1879, xxxiii, 6-33, 2 pl.—**Baker** (F.) Some unusual muscular anomalies. Med. Rec., N. Y., 1887, xxxii, 809–811.—**Baker** (W. N.) Muscular anomaly. Maryland M. & S. J., Balt., 1839-40, i, 200, 1 pl.—**Bardeleben** (K.) Der Musculus sternalis. Ztschr. f. Anat. u. Entwcklngsgesch., Leipz., 1875-6, i, 424–458. *Also* [Abstr.]: Centralbl. f. d. med. Wissensch., Berl., 1875, xiii, 433-435. ——— Ueber das Episternum des Menschen. Jenaische Ztschr. f. Naturw., Leipz., 1879-80, n. F., vi, 2. Supplhft., 146–151.—**Bellamy** (E.) Note on the absence of the quadratus femoris muscle and on a spine possessing a sixth lumbar vertebra, the first rib being rudimentary. J. Anat. & Physiol., Lond., 1874-5, ix, 185.—**Bergeron.** [Variété anatomique du muscle couturier.] Bull. Soc. anat. de Par., 1866, xli, 2.—**Beswick-Perrin** (J.) Record of irregular muscles. Med. Times & Gaz., Lond., 1873, i, 31; 463; 566.—**Bianchi** (S.) Di un muscolo sopranumerario della regione anterolaterale del collo. Bull. d. Soc. tra i cult. d. sc. med. in Siena, 1884, ii, 65–69, 1 pl. ———. Varietà muscolari. Sperimentale, Firenze, 1885, lv, 161: 1886, lviii, 113.—**Bochdalek.** Beitrag zu den anomalen Muskeln in der Augenhöhle. Vrtljschr. f. d. prakt. Heilk., Prag, 1868, c, 1–7.—**Bochdalek** jun. Anomaler Musculus supracostalis anterior. Arch. f. path. Anat., etc., Berl., 1867, xli, 257, 1 pl.—**Bower** (C. L.) An anomalous facial muscle. Polyclinic, Phila., 1883-4, i, 119.—**Bradley** (S. M.) Notes of myological peculiarities. J. Anat. & Physiol., Lond., 1871-2, vi, 420.—**Brizard.** Trois muscles palmaires grêles à l'avant-bras. Lyon méd., 1875, xviii, 374.—**Brooks** (H. St. J.) Variations in the nerve-supply of the flexor brevis pollicis muscle. Tr. Acad. M. Ireland, Dubl., 1886, iv. 434-437.—**Brown** (J. M.) Variations in myology. J. Anat. & Physiol., Lond., 1879-80, xiv, 512.—**Brown** (J. W. D.) On an undescribed muscle of the scapula. Lond. M. Gaz., 1850, n. s., x, 753.—**Brühl.** Ein Extensor hallucis longus accessorius seltenerer Art. Wien. med. Wchnschr., 1871, xxi, 389-391. — **von Brunn** (A.) Varietät des Musc. interosseus dorsal. manus, ii. Arch. f. Anat., Physiol. u. wissensch. Med., Leipz., 1873, 126, 1 pl.—**Budge** (J.) Beschreibung eines neuen Muskels und mehrerer Muskel- und Knochenvarietäten. Ztschr. f. rat. Med., Leipz. u. Heidelb., 1859, 3. R., vii, 273-278, 1 pl.—**Calori** (L.) Varietà di muscoli del tronco e de-

Muscles (*Abnormities of*).

scrizione di una pettorina di fanciullo singolare per varie anomalie. Mem. Accad. d. sc. d. Ist. d. Bologna, 1867, 2. s., vii, 383–393, 3 pl. *Also*, Reprint. ———. Di un muscolo sopranumerario cubito-radio-carpeo e degli usi del muscolo pronatore quadrato. Bull. d. sc. med. di Bologna, 1871, 5. s., xi, 321–331, 1 pl.—**Chiarugi** (G.) Varietà muscolare combinata del grande dorsale e del gran pettorale. Boll. d. Soc. tra i cult. d. sc. med. in Siena, 1884, ii, 56.—**Chudzinski** (T.) Sur une anomalie du muscle adducteur du pouce, observée chez la négresse Louise Zoulou. Bull. Soc. d'anthrop. de Par., 1881, 3. s., iv, 748-751. ———. Contributions à l'étude des variations musculaires dans les races humaines. Rev. d'anthrop., Par., 1882, 2. s., v, 280; 613, 2 pl. ———. Sur un faisceau supplémentaire du muscle grand pectoral. *Ibid*, 446. ———. Anomalie du muscle grand pectoral. *Ibid.*, 446.—**Clason** (E.) Muskelanomalier. Upsala Läkaref. Förh., 1865-6, i, 425-430. ———. Om muskelanomalier. *Ibid.*, 1866-7, ii, 417-430. ———. Muskel-anomalier, observerade på anatomisalen i Upsala. *Ibid*, 1867-8, iii, 104: 1868-9, iv, 244.—**Colucci** (C.) Di una nuova anomalia del muscolo sterno-mastoideo. Osservatore, Torino, 1887, xxxviii, 322–324.—**Cunningham** (D. J.) The musculus sternalis. J. Anat. & Physiol., Lond., 1883-4, xviii, 208–210.—**Curnow** (J.) Notes of some irregularities in muscles and nerves. J. Anat. & Physiol., Lond., 1872-3, vii, 304-311. ———. Notes of some muscular irregularities. *Ibid.*, 1873-4, viii, 377-379.—**Dareste** (C.) Recherches sur la production artificielle des anomalies de l'organisation. Compt. rend. Soc. de biol. 1864, Par., 1865, 4. s., i, 143-146.—**Dawson** (M.) Sketch of two small supernumerary muscles of the arm. Edinb. M. & S. J., 1822, xviii, 82, 1 pl.—**Debierre** (C.) Anomalies des muscles et des nerfs. Compt. rend. Soc. de biol., Par., 1886, 8. s., iii, 176.—**Denucé.** [Anomalie musculaire du grand pectoral.] Bull. Soc. anat. de Par., 1853, xxviii, 15.—**Deshayes.** Absence congénitale des deux pectoraux gauches. *Ibid.*, 1873, xlviii, 305.—**Deville.** [Anomalie musculaire du grand pectoral et du grand dorsal.] *Ibid.*, 1848, xxiii, 319.—**Drachmann** (A. G.) Tilfælde af medfödt mangel af musc. quadriceps femoris. Nord. med. Ark., Stockholm, 1872, iv, no. 6, 7.—**Dubar** (L.) Muscle ansiforme sub-claviculaire; tenseur de l'aponévrose cervicale superficielle. Bull. Soc. anat. de Par., 1880, lv, 388-390. *Also:* Progrès méd., Par., 1881, ix, 147.—**Dwight** (T.) A case of an accessory belly to the second interosseous muscle of a hand. Boston M. & S. J., 1872, lxxxvi, 417. ———. Absence of flexor carpi radialis. J. Anat. & Physiol., Lond., 1887-8, xxii, 96. ———. Notes on muscular abnormalities. *Ibid.*, 96–102.—**Ebstein** (W.) Angeborner Mangel der Portio sterno-costalis musc. pect. major. und des Musc. pect. minor dext. nebst Verkümmerung der Mammilla derselben Seite. Deutsches Arch. f. klin. Med., Leipz., 1869, vi, 283–285.—**Ehlers.** Eine Varietät des M. subcutaneus colli, M. sternocleidomastoideus und M. subclavius. Ztschr. f. rat. Med., Leipz. u. Heidelb., 1864, 3. R., xxi, 297–299.—**Eulenberg** (A.) Ein Fall von angeborener Anomalie der Brustmuskeln. Deutsche med. Wchnschr., Berl., 1877, iii, 413–415.—**Faye** (F. C.) Om nogle Abnormiteter i Muskelsystemet, der undertiden kunne give Anledning til practiske Feiltagelser. Norsk Mag. f. Lægevidensk., Christiania, 1843, vi, 17–31.—**Fenwick** (G. E.) Double pronator quadratus muscle; two cases. Canada M. J., Montreal, 1864-5, i, 7.—**Fleischmann** (J.) Anatomische Wahrnehmungen. Abhandl. d. phys.-med. Soc. zu Erlang., 1810, i, 23–36, 1 pl.—**Fränkel** (B.) Angeborener Mangel der Musculi pectorales der rechten Seite. Berl. klin. Wchnschr., 1885, xxii, 35.—**Fritsch** (G.) Abnorme Muskelbündel der Achselhöhle. Arch. f. Anat., Physiol. u. wissensch. Med., Leipz., 1867–371, 1 pl.—**Gegenbaur** (C.) Ein Fall von mehrfachen Muskelanomalien an der oberen Extremität. Arch. f. path. Anat., etc., Berl., 1861, xxi, 376–385, 1 pl.—[**Giovanardi**] Anomali muscolari. Spallauzani, Modena, 1874, xii, 177.—**Giuria** (P. M.) Di un muscolo gluteo-perineale. Salute: Italia med., Genova, 1885, xix, 690–699, 1 pl.—**Gläser** (I. A.) Anomaler Muskelbruch, die Arteria tibialis postica verdeckend. Berl. klin. Wchnschr., 1867, iv, 306.—**Gromo.** Bifurcation du muscle second radial externe. Lyon méd., 1870, v, 181.—**Gruber** (W. L.) Ueber neue Muskelanomalieen in der Kniekehle. Ztschr. d. k.·k. Gesellsch. d. Aerzte zu Wien, 1846, i, 114–117, 1 pl. ———. Ueber die Nichtexistenz eines Analogon des anomalen Musculus supraclavicularis des Menschen bei Myogale. Arch. f. Anat., Physiol. u. wissensch. Med., Leipz., 1864, 667–671. ———. Neue supernumeräre Schlüsselbeinmuskeln. *Ibid.*, 1865, 703–706, 1 pl. ———. Ueber die Varietäten des Musculus radialis internus brevis (M. radio-carpeus et radiocarpo-metacarpeus, Gruber 1859; M. flexor carpi radialis brevis, Wood 1866.) Mélanges biol. Acad. imp. d. sc. de St.-Pétersb., 1868, vi, 493-508, 1 pl. ———. Ueber eine neue Variante des Musculus thyreo-trachealis und über den Musculus hyo-trachealis. Arch. f. Anat., Physiol. u. wissensch. Med., Leipz., 1868, 642-645, 1 pl. ———. Ueber einen Musculus tibio-astragaleus anticus des Menschen. *Ibid.*, 1871, 663-668, 1 pl. ———. Ueber einen Musculus cubito-carpeus und einen Musculus radio-cubito-carpeus

Muscles (*Abnormities of*).

biceps beim Menschen. Mélanges biol. Acad. imp. d. sc. de St.-Pétersb., 1871-2, viii, 142–149. ———. Ueber einen vom Musculus semitendinosus abgegangenen Musculus tensor fasciæ suralis. *Ibid.*, 437-440, 1 pl. ———. Nachträge zu den Varietäten des Musculus palmaris longus. *Ibid.*, 441-446. ———. Ueber einen Musculus biceps brachii mit einem Caput coracoideum und einem Caput humerale anomalum statt des mangelnden Caput glenoideum. *Ibid.*, 451-456. ———. Ein den mangelnden Musculus palmaris longus durch einen supernumerären Bauch ersetzender Musculus radialis internus longus bicaudatus beim Menschen. *Ibid.*, 457. ———. Nachträge zu den Varietäten des Musculus radialis internus brevis. *Ibid.*, 459-472. ———. Ueber einen Musculus costo-coracoideus supernumerarius beim Menschen. *Ibid.*, 499-505. ———. Ueber einen Musculus sterno-fascialis beim Menschen. *Ibid.*, 563-565. ———. Ein Musculus obliquus abdominis internus mit völligem Defect seiner Inguinalportion. *Ibid.*, 703. ———. Ueber einige supernumeräre Bauchmuskeln des Menschen. *Ibid.*, 719-724, 1 pl. ———. Ueber einen Musculus cleido-hyoideus auf der einen Seite und einen Musculus supra-clavicularis singularis auf der anderen, beim Menschen. *Ibid.*, 725-729. ———. Mangel der mittleren Portion des Musculus deltoideus. Arch. f. path. Anat., etc., Berl., 1872, liv, 184, 1 pl. ———. Ein Spanner der unteren Radio-Cubitalkapsel, Tensor capsulæ radiocubitalis inferioris. *Ibid.*, 186, 1 pl. ———. Zwei neue Fälle eines rudimentären Musculus obliquus externus abdominis ii. *Ibid.*, 1875, lxv, 16. ———. Ein Musculus scapulo-clavicularis. *Ibid.*, 18-21, 1 pl. ———. Ein neuer Fall des Musculus tensor semivaginæ articulationis humero-scapularis. *Ibid.*, 21-23. ———. Ein Musculus extensor digiti ii. pedis longus. *Ibid.*, 23-25, 1 pl. ———. Ein Musculus piso-hamatus beim Menschen. Arch. f. Anat., Physiol. u. wissensch. Med., Leipz., 1875, 202, 1 pl. ———. Ueber den Musculus extensor digitorum communis manus anomalus mit 5 Sehnen zu allen Fingern, und über den Musculus extensor digitorum longus pedis anomalus mit 5 Sehnen zu allen Zehen. *Ibid.*, 204-210, 1 pl. ———. Ein Fall des Vorkommens des Musculus flexor pollicis longus beim Menschen, als Tensor bursæ mucosæ tendinum mm. flexorum, oder als Kopf des M. flexor digitorum profundus manus. *Ibid.*, 211-214. ———. Ueber die Varietäten des Musculus extensor hallucis longus. *Ibid.*, 565-589, 1 pl. ———. Ein Musculus teres minimus scapulæ. *Ibid.*, 593-598, 1 pl. ———. Ein neuer Fall von Musculus extensor hallucis longus tricaudatus. *Ibid.*, 1876, 750-752, 1 pl. ———. Ueber einen anomalen Musculus transversus perinei superficialis. Arch. f. path. Anat., etc., Berl., 1876, lxvii, 353-358, 1 pl. ———. Verlängerung des Musculus spinalis und semispinalis cervicis durch ein gemeinschaftliches Fleischbündel auf das Hinterhaupt. *Ibid.*, 358. ———. Tensor laminæ posterioris vaginæ musculi recti abdominis. *Ibid.*, 1877, lxix, 400-403. ———. Ueber den Musculus radialis externus accessorius. Arch. f. Anat. u. Entwcklngsgesch., Leipz., 1877, 388-397, 1 pl. ———. Ein Musculus præclavicularis subcutaneus. Arch. f. path. Anat., etc., Berl., 1878, lxxii, 496. ———. Ein Nachtrag zum Vorkommen des Musculus interclavicularis anticus digastricus. [2 cases.] *Ibid.*, 497-500. ———. Ueber einen Fall einseitigen Vorkommens zweier den Musculus omohyoideus substituirender Musculi cleidohyoidei. *Ibid.*, lxxii, 342-345. ———. Beobachtungen über den Mangel des Musculus omohyoideus. *Ibid.*, 345. ———. Beobachtungen über den Mangel des Musculus quadratus femoris. *Ibid.*, 346-348. ———. Ein Musculus obturator internus biceps. *Ibid.*, 348-350. ———. Ein den oberen Bauch des Omohyoideus (bei Mangel des unteren Bauches des letzteren) repräsentirender Musculus hyofascialis. (Neu.) *Ibid.*, lxxiv, 454-456. ———. Ueber die ungewöhnlichen Musculi tensores fasciæ suralis beim Menschen. Mélanges biol. Acad. imp. d. sc. de St.-Pétersb., 1879, x, 199 - 209. ———. Nachträge zum Vorkommen des Musculus scapulo-costalis minor (6.-11. Fall eigener Beobachtung) und neuer Musculus scapulo-costoclavicularis. Arch. f. path. Anat., etc., Berl., 1879, lxxvii, 123–128. ———. Nachtrag zum Vorkommen des Musculus extensor digitorum communis manus mit 5 Sehnen zu allen Fingern. *Ibid.*, 129. ———. Ein in der Haut oder Fascie des Gesichtes und mit seiner Endzacke am Mundwinkel als Musculus risorius endender Musculus occipitalis minor. *Ibid.*, 1880, lxxx, 83-86. ———. Ein vom Musculus biceps brachii abgegebener Tensor der Dorsalfascie des Unterarmes. (Vorher nicht gesehen.) *Ibid.*, 86. ———. Tensor laminæ posterioris vaginæ musculi recti abdominis. *Ibid.*, 87. ———. Ein mit seiner Inguinalportion durch die ganze Regio inguinalis sich herab erstreckender Musculus transversus abdominis (vorher nicht gesehen.) *Ibid.*, 88-91. ———. Ueber den Musculus trigastricus maxillæ inferioris. (Vorher nicht gesehen, oder doch neue Varianten.) *Ibid.*, lxxxi, 445-449, 1 pl. ———. Musculus digastricus maxillæ inferioris mit Ursprung seines vorderen Bauches an statt der Mitte des Seitentheiles der Maxilla im Bereiche der Strecke zwischen dem Ansatze des M. masseter und dem Ursprunge des M. depressor anguli oris. (Dritter der im Verlaufe von 127 Jahren beobachteten Fälle.) *Ibid.*, 449-453, 1 pl. ———. Ueber den Musculus myoglossus bei Mangel und Vorkom-

men des M. styloglossus. (3. und 4. der bis jetzt gesehenen Fälle.) *Ibid.*, 453-457, 1 pl. ———. Ueber den Musculus atlantico-basilaris, M. epistropheobasilaris und andere vor den obersten Halswirbeln zwischen den Mm. recti capitis antici majores vorkommende Muskelvarietäten. *Ibid.*, lxxxii, 465-473, 1 pl. ———. Ein bilaminärer Musculus vastus externus biceps. (Vorher nicht gesehen.) *Ibid.*, 473. ———. Ueber den dem constanten Musculus extensor pollicis et indicis gewisser Säugethiere homologen supernumerären Muskel beim Menschen; (16 Fälle eigener Beobachtung; Bestimmung der Häufigkeit seines Vorkommens an 200 Leichen). *Ibid.*, 1881, lxxxvi, 471-490, 2 pl. ———. Musculus sterno-fascialis; zweiter Fall. *Ibid.*, 492. ———. Vorderarmmuskel-Varietäten mit der Bedeutung constanter Muskeln bei Thieren. *Ibid.*, 1882, xc, 88-97, 2 pl. ———. Ein neuer Musculus peroneo-calcaneus externus anterior. *Ibid.*, 1884, xcv, 177-180, 1 pl. ———. Mangel beider Musculi gemelli bei Anwesenheit des Obturator internus; Zurückweisung der Homologie dieser bei dem Menschen anomalen Anordnung mit derselben, bei gewissen Säugethieren normalen, aber bei Abwesenheit des Obturator internus bestehenden Anordnung. *Ibid.*, 180-183. ———. Neuer Musculus retro-clavicularis proprius; Tensor laminæ prufundæ fasciæ colli. *Ibid.*, xcviii, 416-422. ———. Neuer Musculus radialis digiti I. s. pollicis. *Ibid.*, 422-424, 1 pl. ———. Ein Zwischensehnen-Muskelchen am Handrücken. Vorher nicht gesehen. *Ibid.*, 424. ———. Ueber den seltenen Musculus crico-hyoideus medianus oder den wahren supernumerären Musculus crico-hyoideus. 2. Fall. *Ibid.*, 256-259. ———. Monographie über den Musculus ulnaris digiti v. und seine Reductionen auf einen supernumerären Radialbauch und auf eine Handrückensehne des Musculus ulnaris externus und deren Homologie. *In his*: Beobacht. a. d. menschl. u. vergleich. Anat., 4°, Berl., 1884, 5. Hft., 32, 2 l., 2 pl. ———. Der Musculus ulno-carpeus externus (eine neue Variante des Musculus ulnaris externus brevis) und sein Homologon, des Musculus peroneo-cuboideus. Arch. f. path. Anat., etc., Berl., 1885, xcix, 475-478, 1 pl. ———. Mangel des Musculus ulnaris externus bis auf einen Sehnenstreifen. *Ibid.*, 478-480, 1 pl. ———. Zweibäuchiger Extensor digiti v. proprius manus mit Insertion eines seiner Bäuche an die Basis des Metacarpale v, und die ihm homologe Variante des Peroneus iii. (Vorher nicht gesehen.) *Ibid.*, 480-483. ———. Absoluter Mangel des Extensor digiti quinti proprius manus bei Mangel seiner Vagina im Ligamentum carpi dorsale; ganz ausnahmsweise und nur beim Menschen (2. Fall); bei Vorkommen des Muskels dennoch Mangel der Vagina; constant bei den Prosimiæ. *Ibid.*, 484-488. ———. Auftreten der Bäuche des Musculus digastricus maxillæ inferioris als selbständige Muskeln; Musculus mentohyoideus und M. mastoideo-maxillaris; vorher nicht gesehen. *Ibid.*, ci, 253-255. ———. Ein Musculus tensor ligamenti carpi dorsalis; vorher nicht gesehen. *Ibid.*, 259. ———. Duplicität des Musculus extensor digiti quinti et quarti proprius manus; vorher nicht gesehen. *Ibid.*, 260-262, 1 pl. ———. Ein Musculus stylo-pharyngeus biceps durch Auftreten eines vom Processus mastoides entsprungenen Caput accessorium. *Ibid.*, cii, 536-538. ———. Supernumerärer Bauch des Musculus sternocleidomastoideus in der Richtung des hinteren Bauches des M. digastricus maxillæ inferioris und abwärts von diesem zum Os hyoides. Vorher nicht gesehen. *Ibid.*, 538. ———. Ein Musculus cleido-occipitalis mit enorm breiter Endaponeurose; so vorher nicht gesehen. *Ibid.*, 539. ———. Ein Tensor fasciæ femoris posterior digastricus; so vorher nicht gesehen. *Ibid.*, 1886, ciii, 475-477. ———. Wahrer Musculus semitendinosus biceps; vorher nicht gesehen. *Ibid.*, 477-479. ———. Musculus semimembranosus mit zwei bis vier Bäuchen; 4 Fälle eigener Beobachtung. *Ibid.*, 480-483. ———. Vollständiger Mangel des Musculus semimembranosus an der einen Seite und rudimentäres Vorkommen an der anderen Seite; wohl jeder der Fälle der zweite in der Literatur. *Ibid.*, 483. ———. Monographie über den Musculus extensor digiti indicis proprius und seiner Varietäten bei dem Menschen und bei den Säugethieren. *In his*: Beobacht. a. d. menschl. u. vergleich. Anat., 4°, Berl., 1886, 6. Hft., 1-69, 4 pl. ———. Auftreten des Musculus radialis externus accessorius als Musculus supinator longus ii. s. accessorius; vorher nicht gesehen. Arch. f. path. Anat., etc., Berl., 1887, cvii, 476-478, 1 pl. ———. Ein dreibäuchiger Musculus tibialis anticus, zugleich ein Tensor ligamenti cruciati tarsi. *Ibid.*, 485. ———. Ein Musculus peroneus brevis mit Insertion an den Calcaneus, bei Abgabe einer mit einem Fleischbauche versehenen Fussrückensehne zur 5. Zehe (eines auf dem Fussrücken verkürzten Musculus peroneus digiti quinti). *Ibid.*, 487-489. ———. Musculus peroneus longus und brevis zu einem Muskel verschmolzen. *Ibid.*, 485-487. ———. Seltener Extensor proprius digiti quarti manus bei dem Menschen und bei Säugethieren; beim Menschen vor her nicht gesehen. *Ibid.*, 478-480. ———. Ueber einen Musculus gluteus quartus bei dem Menschen (1. u. 2. Fall) und einen homologen Muskel bei Säugethieren. *Ibid.*, 480-484, 1 pl. ———. Dreibäuchiger Musculus peroneus longus; vorher nicht gesehen. *Ibid.*, cix, 5. ———. Ein Musculus flexor brevis digiti ii. pedis; vorher nicht gesehen. *Ibid.*,

Muscles (*Abnormities of*).

6-8. ——. Ein Musculus flexor brevis digiti iv pedis, vorher nicht gesehen. *Ibid.*, 8. ——. Ein Musculus gracilis biceps; vorher nicht gesehen. *Ibid.*, 4. ——. Ein Musculus peroneo-malleolaris als Tensor des Ligamentum internusculare externum posterius fasciæ cruris; vorher nicht gesehen. *Ibid.*, 5. ——. Auftreten des Zeigefingerbauches des Flexor digitorum sublimis als Venter bifissus digastricus biceps. *Ibid.*, cx, 559-561, 1 pl. ——. Eine Reihe neuer Varietäten des Musculus lumbricalis i. manus. *Ibid.*, 555-559. ——. Ein rudimentärer Musculus obliquus abdominis externus accessorius. *Ibid.*, 561.—**Gunn** (M.) Case of deficiency of the stylo-hyoideus muscle. N. York J. M., 1847, ix, 216.—**Halbertsma** (H. J.) Musculus gastrocnemius triceps. Nederl. Tijdschr. v. Geneesk. A.nst., 1862, vi, 609. *Also*: Arch. f. d. holländ. Beitr. z. Nat.- u. Heilk., Utrecht, 1861-4, iii, 233. ——. Musculus pyriformis fissus. Nederl. Tijdschr. v. Geneesk., Amst., 1862, vi, 609. *Also*: Arch. f. d. holländ. Beitr. z. Nat.- u. Heilk., Utrecht, 1861-4, iii, 234-236. ——. Musculus supinator brevis accessorius. Nederl. Tijdschr. v. Geneesk., Amst., 1862, vi, 610. *Also*: Arch. f. d. holländ. Beitr. z. Nat.- u. Heilk., Utrecht, 1861-4, iii, 236. ——. Vena cava superior sinistra. Nederl. Tijdschr. v. Geneesk., Amst., 1862, vi, 610-612. *Also*: Arch. f. d. holländ. Beitr. z. Nat.- u. Heilk., Utrecht, 1861-4, iii, 236-239.— **Hallett** (C. H.) An account of the anomalies of the muscular system, met with in the dissecting-room of the university during the years 1846-7; with general remarks. Edinb. M. & S. J., 1848, lxix, 1-32. ——. An account of the varieties of the muscular system met with in the dissecting-room of the University of Edinburgh during the winter session 1847-8. *Ibid.*, 1849, lxxii, 1-20.—**Handy** (W. R.) An account of a new muscle. Med. Exam., Phila., 1850, n. s., vi, 202.—**Hard.** Anatomical anomaly. West. M.-Chir. J., Keokuk, 1850, i, 360. —**Hervé** (G.) Anomalie du muscle biceps brachial. Bull. Soc. d'anthrop. de Par., 1883, 3. s., vi, 40-46. —**Hesse** (F.) Fall eines Musculus sternalis. Ztschr. f. Anat. u. Entwcklngsgesch., Leipz., 1875-6, i, 459-462.—**Heuston** (F. T.) Complicated muscular anomaly in human arm. Tr. Acad. M. Ireland, Dubl., 1886, iv, 432, 1 pl. *Also*: Dublin J. M. Sc., 1886, lxxxi, 367.—**Hill** (M. B.) On the occasional occurrence of an additional muscle to the subclavius in man. Proc. Roy. M. & Chir. Soc. Lond. (1861-4), 1864, iv, 351.—**Hinterstoisser** (H.) Ueber einige seltene Muskelvarietäten. Med. Jahrb., Wien, 1887, n. F., ii, 407-422, 4 pl.— **Hodges** (R. M.) The rectus sternalis muscle. Boston M. & S. J., 1858, lvii, 321-324. *Also*: Extr. Rec. Bost. Soc. M. Improve. (1856-9), 1859, iii, 143-146.—**Howard** (M.) A singular muscle. Virginia M. J., Richmond, 1858, xi, 354.—**Humphry** (G. M.) On the varieties in the muscles of man. Brit. M. J., Lond., 1873, i, 663; 693: ii, 33; 51; 78; 108. *Also* [Abstr.]: J. Anat. & Physiol., Lond., 1873, vii, 360-368. *Also* [Abstr.]: Med. Times & Gaz., Lond., 1873, i, 633; 663.—**Huntington** (P. K.) Case of arrested muscular development. Med. Exam., Phila., 1850, n. s., vi, 453.—**Hyrtl.** Abnormer Ursprung des Pronator teres. Oesterr. Ztschr. f. prakt. Heilk., Wien, 1862, viii, 418.— **Incoronato.** Contribuzione alla storia delle anomalie dei muscoli. Atti Accad. med. di Roma, 1877, iii, fasc. 2, 89-92, 1 pl.—**Jacquart** (H.) Exemple d'insertion anormale du muscle adducteur du pouce sur une main d'homme, qui prouve que ce muscle n'est en réalité que le premier interosseux palmaire. Compt. rend. Soc. de biol. 1859, Par., 1860, 3. s., i, 252.—**Jansen** (J. H.) Waarnemingen van anomale spieren. Nederl. Lancet, Gravenh., 1849-50, 2. s., v, 431-437.—**Joessel.** Ein besonderer Fall von Musculus sternalis. Arch. f. Anat. u. Physiol., Leipz., 1878, 429-432.—**Jordan** (P.) Respiratory muscle. observations on. Virginia M. J., Richmond, 1857, ix, 363, 1 pl.—**Juppin.** Lettre sur une observation de M. Bourienne, concernant un prolongement du sterno-mastoïdien, dissectée et examinée dans une leçon d'anatomie. J. de méd., chir., pharm., etc., Par., 1773, xxxix, 309-313.—**Kaczander** (J.) Beitrag zur Lehre der Muskel- und Bänderanomalien. Arch. f. path. Anat., etc., Berl., 1881, lxxxv, 173-175, 1 pl.— **Kneeland.** Muscular anomalies. Am. J. M. Sc., Phila., 1853, n. s., xxvi, 77.—**Knott** (J. F.) Muscular anomalies. J. Anat. & Physiol, Lond., 1880-81, xv, 139.—**de Koning** (P.) Beschrijving van een musculus thoracicus. Nederl. Tijdschr. v. Geneesk., Amst., 1879, 2. R., xv, 193.—**Konstantinovski** (M. V.) K kazuist. anomal.; polnii nedostat. prav. bolshoi i maloi grudnich mushtse. [Anomlies; complete absence of right pectoralis major and minor.] Med. Sbornik, Tiflis, 1886, no. 40, 100-112.— **Krause** (W.) Myologische Bemerkungen. Arch. f. Anat. u. Entwcklngsgesch., Leipz., 1881, 419-422.—**Krueg** (G.) Ein accessorischer Palmaris longus mit doppelter Endsehne. Wien. med. Wchnschr., 1872, xxii, 1229.— **Lamont** (J. C.) Note on the nervous supply of the musculus sternalis. J. Anat. & Physiol., Lond., 1886-7, xxi, 514.—**Lane** (W. A.) An interclavicular muscle in the human subject. *Ibid.*, 1885-6, xx, 544. ——. Abnormal muscle of the hand. *Ibid.*, 1886-7, xxi, 674. ——. A coraco-clavicular sternal muscle. *Ibid.*, 673.—**Leboucq** (H.) Note sur deux cas d'anomalies musculaires. Ann. Soc. de méd. de Gand, 1873, li, 106-116. [Rap. de R. Bod-

Muscles (*Abnormities of*).

daert], 117–123.—**Le Double** (A.) Sur le muscle "sternalis brutorum" ou "rectus thoracis" chez l'homme, et de son volume plus considérable à gauche. Bull. Soc. d'anthrop. de Par., 1879, 3. s., ii, 408–415. ——. Muscle sus-claviculaire tenseur de l'aponévrose cervicale superficielle. Bull. Soc. anat. de Par., 1881, lvi, 563. ——. Note sur certains muscles communs aux animaux et à l'homme. Rev. d'anthrop., Par., 1881, 2. s., iv, 635-638. ——. Sur une anomalie musculaire chez une femme (muscle-omo-trachélien). Bull. Soc. d'anthrop. de Par., 1881, 3. s., iv, 111-115. ——. Sur les diverses variations du cléido-occipital chez l'homme. *Ibid.*, 1881, 3. s., iv, 654-657. ——. Sur la question des anomalies musculaires chez l'homme. *Ibid.*, 1883, 3. s., vi, 791-795. ——. Des anomalies du grand pectoral chez l'homme et de leur signification au point de vue de l'anthropologie zoologique. Rev. d'anthrop., Par., 1885, 2. s. viii, 99-106. ——. Anomalies du petit pectoral. *Ibid.*, 282-285. ——. Muscles péri-claviculaires surnuméraires. *Ibid.*, 286-299. ——. Contributions à l'histoire des anomalies musculaires. *Ibid.*, 1886, 3. s., i, 111; 658. ——. Contributions à l'histoire des anomalies musculaires; muscles de la nuque et du dos. *Ibid.*, 1887, 3. s., ii, 551-258 [558].—**Lee** (H.) Case of imperfect development of the circular muscular fibres of the rectum and vagina. Lancet, Lond., 1873, ii, 595.—**Léger** (H.) Anomalie musculaire du triceps huméral. Gaz. méd. de Picardie, Amiens, 1886, iv, 182.—**Legge** (F.) Di alcune anomalie muscolari osservate nella camera Settoria della libera Università di Camerino. Gazz. med. di Roma, 1883, ix, 169-172.—**Linhart.** Ueber einen bisher unbekannten Muskel an der unteren Extremität. Oesterr. med. Wchnschr., Wien, 1846, 12-14.—**Lotze** (K.) Eine Varietät des M. extensor digitorum pedis brevis. Ztschr. f. rat. Med., Leipz. u. Heidelb., 1866, 3. R., xxviii, 99, 1 pl.—**Louge** (P.) Anomalies musculaires; entrecroisement surnuméraire des radiaux externes. Gaz. d. hôp., Par., 1887, lx, 1101.—**Luschka** (H.) Ein Musculus supraclavicularis beim Menschen. Arch. f. Anat., Physiol. u. wissensch. Med., Leipz., 1856, 282 - 285, 1 pl.—**Macalister** (A.) Notes on an instance of irregularity in the muscles around the shoulder joint. J. Anat. & Physiol., Lond., 1866-7, i, 316-319. ——. Variations of the rectus femoris muscle. Med. Press & Circ., Dubl., 1868, v, 131. ——. Variety of the plantaris muscle. *Ibid.*, 305. ——. The varieties of the styloid muscles. J. Anat. & Physiol., Lond., 1870-71, v, 28-31. ——. On the varieties of the pronator quadratus. *Ibid.*, 32-34.—**M'Whinney** (A. M.) On the varieties in the muscular system of the human body. Lond. M. Gaz., 1846, n. s., ii, 184 - 196. *Also*, Reprint. —**Magnanon.** Anomalie du long supinateur. Lyon méd., 1874, xv, 500.—**Maguire.** Congenital absence of pectoral muscles. Brit. M. J., Lond., 1887, i, 1216.—**Malbranc** (M.) In Sachen des Sternalmuskels. Ztschr. f. Anat. u. Entwcklngsgesch., Leipz., 1876-7, ii, 310-316.— **Mathieu.** Statistique sur les muscles grand et petit pectoral. Lyon méd., 1875, xix, 220.—**Mattei.** Sur un muscle surnuméraire de la jambe. J. Soc. de méd.-prat. de Montpel., 1844, xi, 206-213.—**Meckel** (J. F.) Ueber mehrere Abweichungen im Muskelsystem desselben Körpers. Deutsches Arch. f. d. Physiol., Halle, 1819, v, 115-125. ——. Beschreibung einiger Muskelvarietäten. *Ibid.*, 1823, viii, 585-591.—**Merkel** (F.) Ueber eine anomale Verbindung des M. pectoralis major und latissimus dorsi in der Achselgrube. Ztschr. f. rat. Med., Leipz. u. Heidelb., 1867, 3. R., xxix, 158-160, 1 pl.—**Merlin** (H.) Dreiköpfiger Musculus gastrocnemius. Ber. d. naturw.-med. Ver. in Innsbruck, 1884-6, xv, 7. ——. Musculus psoas accessorius. *Ibid*, 3-5. ——. Supernumeräres Fascikel des. M. extensor digitorum pedis communis brevis. *Ibid.*, 8. ——. Verdoppelung des M. peroneus tertius. *Ibid.*, 8.— **Mingazzini** (G) Un musculus extensor atque abductor pollicis accessorius. Gazz. d. osp., Milano, 1886, vii, 243.—**Morton.** Absence of the glutei, gemellus inferior, quadratus femoris, and other muscles. Lancet, Lond., 1836-7, i, 905.—**Moser.** Beschreibung mehrerer im Winterhalbjahr 1820 bis 1821 auf dem anatomischen Saale zu Halle gefundenen Muskelvarietäten. Deutsches Arch. f. d. Physiol., Halle, 1822, vii, 224-231.—**Nelham** (A.) Muscular abnormity. Med. Times & Gaz., Lond., 1852, n. s., iv, 47.—**von Noorden** (C.) Zwei Fälle von angeborenem Mangel der Pectoralmuskeln, nebst Beobachtungen über die Wirkung der Intercostalmuskeln. Deutsche med. Wchnschr., Berl., 1885, xi, 667.—**Nordland** (G.) Muskelanomalier. Upsala Läkaref. Förh.,1877-8, xiii, 160-168.— **Nunn** (T. W.) Drawing of a case of congenital deficiency of the latissimus dorsi, and of the lower portion of the pectoralis major muscles, the pectoralis being wanting below the second rib. Tr. Path. Soc. Lond., 1857-8, ix, 427.—**Palletta** (J. B.) De m. gastrocnemiorum defectu. *In his:* Exerc. pathol., 4º, Mediolani, 1820, 151.—**Parkman** (S.) Anatomical anomaly. Am. J. M. Sc., Phila., 1847, n. s., xiii, 507.—**Paulicky** (A.) Defect der Portio sterno-costalis des Musculus pectoralis major rechterseits. Deutsche mil.-ärztl. Ztschr., Berl., 1882, xi, 207-210. *Also, in his:* Ueber congen. Missbild., 8º, Berl., 1882, 9-12.— **Perrin** (J. B.) Notes on some variations of the pectoralis major, with its associate muscles seen during ses-

Muscles (*Abnormities of*).

sions 1868-9, 1869-70. J. Anat. & Physiol., Lond., 1870-71, v, 233-240, 4 pl. ————. Notes on an aberrant form of the supracostalis of Wood. Med. Times & Gaz., Lond., 1871, i, 600. ————. Record of irregular muscles noticed in the dissecting-room at King's College, London, during the sessions 1868-9, 1869-70, and 1870-71. *Ibid.*, 1872, ii, 622 ; 649 : 1873, i, 31 ; 463 ; 596.—**Pietsch.** Observation anatomique sur un muscle biceps du bras qui avoit une structure singulière. J. de méd., chir., pharm., etc., Par., 1764, xxi, 245-247.—**Pizzetti** (D.) Della duplicità del muscolo omojoideo. Boll. d. Soc. tra i cult. d. sc. med. in Siena, 1884, ii, 100.—**Poland** (A.) Case of deficiency of the pectoral muscles. Guy's Hosp. Rep., Lond., 1841, vi, 191-193, 1 pl.—**Pozzi** (S.) Note sur une variété fréquente du muscle court péronier latéral chez l'homme (anomalie réversive). Bull. Soc. d'anthrop. de Par., 1872, 2. s., vii, 155-161. *Also:* J. de l'anat. et physiol., etc., Par., 1872, viii, 269-274.—**Pye-Smith** [Guy's Hospital, London]. Ein zweiter Fall von Musculus supracostalis anterior anomalus. Arch. f. path. Anat., etc., Berl., 1868, xliii, 142.—**Ramsay** (A.) Account of unusual conformations of some muscles and vessels. Edinb. M. & S. J., 1812, viii, 281-283, 1 pl.—**Ransom** (W. B.) Notes of some variations of the shoulder- muscles. J. Anat. & Physiol., Lond., 1884-5, xix, 508.—**Rea** (R. L.) Muscular anomalies. Ann. Anat. & Surg., Brooklyn, N. Y., 1882, v, 220.—**Redon** & **Coulomb.** Muscle présternal. Lyon méd., 1875, xviii, 484.—**Reid** (R. W.) & **Taylor** (S.) Interesting muscular variations. St. Thomas's Hosp. Rep. 1878, Lond., 1879, n. s., ix. 43-49.—**Reinhardt.** Beobachtung eines Musculus accessorius flexoris hallucis longi superior. Arch. f. Anat., Physiol. u wissensch. Med., Berl., 1846, 298.—**Rennie** (G. E.) On an anomalous muscle in the front of the neck in a human subject; a sterno-petroso-pharyngeus. J. Anat. & Physiol., Lond., 1885-6, xx, 356-358.—**Romiti** (G.) Duplicità del muscolo coraco-brachiale. Boll. d. Soc. tra i cult. d. sc. med. in Siena, 1884, ii, 87.—**Shattock** (S. G.) A "keratothyro-hyoid" muscle as a variation in human anatomy. J. Anat. & Physiol., Lond., 1882-3, xvii, 124.—**Shepherd.** Musculus sternalis in anencephalous fœtus. Med. Press & Circ., Lond., 1885, n. s., xxxix, 309. *Also:* Dublin J. M. Sc., 1885, lxxx, 69. — **de Souza** (A.) Communication sur les anomalies musculaires. Compt. rend. Soc. de biol. 1853, Par., 1854, 2. s., i, 151. — **Sperino** (G.) Sulla mancanza del m. semimembranoso. Gior. d. r. Accad. di med. di Torino, 1886, 3. s., xxxiv, 312–322, 1 pl.—**Streets** (T. H.) Anatomical anomalies. (Flexor sub. digitorum and flex. prof. digitorum.) Am. J. M. Sc., Phila., 1872, n. s., lxiv, 131.—**Symington** (J.) Note on a case of complete absence of both semi-membranosus muscles. J. Anat. & Physiol., Lond., 1883-4, xviii, 461. — **Tafani** (A.) Conformazione variatà e simmetricamente ripetuta di molti muscoli brachiali nell' uomo. Sperimentale, Firenze, 1884, liv, 630-636.—**Tait** (L.) Notes on unusual accessory muscles. J. Anat. & Physiol., Lond., 1869-70, iv, 236-238.—**Taylor** (F.) Chondro-epitrochlearis muscle on each side. (Living subject.) Tr. Path. Soc. Lond., 1883-4, xxxv, 466.—**Tenchini** (L.) Anomalie del muscolo bicipite omerale. Gazz. med. ital. lomb., Milano, 1879, 8. s , i, 31-33, 1 pl. ————. Una anomalia dell' arteria succlavia *Ibid.*, 33.—**Testut** (L.) Sur un nouveau cas de muscle chondroépitrochléen. J. de méd. de Bordeaux, 1881-2, xi, 349. ————. Le muscle omo-hyoïdien et ses anomalies. Gaz. hebd. d. sc. méd. de Bordeaux, 1882, ii, 182 ; 237. *Also,* Reprint. ————. Des variations anatomiques du muscle pyramidal de l'abdomen. *Ibid.*, 362. ————. Sur la reproduction chez l'homme d'un muscle simien ; le scalène intermédiaire des singes anthropoïdes Bull. Soc. d'anthrop. de Par., 1883, 3. s., vi, 65. ————. Recherches sur quelques muscles surnuméraires de la région scapulaire antéro-interne. Rev. d'anthrop., Par., 1883, 2. s., vi, 464-479. ————. Quelques observations d'anomalies musculaires recueillies sur un nègre de l'île de Bourbon. Gaz. hebd. d. sc. méd. de Bordeaux, 1883, iv, 572. ————. Trois muscles surnuméraires de la région fessière. *Ibid.*, 1884, v, 112-115. ————. Le muscle présternal, et sa signification anatomique. J. de l'anat. et physiol., etc., Par , 1884, xx, 71-84.—**Thomson** (A.) Unusual insertion of the brachialis anticus into the orbicular ligament and capsule of the elbow-joint. J. Anat. & Physiol., Lond., 1884-5, xix, 332.—**Tiedemann** (F.) Selteue Verdoppelung mehrerer Muskeln. Deutsches Arch. f. d. Physiol., Halle u. Berl., 1818, iv, 412.—**Tigri** (A.) Delle anomalie muscolari, considerate quali omologie. Gazz. med. ital. feder. tosc., Firenze, 1850–51, 2. s., i, 233-235. ————. Sul torcicollo e sullo strabismo per anomalia muscolare. *Ibid* , 1854, 2. s., iv, 170-174.—**Turner** (W.) On the musculus sternalis. J. Anat. & Physiol., Lond., 1866-7, i, 246–253, 1 pl. *Also* [Abstr.] : Proc. Roy. Soc. Edinb., 1866-9, vi, 65. ————. Note on the occasional occurrence of the musculus rectus thoracis in man. *Ibid.*, 268-270. ————. Case of absence of the semi-membranosus muscle; also case of absence of gemelli and quadratus femoris. J. Anat. & Physiol., Lond., 1883-4, xviii, 463. ————. Absence of extensor carpi ulnaris and presence of an accessory sural muscle. *Ibid.*, 1884-5, xix, 333.—**Uhde.** Partieller ringförmiger Mangel der Muskeln des Oberarms. Arch. f. klin. Chir., Berl , 1876-7, xx, 639.—**Vara-**

Muscles (*Abnormities of*).

glia (S.) Varietà del muscolo piccolo pettorale. Osservatore, Torino, 1883, xix, 593-604. ————. Un muscolo episternale ed una varietà del muscolo triangolare dello sterno. *Ibid.*, 673; 689.—**Verga** (A.) Sul muscolo anomalo dello sterno. R. Ist. Lomb. di sc. e lett. Rendic. Cl. di sc. matemat. e nat., Milano, 1865, ii, 269-273.—**Vlacovich** (G. P.) Intorno alcune anomale muscolari. Atti r. Ist. Veneto di sc., lett. ed arti, Venezia, 1874-5, 5. s., i, 319 - 356, 1 pl.—**Wagstaffe** (W. W.) & **Reid** (R. W.) Third belly to digastric muscle. St. Thomas's Hosp. Rep. 1877, Lond , 1878, n. s., viii, 271. ————. Accessory geniohyoid muscle. [Case.] *Ibid.*, 272. — **Walsham** (W. J.) A two-headed muscle extending from the front of the axis to the basilar process of the occipital bone (rectus capitis anticus medius). J. Anat. & Physiol., Lond., 1883-4, xviii, 461.—**West** (S. H.) On a peculiar digastric muscle ; a variety of the occipito-hyoid. *Ibid.*, 1873-4, viii, 150.—**Wood** (J.) On human muscular variations and their relation to comparative anatomy. *Ibid.*, 1866-7, i, 44-59.—**Wright** (T. H.) A description of an anomalous pectoral muscle. Am. J. M. Sc., Phila., 1829-30, v, 543.—**Yeo** (J.B.) Case of congenital absence of the sternal and costal portions of the pectoralis major and the pectoralis minor. Tr. Clin. Soc. Lond., 1873, vi, 95.—**Zaaijer** (T.) Muscle radio-carpo-méta-carpien (m. fléchisseur radial court de la main). Arch. néerl. d. sc. exactes, etc., La Haye, 1872, vii, 453-456, 1 pl.

Muscles (*Abscess of*).

RŒSELER (L.-H.) * Des abcès phlegmoneux des muscles. 4°. *Paris*, 1875.

Henry (G. R.) Muscular abscesses. Boston M. & S. J., 1853, xlvii, 115-117.—**Michel.** Note sur le diagnostic de la suppuration dans les muscles, à l'aide des données microscopiques. Gaz. méd. de Strasb., 1860, xx, 106-108.—**Ollier.** Observations de suppuration musculaire. Gaz. d. hôp., Par., 1873, xlvi, 411-418.

Muscles (*Atrophy and degenerations of*).

See, *also*, **Atrophy** (*Muscular, Progressive*); **Joints** (*Diseases of, Complications, etc., of*); **Muscles** (*Hypertrophy of*); **Muscles** (*Ossification in*); **Nerves** (*Wounds, etc., of*); **Paralysis**; **Paralysis** *from lead poison.*

BENNDORF (M. E.) * Muskelveränderungen in einem Falle von Erfrierung. 8°. *Leipzig*, 1865.

BERNHEIM (H.) De l'état dit cireux des muscles. 8°. *Strasbourg*, 1870.

BESTELMEYER (W.) * Ueber Muskelatrophie. [Erlangen.] 8°. *Würzburg*, 1871.

BOCQUET (C.-A.) * Contribution au traitement par les courants interrompus de l'atrophie du deltoïde consécutive à l'arthrite scapulo-humérale. 4°. *Paris*, 1878.

BONNEFIN (J.-C.) * De l'atrophie musculaire consécutive aux névralgies. 4°. *Paris*, 1860.

DALHAT (M. M. O.) * Atrophia musculorum lipomatosa. 8°. *Würzburg*, 1875.

DOUAUD (C.-S.) * De la dégénérescence graisseuse des muscles chez les vieillards. 4°. *Paris*, 1867.

FLASHAR (C.) * Die Verfettungen der quergestreiften Muskeln. 8°. *Berlin*, [1869].

GOETZ (R.) * Beiträge zur Atrophia musculorum lipomatosa aus der medicinischen Klinik Würzburg. [Wurtzburg.] 8°. *München*, 1879.
Also, in : Aerztl. Int.-Bl., München, 1879, xxvi, 419 ; 430.

GRELLIÈRE (M.) * Sur l'atrophie musculaire dans la paralysie générale des aliénés. 4°. *Paris*, 1875.

HASSE (J. H.) * De atrophia membrorum particulari. Continens partem alteram anatomes feminæ, pede instar manus utentis. 8°. *Tubingæ*, [1813].
Also, transl. in: WEBER (J. S.) Samml. med.-prakt. Diss , [etc.] 8°. *Tübingen*, 1824, iv, 173-208.

HAYEM (G.) Recherches sur l'anatomie pathologique des atrophies musculaires. 4°. *Paris*, 1877.

KYRIERIS (A.) * Ueber Atrophia musculorum lipomatosa. 8°. *München*, 1879.

LE COARER (L.) * Essai clinique sur quelques atrophies musculaires. 4°. *Paris*, 1878.

LEJEUNE (N.-L.-C.) * De l'atrophie musculaire consécutive aux fractures des os longs chez les adultes et les enfants. 4°. *Paris*, 1859.

Muscles (*Atrophy and degenerations of*).

MAIER (R.) * Eine anatomische Beobachtung über Fettdegeneration und Verknöcherung von Muskeln und Sehnen. 8°. *Freiburg*, 1852.

OLLIVIER (A.) * Des atrophies musculaires. 8°. *Paris*, 1869.

PUGIBET (J.) * De l'amyotrophie en général; essai de classification. 4°. *Paris*, 1875.

ROTHE (I. V.) * De atrophia partiali sive de ariduris. 4°. *Vitembergæ*, [1792].

SCHECH (P.) * Die Atrophia musculorum lipomatosa. 8°. *Würzburg*, 1870.

SEIDEL (M.) Die Atrophia musculorum lipomatosa (sogenannte Muskelhypertrophie). 8°. *Jena*, 1867.

STRAHL (H.) * Zur Lehre von der wachsartigen Degeneration der quergestreiften Muskeln. 8°. *Leipzig*, 1880.

STRAUS (I.) * Essai sur la physiologie de la dégénérescence graisseuse des muscles. 4°. *Strasbourg*, 1868.

Apolinario (B.) Observation d'atrophie musculaire généralisée d'origine saturnine. Montpel méd., 1877, xxxix, 237; 329.—**Bäumler.** Fall von vollständiger Atrophie des rechten Musc. serratus anticus major. Arch. f. Psychiat., Berl., 1879-80, x, 270.—**Bardeleben.** Ueber die Umwandlung von Muskelgewebe in Fett. Jenaische Ann. f. Physiol. u. Med., Jena, 1851, ii, 14-17.—**Baréty** (A.) Observations d'atrophie des muscles interosseux de la main chez deux syphilitiques. Ann. de dermat. et syph., Par., 1873-4, v, 206; 276.—**Barling.** Atrophy of deltoid. Brit. M. J., Lond., 1882, ii, 896.—**Barow** (W. F.) On the atrophy of paralysis and the means of preventing it. Lond. M. Gaz., 1848, n. s., vii, 529-532.—**Barth** (O.) Beiträge zur Kenntniss der Atrophia musculorum lipomatosa. Arch. d. Heilk., Leipz., 1871, xii, 121 133.—**Benedikt** (M.) Atrophia neurotica. Allg. Wien. med. Ztg., 1870, xv, 453.—**Beneke** (R.) Zur Lehre von der hyalinen (wachsartigen) Degeneration der glatten Muskelfasern. Arch. f. path. Anat., etc., Berl., 1885, xcix, 71-98, 1 pl.—**Bennett.** Atrophy of the muscles from disuse. Dublin Q. J. M. Sc., 1869, xlviii, 658-660.—**Béraud.** Sur un cas d'infiltration graisseuse des muscles sans changement de volume. Gaz. d. hôp., Par., 1851, 3. s., iii, 313. *Also:* Compt. rend. Soc. de biol. 1851, Par., 1852, iii, 65-67.—**Berger.** Sur un cas d'atrophie musculaire portant sur les muscles de l'épitrochlée et consécutive à une luxation du coude réduite; guérison par les courants continus. Bull. Soc. clin. de Par., 1877, i, 160-166.—**Bernard** (C.) Note sur deux cas d'atrophie musculaire, consécutive à des phénomènes paralytiques et convulsifs. Gaz. méd. de Par., 1852, 3. s., vii, 620. *Also:* Compt. rend. Soc. de biol. 1852, Par., 1853, iv, 128-131.—**Bidon** (H.) Les amyotrophies. Marseille méd., 1886, xxiii, 465; 525; 594; 671.—**Bizzozero** (G.) Sulle alterazioni prodotte nei muscoli dal taglio dei loro nervi. R. Ist. Lomb. di sc. e lett. Rendic., Milano, 1872, 2. s., v, 449-451.—**Bourceret** (P.) Note sur quelques cas d'atrophie musculaire avec ou sans anesthésie; influence de la faradisation dans certains cas d'anesthésie cutanée. Arch. de physiol., norm. et path., Par., 1876, 2. s., iii, 807-813.—**Brenner.** Hochgradige örtliche Muskelatrophie des rechten Oberarmes. St. Petersb. med. Ztschr., 1863, iv, 197-204.— Ueber Muskelatrophien. *Ibid.*, 1865, viii, 58.—**Broca.** La prétendue transformation fibreuse des muscles. Bull. Soc. anat. de Par., 1851, xxvi, 379.—**Brossard.** Atrophie du trapèze et du rhomboïde. Lyon méd., 1879, xxxii, 78-82. *Also:* Mém. et compt.-rend. Soc. d. sc. méd. de Lyon (1879), 1880, xix, pt. 2, 158-162.—**Buck.** Condition of muscles of a limb long under treatment for fracture. N. York J. M., 1856, [2.] s., xvi, 379.—**Chambers** (T. K.) Case of mollities ossium, preceded by degeneration of the muscles. Med.-Chir. Tr., Lond., 1854, xxxvii, 19-25.—**Chvostek** (F.) Ein Fall von Atrophia musculorum lipomatosa. Oesterr. Ztschr. f. prakt. Heilk., Wien, 1871, xvii, 633; 649; 665.—**Clément.** Amyotrophie secondaire. Lyon méd., 1871, viii, 504; 525.—[**Cognard.**] Cas d'atrophie musculaire. *Ibid.*, 1870, v, 35.—**Debove.** Note sur un cas d'atrophie musculaire protopathique. Progrès méd., Par., 1878, vi, 856.—**Debove & Renaut** (J.) Note sur les lésions des faisceaux primitifs des muscles volontaires dans l'atrophie musculaire progressive et dans la paralysie saturnine. Mouvement méd., Par., 1876. xiv, 135.—**Dejernie** (J.) Atrophie musculaire et paraplégie dans un cas de syphilis maligne précoce. Arch. de physiol. norm. et path., Par., 1876, 2. s., iii, 430-442, 1 pl.—**Desnos & Barié** (E.) Note sur un cas d'atrophie générale du membre droit, consécutive à un traumatisme. Progrès méd., Par., 1875. iii, 557.—**Diemer.** Ueber das Fortschreiten der Atrophie der Muskeln. Ztschr. f. klin. Med., Bresl., 1856, vii, 65-70.—**Dubois.** Observation d'atrophie des muscles moteurs de l'humérus. Gaz. méd.

Muscles (*Atrophy and degenerations of*).

de Par., 1847, 3. s., ii, 926.—**Dupuytren.** Atrophie ancienne du bras droit; fracture à l'humérus de ce côté; consolidation complète. Gaz. d. hôp., Par., 1831-2, v, 324.—**Eisenlohr** (C.) Idiopathische subacute Muskellähmung und Atrophie. Centralbl. f. Nervenh., Coblenz, 1879, ii, 100-102.—**Erb** (W.) Bemerkungen über die sogenannte wachsartige Degeneration der quergestreiften Muskelfasern. Arch. f. path. Anat., etc., Berl., 1868, xliii, 108-124. — . Ueber die wachsartige Degeneration der quergestreiften Muskelfasern. Deutsches Arch. f. klin. Med., Leipz., 1869, vi, 545-560.—**Evans** (G. A.) Fatty degeneration and progressive atrophy of muscle, with microscopic preparations. Proc. M. Soc. County Kings, Brooklyn, 1876, i, 61-63.—**Evans** (J. F.) Cases of muscular atrophy and degeneration. Bristol M.-Chir. J., 1883, i, 212-217, 1 pl.—**Fiddian** (A. P.) Magneto-electricity in the treatment of muscular atrophy. Med. Times & Gaz., Lond., 1872, ii, 66.—**Fischer** (E.) Ueber die Ursachen der verschiedenen Grade der Atrophie bei den Extensoren der Extremitäten gegenüber den Flexoren. Deutsche Ztschr. f. Chir., Leipz., 1877, viii, 1-33.—**Fite** (C. C.) The treatment of muscular degeneration by electricity. Nashville J. M. & S., 1878, n. s., xxii, 94-96.—**Forget.** Atrophie paralytique isolée des deux membres supérieurs. Union méd., Par., 1853, vii, 174.—**Genth** (A.) Vier Fälle von granulöser und fettartiger Entartung sämmtlicher dem Willen unterworfener Muskeln. Allg. med. Centr.-Ztg., Berl., 1854, xxiii, 625-628.—**Greenhow** (E. H.) Case of acute muscular atrophy. Tr. Clin. Soc. Lond., 1873, vi, 149-160, 1 pl.—**Guérin** (J.) Transformation tendineuse des muscles. Bull. Acad. de méd., Par., 1852, 2. s., xi, 237-239.—**Habershon.** General muscular atrophy. Lancet, Lond., 1870, i, 583.—**Haddon** (J.) Acute muscular atrophy. Edinb. M. J., 1870, xv, 1108.—**Hallett.** On steatosis, or adipification of muscle. Edinb. M. & S. J., 1849, lxxi, 257-269.—**Hjort** (J.) Et Tilfælde af circumscript Muskelatrophi. Norsk Mag. f. Lægevidensk., Christiania, 1865, xix, 352-359.—**Ingalls** (W.) A case of progressive muscular sclerosis. Boston M. & S. J., 1870, iv, 321-325.—**Kagan** (A.) Atrophia musculi deltoidei sinistri vsliedstvie utchiba. [From contusion.] Vrach. Vaidom., St. Petersb., 1879, iv, 542.—**Kerlin** (I. N.) & **Mills** (C. K.) Three cases of progressive muscular degeneration. Tr. Am. M. Ass., Phila., 1880, xxxi, 325-337, 1 pl.—**Labadie de Lalande** (J.) Trois cas d'atrophie musculaire. Union méd. de la Gironde, Bordeaux, 1857, ii, 249-253.—**Laure** (P.) Note sur un cas d'atrophie musculaire compliqué de contracture des extrémités. Gaz. d. hôp., Par., 1869, 470.—**Le Gendre.** Atrophie musculaire du bras droit; dégénérescence graisseuse des fibres musculaires; intégrité des cordons nerveux. Compt. rend. Soc. de biol. 1859, Par., 1860, 3. s., i, 115.—**Léger.** Douleurs de nature névralgique du membre abdominal droit, suivies d'atrophie des masses musculaires. Gaz. d. hôp., Par., 1862, xxxv, 154.—**Leggatt.** On a case of progressive fatty degeneration and atrophy of the voluntary muscles. Lancet, Lond., 1857, i, 383.—**Leggatt** (A.) Case of fatty degeneration of the voluntary muscles; softening of the spinal cord. Tr. Path. Soc. Lond., 1873, xxiv, 7, viii, 1-8.—**Le Tual.** Lettre sur l'ouverture d'un cadavre. J. de méd., chir., pharm., etc., Par., 1771, xxxv, 455-461.—**Lucas** (J.) A singular extenuation in the leg: with the method of cure. Med. & Phys. J., Lond., 1803, ix, 231.—**McDonnell** (R.) Case of muscular atrophy and paralysis, consequent on injury to the spine; recovery. Irish Hosp. Gaz., Dubl., 1873, i, 225.—**Macnamara** (C.) Fatty degeneration of muscle. Med. Times & Gaz., Lond., 1867, i, 412.—**Martin** sen. & jun. Observation sur le changement de la fibre musculaire en substance graisseuse. Rec. d. actes Soc. de santé de Lyon, 1798, i, 384-386. *Also, transl.:* Arch. f. d. Physiol., Halle, 1800, iv, 189-200.—**Martini** (E.) Zur Kenntniss der Atrophia musculorum lipomatosa. Centralbl. f. d. med. Wissensch., Berl., 1871, ix, 641.—**Menzel** (A.) Atrofia muscolare all' omero destro. Resoc. san. d. Osp. civ. di Trieste, 1876, ii, 153.—**Meryon** (E.) On granular and fatty degeneration of the voluntary muscles. Med.-Chir. Tr., Lond., 1852, xxxv, 73-84, 1 pl. *Also, transl.* [Abstr.]: Gaz. d. hôp., Par., 1853, xxvii, 506. ——. On granular degeneration of the voluntary muscles. Med.-Chir. Tr., Lond., 1866, xlix, 45-50, 1 pl.—**Miles** (F. T.) Case of extreme muscular atrophy of the lower extremities; neuritis (?); recovery. Maryland M. J., Balt., 1877, i, 234-239.—**Moussous.** Trois observations d'atrophie musculaire. Gaz. d hôp., Par., 1857, xxx, 430.—**Niepce.** Atrophie musculaire. Gaz. méd. de Par., 1853, 3. s., viii, 260-263.—**Onimus** (E.) On professional muscular atrophy. Lancet, Lond., 1876, i, 127.—**Oppolzer.** Ueber Muskelatrophie. Spitals-Ztg., Wien, 1860, 161; 177; 225.—**Partridge.** Fatty degeneration of voluntary muscle. Tr. Path. Soc. Lond., 1846-8, i, 334.—**Pepper** (W.) Clinical lecture on a case of progressive muscular sclerosis. Med. Times, Phila., 1870-71, i, 329; 349. *Also*, Reprint. ——. Atrophy of the pectoral muscles of one side of the chest, associated with functional palpitation of the heart and intercostal neuralgia. Med. Bull., Phila., 1883, v, 1-4.—**Poncet.** Coup de feu sous la clavicule droite; atrophie musculaire envahissant le bras droit, le

Muscles (*Atrophy and degenerations of*).
bras gauche et le tronc. Gaz. méd. de Par., 1875, 4. s., iv,
304.—**Prévost.** Atrophie musculaire produite expérimentalement par lésion de la moelle. Compt. rend. Soc.
de biol. 1872, Par., 1874, 5. s., iv, 105.—**Rakovac** (L.) Ein
Fall von "Atrophia musculorum lipomatosa". Wien.
med. Wchnschr., 1872, xxii, 273–276. — **Ramskill** (J.)
A case of acute muscular atrophy. Lancet, Lond., 1868,
ii, 634.—**Ranvier** (L.) L'atrophie d'un muscle déterminée par l'amaigrissement est en rapport avec l'atrophie
des faisceaux primitifs. Compt. rend. Soc. de biol. 1871,
Par., 1873, 5. s., iii, 186–188. — **Revillout** (V.) Atrophies musculaires consécutives aux affections du système
nerveux. Gaz. d. hôp., Par., 1878, li, 801–803.--**Rhoads**
(E.) Interstitial and necrobiotic degeneration of muscle.
Am. J. M. Sc., Phila., 1865, n. s., l, 107. — **Robin** (C.)
Note sur l'état de la graisse dans les muscles. Compt.
rend. Soc. de biol. 1864, Par., 1865, 4. s., i, 157 – 159. — **Rosenthal** (M.) Ueber einen Fall von Muskel-
atrophie. Wien. Med.-Halle, 1862, iii, 400; 416; 435; 443.—
S. (H.) Congenital want of power, and muscular atrophy
of the lower extremities. Med. Exam.. Phila., 1842, v, 35-
38.—**Schaumont.** Chute d'un lieu élevé; atrophie complète des muscles de l'épaule et incomplète de ceux du
bras. Rec. de mém. de méd. . . . mil., Par., 1870, 3. s.,
xxv, 342–344.—**Scholz.** Ein exquisiter Fall von Muskelatrophie. Wien. Med.-Halle, 1861, ii, 398.—**Schüller**
(M.) Fall von Atrophie der rechtsseitigen Schulter- und
Rückenmusculatur. Deutsche Ztschr. f. Chir., Leipz.,
1877-8, ix, 298–300.—**Shershevski** (M.) O zavisimosti
jyrovaho perejenia myshtz pavalizovanych tchastey ot pre-
krash-tchenia inervatziy. [Of the influence of the innervation of the paralyzed part on the transformation of muscles into fat.] Vojenno-med. J., St.-Petersb., 1867, xcviii,
pt. 2, 87–104.—**Signol.** De la brusque dégénérescence
graisseuse des muscles chez le cheval. Bull. Soc. de méd.
prat. de Par., 1876, 35–37.—[**Soulier.**] Exemple d'atrophie musculaire. Lyon méd., 1870, v, 35.—**Steinert** (B.)
Beitrag zur Kenntniss der Inactivitätsatrophie der Muskelfaser. Verhandl. d. phys.-med. Gesellsch. zu Würzb.,
1887. n. F., xx, 217–227.—**Stuart** (A.) Experimentelle
Studien über die fettige Entartung des Muskelgewebes.
Arch. f. mikr. Anat , Bonn, 1865, i, 415–427, 1 pl.—**Takács**
(E.) Az elöhaladó izomsorvadás egy esete. [Case of progressive atrophy of muscles.] Orvosi hetil., Budapest,
1881, xxv, 825; 848, 1 pl. — **Tillaux.** Atrophie musculaire consécutive aux congélations Bull. gén. de thérap.,
etc., Par., 1871, lxxx, 226–230.—**Tulenburg.** Cas remarquable d'affection musculaire (atrophie ascendante
chronique). Gaz. hebd. de méd., Par., 1863, x, 750–753.—
Valtat (E.) De l'atrophie musculaire dans le cours des
maladies des articulations. Arch. gén. de méd., Par.,
1877, ii, 159–183.—**de Vicq-d'Azyr.** Observation anatomique. [*From:* Mém. Acad. roy. d. sc. de Par., 1772.]
Collect. acad. d. mém., etc., Par., 1787, xv, 311–313.—
Voisin (A.) & **Hanot** (V.) Sur deux cas d'atrophie
musculaire observée dans le cours de la paralysie générale.
Compt. rend. Soc. de biol. 1872, Par., 1874, 5. s., iv, pt. 2,
93–105. *Also:* Gaz. méd. de Par., 1874, 4. s., iii, 136; 164.—
Vulpian (A.) Sur les modifications que subissent les
muscles sous l'influence de la section de leurs nerfs.
Arch. de physiol. norm. et path., Par., 1869, ii, 558–578.—
Webber (S. G.) The relation between lesion of the nervous system and muscular atrophy. J. Psych. M., N. Y.,
1871, v, 242–261.—**Weihl** (W.) Experimentelle Untersuchungen über die "wachsartige Degeneration" der quergestreiften Muskelfasern. Arch. f. path. Anat., etc., Berl,
1874, lxi, 253–267, 1 pl.—**Weiss** (N.) Ueber einen Fall von
progressiver Muskelatrophie. Wien. med. Wchnschr.,
1877, xxvii, 701–703.—**Whitford.** Case of atrophy of
numerous muscles of the upper extremities. Brit. M. J.,
Lond., 1858, 346.—**Wyman** (J.) Transformation of muscular fibre into fat. Boston M. & S. J., 1865, lxxii, 18.

Muscles (*Cancer of*).
KARPOVITCH (J.) * Ke voprosu o razvitii raka
ve mishtsache ve patologo-gistolog. otnoshenii.
[On the development of cancer in muscles.] 8°.
St. Petersburg, 1868.

ROSENBACH (A.) * Der Epithelialkrebs im
quergestreiften Muskel. 8°. *Göttingen*, 1873.

VIGNES (L.) Des tumeurs dites cancéreuses
primitives des muscles de la vie de relation. 4°.
Paris, 1862.

Chevalier (T. W.) General observations on morbid
tumors, and on the different modes in which the muscular
structure is attacked by cancer and medullary sarcoma.
Lond. M. & Phys. J., 1826, lv, 95–103, 1 pl.—**Demarquay.** Sur les tumeurs dites cancéreuses des muscles de
la vie de relation. Union méd., Par., 1861, 2. s., xi, 403;
421. — **Donati** (P.) Carcinoma muscolare primitivo.
Gazz. med. ital., prov. venete, Padova, 1869, xii, 139–141.—
Luzzatto (M.) Cancro primitivo dei muscoli. Gior.
veneto di sc. med., Venezia, 1871, 3. s., xiv, 33–51.—**Popper** (F.) Beiträge zur näheren Kenntniss der Entwick-

Muscles (*Cancer of*).
lung des Krebses in den quergestreiften Muskeln. Med.
Jahrb., Wien, 1865, x, 37–80, 2 pl. *Also* [Abstr.]: Wien.
med. Presse, 1865, vi, 688.—**Sick** (P.) Ein Muskelkrebs.
Arch. f. path. Anat., etc., Berl., 1864, xxxi, 331–335.—
Volkmann (R.) Zur Histiologie des Muskelkrebses.
Ibid., 1870, l, 543–549, 1 pl. — **Weil** (C.) Beiträge zur
Kenntniss des Muskelkrebses. Med. Jahrb., Wien, 1873,
285–291, 1 pl.—**von Wittich.** Krebs der Muskeln. Arch.
f. path. Anat., etc., Berl., 1853, vii, 324–327.

Muscles (*Contraction and spasm of*).
See, also, **Cadaver** (*Attitudes of*); **Chorea** ;
Contractions ; **Cramp** ; **Rigor** *mortis* ; **Risus**
sardonicus ; **Tetanus** ; **Thomsen's** *disease*.

CESBRON (J.) * Étude sur la contracture musculaire syphilitique. 4°. *Paris*, 1879.

GAILLARD (F.-L.) Étude sur la contraction
musculaire à propos du jugement de la croix des
affections simulées et des luxations. 8°. *Poitiers*,
1864.

MAYR (D.) * Ueber Durchschneidung der
Kaumuskeln. 8°. *Erlangen*, 1852.

Aeby (C.) Ueber die Fortpflanzungsgeschwindigkeit
der Muskelzuckung. Arch. f. Anat , Physiol. u. wissensch.
Med., Leipz., 1860, 253. — **Bell** (G. H.) A peculiar convulsive affection of the respiratory muscles. Edinb. M. &
S. J., 1835, xliii, 260–262. — **Bouveret** (L.) Note sur un
spasme fonctionnel du long péronier latéral et des jumeaux.
Mém. et compt.-rend. Soc. d. sc. méd. de Lyon (1881),
1882, xxi, pt. 2, 150–156.—**Ceysens** (E.) Contracture des
muscles fléchisseurs des avant-bras et des mains; emploi
de l'électrisation localisée; guérison. J. de méd., chir. et
pharmacol., Brux., 1858, xxvi, 230–232. — [**Chronic**
spasm of the trapezius resembling fatty tumour; incision;
restoration of the muscle to its normal state.] St. George's
Hosp. Rep. 1877–8, Lond., 1879, ix, 265. — **Desalleurs**
fils. Affection convulsive de la jambe gauche. Clin. d.
hôp., Par., 1829, iv, 55.—**Duchenne.** Note sur le spasme
fonctionnel et la paralysie musculaire fonctionnelle. Bull.
gén. de thérap., etc., Par., 1860, lviii, 145 ; 196 ; 245. —
Fieber (F.) Ein Fall von Muskelcontractur und seine
Reaction gegen electrischen und mechanischen Einfluss.
Arch. f. path. Anat., etc., Berl., 1879, lxxvi, 364–368.—
Fleury. Contracture du muscle couturier; myotomie.
Bull. Soc. de chir. de Par., 1872, 3. s., i, 188–190.—**Friedberg** (H.) Ein Fall von myopathischer Luxation [of
shoulder]. Oesterr. Ztschr. f. prakt., Heilk., Wien, 1857,
iii, 1–10.—**Gairdner** (J.) A peculiar affection of the
organs of respiration. Edinb. M. & S. J., 1835, xliii, 257–
260.—**Itard** (J.-M.-G.) Mémoire sur quelques fonctions
involontaires des appareils de la locomotion, de la préhension et de la voix. Arch. gén. de méd., Par., 1825, viii,
385–407.—**Jackson** (H.) Spasm of the muscles supplied
by the portio dura of the right side for more than thirty
years ; good general health until the age of seventy-one;
then hemiplegia on the left side ; recovery ; subsequent
amaurosis of one eye. Med. Times & Gaz., Lond., 1863,
ii, 11.—**Malgaigne.** Recherches et expériences sur
la rétraction musculaire, considérée sous le point de vue
chirurgical. J. hebd. d. progr. d. sc. et inst. méd., Par.,
1836, iv, 417–438. *Also:* Ann. de méd. belge, Brux., 1837,
i, 55–62. ———. Lettre sur un cas de contracture bornée
au cleïdo-mastoïdien. Gaz. méd. de Par., 1838, 2. s., vi,
255. — **Manouvriez** (A.) Recherches sur les troubles
de la sensibilité dans la contracture idiopathique des extrémités. Bull. méd. du nord, Lille, 1876, xv, 263–296.—
Meyer (M.) Jahre lang bestehender klonischer Krampf
der hinteren linksseitigen Halsmuskeln (Mm. biventer
und complexus) durch Electricität geheilt. Deutsche
med. Wchnschr., Berl., 1876, ii, 205.—**Michel** (M.) Examination of the negro, Thomas, who arrests his heart's
action, and pretends to throw his heart into the abdomen. Boston M. & S. J., 1878, xcix, 551–557. — **Murdoch** (W.) Considérations sur les rétractions musculaires
spasmodiques. J. univ. et hebd. de méd. et chir. prat.,
Par., 1832, viii, 417–426. — **Onimus** (E.) Contractures.
Dict. encycl. d. sc. méd., Par., 1877, xx, 62–95.—**Piollet.**
Observation sur une irritation périodique des jambes.
Clin. d. hôp., Par., 1829, iv, 55. — **Rennes.** Accès de
crampes partielles se succédant rapidement dans la plupart des muscles et produisant dans ceux du larynx une
constriction voisine de la strangulation, chez une malade
gravement atteinte de phlegmasie chronique du poumon.
Gaz. d. hôp., Par., 1861, xxxiv, 294.—**Romberg.** Ueber
den Krampf der Nacken- und Halsmuskeln. Deutsche
Klinik, Berl., 1849, i, 4.—**Werner.** Clonische Krämpfe
der Nackenmuskeln und des Kopfnickers rechterseits;
wiederholte Myotomieen; innerlicher Gebrauch von Arsenik ; sehr bedeutende Besserung. Med. Cor.-Bl. d. württemb. ärztl. Ver., Stuttg., 1860, xxx, 300–303.—**Zuradelli**
(C.) Su varie specie di contratture, che si osservano agli
arti superiori, e specialmente sulla contrattura simultanea
del bicipite e del supinator lungo. Gazz. med. ital. lomb.,
Milano, 1861, 4. s., vi, 25 ; 49 ; 57 ; 65.

Muscles (*Degenerations of*).

See **Muscles** (*Atrophy, etc., of*).

Muscles (*Diseases and pathology of*).

See, also, **Atrophy** (*Muscular, etc.*); **Locomotion** (*Organs of, etc.*); **Muscles** (*Hypertrophy of*); **Muscles** (*Inflammation of*); **Myalgia**: **Paralysis**; **Rheumatism** (*Muscular*); **Tremor**.

BODEN (O.) * De musculorum paralysi ex alienata eorum nutritione. 8°. *Berolini*, [1862].

BOKMA DE BOER (B.) * De sarcogenesi et morbis musculorum organicis. 8°. *Groningæ*, [1834].

CEYSENS (H.-E.) Considérations théoriques et pratiques sur quelques maladies musculaires et surtout sur le rhumatisme musculaire. 12°. *Hasselt*, 1862.

DANNEIL (H.) * Quædam de anatomia musculorum pathologica. 8°. *Halis*, 1859.

HELLERSBERG (F.) * De nonnullis musculorum morbis. 8°. *Berolini*, [1833].

HEPP (L.) * Die pathologischen Veränderungen der Muskelfaser. 8°. *Zürich*, 1853.

HOPMANN (M.) * Ueber die primären Myopathien. 8°. *Berlin*, [1886].

ISENFLAMM (J. F.) Versuch einiger praktischen Anmerkungen über die Muskeln zur Erläuterung verschiedener verborgener Krankheiten und Zufälle entworfen. 8°. *Erlangen*, 1778.

LANTENOIS (A.-P.) * Sur l'influence de l'action musculaire dans le développement et les phénomènes des maladies chirurgicales. 4°. *Paris*, 1826.

LESER (E.) Untersuchungen über ischämische Muskellähmungen und Muskelcontracturen. roy. 8°. *Leipzig*, 1884.

OLTENDORF (H.) * Ueber Tuberkulose quergestreifter Muskeln. [Erlangen.] 8°. *Berlin*, [1885].

DE SCHALLHAMMER (F. L.) * De morbis fibræ muscularis ex materiei animalis mixtura mutata cognoscendis. 4°. *Halæ*, 1799.

Also, transl. in: Arch. f. d. Physiol., Halle, 1800, iv, 222–289, 1 pl.

WEISS (J. J.) * De musculorum pathologia. sm. 4°. *Erlangæ*, [1774].

ZADE (H.) * Ueber Dystrophia musculorum progressiva. 8°. *Würzburg*, 1886.

Bamberger. [Combinirter Fall von Muskelatrophie und Muskelhypertrophie.] Anz. d. k. k. Gesellsch. d. Aerzte in Wien, 1878, 13.—**Benedikt** (M.) Ueber spontane und reflectorische Muskelspannungen. Deutsche Klinik, Berl., 1864, xvi, 281; 297; 309; 317; 327.—**Bennett** (A. H.) Case of remarkable hyper-excitability of all the muscles and tendons of the body to direct mechanical percussion, with clonus of various regions, including the lower jaw; recovery. Brain, Lond., 1886-7, ix, 228–233.—**Berger.** Fall von hochgradiger Pseudohypertrophie der Muskeln. Jahresb. d. schles. Gesellsch. f. vaterl. Kult., Bresl., 1876, liii, 202.—**Blasius** (E.) Ueber Stabilität der Theile und Stabilitätsneurosen. Arch. f. physiol. Heilk., Stuttg., 1851, x, 210–275. *Also*, Reprint.—**Blot** (H.) Examen histologique des muscles gras. Compt. rend. Soc. de biol. 1857, Par., 1858, 2. s., iv, 92.—**Bouilly** (G.) Synovite fongueuse des péroniers latéraux. Gaz. méd. de Par., 1881, 6. s., iii, 437–440.—**Brissaud** (E.) De la myopathie progressive primitive. Gaz. hebd. de méd., Par., 1886, 2. s., xxiii, 582–585.—**Clarke** (J. L.) Muscular system, Diseases of. Syst. Surg. (Holmes), 2. ed., N. Y., 1870, iii, 621–657.—**Conner** (P. S.) Injuries and diseases of the muscles, tendons, and fasciæ. Internat. Encycl. Surg. (Ashhurst), N. Y., 1883, iii, 1–25.—**Dally.** Contributions à la pathologie musculaire. Gaz. hebd. de méd., Par., 1874, 2. s., xi, 622–625.—**Edgren** (J. G.) Om den primära progressiva myopatin dess scapulo-humerala typ jämte en öfversigt af beslägtade kliniska former. Nord. med. Ark., Stockholm, 1887, xix, no. 5, 1-51, 4 pl.—**Endurcissement** des muscles larges de l'abdomen, des muscles des cuisses et de ceux des jambes. J. gén. de méd., chir. et pharm., Par., 1826, xcvii, 35–37.—**Erb** (W.) Zur Casuistik der Nerven- und Muskelkrankheiten. Deutsches Arch. f. klin. Med., Leipz., 1870, vii, 246–255. — **Eulenburg** (A.) Ueber successives Auftreten diffuser Muskelerkrankungen bei Geschwistern. Arch. f. path. Anat., etc., Berl., 1871, liii, 361-370. — **França** (F.) Hypertrophia do musculo recto anterior da coxa, simulando um lipoma. J. Soc. d.

Muscles (*Diseases and pathology of*).

sc. med. de Lisb., 1876, xl, 321.—**Giraudeau** (C.) Des infarctus musculaires. Rev. de méd., Par., 1884, iv, 466–472.—**Gubler** (A.) De la cinésialgie, spécialement dans le diastasis musculaire, et de sa guérison instantanée par la faradisation locale. J. de thérap. Par., 1874, i, 697; 721; 761; 801; 891.—**Hallett** (C. H.) On steatosis; or adipification of muscle. Edinb. M. & S. J., 1849, lxxi, 257–269. *Also*, Reprint. — **Hammond** (W. A.) On a hitherto undescribed form of muscular in-coordination. Tr. Am. Neurol. Ass., N. Y., 1877, ii, 154–158.—**Hayem** (M.-G.) Note sur les altérations des muscles dans les fièvres, et particulièrement dans la variole. Gaz. méd. de Par., 1866, 3. s., xxi, 698; 712. *Also:* Compt. rend. Soc. de biol. 1866, Par., 1867, 4. s., iii, pt. 2, 93–106. ———. Note sur les altérations musculaires qu'on observe dans les maladies chroniques. Gaz. méd. de Par., 1874, 4. s., iii, 54–56. *Also:* Compt. rend. Soc. de biol. 1874, Par., 1875, 6. s., i, 69-78. ———. Musculaire (Tissu). Pathologie. Dict. encycl. d. sc. méd., Par., 1876, 2. s., x, 697–770. — **Hedenius** (P.) Öfversigt af nyarebidrag till de tvärstrimmiga musklernas pathologiska anatomi. Upsala Läkaref. Förh., 1866–7, ii, 342–375.—**Hénocque** (A.) Musculaire (Tissu). Pathologie chirurgicale. Dict. encycl. d. sc. méd., Par., 1876, 2. s., xi, 87–119.—**Hodge** (H. L.) Extensive fatty degeneration of muscle. Tr. Path. Soc. Phila., 1878, vii, 159.—**Hüter** (C.) Ueber Längeninsufficienz der bi- und polyarthroidalen Muskeln; ihre Bedeutung für die Muskelkraft. Arch. f. path. Anat., etc., Berl., 1869, xlvi, 37–52.—**Katischeff** (I.) Sluch. miotonii. Trudi Obsh. Russk. vrach. v. S.-Peterb., 1887, ii, 146-152.—**Labalbary.** Myosclérose sterno-mastoïdienne. Gaz. d. hôp., Par., 1862, xxxv, 591. — **Landouzy** (L.) & **Déjerine** (J.) De la myopathie atrophique progressive: myopathie héréditaire, sans neuropathie, débutant d'ordinaire dans l'enfance, par la face. Rev. de méd., Par., 1885, v, 81; 253. *Also*, Reprint.—**Le Dentu** (A.) Muscle; pathologie chirurgicale. N. dict. de méd. et chir. prat., Par., 1877, xxiii, 357–376.—**Longuet** (R.) Des myopathies progressives primitives. Union méd., Par., 1886, 3. s., xli, 157; 181.—**Lücke.** Ein Fall von Muskelnecrose. Verhandl. d. deutsch. Gesellsch. f. Chir., Berl., 1878, vii, pt. 1, 112–114.—**Luzzatto** (M.) Miopatie progressive primitive. Riv. sintetica. Riv. veneta di sc. med., Venezia, 1885, iii, 615–639.—**Marchand** (F.) Ueber Tuberculose der Körpermuskeln. Arch. f. path. Anat., etc., Berl., 1878, lxxii, 142–144.—**Martini** (E.) Beitrag zur pathol. Histiologie der quergestreiften Muskeln. 1. Wachsige Degeneration. 2. Traumatische Myositis. 3. Muskelregeneration. Deutsches Arch. f. klin. Med., Leipz., 1868, iv, 505–534. *Also*, Reprint.—**Mégnin** (P.) Note sur une prolifération extraordinaire de corpuscules calcaires dans le tissu musculaire d'un cheval. Compt. rend. Soc. de biol., Par., 1884, 8. s., i, pt. 2, 129. *Also:* Gaz. d. hôp., Par., 1884, lvii, 234.—**Meryon** (E.) Case of granular degeneration of the voluntary muscles. Brit. M. J., Lond., 1870. ii, 32.—**Meyer** (S. H.) Mechanische Stase in den Muskeln. Arch. f. physiol. Heilk., Stuttg., 1844, iii, 126–128.—**von Millbacher** (H.) Beitrag zur Pathologie des quergestreiften Muskels. Deutsches Arch. f. klin. Med., Leipz.. 1881-2, xxx, 304–331, 1 pl. *Also:* Arb. a. d. med.-klin. Inst. d. k. Ludwig-Maximilians-Univ. zu München, Leipz., 1884, i, 305–332, 1 pl.—**Müller** (E.) Ueber Muskeltuberkulose. Beitr. z. klin. Chir., Tübing., 1886, ii, 489–494.—**Nevermann.** Crepitatio musculorum, eine neue oder sehr seltene Krankheit. Med. Ann., Heidelb., 1837, iii, 318–320.—**Nicoladoni.** Ueber einen seltenen Fall von Muskel-Erkrankung. Wien. med. Presse, 1878, xix, 738. — **Oppolzer.** Ueber Muskelschwiele. Allg. Wien. med. Ztg., 1861, vi, 217. — **Paget** (J.) On some affections of voluntary muscles. Med. Times & Gaz., Lond., 1858, n. s., xvi, 260. ———. Remarks on stammering with other organs than those of speech. Brit. M. J., Lond., 1868, ii, 437.—**Paulicki.** Zur Entartung der quergestreiften Musculatur in acuten Krankheiten. Central'bl. f. d. med. Wissensch., Berl., 1867, v, 660.—**Perroncito** (E.) Contribuzione alla patologia del tessuto muscolare. Gior. d. r. Accad. di med. di Torino, 1882, 3. s., xxx, 574–602, 1 pl. *Also, transl.:* Arch. ital. de biol., Turin, 1882, i, 367–388, 2 pl.—**Popoff** (L.) Ueber die Veränderung des Muskelgewebes bei einigen Infectionskrankheiten. Arch. f. path. Anat., etc., Berl., 1874, lxi, 322–342, 3 pl.—**Rasmussen** (A. F.) To Tilfælde af akut Ossifikation af Musc. brachiæus int. Hosp.-Tid., Kjøbenh., 1883, i, 3. R., 769–773.—**Rhoads.** Interstitial and necrobiotic degeneration of muscle. Proc. Path. Soc. Phila. (1860-66), 1867, ii, 176 —**Ringer** (S.) & **Sainsbury** (H.) On the nervous or muscular origin of certain spastic conditions of the voluntary muscles. Lancet, Lond., 1884, ii, 767; 815; 860.—**Russell** (C. M.) Case of compound fracture of hand; softening of bones about elbow-joint; conversion of muscles around joint into adipocere; amputation of arm; recovery. Indian M. Gaz., Calcutta, 1876, xi, 331.—**Schottin** (E.) Untersuchungen über den Wassergehalt der Muskeln in verschiedenen pathologischen Zuständen. Arch. f. physiol. Heilk., Stuttg., 1852, xi, 622–625. — **Seidel** (M.) Die Krankheiten der Muskeln. Handb. d. Kinderkr. (Gerhardt), Tübing., 1879, v, 1. Abth., 3-58.— **Singer** (J.) Zur Kenntniss der primären Myopathieen. Ztschr. f. Heilk., Prag, 1887, viii, 229–250, 2 pl.—

Muscles (*Diseases and pathology of*).

Sonnenberg (J.) Example of a periodical myopathy, following a contusion of the thighs. Lancet, Lond., 1832-3, ii, 621-623. — **Staub.** Crepitatio musculorum. Schweiz. Ztschr. f. Nat.- u. Heilk., Zürich, 1841, vi, 26. — **Straus** (I.) Muscle; pathologie. N. dict. de méd. et chir. prat., Par., 1877, xxiii, 263-357. — **Taylor** (F.) Induration of the sterno-mastoid muscle. Tr. Path. Soc. Lond., 1874-5, xxvi, 224-227. — **Thurn.** Veränderungen des Elasticitätsmasses von Muskeln und Bändern. Wien. med. Wchnschr., 1867, xvii, 596; 611. — **Uchastii** (Ob) nervnoi sistemwi v' atrophii myoshits pri golodai. [Part played by the nervous system in atrophy of the muscles from defective nutrition.] Protok. zasaid. Obsh. russk. vrach. v St. Petersb., 1875, 51-58. — **Ughetti** (G. B.) Delle alterazioni dei tessuti da mancata influenza nervose; ricerche sperimentali, a speciale contribuzione della patologia del tessuto muscolare striato. Arch. per le sc. med., Torino, 1880, iv, 190-220, 1 pl. — **W.** (J. A.) Liabilities of the muscle in disease; paralysis. Lancet, Lond., 1845, ii, 669. — **Wagner.** Zur Casuistik chronischer Muskelerkrankung. Berl. klin. Wchnschr., 1866, iii, 185-188. — **Wagner** (E.) Fall einer seltnen Muskelkrankheit. Arch. d. Heilk., Leipz., 1863, iv, 282. — **Waldeyer** (W.) Ueber die Veränderungen der quergestreiften Muskeln bei der Entzündung und dem Typhusprozess, sowie über die Regeneration derselben nach Substanzdefecten. Arch. f. path. Anat., etc., Berl., 1865, xxxiv, 473 - 514, 1 pl. — **Werner.** Untersuchungen über die Folgen der vermehrten und verminderten Thätigkeit der Muskeln; zur Begründung einer wissenschaftlichen Therapie der Skoliosen leitend. Med. Ztg., Berl., 1850, xix, 131-133. — **Wilson** (J. A.) Liabilities of the muscle in disease. Lancet, Lond., 1846, i, 333. — **Wilson** (J. C.) Observations on the hypodermic use of atropia in muscular rigidities, rheumatic and myalgic. Phila. M. Times, 1874-5, v, 81-83. — **Wright** (T. H.) Muscular tissue; calcareous deposit. Am. J. M. Sc., Phila., 1831-2, ix, 89.

Muscles (*Dislocations, ruptures, and injuries of*).

See, also, Biceps (*Dislocation, etc., of*).

ASCHER (S.) * Ueber die subcutanen Muskel-und Nerven-Verletzungen. 8°. *Erlangen*, 1887.

BOUQUET (J.) * De la rupture spontanée des muscles de la vie animale. 4°. *Paris*, 1847.

BOURGOUGNON (G.) * Ruptures et contractures musculaires des ouvriers chargeurs. 4°. *Paris*, 1875.

CAMBON (E.) * Contribution à l'étude des hernies musculaires spontanées et traumatiques. 4°. *Montpellier*, 1878.

DAGOTT (C. A.) * Ueber die Regeneration der quergestreiften Muskeln nach Verletzungen. 8°. *Königsberg*, 1869.

DEVÉMY (P.) * Contribution à l'étude des ruptures musculaires. 4°. *Paris*, 1878.

ERBKAM (R.) * Beiträge zur Kenntniss der Degeneration und Regeneration von quergestreifter Musculatur nach Quetschung. 8°. *Königsberg i. Pr.*, [1879].

HAUSBRAND (J.) * Diss. luxationis sic dictæ musculorum refutationem sistens. 8°. *Berolini*, 1814.

PRAT (C.) * Contribution à l'étude des hernies musculaires. Considérations sur la hernie du jambier antérieur. 4°. *Paris*, 1879.

RÉGEARD (A.) * Étude sur les ruptures musculaires. 4°. *Paris*, 1880.

SCHNELL (B. F.) * De natura reunionis musculorum vulneratorum. 12°. *Tubingæ*, [1804].

Addison (K.) Rupture of the rectus femoris muscle. Canada Lancet, Toronto, 1871-2, iv, 212. — **Alleson** (W.) On contusion of muscles. Prov. M. & S. J., Lond., 1842, iv, 144 - 146. — **Alling** (E.) Injections sous-cutanées de chlorhydrate de morphine dans les ruptures musculaires partielles. Bull. gén. de thérap., etc, Par., 1869, lxxvi, 113 - 117. — **Barlow** (E.) Case of laceration in the fibres of the gastrocnemius muscle, treated without rest or confinement. Edinb. M. & S. J., 1823, xix, 358-360. — **Baudin** (L.) Contribution à l'étude de la hernie musculaire spontanée. Rec. de mém. de méd. . . . mil., Par., 1881, 3. s., xxxvii, 319 - 339. — **Boinet.** Hernie musculaire du moyen adducteur gauche. Lyon méd., 1884, xlvii, 111-117. *Also:* Mém. et compt.-rend. Soc. d. sc. méd. de Lyon (1884), 1885, xxiv, 158-164. — **Bousquet.** Tumeur formée par la rupture du moyen adducteur du côté droit. Bull. et mém. Soc. de chir. de Par., 1881, n. s., vii, 454-456. — **Brachini** (A.) Caso di sutura muscolare e nervosa. Imparziale, Firenze, 1883, xxiii, 141; 189. — **Broca.** Sur

Muscles (*Dislocations, ruptures, and injuries of*).

un cas de luxation du muscle tibial postérieur comparé à celles des péroniers latéraux et de la longue portion du biceps brachial. Bull. Acad. de méd., Par., 1874, 2. s., iii, 7-20. — **Brunzlow.** Zerreissung des schlanken Schenkelmuskels (M. gracilis) der rechten Seite. Med. Ztg., Berl., 1838, vii, 61. — **Bryant.** Rupture of gastrocnemius; hæmorrhage into muscle; recovery after incision. Lancet, Lond., 1880, i, 487. — **Callender** (G. W.) Dislocations of muscles and their treatment. Brit. M. J. Lond., 1878, ii, 51. — **Charvot & Couillault.** Étude clinique sur les ruptures musculaires chez les cavaliers. Rev. de chir., Par., 1887, vii, 325; 448. — **Collins** (S. B.) Rupture of quadriceps tendon from muscular violence. Phila. M. Times, 1876-7, vii, 174. — **Courtaux.** Rupture par contraction spasmodique, de quelques faisceaux du jumeau interne droit, au niveau de leur insertion avec le tendon d'Achille. Rev. de thérap. méd.-chir., Par., 1877, xliv, 286-288. — **Crow** (W. A.) A case of rupture of a muscular attachment followed by a large abscess. South. M. Rec., Atlanta, 1885, xv, 125. — **Dartière** (É.) Déchirure de l'aponévrose fémorale antérieure avec hernie consécutive du muscle crural, et rupture des fibres superficielles de ce muscle. Progrès méd., Par., 1885, 2. s., ii. 517. — **Denis.** Observations sur la lésion des aponévroses. J. d'obs. de méd., chir.et pharm., Calais, [1786?], 278-285. — **Deramé** (M.) Observation sur une rupture de muscle par une violente contraction. Mém. Soc. méd. d'émulat. de Par. (an v), an vi [1798], i, 159-162. — **Elleaume.** Rupture musculaire dite coup de fouet; tumeur sanguine; massage; guérison. Bull. Soc. de méd.-prat. de Par., 1862, 10-12. — **England** (W.) Rupture of the rectus femoris of both thighs. Lond. M. Gaz., 1841-2, xxix, 49. — **Fabrizi.** Application de la ténotomie au traitement chirurgical des anciennes plaies des muscles. Gaz. méd. de Par., 1844, 2. s., xii, 526-528. — **Farabeuf.** Rapport sur une observation de M. le Dr. Larger, intitulée : Hernie du muscle tibial antérieur. Bull. et mém. Soc. de chir. de Par., 1881, n. s., vii, 293-299. — **Forster** (J. C.) Laceration of extensors of thigh at insertion into patella by muscular action. Guy's Hosp. Rep., Lond., 1874, 3. s., xix, 45. — **Frédericq** (A.) Rupture de quelques muscles qui fixent l'omoplate. Ann. Soc. méd. d'émulat. de la Flandre occid., Roulers, 1849, iii, 5-8. — **Gayet.** Rupture des muscles droits de l'abdomen. Mém. et compt.-rend. Soc. d. sc. méd. de Lyon (1864), 1865, iv, 979-98. — **Gies** (T.) Zwei operativ behandelte Fälle von Hernia muscularis. Berl. klin. Wchnschr., 1886, xxiii, 174. — **Gillet de Grandmont.** Observation de luxation des péroniers latéraux. Bull. Soc. de méd. prat. de Par. (1878), 1879, 24-28. — **Graham** (D.) Two cases of muscular rupture in which massage was used. Med. Rec., N. Y., 1876, xi, 233. — **Grantham** (J.) On the diagnosis and treatment of rupture of the tendon of the triceps cruralis muscle. Lond. M. Gaz., 1848, n. s., iii, 670. — — . Oblique laceration of the middle portion of the flexor carpi radialis and palmaris longus. *Ibid.*, 1849, n. s., viii, 1107. — **Gross** (S. D.) Rupture of muscle in lumbar region. Med. & Surg. Reporter, Phila., 1874, xxx, 400. — **Hamon** (L.) Rupture du deltoïde à son insertion acromio-claviculaire, suite de convulsions épileptiques. France méd., Par., 1869, xvi, 309. — **Hill** (J. D.) Notes on sub-cutaneous rupture of muscles and tendons in the upper and lower extremities. Med. Press & Circ., Lond., 1870, n. s., ix, 205; 226. — **Hofmokl.** Ruptura tendinis musculi quadricipitis lateris triusque; Heilung. Ber. d. k. k. Krankenanst. Rudolph-Stiftung in Wien (1885), 1886, 336. *Also:* Med.-chir. Centralbl., Wien, 1887, xxii, 3. — **Holthouse** (C.) Cast of a supposed rupture of the upper and anterior part of the sheath of the rectus abdominis muscle. Tr. Path. Soc. Lond., 1861-2, xiii, 263. — **Jeannel** (M.) Blessures et maladies des muscles, des tendons et des aponévroses. Encycl. internat. de chir. (Ashhurst), Par., 1884, iii, 149-186. — **Lardier.** Du coup de fouet, ou diastasis musculaire, et de sa guérison immédiate par la faradisation. Concours méd., Par., 1883, v, 446; 458. — **Larrey** (H.) Hernie musculaire. Bull. Soc. de chir. de Par. (1871), 1872, 2. s., xi, 51. — **Legouest.** Rupture du muscle droit antérieur de l'abdomen du côté gauche. Gaz. d. hôp., Par., 1860, xxxiii, 301. — **Lemoine.** Des tumeurs hématiques consécutives à la rupture du grand muscle droit de l'abdomen. Rec. de mém. de méd: . . . mil., Par., 1881, 3. s., xxxvii, 285-297. — **Letenneur.** Rupture sous-cutanée du muscle grand pectoral; guérison complète en quinze jours. J. de la sect. de méd. Soc. acad. Loire-Inf., Nantes, 1861, n. s., xxxvii, 202-205. *Also:* Gaz. d. hôp., Par., 1862, xxxv, 54. — **Lionville.** Ruptures musculaires et hématomes dans les muscles. Bull. Soc. anat. de Par. (1869), 1870, xliv, 187. — **Löwenstamm.** Hernia muscularis. Med.-chir. Centrabl., Wien, 1877, xii, 317. — **Malinovski** (I.) Redkii sluchai otriva suchojilija bol. grudnoi mush. (M. pectoralis major) ot miesta prikriep. k spina tuberculi maj. ossis humeri. [Rare case of rupture of the pectoralis major muscle at its attachment with the process of the humerus.] Voyenno-med. J., St. Petersb., 1885, cliii, pt. 3, 136-138. — **Martins** (C.) Sur un cas de luxation du muscle tibial postérieur comparé à celles des péroniers latéraux et de la longue portion du bi-

Muscles (*Dislocations, ruptures, and injuries of*).

ceps brachial. Bull. Acad. de méd., Par., 1874, 2. s., iii, 7–20. *Also*, Reprint. *Also* [Abstr.]: France méd., Par., 1874, xxi, 58; 81.—**Maslowsky** (J.) Ueber die Neubildung und die Heilung des quergestreiften Muskelgewebes nach traumatischen Verletzungen. Wien. med. Wchnschr., 1868. xviii, 192-194.—**Mason** (F.) Ruptured muscle from tetanic spasms. Tr. Path. Soc. Lond., 1867-8, xix, 448.—**Masson.** Diastasis musculaire; guérison immédiate par la faradisation. Bull. Soc. méd. de l'Yonne 1883, Auxerre, 1884, xxiv, 146-148.—**Mastin** (C. H.) A case of rupture of the quadriceps femoris muscle. South. M. & S. J., Augusta, 1849, n. s., v, 714.—**Maydl** (K.) Ueber subcutane Muskel- und Sehnenzerreissungen, sowie Rissfracturen, mit Berücksichtigung der analogen, durch directe Gewalt entstandenen und offenen Verletzungen. Deutsche Ztschr. f. Chir., Leipz., 1882, xvii, 306; 513: 1882-3, xviii, 35.—**Michael** (J. E.) Cast and case of rupture of rectus femoris. Maryland M. J., Balt., 1884-5, xii, 98.—**Mollière** (D.) Nouveau traitement de la luxation du long péronier latéral. Lyon méd., 1879, xxxii, 298-302. *Also:* Mém. et compt.-rend. Soc. d. sc. méd. de Lyon (1879), 1880, xix, pt. 2, 184-189.—**Mothe.** Réflexions sur la luxation des muscles. *In his:* Mélanges de chir., etc., 8°, Par., 1812, i, 289 - 316. ———. Mémoire contre la luxation supposée des muscles. *Ibid.*; 1827, ii, 401-426.—**Mourlon.** Essai sur les hernies musculaires, précédé de quelques considérations sur les autres déplacements des muscles. Rec. de mém de méd. . . . mil , Par., 1861, 3. s., vi, 227-255. *Also:* Monit. d. sc. méd. et pharm., Par., 1861, iii, 970; 980.—**Murphy** (E.) Rupture of the biceps. Brit. M. J., Lond., 1887, ii, 829.—**Neumann** (E.) Ueber den Heilungsprocess nach Muskelverletzungen. Arch. f. mikr. Anat., Bonn, 1868, iv, 323-333.—**Phocas** (G.) Rupture musculaire; épanchement fibrineux; déformations consécutives. Bull. Soc. clin. de Par., 1884, viii, 96-102. *Also:* France méd., Par., 1884, ii, 1359-1364.—**Piorry** (P.-A.) Rupture des muscles jumeaux qu'on aurait pu facilement prendre pour celle du plantaire grêle. Bull. clin., Par., 1835-6, i, 99.—**Pouteau** (C.) Sur la luxation des muscles et sur leur réduction. *In his:* Mélanges de chir., 8°, Lyon, 1760, 405-437.—**Ransohoff** (J.) Hernia of the abductor longus. Cincin. Lancet & Clinic, 1880, n. s., iv, 56.—**Raud** (D.-M.) Observation de rupture du droit antérieur de la cuisse. Bull. gén. de thérap., etc., Par., 1844, xxvii. 60.—**Rawitz** (B.) Zwei Fälle von Muskelhernie. Arch. f. klin. Chir., Berl., 1879, xxiv, 382-386, 1 pl.—**Richardson** (S. B.) Rupture of the right rectus abdominis muscle from muscular efforts; operation and recovery. Am. J. M. Sc., Phila., 1857, n. s., xxxiii, 41-45.—**Richter** (C.) Du traitement du tour de reins par l'électricité. France méd., Par., 1874, xxi, 283.—**Robertson** (C. A.) Rupture and section of the rectus muscle. Med. & Surg. Reporter, Phila., 1873, xxix, 184.—**Roulin.** Du mécanisme des ruptures musculaires. J. de physiol expér., Par., 1821, i, 295-300.—**Rupture** of the muscular fibres of the biceps humeri. Lancet, Lond., 1859, ii, 266.—**Sanson** aîné. Observations de rupture musculaire. Gaz. d. hôp., Par., 1831, viii, 45.—**Schüle** (H.) Ueber hämorrhagische Muskel-Rupturen bei schweren Hirnprocessen. Allg. Ztschr. f. Psychiat., etc., Berl., 1867, xxiv, 569-575.—**Sédillot** (J.) Mémoire sur la rupture musculaire. Mém. Soc. de méd. de Par., 1817, 155-199. *Also* [Abstr.]: J. gén. de méd., chir. et pharm., Par., 1817,lxi, 52-74.—**Segond** (P.) Note sur un cas d'arrachement du point d'insertion des deux languettes phalangettiennes de l'extenseur du petit doigt, par flexion forcée de la phalangette sur la .phalangine. Bull. Soc. anat. de Par., 1879, liv, 724-727. *Also:* Progrès méd., Par., 1880, viii, 534.—**Seydel.** Beitrag zur Casuistik der Muskelhernien. München. med. Wchnschr., 1887, xxxiv, 637.—**Silberstein** (A.) Ein Fall von spontaner Muskelruptur. Wien. med. Presse, 1878, xix, 1513.—**Simon** (G.) Ueber die Heilung verletzter Muskeln. Med. Ztg., Berl., 1843, xii, 169.—**Smart** (A.) Rupture of pectoralis major. Guy's Hosp. Gaz., Lond., 1873, ii, 61.—**Szuman** (L.) Przyczynek do leczenia ran mięśniowych i ściegnowych. [Treatment of wounds of muscles and tendons.] Pam. Towarz. Lek. Warszaw., 1880, lxxvi, 381-387.—**Tartière** (E.) Rupture et contracture de l'un des muscles droits antérieurs de l'abdomen dans les exercices de voltige. Arch. de. méd et pharm. mil., Par., 1886, viii, 41-48.—**Thompson** (H.) Case of pneumonia; delirium tremens; rupture of the recti muscles; atrophy of one kidney, and hypertrophy of the other. Med. Times & Gaz., Lond., 1874, i, 476.—**Trélat.** Rupture des fibres du muscle droit de l'abdomen. Gaz. d. hôp., Par., 1882,lv, 948.—**Uhde** (C. W. F.) Zur Casuistik subcutaner Rupturen der Muskeln und Sehnen. Arch. f. klin. Chir., Berl., 1874, xvi, 202-206.—**Verneuil** (A.) De certaines formes graves du coup de fouet. Arch. gén. de méd., Par., 1877, i, 24; 158.—**Virchow.** Ueber Entzündung und Ruptur des Musculus rectus abdominis. Verhandl. d. phys.-med. Gesellsch. in Würzb., 1857, vii, 213.—**Wardrop** (J.) On the larceration of the fibres of muscles, particularly of the external gastrocnemius. Med.-Chir. Tr., Lond., 1816, vii, 278-283.—**Weber** (O.) Ueber die Neubildung quer-

Muscles (*Dislocations, ruptures, and injuries of*).

gestreifter Muskelfasern, insbesondere die regenerative Neubildung derselben nach Verletzungen. Arch. f. path. Anat., etc., Berl., 1867, xxxix, 216–253, 1 pl. — **Weili.** Observation de hernie musculaire du premier adducteur de la cuisse gauche. Rec. de mém. de méd. . . . mil., Par., 1880, 3. s., xxxvi, 612–614. — **Weinlechner** (J.) Ueber subcutane Muskel - Sehnen- und Knochenrisse. Wien. med. Bl., 1881, iv, 1561; 1589. — **Wells** (T.) Injury of the thigh; rupture of the gracilis muscle; extensive effusion; treated, in a chronic state, by incision; cure. Am. J. M. Sc., Phila., 1844, n. s., viii, 77 – 79. — **Whitehead** (W. R.) Rupture of the posterior tibial muscle. Denver M. Times, 1885-6, v, 169-174. — **Wilkie** (J.) On contusions of the muscles. Indian J. M. & Phys. Sc., Calcutta, 1837, n. s., ii, 248-250. — **Wolff** (W.) Die Innervation der glatten Muskulatur. Arch. f. mikr. Anat., Bonn, 1881-2, xx, 361-372, 1 pl. — **Zambelli** (G.) Due casi di strappamento del muscolo gracile della gamba. Gazz. med. ital., prov. venete, Padova, 1864, vii, 36. — **Zsigmondy.** Hæmorrhagia intermuscul. Aerztl. Ber. d. k. k. allg. Krankenh. zu Wien (1875), 1876, 87.

Muscles (*Exhaustion of*).

See **Fatigue.**

Muscles (*Hypertrophy of*).

See, also, **Paralysis** (*Pseudohypertrophic*).

BASHINSKI (I.) * Razvitie gipertrophii gladkoi mishechnoi tkani. [Hypertrophy of muscular tissues.] 8°. *St. Petersburg*, 1872.

BLUM (K.) * Die wahre Muskelhypertrophie. 8°. *Würzburg*, 1879.

KORWATZKI (A.) * Ueber die Hypertrophie des quergestreiften Muskelgewebes. 8°. *Erlangen*, 1874.

KRAU (A.) * Ein Fall von wahrer Muskelhypertrophie. 8°. *Greifswald*, 1876.

LASER (I.) * Ueber Pseudohypertrophie der Muskeln. 12°. *Berlin*, 1885.

REINACH (O.) * Zur Pseudohypertrophia musculorum lipomatosa. 8°. *Würzburg*, 1885.

Auerbach (L.) Ein Fall von wahrer Muskelhypertrophie. Arch. f. path. Anat., etc., Berl., 1871, liii, 234; 397. — **Bergeron.** Hypertrophie musculaire. Gaz. d. hôp., Par., 1867, xl, 249. *Also, transl.:* J. f. Kinderkr., Erlang.,1868, l, 126. ——. Présentation d'un enfant de 10 ans, remarquable par le développement hypertrophique de ses masses musculaires. Bull. et mém. Soc. méd. d. hôp. de Par. (1867), 1868, iv, 157-160, 1 pl. *Also, transl.:* J. f. Kinderkr., Erlang., 1869, liii, 383-386.—**Bernhardt** (M.) Muskelsteifigkeit und Muskelhypertrophie. (Ein selbstständiger Symptomencomplex.) Arch. f. path. Anat., etc., Berl., 1879, lxxv, 516-537.—**Eulenburg** (A.) Ueber Muskelhypertrophie. Berl. klin. Wchnschr., 1865, ii, 490-496. ——. Ergebnisse des Obductionsbefundes bei Muskelhypertrophie. *Ibid.*, 1866, iii, 364. ——. Wahre Muskelhypertrophie (Hypertrophia musculorum vera). Handb. d. spec. Path. [Ziemssen], Leipz., 1875, xii, 2. Th., 171-175. *Also, transl.:* Cycl. Pract. M. (Ziemssen), N. Y., 1877, xiv, 175 - 179. ——. Pseudohypertrophie der Muskeln. Handb. d. spec. Path. [Ziemssen], Leipz., 1875, xii, 2. Th., 149-170. *Also, transl.:* Cycl. Pract. M. (Ziemssen), N. Y., 1877, xiv, 153-174.—**Griesinger** (W.) Ueber Muskelhypertrophie. Arch. d. Heilk., Leipz., 1865, vi, 1-13, 1 pl. — **Hepp** (L.) Beitrag zur Lehre von der Hypertrophie der Muskeln. Ztschr. f. rat. Med., Heidelb., 1854, 2. R., iv, 257 - 259. — **Legg** (J. W.) Enlargement of the temporal and masseter muscles on both sides. Tr. Path. Soc. Lond., 1879-80, xxxi, 361-366. *Also* [Abstr.]: Lancet, Lond., 1880, i, 405.—**Nothnagel** (H.) Ueber kompensatorische Muskelhypertrophie. Wien. med. Wchnschr., 1885, xxxv, 801-805. *Also:* Wien. med. Bl., 1885, viii, 780-784. *Also:* Wien. med. Presse, 1885, xxvi, 872-877.—**Petrone** (L. M.) Un caso di rigidità muscolare con lieve ipertrofia dei muscoli (Muskelsteifigkeit und Muskelhypertrophie); (nuovo sintoma patologico del sistema nervoso). Riv. sper. di freniat., Reggio-Emilia, 1881, vii, 301-307.—**Pütz** (H.) Ueber fibroide Pseudohypertrophie vieler Skeletmuskeln eines Pferdes bei Anwesenheit Miescher'scher Schläuche. Arch. f. path. Anat., etc., Berl., 1887, cix, 144-175, 3 pl.—**Sakaki.** Fall von wahrer Muskelhypertrophie. Centralbl. f. Nervenh., Leipz., 1885, viii, 10.—**Schrakamp** (F.) Ueber einen Fall von Pseudohypertrophia muscularis. Med. Cor.-Bl. d. württemb. ärztl. Ver., Stuttg., 1886, lvi, 89-92.—**von Stoffella** (E. R.) Demonstrativer Vortrag über eine merkwürdige Muskel-Hypertrophie. Wien. med. Halle, 1863, iv, 256. ——. Ein Fall von Muskelhypertrophie. Med. Jahrb., Wien, 1865, ix, 85-98.—**Weber.** Ein Fall von Pseudohypertrophie der Muskeln. Deutsche mil.-ärztl. Ztschr., Berl., 1886, xv, 232-236.—**Wernich** (A.) Fall von Muskelhy-

Muscles (*Hypertrophy of*).

pertrophie. Deutsches Arch. f. klin. Med., Leipz., 1867, ii, 232–243.—**Westphal** (C.) Zwei Schwestern mit Pseudohypertrophie der Muskeln. Charité-Ann. 1885-6, Berl., 1887, xii, 447–458.—**Zunker.** Ein Fall von Muskelhypertrophie mit Rigidität. Ztschr. f. klin. Med., Berl., 1879, i, 377.

Muscles (*Inflammation of*).

See, *also*, **Muscles** (*Ossification in*); **Psoitis**; **Sterno-mastoid.**

BERGKAMMER (F.) * Beiträge zur Lehre von der Entzündung und Entartung der quergestreiften Muskelfasern. 8°. *Strassburg i. E.,* 1884.

BRUNON (R.) * Contribution à l'étude de la myosite infectieuse primitive. 4°. *Paris,* 1887.

———. The same. 8°. *Paris,* 1887.

DIONIS DES CARRIÈRES (A.-V.-J.) * Études sur la myosite. 4°. *Paris,* 1851.

IPSCHER (G. F. G.) * De myositide. 8°. *Berolini,* 1856.

MARQUET (A.) * Recherches expérimentales sur le processus inflammatoire dans les muscles striés au point de vue de l'anatomie pathologique. 4°. *Nancy,* 1879.

ROY (A.) * I. Des caractères anatomiques de l'inflammation du tissu musculaire. II. [etc.] 4°. *Paris,* 1842.

Alpuente (F.) [Myositis.] N. Orl. J. M., 1869, xxii, 84–88.—**Bellouard** (V.) Myosite du droit antérieur de la cuisse; guérison. Gaz. méd. de Bordeaux, 1872-3, i, 299.—**Buch** (M.) Ein Fall von einseitiger Entzündung der Musculi peronæi in Folge eines Leichdornes. St. Petersb. med. Wchnschr., 1884, n. F., i, 502.—**Castellanos** (J. J.) A case of myositis successfully treated by hydropathy. N. Orl. M. & S. J., 1874-5, ii, 358–360.—**Cattani** (G.) Della miosite lombare interstiziale a corso rapido (miosite purulenta). Gazz. d. osp., Milano, 1883, iv, 197; 210; 219; 243; 267; 275; 282; 323.—**Clark** (F. W.) A case of acute suppurative myositis. Brit. M. J., Lond., 1887, ii, 69.—**Devis** (C. J.) A case of acute myositis of thigh. Tr. Path. Soc. Lond., 1880-81, xxxii, 273–275.—**Fischer** (P.) De la myosite. Union méd. de la Gironde, Bordeaux, 1859, iv,,11; 57.—**Foucault.** Myosite suppurée suraiguë. Bull. Soc. anat. de Par., 1869, xliv, 506–512.—**Fouque.** Myosite du muscle grand pectoral. Gaz. d. hôp., Par., 1884, lvii, 388. *Also:* Abeille méd., Par., 1884, xli, 170.—**Friedberg** (H.) Anatomische Erscheinungen bei der Muskelentzündung. Wchnbl. d. k. k. Gesellsch. d. Aerzte in Wien, 1857, iii, 65–70.—**Gellé.** Myosite suppurée, suite de fatigue musculaire; infection purulente; mort. Bull. Soc. anat. de Par., 1858, xxxiii, 414–417.—**Gies** (T.) Ueber Myositis chronica. Deutsche Ztschr. f. Chir., Leipz., 1878-9, xi, 161–168.—**Gobée** (C.) Uitgebreide (rheumatische?) spierontsteking met ettervorming, en gelijktijdig bestaande dermatitis erysipelatosa; lijkopening. N. pract. Tijdschr. v. de Geneesk., Gorinchem, 1855, n. s., i, 653–662.—**Guermonprez** (F.) Contribution à l'étude de la myosite. J. d. sc. méd. de Lille, 1878-9, i, 849; 969. [Discussion], 973; 1880, ii, 10–32. *Also,* Reprint.—**Guyot.** Myosite suppurée suraiguë. Union méd., Par., 1883, 3. s., xxxvi, 912. *Also:* Bull. et mém. Soc. méd. d. hôp. de Par. (1883) 1884, 2. s., xx, 213.—**Hayem** (G.) Études sur les myosites symptomatiques. Arch. de physiol. norm. et path., Par., 1870, iii, 81; 269; 422; 473; 569.—**Hepp** (P.) Ueber einen Fall von acuter parenchymatöser Myositis, welche Geschwülste bildete und Fluctuation vortäuschte. Berl. klin. Wchnschr., 1887, xxiv, 389–391.———. Ueber Pseudotrichinose, eine besondere Form von acuter parenchymatöser Polymyositis. *Ibid.,* 297 322.—**Jackson** (H.) Myositis universalis acuta infectiosa, with a case. Boston M. & S. J., 1887, cxvi, 498.—**Janovitch-Thainski** (S.) O vospalitelnych izmienieniach myshetchowy tkani. [Of the inflammatory changes of the muscular tissue.] Med. Vestnik, St. Petersb., 1869, ix, 371; 379.—**Jansen** (A.) Observation de myosite suppurée. Arch. méd. belges, Brux., 1874, 3. s., vi, 369–378. — **Kreiss.** Ein Fall von primärer schwieliger Myositis der Wadenmuskeln (rheumatische Muskelschneide Froriep's). Berl. klin. Wchnschr., 1886, xxiii, 877–881.—**Lange** (F.) Specific myositis of the gastrocnemius. N. York M. J., 1884, xxxix, 367.—**Lartigue.** Cas de myosites multiples suppurées observé à la Guadeloupe. Arch. de méd. nav., Par., 1881, xxxv, 67–72.—**Léger.** Deux observations de myosite circonscrites. Soc. méd. d'Amiens. Bull. (1878-9) 1880, xviii-xix, 127–131.—**Myositis** suppurativa; pyæmia. Ber. d. k. k. Krankenh. Wieden 1870, Wien, 1872, 225–228.—**Nicaise.** De la myosite infectieuse. Rev. mens. de méd. et chir., Par., 1877, i, 51–58.—**Niederkorn** (J.) Acute Entzündung des M. biceps brachialis; vollständige Hei-

37

Muscles (*Inflammation of*).

lung. Bull. Soc. d. sc. méd. du gr.-duché de Luxemb., 1869, 165–168.—**Parker** (R.) Acute myositis, simulating acute necrosis; recovery after incision and antiseptic dressing. Brit. M. J., Lond., 1887, ii, 178. — **Rauzier.** Inflammation suppurée du muscle iliaque; symptômes d'état typhoïde avec ataxo-adynamie; mort. Gaz. hebd. d. sc. méd. de Montpel., 1887, ix, 386–388.—**Scriba** (J.) Beitrag zur Aetiologie der Myositis acuta. Deutsche Ztschr. f. Chir., Leipz., 1885, xxii, 497–502.—**Spina** (A.) Untersuchungen über die entzündlichen Veränderungen der quergestreiften Muskelfasern. Med. Jahrb., Wien, 1878, 349–362, 1 pl.—**Treves.** Acute myositis. Brit. M. J., Lond., 1886, ii, 1215. *Also:* Tr. Clin. Soc. Lond. (1886-7), 1887, xx, 84–90.—**Unverricht.** Polymyositis acuta progressiva. Ztschr. f. klin. Med., Berl., 1887, xii, 533–549, 1 pl. ———. Ueber eine eigenthümliche Form von acuter Muskelentzündung mit einem der Trichinose ähnelnden Krankheitsbilde. München. med. Wchnschr., 1887, xxxiv, 488–492. *Also:* Cor.-Bl. d. allg. ärztl. Ver. v. Thüringen, Weimar, 1887, xvi, 207–219.—**Vallin.** De la myocardite et des myosites symptomatiques dans les fièvres palustres graves. Union méd , Par., 1874, xxvii, 293; 316.—**Velpeau.** De la myosite. Gaz. d. hôp., Par., 1853, xxv, 600.—**Wagner** (E.) Ein Fall von acuter Polymyositis. Deutsches Arch. f. klin. Med., Leipz., 1886-7, xl, 241–266.—**Walther** (E.) Ueber idiopathische, acute eiterige Muskelentzündung. Deutsche Ztschr. f. Chir., Leipz., 1886-7, xxv, 260–286. — **Winckel** (F.) Ein eigenthümlicher Fall von Polymyositis parenchymatosa puerperalis mit Neuritis interstitialis. Centralbl. f. Gynäk., Leipz., 1878, ii, 145–150.

Muscles (*Injuries of*).

See **Muscles** (*Dislocations, etc., of*).

Muscles (*Nerves of*).

See, *also*, **Muscle** (*Physiology of*); **Muscular sense**; **Nerves** (*Terminations of*).

CALBERLA (E.) * Ueber die Endigungsweise der Nerven in den quergestreiften Muskeln der Amphibien. [Freiburg i. Br.] 8°. *Leipzig,* 1874.

EMMERT (F. C.) Ueber die Endigungsweise der Nerven in den Muskeln, nach einigen Untersuchungen. 4°. *Bern,* 1836.

ENGELMANN (T. W.) Untersuchungen über den Zusammenhang von Nerv- und Muskelfaser. 4°. *Leipzig,* 1863.

FORGUE (E.) * Distribution des racines motrices dans les muscles des membres. 4°. *Montpellier,* 1883.

Also [Abstr.], *in:* Gaz. hebd. d. sc. méd. de Montpel., 1883, v, 253; 279; 329; 388. *Also* [Abstr.], *in:* Compt. rend. Acad. d. sc., Par., 1884, xcviii, 685–687.

GERLACH (J.) Das Verhältniss der Nerven zu den willkürlichen Muskeln der Wirbelthiere. 8°. *Leipzig,* 1874.

HÉNOCQUE (A.-W.-L.) * Du mode de distribution et de la terminaison des nerfs dans les muscles lisses. 4°. *Paris,* 1870.

Also [Abstr.], *in:* Arch. de physiol. norm. et path., Par., 1870, iii, 397–407. *Also* [Abstr.], *in:* Gaz. hebd. de méd., Par., 1871, 2. s., viii, 11; 63; 82; 117.

JAEGER (E.) * Ueber die Endigung der motorischen Nerven. 8°. *Würzburg,* 1867.

KRAUSE (W.) Die motorischen Endplatten der quergestreiften Muskelfasern. 8°. *Hannover,* 1869.

KÜHNE (W.) Ueber die peripherischen Endorgane der motorischen Nerven. 4°. *Leipzig,* 1862.

See, *also, infra.*

LINNERT (F. L.) * De finibus periphericis nervorum musculorum. 8°. *Gryphiswaldiæ,* 1863.

LIPMANN (H.) * Die Nerven der organischen Muskeln. 8°. *Berlin,* 1869.

MARGÓ (T.) Ueber die Endigung der Nerven in der quergestreiften Muskelsubstanz. 4°. *Pest,* 1862.

SOKOLOVSKI (C.) * Otnoshenie nervov k sosudam v poperechno-polosatich muschitsach i ich okonchanija. [Relation of nerves at their terminations in transverse striated muscle.] 8°. *St. Petersburg.* 1864.

Muscles (Nerves of).

VIALLANES (H.) * Recherches sur les terminaisons nerveuses motrices dans les muscles striés des insectes. 4°. *Paris*, 1881.
See, also, infra.

ZEINEMANN-LANGE (A.) * Materialien zum Gesetz des Muskelnerveneintritts. 8°. *Jena*, 1879.

Arndt (R.) Untersuchungen über die Endigung der Nerven in den quergestreiften Muskelfasern. Arch. f. mikr. Anat., Bonn, 1873, ix, 481-590, 3 pl. — **Arnold** (J.) Ueber die Krause'schen Endkolben. [Eine Antwort auf C. Lüdden's Nachuntersuchungen.] Arch. f. path. Anat., etc., Berl., 1863, xxvii, 399-405. — **Beale** (L. S.) On the distribution of nerves to the elementary fibres of striped muscle. Phil. Tr., Lond., 1860, cl, 611-619. ———. Further observations on the distribution of nerves to the elementary fibres of striped muscle. *Ibid.*, 1862, clii, 889-910, 4 pl.— **Bernstein** (J.) Die Erregungszeit der Nervenendorgane in den Muskeln. Arch. f. Physiol., Leipz., 1882, 329-346. — **Bert** (P.) & **Marcacci.** Studio della distribuzione delle radici motrici nei muscoli degli arti. Gior. internaz. d. sc. med., Napoli, 1881, n. s., iii, 906-908. — **Biedermann** (W.) Ueber das elektromotorische Verhalten des Muschelnerven bei galvanischer Reizung. Sitzungsb. d. k. Akad. d. Wissensch. Math.-naturw. Cl., Wien, 1886, xciii, 3. Abth., 56-98. — **Bizzozero** (G.) & **Golgi** (C.) Ueber die Veränderungen des Muskelgewebes nach Nervendurchschneidung. Med. Jahrb., Wien, 1873, 125-127.— **Bremer** (L.) Ueber die Endigungen der markhaltigen und marklosen Nerven im quergestreiften Muskel. Arch. f. mikr. Anat., Bonn, 1882, xxi, 165-201, 2 pl. — **Brown-Séquard.** Faits relatifs aux voies de communication entre le cerveau et les muscles. Compt. rend. Soc. de biol., Par., 1886, 8. s., iii, 75.— **Cattaneo** (A.) Sugli organi nervosi terminali muscolo-tendinei in condizioni normali e sul loro modo di comportarsi in seguito al taglio delle radici nervose e dei nervi spinali. Gazz. d. osp., Milano, 1886, vii, 586. — **Ciaccio** (G. V.) Nuove osservazioni intorno alla terminazione de' nervi motori nei muscoli striati delle torpedini e delle razze, e intorno alla somiglianza tra la piastra elettrica delle torpedini e la motrice. Spallanzani, Modena, 1877, xv, 501-504. ———. Osservazioni istologiche intorno alla terminazione delle fibre nervose motive ne' muscoli striati delle torpedini, del topo casalingo e del ratto albino conciliati col doppio cloruro d' oro e cadmio. Mem. Accad. d. sc. d. Ist. di Bologna, 1882, 4. s., iv, 821-825. *Also:* Spallanzani, Modena, 1883, 2. s., xii, 10-13. *Also, transl.* [Abstr.]: J. de microg., Par., 1883, vii, 38-41. *Also, transl.* [Abstr.]: Arch. ital. de biol., Turin, 1883, iii, 75-78.— **Cohnheim** (J.) Ueber die Endigung der Muskelnerven. Centralbl. f. d. med. Wissensch., Berl., 1863, i, 865-867. ———. Ueber die Endigung der Muskelnerven. Arch. f. path. Anat., etc., Berl., 1865, xxxiv, 194-207, 1 pl. *Also, in his:* Ges. Abhandl., 8°, Berl., 1885, 51-62, 1 pl. ———. Zur Geschichte der motorischen Nervenendigung. Arch. f. path. Anat., etc., Berl., 1878, lxxiv, 141. — **Cunningham** (D. J.) The relation of nerve-supply to muscle-homology. [Abstr.] J. Anat. & Physiol., Lond., 1881-2, xvi, 1-9. — **[Demarquay.]** Sarcome développé sur le trajet du nerf musculo-cutané. Rev. méd.-phot. d. hôp. de Par., 1875, vii, 17-19. — **Engelmann** (T. W.) Ueber die Endigungen der motorischen Nerven in den quergestreiften Muskeln der Wirbelthiere. Centralbl. f. d. med. Wissensch., Berl., 1863, i, 289-291. ———. Ueber Endigung motorischer Nerven. Jenaische Ztschr. f. Med. u. Naturw., Leipz., 1864, i, 322-324, 1 pl. ———. Bijdrage tot de kennis der zenuw-eindiging in de spier. Onderzoek. ged. in h. physiol. Lab. d. Utrecht. Hoogesch., 1868-9, ii, 121-127. *Also, transl.:* Jenaische Ztschr. f. Naturw., Leipz., 1868, iv, 2. Hft., 307-311. *Also, Reprint.*— **Ewald** (A.) Ueber die Endigung der motorischen Nerven in den quergestreiften Muskeln. Arch. f. d. ges. Physiol., Bonn, 1875-6, xii, 529-548, 2 pl. — **Exner** (S.) Notiz zu der Frage von der Faservertheilung mehrerer Nerven in einem Muskel. *Ibid.*, 1885, xxxvi, 572-576.— **Fischer** (E.) Ueber die Endigung der Nerven im quergestreiften Muskel der Wirbelthiere. Centralbl. f. d. med. Wissensch., Berl., 1876, xiv, 354-356.— **Flesch** (M.) Zur Kenntniss der Nervenendigung in den quergestreiften Muskeln des Menschen: nach Untersuchungen an Querschnitten vergoldeter Präparate der Augenmuskeln. Mitth. d. naturf. Gesellsch. in Bern, 1885, 3-25, 1 pl. — **Foettinger** (A.) Sur les terminaisons des nerfs dans les muscles des insectes. Onderzoek. ged. in h. physiol. Lab. d. Utrecht. Hoogesch., 1878-80, 3. r., v, 293-322, 1 pl. *Also:* Arch. de biol., Gand, 1880, i, 279-304, 1 pl. — **Frankenhäuser** (F.) Die Nervenendungen in den glatten Muskelfasern. Centralbl. f. d. med. Wissensch., Berl., 1866, iv, 865-868.— **Gaskell** (W. H.) On the vasomotor nerves of striated muscles. J. Anat. & Physiol., Lond., 1876-7, xi, 720-753. ———. Preliminary note of further investigations upon the vaso-motor nerves of striated muscle. J. Physiol., Lond., 1878-9, i, 108. — **Gerlach** (J.) Ueber das Verhalten der Nerven in den quergestreiften Muskelfäden der Wirbelthiere. Sitzungsb. d. phys.-med. Soc. zu Erlang., 1872-3,

Muscles (Nerves of).

v, 97-106. ———. Ueber das Verhältniss der nervösen und contractilen Substanz des quergestreiften Muskels. Arch. f. mikr. Anat., Bonn, 1876, xiii, 399-414, 1 pl. — **Gerlach** (L.) Ueber die Nervenendigungen in der Musculatur des Froschherzens. Arch. f. path. Anat., etc., Berl., 1876, lxvi, 187-223, 1 pl. *Also, Reprint.*—**Gessler** (H.) Untersuchungen über die letzten Endigungen der motorischen Nerven im quergestreiften Muskel und ihr Verhalten nach der Durchschneidung der Nervenstämme. Deutsches Arch. f. klin. Med., Leipz., 1883, xxxiii, 42-53, 4 pl. *Also:* Arb. a. d. med.-klin. Inst. d. k. Ludwig-Maximilians-Univ. zu München, Leipz., 1884, i. 517-528, 2 pl. — **Greeff** (R.) Zur Frage über die Endigungen der Muskelnerven. Arch. f. mjkr. Anat., Bonn, 1865, i, 437-439. ———. Ueber einen eigenthümlichen Zusammenhang zwischen Nerven- und Muskelsystem. Verhandl. d. naturh. Ver. d. preuss. Rheinl. u. Westphal., Bonn, 1865, xxii, pt. 2, 33.—**Gscheidlen** (R.) Beiträge zur Lehre von der Nervenendigung in den glatten Muskelfasern. Arch. f. mikr. Anat., Bonn, 1877, xiv, 321-332, 1 pl. ———. Ueber die Nervenendigung in den glatten Muskelfasern. Jahresb. d. schles. Gesellsch. f. vaterl. Kult., Bresl., 1878, lv, 228-230.—**Henry** (W. C.) A critical and experimental inquiry into the relations subsisting between nerve and muscle. Edinb. M. & S. J., 1832, xxxvii, 11-20. *Also, Reprint.* — **Hitzig** (E.) Ueber die Auffassung einiger Anomalieen der Muskelinnervation. Arch. f. Psychiat., Berl., 1872, iii, 312; 601.— **Key** (A.) Bidrag till frågan om nervernas ändningsätt i musklerna. Förh. v. de skandin. Naturf. 1863, Stockholm, 1865, 680-684. — **Klebs** (E.) Die Nerven der organischen Muskeln. Centralbl. f. d. med. Wissensch., Berl., 1863, i, 561-565. ———. Die Nerven der organischen Muskelfasern. Arch. f. path. Anat., etc., Berl., 1865, xxxii, 168-198, 2 pl. — **Kowalewsky** (N.) & **Nawrocki** (J.) Untersuchungen über die sensiblen Nerven der Muskeln. Centralbl. f. d. med. Wissensch., Berl., 1878, xvi, 145-148.— **Krause** (W.) Ueber die Endigung der Muskelnerven. Ztschr. f. rat. Med., Leipz. u. Heidelb., 1863, 3. R., xviii, 136, 2 pl.: xx, 1, 2 pl.: 1864, 3. R., xxi, 77, 1 pl.: 1865, 3. R., xxiii, 157, 3 pl. ———. Die Querlinien der Muskelfasern und ihr Verhalten zu der motorischen Endplatte. Nachr. v. d. k. Gesellsch. d. Wissensch. u. d. Georg-Aug.-Univ., Götting., 1868, 382-384. ———. Ueber die Nerven-Endigung innerhalb der motorischen Endplatten. Arch. f. Anat., Physiol. u. wissensch. Med., Leipz., 1868, 646-648. ———. Die Nervenendigung in den glatten Muskeln. *Ibid.*, 1870, 1-8, 1 pl. ———. Die Entladungshypothese und die motorischen Endplatten. Arch. f. mikr. Anat., Bonn, 1876, xiii, 170-179, 1 pl.—**Kühne** (W.) Ueber die Endigung der Nerven in den Muskeln. Arch. f. path. Anat., etc., Berl., 1863, xxvii, 508-533, 1 pl. ———. Der Zusammenhang von Nerv- und Muskelfaser. *Ibid.*, 1864, xxix, 207-209, 1 pl. ———. Ueber den feineren Bau der peripherischen Endorgane der motorischen Nerven. *Ibid.*, 1863, 433-450. ———. Ueber die Endigung der Nerven in den Nervenhügeln der Muskeln. *Ibid.*, xxx, 187-220, 1 pl. ———. Ueber die Endigungsweise der Nerven in den Muskeln der beschuppten Amphibien, der Säugethiere und des Menschen. Centralbl. f. d. med. Wissensch., Berl., 1864, ii, 369-371. ———. Ueber das Verhalten des Muskels zum Nerven. (Im Auszuge mitgetheilt.) Verhandl. d. naturh.-med. Ver. zu Heidelb. (1877-80), 1880, n. F., ii, 227-246. ———. Widerlegung der Bemerkungen E. Du Bois-Reymond's über mehrfache Nervenendigungen an einer Muskelfaser. Ztschr. f. Biol., München, 1884, xx, 531-539. ———. Neue Untersuchungen über motorische Nervenendigung. *Ibid.*, München u. Leipz., 1886, n. F., v. 1-148, 16 pl. ———. Untersuchung der motorischen Nervenendigung an Durchschnitten und Schnittserien. Verhandl. d. naturh.-med. Ver. zu Heidelb., 1887, n. F., iv, 1-15. — **Lannegrace.** Distribution des racines motrices dans les muscles des membres. Gaz. hebd. d. sc. méd. de Montpel., 1883, v, 448; 457; 472; 495.—**Lavdovski** (M.) O nervnich okonchan. nushtsi kojnago snarjada. [Termination of nerve-fibres in muscles and tissues.] Voyenno-med. J., St. Petersb., 1885, clii, pt. 2, 173; 281: cliii, 1.—**Letzerich** (L.) Ueber die Endigungsweise der motorischen Nerven. Allg. med. Centr.-Ztg., Berl., 1863, xxxii, 289.—**Löwitt** (M.) Die Nerven der glatten Musculatur. Sitzungsb. d. k. Akad. d. Wissensch. Math.-naturw. Cl., Wien, 1875, lxxi, 355-376, 1 pl. — **Lustig** (A.) Ueber die Nervenendigung in den glatten Muskelfasern. *Ibid.*, 1881, lxxxiii, 3. Abth., 186-194, 1 pl. — **Mays** (K.) Histo-physiologische Untersuchungen über die Verbreitung der Nerven in den Muskeln. Ztschr. f. Biol., München, 1884, xx, 449-530, 5 pl. ———. Ueber Nervenfasertheilungen in den Nervenstämmen der Froschmuskeln. *Ibid.*, 1886, n. F., xiv, 354-372, 1 pl.—**Miura** (M.) Untersuchungen über die motorischen Nervenendigungen der quergestreiften Muskelfasern. Arch. f. path. Anat., etc., Berl., 1886, cv, 129-135, 1 pl.—**Munk** (H.) Ueber die Abhängigkeit des Absterbens der Muskeln von der Länge ihrer Nerven. Allg. med. Centr.-Ztg., Berl., 1860, xxix, 57.—**Naunyn** (B.) Ueber die angeblichen peripherischen Endorgane der motorischen Nervenfaser. Arch. f. Anat., Physiol. u. wissensch. Med., Leipz., 1862, 481-496.—**Odenius** (M. V.) Under-

Muscles (*Nerves of*).

sökningar öfver de sensibla muskelnerverna. Nord. Med. Ark., Stockholm, 1872, iv, no. 18, 1–18, 1 pl. — **Onimus.** Recherches expérimentales sur les phénomènes consécutifs à l'ablation du cerveau et sur les mouvements de rotation. J. de l'anat. et physiol., etc., Par., 1870–71, vii, 633–677. *Also* [Abstr.]: Rev. scient., Par., 1872, ix, 871–878. *Also, transl.* [Abstr.]: Pop. Sc. Month., N. Y., 1872, i, 344–356. *Also, transl.* [Abstr.]: Quart. J. Psych. M., N. Y., 1872, vi, 510–529. — **Pogosheff** (L.) Ueber die Nerven in den Enden des Musculus sartorius. Mélanges biol. Acad. imp. d. sc. de St.-Pétersb., 1886, xii, 321–324. — **Poole** (T. W.) On the relations of nerve and muscle. Med. Rec., N. Y., 1880, xvii, 481 ; 511 ; 536 : xviii, 445. — **Ranvier** (L.) De la méthode de l'or et de la terminaison des nerfs dans le muscle lisse. Compt. rend. Acad. d. sc., Par., 1878, lxxxvi, 1142–1144. — **Reid** (J.) On the relation between muscular contractibility and the nervous system. Lond. & Edinb. Month J. M. Sc., 1841, i, 320–329. *Also, Reprint.* — **Rouget** (C.) Mémoire sur la terminaison des nerfs moteurs dans les muscles chez les reptiles, les oiseaux et les mammifères. J. de la physiol. de l'homme, Par., 1862, v, 574–593. ——. Note sur la terminaison des nerfs moteurs dans les muscles. Compt. rend. Acad. d. sc., Par., 1866, lxii, 1377–1381. *Also:* Rev. méd. franç. et étrang., Par., 1866, ii, 81–85. — **Roux** (P.-J.) De l'influence des nerfs cérébraux et de ceux des ganglions sur la contractilité musculaire. J. de méd., chir., pharm., etc., Par., 1802, iv, 316–337. — **Sachs** (C.) Untersuchungen über Quer- und Längendurchströmung des Froschmuskels, nebst Beiträgen zur Physiologie der motorischen Endplatten. Arch. f. Anat., Physiol. u. wissensch. Med., Leipz., 1874, 57–95. — **Sandmann** (G.) Ueber die Vertheilung der motorischen Nervenendapparate in den quergestreiften Muskeln der Wirbelthiere. Arch. f. Physiol., Leipz., 1885, 240–252, 1 pl. — **Schwalbe** (G.) Ueber das Gesetz des Muskelnerveneintritts. Arch. f. Anat. u. Entwcklngsgesch., Leipz., 1879, 167–174. — **Sihler** (C.) On the endings of the motor nerves in the voluntary muscles of the dog. Johns Hopkins Univ. Stud. biol. lab., Balt., 1884–7, iii, 155–164, 1 pl. — **Tergast** (P.) Ueber das Verhältniss von Nerve und Muskel. Arch. f. mikr. Anat., Bonn, 1873, ix, 36–46, 1 pl. — **Tigri** (A.) Lettera sul fatto anatomico della fibra muscolare annessa all' apparecchio nervoso, e sulle sue consequenze fisiologiche. Ann. univ. di med., Milano, 1814, ccxxvii, 104–109, 1 pl. — **Tischer** (E.) Ueber die Endigung der Nerven im quergestreiften Muskel der Wirbelthiere. Arch. f. mikr. Anat., Bonn, 1876, xiii, 365–390, 2 pl. — **Trinchese** (S.) Sulla terminazione periferica dei nervi motori. Liguria med., Genova, 1866, xi, 289–323, 4 pl. *Also, transl.*: J. de l'anat. et physiol., etc., Par., 1867, iv, 485–504, 4 pl. ——. Terminaison des nerfs dans les muscles striés. Arch. ital. de biol., Turin, 1882–3, ii, 343. — **Tschiriew** (S.) Zur Physiologie der motorischen Nervenendplatte. Arch. f. Anat. u. Physiol., Leipz., 1878 (Physiol., Abth.), 137–154, 1 pl. ——. Sur les terminaisons nerveuses dans les muscles striés. Arch. de physiol. norm. et path., Par., 1879, 2. s., vi, 89–116, 2 pl. *Also:* École prat. d. hautes études. Lab. d'histol. du Coll. de France. Trav., Par., 1879–80, v, 1–28, 2 pl. *Also* [Abstr.]: Compt. rend. Acad. d. sc., Par., 1878, lxxxvii, 604–606. ——. Études sur la physiologie des nerfs des muscles striés. Arch. de physiol. norm. et path., Par., 1879, 2. s., vi, 295–329. *Also:* École prat. d. hautes études. Lab. d'histol. du Coll. de France. Trav., Par., 1879–80, v, 64–98. — **Viallanes** (H.) Note sur la structure du nerf et sa terminaison dans les muscles striés chez quelques insectes. Compt. rend. Soc. de biol. 1880. Par., 1881, 7. s., ii, 371. [*See, also, supra.*] — **Vlacovich** (G. P.) Sulla terminazione dei nervi nei muscoli a fibre striate. Gazz. med. ital., prov. venete, Padova, 1875, xviii, 281 ; 289. — **Waldeyer.** Ueber Muskélnervenendigungen. Arch. f. Psychiat., Berl., 1882, xiii, 715. — **Waldeyer** (W.) Ueber die Endigung der motorischen Nerven in den quergestreiften Muskeln. Centralbl. f. d. med. Wissensch., Berl., 1863, i, 369–372. — **Wallace** (D.) Note on the nerve supply of the musculus sternalis. J. Anat. & Physiol., Lond., 1886–7, xxi, 153. — **Weber** (E. H.) Ueber die Abhängigkeit der Entstehung der animalischen Muskeln von der der animalischen Nerven, erläutert durch eine von ihm und Eduard Weber untersuchte Missbildung. Arch. f. Anat., Physiol. u. wissensch. Med., Berl., 1851, 547–566, 1 pl. — **Wolff** (W.) Ueber Nervenendigungen im quergestreiften Muskel. Arch. f. mikr. Anat., Bonn, 1880–81, xix, 331–347, 1 pl.

Muscles (*Ossification in*).

BULHAK (E.) * Ueber Verknöcherung und Verirdung des Muskel- und Sehnengewebes. 8°. [*Dorpat*], 1860.

GERBER (R.) * Ueber Myositis ossificans progressiva. 8°. *Würzburg*, 1875.

GOLDBERG (L.) * Die Myositis ossificans bei Dementia paralytica. 8°. *Berlin*, [1877].

PINTÉR (G.) * Beitrag zur Casuistik der Myositis ossificans progressiva. 8°. *Würzburg*, 1883.

Muscles (*Ossification in*).

Abbe (R.) Osteoplaques of the thigh. N. York M. J., 1887, xlvi. 555. *Also:* Med. News, Phila., 1887, li, 552. — **Billroth** (T.) Ueber den Reiterknochen. Deutsche Klinik, Berl., 1855, vii, 301. — **Broca.** [Ossification du muscle psoas-iliaque s'étendant jusque dans la fosse iliaque interne.] Bull. Soc. anat. de Par., 1850, xxv, 37–40. — **Byers** (W. M.) Almost complete ossification of the human body. N. Orl. J. M., 1870, xxiii, 122. — **Düms.** Ein Exercirknochen im rechten Deltamuskel als Ursache einer Reflexneurose. Deutsche mil.-ärztl. Ztschr., Berl., 1887, xvi, 321–330. — **Giacomini** (C.) Ossificazione della troclea del muscolo grande obliquo dell' occhio. Gior. d. r. Accad. di med. di Torino, 1886, 3. s., xxxiv, 700–713, 1 pl. — **Gibney** (E. P.) Ossification of the latissimus dorsi, scaleni, and erector-spinal muscles. Med. & Surg. Reporter, Phila., 1875, xxxiii, 405. — **Gibney** (V. P.) Myositis ossificans. Med. Rec., N. Y., 1875, x, 747. — **Godlee** (R. J.) A case of myositis ossificans. Tr. Clin. Soc. Lond., 1886, xix, 333–337, 1 pl. — **Hasse.** Verknöcherung im Muskelfleisch durch mechanische Veranlassung. (Der sogenannte Exercirknochen bei Infanteristen.) Med. Ztg., Berl., 1832, i, 12. — **Hawkins** (C.) On a case of ossific formations in muscles. Lond. M. Gaz., 1844, xxxiv, 273–277. *Also, in his:* . . . Path. & Surg. Writings, 8°, Lond., 1874, ii, 193–200. — **Helferich** (H.) Ein Fall von sogenannter Myositis ossificans progressiva. Aerztl. Int.-Bl., München, 1879, xxvi, 485–489. *Also* [Abstr.]: Tagebl. d. Versamml. deutsch. Naturf. u. Aerzte, 1881, liv, pt. 2, 144. *Also* [Abstr.]: Allg. Wien. med. Ztg., 1881, xxvi, 403— 144. — **Huth.** Fall von Myositis ossificans. Allg. med. Centr.-Ztg., Berl., 1876, xlv, 493. — **Josephson.** Ueber Osteome in den Adductions-Muskeln von Cavalleristen. [Reitknochen.] Deutsche mil.-ärztl. Ztschr., Berl., 1874, iii, 53–67. — **Jurasz** (A.) Zapalenie mięsni postępowe kostniejące (Myositis ossificans progressiva). Medycyna, Warszawa, 1873, i, 533; 549. — **Kohts** (O.) Ein Fall von Myositis ossificans progressiva. Jahrb. f. Kinderh., Leipz., 1884, n. F., xxi, 326–333. *Also* [Abstr.]: Arch. f. Psychiat., Berl., 1884, xv, 263–265. — **Kümmell** (H.) Zur Myositis ossificans progressiva. Verhandl. d. deutsch. Gesellsch. f. Chir., Berl., 1883, xii, pt. 2, 221–232, 1 pl. *Also:* Arch. f. klin. Chir., Berl., 1883, xxix, 615–626, 1 pl. — **Legros.** Ossification des muscles psoas iliaque. Bull. Soc. anat. de Par., 1862, xxxvii, 400–404. — **Mays** (K.) Ueber die sogenannte Myositis ossificans progressiva. Arch. f. path. Anat., etc., Berl., 1878, lxxiv, 147–173. — **von Mosetig-Morhof.** Ein Fall von Myositis ossificans. Wien. med. Presse, 1879, xx, 1238. — **Münchmeyer.** Ueber Myositis ossificans progressiva. Ztschr. f. rat. Med., Leipz. u. Heidelb., 1869, 3. R., xxxiv, 9–41, 1 pl. — **Nicoladoni** (C.) Ueber Myositis ossificans progressiva. Wien. med. Bl., 1878, i, 476; 503; 529; 548; 576. — **Partsch.** Ueber einen Fall von Myositis ossificans progressiva. Jahresb. d. schles. Gesellsch. f. vaterl. Kult. 1881, Bresl., 1882, lix, 163–173. *Also:* Breslau. aerztl. Ztschr., 1882, iv, 66–70. — **Pintér** (G.) Einige neue Fälle von Myositis ossificans progressiva. Ztschr. f. klin. Med., Berl., 1884, viii, 155–174. — **Raushoff** (J.) Myositis ossificans. Cincin. Lancet & Clinic, 1878, n. s., i, 146. — **Rogers** (D. L.) A case of ossification of the muscular tissue. Am. J. M. Sc., Phila., 1833, xiii, 386–388. — **Schwarz** (E.) Ein bemerkenswerther Fall von Myositis ossificans progressiva. Deutsche med. Wchnschr., Berl., 1884, x, 807–810. — **Skinner** (W.) Case of ossification of the muscles. Med. Times & Gaz., Lond., 1861, i, 413. — **Sympson** (T.) Case of myositis ossificans. Tr. Clin. Soc. Lond., 1886, xix, 315, 1 pl. *Also:* Brit. M. J., Lond., 1886, ii, 1026. — **Terquem.** Rapport sur le mémoire de M. le docteur Richter, de Dusseldorff, relatif aux formations osseuses anomales dans les muscles. Sommaire d. trav. de la Soc. d. sc. méd. de la Moselle, Metz, 1830–38, 55–59. — **Testelin** & **Danbressi** (C.) Rhumatisme terminé par l'ossification des muscles; observation suivie de réflexions. Gaz. méd. de Par., 1839, 2. s., vii, 170–172.

Muscles (*Pain in*).
    See **Myalgia.**

Muscles (*Parasites in*).
    See **Psorospermia.**

Muscles (*Pathology of*).
    See **Muscles** (*Diseases, etc., of*).

Muscles (*Pseudohypertrophy of*).
    See **Muscles** (*Hypertrophy of*).

Muscles (*Ruptures of*).
    See **Muscles** (*Dislocations, etc., of*).

Muscles (*Semeiology of*).
    See, also, **Myoidema**; **Nervous** *system* (*Diseases of, Diagnosis, etc., of*); **Reflexes.**

COLANÉRI (F.) * Des secousses musculaires; étude critique et seméiologique. 4°. *Paris*, 1884.

Muscles (*Semeiology of*).

Auerbach (L.) Ueber Percussion der Muskeln. Ztschr. f. rat. Med., Leipz. u. Heidelb., 1862, 3. R., xiv, 215–231.—**Brown-Séquard** (C. E.) Vibratory or oscillatory muscular movements and their significance. Arch. Scient. & Pract. M. & S., N. Y., 1875, i, 279.—**Chauveau.** De la valeur de la contractilité électrique comme moyen diagnostic. Mém. et compt.-rend. Soc. d. sc. méd. de Lyon (1862), 1863, ii, 236.

Muscles (*Spasm of*).

See **Muscles** (*Contraction, etc., of*).

Muscles (*Syphilis of*).

BALLIVET (J.) * Quelques considérations sur les tumeurs syphilitiques du muscle sterno-mastoïdien et la myosite des nouveau-nés. 4°. *Lyon*, 1878.

HABERSTOLZ (A.) * Fall von schwerer Muskelgummose. 12°. *Jena*, 1883.

MONGINOT (L.-E.) * Les tumeurs syphilitiques des muscles et des tendons. 4°. *Paris*, 1851.

ROUSSET (G.-A.) * Considérations sur la syphilis musculaire, principalement dans les muscles de la vie de relation. 4°. *Paris*, 1875.

Andronico (C.) La sifilide del sistema muscolare. Gazz. med. di Torino, 1886, xxxvii, 265–275.—**Bouisson** (F.) Mémoire sur les tumeurs syphilitiques des muscles et de leurs annexes. Gaz. méd. de Par., 1846, 3. s., i, 542; 563; 583; 594.—**Courtin.** Myosite syphilitique suppurée et affection cardiaque concomitante. J. de méd. de Bordeaux, 1879–80. ix, 65.—**Dunn** (H. P.) Gummatous tumours of muscles. Lancet, Lond., 1883. ii, 899.—**Duplay.** Deux observations de myosite syphilitique. Arch. gén. de méd., Par., 1880, ii, 218–223.—**Guyot.** Myosite syphilitique. Bull. et mém. Soc. méd. d. hôp. de Par., 1885, 3. s., ii, 244.—**Hennig** (C.) Ererbtes Lues; Muskelleiden. Jahrb. f. Kinderh., etc., Leipz., 1870–71, iv, 230–232.—**Jacobson** (W. H. A.) Syphilitic myositis. Brit. M. J., Lond., 1879, i, 271.—**Jones** (S.) Syphilitic tumors of muscle. Lancet, Lond., 1859, ii, 617. *Also*: Tr. Path. Soc. Lond., 1859–60, xi, 246.—**Lucas** (J. C.) On syphilitic contraction of muscles. Indian M. Gaz., Calcutta, 1878, xiii, 209.—**de Macedo** (L.) Algunas reflexiones sobre la miositis sifilítica. España méd., Madrid, 1863, viii, 729.—**Malloch** (A. E.) Case of syphilitic disease of a portion of the deltoid. Canada M. J., Montreal, 1870, vi, 157.—**Mauriac** (C.) Leçons sur les myopathies syphilitiques. Ann. de dermat. et syph., Par., 1875–6, vii, 250; 339; 425: 1876–7, viii, 5; 137; 182; 269; 339; 452: 1877–8, ix, 33. *Also*, Reprint.—**Nélaton.** Tumeurs syphilitiques des muscles. Gaz. d. hôp., Par., 1851, 3. s., iii, 349. ——. Tumeurs syphilitiques musculaires. *Ibid.*, 1861, xxxiv, 234.—**Neumann** (I.) Ueber syphilitische Muskelentzündung. Anz. d. k. k. Gesellsch. d. Aerzte in Wien, 1883–4, 85–87. ——. Ueber syphilitische Erkrankung der Muskeln. Wien. med. Bl., 1884, vii, 351: 386. *Also*: Aerztl. Ber. d. k. k. allg. Krankenh. zu Wien (1883), 1884, 153–159.—**Notta** (A.) Mémoire sur la rétraction musculaire syphilitique. Arch. gén. de méd., Par., 1850, xxiv, 413–440. ——. Observation de rétraction musculaire syphilitique. Monit. d. hôp., Par., 1853, i, 477.—**Richet.** Tumeurs goumeuses du triceps fémoral. Gaz. d. hôp., Par., 1880, liii, 897.—**Rollet** (J.) Musculaire (Tissu). Affections syphilitiques. Dict. encycl. d. sc. méd., Par., 1876, 2. s., xi, 119–126.—**Tourrel** (G.) Observation de rétraction musculaire syphilitique. Rev. de thérap. du midi, Montpel., 1855, viii, 329–339.—**Van Harlingen** (A.) Three cases of syphilitic muscular contraction. Am. J. M. Sc., Phila., 1880, n. s., lxxix, 399–405.

Muscles (*Tumors of*).

See, also, Sterno-cleido-mastoid.

AUDIAT (C.) * Des kystes hydatiques des muscles. 4°. *Paris*, 1886.

DESPRÉS (A.) * Des tumeurs des muscles. 8°. *Paris*, 1866.

KLEIN (T.) * Ueber Entwicklungs-Kreislaufverhältnisse kleinzelliger Rundzellensarkome der Muskeln. 8°. *Burg*, 1886.

RONCIÈRE (B.-A.) * Kystes hydatiques des muscles. 4°. *Paris*, 1884.

Barling (G.) Alveolar sarcoma of triceps (recurrence); one lymphatic gland infected. Tr. Path. Soc. Lond., 1884–5, xxxvi, 414. ——. Round-celled sarcoma of peroneus longus. *Ibid.*, 414.—**Billroth** (T.) Ueber eine eigenthümliche Geschwulst der Muskeln (Myoma cysticum). Arch f. path. Anat., etc., Berl., 1855, ix, 172–184. 1 pl.—**Cristiani** (J.) Recherches sur les tumeurs malignes des muscles striés. Arch. de physiol. norm et path., Par., 1887, 3. s., x, 107–125, 1 pl.—**Davy** (R.) De-

Muscles (*Tumors of*).

generative cyst in muscles. Proc. M Soc. Lond., 1875–7, iii, 114–116.—**De Morgan** (C.) Remarks on some cases of vascular tumour seated in muscle. Brit. & For. M.-Chir. Rev., Lond., 1864, xxxiii, 187–199.—**Guyon.** Concrétion calcaire dans l'épaisseur du muscle couturier. Bull. Soc. anat. de Par., 1859, xxxiv, 10.—**Hawkins** (C. H.) Case of temporary tumours among muscles. Lond. M. Gaz., 1844, xxxiv, 273. *Also, in his*: . . . Path. & Surg. Writings, 8°, Lond., 1874, ii, 260.—**Jacobson** (W. H. A.) Fibro-chondroma removed from the sheath of the flexor longus pollicis. Brit. M. J., Lond., 1879, i, 227.—**Poläillon.** Des kystes hydatiques des muscles. Paris méd, 1887, xii, 129.—**Richardson** (B W.) Muscular tumours. Dublin Q. J. M. Sc., 1859, xxvii, 275–280.—**Richet.** Observation de kyste hydatique du biceps France méd., Par., 1880, xxvii, 49–51.—**Roloff** (F.) Ueber die Anhäufung von Zellen und Kernen in den Muskeln des Frosches. Arch. f. path. Anat., etc., Berl, 1869, xlvii, 96–102, 1 pl.—**Salomon.** Die bösartige Muskelgeschwulst. Wchnschr. f. d. ges. Heilk., Berl., 1844, 621; 645.—**Saxtorph** (S.) Multipelt idiopatisk Muskelsarkom. Hosp.-Tid., Kjøbenh., 1880, 2. R., vii, 961–965.—**Segond** (P.) Note sur une observation de kyste hydatique développé dans l'épaisseur du muscle grand pectoral. Progrès méd., Par., 1879, vii, 497.—**Seydeler** (R.) Schleifstein - Exsudate der Recruten. Deutsche mil.-ärztl. Ztschr., Berl., 1879, viii, 33–36.—**Sokolow** (A. A.) Ueber die Entwickelung des Sarkoms in den Muskeln. Arch. f. path. Anat., etc., Berl., 1873, lvii, 321–370, 2 pl.—**Teevan** (W. F.) On tumours in voluntary muscles; with an analysis of sixty-two cases, and remarks on the treatment Brit. & For. M.-Chir. Rev., Lond., 1863, xxxii, 504–517. *Also, transl.*: Allg. Wien. med. Ztg., 1864, ix, 89; 105.—**Vincent.** Angiome caverneux intramusculaire. Mém. Soc. d. sc. méd. de Lyon (1877), 1878. xvii, pt. 2, 191–194.

Muscles (*Individual*).

See, also, Biceps, Intercostal, Levator *ani*, Omohyoid, Serratus *anticus*, Sterno-cleido-mastoid, Subscapular, Tensor *tympani*, Transversus *nuchœ*, Trapezius, *muscle*; *and under names of organs and regions, e. g.*, Ciliary body, *etc.*; Extremities; Œsophagus; Pharynx, *etc.*

GRUBER (W.) Ueber den Musculus epitrochleo-anconeus des Menschen und der Säugethiere. Der Akademie vorgelegt am 12. April 1866. 4°. *St. Petersburg*, 1866.

Repr. from: Mém. Acad. imp. d. sc. de St.-Pétersb., 1867, 6. s., x, no. 5.

SIOLI (E.) * Vergleichungen über die Zwischenrippen- und Bauchmuskulatur der Wirbelthiere. 8°. *Halle*, 1875.

Blumenthal (C.) M. extensor triceps als quadriceps. Ztschr. f. rat. Med., Leipz. u. Heidelb., 1869, 3. R., xxxvi, 1–3, 1 pl.—**Clason** (E.) Om musculus adductor brevis och magnus hos menniskan Upsala Läkaref. Förh., 1872, vii, 599–602.—**Colson** (L.) Le muscle supracostal. Ann. Soc. de méd. de Gand, 1887, lxvi, 150–155.—**Cooper** (O. B.) Hyo-epiglottideus muscle. Lond. M. Gaz., 1828–9, iii, 475, 1 pl.—**Cruveilhier** (E.) [Les gaines tendineuses des péroniers latéraux.] Bull. Soc. anat. de Par., 1862, xxxvii, 438.—**Dubar** (L.) Muscle ansiforme sus-claviculaire; tenseur de l'aponévrose cervicale superficielle. *Ibid.*, 1880, lv, 388–390.—**Franks** (K. M.) The chondrocoracoid muscle. Dublin J. M. Sc., 1876, lxi, 19–21.—**Galton** (J. C.) Note on the epitrochleo-anconeus or anconeus sextus (Gruber). J. Anat. & Physiol., Lond., 1874–5, ix, 169–175, 1 pl.—**Gruber** (W.) Ueber die Identität d. Stylo-auricularis (Hyrtl 1840) mit einer Varietät des Caput auriculare m. styloglossi (mihi 1854) und Duverney's Priorität der Entdeckung (1749). Ztschr. f. rat. Med., Leipz. u. Heidelb., 1861, 3. R., x, 368–372. ——. Nachtrag zur Kenntniss des Musculus epitrochleo-anconeus der Säugethiere. Mélanges biol. Acad. imp. d. sc. de St.-Pétersb., 1868, vi, 464–472.—**Halbertsma** (H. J.) Anatomisches und Pysiologisches über den Musculus frontalis. [*Transl. from*: Versl . . . . d. k. Akad. v. Wetensch. Afd. Natuurk., Amst., 1858, vii.] Arch. f. d. holländ. Beitr. z. Nat.- u. Heilk., Utrecht, 1859–60, ii, 49–56. *Also, transl.*: J. de la physiol. de l'homme, Par., 1863, vi 117–123. ——. Musculus gastrocnemius triceps. Nederl. Tijdschr. v. Geneesk., Amst., 1862, vi, 609. *Also, in his*: Ontleedk. Aanteeken., 8°, Amst., 1862, 1–3.—**Henle.** Ueber den Musculus spinalis cervicis des Menschen. Arch. f. Anat., Physiol.u. wissensch. Med., Berl., 1837, 297–303.—**Jacobson** (A.) Zur Lehre vom Bau und der Function des Musculus thyreo-arytænoideus beim Menschen. Arch. f. mikr. Anat., Bonn, 1887, xxix, 617–629, 1 pl.—**Kulaewsky** (M.) Musculi subcrurales et sub anconæi. Arch. f. Anat., Physiol. u. wissensch. Med., Leipz., 1869, 410–421.—**Le Double.** Muscle sus-claviculaire tenseur

Muscles (*Individual*).

de l'aponévrose cervicale superficielle. Bull. Soc. anat. de Par., 1881, lvi, 563. *Also:* Progrès méd., Par., 1882, x, 345.—**von Luschka** (H.) Der lange Halsmuskel des Menschen. Arch. f. Anat., Physiol. u. wissensch. Med., Leipz., 1854, 103-118. 1 pl. ——. Der Musc. hyo- und genio-epiglotticus. *Ibid.*, 1868, 224-230, 1 pl. ——. Der Musc. pubo-transversalis des Menschen. *Ibid.*, 1870, 227-231, 1 pl.—**Merkel** (F.) Der Musculus superciliaris. Anat. Anz., Jena, 1887, ii, 17.—**Perrin** (J. B.) Psoas parvus. Med. Times & Gaz., Lond., 1872, i, 202.—**Theile** (F. W.) Entdeckung von Muskeln, welche die Rücken-wirbel drehen (Rotatores dorsi), beim Menschen und den Säugethieren, nebst Bemerkungen über die Processus transversi und obliqui und über die Rückenmuskeln. Arch. f. Anat., Physiol. u. wissensch. Med., Berl., 1839, 102-138, 1 pl. ——. Ueber den Triceps brachii und den Flexor digitorum sublimis des Menschen. *Ibid.*, 420-430.—**Turner** (W.) Sur le muscle kérato-cricoïde. J. de la physiol. de l'homme, Par., 1862, v, 493. ——. On a rudi-ment of the panniculus carnosus superficial to the trape-zius. J. Anat. & Physiol., Lond., 1870-71, v, 116.—**Williams** (W. R.) The anatomy of the quadriceps extensor cruris. *Ibid.*, 1878-9, xiii, 204-218.

Muscles (*Intercostal*).

See **Intercostal** *muscles*.

Muscles (*Ocular, Paralysis of*).

See **Eye** (*Paralytic affection of*).

Muscles (*Orbital*).

See **Eye** (*Movements, etc., of*).

Muscroft (C. S.) Osteo-sarcoma of superior maxilla. Removal of a large recurrent fibroid tumor from the face, neck, and mouth; return-ing after an operation performed nearly fifteen years previous, for the exsection of a very large "osteo-sarcoma" of the right half of the inferior maxilla. 12 pp. 12°. *Cincinnati, R. Clarke & Co.*, [1875].

Repr. from: Cincin. Lancet & Obs., 1875, xviii.

——. A new, simple, and safe method of pre-venting hemorrhage, treating aneurisms, and ap-plicable to other surgical conditions. Present-ing a case of successful amputation of the hip joint and a case of amputation at the shoulder joint, where the method was put in practice. 7 pp. 8°. *Cincinnati*, 1887.

Repr. from: Cincin. Lancet & Clinic, 1887, n. s., xviii.

Muscular *sense*.

BRACH (B.) *Dè coenæsthesi quædam. 8°. Berolini*, [1826].

DUBUISSON (P.) *Quelques considérations sur les quatre sens du toucher en général et sur la musculation ou sens musculaire en particulier. 4°. Paris*, 1874.

RAUBER (A.) *Vater'sche Körper der Bänder- und Periostnerven und ihre Beziehung zum so-genannten Muskelsinne. [Munich.] 8°. Neu-stadt a. d. Haardt*, 1865.

SACHS (C.) *Physiologische und anatomische Untersuchungen über die sensiblen Nerven der Muskeln. 8°. Berlin*, 1875.

Third part of: Anatomische und physiologische Unter-suchungen [etc.] [*See, infra.*]

STROMEYER (L.) De combinatione actionis nervorum et motoriorum et sensoriorum sive de sensuum impressionibus musculorum actione ef-fectis. 8°. *Erlangæ*, 1839.

Bastian (H. C.) On the "muscular sense" and on the physiology of thinking. Brit. M. J., Lond., 1869, i, 394; 437; 461; 509. ——. The "muscular sense"; its nature and cortical localisation. Brain, Lond., 1887-8, x, 1-137.—**Beaunis** (H.) Une expérience sur le sens mus-culaire. Rev. phil., Par., 1887, xxiii, 328-330.—**Bene-dikt.** Muskel-, rectius Bewegungsbewusstsein und zwar speciell über das Bewusstsein einer zu machenden oder gemachten Leistung. Allg. Wien. med. Ztg., 1869, xiv, 439.—**Bernhardt** (M.) Zur Lehre vom Muskelsinn. Arch. f. Psychiat., Berl., 1872, iii, 618-635.—**Blix** (M.) Ett enkelt förfaringssätt att bestämma muskelsinnets skärpa. Upsala Läkaref. Förh., 1884, xix, 123-128.—**Bloch** (A. M.) Expériences sur les sensations de contraction musculaire. Compt. rend. Soc. de biol., Par., 1884, 8. s., i, pt. 2, 31-33.—**Exner** (S.) Einige Beobachtungen über Bewegungs-nachbilder. Centralbl. f. Physiol., Leipz. u. Wien, 1887-8,

Muscular *sense*.

i, 135-140.—**Galton** (F.) On apparatus for testing the delicacy of the muscular and other senses in different persons. J. Anthrop. Inst., Lond., 1882-3, xii. 469-477.—**George.** Der Muskelsinn. Arch. f. Anat., Physiol. u. wissensch. Med., Leipz., 1870, 251-263.—**Haworth** (T.) On the association of the senses with the muscular feeling. Lond. M. Gaz., 1848, n. s., vi, 935; 977; 1028.—**Landry** (O.) Mémoire sur la paralyse du sentiment d'activité musculaire. Gaz. d. hôp., Par., 1855, xxviii, 262; 269; 282; 318; 334. *Also,* Reprint.—**Lewinski** (L.) Ueber den Kraftsinn. Arch. f. path. Anat., etc., Berl., 1879, lxxvii, 134-146.—**Odenius** (M. V.) Undersökningar öfver de sensibla muskelnerverna. Nord. med. Ark., Stockholm, 1872, iv, no. 18, 1-18. *Also,* Reprint.—**Sachs** (C.) Anatomische und physiologische Untersuchungen über die sensiblen Nerven der Muskeln. Arch. f. Anat., Physiol. u. wissensch. Med., Leipz., 1874, i, 175; 491, 3 pl.; 645, 2 pl. [*See, also, supra.*]—**Sémerie.** Hallucinations de la musculation. Tribune méd., Par., 1883, xv, 232; 256.—**Sklotovski** (P.) K' voprosu o mishechnom chuvstvai. [On the question of a muscular sense.] Med. Vestnik, St. Petersb., 1868, viii, 127-130.—**Sollier** (P.) Le sens musculaire. Arch. de neurol., Par., 1887, xiv, 81-101.—**Teissier** (J.) Sur le sens musculaire. Mém. et compt.-rend. Soc. d. sc. méd. de Lyon (1881), 1882, xxi, pt. 2, 113-115.—**Zernial.** Experimentalbeiträge zur Kenntniss des Muskelsinns. Arch. d. Heilk., Leipz., 1864, v, 546-549.

Musculine.

Aroud (F.) Préparation de la musculine. Gaz. méd. de Lyon, 1868, xx, 564.—**Passot** (P.) Note sur la mus-culine. Ann. Soc. de méd. de Lyon, 1863, 2. s., xi, 292-294. *Also:* Gaz. méd. de Lyon, 1864, xvi, 14.

Musculo-cutaneous *nerve*.

See **Nerve** (*Musculo cutaneous*).

Musculo-spiral *nerve*.

See **Nerve** (*Musculo-spiral*).

Musculo-spiral *nerve* (*Paralysis of*).

See **Extremity** (*Upper, Paralysis of*).

Musculus *sternalis*.

See **Muscles** (*Abnormities of*).

Musculus *venosus*.

Crumpe (F.) Observations on the musculus venosus and on its use in tetanus. Dublin J. M. Sc., 1872, liv, 257-262.

Musée de l'Hôpital St.-Louis. Pièces moulées par M. Baretta. MS. 6 v. 12°. [*Paris*, 1886.]

Musehold (Albert) [1854–]. *Experimen-telle Untersuchungen über das Sehcentrum bei Tauben. 30 pp., 1 l. 8°. *Berlin, G. Schade*, 1878.

Musehold (Carl) [1853–]. *Ein Fall von Echinococcus der Gallenblase und der Leber. 31 pp. 8°. *Berlin, M. Niethe*, [1876].

Musehold (Paul) [1861–]. *Die Bleiver-giftung eine Ursache chronischer Nierenerkran-kung. 28 pp. 8°. *Berlin, O. Francke*, [1883].

Muselier (Paul). *Étude sur la valeur séméio-logique de l'ecthyma. 128 pp. 4°. *Paris*, 1876, No. 130.

Muselli (J.-M.) *De la fistule gastrique; étude pathologique, physiologique et chirurgicale. 164 pp., 1 l. 4°. *Bordeaux*, 1881, 3. s., No. 6.

Museum der Heilkunde. Hrsg. von der helve-tischen Gesellschaft correspondirender Aerzte und Wundärzte. v. 1-4, 1792-7. 8°. *Zürich, Orell, Gessner, Füssli u. Comp.*

Museums.

See, also, **Medicines** (*Classification, etc., of*).

ACLAND (H. W.) The Oxford Museum. Re-marks addressed to a meeting of architectural societies; with letters from John Ruskin and John Phillips. 16°. *Oxford*, 1860.

AMERICAN Museum of Natural History. [Cen-tral Park, New York City.] Annual reports of the trustees and officers of the American Mu-seum of Natural History to the patrons, mem-bers, and subscribers. 3.-4., 1871-2. 8°. *New York*, 1872.

Third report is added as appendix to the fourth.

Museums.

BALK (L.) * Museum Adolpho-Fridericianum. *In:* LINNÆUS. Amœnitates acad. [etc.] 8°. *Lugd. Bat.,* 1749, i, 556-610.

BOITARD. Manuel du naturaliste préparateur, ou l'art d'empailler les animaux et de conserver les végétaux et les minéraux. 3. éd. 16°. *Paris,* 1835.

BRITISH Museum. Catalogue of the specimens of lizards in the collection of the British Museum. sm. 8°. *London,* 1845.

——. Catalogue of shield reptiles in the collection of the British Museum. Part I. Testudinata (tortoises). By John Edward Gray. 4°. *London,* 1855.

——. The same. Part II. Emydosaurians, rhynchocephalia, and amphisbænians. By John Edward Gray. 4°. *London,* 1872.

——. The same. Supplement. Part I. Testudinata (tortoises). With figures of the skulls of 36 genera. By John Edward Gray. 4°. *London,* 1870.

——. The same. Appendix. Part I. Testudinata (tortoises). By John Edward Gray. 4°. *London,* 1872.

——. Catalogue of the acanthopterygian fishes in the collection of the British Museum. By Albert Günther. 8°. *London,* 1859-62.

——. Catalogue of the fishes in British Museum. By Albert Günther. 8°. *London,* 1864-70.

——. Hand-list of the specimens of shield-reptiles in the British Museum, by J. E. Gray. 8°. *London,* 1873.

——. The gigantic land-tortoises (living and extinct) in the collection of the British Museum. By Albert C. L. G. Günther. 4°. *London,* 1877.

——. Catalogue of the Batrachia gradientia s. caudata and Batrachia apoda in the collection of the British Museum. 2. ed., by George Albert Boulenger. 8°. *London,* 1882.

——. Catalogue of the Batrachia salientia s. ecaudata in the collection of the British Museum. 2. ed., by George Albert Boulenger. 8°. *London,* 1882.

——. Guide to the galleries of reptiles and fishes in the department of zoölogy of the British Museum. (Natural history.) 8°. [*London*], 1887.

——. Guide of the shell and starfish galleries (mollusca, echinodermata, vermes) in the department of zoölogy of the British Museum (natural history), Cromwell road, London, S. W. 8°. [*London*], 1887.

CAPE OF GOOD HOPE Association for Exploring Central Africa. Catalogue of the South African Museum, the property of a society entitled "The Cape of Good Hope Association for Exploring Central Africa". 8°. [*London*], 1838.

GEINITZ (H. B.) Mittheilungen aus dem königl. mineralogischen Museum in Dresden für die Jahre 1872 und 1873. 8°. *Dresden,* 1874.

GOODE (G. B.) Classification of the collection to illustrate the animal resources of the United States. A list of substances derived from the animal kingdom, with synopsis of the useful and injurious animals, and a classification of the methods of capture and utilization. 8°. *Washington,* 1876.

HARVARD University. *Museum of Comparative Zoölogy.* Annual reports of the trustees of the Museum of Comparative Zoölogy, at Harvard College, in Cambridge; together with the report of the curator to the committee on the museum, for the years 1864; 1871-6. 8°. *Boston,* 1865-77.

——. Annual reports of the curator of the Museum of Comparative Zoölogy, at Harvard

Museums.

College, to the president and fellows of Harvard College, for the years 1864-6; 1870 to 1878-9; 1881-2. 8°. *Boston,* 1865-82.

——. Bulletins of the Museum of Comparative Zoölogy, at Harvard University, Cambridge, Mass. v. 2, No. 1; v. 3, Nos. 7-14; v. 5, Nos. 1-3, 15-16; v. 6, Nos. 3, 5-9. 8°. *Cambridge,* 1879-80.

——. Illustrated catalogue of the Museum of Comparative Zoölogy, at Harvard College, Cambridge, Mass. 2 pts., Nos. 7-8. 4°. *Cambridge,* 1874-5.

HARVARD University. *Peabody Museum of American Archæology and Ethnology, Cambridge, Mass.* Annual reports of the trustees to the president and fellows of Harvard College. 1.-17., Nov., 1866, to Feb. 18, 1884. v. 1-3. 8°. *Cambridge,* 1868-84.

VAN DER HOEVEN (J.) Eenige aanteekeningen over het kabinet van vergelijkende ontleedkunde te Pariis. 8°. [*n. p., n. d.*]

HULTMAN (D.) * Instructio musei rerum naturalium. *In:* LINNÆUS. Amœnitates acad. [etc.] 8°. *Amstelædami et Lugd. Bat.,* 1756, iii, 446-464.

MARTIN (P. L.) Dermoplastik und Museologie, oder das Modelliren der Thiere und das Aufstellen und Erhalten von Naturaliensammlungen. Unter Mitwirkung von Präparator Bauer, Prof. Dr. G. Jäger, Dr. Steudel, etc. 8°. *Weimar,* 1870.

MILWAUKEE. *Public Museum.* Annual report of the board of trustees to the common council. 2., 1883-4. 8°. *Milwaukee,* 1884.

MUSEUM (Das) Ludwig Salvator in Ober-Blasewitz bei Dresden. 8°. *Dresden,* 1879.

MUSEUM Senckenbergianum. Abhandlungen aus dem Gebiete der beschreibenden Naturgeschichte. 3 v. 4°. *Frankfurt a. M.,* 1833-9.

NEW SOUTH WALES. *Technological, Industrial, and Sanitary Museum.* Report of the committee of management to the governor and executive council. 6., 1885. fol. [*Sydney,* 1886.]

NEW YORK Historical Society. *Museum and Gallery of Art.* Catalogue of the Museum and Gallery of Art. 8°. *New York,* 1886.

NEW YORK State Cabinet of Natural History. Annual reports of the regents of the University of the State of New York on the condition of . . . and the historical and antiquarian collection annexed thereto. 3., 1850; 4., 1851; 20., 1867. 8°. *Albany,* 1850-67.

SMITHSONIAN Institution. Directions for collecting, preserving, and transporting specimens of natural history. Prepared for the use of the Smithsonian Institution. 2. ed. 8°. *Washington,* 1854.

——. The same. 3. ed. 8°. *Washington,* 1867.

UNITED STATES. *Department of the Interior. United States National Museum.* Bulletins. Nos. i-xxxii. 8°. *Washington,* 1875-86.

——. Proceedings. v. 1-10, 1878-86. 8°. *Washington,* 1879-87.

WARD (H. A.) Catalogue of mammals, birds, reptiles, and fishes in skins and mounted specimens. Also alcoholic specimens of reptiles, amphibia, and fishes. 8°. *Rochester,* 1877.

WESLEYAN University. Annual reports of the curators of the museum. 5.-6., 1875-6 to 1876-7; 9., 1879-80. 8°. *Middletown,* 1877-80.

Antiguo (El) Gabinete de historia natural de Madrid. Siglo méd., Madrid, 1858, v, 263.—**Dawkins** (W. B.) The organization of natural history museums. Nature, Lond., 1877, xvi, 137.—**Fatio** (V.) Quelques mots sur la formation de collections locales dans les musées cantonaux de la Suisse. Verhandl. d. schweiz. naturf. Gesellsch. 1872, Freib., 1873, lv, 172-182.—**Peter** (R.) On the mode of

Museums.

collecting and preserving objects of natural history, with a view to the formation of a cabinet, or to their transporta tion. Transylv. J. M., Lexington, Ky., 1834, vii, 133–149. *Also*, Reprint.—**Rau** (C.)—Die Jadeitgegenstände des National-Museums zu Washington. [Mit Bemerkungen von H. Fischer (Freiburg).] Arch. f. Anthrop., Brnschwg., 1882-3, xiv, 157-163, 1 pl.—**Roberts** (M. J.) Museums as educational adjuncts to medical colleges. Am. Vet. Rev., N. Y., 1882-3, vi, 136; 191; 252.—**Tischler** (O.) Bericht über die anthropologisch-prähistorische Abthei lung des Provincial-Museums der physik.-ökonom. Gesell- schaft. Arch. f. Anthrop., Brnschwg., 1879-80, xii (App.), 69-74.—**Wilder** (B. G.) Educational museums of verte- brates. Proc. Am. Ass. Adv. Sc. 1885, Salem, 1886, xxxiv, 263–281. *Also*, Reprint.—**Zittel** (K. A.) Museums of natural history in the United States. [*Transl. from suppl. to:* Allg. Ztg., München, Dec. 16.] Science, Cam- bridge, 1884, iii, 191–196.

Museums (*Anatomical and pathological*).

See, also, **Anatomy** (*Pathological*).

ALBINUS (B. S.) Index supellectilis anatomi- cæ, quam Academiæ Batavæ quæ Leidæ est legavit Johannes Jacobus Rau, qui et vitam ejus et curationem quam calculosis adhibuit in- strumentorumque figuras addidit. 4°. *Lugd. Bat.*, 1725.

——. Index supellectilis anatomicæ, rerum anatomicarum, tum phialis contentarum in li- quore limpido, tum exsiccatarum, quam suos in usus summa cum peritia atque dexteritate con- fecit, [etc.] 8°. *Lugd. Bat.*, 1771.

ALBINUS (F. B.) Suppellex anatomica Bern. Siegfr. Albini. 8°. [*Lugd. Bat.*, 1775.]

BARKOW (J. C. L.) Die angiologische Samm- lung im anatomischen Museum der königlichen Universität zu Breslau, verzeichnet und be- schrieben von dem Director der Anstalt. 4°. *Breslau*, 1869.

BIERMAYER (L.) Musæum anatomico-patho- logicum Nosocomii universalis Vindobonensis, quod ordine systematico descripsit [etc.] 16°. *Vindobonæ et Tergesti*, 1816.

BLANCKEN (G.) Catalogue de ce qu'on voit de plus remarquable dans la chambre de l'ana- tomie publique de l'Université de Leide. 4°. *Leyden*, 1715.

BLEULAND (J.) Descriptio Musei anatomici quod universi Belgii regis augustissimi Guilielmi I. munificentia Academiæ Rheno - Trajectinæ concessit. 4°. *Traj. ad Rhenum*, 1826.

BRITISH Medical Association. Annual meet- ings. 41. (1873); 45. (1877). Museum cata- logues. 8°. *London*, [1873, 1877].

BROOKES (J.) Brookesian Museum. The mu- seum of Joshua Brookes consists of a collection of anatomical and zoological preparations, which has almost wholly occupied Mr. Brookes's time and attention for upwards of thirty years, and is acknowledged to be elegant, extensive, and justly celebrated, being the production of indi- vidual talent and exertion, without regard to trouble or expense. 8°. *London*, 1828.

——. A catalogue of the anatomical and zoological museum of . . . 8°. *London*, 1828.

——. Museum Brookesianum. A descrip- tive catalogue of the remainder of the anatomi- cal and zootomical museum of . . . 8°. *London*, 1830.

CÆSAREÆ Academiæ medico - chirurgicæ Vil- nensis museum anatomicum. 4°. *Vilnæ*, 1842.

CATALOG der pathologisch - anatomischen Sammlung zu Giessen. 4°. *Giessen*, 1851.

CATÁLOGO de los museos y laboratorios de la Facultad de medicina de Madrid. sm. 8°. *Ma- drid*, 1875.

CATALOGUE of preparations, etc , in morbid anatomy and experimental physiology, contained in the museum of the army medical department, Fort Pitt, Chatham. By George Williamson. 8°. *London*, 1845.

Museums (*Anatomical and pathological*).

CERUTTI (F. P. L.) Beschreibung der patho- logischen Präparate des anatomischen Theaters zu Leipzig. 8°. *Leipzig*, 1819.

CHRIST Church Museum. Synopsis of the physiological series in the Christ Church Mu- seum, arranged for the use of students after the plan of the Hunterian collection, and chiefly under the divisions of the Hunterian catalogue. 4°. *Oxford*, 1853.

CIVININI (F.) Indice degli articoli del Museo d' anatomia fisiologica e patologica umano, com- parata dell' I. e R. Università di Pisa a tutto il decembre 1841. 8°. *Lucca*, 1842.

COLLEGE of Physicians of Philadelphia. To the honorable the judges of the court of common pleas, No. 2, of Philadelphia County, March term, 1884, No. 506. The petition of William Hunt, M. D., chairman, S. Weir Mitchell, M. D., and John B. Brinton, M. D., "committee of the Mütter Museum" [of the College of Physicians of Philadelphia, in relation to the disposition of the fund left by Thomas D. Mütter for the sup- port and increase of the museum]. 8°. [*Phila- delphia*, 1884.]

CROSSE (J. G.) An inaugural address deliv- ered at the opening of the Norfolk and Norwich Hospital Museum, September 10, 1845. 8°. *Nor- wich*, [1845].

DEI (A.) Catalogo sistematico del gabinetto di anatomia comparata della R. Università di Siena. 8°. *Siena*, 1880.

DUSSEAU (J.-L.) Musée Vrolik. Catalogue de la collection d'anatomie humaine, comparée et pathologique de MM. G. et W. Vrolik. 8°. *Amsterdam*, 1865.

DZONDI (C. H.) [Pr.] de museo anatomico- pathologico vite colligendo, conservando, dispo- nendo et inspiciendo. Prolusio i–ii, iv–vii. 8°. *Halæ*, 1823-4.

EHRMANN (C.-H.) Musée anatomique de la Faculté de médecine de Strasbourg, ou catalogue méthodique de son cabinet d'anatomie physiolo- gique, avec indication des ouvrages, mémoires et observations, où se trouvent consignées les his- toires des maladies qui se rapportent aux diffé- rentes préparations que renferme cette collection. 8°. *Strasbourg*, 1837.

——. Musée de la Faculté de médecine de Strasbourg. Observations d'anatomie patholo- gique, accompagnées de l'histoire des maladies qui s'y rattachent. 1. fasc. 4°. *Strasbourg*, 1843.

——. Nouveau catalogue du Musée d'ana- tomie normale et pathologique de la Faculté de médecine de Strasbourg. 8°. *Strasbourg*, 1843.

——. Notice sur les accroissements du Mu- sée d'anatomie pathologique de Strasbourg; suivie d'un catalogue, formant le premier sup- plément de celui publié en 1843. 8°. *Strasbourg*, 1846.

Also, in: Gaz. méd. de Strasb., 1846, vi, 33–58.

——. Accroissements du Musée d'anatomie de Strasbourg. 8°. *Strasbourg*, 1857.

ESCHOLA medico-chirurgica de Lisboa. Cata- logo das peças do museu d'anatomia da . . . coor- denado por J. G. Teixeira Marques. 8°. *Lisboa*, 1862.

ESCHOLA medico-cirurgica do Porto. Catalogo do gabinete d'anatomia da . . . pelo professor d'anatomia Luiz Pereira da Fonseca. [With first supplement.] 8°. *Porto*, 1860–61.

——. Segundo supplemento. 8°. *Porto*, 1861.

——. Terceiro supplemento. 8°. *Porto*, 1862.

——. Catalogo do museu anatomico da . . . 8°. *Porto*, 1865.

Museums (*Anatomical and pathological*).

FACULTÉ de médecine de Paris. Muséum d'anatomie pathologique de la Faculté de médecine de Paris, ou musée Dupuytren. Text, 2 v. 8°; atlas, fol. *Paris*, 1842.

——. Livret du musée d'anatomie normale de la Faculté de médecine de Paris. 8°. *Paris*, 1863.

FLORMAN (A. H.) Thesaurus anatomicus complectens præparata anatomica et pathologica ex homine et brutis, quæ, pro publicis prælectionibus in theatro anatomico servata, conquisivit. 16°. *Lundæ*, 1817.

FOWLER (J. K.) & SUTTON (J. B.) A descriptive catalogue of the Pathological Museum of the Middlesex Hospital. 8°. *London*, 1884.

GERMER (E. W) Das Museum der Gesundheitspflege [und das Army Medical Museum (Ford's Theatre)] in Washington.
Cutting from: Erie Tageblatt, Erie, 1886, Jan. 21.

GREAT BRITAIN. *Army Medical Department.* Catalogue of articles contained in the museum of military surgery, attached to the Army Medical School, at Netley. 8°. *London*, 1867.

——. Catalogue of preparations, etc., in morbid, natural, and comparative anatomy, contained in the museum of the army medical department, Fort Pitt, Chatham. 8°. *London*, 1833.

——. Medical School at Netley. Appendix to the catalogue of articles contained in the Museum of Military Surgery, attached to the Army Medical School, at Netley. 8°. *London*, 1875.

——. Medical School Museum. Description of a series of water-colour drawings, executed by the late Sir Charles Bell, illustrative of wounds received at the battle of Waterloo, presented by his widow to the Army Medical School, together with a sketch-book of manuscript notes and some original letters. By Deputy Inspector-General T. Longmore. 8°. [*London, n. d.*]

GREAT BRITAIN. *Parliament.* Medical museums. Return to an order of the House of Commons, dated 17 July. 1856, for "Returns from the Colleges of Physicians of London, Edinburgh, and Ireland, the Colleges of Surgeons of England, Edinburgh, and Ireland, the Faculty of Physicians and Surgeons of Glasgow, the Societies of Apothecaries of London and Dublin, and the Universities in England, Scotland, and Ireland, stating whether any museum for medical purposes is maintained out of the funds of the institution; under what conditions such museum, if any, is open to students or members of the medical profession; the annual cost of such museum in each of the last ten years, distinguishing the expenditure for building, for salaries and wages, for catalogues, and for preserving and increasing the collection; the total number of the catalogued specimens in each of the last ten years; what lectureships for medical purposes are maintained by the funds of the institution, and at what annual cost; under what conditions have the lectures, if any, been open to the public, or to students, or members of the medical profession; whether any expenses have been incurred for medical libraries, botanic gardens, or other objects of medical science, and, if so, at what annual cost for the last ten years, and under what conditions available to the public or to students or members of the medical profession". fol. [*London*, 1857.]

GREW (N.) Musæum Regalis Societatis; or, a catalogue and description of the natural and artificial rarities belonging to the Royal Society and preserved at Gresham Colledge. Whereunto is subjoyned the comparative anatomy of stomachs and guts, by the same author. (Being

Museums (*Anatomical and pathological*).

several lectures read before the Royal Society in the year 1676.) fol. *London*, 1681.

——. The same. fol. *London*, 1681–94.

GUY's Hospital, London. *Anatomical Museum.* A catalogue of the preparations in the anatomical museum of Guy's Hospital. Arranged and edited by desire of the treasurer of the hospital, and of the teachers of the medical and surgical school, by Thomas Hodgkin. 8°. *London*, 1829.

——. Catalogue of the pathological preparations in the museum of Guy's Hospital. Revised and edited by Samuel Wilkes. 2 v. 8°. *London*, 1857–63.

HAHNEMANN Medical College of Philadelphia. Catalogue of the museum and library of the Hahnemann Medical College of Philadelphia. By C. M. Thomas. 8°. *Philadelphia*, 1869.

HARVARD University. *Medical School.* A descriptive catalogue of the Warren Anatomical Museum, by J. B. S. Jackson. 8°. *Boston*, 1870.

HEAVISIDE (J.) Catalogue of the museum of . . . comprising human anatomy, natural and morbid; comparative anatomy, and natural history. With an appendix, including additions to the morbid anatomy, between 1818 and Aug., 1823. 8°. *London*, 1818.

——. A catalogue of the extensive and valuable anatomical museum of the late . . . Part second, comprising morbid anatomy, mummies, models, natural history, comparative anatomy, skeletons, monsters, and worms. Together with instruments, books, minerals, etc., which will be sold by Wheatley & Adlard, Oct. 6, 1829. 8°. [*London*, 1829.]

HERZOGLICHES Collegium anatomico-chirurgicum zu Braunschweig. Catalog der pathologisch - anatomischen Sammlung. 8°. *Braunschweig*, 1854.

HOLST (L.) Das Kriegs-Museum in Washington. 8°. *Würzburg*, 1865.

HOUEL (C.-N.) Manuel d'anatomie pathologique générale et appliquée, contenant la description et le catalogue du musée Dupuytren. 8°. *Paris*, 1857.

——. The same. 2. 6d. 12°. *Paris*, 1862.

——. Catalogue des pièces du Musée Dupuytren, publié sous les auspices de la Faculté de médecine de Paris. v. 1–5 (with atlas). 8°. *Paris*, 1877–80.

——. Catalogue du Musée Orfila, publié sous les auspices de la Faculté de médecine de Paris. 8°. *Paris*, 1881.

HOWSHIP (J.) Practical remarks on the discrimination and appearances of surgical disease; with an appendix, containing the descriptive catalogue of the author's collection in pathological anatomy, and the Hunterian oration for 1833. 8°. *London*, 1840.

HUNTER (W.) Two introductory lectures to his last course of anatomical lectures; to which are added some papers relating to Dr. Hunter's intended plan for establishing a museum in London for the improvement of anatomy, surgery, and physic. 4°. *London*, 1784.

HYRTL (J.) Das vergleichend-anatomische Museum an der Wiener medicinischen Facultät im Jubiläums-Jahre 1865. 8°. *Wien*, 1865.

——. Catalog mikroskopischer Injections-Präparate, welche durch Tausch oder Kauf zu beziehen sind von . . . 8°. *Wien*, 1873.

IMPERATORSKOI Sankt Peterburgiskoi Medico-chirurgicheskoi Akademii. Katalog chirurgicheskago Mouzeja. 8°. *St. Petersburg*, 1867.

INDEX rerum Musei anatomici Ticinensis. Accedit Antonii Scarpa in solemni theatri anatomici Ticinensis dedicatione oratio habita prid. kalend. November an. 1785. 8°. *Ticini*, 1804.

Museums (*Anatomical and pathological*).

JACKSON (J. B. S.) A descriptive catalogue of the anatomical museum of the Boston Society for Medical Improvement. 8°. *Boston*, 1847.

JANCKE (J. G.) Præparata anatomica Lipsiæ d. 18 Nov. 1765, in Vaporario Collegii Rubri auctione publica vendenda. 8°. *Lipsiæ*, [*n. d.*]

KENNEDY (E.) Descriptive catalogue of the museum of Dr. . . . illustrative of his lectures on midwifery and the diseases of women and children. 8°. *Edinburgh*, 1840.

KÖNIGLICH rheinische Friedrich-Wilhelms-Universität zu Bonn. Bericht über das anatomische Institut der . . . entworfen im Jahre 1830 von A. T. J. C. Mayer. 4°. *Bonn*, 1830.

KREUTZBERG (C.) Guide to the European anatomical, pathological, and ethnological museum of . . . 8°. *Buffalo*, 1875.

LANGENBECK (C. J. M.) Novum theatrum anatomicum quod Gottingæ est. 4°. *Gottingæ*, 1829.

LANGSTAFF (G.) Catalogue of the preparations illustrative of normal, abnormal, and morbid structure, human and comparative, constituting the anatomical museum of . . . 8°. *London*, 1842.

LASKEY (J.) A general account of the Hunterian Museum, Glasgow, including historical and scientific notices of the various objects of art, literature, natural history, anatomical preparations, antiquities, etc., in that celebrated collection. 8°. *Glasgow*, 1813.

LOBSTEIN (J.-F.) Compte rendu à la Faculté de médecine de Strasbourg sur l'état actuel de son muséum anatomique, suivi du catalogue des objets qu'il renferme. 8°. *Strasbourg*, 1820.

VON LODER (J. C.) Index præparatorum aliarumque rerum, ad anatomen spectantium, quæ in museo Cæsareæ Universitatis Mosquensis servantur. 8°. *Mosquæ*, 1823.

LOGAN (T. M.) Report on the annual museum for the exhibition of the American Medical Association in Philadelphia, and the contributions from California. 8°. *Sacramento*, 1872.

MANCHESTER Theatre of Anatomy, Marsden street. A catalogue descriptive chiefly of the morbid preparations contained in the museum of the . . . with occasional explanatory remarks. By Thomas Fawdington. 8°. *Manchester*, 1833.

MAYER (A. F. J. C.) Icones selectæ præparatorum musei anatomici Univ. Frid. Wilh. Rhenanæ quæ Bonnæ floret. fol. *Bonnæ*, 1831.

MÉDECINE (La) à l'Exposition universelle de 1867. Guide-catalogue publié par la Société médicale allemande de Paris. 12°. *Paris*, 1867.

MONTGOMERY (W. F.) Catalogue of the preparations in the museum of . . . 8°. *Dublin*, 1830.

———. The same. 8°. *Dublin*, 1834.

MOTT (V.) & MOTT (A. B.) Catalogue of the surgical and pathological museum of Valentine Mott, and of his son, Alexander B. Mott. 8°. *New York*, 1858.

MÜTTER (T. D.) Catalogue of the pathological museum of . . . 8°. *Philadelphia*, 1856.

MUSÆUM Franc. Calceolari jun. Veronensis a Benedicto Ceruto medico incæptum, et ab Andrea Chiocco . . . luculenter descriptum et perfectum, in quo multa ad naturalem moralemque philosophiam spectantia, non pauca ad rem medicam pertinentia erudite proponuntur et explicantur. Non sine magna rerum exoticarum supellectile, quæ artifici plane manu in æs incisæ, studiosis exhibentur. fol. [*Veronæ*, 1622.]

MUSÉE de l'Hôpital St.-Louis. Pièces moulées par M. Baretta. MS. 6 v. 12°. [*Paris*, 1886.]

MUSEUM anatomicum Holmiense, quod auspiciis augustissimi regis Oscaris primi ediderunt

Museums (*Anatomical and pathological*).

professores regiæ Scholæ medico-chirurgicæ Carolinensis. Sectio pathologica. Fasciculus I: s, continens casus x cum xii tabulis. fol. *Holmiæ*, 1855.

MUSSEY (R. D.) Anatomical cabinet belonging to . . . 8°. [*n. p., n. d.*]

NEW YORK (City). *Bellevue Hospital.* Catalogue of the "Wood" Museum of Bellevue Hospital, New York City. Comprising a descriptive and classified list of anatomical and pathological specimens. 12°. *New York*, 1880.

NEW YORK Hospital. *Pathological Cabinet.* A catalogue of the pathological cabinet of the New York Hospital, classified and arranged by Robert Ray, jr. With a memoir of the author [by John Watson]. Edited by H. D. Bulkley. 8°. *New York*, 1860.

OSIANDER (F. B.) Epigrammata in diversas res musei anatomici et pinacothecæ. Ed. altera. 12°. *Gottingæ*, 1814.

OTTO (A. W.) Verzeichniss der anatomischen Präparatensammlung des königlichen Anatomie-Instituts zu Breslau, nebst Nachtrag 1–2. 8°. *Breslau*, 1826–33.

OXFORD Museum. Synopsis of the pathological series in the Oxford Museum, provisionally arranged for the use of students after the plan of the Hunterian collection, and chiefly under the division of the Hunterian catalogue. 8°. *Oxford*, 1867.

PENNSYLVANIA Hospital. *Pathological Museum.* Descriptive catalogue of the pathological museum of the Pennsylvania Hospital. By Wm. Pepper. 8°. *Philadelphia*, 1869.

PHARMACEUTICAL Society of Great Britain. Catalogue of the collections in the museum of the . . . Compiled by E. M. Holmes. 8°. *London*, 1878.

PHILADELPHIA Hospital. *Pathological Museum.* Catalogue of the specimens in the pathological museum of the Philadelphia Hospital, prepared by James Tyson, assisted by R. M. Bertolet. 8°. *Philadelphia*, 1874.

REALE Scuola di ostetricia in Milano. Catalogo del gabinetto anatomo-patologico della R. Scuola di ostetricia in Milano, compilato ed illustrato dall' Assistente Dot. F. Agudio. 4°. *Milano*, 1862.

REALE Università di Pavia. Il gabinetto di anatomia normale della R. Università di Pavia. Descritto dal direttore e professore Giovanni Zoja. Serie B. Osteologia. Serie E. Angiologia. Serie L. Embriologia. Serie M. Anatomia generale. 4°. *Pavia*, 1873–87.

REFERENCES to the anatomical paintings and preparations at the anatomical rooms, Surgeon's Square, Edinburgh. 16°. *Edinburgh*, 1799.

REGIA Università degli studi di Napoli. Catalogo sistematico del gabinetto di anatomia comparata nella Regia Università degli studi di Napoli. 8°. *Napoli*, 1868.

———. The same. Supplemento primo. 8°. *Napoli*, 1872.

RIBKE (C. H.) Verzeichniss einer Sammlung anatomischer Präparate. 8°. *Berlin*, 1819.

DE RIEMER (P.) Beredeneerde beschrijving van het museum anatomico-physiologicum van . . . 4°. *Rotterdam*, 1831.

ROMITI (G.) & LACHI (P.) Catalogo ragionato del museo anatomico della R. Università di Siena, preceduto da una introduzione storica per Guglielmo Romiti. Pt. I. Osteologia e sindesmologia. 8°. *Siena*, 1883.

ROYAL College of Surgeons of Edinburgh. Catalogue of the museum of the . . . Pt. I. Comprehending the preparations illustrative of pathology. 8°. *Edinburgh*, 1836.

Museums (*Anatomical and pathological*).

ROYAL College of Surgeons of England. Synopsis of the arrangement of the preparations in the gallery of the museum of the Royal College of Surgeons. 12°. *London*, 1818.

———. Invitation to surgeons and naturalists for donations to the museum of the Royal College of Surgeons in London, of preparations, casts, models, paintings, drawings, engravings, manuscripts, printed books, and chirurgical instruments; also, directions for preserving animals and extraneous fossils. 8°. [*London*, 1826.]

———. Catalogue of the museum of the Royal College of Surgeons in London. Pt. I. Comprehending the pathological preparations in spirit. 4°. *London*, 1830.

———. The same. Beschreibung von Hunter's anatomisch-pathologischem Museum des Collegiums der Wundärzte in London. Aus dem Englischen für deutsche Aerzte und Wundärzte bearbeitet und mit einigen Anmerkungen begleitet von Dr. Michael Jäger. 8°. *Erlangen*, 1835.

———. Catalogue of the contents of the museum of the Royal College of Surgeons in London. Pt. IV, Fasc. I. Comprehending the first division of the preparations of natural history in spirit. 4°. *London*, 1830.

———. Descriptive and illustrated catalogue of the physiological series of comparative anatomy contained in the museum of the Royal College of Surgeons in London. v. 5. Products of of generation. 4°. *London*, 1840.

———. Description of the skeleton of an extinct gigantic sloth, Mylodon robustus, Owen, with observations on the osteology, natural affinities, and probable habits of the megatherioid quadrupeds in general. By Richard Owen, conservator of the museum. Published by direction of the council. 4°. *London*, 1842.

———. A descriptive and illustrated catalogue of the calculi and other animal concretions contained in the museum of the Royal College of Surgeons in London. [Pt. I, Div. I. Calculi from the urinary organs of man.] 4°. *London*, 1842.

———. The same. [Div. II. Calculi from the urinary organs of the lower animals.] 4°. *London*, 1845.

———. The same. By Thomas Taylor. Supplement No. 1. 4°. *London*, 1871.

———. Descriptive and illustrated catalogue of the fossil organic remains of mammalia and aves contained in the museum of the Royal College of Surgeons of England. 4°. *London*, 1845.

———. Descriptive catalogue of the pathological specimens contained in the museum of the Royal College of Surgeons of England. v. 1. General pathology. 4°. *London*, 1846.

———. The same. v. 2. Pathology of the blood and organs of locomotion. 4°. *London*, 1847.

———. The same. v. 3. Pathology of the organs of digestion, absorption, and circulation. 4°. *London*, 1848.

———. The same. v. 4. Pathology of the respiratory and urinary organs, the nervous system and the organs of the senses, the generative organs, and the mammary glands. 4°. *London*, 1849.

———. The same. v. 5. Specimens preserved in the dry state in cabinets. 4°. *London*, 1849.

———. Descriptive and illustrated catalogue of the histological series contained in the museum of the Royal College of Surgeons of England. v. 1. Elementary tissues of vegetables and animals. 4°. *London*, 1850.

Museums (*Anatomical and pathological*).

———. The same. Prepared for the microscope. v. 2. Structure of the skeleton of vertebrate animals. 4°. *London*, 1855.

———. Descriptive and illustrated catalogue of the physiological series of comparative anatomy contained in the museum of the Royal College of Surgeons of England. v. 1. Including the organs of motion and digestion. 2. ed. 4°. *London*, 1852.

———. Descriptive catalogue of the osteological series contained in the museum of the Royal College of Surgeons of England. v. 1. Pisces, reptilia, aves, marsupialia. 4°. *London*, 1853.

———. The same. v. 2. Mammalia placentalia. 4°. *London*, 1853.

———. Descriptive catalogue of the fossil organic remains of reptilia and pisces contained in the museum of the Royal College of Surgeons of England. 4°. *London*, 1854.

———. Descriptive catalogue of the fossil organic remains of invertebrata contained in the museum of the Royal College of Surgeons of England. 4°. *London*, 1856.

———. Catalogue of the contents of the museum of the Royal College of Surgeons of England. Pt. I. Plants and invertebrate animals in the dried state. 4°. *London*, 1860.

———. Descriptive catalogue of the pathological specimens contained in the museum of the Royal College of Surgeons of England. Supplement I. 4°. *London*, 1863.

———. Descriptive catalogue of the pathological specimens contained in the museum of the Royal College of Surgeons of England. Supplement II. Additional specimens of injuries and diseases of the eye. 4°. *London*, 1864.

———. Synopsis of the contents of the museum of the Royal College of Surgeons of England. 8°. *London*, 1850.

———. Synopsis of the contents of the museum of the Royal College of Surgeons of England. 8°. *London*, 1865.

———. Descriptive catalogue of the dermatological specimens contained in the museum of the Royal College of Surgeons of England. By Erasmus Wilson. 4°. *London*, 1870.

———. The same. 2. ed. 4°. *London*, 1875.

———. Descriptive catalogue of the teratological series in the museum of the Royal College of Surgeons of England. By B. T. Lowne. 8°. *London*, 1872.

———. Catalogue of the specimens illustrating the osteology and dentition of vertebrated animals, recent and extinct, contained in the museum of the Royal College of Surgeons of England. Pt. I. Man. By W. H. Flower. 8°. *London*, 1879.

———. The same. Pt. II. Class mammalia, other than man. By Wm. H. Flower, assisted by John Geo. Garson. 8°. *London*, 1884.

———. Descriptive catalogue of the pathological specimens contained in the museum of the Royal College of Surgeons of England. By Sir James Paget, Bart., with the assistance of James F. Goodhart and Alban H. G. Doran. v. 1. General pathology. 2. ed. 8°. *London*, 1882.

———. The same. v. 2. Morbid conditions of the blood, the organs of motion, and the skeleton. 2. ed. 8°. *London*, 1883.

———. The same. v. 3. Morbid conditions of the teeth, jaws, alimentary tract, liver, and gallbladder, ductless glands, circulatory and respiratory organs. 2. ed. 8°. *London*, 1884.

———. The same. v. 4. Morbid conditions of the urinary organs, of the nervous system and organs of special senses, of the generative organs and breast, and the anatomy of stumps. 2. ed. 8°. *London*, 1885.

Museums (*Anatomical and pathological*).

ROYAL College of Surgeons in Ireland. Descriptive catalogue of the preparations in the . . . By John Houston. v. 1. Anatomy. 8°. *Dublin*, 1834.

RUYSCH (F.) Thesaurus anatomicus primus ad decimum. 4°. *Amstelædami*, 1722–39.

———. Curæ posteriores, seu thesaurus anatomicus omnium præcedentium maximus. 4°. *Amstelodami*, 1724.

———. The same. 4°. *Amstelodami*, 1738.

———. Thesaurus animalium primus. 4°. *Amstelodami*, 1725.

———. Curæ renovatæ, seu, thesaurus anatomicus post curas posteriores, novus. 4°. *Amstelodami*, 1728.

———. Curæ posteriores, seu thesaurus anatomicus omnium præcedentium maximus. 4°. *Amstelodami*, 1738.

———. Museum anatomicum Ruyschianum, sive catalogus rariorum, quæ in authoris ædibus asservantur. 4°. *Amstelodami*, 1691.

SAINT BÁRTHOLOMEW's Hospital. *Anatomical Museum.* A descriptive catalogue of the anatomical museum of . . . 3 v. 8°. *London*, 1846–62.

———. A descriptive catalogue of the anatomical and pathological museum of . . . 2 v. roy. 8°. *London*, 1882–4.

SAINT GEORGE's Hospital. *Pathological Museum.* Catalogue of the pathological museum of Saint George's Hospital, edited by John W. Ogle and Timothy Holmes. 8°. *London*, 1866.

SAINT THOMAS's Hospital. Descriptive catalogue of the preparations in the museum of St. Thomas's Hospital. 3 v. 8°. *London*, 1847–9.

SANDIFORT (E.) Museum anatomicum academiæ Luguno-Batavæ descriptum ab . . . 4 v. roy. fol. *Lugd. Bat.*, 1793; 1827; 1835.

SCHERER (J.) Tabulæ anatomicæ quæ exhibent musæi anatomici Academiæ Cæs. Reg. Josephinæ præparata cerea. Perlustratæ et commentatæ a . . . delineata . . . a P. J. Weindl. 5 v. in 2. fol. *Vindobonnæ*, 1817–20.
Latin and German text.

SCHULTZE (C. A. S.) Die anatomischen Sammlungen und das neue Anatomie-Gebäude zu Greifswald. 1. Hft. Geschichte des Anatomie-Instituts; Beschreibung des neuen Gebäudes und Katalog der Präparate über Krankheiten des Nervensystems. 4°. *Greifswald*, 1856.

SCHUYL (F.) Catalogus rerum memorabilium, quæ in Theatro anatomico Academiæ, quæ Luguduni Batavorum floret, demonstrantur per . . . sm. 4°. *Lugd. Bat.*, 1721.

———. The same. sm. 4°. *Lugd. Bat.*, 1738.

———. The same. Catalogus van alle de principaalste rariteiten die op de Anatomie-Kamer, binnen de stadt Leiden vertoond werden. 16°. *Leyden*, 1748.

———. The same. Catalogue de ce qu'on voit de plus remarquable dans la chambre de l'anatomie publique de l'Université de la ville de Leide. sm. 4°. *Leide*, 1748.

SEIDEL (J. F.) *Index Musei anatomici Kiliensis, quem præfatus est illustris D. Fischer. 4°. *Kiliæ*, 1818.

SHUFELDT (R. W.) Outlines for a museum of anatomy, prepared for the Bureau of Education. 8°. *Washington*, 1885.

SURINGAR (G. C. B.) Pars supellectilis anatomicæ, sive catalogus speciminum pathologico-anatomicorum, quæ in usus privatos a se collecta, præparata et ordine disposita, Academiæ Leidensi vivus donavit. 8°. *Lugd. Bat.*, 1866.

SYSTEMATISCHER Catalog der Präparate des anatomischen Museums der königlich rheinischen Friedrich-Wilhelms-Universität zu Bonn.

Museums (*Anatomical and pathological*).
1. Decenium von den Jahren 1820–30, von A. F. J. C. Mayer. 8°. *Bonn*, [1831].

TALRICH (J.) Catalogue de préparations anatomiques normales et pathologiques en cire, plastique et plâtre; anatomie comparée et zoologie. Expositions universelles de Paris et Londres, 1855–1862. Exposition de 1867, classes xi et xii. 8°. *Paris*, 1866.

THIBERT (F.) Musée d'anatomie pathologique. Bibliothèque de médecine et de chirurgie pratiques, représentant en relief les altérations morbides du corps humain. 8°. *Paris*, 1844.

———. Musée d'anatomie pathologique et normale, fondé par . . . actuellement sous la direction du Dr. E. - V. Léger. 8°. *Paris*, 1860.

TOURTUAL (C. T.) Zweiter anatomischer Bericht, enthaltend die Beschreibung der seit meinem Antritte des Lehramtes der Anatomie im Frühjahre 1830 zum anatomischen Museo zu Münster hinzugekommenen pathologischen Präparate. 4°. *Münster*, 1833.

———. Verzeichniss und kurze Beschreibung einiger seit 1833 für das anatomische Museum zu Münster erworbenen pathologischen Gegenstände. 4°. *Münster*, 1840.

TRINITY College. A descriptive catalogue of the minerals in the systematic collection of the museum of Trinity College, Dublin. 8°. *Dublin*, 1818.

UNITED STATES. *Congress.* An act providing for the erection of a building to contain the records, library, and museum of the Medical Department, United States Army. Approved March 2, 1885. 8°. [*Washington*, 1885.]

———. Joint resolution to provide for the preparation and printing of an illustrated catalogue of the Army Medical Museum. 50. Cong., 1. sess. H. R. 14. Dec. 14, 1887. Introd. by Mr. Dolph. roy. 8°. [*Washington*, 1887.]

UNITED STATES. *War Department. Surgeon-General's Office.* Catalogue of the Army Medical Museum, Surgeon-General's Office, Washington, D. C. 8°. *Washington*, 1863.

———. Catalogue of the surgical section of the United States Army Medical Museum. Prepared under the direction of the Surgeon-General, U. S. Army, by A. A. Woodhull, Asst. Surg., U. S. Army. 4°. *Washington*, 1866.

———. Catalogue of the medical section of the United States Army Medical Museum. Prepared under the direction of the Surgeon-General, U. S. Army, by J. J. Woodward, Asst. Surg., U. S. A., in charge of the medical and microscopical sections of the museum. 4°. *Washington*, 1867.

———. Catalogue of the microscopical section of the United States Army Medical Museum. Prepared under the direction of the Surgeon-General, U. S. Army, by E. Curtis, Asst. Surg., U. S. Army. 4°. *Washington*, 1867.

———. List of skeletons and crania in the section of comparative anatomy of the United States Army Medical Museum, for use during the International Exhibition of 1876, in connection with the representation of the Medical Department, U. S. Army. Prepared by H. C. Yarrow. 8°. *Washington*, 1876.

———. Check list of preparations and objects in the sections of human anatomy of the United States Army Medical Museum for use during the International Exhibition of 1876. By G. A. Otis. 8°. *Washington, D. C.*, 1876.

———. List of the specimens in the anatomical section of the United States Army Medical Museum. By G. A. Otis. 8°. *Washington, D. C.*, 1880.

Museums (*Anatomical and pathological*).

———. The World's Industrial and Cotton Centennial Exposition, New Orleans, La., 1884–5. Medical Department, United States Army, Exhibit, Class 4, No. 5. Description of selected specimens from the medical and surgical sections of the Army Medical Museum, at Washington, D. C. Surg. John S. Billings, U. S. A., curator of Army Medical Museum. Henry McElderry, Asst. Surg., U. S. A., in charge of the representation of the Medical Department, U. S. A. 8°. *New Orleans*, 1884–5.

———. Advertisement and specifications for the erection of a fire-proof building for Army Medical Museum and Library. Text and plans. fol. *Washington*, 1885.

UNIVERSIDAD de Coimbra. Catalogo dos gabinetes de chimica medica e anatomia pathologica na Universidade de Coimbra, coordenado por F. A. Alves. 8°. *Coimbra*, 1865.

———. Supplemento ao catalogo do gabinete de anatomia pathologica da Universidade de Coimbra, coordenado por F. A. Alves. 8°. *Coimbra*, 1866.

UNIVERSITY of Cambridge. *Anatomical Museum.* Catalogue of the osteological portion of specimens contained in the anatomical museum of the University of Cambridge. 8°. *Cambridge*, 1862.

UNIVERSITY College, Liverpool. *Pathological Museum.* Descriptive catalogue of the pathological museum of University College, Liverpool (Royal Infirmary School of Medicine). 8°. *Liverpool*, 1883.

UNIVERSITY College, London. Descriptive catalogue of the specimens illustrating surgical pathology in the museum of University College, London. By Marcus Beck and S. G. Shattock. Pts. i and ii. 8°. *London*, 1881–7.

C. Stonham added as author in pt. ii.

UNIVERSITY of Edinburgh. *Anatomical Museum.* Descriptive catalogue of the anatomical museum of the University of Edinburgh. 8°. *Edinburgh*, 1831.

———. Amended report by the college committee in regard to the anatomical museum. 8°. [*Edinburgh*, 1839.]

UNIVERSITY of Glasgow. *Hunterian Museum.* Catalogue of anatomical preparations in the Hunterian Museum, University of Glasgow. 8°. *Glasgow*, 1840.

UNIVERSITY of Pennsylvania. *Anatomical Museum.* Report on the state of the anatomical museum of the University of Pennsylvania. June 30, 1824. By W. E. Horner. 8°. [*n. p.*], 1824.

———. Catalogue of the anatomical museum of the . . . With a report to the museum's committee of the trustees. Nov., 1832. By William Edmonds Horner. 2. ed. 8°. *Philadelphia*, 1832.

UNIVERSITY of Pennsylvania. *Wistar or Anatomical Museum.* Catalogue of the Wistar or anatomical museum of the Pennsylvania University. By W. E. Horner. 3. ed. 8°. *Philadelphia*, 1850.

VAN DERVEER (A.) Facts in relation to the history of the Albany Medical College Museum, together with a comparative review of the museums of Great Britain. The introductory address of the course of 1879–80, at the Albany Medical College, delivered Oct. 7, 1879. 8°. *Albany*, 1879.

VATER (A.) Regii in academia ad Albim musei anatomici Augustei catalogus universalis præparata anatomica Ruyschiana variorumque celeberrimorum auctorum tam sicca, quam in liquore contenta fœtus, monstra, sceleta et artefacta ex-

Museums (*Anatomical and pathological*).

hibens cum oratione de museis [etc.] 4°. *Wittenbergæ*, [1736].

VERGANGENHEIT und Gegenwart des Museums für menschliche Anatomie an der Wiener Universität. 8°. *Wien*, 1869.

WALTER (J. G.) Anatomisches Museum. Gesammelt von . . . Beschrieben von Friedrich August Walter. 2 Th. in 1 v. 4°. *Berlin*, 1796.

———. Museum anatomicum, per decem, et quod excurrit, lustra maximo studio congestum in defessoque labore perfectum a . . . Tomus i. 4°. *Berolini*, 1805.

WORMIUS (O.) Museum Wormianum seu historia rerum rariorum, tam naturalium quam artificialium, tam domesticarum quam exoticarum, quæ Hafniæ Danorum in ædibus authoris servantur. fol. *Amstelodami*, 1655.

A. (M.) Una visita al museo anatómico del Dr. D. Pedro Gonzalez Velasco. Siglo méd., Madrid, 1856, iii, 81.—**Ager** (J.) & **Macleod** (R.) Hunterian museum. Med.-Chir. Rev., Lond., 1826–7, n. s., vi, 283–289.—**Bell** (C.) Lectures on the Hunterian preparations in the museum of the Royal College of Surgeons, London. Lancet, Lond., 1833–4, i, 279; 313; 486; 912; 962.—**Bérenger-Féraud.** Note sur le catalogue du musée médical, chirurgical et micrographique de l'armée des États-Unis. Gaz. d. hôp., Par., 1870, xliii, 293.—**Brookes** (J.) A description of the anatomical museum of . . . Lond. M., S., & Pharm. Reposit., 1814, i, 116–121.—**Building** (The) for the Army Medical Museum and Library, Washington. Med. News, Phila., 1886, xlix, 330–334 [with cut].—**Carruccio** (A.) Aumenti fatti alle collezioni del museo di zoologia e di anatomia comparata della R. Università di Modena dal gennaio 1872 a tutto dicembre 1873; catalogo metodico. Spallanzani, Modena, 1874, xii, 87; 129; 173; 215.—**Ciniselli** (L.) Sopra il gabinetto anatomo-patologico esistente nello Spedale Maggiore di Cremona. Ann. univ. di med., Milano, 1848, cciv, 520: 1869, ccx, 48; 487. *Also, Reprint.*—**Desgenettes.** Réflexions générales sur l'utilité de l'anatomie artificielle, et en particulier sur la collection de Florence, et la nécessité d'en former de semblables en France. J. de méd., chir., pharm., etc. Par., 1793, xciv, 162; 233.—**Devergie** (A.) Note sur le musée pathologique créé à l'Hôpital St.-Louis. Union méd., Par., 1869, 3. s, vii, 135.—**Dobson** (G. E.) Report on the present condition of the museum of the army medical department, at the Royal Victoria Hospital, Netley, November, 1874. Army M. Dep. Rep. 1873, Lond., 1875, xv, 373.—**Ercolani** (G. B.) Descrizione metodica dei preparati esistenti nel museo di anatomia patologica comparata della R. Università di Bologna. Mem. Accad. d. sc. d. Ist. di Bologna, 1871, 3. s., i, 567–604, 6 pl.—**Eve** (F. S.) Our museum and its associations. St. Barth. Hosp. Rep., Lond., 1881, xvii, 165–184.—**Fabbri** (G.) Antico museo ostetrico di Giovanni Antonio Galli restauro fatto alle sue preparazioni in plastica e nuova conferma della suprema importanza dell' ostetricia sperimentale. Mem. Accad. d. sc. d. Ist. di Bologna, 1872, 3. s., ii, 129–166.—**Fede** (F.) Relazione sul museo anatomo-patologico del grande Ospedale degl' incurabili. Ann. clin. d. osp. incur., Napoli, 1880, v, 181–216.—**Flower** (W. H.) Note on the construction and arrangement of anatomical museums. J. Anat. & Physiol., Lond., 1874–5, ix, 259–262. ———. Museum specimens for teaching purposes. Nature, Lond., 1876–7, xv, 144; 184; 204. ———. The Museum of the Royal College of Surgeons of England. Tr. Internat. M. Cong., 7. sess., Lond., 1881, i, 133–144.—**Gabinete** i museo anatómico de la delegacion universitaria. An. Univ. de Chile, Santiago, 1887, xxix, 554–557.—**Giraldès.** Rapport sur un ouvrage de Ehrmann: "Musée anatomique de la Faculté de médecine" (Strasbourg), folio, 1843, 1850, 1852. Bull. Soc. de chir. de Par., 1852–3, 422–426.—**de Grazia y Alvarez** (A.) Investigaciones anatómicas é históricas sobre los originales y modelos patológicos existentes en el gabinete de la Facultad de medicina y cirugía de Cádiz. Siglo méd., Madrid, 1857, iv, 41.—**Hamilton** (F. H.) The Hyatt's anatomical, pathological, surgical, and microscopical collection. Buffalo M. J., 1854–5, x, 367–371.—**Holst** (F.) Det Kgl. Frederiks Universitets pharmakologiske Museum. Norsk Mag. f. Lægevidensk., Christiania, 1866, 2. R., xx, 481–496. — **Holst** (L.) Zamietki obe ustroistvě voenno-med. chasti ve Sievero-Amerikanskiche Shtatache. [Description of Army Medical Museum in Washington.] Med. pribav. k. morsk. sborniku, St. Petersb., 1865, v, 49–108. *Also, transl.* [Abstr.]: Würzb. med. Ztschr., 1865, vi, 285–318. *Also, Reprint.*—**Hulme** (R. T.) On the formation and arrangement of a dental museum, with a proposed dental classification of the placental mammalia. Tr. Odont. Soc. Gr. Brit., Lond., 1868–9, n. s., i, 73–142.—**Isenflamm** (H. F.) Die Sammlung des Theaters in Dorpat. *In his:* Anat. Untersuch.. 8°, 1822, 321–330.—**Key** (A.) On den nya Patologiskt Anatomiska Institutionen i

Museums (*Anatomical and pathological*).
Stockholm. Nord. med. Ark., Stockholm, 1869, i, no. 6, 1-24, 1 pl. — **Knox** (R.) Anatomical museums; their objects and present condition. Med. Times, Lond., 1846, xiv, 307; 327. — **Leboucq** (H.) Le musée anatomique de l'Université de Gand. Livre jubil. publié p. la Soc. de méd. de Gand, etc., Gand, 1884, 73-97. — **Malcolm** (A. G.) Report on the pathological museum of the Belfast Medical Society. Dublin Q. J. M. Sc., 1851, xi, 207; 471: xii, 471: 1852, xiii, 472. — **Martens** (C.) Revue de quelques musées anatomiques de l'Allemagne, de l'Angleterre et de la France. Rev. méd. franç. et étrang., Par., 1834, iii. 337-350. *Also*, Reprint. — **Mayer** (A. M.) Uebersicht der an der hiesigen Universität aufbewahrten anatomischen und pathologisch-anatomischen Präparate. Med. Jahrb. d. k. k. österr. Staates, Wien, 1829, n. F., i, 148-160. — **Meusel.** Catalogue of the United States Army Medical Museum, prepared under the direction of the Surgeon-General, U. S. Army. [Rev.] Cor.-Bl. d. allg. ärztl. Ver. v. Thüringen, Leipz., 1876, v, 81-96. — **Münz.** Einige Worte über die anatomische Präparaten-Sammlung der vormaligen Universität zu Landshut. Med. Argos, Leipz., 1840, li, 666-670. — **Munaret.** Un musée de médecine à Lyon. Lyon méd., 1877, xxiv, 471-475. — **Musée** Dupuytren. J. hebd. d. progr. d. sc. méd., Par., 1835, iv, 190. — **Musée** d'anatomie comparée à l'École de médecine. Gaz. méd. de Par., 1845, 2. s., xiii, 693 - 705. — **Notice** of the anatomical preparations of Harvey, lately presented to the Royal College of Physicians. Med.-Chir. Rev., Lond., 1823-4, iv, 234. — **Objetos** ingresados en el Museo antropológico durante el año de 1876 y principios de 1877. Anfiteatro anat., Madrid, 1877, v, 110. — **Obstetrical** Society of London. Catalogue of the museum of the Obstetrical Society of London, comprising instruments, anatomical and pathological specimens, casts and models. December, 1875. Tr. Obst. Soc. 1875, Lond., 1878, xvii [app.], 143-151. — **Otis** (G. A.) Notes on contributions to the Army Medical Museum by civil practitioners. Boston M. & S. J., 1878, xcviii, 163-169. — **Pepper** (W.) List of the more important specimens added to the Pathological Museum during the past year; with descriptions. Penn. Hosp. Rep., Phila., 1868, i, 395-416, 1 pl. ——. Descriptive list of the specimens added to the hospital museum during 1868. *Ibid.*, 1869, ii, 298-316. — **Percy** & **Laurent.** Muséum (d'anatomie et de pièces pathologiques). Dict. d. sc. méd., Par., 1819, xxxv, 11-41, 3 pl. — **Pétrequin.** Revue des cabinets d'anatomie pathologique de l'Italie. Gaz. méd. de Par., 1837, 2. s., v, 657-666. — **Pick** (T. P.) Report of the curator of the Pathological Museum. St. George's Hosp. Rep., Lond., 1869, iv, 261-284. — **Power** (D'A.) Specimens added to the museum during the year ending October 1, 1886. St. Barth. Hosp. Rep., Lond., 1886, xxii, 371-430. — **Quelques** détails sur l'établissement du Muséum Dupuytren et de la chaire d'anatomie pathologique. Gaz. méd. de Par., 1835, 2. s., iii, 497-500. — **Quissac** (J.) Le conservatoire de la Faculté de médecine; aperçu sur ses collections. Montpel. méd., 1859, ii, 251; 346. — **Reymond.** (Rapporto a nome della commissione incaricata di una visite al Museo d' anatomia normale dell' Università di Torino.) Gior. d. r. Accad. di med. di Torino, 1870, 3. s., ix, 834-840. — **Storer** (H. R.) The gynæcological cabinet of Harvard University. J. Gynæc. Soc., Bost., 1872, vi, 357-367. — **Tantini** (F.) Brevi cenni sopra alcuni musei anatomico-patologici della Germania. Ann. univ. di med., Milano, 1830, lv, 543-547. — **Van Derveer** (A.) The pathological museums of Great Britain. Med. & Surg. Reporter, Phila., 1879, xli, 390-441. — **Velasco** (P. G.) Breve reseña del Museo de Orfila en la Facultad de medicina de Paris. Siglo méd., Madrid, 1857, iv, 406: 1858, v, 7; 22. — **Vicende** (Delle) e dello stato del gabinetto e laboratorio d' anatomia patologica dell' Università ticinese. Gior. di anat. e fisiol., Milano, 1867, iv, 166; 233. — **Wagner** (J.) Geschichtliche Notizen über das pathologische Museum im k. k. allgemeinen Krankenhause zu Wien; nebst Uebersicht der Leistungen der pathologisch-anatomischen Lehranstalt während des Jahres 1830. Med. Jahrb. d. k. k. österr. Staates, Wien, 1832, xii, 1-17. — **Wigg** (H. C.) Catalogue of specimens recently added to the Melbourne Hospital Museum. Austral. M. J., Melbourne, 1873, xviii, 1; 83. — **Wood** (The) Museum of Bellevue Hospital. [Edit.] Med. Rec., N. Y., 1881, xix, 492.

Museums (*Anthropological and ethnological*).
FISCHER (L. H.) Das Museum für Urgeschichte und Ethnographie an der Albert-Ludwigs Hochschule in Freiburg. 4°. *Freiburg*, 1875.

GADDI (P.) Il museo etnografico-antropologico della r. Università di Modena. 4°. *Modena*, 1870.

Museu (O) d'anthropologia do Dr. Velasco. Correio med. de Lisb., 1876 - 8, vi, 37. — **Pulido** (A.) Reseña del museo antropológico del Dr. Velasco (sito en el paseo de Atocha, Madrid). Anfiteatro anat., Madrid, 1875, iii, 426; 474.

Museux.
G. (O.) Les Museux, chirurgiens rémois. Union méd. et scient. du nord-est, Reims, 1887, xi, 257-268.

Musgrave (Guilhelmus) [1657-1721]. De arthritide anomala, sive interna, dissertatio. 18 p. l., 479 pp., 10 l. 8°. *Exoniæ, T. S. Farley et J. Bliss*, 1707.
——. The same. Ed. nova. 7 p. l., 170 pp. 4°. *Genevæ, apud fratres de Tournes*, 1715.
Bound with: SYDENHAM (Thomas). Opera med. 4°. *Genevæ*, 1715.
——. The same. Ed. nova accuratior. 3 p. l., 168 pp. 4°. *Genevæ, apud fratres de Tournes*, 1736.
Bound with: SYDENHAM (Thomas). Opera med. 4°. *Genevæ*, 1736.
——. The same. Ed. nova. 3 p. l., 168 pp. 4°. *Genevæ, apud fratres de Tournes*, 1749.
Bound with: SYDENHAM (Thomas). Opera med. 4°. *Genevæ*, 1749.
——. The same. Ed. nova. 3 p. l., 168 pp. sm. 4°. *Genevæ, apud fratres de Tournes*, 1757.
Bound with: SYDENHAM (Thomas). Opera med. sm. 4°. *Genevæ*, 1756.
——. The same. 3 p. l., 168 pp. 4°. *Genevæ*, 1769.
Bound with: SYDENHAM (Thomas). Opera med. 2 v. 4°. *Genevæ*, 1769.
——. De arthritide symptomatica dissertatio. Ed. nova. 4 p. l., 88 pp. 4°. *Genevæ, fratres de Tournes*, 1715.
Bound with: SYDENHAM (Thomas). Opera med. 4°. *Genevæ*, 1716.
——. The same. Ed. nova. 3 l., 88 pp. 4°. *Genevæ, G. de Tournes et fil.*, 1723.
——. The same. Ed. nova accuratior. 3 p. l., 88 pp. 4°. *Genevæ, apud fratres de Tournes*, 1736.
Bound with: SYDENHAM (Thomas). Opera med. 4°. *Genevæ*, 1736, ii.
——. The same. Ed. nova accuratior. 3 p. l., 88 pp. 4°. *Genevæ, apud fratres de Tournes*, 1749.
Bound with: SYDENHAM (Thomas). Opera med. 4°. *Genevæ*, 1749.
——. The same. Ed. nova. 3 p. l., 88 pp. sm. 4°. *Genevæ, apud fratres de Tournes*, 1757.
Bound with: SYDENHAM (Thomas). Opera med. sm. 4°. *Genevæ*, 1757.
——. The same. Ed. nova accuratior. 3 p. l., 88 pp. 4°. *Genevæ*, 1769.
Bound with: SYDENHAM (Thomas). Opera med. 2 v. 4°. *Genevæ*, 1769.
——. Dissertatio de dea salute, in qua illius symbola, templa, statuæ, nummi, inscriptiones exhibentur, illustrantur. 2 p. l., 28 pp., 3 pl. 4°. *Oxonii, L. Lichfield*, 1716.

Musgrave (H. B.) Homœopathic pharmacy demonstrated. 7 pp. 8°. [*n. p., n. d.*]
Repr. from: West. Lancet, Cincin., 1853, xiv.

Musgrave (Samuel) [1732-82]. *Apologia pro medicina empirica. 2 p. l., 41 pp. 4°. *Lugd. Bat., S. et J. Luchtmans*, 1763. [*Also, in*: P., v. 1001.]
——. An essay on the nature and cure of the (so-called) worm-fever. 32 pp. 8°. *London, T. Payne*, 1776. [P., v. 723.]
——. Speculations and conjectures on the qualities of the nerves. iv, 146 pp. 8°. *London, P. Elmsly, T. Payne [and others]*, 1776.
——. Gulstonian lectures read at the College of Physicians, [etc.] 3 p. l., 124 pp., 2 l. 8°. *London, T. Payne [and others]*, 1779. [*Also, in*: P., v. 610.]

CONTENTS.
1. On the dyspnœa.
2. On the pleurisy and peripneumony.
3. On the pulmonary consumption.

de Musgrave-Clay (Charles-Réné). *Étude sur la contagiosité de la phthisie pulmonaire. 116 pp. 4°. *Paris*, 1879, No. 464.

Mushard (Christianus Sievers). *De purgatione per alvum. 22 pp., 1 l. 4°. *Helmstadii, typ. H. D. Hammii,* [1721].

Mushard (Franciscus). *De morbis fibrarum in genere. 22 pp., 4 l. 4°. *Lugd. Bat., C. Wishoff,* [1716].

Mushet (William Boyd). A practical treatise on apoplexy (cerebral hemorrhage); its pathology, diagnosis, therapeutics, and prophylaxis; with an essay on (so-called) nervous apoplexy, on congestion of the brain and serous effusion. iv, 194 pp. 8°. *London, J. Churchill,* 1866.

Mushkin (M. M.) K uchen. o proischoj. vrojden. urodstve. Monstrum humanum kyphoscoliosi cum spina bif. consecutivisque ventroschysi seu abdom. hiatu compl. et genitalium extrem. inf. defectu depravatum. 16 pp., 1 pl. 8°. *St. Petersburg,* 1886.

Mushrooms.

See Fungi; Fungi (*Edible, etc.*)

Musiari (G.) Compendio di propedeutica chirurgica. Parte prima. Semejottica generale. 181 pp., 1 l. 8°. *Parma, L. Battei,* 1885.

Music.

See, also, Apoplexy (*Observations, etc., of*); Insanity (*Treatment of, Mental, etc.*)

ABHANDLUNG von dem Einflusse der Musik in die Gesundheit der Menschen. 12°. *Leipzig,* 1770.

ALBRECHT (J. W.) Tractatus physicus de effectibus musices in corpus animatum. 16°. *Lipsiæ,* 1734.

ANCHERSEN (A.) *De medicatione per musicam. sm. 4°. *Hafniæ,* [1720].

ATLEE (E. A.) *On the influence of music in the cure of diseases. University of Pennsylvania. 8°. *Philadelphia,* 1804.

BACH (H. A.) *De musices effectu in homine sano et ægro. 8°. *Berolini,* [1817].

BACHMANN (C. L.) *De effectibus musicæ in hominem. 18°. *Erlangæ,* [1792].

BECKER (J. C.) *De musicæ vi salutari. 8°. *Berolini,* 1821.

VAN DEN BOSCH (R. B.) *De musices effectu in morbis sanandis. 8°. *Lugd. Bat.,* 1837.

BROWN (I.) *De sonorum modulatorum vi in corpora humana. 8°. *Edinburgi,* 1751.

CAMPBELL (D.) *De musices effectu in doloribus leniendis aut fugandis. 8°. *Edinburgi,* 1777.

CHOMET (H.) Effets et influence de la musique sur la santé et sur la maladie. 8°. *Paris,* 1874 [1873].

COLOMBAT (E.) De la musique dans ses rapports avec la santé publique. 8°. *Paris,* 1873.

DELAGRANGE (P.-A.) *Essai sur la musique, considérée dans ses rapports avec la médecine. 4°. *Paris, an XII* [1804].

DENK (J. J.) *De musices vi medicatrice. 8°. *Vindobonæ,* 1822.

DESBOUT (L.) Ragionamento fisico-chirurgico sopra l' effetto della musica nelle malattie nervose. 12°. *Livorno,* 1780.

DÉSESSARTZ (J.-C.) Réflexions sur la musique, considérée comme moyen curatif. 8°. *Paris, an XI* [1803].

Also, in his: Rec. de discours, mém. [etc.] 8°. *Paris,* 1811, 53–73.

DURAND (A.) *Sur l'influence que peut exercer sur l'homme la musique, considérée dans ses rapports avec la médecine, suivie de quelques propositions médicales. 4°. *Paris,* 1819.

ETTMÜLLER (M. E.) & JÖCHER (C. G.) Disp. effectus musicæ in hominem. 4°. *Lipsiæ,* [1714].

FRANCK (F. A.) *De musices effectibus in hominem sanum et ægrotum. 8°. *Berolini,* [1835].

FRANZIUS (J. G. F.) Prolusio de medicorum legibus metricis. sm. 4°. *Lipsiæ,* [1782].

Music.

GUILLAUME (J.-A.) *Sur la musique, appliquée à l'hygiène et à la thérapeutique. 4°. *Paris,* 1817.

HANSEN (J. N.) *De musicæ in corpus humanum vi. 4°. *Berolini,* [1833].

HELMHOLTZ (H.) Die Lehre von den Tonempfindungen als physiologische Grundlage für die Theorie der Musik. 8°. *Braunschweig,* 1863.

HENNEBERG (E.) *De vi soni et musicæ in hominem sanum et ægrotum. 8°. *Jenæ,* 1846.

VON IVÁNCHICH (V.) *Musica medice considerata. 8°. *Pestini,* 1834.

KOPF (J. J.) *De influxu musicæ in animum et corpus. 8°. *Pragæ,* 1845.

KÜNZEL (A.) *De musicæ artis cum medicina connubio. sm. 8°. *Halæ,* [1800].

LAËNNEC (T.-A.) Discours prononcé . . . à la séance annuelle de la Société académique de la Loire-Inférieure. [Étude sur la théorie physiologique de la musique.] 8°. *Nantes,* 1872.

LAMARCHE (J.-B.) *Sur la musique, considérée dans ses rapports avec la médecine. 4°. *Paris,* 1815.

LA TORRE (F.) La musica e l' igiene; studi ed impressioni. Definizione e origine della musica; azione dei suoni; influenza sull' organismo; effetti fisiologici, terapeutici e pathologici. 2. ed. 12°. *Bergamo,* 1886.

LICHTENTHAL (P.) Trattato dell' influenza della musica sul corpo umano e del suo uso in cérte malattie; con alcuni cenni come si abbia ad intendere una buona musica. Tradotto dal tedesco e ricorretto dall' autore medesimo. 8°. *Milano,* 1811.

LOEWENSTEIN (J. J.) *De musices in homines et animalia efficacia. 8°. *Berolini,* 1835.

MARTEAU (L. R.) *An ad sanitatem musice ? [1743.]

In: SIGWART (G. F.) Quæst. med. Paris. 4°. *Tubingæ,* 1789, i, 106–119.

MATHEWS (S.) *On the effects of music in curing and palliating diseases. 8°. *Philadelphia,* 1806.

MERCURIN (L. S.) *De musice seu de influxu musices in corpus humanum. 4°. *Monspelii,* 1782.

MITCHEL. De arte medendi apud priscos musices ope atque carminum epistola ad Antonium Relhan. sm. 8°. *Londini,* 1766.

DE MOELLER (G.) *De musices et sonorum vi salutari. 8°. *Berolini,* 1824.

MOJON (B.) Mémoire sur l'utilité de la musique, tant dans l'état de santé que dans celui de maladie. Trad. de la 2. éd. italienne, avec notes par C.-D. Muggetti. 8°. *Paris,* 1803.

ODIER (L.) *De elementariis musicæ sensationibus. 8°. *Edinburgi,* 1770.

Also, in: SMELLIE. Thesaurus med. [etc.] 8°. *Edinburgi,* 1785, iii, 181–209.

POHL (J. F. B.) *De artis musicæ in sanos et ægrotantes effectu. 8°. *Berolini,* [1818].

POHLE (M. A.) *De curatione morborum per carmina et cantus musicos. 4°. *Vitembergæ in Saxonibus,* [1706].

REFLECTIONS on antient and modern music with the application to the cure of diseases; to which is subjoined an essay to solve the question wherein consisted the difference of antient musick from that of modern times. 8°. *London,* 1749.

RITZ (J.) *Untersuchungen über die Zusammensetzung der Klänge der Streichinstrumente. Physikalisch-musiktheoretische Abhandlungen. 8°. *München,* 1883.

ROBINOT DE LA LANDE (A.) *Sur les effets avantageux de la musique dans les maladies. 4°. *Paris,* 1835.

Music.

SCHMOLZNOP (W. R.) * De musæ Polyhymniæ in sanos et ægrotantes effectu. 8°. *Pragæ*, 1836.

SCHNEIDER (P. J.) Die Musik und Poesie. Nach ihren Wirkungen historisch-kritisch dargestellt, oder: systematisch geordneter Versuch einer genauen Zusammenstellung und möglichst richtigen Erklärung derselben. Eine auf Belehrung und Unterhaltung abzweckende Familien-Lektüre für die gebildete Welt. 2 v. 8°. *Bonn*, 1835.

SMITH (W. L.) A plea for vocal music in public schools. A paper read before the Michigan State Teachers' Association. 8°. *Lansing*, [*n. d.*]

SOULA (H.) * Essai sur l'influence de la musique et son histoire en médecine. 4°. *Paris*, 1883.

STEINBECK (F. A.) * De musices atque poëseos vi salutari operis prodromus. 8°. *Berolini*, [1826].

STEINITZER (M.) Ueber die psychologischen Wirkungen der musikalischen Formen. 8°. *München*, 1885.

VAN SWIETEN (P.) * Spec. inaug. sistens musicæ in medicinam influxum atque utilitatem. 4°. *Lugd. Bat.*, 1773.

UNITED STATES. *Department of the Interior. Bureau of Education.* Circular of information. No. 1, 1886. The study of music in the public schools. 8°. *Washington*, 1886.

VON VOGEL (S. G.) Erinnerungen an den so mächtigen als merkwürdigen Einfluss der Music auf Menschen und Thiere. 4°. *Rostock*, [1807].
Beardsley (G. L.) The medical uses of music. N. Eng. M. Month., Newtown, Conn., 1882-3, ii, 214–216.—**Brierre-de-Boismont** (A.-J.-F.) De la musique dans les asiles d'aliénés et des concerts de la Senavra et de Quatre-Mares. Union méd., Par., 1860, 2. s., vii, 337 - 344.—**Brofferio.** Straordinario e fatale effetto della musica. Bull. d. sc. med. di Bologna, 1834, x, 66.—**Brückmann.** Ueber eine merkwürdige Nervenkrankheit [welche durch Musik geheilt wurde]. Arch. f. med. Erfahr., Berl., 1811, i, 8-10.—**Cramer** (S.) Memorandum concerning the influence of music on the common mouse. Phila. M. & Phys. J., 1804–5, i, 37.—**Dendopoulos** (D. G.) 'H μουσικὴ ἐν τῇ θεραπευτικῇ. Γαληνός, Ἀθῆναι, 1880, Δ', 237-240.—**Dogiel** (J.) Ueber den Einfluss der Musik auf den Blutkreislauf. Arch. f. Physiol., Leipz., 1880, 416-428, 2 pl.—**Duffy** (F.) Nature and use of the musical faculty. North Car. M. J., Wilmington, 1879, iii, 1-9.—**Erdmann.** Ueber den Einfluss der Musik auf Kranke. Arch. f. med. Erfahr., Berl., 1809, n. F., x, 121–134.—**Fournier-Pescay.** Musique. Dict. d. sc. méd., Par., 1819, xxxv, 42–80. — **Girgensohn** (L.) Verhältniss der Musik zur Medicin besonders zur psychischen. Beitr. z. Heilk., Riga, 1849-51, i, 187–236. — **Helmholtz** (H. L. F.) On the physiological causes of harmony in music; a lecture delivered in Bonn during the winter of 1857. *In his:* Pop. Lect. Sc. Sub., 8°, Lond., 1873, 61–106.—**Héricourt.** Essai sur les sensations musicales. Rev. scient., Par., 1882, 3. s., iv, 168–175. *Also, transl.:* Pop. Sc. Month., N. Y., 1882–3, xxii, 225–231.—**von Holberg.** Cur seines Fiebers durch Musik. Aus des Freiherrn von Holberg eigener Lebensbeschreibung. Arzt, Hamb., 1768, vi, 250-255. *Also, in:* New ed., 1769, iii, 535-538.—**Jennings** (O.) Music as a therapeutic agent. Lancet, Lond., 1880, ii, 794.—**Kraus** (A.) Di alcuni strumenti musicali della Micronesia e della Melanesia regalati al Museo nazionale d'antropologia e di etnologia dal Dott. Otto Finsch. Arch. per l' antrop., Firenze, 1887, xvîi, 36–41, 2 pl.—**Laurent** (A.) Quelques observations relatives à l'influence qu'exerce la musique sur les aliénés. Ann. méd.-psych., Par., 1860, 3. s., vi, 331–336.—**Levinstein.** Etwas über Musik als Heilmittel. Med. Alm., Berl., 1838, 72–79.—**Lucas** (J.) An account of the singular effects of music on a patient. Lond. M. J., 1790, xi, 125–130. — **Luzinsky** (A. M.) Die Musik in der Medizin. Allg. Wien. med. Ztg., 1882, xxvii, 271; 283.—**Maso** (A.) Estudio médico de la música. Rev. de cien. méd., Barcel., 1876, ii, 391–394. — **Miraglia** (L.) La musica come mezzo igienico e terapeutico, specialmente in alcune malattie nervose e mentali. Pisani, Palermo, 1885, vi, 87; 165: 1886, vii, 3–50.—**Music** in mind medicine. Virginia M. Month., Richmond, 1877-8, iv, 920–923. — **Prion.** Coup de sang produit par l'effet de la musique. J. de la sect. de méd. Soc. acad. Loire-Inf., Nantes, 1833, ix, 72–74.—**Rambosson.** Spécification des diverses influences de la musique dans ses applications à l'hygiène et à la médecine.

Music.

Bull. Acad. de méd., Par., 1876, 2. s., v, 1041.—**von Reichert** (C.) Versuch einer Richard Wagner-Studie; mit einer culturhistorischen Einleitung von H. Rohlfs. Deutsches Arch. f. Gesch. d. Med. u. med. Geog., Leipz., 1884, vii, 16-43. — **Tanzi** (D.) Sopra alcune leggi biologiche dell' estetica musicale. Psichiatria, Napoli, 1886, iv, 199-201.—**Vasileff** (S.) O vlijanii pienija na zdorove tchelovieka. [Influence of vocal music on the health.] Voyenno-med. J., St. Petersb., 1879, cxxxv, 192; 310; 355. *Also, transl.* [Abstr.]: St. Petersb. med. Wchnschr., 1879, iv, 53. — **Verrier de Villers** (E.) La comédie et la musique dans leurs rapports avec la santé. J. d'hyg., Par., 1878, iii, 325; 337. *Also*, Reprint.—**Vidal y Careta** (F.) La música en sus relaciones con la medicina; estudio especulativo, fisiológico, higiénico y terapéutico. [Tésis.] Gac. méd. catal., Barcel., 1882, ii, 20; 38; 65; 110.—**Vigna** (C.) Sull' importanza fisiologica e terapeutica della musica. Psichiatria, Napoli, 1886, iv, 185–198.—**Walther** (J. A.) Bemerkungen über den Einfluss der Musik auf psychische Zustände, mit einigen besondern, ihre Anwendung heischenden Bestimmungen. Allg. med. Ann., Altenb., 1814, 289 - 301. — **Whittaker** (J. T.) Music as a medicine. Clinic, Cincin., 1874, vi, 289–294.

Musicians.

HAPP (C. F.) De instrumentorum musicorum quæ flatu administrantur incommodis. 4°. *Lipsiæ*, [1778].
Bobillier. De l'influence des instrumens à vent, en cuivre, sur la santé des soldats qui en font usage, notamment de la trompette, du cornet et du clarion, avec quelques modifications à apporter dans la construction de ce dernier. Rec. de mém. de méd. . . . mil., Par., 1825, xvi, 57-67.—**Burq.** De l'influence du chant et du jeu des instruments à vent, chez les chanteurs et les musiciens de profession; de l'avenir des sociétés chorales et des orphéons au point de vue de la phtisie pulmonaire. Cong. internat. d'hyg. 1878, Par., 1880, ii, 408–419.—**Fournier-Pescay.** Musiciens (Maladies des). Dict. d. sc. méd., Par., 1819, xxxv, 41.—**Kellogg** (T. H.) Laryngeal cramp of musicians and speakers. Med. Rec., N. Y., 1887, xxxii, 106–108.—**Krishaber** (M.) Musiciens (Hygiène des). Dict. encycl. d. sc. méd., Par., 1876, 2. s., xi, 129–132.

Musil (Mathias). * De facie humana. 32 pp. 12°. *Viennæ, L. Grund*, [1835].

Musitanus (Carolus) [1635–1714]. Chirurgia theoretico-practica, seu trutina chirurgico-physica. 4 v. in 1. 4°. *Coloniæ Allobrogum, Cramer et Perachon*, 1698.

CONTENTS.

v. 1. De tumoribus. xxiv, 2 l., 327 pp.
2. De ulceribus. 1 p. l., 241 pp.
3. De vulneribus. 3 p. l., 425 pp.
4. De lue venerea. 3 p. l., 197, 30 pp.

————. Ad thesaurum, et armamentarium medicochymicum Hadriani a Mynsicht mantissa, quæ locupletiori penu non adhuc cognita, vulgataque medicamenta congerit, sive conquisita, sive propria industria excogitata et experientia probata, eorumdem usu, atque operandi rationabili energia. 162 pp. 16°. *Venetiis, J. G. Hertz*, 1707.
Bound with: VON MYNSICHT (H.) Thesaurus et armamentarium, [etc.] 16°. *Venetiis*, 1707.

————. De morbis mulierum tractatus, cui quæstiones duæ, altera de semine cum masculo, tum fœmineo, altera de sanguine menstruo . . . sunt præfixæ . . . 3 p. l., 240 pp. 4°. *Coloniæ Allobrogum, Choüet [et al.]*, 1709.

————. The same. 2 p. l., 240 pp., port. 4°. *Coloniæ Allobrogum. sumpt. Choüet [et al.]*, 1709.
With this is bound: RAYSCH (F.) Kurtze Hoch gründliche Erörterung. 4°. *Leipzig*, 1728.

————. The same. Weiber Kranckheiten, worinnen die Erzeugung der Menschen auf das genaueste untersuchet, auch noch zwey curiöse Fragen beygefüget werden, deren die eine von dem Saamen der Männer und Weiber, die andere aber von der monatlichen Zeit handelt, alles nach denen Principiis der neuesten Doctorum Medicinæ abgefasset. Aus dem Lateinischen übersetzet. 2 p. l., 746 pp., 7 l., port 12°. *Leipzig, J. F. Braun's Erben*, 1732.

————. The same. Neue und vermehrte Aufl. 2 p. l., 746 pp., 7 l. 12°. *Leipzig, C. L. Jacobi*, 1743.

————. Opera omnia, seu trutina medica, chirurgica, pharmaceutico-chymica, etc.; omnia juxta

Musitanus (Carolus)—continued.
recentiorum philosophorum principia, et medicorum experimenta, excogitata et adornata. Accesserunt huic novæ editioni tractatus tres, nunquam editi, nempe de morbis infantum, de luxationibus et de fracturis. 2 v. 8 p. l., 636 pp., 10 l. ; 7 p. l., 506 pp., 9 l. fol. *Genevæ, sumpt. Cramer et Perachon,* 1716.

————. The same. Editio omnium operum secunda, cui præter tractatus de morbis infantum, de luxationibus, et de fracturis, accesserunt notæ et observationes D. De Vaux in tractatum de lue venerea, et præfatio de eadem materia, quam Hermannus Boerhaave aphrodisiacis præposuit. 2 v. in 1. 10 p. l., 58 pp., 1 l., 636 pp., 10 l. ; 7 p. l., 506 pp., 9 l. ; 41 pp. fol. *Lugduni, sumpt. Perachon et Cramer,* 1733.

————. The same. Editio prima Veneta, ab antecedentis editionis mendis accuratissime expurgata. 2 v. lxxii, 551 pp.; xvi, 452 pp. fol. *Venetiis, J. Bortoli,* 1738.

For Portrait, see **Collection**—van Kaathoven.

————. See, also :
CELEBERRIMORUM virorum apologiæ pro R. D. Carolo Musitano adversus Petrum Antonium de Martino, medicum Geofonensem, qui trutinam medicam anno 1688 Venetiis typis editam, qua Harveana sanguinis circulatio, aliæque recentiorum medicorum sententiæ statuminantur, temere et inepte impugnare ausus est. fol. [*n. p., n. d.*]

Musk.
BIERKOWSKI (L. J.) *Diss. inaug. sistens moschi historiam, naturalem et medicam. 8°. *Lipsiæ,* [1830].
GROS (B. F.) *De moscho. sm. 4°. *Tubingæ,* [1790].
HEUSINGER (C. F.) Meletemata quædam de antiquitatibus castorei et moschi. fol. *Marburgi Cattorum,* [1852].
KAPP (G. L. C.) Ueber einige Wirkungen des Moschus in den Krankheiten des Menschen. 8°. *Nürnberg,* [1811].
KOCH (G. A.) *De moscho. 8°. *Pestini,* 1829.
KÜHN (C. G.) [Pr.] moschi antiquitates. 4°. [*Lipsiæ,* 1833.]
MILITZER (J. G.) *De nonnullis moschi, muriatis oxyduli hydrargyri mitis et muriatis oxyduli ferri in organismo sano effectibus. 8°. *Erlangæ,* [*n. d.*]
REINICK (G. G.) *Diss. inaug. sistens momenta quædam de moscho naturali et artefacto. 4°. *Jenæ,* [1784].
SCHROECKIUS (L.) De moscho. 4°. *Jenæ,* [1667].
————. Historia moschi. sm. 4°. *Augustæ Vindelicorum,* 1682.
TRALLES (B. L.) De limitandis laudibus et abusu moschi in medela morborum, dissertatio. 8°. *Vratislaviæ,* 1783.
WERNER (J. B.) *De moscho. sm. 4°. *Gottingæ,* [1784].

B. Substitute for the oil of amber in the formation of artificial musk. Boston M. & S. J., 1835, xii, 63.—**Bergrath.** Ueber Castoreum und Moschus, nebst Bemerkungen über Kritik der Arzneimittel. Rhein. Monatschr. f. prakt. Aerzte, Köln, 1850, iv, 623 ; 667.—**Bernatzik** (W.) Ueber Verfälschungen und Prüfungsweise des Moschus auf Reinheit und Güte. Ztschr. d. k.-k. Gesellsch. d. Aerzte zu Wien, 1860, xvi, 369–374.—**Bertherand** (E.) Le musk de gazelle, au point de vue des applications thérapeutiques. Bull. Soc. d. sc. . . . . d'Alger, 1877, xiii *bis,* 81–84.—**Debourge** (J.-B.) De l'emploi du musc contre le délire qui vient compliquer les pleurésies et les pneumonies aiguës ou typhoïdes. Ann. Soc. d. sc. méd. et nat. de Brux., 1842, 53–56.—**Deschamps.** Note sur la préparation de la teinture de musc. Bull. gén. de thérap., etc., Par., 1861, lxi, 219–221.——. Note sur quelques préparations de musc et de castoréum. Ibid., 1866, lxx, 357–359.—**Deutsch.** Etwas über die Wirkung des Moschus. Med. Ztg., Berl., 1850, xix, 127–129.—**Goppert** (H. R.) Ueber die Einwirkung des Moschus auf die Vegetation. Ztschr. f. Physiol., Darmst., 1829, iii, 269 – 273. — **Hannon** (J.) Du musc

Musk.
végétal comme succédané du musc animal. Presse méd. belge. Brux., 1852-3, v, 285 ; 325.—**Hiltscher** (J. A.) Zur Würdigung des Moschus. Med. Jahrb. k. k. österr. Staates, Wien, 1847, lxii, 19, 147, 283. — **Himmelreich** (L.) Ueber die Wirkungen des Moschus. Org. f. d. ges. Heilk., Aachen, 1853, ii, 193–197. ———. Ueber den Moschus. *Ibid.,* 1856, v, 234–236. — **Klein.** Vorzügliche Wirkung des Moschus gegen Schluckkrampf. Allg. med. Centr.-Ztg., Berl., 1851, xx, 449.—**Lailler** (A.) Note sur l'emploi et la préparation des potions au musc. Bull. gén. de thérap., etc., Par., 1866, lxx, 215–218.—**Löwenstein** (M. G.) Ist Moschus ein Specificum ? Med. Ztg. Russlands, St. Petersb., 1847, iv, 289.—**Martin** (S.) Un succédané du musc. Bull. gén. de thérap., etc., Par., 1868, lxxiv, 319.—**Moschus-Mischungen.** Wchnschr. f. d. ges. Heilk., Berl., 1843, 693-695.—**Neligan** (J. M.) A new method for detecting spurious musk-pods. Dublin Q. J. M. Sc., 1846, i, 77.—**O'Brien** (J. E.) [Medical uses of musk.] Chicago M. J., 1870, xxvii, 205–207.—**Parsons** (J.) A remarkable instance of the happy effect of musk in a very dangerous case. Phil. Tr., Lond., 1743–50, xi, 1054–1056.—**de la Peyronie.** Description anatomique d'un animal connu sous le nom de musc. [*From:* Mém. Acad. roy. d. sc. de Par., 1731.] Collect. acad. de mém., etc. Partie franç., Par. et Liége, 1784, vii, 241–255.—**Reid** (A.) A letter concerning the effects of the Tonquinese medicine. Phil. Tr., Lond., 1743–50, xi, 1051 - 1054. — **Sundelin.** Ueber die Wirkungen und Heilanzeigen des Moschus und der Digitalis. Arch. f. med. Erfahr., Berl., 1824, i, 415-440. — **Teplouchoff** (A. E.) Moschusochse. Arch. f. Anthrop., Brnschwg., 1885-6, xvi, 519–521 — **Wall** (J.) Of the extraordinary effects of musk in convulsive disorders. Phil. Tr., Lond., 1743-50, xi, 1044 - 1050. — **Williams** (S. W.) Artificial musk. Boston M. & S. J., 1835, xii, 13–15.

Muskau.
PROCHNOW. Muskau, seine Kur-Anstalten und Umgebungen. 12°. *Muskau,* 1857.
————. Bad Muskau. Eröffnung der Saison am 1. Juni, 1865. Schluss Mitte September. sm. 8°. *Dresden,* [1865].

Haxtrausen (L.) Ueber die Heilkraft des Mineralwassers, besonders des Moor- oder Badeschlammes bei Muskau ; mit einem Vorworte von Dr. J. N. Rust. Mag. f. d. ges. Heilk., Berl., 1826, xxi, 489–542.—**Hermbstüdt.** Einige Notizen über das Hermannsbad bei Muskau, dessen mineralische Trink- und Badequelle und den Moor- oder Badeschlamm daselbst. Allg. med. Ann., Leipz., 1825, 571–576. *Also:* J. d. pract. Heilk., Berl., 1825, lx, 4. st., 65–73. — **Herrmannsbad** Muskau. Deutsche Klinik, Berl., 1854, vi, 181-185.—**Kleeberg** (W.) Auszug aus dem Berichte über das Hermannsbad zu Muskau in der Oberlausitz vom Jahre 1830. Mag. f. d. ges Heilk., Berl., 1831, xxxiv, 305-313.—**Kleemann.** Einige Notizen über das bei Muskau in der Oberlausitz befindliche Herrmannsbad. *Ibid.,* 1824, xvii, 152 - 160. — **Sturm.** Geschichte einiger Kranken, bei welchen sich das Hermannsbad bei Muskau in verschiedenen Graden heilsam erwies. *Ibid.,* 1828, xxvi, 31–42.—**Wendt** (J.) Neueste Dartstellung des Hermannsbades in Muskau im k. preussischen Herzogthume Sachsen ; mit einem Vorworte. *Ibid.,* 1829, xxix, 498–529.

Muskingum *Valley.*
Richards (W. S.) Diseases, climate, and topography of the Muskingum Valley, (portion of) Licking County, Ohio. Proc. Convent. Phys. Ohio, Cincin., 1839, 36–41.

Musnhier-Lariboutie (J.-B.-Jérémie). *I. Établir le diagnostic et le traitement des éphélides. II. [etc.] 26 pp. 4°. *Paris,* 1839, No. 79, v. 347.

Musnier (Olivier). *Sur les hydropisies enkystées des ovaires. 22 pp. 4°. *Paris,* 1820, No. 41, v. 155.

Muspratt (James Sheridan). Untersuchung der schwefligsauren Salze. 36 pp. 8°. [*Heidelberg,* 1844.]   C.
Repr. from : Ann. d. Chem. u. Pharm., Heidelb., 1844, l.

————. On the chemistry of vegetation. 16 pp. 8°. *Glasgow, D. Robertson,* [1846].

————. Chemistry, theoretical, practical, and analytical, as applied and relating to the arts and manufactures. 2 v. 836 pp., 13 port. ; 1186 pp., 18 port. 4°. *Glasgow, Edinburgh, London & New York, W. Mackenzie,* 1860.

Musquetier (H. A.) Wet van den 27. April 1884 (Stbl. No. 96) waarbij met intrekking van de wet van 29. Mei 1841 (Stbl. No. 20), nadere bepalingen worden vastgesteld, betreffende het staatstoezicht op krankzinnigen en krankzinnigen-

Musquetier (H. A.)—continued.
gestichten . . . En aanhangsel. xx, 191 pp.
12°. *'s Gravenhage, gebroeders Belinfante*, 1884.

Muss (Maximilianus Fridericus Alexander) [1828–
]. * De adminiculis diagnosticis eorumque
dignitate. 27 pp., 2 l. 8°. *Berolini, F. G. Nietack*, [1856].

Mussaphia (Imanuel). * De hydrope universali. 31 pp. sm. 4°. *Lugd. Bat., J. et H. Verbeek*, 1730. [P., v. 78.]

Mussat (Albert). * De la trachéotomie préventive dans les fractures du larynx. 33 pp.
4°. *Paris*, 1872, No. 36.

de Mussay (Joannes Baptista Faustus Alliot).
*An spiritus sint ab aëre diversi? 4 pp. 4°.
[*Parisiis, J. Quillau*, 1715.]
See, also, **Thuillier** (Matthæus). An cæna, prandio
uberior, sit salubrior? 4°. *Parisiis*, [1716].

van Musschenbroek (Petrus) [1692–1763].
* De aëris præsentia in humoribus animalibus.
1 p. l., 42 pp., 1 l. 4°. *Lugd. Bat., S. Luchtmans*,
[1715]. [*Also, in :* P., v. 983.]
Also, in : HALLER. Disp. anat. [etc.] 4°. *Gottingæ*,
1749, iv, 561–618.
———. * De mente humana semet ignorante. 1
p. l., 28 pp. 4°. *Lugd. Bat., S. Luchtmans*, 1740.
———. Introductio ad philosophiam naturalem.
2 v. [paged consecutively]. 10 p. l., 1132 pp.,
8 l., 54 pl. 4°. *Lugd. Bat., S. et J. Luchtmans*,
1762.
For Biography, see Nederl. Tijdschr. v. Geneesk., Amst.,
1866, ii, 275–277.
For Portrait, see **Collection** of Portr. of Phys. & Men
of Sc., 137.

Musschl (K.) [1799–1852].
Ostrowski (E.) O życiu i pracach K. Musschl. [Life
and labors of K. Musschl.] Pam. Towarz. Lek. Warszaw.,
1852, xxviii, 3–25.

Musselburgh.
See, also, **Cholera** (*Asiatic, History, etc., of*), *by
localities.*
Stevenson (W.) On the sanitary condition and gen-
eral economy of the town of Musselburgh and parish of
Inveresk, in the county of Mid-Lothian. San Inquiry :
Scotland, Lond., 1842, 130–152. *Also,* Reprint.

Mussels.
de Beunie (J.-B.) Sur une maladie produite par les
moules vénimeuses. Mém. Acad. imp. et roy. d. sc. de
Brux., 1777, i, 229.—**Brooks** (W. K.) Embryology of the
fresh-water mussels. Proc. Am. Ass. Adv. Sc., 1875, Sa-
lem, 1876, xxiv, pt. 2, 238–240.—**Drost** (K.) Ueber das
Nervensystem und die Sinnesepithelien der Herzmuschel
(Cardium edule L.), nebst einigen Mittheilungen über den
histologischen Bau ihres Mantels und ihrer Siphonen.
[Kiel.] Morphol. Jahrb., Leipz., 1886, xii, 163–196. *Also,*
Reprint.—**Möbius** (K.) Mittheilungen über die giftigen
Wilhelmshavener und die nicht giftigen Kieler Mies-
muscheln. Schrift. d. naturw. Ver. f. Schlesw.-Holst.,
Kiel, 1886, vi, 2. Hft., 3–12.—**Moehring** (P. H. G.) My-
tulorum quorundam venenum et ab eo natas papulas cuticulares epistola. Acta Acad. nat. curios., Norimb., 1744,
vii [app.], 113–140.

Mussels (*Poisonous*).
See **Fish** (*Poisonous*).

Musser (*Benjamin*).
Stehman (H. B.) Obituary. Practitioner, Lancaster,
1883, i, 75–77.

Musser (J.)
Co-Editor of : **Allgemeine** Zeitung für Homöopathie,
Augsburg, 1848–9.

Musser (John H.) A modification of the sphygmograph, being a change in the base of the instrument of Pond. 4 pp. 8°. *Philadelphia*,
1884.
Repr. from : Med. & Surg. Reporter, Phila., 1884, l.
———. On idiopathic anæmia. A report of three
cases, with remarks; and an analysis of the
cases hitherto published in America. 31 pp.
8°. *Philadelphia*, 1885.
———. Some statistics of hepatic diseases. An
analysis of cases presented to the Pathological
Society of Philadelphia from 1837 to 1881, inclu-

Musser (John H.)—continued.
sive; with a detailed study of the fatty, the
cancerous, and the cirrhotic liver. 14 pp. 8°.
[*n. p.*, 1885.]
Repr. from : Med. Times, Phila., 1884–5, xv.
———. Notes of thirteen cases of tubercular
meningitis. 8 pp. 12°. [*Philadelphia*, 1886.]
Repr. from : Med. News, Phila., 1886, xlviii.
———. Abscess of the pancreas and thrombosis of
the portal vein. 6 pp. 8°. [*Philadelphia*, 1886.]
Repr. from : Am. J. M. Sc., Phila., 1886, n. s., xci.
———. Notes of a case (1) of Raynaud's disease,
and (2) of gangrene complicating diabetes mel-
litus. 19 pp. 8°. *Philadelphia, W. J. Dornan*,
1886.
Repr. from : Tr. Coll. Phys. Phila , 1886, 3. s., viii.
———. On the influence of age on the dosage of
of nux vomica, with some remarks on its thera-
peutics. 7 pp. 8°. *Detroit, Mich., G. S. Davis*,
1886.
Repr. from : Therap. Gaz., Detroit, 1886, x.
———. Two cases of malignant or ulcerative endocarditis. A clinical lecture. 16 pp. 12°.
Boston, 1886.
Repr. from : Boston M. & S. J., 1886, cxv.
——— & **Keen** (W. W.) Cholecystotomy; with
a report of two cases, a table of all the hitherto
reported cases, and remarks. 59 pp. 8°. [*n. p.*,
1884.]
Repr. from : Tr. Coll. Phys. Phila., 1884, 3. s., vii.
——— & **Piersol** (George A.) Notes of a case of
infectious, so-called ulcerative, endocarditis and
of a case of acute pericarditis. 15 pp. [8 photographic plates.] 8°. *Philadelphia, W. J. Dornan*, 1885.
———. Studies in pathology. 2 photographs. 4°. [*Philadelphia*, 1885.]
Subjects: Gall stones; gall-stone section.
Repr. from : Tr. Coll. Phys. Phila., 1886, 3. s., viii.

Musset (Ch.) Nouvelles recherches expérimentales sur l'hétérogénie, ou génération spontanée.
44 pp., 1 pl. 4°. *Toulouse, Bonnal & Gibrac*, 1862.
See, also, **Joly** (N.) & **Musset** (Ch.) Réfutation de
l'une des expériences capitales de M. Pasteur [etc.] 4°.
Paris, 1862.

Musset (Guillaume-Henri). * Études physiologiques et thérapeutiques sur les eaux thermales
de Plombières. 39 pp. 4°. *Paris*, 1852, No. 90,
v. 530.

Musset (H.-J.-M.-Hyacinthe). * Sur la nostalgie.
41 pp. 4°. *Paris*, 1830, No. 292, v. 237.
———. Traité des maladies nerveuses ou névroses,
et en particulier de la paralysie et de ses variétés,
de l'hémiplégie, de la paraplégie, de la chorée ou
danse de Saint-Guy, de l'épilepsie, de l'hystérie,
des névralgies internes et externes, de la gastralgie, etc. 416 pp. 8°. *Paris, A. Appert*, 1840.

Musset (Pitre). * Des kystes de l'ovaire, de leur
traitement. 51 pp. 4°. *Paris*, 1864, No. 2.

Mussey (Reuben Dimond) [1780–1866]. Experiments and observations on cutaneous absorption.
16 pp. 8°. *Philadelphia, T. & G. Palmer*, 1809.
[*Also, in :* P., v. 823.]
Repr. from : Phila. M. & Phys. J., 1809, 3. suppl.
———. An address read to the medical class at
Dartmouth College, December 1, 1818. 24 pp.
8°. *Hanover, N. H., C. Spear*, 1818.
———. An address on ardent spirit, read before
the New Hampshire Medical Society at their an-
nual meeting, June 5, 1827. 24 pp. 8°. *Hano-
ver, T. Mann*, 1828.
———. The same. 16 pp. 12°. *Boston, Perkins
& Marvin*, 1829.
———. Essay on ardent spirits and its substitutes
as a means of invigorating health. 65 pp. 12°.
Washington, D. Green, 1835.
Also, in : TEMPERANCE prize essays. 12°. *Washington*,
1835, 10–65.

Mussey (Reuben Dimond)—continued.

——. The same. 65 pp. 12°. *Washington, D. Green*, 1837.

——. An essay on the influence of tobacco upon life and health. 48 pp. 12°. *Boston, Perkins & Marvin*, 1836.

——. The same. A new ed., enlarged by the author. 64 pp. 18°. *New York, American Tract Society*, [1836].

——. The same. 3. ed. 48 pp. 12°. *Cincinnati, G. L. Weed*, 1839.

——. Animalcula in the atmosphere of cholera patients. 4 pp. 8°. [*Cincinnati*], 1849.
Repr. from: West. Lancet, Cincin., 1849, x.

——. An introductory lecture delivered at the opening of the thirty-second session of the Medical College of Ohio, October 15, 1851. 23 pp. 8°. *Cincinnati, Marshall & Langtry*, 1852.

——. The trials and rewards of the medical profession; an introductory lecture delivered at the opening of the first session of the Miami Medical College, at Cincinnati, October 3, 1852. 24 pp. 8°. *Cincinnati, T. Wrightson*, 1853. [*Also, in:* P., v. 228.]

——. Surgical cases. Aneurismal tumours upon the ear, successfully treated by the ligation of both carotids. Recto-vaginal fistula cured by operation. 6 pp. 8°. [*n. p.*, 1853.]
Repr. from: Am. J. M. Sc., Phila., 1853, n. s., xxvi.

——. Alcohol in health and disease. A lecture introductory to the fourth annual course of the Miami Medical College, at Cincinnati, October 15, 1855. 19 pp. 8°. *Cincinnati, T. Wrightson & Co.*, 1856.

——. Fracture of the neck of the thigh bone. 19 pp. 8°. [*n. p.*, 1857.]
Repr. from: Am. J. M. Sc., Phila., 1857, n. s., xxxiii.

——. What shall I drink? 35 pp. 16°. *Boston, American Tract Society*, [1863, *vel subseq.*].

——. Health; its friends and its foes. xii, 13–380 pp., 1 pl. 8°. *Boston, Gould & Lincoln*, 1866.

——. Anatomical cabinet belonging to . . . Printed for the use of pupils. 20 pp. 8°. [*Cincinnati, n. d.*]
See, also, **Potter** (J. F.) Letter to Prof. Mussey [etc.] 8°. *Cincinnati*, 1850.*
For Biography, see Cincin. Lancet & Obs., 1866, n. s., ix, 514–517. *Also:* Cincin. M. Obs., 1866, i, 308–316. *Also:* Med. Communicat. Mass. M. Soc., Bost., 1867, xi, 37–39. *Also:* Med. Rec., N. Y., 1866, i, 269. *Also:* N. Hampshire J. M., 1855, v, 31–39. *Also:* N. Jersey M. Reporter, Burlington, 1854, vii, 510–519, port. *Also:* Tr. N. Hampshire M. Soc., 1869, 61–81 *Also,* Reprint (A. B. Crosby). *Also:* Tr. Ohio M. Soc., 1867, 80–82 (W. P. Kincaid).
For Portrait, see **Collection** of Portr. (Libr.)

Mussey (William Heberden) [1818–82]. Anæsthesia. Non-fatal accidents from anæsthetic agents, with observations. 8 pp. 8°. *Cincinnati*, 1853.
Repr. from: West. Lancet, Cincin., 1853, xiv.

——. Vesico-vaginal fistula complicated with vesical calculus, cured by operation. 3 pp. 8°. *Cincinnati*, 1854.
Repr. from: West. Lancet, Cincin., 1854, xv.

——. Surgical cases. Cases of polypi of the larynx cured by operation. 4 pp. 8°. [*Cincinnati*, 1856.]
Repr. from: Cincin. M. Obs., 1856, i.

——. A case of fracture of the os inominatum; and death in connection with the administration of sulphuric ether. 8 pp. 8°. *Cincinnati*, [1861].
Repr. from: Cincin. Lancet & Obs., 1861, iv.

——. Successful double ovariotomy. 7 pp. 8°. [*n. p.*, 1867, *vel subseq.*]

——. Report on surgery. A paper read before the Ohio State Medical Society, at the annual meeting, held at Delaware, June, 1868. 16 pp. 8°. *Cincinnati, A. Abraham*, 1868. [*Also, in:* P., v. 217.]

Mussey (William Heberden)—continued.

——. Death from inhalation of chloroform. 3 pp. 8°. [*Cincinnati*, 1873.]
Repr. from: Cincin. Lancet & Obs., 1873, xvi.
Also, Co-Editor of: **Cincinnati** (The) Lancet and Observer, 1867–73.
For Biography, see **Hartwell** (Edward Mussey). A memorial sketch of W. H. Mussey. 8°. [*Baltimore*, 1883.]
Repr. from: Ann. Soc. Army of Cumberland, 1882.
See, also, Rep. Cincin. Hosp. (1883), 1884, xxiii, 11, port.
For Portrait, see **Collection** of Portr. (Libr.)

Mussmann (Joannes Georgius). *De idealismo sive philosophia ideali. viii, 48 pp., 1 l. 4°. *Berolini, typ. Reimerianis*, [1826].

Musso (Giovanni) **& Bignamini** (Angelo). Le acque potabili della città di Lodi, con nozioni intorno alla scelta delle acque potabili ed alla interpretazione dei risultati annalitici. 46 pp. 8°. *Lodi, C. Dell' Avo*, 1881.

Musso (Victor). *Sur l'étiologie, le diagnostic et les caractères anatomiques des anévrysmes du cœur. 26 pp. 4°. *Paris*, 1827, No. 164, v. 209.

Musson (Achille). *Du torticolis. 50 pp. 4°. *Paris*, 1867, No. 69.

Mussot (Pierre-Alphonse). *Propositions de médecine. 20 pp. 4°. *Paris*, 1833, No. 301, v. 265.

de Mussy (Henry-Guéneau).
See **Murchison** (Charles). La fièvre typhoïde. 8°. *Paris*, 1878.

Mustard.

See Sinapis; Sinapisms.

Mustela.

BISCHOFF [T. L. W.] Ueber die Ei- und Placenta-Bildung des Stein- und Edel-Marders, Mustela foina und martes, und des Wiesels, Mustela vulgaris. 8°. [*München*, 1865.]
Cutting from: Sitzungsb. d. k.-bayer. Akad. d. Wissensch. zu München, 1865, i, 339–348.

Parker (T. J.) On the blood-vessels of Mustelus antarcticus; a contribution to the morphology of the vascular system in the vertebrata. [Abstr.] Proc. Roy. Soc. Lond., 1886, xl, 472–474.

Mustinger (Joh. Casparus). *De articulationibus artuum. 2 p. l., 54 pp. sm. 4. *Argentorati, lit. D. Maagii*, 1712.

Muston (Étienne). *Du goître. 36 pp. 4°. *Paris*, 1845, No. 156, v. 435.

Mustoph (Antonius Fridericus). *De usu aquarum medico. 21 pp., 1 l. 8°. *Gottingæ, H. M. Grape*, [1793].

Musurus (Marcus).
See **Podagra** (De) libellus incerti autoris. fol. [*Francofurti*], 1567.

Musy (Jules-Joseph). *L'acide salicylique et le salicylate de soude. 52 pp., 1 pl. 4°. *Paris*, 1877, No. 113.

Mutamba.

Jaguaribe filho. A mutamba. Progresso med., Rio de Jan., 1876–7, i, 660–667. — **Jaguaribe** filho (D.) A mutamba; noticia sobre uma planta Brazileira. Rev. med., Rio de Jan., 1874–6, ii, 10–12.

Mutchnik (I.) *K voprosu o patologo-anatomicheskich izmenenijach pri uremii. 81 pp., 1 l. 8°. *St. Petersburg, tipo-litog. A. E. Landau*, 1884.

Muteau (Ch.) Du secret professionnel, de son étendue et de la responsabilité qu'il entraine d'après la loi et la jurisprudence. Traité théorique et pratique à l'usage des avocats, avoués, notaires, ministres du culte, médecins, chirurgiens, sages-femmes et de toutes autres personnes dépositaires, par état ou profession des secrets qu'on leur confie. xvi, 565 pp. 8°. *Paris, Maresq aîné*, 1870.

Mutel (Philippe). Des poisons considérés sous le rapport de la médecine pratique et de la médecine légale. xiv, 560 pp. 8°. *Paris, Ferra*, 1830.

——. The same. Dei veleni considerati sotto il rapporto della medicina pratica e della medicina

Mutel (Philippe)—continued.
legale. 3 p. l., 557 pp. 8°. *Milano, P. A. Molina*, 1831.
Imperfect.

——. La guillotine, ou réflexions physiologiques sur ce genre de supplice. 32 pp. 8°. *Paris, Paulin*, 1834.

——. Elementos de higiene militar. Obra escrita en francés por M. . . . y traducida al castellano por Antonio Navarro Zamorano. 2 v. in 1. 6 p. l., 230, 240 pp. 8°. *Madrid, L. Gonzalez & Comp.*, 1846.

Muter (John). The alkaline permanganates and their medicinal uses. 48 pp. 12°. *London, J. Churchill*, 1866.

——. An introduction to pharmaceutical and medical chemistry (theoretical and practical). Arranged on the principle of the course of lectures on chemistry as delivered at the South London School of Pharmacy. xiii, 785 pp., 1 tab. roy. 8°. *London, Simpkin & Marshall*, 1874.

——. A key to organic materia medica, written for the students of the South London School of Pharmacy. 2. ed. lxxxix, 480 pp., 18 l. 8°. *London, Simpkin, & Marshall*, 1878.

——. A manual of analytical chemistry, qualitative and quantitative, inorganic and organic. Arranged on the principle of the course of instruction given at the South London Central Public Laboratory and the South London School of Pharmacy. 3. ed. xii, 200 pp. roy. 8°. *Philadelphia, P. Blakiston, Son & Co.*, 1887.
Also, Co-Editor of: **Analyst** (The), London, 1877.

Muter (Robert). Practical observations on various novel modes of operating on cataract and of forming an artificial pupil. ix, 115 pp., 1 l., 2 pl. 8°. *London, T. Underwood*, 1811.

——. Practical observations on the lateral operation of lithotomy; and on various improved and new modes of performing this operation; together with remarks on the recto-vesical operation. viii, 9–107 pp. 8°. *New York, E. Bliss & E. White*, 1824.

Muter (Robertus). * De hepatitide chronica. 1 p. l., 28 pp. 8°. *Edinburgi, R. Allan*, 1813. [P., v. 864.]

Mutes.

See **Aphonia**; **Deaf-mutes**; **Dumbness**; **Speech**; **Speech** (*Disordered, etc.*)

Muth (Adolf). * Ueber die Resorptionsfähigheit des Uterus im Wochenbett. 32 pp. 8°. *Giessen, W. Keller*, 1882.

Muthwill (Joh. Andreas). * De nutritione. 46 pp. 4°. *Jenæ, lit. Ritterianis*, [1750].
For Biography, see **Hamberger** (Geo. Erh.)

Mutilation.

See, also, **Circumcision**; **Eunuchs**; **Genitals** (*Operations upon, Ceremonial, etc.*); **Genitals** (*Wounds, etc., of*); **Infibulation**; **Insane** (*Injuries, etc., of*); **Skoptzy**; **Testicle** (*Excision of*).

BESNON. Constatation de la nature d'une parcelle microscopique d'acier dans l'os d'un remplaçant soupçonné d'amputation volontaire de l'index droit. 8°. [*Cherbourg*, 1856.]
Cutting from: Mém. Soc. acad. de Cherbourg, 1856, 275-279.

FREYTAG (J. H.) Inest resectio pudendorum melancholici, propria manu sibi facta, ejusque curatio. 4°. *Lipsiæ*, 1779.
Also [Abstr.], *in:* WEIZ (F. A.) Neue Ausz. [etc.] 12°. *Frankf. u. Leipz.*, 1781, xiii, 94-96.

RUGGIERI (C.) Histoire du crucifiement exécuté sur sa propre personne par Mathieu Lovat. Communiqué au public dans une lettre à un médecin. 8°. [*Venice*, 1806.]

Mutilation.

——. The same. Storia della crocifissione di Mattio Lovat, da se stesso eseguita; communicata in lettera ad un medico, suo amico. 4°. *Venezia*, 1814.

Abraham (P. S.) Self-mutilation in a lioness. Tr. Acad. M. Ireland, Dubl., 1885, iii, 301-305. *Also:* Dublin J. M. Sc., 1885, lxxix, 193-197.—**Barthelson** (C. G.) Sjelfamputation under sinnesrubbning. Hygiea, Stockholm, 1866, xxviii, 43.—**Begriff** (Ueber den) der Verstümmelung. Bl. f. gerichtl. Anthrop., Nürnb., 1861, xii, 305-310.—**Begriff** (Ueber den) von Verstümmelung und Verunstaltung. *Ibid.*, 1860, xi, 4. Hft., 291-304.—**Bliss** (H. D.) Self-mutilation by amputation of the genitals. N. York M. J., 1885, xlii, 49.—**Casper** (J. L.) Was ist "Verstümmelung" im Sinne des §193. des Strafgesetzbuchs? Superarbitrium. Vrtljschr. f. gerichtl. u. öff. Med., Berl., 1857, xi, 193-202.—**Channing** (W.) Case of Helen Miller; self-mutilation; tracheotomy. Am. J. Insan., Utica, N. Y., 1877-8, xxxiv. *Also,* Reprint.—[**Chéreau** (A.)] Mutilations ethniques. Dict. encycl. d. sc. méd., Par., 1876, 2. s., xi, 155-167.—**von Fillenbaum.** Ueber einige Formen von Selbstverstümmlung by galizischen Wehrpflichtigen. Allg. Wien. med. Ztg., 1883, xxviii, 162 ; 174.—**Fredericq** (L.) Les mutilations spontanées, ou l'autotomie. Rev. scient., Par., 1886, xxxviii, 613-620.—**Frigerio** (L.) Le automutilazioni negli alienati. Gazz. d. osp., Milano, 1882, iii, 587-590.—**Galt** (J.) Suicidal amputation of the penis. Med. Herald, Louisville, 1884-5, vi, 225-228.—**Hospital.** Des eunuques volontaires. Ann. méd.-psych., Par., 1886, 7. s., iii, 379-393.—**Indemini** (E.) Ferita penetrante nelle vie aeree e contemporanea evirazione completa nel medesimo individuo; guarigione. Gazz. d. osp., Milano, 1885, vi, 395; 403.—**Krahmer** (L.) Die Verstümmelungen nach Par. 193 des Strafrechts. Vrtljschr. f. gerichtl. u. öff. Med., Berl., 1869, x, 87-128.—**Ludwich.** Ein seltener Fall von Selbstverstümmelung. Org. f. d. ges. Heilk., Aachen, 1856, v, 74-76.—**M.** Arrachement des deux yeux par une femme atteinte d'aliénation mentale. Courrier méd., Par., 1868, xviii, 37.—**Magitot** (E.) Essai sur les mutilations ethniques. Cong. internat. d'anthrop. Compt. rend. 1880, Lisbonne, 1884, ix, 549-614. *Also* [Abstr.]: Bull. Soc. d'anthrop. de Par., 1885, 3. s., viii, 21-25.—**Martinenq** (L.) Automutilations répétées chez une mélancholique. Ann. méd.-psych., Par., 1884, 6. s., xii, 425-436.—**Mulvany** (E.) Two cases of self-mutilation. Indian M. Gaz., Calcutta, 1881, xvi, 14.—**Rousseau.** Mutilation volontaire pendant un accès de folie alcoolique et par suite d'une conception délirante hypochondriaque. Ann. méd.-psych., Par., 1882, 6. s., vii, 409-414.—**Rust** (M. A.) Mutilations. Gaillard's M. J., N. Y., 1887, xliii, 538: xliv, 26.—**Santesson** (C.) Fall af sjelfkastration. Förh. Läk.-Sällsk. Sammank., Stockholm, 1883, 136-138.—**del Saz y Lopez** (T.) Herida del muslo y partes genitales ; mania y terror pánico ; castracion por el mismo paciente; majoria en su alienacion mental. Abeja méd., Barcel., 1852, 2. s., vi, 231-233.—**Sinclair** (E.) Case of persistent self-mutilation. Australas. M. Gaz., Sydney, 1885-6, v, 88. *Also:* J. Ment. Sc., Lond., 1886-7, xxxii, 44-46.—**Spencer** (H.) Evolution of ceremonial government. III. Mutilations. Pop. Sc. Month., N. Y., 1878, xii, 641-662.—**Tiling** (F.) Zwei Fälle von Selbstverstümmlung Geisteskranker. St. Petersb. med. Wchnschr., 1881, vi, 10.—**Warrington.** The case of Isaac Brooks. J. Ment. Sc., Lond., 1882-3, n. s., xxviii, 69-74.—**Whiting** (M.) Self-castration; a case. Peoria M. Month., 1884-5, v, 297-300.

Mutillet (Joh. Ephraim). * Diss. qua febris tertiana ob empyema e vomica pulmonis rupta in cavitatem pectoris dextram effusum, indeque pulmonem hujus lateris compressum, penitusque ab officio remotum mortem post se relinquens exponitur. 22 pp., 1 l., 1 pl. 4°. *Vitembergæ, prelo Schlomachiano*, 1731.
Also, in: HALLER. Disp. ad morb. [etc.] 4°. *Lausannæ*, 1747, ii, 403-419, 1 pl.

Mutin (Pierre). * Du pityriasis. 20 pp., 1 pl. 4°. *Strasbourg*, 1860, No. 542, 2. s., v. 30.

Mutina.

PLANCUS (J.) Dissertationes habitæ in academia medica conjecturantium, quæ Mutinæ est.
In: N. rac. d' opusc. scient. e filol. 16°. *Venezia*, 1759, v, pp. i-xix.

Mutinelli (Joannes Baptista). Della generazione dell' uomo, libri tre. 372 pp. 4°. *Verona*, 1769.

Mutiquite.

Roquete (A. P.) Aguas sulphureas thermaes de Mutiquite, districto de Sancul em Moçambique. J. Soc. d. sc. med. de Lisb., 1863, 2. s., xxvii, 70-79.

Mutis (*José* [*Bruno*] *Celestino*) [1732–1808].

de Gregorio (H.) Biografía. Anfiteatro anat., Madrid, 1876, iv, 310; 325.

Mutru (Egide). * Quelques mots sur les maladies de Cayenne. 27 pp. 4°. *Montpellier*, 1835, No. 32. [P., v. 1083.]

Muts (Jacobus). * De morbis gravidarum, et puerperarum. 1766.
In: LOUVAIN Diss. 8°. *Lovanii*, 1795, i, 86–100.

Mutschler (Conrad). Bezoarticum animale verum. Das ist: ein Secretum, oder geheimes Kunst-Stückl, durch welches sich der Mensch vor allem Gifft, gifftigen Kranckheiten, und von der Pest selbsten, etlich Jahr lang præservieren, auch von der allbereits habenden Pest oder Gifft, nächst Gott geschwind liberieren, und das Leben solcher Gestalt erjüngern kan, als wann er jung gebohren wäre. Erstlich durch ... in Druck geben zu Passau Anno 1645. Nach des Authoris Todt aber, nun wiederumben in Druck verfertiget, und mit nutzlichen Anmerckungen sambt einem Appendice, oder Anhang und Zugab underschiedlich - heylsamer Pest - Mitteln vermehrt, und an das Tag-Liecht gebrach durch Franciscum Albertum Hueber. 17 p. 1., 292 pp. 16°. *Freysing, J. C. C. Immel*, 1712.

Mutschler (Ludwig). * Ueber Cyclamin, Primulin u. Primulacamphor. Ein Beitrag zur Kenntniss der Bestandtheile der Primulaceen. 32 pp. 8°. *Erlangen, E. T. Jacob*, 1876.

Mutton.
See **Meats.**

Muttra.
Kastagiri (U. C.) Short notices of Muttra and Brindaban, especially with reference to their topography, people, and prevalent diseases. Calcutta J. M., 1870, iii, 81; 215. — **MacRae** (J.) Topography of Muttra. India J. M. & Phys. Sc., Calcutta, 1837, n. s., ii, 590–597.

Muttray (Joannes Augustus) [1808–   ]. * De cruribus fractis gypso liquefacto curandis. 29 pp., 1 pl. 8°. *Berolini, typ. A. Petschii*, [1831]. [*Also, in*: P., v. 192.]

Muttray (Richard) [1856–   ]. * Totalextirpation des Uterus. 31 pp. 8°. *Berlin, H. S. Hermann*, [1880].

Mutual *aid associations.*
See **Life-insurance.**

Mutual Benefit Life Insurance Company, Newark, N. J. Rules to be observed by medical examiners, in the selection of applicants for insurance, on and after June 1, 1868. 25 pp. 12°. *Newark*, 1868.

———. Mortuary report of the medical board, for the year 1868. 12 pp., 2 tab. 8°. *Newark, Jennings Bros.*, 1869.

———. Mortuary experience of the ... 1845–1879. By Bloomfield J. Miller, actuary. 16 pp., 15 l., 2 diag. 4°. [*Newark*, 1880?]

———. Annual statement, with report of the president to the board of directors. 41., 1885. 52 pp. 16°. *Louisville*, 1886.

Mutual Life Insurance Company of New York. Report of the board of examiners appointed April 15, 1865. 64 pp. 8°. *New York, H. Austice & Co.*, 1856.

———. Report exhibiting the experience, for fifteen years ending Feb. 1, 1858. [By Sheppard Homans, actuary.] vi, 7–34 pp., 5 diag. 4°. *New York*, 1859.

———. Instructions to the medical examiners. 21 pp. 12°. *New York, J. A. Gray & Green*, 1866.

———. The agent's manual of life insurance. 153 pp. 16°. [*New York, Wynkoop & Hallenbeck*, 1867?]

———. Preliminary report of the mortality experience of the ... From 1843 to 1874. By G. S.

Mutual Life Insurance Company [etc.]—cont'd. Winston and E. J. Marsh, of the medical department. 46 pp., 3 diag. 4°. *New York, printed by order of the board of trustees*, 1875.

———. Report of the mortuary experience of the ... From 1843–1874. By Wm. H. C. Bartlett, actuary. 3 p. l., 26 pp., 28 tables, 10 diag. 4°. *New York, printed by order of the board of trustees*, 1875.
Bound with preceding.

———. Mortuary experience, with tabulated reports and an analysis of the causes of death. By G. S. Winston, W. K. Gillette, E. J. Marsh. v. 2. 224 pp., 2 l. 8°. *New York, printed by order of the board of trustees*, 1877.

———. Weekly statements issued by the ... v. 1. No. 10; v. 4, Nos. 14, 23–25; v. 5, Nos. 2, 21, 24. 4°. *New York*, 1885–8.

Mutzenbecher (F. M.) * De hæmorrhagicis. 42 pp. 8°. *Heidelbergæ, C. Groos*, 1841.

Mutzenbecher (L. S. D.) Vorläufige Nachricht von den jezt herrschenden Krankheiten dieser Stadt; über Zeichen, Charakter, Behandlung und Verhütung derselben. 32 pp. 8°. *Altona, J. F. Hammerich*, 1814.

Mutzer (Franciscus). * De nitro. 28 pp., 1 l. 8°. *Vindobonæ, typ. J. Thom. nob. de Trattnern*, [1776].
Also, in: DE WASSERBERG. Op. min. med. et diss. 8°. *Vindob.*, 1776, iv, 433–454.

Mutzig.
See **Cholera** (*Asiatic, History, etc., of, by localities.*

Muybridge (Eadweard). Animal locomotion. An electro-photographic investigation of consecutive phases of animal movements. Published under the auspices of the University of Pennsylvania. Prospectus and catalogue of plates. 18, xxxii pp., 1 tab. 12°. *Philadelphia, J. B. Lippincott & Co.*, 1887.

———. Animal locomotion. An electro-photographic investigation of consecutive phases of animal movements. 1872–1885. Published under the auspices of the University of Pennsylvania. [A selection of 131 pl.] fol. *Philadelphia*, 1887.

van Muyen (Joannes). * De phthisi. 5 l. 4°. *Lugd. Bat., A. Elzevier*, 1685.

van Muyen (Theodorus). * De hydrope febri quartanæ superveniente. 18 pp., 1 l. 4°. *Harderovici, J. Moojen*, 1748.

de Muynck (Jacobus Joannes). * De cordis et ventriculi in producendam apoplexiam actione. 39 pp. 4°. *Gandavi, H. Vandekerckhove*, [1829]. [P., v. 959.]

de Muynk Brevet (Petrus Ludovicus). *See* **Brevet** (Petrus Ludovicus de Muynk).

Muys (Joannes). Praxis chirurgica rationalis seu observationes chirurgicæ secundum solida philosophiæ fundamenta resolutæ. Decas prima et secunda. 2 v. 10 l., 84 pp.; 1 l., 44 pp. 12°. *Lugd. Bat., P. vander Aa*, 1683.
Bound with: STENOSIUS (N.) Observ. anat. 12°. *Lugd. Bat.*, 1680.

———. The same. Quinque decades. 8 p. l., 318 pp. 16°. *Lugd. Bat., P. vander Aa*, 1685.

———. The same. Decas sexta et septima. 7 p. l., 78 pp. 16°. *Lugd. Bat., P. vander Aa*, 1690.

———. The same. Decades duodecim. 419 pp., 8 l., 1 pl. 12°. *Amstelædami, J. Wolters*, 1695.

Muys (Joh. Henr. Gulielmus).
See **Muys** (Wyerus Wilhelmus). Opuscula posthuma [etc.]. 4°. *Leovardiæ*, 1749.

Muys (Wyerus Wilhelmus) [1682–1744]. * De catalepsia. 17 pp., 1 l. 4°. *Traj. ad Rhenum, G. Van de Water*, 1701.

———. Investigatio fabricæ, quæ in partibus musculos componentibus extat. Dissertatio prima

Muys (Wyerus Wilhelmus)—continued.
de carnis musculosæ fibrarumque carnearum structura, quatenus sine vasis sanguiferis, nervis, nervosisque villis, atque membranis spectantur. 75 p. l., 431 pp., 3 pl. 4°. *Lugd. Bat., J. A. Langera*, 1738.

——. The same. Musculorum artificiosa fabrica, observationibus copiosissimis et experimentis physicis demonstrata atque iconibus manu autoris delineatis illustrata. 75 p. l., 431 pp., 3 pl. 4°. *Lugd. Bat., P. Bonk et C. de Becker*, 1751.
This is identical with the preceding, with the exception of the title-page. Some authorities mention an edition of 1741, but of the two copies of what purport to be that edition in this library, each has the figures "41" neatly printed and pasted over the figures "38".

——. Oratio inaug. de theoriæ medicæ usu atque recta illam excolendi ratione. 71 pp. fol. *Franequeræ, F. Halma*, 1714.

——. Dissertatio et observationes de salis am moniaci præclaro ad febres intermittentes usu, una cum epistola præfixa ad regiam Societatem Londinensem missæ. 100 pp., 2 l., 1 tab. 4°. *Franequeræ, F. Halma*, 1716.
Another copy bound with: VALENTINUS (Michael. Bernhardus). Praxeos medicinæ [etc.] 4°. *Francof. a. M.*, 1715.

——. Opuscula posthuma, seu sermones academici de selectis materiis, et dissertatio de distinctione mentis et corporis; cum Hermanni Venema oratione funebri in ejus memoriam; edente Joh. Henr. Gulielmo Muys, W. G. filio. 2 p. l., 72, 269 pp. 4°. *Leovardiæ, G. Coulon; Franequeræ, J. Brouwer*, 1749.

Muys van de Moer (Joannes Henricus Gulielmus). *De scabie. 2 p. l., 44 pp., 2 l. 4°. *Lugd. Bat., Haak et soc.*, 1812.

Muysken (Isaäcus Florus). *Quæstiones medicæ inaugurales. viii, 39 pp. 8°. *Traj. ad Rhenum, C. vander Post jun.*, 1833.

Muzeau (Charles-Albert). *De l'ostéotomie verticale bilatérale du nez pour la cure des polypes naso-pharyngiens. 36 pp., 1 l. 4°. *Montpellier, Boehm et fils*, 1866, No. 8. C.

Muzelius (Fridricus Guilielmus Daniel.) Examen usus chemiæ in medicamentorum scientia. 2 p. l., 30 pp. 4°. *Halæ ad Salam, stanno Hendeliano*, [1772].

Muzell (Friderich Hermann Ludewig) [1716–84]. Medicinische und chirurgische Wahrnehmungen. 1.–2. Samml. 9 p. l., 138 pp., 1 l.; 3 p. l., 149 pp., 1 pl. 16°. *Berlin, A. Haude u. J. C. Spener*, 1754–64.

——. The same. Medical and chirurgical observations. Transl. from the German original. xvi, 131 pp. 8°. *London, A. Linde*, 1755. [Also, in: P., v. 563.]

——. The same. 1. Samml. 3. Aufl. xii, 138 pp., 1 l. 2. Samml. 2. Aufl. 3 p. l., 149 pp., 1 pl. 8°. *Berlin, Haude u. Spener*, 1772–6.
For Portrait, see **Collection**—van Kaathoven.—**Collection** of Portr. of Phys. & Men of Sc., 1–121.

Muzio (Pietro). Lezioni teorico-pratiche di igiene ed umanità. 178 pp. 8°. *Mantova, Seffer, Gozzi & Comp.*, 1871.

——. La salute. Precetti igienici e morali spiegati al popolo. v, 246 pp. 12°. *Milano*, 1875.

——. L' igiene delle professioni, ossia il miglior tesoro per gli operai. 63 pp. 12°. *Mantova, Mondovi*, 1877.

——. Gli ospitali. Almanacco igienico umanitario dell' infermiere. Anno primo, 1878. 132 pp. 18°. *Mantova, Mondovi*, 1878.

Muzzarelli (Alberto).
See **Isfordink** (Joh. Nep.) Polizia medica militare [etc.] 2 v. in 1. 8°. *Venezia*, 1829–30.

Muzzey (Henry W.) Petition of the mayor of Cambridge for leave to fill up the basins of Mil-

Muzzey (Henry W.)—continued.
ler's River and construct a sewer therein. Closing argument for remonstrants. 31 pp. 8°. *Boston, Rand, Avery & Co.*, 1872.

——. John M. Tyler et al., petitioners, vs. John P. Squire et al., respondents. Closing argument in behalf of the respondents before the State board of health, Dec. 29, 1873. 34 pp. 8°. *Cambridge, University Press*, 1874.
See, also, **Massachusetts**. Arguments . . . before the commission on Miller's River. 8°. *Boston*, 1872.

Muzzey (L. M.) The sewerage of the city of Keene, N. H. 7 pp., 1 pl. 8°. *Boston, J. R. Osgood & Co.*, [1883].
Repr. from: Am. Architect.

Muzzi (Luigi). Iscrizioni e sonetto in lode di Girolamo Segato, petrificatore degli animali. 3 l. 12°. *Terni, C. Possena*, 1835. [P., v. 905.]

——. Considerazioni sopra una lettera del Signor Professor Giovanni Rossi Toscano concernente a Girolamo Segato. 20 pp. 8°. *Modena, E. Soliani*, 1836.

My physician, mind. Metaphysics in a nutshell. A concise treatise on mental and spiritual dynamics. Their application as a therapeutic agent in the cure of all diseases, whether in acute or chronic form. In scope it covers the entire domain of man's relations to God, the neighbor, and to the universe of things. 66 pp. 8°. *Topeka, G. W. Crane*, 1886.

Myalgia.

See, also, **Lumbago**; **Pleurodynia**; **Rheumatism** (Muscular); **Spine** (Pain, etc., in).

HAVÁ (J.-G.) *De quelques douleurs musculaires, ou myosalgies, et de leur traitement, principalement à l'aide des courants électriques par induction. 4°. *Paris*, 1859.

INMAN (T.) On certain painful muscular affections simulating inflammatory, neuralgic, or organic disease. 8°. *Liverpool*, 1856.

——. On myalgia; its nature, causes, and treatment; being a treatise on painful and other affections of the muscular system, which have been frequently mistaken for hysterical, inflammatory, hepatic, uterine, nervous, spinal, or other diseases. 2. ed. 8°. *London*, 1860.
Finch (J. E.) Report on myalgia. Tr. Minnesota M. Soc., St. Paul, 1877, 31–50.—**Inman** (T.) Remarks on myalgia, or muscular pain. Brit. M. J., Lond., 1858, 407; 866. ——. Letter on myalgic pain. Ibid., 993. ——. Myalgia and myositis. Ibid., 1860, i, 28–30. ——. The physical condition of the muscles during myalgia. Ibid., 87. ——. Myositis and myalgia, dysphagia and phlegmasia dolens. Ibid., 145.—**Jackson** (J. D.) A case of myalgia. Cincin. Lancet & Obs., 1870, xiii, 257–261.—**Janeway** (E. G.) Remarks on "pain in the side". Hosp. Gaz., N. Y., 1879, vi, 485–487.—**Mattison** (J. B.) Myalgia and its treatment. Med. & Surg. Reporter, Phila., 1872, xxvii, 309–311.—**Parmentier**. Douleurs musculaires violentes, résultant du surmènage; insuffisance et inconvénients des injections de morphine; excellents effets de la faradisation. Rev. de thérap. méd.-chir., Par., 1879, xlvi, 177–179.—**Piorry**. Observation de douleur musculaire très-ancienne, guérie rapidement par le massage. Gaz. d. hôp., Par., 1860, xxxiii, 193.—**Pizzamiglio** (A.) Reumatalgia muscolare, seguita da idrope del peritoneo e del pericardio. Gazz. med. ital. Lomb., Milano, 1861, 4. s., vi, 297.—**Rosenthal** (M.) Ueber rheumatische Myalgie. Oesterr. Ztschr. f. prakt. Heilk., Wien, 1864, x, 931; 954; 967.—**Sieffermann**. Deux cas de cinésialgie consécutive au diastasis musculaire, guéris par les courants continus. Gaz. méd. de Strasb., 1875, xxxiv, 6.—**Smith** (A. H.) Static electricity in myalgia. Arch. Med., N. Y., 1884, xi, 163–167.—**Wilson** (J. C.) Two cases of myalgia following contusions. Phila. M. Times, 1876-7, vii, 199–201. ——. Myalgia. Med. & Surg. Reporter, Phila., 1877, xxxvi, 95–99. Also: Phila M. Times, 1885-6, xvi, 119–123. ——. Myalgia. Syst. Pract. M. (Pepper), Phila., 1886, iv, 529–539.

Myatowitsch (Georg). *Ueber das osteomalacische Becken. Ein klinischer Beitrag. iv, 80 pp., 1 l. 8°. *Zürich, Orell u. Comp.*, 1875.

Mycetoma.

See **Foot** (Fungus disease of).

Mycology.

See Fungi.

Mycosis.

See Actinomycosis; Frambœsia; Fungi (*Parasitic*); Genitals (*Female, Parasites in*); Heart (*Inflammation of, Infectious, etc.*); Kidney (*Parasites in*); Molluscum; Parasites, *etc.*; Scherlievo; Sibbens; Stomach (*Fungi in*).

Mycosis *endocardii.*

See Heart (*Inflammation of, Infectious, etc.*)

Mycosis (*Fungoid*).

See Skin (*Lymphadenoma of*).

Mycosis (*Intestinal*).

See Intestines (*Fungi in*).

Mydorge (Claude) [1585–1647]. Examen du livre des récréations mathématiques et de ses problèmes en géométrie, méchanique, optique, et catoptrique, où sont aussi discutées et restablies plusieurs expériences physiques y proposées. 7 p. l., 280 pp., 5 l. 12°. *Paris, R. Boutonné,* 1638.

Mydriasis *and mydriatics.*

See, also, Atropine (*Physiological, etc., effects of*); Duboisia; Eye (*Accommodation, etc., of, Disordered*); Glaucoma (*Causes of*); Homatropine; Hyoscine; Iritis (*Treatment of*); Mydriasis, *etc.*; Scopoleine; Spine (*Diseases of, Complications, etc., of*).

BÖTTIGER (S.) * De visionis læsionibus, in specie in mydriasi et myosi. sm. 4°. *Vitembergæ,* [1706].

BROCKMANN (C. H.) * De mydriaticis. 4°. *Gottingæ,* [1829].

DONDERS (F. C.) De werking der mydriatica en der myotica. 8°. [*n. p., n. d.*]

FITZ-GERALD (D.-S.) *Recherches expérimentales sur le mode d'action physiologique des principales substances médicamenteuses qui agissent. 4°. *Paris,* 1880.

Also, in: Tribune méd.. Par., 1880, xii, 555; 579; 604; 1881, xiii, 27; 136. *Also, in:* Rev. clin. d'ocul., Bordeaux, 1880–81, i, 85; 118; 133; 232.

HONOLD (C) *Ueber die Erweiterung der Pupille durch Narcotica. 8°. [*Tübingen*], 1837.

KUNHARDT (O.) *Ueber Mydriasis. 8°. *Erlangen,* 1832.

L'ÉTENDART (A.) * De la mydriase. 4°. *Paris,* 1868.

MAUCHART (B. D.) *Mydriasin pupillæ p. n. dilatationem enucleabit. Resp. Phil. Jac. Neuffer. 4°. *Tubingæ,* 1745.

Also, in: HALLER. Disp. chir. [etc.] 4°. *Lausannæ,* 1755, i, 453–473. *Also, in:* DISS. med. select. 12°. *Tubingæ,* 1783, ii, 18–72.

PERCEPIED (E.) * De la mydriase. 4°. *Paris,* 1876.

PETRINUS (E. F.) *Nonnulla de mydriaticis atque mydriasi. 8°. *Lipsiæ,* 1857.

REINHARD (W.) *Vorderkammerdruck und Substanzverluste der Cornea unter Atropin und Eserin. 8°. *Basel,* 1882.

Agnew (C. R.) Two cases of mydriasis with paralysis of accommodation treated by electricity. Phila. M. Times, 1874–5, v, 53.—**Arlt.** Mydriasis spastica oculi sinistri. Allg. Wien. med. Ztg., 1861, vi, 143.—**Bell** (J.) On the physiology and pathology of certain forms of dilated pupil. Edinb. M. J., 1864–5, x, 917–923.—**Bengel.** Ein Fall von Mydriasis. Med. Cor.-Bl. d. württemb. ärztl. Ver., Stuttg., 1851, xxi, 117–120.—**Bérard** (A.) Quelques remarques sur la mydriase, suivies d'une observation de mydriase bornée à l'œil droit. Ann. d'ocul., Brux., 1845, xiv, 149–155.—**Bernstein** (J.) & **Dogiel** (J.) Ueber Versuche über die Wirkung einiger Gifte auf die Iris. Verhandl. d. naturh.-med. Ver. zu Heidelb. (1865-6), 1868, iv, 28–31.—**Bowman.** Cases of mydriasis. Med. Times & Gaz., Lond., 1853, n. s., vii, 91.—**Braun** (H.) Zur Lehre von den Mydriaticis. Arch. f. Ophth., Berl., 1859, v, 2. Abth., 112–126.—**Brière.** Mydriase datant de 14 mois, guérie complètement après 10 jours de traitement. Ann. d'ocul., Brux., 1875, lxxiv, 84–90.—**Bruns** (H. D.) Poisoning by atropia and duboisia sulphates instilled into the eye. N. Orl. M. & S. J., 1885–6, n. s., xiii, 604–608.—**Can-**

Mydriasis *and mydriatics.*

statt (K.) Beiträge zur Pathologie der Mydriasis und anderer Neurosen des Nervus trigeminus und des Nervus oculomotorius. Monatschr. f. Med., Augenh. u. Chir., Leipz., 1839, ii, 97–144.—**de Castro** (A. B.) Mydriase; emprego da fava do Calabar. Escholiaste med., Lisb., 1866, xvii, 295.—**Chevallereau** (A.) Mydriatiques et myotiques. France méd., Par., 1877, xxiv, 817.—**Coc.** Case of syphilitic affection of the third nerve, producing mydriasis with ptosis, followed by facial paralysis and hemiplegia of the same side. Lancet, Lond., 1870, i, 584.—**Consultation** no. 60 pour une mydriase unilatérale. J. d'ocul. et de chir., Par., 1880, viii, 197–199.—**Dehenne** (A.) Sur l'emploi de l'ésérine en ophthalmologie. Médecin, Par., 1879, v, no. 15.—**Delgado.** Midriasis idiopática tratada por el haba del Calabar; curacion. España méd., Madrid, 1864, ix, 4.—**Dickinson** (W.) Mydriasis. St. Louis M. & S. J., 1878, xxxiv, 452–454. ———. Mydriasis. Illinois M. Recorder, Vandalia, 1878–9, i, 189–192. ———. Mydriatics and myotics, and some of the indications for their use. Tr. M. Ass. Missouri, St. Louis, 1879, xxii, 106–115. ———. Mydriasis. St. Louis M. & S. J., 1885, xlix, 18–26.—**Dogel** (I.) Daiistvie maikotorekh laikarstvennikh sredstv na dvizhenie raduzhnoi oboloch ki. [Effect of certain medicaments on the movements of the iris.] Med. Vestnik, St. Petersb., 1866, vi, 481–484.—**Donders** (F. C.) Over de vereischte hoeveelheid sulphas atropini tot dilatatie der pupil. Nederl. Lancet, Gravenh., 1853–4, 3. s., iii, 533–536. ———. De werking der mydriatica en der myotica. Versl. . . . Nederl. Gasth. v. Ooglijders, Utrecht, 1864, v, 187 - 230. *Also:* Nederl. Arch. v. Genees- en Natuurk., Utrecht, 1864–5, i, 83 – 126. *Also, transl.:* Ann. d'ocul., Brux., 1865, liii, 5–50. *Also,* Reprint.—**Dor.** Ueber Behandlung der Midriasis. Cor.-Bl. f. schweiz. Aerzte, Basel, 1875, v, 99–102.—**Doyer.** Sur les agents myotiques et mydriatiques. Cong. périod. internat. d. sc. méd. Compt.-rend., Amst., 1881, vi, pt. 2, 251–253.—**Dupont.** Quelques mots sur la mydriase et sur la fève de Calabar à propos d'une forte contusion de l'œil gauche. Arch. méd. belges, Brux., 1866, 2. s., iii, 309; 325.—**Fano.** Pathologie et thérapeutique de la mydriase idiopathique. Abeille méd., Par., 1862, xix, 198–200. ———. De la paracenthèse de la chambre antérieure dans les cas de mydriase rebelle aux autres médications. J. d'ocul. et chir., Par., 1877–8, iii, 69.—**Fauqué.** De la duboisine, de ses applications dans la thérapeutique oculaire. Rec. d'ophth. Par., 1879, 3. s., i, 234; 280. — **Ferriere** (F.) Mydriatics among the ancients ; a commentary on Prof. J. Reynauld's commentary on Galen and the grayish-eyed ladies of Rome. St. Louis Clin. Rec., 1881-2, viii, 265–267.—**Fieber** (F.) Zur Elektrotherapie der Mydriasis paralytica intoxicativa. Wien. med. Wchnschr., 1864, xiv, 340–343.—**de Fleury** (A.) De la mydriase provoquée et de la mydriase pathologique. Gaz. méd. de Bordeaux, 1874, iii, 393–401.—**Fournet** (F.) Mydriase du côté droit dans un cas d'hypertrophie des ganglions cervicaux du côté correspondant; méningite spinale limitée à la région dorsale. Rec. d'ophth., Par., 1879, 3. s., i, 304 – 307. — **Giraud - Teulon.** Mydriase. Dict. encycl. d. sc. méd., Par., 1876, 2. s., xi, 205–213.—**Gnauck** (R.) Ueber die Wirkungen des Hyoscin. Centralbl. f. d. med. Wissensch., Berl., 1881, xix, 801–806. *Also, transl.* [Abstr.]: Thérap. contemp., Par., 1882, ii, 65–68. *Also:* Rec. d'ophth., Par., 1882, 3. s., iv, 123–127. *Also, transl.* [Abstr.]: Cincin. Lancet & Clinic, 1882, n. s., ix, 295–298. — **Gosselin** (L.) Note sur la mydriase binoculaire spontanée. Bull. Acad. de méd., Par., 1859–60, xxv, 1094–1101.—**von Graefe** (A.) Notiz über die Behandlung der Mydriasis. Arch. f. Ophth., Berl., 1854–5, i, 1. Abth., 315–319. ———. Fall von ephemerer und stets aufs neue auftauchender Mydriasis. *Ibid.*, 1857, iii, 2. Abth., 359–362.—**Green** (J.) Castor-oil as a menstruum for dissolving atrophia for application to the eye. Tr. Am. Ophth. Soc. 1875, N. Y., 1876, ii, pt. 3, 355. — **Harley** (G.) On the physiological action of atropine in dilating the pupil. Edinb. M. J., 1856-7, ii, 431–434. *Also,* Reprint.—**Hart** (E.) Cases of mydriasis treated by the solution of old Calabar bean, a new ophthalmic agent. Lancet, Lond., 1863, i, 604. ———. Substitution of atropized and calabarized gelatine for paper for the purpose of dilating or contracting the iris. *Ibid.*, 1864, i, 65.—**Hirschler** (I.) Zur Kasuistik der Mydriasis spastica. Wien. med. Wchnschr., 1873, xxiii, 387–393. — **Hirschmann** (L.) Zur Lehre von der durch Arzneimittel hervorgerufenen Myosis und Mydriasis. Arch. f. Anat., Physiol. u. wissensch. Med., Leipz., 1863, 309 – 318. — **Jackson** (E.) A comparative study of the action of certain mydriatic alkaloids. Tr. M. Soc. Penn., Phila., 1882, xiv, 157–162. ———. Some practical points in the use of mydriatics. Phila. M. Times, 1882–3, xiii, 894–896. ———. Alarming and dangerous doses of the mydriatics. Tr. M. Soc. Penn., Phila., 1884, xvi, 332–339. ———. Homatropin hydrobromate. Med. News, Phila.,1886, xlix, 88–95.—**Jeaffreson.** Case of mydriasis, with paralysis of the accommodation. Med. Times & Gaz., Lond. 1873, ii, 89.—**Jessop** (W. H.) On the mydriasis produced by the local application of cocaine to the eye. Proc. Roy. Soc. Lond., 1884–5, xxxviii, 432–441. — **Keyser** (P. D.) Mydriasis and paralysis of accommodation permanently cured by use of Calabar bean. Med. & Surg. Reporter,

Mydriasis *and mydriatics.*

Phila., 1865, xiii, 231.—**Kobert** (R.) On the discovery of the mydriatic action of the solanaceæ. Therap. Gaz., Detroit, 1886, 3. s., ii, 445-448. *Also, transl.:* Presse méd. belge, Brux., 1886, xxxviii, 393-396. — **Ladenburg** (A.) Sur les tropéines, alcaloïdes mydriatiques artificiels. Compt. rend. Acad. d. sc., Par., 1880, xc, 921-924. ——. Sur les alcaloïdes à action mydriatique. [Transl. from the German by de Bechi.] Monit. scient., Par., 1882, 3. s., xii, 33-41.—**Lang** (W.) & **Barrett** (J. W.) The action of myotics on the accommodation. Ophth. Hosp Rep., Lond., 1886-7, xi, 136-187, 2 diag. ——. The action of myotics and mydriatics on the accommodation. *Ibid.,* 219-259, 1 diag.—**Laqueur.** Ueber Atropin und Physostigmin und ihre Wirkung auf den intraoculären Druck. Arch. f. Ophth., Berl., 1877, xxiii, 149-176. — **Lehmann** (H.) Mydriasis. Hosp.-Tid., Kjøbenh., 1858, i, 193.—**Lenton** (S.) Idiopathic mydriasis, treated with eserine; good recovery. Brit. M. J., Lond., 1878, ii, 54.—**Lenz.** Beobachtung einer widernatürlich erweiterten Pupille ohne Nachtheil für das Gesicht. Heidelb. klin. Ann., 1828, iv, 302-304.—**McEvers** (J. F.) On the use of ergot of rye in mydriasis. Dublin Q. J. M. Sc., 1848, vi, 484.—**Mackenzie** (F. M.) Traumatic mydriasis. Indian M. Gaz., Calcutta, 1870, v, 108. —**Malvani.** Observation de mydriasis guéri par la cautérisation de la cornée transparente. J. compl. du dict. d. sc. méd., Par., 1832, xlii, 317. — **Mayer** (I.) Az önszenvi látatágulat viszonya az együttérz-éz háromosztatú ideg bántalmaihoz. [Idiopathic mydriasis.] Magy. orv. és term-vizsg., Egerben, 1869, xiii, 173.—**Menjot** (A.) De mydriasi. *In his:* Februm malig. hist., etc . 4°, Par., 1622, 152-171.—**de Méric** (V.) Cases of syphilitic affection of the third nerve producing mydriasis, with and without ptosis. Brit. M. J., Lond., 1870, i, 29; 52. — **Miller** (M. N.) A case of mydriasis, or permanent dilatation of the pupil. Med. Rec., N. Y., 1872, vii, 387.— **del Monte** (M.) Midriasi e miosi. Movimento, Napoli, 1882, 2. s., iv, 429-436.—**Murrell** (T. E.) An unusual case of mydriasis. Nashville J. M. & S., 1878, n. s., xxii, 10-12.—**Nettleship** (E.) Clinical remarks on a case of mydriasis with iritis, and on cases of mydriasis following a blow on the eye. Med. Times & Gaz., Lond., 1885, ii, 865. ——. Mydriasis without cycloplegia, affecting one eye of a man in an early stage of locomotor ataxy. Ophth. Hosp. Rep., Lond., 1886-7, xi, 260. ——. Wide mydriasis of both eyes, for 15 years, with only slight cycloplegia; locomotor ataxy. *Ibid.,* 261. ——. Mydriasis without cycloplegia, affecting one eye and coming on several years after a severe abdominal illness following injury; knee reflexes absent. *Ibid.,* 261-263. ——. Mydriasis without cycloplegia in one eye only, of unknown duration; suspicion of old vasomotor paralysis on same side of face. *Ibid.,* 263. ——. Wide mydriasis without cycloplegia following a severe blow on eye. *Ibid.,* 264.— **Neuhausen** (J.) Heilung der Mydriasis paralytica durch Anwendung der Euphorbia cyparissias. Med. Cor.-Bl. rhein. u. westfäl. Aerzte, Bonn, 1844, iii, 44-46. ——. Ueber Mydriasis artificialis. Org. f. d. ges. Heilk., Aachen, 1854, iii, 278-280.—**Nicholson** (E.) Traumatic mydriasis. Indian M. Gaz., Calcutta, 1871, vi, 15.—**Noël** (L.) De l'atropine en opthalmologie. J. d. sc. méd. de Louvain, 1876, i, 99-119. — **Oehler** (E.) Essentielles Bilsensamen-Extract und Atropin als Augenmittel. Ztschr. f. d. Ophth., Dresd., 1832, ii, 223-229.— **Oliver** (C. A.) The comparative action of daturia and of sulphate of hyoscyamia upon the iris and ciliary muscle. Am. J. M. Sc., Phila., 1882, lxxxiv, 102-108. *Also,* Reprint.—**Panas.** De la mydriase. Tribune méd., Par., 1880, xiii, 185-187. *Also:* Presse méd. de Par., 1880-81, i, 18-20.—**Pettorelli.** De la nitro-atropine et de la nitro-daturine; leurs effets sur l'organe de la vue. Cong. périod. internat. d'opth. Compt. rend. 1880, Milan, 1881, vi, 203-205. — **Pflüger.** 1. Wie Verhalten sich einige Glaukom - Symptome zur Drucktheorie? Ueber die Einwirkung der Mydriatica und Myotica auf den intraoculären Druck unter physiologischen Verhältnissen. Ber. ü. d. Versamml. d. ophth. Gesellsch., Stuttg., 1885, xvii, 91-101. — **Pirocchi** (P.) & **Porlezza** (P. L.) Midriasi da sifilide. Gior. ital. d. mal. ven., Milano, 1872, xiii, 129-132. — **Rampoldi** (R.) Una nuova causa di midriasi. Ann. di ottal., Pavia, 1882, xi, 513-516. ——. Sur une nouvelle cause de mydriase. Rec. d'opth., Par., 1887, 3. s., ix, 147-149. — **Regnauld** (J.) Une recette de Galien, à propos des mydriatiques. J. de pharm. et chim., Par., 1881, 5. s., iii, 534-537. [*See, also, supra,* Ferriere (F.)]—**Regnauld** (J.) & **Valmont.** Étude pharmacologique sur les alcaloïdes mydriatiques. Arch. gén. de méd., Par., 1881, cxlvii, 5-16.— **Ringer** (S.) On the relative action of duboisia and atropia. Practitioner, Lond., 1879, xxiii, 247-249.—**Risley** (S. D.) The comparative value of the mydriatics. Tr. Am. Ophth. Soc., N. Y., 1881, iii, 228-257.—**Romiée** (H.) Atropine; duboisine; gelsémine. Ann. Soc. méd.-chir. de Liége, 1879, xviii, 258-262.—**Roy** (T. P.) On the use of dhatura as a mydriatic. Indian M. Gaz., Calcutta, 1870, v, 187.—**de Ruiter** (G. C. P.) Onderzoekingen over de werking van atropa belladonna op de iris. Nederl. Lancet, Gravenh., 1853-4, 3. s., iii, 433-472. — **Saisset.** Observation sur l'espèce de lésion de la vue, occasionnée par le re-

Mydriasis *and mydriatics.*

trécissement de la pupille; et sur les bons effets de l'extrait de jusquiame blanche, contre cette affection particulière. Ann. Soc. de méd.-prat. de Montpel., 1807, x, 47-53.— **von Schroff.** Ueber Grandval's Extracte der heurigen Pariser Ausstellung, über Mydriatica im Allgemeinen und über das Verhältniss des Hyoscyamins zum Atropin insbesondere. Wchnbl. d. k. k. Gesellsch. d. Aerzte in Wien, 1868, viii, 1; 9; 17. 25.—**Seely** (W. W.) Permanent dilatation of the pupil by atropine and paralysis of ciliary muscle. Clinic, Cincin., 1878, xiv, 206. ——. On the use of duboisine. Arch. Ophth., N. Y., 1879, viii, 79-81.—**Ségalas-D'Etchepare.** De la manière d'agir de la belladone, appliquée sur l'œil. J. de physiol. expér., Par., 1827, vii, 122-126.—**Sichel.** Du mydriasis congénial. Gaz. hebd. de méd., Par., 1859, vi, 308-310. — **Snell** (S.) The effect of general anæsthesia on cucaine mydriasis. Brit. M. J., Lond., 1885, ii, 153.—**Stocker** (F.) Ueber den Einfluss der Mydriatica und Myotica auf den intraoculären Druck unter physiologischen Verhältnissen. Arch. f. Ophth., Berl., 1887, xxxiii, 1. Abth., 105-158. — **Streatfeild.** On the use of atropine paper. Ophth. Hosp. Rep., Lond., 1860-62, iii, 310-314. — **Talko** (J.) Amaurosis ex atrophia papillæ n. optici utriusque oculi post vulnus sclop. Dieistvie kalabara pui mydriasis amaurotica et simulata. Voyenno-med. J., St. Petersb., 1868, ci, pt. 2, 5-11. ——. Urażeniowe rozszerzenie zrenicy (mydriasis traum.) [etc.] Medycyna, Warszawa, 1875, iv, 845. — **Tavignot.** La mydriase artificielle, dans les cas d'opacité centrale de la cornée, peut-elle rétablir la vision? Union méd., Par., 1854, viii, 156.—**Tay** (W.) Unilateral dilatation of the pupil following injury of the head. Med. Times & Gaz., Lond., 1866, i. 8.—**Tonoli** (S.) Ancora sull' azione dello jaborandi nella miosi e midriasi pupillare. Gazz. med. ital. lomb., Milano, 1879, 8. s., i, 334.—**Trousseau** (A.) Note sur le santonate d'atropine. Bull. clin. nat. opht. de l'hosp. d. Quinze-Vingts, Par., 1886, iv, 130-132. — **Tweedy** (J.) On the mydriatic properties of hydro-bromate of hyoscine. Lancet, Lond., 1886, ii, 1065. — **von Wecker** (L.) Ueber den vergleichenden Gebrauch des Eserins, Atropins und Duboisins. Klin. Monatsbl. f. Augenh., Cassel, 1878, xvi, 216-230. ——. Valeur sémiologique de la mydriase et du myosis; traitement. Gaz. d. hôp., Par., 1879, lii, 141.— **Zehender** (W.) Beobachtungen bei artificieller Mydriasis. Arch. f. Ophth., Berl., 1855-6, ii, 2. Abth., 95-103.

van der Mye (Fredericus). De arthritide, et calculo gemino tractatus duo; in quibus universa horum morborum essentia, causæ, differentiæ, signa, et curatio, secundum Hippocratis et Galeni mentem dilucidissime explicantur. Una cum disputatione phylosophica, de lapidum generatione. Ejusdem historia medica. 77 l. 4°. *Hagæ-Comitum, A. Meuris,* 1624.

——. De morbis et symptomatibus popularibus Bredanis tempore obsidionis, et eorum immutationibus pro anni victusque diversitate, deque medicamentis in summa rerum inopia adhibitis, tractatus duo. Ejusdem dissertationes duæ medico-physicæ, de contagio, et cornu monocerotis quondam in aquis circa Bredam reperto. 3 p. l., 160 pp., 1 l. 4°. *Antverpiæ, ex off. Plantiniana,* 1627.

——. The same. Iterum edidit ob raritatem et argumenti gravitatem notulis auxit et præfatus est Christ. Gothf. Gruner. [2. ed.] 104 pp. 4°. *Jenæ,* 1792.

Myelin.

KOEHLER (A.) *De myelini quod vocant constitutione chemica disquisitio. 8°. *Halæ,* 1867.

Arthaud (G.) Note sur l'emploi du sulfate d'indigo comme réactif de la myéline. Compt. rend. Soc. de biol., Par., 1887, 8. s., iv, 252.—**Beneke** (F. W.) Zur Frage über die Entstehung der Myelinformen. Arch. d. Ver. f. wissensch. Heilk., Leipz., 1866, n. F., ii, 379-381.—**Chatin** (J.) De la myéline dans les fibres nerveuses des lamellibranches. Bull. Soc. philomat. de Par., 1881-2, 7. s., vi, 198-200. — **Hoffmann** (H.) Ueber Myelin. Arch. f. path. Anat., etc., Berl., 1863, xxvii, 575.—**Köhler** (H.) Ueber die chemische Zusammensetzung und Bedeutung des sogenannten Myelin's. *Ibid.,* 1867, xli, 265-278. [*See, also, supra.*]—**Liebreich** (O.) Ueber die Entstehung der Myelin-Formen. *Ibid.,* 1865, xxxii, 387-389.—**Mondino** (C.) De la structure des fibres périphériques à myéline. Arch. ital. de biol., Turin, 1884, v, 340-344.— **Neubauer** (C.) Ueber Myelinformen. Arch. f. path. Anat., etc., Berl., 1866, xxxvi, 303.

Myelitis.

See Bones (*Inflammation of*); Marrow (*Diseases of*); Spinal cord (*Inflammation of*).

Myeloid *disease.*
See **Fibula** (*Tumors of*).

Myeloma.
Zahn (F. W.) Ueber das multiple Myelom, seine Stellung im onkologischen System und seine Beziehung zur Anæmia lymphatica. Deutsche Ztschr. f. Chir., Leipz., 1885, xxii, 1–21.

Myeloplaxes.
See **Bone** (*Absorption of*).

Myers (Arthur B. R.) On the etiology and prevalence of diseases of the heart among soldiers. The "*Alexander*" prize essay. 2 p. l., 92 pp., 1 l. 8°. *London, J. Churchill & Sons,* 1870.

Myers (Josephus Hart) [–1823]. *De diabete. 1 p. l., 41 pp. 8°. *Edinburgi, Balfour et Smellie,* 1779.

Myers (*Miles G.*) [1831–80].
Dobson (N. M.) Obituary. Tr. M. Soc. Wisconsin, Milwaukee, 1881, xv, 158.

Myers (William H.) Puerperal pyæmia. 19 pp. 8°. *Chicago, Review Printing Co.,* 1884.
Repr. from: J. Am. M. Ass., Chicago, 1884, iii.

Myèvre (A.)
See **Pouchet** (G.) & **Myèvre** (A.) Contribution à l'anatomie des alcyonaires. 8°. *Paris,* 1870.

Myffant (Guillelmus). *Quæstio med. : An aër spiritu ductus sanguinem fermentet? 5 pp. 4°. *Cadomi, A. Cavelier,* 1711. [P., v. 1218.]

Mygge (Joh.) [1850–]. *Om Ægteskaber mellem Blodbeslægtede med specielt Hensyn til deres Betydning for Døvstumhedens Ætiologi. [Consanguineous marriages with special regard to their effect in producing deaf-mutes.] xiii, 289 pp., 2 tab. 8°. *Kjøbenhavn, V. Tryde,* 1879.

Mygind (Holger). Om Jodoformens Anvendelse til Sårbehandling. En klinisk Undersøgelse. 2 p. l., 192, vii pp. 8°. *Kjøbenhavn, Thaning & Appel,* 1883.

———. Sæby Jærnvand, et Bidrag til Bedømmelsen af dets Egenskaber og til Oplysning om nogle Betingelser for en dansk Jærnvandskuranstalts Anlæggelse her. [The iron waters of Sæby; contribution to define its qualities and to the explanation of some conditions for the establishment of a water-cure there.] 72 pp., 1 pl. 8°. *Kjøbenhavn, B. Lunos Kgl. Hof-Bogtr.,* 1887.
Suppl. to: Ugesk. f. Læger, Kjøbenh., 1887, 4. R., xvi, No. 30.

Myiasis.
See **Skin** (*Larvæ, etc., in*).

Myionnet (Paul-Henri). *De l'allongement des os de la jambe à la suite d'ulcères. 60 pp. 4°. *Paris,* 1879, No. 403.

Mylabris.
See, also, **Blisters** (*Pharmacy, etc., of*); **Cantharides,** *etc.* ; **Hydrophobia** (*Treatment of*).
Chapman (I.) An account of a species of cantharis, found in Buck's Co., Penna. Med. Reposit., N. Y., 1799, ii, 174–177.—**Labbée.** Mouvement méd., Par., 1876, xiv, 661–663.—**Prestat** (E.) Note sur l'emploi du Mylabris interrupta, comme succédané de la cantharide. Rec. de mém. de méd. . . . Mil., Par., 1876, xxxii, 94–96.— **Riley** (C. V.) On the transformations and habits of the blister-beetles. Am. Naturalist, Phila., 1878, xii, 213; 282, 1 pl.—**Young** (D. S.) [*et al.*]. Reports on the Mylabris cichorei, as a substitute for the cantharis. Madras Q. M. J., 1840, iii, 96–103.

Mylæus (Petrus).
See **Varandæus** (Jo.) De morbis et affectibus mulierum [etc.] 8°. *Lugduni,* 1619.

Mylich (Henricus Carolus). *Morborum ad folliculos sebaceos pertinentium, in justum ordinem redigendorum ac describendorum, specimen. [Dorpat.] 62 pp. 8°. *Mitaviæ, ex off. J. F. Steffenhagen et filii,* 1827.

Mylius (Adolphus Theodorus) [1809–]. *De venæsectionis historia. 28 pp., 2 l. 8°. *Berolini, typ. Nietackianis,* [1835].

Mylius (Andreas Christophorus). *De medicamentis selectioribus. 32 pp. 4°. *Halæ Magdeb., typ. G. J. Lehmanni,* [1713].

Mylius (Bernhard). *Ueber Laryngeal-Croup. 20 pp. 8°. *Würzburg, C. J. Becker,* 1868.
For Portrait, see **Collection**—van Kaathoven.

Mylius (Carolus Gottlieb) [1766–]. *De signis fœtus vivi ac mortui. 16 pp., 1 l. sm. 4°. *Jenæ, lit. Gæpferdtianis,* [1789].
Also, in: SCHLEGEL (J. C. T.) Sylloge op. min. [etc.] 8°. *Lipsiæ,* 1796, ii, 507–516.
For Biography, see **Nicolai** (Ern. Ant.)

Mylius (*Friedrich Jacob*).
Portrait in: **Collection**—van Kaathoven.

Mylius (Guilielmus). De glandulis. 4°. *Lugd. Bat.,* 1698.
In: HALLER. Disp. anat. [etc.] 4°. *Gottingæ,* 1747, ii, 709–730, 1 pl.

Mylius (Jacobus). *De dracone volante et igne fatuo. Resp. Benjamine Prætorio. 7 l. 4°. *Lipsiæ, Q. Bauch,* [1653].

Mylius (Joannes Christophorus). *De resolutione noxia. 1 p. l., 20 pp., 2 l. 4°. *Erlangæ, apud J. D. M. Camerarium,* [1765].

Mylius (Joannes Daniel.) Opus medico-chymicum : continens tres tractatus sive basilicas, quorum prior inscribitur basilica medica ; secundus basilica chymica ; tertius basilica philosophica. 3 pts. in 2 v. 4°. *Francofurti, L. Jennis,* 1618.

———. De diarrhœa, cum prosthemate hermetico syncritico.
In: AGONISMATA med. Marpurgensia. 4°. *Marpurgi Cattorum,* 1618, 196–205.

———. Antidotarium medico-chymicum reformatum : continens quatuor libros distinctos, quorum : 1. Generaliora in pharmaciam requisita explicat. 2. Tractat de quibusdam exoticis in nostris basilicis omissis. 3. Tradit præcepta Galenic. et chymicorum de præparatione medicamentorum. 4. Resolvit formas et dividit medicamenta tam Galen. quam chymicorum. 4 p. l., 1044 pp., 36 l., port. 4°. *Francofurti, L. Jennis,* 1620.

———. Complementum operis medico-chymici, continens tres tractatus sive basilicas. Quorum prior inscribitur basilica medica, continens iii libros de medicina antiqua Hippocratica. Secundus inscribitur basilica chymica, continens libros septem de metallis, mineralibus, vegetabilibus et animalibus. Tertius basilica philosophica, tractat de medicina universali, chymicorum instrumentis et obscuritatibus. pp. 185–428 ; 1470 pp., 1 pl. ; pp. 185–271, 7 pl. ; 44 pp., 10 pl. 4°. *Francofurti, L. Jennis,* 1620.
Imperfect.
See, also, **Mercklinus** (George Abraham). Sylloge physico-medicinalium casuum incantationi, etc. 4°. *Norimbergæ,* 1698.—**Petræus** (Henricus). De diarrhœa. Respondente Joh. Daniel Mylius. *In:* NOSOL. harmonica dogmat. et hermet. 4°. *Marpurgi Cattorum,* 1616, ii, 78–90. ——. De epilepsia. Respondente Joh. Daniel Mylius. *In:* NOSOL. harmonica dogmat. et hermet. 4°. *Marpurgi Cattorum,* 1615, i, 89–123.

Mylius (Joh. Fridericus). *Diss. morbos eorumque affinitatem ex incompletis motibus hæmorrhagicis ortos sistens. 26 pp., 2 l. 4°. *Lugd. Bat., C. Wishoff,* [1724]. [*Also, in:* P., v. 72.]

Mylius (Joh. Gottlieb). *De cognoscenda et curanda arthritide. 24 pp. 4°. *Erfordiæ, typ. J. H. Groschir,* [1720].

Mylius (Leonh. Henricus) [1696–1721]. *De anatomia et physiologia in genere. 23 pp. sm. 4°. [*Lipsiæ*], lit. I. Titii, [1715].

———. *De puella monstrosa. 33 pp., 1 pl. sm. 4°. *Lipsiæ, lit. I. Titii,* [1717].
For Biography, see **Paulus** (Joh. Guilielmus).
For Portrait, see **Collection**—van Kaathoven.

Mylius (R.) *Ueber Behandlung der Syphilis mit subcutanen Injectionen von Quecksilber-

Mylius (R.)—continued.
chloridchlornatrium. 38 pp. 8°. *Göttingen, Dieterich*, 1877.

Mylodon.
Burmeister (H.) Hautpanzer bei Mylodon. Arch. f. Anat., Physiol. u. wissensch. Med., Leipz., 1865, 334–336.

Mynors (Robert) [1739–1806]. Practical thoughts on amputations, etc. 91 pp., 1 pl. 12°. *Birmingham, G. Robinson*, 1783.

———. A history of the practice of trepanning the skull, and the after-treatment; with observations upon a new method of cure. xii, 152 pp. 12°. *Birmingham, G. Robinson*, 1785.
Bound with preceding.

von Mynsicht (Hadrianus) [16 –1668]. Thesaurus· et armamentarium medico - chymicum; hoc est, selectissimorum contra quosvis morbos pharmacorum conficiendorum secretissima ratio, propria laborum experientia, multiplici et felicissima praxi confirmata, et nunc una cum remediorum virtute, usu et dosi, doctrinæ et sapientiæ filiis fideliter revelata et communicata; cui in fine adjunctum est testamentum Hadrianeum de aureo philosophorum lapide. 4 p. l., 532 pp., 25 l., 24 pp. 4°. *Lubecæ, A. J. Becker*, 1662.

———. The same. 5 p. l., 525 pp., 27 l.; 22 pp., port. 12°. *Francofurti, typ. B. C. Wustii*, 1675.

———. The same. Accessit etiam D. Caroli Musitani mantissa atque Andreæ Battimelli auctarium, denique Hieronymi Piperi corollarium. Opus hac in novissima impressione variis erroribus expurgatum. 2 p. l., 446 pp., 26 l. 16°. *Venetiis, J. G. Hertz*, 1707.

———. The same. Thesaurus et armamentarium medico chymicum; or, a treasury of physick. With the most secret way of preparing remedies against all diseases. Written originally in Latine, and faithfully rendered into English by John Partridge, physician to his majesty. 7 p. l., 377 pp., 17 l. 8°. *London, A. Churchill*, 1682.

———. Thesauri et armamentarii medico-chymici appendix philosophico-poëtica, videlicet, testamentum Hadrianeum, quo suam de aureo philosophorum lapide sententiam, adeoque ultimæ voluntatis suæ dispositionem, sapientiæ et doctrinæ filiis revelat author. 24 pp. 4°. [*Lubecæ*, 1662.]
Bound with his: Thesaurus [etc.] 4°. *Lubecæ*, 1662.
See, also, de **Sgobbis** (Antonio). Universale theatro farmaceutico, etc. fol. *Venezia*, 1682.
For Portrait, see **Collection**—van Kaathoven.

Mynsinger (Gustavus Benoni). *Diss. sistens methodum curandi pestem. 1 p. l., 40 pp. 4°. *Halæ Magdeb., lit. J. Gruneri*, [1708].

Mynster (Olaus Hieronymus) [1772–1818]. *De carbone ejusdemque præcipuis connubiis, de ætiologia phthiseos Beddoesiana et de remediis alcalinis carbonicis. 3 p. l., 80 pp. 8°. *Havniæ, typ. C. F. Holmii*, [1797].

Mynter (Herman). Aneurism of the innominate artery treated with ligature of the right carotid and subclavian arteries. 12 pp. 12°. *New York, Trow's*, 1887.
Repr. from: Med. Rec., N. Y., 1887, xxxii.

———. Compound dislocation of the ankle joint and its treatment. 7 pp. 8°. [*Buffalo*, 1888.]
Repr. from: Med. Press West. N. York, Buffalo, 1888, iii.

Myocarditis.
See **Heart** (*Inflammation of*).

Myochronoscope.
Czermak (J.) Das Myochronoskop. 8°. [*Wien*, 1861.]
Repr. from: Sitzungsb. d. k. Akad. d. Wissensch. Math.-naturw. Cl., Wien, 1861, xliv.

Myoctonin.
Salmonowitz (S.) *Beiträge zur Kenntniss der Alcaloide des Aconitum iycoctonum. II. Myoctonin. 8°. *Dorpat*, 1885.
Dragendorff (G.) Ueber das Myoctonin. Pharm. Ztschr. f. Russland, St. Petersb., 1886, xxv, 237–344.

Myodesopia.
See **Muscæ** *volitantes*.

Myograph.
See, also, **Graphic** *method*.
Gruenhagen (A.) Beschreibung eines neuen Myographions zur Messung der Geschwindigkeit nervöser Leitungsvorgänge. 4°. *Königsberg i. Pr.*, 1883.
Repr. from: Schrift. d. phys.-ökonom. Gesellsch. zu Königsb., 1883, xxiv.
Jendrássik (J.) A magától sorakoztató esömyographium és alkalmazásának vázlata. [A self-registering myograph.] 4°. *Budapest*, 1881.
Blix (M.) En ny myograf. Upsala Läkaref. Förh., 1879–80, xv, 471–480, 1 pl.—**Czermak** (J.) Das Myochronoskop. [*From:* Sitzungsb. d. Wien. Akad. d. Wissensch.] Untersuch. z. Naturl. d. Mensch. u. d. Thiere, Giessen, 1862, viii, 478–488.—**François-Franck.** Myographes; myographie. Dict. encycl. d. sc. méd., Par., 1876, 2. s., ii, 225–239.—**Fredericq** (L.) Myographe pour l'étude de la période latente. Arch. de biol., Gand, 1882, iii, 275–284.—**Grützner** (P.) Ein neues Myographion. Arch. f. d. ges. Physiol., Bonn, 1887, xli, 281–290, 1 pl.—**Landois** (L.) & **Mosler** (F.) Ein Myographium und dessen Anwendung auf die Untersuchung gesunder und kranker Muskeln bein Menschen. Berl. klin. Wchnschr., 1869, vi, 25; 33.—**Rosenthal** (J.) Ueber ein neues Myographion und einige mit demselben angestellte Versuche. Arch. f. Physiol., Leipz., 1883, Suppl.-Bd., 240–279.—**Thiry** (L.) Ueber ein neues Myographion. Ztschr. f. rat. Med., Leipz. u. Heidelb., 1864, 3. R., xxi, 300–306, 1 pl.

Myoidema.
Labbé (D.) *De la contraction iodio-musculaire, ou myoïdème en clinique. 4°. *Paris*, 1881.
Marcus (C.) *Contribution à l'étude clinique du myoœdème. 4°. *Paris*, 1886.
Jeanselme (E.) & **Lermoyez.** Du myœdème et de ses modifications chez les cholériques. Gaz. hebd. de méd., Par., 1885, 2. s., xxii, 453–456.—**West** (S.) Myoidema. St. Barth. Hosp. Rep., Lond., 1879, xv, 151–155.

Myology.
See **Muscles.**

Myoma.
Arnozan & **Vaillard.** Myômes à fibres lisses, multiples, confluents et isolés de la peau. J. de méd. de Bordeaux, 1880–81, x, 230–233. —**Buhl** (L.) Wahres recidivirendes Myom (Rhabdomyoma Zenker's). Ztschr. f. Biol., München, 1865, i, 263–272.—**Henocque** (A.) Myome (myome strio-cellulaire, rhabdomyome). Dict. encycl. d. sc. méd., Par., 1876, 2. s., xi, 239–241.

Myopia.
See, also, **Eye** (*Accommodation, etc., of, Disordered*); **Eye** (*Diseases of*) *in children*; **Presbyopia**; **Spectacles.**
Abadie (J.-M.-C.) *Étude sur la myopie stationnaire et progressive. 4°. *Paris*, 1870.
Beckh (W.) *Die Hebetudo visus ex insufficientia musculi recti interni oculi bei Myopen, ihre Folgen und Therapie. 8°. *Erlangen*, 1862.
Bergstrand (A.) *Studier öfver myopiens etiologi. 8°. *Lund*, 1877.
Borgmann (H.) *Ueber die Verwendung decentrirter Brillen bei Myopie. 8°. *Berlin*, [1873].
Breiter (G. A.) *De myopia observationes septuaginta cum adnotationibus nonnullis. roy. 8°. *Lipsiæ*, [1861].
Burgl (M.) *Beiträge zur Aetiologie der Kurzsichtigkeit. 8°. *München*, 1874.
Also, in: Aerztl. Int.-Bl., München, 1874, xxi, 240; 247.
Chasanow (J.) *Ueber die Progression der Myopie. 8°. *Königsberg*, [1883].
Collet (M.-J.-T.) *De la myopie et de la presbyopie; des véritables modifications oculaires qui les déterminent. 4°. *Paris*, 1853.

Myopia.

COLSMAN (A.) Die überhandnehmende Kurzsichtigkeit unter der deutschen Jugend, deren Bedeutung, Ursachen, Verhütung. 8°. *Barmen*, 1877.

Also, in: Cor.-Bl. d. nied.-rhein. Ver. öff. Gsndhtspflg., Köln, 1877, vi, 140–155.

COOPER (W. W.) Practical remarks on near sight, aged sight, and impaired vision; with observations upon the use of glasses and on artificial light. 8°. *London*, 1847.

COTY (A. E.) * De la myopie et de l'hypermétropie. 4°. *Paris*, 1862.

DONDERS (F. C.) Myopie en hare behandeling. 8°. *Tiel*, 1866.

DÜRR (E.) Die Entwickelung der Kurzsichtigkeit während der Schuljahre erläutert durch die Refractionstafeln von Schülern des Lyceum II in Hannover. 8°. *Braunschweig*, 1884.

Also [Abstr.], *in:* Tagebl. d. Versamml. deutsch. Naturf. u. Aerzte, Magdeb., 1884, lvii, 117–121.

———. Rathschläge für Kurzsichtige. 12°. *Hannover*, 1886.

DUFRESSE - CHASSAIGNE (J.-E.) Traité du strabisme et du bégaiement, suivi de quelques considérations nouvelles sur la guérison de la myopie, de l'amaurose par rétraction musculaire, et du mouvement convulsif des yeux par la division des muscles de l'œil. 8°. *Paris*, 1841.

HEBERLING (F. G.) * De myopia. 8°. *Berolini*, 1865.

HINRICHSEN (C.) *Accommodationskrampf bei Myopie. 8°. *Kiel*, 1882.

KATZ. Die Kurzsichtigkeit nach Ursache, Wesen und Gefahren, mit besonderer Rücksicht auf Auge und Schule allgemein verständlich dargestellt. 8°. *Berlin*, 1882.

LEININBERG (N.) * Klinisch-statistische Beiträge zur Myopie. [Wurtzburg.] 8°. *München*, 1886.

LÖWEGREN (M. K.) * Om myopi. 4°. *Lund*, 1866.

Also, in: ACTA univ. Lund. 4°. *Lund.*, 1866, ii, 1–86.

MAES (C.) * Ein Beitrag zur Aetiologie der Myopie. 8°. *Kiel*, 1884.

MALLING (L.) * Die mechanischen Momente bei der Entstehung von Myopie. 4°. *Kiel*, 1874.

MIARD (A.) Origine de la myopie, l'accommodation et les défauts. 4°. *Paris*, 1870.

———. Des troubles fonctionnels et organiques de l'amétropie et de la myopie en particulier, de l'accommodation binoculaire et ciliaire dans les vices de la réfraction. Recherches étiologiques des conditions d'existence des divers défauts réfractifs; nature et mécanisme des phénomènes physiologiques qu'ils comportent et des états pathologiques principaux qu'ils engendrent. Traitement de la myopie. 8°. *Paris*, 1872.

NARDO (G. D.) Sopra un semplice e facile mezzo di leggere distinto senza lenti tanto in caso di miopia, come in caso di presbiopia. 8°. *Venezia*, 1855.

NORTHROP (B. G.) Near-sightedness in schools; its causes, prevalence, and preventives. 8°. *New Haven*, 1878.

Repr. from: Rep. State Bd. Education.

PAULSEN (O.) Die Entstehung und Behandlung der Kurzsichtigkeit. 8°. *Berlin*, 1883.

PFLÜGER (E.) La myopie scolaire. 8°. *Paris*, 1887.

REBSTOCK (M.-É.) * De la myopie. 4°. *Strasbourg*, 1859.

RINDFLEISCH (M.) * Ueber die Kurzsichtigkeit (Myopie). 8°. *Neuburg*, 1860.

SCHIESS-GEMUSEUS (H.) Beitrag zur Therapie der Myopie. 8°. *Basel*, 1872.

Also, transl. in: Ann. d'ocul., Brux., 1874, lxxii, 23–34.

Myopia.

SCHMITHAUSEN (A.) * Ueber das Sehen der Myopen mittelst Zerstreuungskreise. 8°. *Greifswald*, 1874.

SCHRÖDER (C.) Ueber Atropinkuren gegen Kurzsichtigkeit. 8°. *Leipzig*, 1874.

SCHÜTZE (H.) * Beitrag zur Statistik der Myopie und der Netzhautpunction. 8°. *Kiel*, 1882.

SONNTAG (G. E.) * Ueber transitorische Myopie. 8°. *Freiburg i. Br.*, 1885.

STILLING (J.) Untersuchungen über die Entstehung der Kurzsichtigkeit. roy. 8°. *Wiesbaden*, 1887.

SULZBERGER (J. C.) * De myopia et presbyopia. 4°. *Rostochii*, [1756].

TUELLMANN (L.) * De myopia. 8°. *Berolini*, [1852].

UNGEFUG (F.) * Ueber Myopie. 8°. *Halle*, [1868].

WEISS (L.) Beiträge zur Entwicklung der Myopie. 1. Ueber eine leicht ausführbare Messung des Augenspiegelbildes und die Bedeutung solcher Messungen für die Beurtheilung des dioptrischen Apparates des Auges. 8°. *Berlin*, 1876.

Also, in: Arch. f. Ophth., Berl., 1876, xxii, 3. Abth. 1–124. [*See, also, infra*, Landolt (E.)]

WELLS (J. S.) On long, short, and weak sight, and their treatment by the scientific use of spectacles. 8°. *London*, 1862.

———. The same. 4. ed. 8°. *London*, 1873.

WERTH (R.) * Ein Beitrag zur Lehre von der Myopie. 4°. *Kiel*, 1874.

WESTHOFF (C. F.) * De myopia. 8°. *Berolini*, [1860].

Abadie. Des complications de la myopie progressive. Bull. et mém. Soc. franç. d'opht., Par., 1885, iii, 247–261.—**Abadie** (J.-M.-C.) De la ténotomie partielle des muscles de l'œil pour combattre le développement de la myopie progressive. Bull. et mém. Soc. de chir. de Par., 1880, n. s., vi, 325–339.—**Adams** (J.) Case of shortsightedness cured by operation. Prov. M. & S. J., Lond., 1841, ii, 470–473.—**Adamuk** (E.) K vopr. o miopii v schkolach. [Myopia in schools.] Vestnik oftalmol., Kieff, 1886, iii, 269; 429.—**Albrecht** (J.) Statistische Beiträge zur Lehre von der Myopie. Klin. Monatsbl. f. Augenh., Stuttg., 1882, xx, 342–346.—**Baas.** Die Ueberhandnahme der Myopie. Med.-chir. Centralbl., Wien, 1883, xviii, 21.—**Bader** (C.) A description of the appearances of the human eye in health and disease as seen by the ophthalmoscope. 7. s. Myopia; region of the yellow spot. Guy's Hosp. Rep., Lond., 1873, 3. s., xviii, 243, 1 l., 1 pl.—**Barrett** (J. W.) The influence of concave glasses on myopia. Austral. M. J., Melbourne, 1887, n. s., ix, 289–291.—**Bartlett** (E. W.) Progressive near-sightedness. Tr. Wisconsin M. Soc., Milwaukee, 1874, viii, 103–108.—**Becker** (O.) Ueber zunehmende und überhandnehmende Kurzsichtigkeit. Ber. ü. d. Versamml. d. ophth. Gesellsch., Stuttg., 1883, xv, 77–89.—**Bendell** (H.) Nearsightedness in our public schools; its causes and prevention. Med. Ann., Albany, 1884, v, 355–363.—**Benkendorf** (E.) A case of myopia complicated with nystagmus. St. Louis M. & S. J., 1883, xliv, 347.—**Berthold** (A. A.) Das Myopodiorthoticon oder der Apparat, die Kurzsichtigkeit zu heilen. Monatschr. f. Med., Augenh. u. Chir., Leipz., 1840, iii, 332–336.—**Bertin-Sans** (É.) Le problème de la myopie scolaire. Ann. d'hyg., Par., 1882, 3. s., vii, 46; 127.—**Bertrand.** Influence des diaphragmes pupillaires sur les effets de la myopie artificielle. Bull. et mém. Soc. franç. d'opht., Par., 1884, ii, 156–165. ———. Expériences sur la myopie et la pupille artificielles. Ann. d'ocul., Brux., 1884, xci, 32–44.—**Binard.** Une variété de la myopie (myopia in distans), importante à connaître pour la visite des conscrits. Arch. belges de méd. mil., Brux., 1850, vi, 336–339.—**Bowen** (W. S.) A portable book-rack for the use of myopic children and adults. Med. Rec., N. Y., 1876, xi, 5.—**Browne** (E. A.) The genesis of short sight. Liverpool M.-Chir. J., 1886, vi, 269–279.—**Burchardt.** Ueber den Einfluss, den Sehschwäche und Kurzsichtigkeit auf die Militair-Diensttauglichkeit haben. Deutsche mil.-ärztl. Ztschr., Berl., 1873, ii, 247–259. [*See, also, infra*, Schmidt (H.)] ———. Ueber die Verhütung der Kurzsichtigkeit. Deutsche med. Wchnschr., Berl., 1878, iv, 6.—**Carl** (T.) Ueber einige anatomische Befunde bei der Myopie. Mitth. a. d. k. Univ.-Augenklin. zu München, 1882, i, 233–246, 1 pl.—**Carreras y Aragó.** Estudios sobre la miopia. Independ. méd., Barcel., 1873–4, v, 206; 228, 299.—**Castañeda** (J. M.) La miopia y las escuelas. Crón.-méd.-quir. de la Habana, 1880, vi, 91–96.—**Chalons.** Beurtheilung und Untersuchung der Kurzsichtigkeit bei dienstpflichtigen

Myopia.

Mannschaften. Preuss. mil.-ärztl. Ztg., Berl., 1861, ii, 152–159.—**Chibret.** Note sur la myopie progressive avec diminution de l'acuité visuelle. Assoc. franç. pour l'avance. d. sc. Compt.-rend. 1876, Par., 1877, v, 876–878. ——. Détermination quantitative de la myopie par la kératoscopie (fantoscopie rétinienne), à l'aide d'un simple miroir plan. Ann. d'ocul., Brux., 1882, lxxx, viii, 238–240.—**Chisolm** (J. J.) Myopia; its increase, some of its causes, and how it may be in a measure prevented. Richmond & Louisville M. J., Louisville, 1869, vii, 361–367. ——. Myopia in its various phases. Virginia M. Month., Richmond, 1880–81, vii, 421–452. *Also*, Reprint. *Also*, Revised reprint.— **Cohn** (H.) Die Augen der Breslauer Studenten. Berl. klin. Wchnschr., 1867, iv, 527. ——. Die Verwechselung von "Kurzsichtigkeit" und "Schwäche" im preussischen Abgeordnetenhause. Deutsche med. Wchnschr., Berl., 1878, iv, 39. ——. Ueber Schrift, Druck, und überhandnehmende Kurzsichtigkeit. Tagebl. d. Versamml. deutsch. Naturf. u. Aerzte, Danzig, 1880, liii, 42–52, 5 tab., 1 pl. *Also*: Mitth. d. Ver. d. Aerzte in Nied.-Oest., Wien, 1880, vi, 245; 262. *Also*: Breslau. aerztl. Ztschr., 1880, ii, 217; 231. *Also*: Wien. med. Wchnschr., 1880, xxx, 1101; 1124. *Also*: Allg. Wien. med. Ztg., 1880, xxv, 412; 424; 433; 452. *Also*: Wien. med. Bl., 1880, iii, 991; 1019; 1045. *Also*: Med.-chir. Centralbl., Wien, 1881, xvi, 86; 99; 111; 122; 134; 146; 158. *Also, transl.*: Rev. scient., Par., 1881, 3. s., xxvii, 290–298. ——. Ueber Kurzsichtigkeit, Bücherdruck und Schulärzte. Deutsche Rundschau, Berl., 1880, lxx, 423–438. ——. Ueber weisse Kunststeintafeln zur Verhütung der Kurzsichtigkeit. Centralbl. f. prakt. Augenh., Leipz., 1882, vi, 334–337. — **Considérations** pratiques sur la myopie et son traitement. Bull. gén. de thérap., etc., Par., 1861, lxi, 464–468. — **Cornwell** (H. G.) The origin and prevalence of myopia among school children. "The Transactions", Youngstown, O., 1880, ii, 10–20. *Also*, Reprint.—**Critchett.** Examination of a globe which presented some features of myopia. Ophth. Hosp. Rep., Lond., 1876–9, ix, 76–78.—**Cuignet.** Exercices avec des verres concaves et convexes pour la simulation de la myopie et de l'hypermétropie. Rec. d'ophth., Par., 1875, 2. s., ii, 230–233.—**Culbertson** (H.) On the value of "prisoptometer" in determining the degree of myopia. Am. J. Ophth., St. Louis, 1884, i, 10–17. ——. On the application of cylindrical glasses in myopic astigmatism. *Ibid.*, 1885, ii, 211–214. ——. A mode of determining the absolute myopia through the aid of glasses with the prisoptometer. *Ibid.*, 1886, iii, 325–327. — **Cutter** (J. C.) Myopia. Rep. Sapporo Agric. Coll., Japan, 1880, 8°, 1881, v, 69–84. — **Deeren.** Étiologie et prophylaxie de la myopie axile chez les écoliers. Rec. d'ophth., Par., 1886, 3. s., viii, 449–458. — **Dehenne** (A.) Un mot sur la mesure de la myopie. *Ibid.*, 1878, 2. s., v, 269–279.— **De Neffe.** La myopie à l'école moyenne de Gand. Ann. Soc. de méd. de Gand, 1886, lxv, 330–334. — **Derby** (H.) On the atropine treatment of acquired and progressive myopia, with a table of cases. Tr. Am. Ophth. Soc., N. Y., 1873–9, ii, 139–154. *Also*, Reprint. ——. I. A report on the percentage of near-sight found to exist in the class of 1880 at Harvard College, with some account of similar investigations. II. An account of the phakometer of Snellen. Boston M. & S. J., 1877, xcvi, 337–343. *Also*, Reprint. ——. On the prevention of near-sight in the young. Boston M. & S. J., 1880, cii, 533–535. *Also*: Extr. Rec. Bost. Soc. M. Improve. (1880–82), 1883, viii, pp. xxv–xxix. ——. Near-sight in the young. Boston M. & S. J., 1880, cii, 620.—**Derby** (R. H.) Progressive myopia, and its operative cure. N. York M. J., 1873, xvii, 577–592. *Also*, Reprint. — **Devot.** Statistique de la myopie en France considérée sous le point de vue de l'exemption du service militaire. Arch. d'ophth., Par., 1855, v, 101. — **Discussion** zur Myopiefrage. Ber. ü. d. Versamml. d. ophth. Gesellsch., Stuttg., 1885, xvii, 170–186. — **Dobrowolsky** (W.) Kazhushchayasya ili lozhnaya blizorukost i lozhnii miopicheskii astigmatizm. [False myopia and myopic astigmatism.] Med. Vestnik, St. Petersb., 1868, viii, 272; 281; 289; 303; 311; 319. ——. K voprosu o prichinach miopii. [Causes of myopia.] Ejened. klin. gaz., St. Petersb., 1885, v, 13–19. *Also, transl.*: Klin. Monatsbl. f. Augenh., Stuttg., 1885, xxiii, 157–162.—**Doneran** (H.) La miopia. Pabellon méd., Madrid, 1874, xiv, 446. — **Dransart** (H.) Guérison de la myopie progressive par l'iridectomie et la sclérotomie; théorie circulatoire de la myopie. Ann. d'ocul., Brux., 1885, xciv, 109–116. — **Dürr.** Ueber die Kurzsichtigkeit in den höheren Schulen Hannovers, die Beleuchtung der Klassenzimmer in denselben und die für den Schutz der Schüleraugen nothwendigen Massregeln. Verhandl. u. Mitth.d. Ver. f. öff. Gsndhtspflg. zu Hannov., 1883, 5. Hft. 73–89. — **Éperon.** De la détermination à l'image droite des degrés élevés de myopie. Arch. d'ophth., Par., 1884, iv, 217–289.—**Erismann** (F.) Vlijanie schkole na proischojdenie blizorukosti. [Influence of the school in producing near-sightedness.] Arch. sudebnoi med., St. Petersb., 1870, vi, pt. 3, 84–160; pt. 4, 202–256. — **Fano.** Ce qu'il faut entendre par myopie acquise, myopie progressive. J. d'ocul et chir., Par., 1877–8, iii, 129–132. — **Fick** (A. E.) Ueber den Zusammenhang zwischen Myopie und Divergenzschielen. Breslau. aerztl. Ztschr., 1879, i, 38.—

Myopia.

Foderà. Observation d'une myopie de l'œil droit et d'une presbyopie de l'œil gauche sur le même individu. Arch. gén. de méd., Par., 1823, iii, 221–224. — **Förster.** Ueber die Entstehungsweise der Myopie. Ber. ü. d. Versamml. d. ophth. Gesellsch., Stuttg., 1883, xv,119–131. ——. Ueber den Einfluss der Concavgläser und der Achsenconvergenz auf die Weiterentwickelung der Myopie. Arch. f. Augenh., Wiesb., 1884–5, xiv, 295–328. *Also, transl.*: Arch. Ophth., N. Y., 1886, xv, 399–435. ——. Ueber Behandlung der Myopie. Breslau. aerztl. Ztschr., 1886, viii, 37–41.—**Foltz.** Note sur le traitement mécanique de la myopie. Gaz. méd. de Par., 1859, 3. s., xiv, 87.—**da Fonseca** (L.) Nova anomalia das papillas opticas; myopia subita e persistente por espasmo d'accomodação derivado de epilepsia. Arch. ophth. de Lisb., 1887, viii, 44. — **Fröbelius** (W.) Der höchste Grad von Kurzsichtigkeit, erworben durch Missbrauch von Concavlinsen, und Mydriasis, geheilt durch zweckmässigen Gebrauch schwächerer Brillen. Med. Ztg. Russlands, St. Petersb., 1854, xi, 235–237.— **Fuchs** (E.) Zur Entstehung der Myopie. Klin. Monatsbl. f. Augenh., Stuttg., 1884, xxii, 14–19. — **Gamba** (A.) Il miope al 3° grado è atto al servizio ordinario della milizia nazionale? Gior. d. r. Accad. med.-chir. di Torino, 1852, 2. s., xiii, 346–354. — **García Calderon** (A.) Consideraciones sobre la miopia. Rev. esp. de oftal., sif., etc., Madrid, 1880–81, i, 210; 288; 337: ii, 65. — **Giraud-Teulon.** De la myopie au point de vue du service militaire. Gaz. hebd. de méd., Par., 1870, 2. s., vii, 514–517. ——. Des troubles fonctionnels de la vision dans leurs rapports avec le service militaire. Bull. Acad. de méd., Par., 1875, 2. s., iv, 729; 775. [Discussion] 1044; 1050; 1075; 1104; 1179; 1217; 1246; 1291; 1315; 1343; 1389; 1419; 1449; 1468: 1876, 2. s., v, 10. ——. Myopie. Dict. encycl. u. sc. méd., Par., 1876, 2. s., xi, 242–307. — **Giudici** (V.) Sulla misurazione obbiettiva della miopia e della ipermetropia. Gior. di med. mil., Roma, 1885, xxxiii, 128–130, 1 pl.—**Guérin** (J.) Sur la cause et le traitement chirurgical de la myopie. Gaz. méd. de Par., 1841, 2. s., ix, 177–185.—**von Graefe** (A.) Ueber Myopia in distans, nebst Betrachtung über das Sehen jenseits der Grenzen unserer Accommodation. Arch. f. Ophth., Berl., 1855–6, ii, 1. Abth., 158. ——. Ueber die Operation des dynamischen Auswärtsschielens, besonders in Rücksicht auf progressive Myopie. Klin. Monatsbl. f. Augenh., Erlang., 1869, vii, 225 – 281. ——. Myopie und Divergenz. Breslau. aerztl. Ztschr., 1879, i, 56–58. — **Hadlow** (H.) Short sight amongst the boys of Greenwich Hospital School. Brit. M. J., Lond., 1883, i, 952–954.—**Hall** (G. P.) A case of temporary near-sightedness, caused by a carious molar. Tr. Texas M. Ass., Fort Worth, 1884, xvi, 175.— **Haltenhoff** (G.) Étiologie et prophylaxie de la myopie. Cong. périod. internat. d. sc. méd. Compt.-rend. 1877, Genève, 1878, v, 749–755.—**Harlan** (G. C.) Rapidly progressive myopia, permanently checked by division of the external rectus. Tr. Am. Ophth. Soc., Bost., 1885, 24–27.—**Hell.** Kurzsichtigkeit in Bezug auf Militairdienstbrauchbarkeit. Deutsche mil.-ärztl. Ztschr., Berl., 1873, ii, 88–92.—**Heren** (N.) La miopia considerada bajo el punto de vista de la oftalmología moderna. Compilador méd., Barcel., 1866–7, ii, 355; 370; 416; 443; 465; 489.—**Hock** (J.) Ueber scheinbare Myopie. Allg. Wien. med. Ztg., 1872, xvii, 114. — **Hofmann** (J.) Ein Erklärungsversuch für die scheinbare Kurzsichtigkeit. *Ibid.*, 1886, xxxi, 410.— **Hogg** (J.) Entoptics; observations on the relatively greater frequency of myodesopia in the myopic eye. Brit. M. J., Lond., 1865, i, 504; 531. — **Horner** (F.) De la myopie congénitale. Rev. méd. de la Suisse Rom., Genève, 1885, 24–1, 4–7, 2 pl.—**Horstmann** (C.) Beiträge zur Myopiefrage. Charité-Ann. 1878, Berl., 1880, v, 408–449. ——. Ueber Myopie. Deutsche med. Wchnschr., Berl., 1878, iv, 218–220. ——. Ueber Myopie. Arch. f. Augenh., Wiesb., 1880, ix, 208–224. — **Hunt** (D.) A new theory regarding myopia. Boston M. & S. J., 1878, xcix, 533. ——. On the causation of myopia. N. York M. J., 1883, xxxvii, 255–259.—**Hutchinson** (J.) Case of extreme myopia. Ophth. Hosp. Rep., Lond., 1871–3, vii, 44.—**Instruction** du conseil de santé des armées à l'effet d'indiquer les mesures qui doivent être prescrites pour empêcher le développement ou l'aggravation de la myopie dans les écoles militaires. Bull. de la méd. et pharm. mil., Par., 1882, xxxi, 979.—**Jacob** (A. H.) The origin of posterior staphyloma and the mechanism of short-sightedness. Med. Press & Circ., Lond., 1878, n. s., xxv, 128–130. — **Javal.** Sur les mesures à prendre pour enrayer l'envahissement de la myopie. Cong. internat. d'hyg. 1878, Par., 1880, ii, 108–122. *Also* [Abstr.]: Ann. Soc. méd.-chir. de Liége, 1879, xviii, 60–64. *Also* [Abstr.]: Art méd., Brux., 1878–9, xiv, 257–260. ——. La myopie progressive dans ses rapports avec la longueur des lignes d'impression. Ann. d'ocul., Brux., 1880, lxxxiv, 60–64. ——. Sur la myopie scolaire. Bull. Acad. de méd., Par., 1887, 2. s., xviii, 443.—**Jeannel** (J.) La myopie dans l'armée. Union méd., Par., 1877, 3. s., xxiii, 1025–1028.—**Juba** (A.) Az iskolai rövidlátás kérdéséhez. [The question of myopia in schools.] Szemészet, Budapest, 1887, 49; 68.—**Just** (O.) Beiträge zur Statistik der Myopie und des Farbensinns. Arch. f. Augenh., Wiesb., 1879, viii, 191–201. *Also transl.* [Abstr.]: Arch. Ophth., N. Y., 1881, x, 23–25.—

Myopia.

Kämpf. Ueber Aetiologie und Prophylaxis der Kurzsichtigkeit. Oesterr. Ztschr. f. prakt. Heilk., Wien, 1870, xvi, 769; 793. ———. Zur Aetiologie und Prophylaxis der Myopie. Allg. Wien. med. Ztg., 1871, xvi, 10; 18. ———. Ueber die Correctur der Myopie. Ibid., 125; 131; 143; 159. Also. transl.: Boston M. & S. J., 1871, viii, 132–136.—**Kennedy** (S. D.) Myopia. N. Orl. M. & S. J., 1883–4, n. s., xi, 657–663.—**Knies** (M.) Ueber Wesen und Therapie der Myopie. Ber. ü. d. Versamml. d. ophth. Gesellsch., Stuttg., 1886, xviii, 2. Hft., 26–43. ———. Ueber Myopie und ihre Behandlung. Arch. f. Ophth., Berl., 1886, xxxii, 3. Abth., 15–72.—**Königstein** (L.) Ueber scheinbare Kurzsichtigkeit. Mitth. d. Ver. d. Aerzte in Nied.-Oest., Wien, 1880, vi, 214–218.—**Krüger** (G.) Untersuchung der Augen der Schüler des Frankfurter Gymnasiums; ein Beitrag zur Entwicklungsgeschichte der Kurzsichtigkeit. Jahresb. ü. d. Verwalt. d. Med.-Wes., d. Krankenanst. . . . d. Stadt Frankf. (1871), 1872, xv, 84–97.—**Kugel** (L.) Ueber acute Entwickelung der Myopie. Arch f. Ophth., Berl., 1870, xvi, 323–328. — **Kuhnt** (H.) Welche Gesichtspunkte müssen bei Verordnung von Brillen für Kurzsichtige beachtet werden? Cor.-Bl. d. allg. ärztl. Ver. v. Thüringen, Weimar, 1881, x, 1; 105.—**Landolt** (E.) Bemerkungen zu dem Artikel: "Beiträge zur Entwicklung der Myopie", von L. Weiss. Arch. f. Ophth., Berl., 1877, xxiii, 263. ———. On myopia. Ophth. Hosp. Rep., Lond., 1879, ix, pt. 3, 345–354. ———. L'état actuel de la question de la myopie. Arch. d'opht., Par., 1884, iv, 1–65.—**von Langenbeck.** Gutachtliche Aeusserung der kgl. wissenschaftlichen Deputation für das Medicinalwesen über das Gesuch des Dr. X. hierselbst, die Behandlung der Schulkurzsichtigkeit betreffend. Vrtljschr. f. gerichtl. Med., Berl., 1878, xxix, n. F., 270–272.—**Leininberg** (N.) Klinisch-statistische Beiträge zur Myopie. München. med. Wchnschr., 1886, xxxiii, 496; 514.—**Leroy.** De la myopie au point de vue du service militaire. Arch. méd. belges, Brux., 1875, 3. s., viii, 241–252. Also: Gaz. hebd. de méd., Par., 1875, 2. s., xii, 710–713.—**Liebreich** (R.) Methode, dem umgekehrten Bilde bei kurzsichtigen Augen eine starke Vergrösserung zu geben. Arch. f. Ophth., Berl., 1860, vii, 2. Abth., 130–133. ———. Scheinbare Kurzsichtigkeit bei übersichtigem Bau und Accommodations-Krampf. Ibid., 1861–2, viii, 1. Abth., 259–270. Also, Reprint.—**Loring** (E. G.), jr. Are progressive myopia and conus (posterior staphyloma) due to hereditary predisposition, or can they be induced by defect of refraction acting through the influence of the ciliary muscle? Tr. Internat. M. Cong. 1876, Phila., 1877, 923–941. ———. "Is the human eye changing its form and becoming near-sighted under the influence of modern education?" Med. Rec., N. Y., 1877, xii, 732–734. — **Ludwig.** Bestimmung der Kurz- und Uebersichtigkeit.mit dem Augenspiegel. Allg. mil.-ärztl. Ztg., Wien, 1875, xvi, 41; 52.—**Magnus** (H.) Die Kurzsichtigkeit ein Schmerzenskind unserer modernen Cultur. Deutsche Rev., Berl., 1882, vii, 81–92. ———. Die neuesten Fortschritte in der Lehre der Kurzsichtigkeit. Ibid., Bresl. u. Berl., 1883, viii, 261–363. — **Mannhardt** (J.) Muskuläre Asthenopie und Myopie. Arch. f. Ophth., Berl., 1871, xvii, 2. Abth., 69–97. — **Mayoral** (D.) Investigaciones sobre la miopia considerada con esencion para el servicio militar y los medios de reconocerla. Bol. de med., cirug. y farm., Madrid, 1846, 3. s., i, 262–264.—**Mittendorf** (W. F.) Myopia and the necessity of its correction by glasses. Med. Gaz., N. Y., 1882, ix, 486–492. Also: Phila. M. Times, 1882–3, xiii, 60–64. — **Müller.** Ueber Kurzsichtigkeit, Uebersichtigkeit und Weitsichtigkeit und deren Correction. Cor.-Bl. f. d. Aerzte u. Apoth. d Grossherz. Oldenburg, 1860–61, i, 22; 25; 36.—**Myopia** in the schools of different nations. [Edit.] Med. Rec., N. Y., 1881, xix, 156.—**Nagel** (A.) Ueber den ophthalmoskopischen Befund in myopischen Augen. Mitth. a. d. ophth. Klin. in Tübing., 1880, 231. — **Nettleship** (E.) Myopia from childhood; rapid increase soon after marriage, to almost total blindness; question of myopic choroiditis. Ophth. Hosp. Rep., Lond., 1886, xi. 73–75.—**Nicati.** La myopie dans les écoles de Marseille. Gaz. hebd. de méd., Par., 1879, 2. s., xvi, 695.—**Niemann** (E.) Die Kurzsichtigkeit mit besonderer Berücksichtigung ihrer Zunahme während der Schulzeit. Verhandl. u. Mitth. d. Ver. f. öff. Gsndhtspflg. in Magdeb., 1878, 6. Hft. 89–104.—**Noel.** Sur la vision au loin chez les myopes non munis de verres. Bull. Acad. roy. de méd. de Belg., Brux., 1875, 3. s., ix, 1207–1215.—**Noyes** (H. D.) Case of extreme myopia. Tr. Am. Ophth. Soc., N. Y., 1873–9, ii, pt. 2, 155–157. — **Nuel** (J. P.) Colobome temporal de la papille du nerf optique; contribution à l'étude de la myopie héréditaire. Livre jubil. publié p. la Soc. de méd. de Gand, etc., Gand, 1884, 335–351. Also: Ann. d'ocul., Brux., 1885. xciii, 174–185. — **Ott.** Myopie und Schule. Cor.-Bl. f. schweiz. Aerzte, Basel, 1878, viii, 456; 487. — **Percy & Laurent.** Myopie. Dict. d. sc. méd., Par., 1819, xxxv, 123–131.— **Perrin** (M.) Rapport sur un travail ayant pour titre: Les livres scolaires et la myopie, par le Dr. Javal. Bull. Acad. de méd., Par., 1880, 2. s., ix, 221–236.— **Pflüger.** Zwei Fälle von plötzlich entstandener Myopie in Folge traumatischer Linsenluxation. Klin. Monatsbl. f. Augenh., Stuttg., 1875, xiii, 109–111. ———. Ueber Pupil-

Myopia.

lendistanz. Ibid., 451–458. — **Pflüger** (E.) La myopie scolaire. Ann. d'hyg., Par., 1886, 3. s., xviii, 113–146.— **Piotrovski** (F.) Blizorukoste i voennaja sleyba. [Myopia and military service.] Voyenno-med. J.. St. Petersb., 1876, cxxvii, 287–300.—**Plagge** (T.) Die Prüfungsmethoden der Kurzsichtigen vom staatsärztlichen Standpunkte aus. Deutsche Ztschr. f. d. Staatsarznk., Erlang., 1857, n. F., x, 29–36. — **Pravaz.** Remarques sur l'action des muscles de l'œil et sur la guérison de la myopie consécutive à la section de ces muscles. Arch. gén. de méd., Par., 1841, 3. s., xi, 86–91.—**Prouff** (J.-M.) Antagonisme entre la myopie progressive et les forts degrés d'astigmatisme conforme à la règle. Rev. clin. d'ocul., Bordeaux, 1883, iii, 100–104.—**Querenghi** (F.) Alcune considerazioni intorno alla eziologia e patogenesi della miopia. Ann. di ottal., Pavia, 1887, xvi, 27–40. — **Reclam** (C.) Die Bekämpfung der Kurzsichtigkeit der Schuljugend. Gesundheit, Frankf. a. M., 1881, vi, 66–68. — **Reich** (M.) Blizorukost v Zakavkazskom dievichem institutie, v Tiflisskoi voennoi gimnazii i junk. uchilitshie. [Myopia in the Transcaucasian Ladies' Institute, etc.] Med. Sbornik, Tiflis, 1882, xviii, no. 34, 33–85, 1 tab. — **von Reuss** (A.) Ein myopisches Auge mit extrem geringer Wölbung der Linsenflächen. Arch. f. Ophth., Berl., 1880, xxvi, 3. Abth., 1–6. ———. Ueber den Einfluss der Schule auf das Entstehen und Wachsen der Kurzsichtigkeit. Oesterr. ärztl. Vereinsztg., Wien, 1885, ix, 220; 244.—**Risley** (S. D.) A contribution to the clinical history of myopia. Am. J. M. Sc., Phila., 1880, n. s., lxxx, 442–450. ———. Three additional cases of hypermetropic refraction, passing while under observation into myopia. Tr. Am. Ophth. Soc., Bost., 1885, 102–106.—**R[oberts]** (P. F.) Miopia alto con espasmo de la acomodacion y otras lesiones sintomáticas, simulando una fuerte ambliopia; ventajosamente tratada con las instilaciones de atropina y el uso metódico de lentes. Rev. méd.-quir., Buenos Aires, 1884–5, xxi, 189–191. ———. Miopia extrema con insuficiencia de los rectos internos y estrabismo concomitante, divergente, relativo. Ibid., 219–221.—**van Roosbroeck** (J.) Considérations sur la myopie. Mém. Acad. roy. de méd. de Belg., Brux., 1857–63, iv, 209–269. Also: Ann. d'ocul., Brux., 1861, xlv, 130–178. Also [Abstr.]: Bull. Acad. roy. de méd. de Belg., Brux., 1861, 2. s., iv, 128–136. [Discussion], 1862, 2. s., v, 458; 803: 1863, 2. s., vi, 38; 277. — **Santos Fernandez** (J.) ¿La miopia es un producto de la civilizacion? Crón. méd.-quir. de la Habana, 1886, xii, 532–539. — **Schiess-Gemuseus.** Traumatische Myopie, langsame spontane Restitution. Klin. Monatsbl. f. Augenh., Stuttg., 1881, xix, 384–386.—**Schiötz** (H.) Om Myopi. Norsk Mag. f. Lægevidensk., Christiania, 1883, xiii, 304–321.—**Schleich.** Klinisch statistische Beiträge zur Lehre von der Myopie. Mitth. a. d. ophth. Klin. in Tübing., 1882, i, 3. Hft., 1–62.— **Schmidt** (H.) Einige Bemerkungen zu dem Vortrage Burchardt's: "Ueber den Einfluss, den Sehschwäche und Kurzsichtigkeit auf die Militair-Diensttauglichkeit haben". Deutsche mil.-ärztl. Ztschr., Berl., 1874, iii, 16–21.—**Schmidt-Rimpler** (H.) Ueber Chorioideal-Colobome mit Berücksichtigung ihrer Beziehungen zur Myopie. Arch. f. Ophth., Berl., 1880, xxvi, 2. Abth., 221–235. ———. Zur Frage der Schulmyopie. Ber. ü. d. Versamml. d. ophth. Gesellsch., Stuttg., 1885, xvii, 146–155. Also: Arch. f. Ophth., Berl., 1885, xxxi, 4. Abth., 115–182. ———. Noch einmal die Myopie am Frankfurter Gymnasium. Ibid., 1886, xxxii, 2. Abth., 301–306.—**Schnabel** (J.) Zur Lehre von den Ursachen der Kurzsichtigkeit. Arch. f. Ophth. Berl., 1874, xx, 2. Abth., 1–70. ———. Ueber den Einfluss der Augenarbeit auf die Entwicklung der Kurzsichtigkeit. Anz. d. k. k. Gesellsch. d. Aerzte in Wien, 1874–5, 9.—**Schneller.** Ueber Entstehung und Entwicklung der Kurzsichtigkeit. Arch. f. Ophth., Berl., 1886, xxxii, 3. Abth., 245–360. — **Schöler** (H.) Acute Entwicklung hochgradiger Myopie unter dem Bilde der Hemeralopie. Deutsche Klinik, Berl., 1874, xxvi, 11–13.—**Seely** (W. W.) Myotics and glaucoma. Cincin. Lancet & Clinic, 1878, xl, 249. ———. Weiteres über die Entstehungsweise der Myopie. Klin. Monatsbl. f. Augenh., Stuttg., 1885, xxiii, 278–282.—**Seggel.** Die objective Bestimmung der Kurzsichtigkeit beim Musterungsgeschäfte. Aerztl. Int.-Bl., München, 1876, xxiii, 127–130. ———. Die Zunahme der Kurzsichtigkeit an den höheren Unterrichtsanstalten. Ibid., 1878, xxv, 341–346. Also: Centr.-Ztg. f. Kinderh., Berl., 1878–9, ii, 312. ———. Ueber Anisometropie, deren Häufigkeit im Allgemeinen und als Uebergangsstadium zur Myopie. Cong. périod. internat. d. sc. méd. Compt.-rend. 1884, Copenh., 1886, iii, sect. d'ophth., 118–129. — **Sigismund** (R.) Untersuchungen über Myopie und Hypermetropie. Berl. klin. Wchnschr., 1881, xviii, 255–258.— **Smith** (P.) On means for the prevention of myopia. Ophth. Rev., Lond., 1886, v, 153–170. — **Solomon** (J. V.) The value of intra-ocular myotomy in myopia. Rep. Internat. Ophth. Cong. 1872, Lond., 1873, iv, 66–69. Also, transl.: Cong. périod. internat. d'ophth. 1872 Par., 1873, iv, 71–75.—**Somonte** (J. M.) Un caso de hipermiopia. Rev. de cien. méd., Barcel., 1885, xi, 249–252. — **Steffan.** Die Myopie am Frankfurter Gymnasium. Arch. f. Ophth., Berl., 1886, xxxii, 1. Abth., 267–274.—**Steinheil** (A.) Einige Notizen über M. Burgl's: "Beiträge zur Aetiologie

Myopia.

der Kurzsichtigkeit ". Aerztl. Int.-Bl., München, 1874, xxi, 467.—**Stellwag von Carion** (K.) Ueber das Verfahren mit Kurzsichtigen auf dem Assentplatze. Wien. med. Wchnschr., 1860, x, 81; 102; 117.—**Stilling** (J.) Eine Studie zur Kurzsichtigkeitsfrage. Arch. f. Augenh., Wiesb., 1885-6, xv, 133-158, 3 diag. *Also, transl.* [Abstr.]: Arch. Ophth., N. Y., 1886, xv, 296-310, 1 pl., 2 tab. ——. Ueber Entstehung der Myopie. Ber. ü. d. Versamml. d. ophth. Gesellsch., Stuttg., 1886, xviii, 2. Hft., 14-26. ——. Ricerche anatomiche sopra l' influenza dei muscoli nella forma dell' occhio, specialmente in riguardo allo sviluppo della miopia. Gior. d. r. Accad. di med. di Torino, 1887, 3. s., xxxv, 237-239.—**Strack.** Observation sur un homme myope d'un œil et præsbyte de l'autre. J. de méd., chir., pharm., etc., Par., 1763, xix, 459.—**Straub** (M.) Ueber die Dehnung des hinteren Bulbustheils bei Myopie. Arch. f. Ophth., Leipz., 1887, xxxiii, 3. Abth., 84-92. *Also, transl.:* Nederl. Tijdschr. v. Geneesk., Amst., 1887, xxiii (2. d.), 357-363.—**Szili** (A.) Szerzett rövidlátóság rendkivüli esetei. [Unusual cases of acquired myopia.] Szemészet, Budapest, 1886, 25-27.—**Tavignot.** Qu'est ce que la brachyopie? Gaz. d. hôp., Par., 1855, xxviii, 110.—**Theobald** (S.) An endeavour to show that insufficiency of the internal recti muscles and myopia have been erroneously associated; and that the muscular asthenopia of myopia is not the result of such insufficiency, but of the anomaly of refraction. Am. J. M. Sc., Phila., 1874, n. s., lxvii, 65-77. *Also,* Reprint. *Also* [Rap. de Bribosia]: Bull. Acad. roy. de méd. de Belg., Brux., 1878, 3. s., xii, 306-349, 1 pl.—**Titeca.** Pathogénie et prophylaxie de la myopie. Mém. couron. Acad. roy. de méd. de Belg., Brux., 1876-8, iv, 1-135.—**Treichler.** Die Kurzsichtigkeit als Folge von Missgriffen in unserer Erziehungsmethode. Tagebl. d. Versamml. deutsch. Naturf. u. Aerzte, Baden-Baden, 1879, lii, 344-347. *Also:* Med.-chir. Centralbl., Wien, 1880, xv, 436; 448.—**Tscherning** (M.) Studien über die Aetiologie der Myopie. Arch. f. Ophth., Berl., 1883, xxix, 1. Abth., 201-272.—**Ulrich** (R.) Untersuchungen über den Zusammenhang von Convergenz und erworbener Myopie. Klin. Monatsbl. f. Augenh., Stuttg., 1885, xxiii, 433-446.—**Unterharnscheidt.** Zur Entstehungsweise der Netzhautablösung bei Myopie. Berl. klin. Wchnschr., 1881, xviii, 585-589. ——. Ein Fall von Zerreissung einer Arteria hyaloidea persistens in Folge von progressiver Myopie. Klin. Monatsbl. f. Augenh., Stuttg., 1882, xx, 449-452.—**Vanden Bergh.** Du développement de la myopie, considéré au point de vue du surmenage scolaire. Clinique, Brux., 1887, i, 163-166.—**Verdese.** Genesi della miopia. Ann. di ottal., Pavia, 1886, xv, 507-521.—**Verhütung** (Zur) der überhandnehmenden Kurzsichtigkeit unter der Schuljugend. Oesterr. ärztl. Vereinsztg., Wien, 1878, ii, 191.—**Veszely** (K. K.) Zur Genese der Myopie. Wien. med. Wchnschr., 1887, xxxvii, 1119; 1150; 1173.—**Waidele** (C.) Ueber Myopie und Presbyopie. Memorabilien, Heilbr., 1861, vi, 31-34.—**Wallace** (W. C.) On myopia. Lond. M. Gaz., 1842-3, xxxi, 412; 444. *Also:* Boston M. & S. J., 1844, xxx, 274; 289; 317.—**Weidlich** (J.) Die quantitativen Beziehungen zwischen der Pupillenverengung und der scheinbaren Abnahme der Kurzsichtigkeit. Arch. f. Augenh., Wiesb., 1885, xv, 175-178.—**Weiss** (L.) Einen neuen ophthalmoskopischen Befund am myopischen Auge und seine Bedeutung. Tagebl. d. Versamml. deutsch. Naturf. u. Aerzte, Baden-Baden, 1879, lii, 339-342. ——. Beiträge zur Anatomie des myopischen Auges. Mitth. a. d. ophth. Klin. in Tübing., 1882, i, 3. Hft., 63-117, 3 pl. ——. Ueber den an der Innenseite der Pupille sichtbaren Reflexbogenstreif und seine Beziehung zur beginnenden Kurzsichtigkeit. Arch. f. Ophth., Berl., 1885, xxxi, 3. Abth., 239-320, 1 pl. ——. Ueber die ersten Veränderungen des kurzsichtigen, bezw. kurzsichtig werdenden Auges. Ber. ü. d. Versamml. d. ophth. Gesellsch., Stuttg., 1885, xvii, 138-146.—**Williams** (H. W.) Near-sightedness a disease, and not merely an infirmity. Boston M. & S. J., 1865-6, lxxiii, 69-72. *Also:* Extr. Rec. Bost. Soc. M. Improve. (1862-6), 1867, v (app.), 201-204. ——. Separation of retina produced by myopia. Boston M. & S. J., 1868, lxxviii, 266. ——. Curious pathological changes in myopic eyes. *Ibid.*, 1874, xci, 412-415.—**Windsor** (T.) Atropine in the treatment of short sight. Liverpool & Manchester M. & S. Rep., 1873, i, 12-15. *Also,* Reprint.—**Wojciechowski.** Projekt eines Apparats zur Erleichterung des Schreibens für Schwachsichtige und Erblindete. Illust. Monatschr. d. ärztl. Polytech., Bern, 1886, viii, 267-269.—**Wright** (C. W.) The true cause of long and short sightedness, together with a few observations on the power to dilate and contract the pupil of the eye at will. N. Am. M.-Chir. Rev., Phila., 1859, iii, 704-707.

Myosin.

Chittenden (R. H.) & **Whitehouse** (H. H.) On some metallic compounds of albumen and myosin. [*From:* Tr. Connect. Acad., 1886, vii.] Stud. Lab. Physiol. Chem. (1885-6), N. Haven, 1887, ii, 95-125.—**Danilewsky** (A.) Myosin, seine Darstellung, Eigenschaften, Umwandlung in Syntonin und Rückbildung aus demselben. Ztschr. f. physiol. Chem., Strassb., 1881, v, 158-184.

Myosis.

See, also, **Mydriasis,** *etc.*

DUBOS (L.) * Du myosis. 4°. *Paris,* 1874. *Also* [Abstr.], *in :* Rec. d'ophth., Par., 1873-4, 2. s., i, 402-430.

KIRN (C. E.) * Bemerkungen über Pupillen-Verengerungen. 8°. *Tübingen,* 1835.

ROBERTSON (D. A.) Four cases of spinal myosis; with remarks on the action of light on the pupil. 8°. *Edinburgh,* 1869.

WEISSENBORN (J. F.) * De pupilla nimis coarctata vel clausa. 4°. *Erfordiæ,* 1773.

Carron (J.) Observation sur un resserrement morbifique de la pupille, guéri par les frictions avec le laudanum liquide de Sydenham sur les paupières, et employé en collyre. Rec. périod. Soc. de méd. de Par., 1802, xiii, 429-431.—**Carson** (W.) [Significance of "contraction of the pupil" as a symptom.] Cincin. Lancet & Obs., 1873, xvi, 112-119.—**Colby** (M. F.) Contraction of the pupil as a symptom of thoracic tumour. Med. Chron., Montreal, 1858-9, vi, 199.—**Dmitrovski** (D.) Myosis spastica u subekta ve pojilome vozrastie, hipermetropia, neupotreblenie ochkove [in an old person]. Med. Vestnik, St. Petersb., 1881, xxi, 121.—**Giraud-Teulon.** Myosis. Dict. encycl. d' sc. méd., Par., 1876, 2. s., ii, 308-311.—**Hempel.** Ueber die Spinalmyosis. Arch. f. Ophth., Berl., 1876, xxii, 1.—**Lindsay** (W. L.) Use of belladonna in various affections marked by contracted pupils; and on the non-susceptibility of the dog to the action of certain poisons. Assoc. M. J., Lond., 1854, 509.—**MacDonnell** (R. L.) Contraction of the pupil a symptom of intra-thoracic tumours. Med. Chron., Montreal, 1858-9, vi, 64-72.—**Reuling** (J.) A case of myosis caused by paralysis of the left side of the cervical portion of the sympathetic, in consequence of a gun-shot wound. Arch. Ophth. & Otol., N. Y., 1874-5, iv, 228-230. *Also:* Virginia M. Month., Richmond, 1875-6, ii, 423-425.—**Robertson** (D. A.) Four cases of spinal myosis, with remarks on the action of light on the pupil. Edinb. M. J., 1869-70, xv, 487-493. —**Russell.** Congenital myosis. Med. Times & Gaz., Lond., 1870, ii, 392. — **Woodman** (W. B.) Enlarged glands in the neck, with well-marked contraction of pupil. Clin. Lect. & Rep. Lond. Hosp., 1864, i, 205-207.

Myositis.

See Muscles (*Inflammation of*).

Myositis ossificans.

See Muscles (*Ossification in*).

Myotics.

See Mydriasis, *etc.* ; Pilocarpus, *etc.*

Myotomy.

See Tenotomy.

Myotonia congenita.

See Thomsen's *disease.*

Myrdacz (Paul) [1847 -]. Sanitäts - Geschichte und Statistik der Occupation Bosniens und der Hercegovina im Jahre 1878; mit Benützung amtlicher und anderer authentischen Quellen. xii, 420 pp. 8°. *Wien u. Leipzig, Urban u. Schwarzenberg,* 1882.

——. Sanitäts-Geschichte der Bekämpfung des Aufstandes in der Hercegovina, Süd-Bosnien und Süd-Dalmatien im Jahre 1882; nach amtlichen und anderen authentischen Quellen dargestellt. 3 p. l., 208 pp., 1 map. 8°. *Wien, L. W. Seidel u. Sohn,* 1885.

——. Ergebnisse der Sanitäts-Statistik des k. k. Heeres in den Jahren 1870-82. Mit vergleichender Berücksichtigung der Jahre 1883-5, sowie der Sanitäts-Statistik fremder Armeen. Mit xxxviii Tabellen und xvii graphischen Beilagen, nach den militär-statistischen Jahrbüchern und anderen authentischen Quellen bearbeitet. vii, 334 pp., 14 ch., 3 diag. 8°. *Wien, L. W. Seidel u. Sohn,* 1887.

Also, Co-Editor of: **Jahrbuch** für Militär-Aerzte, Wien, 1879.

Myréen (Oskar). * Om cirrhos i lefvern. 70 pp. 8°. *Helsingfors, J. C. Frenckell & Son,* 1860.

Myrepsus (Nicolaus). Liber de compositione medicamentorum secundum loca, translatus e

Myrepsus (Nicolaus)—continued.

græco in latinum a Nicolao Rhegino Calabro, ante hac nusquam impressus, cum brevissimis annotationibus locorum difficilium Joannis Agricolæ Ammonij. 266 l. 4°. *Ingolstadii, A. Vueissenhorn,* 1541.

————. The same. De compositione medicamentorum opus.

In: MEDICÆ artis principes. fol. [*Francofurti*], 1567, ii, pt. 2, 337–884.

————. Medicamentorum opus, in sectiones quadraginta octo digestum, hactenus in Germania non visum, omnibus tum medicis tum seplasiariis mirum in modum utile, a Leonharto Fuchsio e græco in latinum recens conversum, luculentissimisque annotationibus illustratum. 7 p. l., 586 col., 4 l. roy. 8°. *Basileæ, per J. Oporinum,* 1549.

Myriapoda.

DE SAUSSURE (H.) Diagnose de divers myriapodes nouveaux. 8°. [*n. p.,* 1859.]

Cutting from: Linnæa entomologica, 1859, xiii, 328–332.

Guldensteeden-Egeling (C.) Ueber Bildung von Cyanwasserstoffsäure bei einem Myriapoden. Arch. f. d. ges. Physiol., Bonn, 1882, xxviii, 576–579. — **Heathcote** (F. G.) On a peculiar sense organ in Scutigera coleoptrata, one of the myriapoda. Quart. J. Micr. Sc., Lond., 1885, n. s., xxv, 253–260, 1 pl.—**Metschnikoff** (E.) Zur Embryologie der Myriapoden. Mélanges biol. Acad. imp. d. sc. de St.-Pétersb., 1872, viii, 739–741.

Myrica *cerifera.*

HALE (E. M.) Pathogenesis of Myrica cerifera. 8°. *Detroit, Mich.,* 1868.

Myringectomy.

See Ear (*Surgery of*).

Myringitis.

See Ear (*Diseases of, Catarrhal, etc.*); Membrana *tympani* (*Diseases of*).

Myringodectomy.

See Membrana *tympani* (*Surgery of*).

Myringomycosis.

See Auditory *canal* (*Parasitic disease of*).

Myristica.

See Nutmeg.

Myrmecophagidæ.

MASSMANN (J. C.) Descriptio osteologica cranii Myrmecophagæ tetradactylæ. 4°. *Berolini,* 1823.

TUCH (J. A.) * Descriptio osteologica capitis Myrmecophagæ jubatæ. 4°. *Berolini,* 1821.

Pouchet (G.) Sur la composition vertébrale du tamanoir (Myrmecophaga jubata L.). J. de l'anat. et physiol., etc., Par., 1872, viii, 539–549.

Myrrh.

BECKER (S. A.) * De myrrha. 4°. *Jenæ,* [1676].

FÜLLEBORN (J. G.) * De eximia myrrhæ genuinæ virtute. 4°. *Francof. ad Viadr.,* [1746].

Also, in: CARTHEUSER (J. F.) Diss. nonn. select. physchym. ac med. 12°. *Francof. ad Viadr.,* 1775, 28–55.

Pavesi (C.) Della gomma resina e suoi preparati e specialmente dell' estratto acquoso di mirra jodo-ferroso. Indipendente, Torino, 1876, xxvii, 190–194. — **Polisius** (G. S.) Myrrhologia seu myrrhæ disquisitio curiosa . . . variisque medicamentis illustrata. Misc. Acad. nat. curios. 1687, Norimb., 1707, decuria 2, vi, 7 p. l., 343 pp. [bound after app.]. — **Rode** (C. N.) Gummi-resina balsamodendri myrrhæ og dets Forbindelser. Norsk Mag. f. Lægevidensk., Christiania, 1866, xx, 43–47. — **de Savignac** (D.) La myrrhe et ses propriétés thérapeutiques. Bull. gén. de thérap., etc., Par., 1871, lxxxi, 481–494.

Myrtle.

LINARIX (E.-C.) * De l'emploi du myrtol, ou essence de myrte, principalement dans les maladies des voies respiratoires et génito-urinaires. 4°. *Paris,* 1878.

Myrtle.

Delioux de Savignac (J.-F.-J.-A.) La myrte et ses propriétés thérapeutiques. Bull. et mém. Soc. de thérap. 1874, Par., 1875, 87–102. *Also:* Bull. gén. de thérap., etc., Par., 1876, xc, 165; 217.

Myrtle (Andrew Scott). On jaded brains. (Read before the Northumberland and Durham Medical Society, December 8, 1864.) 8 pp. 8°. *London, M. & M. W. Lambert,* [*n. d.*]

For Biography, see Prov. M. J., Leicester, 1887, vi, 193, port.

Mysing (Georgius Ernestus Fridericus). * De hæmorrhoidibus mucosis vesicæ urinariæ ab infarctibus ortis. 32 pp. 8°. *Jenæ, lit. Maukianis,* 1795.

Mysophobia.

See, also, Insanity (*Anomalous, etc.*)

Dana (C. L.) Folie du doute and mysophobia. Alienist & Neurol., St. Louis, 1884, v, 512–519.—**Hammond** (W. A.) Mysophobia. Neurol. Contrib., N. Y., 1879, i, 40–54. *Also* [Abstr.]: Med. Rec., N. Y., 1879, xv, 426.—**Russell** (I.) Mysophobia; melancholia with filth dread, mania contaminationis. Alienist & Neurol., St. Louis, 1880, i, 529–533. — **Tamburini** (A.) Sulla misofobia e le idee fisse ed impulsive. Atti Cong. gen. d. Ass. med. ital. 1882, Modena, 1883, x, 329–331.—**Verga** (A.) Sulla rupofobia. Arch. ital. per le mal. nerv., Milano, 1881, xviii, 194: 1882, xix, 101: 1883, xx, 246.

Mysore. Annual medical and sanitary reports; also, reports on hospitals and dispensaries, and special hospitals [the lunatic and leper asylums] in Mysore, for the years 1877–80, and on vaccination for the year 1880–81, by the surgeon to the Mysore government to the chief commissioner. fol. [*Bangalore,* 1878–81.]

————. Annual reports on special hospitals in Mysore [lunatic asylum and leper asylum], for the years 1877–80. fol. [*n. p.,* 1878–81.]

Bound with preceding.

————. Annual reports on hospitals and dispensaries in the province of Mysore, for the years 1877–80. fol. [*Bangalore,* 1878–81.]

Bound with preceding.

————. Report on leprosy in the province of Mysore. By J. Henderson. Bangalore, 10. Jan., 1878. 4 pp. fol. [*Calcutta,* 1879.]

————. Annual reports on vaccination in Mysore, to the chief commissioner, by the surgeon to the commission, for the years 1878–9 to 1880–81. fol. [*Bangalore,* 1879–81.]

1880–81 *bound with:* Annual Med. and San. Rep. for 1880. *See, also,* **India.** *Madras, Mysore.*

Mysore.

See Hospitals (*Descriptions, etc., of*), *by localities.*

Mysteria physico-medica, ob augustissimos suos natales, uberrimamque rerum haud quotidianarum, quibus referta sunt, segetem, curioso obtutu quam maxime veneranda. Multis abhinc seculis Syriace, Arabice, et Græce conscripta; iterata nunc vice e membranis Latinis publicæ luci exposita. 201 pp., 6 l. 16°. *Francofurti, J. J. Erythropilus,* 1681.

Another edition of "Moderante auxilio redemptoris supremi, Kirani Kiranides," etc., Lips., 1638, in 8°, ed. Andr. Rivinis.

Mystery *in medicine.*

See Quacks, *etc.*

Mystics.

See, also, Ecstasy.

Charbonnier. Maladies et facultés diverses des mystiques. Art méd., Brux., 1875-6, xi, 98–103.

Mysz (Martinus). * Diss. sistens viduam xxx. annorum chlorosi laborantem. 20 pp., 2 l. 4°. *Jenæ, lit. Tennemannianis,* [1752].

For Biography, see **Kaltschmied** (Car. Frid.)

Mytilus *edulis.*

See Mussels.

Myxine.

FÜRBRINGER (P.) * Die Muskeln des Kopf-skelets der Myxine glutinosa unter speciel-ler Würdigung der Kaufunction. 8°. *Jena,* 1874.

Blomfield (J. E.) The thread-cells and epidermis of Myxine. Quart. J. Micr. Sc., Lond., 1882, n. s., xxii, 355-361, 1 pl. — **Cunningham** (J. T.) On the struct-ure and development of the reproductive elements in Myxine glutinosa, L. *Ibid.,* 1886-7, n. s., xxvii, 49-76, 2 pl.

Myxœdema.

See, also, **Thyroid** *gland* (*Excision of*).

GIMIÉ (J.-A.) * De la cachexie pachyder-mique (myxœdème des auteurs anglais). 4°. *Montpellier,* 1883.

LANDOUAR (J.-B.) * Une observation de myxœdème. 4°. *Paris,* 1887.

RIDEL-SAILLARD (G.) * De la cachexie pachy-dermique. 4°. *Paris,* 1881.

Abbott (C. E.) A case of myxœdema. Brit. M. J., Lond., 1886, i, 1212. — **Allan** (J.) † Necropsy. *Ibid.,* 1884, i, 267. — **Anderson** (J.) † Tr. Clin. Soc. Lond., 1884-5, xviii, 21-24. *Also* [Abstr.]: Brit. M. J., Lond., 1884, ii, 861. *Also* [Abstr.]: Lancet, Lond., 1884, ii, 776-778. — **Anderson** (McC.) Case of myxœdema, very consider-ably improved by treatment. Glasgow M. J., 1884, [4. s.], xxii, 303-306. — **Atkinson** (J. M.) † Proc. W. Lond. Med.-Chir. Soc. 1884-6, Lond., 1887, ii, 32-35. — **Ball** (A. B.) The possible relation of myxœdema to absence or disease of the thyroid gland. N. York M. J., 1884, xxxix, 253. — **Ballet** (G.) Cachexie pachydermique. Progrès méd., Par., 1880, viii, 605. — **Barling** (G.) † Necropsy. Lan-cet, Lond., 1886, ii, 970. — **Bianchi** (A.) La cachessia pachidermica o missœdema. Sperimentale, Firenze, 1883, lii, 420-435. — **Blaise** (H.) De la cachexie pachyder-mique; observation nouvelle avec aliénation mentale transitoire. Arch. de neurol., Par., 1882, iii, 60 ; 141. — **Botkin** (S. P.) Myxœdema. Ejened. klin. gaz., St. Petersb., 1887, vii, 449 ; 473. — **Bourneville & d'Olier.** Note sur un cas de crétinisme avec myxœdème. Progrès méd., Par., 1880, viii, 709-711. — **Brandes** (L.-J.) Un cas de myxœdème. Cong. périod. internat. d. sc. méd. Compt.-rend. 1884, Copenh., 1886, ii, sect. de méd., 66-69. — **Bry-ant** (W. H.) † Med. Rec., N. Y., 1886, xxx, 545. — **Cam-pana** (R.) Mixœdema. Salute: Italia med., Genova, 1883, 2. s., xvii, 273 ; 297, 1 pl. — **Cavafy** (J.) Two cases of myxœdema. Tr. Clin. Soc. Lond., 1881-2, xv, 87-92, 1 pl. — **Charcot.** Myxœdème, cachexie pachydermique ou état crétinoïde. Gaz. d. hôp., Par., 1881, liv, 73-75. — **Chevallereau** (A.) Myxœdème aigu consécutif à l'extirpation du corps thyroïde. France méd., Par., 1886, ii, 1493 ; 1505. — **Clouston.** † Edinb. M. J., 1880-81, xxvi, 743. — **Coxwell** (C. F.) A child with symptoms resem-bling those of myxœdema. Tr. Clin. Soc. Lond., 1882-3, xvi, 75-79. *Also:* Lancet, Lond., 1883, i, 101. *Also:* Brit. M. J., Lond., 1883, i, 110. — **Cushier** (Elizabeth M.) † Arch. Med., N. Y., 1882, viii, 203-218. *Also,* Reprint. — **Davies** (A.) A case of myxœdema in a male. Tr. Clin. Soc. Lond., 1886-7, xx, 267. ———. † *Ibid.,* 268. — **De Barbieri** (A.) Salute: Italia med., Genova, 1885, xix, 650-657. — **Drewitt** (F. D.) † Tr. Clin. Soc. Lond., 1883-4, xvii, 49-51, 1 pl. *Also* [Abstr.]: Brit. M. J., Lond., 1883, ii, 1072-1074. [Discussion], 1079. *Also:* Med. Press & Circ., Lond., 1883, n. s., xxxvi, 466-468. — **Duckworth** (D.) † Lancet, Lond., 1879, ii, 577. ———. On a case of myxœdema, or a universal mucoid degen-eration of the connective tissue of the body. Tr. Clin. Soc. Lond., 1879-80, xiii, 12-14. *Also* [Abstr.]: Med. Press & Circ., Lond., 1879, n. s., xxviii, 331. ———. Two cases of myxœdema. Med. Press & Circ., Lond., 1880, n. s., xxx, 411. *Also:* Med. Times & Gaz., Lond., 1880, ii, 632. *Also:* Tr. Clin. Soc. Lond., 1880-81, xiv, 53-58. — **Dunlop** (J. D.) † Proc. South. Austral. Branch Brit. M. Ass., Adelaide, 1883, 45. *Also:* Australas. M. Gaz., Syd-ney, 1883, ii, 218. — **E.** O myxœdema. Gaz. d. hosp. mil., Lisb., 1879, iii, 25. — **Edes** (R. T.) † Clinical lecture. Bos-ton M. & S. J., 1884, cx, 385. — **Erb** (W.) Ueber Myxœ-dema. Berl. klin. Wchnschr., 1887, xxiv, 33. — **Féris** (B.) Myxœdème et béribéri, ou hydroparésie névrovasculaire. Gaz. hebd. de méd., Par., 1883, 2. s., xx, 383-389. — **Fies-singer** (C.) Contribution à l'étude de la cachexie pachy-dermique. Rev. méd. de l'est, Nancy, 1881, xiii, 301-304. *Also:* Mém. Soc. de méd. de Nancy (1880-81), 1882, p. lxix, pt. 2, 102-106. — **Fournier** (A.) Un cas de myxœdème et quelques réflexions sur la pathogénie de cette affection. Gaz. hebd. de méd., Par., 1882, 2. s., xix, 55-59. — **Fraser** (D.) A case of myxœdema with recovery, which was marked by profuse perspiration. Med. Times & Gaz., Lond., 1884, ii, 572. — **Fuchs** (A.) Myxödem. Prag. med. Wchnschr., 1887, xii, 125. — **Gimeno** (A.) La pa-quidermia cretinoide. Crón. méd., Valencia, 1881-2, v, 481-486, 1 pl. — **Goodhart** (J. F.) Sporadic cretinism and myxœdema. Med. Times & Gaz., Lond., 1880, i, 474-

Myxœdema.

476. ———. A case which presented the clinical, but not the pathological, characteristics of myxœdema. Tr. Clin. Soc. Lond., 1881-2, xv, 94-98. — **Gordon** (J.) Myxœdema following upon removal of the thyroid gland. Lancet, Lond., 1886, ii, 65-67. [*See, also, infra,* Richardson (B. W.)] — **Gowans** (W.) † Brit. M. J., Lond., 1882, i, 772. — **Grocco** (P.) Il mixœdema e la malattia di Bright. Ann. univ. di med. e chir., Milano, 1883, cclxiii, 3-34. — **Guerlain-Dudon.** Cachexie pachydermique consécutive à un traumatisme du cou. Bull. et mém. Soc. de chir. de Par., 1882, n. s., viii, 783-788. — **Gull** (W. W.) On a cretinoid state supervening in adult life in women. Tr. Clin. Soc. Lond., 1874, vii, 180-185. ———. Sur le myxœdème. Arch. gén. de méd., Par., 1879, 7. s., iii, 677-685. — **Hadden** (W. B.) † Tr. Clin. Soc. Lond., 1880-81, xiv, 58-61. ———. Du myxœdème. Progrès méd., Par., 1880, viii, 603 ; 625. ———. The nervous symptoms of myxœdema. Brain, Lond., 1882, v, 188-196. ———. Fatal cases of myxœdema. St. Thomas's Hosp. Rep. 1885, Lond., 1886, xv, 276. ———. Myxœdema and its pathology. Cong. périod. internat. d. sc. méd. Compt.-rend. 1884, Copenh., 1886, ii, sect. de méd., 61-66. — **Hamilton** (A. McL.) A case of myxœdema, with a consideration of the neurotic origin of the disease. Med. Rec., N. Y., 1882, xxii, 645-651. *Also:* Med. News, Phila., 1882, xli, 694-696. ———. A case of myxœdema in the male. J. Nerv. & Ment. Dis., N. Y., 1885, n. s., x, 180-182. — **Hammond** (W. A.) On myxœdema, with special reference to its cerebral and nervous symptoms. Neurol. Contrib., N. Y., 1881, i, no. 3, 36-43. *Also:* St. Louis Clin. Rec., 1880-81, vii, 97-100. — **Handford** (H.) A case for diagnosis; myxœdema or elephantiasis. Tr. Clin. Soc. Lond., 1886, xix, 327-329. — **Harley** (J.) The pathology of myxœdema as illustrated in a typical case. Med.-Chir. Tr., Lond., 1884, lxvii, 189-204. *Also* [Abstr.]: Proc. Roy. M. & Chir. Soc. Lond., 1883-4, n. s., i, 237-240. *Also* [Abstr.]: Lancet, Lond., 1884, i, 706. *Also* [Abstr.]: Brit. M. J., Lond., 1884, i, 762. — **Hartmann** (H.) Observation de myxœdème. France méd., Par., 1884, i, 867; 881. — **Henrot** (H.) Des lésions anatomi-ques et de la nature du myxœdème. Union méd. et scient. du nord-est, Reims, 1882, vi, 353-365, 2 pl. *Also:* Assoc. franç. pour l'avance. d. sc. Compt. rend. 1882, Par., 1883, xi, 729-737. — **Holland** (J. W.) Remarks upon a case of myxœdema. Am. Pract., Louisville, 1882, xxvi, 129-134. — **Hopkins** (J.) † Lancet, Lond., 1881, ii, 998. ———. Two cases of myxœdema. Tr. Clin. Soc. Lond., 1885, xviii, 332-334. — **Horsley** (V.) A recent specimen of artificial myxœdema in a monkey. Lancet, Lond., 1884, ii, 827. ———. The thyroid gland; its relation to the pathology of myxœdema and cretinism. [Abstr.] *Ibid.,* 1133. ———. Further researches into the function of the thyroid gland and into the pathological state produced by removal of the same. Proc. Roy. Soc. Lond., 1886, xl, 6-9. [*See, also, infra,* Richardson (B. W.)] — **Inglis** (T.) Two cases of myxœdema. Lancet, Lond., 1880, ii, 496. — **Jacob** (E. H.) † *Ibid.,* 1884, i, 976. — **Kielland** (K.) To Tilfælde af Myxœdema chronicum. Norsk Mag. f. Lægevidensk., Christiania, 1887, 4. R., ii, 590; 660. — **Kinnier** (D. F.) The history of myxœdema; with the report of a case. Med. Rec., N. Y., 1885, xxvii, 91-93. — **Kirk** (R.) † Glas-gow M. J., 1883, [4. s.], xx, 452. *Also:* Tr. Glasg. Path. & Clin. Soc., 1883-4, i, 1. ———. † Glasgow M. J., 1884, [4. s.], xxi, 1-10. — **Kuster.** Myxœdema; cachexia pachyder-mica. Med. Vestnik, St. Petersb., 1880, xx, 262. — **Lan-dau** (L.) Ueber Myxœdema. Berl. klin. Wchnschr., 1887, xxiv, 183-185. — **Lane** (J. O.) On a case of myxœ-dema, with remarks upon the etiology of the disease. Lan-cet, Lond., 1883, ii, 56. — **Lattey** (A.) † *Ibid.,* 1882, i, 1031. — **Lediard** (H. A.) † *Ibid.,* 1881, i, 696. — **Legrand du Saulle.** Nouveau cas de myxœdème, ou cachexie pachy-dermique. Progrès méd., Par., 1882, x. 81. — **Lloyd** (R. H.) † Tr. Clin. Soc. Lond., 1880-81, xiv, 111-113. *Also* [Abstr.]: Lancet, Lond., 1881, i, 138: 1882, i, 106. *Also:* Med. Press & Circ., Lond., 1881, n. s., xxxi, 53. *Also:* Brit. M. J., Lond., 1881, i, 123. — **Lunn** (J. R.) Cases of myxœdema. Brit. M. J., Lond., 1881, ii, 1017. *Also:* Tr. Clin. Soc. Lond., 1882-3, xvi, 263, 1 pl. ———. Two cases of myxœ-dema, male and female. Tr. Clin. Soc. Lond., 1881-2, xv, 84-87. ———. A case of myxœdema(?) and want of de-velopment of the genital organs. *Ibid.,* 1886-7, xx, 260. — **Lussana** (F.) Mixœdema o sclerodermia? Ann. univ. di med. e chir., Milano, 1886, cclxxvii, 214-243. — **Mac-kenzie** (S.) A case of myxœdema in a male. Tr. Clin. Soc. Lond., 1882-3, xvi, 260. — **Mahomed** (F. A.) The pathology and etiology of myxœdema. Lancet, Lond., 1881, ii, 1078. ———. Case of myxœdema, improving under treatment. Tr. Clin. Soc. Lond., 1881-2, xv, 98-100. *Also:* Med. Times & Gaz., Lond., 1882, i, 318. — **Mercer** (A. C.) Myxœdema. Med. Rec., N. Y., 1881, xix, 421-425. *Also,* Reprint. — **Merklen** (P.) Cachexie pachydermique (œdème crétinoïde, myxœdème). Ann. de dermat. et syph., Par., 1881, 2. s., 259-265. *Also:* Gaz. hebd. de méd., Par., 1881, 2. s., xviii, 295-298. — **Miller** (W. B.) † Brit. M. J., Lond., 1885, i, 429. — **Morvan.** Contribution à l'étude du myxœdème; du myxœdème en basse Bretagne. Gaz. hebd. de méd., Par., 1881, 2. s., xviii, 542; 557; 573; 590. — **Nixon** (C. J.) † Dublin J. M. Sc., 1887, 3. s., lxxxiii,

Myxœdema.

1-9. — **von Noorden** (C.) Der gegenwärtige Stand der Lehre von der Bedeutung der Schilddrüse. II. Zur Entwicklung der Myxödemfrage. München. med. Wchnschr., 1887, xxxiv, 240–244. — **Oliver** (T.) Clinical lecture on myxœdema. Brit. M. J., Lond., 1883, i, 502–504. — **Ord** (W. M.) Clinical lecture on myxœdema. *Ibid.*, 1878, i, 671. ———. On myxœdema, a term proposed to be applied to an essential condition in the "cretinoid" affection occasionally observed in middle-aged women. Med.-Chir. Tr., Lond., 1878, lxi, 57–78, 3 pl. *Also* [Abstr.]: Proc. Roy. M. & Chir. Soc. Lond., 1875–80, viii, 248–251. *Also* | Abstr.]: Brit. M. J., Lond., 1879, ii, 620. ———. Cases of myxœdema. Tr. Clin. Soc. Lond., 1879–80, xiii, 15–19, 1 l., 1 pl. — **Paton.** Case of myxœdema. Glasgow M. J., 1887, [4. s.], xxviii, 425–429. — **Rabère** (C.) Myxœdème et sclérodermie. J. de méd. de Bordeaux, 1880–81, x, 474; 486. *Also:* Mém. et bull. Soc. de méd. et chir. de Bordeaux (1881), 1882, 243–268. — **de Ranse** (F.) La cachexie pachydermique. Gaz. méd. de Par., 1880, 6. s., ii, 673. — **Reverdin** (J.-L.) Contribution à l'étude du myxœdème consécutif à l'extirpation totale ou partielle du corps thyroïde. Cong. franç. de chir. Proc.-verb., etc., 1886, Par., 1887, ii, 25–49. *Also:* Rev. méd. de la Suisse Rom., Genève, 1887, vii, 275; 318. — **Ribbert.** Die neueren Beobachtungen über die Function der Schilddrüse und das Myxödem. Deutsche med. Wchnschr., Leipz., 1887, xiii, 286. — [**Richardson** (B. W.)] Myxœdema. Asclepiad, Lond., 1886, iii, 281–284. — **Riess** (L.) † Berl. klin. Wchnschr., 1886, xxiii, 881. — **Roberts** (M. J.) † Planet, N. Y., 1883, i, 86. — **Robinson** (A. H.) A case of sporadic cretinism, with myxœdema. Tr. Clin. Soc. Lond., 1886–7, xx, 261–264, 1 pl. — **Robinson** (J. A.) Myxœdema. Chicago M. J. & Exam., 1883, xlvii, 467–473. — **Robinson** (T.) † Tr. Willan Soc. Lond. (1883-4), 1885, i, 56. — **Savage** (G. H.) Myxœdema and its nervous symptoms. J. Ment. Sc., Lond., 1879–80, n. s., xxv, 517–519, 1 pl. — **Savill** (T. D.) Case of myxœdema in a male aged twenty-nine. Lancet, Lond., 1885, ii, 899. *Also:* Brit. M. J., Lond., 1885, ii, 916. ———. † Tr. Clin. Soc. Lond., 1885-6, xix, 306–308. — **Semon** (F.) † Tr. Clin. Soc. Lond., 1880–81, xiv, 61–67. — **Seppilli** (G.) Del mixœdema, o cachessia pachidermica. (Riv. crit.) Riv. sper. di freniat, Reggio-Emilia, 1882, viii, 114–123. *Also, transl.:* Alienist & Neurol., St. Louis, 1883, iv, 14–25. — **Shelswell** (O. B.) Cases of hæmorrhagic tendency in myxœdema. Lancet, Lond., 1887, i, 675. — **Stewart** (J.) Myxœdema appearing during the course of chronic tetany. Canada M. & S. J., Montreal, 1887-8, xvi, 70–75. — **Stokes** (W.) Acute myxœdema following thyroidectomy. Brit. M. J., Lond., 1886, ii, 709–711. — **Suckling** (C. W.) Case of myxœdema. Brit. M. J., Lond., 1883, i, 716. *Also:* Bir-

Myxœdema.

mingham M. Rev., 1884, xv, 156–158. *Also* [Abstr.]: Lancet, Lond., 1883, i, 548. ———. Case of myxœdema in a woman aged seventy-six. Lancet, Lond., 1885, i, 889. ———. Sequel to a case of myxœdema in a woman aged seventy-six. Lancet, Lond., 1886, i, 918. — **Thaon** (L.) Cachexie pachydermique. Rev. mens. de méd. et chir., Par., 1880, iv, 614–631. — **Ujfalusy** (J.) A myxo-œdemáról. Orvosi hetil., Budapest, 1887, xxxi, 1193; 1233. *Also, transl.:* Pest. med.-chir. Presse, Budapest, 1887, xxiii, 868; 881. — **Verriest.** † Bull. Soc. de méd. ment. de Belg., Gand et Leipz., 1886, no. 41, 61–63. *Also:* Rev. méd., Louvain, 1886, v, 193–199. ———. † Art méd., Brux., 1886-7, xxii, 185–190. — **Virchow** (R.) Ueber Myxœdema. Berl. klin. Wchnschr., 1887, xxiv, 121–126. *Also:* Wien. med. Bl., 1887, x, 201–205. — **Wadsworth** (O. F.) A case of myxœdema with atrophy of the optic nerves. Tr. Am. Ophth. Soc. 1884, Bost., 1885, iii, pt. 5, 725–727. *Also:* Boston M. & S. J., 1885, cxii, 5. — **Warfvinge** (F. W.) † Hygiea, Stockholm, 1887, xlix, 85–91. — **West** (E. G.) † Autopsy. Boston M. & S. J., 1884, cxi, 50–55. [Discussion], 60. — **Wewer.** † Frauenarzt, Berl., 1887, ii, 525–531. — **White** (E. W.) A case of myxœdema associated with insanity. Lancet, Lond., 1884, i, 974–976. ———. † Postmortem examination. Tr. Clin. Soc. Lond., 1885, xviii, 159–163. *Also:* Brit. M. J., Lond., 1885, i, 381. — **Zielewicz.** Ein Fall von Myxödem mit starker Stomatitis und Hepatitis interstitialis. Berl. klin. Wchnschr., 1887, xxiv, 400.

Myxoma *and myxosarcoma.*

See **Brain** (*Tumors of*); **Nerve** (*Optic, Tumors of*); **Tumors** (*Myxomatous*).

Myxomycetes.

Kent (W. S.) The myxomycetes or mycetozoa; animals or plants. Pop. Sc. Rev., Lond., 1881, n. s., v, 97–116, 2 pl. — **Krukenberg** (C. F. W.) Ueber ein peptisches Enzym in Plasmodium der Myxomyceten und im Eidotter vom Huhne. Untersuch. a. d. physiol. Inst. d. Univ. Heidelb., 1878, ii, 273–286. — **Stahl** (E.) Zur Biologie der Myxomyceten. [*From:* Bot. Ztg., 1884, No. 10-12.] Biol. Centralbl., Erlang., 1884-5, iv, 353–356.

Myzostoma.

Nansen (F.) Anatomie und Histologie des Nervensystemes der Myzostomen. Jenaische Ztschr. f. Naturw., Jena, 1887, n. F., xiv, 267–321, 1 pl.

M'Zab.

Amat (C.) Les eaux du M'Zab. Arch. de méd. et pharm. mil., Par., 1884, iii, 463–471.

N. (C. A.) De vi naturæ medicatrice. Theses in examine pro licentia. 36 pp. 8°. [*n. p., n. d.*]

N. (C. F.) Homœopathy ; its reason. Compiled by . . . 3. ed. 24 pp. 32°. *Boston, O. Clapp & Son*, [1872, *vel subseq.*].

N. (F. D.) Dedicated to ye tercentenary of Edinburgh University. Sketches of ye seven ages of ye Edinburgh student, with apologies to Shakespeare. 1 l., 7 pl. sm. 4°. *Edinburgh,* 1884.

N. (M.)[1] Medela medicinæ. *See* **Nedham** (Marchmont).

N. (M.)[2] Anatomy epitomized and illustrated, containing: I. A concise and plain description of all the parts of the human body; together with their various uses in the animal œconomy. II. A large and choice collection of sculptures, exhibiting a just idea of the figure, size, situation, connection, and uses of the several parts of the body, in seventeen folio copper-plates. 2 p. l., 182 pp., 17 pl. 8°. *London, J. Noon,* 1737.

N. (N.)[1] Della naturale incorruzione de' cadaveri. *In:* RAC. d' opusc. scient. e filol. 16°. *Venezia,* 1732, vii, 341–409.

———. Riflessioni sopra la relazione dell' infirmità ultimamente accaduta in persona delle N. N., distesa nel primo foglio del suo libro intitolato: Risposte ad alcuni consulti, parte prima. *In:* RAC. d' opusc. scient. e filol. 16°. *Venezia,* 1738, xvi, 477–544.

N. (N.)[2]
See [**Wittmann** (Frans Joseph) & **N.** (N.)] Twee verhandelingen. 8°. *Haarlem,* 1825.

N. (R.) En kärt afhandling om kräftan, hwaruti dess orsaker undersökas, och twänne emot samma sjukdom tjenlige medel, hwilka hitintils blifwit hos oss hemlige hållne, läggas för allmänhetens ögon i bästa wälmening. [On cancer, its causes, and two cases in which a proper remedy was applied which has been kept secret hitherto, etc.] 31 pp. 12°. *Stockholm, C. F. Marquard,* 1800.

N. K. P. S.
See **Edle** (Der) Scharbocks- oder Sieber-Klee. 16°. *Budissin u. Görlitz,* 1725.

Naaldenberg (Albertus). *Specimen sistens observationem de lethali inter parturiendum uteri ruptura. 31 pp., 1 l. 8°. *Leovardiæ, D. v. d. Sluis,* 1801.

Naberschulte (Joseph). * Ueber die Aetiologie der Krämpfe im Kindesalter. 30 pp., 1 l. 8°. *Bonn, C. Georgi,* 1879.   C.

Nabert (Jean). *Sur l'hystérie. 24 pp. 4°. *Paris,* 1820, No. 282, v. 162.

Nabias (Barthélemy-Marie-Napoléon). * Jean Prevost, médecin de la ville de Pau, et son catalogue des plantes du Béarn, de la Navarre, du Bigorre et des côtes de la mer depuis Bayonne jusqu'à Saint-Sébastien (1600–60). 143 pp. 4°. *Bordeaux,* 1886, No. 27, 1885-6.

———. *Les Galles et leurs habitants. vii, 9–144 pp. 8°. *Paris, O. Doin,* 1886.

Nabona (Edmond). Du traitement de l'emphysème pulmonaire par l'air comprimé. (Appareil de Waldenburg.) 46 pp., 1 l. 4°. *Montpellier,* 1884, No. 67.

Nabonne (B.) *Sur la fièvre intermittente simple. 25 pp. 4°. *Paris,* 1835, No. 178, v. 287.

Naboth (Martinus). * De auditu difficili. 30 pp., 1 l. 4°. *Halæ Magdeb., lit. C. Henckelii,* [1703].

———. The same. [Recusa?] 30 pp., 1 l. 4°. *Halæ Magdeb., lit. C. Henckelii,* [1703].

———. De organo auditus. Resp. Georgio Münchenrod. 7 l. sm. 4°. *Lipsiæ, lit. C. Gözi,* [1703].

———. De sterilitate. Resp. Joh. Ernest. Kruschius. 14 l. 4°. *Lipsiæ, typ. A. Zeidleri,* [1707].

———. The same. Recusa. 14 l. 4°. *Lipsiæ,* 1709.
Also, in: HALLER. Disp. anat. [etc.] 4°. *Groningæ,* 1750, v, 232–259.

Naceff (Demeter R.) *Beiträge zur Statistik der künstlich eingeleiteten Frühgeburt. 22 pp. 8°. *Würzburg, F. E. Thein,* 1872.

Nachet (A.) Instruction sur l'application du microscope dans la production de la graine des vers à soie. 12 pp., 1 pl. 8°. *Paris, Nachet & fils,* 1872.

Nachet & fils. Catalogue descriptif des instruments de micrographie. 20 pp. 8°. *Paris, E. Martinet,* 1863.

Nachich (G.) *Alcune idee sulle sale d' asilo del Sig. Cochin, primo fondatore delle stesse a Parigi, applicate alla pubblica igiene da . . . 20 pp. 8°. *Padova, Crescini,* 1834. [P., v. 946.]

Nachricht von dem Emser Mineralwasser. 13 pp. 16°. *Wiesbaden, E. F. C. Enden,* 1833.

Nachricht von der Heil- und Verpflegungsanstalt Sonnenstein bei Pirna. *See* **Heil- und Verpflegungsanstalt** Sonnenstein bei Pirna.

Nachricht von dem Krancken-Spital zur Allerheiligsten Dreyfaltigkeit, worinnen dessen Anordnung und Beschaffenheit beschrieben, zugleich aber alle diejenige Ordnungen und Instructiones zusammen getragen worden, welche die, zur Besorgung der Billiot-Hoffmann- und Kirchnerischen Stiftung, von hoch-löbl. n. Oe. Regierung, bestellte Commission zum Behuf dieses Spitals gemachet, und ertheilet hat. 55 pp. fol. *Wienn, J. P. v. Ghelen,* 1742.

Nachricht an das Publikum, die Gesundbrunnen zu Cudowa, Reinertz, Altwasser, Charlottenbrunn, Salzbrunn und Flinsberg, in Schlesien betreffend. 20 pp. sm. 4°. *Breslau, W. G. Korn,* 1777.

Nachricht, wie sich bey jetzigen besorglichen Zeiten das gemeine Land- und Bauers-Volck in dem sächsischen Lande vor der hin und wieder grassirenden Kranckheit präserviren. *See* **Saxony.**

Nachricht von einem Unglücklichen, der durch einen Schuss seine untere Kinnlade verlor, mit der Abbildung seines Zustandes und der Maschine, deren er sich bedient, um die fehlende Kinnlade dadurch zu ersetzen. 6 pp., 1 l., 1 pl. 4°. *Berlin, J. W. Schmidt,* 1799.

Nachricht von zwey neuentdeckten Mitteln für Schwangere und Gebährende. 109 pp. 12°. *Bern, Haller,* 1780.

Nachrichten über die Cholera morbus und ihre schrecklichen Verheerungen im Jahr 1830, mitgetheilt von zwey evangelischen Pastoren im russischen Gouvernement Saratow, nebst einem

Nachrichten über die [etc.]—continued.
Anhang über die Entstehung und Verbreitung
dieser Krankheit, so wie einige Heilmittel gegen
dieselbe. 52 pp. 8°. *Basel, C. F. Spittler*, 1831.

Nachrichten von dem Leben und den Schriften
jeztlebender teutscher Aerzte, Wundärzte, Thierärzte, Apotheker und Naturforscher; hrsg. von
Johann Kaspar Philipp Elwert. 1. Bd. xii,
690 pp., 1 l. 8°. *Hildesheim, J. D. Gerstenberg*,
1799.

Nachrichten von dem Ludwigsbrunner Mi-
neral-Wasser, dessen Bestandtheilen und Heilkräften, so wie von der Lage des Ludwigsbrun-
nens bei Burggräfenrode, im Grossherzogthum
Hessen. 13 pp., 1 l. 8°. *Frankf. a. M., C. Naumann*, 1836.

Nachrichten von dem Selterser Mineral-Was-
ser, dessen Bestandtheilen und Heilkräften sowie von der Lage des Gesundbrunnens zu Niederselters. 28 pp., 1 pl., 1 l. 8°. *Wiesbaden*, 1834.

Nachtel (Henri). * De l'hématocèle péri-utérine.
59 pp. 4°. *Paris*, 1875, No. 355.

——. Fonctionnement de l'ambulance urbaine
de New York, destinée à porter les premiers
secours sur la voie publique, et utilité qu'il y a
d'établir un service de ce genre à Paris. 14 pp.
8°. [*Paris*], *G. Masson*, 1881.

Nachtigal (Gustav). * Ueber Area Celsi. 31 pp.
8°. *Würzburg, Becker*, 1885.

Nachtigal (Gustavus) [1834–85]. * Nonnulla
de venæ portarum thromboseos ætiologia et
symptomatologia, præmissa morbi historia. 46
pp. 8°. *Gryphiæ, F. G. Kunike*, 1857.

Nachtigal (Jo. Wences.) * De submersis.
In: DE WASSERBERG. Op. min. med. et diss. 8°.
Vindob., 1776, iv, 325–344.

Nachtigal (Richard) [1845–]. Die Pathologie des Lungenemphysems, dargestellt nach
der Cellular - Physiologie. 42 pp. 8°. *Berlin,
G. Lange*, 1870.

Nachtrag zum Rathgeber für alle, [etc.] *See*
Schnitzer (Adolph).

Nachweis der Verbandmittel, Apparate, Laza-
reth-Utensilien, Medicamente und Labemittel,
etc., welche der freiwilligen Krankenpflege theils
als nothwendige, theils als nützliche zur even-
tuellen Beschaffung oder zur Bereithaltung in
Musterdepots zu empfehlen sind. Festgestellt
in der Sachverständigen-Conferenz, Berlin, den
6. November 1875. Und mittels Erlasses des
königl. Kriegs-Ministeriums an den Militair-In-
specteur der freiwilligen Krankenpflege vom 19.
Januar 1876 als Richtschnur für die Vereine der
freiwilligen Krankenpflege empfohlen. 24 pp.
8°. *Berlin, J. F. Starcke*, 1876.

Nacquart (Jean-Baptiste) [1780–1853]. * Sur
les phlegmasies aiguës de la poitrine. 52 pp.
8°. *Paris, an XI* [1803]. [*Also, in:* P., v.
1635.]

de Nadaillac (*Vicomte*). Les trépanations pré-
historiques. 11 pp. 8°. *Paris, J. Gervais*, 1879.
Repr. from: Correspondant.

——. Affaiblissement de la natalité en France,
ses causes et ses conséquences. 2. éd. vi,149 pp.,
1 l. 8°. *Paris, G. Masson*, 1886.

Nadal (J.) * I. Du mécanisme suivant lequel se
produit la fracture du calcanéum, quels en sont
les signes? Des indications que présente cette
fracture. Déterminer si les divers appareils
employés jusqu'à ce jour remplissent ces indications. II. [etc.] 72 pp. 4°. *Paris*, 1843, No.
64, v. 407.

Nadau des Islets (E.-L). * De l'inoculation
du chancre mou à la région céphalique, au point
de vue de la distinction à établir entre les deux
virus chancreux, et de la thérapeutique qui leur
est propre. 83 pp. 4°. *Paris*, 1858, No. 284, v.
622.

Nadaud (J.-F.-Angel-Cyprien). * Étude sur les
gangrènes dans les blessures par armes à feu.
42 pp. 4°. *Paris*, 1873, No. 69.

Nadaud (P.-A.-Hilaire). * Paralysies obstétricales des nouveau-nés. 60 pp. 4°. *Paris*, 1872,
No. 282.

Nadaud (Pierre-Paul-Louis). * Sur les furon-
cles de la face. 46 pp. 4°. *Paris*, 1864, No.
74.

Nadeaud (Jean). * Plantes usuelles des Tahi-
tiens. 52 pp., 1 l. 4°. *Montpellier, J. Martel
aîné*, 1864. [P., v. 46.]

Nader (Joseph). * De morbis potatorum. 22 pp.
8°. *Viennæ, typ. Congregationis Mechitaristicæ*,
1842.

——. Oesterreichischer Medizinal - Schematis-
mus. Verzeichniss aller Civil- und Militär-
Aerzte, Wundärzte und Apotheker der österreichischen Monarchie. 292 pp. 8°. *Wien, Tendler u. Comp.*, 1859.

Nadermann ([Joannes] Josephus) [1808–].
* Quædam de febre intermittente soporosa.
25 pp., 2 l. 8°. *Berolini, typ. Nietackianis*, [1832].

Nadherny (Ignaz Florian) [1789–1867]. * De
febre puerperali. 31 l. 8°. *Pragæ, typ. J.
Diesbach vid.*, [1812].

——. Ueber die Verletzungen in gerichtlich-
medizinischer Beziehung für Gerichtsärzte und
Richter. 5 p. l., 148 pp. 8°. *Prag, G. Haase*,
1818.
For Biography, see Wien. med. Presse, 1867, viii, 1097.

Nadrowski (Gulielmus). * De amenorrhœa.
31 pp. 8°. *Regiomontii Pr., Samter et Rathke*,
1849. c.

Näcke (Paul). * Ueber Darmperforation im
Typhus abdominalis. 30 pp. 8°. *Würzburg,
C. J. Becker*, 1873.

Naef (Georgius). * Diss. continens observationes
de scirrho. 22 pp. 4°. *Gottingæ, H. Dieterich*,
[1802].

Näf (Heinrich). * Ueber den Eintritt der Voll-
lendung bei dem Verbrechen der Brandstiftung.
39 pp. 8°. *Zürich, E. Kiesling*, 1851. c.

Naegele (Emil). * Ueber die angeborene Halsfistel (Halskiemen-Fistel). [Wurtzburg.] 50 pp.
8°. *Speyer, D. Kranzbühler*, 1866.

Nägele (Franz Carl) [1777–1851]. Beytrag
zu einer naturgeschichtlichen Darstellung der
krankhaften Erscheinung am thierischen Körper, welche man Entzündung nennet, und ihrer
Folgen: der Zertheilung, der Eiterung, der Verhärtung und des Brandes. xvi, 158 pp., 1 l. 8°.
Düsseldorf, 1804.

——. Erfahrungen und Abhandlungen aus dem
Gebiethe der Krankheiten des weiblichen Geschlechtes. Nebst Grundzügen einer Methoden-
lehre der Geburtshülfe. viii, 451 pp., 4 pl. 8°.
Mannheim, T. Loeffler, 1812.

——. Schilderung des Kindbettfiebers, welches
vom Juni 1811 bis zum April 1812 in der gross-
herzoglichen Entbindungsanstalt zu Heidelberg
geherrscht hat. 48 pp. 8°. *Heidelberg, Mohr u.
Zimmer*, 1812.
Bound with: PITSCHAFT (J. A.) Unterricht [etc.] 12°.
Heidelberg, 1812.

——. Ueber den Mechanismus der Geburt.
67 pp. 8°. *Heidelberg, Engelmann*, 1822.
Repr. from: Deutsches Arch. f. d. Physiol., Halle,
1819, v, 4. Hft.
Imperfect.

——. The same. An essay on the mechanism
of parturition. From the German, by Edward
Rigby. xxii (1 l.), 166 pp. 12°. *London, Callow
& Wilson*, 1829.

——. Das weibliche Becken betrachtet in Beziehung auf seine Stellung und die Richtung
seiner Höhle, nebst Beyträgen zur Geschichte
der Lehre von den Beckenaxen. viii, 126 pp.,
3 pl. 4°. *Carlsruhe, C. F. Müller*, 1825.

Nägele (Franz Carl)—continued.

——. De jure vitæ et necis quod competit medico in partu. 31 pp. 4°. *Heidelbergæ, typ. A. Osswald,* [1826].

——. Lehrbuch der Geburtshülfe für die Hebammen im Grossherzogthume Baden. xvi, 400 pp. 8°. *Heidelberg, J. C. B. Mohr,* 1830.

——. The same. 4. Aufl. xvi, 406 pp. 8°. *Heidelberg, J. C. B. Mohr,* 1839.

——. The same. 5. Aufl. xvi, 407 pp., 1 pl. 8°. *Heidelberg, J. C. B. Mohr,* 1842.

——. The same. 6. Aufl. xvi, 386, 127 pp., 1 pl. 8°. *Heidelberg, J. C. B. Mohr,* 1844.

——. The same. 8. Aufl. xvi, 411 pp. 8°. *Heidelberg, J. C. B. Mohr,* 1850.

——. The same. Manuel d'accouchements, à l'usage des sages-femmes. Trad. de l'allemand par J.-B. Pigné. 383 pp., 1 pl. 8°. *Paris, Vve. Hildebrand,* [n. d.]

——. Katechismus der Hebammenkunst, als Anhang zur zweiten Auflage seines Lehrbuches der Geburtshülfe für Hebammen. 1 p. l., 127 pp. 8°. *Heidelberg, J. C. B. Mohr,* 1834.

——. The same. 3. Aufl. 1 p. l., 127 pp. 8°. *Heidelberg, J. C. B. Mohr,* 1836.

——. The same. Als Anhang zur vierten Auflage seines Lehrbuches der Geburtshülfe für die Hebammen im Grossherzogthume Baden. iv, 127 pp. 8°. *Heidelberg, J. C. B. Mohr,* 1839.
Bound with his: Lehrbuch der Geburtshülfe für Hebammen. 8°. *Heidelberg,* 1839.

——. Das schräg verengte Becken, nebst einem Anhange über die wichtigsten Fehler des weiblichen Beckens überhaupt. vi (1 l.), 118 pp., 16 pl. fol. *Mainz, V. von Zabern,* 1839.

——. The same. 2. Ausg. vi, 118 pp., 16 pl. 4°. *Mainz, V. von Zabern,* 1850.

——. The same. Des principaux vices de conformation du bassin, et spécialement du rétrécissement oblique. Trad. de l'allemand et augmenté de notes par A.-C. Danyau. viii, 272 pp., 16 pl. 8°. *Paris, J.-B. Baillière,* 1840.

——. The same. The obliquely contracted female pelvis, with an appendix on its most important vices of conformation. Transl. from the German, by John Christie, with the notes and plates of M. Danyau. xiii, 134 pp. 8°. *Manchester, W. Irvin,* 1848-9.
Bound with: CLAY (C.) British record of obstetric medicine and surgery. 8°. *Manchester,* 1848-9, ii.

——. Zur Methodologie der Geburtshülfe. Grundzüge der allgemeinen Pathologie und Therapie der Geburt, als Manuscript für seine Zuhörer. 1. Lfg. 56 pp. 8°. *Heidelberg, J. C. B. Mohr,* 1847.
Also, Co-Editor of: **Heidelberger** klinische Annalen, 1825-34. — **Medicinische** Annalen, Heidelberg, 1835-47.
See, also, **Baltz** (Theodorus Fridericus). De ophthalmia catarrhali bellica [etc.] 4°. *Heidelbergæ,* 1816.— **Puchelt** (Bennone Rudolph). Commentatio de tumoribus in pelvi [etc.] 4°. *Heidelbergæ,* 1840. — **Wigand** (Justus Heinrich). Die Geburt des Menschen, [etc.] 8°. *Berlin,* 1820. ——. The same. 8°. *Berlin,* 1839.
For Biography. see Allg. med. Centr.-Ztg., Berl., 1851, xx, 85. *Also:* Arch. gén. de méd., Par., 1851, i, 494-496 (Raige-Delorme). *Also:* Deutsche Klinik, Berl., 1851, iii, 54. *Also:* Med. Alm., Berl., 1852, ix-x.
For Portrait, see **Collection**—van Kaathoven.

Naegele (Hermann Franz Joseph) [1810-51]. * Mogostocia e conglutinatione orificii uteri externi. iv, 43 pp. 8°. *Heidelbergæ, G. Reichard,* 1835.

——. Die geburtshülfliche Auscultation. xii, 140 pp. 8°. *Mainz, V. von Zabern,* 1838.

——. The same. A treatise on obstetric auscultation. Transl. from the German, by Charles West. ix, 120 pp. 18°. *London, H. Renshaw,* 1839.

——. Die Lehre vom Mechanismus der Geburt, nebst Beiträgen zur Geschichte derselben. xv, 243 pp. 8°. *Mainz, V. von Zabern,* 1838.

Naegele (Hermann Franz Joseph)—continued.

——. The same. The theory of the mechanism of labour. [Abstr.] transl. from the German, by John Christie. 42 pp. 8°. *Manchester, W. Irwin,* [n. d.]
Bound with: CLAY (C.) British record of obstetric medicine and surgery. 8°. *Manchester,* 1849, ii.

——. Commentatio de causa quadam prolapsus funiculi umbilicalis in partu, non rara illa quidem, sed minus nota. 30 pp. 4°. *Heidelbergæ, C. Winter,* 1839.

——. Lehrbuch der Geburtshülfe. 1. u. 2. Theil. ix, 320 pp. ; 207 pp. 8°. *Mainz, V. von Zabern,* 1843-5.
Incomplete.

CONTENTS.
1. Theil. Physiologie und Diätetik der Geburt.
2. Theil. Pathologie und Therapeutik der Geburt. 1. Abth.

——. The same. 4. Aufl., besorgt von Dr. Woldemar Ludwig Grenser. xv, 736 pp. 8°. *Mainz, V. von Zabern,* 1854.

——. The same. 5. Aufl., den Fortschritten der Wissenschaft entsprechend bearbeitet und vermehrt von Dr. Woldemar Ludwig Grenser. xvii, 799 pp. 8°. *Mainz, von Zabern,* 1863.

——. The same. 7. Aufl., den Fortschritten der Wissenschaft entsprechend bearbeitet und vermehrt von Woldemar Ludwig Grenser. xxi, 858 pp. 8°. *Mainz, V. von Zabern,* 1869.

——. The same. 8. Aufl., bearbeitet und vermehrt von Dr. Woldemar Ludwig Grenser. xv, 842 pp. 8°. *Mainz, V. von Zabern,* 1872.

—— **& Grenser** (W. L.) The same. Traité pratique de l'art des accouchements. 2. éd. française, traduite sur la 8. et dernière éd. allemande, annotée et mise au courant des derniers progrès de la science par G.-A. Aubenas ; ouvrage précédé d'une introduction par J.-A. Stoltz. xxxii, 816 pp. 8°. *Paris, J.-B. Baillière & fils,* 1880.

Naegele (*Joseph*).
Portrait in: **Collection**—van Kaathoven.

Naegelé (Ortwin) [1815–]. * Historia partus, post matris mortem ope forcipis absoluti. 30 pp., 1 l. 8°. *Berolini, typ. Nietackianis,* [1838].

——. Diätetik der Schwangerschaft. Die wichtigsten Lebensregeln für schwangere Frauen. vii, 73 pp. 24°. *Düsseldorf, W. Kaulen,* 1853.

——. Wasserheilanstalt Marienberg bei Boppard am Rhein, im Februar 1867. [Circular.] 1 l. 8°. [n. p., 1867.]

Nägeli (Carl). Beiträge zur wissenschaftlichen Botanik. 3. Hft. iv, 198 pp., 11 pl. 8°. *Leipzig, W. Engelmann,* 1863.

CONTENTS.
Die Anwendung des Polarisationsmicroscops auf die Untersuchung der organischen Elementartheile.
Untersuchungen über den Flechtenthallus von S. Schwendener. II. Laub- und Gallertflechten.

——. Die niederen Pilze in ihren Beziehungen zu den Infectionskrankheiten und der Gesundheitspflege. xxxii, 285 pp. 8°. *München, R. Oldenbourg,* 1877.

——. Untersuchungen über niedere Pilze aus dem pflanzenphysiologischen Institut in München. 1 p. l., 285 pp. 8°. *München u. Leipzig, R. Oldenbourg,* 1882.
See, also, **Buchner** (Hans). Die Naegeli'sche Theorie. 8°. *Leipzig,* 1877. — **Pijzel** (E. D.) Een revolutionair op het gebied [etc.] 8°. [*Amersfoort,* 1878.] ——. Naegeli's theorie, etc. 8°. *Amsterdam,* 1878.

—— **& Schwendener** (S.) Das Mikroskop ; Theorie und Anwendung desselben. ix, 628 pp. 8°. *Leipzig, W. Engelmann,* 1867.

Nägeli (Caspar). * Ueber das häufige Vorkommen kleinerer Ausdehnungen der Arterien. 29 pp., 1 l. 8°. *Zürich, E. Kiesling,* 1852.

Nägeli (Heinrich)[1]. * Beiträge zur Entwicklungsgeschichte der Räderthiere. 31 pp., 2 pl. 8°. *Zürich, E. Kiesling*, 1852.

Nægeli (Heinrich)[2]. * Ueber die Beziehungen der Lues zur Tabes dorsalis. [Zurich.] 42 pp. 8°. *Glarus, V. Schmid*, 1887.   c.

Naegeli (Louis Aug.) * Ueber den Einfluss der Pilze auf die Bildung von Riesenzellen mit wandständigen Kernen. [Bern.] 20 pp. 8°. *Leipzig, J. B. Hirschfeld*, 1885.

Nägeli (Wilhelm). Beiträge zur Lehre der elektrischen Muskelreizung. 30 pp., 1 l. 8°. *Zürich, F. Walder u. Sohn*, 1861.

Naeghels. * De phthisi pulmonali. 13 pp. 4°. *Parisiis*, 1808, No. 56, v. 70.

Naether (Carolus Fridericus Ephraim.) * De hernia inguinali incarcerata. 34 pp. 8°. *Jenæ, typ. F. Frommanni*, 1838.

Nævius (Carol. Gottlob.) * De phrenitide. 40 pp. sm. 4°. *Gissæ-Hassorum, E. B. Lammers*, [1742].

Nævius (*Caspar*) [1514–79].

Portrait in: **Collection**—van Kaathoven.—**Collection** of Portr. of Phys. & Men of Sc., pp. 9, 125, and 143, 217[b].

Nævius (*Joannes*) [1499–1574].

Portrait in: **Collection**—van Kaathoven.—**Collection** of Portr. of Phys. & Men of Sc., 217[b].

Nævus.

See, also, **Aneurism** *by anastomosis, etc.*; **Angioma,** *etc.*; **Artery** (*Carotid, Ligature of*); **Conjunctiva** (*Tumors of*); **Eyelids** (*Tumors of, Vascular*); **Fœtus** (*Maternal influence on*); **Scalp, Scrotum,** *Nævus of*; **Tumors** (*Cavernous, etc.*)

ARNDT (M.) * De nævo materno. 4°. *Halæ*, [1839].

BOEHM (L. I.) * De nævo nonnulla. 4°. *Berolini*, [1848].

CHAIGNEAU (G.) * Des tumeurs érectiles. 4°. *Strasbourg*, 1867.

FINELLA (F.) Primo libro de nevi. 16°. *Antverpiæ*, 1632.

HECHTEL (J. L.) De nævis maternis. 4°. *Jenæ*, [1688].

INDISCRÉTIONS (Les) de Lavater. Étude inédite par ce professeur célèbre; lithographiée d'après le dessin original de Lavater, qui nous a été communiqué par M. Schwitzer. 2. éd. 1 pl. fol. [*Paris, n. d.*]

KRAUSE (C. C.) Abhandlung von den Muttermälern, welche mit dem, von der kaiserl. Akademie der Wissenschaften zu St. Petersburg, auf das Jahr 1756 ausgesetzten Preise gekrönt worden; nebst einer andern Abhandlung, welche die gegenseitige Meynung behauptet. Aus dem Lateinischen übersetzt von Christian August Wichmann. 4°. *Leipzig*, 1758.

LABOULBÈNE (J.-J.-A.) * Sur le nævus en général, et sur une modification particulière et non décrite, observée dans un nævus de la paupière supérieure. 4°. *Paris*, 1854.

MANDT (C.) * De teleangiectaseos notione et cura. 8°. *Marburg*, [1837].

MATTHIAS (F.) * De telangiectasia. 8°. *Berolini*, [1850].

RAU (W. T.) * De nævis maternis. 4°. *Altorfii*, [1742].

RICHTER (G. G.) [Pr.] de nævis theoriæ medicæ strictim disserens. 4°. *Gottingæ*, [1741].

ROELVINK (H. J.) * Diss. exhibens teleangiectaseos notionem et curam, observationibus illustratam. 8°. *Traj. ad Rhenum*, 1842.

RUMPF (G. A.) * De nævis maternis. sm. 4°. *Duisburgi*, [1816].

SALOMON (M. G.) * De teleangiectasia. 8°. *Heidelbergæ*, 1839.

SCHERZER (H. A.) * Ueber Telangiectasia. 8°. *Leipzig*, [1867].

Nævus.

SEPTALIUS (L.) De nævis liber. 8°. *Patavii*, 1628.

———. The same. Editio postrema emendatior et indiculo auctior. 16°. *Dordrechti*, 1650.

———. The same. 4°. [*Genevæ*, 1687.]

SOLDAN (C. E.) * Akad. afhand. om teleangiectasi. 8°. *Helsingfors*, [1847].

VRIENS (G. H. L.) Over teleangiectasie. 8°. *Rotterdam*, 1860.

Adams (A. L.) On a few abnormalities and certain morbid conditions met with in recruits. Lancet, Lond., 1874, i, 364. — **Agnew** (D. H.) Nævus. Cincin. Lancet & Clinic, 1879, n. s., iii, 434. — **Amundson** (A. C.) Mother's mark. Med. Age, Detroit, 1886, iv, 111. — **Baerensprung.** Nævus unius lateris. Ann. d. Char.-Krankenh. . . . zu Berl., 1863, xi, 2. Hft., 91-95, 1 pl.— **Barthélemy.** Deux observations de nævus zoniformes lisses, l'un pigmentaire, l'autre vasculaire. Ann. de dermat. et syph., Par., 1882, 2. s., iii, 280-284. — **Bennett** (G.) Case of singular nævus maternus. Lond. M. & Phys. J., 1827, n. s., iii, 48, 1 pl.— **Birkett** (J.) Account of the structure of a nævus. Med.-Chir. Tr., Lond., 1847, xxx, 193-198.— **Boardman** (J.) Nævi. Buffalo M. J., 1858-9, xiv, 577-580. — **Bryant** (T.) On nævus. Guy's Hosp. Rep., Lond., 1860, 3. s., vi, 69-74.— **Buchanan** (G.) Clinical lecture on nævus. Brit. M. J., Lond., 1875, i, 831-833. — **Campana** (R.) Sopra alcuni nei materni; studii clinici. Resoc. Accad. med.-chir. di Napoli, 1875, xxix, 31-49, 1 pl.: 1876, xxx, 50-75, 12 pl. — **Carpenter** (G. W.) [Mother's marks.] Peoria M. Month., 1883-4, iv, 404-406.— **Carter** (W. G.) On nævi materni. Lancet, Lond., 1873, i, 87-89.— [**Cases.**] De nævo materno, nulla arte medicabili. Soc. med. Havn. collect., 1775, ii, 112-115. — Nævus maternus. Lancet, Lond., 1850, i, 127. — More than a hundred nævi on the same infant. *Ibid.*, 1858, i, 63. — Ein merkwürdiger haariger Nævus. (Maria der Orang - Utang.) Wien. med. Presse, 1869, x, 877. — Nævi materni. Anfiteatro anat., Madrid, 1871, i, 49. — **Coote** (H.) On nævi materni and dilatations of the vessels of the integument. Lond. M. Gaz., 1850, n. s., x, 412-416. *Also, transl.:* J. f. Kinderkr., Erlang., 1850, xv, 157-163. — **Curling** (T. B.) Observations on nævi, their structure and treatment. Lond. M. Gaz., 1838, n. s., ii, 791; 833. — **Desprès** (A.) Hétérotopie pileuse cutanée congénitale (nævus pilosus occupant presque tout le corps). Gaz. hebd. de méd., Par., 1874, xxi, 244. — **Dubois.** Tache mélanique circumorbitaire congénitale. Ann. d'ocul., Brux., 1855, xxxiv, 265-267. — **Duncan** (J.) Nævus. Edinb. M. J., 1885-6, xxxi, 697-714.— **Erichsen** (J. E.) On nævus Brit. M. J., Lond., 1858, 869.— **Fayrer** (J.) † Nævus. Indian Ann. M. Sc., Calcutta, 1865, No. xix, 81.— **Fergusson.** Extensive rhinoceros nævus. Lancet, Lond., 1859, i, 32.— **Garretson** (J. E.) Nævus. Med. & Surg. Reporter, Phila., 1871, xxiv, 7-9. ———. Melanoid nævus. *Ibid.*, 366-368.— **Geber** (E.) Ueber eine seltene Form von Nævus der Autoren. Vrtljschr. f. Dermat., Wien, 1874, n. s., i, 3-16.— **Gherini** (A.) Dell' angiectania. *In his:* Contrib. a. chir. sui bambini, 8°. Milano, 1876, 7-19, 1 pl.— **Greiner** (A.) Muttermäler (Nævi materni) betreffend. Allg. Wien. med. Ztg., 1863, viii, 278. — **Griffith** (T. T.) On nævus. Brit. M. J., Lond., 1863, ii, 344.— **Guéniot.** Nævus hypertrophique de la région fronto-sourcillière droite chez un enfant de 2 ans. Bull. Soc. de chir., Par., 1871, 2. s., xi, 249.— **Guersant.** Quelques réflexions pratiques sur les tumeurs et taches vasculaires et sur les nævi materni chez les enfants. Bull. gén. de thérap., etc., Par., 1863, lxiv, 494-502.— **Hawkins** (C. H.) Large nævus of the cheek. Lond. M. Gaz., 1834-5, xv, 815. *Also, in his:* . Path. & Surg. Writings, 8°, Lond., 1874, i, 255-257.— **Hickma** (C.) Vascular nævus. Lancet, Lond., 1834, ii, 111.— **Hofmokl.** Teleangiectasie von ungewöhnlicher Ausdehnung; geheilt. Wien. med. Presse, 1881, xxii, 485-487.— **Horrocks** (P.) A case of facial and ocular nævus. Tr. Ophth. Soc. U. Kingdom, Lond., 1882-3, iii, 106 - 108, 1 pl.— **Hosmer.** Case of nævus in a child five months old. Boston M. & S. J., 1875, xcii, 504. — **Hubbard** (G. H.) The big nævus. Tr. M. Soc. N. Y., Albany, 1870, 135-138, 1 pl.— **Jacquin** (C.) Mémoire et observations sur les marques ou taches de naissance. J. gén. de méd., chir. et pharm., Par., 1812, xliv, 121; 245.— **Johnson** (J.) Cases of, and reflections on, nævi materni. West. & South. M. Recorder, Lexington, Ky., 1841-2, i, 506 - 512. — **Krylovski** (M. G.) K kazuist. sosud. novoobraz. koji u novorojden (nævus vascularis) [in new-born infant]. J. akush. i jensk. boliez., St. Petersb., 1887, i, 792-796.— **Landi** (P.) † † Angectasie. *In his:* Clin. chir. n. spedale di Santa Maria d. Scala di Siena, 8°. Siena, 1862 - 4, pt. 2, 61 - 68.— **Larcher** (O.) Nævus maternus. Dict. encycl. d. sc. méd., Par., 1876, 2. s., xi, 368 - 381. — **Leigh** (R.) Ulcerating post-natal nævus. Lancet, Lond., 1886, ii, 867. — **Leopold** (J. H.) Ungeheurer Nævus lenticularis und über die muthmassliche Ursache desselben, als einer Fötuskrankheit. Monatschr. f. Geburtsk. u. Frauenkr., Berl., 1857, x, 362-365.— **Lord** (A.) Case of nævus maternus. Lond. M. Gaz., 1842, n.

Nævus.

s., ii, 690–692.—**Mandelbaum** (W.) Ein Fall von äusserst zahlreichen Telangiektasien der sämmtlichen Haut. Vrtljschr. f. Dermat., Wien, 1882, ix, 213–219.—**Markoe.** Case of nævus. Annalist, N. Y., 1846–7, i, 487. ——. [Extensive nævus in the sole of the foot.] N. York M. Times, 1855–6, v, 167.— **Martin.** Rapport sur le mémoire du citoyen Desgranges, de Morges, en Suisse, dans lequel il établit, par plusieurs observations, que les taches des enfans, nævi materni, sont produites par l'imagination de la mère. Rec. d. actes Soc. de santé de Lyon, 1801, ii, 83–91.—**Melampus.** De nævis corporis tractatus. *In:* Meletius. De natura structuraque hominis opus, etc., sm. 4°, Venetiis, 1552, 189–191.—**Michaelis.** Ueber Muttermähler. J. f. Chir. u. Augenh., Berl., 1830, xiv, 645–650.—**Mott** (V.) Congenital nævus. Am. M. Times, N. Y., 1860, i, 456.—**Muraltus** (J.) Historia nævi materni. Acad. nat. curios. ephem., Norib., 1715, cent. iii–iv, 304, 2 pl.—**Muttermäler** (Die). N. Mag. f. Aerzte, Leipz., 1791, xiii, 349–351. — **Nævi** (On) Lond. M. & Phys. J., 1824, lii, 303.—**Nævus** vasculaire. Rev. phot. d. hôp. de Par., 1869, i, 141.—**Neumann.** Ueber Nerven-Nævus. Mitth. d. Wien. med. Doct.-Coll., 1877, iii, 315–319.—**van Onscnoort** (A. G.) Waarneming van aanmerkelijke met haar begroeide moedervlekken (nævi materni pilaris), over de geheele oppervlakte des ligchaams verspreid. Nederl. Lancet, Utrecht, 1839–40, ii, 25–30, 1 pl. — **Ornstein** (B.) Sehr ausgedehnter Nævus. Verhandl. d. Berl. Gesellsch. f. Anthrop., Berl., 1884, xvi, 99–106. — **Parker** (W. T.) Four cases of nevus maternus, related from the observation of Benjamin Parker. Arch. Pediat., Jersey City, 1884, i, 84–87.—**Pascalis** (F.) Nævi materni; or, remarks on the respective influence of imagination and disease in the formation and deformities of the human fœtus. Med. Reposit., N. Y., 1815, n. s., ii, 1–14, 1 pl.—**Piffard.** Extensive nævus vascularis. J. Cutan. & Genito-Urin. Dis., N. Y., 1887, v, 149. — **Pollock.** A very extensive nævus on the chest of an infant. Lancet, Lond., 1857, ii, 522.—**Pooley** (J. H.) Nævus. N. York M. J., 1873, xvii, 593–617. *Also,* Reprint.—**Profeta** (G.) Neo vascolare. *In his:* Decen. de clin. dermo-sif. d. Univ. di Palermo, 8°, Palermo, 1878, 52–57, 2 pl. — **Richmond** (J. S.) Mother's marks. Tr. Vermont M. Soc. 1881, St. Albans, 1882, 21–30.—**Riley** (R.) Singular case of nævus maternus. N. Orl. M. & S. J., 1852–3, ix, 471.—**Rivington.** Congenital nævoid growth of the cheek; operation; cure. Brit. M. J., Lond., 1877, i, 481.—**Rustomjee** (B.) Nævus of the parts above the left upper lip, and interior of the mouth, causing deformity of the face. Tr. M. & Phys. Soc. Bombay (1860), 1861, n. s., vi (app.), p. xxv.—**Sayre.** Nævus of foot. N. York M. J., 1877, xxv, 60.—**Schaeffer** (M.) Nævus der Mund.- Schlund-, Larynxschleimhaut. Monatschr. f. Ohrenh., Berl., 1881, xv, 183.—**Schirmer** (R.) Ein Fall von Teleangiektasie. Arch. f. Ophth., Berl., 1860, vii, 1. Abth., 119–121.—**Smith** (J. H.) Mother's marks. Mississippi Valley M. Month., Memphis, 1883, iii, 111.—**Smith** (N. R.) Remarks on the vascular nævus, with a new mode of treatment. Maryland M. & S. J., Balt., 1843, iii, 309–313.—**Smith** (T.) Nævus. Lancet, Lond., 1867, ii, 65; 124; 191.—**Stearns** (J.) Remarks on nævi materni, etc., with a case. U. States M. & S. J., N. Y., 1835–6, ii, 289–291.—**Stocker.** Large nævus, involving the whole of the left labium. Lancet, Lond., 1849, ii, 527. — **Subcutaneous** nævus over the anterior fontanelle. *Ibid.,* 1858, i, 505. — **Succow.** Telangiectasien. Med. Cor.-Bl. rhein. u. westfäl. Aerzte, Bonn, 1843, ii. 31. — **Suesserott** (J. L.) Vascular nævi; with report of an interesting case. Med. & Surg. Reporter, Phila., 1859–60, n. s., iii, 37.—**Sym** (J.) Nævus resembling a fatty tumour; removal by excision. Edinb. M. & S. J., 1836, xlv, 20.—**Tracy** (R. T.) Report of a case of nævus. Austral. M. J., Melbourne, 1861, vi, 201. — **Turner** (C. W.) Extensive nævus maternus; varicose veins. Midland M. & S. J., Worcester, 1830–31, ii, 308–310.—**Tyrrell** (G. G.) On nævus maternus and its treatment. Calif. M. Gaz., San Fran., 1869–70, ii, 9–12.—**Unusual** (An) case of nævus maternus. St. Louis M. & S. J., 1868, n. s., v, 220.—**Uytterhoeven** (V.) Cas remarquable de pathologie chirurgicale. Ann. Soc. d. sc. méd. et nat. de Brux., 1839, 43–46.—**Walker** (B.) On two cases of nævus. Med. Times & Gaz., Lond., 1880, i, 232. — **Warren** (J. M.) Nævus over the knee-joint. Am. J. M. Sc., Phila., 1853, n. s., xxvi, 355.— **Werner.** Fall von Nævus pilosus. Verhandl. d. Berl. med. Gesellsch. (1881–2), 1883, xiii, 187.—**West** (R. U.) Observations on mother's marks. Lond. M. & S. J., 1834, v, 467.—**Westmoreland** (W. F.) Nævus; and report of cases. Tr. M. Ass. Georgia, Augusta, 1881, xxxii, 191–217. *Also:* Atlanta M. & S. J., 1884, n. s., i, 321–336.—**Wordsworth** (J. C.) On nævus. Brit. M. J., Lond., 1858, 1062.—**Zeissl.** Zur Pathologie und Therapie des Gefässmuttermales. Wchnbl. d. k. k. Gesellsch. d. Aerzte in Wien, 1862, xviii, 65–70.

Nævus (*Complications and sequelæ of*).

See, also, **Melanosis,** *etc.*

Benzler (H.) *Die Nævi als Ursprungsstätten melanotischer Geschwülste. 8°. *Berlin,* [1880].

Nævus (*Complications and sequelæ of*).

Armaignac (H.) Sarcome fasciculé de la joue ayant succédé à un nævus maternus écorché avec un peigne. J. de méd. de Bordeaux, 1878–9, viii, 148–150.—**Battistini.** Di nævus pigmentarius lypomatodes, hypertrophicus, pilosus. Atti Accad. med. di Roma, 1877, iii, 92–97, 1 pl.—**Bickersteth** (E. R.) Large subcutaneous nævus in process of undergoing a peculiar transformation. Month. J. M. Sc., Lond. & Edinb., 1853, xvi, 513–517.—**Birkett** (J.) Very large nævus of the right arm; spontaneous atrophy. Guy's Hosp. Rep., Lond., 1850–51, 2. s., vii, 291–294, 1 pl.—**Bryant** (T.) Extensive nævus, involving the whole of the right leg, in different stages of development. Tr. Path. Soc. Lond., 1857–8, ix, 186–188, 1 pl. ——. Large nævus involving the upper lip, flattening the front teeth in both jaws from its pressure. *Ibid.,* 1870, 3. s., xv, 237.—**Cabot** (S.) Death following excision of a nævus. Boston M. & S. J., 1864, lxx, 216.—**Churchill** (F.) Compound pedunculated growths of the skin developed from moles: A. Melanotic; B. Warty. Tr. Path. Soc. Lond., 1871, xxii, 314–316, 1 pl. ——. Melanotic pedunculated growth developed upon a mole; excision; recovery. Med. Times & Gaz., Lond., 1872, i, 160.—**Durante** (F.) Un caso raro di neo materno maligno. Bull. d. r. Accad. med. di Roma, 1882, viii, 389–393. ——. Neo materno maligno pigmentato. *Ibid.,* 1884, x, 280–287.—**Duret** (H.) Note sur un cas de sarcome, développé sur un nævus pigmentaire; aspect carcinomateux d'une partie de la tumeur. Arch. de phys. norm. et path., Par., 1873, v, 319–321.—**Galliard** (L.) Dermatome hypertrophique congénital pigmentaire, plan généralisé; (nævus pigmentaire, lichénoïde généralisé). Ann. de dermat. et syph., Par., 1880, 2. s., i, 498–509, 1 pl.—**Gascoyen.** Case of nævus involving the parotid gland, and causing death from suffocation; nævi of the viscera. Tr. Path. Soc. Lond., 1859–60, xi, 267.—**Gay** (J.) Spontaneous cure of nævi materni. Med. Times & Gaz., Lond., 1857, xiv, 146.—**Groos** (O.) Nævus von enormer Ausdehnung, mit excessiver Pigmentablagerung und Haarbildung längs des Rückens. Berl. klin. Wchnschr., 1870, vii, 396.—**Hutchinson.** Tumour of the face, of nævoid origin. Med. Times & Gaz., Lond., 1879, ii, 690.—**Hutchison.** † Degeneration of a mole into an epithelioma. Brit. M. J., Lond., 1878, i, 485.—**Jordan** (F.) On the nævoid origin of some congenital hypertrophies. *In his:* Surg. Enq., 2. ed., 8°, Lond., [1880], 124–126.—**Kröhlein** (R. W.) Ausgedehntes Angioma cavernosum polyposum der Wange, aus einem Nævus hervorgegangen; Exstirpation; Heilung. Arch. f. klin. Chir., Berl., 1877, xxi (Supplhft.), 96.—**Laboulbène.** Sur une modification particulière observée dans un nævus vasculaire. Compt. rend. Soc. de biol. 1853, Par., 1854, v, pt. 2, 197–210.—**Léger.** Dégénérescence précoce d'un nævus. Gaz. méd. de Picardie, Amiens, 1886, iv, 54.—**McShane** (A.) Large nævus in an unusual location [on the right side of the soft palate]. N. Orl. M. & S. J., 1887, n. s., xvi, 436.—**Mathieu** (A.) Sarcome mélanique de la tempe droite ayant débuté par une tumeur érectile veineuse; récidive ganglionnaire; tumeur cérébrale de même nature. Bull. Soc. anat. de Par., 1880, lv, 544–548. *Also:* Progrès méd., Par., 1881, ix, 343.—**Mazzoni** (C.) Sarcoma fusocellulare della natica destra, sviluppatosi da un neo materno dermoidale; cauterizzazione; guarigione. Clin. chir. (Mazzoni), Roma, 1876, iii, 155–157.—**von Mosengeil** (K.) Ein Fall von sehr weit verbreiteten Nævus mit Hypertrophie aller davon befallenen Gewebstheile. Arch. f. klin. Chir., Berl., 1870, ii, 735.—**Olavide.** Nevus vascularis; úlcera varicosa y callosa de la pierna izquierda. Rev. esp. de oftal., sif., etc., Madrid, 1882–3, i, 107–109.—**Paget.** Cases of tumors under moles. Med. Times & Gaz., Lond., 1864, n. s., i, 58.—**Petit** (A.) Nævus pigmentaire de la jambe; transformation sarcomateuse. Bull. Soc. anat. de Par. 1879, liv, 499–502. *Also:* Progrès méd., Par., 1880, viii, 235.—**von Planner** (R.) Ein Fall von Nævus congenitus mit excessiver Geschwulstbildung. Vrtljschr. f. Dermat., Wien, 1887, xiv, 449–476, 2 pl. **Prewitt.** [Sub-cutaneous nævus undergoing cystic degeneration.] St. Louis M. & S. J., 1879–80, xxxviii, 544.—**Scharf** (W. F.) Exstirpation eines Nævus telangiectodes. Ztschr. d. nordd. Chir.-Ver., Magdeb., 1848, ii, 54–59.—**Verbeeck** (W. J. L.) Guérison spontanée d'un nævus maternus (teleangiectasia congenita). Ann. Soc. méd. d'émulat. de la Flandre occid., Roulers, 1850, iv, 256–260.—**Weinlechner** (J.) Mehrere pigmentirte Nævi, wovon einer an der Brustwirbelsäule Krebsig degenerirte; nach dessen fruchtloser Exstirpation entwickelte sich Carcinom der Achseldrüsen und in Knötchenform an der rechten Brustdrüse in rapider Weise; Tod durch Pleuritis mit Carcinom der Pleura. Ber. d. k. k. Krankenanst. Rudolph-Stiftung in Wien, 1878, 308.—**Wood.** Case of subcutaneous venous nævus of the cheek, with phlebolites in the interior. Med. Times & Gaz., Lond., 1865, ii, 468.

Nævus (*Lipomatous*).

See, also, **Nævus** (*Complications, etc., of*).

Hyde (J. N.) A case of congenital nævus lipomatodes. J. Cutan. & Ven. Dis., N. Y., 1885, iii, 193–198, 1 pl.—**Larcher** (O.) Note sur un cas de nævus lipomatodes. Compt. rend. Soc. de biol. 1866, Par., 1867, 4. s., iii, 58–61.

Nævus (*Lipomatous*).

Also: Gaz. méd. de Par., 1866, 3. s., xxi, 493. ———. Nævus lipomatodes. *In his:* Études clin. et anat. path., Par., 1869, 13–16.—**Torri.** Osservazioni riguardanti uno straordinario lipoma. Bull. d. sc. med. di Bologna, 1837, 2. s., iii, 122–127.

Nævus (*Pigmentary*).

See, also, **Nævus** (*Complications, etc., of*); **Nævus** (*Treatment of*).

Arnold (G. J.) Case of nævus; or hypertrophy, corrugation and discoloration of the skin. Boston M. & S. J., 1866, lxxiv, 371. *Also,* Reprint. — **Budzko** (V. A.) Sluch. obshir. rod. pjatna (nævus pigmentosus permagnus s. nigrismus partialis). Med. Obozr. Mosk., 1887, xxvii, 673–680.—**Burnotte** (J.-B.) Conception pendant l'écoulement des règles; taches maternelles, couleur des cheveux. J. de méd. et chir. prat., Par., 1857, 2. s., xxviii, 167.— **Cutaneous** nævus. Lond. M. & S. J., 1834–5, vi, 539.— **De Schweinitz** (G. E.) Two cases of nævus pigmentosus. Phila. M. Times, 1884–5, xv, 441. — **Harvey** (G.) An account of a very unusual mark (nævus?) on the neck of an infant. Lond. M. Gaz., 1846, n. s., ii, 379. *Also:* Lancet, Lond., 1846, i, 417. — **Hyde** (J. N.) Rare form of congenital, multiple, and monolateral pigmentary nævus, having the disposition of zoster corporis. Chicago M. J. & Exam., 1877, xxxv, 377 – 381. — **Manassei** (C.) Su di un caso di neo verrucoso, pigmentario, peloso congenito. Atti Accad. med. di Roma, 1877, i–ii, 253–263, 1 pl. *Also:* Gior. ital. d. mal. ven., Milano, 1877, xii, 227–234, 1 pl.—**Murray** (J.) Extensive and increasing hairy moles in a child. Tr. Path. Soc. Lond., 1873, xxiv, 257–259, 1 pl.—**Sherwell** (S.) Remarks on and queries as to relative frequency of pathological changes in moles and other tumors on face and head. J. Cutan. & Genito-Urin. Dis., N. Y., 1887, v, 9–12. *Also* [Abstr.]: Med. News, Phila., 1886, xlix, 296. *Also:* Med. Rec., N. Y., 1886, xxx, 305. *Also:* J. Am. M. Ass., Chicago, 1886, vii, 303. — **Variot** (G.) Lésions de la peau dans la mélanodermie congénitale et dans le nævus pigmentaire circonscrit. Compt. rend. Soc. de biol., Par., 1887, 8. s , iv, 257.

Nævus (*Treatment of*).

Appia (L.) * Des tumeurs sanguines érectiles et spécialement de leur traitement par les injections au perchlorure de fer. 4°. *Paris,* 1877.

Colson (A.) * Des taches vineuses et de leur traitement par les scarifications. 8°. *Paris,* 1878.

Drouin (L.) * Traitement des tumeurs érectiles par l'électrolyse. 4°. *Paris,* 1878.

Gravenhorst (G. C. B.) * De teleangiectasia, ejusque curandi ratione. 8°. *Traj. ad Rhenum,* [1835].

Squire (B.) Essays on the treatment of skin diseases. No. III. On port-wine mark and its obliteration without scar. 8°. *London,* 1876.

Adams. On the subcutaneous application of the ligature for deep-seated nævi. Med. Times, Lond., 1851, n. s., ii, 178.—**Albers.** Ueber die Behandlung der Telangiectasie mit Kuhpockenlymphe; Brechweinstein-Salbe, Auflösung und Pflaster. Med. Cor.-Bl. rhein. u. westfäl. Aerzte, Bonn, 1843, ii, 253.—**Appia.** Observations de tumeurs érectiles traitées par le perchlorure de fer. (Extrait d'un travail inédit envoyé à la Soc. de méd. de Bordeaux.) Union méd. de la Gironde, Bordeaux, 1860, v, 155–159, 1 pl.—**Assandri** (G.) Di un caso di neo materno passato allo stato di fungo sanguigno; cura con soluzione di sublimato corrosivo sciolto nel collodion. Gazz. med. ital. lomb., Milano, 1857, 4. s., ii, 161.—**Aubert.** Nævus pigmentaire traité avec succès par le raclage. Mém. et compt.-rend. Soc. d. sc. méd. de Lyon (1879), 1880, xix, pt. 2, 171–173.—**Baker** (W. M.) On the removal, by operation, of a hairy mole occupying half the forehead. [Abstract.] Proc. Roy. M. & Chir. Soc. Lond., 1878, viii, 255–257.—**Barwell** (R.) On scarless eradication of nævi. Lancet, Lond., 1875, i, 642.—**Bateman** (H.) Letter on the treatment of nævus by tartarised antimony plaster. *Ibid.,* 1869, ii, 660.—**Beard** (G. M.) Letter to a surgeon who inquires the best method of treating nævi by electricity. Arch. Electrol. & Neurol., N. Y., 1875, ii, 17. ———. Large mother's marks treated by electrolysis. *Ibid.,* 76. ———. Cases of nævi treated by electrolysis. N. York M. J., 1877, xxvi, 616–619.—**Bellamy.** Large congenital nævus of face; operation; recovery. Brit. M. J., Lond., 1871, ii, 668.—**Bellingham** (O'B.) Cases of nævus treated by the seton. Dublin M. Press, 1848, xx, 97.— **Bérard** (A.) Mémoire sur le traitement des tumeurs érectiles. Gaz. méd. de Par., 1841, 2. s., ix, 689–698. *Also:* Ann. de méd. belge, Brux., 1841, iv, 242–254.— **Bernard** (P. M.) Case of nævus of the eyelid cured by platinum wire heated red hot by galvanism. Med. Times & Gaz., Lond., 1852, n. s., iv, 318.—**Birkett** (J.) Subcutaneous nævus, or growth of erectile tissue on the side of

Nævus (*Treatment of*).

the face, tied with a subcutaneous ligature. Guy's Hosp. Rep., Lond., 1850-51, 2. s., vii, 294–298, 1 pl. ———. Very remarkable case of nævus; operation; recovery. Lancet, Lond., 1855, ii, 226. ———. Venous capillary nævus in cutaneous and subcutaneous tissue of back; removal by excision. Med. Times & Gaz., Lond., 1871, ii, 189.—**Blair** (J.) Nævus treated successfully by local application of liquor arsenicalis. Brit. M. J., Lond., 1884, i, 761.—**Bobbs** (J. S.) Two cases of nævi, in infants, treated by ligation and excision, and exci-ion alone. Indiana J. M., Indianap., 1870–71, i, 33–37.—**Böing.** Zur Behandlung der Telangiectasien. Deutsche med. Wchnschr., Berl., 1886, xii, 290.—**Bradley** (S. M.) Large veno-cutaneous nævus treated successfully by repeated injections with carbolic acid. Brit. M. J., Lond., 1876, i, 443.—**Brandt** (G. H.) A new operation for nævus. Practitioner, Lond., 1870, v, 348.—**Brodhurst** (B. E.) Of the treatment of nævus. Med. Times & Gaz., Lond., 1852, n. s., iv, 474.—**Brown** (J.) Large nævus of the lower lip removed by ligatures. Med. Times, Lond., 1849, xx, 180. — **Browning** (G.) Letter on the treatment of nævus with collodion. Med. Times & Gaz., Lond., 1859, xl, 513.—**Browning** (J. H.) Eradication of nævi by electrolysis. Australas. M. Gaz., Sydney, 1881–2, i, 162.—**Brunton** (J.) Treatment of nævus by sodium ethylate. Lancet, Lond., 1878, ii, 625. ———. Treatment of nævus and other diseases by ethylate of sodium. *Ibid.,* 1881, i, 176.—**Campana** (R.) Sopra alcuni nei materni. Gior. ital. d. mal. ven., Milano, 1876, xi, 257-287.—**Carpenter** (Julia W.) The removal from the skin of papilloma, pigmentary moles, and superfluous hair; with report of cases. Cincin. Lancet & Clinic, 1886, n. s., xvii, 515–520.—**Carter** (R. B.) Case of death following the subcutaneous injection of a nævus. Med. Times & Gaz., Lond., 1863, ii, 262; 1864, i, 683. *Also, transl.:* Ann. d'ocul., Brux., 1864, lii, 214–218.—**del Castillo de Piñeiro** (E.) Nævus del labio inferior; operacion por la sutura elástica; curacion. An. de obst., ginepat. y pediat., Madrid, 1886, 2. ép., vi, 5.—**de Ceulencer** (H.) Études sur le nævus maternus. Ann. Soc. de méd. prat. de la prov. d'Anvers, Malines, 1849, vii, 313–343.— **Chassaignac.** De la destruction chirurgicale des envies, ou taches maternelles de la peau. Union méd. de la Gironde, Bordeaux, 1856, i, 571–575.—**Choisy.** Tumeurs érectiles traitées par des injections de perchlorure de fer. Soc. d. sc. méd. de Gannat. Compt. rend , Gannat, 1860, xiv, 28.—**Christopher** (J. C.) New mode of applying ligatures to nævi. Lancet, Lond., 1845, i, 676. ———. On the removal of nævi. *Ibid.,* 1862, i, 366.—**Clark** (F. LeG.) Cases of nævus treated in various ways. Med. Times & Gaz., Lond., 1862, i, 76.—**Clutton** (H. H.) Nævi of the face treated by electrolysis. St. Thomas's Hosp. Rep. 1881, Lond., 1882, n. s., xi, 49-52.—**Coates** (W. M.) The treatment of nævi. Brit. M. J., Lond., 1883, ii, 318–320.—**Colvan** (J.) Treatment of nævus. Dublin M. Press, 1856, xxxv, 140.—**Coombs** (C.) A new method of treating subcutaneous nævi. Lancet, Lond., 1881, ii, 374.—**Cordier** (F.- S.) Mémoire sur la possibilité de faire disparaitre, par le moyen du tatouage, certaines taches, ou nævi materni, de la peau. Rev. méd.-chir. de Par., 1848, iv, 25–28. — **Costilhes.** Cas rare de nævus maternus guéri par un traitement antisyphilitique. Rev. méd. franç. et étrang., Par., 1851, i, 464-466. *Also:* Ann. de méd. belge, Brux., 1851, iii, 129–131.—**Curling** (T. B.) Observations on the treatment of nævi materni, with cases of removal of these growths from different parts of the face without deformity. Lond. M. Gaz., 1850, xlv, 133–138, 2 pl. — **Cutaneo-subcutaneous** nævus in mastoid region of an infant; operation by ligature (under the care of Mr. Haynes Walton). Med. Times & Gaz., Lond., 1872, i, 96.—**Dawson** (B. F.) On vascular nævi, and their treatment by the actual cautery. Am. J. Obst., N. Y., 1871, iv, 513-532. *Also,* Reprint. ———. Treatment of vascular nævi with the galvanic cautery. Am. J. Obst., N. Y., 1874, vii, 137-140.—**Delore** (X.) Traitement des tumeurs érectiles. Lyon méd., 1879, xxx, 145-155. *Also:* Mém. et compt.-rend. Soc. d. sc. méd. de Lyon (1879), 1880, xix, 2-14, pt. 2. [Discussion], 3. ———. Du traitement des tumeurs érectiles par l'électrolyse. Gaz. méd. de Par., 1884, 7. s., i, 481.—**Denis.** Quelques réflexions sur le traitement des tumeurs érectiles. Arch. de la méd. belge, Brux., 1842, viii, 254–257.—**Dieffenbach** (J. F.) Operation der Angiektasien, Telangiektasien und farbigen Muttermäler. *In his:* Operat. Chir , 8°, Leipz., 1845, i, 234-247. *Also, transl.:* Brit. Rec. Obst. M. & S., Manchester, 1848, i, 32 ; 74 ; 138 ; 169.—**Doubleday** (E.) Case of nævus cured by puncture. Brit. Ann. Med., Pharm., etc., Lond., 1837, i, 49.—**Douglas** (J. R. A.) The actual cautery for nævi. Lancet, Lond., 1866, i, 328. — **Duncan** (J.) On galvano-puncture of nævus. Edinb. M. J., 1870, xv, 777–781. *Also,* Reprint. ———. The treatment of nævus. Edinb. M. J., 1875-6, xxi, 703-710. *Also,* Reprint.—**Durham.** Removal of nævus from behind the ear. Guy's Hosp. Gaz., Lond., 1873, ii, 59.—**Edwards** (S.) Cutaneous nævi cured by the application of iodine paint. Med. Times & Gaz., Lond., 1855, x, 540. — **Effect** (The) of injections of carbolic acid into vascular tumours. N. York M. J., 1879, xxix, 318-321.—**Erichsen** (J. E.) Cases of nævi, with a new mode of

Nævus (*Treatment of*).

applying the ligature to particular forms of these growths. Lancet, Lond., 1851, ii, 31.—**Fagan** (J.) Notes and remarks on the treatment of three cases of nævus. Dublin J. M. Sc., 1881, 3. s., lxxi, 80–83. — **Fawdington** (T.) Cure of subcutaneous nævus by the seton. Lond. M. Gaz., 1834, xv, 157–159.—**Fergusson.** The treatment of nævi by compression, or strangulation by a peculiar knot; cutaneous cancer of the hand; amputation. Lancet, Lond., 1850, n. s., ii, 421.—**Fochier.** Note sur l'ablation des tumeurs érectiles avec le thermo-cautère. Mém. et compt.-rend. Soc. d. sc. méd. de Lyon (1878), 1879, xviii, pt. 2, 165–168.—**Forster** (C.) Treatment of nævus by the injection of perchloride of iron. Med. Times & Gaz., Lond., 1853, n. s., vii, 654.—**Fox** (G. H.) The treatment of wine-mark by electrolysis. Tr. M. Soc. N. Y., Syracuse. 1882, 319–323. *Also:* Arch. Med., N. Y., 1882, vii, 166–171.—**Frölich** (T.) Ueber die Behandlung der Nævi materni vasculares durch Einimpfung von Kuhpocken. Ztschr. f. Wundärzte u. Geburtsh., Stuttg., 1857, x 96–102.—**Gallozzi.** Angioma curato in una bimba facilissimamente colla spilli-pressione Morgagni, Napoli, 1878, xx, 682–684. — **Gamberini** (P.) Il raschiamento nella cura di talune malattie cutanee applicato in un caso di doppio neo sanguigno alla facia. Gior. ital. d. mal. ven., Milano, 1876, xi, 288.—**Gauran.** Tumeur érectile de la région sourcillière gauche opérée par le thermo-cautère et en voie de guérison. Union méd. de la Seine-Inf., Rouen, 1882, xxi 29–31.—**Gazzo** (J. B. C.) Facts, relative to the action of nitrate of silver, and the process of treating nævus with nitric acid. Med. & Surg. Reporter, Phila., 1875, xxxiii, 343–345.—**Giese.** Entfernung eines grossen Nævus. Gen.-Ber. d. k. rhein. Med.-Coll. 1830, Koblenz, 1833, 94.—**Giraldès.** Gefässmutter-mäler im Gesichte und deren Behandlung. J. f. Kinderkr., Erlang., 1863, xli, 104–106. — **Gnocchi** (G.) Note terapeutiche sulla cura di tumori erettili e della guarigione di un caso col metodo del Wardrop. Riv. ital. di terap edig., Piacenza, 1884, iv, 9–15.—**Grose** (S.) Sodium ethylate for nævi. Lancet, Lond., 1879, ii, 220.—**Hall** (M.) On a new and simple mode of operation for nævus. Lond. M. Gaz., 1831, vii, 677. ——. On the treatment of vascular nævus. Lancet, Lond., 1834, ii, 43.—**Hammond** (W. A.) Three cases of the successful treatment of vascular tumors by injection with the fluid extract of ergot. Arch. Clin. Surg., N. Y., 1876, i, 123.—**Hardaway** (W. A.) Note on the treatment of port-wine mark by electrolysis. St. Louis Cour. Med., 1886, xv, 201–206. *Also,* Reprint.—**Harris** (R. P.) Case of venous erectile nævus, cured by subcutaneous vaccination by means of many-eyed needles. Am. J. Obst., N. Y., 1871, iv, 20–27.— **Herrmann** (A.) Das gefärbte Muttermal (Nævus, Spilus). Vrtljschr. f. d. prakt. Heilk., Prag, 1864, lxxxii, 128–133.—**Hewett** (P.) Excision of a bleeding nævus. Lancet, Lond., 1870, ii, 565.—**Hewitt** (C. N.) Hypodermic injection of the solution of per-sulphate of iron for the cure of nævi materni. Cincin. M. Repert., 1868, i, 233–235.—**Heyfelder** (O.) Teleangiektasie am Vorderarme; Écrasement linéaire; Heilung. Med. Ztg., Russlands, St. Petersb., 1860, xvii, 162.—**Hodges.** Injection of a nævus with perchloride of iron. Boston M. & S. J., 1864, lxx, 60.—**Hoffmann.** Salpetersaures Silberoxyd gegen Molenbildung. Med. Ztg., Berl., 1848, xvii, 97.—**Hoggan** (F. E.) Three venous nævi successfully removed by means of the elastic ligature. Med. Exam., Lond., 1876, i, 481.—**Hudson** (S.) A case of hypodermic injection of nevus. Ohio M. J., Columbus. 1881–2, i, 16. *Also:* Brit. M. J., Lond., 1881, ii, 845.—**Hulke.** Operation for the cure of nævus. Med. Times & Gaz., Lond., 1870, ii, 122.—**Jægerschmits.** Nævus maternus traité et radicalement guéri par le caustique de Vienne. Bull. gén. de thérap., etc., Par., 1818, xxxv, 29.—**Jordan** (F.) The piecemeal excision of nævi. Brit. M. J., Lond., 1869. i, 490.—**Joynes** (L. S.) Case of nævus successfully treated by the application of collodion. Richmond & Louisville M. J., Louisville, 1868, v, 170–172.—**Kingston** (S.) Treatment of nævus by adhesive or suppurative inflammation. Lancet, Lond., 1862, i, 420. — **Knott** (S. J.) Forty cases of nævi successfully treated with electrolysis. *Ibid.*, 1875, i, 402.—**Lagout.** Efficacité de l'acide nitrique dans le traitement des nævi-materni. Rap. gén. d. trav. Soc. d. sc. méd. de Gannat, 1856–7, xi, 28.—**Lamoureux** (J.) Observation d'un nævus-maternus, traité d'après le procédé du docteur A. Withe. J. de la sect. de méd. Soc. Acad. Loire-Inf., Nantes, 1830, vi, 14. — **Large** (A.) nævus of the lower lip removed by ligatures. Lancet, Lond., 1849, n. s., i, 174.—**Laroyenne.** De quelques modifications apportées au traitement des tumeurs érectiles, soit par l'excision, soit par la cautérisation. Lyon méd., 1878, xxix, 537–542. *Also:* Mém. et compt.-rend. Soc. d. sc. méd. de Lyon (1878), 1879, xviii, 166–172. — **Lawrence** (W.) On the treatment of nævi materni by ligature. Med.-Chir. Tr., Lond., 1827, xiii, 420–443. — **Legendre** (F.-L.) Sur le traitement des nævi materni vasculaires (tumeurs érectiles) par l'inoculation vaccinale. Arch. gén. de méd., Par., 1856, i, 513–526. — **Legrand** (A.) Nævi materni guéris par la vaccination. Rec. de proc.-verb. . . . Soc. de méd. prat., Par., 1860, 144–146.—**Little** (J. L.) On the treatment of nævus maternus. [Abstr.] Med. News, Phila., 1883, xlii, 551.—**Lloyd** (E. A.) Ob-

Nævus (*Treatment of*).

servations on the treatment of vascular nævi materni. Lond. M. Gaz., 1836, xix, 13–20.—**Losada y Rodriguez** (F.) Tratamiento del onixis y de los tumores eréctiles por el percloruro de hierro. Siglo méd., Madrid, 1878, xxv, 151–153.—**Lucas-Championnière** (P.) Traitement du nævus par les scarifications multiples. J. de méd. et chir. prat., Par., 1878, xlix, 205–208.—**Luke** (J.) On extirpation of "capillary aneurism" by ligature. Lond. M. Gaz., 1848, n. s., vi, 581–583, 1 pl.—**Maclean** (D.) Large nævus of face; electrolysis; good result. Physician & Surg., Ann Arbor, Mich., 1884, vi, 400.—**Makovski** (A.) K' laicheniyu uprugikh opukholei sosudistago storeniya. [Treatment of telangiectasia.] Med. Sbornik, Tiflis, 1867, pt. 2, 13–29.—**Malgaigne.** Observations de nævi materni. traités avec succès par le procédé de M. Fayolle modifié. Gaz. d. hôp., Par., 1848, 2. s., x, 248. *Also:* Rev. méd.-chir. de Par., 1848, iii. 307–311.—**Marjolin.** Vaccination des tumeurs érectiles. [Discussion.] Bull. Soc. de chir. de Par., 1851, i, 641–647.—**Michalski** (A.) Tumeur érectile veineuse de la muqueuse labiale; ligature; guérison. Bull. Soc. méd. de l'Yonne, Auxerre, 1871, xii, 98–104.—**Mitchell** (B. C.) Maternal nævi treated with carbolic acid. Texas Cour.-Rec. Med., Fort Worth, 1884–5, ii, 19–21.—**Monoyer.** Enfant de 11 mois, porteur d'une tumeur érectile de la paume de la main, réduite à moins de moitié de son volume après quatre séances de galvanocaustique chimique. Mém. Soc. de méd. de Nancy (1876–7), 1878, p. lxii.—**Moore** (W.) On the removal of nævi and encysted tumours. Dublin M. Press, 1854, xxxii, 369.— **Murray** (J. J.) Removal by ligature of large subcutaneous nævi without loss of skin. Lancet, Lond., 1864, i, 321–323.—**Nævi** over the angles of the ribs and in the perinæum; successful removal. *Ibid.*, 1861, i, 362.—**Negretto** (A.) La cura degli angiomi col metodo di Macke. Gazz. med. ital. lomb., Milano, 1885, 8. s., vii, 313–316—**Neumann** (I.) Zur Behandlung des Nævus vascularis und des Nævus spilus. Wien. med. Presse, 1865, vi, 599–601.—**Newman** (W.) On the electrolysis of nævi. *In his:* Surg. Cases, 8°, Lond., 1881 (app.), pp. i–x. *Also,* Reprint.—**Notta.** Mémoire sur le traitement des tumeurs érectiles. Année méd., Caen, 1877, ii, 180–190: 1878, iii, 8–10. — **[Nunn.]** New operation for the radical cure of nævus. Lancet, Lond., 1866, i, 456.— **Ormsby** (L. H.) Case of venous nævus on face treated by ligature. Med. Press & Circ., Lond., 1881, n. s., xxxii, 26.— **Owen** (E.) On the treatment of large nævi, Brit. M. J., Lond., 1883, ii, 320.—**Paget** (T.) Fatal convulsion during the injection of nævus. Lond. M. Gaz., 1837. n. s., i, 529.— **Pancoast** (J.) An account of a successful operation for erectile tumour after the manner of Lallemand. Med. Exam., Phila., 1838, i, 92.—**Parker** (R. W.) On the treatment of nævus by excision; to which is appended a clinical analysis of 564 cases of nævus; together with the microscopic nature of this condition. Tr. Clin. Soc. Lond., 1886, xix, 279–289. *Also* [Abstr.]: Med. Press & Circ., Lond., 1886, n. s., xli, 495. *Also:* Lancet, Lond., 1886, i, 1069. — **Partridge** (S. B.) Two cases of vascular tumor treated by injection with a saturated watery solution of tannin. Indian M. Gaz., Calcutta, 1866, i, 36.—**Paul** (C.) Deux cas de guérison de tumeurs érectiles par la vaccination. Courrier méd., Par., 1877, xxvii, 322. *Also:* Bull. et mém. Soc. de thérap. 1877, Par., 1878, 2. s., iv, 65–68. ——. Du traitement des tumeurs érectiles par la vaccination. Bull. Acad. de méd., Par., 1881, 2. s., x, 1157–1165.— **Pauli.** Ueber das Feuermaal und die einzig sichere Methode, diese Entstellung zu heilen. J. f. Geburtsh., Leipz., 1835, xv, 66–72.—**Paxton** (J.) On the treatment of subcutaneous nævus, with a case. Glasgow M. J., 1856–7, iv, 287–289. *Also,* Reprint.—**Penhall** (J.) Treatment of nævus. Lancet, Lond., 1881, i, 530.—**Pinolini** (F.) Il termo-cauterio nella cura delle teleangiectasie. Ann. di ostet., Milano, 1881, iii, 38–44.—**Pitoy** (H.) Traitement des nævi vasculaires par l'électrolyse (monopuncture positive). Union méd. et scient. du nord-est, Reims, 1886, x, 169–177.—**Pols** (E. T.) Electrolyses in the treatment of vascular nævi. Med. Herald, Louisville, 1879–80, i. 457.— **Pujo.** Traitement par les caustiques des maladies désignées sous les noms divers de nævi materni, signes, spili, taches de naissance (envies), tumeurs érectiles, tumeurs fongueuses sanguines, tumeurs variqueuses artérielles, veineuses; angiectasie, fongus hématodes. J. de méd. de Bordeaux. 1857, 2. s., ii, 65; 143; 193.—**Quain** (R.) A case of unusually large nævus successfully treated. Proc. Roy. M. & Chir. Soc. Lond., 1857, i, 124–131, 1 pl.—**Quantin.** Note sur le traitement des tumeurs vasculaires sanguines de la peau. Union méd., Par., 1881, 3. s., xxxii, 103.—**Quelques** remarques sur deux cas de nævi materni, traités avec succès par la vaccination. Bull. gén. de thérap., etc., Par., 1853, xliv, 534–537.—**Ragaine.** Des nævi materni; de leur traitement par l'inoculation vaccinale. J. de méd., chir. et pharmacol., Brux., 1873, lvi, 402; 522.— **Redard** (P.) Du traitement des tumeurs érectiles par l'électrolyse. Gaz. méd. de Par., 1887, 7. s., iv, 517.—**Richardson** (B. W.) On sodium ethylate in the treatment of nævus and other forms of disease. Proc. M. Soc. Lond., 1879–81, v, 257–261. ——. Further researches on ethylate of sodium in the treatment of nævus and other forms of disease, with observations on ethylate of potassium. Lan-

Nævus (*Treatment of*).

cet, Lond., 1881, i, 168; 242. ———. An improvement in the treatment of nævus by sodium ethylate. Asclepiad, Lond., 1885, ii, 253.—**Richardson** (E. S.) Iodine in nevi. Med. Summary, Lansdale, Pa., 1879-80, i, 244-246.—**Sadler.** Vaccination einer Teleangiectasie. Ztschr. f. d. ges. Med., Hamb., 1838, ix, 371.—**de Saint-Germain** (L.-A.) Traitement des tumeurs érectiles chez l'enfant. Gaz. d. hôp., Par., 1883, lvi, 441. ———. Mort à la suite d'une injection de liqueur de Piazza; cautérisation tubulaire des tumeurs érectiles par la pâte de Vienne. Rev. mens. d. mal. de l'enf., Par., 1884, ii, 426-437.—**Santesson** (C.) Om vådan af klorjern-insprutning vid behandling af teleangiektasier, och sättet att densamma förekomma. [Danger of injection of chloride of iron in treatment of telangiectasia.] Hygiea, Stockholm, 1866, xxviii, 53-57. *Also,* Reprint. *Also, transl.:* J. f. Kinderkr., Erlang., 1868, i, 217-225.—**Scharlau.** Behandlung und Heilung der gefässreichen Muttermäler der Kinder. Med. Ztg., Berl., 1848, xvii, 157.—**Schmidt.** Bedeutende Angiectasie durch die Vaccination geheilt. Prov. San.-Ber. d. k. k. Med.-Coll. v. Pommern 1834, Stettin, 1835, 115.—**Schmidtmüller.** Etwas über die Entstehung der Muttermähle u. degl. Lucina, Leipz., 1805, ii, 3. St., 46-75.—**Schütte.** Beitrag zur Heilung der Warzen und Muttermähler. J. f. Chir. u. Augenh., Berl., 1829, xiii, 170-172.—**Secondi** (R.) Sulla cura delle teleangiectasie colla galvano-caustica. N. Liguria med., Genova, 1871, xvi, 113-115.—**Sewell.** Melanotic pedunculated growth developed upon a mole; excision; recovery. Med. Times & Gaz., Lond., 1872, i, 160.—**Sherwell** (S.) Tattooing of nævi. Arch. Dermat., N. Y., 1876-7, iii, 214: Phila., 1879, v, 354. ———. The cutipunctor. Med. Rec., N. Y., 1880, xvii, 23.—**Sigmund** (J.) Ueber die Behandlung kleiner Teleangiektasien bei Kindern mit Acetum lithargyri. Oesterr. med. Wchnschr., Wien, 1842, 437.—**Snell** (S.) Case of orbital nævi treated by electrolysis. Lancet, Lond., 1886, ii, 163.—**Späth.** Plötzlicher Tod durch Injection von Liquor ferri sesquichlorati in eine Teleangiektasie. Med. Cor.-Bl. d. württemb. ärztl. Ver., Stuttg., 1867, xxxvii, 297-299.—**Squire** (B.) Two cases of port-wine mark treated with a view to obliterating the mark without scar. Brit. M. J., Lond., 1878, i, 865. *Also:* Lancet, Lond., 1878, i, 421. ———. An improvement in the treatment of port-wine mark by linear scarification. Brit. M. J., Lond., 1879, ii, 732. *Also, transl.:* Gior. ital. d. mal. ven., Milano, 1879, xiv, 339-341. ———. On oblique linear scarification of the skin in the treatment of port-wine mark. Med. Press & Circ., Lond., 1879, n. s., xxviii, 454.—**Startin.** Cure of nævus by elastic subcutaneous strangulation. Med. Times, Lond., 1852, n. s., v, 22.—**Startin's** (Mr.) new method of applying the ligature to the treatment of nævus. pl. Med. Times, Lond., 1852, n. s., v, 594.—**Steele** (C.) [Nævus maternus over left orbital region; ligature; comatose symptoms; death.] Edinb. M. & S. J., 1849, lxxii, 248.—**Stoeber.** De la galvano-caustique chimique positive dans ses applications au traitement des tumeurs érectiles. Rev. méd. de l'est, Nancy, 1878, x: 1879, xi, 137-145.—**Subcutaneous** ligature of extensive nævi materni. Med. Times & Gaz., Lond., 1858, xvi, 113.—**Talini** (B.) Alcuni casi di angioma curati coll' etilato di sodio (metodo Richardson). Rev. ital. di terap. ed ig., Piacenza, 1885, v, 113-116.—**Tarral** (C.) Du traitement des tumeurs érectiles, et particulièrement du traitement par le caustique. Arch. gén. de méd., Par., 1834, 2. s., vi, 5; 195. *Also:* Abeille, Brux., 1834, iv, 145; 233.—**Tassell** (R.) Operation for nævus. Lancet, Lond., 1862, i, 236.—**Teale** (T. P.), jr. On enucleation of nævus. Med.-Chir. Tr., Lond., 1866-7, l, 57-63. *Also* [Abstr.]: Proc. Roy. M. & Chir. Soc. Lond., 1864-7. v, 241.—**Treatment** (The) and cure of nævi; New York testimony and results. Am. M. Weekly, Louisville, Ky., 1876, iv, 1-3.—**Turnbull** (L.) Case of extensive nævus removed successfully by extirpation. Med. & Surg. Reporter, Phila., 1858, xi, 458-460.—**Tylecote** (L. H.) Removal of nævus by excision. Lancet, Lond., 1862, i, 290.—**Valeriani** (F.) Sulla cura delle angiectasi colla galvano-caustica termica. Ann. univ. di med. e chir., Milano, 1878, ccxliii, 53-71.—**Valette.** Du traitement des tumeurs érectiles. Ann. Soc. de méd. de Lyon, 1868, 2. s., xvi, 91-102.—**Varvelli** (E.) Telangectasia alla regione giugulare destra; cura colla legatura elastica; guarigione. Indipendente, Torino, 1879, xxx, 314.—**Verneuil.** Injections coagulantes dans le traitement des tumeurs érectiles; fièvre accompagnant le développement d'une tumeur. Méd. contemp., Par., 1878, xx, 38-40.—**Voltolini.** Die Anwendung der Elektrolyse zur spurlosen Beseitigung von Muttermälern und Warzen. Deutsche med. Wchnschr., Berl., 1886, xii, 104.—**Walker** (B.) Treatment of nævus. Lancet, Lond., 1880, i, 680.—**Wallace** (W.) Clinical lecture, containing remarks on the structure of subcutaneous nævi; and the effect of diminishing the supply of blood to such tumors. Lancet, Lond., 1834, i, 849-855, 1 pl.—**Walsh.** Case of nævus maternus, treated after the failure of the ligature, by red-hot needles. Med. Press, Dubl., 1865, liv, 266.—**Walton** (H.) The treatment of nævus by injections with tannic acid. Lancet, Lond., 1858, i, 458. ———. Cutaneo-subcutaneous nævus in mastoid region of an infant; operation by ligature. Med. Times & Gaz., Lond., 1872, i, 96.—**Wardrop.** Cases of

Nævus (*Treatment of*).

nævus successfully treated by artificial ulceration. Lancet, Lond., 1834, ii, 715.—**West** (L. T.) On the use of the écraseur for the removal of nævoid growths. *Ibid.,* 1871, i, 302.—**White** (A.) Observations on the surgical treatment of the nævus maternus, with ligature. Med.-Chir. Tr., Lond., 1827, xiii, 444-450.—**Wittlinger.** Fall von Kuhpockenimpfung bei Telangiectasie. Med. Cor.-Bl. d. württemb. ärztl. Ver., Stuttg., 1844, xiv, 7.—**Wood.** Extensive nævi materni cured by operation. Lancet, Lond., 1858, ii, 143.—**Woolcott** (J.) Case of a large sub-cutaneous nævus cured by vaccination. *Ibid.,* 1852, i, 261.—**Worthington** (W. C.) Subcutaneous vascular nævus, cured with an ointment of tartarized antimony. *Ibid.,* 1834, ii, 557.

Nævus (*Verrucose*).

Kaposi (M.) Nævus verrucosus universalis. Anz. d. k. k. Gesellsch. d. Aerzte in Wien, 1884-5, 323-327. ———. Ueber einen Fall von Nævus verrucosus universalis. Wien. med. Bl., 1885, viii, 718. *Also:* Wien. med. Wchnschr., 1885, xxxv, 773.

Naezén (Daniel Ericus) [1752-1808]. *Nova graminum genera. Upsaliæ,* 1779. *In:* LINNÆUS. Amœnitates acad. [etc.] 8°. *Erlangæ,* 1790, x, pt. 2, 1-40.

Nafilyan (Andon-Gomidas). *Opérations de fistules vésico-vaginales par le procédé américain de M. Marion Sims. 79 pp. 4°. Paris,* 1862, No. 102.

Nagamachi Kohei. Jika Shinsatsu. [The modern practice of otology.] 1 p. l., 48 pp., 2 l. 12°. *Tokio,* 1886. Japanese text.

Nagamatsu Tokai. Seiri Gaku. [The science of physiology.] 2 v. 4 p. l., 367, 5 pp., 1 l.; 459, 7 pp., 1 l. 8°. *Tokio,* 1882. Japanese text.

Nagasaki Ken. [Tables of the prevalent diseases of Nagasaki Ken. From Oct. 29 to Dec. 2, 1882. Original reports and translations.] 5 sheets. fol. [*Nagasaki Ken,* 1882.]
———. *See also:* **Van Gogh** (J.) Overzigt van de heerschende winden en daarbij waargenomen barometerstanden te Nagasaki, op het eiland Desima in Japan. Versl. . . . . d. k. Akad. d. Wetensch. Afd. Natuurk., Amst., 1866, i, 400-407.—**Woods** (G. W.) Report on Nagasaki. Rep. Surg.-Gen. Navy, Wash., 1886, 90-92.

Nagasawa Dojiu. I Ho Ko Ketsu Shiu. [The practice of medicine, and a collection of formulæ.] 3 v. 8°. *Kioto,* 1672. Japanese text.

Nagata Tokuhon. Tokuhon wo Jiuku Ho. [Tokuhon's nineteen principal diseases and their treatment.] 2 v. 21, 21 pp. 8°. *Osaca,* 1803. Japanese text.

Nagaty (Soleiman). *Contribution à l'étude de la folie religieuse. 72 pp. 4°. Paris,* 1886, No. 249.

Nagel (Albrecht) [1833-] *Observationes quædam ophthalmoscopicæ. 35 pp., 1 l., 1 pl. 8°. Berolini, typ. fratrum Schlesinger,* [1855].
———. Das Sehen mit zwei Augen und die Lehre von den identischen Netzhautstellen. 2 p. l., 184 pp., 4 pl. 8°. *Leipzig u. Heidelberg, C. F. Winter,* 1861.
———. Die Refractions- und Accommodations-Anomalien des Auges. iv, 217 pp. 8°. *Tübingen, H. Laupp,* 1866.
———. Die Benutzung des Metermaasses zur Numerirung der Brillen. 14 pp. 8°. [*Rostock, C. Boldt,* 1868.] *Repr. from:* Klin. Monatsbl. f. Augenh., Erlang., 1868, vi, 65.
———. Die Reform des ophthalmologischen Universitäts-Unterrichts. 48 pp. 8°. *Tübingen, H. Laupp,* 1870.
———. Die Behandlung der Amaurosen und Amblopieen mit Strychnin. 3 p. l., 141 pp. 8°. *Tübingen, H. Laupp,* 1871.
Also, Editor of: **Jahresbericht** über die Leistungen und Fortschritte im Gebiete der Ophthalmologie, Tübingen, 1870-76.
See, also, **Mittheilungen** aus der ophthalmiatrischen Klinik in Tübingen. 8°. *Tübingen,* 1880.

Nagel (Anton). * Ueber Cholera. 33 pp. 8°. *Würzburg, C. J. Becker*, 1860.

Nagel (Carl). Fragmente aus der gesammten microscopischen Anatomie. 28 pp. 4°. *Wien, gedruckt bei den p. p. Mechitaristen*, 1839.

Nagel (Carl Friedrich) [1794–]. Ueber das Entkräftungsfieber der alten Leute, eine wenig gekannte und bisher noch nicht beschriebene Krankheit. x, 100 pp. 12°. *Altona, P. S. Schönfeldt*, 1829.

——. Nachricht an das Publikum über die zweckmässigsten Verhaltungsmaassregeln bei einer etwanigen Erscheinung der morgenländischen Brechruhr (Cholera morbus). Auf Befehl Sr. Exc. des Herrn Geheime-Conferenzraths und Oberpräsidenten Grafen von Blücher-Altona. 2. Abdruck. 15 pp. 8°. *Altona, K. Aue*, 1831.

Nagel (Carolus Antonius) [1798–]. * De signis ex ventre. 51 pp. 8°. *Berolini, formis Brueschckianis*, 1820.

Nagel (Carolus Henricus) [1810–]. * De tussi convulsiva. 30 pp., 1 l. 8°. *Berolini, typ. Nietackianis*, [1835].

Nagel (Carolus Leopoldus) [1829–]. * Commentatio de anatomia Salernitana per compendium Salernitanum. 3 p. l., 32 pp. 8°. *Vratislaviæ, R. Nischkowsky*, [1852].

Nagel (Eduardus) [1840–]. * De anencephalia quædam, cum descriptione monstri unius. 31 pp., 1 l. 8°. *Gryphiæ, F. Hache*, 1865.

Nagel (*F.*)
Portrait in: **Collection** of Portr. of Phys. & Men of Sc., 217[b].

Nagel (Friedrich Wilhelm) [1841–]. * Ueber Prädispositionen zu Knochenbrüchen. 18 pp., 1 l. 8°. *Marburg, C. L. Pfeil*, [1870].

Nagel (Gunther) [1858–]. * Ueber Athetose. 34 pp. 8°. *Berlin, G. Lange*, [1881].

Nagel (Hermannus Ferdinandus) [1820 –]. * De arthritide. 31 pp. 8°. *Berolini, typ. Nietackianis*, [1844].

Nagel (Karl). * Die Venenentzündung. 20 pp. 8°. *Erlangen, Junge*, 1839.

Nagel (Ludwig) [1864–]. * Ueber Diabetes mellitus mit Hemiplegie. 30 pp., 1 l. 8°. *Berlin, G. Schade*, [1886].

Nagel (Mauritius) [1808–71]. * De renum succenturiatorum in mammalibus structura penitiore. 32 pp. 4°. *Berolini, typ. Nietackianis*, [1834].

Nagel (Mauritius [Ferdinandus]) [1823–]. * De hydronephrosi. 43 pp. 8°. *Berolini, G. Schade*, 1847.

Nagel (Philippus Jacobus). * De vitiis primarum viarum morbisque ex iis oriundis. 39 pp. 4°. *Argentorati, ex prelo J. H. Heitzii*, [1761].

Nagel (Richard Gustav) [1823–]. * De morbis protopathicis quædam. 26 pp., 2 l. 8°. *Berolini, typ. fratrum Schlesinger*, [1848].

——. Das Fleisch-Essen vor dem Richterstuhle des Instinkts, der Vernunft, des Gewissens, der Religions-Geschichte und der Natur-Wissenschaft oder: der Weg zur Gesundheit, zum Wohlstande und Glück, zum Paradiese. 3. Aufl. 120 pp. 12°. *Berlin, T. Grieben*, 1870.

——. Vier Fragen an die Impf-Aerzte. 63 pp. 8°. *Barmen*, 1872.

——. Der wissenschaftliche Unwerth der Vivisektionen in allen ihren Arten. 30 pp., 1 l. 12°. *Berlin, Verfasser*, 1881.

——. Die Vivisektionen, Irrwege der Wissenschaft. 4. u. 5. Tausend. 32 pp. 12°. *Barmen, Verfasser*, 1883.

Nagel (Wilhelm). * Die Entwicklung der Extremitäten der Säugethiere. 41 pp., 3 l., 1 pl. 8°. *Marburg, R. Friedrich*, 1878. S. D.

Naghten (Timotheus). * De peritonitide puerperarum. 28 pp. 8°. *Edinburgi, Creech*, 1803. [P., v. 27.]

Nagl (Mathias). * De morbo scrophuloso. 30 pp. 8°. *Vindobonæ, C. Ueberreuter*, [1838].

Nagle (*Frank O.*) [1857–84].
Obituary. Tr. M. Soc. Penn., Phila., 1885, xvii, 387–390.

Nagle (John T.) Summary of births, marriages, still-births, deaths, etc., in New York City, compared with 352 American and foreign cities, for the year 1878. And also the mortality from some of the most prominent causes which took place in New York City during the past 75 years. 14 pp., 1 tab. 8°. *New York, C. L. Bermingham & Co.*, 1879.
Repr. from: Hosp. Gaz., N. Y., 1879, vi.

——. Table showing the total number of still-births and deaths (with an enumeration of some of the most prominent causes) which occurred in this city during the seventy-five years ending Dec. 31, 1878, and the number of births and marriages reported since the year 1847. 1 sheet. fol. [*New York*, 1879.]

——. Epitome of the births, marriages, still-births, and deaths in New York City during the year 1879. 1 sheet. 4°. [*New York*, 1880.]

——. Suicides in New York City during the eleven years ending Dec. 31, 1880, showing the sex, age, color, nativity, means used for self-destruction, and the season of the year when committed; together with a comparison of the deaths by suicide in two hundred and forty-seven American and foreign cities in the year 1880, obtained from official sources; and the proportion of suicides to the population of New York City from the year 1804 to 1880, inclusive. Read before the American Public Health Association at Savannah, Ga., Nov. 30, 1881. 19 pp. 8°. *Cambridge*, 1882.
Repr. from: Am. Pub. Health Ass. Rep., N. Y., 1880, vii.

——. Summary of births, marriages, still-births, and deaths in New York City during the year 1880. 13 pp. 8°. *New York, M. B. Brown*, 1882.

——. [Application for the position of health-commissioner of the city of New York. Accompanied by testimonials as to qualification. March 23, 1883.] 16 pp. 8°. [*New York*, 1883.]

Nagle (P. E.)
See **Vaughan** (Victor C.) & **Nagle** (P. E.) Contamination of drinking-water by filtration of organic matter through the soil. [Read at the Sanitary Convention in Detroit, Mich., January 7, 1880.] 8°. [*n. p.*, 1880.]

Naglee (Henry M.) & **Bleasdale** (John I.) The report of a jury of experts on brandy made by . . . 48 pp. 8°. *San Francisco, Spaulding, Barto & Co.*, 1879.

Nagorski (Valentin). * Sposob Pettenkofera dlja kolichestvennago opredielenija v vozduchie uglekisloti. [On Pettenkofer's experiments to ascertain the proportion of carbonic acid in the air.] 43 pp., 3 pl., 1 l. 8°. *St. Petersburg*, 1880.

Nagoya Geni. Kin Ki Yo Riyaku Chiu Kai. [The golden books of medicine condensed and explained, with certain additions.] 4 v. 8°. *Osaka*, 1696.
Japanese text.

Nagpur.
See **Education** (*Medical*), etc., *by localities.*

Nagpur School of Medicine. Annual reports on the . . . By the deputy surg. genl. and principal, to the secy. to the chief commissioner. 4.–7., 1871–2 to 1874–5; 9.–15., 1876–7 to 1882–3. fol. *Nagpur*, 1872–83.

Nagrodzki (Eduardus) [1812–]. * De nymphomania ejusque curatione. 31 pp., 2 l. 8°. *Berolini, typ. Nietackianis*, [1834].

Nagura Chibun. Seikotsu Riakusetsu. [Manual of fractures.] 2 v. 19 pp., 6 pl.; 2 p. l., 43 pp. 12°. *Tokio*, 1874.
Japanese text.

Nagy (Georgius). *De peste. 32 pp. sm. 4°. *Jenæ, lit. Croekerianis*, [1740].
For Biography, *see* **Hilscher** (Simon Paulus).

Nagy (Martinus). De potentia et impotentia animæ humanæ in corpus organicum sibi junctum. (Ob und wie weit die Seele in den menschlichen Cörper würcke) disquisitio philosophico-medica, in qua animæ in producendis motibus voluntariis potentia, spontaneis vero impotentia, secundum philosophiæ sanioris et medicinæ rationalis principia explicatur ac demonstratur. 2 p. l., 68 pp. sm. 4°. *Halæ Magdeb., typ. J. C. Hilligeri*, 1729.

Nagy (Nicolaus). *De febri nervosa. 26 pp., 1 l. 8°. *Viennæ, typ. vid. A. Stoeckholzer de Hirschfeld*, [1833].

Nagy de Path (Carolus). *Observata clinica in clinico medico pro chirurgis regiæ scientiarum universitatis Hungaricæ anno scholastico 1828-9. x, 11-53 pp. 8°. *Pesthini, J. M. Trattner*, 1830. [P., v. 1318.]

Nagy Igmand.
von **Verebély** (J.) Die Nagy Igmander kohlensaure Bitterwasser-Quelle in Ungarn und deren pharmazeutische Produkte. Wien. med. Presse, 1865, vi, 409–414.—**Wolf.** Das jüngst aufgefundene Bitterwasser zu Nagy-Igmand. Wien. Med.-Halle, 1864, v, 420.

Nahant.
See, also, **Fever** (*Typhoid, History, etc., of*), by localities.
Bowditch (E. W.) The sanitary aspect of Nahant, Mass. Boston M. & S. J., 1882, cvii, 97–101. ——. The sewerage of Nahant. Rep. Bd Health., etc., Mass. Suppl., Bost., 1883, iv, 227–248. *Also:* San. News, Chicago, 1883–4, iii, 59; 74; 88; 100.—**Channing** (W.) A togographical sketch of Nahant, with comparative meteorological tables for July, Aug., and Sept., 1820, with some observations on its advantages as a watering place. N. Eng. J. M. & S., Bost., 1821, x, 22–37.

Nahke (Carolus). *De elephantiasi arabica adnexis morbi historiis quatuor. 1 p. l., 44 pp. 8°. *Pragæ, T. Haase*, 1839.
——. The same. 1 p. l., 44 pp., 3 pl. 8°. *Pragæ, typ. filiorum T. Haase*, 1839.

von der Nahmer (Frider. Wilh.) [1822-]. *De hydrophobia nonnulla. 1 p. l., 67 pp. 12°. *Gryphiæ, F. G. Kunike*, 1850.

Nahnsen (R.) *Untersuchungen in der Thiophengruppe. [Basel.] 35 pp. 8°. *Schönebeck, T. Wulfert*, 1885.

Nahuys (Alexander Petrus) [1737-94]. Tractatus chemicus continens nova quædam experimenta cum basi salis marini, nitri et aluminis; pars prima. 4 p. l., 48 pp. 8°. *Amstelodami, J. Schreuder et P. Mortier jun.*, 1761.
——. Oratio de quæstione illa: Utrum uroscopus ex folia urinæ inspectione morbos quorumvis ægrotantium rite detegere, iisque ex arte mederi possit? 48 pp. 8°. [*Harderovici*, 1761.]
——. Oratio de anatome chirurgiæ dextra ipsiusque neglectu uberrimo calamitatum et errorum fonte. 3 p. l., 43 pp. 4°. *Harderovici, J. Moojen*, 1772.
——. Quelle est la qualité nuisible que l'air contracte dans les hôpitaux et les prisons, et quels sont les meilleurs moyens d'y remédier? Trad. du latin et commenté par André Uytterhoeven. iv, 48 pp. 8°. *Bruxelles, Tircher & Manceaux*, 1863.
See, also, **Le Cat** (Claude-Nicholas). Parallèle de la taille latérale, etc. 8°. *Amsterdam*, 1766.

Naiad.
Flemming (W.) Studien in der Entwicklungsgeschichte der Najaden. Sitzungsb. d. k. Akad. d. Wissensch., Wien, 1875, lxxi, 81–212, 4 pl.

Naigeon (Alfred-Jules). *Quelques considérations sur la vaccine. 27 pp. 4°. *Paris*, 1818, No. 115, v. 138½.

Nail (*Surgical*).
Motais. Nouvel ongle chirurgical. Bull. et mém. Soc. de chir. de Par., 1875, i, 93.

Naïl (Achille-Pierre-Marie). *Considérations sur le traitement des plaies et des hémorrhagies traumatiques à la main. 40 pp. 4°. *Strasbourg*, 1860, No. 538, 2. s., v. 29.

Naïl (Charles-Jules). *Sur la fièvre puerpérale. 36 pp. 4°. *Paris*, 1846, No. 122, v. 448.

Naila.
See **Fever** (*Cerebro-spinal, History, etc., of*), by localities.

Nail-makers.
Bigg (Ada H.) Female labour in the nail trade. Fortnightly Rev., Lond., 1886, n. s., xxxix, 829–838.

Nails.
See, also, **Hair**; **Skin**.
ANCEL (L.) *Des ongles au point de vue anatomique, physiologique et pathologique. 4°. *Paris*, 1868.
——. The same. 8°. *Paris*, 1868.
BERTHOLD (A. A.) Beobachtungen über das quantitative Verhältniss der Nagel- und Haarbildung beim Menschen. 4°. *Göttingen*, 1850.
BESSERER (A.) *Observationes de unguium anatomia atque pathologia. 8°. *Bonnæ*, [1834].
CHARLES (C.) *Considérations sur les ongles. 4°. *Paris*, 1834.
EPHRAIMSOHN (S.) *De unguibus humanis. 8°. *Berolini*, [1833].
FAYE (C.) *Quelques considérations sur les ongles, suivies d'un nouveau procédé pour la cure de l'ongle incarné. 4°. *Paris*, 1822.
FINELLA (P.) De quatuor signis quæ apparent in unguibus manuum. 16°. *Neapoli*, 1649.
FRANCUS DE FRANKENAU (G. F.) Ὀνυξολογία curiosa, sive de unguibus tractatio physico-medica, non tantum eorum physiologiam ubi et de cornibus, sed et pathologiam ac therapiam tradens, observationibus oppido variis. 8°. *Jenæ*, 1696.
HAASE (J. G.) Experimenta anatomica ad nutritionem unguinum declarandam capta commemorat. 4°. *Lipsiæ*, [1774].
HÉLIOT (J.-M.-G.) *Sur l'ongle et son organe générateur. 4°. *Paris*, 1838.
HEMPEL (C.) & SPIESMACHER (J.) *Ex ungue hominem. 4°. *Lipsiæ*, [1685].
HENLE (J.) Das Wachsthum des menschlichen Nagels und des Pferdehufs. 4°. *Göttingen*, 1884.
Repr. from: Abhandl. d. königl. Gesellsch. d. Wissensch. zu Götting., xxxi.
JARDON (J.-L.-H.) *Considérations anatomiques, physiologiques et pathologiques sur l'ongle et son organe générateur. 4°. *Paris*, 1836.
LEDERER (L. O.) *De unguibus humanis. 8°. *Berolini*, [1834].
VAN LEYDEN (P.) jun. *De unguibus. 8°. *Lugd. Bat.*, [1845].
LUDWIG (C. G.) De ortu et structura unguium. 4°. *Lipsiæ*, [1748].
Also, in: HALLER. Disp. anat. [etc.] 4°. *Gottingæ*, 1751, vii, pt. 2, 17–32.
[NÜRNBERGER (C. F.)] Meletemata super digitorum unguibus. 4°. *Wittebergæ*, [1786].
——. [Pr.] de unguium et pilorum sorte post fata. Parts 1 & 2. 4°. *Vittebergæ*, [1787].
SCHLEGEL (F.) *De unguium structura eorumque physiologia. 8°. *Jenæ*, [1848].
SINDS (J. G. W.) *De unguibus humanis. 4°. *Landishuti Bavarorum*, 1825.
WERNER (P. C. F.) De unguibus humanis varioque modo quo possunt corrumpi. 4°. *Lipsiæ*, [1773].

Nails.

Cooper (A.) Observations on the anatomy and diseases of the nails. Lond. M. & Phys. J., 1827, n. s., ii, 289-291, 1 pl. — Crisis morbi per ungues. Acta med. et phil. Hafn., 1680, v, 87.— Dufour (L.) Observations sur la vitesse d'accroissement des ongles. Bull. Soc. vaudoise d. sc. nat., Lausanne, 1873, xi, 183-211. — Gegenbaur (C.) Zur Morphologie des Nagels. Morphol. Jahrb., Leipz., 1884-5, x, 465-479. — Guldberg (G. A.) Ueber die Nagelmatrix und die Verhornung des Nagels. Monatsh. f. prakt. Dermat., Hamb., 1885, iv, 7-16.— Hebra (H.) Beitrag zur Anatomie des Nagels. Med. Jahrb., Wien, 1880, 59-66, 1 pl.—Heynold (H.) Beitrag zur Histiologie und Genese des Nagels. Arch. f. path. Anat., etc., Berl., 1875, lxv, 270-272, 1 pl.—Humbert (G.) Ongles. Dict. encycl. d. sc. méd., Par., 1881, 2. s., xv, 388-425. — Hutchinson (J.) On the nails and the diseases to which they are liable. Med. Times & Gaz., Lond., 1878, i, 423-426.—Jardon. Anatomie et pathologie de l'ongle. J. d. conn. méd.-chir., Par., 1836-7, iv, pt. 1, 45-54. — Ledentu (A.) Ongles. N. dict. de méd. et chir. prat., Par., 1877, xxiv, 539-576. — Mareschal de Rougeres. Lettre sur la régénération d'un ongle à la suite de la mutilation d'un doigt. J. de méd., chir., pharm., etc., Par., 1767, xxvii, 177.—Ollivier. Mémoire sur l'anatomie et la pathologie de l'ongle. Dict. de méd., 2. éd., Par., 1840, xxii, 80-97. Also, Reprint.—Ormancey (A.-B.) Observation sur la reproduction d'un ongle à la deuxième phalange du doigt du milieu. J. de méd., chir., pharm., etc., Par., 1809, xvii, 218. — Patissier. Ongle. Dict. d. sc. méd., Par., 1819, xxxvii, 321-355. — Pradier (F.) Note sur la reproduction des ongles. Gaz. d. hôp., Par., 1861, xxxiv, 147.—Zander (R.) Die frühesten Studien der Nagelentwickelung und ihre Beziehungen zu den Digitalnerven. Arch. f. Anat. u. Entwcklngsgesch., Leipz., 1884, 103-144, 1 pl. —. Die Histogenese des Nagels beim menschlichen Fötus. Ibid., 1886, 273-306, 1 pl.

Nails (Abnormities and deformities of).

See, also, Nails (Ingrowing); Nails (Semeiology of).

Musæus (C.) * De unguibus monstrosis, et cornuum productione in puella cornigera Lalandiæ. sm. 4°. Hafniæ, [1716].

Broca. Production irrégulière du tissu unguéal. Bull. Soc. de chir., Par., 1867, 2. s., vii, 403.—Cooper (G. L.) On hypertrophy of the toe-nails. Lancet, Lond., 1866, i, 454.—Davidson (H. E.) Incurvation of nails. Boston M. & S. J., 1851, xliv, 14.—Fürst (L.) Allgemeiner Fingernagelwechsel bei einem ⅓jährigen Kinde. Arch. f. path. Anat., etc., Berl., 1884, xcvi, 355-357, 1 pl.— Hamy (E.-T.) Sur les ongles chinois, annamites et siamois. Bull. Soc. d'anthrop. de Par., 1876, 2. s., xi, 80-85.—Henning. Eine eigene Missbildung des Nagels an der grossen Zehe des rechten Fusses. Arch. f. med. Erfahr., Berl., 1823, ii, 205, 1 pl.—Hillingius (G.) De ungue utriusque pedum pollicis monstroso. Misc. Acad. nat. curios. 1682, Norimb., 1683, 2 decur., i, 385, 1 pl.— Kaposi (M. Kohn). Hypertrophie der Nägel. Handb. d. spec. Path. u. Therap. (Virchow), Stuttg., 1876, iii, 2. Abth., 60-73. Also, Reprint. —. Atrophie der Nägel. Handb. spec. Path. u. Therap. (Virchow), Stuttg., 1876, iii, 2. Abth., 179. Also, Reprint.—Leopold. Pathologische Nagelbildung. Wchnschr. f. d. ges. Heilk., Berl., 1849, 113.—Mailliot. [Rhumatisme chronique; extrême courbature des ongles des doigts.] Bull. Soc. anat. de Par., 1846, xxi, 239.—Partridge. Outgrowth of nails in a woman, æt. 84. Tr. Path. Soc. Lond., 1861, xii, 240.—Rehm (P.) Ein Fall von Onychogryphosis. Arch. d. Heilk., Leipz., 1875, xvi, 80-91.—Thorens. Développement exagéré de l'ongle du gros orteil. Bull. Soc. anat. de Par., 1872, 2. s., xvii, 399.

Nails (Diseases of).

See, also, Diabetes (Diagnosis, etc., of); Exostosis (Subungual); Onychia; Paronychia.

Benjamin (L.) * Nonnulla de morbis unguium. 8°. Berolini, [1848].

Blech (E. P. E.) * De mutationibus unguium morbosis. 4°. Berolini, [1816].

Box (C.-A.) * Des ongles. De l'onyxis ulcéreux latéral. 4°. Paris, 1878.

Durlacher (L.) A treatise on corns, bunions, the diseases of nails, and the general management of the feet. 8°. London, 1845.

—. The same. 12°. Philadelphia, 1845.

—. A concise treatise on corns, bunions, and the disorders of nails, with advice for the general management of the feet. 16°. London, 1858.

Esmenard (J.) Considérations anatomiques, physiologiques et pathologiques sur les ongles et

Nails (Diseases of).

de l'onyxis ulcéreuse sous-unguéale rebelle. 4°. Paris, 1861.

Guichenon (S. H.) * De paronichia. 4°. Monspellii, 1788.

von Halem (E.) * De mutationibus unguium morbosis. 8°. Halis, [1835].

L'Herminier (A.) * Du traitement curatif de l'onyxis chronique. 4°. Paris, 1862.

Neumann (C. E. O.) Die Haut, Haare, Nägel und Zähne des Menschen. Deren Bau, Pflege, Krankheiten und naturgemässe Behandlung. 2. Aufl. 12°. Leipzig, [1887 ?].

Unna (P. G.) Beiträge zur Onychopathologie. 8°. [Hamburg, 1881.]

Audry. Note sur une épidémie de tournioles développées par contagion dans une école. Lyon méd., 1886, liii, 235-242. Also: J. d. conn. méd. prat., Par., 1886, 3. s., viii, 354-356. — Boinet. Chute des ongles dans le diabète sucré. Rev. méd. franç. et étrang., Par., 1874, i, 302-304.— Burnett (G. T.) On diseases of the nails. Lond. M. & Phys. J., 1829, n. s., vi, 91-95.—Chassaignac. Rupture de la matrice de l'ongle par l'ongle; ecchymose sous-unguéale. Gaz. d. hôp., Par., 1854, 3. s., xxvii, 26.— Christine (G. M. M.) Curious affection of the nails. Med. & Surg. Reporter, Phila., 1881, xliv, 163.—Colles (A.) Observations on some morbid affections of the nail of the great toe. Dublin J. M. Sc., 1843, xxiii, 240-249.— Cummiskey (J.) Case of psoriasis of the nails, the lepra unguium of Wilson. Am. J. Syph. & Dermat., N. Y., 1872, iii, 313.—Deligny. L'eczéma des ongles. Union méd., Par., 1887, 3. s., xliv, 817-823.—De Sanctis (S.) Sopra un caso di necrosi totale delle unghie in ambedue le mani. Sperimentale, Firenze, 1887, lx, 31-34. — Duarte. Panarizo gangrenoso; consideraciones acerca de su diagnóstico, pronóstico y tratamiento. Clínica, Granada, 1886, ii, 17.—Dupont. Traitement de la turniole. Arch. méd. belges, Brux., 1868, 2. s., viii, 245-247.—Eitner. Chronische Entzündung und Vereiterung der Nägel. Wchnschr. f. d. ges. Heilk., Berl., 1849, 483.— Fagge (C. H.) Cases of ring-worm of the nails. Tr. Path. Soc. Lond., 1870, xxi, 407. —. On some affections of the nails. Guy's Hosp. Rep., Lond., 1870, 3. s., xv, 551-561.— Flajani (G.) Practische Beobachtungen über das Nagelgeschwür. [Osservazioni pratiche supra . . . il panereccio, Roma, 1791.] Ital. med.-chir. Biblioth., Leipz., 1796, ii, 2. St., 50-60.— Foley (J. L.) The morbid changes and surgery of the nails. Boston M. & S. J., 1887, cxvii, 301-303.—Forster (J. C.) Description of a wax model illustrating a case of disease of the finger-nails, arising from arsenic. Guy's Hosp. Rep., Lond., 1859, 3. s., v, 160-162.—Hare. Psoriasis of the matrices of the nails. Lancet, Lond., 1858, i, 119.—Hutchinson (J.) On the nails and the diseases to which they are liable. In his: Lect. on Clin. Surg., 8°, Lond., 1878, i, pt. 1, 137-149. —. Disease of the nails in connection with the psoriasis diathesis (dartrous). Ibid., 150-158.—Hutchinson (J.), jr. Case of epithelioma of the nail. Tr. Path. Soc. Lond., 1884-5, xxxvi, 468, 1 pl. —. Chronic inflammatory disease of many finger-nails, beginning in early childhood, and continuing for ten years; history of syphilis in the father, but no signs whatever of it in the child. Brit. M. J., Lond., 1887, i, 984. —. Psoriasis of the nails; true psoriasis of nails contracted with chronic onychitis attended by fibrous thickening. Ibid., 984.—Joffroy (A.) Chute spontanée de l'ongle des gros orteils chez un malade non ataxique. Union méd., Par., 1882, 3. s., xxxiv, 210-212. Also: Bull. et mém. Soc. méd. d. hôp. de Par. (1882), 1883, 2. s., xix, 115-118.—Kraske (P.) Ueber subunguale Geschwülste. München. med. Wchnschr., 1887, xxxiv, 889-891.—Lélut Études anatomiques et pathologiques sur l'onglade. Répert. gén. d'anat. et physiol. path., Par., 1827, iv, 125-147, 1 pl.—Mettenheimer (C.) Krankheiten der Nägel [im höheren Alter]. Memorabilien, Heilbr., 1873, xviii, 104-108.—Morison (R. B.) Leucopathia unguicum, a peculiar affection of the nails. Med. News, Phila., 1887, li, 430.—Nied (A.) Onychogryposis. In his: Casus pract., 8°, Vindobonæ, 1840, 47-49. — Niezwyczajny przykład choroby paznogci (onychophthora). Gaz. lek., Warszawa, 1878, xxiv, 321.—Ollivier. Altérations pathologiques des ongles. Dict. de méd., 2. éd., Par., 1840, xxii, 84-97.—Ozanam. Remarques sur quelques maladies des ongles. Rev. méd. franç. et étrang., Par., 1823, x, 71-77.— Parsons (J.) Extirpation of nail of thumb under anesthesia by cold. Am. J. M. Sc., Phila., 1867, n. s., liv, 281.—Patissier. Des maladies des ongles. Dict. d. sc. méd., Par., 1819, xxxvii, 326-355.—Paulli (S.) Ungues nigri. Acta med. et phil. Hafn. (1671-2), 1673, i, 64. — Robin. Épithélioma de la racine de l'ongle. Bull. Soc. anat. de Par., 1873, xlviii, 421-423.—Routier (A.) De la dactylite unguéale scrofuleuse chez les enfants. France méd., Par., 1880, xxvii, 41-44. — Royer-Collard (H.) De quelques altérations des ongles et de la peau qui les environne. Répert. gén. d'anat. et physiol. path., Par., 1826,

Nails (*Diseases of*).

ii, 108–136, 2 pl. — **Sachs** (A.) Die Verschwärung des Nagelbettes, in geschichtlicher und practischer Beziehung erörtert. J. d. Chir. u. Augenh., Berl., 1834, xxii, 108–152.—**Sangster** (A.) Disease of the nails; case. Med. Times & Gaz., Lond., 1881, i, 238. ——. A case of exfoliation and suppuration of the nails, of uncertain origin. Tr. Clin. Soc. Lond., 1880, xiii, 149–151, 1 pl. — **Selldén** (H.) Om behandling af panaritium. Eira, Göteborg, 1886, x, 399–403.—**Smith** (H. A.) Psoriasis of the nails. Brit. M. J., Lond., 1883, i, 405. — **Suchard.** Des modifications des cellules de la matrice et du lit de l'ongle dans quelques cas pathologiques. Arch. de physiol. norm. et path., Par., 1882, 2. s., x, 445–456, 1 pl. ——. Lésions histologiques de l'ongle dans les inflammations de cet organe. Progrès méd., Par., 1882, x, 221. *Also:* Compt. rend. Soc. de biol., Par., 1882, 7. s., iv, 217. — **Thin** (G.) A case of interference with nail-growth during illness. Lancet, Lond., 1880, i, 445.—**Unna** (P. G.) Anatomisch-physiologische Vorstudien zu einer künftigen Onychopathologie. Vrtljschr. f. Dermat., Wien, 1881, viii, 3–24. ——. Beiträge zur Onychopathologie. *Ibid.*, 1882, ix, 3–20. — **Vérité** (A.) Du psoriasis superunguéal. Cong. périod. internat. d. sc. méd. Compt.-rend. 1875, Brux. et Par., 1876, 310–312. — **Vimont.** Observation sur une affection dartreuse, compliquée du développement contre-nature des ongles. Ann. Soc. de méd.-prat. de Montpel., 1805, vi, 355–359. — **Virchow.** Zur normalen und pathologischen Anatomie der Nägel und der Oberhaut, insbesondere über hornige Entartung und Pilzbildung an den Nägeln. Verhandl. d. phys.-med. Gesellsch. in Würzb., 1855, v, 83. — **Wilks** (S.) Description of wax models illustrating two cases of inflammation of the roots of the nails, followed by their decay. Guy's Hosp. Rep., Lond., 1859, 3. s., v, 158–160.—**Wordsworth** (J. C.) Removal of the toe-nail. Med. Times & Gaz., Lond., 1857, xv, 295. — **Yemans** (C. C.) Diseases of the nails. Detroit Lancet, 1884–5, n. s., viii, 396–398.

Nails (*Diseases of, Parasitic*).

Bergh (R.) Tilfælde af Negleskurv (favus Onychomycose). [3 cases.] Hosp.-Tid., Kjøbenh., 1869, xii, 89; 93.—**Collas** (A.) Note sur la teigne des ongles (onychomycosis, Purser), indépendante de toute autre manifestation de favus. Arch. de méd. nav., Par., 1867, viii, 453–459.—**Dall' Acqua** (E.) Osservazione di un caso di onicoelcosi settica. Gior. ital. d. mal. ven., Milano, 1882, xxiii, 299–302, 2 pl.—**Duhring** (L. A.) A case of tinea tricophytina unguium. Med. & Surg. Reporter, Phila., 1878, xxxix, 89–92.—**Ercolani** (G. B.) Dell' onychomykosis dell' uomo e dei solipedi. Mem. Accad. d. sc. d. Ist. di Bologna, 1875, 3. s., vi, 363–381, 1 pl. *Also, transl.:* J. de microg., Par., 1880, iv, 131; 187; 337, 1 pl.—**Horand.** Trichophytie des ongles. Compt.-rend. Soc. d. sc. méd. de Lyon (1872), 1873, xii, pt. 2, 19–21. *Also:* Lyon méd., 1872, ix, 468–470.—**Köbner** (H.) Onychomycosis tonsurans. [Herpes unguium.] Arch. f. path. Anat., etc., Berl., 1861, xxii, 411–415.—**Meissner** (G.) Pilzbildung in den Nägeln. Arch. f. physiol. Heilk., Stuttg., 1853, xii, 192–196, 1 pl.—**Neumann** (I.) Ein Fall von Nagelpilzen (Onychomykosis). Wien. med. Wchnschr., 1867, xvii, 822.—**Purser** (J. M.) Two cases of onychomycosis. Dublin Q. J. M. Sc., 1865, xl, 353–361.—**Ripping** (S. H.) Ueber die Therapie der Onychomycosis. Deutsche Klinik, Berl., 1865, xvii, 360–362.—**Vidal.** Onychomycose trichophytique, ou trichophytie unguéale. Gaz. d. hôp., Par., 1880, liii, 227–229.—**Waldenström** (J. A.) Onychomycosis. Upsala Läkaref. Förh., 1869–70, v, 97–104.

Nails (*Ingrowing*).

Albrecht (J.) * Ueber Unguis incarnatus. 8°. *Heiligenstadt*, 1886.

Barbaux (M.) * Considérations sur l'ongle incarné. 4°. *Paris*, 1877.

Barberet (H.) * Contribution à l'étude de l'onyxis. 4°. *Paris*, 1882.

Damée (G.) * De l'ongle incarné et d'un procédé spécial d'opération. 4°. *Paris*, 1881.

Donzel (É.) * Essai sur l'ongle incarné, suivi de la description d'un nouveau procédé opératoire. 4°. *Strasbourg*, 1836.

Dupont (C.-J.) * Étude critique sur le traitement de l'ongle incarné. 4°. *Paris*, 1873.

Felgner (P. G. B.) * Ueber den ins Fleisch gewachsenen Nagel. 8°. *Leipzig*, 1869.

Holder (W.) * De l'ongle incarné. 4°. *Paris*, 1856.

Marianny (V.-M.-J.) * De l'ongle incarné. 4°. *Paris*, 1856.

Moutet (A.-J.) * De l'ongle incarné. 4°. *Strasbourg*, 1863.

Nails (*Ingrowing*).

Negri (L.) Chirurgia conservatrice. Due parole sull' unghia incarnata. 8°. *Milano*, 1868.

Paulinier (J.-P.-L.-T.) * De l'ongle entré dans les chairs. Essai monographique, ou fragment pouvant servir à un traité complet des maladies de l'ongle. 4°. *Beziers*, 1837.

Robbe (L.-É.) * Que l'affection désignée sous le nom d'ongle entré dans les chairs se compose de deux affections entièrement différentes par leurs causes, leur nature, et surtout par leur traitement. 4°. *Paris*, 1826.

Sacreste (E.) * De l'onyxis ulcéreuse latérale. 4°. *Paris*, 1873.

Simmerl (J.) * Ueber den eingewachsenen Nagel (Incarnatio unguis). 8°. *Würzburg*, 1870.

Stilwell (G.) Observations on the surgical treatment of in-growing toe-nail. With a pamphlet by Dr. Cotting. 2. ed. 8°. *London*, 1873.

Vacquerie (A.-L.-F.) * De l'ongle incarné. 4°. *Paris*, 1855.

Agard (A. H.) Ingrown toe nail. Tr. M. Soc. Calif. 1876–7, Sacramento, 1877, 45–54.—**Anderson** (J.) To remove ingrowing toe-nail. Indian M. Gaz., Calcutta, 1877, xii, 23.—**Arlaud** (C.) Évulsion de l'ongle au moyen de la gouge-mousse de . . . Monit. d. sc. méd. et pharm., Par., 1861, 2. s., iii, 661. — **B.** (A.-C.) Traitement de l'ongle entré dans les chairs. Bull. gén. de thérap., etc., Par., 1832, ii, 197–199.—**Babb** (L. P.) Ingrowing nail. Boston M. & S. J., 1868, lxxviii, 362. — **Bailey** (M.) Ingrowing toe nails; an essay. Leavenworth M. Herald, 1867–8, i, 154–156.—**Barbette.** Nouveau traitement de l'ongle incarné. J. d. conn. méd.-chir., Par., 1839–40, vii, pt. 1, 197.—**Barella.** Traitement de l'ongle incarné par la solution normale de perchlorure de fer. Arch. méd. belges, Brux., 1864, xxxiv, 260–262. — **Batchelder** (J. P.) Inverted or imbedded nail. N. York J. M., 1856, 3. s., i, 9–12.—**Baudens** (M.-L.) Nouveau mode opératoire pour la destruction des ongles rentrés dans les chairs. J. univ. et hebd. de méd. et chir. prat, Par., 1832, ix, 24. ——. Ongles incarnés; opération d'après un nouveau mode opératoire. Gaz. d. hôp., Par., 1839, 2. s., i, 446. ——. Ongle incarné opéré sans succès par diverses méthodes, guéri radicalement par le procédé de . . . *Ibid.*, 1843, 2. s., v, 475. — **Beech** (J. H.) Ingrowing toe-nails. Penins. J. M., Ann Arbor, Mich., 1856–7, iv, 78.—**Bertherand** (A.) À propos du traitement de l'ongle incarné. Gaz. méd. de l'Algérie, Alger, 1876, xxi, 39–41.—**Besnchet** (J.-C.) Note sur l'incarnation de l'ongle et sur un procédé de guérison non sanglant. Gaz. méd. de Par., 1846, 3. s., i, 208.—**Bichat** (X.) Ongle du gros orteil entré dans les chairs. J. de chir., Par., 1792, iv, 118–223.—**Biessy** (C.-V.) Méthode très-simple de guérir les ongles rentrés dans les chairs. Rev. méd. franç. et étrang., Par., 1830, ii, 54–58.—**Björkén** (J.) Om behandling af inväxt nagel. Upsala Läkaref. Förh., 1869–70, v, 400–410.—**Black** (J. R.) Inverted toe nail. Cincin. Lancet & Obs., 1860. n. s., iii, 760–762.—**Blaquière.** Sur le traitement de l'ongle entré dans les chairs. J. compl. du dict. d. sc. méd., Par., 1824, xviii, 208–210.—**Bonnal.** Traitement de l'ongle incarné par le perchlorure de fer. Mém. et bull. Soc. de méd. de Bordeaux (1869), 1871, 93. [Discussion], 95–97.—**Bonnet** (A.) De l'emploi de l'éponge préparée dans le traitement de l'ongle rentré dans les chairs. Bull. gén. de thérap., etc., Par., 1834, vi, 339–344.—**Borelli** (G.) Intorno a due casi di unghia incarnata. *In:* Borelli (G.) & Garelli (G.) Racc. di oss. clin.-patol., 8°, Torino, 1853, fasc. ii–iii, 59–65. ——. Sui cenni pratici intorno all' unghia incarnata del Dott. Claire, etc. *Ibid.*, 66–71.—**Bouchaud.** Méthode curative de l'ongle incarné sans opération. Arch. gén. de méd., Par., 1877, xxx, 428; 564.—**Brachet.** Lettre à M. Sédillot, sur l'ongle incarné ou rentrant. J. gén. de méd., chir. et pharm., Par., 1816, lviii, 316–320. — **Brando** (J. A.) Curacion radical de la uña clavada en la carne por el percloruro de hierro. Siglo méd, Madrid, 1877, xxiv, 55–57.—**Breitung** (M.) Ueber den "eingewachsenen Nagel". Deutsche Med.-Ztg., Berl., 1885, ii, 1153; 1165. *Also, transl.:* J. de méd., chir. et pharmacol., Brux., 1886, lxxxiii, 382–394.—**Browne** (J. W.) Treatment of in-growing toe-nail. Brit. M. J., Lond., 1884, ii, 857.—**Caillet.** Nouveau cas de guérison de l'ongle incarné par le perchlorure de fer. Gaz. d. hôp., Par., 1863, xxxvi, 67.—**Campbell** (R.) Inverted toe nail, treated without operation. South. M. & S. J., Augusta, 1857, n. s., xiii, 72–75.—**Chancellor** (J. E.) Treatment of ingrowing toe-nail. Virginia M. Month., Richmond, 1879–80, vi, 813–815.—**Clark** (F. Le G.) In-growing nail. St. Thomas's Hosp. Rep. 1883, Lond., 1884, n. s., xiii, 1.—**Clarkson** (H. M.) Gilman's treatment of in-growing nail. Med. & Surg. Reporter, Phila., 1860, n. s., v, 34.—**Cotting** (B. E.) Infleshed toe-nail; a new operation for radical relief. Boston M. & S. J., 1873,

Nails (*Ingrowing*).

lxxxviii, 5-8. ———. In-grown toe nail. *Ibid.*, 1879, c, 901. ———. A few fragmentary remarks on the radical relief of infleshed toe-nail. *Ibid.*, 1887, cxvi, 324. *Also*, Reprint.— **Da Camino** (F. S.) Sulla cura dell' unghia incarnata. Lettera al Dott. Baffico. Ann. univ. di med., Milano, 1848, cxxvi, 145-160. *Also*, Reprint. ———. Sull' unghia incarnata. Ann. univ. di med., Milano, 1848, cxxvi, 145: 1849, cxxxi, 495. *Also*, Reprint.—**Dammann.** Die Operation der eingewachsenen Nägel. Med. Ztg., Berl., 1844, xiii, 241.—**Dechange** (C.) Note sur le traitement de l'ongle incarné. Arch. de méd. mil., Brux., 1849, iv, 200-203.— **Depas** (C.) Étude sur le traitement de l'ongle incarné. Ann. Soc. de méd. de Liége, 1854, v, 5-58.—**Desault** (P.-J.) Réflexions sur la rentrée de l'ongle du gros orteil dans les chairs. *In his:* Œuvres chirurgicales, [etc.], 8°, Par., 1813, ii, 526-530.—**Després** (H.) De l'ongle incarné. Union méd., Par., 1868, 3. s., v, 645-648.— **Detmold.** Treatment of ingrowing toe-nail. N. York J. M., 1856, n. s., xvi, 386.—**Drake** (B. P.) Inverted toe-nail; a new remedy. West. J. M. & S., Louisville, 1851, 3. s., vii, 104.—**Dugan** (W. C.) Ingrowing toe-nail, and the best method of treatment. Am. Pract. & News, Louisville, 1887, n. s., iv, 295-297.—**Emmert** (C.) Zur Operation des eingewachsenen Nagels. Arch. f. klin. Chir., Berl., 1869, xi, 266-277. ———. Zur Operation des eingewachsenen Nagels. Centralbl. f. Chir., Leipz., 1884, xi, 641.—**Fanning** (W. A.) Ingrowing toe-nail. Med. Rec., N. Y., 1879, xv, 238.—**Finaz.** Ongle incarné, nouveau procédé opératoire. J. de méd., chir., pharm., etc., Par., 1852, xxiii, 261.—**Folts** (D. V.) Infleshed toe-nail. Boston M. & S. J., 1873, lxxxviii, 280. — **Gairal** (J.-V.) De l'ongle incarné et de son traitement au moyen d'un nouveau procédé opératoire. Bull. clin., Par., 1836-7, ii, 108-11G.— **Gallway** (J. B.) An easy and efficient mode of treating inversion of the nail of the great toe. Lancet, Lond., 1856, ii, 160. — **Gautier** (V.) Du traitment de l'ongle incarné. Écho méd., Neuchât., 1857. i, 3-11. — **Gay** (G. W.) Treatment of ingrown toe nail. Boston M. & S J., 1879, c, 631.—**Gerdy.** Ongles incarnés; opération d'après un nouveau procédé. Gaz. d. hôp., Par., 1839, 2. s., i, 369.—**Godman** (J. D.) Remarks on inverted toe-nail. Phila. J. M. & Phys. Sc., 1826, xii, 339-341.—**Gosselin** (L.) Sur le traitement de l'ongle incarné. Gaz. hebd. de méd., Par., 1853, i, 7.—**Gouriet.** Quelques mots sur l'ablation de l'ongle dans le traitement de l'ongle incarné. Gaz. d. hôp., Par., 1859, xxxii, 227. — **Gross** (S. D.) Operation for inverted toe-nail. Phila. M. Times, 1872, ii, 410.—**Guilmot.** De la cure de l'ongle incarné, ou ongle rentrant. Rec. de mém. de méd.... mil., Par., 1815, i, 264-269.—**Gusserow.** Ueber das Einwachsen der Nägel. Med. Ztg., Berl., 1845, xiv, 145; 149.—**Guyon.** Nouveau procédé opératoire pour la cure de l'ongle incarné. Gaz. d. hôp., Par., 1862, xxxv, 498. *Also:* Bull. Soc. de chir. de Par., 1863, 2. s., iii, 463-465.—**Hahn.** Ueber das Einwachsen oder die Verkrümmung des Nagels. Ztschr. f. Wundärzte u. Geburtsh., Stuttg., 1866, xix, 250-270.— **Haindorf** (A.) Vom Ausreissen der Nägel. *In his:* Beytr. z. Culturgesch. d. Med. u. Chir. Frankreichs, [etc.], 8°, Götting., 1815, 437-441.—**Hamilton** (F. H.) Ingrowing of the toe-nail. Buffalo M. & S J., 1873-4, xiii, 361-363.—**van Hasselt** (A. W. M.) Over de exsectio der nagelkootjes. Nederl. Lancet, Gravenh., 1845-6, 2. s., i, 526-534, 1 pl.—**Heylen** (R.) Du traitement de l'ongle incarné. J. de méd., chir. et pharmacol., Brux., 1887, lxxxiv, 648-652.—**Hiard.** Ongle incarné. J. de méd. de Bordeaux, 1861, 2. s., vi, 316.—**Hildebrandt.** Ueber das Einwachsen des Grosszehennagels. Deutsche med. Wchnschr., Berl., 1884, x, 85. — **Hiller.** Ueber das Einwachsen der Nägel. Med. Ztg., Berl., 1844, xiii, 213.— **Hough** (J.S.) Knife for operations on club and inverted nails. Am. J. M. Sc., Phila., 1872, n. s., lxiii, 280.—**Hudson** (J. Q. A.) In-growing toe-nail. South. M. Rec., Atlanta, 1874, iv, 125-133.—**Hukill** (W.) Treatment of inverted toe-nails. Med. & Surg. Reporter, Phila., 1874, xxxi, 105.— **Hunter** (C. T.) Treatment of ingrown toe-nail. Phila. Med. Times, 1879, ix, 201-206. *Also:* Proc. Phila. Co. M. Soc., 1879, i, 34-40.—**In-growing** toe-nail. Lancet, Lond., 1869, i, 747.—**Jacopi** (G.) Osservazioni delle ugne incarnate nei pollici dei piedi. *In his:* Prosp. d. Scuola di chir. prat., 8°, Milano, 1813, ii, 1-7. — **Jardon** (J.-L.-H.) De l'onyxis. J. hebd. d. progr. d. sc. et inst. méd., Par., 1836, iii, 240 ; 276 ; 289.—**Jobert** (*de Lamballe*). De l'onyxis; de l'ongle rentré dans les chairs. Gaz. d. hôp., Par., 1858, xxxi, 469.—**Jones** (H. E.) Ingrowing toe-nail. Ohio M. Recorder, Columbus, 1877, ii, 161. — **Jounia-Raymond.** Traitement de l'ongle incarné par la cautérisation. Gaz. d. hôp., Par., 1864, xxxvii, 35.—**Kelly** (S. B.) Ingrowing toe-nail. Boston M. & S. J., 1868, i, 311.— **King** (T. D.) A new method for the treatment of ingrowing toe-nails. Med. & Surg. Reporter, Phila., 1884, li, 733.— **Küpper.** Behandlung der ulcerirenden Onyxis und des eingewachsenen Nagels durch trockenen Verband mit salpetersaurem Bleioxyd. Allg. med. Centr.-Ztg., Berl., 1867, xxxvi, 73.—**Küster** (F.) & **Küster** (R.) Der eingewachsene Nagel. Wchnschr. f. d. ges. Heilk., Berl., 1847, 273.— **Labarraque** (H.) Note sur un procédé de traitement de l'ongle rentré dans les chairs, sans opération chirurgi-

Nails (*Ingrowing*).

cale. *In his:* *Essai sur la céphalalgie, [etc.], 4°, Par., 1837, 71-94, 1 pl. *Also* [Abstr.]: Gaz. d. hôp., Par., 1837, xi, 201.—**Lawson** (F. B.) New operation for the radical cure of ingrowing toe-nail. Med. Rec., N. Y., 1871, v, 511, 1 pl.— **Legrand** (A.) De l'ongle incarné, de son traitement par une méthode aussi efficace que simple et inoffensive. Gaz. d. hôp., Par., 1861, xxxiv, 295. — **Lélut** (F.) Études anatomiques et pathologiques sur deux observations d'onglade. J. d. progr. d. sc. méd., Par., 1827, iv, 203-219.—**Leonard** (J. P.) On fungous ulcer of the toe, or that disease usually styled inverted toe-nail. Boston M. & S. J., 1846, xxxiv, 76.—**Long.** Nouveau procédé pour l'avulsion de l'ongle incarné. Gaz. méd. de Montpel., 1847-8, viii, 67. — **Long** (J.) On the treatment of in-growing nails. Liverpool M.-Chir. J., 1858, ii, 26. — **Lorinser** (F. W.) Ueber den eingewachsenen Nagel. Oesterr. Ztschr. f. prakt. Heilk., Wien, 1859, v, 329-335.—**Lovegrove** (C.) Treatment of the inversion of the toe-nail. Lancet, Lond., 1856, ii, 250.— **de Luca** (D.) Sulla cura dell' unghia incarnata. Resoc. Accad. med. - chir. di Napoli. 1879, xxxiii, 133-135. — **Luton.** Exostose sous-onguéale. Bull. Soc. méd. de Reims, 1877, no. 15, 84. — **M'Dougal** (H. J.) On "in-growing" of the toe-nail. Med. Times, Lond., 1850, xxi, 195.—**Martin.** Traitement de l'ongle entré dans les chairs (ongle incarné). Rec. de mém. de méd. . . . mil., Par., 1836, xxxix, 207-210. — **Martin** (H. A.) Toe nail ulcer; what it is and its treatment, ancient and modern. Toledo M. & S. J., 1879, iii, 89; 129. *Also*, Reprint. — **Medini** (L.) Pinzetta per l' estirpazione dell' unghia incarnata. Bull. d. sc. med. di Bologna, 1884, 6. s., xiv, 41-45.—**Meigs** (C.) cursory remarks on inverted toe-nail. Phila. J. M. & Phys. Sc., 1821, ii, 265-267. — **Melion** (J. V.) Ueber eingewachsene Nägel. Oesterr. med. Wchnschr., Wien, 1846, 1539-1544.—**Mezger.** Zur Behandlung des eingewachsenen Nagels der grossen Zehe. Mitth. d. badisch. aerztl. Ver., Karlsruhe, 1857, xi. 143.—**Miall** (P.) Treatment of ingrowing toe-nail. Brit. M. J., Lond., 1886, ii, 922. — **Michaelis** (H. S.) Ueber das Einwachsen des Nagels. J. d. Chir. u. Augenh., Berl., 1830, xiv, 234-255. *Also, transl.:* J. compl. du dict. d. sc. méd., Par., 1830, xxxviii, 373 - 385. — **Molard.** Ongle incarné. Gaz. d. hôp., Par., 1850, 3. s., ii, 306.—**Monod** (G.) Sur le traitement de l'ongle incarné par le nitrate d'argent. Union méd., Par., 1880, 3. s., xxx, 763. — **von Mosetig-Moorhof.** Incarnatio unguis. Ztschr. f. Therap. m. Einbzhng. d. Elect.- u. Hydrotherap., Wien, 1885, iii, 1-4.—**Naegeli** (O.) Ein Fall von Onychogryphosis sämmtlicher Zehen. Deutsche Ztschr. f. Chir., Leipz., 1881-2, xvi, 104-106, 1 pl.— **Néret.** Nouveau procédé pour l'arrachement de l'ongle incarné (ongle entré dans les chairs). Arch. gén. de méd., Par., 1838, ii, 202.—**Nicholson** (B.) Rough notes from practice. On a cause of "in-growing toe-nail". Med. Times & Gaz., Lond., 1866, ii, 222. — **Ongle** incarné dans les chairs: opération par le procédé mixte de M. Jobert (*de Lamballe*); guérison. Gaz. d. hôp., Par., 1854. xxvii, 201.—**Ozanam.** Du traitement médical de l'ongle incarné, par les lames de caoutchouc. J. d. conn. méd. prat., Par., 1875, xlii, 49. —**Pancoast** (J.) Inversion of the toe-nail. Phila. M. Times, 1871, i, 258.—**Papillaud** (L.) Lettre sur l'ongle incarné. Union méd., Par., 1868, 3. s., v, 498-500.—**Paterson** (J. L.) Nota sobre o tratamento da unha engravada. Gaz. med. da Bahia, 1876, 2. s., i, 28-30.—**Paulli** (E.) Om Operationen for den nedgroede Negl. Hosp.-Medd., Kjøbenh., 1853, vi, 318-330.—**Payan.** Ongle incarné ; méthode curative simple et facile. J. de méd., chir., pharm., etc., Par., 1840, xi, 453-457. —. Considérations sur la thérapeutique de l'ongle incarné, et son vrai traitement. Rev. méd. franç. et étrang., Par., 1840, iii, 44-57.—**Perrotton** (L.) Notice sur les ongles incarnés. J. gén. de méd., chir. et pharm., Par., 1826, xciv, 343-352. ———. Nouvelle notice sur les avantages de l'emploi du caustique dans le traitement de l'ongle incarné. Tr. méd., Par., 1833, xi, 41-44.—**Pertusio** (G.) Nuova modificazione al metodo di Désault per la cura dell' unghia incarnita. Gior. d. r. Accad. di med. di Torino, 1874, xxxvii, 279-284.—**Petersen** (F.) Zur Operation des eingewachsenen Nagels. Deutsche med. Wchnschr., Berl., 1884, x, 196.—**Pétrequin.** Note sur un nouveau procédé pour le traitement de l'ongle incarné. Arch. de méd. belge, Brux., 1841, iv, 181-189. ———. Note sur un nouveau procédé pour le traitement de l'ongle incarné. Ann. Soc. méd.-chir. de Bruges, 1841, ii, 175-188.—**Pollak** (S.) Case of onychogryphosis. St. Louis Cour. Med., 1881, vi, 398.— **Porcher** (F. P.) Cocaine in the avulsion of ingrowing toe-nails. Med. News, Phila., 1885, xlvii, 34.—**Porter** (I. G.) On incurved toe-nail. Am. J. M. Sc., Phila., 1860, n. s., xxxix, 124-126.—**Quénu.** Des limites de la matrice de l'ongle ; applications au traitement de l'ongle incarné. Bull. et mém. Soc. de chir. de Par., 1887, n. s., xiii, 552-558. ———. Ongle incarné. Réponse à une lettre de M. le Dr. Stocquart, réclamant la priorité pour son procédé de l'ongle incarné. *Ibid.*, 331-333.—**Richter** (H. E.) Du traitement de l'ongle incarné. Ann. méd. de la Flandre occid., Roulers, 1854, iii, 245.—**Ricketts** (B. M.) Onychogryphosis. Cincin. Lancet-Clinic, 1887, n. s., xviii, 302.— **Robbe.** De la cure radicale de l'ongle incarné, par le procédé de M. Dupuytren. Arch. gén. de méd., Par.-

Nails (*Ingrowing*).

1826, xi, 432–438.—**Rothamel.** Heilung des eingewachsenen Nagels. Ztschr. f. d. ges. Heilk., etc., Kassel, 1842, i, 1. Hft. 63.—**Rousse.** Traitement de l'ongle incarné. Gaz. d. hôp., Par., 1859, xxxii, 278.—**de St. Germain.** Ongle incarné; trois modes opératoires. Rev. de thérap. méd.-chir., Par., 1879, xlvi, 563.—**Satterthwaite** (T. E.) Treatment of inverted toe-nail. N.York M. J., 1878, xxvii, 392. — **Schlegtendal.** Zur Behandlung des eingewachsenen Grosszehennagels. Deutsche med. Wchnschr., Berl., 1884, x, 666.—**Schuppert** (M.) The cure of an ingrown nail. Am. M. Weekly, N. Y., 1883, xvi, 30.—**Secretan** (H.) Nouveau procédé pour l'extirpation des ongles incarnés. Rev. méd. de la Suisse Rom., Genève, 1886, vi, 759. — **Senné.** Traitement de l'ongle entré dans les chairs au moyen de la cautérisation par la potasse caustique. Bull. gén. de thérap., etc.. Par., 1832, ii, 378–380.—**Scutin.** Sur l'ongle incarné. [Discussion.] Bull. Acad. roy. de méd. de Belg., Brux., 1860, 2. s., iii, 822–858, 1 pl. *Also:* Arch. belges de méd. mil., Brux., 1861, xxvii, 162–165, 1 pl.—**Shortt** (J.) Ingrowing of the toe-nail. Indian M. Gaz., Calcutta, 1866, i, 255. — **Smith** (J. G.) Ingrowing toe-nail. Bristol M.-Chir. J., 1884, ii, 99–109. — **Sommé.** Du traitement de l'ongle incarné par l'alun calciné. Ann. Soc. de méd. d'Anvers, 1852, ix, 281–283.—**Spediacci** (A.) Operazione dell' unghia incarnata; descrizione d' una pinzetta utile per esguirne lo strappamento. Boll. d. Soc. tra i cult. d. sc. med. in Siena, 1885, iii, 170–173.—**Stewart** (P.) On inverted toe-nail. N. York J. M., 1856, 3. s., i, 367–369. — **Stocquart.** Traitement chirurgical de l'ongle incarné; procédé nouveau pour obtenir la guérison complète et définitive avec reproduction de l'ongle. J. de méd., chir. et pharmacol., Brux., 1885, lxxx, 464–467.—**Suchard** (E.) Note sur les lésions histologiques de l'ongle incarné ou onyxis latéral. Bull. Soc. anat. de Par., 1884, lix, 664–666. *Also:* Progrès méd., Par.. 1885, 2. s., ii, 202.—**Thierry-Mieg.** Observation d'un ongle incarné guéri par l'emploi topique du perchlorure de fer. Bull. gén. de thérap., etc., Par., 1863, lxv, 547–550. — **Thompson** (F.) Inverted nails. Leavenworth M. Herald, 1870–71, iv, 145.—**Trueheart** (C. W.) Radical cure of "ingrowing nail". Med. Rec., N. Y., 1870, v, 196, 1 pl. — **Vanderbach** (P.) Réflexions sur les ongles incarnés et sur l'emploi de la potasse caustique pour les détruire. Rec. de mém. de méd. . . . mil., Par., 1827, xxiii, 226–235.—**Van Hoeter.** Considérations sur l'ongle entré dans les chairs. J. de méd., chir. et pharmacol., Brux., 1848, vii, 27–32. — **Verneuil.** Pansement à la ouate après arrachement de l'ongle incarné. J. de méd. et chir. prat., Par., 1874, xlv, 156.—**van Wageninge** (P.J.) Emploi d'un moyen simple et certain, pour procurer sans douleur la guérison de l'ongle incarné. Ann. Soc. de méd. prat. de la prov. d'Anvers, Boom, 1846, iv, 222–228.—**Wahu.** Nouvelle méthode pour le traitement de l'ongle incarné. Gaz. d. hôp., Par., 1861, xxxiv, 335.—**Wardrop** (J.) Inflammation of the soft parts surrounding the nail of the toes. Med.-Chir. Tr., Lond., 1814, v, 129–135.—**Weber** (B.) Incarnatio unguis, inverted toe nail. Cincin. Lancet & Obs., 1860. n. s., iii, 691–693.—**Weiss** (M.) Behandlung eingewachsener Nägel der grossen Fusszehe mit Lapis caust. chirurg. Memorabilien, Heilbr., 1867, xii, 222. — **Wenz** (R.) Ueber die Behandlung des eingewachsenen Nagels. Ztschr. f. Wundärzte u. Geburtsh., Stuttg., 1865, xviii, 31. — **Wilkins** (J.) On in-growing toe-nail and its cure without an operation. Austral. M. J., Melbourne, 1871, xvi, 10: 1874, xix, 297.—**Younkin** (E.) Inverted toe-nail. Am. M. J., St. Louis, 1876, iv, 539–541. — **Zechmeister.** Ueber eingewachsenen Nagel der grossen Zehe, Onychia halucis. Allg. Wien. med. Ztg., 1867, xii, 45.

Nails (*Semeiology of*).

See, also, **Diabetes** (*Diagnosis, etc., of*); **Fever** (*Complications, etc., of*); **Nails** (*Syphilis of*); **Paralysis** (*Diagnosis, etc., of*).

DOMECQ-TURON (E.) * De la chute et de la dystrophie des ongles chez les ataxiques. 4°. *Bordeaux*, 1883.

FRANZ (G. A.) * De signis ex unguibus. 8°. *Berolini*, [1840].

HAZA (J.) * De la dystrophie des ongles dans l'aliénation mentale et particulièrement dans la paralysie générale progressive. 4°. *Bordeaux*, 1884.

MILITCHÉVITCH (D.) * Considérations sur quelques troubles trophiques des ongles dans quelques maladies des centres nerveux. 4°. *Paris*, 1883.

POUGET (A.-J.-P.) * De la chute des ongles dans les affections nerveuses, et, en particulier, dans l'ataxie locomotrice. 4°. *Paris*, 1882.

ULMO Y TRUFFIN (A.) * Considérations sur les ongles séméiotiques et médecine légale. 4°. *Paris*, 1875.

Nails (*Semeiology of*).

[**Alliot.**] Du sillon des ongles et de sa valeur pronostique. Gaz. d. hôp., Par., 1861, xxxiv, 442. — **Beau** (J.-H.-S.) Note sur certains caractères de séméiologie rétrospective présentés par les ongles. Arch. gén. de méd., Par., 1846, ii, 447–458.—**Bernhardt** (M.) Einige Beobachtungen über das Längenwachsthum der Nägel bei Gesunden und Nervenkranken. Arch. f. path. Anat., etc., Berl., 1881, lxxxvi, 363–368. — **Coutagne** (H.) Des blessures des ongles au point de vue des données chronologiques qu'elles peuvent fournir en médecine légale. Mém. et compt.-rend. Soc. d. sc. méd. de Lyon (1881), 1882, xxi, pt. 2, 64–69, 1 pl. *Also:* Lyon méd., 1881, xxxvii, 381–385, 1 pl.—**Double** (F.-J.) Considérations séméiotiques sur les ongles. J. gén. de méd., de chir. et pharm., Par., 1808, xxxiii, 397–418.—**Down** (L.) Case of markings on the nails after illness. Tr. Path. Soc. Lond., 1870, xxi, 409.—**Falcone** (T.) Caso di caduta spontanea delle unghie in una donna isterica; qualche considerazione sulla crescenza delle unghie. Gior. ital. d. mal. ven., Milano 1887, xxviii, 206–212. *Also:* Gazz. d. osp., Milano, 1887, viii, 156. — **Fohn.** Ein Fall von abnormer, angeborener Nagelbildung. Tagebl. d. Versamml. deutsch. Naturf. u. Aerzte, Graz, 1875, xlviii, 225 – 227. – **Henning.** Eine Crise durchs Abfallen der Nägel. J. d. pract. Arznk. u. Wundarznk., Berl., 1803, xvi, 1. St., 150–160. — **Heridas** (De las) de las uñas bajo el punto de vista médico legal. Encicl. méd.-farm., Barcel., 1881, v, 730. — **Hilbert** (R.) Ein Fall von spontanem wiederholten Nagelwechsel. Memorabilien, Heilbr., 1884, n. F., iv, 462–464. — **Longstreth** (M.) On changes in the nails in fever, and especially in relapsing fever. Tr. Coll. Phys. Phila., 1877, 3. s., iii, 113–125.—**Mader.** Trophische Affection der Zehennägel bei chronischer Myelitis (Tabes); ungeheilt entlassen. Ber. d. k. k. Krankenanst. Rudolph-Stiftung in Wien (1881), 1882, 314.—**Mailliot.** [Déformation des ongles des doigts et des orteils dans un phthisique.] Bull. Soc. anat. de Par., 1850, xxv, 46.—**Mitchell** (S. W.) On the growth of the nails as a prognostic indication in cerebral paralysis. Tr. Coll. Phys. Phila., 1870, n. s., iv, 364–366.—**Ogle** (J. W.) Drawing illustrating a remarkable condition of the nail and end of one finger in connection with neuralgia of the same finger and of the upper arm. Tr. Path. Soc. Lond., 1865, xvi, 268.—**Prioleau** (L.) De quelques cas de dystrophie unguéale dans certaines affections autres que l'ataxie locomotrice. J. de méd. de Bordeaux, 1883–4, xiii, 111. ———. De la croissance des ongles dystrophiés. Bull. Soc. d'anat. et physiol. . . . de Bordeaux, 1883, iv, 195–197. ———. Deux cas nouveaux d'ataxie locomotrice avec dystrophie unguéale. *Ibid.*, 157–165. Dystrophie des ongles chez les ataxiques. *Ibid.*, 32–48, 2 pl. ———. De quelques cas de dystrophie unguéale dans certaines affections autres que l'ataxie locomotrice. *Ibid.*, 179–184. — **Rœser.** Semiotische Bedeutung der Querfurchen auf den Fingernägeln. Memorabilien, Heilbr., 1862, vii, 13.—**Roth.** Ueber Veränderungen der Nägel nach acuten Krankheiten. Allg. Wien. med. Ztg., 1875, xx, 388.—**Royer-Collard** (H.) De quelques altérations des ongles et de la peau qui les entoure. Répert. gén. d'anat. et physiol. path., Par., 1826, ii, 108 – 136, 2 pl. *Also* [Abstr.]: Arch. gén. de méd., Par., 1827, xiii, 89–92.—**Sillon** (Du) des ongles au point de vue séméiologique et physiologique. Gaz. d. hôp., Par., 1860, xxxiii, 506.—**Suchard.** Des modifications des cellules de la matrice et du lit de l'ongle dans quelques cas pathologiques. École prat. d. hautes études. Lab. d'histol. du Coll. de France. Trav., Par., 1882, 161 – 172, 1 pl. — **Thin** (G.) Transverse depressions on the nails. Lancet, Lond., 1880, i, 697. — **Vanoye** (R.) Influence du rhumatisme sur les ongles. Ann. méd. de la Flandre occid., Roulers, 1852 – 3, ii, 500. — **Vernois** (M.) Étude des diverses circonstances qui semblent, pendant le cours des maladies, déterminer la forme recourbée des ongles. Arch. gén. de méd., Par., 1839, iii, 310 – 327. *Also*, Reprint.—**Vogel** (A.) Die Nägel nach fieberhaften Krankheiten. Deutsches Arch. f. klin Med., Leipz., 1870, vii, 333–344, 1 pl.—**Wilks** (S.) On markings or furrows on the nails as the result of illness. Lancet, Lond., 1869, i, 5: 1870, i, 3; 5.

Nails (*Syphilitic diseases of*).

Bergh (R.) Om den syphilitiske Neglelideu og det syphilitiske Panaritium. Hosp.-Tid., Kjøbenh., 1860, iii, 49. ———. Tilfælde af syphilitisk Neglelidelse. [Syphilis of nails.] *Ibid.*, 1880, 2. R., vii, 901; 922.—**Breda** (A.) Perionissi multiple e gomme cutanee precoci. Riv. veneta di sc. med., Venezia, 1887, vi, 159–163.—**Hutchinson.** Diseased conditions of the nails consequent on inherited syphilis. Tr. Path. Soc. Lond., 1862, xiii, 260, 1 pl. ———. Syphilitic psoriasis of the nails. *Ibid.*, 259. — **Kohn** (E.) Bemerkungen zur Pathologie und Therapie der Nagel-Erkrankungen Syphilitischer. Wien. med. Presse, 1870, xi, 457: 537: 562.—**Ratier.** Note sur le traitement de l'onglade syphilitique. J. univ. et hebd. de méd. et chir. prat., Par., 1832, 2. s., viii, 48–53.—**Vajda.** Onyxis hypertrophica syphilitica. Cong. period. internat. d. sc. méd. Compt.-rend. 1884, Copenh., 1886, iii, sect. de dermat. et syph., 63.

Nairne. The description and use of Nairne's patent electrical machine; with the addition of some philosophical experiments and medical observations. 68 pp., 5 pl. 8°. *London*, 1783.

Nairne (*Robert*) [–1886].
Obituary. Lancet, Lond., 1886, ii, 1005.

Naïs (Hugues). * De la dystocie par procidence des membres inférieurs. 59 pp. 4°. *Paris*, 1882, No. 322.

Nakachian (Hampartzoum) [1856–]. * De la maladie de Ménière considérée principalement au point de vue de son traitement (sulfate de quinine et salicylate de soude). 49 pp., 1 l. 4°. *Paris*, 1882, No. 179.

Nakalakeff.
Pantyukhoff (I.) Nakalakevskii mineralinui istochnik. [Mineral spring of Nakalakeff.] Med. Sbornik, Tiflis, 1867, No. iii, pt. 3, 10–13.

Nakanishi Shiusai. Sho Kan Ron Ben Sei. [Commentary on Sho Kan Ron=fever-cold-treatise.] 6 v. 8°. *Kioto*, 1790.
Japanese text.
Sho Kan Ron is a classical work of Chinese medicine, reducing all diseases to the operations of cold or fever.

Nakir *Arabum.*
FABER (J. M.) * Nakir Arabum, seu flatus ambulativus. sm. 4°. *Argentorati*, 1653.

Nakonz (Carolus Guido) [1833 –]. * De nystagmo. 15 pp. 8°. *Lipsiæ, typ. A. Edelmanni*, 1858.

Naldi (Giacomo). Delle acque medicinali dette volgarmente di San Marino. 3 p. l., 140 pp., 1 l. 8°. *Bologna, stamperia di S. Tommaso d'Aquino*, 1792. [P., v. 1213.]

Naleczow.
Weinberg (A. M.) Zdrojowiska żelaziste w Nałęczowie. [Chalybeate springs of Naleczow.] Gaz. lek., Warszawa, 1881, 2. s., i, 605–607.

Nalenz (Carl). * Beiträge zur Kenntniss der Wirkung des Ergotin. 24 pp. 8°. *Greifswald, F. Hache*, [1874].

Nalet (Henri). * Essai sur les fièvres intermittentes masquées. 1 p. l., 14 pp. 4°. *Strasbourg*, 1805, v. 43.

Nalin (Paul). * De l'alimentation vicieuse dans ses rapports avec la mortalité et la pathologie de la première enfance. viii, 9–66 pp., 2 l. 4°. *Montpellier*, 1878, No. 55.

Nallinger (Joh. David). * De chlorosi ab uterinæ purgationis obstructione. 2 p. l., 42 pp. 4°. *Gryphiswaldiæ, lit. Struckianis*, [1747].
See, also, **Westphal** (Andreas). Existentiam ductuum hepatico-cysticorum in homine [etc.] 4°. *Gryphiswaldiæ*, 1742.
For Biography, see **Scheffel** (Christianus Stephanus).

Nallino (G.)
See **Cossa** (A.) & **Nallino** (G.) Intorno ai semi de ricino, etc. 8°. [*Torino*, 1863.]

Nam-Dinh.
Morand (J.-S.-L.) Le poste de Nam-Dinh dans le delta du Fleuve Rouge. Arch. de méd. et pharm. mil., Par., 1887, x, 1; 119.

Namensverzeichniss der Aerzte von Baden. 16, 3, 5 pp. 16°. [*n. p.*, 1877?]
Namensverzeichniss der Aerzte von Braunschweig. 7 pp. 16°. [*n. p.*, 1877?]
Namensverzeichniss der Aerzte von Elsass-Lothringen. 4, 27 pp. 16°. [*n. p.*, 1877?]
Namensverzeichniss der Aerzte von Hessen. 21 pp. 16°. [*n. p.*, 1877?]
Namensverzeichniss der Aerzte von Mecklenburg. 32 pp. 16°. [*n. p.*, 1877?]
Namensverzeichniss der Aerzte von Oldenburg. 4 pp. 16°. [*n. p.*, 1877?]
Namensverzeichniss der Aerzte von Pfalz. 9 pp. 16°. [*n. p.*, 1877?]
Namensverzeichniss der Aerzte von Sachsen. 49 pp., 1 l. 16°. [*n. p.*, 1877?]

Namensverzeichniss der Aerzte von Schleswig-Holstein. 31 pp. 16°. [*n. p.*, 1877?]
Namensverzeichniss der Aerzte von Thüringen. 25 pp. 16°. [*n. p.*, 1877?]
Namensverzeichniss der Aerzte von Württemberg. 34 pp. 16°. [*n. p.*, 1877?]
Namentliche Nachweisung der Aerzte und Officiers de santé in Elsass-Lothringen nach dem Stande vom April 1880. 15 pp. 8°. *Strassburg, C. F. Schmidt*, 1880.

Namias (Giacinto) [1810–74]. Storia di una diatesi scirrosa, con alcune ricerche generali intorno allo scirro ed al cancro. 36 pp., 1 pl. 8°. *Padova, A. Zambeccari*, 1833.

——. Intorno alle malattie che dominarono in Venezia nel primo quadrimestre del 1836; ossia memoria seconda sul colera. 32 pp. 8°. *Venezia, F. Andreola*, [1836]. [P., v. 942.]
Repr. from: Gior. per serv. ai progr. d. patol., Venezia, 1836, iv, fasc. xi.

——. Intorno all' angina del petto e all' uso del ferro ne' morbi cardiaci e vascolari. Lettera al professor Giovanni Maria Zecchinelli. 24 pp. 8°. *Venezia, F. Andreola*, 1837. [P., v. 905.]
Repr. from: Gior. per serv. ai progr. d. patol., Venezia, 1837, vii, fasc. xxi.

——. Osservazioni cliniche intorno al valerianato di zinco. 21 pp. 8°. *Venezia, Andreola*, 1845.
Repr. from: Atti r. Ist. Veneto di sc., lett. ed arti, iii.

——. Sulla tubercolosi dell' utero e degli organi ad esso attinenti. 8 pp., 1 pl. 4°. *Venezia, segreteria dell' I. R. Istituto*, 1858. [P., v. 584.]
Repr. from: Mem. dell' istituto stesso, v. 7.

——. Anno clinico 1863-4 (dal 1°. maggio del 1863 al 30 aprile del 1864). Fattovi precedere il breve discorso, che il dott. . . . tenne ai suoi uditori il dì che ripigliò gli esercizii clinici al cominciare del secondo anno dell' insegnamento nello spedale di Venezia, raccolto pel Dott. Candido Trevisanato. 368 pp. [*Venezia, Antonelli*, 1865.] [P., v. 1144.]
Repr. from: Gior. veneto di sc. med., Venezia, 1865, 3. s., i–iii.

——. Storia naturale e cura del colera; due letture tenute all' Ospitale civile di Venezia. 3. ed. 114 pp. 12°. *Milano, F. Trevers*, 1873.

——. Sulla pellagra; relazione sopra un libro del Dott. Typaldos. 6 pp. 8°. *Venezia, Grimaldo & Comp.*, 1874.
Repr. from: Atti r. Ist. Veneto di sc., lett. ed arti, 1874, iii.
See, also, **Restelli** (Antonio) & **Namias** (Giacinto). [Lettres médicales sur la galvano-puncture, etc.] 8°. *Montpellier*, 1846.—**Trombini** (Antonio). Riposta del dottor Antonio Trombini, etc. 8°. *Venezia*, 1871.
For Biography, see Atti r. Ist. Veneto di sc., lett. ed arti, 1874, 4. s., iii, 1494–1525 (A. Berti). *Also:* Gior. Veneto d. sc. med., Venezia, 1874, lxxxvii, 5–36 (A. Berti).

—— & **Berti** (Antonio). Sulla contagiosità del cholèra. 32 pp. 8°. *Venezia, G. Antonelli*, 1866.

—— & **Tommasi-Crudeli** (C.) Cosa si può fare in tempo di còlera? Tre conferenze. vi, 146 pp., 1 l. 8°. *Milano, fratelli Treves*, 1884.

—— & **Ziliotto** (Pietro). Intorno alla cura del colera. 16 pp. 8°. *Venezia, Andreola*, 1855.

Namin (J.) * Relation des néoplasmes avec l'arthritis. 58 pp. 4°. *Paris, A. Parent*, 1878, No. 469.

Namur.
See, also, **Cholera** (*Asiatic, History, etc., of*), **Fever** (*Typhoid, History, etc., of*), **Fever** (*Typhus, History, etc., of*), **Hospitals** (*Military*), *by localities.*

FALLOT (S.-[L.]-L.) Études cliniques, ou choix d'observations recueillies à l'Hôpital militaire de Namur pendant le deuxième semestre, 1842. 8°. *Bruxelles*, 1843.

de Nánás (Ladisl. Fodor). *See* **Fodor de Nánás** (Ladisl.)

Nance (*James*) [1818–75].
Obituary. Lancet, Lond., 1875, ii, 365.

de Nancel (Nic.) Discours très-ample de la peste, divisé en trois livres; adressant à messieurs de Tours. 367 pp., 4 l. 8°. *Paris, D. du Val*, 1581.

Nancrede (Charles Beylard) [1847–   ]. Some points in the anatomy of the shoulder-joint examined with reference to its luxations. 2 pp. 8°. *Philadelphia*, [1880].
Repr. from: Phila. M. Times (1879–80), 1880, x.

———. An analysis of the principles on which depends the success of the modern methods of treating wounds. 16 pp. 8°. *New York, G. P. Putnam's Sons*, 1881.
Repr. from: Arch. Med., N. Y., 1881, v.

———. Have we any therapeutic means, as proven by experiment, which directly affect the local processes of inflammation? Read before the Am. Surg. Ass., Cincinnati, May 31, 1883. 16 pp. 8°. [*Philadelphia*, 1883.]
Repr. from: Med. News, Phila., 1883, xlii.
See, also, **Henry** (F. P.) & **Nancrede** (Charles B.) Blood-cell counting, etc. 8°. *Cambridge*, 1879.

Nancrede (Joseph G.) Observations on the Cæsarean operation, accompanied by the relation of a case in which both mother and child were preserved. 12 pp. 8°. [*Philadelphia*, 1835.]
Repr. from: Am. J. M. Sc., Phila., 1835, xvi.
See, also, **Legallois** (Cesar Julien Jean). Experiments on the principle of life, [etc.] 8°. *Philadelphia*, 1813. — **Orfila** (P. [Matthieu Joseph Bonaventure]). A general system of toxicology. 8°. *Philadelphia*, 1817.

Nancrede (N. C.)
See **Legallois** (Cesar Julien Jean). Experiments on the principle of life, [etc.] 8°. *Philadelphia*, 1813.

Nancy. Rapport au Conseil municipal sur la réorganisation du service médical municipal et sur la création d'un bureau municipal d'hygiène. Par le Dr. Ed. Lallement. (16 février 1879.) 16 pp. 8°. *Nancy*, 1879.

Nancy. *Bureau d'hygiène.* Bulletin hebdomadaire de statistique démographique et medicale dressé sur les documents officiels. 5e année, 10e semaine (du 4–10 mars 1883). 1 l. 4°. *Nancy*, 1883.

Nancy.
See, also, **Cholera** (*Asiatic, History, etc., of*), **Education** (*Medical*), *etc.*, **Fever** (*Typhoid, History, etc., of*), **Hospitals** (*Description, etc., of*), *by localities*; **Pharmacy** (*Education in, etc.*); **Prostitution** (*History, etc., of*), *by localities.*
GUTTON. Étude sur l'assainissement de la ville de Nancy. 8°. *Nancy*, 1885.
NANCY. Rap. au Conseil municipal sur la ré organisation du service médical municipal et sur la création d'un bureau municipal d'hygiène. Par E. Lallement. (16 février 1879.) 8°. *Nancy*, 1879.
Chautard (J.) Compte rendu météorologique de 1867. Compt. rend. Soc. de méd. de Nancy, 1867, 108–147. ———. Compte rendu météorologique de 1868. *Ibid.*, 1868, 55–101.—**Delcominete** (E.) Statistique de la ville de Nancy pendant l'année 1879. Rap. gén. trav. Cons. d'hyg. pub. de Meurthe-et-Moselle 1880, Nancy, 1881, xvi, 367 – 392. ——. Statistique de la ville de Nancy pendant l'année 1880. *Ibid.*, 395–416.—**Garnier** (L.) Analyse de l'eau de la fontaine Saint-Thiébaut à Nancy. Mém. Soc. de méd. de Nancy (1880 - 81), 1882, pt. 2, 132–140. — **Ritter** (E.) Les eaux qui servent à l'alimentation de Nancy au point de vue hygiénique. Rap. gén. Cons. d'hyg. pub. de Meurthe-et-Moselle 1876-7, Nancy, 1879, xiv, 56–156.—**Simonin** (J.-B.) Sur les égouts de Nancy. *Ibid.*, 1852-3, Nancy, 1854, ii, 29–34. ——. Résumé des observations météorologiques et médicales faites à Nancy pendant l'année 1860. Mém. Acad. de Stanislas 1860, Nancy, 1861, ii, 276–284. ——. Résumé des observations météorologiques et médicales faites à Nancy pendant l'année 1864. *Ibid.*, 1861, Nancy, 1862, iii, 283–292.

de Nancy (Richard). Discours inaugural sur les fonctions du chirurgien en chef de la Charité

de Nancy (Richard)—continued.
de Lyon, prononcé en séance publique et en présence de l'administration le 27 août 1823. 62 pp. 8°. *Lyon, Durand & Perrin*, 1823. [P., v. 1670.]

Nanet (Pierre - Édouard). *Contribution à l'étude des luxations sous-astragaliennes. 54 pp., 1 l. 4°. *Paris*, 1880, No. 178.

Náni (Giacomo D.) Trattato teorico-pratico sul magnetismo animale. lxiii, 305 pp., 1 l. 12°. *Torino, Ferrero & Franco*, 1850.

Nanke (Walter). *Vergleichend-anatomische Untersuchungen über den Bau von Blüten- und vegetativen Axen dikotyler Holzpflanzen. 54 pp., 1 l. 8°. *Königsberg, Hartung*, 1886.

Nankivell.
Co-Editor of: **Monthly** (The) Homœopathic Review, London, 1874-5.

Nankivell (C. B.) South-western Branch of the British Medical Association. President's address; with remarks on medical charities, their evils, and the remedy. Delivered at Torquay, July 20, 1864. 11 pp. 12°. *London, T. Richards*, 1864.
Repr. from: Brit. M. J., Lond., 1864, ii.

Nanninga (Hendrik Dirk). * Over den invloed van de lucht-electriciteit op het heerschend ziekte-karakter vooral met betrekking tot de cholera. 4 p. l, 46 pp. 8°. *Groningen, P. W. van Heijningen Bosch*, 1859. [*Also, in:* P., v. 213; 305.]

Nannius (*Petrus*) [1677–1717].
MEDICI (M.) De vita, et scriptis Petri Nannii anatomici, et medici Bononiensis. 4°. *Bononiæ*, 1848.

Nannizzi (Domenico). Relazione anatomica d' un doppio feto.
In: RAC. d' opusc. scient. e filol. 16°. *Venezia*, 1748, xxxix, 505–532.

Nannoni (Angelo) [1715–90]. Trattato chirurgico sopra la semplicità del medicare i mali d' attenenza della chirurgia. Aggiuntevi varie esperienze, osservazioni e ragionamenti, che molto giovano per lo stabilimento del buon metodo di medicare i mali appartenenti al chirurgo, ed un discorso sopra alcuni fatti seguiti. Si premette in questa edizione il trattato chirurgico sopra le malattie delle mammelle. 184 pp. 4°. *Venezia, A. Zatta*, 1770.

———. Memorie sopra alcuni casi rari di chirurgia. Queste memorie serviranno per compimento del trattato sopra la semplicità del medicare. 1 p. l., 156 pp. 4°. *Firenze, nella stamperia già Albizziniana*, 1776.

Nannoni (Lorenzo) [1749–1812]. Trattato di ostetricia e di lei respettive operazioni di . . . 2 v. 299, 326 pp., 2 pl. 8°. *Siena, L. & B. Bindi*, 1785-6.

———. Trattato di anatomia, fisiologia e zootomia. 3 v. 4°. *Siena, L. & B. Bindi*, 1788.

———. A treatise on the hydrocele. 3 p. l., 9–82 pp. 8°. *London, W. Mackintosh*, [1779]. [*Also, in:* P., v. 562.]

———. Trattato delle materie chirurgiche, e delle operazioni loro respettive. 2. ed., aumentata considerabilmente dall' autore, e corredata di note anatomico - fisiologiche dal Giovanni Gereme' Santerelli. 3 v. 4°. *Pisa, F. Pieraccini*, 1793-4.

Nansot (P.-E.) *Des quarantaines. 30 pp. 4°. *Paris*, 1859, No. 161, v. 634.

de Nansouty (Max). Les laboratoires de chimie. 8°. [*n. p., n. d.*]
Cutting from: Le Génie civil, 1882, ii, 145-148, 2 pl.
See, also, **de Pietra Santa** (Prosper) & **de Nansouty** (Max). La crémation. 8°. *Paris*, 1881.

Nant (A.) *Sur les tumeurs blanches des articulations. 21 pp. 4°. *Paris*, 1817, No. 202, v. 127.

Nantes. Rapports généraux sur les travaux du Conseil de salubrité de Nantes, pendant les années 1826, 1828, 1829. 8°. *Nantes, 1827–30.* [P., v. 1739.]

For continuation, see **Loire-Inférieure** (*Département de la*).

——. Formulaire des hôpitaux de Nantes, rédigé par le Conseil de santé des hospices. 159 pp. 16°. *Nantes, V. Forest, 1851.*

——. L'épidémie cholérique de Nantes et le service sanitaire maritime en 1884. G. Du Bellay. 12 pp. 8°. [*Nantes, C. Mellinet, 1884.*]
Repr. from: Rec. d. trav. cons. salub. de Nantes.

Nantes.

See, also, **Cholera** (*Asiatic, History, etc., of*), **Education** (*Medical*), *etc.,* **Fever** (*Cerebro-spinal, History, etc., of*), **Fever** (*Malarial, History, etc., of*), **Fever** (*Typhoid, History, etc., of*), **Hospitals** (*Descriptions, etc., of*), **Insane** (*Asylums for, etc.*), *by localities;* **Medicine** (*Clinical, Cases of*).

BOBIERRE (A.) Recherches sur les eaux pluviales recueillies à Nantes en 1863. 4°. *Nantes, 1864.*

GAZETTE médicale de Nantes. Bulletin mensuel de statistique météorologique, démographique et sanitaire de la ville de Nantes. Fondé et publié par la Gazette médicale de Nantes. Années 1–5, Oct., 1882, to Sept., 1887; année 6, Oct., 1887, to March, 1888. 4°. [*Nantes, 1882–8.*]

——. Bulletin annuel de statistique météorologique, démographique et sanitaire de la ville de Nantes. Fondé et publié par la Gazette médicale de Nantes. Année 1882–3. 4°. [*Nantes, 1883.*]

HERBELIN (M.) Note sur une source d'eau ferrugineuse (Nantes). 8°. [*Nantes, 1867–76?*]

Boucher de la Villejossy. Rapport sur le service médical du comité de secours mutuels institué par la Société industrielle de Nantes. Trimestre de printemps: mars, avril, mai, 1838. J. de la sect. de méd. Soc. acad. Loire-Inf., Nantes, 1839, n. s., xv, 69–74.—**Cleiftie.** Sur le filtrage des eaux de fleuve ou de rivière et spécialement de la Loire, à Nantes, au moyen de galeries ouvertes dans les graviers des berges. Assoc. franç. pour l'avance. d. sc. Compt.-rend. 1875, Par., 1876, iv, 293–312.—**Laënnec** (T.) Rapport sur l'état sanitaire de la prison de Nantes et sur les modifications à conseiller pour atténuer les causes d'insalubrité de cet établissement. J. de méd. de l'ouest, Nantes, 1882, xvi, 209–221.—**Maître** (L.) L'ancienne Faculté de médecine de Nantes. Gaz. méd. de Nantes, 1882–3, i, 1; 13.—**Mareschal.** Rapport sur les maladies qui ont occasioné la mort à Nantes dans les années 1827 et 1828. J. de la sect. de méd. Soc. acad. Loire-Inf., Nantes, 1829, v, 169–186.—**Moreau.** Fragmens d'une topographie physique et médicale de Nantes. Rec. périod. Soc. de méd. de Par., 1798, iii, 277–291.—**Pihan-Dufeillay.** Sur les épidémies qui ont régné dans l'arrondissement de Nantes en 1862. J. de la sect. de méd. Soc. acad. Loire-Inf., Nantes, 1863, xxxix, 137–212. ——. Étude sur la constitution médicale de 1864, à Nantes, et sur les épidémies qui ont régné dans son arrondissement. *Ibid.*, 1865, xli, 55–106.—**Plan** de travail pour l'établissement de la topographie médicale de Nantes et du département de la Loire-Inférieure. *Ibid.*, 1826, ii, 177.—**Priou.** Constitution médicale, et maladies régnantes de 1824 et 1825 à Nantes (Loire-Inférieure). J. gén. de méd., chir. et pharm. Par., 1826, xcvi, 289–387.

Nanteuil.

See **Cholera** (*Asiatic, History, etc., of*), *by localities.*

Nantucket.

Abbott (S. W.) The sanitary condition of Nantucket. Boston M. & S. J., 1885, cxii, 357–359.—**Lincoln** (D. F.) Notes on the climate of the Isle of Shoals and of Nantucket. *Ibid.*, 1875, xciii, 405–411. *Also,* Reprint.—**Williams** (H.) The sanitary condition of Nantucket. Boston M. & S. J., 1885, cxii, 309–311.

Nantwich.

LEE (W.) Report to the General Board of Health, on a preliminary inquiry into the sewerage, drainage, and supply of water, and the sanitary condition of the inhabitants of the township of Nantwich, in the county of Chester. 8°. *London, 1850.*

Nanu (G.) [1860–]. * Sur les ostéomes sous-périostiques de la mâchoire inférieure. 50 pp., 1 l. 4°. *Paris, 1884, No. 145.*

Nanula (Antonio). Lettera al chiarissimo Ab. Alessandro Casano. 15 pp. 8°. *Palermo, 1839.*

de Nanzio (Ferdinando) [1802–73]. Sul tifo contagioso de' bovi o peste bos-ungarica ingeneratosi il 1837 nelle Puglie; memoria. 58 pp. 8°. *Napoli, A. Della Croce, 1863.*
Repr. from: Le utili conoscenze.
For Biography, see Lavori Accad. d. r. Ist. d' incorag. a sc. nat. . . . di Napoli (1873), 1874, 36–40.

Napa State Asylum for the Insane. Biennial and annual reports of the trustees and resident physician to the governor of the State. 1.–2., 1875–6 to 1878–9. 8°. *Sacramento, 1877–9.*
Opened Nov. 15, 1875. Trustees make biennial reports to the governor, and the resident physician makes an annual report to the trustees.

Napelline.

See, also, **Neuralgia** (*Facial, etc., Treatment of*).

Laborde. La napelline (alcalcide amorphe soluble de l'aconit). J. de thérap., Par., 1883, x, 411–413.—**Laborde & Duquesnel.** La napelline, alcaloïde amorphe soluble de l'aconit; son action physiologique et thérapeutique. Tribune méd., Par., 1881–2, xiii, 472; 499; 520.

Napheys (George H.) [1842–76]. Modern therapeutics; a compendium of recent formulæ and specific therapeutical directions. 390 pp. 12°. *Philadelphia, S. W. Butler, 1870.*

——. The same. 2. ed. vii, 412 pp. 12°. *Philadelphia, S. W. Butler, 1871.*

——. The same. 3. ed. vii, 8–496 pp. 8°. *Philadelphia, S. W. Butler, 1871.*

——. The same. Approved treatment, and specific methods in medicine and surgery, with an appendix on hypodermic medication, inhalation, aeration, and other remedial agents and therapeutic methods of recent introduction. xv, 17–609 pp. 8°. *Philadelphia, D. G. Brinton, 1877.*

——. The same. And specific therapeutical directions, from the practice of eminent contemporary physicians, American and foreign. 6. ed. xvi, 17–607 pp. 8°. *Philadelphia, D. G. Brinton, 1879.*

——. The same. Edited by J. F. Edwards and D. G. Brinton. 8. ed. xv, 17–629 pp. 8°. *Philadelphia, D. G. Brinton, 1885.*

——. The same. Novísima terapéutica médica; compendio de las fórmulas modernas y tratamientos específicos terapéuticos segun la práctica de los más distinguidos médicos contemporáneos, americanos y extranjeros, traducida de la 7ª edicion norte-americana por Federico Toledo. 379 pp., 1 l. 8°. *Madrid, García y Caravera,* 1881[–3].
Signature 31, pp. 265-270 wanting.

——. The transmission of life. Counsels on the nature and hygiene of the masculine function. 9. ed. iv, 346, v–xxxi pp. 8°. *Philadelphia, J. G. Fergus & Co., 1871.*

——. Modern surgical therapeutics. A compendium of current formulæ, approved dressings, and specific methods for the treatment of surgical diseases and injuries. Revised to the most recent date. xv, 16–587 pp. 8°. *Philadelphia, D. G. Brinton, 1878.*

——. The same. 6. ed. xvi, 17–605 pp. 8°. *Philadelphia, D. G. Brinton, 1879.*
Also, Co-Editor of: **Half-Yearly** Compendium of Medical Science, Philadelphia, 1868–74.—**Physician's** (The) Annual, Philadelphia, 1872.
For Biography, see **Biographical** sketch of the late George H. Napheys, with the opinions of various eminent contemporaries on the value of his works to the public. 12°. *Philadelphia, 1878.*
See, also, Tr. M. Soc. Penn., Phila., 1877, xi, pt. 2, 719.

Naphtha.

See, also, **Petroleum; Phthisis** (*Treatment of*).

HENCKEL (G. M.) * Experimenta chymica de naphtha nitri etiam per iguem elaboranda. 4°. *Erfordiæ,* [1761].

Naphtha.

Leclercq (D.) * De ligni distillatione. 4°. *Leodii*, 1829.

Reichel (C. C.) Epistola novam ac succinctam naphthæ petrolei et inde productorum historiam complexa. 4°. *Vitembergæ*, 1746.

Testimonies and cases by eminent physicians and surgeons in favour of the Barbadoes naphtha, from the springs on the Mount Hall estate, in the island of Barbadoes. 8°. [*n. p., n. d.*]

Gulishambaroff (St. O.) Znachenie nefti i eja derivatov. [Value of naphtha and its source.] Med. Sbornik, Tiflis, 1884, no. 38, 90–112.—Leopold (J. H.) Vorsicht bei Anwendung der Naphtha Vitrioli. Monatschr. f. Geburtsk. u. Frauenkr., Berl., 1857, x, 351–353.—de Rovira (J.) Informe sobre deposito de aparatos para el uso del aceite de nafta. Trab. Com. d. med. leg. é hig. púb. de la Acad. de cien. méd. . . . de la Habana, 1873, ii, 251–254.—Watson (L. H.) Naphtha as a disinfectant. Med. & Surg. Reporter, Phila., 1878, xxxix, 239.

Naphthalin.

Bellocq (C.) * Effets physiologiques de naphtaline. 8°. *Toulouse*, 1876.

Fischer (E.) Das Naphtalin in der Heilkunde und in der Landwirthschaft. Mit besonderer Rücksicht auf seine Verwendung zur Vertilgung der Reblaus. 8°. *Strassburg*, 1883.

Guareschi (I.) Nuove ricerche sulla naftalina. 8°. *Torino*, 1885.

Repr. from: Atti d. r. Accad. d. sc. di Torino, 1885, xxi.

Kleiner (C. E.) * Ueber a-Disulfhydrat und Dirhodanat des Naphtalins. 8°. *Bern*, 1877.

Muret (M.) * Ueber die therapeutische Verwerthung des Naphthalins, besonders bei Typhus abdominalis. [Strasburg.] 8°. *Basel*, 1886.

Sauermann (J.) * Ueber Monochlornaphtaline. [Bern.] 8°. *Neustadt*, [1883].

Taylor (T.) Naphthaline as an insecticide, etc.; its effect on seeds, plants, insects, and other animals. 8°. [*Washington*, 1884.]

Weidig (H.) * Studien über das Verhalten einiger Naphtalin- und Naphtolderivate. [Bern.] 8°. *Giessen*, 1883.

Ziegler (J. H.) * Ueber Derivate des Beta-Naphtylamins. 8°. *Frauenfeld*, 1883.

Anschütz. Resultate einiger Versuche mit dem Naphthalinverbande. Centralbl. f. Chir., Leipz., 1882, ix, 521–524.—Bonning (C.) Naphthaline, a new antiseptic. Physician & Surg., Ann Arbor, Mich., 1883, v, 1–4.—Brémond. De la naphtaline. Mém. Soc. d. sc. nat. et méd. de Seine-et-Oise 1874–82, Versailles, 1883, xii, 217–225.—Cagnoli. La naftalina in terapia. Riv. di chim. med. e farm., Torino, 1884, ii, 494–498.—Dejakonoff (P. I.) O perevjazke ran naphtalinom. Vrach, St. Petersb., 1882, iii, 647–649.—Dupasquier (A.) Emploi de la naphtaline comme médicament incisif, expectorant, formules pour son administration. J. de méd. de Lyon, 1842, iii, 476–479. — Eichhorst. Die Züricher Naphthalinbeobachtungen. Centralbl. f. klin. Med., Leipz., 1885, vi, 57.—Evers. Erkrankung, anscheinend hervorgerufen durch Naphthalin. Berl. klin. Wchnschr., 1884, xxi, 593–595.—Fischer (E.) Naphtalin, ein neues Antisepticum. *Ibid.*, 1881, xviii, 710. ———. Untersuchungen über die Wirkung des Naphtalin. *Ibid.*, 1882, xix, 113; 135.—Fronmüller. Das Naphtalin und die Naphtole. Memorabilien, Heilbr., 1883, n. F., iii, 257–267.—Frühauf (H.) Contribuzione allo studio sul uso e azione della naftalina come antisettico. Rivista, Genova, 1882, i. 164–169. — Hoeftman (H.) Versuche über das Naphthalin als Verbandmittel. Centralbl. f. Chir., Leipz., 1882, ix, 697–702.—Klink (E.) Naftalina jako noroy lek do opatrunku owrzodzeń szankrowych i przymiotowych. [Naphthaline in the treatment of chancre and contagious eruptions.] Gaz. lek., Warszawa, 1883, 2. s., iii, 120; 153. — Kovács (A.) Mit Naphthalin behandelte Fälle. [*Transl. from:* Közegészségügyi kalauz, 1885, No. 4. Extr.] Pest. med.-chir. Presse, Budapest, 1885, xxi, 181.—Lehmann (E.) Ueber Phenolharnreaction bei innerlichem Naphthalingebrauch. Berl. klin. Wchnschr., 1885, xxii, 122.—Magnus. Ueber den Einfluss des Naphthalins auf das Sehorgan. Therap. Monatsh., Berl., 1887, i, 387–389. — Matlakowski (W.) Naftalina jako środek opatrunkowy. [Naphthaline for dressing wounds.] Gaz. lek., Warszawa, 1883, 2. s., iii, 333; 351; 381.—Morelli (G. B.) Della naftalina in chirurgia. Gazz. d. osp., Milano, 1883, iv, 347.—Neubauer (H.) A naphtalin mint a jodoform helyettesitöje. [Naphthaline a substitute for iodoform.] Gyógyászat, Budapest,

Naphthalin.

1883, xxiii, 569–571.—Park (R.) Naphthalin as an antiseptic for surgical dressings. Weekly M. Rev., Chicago, 1883, vii, 54.—Pellacani (P.) I balsamici e la naftalina nella medicazione dell' urina. Salute: Italia med., Genova, 1885, xix, 431–437. *Also*, Reprint.—Penzoldt (E.) Ueber einige Erscheinungen am Harn nach Naphtalingebrauch. Arch. f. exper. Path. u. Pharmakol., Leipz., 1886, xxi, 34–40.—Pick (R.) Ueber eine unangenehme Nebenwirkung des Naphthalinum purissimum. Deutsche med. Wchnschr., Berl., 1885, xi, 149.—Popoff. Etshe neskolko slov o lechen. naftalinom. [A few more words on treatment by naphthaline.] Arch. vet. nauk, St. Petersb., 1886, xvi, pt. 3, 153–164.—Raimondi (C.) La naftalina come antisettico. Riv. di chim. med. e farm., Torino, 1883, i, 290–293.—Rasmussen (A. F.) Om Naftalinet. Hosp.-Tid., Kjøbenh., 1885, 3. R., iii, 921–930.—Riley (C. V.) The use of naphthaline as an insecticide. Science, Cambridge, 1884, iii, 455.—Rossbach (M. J.) Ueber eine neue Heilwirkung des Naphthalin. Verhandl. d. Cong. f. innere Med., Wiesb., 1884, iii, 199–203. *Also:* Allg. Wien. med. Ztg., 1884, xxix, 461. ———. Zur Naphthalinfrage. Berl. klin. Wchnschr., 1885, xxii, 213–215. ———. Die Züricher Naphthalinbeobachtungen. Centralbl. f. klin. Med., Leipz., 1885, vi, 1–3.—Rydygier. Zur Naphthalinbehandlung. Berl. klin. Wchnschr., 1883, xx, 239–241.—Schwarz (E.) Klinische Beobachtungen über Naphthalin. Centralbl. f. klin. Med., Leipz., 1884, v, 793–795.—Stewart (J.) The actions and uses of naphthalin. Canad. Pract., Toronto, 1884, ix, 329.—Tashiro Ittoku. [The uses of naphthaline.] Iji Shinbun, Tokei, 1883, no. 99, Oct. 5.—Testa (B.) Ricerche sperimentali sull' azione biologica della naftalina. Riv. clin. di Bologna, 1884, 3. s., iv, 706–719. ———. Naftalina. Gior. di clin. e terap., Messina, 1884, iii, 310–321.

Naphthol.

Allen (C. W.) Naphthol. Med. Rec., N. Y., 1887, xxxi, 565–569.—Bouchard (C.) Sur le naphtol comme médicament antiseptique. Compt. rend. Acad. d. sc., Par., 1887, cv, 702–707. *Also:* France méd., Par., 1887, ii, 1605–1610. *Also:* Union méd., Par., 1887, 3. s., xliv, 676–679.—Jarisch (A.) Chrysarobin, Pyrogallussäure, Naphtol. Centralbl. f. d. ges. Therap., Wien, 1883, i, 14–20: ii, 68–75.—Kaposi. Ueber ein neues Heilmittel gegen Hautkrankheiten. [Naphtol.] Anz. d. k. k. Gesellsch. d. Aerzte in Wien, 1880–81, 247–251.—Kobert (R.) Ueber Naphtol. Therap. Monatsh., Berl., 1887, i, 164.—Mauthner (J.) Ueber das Verhalten des β-Naphtols im Organismus nach Application auf die Haut. Med. Jahrb., Wien, 1881, 201–205.—Neisser (A.) Die Hämoglobinurie erzeugende Wirkung des Naphtols. Centralbl. f. d. med. Wissensch., Berl., 1881, xix, 545–547.—Shoemaker (J. V.) Naphthol; its medicinal uses and value. Proc. Phila. Co. M. Soc., Phila., 1883–4, vi, 37–43. *Also:* J. Am. M. Ass., Chicago, 1883, i, 501–504. *Also:* Boston M. & S. J., 1883, cix, 440–442. *Also:* Cincin. Lancet & Clinic, 1883, n. s., xi, 435–437. *Also:* Med. Bull., Phila., 1883, v, 272–275.—Viñeta Bellaserra (J.) El naftol; su uso en las enfermedades de la piel. Rev. de cien. méd., Barcel., 1881, vii, 385; 565. *Also:* Bol. de med. y cirug. de Jaen, 1881–2, iv, 49–54.

Naphthochinon.

Plimpton (R. T.) * Beiträge zur Kenntniss des Naphtochinons. 8°. *Marburg*, 1880.

Napias (Henri). * Sur la fièvre pernicieuse algide. 64 pp. 4°. *Paris*, 1870, No. 113.

———. Dispositions prises dans les différents pays de l'Europe pour protéger la santé des enfants travaillant dans l'industrie. 16 pp. 8°. *Paris*, *G. Masson*, 1880.

Repr. from: Rev. d'hyg., Par., 1880, ii.

———. Manuel d'hygiène industrielle, comprenant la législation française et étrangère et les prescriptions les plus habituelles des conseils d'hygiène et de salubrité relatives aux établissements insalubres, incommodes et dangereux. viii, 580 pp. 8°. *Paris, G. Masson*, 1882.

——— & Martin (A.-J.) Société de médecine publique et d'hygiène professionnelle. L'étude et les progrès de l'hygiène en France de 1878 à 1882. Avec une préface de Brouardel. xi, 546 pp. 8°. *Paris, G. Masson*, 1882.

Napias (Maxime). La question des odeurs de Paris. Législation et procédure des établissements dangereux insalubres, ou incommodes. 112 pp. 12°. *Paris, A. Rousseau*, 1881

Napier.

Allen (F. H. L.) Napier (New Zealnad) as a health-resort. Brit. M. J., Lond., 1885, ii, 343.

Napier (Alex.)

See **Eulenberg** (A.) Physiology and pathology of the sympathetic system of nerves. 8°. *London*, 1879.—**Guttmann** (Paul). A handbook of physical diagnosis, etc. 8°. *London*, 1879. ——. The same. 8°. *New York*, 1880.

Napier (Duncan). Neurotonics (the art of strengthening the nerves). A new view of health and disease in relation to the nervous system, the influence of mental emotions upon the body and the origin of chronic diseases, with numerous cases and instructions for cure. 32. ed. 96 pp. 8°. *London, Houlston & Stoneman*, 1854.

Napier (James). Report on Mr. Manning's process as carried out at his works at Edinburgh, and on experiments with the Glasgow sewage. 9 pp. 8°. [*n. p.*, 1857.] [P., v. 14*7.]

Napier (William).

See **Taylor** (Thomas). Letter to the Honorable Wm. Napier on the chemical composition of certain waters [etc.] 8°. *London*, 1851.

Napier (William Francis Patrick) [1785–1860]. History of the war in the peninsula and in the south of France, from 1807 to 1814. 5 v. 8°. *New York, W. G. Widdleton*, 1863.

Napiéralski (Érasme). * Du chloral aux points de vue chimique, physiologique et thérapeutique. 56 pp. 4°. *Paris*, 1870, No. 215.

Napione (Carolus Antonius). Memoria sul lincurio. 14 pp., 1 l. 4°. *Roma, A. Fulgoni*, 1795.

Naples. Regolamento per guarentire le provincie del regno dalla diffusione del cholera asiatico, qualora vi penetrasse. 18 pp. 4°. *Napoli, dai tipi di Cataneo*, 1819.

——. Ordinanza della amministrazione militare del regno delle due Sicilie. xviii, 379 pp. fol. *Napoli, dalla reale tipog. della guerra*, 1824.

——. Statuti per lo reale stabilimento degl' incurabili e luoghi riuniti. 247 pp., 4 tab. 8°. *Naples*, 1839.

——. Relazione per le fognature della città di Napoli a Consiglio municipale dell' assessore Giuseppe Buonomo. Sessione straordinaria, giugno 1874. 97, clxxxvii pp. 8°. *Napoli, F. Giannini*, 1874.

——. Pubblicazioni dell' ufficio statistico della città di Napoli. Nos. 43, 46, 47, 49–52 *bis*, 1879 ; Nos. 1–5, 46, 47, 1880. imp. fol. [*Napoli*, 1879–80.] Continued as the following.

——. Bollettino medico demografico del comune di Napoli. No. 5 (Feb. 5), 1881. fol. [*Napoli*, 1881.] Continuation of preceding.

Naples.

See, also, **Cholera** (*Asiatic, History, etc., of*), **Education** (*Medical*), *etc.,* **Fever** (*Typhus, History, etc., of*), **Hospitals** (*Descriptions, etc., of*), **Hospitals** (*Management, etc., of*), *by localities* ; **Medicine** (*Clinical, Cases of*).

ABATE (F.) Proposta di una necessaria riforma del sistema cloacale pel più pronto ed efficace bonificamento della città di Napoli. 8°. *Napoli*, 1884.

BALSAMO (P.) Sul miglioramento igienico de' tre quartieri mercato pendino porto. 8°. *Napoli*, 1884.

BRACALE (F.) Il risanamento della città di Napoli ; esposizione della legge del 15 gennaio 1885, n. 2892 (serie 3ª), coordinata alle leggi sulla espropriazione per causa di utilità pubblica del 25 giugno 1865, n. 2359 e del 18 dicembre 1879, n. 5188 (serie 2ª); nonchè ed altre leggi e disposizioni relative. 8°. *Napoli*, 1887.

BRUNO (G.) Liernur e Waring, ovvero due sistemi tubolari proposti per la fognatura di Napoli. 8°. *Napoli*, 1883.

——. Fognatura della città di Napoli. Ultimi studi e proposte definitive in seguito al parere emesso dal consiglio dei lavori pubblici. 8°. *Napoli*, 1885.

Naples.

CARRELLI (F.) Sulla fognatura cloacale della città di Napoli. Giustifica del parere propugnato. 8°. *Napoli*, 1885.

DEL CARRETTO (G.) Sul sistema di fognature tubolare pneumatico e sulla convenienza di applicarlo alla città di Napoli. Voto ragionato, risposte a questi conclusioni. roy. 8°. *Napoli*, 1874.

CORTESE (F.) Progetto pel sottosuolo di Napoli. 4°. *Napoli*, 1883.

DE CESARE (F.) Fognatura e Napoli risanata seguito delle idee igieniche. roy. 8°. *Napoli*, 1885.

DE DOMINICIS (N.) La febbre da fogne, ovvero la febbre napoletana. 8°. *Napoli*, 1883.

DE RENZI (S.) Topografia e statistica-medica della città di Napoli. 2. ed. 8°. *Napoli*, 1832.

——. Napoli nell' anno 1764, ossia documenti della carestia e della epidemia che desolarono Napoli nel 1764, preceduti dalla storia di quelle sventure. 12°. *Napoli*, 1868.

EAUX (Des) minérales du golfe de Naples. 8°. *Paris*, [*n. d.*]

CONTENTS.

I. La côte de Castellamare.
II. Naples.
III. La côte de Baies et de Pouzzoles.
IV. L'île d'Ischia.

FASANO (T.) Della febbre epidemica sofferta in Napoli l' anno 1764. Libri iii. 8°. *Napoli*, 1765.

FAZIO (E.) Profili sanitarii. Le abitazioni in Napoli e la profilassi del colera. 12°. *Napoli*, 1887.

FLORENZANO (G.) Bisogna sventrare Napoli. 8°. *Napoli*, 1884.

FRANCHINI (M.) & **SELLITTI** (G.) Novello quartiere per la città di Napoli ove allogare la clase operarà. roy. 8°. *Napoli*, 1884.

FRANCO (D.) Guida popolare ai bagni di Napoli e sue vicinanze non che dei più sviluppati nelle altre provincie meridionali. 18°. *Napoli*, 1885.

FUSCO (S.) Sul risanamento di Napoli ; relazione letta nell' adunanza dell' Associazione politica la Sinistra Meridionale, il dì 3 novembre 1884, seguita da altra relazione speciale per la parte igienica del Prof. Enrico De Renzi. Uditi gl' ingegneri Breglia e Vitale. 16°. *Napoli*, 1884.

GIORDANO (F.) Sulle condizioni di Napoli e dei mezzi più adatti a migliorarle. 8°. *Napoli*, 1884.

DEL GIUDICE (F.) Statistica medica dell' Ospedale di S. Maria della Pace per l' anno 1852. 8°. *Napoli*, 1854.

GUIDA (F.) Discorso preliminare sul problema di Napoli. 8°. *Napoli*, 1884.

DI LORENZO (G.) La insalubrità di Napoli in rapporto alla igiene pubblica della città. 8°. *Napoli*, 1875.

MARTINEZ (J.-P.) * Notice sur la topographie médicale de Naples. 4°. *Paris*, 1834.

MAYO (E.) Pel bonificamento dei bassi quartieri della città di Napoli. Saggio di studi e proposte e progetto di massima dell' ingegnere . . . roy. 8°. *Napoli*, 1885.

MELISSENOS (G. C. A.) L' igiene omicida e gli odori di Napoli. 12°. *Napoli*, 1882.

MONTICELLI (T.) Sulla economia delle acque da ristabilirsi nel regno di Napoli ; memoria. 3. ed. 8°. *Napoli*, 1820.

NAPLES. Relazione per le fognature della città di Napoli al consiglio municipale, sessione straordinaria, giugno 1874. roy. 8°. *Napoli*, 1874.

Naples.

O'CONNOR (B.) Ζωοθανάσιον θαυμαστόν, seu mirabilis viventium interitus in Charonea Neapolitana crypta. Dissertatio physica, Romæ in Academia . . . Ciampini proposita. 16°. *Coloniæ Agrippinæ*, 1694.

PALMIERI (L.) Annali del reale osservatorio meteorologico Vesuviano compilati da . . . Anno primo, 1859. roy. 8°. *Napoli*, 1859.

PIGNATARO (D.) Memoria sullo stato attuale della medicina nelle provincie di questo regno di Napoli, su gli ostacoli, che ne impediscono il miglioramento, e intorno a' mezzi per migliorarlo, diretta a . . . Francesco Andrea Miot, ministro dell' interno. 12°. *Napoli*, 1806.

RELAZIONE e voti del Collegio degli ingegneri ed architetti in Napoli intorno al bonificamento ed ampliamento della città di Napoli. 8°. *Napoli*, 1885.

RICHTER & Co. Lo sventramento i nuovi rioni e le ampliazioni della città di Napoli. Secondo i progetti definitivi legalmente approvati. 1 map, 34×48 in. *Napoli*, [*n. d.*]

SANNICOLA (G.) Riflessioni critiche di un medico amante della patria sur un' opera inglese di I. C. Cox, pubblicata in Londra ed intitolata: Avviso agl' infermi che si dispongono a visitare Napoli, contenente la topografia medica di questa città e la descrizione delle acque minerali del golfo napoletano. 2. ed. 8°. *Palermo*, 1850.

SARCONE (M.) Istoria ragionata de' mali osservati in Napoli nell' intero corso dell' anno 1764. 8°. *Napoli*, 1765.

——. The same. 3 v. 8°. *Venezia*, 1802.

SPATUZZI (A.) La statistica medica diretta all' igiene pubblica della città di Napoli. 4°. *Aversa*, 1873.

——. La costituzione sanitaria di Napoli; note statistico-etiologiche in rapporto alla mortalità del sessennio 1873-8. 8°. *Napoli*, 1879.

[TENORE (M.)] Intorno alla proposta di riforma dello statuto della Società reale. 8°. [*Napoli*, 1848.]

TURCHI (M.) Sulle acque e sulle cloache della città di Napoli. 8°. *Napoli*, 1863.

Canovetti. Note sur les travaux d'assainissement de la ville de Naples. Rev. d'hyg., Par., 1887, ix, 10–27.—**Cantani** (A.) Sulle acque di Napoli in rapporto colle malattie da infezione. Morgagni, Napoli, 1885, xxvii, 241–248.—**Casati** (L.) Una visita alle cliniche di Napoli. Raccoglitore med., Forlì, 1878, 4. s., x, 3–15.—**Coco** (D.) Rendiconto della 1° clinica medica diretta dal Prof. S. Tommasi dei due anni scolastici 1873-4 (malattie infettive). Morgagni, Napoli, 1874, xvi, 881–894. *Also:* Osservatore med., Palermo, 1875, v, 18–36.—**Costa** (O. G.) Estratto delle osservazioni meteorologico-economiche e campestri, fatte da aprile a settembre 1827. Esculapio napol., Napoli, 1828, iii, 65–74.—**De Renzi** (S.) Considérations statistiques sur le royaume de Naples. Ann. d'hyg., Par., 1836, xvi, 298–309.—**Diruf.** Medicinische Briefe über Neapel. Deutsche Klinik, Berl, 1861, xiii, 219; 231; 239; 257; 269; 289; 297.—**Diritto** sanitario. Disposizioni per provvedere alla pubblica igiene della città di Napoli. Gior. d. Soc. ital. d'ig., Milano, 1885, vii, 541–569.—**Eaux** (Les) minérales du golfe de Naples; les sources de Castellamare, de Chiatamone et de Sainte-Lucie. Gaz. méd de Par., 1846, 3. s., i, 807; 927.—**Fazio** (E.) Naples. J. d'hyg., Par., 1883, viii, 335; 349.—**Lippert** (H.) Ein Winter in Neapel, 1870-71; medicinische Skizze. Berl. klin. Wchnschr., 1872, ix, 86; 110.—**di Lorenzo** (G.) La insalubrità di Napoli in rapporto alla igiene pubblica della città. Clinica, Napoli, 1874, i, 22; 28; 37; 46; 53; 60; 75; 84; 91: 1875, ii, 14; 22; 27; 39.—**MacLeod** (J.) La station zoologique de Naples. Ann. Soc. de méd. de Gand, 1882, lx, 13–21.—**Macpherson** (J.) Glimpses at the health resorts of the Bay of Naples in ancient and modern times. Edinb. M. J., 1875, xx, 812; 1103: xxi, 46. — **Malatie** reumatiche ch' han dominato in Napoli nell' autunno dell' anno 1833. Esculapio napol., Napoli, 1834, xv, 65–78.—**Medical** institutions of Naples. N. Am. M. & S. J., Phila., 1830, x, 249–278: 1831, xi, 17–61.—**Menzies** (J. A.) Clinical notes on some fevers at Naples. Edinb. M. J., 1876, xxii, 507–512.—**Mordini** (A.) Sul fenomeno della mortalità in Napoli e sulle condizioni sanitarie delle citta'. Gazz. med. pubb., Napoli, 1874, v, 135–141.—**Movimento** della popolazione del comune di Napoli, nell' anno 1875. *Ibid.*

Naples.

1876, vii, 129–133.—**Naples.** The climate and the public health. Med. Times & Gaz., Lond., 1861, ii, 173.—**Naples** (The) waterworks. Lancet, Lond., 1885, ii, 687.—**Osservazioni** meteorologiche pel mese di Ottobre 1835. Esculapio napol, Napoli, 1836, xix, 64; 128; 192; 256; 320; 384: xx, 64; 128; 192; 256; 320; 383 —**Osservazioni** meteorologiche fatte nella R. Specula di Capodimonte, 1827. *Ibid.*, 1827, i, *passim.* — **Osservazioni** meteorologiche fatte nella R. Specula di Marina, 1827–37. *Ibid.*, 1827–37, i–xxi, *passim.* — **Requin** (A.-P.) Notice médicale sur Naples. Gaz. méd. de Par., 1834, 2. s., ii, 161; 177.—**Strange** (R.) On the climate of Naples. Med.-Chir. Rev., Lond., 1839–40, n. s., xxxii, 307–312.—**Valentin** (L.) Medicinische Bemerkungen über die Hauptstadt Neapel. Hospitäler; grosses Arbeits- und Erziehungshaus; Zustand der Arzneywissenschaft; Mineralwasser; Bäder; die Hundsgrotte; das Observatorium; die Akademieen in Neapel. [From L. Valentin's "Voyage en Italie, fait en année 1820 et 1824, 2. éd., Paris, 1826". Transl. by Albers.] Heidelb. klin. Ann., 1828, iv, Suppl., 161–193.—**Ventra** (D.) Note préliminaire sur le sfregio (la balafre) dans le bas peuple napolitain. Actes Cong. internat. d'authrop. crim. 1885, Rome, 1886-7, i, 458–466.

Napoleon I. [1769–1821].

ARNOTT (A.) An account of the last illness, decease, and post mortem appearances of Napoleon Bonaparte. To which is added a letter from Dr. Arnott to Lieutenant-General Sir Hudson Lowe, giving a succinct statement of Napoleon Bonaparte's disease and demise. 8°. *London*, 1822.

Also, in: Phila. J. M. & Phys. Sc., 1822, v, 380–397.

HÉREAU (J.) Napoléon à Sainte-Hélène; opinion d'un médecin sur la maladie de l'empereur Napoléon et sur la cause de sa mort; offerte à son fils au jour de sa majorité. 8°. *Paris*, 1829.

Mask (The) of Napoleon not made by Antommarchi. Lond. M. & S. J., 1835, vii, 785; 826.

Napoleon III. [1808–73].

ROCHON. Des moyens rationnels de guérison immédiate des rétrécissements de l'urètre et de leurs complications. Cinquième éd. augmentée de quelques faits et documents à propos de la maladie de Napoléon III, et d'observation de guérison radicales par le Dr. Rochon [etc.] 8°. *Paris*, 1873.

Emperor (The) Napoleon. [Lithotrity. Edit.] Lancet, Lond., 1873, i, 58 60.—**Fritsche** (G.) Opis ostatniéj choroby Napoleona III-go. [Account of the disease of Napoleon III.] Medycyna, Warszawa, 1873, i, 65–69.—**Sée** (G.) Maladie et mort de Napoléon III. Gaz. d. hôp., Par., 1873, xlvi, 30.

Napp (Richard). The Argentine Republic; written in German by . . . assisted by several fellow-writers for the Central Argentine Commission on the Centenary Exhibition at Philadelphia. 463, xcvii pp., 1 ch., 2 tab., 5 maps. 8°. *Buenos Aires, Sociedad anonima*, 1876.

Napper (Albert). On the advantages derivable to the medical profession and the public from the establishment of village hospitals, with general instructions concerning costs, plans, rules, etc., and an appropriate dietary. 3. ed. 20 pp. 8°. *London, H. K. Lewis*, 1866.

Napper (James). *Observations pratiques sur l'entérite chronique des enfans. 30 pp. 4°. *Paris*, 1825, No. 221, v. 196.

Naquard (Jean - Baptiste - François - Adolphe). *Essai de gérocomie, ou hygiène des vieillards. 1 p. l., 30 pp. 4°. *Strasbourg*, 1830, v. 61.

Naquard (Paul-Emmanuel). *Étude sur les luxations dù cristallin. 40 pp. 4°. *Paris*, 1871, No. 184.

Naquard (Pierre-Louis-Emmanuel). *I. Quelle est la valeur des signes fournis par l'odeur de la bouche? II. [etc.] 39 pp. 4°. *Paris*, 1844, No. 199, v. 421.

Naquet (A[lfred-Joseph]) [1834–]. De l'allotropie et de l'isomérie. 98 pp. 8°. *Paris, J.-B. Baillière fils*, 1860.

Naquet (A[lfred-Joseph])—continued.

——. Principles of chemistry, founded on modern theories. Transl. from the 2. ed. by William Cortis. Revised by Thomas Stevenson, M. D. xxviii, 848 pp. 8°. *London, H. Renshaw, 1868.*

——. Précis de chimie légale. Guide pour la recherche des poisons, l'examen des armes à feu, l'analyse des cendres, l'altération des écritures, des monnaies, des alliages, des denrées et la détermination des taches dans les expertises chimico-légales à l'usage des médecins, pharmaciens, chimistes, experts, avocats, etc. 1 p. l., 191 pp. sm. 8°. *Paris, F. Savy, 1873.*

——. The same. Compendio de química legal, [etc.] Traducida y adicionada con trabajos especiales de los célebres químicos Fressenius, Wurtz, Bolley y Odling, por Vicente Martin de Argenta. Edicion del Semanario farmacéutico. 512 pp. 8°. *Madrid, Taller tip. del Hospicio, 1873.*

See, also, **Marcano** (Vicente). Elementos de filosofia química [etc.] 8°. *Carácas, 1881.*

For Biography, see Rev. de lit. méd., Par., 1876, i, 126 (F. Rado).

Nar (Gustavus). * De diversis iridis inflammationibus. 14 pp. 8°. *Monachii, J. A. Giesser. 1834.*

Naranjo (Ant. José de Jesus). * De l'action physiologique du chloroforme et de son application aux accouchements. 68 pp. 4°. *Paris, 1869, No. 242.*

von Naranowitsch (Paul) [1801–74]. Das Sanitätswesen in der preuss. Armee während des Krieges 1866. Aus dem Russischen. 1 p. l., 54 pp. 8°. *Berlin, Stuhr, 1866.*

Naranzi (Demetrio). Dell' innesto vaccino; lettera all' . . . Francesco Aglietti.

In: RAGGUAGLIO della vaccina [etc.] 8°. *Udine,* [1801], 209–249.

Narbonne.

See, also, **Cholera** (*Asiatic, History, etc., of*), **Fever** (*Malarial, History, etc., of*), *by localities.*

Py. Constitution météorologico-médicale du mois de décembre 1807, du mois de janvier 1808, et des douze premiers jours de février même année. Hist. Soc. de méd.-prat. de Montpel., 1808, xvii, 89–94.

Narbug (S. O.) * K voprosu o vlijanii vysokoi i nizkoi temperatur pitshi i pitja na usvoenie azotistych tchastei u zdorovych loudei. [Effect of high and low temperature of aliments and beverages on nitrogenous assimilation and on health.] 32 pp., 2 l. 8°. *St. Petersburg, tipog. M. M. Stasoulevitcha, 1887.*

Narceine.

BOUCHARDAT (J.) * De la narcéine. 4°. *Paris, 1865.*

LINÉ (C.) * Études sur la narcéine et son emploi thérapeutique. 4°. *Paris, 1865.*

OETINGER (W.) * Das Narcein als Arzneimittel. 8°. *Tübingen, 1866.*

PETRINI (P.) * Des injections hypodermiques de chlorhydrate de narcéine. 4°. *Paris, 1871.*

——. The same. 4°. *Paris, 1871.*

SALAZAR Y MURPHY (A. M.) * Estudio sobre la accion fisiológica y terapeutica de la "narceina". 4°. *México, 1875.*

SICHTING (O.) * Therapeutische Wirkungen des Papaverin und Narcein. 8°. *Bonn,* [1869].

Beckett (G.-H.) & **Wright** (C.-R.-A.) Sur les sulfates de narcéine et sur d'autres dérivés de narcéine. Monit. scient., Par., 1875, 3. s., v, 1048–1051. — **Béhier.** Contribution à l'histoire clinique de la narcéine. Bull. gén. de thérap., etc., Par., 1864, lxvii, 151–158. — **Caspari.** Das Narceïn als Hypnoticum. Deutsche Klinik, Berl., 1872, xxiv, 187. — **Couyba** (L.) Action du chlorhydrate de narcéine. J. de méd. et chir. prat., Par., 1877, xlviii, 401–403.—**Da Costa** (J. M.) Observations on the action of narcein. Penn. Hosp. Rep., Phila., 1868, i, 177–191.—**Debout.** Coup d'œil sur un des alcaloïdes les plus importants de l'opium. la narcéine. Bull. gén. de thérap., etc., Par., 1864, lxvii, 145–151.—**Erlenmeyer.** Weitere Untersuchungen über die "schlafmachende und schmerzstillende" Wirkung des Narcein. Cor.-Bl. d. deutsch. Gesellsch. f. Psychiat., etc., Neuwied, 1866,

Narceine.

xiii, 321–324.—**Eulenburg** (A.) Ueber Narcein als Heilmittel. Deutsches Arch. f. klin. Med., Leipz., 1866, i, 55–66. *Also, transl.:* J. de méd., chir. et pharmacol., Brux., 1866, xlii, 227–230.—**Fronmüller.** Ueber Narcein und dessen angeblich sedative Wirkung. Memorabilien, Heilbr., 1868, xiii, 58–60.—**Gigon.** De la narcéine. Bull et mém. Soc. de thérap., Par., 1886, 2. s., xiii, 123–126.—**Harley** (J.) The action of narceine. Practitioner, Lond., 1868, i, 289–295.—**Heintz** (K.) Ueber die Wirkung des Narceïnum muriaticum bei subcutaner Anwendung. N. Repert. f. Pharmac., München, 1876, xxv, 669–703. — **Injections** (Des) hypodermiques de chlorhydrate de narcéine. Bull. gén. de thérap., etc., Par., 1872, lxxxii, 136–138.—**Insomnie** et agitation nocturne chez une jeune fille atteinte de phthisie pulmonaire tuberculeuse au troisième degré; impuissance du sirop diacode et de l'extrait thébaïque simultanément employés; bons effets de la narcéine. *Ibid.,* 1865, lxviii, 87–89. — **Kersch.** Narceïn. Memorabilien, Heilbr., 1868, xiii, 159–164.—**Laborde** (J.-V.) La narcéine, son action physiologique et médicamenteuse. Compt. rend. Soc. de biol., Par., 1886, 8. s., iii, 265–268.—**Laborde** (S.-V.) Étude sur les effets physiologiques de la narcéine et sur son action thérapeutique dans quelques maladies chez les enfants. Rec. d. trav. Soc. méd. d'obs. de Par., 1865-6, 2. s., i, 51–60. *Also:* Bull. gén. de thérap., etc., Par., 1865, lxix, 224–233. *Also:* Gaz. d. hôp., Par., 1865, 3. s., xxxviii, 149–151. — **Lecout** (C) Note sur l'action thérapeutique et toxicologique de la narcéine. Compt. rend. Soc. de biol. 1852, Par., 1853, iv, 29–31. — **Liné** (C.) Études sur la narcéine et son emploi thérapeutique. Arch. gén. de méd., Par., 1866, i, 358 - 360. — **Petit** (A.) Sur le chlorhydrate de narcéine. Bull. gén. de thérap., etc., Par., 1872, lxxxiii, 507–511.—**Robertson.** Supplément à l'étude de la narcéine. *Ibid.,* 1865, lxix, 216–219.—**Wright** (C.-R.-A.) Sur le chlorhydrate de narcéine. Monit. scient., Par , 1874, 3. s., iv, 845–847.

Narcissus.

Jourdain (C.) Nouvelles considérations sur la propriété vomitive de la narcitine. Arch. de la méd. belge, Brux., 1840, i, 176–179.—**Loiseleur-Deslongchamps** (J.-L.-A.) Cinquième mémoire; recherches et observations sur les propriétés du narcisse des prés ou narcisse-porillon. *In his:* Hist. méd. d. succéd., 8°, Par., 1830, 147–167.—**Martin-Lauzer.** Propriétés thérapeutiques du narcisse des prés. J. d. conn. méd.-chir., Par., 1852, 2. s., ii, 29–33.—**Pfau.** Drastische Wirkung des Narcissus poëticus (weisse Narcisse). Oesterr. med. Wchnschr., Wien, 1844, 813. — **Pourché.** Observations sur l'emploi de l'extrait du narcisse des prés, dans le traitement de quelques maladies nerveuses. Éphém. méd. de Montpel., 1826, iii, 171–183.—**Ringer** (S.) & **Morshead** (E. A.) On the physiological action of narcissia, an alkaloid obtained from the bulb of the common daffodil (Narcissus pseudo-narcissus). J. Physiol., Lond., 1879, i, 437–451.

Narcissus (Ferdinandus Georgius). * Diss. sistens circa nitrum observationes physico-medicas. 20 pp. sm. 4°. *Halæ Magdeb., lit. C. Henckelii,* [1712].

Narcissus (Franc. Jacobus). * Diss. de generatione et receptaculis chyli. 23 pp. 4°. *Lugd. Bat., 1742.*

Also, in: HALLER. Disp. anat. [etc.] 4°. *Gottingæ,* 1746, i, 769–792.

Narcolepsy.

See, also, **Sleep** (*Abnormal, etc.*)

Ballet (G.) Contribution à l'étude du sommeil pathologique; (quelques cas de narcolepsie). Rev. de méd., Par., 1882, ii, 945–957.—**Camuset** (G.) À propos de la narcolepsie. Gaz. d. hôp., Par., 1880, liii, 659.—**Foot** (A. W.) Narcolepsy. [Abstr.] Lancet, Lond., 1887, i, 25.—**Gélineau.** De la narcolepsie. Gaz. d. hôp., Par., 1880, liii, 626 , 635.—**Porter** (R. H.) Narcolepsy; a seventy-two hours' sleep. Med. Rec., N. Y., 1880, xviii, 610.—**Shataloff** (N.) Sluch. narcolepsiæ. Trudi Obsh. Russk. vrach. v Mosk , Moskva, 1885, 1–5.—**Workman** (J.) Narcolepsia. Am. J. Insan., Utica, N. Y., 1880–81, xxxvii, 294–299.

Narcosis.

See **Narcotism.**

Narcotics.

See, also, **Anæsthetics** ; **Belladonna** ; **Chloral** ; **Chloroform** ; **Conium** ; **Datura** *stramonium* ; **Hyoscyamus** ; **Hypodermic** *injections, etc.* ; **Insanity** (*Treatment of*); **Morphine,** *etc.* ; **Narceine** ; **Narcotism** ; **Neurotics** ; **Opium** ; **Stimulants,** *etc.*

ANSTIE (F. E.) Stimulants and narcotics, their mutual relations; with special researches on the action of alcohol, æther, and chloroform on the vital organism. 8°. *Philadelphia, 1865.*

Narcotics.

BÄR (G. S.) * De narcoticorum effectibus, eorumque imprimis opii usu medico. 12°. *Wirceburgi*, [1813].

BEARD (G. M.) Stimulants and narcotics, medically, philosophically, and morally considered. 8°. *New York*, 1871.

VON BIBRA (E.) Die narkotischen Genussmittel und der Mensch. 8°. *Nürnberg*, 1855.

BLUMROEDER (G.) * De hypnoticis. 4°. *Erlangæ*, [1826].

BOLSTER (J. H.) * De hypnoticis et narcoticis. sm. 4°. *Jenæ*, [1748].

BORRICHIUS (O.) De somno et somniferis maxime papavereis dissertatio. sm. 4°. *Hafniæ*, 1680.

———. The same. sm. 4°. *Hafniæ et Francofurti*, 1682.

———. The same. sm. 4°. *Hafniæ*, 1683.

BRAINERD (J.) A lecture upon narcotic stimulants. 8°. *Cleveland*, 1858.

COLLINS (S. B.) Theriaki ; a treatise on the habitual use of narcotic poison. How the habit is formed ; its consequences and cure. 8°. *Laporte, Ind.*, [1887].

COZE (L.) * Histoire naturelle et pharmacologique des médicaments narcotiques fournis par le règne végétal. 4°. *Strasbourg*, 1853. Concours.

DALMAN (J. W.) * De narcoticis observationes. sm. 4°. *Upsaliæ*, [1816].

DOELTZ (J. C.) * Nova experimenta circa quædam venena ex narcoticorum genere. 8°. *Altorfii*, [1793].

FRONMÜLLER (B.) Klinische Studien über die schlafmachende Wirkung der narkotischen Arzneimittel. 8°. *Erlangen*, 1869.

GREINER (G. F. C.) Die narkotischen Mittel. Als Beitrag zur Erkenntniss ihrer Bedeutung und Wirksamkeit und zur Erinnerung an ihren Werth und Gebrauch. 8°. *Leipzig*, 1842.

HEBERDEN (W.) Ἀντιϑηριακά. An essay on mithridatium and theriaca. sm. 8°. [*London*], 1745.

HITCHCOCK (E.) An essay on alcoholic and narcotic substances, as articles of common use. 12°. *Amherst*, 1830.

JESSENIUS À JESSEN (J.) De mithridatio et theriaca. Disputatio pro qua, pridie nonas Augusti, publico loco stabit Stephanus Marcellus, Austrius. 4°. *Witebergæ*, 1598.

KNOX (R.) * Disp. quædam de viribus stimulantium et narcoticorum in corpore sano. 8°. *Edinburgi*, 1814.

KOESTLIN (C. H.) * Diss. sistens animadversiones de materiis narcoticis regni vegetabilis earumque ratione botanica. 8°. *Tubingæ*, [1808].

KONDURA (A.) * De narcoticorum remediorum virtute. 8°. *Halæ*, [1798].

KRAAKMAN (J. P.) * Diss. quædam de narcoticis in genere continens et de opio in specie. 8°. *Alcmariæ*, 1845.

LARACINE (G.-J.-A.) * Quelques considérations sur l'emploi des narcotiques. 4°. *Paris*, 1806.

LESZIG (E.) * De narcoticorum in infantibus usu. 12°. *Dorpati Livonorum*, 1836.

MICHÉA (C.-F.) Recherches expérimentales sur l'emploi comparé des principaux agents de la médication stupéfiante dans le traitement de l'aliénation mentale. 8°. *Paris*, [*n. d.*]

———. The same. 2. éd. 8°. *Paris*, 1857. See, also, infra.

PICKFORD (P.) Quædam de narcoticis. Commentatio. 4°. *Heidelbergæ*, [1844].

VAN PRAAG (J. L.) Proeve eener historischkritische beschouwing der narcotica. 8°. *Tiel*, 1852.

Narcotics.

PREISENDÖRFER (P.) * Zur Lehre von der Wirkung der Narkotika. 8°. *Leipzig*, 1879.

SARPHATI (S.) * Diss. inaug. continens quæstiones duas. I. Quædam de phthisi. II. De extractorum narcoticorum ex herbis recentibus usu. 8°. *Lugd. Bat.*, 1839.

SCHROETER (C. G.) * De actione narcoticorum in fluidum nerveum. sm. 4°. *Halæ Magdeb.*, [1762].

SINAPIUS (M. A.) Tractatus de remedio doloris, sive materia anodynarum nec non opii causa criminali in foro medico. Accessit visio Alethophili advocati de secta et religione empyricorum panacæistarum. 16°. *Amstelædami*, 1699.

THIEMANN (B. F.) * De viis quibus medicamenta narcotica in corpus recepta vim exserant. 8°. *Berolini*, [1846].

WILLUDOVIUS (G. L. H.) * De caussis quibusdam in effectum, per venena narcotica peractum, venientibus. 8°. *Jenæ*, [1809].

Albrecht (H. R.) Ueber die Gefahren der Anwendung narkotischer Mittel bei Neugebornen. Cor.-Bl. f. schweiz. Aerzte, Basel, 1874, iv, 266–269.—Allen (J. R.) Suggestions as to the method of using narcotics in nervous diseases. Iowa M. J., Keokuk, 1855, ii, 332 ; 424.—van Atteveld (N.) Narcotica non semper prosunt in affectionibus spasmodicis ; immo vero interdum nocent ; præcipue ubi hæ affectiones cum spastica tensione et febrarum rigiditate sunt conjunctæ. *In his*: Quæst. med., 4°, Traj. ad Rhen., 1811, 9.—Barbier. Narcotique. Dict. d. sc. méd., Par., 1819, xxxv, 194–215. ———. Stupéfiant. *Ibid.*, 1821, liii, 52–67. —Barnes (H.) On the abuse of narcotics. Brit. M. J., Lond., 1882, ii, 1032.—Bartholow (R.) On the combined administration, chiefly hypodermically, of chloral, morphia and atropia. Leavenworth M. Herald, 1874, viii, 85–91. —Binz (C.) Zur Wirkungsweise schlafmachender Stoffe. Arch. f. exper. Path. u. Pharmakol., Leipz., 1877, vi, 310–317. ———. Aphorismen und Versuche über schlafmachende Stoffe. *Ibid.*, 1880–81, xiii, 157–168.—Bischoff (E.) Ueber den Begriff der sogenannt narkotischen Arzneistöffe überhaupt und der schmerzlindernden, wie krampfstillenden und entzündungswidrigen Erscheinung ihrer Wirkung im Besonderen. Med. Argos, Leipz., 1840, ii, 409 ; 536. — Bischoff (T. L. W.) Ueber die Resorption der narkotischen Gifte durch die Lymphgefässe. Ztschr. f. rat. Med., Heidelb., 1846, iv, 62–70.— Bodiänder (G.) Experimenteller Beitrag zur Theorie der Narkose. Centralbl. f. klin. Med., Leipz., 1884, v, 249–254.— Brunton (T. L.) The influence of stimulants and narcotics on health. *In*: Book of Health (Morris), 8°, Lond., 1883, 183–267. — Capus (G.) Les narcotiques dans l'Asie centrale. Rev. scient., Par., 1883, xxxi, 745–750. — Carter (W.) On the mechanical and physical effects of narcotics on the brain. Liverpool M. & S. Rep., Lond., 1868, ii, 33–38.—Chauffard. Mémoire sur l'emploi et l'abus des médicaments stupéfiants les plus usités. Tr. méd., Par., 1830, i, 18–29.—De Bast. Réflexions sur la préparation des extraits narcotiques. [Rap. de Cales.] Bull. Soc. de méd. de Gand, 1835, i, 122–128.—Dickson (S. H.) On stimulant narcotics. Richmond & Louisville M. J., Louisville, 1871, xii, 119–132.—Dungan (S. A.) On the combination of chloroform with opiates, for the relief of pain. Nashville J. M. & S., 1870, n. s., vi, 14–16.—Fischer. Einige Worte über die narcotischen Extracte als innere Heilmittel. J. d. pract. Heilk., Berl., 1827, lxv, 6. St., 96–104.—Fisher (J.) Medical discourse on several narcotic vegetable substances. Med. Communicat. Mass. M. Soc., Bost., 1783–1808, i, pt. 2, 1–13.—Fristedt (R. F.) Fronmüllers mångåriga studier af hypnotica. Upsala Läkaref. Förh., 1869–70, v, 218–224.— Fröhner. Ueber neuere Narkotica und Kardiaca. Deutsche Ztschr. f. Thiermed., Leipz., 1887, xiii, 237–266.— Fronmüller, sen. Weitere Untersuchungen über die schlafmachende Kraft der Narcotica. Deutsche Klinik, Berl., 1865, xvii, 331 ; 380.—Godefroi (M. J.) Nasporingen omtrent de wijze van werking der narcotica. Boerhaave. Tijdschr., etc., Amst., 1846, n. s., v, 193–226.— Hauff. Einiges über die Anwendung narkotischer Alkaloide. Med. Cor.-Bl. d. württemb. ärztl. Ver., Stuttg., 1836, vi, 53–56.—Hufeland (C. W.) Erfahrungen über die Anwendung narkotischer Mittel in Rauchgestalt. J. d. pract. Heilk., Berl., 1822, lv, 2. St., 85–93.—Ladenburg (A.) Sur les alcaloïdes naturels et mydriatiques de la belladone, du datura, de la jusquiame et de la duboisia. Compt. rend. Acad. d. sc., Par., 1880, xc. 874–876.—Lane (J. S.) Excessive use of narcotics. Boston M. & S. J., 1860, lxiii, 391–393.—Lutz (C.) Physiologischer Erklärungs-Versuch über die Verschiedenheit der Wirkung von Opiaten bei Kindern und Erwachsenen. Aerztl. Int.-Bl., München, 1878, xxv, 504.—de Man (J. C.) De narcotische extracten door alcohol bereid. Nederl. Weekbl. v. Geneesk., Amst., 1853, iii, 59–63.—Mantegazza (P.)

Narcotics.

Degli alimenti nervosi narcotici: il tabacco; la coca; l'oppio. Igea, Milano, 1864, ii, 354; 370: 1865, iii, 3–7.—**Medicinal** (On the) effects and best administered of narcotics. Med. Mag., Bost., 1834, ii, 552–569. — **Meurer** (F.) Noch ein Beitrag zur Lehre von den narcotischen Mitteln, mit besonderer Berücksichtigung eines Aufsatzes des . . . Richter in Dresden über denselben Gegenstand. Wchnschr. f. d. ges. Heilk., Berl., 1844, 377; 405.—**Meyer** (L.) Ueber die temporisirende Anwendung der Hypnotica. Berl. klin. Wchnschr., 1880, xvii, 521 – 523. — **Michéa** (C.-F.) Recherches expérimentales sur l'emploi de l'opium dans le traitement de l'aliénation mentale. Gaz. méd. de Par., 1853, 3. s., viii, 46; 111; 147; 183; 274; 480; 498; 517; 693; 713. [*See, also, supra.*]—**Morawitzky** (S.) Des narcotiques et de quelques autres substances vénéneuses employées par la population de la province de Fergan. [Transl. by S. Artault.] Arch. slaves de biol., Par., 1886, ii, 97–99.—**Parrish** (E.) Notes on the narcotics. Med. & Surg. Reporter, Phila., 1862, vii, 105–107.—**Pickford** (P.) Die Ergebnisse des Experiments in Bezug auf die Lehre von den narkotischen Arzneimitteln im Allgemeinen. Nach fremden und eigenen Untersuchungen. Arch. f. physiol. Heilk., Stuttg., 1844, iii, 347–379.—**Preisendörfer** (P.) Zur Lehre von der Wirkung der Narkotika. Deutsches Arch. f. klin. Med., Leipz., 1879–80, xxv, 40–52.—**Purdy** (G. B) Inquiry into the effects of vegetable acids, in counteracting narcotics. Tr. Phys. Med. Soc. N. Y., 1817, i, 253–266.—**Richardson** (B. W.) Condensation of water on the bronchial surface during narcotism and in disease. Asclepiad, Lond., 1884, i, 253–255.—**Richter** (H. E.) Gegenbemerkung, die narcotischen Mittel betreffend. Wchnschr. f. d. ges. Heilk., Berl., 1844, 669–672. ———. Beitrag zur Lehre von den narkotischen Mitteln. Arch. f. d. ges. Med., Jena, 1844, vi, 189–205. — **Rode** (C. N.) De narkotiske Extrakter. Norsk Mag. f. Lægevidensk., Christiania, 1867, xxi, 145–148.—**Rowling** (C. E.) The abuse of narcotics. Australas. M. Gaz., Sydney, 1885–6, v, 299. — **Schapiro** (B. M.) K vopr. o novych snotvor. sredstavach. [On new specific remedies.] Mejdunar. Klin., St. Petersb., 1887, vi, no. 5, 1–11. — **Shumovski** (V.) O narkoticheskekh veshchestvakh. [On narcotic substances.] Med. Vestnik, St. Petersb., 1863, iii, 127; 133.—**Sibson** (F.) On the narcotic poisons, particularly opium, and their antidotes. Lond. M. Gaz., 1848, n. s., vii, 578; 792.—**Spalding** (V. M.) Commercial distinctions of the narcotic leaves. Therap. Gaz., Detroit, 1880, n. s., i, 62–64. — **Spender** (J. K.) Remarks on analgesics. Brit. M. J., Lond., 1887. i, 819–822. — **Strzemiński** (J.) Antypiryna i antyfebryna, jako środki kojące ból. [Antipyrine and antifebrine as means to assuage pain.] Gaz. lek., Warszawa, 1887, 2. s., vii, 908–911. — **Thomson** (A. T.) Narcotics. Cycl. Pract. M. (Tweedie), Phila., 1845, iii, 362–376.— **Traube** (L.) Zur Lehre von der Wirkung der Narcotica. *In his:* Ges. Beitr. z. Path. u. Physiol., Berl., 1878, iii, 591. — **Trousseau** (A.) Mémoire sur quelques cas de guérison par l'application de médicaments narcotiques sur le derme dénudé. J. univ. et hebd. de méd. et chir. prat., Par., 1831, iv, 61–76. — **Use** (The) of narcotics. Pop. Sc. Month., N. Y., 1875, vii, 611–617.—**Vergiften** (De) van ons denkvermogen; coca, betel en doornappel. Geneesk. Courant, Tiel, 1886, xl, no. 24.

Narcotine.

Blyth (J.) On the composition of narcotine, and some of its products of decomposition by the action of bichloride of platinum. 8°. [*London, n. d.*]

Repr. from: Mem. Chem. Soc. Lond., 1843–5, ii.

Albers (J. F. H.) Ueber Narcotin und Aesculin und ihre Anwendung in Krankheiten. Deutsche Klinik, Berl., 1862, xiv, 144–146.—**Bally** (V.) Mémoire sur les propriétés de la narcotine. Rev. méd. franç. et étrang., Par., 1825, ii, 365 – 384. — **Beckett** (G. H) & **Wright** (C. R. A.) On narcotine, cotarnine, and hydrocotarnine. J. Chem. Soc. Lond., 1875, n. s., xiii, 573–585: 1876, xxix, 461–474.— **Buet.** Dothinentérite et méningo-céphalite suraiguës; durée: cinq jours et demi. Doit-on les attribuer à la narcotine? Clin. d. hôp., Par., 1827–8, ii, 175.—**Matthiessen** (A.) & **Foster** (G. C.) Researches into the chemical constitution of narcotine, and of its products of decomposition. Phil. Tr. 1863, Lond., 1864, cliii. 345: (1867), 1868, clvii, 657: (1869), 1870, clix, 661. — **Tully** (W.) Experiments for the purpose of determining the operation of narcotine upon the human system, in a state of health. Boston M. & S. J., 1833, vii, 37; 56.—**Wormley** (T. G.) Notes on some of the chemical reactions of narcotine and meconic acid. Ohio M. & S. J., Columbus, 1859–60, xii, 277–285. *Also:* Chem. News, Lond., 1860, ii, 158; 170.

Narcotism.

See, also, **Anæsthesia; Narcotics; Opium** (*Toxicology of*).

Bujades (F.) Contribucion al estudio de la narcosis. Encicl. méd.·farm., Barcel., 1877, i, 543; 555.—**Campbell** (W. H.) A case of fatal narcotism in a child fourteen days old; probably induced by a dose of chloral and morphia administered to the mother. Boston M. & S. J., 1873, x, 116. — **Cavalier.** Sur un phénomène singulier, observé pendant le narcotisme par l'opium. Rev. méd. franç. et étrang., Par., 1830, i, 42–53.—**Comegys** (C. G.) Artificial respiration in extreme narcotism. Cincin. Lancet & Obs., 1859, n. s., ii, 581.—**Evans.** Electro-galvanism in narcotism. Tr. Coll. Phys. Phila., 1850, n. s., i, 66.—**Harris** (E. J.) Application of cold water to the head in narcotism from opium. South. M. & S. J., Augusta, 1852, viii, 461–465.—**Jackson** (A. R.) On the efficacy of cold affusion in narcotism. Am. J. M. Sc., Phila., 1859, n. s., xxxviii, 74–78.—**Levin** (P. A.) Ar en morfinsjuk persen juridiskt tillräknelig? Eira, Göteborg, 1883, vii, 569–573.—**Morache** (G.) Relation médico-légale de l'affaire dite des "Scandales de Bordeaux"; narcotisme par la poudre d'opium torréfié; état mental de la principale accusée. Ann. d'hyg., Par., 1882, 3. s., viii, 225–244.—**Pelletan** (G.) Narcotisme par absorption. J. de chim. méd., etc., Par., 1831, vii, 250–252.—**Salone.** Observations de narcotisme. Clin. d. hôp., Par., 1827, i, 3.—**Wade** (W. F.) On alcoholic narcotism. Brit. M. J., Lond., 1867, i, 689; 729.—**Waller** (A.) Further observations on so-called voltaic narcotism. Med. Times & Gaz., Lond., 1859, xl, 107–109.—**Wilson** (J. S.) Cold affusions in narcotism. Savannah J. M., 1859–60, ii, 293–295.—**Young** (J.) Excessive narcotism. Am. J. M. Sc., Phila., 1852, n. s., xxiii, 426–428.

Nardelli (Raffaele). Tre perizie medico-legali. 59 pp., 1 l. 8°. *Avezzano, Angelini & Pietrocola, 1884.*

———. Igiene e medicina curativa. 23 pp. 8°. *Arezzano, Angelini & Pietrocola, 1885.*

Nardin (Charles). * Sur l'électrothérapie dans l'incontinence nocturne de l'urine. 36 pp. 4°. *Paris, 1864, No. 113.*

Nardin (D. F.)
Editor of : **Southern** (The) Botanic Journal, Charleston, S. C., 1837–8.

Nardius (Joannes). Lactis physica analysis. 6 p. l., 342 pp., 9 l. 4°. *Florentiæ, typ. P. Nestij, 1634.*

———. Noctes geniales. Annus primus. [Opus posthumum, a filio Philippo editum.] 5 p. l., 748 pp., 20 l. sm. 4°. *Bononiæ, typ. J. B. Ferronij,* 1656.

Nardius (Philippus).
See **Nardius** (Joannes). Noctes geniales. sm. 4°. *Bononiæ.* 1656.

Nardo (Gio. Demenico). Prospetto analitico rischiarante l' etiologia e la diagnostica dei mali nervosi, specialmente. isterici ed ipocondriaci. 9 pp., 1 tab. 8°. *Venezia, G. Cecchini & Comp.,* 1842.

———. Sopra un semplice e facile mezzo di leggere distinto senza lenti tanto in caso di miopia, come in caso di presbiopia. 18 pp., 1 l., 1 pl. 8°. *Venezia, G. Antonelli,* 1855.

———. Quali sieno i fatti principali che condurrebbero a suppore essere una mucedinea venefica la causa efficiente del cholera-asiatico; ricerche; con note illustrative. 59 pp. 8°. *Venezia, G. Cecchini,* 1865.

Nardo (Luigi) [1806 – 69]. Della vita e degli studi di Francesco Enrico Trois. 28 pp. 4°. *Venezia, P. Naratovich,* 1855.

———. Come si provvegga a migliorare lo spedale civile generale di Venezia in armonia al progresso dei tempi. Cenni del . . . xxvi, 50 pp., 1 tab. 8°. *Venezia, G. Longo,* 1863.

For Biography, see Gior. veneto di sc. med., Venezia, 1869, 3. s., xi, 755–774 (Berti).

Nardon - Durosier (Félix). * Étude sur la péritonite après l'ovariotomie. 138 pp. 4°. *Paris,* 1869, No. 188.

Nardus.
Portrait in : **Collection**—van Kaathoven.

Nardus *Indica.*
Lafite (H.) Ueber die echte indische Narde. Pharm. Ztschr. f. Russland, St. Petersb., 1887, xxvi, 465-468.

Narens (Xaverius). * De peripneumonia chronica ac imprimis illius symptomatum accurata

Narens (Xaverius)—continued.
expositio. 21 pp. 4°. *Parisiis*, 1817, No. 11,
v. 129.

Nares.

See **Nose**, *etc.*

Naret (Georges-Léon). * Des paralysies consécutives à la diphthérie. 44 pp. 4°. *Paris*, 1862,
No. 198.

Nargaud (Arthur-Léon). * Suppuration chronique des voies séminales. 36 pp. 4°. *Paris*,
1873, No. 162.

Narich (Bélisaire-Jacob) [1856–]. * Expériences avec le cranioclaste de Karl Braun (de
Vienne) dans les bassins très rétrécis, et proposition d'un nouveau procédé d'extraction du fœtus
avec le même instrument. 90 pp., 5 l., 4 pl. 4°.
Paris, 1882, No. 3.

————. À propos d'une opération de céphalotrip-
sie sans broiement chez une femme à bassin ob-
lique-ovalaire. Petite modification dans le cranioclaste. 46 pp., 5 pl. 8°. *Paris, A. Delahaye
& E. Lecrosnier*, 1882.

Nařízení, vydané od c. k.-ministerium záleži-
tosti onitřních dne 4. čerona 1881, jímžto se vydává revidovaná instrukce bábám porodním.
[Regulations, issued by the I. R. ministry for the
the interior, June 4, 1881, concerning instructions for midwives.] 19 pp. 12°. [*Prague?*
1881.]

Narodno Zdravje, izdaje sanitetsko odelenje mi-
nistarstva unutrashnich dela. Uprednik Dr. V.
Dchorjevich. [Popular health, issued by medical department of the Ministry of the Interior.]
[Weekly.] v. 1, 3–4, 1881–5. 3v. 4°. *Beograd*.

Narona.

LANZA (F.) Saggio storico statistico-medico
sopra l' antica città di Narona e lo stato presente
del suo territorio; corredato di alcune inedite
antiche iscrizioni e di una carta topografica lito-
grafata. 8°. *Bologna*, 1842.

Narp (Gustave). * De l'eczéma du sein. 30 pp.
4°. *Paris*, 1872, No. 346.

Narr (Joh.) [1802–69]. * Ueber die Natur und
das Wesen des Friesels. 77 pp. 8°. *München,
Leutner*, 1827.

————. De processu hæmorrhoidali. Diss. path.
14 pp. 4°. *Monachii, sumpt. A. Weber*, 1828.

Narrative [of the appearance of cholera at
Kirkintilloch]. 22+pp. 8°. [*n. p., n. d.*] [P.,
v. 1061.]

Narrative of the conduct of Dr. James Gregory,
towards the Royal College of Physicians of Edinburgh, drawn up and published by order of the
college, in consequence of the various printed
papers circulated by him relative to their affairs.
[With appendix.] viii, 98, 42 pp. 4°. *Edinburgh, P. Miller [and others]*, 1809.

Narrative (A) of the late extraordinary cure
wrought in an instant upon Mrs. Eliz. Savage
(lame from her birth), without the using of any
natural means. With the affidavits which were
made before the right honorable the lord mayor;
and the certificates of several credible persons,
who knew her both before and since her cure.
Enquired into with all its circumstances, by
noted divines, both of the Church of England
and others, and by eminent physicians of the
college; and many persons of quality, who have
expres'd their full satisfaction. With an appendix, attempting to prove, that miracles are not
ceas'd. 46 pp., 1 l. 12°. *London, J. Dunton &
J. Harris*, 1694.

Narrative (A) of the method and success of inoculating the small-pox. *See* **Neal** (Daniel).

Narrative of the recent difficulties in the Provincial Lunatic Asylum in Canada West. *See*
Park (Geo. H.)

Narrative (A) of some proceedings in the management of Chelsea Hospital as far as relates to
the appointment and dismission of Samuel Lee,
surgeon. 5–95 pp. 8°. *London, W. Owen*, 1753.

Narrative (A) of the treatment experienced by
a gentleman during a state of mental derangement; designed to explain the causes and nature of insanity, and to expose the injudicious
conduct pursued towards many unfortunate sufferers under that calamity. 278 pp., 1 l. 8°.
London, E. Wilson, 1838.

Narrative of two wonderful cures, wrought in
the Monastery of the Visitation, at Georgetown,
in the District of Columbia, in the month of
January, 1831. Published with the approbation
of the most Rev. Archbishop of Baltimore, by
James Myers. 24 pp. 8°. *Baltimore, W. A.
Francis*, 1831.

Narratives and confessions of Lucretia P. Cannon, who was tried, convicted, and sentenced to
be hung at Georgetown, Del., with two of her
accomplices; containing an account of some of
the most horrible and shocking murders ever
committed by one of the female sex. 24 pp.,
2 pl. 8°. *New York*, 1841.

Narva.

HALLER (P.) * Biostatik der Stadt Narva,
nebst Vorstädten und Fabriken in den Jahren
1860–85, mit einem Anhang über die Morbilität
daselbst. 8°. *Dorpat*, 1886.

Narwhal.

TURNER. Note on a bidental skull of a narwhal. J.
Anat. & Physiol., Lond., 1873–4, viii, 133.—**Wilson** (H.
S.) The rete mirabile of the narwhal. *Ibid.*, 1879–80, xiv,
377–398, 2 pl.

Narzan.

VETTER. Einiges über das Wasser von Narzan. (Vor-
gelesen in der Hufeland. med.-chir. Gesellsch. zu Berlin d.
7. Juli 1837.) J. d. pract. Heilk., Berl., 1837, lxxxv, 1. St.,
82–88.

Nasal *bones, cartilage, fossæ.*
See **Nose** [*and nasal fossæ*].

Nasal *bones* (*Fracture of*).
See **Nose** (*Wounds, etc., of*).

Nasal *catarrh.*
See **Catarrh** (*Nasal, etc.*)

Nasal *douche.*
See **Douche** (*Nasal*).

Nasal *duct.*
See **Lachrymal** *organs.*

Nasal *index.*
COLLIGNON (R.) La nomenclature quinaire de l'indice
nasal du vivant. Rev. d'anthrop., Par., 1887, 3. s., ii, 8–19.

Nasal *neuroses.*
See **Nose** (*Diseases of, Complications, etc., of*).

Nasal *speculum.*
See **Nose** (*Exploration of*).

Nasal *spine.*
See, also, **Evolution.**
HAMY (E.-T.) De l'épine nasale antérieure dans l'ordre
des primates. Bull. Soc. d'anthrop. de Par., 1869, 2. s.,
iv, 13–28.

Nasalli (Giuseppe). Comitato centrale piacen-
tino degli ospizi marini pei fanciulli poveri scro-
fulosi. Relazione sanitaria e resoconto economico amministrativo. 3., 1872. 27 pp. 8°.
Piacenza, F. Solari, 1873.

Nasaroff (D. A.) * Usilennoe kormlenie chacho-
tochnych mjasnymi poroshkami po sposobu Debova. [Overfeeding in phthisis by powdered
meat, according to Debove's method.] 84, iv
pp., 3 l., 10 diag. 8°. *St. Petersburg, tipog. P.
Voshinskoi*, 1887.

Nascivera (Lodovico). Istruzione dei mezzi
conosciuti più efficaci per preservarsi dalla ma-

Nascivera (Lodovico)—continued.
lattia contagiosa chiamata tifo. 16 pp. 8°.
Treviso, dalla tipografia di A. Paluello, 1814.

Nasemann (Joh. Aug. Ferd.) [1824-].
* Quæstiones de rhinoplastice. 29 pp., 1 l., 1 pl.
8°. *Halis Sax., typ. Heynemannianis*, [1849].

Nashua. Annual report of the municipal government of the city of Nashua, for the year
1878-9. 51 pp. 8°. *Nashua*, 1879.

Nashville. *Board of Health.* Condensed weekly
statements of mortality in the city of Nashville,
Tenn. Jan. 2, 1875, to July 1, 1876. 4°. [*Nashville*, 1875-6.]

——. Reports of deaths in Nashville. [Weekly.]
Dec. 8, 1883, to Oct. 25, 1884; Nov. 8, 1884, to Jan.
3, 1885. 18°. [*Nashville*, 1883-5.]

——. Annual and biennial reports to the city
council of the city of Nashville. 1.-3. (1874-8).
8°. *Nashville*, 1875-9.
2. and 3. reports for two years.

——. Condensed monthly statements of mortality in the city of Nashville, Tenn. Accompanied by the daily meteorological observations. July, 1876, to Dec., 1887. 4°. [*Nashville*, 1876-88.]

——. Condensed statements of mortality in the
city of Nashville, Tenn. Accompanied by the
daily meteorological observations. For the
years 1883 to 1886-7. 4°. [*Nashville*, 1884-7.]

Nashville.

See, also, **Blind** (*Asylums, etc., for*); **Cholera**
(*Asiatic, History, etc., of*), *by localities*; **Dentistry** (*Colleges, etc., of*); **Education** (*Medical*),
etc., **Fever** (*Cerebro-spinal, History, etc., of*),
Hospitals (*Descriptions, etc., of*), **Insane** (*Asylums for, etc.*), **Medicine** (*Clinical, Statistics,
etc., of*), *by localities*; **Pharmacy** (*Education in,
etc.*)

CITIZENS' Auxiliary Sanitary Association of
Nashville. Address [to the officers of the Auxiliary Sanitary Association on the importance of
co-operating with the board of health]. 8°.
Nashville, 1879.

[**Bowling** (W. K.)] A reply to the St. Louis Medical
and Surgical Journal by the editor of the Nashville Journal of Medicine and Surgery. [On an editorial in the
former, headed "Nashville *vs.* Philadelphia and the rest of
creation".] Nashville J. M. & S., 1855, viii, 312-329.
Also, Reprint.—**Currey** (R. O.) [Mortality of Nashville,
for the period from 1822-52; drawn from the cemetery reports.] South. J. M. & Phys. Sc., Nashville, 1853, i, 322;
402: 1854, ii, 87.—**Ford** (A. C.) On the climate of Nashville. Rep. Bd. Health Nashville, 1877, 171-181.—**Foster**
(W. F.) The topography of Nashville. *Ibid.*, 133-144, 1
map.— **Lupton** (N. T.) Report on the water supply of
Nashville. *Ibid.*, 153-170.—**Medical** (The) topography
of the city of Nashville and its vicinity. South. J. M. &
Phys. Sc., Nashville, 1854, ii, 88-94.—**Mitchell** (C.) Mortality statistics of the city of Nashville for the years 1879,
1880, 1881, 1882, 1883, and 1884. Rep. Bd. Health Tenn.
1880-84, Nashville, 1885, ii, 472-512.—**Sevier** (J. W.) Report of cases treated at the "City Dispensary", medical
department, University of Nashville. Nashville J. M. &
S., 1856, x, 130-134.

Nashville (The) Journal of Medicine and Surgery. Edited by W. K. Bowling and Paul F. Eve.
[Bi-monthly.] v. 1-21, Feb., 1851, to Nov., 1861.
N. s., v. 1-41, July, 1866-88. 8°. *Nashville,
Tenn.*
Current. v. 2 became monthly, 2 v. annually; v. 3-5,
n. s., 1 v. annually. Nothing between Nov., 1861, and
July, 1866. v. 14, Eve dropped and R. C. Foster and Geo.
S. Blackie added; v.1-40, n. s., edited successively by
Drs. Bowling, Eve, Joseph Jones, G. S. Blackie, W. T.
Briggs, W. L. Nichol, Thomas O. Summers, and C. S.
Briggs.

——. *See, also:*
First (The) decade of the life of the Nashville Journal
of Medicine and Surgery, 1851-1861. [Edit.] Nashville J.
M. & S., 1881, n. s., xxvii, 271-278.

Nashville Medical College, medical department
of the University of Tennessee. Annual an-

Nashville Medical College [etc.]—continued.
nouncements for the sessions of 1877 to 1887-8
(1.-13.). 8°. *Nashville*, 1877-87.
Organized in 1877. In 1879 became the medical department of the University of Tennessee. Held two graduating courses in 1877 and 1878. List of students and graduates for the sessions of 1877 to 1885-6 in announcements
for subsequent years.

——. Announcement of the spring and special
course of instruction for 1881. 2 l. 8°. *Nashville*, 1881.

Nashville (The) Medical News. A semi-monthly
journal, edited by Richard Douglas and John
W. McAlister. Nos. 1-9, v. 1, April 1 to Aug.
1, 1887. 272 pp. 8°. *Nashville*.
Ended.

Nashville (The) Medical Record. *See* **Nashville** (The) Monthly Record of Medical and
Physical Science, v. 2-3, 1859-60.

Nashville (The) Monthly Record of Medical and
Physical Science. Edited by D. F. Wright, R.
O. Currey, John H. Callender, and Thos. L.
Maddin. v. 1-2; Nos. 1-2, v. 3, Sept., 1858, to
Dec. 1, 1860. 8°. *Nashville.*
Ended. Title of v. 2-3 was: **Nashville** (The) Medical
Record. In v. 2, Currey dropped; in v. 3, Wright dropped
and J. J. Abernathy added.

Nasi (Luigi). Dell' ernia ciecale acistica, considerazioni e nota clinica. Dell' erniotomia, suoi
accidenti e relative indicazioni. 25 pp. 8°.
Modena, Moneti & Namias, 1883.

Nasiloff (Ivan). * O vospalenii barabannoi pereponki (myringitis) ve patolog.-anatom. otnoshenii. 34 pp., 1 pl. 8°. *St. Petersburg*, 1867.

Nasmyth (Alexander). Researches on the developement, structure, and diseases of the teeth.
xvi, 165, 3 pp., 7 pl. 8°. *London, J. Churchill*,
1839.
Historical introduction.

——. The same. xii, 13-116 pp. 8°. *Baltimore, published by the American Society of Dental
Surgeons*, 1842. [P., v. 542.]

——. Researches on the developement, structure, and diseases of the teeth. viii, 230 pp.,
10 pl., port. 8°. *London, J. Churchill*, 1849.
This is a posthumous work, of which the foregoing is
the introduction.

——. Three memoirs on the developement and
structure of the teeth and epithelium. xvi, 47
pp., 9 pl. 8°. *London, J. Churchill*, 1841.

Nasmyth (Robert). * On tic douloureux. 2
p. l., 31 pp. 8°. *Edinburgh, Abernethy & Walker*,
1823. [*Also, in :* P., v. 1272.]

Nasmyth (Thomas). * De rachitide. 44 pp.
8°. *Edinburgi, Balfour et Smellie*, 1777.

Nason (John James). On some of the responsibilities of the medical profession in regard to
sanitation, moral as well as general. The presidential address, delivered at the annual meeting
of the Birmingham and Midland Counties Branch
of the British Medical Association, June 19, 1884.
32 pp. 8°. *London, J. & A. Churchill*, [1884].

Nasopalatine *canal.*
Leboucq (H.) Le canal naso-palatin chez l'homme.
Arch. de biol., Gand, 1881, ii, 386-397, 1 pl.

Nasopalatine *gland* (*Disease of*).
Aschenbrandt (T.) Das Ganglion nasopalatinum s.
incisivum der Nagetiere. Verhandl. d. phys.-med. Gesellsch zu Würzb., 1886, n. F., xx, 9-24, 1 pl.—**Clark** (A.)
Nasopalatine gland disease. Clin. Lect. & Rep. Lond.
Hosp., 1864, i, 211.

Nasopharyngeal *polypus.*
See **Nose** (*Tumors of*).

Nass (Paul). * Ueber den Gerbstoff der Castanea
vesca. 39 pp. 8°. *Dorpat, W. Just*, 1884.

Nassall (Leo Laurentius). * De sectione legali.
32 pp. 12°. *Wirceburgi, F. E. Nitribitt*, [1798].

Nassans (Alexandre). * Du traitement du catarrhe vésical, principalement par les injections

Nassans (Alexandre)—continued.
de nitrate d'argent. 34 pp. 4°. *Paris*, 1857, No. 276, v. 608.

Nassau, N. P., Bahamas, with meteorological tables and other statistics of interest to invalids and travelers. 16 pp. 8°. [*Montreal, n. d.*]

Nassau, *Bahamas.*

See, also, **Fever** (*Malarial, History, etc., of*), **Fever** (*Typhus, History, etc., of*), *by localities.*

GENERAL description of the city of Nassau and island of New Providence, Bahamas, West Indies, with meteorological tables and other statistics of interest to invalids and travelers. 12°. *New York*, 1871.

GUIDE to Nassau, island of New Providence, Bahamas, West Indies. 8°. *New York*, 1876.

NASSAU, island of New Providence, Bahamas. A guide to the sanitarium of the western hemisphere, its attractions, and how to get there; with illustrations from photographs, meteorological tables, and other statistics of interest to invalids and travellers; including "An isle of June", republished from Scribner's Monthly for November, 1877; also, St. Augustine, Fla., and Havana, Cuba, with illustrations, descriptions, routes, etc. 8°. *New York*, 1878.

————. The same. 16°. *New York*, 1879–80.

————. The same. West Indies. The Royal Victoria Hotel and the New York, Nassau and Savannah Mail Steamship Line, with meteorological tables and other statistics of interest to invalids and travellers. 8°. *New York*, 1878.

"**Nassau**" (New Providence). Med. Times & Gaz., Lond., 1885, ii, 197–199.—**Osgood** (H.) Notes on Nassau as a winter resort. Boston M. & S. J., 1884, cxi, 555–558.—[**Shrady** (G. F.)] The climate of Nassau. Med. Rec., N. Y., 1877, xii, 88–90.—**Townsend** (P. S.) An account of the topography, weather, and diseases of Nassau, island of New Providence, capital of Bahamas. N. York M. & Phys. J., 1825, iv, 68; 185.

Nassau, *German Empire.*

See, also, **Cholera** (*Asiatic, History, etc., of*), *by localities*; **Cronthal**; **Ems**; **Hospitals** (*Descriptions, etc., of*), **Idiots** (*Asylums, etc., for*), *by localities*; **Langenschwalbach**; **Medicine** (*History, etc., of*), *by nations, etc.*; **Soden**; **Wiesbaden.**

REUTER (C. F. R.) Die Medicinalverfassung des Herzogthums Nassau, beurtheilt nach einem dreissigjährigen Bestande mit Rücksicht auf das Bedürfniss der Gegenwart. 8°. *Wiesbaden*, 1849.

von Franque (J. B.) Witterungsverhältnisse und allgemeiner Krankheitszustand von 1818–41. Med. Jahrb. f. d. Herzogth. Nassau, Wiesb., 1843, i, 1: 1847, vi, 176, 11 tab.—**Menges** (P.) Statistik der Lebens- und Gesundheits-Verhältnisse in Nassau im Allgemeinen und derjenigen der Aerzte im Besonderen. Mitth. d. Ver. nassau. Aerzte, Weilburg, 1855, ii, 1–29.—**Müller** (A.) Ueber die seit 25 Jahren im Herzogthum Nassau vorgekommenen Unglücksfälle. Med. Jahrb. f. d. Herzogth. Nassau, Wiesb., 1843, i, 34–51. ————. Beitrag zur Statistik oder Beleuchtung der Verhältnisse der Geburten und Sterbefälle der Bevölkerung und deren Lebensdauer im Herzogthum Nassau. Ibid., 1847, vi, 1–89. — **Zusammenstellung** der Einwohnerzahl, des Steuerbetrags, der Geborenen und Gestorbenen, der Zahl der Aerzte und der Apotheken im ganzen Herzogthum Nassau vom Jahr 1818–54. Mitth. d. Ver. nassau. Aerzte, Weilburg, 1855, 35–36.

Nassau, *German Empire* (*Mineral waters of*).

FRESENIUS (C. R.) Chemische Untersuchung der wichtigsten Mineralwasser des Herzogthums Nassau. 8°. *Wiesbaden*, 1850–68.

NASSAUISCHEN (Die) Heilquellen Soden, Cronthal, Weilbach, Wiesbaden, Schlangenbad, Schwalbach und Ems; beschrieben durch einen Verein von Aerzten. 8°. *Wiesbaden*, 1851.

————. The same. Traité sur les eaux minérales du duché de Nassau; précédé d'une esquisse et d'une carte géologique du Taunus. par

Nassau, *German Empire* (*Mineral waters of*).

une réunion de médecins de ces eaux; ouvrage traduit de l'allemand par H. Kaula; avec une introduction du Dr. Aronssohn. 8°. *Wiesbade*, 1853.

OSANN (E.) Bemerkungen über die wichtigsten Mineralquellen des Herzogthums Nassau. 8°. *Berlin*, 1824.

Franque (J. B.) Die Heilquellen des Herzogthums Nassau im Jahre 1836-7. Jahrb. f. Deutschl. Heilq. u. Seebäder, Berl., 1837, ii, 305: 1838, iii, 87. ————. Die Kurorte des Herzogthums Nassau im Jahre 1838–39. Ibid., 1839, iv, 2. Abth., 175: 1840, v, 1. Also, Reprint of last article. — **Grossmann** (F.) Statistische Mittheilungen über die Mineralquellen und Badeorte mit Einschluss der Privat-Bade- und Heilanstalten des nassauischen Taunus während des Jahres 1870. Jahrb. f. Balneol., etc., Wien, 1871, i, pt. 1, 71–92.—**Helfft.** Die nassauischen und Taunusbäder. Deutsche Klinik, Berl., 1853, v, 431–433.—**Kastner** (K. W. G.) Ueber Nassau's Thermalquellen; Beobachtungen, Versuche und Bemerkungen. Arch. f. d. ges. Naturl., Nürnb., 1828, xiii, 401: xiv, 66: 1829, xviii, 489. ————. Die vorzüglichsten Heilquellen des Herzogthums Nassau, ihrem physischen Verhalten und chemischem Gehalte nach geprüft und untersucht. J. d. pract. Heilk., Berl., 1841, xcii, 2. St., 67–104.

Nassauischen (Die) Heilquellen Soden, Cronthal, Weilbach, Wiesbaden, Schlangenbad, Schwalbach und Ems; beschrieben durch einen Verein von Aerzten. v (1 l.), 330 pp., 2 l., 1 map. 8°. *Wiesbaden, C. W. Kreidel*, 1851. [P. v., 886.]

————. The same. Traité sur les eaux minérales du duché de Nassau; précédé d'une esquisse et d'une carte géologique du Taunus; par une réunion de médecins de ces eaux; ouvrage traduit de l'allemand par H. Kaula; avec une introduction du Dr. Aronssohn. xii (1 l.), 281 pp., 1 map. 8°. *Wiesbade, C. G. Kreidel*, 1853. [P., v. 876.]

Nassauischer Verein für Naturkunde. Jahrbücher. Jahrg. 15–30 (1860–77). In 7 v. 8°. *Wiesbaden*, 1860–77.
Want 23. and 24., 1869–70.

Nasse ([Karl Friedrich] Werner, [1822–]. *De singularum cerebri partium functionibus ex morborum perscrutatione indagatis. 1 p. l., 62 pp., 1 l. 4°. *Bonnæ, typ. Lechnerianis*, 1845.

————. Vorschläge zur Irrengesetzgebung, mit besonderer Rücksicht auf Preussen. 1 p. l., 48 pp. 8°. *Marburg, N. G. Elwert*, 1850.

————. Statistische Mittheilungen über die grossherzogl. Irrenanstalten [Heilanstalt Sachsenberg und Pflege-Anstalt zu Dömitz] aus dem sechsjährigen Zeitraume von 1856–61, incl. (vom Herrn Dr. Nasse dem statistischen Bureau mitgetheilt). 12 pp. roy. 8°. [*Schwerin*, 1862.]

Nasse (Christianus Fridericus) [1778–1851]. *De neuritide. 67 pp. 8°. *Halæ, in off. Batheana*, [1800].

————. Untersuchungen zur Lebensnaturlehre und Heilkunde. Ersten Bandes erste Abtheilung. Ueber das Verhältniss des Gehirns und Rückenmarks zur Belebung des übrigen Körpers. 1 p. l., 196 pp., 1 l. 8°. *Halle, Curt*, 1818.

————. Leicheneröffnungen. Zur Diagnostik und pathologischen Anatomie. Erste Reihe. 194 pp., 1 l. 8°. *Bonn, A. Marcus*, 1821.

————. Von der Stellung der Aerzte im Staate. iv, 1 l., 408 pp. 8°. *Leipzig, C. Cnobloch*, 1823.

————. Das medicinische Klinikum Bonn [im Jahr 1824 (6.)]. 1 p. l., 36 pp. 4°. *Coblenz, J. Hölscher*, 1825.

————. Anleitung zur Uebung angehender Aerzte in Krankheits-Beobachtung und Beurtheilung. 2 p. l., 142 pp. 8°. *Bonn, T. Habicht*, 1834.

————. Die Behandlung der Gemüthskranken und Irren durch Nichtärzte. 1 p. l., 65 pp., 1 l. 8°. *Bonn, E. Weber*; 1844.

Nasse (Christianus Fridericus)—continued.
——. Verbrennung und Athmen; chemische Thätigkeit und organisches Leben. vi, 154 pp. 8°. *Bonn, E. Weber*, 1846.

Also, *Co-Editor of:* **Archiv** für den thierischen Magnetismus, Altenburg u. Leipzig, 1817–22.—**Archiv** für medizinische Erfahrung im Gebiete der praktischen Medizin, Chirurgie, Geburtshülfe und Staatsarzneikunde, Berlin, 1817–34.—**Zeitschrift** für psychische Aerzte, Leipzig, 1818–22.—**Zeitschrift** für die Anthropologie, Leipzig, 1823–6. Also, *Editor of:* **Jahrbücher** für Anthropologie und zur Pathologie und Therapie des Irrseyns, Leipzig, 1830. Also, *Co-Editor of:* **Zeitschrift** für die Beurtheilung und Heilung der krankhaften Seelenzustände, Berlin, 1838. — **Rheinische** Monatsschrift für praktische Aerzte, Köln, 1847–51.

See, also, **Budge** (Julius). Die Lehre vom Erbrechen. 8°. Bonn, 1840. — **Collin** (V.) Die Untersuchung der Brust mit dem Stethoscop [etc.] 8°. Reutlingen, 1832. — **Knight** (Paul Slade). Beobachtungen über die Ursachen, Symptome und Behandlung des Irrseyns. 8°. Köln am Rhein, 1829. — **Levié** (Leo). Deutsch-lateinisches Wörterbuch, [etc.] 8°. Bonn, 1833.—**Mayer** (A.) Die Krankheiten, [etc.] 8°. Düsseldorf, 1844.—**Negrier** (G.) Die Behandlung der Scrofeln [etc.] 8°. Bonn, 1843.

For *Biography*, see Deutsche Klinik, Berl., 1851, iii, 219–221.

For *Portrait*, see **Collection** of Portr. (Libr.)

——— & **Nasse** (Hermann). Untersuchungen zur Physiologie und Pathologie. 2 v. 486, 302 pp., 1 pl. 8°. *Bonn, J. Habicht*, 1835–9.
All published.

Nasse (Gaston). * Du traitement des rétrécissements spasmodiques de l'œsophage, la dilatation brusque à l'aide de la pince de M. le professeur Broca. 34 pp., 1 l., 1 pl. 4°. *Paris*, 1878, No. 425.

Nasse (Hermann) [1807–]. * De insania commentatio secundum libros Hippocraticos. 3 p. l., 83 pp., 1 l. 4°. *Bonnæ, typ. Thormannianis*, [1829].
——. Das Blut in mehrfacher Beziehung physiologisch und pathologisch untersucht. 2 p. l., viii, 370 pp. 8°. *Bonn, T. Habicht*, 1836.
——. Ueber den Einfluss der Nahrung auf das Blut. 99 pp., 1 l. 8°. *Marburg, Elwert*, 1850.
——. Commentatio de bilis quotidie a cane secreta copia et indole. 24 pp. 4°. *Marburgi, typ. Bayrhofferi Academicis*, [1851].
——. Vorstudien zur Lehre von der Lymphbildung. Untersuchungen über die Verschiedenheiten und Schwankungen in der Absonderung und Zusammensetzung der Lymphe. 40 pp. 4°. *Marburg, N. G. Elwert*, [1862].
——. Untersuchungen über die Einflüsse, welche die Lymphbildung beherrschen. 1 p. l., 72 pp. 4°. *Marburg, N. G. Elwert*, 1871. c.
——. Untersuchungen über den Austritt und Eintritt von Stoffen (Transsudation und Diffusion) durch die Wand der Haargefässe. II. Untersuchungen über die normale Transsudation im allgemeinen Haargefässsystem. pp. 534–614. 8°. *Bonn*, 1879.
Cutting from: Arch. f. d. ges. Physiol., Bonn, 1879, xx.

Also, *Co-Editor of:* **Archiv** des Vereins für gemeinschaftliche Arbeiten zur Förderung der wissenschaftlichen Heilkunde, Göttingen, 1854–67.

See, also, **Nasse** (Friedrich). Untersuchungen zur Physiologie, etc. 8°. Bonn, 1835.

Nasse (Jn.-Julien). * Sur l'opération de la boutonnière appliquée au traitement des fistules urinaires urétrales. 23 pp. 4°. *Montpellier, J. Martel ainé*, 1822.

Nasse (Joannes Christianus). * Diss. sistens mechanicam obstructionis theoriam. 35 pp., 2 l. 4°. *Halæ Magdeb., typ. J. C. Hilligeri*, [1747].

Nasse (Otto [Joh. Friedrich]) [1839–]. * Die Schleimhaut der inneren weiblichen Geschlechtstheile im Wirbelthierreich. 39 pp. 8°. *Marburg, C. L. Pfeil*, 1862.
——. De materiis amylaceis num in sanguine mammalium inveniantur disquisitio. Socio ad respondendum assumpto M. Vogel. 35 pp. 8°. *Halis, typ. orphanotrophei*, 1866. c.

Nasse (Otto [Joh. Friederich])—continued.
——. Beiträge zur Physiologie der Darmbewegung. 1 p. l., 70 pp. 8°. *Leipzig, W. Engelmann*, 1866. [*Also, in :* P., v. 794.]
——. Zur Anatomie und Physiologie der quergestreiften Muskelsubstanz. vi, 106 pp., 1 pl. 8°. *Leipzig, F. C. W. Vogel*, 1882.

Nasser (Constantin). * Recherches sur les modifications de la température par les onctions générales. 50 pp. 4°. *Lyon*, 1884, 1. s., No. 201.

Nassick.
See **Cholera** (*Asiatic, History, etc., of*), *by localities*.

Nassokin (Casimir). * Om ros. [Erysipelas.] 54 pp. 8°. *Helsingfors, J. C. Frenckell & Son*, 1862.

Nassy (D.) Observations on the cause, nature, and treatment of the epidemic disorder prevalent in Philadelphia. 48 pp. 8°. *Philadelphia, Parker & Co.*, 1793.
French and English text and title-pages.

Nastorg (Jean-François-Xavier). I. Des complications en pathologie. II. [etc.] 29 pp. 4°. *Paris*, 1843, No. 81, v. 407.

Nasturtium.
MIEG (J. R.) * Plantarum nasturcinarum, quo vegetabilium horum structura naturalis, qualitates, vires atque usus in vita humana salubris breviter ac dilucide explicantur. sm. 4°. *Basileæ*, [1714].

Vido (L.) Il crescione comune o nasturzio acquatico. Orosi, Firenze, 1882, v, 217–220.

Nasturtius (Philo). Eilfertiges Gutachten . . . Zwelferischen Bundesgenossen, über die hochbedenckliche Attentata, tieff-ersinnte, unbesonnene und ärgerliche Defensions-Schrifft eines Raphaël Schmuz von Poystorff, uhralten Neuburgischen Leib-Medici, so er aufgerichtet zu unsterblichem Lob und ewigwehrenden Siegs-Preiss des Augspurgischen Dispensatorii, wie dann auch zu schändlichem Nachtheil, Hohn und Schimpff des . . . Herrn Joannis Zwelfers, weitberühmten Practici in Wien, erb- und meisterlichen Correctoris des weltbekanten Augustani. Nebenst zu End angehengter Erinnerung an den in Arte pharmaceutica ganz seichtgelehrten Lucam Schrökium Lucis filium. 5 p. l., 59 pp. 18°. [*Grein*], 1673.

Nasu Kotoku. Hon Cho I Dan. [The history of medicine in Japan.] 5, 49 pp. 8°. [*n. p.*], 1823.
Japanese text.

Natal.
See, also, **Cape Colony**; **Maritzburg**; **Medicine** (*Military, etc.*)—*Campaigns, etc.—African.*
Alcock (N.) Report on the climate and diseases of Natal and Zululand. Army M. Dep. Rep. 1878, Lond., 1880, xx, 264–266.

Natal *sore.*
See **Ulcers** (*Endemic*).

Natalucci (Giuseppe). Un raro caso di glandole mammarie succenturiate. 12 pp. 8°. *Civitanova-Marche, D. Natalucci*, 1886.

Natanson (Gregor). * Ueber das Verhalten des Blutdruckes in den Capillaren nach Massenumschnürungen. 1 p. l., 39 pp., 1 l. 8°. *Königsberg i. Pr., E. Erlatis*, [1886].

Natanson (I. M.) * O siemenache polevago kukolja (Agrostemma githago L., S. Lychis githago Lam.). [Chemical analysis of plant.] 18 pp. 8°. *St. Petersburg*, 1867.

Natanson (I. N.) * Materialy k vodolecheniou gorjachechnych. [Hot-water treatment.] 83 pp., 1 l. 8°. *St. Petersburg, tipog. M. M. Stasoulevitcha*, 1887.

Natanson (*Jakób*) [1832–84].
D. (H.) Nekrologia. Medycyna, Warszawa, 1884, xii, 629–631.—**Leppert** (W.) Wspomnienie pośmiertne. [Reminiscences.] Gaz. lek., Warzawa, 1884, 2. s., iv, 757–763.

Natanson (Louis). La circulation des forces dans les êtres animés; essai de psychologie scientifique. 74 pp. 8°. *Paris, Bureau des Deux Revues,* 1886.

Natchez.

See, also, **Cholera** (*Asiatic, History, etc., of*), **Fever** (*Malarial, History, etc., of*), **Fever** (*Yellow, History, etc., of*), **Hospitals** (*Descriptions, etc., of*), *by localities.*

Cartwright (S. A.) Remarks on statistical medicine, contrasting the result of the empirical with the regular practice of physic, in Natchez. West. J. M. & S., Louisville, 1840, ii, 1–21.—**Hogg** (S.) An account of the epidemic fevers of Natchez, Miss., in the years 1837–8. *Ibid.*, i, 401–424.—**Magoun** (C. S.) Natchez; its population; its health; its mortality; Marine Hospital, etc. N. Orl. M. & S. J., 1850–51, vii, 96–98. ———. Natchez; its health, diseases, and mortality. [Dysentery, cholera, and hooping-cough.] *Ibid.*, 249–251. ———. Sanitary condition of Natchez, Miss., with mortuary statistics. *Ibid.*, 1851–2, viii, 444–453. ———. Natchez (Miss.) considered as a winter resort or permanent location for Northern consumptive invalids. *Ibid.*, 1852–3, ix, 23–25.

Nates.

See **Buttock.**

Nath (Friedrich Wilhelm Reinhold) [1830–]. * De pseudarthrosi ex fractura et resectione ossium. 37 pp., 1 l., 1 pl. 8°. *Berolini, typ. fratrum Schlesinger,* [1853].

———. Zur Medicinal-Statistik. Die Geburts- und Sterblichkeitsverhältnisse des Kreises Oberbarnim pro 1876. Anhang: Practische Anleitung zur Gewinnung einer amtlich sicheren und leicht ausführbaren Kreis-Sterblichkeits- resp. Erkrankungs-Statistik nach der im Kreise Oberbarnim bestehenden Organisation. iv pp., 1 l., 92 pp., 11 pl. roy. 8°. *Berlin, G. Reimer,* 1878.

———. Die neue Stellung der preussischen Hebeammen zum Staat und zur Geburtshülfe. Auf Grund der neueren Gesetzgebung und mit besonderer Berücksichtigung des neuen preussischen Hebeammen-Lehrbuches für Aerzte, besonders Medicinal-Beamte, zum Gebrauch bei den gesetzlichen Hebeammen - Nachprüfungen sowie für Hebeammen zum Selbstunterricht in gedrängter Kürze bearbeitet. viii, 96 pp. 8°. *Stuttgart,* 1879.

Nathan (Adolf). * Ueber die Bedeutung des Natron salicylicum als Antipyreticum. 31 pp. 4°. *Kiel, C. F. Mohr,* 1875.

In : SCHRIFT. d. Univ. zu Kiel, xxii, 1875, vii, Med. xvii.

Nathan (Alfons) [1862–]. * Die Complication der Geburt mit Tumoren. 43 pp. 8°. *Berlin, Wilhelm u. Brasch,* [1886].

Nathan (*Charles*) [1807–72].

Obituary notice. N. South Wales M. Gaz., Sydney, 1872–3, iii, 45, port.

Nathan (E.) Zustand oder Richtung und Leistung der deutschen Medicin im Jahre 1837, mit besonderer Beziehung auf Journalistik. Ein literär-historischer Versuch. 71 pp. 8°. *Hamburg, Hartwig u. Müller,* [1838, *vel subseq.*].

Repr. from : Ztschr. f. d. ges. Med., Hamb., 1838, viii, Hft. 3, 245.

———. Beilage. Weitere Bemerkungen über das Wesen und Unwesen der Phrenologie. 26 + pp. 8°. Incomplete.

Repr. from : Hamb. lit. u. krit. Bl. von F. Niebour und Dr. L. Wienbarg, 1844, No. 11, u. ff., als Fortsetzung der "Bemerkungen", etc., auch in dieser Zeitschrift, Bd. 23, S. 269 u. 404.

Nathan (Elias Salomon). * De febre intermittente traumatica. 28 pp. 4°. *Kiliæ, C. F. Mohr,* 1830.

Nathan (Joh. Christianus). * De angina. 32 pp. sm. 4°. *Lipsiæ, lit. Fleischeri,* [1709].

For Biography, see **Rivinus** (Aug. Quirin.) "Certa quædam", etc. 8°. [*Lipsiæ,* 1709.]

Nathan (N.) * Ueber den Mutterblutfluss während der Schwangerschaft und bei der Geburt. 21 pp. 8°. *Würzburg, Becker,* 1839.

Nathanson (Ferdinandus) [1827–]. * De dyscrasia quadam affectionem cordis, strumam, exophthalmum efficiente. 30 pp., 1 l. 8°. *Berolini, B. Schlesinger,* [1850].

Nathhorst (Joh. Theophilus).

See **Murray** (Adolphus). * Descriptio arteriarum [etc.] sm. 4°. *Upsaliæ,* [1780].

Nathhorst (Theoph. Erdm.) Flora Monspeliensis. *Upsaliæ,* 1756.

In : LINNÆUS. Amœnitates acad. [etc.] 8°. *Lugd. Bat.,* 1760, iv, 468–495.

Nathusius (Carolus Henricus Æmilius) [1836–]. * De more humandi et concremandi mortuos apud Græcos usitato. 33 pp., 1 l. 8°. *Halis Sax., formis Ploetzianis,* [1864]. c.

Nathusius (Elias).

See **Oheim** (Joh. Philippus) & **Nathusius** (Elias). Theses physicæ [etc] 4°. *Lipsiæ,* 1651.

Nati da Bibbiena (M. Pietro). Breve discorso intorno alla natura del popone, e sopra il cattivo uso del ber fresco con la neve.

In : RAC. d' opusc. scient. e filol. 16°. *Venezia,* 1730, iv, 373–398.

National Academy of Sciences. Annual report of the . . . for 1863–4. 112 pp. 8°. *Cambridge, Welch, Bigelow & Co.,* 1865. [P., v. 399.]

———. Memoirs. v. 1, 2; pt. 2, v. 3. 4°. *Washington,* 1866–86.

———. Annual reports. 1867; 1879; 1880–81; 1883. 8°. *Washington,* 1868–84. [1867 *in :* P., v. 358.]

———. Biographical memoirs. v. 1. v, 343 pp. 8°. *Washington,* 1877.

———. Proceedings. v. 1. 239 pp. 8°. *Washington,* 1877–84.

———. Constitution and membership, April 21, 1882. 21 pp. 8°. *Washington, Judd & Detweiler,* 1882.

———. The same. April 21, 1883. 24 pp. 8°. *Washington,* 1883.

———. The same. July 10, 1884. 23 pp. 8°. *Washington, Judd & Detweiler,* 1884.

———. The same. June 10, 1885. 23 pp. 8°. *Washington, Judd & Detweiler,* 1885.

———. The same. June 3, 1886. 23 pp. 8°. *Washington, Judd & Detweiler,* 1886.

———. The same. June 7, 1887. 23 pp. 8°. *Washington, Judd & Detweiler,* 1887.

———. Report on glucose, prepared in response to a request made by the Commissioner of Internal Revenue. 108 pp. 8°. *Washington, Government Printing Office,* 1884.

National Almanac and Annual Record for the years 1863–4. 2 v. 8°. *Philadelphia, G. W. Childs.*

National (The) Anti-Compulsory Vaccination Reporter. Mary C. Hume - Rothery, editor. Supplement, Jan. 1, 1878. 16 pp. 4°. [*London.*]

National Association for the Promotion of Social Science. Transactions, 1857–83. 27 v. 8°. *London,* 1858–84.

———. The practice of hiring wet nurses (especially those from the "fallen") considered, as it affects public health and public morals. A paper contributed to the public health department, at the Bradford meeting, Oct., 1859. [Published by permission of the council.] 16 pp. 8°. *London, J. Churchill,* [1860 ?]

———. Quarantine. Return to an address of the House of Commons, dated 22 May, 1860, for "copy of abstract of regulations in force in foreign countries respecting quarantine, communicated to the board of trade". 35 pp. fol. [*London,* 1860.]

———. Return to an order of the House of Commons, dated 18 Aug., 1860, for abstracts "of returns of information on the laws of quarantine which have been obtained by the board of trade".

National Association [etc.]—continued.
[Prepared and presented to the board of trade.]
86 pp. fol. [*London*, 1860.]
Bound with preceding.

——. Return to an order of the House of Commons, dated 5 Aug., 1861, for copy " of the papers relating to quarantine, communicated to the board of trade on the 30th day of July, 1861 ". 48 pp. fol. [*London*, 1861.]
Bound with preceding.

——. Report of the proceedings at the seventh annual congress, held in Edinburgh, October, 1863. xlii, 381 pp. 12°. *Edinburgh, W. P. Nimmo,* 1863.

——. On the evils of overcrowding in the dwellings of the poor, and means suggested for their removal. By William Hardwicke. (Read at a meeting of the health department, June 7, 1865.) 16 pp. 8°. *London,* 1865.

——. Constitution and laws; with list of officers and members. 41 pp. 8°. [*London, W. W. Head,* 1868.]

——. Report of the council to the annual business meeting of members. July 16, 1868. 17 pp. 8°. *London, W. W. Head,* 1868. [P., v. 1432.]

——. Programme of papers. Ed. for Thursday, Oct. 5. 15. annual meeting, Leeds, Oct. 4 to 11, 1871. 15 pp. 8°. *Leeds, C. Goodall,* 1871.

——. Social Science Congress at Leeds, Oct. 4th to 11th, 1871. Report and catalogue of sanitary and other articles, exhibited in the Colored Cloth Hall, prepared by Dr. [William] Hardwicke, medical officer of Paddington. 4. ed. 32 pp. 8°. *Leeds, C. Goodall,* [1871.]

——. Twenty-fifth anniversary. A manual for the congress; with a narrative of past labours and results, by J. L. Clifford-Smith. viii, 190 pp., 2 port. 12°. *London, office of the Assoc.,* 1882.

National Association for the Protection of the Insane and the Prevention of Insanity. Constitution and by-laws. 31 pp. 8°. *Boston, Tolman & White,* 1880.

——. Papers and proceedings at the stated meeting, held in New York City, January 20, 1882. 55 pp. 8°. *New York, G. P. Putnam's Sons,* 1882.

National Association for the Relief of Destitute Colored Women and Children, Washington. Annual reports of the executive committee to the public. 3.–19., 1865–81. 8°. *Washington,* 1866–82.
Incorporated Feb. 14, 1863.

National Association for the Repeal of the Contagious Diseases Acts. A critical summary of the evidence before the royal commission upon the contagious diseases acts, 1866–9. Prepared by Douglas Kingsford. In seven chapters, published and paged separately. 8°. *London, Tweedie & Co.,* [*n. d.*]

CONTENTS.

Chapter I. Proof of being a common prostitute, and the mode of obtaining such proof. 14 pp.
II. Voluntary submission and magistrate's order. 16 pp.
III. Periodical examinations. 19 pp.
IV. Relative advantages and disadvantages of compulsory and voluntary hospitals. 23 pp.
V. Effect of the acts on venereal disease. 36 pp.
VI. Certain alleged benefits resulting from the acts. 23 pp.
VII. Abuses under the acts. 14 pp.

National Association for Sanitary and Rural Improvement. [An invitation to attend a conference of delegates from sanitary and rural improvement societies, to be held July 7, 8, and 10, at Warwick Woodlands, Greenwood Lake, New Jersey.] 1 l. 8°. [*n. p., n. d.*]

——. Objects: To establish local societies for sanitary and rural improvement, [etc.] 1 l. 8°. [*New York,* 1883.]

National Association [etc.]—continued.
——. [Circular announcing issue of a small monthly journal adapted for householders, etc. The first number to appear about May 1, 1883.] 1 l. 4°. [*n. p., n. d.*]

National *Association of Volunteer Medical Officers, Army and Navy of the United States.*
Hood (T. B.) National Association of Volunteer Medical Officers, Army and Navy of the United States. History and constitution. Nat. M. J., Wash., 1870–71, i, 359–366.

National Benevolent Institution, London, W. C. Annual reports of the committee of management to the members of the corporation. 44., 1855–6; 54., 1865–6; 57., 1868–9. 8°. *London,* 1857–70. [44. *in :* P., v. 970; 54. and 57. *in :* P., v. 973.]

——. Rules and bye-laws. 27 pp. 12°. *London,* [*J. Davy & Sons*], 1862. [P., v. 965.]

National *Board of Health.*
See **Hygiene** (*Public, Laws, etc., of*); **United States.** *Treasury Department. National Board of Health.*

National Board of Health Bulletin. [Weekly.] v. 1–3; No. 1, v. 4. June 28, 1879, to July 1, 1882. 4°. *Washington, D. C.*
Ended. v. 2 is paged consecutively with v. 1.

National Board of Trade. Memorial of the . . . accompanying a bill for the prevention of the adulteration of food or drugs. Dec. 31, 1880. 3 l. fol. [*Boston,* 1880.]

——. [Draft of] a bill to prevent the adulteration of food or drugs. [With resolutions adopted by the . . .} 4 pp., 1 l. 8°. [*New York,* 1881.]

National (A) Calendar; containing an official list of all the officers, civil, military, and naval, of the United States of America, [etc.] By Peter Force. v. 1–2, 4–6, 8–9, 12, 1820–34. 8 v. 12°. *Washington, Davis & Force.*
Title of v. 4–12 was: **National** (The) Calendar and Annals of the United States.

National Calendar, or Herrick's Almanac, for the years 1861; 1875. 12°. *New York,* [1860; 1874].

National College of Pharmacy, Washington. Annual circulars for the sessions of 1872–3 to 1884–5 (1.–13.). 8°. *Washington,* 1872–84.
Lists of students and graduates for the sessions of 1872–3 to 1883–4 in circulars for subsequent years. List of alumni, 1873–84, in circular for 1884–5.

——. Circular letter [of subcommittee] to the members of the medical and pharmaceutical professions in the District of Columbia [desiring co-operation towards the establishment of a uniform and reliable formula in the District]. May 1, 1875. 2 pp. 8°. [*Washington,* 1875.]

National Conference of Charities and Correction. Proceedings of the . . . held in connection with the general meeting of the American Social Science Association. 1.–14., 1874–87. Bound in 9 v. 8°. *Boston,* 1874–87.
Volume for 1882 published at Madison, Wis.

——. Charity organization societies, as presented by the " committee on organization of charities in cities ", at the conference in Boston, July 26, 1881. 163 pp. 8°. *Boston, Tolman & White,* 1881.

——. [Announcement of 10th annual meeting at Louisville, Kentucky.] 2 l. 8°. [*Louisville,* 1883.]

——. [Programme of the 10th annual meeting.] 4 pp. 4°. [*Louisville,* 1883.]

——. Report of the standing committee on crimes and penalties. 15 pp. 8°. [*n. p.,* 1883.]

National Conference of Principals of Institutions for Deaf Mutes. Proceedings of . . . at Clark's Institution, Northampton, Mass., May

National Conference [etc.]—continued.
25–28, 1880. 141 pp., 1 l. 8°. *Northampton, Mass.*, 1880.

National Conference of State Boards of Health. [First annual meeting.] 63 pp. 8°. [*Springfield, Ill.*, 1885.]
Repr. from: Rep. Bd. Health Illinois 1884, Springfield, 1885, vii.

——. The same. Third annual meeting. 82, v pp. 8°. *Indianapolis, W. B. Burford*, 1887.

——. The same. Fourth annual meeting. 34 pp. 8°. *Columbus, O., Myers Bros.*, 1888.

——. [Circular letter of the secretary, announcing the annual conference to be held at Washington, D. C., Sept., 1887.] 1 sheet. 4°. [*Concord, N. H.*, 1887.]

——. [Programme of the conference to be held at Washington, D. C., Sept., 1887.] 2 sheets. 4°. [*Concord, N. H.*, 1887.]

National Cottage Hospital for Consumption and Diseases of the Chest, Ventnor, Isle of Wight. *See* **Royal** National Hospital for Consumption and Diseases of the Chest, Ventnor, Undercliff, Isle of Wight.

National Dental Hospital, London, W. Annual reports of the committee of management and medical committee to the governors and subscribers. 15.–20., 1876–81; 22., 1883; 24., 1884. 16°. *London*, 1877–85.
Established in 1861. 1876–81 bound in 1 v.

National Dental Hospital and College, London, W. Prospectuses for the sessions of 1877–8 to 1880–81; 1882–3. 8°. *London*, 1877–82.
The first special dental school in the United Kingdom was the Metropolitan Dental School of Science, which was opened Oct. 5, 1859. Suspended for a few years, but reorganized May 8, 1877, and the present title was adopted.

National disease. Remarks upon the prevailing epidemic of small-pox, its cause and prevention, with notes on public health, eruptive disease, etc. (amongst mankind and the animal world). 2 p. l., 85 pp., 1 tab. 8°. *London, Longmans* [*and others*], [1871].

National (The) Druggist. (Formerly "St. Louis Druggist".) A weekly history of pharmacy, materia medica, chemistry, the kindred sciences, and business interests. [2 v. annually.] v. 5–12, July, 1884, to 1888. 7 v. 4°. *Saint Louis, Druggist Publishing Co.*
Current. Title of v. 1–4 was: **Saint Louis** Druggist.

National Eclectic Medical Association. Transactions at the 3. annual meeting, held at Rochester, N. Y., May 11, 1852; together with the accepted reports presented by the members. x, 173 pp. 8°. *Rochester, E. Darrow*, 1852.

——. Transactions. v. 1–15, 1870–71 to 1887–8. 8°. [*v. p.*], 1872–87.

——. Constitution, by-laws, and standing resolutions, 1879. 16 pp. 8°. [*n. p., n. d.*]

——. [Announcement of meeting to be held at Chicago, June 16, 1880.] 7 pp. 8°. [*n. p., n. d.*]

——. [Announcement of meeting to be held at Topeka, Kansas, June 20, 1883.] 15 pp. 8°. [*n. p., n. d.*]

National (The) hand-book of facts and figures, historical, statistical, documentary, political, from the formation of the Government to the present time. With a full chronology of the rebellion. viii, 9–407 pp., port. 8°. *New York, E. B. Treat & Co.*, 1870.

National Health Society. Annual reports read at the general meetings of the society. 1., 1872–3; 3.–8., 1875–80; 10.–12., 1882–4. 8°. *London*, 1873–85.
Organized in July, 1871.

[——.] Facts concerning vaccination, for heads of families. [Revised by the Local Government Board, and issued with their sanction.] Vacci-

National Health Society—continued.
nation and small-pox. 8 pp. 12°. [*London, Allman & Son*, 1880 ?]

——. How to prevent and oppose the cholera. Plain instructions for heads of families and others, issued by the . . . 8 pp. 12°. [*London*], *Allman & Son*, [1884].
See, also, **Smoke** Abatement Fund.

National *homes for disabled soldiers.*
See **United States**. *National Home for Disabled Volunteer Soldiers.*

National Hospital for Consumption and Diseases of the Chest, Ventnor, Isle of Wight. *See* **Royal** National Hospital for Consumption and Diseases of the Chest, Ventnor, Undercliff, Isle of Wight.

National Hospital for the Deformed, London. *See* **National** Orthopædic Hospital (for the Deformed).

National Hospital for Diseases of the Heart and Paralysis, London, W. Annual reports of the committee to the governors and subscribers. 15., 1870; 26., 1881; 28., 1883; 29., 1884. 8°. *London*, 1871–85.
Established 1857.

——. Balance-sheet for 1879. MS. 2 pp. fol. [*London*, 1880.]

National Hospital for the Paralyzed and Epileptic, Bloomsbury, W. C. Bye-laws for the management of the . . . 23 pp. 8°. *London, Harrison & Sons*, 1864.
Instituted Nov. 2, 1859. The institution comprises: I. An hospital for in and out patients. II. A country convalescent branch. III. A Samaritan society to assist the more destitute sufferers and their families. IV. A pension fund for the incurable. V. An In Memoriam wing for patients able to contribute a portion of the bare cost of their maintenance.

——. Annual reports of the board of management to the governors and subscribers. 11.–13., 1870–72; 15., 1874; 16., 1875; 18., 1877; 19., 1878. 8°. *London*, 1871–9.

——. In testimony; being a selection from recent utterances by distinguished persons, concerning the . . . which is the Albany Memorial Hospital. 36 pp. 8°. [*Bloomsbury*, 1884.]

——. Privileges of governors and members, with rules for admission of patients and system of election. 2 l. 8°. [*London, n. d.*]

National Hotel *disease.*
STONE (R. K.) Letter to Dr. Cornelius Boyle, in regard to the National Hotel sickness. 8°. *Washington, D. C.*, 1857.
Repr. from: National Intelligencer, Washington, D. C.
Barnes (J. O.) The National Hotel disease. Boston M. & S. J., 1857, lvi, 371–376.—**Disease** (On the) affecting the inmates of the National Hotel, at Washington, D. C. Am. M. Month., N. Y., 1857, vii, 347–358. — **Ely** (A. W.) The poisoning at the National Hotel [Washington, D. C.]. N. Orl. M. & S. J., 1856–7, xiii, 796–799. — **Stone** (R. K.) The National Hotel endemic. [A letter to Dr. C. Boyle, published in The States, May 8. 1857.] Virginia M. J., Richmond, 1857, viii, 478–485.—**Waring** (J. J.) National Hotel endemic. Autopsy; with remarks. Am. J. M. Sc., Phila., 1858, n. s. xxxv, 97–104.— **Wynne** (J.) National Hotel disease. N. York J. M., 1857, 3. s., iii, 90–92. ——. On the disease affecting the inmates of the National Hotel, at Washington, D. C. Am. M. Month., N. Y., 1857, vii, 347–358.

National Hygiene, Athletic Sports, and Aquatics. Hydropathy, Turkish - Baths, bath, and bathing. No. 109, v. 2, March 13, 1886. pp. 105–120. 4°. *London, E. Curtice.*

National (The) Independent. Edited by William Y. Leader and Dr. William Paine. [Weekly.] Nos. 4–7, v. 4, Jan. 27 to Feb. 17, 1872. fol. *Philadelphia, C. H. Leader & Co.*
A continuation of: **Medical** (The) Independent.

National Indian Association in Aid of Social Progress and Education in India. Annual report of the council to the subscribers. 14., 1884. 29 pp. 8°. *Bristol, J. W. Arrowsmith*, 1885.

National Industrial Home for Crippled Boys, and Refuge, Kensington, London, W. Annual reports of the committee to the subscribers and supporters. 5.–18., 1870 to 1883. 12°. *London,*1871–84.

National Institute of France. The report made to the . . . in the month of December, 1799, by citizens Portal, Pelletan, Fourcroy, Chaptal, and Vauquelin, respecting the artificial mineral waters prepared at Paris by Nicholas Paul & Co. With extracts from the reports of the Society of Physicians of Paris, and the faculty of Geneva, and other testimonials in favor of the same waters; to which are added some notes and observations, by N. Paul. Transl. from the French. 3 p. l., vii, 64 pp. 8°. *London, N. Paul,* 1802. [P., v. 667; 673.]

National Institute of General Practitioners in Medicine, Surgery, and Midwifery. Report of the council of the National Institute of General Practitioners in Medicine, Surgery, and Midwifery on the present state of the medical reform question. Containing the "Principles" of medical reform promulgated by the conference of delegates at the Royal College of Physicians, London; the draft of the proposed charter to the general practitioners in medicine, surgery, and midwifery; the "Outlines of a bill" furnished to the parliamentary committee by the conference, with the concurrence of the universities and medical corporations of Scotland and Ireland; and other public documents. With re-remarks on the objections which have been recently urged against the proposed measures, August 9, 1848. 84 pp. 8°. *London, W. Davy & Son,* 1848. [*Also, in:* P., v. 38.]

National Institution for the Promotion of Science. Constitution of . . . amended and ordered to be printed, April, 1841. 19 pp. 8°. *Washington, P. Force,* 1841.
    Established May, 1840.

————. Bulletin of proceedings. 1., 2., 1840–42, 220 pp., 5 pl.; 4., 1845–6, 483–567 pp. 8°. *Washington,* 1843–6.

————. Proceedings. Nos. 1, 2, v. 1, 1855–6. 82 pp. 8°. [*n. p., n. d.*]

National Insurance Convention of the United States. Annual report of the proceedings, held in the city of Detroit, Sept., 1874. 5., 1874. iv, 38, 15, 38, 22, 6 pp., 2 l. 8°. *New York, J. F. Trow & Son,* 1875.

National Medical College. *Medical Department of Columbian University, Washington.* Memorial of the professors in the medical department of the Columbian College, in the District of Columbia. 19. Cong., 1. sess., Feb. 13, 1826. 5 pp. 8°. *Washington, printed by order of the Senate of the United States, by Gales & Seaton,* 1826.
    Columbian College was chartered Feb. 9, 1821. The medical department was completed Oct., 1824. In Nov., 1824, an announcement was made that the first course would commence March 20, 1825. List of students for the sessions of 1841–2; 1858–9 to 1861–2; 1868–9; 1869–70; 1871–2 to 1874–5; 1876–7; 1879–80 to 1886–7, in announcements for subsequent years. List of all the graduates from 1822 to 1886 in announcement for 1887.

————. Annual announcements and circulars for the sessions of 1842–3 (21.); 1844–5 (23.); 1846–7 (25.); 1848–9 to 1856–7 (27.–35.); 1858–9 to 1861–2 (37.–40.); 1863–4 (42.); 1865–6 to 1867–8 (44.–46.); 1869–70 (48.); 1870–71 (49.); 1872–3 to 1887–8 (51.–66.). 8° & 4°. *Washington,* 1842–87.
    1856–7 is 4°.

————. Chart of skin diseases, as taught by H. C. Yarrow, M. D. 2 l. 16°. [*Washington,* 1884.]
————. *See, also:*
SAMSON (G. W.) Address at the opening of the hall presented by W. W. Corcoran to the Columbian College for the use of the National Medical College. 12°. *Washington, D. C.,* 1866.

National Medical Convention. *See* **American** Medical Association.

National medical establishment (proposed) for the government of the medical body, [etc.] *See* [**Pidduck** (Isaac)].

National (The) Medical Journal. Edited by C. C. Cox. [Quarterly.] v. 1; Nos. 1–10, v. 2, April, 1870, to Feb., 1872. 8°. *Washington, D. C., Judd & Detweiler.*
    Ended. v. 2 became monthly, commenced May, 1871, and edited by S. C. Busey and Wm. Lee.

National (The) Medical Journal. By A. H. Brown. No. 9, v. 2, March, 1876. 2 l. fol. *New York.*
    An advertisement.

National Medical Review. Walter S. Wells, editor. [Monthly.] v. 1., Dec., 1878, to May, 1879. 280 pp. 8°. *Washington, D. C.*
    Ended.

National Microscopical Congress. Proceedings of the National Microscopical Congress, held at Indianapolis, Aug. 14 to 19, 1878, and of the American Society of Microscopists, held at Buffalo, N. Y., Aug. 19 to 24, 1879. 77 pp., 5 pl., 1 tab. 8°. *Indianapolis, W. B. Burford,* 1880.
    Bound with: AMERICAN Society Microscopists. Proceedings, 1879–82.

————. *See, also:*
    National (The) Microscopical Congress. Am. Q. Micr. J., N. Y., 1878, i, 61–69.

National Orphan Home, Ham Common, Richmond. Office, 9 West Strand, W. C. Annual report of the committee of management to the subscribers. 22., 1870–71. 10 pp., 2 l. 8°. *London,* 1871. [P., v. 973.]

National Orthopædic Hospital (for the Deformed), London. Annual reports of the committee of management to the governors and subscribers. 22.–48., 1878–84. 12°. *London,* 1879–85.
    Founded in 1836, for the treatment of distortions of the spine, club-foot, and all other contractions and deformities.

National Park.
    Heizmann (C. L.) The therapeutical value of the springs in the National Park, Wyoming Territory. Phila. M. Times, 1876, iv, 409–414.

National Pharmaceutical Association. *See* **American** Pharmaceutical Association.

National Philanthropic Association. Employment of the poor. First report of the employment of the poor as street orderlies, in promoting the health and cleanliness of the parishes of St. James, St. Anne's, and St. Martin-in-the-Fields, by the council of the National Philanthropic Association. 16 pp. 8°. *London, T. R. Harrison,* 1848. [P., v. 38.]

————. Sanatory progress; being the fifth report of the National Philanthropic Association, for the promotion of social and saltiferous improvements, street cleanliness, and the employment of the poor, so that able-bodied men may be prevented from burthening the parish rates, and preserved independent of workhouse alms and degradation. 2. ed. xvi, 251 pp., 8 pl. 8°. *London, J. Hatchard & Son,* 1850.

National (The) Philanthropist. [Monthly.] Nos. 1–13, July 1, 1884, to July 1, 1885. fol. *London, F. Pitman.*
    Each number paged separately.

National Political Union. Proceedings at the . . . respecting legislative interference in the study of anatomy, and the supply of bodies for anatomical research. 24 pp. 8°. *London, Barnes,* 1832.

National Quarantine and Sanitary Convention. Minutes and proceedings of the annual meetings. 1.–4., 1857–60. In 2 v. 8°. [*v. p.*], 1857–60. [2. *also, in:* P., v. 357.]

————. Report of the committee on quarantine, appointed at convention held in Baltimore, April 29, 1858. 84 pp. 8°. [*n. p.,* 1859.]

National Quarantine [etc.]—continued.
———. Proceedings and debates 3. meeting, held in the city of New York. Board of councilmen, document No. 9. 728 pp. 8°. *New York*, 1859.
———. Report of the committee on the internal hygiene of cities. Introduction by Thomas Miller, Washington, D. C., [1859 ?] 190 pp. 8°. [*n. p.*, 1859.] [*Also, in :* P., v. 321.]

CONTENTS.
Disinfectants, by W. C. Van Bibber.
Sewerage, by J. H. Griscom.
Importance and economy of sanitary measures to cities, by John Bell.
Sanitary code for cities, by H. G. Clark.

———. Quarantine regulations as approved by the National Quarantine and Sanitary Association of the United States. 39 pp. 8°. *Boston, Rand & Avery*, 1860. [*Also, in :* P., v. 357.]
———. Report of committee of National Quarantine and Sanitary Association on external hygiene. 46 pp. 8°. *New York*, 1860. [*Also, in :* P., v. 231.]
———. Report of the committee on the utility of wet docks in connection with quarantines, and the propriety of placing the entire establishment under the jurisdiction of the United States Government. John W. Sterling, M. D.; Alex. H. Stevens, M. D.; John McNulty, M. D., committee, appointed by the Third National Quarantine and Sanitary Convention. New York, June 1, 1860. 28 pp. 8°. *Boston, Rand & Avery*, 1860. [*Also, in :* P., v. 231.]
———. Report on registration, presented to the Quarantine and Sanitary Convention at its fourth annual meeting, held in the city of Boston, June 14, 1860, by Edwin M. Snow. 24 pp. 8°. [*n. p.*], 1860. [*Also, in :* P., v. 355.]
National Sanatorium for Consumption and Diseases of the Chest, at Bournemouth, Hants. Annual reports of the committee of management to the governor and subscribers. 25., 1879; 29., 1883. 25, 36 pp. 8°. *Bournemouth, E. Offer*, 1880–84.
Founded 1855.
National Sanitary Corporation. Limited [for inspection of houses, sanitary engineering work, etc. Prospectus]. 19 pp. 4°. *London, Crown Printing Co.*, [1881].
National Smoke Abatement Institution. *See* Smoke nuisance acts.

National *Soldiers' and Sailors' Orphans' Home.*
UNITED STATES. *Congress.* A bill to amend the charter of the National Soldiers' and Sailors' Orphans' Home, and in relation to the assets thereof. roy. 8°. [*Washington*, 1884.]
National Temperance Convention. Proceedings of the sixth . . . held at Cleveland, Ohio, July 29th and 30th, 1868 ; containing the papers presented, speeches delivered, resolutions and reports adopted, question drawer, etc. 120 pp. 8°. *New York, Nat. Temper. Soc. and Publ. House*, 1868.
———. Liquor laws of the United States. Prohibitory, license, local option, tax, and civil damage laws. 138 pp. 8°. *New York*, 1877.
National Temperance Society and Publication House. Seventh annual report of the . . . presented at New York, May 8, 1872. With an appendix, containing list of the officers, life patrons, life directors, and life members of the society. 53 pp. 8°. *New York, Nat. Temper. Soc. and Publ. House*, 1872.
National Truss Society, London, E. C. Annual reports of the committee to the subscribers, for the years 1881–3. 12°. *London, Zapp & Bennett*, 1882–4.
Instituted in 1786 for the relief of the ruptured poor of both sexes throughout the kingdom.

National University, Washington, D. C. *Law Department. Medical Department. Dental Department.* Announcements for the sessions of 1884–5 (16.). 26 pp. 8°. *Washington, R. H. Darby*, 1884.
National University, Washington. *Medical and Dental Departments.* Annual announcements for the sessions of 1884–5 to 1887–8 (1.–4.). 8°. *Washington*, 1886.
First announcement in preceding.
National Vaccine Establishment, London. [Circular of the board, relating to indiscriminate inoculation, and the illegal and dangerous exposure of patients suffering under the small-pox.] 1 l. 4°. [*London, J. Brettell, n. d.*]
Bound with : JENNER (E.) An inquiry into the causes and effects of variolæ vaccinæ. 4°. *London*, 1798.
National Vaccine Establishment of London. [Description of the vaccine vesicle, and instructions relating to vaccination ; issued by the . . . and reissued by H. G. Clark, city physician of Boston.] 8 pp. 8°. [*Boston*, 1859.] [P., v. 337.]
National Yellow Fever Relief Commission. A plan for the immediate relief of the orphans of the late yellow fever epidemic. [Being a communication from C. K. Marshall. Read and ordered to be printed Jan. 10, 1879.] 6 pp. 8°. [*Washington*, 1879.]
Nation's (The) Journal of Health. Published by Dr. S. Van Meter & Co. [Monthly.] No. 181, v. 28, n. s., 1873. 4 pp. fol. *Charleston, Ill.*
An advertisement.
Nativel (R.) * De la chylurie intertropicale (lymphurie), en particulier aux îles de la Réunion et Maurice. 76 pp. 4°. *Paris*, 1886, No. 108.
Nativelle (Adolphe). * Sur la résine de jalap et le cnicin, principe amer cristallisable du chardon bénit. 10 pp. 4°. *Paris, Poussielgue*, 1841. [P., v. 1698.]
École de pharmacie.
Natorp (Carolus). * De vi consuetudinis. 35 pp. 4°. *Gottingæ, H. Dieterich*, [1808].
Natorp (Carolus Guilelmus) [1812–]. * Diss. sistens historiam morbi de melanosi, cordis, hepatis totiusque telæ cellulosæ. 35 pp. 8°. *Berolini, typ. Nietackianis*, [1836].
Natorp (Ernestus Julius) [1825–]. * De graviditatis spatio. 28 pp., 1 l. 8°. *Berolini, F. Schlesinger*, [1849].
Natorp (Ernestus Otto Ludovicus) [1813–]. * De spina bifida. 36 pp. 8°. *Berolini, typ. Friedlaenderianis*, [1838].
Natorp (Paul). * Doppelseitiger Pneumothorax in Folge vicariirenden Emphysems. 48 pp. 8°. *Würzburg, Becker*, 1882.
Natu (F.) [1854–]. * Du purpura rhumatismal. 54 pp. 4°. *Paris*, 1882, No. 28.
Natürliche (Das) Friedrichshaller Bitterwasser und sein Gebrauch. 5. Aufl. 46 pp. 8°. *Berlin, Ahrens u. Wolff*, [1879].
Natürliche Vorzeichen verschiedenen Wetters, welche man an der Sonne, am Monde, an den Sternen, der Luft, dem Wasser, der Erde, an Thieren, etc., wahrgenommen hat, allen Landleuten, Gärtnern wie auch Schiffern sehr dienlich vor einem Liebhaber von Zeit zu Zeit in Acht genommen, und durch eigene Erfahrung aufgesetzt. Aus dem Holländischen übersetzt. 64 pp. 12°. *Leipzig, J. G. Löwen*, 1775.
Natürliches Emser Quellsalz in gelöster Form, erzeugt durch die Administration der König Wilhelms-Felsenquellen in Bad-Ems. Unter Leitung des Chemikers Dr. C. F. Thomas. 2 l. 4°. *Ems, J. B. Dorn*, [n. d.]
Natur (Die). Zeitung zur Verbreitung naturwissenschaftlicher Kenntniss und Naturanschauung für Leser aller Stände. Hrsg. von Otto Ule

Natur (Die)—continued.
und Karl Müller [et al.]. [Weekly.] v. 1, 1852. 420 pp. 4°. Halle.

Naturæ (De) aliquot arcanis, sympathiis et antipathiis, insignibusque medicamentis. Libelli duo aurei. 252 pp., 11 l. 16°. Bosphori, apud C. Justinum, 1622.

Natural (The) bitter waters of Friedrichshall, one of the most popular of the numerous mineral waters of Germany. 4 l. 8°. [Naumburg, G. Pätz, 1872.]

——. The same. 17 pp. 8°. Hildburghausen, F. W. Gadow & Son, [n. d.]

Natural bromo-iodine water of the Woodhall spa, Lincolnshire. 1 l., 1 map. 8°. [London, 1868.] [P., v. 1193.]

Natural (The) history of chocolate, being a distinct and particular account of the cocao tree, its growth and culture, and the preparation, excellent properties, and medicinal vertues of its fruit, wherein the errors of those who have wrote upon this subject are discovered, the best way of making chocolate is explained, and several uncommon medicines drawn from it are communicated. Being published with the particular approbation of Mons. Audry, translated from the last edition of the French by a physician. viii, 95 pp. 12°. London, J. Roberts, 1724. [P., v. 1240.]

Natural history and the natural sciences.
See, also, **Anatomy** (Comparative); **Birds**; **Botany**; **Crustaceæ**; **Development**; **Fish**; **Insects**; **Museums**; **Physics**; **Serpents**; **Spiders**; **Vertebræ**; **Worms**; **Zoölogy**.

AGASSIZ (L. J. R.) An introduction to the study of natural history, in a series of lectures delivered in the hall of the College of Physicians and Surgeons, New-York. Illustrated with numerous engravings; also a biographical notice of the author. 8°. New-York, 1847.

——. Importance of the study of natural history as a branch of elementary education. 8°. [n. p., n. d.]
Repr. from: The Massachusetts Teacher, Jan., 1850.

ALDROVANDUS (U.) Opera. 13 v. fol. Bonon., 1646–8.

ALLMAN (G. J.) Introductory lecture delivered to the students of the natural history class in the University of Edinburgh on the opening of the winter session, 1855. 8°. Edinburgh, 1855.

AMOREUX (P. J.) * Tentamen de noxa animalium. 4°. Avenione, 1762.

ANTIGONUS (C.) Historiarum mirabilium collectanea. Joannes Meursius recensuit et notas addidit. 4°. Lugd. Bat., 1619.

ARISTOTELES. Opera omnia. Græce et Latine cum indice nominum et rerum absolutissimo. 5 v. roy. 8°. Parisiis, 1862–74.

VON BAER (K. E.) Berichte über die Zoographia Rosso-Asiatica von Pallas. 4°. Königsberg, 1831.

——. Reden gehalten in wissenschaftlichen Versammlungen und kleinere Aufsätze vermischten Inhalts. 2 v. 8°. St. Petersburg, 1864–76.

BAIRD (W.) A dictionary of natural history. Map. roy. 8°. London & Glasgow, 1860.

BARTON (B. S.) A discourse on some of the principal desiderata in natural history, and on the best means of promoting the study of this science in the United States. 8°. Philadelphia, 1807.

BLUMENBACH (J. F.) Handbuch der Naturgeschichte. 9. Aufl. 8°. Wien, 1876.

——. The same. A manual of the elements of natural history. Transl. from the 10. German ed. by R. T. Gore. 8°. London, 1825.

Natural history and the natural sciences.
BOEHMER (G. R.) Freundschaftliche Beantwortung der im CX. Stücke dieses Jahres in den Götting. gel. Anzeigen befindlichen Recension des ersten Theiles des systematisch-literärischen Handbuches der Naturgeschichte, Oekonomie u. s. f. 8°. Wittenberg, 1786.

BOSTON Society of Natural History. Annual reports of the . . . 1881–2. 8°. Boston, 1882.

BRULLÉ. Quelques observations concernant les polypes d'eau douce. 8°. Dijon, [n. d.]
Repr. from: Mém. Acad. d. sc. de Dijon, 1851-2.

BURTON (A.) *An inaugural essay on physeodesmos; or the tie of creation. 8°. Baltimore, 1813.

CARUS (C. G.) Von den äussern Lebensbedingungen der weiss- und kaltblütigen Thiere . . . Gekrönte Preisschrift. Nebst zwei Beilagen über Entwicklungsgeschichte der Teichhornschnecke, und über Herzschlag und Blut der Weinbergsschnecke und des Flusskrebses. 4°. Leipzig, 1824.

CHANNING (W.) A lecture on the moral uses of the study of natural history, delivered before the American Institute of Instruction. 8°. Boston, 1836.

COCCHI (A.) Discorso sopra l' istoria naturale letto da lui pubblicamente in Firenze in occasione del ristabilimento della Società botanica fiorentina il dì 2 di settembre 1734.
In: DISSERTAZIONI e lett. [etc.] 8°. Firenze, 1750, ii, 81–102. Also. transl. in: PIÈCES intéressantes sur la méd. et la phys. 12°. Paris, 1782, 75-108.

COLQUHOUN (J.) Lecture on the natural history of the British islands. 8°. Edinburgh, 1856.

CORK Cuvierian Society for the Cultivation of the Sciences. Report of the . . . for the session 1854–5; with an account of the conversaziones held at the Athenæum on the 29th and 31st May; and the addresses delivered by the president, Dr. Boole; and by Professor Shaw, and Richard Dowden, esq. 8°. Cork, 1855.

COURS élémentaire d'histoire naturelle à l'usage des colléges, des séminaires et des maisons d'éducation, rédigé conformément au programme de l'université du 14 septembre 1840, par MM. Milne-Edwards, A. De Jussieu et Beudant. Botanique par M. Adrien De Jussieu. 8°. Paris, [n. d.]

CUNNINGHAM (R. O.) Notes on the reptiles, amphibia, fishes, mollusca, and crustacea obtained during the voyage of H. M. S. "Nassau" in the years 1866–9. 4°. London, [n. d.]
Cutting from: Transactions of the Linnean Society of London, xxvii.

DE SÈDE (P.) Conférences sur l'histoire naturelle à l'usage des candidats à la licence et des étudiants en médecine. 8°. Paris, 1887.

DICTIONNAIRE classique d'histoire naturelle. Par MM. Audouin, Isid. Bourdon, Ad. Brongniart, De Candolle, etc. 16 v. & 1 v. of pl. 8°. Paris, 1822–31.

DOEDERLINUS (J. G. Z.) Theses extemporaneæ usum rationemque experimentorum in perficienda historia naturali indicantes. sm. 4°. Altdorfii Noric., [1718].

DUVERNOY (G.-L.) Discours prononcé le 22 décembre 1827, à l'ouverture du cours d'histoire naturelle de la Faculté des sciences de Strasbourg. 8°. [n. p., n. d.]
Cutting from: J. Soc. d. sc. de Strasb., 1828, v, 41-80.

——. Discours de clôture du cours d'histoire naturelle de la Faculté des sciences de Strasbourg, prononcé le 30 juillet 1828. 8°. [Strasbourg, n. d.]

——. Discours d'ouverture du cours d'histoire naturelle de la Faculté des sciences, prononcé le 15 novembre 1831. 8°. Strasbourg, 1832.

41

Natural *history and the natural sciences.*

——. Leçons sur l'histoire naturelle des corps organisés professées au Collége de France. 1.-4. fasc. 8°. [*Paris*, 1839–51.]

EDWARDS (H.-M.) & COMTE (J.-A.) Cahiers d'histoire naturelle à l'usage des colléges et des écoles normales primaires. Six cahiers dans 1 v. 1. cahier, 3. éd. ; 2.-6. cahier, 2. éd. 12°. *Paris*, 1835.

ENGELMANN (W.) Bibliotheca historico-naturalis. Verzeichniss der Bücher über Naturgeschichte, welche in Deutschland, Scandinavien, Holland, England, Frankreich, Italien und Spanien in den Jahren 1700–1846 erschienen sind. v. 1. 8°. *Leipzig*, 1846.

ETHERINGTON (G. F.) Address delivered to the Cuvierian Natural History Society of Edinburgh, upon the occasion of being elevated to the chair of vice-president. 8°. *Edinburgh*, 1841.

FIGUIER (L.) The ocean world; being a descriptive history of the sea and its living inhabitants. Chiefly translated from "La vie et les mœurs des animaux". Illustrated by 427 engravings, chiefly designed under the direction of M. Ch. Bévalet, from specimens in the museums of Paris. roy. 8°. *London*, 1868.

FISHER (T.) Dial of the seasons, or a portraiture of nature. 8°. *Philadelphia*, 1845.

FLEMING (J.) On the different branches of natural history, the chairs which have been instituted for their illustration, and the manner in which they should be subordinated. 8°. [*Edinburgh*, 1856.]
Repr. from: Edinb. N. Phil. J., 1856.

FOGG (F. B.) Barrington's elements of natural science; comprising hydrology, geognosy, geology, meteorology, botany, zoölogy, and anthropology. 8°. *Nashville, Tenn.*, 1858.

FRANCIS (J. W.) A discourse; delivered upon the opening of the new hall of the New York Lyceum of Natural History. 8°. *New York*, 1841.

FYFE (W. W.) Address to the Cuvierian Natural History Society. 8°. *Edinburgh*, 1840.

GEDNER (C.) *Quæstio historico-naturalis, cui bono?
In: LINNÆUS. Amœnitates acad. [etc.] 8°. *Lugd. Bat.*, 1756, iii, 231–255.

GÉRARD. De la zoogénie et de la distribution des êtres organisés à la surface du globe. 8°. *Paris*, 1845.

GODMAN (J. D.) Rambles of a naturalist. To which are added reminiscences of a voyage to India, by Reynell Coates. 8°. *Philadelphia*, 1833.

GOOD (J. M.) The book of nature. 2 v. 8°. *Boston*, 1826.

——. The same. From the last Lond. ed. To which is now prefixed, a sketch of the author's life. 8°. *New York*, 1831.

GOULD (A. A.) Search out the secrets of nature; the annual discourse before the Massachusetts Medical Society, Springfield, June 27, 1855. 8°. *Boston*, 1855.

GRANT (R. E.) Syllabus of four lectures on foraminiferous animalcules, polypiferous animals, insects, and reptiles. 8°. *London*, 1860.

VAN HALL (H. C.) Oratio de Neerlandia, historiæ naturali excolendæ atque amplificandæ, reliquis Europæ partibus non minus idonea. 4°. *Groningæ*, 1837.

HASTINGS (C.) The address of the council of the Worcestershire Natural History Society, delivered at the eleventh anniversary meeting, on Wednesday, October 9, 1844. 8°. *Worcester*, 1844.

HELMHOLTZ (H.) Ueber das Verhältniss der Naturwissenschaften zur Gesammtheit der Wissenschaften. 4°. *Heidelberg*, 1862.

Natural *history and the natural sciences.*

HJELT (O. E. A.) Naturhistoriens studium i Finland under sjuttonde och adertonde seklet. 8°. *Helsingfors*, 1868.

HUXLEY (T. H.) On our knowledge of the causes of the phenomena of organic nature, being six lectures to working men. 8°. *London*, 1863.

JONSTON (J.) Thaumatographia naturalis in decem classes distincta. 18°. *Amsterdami*, 1632.

KWEEKSCHOOL der Natuurkunde. Zijnde verzamelingen en waarneemingen uyt de beste en nieuwste schrijvers getrokken. Ten dienste der geene, die zich in deeze weetenschappen willen oeffenen. 8°. *Amsterdam*, 1773.

LEZCANO (F. L.) Resúmen de los trabajos en que se ha ocupado el Ateneo propagador de las ciencias naturales durante el año económico de 1871 á 1872. Leido en la sesion inaugural celebrada el 28 de octubre. 8°. *Madrid*, 1872.

LINNÆUS (C.) Deliciæ naturæ. Oratio recitata in templo cathedrali Upsaliensi.
In his: Amœnitates acad. [etc.] 8°. *Erlangæ*, 1790, x, 66–99.

LORD (J. K.) The naturalist in Vancouver Island and British Columbia. Illustrated. 2 v. 8°. *London*, 1866.

LYCEUM (The) of Natural History in the City of New-York. Charter, constitution, and bylaws of the Lyceum of Natural History in the City of New-York. Incorporated April 20, 1818. 8°. *New-York*, 1835.

MARTINS (C.) Un hivernage scientifique en Laponie. 8°. *Paris*, 1845.

MONCKTON (S.) The metaphysical aspect of natural history. An address to the Rochester Natural History Society, delivered in the Mathematical School, Rochester, December 10, 1884. sm. 4°. *London*, 1885.

MUSÉUM royal d'histoire naturelle. Instruction pour les voyageurs et pour les employés dans les colonies, sur la manière de recueillir, de conserver et d'envoyer les objets d'histoire naturelle; rédigée sur l'invitation de son excellence le ministre de la marine et des colonies. 3. éd. 8°. *Paris*, 1829.

NEILL (P.) An address to the members of the Wernerian Natural History Society, 1830. 8°. [*Edinburgh*], 1830.

NEMNICH (P. A.) Allgemeines Polyglotten-Lexicon der Naturgeschichte, mit erklärenden Anmerkungen. [2. *title:*] Wörterbücher der Naturgeschichte in der deutschen, holländischen, dänischen, schwedischen, englischen, französischen, italienischen, spanischen und portugisischen Sprache. 3 v. 4°. *Hamburg u. Leipzig*, [1792–3].

NICOL (J.) On the study of natural history as a branch of general education; an inaugural lecture. 8°. *Edinburgh*, 1853.

NITSCHE (A.) *Momenta quædam comparationis regni animalis cum vegetabili. 4°. *Lipsiæ*, [1788].

NOUVEAU dictionnaire d'histoire naturelle, appliquée aux arts, à l'agriculture, à l'économie rurale et domestique, à la médecine, etc. Par une société de naturalistes et d'agriculteurs. Nouv. éd. 36 v. 8°. *Paris*, 1816–19.

OPENINGSPLECHTIGHEID van de Tentoonstelling. 10 Januari 1 uur 's namiddags in de Bibliotheek van het Koninklijk Zoölogisch Genootschap Natura Artis Magistra. 8°. *Amsterdam*, 1878.

ORR. Circle of the sciences. A series of treatises on the principles of science, with their application to practical pursuits. With an introductory treatise on the nature and uses of the great departments of knowledge. 3 v. 8°. *London*, 1859.

Natural *history and the natural sciences.*

PITCAIRN (A.) Dissertatio de legibus historiæ naturalis.
In his: Opusc. med. 4°. *Roterod.*, 1714, 177–229. *Also, in his:* Op. omn. 4°. *Lugd. Bat.*, 1737, 330–369.

PLANCHON (G.) * Les principes de la méthode naturelle appliqués comparativement à la classification des végétaux et des animaux. 8°. *Montpellier*, 1860.

PLINIUS *secundus* (C.) Historiæ naturalis libri xxxvii. Quibus accessere novus index animalium, mineralium, vegetabilium synonymicus, nominumque et rerum quoad cetera enodatio, habita alphabetici ordinis ratione, e notis gallicæ editionis Ajasson de Grandsagne. Quarum auctores exstitere ad zoosophiam, ut plurimum G. Cuvier, passim vero, et in iis quæ zoosophiæ non erant, Doe, E. Dolo, Fée, L. Fouché et al. 4 v. in 2. 8°. *Lipsiæ*, 1836.

——. The same. Cajus Plinius secundus Naturgeschichte. Uebersetzt und erläutert von Ph. H. Külb. [35. Bändchen, 37. Buch, pp. 4249–4380.] 12°. *Stuttgart*, 1856.
Römische Prosaiker in neuen Uebersetzungen. 215 v.

——. The same. The natural history of . . . translated, with copious notes and illustrations, by John Bostock and H. T. Riley. 6 v. 12°. *London*, 1855–6–7.

PORTLAND Society of Natural History. Proceedings of the Portland Society of Natural History. v. 1, pt. 2. 8°. *Portland*, 1869.

PORTLOCK (J. E.) Address delivered at the anniversary meeting of the Geological Society of London, on the 19th of February, 1858, prefaced by the announcement of the award of the Wollaston Palladium medal and proceeds of the donation fund for the same year. 8°. *London*, 1858.

POUCHET (F. A.) The universe, or the infinitely great and the infinitely little. Transl. from the French. Illustrated. 8°. *London*, 1870.

PROBLEMATA Aristotelis, das ist: gründtliche Erörterung und Aufflösung mancherley zweiffelhafftiger Fragen, des hochberühmbten Aristotelis, und vieler anderer bewehrter Naturkündiger, fast nützlich und kurtzweilig, allerley fürgebrachte Fragen eigentlich und scheinbarlich zu entscheiden. 24°. *Hamburg*, 1604.

RAFINESQUE (C. S.) The good book, and amenities of nature, or annals of historical and natural sciences. Containing selections of observations, researches, and novelties in all the branches of physical and historical knowledge, with letters of eminent authors, chiefly on zoölogy, botany, agronomy, geognosy, ethnography . . . or organized beings and fossils, nations and languages. 8°. *Philadelphia*, 1840.

REDI (F.) Opusculorum pars secunda, sive experimenta circa varias res naturales, speciatim illas quæ ex Indiis afferuntur. 16°. *Lugd. Bat.*, 1729.

RENGADE (J.) La création naturelle et les êtres vivants. Histoire générale du monde terrestre des végétaux, des animaux et de l'homme, avec la description des espèces les plus remarquables au point de vue de leur développement, de leur organisation, de leurs mœurs et de leur utilité dans la nature. Zoologie; races humaines. Animaux; zoophytes; vers; mollusques; échinodermes; arthropodes; vertébrés; hommes. roy. 8°. *Paris*, 1885.

ROBIN (C.) Notice sur [ses] travaux d'histoire naturelle, d'anatomie et de pathologie. 4°. [*Paris*, 1852.]

SAGE. Observations sur un écrit qui a pour titre: Vues sur le Jardin royal des plantes et le Cabinet d'histoire naturelle; à Paris, chez Baudouin, imprimeur de l'Assemblée nationale, 1789. 8°. *Paris*, 1790.

Natural *history and the natural sciences.*

SAVORY (W. S.) The relation of the vegetable and animal to the inorganic kingdom. 8°. *London*, 1861.

SCHNEIDER (O.) Naturwissenschaftliche Beiträge zur Kenntniss der Kaukasusländer, auf Grund seiner Sammelbeute. 8°. *Dresden*, 1878.

SCHOTT (P. G.) Physica curiosa, sive mirabilia naturæ et artis libris xii. comprehensa. 4°. *Herbipoli*, 1662.

DE SIEBOLD (P. F.) * De historiæ naturalis in Japonia statu nec non de augmento emolumentisque in decursu perscrutationum exspectandis cui accedunt spicilegia faunæ japonicæ. 8°. *Wirceburgi*, 1826.

——, TEMMINCK (C. J.), SCHLEGEL (H.) & DE HAAN (W.) Fauna japonica, sive descriptio animalium, quæ in itinere per Japoniam, jussu et auspiciis superiorum, qui summum in India Batava imperium tenent, suscepto, annis 1823–30 collegit, notis, observationibus et adumbrationibus illustravit. fol. *Lugd. Bat.*, 1850.
French text.

SMELLIE (W.) The philosophy of natural history. With an introduction and various additions and alterations, intended to adapt it to the present state of knowledge, by John Ware. 8°. *Boston*, 1824.

SOCIÉTÉ d'agriculture de la Haute-Garonne. Rapport fait au nom d'une commission chargée d'examiner les propositions de M. N. Joly, tendant à ce que la . . . se fasse affilier à la Société impériale zoologique d'acclimatation siégeant à Paris. [N. Jolly, rapporteur.] 8°. [*Toulouse*, 1857.]

SPECTACLE de la nature, or nature displayed. Being discourses on such particulars of natural history as were thought most proper to excite the curiosity and form the minds of youth. Transl. from the original French. 2. ed. 8°. *London*, 1735.

STARK (B.) * De animalium et terra natorum similitudine. 8°. *Edinburgi*, 1799.

SYLLABUS of lectures on natural history. 8°. [*Edinburgh, n. d.*]

TELLIAMED; or, the world explain'd. Containing discourses between an Indian philosopher and a missionary on the diminution of the sea, the formation of the earth, the origin of men and animals, and other singular subjects relating to natural history and philosophy. A very curious work. 8°. *Baltimore*, 1797.

VALENTINUS (M. B.) Prodromus historiæ naturalis Hassiæ, quem anno academiæ Gissenæ jubilæo mdccvii. sub præsidio autoris, publicæ curiosorum ventilationi sistebat Joh. Nicolaus Müllerus. 4°. *Gissæ-Hassorum*, [1707].

VALMONT DE BOMARE. Dictionnaire raisonné universel d'histoire naturelle. Éd. augmentée par l'auteur; avec plusieurs articles nouveaux . . . sur l'histoire naturelle, la médecine [etc.], fournies par Mrs. Haller . . . Deleuze . . . [etc.] 12 v. sm. 8°. *Yverdon*, 1768–9.

VIRCHOW (R.) Ueber die nationale Entwickelung und Bedeutung der Naturwissenschaften. Rede gehalten in der zweiten allgemeinen Sitzung der Versammlung deutscher Naturforscher und Aerzte zu Hannover am 20. September 1865. 12°. *Berlin*, 1865.

WARREN (J. C.) Address to the Boston Society of Natural History. 8°. *Boston*, 1853.

WATERHOUSE (B.) Heads of a course of lectures on natural history. 8°. *Cambridge*, 1810.

WILCKE (H. C. D.) * Politia naturæ.
In: LINNÆUS. Amœnitates acad. [etc.] 8°. *Lugd. Bat.*, 1764, vi.

WOLF (C. A. F.) De limitum inter regnum animale et vegetabile constituendorum difficultatibus disserit. 4°. [*Vitebergæ, n. d.*]

Natural *history and the natural sciences.*

WOOD (J. G.) The illustrated natural history. 3 v. roy. 8°. *London*, 1862–3.

WOODWARD (J.) Naturalis historia telluris illustrata et aucta. Una cum ejusdem defensione; præsertim contra nuperas objectiones D. El. Camerarii ad Thomam Pembrochiæ comitem. 8°. *Londini*, 1714.

ZABARELLA (J.) De rebus naturalibus libri xxx, quibus quæstiones, quæ ab Aristotelis interpretibus hodie tractari solent, accurate discutiuntur. 3. ed. 4°. *Coloniæ*, 1597.

Choulant (L.) Die Anfänge wissenschaftlicher Naturgeschichte und naturhistorischer Abbildung im christlichen Abendlande. *In:* Hochverdienten (Ihrem) Collegen [etc.], 4°, Dresden, 1856, 1–46.—**Coldstream** (J.) Additions to the natural history of British animals. Edinb. N. Phil. J., 1830, ix, 234–241. *Also,* Reprint.—**Curran** (W.) The vitality of wild animals under fire. J. Anat. & Physiol., Lond., 1885–6, xx, 596–603, 1 pl.—**Goode** (G. B.) The beginnings of natural history in America. Proc. Biol. Soc. Wash., 1884–6, iii, 35–105.—**Huxley** (M. T. H.) Ueber die Grenze zwischen Thier- und Pflanzenreich. Deutsche med. Wchnschr., Berl., 1878, iv, 239; 251; 267; 279.—**Hyades.** Rapport sommaire sur les recherches d'histoire naturelle faites par la mission du Cap Horn. Monit. scient., Par., 1884, 3. s., xiv, 424–426.—**de Lanessan** (J.-L.) Buffon; ses idées, son rôle dans l'histoire des sciences, son œuvre et le développement des sciences naturelles depuis son époque. Rev. internat. d. sc. biol., Par., 1883, xii, 381; 477.—**Lucae** (J. C. G.) Noch Einiges zum Zeichnen naturhistorischer Gegenstände. Arch. f. Anthrop., Brnschwg., 1873–4, vi, 1–12.—**McClelland.** List of objects in natural history collected in Assam. Tr. M. & Phys. Soc. Calcutta, 1835–42, viii, pt. 2, pp. ccxvi–ccxxiii.—**Maget** (G.) Note sur la faune du Japon. Arch. de méd. nav., Par., 1877, xxviii, 5–22.—**Pouchet.** Instruction pour la récolte des objets d'histoire naturelle à la mer. *Ibid.*, 1887, xlvii, 211–228.—**Ritter** (J. J.) Tentamen historiæ naturalis Ditionis Riedeselio-Avimontanæ in quatuor partes, nempe floram, mineralogiam, faunam et commentatiunctlam de aëre, aquis et locis, etc., divisum. Acta Acad. nat. curios., Norimb., 1754, x (app.), 21; 343.—**Stokvis** (B. J.) Nationalität und Naturwissenschaft. Deutsche med. Wchnschr., Leipz., 1887, xiii, 1124. — **Vallisneri** (A.) Tre lettere sopra alcune cose di storia naturale e di medesimo. *In:* Rac. d' opusc. scient. e filol., 16°, Venezia, 1729, ii, 1–62.—**Zapiski** Kievskago Obshestva Estestvoispitatelei. [Records of Kieff Society of Naturalists.] Zapiski Kievsk. Obsh. Estestvo., Kieff, 1875–87, iv–viii.

Natural *history (Medical).*

See, also, **Botany** *(Medical);* **Materia** *medica;* **Materia** *medica (Animal);* **Materia** *medica (Vegetable);* **Parasites,** *etc.*

BOCQUILLON (H.) Manuel d'histoire naturelle médicale. 2 v. 8°. *Paris*, 1871.

BOURSIN (L.) Leçons d'histoire naturelle médicale. 2 pts. in 1 v. sm. 4°. *Paris*, 1874.

CARLET (G.) Précis de zoologie médicale. 12°. *Paris*, 1881.

CAUVET (D.) Nouveaux éléments d'histoire naturelle médicale. 2 v. 8°. *Paris*, 1869.

ERNDL (C. H.) * De usu historiæ naturalis exotico geographicæ in medicina. 4°. *Lipsiæ*, [1700].

HALBERTSMA (H. J.) Jaarlijksch verslag over de Nederlandsche geneeskundige litteratuur (1854). III. Verslag over de geschriften aangaande de natuurkunde. 8°. [*n. p.*, 1854.]

KUNDMANN (J. C.) Rariora naturæ et artis, item in re medica, oder Seltenheiten der Natur und Kunst des Kundmannischen Naturalien-Kabinets, wie auch in der Artzeney-Wissenschaft. fol. *Bresslau u. Leipzig*, 1737.

DE LANESSAN (J. L.) Manuel d'histoire naturelle médicale. 3 v. 12°. *Paris*, 1879–82.

MOQUIN-TANDON (A.) Éléments de zoologie médicale, contenant la description détaillée des animaux utiles à la médecine et des espèces nuisibles à l'homme, particulièrement des venimeuses et des parasites, précédée de considérations générales sur l'organisation et sur la classification des animaux et d'un résumé sur l'histoire naturelle de l'homme. 12°. *Paris*, 1860.

Natural *history (Medical).*

PETROZ (M.-A.) * Dissertation sur quelques rapports de l'histoire naturelle avec la médecine. 4°. *Paris*, 1808.

WALLERIUS (J. G.) & MALMSTEN (O.) De historiæ naturalis usu medico. 4°. *Upsaliæ*, [1740].

Beaudry (G.-O.) Nécessité des sciences naturelles appliquées à la médecine. Union méd. du Canada, Montréal, 1876, v, 1–11. — **Duparc** (H. M.) De waarde der wetenschappelijke natuur-studien voor de geneeskundige getoest. Boerhaave. Tijdschr., etc., Amst., 1845, n. s., iv, 354; 393. — **Guldberg** (G. A.) Zoologi og Medicin. Norsk Mag. f. Lægevidensk., Christiania, 1883, 3. R., xiii, 185–196.—**Ragazzi** (V.) Cenni medico-zoologici su di un viaggio all' America del Sud. Spallanzani, Modena, 1882, 2. s., xi, 201; 293.—**Riddell** (J. L.) Introductory lecture delivered Nov. 18, 1851, before the medical class, University of Louisiana, New Orleans, on our knowledge of nature, the natural sciences, and on certain truths revealed by the microscope. N. Orl. M. & S. J., 1851–2, viii, 468–480.—**Rodriguez** (P. de Salazar R.) Discurso: [Del influjo de las ciencias naturales sobre las demás y en particular sobre la medicina.] Mem. r. Acad. méd. de Madrid, 1862, ii, pt. 1, 129–138.

Natural (The) History Review. Published quarterly; including the proceedings of the Irish Natural History Societies for the sessions 1855–6. v. 3. 444 pp. 8°. *London, Williams & Norgate*, 1856.

———. The same. A quarterly journal of biological science. Edited by G. Busk, W. B. Carpenter [*et al.*]. v. 1–2, Jan., 1861–2. 8°. *London, Williams & Norgate.*

Natural (The) mineral water of Friedrichshall and its use. 2 l. 8°. *Coburg, A. Rossteutscher*, [*n. d.*]

Natural *philosophy.*

See **Physics.**

Natural *sciences.*

See **Meteorology**; **Natural** *history, etc.*; **Science.**

Natural *selection.*

See **Darwinian** *theory.*

Naturaliste (Le) canadien. Bulletin de recherches, observations et découvertes se rapportant à l'histoire naturelle du Canada. Rédacteur: M. l'abbé Provancher. [Monthly.] Nos. 4, 7, v. 10, April, July, 1878. 8°. *Cap Rouge, Province de Québec.*

Naturalists' (The) directory, containing the names, addresses, special departments of study, etc., of the naturalists, chemists, physicists, astronomers, etc., of the United States and Canada. Arranged alphabetically, also geographically. Edited by Samuel E. Cassino. 1878, 1879, 1880, 1884, 1886. 5 v. 8°. *Boston & Salem*, 1878–86.

Naturarzt (Der). Correspondenzblatt für Freunde naturgemässer Heilmethoden. Hrsg. von Wilhelm Meinert. [Weekly.] v. 2–8, 1863–9; v. 15–25, 1876–86. 18 v. 4° & 8°. *Dresden; Berlin*, 1864–9.

Title of v. 1 was: **Wasserfreund** (Der). In 1867 Theodor Hahn became editor; in 1876 Gustav Wolbold became editor.

Naturarzt (Der). (Früher Volksarzt). Organ des "Central-Verbands" von über 100 Vereinen für naturgemässe Gesundheitspflege und Heilkunde, [etc.] Hrsg. von Dr. Med. Schulze. [Monthly.] v. 4, 1887. 192 pp. 8°. *Berlin.*

Current. Title of v. 1–3; no. 1, v. 4, was: **Volksarzt** (Der).

Nature.

See, also, **Physics.**

BALDOVIUS (J.) * De natura. sm. 4°. *Lipsiæ*, [1637].

BARRA DE H. ALMÁS (S.) * De affinitate elementorum individualium trium naturæ regno

Nature.

rum, et parallela eorundem evolutione. 8°. *Pesten*, 1833.

BOECLER (J.) Theses physicæ de natura, physicæ objecto. sm. 4°. *Argentorati*, [1730].

VAN DER BOON MESCH (H. C.) Oratio de naturæ coutemplatore, tum sui tum alieni commodi adjutore. 4°. *Amstelodami*, 1824.

DEUSINGIUS (A.) Dissertatio de natura.
In his: Sylva-cædua jacens, etc. 16°. *Groningæ*, 1665, 243–367.

VAN DER EYK (S. S.) Carmen de natura. 4°. *Lugd. Bat.*, 1810.

FOERTSCH (P. J.) * De spiritu mundi. sm. 4°. *Jenæ*, [1707].

VAN DER HOEVEN (J.) Oratio de diligenti veritatis studio præcipua naturæ interpretis dote. 4°. [*Lugd. Bat.*, 1826.]

KAESTNER (A. G.) De lege continui in natura. 4°. *Lipsiæ*, 1750.

MIZALDUS (A.) Harmonia superioris naturæ mundi et inferioris; una cum admirabili fœdere et sympatheia rerum utriusque. 8°. *Parisiis*, 1598.

NATURE (De la). 8°. *Amsterdam*, 1761.

NEISSER (J.) * De autocratia naturæ. 8°. *Halæ*, 1836.

PLAZ (A. G.) [Pr.] de natura non fatiscente. 4°. *Lipsiæ*, [1779].

ROSENKRANZ (J. C. F.) De integritate naturæ dissertatio. 8°. *Regiomonti*, 1834.

SCHÜTZE (G.) * De apotheosi naturæ. sm. 4°. *Vitembergæ*, [1698].

VALENTINI (M. B.) De natura et essentia naturæ, ad Robertum Boyle. 1689.
In his: Polychresta exotica, etc. 4°. *Francof. a. M.*, 1700, 115–128.

———. De instinctu naturæ, ad Carolum Patini. 1691.
In his: Polychresta exotica, etc. 4°. *Francof. a. M.*, 1700, 154–166.

———. De legibus artis et naturæ. 1697.
In his: Declamationum panegyricarum δεκάς. 4°. *Francof. a. M.*, 1701, 7–18.

Schaaffhausen (H.) Ueber das Zweckmässige in der Natur. Arch. f. Anthrop., Brnschwg., 1868, iii, 87–100. *Also, in his:* Anthrop. Studien, 8°, Bonn, 1885, 433–454. — **Virey.** Nature. Dict. d. sc. méd., Par., 1819, xxxv, 240–300.

Nature *in disease.*

See, also, **Disease ; Diseases** (*Duration of*) ; **Fever ; Therapeutics** (*Expectant*).

ALBERTUS (M.) Epistola gratulatoria in qua mysterium naturæ in medicina explicatur ad Christ. Berghauer. 4°. *Halæ Magdeb.*, [1707].

———. [Pr.] de falso sensu medico naturæ corpore Hippocratico. 4°. [*Halæ Magdeb.*, 1718.]

———. [Pr.] de natura quatenus idolo et asylo ignorantiæ medicorum. 4°. [*Halæ Magdeb.*, 1723.]

ALBRECHT (G. A. H.) * De natura, se ipsam nunc vindicante, nunc destruente. 4°. *Gottingæ*, [1737].

ALISON (W. P.) * De viribus naturæ medicatricibus. 8°. *Edinburgi*, 1811.

ASENHAMMER (J. C.) * De naturæ viribus earumque ad organismum relatione. sm. 4°. *Wirceburgi*, [1808].

BEEVER (J.) * De natura morborum medicatrice. 4°. *Lugd. Bat.*, 1736.

BENES (B.) * De natura humana sibi ipsi salutifera. 4°. *Groningæ*, 1762.

À BERGEN (J.) * De naturæ humanæ efficacia tam in præsenti sanitate conservanda quam in amissa restituenda. 4°. *Lugd. Bat.*, 1765.

BERGHAUER (C.) * De medicina sine medico. 4°. *Halæ Magdeb.*, [1707].

BIGELOW (J.) Nature in disease; illustrated in various discourses and essays. 2. ed., enlarged. 8°. *Boston*, 1859.

Nature *in disease.*

BONNAIN (O.-G.) * Essai sur la nature médicatrice. 4°. *Paris*, 1836.

BONSDORFF (E. J.) Andra Brefvet, till Herr Alexander af Forselles, om Naturläkekonst och Medicin. 8°. *Helsingfors*, 1862.

BRAUNE (A.) De nisu in morbis salutari therapiæ generalis fundamento. 8°. *Lipsiæ*, [1842].

BURGHARDT (G. E.) * De naturæ lucta cum morbo et medico. sm. 4°. *Halæ Magdeb.*, [1727].

CAPERET (J.) * De la nature médicatrice à propos de l'interprétation de quelques actes morbides. 4°. *Montpellier*, 1877.

CAPPEL (L. C. G.) Disquisitio de viribus corporis humani, quæ dicuntur medicatrices. 4°. *Gottingæ*, [1800].

CASTERMAN (L.) * De viribus naturæ. [Gand.] 4°. *Tornaci*, 1824.

CAVAYÉ (C.) * Essai sur la force médicatrice. 8°. *Montpellier*, 1844.

CHORTET (J.-F.) Réfutation de la doctrine des crises, des métastases, des forces conservatrices et médicatrices de la nature. 8°. *Paris, an XII* [1804].

CLAUSIUS (R.) Ueber die Energievorräthe der Natur, und ihre Verwerthung zum Nutzen der Menschheit. 8°. *Bonn*, 1885.

COLIN (J. J.) * De naturæ humanæ præsidiis, quibus ad morbos præcavendos et curandos utitur. 12°. *Moguntiæ*, [1783].

CONSBRUCH (G. G. C.) * De vi corporis animalis medicatrice. 8°. *Halæ*, [1787].

VAN COOTH (E. E.) * De medico naturæ ministro ejusdemque rectore. 4°. *Hardervici*, [1787].

COTTING (B. E.) Nature in disease. An address. 8°. *Boston*, 1852.
Also, in: Boston M. & S. J., 1852–3, xlvii, 223–231. *Also, in his:* Med. addresses. 8°. *Boston*, 1875, 1–23.

COUTY DE LA POMMERAIS (E.) * Du rôle que joue la nature dans les maladies. 4°. *Paris*, 1854.

COVENTRY (C. B.) Nature and art in the cure of disease. 8°. *Utica*, 1859.

CRAUSIUS (R. W.) [*sometimes called* CRAUSE DE MELLINGEN]. [Pr.] de συνεργοῖς naturæ in curatione necessariis. sm. 4°. *Jenæ*, [1702].

DEESEN (C. H.) * De vi naturæ humanæ medica. 4°. *Jenæ*, [1725].

DOLLEZ (M.-S.-J.) * Quæstio medica. An in morbis acutis soli naturæ crises molienti fidendum? 4°. *Duaci*, 1782.

DUFORT. * De la nature et de l'art dans la guérison des maladies. 4°. *Paris*, 1828.

EDES (R. T.) The part taken by nature and time in the cure of diseases. 8°. *Boston*, 1868.

———, HIBBERD (J. F.) & SPARE (J.) Dissertations on the part performed by nature and time in the cure of diseases; for which prizes were awarded by the Massachusetts Medical Society, 1868. 8°. *Boston*, 1868.

ERASTUS (T.) Morborum naturæ medicatrices. Hippocratis lib. vi. de morb. popul. sect. 5., aphoris. 1.
In his: Varia opuscula. fol. *Francof. a. M.*, 1590, 174–181.

FINOT (P. X.) * Considérations générales sur l'expectation. 4°. *Strasbourg*, 1834.

FLEMMING (J. C. G.) * Natura præstantior in re medica et œconomica. 4°. *Vitebergæ*, [1773].

FORBES (*Sir J.*) Of nature and art in the cure of disease. 8°. *London*, 1857.

———. The same. From the 2. Lond. ed. 8°. *New York*, 1858.

GEIER (G. F.) * Natura medicatrix philosophiæ et physices generalis legibus æstimata. 4°. *Wirceburgi*, [1798].

GRAF (F. C. A. G.) * De viribus naturæ medicatricis. 8°. *Wirceburgi*, 1820.

Nature *in disease.*

GRAVE (J. S.) *De amethodia naturæ. 4°. *Halæ Magdeb.*, [1709].

GRESSENT (J.-É.) *Du rôle de la nature et de celui de l'art dans la guérison des maladies. 4°. *Paris*, 1844.

HAACKE (J. F. G.) *De viribus quæ insunt organismo. 8°. *Gottingæ*, 1811.

HAXTHAUSEN (J. L.) *De vi naturæ medicatrice. 8°. *Berolini*, [1824].

HERZOG (J. G.) *Natura præstantior arte in re medica et œconomica; disputatio prior. 4°. *Vitemburgæ*, [1772].

HIBBERD (J. F.) The part taken by nature and time in the cure of diseases. A dissertation for which a prize was awarded by the Massachusetts Medical Society, 1868. 8°. *Boston*, 1868.

[HICKS (T. F.)] Nature in disease. A lecture. 16°. [*Wilmington, Del.*, 1878.]

HODGKINSON (D.-H.) *Sur le rôle de la nature et de certains moyens simples dans les maladies. 4°. *Paris*, 1864.

HŒNLEIN (C.) *De naturæ vi medicatrice. 4°. *Argentorati*, 1808.

HOFFMANN (C. R.) Kurze Betrachtnng über die verschiedene Art und Weise, in welcher man das Verhältniss des natürlichen Heilungsprozesses zum Krankheitsprozesse aufgefasst hat. 4°. *Würzburg*, [1828].

HOFFMANN (J. F.) *De natura solerte sanitatis conservatrice. 4°. *Jenæ*, [1715].

HOUTH (M. F.) *De natura in medicina dulce. 4°. *Gottingæ*, [1766].

JANOWITZ (M.) *De natura medicatrice. 8°. *Pragæ*, [n. d.]

JOHNSON (G.) Nature and art in the cure of disease. Address in medicine, at the meeting of the British Medical Association, at Plymouth. 8°. *London*, 1871.
Also, in: Brit. M. J., Lond., 1871, ii, 171–175.

JOYET (L.-H.) *I. De la force médicatrice. II. [etc.] 4°. *Paris*, 1842.

KENTLING (J. B.) *De natura medicatrice. sm. 8°. *Berolini*, [1836].

KEYSLER (J. F.) *De natura morborum medicatrice. 4°. *Halæ Magdeb.*, [1729].

KIRCHOF (G.) *De natura morborum medica. 4°. *Lugd. Bat.*, 1692.

KLEIN (M.) *De autocratia naturæ in conservanda et restituenda sanitate. 8°. *Pestini*, 1831.

KLETTE (A. G.) *De motibus naturæ cynosura medici. 4°. *Halæ Magdeb.*, [1716].

KOELMAN (J. J.) *Diss. sistens brevem conspectum virium naturæ humanæ medicatricium. 4°. *Lugd. Bat.*, 1763.

KUNZENDORF (P. E.) *De processibus compensatoriis. 8°. *Berolini*, [1863].

LASIUS (J. A.) *De αὐτοκρατία naturæ, sive spontanea morborum excussione, et convalescentia. sm. 4°. *Halæ Magdeb.*, [1696].

VON LESEN (J.) *De naturæ in conservanda et restituenda sanitate viribus. 4°. *Helmstadii*, [1714].

LION (A.) *Vires naturæ medicatrices. 8°. *Vratislaviæ*, [1833].

LISCHWITZ (J. C.) Oratio inauguralis, de naturæ sollicitudine et energia, in compensandis provideque sublevandis defectubus humanis. 4°. [*Kiliæ*, 1743.]

VAN MAANEN (F. J.) *De natura humana, suæ ipsius conservatrice ac medicatrice. 4°. *Hardervici*, 1801.

MACK (J.) *De vi natura medicatrice. 8°. *Monachii*, 1833.

METZGER (J. C.) *De naturæ et artis effectu in medendo. sm. 4°. *Halæ Magdeb.*, [1708].

Nature *in disease.*

N. (C. A.) De vi naturæ medicatrice. 8°. [*n. p., n. d.*]

NENTER (G. P.) Epistola de motibus naturæ in morbis prudenter tractandis ad B. G. Garmannum de cautelis in hæmorrhoidum curatione observandis disputantem. 4°. *Argentinæ*, [1715].

NOLST (L.) *De viribus naturæ medicatricibus notabili exemplo chirurgico illustratis. 4°. *Lugd. Bat.*, 1779.

ORLAY (J.) *Diss. sistens doctrinæ de viribus naturæ medicatricibus historiam, brevem expositionem, vindicias. 8°. [*Dorpat*], 1807.

PARSONS (C. W.) An essay on the question, Vis medicatrix naturæ, how far is it to be relied on in the treatment of diseases? Fiske fund prize dissertation of the Rhode Island Medical Society. 8°. *Boston*, 1849.
Also, in: Boston M. & S. J., 1849, xl, 189–201.

PAULINI (J.) *De autocratia naturæ in conservanda et restituenda sanitate. 8°. *Pestini*, 1834.

PELLETAN (J.) *De la nature médicatrice. 4°. *Paris*, 1835.

PHILIPPSOHN (P. M.) *De natura medicatrice. 8°. *Halæ*, [1828].

PIDOUX (H.) *Essai sur les lois de la force médicatrice. 4°. *Paris*, 1835.

PLAZ (A. G.) [Pr.] de arte naturam superante. 4°. *Lipsiæ*, [1772].

POKORNY (M. H.) *Analecta quædam ad doctrinam de naturæ vi medicatrice. 8°. *Berolini*, [1838].

PUGH (W. H.) An inaugural essay on the supposed powers of nature in the cure of disease. 8°. *Philadelphia*, 1804.

SARTORIUS (F.) De arte naturæ æmula. 4°. *Lipsiæ*, 1704.

SAUTER (F.) *De natura contra morbos luctante. 8°. *Monachii*, 1834.

SCHLITTE (F. G.) *De natura medicatrice. 8°. *Halæ*, [1801].

SCHMIDT (A. C. F.) *De vi naturæ medicatrice. 8°. *Gottingæ*, [1831].

SEELMATTER (S.) *De natura Hippocratis. 4°. *Argentorati*, [1721].

SILBERT (P.) *Du naturisme chirurgical. 4°. *Paris*, 1843.

SLEVOGT (J. H.) [Pr.] de natura morborum per morbos curatrice. 4°. *Jenæ*, [1700].

———. [Pr.] de natura morborum effectrice. 4°. *Jenæ*, [1700].

SPITZNER (J. A.) *De artis naturam imitandi principiis generalioribus. 4°. *Wittebergæ*, [1783].

STAHL (G. E.) [Pr.] de συνέργεια naturæ in medendo. 4°. [*Halæ Magdeb.*, 1695.]

STEVENS (N.) *De naturæ in morbis curandis efficacia. 4°. *Lugd. Bat.*, 1731.

STRACHAN (J. M.) Nature in the cure of disease; a lecture. 8°. *Edinburgh*, 1861.

SURINGAR (G. C. B.) Commentatio medica de modo quo natura versatur in restituendo omni quod in corpore humano solutum est. Præmio regio ornata. 4°. *Lugd. Bat.*, 1823.

THALHEIM (C. E.) *De salutari vis vitæ in morbis actione. 4°. *Halæ ad Salam*, [1764].

VOELCKER (A. H.) *De vi medicatrice naturæ. 8°. *Berolini*, [1829].

VOIGT (C. F.) *De recta motuum naturæ æstimatione in morbis. sm. 4°. *Francof. ad Viadr.*, [1747].
Also, in: CARTHEUSER (J. F.) Diss. nonn. select. phys.-chym. ac med. 12°. *Francof. ad Viadr.*, 1775, 56–86.

WALLE (J. C.) *De natura morborum medicatrice a medico arte ad juvanda. 4°. *Lugd. Bat.*, 1746.

WEHLE (E. S.) *De veritate paradoxi Hippocratici nullam medicinam interdum esse optimam. sm. 4°. *Vitembergæ*, [1754].

Nature *in disease.*

WEIKARD (M. A.) * Disquirens an et in quibus natura sit medicatrix, medicus vero naturæ minister? 4°. [*Wirceburgi*, 1764.]

WEISBACH (C.) * De intentione et inventione naturæ in administratione œconomiæ vitalis. 4°. *Basileæ*, [1711].

WELZ (J.) * De natura medicatrice. 8°. *Parisiis*, [1831].

WOLFRING (M. C.) *Autokratia naturæ. 8°. *Monachii*, [1834].

WÜRM (W.) Ueber Naturhülfe in Krankheiten. 8°. *Landshut*, 1867.

VAN WYNGAARDEN (H.) * De salutaribus naturæ operibus et quibus ei succurratur. 4°. *Lugd. Bat.*, [1750].

YOUNG (T.) De corporis humani viribus conservatricibus dissertatio. 8°. *Gottingæ*, 1796.

VAN YSENDYK (E.) * De viribus naturæ medicatricibus, quibus etiam, quæ mechanica vi corpori vivo nocent, melius ipsa arte, subinde expellere novit. 4°. *Traj. ad Rhenum*, [1802].

ZIPRIAN (F. V.) * De autocrateia organismi in præcavendis et sanandis morbis. 8°. *Pragæ*, 1820.

ZOPF (C. D.) * De mira naturæ solertia in reparandis damnis corpori animato illatis. 4°. *Wittebergæ*, [1766].

Albee (W. A.) Vis medicatrix naturæ. Tr. Maine M. Ass. 1874–6, Portland, 1876, v, 334–338.—**Anderson** (J. W.) On the vis medicatrix naturæ. Glasgow M. J., 1885, [4.] s., xxiv, 321–331.—**Armor** (S. G.) The natural cure of disease. N. York M. J., 1873, xvii, 51–58.—**Bassols Prim** (A.) Ensayo sobre la interpretacion de la fuerza medicatriz. Encicl. méd. farm., Barcel., 1880, iv, 353; 361.—**Battey** (R.) Nature and art. Atlanta M. & S. J., 1873–4, xi, 323.—**Bayard** (W.) An address upon the power of nature in the cure of disease. Canada M. J., Montreal, 1872, viii, 385–394.—**Beneke** (F. E.) Ueber die Heilkraft der Natur. Ein Versuch zur Lösung des Problemes von einem verwandten Naturgebiete aus. Lit. Ann. d. ges. Heilk., Berl., 1829, xv, 389–411.—**Bottani** (A.) Sulla forza medicatrice della natura. Gior. per serv. ai progr. d. patol., Venezia, 1837, vi, 181–205. *Also*, Reprint.—**Buxton** (H. W.) Does nature cure disease? Pub. Mass. Eclect. M. Soc., Bost., 1860–72, 75.—**Canniff** (W.) Nature's power to heal. Canada M. Rec., Montreal, 1875–6, iv, 1–6. *Also*, Reprint.—**Carril** (A. F.) Importancia del poder de la naturaleza en la curacion de las enfermedades. Anfiteatro anat., Madrid, 1873, i, 22; 45; 68; 98; 116; 138; 175; 213; 236; 259: 1874, ii, 16.—**Choulant** (L.) Die Heilkraft der Natur, als Wurzel der Medizin. Allg. med. Ann., Leipz., 1829, 1–8.—**Christian** (E. P.) The vis medicatrix as a blood-letter. Penins. J. M., Detroit, 1873, ix, 195–202.—**Clark** (F. LeG.) On nature's methods of cure. St. Thomas's Hosp. Rep. 1885, Lond., 1886, xv, 17–29.—**Clark** (J. E.) Vis medicatrix naturæ. Therap. Gaz., Detroit, 1880, n. s., i, 85–87.—**Combe** (A.) On the observation of nature in the study and treatment of disease. Brit. & For. M. Rev., Lond., 1847, xxiii, 257; 592.—**Condie.** Nature and art in the cure of disease. Disc. Phila. Co. M. Soc., 1862, 34–42.—**Criaro y Aguilar.** La naturaleza medicatriz. Clinica, Zaragoza, 1884, viii, 113; 121; 129; 137; 145; 153; 161; 169; 177.—**Davis** (N. S.) Nature and art: their relative influence in the management of diseases. Are they antagonistic or cooperative? Chicago M. Exam., 1861, ii, 129–139.—**Dent** (A. M.) A dissertation on the relative merits of vis medicatrix naturæ and physic. Tr. M. Soc. W. Virg., Wheeling, 1879, ii, pt. 4, 479–487.—**Dickson** (J.) On the vis medicatrix naturæ. Am. J. M. Sc., Phila., 1834–5, xv, 116–120.—**Dime.** Compte-rendu d'un mémoire de Maurin. Caractères et limites du pouvoir de la nature médicatrice. Gaz. méd. de Lyon, 1866, xviii, 223–228. *Also*: Ann. Soc. de méd. de Lyon, 1866, 2. s., xiv, 71–82.—**Dowler** (B.) Speculative and practical researches on the supposed duality, unity, and antagonism of nature and art in the cure of diseases. N. Orl. M. & S. J., 1858–9, xv, 787–805.—**Fallot.** De la maladie et de la force vitale. Presse méd. belge, Brux., 1855–6, viii, 229; 237.—**Farrat** (E.) Étude pour servir à l'histoire du dogme de la force vitale médicatrice. Rev. de thérap. du midi, Montpel., 1852, iii, 33; 76; 141.—**Fauntleroy** (A. M.) Vis medicatrix naturæ. Tr. M. Soc. Virg., Richmond, 1872, iii, 29–34. *Also*: Richmond & Louisville M. J., Louisville, 1873, xvi, 56–66.—**Fernandez** (P.) Poder incalculable de la fuerza medicatriz. Corresp. méd., Madrid, 1876, xi, 325. — **Ferro.** Cenni sulle forze medicatrici della natura e specialmente sull' abuso del salasso. Gior. di. sc. med., Torino, 1839, iv, 257–270.—**Franceschi** (G.) La medicatrice natura. Raccoglitore med di Fano, 1860, 2. s., xxii, 505–519.—**Gonza-**

Nature *in disease.*

lez (Z. B.) Del poder de la naturaleza en la curacion de las enfermedades. Bol. de med., cirug. y farm., Madrid, 1851, 2. ép., i, 292; 298; 308; 314; 361; 369.—**Grant** (C.) The fallacy of a supposed vis medicatrix naturæ. West. Lancet, Cincin., 1850, xi, 348–357.—**Gross** (S. D.) Nature's voice in disease and convalescence. Am. Pract., Louisville, 1870, i, 257–274.—**Günther.** Einige Bemerkungen die Heilkraft der Natur betreffend. J. d. pract. Heilk., Berl., 1823, lvii, 3. St., 18–38.—**Guislain** (J.) La nature, considérée comme force instinctive des organes. À la mémoire de Van Helmont. Ann. Soc. de méd. de Gand, 1846, xvii, 5–204, port.—**Holmes** (W. F.) The vis medicatrix naturæ. Charleston M. J. & Rev., 1850, v, 311–315.—**Jones** (J. W.) "Vis medicatrix naturæ and antistasis". Atlanta M. & S. J., 1855–6, i, 193.—**Kausch.** Ueber die Urkräfte der Natur und die Ableitung der animalischen Kräfte von denselben. J. d. pract. Heilk., Berl., 1810, xxx, 1. St., 22–45.—**Lundt** (O.) Nature, and her medicine. Dublin J. M. Sc., 1875, lix, 1–4.—**Macgowan** (A. T.) The healing power of nature. with cases. Med. Mirror, Lond., 1866, iii, 345–349.—**Mackenzie** (W.) A sketch of the natural cure of diseases. Glasgow M. J., 1829, ii, 1–11.—**Martinet** (L.) Considérations cliniques sur les différens degrés de résistance vitale dans les maladies, déduites des rapports des lésions organiques avec leurs effets. Rev. méd. franç. et étrang., Par., 1824, iv, 45–69.—**de Meis** (A. C.) La natura medicatrice e la storia della medicina. Morgagni, Napoli, 1868, x, 549–572.—**Murdoch** (J. B.) Nature versus art in the cure of disease. J. Am. M. Ass., Chicago, 1885, iv, 337–342.—**Nature** (La) médicatrice étudiée dans ses procédés curatifs. Rev. méd. franç. et étrang., Par., 1876, ii, 129 – 134. — **Nature-worship.** Med. Times & Gaz., Lond., 1872, i, 8. — **Nicolas** (M.) Maladie chronique, guérie par la nature seule. [*Repr. from*: Histoire des mal. épidém. qui ont régné dans la province de Dauphiné, Grenoble, 1786.] J. Soc. de méd. et pharm. de l'Isère, Grenoble, 1883 – 4, viii, 273. — **Nieto.** De la naturaleza medicatriz. Siglo méd., Madrid, 1855, ii, 177.—**Nixon** (A. B.) Nature in disease, or conservative medicine. Pacific M. & S. J., San Fran., 1872–3, xv, 528–535.—**P.** Werden fast alle Kranke, die genesen, durch Hülfe der Natur wieder hergestellt, und sind also die Aerzte wirklich überflüssig? Abhandl. u. Beob. v. einer Gesellsch. v. Aerzten in Hamb., 1776, 18–31.—**Peck** (W. A.) Vis medicatrix naturæ. Penins. J. M., Ann Arbor, Mich., 1856–7, iv, 169; 281.— **Porter** (I. G.) "The self-restorative power", in the light of modern science. Proc. Connect. M. Soc. 1864–7, N. Haven, 1867, ii, 275 – 293. — **Reynolds** [*et al.*]. The place of nature in therapeutics. Pacific M. & S. J., San Fran., 1872–3, xv, 573–592.—**Richardson** (B. W.) Vis medicatrix naturæ. Asclepiad, Lond., 1886, iii, 262–268.—**Richter** (C. A. W.) Rückblicke auf den Einfluss der Begriffe von der Naturheilkraft auf die ärztliche Kunst. Wchnschr. f. d. ges. Heilk., Berl., 1850, 225; 241.—**Stöller.** Von den wirkenden Naturkräften bey Verletzungen des menschlichen Körpers, und diesemal vorzüglich bey wichtigen Kopfverletzungen. J. f. d. Chir., Geburtsh. u. gerichtl. Arznk., Jena, 1797, i, 77–92. *Also*, *transl.*: Verhandel. en Waarn. t. Bevord. d. Genees-, Heel-, Verlos- en Scheik., Leyden, 1803, i, 66–78.—**Summer** (W. J.) On the vis medicatrix naturæ. South. M. & S. J., Augusta, 1851, n. s., vii, 195–203.—**Tommasini** (G.) Sulle forze medicatrici della natura. *In his*: Opere complete di . . . Firenze, 1832, i, 941–956. *Also*: Ann. univ. di med., Milano, 1835, lxxiv, 171–199.—**Valorani** (V.) Delle forze medicatrici della natura. Bull. d. sc. med. di Bologna, 1849, 3. s., xvi, 5–21. *Also*: Raccoglitore med., Forlì, 1849, xxiv, 225–237.—**Vaughan** (S. W.), jr. A thesis on the "vis medicatrix naturæ". Atlanta M. & S. J., 1858–9, iv, 261.—**Will** (J. C. O.) Clinical lecture on the vis medicatrix naturæ in the treatment of wounds. Lancet, Lond., 1881, ii, 819–821.

Nature. A weekly illustrated journal of science. [Edited by J. N. Lockyer.] [2 v. annually.] v. 1–37, November, 1869–88. 4°. *London, Macmillan & Co.*
Current.

Nature (De la). xx, 456 pp., 1 pl. 8°. *Amsterdam, E. van Harrevelt,* 1761.

Nature (La). Revue des sciences et de leurs applications aux arts et à l'industrie. Journal hebdomadaire illustré. Rédacteur en chef: Gaston Tissandier. [2 v. annually.] Année 15, Dec. 4, 1886–7. 2 v. roy. 8°. *Paris, G. Masson.*
Current.

Nature and her agents shown to be more efficient in curing disease [etc.] *See* "**Scrutator Verax**".

Nature (The) and treatment of rabies or hydrophobia. Being the report of the special commission appointed by the Medical Press and Circular, with valuable additions. viii, 9–287 pp. 12°. *London, Baillière, Tindall & Cox,* 1878.

Nature's Arcana. Devoted to medical reform, science, art, literature, and general intelligence. [Bi-monthly.] v. 17–18, 1872–3. fol. *Boston.*

Nature's hygiene and its artificial imitation. 16 pp. 8°. [*London*, 1877.]

Nature's remedy. Endorsed by the medical profession. A representative record of results attending the use of the Bedford alum and iron springs water and moss for the last twenty-seven years. 31 pp. 8°. [*n. p.*, 1878.]

Naturforschende Gesellschaft in Bamberg. Dreizehnter Bericht. Fest-Schrift zur Halbsä-cular-Feier der . . . 1884. 1 p. l., 34, 115, 40, 16, 5 pp. 8°. *Bamberg, Humann'sche Buchdrucke-rei, 1884.*

Naturforschende Gesellschaft in Basel. Festschrift zur Feier des fünfzigjährigen Bestehens. 166 pp., 1 pl. 8°. *Basel, C. Schultze,* 1867.
——. Verhandlungen. 3. u. 4. Hft., 5. Theil; 6. Theil; 7. Theil; 1. Hft., 8. Theil. 8°. *Basel,* 1871–86.

Naturforschende Gesellschaft in Bern. Mit-theilungen. No. 654–1168 in 13 v. 8°. *Bern,* 1869–87.

Naturforschende Gesellschaft in Danzig. Schriften. Neue Folge. Bd. 1–6. 8°. *Danzig,* 1863–87.

Naturforschende Gesellschaft in Emden. Jahresbericht. 52., 1866; 54.–68., 1868 to 1882–3; 71., 1885–6. 8°. *Emden,* 1867–86.
——. Kleine Schriften. No. XVI. "Die Winde in ihrer Beziehung zur Salubrität und Morbi-lität." Von Professor Dr. Prestel. 19 pp. 8°. *Emden, T. Hahn Wwe.,* 1872.
——. The same. No. XVII. Ergebnisse der Witterungs-Beobachtungen von 1864–1873. Von M. A. F. Prestel. 44 pp. 4°. *Hannover, Gebr. Jänecke,* 1875.
——. The same. No. XVIII. Die höchste und niedrigste Temperatur, welche an jedem Tage von 1836 bis 1877 auf dem meteorologischen Observatorium in Emden beobachtet ist. Von Professor Dr. M. A. F. Prestel. xliv, 49 pp. 4°. *Emden,* 1879.

Naturforschende Gesellschaft zu Freiburg i. Br. Berichte über die Verhandlungen. Hft. 1–2, Bd. 5 (1868–69). 8°. *Freiburg i. Br., J. Diernfell-ner,* 1868–9.
——. Berichte der . . . 2. Bd., 1887. 278 pp. 8°. *Freiburg i. Br., J. C. B. Mohr,* 1887.

Naturforschende Gesellschaft zu Halle. Ab-handlungen. Originalaufsätze, aus dem Gebiete der gesammten Naturwissenschaften. Hft. 1–2, Bd. 11; Bd. 12, 13; Hft. 1–3, Bd. 14; Bd. 15, 16. 4°. *Halle,* 1869.
——. Bericht über die Sitzungen in den Jahren 1870–86. 4°. [*Halle,* 1870–86.]
Want 1879.
——. Festschrift zur Feier des hundertjährigen Bestehens. xlvii, 342 pp., 12 pl. 4°. *Halle, M. Niemeyer,* 1879.

Naturforschende Gesellschaft des Oberlandes zu Altenburg. Verzeichniss der Mitglieder, am fünfzigsten Stiftungsfeste, den 9. October 1867. 11 pp. 8°. *Altenburg,* [1867].

Naturforschende Gesellschaft zu Zürich. Vierteljahrsschrift. Redigiert von R. Wolf. 12.–15. Jahrgang. 8°. *Zürich, S. Hohr,* 1867–70.

Naturforschender Verein zu Bamberg. Ue-ber das Bestehen und Wirken. 1. Bericht. 79 pp., 2 tab. 4°. *Bamberg, J. M. Reindl,* 1852.

Naturforschender Verein in Brünn. Ver-handlungen. Bd. 1–7, 1861–8; Hft. 1, Bd. 8, 1869; Bd. 9–13, 1871–4; Bd. 15–18, 1876–9. 8°. *Brünn,* 1861–80.
——. Katalog der Bibliothek. 161 (2 l.), 62 pp. 8°. *Brünn, W. Burkart,* 1875.

Naturforscher (Der). Wochenblatt zur Ver-breitung der Fortschritte in den Naturwissen-schaften. Hrsg. von Wilhelm Sklarek. Nos. 1–26 (Hft. 1–6), Jahrg. 5, Jan. to June, 1872. 4°. *Berlin, F. Dümmler.*

Naturforscherverein zu Riga. Arbeiten. 1. Hft. 191 pp. 8°. *Riga, W. F. Häcker,* 1865.
——. The same. Neue Folge. 5. Hft. 8°. *Riga, W. F. Häcker,* 1873.
——. Register zu den Jahrgängen 1–15 des Cor-respondenzblattes. Angefertigt von E. L. See-gen. 26 pp. 8°. *Riga, W. F. Häcker,* 1866.
——. Correspondenzblatt. 1867, 1869–70. 8°. *Riga, W. F. Häcker,* 1867–70.
——. Denkschrift. Hrsg. in Anlass der Feier seines 25jährigen Bestehens. xxix, 63 pp. 4°. *Riga, W. F. Häcker,* 1870.

Naturgeschichte des Elephanten. 26 pp. 12°. *Wien,* 1776.
Bound with : BETRACHTUNGEN von dem grossen Nutzen und Schaden der vierfüssigen Thiere. 12°. *Bunzlau,* 1776.

Naturhistorische Gesellschaft zu Nürnberg. Abhandlung. 2. Hlfte., 3. Bd.; 4. Bd. 8°. *Nürnberg, W. Schmid,* 1866–8.

Naturhistorischer Verein für Anhalt in Des-sau. Verhandlungen. 28.–29. Bericht, 1869–70. 8°. *Dessau, H. Neuburger,* 1870–71.

Naturhistorischer Verein in Augsburg. Be-richte. 9., 1855; 18.–23., 1865–75. 8°. *Augs-burg,* 1855–75.

Naturhistorischer Verein in Passau. Jahres-bericht. 1.–10., 1857–74. 8°. *Passau,* 1857–75.
Want 3., 1859.

Naturhistorischer Verein der preussischen Rheinlande und Westphalens. Verhandlungen. 3.–28. Jahrg., 1846–71. 8°. *Bonn,* 1846–71.
11.–20. Jahrg., n. F., Bd. 1–10; 21.–28. Jahrg., 3. F., Bd. 1–8.

Naturhistorischer Verein von Wisconsin. Jahres-Bericht, für die Jahre 1876–7; 1878–9. 8°. *Milwaukee, C. Dörflinger,* 1877–9.

Naturhistorisch - medizinischer Verein zu Heidelberg. Verhandlungen. Bd. 2–6, 1859–72; n. F., Bd. 1, 2; Hft. 1, 2, & 5, Bd. 3; Hft. 1, Bd. 4. 8°. *Heidelberg,* 1862–87.

Naturwarme (Das) Stahlbad Szliács (bei Altsohl in Ungarn). Einzige bekannte Eisen-therme reich an Kohlensäure. Saison von 1883. Die Badedirection: Geo. André Lenoir. 4 l. 4°. [*Wien, M. Bettelheim,* 1883.]

Naturwissenschaftliche Gesellschaft zu Chemnitz. Berichte, umfassend die Geschäfts-jahre 1.–8., 1859–80. 8°. *Chemnitz,* 1865–80.

Naturwissenschaftliche Gesellschaft Isis in Dresden. Sitzungs-Berichte der . . . 1868–86. In 7 v. 8°. *Dresden,* 1868–86.
——. Festschrift zur Feier ihres 50jährigen Be-stehens am 14. Mai 1885. iv (2 l.), 178 pp., 1 l., 4 pl. 8°. *Dresden, Warnatz u. Lehmann,* 1885.

Naturwissenschaftlicher Verein zu Ham-burg-Altona. 3. Bolau, H. (und Pansch, Ad.). Ueber die menschenähnlichen Affen des Ham-burger Museums. Den Mitgliedern und Theil-nehmern der 49. Versammlung deutscher Natur-forscher und Aerzte als Festgabe gewidmet vom naturwissenschaftlichen Verein. 2 p. l., 26 pp., 2 pl. 4°. *Hamburg, L. Friederichsen u. Comp.,* 1876.

Naturwissenschaftlicher Verein für Schleswig-Holstein. Schriften. v. 1–6, 1873–86. In 5 v. 8°. *Kiel,* 1873–86.

Naturwissenschaftlicher Verein für Steier-mark. Der 48. Versammlung deutscher Natur-forscher und Aerzte als Festgabe. xvi, 190 pp., 4 pl. 8°. *Graz, Leykam-Josephsthal,* 1875.

Naturwissenschaftlich-medizinischer Verein in Innsbruck. Berichte. Jahrg. 1–5, 1870 to 1884–6. 8°. *Innsbruck,* 1870–86.

Natuur- en geneeskundig Archief voor Neêrlandsch Indië. [Quarterly.] v. 1–3, 1844–6. 8°. *Batavia.*

In no. 1 no editors named; no. 2, P. J. Godefroy, M. J. E. Muller, P. A. Fromm, and P. Bleeker became editors; no. 3, v. 2, Godefroy dropped; no. 4. v. 2, W. Bosch added; no. 2, v. 3, S. L. Heijman an.. J. Munnich added.

Natuur- en geneeskundige Bibliotheek. Bevattende den zaakelijken inhoud van alle nieuwe werken, welke, in de geneeskunde en natuurlijke historie, buiten ons vaterland uitkomen. Door Eduard Sandifort. v. 1–11, 1765–75. 8°. *'s Gravenhage, P. van Cleef.*

v. 11, 1775, is general index to v. 1–10.

Natuur- en geneeskundige Correspondentie-Societeit, in de Vereenigde Nederlanden. Verhandelingen van de . . . opgericht in 's Hage. Behelzende de weêrkundige waarneemingen van het jaaren 1779–1790. 4 v. in 7. 8°. *'s Gravenhage,* 1783–93.

Natuurkundig Tijdschrift voor Nederlandsch Indië. Uitgegeven door de Natuurkundige Vereeniging in Nederlandsche Indië. Hoofredacteur: P. Bleeker. v. 1–45, 1850–86. [Also, general index to v. 1–30.] 8°. *Batavia, Lange & Co.*

In 1882, H. Onnen became editor.

Natuurkundige Vereeniging in Nederlandsch Indie. Verhandelingen der . . . Deel 1–8, 1856–60. 4°. *Batavia, Lange & Co.,* 1856–60.

Natuuronderzoek en humaniteit. Een woord van verzoening gesproken door eenen geneeskundige. Uit het Hoogduitsch vertaald door Dr. J. B. Roll. iv, iv, 1 l., 58 pp. 8°. *Amsterdam, C. G. van der Post,* 1862.

Nau (B. S.) Entwurf einer Polizeiverordnung gegen die weitere Verbreitung der westindischen Pest. xii, 156 pp. 12°. *Frankf. a. M., Andreä,* 1805.

Bound with: PALLONI (C.) Medicinische Bemerkungen etc. 12°. *Salzburg,* 1805.

Nau (François-Georges). *Quelques considérations générales sur l'érysipèle. 39 pp. 4°. *Paris,* 1872, No. 420.

Nau (J.) *Contribution à l'étude de la congestion et de l'apoplexie pulmonaire unilatérale dans les cas de ramollissement du cerveau. 40 pp. 4°. *Paris,* 1877, No. 408.

Nauche (J.-L.) *Sur le catarrhe de la vessie. 23 pp. 4°. *Strasbourg,* 1823, v. 52.

Nauche (Jacques-Louis) [1776–1843]. *Nouvelles recherches sur la rétention d'urine par ré trécissement organique de l'urètre. ii, 3–76 pp. 8°. *Paris, an IX* [1801], v. 3.

——. The same. 2. éd. 109 pp 8°. *Paris, Croullebois, an XI* [1803]. [*Also, in:* P., v. 1692.]

——. The same. . . . et par paralysie de la vessie; suivies de remarques sur la gravelle. 3. éd. 142 pp. 8°. *Paris, Croullebois,* 1806.

——. Des maladies de la vessie et du méat urinaire chez les personnes avancées en âge; pour servir de réponse aux questions proposées en 1807, sur ces maladies, par l'Académie Joséphine de médecine et de chirurgie de Vienne. ii, 3–252 pp. 12°. *Paris, D. Colas,* 1810.

——. Des maladies de l'utérus, ou de la matrice. 461 pp. 8°. *Paris, Gabon,* 1816.

——. De l'application de l'électricité au traitement des maladies, d'après les procédés de Mr. Girardin. 8 pp. 8°. [*Paris, Leblanc,* 1819?]

Repr. from: Rapport fait à la Soc. roy. Acad. d. sc.

——. The same. [With additions.] 8 pp. 8°. [*Paris, Fain,* 1819.]

Repr. from: Rapport fait à la Soc. roy. Acad. d. sc.

Nauck (August). *Ueber eine neue Eigenschaft der Producte der regressiven Metamorphose der Eiweisskörper. 52 pp., 1 l. 8°. *Dorpat, H. Laakmann,* 1886.

Nauck (Georg) [1857–]. *Ueber Gelbfieber. 31 pp. 8°. *Berlin, G. Lange,* [1880].

Nauclerus (Samuel). Descriptio horti Upsaliensis. *Upsaliæ,* 1745.

In: LINNÆUS. Amœnitates acad. [etc.] 8°. *Lugd. Bat.,* 1749, i, 20–59, 4 pl.

Naud (Paul). *D'une forme spéciale d'ostéite, ou ostéite à forme névralgique. 96 pp. 4°. *Paris,* 1868, No. 136.

Naudæana et Patiniana, ou singularitez remarquables, prises des conversations. 2. éd., revuë, corrigée et augmentée d'additions au Naudæana qui ne sont point dans l'édition de Paris. 8 p. l., 256 pp., 132 pp., 5 l., 2 port. 12°. *Amsterdam, F. vander Plaats,* 1703.

Naudain (Arnold). Annual address read before the Northern Medical Association of Philadelphia, Jan. 6, 1848. 14 pp. 8°. *Philadelpbia, S. H. Clark,* 1848. [P., v. 101.]

Naudé (Gabriel) [1600–53]. De antiquitate et dignitate scholæ medicæ Parisiensis panegyris; cum orationibus encomiasticis ad ix iatrogonistas laurea medica donandos. 2 p. l., 150 pp., 1 l. 12°. *Lutetiæ Parisiorum, J. Moreau,* 1628.

Bound with: MATTHIAS (G.) Conspectus historiæ medicorum chronologicus. 12°. *Gottingæ,* 1761.

——. The same. 176 pp. 16°. [*n. p., n. d.*]

Bound with: DECRETA, ritus, usus, [etc.] 16°. *Parisiis,* 1714. *Another copy bound with:* STATUTA facultatis medicinæ Parisiensis. 16°. *Parisiis,* 1751.

——. Quæstio iatrophilologica. An magnum homini a venenis periculum? 29 pp. 12°. *Romæ, G. Facciotti,* 1632.

——. Quæstio secunda iatrophilologica. An vita hominum hodie quam olim brevior? 27 pp. 12°. *Cæsenæ, ex typog. J. Nerii,* 1634.

Bound with preceding.

——. Quæstio tertia iatrophilologica. An ma utina studia vespertinis salubriora? 3 p. l., 45 pp. 12°. *Patavii, ex typog. J. Crivellarij,* 1634.

Bound with preceding.

——. Quæstio quarta iatrophilologica. An liceat medico fallere ægrotum? 51 pp. 12°. *Romæ, J. Facciotti,* 1635.

Bound with preceding.

——. Πέντας quæstionum iatro-philologicarum. 3 p. l., 332 pp., 2 l. 12°. *Genevæ, C. Chouët,* 1647.

   I. An magnum homini a venenis periculum?
   II. An vita hominum hodie quam olim brevior?
   III. An matutina studia vespertinis salubriora?
   IV. An liceat medico fallere ægrotum?
   V. De fato et fatali vitæ termino.

——. Apologie pour les grands hommes soupçonnez de magie. Dernière édition, où l'on a ajouté quelques remarques. 8 p. l., 470 pp., 1 pl. 16°. *Amsterdam, P. Humbert,* 1712.

——. The same. The history of magick by way of apology for all the wise men who have unjustly been reputed magicians, from the creation to the present age. Written in French. English ed. by J. Davies. 7 p. l., 306 pp. sm. 8°. *London, J. Streater,* 1657.

See, also, **Naudæana et Patiniana** [etc.] 12°. *Amsterdam,* 1703.

For Portrait, see **Collection** van Kaathoven.—**Collection** of Portr. of Phys. & Men of Sc., 143.

Naudeau (Athanase-Auguste). *De l'allaitement. 56 pp. 4°. *Paris,* 1858, No. 2, v. 622.

Naudeau (Camille). *I. Du diagnostic et du pronostic de l'hystérie. II. [etc.] 31 pp. 4°. *Paris,* 1839, No. 446, v. 347.

Naudet.

See **Höltschl** (Josef). Die Anéroïde, etc. 8°. *Wien,* 1872.

Naudet (Antoine) [1853–]. *Des périostoses crâniennes dans la période secondaire de la syphilis. 46 pp. 4°. *Paris,* 1882, No. 96.

Naudet (Frédéric-Mathieu). *Du phlegmon périnéphrétique. 108 pp. 4°. *Paris,* 1870, No. 123.

Naudet (S.-V.-Onésipe). *Sur l'hygiène du laboureur. 63 pp. 4°. *Paris,* 1861, No. 90.

Naudier (G.) * De l'obstruction des voies lacrymales. 91 pp. 4°. *Paris*, 1872, No. 335.
——. The same. 91 pp. 8°. *Paris, A. Delahaye*, 1872.

Naudin (Étienne-Nicolas). * Sur la fracture de
jambe. 46 pp. 8°. *Paris, an XI* [1803], v. 38.

Naudin (L.) * Essai sur la tarsotomie. 102 pp.
4°. *Paris*, 1885, No. 27.

Naudin (Louis). * Sur les bubons syphilitiques.
vi, 7–32 pp. 4°. *Paris*, 1822, No. 154, v. 174.

Naudin (Louis-Silvain-Emmanuel). * I. Des
différences entre le sang humain à l'état normal
et le sang des individus atteints de pneumonie.
II. [etc.] 38 pp. 4°. *Paris*, 1841, No. 188, v.
379.

Naudin (Lucien). * Contributions à l'étude des
ulcérations du col de l'utérus. 77 pp. 4°. *Paris*, 1885, No. 245.

Naudin (Pierre). * Sur les polypes utérins. 27
pp. 4°. *Paris*, 1813, No. 13, v. 95.

Naudot. Notice sur les eaux minérales ferrugineuses acidules froides de Provins, précédée d'un
essai sur la topographie médicale de Provins et
de ses environs. 106 pp. sm. 8°. *Provins, Lebeau*, 1841.
——. Influence du climat de Nice sur la marche
des maladies chroniques et particulièrement sur
la phthisie pulmonaire. 82 pp., 1 tab. 8°. *Paris, Allouard*, 1842. [*Also, in :* P., v. 1666.]

Naudot (Alexis). * Considérations sur les hémorrhagies utérines pendant la grossesse. 20
pp. 4°. *Paris*, 1818, No. 142, v. 139.

Naugerius (Andreas).
See **Fracastorius** (Hieronymus). Opera omnia [etc.]
4°. *Veretiis*, 1555. ——. The same. 4°. *Venetiis*, 1584.
——. The same. 12°. *Lugduni*, 1591.

Nauheim.

BAD Nauheim und seine Umgebung. 24°.
Friedberg, 1855.

BODE (F.) Nauheim, seine natürlich warmen
Soolquellen und deren Wirkung, nebst einer
kurzen Nachricht über den Schwalheimer Mineralbrunnen. 2. Aufl. 8°. *Cassel*, 1853.

KOHLENSÄUREHALTIGE (Das) Soolbad Nauheim. Nach den Schriften Sachverständiger zusammengestellt und herausgegeben vom Kur-
und Verschönerungs-Verein zu Bad-Nauheim.
8°. *Frankf. a. M.*, 1872.
   Beneke (F. W.) Ueber das Verhalten des Pulses und
der Respiration beim Gebrauche des warmen Soolbades
(Nauheim). Arch. d. Ver. f. gemeinsch. Arb. z. Förd. d.
wissensch. Heilk., Götting., 1860, iv, 127 - 158. ——. Ueber die Wirkungen der Nauheimer Soolquellen gegen Rheu-
mātismus und dessen Folgezustände. Deutsche Klinik,
Berl., 1863, xv, 128. ——. Nauheim's Soolthermen gegen
Gelenkrheumatismus mit oder ohne Herzaffection. Berl.
klin. Wchnschr., 1870, vii, 269. ——. Neue Erfahrungen
über die Wirkungen der kohlensäurehaltigen Soolthermen
Nauheim's bei Gelenkrheumatismus und den ihm verbundenen Herzkrankheiten. *Ibid.*, 1875, xii, 109; 124.—**Bode.**
Das Soolbad Nauheim. Ber. d. oberhess. Gesellsch. f.
Nat.- u. Heilk., Giessen, 1847, i, 41–44.—**Bode**, jun. Das
Soolbad Nauheim (insbesondere sein Verhältniss zu Kreuznach und Rehme). Deutsche Klinik, Berl., 1870, xxii, 118;
128. ——. Notizen über einen neuen Trinkbrunnen
(Karlsquelle) in Bad Nauheim. *Ibid.*, 245. ——. Bad
Nauheim ohne Spielbank, ein Rückblick in die Vergangenheit. *Ibid.*, 1873, xxv, 117; 137.—**Faye** (F. C.) Sool-
badet "Nauheim". Norsk Mag. f. Lægevidensk., Christiania, 1878, 3. R., viii, 321–328.—**Labat** (A.) Étude sur la
station et les eaux de Nauheim. Ann. Soc. d'hydrol. méd.
de Par., 1867–8, xiv, 409–456. *Also*, Reprint.—**Ludwig.**
Ueber die warmen Soolquellen Nauheim's. Ber. d. oberhess. Gesellsch. f. Nat.- u. Heilk., Giessen, 1853, iii, 2–11.—
Schott (A.) & **Schott** (T.) Die Nauheimer Sprudel- und
Sprudelstrombäder. Berl. klin. Wchnschr., 1884, xxi, 294;
307.

Nauheimer (Joannes Jacobus). * De sobrietate
ejusque insigni ad sanitatem vitamque in seros
usque annos producendam emolumento. 44 pp.
4°. *Erfordiæ, typ. Heringii*, [1741].

Naulin (Louis-Marcel). * Hygiène de la femme
récemment accouchée. 34 pp. 4°. *Paris*, 1870,
No. 48.

Nauman (Joh. Just.) Mus porcellus. *Upsaliæ*,
1754.
   In : LINNÆUS. Amœnitates acad. [etc.] 8°. *Lugd. Bat.*,
1760, iv, 190–209.

Naumann (Alex.) * Ueber Einwirkung von
Brom auf Acetylchlorid, Eigenschaften des dabei sich bildenden Monobromacetylbromids und
daraus sich ableitende Producte; als Beitrag
zur Darstellung substituirter Anhydride. 25 pp.,
1 l. 8°. *Giessen, W. Keller*, 1864.   c.

Naumann (Augustus Fridericus). * De ostitide.
28 pp. 4°. *Lipsiæ, J. B. Hirschfeld*, 1818.
   For Biography, see **Kuehn** (C. G.)

Naumann (Augustus Gottlob.) [1792–   ]. * De
induratione hepatis. 26 pp. 4°. *Lipsiæ, J. B.
Hirschfeld*, [1818].
   For Biography, see **Ludwig** (Christianus Fridericus).

Naumann (Carl Fr.) [1816–   ]. * Om byg-
gnaden af luftrörshufvudet hos den fullväxta
menniskan. 3 pts. 2 p. l., 64 pp., 1 l., 6 pl. 4°.
Lund, Berlingska Boktryck., 1851.
      RESPONDENTES.
   I. Paul Henrik Paulsson.
   II. Fredrik Mauritz Kåhé.
   III. Andreas Larsson.
   Plates wanting.
——. The same. 1 p. l., 64 pp., 6 tab. 4°.
Lund, Berlingska Boktryck., 1851.

Naumann (Carolus Fridericus). * De hexago-
nali crystallinarum formarum systemate. 1 p. l.,
81 pp. 8°. *Lipsiæ, ex off. Glueckii*, 1825.
   Pts. i–ii each with separate title-page.

Naumann (Carolus Otto) [1823–   ]. * De
bronchiectasia. 38 pp., 1 l. 8°. *Halis Sax., typ.
Colbatzkii*, 1847.   c.

Naumann ([Christophorus] Ferdinandus)
[1841 –   ]. * De cordis ictu. 31 pp. 8°.
Berolini, G. Schade, [1865].

Naumann (Fridericus Augustus Guilielmus)
[1825–   ]. * De labiorum pudendi excoriatio-
nibus per explorationem. 16 pp. 8°. *Lipsiæ,
typ. G. Staritzii*, [1849].

Naumann (Friedmarus Gotthelf) [1815–   ].
* De artis gymnasticæ usu medico. 23 pp. 4°.
Lipsiæ, typ. Staritzii, [1842].

Naumann (H.) * De pericarditide. 15 pp. 8°.
Jenæ, typ. A. Neuenhahni, 1851.   c.

Naumann (H[enricus] B[enjaminus] F[erdi-
nandus] Guilelm[us]) [1816–   ]. * Quæstionum de gastromalacia infantium particula. 27
pp., 1 l. 8°. *Halæ, formis Ploetzianis*, [1841].

Naumann (J. Fr.) Taxidermie, oder die Lehre
Thiere aller Klassen am einfachsten und zweckmässigsten für Kabinette auszustopfen und auf-
zubewahren. xii, 180 pp., 5 pl. 8°. *Halle, Hemmerde u. Schwetschke*, 1815.

Naumann (J. G.)
   Portrait in: **Collection**—van Kaathoven.

Naumann (Joan. Godofredus). * De emplas-
trorum usu et abusu. 36 pp. 4°. *Halæ Magdeb., lit. J. C. Hilligeri*, [1739].

Naumann (Joannes Henricus) [1824–   ]. * Adnotationes quædam de herniis incarceratis earumque diagnosi. 26 pp., 3 l. 8°. *Berolini, typ.
fratrum Schlesinger*, [1849].

Naumann (L.) Welche Vortheile bieten con-
servirte Gewürze der Kochkunst? Vortrag mit
praktischen Anleitungen zur Verwendung der
conservirten Gewürze in der Küche, Conditorei,
Bäckerei und Wurstfabrikation, etc. Gehalten
am 10. November 1876 im Dresdner Kochkunst-
Verein. Mit einem Nachtrag : Die Fabrikation
der Liqueure, Doppel- und Einfachbranntweine
und dergleichen geistigen Getränke. 12. Aufl.
77 pp. 8°. *Dresden, R. H. Dietrich*, [1876].

Naumann (Moritz [Ernst] Adolph) [1798 –
1869]. * De signis ex urina. 100 pp. 4°. *Lipsiæ, e typog. Hirschfeldiano*, [1820].

Naumann (Moritz [Ernst] Adolph)—cont'd.

——. Einige Bemerkungen über das Gemein-Gefühl, im gesunden und im krankhaften Zustande. vii, 144 pp. 12°. *Leipzig, A. Wienbrack,* 1824.

——. Skizzen aus der allgemeinen Pathologie. viii (1 l.), 294 pp. 12°. *Leipzig, A. Wienbrack,* 1824.

——. Handbuch der allgemeinen Semiotik. xviii, 456 pp. 12°. *Berlin, A. Hirschwald,* 1826.

——. Theorie der praktischen Heilkunde, ein pathologischer Versuch. xii, 279 pp. 12°. *Berlin, A. Hirschwald,* 1827.

——. De pestibus nonnulla. 16 pp. 4°. *Bonnæ, [ex off. typog. Thormanniana],* 1828.

——. Zur Lehre von der Entzündung. 35 pp. 12°. *Bonn, T. Habicht,* 1828.

——. Handbuch der medicinischen Klinik. 8 v. in 11. 8°. *Berlin, A. Rücker u. Püchler,* 1829–39.
v. 3, Abth. 1, has also title : Darstellung der wichtigsten acuten, epidemisch-contagiösen Krankheiten, besonders der septischen und typhösen Fieber, etc.

——. The same. 1. Bd. 2. völlig umgearbeitete Ausg. 8°. *Berlin, Rücker u. Püchler,* 1848.
Only v. 1, 2. Aufl., was published.

——. Darstellung der wichtigsten acuten, epidemisch-contagiösen Krankheiten, besonders der septischen und typhösen Fieber, [etc.] 8°. *Berlin, A. Rücker,* 1831.
Additional title-page of his : Handbuch der medicinischen Klinik, v. 3, Abth. 1.

——. Grundzüge der Contagienlehre. vi, 73 pp. 8°. *Bonn, E. Weber,* 1833.

——. Elemente der physiologischen Pathologie. 80 pp. 8°. *Bonn, A. Marcus,* 1834.

——. Die Probleme der Physiologie, oder der Gegensatz von Nervenmark und Blut. viii, 198 pp. 8°. *Bonn, E. Weber,* 1835. [*Also, in :* P., v. 1517.]

——. De veterum medicorum Græcorum cognitione morborum uteri nonnulla. 22 pp. 4°. *Bonnæ, typ. C. Georgii,* 1838.

——. Pathogenie. 2 v. xxii, 690, viii, 160 pp.; x, 438, xvi, 589 pp. 8°. *Berlin, Rücker u. Püchler,* 1840–44.

——. Spezielle Pathologie und Therapie der entzündlichen Brust- und Unterleibskrankheiten. 8°. *Berlin, Rücker u. Püchler,* 1848.
Additional title-page of his : Handbuch der medicinischen Klinik, v. 1.

——. Metaphysisches in der Physiologie. 53 pp. 8°. *Bonn, E. Weber,* 1848.

——. Vermischte Schriften physiologischen und psychologischen Inhalts. 1 p. l., 132, viii, 198 (1 l.), 73 pp. 8°. *Bonn, E. Weber,* 1850.

CONTENTS.
Versuch eines Beweises für die Unsterblichkeit der Seele aus dem physiologischen Standpunkte, zugleich als Einleitung in die Lehre von den sogenannten Geisteskrankheiten.
Die Probleme der Physiologie, oder der Gegensatz von Nervenmark und Blut.
Grundzüge der Contagienlehre.

——. Allgemeine Pathologie und Therapie. 1. Theil. xvi, 890 pp. 8°. *Berlin, G. Reimer,* 1851.
No more published.

——. Ergebnisse und Studien aus der medicinischen Klinik zu Bonn. 2 v. xxx, 408 pp.; xxviii, 645 pp. 8°. *Leipzig, W. Engelmann,* 1858–60.

——. Zur Lehre von der Entzündung. 14 pp. 8°. [*Berlin, J. Sittenfeld, n. d.*]
Repr. from : Berl. klin. Wchnschr., 1865, xxii.
For Biography, see **Kühn** (Carolus Gottlob).
For Portrait, see **Collection**—van Kaathoven.

Naumann (Oswald) [1833–]. * Oleum jecoris aselli ad membranas animalium affinitatem habere multo majorem quam alia pinguia defendet. 20 pp., 2 pl. 8°. *Lipsiæ, typ. A. Edelmanni,* 1858.

Naumann (Oswald)—continued.

——. Beiträge zur Lehre vom Puls, insbesondere vom doppelschlägigen. 24 pp. 8°. *Leipzig u. Heidelberg, C. F. Winter,* 1863.

Naumann (Solomo Daniel). * De partu difficili ex hydrope fœtus. 1 p. l., 32 pp. 4°. *Lipsiæ, ex off. Langenhemi,* [1762].
For Biography, see **Ludwig** (Christ. Gott.)

Naumburg.

Drechsler. Beiträge zu einer medizinischen Topographie von Naumburg. Med. Nat.-Ztg. f. Deutschl., Altenb., 1799, ii, 101–110.

Naumburg (Isaacus). * De pruritu senili. 28 pp. 8°. *Halæ, typ. J. C. Dietleinii,* [1803].

Naumburg (Joh. Samuel). * Diss. botanica sistens delineationes Veronicæ Chamædryos, Dianthi Carthusianorum, Lamii maculati et purpurei, Arabis alpinæ, Violæ grandifloræ, Zanichelliæ palustris ac Polymorphi tremelloidis. viii, 9–35 pp. 12°. *Erfordiæ, lit. I. C. Goerling,* [1792].

Naumoff (J.) Kratkii uchebnik anatomii i fiziologii cheloveka. Kurs srednich ucheb. zavedenii. [Short instruction on the anatomy and physiology of man. Course of lectures for the middle classes of schools.] iii, 105 pp. 8°. *St. Petersburg, J. N. Erlich,* 1886.

Naundorff (Julius). Unter dem rothen Kreuz. Fremde und eigene Erfahrungen auf böhmischer Erde und den Schlachtfeldern der Neuzeit gesammelt. x, 519 pp. 8°. *Leipzig, Veit u. Comp.,* 1867.

Naunyn (Bernard) [1839–]. * De echinococci evolutione. 35 pp. 8°. *Berolini, G. Lange,* [1862].

——. Zum derzeitigen Standpunkt der Lehre von den Schutzimpfungen. Rede gehalten beim Protectoratswechsel der Albertina zu Königsberg i. Pr. 18 pp. 8°. *Leipzig, F. C. W. Vogel,* 1886.
Also, Co-Editor of : **Archiv** für experimentelle Pathologie und Pharmakologie, Leipzig, 1873.
See, also, **Handbuch** d. spec. Path. (Ziemssen), Leipz., 1876, xv. — **Cyclopædia** Pract. M. (Ziemssen), N. Y., 1878, xvii. — **Nothnagel** (H.) & **Naunyn** (B.) Ueber die Localisation der Gehirnkrankheiten. 8°. *Wiesbaden,* 1887.
For Biography, see Cycl. Pract. M. (Ziemssen), N. Y., 1878, pp. iii–v.

—— & **Quincke** (H.) Ueber den Einfluss des Centralnervensystems auf die Wärmebildung im Organismus. [In two parts, each with separate title-page and pagination.] 28, 15 pp. 8°. *Berlin, Gebr. Unger,* 1869.
Repr. from : Arch. f. Anat., Physiol. u. wissensch. Med., Berl., 1869, xxxvi, Hft. 2 & 5.

—— & **Schreiber** (J.) Ueber Gehirndruck. 112 pp., 7 pl. 8°. *Leipzig, F. C. W. Vogel,* 1881.

Nauplia.

See **Fever** (*Cerebro-spinal, History, etc., of*), *by localities.*

Naurath (Martinus). Tractatus politico-juridicus ad usum horum temporum accomodatus, de vita et morte hominis, in quo ex universo jure, ejusdemque interpretibus, tam veteribus quam recentioribus, ad hanc materiam spectantia, centum theorematibus compendiose evolvuntur. Accesserunt ejusdem additamenta miscellanea practica. 6 p. l., 456 pp., 12 l. 12°. *Gissæ Hassorum, ex off. J. G. Seyler,* 1673.

Naurath (Lud. Jul. Ern.) [1804–]. * De manuum morphologia et physiologia, xii, 131 pp. 8°. *Berolini, typ. A. G. Schadii,* [1835].

Naury. * Essai sur les fistules urinaires ombilicales par persistance de l'ouraque et sur leur traitement. 76 pp. 4°. *Paris,* 1881, No. 253.

Nausea *and nauseants.*

See, also, **Anæsthetics** (*Accidents, etc., in*); **Emetics**; **Pregnancy** (*Vomiting in*); **Sea-sickness**; **Vomiting.**

FRIEDRICH (S. F.) * De nausea et vomitu. 8°. *Traj. ad Viadr.,* 1794.

Nausea *and nauseants.*

HAFNER (D. G.) * De effectu nauseantium. 8°. *Gottingæ,* 1817.

HALLANER (P. J. C.) * De nausea. 4°. *Jenæ,* 1765.

RENTZ (C. H. J.) * Nonnulla de nauseosis. 4°. *Kiliæ,* 1827.

SCHNIZLEIN (C. H.) * De nausea. 4°. *Erlangæ,* [1785].

ZWEIGEL (J. C.) * De spasmis gulæ inferioris et de nausea. Oder: vom Krampff des Unterschlundes und vom Eckel. 4°. *Halæ Magdeb.,* [1733].

Brochin. Nausées. Dict. encycl. d. sc. méd., Par., 1876, 2. s., xi, 543–556.—**Peare** (R. J.) Buttermilk in sick stomach. Therap. Gaz., Detroit, 1885, 3. s., i, 221.—**Stich** (A.) Ueber das Ekel-Gefühl. Ann. d. Char.-Krankenh. . . . zu Berl., 1858, viii, 2. Hft., 22–43.

Nauss (Carl Eberhard) [1849–]. * Ueber Complication von Schwangerschaft, Geburt u. Wochenbett mit Myomen des Uterus. 1 p. l., 35 pp., 2 l. 8°. *Halle, O. Hendel,* [1872]. c.

Naussac (Henri). * Considérations sur la saignée. 34 pp. 4°. *Paris,* 1868, No. 62.

Nauta (Hemmo Hyleco). * Twaalf ovariotomiën. 2 p. l., 3–46 pp. 8°. *Groningen, P. Noordhoff,* 1881.

Nauta (Stephanus Sybrandus). * De corporibus peregrinis ex œsophago removendis. 53 pp. 8°. *Workumi Frisiorum, I. Verwey,* 1803.

Nauthonier (A.) * Essai sur le rhumatisme articulaire aigu; suivi de quelques propositions de médecine. 24 pp. 4°. *Paris,* 1835, No. 74, v. 284.

Nautilus.

ROYAL College of Surgeons of England. Memoir on the pearly nautilus (Nautilus pompilius, Linn.), with illustrations of its external form and internal structure. Drawn up by Richard Owen, asst. conservator of the museum of the college. Published by direction of the council. 4°. *London,* 1832.

Lankester (E. R.) & **Bourne** (A. G.) On the existence of Spengel's olfactory organ and of paired genital ducts in the pearly nautilus. Quart. J. Micr. Sc., Lond., 1883, n. s., xxiii, 340–348.

Nauwerck (Gustav Adolf Friedrich) [1862–]. * Studien über die Pharynx-Mucosa. 23 pp., 1 l. 8°. *Halle a. S., E. Karras,* 1887.

Nauwerck (Robert). * Zur Casuistik der Tumoren des Bulbus. 28 pp. 8°. *Zürich, J. Herzog,* 1866. c.

Nauzais (J.-E.) * De la colite aiguë. 19 pp. 4°. *Paris,* 1830, No. 101, v. 232.

Nava (David) & **Selmi** (Geo. Francesco). * Sul caglio vitellino; memorie. 95 pp. 8°. *Milano, R. Istituto Lombardo,* 1857.

Navailles (Louis). * De l'ictère. 26 pp. 4°. *Paris,* 1845, No. 54, v. 436.

Navajas.

Vazquez (F.) Apuntes físico-médicos de las aguas de dos fuentes de Navajas (provincia de Castellon), conocidas por la del Baño y la de Mosen Miguel. Telégrafo méd., Barcel., 1850–51, iv, 91–96.

Navajos.

See Indians (*North American*).

Naval Medical Society Proceedings. Nos. 1–6, v. 1; No. 1, v. 2; 243, 41 pp. 8°. *Washington, D. C., Judd & Detweiler,* 1883.

Naval staff rank. By a naval staff officer. 11 pp. 8°. [*n. p., n. d.*]

Navalcarnero.

BAUSA Y MONTES (J.) Estudio médico-topográfico de la villa de Navalcarnero. 8°. *Madrid,* 1886.

Navarini (Andrea). Ricerche, meditazioni e conclusioni sul colèra-morbus. 30 pp. 8°. *Bassano,* 1886.

Navarra (Antonio). Bollettino del Istituto medico Valenziano. Mese di novembre dell' anno 1856. Lettere sulla febbre gialla. 16 pp. 8°. [*n. p.*, 1856.] [P., v. 1132.]

Repr. from: Gior. Arcadico, cxlviii.

Navarre.

See Fever (*Malarial, History, etc., of*), *by localities.*

Navarre (Auguste). * De quelques lésions pulmonaires consécutives aux traumatismes du crâne et de l'encéphale. 52 pp. 4°. *Paris,* 1876, No. 31.

Navarre (Charles-Clément). * Aperçu sur le toucher et sur son utilité dans la médecine. 24 pp. 4°. *Paris,* 1836, No. 207, v. 300.

Navarre (Pierre-Just). * Étude médicale de la presqu'île Ducos. 52 pp. 4°. *Paris,* 1879, No. 527.

——. L'homéopathie et les homéopathes. Étude spécialement adressée aux gens du monde. 27 pp. 8°. *Lyon, H. Georg,* 1887.

Navarrette y Romay (Emilio). Étude des abcès du foie dans la dysenterie chronique. Étiologie; anatomie pathologique; terminaisons et traitement chirurgical. 76 pp., 3 tab. 4°. *Paris,* 1872, No. 216.

Navarro (Francisco de Paula). * Étude sur la fève de Calabar. 115 pp. 4°. *Paris,* 1869, No. 250.

Navarro y Albero (Vicente).

See Sanchez Palacio (C.) & **Navarro y Albero** (V.) Una residencia de invierno . . . Alicante, [etc.] 8°. *Alicante,* 1882.

Navarro y Rodrigo (*Francisco*) [– 1882].

Campa. Necrología. Crón. méd., Valencia, 1881–2, v, 545–551.—**Cantó.** Necrología. Gac. de l. hosp., Valencia, 1882, i, 169–175.

Navault (Ferdinand). * Observations cliniques sur les effets physiologiques de l'acide arsénieux. 39 pp. 4°. *Paris,* 1878, No. 307.

Nave (F.-G.-Édouard). * Quelques considérations sur la dyspepsie stomacale envisagée surtout au point de vue des sympathies qu'elle détermine. 38 pp. 4°. *Paris,* 1866, No. 61.

Nave (Franz). * Die Ménièresche Krankheit. 3 p. l., 42 pp., 1 l. 8°. *Breslau, F. W. Jungfer,* 1877.

Naveau (Joann. Ludov. Theophil.) * Diss. sistens experimenta quædam circa urinæ secretionem. viii, 48 pp. 8°. *Halæ, typ. F. A. Grunerti patris filiique,* [1818].

Naveau (Josephus). * De febribus in genere. 28 pp. 4°. *Lugd. Bat., H. W. Hazenberg,* 1814.

Navel.

See Umbilicus.

Navet (Stanislas-Victor-Amédée). * Propositions sur le tempérament de la femme, sur sa menstruation et sur son âge critique. vi, 7–19 pp. 4°. *Paris,* 1830, No. 267, v. 236.

Navez (Joan. Car. Jos.) De corpore humano ut mixto. 1788.

In: LOUVAIN Diss. 8°. *Lovanii,* 1796, iv, 161–166.

a Navibus (Jacobus).

See Venustus (Ant. Maria). Consilium de febre pestilenti. 4°. *Venetiis,* 1574.

Navier (Jean-Claude). Quæstio medica, an cutis, gummosæ sanguinis materiæ, organum secretorium? Præs.: Ludovico Hieronymo Raussin, 8 pp. 4°. [*Reims*], *Jeunehomme,* 1776. [P., v. 1397.]

——. Sur l'usage du vin de champagne mousseux contre les fièvres putrides et autres maladies de même nature. ix, 10–64 pp. 8°. *Paris & Reims, Méquignon l'aîné,* 1778.

Navier (Pierre-Toussaint) [1712–79]. Réflexions sur les dangers des exhumations précipitées, et sur les abus des inhumations dans les églises;

Navier (Pierre-Toussaint)—continued.
suivies d'observations sur les plantations d'arbres dans les cimetières. viii, 79 pp. 12°. *Amsterdam & Paris, B. Morin*, 1775.

———. Contre-poisons de l'arsenic, du sublimé corrosif, du verd-de-gris et du plomb. Suivis de trois dissertations intitulées: 1. Recherches médico-chymiques sur différens moyens de dissoudre le mercure, etc. 2. Exposition de différens moyens d'unir le mercure au fer. 3. Nouvelles observations sur l'éther, etc. 2 v. xxv, 30, 360 pp.; xxi, 389 pp. 12°. *Paris, la veuve Méquignon & fils & Didot jeune*, 1777.

For Biography, see Hist. de la Soc. roy. de méd., Par., 1779, 52-73.

Navières (P.-M.) * Sur une épidémie de fièvres inflammatoires (angioténiques), observée et décrite pendant l'automne de l'an X (1802) dans une commune près de Mantes, département de Seine-et-Oise. 22 pp. 4°. *Paris, an XII* [1804], No. 174, v. 47.

Navies.

See, also, **Hospitals** (*Naval, etc.*); **Hygiene** (*Naval*); **Medicine** (*Naval*); **Navy** (*Austrian*), *et seq.*; **Sailors**; **Surgery**; **Travels**, *etc.*

BOYNTON (C. B.) The navies of England, France, America, and Russia. Extract from a work on English and French neutrality and the Anglo-French alliance. 8°. *New York*, 1865.

Naville (E.)
See **Hemmann** (August). Notes et observations nouvelles relativement à l'établissement thermal de Schinznach [etc.] 8°. *Genève*, 1867.

Naville (Georg. Const.) Diss. psychologica in qua facultates hominis ad præsentem futurumque statum referri evincitur. 31 pp. 8°. *Genevæ, J. P. Bonnant*, 1774.

Navonus (Bernardus). * I. Ex botanica. De succis concretis. Acacia, manna et opium. II. [etc.] 8 pp. sm. 4°. *Augustæ Taurinorum, P. J. Zappatæ et fil.*, 1748. [P., v. 979.]

Navratil (Emerich) [1834–]. Laryngologische Beiträge. Bericht über die Abtheilung für Kehlkopfkranke im St. Rochus-Spitale zu Pest, umfassend die Krankenbewegung vom 12. Mai 1868 bis 31. December 1870. 1 p. l., 80 pp., 3 pl. 8°. *Leipzig, B. Zechel*, 1871.

———. Chirurgische Beiträge. iv, 126 pp., 3 pl. 8°. *Stuttgart, F. Enke*, 1882.

Navrátil (Franz). Prof. Dr. Oertel's (München) Heilverfahren bei Herzkrankheiten, Wassersucht und Fettleibigkeit; allgemein verständlich dargestellt. 1 p. l., 36 pp. 8°. *Wien, W. Braumüller*, 1885.

Navrotski (F.) * O vlijanii davlenija krovi na tsentri blujdaioushich nervov. [Effect of pressure of blood in centre of vagus.] 24 pp. 8°. *St. Petersburg*, 1870.

Navrotski (Ivan). * Materiali ke morphologii nervnoi sistemi nasiekomiche se nepolnime prevrashenieme. [Morphology of nervous system of insects and their metamorphoses.] 36 pp. 8°. *St. Petersburg*, 1876.

Navy (*Austrian*).

AUSTRIA. Die Krankheits- und Sterblichkeitsverhältnisse in Sr. Maj. Kriegsmarine während des Quinquenniums 1863-7. Im Auftrage der Marine-Section des Reichs-Kriegs-Ministeriums statistisch zusammengestellt von Dr. Robert Kolaczek. roy. 8°. *Wien*, 1870.
Also [Rev.], *in:* Monatsbl. f. med. Statist. u. öff. Gsndhtspflg., Berl., 1871, xxiii, 70; 86.

AUSTRIA. *Kaiserliche königliche Kriegs-Marine.* Statistische Sanitäts-Berichte für die Jahre 1870-84. Im Auftrage des k. k. Reichs-Kriegs-Ministeriums (Marine-Section) zusammengestellt von Drs. Robert Kolaczek, Adolph Altschul, Alexius

Navy (*Austrian*).

Uhlik, Josef Potočnik und Hans Krumpholz. roy. 8°. *Wien*, 1872-85.
Kirchenberger. Die Sanitäts-Verhältnisse der k. k. Kriegsmarine im Jahre 1875. Prag. med. Wchnschr., 1877, ii, 1055; 1077. — **Winternitz** (W.) Die Morbilität in Sr. Maj. Kriegsmarine. Wchnbl. d. k. k. Gesellsch. d. Aerzte in Wien, 1864, xx, 71; 85; 97; 114; 125; 469.

Navy (*Austrian, Medical department of*).

AUSTRIA. *Kaiserliche königliche Kriegs-Marine.* Vorschrift über die Gebarung mit dem Sanitäts-Materiale auf S. M. Schiffen. 4°. *Wien*, 1886.
Beilage zum Marine-Normal-Verordnungsbl., Wien, 1886.

———. Vorschrift zur Verfassung der ärztlich-statistischen Eingaben. [Including blank forms.] 4°. *Wien*, [*n. d.*]
Repr. from: Marine-Normal-Verordnungsbl., Wien, 1873, xxxii. Stück.

———. [Blank forms used by the medical department.] v. s. [*Wien, n. d.*]

———. Gebürs- und Anweisungsbogen. [Blank forms used by the medical department.] fol. [*Wien, n. d.*]
[**Kovanitzky.**] Note sur le service de santé de la marine autrichienne. Arch. de méd. nav., Par., 1881, xxxv, 72-74. — **Reorganisation** (Zur) der marineärztlichen Branche. Allg. mil.-ärztl. Ztg., Wien, 1871, 30-32. — **Schiffsärzte** in der österreichischen Handelsmarine. Wchnbl. d. k. k. Gesellsch. d. Aerzte in Wien, 1864, xx, 63. — **Weiser** (M. E.) Der Marinearzt—wie der Seeoffizier. Allg. mil.-ärztl. Ztg., Wien, 1868, 233; 242.

Navy (*Brazilian, Medical department of*).

BRAZIL. *Navy. Medical Départment.* Decreto N. 9579 de 10 abril 1886. Manda por em execução as novas tabellas para a distribuição das rações diarias aos officiaes e guarnições dos navios da armada e praças dos corpos de marinha e das escolas de aprendizes marinheiros e dietas a bordo, nos hospitaes e enfermarias de marinha. 8°. *Rio do Janeiro*, 1886.

———. Mappa do movimento dos doentes do Hospital de Marinha. 4°. [*Rio de Janeiro*, 1886.]

Navy (*British*).

BLANE (G.) A brief statement of the progressive improvement of the health of the royal navy at the end of the eighteenth and beginning of the nineteenth century. 8°. *London*, 1830.

BRYSON (A.) Report on the climate and principal diseases of the African station. Compiled . . . under the immediate direction of Sir William Burnett, M. D. 8°. *London*, 1847.

FRIEDEL (C.) Die Krankheiten in der Marine. Geographisch und Statistisch nach den Reports on the health of the Royal Navy, dargestellt von . . . roy. 8°. *Berlin*, 1866.

———. Bolaizni na flotai. Geographicheskii i statisticheskii obsor. "Reports on the health of the Royal Navy" [British]. Perevedeno i izdano po rasporyazheniyu Morskago Ministerstva. [Diseases in the navy; a geographical and statistical review. Transl. and published by the order of the navy department.] 8°. *St. Petersburg*, 1869.

GREAT BRITAIN. *Navy.* Regulations and instructions relating to his majesty's service at sea. 13. ed. 4°. *London*, 1790.

———. Instructions for the conduct of ships of war, explanatory of, and relative to, the signals contained in the signal-book herewith delivered, 1796. fol. [*London*, 1796.]

———. The navy list, corrected to Sept. 20, 1866. By authority. 12°. *London*, 1866.

———. The same. To Dec. 20, 1867. 12°. *London*, 1867.

———. The same. Jan., 1874. 12°. *London*, 1874.

GREAT BRITAIN. *Navy Medical Department.* Return to an order of the House of Commons, dated March 20, 1840, for statistical reports on

Navy (*British*).

the health of the navy, for the years 1830–36. Part I. South American, West Indian and North American, Mediterranean and Peninsular commands. fol. [*London*, 1840.]

——. The same. [Without appendices.] 8°. *London*, 1841.

——. The same. (In continuation of Parliamentary paper No. 159, March 24, 1840.) Part II. Cape of Good Hope and West Coast of Africa, and East India commands, home and various forces, together with the totals for seven years throughout the service. fol. [*London*, 1841.]

——. The same. Health of the navy. Return to an order of the House of Commons, dated May 17, 1849, for copies "of statistical reports on the health of the navy (in continuation of Parliamentary paper No. 53, sess. 1841)" for the years 1837–43. Part I. South American station, North American and West Indian station, and Mediterranean station. fol. [*London*, 1849.]

——. The same. (In continuation of Parliamentary paper No. 436, of sess. 1849.) Part II. East India station. fol. [*London*, 1853.]

——. The same. (In continuation of Parliamentary paper No. 555, of sess. 1853.) Part III. North Coast of Spain station, Cape station, West Coast of Africa station, packet service, home station, ships employed variously. fol. [*London*, 1854.]

——. Baltic and Black Sea fleets. A copy of the medical and statistical returns of the Baltic and Black Sea fleets, during the years 1854 and 1855. fol. [*London*, 1857.]

——. Navy (health). Statistical reports of the health of the navy. By the director-general, to the lords commissioners of the admiralty. For the years 1856–85. 8°. *London*, 1857–87.

GREAT BRITAIN. *Navy. Royal Naval College, Greenwich.* Annual report of the president to the secretary of the admiralty, for the year 1875–6. fol. [*London*, 1876.]

Blane (*Sir* G.) Statements of the comparative health of the British navy, from the year 1799 to the year 1814, with proposals for its farther improvement. Med.-Chir. Tr., 2. ed. Lond., 1819, vi, 490–573, 3 pl. *Also*, Reprint. *Also, in his:* Select dissertations, 8°, Lond., 1822, 1–64.—**Bulletin** of the health of her majesty's fleet in the Euxine during the quarter ending June 31—the first quarter of the war. Med. Times & Gaz., Lond., 1854, n. s., ix, 156.—**Fisher** (A.) Remarks on the physical examination of men and boys for the navy, and recruits for the royal marines, in the London district, during the year 1876. Statist. Rep. Health Navy, Lond., 1876, App., 171–183.—**Gillespie** (L.) Copy of a letter to Vice-Admiral Lord Nelson, from . . . physician to the fleet, dated Aug. 14, 1805, Victory at Sea. [Report of the number of men on sick list, diseased, and sent to general hospitals.] Med. & Phys. J., Lond., 1805, xiv, 413–416.—**Rattray** (A.) Influence du régime, du climat et des longs voyages sur la santé et les maladies des marines. Déduite des variations de leurs poids d'après les expériences instituées de 1864 à 1866 sur le navire H. M. S. Salamander. Analyse et traduction par Ad. Nicolas. Arch. de méd. nav., Par., 1869, xii, 321–331.—**Shoveller** (W.) Remarks at the end of the journal for the Sybille, between Oct. 28, 1818, and June 22, 1819. Lond. M. Reposit., 1820, xiv, 10–15

Navy (*British, Medical department of*).

BROWN (F. J.) Requisitions of the naval medical officers, based on the principle of equality with the army. 8°. *London*, 1865.

EXPOSITION (An) of the case of the assistant surgeons of the royal navy. By a naval medical officer. 8°. *London*, 1849.

——. The same. 8°. *London*, 1850.

GREAT BRITAIN. *Navy. Naval Medical Supplemental Fund Society.* Return to an address of the House of Commons, dated 21 June, 1861; for a "copy of the order in council of the 13th day of August, 1817, establishing the Naval Medical Supplemental Fund Society". fol. [*London*, 1861.]

Navy (*British, Medical department of*).

GREAT BRITAIN. *Navy Medical Department.* Regulations and instructions for the medical officers of his majesty's fleet. 4°. [*London*], 1825.

——. [Blank forms used in the medical department of the navy.] v. s. [*London*, 1866–85.]

——. [Blank forms used in hospital service and service afloat.] v. s. [*London*, 1866–87.]

——. Medical and surgical handbook for the guidance of officers in command of those vessels in her majesty's service in which no medical officer is borne. 12°. *London*, 1878.

——. Regulations and instructions for the surgeons and agents of sick quarters. 8°. *London*, 1884.

——. Royal marine infirmaries. Orders for the behaviour of patients in the infirmaries. No. 80. (Rev. Oct., 1885.) broadside, 17×23 in. *London*, [1885].

——. Royal Marine Infirmary. Regulations for nurses. No. 81. (Rev. Oct., 1885.) broadside, 17×22 in. *London*, [1885].

GREAT BRITAIN. *Parliament. House of Commons.* Minutes of evidence taken before the select committee on the Naval Medical Supplemental Fund Society bill; with the proceedings of the committee, and appendix. fol. [*London*, 1861.]

Disabilities of the naval medical service. [Edit.] Brit. M. J., Lond., 1880, i, 57; 144; 179.—**Dismissal** of a naval surgeon from the service. Med. Times & Gaz., Lond., 1853, n. s., vi, 577–579.—**Dundas** (W.) Improving the situation of the medical officers of the navy. Edinb. M. & S. J., 1805, i, 241–243.—**F.** (T.) Sketch of a plan for improving the medical department of the navy. *Ibid.*, 1811, vii, 25–29.—**Medical** (The) officers in the English and French navies. Med. Times & Gaz., Lond., 1854, n. s., ix, 166.—**Naval** medical reform warrant. [Edit.] Lancet, Lond., 1880, i, 306; 408.—**Naval** surgeons. *Ibid.*, 1838, ii, 189.—**Navy** victualling, and our navy medical officers. Med. Times & Gaz., Lond., 1852, n. s., iv, 39.—**Peel** (C. L.) The naval medical service. Lancet, Lond., 1881, i, 598–600.—**Reynolds** (T.) Proposals for a regulation of the œconomy of the sick, and preservation of life on board of his majesty's ships of war at sea. Presented to Lord Anson, first commissioner of the admiralty. Gent's Mag. & Hist. Chron., Lond., 1758, xxviii, 61; 105; 157; 207.—**Scott** (R. T. C.) New mode of punishment in the navy. Lancet, Lond., 1838, ii, 317.—**Smart** (W. R. E.) Notes on the institutions for the relief of the sick, wounded, and disabled of the royal navy. Brit. M. J., Lond., 1871, ii, 487–490.—**Statement** of yearly pay of naval and army medical officers. *Ibid.*, 1880, i, 222.—**Stratton** (T.) Naval medical department of Great Britain and the United States. Edinb. M. & S. J., 1852, lxxvii, 58–62. ——. Mortality in the medical department of the British navy. *Ibid.*, 1861, vi, 813, 1 tab. ——. On the rate of mortality in the medical department of the British navy for the ten years ending December, 1870. *Ibid.*, 1870–71, xvi, 795, 1 tab. ——. On the rate of mortality in the medical department of the British navy for the ten years ending in December, 1880. *Ibid.*, 1880–81, xxvi, 1099.—**Thompson** (*Sir* R.) Naval and military medical services; relative rank. Brit. M. J., Lond., 1887, i, 851.

Navy (*Chilian*).

CHILE. Memoria que el ministro de estado en el departamento de marina presenta al Congreso nacional de 1870. 8°. *Santiago*, 1870.

Navy (*Danish, Medical department of*).

DENMARK. *Marineministerium.* Bestemmelser angaaende de fra Orlogskibene efter endt Togt tilbageleverede Medikamenter med tilhørende Rekvisiter. 8°. [*Kjøbenhavn*, 1885.]

——. [Blank forms used by the medical department of the navy.] fol. [*Kjøbenhavn*, 188-.]

Navy (*French*).

AUDE. Extraits du rapport d'ensemble sur le service médical de l'escadre d'évolutions. (Du 1er août 1883 au 1er août 1884.) 8°. *Paris*, [1886]. *Repr. from:* Arch. de méd. nav., Par., 1886, xlv.

Rapports médicaux et statistiques de la marine française. Ann. d'hyg., Par., 1859, 2. s., xi, 218–222.

Navy (*French, Medical department of*).

AUDE (P.) Code des officiers du corps de santé de la marine. 8°. *Paris*, 1877.

COUP d'œil sur l'organisation du service de santé de la marine. [Mémoire discuté et adopté par la majorité des chirurgiens de la marine présens au port de Brest. Signé: Eug. Fatou, Sagot, Berdelo, etc.] 8°. *Brest*, [*n. d.*]

FRANCE. *Département de la marine.* Ordonnance du roi. Composition du corps des officiers de la marine. 8°. *Paris*, 1835.

————. Manuel de l'infirmier marin, ou instruction sur le service des infirmiers maritimes auprès des malades, dans les hôpitaux des ports, à bord des navires de la flotte et dans les postes de la chirurgie. 12°. *Paris*, 1857.

————. Programmes des questions auxquelles les candidats ont à répondre dans les concours pour les différents grades et emplois du corps de santé de la marine. (Publiés par ordre du ministre de la marine et des colonies.) 8°. *Paris*, 1875.

MALESPINE (A.) Le corps de santé de la marine; ses besoins; ses revendications; assimilation; pondération des grades. 8°. *Paris*, 1879.

PEZZONI (A.) Un mot sur le rapport de la commission créée en 1849 par le Conseil général de santé maritime siégeant à Gênes, par Angelo Bo, rapporteur de la commission. 8°. *Smyrne*, 1850.

PROJET de réformes dans le service de santé de la marine. 8°. *Toulon*, 1882.

Authenac (E.) Les médecins de la marine. Concours méd., Par., 1881, iii, 17–19.—**Barnier.** Le contre-projet de M. Georges Roche et le corps de santé de la marine. Gaz. méd.-chir. de Toulouse, 1887, xix, 129; 137; 149.—**Caradec** (T.) fils. Le corps de santé de la marine au xviie et xviiie siècles. Rev. scient., Par., 1876, 2. s., x. 180–185.—**de Chasseloup-Laubat** (P.) Réorganisation du service de santé de la flotte. Rapport à l'empereur. Rev. scient. d. méd. d. armées, Par., 1870, viii, 59–65.—**Corps** de santé de la marine; rapport au président de la République française. Gaz. d. hôp., Par., 1875, xlviii, 609–611.—**Décret** introduisit des réformes dans l'organisation du corps de santé de l'armée de mer. Arch. gén. de méd., Par., 1865, ii, 369–371.—**Décret** du 24 juin 1886 portant organisation du service de santé de la marine; règlement ministériel annexé. Arch. de méd. nav., Par., 1886. xlvi, 161–209.—**Didiot** (P.-A.) Service de santé de la marine en France. Rev. scient. d. méd. d. armées, Par., 1865, vii, 305–319.—**Latour** (A.) Réorganisation du service de santé de la marine. Union méd., Par., 1865, 2. s., xxvii, 401–408.—**Layet.** Le corps de santé de la marine. Gaz. hebd. d. sc. méd. de Bordeaux, 1880–81, i, 415; 443; 503, 1 tab.—**Lefèvre** (A.) Histoire du service de santé de la marine et des écoles de médecine navale étudiée plus particulièrement au port de Rochefort. Arch. de méd. nav., Par., 1864, i, 100; 417: ii, 229: 1865, iii, 62; 256; 627: 1866, v, 119; 300; 500, 1 pl.: vi, 118, 3 pl.; 271; 453, 2 pl.: 1867, vii, 96; 274, 2 pl. *Also*, Reprint. — **Lereboullet** (L.) La nouvelle organisation du service de santé de la marine. Gaz. de méd., Par., 1886, 2. s., xxiii, 437–439. — **Montaignac.** Rapport au président de la République française, suivi d'un décret portant modification dans l'organisation du corps de santé de la marine. Arch. de méd. nav., Par., 1875, xxiv, 325–379.—**Ollivier.** Le médecin de la marine dans les voyages de découvertes autour du monde. *Ibid.*, 1864, ii, 489–528.—**Rapport** au président de la République par le ministre de la marine et décret relatifs à des modifications dans le service des hôpitaux de la marine. Rev. scient. d. méd. d. armées, Par., 1882, x, 2112–2115. — **Rapport** au président de la République française. [Un projet de décret portant réorganisation du service de santé de la marine.] Nederl. mil. geneesk. Arch., etc., Utrecht, 1886, x, 800–810. — **Règlement** ministériel concernant le mode d'admission, d'enseignement et de concours dans le corps de santé de la marine. Arch. de méd. nav., Par., 1866, v, 421–448. *Also* [Abstr.]: Gaz. hebd. de méd., Par., 1866, 2. s., iii, 317–319.—**Réorganisation** du service de santé de la marine. Gaz. d. hôp., Par., 1885, lviii, 297: lix, 597–600.—**Réorganisation** du corps de santé de la marine française. Rev. scient. d. méd. d. armées, Par., 1887, x, 481–486. — **Rey** (H.) Du service médical des compagnies de débarquement. Arch. de méd. nav., Par, 1868, ix, 124; 195.

Navy (*German*).

GERMANY. *Kaiserlich deutsche Marine.* Statistische Sanitätsberichte über die . . . für die

Navy (*German*).

Jahren 1874–5; 1875–6; 1879–80 bis 1881–2; 1883–4 u. 1884–5. Zusammengestellt vom Generalarzt der Marine. 8°. *Berlin*, 1875–85.

Navy (*German, Medical department of*).

GERMANY. *Kaiserlich deutsche Marine.* Instruction für Marine-Aerzte zur Untersuchung und Beurtheilung der Dienstbrauchbarkeit oder Unbrauchbarkeit der in die königliche Marine einzustellenden, resp. der in derselben dienenden Mannschaften, so wie zur Beurtheilung der Invalidität in Dienst befindlicher oder entlassener versorgungsberechtiger Mannschaften der Marine vom 5. November 1860. 8°. *Berlin*, 1861.

————. Dienstanweisung für Marineärzte zur Beurtheilung der Dienstfähigkeit und zur Ausstellung von Attesten. Vom 10. April 1884. 8°. *Berlin*, 1884.

JAHN (B.) Vollständiges Verzeichniss der activen Sanitäts-Offiziere des deutschen Reichs-Heeres und der kaiserlichen Marine, mit genauer Angabe der Beförderungen in die einzelnen Rangstufen. 1. Jahrg. 8°. *Burg*, 1882.

Holbeck. Sanitarnaya chast Germanskago flota. [Sanitary department of the German navy.] Med. pribav. k morsk. sborniku, St. Petersb., 1876, 160–201.—**Steinberg.** Ueber den Etat der Marineärzte. Preuss. mil.-ärztl. Ztg., Berl., 1860, i, 189; 206.—**Stellung** (Die) der preussischen Marineärzte. Deutsche Klinik, Berl., 1860, xii, 93; 105; 113; 131.—**Uebersicht** der im 2. Semester 1872 bei der Marine am Lande und an Bord der Schiffe vorgekommenen Krankheits-, Unbrauchbarkeit-, Invaliditäts- und Todesfälle. Monatsbl. f. med. Statist. u. öff. Gsndhtspflg., Berl., 1873, 30; 89.

Navy (*Italian*).

ITALY. *Navy Medical Department.* Relazione sulle condizioue sanitarie dei corpi della regia marina durante gli anni 1873–82. roy. 8°. *Roma*, 1877–83.

Sormani (G.) Relazione sulle condizioni sanitarie dei corpi della regia marina durante il biennio 1877–78. Ann. di statist., Roma, 1881, 2. s., xxi, 9–13.

Navy (*Italian, Medical department of*).

Décret d'organisation du corps de santé de la marine italienne. Rev. scient. d. méd. d. armées, Par., 1865, vii, 113–143.

Navy (*Japanese*).

JAPAN. *Navy Medical Department.* First special report upon the improvement in the scale of diet in the imperial Japanese navy. For the 17th year of Meiji (1884). 8°. [*Tokyō*, 1885.]

————. Second special report upon the improvement in the scale of diet in the imperial Japanese navy. For the 18th year of Meiji (1885). 8°. [*Tokyō*, 1886.]

Navy (*Netherlands*).

Bouvin (M. J.) Het onlangs gewijzigde keurings-reglement, hoofdzakelijk beschouwd in verband met de eischen voor het gezichtsvermogen van het personeel bij de marine. Nederl. Tijdschr. v. Geneesk., Amst., 1881, 2. R., xvii, 881–886. — **Geneeskundig** jaarverslag nopens den gezondheidstoestand bij de Kon. Nederlandsche Marine (1876–83). Nederl. mil. geneesk. Arch., etc., Utrecht, 1878, ii, 528: 1879, iii, 517: 1880, iv, 607: 1881, v, 503: 1882, vi, 439: 1883, vii, 431: 1884, viii, 555: 1885, ix, 387.—**Geneeskundige** dienst bij de marine. Geneesk. Courant, Tiel, 1880, xxxiv, no. 9.—**Pop** (G. F.) & **Slot** (H.) Overzigt der ziekten en gebreken, onder behandeling gekomen bij de geneeskundige dienst der zeemagt [for the years 1860–68]. Geneesk. Tijdschr. v. de Zeemagt, Gravenh., 1862–3, i, 309: 1864, ii, 369: 1865, iii, 337: 1866, iv, 306: 1867, v, 313: 1868, vi, 305: 1869, vii, 209: 1870, viii, 335: 1871, ix, 291.—**Uittreksel** uit het algemeen rapport van den inspecteur van de geneeskundige dienst der zeemagt aan den minister van marine, betreffende de geneeskundige dienst, over het jaar 1854. Pract. Tijdschr. v. de Geneesk., Gorinchem, 1856, n. s., ii, 300–323.—**Underdänigt** betänkande med förslag angående ordnande af flottans sanitetsväsende afgifvet af militära helsovårdskomitén den 18. December 1882. Tidskr. i mil. Helsov., Stockholm, 1883, viii, 33–140.

Navy (*Netherlands, Medical department of*).

NETHERLANDS. *Koninklijke Nederlandsche Marine.* Reglement voor het Hospitaal der marine te Willemsoord. 8°. *'s Gravenhage*, 1880.

Navy (*Netherlands, Medical department of*).

——. [Blank forms used by the medical department of the navy.] v. s. [*'s Gravenhage*], 1880–86.

——. VI^de Hoofdstuk. Reglement op den geneeskundigen dienst bij de zeemacht. Vastgesteld bij Zr. Ms. besluit van 27. Juli 1884, No. 36. 2. deel. 8°. [*'s Gravenhage*, 1884.]

——. Geneeskundig jaarverslag nopens den gezondheidstoestand gedurende het jaar 1884, medegedeeld door J. D. Sachse. 8°. *Utrecht*, 1886.

——. The same. ... het jaar 1885 medegedeeld door J. D. Sachse. 8°. *Utrecht*, 1887.

VAN STOCKUM (H.) Denkbeelden over re-denen van het tegenwoordig gebrek aan officieren van gezondheid bij 's rijks zeedienst en der middelen die aangewend kunnen worden om in dien toestand verbetering te brengen. 8°. *Nieuwediep*, 1875.

Kön. Niederl. Marine. Zulassung fremder Aerzte als temporäre Militär-Aerzte der 2ten Classe bei der kön. Niederl. Marine. Tidskr. i mil. Helsov. Stockholm, 1883, viii, 159.—**Pop** (G. F.) De geneeskunde bij het Nederlandsche zeewezen. Geneesk. Tijdschr. v. de Zeemagt, Gravenh., 1867, v, 1; 103; 199: 1868, vi, 1; 97; 207: 1869, vii, 1; 85.

Navy (*Portuguese, Medical department of*).

PORTUGAL. Serviço sanitario a bordo dos navios do estado, extrahido do regulamento de saude naval decretado em 17 de maio de 1837, e outros documentos posteriores relativos ao mesmo serviço. 8°. *Lisboa*, 1845.

——. Quadros estatisticos do hospital da marinha e outros documentos para a estatistica das doenças e mortalidade na armada referidos ao annos 1867–76. 4°. *Lisboa*, 1868–78.

——. Decreto ácerca dos aspirantes a facultativos da armada e do ultramar promulgado em 23 de dezembro de 1869. 8°. *Lisboa*, 1869.

——. Regulamento do serviço de saude naval. [Including blank forms, Nos. 1–46.] 8°. *Lisboa*, 1886.

Ministerio de la gobernacion. Real decreto organizando la sanidad marítima. Correo méd. castellano, Salamanca, 1886, iii, 519; 537.

Navy (*Russian*).

RUSSIA. Medisinskiya pribavleniyo k morskomu sborniku. [Medical supplements to the "Russian Naval Archives", published under the supervision of the chief medical inspector of the navy.] v. 1–24, 1861–86. 16 v. 8°. *St. Petersburg*, 1861–86.

Russian text. Current.

——. Otchete o sostojaniĭ zdorovja na flotie g. Flota Generale Tshtabe Doktora. [Reports of the state of health of the navy, for the years 1863–83.] 14 v. 8°. *St. Petersburg*, 1864–86.

Gumileff. O phisicheskom izsliedovaniĭ rekrutov v 1869 i 1870 g. v Kronstadté. [Examination of recruits for navy.] (Ib. for 1870.) Med. pribav. k morsk. sborniku, St. Petersb., 1871, xii, 175; 187. — **Kovaleva-Runski.** Otchet o viboré rekrutov v gvardeiskii ekipaje. [Examination of recruits for navy.] Ibid., 122–160. — **Levandovski** (G.) O normalnom sostavie pitchi, vs primienenii ke bitu njiniche tchinove morskago viedomstva, i obe iztochnikache nichechnoi sili. [Quality of rations in Russian navy.] Ibid., 1870, ix, 372–444. — **Loubinski** (A.) Rezultati izcliedovanija zrienija i phyzycheskago sostojanija u 957 chelovieke njinich chinove. [Examination of naval recruits.] Protok. zasaid. Obsh. Morsk. vrach. v Kronstadt, 1880, xvii, 71–79.—**Marine** (La) russe. Rev. scient., Par., 1876. 2. s., xi, 337–348.—**Michell** (J.) Report of the medical director-general of the Russian navy, for ten months in the year 1857, viz, January 1 to October 31, 1857. Med. Times & Gaz., Lond., 1858, n. s., xvii, 495–497. ——. Report of the medical director-general of the Russian navy, for the period between Nov. 1, 1857, and Oct. 31, 1858. Ibid., 1859, n. s., xix, 400; 427. — **Rosenberger.** Jahresberichte der Medicinal-Verwaltung des k. russischen Marine-Ministeriums für die Jahre 1860–62. Monatsbl. f. med. Statist. u. öff. Gsndhtspflg., Berl., 1861, 60–71: 1863, 1; 12: 1865, 1; 17; 25; 33.—**Sanitarnœ** sostoyanie russkago flota. [Sanitary condition of

Navy (*Russian*).

the Russian navy.] Vrach. Vaidom., St. Petersb., 1876, i, no. 34, 1; no. 35, 1.—**Schulz** (H.) Bericht über den Gesundheitszustand des Commandos derjenigen russischen Schiffe. welche in den Jahren 1862 und 1863 in ausländischen Meeren segelten. Monatsbl. f. med. Statist. u. öff. Gsndhtspflg., Berl., 1865, 43; 46; 63.

Navy (*Spanish, Medical department of*).

SPAIN. *Ministerio de la gobernacion.* Direccion general de beneficencia y sanidad. Disposiciones reglamentarias sobre sanidad marítima dictadas desde el 14 de junio de 1879 al 21 de mayo de 1880. Coleccion oficial publicada por la direccion del ramo. 8°. *Madrid*, 1880.

——. *Navy Medical Department.* Escalafon general de los sres. jefes y oficiales del cuerpo de sanidad de la armada. 1882–84. 16°. [*San Fernando*, 1882–4.]

——. Escalafon de practicantes de la armada. 1882–84. 16°. *San Fernando*, [1882–4].

——. Reglamento del cuerpo de sanidad de la armada. 8°. *Madrid*, 1885.

——. Reglamento del cuerpo de practicantes de la armada. roy. 8°. [*Madrid*, 1886.]

DE VEGA (L.) Pharmacopea de la armada ó real catálogo de medicamentos pertenecientes á las enfermedades médicas, trabajado para el uso de los médicos, y cirujaros de la real armada que sirven á nuestro muy poderoso rey de España en este real hospital, y en los navios, así de guerra come marchantes. 4°. *Cádiz*, 1759.

Latin and Spanish text.

Cabello (E.) Memoria acerca del movimiento sanitario de la división naval de Algeciras en el bienio de 1879 á 81, procedida de unos ligeros apuntes para la topografía médica de la localidad. Confer. cient. d. Cuerpo de sanid. de la Armada, San Fernando, 1882–6, i, 349–370.—**Cabello** (V.) Estado sanitario de los hospitales y enfermerías de nuestra armada, durante el quinquenio de 1877 á 1882. Bol. de med. nav., San Fernando, 1882, v, 80; 112; 134; 190: 1883, vi, 158. ——. De la mortalité dans les hôpitaux de la marine espagnole. Cong. internat. d'hyg. et de démog. Compt. rend. 1882, Genève, 1883, ii, 162–171.—**de Erostarbe** (J.) De las enfermedades observadas en los individuos de marina asistidos en los hospitales de San Francisco y San Carlos de la Habana, desde el 15 agosto de 1855 al 15 diciembre del mismo año. Siglo méd., Madrid, 1856, iii, 257; 267; 275; 291; 306; 316: 1857, iv, 211; 221; 243. ——. Sanidad de la armada. Ibid., 1861, viii, 391; 436.—**Espagne.** Décret royal réorganisant le corps de santé de la flotte. Rev. scient. d. med. d. armées, Par., 1865, vii, 215.—**Reales** órdenes concernientes á sanidad de la armada expedidas por el ministerio de marina, durante el mes de abril de 1882. Bol. de med. nav., San Fernando, 1882, v, 142.—**Reformas** necesarias para el mejor servicio sanitario de la armada. Ibid., 5; 33.—**Reglamento** al cual han de sujetarse los ejercicios de oposicion pública para el ingreso en el cuerpo de sanidad de la armada. Corresp. méd., Madrid, 1886, xxi, 66–71.— **Reglamento** orgánico provisional de la sanidad marítima para los servicios de las dependencias. Jurado méd.-farm., Madrid, 1887, viii, 200; 207; 214; 221; 231; 238; 245; 253; 261; 269; 277. Also: Diario méd.-farm., Madrid, 1887, iv, nos. 1013–1030.—**Sanidad** de la armada. Siglo med., Madrid, 1865, xii, 744; 762; 803 818.—**X. X.** Sanidad de la armada. Ibid., 1877, xxiv, 664.

Navy (*United States*).

BARTLEY & SOUTHARD. Argument before the Secretary of the Navy on the question of inserting the "title and grade" of staff officers of the Navy in their commissions. 8°. [*n. p., n. d.*]

BARTON (C. C.) Manifest of the charges preferred to the Navy Department, and subsequently to Congress, against J. D. Elliott, a captain in the Navy of the United States, for unlawful conduct while commodore of the late Mediterranean squadron, [etc.] 8°. [*n. p.*], 1839.

BOYNTON (C. B.) The history of the Navy during the rebellion. 2 v. 8°. *New York*, 1867–8.

HAMERSLY (L. R.) The records of living officers of the U. S. Navy and Marine Corps; with a history of naval operations during the rebellion of 1861–5, and a list of the ships and officers participating in the great battles. 8°. *Philadelphia*, 1870.

Navy (*United States*).

HAMERSLY (T. H. S.) Complete general Navy register of the United States of America, from 1776 to 1887. Arranged in alphabetical order. Containing the names of all officers of the Navy, volunteer and regular, who have entered the service from the time of the revolutionary war to the present time (1776–1887), containing the official record of each officer as on file at the Navy Department, showing the dates of their original entry, of their progressive rank, and in what manner they left the service if not now in it. Compiled from the official records. 8°. *New York,* 1884.

JENKINS (T. A.) Paper read before the Naval Committee of the House of Representatives January 21, 1868, in reply to Rear Admiral Goldsborough's claim to be continued on the active list of the Navy. 8°. *Washington,* [*n. d.*]

MECHLIN (A. H.) & WINDER (C. H.) A general register of the Navy and Marine Corps of the United States, alphabetically arranged, containing the names of all officers of the Navy and Marine Corps, military and civil, commissioned and warrant, who have entered the service since the establishment of the Navy Department in 1798, [etc.] Compiled from the official records of the Navy Department, by authority of the Secretary of the Navy. 8°. *Washington,* 1848.

MEMORIAL (A) by certain line officers of the Navy, intended to reopen a dispute which was settled by Congress in 1871, after full discussion and deliberation. With notes, comments, and an appendix. 8°. [*n. p.*], 1879.

STEVENS (A. F.) Rank in the Navy. Speech delivered in the House of Representatives January 23, 1871. 8°. *Washington,* 1871.

[TURNER (T. J.)] Relative number of cubic feet of space allotted to officers and men on berth-decks of the U. S. S. Swatara, U. S. S. Richmond, and U. S. S. Miantonomoh, which represent the different classes of vessels in the Navy. broadside 4°. [*n. p.*, 1876.]

UNITED STATES. *Congress.* A bill to reorganize and render more efficient the administration of the Navy Department. roy. 8°. [*Washington,* 1876.]

——. A bill to reduce, reorganize, and render more efficient the Navy of the United States. roy. 8°. [*Washington,* 1876.]

——. A bill defining sea-service. roy. 8°. [*Washington,* 1884.]

——. A bill to equalize the rank and pay of certain staff officers of the Navy. roy. 8°. [*Washington,* 1884.]

——. A bill to fix the positions of the assistant astronomers at the Naval Observatory. roy. 8°. [*Washington,* 1884.]

——. A bill to prevent the retroactive operation of the portion of the naval appropriation act of August 5, 1882, limiting the number of graduates of the Naval Academy to be retained in the service. Printed on page 285 of volume 22 of the United States Statutes at Large. roy. 8°. [*Washington,* 1884.]

——. Amendment intended to be proposed by Mr. Groome to the bill (S. 341) to regulate the rank of engineer officers in the United States Navy. roy. 8°. [*Washington,* 1884.]

——. Amendment intended to be proposed by Mr. Miller to the bill (S. 697) to promote the efficiency of the Navy. roy. 8°. [*Washington,* 1884.]

——. Amendment intended to be proposed by Mr. Sewell to the bill (S. 698) to authorize the construction of additional steel vessels for the Navy. roy. 8°. [*Washington,* 1884.]

——. An act making appropriations for the naval service for the fiscal year ending June 30,

Navy (*United States*).

1885, and for other purposes. roy. 8°. [*Washington,* 1884.]

——. Report from the committee on naval affairs, to which was referred the bill (S. 1039) for the relief of the survivors of the exploring steamer Jeannette and the widows and children of those who perished in the retreat from the wreck of that vessel in the Arctic seas. 8°. [*Washington,* 1884.]

——. Report from the Committee on Naval Affairs, to whom was referred the bill (S. 698) to authorize the construction of additional steel vessels for the Navy. 8°. [*Washington,* 1884.]

——. A bill relating to the bureaus of the Navy Department. 49. Cong., 1. sess. S. 672. Dec. 18, 1885. Introd by Mr. Frye. roy. 8°. [*Washington,* 1885.]

——. A bill limiting a portion of an act entitled "An act making appropriations for the naval service for the fiscal year ending June 30, 1883 [views of the minority No. 108. Pts. 1 & 2], and for other purposes. 49. Cong., 1. sess. S. 371. Dec. 10, 1885. Introd. by Mr. Cockrell. Committee discharged February 15, 1886. 8°. [*Washington,* 1886.]

——. A bill to provide for the retirement of a certain class of officers in the United States Navy. 49. Cong., 1. sess. S. 2815. July 7, 1886. Introd. by Mr. Hale. roy. 8°. [*Washington,* 1886.]

——. A bill to provide for the retirement of a certain class of officers in the United States Navy. 49. Cong., 2. sess. S. 2815. Introd. by Mr. Hale June 7, 1886. Reported by same Feb. 10, 1887. roy. 8°. [*Washington,* 1887.]

UNITED STATES. *Naval Academy.* Annual register of the United States Naval Academy, at Annapolis, Md. For the academic years 1874–5 (24.); 1875–6 (26.). 8°. *Washington,* 1874–5.

——. A catalogue of specimens added to the cabinet of the . . . 8°. *Washington,* 1881.

UNITED STATES. *Navy Department.* Rules, regulations, and instructions for the naval service of the United States; prepared by the Board of Navy Commissioners of the United States, with the consent of the Secretary of the Navy, in obedience to an act of Congress passed February 7, 1815, entitled "An act to alter and amend the several acts for establishing a navy department, by adding thereto a board of commissioners". 12°. *Washington,* 1818.

——. Registers of the commissioned and warrant officers of the Navy of the United States and of the officers of the Marine Corps for the years 1834, 1836, 1857, 1862, 1863, 1865, 1866, 1867, 1868, 1870, 1871, 1873, 1875, 1878, 1882, 1883, 1884, 1886. 8°. *Washington,* 1834–86.

——. (Regulations for the uniform and dress of the U. S. Navy) 1841. 8°. *Washington,* [*n. d.*]

——. Allowances established for vessels of the United States Navy, 1864. Issued by the Navy Department. 8°. *Washington,* 1865.

——. Message of the President of the United States and accompanying documents to the two Houses of Congress at the commencement of the 2d session of the 39th Congress. [Containing the report of the Secretary of the Navy for 1865–6.] 8°. *Washington,* 1866.

——. Annual reports of the Secretary of the Navy on the operations of the Department for the years 1866–7, 1872–3, 1875–6. 8°. *Washington,* 1867–76.

——. Regulations for the Government of the United States Navy, 1870. 12°. *Washington,* 1870.

——. United States International Centennial Exhibition of 1876. Catalogue of the articles and objects exhibited by the United States Navy Department in the United States Govern-

Navy (*United States*).

ment Building, Fairmount Park, Philadelphia, Pa. 4°. *Philadelphia*, 1876.

——. Letter from the Secretary of the Navy in answer to a Senate resolution of June 17, 1879, accompanying a copy of the report of the Board of Naval Engineer Officers in relation to plans and specifications of refrigerating ship and machinery. 8°. [*Washington*, 1879.]

——. Letter from the Secretary of the Navy, transmitting letter from the Superintendent of the Naval Observatory, relating to the status of assistant astronomers thereat. 8°. [*Washington*, 1884.]

——. Regulations governing the admission of candidates into the Naval Academy. [Signed Geo. M. Robeson, Secretary of the Navy.] 8°. [*n. p., n. d.*]

UNITED STATES. *Treasury Department.* Letter from the Secretary of the Treasury, transmitting, in compliance with Senate resolution, Jan. 16, 1884, the opinion of the Attorney-General of June 22, 1883, on the so-called longevity clauses of the naval appropriation acts of Aug. 5, 1882, and March 3, 1883. 8°. [*Washington*, 1884.]

Cleborne (C. J.) Recruiting in the Navy. San. & M. Rep. U. S. Navy 1873–4, Wash., 1875, 491–498. — **Maccoun** (R. T.) Sanitary condition of the U. S. Asiatic squadron during the period of two years from April 1, 1868, to March 31, 1870. Med. Essays, Bureau M. & S., U. S. Navy, Wash., 1872–3, i, 223–232.—**Walton** (T. C.) Report on the U. S. Naval Academy. Rep. Surg.-Gen. Navy, Wash., 1886, 122, 4 diag.

Navy (*United States, Medical Department of*).

ACT (An) to reorganize and increase the efficiency of the Medical Department of the Navy. fol. [*n. p., n. d.*]

BARTON (W. P. C.) A polemical remonstrance against the project of creating the new office of Surgeon-General in the Navy of the United States. 8°. *Philadelphia*, 1838.

——. Report [to the Secretary of the Navy, on the condition of the Medical Department of the Navy]. 8°. *Navy Department*, [*n. p.*], 1842.

——. Appeal [to the U. S. Senate, through the Hon. George Evans, chairman of the Committee of Finance]. 8°. [*n. p.*, 1843.]

BRIEF showing that it is contrary to law and wrong in principle to appoint a medical inspector, an officer of the second grade in the Medical Corps, to the office of Chief of Bureau of Medicine and Surgery in the Navy Department, instead of a medical director, an officer of the first grade, with the relative rank of captain in the Navy. 8°. [*Washington*, 1879?]

CASE (The) of Surgeon Green. [A conflict of authority between Dr. Green and Lieut. Commander Selfridge, of the U. S. steamer Nipsic.] 8°. [*n. p., n. d.*]

[CHLOROFORM.] Assimilated rank of the civil branch of the Navy. Jan. 17, 1848. 8°. [*n. p.*, 1848.]

[CLYMER (G.)] The principles of naval staff rank, with its history in the United States Navy for over half a century. [By a surgeon in the U. S. Navy.] 8°. [*n. p.*], 1869.

DISCIPLINE (The), harmony, and efficiency of the Navy. [Signed, A Senior Surgeon, U. S. Navy, Dec. 1, 1870.] 8°. [*Washington*, 1870?]

GIHON (A. L.) Thirty years of sanitary progress in the Navy; its present needs. The annual address before the Naval Medical Society, at the Museum of Hygiene, Washington, D. C., Jan. 4, 1884. 8°. *New York*, 1884.

Repr. from: United Service Mag., Feb., 1884.

LIST of the present medical directors of the Navy, on the active list (or officers of the first grade of the Medical Corps with the relative

Navy (*United States, Medical Department of*).

rank of captain), with a brief sketch of the service of each. 8°. [*Washington*, 1879?]

MEMBER (A). An exposition of the unjust and injurious relations of the U. S. Naval Medical Corps. 8°. *Baltimore*, 1842.

NAVAL staff rank. By a [U. S.] naval staff officer. 8°. [*n. p., n. d.*]

[RUSCHENBERGER (W. S. W.)] The Navy. Hints on the reorganization of the Navy, including an examination of the claims of its civil officers to an equality of rights. 8°. *New York*, 1845.

——. Naval. An examination of the legality of the general orders which confer assimilated rank on officers of the civil branch of the United States Navy. 8°. *Philadelphia*, 1848.

——. Naval. A brief history of an existing controversy on the subject of assimilated rank in the Navy of the United States. 8°. *Philadelphia*, 1850.

SHIPPEN (E.) Some account of the origin of the Naval Asylum at Philadelphia. 8°. [*Philadelphia*, 1883.]

UNITED STATES. *Congress. Senate.* A bill authorizing the appointment and retirement of John A. Lockwood as surgeon in the Navy of the United States. 48. Cong., 1. sess. S. 2317. June 16, 1884. Introd. by Mr. Miller. roy. 8°. [*Washington*, 1884.]

——. A bill to provide for the enlistment of apothecaries in the Navy and for other purposes. 48. Cong., 1. sess. S. 1637. Feb. 26, 1884. Introd. by Mr. Conger. roy. 8°. [*Washington*, 1884.]

UNITED STATES. *Navy Department. Bureau of Medicine and Surgery.* Instructions for the government of the medical officers of the Navy of the United States. 8°. *Washington*, 1844.

——. Instructions for the government of the medical officers of the Navy of the United States. 8°. *Washington*, 1864.

——. Extracts from the reports of the Chief of the Bureau of Medicine and Surgery, Navy Department, for 1863 and 1864. 8°. [*Washington*, 1865?]

——. Instructions to medical officers of the United States Navy. 8°. *Washington*, 1867.

——. The same. 8°. *Washington*, 1873.

——. The same. 12°. *Washington*, 1878.

——. The same. 8°. *Washington*, 1881.

——. The same. 8°. *Washington*, 1886.

——. Annual reports of the Surgeon-General of the Navy, for the years 1866–7; 1871–2; 1872–3; 1874–5 to 1878–9; 1880–81 to 1886–7. 8°. *Washington*, 1872–87.

1866–7, 1872–3, and 1874–5 in Reps. of the Secretary for the same years.

——. Medical essays; compiled from reports to the Bureau of Medicine and Surgery by medical officers of the U. S. Navy. 8°. *Washington*, 1872.

——. The same. 2. ed. 8°. *Washington*, 1873.

——. Special report of the Chief of Bureau of Medicine and Surgery of the Navy Department, on the difficulty of officering the Medical Corps of the Navy, its causes and the remedy. 8°. [*n. p., n. d.*]

——. [Blank forms in use.] v. s. [*Washington*, 188–.]

——. Circular for the information of persons desiring to enter the Medical Corps of the U. S. Navy. 8°. [*Washington*, 188–.]

VIEWS (The) of the Navy afford a strong argument for adhering to the "seniority rule" in filling the office of Surgeon-General. 8°. [*Washington*, 1879?]

Navy (*United States, Medical Department of*).

Davis (N. S.) On the rank and regulations of the medical staff of the U. S. Navy. Tr. Am. M. Ass., Phila., 1868, xix, 83.—**Horner** (F.), jr. The U. S. naval medical service Med. & Surg. Reporter, Phila., 1875, xxxii, 267. ———. The American naval medical service. *Ibid.*, 1877, xxxvii, 203-205.—**Kersey** (V.) Medical rank in the United States Navy. Tr. Indiana M. Soc., Indianap., 1870, 133-136.—**Report** of the committee on the rank of the medical officers of the Navy. Tr. Am. M. Ass., Phila., 1865, xvi, 583.—**Ruschenberger** (W. S. W.) The Naval Laboratory; error corrected. J. Am. M. Ass., Chicago, 1883, i, 279.—**Turner** (T. J.) Some considerations upon the Naval Retiring Board in its medico-legal relations. Rep. Surg.-Gen. Navy 1884, Wash., 1885, 268-275. *Also*, Reprint.—**Wood** (W. M.) Report upon the rank of the naval medical staff. Tr. Am. M. Ass., Phila., 1867. xviii, 285-295. *Also*, Reprint.—**Wood** (W. M.) & **Pinkney** (N.) Statement in relation to the United States Naval Medical Corps. Tr. Am. M. Ass., Phila., 1848, i, 301-304.

Nawrocki (Felix) [1838–]. * De Claudii Bernardi methodo oxygenii copiam in sanguine determinandi. 15 pp. 4°. *Vratislaviæ, typ. A. Neumanni*, [1863].
Bound with: HEER (H. C.) De ossium concretione, [etc.] 4°. *Vratislaviæ*, [1836].

———. Beiträge zum Stoffwechsel im Muskel. 1 l. 8°. [*Berlin, H. S. Hermann*, 1866.] [P., v. 794.]
Repr. from: Centralbl. f. d. med. Wissensch., Berl., 1866, iv.

———. Zur Kreatinfrage. 2 l. 8°. [*Berlin, H. S. Hermann*, 1866.] [P., v. 794.]
Repr. from: Centralbl. f. d. med. Wissensch., Berl., 1866, iv.

———. Beitrag zur Kenntniss des Blutfarbstoffs. 1 l. 8°. [*Berlin, H. S. Hermann*, 1867.] [P., v. 802.]
Repr. from: Centralbl. f. d. med. Wissensch., Berl., 1867, v.

———. Ueber die optischen Eigenschaften des Blutfarbstoffes. 3 l. 8°. [*Berlin, H. S. Hermann*, 1867.] [P., v. 794.]
Repr. from: Centralbl. f. d. med. Wissensch., Berl., 1867, v.

———. Raboti proizvedennija v phiziologicheskoi laboratorii Imper. Varshavskago Universiteta. 2 v. 198 pp., 1 l. 8°. *Warsaw*, 1873.

———. Ueber die quantitative Bestimmung des Kreatins in den Muskeln. 18 pp. 8°. [*n. p.*, 1876.] [P., v. 794.]
Repr. from: Ztschr. f. anal. Chem., Wiesb., 1876, xv.

Nayel (Charles). * De la néphrite. 27 pp. 4°. *Paris*, 1835, No. 297, v. 291.

Nayler (George). A practical and theoretical treatise on the diseases of the skin. xv, 292 pp., 7 pl. 8°. *London, J. Churchill & Sons*, 1866.
See, also, **Cottle** (E. Wyndham). The hair in health and disease. 12°. *London*, 1867.

Nayler (Richard). A cursory view of the treatment of ulcers, more especially those of the scrofulous, phagedænic, and cancerous description. With an appendix, on Baynton's new mode of treating old ulcers of the leg. ix (1 l.), 180 pp. 8°. *Glocester, R. Raikes*, 1800. [P., v. 705.]

Nayme (J. B. Y.) * Vox indicium in morbis. 11 pp. 4°. *Parisiis, an. XII* [1804], No. 144, v. E.

Nayrand (Auguste). * Des adénites inguinales et de leur importance dans l'étude des maladies vénériennes. 59 pp. 4°. *Paris*, 1862, No. 93.

Nayrod (F.-M.) * Sur la fièvre pernicieuse. vi, 7-33 pp. 4°. *Paris*, 1811, No. 52, v. 83.

Nazair (Gabriel). * Contributions à l'étude de l'ulcère simple de l'estomac. 55 pp. 4°. *Paris*, 1878, No. 344.

Nazaret (Garabet). * Essai de traitement chirurgical de la contracture permanente infantile. 34 pp., 1 pl. 4°. *Lyon*, 1885, No. 273.

Nazareth House, Hammersmith. Home of the aged poor, incurable orphans, and deserted infants. [Circular to the public.] 1 sheet. 8°. [*London, n. d.*]

Nazarre (Alberto). * Contribucion al estudio de la viruela hemorrágica y su tratamiento. 62 pp., 1 l. roy. 8°. *Buenos Aires, imp. del Porvenir*, 1884.

Neal (Daniel) [1678–1743]. A narrative of the method and success of inoculating the small-pox in New England, by Mr. Benj. Colman. With a reply to the objections made against it from principles of conscience in a letter from a minister at Boston [Rev. Wm. Cooper]. To which is now prefixed an historical introduction. 48 pp. 8°. *London, E. Matthews & R. Ford*, 1722.

Neal (E.) Diet for the sick and convalescent. viii, 59 pp. 8°. *Philadelphia, J. Challen & Son*, 1861.

———. The same. 52 pp. 8°. *Philadelphia, J. Challen & Son*, 1864.

Neal (Stephen). Special report on the state of juvenile education and delinquency in the borough of Salford. Dedicated, by permission, to Thos. Agnew, esq., mayor of that borough. To which is added an appendix, containing observations on the state of crime in Salford, and in the country generally; on ragged or industrial schools, and on reformatory institutions for criminals; and in which are also noticed the schemes of education proposed by the National Public School Association, and the committee of the Manchester and Salford municipal boroughs' educational bill. 29 pp. 8°. *Salford, W. F. Jackson*, 1851.

Neal (*Thomas L.*) [1830–85].
Conn (G. P.) Obituary. Am. Pub. Health Ass. Rep. 1885, Concord, N. H., 1886, xi, 399.—**Obituary.** Tr. Ohio M. Soc., Columbus, 1885, 209.

Neale (A. J.) Facts about the skin. 19 pp. 12°. *Manchester & London, Deansgate & Ridgefield*, 1884.

Neale (Adam) [–1832]. * De acido nitrico, ejusque in medicina usibus. 24 pp. 8°. *Edinburgi, excud. A. Neill et socii*, 1802. [P., v. 23.]

———. Researches respecting the natural history, chemical analysis, and medicinal virtues of the spur, or ergot of rye, when administered as a remedy in certain states of the uterus viii, 105 pp., 1 l., 1 pl. 8°. *London, H. Phillips*, 1828.

———. Researches to establish the truth of the Linnæan doctrine of animate contagions; wherein the origin, causes, mode of diffusion, and cure of epidemic diseases, spasmodic cholera, dysentery, plague, small-pox, hooping cough, leprosy, etc., are illustrated by facts from the natural history of mankind, of animals, and of vegetables, and from the phenomena of the atmosphere. 1 p. l., viii, 258 pp., 1 pl. 8°. *London, Longman* [*and others*], 1831.

———. A letter to a professor of medicine, in the University of Edinburgh, respecting the nature and properties of the mineral waters of Cheltenham. viii, 9-40 pp. 8°. *London, J. Swan*, [*n. d.*]
See, also, **Assalini** (Paul). Observations on the disease called plague, [etc.] 8°. *New York*, 1806.—**Halpin** (Wm. Henry), jr. Fact versus assertion, [etc.] 8°. *London*, 1820.

Neale (George). Some observations on the use of the agaric, and its insufficiency in stopping hæmorrhages after capital operations, in a letter to a surgeon in the country. 50 pp. 8°. *London, J. Robinson*, 1757.
See, also, **Memoirs** of the Royal Academy of Surgery at Paris. 3 v. sm. 8°. *London*, 1759.

Neale (Henry St. John). Practical observations on venereal complaints, or a plain, easy, safe, and certain method of cure, without endangering the constitution with mercury. An efficacious mode of curing gleets, seminal or venereal, and every other malady of the urinary passage; with a new remedy, [etc.] viii, 133 pp. 8°. *London, G. Burnett*, 1786.

Neale (Henry St. John)—continued.

———. The same. 6. ed. xiv (1 l.), xiii, 259 pp. 8°. *London, the author*, 1793. [P., v. 815.]

———. Practical dissertations on nervous complaints, and other diseases incident to the human body; with an historical investigation of their causes and cure; in which are interspersed some singular cases. 1 p. l., x, 68 pp. 8°. *London, printed for the author*, 1788. [*Also, in :* P., v. 711.]

———. The same. Practische Abhandlung über die Nervenkrankheiten. Aus dem Englischen übersetzt. xvi, 72 pp. 16°. *Berlin, Petit u. Schöne*, 1790.

———. Practical essays and remarks on that species of consumption incident to youth, and the different stages of life, commonly called tabes dorsalis; with an account of the nature, causes, and cure of that distemper and the diseases arising therefrom, especially the nervous atrophia and the phthisis, or consumption in general. To which are added, extracts from the works of the most distinguished practitioners of the present and former ages, coinciding with the author's own practice and experience, demonstrating the baneful effects of unnatural venery on the finest functions in the animal œconomy. xiii, 223 pp. 8°. *London*, 1800.

———. Chirurgical institutes, drawn from practice, on the knowledge and treatment of gunshot wounds. Illustrated with some singular cases and cures of gallant warriors. xxii, 295 pp. 8°. *London, T. Jones*, 1804.

———. The same. 2. ed. xxii, 295 pp. 8°. *London, T. Egerton*, 1805.

Neale (Richard). The medical digest, being a means of ready reference to the principal contributions to medical science during the last thirty years. xiii, 650 pp. 8°. *London, New Sydenham Society*, 1877.

———. The same. 2. ed. 5 p. l., 643, lxxxii pp. 8°. *London, Ledger, Smith & Co.*, 1882.

———. The chemical lung, as adapted to purify the air of large buildings, without causing draught, by fan and tank. 1 sheet. fol. [*London*, 1882.]

———. The same. Chemical lung and punkah. For sick rooms, hot climates, crowded buildings, and railway tunnels. 2 l. fol. [*London*, 1882.]

———. The first appendix to the Medical digest, including the years 1882–5, and early part of 1886. 2 p. l., 218, xxxiii pp. 8°. *London, Ledger, Smith & Co.*, 1886.

Neander (Jean) [1596–]. Tabacologia: hoc est tabaci, seu nicotianæ, descriptio medico-chirurgico - pharmaceutica, vel ejus præparatio et usus in omnibus ferme corporis humani incommodis. 16 p. l., 256 pp., 9 pl. 4°. *Lugd. Bat., ex off. J. Elzeviri*, 1626.

———. The same. Traicté du tabac, ou nicotiane, panacée, petun: autrement, herbe à la reyne, avec sa préparation et son usage pour la plus part des indispositions du corps humain; ensemble les diverses façons de le falsifier, et les marques pour le recognoistre; composé première-ment en latin . . . et mis de nouveau en françois, par I. V. 3 p. l., 342 pp., 9 pl. 12°. *Lyon, B. Vincent*, 1626.

For Biography, see Biogr. Skizzen verstorb. Bremisch. Aerzte, Bremen, 1844, 95–98.

Neander (Michael) [1529–81]. Lapidis indago totius philosophiæ et magiæ naturalis unica et præcipue margarita. MS. 81. 4°. [*n. p., n. d.*]

Neanderthal *skull.*
  See **Craniology.**

Neatby (T.) Homœopathy; a lecture delivered in Myddelton Hall, Islington, August 19, 1862, entitled "The social importance of homœopathy". 32 pp. 8°. *London, Leath & Ross*, [1862]. [*Also, in :* P., v. 1187.]

Neath.

AIRY (H.) Report to the Local Government Board on the sanitary state of the Neath registration district. Aug. 11, 1877. fol. [*London*, 1877.]

Nebe (Franciscus Carolus) [1823–]. * De gangræna pulmonum. 32 pp. 8°. *Berolini, G. Schade*, [1846].

Nebe (Franciscus Jos.) [1796–]. * De psychica dignitate cutis. 82 pp. 8°. *Bonnæ, ex off. Thormannia*, 1823.

Nebel. Ueber einige im allgemeinen Krankenhause in Hamburg mittelst der Sayre'schen Behandlungsmethode erzielte Resultate. 8 pp. 8°. *Berlin, G. Reimer*, [1886].

  Repr. from : Deutsche med. Wchnschr., Berl., 1886, xl.

Nebel (Christophorus Ludovicus) [1738–90]. * De mola seu conceptu fatuo. 40 pp. 4°. *Giessæ, ex off. Brauniana*, [1761].

———. [Pr.] dissertationem suam de secali cornuto a temerariis et contumeliosis objectionibus D. D. Schlegeri vindicat. 16 pp. 4°. *Giessæ, typ. Schroederianis*, [1772].

———. [Pr.] de aëris effectu in morbis chirurgicis disserit et observationes suas proponit. [Cum vita candidati Ludovici Gustavi Wagner.] 12 pp. 4°. *Giessæ, ex off. Brauniana*, 1780.

Nebel (Conrad David). * Hippocratis doctrina semiotica de spasmis atque convulsionibus. 40 pp., 1 l. 12°. *Marburgi Cattorum, ex off. nova typogr. academica*, [1791].

Nebel (Daniel) [1664–1733].

  Memoria Nebeliana. Acta Acad. nat. curios., Norimb., 1742, vi (app.), 159–179, port.

  Portrait in : **Collection**—van Kaathoven.

Nebel (Daniel) & **Wepfer** (Bernardinus). De medicamentis chalybeatis. *Heidelbergæ*, 1711.

  In : HALLER. Disp. ad morb. [etc.] 4°. *Lausannæ*, 1760, vii, 165–180.

Nebel (Daniel. Guilielmus Henricus). * Diss. exhibens observationem duorum aneurysmatum rariorum, quorum alterum ex arcu aortæ, alterum ex arteria corporis callosi ortum est. 46 pp., 5 pl. 4°. *Heidelbergæ, G. Reichard*, 1834.

Nebel (Daniel. Wilhelmus) [1735–1805]. * De electricitatis usu medico. 2 p. l., 58 pp. 4°. *Heidelbergæ, J. J. Haener*, [1758].

———. Fœtus ossei per quinquaginta quatuor annos extra uterum in abdomine detenti historia. pp. 403–422, 6 pl. 4°. [*Heidelbergæ*, 1767.] Cutting.

———. [Pr.] de paralysi artuum tum superiorum tum inferiorum electricitatis ope sanata. [Cum vita candidati Francisci Jacobi Schwarz.] 3 l. 4°. [*Heidelbergæ*, 1778.]

———. [Pr.] de ulcere prope umbilicum sinnoso, in ventriculum penetrante, ex quo alimenta effluebant. [Cum vita candidati Guilielmi Ludovici Hoffmann.] 3 l. 4°. [*Heidelbergæ*, 1782.]

———. [Pr.] de apoplexia ex abscessu cerebri lethali. [Cum vita candidati Michael Joseph. Wolfg. Steinbach.] 3 l. 4°. [*Heidelbergæ*, 1790.]

———. [Pr.] ad nuper editam observationem de apoplexia ex abscessu cerebri lethali continuatio ii. de abscessibus cerebri a causa externa ortis. [Cum vita candidati Ferdinandi Henrici Schmitt.] 3 l. 4°. [*Heidelbergæ*, 1790.]

———. The same. Continuatio iii. [Cum vita candidati Ferdin. Antonii Bernard. Heuser.] 3 l. 4°. [*Heidelbergæ*, 1791.]

Nebel (Ernestus Ludovicus Wilhelmus) [1772–1854]. Antiquitates morborum cutaneorum. 32 pp. 4°. *Giessæ, J. W. Braun*, [1793].

———. De morbis veterum obscuris. 47 pp. 8°. *Giessæ*, 1794.

———. De nosologia brutorum cum hominum morbis comparata. 80 pp., 1 l. 8°. *Giessæ, J. W. Braun*, [1798].

Nebel (Ernestus Ludovicus Wilhelmus)—cont'd.
———. [Professores Giessenses.] 26 pp. 4°. *Giessæ, J. W. Braun*, 1802.

Nebel (F.) Die Muskeln, Knochen und Bänder des menschlichen Körpers. Vorwort, Revision und Neuordnung des Textes von Dr. J. Herm. Baas. 2. Aufl. 7 l., 6 pl. imp. fol. *Tübingen*, 1885.

Nebel (*Guilielmus Bernardus*) [1699–1748].
Memoria. Acta Acad. nat. curios., Norimb., 1752, ix (app.), 209–226, port.

Nebel (Hermann) [1853–]. * Ueber die desmoiden und adenoiden Geschwülste der Mamma. 26 pp., 1 l. 8°.. *Bonn, C. Georgi*, 1877.

———. Die Behandlung der Rückgratsverkrümmungen mittelst des Sayre'schen Gypscorsets und "Jury-masts" und im "Holzcuirass" des Dr. Phelps.
In: SAMML. klin. Vortr., Leipz., 1886, No. 277–278 (Chir., No. 86, 2511–2604).

———. Ueber Heilgymnastik und Massage.
In: SAMML. klin. Vortr., Leipz., 1886, No. 286 (Innere Med., No. 98, 2641–2660).

———. Briefe aus Schweden. 17 pp. 8°. *Berlin u. Leipzig, G. Thieme*, 1887.
Repr. from: Deutsche med. Wchnschr., Berl., 1887, xiii.

Nebel (Joh. Henricus). Physiologiæ biblicæ selecta quædam capita breviter ac strictim illustrata. 34 pp. 4°. *Giessæ Hassorum, lit. vid. B. J. R. Vulpii*, [1711].

Nebel (*N.*) [1785–1841].
Portrait in: **Collection**—van Kaathoven.

Nebel (Wilhelm).
See **Wernher** (Adolph). Die angeborenen Kysten-Hygrome und die ihnen verwandten Geschwülste, etc. Denkschrift zur Feier des 50jährigen Doctor-Jubiläums des . . . 4°. *Giessen*, 1843.

Nebelung (Henricus Otto) [1831–]. * De functionum perturbationibus per hemiplegiam nervorum systemati illatis et exemplo demonstratis. 28 pp., 2 l. 8°. *Berolini, typ. fratrum Schlesinger*, [1855].

Neber (Heinrich). * Beitrag zur spontanen Aortenruptur. 20 pp.; 1 tab., 1 pl. 4°. *Kiel, C. F. Mohr*, 1879.
In: SCHRIFT. d. Univ. zu Kiel, xxvi, 1879, vii, Med. ix.

Nebinger (Andrew) [1819–86]. Variola; its nature and treatment. With an addendum. [Discussion.] (Read before the Phila. Co. Med. Society, Nov., 1857.) 35 pp. 8°. *Philadelphia, Collins*, 1862.

———. Small-pox; its pathology and treatment. 25 pp. 8°. *Philadelphia, Collins*, 1865.
Repr. from: Tr. Am. M. Ass., Phila., 1865, xvi.

———. Biography of William Darrach, M. D. 24 pp. 8°. *Philadelphia, Collins*, 1867.

———. Criminal abortion; its extent and prevention. 32 pp. 8°. *Philadelphia, Collins*, 1870.

———. An address delivered before the Medical Society of the State of Pennsylvania at its annual meeting held at Altoona, May, 1880. 19 pp. 8°. *Philadelphia*, 1880.
Repr. from: Tr. M. Soc. Penn , Phila., 1880, xiii, pt. 1.
For Biography, see **Grove** (J. H.) Biography of Andrew Nebinger. 12°. *Philadelphia*, 1887. *See, also,* Med. & Surg. Reporter, Phila., 1886, liv, 584.

Nebinger (Lothar). * Ueber Brüche der Patella. 28 pp. 8°. *Würzburg, F. E. Thein*, 1870.

Nèble (E.) [1852–]. * Considérations sur les causes, le siège et la classification des coxalgies. 34 pp. 4°. *Paris*, 1881, No. 368.

Nebler (Carl) [1856–]. * Ueber Varicocele und deren chirurgische Behandlung. 43 pp. 8°. *Breslau, Lindner*, 1880.

Nebout (Adolphe). * Sur le scorbut observé à bord de la frégate la Vénus, pendant la cam-

Nebout (Adolphe)—continued.
pagne qu'elle a faite autour du monde dans les années 1837, 1838 et 1839. 42 pp., 1 tab. 4°. *Paris*, 1840, No. 142, v. 363.

Nebout (Georges). * De l'action des moyens considérés comme préventifs de la pyohémie. 55 pp. 4°. *Paris*, 1873, No. 190.

Nebout (Joseph). * Étude sur la grippe. 71 pp. 4°. *Paris*, 1876, No. 185.

Nébout-Lapinolie (François-Louis). * Sur le catarrhe pulmonaire aigu. 17 pp. 4°. *Paris*, 1822, No. 6, v. 170.

Neboux. Projet d'organisation de l'assistance publique dans la ville de Paris limité au service des secours à domicile, service dirigé actuellement par l'administration des bureaux de bienfaisance; suivi d'un projet d'une nouvelle organisation du service médical des indigents dépendant de la même administration. 47 pp. 8°. *Paris, N. Chaix & Cie.*, 1850.

Neboux (Jean-Simon). * Sur la phthisie en général, ou les maladies de consomption; avec une nouvelle méthode de classification par ordres, genres et espèces de ces maladies. 69 pp. 4°. *Paris, an XII* [1804], No. 325, v. 51.

Nebraska.

UNITED STATES. *Department of the Interior. Land Office.* Final report of the United States Geological Survey of Nebraska and portions of the adjacent Territories, made under the direction of the Commissioner of the General Land Office. By F. V. Hayden, United States geologist, March 23, 1871. Ordered to be printed. H. of Rep. 42. Cong., 1. sess. Ex. Doc. No. 19. 8°. *Washington*, 1871.
Peabody (J. H.) Climatology and diseases of Nebraska. Tr. Am. M. Ass., Phila., 1875, xxvi, 357–369.—
Report of committee on climatology and prevailing diseases of Nebraska. Tr. Nebraska M. Soc., Lincoln, 1877, 207–221.

Nebraska. *Nebraska Institution for the Blind, Nebraska City.* Biennial report of the principal to the governor of the State. 2., 1877–8. 13 pp. 8°. *Lincoln, Neb., Journal Co.*, 1879.

Nebraska. *Nebraska Institute for the Deaf and Dumb, Omaha.* Biennial report of the board of directors and officers to the governor of State. 4.–5., 1873–6. 8°. *Omaha, by the pupils*, 1875–7.

Nebraska. *University of Nebraska. College of Medicine, Lincoln.* Annual announcement and catalogue for the session of 1886–7 (4.). 16 pp. 12°. *Lincoln, King & Dobbins*, 1886.

Nebraska. *University of Nebraska. Patho-Biological Laboratory.* [Circular letter of the director, calling attention to the objects of the laboratory. Established for original research into the nature and causes of contagious and infectious diseases of animals. Nov. 28, 1887.] 1 sheet. 4°. [*Lincoln*, 1887.]

Nebraska Medical Journal. An eclectic monthly. W. S. Latta, editor; associate editors, E. B. Guild and J. M. Keys. v. 1, Jan. to Dec., 1884. 288 pp. 8°. *Lincoln*.

Nebraska State Medical Society. Proceedings of the convention for the organization of . . . held in Omaha, June 24, 1868. 28 pp. 8°. *Omaha*, 1868.
Bound with: Transactions.

———. Transactions. 1.–19., 1869–87, in 7 v. 8°. *Lincoln & Omaha*, 1869–87.

Nebreda y Lopez (Carlos). Memoria relativa á las enseñanzas especiales de los sordo-mudos y de los ciegos, premiada con medalla de plata en la exposicion Aragonesa de 1868. viii p. l., 218 pp., 5 l. 8°. *Madrid, imp. del Colegio nacional de sordo-mudos y de ciegos*, 1870.

Nebykoff (V. I.) O trichinach i trichinozno bolezni. [On trichinæ and trichinous diseases.]

Nebykoff (V. I.)—continued.
ii, 72 pp., 2 pl. 8°. *Charkoff, tip. A. Lappe,* 1886.

Neccerus (Carolus Ludovicus). * De fame canina. 24 pp. 4°. *Francof. ad Viadr., C. Zeitlen,* [1691].

Neck.

See, also, **Artery** (*Subclavian*); **Fascia**.

Ask (C. J.) * Halsens chirurgiska Anatomi. 8°. *Lund,* 1858.

Burns (A.) Observations on the surgical anatomy of the head and neck . . . and additional cases and observations by Granville S. Pattison. 8°. *Glasgow,* 1824.

———. The same. Bemerkungen über die chirurgische Anatomie des Kopfes und Halses. Aus dem Englischen übersetzt und mit Anmerkungen begleitet von Georg Eduard Dohlhoff. Nebst einer Vorrede von Johann Friedrich Meckel. 8°. *Halle,* 1821.

Cunningham (D. J.) The dissector's guide; being a manual for the use of students. Head and neck. 8°. *Edinburgh,* 1887.

Degrusse (C.-G.) *Aponévrologie du cou. 4°. *Paris,* 1849.

Dittel (L.) Die Topographie der Halsfascien. 8°. *Wien,* 1857.

Dotter (A.) * Die Regio thyreo-hyoidea des menschlichen Halses. 8°. *Tübingen,* 1871.

Gimelle (L.-L.-J.) *Anatomie chirurgicale de la région sus-hyoïdienne. 4°. *Paris,* 1848.

Michel (M.) Effects consequent upon the section of the posterior muscles on the neck, with a short history of the cerebro-spinal fluid. 8°. [*n. p., n. d.*]

Poulsen (K.) * Om Fascierne og de interfasciale Rum på Halsen. 4°. *Kjøbenhavn,* 1884.

Robert (A.-A.-J.) * Recherches anatomiques sur le cou. 4°. *Strasbourg,* 1840.

Zuckerkandl (E.) Ueber eine bisher noch nicht beschriebene Drüse in der Regio suprahyoidea. 8°. *Stuttgart,* 1879.

Brown-Séquard. Sur divers effets d'irritation de la partie antérieure du cou et, en particulier, la perte de la sensibilité et la mort subite. Compt. rend. Acad. d. sc., Par., 1887, civ, 951–954. *Also, transl.:* Wien. med. Bl., 1887, x, 495.—**Colson.** Le muscle tenseur de l'aponévrose cervicale superficielle. Ann. Soc. de méd. de Gand, 1887, lxvi, 63–66.—**Foltz.** Note sur les fonctions des muscles peauciers du cou. Rev. méd. franç. et étrang., Par., 1852, i, 138–148.—**Froriep** (A.) Ueber den Hautmuskel des Halses und seine Beziehung zu den unteren Gesichtsmuskeln. Arch. f. Anat. u. Physiol., Leipz., 1877, 46–62.—**Gillette.** Cou (anatomie). Dict. encycl. d. sc. méd., Par., 1877, xxi, 140–165.—**Gruber** (V.) Ligamentum hyo-thyreoideum accessorium. Med. Vestnik, St. Petersb., 1868, viii, 222. —— O mishtsakh nizhnyago kraya shchitovidnago khryashcha. [On the inferior marginal thyroid muscles.] *Ibid.,* 244. —— Ueber den Musculus atlantico-mastoideus. Arch. f. Anat., Physiol. u. wissensch. Med., Leipz., 1876. 733–738, 1 pl. —— Ein Musculus cleido-epistrophicus bei Existenz des Musculus cleido-mastoideus der Norm. *Ibid.,* 739–745, 1 pl. ——. Ein Musculus cleido-cervicalis s. trachelo-clavicularis imus. *Ibid.,* 757. ——. Vorkommen des Musculus cleido-mastoideus als Musculus cleido-epistrophicus. *Ibid.,* 759. ——. Ein Musculus cleido-atlanticus. *Ibid.,* 761.—**His.** Zur Entwicklungsgeschichte des menschlichen Halses. Cor.-Bl. d. deutsch. Gesellsch. f. Anthrop., etc., München, 1886, xvii, 23; 27. *Also:* Memorabilien, Heilbr., 1886, n. F., vi, 193–198. —— Ueber den Sinus præcervicalis und über die Thymusanlage. Arch. f. Anat. u. Entwicklngsgesch., Leipz., 1886, 421–433, 1 pl.—**Jannuzzi** (G.) Indagare e descrivere quale sia la reale disposizione delle fasce (aponevrosi) nella regione anterolaterale del collo, deducendone le possibili conseguenze fisiologiche e pratiche. Spallanzani, Modena, 1879, 2. s., viii, 193–231.—**Kadyi** (H.) O grucz łach tarczykowych dodatkowych w okolicy gnykowéj (glandulæ præhyoideæ et suprahyoideæ). Rozpr. . . . wydz. matemat.-przyr. Akad. Umiej. w Krakow., 1880, vi, 129–142, 1 pl. — **de Koning** (P.) Een nieuw ontdekte klier. Nederl. Tijdschr. v. Geneesk.. Amst., 1879, 2. R., xv, 267–269. — **Krause** (W.) Der M. coracocervicalis. Internat. Monatschr. f. Anat. u. Histol., Berl., 1885, ii, 262. — **Lemoigne** (A.) Fisiologia; intorno ai fenomeni di alterata locomozione in conseguenza del taglio dei muscoli della

Neck.

nuca. R. Ist. Lomb. di sc. e lett. Rendic., Milano, 1870, 2. s., iii, 386–394.—**Peli** (G.) Sulla relativa lunghezza del collo in ambo i sessi, e sulla disposizione da darsi al capo nelle ricerche antropometriche. Mem. Accad. d. sc. d. Ist. di Bologna, 1882, 4. s., iv, 377–393.—**Pilcher** (L. S.) The anatomy of the anterior median region of the neck, with especial reference to the operation of tracheotomy in children. Ann. Anat. & Surg., Brooklyn, 1881, iii, 145–175, 1 pl.—**Poulsen** (K.) Ueber die Fascien und die interfascialen Räume des Halses. Deutsche Ztschr. f. Chir., Leipz., 1885-6, xxiii, 223–272, 2 pl. — **Rabl** (C.) Zur Bildungsgeschichte des Halses. Prag. med. Wchnschr., 1886, xi, 497–499; 1887, xii, 3. *Also:* Wien. med. Wchnschr., 1887, xxxvii, 43.—**Ruge** (G.) Die vom Facialis innervirten Muskeln des Halses, Nackens und des Schädels eines jungen Gorilla (Gesichtsmuskeln). Morphol. Jahrb., Leipz., 1887, xii, 459–529, 1 pl.—**Sarazin** (C.) Cou. N. dict. de méd. et chir. prat., Par., 1869, ix, 597–666 . — **Schadewaldt.** Ueber die Localisation der Empfindungen in den Halsorganen. Deutsche med. Wchnschr., Leipz.. 1887, xiii, 709; 733. — **Schmidtmüller.** Beschreibung eines seltenen Halsmuskels. Arch. f. d. Physiol., Halle, 1807-8, viii, 269.—**Törnblom** (P. A.) En ny muskel på halsen hos menniskan (M. transversalis cervicis medius). Förh. v. de skandin. Naturf., Stockholm, 1865, 603–605.—**Zuckerkandl** (E.) Beitrag zur descriptiven und topographischen Anatomie des unteren Halsdreieckes. Ztschr. f. Anat. u. Entwcklngsgesch., Leipz., 1876, ii, 54–68, 1 pl.

Neck (*Abnormities of*).

See, also, **Fistula** (*Cervical*).

Buttersack (P.) Congenitale Knorpelreste am Halse. Arch. f. path. Anat., etc., Berl., 1886, cvi, 206–208.—**Chiarugi** (G.) Varietà muscolari della nuca e del dorso. Boll. d. Soc. tra i cult. d. sc. med. in Siena, 1886, iv, 68–77. — **Fernandez Osuna** (L.) Un caso notable de vitia congénita. Prensa méd. de Granada, 1882, iv, 8–13.—**Kobylinski** (O.) Ueber eine flughautähnliche Ausbreitung am Halse. Arch. f. Anthrop., Brnschwg., 1883, xiv, 343–348, 1 pl. — **Muirhead** (J. B.) Abnormality of neck. Brit. M. J., Lond., 1887, ii, 177.—**Paulicky** (A.) Angeborner, kiemendeckelähnlicher Hautanhang an der rechten Halsseite. Deutsche mil.-ärztl. Ztschr., Berl., 1882, xi, 270–273. *Also, in his:* Ueber congen. Missbild., 8°, Berl., 1882, 48–51. — **Sangalli** (G.) Patologia; altro fatto di cattiva conformazione dell' atlante, qual causa di torcicollo congenito. R. Ist. Lomb. di sc. e lett. Rendic., Milano, 1870, 2. s., iii, 515–518.

Neck (*Abscess, cellulitis, and phlegmon of*).

See, also, **Abscess** (*Pharyngeal, etc.*); **Abscess** *connected with blood-vessels*; **Arteries** (*Carotid, Ligature of*); **Glottis** (*Œdema of*); **Laryngotomy,** *etc.*; **Scarlatina** (*Complications, etc., of*).

Boehler (G.) * Étude critique sur l'angine de Ludwig. 4°. *Paris,* 1885.

Castelain (F.) *Phlegmasies et abcès sous le muscle sterno-mastoïdien. 4°. *Paris,* 1869.

Caulet (E.-E.-J.) Remarques sur un cas de périœsophagite. 4°. *Paris,* 1864.

Charbol. * De l'angine dite de Ludwig. 4°. *Paris,* 1887.

Delobel (J.) * Contribution à l'étude de abcès chroniques de la région sous-hyoïdienne. 4°. *Paris,* 1887.

Descubes (M.-É.) *Phlegmons diffus cervicaux d'origine dentaire. 4°. *Paris,* 1881.

Dumesthé (V.) * Abcès sous le sterno-cléidomastoïdien. 4°. *Paris,* 1864.

Follet (A.) * De l'adénite cervicale considérée chez les militaires. 4°. *Paris,* 1844.

Hernandes (D.) * Des abcès du cou. 4°. *Paris,* 1870.

Houllion (C.) * Contributions à l'étude de l'angine de Ludwig. 8°. *Strasbourg,* 1875.

Jacquey (V.-E.) * Des complications des phlegmons de la région carotidienne. 4°. *Paris,* 1876.

Kurzwelly (T.) * De angina sic dicta Ludwigii. 8°. *Lipsiæ,* 1856.

Landauer (I.) * Die brandige Zellgewebsverhärtung am Halse. 8°. *Tübingen,* 1849.

Levin (J.) *Paristhmitidis acutæ seu anginæ externæ Ludvigii historia. 8°. *Berolini,* [1839].

Neck (*Abscess, cellulitis, and phlegmon of*).

SCHÜTZENMEISTER (C. T. F.) * De phlegmone colli typhosa. 8°. *Lipsiæ*, 1847.

SCHULTZ (A.) * De angina Ludovici, addita morbi historia. 24 pp. 8°. *Gryphiæ*, 1865.

SICARD (M.-J.) * Étude sur les phlegmons et abcès de la région sterno-mastoïdienne. 4°. *Montpellier*, 1879.

STANZL (A.) * Ueber Ludwig'sche Halsbinde-gewebsentzündung. 8°. *München*, 1880.

Adams (C.) Deep cervical abscess. Med. Era, Chicago, 1883–4, i, 292–296.—**Advena.** Zellgewebeverhärtung des Halses (Induratio telæ cellulosæ colli, auch Pseudo-erysipelas subtendinosum colli Ludwigi genannt). Med. Ztg., Berl., 1842, xi, 209.—**Agnew.** Abscess simulating aneurism. Med. & Surg. Reporter, Phila., 1867, xvii, 374.—**Ascesso** acuto profondo della regione laterale sinistra del collo; doppia incisione; guarigione. Clin. chir. (Mazzoni), Roma, 1884, viii-x, 2.—**Ascesso** profondo flemmoso nella fossa sopra claviculare sinistra; apertura e contro apertura dell'ascesso; guarigione. *Ibid.*, 5.—**Atlee** (W. F.) Deep-seated abscess in the neck. Tr. Coll. Phys. Phila. (1863-74), 1874, n. s., iv, 463. *Also*: Am. J. M. Sc., Phila., 1873, n. s., lxvi, 140.—**Barker** (A.) Two cases of angina Ludovici. Lancet, Lond., 1885, ii, 571.—**Bauche.** Observation d'un flegmon sous-cutané par cause traumatique, développé au niveau de la région antérieure et latérale droite du cou. Bull. Soc. méd.-prat. de Par., 1851-2, 136–141.—**Becker.** Phlegmone colli. Med. Ztg., Berl., 1860, n. F., iii, 166.—**Bermann.** Fall einer tödtlich abgelaufenen Halsentzündung eigenthümlicher Art. Wchnschr. f. d. ges. Heilk., Berl., 1840, 740–744.—**Bertels** (E.) Phlegmone diffusum colli, s. cynanche sublingualis, s. angina Ludwigii. Protok. zasaid. Obsh. russk. vrach. v St. Petersb., 1874, xli, 319–321. *Also, transl.* [Rhst.]: Gaz. lek., Warszawa, 1875, xix, 4.—**Bertherand** (A.) Adénites cervicales idiopathiques, suppurées, traitées avec succès au moyen de l'injection iodée. Gaz. méd. de l'Algérie, Alger, 1876, xxi, 85–87.—**Bickersteth** (E. R.) [Abscess of the neck mistaken for tumor.] Assoc. M. J., Lond., 1863, i, 225. ———. Clinical observations on sub-maxillary cellulitis. Liverpool M. & S. Rep., Lond., 1869, iii, 96–111. *Also, Reprint.*—**Binaut.** Abcès profond du cou ouvert spontanément dans la trachée-artère et artificiellement par la peau; phénomènes asphyxiques très graves survenant consécutivement au développement de végétations à la partie supérieure de la trachée et nécessitant la trachéotomie. Prodige homœopathique! Bull. méd. du nord, Lille, 1863, 2. s., iv, 191–212.—**Blasberg.** Einige Fälle von sogenannter Cynanche typhodes (Dr. von Ludwig), die auf eine eigenthümliche Weise glücklich behandelt wurden. Wchnschr. f. d. ges. Heilk., Berl., 1846, 752–760.—**Bœhler.** Des phlegmons du cou appelés angines de Ludwig. Paris méd., 1886, 2. s., xi, 241.—**Bouqué** (E.-F.) [Un abcès du cou qui s'est terminé par la mort.] *In his*: Clin. chirurg. de l'Univ. de Gand, 8°, 1877, 25.—**Breithaupt.** Ueber die tiefliegenden Abscesse hinter dem Winkel des Unterkiefers. Med. Ztg., Berl., 1859, n. F., ii, 151; 167; 175.—**Brinton** (J. H.) Deep cervical abscess. Med. & Surg. Reporter, Phila., 1873, xxviii, 439–441.—**Broca.** Phlegmon du cou développé autour de ganglions cancéreux; œdème et couleur rosée de la peau; signe de suppuration profonde; nécessité d'inciser de très-bonne heure. J. de méd. et chir., Par., 1874, xlv, 446.—**Bucerius.** Brand des Zellgewebes am Hals. Wchnschr. f. d. ges. Heilk., Berl., 1839, 842.—**Burg** (J.) Von einem mit Wind erfüllten Schwamme am Hals. Auserl. med.- chir. . . . Abhandl. d. röm.-kais. Akad. d. Naturf, Nürnb., 1770, xix, 241.—**Camerer.** Ein Beitrag zur Geschichte derjenigen Form von Halsentzündung, welche Herr Leibmedicus v. Ludwig zuerst beschrieben hat. Med. Cor.-Bl. d. württemb. ärztl. Ver., Stuttg., 1837, vii, 73–78.—**Campbell** (F. R.) A case of cervical abscess. Buffalo M. & S. J., 1883-4, xxiii, 221.—**Cantani.** Meningo-mielite consecutiva ad ascesso della nuca. Morgagni, Napoli, 1878, xx, 308–315.—**Cartouli** (É.) Κακοήθης κυνάγχη. Angina Ludovici; cynanche cellularis maligna. Γαληνός, Ἀθῆναι, 1880, Γ', 113–117. *Also, transl.*: Paris méd., 1879-80, 2. s., v, 385–387.—**Charcellay.** Abcès du cou communiquant à l'intérieur avec les voies aériennes. Gaz. d. hôp., Par., 1855, xxviii, 255.—**Chassaignac.** Abcès profonds à la partie inférieure du cou; abcès qui siégent derrière le corps thyroïde; guérison; quelques principes pour l'ouverture de ces abcès; considérations pratiques sur le diagnostic et la marche de ces abcès. *Ibid.*, 1843, 2. s., v, 535.—**Cheever** (D. W.) Deep abscess of the neck. Boston M. & S. J., 1880, ciii, 390. *Also*: Extr. Rec. Bost. Soc. M. Improve. (1880-82), 1883, viii, pp. xlvi-xlviii.—**Cholshevnikoff.** Sluchai anginæ Ludovici. Protok. zasaid. Obsh. Morsk. vrach. v Kronstadt, 1883, 56-61.—**Cless,** jun. Ein Beitrag zur Ludwig'-schen Halsentzündung. Med. Cor.-Bl. d. württemb. ärztl. Ver., Stuttg., 1839, ix, 28.—**Cnopf.** Ein Fall von Cynanche sublingualis rheumatico-typhoides. Deutsche Klinik, Berl., 1849, i, 45.—**Crean** (R.) Treatment of

Neck (*Abscess, cellulitis, and phlegmon of*).

superficial abscess in the neck. Med. Press & Circ., Lond., 1871, xii, 362.—**Croly** (H. G.) Observations on diffuse inflammation of the areolar tissue of the neck (cellulitis); importance of early, free, and deep incisions; with practical reference to the surgical anatomy of that region. Dublin Q. J. M. Sc., 1873, lv, 401–412, 4 pl. *Also, Reprint.* ———. Cellulitis of the neck. Lancet, Lond., 1883, ii, 327.—**Curling.** Cervical abscess; autopsy. *Ibid.*, 1850, ii, 485.—**Dariste.** Observation d'un abcès développé entre la colonne vertébrale et le pharynx. [Rap. de Forget] Bull. Soc. anat. de Par., 1836, xi, 251–259.—**Demarquay.** Phlegmon gangréneux de la région cervicale. Gaz d. hôp., Par., 1852, xxv, 469. — **Desplats** (H.) Fonte purulente des ganglions cervicaux simulant un mal de Pott; vaste abcès comprimant les deux plexus brachiaux et s'ouvrant dans le pharynx, sur les parties latérales du cou et à la nuque; paralysie des deux membres supérieurs. Rev. méd. franç. et étrang., Par., 1879, ii, 40–47.—**Doig** (A.) Angina Ludovici. Brit. M. J., Lond., 1876, i, 475.—**Dumaz.** Phlegmon diffus du cou. Bull. Soc. méd. de Chambéry. 1875-7, no. 5, 99–103.—**Duplay.** Adéno-phlegmon syphilitique du cou. Gaz. d. hôp., Par., 1880, liii, 180.—**Dupré** (G.) Un cas de phlegmon de la région sus-hyoïdienne. J. de méd., chir. et pharmacol., Brux., 1886, lxxxiii, 704–706.—**Duret.** Phlegmon du cou; trachéotomie; cause de la mort. J. d. sc. méd. de Lille, 1885, vii, 382–384.—**Englisch.** Angina Ludovici; Tracheotomia; Tod. Ber. d. k. k. Krankenanst. Rudolph-Stiftung in Wien (1881), 1882, 367. — **Ferraton.** Abcès du tissu cellulaire périphérique de la glande sous - maxillaire; inflammation phlegmoneuse; abcès consécutif de l'intérieur de la gaine d'enveloppe; ouverture au 8e jour; guérison complète au 22e. Gaz. méd. de l'Algérie, Alger, 1865, x, 50–54.—**Finger.** Klinische Mittheilungen. Vrtljschr. f. d. prakt. Heilk., Prag, 1861, lxxi, 82.—**Flecken.** Zwei Fälle von Cynanche sublingualis rheumatico-typhoïdes, als Beiträge zu den im General-Berichte des Rh. Med.-Colleg. pro 1838, S. 67, und 1842, S. 83, aufgeführten Fällen. Rhein. Monatschr. f. prakt. Aerzte, Köln, 1849, 228–230. — **Fournier.** Traumatic abscess of the neck, opening into the pleural cavity; death. Virginia M. Month., Richmond, 1875-6, ii, 744.—**Frazer** (J.) Case of extensive scrofulous ulceration, with abscess bursting into the trachea. Month. J. M. Sc., Lond. & Edinb., 1847-8, viii, 476-478. — **Frölich** (H.) Das königl. sächsische Collegium medico-chirurgicum. Feldarzt, Wien, 1877, 33.—**Froriep** (R.) Einige Fälle zur Erläuterung der übelen Folgen der Abscesse an der Oberfläche des Halses. Med. Ztg., Berl., 1834. iii, 129–132. *Also, transl.*: Dublin J. M. & Chem. Sc., 1835, vii, 84–96. — **Garcia** (M.) Abceso submaxilar al exterior del cuello y al interior de la faringe. Rev. méd.-quir., Buenos Aires, 1865-6, ii, 363.—**Gómez y Ferrer** (A.) Caso raro de flegmon profundo del cuello. Crón. méd., Valencia, 1883-4, vii, 425; 554; 586.—**Gorjacheff** (I. A.) Sluchai anginæ Ludovici. Laitop. khirurg. Obsh. v Morsk., 1881, iv, 417–419.—**Gregory** (G.) Case of cynanche cellularis. Med. & Phys. J., Lond., 1822, xlviii, 287–290.—**Gundrim** (F.) A clinical study of deep, acute and chronic abscess of the neck. Detroit Lancet, 1884–5, n. s., viii, 529–537.—**Halton** (R. J.) Acute rheumatism; typhoid symptoms and dyspnea, due to deep-seated abscess in neck. Dublin Q. J. M. Sc., 1869, xlvii, 368.—**Hanna.** Case of cervical abscess communicating with the lung. Tr. Belfast Clin. & Path. Soc., 1854, 63.—**Hargrave** (W.) On cervical abscesses, the accidents which sometimes attend their treatment in reference to hæmorrhage, and a new operation for securing the common carotid artery. Dublin Q. J. M. Sc., 1849, viii, 86–98.—**Hashimoto.** Ein Fall von Angina Ludovici. Arch. f. klin. Chir., Berl., 1885, xxxii, 42.—**Hawkins** (C.) Abscess in the cervical region after scarlet fever; hæmorrhage; recovery. Lancet, Lond., 1851, i, 13.—**Heim.** Zur Geschichte der Metaphlogose des Zellgewebes am Halse. Med. Cor.-Bl. d. württemb. ärztl. Ver., Stuttg., 1836, vi, 69–73.—**Henrich.** Angina gangrænosa Ludovici (gangræna telæ cellulosæ colli, lateris dextri). Wchnschr. f. d. ges. Heilk., Berl., 1851, 97–106.—**Heyfelder.** Cynanche sublingualis typhodes. Med. Ann., Heidelb., 1838, iv, 245. — **Hill** (B.) Two cases of inflammation of the deep cellular tissue of the neck (angina Ludovici). Brit. M. J., Lond., 1882, ii, 683.—**Hirsch** (G.) Scirrhöse Halsverhärtungen nach vergeblichen Gebrauch der Inunctionskur durch die äussere Anwendung der Jodine geheilt. J. d. pract. Heilk. Berl., 1826, lxii, 1. St., 101–106.—**Hofmokl.** Angina Ludovici; Septicopyæmia; Tod. Ber. d. k. k. Krankenanst. Rudolph-Stiftung in Wien (1883), 1884, 349. — **Hopkins** (B. S.) Abscess of the neck. Nashville J. M. & S., 1854, vi, 208.—**Horner** (W. E.) An anomalous case. [Complicated abscess of neck probably of syphilitic origin, resulting in death.] Am. M. Recorder, Phila., 1818, i, 22–29. — **Houston.** Abscess in the neck caused by a piece of hay-stalk getting into the throat. Dublin M. Press, 1839, ii, 134.—**Hue** (J.) Angine phlegmoneuse et abcès de la base du cou consécutifs à la carie syphilitique des cornets moyen et inférieur et de la première côte gauches; autopsie. Union méd. de la Seine-Inf., Rouen, 1879, xviii, 50–67.—**Hutchinson.** Tracheal abscess in

Neck (*Abscess, cellulitis, and phlegmon of*). the neck, with phthisis and laryngeal disease. Med. Times & Gaz., Lond., 1863, ii, 196.—**Jackson** (S.) Case of pulmonary disease, attended with some anomalous symptoms. Phila. J. M. & Phys. Sc., 1823, vii, 99–103.—**Jeffrey** (W.) Cervical abscess in an infant, caused by the swallowing of a piece of glass. Edinb. M. J., 1866–7, xii, 794–797, 1 cut.—**Jordon** (F.) Cellulitis of the neck. Birmingh. M. Rev., 1872, i, 202–204. *Also, in his:* Surg. Enq., 2. ed., 16°, Lond., [1880], 206–211.—**Jourdain.** Réponse à la lettre de M. Poulain, sur la manière d'ouvrir les dépôts purulens, qui avoisinent la mâchoire inférieure. J. de méd., chir., pharm., etc., Par., 1771, xxxvi, 448–464.—**K.** Phlegmone des Halses; Perforation in die Luftwege; Heilung. Cor.-Bl. f. schweiz. Aerzte, Basel, 1873, iii, 589–593.—**Kempen.** Adéno-phlegmon profond du cou suppuré; ouverture de l'abcès dans le pharynx. Arch. méd. belges, Brux., 1884, 3. s., xxvi, 307–311.—**Klatten.** Abscess am Halse und in der Brusthöhle. Med. Ztg., Berl., 1859, n. F., ii, 29.—**Kleijnenberg** (A. P.) Phlegmone in de ondertongbeenstreek; opvolgende verschijnselen van etteropslorping (pyaemie), [benevens suikergisting in de urine, herstelling met voortduring der gisting en schimmelvorming in de urine]. Kliniek, Utrecht, 1847, iii, 1–15.—**Klein** (A.) Ueber Angina Ludovici. Med.-chir. Centralbl., Wien, 1880, xv, 193; 205; 217; 229; 241.—**Kreitner** (L.) Ein Fall von ausgedehnter jauchiger Zellgewebsvereiterung am Halse. Allg. Wien. med. Ztg., 1880, xxv, 293.—**Lannelongue.** Phlegmon large du cou; trachéotomie; mort. Bull. Soc. anat. de Par., 1865, xl, 12–15.—**Legrand.** Phlegmon diffus de la région cervicale. Bull. Soc. anat. de Par., 1849, xxiv, 162–167.—**Leube.** Beobachtung einer Cynanche sublingualis rheumatico-typhodes. Med. Cor.-Bl. d. württemb. ärztl. Ver., Stuttg., 1836, vi, 165–168.—**Lidell** (J. A.) On certain abscesses of the neck which may cause sudden death, and how to treat them with success. Am. J. M. Sc., Phila., 1883, n. s., lxxxvi, 321–341.—**Long** (B. G.) Deep abscess of the post cervical region, with sudden death. Buffalo M. & S. J., 1883–4, xxiii, 301.—**Lucas-Championnière.** Obstruction de la veine pulmonaire et de ses branches, consécutive à un phlegmon du cou. Bull. Soc. anat. de Par., 1868, xliii, 342–344.—**Ludwig** (D.) [Ueber eine in neuerer Zeit wiederholt hier vorgekommene Form von Halsentzünd·ng.] Med. Cor.-Bl. d. württemb. ärztl. Ver., Stuttg., 1836, vi, 21–25.—**Luzzatto** (M.) Storia di un ascesso pulsante alla regione antero-inferiore del collo. Gior. veneto di sc. med., Venezia, 1862, 2. s., xix, 657–684.—**Lyall** (A.) A case of inflammation of the deep cellular tissue of the neck. Edinb. M. J., 1886–7, xxxii, 715. — **Lydston** (G. F.) Cellulitis of neck accompanied by œdema glottidis; difficult laryngotomy. Chicago M. J. & Exam., 1881, xlii, 47–51.—**Macfarlane** (J.) Chronic abscess in the neck; cured by puncture. *In his:* Clin. Rep. Surg. Pract. Glasg. Roy. Infirm., 8°, Glasg., 1832, 32. —**Malassez.** Angine gangréneuse et tumeur ganglionnaire du cou; rate volumineuse avec symptômes du cancer de l'estomac. Bull. Soc. anat. de Par. (1870), 1874, xlv, 119.—**Mauly** (B. S.) Notes of an unusual case. Med. & Surg. Reporter, Phila., 1864–5, xii, 250–252.—**Marshall** (J.) Epithelioma of tongue; excision of part of tongue; cellulitis of neck extending beneath deep fascia into neck; œdema glottidis; tracheotomy; death. Med. Times & Gaz., Lond., 1876, i, 112. ——. Clinical lecture on subfascial suppuration in the neck, and its treatment by a median incision in front. Lancet Lond., 1879, i, 217–219. — **Maunder.** Abscess of the neck, involving the tonsil; hæmorrhage from the latter; recovery. *Ibid.*, 1861, ii, 349.—**Mayor.** Phlegmon de la partie postérieure du cou à la suite d'altération des côtes; pleurésie purulente. Bull. Soc. anat. de Par., 1878, liii, 353–358. *Also:* Progrès méd., Par., 1879. vii, 7–9.—**Meinel** (E. A.) Phlegmonöse Zellgewebsentzündung der Unterkiefergegend. Deutsche Klinik, Berl., 1851, iii, 407.—**Melchiori** (G.) Flemmone e marcimento, diffuso del tessuto cellulare della regione anteriore profonda del collo, da periostitide della mascella inferiore. Gazz. med. di Milano, 1843, ii, 125 - 127. — **Metzler von Andelberg** (J. B.) Der sporadische Halszellgewebs-Brand. Ztschr. d. k.-k. Gesellsch. d. Aerzte zu Wien, 1846, ii, 319 – 344.— **Michel.** Phlegmon profond du cou avec perforation du pharynx. Arch. méd. belges, Brux., 1885, 3. s., xxviii, 369–378.—**Mollière** (D.) Du phlegmon sus-hyoïdien septique. Province méd., Lyon, 1887, ii, 515–517.—**Monnier** (L.) Abcès préthyroïdien déterminant des accès de suffocation. Rev. mens. d. mal. de l'enf., Par., 1883, i, 469.—**Mordret** (J.) Phlegmon diffus à la région cervicale; anémie; marche lente; mort. Bull. Soc. de méd. de la Sarthe 1872–3, Le Mans, 1874, 26–31.—**Murchison** (F.) A note on angina Ludovici. Brit. M. J., Lond., 1875, ii, 778.—**Narbonne.** Phlegmon diffus occupant la presque totalité des parties molles du cou et de l'isthme du gosier. Bull. Soc. anat. de Par., 1849, xxiv, 167–170. — **Nevitt** (R. B.) Cervical cellulitis and abscess. Canad. Pract., Toronto, 1887, xii, 36–40.—**Noquet.** Abcès résiduaux du cou ressemblant à un kyste; guérison après une seule ponction aspiratrice suivie d'une légère compression. Bull. méd. du nord, Lille, 1879, xviii, 157–167. *Also,* Reprint.—**Obissier** (H.) Du traitement des adénites suppurées du cou. Bordeaux méd., 1878, vii, 193; 201; 209; 225; 234.—**[Op-**

Neck (*Abscess, cellulitis, and phlegmon of*). **polzer.**] Ueber Cynanche cellularis maligna, oder Angina Ludwigii. Allg. Wien. med. Ztg., 1873, xviii, 482; 491; 500; 508.—**Paasch.** Vorübergehender theilweiser Verlust des Sehvermögens nach einer Halsentzündung. Allg. med. Centr.-Ztg., Berl., 1854, xxiii, 113–115.—**Parker** (R. W.) Remarks on cellulitis of the neck (angina Ludovici). Lancet, Lond., 1879, ii, 570; 607. — **Picqué.** Abcès froid périlaryngien simulant un kyste médian du cou. Gaz. méd. de Par., 1882, 6 s., iv, 537.—**Polack.** Ueber den Zellgewebsabscess am Halse. Memorabilien, Heilbr., 1867, xii, 166–170.—**Pollak** (S.) Abcesses on the forepart of the neck. St. Louis M. & S. J., 1845–6, iii, 49–54.—**Popper.** Extractum Belladonnæ gegen Halsentzündungen. Oesterr. med. Wchnschr., Wien, 1844, 1317 – 1319.—**Post** (A. C.) Inflammation of the cellular tissue of the throat. N. York J. M. & S., 1841, iv, 105.—**Poulain.** Lettre contenant quelques remarques sur la manière d'ouvrir les dépôts purulens qui avoisinent la mâchoire inférieure et le col. J. de méd., chir., pharm., etc., Par., 1771, xxxvi, 334–348.—**Pretty** (W.) A case of gangrenous inflammation in the neck. Med. Times & Gaz., Lond., 1858, xvii, 5–7.—**Quinlan** (F. J. B.) On the cure of abscesses about the neck without cicatrix or other deformity. [Abstr.] Lancet, Lond., 1883, i, 94.—**Raeis** (E.) Phlegmon diffus du cou; incisions profondes; guérison. Gaz. méd. de Strasb., 1874, xxxiii, 101–103.—**Ranking** (W. H.) Death from the impaction of a portion of the beard of barley under the tongue. Prov. M. & S. J., Lond., 1844, 462. — **Renaut.** Phlegmon péri-laryngien. Bull. Soc. anat. de Par., 1870, xlv, 139. — **Rieger.** Krankheitsgeschichte einer Halsentzündung, nach welcher der linke Fortsatz des Zungenbeines ausgeschieden worden ist. Mag. f. d. ges. Heilk., Berl., 1831, xxxiv, 211–214.—**Rösch.** Halszellgewebsbrand. Med. Cor.-Bl. d. württemb. ärztl. Ver., Stuttg., 1841, xi, 76. ——. Ueber den Halszellgewebsbrand. Wchnschr. f. d. ges. Heilk., Berl., 1844, 653; 673; 688.—**Roser** (W.) Die Ludwig'sche Angina. Deutsche med. Wchnschr., Berl., 1883, ix, 153–155.—**Rudnik** (M.) Ueber einen seltenen Fall von Zellgewebs-Entzündung am Halse. Allg. Wien. med. Ztg., 1877, xxii, 167; 179; 190. *Also* [Abstr.]: Mitth. d. Wien. med. Doct.-Coll., 1877, iii, 81–83. — **Savory** (W. S.) A case of abscess in the neck, which in its course destroyed a large portion of the carotid artery, jugular vein, and pneumogastric nerve. Med.-Chir. Tr., Lond., 1881, 2. s., xlvi, 21–29, 1 pl. *Also* [Abstr.]: Med. Times & Gaz., Lond., 1880, ii, 577. *Also* [Abstr.]: Lancet, Lond., 1880, ii, 696.—**Schmetzer.** Drei Fälle von Zellgewebs-Metaphlogose am Halse. Med. Cor.-Bl. d. württemb. ärztl. Ver., Stuttg., 1836, iv, 124; 133.—**Schützenberger** (C.) Phlegmon du cou; phlébite de la jugulaire interne; polyarthrite suppurée. Gaz. méd. de Strasb., 1866, xxi, 43 – 46. *Also, in his:* Fragments d'études path. et clin., 8°, Par., 1879, 363–374.—**Schützenmeister.** Eine seltener vorkommende Krankheit am Halse. Ztschr. d. nordd. Chir.-Ver., Magdeb., 1847, i, 315 – 329. — **Semeleder** (F.) Ueber Entzündung und Brand des Halszellgewebes. Wien. Med.-Halle, 1863, iv, 265; 275.—**Skibnevski** (A.) Dva sluchaja anginæ Ludovici; parenchimatoznija vpriskivanija karbol. kisloti. Vrach, St. Petersb., 1883, iv, 4.—**de la Sota y Lastra** (R.) Angina de Ludwig. Rev. med. de Sevilla, 1887, xi, 169–173.—**Sourris** (J.) Contribution à l'histoire des inflammations phlegmoneuses du cou. Rec. de mém. de méd. . . . mil., Par., 1878, 3. s., xxxiv, 591–607.—**Spengler** (L.) Brandige Zellgewebsentzündung um die Unterkiefer-Speicheldrüse. Deutsche Klinik, Berl., 1851, iii, 35.—**Stanelli.** Cynanche sublingualis rheumatico-typhoides. Deutsche Klinik, Berl., 1850, ii, 46 - 48. — **Stilmant** (L.) Adénite cervicale; phlegmon diffus consécutif; accidents graves; ponction et incision; application des principes de la méthode amovo-inamovible; guérison. Presse méd. belge, Brux., 1877–8, xxx, 249 – 251. — **von Stoffela** (E.) Angina Ludwigii. Oesterr. Ztschr. f. prakt. Heilk., Wien, 1871, xvii, 745; 761.—**Storks** (R.) Abscess in the neck, requiring the operation of tracheotomy. Lancet, Lond., 1847, ii, 13.—**Strathy** (F. R. L.) Case of ante-laryngeal abscess. Canada Lancet, Toronto, 1872–3, v, 1–4.—**Stuart** (J. A. E.) Case of "angina Ludovici". Brit. M. J., Lond., 1879, ii, 937.—**Stunde.** Ueber einen Fall von Phlegmone diffusa submentalis. St. Petersb. med. Ztschr., 1865, ix, 176.—**Taberlet.** Abcès profonds du cou; opération par la méthode d'écartement. Nice-méd., 1881–2, vi, 401–403.—**Timpe.** Fall von typhöser rheumatischer Hals Entzündung. Wchnschr. f. d. ges. Heilk., Berl., 1841, 285–289.—**Trélat.** Formes graves et compliquées des phlegmons de la région sus-hyoïdienne. Gaz. d. hôp., Par., 1869, xlii, 289. ——. Abcès froid du cou; incision; rugination de la poche purulente; suture; pansement de Lister; réunion par première intention. Bull. et mém. Soc. de chir. de Par., 1880, n. s., vi, 672. — **Triponel.** Gonflement œdémateux et emphysémateux de la partie antérieure du cou et qui entraîna la mort par asphyxie. Gaz. méd. de Strasb., 1845, v, 311. — **Uhde** (C. W. F.) Brandige Zellgewebs-Verhärtung am Halse. Deutsche Klinik, Berl., 1854, vi, 44; 65; 76.—**Vallescá** (P.) Absceso frio cervical de gran volúmen; tratamiento por las punciones evacuadoras seguidas de la inyeccion de Lugol; empleo de los tubos de

Neck (*Abscess, cellulitis, and phlegmon of*).

drenage; curacion. Independ. méd., Barcel., 1873-4, v, 151-153. — **Velpeau.** Abcès dans la région sous-hyoïdienne; opération. Gaz. d. hôp., Par., 1835, ix, 158. — **Verneuil.** Des phlegmons profonds du cou ou des adénites qui ont pour point de départ les ganglions carotidiens. Mouvement méd., Par.. 1875, xiii, 784.—**Voltolini** (R.) Die acute Zelihautentzündung in der Supra- und Post-auricular-Gegend. Monatschr. f. Ohrenh., Berl., 1875, ix, 139-143. — **Weber** (F.) Zur Casuistik der Ludwig'schen Krankheit. Allg. med. Centr.-Ztg., Berl., 1870, xxxix, 49. St., 581-584.—**Weteling** (J.) Ueber die Anwendung des Alumen ustum mit Crocus in acuten Hals-Entzündungen; nach dem Holländischen von Jac. Moleschott. Rhein. Monatschr. f. prakt. Aerzte, Köln, 1849, iii, 435-440.—**Wilmot** (S. G.) Idiopathic diffuse inflammation of the sub-cutaneous areolar tissue of the anterior and lateral parts of the neck. Dublin Hosp. Gaz., 1855-6, ii, 5.—**Younge** (G. H.) Pathology, symptoms, and treatment of cellulitis of the neck. Brit. M. J., Lond., 1884, i, 1141.—**Zillner** (F.) Sechs Fälle von Zellgewebsentzündung in der Hals- und Kiefergegend. Oesterr. med. Wchnschr., Wien, 1845, 1049-1053.

Neck (*Broken*).
See Spine (*Dislocation of*).

Neck (*Cellulitis of*).
See Neck (*Abscess, etc., of*).

Neck (*Cysts and cystic tumors of*).
See, also, **Goitre**; **Thyroid** gland (*Tumors of*).
AFFRE (V.) * Des kystes thyro-hyoïdiens. 4°. *Paris*, 1875.
BAENA (J.-L.) * Des kystes séreux congénitaux du cou. 4°. *Paris*, 1884.
BAGGERD (F.) * Blutcysten der seitlichen Halsgegend. 12°. *Berlin*, [1883].
BOOCKHOLTZ (J. H.) * Ueber Atheromcysten auf den Gefässscheiden des Halses und deren Radicalheilung durch Punktion mit nachfolgender Injection von Jodflüissigkeit. 4°. *Kiel*, 1869.
BOUCHER (P.) * Étude sur les kystes congénitaux du cou. 4°. *Paris*, 1868.
———. The same. 8°. *Paris*, 1868.
FAUVEL (J.) * Contribution à l'étude des kystes dermoïdes médians du cou situés dans l'espace thyrohyoïdien. 4°. *Paris*, 1887.
GÉRONNE (T.) * Zur Casuistik der Cystengeschwülste des Halses. 8°. *Greifswald*, 1872.
GÜNTHER (O.) * Ueber die Blutcysten des Halses, anschliessend an einen in der Greifswalder Klinik beobachteten Fall. 8°. *Leipzig*, 1877.
GUÉRIN (L.-F.) * Des kystes congénitaux du cou, et de leur traitement. 4°. *Paris*, 1876.
GURLT (E.) Ueber die Cystengeschwülste des Halses. 8°. *Berlin*, 1855.
HELLER (H.) * Over hygroma colli cysticum congenitum. 8°. *Leiden*, 1881.
LARONDELLE DE VERVIERS (N.) * Des kystes du cou. 8°. *Liége*, 1865.
LÜSSE (W.) * Ueber atheromatöse Cysten am Halse. 8°. [*Soest, n. d.*]
MOSSEL (É.) * Des kystes séreux du cou. 4°. *Paris*, 1868.
PILON (G.) * Des kystes dermoïdes du cou. 4°. *Nancy*, 1883.
ROBERT (L.) * Quelques considérations sur le traitement des hydrocèles du cou. 4°. *Strasbourg*, 1864.
SEIDMANN (M.) * Beitrag zur Casuistik und Kenntniss der Dermoidcysten in der Halsgegend. 8°. *Würzburg*, 1886.
TIETZE (Æ. E. C. J.) * De tumoribus colli et thoracis quibusdam sanguinolentis. 8°. *Berolini*, [1853].
TRENDELENBURG (F.) Mittheilungen aus der Klinik des Herrn Geh.-Rath von Langenbeck. Vier Fälle von congenitalen Halscysten, mit Injection von Jodtinctur behandelt. 8°. [*n. p., n. d.*]
ULLIAC (H.) * Étude sur les hygromas de la région cervicale antérieure. 4°. *Paris*, 1878.

Neck (*Cysts and cystic tumors of*).
VIALA (J.) * Des kystes séreux du cou. 4°. *Paris*, 1859.
VIRLET (N.-F.) * Des kystes congénitaux du cou. 4°. *Paris*, 1854.
VISCARO (S.) * Des tumeurs ganglionnaires du cou. 4°. *Paris*, 1852.
VOILLEMIER (L.) * Des kystes du cou. 4°. *Paris*, 1851.
Agnew (D. H.) [Hydrocele of the neck.] Phila. M. Times, 1870-71, i, 322. ——. Cystomata. Med. & Surg. Reporter, Phila., 1871, xxiv, 411-414. — **Albarran** (J.) Kyste ganglionnaire du cou. Arch. de physiol. norm. et path., Par., 1885, 3. s., vi, 168-178, 1 pl. — **Amussat** (A.) Kyste hématique occupant le côté droit du cou, depuis la clavicule jusqu'à l'angle de la mâchoire inférieure; cautérisation; guérison. Gaz. d. hôp., Par., 1855, xxviii, 174. *Also*, Reprint. ——. Traitement des kystes séro-sanguins du cou par l'électricité. Bull. gén. de thérap., etc., Par., 1872, lxxxiii, 321-324. — **Arnold** (J.) Zwey Fälle von Hygroma colli cysticum congenitum und deren fragliche Beziehung zu dem Ganglion intercaroticum. Arch. f. path. Anat., etc., Berl., 1865, xxxiii, 209-228, 1 pl.—**Ashhurst** (J.), jr. Sebaceous cyst of the neck; removal. North Car. M. J., Wilmington, 1884, xiii, 113. — **Atlee** (W. F.) Encysted tumor of the neck. Tr. Col. Phys. Phila., 1863-74, n. s., iv, 398.—**Baiardi** (D.) Ciste sanguigna della regione laterale destra del collo; estirpazione; guarigione. Osservatore, Torino, 1878, xiv, 257-260.—**Balassa.** Beiträge zur Geschichte der extrathyreoidalen Cystengeschwülste am Halse. Wien. med. Wchnschr., 1859, ix, 737; 753. — **Barthez** (E.) Kystes du col. Union méd., Par., 1857, xi, 535.—**Bartlett** (E.) Hydrocele of the neck cured by an operation. Med. Mag., Bost., 1835, iii, 568-570. — **Barton** (J. M.) Cystic papillary adenoma of the neck. Tr. Path. Soc. Phila. (1883-5), 1886, xii, 249.—**Barwell.** Hæmatocele of neck. Lancet, Lond., 1879, i, 880.—**Bary.** Observation d'un kyste volumineux à la région thyroïdienne simulant un goitre; opération. Presse méd. belge, Brux., 1850, ii, 364.—**Beck** (M.) Blood-cyst in the neck; tapping; subsequently laid open; healing by granulation. Med. Times & Gaz., Lond., 1882, ii, 472.—**Benoit** (J.) Extirpation d'une tumeur volumineuse formée par un kyste développé dans la région du cou. Rev. de thérap. du midi, Montpel., 1850, i, 132-141. — **Berend** (H. W.) Seröse Cysten am Halse. Ztschr. d. deutsch. Chir.-Ver., Magdeb., 1852, v, 160-165. ——. Hygroma cysticum colli congenitum. *Ibid.*, 165. — **Bidder** (A.) Zur Casuistik und Behandlung der tiefen Atheromcysten des Halses. Arch. f. klin. Chir., Berl., 1876, xx, 434-439.—**Bigler.** Drei Cystenbildungen in der vordern Halsgegend. Wien. med. Wchnschr., 1853, iii, 545; 561. — **Birkett** (J.) [Cysts in the neck; 9 cases.] Guy's Hosp. Rep., Lond., 1860, 3. s., vi, 453-466, 1 pl. ——. A contribution to the surgical pathology of serosanguineous cysts in the neck and axilla. Proc. Roy. M. & Chir. Soc. Lond. (1867-71), vi, 94.—**Blachez.** Kyste congénital du cou chez un fœtus. [Rap. de Charrier.] Bull. Soc. anat. de Par., 1856, xxxi, 286-293.—**Blockman** (G. C.) Hydrocele of the neck. Cincin. Lancet & Obs., 1870, n. s., xiii, 23-25.—**Blocq** (P.) D'une variété nouvelle de kystes du cou (kyste crico-thyroïdien). Gaz. méd. de Par., 1886, 7. s., iii, 135; 147; 184; 196.—**Broca.** Un lipôme offrant une cavité centrale. Bull. Soc. anat. de Par., 1851, xxvi, 234. — **Broca.** Kystes congénitaux et fistules du cou. J. de méd. et chir. prat., Par., 1872, 3. s., xliii, 106-110.—**Brodie.** Encysted tumor of the neck. Lond. M. & S J., 1834, iv, 639. — **Bryck** (A.) Das sublinguale Atherom; ein Beitrag zu den Cystengeschwülsten des Halses. Wien. med. Wchnschr., 1864, xiv, 337; 357. — **Campenon** & **Albarran** (J.) Kyste ganglionnaire du cou. Bull. Soc. anat. de Par., 1885, lx, 298-306. — **Carnochan** (J. M.) A case of encysted sanguineous tumor of the neck, successfully removed. Am. M. Gaz., N. Y., 1856, vii, 65-70. *Also*, Reprint.—[Cases.] Des kystes séreux congénitaux du cou et de leur traitement par les badigeonnages et les injections de teinture d'iode. Bull. gén. de thérap., etc., Par., 1856, li, 447-459.—Cystic tumor of the neck. Dublin Hosp. Gaz., 1858, v, 171.—Cyste der r. Supraclaviculargrube. Jahresb. ü. d. chir. Abth. d. Spit. zu Basel (1883) 1884, 53.—**Chapin** (H. D.) Two cases of branchial cyst. Med. Rec., N. Y., 1885, xxviii, 87-89.—**Chiarugi** (G.) Contributo alla conoscenza dei tumori congeniti del collo e allo studio della loro genesi. Arch. med. ital., Torino, 1883, ii, 441-453.—**Cloquet.** Hydrocèle du cou; ponction; guérison incertaine. Gaz. d. hôp., Par., 1837, xi, 119.—**Clutton** (H. H.) Congenital hydrocele of the neck. St. Thomas's Hosp. Rep. 1881, Lond., 1882, n. s., xi, 52-54.—**Cooper** (B.) Case of hydrocele of the neck, cured by the introduction of a seton. Guy's Hosp. Rep., Lond., 1836, i, 105-110. — **Coote** (H.) Large sanguineous cyst of the neck, connected with the thyroid body, successfully treated by injection with the tincture of iodine. Med. Times & Gaz., Lond., 1854, n. s., ix, 464.—**Deane** (J.) Hydrocele of the neck. Boston M. & S. J., 1852, xlvi, 401. — **Debout.** Des kystes séreux congéni-

Neck (*Cysts and cystic tumors of*).

taux du cou et de leur traitement par les badigeonnages et les injections de teinture d'iode. *In his:* De l'état de la thérap., etc., 8°, Par., 1858, 71–82. — **Délie.** Kyste de la région sous-hyoïdienne. Rev. mens. de laryngol., etc., Par., 1886, vi, 551. — **Demeaux.** Kyste gélatiniforme situé à la partie antérieure du cou. Ann. de la chir. franç. et étrang., Par., 1841, ii, 323–326. — **Devalz.** Kyste congénital du tissu cellulaire du cou guéri après deux ponctions successives par le trocart capillaire. Bull. et mém. Soc. de chir. de Par., 1876, n. s., ii, 762–764.— **Dieulafoy** (P.) Observation d'hydrocèle du cou; guérison. Gaz. d. méd.-prat., Par., 1840, ii, 49.— **Dittl.** Cystoid in der vordern Halsgegend eines 2jährigen Kindes; Exstirpation; Heilung; anatomische Beschreibung der Geschwulst von Rokitansky. Oesterr. Ztschr. f. prakt. Heilk., Wien, 1859, v, 81–86.— **Droste** (A.) Hygroma celluloso-cysticum am Halse eines Neugebornen. Hannov. Ann. f. d. ges. Heilk., 1839, iv, 295–303.— **Dubrueil** (A.) Tumeur du cou; sarcome de l'œsophage. Gaz. méd. de Par., 1885, 7. s., ii, 277–279.— **Dupin.** Kyste séreux du cou; ponction iodée; guérison. Gaz. méd.-chir. de Toulouse, 1886, xviii, 25–27, 2 pl.— **Dupuy.** Kyste séreux du cou; injection iodée; guérison. Union méd. de la Gironde, Bordeaux, 1857, ii, 201. *Also:* Monit. d. hôp., Par., 1857, v, 524. *Also:* Gaz. d. hôp., Par., 1857, xxx, 506.— **Dupuytren.** Kystes séreux développés au cou entre l'os hyoïde et le cartilage thyroïde. Gaz. d. hôp., Par., 1831, v, 101. ———. Hydrobroncocèle, ou hydrocèle du cou. Rev. méd. franç. et étrang., Par., 1834, i, 379–385.— **Ebermaier.** Eigenthümliche Blutgeschwulst am Halse eines Neugebornen. Wchnschr. f. d. ges. Heilk., Berl., 1836, 13–15.— **Englisch** (J.) Halscysten. Wien. med. Presse, 1867, viii, 765.— **Esmarch** (F.) Zur Behandlung der tiefen Atheromcysten des Halses. Verhandl. d. deutsch. Gesellsch. f. Chir. 1875, Berl., 1876, iv, pt. 2, 129–132, 1 pl. *Also:* Arch. f. klin. Chir., Berl., 1876, xix, 224–227, 1 pl.— **Fabre** (P.) Contribution à l'étude des tumeurs gazeuses de la région antérieure du cou. Gaz. méd. de Par., 1886, 7. s, iii, 373–376. — **Fano.** Observation de kystes séreux du cou. Union méd., Par., 1861, 2. s., x, 122.— **Fergusson.** Removal of a large sebaceous cyst from the neck. Lancet, Lond., 1869, i, 46. — **Fifield** (W. C. B.) Congenital cyst. Boston M. & S. J., 1860, lxii, 62. ———. Congenital cyst of the neck. *Ibid.*, 1873, x, 317–319. — **Fitz Patrick** (L.) Large cystic tumour of the neck; complete removal by operation; recovery. Australas. M. Gaz., Sydney, 1886–7, vi, 274.— **Fleming.** Hydrocele of the neck. Med. Press & Circ., Dubl., 1867, iii, 304. — **Fleury** (L.) Observations pour servir à l'histoire de l'hydrocèle du cou. J. d. conn. méd.-chir., Par., 1843–4, xi, pt. 2, 101–103.— **Fleury** (L.) & **Marchessaux** (L.) De quelques tumeurs enkystées du cou désignées par les noms de: struma aquosa, kystes cystiques, hydrocèles du cou; de leur siége, de leur nature, de leur traitement. Arch. gén. de méd., Par., 1839, ii, 269; 429. *Also,* Reprint. — **French** (J. G.) Hæmatoma, or sanguineous cyst in neck. Indian Ann. M. Sc., Calcutta, 1876, xviii, 43.— **Fröbelius.** Fall von angeborener Halscyste; Heilung durch Jodinjectionen. St. Petersb. med. Ztschr., 1865, ix, 173. — **Gamgee** (S.) On hydrocele of the neck. Lancet, Lond., 1875, i, 301.— **Gautier.** Deux observations de kystes séreux du cou traités par l'injection iodée et guéris. Echo méd., Neuchât., 1858, ii, 85.— **Gay** (J.) Cyst removed from the neck of a woman aged fifty-two. Tr Path. Soc. Lond., 1871–2, xxiii, 273. ———. Blood cyst removed from the neck. *Ibid.*, 1878–9, xxx, 435–438. ———. Removal of a large cyst from the neck. Lancet, Lond., 1872, i, 358. — **Giraldès.** Observation de kyste congénital du cou; autopsie. Gaz. d. hôp., Par., 1860, xxxiii, 13–15. *Also* [Abstr.]: Bull. Soc. de chir. de Par. (1859), 1860, x, 221; 272. ———. Kystes congénitaux du cou. Bull. Soc. de chir. de Par. (1860), 1861, 2. s., i, 107–112.— **Gluck.** Ueber Blutcysten der seitlichen Halsgegend. Deutsche med. Wchnschr., Berl., 1886, xii, 70 – 72. — **Godard.** Observation de tumeur enkystée du col; ouverture de la tumeur; injection avec la teinture d'iode; guérison. Rec. de mém. de méd. . . . mil., Par., 1842, liii, 198-200.— **Gœbel** (Anna M.) Case of hydrocele of the neck. Physician & Surg., Ann Arbor, Mich., 1885, vii, 243–245.— **Goodeve** (H. H.) Case of encysted tumor [of neck] cured by iodine injection. Tr. M. & Phys. Soc. Calcutta, 1835–42, viii, p. clxxxiv.— **Gosselin.** Kyste congénital composé du cou. France méd., Par., 1875, xxii, 761–763. — **Gross** (S. D.) Serous cyst of the neck, cured by palpation. N. Am. M.-Chir. Rev., Phila., 1860, iv, 81. ———. Congenital cystic tumor. Phila. M. Times, 1873, iii, 422.— **Gross & Vautrain.** Kyste congénital du cou; traitement palliatif par les ponctions capillaires. Rev. méd. de l'est, Nancy, 1886, xviii, 244.— **Gruber** (W.) Ein seltenes Beispiel von Hygroma ante-thyreoideum subfasciale. Arch. f. path. Anat., etc., Berl., 1879, lxxvii, 105-109, 1 pl. ———. Hygroma ante-hyoideum subfasciale. *Ibid*, lxxviii, 84–91, 1 pl. ———. Cystis atheromatosa præhyoidea submuscularis. *Ibid.*, 1880, lxxxi, 442–445, 1 pl.— **Günther** (O.) Ueber die Blutcysten des Halses. Deutsche Ztschr. f. Chir., Leipz., 1877, viii, 451 - 470. — **Guersant.** Tumeur du cou. Bull. Soc. de chir. de Par., 1856-7,

Neck (*Cysts and cystic tumors of*).

vii, 548-550. ———. Des kystes sérenx congénitaux du cou. J. de méd. et chir. prat., Par., 1859, 2. s., xxx, 545–548.— **Guillaumet.** Kyste séreux congénital de la nuque et du cou chez un fœtus de quatre mois et demi. Bull. Soc. anat. de Par., 1874, xlix, 582–585.— **Guitéras** (D. M.) Congenital cyst of the neck. Phila. M. Times, 1878, ix, 134.— **Hamilton** (F. H.) Superlaryngeal encysted tumors; or encysted bursal tumors in front of the larynx. N. York M. J., 1870, xi, 50–55.— **Hannay** (A. J.) Bloody cyst in neck. Edinb M. & S. J., 1843, lx, 319. ———. Serous cyst in neck. *Ibid*, 320.— **Hardie** (J.) Congenital cystic tumor in the neck, successfully extirpated. Lancet, Lond., 1872, ii, 667. — **Hawkins** (C. H.) On a peculiar form of congenital tumour of the neck. Med.-Chir. Tr., Lond., 1838–9, xxii, 231–244. ———. Clinical remarks on serous or aqueous cysts of the neck. Lond. M. Gaz., 1841, xxviii, 841–844. *Also, in his:* . . . Path. & Surg. Writings, 8°, Lond., 1874, i, 270–276.— **Heiberg** (J.) Pfropfung der Wand einer Atheromcyste vom Halse. Centralbl. f. d. med. Wissensch., Berl., 1872, x. 177.— **Hennig.** Hæmatocele colli connata. Wien. Med.-Halle, 1864, v, 542.— **Heusinger** (C. F.) Zu den Halskiemenbogen-Resten. Arch. f. path. Anat., etc., Berl., 1865, xxxiii, 177; 441.— **Hewett** (P. G.) Hydrocele of the neck. Brit. M. J., Lond., 1858, 446. *Also:* Lancet, Lond., 1858, i, 605. ———. Cystic tumor of the neck. Brit. M. J., Lond., 1858, 863. — **Hogg** (J.) Congenital multilocular serous cyst in the neck of a child. Med. Press & Circ., Lond., 1875, xvi, 50l. — **Holt.** Cystic tumor removed from the side of the neck. Tr. Path. Soc. Lond., 1853–4, v, 328.— **Houel.** Kyste congénital du cou, paraissant développé aux dépens du corps thyroïde. Bull. Soc. anat. de Par., 1873, xlviii, 632.— **Hueter.** Ein Fall von Blutcyste der seitlichen Halsgegend. Verhandl. d. deutsch. Gesellsch. f. Chir., Berl., 1877, vi, 30–32. *Also:* Berl. klin. Wchnschr., 1877, xiv. 466 — **Hunt** (W.) Two cases of large cystic tumors of the neck. Surg. Penn. Hosp., Phila., 1880, 298.— **Jackson** (A. R.) Hydrocele of the neck, and its treatment by excision, with two cases. Am. J. M. Sc., Phila., 1861, n. s., xli, 101–108.— **Jaksch** (R.) Ein Beitrag zur Entwicklung der cystischen Geschwülste am Halse. Ztschr. f. Heilk., Prag, 1885, vi, 131–142, 1 pl.— **Johnson** (T. G.) Removal of a deep-seated cystic tumor of the neck. Canada M. J., Montreal, 1870–71, vii, 65–67.— **Joüon.** Kyste du cou muni d'épithélium vibratile. J. de la sect. de méd. Soc. acad. Loire-Inf., Nantes, 1864, xl, 23–28. ———. Tumeur kystique de la région sous-maxillaire (épithéliome tubulé). J. de méd. de l'ouest, Nantes, 1882, xvi, 143.— **Kebler** (F.) Cystic degeneration of a cervical gland. Cincin. Lancet & Clinic, 1881, n. s., vii, 69.— **Kiatibian.** Kyste sanguin du cou; guérison. Gaz. méd. d'Orient, Constantinople, 1867–8, xi, 183–185.— **Koch** (O.) Eine branchiogene Halscyste von ungewöhnlicher Grösse. Mitth. a. d. chir. Klin. zu Tübing., 1884, 2. Hft., 373–376.— **Koester** (K.) Ueber Hygroma cysticum colli congenitum. Verhandl. d. phys.-med. Gesellsch. in Würzb., 1872, iii, 44–61.— **Krabbel.** Hygroma colli cysticum congenitum. Arch. f. klin. Chir., Berl, 1878, xxiii, 371.— **Küster** (E.) Kystenscheides des Halses. [4 cases.] *In his:* Ein chir. Trienn. 1876–8, 8°, Kassel u. Berl., 1882, 104–106. — **Lafosse.** Kyste extrêmement étendu, situé dans la région cervicale, oblitéré par la voie de la suppuration. Mémor. d. hôp. du midi, Par., 1830, ii, 482–487.— **Larghi** (B.) Gozzo cistico, mediano, comunicante col mediastino posteriore. Ann. univ. di med., Milano, 1867, cci, 493-499.— **Larondelle.** Des kystes du cou. [Rap. de Verhaeghe.] Bull. Acad. roy. de méd. de Belg., Brux., 1865, 2. s., viii, 447–451.— **Larrey.** Kyste canaliculé de la région antérieure du cou. Bull. Soc. de chir. de Par., 1852–3, iii, 489; 503; 607.— **Lawrence** (W.) Thick and vascular cyst in the neck connected with the thyroid body; exposure of the cavity by free incision; cure. Med. Times, Lond., 1851; n. s., ii, 28.— **Lee** (N.) Suppurating cyst of neck. Brit. M. J., Lond., 1858, 223. — **Lejars.** Épithéliome kystique de la région sus-hyoïdienne gauche; ulcération de l'artère faciale; ligature de la carotide primitive. Bull. Soc. anat. de Par., 1886, lxi, 732–735. *Also:* Progrès méd., Par., 1887, 2. s., vi, 48.— **Lelong.** Kyste congénitale de la partie médiane et postérieure du cou. Bull. Soc. anat. de Par., 1866, xli, 59–61. — **Lépine** (R.) De la valeur de la cautérisation dans le traitement des goîtres cystiques. [Avec 17 observations.] Mém. et compt.-rend. Soc. d. sc. méd. de Lyon, 1861–2, i, 335–356.— **Lesueur.** Observation d'une tumeur cystique du cou. Ann. Soc. méd. d'émulat. de la Flandre occid., Roulers, 1850, iv, 156–162.— **Levis** (R. J.) Enormous hydrocele of the neck in a child; paracentesis of the cysts, and removal of the solid portion by the écraseur. Phila. M. Times, 1874-5, v, 373.— **Linares** (A. R.) Quiste sanguinolento, situado en la parte anterior del cuello; extirpacion total; curacion completa á los 49 dias. Corresp. méd., Madrid, 1879, xiv, 197.— **Lorain** (P.) Mémoire sur les kystes congénitaux du cou. Compt. rend. Soc. de biol. 1854, Par., 1855, i, pt. 2, 134–141. *Also:* Gaz. méd. de Par., 1855, 3. s., x, 173–176.— **Loumeau.** Kyste du cou traité et guéri par la ponction suivie d'injection iodée. Mém. et bull. Soc. de méd. et chir. de Bordeaux (1885), 1886, 221-228. *Also:* J. de méd. de

Neck (*Cysts and cystic tumors of*).

Bordeaux, 1885-6, xv, 1.—**Luschka** (H.) Das Hygroma hyo-epiglotticum. Arch. f. path. Anat., etc., Berl., 1864, xxx, 234–239.—**McCraith.** Melanotic (?) encysted tumor simulating bronchocele. Med. Times & Gaz., Lond., 1861, ii, 577.—**MacDonald** (K. N.) Case of large congenital cystic tumour of the left side of the neck, simulating encephalocele; death after the third month, from suppuration of its contents and meningitis Edinb. M. J., 1880-81, xxvi, 690–695.—**McGraw** (T. A.) Congenital cyst of the neck; operation and recovery. Detroit Rev. Med. & Pharm., 1874, ix, 532.—**Mackenzie** (M.) Traitement des kystes et des fibro-kystes du cou. Progrès méd., Par., 1874, ii, 543.—**Maclean** (D.) Case of hydrocele of the neck. Penins. J. M., Detroit, 1875, xi, 547–550. *Also* [Abstr.]: Canada Lancet, Toronto, 1875-6, viii, 136.—**McMahon** (W. R.) Congenital cyst of the neck; or the "hygromatous cyst" of von Ammon. Med. & Surg. Reporter, Phila., 1872, xxvii, 76.—**Malherbe** (A.) Kyste du cou à contenu huileux; guérison par une injection d'alcool pur après évacuation partielle du contenu au moyen d'une aiguille capillaire; remarques sur la nature de ce kyste et sur le traitement de diverses collections liquides par l'injection d'alcool pur. Bull. et mém. Soc. de chir. de Par., 1878, n. s., iv, 257–263. *Also:* J. de méd. de l'ouest, Nantes, 1878, xii, 9-19. *Also,* Reprint.—**Marduel.** Hématome du cou. [Rap. de Sérullaz.] Mém. et compt.-rend. Soc. d. sc. méd. de Lyon, 1863-4, iii, pt. 2, 169–174.—**Martin.** Ueber ein todtgebornes reifes männliches Kind mit mehrfachen Kysten am Halse, unter beiden Achseln und in der Gegend der Brustdrüse, nebst Verunstaltung der Fusszehen und Finger und blaurother Färbung der Oberschenkel und Bauchdecken. Verhandl. d. Gesellsch. f. Geburtsh. in Berl. (1861–2), 1863, xv, 155–159. *Also:* Monatschr. f. Geburtsk. u. Frauenkr., Berl., 1862, xx, 170–174.—**Martinez** (F. R.) Diagnóstico i tratamiento de los quistes del cuello. An. Univ. de Chile, Santiago, 1869, xxxii, 245–265.—**Martinez del Rio.** Tumor enquistado [del cuello] operado por puncion é inyeccion. Periód. Acad. de med. de Mégico, 1837-8, ii, 156–158.—**Martone** (V.) Cisti sierose multiple congenite del collo; estirpazione con allaccitura della gingulare interna; vasta eresipela consecutiva; guarigione. Resoc. Accad. med.-chir. di Napoli, 1876, xxx, 143–145. *Also:* Ann. clin. d. osp. incur., Napoli, 1877, n. s., ii, 156–159.—**Marzuttini** (G. B.) Idrocele del collo. Mem. d. Soc. med.-chir. di Bologna, 1844, 2. s., iii, 319–333, 1 pl.—**Maunoir** (J.-P.) Mémoire sur l'hydrocèle du cou. *In his:* Mémoires sur les amputations, etc., 8°. Genève, 1825, 93–134.—**Michaux.** Note sur l'hématocèle ou les kystes sanguins du cou. Bull. Acad. roy. de méd. de Belg., Brux., 1851-2, xi, 668: 1852-3, xii, 247. [Discussion], 1854-5, xiv, 464–474 *Also :* Gaz. d. hôp., Par., 1853, xxvi, 136; 144; 147.—**Miller** (N.) Encysted gelatinous tumour of the neck. Extr. Rec. Bost. Soc. M. Improve., 1854-6, ii, 85.—**Miner** (J. F.) Cystic tumor of the neck. Buffalo M. & S. J., 1864, iii, 379.—**Moitessier** (A.) Kyste du cou. Montpel. méd., 1863, xi, 228-230.—**Monti** (L.) Di un voluminoso ematoma congenito al collo in un bambino; spaccatura del tumore; guarigione. Bull. d. sc. med. di Bologna, 1873, 5. s., xv, 250–255.—**Mootoosamy** (P. S.) Hydrocele of the neck. Indian M. Gaz., Calcutta, 1877, xii, 69.—**Morgan** (J. H.) Cysts of the neck. Med. Times & Gaz., Lond., 1884, ii, 878-880.—**Morris.** Inflamed cystic tumour in anterior triangle of the left side of the neck. Med. Times & Gaz., Lond., 1873, i, 248.—**Mott.** Case of hydrocele of the neck. N. York M. & S. Reporter, 1846, i, 151.—**Muret** (C.) Quelques mots sur une énorme tumeur de la région latérale du cou. Écho méd., Neuchât., 1861, v, 297–304.—**Musser** (J. H.) Case of congenital cyst of the neck. Tr. Path. Soc. Phila. (1881-3), 1884, xi, 243. *Also:* Phila. M. Times, 1881-2, xii, 541.—**Musset** (H.) Observation d'un kyste séreux du cou, à fond vasculaire, traité avec succès par les caustiques. J. de méd. de Bordeaux, 1860, 2. s., v, 201–210.—**Mutter** (T. D.) Hydrocele of the neck. Med. Exam., Phila., 1850, n. s., vi, 257–275.—**Nagel** (E.) Zur Behandlung umfangreicher Halscysten. Wien. med. Wchnschr., 1867, xvii, 305; 321.—**Nélaton.** Kyste énorme de la région cervicale chez un enfant nouveau-né; évacuation par la ponction, et excision de la poche après suture préalable. Gaz. d. hôp., Par., 1854, xxvii, 310. ——. Kyste séro-purulent à parois fibro-cartilagineuse, situé dans la région du cou. *Ibid.*, 1861, xxxiv, 265.—**O'Beirne** (J.) On hydrocele of the neck. Dublin J. M. & Chem. Sc., 1834, vi, 1–22, 2 pl.—**Packman** (J. D. V.) Case of encysted tumour, treated by puncture and injection. Madras Q. M. J., 1840, ii, 319.—**Panas.** Kyste séro-muqueux du cou (hygroma) guéri par l'injection de chlorure de zinc. Paris méd., 1875-6, i, 225–227.—**Parrot.** Kyste séreux multiloculaire congénital; curieuses attaques de cyanose. Gaz. d. hôp., Par., 1880, liii, 34.—**Pécot.** Excision d'un kyste volumineux, situé sur l'artère carotide. Bull. Acad. de méd., Par., 1836-7, i, 97.—**Phillips** (B.) Observations on a particular form of encysted tumour, which occurs in the neck, but is not necessarily connected with the thyroid body. Med.-Chir. Tr., Lond., 1841-2, xxv, 297–303.—**Pilcher** (L. S.) The galvano-cautery in the treatment of hydrocele of the neck. Med. Rec., N. Y., 1875, x, 190.—**Plath.** Ueber einen Fall von operativer Beseitigung eines Cysten-

Neck (*Cysts and cystic tumors of*).

hygroms des Halses. Jahrb. f. Kinderh., Leipz., 1884, n. F., xxi, 417–419. — **Pooley** (J. H.) Cyst of the neck. Ohio M. & S. J., Columbus, 1878, iii, 171–177. *Also,* Reprint.—**Porter** (G. H.) A large encysted tumour of the neck treated by drainage and injection; long-continued suppuration; recovery. Dublin Q. J. M. Sc., 1870, xlix, 58–61, 1 pl.—**Preiss.** Von einem glücklich operirten und geheilten Fröschlein, welches mit einem Hygrom am Halse vergesellschaftet war. J. f. d. Chir., Geburtsh. u. gerichtl. Arznk., Jena, 1802, iii, 468–472.—**Rampond** [*et al.*]. Observation d'un kyste séreux très-considérable, occupant la plus grande partie du cou. Ann. clin., Montpel., 1814, xxxiii. 339–354. — **Ransohoff** (J.) Sanguineous cyst of the neck. Tr. Ohio M. Soc. 1883, Columbus, 1884, xxxviii, 171–177. *Also:* Cincin. Lancet & Clinic, 1884, n. s., xiii, 1–4.—**Rendu.** Kyste du cou. Bull. Soc. anat. de Par. (1871), 1873, xlvi, 171.—**Reyes** (A.) Tumor quístico unilocular implantado en el lado izquierdo del cuello sobre la carótida. Gac. méd., México, 1887, xxii, 41. — **Richard** (A.) Note sur un hydrocèle du cou et le siège présumé de ces sortes de tumeurs. Mém. Soc. de chir. de Par. (1851–2), 1853, iii, 38-44, 1 pl. [Rap. de Lebert], 45–53.—**Richardson** (B. W.) Hematic cyst of the neck; rapid subsidence of the swelling after partial tapping, followed by the injection of a few drops of the solution of perchloride of iron. Dublin Q. J. M. Sc., 1869, xlviii, 462–465, 1 pl.—**Richardson** (E.) Hydrocele of the neck. Tr. Path. Soc. Phila. (1871–3), 1874 iv, 220. — **Robin.** Sur un enfant qui présentait, au moment de la naissance, des kystes multiples du cou. Compt. rend. Soc. de biol. 1853, Par., 1854, v, 62–67.—**Romero** (A.) Quiste sanguinolento, situado en la parte anterior del cuello; estirpacion total; curacion completa á los 41 dias. Bol. de med., cirug. y farm., Madrid, 1850, 3. s., v, 83.—**Roser.** Mittheilungen über Kiemengangcysten. Verhandl. d. deutsch. Gesellsch. f. Chir. 1875, Berl., 1876, iv, pt. 1, 25.—**Roux** (J.) Des kystes séreux du cou. Bull. Acad. de méd., Par., 1854-5, xx 1110-1123. *Also:* Rev. méd.-chir. de Par., 1855, xviii, 79–87. ——. Injections iodées dans deux kystes congénitaux du cou. Bull. Acad. de méd., Par., 1855-6, xxi, 1057–1064. *Also:* Monit. d. hôp., Par., 1856, iv, 994–996. *Also:* Gaz. d. hôp., Par., 1856, x, 409. *Also :* Rev. de thérap. du midi, Montpel., 1856, x, 551–557. ——. Des kystes séreux du cou au point de vue opératoire. Marseille méd., 1877, xiv, 663–670.— **Royer** (A.) Kyste du cou contenant de la cholestérine; guérison par la ponction et l'injection iodée. Gaz. d. hôp., Par., 1856, xxix, 198.—**Ruchmore.** Cystic tumors of neck. Med. & Surg. Reporter, Phila., 1878, xxxviii, 418. — **Savory** (W. S.) Large cyst in the neck, opening into the pharynx. Lancet, Lond., 1866, ii, 573. ——. Cystic tumour of neck; incision; suppuration; sudden hæmorrhage; death. Med. Times & Gaz., Lond., 1882, ii, 579.—**Schede** (M.) Ueber die tiefen Atherome des Halses. Arch. f. klin. Chir., Berl., 1872, xiv, 1–22 —**Scholz** (W.) Angeborene Halscyste; Versuch der Extirpation; Abbinden der vordern Wand; Heilung. Wien. med. Wchnschr., 1863, xiii, 612; 628 —**Schwerin** (E.) Ein Fall von Tumor cystoides colli congenitus. Arch. f. klin. Chir., Berl., 1878, xxiii, 430.—**Senn** (N.) On branchial cysts of the neck. J. Am. M. Ass., Chicago, 1884, iii, 197–209.—**Seutin.** Mémoire et observations sur les kystes du cou. Bull. Acad. roy. de méd. de Belg., Brux., 1852-3, xii, 257–293, 1 pl. [Discussion], 1854–5, xiv, 464–474. *Also:* Presse méd. belge, Brux., 1853, v, 93; 101; 109; 117. *Also:* Arch. belges de méd. mil., Brux., 1853, xi, 177; 292. *Also* [Abstr.]: Union méd., Par., 1853, vii, 131.—**Silcock** (Q.) Cystic epithelioma of the neck. Brit. M. J., Lond., 1887, i, 620.—**Söderbaum** (P.) Ett fall af lymphangioma cysticum congenitum colli. Eira, Göteborg, 1887, xi, 483.—**Soulé** (E.) Réflexions sur le traitement des kystes du cou. Gaz. d. hôp., Par., 1854, xxvii, 90. ——. Kyste séreux du cou; injection iodée; guérison. Union méd. de la Gironde, Bordeaux, 1857, ii, 201.—**Spence.** Cystic tumour of neck. Edinb. M. J., 1879, xv, 397.—**Stoltz.** Observation sur un enfant nouveau-né portant un kyste congénital volumineux au côté droit du cou, suivie de réflexions. Rev. méd. de l'est, Nancy, 1878, x, 161–173.—**Stone** (J. O.) Hydrocele of the neck cured by the seton. *In his:* Clinical cases, 8°, N. Y., 1878, 220.—**Storch** (O.) Hygroma colli congenitum. Hosp.-Tid., Kjøbenh., 1860, iii, 125–128. *Also, transl.:* J. f. Kinderkr., Erlang., 1861, xxxvii, 68–84.—**Syme** (J.) Encysted or rather cystic tumour of the neck. Month. J. M. Sc., Lond. & Edinb., 1846, vi, 84.—**Terrillon.** Note à propos d'une observation de kyste congénital du cou. France méd., Par., 1878, xxv, 49. ——. Kystes de la région latérale droite du cou, situés sous le sterno-mastoïdien et probablement d'origine ganglionnaire; examen histologique des kystes; extirpation; guérison. Bull. et mém. Soc. de chir. de Par., 1883, n. s., ix. 598–604.—**Thevenot** (A.) Apuntes sobre los quistes del cuello i su tratamiento por el drenaje quirúrjico. Rev. méd. de Chile, Sant. de Chile, 1872-3, i, 44; 85; 141.—**Thomas** (L.) Kyste sanguin uniloculaire du cou; ablation incomplète; blessure de la jugulaire interne; forcipressure; récidive; kyste sanguin multiloculaire. Bull. et mém. Soc. de chir. de Par., 1887, n. s., xiii, 142–147.—**Thornton** (W. P.) Cervical hydrocele. Lancet, Lond.,

Neck (*Cysts and cystic tumors of*).

1882, i, 420.—**Tillaux.** Kyste séreux du creux sus-claviculaire droit présentant des signes insolites; injection iodée; guérison. Bull. gén. de thérap., etc., Par., 1868, lxxx, 556. ———. Kyste dermoïde de la région sus-hyoïdienne. Gaz. d. hôp., Par., 1885, lviii, 569.—**Toland** (H. H.) Cystic tumors of the neck. West. Lancet, San Fran., 1872, i, 385–387, 2 pl.—**Tonoli** (S.) Igroma del collo. Gazz. med. ital. lomb., Milano, 1880, 8. s., ii, 310.—**Tourneret.** Kyste sanguin congénital du cou; extirpation; mort. Gaz. méd. de Strasb., 1876, xxxv, 116. ———. Kyste hydatique du cou; extirpation partielle; guérison. *Ibid.*, 117. — **Townsend** (R. M.) Congenital multilocular cystic tumor, removed from the neck of a boy aged ten years. Phila. M. Times, 1870–71, i, 302.—**Travers** (B.) & **Stratham.** Removal of a large tumor from the neck. Lancet, Lond., 1851, ii, 561.—**Trendelenburg** (F.) Sehr grosses Hygroma cysticum colli congenitum; Jodinjectionen; Tod. Arch. f. klin. Chir., Berl., 1872, xiii, 404–411.—**Treves** (F.) Dissection of a congenital hydrocele of the neck. Tr. Path. Soc. Lond., 1880–81, xxxii, 194–197, 1 l., 1 pl.—**Valenta.** Colossales congenitales Cystenhygrom des Halses, combinirt mit cavernösem Angiome und Makroglossie. Oesterr. Jahrb. f. Paediat., Wien, 1871, i, 35–40—**Van Buren.** A mass of serous cysts, originally double the size of the closed fist, removed from the side and root of the neck of a boy 14 years of age. Am. M. Month., N. Y., 1857, vii, 227.—**Velpeau.** Kyste situé au devant du larynx; kystes thyroïdiens de formes diverses. J. de méd. et chir. prat., Par., 1850, 2. s., xxi, 298–300.— **Verneuil.** Recherches anatomiques pour servir à l'histoire des kystes de la partie supérieure et médiane du cou. Arch. gén. de méd., Par., 1853, 5. s., i, 185; 450.—**Virchow** (R.) Ein tiefes auriculares Dermoid des Halses. Arch. f. path. Anat., etc., Berl., 1866, xxxv, 208–210.—**Völckers** (C.) Hygroma cellulosum am Halse eines Neugebornen. Wchnschr. f. d. ges. Heilk., Berl., 1837, 704–707.—**Walker** (B. M.) † Cystic tumor of the neck treated with ergot. South. M. Rec., Atlanta, 1878, viii, 161–163.—**Warren** (J. W.) Sero-cystic tumor of the neck, adherent to the internal jugular vein; dissection of the vein; union by adhesive inflammation; cure in one week. Boston M. & S. J., 1843, xxviii, 157. ———. Hydrocele of the neck; inflammation; suppuration; removal of the sac. *In his:* Surg. Obs., 8°, Bost., 1867, 509.—**Werner.** Hydrocele colli. Med. Cor.-Bl. d. württemb. ärztl. Ver., Stuttg., 1837, vii, 246.—**West** (J. F.) Notes of a case of fibro-cystic tumour, or hydrocele of the neck. Birmingh. M. Rev., 1875, 104–109.—**Whitehead** (W.) Two cases in which cystic tumours were removed from the anterior triangle of the neck; recovery in both cases. Brit. M. J., Lond., 1881, ii, 13.—**Whitson** (J.) Case of hydrocele of the neck. Lancet, Lond., 1882, i, 268.—**Wölfler** (A.) Zur operativen Behandlung des Hygroma colli congenitum (Wernher); Lymphangioma colli cysticum (Wegner). Wien. med. Presse, 1886, xxvii, 905; 937.—**Wutzer.** Hygroma cellulosum am Halse eines Neugebornen. Wchnschr. f. d. ges. Heilk., Berl., 1836, 257–260.—**Zsigmondy.** Cystis atheromatosa in der Medianlinie des Halses. Aerztl. Ber. d. k. k. allg. Krankenh. zu Wien (1876), 1877, 165.

Neck (*Deformities of*).

Bobichon (C.-L.) *Contribution à l'étude du torticolis postérieur d'origine musculaire. 8°. *Lyon,* 1886.

Couete (C. F.) *De capite obstipo. 4°. *Jenæ,* [1817].

Couillard - Labonnote (G.-M.) *Du torticolis. 4°. *Paris,* 1869.

Drissen (A.) *De capitis obstipitate. sm. 8°. *Berolini,* [1859].

Elsner (C. F.) [Pr.] complectitur colli curvi atque inclinati historiam. Quæ sit testulæ meæ suffragium de magnetismo animali. 4°. *Regiomonti,* 1787.

Gautiez (A.-H.) *Contribution à l'étude des spasmes du cou. 4°. *Paris,* 1884.

Greeve (G.) *De capite obstipo. 4°. *Traj. ad Rhenum,* 1786.

Gürleth (H.) *Ueber Verkrümmung des Halses. 8°. *Erlangen,* 1840.

Hopf (L.) *Zur Therapie des Caput obstipum. 8°. *Tübingen,* 1865.

Jæger (G. F.) *Caput obstipum affectum rariorem in libris et praxi. 4°. *Tubingæ,* [1737].

Krug (A.) *De capite obstipo. 8°. *Halæ,* 1865.

Musson (A.) *Du torticolis. 4°. *Paris,* 1867.

Nègre (C.) *Du torticolis fonctionnel. 4°. *Montpellier,* 1883.

Neck (*Deformities of*).

Rettig (F. X.) *Caput obstipum. 12°. *Budæ,* [1783].

Vonck (A.) *Studie over het caput obstipum musculare. 8°. *Amsterdam,* 1887.

Zillich (J. H. T.) *De contractura musculi sterno-cleidomastoidei ejusque curandi ratione. 4°. *Lipsiæ,* 1843.

Althaus (J.) Two cases of wry-neck treated successfully by electricity. Med. Times & Gaz., Lond., 1861, i, 544. ———. Disease of the lateral columns of the medulla; double histrionic spasm and torticollis. Brit. M. J., Lond., 1872, i, 48. ———. Case of spasmodic torticollis. Tr. Clin. Soc. Lond., 1878–9, xii, 85–89.—**von Ammon** (F. A.) Bemerkungen über die angeborene Obstipitas capitis. Monatschr. f. Med., Augenh. u. Chir., Leipz., 1839, ii, 577–580.— **Ballance** (C. A.) A case of spasmodic wry-neck, treated by excision of a portion of the spinal accessory nerve. St. Thomas's Hosp. Rep. 1884, Lond., 1886, n. s., xiv, 95–104.— **Banham** (H. F.) Unrhythmical spasmodic torticollis. Med. Press & Circ., Lond., 1884, n. s., xxxviii, 392.—**Bartscher.** Angeborener Schiefhals [Caput obstipum congenitum]. J. f. Kinderkr., Erlang., 1863, xl, 14–16.—**Bauer** (L.) Deformities of the neck. Med. & Surg. Reporter, Phila., 1863, x, 293; 329; 441, 1 pl.—**Baumgarten.** Ein Blick auf den heutigen Standpunkt der Orthopädie, nebst Beiträgen zur operativ-mechanischen Heilung des Caput obstipum. Monatschr. f. Med., Augenh. u. Chir., Leipz., 1840, iii, 337–358, 1 pl.—**Bellingham** (O'B.) Case of wryneck; subcutaneous section of the right sterno-mastoid muscle. Dublin M. Press, 1848, xx, 161. ———. Case of wry-neck; division of the sternal origin of the sterno-mastoid muscle; cure. *Ibid.*, 1850, xxiii, 273.—**Bennet** (J.) Case of spasmodic wryneck successfully treated by division of the spinal accessory nerve, after failure of stretching. Lancet, Lond., 1879, i, 555.—**Birch** (D. B.) On the operation of dividing the sterno-cleido mastoideus muscle for the cure of wry neck. Madras Q. M. J., 1842, iv, 173–177.—**Björnström** (F.) Om torticolis muscularis-rheumatica. Upsala Läkaref. Förh., 1868–9, iv, 251–257.— **Bottini** (E.) Torticollo congenito destro; tenotomia dello sterno-cleido-mastoideo; guarigione. Osservatore, Torino, 1880, xvi, 135.—**Bouland.** Torticolis articulaire avec contracture de l'angulaire et du trapèze droits; vésicatoires; manipulations; courants continus; guérison. Bull. Soc. de méd. prat. de Par., 1879, 103–110. *Also:* France méd., Par., 1879, xxvi, 666–668.—**Bouvier.** Réclamation contre les articles de J. Guérin, relatifs au traitement du torticolis ancien. Gaz. méd. de Par., 1838, 2. s., vi, 318; 382. ———. Section du sterno-mastoïdien pour un torticolis musculaire ancien. Bull. Acad. de méd., Par., 1839–40, iv, 518. *Also:* Bull. gén. de thérap., etc., Par., 1840, xviii, 163–168.—**Bradford** (E. H.) A case of posterior torticollis, treated successfully by Delore's method. N. York M. J., 1880, xxxi, 24–29. ———. Cases of wry neck. Boston M. & S. J., 1882, cvi, 513–516.—**Brandt.** D'une nouvelle espèce de tortico is et de son traitement. Bull. gén. de thérap., etc., Par., 1840, xix, 297–300.—**Briddon.** Chronic torticollis; unsuccessful attempt to stretch the spinal accessory nerve. Med. Rec., N. Y., 1882, xxii, 46.—**Broca** (P.) De la déformation du crâne sous l'influence du torticolis chronique. Bull. Soc. d'anthrop. de Par., 1872, 2. s., vii, 21–25. ———. Du torticolis. Rev. phot. d. hôp. de Par., 1872, iv, 65–70, 3 pl.—**Brooks** (F. D.) Congenital torticollis. Med. Rec., N. Y., 1886, xxix, 257.—**Brosius.** Caput obstipum spasticum. Med. Ztg., Berl., 1856, xxv, 39; 45.— **Brown** (J. B.) Torticollis successfully treated at the Boston Orthopedic Infirmary. Boston M. & S. J., 1842, xxvi, 58–60.—**Buck** (G.) Wry neck cured without cutting. N. York M. Times, 1852, ii, 131–134.—**Busey** (S. C.) Anæsthesia and hot water in the treatment of torticollis. Med. Rec., N. Y., 1879, xvi, 295.—**Caire** (P.) Osservazioni teorico-pratiche sopra alcuni casi di strabismo e torticollo. Gior. d. sc. med., Torino, 1846, xxv, 170–194. —**Carron du Villards** (C.-J.-F.) Observation relative à un cas de torticolis ancien, très-compliqué, guéri par la section sous-cutanée du sterno-mastoïdien et du peaucier. Gaz. méd. de Par., 1852, 3. s., vii, 451.—**Curling.** Torticollis following rheumatic fever. Lancet, Lond., 1860, i, 348.— **Dally.** Du torticolis occipito-atloïdien. Bull. gén. de thérap., etc., Par., 1875, lxxxix, 354; 388; 438. — **Daly** (P.) Case of wry neck relieved by operation. Dublin M. Press, 1839, i, 245.—**Daviers** (E.-J.) Torticolis congénital; section sous-cutanée du sterno-mastoïdien. Bull. Soc. de méd. d'Angers, 1841–2, i, 60–65.—**Davis** (J. D. S.) A case of congenital torticollis, with fissure of upper lip. Atlanta M. & S. J., 1884–5, n. s., i, 516–518.—**Debout.** Remarques sur un cas de torticolis dû à la contracture des muscles splénius droit et sterno-mastoïdien gauche, guéri par l'excitation électrique localisée dans les muscles antagonistes. Bull. gén. de thérap., etc., Par., 1855, xlix, 61–71. *Also* [Abstr.]: Bull. Soc. de chir. de Par., 1854–5, v, 200. *Also, transl.:* Allg. med. Centr.-Ztg., Berl., 1856, xxv, 225; 233; 241.—**De-Giovanni** (A.) Sopra un caso di torticollo a contribuzione della dottrina sul trasporto delle influenze spinali e a fondamento d' una ipotesi per la

Neck (*Deformities of*).

loro spiegazione. R. Ist. Lomb. di sc. e lett. Rendic., Milano, 1880, 2. s., xiii, 682–685.—**Delore.** Du torticolis postérieur et de son traitement par le redressement forcé et le bandage silicaté. Gaz. hebd. de méd., Par., 1878, 2. s., xv, 167 ; 178.—**Dieffenbach.** Durchschneidung des Musculus sternocleidomastoideus zur Heilung des schiefen Halses. Med. Ztg., Berl., 1838, vii, 135–138. *Also, transl.*: Lancet, Lond., 1838–9, i, 30 ; 47.—**Dollinger** (G.) Testegyenészeti közlemények. Adatok a ferdenyak (torticollis) kórokahoz és gyogykezel. [Pathology and therapeutics of torticollis.] Orvosi hetil., Budapest, 1885, xxix, 1219–1225. *Also, transl.*: Pest. med.-chir. Presse, Budapest, 1885, xxi, 957 ; 977.—**Dubrueil** (A.) Torticolis dû à la rétraction des scalènes. Gaz. hebd. d. sc. méd. de Montpel., 1886, viii, 457. — **Duchenne de Boulogne.** Torticolis de la portion claviculaire du trapèze. Rev. méd. franç. et étrang., Par., 1853, i, 394–398.—**Ebert.** Das krampfhafte Kopfnicken der Kinder. [7 cases.] Ann. d. Char.-Krankenh. . . . zu Berl., 1850, i, 752–769.—**Eidenmuller** (G.) Case of Torticollis. San Francisco M. Press, 1860, i, 73.—**Ekeroth** (E.) & **Tengstrand** (E. U.) Tvenne händelser af caput obstipum ; myotomi. *In*: Bergström (C. H.) Chir. Iakttagelser, 8°, Upsala, [n. d.], 176–201.—**Eulenburg.** Bruchstück aus einer noch unveröffentlichten Abhandlung "Ueber Verdrehung des Kopfes durch Krampf einzelner Halsmuskeln". Allg. med. Centr.-Ztg., Berl., 1856, xxv, 623–627. ——. Fall von Torticollis (Scoliosis cervicalis) nach Suppuration des Zellgewebes im Nacken ; Heilung. Arch. f. klin. Chir., Berl., 1863, iv, 301–303. ——. Apparat gegen Torticollis. Verhandl. d. Berl. med. Gesellsch. (1867–8), 1871, pp. xxxiv-xl. *Also*: Berl. klin. Wchnschr., 1867, iv, 350–352. ——. Einige Bemerkungen zur Diagnose und Behandlung des Torticollis. Verhandl. d. Berl. med. Gesellsch. (1869–71), 1872, pt. 1, 289–296. *Also*: Berl. klin. Wchnschr., 1871, viii, 479–481. — **Fisher** (F. R.) Wry neck of infantile origin in an adult ; tenotomy ; recovery. Lancet, Lond., 1877, ii, 609.—**Fisher** (W. R.) A case of torticollis ; illustrating some principles of treatment. Med. Rec., N. Y., 1873, viii, 588–591.—**Fleury** (L.-J.-D.) Mémoire sur un cas de torticolis permanent, déterminé par la contraction du faisceau sternal du muscle sternocléido-mastoïdien, et guéri par la section sous-cutanée du tendon inférieur de ce faisceau charnu. Arch. gén. de méd., Par., 1838, 3. s., ii, 78–96. *Also*, Reprint.—**García** y **Frutos** (J. M.) Historia clínica de un torticolis. Anfiteatro anat., Madrid, 1873, i, 144.—**Geraldes** (M. J.) Congenital torticollis. Med. & Surg. Reporter, Phila., 1871, xxiv, 323–329.—**Germain** (J.) Section sous-cutanée du muscle sternomastoïdien dans le torticolis ; nouvel instrument du . . . Arch. de la méd. belge, Brux., 1842, ix, 25–29.—**Gilby** (W.) Efficacy of electricity in contraction of the muscles of the neck. Lancet 1825, 2. ed., Lond., 1826, viii, 280.—**Girbal** (A.) Observation de torticolis congénital ancien, guéri par la section sous-cutanée des deux tendons du sterno-cléido-mastoïdien. Bull. gén. de thérap., etc., Par., 1860, lix, 307–309.—**Gottschalk** (A.) Zur Operation des schiefen Halses. Org. f. d. ges. Heilk., Bonn, 1840–41, i, 421–428.—**Grohnert** (F.) Un caso de torticolis intermitente. Rev. méd. de Chile, Sant. de Chile, 1877, vi, 145–150.—**Gross** & **Vautrain.** Torticolis congénital ; ténotomie du muscle sterno-mastoïdien droit ; traitement orthopédique consécutif par l'extension continue et par un collier redresseur ; guérison. Rev. méd. de l'est, Nancy, 1886, xviii, 245–247.—**Gross** (S. D.) Torticollis. Med. & Surg. Reporter, Phila., 1868, xix, 418. ——. Torticollis. Phila. M. Times, 1871–2, ii, 89. ——. Myotomy in a case of torticolis. *Ibid.*, 1873–4, iv, 4. — **Guérin** (J.) Mémoire sur une nouvelle méthode de traitement du torticolis ancien. Gaz. méd. de Par., 1838, 2. s., vi, 209–216. *Also*, Reprint. ——. Observations de torticolis ancien traité par la section sous-cutanée du muscle sterno-mastoïdien. Gaz. méd. de Par., 1838, 2. s., vi, 259–264. ——. Résumé d'un mémoire sur le torticolis ancien et le traitement de cette difformité par la section sous-cutanée des muscles rétractés. *Ibid.*, 1840, 2. s., viii, 465. ——. Nouvelles recherches sur le torticolis ancien, et sur le traitement de cette difformité par la section sous-cutanée des muscles retractés. *Ibid.*, 1841, 2. s., ix, 353 ; 417. ——. Torticolis ancien. Rap. sur les traitements orthiopéd. 1843–5, Par., 1848, 24–40. ——. Variations thermiques dans les maladies ; déformations de la face et du crâne dans le torticolis ancien. Bull. Acad. de méd., Par., 1880, 2. s., ix, 27–36.—**Guersant** (P.) Du torticolis chez les enfants. Bull. gén. de thérap., etc., Par., 1865, lxviii, 448–452. — **Hadra** (B. E.) Two cases of congenital torticollis. Med. Rec., N. Y., 1886, xxix, 91.—**Hall** (C. R.) Case of spasmodic wry-neck cured by practure. Prov. M. & S. J., Lond., 1841, ii, 129.—**Hall** (M.) On epileptic torticollis. Lancet, Lond., 1852, ii, 463. —**Hambursin.** Note sur une variété de torticolis, simulant la tumeur blanche des deux premières vertèbres cervicales à sa première période, et paraissant avoir été confondue jusqu'aujourd'hui avec cette dernière affection. Bull. Acad. roy. de méd. de Belg., Brux., 1861, 2. s., iv, 51–58. [Rap. de Michaux], 19.—**Hamilton** (A. McL.) The physiological treatment of wry-neck. N. York M. J.,

Neck (*Deformities of*).

1880, xxxi, 140–144.—**'Hancock** (H.) Division of contraction of the neck from a burn. Lancet, Lond., 1857, ii, 141. ——. Torticollis from carious tooth. *Ibid.*, 1859, i, 80.—**Heyfelder** (J. F.) Subcutane Durchschneidung des M. sternocleido-mastoideus. Deutsche Klinik, Berl., 1858, x, 227.—**Hilton.** Severe burn of the neck treated by extension from the beginning. Lancet, Lond., 1859, ii, 662.—**Hugman** (C.) Subcutaneous incision for wry-neck. Med. Times, Lond., 1850, i, 85.—**James** (J. H.) Treatment of contracted neck after burns; the advantages of the screw collar in this and other maladies. Assoc. M. J., Lond., 1856, ii, 667. —**Jobert** (*de Lamballe*). Torticolis musculaire chronique ; section sous-cutanée de la portion claviculaire du sterno - mastoïdien. Gaz. d. hôp., Par., 1863, xxxvi, 314.—**Kersch** (S.) Tenotomie zur Heilung des Torticollis und dessen Nachbehandlung. Memorabilien, Heilbr., 1868, xiii, 5–7.—**Kirby** (J.) Wry-neck. Dublin M. Press, 1853, xxix, 259–261.—**Labatt** (H.) Wry-neck, depending on a tetanic condition of the right sterno-mastoid muscle ; together with a spastic state of the trapezius and abdominal muscles of the same side, consequent on severe strain of the spine. *Ibid.*, 1844, xi, 117–119.—**Legouest.** Torticolis intermittent. Bull. Soc. de chir. de Par. (1861), 1862, 2. s., ii, 234 ; 420. — **Lehmann.** Fall von Durchschneidung des Musculus sternocleidomastoideus unter der Haut beim schiefen Halse. Med. Ztg., Berl., 1839, vii, 245. — **Leszynsky** (W. M.) Treatment of wry-neck by sulphate of atropia. Med. Rec., N. Y., 1884, xxv, 288–290.—**Leva.** Torticolis intermittent; sulfate de quinine; guérison. Ann. Soc. de méd. d'Anvers, 1844, 249–251.—**Louis.** Torticolis. Gaz. d. hôp., Par., 1846, 2. s., viii, 390.—**Meyer.** Beobachtung eines Falles von krampfhaftem Schiefhals, Torticollis spasmodica, geheilt durch subcutane Tenotomie. Med. Cor.-Bl. rhein. u. westfäl. Aerzte, Bonn, 1843, ii, 49 ; 61 ; 83.—**Middel** (P.) Onderhuidsche doorsnijding (Teneotomia subcutanea) van den musculus sternocleidomastoideus bij den scheeven hals (Caput obstipum). Pract. Tijdschr. v. de Geneesk., Gorinchem, 1840, xix, 34–36.—**Mills** (C. K.) Spasm of the muscles supplied by the spinal accessory nerve. Am. J. M. Sc., Phila., 1877, n. s., lxxiv, 425–433.—**Mosetig von Moorhof.** Collum obstipum spasticum ; Dehnung beider Nervi recurrentes Willisii ; Heilung. Wien. med. Presse, 1881, xxii, 853–855. — **Nottingham** (J.) Wry-neck ; division of the sternomastoid. Lancet, Lond., 1841–2, i, 187.—**Ormsby.** Clonic torticollis. Dublin J. M. Sc., 1882, 3. s., lxxii, 248–250.—**Owen** (E.) Notes on a case of wry neck. Prov. M. J., Leicester, 1885, iv, 371.—**Par** (Et) Tilfælde af spastisk Torticollis. Hosp.-Tid., Kjøbenh., 1866, ix, 161; 165.—**Petersen** (F.) Caput obstipum. (Zur Aetiologie und Behandlung.) Arch. f. klin. Chir., Berl., 1884, xxx, 781–798.—[**Poore.**] Case of clonic torticollis treated by the continuous galvanic current and the rhythmical exercise of the affected muscles. Lancet, Lond., 1873, ii, 520.—**Post** (A. C.) A case of torticollis cured by division of the sterno-cleido-mastoid muscle followed by elastic traction of the head. Tr. Am. M. Ass., Phila., 1880, xxxi, 837–839. *Also* [Abstr.]: Med. Rec., N. Y., 1881, xix, 23.—**Price** (P. G.) Wry-neck; division of the sterno-mastoid muscle. Lancet, Lond., 1840–41, ii, 583. — **Regimbeau.** Torticolis; affection rhumatismale occupant les articulations des vertèbres cervicales et produisant une contracture réflexe des scalènes et du splénius. Gaz. hebd. d. sc. méd. de Montpel., 1881, iii, 25 ; 49. — **Remak.** Ueber Torticollis und Chorea. Oesterr. Ztschr. f. prakt. Heilk., Wien, 1863, ix, 224. — **Reynier** (J.-B.) Contribution au traitement des déviations de la taille et du torticolis. Ann. Soc. méd.-chir. de Liége, 1878, xvii, 129 ; 313 ; 405 ; 474.—**Reynolds** (J. R.) Torticollis. Syst. Med. (Reynolds), Lond., 1868, ii, 774–780. — **Richet** (P.) Notes sur deux maladies opérées de torticolis congénital. Rev. méd.-phot. d. hôp. de Par., 1874, vi, 163, 2 pl.—**Rivington** (W.) Spasmodic wry-neck ; excision of a portion of the spinal accessory nerve; death from erysipelas. Brain, Lond., 1881–2, iv, 257–263.—**Robert.** Cas remarquable de torticolis accompagnés de circonstances assez rares, dont un suivi de mort après l'opération; réflexions cliniques sur ce dernier. Gaz. d. hôp., Par., 1846, 2. s., viii, 174.—**Roth** (B.) The treatment of non-spasmodic wry-neck (torticollis). Brit. M. J., Lond., 1884, i, 1139–1141.—**Roux.** Torticolis congénital ; considérations générales. Gaz. d. hôp., Par., 1841, 2. s., iii, 15.—**Ryan** (G. W.) Report and presentation of two cases of torticollis. Cincin. Lancet-Clinic, 1886, n. s., xvi, 395–397. — **de Saint-Germain.** Du torticolis chez les enfants. J. de méd. et chir. prat., Par., 1876, xlvii, 304–308. ——. Du torticollis. Gaz. d. hôp., Par., 1881, liv, 339; 347. — **Salter** (J. A.) Wry neck from carious teeth of lower jaw. Guy's Hosp. Rep., Lond., 1868, 3. s., xiii, 89.—**Sands** (H. B.) Excision of a portion of the spinal accessory nerve for spasmodic torticollis. Ann. Anat. & Surg., Brooklyn, N. Y., 1883, viii, 277–279. *Also*: N. York M. J., 1883, xxxviii, 555. *Also*: Med. News, Phila., 1883, xliii, 572.—**Sangalli** (G.) Sopra una causa non ben conosciuta di torcicollo. R. Ist. Lomb. di sc. e lett. Rendic., Milano, 1870, 2. s., iii, 31–36.—**Séguin.** Torticolis datant de sept mois, avec déviation de l'épine, guéri par l'extension, le massage et la percussion cadencée.

Neck (*Deformities of*).

Rev. méd. franç. et étrang., Par., 1838, ii, 75–79.—**Siegen** (C.) Du torticollis chez le cheval. Bull. Soc. d. sc. méd. du gr.-duché de Luxemb., 1869, 172–174. [Rap. de E. Fischer], 175.—**Siredey.** Torticolis rhumatismal à accès répétés. Gaz. d. hôp., Par., 1867, xl, 69. — **Smith** (L.) Case of congenital wry-neck. Canada M. Rec., Montreal, 1886-7, xv, 5.—**Snaith** (F.) Division of the sterno-cleido-mastoid muscle for the cure of wry-neck. Lancet, Lond., 1840–41, i, 227.—**Southam** (F. A.) Abstract of a clinical lecture on torticollis, and its treatment by tenotomy and neurectomy. Brit. M. J., Lond., 1885, ii, 59–61. — **Steele** (A. J.) Torticollis. Tr. M. Ass. Missouri, St. Louis, 1876, x, 37–49.—**Stephenson** (M.) Case of torticollis. N. York M. Times, 1855, iv, 46–48.—**Steudel.** Torticollis spastica. Med. Cor.-Bl. d. württemb. ärztl. Ver., Stuttg., 1848, xviii, 333. — **Stromeyer** (L.) Habitueller Krampf des Kopfnickers. Wchnschr. f. d. ges. Heilk., Berl., 1837, 489; 511; 527.—**Swan** (R. L.) Wry neck; its phases and treatment. Dublin J. M. Sc., 1879, 3. s., lxviii, 114–119, 1 pl. — **Talko** (J.) Udawane kręcenie głową przerwane zawłoką na karku. [Twisting of the head (m. sterno-cleido-mastoideus) treated by seton to nape of neck.] Medycyna, Warszawa, 1873, i, 661–663.—**Testelin.** Contracture des muscles de l'œil: torticolis. Bull. méd. du nord, Lille, 1874, xiv, 21.—**Tillaux.** Torticolis fonctionnel; résection du nerf spinal. Tribune méd, Par., 1882, xiv, 77–80.—[**do Valle** (A. G.)] Torcicollo intermittente; cura na presença do tratamento pelo sulphato de quinina. Escholiaste méd., Lisb., 1862, xiii, 153.—**Vallin.** Observation d'une forte contracture du muscle sterno-mastoïdien gauche, avec rotation de la tête, inflexions et torsions de l'épine; guérison sans opération. J. de la sect. de méd. Soc. acad. Loire-Inf., Nantes, 1838, xiv, 94–103, 1 pl. ———. Torticolis de naissance; section sous-cutanée des deux muscles sterno et cléido-mastoïdiens droits; guérison. *Ibid.*, 1842, xviii, 192–207.—**Volkmann** (R.) Das sogenannte angeborene Caput obstipum und die offene Durchschneidung des M. sternocleido-mastoides. Centralbl. f. Chir., Leipz., 1885, xii, 233–236.— **Warren** (J. M.) Division of the sterno-mastoid muscle for wry-neck. Boston M. & S. J., 1841-2, xxv, 121–126. *Also, in his*: Surg. Obs. 8°, Bost., 1867, 601–609.—**Weiss** (T.) Torticolis. N. dict. de méd. et chir. prat., Par., 1883, xxxv, 644–671.—**Witzel** (O.) Beiträge zur Kenntniss der secundären Veränderungen beim muskulären Schiefhalse. Deutsche Ztschr. f. Chir., Leipz., 1882-3, xviii, 534–578.— **Wood.** Congenital torticollis in a young girl. Lancet, Lond., 1857, ii, 498. ———. Torticollis; new method of operating. Med. Press & Circ., Lond., 1871, xi, 351.

Neck (*Diseases and surgery of*).

See, also, **Spine** (*Cervical diseases of*); **Sterno-cleido-mastoid.**

ACADÉMIE royale de chirurgie. Observations on surgical diseases of the head and neck. Selected from the memoirs of the Royal Academy of Surgery of France. Transl. and edited by Drewry Ottley. 8°. *London,* 1848.

ALBERT (E.) Lehrbuch der Chirurgie und Operationslehre. 1. Bd. Die chirurgischen Krankheiten des Kopfes und Halses. 8°. *Wien,* 1877. ———. The same. 3. Aufl. 8°. *Wien u. Leipzig,* 1884.

DEMETRIADES (A.) * Ueber Spasmen der Kopfrotatoren und deren Therapie. 8°. *Erlangen,* 1874.

FISCHER (G.) Krankheiten des Halses; topographische Anatomie; angeborne Krankheiten; Unterbindungen; Verletzungen. 8°. *Stuttgart,* 1880. ———. The same. Malattie del collo. Anatomia topografica. Malattie congenite, allacciature. Lesioni violente. Traduzione (dal tedesco) pel Dott. Ferdinando Massei. 8°. *Napoli,* 1881.

HAESEMANN (H. L.) Geschichte und Heilung eines Spekgeschwürs. Eine Streitschrift. 12°. *Kopenhagen,* [1775]. ———. Bemerkung von einer Halsentzündung. 12°. *Kopenhagen,* [1779].

HALLER (A.) [Pr.] de morbis colli observationes adjicit. 4°. *Gottingæ,* 1753.

HECKER (A. F.) Von den Entzündungen im Halse, besonders von der Angina polyposa und dem Asthma Millari. 8°. *Berlin,* 1809.

HONCAMP (E.) * Ein Fall von spontaner Gangrän der linken Halsgegend mit besonderer Berücksichtigung der consecutiven pathologischen

Neck (*Diseases and surgery of*).

Felsenbeinveränderungen. [Wurtzburg.] 8°. *München,* 1885.

LINDPAINTNER (J.) * Ueber die Gefahren bei Operationen am Halse. 8°. *München,* 1873.

MAEDGE (C. F. G. L.) * De induratione telæ colli cellulosæ gangrænosa. 4°. *Brunsvigæ,* 1848.

PEYROT (J.-J.) Maladies des régions; cou, poitrine, abdomen. 8°. *Paris,* 1887.

Arnheimer. Sehr hartnäckige Convulsibilitas colli, durch Seebäder verscheucht. Med. Ztg., Berl., 1837, vi, 18 - 20. - **Bourguet.** Observation d'extraction d'une chaine disparue à travers la peau, dans le tissu cellulaire sous-cutané du cou. Lyon méd., 1879, xxxii, 339–342.— **Braid** (J.) Case of a peculiar ulcerous affection, successfully treated. Edinb. M. & S. J., 1825, xxiii, 42–49.— **Caponotto** (A.) Malattie del collo e della nuca; casi 21 (M. 14, F. 7), di cui morti 2 M. Osservatore, Torino, 1883, xix, 289–300.—**De Morgan.** Case of severe spasmodic contraction of cervical muscles produced by movement. Lancet, Lond., 1867, ii, 128.—**Faucon** (A.) Ulcère scrofuleux du cou, respiration difficile; cornage; accès de suffocation; trachéotomie par le thermo-cautère. *In his*: Leç. de clin. chir., 8°, Par., 1879, 109–120.—**Fosbroke** (J.) Cellular hypertrophy of the throat and neck, with chronic affection of the pharynx and larynx. Lancet, Lol d., 1835, ii, 247 – 250. — **Gillette.** Cou (pathologie chirurgicale). Dict. encycl. d. sc. méd., Par., 1877, xxi, 165–387.—**Hall** (M.) On the neck as a medical region, and on paroxysmal paralysis Lancet, Lond., 1849, i, 174; 285; 394; 506; 687: ii, 66: 1850, ii, 75.—**Hancock** (H.) Case of ulceration of the neck, apparently malignant, probably syphilitic. Med. Times & Gaz., Lond., 1869, ii, 540.—**Hoering.** Beiträge zu der in No. 4 dieser Zeitschrift mitgetheilten Halskrankheit. Med. Cor.-Bl. d. württemb. ärztl. Ver., Stuttg., 1836, vi, 109–112. — **Jaccoud.** Arthrite rhumatismale de la région cervicale, compliquée de méningite; paraplégie. Gaz. d. hôp., Par., 1884, lvii, 1170.—**Kumar** (A.) Spasmus der Halsmuskeln. Wien. med. Bl., 1882, v. 1440.—**Laugier** (S.) Des maladies du cou et des opérations qui se pratiquent sur cette région. Dict. de méd., 2. éd., Par., 1835, ix, 162 – 186. — **Mears** (J. E.) Specimen of large ulcer of the neck, involving the sub-maxillary gland, removed by operation. Tr. Path. Soc. Phila. (1878), 1879, viii, 144. — **Ogle** (J. W.) Clonic spasmodic contraction of the muscles of the neck, possibly having its origin in some affection of the contents of the spinal canal. Tr. Clin. Soc. Lond., 1873, vi, 114–120. — **Oldman** (C.) Case of diffuse hypertrophy of the adipose tissue of the neck. Lancet, Lond., 1873, i, 768. — **Palmer** (A. C.) Sponge dressings in operations upon the neck. Atlantic J. M., Richmond, 1883, i, 257.—**Parrish** (J.) Singular case of swelling of the neck. N. Jersey M. Reporter, Burlington, 1848, i, 187–189.—**Purdy** (G. L.) An anomalous case. Cincin. Lancet & Obs., 1860, n. s., iii, 399–402.—**Schaffer** (L.) Beitrag zur Heilung von Adenitiden am Halse. Allg. Wien. med. Ztg , 1883, xxviii, 58. — **Schmigelow** (E.) Anden Beretning fra Kommune-hospitalets Klinik for Øre-, Næse- og Hals-Sygdomme. Hosp.-Tid., Kjøbenh., 1887, 3. R., v, 512; 537; 561; 586; 607. — **Theurer.** Zwei Fälle von einer bis jetzt noch ohne Namen befindlichen Halskrankheit. Med. Cor.-Bl. d. württemb. ärztl. Ver., Stuttg., 1836, vi, 33–35.—**Trendelenburg** (F.) Die chirurgischen Erkrankungen und Operationen am Halse. Handb. d. Kinderkr. (Gerhardt), Tübing., 1880, vi, 2. Abth., 225–315.

Neck (*Dislocations of*).
See **Spine** (*Cervical, Dislocations of*).

Neck (*Fistula of, Congenital*).
See **Fistula** (*Cervical*).

Neck (*Glands of, Diseases of*).
See, also, **Neck** (*Tumors of*).

ALLBUTT (T. C.) & TEALE (T. P.) Clinical lectures. On scrofulous neck and on the surgery of scrofulous glands. 8°. *London,* 1885.

BARCHEWITZ (P. E. O.) * Zur Behandlung scrophulöser Halsdrüsen-Geschwülste. 8°. *Berlin,* [1886].

BERTHERAND (A.) Traité des adénites idiopathiques et spécialement de celles du col. 8°. *Paris,* 1852.

BRUHN (T.) * Beitrag zur Statistik der Exstirpation tuberknlöser Lymfdrüsentumoren. 8°. *Kiel,* 1887.

DELIGNY (L.) * De l'adénopathie cervicale chez les scrofuleux. 4°. *Paris,* 1876.

Neck (*Glands of, Diseases of*).

DUNKELBERG (H.) * Lymphadenitis colli und ihre Folgen bei Diphtherie und Scarlatina. 8°. *Berlin*, [1884].

ÉCOT (F.) * Contribution à l'étude de l'ablation des ganglions tuberculeux du cou. 4°. *Paris*, 1886.

GEY (S.-A.) * De l'adénite cervicale envahissante. 4°. *Strasbourg*, 1852.

JUERGENS (J. F.) * De scirrhis glandularum colli maximis feliciter extirpatis. 4°. *Helmstadi*, [1777].

KÜCHLER (J. C.) * De glandulis colli puerorum tumefactis. 4°. *Lipsiæ*, [1723].

LAMBRY (P.) * Du traitement chirurgical des tumeurs ganglionnaires du cou. 4°. *Paris*, 1872.

LAUZERAL (A.) * De l'adénite cervicale chez les militaires considérée surtout au point de vue de l'étiologie. 4°. *Paris*, 1874.

LEGALLOIS (A.) * De lymphadénome du cou, ou de l'hypertrophie ganglionnaire idiopathique de la région cervicale. 4°. *Paris*, 1873.

MONART (H.) * Considérations sur l'adénite cervicale chez les soldats. 4°. *Paris*, 1875.

OBISSIER (H.) Du traitement des adénites suppurées du cou. 8°. *Bordeaux*, 1878.

OCKEL (A. F. R.) * Zur Casuistik der Strumectomie und der Cachexia strumipriva. 8°. *Berlin*, [1887].

TIXIER (J.-E.) * Étiologie de l'adénite cervicale du soldat. 4°. *Paris*, 1877.

Ashhurst (J.), jr. Hypertrophied cervical and bronchial glands. Proc. Path. Soc. Phila. (1860–66), 1867, ii, 155–157. *Also*: Am. J. M. Sc., Phila., 1865, n. s., xlix, 128.—**Banon.** Hæmorrhage in a case of strumous disease of the glands of the neck. Dublin M. Press, 1854, xxxi, 177.—**Barudel.** Traitement de l'adénite chronique cervicale et sous maxillaire par les bains de mer. Rec. de mém. de méd. . . . mil., Par., 1862, 3. s., vii, 474–483.—**Blaschko.** Gutartige kontagiöse Drüsen- und Zellgewebsaffektion am Halse. J. f. Kinderkr., Erlang., 1869, liii, 302–304.—**Bottomley** (T. A.) Report of an operation for removal of a tumor from a child's neck. Lancet, Lond., 1853, ii, 95.—**Boulu.** Traitement de l'adénite cervicale au moyen de l'électricité localisée. [Rap. de Bouvier.] Bull. Acad. de méd., Par., 1855–6, xxi, 678–687. *Also*, Reprint. *Also* [Abstr.]: Union méd., Par., 1856, x, 256. ——. Lettres sur le traitement de l'adénite cervicale par l'électricité localisée. Monit. d. hôp., Par., 1857, v, 921; 2032: 1858, vi, 1228.—**Braun** (M.) Beitrag zur Therapie von Halsdrüsentumoren. Wien. med. Bl., 1887, x, 976.—**Broca.** Hypertrophie ganglionnaire cervicale multiple ayant envahi toute une moitié du cou, chez un jeune homme de 18 ans. Bull. Soc. de chir. de Par. (1871), 1872, 2. s., xi, 184–186.—**Brunelli** (C.) Adenite cervicale multipla d' indole scrofolosa con principio di suppurazione in qualche glandola; cura elettrica. Gior. med. di Roma, 1865, i, 632.—**Cheever** (D. W.) Large glandular tumor removed from the neck of a boy, eight years of age. Boston M. & S. J., 1863, lxviii, 259.—**Clark** (A.) Enlarged glands surrounding the carotid artery and simulating aneurism. Lancet, Lond., 1882, ii, 703.—**Cody** (J.) Case of glandular tumor of neck; successful operation. Chicago M. J., 1859, n. s., ii, 658–661.—**Cramer** (F.) Beitrag zur Kenntniss der Struma maligna. Arch. f. klin. Chir., Berl., 1887, xxxvi, 259–282, 1 pl.—**Creath** (L. B.) Scrofulous glands in the neck; their removal with some remarks on their nature and treatment. Tr. Texas M. Ass., Austin, 1887, 263–275.—**Curling.** Enlargement of the glands of the neck in an adult. Med. Times & Gaz., Lond., 1861, ii, 109.—**Davies** (J. R.) Removal of glandular enlargements in the neck pressing upon the trachea. Brit. M. J., Lond., 1858, 677.—**Deligny** (L.) Contribution à l'étude du traitement de l'adénopathie cervicale chez les scrofuleux. Ann. Soc. méd.-chir. de Liége, 1878, xvii, 52–59.—**Dolbeau.** Lymphosarcome du cou; extirpation; guérison. France méd., Par., 1874, xxi, 89.—**Duplay** (S.) Des tumeurs ganglionnaires de la région cervicale; lymphadénôme, lymphosarcôme. Progrès méd., Par., 1876, iv, 689.—**Fagan** (J.) On the treatment of scrofulous cervical glands by excision. Dublin J. M. Sc., 1884, 3. s., lxxvii, 495–502. — **Fenwick** (G. E.) Scrofulous or tuberculous glands of the neck. Canada M. & S. J., Montreal, 1886–7, xv, 207–215.—**Follet** (A.) Mémoire sur l'adénite cervicale considérée chez les militaires. Gaz. méd. de Par., 1844, 2. s., xii, 540–545.—**Forestier.** Tumeurs glanduleuses du cou et des aisselles, et leur extirpation. J. de méd., chir., pharm., etc., Par., 1791, lxxxviii, 67–81.—**Franks** (K.) On the nature of scrofulous glands in the neck, and their surgical treatment. Tr. Acad. M. Ireland, Dubl., 1886, iv, 160–

Neck (*Glands of, Diseases of*).

180. *Also*: Lancet, Lond., 1886, i, 1155; 1214. *Also* [Abstr.]: Med. Press & Circ., Lond., 1886, n. s., xli, 539.—**Gibb** (W. F.) On scrofulous neck and its surgical treatment, with illustrative cases. Glasgow M. J., 1888, [4.] s., xxix, 27–35.—**Gilbert.** Adénite cervicale chronique avec production de corpuscules crétacés. Presse méd. belge, Brux., 1887, xxxix, 266.—**Grünfeld** (E.) Erfahrungen über die Exstirpation tuberculöser Halslymphdrüsen. Ztschr. f. Heilk., Prag. 1887, viii, 191–228.—**Guersant.** Des adénites cervicales chez les enfants. Bull. gén. de thérap., etc., Par., 1863, lxiv, 348–352.—**Howard** (W.) A case of lymphadenoma. Tr. Clin. Soc. Lond., 1876, ix, 40–44.—**Larrey** (H.) Mémoire sur l'adénite cervicale observée dans les hôpitaux militaires, et sur l'extirpation des tumeurs ganglionnaires du cou. Mém. Acad. de méd. 1850–51, Par., 1852, xvi, 273–365. *Also*, Reprint. *Also* [Abstr.]: Bull. Acad. de méd., Par., 1848–9, xiv, 834. *Also* [Rap. de Gimelle], 1849–50, xv, 619–632. — **Larzelere** (J. R.) Adenitis, acute and chronic. Buffalo M. & S. J., 1878, xvii, 204–207.—**Leube.** Ueber epidemische Erkrankung der Halslymphdrüsen. Sitzungsb. d. phys.-med. Soc. zu Erlang., 1870–71, 3. Hft., 5–8.—**Mackenzie** (M.) On the hypodermic treatment of indolent enlargements of the cervical glands. Med. Times & Gaz., Lond., 1875, i, 577.—**Magnier.** Observation sur l'extirpation des glandes du cou. J. de méd. mil., Par., 1784, iii, 371–378.—**Marjolin.** Adénopathie cervicale; diagnostic douteux. Bull. et mém. Soc. de chir. de Par., 1877. iii, 344.—**Marston** (C. H.) An hypertrophied cervical gland treated by injections of iodine. Med. Times & Gaz., Lond., 1867, ii, 87.—**Martin** (E.) Note sur l'adénopathie cervicale, suivie de relation de deux opérations. Rec. de mém. de méd. . . . . mil., Par., 1863, 3. s., x, 109–112.—**Mazzoni** (C.) Adenite cronaca cervicale; piaghe scrofolose; estirpazione del tumore scrofoloso; pennellazioni di tintura di jodio; guarigione. Clin. chir. (Mazzoni), Roma, 1876, iii, 149.—**Mollière** (D.) Des tumeurs ganglionnaires du cou. Province méd., Lyon, 1887, ii, 627–631.—**Obissier** (H.) Traitement de l'adénite cervicale suppurée. Bordeaux méd., 1877, vi, 377–379.—**Ogle** (J. W.) Enlarged cervical glands affected by a peculiar deposit. Tr. Path. Soc. Lond., 1859–60, xi, 255.—**Panck** (J.) Ueber Zellgewebsverhärtung am Halse. Ztschr. f. d. ges. Med., Hamb., 1842, xx, 1–17.—**Pauffard.** Leucémie; lymphadénôme (?) énorme du cou; extirpation suivie de guérison; récidive; mort. Progrès méd., Par., 1877, v, 32–34.—**Persichetti-Antonini** (C.) Dell' adenopatia cervico-ascellare e sua etiogenesi. Gior. di med., farm. e vet. mil., Firenze, 1874, xxi, 99–143.—**Philipeaux** (R.) De la résolution des adénites cervicales chroniques par le galvanisme. Gaz. méd. de Lyon, 1858, x, 321–325.—**Picot.** Hypertrophie ganglionnaire cervicale (adénite chronique); traitement par les courants continus; guérison. Gaz. d. hôp., Par., 1870, xliii, 199.—**Pollosson** (M.) Des tumeurs ganglionnaires du cou. Province méd., Lyon, 1887, ii, 547–551.—**Report** on the treatment of scrofulous abscess of the cervical glands. Brit. M. J., Lond., 1871, ii, 726; 756.—**Smith** (T.) A clinical lecture on disease of the glands of the neck in children. Lancet, Lond., 1852, i, 464. — **Storchi** (F.) Glandule linfatiche cervicali affette da degenerazione caseosa; estirpazione; guarigione. Spallanzani, Roma, 1886, 2. s., xv, 461.—**Tait** (L.) On the treatment of suppurating glands of the neck by frequently repeated tapping. Brit. M. J., Lond., 1871, i, 117.—**Texier.** Observation sur une tumeur lymphatique d'un volume considérable, accompagnée d'une fistule située à la partie antérieure du col. Rec. périod. Soc. de méd. de Par., an ix [1800–1], xi, 190–193.—**Treves** (F.) Rest in the treatment of scrofulous neck. Lancet, Lond., 1886, i, 1060–1062.—**Varges** (A. W.) Exstirpation von Drüsen-Geschwülsten am Halse. Ztschr. f. Med., Chir. u. Geburtsh., Magdeb. u. Leipz., 1858, xii, 353–359.—**Vincent** (J. P.) Case of a large glandular tumor in the neck. Med.-Chir. Tr., Lond., 1821–3, xii, 247–249.—**Wyeth** (J. A.) Tuberculous degeneration of the lymphatic glands of the neck. Bull. N. York Path. Soc., 1881, 2. s., i, 320.

Neck (*Hydatids in*).

A. (J. A.) Quistes hidatídicos en la region del cuello. Rev. méd.-quir., Buenos Aires, 1878, xv, 116–118.—**Albert** (E.) Ein vereiternder Echinococcus unter der Haut des Halses. Wien. med. Presse, 1871, xii, 1191.—[**Erichsen.**] Large acephalocyst at the back of the neck; successful removal. Lancet, Lond., 1866, i, 257.—**Hewnden** (A.) A tumour on the neck, full of hydatides. Phil. Tr., Lond., 1700–20, v, 214.—**Lindpaintner.** Ein Fall von Echinococcus am Halse. Festschr. d. ärztl. Ver. München, etc., 1883, 342–345.—**Tourneret.** Kyste hydatique du cou; extirpation partielle; guérison. Gaz. méd. de Strasb., 1876, xxxv, 117.

Neck (*Hydrocele of*).

See **Neck** (*Cysts, etc., of*).

Neck (*Inflammation of*).

See **Neck** (*Abscess, etc., of*); **Parotid** *gland* (*Inflammation, etc., of*).

Neck (*Phlegmon of*).

See **Neck** (*Abscess, etc., of*).

Neck (*Tumors of*).

See, also, **Aneurism** *by anastomosis* (*Cases of*); **Aneurisms** (*Carotid*); **Artery** (*Carotid, Abnormities of*); **Artery** (*Carotid, Ligature of*); **Clavicle** (*Tumors of*); **Goitre**; **Neck** (*Cysts, etc., of*); **Parotid region** (*Tumors of*); **Sternomastoid** (*Tumors of*); **Submaxillary** *region* (*Tumors of*); **Thyroid** *gland* (*Tumors of*); **Varix** *of neck*.

BERGERON (H.) Sur les tumeurs ganglionnaires du cou. 8°. *Paris*, 1872.

BONNAUD (J.-C.) * Des accidents produits par certaines tumeurs du cou; traitement par la méthode de déplacement (Bonnet). 4°. *Paris*, 1855.

BRÜNNINGHAUSEN (H. J.) Ueber die Exstirpation der Balggeschwülste am Halse und über eine neue Methode dieselbe mit Sicherheit zu verrichten. Nebst einem Anhange über die verbesserte Geburts-Zange. 8°. *Würzburg*, 1805.

HIEROKLES (K. X.) * Ein Fall von Tumor colli congenitus. 8°. *Berlin*, [1886].

KELL (J. P.) * Diss. sistens casum tumoris tunicati membranacei. 4°. *Argentorati*, [1721].

Also, in: HALLER. Disp. chir. [etc.] 4°. *Lausannæ*, 1756, v, 388-405.

KLINGER (F.) * Ueber die Behandlung der Lymphome am Halse. 8°. *Berlin*, 1876.

KÖLPIN (F. C.) Heilungsgeschichte von einer beträchtlichen, in Vereiterung übergegangenen Hals-Drüsengeschwulst. 12°. *Kopenhagen*, [1780].

KÖNIG (F.) & RIEDEL. Die entzündlichen Processe am Hals und die Geschwülste am Hals. 8°. *Stuttgart*, 1882.

KRISCH (G.) * Beitrag zur Statistik der Operation der Lymphomata colli. 8°. *Breslau*, [1883].

KROELL DE GRIMMENSTEIN (P. C.) * De tumore albo nuchæ psorico. 12°. *Tubingæ*, 1821.

LAENNEC (T.-A.) Tumeur complexe; observation et examen. 8°. *Nantes*, 1869.

Repr. from: J. de méd. de l'ouest, Nantes, 1869, iii.

LE BRETON (C.-A.-J.) * Étude sur une variété de tumeurs du cou chez les nouveau nés. 4°. *Paris*, 1883.

Also [Abstr.], *in:* Paris méd., 1883, viii, 542-544.

PIEPER (C. F. W.) * Ueber Lymphangiectasia colli congenita. 8°. *Halle a. S.*, 1887.

PORTALUPI (F. G. L.) Storia ragionata dell' enorme tumore del Luigi Tedeschi di Verona estirpato nel giorno 26 giugno 1823. 8°. *Venezia*, 1823.

REY (L.) * Des déformations de la trachée par les tumeurs du cou et des moyens propres à combattre l'asphyxie qui en résulte. 4°. *Paris*, 1875.

SALINIER (J.) * Étude sur les causes et symptômes de l'asphyxie provoquée par les tumeurs du cou. 4°. *Paris*, 1876.

WHITE's (Dr. S. P.) vindication. 8°. [*New York, n. d.*]

Adams (R.) Two cases of successful removal of tumours from the neck. Tr. Ass. King's & Queen's Coll. Phys. in Ireland, Dubl., 1824, iv, 222 - 254. — **Agnew** (D. H.) Fatty tumor of neck. Phila. M. Times, 1871-2, ii, 227.—**Aguilar.** Encondroma del cuello; estirpacion por el bisturi; curacion. Ann. d. Circ. méd. argent., Buenos Aires, 1882-3, vi, 293 - 297. — **Albarrán** (J.) Quiste ganglionar del cuello. Crón. méd.-quir. de la Habana, 1885, xi, 410-416.—**Albert** (E.) Exstirpation einer Struma mit Anwendung eines Lappenschnittes; Heilung in vier Wochen. *In his:* Beitr. z. operat. Chir., 8°, Wien, 1878, 21-24.—**Allen** (H.) Fatty tumor of the neck. Phot. Rev. M. & S., Phila., 1871-2, ii, 48, 1 pl —**Anderson** (A. D.) † Glasgow M. J., 1855-6, iii, 270 - 279. — **Andrews** (T. H.) Encephaloid tumor of the neck; removal; recovery. Phot. Rev. M. & S., Phila., 1871-2, ii, 34 - 36, 1 pl. — **Appenrodt.** Exstirpation einer strumösen Geschwulst. Ztschr. f. Chir. v. Chir., Osterode, 1841, i, pt. 3, 15 - 17. — **Atkinson** (J.) † Med. & Phys. J., Lond., 1813, xxx, 353- 355, 1 pl.—**Atlee** (W. F.) Encysted tumour of neck. Tr.

Neck (*Tumors of*).

Coll. Phys. Phila., 1863-74, n. s., iv, 398. *Also:* Am. J. M. Sc., Phila., 1872, n. s., lxiii, 411. — **Attimont.** Sarcome alvéolaire des muscles de l'épaule et du cou. Bull. Soc. anat. de Nantes 1881, Par., 1882, v, 31. — **Auchincloss** (W.) Mammary sarcoma of neck. Glasgow M. J., 1830, iii, 218.—**Audouin de Chaignebrun** (H.) Tumeur singulière par son origine, sa figure, sa grosseur. J. de méd., chir., pharm., etc., Par., 1779, lii, 515-517.—**Bacqua.** Tumeur anévrismale à la partie antérieure du cou, guérie par les moyens débilitans. Bull. Fac. de méd. de Par., 1809-11, ii (6. année), 136-141.—**Bailhéron.** Observation sur une tumeur froide énorme, située le long de la jugulaire externe d'une jeune fille qui étoit obligée d'appuyer son menton sur l'épaule droite, laquelle tumeur a été guérie par l'application des boues de Balaruc. J. de méd., chir., pharm., etc., Par., 1781, lv, 490-493. — **Baker** (W. M.) Lymphadenomatous tumours of scalp and neck. Tr. Path. Soc. Lond., 1879, xxx, 417-419.—**Ballingall** (G. R.) † Tr. M. & Phys. Soc. Bombay (1853-4), 1855, n. s., ii, 281.—**Banon.** Ulcerated tumor of the neck, proving fatal from hemorrhage. Dublin Hosp. Gaz., 1854, n. s., i, 45-47. — **Bardenheuer** (B.) Lymphomata colli. *In:* Jahresb. ü. d. Thätigk. im Cölner Städt. Bürger-Hosp. (1875), Cöln, 1876, 150. — **Barker** (A. E.) On the removal of deep-seated tumours of the neck. Lancet, Lond., 1886, i, 194; 1011. — **Barrier.** Tumeur ganglionnaire de nature squirrheuse siégeant au côté gauche du cou, et envoyant de profondes racines entre les gros vaisseaux artériels et veineux; opération; guérison. Gaz. méd. de Lyon, 1850, ii, 273-275.—**Barton.** [Fibrous tumour, taken from the back of the neck of an infant.] Dublin Q. J. M. Sc., 1870, n. s., l, 201.—**Bassini** (E.) Fibro-condro-sarcoma alla regione soprajoidea, lato sinistro. *In his:* Clin. operat., 8°. Genova, 1878, 85-87.—**Batchelder** (J. P.) † N. York J. M., 1846, vii, 27-33. ———. Case of tumor. *Ibid.*, 200-206. *Also*, Reprint. ———. Case of tumor at the angle of the jaw. N. York J. M., 1847, viii, 27-35.— **Battey** (R.) Fibro-cystic tumor of the neck. Arch. Clin. Surg., N. Y., 1877, i, 293-299.—**Beauregard.** Lymphosarcome de la région sus-claviculaire; extirpation. J. d. conn. méd. prat., Par., 1881, 3. s., iii, 331. — **Bégin.** Extraction d'une tumeur très-volumineuse enveloppée dans la région cervicale. Bull. Acad. de méd., Par., 1840, v, 482-484.—**Bellhomme.** Observation d'une énorme tumeur du cou. [Rap. de Velpeau.] *Ibid.*, 1841-2, vii, 598.—**Bell** (B.) Extirpation of a tumour in the neck, which was situated beneath the digastric fascia, and behind the submaxillary gland. Edinb. J. M. Sc., 1827, iii, 311-313.—**Bell** (G.) Case of extensive tumour successfully extirpated from the muscular fascia of the neck. *Ibid.*, 1826, i, 61-68, 1 pl.—**Bellini** (G. B.) Tumori glandulari al collo e sotto l' ascella, guariti colla adustione mediante potassa caustica. Gior. d. r. Accad. med.-chir. di Torino, 1852, 2. s., xv, 262-264. — **Bellouard** (V.) Hypertrophie des ganglions lymphatiques du cou; électrisation; érysipèle fugace; inflammation de toutes les glandes séreuses; mort. Gaz. méd. de Bordeaux, 1873, ii, 222-225. — **Bergeron** (J.-E.) Un adénome à la région cervicale. Abeille méd., Montréal, 1880, ii, 7.—[**Bigelow.**] † Boston M. & S. J., 1875, xcii, 170-172. — **Binet.** [Tumeur chondroïde de la région parotidienne.] Bull. Soc. anat. de Par., 1857, xxxii, 250.— **Birkett.** Fibrous tumour of the neck and pharynx, threatening suffocation; survival seventy-seven days after tracheotomy. Lancet, Lond., 1858, i, 339.— **Blake** (J. M.) Removal of an encysted tumor from the neck. Maine M. & S. Reporter, 1858-9, i, 151-153.—**Blandin.** Tumeur fibreuse très-considérable de la partie postérieure et latérale gauche du col. Bull. Acad. de méd., Par., 1842-3, viii, 636.—**Bloxam** (J. A.) Adenoma of the neck; removal; recovery. Med. Times & Gaz., Lond., 1879, ii, 396.— **Bock.** Skirrhöse Geschwulst am Halse. Med. Ztg., Berl., 1854, xxiii, 146. — **Bœckel** (E.) Extirpation des tumeurs profondes du cou avec pansement antiseptique. Bull. gén. de thérap., etc., Par., 1879, xcvii, 289–301. *Also:* Gaz. méd. de Strasb., 1880, xxxix, 37–40. ———. Sarcome du cou; extirpation; lésion de l'artère vertébrale; ligature du vaisseau; guérison. Gaz. méd. de Strasb., 1884, 4. s., xiii, 13.—**Bœckel** (J.) Lymphomes malins du cou (132); extirpation sans section du muscle sternocléido-mastoïdien et sans déviation consécutive de la tête; pansement de Lister; guérison; récidives nécessitant trois nouvelles opérations. Mém. Soc. de méd. de Strasb., 1877, xiii, 81–89.— **Bolling.** Lymphoma colli; extirpation; död. Hygiea, Stockholm, 1886, xlviii, 759. — **Bose** (M. L.) Fibrous tumour of the neck and face; removal. Indian M. Gaz., Calcutta, 1874, ix, 16, 1 pl. — **Bottini** (E.) Cospicuo mixoma delle regioni profonde del collo rimosso con felice successo. Ann. univ. di med., Milano, 1872, ccxix, 534–541, 1 pl. *Also*, Reprint. ———. Vasto sarcoma del collo esportato con felice successo. Gior. d. r. Accad. di med. di Torino, 1874, 3. s., xv, 55–63, 2 pl. *Also, transl.* [Abstr.]: Presse méd. belge, Brux., 1874, xxvi, 301. *Also, transl.* [Abstr.]: Lond. M. Rec., 1874, ii, 230.—**Bouyer.** Tumeur sous-maxillaire (côté droit); ligature préalable de la carotide primitive; ablation de la tumeur douze jours après par l'écrasement linéaire; mort. Bull. Soc. de chir. de Par. (1864), 1865, 2. s., v, 2–5.—**Br.** Glückliche Operation einer 25 Pfund schweren Speckgeschwulst. Ἀσκληπίειον, Berl.,

Neck (*Tumors of*).

1811, i, 845–847. — **Bradbury** (J. C.) Encysted tumor of the neck. Boston M. & S. J., 1852, xlvi, 69–72.—**Bradley** (S. M.) Large myxomatous tumour successfully removed from the neck of an infant. Lancet, Lond., 1877, i. 680.— **Braun** (H.) Topographisch-anatomische Verhältnisse bei malignen Lymphomen am Halse. Verhandl. d. deutsch. Gesellsch. f. Chir., Berl., 1882, xi, pt. 2, 66–75, 1 pl. *Also:* Arch. f. klin. Chir., Berl., 1882, xxviii, 356–365, 1 pl.—**Bray.** Fibrous tumor successfully removed. Proc. Indiana M. Soc., Indianap., 1853, iv. 94–96.—**Breitenstein** (H.) Tumoren aan den hals. Nederl. mil. geneesk. Arch., etc., Utrecht, 1879, iii, 613–615.—**Brent** (J. C.) Removal of a large steatomatous tumor from the neck. West. J. M. & Phys. Sc., Cincin., 1831, iv, 487–489. — **Briggs** (W. T.) Large glandular tumor of the neck. Nashville J. M. & S., 1876, xviii, 204. ———. Large fatty tumor of the neck; removal; death. *Ibid.*, 1881, n. s., xxviii, 259–261. ———. Large glandular tumor of neck; removal. *Ibid.*, 1882, n. s., xxix, 10–12.—**Broca.** [Tumeur dans la région cervicale gauche chez un nouveau-né; ablation.] Bull. Soc. anat. de Par., 1855, xxx, 240. — **Brooks** (B.) Extirpation of tumors from the neck. N. Orl. M. & S. J., 1854–5, xi, 457–460.—**Brooks** (J.) Malignant tumor of the neck; cure. Boston M. & S. J., 1846, xxxiv, 361.—**Browne.** Large fibrous tumour of the neck. Dublin Q. J. M. Sc., 1857, xxiv, 464–468.—**Browne** (L.) Cast, photographs, and drawings of a case of lymphoma displacing the trachea. Tr. Path. Soc. Lond., 1873–4, xxv, 255–258.—**Buchanan** (G.) Large sarcomatous tumour of neck; operation; recovery. Glasgow M. J., 1882, xvii, 54–56.—**Burow.** Durchschneidung des Facialis bei Excision einer Balggeschwulst. Wchnschr. f. d. ges. Heilk., Berl., 1844, 177–179.—**Busch.** Ueber einen eigenthümlichen Vorgang bei einem harten Drüsensarcome des Halses. Verhandl. d. natu h. Ver. d. preuss. Rheinl. u. Westphal., 1866, xxiii, 30–33. ———. Eigenthümliche Heilung eines bösartigen Lymphosarkomes am Halse. Sitzungsb. d. nied.-rheu. Gesellsch. f. Nat.- u. Heilk. zu Bonn, 1880, 292–295.—**Byrd** (W. A.) Successful extirpation of twenty-five adenoid growths from the left posterior cervical triangle, exposing the great vessels and nerves. St. Louis Clin. Rec., 1878–9, v, 213. ———. Two cases of successful ligation of the jugular vein during operations for the removal of tumors from the neck. Gaillard's M. J., N. Y., 1885, xxxix, 125.—**Caccioppoli** (D.) Estirpazione di un tumore grossissimo dal collo di un uomo. Rendic. Accad. med.-chir. di Napoli, 1862, xvi, 11.—**Cantó.** Sifiloma del cuello. Gac. de l. hosp., Valencia, 1883, ii, 424–426.—**Cardenal.** Linfo-sarcoma múltiple de los gánglios cervicales. Arch. de la cirug., Barcel., 1877, i, 21–25.—**Carlisle** (A.) Malignant fungus of the neck; exploratory incisions. Lancet, Lond., 1833–4, i, 419.—**Carnochan** (J. M.) Case of encysted sanguineous tumor of the neck; successful removal. Am. M. Gaz. & J. Health, N. Y., 1856, vii, 55–70.—**Casaubon.** Enchondrome de la région parotidienne; opération. Bull. Soc. anat. de Par., 1867, xlii, 363.—[**Cases.**] Extirpation d'une tumeur à la région parotidienne. Clin. d. hôp., Par., 1827–8, ii, 196.—Tumeur située à la partie supérieure et latérale gauche du cou, faisant saillie au dessous de la langue, et simulant une grenouillette; extirpation; mort. J. compl. du dict. d. sc. méd., Par., 1831, xli, 107–110.— Tumor del cuello á consecuencia de una afeccion de la médula espinal producida por el abuso de la Venus. Bol. de med., cirug. y farm., Madrid, 1843, 2. s., iv, 29.—Tumor de la parte anterior del cuello; ulceracion despues de muchos meses; operacion. *Ibid.*, 181.—Fatal result of an operation for the removal of a tumor from the neck. Tr. M. Soc. N. Y., Albany, 1855, 158–164.—Three examples of fibro-cartilaginous and gelatino sarcomatous tumours of the neck successfully removed; microscopical examination. Lancet, Lond., 1857, i, 32–34.—Tumour above the clavicle; pulsation of subclavian artery abnormally evident; obliteration of brachial artery and distal branches. Brit. M. J., Lond., 1870, i, 519.—Lymphoma of neck. Abstr. M. & S. Cases Gen. Hosp. Sick Children 1882, Pendlebury, Manchester, 1883, ii, 113.—Lympho-sarcoma on the right side of the neck. North Lond. or Univ. Coll. Hosp. Rep. 1885, Lond., 1886, 37.—**Castellarnau.** Lipoma de la region supraioidea extirpado entero sin operacion. Gac. méd. de Cataluña, Barcel., 1879, ii, 550–553.— **Casuso** (G.) Adenoma del cuello. Crón. méd.-quir. de la Habana, 1886, xii, 577–581, 2 pl.—**Caytan.** Note sur un cas de tumeur enkystée du cou. Ann. Soc. méd.-chir. de Bruges, 1858, 2. s., vi, 20.—**Chamart.** Tumeur de la région thyrohyoïdienne. Bull. Soc. de chir. de Par., 1851–2, ii, 584–587.—**Chambers** (J. W.) Surgical treatment of tubercular disease of the glands of the neck. Tr. M. & Chir. Fac. Maryland, Balt., 1886, 89–97.—**Charrier.** [Enchondrome de la région parotidienne.] Bull. Soc. anat. de Par., 1860, xxxv, 346.—**Chassaignac.** Tumeur érectile. Bull. Soc. de chir. de Par., 1882, 2. s., i, 341.— **Chavasse** (T. F.) The diagnosis of cervical tumours. Birmingh. M. Rev., 1882, xii, 241–248. — **Chédevergne.** [Tumeur cutanée du cou et du dos.] Bull. Soc. anat. de Par., 1864, xxxix, 505. — **Chiralt** (V.) Gran neoplasma situado sobre la region cervical lateral derecha invadiendo

la anterior y la posterior; dolores intensisimos que amenazaban acabar con la enferma; estirpacion practicada por F. Rubio, de Sevilla; rápida y completa curacion. Compilador méd., Barcel., 1867–8, iii, 544; 577.—**Chrétien** (H.) De l'extirpation des grosses tumeurs ganglionnaires de nature strumeuse et non ulcérées du cou. Gaz. hebd. de méd., Par., 1886, 2. s., xxiii, 23–25. — **Clark** (A.) Lymphoma affecting cervical glands and connective tissue between the larynx and œsophagus. Tr. Path. Soc. Lond. 1874, xxv, 253–255.—**Clarke** (J. F.) Case of congenital cervical tumor. Med. Times & Gaz., Lond., 1865, i, 318.— **Clot.** Extirpation d'une tumeur squirrheuse du cou. Gaz. d. hôp., Par., 1831, v, 213. *Also:* Ann. de la méd. physiol., Par, 1832, xxii, 350–357. — **Clutton** (H. H.) Large vascular growth in the neck. St. Thomas's Hosp. Rep. 1881, Lond., 1882, n. s., xi, 48.—**Cock.** Large solid glandular tumour in the neck; excision; recovery. Med. Times & Gaz., Lond., 1853, n. s., vii, 191. ———. Fatty tumors encircling the neck. Lancet, Lond., 1860, ii, 188.— **Cockle** (J.) On aneurismal tumors involving the neck. Med. Times & Gaz., Lond., 1863, i, 504; 530; 557. ———. Contributions to the pathology of aneurisms and tumors involving the chest and root of the neck. Med.-Chir. Tr., Lond., 1866–7, 2. s., xxxii, 459–475, 3 pl. *Also* [Abstr.]: Proc. Roy. M. & Chir. Soc. Lond., 1864–7, v, 328–330. ———. Further contributions to the pathology and treatment of aneurismal tumours of the neck and chest. Lancet, Lond., 1869, i, 422; 489; 1870, i, 6; 43. ———. Contributions to the pathology of tumours of the neck. Med. Times & Gaz., Lond., 1873, i, 5; 30.—**Conant.** Removal of an inch and a half of common carotid artery from the substance of a cancerous tumor; ligation of jugular vein; recovery of the patient. Am. M. Times, N. Y., 1864, viii, 28. — **Cooper.** Clinical remarks on a case of medullary sarcoma. Lond. M. & S. J., 1836, viii, 702.— **Cornillon** (J.) Sarcome ganglionnaire primitif. Rev. phot. d. hôp. de Par., 1871, iii, 257–262, 1 pl. — **Coskery** (O. J.) Tumor in the neck. Maryland M. J., Balt., 1881–2, viii, 8.—**Costetti** (E.) Relazione di un tumore nel collo curato coll' agopuntura. Bull. d. sc. med. di Bologna, 1845, 3. s., viii, 217–221.—**Coulson.** Case of non-malignant tumour, of considerable size, situated on the lateral part of the neck. Lancet, Lond., 1854; ii, 101. — **Cox** (A. L.) Large tumor on the right side of the neck, successfully removed. N. York M. & S. Reporter, 1846, i, 221–223.— **Critchett.** Tumor of the neck, consisting of a mass of hypertrophied glands; successful removal. Lancet, Lond., 1862, i, 120. — **Croft** (J.) Fibro cystic tumour of neck. Tr. Path. Soc. Lond., 1874–5, xxvi, 180–182. — **Croly** (H. G.) Enormous pendulous tumour of (14 years' growth) occupying the right parotidean space, and side of the neck; excision; complete recovery. without deformity. Dublin Q. J. M. Sc., 1868, xlvi, 258–261, 2 pl.—**Crooke** (E. G.) Removal of a fibrous tumour from the left neck. Lancet, Lond., 1855, i, 64.—**Cruveilhier** (E.) [Enchondrome de la région parotidienne.] Bull. Soc. anat. de Par., 1860, xxxv, 177.—**Cullerier.** Observation sur l'extirpation de plusieurs glandes lymphatiques très-volumineuses, situées à la partie supérieure du cou et à la partie latérale de la face. J. gén. de méd., chir. et pharm., Par., 1806, xxvi, 279 – 300. — **Curling.** Tumor in the cervical region; pressure upon the great blood-vessels; coma; death. Med. Times & Gaz., Lond., 1862, ii, 7.—**Curran** (R. H.) Enormous pendulous tumor, occupying the whole of the left side of the neck and parotid space; weight, three pounds eight ounces; removed successfully. Indian M. Gaz., Calcutta, 1872, vii, 160. — **Daly** (P.) A case of extirpation of an unusually large steatomatous tumor from the neck. Tr. Ass. King's & Queen's Coll. Phys. Ireland, Dubl., 1828, v, 84–95.—**Danzel.** Ein Beitrag zur Exstirpation grosser Halstumoren. Arch. f. klin. Chir., Berl. 1866, vii, 887–890.—**Davis** (J. S.) Removal of an encysted tumour of the neck weighing over one and a half pounds; recovery. Am. J. M. Sc., Phila., 1873, n. s., lxv, 568.— **Davis** (M. M.) Tumor of the neck, successfully treated by hypodermic injections of nitrate of silver. Tr. Wisconsin M. Soc., Milwaukee, 1877, 145.—**Dehler** (A.) Ein Beitrag zu den Geschwülsten am Halse. Würzb. med. Ztschr., 1861, ii, 97–102, 1 pl.—**De Lavacherie.** De l'opportunité de l'extirpation des tumeurs du cou non susceptibles de résolution; réflexions sur l'introduction de l'air dans le cœur par des veines ouvertes accidentellement. Bull. Acad. roy. de méd. de Belg., Brux., 1847–8, vii, 788–802. [Rap. de Gouzée], 1848–9, viii, 15.— **Diaz** (J. G.) Extirpacion de un tumor supra-parotideo. An. Acad. de cien. méd. . . . de la Habana, 1867–8, iv, 242–247.—**Dichiara** (F.) Adenoma alla regione laterale destra del collo, curata con la corrente continua. Gazz. clin. di elettroter., Palermo, 1883, i, 104.—**Dodge.** Cervical tumor; recovery. Ann. Anat. & Surg. Soc., Brooklyn, N. Y., 1880, ii, 336. ———. Cervical tumor; extirpation; recovery. *Ibid.*, 383. — **Dohlhoff.** Exstirpation einer grossen Balggeschwulst am Halse. Med. Ztg., Berl., 1838, vii, 256.— **Douglas** (J.) A large tumour in the neck, with a boney substance. Phil. Tr., Lond., 1700–20, v, 211–214, 1 pl.— **Draper** (F. W.) Large tumor of the neck. Boston M. & S. J., 1868, i, 410.—**Duffy** (C. C.) Successful extirpa-

Neck (*Tumors of*).

tion of tumor over the external jugular veins. Virginia M. Month., Richmond, 1883-4, x, 536. — **Dugas** (L. A.) Remarks on tumours of the neck; with cases. South. M. & S. J., Augusta, 1846, n. s., ii, 513-517. ———. Extirpation of a cervical tumor. *Ibid.*, 1853, ix, 42-44. — **Duplay** (S.) Des tumeurs ganglionnaires de la région cervicale; lymphadénôme; lymphosarcôme. *In his:* Confér. de clin. chir., 8°, Par., 1877, 73-77. — **Dupuy** (L.-E.) Lipome sous-parotidien; extirpation. Bull. Soc. anat. de Par., 1873, xlviii, 50. — **Dupuytren.** Plötzlich erfolgter Tod während der Ausschälung einer fibröszelligen Geschwulst aus dem Halse. J. d. Chir. u. Augenh., Berl., 1825. viii, 469-472. ———. Tumeur mélanique développée derrière l'angle maxillaire du côté droit. Rev. méd. franç. et étrang., Par., 1829, i, 353-358. ———. Tumeur érectile accidentelle du volume d'une grosse noisette, développée à la partie antérieure et latérale droite du cou; opération. Gaz. d. hôp., Par., 1833, vii, 18. — **Durham** (A. E.) Extensive sloughing of the neck, "nondescript," lymphosarcomatous tumour. Tr. Path. Soc. Lond., 1882-3, xxxiv, 245, 1 pl. — [**Eberl.**] Dartre dégénérée, guérie par l'extirpation. Clin. d. hôp., Par., 1828-9, iii, 168. — **Eddison** (B.) Tumour on the neck. Lond. M. Reposit., 1828, xxix, 228. — **Eder** (A.) Lymphoma colli lateris sinistri. *In his:* Aerztl. Ber. 1884, 8°, Wien, 1885, 17. — **Ellis.** Tumor of the neck, composed of a large number of caseous nodules; same disease in the abdomen; paraplegia, without lesion of the nervous centres. Boston M. & S. J., 1860-61, lxiii, 362. — **Ellsworth** (P. W.) Tumor in the neck. *Ibid.*, 1859, lx, 418-420. — **Encinas** (S. G.) Linfo-sarcoma del cuello; extirpación; muerte. Génio méd.-quir., Madrid, 1884, xxx, 421. — **Englisch.** Lymphoma colli; Exstirpation, nachdem Tinctura Fowleri zuerst ohne Erfolg angewendet wurde; Heilung. Ber. d. k. k. Krankenanst. Rudolph-Stiftung in Wien (1878), 1879, 300 — **Eschenbach** (C. E.) Sarcoma in jugulo lethale. *In his:* Obs. anat.-chir.-med. rariora, 12°, Rostoch., 1769, 244-250. — **Eve** (P. F.) Successful removal of a large schirrous tumour from the neck, attached to the left tonsil. South. M. & S. J., Augusta, 1837-8, ii, 643. — **Fardeau.** Observation sur une tumeur pneumato-lymphatique située à la partie antérieure du col. J. gén. de méd., chir. et pharm., Par., 1803, xvi, 62-65. — **Fawcett** (E.) A case of fibroplastic tumor of the neck of ten years' standing, successfully removed by operation. Madras Month. J. M. Sc., 1871, iii, 412. — **Ferreri** (G.) Lipoma missomatoso della nuca; estirpazione; medicatura alla Lister; guarigione di prima intenzione. Sperimentale, Firenze, 1881, xlvii, 153-157. — **Ferrero** (E.) Voluminoso plasmoma della parte anteriore del collo; estirpazione seguita da guarigione per prima intenzione; medicatura all' acqua calda sterilizzata. Osservatore, Torino, 1887, xxxviii, 361-363. — **Fischer.** Beobachtung und Heilung einer Geschwulst am Halse. Allg. med. Ann., Altenb., 1811, pt. 2, 1084-1094. — **Fischer** (E.) Ein mannskopfgrosses Cystosarkom am Halse. Deutsche Ztschr. f. Chir., Leipz., 1878, x, 478-486, 1 pl. — **Flint** (A.) Death from suffocation produced by enlargement of the glandular adipose substance posterior to larynx. Boston M. & S. J., 1841, xxiv, 69. — **Forster** (J. C.) Follicular sarcoma of neck; excision. Guy's Hosp. Rep., Lond., 1875, 3. s., xx, 12. — [**Fosse** (L.)] Kyste fibro-séreux considérable à parois squirrheuse sur un point; extirpation; guérison. Ann. clin. de Montpel., 1857-8, v, 41. — **Foucault.** Hypertrophie ganglionnaire de la région sous-maxillaire. Bull. Soc. anat. de Par. (1871), 1873, xlvi, 131. — **Fouilloux.** Tumeur de la région maxillo-pharyngienne droite. *Ibid.*, 273. — **Fraenkel** (A.) Zur Histologie, Aetiologie und Therapie der Lymphomata colli. Ztschr. f. Heilk., Prag, 1885, vi, 193-275. — **Freeman** (H. W.) On recurrent fibromata of the neck, and their relation to the branchial arches. Brit. M. J., Lond., 1884, i, 1083. — **Gärtner.** Fibromyxosarcoma colli; Exstirpation; Heilung nach 4 Wochen. Med. Cor.-Bl. d. württemb. ärztl. Ver., Stuttg., 1871, xli, 91. — **Galliet.** Tumeur au cou du volume d'un petit œuf de poule, occupant les parties profondes de cette région et s'accompagnant d'un développement considérable du corps thyroïde. Bull. Soc. méd. de Reims, 1871, No. x, 40-45. — **Gay** (C. C. F.) Tumors of the neck. Buffalo M. & S. J., 1872-3, xii, 88. — **Gayet.** Tumeur dans la région sus-hyoïdienne; ablation; résection d'une portion du maxillaire; examen anatomique de la pièce. Mém. et compt.-rend. Soc. d. sc. méd. de Lyon, 1863-4, iii, 18-22. — **Gerster.** Melanotic lympho-sarcoma removed from the neck. Ann. Anat. & Surg., Brooklyn, N. Y., 1883, viii, 32. — **Gibson** (W.) Case of extirpation of a tumor of the neck, in which the carotid artery and internal jugular vein were tied; with remarks. Am. J. M. Sc., Phila., 1833-4, xiii, 305-309, 1 pl. — **Giné** (J.) Linfomas de las regiones laterales del cuello; médicacion expoliativa local; compresion de las venas yugulares; congestion meningea con edema cerebral; muerte. Independ. méd., Barcel., 1874-5, vi, 116; 128. — **Godlee** (R. J.) A case of removal of a tumour of the neck causing injury to the cervical sympathetic. Tr. Clin. Soc. Lond., 1886, xix, 321. — **Golding-Bird** (C. H.) & **Mahomed** (F. A.) Two cases of pulsatile tumour at the root of the neck. Guy's Hosp. Rep., Lond., 1883, 3. s.,

Neck (*Tumors of*).

xxvi, 83-99. — **Gordon.** Cartilaginous tumor removed from the region of the parotid gland. Dublin Hosp. Gaz., 1858. v, 121. — **Gosselin.** Lipôme mou sus, sous et rétro-claviculaire, ablation par énucléation avec les doigts. Gaz. d. hôp., Par., 1869, xlii, 581. — **Greene** (W. W.) Encysted tumor of neck. Boston M. & S. J., 1864, lxx, 455-457. ———. Deep cervical tumor, the removal of which involved the exsection of a portion of the internal jugular vein, with some remarks upon the ligation of veins in general. Med. Rec., N. Y., 1867-8, ii, 173. — **Greensward** (M. P.) Removal of a tumor from the throat. Med. Summary, Lansdale, 1879-80, i, 97. — **Grilli** (F.) Ciste fibrosa al collo. Sperimentale, Firenze, 1873, xxxii, 177 - 182. — **Gross.** Sebaceous tumour of neck and shoulder. Med. Rec., N. Y., 1867-8, ii, 343. ———. Large venous tumor. Med. & Surg. Reporter, Phila., 1868, xviii, 508. — **Günther** (O.) O krwawych torbielach szyi. [Hæmatocele of neck.] Gaz. lek., Warszawa, 1877, xxiii, 215; 292. — **Güntner** (W.) Atherom der rechten Supraclaviculargegend unter dem Bilde eines Lipoms. Vrtljschr. f. d. prakt. Heilk., Prag, 1859, lxiii, 45. ———. Atherom an der linken Seite des Halses in Form einer Drüsengeschwulst. *Ibid.*, 45. — **Guersant** fils. Tumeur du cou d: nature douteuse. Gaz. d. hôp., Par., 1845, 2. s., vii, 479. ———. Tumeur énorme occupant toute la partie antérieure et latérale droite du cou. *Ibid.*, 1846, 2. s., viii, 255. — **Guillemet.** Verrue du cou (angiôme caverneux). Bull. Soc. anat. de Nantes 1878 - 9, Par., 1879, ii, 100. — **Guthrie** (C. G.) Enormous pendulous and fatty tumor in the clavicular region; removal; recovery. Lancet, Lond., 1851, ii, 227. — **Guyon.** Tumeur fibro-plastique du cou. Bull. Soc. chir. de Par., 1870. 2. s., x, 37-40. — **Haartmann.** Halsgeschwulst. Verm. Abhandl. . . . v. einer Gesellsch. pract. Aerzte zu St. Petersb., 1830, iv, 248, 1 pl. — **Hadra** (B. E.) Scrofulous glands beneath the sterno-cleido-mastoid muscle. N. Orl. M. & S. J., 1875, iii, 329-334. — **Hahn** (E.) Ein durch Operation entferntes 17 Pfund schweres Lipoma fibrosum petrificum polyposum mit Elephantiasis der Haut. Berl. klin. Wchnschr., 1884, xxi, 553. — **Haig** (W.) On a case of tumour in the neck. Austral. M. J., Melbourne, 1874, xix, 53, 1 pl. *Also*, Reprint. — [**Hamilton.**] Encysted tumour. Dublin Q. J. M. Sc., 1864, xxxvii, 174. — **Hancock.** Two cases of deep seated tumours of the neck; removal of the growth; severe hæmorrhage; recovery. Lancet, Lond., 1853, i, 449. — **Harris** (C.) Account of the successful extirpation of tumours from the neck. Med. Reposit., N. Y., 1808, v, 246-249. — **Hawkins** (C.) On a peculiar form of congenital tumor of the neck. Med.-Chir. Tr., Lond., 1838-9, xxii, 231-244. *Also :* Lancet, Lond., 1839, ii, 406-408. *Also, in his :* . . . Path. & Surg. Writings, 8°, Lond., 1874, i, 278-284. — **Helmuth** (W. T.) Removal of a large recurrent fibroid (spindle-shaped sarcoma) from the neck; recurrence in three localities. *In his :* A dozen cases clin. surg. 8°, Albany, 1876, 10-15. — **Henry.** Tumeur considérable du cou, faisant saillie dans le pharynx et sous la base de la langue. Rec. de mém. de méd. . . . mil., Par., 1840, xix, 336-342. — **Hervez de Chégoin.** Tumeur du poids de quinze livres, à l'instant de son ablation. Bull. Acad. de méd., Par., 1845-6, xi, 82-84. — **Heurtaux.** Sarcome mélanique de la région sous-maxillaire. J. de méd. de l'ouest, Nantes, 1886, xx, 298. — **Hewitt** (G. A.) Lympho-sarcoma of neck; excision. Northwest. Lancet, St. Paul, 1884-5, iv, 28-32. — **Hicks** (J. B.) & **Gervis** (H.) Report on neck-tumour in a fœtus. Tr. Obst. Soc. Lond. (1863), 1864, v, 290. — **Hill** (G. N.) Case of tumour of the neck, which terminated fatally. Lond. M. Reposit., 1815, iv, 186 - 191. — **Hilton.** Fibro-plastic tumour of the neck. Lancet, Lond., 1859, i, 611. — **Hodges** (R. M.) Tumor of neck. Boston M. & S. J., 1867-8, lxxvii, 525. — **Hofmokl.** Grosse lipomatöse Gefässgeschwulst am Halse bei einem achtmonatlichen Kinde; Entfernung durch elastische Ligatur auf zwei Mal; Tod durch Pyämie am 30. Tage. Wien. med. Presse, 1874, xv, 571. — **Hogner** (R.) Plötsligt försvinnande af en tumör. [Sudden disappearance of a tumor of neck.] Eira, Göteborg, 1883, vii, 110. — **Holloway** (J. M.) Cervical lymphomata. Med. Herald, Louisville, 1880-81, ii, 110-114. — **Holmes** (T.) Congenital tumour of the neck. Tr. Path. Soc. Lond., 1860-61, xii, 206-208. ———. Congenital tumour beneath the sterno-mastoid. *Ibid.*, 1863 - 4, xv, 215 - 217. ———. Fibro-fatty tumour of the neck, in a child, successfully removed. *Ibid.*, 1864-5, xvi, 236. *Also :* Lancet, Lond., 1864, ii, 548. — **Holthouse.** Tumor beneath the lower jaw; successful removal. Lancet, Lond., 1861, ii, 207. — **Hontañon** (P. T.) Tumores en el cuello de difícil diagnóstico; degeneracion especial de los tejidos de la ingle formando igualmente tumores imposibles de diagnosticar. Crón. de l. hosp., Madrid, 1854, ii, 452 - 467. — **Hryniewicz** (F.) Balggeschwulst am Halse, die ihren Sitz in dem Triangulum omo-hyoideum unter dem Kopfnicker hatte. Med. Jahrb. d. k. k. österr. Staates, Wien, 1840, n. F., xxi, 55-63, 1 pl. — **Huguier.** Tumeur située dans la région cervicale. Bull. Soc. de chir. de Par., 1852 - 3, iii, 560 - 562. ———. Tumeur ganglionnaire de la région cervicale; ablation. *Ibid.*, 1853-4, iv, 368. ———. Tumeur fibreuse de la région latérale du cou; extirpation; caractères de cette tumeur.

Neck (*Tumors of*).

Ibid. (1862), 1863, 2. s., iii, 501.— **Hutchinson.** Symmetrical fatty tumour of the neck. Brit M. J., Lond. 1883, i, 623.— **Ilinski** (A. I.) Sluch. postepen. (po chastjam) otnjat. ogrom. lipomy na sheil. [Gradual removal of an immense lipoma of neck.] Med. Obozr., Mosk., 1887, xxviii, 596–600.— **Isaacs** (C. E.) Large encysted tumor removed from the anterior region of the neck. Tr. M. Soc. County Kings 1858–64, Brooklyn, 1865, i, 3–6. *Also*: N. York J. M., 1859, 3. s., vii, 35–38.— **Jamieson** (A.) Glandular tumour of neck; operation; entrance of air into veins; death. China. Imp. Customs. Med. Rep., Shanghai, 1879–80, No. xix, 19–21. ——. Front, side. and back view of adenoid tumour of neck and side of head in a woman of 44. *Ibid.*, 1885–6, No. xxxi, 35, 2 pl.— **Jessett** (F. B.) On the surgical treatment of certain tumours of the neck. Brit. M. J., Lond., 1886, ii, 712–715. ——. Lectures on tumours of the neck, their pathology, symptoms, and treatment. Med. Press & Circ., Lond., 1887, n. s., xliii, 487; 518; 542; 564. *Also*: Med. Reg., Phila., 1887, i, 601; ii, 1; 25; 49.— **Johnson** (H. J.) Tumour in the neck; new exploring instrument. Lancet, Lond., 1841–2, ii, 60.— **Journez.** Contribution à l'observation d'une tumeur siégeant au côté gauche du cou chez un vieux soldat. Arch. méd. belges, Brux., 1877, 3. s., xi, 468.— **Keen** (W. W.) Removal of a lymphoma from the neck; recovery. Med. & Surg. Reporter. Phila., 1885, liii, 66. *Also*: N. York M. J., 1885, xlii, 217.— **Keister** (B. C.) Spasmodic asthma due to fatty tumor of the neck; removal; cure. Virginia M. Month., Richmond, 1885–6, xii, 272.— **Kempf** (M.) Excision of a deep-seated tumor of the neck. Louisville M. News, 1877, iii, 274.— **Kennedy** (N. B.) Removal of a fibro-cellular tumor from the left carotid triangle. Med. & Surg. Reporter, Phila., 1879, xli, 68.— **Kerr** (J. G.) † Rep. Med. Miss. Soc. in China 1860, Canton, 1861, xxii, 10.— **Kilgarriff** (M. J.) Cervical lymphosarcoma. Tr. Acad. M. Ireland, Dubl, 1885, iii, 360.— **Klose** (C. W.) & **Paul** (J.) Medullarsarcom der Halsdrüsen. Ztschr. f. klin. Med., Bresl., 1852, iii, 53.— **Knight** (F. I.) Lympho-sarcoma of the neck involving the lung. Boston M. & S. J., 1878, xcix, 498. *Also*: Extr. Rec. Bost. Soc. M. Improve. (1874–9), 1880, vi, 120–122.— **Köhler.** Scrophulöses Sarcom der Lymphdrüsen (Lobstein) des Halses. [3 cases.] Charité-Ann. 1876, Berl., 1878, iii, 435.— **Koller** (F. S.) Die Exstirpation eines voluminösen Halstumors. Med.-chir. Centralbl., Wien, 1882, xvii, 533.— **Kramoling** (H. S.) Steatom am Halse. Ztschr. f. Nat.- u. Heilk. in Ungarn, Oedenburg, 1856, vii, 260.— **Kranefuss** (B. G.) Glücklich vollbrachte Heilung einer anscheinend bösartigen Geschwulst im Halse. Org. f. d. ges. Heilk., Aachen, 1856, v, 12–21.— **Kraus** (F.) Kritisch-etymologische Betrachtungen über einige am Halse vorkommende Geschwülste. Vrtljschr. f. d. prakt. Heilk., Prag, 1846, ii, 63–86.— **Küchler** (H.) Zur Ausschälung der Geschwülste in der Augenhöhle und am Halse. Deutsche Klinik, Berl., 1854, vi, 543.— **Küster** (E.) Ausgedehntes Lymphosarcom r. am Halse; Exstirpation; Tod an Lufteintritt in die V. jugul. int. *In his*: Ein chir. Trien. 1872–8, 8°, Kassel u. Berl., 1882, 103. *Also*: Med.-chir. Centralbl., Wien, 1882, xvii, 448. ——. Lymphangioma cavernosum colli; Exstirpation; Heilung. *In his*: Ein chir. Trienn. 1876–8, 8°, Kassel u. Berl., 1882, 104.— **Labat** (L.) Extirpation d'une tumeur squirrheuse, accompagnée d'un kyste séreux, occupant tout le côté gauche du cou, depuis l'apophyse mastoïde jusqu'à la clavicule; opération qui a nécessité la ligature de l'artère carotide, celle de la veine jugulaire interne et la section de la huitième paire de nerfs. Ann. de la méd. physiol., Par., 1834, xxvi, 297–317. *Also*, Reprint.— **Labbé** (L.) [Tumeur cartilagineuse dans la région parotidienne.] Bull. Soc. anat. de Par., 1860, xxxv, 353.— **Lafauric.** [Tumeurs mélaniques développées dans la région parotidienne.] *Ibid.* (1845), 1846, xx, 266. ——. Tumeurs mélaniques du cou. *Ibid.*, 1846, xxi, 23–25.— **Lafosse.** Cérébroïde énorme occupant la région jugulaire gauche, énuclée avec succès. Mémor. d. hôp. du midi, Par., 1830, ii, 487–491.— **Lanelongue.** Tumeurs branchiales du cou. J. de méd. de Bordeaux, 1886–7, xvi, 374–376.— **Langenbeck** (B.) Ueber eine seltnere Geschwulst am Halse; eine Jodschmierkur; Electropunctur. Deutsche Klinik, Berl., 1855, vii, 175–180.— **Lankford** (A. P.) A tumor successfully removed from beneath the sterno-mastoid muscle. St. Louis M. & S. J., 1872, ix, 65–73.— **Lassing** (H.) Case of encysted cervical tumor. Am. M. Times, N. Y., 1862, v, 34.— **Latouche.** Kystes et tumeur fibro-kystique congénitale du cou. Rev. mens. d. mal. de l'enf., Par., 1885, iii, 415–419.— **de Lavacherie.** De l'opportunité de l'extirpation des tumeurs du cou non susceptibles de résolution. Gaz. d. hôp., Par., 1849, 3. s., i, 10.— **Lawrence** (W.) Encysted tumour of the neck on the left side of the larynx. Med. Times, Lond., 1851, n. s., ii, 28. ——. Large anomalous tumour in the neck, with great distension and varicose enlargement of closely adjacent veins; operation; autopsy. Med. Times & Gaz., Lond., 1853, vi, 213–215.— **Lawrie** (J. A.) Two cases of deep seated tumour in the neck. Glasgow M. J., 1856–7, iv, 61–68.— **Leasure** (D.) A tumor of the neck (probably malignant) treated by injection of chromic acid. Med. & Surg. Re-

Neck (*Tumors of*).

porter, Phila., 1870, xxii, 507–510. — [**Legie** (E.)] Ein reines Enchondrom mit sehr raschem Wachsthum; Operation: Tod. Wien. med. Wehnschr., 1868, xviii, 1097–1099.— **Legrande.** [Tumeur osseuse ganglionnaire du cou.] Bull. Soc. de chir. de Par. (1860), 1861, 2. s., i, 223.— **Leisrink** (H.) Spindelzellensarcom. [Neck.] *In his*: Ber. d. chir. Poliklin. d. Frauen-Hülfs-Ver. zu Hamb. (1872–8), 4°, 1879, 26.— **Letenneur.** Tumeur fibro-plastique du cou extirpée avec succès; récidive sous forme de cancer encéphaloïde; anévrysme diffus par l'ulcération de l'artère dentaire inférieure; ligature de l'artère carotide primitive; hémiplégie du côté opposé; mort par suite des progrès du cancer. Monit. d. hôp., Par., 1859, vii, 658–660. *Also*: J. de la sect. de méd. Soc. acad. Loire-Inf., Nantes. 1859, xxxv, 13–22.— **Létiévant.** Enchondrome volumineux du côté gauche du cou; ablation; guérison rapide. Mém. et compt.-rend. Soc. d. sc. méd. de Lyon, 1864, iii, 249. *Also*: Gaz. méd. de Lyon, 1864, xvi, 367.— **Lévêque.** Extirpation d'une glande située au bas de l'oreille. J. de méd.. chir., pharm., etc., Par., 1817, xl, 61–65.— **Lindh** (A.) Plötsligt försvinnande af en tumör. [Sudden disappearance of a tumor.] Eira, Göteborg, 1882, vi, 367–369.— **Link** (I.) Chrzestniak wielkości główki dziecięcéj wychodzący z kości gnykowéj. [Large sarcoma on the neck of a child, involving the hyoid bone.] Przegl. lek., Krakow., 1886, xxv, 385–387.— **Lisenko** (A. V.) Sluch. vilosh. sarkomi shei. [Extirpation of sarcoma of neck.] Chir. Vestnik, St. Petersb., 1886, ii, 632–634.— **Lopez Alonso** (J.) Linfo-sarcoma voluminose del cuello. Correo méd. castellano, Salamanca, 1885, ii, 713–717.— **Lücke.** Entfernung des N. vagus mit einer Halsgeschwulst; Heilung. Centralbl. f. Chir., Leipz., 1880, vii, 577.— **Luke.** Deep-seated tumor of the neck; extirpation; recovery. Lond. M. Gaz., 1830–31, vii, 606.— **Lumniczer.** Extirpation eines kindskopfgrossen Fibrosarkoms. Pest. med.-chir. Presse, Budapest, 1880, xvi, 130.— **Lyon** (I.) Tumor on the carotid, removed. Lond. M. Gaz., 1833–4, xiii, 45.— **M'Clellan** (G.) Three cases of specific tumours in the neck, which were successfully extirpated. Am. M. Rev., Phila., 1826, iii, 377–386. ——. Extirpation of a tumour in the neck. St. Louis M. & S. J., 1847–8, v, 437–442.— **M'Clellan** (J.) A large tumor taken from the neck. Med. & Surg. Reporter, Phila., 1862–3, ix, 129.— **MacConnell** (W. G.) Myxomatous tumor of the posterior cervical region. Tr. Path. Soc. Phila. (1881–3), 1884, xi, 247–249. *Also*: Med. News, Phila., 1882, xli, 611. *Also*: Boston M. & S. J., 1882, cvii, 496. *Also*: Med. & Surg. Reporter, Phila., 1882, xlvii, 629. *Also*: Phila. M. Times, 1882–3, xiii, 169. *Also*: St. Louis M. & S. J., 1883, xliv, 79.— **MacCormac** (W.) Four cases of symmetrical development of fat at the back of the neck. St. Thomas's Hosp. Rep. 1883, Lond., 1884. n. s., xiii, 287–297.— **McIntyre** (J.) A successful operation for lymphoma of the neck, with ligation of common and external carotid arteries and external jugular vein. St. Louis M. & S. J., 1883, xlv, 174–178.— **McKay** (A.) Removal of a lipomatous tumour from the left side of the neck. Canada Lancet, Toronto, 1876–7, ix, 290.— **Mackinton.** A tumour extirpated from the neck and face of a native. India J. M. & Phys. Sc., Calcutta, 1836, n. s., i. 500.— **Maclean** (D.) Tumor in superior carotid triangle; removal; secondary hæmorrhage; recovery. Penins J. M., Detroit, 1876, n. s., i, 634.— **McLeod** (K.) Case of glandular sarcoma of the neck; removal; death from pyæmia. Indian M. Gaz., Calcutta, 1879, xiv, 161–164. ——. Cartilaginous tumour of the neck. *Ibid.*, 1882, xvii, 250. *Also*: Tr. Calcutta M. Soc., 1882, iii, 116–119.— **McReddie.** Sarcomatous tumour of neck; operation; necropsy. Indian M. Gaz., Calcutta, 1884, xix, 327.— **M'Whinnie** (A. M.) Observations on certain tumours of the neck, with notes relating to its surgical anatomy. Lancet, Lond., 1862, i, 33; 95; 143; 596. ——. Observations on certain tumours of the neck, with notes relating to its surgical anatomy. *Ibid.*, 1864, ii, 35–37.— **Maddux** (T. C.) Fibro-cystic tumor of the neck. Tr. M. & Chir. Fac. Maryland, Balt., 1879, lxxxi, 188–193.— **Magnier.** Mémoire sur l'extirpation des tumeurs glanduleuses du cou et autres, pratiquée avec succès sur les soldats envoyés par le roi, à l'Hôpital de la ville de Saint-Quentin, depuis 1772 jusqu'en 1783. J. de méd. mil., Par., 1784, 'ii, 87–111.— **Maisonneuve.** Note sur l'extirpation des tumeurs fibreuses profondes, par la méthode de morcellement. Compt. rend. Acad. d. sc., Par., 1854, xxxix, 267–270. *Also*: Monit. d. hôp., Par., 1854, ii, 767. *Also*: Gaz. d. hôp., Par., 1854, xxvii, 383. *Also, transl.*: St. Louis M. & S. J., 1855, xiii, 122–125.— **Malle.** Mémoire sur les tumeurs ganglionnaires de la région cervicale. Arch. méd. de Strasb., 1836, ii, 365–395.— **Marcacci** (G.) Voluminosi tumori al lati della base del collo; estirpazione di quello del lato destro; comparsa successiva di emiplegia a destra; afasia; neoplasmi nell' apparecchio otto striato. Raccoglitore med., Forlì, 1874, xxxvii, 281; 313.— **Marfan** & **Marfan** (A.) Énorme lipome de la région latérale droite du cou coexistant avec des néoplasies diverses; enkystement complet de la tumeur graisseuse. Bull. Soc. anat. de Par., 1885, lx, 296–298.— **Martin** (J. R.) Excision of two enormous tumors from the neck. Quart. J. Calcutta M. & Phys. Soc., 1838, ii,

Neck (*Tumors of*).

104–106.—**Martone** (V.) Estirpazione di vasto sarcoma al collo; guarigione. Ann. clin. d. osp. incur., Napoli, 1881, vi, 287–290.—**Mascaró** (A.) Tumor indolente en la parte anterior del cuello. Anfiteatro anat., Madrid, 1873, i, 95.—**Mastin** (C. B.) Deep-seated fibrous tumor of neck. Nashville J. M. & S., 1867, n. s., ii, 257–259.—**Mayer.** Tumeur adénoïde volumineuse de la nuque; nécropsie. Ann. Soc. de méd. d'Anvers, 1862, xxiii, 616–624, 1 pl.—**Mayo** (C.) Encysted tumor on the right side of the neck. Lancet, Lond., 1847, i, 667.— **Michaux.** Tumeur située entre l'artère carotide et la veine jugulaire interne, s'étendant de l'angle de la mâchoire inférieure à deux travers de doigt au-dessus de la clavicule; extirpation sans aucun accident; guérison radicale. Bull. Acad. roy. de méd. de Belg., Brux., 1848-9, viii, 1294–1302. — **Middlemist.** Fibrous tumor over the carotid artery; successful removal. Lancet, Lond., 1862, i, 355.—**Miller** (N.) Encysted gelatinous tumour of the neck. Am. J. M. Sc., Phila., 1854, n. s., xxviii, 110.—**Miller** (T.) Case of a large fibro-cartilaginous tumour successfully removed from the neck. Med. Exam , Phila., 1839, ii, 761.— **Minkiewicz** (J.) Pomyślne wyłuszczenie przerodzonego gruczołu przyusznego przez odgniecenie ekrazerem bez podwiązania głownych tętnic szyjowych. [Successful removal of an enlarged ganglion of nori.] Gaz. lek., Warszawa, 1867, iii, 89–94.—**Minor** (P. B.) Removal of a tumor from the neck. N. Orl. M. & S. J., 1861, xviii, 13.—**Mörner** (K. A. H.) Undersökning af en vätska, erhållen genom punktion af en vätskeansamling på halsen. [Examination of a fluid obtained by puncture from tumor of neck.] Hygiea, Stockholm, 1887, xlix, 381–386. — **Monod.** [Extirpation des ganglions lymphatiques du cou hypertrophiés.] Bull. Soc. anat. de Par., 1835, 3. s., i, 13.—**Morejon** (A.) Cystosarcomatous tumor of the neck; tying of the internal jugular vein. Phila. M. Times, 1878, ix, 37. — **Morelot.** Une opération d'une tumeur enkystée, située à la partie antérieure du cou. [Rap. de Laurent.] J. gén. de méd., chir. et pharm., Par., 1818, lxv, 208–214.—**Moreschi** (A.) Sopra tre casi di tumori del collo e sopra una rara complicazione in uno di essi. Raccoglitore med., Forlì, 1886, ii, 401–412. — **Morgan.** Tumor in the neck. Lond. M. Gaz., 1828, ii, 380–382.—**Mori** (G.) Caso di linfosarcoma al collo con nevromi multipli nei nervi periferici. Ann. univ. di med. e chir., Milano, 1880, ccliii, 297–307. — **Morris** (A. B.) Excision of fibroid tumour of the neck, weighing five pounds and a quarter; recovery. Lancet, Lond., 1881, ii, 363. *Also:* Indian M. Gaz., Calcutta, 1881, xvi, 79.— **Mott** (V.) A large tumor on the side of the neck, below the posterior angle of the lower jaw; subject, a little boy not quite five years old. N. York J. M., 1851, vii, 14–17. ———. A lobulated tumor upon the right side of the neck, in a delicate boy five and a half years of age. *Ibid.*, 18–21. ——— [Two cases of tumor of neck; operation; chloroform in.] Tr. N. York Acad. M., 1857, i, 86–93, 2 pl.— **Moulinié.** Mort par asphyxie, occasionnée par une tumeur strumeuse du cou. Gaz. d. hôp., Par., 1833, vii, 600.—**de Moura** (J. R.) Lipoma do volume de uma maçã, bilobado, occupando parte do tumor a região parotidiana do lado direito, e parte prolongandose para a região carotidiana do mesmo lado; estirpação; emprego da costura metallica, e união da ferida por primeira intenção no fim de 3 dias. Gaz. med. da Bahia, 1867-8, ii, 93.—**Moutard-Martin.** Myxome hémorrhagique. Progrès méd., Par., 1877, v, 88.—**Müller** (E.) Extirpation d'une tumeur ganglionnaire du cou (région carotidienne); guérison en huit jours. Mém. Soc. de méd. de Strasb. (1882-3), 1884, xx, 40–43. *Also:* Gaz. méd. de Strasb., 1883, 3. s., xii, 49. ———. Extirpation de ganglions sous-sterno-mastoïdiens; suture profonde absolue, sans drainage; guérison par première intention. Gaz. méd. de Strasb., 1883, 3. s., xii, 101.—**Mütter.** Tumour of the nape of the neck. Med. Exam., Phila., 1843, vi, 289.—**Muret** (E.) A short account of an immense tumour of the lateral region of the neck and its removal. Dublin Q. J. M. Sc., 1863, xxxv, 492–497.—**Murray** (J.) Tumour at lower part of the left side of the neck. Indian Ann. M. Sc., Calcutta, 1857, iv, 652.—**Mussey** (R. D.) Case of apparently malignant disease. Am. J. M. Sc., Phila., 1837, xxi, 396. ———. Excision of a large tumor upon the neck. West. Lancet, Cincin., 1842-3, i, 8–11.—**Nasi** (L.) Voluminoso tumore del collo asportato col termo-cauterio di Paquelin. Spallanzani, Modena, 1878, 2. s., vii, 174.—**Naudin.** Observation sur l'extirpation d'une tumeur squirrheuse qui avoit son siège à la partie latérale gauche et supérieure du cou. J. gén. de méd., chir. et pharm., Par., 1813, xlvii, 367–374.— **Navratil** (L.) (Nyakow előforduló daganatok.) [Strumous swelling of neck.] Orvosi hetil., Budapest, 1881, xxv, 229; 249; 273; 325; 369; 397.—**Nélaton** (E.) [Tumeur fibro-graisseuse du cou.] Bull. Soc. anat. de Par., 1858, xxxiii, 489–492. *Also:* J. de méd. et chir. prat., Par., 1859, 2. s., xxx, 255–260. *Also:* Gaz. d. hôp., Par., 1859, xxxi, 129. *Also, transl.:* Allg. Wien. med. Ztg., 1859, iv, 11. — **Novaro** (G. F.) Sarcoma voluminoso delle ghiandole linfatiche profonde del lato destro del collo; estirpazione; pronta recidiva locale; morte per esaurimento. Osservatore, Torino, 1877, xiii, 1; 17; 33; 49; 88.—**Nunneley.** Part of a large medullary tumour

Neck (*Tumors of*).

from the neck of a woman. Tr. Path. Soc. Lond., 1859-60, xi, 265.—**Obalinski** (A.) W sprawie chirurgicznego leczenia wola. [Surgical treatment of parenchymatous struma of neck.] Medycyna, Warszawa, 1884, xii, 77–80.— **O'Ferrall.** Pendulous tumor. Dublin Q. J. M. Sc., 1846, ii, 536.—**de Oliveira** (M. J.) Observação sobre um tumor da região cervical; operação e morte. Ann. Brasil. de med., Rio de Jan., 1883-4, xxxv, 345–853.—**Ollier.** [Tumeur fibro-plastique, pesant environ 3,500 gr.] Mém. et compt.-rend. Soc. d. sc. méd. de Lyon, 1865-6, v, pt. 2, 134.—**O'Shaughnessy.** Removal of a tumour behind the angle of the jaw, and which occupied the cervical region to within an inch of the clavicle, necessitating the division and ligature of the internal jugular vein; the patient under the influence of chloroform. Lancet, Lond., 1849, i, 661.—**Osler** (W.) Lympho-sarcoma of deep cervical glands, involving the thyroid and simulating goitre. Montreal Gen. Hosp. Rep., 1880, i, 340–342.—**Ostertag** (A.) Adenoid tumor of the neck; cured by the internal use of arsenic. St. Louis Cour. Med., 1879, ii, 567–569.— **Paci** (A.) Enorme mixoma sarcomatoso del collo e del torace; estirpazione; guarigione. Sperimentale, Firenze, 1876, xxxvii, 284–290, 1 pl.—**Palletta** (J. B.) De duobus rarioribus cervicis tumoribus. *In his:* Exercitationes pathol., 4°, Mediolani, 1820, 62.—**Palm.** Geschichte der Extirpation einer drei Fäuste grossen Balggeschwulst. Med. Cor.-Bl. d. württemb. ärztl. Ver., Stuttg., 1838, viii, 117.—**Palmer** (E.) Case of suddenly-formed enormous tumour of the neck. Am. J. M. Sc., Phila., 1846, n. s., xi, 259.—**Pamard.** Tumeur de la région parotidienne simulant l'enchondrome. [Rap. de Dolbeau.] Bull. Soc. anat. de Par., 1860, xxxv, 450–457.—**Pancoast** (J.) Encephaloid tumor of the neck; extirpation; recovery. Phot. Rev. M. & S., Phila., 1870–71, i, 35–37, 1 pl.—**Parker.** Tumour of the face and neck; excision; recovery. Month. J. M. Sc., Lond. & Edinb., 1846, vi, 393.—**Parker** (R.) Excision of a tumour from the stylo-hyoid region; ligature of the common, external, and internal carotid arteries; absence of internal jugular vein; recovery; sudden death three months later from dyspnœa. Lancet, Lond., 1883, ii, 499.—**Parker** (R. W.) Congenital tumour in the right side of the neck, rising and falling with respiration. Tr. Clin. Soc. Lond., 1886, xix, 322.—**Parkman.** Colloid tumour of the neck; several operations; frequent recurrence; death. Am. J. M. Sc., Phila., 1854, n. s., xxviii, 386. *Also:* Extr. Rec. Bost. Soc. M. Improve., 1854-6, ii, 114–117.—**Parrish.** A small tumor removed from the neck. Tr. Coll. Phys. Phila., 1850-53, n. s., i, 85.—**Parrot.** Tumeur du cou chez un nouveau-né, simulant l'hydrocèle congénitale du cou. Gaz. méd. de Par., 1880, 6. s., i, 586; 598. *Also:* Abeille méd., Par., 1880, xxxvii, 442–444.— **Partridge** (R.) Half of a fibrous tumour removed from the left side of the back of the neck of a healthy woman, twenty-six years of age. Tr. Path. Soc. Lond., 1859-60, xi, 260.—**Partridge** (S. B.) A case of large fibrous tumour connected with the upper part of the ligamentum nuchæ; excision; recovery. Med. Times & Gaz., Lond., 1867, ii, 318.—**Passaquay.** Tumeur du cou, accompagnée d'accidens graves vers les organes respiratoires; guérison. Gaz. méd. de Par., 1833, 2. s., i, 407.—**von Patruban.** Exstirpation eines subfascialen Lipoms aus dem Trigonum colli superius. Oesterr. Ztschr. f. prakt. Heilk., Wien, 1858, iv, 509–512.—**Pauffard.** Leucémie; lymphadénome (?) énorme du cou; extirpation suivie de guérison; récidive; mort. Bull. Soc. anat. de Par., 1877, lii, 663–667.—**Paulicki** (A.) Sarcomatöse Tumoren am Hals mit Compression der Trachea und des Oesophagus; Thrombose beider Venæ jugulares internæ; Sarcombildungen in den Lungen, im Herzen, der Leber und den Nieren; amyloide Degeneration; Echinococcus hepatis. Berl. klin. Wchnschr., 1867, iv, 347.—**Pennel & Leprévost.** Tumeur ganglionnaire du cou chez un nouveauné, prise pour une trachéocèle. France méd., Par., 1884, i, 771–774. *Also:* Bull. Soc. clin. de Par., 1884, viii, 77–81.—**Pézerat** (P.) Observation d'une tumeur fibreuse, située au cou et extirpée. J. compl. du dict. d. sc. méd., Par., 1827, xxvii, 82–86.—**Phillips** (B.) Curious tumor of the neck. Lond. M. Gaz., 1846, n. s., ii, 51.— **Picard** (P.) Observation de ganglion carotidien squirrheux occupant les régions carotidienne et sus-hyoïdienne gauches; extirpation de la tumeur; hémorrhagie grave; ligature de la carotide primitive au-dessous de l'omoplathyoïdien; pneumonie intercurrente à droite; mort sept jours après l'opération. Marseille méd., 1870, vii, pt. 1, 342–348.—**Piogey.** [Lipome volumineux de la région cervicale postérieure.] Bull. Soc. anat. de Par., 1857, xxxii, 162.—**Pirovano.** Linfo-adenoma del cuello, extirpacion á colgajo; curacion. Rev. méd.-quir., Buenos Aires, 1879-80, xvi, 268–271, 1 pl. *Also, transl.:* Canada Lancet, Toronto, 1879-80, xi, 132–134.—**Pitha.** Zur Diagnose und Therapie der am Halse vorkommenden Geschwülste. Oesterr. Ztschr. f. prakt. Heilk., Wien, 1859, v (Beilage), 1–17.—**Plasencia** (L.) Lipoma enorme de la region lateral superior del cuello; excision; curacion. Crón. méd.-quir. de la Habana, 1887, xiii, 231–234.—**Plouviez.** Extirpation de deux tumeurs situées au menton et à la région du cou; suites d'abord heureuses; récidive au bout

Neck (*Tumors of*).

d'un an; mort. Bull. Soc. de chir. de Par., 1854–5, v, 65.—
Post (G. E.) Extirpation of large fibro-cellular tumor of neck, with removal of portions of primitive carotid artery, internal jugular vein, descendens noni, pneumogastric, recurrent laryngeal and sympathetic nerves. Med. Rec., N. Y., 1878, xiv, 385.—**Pradel** (N. A.) Estirpacion de un tumor del cuello. Rev. méd. de Chile, Sant. de Chile, 1874–5, iii, 158–161.—**Prato** (D.) Raro caso di tumore aereo (?) alla regione superiore laterale sinistra del collo. Gior. di med. mil., Roma, 1875, xxiii, 97–103.—**Prewitt** (T. F.) Tumor of the neck; epulis. St. Louis M. & S. J., 1881, xli, 280–282. ———. Lympho-sarcoma of neck; extirpation; ligation internal jugular vein; recovery. St. Louis Cour. Med., 1884, xii, 517–520.—**Pulido** (A.) Tumores adenoplásticos del cuello. Anfiteatro anat., Madrid, 1873, i, 142.—**Raleigh** (W. W.) † Operation. India J. M. Sc., Calcutta, 1834, i, 33, 1 pl.—**Ramos** (T. M.) Sarcoma del cuello; operacion; muerte. Rev. méd. de Chile, Sant. de Chile, 1877–8, vi, 183–186.—**Reade** (H. C.) Removal of a large tumour from the neck. Med. Times, Lond., 1850, n. s., i, 113.—**Redfern** (P.) On the nature and primary changes of cancerous exudations, and on the development of fibrous structure in cancerous formations; with remarks on the diagnosis of tumours of the neck. Month. J. M. Sc., Lond. & Edinb., 1850, xi, 507–525.—**Regnaud.** Tumeur fibro-plastique de la région parotidienne. Bull. Soc. anat. de Par., 1865, xl, 175.—**Remedi** (V.) Contributo ai tumori sanguigni profundi del collo. Boll. d. Soc. tra i cult. d. sc. med. in Siena, 1886, iv, 248–259.—**Rendu.** Tumeur du cou; épithélioma des ganglions. Bull. Soc. anat. de Par. (1869), 1870, xliv, 206–209.—**Reverdin** (J. L.) & **Mayor** (A.) Appendices congénitaux de la région auriculaire et du cou (fibrochondrômes branchiaux de Lannelongue). Rev. méd. de la Suisse Rom., Genève, 1887, vii, 458–466.—**Rey** (P. F.) Extirpation d'une tumeur volumineuse à la région jugulaire et sur le trajet de la carotide. J. compl. du dict. d. sc. méd., Par., 1821, ix, 184–188.—**Richardson** (E.) Fatty tumour of the neck. Phot. Rev. M. & S., Phila., 1871–2, ii, 13–15, 1 pl.—**Robertson** (E. B.) Encysted tumor of the neck; extirpation and recovery. Tr. M. Soc. Calif., Sacramento, 1872–3, 55.—**Robinson** (B.) Tumor of neck; sudden death. N. York M. J., 1875, xxii, 529.—**Rochs.** Heilung eines Falles von Struma durch Unterbindung der Arteria thyreoidea superior. Therap. Monatsh., Berl., 1887, i, 346.—**Rockwell** (F. W.) Glandular tumor of the neck. Proc. M. Soc. County Kings, Brooklyn, 1879, iv, 91.—**Rodriguez** (S.) Quiste voluminoso en la parte anterior del cuello. Gac. méd., Madrid, 1848, iv, 281.—**Röcker.** Ungewöhnlich grosses Lipom am Halse und an der Brust einer 62 Jahre alten Frauensperson. Med. Cor.-Bl. d. württemb. ärztl. Ver., Stuttg., 1836, vi, 117–119, 1 pl.—**Rogers** (D. L.) Case of a tumour successfully extirpated. Phila. J. M. & Phys. Sc., 1826, xiii, 161. *Also, in his:* Surg. Essays & Cases in Surg., 8°, Newark, 1849, 143–145, 1 pl. *Also: Ibid.,* N. Y., 1850, 152–154, 1 pl.—**Rohrer** (C. F.) Fungus hæmatodes in der Fossa jugularis et suprascapularis; Perforation in den Larynx. Cor.-Bl. f. schweiz. Aerzte, Basel, 1873, iii, 621–624.—**Roose** (R.) Case of bony growth projecting into the posterior triangle of the left side of the neck, causing displacement of the subclavian artery and some laryngeal disturbance. Arch. Laryngol., N. Y., 1881, ii, 223–225.—**Ropes** (F. C.) Removal of sarcomatous tumor of neck. Boston M. & S. J., 1869, ii, 40 —
Rouault. Observation d'une tumeur probablement de nature bénigne, d'un volume énorme, chez une femme de 58 ans; extirpation; guérison. Union méd., Par., 1858, xii, 143.—**Roux.** Tumeur scrofuleuse d'un grand volume au col; extirpation. Gaz. d. hôp., Par., 1831–2, i, 394. ———. Tumeur du poids de quatre livres et demie développée au cou; extirpation. *Ibid.,* 1833, vii, 603. ———. Ablation d'une tumeur; entrée de l'air dans les veines; accidents consécutifs; mort. J. univ. et hebd. de méd. et chir. prat., Par., 1833, xi, 165–172. ———. Ablation d'une tumeur du cou; mort pendant l'opération; autopsie. Bull. Soc. de chir. de Par., 1853, iv, 82–85.—**Ruchmore.** Sarcoma of neck; galvano-cautery. Med. & Surg. Reporter, Phila., 1878, xxxviii, 418.—**Rudderow** (B. J.) † Tr. Path. Soc. Phila. (1876–7), 1878, vii, 150. *Also:* Phila. M. Times, 1876, vii, 150.—**Ruggi.** Relazione intorno a varii operati per tumori alla testa ed al collo e più specialmente intorno ad alcuni casi di nevroma cirsoideo. Arch. ed atti d. Soc. ital. di chir. 1886, Roma, 1887, iii, 59–72.—**Rutz** (E.) Observation d'extirpation d'une tumeur volumineuse du cou, et réflexions sur la nature de cette tumeur et sur l'opération. Arch. gén. de méd., Par., 1839, 3. s., iv, 479–483.—**Sacchi** (C.) Istoria di voluminoso tumore alla nuca felicemente estirpato. Ann. univ. di med., Milano, 1833, lxvii, 317–342.—**Sanders** (R. C.) Removal of a large fibro-cystic tumour from the neck. Indian M. Gaz., Calcutta, 1879, xiv, 199.—**Sandifort** (E.) De singulari membranæ cellulosæ degeneratione. *In his:* Obs. anat.-patol., 4°, Lugd. Bat., 1781, iv, 21–29.—**Sands** (H. B.) Congenital tumor of neck; removal. N. York M. J., 1878, xxvii, 197.—**Santesson** (C.) Fibrös svulst på halsen; underbindning af arteria carotis communis och carotis cerebralis; gangren uti svulsten; helsa. Hygiea, Stockholm,

Neck (*Tumors of*).

1854, xvi, 348–352.—**Savory.** Sanguineous tumour of the neck; hæmorrhage from rupture of the external carotid artery; death. Lancet, Lond., 1871, ii, 467.—**Schede** (M.) Ueber die tiefen Atherome des Halses. Arch. f. klin. Chir., Berl., 1872, xiv, 1–22. *Also,* Reprint.—**af Schultén** (M. W.) Fall af sarcoma colli, vid hvars exstirpation vena jugularis comm. Finska läk.-sällsk. handl., Helsingfors, 1884, xxvii, 131.—**Scott.** Removal of a large tumor from the neck; hæmorrhage; death. Lancet, Lond., 1833–4, i, 224. *Also, transl.:* Gaz. d. hôp., Par., 1833, vii, 519 [619].—**Sédillot** (C.) Des tumeurs cervicales ganglionnaires et de leur ablation sans section du muscle sterno-cléidomastoïdien et sans déviation consécutive de la tête. Mém. Soc. de méd. de Strasb., 1867, vi, 251–260. *Also:* Gaz. méd. de Strasb., 1868, xxviii, 61–63.—**Seeger.** Glücklich ausgeführte Exstirpation eines sehr grossen Lipoms. Ztschr. f. Wundärzte u. Geburtsh., Stuttg., 1851, iv, 203–205, 1 pl.—**Seiler** (C.) Sarcoma of the neck. Tr. Path. Soc. Phila. (1878–9), 1880, ix, 173. *Also:* Phila. M. Times, 1879, ix, 238.—**Senn** (N.) A case of glandular sarcoma of the neck. Tr. Wisconsin M. Soc., Milwaukee, 1876, x, 107–109, 1 pl. ———. Case of patient with cysto-chondro-adenoma. *Ibid.,* 1884, xviii, 35–38.—**Seymour** (F. A.) A contribution to the surgery of tumors of the neck. South. Calif. Pract., Los Angeles, 1886, i, 18–22.—**Shattock** (S. G.) Congenital tumour of the neck. Tr. Path. Soc. Lond., 1881–2, xxxiii, 289.—**Shaw** (A.) Extirpation of a tumor from the neck. Lancet, Lond., 1844, i, 263–265 —**Shillitoe** (B.) Fibrous tumour from near the angle of the lower jaw. Tr. Path. Soc. Lond., 1864–5, xvi, 223, 1 pl.—**Siddall** (H. W.) Case of bleeding tumor. West. Lancet, Cincin., 1849, ix, 81.—**Simon.** Removal of a solid tumour from the neck, possessing peculiar characters. Med. Times & Gaz., Lond., 1853, vi, 160.—**Smith** (H.) Case of sarcomatous tumor of the neck. Lond. M. Gaz., 1847, xl, 975–978.—**Smith** (N. R.) Tumors of the neck. Balt. M. & S. J. & Rev., 1834, ii, 370–375. ———. Extirpation of tumors of the neck. N. Am. Arch. M. & S. Sc., Balt., 1835, ii, 73–75.—**Smith** (R. W.) Glandular tumor of the neck. Dublin Q. J. M. Sc., 1854, xvii, 232. *Also:* Dublin Hosp. Gaz., 1854, n. s., i, 15.—**Smith** (S.) Lympho-sarcoma of the cervical glands; ulceration; hæmorrhage; death. Med. Press & Circ., Lond., 1877, n. s., xxiv, 318.—**Smith** (T. S.) Operation for the removal of a single goitrous tumor of the neck. Am. M. Times, N. Y., 1863, vii, 168.—**Socin** (A.) Rundzellensarcom der linken seitlichen Halsgegend. Jahresb. ü. d. chir. Abth. d. Spit. zu Basel, 1876, 29.—**Soler.** Estirpacion de un gran tumor adenitico situado en la parte lateral izquierda del cuello, llavada felizmente á cabo el dia 11 de junio de 1858. Siglo méd., Madrid, 1858, v, 195–197.—**Soulé** fils. Tumeur cervicale; discussion sur le diagnostic. J. de méd. de Bordeaux, 1852, x, 242–246.—**Sparham** (E. B.) Observations on tumors; cystic sarcoma of the neck, successfully removed by extirpation. Med. Chron., Montreal, 1853–4, i, 12–15.—**Spence** (J.) Case of enormous deep-seated tumour of the face and neck, successfully removed by operation. Dublin Q. J. M. Sc., 1863, xxxvi, 272; 283, 4 pl. ———. Large deep-seated tumor of the neck; removal; recovery. Edinb. M. J., 1867–8, xiii, 393–398, 1 pl.—**Spencer** (P. C.) Tumor of the neck of extraordinary size successfully removed. Am. J. M. Sc., Phila., 1845, n. s., ix, 98–103. *Also:* N. Orl. M. J., 1844–5, i, 302–305.—**Stanley.** Large tumour on the side of the neck; operation; subsequent very rapid growth of the disease; death; dissection of the parts concerned. Med. Times, Lond., 1850, xxi, 18.—**Staples** (F.) A large adenoid tumor of the neck of a child. Tr. Minnesota M. Soc., St. Paul, 1876, 37–39. ———. Lymphatic tumor in the right cervical region. *Ibid.,* 1879, 33–35.—**Steele.** Tumour of the neck. Brit. M. J., Lond., 1862, ii, 572.—**Stevens** (A. H.) A case of an extraordinary tumour successfully extirpated. Med. & Surg. Reg., N. Y., 1818–20, i, 165–170, 2 pl. ———. Account of a case of encysted tumor successfully removed by an operation. N. York M. & Phys. J., 1826, v, 311–314, 1 pl.—**Storchi** (J.) Linfoma profondo della regione carotidea sinistra; estirpazione; guarigione. Spallanzani, Roma, 1886, 2. s., xv, 456–460.—**Suñer** (E.) Fibro-lipoma en la region cervical posterior. Génio méd.-quir., Madrid, 1883, xxix, 102.—**Syme** (J.) Anomalous tumour of the neck; treatment by seton and caustic; recovery. Edinb. M. & S. J., 1835, xliv, 11. ———. Large tumour of the neck removed with success at an advanced age. *Ibid.,* 1838, l, 384. ———. Case of tumour of the neck, simulating aneurism of the carotid artery. Month. J. M. Sc., Lond. & Edinb., 1848, viii, 449–451.—**Tafani** (A.) Di un tumoretto congenito composto di cartilagine reticolata. Sperimentale, Firenze, 1879, xliv, 484–488.—**Tannahill.** A remarkable congenital tumour of the neck. Glasgow M. J., 1871–2, 4. s., iv, 6–11.—**Tansini** (I.) Estirpazione di voluminoso linfo-sarcoma al collo; resezione della carotide primitiva e della giugulare profonda; guarigione. Gazz. med. ital. lomb., Milano, 1887, xlvii, 3.—**Taramelli** (C.) Estirpazione di un tumore adiposo al lato destro della faccia estendentesi a tutta la parte corrispondente del collo. Ann. univ. di med., Milano, 1835, lxxv, 425–430, 1 pl.—**Terrillon.** Lymphadénome du cou. Progrès méd., Par., 1883, xi, 1027.—**Thiele.** Fall eines glücklich exstirpirten

Neck (*Tumors of*).

Tumor cysticus von bedeutender Grösse, der in der Tiefe an der linken Seite des Halses, zwischen dem Larynx und dem Sterno-cleydo-mastoideus seinen Sitz hatte, und mit der Carotis cerebralis und Vena jugularis interna unmittelbar verwachsen war. Mag. f. d. ges. Heilk., Berl., 1821, ix, 72–79.—**Thompson** (H.) Suffocation from a tumor in the throat, in a case of pleuritis and bronchitis. Lancet, Lond., 1859, ii, 237.—**Thompson** (J. H.) Enchondromatous tumor. Nat. M. J., Wash., 1871–2, ii, 449–454, 1 pl.—**Tilanus.** Colloid-cyste met endogene vorming onder de fascia profunda van den hals. Nederl. Weekbl. v. Geneesk., Amst., 1851, i, 81.—**Tirman.** [Tumeur du cou.] Bull. Soc. anat. de Par., 1861, xxxvi, 162–164.—**Toland** (H. H.) Two cases in which tumours were removed from the neck. Charleston M. J., 1855, x, 145–150.—**Torrey** (W. S.) Lymphadeno-sarcoma of the neck; removal; sarcomatous periostitis of petrous portion of temporal bone; death. Med. Rec., N. Y., 1886, xxx, 459.—**Traube.** Sarcomatöse Drüsengeschwülste am Halse, welche durch die Löcher der mittleren Schädelgrube in den Schädel hineingewachsen sind. Ann. d. Char.-Krankenh. zu Berl., 1862–3, x, 2. Hft., 213–220.—**Treves** (F.) Congenital cartilaginous tumour of neck. Brit. M. J., Lond., 1887, ii, 993. *Also:* Lancet, Lond., 1887, ii, 914.—**Ure** (A.) An account of a tumour removed from the neck. Med. Times, Lond., 1850, n. s., i, 226.—**Vacher** (L.) Observation de lympho-sarcome bilatéral du cou et du creux sus-claviculaire. Mém. et compt.-rend. Soc. d. sc. méd. de Lyon (1878), 1879, xviii, pt. 2, 176–182. *Also:* Lyon méd., 1879, xxx, 73–75.—**Vance** (J. W.) Excision of a large cervical glandular tumor. Atlanta M. & S. J., 1871–2, ix. 17–19.—**Vanini** (P.) † Gazz. med. ital. lomb., Milano, 1848, 2. s., i, 327.—**Velpeau.** Tumor, from engorgement of cervical lymphatic ganglia. Lancet, Lond., 1834, ii, 593–595.—**Venables** (T.) [Fatty tumor of the neck.] Canada M. J., Montreal, 1871–2, viii, 164.—**Verneuil.** Tumeur fibro-plastique du cou. Bull. Soc. anat. de Par., 1854, xxix, 344. ———. Tumeur ganglionnaire récidive. Bull. Soc. de chir. de Par. (1864), 1865, 2. s., v, 289–292. ———. Du peloton adipeux, ou pseudo-lipome sus-claviculaire. Gaz. hebd. de méd., Par., 1879, 2. s., xvi, 745–748. ———. Extirpation d'une énorme tumeur ganglionnaire du côté droit du cou; dénudation de la carotide primitive; hémorragie secondaire; ligature de l'artère; accidents cérébraux; mort. Médecin, Par., 1883, ix, no. 52, 1: 1884, x, no. 1, 3.—**Vesey** (J. S.) † Med. Press & Circ., Dubl., 1868, iii, 132.—**Voelker.** Tumeurs ganglionnaires du cou traitées et guéries par les injections intra-parenchymateuses d'acide acétique. Union méd., Par., 1879, 3. s., xxvii, 727–732. *Also:* Paris méd., 1879, v, 360–367.—**Voisin.** Extirpation d'une tumeur ostéo-fibreuse située au côté gauche du cou sur l'artère carotide primitive; guérison. Gaz. méd. de Par., 1835, 2. s., iii, 446.—**Waldenström** (J. A.) Phlegmone granulosum à halsen. Upsala Läkaref. Förh., 1877–8, xiii, 179.—**Walker.** Encysted tumor of the neck. Lond. M. & S. J., 1835, vi, 665.—**Walsham** (W. J.) On the removal of a deep sebaceous cyst of the neck through the mouth, avoiding an external scar. Lancet, Lond., 1883, i, 767.—**Walter.** Geschichte eines Markschwamms. Med. Cor.-Bl. d. württemb. ärztl. Ver., Stuttg., 1837, vii, 86–88.—**Walter** (P. U.) Eigenthümliche Art der Ausrottung scirrhöser Drüsen am Winkel der untern Kinnlade. J. d. Chir. u. Augenh., Berl., 1831, xv, 384–394.—**Walton** (H. H.) Removal of a large tumor from the neck. Med. Times, Lond., 1847–8, xvii, 275–280. *Also* [Abstr.]: Tr. Path. Soc. Lond., 1846–50, i, 130. ———. † Removal. Med. Times, Lond., 1849, xx, 423–425. ———. A large, round, circumscribed, accumulation of fat on the neck having all the outward appearance of a fatty tumor, but without the structural arrangement of such a growth. Med. Times & Gaz., Lond., 1862, ii, 571. ———. Fatty tumour of the neck; operation. Med. Press & Circ., Dubl., 1867, iii, 74.—**Warren** (J. C.) Large tumor of the neck. Boston M. & S. J., 1828–9, i, 367.—**Warren** (J. M.) Tumor of the neck; operation; internal jugular vein cut and tied; recovery. *In his:* Surg. Obs., 8°, Bost., 1867, 502–504. ———. Large tumor of face and neck; removal; recovery; recurrence after three years; operation; death. *Ibid.*, 504–506. ———. Tumor of the neck, involving the axillary plexus of nerves; removal. *Ibid.*, 508.—**Watson** (J.) Deep glandular tumour on the side of the neck; extirpated. N. York J. M. & S., 1840, iii, 358.—**Weikard** (M. A.) Tumor strumosus colli post vomitorium imminutus. *In his:* Obs. med., 12°, Francof. a. M., 1775, 88.—**Weinlechner** (J.) Lymphome am Halse; Oncotomie; Erysipel; Glottisödem; Laryngotomie; Tod. Ber. d. k. k. Krankenanst. Rudolph-Stiftung in Wien (1874), 1875, 425. ———. Lymphome im oberen rechten Halsdreiecke und im Verlaufe der grossen Halsgefässe und in der Nackengegend; mit Blosslegung aller daselbst befindlichen wichtigen Gefässe und Nerven exstirpirt und per primam geheilt. *Ibid.* (1878), 1879, 299. — **Weir** (R. F.) Extirpation of a sub-hyoid bursa. Ann. Surg., St. Louis, 1887, v, 512.—**Weiss** (W.) Lipoma nuchæ. Aerztl. Ber. d. k. k. allg. Krankenh. zu Prag (1881), 1883, 190.—**West** (B. H.) Excision of a fibro-cartilaginous tumor of the neck. Boston M. & S. J., 1845–6, xxxiii, 60–63 —

Neck (*Tumors of*).

Wheaton (C. A.) [Fibro-sarcoma in the right side of the neck; extirpated, and the right common carotid subsequently ligated.] Tr. Minnesota M. Soc., St. Paul, 1881, 55.—**Willmott** (J. E.) Case of obscure tumour in neck; death. Austral. M. J., Melbourne, 1882, n. s., iv, 481–486.—**Winslow** (R.) Lymphoma colli; ablation. Maryland M. J., Balt., 1886, xv, 305.—**Wood** (J.) Removal of a large fibro-glandular tumour from the neck, of seventeen years' growth. Med. Times & Gaz., Lond., 1865, ii, 467.—**Woodward** (W.) Extirpation of a medullary tumor. N. Orl. M. & S. J., 1860, xvii, 318–323.—**Wyeth** (J. A.) Myxo-sarcoma of the neck; ligation of the common, internal, and external carotid, superior thyroid, lingual, facial, and occipital arteries, and of the external jugular vein. Bull. N. York Path. Soc., 1881, 2. s., i, 318–320. [*Also* Med. Rec., N. Y., 1881, xx, 720. — **Wylie** (J. R.) A strange tumour and its cure. Austral. M. J., Melbourne, 1871, xvi, 36, 1 pl.—**Zahn** (J.) Ein Sarkoma alveolare epithelioides der Lymphdrüsen des Halses. Arch. d. Heilk., Leipz., 1874, xv, 143–149. 1 pl.—**Zamponi** (H.) Atherom von seltener Grösse; Ausschälung desselben; Heilung per primam intentionem. Med.-chir. Centralbl., Wien, 1877, xii, 330.

Neck (*Tumors of, Cancerous and malignant*).

Andrews. [Encephaloid tumor of the neck.] Med. Times, Phila., 1870–71, i, 181. — **Andrews** (E.) Malignant sarcoma. Chicago M. J. & Exam., 1879, xxxix, 484–486. — **Arendt.** Kurze Beschreibung einer glücklich verrichteten Exstirpation einer carcinomatösen Halsgeschwulst. J. d. Chir. u. Augenh., Berl., 1822, iv, 459.—**Arnes** (M.) Cancer of the lymphatic glands of the neck in a lad aged fourteen; rapid progress; exophthalmia; convulsions; autopsy. Med. Press & Circ., Lond., 1870, n. s., ix, 207.—**d'Auriol.** Tumeur encéphaloïde du cou; diagnostic rendu impossible par la ponction explorative. Rev. méd. de Toulouse, 1871, v, 112–117.—**Banon.** Case of secondary cancerous and encephaloid disease. Dublin M. Press, 1851, xxv, 226.—**Bardinet.** Tumeurs cancéreuses du cou; ablation; mort par phlébite consécutive à la ligature d'une veine; nécropsie. Rev. méd. de Limoges, 1867–8, i, 120–122.—**Battersby** (F.) Malignant tumour in an infant. Dublin M. Press, 1849, xxii, 53.—**Bérard.** [Tumeur cancéreuse au niveau de la veine jugulaire interne.] Bull. Soc. anat. de Par., 1843, xviii, 39. — **Blache** (R.) Epithélioma de la région cervicale. *Ibid.*, 1865, xl, 177. — **Bock.** Tumeur squirrheuse occupant le cou et la base du crâne. Presse méd. belge, Brux., 1881, xxxiii, 377–379.—**Bourdon** (E.) Carcinome primitif des ganglions du cou. Bull. Soc. anat. de Par. (1872), 1874, xlvii, 310–313.—**Brinton** (W.) A case of peri-tracheal deposit, with secondary disease of the lungs. Lancet, Lond., 1857, i, 209–211. — **Bruns** (P.) Das branchiogene Carcinom des Halses. Mitth. a. d. chir. Klin. zu Tübing., 1884, 2. Hft., 369–373. — **Budd.** Cancerous tumour in the groove between the trachea and œsophagus, on the left side, eating into the trachea just below the larynx and into the œsophagus; death from dyspnœa, occasioned probably by destruction of the left recurrent nerve. Tr. Path Soc. Lond., 1858–9, x, 62.—**Capitan** (L.) Épithélioma de la nuque et du dos. Bull. Soc. anat. de Par., 1877, lii, 633. *Also:* Progrès méd., Par., 1878, vi, 165.—[**Cases.**] Tumeur cancéreuse du col; trachéotomie; mort. Clin. d. hôp., Par., 1827–8, ii, 379.—Medullarcarcinom der r. Halsseite, ausgegangen vom r. Schilddrüsenlappen; Tod. Jahresb. ü. d. chir. Abth. d. Spit. zu Basel (1879), 1880, 32.—**Chaillou.** Cancer nucléaire développé dans les plexus veineux thyroïdéens et le système des veines cervicales gauches; déviation du larynx et atrophie de la thyroïde; tumeurs des côtes et de la cuisse; altération de même nature que les précédentes; tumeurs dans l'intérieur du poumon droit. Bull. Soc. anat. de Par., 1863, xxxviii, 189–195.—**Cleemann** (R. A.) Encephaloid cancer of the lymphatic glands of the neck. Tr. Path. Soc. Phila. (1876–7), 1878, vii, 154. *Also:* Phila. M. Times, 1876–7, vii, 475.—**Cooper** (B.) Encephaloid tumor on the side of the neck; fatal result. Lancet, Lond., 1853, ii, 461.—**Corrochano** (M. M.) Caso notable de cáncer encefaloideo situado en la region carotidea izquierda, operado en 11 de enero de 1870. Siglo méd., Madrid, 1870, xvii, 103; 184. — **Corse.** Cancer of the neck. Tr. Coll. Phys. Phila. (1856–62), 1863, n. s., i, 227.—**Coulson.** Medullary tumor of large size in a boy fourteen years old; autopsy. Lancet, Lond., 1853, ii, 460. — **Crespo** (A. L. P.) Hum carcinoma no pescoço. J. Soc. d. sc. med. de Lisb., 1848, 2. s., iii, 5–12. — **Demarquay.** Tumeur encéphaloïde sous-maxillaire; élimination spontanée. Gaz. d. hôp., Par., 1860, xxxiii, 230.—**Deroubaix** (L.) Tumeur encéphaloïde du cou. Ann. de l'Univ. de Brux. Fac. de méd., 1881, ii, 89.—**Dufour** (L.) Observation d'un fongus hématode du cou. J. gén. de méd., chir. et pharm., Par., 1821, lxxv, 52–57.—**von Dumreicher** (H.) [Carcinom der seitlichen Halsdrüsen.] *In his:* Jahresb. d. chir. Klin. in Wien 1869–70, 8°, 1871, 27. — **Duplay** (S.) Tumeur (cancéreuse) ganglionnaire du cou. Progrès méd., Par., 1877, v, 561–563. — **Englisch** (J.) Lym-

Neck *(Tumors of, Cancerous and malignant).*

phadenoma malignum. Ber. d. k. k. Krankenanst. Rudolph-Stiftung in Wien (1876), 1877, 296. — **Fornari** (F.) Estirpazione di un epitelioma dalla regione carotidea. Indipendente, Torino, 1879, xxx, 625.—**Forster** (J. C.) Malignant growth in neck; necrosis of jaw; exploratory operation; erysipelas. Guy's Hosp. Rep., Lond., 1874, 3. s., xix, 4.—**Frissell** (J.) Encephaloid tumor of the jaw and neck. Tr. M. Soc. W. Virg., Wheeling, 1875, 116. — **Gerster.** Malignant lympho-sarcomata of the neck. Med. Rec., N. Y., 1882, xxi, 328–331.—**Gibb** (G. D.) Cancerous tumour of the neck, simulating scrofula; hypertrophy of the spleen; autopsy. Brit.-Am. M. & Phys. J., Montreal, 1850-51, vi, 477–481.—**Godfray** (A. C.) Removal of cancerous cervical glands by axillary incision. Brit. M. J., Lond., 1886, i, 202.— **Gorré.** Tumeur cancéreuse de la partie latérale gauche du cou; extirpation; ouverture accidentelle de la veine jugulaire interne; introduction spontanée de l'air; mort instantanée; examen cadavérique. Expérience, Par, 1842, x, 309.—**Gougenheim.** [Tumeur du cou, probablement de nature cancéreuse; asphyxie.] Bull. Soc. anat. de Par., 1864, xxxix, 6.—**Gross** (S. D.) Medullary round-celled sarcoma. Phila. M. Times, 1871-2, ii, 89; 116.—**Harley** (G.) Malignant tumour in the neck; stricture of œsophagus; aphonia; perforation of œsophageal (?) artery, and death from hæmorrhage. Tr. Path. Soc. Lond., 1862-3, xiv, 167–169.—**Heurtaux.** Tumeur de la paupière et du cou; épithéliome tubulé. Bull. Soc. anat. de Nantes 1881, Par., 1882, v, 96–98.—**Hume** (G. H.) Removal of malignant tumour of the neck, involving the sterno-mastoid muscle and internal jugular vein. Lancet, Lond., 1882, ii, 888. — **Hutchinson** (J.) Development of cancer in an innocent glandular tumour. *Ibid.*, 1862, ii, 618.—**Hutchison** (A. C.) Some account of a case of fungus hæmatodes. Lond. M. Gaz., 1829-30, v, 663.—**Jaksch.** Carcinoma glandularum. Vrtljschr. f. d. prakt. Heilk., Prag, 1862, lxxiii, 103.—**Jarjavay.** ʼTumeur encéphaloïde du cou; compression de la trachée et de l'œsophage; perforation du pharynx. Bull. Soc. anat. de Par., 1846, xxi, 44–46.—**Johnson** (H. C.) Encephaloid deposit in the parotid and chain of cervical glands. Lancet, Lond., 1854, ii, 102.— **Johnston** (D.) Removal of large cancerous sub-lingual tumor, along with part of the lower jaw. Edinb. M. J., 1867-8, xiii, 436–439.—**Jones** (S.) Tumour, weighing between six and seven pounds, formed by encephaloid disease of the cervical glands. Tr. Path. Soc. Lond., 1856-7, viii, 369–371.—**Kalindéro.** Tumeur épithéliale de la région carotidienne droite; début probable par les ganglions; perforation du pharynx; hémorrhagie; mort. Bull. Soc. anat. de Par., 1865, xl, 273–277.—**Kiose** (C. W.) & **Paul** (J.) Carcinom der Halsdrüsen. Ztschr. f. klin. Med., Bresl., 1852, iii, 53.—**Krabbel.** Zwei Fälle von malignem Lymphosarcom des Nackens. Arch. f. klin. Chir., Berl., 1878, xxiii, 368.—**Küchler.** Carcinoma colli. Deutsche Klinik, Berl., 1866, xviii, 465.—**Kumar.** Primärer Markschwamm der Hals- und Achseldrüsen, welcher in kurzer Zeit rapid um sich greift, die sämmtlichen Weichtheile, endlich auch die Rippen der betreffenden Seite zerstörte, und durch Pleuritis tödtlich endet. Ber. d. k. k. Krankenanst. Rudolph-Stiftung in Wien (1875), 1876, 338.— **Langenbeck** (B.) Carcinom am Halse; Resection der Geschwulst wegen bedeutender Athem- und Schlingbeschwerden; vorübergehende Besserung; Rückkehr und Steigerung der Athembeschwerden bis zu drohender Erstickung; Tracheotomie mit glücklichem Erfolg. Deutsche Klinik, Berl., 1852, iv, 151–153.—**Le Teinturier.** [Dégénérescence épithéliale des glandes sudoripares de la nuque. Rap. de L. Leroy.] Bull. Soc. anat. de Par., 1867, xlii, 560–565.—**Lowe** (T.) Case of melanotic cancerous tumor in the neck. Madras Q. J. M. Sc., 1862, v, 437.— **Mackenzie** (M.) Primary carcinoma in the cervical glands; secondary affection of the larynx. Brit. M. J., Lond., 1870, ii, 682.—**Maclean** (D.) Malignant tumor of the neck, involving the large blood-vessels; removal; death. Physician & Surg., Ann Arbor, Mich., 1881, iii, 164–166.—**Madruzza** (G.) Sulla estirpazione di uno scirro cistico sviluppatosi nella regione anteriore del collo. Raccoglitore med. di Fano, 1856, xiv, 404–409.— **Martinez** (A. S.) Cáncer encefaloideo situado en la parte lateral izquierda del cuello; estirpacion. Bol. de med., cirug. y farm., Madrid, 1851, 2. s., i, 113.—**Martini.** Geschichte einer ungemein rapide verlaufenen carcinomatösen Metamorphose der drüsigen Gebilde des Halses. Ztschr. f. d. ges. Med., Hamb., 1836, i, 265–272.—**Mathieson** (J. H.) Removal of deep seated malignant tumor of the neck. Canada M. J., Montreal, 1870–71, vii, 10.— **Maylard** (A. E.) A case of malignant growth in the neck, implicating the cervical spinal nerves and the cervical sympathetic. Glasgow M. J., 1883, [4.] s, xx, 406–414. — **Menzel** (A.) Linfoma maligno. Resoc. san. d. Osp. civ. di Trieste, 1876, ii, 96.—**Middeldorpf.** Carcinom der rechten Halsseite; Kehlkopf und Luftröhre dislocirend und comprimirend; Laryngo-Tracheotomie; Tod nach 5 Stunden; Section: Zerstörung des Vagus in der Geschwulst; spaltförmige Compression der Luftröhre; Verwachsungen der Geschwulst. Ausz. a. d. Uebers. d.

Neck *(Tumors of, Cancerous and malignant).*

Arb. u. Veränd. d. schles. Gesellsch. f. vaterl. Kult. Jahresb. d. med. Sect., Bresl., 1853, 2.—**Morris** (H.) On a case of epithelioma of the neck following a patch of chronic skin disease, in which the cancer was twice excised and the external and internal jugulars were ligatured. Med.-Chir. Tr., Lond., 1879-80, lxiii, 323–332. *Also* [Abstr.]: Proc. Roy. M. & Chir. Soc., Lond., 1875-80, viii, 515–517.— **Morris** (H.) & **Lawson.** Two cases of strangulating cancer of the neck. Med. Press & Circ., Lond., 1884, n. s., xxxviii, 374.—**Nancrede** (C. B.) Recurrent epithelioma of neck. Tr. Path. Soc. Phila. (1877–8), 1879, viii, 148–150. *Also:* Phila. M. Times, 1877-8, viii, 353. — **Ormerod** (J. A.) Case of cancerous tumour of the neck simulating myelitis. St. Barth. Hosp. Rep., Lond., 1879, xv, 257–262.— **Parker** (W.) Malignant tumor on the neck. Med. & Surg. Reporter, Phila., 1862-3, ix, 74.—**Pasquier.** Tumeur cancéreuse de la région cervicale; extirpation; guérison. Gaz. d. hôp., Par., 1838, xii, 452.—**Piedvache.** Épithélioma ulcéré des ganglions du cou, consécutif à un cancroïde opéré de la lèvre supérieure; dyspnée; accès de suffocation; mort; destruction partielle des nerfs pneumogastrique et phrénique, et de la veine jugulaire interne du côté gauche. Bull. Soc. anat. de Par., 1861, xxxvi, 408–411.—**Pollard** (G. W.) Successful removal of malignant tumor from the neck. Virginia M. Month., Richmond, 1879-80, vi, 817.—**Post** (A. C.) Malignant tumour of the neck, containing scirrhus, encephaloid and melanosis; operation; rapid reproduction of the morbid deposits. N. York J. M. & S., 1841, iv, 117.—**Ransom.** A cancerous growth in the antrum mediastinum. Brit. M. J., Lond., 1873, i, 199.—**Richard.** [Tumeur circonscrite et de nature encéphaloïde, développée dans la région sus-claviculaire; difficultés du diagnostic.] Bull. Soc. anat. de Par., 1843, xviii, 199–201.—**Riedinger.** [Fall von Carcinoma colli.] Chir. Klin. im k. Juliushosp. zu Würzb. (1877-8), 1879, 43–47, 1 pl.—**Ripley.** Epithelioma of the neck. Tr. N. York Path. Soc. (1881), 1882, iv, 285–288. *Also:* Med. Rec., N. Y., 1881, xx, 691.—**Robertson** (E. B.) A case of epithelioma; extirpation; recovery. Tr. M. Soc. Calif., Sacramento, 1880, x, 116.—**Rombeau.** [Tumeur sur les parties latérales de la région cervicale; elle a envahie la région parotidienne, la base de la mâchoire, l'aisselle, les fosses nasales et l'arrière-gorge; asphyxie.] Bull. Soc. anat. de Par., 1852, xxvii, 82–84.—**Salva** (E.) Note pour servir à l'histoire des tumeurs cancéreuses du cou. Gaz. méd. de Par., 1861, 3. s., xvi, 92–95.—**Sands** (H. B.) Carcinoma of the neck. Med. Gaz., N. Y., 1882, ix, 591.—**Schuh.** Cancer medullare in omnibus glandulis lymphat. colli. Spitals-Ztg., Wien, 1864, 115.—**Shaffner** (J. F.) Excision of fibro-malignant tumour from right side of neck. Am. J. M. Sc., Phila., 1867, n. s., liv, 279.—**Sick** (P.) Medullarcarcinom des Rachens und oberen Theiles vom Schlundkopf; Tracheotomie; Tod; Venenkrebs am Halse; Krebsknoten in den Lungen. Arch. f. path. Anat., etc., Berl., 1864, xxxi, 316–331.—**Smyth** (J. S.) Encephaloid cancer; removal by operation; ligature of the carotid; recovery. Brit. M. J., Lond., 1857, ii, 863. — **Sociu** (A.) Carcinom der Lymphdrüsen des Halses. Jahresb. ü. d. chir. Abth. d. Spit. zu Basel, 1876, 28. ———. Faustgrosses Melanosarcom des Nackens. *Ibid.*, 28.—**Stanley.** Encephaloid tumor in the cervical region; operation. Lancet, Lond., 1853, ii, 462.—**Stilwell** (H.) Cancerous infiltration of the lymphatic glands and areolar tissue of the neck. Med. Times & Gaz., Lond., 1858, xvi, 348.—**Teinturier.** Épithélioma des glandes sudoripares de la nuque: ablation. Bull. Soc. anat. de Par., 1867, xlii, 558 - 560. — **Toner** (J. M.) Cancerous tumor of neck, compressing trachea and œsophagus. Tr. M. Soc. Dist. Columb., Wash., 1874, i, 28–31. — **Torre** (P. M.) Tumor escirroso masiforme en la parte lateral derecha del cuello; estirpacion; curacion. Crón. de l. hosp., Madrid, 1857, v, 50–56. *Also:* Siglo méd., Madrid, 1857, iv, 44.—**Treuberg** (J.) K kazuistike per vichnago raka tshei. [.arcinoma of neck.] Vrach, St. Petersb., 1883, iv, 129. *Also, transl.:* St. Petersb. med. Wchnschr., 1883, viii, 125. — **Ulrich** (F.) Medullarer Krebs am Halse; Erstickungsgefahr; Laryngo-Tracheotomie; Rothlauf; Tod. *In his:* Erfahr. u. d. künstliche Eröffnung d. Luftwege, 8°, Berl., 1860. 14 - 19. — **Valude** (E.) Sarcôme de la région sus-hyoïdienne; opération; mort rapide; généralisation du néoplasme aux poumons. Bull. Soc. anat. de Par., 1884, lix, 52 - 56. *Also:* Progrès méd., Par., 1884, xii, 617.—**Van Buren** (W. H.) Case of encephaloid tumor of the right side of the neck; unsuccessful attempt at removal. N. York J. M., 1850, v, 347–351.—**Velasco** (P. G.) Adenomas con degeneracion cancerosas. Anfiteatro anat., Madrid, 1873, i, 48.—**Volkmann** (R.) Das tiefe branchiogene Halskarcinom. Centralbl. f. Chir., Leipz., 1882, ix, 49-51.—**Wey** (W. C.) Case of encephaloid tumor of the neck. Tr. M. Ass. South. Central N. Y., Auburn, 1852, 77-85.

Neck *(Wounds and injuries of).*

See, also, **Artery** *(Carotid, Ligature of);* **Artery** *(Carotid, Wounds, etc., of);* **Cadaver** *(Jurisprudence of);* **Emphysema** *(Traumatic);* **Hyoid**

Neck (*Wounds and injuries of*).

1one (*Fracture of*); **Larynx, Œsophagus, Parotid** *glands*, **Spine, Thyroid** *gland*, **Trachea, Veins** (*Jugular*), *Wounds, etc., of*.

BERNARD (J.-B.) * I. Des accidents qu'entraînent les plaies des régions latérales du cou; comment doit-on les traiter? II. [etc.] 4°. *Paris*, 1838.

BOEY (J.) * Historia vulneris tracheam et œsophagum totum perscindentis feliciter sanati, cum aliorum observationibus et epicrisi. sm. 4°. *Kiliæ*, 1827.

CHAUVET (A.-F.-L.) * Des blessures de guerre intéressant les artères du cou. 4°. *Strasbourg*, 1860.

DIAZ (J.-A.) * Considérations sur certaines plaies de la région antérieure du cou chez les suicidés. 4°. *Paris*, 1883.

HORTELOUP (P.) * Plaies du larynx, de la trachée et de l'œsophage; leurs conséquences, leur traitement. 8°. *Paris*, 1869.

NÖTLING (W.) * Ueber Halswunden im Allgemeinen, insbesondere aber über Wunden der Luftröhre. 8°. *Mannheim*, 1845.

PEYRE (M.-J.) * Des plaies du conduit laryngo-trachéal et de leur traitement. 4°. *Paris*, 1865.

POHL (O.) * Ein seltener Fall von Halsverletzung mit Bildung einer Trachealfistel und einer Oesophagusfistel. 4°. *Greifswald*, 1875.

RAABE (L. C.) * De læsionibus colli in foro recte dijudicandis. 8°. *Halæ*, [1824].

SCHATTENHOFER (M.) * De colli vulneribus. 12°. *Monachii*, 1843.

TSCHIERSCHKI (C. F.) * De colli læsionibus. 8°. [*Berlin*, 1823.]

ZIEGLER (O. G. J.) * De lethalitate vulnerum colli. 8°. *Berolini*, [1844].

Acrel (O.) Vulnera colli et asperæ arteriæ. *In his:* Heelk. Waarn. [etc.], 8°, Gravenh., 1771, 151–154.—**Adams.** Case of cut throat. Dublin Hosp. Gaz., 1855-6, ii, 45.—**Allen** (E. L.) Case of gun-shot wound in Major-General Ripley. Tr. Phys.-Med. Soc. N. Y., 1817, i, 85–90.—**Allen** (H.) Gunshot wound of neck; paralysis of left upper extremity; probable reflex paralysis of both lower extremities; partial recovery; death from phthisis three years afterwards. Am. J. M. Sc., Phila., 1870, n. s., lix, 411–414.—**Alston** (W.) Division of larynx and œsophagus without wounding the jugulars or carotids. Richmond & Louisville M. J., Louisville, 1871, xii, 683–686.—**Anderson** (A. M.) Two remarkable cases of suicidal cut-throat. Glasgow M. J., 1867-8, 3. s., ii, 309–312. ——. Suicidal cut-throat; complete division of the larynx above the pomum Adami; perfect recovery. Lancet, Lond., 1868, i, 559.—**Arming** (F. W.) Heilung einer Halswunde mit grösstentheils durchschnittener Luftröhre. Med. Jahrb. d. k. k. österr. Staates, Wien, 1837, xxii, 441–453.—**Arpal** (F.) Herida por arma de fuego; ligadura de la arteria carótida primitiva; curacion. Siglo méd., Madrid, 1885, xxxii, 675–677.—**Bach** (N. E.) & **Dorhauer** (E. O.) Obduction eines mit einer Halswunde todtgefundenen Mannes. Aufsätze u. Beob. a. d. gerichtl. Arzneyw., Berl., 1791, vii. Samml., 178–187.—**Bannister** (H. M.) Gunshot wound of neck followed by paralysis of cervical sympathetic; insanity. J. Nerv. & Ment. Dis., Chicago, 1879, n. s., iv, 434–440. *Also* [Abstr.]: Med. Rec., N. Y., 1879, xvi, 15.—**Barbosa** (A. M.) Tentativa de suicidio por degolação; divisão completa da trachea; melhora consideravel. Gaz. med. de Lisb., 1856, iv, 78–80.—**Bardeleben.** Penetrirende Schnittwunde zwischen Zungenbein und Schildknorpel; Durchschneidung der Epiglottis, vollkommene quere Trennung des Pharynx; Tod nach 48 Stunden. Charité-Ann. 1883, Berl., 1885, x, 389–392.—**Bartlett** (J.) Account of the effect of a thread round a child's neck. Med. Communicat. Mass. M. Soc., Bost., 1790-1808, i, no. 2, pt. 2, 19–22.—**Bartrum** (J. S.) Case of suicide by cut throat. Assoc. M. J., Lond., 1855, ii, 1052.—**Beaupoil** (A.) Plaie pénétrante de la gorge; guérison. J. de méd., chir. et pharmacol., Brux., 1873, lvi, 227.—**Beck** (J. H.) Gutachten über einen Erschossenen. Ztschr. f. d. Staatsarznk., Erlang., 1831, xxi, 122–140.—**Béclère.** Tentative de suicide au moyen d'un rasoir; division de toute la région antérieure du cou, y compris la trachée-artère, et guérison radicale en douze jours. Gaz. d. hôp., Par., 1862, xxxv, 423.—**Bell** (J.) Suicide by cut-throat; death from intra-lobular suppurative

Neck (*Wounds and injuries of*).

pneumonia. Edinb. M. J., 1874-5, xx, 213. ——. Case of cut-throat; death from suppurative pneumonia. *Ibid.*, 214. ——. Accidental wound of neck and larynx; recovery. *Ibid.*, 216.—**Bennett** (W. H.) Cut-throat; seven cases, three of which died. St. George's Hosp. Rep. 1879, Lond., 1880, x, 128–130.—**Benoît** (E.) & **Carle** (A.) Assassinat par plaie du cou; mutilations cadavériques pratiquées pour faire disparaître les traces d'un viol. Arch. de l'anthrop. crim., Par., 1886, i, 144–147.—**Bergtold** (W. H.) Cut-throat with peculiar attending circumstances. Med. Press West. N. York, Buffalo, 1887, ii, 449.—**Bernt** (J.) Verletzungen des Halses. *In his:* Visa reperta u. gerichtl.- med. Gutachten, Wien, 1827, i, 216–238: 1838, ii, 254–265: 1845, iii, 209–221.—**Bertherand** (A.) De la suture dans le traitement des plaies du col. Rec. de mém. de méd. .-. mil., Par., 1845, lix, 232–245. *Also*, Reprint.—**Bett** (H. S.) Wound of trachea and œsophagus. Stethoscope & Virg. M. Gaz., Richmond, 1853, iii, 329.—**Bianchetti** (V.) Gravi ferimenti al collo e al testicolo; semicastrazione; laringoplastia. Bull. d. sc. med. di Bologna, 1842, 3. s., ii, 89–92.—**Bland** (G.) Case of attempted suicide by cutting the throat; asphyxial attack; recovery; remarks. Lancet, Lond., 1883, i, 863.—**Blandin.** Tentative de suicide; plaie grave à la région cervicale; autre plaie pénétrante à la partie externe gauche de la région précordiale. Gaz. d. hôp., Par., 1839, 2. s., i, 41.—**Blümlein.** Zur Casuistik der penetrirenden Halswunden. Vrtljschr. f. gerichtl. u. öff. Med., Berl., 1867, n. F., vi, 177–184.—**Böhm.** Suicidium tentatum; Vulnera scissa glandulæ thyreoideæ et tracheæ; Heilung. Ber. d. k. k. Krankenanst. Rudolph-Stiftung in Wien (1866), 1867, 179.—**Bonhoure** (G.-J.-A.) Blessures profondes au cou, suites de tentatives de suicide pendant une aliénation mentale; observation suivie de réflexions relatives au traitement de l'hydrophobie rabique. Ann. de la méd. physiol., Par., 1826, x, 568–588.—**Bonnevie.** Plaies au cou; suffocation imminente; trachéotomie. Arch. de la méd. belge, Brux., 1851, xxxvi, 90–94.—**Bork** (J.) Heilung einer durch Schnitt verursachten grossen Halswunde, verbunden mit Durchschneidung der Speiseröhre. J. d. Chir. u. Augenh., Berl., 1847, xxxvii, 256–259.—**Boys de Loury.** Rapports sur un cas d'empoisonnement et d'assassinat. Ann. d'hyg., Par., 1833, ix, 336–379. ——. Affaire de l'assassinat de la dame Renaud. *Ibid.*, 1839, xxii, 170–182.—**Brach.** Befund einer Halswunde nach dem Sturze in einen Brunnen. Med. Ztg., Berl., 1845, xiv, 255.—**Brigham** (C. B.) Gunshot wound of the neck; recovery. West. Lancet, San Fran., 1875, iv, 515–517. *Also, in his:* Surg. Cases, 8°, Cambridge, 1876, 41–43.—**Brown** (T. E. B.) A case of cut throat. Indian M. Gaz., Calcutta, 1876, xi, 73.—**Bryant** (T.) On wounds of the throat. Guy's Hosp. Rep., Lond., 1860, 3. s., vi, 32–35. ——. Lacerated wound of the throat into the larynx and pharynx by broken crockery; recovery. Brit. M. J., Lond., 1884, i, 164.—**Bryce** (S. P.) [Section of trachea and left jugular vein.] Med. & Phys. J., Lond., 1800, iii, 228.—**Buchner** (E.) Tödtliche Halsstichwunde. Friedreich's Bl. f. gerichtl. Med., Nürnb., 1869, xx, 137–142.—**Buot** (P.) Observation de blessure par arme à feu de la région cervicale suivie de méningo-myélite au vingtième jour. Arch. de méd. et pharm. mil., Par., 1886, viii, 290–393.—**Burger** (C. P.) Geval eener diepe halsverwonding met genezing. Nederl. Tijdschr. v. Geneesk., Amst., 1883, xix, 197.—**Burggraeve** (A.) Plaies du cou par suite de tentatives de suicide. Ann. Soc. de méd. de Gand, 1851, xxviii, 36–40.—**Butcher** (R. G.) Suicidal wound of throat, implicating the trunk of the common carotid; successfully ligatured above and below the wound, perfect recovery. Dublin J. M. Sc., 1881, 3. s., lxxii, 386–392.—**de Caisne.** Plaie pénétrante du cou par arme à feu; guérison. Arch. méd. belges, Brux., 1870, xi, 253–259.—**Calori** (V.) Ferita trasversale della trachea per tentato suicidio. Ippocratico, Fano, 1872, 3. s., xxii, 489–497.—**Cameron** (H. C.) Stab in the neck, by which the right hypoglossal nerve was divided. Lancet, Lond., 1884, i, 885 —**Canella** (G.) Osservazione di una ferita dell' esofago e della trachea accompagnata da circostanze aggravanti felicemente trattata. Gior. di chir.-prat., Trento, 1829, vii, 115–120.—[**Cases.**] Casus vom einem, der sich den Hals halb abgeschnitten, und doch glücklich wieder geheilet worden. Med. u. chir. Berl. wchntl. Nachr. (1739), 1742, ii, 83–90.—Case of a fatal wound of the trachea. Lancet, 2. ed., Lond., 1825, vii, 223. — Visum repertum über eine in ihrem Bette durch zwei Halswunden ermordet gefundene junge Frau. Mag. f. d. gerichtl. Arzneiw., Berl., 1832, ii, 60–70.—Plaie à la partie antérieure du col; tentative de suicide; réflexions pratiques sur ces sortes de blessures. J. de méd. et chir. prat., Par., 1834, v, 518–522.—Case of cut throat. Lond. M. & S. J., 1834-5, vi, 766.—Cut throat; division of the trachea, œsophagus, etc. Lond. M. & S. J., 1836, i, 604.—Begutachtung eines Falles, bei welchem in Folge roher Verletzungen mit dem Schlundstösser der Tod eintrat. Ann. d. Staatsarznk., Freib. i. Br., 1842, vii, 297–327.—Severe wound of the throat; division of the larynx and anterior wall of the pharynx; recovery. N. Orl. M. & S. J., 1851-2, viii, 676.—Fall von Tödtung. Bl. f. gerichtl. Anthrop., Nürnb., 1855, vi, 6. Hft., 21–26.—Case

Neck (*Wounds and injuries of*).

of homicide, by severing the atlas from the head. Virginia M. J., Richmond, 1856, vii, 485–490.—Unglücksfall, Mord oder Selbstmord? Bl. f. gerichtl. Anthrop., Nürnb., 1857, viii, 1. Hft., 73–79.—Schnittwunde am Halse; Gutachten der Gerichtsärzte; Zufügung durch einen Andern; unbestimmtes Gutachten der Facultät, jedoch mit Möglichkeit, ja selbst mit Wahrscheinlichkeit eines Selbstmordes. Samml. gerichtsärztl. Gutacht. d. Prag. med. Fak., 1858, 2. F., 79–85.—Schnittwunde am Halse. Aerztl. Ber. d. k. k. allg. Krankénh. zu Wien (1861), 1862, 41.—Selbstmord oder Mord? Bl. f. gerichtl. Anthrop., Nürnb., 1862, xiii, 1. Hft., 116–125. — [Schnittwunden am Halse, beigebracht mit einem Rasirmesser in einem Anfalle von Melancholie.] Aerztl. Ber. d. k. k. allg. Krankenh. zu Wien (1866), 1867, 309–311. — Schläge gegen den Nacken; nachgefolgte Lähmung der linken Körperhälfte mit Contractur im Kniegelenke; schwere und lebensgefährliche Verletzung. Samml. gerichtsärztl. Gutacht. d. Prag. med. Fak., 1867, 3. F., 43–49. — Halsschnittwunde; Mord oder Selbstmord? *Ibid.* Leipz., 1874, 4. F., 170–173. — **Casper.** Ein unerklärlicher, und dennoch leicht erklärter Mord. Vrtljschr. f. gerichtl. u. öff. Med., Berl., 1852, ii, 85–99. *Also* [Abstr.]: Bl. f. gerichtl. Anthrop., Ansbach, 1853, iv, 1. Hft., 31–35.—**Cavalier.** Observation d'une plaie transversale du cou, qui, en 1776, donna lieu à la découverte d'un nouveau bandage. J. gén. de méd., chir. et pharm., Par., 1815, liv, 105–116, 1 pl.—**Cayley** (H.) Case of cut throat. Indian M. Gaz, Calcutta, 1873, viii, 14.—**Chadwick** (S T.) Case of severe gunshot wound in the cervical region. Lancet, Lond., 1851, ii, 369.—**Charles** (D. A.) Case of gunshot wound of neck, with perforation of œsophagus: recovery. Brit. M. J., Lond., 1883, i, 611.—**Chassaignac.** Plaies graves et profondes du cou; trachéotomie; mode particulier de suture. Gaz. d. hôp., Par., 1852, xxv, 365.—**Chauvel** (J.) Plaie du cou par instrument tranchant; tentatives de réunion; mort. Rec. de mém. de méd. . . . mil., Par., 1871, 3. s., xxvi, 136–141.—**Cheever** (D. W.) Three cases of cut throat. Boston M. & S. J., 1865–6, lxxiii, 229–234. *Also*: Med. & Surg. Rep. Bost. City Hosp. (1864–9), 1870, i, 486–499. ———. Partial asphyxia by hanging; incised wounds of trachea and œsophagus; stricture of larynx; secondary tracheotomy; forcible dilatation of the rima glottidis. Boston M. & S. J., 1882, cvii, 577.—**Chisolm** (J.J.) Singular injury to the nerves of the throat from a pistol shot. Balt. M. J. & Bull., 1871, ii, 466–470. — **Clark** (A.) [Case of supposed murder.] Bull. N. York Acad. M., 1860–62, i, 320–344. *Also*: Am. M. Times, N. Y., 1862, iv, 48; 62; 76; 91.—**Coindet.** Quelques réflexions pratiques sur un cas de vaste plaie transversale de la région thyro-hyoïdienne. Rec. de mém. de méd. . . . mil., Par., 1859, 3. s., ii, 416–427. *Also*, Reprint.—**Cooke** (W.) Case of cut-throat, with division of the larynx and pharynx. Lancet, Lond., 1860, ii, 56.—**Cooper.** Cut-throat. Lond. M. & S. J., 1836, i, 905.—**Cotronei** (G.) Ferita da taglio della regione laterale e superiore del collo; flemmone profondo; infiltramento purulento; empiema; morte. Ann. clin. d. osp. d. Pellegr. di Napoli, 1872, ii, 110–114.—**Cotting** (B. E.) Cut-throat; complete division of the cricoid cartilage and œsophagus. Extr. Rec. Bost. Soc. M. Improve., 1848–53, i, 280–282.—**Coulson.** Cut-throat followed by delirium tremens; autopsy. Med. Times & Gaz., Lond., 1855, n. s., x, 543. ———. Wound of the throat between the hyoid bone and the thyroid cartilage; free hæmorrhage; recovery. Lancet, Lond., 1862, i, 277.—**Couper.** Fracture of thyroid cartilage; lacerated wound of throat; broncho-pneumonia; death. Med. Times & Gaz., Lond., 1880, ii, 695.—**Cras.** Ligature de la carotide primitive droite pratiquée à la suite d'hémorragies secondaires consécutives à un coup de corne de vache reçu dans la région des carotides secondaires. Bull et mém. Soc. de chir. de Par., 1884, n. s., x, 734–737.—**Cripps** (W. H.) Treatment of hæmorrhage from punctured wounds of the throat and neck, especially considered with regard to ligature of the external carotid artery. Med.-Chir. Tr., Lond., 1877–8, lxi, 229–241.—**Croly.** Case of extensive suicidal wound of the throat. Med. Press & Circ., Dubl., 1868, v, 352.—**Curling.** Cut-throat, with division of the thyro-hyoid membrane; closure of the wound by sutures; recovery. Med. Times & Gaz., Lond., 1853, n. s., vii, 680. ———. Case of incised throat (suicidal) in which a large opening remained permanently. Clin. Lect. & Rep. Lond. Hosp., 1866, iii, 196–198. ———. Incised throat (attempted murder); complete division of the trachea; recovery with membranous stricture of the trachea; subsequent death from contraction of the fistula. *Ibid.*, 198–200.—**Daniel** (C. F.) Von einer schlechterdings tödtlichen Halswunde eines Kindes von fünf Wochen, dem durch Schnitte die Luftröhre, der Schlund, etc., verletzt worden. *In his*: Samml. med. Gutacht. [etc.], 8°, Leipz., 1776, 28–30.—**Davies** (R.) Case of injury of the neck. Am. J. M. Sc., Phila., 1863, n. s., xlv, 79. — **Davies-Colley.** Transfixion of neck by a walking-stick; recovery. Lancet, Lond., 1882, i, 986.—**Davis** (J. T.) Case of severe injury of the neck; recovery with loss of use of the left shoulder joint. Cincin. Lancet & Obs., 1870, n. s., xiii, 210. — **Debendra** (N. R.) Case of incised wound (transverse) on the nape of the

Neck (*Wounds and injuries of*).

neck. Indian M. Gaz., Calcutta, 1880, xv, 72.—**Dejacghere** (G.) Section transversale complète de l'artère carotide et de la veine jugulaire, mort 26 heures après; le prévenu se blesse volontairement pour détourner les soupçons. Ann. méd.-lég. belges, Brux., 1843, ii, 24.—**Dieffenbach** (J. F.) Beobachtungen über Halswunden. Mag. f. d. ges. Heilk., Berl., 1834, xli, 395–432. *Also, transl.*: Abeille, Brux., 1834, iv, 239–246.—**Djakonoff** (P. I.) Tri sluchaja glubokich rane shei. [Three cases of deep wounds of neck.] Vrach, St. Petersb., 1880, i, 865.—**Dock** (G.) Case of wound of the throat, in a maniac, in which the epiglottis was nearly severed. Med. Exam., Phila., 1855, xi, 476–478.—**Donovan** (D.) Case of extensive wound of the throat. Dublin M. Press, 1862, xlviii, 277.—**Dressel.** Durchschneidung des Halses in einem Anfalle von Wahnsinn. J. d. Chir. u. Augenh., Berl., 1833, xx. 319–322. — **Dujardin - Beaumetz.** Coup de feu à l'angle de la mâchoire inférieure; fracture de cet os; trachéotomie; fistule salivaire; extraction d'un biscaïen pesant 215 grammes. Bull. Soc. de chir. de Par. (1871), 1872, 2. s., xii, 214–217.—**Dupuytren.** Blessure profonde du cou, pénétrant jusqu'au pharynx, s'étendant de l'une à l'autre artère carotides, sans lésion de ces artères; réunion au moyen de quatre points de suture. Gaz. d. hôp., Par., 1828–9, i, 321. ———. Fistule laryngo-pharyngienne. à la suite d'une blessure au cou; expériences sur la voix faites par MM. Magendie, Savard et Cagniard-Latour; opération. *Ibid.*, 1831–2, v, 309; 314.—**Durham** (A. E.) Injuries of the neck. Syst. Surg. (Holmes), 2. ed., N. Y., 1870, ii, 436–551.—**Dutertre.** Observation sur une très-grande plaie du cou. J. de méd., chir., pharm., etc., Par., 1805, x, 136–139.—**Easley** (E. P.) A case of cut-throat; marked effect of opium on the respiratory mucous membrane. Am. Pract., Louisville, 1876, xiv, 73–75.—**Ebel.** Sectionsbefund und Gutachten über eine tödtlich gewordene Stichwunde. Deutsche Ztschr. f. d. Staatsarznk., Freib. i. Br., 1852, xii, 313–335.—**Ellerman.** Bijdrage tot de behandeling van dwarse halswonden. Nederl. Lancet, Gravenh., 1845–6, 2. s., i, 279–282.—**Englisch.** Schnittwunden an verschiedenen Körperstellen mit Eröffnung des Kehlkopfes; Tod in Folge consecutiv aufgetretener Pleuritis sinistra. Ber. d. k. k. Krankenanst. Rudolph-Stiftung in Wien (1878), 1879, 326.—**España y Martin** (T.) Medicina forense [lesion mortal del cuello]. Corresp. méd., Madrid, 1879, xiv, 75.—**Eves** (A.) Case of suicidal wound of the throat. Lancet, Lond., 1852, i, 36–38. — **F.** Extraordinary case of suicide. Med. Mag., Bost., 1834–5, iii, 117–119.—**Faber.** Legalfall; Tod 12–13 Stunden nach zwei tiefen Messerstichen in den Hals, welche nicht tödtlich waren. Med. Cor.-Bl. d. württemb. ärztl. Ver. Stuttg., 1847, xvii, 65–71. ———. Tödtung durch Stich in den Hals. Deutsche Ztschr. f. d. Staatsarznk., Erlang., 1865, n. F., xxiii, 378–383. ———. Tödtung durch Stich in den Hals. Wien. med. Wchnschr., 1866, xvi, 304–306. — **Faure** (L.) Coup de feu de la région cervicale; balle perdue dans le rachis; paralysie progressive des membres inférieurs, du tronc et des bras; intégrité de l'intelligence. Gaz. méd. de l'Algérie, Alger, 1869, xiv, 108.—**Fayrer** (J.) Case of self-inflicted gunshot wound of the throat; recovery. Med. Times & Gaz., Lond., 1871, ii, 404. *Also, in his*: Clin. & Path. Obs. in India, 8°, Lond., 1873, 207–209.—**Fazio** (E.) Ferite portanti pericolo di vita; giudizio medico-legale. Gior. internaz. di sc. med., Napoli, 1879, n. s., i, 654–664.—**Fine.** Observation sur une plaie de la gorge. J. de méd., chir., pharm., etc., Par., 1790, lxxxiii, 64–77.—**Finlay** (W. A.) Wound of the larynx and œsophagus; tracheotomy. Edinb. M. J., 1879–80, xxv, 211.—**Finnel** (T. C.) Suicide, with pathological specimen. Tr. M. Soc. N. Y., Albany, 1861, 81.—**Fithian** (J.) Penetrating wound of the neck. Med. & Surg. Reporter, Phila., 1859, n. s., i, 419.—**Freer** (J. H.) Tobacco-pipe in the neck. Lancet, Lond., 1861, ii, 486. — **French** (W. W.) A case of cut throat involving the larynx. Weekly M. Rev., St. Louis, 1886, xiv, 455. — **Frey** (L.) Ueber Tödtung durch Halsumdrehen. Deutsche Ztschr. f. d. Staatsarznk., Erlang., 1863, n. F., xxi, 138–145.—**Friedel** (C.) [Säbelhieb quer durch die Kehle, horizontal den Kehlkopf vom Zungenbein abtrennend und die vordere Wand des Pharynx durchschneidend.] Arch. f. path. Anat., etc., Berl., 1862, xxiii, 438. ———. [Anderthalb Zoll lange Stichwunde an der rechten Halsseite schmal vorm Rande des Kopfnickers anfangend, und schräg nach unten und vorn sich verbreitend und vertiefend, mit einer Partisane vom Pferde aus beigebracht.] *Ibid.*, 439. ———. [Noch ein Köpfungsversuch; 3 parallele tiefe Schwerthiebe im Nacken.] *Ibid.*, 440.—**Fritz** (T.) Zur gerichtsärztlichen Lehre über Halsverletzungen. Oesterr. med. Wchnschr., Wien, 1844, 1261–1265. — **Fürstenau** (J. F.) De autochiria juguli dissectione tentata. Acta Acad. nat. curios., Norimb., 1752, ix, 202. — **Gairdner** (J.) Case of wound in the throat, in which the trachea and œsophagus were divided across, and which did not terminate fatally, although the parts have not reunited. Edinb. M. & S. J., 1820, xvi, 353–359.—**Gallicier.** Observation d'une blessure des plus graves produite par la traverse d'une vergue de moulin. J. de la sect. de méd. Soc. acad. Loire-Inf., Nantes, 1862, n. s., xxxviii, 173.—**Gallozzi.** Vasta ferita alla gola, per ten-

Neck (*Wounds and injuries of*).

tato suicidio od omicidio? Riv. clin. d. Univ. di Napoli, 1883, iv, 75. — **Garde** (H. C.) Case of suicidal wound of throat. Dublin M. Press, 1861, xlv, 121. — **Garlick** (F. S.) Suicidal cut-throat successfully treated. Lancet, Lond., 1846, i, 648.—**Gay** (G. W.) Bullet-wound of neck; tracheotomy; hæmorrhage from the vertebral artery; death. Med. News, Phila., 1882, xl, 489.—**Gay** (J.) Case of cut throat; wound of left internal jugular vein treated by ligature; recovery; remarks. Lancet, Lond., 1877, i, 126. — **Getz** (H. L.) Incised injuries of the pharynx, œsophagus, and trachea, and their treatment. J. Am. M. Ass., Chicago, 1885, iv, 342. — **Gilland** (L. W.) A case of cut throat. N. Orl. M. & S. J., 1877, v, 297–300.—**Gillbee** (W.) Gunshot wound of the neck. Austral M. J., Melbourne, 1862, vii, 258 – 261. — **Gilmore** (A.) Case of incised wound of the throat. Tr. M. & Phys. Soc. Calcutta, 1833, vi, 478. *Also*: Proc. M. & Phys. Soc. Calcutta, 1833, i, 5. — **Gioffredi** (L.) Grave ferita alla regione anteriore del collo per tentato suicidio completamente guarita. Morgagni, Napoli, 1872, xiv, 429–433.—**Godwin** (I. R.) Severance of the trachea and œsophagus without injury to the carotids or jugulars. Richmond & Louisville M. J., Louisville, 1871, xi, 504 – 507. — **Gozalves** (V.) Algunas consideraciones acerca del tratamiento de las heridas de la región suprahioidea. Gac. de l. hosp., Valencia, 1882, i, 341 – 345. — **Greuling.** Krankheits-Geschichte einer geheilten grossen Halsverwundung. als Versuch einer Selbstermordung. Mag. f. d. ges. Heilk., Berl., 1833, xxxix, 560–564. — **Gross** (S. D.) Case of gunshot wound of the neck, involving the trachea, œsophagus, the right internal jugular vein, and the right subclavian artery, and terminating fatally on the fourteenth day, in consequence of the formation of an abscess in front of the spine. Am. J. M. Sc., Phila., 1848, n. s., xv, 355 – 357. — **Güterbock** (P.) Die Verletzungen des Halses in forensischer Beziehung. Vrtljschr. f. gerichtl. Med., Berl., 1873, n. F., xix, 1 – 88. *Also*, Reprint. — **Gunning** (A. T.) On a case of suicidal cut-throat. Austral. M. J., Melbourne. 1864, ix, 65 —**Guttenberg.** Ueber Halswunden mit Eröffnung der Luftwege. Aerztl. Mitth. a. Baden, Karlsruhe, 1865, xix, 142–144.—**H.** (A.) Plaie du cou par arme à feu; abcès; pleurésie purulente; autopsie. Rev. méd. franç. et étrang., Par., 1881, ii, 729–731.—**Haden** (C. T.) Case of cut throat, successfully treated. Tr. Ass. Apoth., etc., Lond., 1823, i, 351 – 361. — **Hamilton.** Suicidal wounds of throat. Dublin Hosp. Gaz., 1856, iii, 60.—**Hammond** (D. W.) Cutting throat; operation unsuccessful as performed by the patient. Tr. M. Ass. Georgia, Atlanta, 1873, xxiv, 69 – 72. *Also*: Atlanta M. & S. J., 1873-4, xi, 148 – 151.—**Handyside** (P. D.) Account of a remarkable case of suicide, with observations on the fatal issue of the rapid introduction of air in large quantities into the circulation during surgical operations. Edinb. M. & S. J., 1838, xlix, 209–221. 1 pl. *Also*, Reprint.—**Harrison** (R.) Suicidal wound of neck treated by tracheotomy and the insertion of deep sutures. Lancet, Lond., 1885, i, 842. — **Hathaway** (H.) A peculiar case of suicidal cut-throat. Brit. M. J., Lond., 1887, i, 933.—**Hathorn** (R.) Case of extensive wound of the throat. Edinb. M. & S. J., 1815, xi, 194. — **Havá** (J. G.) Informe para determinar si D. F. . . P. . . con una herida grave del cuello, pudo dar ayes que, traspasando el espesor de las paredes de una casa completamente cerrada, se oyeran á una distancia de cerca de doscientas varas. Trab. Com. d. med. leg. é hig. púb. de la r. Acad. de cien. méd. . . . de la Habana, 1872–3, i, 283–289. — **Hawkins** (J.) Cases of injury of neck resembling dislocation of vertebræ. Lond. M. Gaz., 1847, xl, 236–238.—**Hening** (W. H.) Case of gun-shot wound, where a musket ball was lodged in the posterior part of the neck, and subsequently discharged per anum. Eclect. Report., Phila., 1817, vii, 246. — **Henrich.** Ein mit einem zinnernen Suppenlöffel auf den Hals einer bejahrten Frau geführter Schlag bewirkt deren alsbaldigen Tod. Als Berichtigung des unter demselben Titel von Dr. Simeons angeführten Kriminalfalles. Zts hr. f. d. Staatsarznk., Erlang., 1848, lv, 356–413.—**Heuschen** (S.) Fall of läkning efter fullständigt genomskärande af luft- och matstrupe. [Recovery after complete division of trachea and œsophagus.] Upsala Läkaref. Förh., 1874–5, x, 152–155.—**Herbert.** Cas intéressant de médecine légale. Soc. méd. d'Amiens. Bull. (1869–72), 1873, ix–xii, 179–191.—**Heredia** (J. C.) Observacion de un caso de herida por arma de fuego. Gac. méd. de Lima, 1865–6, x, 194– 96.—**Hill** (J. D.) Punctured wound of neck; severe arterial hemorrhage; autopsy. Med. Press & Circ., Dubl., 1867, iv, 316.—**Hilton** (J.) Gunshot wound [in neck]. Lancet, Lond., 1850, ii, 344. ———. Injury to the neck near the second cervical vertebra. *Ibid.*, 1866, ii, 629. — **Hirn.** Sur les plaies du cou. Rec. de mém. de méd. . . . mil., Par., 1820, vii, 226–229. — **Hoar** (C. E) Peculiar wound by a knife, causing speedy death. Brit. M. J., Lond., 1877, i, 324.—**Hodgen** (J. T.) Pistol shot wound; ligation of carotid. St. Louis Cour. Med., 1882, viii, 424–428. — **Höring.** Schussverletzung des Halses. Med. Cor.-Bl. d. württemb. ärztl. Ver., Stuttg., 1851, xxi, 226.—**Holmgren** (F.) Nya iakttagelser vid halshuggning. [On incised wounds of neck.] Upsala Läkaref. Förh., 1882–3, xviii, 68–

Neck (*Wounds and injuries of*).

79.—**Horlacher.** Merkwürdige Heilung einer Rachen-Schusswunde. Mag. f. d. ges. Heilk., Berl., 1819, vi, 62– 67.—**Horsch.** Obduktionsbericht und Gutachten über eine Frau, die durch eine absoluttödliche Halswunde umkam; wobei die Frage entstand: ob die Verletzung von ihr selbst oder von andern beigel racht worden sei. Jahrb. d. Staatsarznk., Frankf. a. M., 1809, ii. 94 – 101. — **Houston** (J.) Case of attempt at suicide, with danger of suffocation by the falling down of the epiglottis. Dublin Hosp. Rep., 1830, v, 315.—**Howden** (T.) Case of cut-throat. Lancet, Lond., 1842–3, ii, 402. — **Janikowski** (S.) Przypadek samobójstwa przez poderznięcie gardła. [Suicide by cutting the throat.] Pam. Towarz. Lek. Warszaw., 1866, lv, 197–200. — **Jas** (F.) Verzameling van waarneemingen over de aangezichts- en hals-wonden. Verhandel. d. Genootsch. t. Bevord. d. Heelk. te Amst., 1799, v, 60 – 212.— **Jasser.** Vom Durchschneiden des Laryngis, wo zugleich der Pharynx verletzet war, und der Patient beym Leben erhalten wurde. Verm. chir. Schrift., Berl. u. Stettin, 1782, iii, 162–169. — **Jeaffreson** (C. S.) Case of severe suicidal wound of the neck. St. Barth. Hosp. Rep., Lond., 1873, ix, 90–96.—**Jeannel** (M.) Blessures et maladies chirurgicales du cou. Encycl. internat. de chir. (Ashhurst), Par., 1886, v, 745–868.—**Joly.** Plaie du col causée par les bourres d'un pistolet chargé à poudre; mort instantanée; éjaculation spermatique. Gaz. méd. de Par., 1836, 2. s., iv, 719.—**Jung.** Versuchter Selbstmord durch Halsverletzung. Gen.-Ber.d.k.rhein. Med.-Coll. 1834, Koblenz, 1837, 140.—**Kelso.** History of a case of an attempt to commit suicide. Phil., M. Museum, 1810–11, n. s., i, 137–140.— **Kenan** (T. H.) Case of cut throat; attempted suicide. Tr. M. Ass. Georgia, Augusta, 1881, xxxii, 105–107.—**Kendall** (J. C.) Prophylactic use of the tracheal tube in injuries of the neck about the region of the larynx. Proc. Connect. M. Soc., Hartford, 1882, n. s., ii, 66–71. — **Key** (C. A.) Abstract of a clinical lecture on wounds of the throat. Lond. M. Gaz., 1829, iv, 229–233. — **Kirby.** Interesting case of attempted suicide, in which a large portion of the thyroid cartilage was removed. Dublin M. Press, 1846, xv, 2. — **Kitchen** (J. M.) A case of cut-throat. Nashville J. M. & S., 1859, xvi, 404–406.—**Kölpin** (A. B.) Obduktion einer ertrunkenen Weibesperson, welche zuglcich eine Wunde am Halse hatte. Aufsätze u. Beob. a. d. gerichtl. Arzneyw., Berl., 1785, 3. Samml., 50– 52.—**Krügelstein** (F. C. K.) Besichtigungs- und Sectionsbericht über eine an einer Halswunde plötzlich gestorbene Frau. Mat. f. d. Staatsarzneiw. u. prakt. Heilk., Meiningen, 1819, i, 155–161.—**Kuby.** Mord- oder Selbstmord-Versuch durch einen Schnitt in den Hals. Friedreich's Bl. f. gerichtl. Med., Nürnb., 1878, xxix, 224–230.—**Kurtzwig.** Geschichte einer glücklich geheilten Hals-Wunde, mit gänzlicher Durchschneidung der Luftröhre und Verletzung des Schlundes. J. f. d. Chir., Geburtsh. u. gerichtl. Arznk., Jena, 1800, ii. 725–732.—**Labarrière.** Perforation du cou de droite à gauche par un échalas. Bull. Soc. méd. de Reims, 1873, xii, 85–87.—**Laidlaw** (J.) Wound of the throat. Lond. M. & Phys. J., 1832, n. s., xii, 93–96.— **Landsberg.** Geschichte eines Selbstmordversuches durch (sogenanntes) Halsabschneiden, nebst einigen Bemerkungen über die Behandlung der Halswunden. Med. Ztg., Berl., 1852. xxi, 85–87.—**Larrey** (H.) Plaie par instrument piquant et tranchant, au cou, avec lésion partielle d'une des moitiés de la moelle épinière. Rec. de mém. de méd. . . . mil., Par., 1840, xlix, 325–336.—**Lawrie** (E.) Wound of the external carotid and vertebral arteries; ligature of the common carotid; death. Indian M. Gaz., Calcutta, 1883, xviii, 251.—**Lawson.** Extensive wound of the neck from falling through a sky-light, opening the carotid sheath, and dividing some of the cervical nerves, followed by a severe attack of erysipelas. Lancet, Lond., 1869, i, 459.—**Lefferts** (G. M.) Stab wound of the neck and division of the right recurrent laryngeal nerve, followed immediately by absolute aphonia. Am. J. M. Sc., Phila. 1881, n. s., lxxxii, 155.—**Legendre.** Plaie transversale de la région antérieure du cou, faite avec un rasoir; ouverture de la trachée; réunion immédiate par la suture entortillée; guérison. Gaz. méd. de Par., 1857, 3. s., xii, 365.—**Letenneur.** Plaie par arme à feu de la région sous-claviculaire. Bull. Soc. de chir. de Par. (1865), 1866, 2. s., vi, 367–374. — **Levis** (R. F.) A case of cut throat in which the pharynx was almost completely divided. Phila. M. Times, 1879, ix, 570.—**Linsmayer** (L.) Selbstmordversuch durch Schnitt in die Kehlkopfgegend; Tod nach 4 Stunden durch Glottisödem, welches durch eine erst bei der Obduction gefundene, sondenknopfgrosse Perforationsöffnung in den einen Ventriculus Morgagnii veranlasst worden war; im Leben keine auffälligen laryngostenotischen Erscheinungen. Ber. d. k. k. Krankenanst. Rudolph - Stiftung in Wien (1876), 1877, 337.— **Llewellyn** (C.) Remarkable case of division of the trachea and œsophagus. India J. M. & Phys. Sc., Calcutta, 1839, n. s., iv, 711.—**Lloyd** (J.) Case of ligature of the left common carotid artery for gunshot wound at the root of the neck. Birmingh. M. Rev., 1882. xi, 24–34.— **Longet.** Sur les troubles qui surviennent dans l'équilibration, la station et la locomotion des animaux. après la section des parties molles de la nuque. Gaz. méd. de Par.,

Neck (*Wounds and injuries of*).

1845, 2. s., xiii, 565–567.—**Lüders.** Heilung einer completen Zerschneidung der Luft- und Speiseröhre, mit Nachbleiben eines künstlichen Respirationsweges. J. d. Chir. u. Augenh., Berl., 1829, xiii, 261–289. *Also, transl.* [Abstr.]: J. compl. du dict. d. sc. méd., Par., 1830, xxxvi, 169–182.— **Luke.** Wound of the throat inflicted by a suicide; autopsy. Lancet, Lond., 1850, ii, 422.—**Macfie** (J.) Case of cut-throat, vertical; recovery. Glasgow M. J., 1877, n. s., ix, 206–212.—**Macgregor** (J. S.) Extensive wound of trachea and œsophagus: recovery. Austral. M. J., Melbourne, 1863, viii, 126.—**Mackenzie** (M.) Stabbing wounds in the neck, with injury of several of the cerebral nerves and probably of branches of the superior cervical ganglion. Brit. M. J., Lond., 1870, ii, 682.—**Macleod** (G. H. B.) Injuries and diseases of the neck. Internat. Encycl. Surg. (Ashhurst). N. Y., 1885, v, 573–623.—**Macleod** (M. D.) Case of severe cut throat; nourishment of patient by enemata; recovery. J. Ment. Sc. Lond., 1875, xxi, 277–279.—**Macnamara** (G. H.) Case of extensive cut-throat. Lancet, Lond., 1854, ii, 122.—**McWhinnie** (A. M.) Observations on severe wounds of the throat, inflicted for the purpose of self-destruction. *Ibid.*, 1846, ii, 267–270.—**Mair** (I.) Schnittwunden an den obersten hinteren Seitentheilen des Halses mit nachfolgender Anästhesie; ob bleibender Nachtheil? Deutsche Ztschr. f. d. Staatsarznk., Erlang., 1871–2, n. F., xxix, 261–269 — **Marchionneschi** (O.) Suicidio tentato con colpi di rasoio; innesto epidermico; guarigione. Indipendente, Torino, 1878, xxix, 401–403.—**Marsden** (A.) Wound of the neck and exposure of the carotid artery: recovery. Lancet, Lond., 1859, ii, 366.—**Martin.** Lettre contenant une observation sur une plaie de la gorge. J. de méd., chir., pharm., etc., Par., 1764, xxi. 148–151. ———. Observation sur une plaie de la gorge. *Ibid.*, 1766, xxv, 174–177.—**Martinet.** Plaie de la région hyoïdienne; sonde œsophagienne laissée à demeure; œdème de la glotte; trachéotomie; infection purulente; ulcérations de l'œsophage. Bull. Soc. anat. de Par., 1875, l, 432–434.—**Maschka.** Verletzung am Halse mittelst eines Taschenmessers; leichte Verletzung; Gutachten. Allg. Wien. med. Ztg., 1857, ii, 145. ———. Schlag in die Nackengegend; schwere Erkrankung mit Erblindung und tödtlichem Ausgange; nicht mit Bestimmtheit nachweisbarer Zusammenhang. Ztschr. f. gerichtl. Med., Wien. 1868, iv, 279. *Also*: Samml. gerichtsärztl. Gutacht. d. Prag. med. Fak., Leipz., 1874, 4. F., 30–34. ———. Stichwunde am Halse eines neugeborenen Kindes. Vrt jschr. f. gerichtl. u. öff. Med., Berl., 1871, xv, 235–244. ———. Stich in die Nackengegend; Septicämie; Tod; Beantwortung der Frage bezüglich des ursächlichen Zusammenhanges. Allg. Wien. med. Ztg., 1881, xxvi, 411. ———. Stichwunde am Halse mit tödtlichem Ausgange; nicht nachweisbarer Zusammenhang des letzteren mit der Verletzung wegen mangelhafter Behandlung. Vrtljschr. f. gerichtl. Med., Berl., 1882, n. F., xxxvii, 261–265.—**Mason** (F.) Case of extensive cut throat, with recovery. Tr. M. Soc. King's Coll.. Lond., 1837–8, ii, 200–202. – **Mezger** (P.) Verwundung mit tödtlichem Erfolg. Deutsche Ztschr. f. d. Staatsarznk., Erlang., 1854, n. F., iii, 401–415.— **Michael** (J. E.) A case of cut throat and other wounds inflicted with suicidal intent; death. Maryland M. J., Balt., 1883–4, x, 585.—**Michaelsen.** Vollkommene Heilung einer completen Zerschneidung des Kehlkopfs in Verbindung mit fast vollständiger Zerschneidung der Speiseröhre. Mitth. a. d. Geb. d. Med., etc., Altona, 1836, iv, 11.–12. Hft., 53–67.—**Miller** (W. C.) A case of gunshot wound of the neck, attended by an interesting train of phenomena. Charleston M. J., 1852, vii, 668.—**Moffatt** (J. E.) Remarks on cut-throat, illustrated by a case. Indian M. Gaz., Calcutta, 1876, xi, 211.—**Moon** (W. P.) Gunshot wound of neck. [Presenting apertures of entrance and exit, but with the bullet lodged.] Am. J. M. Sc., Phila., 1868, n. s., lv, 55.—**Morrison** (J.) Case in which the epiglottis was divided in an attempt to commit suicide. Dublin J. M. & Chem. Sc., 1836, ix, 102–105. *Also*: Lond. M. Gaz., 1835–6, xvii, 900.—**Morton** (T. G.) Incised wound of the neck, involving the larynx and œsophagus; food introduced into the stomach by hydrostatic pressure. Phila. M. Times, 1874–5, v, 71.—**Munro** (W.) Notes of a curious case of accidental death. Edinb. M. J., 1870–71, xvi, 1066–1073.—**Neill** (J.) Traumatic hæmorrhage into the posterior mediastinum. Tr. Coll. Phys. Phila., 1857, n. s., iii, 133–135.—**Neumann** (A. C.) Durchschneidung der Luft- und Speiseröhre, wobei die Hämorrhagie ohne Zutritt der Kunst sistirte. J. d. Chir. u. Augenh., Berl., 1833, xx, 133–136.—**Niemann** (A.) Verletzungen am Halse; gerichtliche Leichenöffnungen. Ztschr. f. d. Staatsarznk., Erlang., 1856, lxxii, 321–330.—**Nötling.** Stichwunde in den Nacken; Verletzung des linken Plexus brachialis und der linken Halslymphdrüsen. Mitth. d. badisch. aerztl. Ver., Karlsruhe, 1858, xii, 78.—**von Nussbaum.** Stich in den Hals und in den Rücken; zurückbleibendes Aneurysma und halbseitige Lähmung. *Ibid.*, 1871, xxii, 81–87.—**Obertenffer** (J. G.) & **Tanner** (G.) Obduktion eines Mannes, der sich in der Melancholie einige Stiche in den Hals beybrachte. Museum d. Heilk., Zürich, 1792, i, 174–177.—**Ogston** (F.) A case of suicide attempted by cut-throat, and terminated

Neck (*Wounds and injuries of*).

by drowning. Edinb. M. J., 1884–5, xxx, 689–691, 2 pl.— **Olivieri** (C.) Ferite del collo. Ann. clin. d. osp. d. Pellegr. di Napoli, 1872, ii, 265–281. – **Orsolini** (G.) Di una profonda ed estesa ferita da taglio orizzontale allo spazio tiro-ioideo per tentato suicidio. Comment. clin. di Pisa, 1877, i, 177–183, 1 pl.—**P.** (M.) Plaies du cou. Dict. d. sc. méd., Par., 1820, xliii, 77–80.—**Pacher.** In selbstmörderischer Absicht beigebrachte Schnittwunde am Halse zwischen Zungenbein und Schildknorpel; Doppelnaht an der Membrana hyothyreoidea und der Haut nach vorausgegangener Laryngotomie; Tod an Pneumonie. Ber. d. k. k. Krankenanst. Rudolph-Stiftung in Wien (1879), 1880, 367.—**Pätsch** (A.) Geheilte Durchschneidung der Luft- und Speiseröhre. Wchnschr. f. d. ges. Heilk., Berl., 1835, 556–560.—**Park** (M.) Instance of severe wound of the throat; speedy recovery, and union by the first intention. Lancet, Lond., 1846, ii, 526.— **Payne** (T.) Case of wound of the throat successfully treated. Lond. M. J., 1785, vi, 28–32.—**Penna** (J. M.) Herida del cuello; edema de la glótis (traqueotomia. An. Asoc. Circ. méd. argent., Buenos Aires, 1877–8, i, 491–493.—**Perkowski** (S.) Godné uwagi nastepcze objawy rany postrzałowéj kręgosłupa w okolicy szyjowéj. [Remarkable course of a gunshot wound of neck.] Gaz. lek., Warszawa, 1878, xxv, 173; 181; 189; 199.—**Petrali** (G.) Ferita della gola; divisione totale della lingua e del palato molle sino all' ugola; guarigione in molta parte per prima intenzione. Ann. univ. di med., Milano, 1838, lxxxv, 115–117.—**Piana** (A.) Storia d' una ferita della carotide e della gingulare nel lato sinistro del collo prodotta da arma tagliente e guarita colla sola compressione. Raccoglitore med., Forlì, 1880, 4. s., xiii, 41–52.—**Pick.** Suicidal penetrating wound of the neck; recovery. Lancet, Lond., 1886, ii, 816.—**Pitt** (W.) A report of a wound in the neck. San Francisco M. Press, 1861, ii, 8.—**Podrazki.** Den Hals durchdringende Schusswunde; Heilung. Wien. Med.-Halle, 1864, v, 51.—**Poncet.** Plaie de la région thyro-hyoïdienne; guérison sans suture; trachéotomie. Gaz. hebd. de méd., Par., 1869, 2. s., vi, 644.— **Porter** (I. G.) Case of complete division of the pharynx above the larynx; loss of the os hyoides, and a portion of the epiglottis cartilage by sloughing; recovery. Am. J. M. Sc., Phila., 1837–8, xxi, 303–308. — **Pretty** (W.) An instance of the loss of irritability in the glottis following a wound of the throat. Lond. M. Gaz., 1843, n. s., ii, 742.— **Preuss.** Heilung einer, die Luftwege völlig und die Speiseröhre zum Theil trennenden Halswunde. Med. Ztg., Berl., 1840, ix, 121.—**P[yl** (J. T.)] Obduction eines im Wasser gefundenen Kindes, dem die Luftröhre abgeschnitten war. Aufsätze u. Beob. a. d. gerichtl. Arzneyw., Berl., 1783, 1. Samml., 128–130. — Von einem Kinde, so an einer ihm zugefügten Halswunde verstorben. *Ibid.*, 1784, 2. Samml., 97–100. — **Pyl** (J. T.) & **Minter** (J. G.) Obduktion eines plötzlich verstorbenen Mannes, wo man eine Vergiftung vermuthete. *Ibid.*, 1785, 3. Samml., 91–94.—**Quissac** (J.) Tentative de suicide; vaste plaie du cou avec séparation complète de l'hyoïde et du larynx; suture entrecoupée; guérison. Gaz. méd. de Par., 1840, 2. s., viii, 555–557. *Also*: Gaz. méd. de Montpel., 1840–41, i, no. 25.—**R.** Considérations pratiques sur les blessures du cou, par armes piquantes. Bull. gén. de thérap., etc., Par., 1836, x, 370–376.—**Raimbert.** Coup de feu à poudre sous la mâchoire inférieure; inflammation œdémateuse très-étendue autour de la partie contuse; symptômes d'empoisonnement; mort. Bull. Soc. de chir. de Par. (1862) 1863, 2. s., iii, 351–356. *Also*: Gaz. d. hôp., Par., 1862, xxxv, 386.—**Rainey** (J. B.) Two cases of cut-throat; recovery. Texas Cour.-Rec. Med., Fort Worth, 1883–4, i, no. 10, 9.—**Rauscher** (J.) Tödtliche Stichwunde in den Hals. Friedreich's Bl. f. gerichtl. Med., Nürnb., 1886, xxxvii, 216.—**Reid** (A. G.) Laryngeal fistula from cut throat. Customs Gaz. Med. Rep., Shanghai, 1872, iii, 51.—**Rennie** (S. J.) Case of severe cut throat; with some remarks on the administration of nutritive enemata. Lancet, Lond., 1881, ii, 703.—**Richter** (J. F.) & **Schade.** Obduktion eines an einer Halswunde verstorbenen Kindes. Aufsätze u. Beob. a. d. gerichtl. Arzneyw., Berl., 1786, 4. Samml., 80–83.—**Ringer** (B. S.) Suicide. China. Imp. Customs. Med. Rep., Shanghai, 1883, no. 2, 3–5, 1 pl.— **Ripoll.** Plaie transversale du cou; mort. Gaz. méd.-chir. de Toulouse, 1874. vi, 169.—**Rodd** (G. H.) Case of hæmorrhage occasioned by a portion of a tobacco pipe sticking in the throat. Lond. M. Reposit., 1815, iv, 115.— **Roddick** (T. G.) A brief account of the recent Longue Pointe murder case; [injury to the glosso-pharyngeal nerve and pharyngeal plexus]. Canada M. & S. J., Montreal, 1882–3, xi, 394 – 397. — **Rodolfi** (R.) Palla d' arma da fuoco penetrata nella base laterale destra del collo e nascosta sotto la scapola corrispondente; guarigione. Gazz. med. ital. lomb., Milano, 1859, 4. s., iv, 440.—**Roe** (J. O.) A stab in the neck, severing internal jugular vein and recurrent laryngeal nerve; complete paralysis of the right vocal cord; recovery from the injury, and, finally, complete restoration of the voice. Med. & Surg. Reporter, Phila., 1881, xlv, 641.—**Rohmer.** Considérations sur certaines plaies de la région sus-hyoïdienne. Rev. méd. de l'est, Nancy, 1881, xiii, 136–143. — **Rooker** (J. J.) A

Neck (*Wounds and injuries of*).

case of cut-throat, with divided trachea and œsophagus. Cincin. Lancet & Obs., 1858, n. s., i, 23–25.—**Rosenbaum** (E.) Ein merkwürdiger Fall von Halsverletzung; horizontale Durchtrennung der Trachea im 2 Ringknorpel bis zur hinteren knorpellosen Wand und dessen Heilung. Wien. med. Wchnschr., 1867, xvii, 568. — **Roy** (G. C.) A new source of danger in wounds of the throat and neck. Indian M. Gaz., Calcutta, 1886, xxi, 42.—**Rudall.** Cut throat; severe secondary hæmorrhage; unsuccessful searches for the bleeding vessel; arrest of hæmorrhage; recovery. Austral. M. J., Melbourne, 1866, xi, 362–364.—**Rüdiger.** Von einer seltenen Schusswunde durch den Hals. Verm. chir. Schrift., Berl. u. Stettin, 1779, ii, 220–223. — **Rust** (J. N.) Einige Beobachtungen über die Wunden der Luft- und Speiseröhre, mit Bemerkungen in Bezug auf ihre Behandlung und ihr Lethalitäts-Verhältniss. Mag. f. d. ges. Heilk., Berl., 1820, vii, 262–288.—**Ryan** (D.) The history of a case, where the pharynx was wounded through the muscles and membranes which connect the larynx and os hyoides, without proving fatal. Med. Comment. 1781–2, 2. ed., Lond., 1787, viii, 319–321.— **Sassard.** Observation d'une plaie transversale de la gorge. J. de méd., chir., pharm., etc., Par., 1777, xlviii, 249–252.—**Sawas.** Application de la suture dans un cas de blessure profonde au cou. Gaz. méd. d'Orient, Constantinople, 1861–2, v, 102–105. [Discussion]. 122; 137; 155.—**Sawtelle** (H. W.) Gun-shot wound of the neck. Boston M. & S. J., 1872, lxxxvii, 335. — **Schade.** Ebenfalls von einem Kinde, so an einer Halswunde verstorben. Aufsätze u. Beob. a. d. gerichtl., Arzneyw., Berl., 1784, 2. Samml., 101–106.—**Schilling.** Sections-Protocoll und Gutachten über die Todesart der, nach erlittenem Wurfe mit einer Sichel an den Hals, plötzlich verstorbenen 15jährigen Christina Siemon. Ztschr. f. d. Staatsarznk., Erlang., 1842, 31. Ergnzngshft., 230–235. — **Schreyer** (F.) Glückliche Heilung einer Halswunde, bei welcher die Luftröhre gänzlich und die Speiseröhre bis auf einen kleinen Theil der hinteren Wand durchschnitten war. Deutsche Klinik, Berl., 1860, xii, 98. *Also, transl.* [Abstr.]: Gaz. d. hôp., Par., 1863, xxxvi, 155.— **Schubert** (A.) Naturheilkraft; ein abgeschnittener Hals. Med. Ztg., Berl., 1858, i, 211.—**Schütz.** Schnittwunde am Halse (Selbstmordversuch) mit nachfolgender Kehlkopfnecrose. Ber. d. k. k. Krankenh. Wieden 1871, Wien, 1873, 132–135. — **Scofield** (D.) A wound severing the larynx and œsophagus; complete recovery, and subsequent death from hanging. Med. Rec., N. Y., 1879, xvi, 284. — **Scriven** (J. B.) On wounds of the throat. Indian M. Gaz., Calcutta, 1872, vii, 106.— **Seeligmüller** (A.) Ueber die traumatischen Läsionen des Halssympathicus. Allg. Wien. med. Ztg., 1876, xxi, 369. — **Seidler.** Beobachtung einer Halsverletzung, durch den Stich eines Bajonnetts veranlasst. Mag. f. d. ges. Heilk., Berl., 1821, ix, 379–385. — **Siemerling & Hagen.** Obduktion eines im Wasser gefundenen Körpers, der zugleich eine Wunde am Halse hatte. Aufsätze u. Beob. a. d. gerichtl. Arzneyw., Berl., 1785, 3. Samml., 130–139.—**Simeons.** Ein mit einem zinnernen Suppenlöffel auf den Hals einer bejahrten Frau geführter Schlag bewirkt deren alsbaldigen Tod; gerichtsärztliches Gutachten. Ztschr. f. d. Staatsarznk., Erlang., 1848, lv, 72–102. [*See, also, supra*, Henrich.] —— Raubmord und Entdeckung des Thäters durch den Zustand der Leiche und die Untersuchung des vermeintlichen Mörders. Ztschr. f. d. Staatsarznk., Erlang., 1853, lxv, 334–367. *Also* [Abstr.]: Bl. f. gerichtl. Anthrop., Ansbach, 1853, iv, 6. Hft., 47–61.—**Sinclair** (A.) Pharynx and upper part of œsophagus of a patient who had died from hæmorrhage. Edinb. M. J., 1875, xx, 642. — **Socin** (A.) Tiefe Schnittwunde am Halse in Folge von Selbstmordversuch; Tracheotomie. Jahresb. u. d. chir. Abth. d. Spit. zu Basel, 1876, 23. —— Messerstichwunde am Halse. *Ibid.*, 23. ——. Schussverletzung der oberen Halsgegend l.; Heilung. *Ibid.* (1878), 1879, 23. —— Perforation des Oesophagus und der Trachea durch ein verschlucktes Knochenstück. *Ibid.*, 28.—**Solly** (S.) Bad case of suicidal cut-throat, between the hyoid bone, and thyroid cartilage; hæmorrhage; recovery. Lancet, Lond., 1864, i, 94.— **Spalding** (J.) Case of a wound in the trachea arteria and œsophagus. Cases & Obs. M. Soc. N.-Haven County. N.-Haven, 1788, 75–77.—**Spiczer** (E.) Zur Casuistik der Halsverletzungen; Schnittwunde des Halses; Durchtrennung der Membr. hyothyreoidea. Allg. Wien. med. Ztg., 1881, xxvi, 41.—**Spittal** (R.) Case of suicide, in which death resulted from a wound in the neck by an earthenware jug. Lond. & Edinb. Month. J. M. Sc., 1842, ii, 493–498.—**Spurway** (C.) A case of cut throat, followed by secondary hæmorrhage, successfully treated by deligation of the common carotid artery. Army M. Dep. Rep. 1836, Lond., 1838, viii, 522.—**Stafford** (R. A.) Case of recovery from cut throat, in which both the larynx and pharynx were extensively opened. Med.-Chir. Tr., Lond., 1839–40, xxiii, 221–223.—**Stark** (J.) The history of a remarkable wound in the trachea and neighbouring parts. Med. & Phil. Comment., Lond., 1776, iv, 434–444.—**Steinberger.** Schnittwunde am Halse, den Kehlkopf eröffnend (Selbstmordversuch); Heilung. Ber. d. k. k. Krankenanst. Rudolph-Stiftung in Wien (1868), 1869, 246. —— Selbst-

Neck (*Wounds and injuries of*).

mordversuch durch Schnitt; Heilung. *Ibid.* (1869), 1870, 188–190.—**Stewart** (C.) On wound of the neck. Austral. M. J., Melbourne, 1860, v, 274–276. — **Stokes** (G.) On asphyxia, resulting from wounds in the neck. Dublin J. M. Sc., 1841, xix, 28–34.—**Stone** (J. O.) Attempted suicide of an insane man; death from œdema of the larynx. *In his:* Clin. Cases. 8°, N. Y., 1878, 104–106.—**Stone** (R. M.) A unique glass wound; successful ligation of the left common carotid artery and internal jugular vein. Med. Rec., N. Y., 1884, xxvi, 456–458. *Also, transl.:* J. de méd., chir. et pharmacol., Brux., 1885, lxxx, 355–360.—**Sullivan** (W. P.) Severe wound of the throat in an aged woman; violent traumatic delirium; recovery. Lancet, Lond., 1869, ii, 673.—**Swinburne** (J.) A review of the case of the people against Rev. Henry Budge, indicted for the murder of his wife, Priscilla Budge, containing an examinating of the medico-legal questions involved in the case, etc. Tr. M. Soc. N. Y., Albany, 1862, 23–124. *Also*, Reprint.—**Switzer** (B. W.) Suicidal cut-throat. Med. Times & Gaz., Lond., 1865, ii, 252. — **Tachard** (E.) Note relative à un cas de déformation remarquable d'une balle de révolver. Rev. méd. de Toulouse, 1878, xii, 355–357.—**Tacheron.** Observation remarquable de plaie du cou, avec lésion de la veine jugulaire interne. Arch. gén. de méd., Par., 1837, 2. s., xiii, 162–172. *Also:* Ann. de méd. belge, Brux., 1837, i, 219–223.—**Tassi** (E.) Nevropatia a forma spinale e vasomotoria per ferita alla regione antero-laterale del collo. Bull. d. r. Accad. med. di Roma, 1886, xii, 305–310.—**Taylor** (A. S.) On homicidal and suicidal wounds of the throat. The power of locomotion or struggling after wounds of the trachea, the common carotid artery, and the internal jugular vein; inference of the time of death from the condition of the dead body; remarks on the case of John Wiggins. Guy's Hosp. Rep., Lond., 1869, 3. s., xiv, 112–144. — **Teubern.** Tödtung eines neugeborenen Kindes durch Halsschnittwunde. Vrtljschr. f. gerichtl. u. öff. Med., Berl., 1870, xii, 98–112.— **Terry** (C. C.) Severe cut of throat, followed by recovery; tracheotomy. Detroit Lancet, 1880–81, n. s., iv, 151.—**Thoman** (E.) Durchdringende Schnittwunde am Halse, dicht über dem oberen Rande des Kehlkopfes; Heilung bis auf eine rundliche Fistelöffnung; Verschluss derselben; Heilung per primam intentionem. Wien. Med.-Halle, 1863, iv, 510.—**Thurnall** (W.) Case of cut-throat; recovery. Brit. M. J., Lond., 1857, ii, 926.— **Todd** (G.) On wounds of the throat inflicted for the purpose of self-destruction. Lancet, Lond., 1846, ii, 477.— **Toogood** (J.) Wound of the trachea and œsophagus. *Ibid.*, 1837–8, ii, 735. ——. Wound of the throat. Prov. M. & S. J., Lond., 1843, v, 315.—**Troy.** Observation d'une plaie transversale du cou, produite par un instrument tranchant, et ayant divisé plus de la moitié de l'espace hyo-thyroïdien, suivie de guérison. Rec. de mém. de méd. . . . mil., Par., 1853, 2. s., x, 298–302.—**Tyerman** (D. F.) Case of wound of the neck, implicating the larynx, pharynx, and superior thyroid artery, and puncture of the abdomen, in attempted suicide by a lunatic. Med. Times & Gaz., Lond., 1853, n. s., vii, 219. —. Case of extensive wound of the throat, implicating the external carotid artery and its branches; ligature of the common carotid artery. *Ibid.*, 1854, n. s., ix, 366. — **Upham** (J. B.) Report of a case of incised wound of the throat, resulting in closure of the larynx by the cicatrix. Boston M. & S. J., 1852, xlvi, 49–53. *Also:* N. Hampshire J. M., 1851–2, ii, 206–210.—**Valera y Jimenez** (T.) Herida penetrante del cuello; curacion. Anfiteatro anat., Madrid, 1877, v, 79.—**Van Buren** (W. H.) Gunshot wound of the neck; severe venous hæmorrhage; recovery. N. York M. Press, 1859, n. s., i, 42.—**Vancleve** (J.) Case of death from a wound of the trachea and œsophagus, with a hot iron. Phila. M. Museum, 1808, iv, 24. — **Van Hook** (W. R.) Complete division of the trachea and wounding of the œsophagus in attempted suicide; recovery. Am. J. M. Sc., Phila., 1870, n. s., lx, 576.—**Velpeau.** Sur les plaies transversales du cou. Monit. d. hôp., Par., 1854, ii, 218–220.— **Verdier.** Sur une plaie à la gorge, avec des remarques intéressantes à ce sujet. Mém. Acad. roy. de chir., Par., 1757, iii, 78–83.—**Vignolo.** Traitement et guérison d'un coup de feu qui a traversé le cou d'avant en arrière. Rev. méd. franç. et étrang., Par., 1839, iii, 59–74.—**Vite** (J.) Case of cut throat; attempted suicide. Proc. M. Soc. Oregon, Portland, 1876, iii, 49–55.—**van Wageninge** (P. J.) Halsverwonding met doorklieving van de aspera arteria; doordringende buikwond; dyspnœa; tracheotomie; ademhaling langs een' kunstmatigen weg; levensbehoud met stemverlies. Nederl. Lancet, Gravenh., 1846–7, 2. s., ii, 42–56.—**Walker** (J.) Case of an extensive wound of the neck. Med. Recorder, etc., Phila., 1824, vii, 718–721.— **Wedemeyer** (G.) Rechtfertigung gegen ein Gutachten der medicinischen Facultät zu Göttingen. Mag. f. d. ges. Heilk., Berl., 1829, xxviii, 318–352. — **Weinlechner** (J.) Selbstmordversuch durch Schnitt zwischen Zungenbein und Kehlkopf; tiefe und oberflächliche Naht; gestorben an Pleuropneumonie. Ber. d. k. k. Krankenanst. Rudolph-Stiftung in Wien (1874), 1875, 465. ——. Selbstmordversuch durch Schnitt zwischen Zungenbein und Kehlkopf und am letzteren selbst mit Verletzung des linken Stimmbandes; Doppelnaht; Heilung grösstentheils

Neck (*Wounds and injuries of*).

per primam; theilweise Necrose des Schildknorpels und bleibende Heiserkeit. Aerztl. Ber. d. k. k. allg. Krankenh. zu Wien (1881), 1882, 226.—**White.** Punctured wound of neck, perforating pharynx. Brit. M. J., Lond., 1876, ii, 146.— **W[ildberg** (C. F. L.)] Obductionsbericht und Gutachten über einen durch eine Halsverletzung um das Lebengebrachten Mann. Mag. f. d. gerichtl. Arzneiw.. Berl., 1831-2, i, 408-413.—**Wirth.** Geschichte und Heilung einer gefährlichen Halsverlezung. Denkschr. d. vaterl. Gesellsch. d. Aerzte u. Naturf. Schwabens, Tübing.. 1805, i, 93-96.—**Wistrand** (A. T.) Statsmedicinska notiser ur egen och andras erfarenhet. [Blood stains on neck.] Hygiea, Stockholm, 1840, ii, 246-251.—**Woodman** (J.) Case of cut-throat wound of internal jugular vein; ligature; recovery. Brit. M. J., Lond., 1873, ii, 459.—**Wornum** (G. P.) Notes on a case of determined suicide, involving points of medico-legal interest. *Ibid.*, 1887, ii, 717.—**Wuth** (E. M.) A case of cut throat. Austral. M. J., Melbourne, 1879, n. s., i, 364-366.—**Yates** (G) Severe wound of throat; recovery. Med. Times, Lond., 1852, n. s., v, 515.— **Young** (D. S.) A new treatment for incised wounds of the throat, penetrating the air passages. Cincin. Lancet-Clinic. 1887, n. s., xviii, 296 - 301. — **Zandyck.** Deux tentatives de suicide par section transversale de la région antérieure du cou; traitements différents; réflexions générales sur le mode de réunion des plaies par instruments tranchants. Bull. méd. du nord, Lille, 1862, iii, 82-90.— **Ziino** (G.) In causa di ferimento al collo; consultazione medico-legale. Morgagni, Napoli, 1882, xxiv, 330-335.— **Zsigmondy** (A.) Grosse penetrirende Halsschmittwunde zwischen Zungenbein und Schildknorpel von einem Selbstmordversuch; vollständige Heilung. Wien. Med.-Halle, 1861, ii, 122.

van Neck (Abrahamus). *De tortura. 30 pp., 4 l. 4°. *Lugd. Bat., apud S. Luchtmans et filios,* 1754. [P., v. 996.]

de Necker (Noël-Joseph) [1729-93]. Physiologie des corps organisés, ou examen analytique des animaux et des végétaux comparés ensemble, à dessein de démontrer la chaine de continuité qui unit les différens règnes de la nature. Édition françoise du livre publié en latin à Manheim sous le titre de Physiologie des mousses . . . xii, 13-340 pp., 1 l., 1 pl. 12°. *Bouillon,* 1775.

de Neckere (Carolus Cælestinus). *De colica pictonum. [Gand.] 23 pp. 4°. *Roularii, D. Van Hee,* [1828]. [P., v. 959.]

Nécrologie de Charles-Auguste Van Coetsem [1788-1865]. 16 pp., port. 8°. *Gand,* 1865.

Repr. from: Bull. Soc. de méd. de Gand, 1865, xxxi.

Necrology.

See Biography.

Necrosis.

See, also, **Bones** (*Absorption of*); **Caries**; **Embolism**; **Erysipelas** (*Complications, etc., of*); **Osteomyelitis**; **Pyæmia**; **Pyæmia** (*Cases, etc., of*); *and under the names of the several bones and joints.*

ABRAMOVICH (J.) *De necrosi ossium. 8°. *Vindobonæ,* [1836].

BELLE (E.) *Nécrose. Trépanation sur la continuité des os longs. 4°. *Paris,* 1865.

BERGER (J.) *Necroseos per necrotomiam sanatæ exempla duo. 8°. *Gryphiswaldiæ,* 1853.

Also, transl. [Abstr.], *in:* Deutsche Klinik, Berl., 1854, vi, 325; 387.

BISCHOFF (H. H.) *Ein Beitrag zur Lehre von der Necrose mit specieller Berücksichtigung der Humerusnecrosen. 4°. *Kiel,* 1878.

BLAISE (L.-N.) *Essai sur la nécrose. 4°. *Paris,* 1815.

BÖDECKER (C. F. W.) .Necrosis. 8°. [*New York,* 1878.]

BONTEMPO (C.) *De necrosi. 8°. *Patavii,* 1842.

TER BORGH (F. J.) Verhandeling over de necrosis, gevolgt van eenige waarnemingen. 8°. *Groningen & Amsterdam,* 1821.

BOULAY DE MONTERU (P.) *Sur l'exfoliation des os. 4°. *Paris,* 1814.

BOUNIOL (L.-A.) *Sur la nécrose. 4°. *Paris,* 1817.

BOYER (F.) *Sur la nécrose. 4°. *Paris,* 1806.

Necrosis.

BRAUMANN (J. G.) * De necroseos operatione. 8°. *Wirceburgi,* 1855.

VON BREUNING (G.) Heilart des Beinfrasses auf arzeneilichem Wege. Zur Vermeidung operativer Verstümmlungen. 12°. *Wien,* 1852.

COLOMBE (F. M. L.) * De ossium necrosi. 4°. *Parisius,* 1827.

DANO (F.) *Sur la nécrose. 4°. *Paris,* 1810.

DAVID (J.-P.) Observations sur une maladie d'os, connue sous le nom de nécrose. 12°. *Paris,* 1782.

DEGIVRY (P.) * I. Caractères anatomiques de la nécrose sous ses différentes formes, à ses différents degrés, et dans les différentes pièces du squelette où elle présente des différences importantes sous le rapport des applications chirurgicales. II. [etc.] 4°. *Paris,* 1838.

DESRUELLES (H.-M.-J.) *Sur la nécrose, à la suite des amputations dans la continuité des membres. 4°. *Paris,* 1814.

ESTLANDER (J. A.) *Nekros i ben. 8°. *Helsingfors,* 1858.

FENAUT (N.) *De necrosi invaginata, seu de necroseos invaginatæ natura, causis, symptomatibus et therapeia. 4°. *Parisiis, an. XII* [1804].

FOURÉ (M.) *Sur la nécrose des os. 8°. *Paris, an XI* [1802].

GALLETTE (J.-B.) *Sur la nécrose. 4°. *Paris,* 1806.

GMELIN (M.) * Kann todter Knochen resorbirt werden ? 8°. *Tübingen,* 1862.

GUERTLER (A.) *De necrosi totali. 8°. *Gryphiswaldiæ,* 1866.

GUYTON (M.) *Quelques observations sur la nécrose. 4°. *Paris,* 1850.

HANCKEL (G. A.) * Quædam de necrosi ossium, adjecto casu ejus morbi commemoratu digno. 8°. *Jenæ,* [1834].

HEGENER (F.) *De necrosi cum epiphyseos solutione conjuncta, addita historia morbi. 8°. *Gryphiæ,* 1862.

HENNEN (J.) *De ossium necrosi. 8°. *Edinburgi,* 1821.

HERBSTMANN (P.) *Ueber den Knochenbrand. 8°. *Erlangen,* 1839.

HINDERNACHT (P.) *Ueber die Erkenntniss und Behandlung des Knochenbrandes. 8°. *Würzburg,* 1827.

HONNERLAG (J. C.) *De necrosi ossium. 8°. *Jenæ,* [1794].

JANSON (L. J.) *De necrosi. 4°. *Gandavi,* [1830].

JUNG (P. A. G.) *De necrosi. 8°. *Berolini,* [1853].

KLEEMANN (G. C. A.) .* De ossium necrosi. sm. 4°. *Berolini,* [1821].

KLEINDIENST (C. A. V.) *De necrosi. 8°. *Erlangæ,* 1828.

KLEMENT (A. J.) *De osteonecrosi. 8°. *Pragæ,* 1831.

KLINGELHÖFFER (W.) *Beitrag zur Lehre der Necrose. 8°. *Giessen,* 1862.

KOHN (J.) * De necrosi ossium nonnulla. 8°. *Berolini,* [1833].

KRUG (J.) *Die Absorption todter Knochen durch lebende Gewebe. 8°. *Giessen,* 1865.

LANNES (J.) *Sur la nécrose en général. 4°. *Paris,* 1815?

LE NOIR (C.) *De la nécrose traumatique dans les fractures et dans les amputations et de son traitement par la cautérisation ponctuée. 4°. *Paris,* 1878.

LIMPER (F. J.) *De osteonecrosi. 8°. *Berolini,* 1859.

MACDONALD (A. H.) *De necrosi ac callo. 8°. *Edinburgi,* 1799.

Necrosis.

Michon (L.-M.) * De la carie et de la nécrose. 4°. *Paris*, 1832.

Morbieu (A.) * Quelques considérations sur la nécrose. 4°. *Paris*, 1857.

Muenzel (A.) * De necrosi ossium. 8°. *Jenæ*, 1853.

Noth (A. J.) * De necrosi ossium. 8°. *Halis Sax.*, [1854].

Pécaut (J.-E.) * Du drainage des os appliqué au traitement de la nécrose centrale des os longs. 4°. *Paris*, 1880.

Pentenrieder (B.) * Beitrag zu Lehre der Necrosen. 8°. *München*, 1878.

Peride (A.) * Étude sur les séquestres profonds des os. 4°. *Paris*, 1874.

Poisson (G.) * Traction continue appliquée à l'extraction des séquestres. 4°. *Paris*, 1875.

Rudolph (C. C. G.) * De necrosi. 8°. *Berolini*, [1827].

Russell (J.) A practical essay on a certain disease of the bones, termed necrosis. 8°. *Edinburgh*, 1794.

Steinbaur (F. X.) * De necrosi. 8°. *Landishuti*, 1843.

Streck (A. F. F.) * De exfoliatione ossium præcavenda vel acceleranda. 4°. *Parisiis*, 1770.

Strigelius (F. G.) * De necrosi ossium. sm. 8°. *Lipsiæ*, [1837].

Suessenguth (G.) * De necrosi ossium. 8°. *Herbipoli*, 1842.

Syme (J.) A probationary essay on necrosis. 8°. *Edinburgh*, 1823.

Thomsen (M.) * De necrotomia. 4°. *Kiliæ*, [1864].

Tricot. * Considérations sur la nécrose. 4°. *Paris*, 1836.

Weidmann (J. P.) De necrosi ossium adnotatio. *Moguntiæ*, 1784.

In: Frank (J. P.) Delect. opusc. med. 8°. *Ticini*, 1787, iv, 124–143.

———. De necrosi ossium. fol. *Francof. ad Mœnum*, 1793.

Weiglein (J. E.) * De necrosi. 8°. *Viennæ*, [1824].

Zucchelli (P. A.) * I. De necrosi. II. [etc.] 4°. *Augustæ Taurinorum*, [1818].

Agnew (D. H.) Necrosis of several bones. Med. Times, Phila., 1870–71, i. 357. — **Avery** (J.)[1] Necrosis of the bones of both legs after injury. Tr. Path. Soc. Lond., 1848–50, ii, 259.—**Avery** (J.)[2] Necrosis, with illustrative cases. Penins. J. M., Detroit, 1876, n. s., i. 83–91. — **Béclard.** Réflexions sur la nécrose. Bull. Fac. de méd. de Par., 1812–13, iii (9. année), 426–430.—**Bettinger.** Ueber Necrosis ossium mit neuer Knochenbildung, und eine Operationsmethode zur Beseitigung dieses Leidens. Verhandl. d. Ver. pfälz. Aerzte 1841, Kaiserslautern, 1842, 19 – 22. — **Blake** (J. E.) Disease of the bones of the leg and foot. Boston M. & S. J., 1862, lxvi, 465. — **Blasius.** Necrosis tabulata. Med. Ztg., Berl., 1854, xxiii, 101. — **Bousselin.** Observation sur la nécrose. Hist. Soc. roy. de méd. 1780 – 81, Par., 1785, iv, pt. 1, 295 – 310. *Also, transl.:* Lond. M. J., 1786, vii, 263 – 279. — **Briggs** (W. T.) Sequestrotomy. Nashville J. M. & S., 1876, xviii, 200 – 202. — **Bristowe** (J. S.) Seven cases of acute necrosis, complicated by pyæmia. Tr. Path. Soc. Lond., 1861–2, xiii, 188–210.—**Bryant** (T.) Exanthematous necrosis. Guy's Hosp. Rep., Lond., 1870, 3. s., xv, 233. ———. On the treatment of necrosis. *Ibid.*, 251. ———. Cases of acute necrosis. Lancet, Lond., 1883, i, 12. — **Buntzen.** Den traumatiske (primære, acute) necrose, osteomyelitis Chassaignac. Hosp.-Tid., Kjøbenh., 1858, i, 145; 149; 153. — **Busch** (F.) Ueber die Nekrose der Knochen. Arch. f. klin. Chir., Berl., 1878, xxii, 795–841.— **Cartier** (L.-V.) De la nécrose. *In his:* Précis d'obs. de chir., 8°. Lyon, 1802, 210 – 218. — **Cases** of necrosis in bone. Med. Times & Gaz., Lond., 1854, viii, 572 – 574. — **Ciniselli** (L.) Delle amputazione nei casi di necrosi invaginata. Gazz. med. ital. lomb., Milano, 1869, 6. s., ii, 49.—**Ciriello.** Necrosi diffusa da causa reumatica. Boll. d. clin., Napoli, 1885, ii, 325.—**Clark** (Le G.) Two cases of necrosis in young subjects, one of the shaft of the humerus, the other of the shaft of the tibia; recovery by the efforts of nature in the first, and by amputation in the second case. Lancet, Lond., 1853, i, 448.—**Cloquet** (J.) & **Bérard** (A.) Nécrose. Dict. de méd., 2. éd., Par.,

1839, xx, 385–409.—**Coffin.** [Nécrose des os du carpe; un séquestre dans l'intérieur du second métacarpien.] Bull. Soc. anat. de Par., 1847, xxii, 283. — **Colles** (W.) Necrosis without suppuration. Dublin J. M. Sc., 1878, 3. s., lxvi, 453 – 455. — **Corley** (A. H.) Treatment of necrosis. Med. Press & Circ., Lond., 1875, i, 335.—**Cutter** (E.) The use of aromatic sulphuric acid in necrosis. Boston M. & S. J., 1876, xcv, 191.—**Deroubaix** (L.) Caries; nécroses. Ann. de l'Univ. de Brux. Fac. de méd., 1880, i, 29–35.— **Donovan** (J. A.) Necrosis of bone. Tr. Maine M. Ass., Portland, 1877–9, vi, 97–103.—**Duffield** (W.) Case of necrosis. Eclect. Repert., Phila., 1814, iv, 126 - 130. — **Eve** (F. S.) On necrosis at the extremity of the diaphysis, and in the epiphysis of growing bones. St. Barth. Hosp. Rep., Lond., 1879, xv, 129 - 137. — **Fischer** (G.) Necrose. *In his:* Mitth. a. d. chir. Univ.-Klin. zu Götting., 8°, 1861, 147 – 151. — **Flecchia** (G. M.) Sulla necrosi, e sovra un raro osseo processo. Ann. univ. di med., Milano, 1821, xvii, 172–192.—**Frayer.** On reproduction and repair of bone in necrosis and after loss of substance from accident or operation. *In his:* Clin. Obs. in Surg., 8°, Calcutta, [n. d.], 23–29.—**Fréteau.** Quelques considérations sur la doctrine des nécroses, suivies d'une observation de nécrose du tibia. J. gén. de méd., chir. et pharm., Par., 1815, liii, 46–62.— *Also:* Ann. clin., Montpel., 1815, xxxvii, 215–230.—**Fulton.** Central necrosis. Canada Lancet, Toronto, 1876–7, ix, 96.—**Gaillard.** Nouveau procédé pour l'extraction des séquestres; section des parties molles par une traction continue. Gaz. hebd. de méd., Par., 1867, 2. s., iv, 538.— **Gauderon.** Séquestre invaginé du fémur droit; amputation de la cuisse: mort à la suite de péritonite suppurée; séquestre invaginé du radius gauche sans suppuration dans la cavité du séquestre. Bull. Soc. anat. de Par., 1875, l, 763–766. — **Gayet.** [Présentation d'un pièce osseuse, retirée de l'extrémité inférieure du tibia d'un jeune homme de 19 ans.] Mém. et compt.-rend. Soc. d. sc. méd. de Lyon, 1865–6, v, pt. 2, 52–54. — **Gerdy.** Recherches sur la nécrose. Gaz. hebd. de méd., Par., 1853–4, i, 688; 704; 719. — **Giacopetti** (L.) Du drainage comme moyen de traitement de la carie et de la nécrose. Bull. gén. de thérap., etc., Par., 1872, lxxxii, 446–452. — **Godlee** (R. J.) Case of acute necrosis, with extensive necrotic patches in the heart. Tr. Path. Soc. Lond., 1884–5, xxxvi, 349–351.— **Grant** (G.) Case of necrosis of the upper and lower jaw, and operation. Tr. N. Jersey M. Soc., Newark, 1859, 45– 47, 2 pl. *Also,* Reprint. — **Grellet** (C. J.) Necrosis; pyæmia; amputation; albuminuria; recovery. Lancet, Lond., 1880, i, 836.—**Güterbock** (P.) Ueber Totalnecrosen langer Röhrenknochen. Arch. f. klin. Chir., Berl., 1872, xiv 208–222.—**Guhman.** Congenital necrosis. St. Louis M. & S. J., 1880, xxxviii, (St. Louis M. Soc.), 211. — **Gulliver** (G.) On necrosis; being an experimental inquiry into the agency ascribed to the absorbents, in the removal of the sequestrum; with some observations concerning the adhesion of living to dead bone. Med.-Chir. Tr., Lond., 1836–8, xxi, 1–19.—**Hamilton** (J.) Remarks on the removal by operation of the sequestrum in necrosis; with cases. Dublin Q. J. M. Sc., 1854, xviii, 73–86. — **Hartmann** (F.) Nekrose, herbeigeführt durch Verstopfung des Foramen nutritium. Arch. f. path. Anat., etc., Berl. 1854, viii, 114–125, 2 pl.—**Heineke** (W.) Ueber die Nekrose der Knochen. Samml. klin. Vortr., Leipz., 1873 No. 63 (Chir., No. 21), 401–406.—**Helferich** (H.) Ueber die nach Nekrose an der Diaphyse der langen Extremitätenknochen auftretenden Störungen im Längenwachsthum derselben. Deutsche Ztschr. f. Chir., Leipz., 1878, x, 325– 368, 2 pl. *Also,* Reprint.—**Henderson** (R. T.) Necrosis. St. Louis Cour. Med., 1879, i, 630–639.—**Henry** (M.) On necrosis. Lancet, Lond., 1859, ii, 477.—**Howse** (H. G.) On certain points connected with the treatment of cases of necrosed bone. Brit. M. J., Lond., 1874, i, 475–477.—**Hubbauer.** Wanderung von nekrotisch abgestossenen Knochenstücken. Ztschr. f. Wundärzte u. Geburtsh., Stuttg. 1865, xviii, 184–188. — **Hutchison** (A. C.) On necrosis *In his:* Pract. Obs. in Surg., 8°, Lond., 1816, 130–144, pl. ——. Some remarks on necrosis, illustrated by case. Med. & Phys. J., Lond., 1821, xlvi, 356–359.—**Jacquin.** Sur les nécroses. J. gén. de méd., chir. et pharm. Par., 1807, xxviii, 222–225.—**Jobert** (A.-J.) [*de Lamballe*] Recherches sur la nécrose et la trépanation des os. J hebd. d. progr. d. sc. et inst. méd., Par., 1836, iii, 353 385: iv. 16; 49; 73. ——. Nécrose (séquestre). Gaz. d hôp., Par., 1860, xxxiii, 381. — **Kelly.** Necrosis of bone Med. Press & Circ., Lond., 1872. xiv, 343–345.—**King** (W.) Necrosis occurring in the neighborhood of joints or othe important parts; with three illustrative cases. Brit. M J., Lond., 1857, i, 521 – 524. — **Klose** (C. W.) Revisio der Lehre von dem Knochenbrande und dem Knochenwie derersatze vom klinischen Standpunkte vorgenommen. Vrtljschr. f. d. prakt. Heilk., Prag, 1855, xlviii, 1–50.— **Knox** (R.) Observations and cases, illustrative of th pathology and treatment of necrosis. Edinb. M. & S. J 1822, xviii, 62–73. *Also,* Reprint. — **Koch** (W.) Uebe embolische Knochennekrosen. Verhandl. d. deutsch. Ge sellsch. f. Chir., Berl., 1878, vii, pt. 2, 110–120. *Also:* Arch f. klin. Chir., Berl., 1878, xxiii, 315–325. — **Kolaczek** Ein Fall von symmetrischer Knochennecrose. Deutsch

Necrosis.

med. Wchnschr., Berl., 1875-6, i, 166. — **Korteweg** (J. A.) Over versterving en aseptische beennekrose. Nederl. Tijdschr. v. Geneesk., Amst., 1879, xv, 177-185. *Also, transl.:* Rev. mens. de méd. et chir., Par., 1879, iii, 929-936.—**Krackowizer.** Necrosis in popliteal space; necessity of early probing. Med. Rec., N. Y., 1867-8, ii, 545.— **Krassnogliadoff** (E.) Zwei Fälle von Ablösung nekrotischer Knochen bei Behandlung mit warmen schwefeligen Mineral-Wassern. Med. Ztg. Russlands, St. Petersb., 1858, xv, 361-363. — **Küchler** (H.) Beobachtungen und Bemerkungen zur örtlichen Behandlung der Necrose, und vorzugsweise der eingekapselten Neciosc. [10 cases.] Deutsche Klinik, Berl., 1858, x, 49; 57; 70.— **Küster** (E.) Multiple Nekrosen der r. Tibia, des l. Oberschenkels, des l. Humerus, des Olecranon auf beiden Seiten, der 5. Rippe; doppelseitige Ellenbogengelenksresection, zahlreiche Nekrotomien; Heilung. *In his:* Ein chir. Trienn. 1876-8, 8°, Kassel u. Berl., 1882, 278. *Also:* Med.-chir., Centralbl., Wien, 1882, xvii, 567. ———. Nekrose. [16 cases.] *In his:* Ein chir. Trienn. 1876-8, 8°, Kassel u. Berl., 1882, 278-284.—**Lancereaux.** Nécroses et gangrènes. Gaz. méd. de Par., 1872, 4. s., i, 519; 545.— **Landi** (P.) [Necrosi.] *In his:* Clin. chir., 8°, Siena, 1864, 133-137.—**Larsen.** Praktiske Bemærkninger om Necrose i Benene. Hosp.-Medd., Kjøbenh., 1850, iii, 63-71.—**Ledeganck** (K.) Du rôle des o ganismes parasitaires dans la production de la nécrose. Presse méd. belge, Brux., 1874, xxvi, 89. — **Léveillé.** Réponse à la lettre de M. Jacquin: "Sur les nécroses". J. gén. de méd., chir. et pharm., Par., 1807, xxviii, 339-347. — **Litten.** Ueber den hämorrhagischen Infarct und die durch arterielle Anämie erzeugten Necrosen. Deutsche med. Wchnschr., Berl., 1879, v, 21.—**Lorinser** (F. W.) Periostitis acuta; Necrose; Heilung. Wien. med. Wchnschr., 1856, vi, 733.—**Malespine.** Quelques remarques sur l'élimination des séquestres. Rev. méd. franç. et étrang., Par., 1843, ii, 196-207.—**Mason** (E.) Necrosis of the bone without involucrum. N. York M. J., 1875, xxii, 528.—**Mayor** (F.-I.) Sur l'époque à laquelle on doit extirper les séquestres. Compt. rend. Soc. de biol. 1850, Par., 1851, ii, 8-12. ———. Mémoire sur la nécrose. Rev. méd.-chir. de Par., 1855, xvii, 339-353. *Also,* Reprint.—**Muhr.** Ueber das Ausschneiden einzelner Knochentheile. J. d. Chir. u. Augenh., Berl., 1824, vii, 139-156, 1 pl.—**Necrosis.** Med. Rec., N. Y., 1873, viii, 256.—**Nicaise.** Nécrose aseptique et réunion immédiate. Rev. de chir., Par., 1882, ii, 43-50.—**Oke** (W. S.) Practical observations on necrosis in the long bones. Prov. M. & S. J., Lond., 1844, 248-250 — **Paget.** Three cases of necrosis. Lancet. Lond., 1867, ii, 734.—**Pétrequin** (J.-E.) De l'opération de la nécrose, au point de vue de ses principes et de sa valeur intrinsèque; et rapport sur ce travail. Ann. Soc. de méd. de Gand, 1857, xxxv, 181-198. [Rap. de Van Leynseele], 199-207. — **Pitha.** Eine durch ihre Ausdehnung über eine grössere Partie des Skelettes merkwürdige Nekrose. Vrtljschr. f. d. prakt. Heilk., Prag, 1848, iii, 148-150. ———. Ueber die operative Behandlung der Nekrose. Allg. Wien. med. Ztg., 1863, viii, 73; 81; 89; 97; 105; 113.—**Pitts** (B.) On subperiosteal resection for acute necrosis, and exhibition of a living specimen. Lancet, Lond., 1886, i, 303. — **Pollock** (G.) On the local application of sulphuric acid in the treatment of carious and necrosed bone. Lancet, Lond., 1870, i, 762-764. — **Poncet** (F.) Des cloaques dans la nécrose et de leur mode de formation; régénération osseuse. Rec. de mém. de méd. . . . mil., Par., 1861, 3. s., vi, 390-399.—**Post.** Rapid exfoliation of bone; non-formation of involucrum. Med. Rec., N. Y., 1867, ii, 208.—**Ribes** (F.) Nécrose. Dict. d. sc. méd., Par., 1819, xxxv, 343-375.—**Richter.** Die Necrose, pathologisch und therapeutisch gewürdigt. J. d. Chir. u. Augenh., Berl., 1825, vii, 403; 612: viii. 111; 286; 473; 554. *Also,* Reprint.—**Rigal** (J.-J.) Observation sur la nécrose. Ann. clin., Montpel., 1812, xxviii, 152-155.—**Robertson** (E. B.) Case of necrosis in a child 2 years and 5 months old. Tr. M. Soc. Calif., Sacramento, 1875, 52-56.—**Roche** (E. B.) Necrosis following injury; removal of dead bone. Med. Times & Gaz., Lond., 1871, ii, 408.— **Roux.** De la nécrose des parties spongieuses des os. J. d. conn. méd.-chir., Par., 1836-7, iv, pt. 2, 187-191.—**Roux** (J.) De la carie chez les enfants. Marseille méd., 1879, xvi, 669-677. — **Savory.** Clinical remarks on cases of acute necrosis. Med. Times & Gaz., Lond., 1876, i, 250.— **Schnyder.** Ueber die Knochennekrose. Schweiz. Ztschr. f. Med., Chir. u. Geburtsh., Zürich, 1856, 314.— **Senftleben** (H.) Ueber die Prädilectionsstellen partieller Nekrosen. Arch. f. path. Anat., etc., Berl., 1861, xxi, 289-293, 1 pl. — **Senn** (N.) Necrosis, and its treatment. Tr. Wisconsin M. Soc., Milwaukee, 1872, vi, 33-51.—**Servier.** Nécrose. Dict. encycl. d. sc. méd., Par., 1877, 2. s., xii, 13-41. — **Simon** (G.) Zur Operation der Knochennecrosen. Deutsche Klinik, Berl., 1866, xviii, 334; 342.— **Smith** (H.) On some cases of necrosis, with remarks on the pathology and treatment of this disease. Med. Times & Gaz., Lond., 1862, i, 290-292.—**Smith** (N.) Observations on the pathology and treatment of necrosis. Phila. Month. J. M. & S., 1827, i, 11; 66.—**Smith** (T.) A lecture on the acute necrosis of growing bones. Brit. M. J.,

Necrosis.

Lond., 1863, ii, 51; 78; 107.—**Smith** (T. M.) Cases of necrosis illustrating the practice of exposing and perforating the diseased bone at an early period in the progress of the malady. Am. J. M. Sc., Phila., 1838-9, xxiii, 93-96.— **Spence** (J.) On necrosis and its relation to caries. Edinb. M. J., 1856-7, ii, 289-294.—**Syme** (J.) Necrosis and caries. Lancet, Lond., 1855, i, 84-86.—**Tapret** & **Chenet.** Séquestres osseux invaginés. Bull. Soc. anat. de Par., 1875, l, 26.—**Tédenat.** Du traitement de la nécrose superficielle des os. Montpel. méd., 1883, l, 330-349.—**Vandenbroeck** (J.-B.) Mémoire sur les effets salutaires du baume opodeldoch dans la carie des os. Observateur, Courtrai, 1853, iii, 137-142.—**Volkmann** (R.) Zur Operation der eingekapselten Necrose. (Case and "Tabellarische Uebersicht von 18 Operationen".) Deutsche Klinik, Berl., 1857, ix, 44; 57. — **Walker.** Cases and remarks relative to diseases of the bones. Med. Tr. Roy. Coll. Phys. Lond., 1772-85, iii, 25-99.—**Ward** (O.) Necrosis of the shaft of the humerus, and of the head of the femur. Tr. Path. Soc. Lond., 1846-8, i, 143.—**Wenzel** (J.) & **Wenzel** (C.) Bemerkungen über die mit dem Knochenbrand verbundenen Geschwüre. Mag. f. d. Wundarzneiw., Götting., 1798-9, ii, 459-464. — **Wiseman** (R.) A case of necrosis, with some physiological and pathological observations on the organic life of the bones, etc. Edinb. J. M. Sc., 1826-7, ii, 315-325.

Necrosis *from phosphorus.*

See **Jaws** (*Diseases of*) *from phosphorus* ; **Phosphorus** (*Accidents from, etc.*)

Nectandra.

Maclagan (D.) & **Gamgee** (A.) On the alkaloids contained in the wood of the bebeeru, or greenheart tree (Nectandra Rodiæi, Schomb.). Tr. Roy. Soc. Edinb., 1868-9, xxv, pt. 2, 567-573.

Necturus.

Gage (S. H.) Observations on the fat cells and connective-tissue corpuscles of necturus (Menobranchus). Proc. Am. Soc. Micr., Buffalo, 1882, v, 109-126, 1 pl. *Also,* Reprint. — I. Notes on the epithelium lining the mouth of necturus and menopoma. II. Notes on the blood-corpuscles of necturus. Proc. Am. Soc. Micr., Buffalo, 1885, viii, 126. *Also,* Reprint.

Nedatz (Konstantin). *O predlejanii i vipadenii pupovini vo vremja rodov. [Prolapse of umbilical cord in delivery.] vi, 124 pp. 8°. *St. Petersburg*, 1862.

———. Tableaux comparatifs de la composition approximative chimique des différents aliments et des boissons les plus usuels. 2 l., 2 pl. 8°. *Bruxelles, J. Fuytynck-Bajart*, 1876.

zur Nedden (Ad.) Die Verderbniss der Zähne und ihre Behandlung. vi, 48 pp., 3 pl. 8°. *Erlangen, F. Enke*, 1858.

———. Zwei Fälle von Erkrankungen der High-morshöhle. 11 pp. 8°. [*n. p.*, 1871.] C. *Repr. from:* Deutsche Vrtljschr. f. Zahnh., Nürnb., 1871, xi.

Nedel (Friedrich Wilhelm). Vorschlag einer neuen Verfahrungsart die Ruptur des Perinæi bey der Geburt zu verhüten, und die erfolgte zu heilen. 92 pp. 12°. *Magdeburg, F. Matthias*, 1806.

———. Inbegriff aller anatomischen und chirurgischen Wissenschaften zum Nutzen und Gebrauch derer, welche sich der Heilkunde befleissigen und etwas Gründliches lernen oder sich zum Examen vorbereiten wollen. x, 470 pp. 8°. *Berlin u. Stettin, Nicolai*, 1817.

Nédelec (Auguste-Edmond). *Quelques considérations pratiques sur la trachéotomie dans le croup chez l'enfant. 94 pp. 4°. *Montpellier, Hamelin frères*, 1879, No. 7.

van Nederhasselt (Joannes Adrianus Josephus). *Specimen sistens observationes tres aneurysmatum arteriæ popliteæ, cum annexa epicrisi. [Leyden.] 1 p. l., 50 pp. 8°. *Amstelodami, C. A. Spin*, 1844.

Nederlandsch Archief voor Genees- en Natuurkunde. Onder medewerking van P. Q. Brondgrest [*et al.*]. Uitgegeven door F. C. Donders en W. Koster. Jaarg. 1-5, 1865-70. 8°. *Utrecht, W. F. Dannenfelser.*

Nederlandsch Gasthuis voor Ooglijders, te Utrecht. De vestiging van het Nederlandsch

Nederlandsch Gasthuis [etc.]—continued.
Gasthuis voor behoeftige en minvermogende
ooglijders te Utrecht, 1858–59. viii, 54 pp. 8°.
Utrecht, P. W. van de Weijer, [1859].

——. Jaarlijksch verslag betrekkelijk de verpleging en het onderwijs in het . . . Uitgebracht
door Geneesheer-Directeur der Inrichting. 1.-
21., 1858–9 to 1879; 24., 1882; 26., 1884. 8°.
Utrecht, 1860–85.

   1858-9 to 1882, by Fran. Corn. Donders; 1884, by H.
Snellen.

——. Jaarlijksch verslag betrekkelijk de verpleging en het onderwijs in het . . . Uitgebracht
door F. C. Donders, Directeur der Instelling.
Met wetenschappelijke bijbladen. 1.–7., 1859–
65; 10., 1868; 11., 1869; 13.–15., 1871–73; 17.–19.,
1875–77; 22.–25., 1880–83; 27., 1885. 8°. *Utrecht,*
1860–86.

——. Album van het Nederlandsch Gasthuis
voor behoeftige en minvermogende ooglijders te
Utrecht. 46 pp. 8°. *Utrecht, P. W. van de
Weijer,* [1865].

   Bound with 6. report (1864).

Nederlandsch Lancet. Tijdschrift aan de
praktische chirurgie en oogheelkunde gewijd
door A. G. van Onsenoort. [Monthly.] v. 1–7,
Aug. 12, 1838–45; 2. serie, v. 1–6, 1845–51; 3.
serie, v. 1–5, 1851, to June, 1856. 18 v. 8°.
Utrecht, 1838–45; *Gravenhage,* 1845–56.

   Edited successively by F. S. Alexander, J. P. Domhel-
ing, F. C. Donders, G. L. H. Ellerman, J. H. Jansen, and
M. Imans. In 1846 **Archief** voor Geneeskunde merged
in this journal.

Nederlandsch militair geneeskundig Archief
van de Landmacht, Zeemacht, het Oost- en West-
Indisch Leger, onder redactie van J. H. Gentis
en A. E. Post. [Quarterly.] v. 1–11, 1877–87.
8°. *Utrecht, Dannenfelser & Co.*
Current.

Nederlansch Tijdschrift voor Geneeskunde,
tevens Orgaan der Nederlandsche Maatschappij
tot Bevordering der Geneeskunst. Comité van
redactie: C. Gobée [*et al.*]. [Weekly.] v. 1–8,
1857–64; 2. Reeks, v. 1–24, 1865–88. 32 v. 8°.
Amsterdam.

   Current. A continuation of: **Tijdschrift** der Nederlandsche Maatschappij tot Bevordering der Geneeskunst.
v. 18, 2. series, contains "Feestnummer" (25 years' review). Index to v. 1–12, 2. series, 1865–76.

Nederlandsch Tijdschrift voor Heel- en Verloskunde, Ziekten der Vrouwen en der Kinderen.
Nieuwe serie, v. 1–11, 1854–69. 8°. *Utrecht.*

   See **Nederlandsch** Tijdschrift voor Verloskunde,
Ziekten der Vrouwen en der Kinderen, v. 6–16, 1854–69.

Nederlandsch Tijdschrift voor Verloskunde,
Ziekten der Vrouwen en der Kinderen; door H.
J. Broers. (Onder medewerking van verschil-
lende kunstgenooten.) v. 1–16, 1846–69. 8°.
Utrecht.

   In v. 3 L. C. van Goudoever added as editor. v. 6–16,
1854–69, are also called v. 1–11, new series, title: **Nederlandsch** Tijdschrift voor Heel- en Verloskunde, Ziekten
der Vrouwen en der Kinderen.

Nederlandsch Weekblad voor Geneeskundigen. Onder redactie van Dr. J. C. Gildemeester
[*et al.*]. v. 1–6, 1851–6. 8°. *Amsterdam, C. G.
van der Post.*

   Want pp. 33–48, v. 3, 1853. v. 6 contains general index
to v. 1–6.

Nederlandsche bibliographie voor genees-,
heel- en verloskunde, veeartsenijkunde en artse-
nijbereidkunde. Eerste deel. 19 pp. 8°. *Leyden, J. Hazenberg,* 1852.

   No more published.

Nederlandsche Maatschappij tot Bevordering
der Geneeskunst. Verslag omtrent de ziekten,
welke in het jaar 1849 in Nederland hebben geheerscht; namens de Commissie voor geneeskundige plaatsbeschrijving en volksziekten, uitgebragt der derde algemeene vergadering der . . .

Nederlandsche Maatschappij [etc.]—cont'd.
door Dr. N. D. Sijbrandi. 168 pp. 8°. [*n. p.,*
1850.]

——. Verschil tusschen de Pharmacopoea belgica en de Pharmacopoea neerlandica (opgemaakt door eene commissie uit de afdeeling:
Leyden en omstreken der Nederlandsche Maatschappij tot Bevordering der Geneeskunst en de
Leydsche Afdeeling der Nederlandsche Maatschappij tot Bevordering der Pharmacie). 36 pp.
12°. *Leijden, D. Noothoven van Goor,* 1853.

——. Catalogus van de bibliotheek der . . .
55 pp. 8°. [*Amsterdam,* 1856.]

——. Catalogus der boekerij der . . . Voor-
looper eener Nederlandsche geneeskundige bibliographie. iv (5 l.), 294 pp., 2 l. 8°. *Amsterdam,* 1861.

——. Catalogus der boekerij der . . . Voor-
looper eener Nederlandsche geneeskundige bibliographie. Eerste supplement. iv (5 l.), 100
pp. 8°. *Amsterdam,* 1867.

——. Catalogus van de boekerij der . . . Tweede
supplement. 5 p. l., 183 pp. 8°. *Amsterdam,*
[*Stads-Drukkerij*], 1882.

——. Iets over Domburg en zijne badinrigting.
(Rapport uitgebragt door de commissie uit de
Afdeeling "Zeeland" der . . . in die vergadering
van April 1867.) 15 pp. 8°. [*'s Gravenhage,*
1867.]

   Repr. from: Tijdschr. v. Gezondhdsl., Gravenh., 1867, i.

——. Handelingen der . . . 1878–81. 4 v. 8°.
[*Amsterdam*], 1878–81.

——. Rapport van de commissie, in de algemeene vergadering van de . . . gehouden te
Leiden den 20 Junij 1851, benoemd tot het geven
van inlichtingen over de beste methode van
onderzoek omtrent werking der geneesmiddelen.
[Signed G. C. B. Suringar and J. D. Frenaij.]
42 pp. 8°. [*n. p., n. d.*]

——. *See, also:*

   Handelingen van de Algemeene Vergaderingen der
. . . 1.–5.; 7.–38., 1849–87. Tijdschr. d. Nederl. Maatsch. t.
Bevord. d. Geneesk., Gravenh., 1850, i 54; 101: 1851, ii,
51: 1852, iii, 45: 1853, iv, 162: 1855, vi, 69: 1856, vii, 145.
Continued in: Nederl. Tijdschr. v. Geneesk., Amst., 1857-
64, i–viii: 1865–87, 2. R., i–xxiii *passim.*

Nederlandsche Maatschappij ter Bevordering
der Pharmacie. Compendium op de Pharmacopoea neerlandica, of bereiding en beproeving van
geneesmiddelen, niet in de Pharmacopoea neerlandica opgenomen. Uitgegeven door het departement "Rotterdam" der . . . vii, 144 pp.
8°. *Voorburg, wed. A. M. Broedelet,* 1861.

——. Supplement op de Pharmacopoea neerlandica, of bereiding en beproeving van geneesmiddelen, niet in de Pharmacopoea neerlandica
opgenomen. Uitgegeven door het departement
"Rotterdam" . . . viii, 160 pp. 8°. *'s Gravenhage, Gebroeders van Cleef,* 1865.

   See, also, **Nederlandsche** Maatschappij tot Bevordering der Geneeskunst. Verschil tusschen de Pharmacopoea belgica en de Pharmacopoea neerlandica. 12°. *Leijden,* 1853.

Nederlandsche Vereeniging van het Roode
Kruis. Hoofd-Comité der . . . Bulletins van
het . . . Nos. 1–38, Aug. 14 1870 te 20 Mei 1871.
8°. [*'s Gravenhage,* 1870–71.]

CONTENTS.

No. 1. Rapporten van den gedelegeerde van het Hoofd-
Comité te Luxemburg. 8 pp.
No. 2. Kort overzicht van het tot 24. Aug. verrichte.
8 pp.
No. 3. Erste rapport van den gedelegeerde uit Dussel-
dorp. 8 pp.
No. 4. Rapport no. 4 van den Commissaris van het Hoofd-
Comité te Luxemburg. 8 pp.
No. 5. Tweede rapport van den Gecommitteerde te Dus-
seldorp. 8 pp.
No. 6. Rapport van den Commissaris in Luxemburg.
8 pp.
No. 7. Uit het 2de rapport van den Commissaris te Dus-
seldorp aan het Hoofd-Comité. 8 pp.

Nederlandsche Vereeniging [etc.]—cont'd.

No. 8. Uit de rapporten van den Commissaris van het Hoofd-Comité te Mannheim. 8 pp.

No. 9 en 10. Rapport van den gedelegeerde to Dusseldorp. 16 pp.

No. 11 en 12. Uit het rapport van den Commissaris te La Chapelle aan het Hoofd-Comité. 16 pp.

No. 13 en 14. Uit het rapport van den gedelegeerde te Versailles. 12 pp.

No. 15 en 16. Uit het rapport van den gedelegeerde te Sedan. 14 pp.

No. 17 en 18. Uit het rapport van den gedelegeerde te Mannheim. 16 pp.

No. 19 en 20. Verslag van de handelingen der "Ambulance néerlandaise". 16 pp.

No. 21 en 22. Uit het rapport van den gedelegeerde te Metz. 16 pp.

No. 23 en 24. Uit het rapport van den gedelegeerde te Versailles. 16 pp.

No. 25 en 26. Uit het rapport van Dr. Arntzenius te Metz. 16 pp.

No. 27 en 28. Uit het rapport van den Heer Louran te Dusseldorp. 16 pp.

No. 29 en 30. Missive van den Heer F. H. Ferguson te Arnba. 16 pp.

No. 31 en 32. Uit het rapport van den Heer Baron van Tuyll van Serooskerken. 16 pp.

No. 33 en 34. Uit het rapport van den gedelegeerde den Heer Mascheck. 16 pp.

No. 35 en 36. Rapport van den gedelegeerde van het Hoofd-Comité, den Heer Mr. D. Baron Mackay. 16 pp.

No. 37 en 38. Algemeene lijst der verzendingen van materiëel. 16 pp.

——. Handelingen der Nederlandsche Vereeniging tot het verleenen van hulp aan zieke en gewonde krijgslieden, in tijd van oorlog. ii, 371 pp., 1 l., 2 maps. 8°. *Haag, J. & H. van Langenhuysen,* 1872.

Nederlandsche Vereeniging tot afschaffing van sterken drank. Jaarverslag. 1., 1844; 3.–22., 1846–65. 8°. *Amsterdam,* 1845–66.

Nederlandsche (Het) volkskarakter, tegenover de graauwet en de wetten op het geslagt en gemaal. 4 pp. 8°. [*n. p., n. d.*] [P., v. 1614.]

Nédey (Gaspard). * Observation sur un polype utérine d'un volume extraordinaire, suivie de réflexions sur cette tumeur et son traitement. 1 p. l., 15 pp. 4°. *Strasbourg,* 1805, v. 43.

N[edham] [*or* **Needham**] (M [archmont]). Medela medicinæ. A plea for the free profession and a renovation of the art of physick, out of the noblest and most authentick writers, shewing the publick advantage of its liberty, the disadvantage that comes to the publick by any sort of physicians imposing upon the studies and practise of others, the alteration of diseases from their old state and condition, the causes of that alteration, the insufficiency and uselesness of meer scholastick methods and medicines, with a necessity of new, tending to the rescue of mankind from the tyranny of diseases, and of physicians themselves, from the pedantism of old authors and present dictators. The author, M. N., Med. Londinens. 10 p. l., 516 pp. 16°. *London, R. Lownds,* 1665.

See, also, **Sylvius** (Franciscus Deleboe). A new idea of the practice of physic, etc. sm. 8°. *London,* 1675.

——. *See, also :*

SPRACKLING (R.) Medela ignorantiæ; or a just and plain vindication of Hippocrates and Galen from the groundless imputations of M. N. Wherein the whole substance of his illiterate plea, intituled Medela medicinæ, is occasionally considered. 16°. *London,* 1665.

Nedswetzky (Eduard). Zur Mikrographie der Cholera. 82 pp., 1 pl. 8°. *Dorpat, H. Laakmann,* 1874.

Née (Pierre-Éléonore). * Sur le rhumatisme musculaire. 23 pp. 4°. *Paris,* 1835, No. 250, v. 289.

Neeb (Joh. Fredericus Guilielmus). * Diss. continens duas observationes de carcinomate epitheliali, adjecta descriptione operationis cheiloplasticæ cum epicrisi. 1 p. l., 41 pp., 1 pl. 8°. *Lugd. Bat., J. Hazenberg, Cornelii fil.,* [1849].

Neebauer (Aloysius). * De examine ægri rite instituendo. 17 pp., 1 l. 12°. *Landishuti, F. S. Storno,* [1819].

Neebe (Conrad Henry). * Geistesstörung bei Tabes dorsalis. [Strasburg.] 48 pp., 1 l. 8°. *Stuttgart, Greiner u. Pfeiffer,* 1885.

Neebe (Conrad Wiegand). * Versuche über die Wirkungen des essigsauren Kupferoxyds und einiger andern organisch-sauren Kupferoxyde. 46 pp., 1 l. 8°. *Marburg, J. A. Koch,* [1857]. c.

Needham (Frederick). Brain exhaustion. 14 pp. 8°. *London, Odell & Ives,* 1871.

Repr. from: St. Andrew's M. Grad. Ass. Tr. 1870, Lond., 1871, iv.

——. Licensing System Amendment Association. Habitual Drunkards Bill. Remarks on the necessity for legislation in reference to habitual drunkards. Together with a reprint of the Habitual Drunkards Bill, and list of donations. 24 pp. 8°. [*London,* 1871, *vel subseq.*]

Needham (Gualterus) [–1691]. Disquisitio anatomica de formato fœtu. 12 p. l., 205 pp., 7 pl., 8 l. 8°. *Londini, G. Godbid,* 1667.

Needham (J. P.) Facts and observations relative to the disease commonly called cholera, as it has recently prevailed in the city of York. xvi, 17–138 pp. 8°. *London, Longman & Co.,* 1833.

Needham (John Turberville) [1713–81]. An account of some new microscopical discoveries founded on an examination of the calamary, and its wonderful milt-vessels (each of which, tho' they exceed not an horse-hair in diameter, contains a minute apparatus analogous to that of a pump, with a fine spiral spring, sucker, barrel, etc.), tending to prove by an accurate description of their motion, action, etc., that the hitherto supposed animalcules in the semen of animals are nothing more than machines similar, tho' inconceivably less, to those discovered in this sea-production. Also, observations on the farina fœcundans of plants; with a new discovery and description of the action of those minute bodies, analogous to that of the calamary's milt-vessels. And an examination of the pistil, uterus, and stamina of several flowers, with an attempt to shew how the seed is impregnated. Likewise observations on the supposed embryo sole-fish fixed to the bodies of shrimps; with a new discovery of a remarkable animalcule found single on the tail-part of each embryo. A description of the eels or worms in blighted wheat; and other curious particulars relating to the natural history of animals, plants, etc. viii, 126 pp., 6 pl. 8°. *London, F. Needham,* 1745.

——. The same. Nouvelles découvertes faites avec le microscope. Traduites de l'anglois, avec un mémoire sur les polypes à bouquet et sur ceux à entonnoir, par A. Tremblay. 7 p. l., 179 pp., 7 pl. 16°. *Leide, E. Luzac fils,* 1747.

Repr. from : Tr. philosophiques.

——. Nouvelles observations microscopiques, avec des découvertes intéressantes sur la composition et la décomposition des corps organisés. xviii, 524 pp., 2 l., 7 pl. 16°. *Paris, L.-É. Ganeau,* 1750.

——. Mémoire sur la maladie contagieuse des bêtes à cornes. 21 pp. 4°. *Bruxelles, imp. royale,* 1770.

See, also, **Spalanzani** (Lazare). Nouvelles recherches sur les découvertes microscopiques, etc. 8°. *Londres & Paris,* 1769.

Needham (Marchmont). *See* **Nedham** (Marchmont).

Needle-holders.

See, also, **Forceps** (*Surgical*).

Cousins (J. W.) A new needle-holder. Lancet, Lond., 1884, ii, 951. *Also :* Brit. M. J., Lond., 1885, i, 336. ——. New needle holder and surgical needle and thread. Liv-

Needle-holders.

erpool M.-Chir. J., 1885, v, 1-3.—**Fischer** (O.) Wutzer's Nadelhalter, nebst einer historisch-kritischen Uebersicht der Nadelhalter älterer und neuerer Zeiten. Org. f. d. ges. Heilk., Bonn, 1840-41, i, 546-581, 2 pl. — **Fowler** (G. R.) An aseptic universal needle forceps. N. York M. J., 1887, xlvi, 727. — **Hagedorn.** Ein neuer Nadelhalter, nebst neuen Nadeln. Verhandl. d. deutsch. Gesellsch. f. Chir., Berl., 1881, x, pt. 2, 54-56, 1 pl. *Also:* Arch. f. klin. Chir., Berl., 1881, xxvi, 783-785, 1 pl. ———. Ein neuer Nadelhalter für platte Nadeln. Verhandl. d. deutsch. Gesellsch. f. Chir., Berl., 1882, xi, pt. 2, 172-175, 1 pl. *Also:* Arch. f. klin. Chir., Berl., 1882, xxviii, 522-525. 1 pl. ———. Description of the flat-curved needle and of a suitable needle-holder. Med. News, Phila., 1885, xlvi, 305–307. — **de la Harpe.** Verbesserter Wutzer'scher Nadelhalter. Schweiz. Ztschr. f. Med., Chir. u. Geburtsh., Zürich, 1851, 298.— **Jarvis** (W. C.) A novel needle-director to facilitate transfixion of the turbinated tissues. N. York M. Month., 1886-7, i, 103.—**Jones** (G. E.) A new needle-holder. Med. Rec., N. Y., 1881, xx, 528.—**Jurasz** (A.) Ein neuer Kehldeckelnadelhalter. Berl. klin. Wchnschr., 1877, xiv, 342.—**Küster** (E.) Der Schwan, ein Nadelhalter für Höhlennähte. Centralbl. f. Chir., Leipz., 1881, viii, 113–115.—**Mathis** (J. T.) A new forceps for holding curved surgical needles. Med. Rec., N. Y., 1880, xviii, 193.—**Nevins** (A. E.) A new needle holder for vaginal operations. Lancet, Lond., 1885. i, 1169. *Also:* Brit. Gynæc. J., Lond., 1885, i, 241-243.—**Skene** (A. J. C.) Imp oved needle forceps. Am. J. Obst., N. Y., 1880, xiii, 880.

Needles.

See, also, **Acupuncture**; **Arteries** (*Ligature of*); **Sutures** (*Metallic*).

Beschorner (O.) Modification von Dr. A. Fiedler's gedeckter Hohlnadel zur Punction der verschiedenen Körperhöhlen. Deutsche med. Wchnschr., Berl., 1881, vii, 201.— **Boyer** (A.) Mémoire sur la meilleure forme des aiguilles propres à la réunion des plaies et à la ligature des vaisseaux; et sur la manière de s'en servir dans les cas où leur usage est indispensable. Mém. Soc. méd. d'émulat. de Par. (an vii), an viii [1800], iii, 79–150. *Also,* Reprint. — **Brooke** (C.) Spiral surgical needle. Lancet, Lond., 1845, ii, 368.— **von Bruns** (V.) Eine neue Nadel zur Anlegung der blutigen Naht. Centralbl. f. Chir., Leipz., 1878, v, 441-444. ———. Meine verbesserte Wundnadel. *Ibid.*, 1880, vii, 81–84.— **Bryant** (G. S.) A new canulated needle for introducing the wire in operations for vaginal fistules. St. Louis M. & S. J., 1866. n. s., iii, 511-513.— **Bulloch** (W. G.) Kinloch's needle for metallic sutures. Savannah J. M., 1860-61, iii, 51.—**Burge** (J. A. H.) A post-mortem needle. Med. Rec., N. Y., 1867, ii, 238.— **Charrière.** Aiguilles destinées à simplifier les sutures métalliques. Bull. Acad. de méd., Par., 1865-6, xxxi, 248.— **Cloquet** (J.) Nouvelle forme d'aiguilles à suture. *Ibid.*, 1854-5, xx, 328.—**Cole** (S.) A new needle for carrying silver wire. Denver M. Times, 1884-5. iv, 326-329.—**Cousins** (J. W.) New surgical needle and thread. Med. Press & Circ., Lond., 1884, n. s., xxxvii, 326.—**Currie** (D. A.) A double canulated needle. Med. Rec., N. Y., 1879, xv, 406.— **De Mooij** (C.) Note sur une nouvelle aiguille à suture. Ann. Soc. de méd. d'Anvers, 1874, xxxv. 380-385, 1 pl.— **Doctor Hagedorn's** needle and needle-holder. Brit. M. J., Lond., 1885, i, 899.—**Eve** (P. F.) A new needle for sutures. Nashville J. M. & S., 1860, xix, 295-297. *Also:* Chicago M. J., 1860. n. s., iii, 629. ———. A canula needle for applying ligatures and stitches. Tr. Am. M. Ass., Phila., 1869, xx, 435-437.—**Fahrnholz.** Eine Abänderung der chirurgischen Nadel. Aerztl. Int.-Bl., München, 1866, xiii, 715.—**Ferguson's** fissure needle. Med. Times & Gaz., Lond., 1858, xvii, 537.—**Fuentes** (F. V.) Puntos de sutura practicados en la lengua de un niño de cuatro meses de edad. Siglo méd., Madrid, 1860, vii, 406.—**Goez** (A.) Eine neue chirurgische Nadel mit endlosem desinficirtem Faden. Berl. klin. Wchnschr., 1883, xx, 147.— **Hodder** (F. W. L.) A guarded aspirating-needle. Brit. M. J., Lond., 1885, ii, 920.—**Holden** (E.) Another post-mortem needle. Med. Rec., N. Y., 1867, ii, 333. — **Lead** (The) wire suture. Med. Times & Gaz., Lond., 1857, xiv, 540. — **Levis** (R. J.) Needle for the wire suture. Med. & Surg. Reporter, Phila., 1859-60, n. s., iii, 223. *Also:* Chicago M. J., 1860, n. s., iii, 51.—**Maclaren** (P. H.) On a needle for fissure operations. Glasgow M. J., 1867, 3. s., ii, 102.—**Martin** (G.) Enfilure solide des aiguilles à sutures. Ann. d'ocul., Brux., 1876, lxxv, 117-119.—**van de Mooy.** De hechtingsnaald. Nederl. mil. geneesk. Arch., etc., Utrecht, 1887, xi, 451-454.—**New** needle with opening eye. Med. Times & Gaz., Lond., 1857, xiv. 540.—**New** (A) open-eyed surgical needle. Med. Rec., N. Y., 1886, xxx, 390.— **Packard** (J. H.) Suture-needle with the eye near the point, for the purpose of introducing wire sutures. Proc. Phila. Co. M. Soc., 1879, i, 18.—**Passavant.** Eine neue Nadel. Deutsche Ztschr. f. Chir., Leipz., 1873, ii, 513-517.— **Post** (A. C.) Needle director. Med. Rec., N. Y., 1866, i, 195.— **Reverdin.** Modification de l'aiguille de Bruns. Bull. et mém. Soc. de chir. de Par., 1879, n. s., v, 739-741.— **Shrady** (G. F.) A new open-eyed needle. Med. Rec.,

Needles.

N. Y.. 1877, xii, 782.—**Skene** (A. J. C.) A new needle for introducing the sutures in rupture of the perinæum. *Ibid.*, 1871, v, 573. — **Theobald** (S.) On a new form of needle-holder. Lancet, Lond., 1871, ii, 575.—**Tyrrell** (H. J.) Description of a needle guard, for use in operations for harelip and other plastic operations on the lips and face. Dublin J. M. Sc., 1874, lviii, 223. — **Wackerhagen** (G.) A new needle for continuous or interrupted suture. Med. Rec., N. Y., 1884, xxvi, 419.—**Williams** (U. V.) A surgeon's needle. Richmond & Louisville M. J., Louisville, 1879, xxvii, 75.

Needles (*Aneurismal*).

See **Aneurism** (*Treatment of, Operative*).

Needles (*Manufacture of*).

Johnstone (J.) Some account of a species of phthisis pulmonalis, peculiar to persons employed in pointing needles in the needle manufacture. Mem. M. Soc. Lond., 1799, v, 89-93.—**Pappenheim** (L.) Ueber das Schleifen der Nähnadeln im Regierungsbezirk Arnsberg. Monatschr. . . . d. San.-Pol., Berl., 1860, ii, 68–76.—**Villermé** fils. Note sur la santé de certains ouvriers en aiguilles, et, à cette occasion, sur la tenure des registres de l'état civil. Ann. d'hyg., Par., 1850, xliii, 82–88.—**Vondalovski** (V. A.) Kolentsevskaja igolnaja fabrika v gigienicheskom otnoshenii. [Hygienic influences of needle-making.] Vrach, St. Petersb., 1880, i, 412-416.

Needles *and pins in the body, swallowed, etc.*

See, also, **Heart**, **Intestines**, *Foreign bodies in.*

HERHOLDT (J. D.) Observatio de affectibus morbosis virginis Havniensis, cui plurimæ acus e variis corporis partibus excisæ et extractæ sunt. 8°. *Haviniæ,* 1822.

Also, transl. [Abstr.], *in:* Biblioth. f. Læger, Kjøbenh., 1822, ii, 134-145. *Also, transl.* [Abstr.], *in:* Med. & Phys. J., Lond., 1822, xlviii, 389-392. *Also, transl.* [Abstr.], *in:* Lit. Ann. d. ges. Heilk., Berl., 1825, ii, 257-272. *Also, transl.* [Abstr.], *in:* Clin. d. hôp., Par., 1827, i, no. 97, 3; no. 99, 2: 1827-8, ii, 15.

SMEE (A.) On the detection of needles and other steel instruments impacted in the human body. 8°. *London,* 1845.

Also, in: MEMOIR, etc., by his daughter. 8°. *London,* 1878, 221-225.

Ady (A.) A pin retained in the throat fourteen months; removal. Am. J. M. Sc., Phila., 1872, n. s., lxiv, 575.— **Anderson** (N. B.) Remarkable migrations of a pin and needle through the body of a young lady. West. J. M. & S., Louisville, 1851, 3. s., viii, 200.—**Aveling** (J. H.) On the detection by the aid of magnetism of needles imbedded near the surface of the body. Lancet, Lond., 1851, i, 149.— **B.** (J. R.) An infantine pin-swallower. Med. Times & Gaz., Lond., 1873, i, 457.—**Bate** (H.) A remarkable case [the result of swallowing a needle]. Lancet, Lond., 1874, i, 253.—**Baur.** Verschlucken von Nadeln. Med. Cor.-Bl. d. württemb. ärztl. Ver., Stuttg., 1861, xxxi, 301.—**Bell** (J.) Fatal hæmorrhage from swallowing a needle. Lond. M. Gaz., 1842-3, xxxi, 694.—**Bérenger-Féraud.** Extraction d'une aiguille à coudre logée dans le sein depuis plusieurs années. Bull. gén. de thérap., etc., Par., 1864, lxvii, 544. ———. Extraction d'une aiguille à coudre logée depuis longtemps dans le bras. Gaz. d. hôp., Par., 1867, xl, 392.—**Binswanger** (L.) Tod durch eine Nähnadel. Schweiz. Ztschr. f. Med., Chir. u. Geburtsh., Zürich, 1853, 326.—**Bonzel.** Wanderung verschluckter Nadeln, zur Beruhigung mancher erschrockenen Mutter und zugleich ein Wink für angehende Aerzte. J. d. pract. Heilk., Berl., 1815, xli, 5. St., 112-114.—**Boucher.** Histoire d'une fille des environs de Lille en Flandre, à qui l'on a tiré pendant dix à douze ans des aiguilles de toutes les parties du corps Rec. périod. d'obs. de méd., de chir. et pharm., Par., 1757, vi, 163-173.—**Boudant.** Ingestion d'une grosse et longue épingle dans les organes digestifs; sortie par les voies urinaires. Soc. d. sc. méd. de Gannat. Compt. rend., 1859, xiii, 15-19. *Also:* Monit. d. sc. méd. et pharm., Par., 1859, vii, 380.—**Boult** (E.) On the passage of a needle through the tissues of the body. Lancet, Lond., 1846, i, 9.—**Bouteiller** fils. Note pour servir à l'histoire des corps étrangers avalés; aiguille avalée; mort 29 jours après; autopsie. Monit. d. hôp., Par., 1854, ii, 151. ———. Aiguille avalée; autopsie. Gaz. d. hôp., Par., 1857, xxx, 398.—**Braun.** Verschluckte Nadeln. Rhein. Monatschr. f. prakt. Aerzte, Köln, 1851, v, 487-489.—**Bredow** (C. A.) Intermittirende Krämpfe in Folge einer im Körper herumwandelnden Nadel. Med. Ztg. Russlands, St. Petersb., 1844, i, 93.—**Broca.** [Aiguille à coudre engagée dans l'épiploon et n'ayant déterminé aucun accident.] Bull. Soc. anat. de Par., 1850, xxv, 6.—**Brodie** (B. C.) Needles extracted from various parts of the body. Lond. M. Gaz., 1827-8, i, 148. — **Buchmüller** (F.) Glücklich abgelaufener Fall von verschluckten Nähna-

Needles *and pins in the body, swallowed,* etc.

deln. Oesterr. med. Wchnschr., Wien, 1843, 851.—**Budd.** The mania of thrusting needles into the flesh. Lancet, Lond., 1850, ii, 676.—**Büchner** (E.) Versuchter Selbst-mord durch Verschlucken von Stecknadeln. Ztschr. f. d. Staatsarznk., Erlang., 1823, vi, 305-348.—**Buist** (J. S.) Two interesting cases of needles in the body for a considerable time. Med. & Surg. Reporter, Phila., 1883, xlix, 529.—**Callender & Baker** (M.) Hysteria; a number of needles and pins removed from the arms and legs. Lancet, Lond., 1872, ii, 78.—**da Camara Cabral** (J. C.) Mais um caso notavel de corpos estranhos no organismo; oitenta agulhas extrahidas do corpo de uma rapariga. em quem produziram variados accidentes nervosos. J. Soc. d. sc. med. de Lisb., 1874, 2. s., xxxviii, 47-59. *Also:* Correio med. de Lisb., 1873-4, iii, 123 ; 134 ; 149.—**Campbell** (I.) Account of a sewing needle lodged in the breast of a woman being removed by incision. Med. Comment. 1783-4, Lond., 1785, ix, 275-277.—**Carmichael** (R.) Case of incurable disease of the arm arising from extraordinary circumstances. [Amputation at shoulder.] Tr. Ass. King's & Queen's Coll. Phys. Ireland, Dubl., 1818, ii, 377-382.—**Caruthers** (H.) & **Caruthers** (W. A.) Needles. pins, etc., in body. Gaillard's M. J., N. Y., 1880, xxix, 547-550.—[**Cases.**] The case of Mary Howell, who had a needle run into her arm and came out at her breast. Phil. Tr. 1732-44, Lond., 1747, ix, 238.—Exposé de l'effet et des suites d'une épingle avalée. J. de méd., chir., pharm., etc., Par., 1771, xxxv, 439-443.—[Avalement d'une aiguille à coudre; expulsion par l'anus.] Collect. Acad. d. mém., etc. Partie franç., Par. et Liége, 1786, xi, 410.—Verschluckung und Abgang von Nadeln. Mag. f. d. ges. Heilk., Berl., 1824, xvii, 556-558.—†† Pin swallowing. Lond. M. & S. J., 1836-7, ii, 907.—Emergence at the surface of the body of pins and needles that had been swallowed. Lancet, Lond., 1851, i, 30 —Nadeln in Brust- und Baucheingeweiden; plötzlicher Tod. Allg. Wien. med. Ztg., 1863, viii, 266.—A case in which a common sewing-needle caused death by hæmorrhage from the aorta into the pericardium. Lancet, Lond., 1867, i. 298.—The travelling of needles under the skin. Med. Press & Circ., Lond., 1870, x, 193.—**Chappet.** [Une grosse épingle d'acier de plus de 6 centimètres de long, avec une tête en verre noir, avalée par un enfant.] Lyon méd., 1878, xxviii, 492-497.—**Cheatham** (A.) A needle swallowed removed from arm. Virginia M. Month., Richmond, 1886-7, xiii, 4c6.—**Clemens** (A.) Eine für einen Knochenbruch gehaltene Nähnadel, die aus dem Schenkel eines Kindes geschnitten wurde. J. f. Kinderkr., Erlang., 1861, xxxvii, 355-357. ——. Eine Nähnadel aus der Magengegend eines Knaben geschnitten. *Ibid.*, 357. ——. Eine Nähnadel in dem Oberschenkel eines Kindes, für einen Knochenbruch gehalten. Deutsche Klinik, Berl., 1863, xv, 314. ——. Eine Nähnadel aus der Magengegend eines Knaben geschnitten. *Ibid.*, 315.—**Closmadeuc** (G.) Aiguille avalée dans un peloton de fil et extraite de la cuisse six mois après. Union méd., Par., 1874, xxviii, 917.—**Cooper** (G. L.) A cravat-pin swallowed; favorable result. Lancet, Lond., 1863, i, 82.—**Corbett** (R. de la C.) Transit of a needle from the stomach to the hand. Brit. M. J., Lond., 1879, ii, 614.—**Cramer.** Eine verschluckte Nähnadel aus dem Beine ausgeschnitten. Wchnschr. f. d. ges. Heilk , Berl., 1848, 623.—**Cregeen** (J. J.) Removal of needles from the abdomen. Lancet, Lond., 1861, ii, 580.—**Davis** (W. G.) On emergence from the surface of the body of pins and needles formerly swallowed. *Ibid.*, 1851, i, 83.—**Davy** (R.) Case illustrating the value of the induction balance for detecting a needle in the thumb. *Ibid.*, 1887, ii, 215.—**Desprès** (A.) Des aiguilles introduites dans les tissus ; de la manière de les extraire. Gaz. méd. de Par., 1884, 7. s., i, 229-231.—**Dickinson** (W. H.) A pin which had been swallowed and discharged from the bowels. Tr. Path. Soc. Lond., 1870, xxi, 169 —**Dix** (J.) Death from a wound by a needle. Brit. M. J., Lond., 1858, 847.—**Dolbeau.** [Une aiguille très fine, longue d'environ 3 centimètres, retirée du sein d'une femme.] Bull. Soc. anat. de Par., 1860, xxxv, 349.—**Dugan.** A large needle swallowed and passed by an infant. Med. Rec., N. Y., 1885, xxviii, 204.—**Durand.** Observation sur un abcès à la cuisse, à l'ouverture duquel est sorti une épingle, d'un pouce deux lignes, et incrustée du côté de sa pointe. Rec. périod. d'obs. de méd., de chir. et pharm., Par., 1757, vi, 296-299.—**Duret.** Observation sur des aiguilles introduites à travers la peau et expulsées par l'anus. J. univ. d. sc. méd., Par., 1825, xxxviii, 108-110.—**Fearing** (E. P.) Extraction of needles, etc., from the human body. Boston M. & S. J., 1856-7, lv, 29-31.—**Ferrario** (E.) Uno spillo trangugiato. Gazz. med. ital. lomb., Milano, 1867, 5. s., vi, 61.—**Fló** (J.) Estraccion de las agujas de trabajar crochet sin el uso de instrumento cortante. Encicl. méd.-farm., Barcel., 1877, i, 351; 399.—**Fryer** (H.) Case of pins extracted from the breast of a woman, after remaining there sixty years. Med. Facts & Obs., Lond., 1797, vii, 86-89.—**Garratt.** Needle in the foot detected by a magnetic needle. Boston M. & S. J., 1862, lxvi, 537.—**Gastgeber** (F.) Eine verschluckte Nähnadel ; Entfer-

Needles *and pins in the body, swallowed,* etc.

nung derselben durch spontanes Erbrechen nach reichlichem Genusse breiiger Nahrung. Med.-chir. Centralbl., Wien, 1877, xii, 258.—**Gibb** (G. D.) Removal of a needle from beneath the skin of the abdomen of a child. Lancet, Lond., 1861, ii, 347. ——. Transfixion of the base of the tongue by a needle; diagnosis and removal with the aid of the laryngoscope. *Ibid.*, 1866, i, 710.—**Gillette.** Aiguille retrouvée dans les parois du gros intestin. Bull. Soc. anat. de Par. (1869), 1870, xliv, 20.—**Govorliywi** (Z.) Oblomki igol i bulavok v tailai. [Fragments of needles and pins found in the flesh.] Med. Vestnik. St. Petersb., 1863, iii, 386.—**Gräfe** (E.) Die Donna d' agli Aghi; eine merkwürdige Krankheitsgeschichte. J. d. Chir. u. Augenh., Berl., 1830, xiv, 509-517, 1 pl.—[**Hachin & Gellé.**] Une épingle trouvée dans l'uretère. [*From:* J. d. sç, 1686.] Collect. acad. d. mém., etc., Dijon, 1755, i, 309.—**Hamilton** (J. W.) The removal of needles, pins, etc. Ohio M. Recorder, Columbus, 1878, ii, 498-500. — **Hasbach.** Folgen verschluckter Nähnadeln. Org. f. d. ges. Heilk., Aachen, 1852, i, 28.—**Heddens** (W. J.) Removal of a needle after a sojourn in the body for twenty years. N. Orl. M. & S. J., 1859, xvi, 336.—**Hering** (T.) Extraktion einer Nähnadel aus der linken Fossa pyriformis. Wien. med. Presse, 1879, xx, 338.—**Hewit** (H. D.) Hysteria and erotomania; voluntary introduction of sewing-needles into the knee-joint; amputation; recovery. Med. Rec., N. Y., 1871-2, vi, 570.—**Hodge** (H. L.) A needle found post-mortem within the cranium. Tr. Path. Soc. Phila. (1876-7), 1878, vii, 163. — **Holst** (L.) Eine verschluckte Nadel. St. Petersb. med. Wchnschr., 1884, n. F., i, 29.—**Houts** (S. B.) Extraction of a needle after twenty years' sojourn in the body. St. Louis Clin. Rec., 1879-80, vi, 237.—**Huppert** (M.) Eine Nadel im lebenden Herzen. Arch. d. Heilk., Leipz., 1878, xix, 516-526.—**Hutchison** (G. W.) Extraordinary case of pin-vomiting, etc.; recovery. Lancet, Lond., 1873, i, 91.—**Jones** (H. B.) On a ready method of determining the presence, position, depth, and length of a needle broken into the foot. Proc. Roy. M. & Chir. Soc. Lond., 1856-7, i, 71-74.—**Jones** (J. F.) Case of discharge from the urethra of a pin, which had been taken into the stomach. Med. Reposit., N. Y., 1808, v, 236.—**K.** Geschichte von einer Frau, welcher mehrere Nadeln aus der Haut geschnitten wurden. N. Mag. f. Aerzte, Leipz., 1783, v, 447-453.—**Keating** (J. M.) A pin extracted from the throat of a child 3 years old. Maryland M. J., Balt., 1879-80, vi, 389 - 391. — **Klein** (A.) jun. Wanderung einer 4 Zoll langen Stopfnadel in der Bauchhöhle. Memorabilien, Heilbr., 1871, xvi, 292.—**Kocher** (T.) Nachweis einer Nadel. Cor.-Bl. f. schweiz. Aerzte, Basel, 1884, xiv, 208.—**Kohn** (S.) Removal of a double-pointed needle from the submaxillary connective tissue, by the aid of manipulation. Med. Rec., N. Y., 1881, xix, 705.—**Kottmann** (A.) Die Sehnennaht an der Hand. Cor.-Bl. f. schweiz. Aerzte, Basel, 1878, viii, 513; 545.—**Lawrence.** A needle mistaken for splintered fracture of the humerus. Lancet, Lond., 1859, i, 8; 318.—**Le Double** (A.) Migration des aiguilles à travers les tissus de l'économie. Union méd., Par., 1878, 3. s., xxv, 907.—**Lente** (F. D.) A needle swallowed. Am. M. Times, N. Y., 1863, vii, 299. — **Littlewood** (H.) On a method of detecting and removing needles embedded in the tissues. Lancet, Lond., 1887, ii, 412.—**Lowicki.** Wanderung einer Nähnadel durch den Unterleib. Allg. med. Centr.-Ztg., Berl., 1858, xxvii, 633.—**Lukin** (M. A.) Schveinaja igla v serdtse. [Sewing-needle in heart.] Med. pribav. k morsk. sborniku, St. Petersb., 1887, 12-18. — **Luton.** Aiguille avalée retrouvée sous la peau de l'avant bras. Bull. Soc. méd. de Reims, 1873, xii, 172. — **Luxardo** (E.) Dreiundsiebzig Nadelspitzen herausgezogen aus der rechten Hand und dem Vorderarm. Centralbl. f. d. ges. Therap., Wien, 1887, v, 431.—**McElvoy** (F.) A curious exit for a pin, which was swallowed fourteen months previously. Med. Press & Circ., Lond., 1869, viii, 97. — **Maffett** (R.) Case in which a needle lodged in the throat, and afterwards passed out through the submaxillary gland. Dublin M. Press, 1840, iv, 394.—**Magistel.** Histoire d'une fille qui s'implantait des aiguilles et des épingles dans diverses parties du corps. J. gén. de méd., chir. et pharm., Par., 1823, lxxxiii, 314 - 330. — **Malagodi** (L.) Come si possano estrarre pezzi d' aghi infitti nella palma della mano. Raccoglitore. Fano, 1841, vii, 225-230.—**M[andillon].** Aiguille à tricoter de 9 centimètres de longueur, séjournant dans le cou et simulant une fracture du cartilage thyroïde; sortie spontanée de l'aiguille après la formation préalable d'un abcès. Bordeaux méd., 1878, vii, 9-11.—**Marinus** (J.-R.) Aiguille entrée dans les chairs, et extraite des parois du ventre, chez un enfant âgé de treize mois. Ann. Soc. d. sc. méd. et nat. de Brux., 1837, 7. *Also:* Ann. de méd. belge, Brux., 1837, i, 94.—**Martsinovski** (V. I.) Sluch. smerti ot schveinoi igly v gortani. [Death from swallowing a needle.] Protok. i trudi Obsh. Archangel. vrach., 1886, i, 95-99. — **Marx** (M. J.) Berichtigung der Geschichte einer Frau, welcher mehrere Nadeln aus der Haut geschnitten wurden. N. Mag. f. Aerzte, Leipz.,

Needles *and pins in the body, swallowed, etc.*

1784, vi, 74–76.—**Massa** (G.) Efetti dell' ingestione d' un ago, comparsa ed estrazione del medesimo nell' epigastrio. Riv. clin. di Bologna, 1869, viii, 365–369.—**Maurant.** Observation sur une aiguille à coudre trouvée dans une tumeur. J. de méd., chir., pharm., etc., Par., 1762, xvi, 171–174.—**Mayer.** Geschichte einer verschluckten Nadel. Aerztl. Int.-Bl., München, 1870, xvii, 96.—**Miller** (W.) Removal of a pin from the pharynx of a little girl. Nashville J. M. & S., 1879, n. s., xxiv, 13.—**Milliot.** Des aiguilles introduites dans le corps humain et de leur migration; du diagnostic des aiguilles et de leur extraction. Assoc. franç. pour l'avance. d. sc. Compt.-rend. 1879, Par., 1880, viii, 950–953.—**Mills** (S. G.) Case of a young lady who swallowed a pin. Lond. M. J., 1785, vi, 36–52. *Also, transl.:* Samml. auserl. Abhandl. z. Gebr. prakt. Aerzte, Leipz., 1785, xi, 102–118.—**Moises** (H.) [Extraordinary case of the extraction of needles, etc.] Med. & Phys. J., Lond., 1802, vii, 18–30.—**Moreau** (P.) Migration d'une longue aiguille à tricoter à travers les organes splanchniques. Encéphale, Par., 1881, i, 742–745.—**Müller.** Geschichte einer convulsivischen Krankheit, in deren Verlauf mehrere Nadeln auf der Körperoberfläche zum Vorschein gekommen sind. Ann. f. d. ges. Heilk., Karlsruhe, 1828, 54–62.—**Murray** (J. J.) Remarks on a case of extraction from the pharynx of a needle which had penetrated the neck. Med. Times & Gaz., Lond., 1859, xviii, 468–470. *Also, Reprint.*—**Nancrede** (C. B.) Case of needle removed from os calcis. Phila. M. Times, 1872–3, iii, 237.—**Neuber** (A. W.) Verschluckte Stecknadel. Mitth. a. d. Geb. d. Med., Chir. u. Pharm., Altona, 1837–8, v, Hft. 11–12, 12–14.—**Oettinger.** Ueber die Wirkung verschluckter Nadeln. Jahrb. d. ärztl. Ver. zu München, 1841, iii, 142–145.—**Ollivier.** Mémoire et consultation médico-légale sur les effets qui peuvent résulter de l'introduction des épingles dans les voies digestives. Ann. d'hyg., Par., 1839, xxi, 178–197.—**Ortiz de Laredo** (A.) Aguja en una mano. Corresp. méd., Madrid, 1872, vii, 205.—**Otto** (C.) Verschluckte Nadeln. Mag. f. d. ges. Heilk., Berl., 1822, xii, 535.—**Paris.** Sur la migration facile des aiguilles dans les tissus de l'économie. Union méd., Par., 1878, 3. s., xxv, 798.—**Pergami** (E.) Aghi e spilli nel corpo umano; mistificazione od aberrazione? cacostesia. Bull. d. Comit. med. cremonese, Cremona, 1882, ii, 97–102. *Also:* Gazz. d. osp., Milano, 1882, iii, 818–820.—**Phelippeaux.** Considérations sur l'exérèse des hameçons et des aiguilles; aiguille à repriser disparue dans la fesse d'un enfant; extraction impossible; nouvel instrument proposé. Bull. gén. de thérap., etc., Par., 1879, xcvi, 214–224. — **Pinctus.** Aciculæ per anum emissæ. Zodiacus med.-gall. 1680, Geneva, 1682, ii, 88.—**Ponder** (A. V.) Pin-cushion in the living body. Am. M. J., St. Louis, 1880, viii, 266.—**Pooley** (J. H.) Needles, pins, etc , in the tissues of the body. Gaillard's M. J., N. Y., 1880, xxx, 357–375.—**Popta** (S.) Beobachtung über das Verschlucken einiger Stecknadeln und ihre Ausleerung durch die Brust. [*Transl. from:* Allg. Vaderl. Letter-Oefeningen, 1804, No. 9, Mengelwerk., pag. 393–396.] Chiron, Nürnb. u. Sulzbach, 1805–6, i, 591–596.—**Rake** (B.) Swallowing a pin; solid diet treatment. Lancet, Lond., 1881, ii, 263.—**Revillout** (V.) Aiguille séjournant pendant plusieurs jours dans l'articulation du genou sans provoquer aucun accident. Gaz d. hôp., Par., 1876, xlix, 787.—**Richaud.** [Aiguille cheminant dans les tissus.] Bull. Soc. anat. de Par., 1850, xxv, 80.—**Richardson** (R.) Removal of a needle from the cavity of the abdomen of a child, the magnet proving advantageous in discovering it. Lancet, Lond., 1861, ii, 403.—**Romei** (F.) Caso singolare di un ago insinuatosi nella regione sopraioidea, e di un' altro rinvenuto nella regione ipotenare della mano destra. Bull. d. sc. med. di Bologna, 1868, 5. s., vi, 314–316.—**Roncalli** *Parolino* (F. R.) De ferreis multisque acubus anatomica inspectione in cadavere repertis. *In his:* Diss. quatuor, 4°, Brixiæ, 1740, 95–130. *Also, in his:* Rac. d' opusc. scient. e filol., 16°, Venezia, 1745, xxxii, 99–148.—**Sauvé.** Szpilka zpokarmen polknięta. [A pin swallowed in food.] Pam. Towarz. Lek. Warszaw., 1851, xxv, 128–132.—**Saviard.** Sur une épingle trouvée dans le testicule d'un enfant de douze ans. [*From:* J. d. sçavans, 1691.] Collect. acad. d. mém., etc., Dijon, 1766, vii, 13.—**Schmit** (P.) Aiguille avalée par la bouche et extraite ½ heure après à l'épigastre. Bull Soc. d. sc. méd. du gr.-duché de Luxemb., 1867, 127.—**Schmitt** (F. A.) Freaks of a swallowed needle. Texas Cour.-Rec. Med., Dallas, 1886–7, iv, 208.—**Schrag.** Abnehmung einer Brust, in welcher drey Nadeln befindlich waren. J. f. d. Chir., Geburtsh. u. gerichtl. Arznk., Jena, 1802, iii, 85–91.—**Seerig.** Eine vor drei Jahren verschluckte Stopfnadel kommt in der Gegend der Herzgrube zum Vorschein. Mag. f. d. ges. Heilk., Berl., 1835, xliv, 151.—**Sheppard.** On a case of needle travelling. Lancet, Lond., 1855, i, 583.—**Shipman** (A. B.) On extraction of needles. Boston M. & S. J., 1851, xliv, 153.—**Siegmund** (G.) Verschlucken einer Nähnadel; Durchtritt derselben durch die Thoraxwand. Arch. f. path. Anat., etc., Berl., 1858, xiv, 189.—**Silvy.** Observation sur une quantité prodigieuse d'épingles et

Needles *and pins in the body, swallowed, etc.*

d'aiguilles avalées. Mém. Soc. méd. d'émulat. de Par., 1803, v, 181–188.—**Smith** (J. A.) On emergence from the surface of the body of pins and needles formerly swallowed. Lancet, Lond., 1851, i, 53.—**Smith** (J. R.) Removal of two pieces of a large sewing-needle from the thigh, after remaining there forty-five years. N. Orl. M. & S. J., 1855–6, xii, 774.—**Sörman** (H.) En stoppnals vandring. [Wanderings of a darning-needle.] Upsala Läkaref. Förh., 1884, xix, 141–143.—**Soulé.** Extraction d'un fragment d'aiguille après une migration de trois ans. Ann. Soc. de méd. de St.-Étienne et de la Loire (1876), 1875, v, 546.—**Spencer** (H. G. P.) Account of a case in which sixteen sewing needles and four pins were extracted from the wrist. Med. Exam., Phila., 1845, n. s., i, 146.—**Stahmann** (F.) Eine Nähnadel unter der Haut. Ztschr. f. Chir. v. Chir., Osterode, 1845, iii, 113.—**Stephenson** (A. H.) A pin after a sojourn of 42 years in the body of a lady is at last voided through the bladder. Detroit M. J., 1877, i, 895.—**Storck.** Pins and needles passed through the digestive system. Buffalo M. J., 1859–60, xv, 293–296.—**Thompson** (H.) Pins swallowed accidentally and subsequently removed from various parts of the body. Tr. Path. Soc. Lond., 1853–4, v, 334–336. ——. Case of thrombosis, with a needle found imbedded in the thrombus. Tr. Clin. Soc. Lond., 1875, viii, 19–26. *Also, in his:* Clin. Lect., 8°, Lond., 1880. 186–190, 1 ch.—[**Tscherner.**] Verschluckte Stecknadeln. Mag. f. d. ges. Heilk., Berl., 1832, xxxvii, 286.—**Ungar.** Eine verschluckte Nadel aus dem Beine herausgeschnitten. Rhein. Monatschr. f. prakt. Aerzte, Köln, 1848, ii, 591–593.—**Vander Poel** (J.) A case of wandering needles. Med. Rec., N. Y., 1883, xxiii, 587.—**Ward** (R.) An interesting case of needle-swallowing in a dog. Vet. J. & Ann. Comp. Path., Lond., 1881, xii, 381–383.—**Warren** (J. M.) Extraction of needles. *In his:* Surg. Obs., 8°, Bost., 1867, 590–593.—**White** (A. D.) Swallowing a needle and thread. Lancet, Lond., 1847, ii, 31.—**Wide** (A.) Nedsväljda synålar. [Swallowing of pins.] Upsala Lakaref. Förh., 1883–4, xix, 132–141.—**Wight.** Needle extracted from femur. Ann. Anat. & Surg. Soc. Brooklyn, N. Y., 1880, ii, 288.—**Zoja** (G.) Sulla possibilità di deglutire ed evacuare aghi. [9 experiments.] Gazz. med. ital. lomb., Milano, 1867, 5. s., vi, 200; 217; 283; 329: 1868, 6. s., i, 49.

Needlewoman's Friend Society, Boston. Annual reports of the managers to the subscribers. 2.–3., 1848–9 to 1850–51; 6., 1852–3; 10., 1856–7; 35., 1881–2; 38., 1884–5. 8°. *Boston*, 1849–86.

Needlewomen.

See, also, Sewing-machines.

Lucas (R. C.) A needlewoman's bursa of the second finger of the left hand. Guy's Hosp. Rep. 1884–5, Lond., 1886, 3. s., xxviii, 143–146, 1 pl.—**Ord** (W.) Report on the sanitary circumstances of dressmakers and other needlewomen in London. Rep. Med. Off. Privy Council 1863, Lond., 1864, vi, 362–382.

Needon (Carolus Henricus). * De febri puerperarum. 19 pp. 8°. *Jenæ, typ. Neuenhahni*, 1862. C.

Neefe (Joannes Christianus Augustus). * De medico platonico. xxxvi pp. 4°. *Wittenbergæ, ex off. J. S. Gerdesii*, [1759].

For Biography, see **Langguth** (Geo. Aug.)

Neeff (*Christian Ernst*) [1782–1849].

Stricker (W.) Nekrolog. Allg. med. Centr.-Ztg., Berl., 1849, xviii, 590 : 599.

Neeffen (Joh.) Ein kurtzer Bericht: wie man sich in denen itzo vorstehenden Sterbensleufften, mit der Præservation oder Vorwahrungen, dornach auch der Curation der Pestilentz, und etzlicher irer Accidentien, oder Zufellen, verhalten sol. Zu Dienste den Einwohnern der churfürstlichen Stadt Dressden, und andern, so Berichts nottürfftig, zusammen getragen. 62 l. sm. 4°. [*Dresden, M. Stöckel*], 1566.

——. The same. 55 l. 4°. *Dressden,* [*M. Stöckel*], 1597.

Néel (P.) * Considérations sur les causes de l'affection scrophuleuse. 19 pp. 4°. *Paris*, 1811, No. 57, v. 83.

Neelsen (F.)

See **Perl** (M.) Lehrbuch der allgemeinen Pathologie, [etc.] roy. 8°. *Stuttgart*, 1886.

Neem.

See **Margosa.**

Neemuch.
See **Cholera** (*Asiatic, History, etc., of*), *by localities.*

Neergaard (Jano Weibel) [1776–]. Comment. anat.-physiol. sistens disquisitionem an verum organorum digestioni inservientium discremen inter animalia herbivora, carnivora et omnivora reperiatur. x, 82 pp., 3 pl. 4°. *Gottingæ, typ. H. Dietericii*, 1804.

Neerincx (Vincentius). *De melancholia. 31 pp. sm. 4°. *Lugd. Bat., J. et H. Verbeek*, 1727. [P., v. 79.]

Nees ab Esenbeck (Christian Gottfried) [1786–1858]. Academiæ Cæsareæ Leopoldino-Carolinæ Naturæ Curiosorum novi protectoratus a principe et domino Carolo ab Hardenberg, . . . indicit. 18 pp. 4°. *Bonnæ, typ. Kupferbergianis,* 1819.

Nees ab Esenbeck (Theodorus Fridericus Ludovicus) [1787–1837]. Radix plantarum mycetoidearum. vi (1 l.), 19 pp., 1 pl. 4°. *Bonnæ, A. Marcus,* 1820.

—— **& Ebermaier** (Carl Heinrich). Handbuch der medicinisch-pharmaceutischen Botanik. Nach den natürlichen Familien des Gewächsreiches bearbeitet. 3 Theile. 8°. *Düsseldorf, Arnz u. Comp.,* 1830–32.

Neff (Joannes). *Propositionum et meditationum physico-medicarum sylloge. xxviii pp. sm. 4°. *Erlangæ, typ. Kunstmannianis,* 1784.
Also, in: Delius (H. F.) Adversaria. Fasc. iv. 4°. *Erlangæ*, 1785.

Neff (Joseph S.) Cupric test pellets. 5 pp. 12°. *Philadelphia,* 1880.
Repr. from: Med. & Surg. Reporter, Phila., 1880, xlii.

——. Pyridine in the treatment of asthma. 9 pp. 12°. [*New York,* 1886.]
Repr. from: N. York M. J., 1886, xliii.

Neftel (William Basil) [1830–]. Galvanotherapeutics. The physiological and therapeutical action of the galvanic current upon the acoustic, optic, sympathetic, and pneumogastric nerves. 161 pp. 12°. *New York, D. Appleton & Co.,* 1871.

——. Die electrolytische Behandlung bösartiger Geschwülste. 45 pp. 8°. [*Berlin, G. Reimer,* 1872.]
Repr. from: Arch. f. path. Anat., etc., Berl., 1872, lvii.

——. On periodical melancholia. 22 pp. 8°. *New York, J. F. Trow & Son,* 1875.
Repr. from: Med. Rec., N. Y., 1875, xii.

——. Contribution to the etiology of epilepsy. 11 pp. 8°. *Philadelphia,* 1877.
Repr. from: Tr. Internat. M. Cong., Phila., 1876.

——. The same. Ein Beitrag zur Aetiologie der Epilepsie. 16 pp. 8°. [*Berlin, G. Bernstein,* 1877.]
Repr. from: Arch. f. Psychiat., Berl., 1876-7, vii.

Nega (Julius). *Ein Beitrag zur Frage der Elimination des Mercurs mit besonderer Berücksichtigung des Glycocollquecksilbers. 50 pp. 8°. *Strassburg, K. J. Trübner,* 1882.

——. Vergleichende Untersuchungen über die Resorption und Wirkung verschiedener zur cutanen Behandlung verwandter Quecksilberpräparate. 102 pp. 8°. *Strassburg, K. J. Trübner,* 1884.

Nega (Victor Julius) [1816–]. *De congenitis genitalium fœmineorum deformitatibus. 1 p. l., 20 pp., 1 l., 1 pl. 4°. *Vratislaviæ, typ. off. Kupferianæ,* [1838].

——. Beiträge zur Kenntniss der Funktion der Atrioventrikular-Klappen des Herzens, der Entstehung der Töne und Geräusche in demselben und deren Deutung. Respondent G. Joseph. 42 pp. 4°. *Breslau, Grass, Barth u. Comp.,* 1852.

Négadelle (Charles) [1852–]. *De la composition d'un sac obstétrical. 32 pp. 4°. *Paris,* 1881, No. 171.

Negdi (Mustapha). *Die in Aegypten endemische Angenentzündung. 34 pp. 8°. *München, C. Wolf u. Sohn,* 1854.

Négel (Vassile-G.) *De la syphilis rénale. 190 pp., 1 l. 4°. *Paris,* 1882, No. 354.

Negelein (Gustavus Philippus). * De peste. 4 p. l., 37 pp., 1 l. 4°. *Helmstadii, typ. P. D. Schnorrii,* [1744].

Negenborn (Otto [Paulus Joachimus]) [1833–]. * De rachitidis natura. 29 pp., 1 l. 8°. *Berolini, B. Schlesinger,* [1855].

Neglein (Hugo). * Ueber chirurgische Plastik bei Geschwüren. [Wurtzburg.] 20 pp. 8°. *München, B. Friederich,* 1885.

Nègre (Camille). * Du torticolis fonctionnel. 51 pp. 4°. *Montpellier, Boem & fils,* 1883, No. 37.

Nègre (Henri). * Étude sur le chlorhydrate de cocaïne. 86 pp., 3 l. 4°. *Montpellier,* 1885, No. 7.

Nègre (Jean). * Essai sur la généralisation du cancer par embolie. 1 l., 34 pp. 4°. *Strasbourg,* 1868, 3. s., No. 90.

Nègre (Joseph). * Contribution à l'étude de la rétention du placenta. 60 pp. 4°. *Paris,* 1880, No. 190.

Nègre (Léopold). * Des exagérations que peut offrir l'état dyspeptique flatulent chez les matelots dans les pays chauds. 56 pp. 4°. *Paris,* 1871, No. 164.

Negré (Philoctète). * Sur le délire en général. 58 pp. 4°. *Paris,* 1862, No. 175.

Negretti & Zambra. A treatise on meteorological instruments. xii, 152 pp. 8°. *London, Strahan & Williams,* 1864.

—— ——. Encyclopædic illustrated and descriptive reference catalogue of optical, mathematical, philosophical, photographic, and standard meteorological instruments, manufactured and sold by them. viii, 563 pp. 8°. *London,* [1879].

Negretto (Angelo). Rendiconto biennale di clinica chirurgica. 158 pp., 1 l. 8°. *Treniglio, stabilimento sociale tipog. editore,* 1886.

Negri (Luigi). Sul cholera morbus. Lettera a Carlo Cioccari. 8 pp. 8°. *Milano, tipog. dell P[io] I[stituto] Patronato,* 1836. **c.**

——. Un rimedio nuovo nutritivo ricostituente. Lettera a Giovanni Guaineri. 7 pp. 8°. [*n. p.,* 1867.]

——. Sulla chirurgia conservatrice. Lettera al Ettore Piccinini. 7 pp. 8°. [*n. p.,* 1867.] **c.**

——. Chirurgia conservatrice. Due parole sull' unghia incarnata. 8 pp. 8°. *Milano, tipog. del P[io] I[stituto] di Patronato,* 1868. **c.**

——. Considerazioni teorico-pratiche sulle malattie sifilitiche delle vie respiratorie. 36 pp. 8°. *Milano, tipog. del P[io] I[stituto] di Patronato,* 1868. **c.**

——. Considerazioni teorico-pratiche su la paralisi della gamba sinistra con anestesia del lato sinistro del corpo guarita coll' elettricità, pubblicata nell' Appendice Elettrojatrica, serie 2ª, tomo 1°, 1868. 14 pp. 8°. *Milano, tipog. del Pio Istituto di Patronato,* 1868. **c.**

——. Arnaldo Cantani. Due parole in merito. 8 pp. 8°. [*Milano,* 1868.] **c.**

——. Sul farmaco cerotto-Briziano. Due parole al dottor cavaliere Melchiori Giovanni. 28 pp. 8°. *Milano, tipog. del P[io] I[stituto] di Patronato,* 1869.

Négrié (Georges-Frédéric). * De la mort subite dans la pleurésie. 52 pp. 4°. *Paris,* 1864, No. 13.

——. Compte-rendu général des services de médecine, de chirurgie et d'accouchements de l'Hôpital Saint-André de Bordeaux, pendant l'année 1877. 74–125 pp. 4°. *Bordeaux, A. Bellier,* 1878.
Cutting from: Hôpital Saint-André de Bordeaux, 1877.

Négrié (Jean-Baptiste). * Propositions de médecine et de chirurgie. 14 pp. 4°. *Paris*, 1832, No. 263, v. 256.

Négrier (Charles) [1792–1862]. * Sur l'emploi des bandelettes agglutinatives dans le traitement des ulcères atoniques des jambes. vi, 7–27 pp., 1 pl. 4°. *Paris*, 1817, No. 23, v. 129.

——. Recherches anatomiques et physiologiques sur les ovaires dans l'espèce humaine, considérés spécialement sous le rapport de leur influence dans la menstruation. xix, 131 pp., 11 pl. 8°. *Paris, Bechet jeune & Labé*, 1840.

——. Mémoire sur le traitement des affections scrofuleuses par les préparations de feuilles de noyer. 45 pp. 12°. *Paris, F. Locquin*, 1840.
Repr. from: Arch. gén. de méd., Par., 1841, 3. s., x: 1841, 3. s., xi.

——. The same. Du traitement des affections scrophuleuses par les préparations de noyer. Mémoires publiés dans les Archives générales de médecine de 1841 à 1850. Auxquels ont été ajoutés de nouveaux faits recueillis tant en France qu'à l'étranger. 122 pp. 8°. *Paris, Labé*, 1856.

——. The same. Die Behandlung der Scrofeln mit Wallnussblättern. Nach dem Französischen des . . . mit Beifügung eigener Beobachtungen von M. J. Kreutzwald. Hrsg. von Fr. Nasse. iv, 72 pp. 8°. *Bonn, A. Marcus*, 1843.

——. The same. Weitere Erfahrungen über den Nutzen der Wallnussblätter gegen die Scrofeln. Uebersetzt von M. J. Kreutzwald. 37 pp. 8°. *Bonn, A. Marcus*, 1844.

——. Recherches et considérations sur la constitution et les fonctions du col de l'utérus, dans le but d'éclairer l'étiologie des insertions placentaires sur cette région, et de conduire à un choix de moyens propres à combattre les hémorrhagies qui en sont les conséquences. 172 pp. 8°. *Angers, Cosnier & Lachèse*, 1846.

——. Recueil de faits pour servir à l'histoire des ovaires et des affections hystériques de la femme. Ouvrage couronné par l'Académie des sciences (prix Monthyon, 1858). viii, 176 pp. 8°. *Angers, Cosnier & Lachèse*, 1858.

Negritos.

See, also, **Andaman** *Islands* ; **Formosa** ; **Malacca** ; **Malays** ; **Nicobar** *Islands* ; **Philippine** *Islands.*

HARTMANN (R.) Die Nigritier; eine anthropologisch-ethnologische Monographie. 8°. *Berlin*, 1876.

Allen (F. A.) The original range of the Papuan and Negritto races. J. Anthrop. Inst., Lond., 1878–9 viii, 38–50.—**Baer** (G. A.) Schädel und Skelette von den Philippinen, namentlich von Negritos. Verhandl. d. Berl. Gesellsch. f. Anthrop., 1879, 426–428.—**Flower** (W. H.) Stature of the Andamanese. J. Anthrop. Inst., Lond, 1880–81, x, 124.—**Giglioli** (E. H.) Nuove notizie sui popoli negroidi dell' Asia e specialmente sui Negriti. Arch. per l' antrop., Firenze, 1879, ix, 173: 1880, x, 404.—**Hamy** (E.-T.) Les négritos à Formose et dans l'archipel japonais. Bull. Soc. d'anthrop. de Par., 1872, 2. s., vii, 843–858.—**Jagor.** Ueber die Andamanesen oder Mincopies. Verhandl. d. Berl. Gesellsch. f. Anthrop., 1877, 41–65, 3 pl. —**Lesson** (P.-A.) Quelques mots sur les races noires de Timor. Rev. d'anthrop., Par., 1877, vi, 256–264.—**Man** (E. H.) On the Andamanese and Nicobarese objects presented to Maj.-Gen. Pitt Rivers, F. R. S. J. Anthrop. Inst., Lond., 1881–2, xi, 268–294, 4 pl.—**Meyer** (A. B.) Notiz über den Fundort der von ihm überbrachten Skelete und Schädel von Negritos, sowie über die Verbreitung der Negritos der Philippinen. Verhandl. d. Berl. Gesellsch. f. Anthrop., 1873, v, 90–93.—**de Morgan** (J.) Négritos de la presqu'île Malaise. L'Homme, Par., 1885, ii, 545; 577; 609; 641; 713: 1886, iv, 40–44.—**Negritos** (The) of the Philippines, by Dr. C. Semper. [Review.] J. Anthrop., Lond., 1870–71, i, 131; 296.—**Nicolas** (A.) Des cicatrices du tatouage chez les nègres. Arch. de méd. nav., Par., 1869, xii, 68–70. — **Noirs** (Les) de l'Inde. Rev. d'anthrop., Par., 1875, iv, 567.—**Pihan-Dufeillay.** Sur les îles Andaman. Bull. Soc. d'anthrop. de Par., 1862, iii, 55–63.—**de Quatrefages** (A.) Étude sur les Mincopies et la race négrito en général. Rev. d'anthrop., Par., 1872, i, 36; 193, 1 pl. ——.

Negritos.

Nouvelles études sur la distribution géographique des Négritos et sur leur identification avec les Pygmées asiatiques de Ctésias et de Pline. Rev. d'ethnog., Par., 1882, i, 177–225.—**Reclus** (E.) Studies in ethnology; the Andamans, or Mincopies. Internat. Rev., N. Y., 1882, xii, 365–381.—**de Roepstorff** (F. A.) Ueber die Bewohner der Nicobaren. Ztschr. f. Ethnol., Berl., 1882. xiv, 51–68, 1 pl.—**Schadenberg** (A.) Ueber die Negritos der Philippinen. *Ibid.*, 1880, xii, 133–174, 2 pl.—**Virchow** (R.) Ueber die Andamanen und ihre Bewohner. Verhandl. d. Berl. Gesellsch. f. Anthrop., 1876, 101–109, 3 pl.

Negroes.

See, also, **Craniology** ; **Face** ; **Fever** (*Yellow*) *and the slave trade* ; **Hymen** ; **Skin** (*Color of*).

ERNAULT (L.) * Des conditions étiologiques de la pathologie de la race nègre. 4°. *Paris*, 1882.

GIACOMINI (C.) Annotazioni sulla anatomia del negro. Appendice alle tre prime memorie. VIII. Esistenza della ghiandola d' Harder in un Boschimane. Duplicità della cartilagine della plica semilunaris. Muscolo ciliare nei negri. Distribuzione del pigmento del globo oculare. 8°. *Torino*, 1887.
Repr. from: Atti d. r. Accad. d. sc. di Torino, 1887, xxii.
See, also, infra.

LE CAT (C.-N.) Traité de la couleur de la peau humaine en général, de celle des nègres en particulier, et de la métamorphose d'une de ces couleurs en l'autre, soit de naissance, soit accidentellement. 8°. *Amsterdam*, 1765.

LEVACHER (G.) Guide médical des Antilles et des régions intertropicales, à l'usage de tous les habitans de ses contrées, renfermant des études spéciales sur les maladies des colonies en général, et en particulier sur celles qui sont propres à la race noire, avec le traitement qui convient à chacune de ses affections et un formulaire approprié à la médecine pratique de ses pays. 2. éd. 8°. *Paris*, 1840.

LUCANUS (M. E.) Disputatio de colore Æthiopum qui vulgo Nigritæ. 4°. *Marburgi Cattorum*, [1683].

MULDER (G. J.) De voeding van den neger in Suriname. 8°. *Rotterdam*, 1847.

NORDHOFF (C.) Papers of the day. No. 1. The freedmen of South Carolina; some account of their appearance, character, condition, and peculiar customs. 8°. *New York*, 1863.

PASSAVANT (C.) * Craniologische Untersuchung der Neger und der Negervölker. Nebst einem Bericht über meine erste Reise nach Cameroons (West-Afrika) im Jahre 1883. 8°. *Basel*, 1884.

PECHLINUS (J. N.) De habitu et colore Æthiopum, qui vulgo Nigritæ, liber. 12°. *Kiloni*, 1677.

RAMAER (J. N.) * De æthiopica generis humani varietate. 4°. *Groningæ*, [1839].

REED (J.) An appeal to the British nation to think for themselves, instead of allowing Wilberforce, Buxton, and others to think for them, with a true statement of the condition of the negroes in the island of Jamaica. 8°. *Liverpool*, 1823.

RUFZ. Recherches sur les empoisonnemens pratiqués par les nègres à la Martinique. 8°. *Paris*, 1844.

SÖMMERRING (S. T.) Ueber die körperliche Verschiedenheit des Negers vom Europäer. 8°. *Frankfurt u. Mainz*, 1785.

STUBNER (G. A.) * Diss. phys. de nigritarum affectionibus. sm. 4°. [*Vitembergæ*, 1699.]

THOMPSON (C. B.) The Nachash origin of the black and mixed races. 8°. *St. Louis*, 1860.

UNITED STATES. *Congress.* A bill to prevent the intermarriage of white and negro races in

Negroes.

the District of Columbia. roy. 8°. [*Washington*, 1884.]

VERDELHAN DES MOLES (J.) *An a globulosa sanguinis, ad cutem adpellentis, parte Aethiopum color?

In: SIGWART (G. F.) Quæstiones med. Par. 4°. *Tubingæ*, 1789, ii, 293–300.

Acclimation; and the liability of negroes to the epidemic fevers of the South. N. Orl. M. News & Hosp. Gaz., 1858–9, v, 78–87.—**Alcock** (N.) Why tropical man is black. Nature, Lond., 1884, xxx, 401–403.—**Amat** (C.) L'esclavage au M'zab; étude anthropologique des nègres. Bull. Soc. d'anthrop. de Par., 1884, 3. s., vii, 689–698. ——. Les nègres du M'zab. Rev. scient., Par., 1885, xxxv, 33–38.—**Armstrong** (S. C.) The future of the American negro. Proc. Nat. Confer. Char., Bost., 1887, xiv, 167–170.—**Atkinson** (T. P.) Report on the anatomical, physiological, and pathological differences between the white and black races, and on the modifications of the treatment of diseases of the latter rendered necessary thereby. Tr. M. Soc. Virg., Richmond, 1872, 105: 1873, 65.—**Bäck** (A.) De zwarte huid der mooren onderzogt. Geneesk. Verhandel. a. de k Sweed. Acad. (Sandifort) 1739–53, Leiden, 1775, i, 206–213.—**Baldwin** (H. R.) Unity of the human race. Med. & Surg. Reporter, Phila., 1858, xi, 141–151.—**Bérenger-Féraud.** Note sur la fécondité des mulâtres au Sénégal. Rev. d'anthrop., Par., 1879, 2. s., ii, 577–588.—**Bertillon** (J.) Rapport sur l'examen d'un nègre au point de vue de l'implantation des cheveux. Bull. Soc. d'anthrop. de Par., 1878, 3. s., i, 94–98.—**Binns** (E.) A few facts preliminary to a philosophical examination of negro intellect. Lond. M. & S. J., 1836, i, 137–142.—**Bonfanti** (M.) L' incivilimento dei negri nell' Africa intertropicale. Arch. per l' antrop., Firenze, 1885, xv, 127–138.—**Boudin.** Sur le prétendu acclimatement du nègre blanc et du nègre aux Antilles. Bull. Soc. d'anthrop. de Par., 1864, v, 828–845. — **Broca** (P.) Capsules surrénales d'un nègre. *Ibid.*, 1860, i, 30. ——. Études sur le cerveau d'un nègre. *Ibid.*, 53–55. ——. Sur les proportions relatives du bras, de l'avant-bras et de la clavicule chez les nègres et les européens. *Ibid.*, 1862, iii, 162–172. — **Broca & Verneuil.** [Sur la structure de la peau du nègre.] Bull. Soc. anat. de Par., 1854, xxix, 166; 197.—**Brück** (A.T.) Bildungsfähigkeit der Neger. Wchnschr. f. d. ges. Heilk., Berl., 1846, 357. — **Burt** (W. J.) Report on the anatomical and physiological differences between the white and negro races; the modification of their respective diseases and difference in the treatment resulting therefrom. Tr. Texas M. Ass., Marshall, 1876, viii, 115–123. — **Byrd** (H. L.) An ethnological phenomenon. Independ. Pract., Balt., 1880, i, 375.—**Cartwright** (S. A.) Report on the diseases and physical peculiarities of the negro race. N. Orl. M. & S. J., 1850–51, vii, 691 : 1851–2, viii, 187 ; 361. ——. Philosophy of the negro constitution, elicited by questions propounded by C. R. Hall, of Torquay, England, through Prof. Jackson, of Massachusetts Medical College, Boston. *Ibid.*, 1852–3, ix, 195–208. ——. Alcohol and the Ethiopian; or, the moral and physical effects of ardent spirits on the negro race, and some account of the peculiarity of that people. *Ibid.*, 1853–4, x, 150–165. ——. Ethnology of the negro or prognathous race. *Ibid.*, 1858, xv, 149–163. *Also*, Reprint.—**Chudzinski** (T.) Contribution à l'anatomie du nègre. Rev. d'anthrop., Par., 1873, ii, 398–415, 1 pl. ——. Nouvelles observations sur le système musculaire du nègre. *Ibid.*, 1874, iii, 21–41, 1 pl. ——. Quelques notes sur l'anatomie de deux nègres. *Ibid.*, 1884, 2. s., viii, 603–616. ——. L'extenseur accessoire de l'index et propre du médius observé chez une négresse. Bull. Soc d'anthrop. de Par., 1885, 3. s., viii, 297.—**Colenso** (*Bishop J. W.*) On the efforts of missionaries among savages. J. Anthrop. Soc. Lond., 1865, iii, pp. ccxlviii-cclxxxix.—**Coles** (A.) The unity of the origin of mankind, supported by reason, Scripture and the investigations of science. Med. & Surg. Reporter, Burlington, N. J., 1857, x, 582–590.—**Corre** (A.) De l'acclimatement dans la race noire africaine. Rev. d'anthrop., Par., 1882, 2. s., v, 31–97.—**Corson** (E. R.) The future of the colored race in the United States from an ethnic and medical standpoint. N. York M. Times, 1887-8, xv, 193; 255.—**Crevaux** (J.) Mémoire sur les nègres bosh ou nègres marrons des Guyanes. Mém. Soc. d'anthrop. de Par., 1875-82, 2. s., ii, 259–280.—**Davis** (J. B.) On the weight of the brain in the negro. Anthrop. Rev., Lond., 1869, vii, 190–192.—**Davy** (J.) On the character of the negro, chiefly in relation to industrial habits. J. Anthrop. Soc. Lond., 1869, vii, pp. clvi-clxix.—**Dorrance** (G.) The mulatto a hybrid. Boston M. & S. J., 1843, xxix, 81.—**Douglass** (F.) The future of the colored race. N. Am. Rev., N. Y., 1886, cxli, 436–440.—**Dowler** (B.) The vital statistics of negroes in the United States. N. Orl. M. & S. J., 1856-7, xiii, 164–175.—**Easley** (E. T.) The sanitary condition of the negro. Am. M. Weekly, Louisville, 1875, iii, 49–51.—**Ewcorstart** (J. K.) The negro not a distinct species. Med. & Surg. Reporter, Burlington, N. J., 1857, x, 577 :

Negroes.

1858, xi, 264.—**Fort** (C. H.) Some corroborative facts in regard to the anatomical difference between the negro and white races. Am. J. Obst., N. Y., 1877, x, 258.—**Forwood** (W. S.) The négro a distinct species. Med. & Surg. Reporter, Burlington, N. J., 1857, x, 225 : xi, 69.—**Furniss** (J. P.) Extract from an essay on "The anatomical and physiological peculiarities of the negro". N. Orl. M. & S. J., 1873–4, n. s., i, 168–170, 3 maps. *Also*, Reprint.—**Gannett** (H.) Are we to become Africanized? Pop. Sc. Month., N. Y., 1885, xxvii. 145–150.—**Garner** (R.) On the brain of a negro. Med. Times & Gaz., Lond., 1869, ii, 292.—**Giacomini** (C.) Annotazioni sull' anatomia del negro. Gior. d. r. Accad. di med. di Torino, 1878, 3. s., xxiv, 454 ; 506, 2 pl.: 1882, 3. s., xxx, 729 : 1884, 3. s., xxxii,462: 501, 2 pl. *Also*, Reprint. *Also,transl.:* Arch. ital. de biol., Turin, 1883, iii, 331–361 : 1884, vi, 247, 2 pl. *Also* [Abstr. of 1. mémoire] : Assoc. franç. pour l'avance. d. sc. Compt.-rend. 1878, Par., 1879, vii, 855–858.—**Gibb** (G. D.) Drapetomania and dysæsthesia Æthiopis. Lancet, Lond., 1857, ii, 407. [*See, also, supra.*] ——. Essential points of difference between the larynx of the negro and that of the white man. Mem. Anthrop. Soc. Lond., 1865-6, ii, 1–13.—**Giglioli** (E. H.) Studi sulla razza negrita. Arch. per l' antrop., Firenze, 1876, vi, 293–335, 1 pl.—**Gilliam** (E. W.) The African in the United States. Pop. Sc. Month., N Y., 1882-3, xxii, 433–444.—**Granjux.** L'hygiène de la première enfance chez les nègres de la Côte des esclaves. Gaz. obst., Par., 1880, ix, 81–84.—**Grier** (S. L.) The negro and his diseases. N. Orl. M. & S. J., 1852-3, ix, 752-763.—**Guppy** (H. F. J.) Notes on the capabilities of the negro for civilisation. J. Anthrop. Soc. Lond., 1864, ii, pp. ccix-ccxvi.—**H.** (J. A.) Parturition in the negro. Phila. M. Times, 1885-6, xvi, 296.—**Harris** (J.) What constitutes unsoundness in the negro? Savannah J. M., 1858–9, i, 145 ; 217 ; 289 : 1859-60, ii, 10.—**Herrick** (S. S.) Comparative vital movement of the white and colored races in the United States. N. Orl. M. & S. J., 1881-2, n. s., ix, 677–683, 1 tab. *Also:* San. News, Hamilton, Ohio, 1882, ii, 33–38.—**Hillary** (M.) Some observations on the peculiarities of the capillary circulation of the negro. Med. Press & Circ., Lond., 1879, n. s., xxvii, 400.—**Hille.** Das Gebären bei Negerinnen. Wchnschr. f. d. ges. Heilk., Berl., 1843, 86.—**van der Hoeven** (J.) Aanteekeningen over den negerstam in het algemeen, benevens eenige afmetingen van het beenig hoofd bij denzelven. Tijdschr. v. nat. Geschied. en Physiol., Amst., 1835, ii, 356–371. ——. Over de geographische verbreiding van den Aethiopischen menschenstam. *Ibid.*, 1836, iii, 89–114. ——. Nadere aanteekeningen over den negerstam. *Ibid.*, Leiden, 1839, vi, 248–256.—**Horner** (W. E.) On the odoriferous glands of the negro. Am. J. M. Sc., Phila., 1846, n. s., xi, 13–16.—**Houzé.** Les nègres du haut Congo, tribu Baroumbé. Bull. Soc. d'anthrop. de Brux., 1885-6, iv, 67–83.—**Hunt** (J.) On the negro's place in nature. Mem. Anthrop. Soc. Lond. (1863–4), 1865, i, 1–64. [Discussion.] J. Anthrop. Soc. Lond., 1864, ii, pp. xv-lvi.—**Hunt** (S. B.) The negro as a soldier. Quart. J. Psych. M., N Y., 1867, i, 161–186. *Also:* Anthrop. Rev., Lond., 1869, vii, 40–54.—**Hyatt** (H. O.) Note on the normal anatomy of the vulvo-vaginal orifice. Am. J. Obst., N. J., 1877, x, 253 ; 635.—**Jackson** (R. I.) Unity of the human race. Med. & Surg. Reporter, Phila., 1858, xi, 301–307. — **Jacquart.** Sur quelques-uns des caractères anatomiques spéciaux de la race nègre, et en particulier sur l'obliquité des apophyses ptérygoïdes. Gaz. méd. de Par., 1852, 3. s., vii, 437–439.—**Johnson** (J. T.) On some of the apparent peculiarities of parturition in the negro race, with remarks on race pelvis in general. Am. J. Obst., N. Y., 1875-6, viii, 88–123. — **Johnston** (H. H.) The people of eastern equatorial Africa. J. Anthrop. Inst., Lond., 1885-6, xv, 3–15.—**Joyenes** (L. S.) Remarks on the comparative mortality of the white and colored populations of Richmond. Virginia M. Month., Richmond, 1875, ii, 153–167.—**Kilpatrick** (A. R.) [An account of the colored population of Grimes County, Texas. A comparison between their present and former condition] Richmond & Louisville M. J., Louisville, 1872, xiv, 606–623.—**Kopernicki** (I.) Anatomicz no-antropologiczne postrzeżenia nad murzynem. Rocznik Ces. Król. Towarz. nauk. krakow., Kraków, 1871, xix,75–100. *Also,transl.:* J. Anthrop.,Lond., 1870–71, 245–258.—**Langer** (C.) Negerschädel mit überzähligen Zähnen. Mitth. d. anthrop. Gesellsch. in Wien, 1871, i, 118.—**Larcher** (J.-F.) Du pigmentum de la peau dans les races humaines et, en particulier, dans la race nègre. J. de l'anat. et physiol., etc., Par., 1867, iv, 421–437.—**Lehlbach** (C. F. J.) Is the negro a distinct species? Med. & Surg. Reporter, Burlington, N. J., 1857, x, 532 : 1858, xi, 250.—**McCoy** (A.) Voodooism in the South. Louisville M. News, 1884, xviii, 380.—**McKie** (T. J.) The negro and some of his diseases, as observed in the vicinity of Woodlawn, S. C. Tr. South Car. M. Ass., Charleston, 1881, xxxi, 85–90. — [**de Maupertuis** (P.-L.-M.)] Sur l'origine des noirs. *In his:* Vénus physique, 16°, La Haye, 1746, 111 - 152. — **Meckel.** Recherches anatomiques. I. Sur la nature de l'épiderme et du réseau, qu'on appelle Malpighien. II. Sur la diversité de couleur dans la substance médullaire des nègres. III. Sur la maladie du nè-

Negroes.

gre qui a fourni les observations des deux premiers articles, causée par un endurcissement stéatomateux du péritoine. Mém. Acad. roy. de Prusse 1751-3, Avignon, 1768, iii, 320-388. *Also:* Collect. acad. d. mém., etc., Par., 1770, viii, 414-438. ———. Nouvelles observations sur l'épiderme et le cerveau des nègres. Mém. Acad. roy. de Prusse 1757-8, Avignon, 1768, vi, 59-79. *Also:* Collect. acad. d. mém., etc., Par., 1770, ix, 288-295. — **Médecine** (La) et la religion du nègre, d'après un manuscrit ancien écrit par un étranger ayant longtemps habité l'Afrique centrale. J. de méd. de Par., 1887, xiii, 107-117. — **Medical** (The) education of the African race. Med. & Surg. Reporter, Phila., 1882, xlvi, 643. — **Merrill** (A. P.) An essay on some of the distinctive peculiarities of the negro race. Memphis M. Recorder, 1856, iv, 1; 65; 129; 321. — **Mondière** (A.-T.) Les nègres chez eux, ou études ethnographiques sur les populations de la Côte-d'Or (côte occidentale d'Afrique). Rev. d'anthrop., Par., 1880, 2. s., iii, 621: 1881, 2. s, iv, 73.—**Montané.** Informe acerca de un obra intitulada: Antropologia y patologia comparadas de los hombres de color africanos que viven en la isla de Cuba. An. r. Acad. de cien. méd. . . . de la Habana, 1876-7, xiii, 122-136.—**Morgan** (J. H.) An essay on the causes of the production of abortion among our negro population. Nashville J. M. & S., 1860, xix, 117-123.—**Morton** (W. S.) Causes of mortality amongst negroes. Month. Stethoscope & M. Reporter, Richmond, 1856, i, 289-292.—**Nasse.** Zur Physiologie des Negerkörpers. Ztschr. f. d. Anthrop., Leipz., 1823, 3. Vrtljschr., 242-254.—**Negro** mortality in the South. [*From:* The Nation, Aug. 15, 1872] Clinic, Cincin., 1872, iii, 107.—**Neill** (J.) Observations on the occipital and superior maxillary bones of the African cranium. Am. J. M. Sc., Phila., 1850, n. s., xix, 78-83. *Also.* Reprint.—**Nott** (J. C.) The mulatto a hybrid; probable extermination of the two races if the whites and blacks are allowed to intermarry. *Ibid.*, 1843, n.s., vi, 252-256. ———. The negro race. Pop. Mag. Anthrop., Lond., 1866, i, 102-118.—**Owen** (H. B.) Missionary success and negro converts. J. Anthrop. Soc. Lond., 1865, iii, pp. clxxxiv-ccxlvi.—**Parker** (A. J.) Cerebral convolutions of the negro brain. Proc. Acad. Nat. Sc., Phila., 1878, pt. 1, 11-15. ———. Simian characters in negro brains. *Ibid.*, 1879, 339.—**Pathological** (The) future of the negro. Med. Rec., N. Y., 1886, xxix, 485.—**Patterson** (J. S.) Increase and movement of the colored population. Pop. Sc. Month., N. Y., 1881. xix, 665; 784.—**Payn.** Les nègres du Soudan à la Maison centrale de l'Harroch. J. de méd. et pharm. de l'Algérie, Alger, 1881, vi, 289-292.—**Peacock** (T. B.) On the weight of the brain in the negro, and capacity of the cranial cavity of a negro. Mem. Anthrop. Soc. Lond. (1863-4), 1865, i, 65; 520.—**Pendleton** (E. M.) On the comparative fecundity of the Caucasian and African races. Charleston M. J., 1851, vi, 351-356.—**Penick** (C. C.) The colored race as a problem in sanitation. Proc., addr. & disc. Pub. Health Confer., Frankf., Ky., 1887, 130-136.—**Pruner-Bey.** Mémoire sur les nègres. Mém Soc. d'anthrop. de Par., 1860-63, i, 293-336. — **Pusey** (S. E. B. B.) The negro in relation to civilized society. J. Anthrop. Soc. Lond., 1864, ii, pp. cclxx v-ccxc. — **de Quatrefages** (A.) Craniologie des races nègres africaines; races non dolichocéphales. Compt. rend. Acad. d. sc., Par., 1880, xc, 1390-1396.—**Ramsay** (H. A.) The Southern negro, etc. Phila. M. & S J., 1852-3, i, 293-297. *Also,* Reprint. ———. The pulse, cranial dimensions, etc., of the Southern negro child; with some remarks upon infantile therapeutics. Boston M. & S. J., 1853, xlviii, 396-402.—**Reade** (W. W.) Efforts of missionaries among savages. J. Anthrop. Soc. Lond., 1865, iii, pp. clxiii-ccxciv.—**Régis** (E.) Un mot sur la superstition et sur la folie chez les nègres de Zambèze, d'après les notes de voyage de R. Gaffard. Encéphale, Par., 1882, ii, 76-87.—[**Rei** (G.)] Dissertation sur l'origine des nègres. Rev. d'anthrop., Par., 1883, 2. s., vi, 566-572. — **Reichenbach** (O.) On the vitality of the black race, or the coloured people in the United States, according to the census. J. Anthrop. Soc. Lond., 1864, ii, pp. lxv-lxxii.—**Roberton** (J.) On the period of puberty in negro women. Edinb. M. & S. J., 1842, lviii, 112-120.—**de Rochas** (V.) Nègres. Dict. encycl. d. sc. méd., Par., 1877, 2. s., xii, 60-77.—**Rogers** (T. C.) The negro a distinct species. Med. & Surg. Reporter, Phila., 1858, xi, 448-458.—**Romiti** (G.) La cartilagine della piega semilunare ed il muscolo pellicciaio nel negro. Boll. d. Soc. tra i cult. d. sc. med. in Siena, 1885, iii, 3-7.—**de Saporta.** Sur les descendants d'un européen blond et d'une mulâtresse. Bull. Soc. d'anthrop. de Par., 1885, 3. s., viii, 257-277.—**Schaaffhausen** (H.) Ueber die Hautfarbe des Negers und über die Annäherungen der menschlichen Gestalt an die Thierformen. Amtl. Ber. ü. d. Versamml. deutsch. Naturf. u. Aerzte, Götting., 1860, xxxi, 103-114. *Also, in his:* Anthrop. Studien, 8°, Bonn, 1885, 165-183.—**von Schlagintweit-Sakünlünski** (H.) Angaben zur Characteristik der Kru-Neger. Sitzungsb. d. math.-phys. Cl. d. k.-bayer. Akad. d. Wissensch. zu München, 1879, v, 183-201, 1 pl.—**Senex.** Is the negro a distinct species? Answered in the negative. In reply to an article by W. S. Forwood. Med. & Surg. Reporter, Burlington, N. J., 1857, x, 288; 375.—**Simonot.**

Negroes.

Sur la coloration de la peau du nègre. Bull. Soc. d'anthrop., Par., 1862, iii, 140-152.—**Smith** (W.) Some particulars respecting the negro of the neighbourhood of the Congo, West Africa. Proc. Lit. & Phil. Soc. Manchester, 1874-5, xiv, 54-64.—**Smythe** (A. G.) The position of the hymen in the negro race. Am. J. Obst., N. Y., 1877, x, 638.—**Stassano** (E.) Studii antropologici su trentuno negri della Guinea Superiore, costa della Liberia. Arch. per l' antrop., Firenze, 1886, xvi, 413-429.—**Structural** peculiarities of texture in the negro, except in the skin. Month. J. M. Sc., Lond. & Edinb., 1852, xv, 52-54.—**Sutton** (W. L.) A case of doubtful paternity. What distinguishes a child of pure white blood from one tainted with that of a negro? West. J. M. & S., Louisville, 1852, 3. s., x, 308-313.—**Testut** (L.) Dissection d'une jeune négresse d'origine sénégalienne; myologie. Gaz. méd. de l'Algérie, Alger, 1884, xxix, 12-14. — **Thornton** (S. C.), jr. The ethnological question. Med. & Surg. Reporter, Burlington, N. J., 1857, x, 541-546. — **Tiedemann** (F.) On the brain of the negro, compared with that of the European and the orang-outang. Phil. Tr., Lond., 1836, cxxvi, 497-527, 6 pl. *Also, transl.:* Presse méd., Par., 1837, i, 425-428. — **Tipton** (F.) The negro problem from a medical standpoint. N. York M. J., 1886, xliii, 569-572. *Also,* Reprint. — **Topinard** (P.) Sur l'insertion en touffes des cheveux des nègres. Bull. Soc. d'anthrop. de Par., 1878, 3. s., i, 61-66. — **Tulloch** (A. M.) On the statistics of the negro slave population in the West Indies. Brit. Ann. Med., Pharm., etc., Lond., 1837, i, 392; 447.—**Turner.** Notes on the dissection of a negro. J. Anat. & Physiol., Lond., 1878-9, xiii, 382-386. ———. Notes on the dissection of a second negro. *Ibid.*, 1879-80, xiv, 244-248.—**Turnipseed** (E. B.) [Hymen of the negro woman.] Richmond & Louisville M. J., Louisville, 1868, vi, 194. ———. Some facts in regard to the anatomical differences between the negro and white races. Am. J. Obst., N. Y., 1877, x, 32. — **Valdés Aguirre** (F.) Causas que contribuyen á la disminucion de los esclavos en Cuba, y medios de destruirlos. Trab. Com. de med. leg. é hig. púb. de la r. Acad. de cien. méd. . . . de la Habana, 1873, ii, 8-23.—**Virchow** (R.) Neger von Darfur. Verhandl. d. Berl. Gesellsch. f. Anthrop., 1885, 488-497. ———. Schädel von Baluba und Congonegern. *Ibid.*, 1886, 752-767.—**Virey** (J.-J.) Nègre. Dict. d. sc. méd., Par., 1819, xxxv, 378-432.—**Wallace** (J.) & **Prichard** (J. C.) On the supposed want of the sagital suture in certain tribes of negroes. *In:* Graves (R. J.) Studies in Physiol. & Med., 8°, Lond., 1863, 344-346.—**Wolff** (W.) Einige Beobachtungen an den Negern und Buschmännern Afrika's. Arch. f. mikr. Anat., Bonn, 1886, xxviii, 421-424.—**Zintgraff.** Forschungen und Messungen in Kamerun. Verhandl. d. Berl. Gesellsch. f. Anthrop., 1886, 644-646.

Negroes (*Change of color in*).

See, also, **Skin** (*Discoloration, etc., of*).

Bate (J.) An account of the remarkable alteration of colour in a negro woman. Phil. Tr. 1759, Lond., 1760. li, pt. 1, 175-178. — **Bird** (F.) Ueber die Veränderung der Hautfarbe beim Neger. J. d. Chir. u. Augenh., Berl. 1829, xiii, 475-478.—**Catlin** (A.) Another Ethiopian turning to a white man. Med. Reposit., N. Y., 1802, v, 83.— **Hammer** (A.) Change of color in an adult negro. St. Louis M. & S J., 1853, xi, 63-68. *Also, transl.:* Compt. rend. Soc. de biol., Par., 1854. 2. s., i, pt. 1, 148-152.—**Hood** (E. C.) Another white African. South. M. & S. J., Augusta, 1853, n. s., ix, 461.—**Hutchison** (J.C.) A remarkable case of change of complexion with loss of the sense of smell. Am. J. M. Sc., Phila., 1852, n. s., xxiii, 146-148. — **Pozzi** (S.) Sur la décoloration de la peau chez les nègres sous l'influence du climat et de la maladie. Bull. Soc. d'anthrop. de Par., 1872, 3. s., vii, 815-817.

Negroes (*Diseases of*).

See, also, **Ainhum;** **Appetite** (*Abnormal*); **Chorea** *in negroes;* **Frambœsia;** **West Indies.**

DAZILLE. Observations sur les maladies des nègres, leurs causes, leurs traitements et les moyens de les prévenir. 8°. *Paris,* 1776.

———. The same. 2. éd. v. 1. 8°. *Paris,* 1792.

FRANK (L.) Mémoire sur le commerce des nègres au Kaire et sur les maladies auxquelles ils sont sujet en y arrivant. 12°. *Paris,* 1802.

LEVACHER (M.-G.) Guide médical des Antilles, ou études sur les maladies des colonies en général, et sur celles qui sont propres à la race noire. 8°. *Paris,* 1834.

MOULIN (C.-F.-C.) * Introduction à la pathologie de la race nègre dans les pays chauds. 4°. *Paris,* 1866.

Negroes (*Diseases of*).

PRACTICAL rules for the management and medical treatment of negro slaves, in the sugar colonies. By a professional planter. 8°. *London*, 1811.

SEBASTIAN (A. A.) Over de ziekten der negers. (Voorgedragen in de gewone vergadering der Akademie van den 24sten Sept. 1853.) 8°. [*n. p., n. d.*]

SHANNON (R.) Practical observations on the effects of certain medicines in the prevention and cure of diseases to which Europeans are subject in hot climates, and observations on the diseases and diet of negroes. 8°. *London*, 1794.

STUBNERUS (G. A.) & WOLFFIUS (J. C.) *De nigritarum affectionibus. 4°. [*Vitembergæ*, 1699.]

THOMSON (J.) A treatise on the diseases of negroes as they occur in the island of Jamaica; with observations on the country remedies. 8°. *Jamaica*, 1820.

Affleck (T.) On the hygiene of cotton plantations and the management of negro slaves. South. M. Rep. (Fenner) 1850, N. Orl., 1851, ii, 429-436.—**Armstrong** (S. T.) Frequency of disease in the white and colored races; a comparison of the frequency of disease in the white and colored races at the United States Marine Hospital, Memphis, Tenn., during the quinquennium 1881-6. Rep. Superv. Surg.-Gen. Mar. Hosp., Wash., 1885-6, 123-130. — **Atkinson** (I. E.) Early syphilis in the negro. Maryland M. J., Balt., 1877, i, 135-146.—**Baldwin** (B. I.) The immunity of the negro from trachoma. Med Rec., N. Y., 1884, xxvi, 704. — **Bennett** (J.) An account of a fatal case of acute negro consumption, with the appearances on dissection. West. J. M. & Phys. Sc., Cincin., 1830, iii, 193-206.— **Bowman** (J. A.) A case of disease, with autopsy. Nashville J. M. & S., 1853, iv, 15.—**Buchanan** (A. H.) Remarks on negro-consumption. West. J. M & S., Louisville, 1840, 2. s., ii, 405-418.—**Buchanan** (J. M.) Insanity in the colored race. N. York M. J., 1886, xliv, 67-70. — **Burnett** (S. W.) The comparative frequency of eye diseases in the white and colored races in the United States. Arch. Ophth., N. Y., 1884, xiii, 187-200. — **Carpenter** (W. M.) Observations on the cachexia africana, or the habits and effects of dirt-eating in the negro race. N. Orl. M. J., 1844-5, i, 146-168. — **Carter** (H. R.) Manifestations of syphilis among negroes; a statistical inquiry. Rep. Superv. Surg.-Gen. Mar. Hosp., Wash., 1883, 131-135. — **Cartwright** (S. A.) The diseases and physical peculiarities of the negro race. South. M. Rep. (Fenner) 1850, N. Orl., 1851, ii, 421-429. *Also:* Charleston M. J., 1851, vi, 643-652. — **Chassaniol.** Contributions à la pathologie de la race nègre. Arch. de méd. nav., Par., 1865, iii, 505-520. — **Clark** (J.) Account of the good effects derived from the terra ponderosa muriata, in a peculiar species of scrophula, occurring among negroes in the West Indies. Med. Comment. 1791, Edinb., 1792, 2. decade, 267-270.—**Conrad** (H. W.) The health of the negroes in the South; the great mortality among them; the causes and remedies. Sanitarian, N. Y., 1887, xviii, 502-510.—**Davidson** (G.) Account of the cachexia africana, a disease incidental to negro slaves lately imported into the West Indies. Med. Reposit., N. Y., 1799, ii, 282-284.— **Dugas** (L. A.) Remarks upon some of the pathological peculiarities of the negro race. Tr. M. Ass. Georgia, Atlanta, 1876, xxvii, 73-81.—**Emerson** (G.) An account of an epidemic fever which prevailed among the negroes of Philadelphia in the year 1821. Phila. J. M. & Phys. Sc., 1821, iii, 193-216.—**Goldsmith** (R. H.) Tetanus, epidemic or constitutional among negroes? Practitioner, Balt., 1880, i, 22-24.—**Gray** & **Ellis** (H.) On certain diseases of the African slaves. Med.-Chir. J. & Rev., 1816, i, 373-377.— **Hicks** (J. R.) African consumption. Stethoscope & Virg. M. Gaz., Richmond, 1854, iv, 625-629. — **Jordan** (C. H.) Thoughts on cachexia africana, or negro consumption. Transylv. J. M., Lexington, Ky., 1832, v, 18-30.— **McDowell** (A. W.) Hospital observations upon negro soldiers. Am. Pract., Louisville, 1874, x, 155-158.—**Martin de Moussy.** [Les nègres et le scorbut.] Bull. Soc. d'anthrop. de Par., 1867, 2. s., ii, 37-39.—**Maxwell** (J.) Pathological inquiry into the nature of cachexia africana, as it is generally connected with dirt-eating. Jamaica Phys. J., Kingston, 1835, ii, 409-435.—**Nott** (J. C.) Liability of negroes to the epidemic diseases of the South. South. M. & S. J., Augusta, 1858, n. s., xiv, 253.—**Reyburn** (R.) Remarks concerning some of the diseases prevailing among the freed people in the District of Columbia (Bureau Refugees, Freedmen, and Abandoned Lands). Am. J. M. Sc., Phila., 1866, n. s., li, 364-369.—**Reynes** (J. A.) Algunas consideraciones generales sobre la raza negra, su patología y terapéutica. An. r. Acad. de cien. méd. . . . de la Habana, 1868-9, v, 139; 180.—**Roberts**

Negroes (*Diseases of*).

(J. D.) Insanity in the colored race. North Car. M. J., Wilmington, 1883, xii, 249-259.—**Speranza.** Sulla uniforme organizzazione del cranio e del cervello nel negro e nell' europeo. Gior. per serv. ai progr. d. patol., Venezia, 1837, vii, 391-395.—**Tidyman** (P.) A sketch of the most remarkable diseases of the negroes of the Southern States, with an account of the method of treating them, accompanied by physiological observations. Phila. J. M. & Phys. Sc., 1826, xii, 306-338.—**Tiffany** (L. McL.) Comparison between the surgical diseases of the white and colored races. Tr. Am. Surg. Ass., Phila., 1887, v. 262-273, 1 pl. *Also*, Reprint. *Also:* North Car. M. J., Wilmington, 1887, xx, 340-343.—**Yandell** (L. P.) Remarks on struma africana, or the disease usually called negro-poison, or negro-consumption. Transylv. J. M., Lexington, Ky., 1831, iv, 83-103.

Negroni (M.-L.) *Aperçu sur l'ovariotomie, suivi de tableaux analytiques et synoptiques fondés sur 645 observations. 38 pp., 4 tab. 4°. *Paris*, 1866, No. 17.

———. The same. 34 pp., 5 tab. 8°. *Paris, A. Delahaye*, 1866.

Negura (Nicolaus) [1830-]. *De febre Moldaviensi. 28 pp., 2 l. 8°. *Berolini, F. G. Nietack*, [1856].

Nehr. *Ueber Cachexie. 68 pp. 8°. *Würzburg, C. W. Becker*, 1821.

Nehr (Joh. Joseph) [1757-1820]. Quare plerique moriuntur infantes, et eorum, qui adolescunt, quare plures sunt morbosi? [1778.]

In: KLINKOSCH. Diss. med. [etc.] 4°. *Pragæ et Dresdæ*, 1793, ii, 162-184.

———. Beschreibung der mineralischen Quellen zu Marienbad auf der Stiftsherrschaft Tepl, nahe bei dem Dorfe Auschowitz. 5 p. l., 84 pp. 12°. *Karlsbad, J. Franieck*, 1813.

———. The same. Zweite mit 25 Krankengeschichten vermehrte Aufl. 5 p. l., 209 pp., 1 pl. 8°. *Karlsbad, Wittwe J. Franieck*, 1817.

Nehr (Leonardus). *De syphilide. 40 pp. 8°. *Budæ, typ. Reg. Univ. Hung.*, 1829. [P., v. 1317.]

Nehse (Albertus [Eduardus Henricus]) [1816-]. *De melanosi. 29 pp., 1 l. 8°. *Berolini, typ. Nietackianis*, [1839].

Nehse (Hermann) [1846-]. *Ueber Transplantation. 30 pp. 8°. *Berlin, G. Schade*, [1872].

Neichel (Carolus). *De pollinctura cadaverum humanorum juxta antiquos et recentes. 44 pp. 8°. *Pestini, L. Landerer*, [1821]. [P., v. 1309.]

Neide (Augustus)[1]. *De hæmorrhagiis uteri gravidi. [Breslau.] 1 p. l., 32 pp., 2 l. 8°. *Lublinitii, typ. Plessneri*, [1845].

Neide (Augustus)[2]. *De morbis animi. 35 pp. 8°. *Halæ, in off. Batheana*, [n. d.]

Neide (Fridericus Augustus). *Diss. sistens casum quendam memorabilem vitii cordis. 31 pp., 4 pl. 4°. *Halæ, typ. Bœntschianis*, [1830].

Neide (Joh. Christoph). *De tussi. 13 l. 4°. *Vitembergæ, prelo Gerdesiano*, [1708].

Neidenstein.

Erggelet (F.) Die Brunnen in Neidenstein. Deutsche Vrtljschr. f. öff. Gsndhtspflg., Brnschwg., 1880, xii, 286-291.

Neider (Joannes Christianus). *De medicina morbos faciente. 36 pp. sm. 4°. *Lipsiæ, ex off. Langenhemia*, [1776].

For Biography, see **Bose** (Ernestus Gottlob).

Neidert (Karl). * Ueber die Bedeutung des spec. Gewichtes von Pleuratranssudaten in Bezug auf die Prognose bei operativer Behandlung. [Wurtzburg.] 35 pp. 8°. *München, F. Straub*, 1879.

Neidhard (Charles). An answer to the homœopathic delusions of Dr. Oliver Wendell Holmes. 36 pp. 8°. *Philadelphia, J. Dobson*, 1842.

———. Homœopathy in Germany and England in 1849, with a glance at allœopathic men and things. Being two preliminary discourses, delivered in the Homœopathic Medical College of

Neidhard (Charles)—continued.
Pennsylvania. 45 pp. 8°. *Boston, O. Clapp,*
1850.

———. An address delivered before the Rhode
Island Homœopathic Society, at its annual meet-
ing, May 7, 1851. 28 pp. 8°. *Providence, Sayles
& Miller,* [1851]. [P., v. 1400.]

———. On the efficacy of Crotalus horridus in
yellow fever; also in malignant, bilious, and
remittent fevers. With an account of Humboldt's prophylactic inoculation of the venom of
a serpent, at Havana, Cuba. 82 pp. 8°. *New
York, W. Radde,* 1860.

———. The same. Crotalus horridus; its analogy
to yellow fever, malignant, bilious, and remittent fevers, demonstrated by the action of the
venom on man and animals. With an account
of Humboldt's prophylactic inoculation [etc.]
2. ed. xvi, 9–87 pp. 8°. *New York, W. Radde,*
1868.

———. Diphtheria, as it prevailed in the United
States from 1860 to 1866, preceded by an historical account of its phenomena, its nature and
homœopathic treatment. 176 pp. 8°. *New York,
W. Radde,* 1867.

———. On the universality of the homœopathic
law of cure. 2. ed. 37 pp. 8°. *New York &
Philadelphia, Boericke & Tafel,* [1874].

See, also. **Croserio** (C.) On homœopathic medicine,
[etc.] 12°. *Philadelphia,* 1837.—**Materia** medica of
American provings. 4. ed. 12°. *New York,* 1866.

Neidhart (Joannes Fridericus). * De affectibus
dentium. 36 pp., 2 l. 4°. *Halæ Magdeb., typ.
J. C. Hilligeri,* 1740.

Neidhart (Karl). * Ueber die Veränderungen
der Zunge in Krankheiten. 2 l., 71 pp. 8°.
Giessen, W. Keller, 1860.

Neidl (Michael). * De ligandis arteriis læsis et
dissectis. 42 pp. 8°. *Landishuti, typ. J. Tho-
manni,* 1816.

Neidthardt (Martin). * Beiträge zur Behandlung des acuten Gelenkrheumatismus. 22 pp.
8°. *München, C. Wolf u. Sohn,* 1878.

Neifeld (Ernestus Conradus). * De noxia re-
tinendorum excretione et excernendorum retentione voluntaria.
In: CARTHEUSER (J. F.) Diss. nonn. select. phys.-chym.
ac med. 12°. *Francof. ad Viadr.,* 1775, 260–295.

Neifeld (Ernestus Jeremias) [1721–72]. * De
genesi caloris febrium intermittentium. 32 pp.
4°. *Lipsiæ, ex off. Langenhemiana,* [1744].

———. Specimen i. physico-medicum de secretione humorum in genere, ex mechanica solidorum structura, fluidorumque genio demonstrata.
20 p. l., 168 pp., 4 l., 1 pl. 8°. *Züllichoviæ, apud
J. I. Dendelerum,* 1751.

For Biography, see **Walther** (Aug. Fridericus).
For Portrait, see **Collection**—van Kaathovon.—**Collection** of Portr. of Phys. & Men of Sc., 126.

Neigefind (Godofredus). * De noxiis effectibus
frigoris in humanum corpus. 32 pp. 4°. *Erfordiæ, typ. J. C. Herringii,* [1740].
See, also, **Puscher** (Jo. Carolus) & **Neigefind** (Godofredus). De medicina scientia [etc.] 4°. [*Gottingæ,* 1740.]

Neigefind (Theodosius Gottlieb). * De cortice
peruviano speciebus debilitatis magis accommo-
dando. 1–8, 17–22+ pp. 4°. *Halæ ad Salam,
typ. J. H. Hessii,* [1775].
Incomplete; pp. 9–16 and all after p. 22 missing.

Neikter (Jac. Fr.) Diss. de medicina per incantationem. Cujus partem priorem . . . subjicit
Jacobus Lindblad; partis posterioris primam
sectionem sistit Carolus Magnus Crælius; secundam sectionem sistit Carolus Gustavus Wess-
man; tertiam sectionem offeret Gustavus A. Ju-
ringius. 48 pp. 4°. *Upsaliæ, lit vid. direct.
J. Edman,* 1792–3.

Neild (J.)
Portrait in: **Collection**—van Kaathoven.

Neild (James Edward). On the advantages of
burning the dead. 10 pp. 8°. [*Melbourne, Stillwell & Knight,* 1873.]

———. Address delivered at the annual meeting
of the Victorian branch of the British Medical
Association, July 28, 1882. 12 pp. 8°. *Melbourne, Stillwell & Co.,* 1882.

Neild (Joannes Cash) [1814–]. * De pseudarthrosi quæ ossium fracturas sequitur. 28 pp.
8°. *Berolini, typ. Nietackianis,* 1839.

Neilgherries.

MADRAS Presidency. Report on the medical
topography and statistics of Neilgherry Hills.
(Compiled from the records of the medical board
office. Published by order of government.) 8°.
Madras, 1844.
Birch (De B.) Topographical report on the Neilgher-
ries. India J. M. & Phys. Sc., Calcutta, 1838, n. s., iii,
713: 1839, n. s., iv, 11; 79.—**Mackay** (G.) Remarks on
the climate of the Neilgherry hills. Madras Q. J. M.
Sc., 1861, iii, 13–32.— **Young** (D. S.) An account of the
general and medical topography of the Neelgerries. Tr.
M. & Phys. Soc. Calcutta, 1829, iv, 36–78, 1 pl., 1 map.

Neiling ([Joh.] Michael) [1854–]. * Ein Beitrag zur Lehre von der Trepanation des Processus mastoideus. 20 pp. 4°. *Kiel, C. F. Mohr,*
1878.
In: SCHRIFT. d. Univ. zu Kiel, xxv, 1878, vii, Med. xviii.

Neill (Edward D.) Biographical sketch of Doctor Jonathan Potts, with extracts from his
correspondence. 18 pp. 8°. *Albany, J. Munsell,* 1863. [*Also, in:* P., v. 161.]
Repr. from: N. Eng. Historic & Gen. Register.

Neill (*Henry*) [1783–1845].
Paul (J. M.) Obituary notice. Tr. Coll. Phys. Phila.,
1848, ii, 320–323.

Neill (Hugh). The practice in the Liverpool
Ophthalmic Infirmary, for the year 1834; being
the first special report. iv, 55 pp., 1 tab., 1 pl.
8°. *London, Longman [and others],* 1835.

———. A report upon deafness when resulting
from diseases of the Eustachian passages; with
the modern methods of cure. 2. ed. 3 p. l., viii,
9–39 pp., 1 pl. 8°. *Liverpool, J. Walmsley,*
1840.

———. The same. 3. ed. xx, 21–51 pp. 8°.
Liverpool, J. Walmsley, 1840. [P., v. 35.]

———. The same. 4. ed. 44 pp. 8°. *Liverpool,
J. Walmsley,* 1841. [P., v. 362.]

———. On the cure of cataract, with a practical
summary of the best modes of operating (Conti-
nental and British). 1 p. l., x, 5–224 pp. 8°.
London, J. Churchill, 1848.

———. The same. 2. ed. 1 p. l., x, 5–224 pp.
8°. *London, C. Mitchell; Liverpool, Deighton &
Laughton,* 1850.

Neill (John) [1819–80]. Outlines of the arteries; with short descriptions. 30 pp., 6 pl. 8°.
Philadelphia, E. Barrington & G. D Haswell,
1845.

———. The same. 2. ed. 28 pp., 7 col. pl. 8°.
Philadelphia, E. Barrington & G. D. Haswell,
1852.

———. Outlines of the nerves; with short descriptions. 30 pp., 9 pl. 8°. *Philadelphia, E.
Barrington & G. D. Haswell,* 1845.

———. Outlines of the veins and lymphatics;
with short descriptions. Designed for the use of
medical students. 29 pp., 8 pl. 8°. *Philadelphia, E. Barrington & G. D. Haswell,* 1847.

———. Observations on the occipital and superior maxillary bones of the African cranium. 5
pp. 8°. [*Philadelphia,* 1850.]
Repr. from: Am. J. M. Sc., Phila., 1850, n. s., xix.

———. New means for making extension and
counter-extension in fractures of the leg and
thigh. 7 pp. 8°. *Philadelphia, Merrihew &
Thompson,* 1855.

Neill (John)—continued.

———. On the structure of the mucous membrane of the human stomach. 16 pp., 1 pl. 8°. [*Philadelphia*, 1857.]

   Repr. from: Am. J. M. Sc., Phila., 1851, n. s., xxi.

———. Valedictory address before the medical department of Pennsylvania College, March 6, 1858. (With a list of graduates.) 19 pp. 8°. *Philadelphia, Sherman & Son*, 1858.

   For Biography, see Clin. News, Phila., 1880, i, 92. *Also:* Phila. M. Times, 1879-80, x, 288. *Also:* Proc. Am. Phil. Soc., Phila., 1880, xix, 161 (Brinton). *Also:* Tr. Coll. Phys. Phila., 1881, 3. s., v, pp. cxli–clvi (E. Shippen). *Also*, Reprint.

——— **& Smith** (Francis Gurney). A handbook of anatomy . . . Being a portion of an analytical compend of the various branches of medicine. viii, 14–180 pp. 8°. *Philadelphia, Lea & Blanchard*, 1848.

——————. A handbook of chemistry . . . Being a portion of an analytical compend of the various branches of medicine. viii, 15–115 pp. 8°. *Philadelphia, Lea & Blanchard*, 1848.

——————. A handbook of surgery; being a portion of an analytical compend of the various branches of medicine. 122 pp. 12°. *Philadelphia, Lea & Blanchard*, 1848.

——————. Analytical compendium of the various branches of medical science. A new ed., revised and improved. xxiv, 25–974 pp. 12°. *Philadelphia, Blanchard & Lea*, 1864.

Neill (Patrick). Some account of the habits of a specimen of Siren lacertina, which has been kept alive at Canonmills, near Edinburgh, for more than two years past. 10 pp. 8°. [*Edinburgh*, 1828.] [*Also, in:* P., v. 678.]

   Repr. from: Edinb. N. Phil. J., 1828.

———. An address to the members of the Wernerian Natural History Society, 1830. 26 pp. 8°. [*Edinburgh*], 1830.

Neilson (John). *On the utility of dispensaries, their importance to the community; with hints to their further beneficial effects in attaching small hospitals to each. 32 pp. 8°. *Edinburgh, Neill & Co.*, 1836. [*Also, in:* P., v. 698.]

Neilson (William). Mesmerism in its relation to health and disease and the present state of medicine. xi, 13–250 pp. 8°. *Edinburgh, Shepherd & Elliot*, 1855.

Neilston.

   Ritchie (C.) Remarks on the medical topography of the parish of Neilston. Glasgow M. J., 1828, i, 286; 371.

Neinstedt.

   See **Idiots** (*Asylums, etc., for*), *by localities.*

Neinstedter Erziehungs-Haus für schwachsinnige und blödsinnige Knaben in Neustadt am Harz. *See* **Elizabethstift**. Erziehungs-Haus für blödsinnige und schwachsinnige [etc.]

Neipce (Étienne-Bernard). *I. Quelle est la valeur des signes fournis par la présence des gaz dans les voies digestives? II. [etc.] 36 pp. 4°. *Paris*, 1840, No. 138, v. 364.

Neis (Christian). * De l'anesthésie locale par la pulvérisation de l'éther. 34 pp. 4°. *Paris*, 1870, No. 143.

Neis (Paul). * Observation d'un cas de luxation du maxillaire inférieur en haut ou dans la fosse temporale. 34 pp. 4°. *Paris*, 1879, No. 252.

Neish (James).

   Editor of: **Canadian** (The) Medical Times, Kingston, 1873.

Neison (F. G. P.) Contributions to vital statistics; being a development of the rate of mortality and the laws of sickness, from original and extensive data procured from friendly societies, showing the instability of friendly societies "Odd Fellows," "Rechabites," etc., with an inquiry into the influence of locality on health. vii, 148 pp. 4°. *London, H. Cunningham*, 1845.

Neison (F. G. P.)—continued.

———. The same. With an inquiry into the influence of locality, occupations, and habits of life on health; an analytical view of railway accidents; and an investigation into the progress of crime in England and Wales. 3. ed. 1 p. l., xliv, 630 pp. 4°. *London, Simpkin, Marshall & Co.*, 1857.

———. On the rate of mortality among persons of intemperate habits; read before the Statistical Society of London, 16th June, 1851. 20 pp. 8°. [*London*, 1851.] [P., v. 1189.]

   Repr. from: J. Statist. Soc. Lond., 1851, xiv.

———. The rates of mortality and sickness, according to the experience for the five years 1871–5, of the Ancient Order of Foresters Friendly Society. 217 pp. roy. 8°. *London, Harrison & Sons*, 1882.

Neiss (Carolus Augustus) [1824–]. *De morborum medullæ spinalis symptomatibus. 31 pp. 8°. *Berolini, G. Schade*, [1848].

Neiss (Fridericus Hubertus) [1792–]. *De fistula et polypo sacci lachrimalis. 61 pp., 1 l. 8°. *Bonnæ, typ. Bueschlerianis*, [1822].

Neisse.

   See, also, **Fever** (*Typhoid, History, etc., of*), *by localities.*

   Finkelnburg. Gutachten der königl. wissenschaftlichen Deputation für das Medicinalwesen über den Umbau der städtischen Cloakencanäle in Neisse. Deutsche Vrtljschr. f. öff. Gsndhtspflg., Brnschwg., 1881, xiii, 177–185. — **Lent.** Der Abfluss der Cloakenwässer der Stadt Neisse in den Bielecanal und die Neisse. Cor.-Bl. d. nied.-rhein. Ver. f. öff. Gsndtspflg., Köln, 1881, x, 113; 127.

Neisser (Albert) [1855–]. Versuche über den Vorgang der Harnabsonderung. (Angestellt von R. Heidenhain.) 27 pp., 1 pl. 8°. *Breslau*, 1874. [P., v. 795.]

———. *Die Echinococcen-Krankheit. [Breslau.] 2 p. l., 76 pp. 8°. *Berlin, G. Bernstein*, [1877].

———. The same. [With additions.] 3 p. l., 288 pp. 8°. *Berlin, A. Hirschwald*, 1877.

———. Klinisches und Experimentelles zur Wirkung der Pyrogallussäure. 21 pp. 8°. *Berlin, L. Schumacher*, 1879.

   Repr. from: Ztschr. f. klin. Med., Berl., 1879, i.

———. Ueber eine der Gonorrhöe eigenthümliche Micrococcusform. 2 l. 8°. *Berlin, L. Schumacher*, 1879.

   Repr. from: Centralbl. f. d. med. Wissensch., Berl., 1879, xiii.

———. Zur Aetiologie des Aussatzes. 8 pp. 8°. *Breslau, W. Friedrich*, 1879.

   Repr. from: Breslau. ärztl. Ztschr., 1879, i.

———. Die gegenwärtig für die Behandlung der Syphilis maassgebenden Grundsätze und Methoden. 2 l. 4°. *Leipzig, Ackermann u. Glaser*, 1881.

   Repr. from: Aerztl. Vereinsbl. f. Deutschl., Leipz., 1881, x.

———. Die Hämoglobinurie erzeugende Wirkung des Naphtols. 1 l. 8°. *Berlin, L. Schumacher*, 1881.

   Repr. from: Centralbl. f. d. med. Wissensch., Berl., 1881, xiv.

———. Die chronischen Infectionskrankheiten der Haut.

   In: HANDB. d. spec. Path. (Ziemssen), Leipz., 1883, xiv, 1. Hlft., 553–724.

Neisser (Clemens). Ueber die Katatonie. Ein Beitrag zur klinischen Psychiatrie. 2 p. l., 85 pp., 4 pl. roy. 8°. *Stuttgart, F. Enke*, 1887.

Neisser (Joseph). *Diss. sistens nonnulla de autocratia naturæ. 26 pp., 1 l. 8°. *Halæ, formis Hendelii*, [1836].

———. Die acute Entzündung der serösen Häute des Gehirns und des Rückenmarks. Nach eigenen Beobachtungen am Krankenbett geschrie-

Neisser (Joseph)—continued.

ben. 2 p. l., 454 pp. 8°. *Berlin, A. Hirschwald,* 1845.

———. Fundamenta generalia ad inflammationis, qua morbi generis, rationem et naturam spectantia. 1 p. l., 24 pp., 1 l. 8°. *Vratislaviæ, typ. Grassii, Barthii et soc.,* [1849].

———. Das Wesen der Entzündung vom theoretischen und practischen Standpunkt, insbesondere in Rücksicht auf die Henle'sche Entzündungslehre untersucht. 39 pp. 8°. *Berlin, A. Förstner,* 1849.

———. Die physiologische Diagnostik als Basis für rationelle Therapie. Systematisch bearbeitet. 2 p. l., 68 pp. 8°. *Berlin, A. Hirschwald,* 1879.

Neisske (Bernhardus Joachimus). * Diss. sistens calculorum in corpore humano reperiundorum genesin et curam. 31 pp. sm. 4°. *Gotingæ, A. Vandenhoeck,* [1737].

For Biography, see **Segner** (Joannes Andreas).

Neithard (Bernhardus Albrechtus). * De asthmate consensuali. 20 pp. 4°. *Altorfii, ex off. J. P. Meyeri,* [1797].

Neithardt (F.) Die Thierseuchen, welche in veterinär-polizeilichem Interesse zu beachten sind. Ihre Erkennung, Entstehung, Verhütung und Behandlung, sowie die dagegen zu ergreifenden polizeilichen Massregeln. 1 p. l., 116 pp. 8°. *Berlin, Wiegandt u. Hempel,* 1868.

Neithardus (Petrus). * De tributo lunari fœminarum intercepto, in certo quodam casu. 12 pp. 4°. *Altdorfi, H. Meyer,* [1681].

Neithart (Richardus [Henricus]) [1824–]. * De tetano traumatico. 31 pp. 8°. *Berolini, G. Schade,* [1848].

Neithrop.

RAMMELL (T. W.) Report to the General Board of Health, on a preliminary inquiry into the sewerage, drainage, and supply of water, and the sanitary condition of the inhabitants of the borough and parish of Banbury and township of Neithrop, in the counties of Oxford and Northampton. 8°. *London,* 1850.

Nekkach (Mohamed Ben Si-El Hadj-Benamar). See **Mohamed Ben Si-El-Hadj-Benamar Nekkach.**

Nekrasovoi (E.) Iz proshlago jenskich kursov. [The course (of lectures) for women.] 99 pp. 8°. *Moskva, tip. A. A. Kartsera,* 1886.

Nekrolog des Hofraths und Professors Dr. Carl Himly. 12 pp., 2 l. 8°. *Hannover, Helwing,* 1838.

Repr. from: Ann. f. d. ges. Heilk., Karlsruhe, 1857, ii.

Nekrolog des Geheimen Medicinal-Raths und Professors Ludwig Böhm. 12 pp. 12°. *Berlin,* 1869.

Nekrologie des chirurg. Instrumentenfabricanten Johann Caspar Schnetter in München. 24 pp. 12°. *München, E. Wolf u. Sohn,* 1860.

Nekrosozoic or embalming process. Reports of Dr. Francis Delafield, J. R. Wood, R. Ogden Doremus, A. Flint, jr., and extracts from the press. 32 pp. 8°. *New York, Clark & Co.,* [1868].

Nel (J.-B.-Généreux). * Sur la dysenterie simple ou sans complications. vi, 7–25 pp. 4°. *Paris,* 1825, No. 14, v. 190.

Nélaton (Auguste) [1807–73]. * Recherches sur l'affection tuberculeuse des os. 50 pp., 2 pl. 4°. *Paris,* 1836, No. 376, v. 305.

———. The same. 70 pp., 1 l., 2 pl. 8°. *Paris, Méquignon-Marvis & fils,* 1837. [P., v. 907.]

———. * Sur la question des tumeurs de la mamelle. 135 pp. 4°. *Paris, F. Locquin & Cie.,* 1839. [*Also, in* : P., v. 933.]
Concours.

Nélaton (Auguste)—continued.

———. Élémens de pathologie chirurgicale. 5 v. (v. 4 and 5 publié sous sa direction par A. Jamain.) 8°. *Paris, Germer-Baillière,* 1844–59.

———. The same. 2. éd. 6 v. 8°. *Paris, Germer-Baillière & Cie.,* 1868–84.

v. 1 publié sous sa direction par Jamain; v. 2-4 par J. Péan; v. 5 revu par Armand Després; v. 6 revu par Després, Gillette et Horteloup.

———. * Parallèle des divers modes opératoires employés dans le traitement de la cataracte. 139 pp. 8°. *Paris, Germer-Baillière,* 1850. [*Also, in* : P., v. 938 ; 1660.]

———. * De l'influence de la position dans les maladies chirurgicales. 123 pp. 8°. *Paris, Germer-Baillière,* 1851. [P., v. 464 ; 1660.]

———. The same. Die Körperlage bei chirurgischen Krankheiten, nach ihrer diagnostischen und therapeutischen Bedeutung, ihrem Einflusse und ihrer rationellen Anwendung, durch Beobachtungen, Thatsachen und eigene Operationen erfahrungsmässig belegt, in's Deutsche übertragen von Dr. Hugo Hartmann. iv, 127 pp. 12°. *Grimma u. Leipzig, Verlags-Comptoir,* 1852.

———. Clinical lectures on surgery, from notes taken by Walter F. Atlee, M. D. xii, 17–755 pp. 8°. *Philadelphia, J. B. Lippincott & Co.,* 1855.

See, also, **Ferrier** (Léon-Alexis). * De l'opération nouvelle pratiquée par . . . 4°. *Paris,* 1855.

For Biography, see **Béclard** (J.) Notice historique sur la vie et les travaux de . . . In his : Notices et portraits, 8°, Par., 1878, 289–321. See, also, Bull. et mém. Soc. de chir. de Par., 1876, ɐ. s., ii, 76-95 (F. Guyon). Also: Chicago M. J. & Exam., 1884, xlix, 388–413 (J. E. Owens). Also: Gaz. d. hôp., Par., 1876, xlix, 97–103 (F. Guyon). Also: Gaz. méd de Par., 1876, 4. s., v, 61 ; 73 ; 85 ; 97 (F. Guyon). Also: Ibid., 1878, 4. s., vii, 273; 285; 321 (Béclard). Also: Gaz. méd.-chir. de Toulouse, 1877, ix, 196 ; 204 ; 211 (F. Guyon). Also: Lancet, Lond., 1873, ii, 472. Also: Lyon méd., 1873, xiv, 193–197 (P. Diday). Also: Med. Times & Gaz., Lond., 1873, ii, 445 (Desprès). Also: Mém. Acad. de méd., Par., 1879, xxxii, pp. xxi-xl (J. Béclard). Also: Moniteur, Par., 1876, i, 17; 33; 49 ; 65 (F. Guyon). Also: Progrès méd., Par., 1878, vi, 467 ; 487 ; 506 (J. Béclard). Also: Rev. de lit. méd., Par., 1876, i, 159 (F. R.). Also: Tribune méd., Par., 1876, ix, 61; 89 (F. Guyon). Also: Union méd., Par., 1876, i, 169; 205 ; 245 (F. Guyon). For Portrait, see **Collection** — van Kaathoven. — **Richmond** & Louisville M. J., Louisville, 1870, ix, 375.

Nélaton (Charles). *Des épanchements de sang dans les plèvres consécutifs aux traumatismes. 3 p. l., iii, 192 pp. 4°. *Paris, G. Chamerot,* 1880, No. 95.

———. * Le tubercule dans les affections chirurgicales. iv, 179 pp. 4°. *Paris, G. Chamerot,* 1883.

———. Rapports du traumatisme avec les affections cardiaques. ix, 234 pp. 8°. *Paris, G. Masson,* 1886.

Nélaton (Eugène). * Mémoire sur une nouvelle espèce de tumeurs à myéloplaxes. 375 pp. 4°. *Paris,* 1860, No. 58.

———. The same. 373 pp., 3 pl. 8°. *Paris, A. Delahaye,* 1860.

Nelaton (P.-F.) * Sur la leucorrhée. 16 pp. 4°. *Paris,* 1815, No. 230, v. 115.

Nélaton's *probe.*
See **Missiles,** etc.

Nelavan.

Déclat. Sur les analogies qui semblent exister entre le choléra des poules et le nélavan, ou maladie du sommeil. Compt. rend. Acad. d. sc., Par., 1880, xc, 1088–1090.— **Nicolas** (A.) Sur les analogies et les différences qui existent entre la maladie du sommeil et le nélavan. Ibid., 1128–1131.

Neldelius (Joannes).

See **de Ripa** (Joannes Franciscus). Illustris de peste tractatus [etc.] 4°. *Lipsiæ,* 1598.

Nelet (Alexandre-François). * Essai et observations sur la fièvre intermittente simple. 25 pp. 4°. *Paris,* 1833, No. 281, v. 264.

Neligan (John Moore) [1815–63]. The diagnosis and treatment of eruptive diseases of the scalp. 55 pp. 8°. *Dublin, Hodges & Smith*, 1848.

——. Medicines; their uses and mode of administration, including a complete conspectus of the three British pharmacopœias, an account of all the new remedies, and an appendix of formulæ. 3. ed. xxvii, 555 pp. 8°. *Dublin, Fannin & Co.*, 1851.

——. The same. 5. ed. xxi, 620 pp. 8°. *Dublin, Fannin & Co.*, 1858.

——. The same. With notes and additions conforming it to the Pharmacopœia of the United States, by D. M. Reese. xxi, 22–453 pp. 8°. *New York, Harper & Bros.*, 1844.

——. The same. 3. ed. xxi, 22–453 pp. 8°. *New York, Harper & Brothers*, 1851.

——. Contributions to the pathology and treatment of eruptive diseases of the skin. 15 pp. 8°. [*n. p.*, 1852, *vel subseq.*] [P., v. 39; 1022.]

——. A practical treatise on diseases of the skin. x, 439 pp. 8°. *Dublin, Fannin & Co.*, 1852.

——. The same. 2. ed., revised and enlarged by T. W. Belcher. xxiv, 526 pp. 8°. *Dublin, Fannin & Co.*, 1866.

——. The same. xii, 333 pp. 8°. *Philadelphia, Blanchard & Lea*, 1852.

——. The same. 3. Am. ed. xii, 13–333 pp., 8°; atlas, 16 pl., 4°. *Philadelphia, Blanchard & Lea*, 1859–60.

——. The same. 4. Am. ed. xii, 13–333 pp. 8°. *Philadelphia, Blanchard & Lea*, 1854.

——. The same. 5. Am. from the 2. revised and enlarged Dublin ed., by T. W. Belcher. xvi, 25–462 pp. 8°. *Philadelphia, H. C. Lea*, 1866.

——. Atlas of cutaneous diseases. 19 l., 16 pl. roy. 8°. *Dublin, Fannin & Co.*, 1855.

——. An unusual abnormal condition of the tongue and cheeks, considered in connexion with life assurance. 8 pp. 8°. *Dublin, J. Falconer*, 1862. [P., v. 1025.]
Repr. from: Dublin Q. J. M. Sc., 1862, xxxiv.
See, also, **Graves** (Robert J.) Clinical lectures [etc.] 8°. *Dublin*, 1848.
For Biography, see Dublin Q. J. M. Sc., 1863, xxxvi, 255–258.

Neligan (Laurentius B.) * De morbis respirationis. 1 p. l., 36 pp. 8°. *Edinburgi, C. Stewart*, 1805.

Neligan (Mauricius). * De ferro. 1 p. l., 26 pp. 8°. *Edinburgi, J. Ballantyne*, 1805.

Nelke (Joh.) [1854–]. * Untersuchungen über parenchymatöse und subcutane Alkohol-Injectionen. 24 pp., 1 l. 8°. *Greifswald, C. Sell*, 1880.

Nelken (Michel) [1811–61]. * Des fistules à l'anus. 22 pp., 1 pl. 4°. *Paris*, 1847, No. 148, v. 462.

——. Sea-sickness; its cause, nature, symptoms, and treatment, derived from experience and strict observation. 32 pp. 8°. *New York, Stringer & Townsend*, 1856.
For Biography, see Am. M. Times, N. Y., 1861, iii, 160.

Nellen (Georg. Ludov. Henric.) * De vulnerum quæ sclopetis inferuntur curandorum methodis. 63 pp. 8°. *Halæ, in off. Bathcana*, [1804].

Nellessen (Joh.) [1849–]. * Casuistische Beiträge zur Kenntniss des Glioms der Netzhaut. 30 pp., 1 l., 1 pl. 8°. *Halle, Plötz*, [1872]. c.

Nels (Ludovicus) [1826–]. * De hebetudine visus. 29 pp. 8°. *Berolini, G. Schade*, [1852].

Nelson.
See **Bischoff** (Th. L. W.) Widerlegung des von Dr. Keber bei Najaden und Dr. Nelson bei den Ascariden [etc.] 4°. *Giessen*, 1854.

Nelson (A. W.) Veratrum viride in typhoid fever; its lowering of the pulse and tempera-

Nelson (A. W.)—continued.
ture; twenty-eight successive cases in private practice, all recovering, 1873–82. 17 pp. 8°. [*New York*, 1883.]
Repr. from: Arch. Med., N. Y., 1883, ix.

Nelson (Alfred).
Editor of: **Nelson's** American Lancet, Plattsburgh, N. Y., 1853–6.

Nelson (*Charles Eugene*) [1837–].
Editor of: **Eastern** Medical Journal, Worcester, 1885–7.
Also, Editor of: **Planet** (The), New York, 1883–4.
For Biography, see Eastern M. J., Worcester, 1886, vi, 25.

Nelson (David). * On the principles of health and disease. [Edinburgh.] 2 p. l., vii, 113 pp. 8°. *London, J. Churchill*, 1850. [P., v. 1024.]

——. The same. 2. ed. vii, 113 pp. 8°. *London, J. Churchill*, 1859.

Nelson (Gilbert). A short account of certain remedies used in the cure of the gout. 32 pp. 8°. *London*, 1728.

——. The nature, cause, and symptoms of the gout, as stated by Dr. Sydenham, Cheyne, etc., from which is rationally deduced its direct and perfect cure. To which is added, an account of the action of certain remedies that can effect the same. 2. ed. viii, 85 pp. 12°. *London, T. Warner*, 1728.

Nelson (Horace).
Co-Editor of: **Northern** Lancet and Gazette of Legal Medicine, Plattsburgh, N. Y., 1850–56.

Nelson (Joshua).
See **Douglas** (J.) Descriptio peritonæi, etc. 12°. *Lugd. Bat.*, 1737.

Nelson (Robert)[1] [1794–1873]. Gastrotomy, for the removal of non-malignant tumors from the abdominal cavity. 32 pp. 8°. *New York, J. H. Tobitt*, 1864.

——. Asiatic cholera, its origin and spread in Asia, Africa, and Europe, introduction into America through Canada, remote and proximate causes, symptoms, and pathology, and the various modes of treatment analyzed. xi, 206 pp. 12°. *New York, W. A. Townsend*, 1866.
For Biography, see Canada M. Rec., Montreal, 1880–81, ix, 68.

Nelson [Robert][2].
See **Jenkins** (James). On three fatal cases of cerebro-spinal or tetanoid fever, [etc.] 8°. *London*, 1876.

Nelson (Samuel N.) Plastic splints in surgery. 18 pp. 8°. *Brooklyn*, 1882.
Repr. from: Ann. Anat. & Surg. Soc., Brooklyn, N. Y., 1882, vi.

Nelson (T.) *See* **Vaccine-Pock** Institution.

Nelson (Thomas)[1]. * De frigoris effectibus in morbis medendis. 56 pp. 8°. *Edinburgi, A. Neill et socii*, 1799. [P., v. 9.]

Nelson (*Thomas*)[2].
Portrait in: **Collection** of Portr. (Libr.) — **Stethoscope**, Richmond, 1854, iv, 688.

Nelson (W.), **MacDonnell** (R. L.) & **Perrault** (Zephirin). Report of . . . of the Quebec Marine and Emigrant Hospital. [With documents having reference to the inquiry held by the said gentlemen, concerning the institution.] 124 pp. 8°. *Quebec, J. Lovell*, 1853.

Nelson (William). * Observations on the management of Peruvian bark. 30 pp. 8°. *Philadelphia, J. Geyer*, 1802.

[**Nelson** (Wolfred).] Practical views on cholera, and on the sanitary, preventive, and curative measures to be adopted in the event of a visitation of the epidemic; with an appendix. 19 pp. 8°. *Montreal, B. Dawson*, 1854.

Nelson's American Lancet.
Was title of v. 7–12 of: **Northern** (The) Lancet and Gazette of Legal Medicine, April, 1853–6.

Nelson's Northern Lancet and American Journal of Medical Jurisprudence.
Was title of v. 4–6 of: **Northern** (The) Lancet and Gazette of Legal Medicine, Oct., 1851, to March, 1853.

Nelsson (*Sven*) [1787–1883].
Obituary. Eira, Göteborg, 1883, vii, 766.

Nelz (Josephus Augustus) [1841–   ]. * De carcinomate ventriculi. 8°. *Berolini, G. Lange,* 1866.

Nemann (Julius). * Beiträge zur Pathologie und Therapie der corticalen Sprachstörungen. 43 pp. 8°. *Berlin, G. Schade,* [1884].

Nemann (Michael). * Expositio neurologiæ Galenicæ. 28 pp., 2 l. 8°. *Berolini, typ. fratrum Schlesinger,* [1847].

Nematoid *worms.*
See, also, **Parasites**, *etc.*
CLAPARÈDE (E.) De la formation et de la fécondation des œufs chez les vers nématodes. 4°. *Genève,* 1859.
GABRIEL (B.) * De cucullani elegantis vivipari evolutione. Fragmentum operis majoris. 4°. *Berolini,* [1853].
Babesiu (V.) Ueber einen im menschlichen Peritonäum gefundenen Nematoden. Arch. f. path. Anat., etc., Berl., 1880, lxxxi, 158–165, 1 pl. — **Chatin** (J.) Sur une forme rare des éléments musculaires chez les né.natoïdes. Compt. rend. Soc. de biol. 1877, Par., 1879, 6. s., iv, 278.— **Joseph** (G.) Ueber die in den Krainer Tropfsteingrotten einheimischen, freilebenden Rundwürmer (Nematoden). Jahresb. d. schles. Gesellsch. f. vaterl. Cult. 1878, Bresl., 1879, lvi, 76–78.—**de Magalhães** (P. S.) Nota sobre os nematoides encotrados no sedimento deposto pela agua (potavel) da Carioca. Gaz. med. da Bahia, 1878, 2. s., iii, 503–506.—**Perroncito.** Genesi delle malattie prodotte da nematoelminti le cui larve passano un periodo di vita libera. Gior. internaz. d. sc. med., Napoli, 1881, n. s., iii, 350 ; 461, 1 pl.—**Pouchet** (G.) & **Bergé** (A.) Note préliminaire sur le fonctionnement des nématocystes. Compt. rend. Soc. de biol., Par., 1883, 7. s., iv, 22.—**Schneider** (A.) Ueber die Muskeln und Nerven der Nematoden. Arch. f. Anat., Physiol. u. wissensch. Med., Leipz., 1860, 224–242, 1 pl. ———. Neue Beiträge zur Anatomie und Morphologie der Nematoden. *Ibid.,* 1863, 1–25, 2 pl.

Nemerowsky (Ludmilla). * Ueber das Phänomen der Lücke bei elektrischer Nervenreizung. 24 pp., 1 pl. 8°. *Bern, R. F. Haller-Goldschach,* 1883.

Nemertians.
See, also, **Nervous** *system* (*Comparative anatomy of*).
DESOR (E.) Embryology of Nemertes; with an appendix on the embryonic development of Palynöe. 8°. *Boston,* 1848.
Graff (L.) Geonemertes chalicophora, eine neue Landnemertine. Morphol. Jahrb., Leipz., 1879, v, 430–449, 3 pl.—**Hubrecht** (A. A. W.) Contribution to the embryology of the Nemertea. Quart. J. Micr. Sc., Lond., 1885–6, n. s., xxvi, 417–448, 1 pl. ———. The relation of the Nemertea to the vertebrata. *Ibid.,* 1886–7, n. s., xxvii, 605–644, 1 pl.—**Oudemans** (A. C.) The circulatory and nephridial apparatus of the Nemertea. *Ibid.,* 1885, n. s., xxv (suppl.), 1–80, 3 pl.—**Vaillant** (L.) Remarques sur l'appareil stylifère de quelques némertiens. Compt. rend. Soc. de biol. 1871, Par., 1873, 5. s., iii, 89–97.

Nemesius. Von der Natur des Menschen, nach dem Urtheile der Gelehrten. Eine der scharfsinnigsten Schriften des ganzen christlichen Alterthumes. Aus dem Griechischen zum ersten Male in das Deutsche übersetzt, mit einzelnen Text-Berichtigungen, einer Parallele der alten und neuen Physik, und mit Erläuterungen versehen, worunter ein ganz neuer, in der Geschichte der Heilkunde bisher unbekannter, durch zehnjährige Erfahrung als zuverlässig befundener Heilplan, den Typhus in wenigen Tagen zu heben, und sich gegen Ansteckung durchaus zu bewahren, kürzlich und bestimmt vorgetragen wird von Dr. Osterhammer. viii, 9–166 pp. 8°. *Salzburg, F. X. Duyle,* 1819.

Nemetschke (Franciscus). * Diss. sistens conspectum morborum pharyngis, in nosocomio generali anni scholast. 1842 primo semestri tractatorum. 21 pp., 1 l. 8°. *Pragæ, A. viâ. Špinka,* 1842.

Nemnich (Philipp Andreas). Lexicon nosologicum polyglotton omnium morborum sympto-

Nemnich (Philipp Andreas)—continued. matum vitiorumque naturæ et affectionum propria nomina decem diversis linguis explicata continens. 77 l. fol. *Hamburgi, C. Müller,* 1801.

Nemours, *Algeria.*
Warner. Note sur le climat, la flore et la météorologie de Nemours (Algérie). Rec. de mém. de méd. . . . mil., Par., 1875, 3. s., xxxi, 615–626.

Nemours, *France.*
Rose. Topographie de la ville et de l'hôpital de Nemours. J. de méd., chir., pharm., etc., Par., 1786, lxvi, 193–223.

von Nencki (Marcellus) [1847–   ]. * Die Oxydation der aromatischen Verbindungen im Thierkörper. 28 pp., 2 l. 8°. *Berlin, Gebr. Unger,* [1870].
———. Ueber die Zersetzung der Gelatine und des Eiweisses bei der Fäulniss mit Pankreas. 1 p. l., 38 pp., 1 pl. 4°. *Bern, J. Dalp,* 1876.

Nendtvich (Carolus Max.) * Diss. exhibens enumerationem plantarum in territorio Quinqueecclesiensi sponte crescentium præmisso tractatu generali de natura geognostica montium, deque situ, climate et vegetatione ejusdem regionis. viii, 28 pp., 2 pl. 8°. *Budæ, typ. reg. scient. univ. Hungariæ,* [1836]. [P., v. 1328.]

Nendtvich (Károly). Az életmütlen müipari vegytannak alapismeretei. Mesteremberek, iparüzök, mindennemü vegyészek és tudomány kedvelök számára irta és az iparegyesületi felolvasásokhoz alkalmazta. Számos fába metszett rajzokkal. [Elements of inorganic and industrial chemistry.] vi (1 l.), 409, xvi pp., 1 l. 8°. *Pesten, K. A. Hartleben,* 1844.

Nenndorf.
EWE (E.) Bad Nenndorf. Ein Führer für Kurgäste. 5. Aufl. 16°. *Berlin,* 1887.
GRANDIDIER (L.) Bad Nenndorf. Physicalisch, chemisch und medicinisch dargestellt. 2. Aufl. 8°. *Berlin,* 1868.
RIGLER (J.) Bad Nenndorf. Denkschrift zum hundertjährigen Bestehen des Bades. 8°. *Berlin,* 1887.
WURZER (F.) Physikalisch-chemische Beschreibung der Schwefelquellen zu Nendorf, nebst vorangeschickten Bemerkungen über die Zerlegung der Mineralwasser im Allgemeinen. 8°. *Cassel u. Marburg,* 1815.
———. Das Neueste über die Schwefelquellen zu Nendorf, in der kurhessischen Grafschaft Schaumburg. 8°. *Leipzig,* 1824.
Baldinger (E. G.) Nenndorfs Mineralwässer, aus der Quelle selbst geschöpft und getrunken. N. Mag. f. Aerzte, Leipz., 1790, xii, 289–293.—**Grandidier.** Bad Nenndorf bei Hautkrankheiten. Allg. med. Centr.-Ztg., Berl., 1863, xxxii, 25–30. — **Neussel.** Mittheilung aus Bad Nenndorf. *Ibid.,* 1875, xliv, 377.—**d'Oleira.** Bemerkungen über die Schwefelwasserstoff-Gasbäder in Nenndorf. Jahrb. f. Deutschl. Heilq. u. Seebäder, Berl., 1836, i, 375–382.—**Schröter** (L. P.) Das Neueste von den asphaltischen kalten Schwefelquellen zu Nenndorf in der Grafschaft Schaumburg. N. Mag. f. Aerzte, Leipz., 1789, xi, 193–228, 1 map. ———. Versuch einer historischen Nachricht von den Anlagen und Einrichtungen bey den Schwefelquellen zu Nenndorf. *Ibid.,* 1791, xiii, 289–316. ———. Nenndorfer Brunnen-Nachricht. *Ibid.,* 1793, xv, 487 : xvi, 193. ———. Ueber die bestätigte Wirkung des Nenndorfer Schwefelwassers, nebst einigen Bemerkungen über die künstlichen Schwefelbäder. J. d. pract. Arznk. u. Wundarznk., Jena, 1800, ix, 3. St., 26–51.—**Tünnermann** (J.) Chemisch-physikalische Untersuchung der Schwefelquellen zu Nenndorf. Ein Beleg für eine neue Methode den Schwefelwasserstoff der Schwefelwässer qualitativ und quantitativ zu bestimmen. Arch. f. Chem. u. Meteor., Nürnb., 1832, vi, 1; 129.—**Waitz** (A. C.) Ueber die Bäder zu Nenndorf. N. Mag. f. Aerzte, Leipz., 1790, xii, 52–60. ———. Ueber Erfahrungen in Bädern, mit besonderer Hinsicht auf Nenndorf. J. d. pract. Arznk. u. Wundarznk., Berl., 1803, xvi, 2. St., 5–102. ———. Neue Beobachtungen über die Bestandtheile und Würkungen des Nenndorfer Bades. *Ibid.,* 1804, xviii, 1. St., 87–94. ———. Ueber die Schlammbäder zu Nenndorf, mit Beziehung auf die dortigen Schwefelwasserbäder und deren Wirkungen. J. d. pract. Heilk., Berl., 1830, lxx, 1 St., 7–122.

Nenter (Georgius Philippus) [–1721]. Epistola de motibus naturæ in morbis prudenter tractandis ad B. G. Garmannum de cautelis in hæmorrhoidum curatione observandis disputantem. 3 l. 4°. [*Argentinæ*, 1715.]

——. Theoriæ hominis ægroti sive pathologiæ medicæ pars generalis, quæ remotis inutilibus ea tantum quæ ad praxin vere medicam necessaria sunt tradit. Præmissa est introductio de nævis pathologiæ modernæ et activo in morbis. 3 p. l., 255 pp., 10 l. 12°. *Argentorati, typ. J. Beckii*, 1716.

——. Fundamenta medicinæ theoretico-practica, secundum ... Stahlii potissimum, aliorumque ... medicorum placita conscripta, et propria experientia confirmata, in forma tabularum universam theoriam medicam, praxin generalem et specialem omnium morborum internorum, cum signis, differentiis, prognosi, remediis polychrestis, selectis et specificis, methodo medendi planissima, formulis necessariis et cautelis practicis continentium, exhibita. 24 p. l., 443, 408 pp. 4°. *Argentorati, sumpt. J. R. Dulssckeri*, 1718.

——. The same. 2. ed. xx, 406 pp. fol. *Venetiis, S. Coleti*, 1753.

Nentwig (Ferdinandus Amandus) [1800–]. * Diss. chirurgico-pathologica sistens casus post amputationem artuum majorum secundarios. vi, 31 pp., 1 l. 8°. *Vratislaviæ, typ. Kupferianis*, [1825].

——. Cudowa und seine Heilquellen. iv, 136 pp. 8°. *Breslau, A. Gosohorsky*, 1861.

Neo (Cirillo). Gli amori delle donne. Saggio di critica erotico-femminile ... che può far seguito agli amori degli uomini del Prof. Paolo Mantegazza. 60 pp., 1 l. 12°. *Milano*, 1886.

Neoplasms.
See **Pathology**; **Tumors**.

Neovin (Ott. Jo. Michaele). Cœcus de colore judicans. 11 l. 4°. *Jenæ, typ. J. J. Bauhoferi*, [1682].

Nepal.
See **Cholera** (*Asiatic, History, etc., of*), by localities.

Nepaline.
See **Aconite**, etc.

Nepaul.
Wright (D.) A few notes from Nepaul. Indian M. Gaz., Calcutta, 1867, ii, 170; 194.

Nepentha destillatoria.
Slevogtius (J. H.) [Pr.] de bandura Ceylonensium. 4°. *Jenæ*, [1719].

Nepenthe.
Gregorius (I. F.) Νηπενθὴς ἀθανασίας veterum strictim exponit. 4°. *Laubæ*, [1756].
Marquis. Recherches sur le népenthès d'Homère. Ann. clin., Montpel., 1815, xxxvii, 242–257.

Nepeta cataria.
Antony (M.) Observations on Nepeta cataria (nep, catnep, catmint, mentha felina, seu cataria). South. M. & S. J., Augusta, 1838, ii, 74–77.

Nephelis Mexicana.
See **Leeches**.

Nephralgia.
Basham (W. R.) Nephralgia, lithuria (lithiasis), and oxaluria. Practitioner, Lond., 1874, xiii, 255–261. ——. Nephralgia. Syst. Med. (Reynolds), Lond., 1879, v, 435–445.—**Bornhaupt** (T.) Zur Pathogenese von chirurgischen Nierenleiden. St. Petersb. med. Wchnschr., 1879, iv, 405; 413.—**Brown** (A. P.) Two cases of nephralgia with calculus. Med. & Surg. Reporter, Phila., 1875, xxxii, 361.—**Cramer** (J. A.) De nephralgia. *In:* Fasc. diss. med. select (Zvingerus), 12°, Basil., 1710, 600–649. —**Hulke.** Nephralgia; simulation of renal calculus; exploration of kidney. Lancet, Lond., 1887, ii, 1064.—**Kirkham** (F. W.) Nephralgia due to malarial poisoning. Med. Times & Gaz., Lond., 1885, i, 443.—**Lauder** (R.)

Nephralgia.
Acute nephralgia; cause, malaria. Proc. Connect. M. Soc., Hartford, 1886, n. s., iii, no. 3, 199–201.—**Malécot** (A.) De la néphralgie simulant la colique rénale. France méd., Par., 1887, ii, 1509–1511.—**de Mignot** (P.) Observations de néphralgie essentielle guérie par le sulfate de quinine. J. de méd. et chir. prat., Par., 1846, xvii, 155–159.—**Texier** (H.) Note sur la néphralgie. Monit. d. sc. méd. et pharm., Par., 1860, 2. s., ii, 121; 131.

Nephrectomy.
See **Kidney** (*Surgery of*).

Nephria.
See **Bright's** *disease*.

Nephritis.
See **Bright's** *disease*; **Calculus** (*Renal*); **Kidney** (*Abscess in*); **Kidney** (*Inflammation of*).
Nephrologia nova et curiosa. *See* **Tiling** (Matthæus).

Nephrops.
Bellonci (G.) Sui lobi olfactorî del Nephrops norwegicus. Mem. Accad. d. sc. d. Ist. di Bologna, 1880, 4. s., i, 429–431, 1 pl.

Nephrorrhagia.
See **Kidney** (*Hæmorrhage in or from*).

Nephrotomy.
See **Kidney** (*Surgery of*).

Nepi.
Ratti (F.) Analisi chimica delle acque minerali di Nepi. Idrologia, Firenze, 1884, vi, 88.

Nepilly (Carl) [1838–]. * Die Blasenscheidenfistel und ihre Operation. 1 p. l., 30 pp., 1 l. 8°. *Breslau, F. W. Jungfer*, [1868].

Nepple (P.-Frédéric) [1787–]. * Diss. de physiologie pathologique sur les fausses membranes et les adhérences. vi, 7–27 pp. 4°. *Paris*, 1812, No. 56, v. 88.

——. Essai sur les fièvres rémittentes et intermittentes des pays marécageux tempérés. 307 pp. 8°. *Paris, Gabon*, 1828.

——. The same. Traité sur les fièvres rémittentes et intermittentes, leurs symptômes et leur traitement. 307 pp. 8°. *Paris, J. Rouvier & E. Le Bouvier*, 1835.

Nepveu (Gustave). * Des gangrènes dans les fractures. 52 pp. 4°. *Paris*, 1870, No. 273.

——. Contribution à l'étude des tumeurs du testicule. 60 pp., 2 pl. 8°. *Paris, A. Delahaye*, 1872.

——. Contribution à l'étude des tumeurs mélaniques. 16 pp., 1 pl., 2 l. 8°. *Paris*, 1872. [P., v. 797.]
Repr. from: Gaz. méd. de Par., 1872, 4. s., i.

——. Du rôle des organismes inférieurs dans les lésions chirurgicales. 52 pp. 8°. *Paris*, [*Cusset & Cie.*], 1875. [P., v. 797.]
Repr. from: Gaz. méd. de Par., 1875, 4. s., iv.

——. De l'emploi du chloral en injections souscutanées dans le traitement de la cholérine et du choléra à la période algide. 7 pp. 8°. *Paris, E. Rousset & Cie.*, 1882.
Repr. from: Gaz. méd. de Par., 1873, 4. s., ii.

——. Des bactéries dans l'érysipèle. 8 pp. 8°. *Paris, P. Larousse & Cie.*, 1885.
Repr. from: Compt. rend. Soc. de biol., Par., 1870, xxii.

——. Exposé des titres et travaux scientifiques. 23 pp. 4°. *Paris*, 1887.

Nepveu (Pierre-Ferdinand). * Sur le cancer de l'estomac, considéré comme l'une des terminaisons de la gastrite chronique. 24 pp. 4°. *Paris*, 1821, No. 139, v. 167.

Nerac.
Mondineu (L.-G.) * De quelques considérations sur la pathogénie et l'hygiène des Landes de l'arrondissement de Nérac. 4°. *Paris*, 1867.

Nérard (Jean-Baptiste). * Des indications de l'accouchement prématuré artificiel et d'un nouvel instrument pour exciter les contractions uté-

Nérard (Jean-Baptiste)—continued.
rines et dilater le col. 48 pp., 1 l. 4°. *Montpellier, Boehm & fils*, 1867, No. 43. c.

Nerat (Octave). *De la grippe, considérée dans ses rapports avec la climatologie. 34 pp. 4°. *Paris*, 1851, No. 127, v. 512.

Nerbonneau (Auguste). *Sur la constipation. 17 pp. 4°. *Paris*, 1818, No. 160, v. 140.

Nercam (I.) [1857–   ]. *Action hypnotique et sédative de la paraldéhyde dans les différentes formes d'aliénation mentale. 108 pp., 1 l. 4°. *Paris*, 1884, No. 363.

Neret (Charles-Severin). * Sur le typhus contagieux. 39 pp. 4°. *Paris*, 1814, No. 110, v. 104.

Nerf (Joannes Baptista).
See **Morasch** (Joannes Adamus). Nucleus physiologicus, etc. 16°. *Eustadii*, 1711.

Nerfs (Les) et les eaux de Vichy, dosage dermoscopique, méthode du Dr. Collongues, médecin consultant à Vichy. 23 pp. 18°. *Paris, L. & J. Rainal frères*, [*n. d.*]

Neri (Giuseppe). Il colera a S. Miniato nell' estate del 1855. 35 pp. 8°. *Bastia, Fabiani*, [1856].
Repr. from : Raccoglitore med. di Fano, 1856, 2. s., xiv.

Nerici (Ugo). Correzione di alcune deformità dei piedi. 15 pp., 2 pl. 8°. *Lucca, tip. Canovetti*, 1885.

———. Un pezzo di siringa elastica in vescica estratta con litrontritore. 4 pp. 8°. [*Milano*], *F. Vallardi*, 1885.
Repr. from : Gazz. d. osp., Milano, 1885, vi.

Néris.
BAYARD (P.-L.-E.) *Étude sur Néris-les-Bains et ses eaux thermales. 4°. *Paris*, 1873.

BONNET DE MALHERBE. Guide médical aux eaux de Néris. 12°. *Paris*, 1872.

DE LAURÈS (C.) & BECQUEREL (A.) Recherches sur les conferves des eaux thermales de Néris, sur leur développement, leur structure intime, leurs usages en thérapeutique, etc. 8°. *Paris*, 1855.

MAURIN (A.) Étude historique et clinique sur les eaux minérales de Néris. 12°. *Paris*, 1858.

Becquerel (A.) & de Laurès. Mémoire sur les conferves des eaux thermales de Néris. Ann. Soc. d'hydrol. méd. de Par. Compt.-rend., 1854–5, i, 205–244.—Boirot-Desserviers (P.) Recherches historiques et observations médicales sur les eaux thermales et minérales de Néris en Bourbonnais, département de l'Allier. N. Jour. de méd., chir., pharm., etc., Par., 1822, xiv, 52–55. Also, Reprint.—Bonnet de Malherbe. Eaux minérales de Néris. Tic rotatoire de la tête et du cou, ou hyperkinésie de l'accessoire de Willis. Union méd., Par., 1876, 3. s., xxi, 640–642.—Bouchet. Souvenirs de Néris. Ann. Soc. de méd. de Lyon, 1855, 2. s., iii, 239–247. — de Faivard-Montluc. Précis sur l'aménagement des eaux thermales de Néris (Allier), précédé de quelques réflexions sur les eaux minérales en général, et d'un énoncé sommaire des propriétés physiques, chimiques et médicales de celles de Néris. Rev. méd. franç. et étrang., Par., 1841, ii, 161–212.—Greffier (L.) Communication sur les eaux minérales de Néris. J. de méd. et pharm. de l'Isère, Grenoble, 1885–6, x, 217–220.—Lefort (J.) Étude pour servir à l'histoire des gaz des eaux minérales en général et des eaux thermales de Néris en particulier. Ann. Soc. d'hydrol. méd. de Par. Compt.-rend., 1865–6, xii, 155–162. ———. Études chimiques sur les eaux minérales et thermales de Néris (Allier). *Ibid.*, 1867–8, xiv, 316–383.—Michel. Description et analyse des eaux minérales de Néris, près Montluçon ; leurs vertus, et les maladies auxquelles elles conviennent. J. de méd., chir., pharm., etc., Par., 1766, xxv, 159–174.—Nicolas (J.) Néris-les-Bains et ses eaux minérales. Soc. d. sc. méd. de Gannat. Compt. rend. 1883–4, Par., 1884, xxxviii, 129–131.—Philippe. Mémoire sur les eaux thermales de Néris en Bourbonnois. J. de méd., chir., pharm., etc., Par., 1786, lxvi, 94–113.—de Ranse (F.) Aperçu général des indications et des contre-indications des eaux de Néris. Gaz. méd. de Par., 1875, 4. s., iv, 129 ; 138 ; 164 ; 189. ———. De l'action des eaux de Néris dans le traitement des maladies des femmes. *Ibid.*, 1877, 4. s., vi, 107 ; 121 ; 131 ; 157 ; 168 ; 180 ; 208 ; 219 ; 230. ———. De l'action thérapeutique des eaux de Néris dans le traitement des maladies du système nerveux. Ann. Soc. d'hydrol. méd. de Par. Compt.-rend., 1882–3, xxviii, 512–528.—Robiquet. Réflexions sur les eaux thermales de Néris. J. de chim. méd., etc., Par., 1835, 2. s., i, 617–621.

Néris-Mondesir (Jean-Joseph-Rémy). * Sur le tétanos. 42 pp. 4°. *Paris*, 1842, No. 63, v. 393.

Nerium *Oleander* [*and odorum*].
Broughton (F.) Case of vegetable poisoning. Tr. M. & Phys. Soc. Bombay (1857–8), 1859, n. s., iv (app.), pp. iv–vi.—Empoisonnement par la cigue des jardins et par le laurier-rose. J. de chim. méd., etc., Par., 1843, 2. s., ix, 392–394.—Finocchi (E.) Considerazioni sopra un importante argomento tossicologico. [Oleander.] Orosi, Firenze, 1881, iv, 257–260.—Kohlmann. Vergiftung durch Oleanderblätter bei Thieren. Centralbl. f. klin. Med. Bonn, 1880, i, 161.—Kurzak. Die giftigen Wirkungen des Oleanders (Nerium oleander L.). Ztschr. d. k.-k. Gesellsch. d. Aerzte zu Wien, 1859, xv, 690 ; 785 ; 801. — Larue du Barry (J.) Empoisonnement par le nérion, laurier-rose. J. de chim. méd., etc., Par., 1843, 2. s., ix, 535–538.—Murray (T.) Case of poisoning from the oleander root (Nerium odorum). Indian M. Gaz., Calcutta, 1877, xii, 319.—Pelikan (E.) K' toksikologii oleandra. [Toxicology of the oleander.] Med. Vestnik, St. Petersb., 1866, vi, 1–4. Also, transl.: Gaz. d. hôp., Par., 1866, xxxix, 70. Also, transl.: Compt. rend. Acad. d. sc., Par., 1866, lxii, 237–241. — Sibthorpe (C.) Case of poisoning by Nerium odorum. Indian M. Gaz., Calcutta, 1881, xvi, 15.—Wessinger (J. A.) Nerium oleander ; its poisonous properties. Detroit Clinic, 1882, i, 389.

Nero.
Lisic. Quelques applications de la physiologie et de la médecine à l'étude de l'histoire. Gaz. méd. de Par., 1838, 2. s., vi, 97 ; 145.

Neron (P.) * Sur la bile, comme cause de maladies, et sur ses usages dans l'économie animale. 19 pp. 4°. *Paris, an XII* [1803], No. 130, v. E.

Neroni (Vincenzo). Sopra alcuni punti della terapia delle fratture e più particolarmente del metodo inamovibile. 34 pp. roy. 8°. *Reggio nell' Emilia, L. Bondavalli & Comp.*, 1870.

Neroutsos (Tassos D.) Ἡ χολέρα ἐν Αἰγύπτῳ κατὰ τὰ ἔτη 1865 καὶ 1866. 304 pp. 8°. Ἀλεξάνδρεια, 1867.

Nerve (*Accessory*) *of Willis.*
See **Nerve** (*Spinal accessory*).

Nerve (*Anterior tibial*).
Cunningham (D. J.) Note on the distribution of the anterior tibial nerve on the dorsum of the foot. J. Anat. & Physiol., Lond., 1878–9, xiii, 398.

Nerve (*Auditory*).
See, also, **Cochlea**; **Labyrinth.**
CZERMAK (J. N.) Verästelung der Primitivfasern des Nervus acusticus. 8°. *Breslau*, 1849.

HORBACKZEWSKI (J.) Ueber den Nervus vestibuli. 8°. [*n. p., n. d.*]

LAVDOVSKI (M.) *Gistologija kontsevago apparata ulitkovago nerva. [Histology of terminal apparatus of acoustic nerves.] 8°. *St. Petersburg*, 1874.

Baginsky (B.) Ueber den Ursprung und den centralen Verlauf des Nervus acusticus des Kaninchens. Arch. f. path. Anat., etc., Berl., 1886, cv, 28–46, 1 pl. — Blake (C. J.) Summary of observations on the effect of the galvanic current upon the auditory nerve. Arch. Scient. & Pract. M. & S., N. Y., 1873, i, 326–332.—Brenner. Untersuchungen über die physiologische Reaction des Nervus acusticus bei Einwirkung des constanten (galvanischen) Stromes. St. Petersb. med. Ztschr., 1863, iv, 315–319. ———. Zur Geschichte der Reizung des Hörnerven durch elektrische Ströme. Deutsches Arch. f. klin. Med., Leipz., 1868, iv, 436–448.—Brown-Séquard (E.) The auditive nerve is a nervous centre. Med. Exam., Phila., 1853, ix, 490. —. Remarques sur la physiologie du cervelet et du nerf auditif. J. de la physiol. de l'homme, Par., 1862, v, 484–492. — Cyon (E.) Les organes périphériques du sens de l'espace. Compt. rend. Acad. d. sc., Par., 1877, lxxxv, 1284. — Duval. Sur le nerf acoustique et le sens de l'espace. Compt. rend. Soc. de biol. 1881, Par., 1881, 7. s., ii, 91.—Edinger (L.) Notiz, die Striæ acusticæ betreffend. Nachtrag zu : Ueber die Verbindung der sensibelen Nerven mit dem Zwischenhirn. Anat. Anz., Jena, 1887, ii, 239.—Erlitski (A.) O stroenii stvola sluchovago nerva. [Structure of auditory nerve.] Vrach. Vaidom., St. Petersb., 1881, vi, 2419 ; 2433. Also, transl.: Pam. Towarz. Lek. Warszaw., 1882, lxxviii, 63–77, 1 pl. Also, transl.: Arch. de neurol., Par., 1882, iii, 36–53, 1 pl.—Ferré (G.) Des ganglions intra-rocheux du nerf auditif chez l'homme. Compt. rend. Acad. d. sc., Par., 1885, c, 862–865. — Forel (A.) Vorläufige Mittheilung über den Ursprung des Nervus acusticus. Neurol. Centralbl., Leipz.,

Nerve (*Auditory*).

1885, iii, 101–103. — **Forel** (A.) & **Onufrowicz** (B.) Weitere Mittheilung über den Ursprung des Nervus acusticus. *Ibid.*, iv, 193. — **Freud** (S.) Ueber den Ursprung des N. acusticus. Monatschr. f. Ohrenh., Berl., 1886, xx, 245; 277. — **Katolinsky** (A.) Recherches sur les phénomènes physiologiques dus à l'irritation du nerf auditif par le courant galvanique continu et sur l'emploi de ce courant comme moyen diagnostique dans les maladies de l'oreille. J. de la physiol. de l'homme, Par., 1863, vi, 193 - 203.— **Kiesselbach** (W.) Ueber die galvanische Reizung des Acusticus. Arch. f. d. ges. Physiol., Bonn, 1883, xxxi, 95; 377. — **Onufrowicz** (B.) Experimenteller Beitrag zur Kenntniss des Ursprungs des Nervus acusticus des Kaninchens. Arch. f. Psychiat., Berl., 1885, xvi, 711–742, 2 pl. *Also:* Centralbl. f. Vet.-Wissensch., Leipz., 1886, iv, 81. — **Pierret.** Des origines centrales du nerf auditif. Bull. Soc. anat. de Par., 1876, li, 553–556. *Also:* Progrès méd., Par., 1877, v, 52. — **Retzius** (G.) Ueber die peripherische Endigungsweise des Gehörnerven. Biol. Untersuch., Stockholm, 1881, i, 51–60, 1 pl. — **Roller** (C. F. W.) Eine aufsteigende Acusticuswurzel. Arch. f. mikr. Anat., Bonn, 1880, xviii, 403–408, 1 pl. ——. In Sachen der aufsteigenden Acusticuswurzel. Arch. f. Psychiat., Berl., 1883, xiv, 458–460. — **Sandifort** (E.) De dure quodam corpusculo, nervo auditorio adhærente. *In his:* Obs. anat.-patol., 4°, Lugd. Bat., 1777, i. 116–120. — **Schultze** (M.) Ueber die Endigungsweise der Hörnerven im Labyrinth. Arch. f. Anat., Physiol. u. wissensch. Med., Berl., 1858, 343–381, 1 pl — **Sitsyanko** (I.) Opiti nad vliyaniem galvanicheskago toka na slukhovie nervi. [Experiments on the effect of galvanic current on the auditory nerves.] Med. Vestnik, St. Petersb., 1867, vii, 177; 185.— **Winkler** (C.) Over den oorsprung van den nervus acusticus. Nederl. Tijdschr. v. Geneesk., Amst., 1886, 2. R., xxii, 1. d., 526–529. — **Wolf** (O.) Ligation of the common carotid artery, after a gun shot wound, on account of copious hemorrhage; tinnitus aurium and deafness; diagnosis of the position of the ball from the condition of the ear; accoustic and physiological remarks. Arch. Ophth. & Otol., N. Y., 1871–2, ii, 58–75.— **Zaufal** (E.) Ueber eine eigenthümliche Reflexübertragung auf den Nervus acusticus. Wien. med. Wchnschr., 1872, xxii, 517–520.

Nerve (*Auditory, Pathology of*).

Boettcher (A.) Ueber die Veränderungen der Netzbaut und des Labyrinths in einem Fall von Fibrosarcom des Nervus acusticus. Arch. f. Augen- u. Ohrenh., Carlsruhe, 1871–2, ii, pt. 2, 87–115, 2 pl. *Also, transl.:* Arch. Ophth. & Otol., N. Y., 1873–4, iii, 134–172, 2 pl.— **Brenner.** Zur Elektrophysiologie und Elektropathologie des Nervus acusticus. St. Petersb. med. Ztschr., 1863, iv, 286–296. *Also, Reprint.* — **Eulenburg** (A.) Eine ungewöhnliche Anomalie der galvanischen Reaction des N. acusticus. Berl. klin. Wchnschr., 1869, vi, 408. ——. Ueber eine noch nicht beobachtete Modification der galvanischen Reaction des N. acusticus. Deutsches Arch. f. klin. Med., Leipz., 1869,[v, 547–552.— **Foerster** (A.) Sarkom des linken Acusticus, Hydrocephalus internus, Typhus. Würzb. med. Ztschr., 1862, iii, 199. — **Malassez.** Névromes des nerfs auditifs, chez une femme syphilitique. Bull. Soc. anat. de Par., 1868, xliii, 317–320.— **Moos** (S.) Zur Diagnose der absoluten Acusticuslähmung; Beitrag zur Pathologie der Medulla oblongata. Arch. f. Augen- u. Ohrenh., Carlsruhe, 1871–2, ii, pt. 1, 115–119. *Also, transl.:* Arch. Ophth. & Otol., N. Y., 1871, ii, 199–203. ——. Ein Fall von Sarcom des linken Gehörnerven mit fettiger Metamorphose und theilweisen Untergang des Corti'schen Organs. Arch. f. Augen- u. Ohrenh., Wiesb., 1874–5, iv, 179–191. *Also, transl.:* Arch. Ophth. & Otol., N. Y., 1875, iv, 483–496. ——. Ueber das Vorkommen und die Bedeutung phosphorsaurer Kalkconcremente im Stamme des Gehörnerven. Arch. f. Psychiat., Berl., 1878, ix, 122–128.— **Moos** (S.) & **Steinbrügge** (H.) Ueber Nervenatrophie in der ersten Schneckenwindung; physiologische und pathologische Bedeutung derselben. Ztschr. f. Ohrenh., Wiesb., 1880–81, x, 1–15, 1 pl. *Also, transl.:* Arch. Otol., N. Y., 1881, x, 1–16, 1 pl. ——. Ueber acute Degenerationen der Hörnerven im Gefolge einer mit Pyämie complicirten Pachymeningitis hämorrhagica, sowie über gleichzeitig vorhandene Verstopfung der rechten Art. auditiva int. Ztschr. f. Ohrenh., Wiesb., 1881–2, xi, 287–293. *Also, transl.:* Arch. Otol., N. Y., 1882, xi, 322–327.— **Neftel** (W. B.) Abnormal galvanic reaction of the acoustic nerve in chlorosis and Bright's disease. Arch. Scient. & Pract. M. & S., N. Y., 1873, i, 26–29.— **Robert** (J.) Nuevo tratamiento de la parálisis de los nervios auditivos. Rev. de med. y cirug. práct., Madrid, 1879, v, 97–99.— **Roosa** (D. B. St.-J.) A case of syphilitic disease of the auditory nerves (or cochlea). Arch. Dermat., N. Y., 1875, i, 228. ——. The clinical diagnosis of acoustic neuritis and of atrophy of the acoustic nerve. Arch. Otol., N. Y., 1881, x, 210–219. *Also, transl.:* Ztschr. f. Ohrenh., Wiesb., 1881–2, xi, 9–17.— **Stevens** (G. T.) A case of tumor of the auditory nerve occupying the fossa for the cerebellum. Arch. Otol., N. Y., 1879, viii, 171–176. *Also, transl.:* Ztschr. f. Ohrenh., Wiesb., 1879, viii, 290–294.— **Toynbee.** Neuroma of the auditory nerve. Tr. Path. Soc. Lond., 1850–52,

Nerve (*Auditory, Pathology of*).

iii, 49: 1852-3, iv, 259, 1 pl.— **Urbantschitsch** (V.) Beobachtungen über centrale Acusticusaffectionen. Arch. f. Ohrenh, Leipz., 1880–81, xvi, 171–187.— **Zaufal** (E.) Ueber eine eigenthümliche Reflexübertragung auf den Nervus acusticus. Wien. med. Wchnschr., 1872, xxii, 517–520.

Nerve (*Circumflex*).

Nicaise. Névrite du nerf circonflexe. France méd., Par., 1874, xxi, 51.

Nerve (*Ethmoid*).

See **Neurotomy**, *etc.*

Nerve (*Facial*).

See, also, **Chorda** *tympani*; **Face** (*Nerves of*); **Nerve - stretching**; **Neuralgia** (*Facial, etc.*); **Neurotomy**, *etc.*; **Paralysis** (*Facial*).

BERNARD (C.) On the alteration of the taste in paralysis of the facial nerve. [Transl. by H. L. Thomas.] 8°. *Richmond*, 1853.

GAEDECHENS (B.) * Nervi facialis physiologia et pathologia. 4°. *Heidelbergæ*, [1832].

LIÉGEOIS (A.-T.) * Physiologie du nerf facial. 4°. *Paris*, 1858.

MASSALIEN (H. O.) * De nervo faciali. 4°. *Berolini*, [1836].

RUEHLE (H.) * Experimentorum de nervi facialis functionibus factorum expositio critica. 8°. *Berolini*, [1846].

Beaunis. Présentation d'un lapin (arrachement du facial). Compt. rend. Soc. de biol., Par., 1887, 3. s., iv, 205.— **Bell** (C.) On the origin and compound functions of the facial nerve, or portio dura of the seventh nerve. Tr. Roy. Soc. Edinb., 1836, xiv, 229–236. *Also, in his:* Three papers on the nerves, 4°, Edinb., 1838, 7–14.— **Bérard.** Sur les fonctions du nerf facial et la paralysie de la face. J. d. conn. méd.-chir., Par., 1834–5, ii, 354: 1835–6, iii, 6.— **Bernard** (C.) Nouvelles expériences sur le nerf facial. Compt. rend. Soc. de biol. 1857, Par., 1859, 2. s., iv, 59.— **Bochefontaine.** Sur un procédé pour la section intra-crânienne du nerf facial chez le chien. *Ibid.*, 1879, Par., 1880, 7. s., i, pt. 2, 165–180. *Also:* Gaz. méd. de Par., 1880, 6. s., ii, 314; 547.— **Boudant.** [Note sur les fonctions du nerf facial.] Bull. Soc. anat. de Par. 1829, 2. éd., 1846, vi, 33.— **Dalby** (W. B.) Case of wound of the portio dura, causing facial palsy. Tr. Clin. Soc. Lond., 1872–3, iv, 67.— **Exner** (S.) & **Paneth** (J.) Das Rindenfeld des Facialis und seine Verbindungen bei Hund und Kaninchen. Arch. f. d. ges. Physiol., Bonn, 1887, xli, 349–358. — **Franck** (F.) Sur le rôle du nerf facial dans l'innervation vasculaire des organes glandulaires. Cong. période. internat. d. sc. méd. Compt.-rend. 1875, Brux. & Par., 1876, iv, 483–488. *Also:* Gaz. hebd. de méd., Par., 1875, 2. s., xii, 691–694. — **Frühwald** (F.) Ueber die Verbinduug des Nervus petrosus superficialis major mit dem Genu nervi facialis. Sitzungsb. d. k. Akad. d. Wissensch. Math.-naturw. Cl., Wien, 1877, lxxiv, 9–12, 1 pl.— **Gowers** (W. R.) Ueber den sogenannten Facialis-Abducenskern. Centralbl. f. d. med. Wissensch., Berl., 1878, xvi, 417.— **Graves** (R. J.) On the prognosis to be derived from affections of the portio dura of seventh pair of nerves. Dublin J. M. Sc., 1841–2, xx, 399–404.— **Gros.** [Rameau lingual du nerf facial.] Bull Soc. anat. de Par., 1846, xxi, 111–113.— **Gruber** (J.) Zur Casuistik der Entzündung des Nervus facialis innerhalb des Canalis Fallopiæ. Wien. Med.-Halle, 1869, iv, 377.— **Gruber** (W.) Ungewöhnliche Lage des Nervus facialis in der Parotis zu den Gefässen. Arch. f. path. Anat., etc., Berl, 1872, liv, 190.— **Hallopeau.** Recherches qui peuvent servir à déterminer partiellement le trajet intra-cérébral du rameau supérieur du facial. Compt. rend. Soc. de biol. 1879, Par., 1880, 7. s., i, 244–246. *Also:* Rev. méd. franç. et étrang., Par., 1879, ji, 161–163.— **Jobert** (*de Lamballe*). Origine du nerf facial au-dessous de l'entrecroisement des pyramides; explication anatomique de la paralysie croisée de ce nerf. Compt. rend. Soc. de biol. 1850, Par., 1851, ii, 5.— **Jolyet** & **Laffont.** Nouveau procédé de section du facial dans le crâne. *Ibid.* (1879), 1880, 7. s., i, 334–336.— **Krenchel** (V.) Onderzoekingen over de gevolgen van gezichtszenuw-doorsnijding bij den kikvorsch. Versl. . . . Nederl. Gasth. v. Ooglijders, Utrecht, 1874, xv, 28–35.— **Le Bidois** fils. Observations et réflexions sur les maladies du nerf facial. J. hebd. de méd., Par., 1829. v, 114–117.— **Longet** (A.) Documents et recherches sur quelques points douteux de l'anatomie et de la physiologie du nerf facial. Ann. méd.-psych., Par., 1843, i, 232 - 255. — **Martin-Magron** & **Brown-Séquard.** Du tournoiement et du roulement consécutifs à l'arrachement du nerf facial. Compt. rend. Soc. de biol. 1849, Par., 1850, i, pt. 1, 133.— **Pini** (G.) Ricerche sul nervo facciale. Ann. univ. di med., Milano, 1870, ccxiv, 421–428.— **Rabl** (K.) Ueber

Nerve (*Facial*).

das Gebiet des Nervus facialis. Anat. Anz., Jena, 1887, ii, 219–227.—**Raymond.** Sur l'origine corticale du facial inférieur. Gaz. méd. de Par., 1884, 7. s., i, 241; 253.—**Schmid.** Fall von Verletzung des Ramus superior nervi facialis. Deutsche Klinik, Berl., 1852, iv, 444.—**Stowell** (T. B.) The facial nerve in the domestic cat. Proc. Am. Phil. Soc., Phila., 1887, xxiv, 8–18, 1 diag. *Also,* Reprint.

Nerve (*Glosso-pharyngeal*).

See, also, **Nerves** (*Cranial, Eighth pair of*).

KILIAN (H. F.) Anatomische Untersuchungen über das neunte Hirnnervenpaar, oder den Nervus glossopharyngeus. 4°. *Pesth,* 1822.
Barbarisi (G.) Sulla triplice potenza del nervo glosso faringeo. Rendic. Accad. med.-chir. di Napoli, 1851, v, 31–39, 1 pl. [Relat. de A. de Martini], 92.—**Coyne.** Le nerf glosso-pharyngien. Dict. encycl. d. sc. méd., Par., 1883, 4. s., ix, 273–286.—**Obersteiner** (H.) Der centrale Ursprung des Nervus glossopharyngeus. Biol. Centralbl., Erlang., 1881–2, i, 470–472.—**Roller** (C. F. W.) Der centrale Verlauf des Nervus glossopharyngeus; der Nucleus lateralis medius. Arch. f. mikr. Anat., Bonn, 1880–81, xix, 347–383, 2 pl.

Nerve (*Gustatory*).

See Tongue (*Nerves of*).

Nerve (*Gustatory, Section of*).

See Tongue (*Surgery of*).

Nerve (*Hypoglossal*).

BOEHMER (J. F. W.) * De nono pare nervorum cerebri. 4°. *Gottingæ,* 1777.
Also, in: SCRIPT. neurol. minores selecti. 4°. *Lipsiæ,* 1791, i, 279–309, 1 pl.
Ballard (E.) Case of paralysis of the hypoglossal nerve, followed by sloughing of the tongue. Med. Times & Gaz., Lond., 1869, i, 296.—**Brinton.** Abnormal communication between the two hypoglossal nerves. Tr. Path. Soc. Lond., 1848–9, ii, 30.—**Friedlowsky** (A.) Ueber einen Fall von anormalem Verlauf des Nervus hypoglossus, mit besonderer Berücksichtigung der Unterbindung der Arteria lingualis. Allg. Wien. med. Ztg., 1868, xiii, 131.—**Gerlach** (J.) Ueber die Kreuzungsverhältnisse in dem centralen Verlaufe des Nerv. hypoglossus. Ztschr. f. rat. Med., Leipz. u. Heidelb., 1869, 3. R., xxxiv, 1–8, 1 pl.—**Habershon** (S. O.) Cancerous disease of the breast and vertebræ; enlargement of the glands; paralysis of the right hypoglossal nerve; wasting of one side of the tongue and of the muscles of the neck. Guy's Hosp. Rep., Lond., 1872, 3. s., xvii, 423–428.—**Holl** (M.) Beobachtungen über die Anastomosen des Nervus hypoglossus. Ztschr. f. Anat. u. Entwcklngsgesch., Leipz., 1876, ii, 82–97, 1 pl.—**Iversen** (M.) Bemerkungen über die dorsalen Wurzeln des Nervus hypoglossus. Ber. d. naturf. Gesellsch. zu Freib. i. Br., 1887, ii, 33–36.—**Koch** (P. D.) Untersuchungen über den Ursprung und die Verbindungen des Nervus hypoglossus in der Medulla oblongata. Arch. f. mikr. Anat., Bonn, 1887–8, xxxi, 54–71, 1 pl.—**McMurrich** (J. P.) The ontogeny and phylogeny of the hypoglossal nerve. Science, Cambridge, 1885, v, 374.—**Neussel.** Glossoplegia articulatoria (Lähmung des N. hypoglossus). Allg. med. Centr.-Ztg., Berl., 1852, xxi, 213.—**Phillips** (J.) Section du nerf grand-hypoglosse. Gaz. d. hôp., Par., 1841, 2. s., iii, 461.—**Pierret.** Étude sur le noyau d'origine du nerf hypoglosse. Bull. Soc. anat. de Par., 1876, li, 556–558. *Also:* Progrès méd., Par., 1877, v, 53.—**Remak** (E.) Ein Fall von Hypoglossuskrampf. Verhandl. d. Berl. med. Gesellsch. (1882 3), 1884, xiv, pt. 2, 227–234. *Also:* Berl. klin. Wchnschr., 1883, xx, 513–515.—**Roller** (C. F. W.) Ein kleinzelliger Hypoglossuskern. Arch. f. mikr. Anat., Bonn, 1880–81, xix, 383–395, 2 pl.—**Vulpian** (A.) Sur la racine postérieure ou ganglionnaire du nerf hypoglosse. J. de la physiol. de l'homme, Par., 1862, v, 5–35. *Also,* Reprint.—**Wertheimer** (E.) Des anastomoses de l'hypoglosse avec les nerfs cervicaux; origine et rôle de sa branche descendante. Compt. rend. Soc. de biol., Par., 1884, 8. s., i, pt. 2, 589–591.

Nerve (*Inferior dental, Section of*).

See Neuralgia (*Dental*), *etc.*

Nerve (*Infraorbital*).

See, also, Neurotomy, *etc.*
Nawrocki (F.) O nerwach potowych glowy. [On n. infraorbitalis.] Medycyna, Warszawa, 1886, viii, 817–819.—[**Panas**.] Paralysie traumatique du nerf sousorbitaire. Gaz. d. hôp., Par., 1868, xli, 73.

Nerve (*Lachrymal*).

Manec. [Origine du nerf lachrymal.] Bull. Soc. anat. de Par., 2. éd., 1826, i, 18.

Nerve (*Lingual*).

See, also, **Neuralgia** (*Lingual*); **Tongue** (*Nerves of*).

SCHIFF (M.) Sopra due novi nervi arrestatori. Nota presentata al presidente dal socio Pietro Blaserna nel settembre 1877. 4°. [*Roma,* 1877.]
Repr. from: Atti d. r. Accad. d. Lincei. Cl. di fis., matemat. e nat., Roma, 1876–7, cclxxiv.
Bidder (F.) Beobachtung doppelsinniger Leitung im N. lingualis nach Vereinigung desselben mit dem N. hypoglossus. Arch. f. Anat., Physiol. u. wissensch. Med., Leipz., 1865, 246–260.—**Cazalis.** [Fonction des nerfs de la langue.] Bull. Soc. anat. de Par., 1838, xiii, 265.—**Cusco.** [Un filet anastomotique du nerf mylo-hyoïdien envoyé au nerf lingual.] *Ibid.,* 1847, xxii, 5.—**von Graefe** Ueber die Geschmacksfunction des Nervus lingualis beim Menschen. Berl. klin. Wchnschr., 1868, v, 485. — **Guttmann** (P.) Ueber die Function des Nervus lingualis als Geschmacksnerv. *Ibid.,* 521. — **Hutchinson.** Stab under the jaw followed by symptoms of paralysis of the lingual nerve. Med. Times & Gaz., Lond., 1872, i, 431.—**Prevost** (J.-L.) Note relative aux fonctions gustatives du nerf lingual. Compt. rend. Soc. de biol. 1868, Par., 1869, 4 s., v, 234: (1869), 1870, 5. s., i, 76. ——. Nouvelles expériences relatives aux fonctions gustatives du nerf lingual. Arch. de physiol. norm. et path., Par., 1873, v, 253; 375.—**Rosenthal** (J.) Ueber die Vereinigung des N. lingualis mit dem N. hypoglossus. Centralbl. f. d. med. Wissensch., Berl., 1864, ii, 449–452. — **de Souza** (M. B.) Resumo da communicação scientifica ácerca dos nervos do gosto. J. Soc. d. sc. méd. de Lisb., 1871, 2. s., xxxv, 13–24, 1 pl.—**Vogt** (C.) Ueber die Function des Nervus lingualis und Glosso-pharyngeus. Arch. f. Anat., Physiol. u. wissensch. Med., Berl., 1840, 72–75.—**Vulpian.** Remarques nouvelles sur l'anastomose du nerf lingual avec la corde du tympan. Compt. rend. Soc. de biol. 1873, Par., 1875, 5. s., v, 22. ——. Sur les effets vaso-moteurs produits par l'excitation du segment périphérique du nerf lingual. Compt. rend. Acad. d. sc., Par., 1882, xcv, 365–367.

Nerve (*Lingual, Section of*).

See Neurotomy, *etc.*

Nerve (*Median*).

See, also, **Nerve** (*Musculo-cutaneous*); **Neuroma; Neurotomy,** *etc.*

STRUCK (E. H.) * Diss. sistens observationem fungi medullaris nervi mediani. 4°. *Gryphiæ,* [1836].
Boeckel. Division accidentelle du nerf médian, des tendons fléchisseurs, de l'artère radiale; guérison avec retour des fonctions de la main. Gaz. méd. de Strasb., 1867, xxvii, 293.—**Calori** (L.) Sul variato rapporto vascolare delle due radici del nervo mediano e sulle condizioni atte a produrlo. Mem. Accad. d. sc. d. Ist. di Bologna, 1877, 3. s., viii, 443–456, 2 pl.—**Duret** (H.) Plaie contuse du nerf médian; troubles trophiques; escharres aux extrémités des doigts. Compt. rend. Soc. de biol. 1875, Par., 1876, 6. s., ii, 410–414. *Also:* Gaz. méd. de Par., 1876, 4. s., v, 7.—**Ferret.** Plaie par arrachement du coude; perte de substance du médian et sa suppléance fonctionnelle par le cubital. Progrès méd., Par., 1887, 2. s., v, 375.—**von Fragstein.** Zur Aetiologie der Sensibilitätsneurosen im Gebiete des Nervus medianus. Berl. klin. Wchnschr., 1879, xvi, 181–183.—**Gillette.** Nerf médian. Dict. encycl. d. sc. méd., Par., 1873, 2. s., vi, 210–229.—**Giovanardi** (E.) Ferita del nervo mediano. Rassegna di sc. med., Modena, 1886, i, 49–54. — **Gruber** (W.) Bemerkenswerthe Abweichung des Nervus medianus. Oester. Ztschr. f. prakt. Heilk., Wien, 1866, xii, 125. *Also. transl.:* Med. Vestnik, St. Petersb., 1867, vii, 458–460.—**Lawrie** (E.) Gunshot wound of the median nerve. Lancet, Lond., 1880, ii, 575.—**Le Fort** (L.) Blessure du nerf médian par un plomb de chasse; atrophie marquée des muscles; insomnie; névralgie permanente avec exacerbation dans l'avant-bras correspondant; dissection et élongation du médian à la partie inférieure du bras; guérison. Bull. et mém. Soc. de chir. de Par., 1882, n. s., viii, 574–577. — **Lothrop** (J. R.) A case of injury to the median nerve. Buffalo M. & S. J., 1868–9, viii, 10–18.—**Merlin** (H.) Abnorme Lagerung der Gabel des N. medianus. Ber. d. naturw.-med. Ver. in Innsbruck, 1884-6, xv, 2.—**Moorman** (J. W.) Case of paralysis of the median nerve. Am. J. M. Sc., Phila., 1866, n. s., li, 280.—**Nichell** (C. F. A.) Case of a section of the median nerve, showing in its centre an enlarged condition, the result of a gun-shot wound. Buffalo M. & S. J., 1867–8, vii, 175.—**Ormerod** (J. A.) Enlargement of median nerve; congenital syphilis. Tr. Path. Soc. Lond., 1881, xxxii, 14.—**Potain.** Paralysie rhumatismale du nerf médian. Gaz. d. hôp., Par., 1878, li, 609; 625.—**Rayner** (H.) Case of injury to the median nerve; operation four months afterwards; complete recovery. Lancet, Lond., 1884, i, 467. — **Richelot** (L.-G.) Note sur un cas de blessure du nerf médian. Union méd., Par., 1877, 3. s., xxiv, 474–476. ——. Plaie du nerf médian; cicatrice ad-

Nerve (*Median*).

hérente; anesthésie et troubles trophiques. *Ibid.*, 476.
——. Note sur un cas de blessure incomplète du nerf
médian. *Ibid.*, 1879, 3. s., xxvii, 345; 362.—**Sander** (W.)
Tropische Störungen nach Verletzung des linken Nervus
medianus. Berl. klin. Wchnschr., 1877, xiv, 546.—
Shewen (A.) Peculiar tremor of hand and forearm,
produced by pressure on median nerve after injury.
Australas. M. Gaz., Sydney, 1884–5, iv, 83.—**Voituriez**
(J.) Blessure du nerf médian: lésions trophiques. J. d.
sc. méd. de Lille, 1886, viii, 478–481.—**Vrabie** (V. G.)
Corp străin in nervul median stâng, in regiunea radiocar-
piena. [Foreign body in left median nerve in radiocarpal
region.] Spitalul, Bucurescí, 1887, vii, 133.—**Warren** (J.
M.) Severe neuralgic affection following a gunshot injury
of the median nerve; subcutaneous injection of morphia;
operation; injectiou continued for nine months; recovery.
In his: Surg. Obs., 8°, Bost., 1867, 468–470.—**Webber** (S.
G.) A case of lesion of the median nerve, with reference
to the distribution of that nerve. Boston M. & S. J., 1875,
xciii, 631–633.—**Williams** (J. W.) A peculiarity in the
median nerve and in the jaternal jugular vein. J. Anat.
& Physiol., Lond., 1886–7, xxi, 333.

Nerve (*Musculo-cutaneous*).

Bianchi (S.) Sull' anastomosi fra il nervo muscolo
cutaneo ed il mediano. Gazz. d. osp., Milano, 1886, vii,
266; 372.—**Gegenbaur** (C.) Ueber das Verhältniss des
N. musculocutaneus zum M. medianus. Jenaische Ztschr.
f. Med. u. Naturw., Leipz., 1867, iii, 258–263. — **Hélie.**
Note sur le nerf musculo-cutané. J. de la sect. de méd.
Soc. acad. Loire-Inf., Nantes, 1841, n. s., xvii, 45–50.—
Testut (L.) Mémoire sur la portion brachiale du nerf
musculo-cutané. Mém. Acad. de méd., Par., 1884, xxxiv,
199–237. *Also:* Internat. Monatschr. f. Anat. u. Histol.,
Berl., 1884, i, 305–341.

Nerve (*Musculo-spiral*).

See, also, **Neurotomy,** *etc.*

Cheever. Wound of musculo-spiral nerve. Boston
M. & S. J., 1875, xcii, 113. — **Owen** (E.) Gunshot injury
to the musculo-spiral nerve. Lancet, Lond., 1876, ii, 709.—
Savory (W. S.) A case in which, after the removal of
several inches of the musculo-spiral nerve, the sensibility
of that part of the skin of the hand which is supplied by
it was retained. *Ibid.*, 1868, ii, 142.

Nerve (*Nasal*).

See, also, **Neuralgia** (*Facial, etc., Treatment of*);
Neuralgia (*Nasal*): **Neurotomy,** *etc.*

Abadie (C.) De l'élongation et de l'arrachement du
nerf nasal. Ann. d'ocul., Brux., 1883, lxxxix, 234–242.—
Badal. De l'élongation du nerf nasal externe. *Ibid.*,
231–234.—**Lagleyze** (P.) Estiramiento del nérvio nasal
externo. Rev. argent. de oftal. práct., Buenos Aires, 1883–4,
i, 73–75. —. Arrancamiento del nérvio nasal externo.
Ibid., 93.—**Lagrange.** L'opération de Badal. Gaz. hebd.
d. sc. méd. de Bordeaux, 1886, vii, 115; 293; 307; 317; 329.

Nerve (*Obturator*).

Rosenmueller (J. C.) [Pr.] nervi obturatorii monographia. 4°. [*n. p.*, 1815.]
Styx (M. E.) *Descriptio anatomica nervi
cruralis et obturatorii icone illustrata. 4°. *Jenæ*, [1782].
——. The same. 4°. *Jenæ*, 1784.
Pasquet. Branche du nerf obturateur passant par-
dessus le pubis. Lyon méd., 1874, xv, 498.—**Thomson**
(A.) Discovery of the true distribution of the obturator.
nerve. Lond. M. & S. J., 1834, iv, 463; 496; 529.

Nerve (*Oculo-motor*).

See, also, **Eye** (*Nerves of*); **Eye** (*Paralytic affections of*); **Mydriasis,** *etc.*

Jäger (W.) *Die Varietäten der Oculomo-
toriusgruppe, des Trigeminus und Vagus. 8°.
Giessen, 1864.
Adamük (E.) Zur Physiologie des N. oculomotorius.
Centralbl. f. d. med. Wissensch., Berl., 1870, viii, 177–180.—
Barbarisi (G.) Su di un nuovo rametto nervoso della
branca inferiore del terzo pajo dei nervi encefalici. Rendic. Accad. med.-chir. di Napoli, 1849, iii, 18–21.—**Bell** (C.)
On the third pair of nerves; being the first of a series of
papers in explanation of the difference in the origins of the
nerves of the encephalon, as compared with those which
arise from the spinal marrow. Tr. Roy. Soc. Edinb., 1836,
xiv, 224–228. *Also, in his:* Three papers on the nerves, 4°,
Edinb., 1838, 1–5.—**Bertolet** (R. M.) A psammome, situated upon the left motor oculi nerve, attended with ptosis
and strabismus. Tr. Path. Soc. Phila. (1871–3), 1874, iv,
196–200.—**Hensen** (V.) & **Völckers** (C.) Ueber den Ursprung der Accommodationsnerven, nebst Bemerkungen
über die Function der Wurzeln des Nervus oculomotorius.
Arch. f. Ophth., Berl., 1878, xxiv, 1–26, 1 pl.—**Legendre.**
Chute; plaie à la région frontale droite; encéphaloïde des

Nerve (*Oculo-motor*).

nerfs moteurs occulaires communs et de la glande pituitaire. Bull. Soc. anat. de Par., 1838, xiii, 330–336.—**Mendel** (E.) Ueber den Kernursprung des Augen-Facialis.
Berl. klin. Wchnschr., 1887, xxiv, 913. [Discussion], 913–
916. *Also:* Neurol. Centralbl., Leipz., 1887, vi, 537–542.—
More (J.) Concussion of the brain, followed by paralysis of the third cranial nerve. Lancet, Lond., 1877, ii, 762;
799.—**Parinaud.** Paralysie dissociée de la 3ᵉ paire dans
la syphilis cérébrale. Progrès méd., Par., 1880, viii, 130.—
Spitzka (E. C.) A second origin of the abducens. Am.
Psych. J., N. Y., 1875–6, n. s., iii, 205–209.—**Toribio
González.** Parálisis del nervio del tercer par ó del nervio motor ocular comun, por congestion activa del punto
de orígen en la base del cerebro, borde interno de los pe-
dúnculos anteriores. Union méd., Carácas, 1882, ii, 23.—
Vulpian. Expériences sur les effets de la galvanisation
du nerf oculo-moteur commun chez les mammifères. Compt.
rend. Soc. de biol. 1860, Par., 1861, 3. s., ii, 160.

Nerve (*Olfactory*).

See, also, **Anosmia.**

Erichsen (J.) * De textura nervi olfactorii
ejusque ramorum. 8°. *Dorpati Livonorum*, 1857.
Gourewitsch (A.) *Ueber die Beziehung des
Nervus olfactorius zu den Athembewegungen.
8°. *Bern*, 1883.
Hoffmann (C. K.) *Onderzoekingen over den
anatomischen bouw van de membrana olfactoria
en het peripherische uiteinde van den nervus olfactorius. 8°. *Amsterdam*, 1866.
Horstius (J. O.) * Diss. qua processus cerebri mammillares ex nervorum olfactoriorum numero exemtos submittet. 4°. *Jenæ*, [1715].
In: Haller. Disp. anat. [etc.] 4°. *Gottingæ*, 1747,
ii, 849–869.
Liboschitz (J.) * De morbis primi paris nervorum. 8°. *Dorpati Livonorum*, [1806].
Metzger (J. D.) * Nervorum primi paris historiam defendet. 4°. *Argentinæ*, [1766].
Also, in: Script. neurol. minores selecti. 4°. *Lipsiæ*,
1791, i, 108–126. *Also, in:* Sandifort. Thesaurus diss.
[etc.] 4°. *Lugd. Bat.*, 1778, iii, 457–476.
Pressat (J.-E.) * Observation sur un cas
d'absence du nerf olfactif. 4°. *Paris*, 1837.
Rosenmüller (J. C.) * De nervorum olfactoriorum defectu. 8°. *Lipsiæ*, [1816].
Scarpa (A.) De organo olfactus præcipuo
deque nervis nasalibus interioribus e pari quinto
nervorum cerebri. Liber ii, de anatomicarum
annotationum. 4°. *Ticini Regii*, 1785.
Slevogt (J. H.) [Pr.] de processibus cerebri
mammillaribus ex nervorum olfactoriorum numero exemtis. 4°. *Jenæ*, 1715.
Althaus (J.) A lecture on the physiology and pathology of the olfactory nerve. Lancet, Lond., 1881, i,
771; 813. *Also. transl.:* Arch. f. Psychiat., Berl., 1881,
xii, 122–140. — **Bidloo** (G.) De osse cribroso et nervis
olfactoriis læsis. *In his:* Exercitat. anat.-chir., dec. duæ,
4°, Lugd. Bat., 1708, 180–193.—**Blandin.** [Crâne d'un
fœtus sur lequel il n'existait aucune trace de nerfs olfactifs.] Bull. Soc. anat. de Par. 1827, 2. éd., 1844, ii, 18.—
Colasanti (G.) Untersuchungen über die Durchschneidung des Nervus olfactorius bei Fröschen. [2. Mittheil.]
[*Transl. from:* Atti d. r. Accad. d. Lincei, 2. s., pt. 2, 1875.]
Arch. f. Anat., Physiol. u. wissensch. Med., Leipz., 1875,
469–476.—**Després.** [Absence des nerfs olfactifs.] Bull.
Soc. anat. de Par., 1841, xvi, 140.— **Dubreuil.** Bec-de-
lièvre double; séparation complète de la voûte palatine;
absence des nerfs olfactifs, du trigône cérébral et du
corps calleux. Gaz. méd. de Par., 1835, 2. s., iii, 243.—**Duval** (M.) Du degré de l'atrophie des nerfs olfactifs com-
patible avec la persistance de l'olfaction. Bull. Soc. d'anthrop. de Par., 1884, 3. s., vii, 829–835. — **Eckhard** (C.)
Ueber die Endigungsweise des Geruchsnerven. Beitr. z.
Anat. u. Physiol. (Eckhard), Giessen, 1858, i, 77–84. —
Eschricht (D. F.) De functionibus primi et quinti
paris nervorum in olfactorio propriis. J. de physiol. expér., Par., 1826, vi, 339–361. — **Exner** (S.) Weitere Studien über die Structur der Riechschleimhaut bei Wirbelthieren. [Second paper.] Sitzungsb. d. k. Akad. d. Wissensch. Math.-naturw. Cl., Wien, 1872, lxv, 7–41, 3 pl.
——. Fortgesetzte Studien über die Endigungsweise des
Geruchnerven. Dritte Abhandlung. *Ibid.* (1877), 1878,
lxxvi, 17f–221, 2 pl.—**Golgi** (C.) Sulla fina struttura dei
bulbi olfattorii. Riv. sper. di freniat., Reggio-Emilia, 1875,
i, 405–425, 1 pl. ——. Origine del tractus olfactorius e
struttura dei lobi olfattorii dell' nomo e di altri mammiferi.
Gazz. d. osp., Milano, 1882, iii, 210; 218. *Also, transl.:*
Arch. ital. de biol., Turin, 1882, i, 454–462.—**Harless** (E.)

Nerve (*Olfactory*).

& **von Hessling** (T.) Ueber die Verästelung der Endfasern des Olfactorius. Jenaische Ann. f. Physiol. u. Med., 1851, ii, 275–282, 1 pl.—**Heschl.** Defect der beiden Riechnerven mit Verkümmerung der Genitalien. Oesterr. Ztschr. f. prakt. Heilk., Wien, 1861, vii, 177–179.—**Heyfelder.** Mangel des Nervus olfactorius und des Ramus nasopalatinus paris quinti bei einem Kinde mit Wolfsrachen. Med. Ztg., Berl., 1836, v, 10.—**Horn** (H.) Ueber die Endschlingen des Geruchsnerven. Arch. f. Anat., Physiol. u. wissensch. Med., Berl., 1850, 74, 1 pl. — **Huguenin.** Ueber Neuritis olfactoria. Cor.-Bl. f. schweiz. Aerzte, Basel, 1882, xii, 257 : 295.—**Kneeland.** Case of an affection of the olfactory nerve, with total loss of smell and taste ; with remarks upon the probable identity of these two senses. Am. J. M. Sc., Phila., 1851, n. s., xxi, 41–46.—**Kölliker** (A.) Ueber den Bau der grauen Nervenfasern des Geruchsnerven. Verhandl. d. phys.-med. Gesellsch. in Würzb., 1854, iv, 60. ——. Der Lobus olfactorius und die Nervi olfactorii bei jungen menschlichen Embryonen. Sitzungsb. d. phys.-med. Gesellsch. zu Würzb., 1882, 68–72.—**Magendie.** Le nerf olfactif est-il l'organe de l'odorat ? Expériences sur cette question. J. de physiol. expér., Par., 1824, iv, 169–176.—**Mollière** (D.) Note pour servir à l'histoire de la pathologie du nerf olfactif. Mém. et compt.-rend. Soc. d. sc. méd. de Lyon (1871), 1872, xi, 133–139. *Also:* Lyon méd., 1871, viii, 385–391.—**Obersteiner** (H.) Ursprung und centrale Verbindungen der Riechnerven. Biol. Centralbl., Erlang., 1882–3, ii, 464–468.—**Oehl** (E.) Su la terminazione apparente del nervo olfattorio. Gazz. med. ital. lomb., Milano, 1857, 4. s., ii, 317–320. ——. Su 'l nervo e su l' organo olfattorio. *Ibid.*, 1858, 4. s., iii, 1 ; 11, 1 pl. — **Owsiannikow** (P.) Ueber die feinere Structur der Lobi olfactorii der Säugethiere. Arch. f. Anat , Physiol. u. wissensch. Med., Leipz., 1860, 469–477.—**Prevost** (J. L.) Cas d'atrophie des nerfs olfactifs et d'hypertrophie des racines des nerfs optiques; diminution manifeste de l'odorat. Compt. rend. Soc. de biol. 1865, Par., 1866, 4. s., ii, 37–42. ——. Atrophie des nerfs olfactifs fréquente chez le vieillard et correspondant avec la diminution ou la perte du sens. *Ibid.* (1866), 1867, 4. s., iii, pt. 2, 69–76.—**Randacio** (F.) On the relations of the nucleus tæniæformis with the olfactory nerve. Tr. Internat. M. Cong., 7. sess., Lond., 1881, i, 169. ——. Dell' antimuro o claustrum col nervo olfattorio nell' uomo. Spallanzani, Modena,1881, 2. s., x, 617–625.—**de San Juan** (A. M.) Falta total de los nervios olfatorios con anosmia en un individuo en quien existia una atrofia congénita de los testiculos y miembro viril. Siglo méd., Madrid, 1856, iii, 211 ; 218.—**Schiff** (J. M.) Der erste Hirnnerv ist der Geruchsnerv. Untersuch. z. Naturl. d. Mensch. u. d. Thiere, Giessen, 1860, vi, 254–267.—**Smith** (W.) Note on a reflex action of the olfactory nerves upon the nerves of the palate and stomach. Med. Chron , Manchester, 1886–7, v, 463.—**Wallmann** (H.) Cysticercusblase am rechten Riechnerven. Allg. Wien. med. Ztg., 1858, iii, 182.—**Walter** (G.) Ueber den feineren Bau des Bulbusolfactorius. Arch. f. path. Anat., etc., Berl., 1861, xxii, 241–259, 2 pl.

Nerve (*Ophthalmic*).

Myrtle (A. S.) Neuralgia of ophthalmic nerve, where local symptoms were similar to those resulting from gout and rheumatism. Practitioner, Lond., 1881, xxvii, 198–200. — **Nuel.** Nerf ophthalmique. Dict. encycl. d. sc. méd., Par., 1881, 2. s., xvi, 30–36.

Nerve (*Optic*).

See, also, Amaurosis (*Cases of*) ; Eye ; Hemiopia ; Nerve-stretching ; Ophthalmoscopy ; Retina.

Beck (B.) Ueber die Verbindungen des Sehnerven mit dem Augen- und Nasenknoten, sowie über den feinern Bau dieser Ganglien. 8°. *Heidelberg*, 1847.

Brunner (G. B.) Ein Beitrag zur electrischen Reizung des Nervus opticus. Experimentaluntersuchung. 8°. *Leipzig*, 1863.

Friant (A.) * Recherches sur le chiasma des nerfs optiques dans les différentes classes d'animaux vertébrés. 4°. *Nancy*, 1874.

Goebel (O.) * Einiges über die Eintrittsstelle des Sehnerven und die Entwickelung des Auges. 8°. *Hirschberg i. Schl.*, 1883.

Jaboulay. Relations des nerfs optiques avec le système nerveux central. 8°. *Paris*, 1886.

Lehmann (A.) * Experimenta quædam de nervi optici dissecti ad retinæ texturam vi et effectu. 8°. [*Dorpat*], 1857.

Michaelis (P.) Ueber die Durchkreuzung der Sehenerven. Mit einigen Anmerkungen vom Herrn Hofrath Soemmering. 16°. *Halle*, 1790.

Nerve (*Optic*).

Nicati (W.) * Des fibres nerveuses dans les nerfs optiques et dans la rétine. 4°. *Paris*, 1875.

Also, transl. in : Arch. de physiol. norm. et path., Par., 1875, 2. s., ii, 521–529, 1 pl.

Noethig (F. N.) * De decussatione nervorum opticorum. 8°. *Moguntiæ*, 1786.

Reddingius (R. A. B.) * De nervo optico. 8°. *Groningæ*, 1824.

Russi (A.) * Die Umschnürung des Nervus opticus und deren Folgen für's Auge. 8°. *Bern*, 1880.

Sahmen (H.) * Disquisitiones microscopicæ de chiasmatis optici textura. 8°. *Dorpati Livonorum*, 1854.

Scheel (L.) * Ueber das Chiasma nervorum opticorum bei den Wirbelthieren und beim Menschen. 8°. *Erlangen*, 1874.

Snellen (H.) * De invloed der zenuwen op de ontsteking proefondervindelijk getoetst. 8°. *Utrecht*, 1857.

Swan (J.) On the origins of the visual powers of the optic nerve. 4°. *London*, 1856.

Wagner (J.) * Ueber den Ursprung der Sehnervenfasern im menschlichen Gehirn. 4°. *Dorpat*, 1862.

Adamük (E.) Zur Frage über die Kreuzung der Nervenfasern im Chiasma nervorum opticorum des Menschen. Arch. f. Ophth., Berl., 1880, xxvi, 2. Abth., 187–190, 1 pl.—**von Ammon.** Zur genaueren Kenntniss des Nervus opticus, namentlich dessen intraocularen Endes. Vrtljschr. f. d. prakt. Heilk., Prag, 1860, lxv, 132–167, 2 pl.—**Baumgarten** (P.) Zur sog. Semidecussation der Opticusfasern. Centralbl. f. med. Wissensch., Berl., 1878, xvi, 561. ——. Zur Semidecussation der Opticusfasern. Arch. f. Ophth., Berl., 1881, xxvii, 1. Abth., 342–344. — **Beauregard** (H.) Recherches sur le mode d'entrecroisement des nerfs optiques chez les oiseaux. Compt. rend. Soc. de biol. 1875, Par., 1876, 6. s., ii, 344. — **Bechterew** (W.) Experimentelle Untersuchungen über die Kreuzung der Sehnerven-Fasern im Chiasma nn. opticorum. Neurol. Centralbl., Berl., 1883, ii, 53–58. *Also, transl.:* Ejened. klin. gaz., St. Petersb., 1883, iii, 22 ; 38. ——. Experimentelle Ergebnisse über den Verlauf der Sehnervenfasern auf ihrer Bahn von den Kniehockern zu den Vierhügeln. Neurol. Centralbl., Leipz., 1883, ii, 265–268.—**Bellonci** (G.) La terminaison centrale du nerf optique chez les mammifères. Arch. ital. de biol , Turin, 1884–5, vi, 405–412, 1 pl. — **Berger** (E.) Ueber Bindegewebsbildungen in der Sehnervenpapille und der Netzhaut. Klin. Monatsbl. f. Augenh., Stuttg., 1882, xx, 269–276. ——. Zur feineren Baue des Sehnerven. Arch. f. Augenh., Wiesb., 1882, xi, 314–323.—**Bernoulli** (D.) Versuch in Anseßung des Sehnervens. Phys. u. med. Abhandl. d. k. Akad. d. Wissensch. in Petersb., Riga, 1782, i, 28–32. — **von Biesiadecki** (A.) Ueber das Chiasma nervorum opticorum des Menschen und der Thiere. [*From:* Sitzungsb. d. k. Akad. d. Wissensch., Wien, xlii.] Untersuch. z. Naturl. d. Mensch. u. d. Thiere, Giessen, 1862, viii, 156–173, 1 pl.— **Brücke** (M. E.) Ueber einige Empfindungen im Gebiete der Sehnerven. Sitzungsb. d. k. Akad. d. Wissensch., Wien, 1878, lxxvii, 39–71. — **Calori** (L.) Annotazioni storico-critiche sulle origini dei nervi ottici. Mem. Accad. d. sc. d.Ist. di Bologna, 1870–71, 3. s., i, 513–527, 1 pl. — **Campbell** (H. F.) Remarkable case of amaurosis, illustrating the anatomy of the optic nerves. Tr. Am. M. Ass., Phila., 1851, iv, 75–78. *Also :* South. M. & S. J., Augusta, 1851, n. s., vii, 73–76.—**Chodin** (A.) Ueber die chemische Reaction der Netzhaut und des Sehnerven. Sitzungsb. d. k. Akad. d. Wissensch. 1877, Wien, 1878, lxxvi, 121–137.—**Dogiel** (A.) W kwestyi skrzyżowania się nerwów wzrokowych u człowieka. [The question of chiasma nervorum opticorum in man.] Gaz. lek., Warszawa, 1883, 2. s., iii, 465.— **Dreschfeld** (J.) Pathologisch-anatomische Beiträge zur Lehre von der Semidecussation der Sehnervenfasern. Centralbl. f. prakt. Augenh., Leipz., 1880, iv, 33–36. ——. Pathological contributions on the course of the optic nerve fibres in the brain. Brain, Lond., 1881–2, iv, 543 : 1882–3, v, 118.—**Duwez.** Nerf optique. Dict. encycl. d. sc. méd., Par., 1881, 2. s., xvi, 272–370. — **Erdl.** Ursprung der Sehnerven. N. med.-chir. Ztg., Augsburg, 1843, n. F., i, 113–117. — **Ewetsky** (T.) Ein Fall von Endotheliom der äusseren Sehnervenscheide. Arch. f. Augenh., Wiesb., 1882, xii, 16–29. — **Exner** (S.) Ueber den Erregungsvorgang im Sehnervenapparate. Sitzungsb. d. k. Akad. d. Wissensch., Wien, 1872, lxv, 59–70, 1 pl. ——. Die Empfindungszonen des Sehnervenapparates. Arch. f. d. ges. Physiol., Bonn, 1875, xi, 581–602.—**Falchi** (F.) Sull' istogenesi della retina e del nervo ottico ; nota preventiva. Ann. di ottal., Pavia, 1886, xv, 528–530. *Also:* Gazz. d. clin., Torino, 1886, xxiii, 17.

Nerve (*Optic*).

Also: Spallanzani, Roma, 1887, 2. s., xvi, 460-465.—**Gabriolet.** Su l' espansioni delle radici cerebrali del nervo ottico, e sulla lòro terminazione in una regione determinata dallo strato corticale degli emisferi. Gior. veneto di sc. med., Venezia, 1854, 2. s., iii, 700-702.—**Ganser** (S.) Ueber die periphere und centrale Anordnung der Sehnervenfasern und über das Corpus bigeminum anterius. Arch. f Psychiat., Berl., 1882, xiii, 341-381, 2 pl.—**Gowers** (W. R.) Pathologischer Beweis einer unvollständigen Kreuzung der Sehnerven beim Menschen. Centralbl. f. d. med. Wissensch., Berl., 1878, xvi, 562.—**Gratiolet** (P.) Note sur les expansions des racines cérébrales du nerf optique et sur leur terminaison dans une région déterminée de l'écorce des hémisphères. Arch. d'ophth., Par., 1855, iv, 5-9.—**von Gudden.** Ueber die Kreuzung der Nervenfasern im Chiasma nervorum opticorum. Arch. f. Ophth., Berl., 1874, xx, 2. Abth., 249-268, 2 pl.: 1875, xxi, 3. Abth., 199, 1 pl.: 1879, xxv, 1, Abth., 1, 4 pl.; 4. Abth., 237, 1 pl. ———. Demonstration der Sehfasern und Pupillarfasern des Nerv. opticus. Sitzungsb. d. Gesellsch. f. Morphol. u. Physiol. in München, 1885-6, i, 169.—**Hamilton** (D. J.) On the cortical connexions of the optic nerves. Proc. Roy. Soc. Lond., 1884, xxxvii, 1-3.—**Hiltner** (R.) Ueber die Entwicklung des Nervus opticus der Säugetierë. Biol. Centralbl., Erlang., 1885-6, v, 38-40.—**von Hippel.** Präparate zur Sehnervenkreuzung. Ber. ü. d. Versamml. d. ophth. Gesellsch., Rostock, 1878, xi, 180.—**Hirschberg** (J.) Zur Semidecussation der Sehnervenfasern im Chiasma des Menschen. Arch. f. path. Anat., etc., Berl., 1875, lxv, 116-119. ———. Zur Frage der Sehnervenkreuzung. Arch. f. Augen- u. Ohrenh., Wiesb., 1876, v, 137-139. *Also, transl.:* Arch. Ophth. & Otol., N. Y., 1876, v, 188-190. ———. Ein schwarzer Sehnerv. Centralbl. f. prakt. Augenh., Leipz., 1881, v, 137.—**Hoffmann** (C. K.) Zur Entwicklungsgeschichte des Nervus opticus. Morphol. Jahrb., Leipz., 1885-6, xi, 200, 1 pl.—**Hoffmann** (F. W.) Zur vergleichenden Anatomie der Lamina cribosa nervi optici und einiger angrenzenden Verhältnisse. Arch. f. Ophth., Berl., 1883, xxix, 45-72, 2 pl.—**Holmgren** (F.) Genomskärning af synnerven hos kaninen. Upsala Läkaref: Förh., 1875-6, xi, 231-243.—**Hosch** (F.) Zur Lehre von der Sehnervenkreuzung. Klin. Monatsbl. f. Augenh., Cassel, 1878, xvi, 281-287, 2 pl.—**Krause** (W.) Ueber die Endigung des N. opticus. Arch. f. Anat., Physiol. u. wissensch. Med., Leipz., 1867, 243; 643: 1868, 256. ———. Ueber die Fasern des Sehnerven. Arch. f. Ophth., Berl., 1880, xxvi, 2. Abth., 102-110, 1 pl.—**Kuhnt** (H.) Zur Kenntniss des Sehnerven und der Netzhaut. *Ibid.*, 1879, xxv, 3. Abth., 179-288, 1 pl. *Also,* Reprint. ———. Ueber die physiologische Sehnervenexcavation. Ber. ü. d. Versamml. d. ophth. Gesellsch., Stuttg., 1881, xiii, 138-141.—**Landesberg** (M.) Is the mechanical irritation of the optic nerve always followed by a sensation of light? Phila. M. Times, 1882-3, xiii. 359-361.—**Leber** (T.) Bemerkungen über die Circulations-Verhältnisse des Opticus und der Retina. Arch. f. Ophth., Berl., 1872, xviii, 2. Abth., 25-37.—**Lewis** (R. A.) A dissertation on the function of the chiasma nervorum opticorum; or the reason why we do not see objects in an inverted and reversed position. Stethoscope & Virg. M. Gaz., Richmond, 1852, ii, 144-153.—**Longet** (A.) Faits pathologiques pouvant servir à déterminer le lieu d'origine et le mode d'entrecroisement des nerfs optiques. Ann. méd.-psych., Par., 1843, i, 61-71.—**Maklakoff** (A. N.) O perekresti zutelenikh nervov. [On the intercrossing of the optic nerves.] Laitop. khirurg. Obsh. v Mosk., 1873-5, i, 72.—**Marckwort** (E.) Experimentelle Studien über Läsionen des Nervus opticus. Arch. f. Augenh., Wiesb., 1881, x. 269-307.—**Méry** (J.) Observations sur le nerf optique. [*From:* Mém. Acad. r. d. sc. de Par., 1712.] Rec. d. mém., Dijon, 1769, iii, 546-548.—**Michel** (J.) Ueber den Bau des Chiasma nervorum opticorum. Arch. f. Ophth., Berl., 1873, xix, 2. Abth., 59, 2 pl.; 3. Abth., 375. ———. Zur Frage der Sehnerven-Kreuzung im Chiasma. *Ibid.*, 1877, xxiii, 2. Abth., 227-254, 1 pl.—**Mohr** (A.) Ein Beitrag zur Frage der Semidecussation im Chiasma nervorum opticorum. *Ibid.*, 1879, xxv, 1 Abth., 57-78.—**von Monakow.** Einiges über die Ursprungscentren des N. opticus und über die Verbindungen derselben mit der Sehsphäre. Arch. f. Physiol., Leipz., 1885, 329-331.—**Moullin** (C. W. M.) The chiasma of the optic nerves. St. Barth. Hosp. Rep., Lond., 1879, xv, 277-281.—**Nicati** (W.) Entrecroisement des fibres nerveuses dans la papille de l'œil de la grenouille. Compt. rend. Soc. de biol. 1875, Par., 1876, 6. s., ii, 69. ———. De la distribution des fibres nerveuses dans le chiasma des nerfs optiques. Arch. de physiol. norm. et path., Par., 1878, 2. s., v, 658-678. *Also:* Marseille méd., 1878, xv, 416; 547. ———. Preuve expérimentale du croisement incomplet des fibres nerveuses dans le chiasma des nerfs optiques; section longitudinale et médiane du chiasma non suivie de cécité. Compt. rend. Acad. d. sc., Par., 1878, lxxxvi, 1472-1474. *Also, transl.:* Centralbl. f. d. med. Wissensch., Berl., 1878, xvi, 449.—**Nicolucci** (G.) Sul chiasma de' nervi ottici; ricerche anatomiche. Filiatre-sebezio, Napoli, 1845, xxix, 321-329.—**Nieden.** Drusenbildung auf der Papilla nervi optici. Ber. ü. d. Versamml. d. ophth. Gesellsch., Rostock,

Nerve (*Optic*).

1878, xi, 194-198.—**Norton** (G. S.) A case of tumor at the base of the brain, which serves to prove semi-decussation of the optic nerve fibres. N. Am. Homœop. J., N. Y., 1878, xxvi, 305-312.—**Onodi** (A. D.) Ueber die Verbindung des Nervus opticus mit dem Tuber cinereum. Internat. Monatschr. f. Anat. u. Histol., Leipz., 1886, iii, 247-249.—**Panas.** Note sur la structure de l'espace vaginal du nerf optique. Bull. et mém. Soc. de chir. de Par., 1876, n. s., ii, 668-670.—**Parinaud** (H.) Des rapports croisés et directs des nerfs optiques avec les hémisphères cérébraux. Compt. rend. Soc. de biol. 1882, Par., 1883, 7. s., iv, 179. *Also:* Gaz. d. hôp., Par., 1882, lv. 259.—**Pflüger.** Ligature des nerfs optiques de deux lapins. Cong. périod. internat. d'ophth. Compt.-rend. 1880, Milan, 1881, vi, 48-55.—**Power** (J. H.) Observations on the arrangement of the fibres in the optic nerve of the loligo, and other animals. Dublin J. M. Sc., 1842-3, xxii, 350-364. *Also,* Reprint.—**Purtscher** (O.) Traité sur le croisement et l'atrophie des nerfs et des tractus visuels. Cong. périod. internat. d'ophth. Compt.-rend. 1880, Milan, 1881, vi, 320-327.—**Radwaner** (J.) Ueber die Entwicklung der Sehnervenkreuzung. Mitth. a. d. embryol. Inst. d. k. k. Univ. in Wien, 1877, i, 21-36, 2 pl.—**Reich** (M.) O polnome i nepolnome perekretchivanii epitelniche nervove. [On the complete and incomplete crossing of nervous filaments (in chiasma nerv. opticorum).] Protok. zasaid. Obsh. russk. vrach. v St. Petersb., 1874, xli, 351-361, 2 pl.—**Rousseau.** Un cas de tumeur cérébrale pouvant éclairer la physiologie de la couche optique. Bull. Soc. méd. de l'Yonne 1883, Auxerre, 1884, xxiv, 89-99.—**Rozoff** (V.) Opwiti s' pereraiivaniem zritelnago nerva u krolikof. [Experiments on the section of the optic nerve in rabbits.] Med. Vestnik, St. Petersb., 1865, v, 285; 293; 301.—**Sala** (L.) Ricerche sulla struttura del nervo ottico. Arch. per le sc. med., Torino, 1887, xi, 123-128.—**Samelsohn** (J.) Zur Topographie des Faserverlaufes im menschlichen Sehnerven. Centralbl. f. d. med. Wissensch., Berl., 1880, xviii, 418-420. ———. Ein menschliches Chiasma nervorum opticorum. Sitzungsb. d. nied.-rhein. Gesellsch. f. Nat.- u. Heilk. zu Bonn, 1880, 7. *Also:* Berl. klin. Wchnschr., 1880, xvii, 334.—**Schmidt-Rimpler** (H.) Doppelcontourirte Nervenfasern auf der Papille. Arch. f. Ophth., Berl., 1877, xxiii, 180. ———. Demonstration zur Sehnervenkreuzung. Ber. ü. d. Versamml. d. ophth. Gesellsch., Rostock, 1877, x, 44-52. ———. Zur specifischen Reaction der Sehnerven auf mechanische Reize. Centralbl. f. d. med. Wissensch., Berl., 1882, xx, 1-4.—**Sous** (G.) Anatomie de la papille du nerf optique. Gaz. méd. de Bordeaux, 1876, v, 196-198.—**Stilling** (J.) Ueber eine neue Ursprungsstelle des Sehnerven. Centralbl. f. d. med. Wissensch., Berl., 1878, xvi, 385. ———. Centraler Ursprung des Sehnerven. Ber. ü. d. Versamml. d. ophth. Gesellsch., Stuttg. 1879, xii, 203-208. *Also:* Centralbl. f. prakt. Augenh., Leipz., 1880, iv, 40. ———. Das Chiasma nervorum opticorum. Arch. f. Psychiat., Berl., 1880, xi, 274-276. ———. Ueber einige neue Opticusverbindungen. Centralbl. f. prakt. Augenh., Leipz., 1880, iv, 377. ———. Ueber die centralen Endigungen des Nervus opticus. Arch. f. mikr. Anat., Bonn, 1880, xviii, 468-480, 1 pl.—**Szili** (A.) Zur Morphographie der Papilla nervi optici. Centralbl. f. prakt. Augenh., Leipz., 1881, xi, 1-6.—**Szokalski.** Obecny stan wiedzy o skrzyżowaniu nerwów wzrokowych. [The present state of knowledge on the decussation of the optic nerves.] Medycyna, Warszawa, 1876, iv, 97-105. ———. Sovremennoe polozhenie nauki o perekrestai zritelnikh nervov. [On the intersection of the optic nerves.] Sovrem. med., Warszawa, 1876, xvii, 70; 85; 102; 183. ———. Skutki podrażnień pnia nerwu wzrokowego. [On the effect of irritating the trunk of the optic nerve.] Przegl. lek., Krakow, 1881, xx, 441.—**Türck** (L.) Ueber Compression und Ursprung des Sehnerven. Ztschr. d. k.-k. Gesellsch. d. Aerzte zu Wien, 1852, ii, 299-304.—**Uhthoff.** Zum Sehnervenfaserverlauf. Ber. ü. d. Versamml. d. ophth. Gesellsch., Stuttg., 1884, xvi, 13-27.—**Varolius** (C.) & **Mercurialis** (H.) De nervis opticis, nonnullisque aliis, præter communem opinionem in humano capite observatis epistolæ. *In:* Varolius (C.) Anatomiæ . . . libri iv, 8°, Francof., 1591, 119-172.—**Vossius** (A.) Beiträge zur Anatomie des N. opticus. Arch. f. Ophth., Berl., 1883, xxix, 4. Abth., 119-150, 1 pl.—**Wedemeyer.** Ueber einen muthmasslichen Kanal im Sehnerven des menschlichen Fötus. J. d. Chir. u. Augenh., Berl., 1826, ix, 115-118.—**Woinow.** Ueber Kreuzung des Sehnerven. Klin. Monatsbl. f. Augenh., Stuttg., 1875, xiii, 424-429.—**Wollaston** (W. H.) On semi-decussation of the optic nerves. Phil. Tr., Lond., 1824, 222-231.

Nerve (*Optic, Abnormities of*).

SVITZER (E.) Bericht von einigen nicht häufig vorkommenden und einigen noch nicht beobachteten Variationen der Verzweigung der Augennerven und ihrer Verbindung mit einander. 4°. *Kopenhagen,* 1845.

WULFFERT (F.) * Eine neue Form von Missbildung der Papilla nervi optici. 8°. *Bonn,* 1877.

Nerve (*Optic, Abnormities of*).

Bader (C.) Description of the appearances of the human eye in health and disease as seen by the ophthalmoscope. 6. s. Congenital anomalies. Guy's Hosp. Rep., Lond., 1872, 3. s., xvii, 473–476, 1 pl.—**Brière.** Absence des papilles; cécité absolue. Ann. d'ocul., Brux., 1877, lxxviii, 41.—**Eversbusch** (O.) Eine neue Form von Missbildung der Papilla nervi optici, verbunden mit ausgedehnter Verbreitung markhaltiger Sehnervenfasern und congenitaler hochgradiger Kurzsichtigkeit. Klin. Monatsbl. f. Augenh., Stuttg., 1885, xxiii, 1–24, 1 pl.—**Fano.** De l'arrêt de développement de l'appareil nerveux optique. Union méd., Par., 1864, 2. s., xxi, 162–165.—**Fuchs** (E.) Beitrag zu den angeborenen Anomalien des Sehnerven. Arch. f. Ophth., Berl., 1882, xxviii, 1. Abth., 139–169, 1 pl.—**Gowers** (W. R.) Pathologischer Beweis einer unvollständigen Kreuzung der Sehnerven beim Menschen. Centralbl. f. d. med. Wissensch., Berl., 1878, xvi, 562. *Also*, Reprint.—**von Hebra** (H.) Ueber angebornen Defect des Papillarkörpers. Allg. Wien. med. Ztg., 1881, xxvi, 247.—**Lopez** (J.) Anomalia congénita del nervio óptico. Bol. de benef. y sanid. municip., Madrid, 1881, i, 36.—**Magnus** (H.) Zur Casuistik der angeborenen Sehnerven-Missbildungen. Klin. Monatsbl. f. Augenh., Stuttg., 1884, xxii, 85–87.—**Nieden** (A.) Vier Fälle von Coloboma vaginæ nervi optici, ohne weitere Spaltbildung im Uvealtractus. Arch. f. Augenh., Wiesb., 1879, viii, 292–305.—**Pooley** (T. R.) Un cas de colobome du vagin du nerf optique. Cong. périod. internat. d'ophth. Compt.-rend. 1880, Milan, 1881, vi, 309–311.—**Purtscher** (O.) Eine eigenthümliche Anomalie des Sehnerven. Arch. f. Augenh., Wiesb., 1882–3, xii, 421–423, 1 pl. *Also, transl.*: Arch. Ophth., N. Y., 1883, xii, 419–421, 1 pl.—**Randall** (B. A.) The underlying conus. Am. J. Ophth., St. Louis, 1886, iii, 319–321.—**Remak.** Ein Fall von Colobom der Sehnerven. Centralbl. f. Augenh., Leipz., 1884, viii, 225–229.—**Stood** (W.) Zwei Fälle über Drüsenbildungen am intraocularen Sehnervenende. Klin. Monatsbl. f. Augenh., Suttg., 1883, xxi, 506–514. ———. Zur Casuistik der Missbildungen an der Sehnervenpapille. *Ibid.*, 1884, xxii, 285–294.—**Van Duyse.** Contribution à l'étude des anomalies congénitales du nerf optique. Ann. Soc. de méd. de Gand, 1884, lxii, 89–119. *Also*: Ann. d'ocul., Brux., 1884, xci, 117–144.—**Wiethe** (T.) Ein Fall von angeborener Difformität der Sehnervenpapille. Arch. f. Augenh., Wiesb., 1881–2, xi, 14–19, 1 pl. *Also, transl.*: Arch. Ophth., N. Y., 1882, xi, 70–73, 1 pl.

Nerve (*Optic, Atrophy of*).

See, also, **Erysipelas** (*Facial*), *etc.*

DESCAYS (J.) *Essai sur l'atrophie papillaire et son traitement, spécialement par les courants continus. 4°. *Montpellier*, 1884.

HECQUIN (H.-A.) *De l'atrophie traumatique de la papille. 4°. *Paris*, 1874.

HOLZ (R.) *Drei Fälle von genuiner Atrophia nervorum opticorum simplex progressiva bei Geschwistern. 8°. *Greifswald*, 1885.

KELLERMANN (M.) Anatomische Untersuchungen atrophischer Sehnerven, mit einem Beitrag zur Frage der Sehnervenkreuzung im Chiasma. 8°. *Stuttgart*, 1879.

LEBRIS (L.) *Des différentes formes cliniques des atrophies papillaires. 4°. *Paris*, 1878.

MICHEL (J.) Ueber Sehnerven-Degeneration und Sehnerven-Kreuzung. Fest-Schrift der medizinischen Fakultät der Universität Würzburg zur Feier des lxx. Geburtstages des Dr. Albert von Kölliker. fol. *Wiesbaden*, 1887.

PERREYMOND (F.) *De l'atrophie du nerf optique et de sa papille chez les tabétiques. 4°. *Paris*, 1874.

PROUFF (M.) *Sur une forme d'atrophie papillaire observée chez plusieurs membres d'une même famille. 4°. *Paris*, 1873.

RAOULT (J.) *Des atrophies papillaires. 4°. *Paris*, 1877.

ROUIRE (F.) *De l'atrophie papillaire tabétique et de son traitement. 4°. *Paris*, 1878.

Abadie (C.) De l'atrophie des nerfs optiques dans le mal de Pott. [Rap. de Terrier.] Bull. et mém. Soc. de chir. de Par., 1876, n. s., ii, 16–20. ———. Des atrophies interstitielles et parenchymateuses des nerfs optiques. Ann. d'ocul., Brux., 1878, lxx, 191–201. ———. Sur la pseudo-atrophie de la papille; rapport sur le mémoire du docteur Trousseau. Rec. d'ophth., Par., 1887, 3. s., ix, 174–177.—**Alba Carreras** (J.) Atrófia progresiva de la papila. Rev. argent. de oftal. práct., Buenos Aires, 1883–4, i, 83–85, 1 pl.—**Alt** (A.) One hundred and twenty cases of anæmic and atrophic condition of the optic nerve and retina. Am. J. Ophth., St. Louis, 1886, iii, 201; 264.—

Nerve (*Optic, Atrophy of*).

von Ammon (F. A.) Zur Lehre derjenigen Art von Amaurose, welche durch Degeneration des Neurilyma nervi optici entsteht und zur Lehre von den Krankheiten jener Membran überhaupt. Ztschr. f. d. Ophth., Dresd., 1832, ii, 283–294.—**Armaignac** (H.) Atrophie des deux papilles chez une enfant de quatre mois née avant terme et atteinte d'hydrocéphalie; cécité paraissant complète. Rev. clin. d'ocul., Bordeaux, 1881, ii, 205–207. ———. Du traitement de l'atrophie simple, commençante du nerf optique par la strychnine et les courants continus. *Ibid.*, 1886, vi, 25–32.—**Atwood** (F.) Atrophy of optic nerve, treated by subcutaneous injection of strychnine. Tr. Minnesota M. Soc., St. Paul, 1877, ix, 116–120.—**Bacchi.** Note sur le traitement des atrophies du nerf optique. Bull. clin. nat. opht. de l'hosp. d. Quinze-Vingts, Par., 1884, ii, 119–134.—**Bastien.** Atrophie des nerfs optiques. Bull. Soc. anat. de Par., 1854, xxix, 378–383. *Also*: Arch. d'ophth., Par., 1855, iv, 49–54.—**Benson** (A. H.) On the causes of atrophy of the optic nerve, other than glaucomatous. Brit. M. J., Lond., 1885, ii, 685–688.—**Brailey** (W. A.) Examination of the optic discs in the case of optic atrophy from lead poisoning. Ophth. Hosp. Rep., Lond., 1874–6, viii, 549.—**Bull** (C. S.) A contribution to the etiology of optic nerve atrophy. Am. J. M. Sc., Phila., 1877, n. s., lxxiii, 403–411.—**Burnett** (S. M.) Atrophy of the optic nerve following cerebral disease. Nashville J. M. & S., 1872, n. s., x, 76–83.—**Calhoun** (A. W.) Opaqueness of both vitreous tumors and atrophy of optic nerve. Atlanta M. & S. J., 1874–5, xii, 25.—**Callan** (P. A.) Atrophy of both optic nerves as a sequel of whooping cough. Am. J. Ophth., St. Louis, 1884–5, i, 219.—**Carl** (A.) Zur specielleren Aetiologie der nach Erysipelas faciei auftretenden Sehnervenatrophie. Klin. Monatsbl. f. Augenh., Stuttg., 1884, xxii, 113–128, 2 pl.—**Carreras-Aragó.** Atrofia incipiente en el nervio óptico, principalmente izquierdo con parésis de las extremidades derechas antecedentes sifilíticos hereditarios; curacion. Rev. de cien. méd., Barcel., 1882, viii, 619–623. —**Cheatham** (W.) Atrophy of optic nerves from a slight fall. Am. Pract., Louisville, 1877, xvi, 336.—**Chisolm** (J. J.) Method of using strychnia in the treatment of optic nerve atrophy and allied nervous affections. Am. J. M. Sc., Phila., 1873, n. s., lxv, 342–346. ———. Cases showing the value of strychnia in optic nerve atrophy. Lancet, Lond., 1873, i, 732.—**Debrou.** [Nerf optique atrophié dans un individu aveugle depuis son enfance.] Bull. Soc. anat. de Par., 1836, 3. s., ii, 298.—**De Keersmaecker.** De l'atrophie axiale du nerf optique observée chez plusieurs membres d'une même famille. Rec. d'ophth., Par., 1883, 3. s., v, 193–203.—**Delacroix.** Atrophie partielle du nerf optique et infiltration pigmentaire de la rétine, consécutives à un coup de fusil reçu à bout pourtant dans toute la moitié droite de la face. Bull. Soc. méd. de Reims, 1873, xii, 222–226.—**De Schweinitz** (G. E.) Notes of a case of optic atrophy and temporal hemianopsia; suspected tumor of the pituitary body. Med. & Surg. Reporter, Phila., 1887, lvii, 475–477.—**Dickinson** (W.) Gray atrophy of the optic nerve and its relation to facial erysipelas. Tr. M. Ass. Missouri, St. Louis, 1887, 113–119.—**Dixon.** Case of prominence of the globes, with blindness, in a child; atrophy of the optic nerves. Med. Times & Gaz., Lond., 1860, ii, 81. ———. Amaurosis from white atrophy of the optic nerves. *Ibid.*, 1862, i, 350.—**Dmitrovki** (D. I.) Atrophija zritelnich nervov; ambliopija; zamiechatelnija izmienenija v podie zrienia. [Case of atrophy of optic nerve.] Med. Vestnik, St. Petersb., 1880, xx, 163.—**Drummond.** Case of double optic atrophy with cerebral symptoms the result of gazing at the sun. Med. Press & Circ., Lond., 1883, n. s., xxxvi, 67.—**Duboys de Lavigerie.** Commencement d'atrophie de la papille d'origine centrale et probablement consécutive à une embolie; amélioration. Rev. clin. d'ocul., Bordeaux, 1881, ii, 127, 1 pl.—**Dufaud** (G.) Contribution à l'étude de l'atrophie du nerf optique à la suite de l'érysipèle de la face. Union méd., Par., 1886, 3. s., xlii, 1002; 1014.—**Dumont.** Atrophie papillaire, suite de névrorétinite albuminurique. Bull. clin. nat. opht. de l'hosp. d. Quinze-Vingts, Par., 1886, iv, 142. ———. Atrophie nicotique; dyschromatopsie; champ visuel normal. *Ibid.*, 142.—**Fano.** Traitement de l'amaurose par atrophie des nerfs optiques au moyen du badigeonnage de l'orbite avec un liniment iodo-strychné. France méd., Par., 1873, xx, 10–12. ———. Antécédents d'alcoolisme et de nicotinisme; atrophie partielle du nerf optique droit; persistance de la faculté chromatique des deux yeux; champs visuels intacts. J. d'ocul. et chir., Par., 1880, viii, 231.—**Ferret.** Note sur les caractères cliniques de l'atrophie papillaire qui a pour cause l'intoxication alcoolique. Bull. clin. nat. opht. de l'hosp. d. Quinze-Vingts, Par., 1885, iii, 235–237.—**Friedenwald** (A.) Atrophy of the optic disc following post partum hemorrhage. Virginia M. Month., Richmond, 1876, ii, 739.—**Fuchs** (E.) Sur les lésions anatomiques dans l'atrophie des nerfs optiques. Bull. et mém. Soc. d'opht., Par., 1885, iii, 116–120, 1 pl. ———. Die periphere Atrophie des Sehnerven. Arch. f. Ophth., Berl., 1885, xxxi, 1. Abth., 177–200, 1 pl.—**Galezowski** (X.) Aperçu sur les

Nerve (*Optic, Atrophy of*).

atrophies de la papille du nerf optique et sur leur étiologie. J. d'ophth., Par., 1872, i, 43; 108; 138. ———. Pathologie et thérapeutique de l'atrophie de la papille
du nerf optique et des amblyopies dans certaines affections gastriques. Abeille méd., Par., 1876, xxxiii, 97-99.
Also: Union méd., Par , 1876, 3. s., xxi, 365-372. *Also:*
École de méd., Par., 1876, iii, 1-7. ———. De l'atrophie
progressive de la papille du nerf optique. Mouvement
méd., Par., 1877, xv, 336; 352; 366. ———. Sur les atrophies
traumatiques des papilles optiques. Compt. rend. Soc. de
biol. 1879, Par., 18-0, 7. s., i, 330-334. *Also:* Gaz. hebd. de
méd., Par., 1880, 2. s., xvii, 54-56. ———. Du traitement
des atrophies des papilles ataxiques, par les injections
hypodermiques de cyanure d'or, de cyanure de platine
et de cyanure d'argent. Rec. d'ophth., Par., 1883, 3. s., v,
287-290. ———. De l'atrophie de papille ataxique. *Ibid.*,
1884, 3. s., vi, 255-263.—**Gayat.** Vision persistante avec
les signes d'atrophie du nerf optique. Mém. et compt.
rend. Soc. d. sc. méd. de Lyon (1873), 1874, xiii, pt. 2,
76-79. *Also:* Lyon méd., 1873, xiii, 372; 377.—**Godin.**
[Atrophie du chiasma des nerfs optiques.] Bull. Soc. anat.
de Par., 1835, 3. s., i, 5.—**Goupil.** [Nerfs optiques atro-
phiés dans une femme amaurotique depuis deux ans.]
Ibid., 1853, xxviii, 247.—**Guépin.** Atrophie des papilles
des nerfs optiques, symptomatiques d'une affection cérébrale; congestions épileptiformes. J. de méd. de Bordeaux, 1861, 2. s., vi, 119-121.—**Gunn** (R. M.) On the
continuous electrical current as a therapeutic agent in
atrophy of the optic nerve and in retinitis pigmentosa.
Ophth. Hosp. Rep., Lond., 1880-82, x, 161-192.—**Harlan**
(G. C.) Strychnia in atrophy of the optic nerve. Phila.
M. Times, 1874-5, v, 194-197.—**Heiberg** (J.) [Atrophia
nervi optici; chorioiditis atrophica.] *In his:* Prøvefore-
læsning, 8°, Christiania, 1873, 3-11.—**Hermann** (H. W.)
Atrophy of the optic nerve; multiple sclerosis or spastic
paral\sis; differential diagnosis. Am. J. Ophth., St. Louis,
1884-5, i, 48-51.—**Herschell.** Observation d'atrophie de
la papille optique, symptomatique d'une ataxie locomotrice
traitée avec succès par le nitrate d'argent à l'intérieur,
d'après la méthode de Charcot et Vulpin. Cong. périod.
internat. d'ophth. 1862, Par., 1863, ii, 144-148.—**Higgens**
(C.) Atrophy of optic nerves occurring about puberty.
Med. Times & Gaz., Lond., 1880, i, 450. ———. Three cases
of simple atrophy of the optic nerves, occurring in members of the same family. Lancet, Lond., 1881, ii, 869. *Also,
transl.:* Rev. clin. d'ocul., Bordeaux, 1882, iii, 154.—**Hilbert** (R.) Ein Fall von Atrophia nervorum opticorum
bei einer Ente. Ztschr. f. vergleich. Augenh., Wiesb.,
1886, iv, 71-74.—**Hirschberg** (J.) Atroph. n. opt. sta-
tionar. e neuritide. Arch. f. Augenh., Wiesb., 1879, viii,
181. *Also, transl.:* Arch. Ophth., N. Y., 1879-80, viii,
364.— **Hogg** (J.) On certain forms of atrophy of the
optic nerve. Rep. Internat. Ophth. Cong. 1872, Lond.,
1873, iv, 166-169. ———. Clinical remarks on the value of
strychnia in white atrophy of the optic nerve. Med.
Press & Circ., Lond., 1873, xv, 41; 155.—**Huidicz.** Atrophie des nerfs optiques; examen microscopique. Bull.
méd. du nord, Lille, 1875, xiv, 461-464.—**Hunicke** (W.)
A case of anomalous central retinal blood vessels; atrophy
of the optic nerves. J. Ophth., St. Louis, 1885, ii,
27-31.— **Lagleyze** (P.) Atrofia de la papila; esclero-
coroiditis posterior; rama arterial varicosa terminando en
un aneurisma; anastómosis entre dos ramas de la arteria
central; desprendimiento de la retina; coroiditis atrófica.
Rev. argent. de oftal. práct., Buenos Aires, 1883-4, i, 2,
1 pl.—**Landesberg** (M.) Genuine atrophy of the optic
nerve, and tabes dorsalis, dependent upon syphilis. Proc.
Phila. Co. M. Soc. 1882-3, Phila., 1883, v, 163-165. *Also :*
Phila. M. Times, 1882-3, xiii, 827-829.—**Langlet.** Hémiplégie avec contracture; lésion de la capsule externe et
de la capsule interne; atrophie du bulbe. Union méd. et
scient. du nord-est, Reims, 1877, i, 394-396.—**Lanos** (R.)
Un caso de atrofia de la papila óptica. Encicl. méd.-farm.,
Barcel., 1877, i, 53.—**Leber** (T.) Beiträge zur Kenntniss
der atrophischen Veränderungen des Sehnerven, nebst Bemerkungen über die normale Structur des Nerven. Arch.
f. Ophth., Berl., 1868, xiv, 2. Abth., 164-220, 3 pl.—**Liebreich** (R.) Atrophy of the optic disc. Brit. M. J.,
Lond., 1871, ii, 552.—**Lippincott** (J. A.) A case of atro-
phy of the optic nerves; recovery. Med. & Surg. Reporter,
Phila., 1879, xli, 137-139.—**Loring** (F. B.) Atrophy of
the optic nerve; use of strychnia and the artificial leech.
Nat. M. Rev., Wash., 1879, i, 89-92.—**M'Hardy** (M. M.)
Optic nerve atrophy. St. George's Hosp. Rep. 1877-8,
Lond., 1879, ix, 491.—**Mackenzie** (F. M.) White atro-
phy of the right optic disc, probably caused by smoking.
Indian M. Gaz., Calcutta, 1872, vii, 207.—**McKeown** (D.)
A case of atrophy of the optic nerves treated by hypodermic injections of nitrate of pilocarpine. Brit. M. J.,
Lond., 1884, ii, 905.—**Maunsell** (S. E.) Pigmentary retinitis; optic nerve atrophy. Indian M. J., Allahabad,
1884, iii, 513-516. ———. Atrophy of the optic nerve following severe pain, of a neuralgic nature, in the brow. Indian
M. Gaz., Calcutta, 1884, xix, 15.—**Mengin.** Atrophie des
deux papilles à la suite de méningite aiguë, complète d'un
côté avec cécité, incomplète de l'autre avec conservation
de l'acuité visuelle normale. Rec. d'ophth., Par., 1880,

Nerve (*Optic, Atrophy of*).

3. s., ii, 385-391.—**Müller** (H.) Anatomischer Befund
bei einem Fall von Amaurose mit Atrophie des Sehnerven.
Arch. f. Ophth., Berl., 1857, iii, 1. Abth., 92-98, 1 pl.—
• **Nettleship** (E.) Atrophy of one optic nerve after papil-
litis from erysipelas affecting orbit during convalescence
from scarlet fever. Ophth. Hosp. Rep., Lond., 1886, xi, 65.—
Nieden (A.) Ein Fall von Atrophie des einen Sehner-
venstammes mit nahezu gleichmässigem und normalem
Dickendurchmesser der beiden Tractus optici. Centralbl.
f. prakt. Augenh., Leipz., 1879, iii, 136.—**Norris** (W. F.)
Hereditary atrophy of the optic nerves. Tr. Am. Ophth.
Soc., 18. meeting. N. Y., 1882, iii, 355: 20. meeting, 1884,
Bost., 1885, iii, 662, 4 pl. — **Odevaine** (F.) Disease of
fundus with opacity of lens, in both eyes. Indian M. Gaz.,
Calcutta, 1877, xii, 93. ———. Atrophy of the optic papillæ.
Ibid., 1878, xiii, 213.—**von Oettingen** (G.) Formen progressiver Amblyopie von der Sehnerven-Scheide ausgehend. [3 cases.] Dorpat. med. Ztschr., 1877, vi, 344.—
Ogle (J. W.) Atrophy of the optic nerves and tracts of
both sides and of the optic commissure; total blindness for
twelve or fourteen years. Tr. Path. Soc. Lond., 1855-6,
vii, 334, 1 pl.—**Oglesby** (R. P.) On the recovery of sight
after atrophy of the optic discs. Ophth. Hosp. Rep., Lond.,
1867-9, vi, 190-196. *Also:* Dublin Q. J. M. Sc., 1869, xlviii,
529-531.—**Pagenstecher** (H.) Atrophy of the optic
nerve after erysipelas of the face. Ophth. Hosp. Rep.,
Lond., 1871-3, vii, 32-34.—**Paoli** (C.) Dell' atrofia interstiziale e parenchimatosa del nervo ottico. Sperimentale,
Firenze, 1879, xliv, 164-168.—**Parinaud.** Atrophie des
nerfs optiques dans l'érysipèle de la face. Arch. gén. de
méd., Par., 1879, 7. s., iii, 641-660.—**Parisotti** (O.) &
Melotti (J.) Un cas d'atrophie des deux papilles par
intoxication saturnine. Rec. d'ophth., Par., 1885, 3. s.,
vii, 520-539.—**Peltesohn** (N.) Ursachen und Verlauf
der Sehnervenatrophie. Centralbl. f. prakt. Augenh.,
Leipz., 1886, x, 45; 75; 106.—**Purtscher** (O.) Ueber
Kreuzung der Nervi und Tractus optici; pathologisch-anatomische Untersuchungen. Arch. f. Ophth.,
Berl., 1880, xxvi, 2. Abth., 191-220, 4 pl.—**Quaglino.** De
l'atrophie progressive du nerf optique. Cong. périod. internat. d'ophth. 1862, Par., 1863, ii, 229-235.—**Rampoldi**
(R.) Della stricnina nella cura della atrofia dei nervi
ottici. Ann. di ottal., Pavia, 1882, xi, 390-403. ———. Osservazioni di atrofia progressiva dei nervi ottici. *Ibid.*,
1883, xii, 422-424.—**Rankin** (F. H.) A case of syphilitic
atrophy of both optic nerves. Med. Rec., N. Y., 1875, x,
180.—**Rechtseitiger** Gesichtsschmerz, Vertreibung des
Bulbus, beginnende Atrophie des Nerv. opticus; Parese
des N. oculomotorius; rasche Heilung durch Jodkali.
Ber. d. k. k. Krankenanst. Rudolph-Stiftung in Wien
(1870), 1871, 173-176.—**Reid** (T.) Atrophy of optic nerve;
improvement by galvanism. Brit. M. J., Lond., 1874, i,
517.—**Rullier** (G.) Observation d'atrophie du nerf optique d'origine traumatique (coup de fleuret). Arch. de
méd. et pharm. mil., Par., 1886, viii, 209-211 —**Rumszewicz** (K.) Jednostronny zanik tarczy nerwu wzrokowego z zabarwieniem. [Unilateral atrophy of papilla.]
Gaz. lek., Warszawa, 1882, 2. s., ii, 280-283. *Also, transl.:*
Klin. Monatsbl. f. Augenh., Stuttg., 1882, xx, 279-283.—**von
Russdorf** (E.) Atrophie des Opticus. Deutsche Klin.,
Berl., 1866, xviii, 250-252.—**Schmidt** (H.) Cerebrale
Sehnerven-Atrophie, mit Druck-Excavation der Papilla
optica. Arch. f. Ophth., Berl., 1871, xvii, 1. Abth., 117-
122.--**Schmidt-Rimpler** (H.) Progressive Sehner-
ven-Atrophie und Fehlen des Knie-Phänomens. Klin.
Monatsbl. f. Augenh., Cassel, 1878, xvi, 265-270.—**Seely**
(W. W.) Atrophy of the optic nerve. Cincin. Lancet &
Clinic, 1883, n. s., x, 263.—**Smith** (P.) Persistent dropping of fluid from the nostril, associated with atrophy of
the optic nerves and other brain symptoms. Ophth.
Rev., Lond., 1883, ii, 4-11. — **Stroppa** (L.) Ambliopia;
poscia amaurosi; fenomeni di paralisi spinale; segni mani-
festi di atrofia della papilla; atrofia dei nervi ottici e del
chiasma; rammollimento della parte inferiore del midollo
spinale. Ann. di ottal., Milano, 1872-3, ii, 177-179.—
Trousseau (A.) Pseudo atrophies de la papille. Bull.
clin. nat. opht. de l'hosp. d. Quinze-Vingts, Par., 1887, v,
45-47. *Also:* Union méd., Par., 1887, 3. s., xliii, 401-404.—
Uhthoff (W.) Beitrag zur Sehnervenatrophie. Arch. f.
Ophth., Berl., 1880, xxvi, 1. Abth., 244-282.—**Vieusse.**
De l'atrophie et de la névrite traumatique de la papille.
Rec. d'ophth., Par., 1875, 2. s., ii, 334-349. — **Vossius**
(A.) Beiderseits Atrophia optici nach Embolie der Art.
centralis retinæ; Insufficienz der Valvula mitralis; l. totale
Amaurose; r. Amblyopie. Klin. Monatsbl. f. Augenh.,
Stuttg., 1883, xxi, 298-301. ———. Ein Fall von neuritischer
Sehnervenatrophie mit eigenthümlicher Anomalie der Ve-
nen auf der Papille beiderseits bei angeborener Schädel-
difformität. *Ibid.*, 1884, xxii, 172-178.—**Webster** (D.) A
case of apparent atrophy of the optic nerve, in which recovery of eyesight followed the use of hypodermic injections of nitrate of strychnia. Tr. Am. Ophth. Soc., N. Y.,
1872-9, ii, 573. ———. Cases of atrophy of the optic nerve
apparently benefited by hypodermic injections of strychnia.
N. Eng. M. Month., Sandy Hook, Conn., 1883-4, iii, 199.—
Wendt (H.) Sehnervenatrophie bei Geisteskranken.
Allg. Ztschr. f. Psychiat., etc., Berl., 1868, xxv, 137-161.—

Nerve (Optic, Atrophy of).

Wicherkiewicz (B.) Wsprawie wzroku mniej lubwięcej prawidłowego przy wziernikowych zmianach zanikowych tarczy nerwu wzrokowego. [Function of sight considered in connection with atrophy of the papilla of the optic nerve.] Medycyna, Warszawa, 1886, xiv, 265-269.—**Wick** (D. M.) & **Alt** (A.) A case of rapidly growing tumor of the brain; atrophy of both optic nerves without optic neuritis. Am. J. Ophth., St. Louis, 1886, iii, 331-335.—**Wyman** (J.) Blindness in one eye attended with atrophy of the optic nerve and optic lobe. Am. J. M. Sc., Phila., 1852, n. s., xxiv, 369-371.—**Zehery** I.) Atrophia nervi optici traumatica egy ritka esete. Szemészet, Budapest, 1884, 108-111. Also, transl.: Pest. med.-chir. Presse, Budapest, 1884, xx, 968.

Nerve (Optic, Inflammation of).

See, also, **Brain** (Tumors of); **Nerve** (Optic, Pathology of); **Nose** (Foreign bodies in); **Retinitis.**

AUGSTEIN (C.) * Ueber Störung des Farbensinns bei Neuritis. 8°. Danzig, [1883].

Also, in: Arch. f. Augenh., Wiesb., 1884-5, xiv, 347-359, 1 pl. Also, transl. in: Arch. Ophth., N. Y., 1885, xiv, 435-446, 1 pl.

DEDOME (P.) * Étude sur la névrite optique. 4°. Paris, 1875.

DEUTSCHMANN (R.) Ueber Neuritis optica besonders die sogenannte "Stauungspapille" und deren Zusammenhang mit Gehirn-Affectionen. 8°. Jena, 1887.

HÄNDEL (M.) * Beiträge zur Casuistik der acuten genuinen Neuritis optica. 8°. Berlin, [1885].

PARINAUD (H.) Étude sur la névrite optique dans la méningite aiguë de l'enfance, avec vingt observations suivies d'autopsie, recueillies à l'Hôpital des enfants. 8°. Paris, 1877.

REYNAUD-LACROZE (C.) * De la névrite et de la périnévrite optiques considérées dans leurs rapports avec les maladies cérébrales. 4°. Paris, 1870.

ROI (V.) * De la névrite optique rhumatismale. 4°. Paris, 1886.

SCHLÜTER (F.) * Ueber Neuritis optica. 8°. Berlin, 1882.

Abadie (C.) De la névrite optique produite par des néoplasmes intra-crâniens qui déterminent la cécité sans entraîner la mort. Arch. d'opht., Par., 1880-81, i, 145-151. ———. Sur quelques particularités de la névrite optique des tumeurs cérébrales. Union méd., Par., 18-6, 3. s., xli, 857-860.—**Agnew** (C. R.) Two cases of neuro-retinitis albuminurica. Planet, N. Y., 1883, i, 8.—**Alexander.** Neuritis des Sehnervenstammes; Heilung. Deutsche med. Wchnschr., Berl., 1881, vii, 547. ———. Doppelseitige Papillitis bei Gehirnabscess. Ibid., 1883, ix, 338.—**Allbutt** (T. C.) On "optic neuritis" as a symptom of disease of the brain and spinal cord. Med. Times & Gaz., Lond., 1868, i, 495; 521; 574; 628: ii, 61; 116.—**Alt** (A.) A case of endothelioma of the intervaginal space of the optic nerve; removal, with attempt to preserve the eyeball; subsequent enucleation on account of uncontrollable hemorrhage; remarks. Arch. Ophth. & Otol., N. Y., 1877-8, vi, 367-375. Also, transl.: Arch. f. Augen- u. Ohrenh., Wiesb., 1878, vii, 46-54. ———. A case of sympathetic neuro-retinitis; remarks on sympathetic ophthalmia. Am. J. Ophth., St. Louis, 1884-5, i, 28; 57; 97.—**Annuske.** Die Neuritis optica bei Tumor cerebri. Arch. f. Ophth., Berl., 1873, xix, 3. Abth , 165-300.—**Bader** (C.) The human eye in health and disease, as seen with the ophthalmoscope. Third series. Plates illustrating morbid changes in the optic nerve (optic disc). Guy's Hosp. Rep., Lond., 1869, 3. s., xiv, 456-462, 2 pl. Also, Reprint.—**Barck** (C.) Two cases of disease of the optic nerves, due to cerebral affections. Am. J. Ophth., St. Louis, 1886, iii, 46-49.—**Beck** (K. J.) Amaurose bedingt durch abnorme Beschaffenheit der Sehnerven. Ztschr. f. d. Ophth., Heidelb., 1834-5, iv, 90-94.—**Blessig.** Klinische Beiträge zur Lehre von der Sehnerven-Entzündung. St. Petersb. med. Ztschr., 1866, x, 65-80. ———. Neuritis descendens. Klin. Monatsbl. f. Augenh., Stuttg., 1875, xiii, 420-424.—**Bouchut** (E.) Névro-rétinite en rapport avec une lésion de l'oreille interne et du facial dont l'origine était comprimée par une tumeur de la protubérance. Cong. périod. internat. d'opth. Compt.-rend. 1880, Milan, 1881, vi, 82-86. ———. De la névrite optique dans ses rapports avec les maladies intra-crâniennes. Tr. Internat. M. Cong. 7. sess., Lond., 1881, iii, 58. Also: Paris méd., 1881, vi, 265-267.—**Bousseau.** Névrite optique dans la méningite tuberculeuse et la paralysie générale. Bull. Soc. anat. de Par., 1867, xlii, 681; 753, 1 pl.—**Bouviu** (M.

Nerve (Optic, Inflammation of).

J.) Neuritis optica ten gevolge van tumor cerebri. Nederl. Tijdschr. v. Geneesk., Amst., 1884, 2. R., xx, 45-51.—**Bowen** (A.) Report of a case of albuminuric neuro-retinitis, occurring during pregnancy, and presenting some unusual features. Austral. M. J., Melbourne, 1883, n. s., v, 448.—**Brailey** (W. A.) Examination of an eye excised 6 weeks after a wound, the optic disc of which presents the appearance of optic neuritis. Opth. Hosp. Rep., Lond., 1874-6, viii, 547. ———. Sympathetic neuritis without other visible structural change. Tr. Ophth. Soc. U. Kingdom, Lond., 18-3-4, iv, 87.—**Brière.** Névrite optique double syphilitique; cécité complète pendant trois jours; guérison rapide. Ann. d'ocul , Brux., 1879, lxxxi, 37-39.—**Bristowe** (J. S.) Hæmorrhage into the brain attended with optic neuritis. Tr. Ophth. Soc. U. Kingdom. Lond., 1886, vi, 363-368.—**Brudenell** (R.) Three cases of optic neuritis. Tr. Clin. Soc. Lond., 1870-71, iv, 32-37.—**Bruns** (H. D.) Hemorrhagic neuro-retinitis; incipient atrophy of optic nerves. N. Orl. M. & S. J., 1886-7, n. s., xiv, 760.—**Bull** (C. S.) Analysis of one hundred and three cases of exudative neuro-retinitis, associated with chronic Bright's disease. Tr. Am. Ophth. Soc., Bost., 1886, iv, pt. 2, 184-194. Also: N. York M. J., 1886, xliv, 119-122. Also, Reprint.—**Buller** (F.) Remarks on optic neuritis. Canada M. & S. J., Montreal, 1881-2, x, 641-649.—**Burnett** (S. M.) Double optic neuritis (choked disc) and sloughing of the right cornea, accompanying a sarcomatous tumor on the right side of the brain. Arch. Ophth. & Otol., N. Y., 1877-8, vi, 469-476. Also, transl.: Arch. f. Augen- u. Ohrenh., Wiesb., 1878, vii, 472-478. ———. Clinical contributions to the study of retro-bulbar affections of the optic nerve. Am. J. Ophth., St. Louis, 1885, ii, 62-67.—**Carter** (R. B.) Case of swollen optic disc, in which the sheath of the optic nerve was incised behind the eyeball. Brit. M. J., Lond., 1887, i, 679. Also: Lancet, Lond., 1887, i, 626. ———. On retrobulbar incision of the optic nerve in cases of swollen disc. Brain, Lond., 1887-8, x, 199-209.—**Caudron** (V.) Névro-rétinite intense; retour de la vision normale malgré la persistance de lésions ophthalmoscopiques très notables. Rev. clin. d'ocul., Bordeaux, 1881, ii, 130-133.—**Chauvel** (J.) Névrite optique double avec myélite aiguë temporaire. Bull. et mém. Soc. de chir. de Par., 1880, n. s., vi, 512-515.—**Cheatham** (W.) Neuro-retinitis albuminurica. J. Am. M. Ass., Chicago, 1885, v, 150.—**Chisolm** (J. J.) An obscure case in nerve pathology accompanying optic neuritis. Arch. Ophth., N. Y., 1882, xi, 239-242.—**Clerval.** Névrite optique double d'origine cérébrale. Bull. clin. nat. opht. de l'hosp. d. Quinze-Vingts, Par., 1887, v, 107.—**Connor** (L.) Optic neuritis, considered in some of its relations to cerebral tumors. Tr. M. Soc. Mich., Lansing, 1882, viii, no. 2, 200-215.—**Coomes** (M. F.) A case of optic neuritis, the result of cerebral glioma. Med. Herald, Louisville, 1885-6, vii, 391-393.—**Coupland** (S.) Case of neuro-retinitis following contusion of the brain, with meningitis; death five months after the injury. Tr. Ophth. Soc. U. Kingdom, Lond., 1881-2, ii, 73-82.—**Critchett** (G. A.) Neuro-retinitis of right eye in secondary syphilis. Tr. Ophth. Soc. U. Kingdom, Lond., 1881-2, ii, 59.—**Critchett** (G. A.) & **Sturge** (W. A.) Case of optic atrophy after neuritis, three years; detachment of retina in right eye; hæmorrhage into vitreous; increased tension; probable growth beneath retina. Ibid., 18-0 81, i, 136.—**Daguenet.** Quelques remarques sur la pathogénie de la névrite optique. Rec. d'ophth., Par., 1879, 3. s., i, 705-709.—**De Mets.** Observation d'un cas de névrite optique suivie de guérison. Ann. Soc. de méd. d'Anvers, 1886, xlvii, 365-373. ———. Périnévrite optique droite; paralysie de la troisième paire; syphilis. Rec. d'ophth., Par., 1882, 4. s., iv, 35.—**Dickinson** (W.) Optic neuritis. St. Louis M. & S. J., 1879, xxxvii, 535-542.—**Dickinson** (W. H.) Optic neuritis. Tr. Path. Soc. Lond., 1871-2, xxiii, 214.—**Dowse** (T. S.) The contiguity of neuro-retinitis with descending retinitis from intra-cerebral disease. Med. Press & Circ., Lond., 1879, n. s., xxvii, 519.—**Edmunds** (W.) Contribution to pathology of double optic neuritis. St. Thomas's Hosp. Rep. 1880-81, Lond., 1882, n. s., xi, 71-74, 1 pl.—**Edmunds** (W.) & **Lawford** (J. B.) Examination of the optic nerves in cases of intra-cranial disease, with remarks on the immediate causation of optic neuritis. Tr. Ophth. Soc. U. Kingdom, Lond., 1882-3, iii, 138-158, 3 pl.—Also [Abstr.]: Brit. M. J., Lond., 1883, i, 963. ———. An analysis of cases of intracranial tumour with respect to the existence of optic neuriris. Tr. Ophth. Soc. U. Kingdom, Lond., 1883-4, iv, 172-186. ———. Remarks on Prof. Deutschmann's views on optic neuritis. Ophth. Rev., Lond., 1887, vi, 134-136.—**Erb** (W.) Ueber das Zusammenvorkommen von Neuritis optica und Myelitis subacuta. Arch. f. Psychiat., Berl., 1879, x, 146-157.—**Evans** (T.) A case of double optic neuritis. Australas. M. Gaz., Sydney 1881-2, i, 19.—**Fano.** Névrite optique et névro-rétinite exsudatives, suivies promptement d'une atrophie du nerf optique. J. d'ocul. et chir., Par., 1875-6, ii, 224. ———. Névrite optique et névro-rétinite ponctuée de l'œil droit; iodure de potassium à l'intérieur et en onctions sur l'orbite; guérison. Ibid., 229-231.—**Flarer** (G.) Sullo sviluppo della neurite ottica da affezione cere-

Nerve (*Optic, Inflammation of*).

brale. Riv. di med., di chir. e di terap., Milano, 1870, ii. 285–289. *Also:* Ann. di ottal., Milano, 1871–2, i, 41–46.—**Forlanini** (C.) Osservazioni ed esperienze. Ann. di ottal., Milano, 1871–2, i, 41–56. [*See, also, supra,* Flarer (G.).]—**Foucher.** Névrite optique et maladies cérébrales. Union méd. du Canada, Montréal, 1883, xii, 337–343.—**Fox** (L. W.) Acute uni-ocular neuritis. Am. J. Ophth., St. Louis, 1884–5, i, 113–115.—**Francotte** (X.) Contribution à l'étude de la névrite multiple. Rev. de méd., Par., 1886, vi, 377–408.—**Friedenwald** (A.) Optic neuritis. Maryland M. J., Balt., 1881–2, viii, 145; 171. ——. A case of optic neuritis, with brain symptoms; recovery; with remarks. N York M. J., 1887, xlv, 147–149.—**Fuchs** (E.) Neuritis in Folge hereditärer Anlage. Klin. Monatsbl. f Augenh., Stuttg., 1879, xvii, 332–337.—**Gairdner** (W. T.) Optic neuritis with cerebral symptoms. Brit. M. J., Lond., 1876, i, 194.—**Galezowski.** Névrite optique double avec cécité absolue: accidents cérébraux; guérison complète. Rec.d'ophth., Par., 1875, 2. s., ii, 80–82. ——. Atrophie double des deux papilles par névrite optique. *Ibid.*, 1877, 2. s., iv, 361. ——. De la névrite optique. Mouvement méd., Par., 1877, xv, 402. ——. Quelques mots sur la névrite optique et sur sa curabilité. *Ibid.*, 1881, 3. s., iii, 214; 272. ——. Des thromboses vasculaires amenant des névrites optiques ou des signes d'embolie. Tr. Internat. M. Cong., 7. sess., Lond., 1881, iii, 58–60.—**Gillet de Grandmont.** Névrite optique et condylome de l'iris traités par les injections de peptonate d'hydrargyre et suivis de guérison. Rec. d'ophth., Par., 1886, 3. s., viii, 230–232. —**Goodhart** (J F.) A case of headache and double optic neuritis with almost complete amaurosis, followed by recovery with partial restoration of sight. Tr. Clin. Soc. Lond., 1875–6, ix, 127–134.—**Gowers** (W. R.) The relation of optic neuritis to encephalic disease. *In his:* Manual and atlas of medical ophthalmoscopy, 8°, Lond., 1879, 63–81. *Also, transl. in:* Ann. d'ocul., Brux., 1879, lxxxii, 143–158. ——. Optic neuritis in chlorosis. Brit. M. J., Lond., 1880, ii, 780. ——. Case of slight optic neuritis, with paresis of sixth nerves, probably due to transient meningitis. Tr. Ophth. Soc. U. Kingdom, Lond., 1880–81, i, 115–117. ——. Case of intracranial disease with optic neuritis and paralysis of the upward movement of both eyes. *Ibid.*, 117: 1881–2, ii, 84. ——. Optic neuritis in chlorosis. Brit. M. J., Lond., 1881, i, 796.—**von Gräfe** (A.) Ueber Complication von Sehnervenentzündung mit Gehirnkrankheiten. Arch. f. Ophth., Berl., 1860, vii, 2. Abth., 58–71.— **Grossmann** (L.) Doppelseitige Neuroretinitis descendens mit consecutiv eingetretener Amaurose nach Diabetes mellitus. Berl. klin. Wchnschr., 1879, xvi, 138–142. ——. Beiderseitige Neuritis optica in Folge Schläfenbeinfissur. Wien. med Presse, 1887, xxviii, 1742–1744.—**Guéneau de Mussy** (N.) Périnévrite optique double; apoplexies de la rétine liées probablement à une fièvre larvée; guérison par le sulfate de quinine. J. d'ophth., Par., 1872, i, 5–9.—**Hansell** (H. F.) Acute optic neuritis of rheumatic origin; two cases, one monocular. Med. News, Phila., 1886, xlix, 144–146.—**Harlan** (G. C.) Descending neuritis. Phila. M. Times, 1872, ii, 169.—**Herter.** Fall von retrobulbärer, vielleicht entzündlicher Sehnerven-Affection. Charité-Ann. 1875, Berl., 1877, ii, 521–523. ——. Amaurose nach Blutverlust (Neuroretinitis). *Ibid.*, 525–527.—**Hirschberg** (J.) Stauungspapille und Neuritis optica. Deutsche Ztschr. f. prakt. Med., Berl., 1876, 37. ——. Neuritis specifica. Arch. f. Augenh., Wiesb., 1879, viii, 179. *Also, transl.:* Arch. Ophth., N. Y., 1879–80, viii, 361. ——. Ueber selbstständige Sehnervenentzündung. Centralbl. f. prakt. Augenh., Leipz., 1887, xi, 321–327.—**Hock** (J.) Beiträge zur Lehre von der Neuritis retrobulbaris. Wien. med. Bl., 1883, vi, 595; 631; 664; 700; 794. ——. Neuere Beobachtungen über Neuritis retrobulbaris peripherica (acuta et subacuta). Centralbl. f. prakt. Augenh., Leipz., 1884, viii, 107–111. *Also, transl.:* Rec. d'ophth., Par., 1884, 3. s., vi, 461–468.—**Horstmann** (C.) Ueber Neuritis optica. Deutsche med. Wchnschr., Berl., 1880, vi, 421; 436.—**Hotz** (F. C.) Two cases of retro-bulbar neuritis (amblyopia centralis). Am. J. Ophth., St. Louis, 1884–5, i, 167. — **Hubbard** (C. G.) Neuro-retinitis, from inflammation of the dura-mater. N. York M. J., 1878, xxviii, 292–295.—**Hulke** (J.W.) Four cases of neuro-retinitis associated with kidney disease. Ophth. Hosp. Rep., Lond., 1865–6, v, 16–26, 1 pl. ——. Cases of neuritis optica, neuro-retinitis and retinitis. *Ibid.*, 1867–9, vi, 89–118. ——. Cases of optic neuritis and neuro-retinitis. Lancet, Lond., 1881, i, 210.—**Hutchinson** (J.) Clinical lectures on cases of inflammation of the optic nerves. Ophth. Hosp. Rep., Lond., 1865–6, v, 94; 163. ——. On a group of cases of optic neuritis in children. *Ibid.*, 307–317. ——. Optic neuritis in a child, following severe cerebral symptoms. *Ibid.*, 1867–9, vi, 43–47. ——. Neuro-retinitis in connection with albuminuria and disease of the heart. *Ibid.*, 1871–3, vii, 44. ——. Double optic neuritis during an illness with cerebral symptoms in a child; recovery of perfect health with atrophied discs and great defect of sight. *Ibid.*, 1874–6, viii, 493. ——. Double optic neuritis ending in partial atrophy, but with great improvement of sight; history of failure of sight for a time some years before, and of several

Nerve (*Optic, Inflammation of*).

attacks of hemiplegia: sun-stroke? syphilis? *Ibid.*, 495. ——. Failure of left eye from neuritis, coming on a few days after an attack of slight right hemiplegia; subsequent improvement of sight. *Ibid.*, 496. ——. Optic neuritis of one eye only, with severe pain on same side of face; atrophy of disc, with improvement of sight; no clue to cause; condition 5½ years later. *Ibid.*, 497. ——. Neuritis with cerebral illness in children ending in perfect recovery of health. *Ibid.*, 1876–9, ix, 124–130. ——. Relapsing optic neuritis, with development of new vessels in front of the papilla. *Ibid.*, 1883–6, xi, 191–195, 1 pl. ——. Two cases of double optic neuritis, without impairment of vision and without atrophy resulting, after injury to the head. Lancet, Lond., 1882, i, 485.—**Jackson** (J. H.) Lecture on optic neuritis from intracranial disease. Med. Times & Gaz., Lond., 1871, ii, 241; 341; 581. ——. On a case of recovery from double optic neuritis. West. Riding Lun. Asyl. Rep., Lond., 1874, iv, 24–29, 1 pl. ——. On the relation between optic neuritis and intra-cranial disease. Tr. Ophth. Soc. U. Kingdom, Lond., 1880–81, i, 60–115. *Also:* Med. Times & Gaz., Lond., 1881, i, 311; 460. *Also* [Abstr.]: Lancet, Lond., 1881, i, 620–622.—**Jacobi** (J.) Zwei verschiedenartige Fälle von Neuritis optici. Arch. f. Ophth., Berl., 1868, xiv, 1. Abth., 149–158.—**Jany** (L.) Ein Fall von rechtseitiger Hemianopie und Neuroretinitis in Folge eines Gliosarcoms im linken Occipitallappen. Arch. f. Augenh., Wiesb., 1882, xi, 190–198.—**Knapp** (H.) A case of neuro-retinitis resulting from a gummy tumor of the dura mater. Arch. Ophth. & Otol., N. Y., 1874, iv, 245–249. *Also, in his:* Ophthal. Contrib., 8°, N. Y., 1875, 11–15. *Also, transl.:* Arch. f. Augen- u. Ohrenh., Wiesb., 1874–5, iv, 205–209. ——. Neuro-retinitis, with almost sudden loss of sight in both eyes. Tr. Am. Ophth. Soc. 1884, Bost., 1885, iii, pt. 5, 654–662. —**von Kries** (N.) Zwei Fälle von retrobulbärer Neuritis. Arch. f. Ophth., Berl., 1878, xxiv, 153–156.—**Krohn** (L.) Tvenne fall af neuritis optica. Finska läk.-sällsk. handl., Helsingfors, 1871, xiii, 81–102, 2 pl. *Also, transl.:* Klin. Monatsbl. f. Augenh., Erlang., 1872, x, 93–108.—**Kuhnt** (H.) Zur Genese der Neuritis. Ber. ü. d. Versamml. d. ophth. Gesellsch., Stuttg., 1879, xii, 159–170. — **Landesberg** (M.) Neuro-Retinitis descendens beiderseits in Folge hochgradigen Blutverlustes. Klin. Monatsbl. f. Augenh., Stuttg., 1879, xvii, 283–288. ——. Ein Fall von Neuritis retrobulbaris peripherica acuta beiderseits. Centralbl. f. prakt. Augenh., Leipz., 1884, viii, 280.—**Lang** (W.) Specimen of optic neuritis in an eye lost by corneal ulcer, with hypopyon. Tr. Ophth. Soc. U. Kingdom, Lond., 1880–81, i, 123. — **Lawford** (J. B.) Case of double optic neuritis following purpura, *Ibid.*, 1881–2, ii, 86–89. — **Lawson** (G.) On a case of tumour of the brain; optic neuritis; necropsy. Ophth. Hosp. Rep., Lond., 1880–82, x, 311–315.—**Leber** (T.) Beiträge zur Kenntniss der Neuritis des Sehnerven. Arch. f. Ophth., Berl., 1868, xiv, 2. Abth.; 333–378. ——. Ueber Neuritis optica. Klin. Monatsbl. f. Augenh., Erlang., 1868, vi, 302–315. ——. On the connection between optic neuritis and intra-cranial diseases. Tr. Internat. M. Cong., 7. sess., Lond., 1881, iii, 52–57.—**Lowne** (B. T.) A case of neuro-retinitis followed by partial atrophy of the optic disc, with observations on the perception of colour. Tr. Clin. Soc. Lond., 1877, x, 117–121, 1 pl. — **Lundy** (C. J.) Optic neuritis, with notes of three cases. Detroit Lancet, 1878, i, 890–906. *Also,* Reprint. ——. A case of marked neuro-retinitis with complete recovery of vision. Michigan M. News, Detroit, 1880, iii, 331. — **Mackenzie** (S.) A case of double optic neuritis, without gross cerebral lesion, with remarks upon the immediate causation of optic neuritis. Brain, Lond., 1879, ii, 257–272. ——. Microscopical specimens showing neuro-retinitis with large hæmorrhagic extravasation into retina, from a case of idiopathic (progressive pernicious) anæmia. Tr. Ophth. Soc. U. Kingdom, Lond., 1881–2, ii, 40. ——. Double neuro-retinitis; total loss of vision. Brit. M. J., Lond., 1882, i, 617.—**Macnamara** (C. N.) Optic neuritis, the result of malarial toxæmia. Indian M. Gaz., Calcutta, 1870, v, 28. — **Magni.** Della infiammazione e dell' atrofia del nervo ottico; regole generali per la cura delle affezioni della retina e del nervo ottico. Riv. clin. di Bologna, 1865, iv, 358–368.—**Malmsten.** Amaurosis, ex inflammatione chiasmatis nervorum opticorum. Förh. v. Svens. Läk.-Sällsk. Sammank. 1863–4, Stockholm, 1865, 58–60. — **Mauthner** (L.) Die Sehnerven-Netzhaut-Entzündung bei Hirnerkrankungen. Wien. med. Bl., 1881, iv, 289; 321; 357; 390; 425; 453; 520, 553.—**van Milligen.** Ein seltener Fall von Neuritis optica retrobulbaris. Centralbl. f. prakt. Augenh., Leipz., 1884, viii, 14–17.—**Montgomery** (W. T.) Double optic neuritis from a violent fit of anger; recovery. Tr. Illinois M. Soc., Chicago, 1880, xxx, 159–162.—**Morton** (A. S.) Two cases of double optic neuritis. Tr. Ophth. Soc. U. Kingdom, Lond., 1880–81, i, 121: 1882–3, iii, 136. *Also* [Abstr.]: Brit. M. J., Lond., 1882, ii, 1253.—**Nettleship** (E.) Optic neuritis in an eye lost by ophthalmia neonatorum. Ophth. Hosp. Rep., Lond., 1874–6, viii, 507. ——. Changes left by past neuro-retinitis, probably caused by erysipelas invading the orbits; patient, an old woman. *Ibid.*, 1876–9, ix, 193. ——. Relapsing hæmor-

Nerve (*Optic, Inflammation of*).

rhagic neuro-retinitis and choroiditis, with disease of vitreous and keratitis punctata; only one eye affected; remarkable recovery of sight after repeated attacks; liability to dimness of sight of same eye with dyspepsia, etc. (?functional); influence of neuralgia of 5th in determining one of the hæmorrhagic attacks; rheumatism and perhaps gout in family. *Ibid.*, 194 – 198. ——. Optic nerve from a case of optic neuritis with good sight. Tr. Path. Soc. Lond., 1879–80, xxxi, 252, 1 pl. ——. Case of double optic neuritis, following purpura. Brit. M. J., Lond., 1882, i, 119. ——. Case of optic neuritis followed by dropping of fluid from the nostril. Ophth. Rev., Lond., 1883, ii, 1–3. ——. On cases of retro-ocular neuritis. Tr. Ophth. Soc. U. Kingdom, Lond., 1883–4, iv, 186–226. ——. Clinical lecture on a case of syphilitic optic neuritis. Med. Times & Gaz., Lond., 1885, ii, 276. ——. Single optic neuritis, ending in complete atrophy during the delirium of fever (?typhoid); old nebulæ and high hypermetropia in both eyes. Ophth. Hosp. Rep., Lond., 1883–6, xi, 66.—**Neuroretinitis** optica. J. Comp. M. & S., N. Y., 1884, v, 153–162, 1 pl.—**Norris** (W. F.) Cases of optic neuritis. Tr. Am. Ophth. Soc., 10. meeting, N. Y., 1874, ii, pt. 2, 163–169. *Also*, Reprint.—**Norton** (G. S.) Optic neuritis from intra-cranial diseases. Tr. Am. Homœop. Ophth. & Otol. Soc., Phila., 1879, iii, 67–79.—**Noyes** (H. D.) Acute myelitis with double optic neuritis. Arch. Ophth., N. Y., 1880, ix, 199–206. *Also, transl.:* Arch. f. Augenh., Wiesb., 1881, x, 331–337. — **Odevaine** (F.) Optic neuritis. Indian M. Gaz., Calcutta, 1877, xii, 94.—**Oglesby.** Case of double optic neuritis. Brit. M. J., Lond., 1877, ii, 478. ——. Case of inflamed optic discs. *Ibid.*, 1879, i, 853.—**Owen** (D. C. L.) Brief notes of the ophthalmoscopic appearances and the state of vision in a case of double optic neuritis. Birmingh. M. Rev., 1874, iii, 169–171.—**Parinaud** (H.) De la névrite optique dans les affections cérébrales. Ann. d'ocul., Brux., 1879, lxxxii, 5–47.—**Perlia.** Zur acuten rheumatischen Neuritis retrobulbaris. Klin. Monatsbl. f. Augenh., Stuttg., 1886, xxiv, 132–138.—**Pflüger** (E.) Neuritis optica. Arch. f. Ophth., Berl., 1878, xxiv, 169–189.—**Pooley** (T. R.) A case of sympathetic neuro-retinitis. Am. J. Ophth., St. Louis, 1884–5, i, 69. ——. Double optic neuritis and Ménière's disease. N. York M. J., 1887, xlv, 31–34. — **Power** (H.) Case of optic neuritis. St. Barth. Hosp. Rep., Lond., 1871, vii, 196–198. ——. Case of optic neuritis; both eyes affected; Wecker's operation; relief of symptoms. *Ibid.*, 1872, viii, 171–177. ——. Four cases of double optic neuritis. *Ibid.*, 1873, ix, 181–198. ——. Optic neuritis without evident cause. Tr. Ophth. Soc. U. Kingdom, Lond., 1886, vi, 361–363. — **Rampoldi** (R.) Un notevole caso di neurite retrobulbare. Ann. di ottal., Pavia, 1885, xiv, 202 – 209. ——. Osservazione di neurite ottica coincidente con morbo di Aran. *Ibid.*, 1886, xv, 116 – 118, 1 pl. — **Reich** (M.) Zur Statistik der Neuritis optica bei intra-craniellen Tumoren. Klin. Monatsbl. f. Augenh., Stuttg., 1874, xii, 274. ——. Fall auf den Hinterkopf; scharfer Gesichtsdefect; Neuroretinitis partialis; Heilung. Centralbl. f. prakt. Augenh., Leipz., 1881, v, 100–105. *Also, transl.:* Ejened. klin. gaz., St. Petersb., 1881, i, 300–304.—**Reuling** (G.) A case of retrobulbar- neuritis with only quantitative perception of light, ending in the restoration of perfect vision. N. York M. J., 1877, xxvi, 393–398.—**Reynolds** (D. S.) Circumscribed cortical optic neuritis. Med. Herald, Louisville, 1880–81, ii, 22–25.—**Ricciardi** (E.) Il bromuro di potassio nella nevrite ottica discendente e nella meningite. Indipendente, Torino, 1876, xxvii, 209; 220.—**Risley** (S. D.) A case of sympathetic neuro-retinitis with consecutive serous iritis. J. Am. M. Ass., Chicago, 1885, iv, 43. — **Romiée.** Névro-rétinite, avec phénomènes cérébraux, suivie de guérison. Gaz. d'ophth., Par., 1880, ii, 1–6. — **Samelsohn** (J.) Anatomischer Befund von sogenannter retrobulbärer Neuritis. Sitzungsb. d. nied.-rhein. Gesellsch. f. Nat.- u. Heilk. zu Bonn, 1880, 108–110. ——. The pathological changes in retro-bulbar neuritis (central amblyopia). Tr. Internat. M. Cong., 7. sess., Lond., 1881, iii, 60. ——. Zur Anatomie und Nosologie der retrobulbären Neuritis (Amblyopia centralis). Arch. f. Ophth ., Berl., 1882, xxviii, 1, 2 pl. : 1884, xxx, 1. Abth., 290. — **Saundby** (R.) Note on optic neuritis in children. Birmingh. M. Rev., 1885, xviii. 222–225.—**Schiess-Gemuseus.** Acute Neuritis optici bei Gehirntumor; Section. Klin. Monatsbl. f. Augenh., Erlang., 1870, viii, 100–106. ——. Neuroretinitis beiderseits mit ausgedehnten Netzhauthämorrhagien; Section. *Ibid.*, Stuttg., 1880, xviii, 380–383.—**Schmidt.** [Neuritis optica intraocularis occurring in tumours of the brain, and the consequent œdema of the optic-nerve sheath.] Internat. Ophth. Cong. 1872, Lond., 1873, iv, 150–152. *Also, transl.:* Cong. périod. internat. d'ophth. 1872, Par., 1873, iv, 166–169.—**Schmidt** (E. E.) K vopr. o vospalenii zriteln. nerva. [Inflammation of the optic nerve.] Vestnik oftalmol., Kieff, 1885, ii, 273–289. — **Schmidt** (H.) Zur Entstehung der Stauungspapille (Neuritis optica intraocularis) bei Hirnleiden. Arch. f. Ophth., Berl., 1869, xv, 2. Abth., 193–198, 1 pl.— **Schweigger.** Hyperämie und Entzündung des Sehnerven in seinem orbitalen Theile. (6 Fälle.) Klin. Monatsbl. f. Augenh., Berl., 1874, xii, 18–25.—**Seely** (W. W.) Optic

Nerve (*Optic, Inflammation of*).

neuritis as a sequela of diphtheria. Clinic, Cincin., 1876, xi, 277.—**Seguin** (E. C.) On the coincidence of optic neuritis and subacute transverse myelitis. J. Nerv. & Ment. Dis., Chicago. 1880. n. s., v, 177–188. *Also*, Reprint.—**Sharkey** (S. J.) Double optic neuritis in the early stage of dissemin\ated sclerosis; incomplete atrophy of optic discs. Tr. Ophth. Soc. U. Kingdom. Lond., 1882 - 3, iii, 225.—**Sharkey** (S. J.) & **Lawford** (J. B.) On a case of acute optic neuritis associated with acute myelitis. *Ibid.*, 1883–4, iv, 232–243. *Also:* Brit. M. J., Lond., 1884, i, 1151.—**Silk.** Optic neuritis. Brit. M. J., Lond., 1881, i, 1007.—**Simi** (A.) Sopra un caso di nevrite ottica. Boll. d' ocul., Firenze, 1884–5, vii, 2–14, 1 pl. *Also, transl.:* Rec. d'ophth., Par., 1884. 3. s., vi, 603–616.—**Smith** (J. H.) A case of neuro-retinitis; total loss of vision in both eyes, followed by complete restoration in the right eye, and a partial one in the left. Tr. Texas M. Ass., Austin, 1887, 309 – 311. — **Smith** (T.) Bullet-wound of forehead; optic neuritis; partial recovery. Lancet, Lond., 1886, i, 970.—**Sorokin** (S.) Pilokarpin pri vospalenii zritelnago nerva. [Pilocarpin in inflammation of optic nerve.] Vestnik oftalmol., Kieff, 1885, ii, 222.—**Spalding** (J. A.) A case of sympathetic neuro-retinitis. Tr. Am. Ophth. Soc., N. Y., 1883, iii, 486–497.—**Story** (J. B.) Double optic neuritis, with paralysis of olfactory nerves, and sensory division of right fifth nerve. Tr. Acad M. Ireland 1883–4, Dubl., 1884, ii, 79–86. *Also:* Brit. M. J., Lond., 1884, i, 1153. *Also:* Med. Times & Gaz., Lond., 1884, ii, 95.—**Streatfeild** (J. F.) Double optic neuritis, with bony enlargement in the left frontal region. Tr. Ophth. Soc. U. Kingdom, Lond., 1880–81, i, 119.—**Styan** (T. G.) Cases of optic neuritis from intracranial disease. St. Barth. Hosp. Rep., Lond., 1885, xxi, 223–230.—**Swanzy.** Neuroretinitis in connection with disturbances of menstruation. Irish Hosp. Gaz., Dubl., 1873, i, 46.—**Tay** (W.) Two cases of optic neuritis, without impairment of vision, after injury to the head. Tr. Ophth. Soc. U. Kingdom, Lond., 1881–2. ii, 66–73.—**Thilesen.** Neuritis optica (Hyperæmia et inflammatio papillæ nervi optici, Neuritis retro bulbaris, Neuritis descendens [Perineuritis et Neuritis interstitialis]). Norsk Mag. f. Lægevidensk., Christiania, 1868, xxii, 385–401.—**Thorowgood** (J. C.) Case of optic neuritis, with complete loss of vision; recovery under treatment. Tr. Clin. Soc. Lond., 1874–5, viii, 80 – 83. — **Treitel** (T.) Neuroretinitis in Folge von Tumor cerebri ohne Hydrops der Sehnervenscheide. Arch. f. Ophth., Berl., 1880, xxvi, 3. Abth., 105–109.—**Uhthoff** (W.) Ueber Neuritis optica bei multipler Sklerose. Berl. klin. Wchnschr., 1885, xxii, 244–246. ——. Ueber weitere Fälle anatomischer Sehnervenveränderungen in Folge von Alkoholismus, nebst Bemerkungen über Intoxicationsamblyopie und retrobulbäre Neuritis. Deutsche med. Wchnschr., Leipz., 1887, xiii, 555.—**Ushakoff** (N. V.) K' voprosu o vospalenii zritelenekh nervov pri vnutrecherepnekh stradaniyakh. [Inflammation of the optic nerve from intracranial disease.] Laitop. khirurg. Obsh. v. Mosk. (1873–5), 1876, i, 590–594.] **Vernon.** Double optic neuritis and detached retina, following a fall upon the head. Med. Exam., Lond., 1876, i, 30.—**Vossius** (A.) Ein Fall acuter einseitiger Neuritis optici. Klin. Monatsbl. f. Augenh., Stuttg., 1883, xxi, 292–294. ——. Beiderseits Neuritis nach Erysipelas capitis et faciei. *Ibid.*, 294–298.—**Wadsworth** (O. F.) Double optic neuritis and ophthalmoplegia from lead-poisoning, complicated by typhoid fever. Tr. Am. Ophth. Soc., Bost., 1885, 50–54 — **Warlomont** & **Duwez.** Étiologie de la névro-rétinite. Ann. d'ocul., Brux., 1877, lxxvii, 114–139.—**Watson** (W. S) A case of optic nerve neuritis, with subsequent atrophy, associated with cyst of the antrum. Brit. M. J., Lond., 1880, i, 849. — **Webster** (D.) Sympathetic neuro-retinitis. Tr. M. Soc. N. Y., Syracuse, 1881, 115-123. *Alsc:* Med. Rec., N. Y., 1881, xix, 258–260. ——. A case of neuroretinitis albuminurica terminating in death. Planet, N. Y., 1883, i, 70. ——. A case of double optic neuritis from chronic cerebral meningitis; autopsy. Am. J. Ophth., St. Louis, 1884–5, i, 267 – 270. — **de Wecker** (L.) On incision of the optic nerve in cases of neuro-retinitis. Rep. Internat. Ophth. Cong. 1872, Lond., 1873, iv, 11–14. *Also, transl.:* Cong. périod. internal. d'ophth. Compt.-rend. 1872, Par., 1873, iv, 11 – 16. — **Weiland** (A.) Retrobulbäre Neuritis nach Erysipelas faciei; Heilung. Deutsche med. Wchnschr., Berl., 1886, xii, 677.—**Weir** (J.) Acute neuritis. Louisville M. News, 1885, xix, 19. — **West** (S.) Case of double optic neuritis after a fall, with perfect vision throughout, the neuritis for a long time being the only evidence of mischief; recovery complete. Tr. Ophth. Soc. U. Kingdom, Lond., 1886, vi, 368–371. — **Wilbrand** (H.) Ueber Neuritis axialis [of optic nerve]. Klin. Monatsbl. f. Augenh., Cassel, 1878, xvi, 505–520, 1 pl. — **Williams** (E.) The symptomatology of optic neuritis. St. Louis M. & S. J., 1880, xxxix, 281–292. — **Williams** (R.) Neuroretinitis from blow on the forehead. Brit. M. J., Lond., 1882, i, 157. ——. A case of double neuro-retinitis, apparently due to simple anæmia. *Ibid.*, 1884, i, 10.—**Woods** (H.) Optic neuritis with consecutive atrophy in a child of five years. Maryland M. J., Balt., 1882–3, ix, 552.— **Workman.** Violent headache and symptoms of optic neuritis, probably of syphilitic origin. Glasgow M. J.,

Nerve (*Optic, Inflammation of*).

1887, [4.] s., xxvii, 304–308.—**Wurst.** Kilka słów o obrz-
mieniu zastoinowém tarczy nerwu wzrokowego. [Remarks
on inflammation of the optic nerves.] Przegl. lek , Krakow., 1877, xvi, 385; 393.

Nerve (*Optic, Pathology of*). [*Including
the semeiology of the optic papilla.*]

See, also, **Amaurosis**; **Glaucoma**; **Nerve**
(*Optic, Atrophy of*); **Nerve** (*Optic, Inflammation
of*); **Ophthalmoscopy.**

GALEZOWSKI (X.) *Étude ophthalmoscopique
sur les altérations du nerf optique et sur les
maladies cérébrales dont elles dépendent. 4°.
Paris, 1865.

———. The same. 8°. *Paris*, 1866.
Also, transl. [Abstr.] *in :* Wien. med. Wchnschr., 1866,
xvi, 988–990.

KALTSCHMIED (C. F.) [Pr.] de nervis opticis
in cadavere latis inventis a compressione per
undas facta causa ante mortem subsecutæ guttæ
serenæ. 4°. *Jenæ*, [1752].

KIESSELBACH (W.) *Beitrag zur näheren
Kenntniss der sogenannten grauen Degeneration
des Sehnerven bei Erkrankungen des Cerebro-
spinalsystems. 8°. *Erlangen*, 1875.

MAGNUS (H.) Die Sehnerven-Blutungen. 4°.
Leipzig, 1874.

MALGAT (J.) *De la papille optique; étude
sur les modifications de la papille suivant les
âges, les sexes, certains états physiologiques et
pathologiques. 4°. *Paris*, 1877.

SCHÜLLER (G.) *Beiträge zur Pathologie des
Sehnerven. 8°. *Berlin*, [1881].
Also, in : Centralbl. f. prakt. Augenh., Leipz., 1881, v,
236–244.

Alexander. Drei Fälle von hereditärem Sehnervenleiden. Klin. Monatsbl. f. Augenh., Erlang., 1874, xii, 62–
66.—**Allbutt** (T. C.) On the causation and significance
of the choked disc in intracranial diseases. Brit. M. J.,
Lond., 1872, i, 443–445. — **von Ammon.** Zur genaueren
Kenntniss des Nervus opticus, namentlich dessen intraocularen Endes. Vrtljschr. f. d. prakt. Heilk., Prag, 1860,
lxv, 140–167, 2 pl. *Also, transl. :* Ann. d'ocul., Brux., 1860,
xliv, 157–188. ———. Beiträge zur pathologischen Anatomie des intraocularen Sehnervenendes behufs der ophthal-
moscopischen Diagnose von Krankheiten des Augengrun-
des. Arch. f. Ophth., Berl., 1860, vi, 1. Abth., 1–61, 2 pl.
Also, transl. : Ann. d'ocul., Brux., 1861, xlv, 5–42.—**Bader**
(C.) The human eye in health and disease as seen with
the ophthalmoscope. Guy's Hosp. Rep., Lond., 1865, 3. s.,
xi, 446, 1 pl. : 1867–8, 3. s., xiii, 510, 2 pl. : 1869, 3. s., xiv,
456, 2 pl.—**Biermann.** Glückliche Heilung einer plötzlich eingetretenen Erblindung mit Unbeweglichkeit der
Pupille, in Folge einer Lähmung der Retina und der
Ciliar-Nerven. J. d. pract. Heilk., Berl., 1836, lxxxiii, 1.
St., 85–98.—**Bono** (G. B.) Il cloridrato de tebaina nella
terapia di alcune affezioni del nervo ottico. Osservatore,
Torino, 1884, xx, 609–612.—**Broadbent** (W. H.) On the
causation and significance of the choked disc in intracranial diseases. Brit. M. J., Lond., 1872, i, 633–635. — **Carrier** (F. H.) A case of choked disc. Phila. M. Times,
1880–81, xi, 264–266.—**Chiari** (H.) Ein Fall von Tuberculose des N. opticus dexter. Med. Jahrb., Wien, 1877,
559–563, 1 pl.—**Cornwell** (H. G.) On the value of
ophthalmoscopic examinations in disease of the nervous
system ; together with remarks of hyperæmia of the fundus oculi and pressure-atrophy of the optic nerve in diseases of the brain. Med. Rec., N. Y., 1884, xxv, 635–638.—
Csapodi (S.) Ideghartya-levállás sajátszerü esete. [Pe-
culiar case of separation of optic nerve.] Szemészet,
Budapest, 1883, 61–63. — **Dianoux.** De l'anesthésie du
nerf optique. Gaz. méd. de Nantes, 1883–4, ii, 65–69. *Also :*
Bull. et mém. Soc. franç. d'opth., Par., 1884, ii, 87–100.—
Dobrowolsky (W.) Amaurosis uræmica in Folge von
Sehnervenödem. Klin. Monatsbl. f. Augenh., Stuttg.,
1881, xix, 121–123.—**Förster** (R.) Bemerkungen über
Excavationen der Papilla optica. Arch. f. Ophth., Berl.,
1857, iii, 2. Abth., 81–86. ———. Rapport de ses mensurations du champ visuel monoculaire, dans diverses maladies de la rétine et du nerf optique. Cong. périod. internat.
d'ophth. 1867, Par., 1868, iii, 125–132.—**Gallereux.** Observations relatives à deux modes d'altération du nerf
optique, et qui paroissent avoir été jusqu'à présent con-
fondus avec l'amaurose ou goutte sereine. J. gén. de méd.,
chir. et pharm., Par., 1814, i, 380–383. — **Graefe** (A.)
Eigenthümlicher Fall von Sehnervenexcavation. Arch. f.
Ophth., Berl., 1860, vii, 2. Abth., 113–118.—**von Graefe**
(A.) Sur les excavations et les saillies de la papille du
nerf optique. Compt. rend. Soc. de biol. 1860, Par. 1861,
2, s., ii, pt. 1, 151–154.—**Gray** (W. B.) Hypodermic use

Nerve (*Optic, Pathology of*).

of sulphate of strychnia as an optic nerve stimulant. Tr.
M. Soc. Virg. 1872, Richmond, 1873, iii, 115.—**Harlan**
(G. C.) Two cases of swelling of the optic papilla, pos-
sibly congenital. Tr. Am. Ophth. Soc. 1884, Bost., 1885,
iii, pt. 5, 721–723.—**Heymann.** Oedema nerv. opticorum.
Klin. Monatsbl. f. Augenh., Erlang., 1864, ii, 273–275.—
Hirschberg (J.) Krankheiten des Sehnerven und der
Netzhaut. (Sehnervenkrankh. durch Schädeldeformation,
Retin. syphil.) *In his :* Beitr. z. prakt. Augenh., 8°, Berl.,
1876, 37–42. ———. Staauungspapille durch Hirntumor.
Arch. f. Augenh., Wiesb., 1879, viii, 51–53, 1 pl. *Also,
transl. :* Arch. Ophth., N. Y., 1879, viii, 226–228, 1 pl.
———. Staauungspapille durch Nierenleiden. Arch. f.
Augenh., Wiesb., 1879, viii, 177. ———. Sehnervenleiden
bei Schädelmissbildung. Centralbl. f. prakt. Augenh.,
Leipz., 1883, vii, 1–6.—**Hoppe** (F.) Chemische Untersuchung eines nach aufgehobener Function atrophirten
Seh-Nerven. Arch. f. path. Anat., etc., Berl., 1854, viii,
127.—**Hulke.** Slow failure of sight; complete blindness
two years ; acute glaucomatous inflammation ; deep exca-
vation of the optic nerve-entrance. Ophth. Hosp. Rep.,
Lond., 1860–61, iii, 70.—**Jüngken** (J. C.) Paralysis nervi
optici in utroque oculo, per vitium organicum in basi
cranii. Deutsche Klinik, Berl., 1850, ii, 166.—**von Kries**
(J.) Ueber Ermüdung des Sehnerven. Arch. f. Ophth.,
Berl., 1877, xxiii, 2. Abth., 1–43.—**Lagleyze** (P.) Exca-
vacion glaucomatosa de la papilla. Rev. argent. de oftal.
práct., Buenos Aires, 1883–4, i, 13, 1 pl.—**Landolt.** De
l'influence de la strychnine sur certaines affections du nerf
optique. Bull. Soc. de méd. prat. de Par., 1877, 49–54.—
Also : France méd., Par., 1877, xxiv, 210–212.—**Laskiewicz-Friedensfeld** (A. J.) Przypadek gruźliczego
przeistoczenia gruczołów oskrzelowych i nerwu wzrokowego. [Congestion of the ophthalmic ganglion and the
optic nerve.] Przegl. lek., Krakow., 1878, xvii, 481 ; 496.—
Leber (T.) Ueber hereditäre und congenital-angelegte
Sehnervenleiden. Arch. f. Ophth., Berl., 1871, xvii, 2.
Abth., 249–291. ———. Ueber ein eigenthümliches Verhalten des Corpuscula amylacea im atrophischen Sehnerven. *Ibid.*, 1873, xix, 1. Abth., 191–201, 1 pl. ———. Die
Krankheiten der Netzhaut und des Sehnerven. Handb.
d. ges. Augenh., Leipz., 1875–7, v, 521–1048.—**Leber** (T.)
& **Deutschmann** (R.) Beobachtungen über Sehnerven-
affectionen und Augenmuskellähmungen bei Schädelverletzungen. Arch. f. Ophth., Berl., 1881, xxvii, 1. Abth.,
272–308. *Also, transl. :* Rec. d'ophth., Par., 1881, 3. s., iii.
526–534.—**Lélut** (F.) Observations de maladies du nerf
optique. J. univ. et hebd. de méd. et chir. prat., Par.,
1833, xiii, 401–421.—**Liebreich** (R.) Ueber Veränderungen an der Papille bei Sclerectasia posterior. Arch. f.
Ophth., Berl., 1860, vii, 2. Abth., 124–130. ———. Pigment
in der Papilla nervi optici. Klin. Monatsbl. f. Augenh.,
Erlang., 1864, ii, 229–233. *Also, transl. :* Ann. d'ocul.,
Brux., 1864, lii, 31–35.—**Loring** (E. G.) Remarks on the
etiology of choked disk in brain disease. Am. J. M. Sc.,
Phila., 1875, n. s., cxl, 361–371. ———. A new nervous connection between intra-cranial disease and choked disc.
N. York M. J., 1882, xxxv, 561–575.—**Magnan.** Note
sur la sclérose du nerf optique et des nerfs moteurs de
l'œil (3e, 4e, et 6e paires) dans la paralysie générale. Compt.
rend. Soc. de biol. 1877, Par., 1879, 6. s., iv, 292–299.—
Manz (W.) Experimentelle Untersuchungen über Er-
krankungen des Sehnerven in Folge von intracraniellen
Krankheiten. Arch. f. Ophth., Berl., 1870, xvi, 265–296.
———. Ueber Sehnerven-Erkrankung bei Gehirnleiden
(Hydrops vaginæ n. optici). Deutsches Arch. f. klin.
Med., Leipz., 1872, ix, 339–357. ———. Ueber Veränderungen am Sehnerven bei acuter Entzündung des Gehirns.
Klin. Monatsbl. f. Augenh., Stuttg., 1874, xii, 447–460.
———. Ueber endotheliale Degeneration des Sehnerven.
Ber. ü. d. Versamml. d. ophth. Gesellsch., Stuttg., 1882, xiv,
162. *Also :* Arch. f. Ophth., Berl., 1882, xxviii, 3. Abth.,
93–107, 1 pl. *Also :* Arch. f. Psychiat., Berl., 1882, xiii,
723.—**Maseras** (A.) Breves consideraciones relativas á
algunas alteraciones de la retina y del nervio óptico. Gac.
méd. catal., Barcel., 1883, vi, 33–43.—**Masselon.** Infiltration vitreuse de la rétine et de la papille. Bull. et mém. Soc.
franç. d'opht., Par., 1884, ii, 1–8.—**Meyer** (E.) Contribution à l'étude clinique des maladies du nerf optique de cause
intracrânienne. Rev. clin. d'ocul., Bordeaux, 1881, i, 102–
115.—**Michel** (J.) Beitrag zur Kenntniss der Entstehung
der sog. Staauungspapille und der pathologischen Veränderungen in dem Raume zwischen äusserer und innerer Op-
ticusscheide. Arch. d. Heilk., Leipz., 1873, xiv, 39–60, 1
pl. ———. Ueber eine Hyperplasie des Chiasma und des
rechten Nervus opticus bei Elephantiasis. Arch. f. Ophth.,
Berl., 1873, xix, 3. Abth., 145–164, 1 pl. ———. Ueber einige Erkrankungen des Sehnerven. *Ibid.*, 1877, xxiii, 2.
Abth., 213–216, 1 pl. ———. Blutungen in die Pialscheide
und die Pialfortsätze des Opticus. *Ibid.*, 216–220. ———.
Zur Casuistik der sog. Staauungs-Papille. *Ibid.*, 220–225.
———. Ueber die Erkrankungen der Umhüllungshäute
des Sehnerven. Sitzungsb. d. phys.-med. Gesellsch. zu
Würzb., 1881, 105–107.—**Müller** (H.) Ueber Niveau-Ver-
änderungen an der Eintrittsstelle des Sehnerven. Arch.
f. Ophth., Berl., 1858, iv, 2. Abth., 1–39. — **Nettleship.**
Cases of temporary affection of one optic nerve, compara-

Nerve (*Optic, Pathology of*).

ble to Bell's paralysis of the facial. Lancet, Lond., 1880, i, 765.—**Norris** (W. F.) On the relation between the earlier stages of gray degeneration of the optic nerves, and the increase or diminution of the patellar-tendon reflex (knee-jerk). Tr. Am. Ophth. Soc., Bost., 1885, 158-167, 1 pl. *Also* [Abstr.]: Med. News, Phila., 1885, xlvii, 205.—**Odevaine** (F.) Ischæmia of both optic discs. Indian M. Gaz., Calcutta, 1877, xii, 125.—**Oglesby.** Remarks on a case of hyperæmia of the optic disk. Me.l. Times & Gaz., Lond., 1873, i, 88.—**Owen** (L.) Perineuritis with sudden loss of sight. Lancet, Lond., 1874, i, 639.—**Pinching** (C. J. W.) Reports of cases of anæmia of optic nerve treated with the hypodermic injection of strychnia. Brit. M. J., Lond., 1872, ii, 466.—**Pye-Smith** (R. J.) Anæmia of the optic nerves treated by galvanism. *Ibid*., i, 521-523.—**Randall** (B. A.) Coloboma of the optic nerve and sheath. Tr. Am. Ophth. Soc., Bost., 1887, iv, 558-564.—**Reich** (M.) Zur Pathologie des Sehnerven. Arch. f. Ophth., Berl., 1876, xxii, 1. Abth., 103, 2 pl.—**Rousseau.** Hémorrhagie et ramollissement de la couche optique; a esthésies sensorielles. Bull. Soc. méd. de l'Yonne 1883, Auxerre, 1884, xxiv, 137-141.—**Rumszewicz** (K.) Kilka przypadków prawidłowego wzroku przy wziernikowych zmianach zanikowych w tarczy nerwu wzrokowego. [Some accidents in normal vision caused by alterations in the papilla of optic nerve.] Medycyna, Warszawa, 1886, xiv, 123-126.—**Sachs** (T.) Ueber Scotome bei glaucomatösem Sehnervenleiden. Centralbl. f. prakt. Augenh., Leipz., 1887, xi, 161-169. ———. Anatomisch-klinischer Beitrag zur Kenntniss des Centralscotoms bei Sehnervenleiden. Arch. f. Augenh., Wiesb., 1887, xviii, 21-50.—**Santos Fernandez** (J.) De las enfermedades del nervio óptico por causa cerebral. Crón. méd.-quir. de la Habana, 1879, v, 351-357. *Also, in his:* Clin. de enfermed. de l. ojos, 8°. Par., 1879, 48-60.—**Sattler** (H.) Ueber eine tuberkulöse Erkrankung des Sehnerven und seiner Scheiden und über Netzhauttuberculose. Arch. f. Ophth., Berl, 1878, xxiv, 3. Abth., 127-162, 1 pl.—**Savary.** De l'emploi de la strychnine dans l'atrophie des nerfs optiques. Ann. d'ocul., Brux., 1876, lxxvi, 158-160.—**Schott.** Mittheilungen über Erkrankungen des Opticus. Arch. f. Augen- u. Ohrenh., Wiesb., 1876, v, 409, 3 pl.: 1877, vi, 21, 1 pl. *Also, transl.:* Arch. Ophth. & Otol., N. Y., 1877-8, vi, 262-283, 4 pl.—**Silcock** (A. Q.) Case of hæmorrhage into the sheaths of both optic nerves after a fracture of the skull. Tr. Ophth. Soc. U. Kingdom, Lond., 1883-4, iv, 274. *Also:* Brit. M. J., Lond., 1884, i, 108.—**Smith** (P.) Cerebral hæmorrhage with passage of blood into both optic nerves. Tr. Ophth. Soc. U. Kingdom, Lond., 1883-4, iv, 271-274, 1 pl.—**Sous** (G.) De l'anémie de la papille du nerf optique. Ann. d'ocul., Brux., 1861, xlv, 106-113. ———. Coloration de la papille du nerf optique. Cong. méd. de France 1865, Par., 1866, iii, 723-725. ———. De l'anémie de la papille du nerf optique. France méd., Par., 1865, xii, 673-675.—**Talko** (J.) Wynaczynieniekrwi (extravasatio) miedzy nerwami wzrokowemi i ich pochwami, oraz do ciała szklistego lewéj gałki w skutek pęknięcia czaszki i rozerwania tętnicy osłonowéj średniéj lewéj (art. meningeæ mediæ sinistræ). [Hæmorrhage into sheath of optic nerve and into vitreous body resulting from fracture of cranium and rupture of middle meningeal artery.] Medycyna, Warszawa, 1873, i, 470-472. *Also, transl.:* Klin. Monatsbl. f. Augenh., Erlang., 1873, xi, 341-344. — **Treitel** (T.) Eine eigenthümliche Configuration der Papille in einem phthisischen Augapfel. Arch. f. Ophth., Berl., 1876, xxii, 2. Abth., 223-231. ———. Ueber den Werth der Gesichtsfeldmessung mit Pigmenten für die Auffassung der Krankheiten des nervösen Sehapparates. *Ibid.*, 1879, xxv, 2. Abth., 29; 3. Abth., 1. — **Ulrich.** Ueber Stauungspapille. Tagebl. d. Versamml. deutsch. Naturf. u. Aerzte, Strassb., 1885, lviii, 504. ———. Ueber Stauungspapille. Ber. ü. d. Versamml. d ophth. Gesellsch., Stuttg., 1886, xviii, 2. Hft., 93-99.—**Wanstall** (A.) Engorged papilla with periodic objective bubbling noise in the temporal fossæ. Tr. Am. Homœop. Ophth. & Otol. Soc., Buffalo, 1882, vi, 81. — **Wecker.** Blutergüsse im Sehnerven und pathologische Pigmentablagerung in der Sehnervenscheibe. Klin. Monatsbl. f. Augenh., Erlang., 1868, vi, 204-207. — **Weiss** (L.) Ein Fall von Sehnervenblutung. *Ibid.*, 1875, xiii, 114-123.—**Wells** (S.) Case of opaque optic nerve-fibres. Lancet, Lond., 1871, ii, 12.—**Westrum** (R.) Beobachtungen über sogenannter Stauungspapille beim Hunde. Ztschr. f vergleich. Augenh., Leipz., 1882, i, 37, 1 pl.; 125, 1 pl.—**Wicherkiewicz** (B.) Einige Betrachtungen über sogenannte Bulbuswarzen. Centralbl. f. prakt. Augenh., Leipz., 1882, vi, 13-18. — **Wilson** (H.) Pigmentation of the optic disc. Irish Hosp. Gaz., Dubl., 1873, i, 229. — **Wolfring.** Uwagi nad cierpieniami nerwu wzrokowego, zaleźnemi od budowy blaszki sitowéj (lamina cribrosa scleræ). [On nervous affections of the eye, dependent on the construction of the lamina cribrosa scleræ.] Gaz. lek., Warszawa, 1871, xi, 305; 321.

Nerve (*Optic, Section of*).

Castiaux. Section du nerf optique. Bull. Soc. anat. de Par. (1871), 1873, xlvi, 359. — **von Gräfe** (A.) Ueber Durchschneidung des Opticus. Wien. med. Presse, 1867,

viii, 788. *Also:* Berl. klin. Wchnschr., 1867, iv, 320. — **Krenchel** (V.) Onderzoekingen over de gevolgen van gezichtszenuw-doorsnijding bij den kikvorsch. Onderzoek. ged. in h. physiol. Lab. d. Utrecht. Hoogesch., 1874-5, 3. R., iii, 14-21. *Also, transl.:* Arch. f. Ophth., Berl , 1874, xx, 1. Abth., 127-134.—**Redard** (P.) Recherches expérimentales sur la section des nerfs ciliaires et du nerf optique. Arch. d'ophth., Par., 1880-81, i, 260, 1 pl. ; 318.—**Rosow.** Experimente über die Durchschneidung des Sehnerven. Wien. Med.-Halle, 1864, v, 201.—**Schweigger** (C.) Resection des Nervus opticus. Ber. ü. d. Versamml. d. ophth. Gesellsch., Stuttg., 1884, xvi, 63-77. ———. Ueber Resection der Sehnerven. Arch. f. Augenh., Wiesb., 1885-6, xv, 50-67. *Also, transl.:* Arch. Ophth., N. Y., 1885, xiv, 223-242.

Nerve (*Optic, Tumors of*).

Huc (E.) *Essai sur les tumeurs du nerf optique. 4°. Paris, 1882.

Jacqs (R.) *Des tumeurs du nerf optique. 4°. Paris, 1887.

Lidell (J. A.) A case of neuroma of the optic nerve. 2. ed. 8°. New York, 1863.

Loch (R.) *Ein Fall von Neuroma verum nervi optici. 8°. Danzig, [1874].

Willemer (W.) *Ueber eigentliche, d. h. sich innerhalb der äusseren Scheide entwickelende Tumoren des Sehnerven. 8°. Berlin, 1879.

Also, in: Arch. f. Ophth., Berl., 1879, xxv, 1. Abth., 161-247, 3 pl.

Alt (A.) A case of an intraocular granuloma traumaticum of the optic nerve. Arch. Ophth. & Otol., N. Y., 1877-8, vi, 356-358, 1 pl. *Also, transl.:* Arch. f. Augen- u. Ohrenh., Wiesb., 1877, vi, 455, 1 pl.—**Arcoléo.** Tumeur gommeuse dans le chiasma des nerfs optiques. Cong. period. internat. d'ophth. 1867, Par., 1868, iii, 183-188. — **Brailey** (W. A.) Fibrous tumour of the optic nerve. Ophth. Hosp. Rep., Lond., 1876-7, ix, 231-233. ———. Case of sarcoma growing from the dural sheath of the optic nerve. Lancet, Lond., 1886, ii, 1024. — **Buller.** Tumor of the optic nerve. Med. News, Phila., 1886, xlix, 555.—**Chenantais.** Tumeur du nerf optique et de l'orbite (névrôme médullaire, ou sarcôme à cellules nerveuses). Bull. Soc. anat. de Nantes 1879, Par., 1880, 48-52.—**Christensen.** Tumor nervi optici. Hosp.-Tid., Kjøbenh., 1875, 2. R., ii, 817-820.—**Cobb** (J.) Notes of case of gutta serena of the right eye, from the pressure of a tumor on the optic nerve. West. J. M. & Phys. Sc., Cincin., 1836, iii, 33.—**Duboué.** Névrome du nerf optique droit. Bull. Soc. anat. de Par., 1859, xxxiv, 178-181. — **Dusaussay.** Sarcôme angiolithique du nerf optique gauche; ablation; méningite de la convexité; contracture; mort. *Ibid.*, 1875, l, 211-217. *Also* [Abstr.]: Rev. méd.-phot. d. hôp. de Par., 1875, vii, 49.—**Frothingham** (G. E.) Two cases of tumor of the optic nerve. J. Am. M. Ass., Chicago, 1887, ix, 741-743. — **Goldzieher** (W.) Die Geschwülste des Sehnerven. Arch. f. Ophth., Berl., 1873, xix, 3. Abth., 119-144, 2 pl.—**Gruening** (E.) A case of myxoma of the optic nerve; removal of the growth with preservation of the eyeball. Arch. Ophth. & Otol., N. Y., 1876, v, 508-512. *Also,* Reprint. *Also, transl.:* Arch. f. Augen- u. Ohrenh., Wiesb., 1877, vi, 35-38. — **Hulke** (J. W.) On a case of spurious neuroma of the optic nerve. Ophth. Hosp. Rep., Lond., 1880-82, x, 293-295.—**Jacobson** (P. J.) Tumoren-Bildung im Nervus opticus und im Fettzellgewebe der Orbita. Arch. f. Ophth., Berl., 1864, x, 2. Abth., 55-61. — **Johnson** (W. B.) & **Prudden** (T. M.) Myxo-sarcoma of the optic nerve with hyalin degeneration. Arch. Ophth., N. Y., 1885, xiv, 151-160. — **Knapp** (H.) A case of carcinoma of the outer sheath of the optic nerve removed with preservation of the eye ball. Arch. Ophth. & Otol., N. Y., 1874-5, iv, 323-354, 4 pl. *Also, transl.:* Arch. f. Augen- u. Ohrenh., Wiesb., 1874-5, iv, 209-238, 4 pl. *Also, transl.:* Klin. Monatsbl. f. Augenh., Stuttg., 1874, xii, 439-447. ———. On tumors of the optic nerve. Tr. Internat. M. Cong. 1876. Phila., 1877, 905-911. ———. Tumor of the optic nerve. Tr. Am. Ophth. Soc., 15. meeting, N. Y., 1879, ii, 557-560.—**Kollock** (C. W.) A peculiar growth of the optic papilla. Med. News, Phila., 1886, xlix, 456.—**Kunachovich** (K. L.) Miksoma zriteln. nerva. [Myxoma of optic nerve.] Med. Obozr., Mosk., 1885, xxiv, 293-295.—**Manfredi** (N.) Missoma del nervo ottico; esame anatomico. Ann. di ottal., Milano, 1871-2, i, 337-341.—**Mauthner** (L.) Gliosarcoma nervi optici et cerebri. Wien. med. Presse, 1878, xix, 111.—**Pana.** [Tumeur fibrense de chiasma des nerfs optiques et de tuber cinereum.] Bull. Soc. anat. de Par., 1858, xxxiii, 279-281. — **Parisotti** (O.) & **Despagnet** (F.) Fibrome du nerf optique. Rec. d'ophth., Par., 1884, 3. s., vi, 720, 1 pl. : 1885, 3. s., vii, 218.—**Peabody** (G. L.) Sarcoma of the right optic nerve. Med. Rec., N. Y., 1883. xxiii, 216. — **Perls** (M.) Beschreibung eines wahren Neuroms des Nervus opticus. Arch. f. Ophth., Berl , 1873, xix, 2. Abth., 287-302, 2 pl. — **Poncet** (F.) Myxome fasciculé du nerf op-

Nerve (*Optic, Tumors of*).

tique. Arch. d'opht., Par., 1880-81, i, 616-631.—**Quaglino**
(A.) Strabismo convergente paralitico con diplopia; consecutiva atrofia della papilla ed amaurosi completa con
midriasi; più tardi esoftalmo; enucleazione del bulbo ed
estirpazione del tumore; missoma del nervo ottico. Ann.
di ottal., Milano, 1871-2, i, 27-32.—**Rampoldi** (R.) Gliosarcoma del nervo ottico. Ann. di ottal., Pavia, 1881, x,
121-128, 1 pl. *Also, transl.* [Abstr.]: Cong. période. internat. d'ophth. Compt.-rend. 1880, Milan, 1881, vi, 333, 1
pl.— **Richet.** Sarcôme angiolitique du nerf optique
gauche; ablation; méningite de la convexité; contracture; mort. Rec. d'ophth., Par., 1875, 2. s., ii, 295-302.
——. Fibro-sarcome du nerf optique; névro-rétinite et
atrophie; extirpation; méningite consécutive; mort.
Paris méd., 1882, vii, 529-531. — **Rothmund** (A.) jun.
Neurom (cystöse Degeneration) des Sehnerven. Klin.
Monatsbl. f. Augenh., Erlang., 1863, i, 261-264.—**Schott.**
Endotheliome an beiden Sehnerven. Arch. f. Augen- u.
Ohrenh., Wiesb., 1877, vi, 21-27, 1 pl. *Also, transl.*: Arch.
Ophth. & Otol., N. Y., 1877-8, vi, 276-283, 1 pl. ——.
Gliosarcom des rechten Opticus. Arch. f. Augen- u.
Ohrenh., Wiesb., 1878, vii, 81-94, 1 pl. *Also, transl.*:
Arch. Ophth. & Otol., N. Y., 1878-9, vii, 159-174, 1 pl.—
Strawbridge (G.) Tumor of the optic nerve; its re-
moval without enucleation of the eyeball. Tr. Am. Ophth.
Soc., 12. - 14. meeting, N. Y., 1876-8, ii, 383 - 385. — **Szokalski** (W.) Neuroma w nerwie optycznajm. [Neuroma
of optic nerve.] Pam. Towarz. Lek. Warszaw., 1855,
xxxiii, 121-128. ——. Tumeur squirrho-cancéreuse du
nerf optique. Ann. d'ocul., Brux., 1861, xlvi, 43 - 50.
——. Tumeur énorme du nerf optique. Cong. période.
internat. d'ophth. 1862, Par., 1863, ii, 245. — **Teillais.**
Tumeur de la partie postérieure de l'œil (gliôme du nerf
optique). Bull. Soc. anat. de Nantes 1876-8, Par., 1879, i,
82-84. ——. Gliôme du nerf optique. J. de méd. de
l'ouest, Nantes, 1881, xv, 74-78. — **Tillaux.** Tumeur
primitive du nerf optique. Gaz. d. hôp., Par., 1887, lx,
161-163. *Also*: Rec. d'ophth., Par., 1887, 3. s., ix, 65-72.—
Véron (L.) Myxo-fibrome du nerf optique; considérations générales sur les tumeurs du nerf optique. Rec.
d'ophth., Par., 1887, 3. s., v, 32-44.—**Vossius** (A.) Das
Myxosarkom des Nervus opticus; Beitrag zur Lehre von
den wahren d. h. innerhalb der äusseren Scheide sich
entwickelnden Sehnervengeschwülsten. Arch. f. Ophth.,
Berl., 1882, xxviii, 3. Abth., 33, 4 pl.; 283. ——. Ueber
Sehnervengeschwülste. Berl. klin. Wchnschr., 1885, xxii,
199-201. ——. *Also, transl.* [Abstr.]: Phila. M. Times,
1885-6, xvi, 46.

Nerve (*Optic, Wounds and injuries of*).

See, also, **Nerve** (*Optic, Section of*).

Benson (A.) Injury to the optic nerve, without injury to the globe, followed by sudden amaurosis, with
subsequent optic atrophy. Brit. M. J., Lond., 1882, ii,
1085. — **Berlin** (R.) Ein Fall von Verletzung des Sehnerven bei Fractur des Canalis opticus. Ber. ü. d. Versamml. d. ophth. Gesellsch., Stuttg., 1881, xiii, 81 - 100.
Also, transl., Tr. Internat. M. Cong., 7. sess.,
Lond., 1881, iii, 115.—**Carter** (R. B.) Permanent injury
to the optic nerves from the effects of a railway collision.
Tr. Ophth. Soc. U. Kingdom, Lond., 1886, vi, 371. —
Hubsch. Blessure par une baïonnette; section du nerf
optique; blépharoptose; cécité. Gaz. d. hôp., Par., 1854,
xxvii, 14.—**Lawson** (G.) Wound of the optic nerve
from a stab with a knife, without injury to the globe.
Lancet, Lond., 1875, i, 13.—**Nettleship** (E.) On cases of
injury to the optic nerve. St. Thomas's Hosp. Rep. 1881,
Lond., 1882, n. s., xi, 113-122.—**Pagenstecher** (A.) Ein
Fall von Verletzung des Nervus opticus mit Zerreissung
der centralen Gefässe und der dadurch bewirkten Veränderungen des Augenhintergrundes. Arch. f. Ophth.,
Berl., 1869, xv, 1. Abth., 223-243, 2 pl.—**Schweigger** (C.)
Verletzung des Sehnerven. Klin. Monatsbl. f. Augenh.,
Stuttg., 1874, xii, 25-29. ——. Fälle von Erschütterung
des Sehnerven. Arch. f. Augenh., Wiesb., 1883 - 4, xiii,
244-247. *Also, transl.*: Arch. Ophth., N. Y., 1885, xiv, 98-
100.—**Treitel** (T.) Verletzung des Nervus opticus in der
Orbita bei intactem Bulbus mit vollkommenem Verlust
des Sehvermögens. Arch. f. Augenh., Wiesb., 1881, x,
464-468, 1 pl.—**Williams** (E.) Probable trauma of the
optic nerve. Cincin. Lancet & Obs., 1861, n. s., iv, 401.

Nerve (*Petrosal*).

Garibaldi (G.) Studi sul piccolo nervo petroso. Speri-
mentale, Firenze, 1877, xxxix, 118-120. — **Krause** (W.)
Bemerkung über den N. petrosus superficialis minor.
Ztschr. f. rat. Med., Leipz. u. Heidelb., 1867, 3. R., xxix, 165.

Nerve (*Phrenic*).

See, also, **Asphyxia** (*Treatment of*); **Diaphragm**
(*Atrophy of*); **Diaphragm** (*Neuralgia, etc., of*).

HAASE (J. G.) [Pr.] de nervo phrenico dextri
lateris duplici parisque vagi per collum decursu.
sm. 4°. *Lipsiæ*, 1790.

Also, in: SCRIPT. neurol. minores selecti [etc.] 4°. *Lipsiæ*, 1793, iii, 112-116.

Nerve (*Phrenic*).

KRÜGER (E.) * De nervo phrenico. 4°. *Lipsiæ*, 1758.

Also, in: SANDIFORT. Thesaurus diss. [etc.] 4°. *Lugd.
Bat.*, 1778, iii, 501-523.

VON LUSCHKA (H.) Der Nervus phrenicus des
Menschen. 4°. *Tübingen*, 1853.

WRISBERG (H. A.) De nervo phrenico quædam animadversiones. *Gottingæ*, 1763.

In: SCRIPT. neurol. minores selecti. 4°. *Lipsiæ*, 1795,
iv, 16.

von Anrep (B.) & **Cybulski** (N.) Ein Beitrag zur
Physiologie des Nervi phrenici. Arch. f. d. ges. Physiol.,
Bonn, 1883-4, xxxiii, 243-248, 1 diag.—**Bochmer** (J. B.)
An a nervi phrenici alterna compressione alternus quoque
thoracis motus? *In*: Ludwig (C. G.) Decas quæst. med.,
4°, Lips., 1740, 25-28.—**Célarier.** Névralgie et hyperkinésie du nerf phrénique gauche. Arch. méd. belges,
Brux., 1879, 3. s., xv, 368-386.—**Colomiatti** (V. F.) La
tubercolosi nel nervo frenico sinistro. Gior. d. r. Accad.
di med. di Torino, 1875, 3. s., xvii, 450-466, 1 pl. *Also, Reprint.*—**De Bisogno** (O.) Nevrosi del frenico; guarigione. Eco d. osp., Napoli, 1883, i, 5-10.—**Gruber** (W.)
Verlauf des Nervus phrenicus durch eine sehr enge Insel
der Vena subclavia. Arch. f. path. Anat., etc., Berl., 1872,
lvi, 436.—**Hawkins** (C.) Concretion round the phrenic
nerve. Lond. M. Gaz., 1827-8, i, 272.—**Hénocque** (A.)
& **Éloy.** Études expérimentales sur les fonctions des
nerfs phréniques. Gaz. hebd. de méd., Par., 1882, 2. s.,
xix, 638-640. *Also* [Abstr.]: Assoc. franç. pour l'avance.
d. sc. Compt.-rend. 1882, Par., 1883, xi, 802.—**Hollister**
(J. H.) Death from prolonged irritation of the left phrenic
nerve. Chicago M. Exam., 1861, ii, 327-330. — **Hunter**
(C. T.) Anomaly of the phrenic nerve. Phila. M. Times,
1873-4, iv, 630. — **Luschka** (H.) Du nerf diaphragmatique chez l'homme. Arch. gén. de méd., Par., 1854, ii,
284-290.—**Moroni** (E.) Sulla origine e sito ove formasi
il tronco dei nervi frenici nella specie equina. Bull. d.
sc. med., Bologna, 1865, 4. s., xxiii, 349 - 355. — **Panizza**
(B.) Sul nervo frenico e sulla bolsaggine. Arch. ital.
per le mal. nerv., Milano, 1865, ii, 28 - 36. *Also*: Gazz.
med. ital. lomb., Milano, 1865, 5. s., iv, 62-64. *Also*: Gior.
di med. mil., Torino, 1865, xiii, 739-746. — **Robert** (B.)
Lesion del nervio frénico. Rev. de med. y cirug. práct.,
Madrid, 1887, xx, 393-399. — **Schreiber** (J.) Ueber die
Functionen des Nervus phrenicus. Arch. f. d. ges. Physiol., Bonn, 1883, xxxi, 577-600, 1 diag.—**Spedi** (A.) De
nervo phrenico. Arch. f. Anat., Physiol. u. wissensch.
Med., Leipz., 1872, 307 - 311. — **Walsham** (W. J.) Abnormal course of the phrenic nerve. St. Barth. Hosp.
Rep., Lond., 1880, xvi, 100.—**Ziemssen** (H.) Die rhythmische Faradisirung der Nervi phrenici und ihrer Genos-
sen bei Asphyxien und Hr. Remak als Kritiker. Deutsche Klinik, Berl., 1865, xvii, 159-161.

Nerve (*Pneumogastric*).

See, also, **Asthma**; **Blood** (*Pressure of*); **Deglutition**; **Diaphragm**; **Digestion**; **Heart**, **Intestines**, **Larynx**, *Nerves of*; **Nerve** (*Recurrent
laryngeal*); **Nerves** (*Cranial, Eighth pair of*);
Nerves (*Degeneration, etc., of*); **Nervous** *system*
(*Ganglionic*) [*etc.*]; **Nux romica** (*Toxicology of*);
Œsophagus (*Nerves of*); **Urea**.

AMMON (E.) * Ueber den Einfluss der verminderten Geschwindigkeit des Blutumlaufes und
des herabgesetzten Blutdruckes durch Reizung
des peripheren Vagusstumpfes auf die Körpertemperatur. 8°. *Greifswald*, 1878.

ANDRIEU (A.) * Recherches sur les fonctions
des nerfs pneumogastriques. 4°. *Strasbourg*, 1837.

BARKOW (J. C. L.) Bemerkungen über die
Bestimmung der Nerven im Allgemeinen und
über den Nervus vagus insbesondere. 8°. *Breslau*, [1845].

BLANKE (B.) * Eine Schussverletzung des linken Nervus vagus und eine dadurch bedingte
paralytische Pneumonie der linken Lunge. 8°.
Göttingen, 1871.

BODDAERT (R.) Recherches expérimentales
sur les lésions pulmonaires consécutives à la section des nerfs pneumogastriques. 8°. *Gand*, 1862.

FINATO (S.) * Cenni fisiologici sulle funzioni
del nervo vago o pneumogastrico. 12°. *Pavia*,
1857.

FORSBLOM (G.) * Vagus tamen nervus inhi-
bens. 8°. *Jenæ*, 1862.

FOWELIN (C.) * De causa mortis post nervos
vagos dissectos instantis. 8°. [*Dorpat*], 1851.

Nerve (*Pneumogastric*).

HARTUNG (W.) * Ueber den Einfluss des Nervus vagus auf die Bewegungen des Magens der Wiederkäuer. 4°. *Giessen*, 1858.

HEINEMANN (C. U.) * Nonnulla de nervo vago ranarum experimenta. 8°. *Berolini*, [1858].

HEINRICI (L. O.) * Quænam sit causa mortis animalium nervis vagis dissectis. 8°. *Berolini*, [1843].

VON HELMOLT (A.) * Ueber die reflectorischen Beziehungen des Nervus vagus zu den motorischen Nerven der Athemmuskeln. sm. 8°. *Giessen*, 1856.

HOFFMANN (C. E. E.) Beiträge zur Anatomie und Physiologie des Nervus vagus bei Fischen. 4°. *Giessen*, 1860.

VAN KEMPEN (E.-M.) Essai expérimental sur la nature fonctionnelle du nerf pneumogastrique, précédé de considérations sur les mouvements réfléchis. 8°. *Louvain*, 1842.

KNAUT (A.) * De vitali, quæ dicitur, pulmonum contractilitate, nervis vagis irritatis. 8°. *Dorpati Livonorum*, 1859.

LANGENBACHER (L.) * Materialy dlja sravnitelnoi anatomii blujdajoushich nervov u domashnich jivotnych. [Materials for comparative anatomy of nervus vagus in domestic animals.] 8°. *St. Petersburg*, 1877.

LEOPOLD (J. H.) * De phænomenis post dissectos nervos sympathicum et vagum in oculo observatis. 4°. *Lipsiæ*, [1840].

LÖWINSOHN (J.) * Experimenta de nervi vagi in respirationem vi et effectu. 8°. *Dorpati Livonorum*, 1858.

MOLESCHOTT (J.) Sugli effetti emodinamici della recisione dei nervi pneumogastrici. 8°. *Torino*, 1873.

NAVROTSKI (F.) * O vlijanii davlenija krovi na tsentri blujdaioushich nervov. [Effect of pressure of blood on vagus.] 8°. *St. Petersburg*, 1870.

OŻEGOWSKI (A.) * Ueber die Folgen der doppelseitigen Vagusdurchschneidung bei Tauben. 8°. *Greifswald*, 1879.

PAETSCH (A. F. T.) * Diss. physiologica sistens experimenta quædam de nervi vagi in digestionem vi atque potentia. 8°. *Gottingæ*, 1822.

PINEL (A.-C.) * De l'asthme. Recherches sur la pathogénie de cette affection, considérée principalement au point de vue de ses rapports avec l'histoire physiologique et pathologique des nerfs pneumogastriques. 4°. *Paris*, 1858.

PREYER (W.) [Ueber telephonische Vagus-Reizung.] 8°. *Jena*, 1881.
Repr. from: Sitzungsb. d. Jenaisch. Gesellsch. f. Med. u. Naturw., 1881.

QUELLHORST (T.) * Beiträge zur Physiologie des Vagus. 8°. *Würzburg*, 1875.

RIU (E.) * Étude expérimentale et clinique sur les nerfs pneumo-gastriques. 4°. *Paris*, 1882.

ROSENBACH (O.) Studien über den Nervus vagus. Ein Beitrag zur Lehre von den automatischen Nervencentren und den Hemmungsnerven. 8°. *Berlin*, 1877.

ROSENTHAL (J.) Die Athembewegungen und ihre Beziehungen zum Nervus vagus. 8°. *Berlin*, 1862.

SÉDILLOT (C.) * Du nerf pneumo-gastrique et de ses fonctions. 4°. *Paris*, 1829.

SOLINVILLE (A.) *Anatomica disquisitio et descriptio nervi pneumogastrici in corpore humano. 4°. *Turici*, 1838.

WALTHER (A. F.) [Pr.] quo paris intercostalis et vagi corporis humani nervorum et ab utroque ejus latere obviorum anàtomen exhibet. 4°. [*Lipsiæ*, 1733.]
Also, in: HALLER. Disp. anat. [etc.] 4°. *Gottingæ*, 1747, ii, 911-926.

Nerve (*Pneumogastric*).

WARWINSKY (J.) * De nervi vagi physiologia et pathologia. 8°. [*Dorpat*], 1838.

WOLFF (E.) * De functionibus nervi vagi. 8°. *Berolini*, [1856].

Adams (J. F. A.) Notes on the pneumogastric. Boston M. & S. J., 1873, lxxxix, 55; 75; 97.—**Ainser** (T.) & **Lohe** (A.) Versuche über die Kreislaufsdauer bei Reizung und Durchschneidung der Nervi vagi. Ztschr. f. rat. Med., Leipz. u. Heidelb., 1868, 3. R., xxxi, 33–37.— **Albers** (J. T. H.) Anatomisch-pathologische Beobachtungen über den Nervus vagus. Mag. f. d. ges. Heilk., Berl., 1834, xli, 120–124. *Also, transl.:* Abeille, Brux., 1834 iv, 86–91.—**von Anrep** (B.) Die Ursache des Todes nach Vagusdurchschneidung bei Vögeln. Verhandl. d. phys.-med. Gesellsch. in Würzb., 1880, n. F., xiv, 35–43.— **Arloing** (S.) & **Tripier** (L.) Contribution à la physiologie des nerfs vagues. Arch. de physiol. norm. et path., Par., 1871–2, iv, 411; 588; 732: 1873, v, 157. ———. Étude comparative de l'action physiologique des deux nerfs pneumogastriques. Compt. rend. Soc. de biol. 1876, Par., 1877, 6. s., iii, 373–376.—**Arnold.** Observations et expériences sur les fonctions du nerf pneumo-gastrique et du nerf accessoire de Willis. [Extrait.] Arch. gén. de méd., Par., 1840, ii, 445–462.— **Aubert** (H.) & **von Tschischwitz** (A.) Versuche über den Stillstand des Zwerchfells durch Reizung des Nervus vagus in Contraction und in Erschlaffung. Untersuch. z. Naturl. d. Mensch. u. d. Thiere, Frankf. a. M., 1857, iii, 272–293.—**Bernard.** Paralysie de l'œsophage par la section des deux nerfs pneumogastriques. Compt. rend. Soc. de biol. 1849, Par., 1850, i, 14.—**Bernstein** (J.) Vagus und Sympathicus; vorläufige Mittheilung. Centralbl. f. d. med. Wissensch., Berl., 1864, ii, 241–243.—**Bert** (P.) Effets de la section et de la galvanisation des nerfs pneumogastriques chez les oiseaux. Compt. rend. Soc. de biol. 1868, Par., 1869, 4. s., v, 39–41. ———. Sur l'élasticité et la contractilité pulmonaires; sur les rapports de celle-ci avec les nerfs pneumogastriques. *Ibid.*, 1869, xvi, 433–464. —**Boddaert** (R.) Observation d'un cas remarquable de prolongation de la vie chez un chien, à la suite de la section simultanée des pneumogastriques à la région cervicale. Ann. Soc. de méd. de Gand, 1877, lv, 197–200. — **Bouley** (H.) Recherches expérimentales sur l'influence que la section des pneumogastriques exerce sur l'absorption stomacale dans le cheval, le chien et le bœuf. Bull. Acad. de méd., Par., 1851–2, xvii, 647. [Rap de Bérard], 763–775. *Also:* Union méd., Par., 1852, vi, 310.—**Brodie** (B. C.) Experiments and observations on the influence of the nerves of the eighth pair on the secretions of the stomach. Phil. Tr., Lond., 1814, civ, 102–106.—**Brown-Séquard** (C. E.) [Two important facts relative to the physiology of the pneumogastric nerves.] Virginia M. & S. J., Richmond, 1855, iv, 161. ———. Étude comparative de l'action physiologique des deux nerfs pneumogastriques. Compt. rend. Soc. de biol. 1872, Par., 1874, 5. s., iv, 181–186.—**Budge** (J.) Ueber den Einfluss der Reizung des N. vagus auf das Athemholen. Arch. f. path. Anat., etc., Berl., 1859, xvi, 433–464. ———. Neuere Untersuchungen über den Einfluss des N. vagus auf die Athembewegungen. Ztschr. f. rat. Med., Leipz. u. Heidelb., 1864, 3. R., xxi, 269–289, 2 pl.—**Burkart** (R.) Ueber den Einfluss des N. vagus auf die Athembewegungen. Arch. f. d. ges. Physiol., Bonn, 1868, i, 107–126. — **Chauveau** (A.) Du nerf pneumogastrique considéré comme agent excitateur et comme agent coordinateur des contractions œsophagiennes dans l'acte de la déglutition. J. de la physiol. de l'homme, Par., 1862, v, 190; 323. — **Cock** (E.) Observations on the ganglionic enlargement of the pneumogastric nerve; the probable function of that ganglion; and the position which it occupies in the human subject and in several of the lower animals. Guy's Hosp. Rep., Lond., 1837, ii, 311–317, 1 pl.—**Cruveilhier.** Section du pneumo-gastrique sur des chiens. Bull. Soc. anat. de Par., 1831, vi, 110.—**Cuniculus.** On experiments on the par vagum. Lond. M. Reposit., 1820, xiii, 467–471.—**Czermak** (J.) Ueber mechanische Vagus-Reizung beim Menschen. Jenaische Ztschr. f. Med. u. Naturw., Leipz., 1865-6, ii, 384–386. ———. Ueber mechanische Reizung des N. vagus beim Menschen. Vrtljschr. f. d. prakt. Heilk., Prag, 1868, c, 30–39, 4 pl.—**van Deen** (I.) Over de zijdelingsche takken der zwervende zenuw (nervus vagus) van den proteus anguineus. Tijdschr. v. nat. Geschied. en Physiol., Amst., 1834, i, 112–129, 1 pl.—**Desmoulins** (A.) Mémoire sur le rapport qui unit le développement du nerf pneumogastrique à celui des parois du quatrième ventricule, et sur la composition de la moelle épinière. J. de physiol. expér., Par., 1823, iii, 362–375. *Also,* Reprint.— **Donders** (F. C.) Zur Physiologie des Nervus vagus. Arch. f. d. ges. Physiol., Bonn, 1868, i, 331–361, 3 pl. ———. De werking van den constanten stroom op den nervus vagus. Versl. . . . k. Akad. v. Wetensch. Afd. Natuurk., Amst., 1871, 2. R., v, 80–93, 3 pl. *Also,* Reprint. *Also:* Onderzoek. ged. in h. physiol. Lab. d. Utrecht. Hoogesch., 1872, 3. R., i, 1–26. *Also, transl.:* Arch. f. d. ges. Physiol., Bonn, 1871-2, v, 1–19, 1 pl. *Also, transl.:* Arch. néerl. d. sc. exactes, etc., La Haye, 1872, vii, 328–350. ——— De duur van de latente werking, bij vagusprikkeling, in be.

Nerve (*Pneumogastric*).

trekking tot dien der harts-perioden. Onderzoek. ged. in
h. physiol. Lab. d. Utrecht. Hoogesch., 1872, 3. R., i, 272–
281. — **Dürr.** Eigenthümliche Neurose des Vagus und
Accessorius durch Ueberfütterung bei einem Kinde.
Med. Cor.-Bl. d. württemb. ärztl. Ver., Stuttg., 1852, xxii,
376.—**Du Moulin.** Observation destinée à l'histoire du
grand-sympathique et du pneumogastrique. Bull. Acad.
roy. de méd. de Belg., Brux., 1872, 3. s., vi, 587–610. *Also,*
Réprint. *Also* [Rev.]: Bull. Soc. de méd. de Gand, 1873, xl,
486–490.—**Dupuy.** Expériences sur la section, la ligature et la compression des nerfs pneumogastriques, ou huitième paire, du cheval et la brebis. J. de méd., chir.,
pharm., etc., Par., 1816, xxxvii, 351–366. ———. De l'effet
de la compression des nerfs pneumo-gastriques, ou de la
huitième paire sur la voix du cheval. J. gén. de méd.,
chir. et pharm., Par., 1821, lxxv, 3–19. ———. Nouvelles expériences sur la section des nerfs pneumogastriques. *Ibid.,*
1827, c, 39–48. *Also,* Réprint.—**Eckhard** (C.) Zur Theorie der Vagus-Wirkung. Arch. f. Anat., Physiol. u. wissensch. Med., Berl., 1851, 205–208. *Also, transl. :* Edinb.
M. & S. J., 1853, lxxix, 145–147. ———. Versuche über die
Wirkung des Vagus einer Seite nach vorausgegangener
Erregung des der andern Seite. Beitr. z. Anat. u. Physiol. (Eckhard) 1876–8, Giessen, 1879, viii, 177–182.— **Fano.**
Observation de résection d'un des nerfs pneumogastriques
pratiquée accidentellement chez l'homme. Arch. gén. de
méd., Par., 1856, i, 183–189. — **Fearn** (S. W.) Case of
wound of the internal carotid artery, and division of the
par vagum, in which the common carotid artery was tied.
Prov. M. & S. J., Lond., 1847, xi, 482–485.—**Finkelstein**
(A.) Der Nervus depressor beim Menschen, Kaninchen,
Hunde, bei der Katze und dem Pferde. Arch. f. Anat. u.
Entwcklngsgesch., Leipz., 1880, 245–252, 1 pl.—**Forgues.**
Contribution à l'étude physiologique comparée des deux
pneumogastriques. Gaz. hebd. d. sc. méd. de Montpel.,
1882, iv, 409; 422.—**Fourcade.** Résultat d'expériences
qu'il a tentées sur les usages du nerf pneumogastrique.
Bull. Soc. anat. de Par., 1830, v, 49.— **François-
Franck.** Ligature et contusion du pneumogastrique;
névrotomie électrique; restitution des fonctions d'un nerf
comprimé. Compt. rend. Soc. de biol. 1879. Par., 1880, 7.
s., i, 293–296. *Also :* Gaz. méd. de Par., 1879, 6. s., i, 578.
———. Recherches sur les effets produits par l'excitation
du bout central du pneumogastrique et de ses branches
sur la respiration, le cœur et les vaisseaux. *In :* Marey
(E.-J.) Physiol. expér., 8°, Par., 1880, 381–386. ———.
Remarques sur une communication de M. Laffont ayant
pour titre: Différence des effets produits sur la pression
vasculaire et les battements du cœur par les excitations
des deux nerfs vagues. Compt. rend. Soc. de biol., Par.,
1886, 8. s., iii, 214. — **Fredericq** (L.) Excitation du
pneumogastrique chez le lapin empoisonné par CO².
Arch. de biol., Gand, 1884, v, 573–579.—**Frey** (O.) Kurze
Mittheilung der Ergebnisse einer Untersuchung über die
pathologischen Lungenveränderungen nach Lähmung der
Nervi vagi. Arch. f. d. ges. Physiol., Bonn, 1876–7, xiv,
487–491.—**Friedleben.** Ueber das Verhalten des Vagus
recurrens zu den Tracheal- und Bronchialdrüsen in
Krankheiten der Kinder. Amtl. Ber. ü. d. Versamml.
deutsch. Naturf. u. Aerzte 1858, Carlsruhe, 1859, xxxiv,
232–234.—**Generali** (G.) Intorno una straordinaria disposizione del nervo pneumogastrico. Ann. univ. di med.,
Milano, 1841, xcvii, 53–60.—**Genzmer** (A.) Gründe für
die pathologischen Veränderungen der Lungen nach doppelseitiger Vagusdurchschneidung. Arch. f. d. ges.
Physiol., Bonn, 1873–4, viii, 101–121. — **Gilchrist** (W.)
On the influence of the vagus upon respiration. Brit. &
For. M.-Chir. Rev., Lond., 1858, xxii, 495–501.—**Gratia.**
Une curieuse anomalie anatomique, constituée par la présence de tissu musculaire strié dans la substance du nerf
pneumogastrique. Ann. de méd. vét., Brux., 1884, xxxiii,
649–652.—**Gurbski** (K.) Nerw błędny (n. vagus) jest
nerwem czuciowym serca. [On the sensibility of the
nervus vagus.] Gaz. lek., Warszawa, 1870, viii, 745;
766.—**Habershon** (S. O.) Clinical observations illustrating the effects produced by the implication of branches
of the pneumogastric nerve in aneurismal tumours and in
some morbid growths. Proc. Roy. M. & Chir. Soc. Lond.,
1864, iv, 281–283. ———. Some clinical facts connected
with the pathology of the pneumogastric nerve. Guy's
Hosp. Rep., Lond., 1875, 3. s., xx, 127–144.—**Hoppe** (J.)
Ueber das spontane Erbrechen nach der Durchschneidung
der N. vagi. Wchnschr. f. d. ges. Heilk., Berl., 1840, 733–
740.—**Jacquart** (H.) De la distribution des nerfs pneumogastriques dans les poumons des ophidiens. J. de
l'anat. et physiol., etc., Par., 1864, i, 371–377, 1 pl.—**Johnson** (G.) On the laryngeal symptoms which result from
the pressure of aneurismal and other tumours upon the
vagus and recurrent nerves. Med.-Chir. Tr., Lond., 1875,
lviii, 29–48. *Also, transl.* [Abstr.]: Lyon méd., 1877,
xxvi, 593–600.—**Jolyet** (F.) Les fibres du nerf pneumogastrique, dont l'excitation a pour résultat de donner naissance au phénomène réflexe qui constitue la toux, ont une
tendance à s'isoler en nerf distinct, séparé du tronc du
nerf pneumogastrique. Compt. rend. Soc. de biol. 1876,
Par., 1877, 6. s., iii, 409–411. ———. Nouvelles recherches
sur le nerf pneumogastrique, démontrant que les filets

Nerve (*Pneumogastric*).

originaires de ce nerf, avant toutes anastomoses, possè-
dent, chez le chien, une fonction motrice propre sur l'œsophage et l'estomac. *Ibid.,* 1878, Par., 1880, 6. s., v, 274–
279. *Also :* Gaz. méd. de Par., 1879. 6. s., i, 72.—**Joseph**
(L.) Beitrag zur Geschichte der Physiologie des Vagus.
Arch. f. path. Anat., etc., Par., 1860, xviii, 368.—**Kappeler** (O.) Excision eines ½ Zoll langen Stückes aus dem
Nervus vagus bei Exstirpation einer grossen Geschwulst
am Halse; Genesung; laryngoscopischer Befund. Arch.
d. Heilk., Leipz., 1864, v, 271–275. — **Kehrer** (F. A.)
Ueber angebliche reflectorische Beziehungen des N. vagus
zur Harnblase. Ztschr. f. rat. Med., Leipz. u. Heidelb.,
1867, 3. R., xxix, 144–148.—**van Kempen** (E.-M.) Nouvelles recherches sur la nature fonctionnelle des racines du
nerf pneumo-gastrique et du nerf spinal. Mém. Acad. roy.
de méd. de Belg., Brux., 1857, iv, 323–349.—**Kohts** (O.)
& **Tiegel** (E.) Ueber die Vagusdurchschneidung auf
Herzschlag und Athmung. Arch. f. d. ges. Physiol.,
Bonn, 1876. xiii, 84–92, 1 pl.—**Krishaber.** Phénomènes
provoqués par l'inhalation du chloroforme après la section
des nerfs pneumogastriques. Arch. de physiol. norm. et
path., Par., 1869, ii, 542. — **Laborde** (J.-V.) Note préliminaire sur le noyau d'origine dans le bulbe rachidien des
fibres motrices ou cardiaques du nerf pneumogastrique;
noyau cardiaque. Tribune méd., Par., 1887, xix, 212.
Also : Compt. rend. Soc. de biol., Par., 1887, 8. s., iv, 240–
242.—**Laffont.** De l'effet des excitations du nerf vague
chez les animaux anesthésiés par le chloroforme ou par
injection intraveineuse d'hydrate de chloral; différence
d'effets produits sur la pression vasculaire et les battements du cœur, par les excitations des deux nerfs vagues.
Compt. rend. Soc. de biol., Par., 1886, 8. s., iii, 193–195.—
Langendorff (O.) Der Einfluss des Nervus vagus und
der sensiblen Nerven auf die Athmung. Mitth. a. d.
Königsb. physiol. Lab., 1878, 33–67. ———. Ueber den
Nervus vagus neugeborener Thiere. Breslau. aerztl.
Ztschr., 1879, i, 247–249.—**Legros** (C.) & **Onimus.** Recherches expérimentales sur la physiologie des nerfs pneumogastriques. J. de l'anat. et physiol., etc., Par., 1872,
viii, 561–592. *Also* [Abstr.]: Compt. rend. Acad. d. sc.,
Par., 1872, lxxv, 1192–1194.—**Ley** (H.) Observations on
the attributes of the pneumogastric or eighth pair of
nerves in their natural and diseased conditions, as illustrative of the general principles of the pathology of nerves.
Lond. M. Gaz., 1835, xvi, 407; 440; 474; 503; 535; 567.—
Livon (C.) Effets de l'arrachement du spinal sur l'action
modératrice du pneumogastrique. Marseille méd., 1886,
xxiii, 205–208.—**Longet** (F.-A.) Sur la véritable nature
des nerfs pneumo-gastriques et les usages de leurs anastomoses. Arch. gén. de méd., Par., 1849, iii. 253–284. *Also,*
Réprint.—**Lussana** (F.) & **Ciotto** (F.) Risultanze
ottenute dal taglio dei due nervi vaghi in un cane, soprav-
vissuto per diecisette giorni. Gazz. med. ital., prov.
venete, Padova, 1877, xx, 219–221.—**Macalister** (A.)
Abnormal position of the pneumogastric nerve. Med.
Press & Circ., Dubl., 1868, v, 132.—**Malerba** (P.) Osservazioni sulla fisiologia del par vago fatte nell' uomo
vivente. Morgagni, Napoli, 1874, xvi, 898–904. — **Masz-
kowski** (M.) Przypadek natural. doświadczalnego
drażnienia nerwów błędnych na szyi u człowieka. [Ex-
periments in a case of natural irritation of pneumogastric
nerve.] Medycyna, Warszawa, 1884, xii, 709–712. —
Mayer. Neue Untersuchungen über die Folgen und
insbesondere über die Ursache des Todes der Thiere nach
Unterbindung des Nervus vagus. Ztschr. f. Physiol.,
Darmstadt, 1827, ii, 62–78. *Also, transl. :* J. compl. du
dict. d. sc. méd., Par., 1827, xxvi, 110–123. — **Michael-
son.** Beiträge zur Untersuchung des Einflusses beiderseitiger Vaguslähmung auf die Lungen. Mitth. a. d.
Königsb. physiol. Lab., 1878, 85–119.—**Moreau.** Régénération en 30 jours du nerf pneumogastrique séparé de son
centre nerveux avec rétablissement complet des fonctions
de ce nerf chez les jeunes rats albinos. Compt. rend. Soc.
de biol. 1876, Par., 1877, 6. s., iii. 376.—**Münzel** (E.) Puls-
folge und Blutdruck nach der Durchschneidung der Nervi
vagi. Arch. f. Physiol., Leipz., 1887, 120–137.—**Munk**
(H.) Ueber Functionen des N. vagus von J. Steiner.
Deutsche med. Wchnschr., Berl., 1876, ii, 349.—**Munson**
(W. W.) The pneumogastric nerve; a study chiefly
physiological. N. York M. J., 1878, xxviii, 243–253. —
Nasse (H.) Einige Versuche über die Wirkung der
Durchschneidung der Nervi vagi bei Hunden, besonders
in Hinsicht auf den Stoffwechsel. Arch. d. Ver. f. gemeinsch. Arb. z. Förd. d. wissensch. Heilk., Götting., 1856,
ii, 327–384.—**Ochl** (E.) Della innervazione motoria del
pneumogastrico sugli organi addominali. Morgagni, Napoli, 1864, vi, 215; 323; 410; 556; 718; 777. *Continued in :*
Gazz. med. ital. lomb., Milano, 1867, 5. s., vi, 342; 368: 1868.
6. s., i, 65; 78; 81; 89; 129; 143; 149; 201. ———. Contribuzione alla fisiologia del ramo simpatico al vago. Gior.
di r. Accad. di med. di Torino, 1885, 3. s., xxxiii, 28–38.—
Onodi (A. D.) A bolygó idegcsoport (nervus vagus)
alaktani jelentöségéröl. [Morphology of nervus vagus.]
Orvosi hetil., Budapest, 1886, xxx, 896–898.—**Paladino**
(G.) Alcuni effetti singolari consecutivi alla recisione del
vago. Movimento, Napoli, 1875, vii, 417–428. — **Péter.**
Cancer latent du poumon et du foie; cancer consécutif

Nerve (*Pneumogastric*).

des ganglions bronchiques; lésion de voisinage d'un des pneumogastriques; dyspnée et fréquence excessive du pouls. Bull. Soc. clin. de Par., 1877, i, 241-246.—**Philipeaux.** Expériences relatives à l'action de l'électrisation des bouts centraux des nerfs pneumogastriques. Compt. rend. Soc. de biol., Par., 1872, 5. s., iv, 31. ———. Régénération en 30 jours du nerf pneumogastrique séparé de son centre nerveux avec rétablissement complet des fonctions de ce nerf chez les jeunes rats albinos. *Ibid.*, 1876, Par., 1877, 6. s., iii, 376.—**Quincke** (H.) Ueber Vagusreizung beim Menschen. Berl. klin. Wchnschr., 1875, xii, 189; 203.—**Ravitsch** (J.) Ueber den Einfluss des Vagus auf die Magenbewegung. Arch. f. Anat., Physiol. u. wissensch. Med., Leipz., 1861, 770-781. — **Remack.** Des ganglions microscopiques sur le trajet des filets du nerf pneumogastrique dans la paroi de l'estomac. Compt. rend. Soc. de biol. 1852, Par., 1853, iv, 153-155.—**Roddaert** (R.) Recherches expérimentales sur les lésions pulmonaires consécutives à la section des nerfs pneumogastriques. J. de la physiol. de l'homme, Par., 1862, v, 442; 527.—**Rosenbach** (O.) Zur Physiologie des Nervus vagus. Centralbl. f. d. med. Wissensch., Berl., 1877, xv, 97-99.—**Rosenthal** (I.) Ueber Vagusreizung. Sitzungsb. d. phys.-med. Soc. zu Erlang., 1879-80, xii, 45-47.—**Rosenthal** (J.) Ueber den Einfluss des Vagus auf die Athembewegungen. Arch. f. Anat., Physiol. u. wissensch. Med., Leipz., 1862, 226-229.—**Rossbach** (M. J.) Weitere Untersuchungen über die physiologischen Wirkungen des Atropin und Physostigmin, mit einem Beitrag zur Physiologie des Vagus. Arch. f. d. ges. Physiol., Bonn, 1875, x, 383-464, 2 pl.— **Rossbach** (M. J.) & **Quellhorst** (T.) Beiträge zur Physiologie des Vagus. Verhandl. d. phys.-med. Gesellsch. in Würzb., 1876-7, n. F., ix, 13-31. *Also:* Pharmakol. Untersuch., Würzb., 1876-7, ii, 59-77. [*See, also, supra,* Quellhorst.]—**Rutherford** (W.) Influence of the vagus upon the vascular system. J. Anat. & Physiol., Lond., 1869, iii, 402-416. *Also, Reprint. Also* [Abstr.]: Proc. Roy. Soc. Edinb., 1866-9, vi, 538. ———. Influence of the vagus upon the vascular system. Tr. Roy. Soc. Edinb., 1869-70, xxvi, 107-148.—**Schiff** (M.) Die Ursache der Lungenveränderung nach Durchschneidung der pneumogastrischen Nerven. Arch. f. physiol. Heilk., Stuttg., 1847, vi, 690: 769. ———. Ueber den Einfluss der Vagusdurchschneidung auf das Lungengewebe. *Ibid.*, 1850, ix, 625-662. ———. Einfluss des Vagus auf die Lungenbläschen. Arch. f. d. ges. Physiol., Bonn, 1871, iv, 226.— **Schmitt** (F. C.) Verwonding van den nervus vagus. Tijdschr. d. Vereen. t. Bevord. d. geneesk. Wetensch. in Nederl. Indië. Batav., 1855, iv, 72-74.—**Schou** (J.) Om behandlingen af de travmatiske vagusläsioner med permanent tamponade af trachea. (C. r. Le traitement des lésions traumatiques du nerf pneumogastrique par le tamponnement permanent de la trachée.) Nord. med. Ark., Stockholm, 1886, xviii, no. 5, 1-8.—**Schweig.** Ueber ein neues und merkwürdiges Respirationssymptom, welches bei mit einseitiger Stenose des Foramen jugulare begleiteter Schädelverdickung beobachtet, und wahrscheinlich durch Druck auf den Vagus hervorgerufen wurde. Mitth. d. badisch. aerztl. Ver., Karlsruhe, 1857, xi, 49-61.—**Scott** (J. A.) Experiments on the central end of the pneumogastric nerve. Tr. Acad. M. Ireland 1883-4, Dubl., 1884, ii, 492-494.—**Sharp** (H. J.) The pneumogastric nerves. Ohio M. Recorder, Columbus, 1878-9, iii, 385-398.—**Spence** (J.) Recherches anatomiques sur les nerfs pneumogastrique et spinal. Ann. méd.-psych., Par., 1843, ii, 46-54.— **Stefani** (A.) Sulla eccitazione del nervo vago. Sperimentale, Firenze, 1876, xxxvii, 268-274.—**Steiner** (J.) Ueber partielle Nervendurchschneidung und die Ursachen der Lungenaffection nach doppelseitiger Vagustrennung am Halse. Arch. f. Anat. u. Physiol., Leipz., 1878 (Physiol. Abth.), 218-245.—**Stockmann** (A.) Dzialanie odruchowe jednego z nerwów czuciowych serca na cisnienie krwi w naczyniach (nervus depressor cyoni et Ludwigii). [Action of reflex motion on sensory nerve of heart by blood pressure.] Gaz. lek., Warszawa, 1889, vii, 1; 24; 36.—**Stowell** (T. B.) The vagus nerve in the domestic cat (Felis domestica). Proc. Am. Phil. Soc., Phila., 1881-2, xx, 123-138. *Also, Reprint.*—**Talamon** (C.) Compression du pneumo-gastrique droit par un anévrysme du tronc brachio-céphalique; broncho-pneumonie suppurée du poumon droit. Progrès méd., Par., 1880, viii, 487-489.—**von Thanhoffer** (L.) Die beiderseitige mechanische Reizung des Nv. vagus beim Menschen. Centralbl. f. d. med. Wissensch., Berl., 1875, xiii, 403-406.—**Traube** (L.) Die Ursachen und die Beschaffenheit derjenigen Veränderungen, welche das Lungenparenchym nach Durchschneidung der Nn. vagi erleidet. Beitr. z exper. Path. u. Physiol., Berl., 1846, i, 65-200. ———. Entgegnung auf die Einwürfe gegen meine Theorie über die Ursachen der nach Durchschneidung der Nn. vagi eintretenden Lungenaffection. Arch. f. physiol. Heilk., Stuttg., 1848, 454-471. ———. Zur Physiologie des Nervus vagus. *In his:* Ges. Beitr. z. Path. u. Physiol., 8°, Berl., 1871, i, 184-189. ———. Versuche über den Einfluss des Lungen-Gaswechsels auf das dem Einfluss der Nn. vagi entzogene Herz. *Ibid.*, 310-320.—**Van Biervliet** (L.) Cas de section des pneumo-gastriques. Bull.

Nerve (*Pneumogastric*).

Acad. roy. de méd. de Belg., Brux., 1857-8, 2. s., i, 471-474. [Rap. de Fossion], 418. — **Van Kempen** (E.-M.) Nouvelles recherches sur la nature fonctionnelle des racines du nerf pneumogastrique et du nerf spinal. Bull. Acad. roy. de méd. de Belg., Brux., 1862, 2. s., v, 668-679. [Rap. de Thiernesse], 1863, vi, 184-192.—**Vincenzi** (L.) Sull' origine reale del nervo pneumogastrico. Gazz. d. clin., Torino, 1885, xxi, 209-211.—**Vogel** (A.) Zur Prognose der Vagusresection. Cor.-Bl. f. schweiz. Aerzte, Basel, 1883, xiii, 469-476. *Also:* Wien. med. Bl., 1883, vi, 1227; 1254.—**Wagner** (J.) Beiträge zur Kenntniss der respiratorischen Leistungen des Nervus vagus. Sitzungsb. d. k. Akad. d. Wissensch. Math.-naturw. Cl. 1879, Wien, 1880, lxxx, 3. Abth., 177-187. *Also:* Med. Jahrb., Wien, 1880, 239-249. —**Waller** (A.) Expériences sur les nerfs pneumogastriques et accessoires de Willis. Compt. rend. Soc. de biol. 1856, Par., 1857, 2. s., iii, 55-57. ———. On the effects of compression of the vagus nerve in the cure or relief of various nervous affections. Practitioner, Lond., 1870, iv, 193-206. ———. On the compression of the vagus nerve, considered as a means of producing asthenia or anæsthesia in surgical operations. *Ibid.*, v, 321-326. *Also, transl.:* Allg. Wien. med. Ztg., 1871, xvi, 65; 74.—**Ware** (E. R.) Experimental inquiry on the influence of the pneumo-gastric nerves. N. Am. M. & S. J., Phila., 1828, v, 264-268.—**Wasylewski** (T.) Ueber Vagusreizung beim Menschen. Vrtljschr. f. d. prakt. Heilk., Prag, 1878, cxxxviii, 69-82.—**Weber** (E.) & **Weber** (E.-H.) Expériences qui prouvent que les nerfs vagues, stimulés par l'appareil de rotation galvanomagnétique, peuvent retarder et même arrêter le mouvement du cœur. Arch. gén. de méd., Par., 1846, Suppl. 12.—**Wood** (H. C.), jr. Suspension of intestinal secretion and failure to produce purgation after section of the par vagum. Tr. Coll. Phys. Phila. (1863-74), 1874, n. s., iv, 317-320. *Also:* Am. J. M. Sc., Phila., 1870, n. s., lix, 395-398. ———. On the influence of section of the cervical pneumogastrics upon the action of emetics and cathartics. Am. J. M. Sc., Phila., 1870, n. s., lx, 75-100. *Also,* Reprint. — **Wundt** (W.) Versuche über den Einfluss der Durchschneidung der Lungenmagennerven auf die Respirationsorgane. Arch. f. Anat., Physiol. u. wissensch. Med., Leipz., 1855, 269-313. — **Zander** (R.) Folgen der Vagusdurchschneidung bei Vögeln. Arch. f. d. ges. Physiol., Bonn, 1878-9, xix, 263-334. *Also* [Abstr.]: Centralbl. f. d. med. Wissensch., Berl., 1879, xvii, 99; 113.— **Zybulsky** (N.) & **Wartanow** (W.) Ueber die Beziehung des N. depressor zum N. vagus. St. Petersb. med. Wchnschr., 1883, viii, 201-203. *Also, transl.:* Ejened. klin. gaz., St. Petersb., 1883, iii, 49-52.

Nerve (*Pneumogastric, Pathology of*).

See, also, Aneurisms (*Aortic*); Aneurisms (*Subclavian*); Hysteria; Neuralgia.

BILLROTH ([C. A.] T.) *De natura et causa pulmonum affectionis quæ nervo utroque vago dissecto exoritur. 4°. *Berolini*, [1852].

HABERSHON (S. O.) On the pathology of the pneumogastric nerve. [Lumleian lectures.] 8°. *London* 1877.

——. The same. Also, cold shock in its action on the pneumogastric nerve. 2. ed. 8°. *London*, 1885.

See, also, infra.

KOHOS (M.) * Die Erscheinungen bei Verletzungen des Nervus vagus. 8°. *Würzburg*, 1883.

LETULLE (M.) * Troubles fonctionnels du pneumogastrique. 4°. *Paris*, 1883.

MANCINI (F.) Sopra un raro caso di neurosi del vago. 8°. *Osimo*, 1884.

MONDRAGON (J.) * Valor semiotico de las alteraciones del dynamismo neümocardiaco. 8°. *México*, 1874.

SCHWARZENBERG (C. G. L.) * Diss. sistens casum rariorem adfectus spasmodico-convulsivi vagi. sm. 4°. *Halæ Magdeb.*, [1764].

SOUDÉE (L.) * Des troubles fonctionnels du pneumogastrique chez les femmes hystériques. 4°. *Paris*, 1875.

TILGEN (M. J.) * Diss. sistens observationem fungi medullaris nervi vagi et partium adjacentium cum epicrisi. 4°. *Bonnæ*, [1830].

VALENTIN (G.) Die Einflüsse der Vaguslähmung auf die Lungen- und die Hautausdünstung. 8°. *Frankf. a. M.*, 1857.

Also [Rev.], *in:* Ztschr. d. k.-k. Gesellsch. d. Aerzte zu Wien, 1857, xiii, 359-362.

Nerve (*Pneumogastric, Pathology of*).

Albers (J. T. H.) Anatomisch-pathologische Beobachtungen über den Nervus vagus. Mag. f. d. ges. Heilk., Berl., 1834, xli, 120–124. — **Anderson** (W. H.) Pneumogastric nerve. [Burning pain in fauces relieved by atropia.] Tr. M. Ass. Alabama, Montgomery, 1874, 349–354. — **Asthma ;** aneurism of the arch of the aorta; disease of the pneumogastric and phrenic nerves; large glandular tumours compressing them; hepatization of the lower part of both lungs; death from small-pox. N. Am. Arch. M. & S. Sc., Balt., 1835, ii, 172–175. — **Bignardi.** Renflements gangliformes le long des nerfs pneumogastriques. Bull. Soc. anat. de Par., 1830, v, 146. — **Blake** (J. H.) Wound of the neck; apparent recovery; sudden death. Boston M. & S. J., 1865, lxxi, 73. — **Bleifus.** Eine Neurose des Vagus. Med. Cor.-Bl. d. württemb. ärztl. Ver., Stuttg., 1842, xii, 70. — **Bufalini** (L.) Una nervosi del vago (angina pectoris?) di origine periferica. Morgagni, Napoli, 1881, xxiii, 762–774. — **Burggraeve.** Cas remarquable de compression traumatique des nerfs vagues et grands sympathiques, suivie de mort par asphyxie pulmonaire. Bull. Acad. roy. de méd. de Belg., Brux., 1851–2, xi, 859–864. — **Campbell** (J.) Essay on the pathology of the pneumogastric nerve. Proc. Connect. M. Soc., Hartford, 1877, 107–120. — **Chapin** (H. D.) A case of sudden death from pressure on an inflamed pneumogastric nerve. N. York M. J., 1884, xxxix, 294. — **Coiffier.** Paralysie du pneumogastrique. Courrier méd., Par., 1882, xxxii, 35–39. — **Couty.** Sur l'état du pneumogastrique appelé épuisement. Compt. rend. Soc. de biol., Par., 1883, 7. s., iv, 82–87. — **Cruveilhier.** Renflemens gangliformes le long des nerfs pneumogastriques. Rev. méd. franç. et étrang., Par., 1831, ii, 55–57. — **De Renzi** (E.) Il cardiopalmo da paresi dello pneumagastrico. Rivista, Genova, 1882, i, 105–108. — **Dix** (T. L.) Functional disturbance of pneumogastric nerve following the removal of a tumor from the inferior carotid triangle. Richmond & Louisville M. J., Louisville, 1872, xiv, 21. — **Fantonetti** (G.) Di alcune malattie del nervo pneumogastrico. Effem. d. sc. med., Milano, 1838, vii, 5–22. — **Gull** (W.) On destructive changes in the lung from diseases in the mediastinum invading or compressing the pneumogastric nerves and pulmonary plexus. Guy's Hosp. Rep., Lond., 1859, 3. s., v, 307–309. — **Guttmann** (P.) Zur Kenntniss der Vagus-Lähmung im Menschen. Arch. f. path. Anat., etc., Berl., 1873, lix, 51–64. — **Habershon** (S. O.) Clinical observations illustrating the effects produced by the implication of branches of the pneumogastric nerve in aneurismal tumours. Med.-Chir. Tr., Lond., 1864, xlvii, 35–53. ——. Some clinical facts connected with the pathology of the pneumogastric nerve. Guy's Hosp. Rep., Lond., 1875, 3. s., xx, 127–144. ——. Lumleian lectures on the pathology of the pneumogastric nerve. Brit. M. J., Lond., 1876, i, 465; 497; 557; 587; 651. *Also* [Abstr.]: Med. Times & Gaz., Lond., 1876, i, 433; 489; 515; 679. — **Hankel.** Erweichung des linken Nervus vagus und des Rückenmarkes; leichte Zerreissbarkeit des Magens. Mag. f. d. ges. Heilk., Berl., 1833, xxxix, 248–259. ——. Langwierige Krankheit des Nervus vagus; Ueberfüllung der Nervenscheiden mit Blutgefässen, vermehrte und verhärtete Nervensubstanz des rechten, Erweichung des linken Nervus vagus und einiger Ganglien des Nervus sympathicus. *Ibid.*, 259–273. — **Hérard.** [Le nerf pneumogastrique droit en rapport avec une tumeur qui a perforé la bronche droite; compression du nerf.] Bull. Soc. anat. de Par., 1846, xxi, 268. — **Hittner** (H. M.) Tumor, involving the pneumogastric; peripheral and reflex pains. Cincin. Lancet & Obs., 1865, viii, 738–740. *Also*: Canada M. J., Montreal, 1866, ii, 315. — **Huchard** (H.) Les synergies morbides du nerf pneumogastrique. Union méd., Par., 1883, 3. s., xxxv, 97–104. — **Kirchner** (J.) Entzündung des Nervus vagus. Med. Jahrb. d. k. k. österr. Staates, Wien, 1838, xxv, 212–214. — **Kredel** (L.) Zur Lehre von den Vagusneurosen. Deutsches Arch. f klin. Med., Leipz., 1881–2, xxx, 547–568. — **Kurtz.** Tödtliche Affection des Nervus vagus. Mag. f. d. ges. Heilk., Berl., 1832, xxxvi, 89–97. — **Langer** (L.) Ueber Vaguslähmung. Wien. med. Wchnschr., 1881, xxxi, 861; 885. — **Larenas** (E.), **Ortíz** (P.) & **Carvallo** (D.) ¿ Perturbacion del pneumogástrico? Rev. méd. de Chile, Sant. de Chile, 1882–3, xi, 68; 106. — **Lederer** (C.) Eine seltene Neuralgie des Vagus, hervorgerufen durch Reizung des Ganglion Bochdaleki. Allg. Wien. med. Ztg , 1861, vi, 197. ——. Neurose des Vagus, hervorgerufen durch Reizung des Ganglion Bochdaleki. Wien. med. Presse, 1866, vii, 628. — **Löwit** (M.) Ueber einen, einer einseitigen Vaguslähmung ähnlichen Symptomencomplex. Vrtljschr. f. d. prakt. Heilk., Prag, 1879, n. F.. iii, 27–46. — **McCollom** (J. H.) Cancerous disease of the neck, and infiltration of the pneumogastric nerve. Boston M. & S. J., 1869, lxxix, 308–310. — **Möser** (H.) Das laryngoskopische Bild bei vollkommener einseitiger Vagusparalyse. Mitth. a. d. med. Klin. zu Würzb., Wiesb., 1885, i, 201–217. — **Montault** (H.) Névralgie pneumo-gastrique, ou symptômes d'asthme, d'affection organique du cœur, d'aphonie, de ramollissement de l'estomac, produit par la présence de tumeurs encéphaloïdes qui comprimaient la huitième paire de nerfs. J. univ. et hebd. de méd. et chir. prat., Par., 1831, ii, 73–76. — **Parises** (N. P.) Ἀτελεκτασία ἐκ παρέσεως τοῦ πνευ-.

Nerve (*Pneumogastric, Pathology of*).

μονογαστρικοῦ συνεπεία ψύξεως εἰς ἔφηβον. Γαληνὸς, Ἀθῆναι, 1883, Θ´, 28. — **Pinel.** Note sur une névralgie des nerfs pneumo-gastriques guérie par les pilules de Méglin. J. gén. de méd., chir. et pharm., Par., 1828, cii, 332 – 334. — **Potain.** [Le pneumogastrique droit comprimé contre le rachis par un ganglion bronchique hypertrophié.] Bull. Soc. anat. de Par., 1861, xxxvi, 96 – 98. — **Preisendörfer** (P.) Ueber reflectorische Vagusneurose. Deutsches Arch. f. klin. Med., Leipz., 1880–81, xxvii, 387. — **Prus** (R.) Observations sur une névralgie de la huitième paire, simulant une affection hystérique. J. gén. de méd., chir. et pharm., Par., 1829, cvi, 31–36. — **Pupier.** Vomissements incoercibles dus à une lésion probable des pneumogastriques vers leur origine cérébrale. Mém. et compt.-rend. Soc. d. sc. méd. de Lyon, 1866–7, vi, 303–306. — **Riedel** (B.) Zur Casuistik der Vagusverletzung. Berl. klin. Wchnschr., 1883, xx, 343. — **Riegel** (F.) Ueber Vaguslähmung. *Ibid.*, 1875, xii, 425 – 428. *Also, transl.*: Chicago J. Nerv. & Ment. Dis., 1875, ii, 556 - 565. — **Rösch** (C.) Ueber die Inflammatio nervi vagi. J. d: pract. Heilk., Berl., 1837, lxxxv, 4. St., 105–115. — **Schupmann** (A.) Neuralgie des Nervus vagus mit allgemeinen Krämpfen. *Ibid.*, 1840, xc, 5. St., 18–28. — **Seeligmüller** (A.) Typische Neurose des Nervus vagus. *In his:* Neuropathol. Beobacht., 8°, Halle, 1873, 27–41. — **Serres.** Affection des nerfs pneumo-gastrique et diaphragmatique. Gaz. d. hôp., Par., 1828–9, i, 65. — **Sherman** (C. J.) On neurosis of the vagus, an idiopathic disease. Med. Times & Gaz., Lond., 1856, n. s., xiii, 281–284. — **Stackler** (A.) Contribution à l'étude de la pathologie du pneumogastrique à propos d'un cas de compression de ce nerf avec pouls lent permanent, crises épileptiformes et syncopales. Rev. de méd., Par., 1882, ii, 404–423. — **Torres** (B.) Neurósis del pneumogástrico; complicaciones; lesiones funcionales consecutivas; muerte. Progreso méd., Madrid, 1877, ii, 375; 384; 395. — **Tuczek** (F.) Ueber Vaguslähmung. Deutsches Arch. f. klin. Med., Leipz., 1877-8, xxi, 102–107. — **Weiss** (C. A.) Over de inflammatio nervi vagi. Pract. Tijdschr. v. de Geneesk., Gorinchem, 1842, xxi, 359–363. — **Worthington** (W. H.) A case of death produced by tumors pressing on the par vagum nerves. Med. Reporter, W. Chester, Pa., 1855, ii, 108–111. — **Zurhelle.** Secundärerkrankung beider Nervi vagi im Verlaufe eines Typhoids. Berl. klin. Wchnschr., 1873, x, 339.

Nerve (*Radial*).

See, also, **Extremity** (*Upper, Paralysis of*).

Bathiat (L.) * Étude sur le pronostic et le traitement de la paralysie à frigore du nerf radial. 4°. *Paris*, 1879.

Lablancherie (O.) * De l'enclavement du nerf radial dans le col de l'humérus. 4°. *Paris*, 1880.

Dagrève. Observation de névrite du radial. Assoc. franç. pour l'avance. d. sc. Compt.-rend. 1877, Par., 1878, vi. 891. — **Dieulafoy.** Paralysie du nerf radial. Bull. Soc. clin. de Par. (1878), 1879, ii, 143–145. — **Farabeuf** (L.-H.) Trajet du nerf radial autour de l'humérus. Progrès méd., Par., 1886, 2. s., iii, 174. — **Gillette.** Morsure du bras droit par la bouche d'un cheval; paralysie traumatique du nerf radial. Union méd., Par., 1875, 3. s., xix, 913–915. — **Giovanardi.** Ferita del nervo radiale e sue conseguenze. Soc. med.-chir. in Modena. Resoc., 1875, 3. — **Gosselin.** Morsure de cheval; lésion du nerf radial. Rev. méd. franç. et étrang., Par., 1880, i, 437–442. — **Gruber** (W.) Verästelung des Ramus superficialis des Nervus radialis in der Haut des Rückens der ganzen Hand und aller Finger bei nur verkümmert vorhandenem Ramus dorsalis des Nervus ulnaris. 2. Fall eigener Beobachtung. Arch. f. path. Anat., etc., Berl., 1885, cii, 5-7. — **Hérard.** Paralysie des extenseurs de l'avant-bras et de la main, survenue à la suite de la compression du nerf radial par une béquille. Gaz. d. hôp., Par., 1865, xxxviii, 381. — **Icard.** Observation pour servir à l'histoire des paralysies traumatiques du nerf radial ; guérison par l'électrisation localisée. Mém. et compt.-rend. Soc. d. sc. méd. de Lyon, 1864, iii, 117–123. — **Krause** (W.) Ueber einen Ast des N. radialis ; historische Bemerkung. Arch. f. path. Anat., etc., Berl., 1881, lxxxvi, 370. — **Ollier** (L.) Paralysie traumatique du nerf radial consécutive à une fracture de l'humérus. Mém. et compt.-rend. Soc. d. sc. méd. de Lyon, 1864, iii, 99. ——. Nerf radial comprimé dans un canal osseux accidentel, à la suite d'une fracture de l'humérus ; dégagement du nerf par une opération chirurgicale ; guérison de la paralysie. Gaz. hebd. de méd., Par., 1865, 2. s., ii, 515–518. — **Onimus.** Sur la paralysie du nerf radial. *Ibid.*, 1878, 2. s., xv, 393. — **Oppolzer.** Entzündung des Radialnerven; subkutane Injektion von Atropin; Heilung. Wien. Med.-Halle, 1861, ii, 199. — **Panas.** Paralysie du nerf radial. Bull. Acad. de méd., Par., 1882, 2. s., xi, 239–241. — **Peter.** Paralysie radiale gauche à frigore; névrite ascendante avec phénomènes de trémulation convulsive du membre supérieur et périarthrites de la main. Bull. Soc. clin. de Par. (1878), 1879, ii, 180–183. — **San Martin** (J.) Parálisis agitante consecu-

46

Nerve (Radial).

tiva á una herida del nervio radial en el brazo izquierdo; breves consideraciones diagnóstico-etiológicas. Crón. méd.-quir. de la Habana, 1880, vi, 276–282. — **Villette.** Anomalie de distribution du nerf radial. Bull. méd. du nord, Lille, 1878, xviii, 72–74.—**Weinlechner** (J.) Traumatische Lähmung des Nerv. radialis, welche auch nach der behufs Loslösung von etwaigen Narbensträngen vorgenommenen Isolirung des Nerven, wegen Atrophie desselben unverändert blieb. Aerztl. Ber. d. k. k. allg. Krankenh. zu Wien (1881), 1882, 228.

Nerve (Recurrent laryngeal).

See, also, **Glottis.**

ANDRÉ (C.-J.-S.) * Influence du nerf récurrent sur le larynx. 4°. *Strasbourg,* 1854.

JOLIVET (A.) * Essai sur les accidents déterminés par l'altération des nerfs récurrents. 4°. *Paris,* 1868.

MOUVEROUX (F.) * Compression des nerfs recurrents ; trachéotomie. 4°. *Paris,* 1880.

Anévrysme de l'aorte comprimant le nerf récurrent; altération particulière de la voix ; atrophie des muscles laryngiens animés par ce nerf. Bull. gén. de thérap., etc., Par., 1852, xliii, 132–134.—**Budd.** Tumour involving the recurrent laryngeal nerve; death from spasm of the glottis. Med. Times & Gaz., Lond., 1859, n. s., xviii, 138.—**Chaput** (H.) Note sur un rapport peu connu du récurrent gauche. Bull. Soc. anat. de Par., 1884, lix, 467–470.—**Cohen** (J. S.) Three cases of pressure upon the recurrent laryngeal nerve from different causes, with fixation of the left vocal band in the phonatory position. Tr. Coll. Phys. Phila., 1886, 3. s., viii, 423–439. *Also,* Reprint. *Also* [Abstr.] : Coll. & Clin. Rec., Phila., 1886, vii, 129–131. *Also, transl.:* Ann. d. mal. de l'oreille, du larynx, etc., Par., 1886, xii, 355–365.—**Dehio** (K.) Fehlschlucken in Folge einer Lähmung des linken Nervus laryngeus recurrens. St. Petersb. med. Wchnschr., 1883, viii, 177–179.—**Donaldson** (F.) The function of the recurrent laryngeal nerve. Brit. M. J., Lond., 1886, ii, 447.—**Donaldson** (F.), jr. The function of the recurrent laryngeal nerve; from experimental studies in the biological laboratory of the Johns Hopkins University. Am. J. M. Sc., Phila., 1886, n. s., xcii, 93–103. *Also,* Reprint. *Also :* Tr. Am. Laryngol. Ass. 1886, N. Y., 1887, viii, 213–225. ———. Further researches upon the physiology of the recurrent laryngeal nerve. N. York M. J., 1887, xlvi, 146 ; 173. *Also,* Reprint. *Also* [Abstr.] : Med. News, Phila., 1887, l, 633.—**Dwight** (T.) The relations of the inferior thyroid artery and the recurrent laryngeal nerve. Boston M. & S. J., 1886, cxv, 173. *Also :* Anat. Anz., Jena, 1886, i, 204.—**François-Franck.** Recherches sur le rôle des filets nerveux contenus dans l'anastomose qui existe entre le nerf laryngé supérieur et le nerf laryngé récurrent. Compt. rend. Acad. d. sc., Par., 1879, lxxxix, 449–451.—**Hérard.** [Anomalie du nerf récurrent droit.] Bull. Soc. anat. de Par., 1846, xxi, 111.—**Hilton** (J.) On the distribution and probable function of the superior and recurrent laryngeal nerves ; as demonstrated, by dissection, in the human subject. Guy's Hosp. Rep., Lond., 1837, ii, 514–518.—**Hirshfelder** (J. O.) Paralysis of the recurrent laryngeal nerve from peripleuritis. Pacific M. & S. J., San Fran., 1887, xxx, 278–281.—**Hooper** (F. H.) The anatomy and physiology of the recurrent laryngeal nerves. N. York M. J., 1887, xlvi, 29 ; 63 ; 99 ; 150. *Also,* Reprint. *Also* [Abstr.] : Med. News, Phila., 1887, l, 634. *Also, transl.:* Ann. d. mal. de l'oreille, du larynx, etc., Par., 1887, xiii, 475; 556 : 1888, xiv, 22–41. ———. Effects of varying rates of stimulation on the action of the recurrent laryngeal nerves. [Preliminary communication.] N. York M. J., 1887, xlvi, 591. *Also,* Reprint. — **Lee** (R. J.) Changes produced in the recurrent laryngeal nerves in cases of thoracic aneurism. Lancet, Lond., 1873, i, 129.—**Mackenzie** (M.) Laryngeal growths pressing upon the left recurrent laryngeal nerve, and causing paralysis and atrophy of the abductor of the left vocal cord. Tr. Path. Soc. Lond., 1867–8, xix, 84–86.—**Martin** (G.) The experiment of cutting the recurrent nerves carried on farther than has hitherto been done. Med. Essays & Obs. Soc. Edinb., 1734, ii, 114–121.—**Newman** (D.) Some points in relation to the diagnostic significance and therapeutic indications of laryngeal symptoms, resulting from pressure of aneurisms upon the vagus and recurrent laryngeal nerves. Glasgow M. J., 1887, [4.] s., xxviii, 214–221.—**Philipeaux** (J.-M.) & **Vulpian** (A.) Sur l'anastomose qui existe entre le nerf laryngé supérieur et le nerf récurrent. Arch. de physiol. norm. et path., Par., 1869, ii, 666.—**Porter** (W.) Pressure upon the recurrent nerve. Arch. Laryngol., N. Y., 1880, i, 66.—**Rainey** (G.) The recurrent laryngeal nerve. Lond. M. Gaz., 1828–9, iii, 11.—**Rossi** (C.) Effetti diversi che ottengonsi sugli animali domestici, delle diverse specie, in conseguenza della recisione o di uno o di ambi i ricorrenti laringei. Gior. di anat., fisiol. e patol. d. anamali, Pisa, 1870, ii, 78–80.—**Semon** (F.) Clinical remarks on the proclivity of the abductor fibres of the recurrent laryngeal nerve to become

Nerve (Recurrent laryngeal).

affected sooner than the adductor fibres, or even exclusively, in cases of undoubted central or peripheral injury or disease of the roots or trunks of the pneumogastric, spinal accessory, or recurrent nerves. Arch. Laryngol., N. Y., 1881, ii, 197–222.—**Verstræten.** Lipome du nerf récurrent gauche. Ann. Soc. de méd. de Gand, 1876, liv, 73–76.—**White** (W. H.) On atrophy of the thyroid body, following pressure on the recurrent laryngeal nerve. Brit. M. J., Lond., 1885, ii, 342. ———. Further communication on the function of the recurrent laryngeal nerve with regard to the thyroid body. *Ibid.,* 1014.—**Wilson** (E. T.) Case of aneurism, with paralysis of the left recurrent laryngeal nerve. Brit. M. J., Lond., 1874, ii, 30.

Nerve (Sciatic).

See, also, **Nerve - stretching ; Neurotomy,** *etc.* ; **Sciatica.**

JOERDENS (J. H.) Descriptio nervi ischiadici iconibus illustrata. fol. *Erlangæ,* 1788.

Bacchi (A.) Storia di singolare simpatia fra le ultime diramazioni del nervo sciatico e l' organo uditivo. Bull. d. sc. med. di Bologna, 1853, 3. s., xxiv, 128–137.—**Brown-Séquard** (C.-É.) Causes des altérations de nutrition qui suivent la section du nerf sciatique et du nerf crural, chez les cobayes. Compt. rend. Soc. de biol., Par., 1885, 8. s., ii, 146.—**Calori** (L.) Sull' alta divisione del nervo grande ischiatico considerata come differenza nazionale e sulla varietà del muscolo piriforme. Mem. Accad. d. sc. d. Ist. di Bologna, 1880, 4. s., ii, 623–633, 1 pl.—**Charvot.** Sciatique (grand nerf). Dict. encycl. d. sc. méd., Par., 1879, 3. s., vii, 595–647.—**Erichsen.** Untersuchungen über den Nervus ischiadicus. St. Petersb. med. Ztschr., 1869, xvii, 40.—**Féré** (C.) Note sur un point de l'anatomie du nerf sciatique. Bull. Soc. anat. de Par., 1879, 4. s., iv, 110–112. *Also :* Progrès méd., Par., 1879, vii, 649.—**Giommi** (M.) Di un' anomalia anatomica del nervo sciatico. Raccoglitore med., Forlì, 1881, 4. s., xvi, 490–492.—**Gley** (E.) De l'action réflexe du nerf sciatique sur la glande sous-maxillaire. Compt. rend. Soc de biol., Par., 1886, 8. s., iii, 79–81.—**Gros-Jean.** Anomalie du nerf grand sciatique et de quelques unes de ses branches. Lyon méd., 1870, v, 182.—**Isenschmid.** Affection des linken Nervus ischiadicus. Aerztl. Int.-Bl., München, 1882, xxix, 360.—**Lépine** (R.) De l'influence qu'exercent les excitations du bout périphérique du nerf sciatique sur la température du membre correspondant. Compt. rend. Soc. de biol. 1876, Par., 1877, 6. s., iii, pt. 2, 21–37. *Also :* Gaz. méd. de Par., 1876, 4. s., v, 147 ; 230. ———. Note additionnelle, relative à l'influence de l'échauffement et du refroidissement artificiels du cœur sur les effets de l'excitation du nerf vague; par MM. Lépine et Tridon. Gaz. méd. de Par., 1876, 4. s., v, 243 ; 278.—**Lereboullet** (L.) Sciatique (pathologie médicale). Dict. encycl. d. sc. méd., Par., 1879, 3. s., vii, 600–616.—**Letiévant.** Motilité et sensibilité suppléées après la section du grand nerf sciatique. Gaz. méd. de Par., 1873, 4. s., ii, 423 ; 435.—**Meissner** (E. A.) jun. Ueber die Mitleidenschatt der Nervi ischiadici in den verschiedenen physiologischen und pathologischen Zuständen des Uterus. Vrtljschr. f. d. prakt. Heilk., Prag, 1856, xlix, 33–42.—**Mitchell** (S. W.) Specimen of the sciatic nerve of a rabbit, in the sheath of which were developed, under irritation, multiple abscesses. Tr. Path. Soc. Phila. (1871-3) 1874, iv, 240. *Also :* Med. Times, Phila., 1870–71, i, 202.—**Philipeaux.** De la non difformité chez les jeunes cochons d'Inde et les jeunes rats albinos après la section du nerf sciatique. Compt. rend. Soc. de biol. 1876, Par., 1877, 6. s., iii, 128.—**Puelma** (F.) & **Luchsinger** (B.) Zum Verlauf der Gefässnerven im Ischiadicus der Katze. Arch. f. d. ges. Physiol., Bonn, 1878, xvii, 489–493.—**Stricker** (S.) Untersuchungen über die Gefässnerven-Wurzeln des Ischiadicus. Sitzungsb. d. k. Akad. d. Wissensch. Math.-naturw. Cl. 1876, Wien, 1877, lxxiv, 173–185. *Also :* Arch. de physiol. norm. et path., Par., 1876, 2. s., iii, 832–844. *Also :* Med. Jahrb., Wien, 1877, 279–290.—**Trélat.** Fibro-myxôme du nerf sciatique. Bull. et mém. Soc. de chir. de Par., 1876, n. s., i, 441–443.—**Vulpian** (A.) Sur la provenance des fibres nerveuses excito-sudorales contenues dans le nerf sciatique du chat. Compt. rend. Acad. d. sc., Par., 1878, lxxxvi, 1308–1310.

Nerve (Sciatic, Tumors of).

HOLZSCHNEIDER (W. H.) * Ein Fall von Myxoneurom des Nervus ischiadicus. 8°. *Greifswald,* [1874].

Balding (D.) Recurrent tumour of sciatic nerve; extensive secondary growth in mediastinum and pleura. Tr. Path. Soc. Lond. (1876-7) 1877, xxviii, 23–31, 1 pl.—**Bardeleben.** Ueber Sarcome des Nervus ischiadicus und seiner Aeste. Verhandl. d. deutsch. Gesellsch. f. Chir., Berl., 1883, xii, 96–98. ———. Sarcome des Nervus ischiadicus. Charité-Ann. 1883, Berl., 1885, x, 481.—**Bernays** (A. C.) Tumor removed from the sciatic nerve. Proc. St. Louis M. Soc. Missouri, 1881, iii, 111.—**Camperon** & **Cornil** (V.) Fibro-myxome du nerf sciatique. Bull. Soc. anat. de Par., 1875, l, 698–708.—**Coupland** (S.)

Nerve (*Sciatic, Tumors of*).

Tumour of the sciatic nerve. Tr. Path. Soc. Lond., 1875-6, xxvii, 23.—**De Schweinitz** (G.) Tumor of the sciatic nerve. Phila. M. Times, 1882-3, xiii, 770. *Also:* Med. News, Phila., 1883, xliii, 215. *Also:* Tr. Path. Soc. Phila. (1881-3), 1884, xi, 234.—**Duncan** (J.) Case of fibrous tumor surrounding the right sciatic nerve. Lond. & Edinb. Month. J. M. Sc., 1841, i, 87-90, 1 pl.—**Flower** (W. H.) Epithelial tumour in the sheath of the sciatic nerve. Tr. Path. Soc. Lond., 1857-8, ix, 11-13, 1 pl.—**Gregory.** Tumor of sciatic nerve. St. Louis M. & S. J., 1879-80, xxxviii, 545.—**Le Dentu.** Tumeur myxomateuse du nerf sciatique. Gaz. d. hôp., Par., 1880, liii, 473.—**Little** (W. B.) Removal of a tumor of the left thigh, adherent to the sciatic nerve, with excision of a portion of the nerve. Boston M. & S. J., 1885, cxiii, 533.—**Marchand.** Lecture sur un cas de sarcôme kystique du nerf sciatique. Bull. et mém. Soc. de chir. de Par., 1879, n. s., v, 677; 683.—**Page** (F.) Large vascular sarcoma of the sciatic nerve; amputation; recovery. Brit. M. J., Lond., 1884, i, 104.—**Tiffany** (L. McL.) Tumor of sciatic nerve; excision, together with five and three-quarter inches of nerve. Maryland M. J., Balt., 1880, vii, 175-177. ———. Specimen of sarcoma developed from sciatic nerve. Virginia M. Month., Richmond, 1880-81, vii, 557-559.—**Trélat.** Myxome du nerf sciatique. Bull. et mém. Soc. de chir. de Par., 1875, n. s., i, 777. ———. Fibro-myxôme du nerf sciatique. *Ibid.*, 1876, n. s., ii, 264-277, 2 pl. — **Tuffier.** Sarcome du creux poplité siégant dans le nerf sciatique; résection du nerf. Bull. Soc. anat. de Par., 1884, lix, 29-31.—**Verneuil.** Un névrôme qui siégeait sur le nerf sciatique poplité externe. *Ibid.*, 1854, xxix, 22.—**Waldenström.** Sarcoma fibrosum nervi ischiadici sinistri. Upsala Läkaref. Förh., 1877, xii, 651-653.

Nerve (*Sciatic, Wounds of*).

See, also, **Neurotomy**, etc.

RYNDSJUN (J.) * Diabetes mellitus bei Ischias und Ischiadicus-Verletzung. 8°. *Jena*, 1877.

Annequin. Section traumatique du grand nerf sciatique gauche à son émergence du bassin. Rec. de mém. de méd. . . . mil., Par., 1878, 3. s., xxxiv, 566-578.—**Banner** (J. M.) Injury of the great ischiatic nerve. Lond. M. Gaz., 1832, x, 253-255.—**Bouilly** (G.) De la contusion du nerf sciatique et de ses conséquences. Arch. gén. de méd., Par., 1880, cxlvi, 655-670.—**Charcot.** Exemple d'affection spinale consécutive à une contusion du nerf sciatique. Progrès méd., Par., 1883, xi, 157; 185.—**Deleau.** Blessure du nerf sciatique, suivie de graves accidents. Rev. méd.-chir. de Par., 1849, vi, 117-119.—**Gaultier de Claubry.** Observation d'une blessure du nerf sciatique poplité externe; paralysie des muscles fléchisseurs du pied; guérison après quelques mois. J. hebd. de méd., Par., 1829, iv, 59-61.—**Heller** (A.) Bleistückchen im Nervus ischiadicus. Arch. f. path. Anat., etc., Berl., 1870, li, 357-361.—**Krönlein** (R. U.) Paralyse des rechten Unterschenkels und Fusses nach einer 2½ Jahre früher stattgehabten Durchschneidung des N. ischiadicus; directe späte Nervennaht; theilweise Besserung der Sensibilitätsstörung. Arch. f. klin. Chir., Berl., 1877, xxi (Supplhft.), 272-274.—**Morat.** Section du nerf sciatique poplité interne par un éclat d'obus; mal perforant des deux premiers orteils. Mém. et compt.-rend. Soc. d. sc. méd. de Lyon (1876), 1877, xvi, 53-59.—**Panas.** Élongation du nerf sciatique devenu névromateux et provoquant des douleurs vives, accompagnées d'épilepsie spinale, à la suite d'un coup de couteau qui avait divisé ce nerf; guérison. Bull. Acad. de méd., Par., 1881, 2. s., x, 1551-1556.—**Park** (R.) Rupture of the sciatic nerve; immediate union; restoration of function. J. Am. M. Ass., Chicago, 1884, ii, 323. — **Rösch.** Verletzung des ischiadischen Nerven; Tod durch Gehirn- und Rückenmarksreizung. Med. Cor.-Bl. d. württemb. ärztl. Ver., Stuttg., 1851, xxi, 107.—**Tassi.** Caso importantissimo di grave ferita del nervo sciatico, seguita da alterazioni nevro-paralitiche immediate e tardive. Bull. d. r. Accad. med. di Roma, 1881, vii, 327-333.—**Van Buren** (W. H.) Partial paralysis of right leg from wound of great sciatic nerve; with circular callous ulcer of sole of the foot. N. York J. M., 1851, vi, 47-49.—**Warren** (J. M.) Gunshot wound of the thigh, implicating the sciatic nerve. *In his:* Surg. Obs., 8°, Bost., 1867, 470.

Nerve (*Spermatic*).

Obolensky (J.) Die Durchschneidung des Nervus spermaticus und deren Einfluss auf den Hoden. Centralbl. f. d. med. Wissensch., Berl., 1867, v, 497-500.

Nerve (*Spinal accessory*).

See, also, **Heart** (*Nerves of*); **Nerves** (*Cranial, Eighth pair of*).

CALORI (A.) Annotationes anatomicæ de origine et connexionibus nervi accessorii Willisii cum posticis nervorum cervicalium superiorum radicibus et cum nervo vago. 4°. *Bononiæ*, 1849.

Nerve (*Spinal accessory*).

ROLLER (C. F. W.) * Der centrale Verlauf der Nervus accessorius Willisii. 8°. *Berlin*, 1880.

Also, in: Allg. Ztschr. f. Psychiat., etc., Berl., 1881, xxxvii, 469-489, 1 pl.

Althaus. A case of disease of the spinal accessory nerve. Brit. M. J., Lond., 1879, i, 171. *Also:* Lancet, Lond., 1879, i, 160.—**Arloing** (S.) Spinal (nerf). Dict. encycl. d. sc. méd., Par., 1884, 3. s., xi, 229-252.—**Bernard** (C.) Recherches expérimentales sur les fonctions du nerf spinal, étudié spécialement dans ses rapports avec le pneumogastrique. Arch. gén. de méd., Par., 1844, 4. s., iv, 397; 851. *Also*, Reprint. *Also, transl.:* Month. M News, Louisville. 1860, ii, 217, 1 pl., 289: iii, 1; 73.—**Darkschewitsch** (L.) Ueber den centralen Ursprung des N. accessorius Willisii. Neurol. Centralbl., Leipz., 1885, iv, 134. ———. Ueber den Ursprung und den centralen Verlauf des Nervus accessorius Willisii. Arch. f. Anat u. Entwcklngsgesch., Leipz., 1885, 361-378, 1 pl.—**Dees** (O.) Ueber den Ursprung und den centralen Verlauf des Nervus accessorius Willisii. Allg. Ztschr. f. Psychiat., etc., Berl., 1887, xliii, 453-470, 1 pl.—**De Morgan** (C.) Case of excision of a part of the spinal accessory nerve for spasmodic wry neck. Brit. & For. M.-Chir. Rev., Lond., 1866, xxxviii, 218-225. — **De Renzi** (E.) Spasmo ritmico dell' accessorio. Boll. d.clin., Napoli, 1885, ii, 291.—**Eckhard** (C.) Geschichte der Experimentalphysiologie des Nervus accessorius Willisii. Beitr. z. Anat. u. Physiol. (Eckhard), Giessen, 1883, x, 171-203.—**Hewer** (J. L.) A case of damage to the spinal accessory nerve. Lancet, Lond., 1885, ii, 431.—**Holl** (M.) Ueber den Nervus accessorius Willisii. Arch. f. Anat. u. Entwcklngsgesch., Leipz., 1878, 491-518, 1 pl.—**Scarpa** (A.) De nervo spinali ad octavum cerebri accessorio commentarius. Acta Acad. Cæs. reg. Joseph. med.-chir. Vindob., 1878, i, 337 - 374, 1 pl. *Also, transl.:* Actes Acad. c. r. Joséphine méd.-chir. de Vienne, Montpel., 1792, i, 409-445. — **Tremaine** (W. S.) Physiological action of spinal accessory demonstrated by injury of its filaments. Buffalo M. & S. J., 1882-3, xxii, 218.

Nerve (*Splanchnic*).

See **Nervous** *system* (*Ganglionic*).

Nerve (*Superficial petrosal*).

See **Nerve** (*Facial*).

Nerve (*Superior maxillary*).

See **Neurotomy**, etc.

Nerve (*Supraorbital*).

See, also, **Eyebrow** (*Wounds of*); **Neuralgia** (*Supra-orbital*); **Neurotomy**, etc.

TARDIF (A.) * Contribution à l'étude des accidents consécutifs aux lésions du nerf sus-orbitaire. 4°. *Paris*, 1885.

Bechtereff (V. G.) Trophicheskoe razstroistvo v oblasti razvet. levago nadglaz. nerva. Hemiatrophia facialis incompleta. [Trophical lesion in ramification of left supraorbital nerve.] Vestnik klin. i sudebnoi psichiat. i nevropatol., St. Petersb.. 1886, iv, pt. i, 97-117.—**Erlenmeyer.** Ueber den Einfluss der Verletzungen des Nervus supraorbitalis auf das Auge. Med. Ztg., Berl., 1847, xvi, 145-147.—**von Graefe** (A.) Fall von Durchschneidung des Supraorbitalnerven und sonstige Ergebnisse über die Heilwirkung dieser Operation. Arch. f. Ophth., Berl., 1859, v, 2. Abth., 184-200. — **Karewski** (F.) Ueber einen Fall von Trophoneurose im Bereiche des Nervus supraorbitalis. Berl. klin. Wchnschr., 1883, xx, 549-551. *Also:* Verhandl. d. Berl. med. Gesellsch. (1882-3), 1884, xiv, pt. 2, 235-238. — **Sharp** (H.) Case of tic douloureux cured by the excision of a mass of phosphate of lime, adhering to the supra-orbital nerve. Edinb. M. J., 1855-6, i, 931. —**Strawbridge** (G.) Some curious reflex conditions following section of the supra-orbital nerve. Arch. Ophth. & Otol., N. Y., 1874-5, iv, 403-407. *Also, transl.:* Arch. f. Augen- u. Ohrenh., Wiesb., 1876, v, 168-172.

Nerve (*Sympathetic*).

See **Meckel's** *ganglion*; **Nervous** *system* (*Ganglionic*).

Nerve (*Thoracic*).

Bowditch. Paralysis of long thoracic nerve. Am. J. M. Sc., Phila., 1848, n. s., xvi, 302. — **Werner.** Die Durchschneidung des Nervus thoracicus posterior (an Kaninchen) und deren Folgen. Wchnschr. f. d. ges. Heilk., Berl., 1850, 753; 769; 791.

Nerve (*Trochlear*).

Exner (S.) Ein Versuch über Trochleariskreuzung. Sitzungsb. d. k. Akad. d. Wissensch., Wien, 1874, lxx, 151-153.

Nerve (*Tympanic*).

Krause (W.) Ueber den N. tympanicus und N. petrosus superficialis minor. Ztschr. f. rat. Med., Leipz. u. Heidelb., 1866, 3. R., xxviii, 92–98, 2 pl.

Nerve (*Ulnar*).

See, also, **Nerve-stretching**; **Neurotomy**, *etc.*

Fèvre (E.-P.) * Étude sur les paralysies du nerf cubital. 4°. *Paris*, 1878.

———. The same. 8°. *Paris*, 1879.

Ledoux (L.) * Des atrophies de la main consécutives aux lésions du nerf cubital. 4°. *Paris*, 1878.

Ashhurst (J.), jr. Incised wound of wrist, with lesion of ulnar nerve; observations of temperature in affected parts. Am. J. M. Sc., Phila., 1868, n. s., lv, 47. — **Ballet** (G.) Accidents consécutifs à la compression habituelle du cubital chez un ouvrier employé à ouvrager le verre. Rev. de méd., Par., 1884, iv, 484–486. — **Bellamy.** Injury to ulnar nerve; paralysis; recovery. Lancet, Lond., 1877, ii, 570.— **Biddon.** Sarcoma of ulnar nerve, ending in amputation of shoulder-joint and exsection of scapula. Med. Rec., N. Y., 1878, xiii, 116.— **Blailock** (W. R.) Wound of digital branch of ulnar nerve, followed by paroxysmal mental aberration; relieved by an operation. Tr. Mississippi M. Ass., Jackson, 1882, xv, 135. — **Blattmann** (A.) Beobachtung einer Dislocation des Nervus ulnaris. Deutsche Klinik, Berl., 1851, iii, 435–437. — **Bossuet.** Lésion traumatique du nerf cubital; névralgie; paralysie; guérison. Mém. et bull. Soc. méd.-chir. d. hôp. de Bordeaux, 1871, v–vi, 72. — **Bouchaud** (J.-B.) Plaie du nerf cubital. Progrès méd., Par., 1876, iv, 35. — **Calder** (F. W. G.) Effects of a division of the ulnar nerve. Lancet, Lond., 1832-3, i, 489.—**Cénas** (L.) Troubles nerveux complexes des extrémités consécutifs à une blessure du nerf cubital. Rev. de méd., Par., 1884, iv, 479–483.—**Chalot** (V.) Lésion traumatique du nerf cubital; troubles trophiques consécutifs. Montpel.méd., 1876, xxxvi, 489–508.—**Charvot** (D.) Cubital (nerf); pathologie chirurgicale. Dict. encycl. d. sc. méd., Par., 1880, xxiv, 99–130.—**Duret** (H.) Griffe consécutive à une lésion traumatique du nerf cubital. Rev. phot. d. hôp. de Par., 1872, iv, 71–77, 1 pl.—**Duvernoy** (É.) Piqûre du nerf cubital droit chez une névropathe; accidents névralgiques persistants. France méd., Par., 1880, xxvii, 418. *Also:* Bull. Soc. clin. de Par. (1880), 1881, iv, 68–73.—**Eulenburg** (A.) Neuritis des N. ulnaris im Zusammenhange mit "Strangcontracturen" der Finger. Neurol. Centralbl., Berl., 1883, ii, 49–53. — **Gruber** (W.) Ob anomalnom khodai loktevago nerva speredi mishchelka. [Anomalous course of the ulnar nerve.] Med. Vestnik, St. Petersb., 1867, vii, 391. — Abgang eines supernumerären Nervus cutaneus ulnaris antibrachii vom Nervus ulnaris am Oberarm über dem Epitrochleus humeri, der einen Kanal an der Spitze des letzteren passirt; so vorher nicht gesehen. Arch. f. path. Anat., etc., Berl., 1885, cii, 7–9.— **Jones** (S.) Traumatic neuroma of ulnar nerve, with loss of power of parts supplied. Lancet, Lond., 1882, ii, 487.— **Lutz** (F. J.) Habitual dislocation of the left ulnar nerve. St. Louis M. & S. J., 1879–80, xxxviii, 550. *Also:* Proc. St. Louis M. Soc. Missouri, 1881, iii, 116.—**Nunn.** Drawing of hand after injury to ulnar nerve, and observations of the temperature, etc., of the hand. Tr. Path. Soc. Lond., 1865-6, xvii, 6.—**Putnam** (J. J.) Injury to ulnar nerve. Extr. Rec. Bost. Soc. M. Improve., 1880, vii, 140.— **Raymond** (P.) Contusion du nerf cubital; troubles trophiques. France méd., Par., 1885, i. 565–568.—**Sabourin.** Paralysie du nerf cubital. Bull. Soc. clin. de Par. (1878), 1879, ii, 292–294. *Also:* France méd., Par., 1879, xxvi, 91.—**Seeligmüller.** Lähmung des Sympathicus neben Lähmung des Nervus ulnaris durch Schussverletzung. Berl. klin. Wchnschr., 1872, ix, 43.—**Straurenghi** (C.) Osservazioni sull' anatomia descrittiva del nervo ulnare ed in particolare della topografia del medesimo nella regione brachiale. Boll. scient., Pavia, 1886, viii, 36.—**Weinlechner** (J.) Neuritis ulnaris; Beugecontractur im Elbogengelenke. Ber. d. k. k. Krankenanst. Rudolph-Stiftung in Wien (1878), 1879, 352. *Also:* Med.-chir. Centralbl., Wien, 1881, xvi, 171.—**Whittaker** (J. T.) Trauma of the ulnar nerve simulating progressive muscular atrophy. Med. Rec., N. Y., 1880, xvii, 588.

Nerve (*Vidian*).

See, also, **Meckel's ganglion.**

Sapolini (G.) Bozzetto neurologico circa il nervo vidiana o ricorrente di Meckel. Ann. univ. di med., Milano, 1871, ccxvii, 591. *Also,* Reprint.

Nerve of *Wrisberg.*

Barbarisi (G.) Ricerche anatomiche sulla corda del timpano e sullo intermediario di Wrisberg. Rendic. Accad. med.-chir. di Napoli, 1853, vii, 121–145, 1 pl.—**de Garay** (A.) Funciones del nervio intermediario de Wrisberg. Escuela de med., México, 1879-80, i, no. 18, 5; no. 22, 8.—**Sapolini** (G.) Studj anatomici sul nervo di Wrisberg e su la corda del timpano o tredicesimo nervo craniale. Ann. univ. di med. e chir., Milano, 1881, cclv,

Nerve of *Wrisberg.*

3–27.—**Tavares** (C.) Contribuição para o estudo anatomico do nervo de Wrisberg. Med. contemp., Lisb., 1883, i, 2; 20; 29; 53; 70; 86; 101; 118; 134; 159; 181; 197; 296; 230; 287; 320; 368. — **Varaglia** (S.) Sull' esistenza di cellule nervose nell' uomo, lungo il decorso del nervo intermediario del Wrisberg e del facciale tra la loro origine apparente ed il ganglio genicolato. Osservatore, Torino, 1883, xix, 789.—**Velits** (A.) A járulékos ideghez (n. accessorius) tartozó izmok görcsének egy esete. [Cramp of . . .] Orvosi hetil., Budapest, 1883, xxvii, 188–190. *Also, transl.* [Abstr.]: Pest. med.-chir. Presse, Budapest, 1883, xix, 381.—**Vulpian.** Recherches sur les fonctions du nerf de Wrisberg. Compt. rend. Acad. d. sc., Par., 1885, ci, 1037; 1447.

Nerve-cell.

See **Nervous** *system* (*Histology of*).

Nerve-currents (*Velocity of*).

See, also, **Thought** (*Rapidity of*).

Camerer (W.) * Versuche über den zeitlichen Verlauf der Willensbewegung. 8°. *Tübingen*, 1866.

von Bezold (A.) Ueber die zeitlichen Verhältnisse, welche bei der elektrischen Erregung der Nerven in's Spiel kommen. [*Repr. from:* Monatsber. d. k. preuss. Akad. d. Wiss. zu Berl., 22. Nov. 1860.] Untersuch. z. Naturl. d. Mensch. u. d. Thiere, Giessen, 1860, vii, 581–589.—**Bloch** (A.-M.) Expériences sur la vitesse du courant nerveux sensitif de l'homme. Compt. rend. Soc. de biol. 1875, Par., 1876, 6. s., ii, 181–199. *Also:* Gaz. méd. de Par., 1875, 4. s., iv, 279; 289. *Also:* Arch. de physiol. norm. et path., Par., 1875, 2. s., ii, 588–623. — Expériences nouvelles sur la vitesse du courant nerveux sensitif chez l'homme. J. de l'anat. et physiol., etc., Par., 1884, xx, 284–290. *Also* [Abstr.]: Compt. rend. Soc. de biol., Par., 1884, 8. s., i, pt. 2, 343. ———. La vitesse comparative des sensations. Rev. scient., Par., 1887, xxxix, 585–589. — **Brown-Séquard** (C.-E.) Recherches démontrant la non-nécessité de l'entrecroisement des conducteurs servant aux mouvements volontaires, à la base de l'encéphale ou ailleurs. France méd., Par., 1878, xxv, 305–307. ——. Recherches montrant la puissance, la rapidité d'action et les variétés de certaines influences inhibitoires (influences d'arrêt) de l'encéphale sur lui-même ou sur la moelle épinière et de ce dernier centre sur lui-même ou sur l'encéphale. Compt. rend. Acad. d. sc., Par., 1879, lxxxix, 657–659.—**Chauveau** (A.) Procédés et appareils pour l'étude de la vitesse de propagation des excitations dans les différentes catégories de nerfs moteurs chez les mammifères. *Ibid.*, 1878, lxxxvii, 95–99. ———. Vitesse de propagation des excitations dans les nerfs moteurs des muscles de la vie animale, chez les animaux mammifères. *Ibid.*, 138–142.—**Frédéricq** (L.) & **Vandevelde** (G.) Vitesse de transmission de l'excitation motrice dans les nerfs du homard. *Ibid.*, 1880, xci, 239.— **Gad** (J.) Zur Methodik der Zeitmessung von Erregungsleistungen. Arch. f. Physiol., Leipz., 1886, 263–266.— **Lautenbach** (B. F.) On the velocity of nervous action. Phila. M. Times, 1876-7, vii, 346–348.—**Marey** (J.) Nouvelles expériences pour la détermination de la vitesse du courant nerveux. Compt. rend. Soc. de biol. 1866, Par., 1867, 4. s., iii, 21–24.—**Ott** (I.) Rapidity of transmission of nerve force in normal and stretched nerves; extra-polar katelectrotonus. J. Nerv. & Ment. Dis., Chicago, 1878, n. s., iii, 94–98.— **Piotrowski** (G.) & **Widmann** (O.) O chyzości z jaka się stan czynny w nerwach udziela. [The velocity of transmission by the irritated nerve.] Przegl. lek., Krakow., 1863, ii, 289–293. — **Place** (T.) Over de geleidingssnelheid in de beweegzenuwen van den mensch. Onderzoek. ged. in h. physiol. Lab. d. Leidsche Hoogesch., 1870, ii, 101–120. *Also.transl.:* Arch. néerl. d. sc. exactes, etc., La Haye, 1871, vi, 80–94.—**Regnard** (P.) Influence des hautes pressions sur la rapidité du courant nerveux. Compt. rend. Soc. de biol., Par., 1887, 8. s., iv, 406–408.— **René** (A.) Étude expérimentale sur la vitesse de transmission nerveuse chez l'homme; durée d'un acte cérébral et d'un acte réflexe, vitesse sensitive, vitesse motrice. Gaz. d. hôp., Par.,1882, lv, 276; 283; 307; 363; 373.—**Waller** (A.) Sur le temps perdu de la contraction d'ouverture. Arch. de physiol. norm. et path., Par., 1882, 2. s., ix, 383–385. — **Wedenskii** (N.) Wie rasch ermüdet der Nerv? Centralbl. f. d. med. Wissensch., Berl., 1884, xxii, 65–68.—**von Wittich.** Untersuchung des zeitlichen Verlaufes der motorischen Action bei dem Kranken Damerau. Arch. f. path. Anat., etc., Berl., 1869, xlvi, 483–493.

Nerve-fibre.

See **Nervous** *system* (*Histology of*).

Nerve-stretching.

See, also, **Leprosy** (*Treatment of*); **Nerve** (*Nasal*); **Nerves** (*Surgery of*); **Neuralgia** (*Facial, etc., Treatment of*); **Neuralgia** (*Inter-*

Nerve-stretching.

costal); **Neuralgia** (*Supraorbital*); **Tetanus** (*Treatment of*).

CONRAD (T.) * Experimentelle Untersuchungen über Nerven-Dehnung. 8°. *Greifswald*, 1876.

DUVAULT (A.) * De la distension des nerfs comme moyen thérapeutique. 4°. *Paris*, 1876.

HESSLER (P.) * Zur Casuistik der Nervendehnung. [Berlin.] 8°. *Greiz*, 1881.

LAGRANGE (F.) Valeur thérapeutique de l'élongation des nerfs. Mémoire couronné par la Société de chirurgie de Paris. 8°. *Paris*, 1886.

LAURENT (G.) * Du traitement de la névralgie sciatique par l'élongation non sanglante du nerf. 4°. *Lyon*, 1885.

MARSHALL (J.) Neurectasy, or nerve-stretching for the relief or cure of pain, being the Bradshaw lecture delivered at the Royal College of Surgeons of England on the 6th December, 1883, with an appendix by the author, dated March, 1887, and 12 illustrations by Victor A. H. Horsley. 8°. *London*, 1887.

NICOLAS (J.) * Du traitement de la névralgie sciatique par l'élongation du nerf. 4°. *Paris*, 1881.

NOCHT (B.) * Ueber die Erfolge der Nervendehnung. 8°. *Berlin*, 1881.

SCHEVING (F.) * De l'élongation des nerfs. 4°. *Paris*, 1881.

SCHUBERT (O.) * Ueber den Einfluss der Dehnung auf die Erregbarkeit der Nerven. 8°. *Königsberg i. Pr.*, 1883.

SCHUTTER (W.) * Over zenuwrekking. 8°. *Groningen*, 1880.

STINTZING (R.) Ueber Nervendehnung. Eine experimentelle und klinische Studie. 8°. *Leipzig*, 1883.

TIGERSTEDT (R.) Studien über mechanische Nervenreizung. Erste Abtheilung. 4°. *Helsingfors*, 1880.
Repr. from: Acta Soc. scient. fenicæ, xi.

VOGT (P.) Die Nerven-Dehnung als Operation in der chirurgischen Praxis; eine experimentelle und klinische Studie. 8°. *Leipzig*, 1877.

WIET. * Contribution à l'étude de l'élongation des nerfs. 4°. *Paris*, 1881.

ZEDERBAUM (A.) * Nervendehnung und Nervendruck. 8°. *Leipzig*, 1883.

Armstrong (H. G.) Nerve-stretching in case of spinal meningitis with ataxic symptoms due to injury. St. Thomas's Hosp. Rep. 1881, Lond., 1882. n. s., xi, 109-112.—**Artaud** (G.) & **Gilson** (H.) De l'élongation des nerfs. Rev. de chir., Par., 1882, ii, 134; 207.—**Ashhurst** (J.), jr. Nerve-stretching; stretching of the musculocutaneous, median, ulnar, internal cutaneous, lesser internal cutaneous, and musculo-spiral nerves for traumatic neuralgia of the fore-arm and hand. Phila. M. Times, 1881-2, xii, 307-309.—**Atherton** (A. B.) Nerve-stretching for sciatica. Canad. Pract., Toronto, 1885, x, 1 —**Auerbach** (B.) Zur Casuistik der Nervendehnung. Deutsche med. Wchnschr., Berl., 1882, viii, 37.—**Bartleet** (T. H.) Nerve-stretching. Birmingh. M. Rev., 1880, n. s., iii, 130-141.—**Baum.** Mimische Gesichtskrampf; Dehnung des Facialis; Heilung. Berl. klin. Wchnschr., 1878, xv, 595.—**Benedikt** (M.) Ueber Nervendehnung. Wien. med. Presse, 1881, xxii, 941-945. ——. Weitere vorläufige Mittheilungen über Nervendehnung. *Ibid.*, 1216; 1245; 1277; 1309; 1409; 1477.—**Berg** (J.) Om nervsträckning. Hygiea, Stockholm, 1883, xlv. 176-189. — **Bernhardt** (M.) Zur Frage von den Erfolgen der Dehnung des N. facialis bei tic convulsif. Deutsche med. Wchnschr., Berl., 1882, viii, 403. — **Berridge** (W. A.) Nerve-stretching. Brit. M. J., Lond., 1881, i, 510. — **Blum** (A.) De l'élongation des nerfs. Arch. gén. de méd., Par., 1878, 7. s., i, 22; 196. ——. Tremblement hystérique d'origine traumatique du membre inférieur droit; élongation du sciatique; guérison. France méd., Par., 1882, i, 121-126. ——. Deux cas d'élongation du sciatique pour névralgie rebelle. [Rap. de Gillette.] Bull. et mém. Soc. de chir. de Par., 1882, n. s., viii, 162-169.—**Bolis** (V.) Intorno allo stiramento dei nervi a scopo terapeutico; casuistica e considerazioni. Raccoglitore med., Forlì, 1882, 4. s., xvii, 47; 129; 185; 289.—**Bramwell** (J. P.) On nerve-stretching as a remedy

Nerve-stretching.

for sciatica. Brit. M. J., Lond., 1880, i, 920. *Also :* Tr. Perthshire M. Ass. 1879-81, Perth, 1882, i, 1-5.—**Braun** (J. P.) Ueber den mechanischen Effect der centrifugalen Nervendehnung auf das Rückenmark. Prag. med. Wchnschr., 1882, vii, 162; 174; 185.—**Brown-Séquard** (C. É.) On certain physiological effects of stretching of the sciatic nerve. Lancet, Lond., 1881, i, 206. ——. Nouveaux faits relatifs à l'élongation du nerf sciatique. Compt. rend. Soc. de biol. 1881, Par., 1882, 7. s., iii, 54. ——. Recherches sur les effets de l'élongation du nerf sciatique chez des animaux ayant eu une hémisection de la moelle épinière. *Ibid.*, pt. 2, 1-3.—**Callender** (G. W.) Neuralgia treated by stretching the median nerve. Tr. Clin. Soc. Lond., 1874, vii, 100-104. ——. On a case of neuralgia treated by nerve stretching. Lancet, Lond., 1875, i, 883-885.—**Cameron** (H. C.) Sciatica treated by nerve stretching. Glasgow M. J., 1884, [4.] s., xxi, 401.— **Carafi.** Tremblement hystérique d'origine traumatique du membre inférieur droit; élongation du sciatique; guérison. France méd., Par., 1882, i, 121-126. *Also :* Bull. Soc. clin. de Par. (1882), 1883, vi, 24 - 30. — **Carpenter** (J. G.) Nerve stretching of the great sciatic nerve for sciatica; recovery. St. Louis M. & S. J., 1883, xliv, 19-22. — **Cattani** (G.) Studio sperimentale sulla distensione dei nervi. Gazz. d. osp., Milano, 1884, v, 410-412. ——. Studio sperimentale intorno alla distensione dei nervi. Arch. per le sc. med., Torino, 1884-5, viii, 365-416, 1 pl. ——. Sulla dis tensione incruenta dei nervi; ricerche sperimentali. *Ibid.*, 1885-6, ix, 261-281, 1 pl.—**Cavafy** (J.) A case of sciatic nerve-stretching in locomotor ataxy. Brit. M. J., Lond., 1881, ii, 928; 973.—**Chambers** (J. W.) Stretching of the sciatic nerve in locomotor ataxia. Maryland M. J., Balt., 1881-2, viii, 289-291. ——. Subcutaneous nerve-stretching in the treatment of sciatic neuralgia. Tr. M. & Chir. Fac. Maryland, Balt., 1883, 183-186.—**Chandler** (W. J.) Nerve stretching. Tr. M. Soc. N. Jersey, Newark, 1882, 100-156. *Also :* Cincin. M. News, 1882, n. s., xi, 598 ; 664. *Also :* Med. Rec., N. Y., 1882, xxii, 253; 282.—**Chauvel** (J.) Élongation des branches terminales du plexus brachial dans un cas de trépidation épileptoïde d'origine traumatique, par M. le Dr. Poulet. [Rap.] Bull. et mém. Soc. de chir. de Par., 1884, n. s., x, 939-947. ——. De l'élongation des nerfs. Arch. gén. de méd., Par., 1885, i, 711 - 723. — **Chiene** (J.) Nerve-stretching in sciatica. Practitioner, Lond., 1877, xviii, 417 - 420. — **Chvostek** (F.) Dehnung der Nn. ischiadici bei herd weiser Sclerose. Wien. med. Bl., 1881, iv, 1325 ; 1356.— **Ciceri** (B.) Distrazione del nervo mediano per nevralgia della mano e del braccio sinistro. Gazz. med. ital. lomb., Milano, 1887, 8. s., vii, 427.—**Dana** (C. L.) The mechanical effect of nerve-stretching upon the spinal cord. Med. Rec., N. Y., 1882, xxii, 113-115. *Also, transl.:* Ann. Soc. méd.-chir. de Liége, 1882, xxi, 241.—**Davidson.** Cases of nerve-stretching. Lancet, Lond., 1882, i, 142.—**Debove** & **Laborde.** Recherches sur la détermination expérimentale des effets de l'élongation des nerfs, et du mécanisme de ces effets dans l'état pathologique et dans l'état physiologique. Compt. rend. Soc. de biol. 1881, Par., 1882, 7. s., iii, 36-38. *Also :* Tribune méd., Par., 1881, xiv, 66; 88. *Also :* Gaz. méd. de Par., 1881, 6. s., iii, 96.—**Discussion** (Die) über Nervendehnungen in der medizinischen Gesellschaft in Berlin. Wien. med. Bl., 1882, v, 174-176.— **Discussion** on the stretching of the infra-trochlear nerve. Quart. Bull. Clin. Soc. N. Y. Post-Grad. M. School & Hosp., N. Y., 1885-6, i, 200.—**Donkin** (H. B.) Nerve-stretching for sciatica. Med. Times & Gaz., Lond., 1883, ii, 707.—**Dorland** (J.) Nerve-stretching for sciatica. Canada M. & S. J., Montréal, 1881-2, x, 541-543.—**Doutrelepont.** Ueber Nervendehnung. Sitzungsb. d. nied.-rhein Gesellsch. f. Nat.- u. Heilk. zu Bonn, 1881, 233-238.— **Duchnovski.** Operatsii rastjajenija siedalishnich nervov. [Stretching the sciatic nerve; two cases.] Vrach. Vaidom., St. Petersb., 1883, viii, 4099.—**Duplay.** Paralysie du nerf radial, consécutive à une plaie de l'avant-bras; troubles dans la zone d'innervation du médian; élongation du nerf radial et du médian; suivi d'une observation personnelle de compression du nerf cubital par un fibrome cicatriciel, guéri par l'ablation du nodus cicatriciel et l'élongation du nerf. Bull. et mém. Soc. de chir. de Par., 1878, n. s., iv, 773 - 778. — **Eder** (A.) Nervendehnung. *In his :* Aerztl. Ber. 1882, 8°, Wien, 1883, 85.—**Elias** (G.) Ueber eine doppelseitige Dehnung des Nervus ischiadicus bei vorgeschrittener Tabes. Breslau. aerztl. Ztschr., 1881, iii, 254 - 256. — **Élongation** (De l') des nerfs dans les névralgies et dans les douleurs fulgurantes de l'ataxie locomotrice. [Edit.] Tribune méd., Par., 1881, xiv, 3; 16.—**Eulenburg** (A.) Zum Verhalten des Kniephänomens bei Cruralis - Dehnung. Neurol. Centralbl., Leipz., 1882, i, 33. — **Farrar** (S. F.) On Professor Nussbaum's operation of nerve-stretching. Chicago M. J. & Exam., 1878, xxxvi, 225-239.—**Fede** (F.) Sulla distensione de' nervi. Resoc. Accad. med.-chir. di Napoli (1883), 1884, xxxvii, 317. — **Fenger** (C.) & **Lee** (E. W.) Nerve-stretching; illustrated by cases from the hospital service and private practice. J. Nerv. & Ment. Dis., N. Y., 1881, n. s., vi, 263-304. — **Fenwick** (G. E.) Two cases of sciatica; nerve-stretching; cured. Canada

Nerve-stretching.

M. & S. J., Montreal, 1866–7, xv, 149–151. — **Fifield** (W. C. B.) Sciatica cured by stretching the sciatic nerve. Med. News, Phila., 1883, xlii, 10.—**Finlay** (W. A.) Case of nerve-stretching for sciatica. Edinb. M. J., 1879–80, xxv, 210. — **Fiorani** (G.) Sullo stiramento dei nervi. Gazz. med. ital. lomb., Milano, 1882, 8. s., iv, 323–333.— **Gena** (A.) O vitjajenii nervov. [Nerve-stretching.] Voyenno-med. J., St. Petersb., 1879, cxxxvi, pt. 2, 7–84.—**Giberson** (C. H.) Nerve-stretching for sciatica. Tr. M. Soc. N. Y., Syracuse, 1878, 189. — **Gillet de Grandmont.** Deux observations d'élongation du nerf optique. J. de méd. de Par., 1883, v, 343–346. *Also:* Bull. Soc. de méd. prat. de Par. (1883), 1884, 91–95. ———. Élongation du nerf occipital interne comme traitement de névralgies rebelles. J. de méd. de Par., 1883, v, 270. *Also:* Bull. Soc. de méd. prat. de Par. (1883), 1884, 97–99.—**Godlee** (R. J.) Stretching of facial nerve for spasmodic tic. Lancet, Lond., 1881, i, 914. ———. Cases of stretching of the facial nerve Tr. Clin. Soc. Lond., 1882–3, xvi, 220–231.—**Golding-Bird.** A case of stretching and subsequent section of the great sciatic nerve. Brit. M. J., Lond., 1880, i, 969.—**Gray** (L. C.) Nerve-stretching. Am. J. Neurol. & Psychiat., N. Y., 1882, i, 198–220. ———. Two cases of stretching of facial nerve. *Ibid.*, 514–516. *Also:* Proc. M. Soc. County Kings, Brooklyn, 1882–3, vii, 127–131.—**Gussenbauer** (C.) Ueber Nervendehnung. Prag. med. Wchnschr., 1882, vii, 1; 13; 24. *Also,* Reprint.—**Hammond** (G. M.) Nerve-stretching as a radical cure for pain. Med. Rec., N. Y., 1881, xx, 180.—**Hammond** (W. A.) A clinical lecture on the treatment of locomotor ataxia; operation for elongation of the sciatic nerve performed. St. Louis Clin. Rec., 1881–2, viii, 193–195.—**Hansen** (T.) Tvende Tilfælde af Nervestrækning af Nervus accessorius. Hosp.-Tid., Kjøbenh., 1878, 2. R., v, 705–712.—**Hegar** (A.) Die Rückenmarksdehnung; ein Beitrag zur mechanischen Behandlung der Nervenkrankheiten. Samml. klin. Vortr., Leipz., 1884, No. 239 (Gynäk., No. 65, 1699–1714). *Also, transl.:* Encéphale, Par., 1884, iv, 590–613.—**Helmuth** (W. T.) Nerve-stretching. N. Engl. M. Gaz., Bost., 1879, n. s., i, 49; 73; 97. *Also,* Reprint. ———. Nerve-stretching; reflex epilepsy, spasms, and neuralgia cured by stretching the ulnar nerve at the condyle of the humerus. Am. J. Electrol. & Neurol., N. Y., 1879, i, 13–21. ———. Stretching of the sciatic nerve for sciatica and reflex tetaniform convulsions. Month. Homœop. Rev., Lond., 1879, xxiii, 459–464. — **Higgens** (C.) Two cases of nerve-stretching. Brit. M. J., Lond., 1879, i, 893.—**Hildebrandt.** Beitrag zur Nervendehnung. Deutsche med. Wchnschr., Berl., 1880, vi, 487. ———. Beiträge zur Nervendehnung. Deutsche Ztschr. f. Chir., Leipz., 1883, xix, 329–332.—**Homberg** (A.) Nervsträckningars användning vid sjukdomar uti det inre nervsystemet. [Nerve-stretching in diseases of internal nervous system.] Eira, Göteborg, 1882, vi, 2–18.— **Isenschmid.** Tabes; subcutane Dehnung des Ischiadicus; neue Methode der Nervendehnung. Aerztl. Int.-Bl., München, 1882, xxix, 401. — **Johnson** & **Wright.** Nerve-stretching. J. Am. M. Ass., Chicago, 1883, i, 504. ———. Sciatica of long standing cured by nerve-stretching. Med. & Surg. Reporter, Phila., 1883, xlviii, 256–258.— **Katsauroff** (I. N.) Tri sluchaja vitjajenija podblokovago nerva. [Three cases of stretching of pathetic nerve.] Vrach, St. Petersb., 1883, iv, 689–707.—**Kaufmann** (C.) Zur Dehnung des Nervus facialis. Centralbl. f. Chir., Leipz., 1885, xii, 33–36. — **Keegan.** A case of sciatica treated by nerve-stretching. Indian M. Gaz., Calcutta, 1882, xvii, 181.—**Keen** (W. W.) Stretching of the facial nerve. N. York M. J., 1886, xliii, 563. ———. Stretching of the facial nerve; report of a new case, with remarks, and a summary of previously reported cases. Tr. Am. Surg. Ass., Phila., 1886, iv, 275–296. *Also,* Reprint. *Also:* Ann. Surg., St. Louis, 1886, iv, 1–19. — **Kinnaird** (J. B.) Nerve-stretching as a therapeutic measure, with special reference to statistics. Louisville M. News, 1883, xv, 113–116.—**van Kleef** (L. T.) Ein Fall von Dehnung der Interkostalnerven. Wien. med. Wchnschr., 1880, xxx, 1098; 1120; 1146.—**Kümmell** (H.) Ueber Dehnung des Nervus opticus. Deutsche med. Wchnschr., Berl., 1882, viii, 4–7.—**Lagrange.** Valeur thérapeutique de l'élongation des nerfs [Abstr.] Gaz. hebd. d. sc. méd. de Montpel., 1886, viii. 579–582.—**de La Harpe** (E.) Un cas de sciatique rebelle; élongation; guérison. Rev. méd. de la Suisse Rom., Genève, 1884, iv, 140–142.— **Landesberg** (M.) Stretching the optic nerve. Phila. M. Times, 1882–3, xiii, 818–822. *Also:* Proc. Phila. Co. M. Soc. 1882–3, Phila., 1883, v, 154–157. *Also, transl.:* Arch. f. Ophth., Berl., 1883, xxix, 4. Abth., 101–118.—**Lawrie** (E.) Nerve stretching in anæsthetic leprosy. Indian M. Gaz., Calcutta, 1878, xiii, 229; 270. — **Lépine** (R.) Sur les effets de l'élongation très modérée du nerf sciatique (par la méthode sous-cutanée) chez les ataxiques. Compt. rend. Soc. de biol., Par., 1883, 7. s., iv, 194–197.—**von Lesser** (L.) Ein Fall von Dehnung der Intercostal-Nerven. Deutsche med. Wchnschr., Berl., 1884, x, 306–308.—**Leyden** (E.) Ueber Nervendehnungen. Wien. med. Bl., 1882, v, 801; 842; 874.—**Loreta** (P.) Intorno allo stiramento dei nervi. Mem. Accad. d. sc. d. Ist. di Bologna, 1880, 4. s., ii, 235–237. *Also:* Raccoglitore med., Forlì, 1881, 4. s., xv, 233–

Nerve-stretching.

237.—**Lumniczer.** Ueber Nervendehnung. Pest. med.-chir. Presse, Budapest, 1880, xvi, 130.—**M'Craith** (J.) Nerve-stretching for cure of lumbago and sciatica without any cutting operation. Med. Times & Gaz., Lond., 1880, ii, 266.—**M'Culloch** (H. D.) Case of nerve-stretching. Lancet, Lond., 1885, ii, 433.—**Macfarlane** (A. W.) Case of sciatica, treated by nerve-stretching. *Ibid.*, 1878, ii. 6.— **Macleod.** Case of nerve stretching in sciatica. Glasgow M. J., 1882, xviii, 376–378.—**McLeod** (K.) Nerve-stretching. Indian M. Gaz., Calcutta, 1880, xv, 129.— **McReddie** (G. D.) Case of sciatica; nerve-stretching. Proc. Allahabad M. Soc., 1882, i, 4.—**Marcus.** Contribution à l'étude de l'élongation des nerfs. Compt. rend. Soc. de biol. 1881, Par., 1882, 7. s., iii, 110.—**Marshall** (J.) Bradshawe lecture on nerve-stretching for the relief or cure of pain. Lancet, Lond., 1883, ii, 1029–1036. *Also:* Brit. M. J., Lond., 1883, ii, 1173–1179.—**Masing** (E.) Zur Casuistik der Nervendehnung. St. Petersb. med. Wchnschr., 1878, iii, 281–285. *Also, transl.* [Abstr.]: Lond. M. Rec., 1879, vii, 5.—**Masse** (E.) De l'élongation des nerfs. *In his:* Mém. de méd. et chir., 8°, Par., 1885, 17–24.—**Medini** (L.) Ulteriore contributo allo stiramento dei nervi e raccolta di casi spettanti a chirurgi italiani. Bull. d. sc. med. di Bologna, 1883, 6. s., xi, 145–177.—**Melchior** (R.) Ein Beitrag zur subcutanen Nervendehnung. Prakt. Arzt, Wetzlar, 1882, xxiii, 169.—**Mikulicz** (J.) Ueber Nervendehnung. Mitth. d. Wien. med. Doct.-Coll., 1882, viii, 117–122.—**Miles** (F. T.) A case of accidental intravertebral nerve stretching. N. Orl. M. & S. J., 1886–7, n. s., xiv, 354–359.—**Minor** (L.) Contribution à l'étude expérimentale de l'élongation des nerfs. Compt. rend. Acad. d. sc., Par., 1883, xcvi, 1159–1162.—**Moeli.** Die Discussion über Nervendehnung in der Berliner medicinischen Gesellschaft. Neurol. Centralbl., Leipz., 1882, i, 76–83.— **Morini** (V.) Sullo stiramento dei nervi a scopo terapeutico. Tesi di laurea. Gazz. med. di Roma, 1885, xi, 265; 337; 409; 433. —**Morton** (T. G.) Two cases of nerve stretching. Am. J. M. Sc., Phila., 1878, n. s., lxxv, 150–152.—**Morton** (W. J.) A contribution to the subject of nerve-stretching; in 1. Lateral sclerosis; 2. Paralysis agitans; 3. Athetosis; 4. Chronic transverse myelitis; 5. Sciatica; 6. Reflex epilepsy. J. Nerv. & Ment. Dis., N. Y., 1882, n. s., vii, 133–163. *Also,* Reprint. *Also:* Med. Rec., N. Y., 1882, xxi, 240–243.—**Müller** (F.) & **Ebner** (L.) Ueber Nervendehnung bei peripheren und centralen Leiden, insbesondere bei Tabes dorsalis. Wien. Klinik, 1881, vii, 151–184.—**Naismith** (W. J.) Nerve-stretching. Lancet, Lond., 1881, i, 782.—**Negretto** (A.) Due casi di ischialgia guariti mercè lo stiramento incruento dello sciatico. Gazz. med. ital., prov. venete, Padova, 1884, xxvii, 257–259.—**Nicoladoni** (C.) Dehnung des N. ulnaris. Wien. med. Presse, 1882, xxiii, 885–888.—**von Nussbaum.** Blosslegung und Dehnung der Rückenmarksnerven; eine erfolgreiche Operation. Deutsche Ztschr. f. Chir., Leipz., 1872, i, 450–465. *Also, transl.:* Lancet, Lond., 1872, ii, 783. ———. Nervendehnung bei centralem Leiden. Aerztl. Int.-Bl., München, 1876, xxiii, 75–77. *Also, in his:* Klinische Mittheilungen, 8°, München, 1876, 21–29. ———. Nervendehnungen. Ann. d. städt. allg. Krankenh. zu München, 1878, i, 451–453. *Also, in his:* Sonst und Jetzt, etc., drei Abhandl., 8°, München, 1878, 21–23. ———. Neuere Erfahrung über subcutane Nervendehnung, auch bei Hautkrankheiten. Aerztl. Int.-Bl., München, 1883, xxx, 381.— **Omboni** (V.) Contribuzione allo stiramento e sbrigliamento dei nervi quale nuovo mezzo terapeutico. Ann. univ. di med. e chir., Milano, 1883, ccli, 43–51. ———. Nuova contribuzione allo stiramento dei nervi nella terapeutica. *Ibid.*, 1883, cclxiii, 62–74. ———. Uno sguardo allo stiramento dei nervi, sì nella parte sperimentale come nella clinica. *Ibid.*, 177–249.— **Ott** (I.) Nerve-stretching; its physiological action. Ohio M. & S. J., Columbus, 1878. iii, 8–12.—**Park** (R.) Chronic sciatica; elongation; recovery. Chicago M. J. & Exam., 1884, xlviii, 636. ———. Paræsthesia and dysæsthesia of unknown origin; elongation of sciatic, and later of crural nerves; no result. *Ibid.*, 637. ———. Elongation of nerves. J. Am. M. Ass., Chicago, 1884, ii. 324. — **Pasini** (D.) Ischialgia destra cronica e ribelle; stiramento cruento del nervo sciatico dietro alla metà della coscia; guarigione. Raccoglitore med., Forlì, 1882, 4. s., xviii, 374–379. — **Patruban.** Blosslegung und Dehnung des grossen Hüftnerven behufs der Heilung der Ischialgie. Allg. Wien. med. Ztg., 1872, xvii, 509; 525; 541 573; 672. *Also, transl.:* Clinic, Cincin., 1872, iii, 234; 244; 259; 297; 1873, iv, 54.—**Petersen** (F.) Zur Nervendehnung. Centralbl. f. Chir., Leipz., 1876, iii, 769–771.—**Pitts** (B.) Two cases of nerve stretching for neuralgia of the inferior dental nerve. St. Thomas's Hosp. Rep. 1885, Lond., 1886, xv. 207–211.—**Pooley** (J. H.) Nerve-stretching. Med. Rec., N. Y., 1880, xviii, 172–175.— **Prevost** (J.-L.) Expériences relatives à l'élongation des nerfs et aux névrites. Rev. méd. de la Suisse Rom., Genève, 1881, i, 469–489.—**Quinquaud.** Recherches sur l'élongation des nerfs. Compt. rend. Soc. de biol. 1881, Par., 1882, 7. s., iii, 119. ———. Élongation des nerfs aux troubles trophiques. *Ibid.*, 120. *Also:* Gaz. méd. de Par., 1881, 6. s., iii, 208.—**Ramaugé.** Estiramiente de nérvios. Rev. méd.-quir., Buenos Aires, 1882–3, xix, 127–

Nerve-stretching.

134.—**Ranke** (H.) "Dehnung" des Nervus cutaneus medius und minor brachii dext. Samml. klin. Vortr., Leipz., 1878, 1078.—**Redard** (P.) Recherches expérimentales sur la température locale des membres après l'élongation des nerfs périphériques. Compt. rend. Soc. de biol., Par., 1883, 7. s., iv, 62-64.—**Remy.** Dreifache blutige Nervendehnung, eine selbsterlittene Operation. Allg. med. Centr.-Ztg., Berl., 1885, liv, 273.—**Riedel.** Zur Nervendehnung nach Wirbelläsion. Deutsche med. Wchnschr., Berl., 1882, viii, 3.—**Robins** (R. P.) Notes of three cases of nerve-stretching for sciatica. Med. News, Phila., 1883, xliii, 339.—**Rogovich.** Vlijanie vitjajenija nerva na ego provodimost i vozbudimost. [On the effect of nerve-stretching.] Univ. Izviestija, Kieff, 1884, xxiv, pt. 4, 1-42.—**Saylor** (W. H.) Nérve stretching for sciatica. Proc. Oregon M. Soc., Portland, 1882, ix, 62.—**Scarenzio** (A.) Stiramento cruento del nervo grande ischiatico per nevralgia datante da più di quattro anni; esito felice. Ann. univ. di med. e chir., Milano, 1885, cclxxi. 134-141.—**Schleich** (G.) Versuche über die Reizbarkeit der Nerven im Dehnungszustand. Ztschr. f. Biol., München, 1871, vii, 379-394.—**Schmid** (H.) Zur Nervendehnung. Centralbl. f. Chir., Leipz., 1883, x, 489.—**Schooler** (L.) Nerve stretching; with a case. Iowa State M. Reporter, Des Moines, 1887-8, n. s., iv, 418-420.—**Schüssler** (H.) Mimischer Gesichtskrampf; Dehnung des Facialis; Heilung. Berl. klin. Wchnschr., 1879, xvi, 684. ———. Neuralgie des Occipitalis major; Nervendehnung; Heilung. Ibid., 1880, xvii, 554.—**Serebrennikoff** (E.) K vopr. o vitjajenii zritel. nerva. [Stretching of the optic nerve.] Vrach, St. Petersb., 1886, vii, 545.—**Shepherd** (F. J.) Case of sciatica; nerve-stretching; cured. Canada M. & S. J., Montreal, 1886-7, xv, 148.—**Solecki.** Nerwoból twarzy w obwodzie iii gałęzi n. troistego; wycięcie całej trzeciej gałęzi n. troistego túz przy dworze jajowatym sposobem Krönleina. [Stretching of third branch of n. trigeminus; cutting of entire third branch of n. trigeminus close to oval aperture by Krönlein's method.] Przegl. lek., Krakow, 1887, xxvi, 115.—**Sonnenburg.** Dehnung des Nervus ischiadicus und des N. peroneus. Berl. klin. Wchnschr., 1884, xxi, 75. Also: Verhandl. d. Berl. med. Gesellsch. (1883-4), 1885, xv, 76-78.—**Southam** (F. A.) On nerve-stretching; with particulars of three cases. Lancet, Lond., 1881, ii, 629. ———. Cases of nerve-stretching. Ibid., 627. ———. Notes on a case of nerve-stretching for facial spasm, operated on five years since. Ibid., 1886, i, 685.—**Spence.** Stretching of sciatic, digital, and infra-orbital nerves. Ibid., 1880, i, 249.—**Stewart** (J.) An account of three cases of sciatica and one of painful stump treated by nerve-stretching. Canada M. & S. J., Montreal, 1882-3, xi, 193-195.—**Stilmant** (L.) De l'élongation des nerfs; physiologie thérapeutique; recherches nouvelles. Presse méd. belge, Brux., 1882, xxxiv, 265; 289; 313; 337; 361.—**Stintzing** (R.) Ueber Nervendehnung; eine experimentelle und klinische Studie. Arb. a. d. med.-klin. Inst. d. k. Ludwig-Maximilians-Univ. zu München, Leipz., 1884, i, 345-516.—**Storchi** (F.) Distensione cruenta del nervo ischiatico per cronica nevralgia da nevrite ascendente; processo Loreta; miglioramento. Spallanzani, Roma, 1886, 2. s., xv, 455.—**Stroug** (A. B.) Flexion of the thigh, with the leg in the straight position, for sciatica. Peoria M. Month., 1885-6, vi, 427-429.—**Struckmann.** Tre Tilfælde af Nerve-Strækning. Hosp.-Tid., Kjøbenh., 1878, 2. R., v, 689-692.—**Sturge** (A.) & **Godlee.** Stretching the facial nerve for the relief of the facial muscles. Brit. M. J., Lond., 1880, ii, 810.—**Svensson** (I.) Nervsträckning. Nord. med. Ark., Stockholm, 1883, xv, no. 14, 7-16.—**Symington** (J.) The physics of nerve-stretching. Brit. M. J., Lond., 1882, i, 770.—**Tarnowski** (P. N.) Ob izmenenijach spinnago mozga pri vitjajenii siedalishnago nerva. [Changes in spinal cord from stretching the gluteal nerve.] Vestnik klin. i sudebnoi psichiat. i nevropatol., St. Petersb., 1884, ii, no. 1, 98-154, 2 pl. Also, transl.: Arch. de neurol., Par., 1885, ix, 289: x, 35, 1 pl.—**Trombetta** (F.) Nerve-stretching. Lancet, Lond., 1882, i, 250.—**Ullersperger** (J. B.) Studie über den vom Prof. v. Nussbaum im Aerztl. Intelligenzblatt 1872 No. 9 mitgetheilten Fall: "Bloslegung und Dehnung der vier unteren Halsnerven am Rückenmarke". Bl. f. Heilwissensch., München, 1872, iii, 169; 177.—**Underwood** (A. S.) On nerve stretching in neuralgia. Tr. Odont. Soc. Gr. Brit., Lond., 1880, n. s., xii, 217-233. [Discussion], 234-238.—**Ustimovich** (K. N.) Kriticheskii obzore izsliedovanii o sosudoraschirjaioutchich nervache. [On stretching of nerves and blood-vessels.] Voyenno-med. J., St. Petersb., 1878, cxxxi, 1-28.—**Veljaminoff** (N. A.) Dva sluchaja rastjajenija nervov i odin sluchai resektsii nerva. [Two cases of nerve-stretching and a case of nerve-resection.] Med. Vestnik, St. Petersb., 1882, xxi, 687.—**Wales** (P. S.) Nerve-stretching. Med. Rec., N. Y., 1882, xxii, 26.—**Wallace.** Nerve stretching, with special reference to its use in anæsthetic leprosy. Indian M. Gaz., Calcutta, 1882, xvii, 220. Also: Tr. Calcutta M. Soc., 1882, iii, 105-112.—**Walsham** (W. J.) Sequel to a case of epileptiform neuralgia treated by nerve-stretching. Brit. M. J., Lond., 1883, ii, 1234.—**Warnots** (L.) De l'élongation des nerfs. J. de méd., chir. et pharmacol., Brux., 1882, lxxiv, 438:

Nerve-stretching.

lxxv, 34; 105; 222.—**Webber** (S. G.) Nerve stretching. Cycl. Pract. M. (Ziemssen), N. Y., 1881, suppl., 518-521.—**de Wecker** (L.) De la distension de los nervios aplicada á la cirujía ocular. Siglo méd., Madrid, 1881, xxviii, 147-149. Also, transl.: Klin. Monatsbl. f. Augenh., Stuttg., 1881, xix, 235-243.—**von Weltrubsky** (G.) Erfahrungen über Nervendehnung. Prag. med. Wchnschr., 1882, vii, 101; 114; 122; 144; 166; 207; 219; 227; 234; 244.—**Westphal** (C.) Unterschenkelphänomen und Nervendehnung. Arch. f. Psychiat., Berl., 1877, vii, 666-670.—**Wilheim.** Kritische Betrachtungen zur sogenannten unblutigen Nervendehnung. Wien. med. Presse, 1882, xxiii, 208-210.—**Winslow** (R.) Nérve stretching in sciatica, with a successful case. Maryland M. J., Balt., 1882-3, ix, 313-316.—**Witkowski** (L.) Zur Nervendehnung. Arch. f. Psychiat., Berl., 1880, xi, 532-537, 1 pl.—**Wyeth** (J. A.) Three cases of nerve stretching for the relief of persistent fulgurating pains in the lower extremities. Am. J. Neurol. & Psychiat., N. Y., 1882, i, 465-467.—**Zederbaum** (A.) Nervendehnung und Nervendruck. Arch. f. Physiol., Leipz., 1883, 161-189. Also, in: Arb. a. d. spec. physiol. Abth. d. physiol. Inst. d. Univ. Berl., 1883, [No 9].—**Zesas** (D. G.) Ueber die Erfolge der Dehnung des Nervus facialis bei Facialiskrampf. Wien. med. Wchnschr., 1885, xxxv, 853; 883.

Nerve-vibration.

GRANVILLE (J. M.) Nerve-vibration and excitation as agents in the treatment of functional disorder and organic disease. 8°. London, 1883.
    Granville (J. M.) Nerve-vibration as a therapeutic agent. Lancet, Lond., 1882, i, 949-951.—**Pattee** (A. F.) Résumé of Dr. J. M. Granville's book on nerve vibration and excitation, with notes of clinical experience with the percuteur. J. Am. M. Ass., Chicago, 1885, v, 113-121.

Nerves.

See, also, **Ear** (Nerves of); **Frog**; **Grafting**; **Myelin**; **Nervous** system (Electro-physiology of); **Nervous** system (Histology of); **Neurology**; and under names of organs and regions.

BLANCK (H. P.) * De resolutione nervorum. 8°. Berolini, [1841].
    BUDGE (J.) Ueber die verschiedene Reizbarkeit eines und desselben Nerven an verschiedenen Stellen desselben. 8°. [n. p., n. d.]
    FICK (A.) * Ueber quere Nervendurchströmung. 8°. Würzburg, 1876.
    GRILLO (F.) Breve saggio sui nervi in genere con l'applicazione al tetano. 8°. Avellino, 1887.
    HOME (E.) On the irritability of nerves. 4°. London, 1801.
    KÜHNE (W.) Note sur l'irritation chimique des nerfs et des muscles. 4°. [Paris, 1859.]
    Repr. from: Compt. rend. Acad. d. sc., Par., 1859, xlviii.
    VON LANGER (C.) * Diss. sistens structuram nervorum. 8°. Viennæ, [1842].
    LENT (E. O. B.) * De nervorum dissectorum commutationibus ac regeneratione. 4°. Berolini, 1855.
    LE THIEULLIER (J.) * An nervi canales? 4°. Parisiis, 1743.
    LÜDERITZ (C.) * Versuche über die Einwirkung des Druckes auf die motorischen und sensiblen Nerven. Habilitationsschrift. 8°. Berlin, 1880.
    MOLESCHOTT (J.) Sugli attributi generali dei nervi. Introduzione al corso di fisiologia sperimentale letta il 16 gennaio 1881. 8°. Torino, 1881.
    NEUMANN (G. C.) * Diss. inaug. sistens rationem inter nervorum vires et imponderabilium indolem. 8°. Berolini, [1828].
    PANIZZA (B.) Ricerche sperimentali sopra i nervi. Lettera al Maurizio Bufalini. 8°. Pavia, 1834.
    PFEFFINGER (J.) * De structura nervorum, cujus sectionem primam defendet. 4°. Argentorati, [1782].
    ———. * De structura nervorum, cujus alteram sectionem submittit. 4°. Argentorati, [1783].
    POHLIUS (J. C.) [Pr.] quasdam de nervis animadversiones proponit. 4°. Lipsiæ, [1774].
    WAGNER (R.) Neue Untersuchungen über den Bau und die Endigung der Nerven und die Struk-

Nerves.

tur der Ganglien. Supplement zu den Icones physiologicæ. fol. *Leipzig*, 1847.

WALTER (J. G.) Tabulæ nervorum thoracis et abdominis. fol. *Berolini*, 1783.

————. The same. Plates on the thoracic and abdominal nerves, reduced from the original, as published by order of the Royal Academy of Sciences at Berlin; accompanied by coloured explanations, and a description of the par vagum, great sympathetic and phrenic nerves. 4°. *London*, 1-19.

WEBER (E. H.) [Pr.] epistola Scarpæ de gangliis nervorum deque origine et essentia nervi intercostalis. 4°. [*Lipsiæ*], 1831.

RAUBER (A.) Ueber die Nerven der Knochenhaut und Knochen des Vorderarmes und Unterschenkels. 8°. *München*, 1868.

TARCHANOFF (I.) * O vlijanii teploti na chuvstvuioushie nervi . . . ljagusheke. [Influence of heat upon sensitive and motor nerves in frog.] 8°. *St. Petersburg*, 1871.

TILANUS (C. B.) * De nervis eorumque actione. 8°. *Traj. ad Rhenum*, 1818.

Arnstein (C.) Die Nerven der behaarten Haut. Sitzungsb. d. k. Akad. d. Wissensch. Math.-naturw. Cl. 1876, Wien, 1877, lxxiv, 3. Abth., 203-232, 3 pl. *Also,* Reprint.—**Bakowiecki.** Zur Frage vom Verwachsen der peripherischen Nerven. Arch. f. mikr. Anat., Bonn, 1876, xiii, 420-426, 1 pl.—**Beale** (L. S.) Observations générales sur la distribution périphérique des nerfs. J. de la physiol. de l'homme, Par., 1862, v, 288-292.—**Bidloo** (G.) De nervis. *In his:* Exercit. anat.-chir., 4°, Lugd. Bat., 1708, 1-9.—**Blix** (M.) Experimentela bidrag till lösning af frågan om hudnervernas specifika energi. [The specific energy of cutaneous nerves,] Upsala Läkaref. Förh., 1882-3, xviii, 427-440.—**Bogros** (J.-A.) Mémoire sur la structure des nerfs. Répert. gén. d'anat. et physiol. path., Par., 1827, iv, 63-73, 3 pl.—**Budge** (A.) Einige Untersuchungen über das Verhalten der Nerven in den Pacinischen Körperchen, den quergestreiften Muskeln und den sympathischen Ganglien. Centralbl. f. d. med. Wissensch., Berl., 1873, xi, 594-597.—**Busch** (W.) Ueber die Innervation einiger am Beckenausgang gelegenen Organe. Arch. f. klin. Chir., Berl., 1863, iv, 44-47.—**Cabadé** (E.) Étude critique sur les propriétés des cordons nerveux. Tribune méd., Par., 1875, viii, 213; 281; 304; 318.—**Filehne** (W.) Ueber die Erregbarkeit degenerirender Nerven. Verhandl. d. Berl. med. Gesellsch. (1869-71), 1872, pt. i, 54-56.—**Fürbringer** (M.) Zur Lehre von den Umbildungen der Nervenplexus. Morphol. Jahrb., Leipz., 1879, v, 324-394, 2 pl.—**Hache** (M.) Sur la génération des nerfs et la suture nerveuse. Médecin clin., Par., 1886, ii, 313; 337.—**Hällstén** (K.) Studier i väfnadselelementens fysiologi. (C. r. Contributions à la connaissance de l'excitation mécanique des nerfs.) Nord. med. Ark., Stockholm, 1881, xiii, no. 6, 1-16. *Also, transl.:* Arch. f. Physiol., Leipz., 1881, 90-104, 1 pl.—**Halbertsma** (H. J.) Ueber einen in der Membrana interossea des Unterschenkels verlaufenden Nerven. Arch. f. Anat., Physiol. u. wissensch. Med., Berl, 1847, 303-312, 1 pl. *Also,* Reprint.—**Harless** (E.) Wirkungen des Ammoniak auf die Nervenstämme. Ztschr. f. rat. Med., Leipz. u. Heidelb., 1861, 3. R., xii, 68-125, 1 pl.—**Lewes** (G. H.) Action of poisons on the nerves. Lancet, Lond., 1859, ii, 471. ————. The sensory and motor functions of nerves. Nat. Hist. Rev., Lond., 1861, i, 176-185.—**Ludwig** (C.) Ueber die Kräfte des Nervenprinitivrohrs. Wien. med. Wchnschr., 1861, 729; 745.—**Meyer** (C.) Ueber die Nervenverbreitung in den hinteren Extremitäten. Ztschr. f. rat. Med., Leipz. u. Heidelb., 1869, 3. R., xxxvi, 164-184, 1 pl.—**Monfalcon.** Nerf. Dict. d. sc. méd., Par., 1819, xxxv, 466-493.—**Nacquart.** Structure et origine des nerfs. J. gén. de méd., chir. et pharm, Par., 1827, c, 153-155.—**Negro** (C.) De l'action que l'acide chlorhydrique dilué exerce sur la sensibilité et la motilité des nerfs. [*Transl. from:* Atti d. r. Accad. d. sc. di Torino, 1884, Nov. 30.] Arch. ital. de biol., Turin, 1884-5, vi, 357-365.—**Parkes** (C. T.) [Experiments upon the tensile strength of nerve trunks.] Tr. Illinois M. Soc., Chicago, 1881, xxxi, 115-119.—**Petrone** (L.-M.) Sur la structure des nerfs cérébro-rachidiens. Internat. Monatschr. f. Anat. u. Physiol., Leipz., 1888, v, 39-47, 2 pl.—**Rosenthal** (J.) Die spezifischen Energien der Nerven. Biol. Centralbl., Erlang., 1884-5, iv, 116; 154.—**Schmidt** (H. D.) On the influence of the structure of the nerve-fibres upon the production and conduction of nerve-force. Proc. Am. Ass. Adv. Sc. 1881, Salem, 1882, xxx, 223-240.—**Smith** (R. M.) Note on the effects of pressure on the irritability of nerve-trunks. Phila. M. Times, 1877-8, viii, 457-462.—**Sokoloff** (A. A.) O dvigatlenikh chuvstvuyushchikh, i trophicheskikh nervakh mishts. [Nerves of sensation and nutrition.] Med.

Nerves.

Vestnik, St. Petersb., 1876, xvi, 167-170.—**Tschirjew** (S.) Ueber die Fortpflanzungsgeschwindigkeit der elektrotonischen Vorgänge im Nerven. Arch. f. Physiol., Leipz., 1879, 525-552, 1 pl.—**Vanlair** (C.) De la dérivation des nerfs. Arch. de physiol. norm. et path, Par., 1885, 3. s., vi, 160-167.—**Vierordt** (H.) Ueber künstliche Bewegungserscheinungen in der Nervenfaser. Arch. f. Heilk., Leipz., 1877, xviii, 179-184.—**Vignal.** Note sur le développement des nerfs chez les embryons des mammifères. Compt. rend. Soc. de biol., Par., 1883, 7. s., v, 139-145. *Also* [Abstr.]: Progrès méd., Par., 1883, xi. 190.—**Villars.** Sur l'organisation des nerfs. [Extrait du rap. de Dupuytren.] Bull. Fac. de méd. de Par. (1804-8), 1812, i, 104-107.—**Wilson** (A.) The origin of nerves. [*From:* Gentleman's Mag.] Pop. Sc. Month. Suppl., N. Y., 1879, n. issue, no. 1, 149-159.—**Wolf.** Ueber die Liquidität der Nerven. Med.-chir. Ztg., Salzb., 1813, iv, 253-256.—**Zinn.** De l'enveloppe des nerfs. Trad. du latin. Mém. Acad. roy. de Prusse, Avignon et Par., 1768, iii, 389-418. *Also:* Collect. acad. d. mém, etc., Par., 1770, viii, 438-448. *Also, transl.:* Phys. u. med. Abhandl. d. k. Acad. d. Wissensch. zu Berl., Gotha, 1786, iv, 316-329.

Nerves (*Abnormities of*).

See, also, **Nerve** (*Median*); **Nerve** (*Optic, Abnormities of*); **Nerve** (*Phrenic*).

BLAWROCK (F. J. J.) * De nervorum sensuum defectu. 8°. *Berolini*, 1828.

KRAUSE (W.) & TELGMANN (J.) Die Nerven-Varietäten beim Menschen. 8°. *Leipzig*, 1868.

OPPERT (C.) * De vitiis nervorum organicis. 4°. *Berolini*, [1815].

Antonelli (G.) Di una rara anomalia nella composizione del plesso brachiale e di alcuni ganglii soprannumerarii nel corso dei sette ultimi nervi intercostali. Resoc. Accad. med.-chir. di Napoli, 1879, xxxiii, 195-201, 1 pl.—**Bianchi** (S.) Varietà del nervo e del canale sottorbitale. Boll. d. Soc. tra i cult. d. sc. med. in Siena, 1884, ii, 228-232.—**Blain des Cormiers.** Anomalie du nerf médian. Bull. Soc. anat. de Par., 1848, xxiii, 129.—**Breglia** (A.) Di una rara anomalia del plesso brachiale. Riv. internaz. di med. e chir., Napoli, 1886, iv. 337-344.—**Calori** (L.) Cinque anomalie dei nervi dell' avambraccio e della mano osservate e descritte dal Prof.... Bull. d. sc. med. di Bologna, 1871, 5. s., xii, 39-48, 1 pl. ————. Sulle anomalie del canale e del nervo sottorbitale e sul punto in cui può tagliarsi questo nervo con maggiore speranza di buon successo nella prosopalgia. Riv. clin. di Bologna, 1874, 2. s., iv, 289-298, 1 pl.—**Chaput.** Note sur deux variétés d'anastomoses nerveuses de l'avant-bras. Bull. Soc. anat. de Par., 1886, lxi, 427-429.—**Chiarugi** (G.) Varietà dell' ansa dell' ipoglosso. Boll. d. Soc. tra i cult. d. sc. med. in Siena, 1884, ii, 275.—**Clason** (E.) Nerv- och kärl-anomalier, præparatet efter van Vetters och Brunettis methoder. Upsala Läkaref. Förh., 1867-8, iii, 492-508. — **Deville.** [Anomalie du plexus brachial.] Bull. Soc. anat. de Par., 1849, xxiv, 8.—**Gaillet.** [Anomalie du nerf brachial.] *Ibid.*, 1853, xxviii, 109.—**Garibaldi** & **Giovanardi.** Sovra un ramo del nervo radiale al muscolo bracciale anteriore. Spallanzani, Modena, 1876, xiv, 233-237.—**Giacomini.** Anomalia dei nervi della mano. Gior. d. r. Accad. di med. di Torino, 1872, 3. s., xi, 210-217, 1 pl.—**Giura** (P. M.) Anomalie dei nervi dorsali della mano. Salute: Italia med., Genova, 1885, xix, 505-508.—**Gros.** [Un petit filet du nerf nasal qui se parte au nerf optique avec lequel il s'anastomose.] Bull. Soc. anat. de Par., 1847, xxii, 84.—**Gruber** (W.) Anomaler Verlauf des Nervus medianus vor dem Musculus pronator teres, bei Durchbohrung des letzteren durch die hoch oben am Oberarme von der Arteria brachialis entsprungene Arteria interossea. Arch. f. Anat., Physiol. u. wissensch. Med., Leipz., 1867, 552-559, 1 pl. ————. Ueber den anomalen Verlauf des Nervus ulnaris vor dem Epitrochleus. *Ibid.*, 1867, 560-564, 1 pl. ————. Abgang des Ramus volaris digitorum communis iii des Nervus medianus hoch am Unterarme. Oesterr. Ztschr. f. prakt. Heilk., Wien, 1869, xv, 432. ————. Ungewöhnliche Anordnung der Hautnerven am Handrücken. Arch. f. path. Anat., etc.. Berl., 1872, liv, 190. ————. Ein Nachtrag zu den Anomalien des Nervus perforans Casserii. *Ibid.*, 1875, lxv, 25. ————. Starker Nervus intercosto-humeralis von N. intercostalis i. *Ibid.*, 1880, lxxx, 92. ————. Inselförmige Spaltung des Nervus peroneus profundus. (Bestätigung der Vorkommens.) *Ibid.*, 93. ————. Ungewöhnlicher Verlauf des Nervus cutaneus anterior externus femoris. (Vorher nicht gesehen.) *Ibid.* ————. Zu den Varietäten des Nervus peroneus profundus et superficialis. (Grösstentheils vorher nicht gesehen.) *Ibid.*, lxxxi, 471-475.—**Hepburn** (D.) Some variations in the arrangement of the nerves of the human body. J. Anat. & Physiol., Lond., 1886-7, xxi, 511-513.—**Hirshfeld** (L.) Anomalie dans la distribution du nerf radial à la main. Compt. rend. Soc. de biol. 1853, Par., 1854, v, 16.—**Hyrtl.** Abnormes Verhalten des Nervus medianus und Cutaneus brachii externus. Oesterr. Ztschr. f. prakt. Heilk., Wien, 1862, viii, 382.—**Leuf** (A. H. P.) Note on

Nerves (*Abnormities of*).

abnormal distribution, hitherto unobserved, of the supra-orbital and infra-orbital nerves, explanatory of the recurrence of certain neuralgias. Arch. Med., N. Y., 1880, iii, 340-344. ———. Further note concerning accessory facial foramina. *Ibid.*, 1881, v, 113.—**Lydston** (G. F.) Anomalous origin of the descendens noni. Chicago M. J. & Exam., 1880, xl, 263-265.—**Macalister** (A.) Variety of arrangement of the nasal nerve. Med. Press & Circ., Dubl., 1868, v, 305.—**Merlin** (H.) Tief herabreichender Bogen des Nervus hypoglossus. Ber. d. naturw.-med. Ver. in Innsbruck, 1884-6, xv, 2, 1 pl. ———. Perforation des N. sartorius durch den N. saphenus major. *Ibid.*, 3.—**Meyer** (G. H.) Zwei Nerven-Varietäten. Arch. f. Anat.. Physiol. u. wissensch. Med., Leipz., 1870, 395-398.—**Mingazzini** (G.) Anomalia di alcuni rami del plexus brachialis. Gazz. d. osp., Milano, 1886, vii, 242.—**Ozenne.** Anomalie du nerf radial portant sur le nombre des rameaux terminaux de sa branche antérieure. Bull. Soc. anat. de Par., 1883, lviii, 108. *Also:* Progrès méd., Par., 1883, xi, 734.—**Sargent** (L. M.) Passage of one of the brachial nerves through a vein. Boston M. & S. J., 1855-6, liii, 102.—**Streets** (T. H.) Anatomical anomalies. (Musculo-cutaneous, and nerve of Wrisberg.) Am. J. M. Sc., Phila., 1872, n. s., lxiv, 133.—**Thomson** (A.) Accessory obturator nerve joined by branch from anterior crural supplying the adductor longus. J. Anat. & Physiol., Lond., 1884-5, xix, 331. ———. Irregularity in the origin and nerve supply of the adductor longus. *Ibid.*—**Turner.** Some additional variations in the distribution of the nerves of the human body. *Ibid.*, 1871-2, vi, 101-106. ———. Further examples of variations in the arrangement of the nerves of the human body. *Ibid.*, 1873-4, viii, 297-299.

Nerves (*Anastomoses of*).

See, also, **Nerve** (*Hypoglossal*); **Nerve** (*Musculo-cutaneous*).

BENDZ (H. C. B.) * De anastomosi Jacobsonii et ganglio Arnoldi. 4°. *Havniæ*, 1833.

FILHOL (H.) * De la sensibilité récurrente dans la main. 4°. *Paris*, 1873.

Arloing & **Tripier** (L.) Des conditions de la persistance de la sensibilité dans le bout périphérique des nerfs sectionnés. Arch. de physiol. norm. et path., Par., 1876, 2. s., iii, 11; 105, 5 pl. *Also,* Reprint.—**Billroth** (T.) Einige Beobachtungen über das ausgedehnte Vorkommen von Nervenanastomosen im Tractus intestinalis. Arch. f. Anat., Physiol. u. wissensch. Med., Berl., 1858, 148-158, 1 pl.—**Dwight** (T.), jr. An instance of a so-called "endless" nerve, with remarks. Boston M. & S. J., 1871, lxxxiv, 126.—**Fearn** (S. W.) Discovery of an anastomosis between the fourth and fifth pair of nerves. Lancet, Lond., 1831-2, i, 828.—**Jacobsen** (C.-L.) Notice sur une nouvelle anastomose nerveuse dans l'oreille interne. J. compl. du dict. d. sc. méd., Par., 1820, vii, 182-185.—**Jacobson** (L.) Description anatomique d'une anastomose entre le nerf pharyngo-glossien, le trifacial et le trisplanchnique. [Avec des notes additionnelles à ce mémoire par G. Breschet.] Répert. gén d'anat. et physiol. path., Par., 1826, ii, 197-215, 1 pl.—**Lacroix** (E.) Mémoire sur les anastomoses des nerfs, considérées comme servant à coordonner les mouvemens involontaires à la sensibilité dans l'accomplissement des fonctions organique : et sensoriales. J. hebd. d. progr. d. sc. méd., Par., 1836, i, 97; 129.—**Richet** (A.) De la sensibilité récurrente. Gaz. d. hôp., Par., 1874, xlvii, 401-403. ———. Sur la sensibilité récurrente des nerfs périphériques de la main. Compt. rend. Acad. d. sc., Par., 1875, lxxxi, 217-220.—**Rosenthal** (L.) Ueber Nervenanastomosen im Bereiche des Sinus cavernosus. Sitzungsb. d. k. Akad. d. Wissensch. Math.-naturw. Cl., Wien, 1878, lxxviii, 93-102, 1 pl.—**Sharpe** (J. B.) The discovery of an anastomosis between the fourth and fifth pairs of nerves not of modern date. Lancet, Lond., 1831-2, i, 866.—**Stricker** (S.) Ueber die collaterale Innervation. Med. Jahrb., Wien, 1877, 415-424.—**Verdon** (W.) On the intercommunication of nerves and the physiological advantages gained thereby. St. Thomas's Hosp. Rep., Lond., 1874, n. s., v, 285-293.—**Volkmann** (A. W.) Beobachtungen und Reflexionen über Nerven-Anastomosen. Arch. f. Anat., Physiol. u. wissensch. Med., Berl., 1840, 510-532, 1 pl.—**Wyman** (J.) A description of some instances of the passage of nerves across the middle line of the body. Am. J. M. Sc., Phila., 1864, n. s., xlvii, 343-352. *Also,* Reprint.

Nerves (*Compression and ligature of*).

See, also, **Nerve** (*Pneumogastric*).

BOINET (É.) * Contribution à l'étude de la compression des nerfs. 4°. *Paris*, 1880.

A BRUNN (J. H.) * Experimenta quædam circa ligaturas nervorum in vivis animalibus instituta. sm. 4°. *Gottingæ*, [1753].

Also, in: SCRIPT. neurol. minores selecti. 4°. *Lipsiæ*, 1792, ii, 271-290. *Also* [Abstr.], *in:* WEIZ (F. A.) Neue Ausz., [etc.]. 12°. *Leipzig*, 1776, v; 47-49. *Also* [Abstr.], *in:* Acta Helvet., Basileæ, 1755, ii, 113-122.

Nerves (*Compression and ligature of*).

Brinton. Aneurism of the aorta; with a description of the morbid anatomy of the recurrent nerve compressed by it. Tr. Path. Soc. Lond., 1850-52, iii, 304-307.—**François-Franck.** Note sur un appareil pour la compression et la décompression graduées des nerfs. Compt. rend. Soc. de biol. 1880, Par., 1881, 7. s., ii, 86-88. *Also:* Progrès méd., Par., 1880, viii, 151. *Also:* Gaz. méd. de Par., 1880, 6. s., ii, 164.—**Lüderitz** (C.) Versuche über die Einwirkung des Druckes auf die motorischen und sensiblen Nerven. Ztschr. f. klin. Med., Berl., 1880, ii, 97-120. *Also,* Reprint.

Nerves (*Degeneration and regeneration of*).

See, also, **Nerves** (*Suture of*); **Nerves** (*Wounds of*); **Neurotomy,** *etc.*

COLASANTI (G.) Sulla degenerazione dei nervi recisi. 4°. *Roma*, 1878.

Repr. from: Atti d. r. Accad. d. Lincei. Cl. di sc. fis., matemat. e nat., Roma, 1877-8, cclxxv.

DRUMMOND (H. P.) * De regeneratione nervorum. 8°. *Turici*, 1839.

EICHHORST (H. L.) * Ueber Nervende- und Nervenregeneration. 8°. *Königsberg*, 1873.

EINSIEDEL (L.) * Ueber Nervenregeneration nach Ausschneidung eines Nervenstücks. 8°. *Giessen*, 1864.

FLIES (A.) * De degeneratione et regeneratione nervorum, necnon de vi gangliorum trophica. 8°. *Berolini*, [1858].

HJELT (O. E. A.) Om nervernas regeneration och dermed sammanhängande förändringar af nervrören. 8°. *Helsingfors*, 1859.

Also, transl. [Abstr.], *in:* Arch. f. path. Anat., etc., Berl., 1860, xix, 352-367, 3 pl.

LAVERAN (A.) * Recherches expérimentales sur la régénération des nerfs. 4°. *Strasbourg*, 1867.

LENT (E. O. B.) * De nervorum dissectorum commutationibus ac regeneratione. 4°. *Berolini*, [1855].

MARCIGUEY (H.) * Contribution à l'étude de la régénération des nerfs périphériques. 4°. *Paris*, 1885.

———. The same. 8°. *Paris*, 1886.

OEHL (E.) Sul processo di regenerazione dei nervi recisi; studj sperimentali. 8°. *Pavia*, 1864.

PEN (C.) * De nervorum regeneratione. 8°. *Traj. ad Rhenum*, 1834.

SCHRADER (L. A.) * Experimenta circa regenerationem in gangliis nerveis vulneribus illatis, in animalibus instituta. Quibus accedunt: nonnullæ commutationes morbosæ in gangliis nerveis observatæ. 4°. *Gottingæ*, 1850.

STEINRUECK (C. O.) * De nervorum regeneratione. 4°. *Berolini*, [1838].

VERGEZ (H.) Coup-d'œil historique et recherches expérimentales sur les régénérations nerveuses. 8°. *Montpellier*, 1842.

Arloing (S.) Dégénération et centre trophique des nerfs; examen critique des opinions émises sur leur nature; applications. Compt. rend. Soc. de biol., Par., 1886, 8. s., iii, 553-556.—**Arnemann.** Ein Paar Worte über die Wiedererzeugung der Nerven. Arch. f. d. Physiol., Halle, 1799, iii, 100 - 105.—**Bert** (P.) Sur la régénération des nerfs pneumogastriques. Compt. rend. Soc. de biol., Par., 1885, 8. s., ii, 100.—**Bertolet** (R. M.) Regeneration of human nerves after excision. Phila. M. Times, 1875-6, vi, 258-260.—**Brown-Séquard.** On the regeneration of nerve-tissue and nerve function in the case of tumors involving the 7th pair of nerves. Med. Rec., N. Y., 1872, vii, 517. ———. Régénération du nerf sciatique dans une longueur de douze centimètres, dans l'espace de dix semaines chez un petit singe. Compt. rend. Soc. de biol., Par., 1882, 7. s., iv, 30.—**Bruch** (C.) Ueber die Regeneration der Nerven. Arch. d. Ver. f. gemeinsch. Arb. z. Förd. d. wissensch. Heilk., Götting., 1856, ii, 409-419.—**Cattani** (Giuseppina). Sulla degenerazione e neoformazione delle fibre nervose midollari periferiche. Arch. per le sc. med., Torino, 1887, xi, 175-194, 2 pl.—**Colasanti** (G.) Sulla degenerazione dei nervi recisi. Atti Accad. med. di Roma, 1877, iii, 43-47. *Also:* Atti d. r. Accad. d. Lincei. Cl. di sc. fis., matemat. e nat., Roma, 1877-8, p. cclxxv. *Also,* Reprint. *Also, transl.:* Arch. f. Physiol., Leipz., 1878, 206-214, 1 pl.—**Cossy** (A.) & **Dejérine** (J.) Recherches sur la dégénérescence des nerfs séparés de leurs centres trophiques. Arch. de physiol. norm. et path., Par., 1875, 2. s., ii, 567-587, 1 pl.—

Nerves (*Degeneration and regeneration of*).

Cruikshank (W.) Experiments on the nerves, particularly on their reproduction, and on the spinal marrow of living animals. Phil. Tr., Lond., 1795, lxxxv, 177–189, 1 pl. — **Dejérine** (J.) & **Mayer** (A.) Recherches sur les altérations de la moelle épinière et des nerfs du moignon chez les amputés d'ancienne date. Gaz. méd. de Par., 1878, 4. s., vii, 478 ; 490.—**Eichhorst** (H.) Ueber Nervendegeneration und Nervenregeneration. Arch. f. path. Anat., etc., Berl., 1873, lix, 1–25, 2 pl.—**Engelmann** (T. W.) Ueber Degeneration von Nervenfasern ; ein Beitrag zur Cellularphysiologie. Onderzoek. ged. in h. physiol. Lab. d. Utrecht. Hoogesch., 1876–7, 3. R., iv, 181–204, 1 pl.— **Fontana** (F.) Expériences faites à Londres en 1778 et 1779, sur la reproduction des nerfs. *In his:* Traité sur le venin de la vipère, 4°, Florence, 1781, ii, 177–186. *Also, transl.:* 8°, Napoli, 1787, iii, 136–147. *Also, transl. :* 8°, Lond., 1787, ii, 203–214. — **Frankl von Hochwart** (L.) Ueber De- und Regeneration von Nervenfasern. Med. Jahrb., Wien, 1887, n. s., ii, 1–20. *Also:* Centralbl. f. klin. Med., Leipz., 1887, viii, 817. — **Friedberg** (H.) Ueber die Innervation der durch Ueberpflanzung gebildeten Nase. Arch. f. path. Anat., etc., Berl., 1859, xvi, 540–545.—**Gena** (A. A.) O nervnom shvie. [On regeneration of nerves.] Vrach, St. Petersb., 1880, i, 358 ; 373.—**Gluck** (T.) Experimentelles zur Frage der Nervennaht und der Nervenregeneration. Arch. f. path. Anat., etc., Berl., 1878, lxxii, 624–642, 1 pl. — **Guenther.** Versuche und Bemerkungen über Regeneration der Nerven und Abhängigkeit der peripherischen Nerven von den Centralorganen. Arch. f. Anat., Physiol. u. wissensch. Med., Berl., 1840, 270–286. — **Haighton** (J.) An experimental inquiry concerning the reproduction of nerves. Phil. Tr., Lond., 1795, 190–201, 1 pl. *Also,* Reprint. *Also:* Arch. f. d. Physiol., Halle, 1797, ii, 71–86, 1 pl.—**Hayem** (G.) Lésions des nerfs des membres consécutives à l'amputation. Bull. Soc. anat. de Par., 1875, l, 684–687. ———. Seconde communication sur l'état des nerfs des membres qui ont subi une amputation ancienne. *Ibid.*, 1876, li, 230–232. *Also:* Progrès méd., Par., 1876, iv, 548. — **Hayem** (G.) & **Gilbert** (J.) Note sur les modifications du système nerveux chez un amputé. Arch. de physiol. norm. et path., Par., 1884, 3. s., iii, 430–443, 1 pl. — **Hertz** (H.) Ueber Degeneration und Regeneration durchschnittener Nerven. Arch. f. path. Anat., etc., Berl., 1869, xlvi, 257–285.—**Hill** (J. D.) Cases showing restoration of motion and sensation after traumatic lesions of large nerves with loss of substance. Med. Times & Gaz., Lond., 1868, ii, 212.—**Hoggan** (G.) & **Hoggan** (Frances-Élisabeth). De la dégénération et de la régénération du cylindre-axe, et des autres éléments des fibres nerveuses dans les lésions non traumatiques. J. de l'anat. et physiol., etc., Par., 1882, xviii, 27–59, 2 pl. — **Holman** (H. W.) Case of restoration of nerve-force after division of a large nerve (the ulnar). Med. Times & Gaz., Lond., 1872, ii, 133.— **Horteloup** (B.) Mémoire et observations sur la non-régénération des nerfs de la vie animale. J. d. conn. méd.-chir., Par., 1834–5, ii, 144–147. — **Jobert** (A.-J.) [*de Lamballe*]. Du rétablissement de l'action nerveuse dans les lambeaux autoplastiques. Compt. rend. Acad. d. sc., Par., 1845, xx, 344. *Also, transl.:* Med. Times, Lond., 1845, xii, 98–100. — **Köster** (H.) Om nervdegeneration och nervatrofi, jemte några ord om varikositernas förekomst och betydelse i de periferiska nerverna. Upsala Läkaref. Förh., 1887–8, xxiii, 31 ; 145. — **Korybutt - Daszkiewicz.** O zwyrodnieniu i odradzaniu się nerwów przeciętych. [The degeneration and regeneration of bisected nerves.] Medycyna, Warszawa, 1879, vii, 67 ; 81. — **de Lacrousille.** Leçons sur la dégénération et régénération des nerfs. Union méd., Par., 1864, 2. s., xxiii, 356 ; 371.—**Lominski** (F. I.) K ucheniou o degeneratsii nervnich klietok. [On the cellular degeneration of nerves.] Vrach, St. Petersb., 1884, v, 635.—**Mayer** (S.) Ueber Degenerations- und Regenerationsvorgänge im normalen peripherischen Nerven. Sitzungsb. d. k. Akad. d. Wissensch. Math.-naturw. Cl., Wien, 1878, lxxvii, 80–92, 1 pl. ———. Nachträgliche Bemerkungen zu meinem Aufsatze : Ueber Degenerations- und Regenerationsvorgänge im normalen peripherischen Nerven. Prag. med. Wchnschr., 1878, iii, 289. ———. Ueber Degenerations- und Regenerationsvorgänge im unversehrten peripherischen Nerven. [*Repr. from :* Anz. d. k. Akad. d. Wissensch., 1879, No. xxv (Sitzungsb. d. mathem.-naturw. Classe, v, 4. December).] *Ibid.*, 1879, iv, 504.— **Meyer** (J. C. H.) Ueber die Wiedererzeugung der Nerven. Arch. f. d. Physiol., Halle, 1797, ii, 449–467, 1 pl.— **Neumann** (E.) Ueber Degeneration und Regeneration zerquetschter Nerven. Arch. f. mikr. Anat., Bonn, 1880, xviii, 302–344, 1 pl.—**Notta.** Sur un cas de régénération des nerfs du bras à la suite de leur destruction dans une étendue de cinq centimètres ; phénomènes physiologiques remarkables; conséquences graves au point de vue médico-légal. Arch. gén. de méd., Par., 1872, ii, 5–10.—**Petrone** (A.) Contribuzione alla rigenerazione dei nervi in un caso raro di spondilite deformante assoido-atlantoidea con lenta compressione spinale. Morgagni, Napoli, 1878, xx, 97–121, 1 pl.—**Philipeaux.** De la régénération en quinze jours du nerf pneumogastrique chez les jeunes rats albinos et chez les jeunes cobayes. Compt. rend. Soc. de biol., Par.,

Nerves (*Degeneration and regeneration of*).

1885, 8. s., ii, 1. — **Philipeaux** (J.-M.) & **Vulpian** (A.) Recherches expérimentales sur la régénération des nerfs séparés des centres nerveux. *Ibid.*, 1859, Par., 1860, 3. s., 343–415. *Also,* Reprint.—**Ranvier** (L.) De la régénération des nerfs de l'épithélium antérieur de la cornée et de la théorie du développement continu du système nerveux. Compt. rend. Acad. d. sc., Par., 1879, lxxxviii, 979–981.— **Reichert** (E. T.) Observations on the regeneration of the vagus and hypoglossal nerves. Am. J. M. Sc., Phila., 1885, n. s., lxxxix, 146–159. *Also,* Reprint.—**Remak.** Ueber die Wiederzeugung von Nervenfasern. Arch. f. path. Anat., etc., Berl., 1862, xxiii, 441–444. — **Schuster** (H.) Hyaline (wachsartige) Degeneration der Fasern des Nervus medianus sin. bei Carcinom des lateralen Myxofibroms an demselben. Ztschr. f. Heilk., Prag, 1886, vii, 73–85, 1 pl.—**Sokolow** (A.) Sur les transformations des terminaisons des nerfs dans les muscles de la grenouille après la section des nerfs. Arch. de physiol. norm. et path., Par., 1874, vi, 300–315, 1 pl. — **Tangl** (F.) Az idegelfajulás- s újraképződésről. [On regeneration of nerve-fibres.] Orvosi hetil., Budapest, 1887, xxxi, 27 ; 62 ; 124 ; 289 ; 326. — **Tiedemann** (F.) Ueber die Regeneration der Nerven. Ztschr. f. Physiol., Heidelb. u. Leipz., 1831, iv, 68–77, 1 pl. *Also, transl. :* J. compl. du dict. d. sc. méd., Par., 1831, xli, 289–295. *Also, transl. :* J. univ. et hebd. de méd. et chir. prat., Par., 1832, vi, 389–440.— **Tizzoni** (G.) Degeneration durchschnittener Nerven ; zur Pathologie des Nervengewebes. Centralbl. f. d. med. Wissensch., Berl., 1878, xvi, 225. — **Vaulair** (C.) De la régénération des nerfs périphériques par le procédé de la suture tubulaire. France méd., Par., 1882, ii, 99–101. ———. Nouvelles recherches sur la régénération des nerfs périphériques. Compt. rend. Acad. d. sc., Par., 1885, c, 1605 - 1607. ———. Nouvelles recherches expérimentales sur la régénération des nerfs. Arch. de biol., Gand, 1885, vi, 127–235, 1 pl. ———. De la distribution périphérique des nerfs régénérés comparée à celle des nerfs primitifs. Bull. Acad. roy. d. sc. de Belg., Brux., 1886, 3. s., xii, 35–38. ———. Sur le trajet et la distribution périphérique des nerfs régénérés. Arch/ de physiol. norm. et path., Par., 1886, 3. s., viii, 97–105.—**Vulpian** (A.) Note sur la régénération dite autogénique des nerfs. *Ibid.*, 1874, 2. s., i, 704–714.—**Waller** (A.) Experiments on the section of the glosso-pharyngeal and hypoglossal nerves of the frog, and observations of the alterations produced thereby in the structure of their primative fibres. Edinb. M. & S. J., 1851, lxxvi, 369–376. ———. Sur la reproduction des nerfs et sur la structure et les fonctions des ganglions spinaux. Arch. f. Anat., Physiol. u. wissensch. Med., Berl., 1852, 392–401. ———. Expérience sur les sections des nerfs et les altérations. Compt. rend. Soc. de biol. 1856, Par., 1857, 2. s., iii, 6–8.—**Wolski** (J.) Czy wlokna nerwowe, czuciowe i odruchowe są też same, czy też różne ? [Do excito-motor nerve-fibres remain unchanged under irritation ?] Gaz. lek., Warszawa, 1869, vii, 118–121.

Nerves (*Diseases of*).

See **Nervous** system (*Diseases of*).

Nerves (*Ganglia and plexuses of*).

See, also, **Ciliary** *ganglion* ; **Intercarotid** *ganglion* ; **Meckel's** *ganglion* ; **Nervous** *system* (*Ganglionic*) ; **Ophthalmic** *ganglion* ; **Otic** *ganglion.*

CRANE (G.) * De gangliis nervorum. 8°. *Edinburgi*, 1813.

EVERSMANN (E. F.) * De systemate gangliorum et cerebrali. 8°. [*Dorpat*], 1816.

GIETL (F. X.) * Fragmenta pathologica de neurogangliis. 8°. *Monachii*, 1829.

HAASE (J. G.) De gangliis nervorum. 4°. *Lipsiæ*, [1772].

Also, in: SCRIPT. neurol. minores selecti. 8°. *Lipsiæ*, 1791, i, 61–88.

JOHNSTONE (J.) An essay on the use of the ganglions of the nerves. 8°. *Shrewsbury*, 1771.

Also, in his: Med. essays and obs. 8°. *Evesham*, 1795, 1–96. *Also, in :* Phil. Tr., Lond., 1764, liv, 177 : 1767, 120 : 1770, lx, 30.

———. The same. Versuch über den Nutzen der Nervenknoten. Aus dem Englischen übersetzt. 8°. *Stettin*, 1787.

KRONENBERG (H.) Plexuum nervorum structura et virtutes. 8°. *Berolini*, 1836.

LANCISI (J. M.) De gangliis nervorum. *In :* MORGAGNI (J. M.) Adversaria anatomica quinta. 4°. *Lugd. Bat.*, 1723, 101–119, 1 pl.

MECKEL (J. F.) De ganglio secundi rami quinti paris nervorum cerebri nuper detecto, de-

Nerves (*Ganglia and plexuses of*).

que vera gangliorum nervosorum utilitate. *Berolini*, 1749.

In : SCRIPT. neurol. minores selecti. 8°. *Lipsiæ*, 1795, iv, 7–9, 1 pl.

POLAILLON (J.-F.-B.) * Étude sur les ganglions nerveux périphériques 4°. *Paris*, 1865.

Also, in : J. de l'anat. et physiol., etc., Par., 1866, iii, 43 ; 130 ; 243, 2 pl.

SCARPA (A.) Anatomicarum annotationum liber primus. De nervorum gangliis et plexubus. 8°. *Mutinæ*, 1779.

——. The same. 4°. *Ticini Regii*, 1785.

SCHRAMM (J.) * Neue Untersuchungen über den Bau der Spinalganglien. 8°. *Würzburg*, 1864.

SCHUMANN (P. G. P.) * De gangliis. 4°. *Berolini*, [1847].

WALTER (G.) * De regeneratione gangliorum. 8°. *Bonnæ*, 1853.

WEBER (E. H.) [Pr.] de gangliis nervorum, deque origine et essentia nervi intercostalis. 4°. [*Lipsiæ*, 1831.]

WUTZER (C. G.) De corporis humani gangliorum fabrica atque usu, monographia. 4°. *Berolini*, 1817.

Arnold (J.) Ein Beitrag zu der feineren Structur der Ganglienzellen. Arch. f. path. Anat., etc., Berl., 1867, xli, 178–220, 2 pl.—**Bischoff** (E.) Ueber die angebliche Anastomose zwischen dem Ganglion geniculi N. facialis und dem N. petrosus superficialis minor. Ztschr. f. rat. Med., Leipz. u. Heidelb., 1867, 3. R., xxix, 161–164, 1 pl.—**Celoni** (P.) Storia di un tubercolo in corrispondenza del ganglio destro di Gasser. Sperimentale, Firenze, 1869, xxiv, 3–15.—**Civinini** (F.) Alcuni casi di abnormi rigonfiamenti nervosi gangliari. Bull. d. sc. med. di Bologna, 1837, 2. s., iv, 113–117. — **Cloquet** (H.) Mémoire sur les ganglions nerveux des fosses nasales, sur leurs communications et sur leurs usages. N. Jour. de méd., chir., pharm., etc., Par., 1818, ii, 211–226.—**Cunningham** (D. J.) Notes on the great splanchnic ganglion. J. Anat. & Physiol., Lond., 1874–5, ix, 303–305.—**van Deen.** Eenige aanteekeningen over de zenuwen, bijzonder over de zenuw-vlechten. Tijdschr. v. nat Geschied. en Physiol., Leiden, 1838–9, v, 294–320.—**François-Franck.** Ganglions nerveux. Dict. encycl. d. sc. méd., Par., 1880, 4. s., vi, 629–653. — **Gad** (J.) Zur Anatomie und Physiologie der Spinalganglien. Deutsche med. Wchnschr., Leipz., 1887, xiii, 927–929. *Also,* Reprint. — **Guarini** (L.) Del ganglio genicolare. Ann. univ. di med., Milano, 1841, xcvii, 255–260, 1 pl.—**Holl** (M.) Ueber den Bau der Spinalganglien. Sitzungsb. d. k. Akad. d. Wissensch. 1875, Wien, 1876, lxxii, 31–37.—**Jewell.** Structure and functions of the ganglia on the posterior roots of the spinal, and also of the corresponding part of the cranial nerves. [Discussion.] Tr. Am. Neurol. Ass., N. Y., 1877, ii, pp. xvii–xxi.—**Joseph** (M.) Zur Physiologie der Spinalganglien. Arch. f. Physiol., Leipz., 1887, 296 – 315. *Also :* Neurol. Centralbl., Leipz., 1887, vi, 172–175.—**Maher & Payen.** Observations sur la transformation ganglionnaire des nerfs de la vie animale et de la vie organique. Compt. rend. Acad. d. sc., Par., 1845, xxi, 1171–1177.—**Meckel.** Examen physiologique du véritable usage des nœuds, ou ganglions des nerfs. [Trad. du latin.] Mém. Acad. roy. de Prusse, Avignon, 1768, ii, 62–86.—**Reil.** Ueber die Eigenschaften des Ganglien-Systems und sein Verhältniss zum Cerebral-Systeme. Arch. f. d. Physiol., Halle, 1807, vii, 189–254.—**Scarpa** (A.) De gangliis nervorum, deque origine et essentia nervi intercostalis ad ill. vir. Henricum Weber. Ann. univ. di med., Milano, 1831, lviii, 474 : lx, 5. — **Schenk** (S. L.) Die Entwicklungsgeschichte der Ganglien und des Lobus electricus. Sitzungsb. d. k. Akad. d. Wissensch., Wien, 1877, lxxiv, 13–36, 2 pl. ——. Zur Entwickelung der Ganglien der Cerebrospinal-Nerven. Allg. Wien. med. Ztg., 1878, xxiii, 365.—**Schiff** (M.) Ueber die angeblich ästhesodische Natur der Spinalganglien. Untersuch. z. Naturl. d. Mensch. u. d. Thiere, Frankf. a. M., 1857, ii, 56 – 61. — **Valentin** (G.) Ueber eine gangliöse Anschwellung in der Jacobsonschen Anastomose des Menschen. Arch. f. Anat., Physiol. u. wissensch. Med., Berl., 1840, 287–290.—**Will** (F.) Vorläufige Mittheilung über die Structur der Ganglien und den Ursprung der Nerven bei wirbellosen Thieren. *Ibid.*, 1844, 76–93.- **Wutzer** (C. W.) Notiz über die Verbindung der Intervertebral-Ganglien und des Rückenmarkes mit dem vegetativen Nervensystems. *Ibid.*, 1842, 424.

Nerves (*Grafting of*).

See **Nerves** (*Suture of*).

Nerves (*Gustatory*).

See **Nerves** of taste.

Nerves (*Hypertrophy of*).

See, also, **Neuroma.**

Moxon (W.) Description of a remarkable enlargement of the nerves. Guy's Hosp. Rep., Lond., 1862, 3. s., viii, 257–261, 1 pl.

Nerves (*Inflammation of*).

See **Neuritis.**

Nerves (*Ligature of*).

See **Nerves** (*Compression, etc., of*).

Nerves (*Nævus of*).

See **Skin** (*Tumors, etc., of*).

Nerves (*Pathology of*).

See **Nervous** system (*Pathology, etc., of*).

Nerves (*Physiology of*).

See **Nerve-currents** (*Velocity of*) ; **Nervous** system.

Nerves (*Regeneration of*).

See **Nerves** (*Degeneration, etc., of*).

Nerves (*Sections of*).

See **Neurotomy,** etc.

Nerves (*Surgery of*)

See, also, **Nerves** (*Suture of*); **Nerve-stretching** ; **Neurotomy,** etc. ; **Sciatica** (*Treatment of*).

BOUVEROT (L.) * Théorie de la suppléance sensitivo-motrice et ses conséquences pratiques relatives à la névrotomie et aux sutures nerveuses. 4°. *Lyon*, 1879.

HILDEBRANDT. Nervendehnung, Neurektomie und Nervennaht. Ein Beitrag zur Nervenchirurgie. 8°. *Berlin*, 1884.

KLOTZ (T.) * Beitrag zur Casuistik der operativen Loslösung und Dehnung von Nervenstämmen. 8°. *Greifswald*, 1874.

TILLAUX (P.) Des affections chirurgicales des nerfs. 8°. *Paris*, 1866.

Albrecht (J.) Klinische Beiträge zur Nervenchirurgie. Deutsche Ztschr. f. Chir., Leipz., 1887, xxvi, 430–497.— **Brun** (P.) Quelques réflexions sur les maladies chirurgicales des cordons nerveux. J. de méd. de Lyon, 1842, iii, 258–284.—**Czerny.** Beiträge zur Nervendehnung und Nerven-Resection. Arch. f. Psychiat., Berl., 1879, x, 284–288.— **Duret** (H.) Griffe consécutive à une lésion traumatique du nerf cubital. Compt. rend. Soc. de biol. 1872, Par., 1874, 5. s., iv, 26–31.—**Fulton** (F. S.) Stretching of the supra- and infra-orbital, and neurotomy of the nasal nerve for neuralgia. N. Am. J. Homœop., N. Y., 1887, 3. s., ii, 289–292.—**Gerster** (A. G.) Pes plano-valgus cured by resection of wedge-shaped portion of the tarsus ; consecutive paralysis of musculo-spiral nerve due to the use of crutches ; dissection of the nerve, found to be adherent to an old callus from comminuted fracture of the humerus. Med. News, Phila., 1886, xlviii, 355.—**Gluck** (T.) Ueber Neuroplastik auf dem Wege der Transplantation. Arch. f. klin. Chir., Berl., 1880, xxv, 606–616, 1 pl. *Also :* Verhandl. d. deutsch. Gesellsch. f. Chir. 1880, Berl., 1881, ix, pt. 2, 22–32, 1 pl.—**Grisson.** Beobachtungen über Neurectomien an der Schädelbasis. Berl. klin. Wchnschr., 1887, xxiv, 982.—**Leisrink** (H.) Beiträge zur Casuistik der Nerven-Chirurgie, speciell der Nervendehnung. Arch. f. klin. Chir., Berl., 1882, xxviii, 569–577.—**M'Leod** (K.) Case of nerve-splitting. Brain, Lond., 1880–81, iii, 117– 120. ——. Nerve splitting. [Case.] Indian M. Gaz., Calcutta, 1887, xxii, 264.—**Medini** (L.) Note ed osservazioni sullo stiramento cruento dei nervi. Bull. d. sc. med. di Bologna, 1882, 6. s., ix, 310–323.—**Nicoladoni** (C.) Beiträge zur Nervenchirurgie. Wien. med. Presse, 1882, xxiii, 853 ; 885 ; 921 ; 952 ; 1013.—**Page** (H. W.) Some cases of nerve resection and nerve stretching. Brain. Lond., 1879–80, ii, 128–133.—**Richardson** (M. H.) Operations on nerves. Boston M. & S. J., 1886, cxv, 368 – 373. ——. Cases of nerve stretching, nerve section and nerve suture, and operation to relieve pressure on nerve trunks. *Ibid.*, 1888, cxviii, 139–141. — **Sands.** Division of the brachial plexus ; suture of the divided ends. N. York M. J., 1888, xlvii, 215. — **Schuh.** Mittheilungen über Resection und andere Operationen an Nerven. Wien. med. Wchnschr., 1863, xiii, 1 ; 17 ; 33 ; 49 ; 65 ; 129 ; 145 ; 161. *Also,* Reprint.—**Szeparowicz** (J.) Statystyka wycięcia nerwu dolnoszczękowego wedlug sposobu Paravciniego, ocena metody. [Statistics of surgical operations on nerves, according to Paravicini's method.] Przegl. lek., Krakow., 1877, xvi, 546 ; 559.—**Tscherning** (E A.) Tra den moderne Nervechirurgies Omvaade. Oversigter. Biblioth. f. Læger, Kjøbenh., 1882, xii, 437 ; 582.—**Vogt** (P.) Beitrag zur Neurochirurgie. Deutsche Ztschr. f. Chir., Leipz., 1876–7, vii, 144–151. ——. Lösung des

Nerves (*Surgery of*).

Plexus brachialis aus einer Callussmasse durch Resektion des Oberarmes. *Ibid.*, 152–154.—**Wolberg** (L.) O zszywaniu, odtwarzaniu się i naciąganiu nerwów. [Nerve-section, suture, and stretching.] Medycyna, Warszawa, 1880, viii, 545; 562; 593; 609.

Nerves (*Suture of*).

ASSAKY (G.) * De la suture des nerfs à distance. 4°. *Paris*, 1886.

Also, in : Arch. gén. de méd., Par., 1886, ii, 529–553.

DIETERICH (M.) * Zur Casuistik der Sehnen- und Nervennaht. 12°. *Greifswald*, 1883.

FALKENHEIM (H.) * Zur Lehre von der Nervennaht und der Prima intentio nervorum. 8°. *Königsberg i. Pr.*, 1881.

GLUGE (G.) & THIERNESSE (A.) Sur la réunion des fibres nerveuses sensibles avec les fibres motrices. 8°. *Bruxelles*, [1864].

Repr. from : Bull. Acad. roy. de Belg., Brux., 1859, 2. s., vii, 415–437. [*See, also, infra,* Gluge.]

JOHANNES (K.) * O nervnome shvie. [On suture of nerves.] 8°. *St. Petersburg*, 1868.

KETTLER (A.) * Ueber einen Fall von Nervennaht. 4°. *Kiel*, 1878.

KRECKE (A.) * Ueber Nervennaht. 8°. *Erlangen*, 1885.

LANGERFELDT (O.) * Die Nervennaht. 8°. *Berlin*, [1877].

LEMKE (F.) * Ueber Nervennaht. 8°. *Berlin*, 1876.

ORELINE (A.) * Ueber Nervennaht. 8°. *Würzburg*, 1886.

PHILIPEAUX (J.-W.) & VULPIAN (A.) Recherches sur la réunion bout à bout des fibres nerveuses sensitives avec les fibres nerveuses motrices. 4°. *Paris*, [1863].

Repr. from : Compt. rend. Acad. d. sc., Par., 1863.

WEISSENSTEIN (R.) Ueber sekundäre Nervennaht, nebst Mittheilung zweier erfolgreicher Fälle. 8°. *Tübingen*, 1884.

WLAZLOWSKI (J.) * Zur Casuistik der Nervennaht. 8°. *Greifswald*, 1875.

Abraham (P. S.) On the suture of nerves. Ann. Surg., St. Louis, 1887, vi, 339–348.—**Ambrosoli** (C.) Sulla riunione dei nervi senzienti coi motori e sugli effetti che ne derivano. Gazz. med. ital. lomb., Milano, 1860, 4. s., v, 229; 237.—**Bernhardt** (M.) & **Treibel** (M.) Ein Fall von (secundärer) Nervennaht am Nervus ulnaris. Berl. klin. Wchnschr., 1881, xviii, 676.—**Bidder** (F.) Versuche über die Möglichkeit des Zusammenheilens functionell verschiedener Nervenfasern. Arch. f. Anat., Physiol. u. wissensch. Med., Berl., 1842, 102–120.—**Bouisson.** Présentation d'un malade ayant subi la suture primitive et directe du nerf médian. Compt. rend. Soc. de biol., Par., 1886, 8. s., iii, 571–574.—**Brown-Séquard** (C.-E.) Du rôle de certaines influences dynamogéniques réflexes dans des cas de suture de nerfs récemment publiés. *Ibid.*, 1884, 8. s., i, pt. 2, 423–425.—**Bruns** (P.) Ueber die Nervennaht. Med. Cor.-Bl. d. württemb. ärztl. Ver., Stuttg., 1884, liv, 17–21.—**Busch** (W.) Ueber Nervennaht. Verhandl. d. deutsch. Gesellsch. f. Chir., Berl., 1881, x, pt. 2, 465–473. *Also :* Arch. f. klin. Chir., Berl., 1881-2, xxvii, 327–335.—**Cerné.** De la suture des nerfs. Normandie méd., Rouen, 1885-6, i, 257–263.—**Chaput.** De la suture des nerfs. [Rev. crit.] Arch. gén. de méd., Par., 1884, ii, 205; 333.—**Chrétien** (J.) Plaie du nerf médian ; suture des deux bouts ; régénération et restauration fonctionnelle. Bull. et mém. Soc. de chir. de Par., 1883, n. s., ix, 879–882.—**Clark** (H. E.) Nerve suture ; recovery of function. Glasgow M. J., 1881, [4.] s., xvi, 62. ——. On the immediate suture of divided nerves. *Ibid.*, 1883, [4.] s., xx, 241–250.—**Dabney** (W. C.) Sutural re-union of divided nerves. Virginia M. Month., Richmond, 1879-80, vi, 757–763.—**Di Fede** (R.) Un caso di neurorafia per lesione del nervo radiale. Bull. d. r. Accad. med. di Roma, 1885, xi, 131–146. *Also :* Gior. di med. mil., Roma, 1885, xxxiii, 721–734.—**Dubrueil** (A.) Cicatrisation des nerfs et des muscles. Bull. Soc. anat. de Par., 1865, xl, 168. ——. Suture des nerfs. Gaz. hebd. de méd., Par., 1865, 2. s., ii, 124.—**Dunn** (H. P.) Suture of tendons and of the median nerve. Proc. W. Lond. Med.-Chir. Soc. 1884-6, Lond., 1887, ii, 85.—**Ehrmann** (J.) Observation de suture secondaire du nerf radial suivie de restauration fonctionnelle. Rev. de chir., Par., 1887, vii, 501–518. *Also :* Bull. et mém. Soc. de chir. de Par., 1887. n. s., xiii, 309–314.—**Eulenburg** (A.) & **Landois** (L.) Die Nerven-Naht. Berl. klin. Wchnschr., 1864, i, 441; 453; 466. ——. Ueber Nervenregeneration bei Anwendung der Sutur. *Ibid.*, 1865, ii, 96. *Also,*

Nerves (*Suture of*).

transl. : Gaz. méd. de Par., 1865, 3. s., xx, 170. — **Falkenheim** (H.) Zur Lehre von der Nervennaht und der Prima intentio nervorum. Deutsche Ztschr. f. Chir., Leipz., 1881-2, xvi, 31–103.—**Fux.** Ein Beitrag zur Nervennaht. Wien. med. Wchnschr., 1884, xxxiv, 1425–1429.—**Gluge** (G.) & **Thiernesse** (A.) Sur la réunion des fibres nerveuses sensibles avec les fibres motrices. Presse méd. belge, Brux., 1858-9, xi, 311; 319. *Also : J.* de la physiol. de l'homme, Par., 1859, ii, 686–695.—**Gunn** (M.) The union of nerves of different function considered in its pathological and surgical relations. Tr. Am. Surg. Ass., Phila., 1886, iv, 1–13. *Also :* Med. News, Phila., 1886, xlviii, 511–515.—**Harrison** (R.) Wound of wrist, with division of median and ulnar nerves ; complete paralysis of motion and sensation ; suture of nerves eighteen months afterwards ; recovery. Brit. M. J., Lond., 1886, i, 443.—**Hoffmann** (E.) Einige Fälle von Nervenlähmungen und Nervennaht. Mitth. a. d. chir. Klin. in Greifswald 1882-3, Wien u. Leipz., 1884, 118–124.—**Holmes** (T.) On a case of suture of the musculo-spiral nerve five months after its complete division, with ultimate restoration of its functions. Lancet, Lond., 1883, i, 1034.—**Holz.** Krankheitsfall ; Nervennaht. Berl. klin. Wchnschr., 1879, xvi, 50.—**Hulke** (J. W.) Case of sutural junction of the ulnar nerve fifteen weeks after its complete severance by a roofing-slate ; early restoration of function. Tr. Clin. Soc. Lond., 1879, xii, 207–210. *Also :* Brit. M. J., Lond., 1879, i, 819. *Also :* Med. Times & Gaz., Lond., 1879, i, 603. ——. A case of sutural union of the medium nerve in the lower part of the forearm five weeks after its division by a broken glass bottle, followed by return of function. Tr. Clin. Soc. Lond., 1880, xiii, 147–149. *Also :* Lancet, Lond., 1880, i, 288.—**Jencken** (F. J.) Suture of divided ulnar nerve after six months. Brit. M. J., Lond., 1887, ii, 1274.—**Johnson** (E. G.) Bidrag till kännedomen om nervsutur och nervtransplantation. Nord. med. Ark., Stockholm, 1882, xiv, no. 27, 1–73.—**Johnston** (W.) Union of nerves by sutures. St. Louis M. & S. J., 1865, n. s., ii, 289–293.—**Kraussold** (H.) Ueber Nerven- und Sehnennaht. Centralbl. f. Chir., Leipz., 1880, vii, 753–757. ——. Beitrag zum Kapitel der Nervennaht. *Ibid.*, 1882, ix, 201–203.—**Landois** (L.) & **Eulenburg** (A.) Ueber Nervenregeneration bei Anwendung der Sutur. Berl. klin. Wchnschr., 1865, ii, 96. — **von Langenbeck** (B.) Ueber Nervennaht. Verhandl. d. deutsch. Gesellsch. f. Chir. 1876, Berl., 1877, v, pt. 1, 106–115. ——. Ueber Nervennaht mit Vorstellung eines Falles von secundärer Naht des N. radialis. Berl. klin. Wchnschr., 1880, xvii, 101–103. *Also :* Verhandl. d. Berl. med. Gesellsch. (1879–80) 1881, xi, pt. 2, 86–93. *Also* [Abstr.] : Verhandl. d. deutsch. Gesellsch. f. Chir. 1880, Berl., 1881, ix, 50–53. *Also* [Abstr.] : St. Louis Cour. Med., 1881, v, 405.—**Langton** (J.) Operation for the union of a divided ulnar nerve. St. Barth. Hosp. Rep., Lond., 1881, xvii, 192.—**Laugier.** Note sur la suture du nerf médian. Rev. de thérap. méd.-chir., Par., 1864, xxxi, 396 ; 424. *Also :* France méd., Par., 1864, ii, 426 ; 484. *Also :* Bull. gén. de thérap., etc., Par., 1864, lxvii, 36; 136. —— Note sur la suture du nerf médian. Gaz. d. hôp., Par., 1864, xxxvii, 358.—**Létiévant.** Persistance de la motilité et de la sensibilité après la section des nerfs des membres. (Motilité et sensibilité suppléces.) Assoc. franç. pour l'avance. d. sc. Compt. rend. 1872, Par., 1873, i, 886–893.—**MacCormac** (W.) On some cases of neuroraphy or nerve suture. St. Thomas's Hosp. Rep. 1885, Lond., 1886, xv, 45–57.—**Mailer** (M.) Cases of suturing divided nerves and tendons. Austral. M. J., Melbourne, 1886, viii, 76.—**Markoe** (T. M.) Secondary nerve suture. N. York M. J., 1885, xli, 295–301. [Discussion], 310. *Also :* Med. News, Phila., 1885, xlvi, 285–291. [Discussion], 302. *Also :* Ann. Surg., St. Louis, 1885, ii, 181–197.—**Merriam** (L. A.) The union of divided nerves and the restoration of their function. St. Louis Cour. Med., 1882, viii, 398–401.—**Monod** (C.) Suture du nerf médian ; réunion. Bull. et mém. Soc. de chir. de Par., 1886, n. s., xii, 933–935.—**Morse** (J. F.) Successful union of a severed nerve by the catgut ligature. Pacific M. & S. J., San Fran., 1879-80, xxii, 465–467.—**Müller** (W.) Beitrag zur Frage der Nervennaht. Deutsche Ztschr. f. Chir., Leipz., 1884, xx, 305–313.—**Nicaise.** Suture des nerfs. Rev. de chir., Par., 1885, v, 373; 566. *Also :* Cong. franç. de chir. Proc.-verb., etc., 1885, Par., 1886, i, 330–335.—**Ogston** (A.) Suture of the ulnar nerve. Brit. M. J., Lond., 1881, i, 391.—**Page** (H. W.) The immediate suture of divided nerves. *Ibid.*, 717–719. ——. Case of secondary suture of ulnar nerve six months after its division. *Ibid.*, 1883, i, 1223.—**Park** (R.) Rupture of the sciatic nerve ; immediate union ; restoration of function. Chicago M. J. & Exam., 1884, xlviii, 632. ——. Division of the radial nerve and certain tendons ; suture of same after two weeks ; restoration of function. *Ibid.*, 633–635.—**Parker** (F. L.) Paralysis of extensor muscles of the hand and forearm from division of the posterior interosseous nerve ; complete recovery by resection and reunion of the ends of divided nerve with carbolized cat-gut sutures. Tr. South. Car. M. Ass., Charleston, 1881, xxxi, 101–104. ——. Primary and secondary reunion of divided nerves by suture. *Ibid.*, 1882, xxxii, 40–59.—**Philipeaux**

Nerves (*Suture of*).

(J.-M.) & **Vulpian** (A.) Recherches expérimentales sur la réunion bout à bout de nerfs de fonctions différentes. J. de la physiol. de l'homme, Par., 1863, vi, 421 ; 474. *Also*, Reprint. ———. Note sur des essais de greffe d'un tronçon du nerf lingual entre les deux bouts du nerf hypoglosse, après excision d'un segment de ce dernier nerf. Arch. de physiol. norm. et path., Par., 1870, iii, 619.—**Pick.** Suture of the musculo-spiral nerve six months after its complete division, with entire restoration of its functions about twelve months after operation. Lancet, Lond., 1883, ii, 184. *Also, transl.*: Union méd., Par., 1883, 3. s., xxxvi, 966–968. *Also, transl*: Bull. et mém. Soc. de chir. de Par., 1883, n. s., ix, 882–884.—**Pilcher** (L. S.) Suturing divided nerve trunks. Ann. Anat. & Surg. Soc., Brooklyn, N. Y., 1880, ii, 275–278.—**Polaillon.** Sur le retour immédiat de l'innervation après la suture des nerfs. Gaz. méd. de Par., 1887, 7. s., iv, 349 ; 361 ; 373 ; 385. ———. Suture secondaire du médian; retour très immédiat de la sensibilité. Bull. et mém. Soc. de chir. de Par., 1887, n. s., xiii, 339 – 346. [Disc.], 347–350.— De la suture des nerfs avec retour immédiat de l'innervation. J. de méd. de Par., 1887, xiii, 580–582. *Also*: Clinique, Brux., 1888, ii, 6–8.— **Pye** (W.) Nerve suture; strangulation at point of junction; operation ; rapid recovery of sensation and motion. Brain, Lond., 1885-6, viii, 255–258.—**Rawa.** Ueber das Zusammenwachsen von Nerven verschiedenster Bestimmung und verschiedenster Functionen. Arch. f. Physiol., Leipz., 1885, 296–328, 1 diag. *Also, transl.*: Zapiski Kievsk. Obsh. Estestvo., Kieff, 1884, vii, 433–474, 1 pl. *Also, transl.*: Voyenno-med. J., St. Petersb., 1884, cli, pt. 2, 1–40. ———. Ueber die Nervennaht. Wien. med. Wchnschr., 1885, xxxv, 321 ; 357.—**Reclus** (P.) De la suture et de la régénération des nerfs. Gaz. hebd. de méd., Par., 1884, 2. s., xxi, 447–449. — **Reger.** Ein Fall von secundärer Nervennaht des N. radialis dexter mit vollkommenem Erfolge. Berl. klin. Wchnschr., 1884, xxi, 327.—**Riedinger.** Ueber Nervenchirurgie. Sitzungsb. d. phys.-med. Gesellsch. zu Würzb., 1886, 43–46.—**Schramm** (H.) Beiträge zur Kasuistik und Technik der Nervennaht. Wien. med. Wchnschr., 1883, xxxiii, 1161 ; 1194. —**Schwartz** (E.) Plaie du poignet; section du nerf médian ; suture immédiate ; insuccès immédiat. Bull. et mém. Soc. de chir. de Par., 1886, n. s., xii, 942–944. — **Scott** (J. H.) Secondary suture of ulnar and median nerves. Lancet, Lond., 1887, i, 1091.—**Shepherd** (F. J.) Secondary suture of the ulnar nerve, with rapid restoration of sensation. Canada M. & S. J., Montreal, 1886-7, xv, 350–353. *Also*: Med. News, Phila., 1886, xlix, 697.—**Snamensky** (N. N.) Ein Fall von Nervennaht bei frischem Trauma. Deutsche Ztschr. f. Chir., Leipz., 1883-4, xix, 519–522. — **Sutton** (J. B.) Suture of the median nerve ten weeks after division, with recovery of function. [Abstr.] Proc. Roy. M. & Chir. Soc. Lond., 1885-7, n. s., ii, 170–176. *Also*: Lancet, Lond., 1887, i, 124.—**Tillaux.** Sur deux cas de suture secondaire du nerf médian avec rétablissement rapide de l'innervation dans les parties paralysées. Compt. rend. Acad. d. sc., Par., 1884, xcviii, 1516-1519. *Also*: Gaz. d. hôp., Par., 1884, lvii, 595. *Also*: Courrier méd., Par., 1884, xxxiv, 262–264. ———. Du traitement des sections nerveuses par la suture. Cong. franç. de chir. Proc.-verb., etc., 1886, Par., 1887, ii, 510–514. ———. Suture secondaire du nerf médian. Bull. et mém. Soc. de chir. de Par., 1887, n. s., xiii, 193–196.—**Tillmanns** (H.) Ueber Nervenverletzungen und Nervennaht. Verhandl. d. deutsch. Gesellsch. f. Chir., Berl., 1881, x, pt. 2, 197–298, 1 pl. ———. Ueber die operative Behandlung von Substanzverlusten an peripheren Nerven. Arch. f. klin. Chir., Berl., 1885, xxxii, 923–946. *Also*: Verhandl. d. deutsch. Gesellsch. f. Chir., Berl., 1885, xiv, pt. 2, 213–236.—**Vanlair** (C.) De la névrotisation du cartilage osseux dans la suture tubulaire des nerfs. Arch. de physiol. norm. et path., Par., 1882, 2. s., v, 595-614, 1 pl. ———. De la régénération des nerfs périphériques par le procédé de la suture tubulaire. Arch. de biol., Gand, 1882, iii, 379-496, 4 pl. *Also* [Abstr.]: Compt. rend. Acad. d. sc., Par., 1882, xcv, 99–101. ———. De l'organisation des drains de caoutchouc dans la suture tubulaire des nerfs. Rev. de chir., Par., 1886, vi, 649–655.—**Vulpian** (A.) Note sur de nouvelles expériences relatives à la réunion bout à bout du nerf lingual et du nerf hypoglosse. Arch. de physiol. norm. et path., Par., 1873, v, 597–602.— **Weissenstein** (R.) Ueber die sekundäre Nervennaht; nebst Mittheilung zweier erfolgreicher Fälle. Mitth. a. d. chir. Klin. zu Tübing., 1884, 2. Hft., 310–359.—**Wolberg** (L.) Igła do zszywania nerwów. [Needle-holder for sutures of nerves.] Medycyna, Warszawa, 1880, viii, 758–762. *Also, transl.* [Abstr.]: Centralbl. f. Chir., Leipz., 1880, vii, 705-707. ———. Krytyczne i doświadczalne badania nad zszywaniem i odt warzaniem się nerwów. [Experiments on nerve sutures.] Gaz. lek., Warszawa, 1881, 2. s., i, 749–751. *Also, transl.*: Centralbl. f. Chir., Leipz., 1881, viii, 593–595. ———. Kritische und experimentelle Untersuchungen über die Nervennaht und Nervenregeneration. Deutsche Ztschr. f. Chir., Leipz., 1882-3, xviii, 293 ; 485, 1 pl. : 1883, xix, 82–117.—**Zagórski** (K.) Przyczynek do kazuistyki szwów nerwowych. [On nerve sutures.] Gaz. lek., Warszawa, 1884, 2. s., iv, 897–901.— **Zesas** (D. G.) Durchtrennung des Nervus ulnaris, pa-

Nerves (*Suture of*).

raneurotische Naht 164 Tage nach der Durchtrennung; Heilung. Wien. med. Wchnschr., 1883, xxxiii, 1399.— **Znamenski** (M. N.) Sluchai nalojenija nervnago shva, vskore posle poranenija. [Suture of median nerve.] Laitop. khirurg. Obsh. v Mosk., 1882, v, 48–60.

Nerves (*Syphilis of*).

See **Nervous** system (*Syphilis of*).

Nerves (*Terminations of*).

See, *also*, **Conjunctiva** ; **Cornea** ; **Epidermis** ; **Muscles** (*Nerves of*) ; **Nerve** (*Olfactory*) ; **Pacinian** bodies.

AMANS (P.) * Des divers modes de terminaisons nerveuses. 4°. *Montpellier*, 1880.

ARONSON (H.) * Beiträge zur Kenntniss der centralen und peripheren Nervenendigungen. 8°. *Berlin*, [1886].

FINKAM (O.) * Ueber die Nervenendigungen im grossen Netz. 8°. *Göttingen*, 1873.

Also [Abstr.], *in*: Arch. f. Anat., Physiol. u. wissensch. Med., Leipz., 1873, 721–731.

IZQUIERDO (V.) * Beiträge zur Kenntniss der Endigung der sensiblen Nerven. 8°. *Strassburg*, 1879.

KRAUSE (W.) Die terminalen Körperchen der einfach sensiblen Nerven. 8°. *Hannover*, 1860.

REICH (B.) * Disquisitiones microscopicæ de finibus nervorum in glandulis salivalibus. 8°. *Vratislaviæ*, 1864.

SAZEPIN (B.) Ueber den histologischen Bau und die Vertheilung der nervösen Endorgane auf den Fühlern der Myriopoden. 4°. *St. Petersburg*, 1884.

Repr. from: Mém. Acad. imp. d. sc. de St.-Pétersb., 7. s., xxxii, no. 9.

SHVABOFF. * O nervach grudnoi plevi i ob ich okonchanii. [On thoracic nerves and their terminations.] 8°. *St. Petersburg*, 1873.

SUCHARD (E.) * Recherches sur la structure des corpuscules nerveux terminaux de la conjonctive et des organes génitaux. 4°. *Paris*, 1885.

Also, in: Arch. de physiol. norm. et path., Par., 1884, 3. s., iv, 337–347, 1 pl.

Arnold (J.) Ueber die Endigung der Nerven in der Bindehaut des Augapfels und die Krause'schen Endkolben. Arch. f. path. Anat., etc., Berl., 1862, xxiv, 250–286, 1 pl.— **Asp** (G.) Om nervernas ändningssätt i spottkörtlarna. Nord. med. Ark., Stockholm, 1873, v, no. 5, 1–9. ———. Bidrag till läran om nervändorganens utveckling. Nord. med. Ark., Stockholm, 1883, xv, no. 23, 1–30, 2 pl ———. Zur Lehre über die Bildung der Nervenendigungen. Mitth. a. d. embryol. Inst. d. k. k. Univ. in Wien, 1885, n. F., i, 1–16, 1 pl.—**Burkart** (R.) Ueber Nervenendigungen in den Tasthaaren der Säugethiere. Centralbl. f. d. med. Wissensch., Berl., 1870, viii, 514.—**Ditlevsen** (J. G.) Fölenervernes endelser hos mennesket og hvirveldyrene. Nord. med. Ark., Stockholm, 1876. viii, no. 11, 36. *Also, Reprint*.— **Dönitz** (W.) Ueber das Remak'sche Sinnesblatt. Arch. f. Anat., Physiol. u. wissensch. Med., Leipz., 1869, 600– 622, 1 pl.—**Eberth** (C. I.) Die Endigung der Hautnerven. Arch. f. mikr. Anat., Bonn, 1870, vi, 225 – 228.— **Eimer** (T.) Ueber die Nervenendigung in der Haut der Kuhzitze. *Ibid.*, 1872, viii, 643–646.—**Engelmann** (T. W.) Ueber die Endigungsweise der Geschmacksnerven des Frosches. Centralbl. f. d. med. Wissensch., Berl., 1867, v, 785-788.—**Flemming** (W.) Zur Kenntniss der sensiblen Nervenendigung; nach Arbeiten Ernst Fischer's. Arch. f. mikr. Anat., Bonn, 1880–81, xix, 513–522, 1 pl.—**Goujon** (E.) Sur un appareil de corpuscules tactiles situé dans le bec des perroquets. J. de l'anat. et physiol., etc., Par., 1869, vi, 449-455, 1 pl.—**Grandry.** Recherches sur la terminaison des nerfs cutanés chez l'homme. *Ibid.*, 1869, vi, 449-455, 1 pl.—**Hartmann** (R.) Ueber die Endigungsweise der Nerven in den Papillæ fungiformes der Froschzunge. Arch. f. Anat., Physiol. u. wissensch. Med., Leipz., 1863, 634 ; 710, 2 pl.—**Hensen.** Das Verhalten der Nerven an den Endapparaten von Sinnesorganen. Anat. Anz., Jena, 1887, ii, 375.—**Hoisholt** (A. W.) Is the nervous impulse delayed in the motor nerve terminations? J. Physiol., Lond., 1885 – 6, vi, 1– 21.—**Ihlder.** Die Nerven-Endigung in der Vogelzunge. Arch. f. Anat., Physiol. u. wissensch. Med., Leipz., 1870, 238–250, 1 pl.—**Inzani** (G.) Recherches sur la terminaison des nerfs dans les muqueuses des sinus frontaux et maxillaires. Lyon méd., 1872, x, 27–34, 2 pl.—**Izquierdo** (V.) Ueber die Endigungsweise der sensiblen Nerven. Nach Untersuchungen von Dr. . . . mitgetheilt von Prof.

Nerves (*Terminations of*).

Waldeyer. Arch. f. mikr. Anat., Bonn, 1879–80, xvii, 367–382.—**Kraus** (M.) Ueber den feineren Bau der Meissner'schen Tastkörperchen. Sitzungsb. d. k. Akad. d. Wissensch., Wien, 1878, lxxviii, 55–63, 1 pl. *Also*, Reprint.—**Krause** (W.) Ueber Nervenendigungen. Ztschr. f. rat. Med., Leipz. u. Heidelb., 1859, 3. R., v, 28–43, 2 pl. ——. Die Nervenendigung im Greifschwanz eines Affen der neuen Welt. *Ibid.*, 1866, 3. R., xxviii, 89–91, 1 pl. ——. Ueber die Nerven-Endigung am Anus des Menschen. Nachr. v. d. k. Gesellsch. d. Wissensch. u. d. Georg-Aug.-Univ., Götting., 1868, 191. ——. Ueber Nerven-Endigungen. *Ibid.*, 1869, 405. ——. Ueber die Endigungen der Drüsennerven. Arch. f. Anat., Physiol. u. wissensch. Med., Leipz., 1870, 9–27, 1 pl. ——. Die Nervenendigung innerhalb der terminalen Körperchen. Arch. f. mikr. Anat., Bonn, 1880–81, xix, 53–136, 3 pl. ——. Zur Pathologie der motorischen Endplatten. Deutsches Arch. f. klin. Med., Leipz., 1883, xxxiii, 435. ——. Die Nervenendigung in der äussern Haut und den Schleimhäuten. Biol. Centralbl., Erlang., 1884–5, iv, 161; 205—**Kühne** (W.) Vorläufige Bemerkungen zu einer vorläufigen Mittheilung des Hrn. A. Kölliker [betreffend dessen Erwiederung auf Dr. W. Kühne's Schrift, "Ueber die peripherischen Endorgane der mortorischen Nerven"]. Arch. f. path. Anat., etc., Berl., 1862, xxiv, 462. ——. Zur Lehre von den Endplatten der Nervenhügel. *Ibid.*, 1865, xxxiv, 412–422. ——. Zur Histologie der motorischen Nervenendigung. Untersuch. a. d. physiol. Inst. d. Univ. Heidelb., 1878, ii, 187–214. ——. Ueber motorische Nervenendigung. Verhandl. d. naturh.-med. Ver. zu Heidelb., 1882, n. F., iii, 97; 212.—**Langerhans** (P.) Zur pathologischen Anatomie der Tastkörper. Arch. f. path. Anat., etc., Berl., 1869, xlv, 413–417.—**Lavdovsky** (M.) Ueber die Endigung der Nerven in der Harnblase des Frosches. Centralbl. f. d. med. Wissensch., Berl., 1871, ix, 33–35.—**Leydig** (F.) Ueber die Schwanzflosse, Tastkörperchen und Endorgane der Nerven bei Batrachiern. Arch. f. mikr. Anat., Bonn, 1876, xii, 513–527, 1 pl.—**Lipmann** (H.) Ueber die Endigung der Nerven im eigentlichen Gewebe und im hinteren Epithel der Hornhaut des Frosches. Arch. f. path. Anat., etc., Berl., 1869, xlviii, 218–227, 1 pl.—**Luchsinger** (B.) Ueber Reizgifte peripherer Nervenenden. Arch. f. d. ges. Physiol., Bonn, 1882, xxviii, 80–84.—**Marchi** (V.) Sulle terminazioni periferiche dei nervi. Riv. sper. di freniat., Reggio-Emilia, 1882, viii, 477–489.—**Merkel** (F.) Bemerkungen zu Herrn Krause's Aufsatz über "die Nervenendigungen innerhalb der terminalen Körperchen". Arch. f. mikr. Anat., Bonn, 1880–81, xix, 523–528.—**von Mojsisovics** (A.) Ueber die Nervenendigung in der Epidermis der Säuger. Sitzungsb. d. k. Akad. d. Wissensch. Math.-naturw. Cl., Wien, 1875, lxxi, 242–248, 1 pl.—**Peyer** (J.) Ueber die peripherischen Endigungen der motorischen und sensiblen Fasern der in den Plexus brachialis des Kaninchens eintretenden Nervenwurzeln. Ztschr. f. rat. Med., Heidelb., 1854, 2. R., iv, 52–77.—**Pfitzner** (W.) Nervenendigungen im Epithel. Morphol. Jahrb., Leipz., 1882, vii, 726–745, 1 pl.—**Podcopaëw.** Ueber die Endigung der Nerven in der epithelialen Schicht der Haut. Arch. f. mikr. Anat., Bonn, 1869, v, 506–508.—**Ranvier** (L.) De la terminaison des nerfs dans les corpuscules du tact. Compt. rend. Acad. d. sc., Par., 1877, lxxxv, 1020–1023. ——. On the terminations of nerves in the epidermis. Quart. J. Micr. Sc., Lond., 1880, n. s., xx, 456–458, 1 pl.—**Remak** (R.) Ueber die Enden der Nerven im elektrischen Organ der Zitterrochen. Arch. f. Anat., Physiol. u. wissensch. Med., Leipz., 1856, 467–472.—**Robinson** (A. R.) Preliminary note on the mode of termination of the nerve entering into the formation of the "tactile corpuscle". Arch. Dermat., Phila., 1880, vi, 53.—**Rossi** (A.) Sul modo di terminare dei nervi nei muscoli dell' organa sonoro della cicala comune. Mem. Accad. d. sc. d. Ist. di Bologna, 1880, 4. s., i, 661–665, 1 pl.—**Rouget** (C.) Note sur la terminaison des nerfs dans les corpuscules de Pacini, dans les organes électriques et dans la peau. Bull. Acad. de méd., Par., 1865–6, xxxi, 802–808. ——. Mémoire sur les corpuscules nerveux qui se rencontrent à l'origine des nerfs sensitifs, dans les papilles de la peau et des muqueuses. Arch. de physiol. norm. et path., Par., 1868, i, 591–609, 2 pl.—**Rubio.** Sur une terminaison spéciale des nerfs. Assoc. franç. pour l'avance. d. sc. Compt. rend., Par., 1872–3, i, 930–932.—**Rudanovski** (P. W.) O prysutstvi sokratitelnych dementov v pervitelnych trubkach perefericheskich nervov. [On the final termination of the nerves in the texture of the organs.] Med. Vestnik, St. Petersb., 1869, ix, no. 18, 141–144.—**Schöbl** (J.) Die Flughaut der Fledermäuse, namentlich die Endigung ihrer Nerven. Arch. f. mikr. Anat., Bonn, 1871, vii, 1–31. ——. Ueber die Nervenendigung an den Tasthaaren der Säugethiere sowie über die feinere Struktur derselben. Abhandl. d. math.-naturw. Cl. d. k. böhm. Gesellsch. d. Wissensch. 1871–2, Prag, 1872, 1–16. ——. Ueber die Nervenendigung an den Tasthaaren der Säugethiere, sowie über die feinere Structur derselben. Arch. f. mikr. Anat., Bonn, 1873, ix, 197–219, 2 pl.—**Schultze** (M.) Ueber die Nervenendigungen in den Sinnesorganen. Verhandl. d. naturh. Ver. d. preuss. Rheinl. u. Westphal.,

Nerves (*Terminations of*).

1862, xix, 121–123.—**Schulze** (F. E.) Ueber die Nervenendigung in den sogenannten Schleimkanälen der Fische und über entsprechende Organe der durch Kiemen athmenden Amphibien. Arch. f. Anat., Physiol. u. wissensch. Med., Leipz., 1861, 759–769, 1 pl.—**Sertoli** (E.) Anatomia; sulla terminazione dei nervi nei peli tattili. R. Ist. Lomb. di sc. e lett. Rendic., Milano, 1872, 2. s., v, 565–567.—**Stirling** (W.) & **Macdonald** (J. F.) The minute structure of the palatine nerves of the frog, and the termination of nerves in blood-vessels and glands. J. Anat. & Physiol., Lond., 1882–3, xvii, 293–307, 1 pl.—**Thin** (G.) On the structure of the tactile corpuscles. *Ibid.*, 1873–4, viii, 30–38, 2 pl. *Also*, Reprint. *Also, transl.:* Sitzungsb. d. k Akad. d. Wissensch. Math.-naturw. Cl., Wien, 1873, lxvii, 130–134, 1 pl.—**Valentin** (G.) Ueber den Verlauf und die letzten Enden der Nerven. Nova acta phys.-med. Acad. nat. curios., Vratisl. et Bonnæ, 1836, xviii, pt. 1, 51; 541, 8 pl. *Also*, Reprint.—**Viallanes** (H.) Sur les terminaisons nerveuses sensitives dans la peau de quelques insectes. Compt. rend. Acad. d. sc., Par., 1880, xci, 1089–1091. ——. Note sur les terminaisons nerveuses sensitives des insectes. Bull. Soc. philomat. de Par., 1881–2, 7. s., vi, 94–98.—**Virchow** (R.) Ueber neurotische Atrophie. Verhandl. d. Berl. med. Gesellsch., 1879–80, xi, 169–180. *Also:* Berl. klin. Wchnschr., 1880, xvii, 409–412.—**Wolff** (W.) Ueber freie sensible Nervenendigungen. Arch. f. mikr. Anat., Bonn, 1881–2, xx, 377–381, 1 pl.

Nerves (*Tumors of*).

See, also, **Nerve** (*Brachial, Diseases, etc., of*); **Nerve** (*Sciatica, Tumors of*); **Nerve** (*Ulnar*); **Nerves** (*Hypertrophy of*); **Neuroma.**

ALEXANDER (F. S.) * De tumoribus nervorum. 8°. *Lugd. Bat.*, 1810.

ARONSSOHN (J.-L.) Observations sur des tumeurs développées dans les nerfs. 4°. *Strasbourg*, 1822.

BAUMEISTER (T.) * De tumoribus nervorum, adjecto eorum casu novo. 8°. *Bonnæ*, [1833].

DUNCAN (J.) Case of fibrous tumour surrounding the right sciatic nerve. 8°. [*Edinburgh, n. d.*]

FOUCAULT (P.) * Sur les tumeurs des nerfs mixtes. 4°. *Paris*, 1872.

GIRARDIN (E.) * Des tumeurs des nerfs en général et des nerfs du creux poplité en particulier. 4°. *Paris*, 1876.

GIRAUDET (L.-E.) * Des diverses tumeurs des nerfs. 4°. *Paris*, 1852.

KUPFERBERG (F.) * Ein Beitrag zur pathologischen Anatomie der Geschwülste im Verlaufe der Nerven. 4°. *Mainz*, 1854.

POMORSKI (J.) * Ein Fall von Rankenneurom der Intercostalnerven, Fibroma molluscum und Neurofibroma. 8°. *Greifswald*, 1887.

TOUREN (T.-B.) * Observation d'un fibrome généralisé des nerfs de la vie de relation et de la vie organique. 4°. *Montpellier*, 1885.

Bard (L.) Des tumeurs du type nerveux, neurosarcomes et névromes adultes. Arch. de physiol. norm. et path., Par., 1885, 3. s., v, 385–397, 1 pl.—**Barkow** (H. C. L.) Bemerkungen über Nervenanschwellungen. Nova acta. phys.-med. Acad. nat. curios., Bonnæ. 1829, xiv, 517–544, 1 pl. *Also*, Reprint.—**Barrett** (J. W.) Two cases of neuro-fibromata. Med. Times & Gaz., Lond., 1883, ii, 7.—**Bauchet.** Tumeur fibro-plastique de la gaine du nerf médian. Bull. Soc. de chir. de Par. (1864), 1865, 2. s., v. 429–431.—**Bellamy** (E.) A communication on the removal of a growth from the brachial plexus, affecting the roots of the eighth cervical and first dorsal nerves at their emergence from the intervertebral foramina. Med.-Chir. Tr., Lond., 1886, lxix, 211–216.—**Berger** (P.) Gliomes développés sur le trajet des branches du nerf de la cinquième paire chez la peuti. Arch. de physiol. norm. et path., Par., 1873, v, 235–237.—**Bergeron** (A.) Myxôme du nerf tibial postérieur gauche. Bull. Soc. anat. de Par. (1872), 1874, xlvii, 5.—**Bertolet** (R. M.) Myxomatous neurome of the brachial plexus. Tr. Path. Soc. Phila., 1876, v, 188.—**Bouvier.** Tumeurs fusiformes des nerfs. Bull. Acad. de méd., Par., 1846–7, xii, 216–221.—**Bruce** (J.) Case of tumours on the branches of the spinal nerves. Edinb. M. & S. J., 1844, lxii, 128.—**Bruce** (J. M.) & **Bellamy** (E.) On a case of removal of a tumour from the roots of the last cervical and first dorsal nerves. [Abstr.] Proc. Roy. M. & Chir. Soc. Lond., 1885–6, n. s., ii, 40–43. *Also:* Lancet, Lond., 1886, i, 107.—**Bruce** (J. M.) & **Mott** (F. W) Case of myxo-fibroma of the fifth dorsal nerve, extending on to the spinal cord. Brain, Lond., 1887–8, x, 210–217.—**Brun**

Nerves (*Tumors of*).

(P.) Trois tumeurs sur le trajet du nerf médian. J. de méd. de Lyon, 1842, iii, 274. *Also, transl.:* Lancet, Lond., 1842-3, ii, 141.—**Chvostek.** Ein Fall von Sarkom des rechten N. facialis an der Schädelbasis. Wien. med. Presse, 1883, xxiv, 1057-1060.—**Colborne** (W. H. Y.) Case of bony tumour in a nerve. Prov. M. & S. J., Lond., 1845, 649.—**Cornil** (V.) Sur la production de tumeurs épithéliales dans les nerfs. J. de l'anat. et physiol., etc., Par., 1864, i, 183-198, 1 pl. *Also,* Reprint.—**Cornil & Martineau.** Tumeur à myélocytes des nerfs de la queue de cheval; altération de ces nerfs et dégénération secondaire des cordons postérieurs de la moelle dans toute sa hauteur. Compt. rend. Soc. de biol. 1865, Par., 1866, 4. s., ii, 88-90.—**Coze** (F.-M.) Observations sur les tumeurs cancéreuses des nerfs et sur la résorption du crystallin. J. univ. d. sc. méd., Par., 1820, xix, 98-105.—**Crocker** (H. R.) A case of papillary growths in the course of nerves. Med. Times & Gaz., Lond., 1880, i, 633.—**Duplay** (S.) Sarcome du nerf cubital. Progrès méd., Par., 1877, v, 383.—**Exchaquet.** Chondrome du nerf radial. Bull. Soc. anat. de Par., 1874, xlix, 307-309.—**Foucault.** Fibro-sarcome du nerf spinal. *Ibid.*, 1871, xlvi, 362.—**Garretson** (J. E.) Nerve-tumor. Phila. M. Times, 1880-81, xi, 181. *Also:* Tr. Path. Soc. Phila. (1879-81), 1882, x, 176. . Nerve-tumor removed from the centre of the posterior tibial. Tr. Path. Soc. Phila. (1879-81), 1882, x, 176.—**Gibbs** (H. L.) Case of a tumor of the radial or spiral nerve of the right arm. Lond. M. Gaz., 1829, iv, 269-271.—**Gutteridge** (T.) Tumor of the peritoneal nerve. *Ibid.*, 1840-41, xxvii, 282.—**Hare** (E. S.) Tumor implicating the nerves of the left side. *Ibid.*, 1838-9, xxiii, 16-18.—**Howard** (R. L.) Tumor of a nerve. Ohio M. & S. J., Columbus, 1851-2, iv, 286-288.—**Hueter** (C.) Myxom des N. tibialis; zur Anatomie der Nervenmyxome; Verhalten des Fusses nach Lähmung des N. tibialis. Arch. f. klin. Chir., Berl., 1866, vii, 827-841.—**Hugnier.** A case of cancerous encephaloid neuroma developed in the course of the tibial nerve. Lancet, M. & S., Louisville, 1848, 3. s., ii, 1-5.—**Hume** (G. H.) A case of sarcoma of the internal popliteal nerve. Lancet, Lond., 1886, ii, 344.—**Key** (A.) Om svulstmetastaser inom centrala nervsystemets serösa banor och särskildt om araknoidalfransarnas rol därvid. [On metastatic tumors of the nervous . system.] Skrift. til. Univ. i Kjøbenh. v. d. Fyrahundra-Års-Fest af Karol. med.-kir. Inst. i Stockholm, 1879, 1-88, 4 pl. *Also:* Nord. med. Ark., Stockholm, 1879, xi, no. 15, 1-20, 1 pl.; no. 20, 1-40, 2 pl.; no. 29, 1-19. . Neuroganglioma verum periphericum. Förh. v. Svens. Läk.-Sällsk. Sammank., Stockholm, 1879, 140-143. *Also, transl.:* Physician & Surg., Ann Arbor, Mich., 1881, iii, 35.—**Kraussold** (H.) Beitrag zur Nervenchirurgie; Sarcom des N. medianus; Resection eines 11 cm. langen Stückes; keine Sensibilitätsstörungen. Arch. f. klin. Chir., Berl., 1877, xxi, 448-462.—**Lenoir.** Tumeur du volume d'un œuf de pigeon développée dans l'aisselle dans l'épaisseur du nerf median. Bull. Soc. anat. de Par., 1838, xiii, 133. . Tumeur développée dans l'épaisseur du nerf médian à deux pouces au-dessous du coude. *Ibid.*, 133.—**McBurney** (C.) Fibro sarcoma of the median nerve. N. York M. J., 1886, xliii, 504. . Fibro-sarcoma of the median nerve; excision. *Ibid.*, 1887, xlvi, 692.—**McGraw** (T. A.) Cystic tumor of the popliteal nerve. Detroit Rev. Med. & Pharm., 1871, vi, 304-306.—**Maclean** (D.) Fibroid tumor in the sheath of the median nerve. Louisville M. News, 1877, iii, 148.—**Moore** (C. H.) Account of an arterio-venous cyst in the popliteal nerve, for which the limb was amputated. Med.-Chir. Tr., Lond., 1866, xlix, 29-38.—**Nancrede** (C. B.) A tumor composed of miliary tubercles of the subcutaneous adipose tissue connected with one of the anterior cutaneous branches of the lumbar nerves. Proc. Path. Soc. Phila., 1881-3, xi, 81-83. *Also:* Boston M. & S. J., 1883, cviii, 324. *Also:* St. Louis M. & S. J., 1883, xliv, 511-513.—**Neumann** (E.) Secundäre Cancroïdinfiltration des Nervus mentalis bei einem Fall von Lippencancroïd. Arch. f. path. Anat., etc., Berl., 1862, xxiv, 201.—**Nicoladoni** (C.) Spindelzellensarkom am Nervus ischiadicus sin. Deutsche Ztschr. f. Chir., Leipz., 1873, ii, 531-537.—**Ormerod.** Enlargement of the median nerve. Brit. M. J., Lond., 1881, i, 88.—**Patterson.** Oblong tumour (false neuroma) removed from median nerve in the upper arm. Glasgow M. J., 1875, [4.] s., vii, 283.—**Pomorski** (J.) Ein Fall von Rankenneurom der Intercostalnerven mit Fibroma molluscum und Neurofibromen. Arch. f. path. Anat., etc., Berl., 1888, cxi, 60-75, 1 pl.—**Renaut** (J.) Note sur le gliome neuroformatif et l'équivalence nerveuse de la névroglie. Gaz. méd. de Par., 1884, 7. s., i, 614-616.—**Rivington** (W.) Neuroma of the median nerve removed by operation. Brain, Lond., 1881-2, iv, 552.—**Satterthwaite** (T. E.) Multiple tumors of the cranial, spinal, and sympathetic nerves with remarkably few symptoms. Med. Rec., N. Y., 1880, xvii, 239.—**Schäffer.** Tumor nervorum. Gen.-Ber. d. k. rhein. Med.-Coll. 1838, Koblenz, 1840, 139.—**Shepherd.** Small tumor on nerve; intense brachial neuralgia; removal. Canada M. Rec., Montreal, 1883-4, xii, 80. *Also:* Canada M. & S. J., Montreal, 1883-4, xii, 355.—**Spangenberg.** Ueber Nervenanschwellungen. Arch. f. med.

Nerves (*Tumors of*).

Erfahr., Berl., 1804, v, 306-312.—**Syme** (J.) Tumour of the median nerve. Lond. & Edinb. Month. J. M. Sc., 1841, i, 9.—**Testut** (L.) Destruction progressive du nerf médian par une tumeur, et suppléance de ce dernier par le nerf cubital; observation clinique suivie d'autopsie. Gaz. méd. de Bordeaux, 1875, iv, 121; 150; 183, 1 pl.—**Tillaux.** Tumeur du plexus brachial. Semaine méd., Par., 1887, vii, 121.—**Van Imschoot** (F.) Fibrosarcome caverneux du nerf radial (propagé au triceps brachial). Ann. Soc. de méd. de Gand, 1887, lxvi, 14-26.—**Van Santvoord** (R.) A case of mixed round- and spindle-celled sarcoma of retro-peritoneal glands, corda equina, nerveroots, dura of spine and brain, pons, medulla and corpora striata. Med. Rec., N. Y., 1887, xxxi, 10.—**Velpeau.** Tumeur de la gaine du nerf médian. Gaz. d. hôp., Par., 1864, xxxvii, 458.—**Verstraeten.** Lipôme du nerf récurrent gauche. Presse méd. belge, Brux., 1875-6, xxviii, 329-332.—**Völker** (O.) & **Schulz** (R.) Ein Fall von Neurom des Nervus peronæus profundus. Deutsche Ztschr. f. Chir., Leipz., 1878-9, xi, 77-86, 2 pl.—**Webber** (S. G.) Neuromata and neuroplastic formations. Cycl. Pract. M. (Ziemssen), N. Y., 1881, Suppl., 532.—**Weber** (O.) Ueber eine Nervengeschwulst. Verhandl. d. naturh.-med. Ver. zu Heidelb., 1865-8, iv, 99-101. . Exstirpation eines Gliosarcoms vom Nervus cruralis mit einem Stücke der Arteria und Vena femoralis; Perforation der Vene durch die Geschwulst; ungestörte Ernährung des Beins; Wiederherstellung der Nervenleitung. Deutsche Klinik, Berl., 1867, xix, 285. — **Werner.** Medullarkrebs des Nervus radialis; Exstirpation; Tod an Krebsrecidiv. Med. Cor.-Bl. d. württemb. ärztl. Ver., Stuttg., 1858, xxviii, 225.—**von Winiwarter** (A.) Plexiformes Fibro-Neurom der Armnerven mit circumscripter Hauthypertrophie und Sarcomentwickelung; ein Beitrag zur Geschwulstlehre. Arch. f. klin. Chir., Berl., 1875-6, xix, 595-643, 2 pl.—**Wutzer.** Ueber Nervengeschwülste. Verhandl. d. naturh. Ver. d. preuss. Rheinl. u. Westphal., Bonn, 1854, xi, 198-200.

Nerves (*Wounds and injuries of*).

See, also, **Epilepsy** (*Causation of*); **Extremity** (*Upper, Wounds, etc., of*); **Eyebrow** (*Wounds of*); **Fingers** (*Gangrene of*); **Humerus** (*Fracture of, Complications, etc., of*); **Nerves** (*Brachial, Diseases, etc., of*); **Nerves** (*Compression, etc., of*); **Nerves** (*Degeneration, etc., of*); **Nerves** (*Surgery of*); **Nerves** (*Suture of*); **Neuralgia** (*Traumatic*); **Neuritis**; **Neurotomy,** *etc.*; **Paralysis**; **Skin** (*Diseases of, Neurotic*); **Stumps**; **Tetanus** (*Causes of*), *and under individual nerves, as:* **Nerve** (*Facial*), **Nerve** (*Median*), *etc.*

BANKS (W. M.) On some peculiar results of injury to digital nerves. 8°. [*Liverpool, n. d.*]

BASILE (G.) Esito delle varie lesioni violente dei nervi motori in ordine ai debilitamenti dimostrati sperimentalmente su diversi animali. 8°. *Trani,* 1885.

BEAUGRAND (G.) * Des lésions traumatiques des nerfs. 4°. *Strasbourg,* 1864.

BÉGUÉ. * Du spasme traumatique consécutif aux déchirures incomplètes des nerfs. 4°. *Paris,* 1885.

BELLEAU (C.) * Essai sur les lésions des nerfs par coup de feu. 4°. *Paris,* 1872.

CAUSARD (V.-A.) * Essai sur la paralysie suite de contusion des nerfs. 4°. *Paris,* 1861.

COUYBA (L.) * Des troubles trophiques consécutifs aux lésions traumatiques de la moelle et des nerfs. 4°. *Paris,* 1871.

CUNIN (L.) * Des blessures de nerfs par coups de feu. 4°. *Paris,* 1873.

DOBBERT (G. A.) * Ueber Nervenquetschung. 8°. *Königsberg,* 1878.

EICHEL (J.) * De punctura nervorum. 4°. *Jenæ,* [1689].

GOLDSCHMIDT (H.) * Untersuchungen über den Einfluss von Nerven-Verletzungen auf die elektrische Erregbarkeit von Nerv und Muskel. [Strasburg.] 8°. *Berlin,* 1877.

GUENOT (F.-M.-É.) * Sur la paralysie consécutive à la compression des nerfs. 4°. *Paris,* 1872.

LARNE (P.-E.) * Des blessures des nerfs par les armes à feu. 4°. *Paris,* 1871.

LONDE (C.) * Recherches sur les névralgies consécutives aux lésions des nerfs. 4°. *Paris,* 1860.

Nerves (*Wounds and injuries of*).

LOZES (P.) *Propositions sur les lésions des nerfs par cause extérieure, suivies de quelques observations de chirurgie pratique. 4°. *Paris, an XII* [1804].

MIE (E.) *De functionibus læsione nervorum alienatis. 8°. *Halæ*, [1818].

MITCHELL (S. W.) Injuries of nerves and their consequences. 8°. *Philadelphia*, 1872.

———. The same. Des lésions des nerfs et de leurs conséquences. Trad. et annoté . . . par M. Dastre et precédé d'une préface par M. Vulpian. 8°. *Paris*, 1874.

MOREHOUSE (G. R.) & KEEN (W. W.) Gunshot wounds and other injuries of nerves. 12°. *Philadelphia*, 1864.

DE PARADES (É.) *Étude sur les lésions traumatiques des nerfs et leurs suites. 4°. *Paris*, 1873.

PETSCHULL (O.) *Ueber Schussverletzungen des Nervensystems. 8°. *Berlin*, [1881].

PINEAU (E.-J.-M.) *De quelques accidents névropathiques à distance observés tardivement à la suite de lésions des nerfs. 4°. *Paris*, 1877.

PORSON (L.) *Étude sur les troubles trophiques consécutifs aux lésions traumatiques des nerfs. 4°. *Paris*, 1873.

ROCHÉ (E.-H.-L.) *Des accidents nerveux traumatiques. 4°. *Paris*, 1861.

WALB (H.) *Ueber die Schussverletzungen der Nerven. 8°. *Bonn*, [1871].

WEIGERT (C.) *De nervorum læsionibus telorum ictu effectis. sm. 8°. *Berolini*, 1866.

WOLFF (G. F.) *Experimenta quædam de nervorum læsionibus. 8°. *Halæ*, [1818].

Bailhache (P. H.) A needle prick and its consequences. Maryland M. J., Balt., 1878-9, iv, 5-8. — **Balling** (F. A.) Ueber Nervenwunden. J. d. Chir. u. Augenh., Berl., 1837, xxvi, 64-69. — **Banks** (W. M.) On some peculiar results of injury to digital nerves. Liverpool M. & S. Rep., 1869, iii, 64-72.— **Bell** (G.) Case of a wounded nerve, followed by severe consequences, and cured by removing the wounded portion of the nerve. Edinb. J. M. Sc., 1826, i, 325-331. — **Benedikt.** Ueber traumatische Reflexneurosen. Wchmbl. d. k. k. Gesellsch. d. Aerzte in Wien, 1867, 108-110. *Also:* Allg. Wien. med. Ztg., 1867, xii, 78.— **Bérard** (A.) Note sur les accidents qui suivent la piqûre des nerfs. J. d. conn. méd.-chir., Par., 1845-6, xiii, pt. 2, 89-92.— **Bergeron** (A.) Plaies complètes des nerfs. France méd., Par., 1874, xxi, 313; 330; 457.—**Beurtheilung** (Zur) der Verletzungen der Nerven. Bl. f. gerichtl. Anthrop., Ansbach, 1854, v, 2. Hft., 45-56.— **Bowlby** (A. A.) Lectures on injuries of nerves. Lancet, Lond., 1887, i, 863; 921; 968; 1021; 1121; ii, 53; 99. — **Brambilla** (A.) Observatio de spasmo cynico fortuitam nervi læsionem insecuto. Acta Acad. Cæs. reg. Joseph. med.-chir. Vindob., 1788, i, 189-195. *Also, transl.:* Actes Acad. c. r. Joséphine méd.-chir. de Vienne, Montpel.. 1792, i, 236-242.—**Brenner.** Fall von traumatischer Lähmung sämmtlicher Nervenstämme der einen oberen Extremität. St. Petersb. med. Ztschr., 1871, n. F., ii, 273. — **Bresgen.** Traumatische Reflexneurose oder Simulation? Allg. med. Centr.-Ztg., Berl., 1874, xl, 1033-1036. — **Broadbent** (W. H.) Cases of local paralysis, etc., from injury or disease of nerves. Brit. M. J., Lond., 1870, i, 434-436.—**Brown-Séquard** (C. E.) Remarks on some interesting effects of injuries of nerves, as shown in three cases. Arch. Scient. & Pract. M & S., N. Y., 1873, i, 54-59. — **Callender** (G. W.) Injuries to nerves, tendons, and ligaments, complicating joint fractures. St. Barth. Hosp. Rep. Lond., 1870, vi, 37. ———. Nutrition spoiled after hurts to nerves. *Ibid.*. 42-47.— **Charvot.** De la névrite traumatique et de ses conséquences en chirurgie. Arch. gén. de méd., Par., 1885, ii, 151; 440; 572; 669. — **Chouppe.** Troubles trophiques à la suite de lésions traumatiques des nerfs de la jambe. Compt. rend. Soc. de biol., Par., 1875, 6. s., ii, 322.—**Clarke** (J. L.) & **Brown-Séquard** (C. E.) Nerves (Injuries of). Syst. Surg. (Holmes), 2. ed., N. Y., 1870, iv, 159-208.— **Clemens** (T.) Ueber partiellen Nerventod, durch traumatische Momente hervorgebracht. Deutsche Klinik, Berl., 1850, ii, 552.—**Coup** d'œil sur la valeur de l'électricité dans le traitement des paralysies de cause traumat-que Bull. gén. de thérap., etc., Par., 1852, xliii, 299; 450.—**Croft.** Punctured wound of the leg, with wound of the posterior tibial and peroneal arteries and posterior tibial nerve; ligature; neuroraphy; recovery. Brit. M. J., Lond., 1887, ii, 774.—**Crummer** (B. F.) The trophic effects of nerve injury. Tr. Illinois M. Soc., Chicago, 1883, xxxiii, 148-151. ———. A case of nerve injury followed by

Nerves (*Wounds and injuries of*).

trophic changes. Weekly M. Rev., Chicago, 1883, vii, 419.—**D.** De l'emploi de électricité d'induction dans le traitement des paralysies de traumatiques. Bull. gén. de thérap., etc., Par., 1852, xliii, 491; 534.—**Dastre & Morat.** Dilatation sympathique croisée, à la suite de l'ablation du ganglion cervical supérieur. Compt. rend. Soc. de biol. 1880, Par., 1881, 7. s., ii, 303. *Also:* Progrès méd., Par., 1880, viii, 867.—**Dickman** (F. F.) A rare case of peri-neuritis following nerve lesion. St. Louis M. & S. J., 1879, xxxvii, 543-549.—**Dresbach** (E.) A case of severe nervous affection resulting from injury of the fibrillæ of the musculo-cutaneous nerve, produced by the introduction of a seton over the cephalic brain. Transylv. J. M., Lexington, Ky., 1837, x, 630-634. ———. Two cases of severe nervous affection, resulting from injury. West. Lancet, Cincin., 1850, xi, 210-215. — **Duménil.** Paralysie traumatique; guérison spontanée. Bull. Soc. de chir. de Par., 1872, 3. s., i, 172-174. — **Dwight** (T.) Injury of the posterior tibial nerve. Boston M. & S. J., 1867, lxxvi, 129.—**Eigenthümliche** Sensibilitätsstörung nach traumatischer Läsion eines peripheren Nerven. Berl. klin. Wchnschr., 1874, xi, 443.—**Eulenburg** (A.) Ueber traumatische Lähmung des N. peronæus, und die daraus entspringenden Deformitäten des Fusses. Greifswalder med. Beitr., Danzig, 1864, ii, 178-199. — **Fischer.** Ueber trophische Störungen nach Nervenverletzungen an den Extremitäten. Berl. klin. Wchnschr., 1871, viii, 145-147. *Also,* Reprint. *Also:* Verhandl. d. Berl. med. Gesellsch. (1869-71), 1872, pt. 1, 244-251. — **Fox** (T.) Constant and severe pain in the stomach, with vomiting after taking food, caused by implication of a divided nerve in cicatrix. St. Louis M. & S. J., 1870, n. s., vii, 136.—**Gilbert** (D. D.) Neuralgic affections after injuries of nerves. Boston M. & S. J., 1864, lxx, 340-342. — **Gillette.** Blessure du nerf tibial postérieur gauche par une lame de canif restée dans la plaie; accidents hystéro-épileptiformes; extraction du corps étranger. Union méd., Par., 1873, 3. s., xvi, 801-803.—**Giovanardi** (E.) Perizia medico-legale intorno ad una ferita di un ramo del nervo radiale. Spallanzani, Modena, 1876, xiv, 296-301.—**Gower.** Secondary arthritic changes in nerve-lesion. Brit. M. J., Lond., 1878, i, 753.—**Graefe** (E.) Bemerkungen über einige pathologische Erscheinungen bei Verletzungen der Nerven und ihrer Wiedervereinigung. J. f. Chir. u. Augenh., Berl., 1825, vii, 299-305.—**Gregory** [*et al.*]. Cases of injuries to nerves. St. Louis M. & S. J., 1880, xxxix, 747-752. — **Hamilton** (J.) On some effects resulting from wounds of nerves. Dublin J. M. Sc., 1838, xiii, 38-55. ———. On partial rupture of nerves. *Ibid.*, 1841-2, xx, 102-118. — **Hanken** (J. H.) Ueber die Folgen von Quetschung peripherischer Nerven. Internat. Monatschr. f. Anat. u. Histol., Leipz., 1886, iii, 265-284, 1 pl. — **Hannen** (H. S.) Gunshot wound of the neck, severing the cervical plexus of nerves. Boston M. & S. J., 1862-3, lxvii, 215. — **Harris** (T.) Wounds of nerves. Med. Exam., Phila., 1838, i, 1.—**Hawkins** (C.) Abstract of a lecture on injuries of the nerves. Med.-Chir. Rev., Lond., 1834-5, xxii, 234-241.— **Hayem** (G.) Nouvelle communication sur les altérations de la moelle consécutives aux lésions des nerfs. Compt. rend. Soc. de biol. 1874, Par., 1875, 6. s., i, 157. ———. Note sur un cas de troubles trophiques avec élévation de la température, consécutifs à une plaie intéressant plusieurs branches nerveuses. Arch. de physiol. norm. et path., Par., 1878, 2. s., v, 90-106. — **Helfft** (J.) Verletzung der Nerven. Wien. med. Wchnschr., 1853, iii, 134.— **Hélie** (T.) Blessure du nerf radial; réflexions sur les blessures des nerfs. J. de la sect. de méd. Soc. acad. Loire-Inf., Nantes, 1837, xiii, 23-37.—**Henriet** (L.) Des paralysies traumatiques des nerfs à propos d'un cas de paralysie traumatique du nerf médian. Tribune méd., Par., 1874, viii, 87; 111.—**Huguier.** Névralgie traumatique; plaie par arme à feu. Bull. Soc. de chir. de Par., 1851-2, ii, 498.— **Jayakar** (A. S. G.) Local anæsthesia of the foot from fracture of the tibia; hypodermic injections of strychnia; recovery. Med. Times & Gaz., Lond., 1871, ii, 347.— **Keen** (W. W.) Gunshot wounds and other injuries of nerves. Proc. Path. Soc. Phila. (1866-70), 1871, iii, 145.— **Kennedy** (J.) [Case of acute pain in arm from shot wound of neck.] Med. Essays & Obs. Soc. Edinb., 1733, i, 206-209.—**Key** (C. A.) Elbow and forearm of a man amputated two years after a gun-shot wound. Tr. Path. Soc. Lond., 1846-8, i, 313. — **Klaatsch.** Ueber Reflexneurosen nach Verletzungen. Wien. med. Wchnschr., 1857, vii, 3; 20.—**Laborde.** Présentation et description anatomique des altérations survenues chez un lapin à la suite de la section du nerf sciatique, datant de dix mois. Compt. rend. Soc. de biol. 1869, Par., 1870, 5. s., i, 344-346.— **Larrey.** Sur quelques phénomènes pathologiques observés dans la lésion des nerfs, et dans leur cicatrisation. Rev. méd., Par., 1824, i, 406-412.—**Lauth.** Note sur un cas de contusion du plexus cervical superficiel et du plexus brachial. Rev. de chir., Par., 1884, iv, 560-563.— **Lésions** (Des) traumatiques des nerfs et de leur influence sur la nutrition. Arch. gén. de méd., Par., 1865, i, 186-202.—**Lorinser** (F. W.) Ueber Quetschung des grossen Hüftnerven. Allg. Wien. med. Ztg., 1871, xvi, 345.— **Mantegazza** (P.) Delle alterazioni istologiche pro-

Nerves (*Wounds and injuries of*).

dotte dal taglio dei nervi. Gazz. med. ital. lomb., Milano, 1867, 5. s., vi, 149–152.—**Mascarel** (J.) Un nerf démis. France méd., Par., 1883, i, 703–705.—**May** (G.) Atrophy of the right deltoid muscle from injury of the circumflex nerve. Lond. M. Gaz., 1841–2, xxix, 50. — **Mitchell** (S. W.) The influence of nerve lesions upon temperature, as illustrating the mode in which nerves act to control thermal conditions. Arch. Scient. & Pract. M. & S., N. Y., 1873, i, 351–353. ———. Cases illustrating local injuries of nerves and their trophic consequences, with comments. Tr. Coll. Phys. Phila., 1875–6, 3. s., ii, 115–138, 1 pl. ———. Local injuries of nerves and their trophic consequences. Med. & Surg. Reporter, Phila., 1876, xxxv, 129. ———. Cases of lesions of peripheral nerve-trunks. Am. J. M. Sc., Phila., 1883, n. s., lxxxvi, 17–31.—**Moon** (W. P.) Gunshot wound of arm and forearm. (Neuralgia from lesion of nerves; excision of radial nerve; amputation.) *Ibid.*, 1868, n. s., lv, 54–62.—**Munro** (W. S.) Loss of a large portion of the right peroneal nerve and recovery of the patient without amputation. Lancet, Lond., 1865, i, 476.—**Nepveu.** Contribution à l'étude de la dénudation des nerfs. Gaz. hebd. de méd., Par., 1878, 2. s., xv, 68–72.—**Neumann** (E.) Degeneration und Regeneration nach Nervendurchschneidungen. Arch. d. Heilk., Leipz., 1868, ix, 193–218.—**Nicaise** (M.) Injuries and diseases of nerves. Transl. by J. H. C. Simes. Internat. Encycl. Surg. (Ashhurst), N. Y., 1883, iii, 545–641, 1 col. pl.—**Padieu** fils. Plaie par arme à feu à la région postérieure gauche du bassin ; paralysie consécutive du sentiment et du mouvement dans les parties auxquelles se distribue le nerf sciatique poplité externe. Soc. méd. d'Amiens. Bull., 1873, ix–xii, 153–157.—**Parker** (W.) Practical remarks on concussion of the nerves. N. York J. M., 1856, 3. s., i, 189–201.—**Parkhill** (C.) Injuries to the superior laryngeal nerve. Tr. Colorado M. Soc., Denver, 1887, 42.—**Parsons** (C. W.) On some of the remote effects of injuries of nerves. Am. J. M. Sc., Phila., 1851, n. s., xxi, 306–319.—**Paulet** (V.) Étude sur les suites immédiates ou éloignées des lésions traumatiques des nerfs. Mém. Soc. de chir. de Par., 1869, vii, 149–212. [Rap. de Tillaux]: Bull. Soc. de chir. de Par. (1868), 1869, 2. s., ix, 103–111.— **Philipeaux** (J.-M.) & **Vulpian** (A.) Recherches expérimentales sur la régénération des nerfs séparés des centres nerveux. Gaz. méd. de Par., 1860, 3. s., xv, 420; 446; 460; 476; 495; 526; 538; 575; 602. **Poinsot** (G.) Pathologie chirurgicale des nerfs. N. dict. de méd. et chir. prat., Par., 1877, xxiii, 624–698.— **Polaillon.** Plaie des nerfs; plaie intéressant les tendons de la face antérieure du poignet, les deux artères radiale et cubitale et les nerfs médian et cubitale; suture des tendons et des nerfs; retour de la mobilité des doigts; perte complète de la sensibilité malgré la suture nerveuse. Bull. et mém. Soc. de chir. de Par., 1887, n. s., xiii, 186–188.— **Pooley** (J. H.) Clinical notes on nerve injuries. Ohio M. Recorder, Columbus, 1880–81, v, 193–206. *Also,* Reprint.— **Poore** (G. V.) On the trophic changes which follow lesions of the nervous apparatus. Lancet, Lond., 1877, i, 713; 751.— **Prévost.** Régénération comparative des nerfs comprimés entre les mors d'une pince et des nerfs sectionnés. Compt. rend. Soc. de biol. 1871, Par., 1873, 5. s., iii, 143.— **Richelot** (L.-G.) Remarques sur la sensibilité collatérale, à propos de quelques observations de plaies nerveuses. France méd., Par., 1881, xxviii, 570; 581. *Also :* Bull. Soc. clin. de Par. (1881), 1882, v, 120–127.—**Richet.** Des plaies des nerfs et de la sensibilité récurrente. École de méd., Par., 1876, iii, 48–53.—**Romberg** (M. H.) Ein Fall von isolirter Lähmung der Extensoren des rechten Armes in Folge anhaltender mechanischer Compression. Deutsche Klinik, Berl., 1850, ii, 256.—**Ronflette.** Plaie par arme à feu; atrophie du deltoïde consécutive à la lésion du nerf circonflexe. Arch. méd. belges, Brux., 1882, 3. s., xxii, 117–125.—**Roonhuyse** (H.) Of a wounded nerve and its cure. *In his:* Med.-Chir. Obs., 12°, Lond., 1676, 193–195.—**Rosenthal** (M.) Ueber traumatische Nervenläsionen. Wien. med. Presse, 1868, ix, 221 : 1869, x, 966; 985; 1012.—**Ruhe.** Eine Verletzung des Plexus cruralis durch Fall. Deutsche Ztschr. f. prakt. Med., Leipz., 1877, iv, 598. — **Rumpf** (T.) Zur Degeneration durchschnittener Nerven. Untersuch. a. d. physiol. Inst. d. Univ. Heidelb., 1878, ii, 307–323.—**Salomon** (G.) Quetschung des N. peronæus. Charité Ann. 1878, Berl., 1880, v, 149–152.—**Schiefferdecker** (P.) Trophische Störungen nach peripheren Verletzungen. Berl. klin. Wchnschr., 1871, viii, 160–163.—**Sherwen** (J.) Case of the puncture of a nerve in phlebotomy. Med. & Phil. Comment., Lond., 1776, iv, 210–227.—**Terrillon.** Contribution à l'étude de la contusion des nerfs mixtes. Arch. de physiol. norm. et path., Par., 1877, 2. s., iv, 265–273. ———. De l'influence des lésions traumatiques des troncs des nerfs mixtes sur la calorification. Compt. rend. Soc. de biol. 1877, Par., 1879, 6. s., iv, 88–92.—**Tiffany** (L. McL.) Deformity of shoulder following nerve injury. Am. J. M. Sc., Phila., 1879, n. s., lxxviii, 85–88.—**Tillaux.** Des troubles de la sensibilité dans les lésions physiques des nerfs. France méd., Par., 1866, xiii, 453; 462.—**Tillmanns** (H.) Ueber Nervenverletzungen und Nervennaht. Arch. f. klin. Chir., Berl., 1881–2, xxvii, 1–102, 1 pl. — **Townsend**

Nerves (*Wounds and injuries of*).

(W. E.) Gun-shot wounds of the arm, followed by anæsthesia of part of hand. Boston M. & S. J., 1858, lviii, 37.— **Traumatic** paralysis of motion and sensation of the arms. N. Orl. M. & S. J., 1855–6, xii, 356 – 360.—**Teevan** (W.) Painful affection of the radial nerve following a trifling wound of the ball of the thumb. Lancet, Lond., 1832–3, i, 653–655. — **Tripier** (L.) Nerfs (pathologie chirurgicale). Dict. encycl. d. sc. méd., Par., 1877, 2. s., xii, 241–313.—**Vallez.** Observation d'atrophie traumatique consécutive à une lésion du nerf maxillaire supérieur droit (branche de la cinquième paire). J. de méd., chir. et pharmacol., Brux., 1846, iv, 22–25. — **Verpinet** (J. B.) History of an injury of a nervous filament of the fore-arm. Edinb. M. & S. J., 1807, iii, 14–16.—**Vitrac.** Exemples de troubles trophiques consécutifs aux sections incomplètes des nerfs. Rev. phot. d. hôp. de Par., 1871, iii, 222.—**Vulpian** (A.) Recherches relatives à l'influence des lésions traumatiques des nerfs sur les propriétés physiologiques et la structure des muscles. Arch. de physiol. norm. et path., Par., 1871–2, iv, 245; 3C0; 639, 1 pl.; 743, 1 pl.— **Wardrop** (J.) Case of a wounded nerve of the thumb, followed by severe symptoms, which were relieved by a division of the nerve. Med.-Chir. Tr., Lond., 1823, xii, 205–212.—**Westphal** (C.) Verlangsamung der Empfindungsleitung bei Verletzungen peripherischer Nerven. Neurol. Centralbl., Berl., 1883, ii, 59.

Nerves (*Brachial*) [*and brachial plexus*].

See, also, **Nerve** (*Median*); **Nerve** (*Musculocutaneous*); **Nerve** (*Musculo-spiral*); **Nerve** (*Radial*); **Nerve** (*Ulnar*); **Nerves** (*Abnormities of*); **Neurotomy,** etc.

KAUFMANN (F.) * Die Varietäten der Nerven des Plexus brachialis. 8°. *Giessen,* 1864.

KLINT (J. J.) * De nervis brachii. 4°. *Gottingæ,* 1784.

Also, in : SCRIPT. neurol. minores selecti. 4°. *Lipsiæ,* 1793, iii, 122–147.

KRAUSE (W.) Beiträge zur Neurologie der oberen Extremität. 4°. *Leipzig u. Heidelberg,* 1865.

Antonelli (G.) Sulla partecipazione del secondo nervo dorsale alla formazione del plesso brachiale nell' uomo. Resoc. Accad. med.-chir. di Napoli, 1882, xxxvi, 95–97.— **Forgue & Lannegrace.** Sur la distribution spéciale des racines motrices du plexus brachial. Compt. rend. Acad. d. sc., Par., 1884, xcviii, 829–831.—**Gruber** (W.) Geschichtliches über den an den Nervus ulnaris angeschlossenen Ast des Nervus radialis zum Musculus anconeus internus; J. Cruveilhier, 1837. (Ramus collateralis ulnaris nervi radialis; W. Krause, 1864.) Arch. f. Anat., Physiol. u. wissensch. Med., Leipz., 1869, 30–37. ———. Ueber die Verbindung des Nervus medianus mit dem Nervus ulnaris am Unterarme des Menschen und der Säugethiere. *Ibid.*, 1870, 501–522, 1 pl. — **Herringham** (W. P.) The minute anatomy of the brachial plexus. Proc. Roy. Soc. Lond., 1886, xli, 423–441.—**Krause** (W.) Beiträge zur systematischen Neurologie des menschlichen Armes. Arch. f. Anat., Physiol. u. wissensch. Med., Leipz., 1864, 349–357, 1 pl. ———. Ueber den Ramus collateralis ulnaris nervi radialis. *Ibid.*, 1868, 134–136. ———. Noch einmal der Ramus collateralis ulnaris nervi radialis. *Ibid.*, 1869, 422. — **Létiévant.** Phénomènes physiologiques et pathologiques consécutifs à la section des nerfs principaux du bras [nouvelle interprétation]. Lyon méd., 1869, iii, 150; 177; 225; 243, 6 pl. *Also :* Mém. et compt.-rend. Soc. d. sc. méd. de Lyon (1869), 1870, ix, 80, 6 pl. ; pt. 2, 217.— **Lucas** (R. C.) On the normal arrangement of the brachial plexus of nerves. Guy's Hosp. Rep., Lond., 1875, 3. s., xx, 539–546, 1 pl.—**Putnam** (J. J.) A contribution to our knowledge of the cutaneous distribution of the brachial and cervical plexuses. Boston M. & S. J., 1879, c, 118, 1 pl.—**Richelot** (L.-G.) Note sur la distribution des nerfs collatéraux des doigts et sur les sections nerveuses du membre supérieur. Arch. de physiol. norm. et path., Par., 1875, 2. s., ii, 177–194, 1 pl.— **Walsh** (J. F.) The anatomy of the brachial plexus. Am. J. M. Sc., Phila., 1877, n. s., lxxiv, 387–399.

Nerves (*Brachial, Diseases and injuries of*).

See, also, **Extremity** (*Upper, Paralysis of*); **Nerve** (*Circumflex*); **Nerves** (*Tumors of*); **Neuralgia** (*Brachial*).

Althaus (J.) On neuritis of the brachial plexus. Proc. Roy. M. & Chir. Soc. Lond. (1867–71), 1871, vi, 328.— **Arnozan** (X.) Plaie du nerf médian et du nerf cubital; troubles trophiques de la peau, des ongles, des poils, de la sécrétion sudorale. J. de méd. de Bordeaux, 1883–4, xiii, 308; 316. *Also :* Bull. Soc. d'anat. et physiol. . . . de Bordeaux, 1883, iv, 121–130.—**Cheever** (D. W.) Neuroma in the formative trunks of the brachial plexus. Med. & Surg.

Nerves (*Brachial, Diseases and injuries of*).

Rep. Bost. City Hosp., 1882, 3. s., 148-151.—**Chouppe.** Examen anatomique d'une tumeur développée au niveau de l'extrémité externe du plexus brachial. Bull. Soc. de chir. de Par. (1874), 1875, 3. s., iii, 724.—**Dwight** (T.) Rupture of the musculo-spiral nerve. Boston M. & S. J., 1867, lxxvi, 130.—**Effects** of injury to the median nerve. Med. Times & Gaz., Lond., 1876, i, 224.— **Farabeuf.** Note sur un cas d'invagination à trois cylindres du nerf médian dans sa gaine à la suite d'un arrachement. Bull. Soc. anat. de Par., 1868, xliii, 610-612.—**Fayrer** (J.) Injury to the musculo-cutaneous, "perforans casserii", and other nerves of the right arm. Med. Times & Gaz., Lond., 1867, i, 278.—**Gay** (C. C. F.) Injury to the brachial plexus resulting in gangrene of the arm and fore-arm; amputation. Buffalo M. & S. J., 1873-4, xiii, 17.—**Guéniot.** Paralysie des muscles du bras, consécutive à une compression du cou. Bull. Soc. de chir. de Par., 1872, 3. s., i, 348.—**Hawkins** (C.) Curious appearance of the median nerve. Lond. M. Gaz., 1827-8, i, 271.—**Hutchinson** (J.) A case of supposed rupture of most of the roots of the brachial plexus. Tr. Path. Soc. Lond., 1879-80, xxxi, 27-29. *Also:* Brit. M. J., Lond., 1880, i, 14. *Also:* Med. Times & Gaz., Lond., 1880, i, 23.—**Kraiss** (C.) Ueber eine vollständige Continuitäts-Trennung d. N. radialis, medianus, und eine unvollständige d. N. ulnaris. Med. Cor.-Bl. d. württemb. ärztl. Ver., Stuttg., 1869, xxxix, 259-262.—**Letenneur.** Coup de couteau dans la région axillaire gauche; section probablement complète des troncs vasculaires et du plexus brachial, phlébartérie, paralysie de la sensibilité et de la motilité; emploi de l'électricité, retour de la sensibilité, retour incomplet des mouvements. Bull. Soc. de chir. de Par. (1870), 1871, 2. s., xi, 314-320.—**Lindwurm.** Stich in den Oberarm mit Durchschneidung des Armnerven. Friedreich's Bl. f. gerichtl. Med., Nürnb., 1871, xxii, 231-235.—**Mader.** Eigenthümliche Neurose der Armnerven mit Trophoneurose. Ber. d. k. k. Krankenanst. Rudolph-Stiftung in Wien (1878), 1879, 359. ———. Neuritis ascendens brachial. ex traumata; Behandlung ohne Erfolg. *Ibid.* (1880), 1881, 343.—**Mauriac** (E.) Note sur un cas de paralysie des nerfs du plexus brachial et principalement du nerf radial résultant de l'usage des béquilles. Gaz. méd. de Bordeaux, 1876, v, 231-234.— **Meursinge** (N.) Contusio humeri dextri, met opvolgende anæsthesia plexus brachialis en atrophia muscularis totius extremitatis, volkomen genezen na eene behandeling van ruim 6 maanden. Nederl. Tijdschr. v. Geneesk., Amst., 1870, 2. R., vi, 49.—**Mills** (C. K.) Traumatic neuritis involving the brachial plexus. Phila. M. Times, 1876-7, vii, 564. ———. Neuritis and peri-neuritis of the brachial plexus. Med. & Surg. Reporter, Phila., 1881, xlv, 589-591.—**Mursick** (G. A.) Case of gun-shot injury of the median and internal cutaneous nerves of the right upper extremity; amputation after unsuccessful treatment by subcutaneous injections of morphia, etc. N. York M. J., 1866, ii, 174-180.—**Neuritis** of the brachial plexus. *Ibid.*, 1878, xxviii, 178.—**Pozzi** (S.) Névrite traumatique du plexus brachial droit; atrophie musculaire du membre blessé; troubles trophiques (éruption vésiculeuse) de la main droite; lésion trophique symétrique du côté sain (main gauche). Gaz. méd. de Par., 1883, 6. s., v, 486-489.—**Putnam** (J. J.) Case of injury of the brachial plexus. Tr. Am. Neurol. Ass., N. Y., 1875, i, 19-22. *Also:* Med. Rec., N. Y., 1875, i, 413. ———. A case of section of the median and ulnar nerves. Boston M. & S. J., 1877, xcvi, 333-337.—**Ross.** Rupture of brachial plexus. Brit. M. J., Lond., 1883, i, 868.—**Sawtelle** (H. W.) An interesting surgical case. Med. Exam., Chicago, 1875, xvi, 209.—**Scott.** Injury to the brachial plexus consequent on a fall. Lancet, Lond., 1844, i, 645.—**Seeligmüller.** Ueber Sympathicusaffectionen bei Verletzungen des Plexus brachialis. Berl. klin. Wchnschr., 1870, vii, 313-316.—**Straus** (L.) Sur un cas de paralysie spontanée du plexus brachial (avec intégrité du nerf médian), et sur quelques localisations rares de paralysie du plexus brachial. Gaz. hebd. de méd., Par., 1880, xvii, 244-248. *Also,* Reprint.—**Symonds** (C. J.) Rupture of the left brachial plexus and subclavian artery. Tr. Clin. Soc. Lond., 1884, xvii, 239-242.—**Warren** (J. M.) Injury of the ulnar and musculo-spiral nerves, from a bullet. *In his:* Surg. Obs., 8°, Bost., 1867, 471.

Nerves (*Cardiac*).

See **Heart** (*Nerves of*); **Nerve** (*Pneumogastric*).

Nerves (*Cranial*).

See, also, **Eye, Face,** *Nerves of*; **Nervous system** (*Ganglionic*); **Paralysis** *of cranial nerves*; **Tongue** (*Nerves of*).

ÅKERMAN (J.) *Sciagraphica nervorum capitis descriptio. 4°. *Upsaliæ,* [1793].

AMICK (M. L.) Cranial nerves. fol. *Cincinnati,* 1883.

Suppl. to: Clin. Brief & San. News, Cincin., 1883, iii, no. 1.

Nerves (*Cranial*).

ARNOLD (F.) Icones nervorum capitis. fol. *Heidelbergæ,* 1834.

BECK (B.) Anatomische Untersuchungen über einzelne Theile des vii. und ix. Hirnnervenpaares. 4°. *Heidelberg,* 1847.

VON BECKER (F. J.) *Anatomisk beskrifning öfver de sex första cerebralnervparen hos sus scrofa, Linn. 4°. *Helsingfors,* 1852.

À BERGEN (C. A.) Programmate de nervis quibusdam cranii ad novem paria hactenus non relatis disserit. 4°. *Francof. ad Viadr.,* 1738.

Also, in: HALLER. Disp. anat. [etc.] 4°. *Gottingæ,* 1751, vii, pt. 2, 471-478.

BISCHOFF (E. P. E.) Mikroskopische Analyse der Anastomosen der Kopfnerven. 4°. *München,* 1865.

COOKE (T.) Tablets of anatomy and physiology. Anatomy; cranial nerves. 4°. *New York,* 1874.

ESCHRICHT (D. F.) *De functionibus nervorum faciei et olfactus organi. 8°. *Hafniæ,* 1825.

FÄSEBECK (G. F.) Die Nerven des menschlichen Kopfes. 4°. *Braunschweig,* 1840.

FRANÇOIS-FRANCK (C.-É.) *Recherches sur l'anatomie et la physiologie des nerfs vasculaires de la tête. 4°. *Paris,* 1875.

GRANDAUR (F.) *Aphorismen über die specifische Energie der Sinnesnerven. sm. 8°. *München,* 1848.

VON HAARTMAN (C. F. G.) *Anatomisk beskrifning öfver de sex första cerebralnervparen hos hunden. 4°. *Helsingfors,* [1846].

HAUSKA (F.) *De nervorum cerebralium functione. 8°. *Pragæ,* [1847].

HEIBERG (J.) Schema der Wirkungsweise der Hirnnerven. Ein Lehrmittel für Aerzte und Studirende in Farbendruck dargestellt. 8°. *Wiesbaden,* 1885.

MATTHEI (A.) *De nervis in genere, accedente i., ii., iii. et quarti nervorum paris descriptione, cum nonnullis in Cl. Meckellii dissertationem. De quinto pari annotationibus. 4°. *Lugd. Bat.,* 1758.

NORAEUS (J.) *Sciagraphica nervorum capitis descriptio, et quidem paris 6:ti, 7:mi, 8:vi, 9:ni, 10:mi et 11:mi. 4°. *Upsaliæ,* [1793].

PAASCH (R.) *Ueber Betheiligung der Gehirnnerven, insbesondere des Nervus trigeminus, bei Tabes dorsualis. 8°. *Berlin,* 1877.

PEIPERS (G. F.) *Diss. inaug. sistens tertii et quarti nervorum cervicalium descriptionem, cui accedit succincta eorundem nervorem quinti; nervi phrenici, præsertim ratione originis; nervi accessorii Willisii; nervi duri, ejusque præcipue rami inferioris; nervi hypoglossi et occipitalis maximi a secundo cervicalium nervo, adumbratio. 4°. *Halæ,* [1793].

Also, in: SCRIPT. neurol. minores selecti. 4°. *Lipsiæ,* 1795, iv, 18-49, 1 pl.

PELLETAN (P.-G.) Mémoire sur la spécialité der nerfs des sens. 8°. *Paris,* 1837.

PELOUX (A.) *Des anastomoses du ganglion cervical supérieur. 4°. *Paris,* 1840.

PHILIPEAUX (J.-M.) & VULPIAN (A.) Essai sur l'origine de plusieurs paires des nerfs crâniens (3e, 4e, 5e, 6e, 7e, 9e et 10e). 4°. *Paris,* 1853.

ROTGANS (J.) *Bijdrage tot de kennis van het halsgedeelte der laatste vier hersenzenuwen. [Amsterdam.] 8°. *Meppel,* 1886.

RÜDINGER (N.) Die Anatomie der menschlichen Gehirnnerven. 8°. *München,* 1868.

SAPOLINI (G.) Un tredicesimo nervo craniale. 8°. *Milano,* 1881.

STAUDINGER (J. J.) *Anatomist beskrifning öfver de sex första cerebralnervparen hos gråa hafsskälen (Halichoerus grypus). 4°. *Helsingfors,* [1847].

Nerves (*Cranial*).

STIECK (N. U.) *De quinque prioribus encephali nervis. 8°. *Gottingæ*, [1791].

STIEDA (L.) Ueber den Ursprung der spinalartigen Hirn-Nerven. 8°. *Dorpat*, 1873.

STUMPFF (F. G. A.) Historia nervorum cerebralium ab antiquissimis temporibus usque ad Willisium necnon Vieussenium. 8°. *Berolini*, [1841].

VULPIAN (E.-F.-A.) *Essai sur l'origine de plusieurs pairs des nerfs crâniens (3e, 4e, 5e, 6e, 7e, 8e, 9e et 10e). 4°. *Paris*, 1853.

Allen (H.) A clinical study of the cranial nerves. Tr. Coll. Phys. Phila., 1881-3, 3. s., vi, 429-436. *Also* [Abstr.]: Med. & Surg. Reporter, Phila., 1883, xlix, 179-181. *Also* [Abstr.]: Med. News, Phila., 1883, xliii, 49.—**Beck** (B.) Eine pathologische Beobachtung über die Verrichtung des 3ten, 4ten, 5ten und 6ten Hirnnervenpaares. Arch. f. path. Anat., etc., Berl., 1856, x, 449-473.—**Bell** (C.) Of the fourth and sixth nerve of the brain; being the concluding paper on the distinctions of the nerves of the encephalon and spinal marrow. Tr. Roy. Soc. Edinb., 1836, xiv, 237-241. *Also, in his:* Three papers on the nerves, 4°, Edinb., 1838, 15-19. — **Bellingeri** (C. F. J.) Quinti, et septimi paris functiones. *In his:* Diss. inaug., 8°, Augustæ Taur., 1818, 119-189. — **Benedict.** "Die Erkrankungen des achten Gehirnnerven." Monatschr. f. Ohrenh., Berl., 1875, ix, 25; 67; 80.—**Bennett** (J.-H.) Note sur le développement de nerfs particuliers, à la surface du cervelet. Bull. Soc. anat. de Par., 1841-2, xvi, 89-92. [Rap. de Giraldès], 93-95. *Also*, Reprint.—**Broadbent** (W. H.) Case of paralysis of the ophthalmic and superior maxillary divisions of the fifth nerve, of the fourth nerve, and of the branch of the third to the levator palpebræ on the right side, from syphilitic disease of the base of the cranium. Tr. Clin. Soc. Lond., 1871, iv, 102-106.—**Broughton** (S. D.) Experiments and observations upon the fifth, seventh, and eighth pairs of nerves. Lond. M. & Phys. J., 1823, xlix, 463-467. — **Chauveau** (A.) Recherches physiologiques sur l'origine apparente et sur l'origine réelle des nerfs moteurs crâniens; détermination expérimentale de cette dernière. J. de la physiol. de l'homme, Par , 1862, v, 272-282. *Also :* Mém. et compt.-rend. Soc. d. sc. méd. de Lyon (1862), 1863, ii, 42-54.—**Cunningham** (D. J.) Observations on the distribution of some of the nerves of the head and neck. J. Anat. & Physiol., Lond., 1872-3, vii, 94-97. — **Dalton** (J. C.) On the physiology of the cranial nerves. Am. M. Times, N. Y., 1861, ii, 73 ; 91 ; 107 ; 123 ; 139 ; 155 ; 171.—**Dupré.** Les nerfs crâniens. Mouvement méd., Par., 1872-3, x, 39. *Also :* Lyon méd., 1872, xi, 284.—**Duval** (M.) Recherches sur l'origine réelle des nerfs crâniens. J. de l'anat. et physiol., etc., Par., 1876, xii, 496-524, 2 pl. : 1877, xiii, 181 ; 571, 4 pl. : 1878, xiv, 1 ; 451, 4 pl. : 1879, xv, 492-514, 2 pl. : 1880, xvi, 285-312, 2 pl. ; 535-555, 2 pl.—**Edinger** (L.) Ueber die Verbindung der sensibeln Nerven mit dem Zwischenhirn. Anat. Anz., Jena, 1887, ii, 145-153.—**Eschricht** (D. F.) De functionibus septimi et quinti paris nervorum in facie propriis. J. de physiol. expér., Par., 1826, vi, 228-259.—**Faescbeck** (F.) Beitrag zur Anatomie der Hirnnerven und des Sympathicus. Arch. f. Anat., Physiol. u. wissensch. Med., Berl., 1840, 69-71.—**Féréol.** Note sur la communication anatomique existant entre les noyaux d'origine de la troisième et de la sixième paires. Union méd., Par., 1873, 3. s., xvi, 286-831. *Also :* Bull. et mém. Soc. méd. d. hôp. de Par. (1873), 1874, 2. s., x, 370.—**Fournier** (A.) Triple paralysie oculaire d'origine syphilitique. (Paralysie des 3e et 6e paires droites ; paralysie de la 6e paire gauche.) Ann. de dermat. et syph., Par., 1873-4, v, 190-196.—**Godman** (J. D.) Neurological table exhibiting a view of the nerves of the head. West. Q. Reporter M. & S. & Nat. Sc., Cincin., 1822, i, 209.—**Günsburg** (F.) Zur Pathologie der Hirnnerven. Ztschr. f. klin. Med., Bresl., 1859, x, 1-8.—**Laura** (E.) Des origines profondes de quelques nerfs crâniens. Tr. Internat. M. Cong., 7. sess., Lond., 1881, i, 182-184.—**Lautenbach.** Paresis of the right oculo-motorius and facial nerves, following trauma. Phila. M. Times, 1875-6, vi, 582.—**Luschka** (H.) Ueber die Nervenzweige, welche durch das Foramen condyloideum anticum in den Hirnschädel eintreten. Ztschr. f. rat. Med., Leipz. u. Heidelb., 1863, 3. R., xvii, 318-320.—**Marshall** (A. M.) The segmental value of the cranial nerves. J. Anat. & Physiol., Lond., 1881-2, xvi, 305-354, 1 pl. *Also :* Stud. Biol. Lab. Owens Coll., Manchester, 1886, i, 125-169, 2 pl.—**Mayo** (H.) Note sur les nerfs cérébraux considérés dans leur rapport avec le sentiment et le mouvement volontaire. J. de physiol. expér., Par., 1823, iii, 345-361.—**Nawrocki** (F.) O nerwach czuciowych mięsni. [On the cranial nerves.] Medycyna, Warszawa, 1878, vi, 81-84.—**Negri** (G.) On the comparative merits of Dr. Bellingeri's and Sir C. Bell's writings and opinions on the functions of the fifth and seventh pairs of cerebral nerves. Lond. M. Gaz., 1834, xiv, 845 ; 881 ; 913 : 1834-5, xv, 41 ; 160.—**Obersteiner.** Ueber einige neuere Entdeckungen, den Ursprung der Hirnnerven betreffend. Wien. med. Bl., 1880, iii, 687.—**Partridge.**

Nerves (*Cranial*).

Wasting of the second and fifth pairs of cerebral nerves on the left side. Tr. Path. Soc. Lond., 1848-50, ii, 166.—**Phisalix** (C.) Sur les nerfs crâniens d'un embryon humain de trente-deux jours. Compt. rend. Acad. d. sc., Par., 1887, civ, 242-244.—**Rattone** (G.) Sull' esistenza di cellule ganglionari in diversi nervi craniani. Osservatore, Torino, 1883, xix, 806.—**Retzius** (A.) Om 5:te och 7:de nervparens ursprung. Tidskr. f. Läk. o. Pharm., Stockholm, 1835, iv, 247. *Also, transl.:* Arch. f. Anat., Physiol. u. wissensch. Med., Berl., 1836, 362-364, 1 pl.—**Roller** (C. F. W.) Die cerebralen und cerebellaren Verbindungen des 3.-12. Hirnnervenpaares ; die spinalen Wurzeln der cerebralen Sinnesnerven. Allg. Ztschr. f. Psychiat., etc., Berl., 1881, xxxviii, 228-264.—**Sapolini** (G.) Sur un treizième nerf cérébral. Tr. Internat. M. Cong., 7. sess., Lond., 1881, i, 181. ———. Études anatomiques sur le nerf de Wrisberg et la corde du tympan ou un treizième nerf crânien. J. de méd., chir. et pharmacol., Brux., 1883, lxxvii, 337 ; 460 ; 570.—**Sloane** (J.) Cases of disease affecting the cranial nerves. Assoc. M. J., Lond., 1857, ii, 959-962.—**Stieda** (L.) Ueber den Ursprung der spinalartigen Hirn-Nerven. Dorpat. med. Ztschr., 1871, ii, 49-61.—**Thomsen** (R.) Ueber eigenthümliche aus veränderten Ganglienzellen hervorgegangene Gebilde in den Stämmen der Hirnnerven des Menschen. Arch. f. path. Anat., etc., Berl., 1887, cix, 459-465, 1 pl.—**Türck** (L.) Mittheilungen über Krankheiten der Gehirnnerven. Ztschr. d. k.k. Gesellsch. d. Aerzte zu Wien, 1855, xi, 517-532.—**Varaglia** (S.) Cellule ganglionari dei nervi facciale, intermediario del Wrisberg, grande e piccolo petrosi superficiali. Arch. di psichiat., etc., Torino, 1885, vi, 141, 1 pl.—**Vincenzi** (L.) Note istologiche sull' origine di alcuni nervi cerebrali (ipoglosso, facciale, oculo-motore esterno, trigemino, acustico, oculo-motore comune). Gior. d. r. Accad. di med. di Torino, 1883, 3. s., xxxi, 646-650. *Also :* Osservatore, Torino, 1883, xix, 519-523. *Also, transl.:* Arch. ital. de biol., Turin, 1884, v, 109-130. ———. Note istologiche sull' origine reale di alcuni nervi cerebrali. Arch. per le sc. med., Torino, 1883-4, vii, 319-346.—**Volkmann** (A. W.) Ueber die motorischen Wirkungen der Kopf- und Halsnerven. Arch. f. Anat., Physiol. u. wissensch. Med., Berl., 1840, 475-509.—**Vulpian.** Nouvelles recherches sur l'origine des fibres nerveuses glandulaires et des fibres nerveuses vaso-dilatatrices qui font partie de la corde du tympan et du nerf glosso-pharyngien. Compt. rend. Acad. d. sc., Par., 1885, ci, 851-855.—**Vulpian** & **Philipeaux.** Sur l'origine profonde des nerfs de la sixième et de la septième paire. Compt. rend. Soc. de biol. 1853, Par., 1854, v, 99-102.—**Weber** (E. H.) Ueber vier Längennerven bei einigen Fischen, von denen zwei von dem Trigeminus und zwei vom Vagus entspringen, die die ganze Länge des Rumpfes durchlaufen. Arch. f. Anat. u. Physiol., Leipz., 1827, 303-308, 1 pl.

Nerves (*Cranial, First pair of*).
See **Nerve** (*Olfactory*).

Nerves (*Cranial, Second pair of*).
See **Nerve** (*Optic*).

Nerves (*Cranial, Third pair of*).
See **Mydriasis**, *etc.* ; **Nerve** (*Oculo-motor*).

Nerves (*Cranial, Fourth pair of*).
See **Eye** (*Nerves of*).

Nerves (*Cranial, Fifth pair of*).
See, also, **Amaurosis** (*Causes of*) ; **Eye, Face, Nerves of**; **Head** (*Injuries of, Sequelæ of*) ; **Nerve** (*Lingual*) ; **Nerve** (*Supraorbital*) ; **Nervous system** (*Vasomotor*) ; **Neuralgia** (*Facial, etc.*) ; **Neuritis** ; **Neurotomy**, *etc.*

BOCK (A. C.) Beschreibung des fünften Nervenpaares und seiner Verbindungen mit anderen Nerven vorzüglich mit dem Gangliensysteme. fol. *Meissen*, 1817-21.

CALORI (A.) Animadversiones historico-criticæ et observationes anatomicæ de portione minore paris quinti nervorum cerebri hominis et nonnullorum mammalium domesticorum. 4°. [*Bologna*, 1847.]

DUMAS-LAMOTHE (C.-E.) *Des fonctions de la cinquième paire des nerfs encéphaliques. 4°. *Paris*, 1827.

FITZAU (A. F. L.) *De tertio ramo paris quinti nervorum cerebri, sive nervo maxillari inferiore. sm. 4°. *Lipsiæ*, [1811].

FRANK (J. C.) *Diss. sistens delineationem anatomicam et physiologico-pathologicam consensus nervi trigemini. 8°. *Jenæ*, [1799].

Nerves (Cranial, Fifth pair of).

GALLO (G.) Dichiarazione delle tre tavole neurologiche alligate nelle annotazioni sul terzo ramo del nervo trigemello nel corpo umano. fol. *Napoli*, 1843.

GRUBER (W.) Menschliches Analogon der thierischen Vagina nervi trigemini ossea am Felsenbeine. 4°. *St. Petersburg*, 1859. *Repr. from:* Mém. Acad. imp. d. sc. de St.-Pétersb. Sc. math., phys. et nat., 7. s., i, no. 4.

HAASE (J. G.) [Pr.] de nervo maxillari superiore sive secundo ramo quinti paris nervorum cerebri exponit. 4°. *Lipsiæ*, 1793.

HIRSCH (A. B. R.) Paris quinti nervorum encephali disquisitio anatomica, in quantum ad ganglion sibi proprium semilunare, et ad originem nervi intercostalis pertinet. *In:* SANDIFORT. Thesaurus diss. [etc.] 4°. *Roterodami*, 1778, iii, 477-500. *Also, in:* SCRIPT. neurol. minores selecti. 4°. *Lipsiæ*, 1791, i, 244-262.

JACOBSON (L.) * De quinto nervorum pari animalium. sm. 4°. *Regiomonti*, 1818.

LEGRAND (F.) * Contributions à la physiologie de la cinquième paire crânienne. 4°. *Paris*, 1875.

MECKEL (J. F.) * De quinto pare nervorum cerebri. 4°. *Gottingæ*, 1748. *Also, in:* SCRIPT. neurol. minores selecti. 4°. *Lipsiæ*, 1791, i, 145-243, 1 pl.

MOLLIÈRE (D.) * Du nerf dentaire inférieur; anatomie et physiologie. Anatomie comparée. 4°. *Paris*, 1871.

MÜLLER (J.) Ueber das Ganglion oticum Arnoldi. 8°. [*Leipzig*, 1832.] *Cutting from:* Arch. f. Anat. u. Physiol., Leipz., 1832, vi.

NIEMEYER (G. H.) * De origine paris quinti nervorum cerebri. 8°. *Halæ*, [1810].

———. The same. 8°. *Halæ*, 1812. *Also, transl. in:* Arch. f. d. Physiol., Halle, 1812, xi, 1-88, 1 pl.

PALLETTA (J. B.) De nervis crotaphitico et buccinatorio. 4°. *Mediolani*, 1784. *Also, in:* SCRIPT. neurol. minores selecti. 4°. *Lipsiæ*, 1793, iii, 63-77, 1 pl.

RAPP (W.) Die Verrichtungen des fünften Hirnnervenpaars. 4°. *Leipzig*, 1832.

STOWELL (T. B.) The trigeminus nerve in the domestic cat (Felis domestica). Read before the American Philosophical Society, May 21, 1886. 8°. [*Philadelphia*], 1886.

WATSON (J. W.) * De quinto nervorum pari. 8°. *Edinburgi*, 1822.

WRISBERG (H. A.) Observationes anatomicæ de quinto pare nervorum encephali, et de nervis qui ex eodem duram matrem ingredi falso dicuntur. 4°. *Gottingæ*, 1777. *Also, in:* SCRIPT. neurol. minores selecti. 4°. *Lipsiæ*, 1791, i, 263-278, 1 pl. *Also, in his:* Comment. med. physiol., etc. 8°. *Gottingæ*, 1800, i, 98-126, 1 pl.

ZAPFF (J. T. C. F.) * De symptomatibus sympathicis quibusdam, quæ ex ramis nervi trigemini, inter se et cum magno nervo sympathico conjunctis, prodeunt. 4°. *Jenæ*, 1829.

Alcock (B.) Account of some particulars in the anatomy of the fifth nerve in the human subject, and in fish, not hitherto observed. Dublin J. M. Sc., 1836, x, 323-327.—Althaus (J.) On certain points in the physiology and pathology of the fifth pair of cerebral nerves. Med.-Chir. Tr., Lond., 1869, lii, 27-42. *Also* [Abstr.]: Proc. Roy. M. & Chir. Soc. Lond. (1867-71), 1871, vi, 122-125. ———. Zur Physiologie und Pathologie des Trigeminus. Deutsches Arch. f. klin. Med., Leipz., 1870, vii, 563-574.—Bankart (J.) On the functions of the buccal branch of the fifth nerve. J. Anat. & Physiol., Lond., 1868, ii, 325-328.—Bechterew (W.) Ueber die Trigeminuswurzeln. Neurol. Centralbl., Leipz., 1887, vi, 289. — Bell (C.) On the nerves [etc.] Of the nerves of the face, in which it is shown that the two sets of nerves, hitherto supposed to be similar, differ in structure, sensibility, and function. Phil. Tr., Lond., 1821, 408-424, 1 pl. ———. On the nerves of the face; being a second paper on that subject. *Ibid.*, 1829, 317-330, 2 pl. *Also, transl.:* J. de physiol. expér., Par., 1830, x, 1; 189, 2 pl. *Also* [Rev.]: Lond. M. & Phys. J., 1829, n. s., vii, 525-537. ———. A reply to some remarks contained in a critical analysis of C. Bell's paper on the nerves

Nerves (Cranial, Fifth pair of).

of the face. Lond. M. & Phys. J., 1830, n. s., viii, 27-44. ———. Clinical lecture on diseases of the fifth pair of nerves. Lond. M. Gaz., 1833-4. xiii, 759-767. — Bernard (C.) La physiologie du nerf trijumeau. Compt. rend. Soc. de biol. 1874, Par., 1875, 6. s., i, 150-152. — Beveridge (R.) Case of disease of the trifacial nerve, and of the Gasserian ganglion. Med. Times & Gaz., Lond., 1868, i, 199. — Bishop (J.) Physiology of the fifth pair of nerves, illustrated by a case of carcinomatous tumor destroying the whole of the left nervus trigeminus. Lond. M. Gaz., 1834-5. xv, 387-389. — Bochdalek (V.) Neue Untersuchung und genauere Würdigung der Nerven des Ober- und Unterkiefers. Med. Jahrb. d. k. k. österr. Staates, Wien, 1836, xix, 223-240.—Bottu-Desmortiers (T.) Examen comparatif de l'influence de chacun des deux nerfs de la face, sur la production de la sensibilité et des mouvemens de cette partie, pour servir à l'histoire des paralysies locales. J. hebd. d. progr. d. sc. méd., Par., 1834. iv, 385-400.—Brinton. Tumour of the fifth nerve. Tr. Path. Soc. Lond., 1848-50, ii, 29.—Budge. Reizung eines Trigeminuszweiges an seinem Centralende. Wchnschr. f. d. ges. Heilk., Berl., 1840, 637; 656.—Büttner (C.) Ueber die nach der Durchschneidung des Trigeminus auftretenden Ernährungsstörungen am Auge und andern Organen. Ztschr. f. rat. Med., Leipz. u. Heidelb., 1862, 3. R., xv, 254-278, 1 pl.—Cerminara (G.) Cecità monoculare in seguito a ferita del ramo frontale del trigemino. Riv. clin. e terap., Napoli, 1886, viii, 609.—Dixon (J.) Case in which a large tumour was developed in the substance of the fifth nerve and its ganglion. Med.-Chir. Tr., Lond., 1846, xxix. 131-136, 1 pl.—Duval (M.) & Laborde (J.-V.) Le trijumeau et sa racine bulbaire sensitive; étude anatomique et expérimentale. Trav. lab. physiol. Fac. de méd. de Par. (1884), 1885, i, 137-166, 2 pl. — Espina y Capo (A.) Lesion del ganglio de Gasser ó Gasserio. Rev. de med. y cirug. práct., Madrid, 1887, xx, 5-9.—Faesebeck. Ueber die motorische Portion des Trigeminus. Tr. Internat. M. Cong., 7. sess., Lond., 1881, i, 167. — Filehne (W.) Trigeminus und Gesichtsausdruck. Arch. f. Physiol., Leipz., 1886, 432-442.—Fleury. Paralysie de la deuxième et de la troisième paire consécutive à une lésion de la cinquième paire survenue à la suite d'une chute sur la tête. Bull. Soc. de chir. de Par. (1862), 1863, 2. s., iii, 575-577.—Gerhardt (C.) Zur Therapie der Erkrankungen des fünften Hirnnerven. Deutsches Arch. f. klin. Med., Leipz., 1880, xxvi, 1-9.—Gowers (W. R.) A case of loss of taste from disease of the fifth nerve. J. Physiol., Lond., 1880-82, iii, 229-231.—Howard (H.) Physiology of the fifth pair of nerves but more particularly of the opthalmic branch. Brit. Am. J. M. & Phys. Sc., Montreal, 1847, iii, 197-199.—Hunter (J.) A description of some branches of the fifth pair of nerves. *In his:* Observ. on cert. parts of the animal œconomy, 4°, Lond., 1786, 219-221.—Jolyet. Note sur l'existence, dans le nerf maxillaire supérieur, de fillets vasodilatateurs pour la muqueuse des fosses nasales, pour la peau des ailes du nez, des lèvres supérieure et inférieure, la muqueuse de ces mêmes parties ainsi que celle des gencives. Compt. rend. Soc. de biol. 1878, Par., 1880. 6. s., v, 223-227.—Kramer (W.) Ueber die Beziehungen des Nervus quintus zum Gehörsinn. Wchnschr. f. d. ges. Heilk., Berl., 1848, 40-48.—Létiévant (E.) Persistance de la sensibilité après la section des nerfs sensitifs de la face; sensibilité suppléée; ses caractères. Cong. méd. de France (Lyon, 1872), Par., 1873, iv, 664-674.—Little (T. E.) Intracranial tumour; glioma of the fifth nerve. Dublin J. M. Sc., 1873, lv, 94-96.—Longet. Quelques points d'anatomie et de physiologie de la branche maxillaire inférieure du trifacial. Bull. Soc. anat. de Par., 1839-40, xiv, 65.—Luschka (H.) Der Nervus spinosus. Arch. f. Anat., Physiol. u. wissensch. Med., Berl., 1853, 445-448. ———. Die Nervi spheno-ethmoidales. *Ibid.*, 1857, 313-326, 1 pl.—Meckel. Observation anatomique sur un nœud, ou ganglion, du second rameau de la cinquième paire des nerfs du cerveau, nouvellement découvert. Traduit du latin. Mém. Acad. roy. de Prusse, Avignon, 1768, ii, 50-62, 1 pl. *Also:* Collect. acad. d. mém., etc., Par., 1770, viii, 171-183, 1 pl. *Also, transl.:* Phys. u. med. Abhandl. d. k. Acad. d. Wissensch. zu Berl., Gotha, 1783, iii, 527-547.—Merkel (F.) Die trophische Wurzel des Trigeminus. Untersuch. a. d. anat. Inst. zu Rostock, 1874, 1, 1 pl.; 98.—Montault. Observation sur une maladie du nerf de la 5e paire, dont le sujet a été présenté au cours de M. Magendie, au Collège de France, les 12 février et 2 mars 1836. J. hebd. d. progr. d. sc. méd., Par., 1836, i, 368-374.—Paulicki & Loos. Schussverletzung des Stammes des linken Nervus trigeminus. Deutsche Ztschr. f. Chir., Leipz., 1880-81, xiv, 151-158.—Piorry. Tumeur survenue après l'évulsion d'une dent molaire; compression du nerf dentaire inférieur; paralysie locale de la peau du menton; preuve du rôle exclusivement sensitif du nerf mentonnier; guérison par l'électricité. Gaz. d. hôp., Par., 1857, xxx, 105. — Poncet (F.) De la section du trijumeau dans ses rapports avec l'œil. Arch. d'opht., Par., 1880-81, i, 400-418, 1 pl.—Robinson (R. R.) Meningitis; tumor of the brain; pressure on the fifth nerve on the left side; sloughing of left cheek; caries of

Nerves (*Cranial, Fifth pair of*).

the bones of this side of the face. Lond. M. Gaz., 1834, xiv, 363.—**Sapolini** (G.) Studii anatomici sul nervo dentario inferiore, d'onde la sua divisione in piccolo e grande dentario. Ann. univ. di med., Milano, 1869, ccix, 346-365. *Also*, Reprint.—**Stowell** (T. B.) The trigeminus nerve in the domestic cat (Felis domestica). Proc. Am. Phil. Soc., Phila., 1886, xxiii, 459-478. *Also*, Reprint.—**Tavignot.** De l'action de la cinquième paire sur l'œil. Expérience, Par., 1844, xtv, 157-161. — **Theviranus** (G. R.) Sur les nerfs de la cinquième paire, considérés comme organes ou conducteurs de sensations. J. compl. du dict. d. sc. méd., Par., 1823. xv, 207-215.—**Urbantschitsch** (V.) Ueber den Einfluss von Trigeminus-Reizen auf die Sinnesempfindungen, insbesondere auf den Gesichtssinn. Arch. f. d. ges Physiol., Bonn, 1882-3. xxx, 129-175.—**Vicq d'Azyr.** Lésion du nerf frontal. Hist. Soc. roy. de méd. 1776, Par., 1779, i, 316. — **Wolff** (P. H.) Ueber die Beziehungen des Nervus quintus zum Gehörsinn; Entgegnungan . . . Kramer. Wchnschr. f. d. ges. Heilk., Berl., 1848. 727-733.—**Zlobikowski** (T.) Nouvelles recherches sur le filet dento-lingual du professeur Sappey. Traduit par l'auteur de la Gazette médicale (polonaise) de Varsovie. J. de l'anat. et physiol., etc., Par., 1870-71, vii, 602-610.

Nerves (*Cranial, Fifth pair of, Paralysis of*).

See, also, **Cornea** (*Neuroparalytic disease of*); **Eye** (*Anæsthesia of*); **Paralysis** (*Facial*).

DAVIDSON (A.) On the sense of taste and its relation to facial paralysis and anæsthesia. 8°. [*Liverpool*, 1874.]

FÜRST (H.) *Ueber Trigeminuslähmung. [Wurtzburg.] 8°. *Neustadt a. d. H.*, 1858.

GALEWSKI (H.) *De anæsthesia faciei. 8°. *Berolini*, [1837].

JAMES (C.) *Observation de paralysie complète de la cinquième paire, suivie de considérations théoriques et pratiques. 4°. *Paris*, 1840. *Also* [Abstr.], *in :* Bull. Acad. de méd., Par., 1840-41, vi, 150-163.

ORTEL-ÉBRARD (P.) *Études sur les paralysies du trijumeau. 4°. *Paris*, 1867.

ROUX (D.-H.) *Anesthésie du nerf trijumeau. 4°. *Montpellier*, 1874.

STEFFEN (C. F. G. Æ.) *Anæsthesiæ cutaneæ, muscularis nervi quinti specimen singulare. 8°. *Berolini*, [1855].

Azam (E.) Observation de paralysie de la 5e paire crânienne; guérison par l'iodure de potassium. J. de méd. de Bordeaux, 1861. 2. s., vi, 49-55. — **Bärwinkel.** Halbseitige Lähmung der Nn. trigemin., abducens olfactorius und petros. superfic. major; anæsthesia dolorosa. Arch. f. physiol. Heilk., Stuttg., 1859, n. F., iii, 238-245.—**Barrier.** Sur la paralysie du nerf trijumeau. Gaz. méd. de Lyon, 1858, x, 479-483. — **Bezold** (F.) Ein Fall von Anästhesie des Trigeminus und dessen Einfluss auf die Ernährung der Hornhaut. Deutsche Klinik. Berl., 1867, xix, 223; 237; 246; 258. — **Blandin.** Lésions du nerf sous-orbitaire, perte de la sensibilité dans les parties où il se distribue; motilité intacte. Gaz. d. hôp., Par., 1840, 2. s., ii, 59.—**Coursserant** (H.) & **Decaisne** (G.) Paralysie complète et douloureuse du trijumeau ; troubles trophiques graves et périodiques Gaz. hebd. de méd., Par., 1876, 2. s., xiii, 678-680.—**Cowan** (J. B.) On facial anæsthesia. Glasgow M. J., 1853-4. [2.] s., i, 146-158. ———. Case of partial facial anæsthesia. *Ibid.*, 1858-9, [2.] s , vi, 183.—**Cras.** Sur un cas de paralysie traumatique des cinquième et sixième paires crâniennes. Arch. de méd. nav., Par., 1873, xix, 132-141.—**Dixon.** Case of partial paralysis of the left fifth nerve, both of its motor and sensory functions; history of epileptic fits and of pain in the parts supplied by the nerve now paralysed; impaired taste and smell; ulceration of the cornea; doubtful diagnosis of syphilis. Ophth. Hosp. Rep., Lond., 1866, v, 354. — **Fagge** (C. H.) A case of paralysis due to partial disease of the nuclei of the motor roots of the fifth nerves. Tr. Clin. Soc. Lond., 1881, xiv. 128-131.—**Fieuzal.** Anesthésie complète du trijumeau du côté droit; hémianesthésie de la face. Progrès méd., Par., 1877, v, 700. *Also:* Tribune méd., Par., 1877, ix, 219-222 —**von Graefe.** Paralysis nervi v. dextri traumatica ; Ophthalmia neuroparalytica; Heilung. Berl. klin. Wchnschr., 1868, v, 486.—**Harlan** (G. C.) Neuroparalytic ophthalmia. Am. J. M. Sc., Phila., 1874, n. s., lxvii. 371-378.—**Henry** (F. P.) Cases of paralysis of the fifth cranial nerve. Phila. M. Times, 1874-5, v, 577. — **Jaccoud.** Paralysie du nerf trijumeau. Gaz. d. hôp., Par., 1867, xl, 214. — **Jacquart** (H.) Observation d'une paralysie du trijumeau droit. Compt. rend. Soc. de biol. 1856, Par., 1857, 2. s., iii, 238; 241.—**James** (C.) Note relative à

Nerves (*Cranial, Fifth pair of, Paralysis of*).

une paralysie complète de la cinquième paire, du côté droit. Gaz. méd. de Par., 1840, 2. s., viii, 622. — **Lücke.** Ein Fall von Trigeminuslähmung. Berl. klin. Wchnschr., 1868, v, 105; 117. — **Martin** (J. F.) Paralysis of the branches of the fifth pair of nerves of the right side of the face. Med. Times, Lond., 1847, xvi, 200. — **Melotti** (N.) Istoria di una paralisi del quinto paio dei nervi cerebrali narrata dal Dott. . . . Bull. d. sc. med. di Bologna, 1854, 4. s., i, 51-53.—**Noyes** (H. D.) Paralysis of the 5th cerebral nerve and its effects. Med. Rec., N. Y., 1871, vi, 231-234. *Also:* N. York M. J., 1871, xiv, 163-177.—**Romberg** (M.-H.) Anästhesie im Gebiete des Quintus. Arch. f. Anat., Physiol. u. wissensch. Med., Berl., 1838, 305-315. *Also, transl.:* Gaz. méd. de Par., 1838, 2. s., vi, 625-628. ———. Anæsthesia n. trigemini. Deutsche Klinik, Berl., 1850, ii, 422. — **Stricker.** Anæsthesia nervi trigemini. Org. f. d. ges. Heilk., Aachen, 1855, iv, 228-234.—**Taylor** (R.) Case of facial anæsthesia, with simultaneous destruction of the eye. Med. Times & Gaz., Lond., 1854, n. s., ix, 54.—**Vogt.** Observation relative à un cas de paralysie du nerf trijumeau. Gaz. méd. de Par., 1840, 2. s., viii, 584.—**Warner.** Atrophy of the muscles supplied by the fifth cranial nerve, with atrophy of the orbital fat on the same side. Lancet, Lond , 1882, i, 13.

Nerves (*Cranial, Sixth pair of*).

Woods (G. A.) The anatomy, etc., of the sixth nerve, with a collection of cases from various sources in which the region of its nucleus has been injured, with the symptoms of ocular derangements, especially those relating to conjugate deviation of the eyes, likewise the symptoms induced by disease attacking this nerve from its apparent origin to its termination ; opinions relating to a connection between the sixth and third nerve nuclei. Liverpool M.-Chir. J., 1883, iii, 304 : 1884, iv, 1.

Nerves (*Cranial, Seventh pair of*).

See, also, **Chorda** *tympani* ; **Ear** ; **Nerve** (*Auditory*) ; **Nerve** (*Facial*).

MECKEL (J. F.) Observationes anatomicæ de glandula pineali, septo lucido, et origine paris septimi nervorum cerebri. *Berolini*, 1765. *In :* SCRIPT. neurol. minores selecti. 4°. *Lipsiæ*, 1795, iv, 9, 1 pl.

Bernard (C.) Recherches expérimentales sur les fonctions du nerf spinal, étudié spécialement dans ses rapports avec le pneumogastrique. Arch. gén. de méd., Par., 1844, i, 397 : ii, 51.—**Davaine** (C.) De la paralysie générale ou partielle des deux nerfs de la septième paire. Gaz. méd. de Par., 1852, 3. s., vii, 716 ; 733 ; 744 ; 780 : 1853, 3. s., viii, 16 ; 30. *Also*, Reprint.—**Gaston** (J.) On the intermediary nerve between the portio dura and portio mollis of the seventh pair. Dublin M. Press, 1853, xxix, 373.—**Morganti** (G.) Anatomia del ganglio ginicolato. Ann. univ. di med., Milano, 1845, cxiv, 449-528. — **Rüdinger.** Ueber den Canalis facialis in seiner Beziehung zum siebenten Gehirnnerv beim Erwachsenen. Monatschr. f. Ohrenh., Berl., 1873, vii, 69-71.—**Wolski** (B.) O wpływie nerwu przydatkowego Willis'a (n. accessorius Willisii) na serce. [Its function with the heart.] Gaz. lek., Warszawa, 1870, viii, 801-804.

Nerves (*Cranial, Seventh pair of, Paralysis of*).

See **Paralysis** (*Facial*).

Nerves (*Cranial, Eighth pair of*).

See, also, **Neck** (*Tumors of*); **Nerve** (*Pneumogastric*); **Nerve** (*Recurrent laryngeal*); **Nerve** (*Spinal accessory*).

BENDZ (H. C. B.) *Tractatus de connexu inter nervum vagum et accessorium Willisii. 4°. *Harniæ*, 1836.

———. Bidrag til den sammenlignende Anatomie af Nervus glossopharyngeus, vagus, accessorius Willisii og hypoglossus hos Reptilierne. 4°. *Kjøbenhavn*, 1843.

BERNARD (C.) Recherches expérimentales sur les fonctions du nerf spinal ou accessoire de Willis. 4°. *Paris*, 1851.

VON BISCHOFF (T. L. W.) *Nervi accessorii Willisii anatomia et physiologia. 4°. *Heidelbergæ*, 1832.

———. The same. 4°. *Darmstadii*, 1832.

BURCHARD (A. A.) *Verlauf des Accessorius Willisii im Vagus. 8°. *Halle*, 1867.

KROPFF (A.) *Beobachtungen über Krampf im Bereiche des Accessorius und der oberen Cer-

Nerves (*Cranial, Eighth pair of*).
vicalnerven. [Gottingen.] 8°. *Heiligenstadt*, 1875.

LOBSTEIN (J. F.) * De nervo spinali ad par vagum accessorio. 4°. *Argentorati*, [1760].
Also, in: SCRIPT. neurol. minores selecti. 4°. *Lipsiæ*, 1792, ii, 219-242, 2 pl. *Also, in*: SANDIFORT. Thesaurus diss. [etc.] 4°. *Roterodami*, 1768, i, 325-354, 2 pl.

Bechterew (W.) Ueber die innere Abtheilung des Strickkörpers und den achten Hirnnerven. Neurol. Centralbl., Leipz., 1885, iv, 145-147.—**Benedict.** "Die Erkrankungen des achten Gehirnnerven". Monatschr. f. Ohrenh., Berl., 1875, ix, 25; 67; 80.—**Bernard.** De l'influence des nerfs de la huitième paire sur les phénomènes chimiques de la digestion. Compt. rend. Acad. d. sc., Par., 1844, xviii, 995-998.—**Biffi** & **Morganti.** Versuche am Nervus glossopharyngeus. Arch. f. Anat., Physiol. u. wissensch. Med., Berl., 1847, 357-362. — **Broughton** (S. D.) Experiments and remarks, illustrating the influence of the eighth pair of nerves over the organs of respiration and digestion. Lond. M. Reposit., 1821, xv, 155; 240; 330. *Also, transl.* [Abstr.]: J. de physiol. expér., Par., 1821, i, 120-131.—**Cruse** (W.) Degeneration des Nervus glosso-pharyngeus durch eine entartete Drüse in der Fossa mastoidea. Wchnschr. f. d. ges. Heilk., Berl., 1839, 695 - 699. — **Dulieu.** Nouvelles observations sur la section des deux nerfs de la huitième paire au milieu du col dans le cheval. J. gén. de méd., chir. et pharm., Par., 1820, lxxi, 62-70.—**Dumas.** Exposé de quelques expériences propres à déterminer quelle est l'influence des nerfs de la huitième paire sur la coloration du sang. *Ibid.*, 1808, xxxiii, 353-361.—**Fleischmann.** Das Vorkommen wandelbarer Ganglien am Nerv. accessor. Willis. bei Stotternden. J. d. pract. Heilk., Berl., 1840, xc, 1. St., 113-115.—**Fränkel** (B.) Fall von Lähmung des rechten Nervus accessorius. Berl. klin. Wchnschr., 1876, xiii, 10. *Also*: Verhandl. d. Berl. med. Gesellsch. (1875-6), 1877, vii, pt. 1, 25.—**Garibaldi** (G.) Di un nuovo ramoscello del glosso faringeo. Liguria med., Genova, 1868, xiii, 212-222, 1 pl.—**Haighton** (J.) Experiments made on the laryngeal and recurrent branches of the eighth pair of nerves, with a view to determine the effects of the division of those nerves on the voice. Mem. M. Soc. Lond., 1792, iii, 422-439.—**Harriss** (J.) Physiology of the pneumogastric nerve and spinal accessory of Willis. South. M. & S. J., Augusta, 1851, n. s., vii, 451; 587.—**Heidenhain** (R.) Ueber die Verbreitung der Fasern des Nerv. accessorius Willisii in den Aesten des Nerv. vagus. Stud. d. physiol. Inst. zu Bresl., Leipz., 1868, iv, 250.—**van Kempen** (E.-M.) Nouvelles recherches sur la nature fonctionnelle des racines du nerf pneumo-gastrique et du nerf spinal. J. de la physiol. de l'homme, Par., 1863, vi, 284-305.—**Little** (T. E.) Case of syphilitic disease of the eighth and ninth nerves at the base of the skull; phthisis. Irish Hosp. Gaz., Dubl., 1874, ii, 117-120.—**Macdonald** (J. D.) Remarks on the physiological connection of the spinal accessory nerve with the posterior roots and ganglia of the spinal nerve. Lond. M. Gaz., 1848, n. s., vii, 246-248.—**de Martini** (A.) Osservazioni sugli effetti della recisione dell' ottavo paio dei nervi. [With report by G. Lucarelli, G. Semmola, and S. Tommasi.] Rendic. Accad. med.-chir. di Napoli, 1851, v. 61; 94.—**Morganti** (G.) Studii sul nervo accessorio del Willis. Ann. univ. di med., Milano, 1843, cvii, 5 - 23. — **Müller** (J.) Ueber ein bisher unbeachtetes kleines Knötchen an der Wurzel des Nervus glossopharyngeus beim Menschen. Med. Ztg., Berl., 1833, ii, 235.—**Philip** (A. P. W.) Some positions respecting the influence of the voltaic battery in obviating the effects of the division of the eighth pair of nerves. Phil. Tr., Lond., 1822, cxii, 22.—**Reid** (J.) An experimental investigation into the functions of the eighth pair of nerves, or the glosso-pharyngeal, pneumogastric, and spinal accessory. Edinb. M. & S. J., 1838, xlix, 109: 1839, li, 269. *Also*, Reprint. *Also, in*: Essays on Phys. & Hyg., 8°, Phila., 1838, 5 - 66. — **Sichel.** Névrose de la septième paire droite; guérison au bout de trois jours par la compression réitérée du nerf à sa sortie du trou stylo-mastoïdien. Union méd., Par., 1864, 2. s., xxii, 69-71.—**Spence** (J.) An inquiry into the anatomy of the par vagum and spinal accessory of the eighth pair of nerves. Edinb. M. & S. J., 1842, lviii, 397-403, 1 pl. *Also*, Reprint. — **Vulpian** (A.) De l'action vaso-dilatatrice exercée par le nerf glosso-pharyngien sur les vaisseaux de la membrane muqueuse de la base de la langue. Compt. rend. Acad. d. sc., Par., 1875, lxxx, 330 - 333. ——. Note sur l'action vaso-dilatatrice exercée sur les vaisseaux de la base de la langue par les nerfs glosso-pharyngiens. Compt. rend. Soc. de biol. 1874, Par., 1875, 6. s., i, 391-394. *Also*: Gaz. méd. de Par., 1875, 4. s., iv, 3.

Nerves (*Cranial, Ninth pair of*).
See **Nerve** (*Hypoglossal*).

Nerves (*Cranial, Tenth pair of*).
Falk (F.) Zur experimentellen Pathologie des x. Gehirnnerven. Arch. f. exper. Path. u. Pharmakol., Leipz., 1877, vii, 183-192.

Nerves (*Cutaneous*).
See **Skin** (*Nerves, etc., of*).

Nerves (*Dental*).
See **Nerves** (*Cranial, Fifth pair of*); **Teeth** (*Diseases of*).

Nerves (*Excito motor*).
See **Nervous** system (*Reflex action of*).

Nerves (*Excito secretory*).
See **Nervous** system (*Reflex action of*).

Nerves (*Inhibitory*).
See **Nervous** system (*Inhibitory*).

Nerves (*Intercostal*).
See, also, **Neuralgia** (*Intercostal*).
À BERGEN (C. A.) * De nervo intercostali. 4°. *Francof. ad Viadr.*, 1731.
Also, in: HALLER. Disp. anat. [etc.] 4°. *Gottingæ*, 1747, ii, 871-909.

GEROLD (J.) * De nervo intercostali. 4°. *Erlangæ*, [1754].

GIRARDI (M.) De nervo intercostali. *Florentiæ*, 1791.
In: SCRIPT. neurol. minores selecti. 4°. *Lipsiæ*, 1793, iii, 78-88.

HALLER (A.) * De vera nervi intercostalis origine. 4°. *Gottingæ*, 1743.
Also, in his: Disp. anat. [etc.] 4°. *Gottingæ*, 1747, ii, 941-951.

IWANOFF (D.) * De origine nervorum intercostalium. 4°. *Argentorati*, [1780].
Also, in: SCRIPT. neurol. minores selecti. 4°. *Lipsiæ*, 1793, iii, 89-104.

MEDICI (M.) Disquisitiones anatomicæ et physiologicæ de nervo intercostali. 4°. *Bononiæ*, 1840.

——. The same. Richerche anatomiche e fisiologiche sopra il nervo intercostale. 8°. *Bologna*, 1843.

MITTIÉ (J. S.) * Utrum a gangliis nervi intercostalis partium omnium consensus? 4°. *Parisiis*, 1764.

MURRAY (A.) Observationes anatomicæ de infundibulo cerebri et variationibus quibusdam in parte cervicali nervi intercostalis. *Upsaliæ*, 1772.
In: SCRIPT. neurol. minores selecti. 4°. *Lipsiæ*, 1792, ii, 242-250.

NEUBAUER (J. E.) Descriptio anatomica nervorum cardiacorum. Sectio prima de nervo intercostali cervicali, dextri imprimis lateralis. 4°. *Francofurti et Lipsiæ*, 1772.

——. The same. 4°. *Lipsiæ et Jenæ*, 1772.

SCHMIDEL (C. C.) Epistola anatomica, qua de controversa nervi intercostalis origine quædam disseruntur. 4°. *Erlangæ*, [1747].

TAUBE (H. W. L.) * De nervi intercostalis origine. 4°. *Gottingæ*, [1743].

VARNIER (C. L.) * Utrum a gangliis nervi intercostalis partium omnium consensus? Præses B. P. de la Noue. 4°. [*Paris*, 1770.]

WALTHERUS (A. F.) [Pr.] paris intercostalis et vagi corporis humani nervorum et ab utroque ejus latere obviorum anatomen exhibet. 4°. [*Lipsiæ*, 1733.]

Des Genettes. Précis d'une dissertation de M. Girardi, et des recherches de M. Fontana, sur l'origine du nerf intercostal J. de méd., chir., pharm., etc., Par., 1793, xciii, 43-70.—**Hénocque** & **Éloy.** Étude comparative de l'action des nerfs intercostaux et des diverses racines du nerf phrénique. Compt. rend. Soc. de biol., Par., 1882, 7. s., iv, 578-585. —**Munniks** (J.) Qua, ad illustrandam artem medicam ostenditur origo nervi intercostalis, ejusque commercium cum aliis nervis, ab ejus origine ad exitum usque e calvaria, cum autopsia, tum observatis medicis confirmata. *In his*: Obs. variæ. 4°, Groningæ, 1805, 19-32, 2 pl.—**Scarpa.** Lettre sur des ganglions nerveux et sur l'origine et la nature du nerf intercostal. Tr. méd., Par., 1831, v, 264-274.

Nerves (*Laryngeal*).

See **Larynx** (*Nerves of*); **Nerve** (*Recurrent laryngeal*).

Nerves (*Lumbar*).

See **Nerves** (*Spinal*).

Nerves (*Motor*).

See, also, **Muscles** (*Nerves of*).

BRÜCKE (E.) Ueber die Reizung der Bewegungsnerven durch elektrische Ströme. 8°. [*Wien*, 1868.]

Repr. from: Sitzungsb. d. k. Akad. d. Wissensch. Math.-naturw. Cl., Wien, 1868, lviii, 2. Abth.

Bert (P.) & **Marcacci** (A.) Comunicazione preventiva sulla distribuzione delle radici motrici nei muscoli degli arti. Sperimentale, Firenze, 1881, xlviii, 356–358.— **Brach.** Die motorischen Nerven sind keinesweges unempfindlich, vielmehr sind sie selber wahrhafte, nur auf besondere Weise wirkende Empfindungs- und Sinnesnerven. Med. Ztg., Berl., 1842, xi, 9; 13. — **Brown-Séquard.** Sur l'indépendance des propriétés vitales des nerfs moteurs. J. de la physiol. de l'homme, Par., 1860, iii, 160–163. ———. Faits montrant que l'excitabilité des nerfs moteurs et l'irritabilité musculaire, loin d'avoir des relations constantes, peuvent varier en sens inverse l'une de l'autre. Compt. rend. Soc. de biol. 1881, Par., 1882, 7. s., iii, 206–208. ———. De l'influence dynamogénique de certaines excitations des nerfs moteurs. *Ibid.*, 208–210.— **Chauveau** (A.) Procédés et appareils pour l'étude de la vitesse de propagation des excitations dans les différentes catégories de nerfs moteurs chez les mammifères. Compt. rend. Acad. d. sc., Par., 1878, lxxxvii, 95. *Also:* Gaz. hebd. de méd., Par., 1878, 2. s., xxv, 523. ———. Vitesse de propagation des excitations dans les nerfs moteurs des muscles rouges de faisceaux striés, soustraits à l'empire de la volonté. Compt. rend. Acad. d. sc., Par., 1878, lxxxvii, 238–242. *Also:* Gaz. hebd. de méd., Par., 1878, 2. s., xv, 558.— **Eckhard** (C.) Ueber die Einwirkung der Temperaturen des Wassers auf die motorischen Nerven des Frosches. Ztschr. f. rat. Med., Heidelb., 1851, x, 165–190, 1 pl.— **Eulenburg** (A.) Bemerkungen über die Wirkung der Metallsalze auf die motorischen Froschnerven. Allg. med. Centr.-Ztg., Berl., 1860, xxix, 521–523.— **Eulenburg** (A.) & **Ehrenhaus** (S.) Ueber die Einwirkung concentrirter Metallsalzlösungen auf die motorischen Froschnerven. *Ibid.*, 1859, xxviii, 809–812.— **Ferrier** (D.) The functional relations of the motor roots of the brachial and lumbo-sacral plexuses. Proc. Roy. Soc. Lond., 1881, xxxii, 12–20. ———. Note on the motor roots of the brachial plexus, and on the dilator nerve of the iris. *Ibid.*, 1883, xxxv, 229–232. — **Harless** (E.) Ueber den Einfluss der Temperaturen und ihrer Schwankungen auf die motorischen Nerven. Ztschr. f. rat. Med., Leipz., 1860, 3. R., viii, 122–184.— **Holmgren.** Föredrag om centripetal ledning af nervretning i motoriska nerver. Upsala Läkaref. Förh., 1865–6, i, 76–84.— **Kossecki** (W.) O powstrszymaniu odruchów u żaby. [Mechanism of motor nerves in the frog.] Gaz. lek., Warszawa, 1870, ix, 129; 148.— **Lamansky** (S.) Ueber Erregung der motorischen Nerven der Frösche durch den kurzdauernden electrischen Strom. Centralbl. f. d. med. Wissensch., Berl., 1867, vii, 577–580.— **Lewes** (G. H.) Motor-feelings and the muscular sense. Brain, Lond., 1878, i, 14–28.— **Moleschott** (J.) Der bewegungvermittelnde Vorgang im Nerven kann auch von einer positiven Schwankung des Nervenstroms begleitet sein. Untersuch. z. Naturl. d. Mensch. u. d. Thiere, Giessen, 1862, viii, 1–35. *Also,* Reprint.— **Place** (T.) Ueber die Fortpflanzungsgeschwindigkeit des Reizes in den motorischen Nerven des Menschen. Arch. f. d. ges. Physiol., Bonn, 1870, iii, 424–436. — **Plugge** (P.-C.) Quelques réflexions sur les modifications de la motricité dans les nerfs moteurs et les muscles à propos de la monographie de MM. Laborde et Duquesnel. (Des aconits et de l'aconitine.) Rev. de méd., Par., 1883, iii, 1045–1053.— **Rosenthal** (J.) Ueber den Einfluss höherer Temperaturgrade auf motorische Nerven. Allg. med. Centr.-Ztg., Berl., 1859, xxviii, 761. — **Volkmann** (A. W.) Beitrag zur nähern Kenntniss der motorischen Nervenwirkungen. Arch. f. Anat., Physiol. u. wissensch. Med., Berl., 1845, 407–429.—**Zenker** (F.) Ein Beitrag zur Anatomie der motorischen Nervenfasern. Ztschr. f. rat. Med., Heidelb., 1847, vi, 298, 1 pl.

Nerves (*Ocular*).

See **Eye** (*Nerves of*); **Iris** (*Anatomy of*); **Nerve** (*Oculo-motor*) ; **Nerve** (*Optic*).

Nerves (*Orbital*).

See **Eye** (*Nerves of*).

Nerves (*Plexuses of*).

See **Nerves** (*Spinal*).

Nerves (*Pulmonary*).

See **Lungs** (*Nerves of*).

Nerves (*Sensory*).

BAUDRIMONT (A.) * Quelles sont les parties sensibles du corps des animaux? La présence des nerfs dans les tissus est-elle une condition de leur faculté de sentir? L'action nerveuse peut-elle être éclairée par l'étude de la composition chimique et de la texture des nerfs? 4°. *Paris*, 1835.

Concours.

ZURHELLE (A.) * De nervorum sensitivorum irritabilitate in statu electrotoni. 8°. *Berolini*, [1864].

Bert (P.) Propriété de transmission des nerfs sensitifs. Compt. rend. Soc. de biol. 1876, Par., 1877, 6. s., iii, 387–390. — **Bocci** (B.) I nervi di senso specifico. Bull. d. r. Accad. med. di Roma, 1886–7, xiii, 122–148. — **Brown-Séquard** (C.-E.) Rapport sur un mémoire de M. le docteur Oré (de Bordeaux) sur la transmission croisée des impressions sensitives. Compt. rend. Soc. de biol. 1853, Par., 1854, v, pt. 2, 301–305. ———. Experimental and clinical researches upon the channels of transmission of the sensitive impressions through the spinal cord and medulla oblongata. Med. Times & Gaz., Lond., 1856, n. s., xii, 407; 432.— **Dahlin** (N.) Betraktelser öfver den sensitiva nerv-verksamheten. Hygiea, Stockholm, 1839, i, 161–166. — **Danilevski** (A.) Zamaitka o yavlenii refleksa v' spherai chuvstvitelnikh nervof. [Remarks on the reflex action of nerves of sensation.] Med. Vestnik, St. Petersb., 1863, iii, 381–384. — **van Deen.** Over de gevoelszenuwen en het verband tusschen de gevoels- en bewegings-zenuwen. Tijdschr. v. nat. Geschied. en Physiol., Leiden, 1839, vi, 275–288. — **Eichholtz** (H.) Das sensitive Nervensystem. Med. Ztg., Berl., 1852, xxi, 51; 55; 99; 105.— **Gubler.** Sur la propriété de transmission des nerfs sensitifs. Compt. rend. Soc. de biol. 1876, Par., 1877, 6. s., iii, 393–396.— **Jobert.** Contribution à l'étude du système nerveux sensitif. J. de l'anat. et physiol., etc., Par., 1870–71, vii, 611–632, 2 pl.—**Lautenbach** (B. F.) On a new method for determining the presence of sensory nerves. J. Physiol., Lond. & Cambridge, 1879–80, ii, 14–18. — **Pierret** (A.) Recherches sur l'origine réelle des nerfs de sensibilité générale dans le bulbe rachidien et la moelle épinière. Compt. rend. Acad. d. sc., Par., 1876, lxxxiii, 1047–1049.— **Richet** (C.) Recherches sur le sentiment comparé au mouvement. *Ibid.*, 1106–1109. ———. Expériences sur les fonctions des nerfs sensitifs. Gaz. méd. de Par., 1876, 4. s., v, 279. *Also:* Compt. rend. Soc. de biol. 1876, Par., 1877, 6. s., iii, 160–165.

Nerves (*Spinal*).

See, also, **Nerves** (*Ganglia, etc., of*) ; **Nervous system** (*Reflex action of*) ; **Spinal cord**.

AHLSTEDT (G. H.) * Sciagraphica nervorum spinalium descriptio, et quidem parium dorsalium atque lumbalium. sm. 4°. *Upsaliæ*, [1796].

ASCH (G. T.) * De primo pare nervorum medullæ spinalis. 4°. *Gottingæ*, [1750].

BOCK (A. C.) Die Rückenmarksnerven nach ihren ganzen Verlaufe, Vertheilungen und Verbindungen, nebst Abbildungen derselben auf 7 Kupfertafeln, gez. von Dr. Martini und gest. von Schröter. 8°; atlas, fol. *Leipzig*, 1827–8.

BOSSE (C. H.) * De gangliorum spinalium vi in mutriendas radices posteriores nervorum spinalium. 8°. *Dorpati Livonorum*, 1859.

BROWN-SÉQUARD (C.-E.) Recherches expérimentales sur les voies de transmission des impressions sensitives et sur des phénomènes singuliers qui succèdent à la section des racines des nerfs spinaux. 8°. *Paris*, 1856.

DRIESSEN (P.) * Diss. exhibens et icone illustrans nervos musculorum abdominalium et superficiei inguinis. 4°. *Groningæ*, 1775.

Also, in: JANSEN (W. X.) Collect. diss. [etc.] 4°. *Dusseldorpii*, 1792, ii, 271–290, 1 pl.

EKMAN (J. J.) * Sciagraphica nervorum spinalium descriptio, et quidem nervi intercostalis s. sympathetici. 4°. *Upsaliæ*, [1796].

FISCHER (J. L.) Descriptio anatomica nervorum lumbalium sacralium et extremitatum inferiorum. imp. fol. *Lipsiæ*, 1791.

GUDENDORF (A.) * Ob izmenenijach v mjakotnych voloknach pererezannago nerva. [On alterations produced by section of spinal nerves.] 8°. *St. Petersburg*, 1882.

Nerves (Spinal).

HARRISON (E.) An essay on the powerful influence of the spinal nerves over the sexual organs, and through them upon the general state of the body. Being an appendix to the first number of the Monthly Gazette of Practical Medicine. 8°. *London*, 1831.

HILBERT (R.) * Zur Kenntniss der Spinalnerven. 8°. *Königsberg i. Pr.*, 1878.

NORÆUS (O.) * Sciagraphica nervorum spinalium descriptio, et quidem parium cervicalium, cum plexu brachiali. 4°. *Upsaliæ*, 1794.

PEIPERS (G. F.) Tertii et quarti nervorum cervicalium descriptio, cui accedit succinta eorumdem nervorum quinti; nervi phrenici, præsertim ratione originis; nervi accessorii Willisii; nervi duri, ejusque præcipue rami inferioris; nervi hypoglossi et occipitalis maximi a secundo cervicalium nervo adumbratio. 4°. *Halæ*, 1793.

Also, in: SCRIPT. neurol. minores selecti. 4°. *Lipsiæ*, 1795, iv, 18-49, 1 pl.

POTOTSKI (S.) * Pojasnichno-kresttsovoe spletenie (plexus lumbo-sacralis) otnoshenie ego k nervam nichnei konechnosti i taza. [Lumbosacral plexus; its relation to final termination of nerves in pelvis.] 8°. *St. Petersburg*, 1887.

ROUDANOVSKY (P.) De la structure des racines des nerfs spinaux et du tissu nerveux dans les organes centraux de l'homme et de quelques animaux supérieurs. Ouvrage traduit du russe par Mlle. Olga Padonovsky. Avec atlas de viii planches contenant 72 photographies. 8°. *Paris*, 1876.

RÜDINGER (N.) Die Anatomie der menschlichen Rückenmarks-Nerven für Studirende und Aerzte. Zweite Abtheilung. 4°. *Stuttgart*, 1870.

SAGEMEHL (M.) * Untersuchungen über die Entwickelung der Spinalnerven. roy. 8°. *Dorpat*, 1882.

SCHMIDT (J. A.) Commentarius de nervis lumbalibus eorumque plexu anatomico-pathologicus. Adjecta est duorum, qui in plexu brachiali majori continentur nuperque inveniebantur, plexuum minorum descriptio et adumbratio. 4°. *Vindobonæ*, 1794.

SEUBERT (M. C. G.) De functionibus radicum anteriorum et posteriorum nervorum spinalium commentatio. 8°. *Carlsruhæ et Badæ*, 1833.

Amidon (R. W.) Note on the structure and arrangement of the medullated nerve-fibres in the ganglia of the posterior roots of spinal nerves. J. Nerv. & Ment. Dis., Chicago, 1876, iii, 391-394.—**Arnold** (F.) Ueber den vermeintlichen Ursprung der hinteren Wurzel des ersten Halsnerven aus dem 11ten Paar der Hirnnerven. Ztschr. f. Physiol., Heidelb., 1835, v, 177-180.—**Balfour** (F. M.) On the spinal nerves of amphioxus. J. Anat. & Physiol., Lond., 1875-6, x, 689-692.—**Bert** (P.) & **Marcacci.** Étude sur la distribution des racines motrices du plexus lombaire dans les muscles du membre inférieur. Compt. rend. Soc. de biol. 1881, Par., 1882, 7. s., iii, 267-269.—**Brown** (T.) On irritation of the spinal nerves. Glasgow M. J., 1828, i, 131-160.—**Bruce** (J.) Tumors on the branches of the spinal nerves. Dublin J. M. Sc., 1844-5, xxvi, 120.—**Cunningham** (D. J.) Note on a connecting twig between the anterior divisions of the first and second dorsal nerves. J. Anat. & Physiol., Lond., 1876-7, xi, 539.—**van Deen** (I.) Microscopische waarneming over de wijze waarop zich bij de hoogere dieren de vezels der zenuwen in het ruggemerg, tot de vezels van het ruggemerg zelf verhouden. Tijdschr. v. nat. Geschied. en Physiol., Leiden, 1844, xi, 118-122, 1 pl.—**Delafield** (F.) A case of syphilitic tumors of the spinal nerves. Am. J. Syph. & Dermat., N. Y., 1873, iv, 26.—**Eckhard** (C.) Geschichte der Leitungsverhältnisse in den Wurzeln der Rückenmarksnerven. Beitr. z. Anat. u. Physiol. (E k-hard), Giessen, 1883, x, 135-169.—**Ellis** (G. V.) On the posterior divisions of the spinal nerves. Lond. M. Gaz., 1842-3, xxxi, 697-699.—**Expériences** sur les fonctions des racines des nerf rachidiens. J. de physiol. expér., Par., 1822, ii, 276-279.—**Féré** (C.) Étude anatomique et critique sur les plexus des nerfs spinaux. Arch. de neurol., Par., 1883, v, 332-345.—**Flint** (A.), jr. Historical considerations concerning the properties of the roots of the spinal nerves. Quart. J. Psych. M., N. Y., 1868, ii, 625-660. *Also, transl.:* J. de l'anat. et physiol., etc., Par., 1868, v, 520-538.—**Forgue**

Nerves (Spinal).

& Lannegrace. Distribution spéciale des racines motrices du plexus lombo-sacré. Compt. rend. Acad. d. sc., Par., 1884, xcviii, 1068.—**Gros.** [Recherches sur l'origine du nerf spinal.] Bull. Soc. anat. de Par., 1846, xxi, 38.—**Hawkins** (C. H.) Sir Charles Bell and M. Magendie on the functions of the spinal nerves. Brit. M. J., Lond., 1869, i, 21-23. *Also, in his:* . . . Path. & Surg. Writings, 8°, Lond., 1874, i, 31-38.—**Holl** (M.) Ueber die Lendennerven. Med. Jahrb., Wien, 1880, x, 141-150.—**Kuchin** (K.) K' stroeniyu spinnakh nervnikh uzlov. [Structure of the spinal ganglia.] Med. Vestnik, St. Petersb., 1867, vii, 305-307.—**Kühlwetter** (E.) Zur Lehre von der Lagerung der Gefässnerven in den Wurzeln der Rückenmarksnerven. Beitr. z. Anat. u. Physiol. (Eckhard), Giessen, 1885, xi, 23-41.—**von Lenhossék** (M.) Untersuchungen über die Spinalganglien des Frosches. Arch. f. mikr. Anat., Bonn, 1885-5, xxvi, 370-453, 2 pl.—**Luschka** (H.) Die Faser-Kern-Geschwulst an Wurzeln von Rückenmarksnerven. Arch. f. path. Anat., etc., Berl., 1856, xi, 384-387.—**Magendie.** Expériences sur les fonctions des racines des nerfs qui naissent de la moelle épinière. J. de physiol. expér., Par., 1822, ii, 366-371.—**Monod.** Tumeur fibreuse développée sur le trajet des racines antérieurs de la neuvième paire dorsale des nerfs rachidiens. Bull. Soc. anat. de Par., 2. éd., 1827, ii, 59-65.—**Müller** (J.) Bestätigung des Bell'schen Lehrsatzes, dass die doppelten Wurzeln der Rückenmarksnerven verschiedene Functionen haben, durch neue und entscheidende Experimente. Notiz. a. d. Geb. d. Nat.- u. Heilk., Weimar, 1831, xxx, 113; 129.—**Pützner** (W.) Ein Fall von accessorischen Spinalnerven. Morphol. Jahrb., Leipz., 1882-3, viii, 681-683.—**Pflüger** (E.) Vorläufige Mittheilung über die Einwirkung der vorderen Rückenmarkswurzeln auf das Lumen der Gefässe. Allg. med. Centr.-Ztg., Berl., 1855, xxiv, 537; 601.—**Poletti** (L.) Intorno all' ufficio dei nervi spinali. Ann. univ. di med., Milano, 1825, xxxvi, 112.—**Pregaldino.** Contribution à l'étude des ganglions intervertébraux. Bull. Acad. roy. de méd. de Belg., Brux., 1887, 4. s., i, 671-683. [Rap. de R. Boddaert], 657-660.—**Rattone** (G.) Sull' esistenza di cellule ganglionari nelle radici posteriori dei nervi spinali nell' uomo. Arch. di psichiat., etc., Torino, 1884, v, 167-181, 2 pl. *Also:* Arch. per le sc. med., Torino, 1884-5, viii, 67-82, 2 pl.—**Rauber** (A.) Die letzten spinalen Nerven und Ganglien. Morphol. Jahrb., Leipz., 1877, iii, 602-624, 1 pl.—**Roudanovski** (P.) Anatomicheskaya ottichiya chuvstvitelnikh i dvigatelnikh nervof spinnago mozga. [Anatomical characters of the sensitive and motor nerves of the spinal cord.] Med. Vestnik, St. Petersb., 1866, vi, 27. [*See, also, supra.*]—**Rutherford** (W.) On the relative excitability of different parts of the trunk of a spinal nerve. J. Anat. & Physiol., Lond., 1871, v, 327-338.—**Salter.** Case of exalted reflex irritability of the spinal nerves of the left side of the body. Lancet, Lond., 1868, i, 656.—**Schlemm.** Anatomische Beobachtungen über die Anzahl der Steissbeinnerven, ihren Ursprung und über die an ihnen befindlichen, neu entdeckten Knoten. Arch. f. Anat., Physiol. u. wissensch. Med., Berl., 1834, 91-94. —**Seubert** (M.) Versuche über die Verrichtungen der vordern und hintern Wurzeln der Rückenmarks-Nerven. Ztschr. f. Physiol., Heidelb., 1835, v, 35-57.—**Vicq-d'Azyr.** Sur la description des nerfs de la seconde et troisième paire cervicale. [*From:* Mém. Acad. roy. d. sc. de Par., 1777.] Collect. acad. d. mém., etc., Par., 1787, xvi, 409-422.

Nerves (Trophic).

See, also, Face (*Atrophy of*); Nerve (*Median*); Nerves (*Cranial, Fifth pair of*); Nerves (*Wounds, etc., of*); Neuralgia (*Complications, etc., of*).

FIGUEIREDO (F. do R. B.) * Dos nervos trophicos. 8°. *Rio de Janeiro*, 1883.

HAUSER (P.) * Nouvelles recherches relatives à l'influence du système nerveux sur la nutrition. [Berne.] 8°. *Paris*, 1858.

HOLLMANN (O. H. R.) * De nervorum in nutritionem efficacitate. 8°. *Berolini*, [1863].

KAULBARS (F.) * Trophische und vasomotorische Störungen peripherer Nervenverletzungen. [Erlangen.] 8°. *Jena*, 1874.

KRASKE (P.) * Beiträge zur Lehre von dem Einflusse der Nerven auf die Ernährung der Gewebe. 8°. *Halle*, [1874].

LAURENS (J.-M.-G.) * Des troubles trophiques consécutifs aux maladies des centres nerveux. 4°. *Toulouse*, 1875.

MOUGEOT (J.-B.-A.) * Recherches sur quelques troubles de nutrition consécutifs aux affections des nerfs. 4°. *Paris*, 1867.

Also, in: J. de l'anat. et physiol., etc., Par., 1867, iv, 276-300.

Nerves (Trophic).

STOOD (W.) * Ueber trophische Nerven, nebst einigen einschlägigen Versuchen an Kaninchen. 8°. *Halle a. S.*, 1881.

STUTE (T. L.) * De usu nervorum telæque cellulosæ in nutriendis corporis humani partibus. 4°. *Halæ Magdeb.*, [1766].

TOBIAS (G.) * De nervis trophicis. 8°. *Berolini*, [1863].

VOS (C. J.) De nutritione imprimis nervosa. *Traj. ad Rhenum*, 1789.

In: SCRIPTORES neurol. minores selecti. 4°. *Lipsiæ*, 1795, iv, 202-251.

Albini (D. G.) Sui fenomeni trofici dei centri nervosi, degli organi periferici e lungo i nervi. Movimento, Napoli, 1869, i, 45-52.—**Brown-Séquard** (C. E.) Remarks on some of the physiological and pathological influences of the nervous system on nutrition. Brit. M. J., Lond., 1880, ii, 915.—**Couty.** Quelques expériences sur le rôle trophique des racines postérieures médullaires. Gaz. méd. de Par., 1876, 4. s., v, 254-256.—**Fano** (G.) & **Lourie** (S.) Sulla presenza di un centro-trofico nel sistema bulbo spinale. Salute: Italia med., Genova, 1885, xix, 501-503.—**Jewell** (J. S.) Remarks on trophic action of the nervous system. Tr. Illinois M. Soc., Chicago, 1877, xxvii, 223-232.—**Jones** (H.) Are there special trophic nerves? St. George's Hosp. Rep., Lond., 1868, iii, 89-109.—**Joseph** (M.) Beiträge zur Lehre von den trophischen Nerven. Arch. f. path. Anat., etc., Berl., 1887, cvii, 119-159, 1 pl.—**Laborde.** Troubles trophiques et de la sensibilité à la suite de la lésion expérimentale de la racine descendante du trijumeau dans le bulbe. Gaz. d. hôp., Par , 1878, li, 13.—**Lewaschew** (S. W.) Zur Lehre von den trophischen Nerven. Centralbl. f. d. med. Wissensch., Berl., 1883, xxi, 193 - 201. *Also, transl.*: Ejened. klin. gaz., St. Petersb., 1883, iii, 148-152.—**Mayet.** Des troubles de nutrition de la peau et du tissu conjonctive liés aux lésions du système nerveux. Mém. et compt.-rend. Soc. d. sc. méd. de Lyon (1867), 1868, vii, 209-230. *Also*: Gaz. méd. de Lyon, 1868, xx, 2 0; 214 ; 237.—**Rosanelli** (C.) Su alcune recenti esperienze di Cl. Bernard, tendenti a dimostrare la influenza che hanno le lesioni dei nervi sulla nutrizione degli organi. Gazz. med. ital., prov. venete, Padova, 1863, vi, 213-215. — **Samuel.** Grundzüge zur Lehre vom trophischen Nervensysteme. Schmidt's Jahrb., Leipz., 1859, civ, 224-233. *Also, transl.*: J. de la physiol. de l'homme, Par., 1860, iii, 572 - 596. — **Stewart** (T. G.) On atrophy or gangrene from disease of nerves. Dublin M. Press & Circ., 1866, i, 24 - 27. — **Stiller** (B.) Zur Frage der trophischen Nerven. Wien. med. Wchnschr., 1881, xxxi, 113 ; 152. — **Tobias** (W.) Bericht einer Controle von drei Versuchen des Herrn Samuel zur Constatirung trophischer Nerven. Arch. f. path. Anat., etc., Berl., 1862, xxiv, 579-600.—**Urbantschitsch** (V.) Trophische Störungen im Gebiete des Nervus auriculo-temporalis trigemini. Wien. med. Presse, 1874, xv, 737 ; 765.—**Weiss** (M.) Ein Beitrag zur Casuistik der Trophoneurosen. Allg. Wien. med. Ztg., 1887, xxxii, 237 ; 252.—**Wight** (J. S.) Some points in regard to trophic nerve cells. Med. & Surg. Reporter, Phila., 1882, xlvi, 33 ; 61 ; 89.

Nerves (Vaso-dilator).

See **Mouth** (*Nerves of*).

Nerves (Vasomotor).

See **Nervous** *system* (*Vasomotor*).

Nerves of nerves.

Horsley (V.) Preliminary communication on the existence of sensory nerves and nerve endings in nerve trunks, true "nervi nervorum". [Abstr.] Proc. Roy. M. & Chir. Soc. Lond., 1883-4, n. s., i, 196-198.—**Prus** (J.) O nerwikach wykrytych w osłonce pni nerwowych (nervi nervorum periphericorum). Przegl. lek., Krakow., 1886, xxv, 413 ; 421 ; 429.

Nerves in skin diseases.

See **Skin** (*Diseases of, Neurotic*).

Nerves of taste.

See, also, **Nerve** (*Lingual*); **Taste**; **Tongue** (*Nerves of*).

MENGER (H.) * Die Nervenendigungen und Epithelien der Geschmackspapillen. 8°. *Berlin*, [1869].

Alcock (B.) Determination of the question, which are the nerves of taste. Dublin J. M. Sc., 1836, x, 256-279.—**Festler** (F. S.) Sui nervi dei sensi specifici in generale, e del gusto in particolare. Gazz. med. ital., prov. venete, Padova, 1869, xii, 189-193. ——. Risposta ai rimarchi del Prof. F. Lussana alla mia memoria; sui nervi dei sensi specifici. *Ibid.*, 225-228. [*See, also, infra,* Lussana (F.)]—**Inzani** (G.) & **Lussana** (F.) Sui nervi del gusto. Ann. univ. di med., Milano, 1862,clxxxi,282.—**Key** (E. A.) Ueber

Nerves of taste.

die Endigungsweise der Geschmacksnerven in der Zunge des Frosches. Arch. f. Anat., Physiol. u. wissensch. Med., Leipz., 1861, 329-349, 1 pl.—**Letzerich** (L.) Ueber die Endapparate der Geschmacksnerven. Arch. f. path. Anat., etc., Berl., 1869, xlv, 9-19, 1 pl. *Also* [Abstr.]: Centralbl. f. d. med. Wissensch., Berl., 1868, vi, 499.—**Lussana** (F.) Sui nervi del gusto. Gazz. med. ital., prov. venete, Padova, 1869, xii, 105 ; 113 ; 121 : 1870, xiii, 345 ; 361 : 369 ; 380. *Also, transl.*: Arch. de physiol. norm. et path., Par., 1869, ii, 20 ; 197 : 1871-2, iv, 150 ; 334. ——. Rimarchi alla memoria del Sig. Dott. F. S. Festler, sui nervi dei sensi specifici in generale e del gusto in particolare. Gazz. med. ital., prov. venete, Padova, 1869, xii, 209 - 213. — **Merkel** (F.) Tastzellen und Tastkörperchen bei den Hausthieren und beim Menschen. Arch. f. mikr. Anat., Bonn, 1875, xi, 636 - 652, 2 pl. — **Nervio** (Del) craneano intermediario de Wrisberg. [Discussion.] Gac. méd. de México, 1871, vi, 47-49.—**Randacio** (F.) Sui nervi del gusto. Movimento, Napoli, 1870, ii, 121-125.—**Schiff** (M.) *Intorno ai nervi del gusto ed alla eterotopia tattile. Morgagni, Napoli, 1870, xii, 47-68.—**von Vintschgau.** Vortrag über die Geschmacksnerven. Ber. d. naturw.-med. Ver. in Innsbruck (1877), 1879, viii, 2. Hft., pp. xiii-xv.—**Vizioli** (F.) Intorno ai nervi del gusto ed alla eterotopia tattile. Morgagni, Napoli, 1870, xii, 122-130.—**Vizioli** (F.) & **Lussana.** Intorno ai nervi del gusto. Movimento, Napoli, 1869, i, 271-273.

Nervi, Italy.

Haughton (E.) On Nervi, near Genoa, as a winter health resort. Lancet, Lond., 1884, ii, 1046.—**Italian** health resorts. IV. Nervi and Rapallo. Med. Times & Gaz., Lond., 1877, ii, 361-363.—**Schetelig.** Notes on the climate of Nervi. *Ibid.*, 1875, ii, 493.—**Wissing** (I. V. R.) Nervi som Kursted for Brystsyge. Ugesk. f. Læger, Kjøbenh., 1877, xxiv, 185; 201.

Nervia (Valley of the).

FARINA (J.-F.) La vallée de la Nervia et ses eaux thermales sulfureuses (Pigna, Castel-Vittorio). 12°. *Paris*, 1874.

Nervines.

See **Sedatives**.

Nervous fluid or force.

See, also, **Magnetism** (*Animal*); **Nerve-currents** (*Velocity of*).

ARNOLD (G. C.) * De motu fluidi nervei per fibras medullares nervorum. 4°. *Lipsiæ*, [1768].

VAN BERKMAN (J. M.) * De actione secretoria cerebri, cerebelli, medullæ spinalis. 4°. *Lugd. Bat.*, 1731.

Also, in: DE OBERKAMP (F. J.) Collect. diss. 4°. *Francof. a. M.*, 1767, i, 233-274.

BURGGRAVIUS (J. P.) De existentia spirituum nervosorum eorumque vera origine, indole, motu, effectibus et affectibus in corpore humano vivo, sano et ægro, commentatio medica, Andr. Ottom. Goelicke opposita. sm. 4°. *Francof. a. M.*, 1725.

CLEVENGER (S. V.) Neurility; correlated, converted physical forces. 12°. [*Chicago*, 1879.]

CREUZÉ (G.) * Des principales opinions émises sur la force nerveuse. 4°. *Paris*, 1872.

DAVID (I.-B.) * Identité du fluide nerveux et du fluide électrique. 4°. *Paris*, 1830.

FLEMYNG (M.) The nature of the nervous fluid, or animal spirits, demonstrated ; with an introductory preface. 8°. *London*, 1751.

DE FRANKENAU (G. F.) Disquisitio epistolaris succi nutricii per nervos transitum ejusque effectus in corpore humano expendens : dicata Joh. Gothofredo Bergero. 16°. *Lipsiæ*, 1696.

HEIDLER (C. J.) Die Nervenkraft im Sinne der Wissenschaft, gegenüber dem Blutleben in der Natur. Rudiment einer naturgemässern Physiologie, Pathologie und Therapie des Nervensystems. 8°. *Braunschweig*, 1845.

HENSEY (F.) * Diss. de existentia vanaque liquoris nervosi ad quosdam explicandos morbos necessitate. 4°. *Lugd. Bat.*, 1749.

IDELER (K. W.) * De principio nervorum activo imponderabili. 8°. *Berolini*, [1820].

KUTTENBERG (G. F.) & GRIEBNER (J. S.) Summi spirituum moderatoris auxilio pneumatosin sistit. 4°. *Lipsiæ*, [1709].

Nervous *fluid or force.*

LE CAT (C.-N.) Mémoire qui a remporté le prix sur la question proposée par l'Académie pour le sujet du prix de l'année 1753. 4°. [*Paris*, 1753.]

———. Traité de l'existence, de la nature et des propriétés du fluide des nerfs, et principalement de son action dans le mouvement musculaire. Ouvrage couronné en 1753, par l'Académie de Berlin; suivi des dissertations sur la sensibilité des méninges, des tendons, etc., l'insensibilité du cerveau, la structure des nerfs, l'irritabilité hallérienne, etc. 8°. *Berlin*, 1765.

LOESCHER (M. G.) & URSIN (S. C.) Tentamen de novo succi nervei motu. 4°. *Wittenbergæ*, [1710].

MARBURG (T. W.) *Succi nervei secretio mechanica. sm. 4°. *Vitembergæ*, [1711].

MICHELITZ (A.) Scrutinium hypotheseos spirituum animalium. *Pragæ*, 1782.

In: SCRIPT. neurol. minores selecti. 4°. *Lipsiæ*, 1793, iii, 209-239.

PLANE (J.) *De l'influence nerveuse. 4°. *Paris*, 1823.

PLATNER (E.) [Pr.] præmissa exercitatiuncula litteraria in qua demonstratur vulgarem de fluido nerveo sententiam non antiquam esse sed novam. 4°. [*Lipsiæ*, 1786.]

QUALINI (F.) Accademia e discorso filosofico-medico intorno lo spiritoso liquor de' nervi. 4°. *Pavia*, 1763.

RICHTER (A. J.) *De universi vis nervosæ prægnantium corporis mutationibus nec non de illis ad animum spectantibus seu psychicis. 8°. *Berolini*, [1828].

SCHREIBER (J. C.) *De fluidi nervei existentia improbabili. 4°. *Halæ*, [1771].

SOEMMERRING (S. T.) Ueber den Saft, welcher aus den Nerven wieder eingesaugt wird, im gesunden und kranken Zustande des menschlichen Körpers. Eine Abhandlung, welche zu Amsterdam den Preis des Monnikhosschen Legats im Jahre 1810 erhielt. 8°. *Landshut*, 1811.

STYRIUS (C. B.) *De liquidi nervei ratione ad vitam et sanitatem. 4°. *Halæ Magdeb.*, [1765].

VEHR (C. F.) *De læta ac læsa spiritus mundi parvi in cerebro generatione. sm. 4°. *Francof. ad Viadr.*, [1698].

VILLEFLOSE (L.) *De vi nervea. 4°. *Parisiis*, 1819.

Baréty. Des propriétés physiques d'une force particulière du corps humain (force neurique rayonnante), connue vulgairement sous le nom de magnétisme animal. Gaz. méd. de Par., 1881, 6. s., iii, 502; 520; 532; 544; 599. *Also*, Reprint.—**Barrett** (W. C.) The origin and physiology of nervous force. Tr. Am. Dent. Ass. 1881, Phila., 1882, xxii, 95-107. *Also*: Ohio State J. Dent. Sc., Toledo, 1882, ii, 517-531. *Also*: Am. J. Dent. Sc., Balt., 1882, 3. s., xvi, 337-354. *Also*, Reprint.—**Baxt** (N.) Ueber die Zeit, welche nöthig ist, damit ein Gesichtseindruck zum Bewusstsein kommt und über die Grösse (Extension) der bewussten Wahrnehmung bei einem Gesichtseindrucke von gegebener Dauer. Arch. f. d. ges. Physiol., Bonn, 1871, iv, 325-336.—**Bevan** (W.) An inquiry into the truth of the electric nature of the nervous principle. Dublin M. Press, 1841, vi, 292-294.—**Bidloo** (G.) De nervis qua statuitur non dari spiritus animales. *In his*: Exercit. anat.-chir., 4°, Lugd. Bat., 1708, 119-128.—**Bird** (R.) Remarks on the nature of nerve motion or force. Indian M. Gaz., Calcutta, 1885, xx, 241-248.—**Bowditch** (H. P.) Note on the nature of nerve-force. J. Physiol., Lond., 1885-6, vi, 133-135. *Also*, Reprint. ———. What is nerve-force? Proc. Am. Ass. Adv. Sc., Salem, 1887, xxxv, 237-246. *Also*, Reprint.—**Caldwell** (J. J.) Is nerve and electric force one and the same? Maryland M. J., Balt., 1880-81, vii, 484-486. ———. The similarity of electric and nerve forces. J. Am. M. Ass., Chicago, 1885, v, 225-229.—**Greding** (J. E.) An fluidum nerveum nutrire possit? *In*: Ludwig (C. G.) Decas quæst. med., 4°, Lips., 1740, 33-36.—**Hughes** (R.) On the generation of nerve-force. Brit. M. J., Lond., 1860, i, 456.—**Levison** (J. L.) Remarks on Mr. Stevenson's comment on Dr.

Nervous *fluid or force.*

Marshall Hall's view of the vis nervosa, and on a case of great loss of nervous power resulting from a carious tooth. Lancet, Lond., 1850, ii, 112.—**Ludwig** (C. G.) An motus fluidi nervei cum motu materiæ lucis et ætheris comparari possit? *In his*: Decas quæst. med., 4°, Lips., 1740, 9-12. ———. An fluidum nerveum nutrire possit? *Ibid.*, 33-36.—**Maire.** Mémoire sur la circulation nerveuse. Cong. méd. de France, Par., 1863, i, 15-25.—**N. S.** (M.) ¿Es admisible una fuerza física especial con el nombre de fuerza néurica? Siglo méd., Madrid, 1881, xxviii, 737; 770.—**Nervenkraft** (Ueber) und ihre Wirkungsart. Arch. f. d. Physiol., Halle, 1796, i, 2. Hft., 3-20.—**Philip** (A. P. W.) A concise summary of the facts relating to the nature of the nervous influence. Lond. M. Gaz., 1835-6, xvii, 738.—**Purton** (T.) On the physiology of the brain and nerves. Med. & Phys. J., Lond., 1800, iv, 334-336. ———. A few additional remarks on the identity of the electric and nervous fluids. *Ibid.*, 1802, vii, 324-328.—**Richardson** (B. W.) A theory of a nervous atmosphere. Med. Times & Gaz., Lond., 1871, i, 507-509.—**Rudolphi** (C. A.) Etwas über die sensible Atmosphäre der Nerven. Arch. f. d. Physiol., Halle, 1797, iii, 188-201.—**Searle** (C.) On the nature, source, and distribution of the nervous fluid, or electricity, of the animal system; and the connection between the mind and the body, and of vital temperature. Lancet, Lond., 1830-31, ii, 299-305.—**Stark** (J.) On the nature of the nervous agency. Edinb. M. & S. J., 1844, lxii, 285-311. *Also*, Reprint.—**Stieff** (J. E.) An motus fluidi nervei cum motu materiæ lucis et ætheris comparari possit? *In*: Ludwig (C. G.) Decas quæst. med., 4°, Lips., 1740, 9-12.—**Strachan** (J. M.) On the origin and circulation of nerve force. Edinb. M. J., 1865-6, xi, 114-120.—**Stuart** (A.) Experiments to prove the existence of a fluid in the nerves. Phil. Tr., Lond., 1719-33, vii, 585.—**Turck.** De la nature du fluide nerveux et des sécrétions organiques. Gaz. méd. de Lyon, 1859, xi, 233, 404.—**White** (W. H.) On neurorheuma, or nervous energy. Lancet, Lond., 1886, ii, 161.

Nervous *mimicry.*

See **Miryachit**; **Nervous** *system* (*Diseases of, Diagnosis, etc., of*).

Nervous *system.*

See, also, **Automatism**; **Blood** (*Circulation of*); **Bones** *and nervous system*; **Brain**; **Cerebellum**; **Cerebro-spinal** *fluid*; **Co-ordination** *of movements*; **Embryology**; **Frog**; **Glands** (*Nerves of*); **Heat** (*Animal*); **Heat** (*Effects of*); **Inflammation** (*Nervous influence on*); **Insects** (*Nervous system of*); **Medulla** *oblongata*; **Muscle** (*Physiology of*); **Nerves**; **Nervous** *fluid, etc.*; **Neurology**; **Pacinian** *bodies*; **Pons** *Varolii*; **Pressure** (*Sense of*); **Psychology** (*Physiological*); **Reflexes**; **Respiration**; **Secretion**; **Sensation**, *etc.*; **Somnambulism**; **Spinal** *cord*; **Sympathy**; **Temperature**; **Time** (*Perception, etc., of*).

ADAMUCCI (A.) Système mécanique des fonctions nerveuses. 2 v. 8°. *Paris*, 1808.

ADOLF (J. T.) *De nervorum longitudine in compensationem multitudinis et vice versa. *Altorfii*, 1769.

In: SCRIPT. neurol. minores selecti. 4°. *Lipsiæ*, 1795, iv, 181-188.

AEBY (C.) Schema des Faserverlaufes im menschlichen Gehirn und Rückenmark. 3. Aufl. 8°. *Bern*, 1885.

ALAVOINE (J.) Tableaux d'anatomie. Le système nerveux. I. Nerfs rachidiens. II. Nerfs crâniens et système nerveux périphérique. fol. *Paris*, 1878.

AMMERMÜLLER (C. F.) *Ist als Bildungs-Typus für den menschlichen Organismus das Nerven- oder das Gefäss-System anzusehen? 12°. *Tübingen*, 1832.

ANDERSCH (C. S.) Tractatio anatomico-physiologica de nervis humani corporis aliquibus, quam edidit Ernst. Ph. Andersch. 8°. *Regiomonti*, 1797.

ARNOLD (F.) Bemerkungen über den Bau des Hirns und Rückenmarks, nebst Beiträgen zur Physiologie des zehnten und eilften Hirnnerven, mehrern kritischen Mittheilungen sowie verschiedenen pathologischen und anatomischen Beobachtungen. 8°. *Zürich*, 1838.

Nervous *system.*

ASCH (M.) * Ueber das Verhältniss des Temperatur- und Tastsinns zu den bilateralen Functionen. 12°. *Berlin*, [1879].

ASTRUC (J.) * An sympathia partium a certa nervorum positura in sensorio interno? [1743.]
In: SIGWART (G. F.) Quæst. med. Par. 4°. *Tubingæ*, 1789, i, 212-219.

AUERBACH (L.) * De irritamentis nervorum studia critica. 8°. *Berolini*, [1849].

BACKER (G.) * Commentatio ad quæstionem physiologicam propositam: "Succincte enarrentur præcipua recentiorum experimenta Bell, Magendie, Eschricht, Schöps et Bellingeri, de actione nervi olfactorii, trigemini, facialis, nec non de utriusque radicis nervorum spinalium officio, ut denique e disputatis concludatur, quænam probabiliter sit actio horum nervorum". 8°. *Traj. ad Rhenum*, 1830.
Also, in: Ann. Acad. Rheno-Traject. (1728-9), 1830, 1-154.

BAILLARGER (J.) Recherches sur l'anatomie, la physiologie et la pathologie du système nerveux. 8°. *Paris*, 1872.

BANG (J.) Nervorum cervicalium anatome. *Havniæ.*
In: SCRIPT. neurol. minores selecti. 4°. *Lipsiæ*, 1791, i, 343-348, 4 pl.

BARKOW (J. C. L.) * Disquisitiones neurologicæ. 4°. *Vratislaviæ*, [1836].

BARRAL (E.-A.) * Observations et réflexions sur quelques points de la pathologie et de la physiologie des centres nerveux. 4°. *Paris*, 1838.

BATAILLEY (P.-D.) * Considérations sur les phénomènes de la vie nutritive (physiologie et pathologie) et leurs rapports avec le système nerveux. 4°. *Paris*, 1854.

BAUR (C. J.) Tractatus de nervis anterioris superficiei trunci humani, thoracis præsertim abdominisque. 4°. *Tubingæ*, 1818.

BAZIN (A.) Thèse sur l'unité propre an système nerveux de la vie animale et à celui de la vie organique, et sur les rapports physiologiques et zoologiques qui existent entre eux. 4°. *Paris*, 1839.

———. Du système nerveux de la vie animale et de la vie végétative; de leurs connexions anatomiques, et des rapports physiologiques, psychologiques et zoologiques qui existent entre eux. 4°. *Paris*, 1841.

BELL (C.) A series of engravings explaining the course of the nerves. 4°. *London*, 1803.

———. The same. With an address to young physicians on the study of the nerves. 2. ed. 4°. *London*, 1816.

———. The same. 2. Am. ed. 4°. *Philadelphia*, 1834.

———. An exposition of the natural system of the nerves of the human body, with a republication of the papers delivered to the Royal Society on the subject of nerves. 8°. *London*, 1824.

———. The same. 8°. *Philadelphia*, 1825.

———. Appendix to the papers on the nerves, republished from the Royal Society's Transactions; containing consultations and cases illustrative of the facts announced in those papers. 8°. *London*, 1827.

———. The nervous system of the human body, embracing the papers delivered to the Royal Society on the subject of the nerves. [With] appendix, containing cases and letters of consultation on nervous diseases, submitted to the author since the publication of his papers on the functions of the nerves, in the Transactions of the Royal Society, and illustrative of the facts announced in the preceding pages. 4°. *London*, 1830.

———. The same. 8°. *Washington*, 1833.

Nervous *system.*

———. The same. 3. ed., with three additional papers on the nerves of the encephalon. 8°. *London*, 1844.

———. The same. Physiologische und pathologische Untersuchungen des Nervensystems. Aus dem Englischen übersetzt von Moritz Heinrich Romberg. Neue mit der ersten Aufl. gleichlautende Ausgabe. 8°. *Berlin*, 1836.

BELLINGERI (C. F.) Ragionamenti, sperienze ed osservazioni patologiche comprovanti l'antagonismo nervoso. 8°. *Torino*, 1833.

BELLMUND (F. C.) * Diss. exhibens theoriam nervorum. 4°. *Wirceburgi*, [1737].

BERENDT (G. C.) * De atmosphæra nervorum sensitiva commentatio. 4°. *Gottingæ*, [1813].

BERNARD (C.) Leçons sur la physiologie et la pathologie du système nerveux. 2 v. 8°. *Paris*, 1858.

BIANCHI (G.) Saggio riguardante l'impressioni sui nervi in generale. 8°. *Pisa*, 1795.

BIDDER (F. H.) Neurologische Beobachtungen. 4°. *Dorpat*, 1836.

BIEGLER (A. P.) Anatomy and physiology of the brain and nervous system. 8°. *Albany*, 1840.

BINDSCHEDLER (R. G.) * Experimentelle Beiträge zur Lehre von der Nervenreizbarkeit. 8°. *Zürich*, 1865.

BIRKNER (G.) Das Wasser der Nerven in physiologischer und pathologischer Beziehung. Mit einem Vorwort von Dr. Emil Harless. 2. Aufl. 8°. *Augsburg*, 1858.

BLANC (C.-M.) * Quelques propositions sur le système nerveux. 4°. *Paris*, 1829.

BOCK (A. C.) Darstellung des Gehirnes, des Rückenmarkes, und der Sinnes-Werkzeuge, sowie auch des menschlichen Körpers überhaupt nach seinem äussern Umfange. 8°; atlas, 4°. *Leipzig*, 1824.

BOGROS (J.-A.) Mémoire sur la structure des nerfs. Précédé d'une notice historique sur ce médecin par le Dr. Vernière. 4°. *Paris*, 1827.

BOICESCU (A.) Centrii nervosi creerul din puntul de vedere anatomiccu óre care considerațiuni asupra fisiologii și patologii lui. 8°. *Bucuresci*, 1882.
Suppl. to: Spitalul, Bucuresci, 1881, i.

BORRELLI (D.) I nervi e la vita; prolusione al corsa di patologia interna, letta nella R. università di Napoli il dì 29 genn. 1873. 8°. *Napoli*, 1873.

BORREMANS. Neurology of the human body, revised by T. King. Explanation of the plates. 8°. [*London, n. d.*]

BOSE (E. G.) De nervorum actione ex collisione. *Lipsiæ*, 1762.
In: SCRIPT. neurol. minores selecti. 4°. *Lipsiæ*, 1792, ii, 251-265.

BROWN-SÉQUARD (C. E.) Course of lectures on the physiology and pathology of the central nervous system. Delivered at the Royal College of Surgeons, of England, in May, 1858. 8°. *Philadelphia*, 1860.

———. Dual character of the brain. 8°. *Washington*, 1877.
Being No. 291 Smithsonian Miscellaneous Collections, and Lecture 2 of the Toner lectures.

BRÜCKE (E.) Vorlesungen über Physiologie. 2. Bd. Physiologie der Nerven und der Sinnesorgane und Entwickelungsgeschichte. 3. Aufl. 8°. *Wien*, 1884.

BUDGE (J.) Untersuchungen über das Nervensystem. 2 v. 8°. *Frankfurt a. M.*, 1841-2.

BURDACH (C. F.) Umrisse einer Physiologie des Nervensystems. 8°. *Leipzig*, 1844.

CAIRNS (J.) * Considérations physiologiques sur le système nerveux. 4°. *Paris*, 1824.

Nervous *system.*

CALDWELL (J. J.) Involuntary action of the nervous system; read before the American Dental Convention, August 17, 1877, at Oakland, Maryland. 8°. *Cincinnati,* 1877.

CARBUTT (E.) *De systematis nervosi physiologia. 8°. *Edinburgi,* 1814.

CARLETON (*Mrs.*) Enquiry into the nature and effects of the nervous influence and its connexion with the vital, moral, and intellectual operations. A physiological, metaphysical, and moral essay. In three parts. 8°. *Paris,* 1836.

CARPENTER (W. B.) Inaugural dissertation on the physiological inferences to be deduced from the structure of the nervous system in the invertebrate classes of animals. 8°. *Edinburgh,* 1839.

CARUS (C. G.) Versuch einer Darstellung des Nervensystems und insbesondere des Gehirns nach ihrer Bedeutung, Entwickelung und Vollendung im thierischen Organismus. 4°. *Leipzig,* 1814.

CASTEL [A.-L.] Les bases physiologiques de la médecine. Première partie, contenant la réfutation de la doctrine de Charles Bell, et l'explication des phénomènes de la paralysie. 8°. *Paris,* 1842.

———. Exposition des attributs du système nerveux; réfutation de la doctrine de Charles Bell et explication des phénomènes de la paralysie. 2. éd., augmentée. 8°. *Paris,* 1845.

CHADWICK (C.) *Inaugural dissertation on the question: How far are secretion and nutrition dependent on nervous influence? 8°. *Edinburgh,* 1837.

CHEVILLARD (A.) Études expérimentales sur certains phénomènes nerveux et solution rationnelle du problème dit spirite. Quatrième édition, revue, corrigée et précédée d'un aperçu sur le magnétisme animal. 8°. *Paris,* 1882.

CLARK (F. Le G.) The practical anatomy and elementary physiology of the nervous system; designed for the use of students in the dissecting room. 8°. *London,* 1836.

COOPMANS (G.) Neurologia, et observatio de calculo, ex urethra excreto, tabulis illustrata. 8°. *Franequeræ,* 1789.

CORBUTT (E.) *De systematis nervosi physiologia. 8°. *Edinburgi,* 1814.

CORLEO (S.) Ricerche su la natura della innervazione, con applicazione fisiologiche, patologiche et terapeutiche. 8°. *Palermo,* 1857.

CROS (A.) Les fonctions supérieures du système nerveux; recherches des conditions organiques et dynamiques de la pensée. 8°. *Paris,* 1874.

CROUS Y CASELLAS (J.) Tratado elemental de anatomía y fisiología normal y patológica del sistema nervioso. 8°. *Valencia,* 1878.

CRUSEN (C. B.) *De tensione nervorum. 4°. *Gottingæ,* [1765].
Also, in: SCRIPT. neurol. minores selecti. 4°. *Lipsiæ,* 1795, iv, 189–201.

CURTIUS (C. L.) *De explicando consensu partium qui nervis debetur. 4°. *Halæ,* [1770].

VAN DEEN (I.) *Disquisitio physiologica de differentia et nexu inter nervos vitæ animalis et vitæ organicæ. 8°. *Lugd. Bat.,* 1834.

DELAROCHE (D.) Analyse des fonctions du système nerveux, pour servir d'introduction à un examen pratique des maux de nerfs. 2 v. 8°. *Genève,* 1778.

DERMOTT (G. D.) A description of the distribution of the nerves of the human body, with elementary physiological and surgical observations, including Mr. Brooke's nomenclature of the nervous system. 8°. *London,* 1830.

Nervous *system.*

DOWLER (B.) Experimental researches, illustrative of the functional oneness, unity, and diffusion of nervous action, of four sets of nerves, and a fourfold set of functions, and transmitted impressions; with a brief exposition of the philosophy of vivisection and of sensation. 8°. *New Orleans,* 1851.
Also, in: N. Orl. M. & S. J., 1851–2, viii, 37–66.

DU BOIS-REYMOND (E.) Gesammelte Abhandlungen zur allgemeinen Muskel- und Nervenphysik. 2 v. 8°. *Leipzig,* 1875–7.

DUCHENNE. Iconographie photographique pour servir à l'étude de la structure intime du système nerveux de l'homme. Note communiquée à la Société de médecine de Paris dans la séance du 16 octobre 1868. 8°. *Paris,* 1869.

DUNBAR (J. R. W.) *An essay on the structure, functions, and diseases of the nervous system. 8°. *Philadelphia,* 1828.

DUPRÉ (S.) *Développement et structure du système nerveux. 4°. *Paris,* 1856.

DURAND (F.-A.) Trois nouveaux mémoires sur l'action nerveuse: 1° Recherches sur la qualité électrique du sang; 2° Lois synthétiques du mouvement vital; 3° Lois synthétiques des mouvements morbides. 8°. *Paris,* 1845.

———. Nouvelle théorie de l'action nerveuse et des principaux phénomènes de la vie. 8°. *Paris,* 1845.

DUVAL (M.) Leçons sur la physiologie du système nerveux (sensibilité) professées à la Faculté de médecine de Paris, recueillies par F. Dassy. 8°. *Paris,* 1883.

EARLE (J. W.) A new exposition of the functions of the nerves. 8°. *London,* 1833.

ECKER (A.) Physiologische Untersuchungen über die Bewegungen des Gehirns und Rückenmarks, insbesondere den Einfluss der Cerebrospinalflüssigkeit auf dieselben. 8°. *Stuttgart,* 1843.

ECKHARD (C.) Grundzüge der Physiologie des Nervensystems. 8°. *Giessen,* 1854.

———. Experimentalphysiologie des Nervensystems. roy. 8°. *Giessen,* 1867.

———. Ueber das Nervenleben. Akademische Festrede. 4°. *Giessen,* [1874].

EDINGER (L.) Zehn Vorlesungen über den Bau der nervösen Centralorgane. 8°. *Leipzig,* 1885.

EDWARDS (W.-F.) Note sur les contractions musculaires produites par le contact d'un corps solide, avec les nerfs, sans arc galvanique. 8°. [*Paris,* 1825.]
Repr. from: Ann. d. sc. nat., Par., 1825.

EGGER (G.) *De consensu nervorum. 8°. *Vindobonæ,* 1775.
Also, in: DE WASSERBERG (F. X.) Op. min. med. et diss. 8°. *Vindobonæ,* 1775, ii, 159–187.

EHRENBERG (C. G.) Observations on the structure hitherto unknown of the nervous system in man and animals. Transl., with additions and notes, by David Craigie, M. D. 8°. *Philadelphia,* 1838.

EKMAN (J. J.) *Sciagraphica nervorum spinalium descriptio, et quidem nervi intercostalis s. sympathetici. 4°. *Upsaliæ,* [1796].

FÉRÉ (C.) Traité élémentaire d'anatomie du système nerveux. 8°. *Paris,* 1886.

FERRAND (E.) *Considérations générales sur l'innervation. 4°. *Strasbourg,* 1836.

FLECHSIG (P. E.) Die Leitungsbahnen im Gehirn und Rückenmark des Menschen auf Grund entwickelungsgeschichtlicher Untersuchungen. 8°. *Leipzig,* 1876.

FLOURENS (P.) Recherches expérimentales sur les propriétés et les fonctions du système nerveux dans les animaux vertébrés. 8°. *Paris,* 1824.

———. The same. 2. éd. 8°. *Paris,* 1842.

Nervous *system.*

———. Expériences sur le système nerveux, faisant suite aux : Recherches expérimentales sur les propriétés et les fonctions du système nerveux dans les animaux vertébrés, du même auteur. 8°. *Paris*, 1825.

FLOWER (W. H.) Diagrams of the nerves of the human body, exhibiting their origin, divisions, and connections, with their distribution to the various regions of the cutaneous surface and to all the muscles. In an atlas of six plates. fol. *London*, 1861.

———. The same. Edited, with additions, by W. W. Keen, M. D. 4°. *Philadelphia*, 1872.

FOERG (A.) Grundlinien zu einer morphologischen Betrachtung des Gehirns. Als Programm zu seiner demnächst erscheinenden morphologischen Darstellung des Cerebrospinalorgans des Menschen. 12°. *München*, 1839.

FORT (A.-J.-A.) Leçons sur les centres nerveux, professées à l'école pratique de la Faculté de médecine de Paris. Publiées par Eug.-A. Poncy, 1877. 8°. *Paris*, 1878.

FOURNIE (É.) Physiologie du système nerveux cérébro-spinal d'après l'analyse physiologique des mouvements de la vie. 8°. *Paris*, 1872.

FOVILLE (A.-L.) Traité complet de l'anatomie, de la physiologie et de la pathologie du système nerveux cérébro-spinal. 1e partie. Anatomie. 8°. Avec atlas, 4°. *Paris*, 1844.

FRAENZEL (F. L.) * Hodiernæ doctrinæ de nervorum cerebralium spinaliumque functionibus epitome. 8°. *Dresdæ*, 1832.

———. The same. 8°. *Dresdæ*, 1833.

FROMENT (J.-B.-F.) Traité d'anatomie humaine, ou description méthodique de toutes les parties du corps humain [etc.] Névrologie. 2 v. 8°. *Paris*, 1846.

GALEN (C.) Lehre vom gesunden und kranken Nervensysteme. Von Dr. Friedrich Falk. 8°. *Leipzig*, 1871.

GALL (F.-J.) & SPURZHEIM (G.) Anatomie und Physiologie des Nervensystemes im Allgemeinen, und des Gehirnes insbesondere. Mit Beobachtungen über die Möglichkeit, die Anlagen mehrerer Geistes- und Gemüthseigenschaften aus dem Baue des Kopfes der Menschen und der Thiere zu erkennen. 1. Bd. 8°. *Paris*, 1810.

——— ———. The same. Anatomie et physiologie du système nerveux en général, et du cerveau en particulier. Avec des observations sur la possibilité de reconnoître plusieurs dispositions intellectuelles et morales de l'homme et des animaux par la configuration de leurs têtes. Avec atlas de cent planches, fol. 4 v. 4°. *Paris*, 1810–19.

GAMA (J.-P.) Discours prononcé à l'Hôpital militaire d'instruction du Val-de-Grâce, le 16 octobre 1827, dans la séance publique destinée à la distribution des prix. 8°. *Paris*, 1827.

GAUTIER D'AGOTY (J.) Exposition anatomique des organes des sens jointe à la neurologie entière du corps humain et conjectures sur l'électricité animale et le siége de l'âme. fol. *Paris*, 1775.

GINTRAC (É.) Traité théorique et pratique de l'appareil nerveux. 4 v. 8°. *Paris*, 1869.

GODDARD (P. B.) Plates of the cerebro-spinal nerves, with references; for the use of medical students. 4°. *Philadelphia*, 1837.

GOURDON (V.-P.) * Considérations physiologiques et pathologiques sur les deux ordres de nerfs, sur la cause principale des affections dites nerveuses, et sur les moyens thérapeutiques propres à combattre ces maladies avec plus de succès. 8°. *Paris*, 1837.

GRANDCHAMP (F.) & GRANDCHAMP (P.) Recherches sur le siège spécial de différentes fonctions du système nerveux. 8°. [*Paris*], 1823.

Nervous *system.*

GROSSMANN (A. T.) * De specifica nervorum sensibilium energia. 4°. *Lipsiæ*, [1842].

GRUENHAGEN (A.) * De novo schemate fluminis nervorum et musculorum galvanici. 8°. *Regimonti Pr.*, 1863.

GUÉRARD (J. A.) * Num a pathologicis observationibus confirmata vel infirmita sunt, de nervosi systematis functionibus physiologorum experimenta. 4°. *Parisiis*, 1829.

HAASE (J. G.) Cerebri nervorumque corporis humani anatome repetita. 8°. *Lipsiæ*, 1781.

HALL (M.) New memoir on the nervous system. 4°. *London*, 1843.

HANDBUCH der Physiologie, bearb. von H. Aubert [*et al.*]. Hrsg. von L. Hermann. v. 2. Physiologie des Nervensystems. 8°. *Leipzig*, 1879.

HARRISON (J. H.) An essay towards a correct theory of the nervous system. 8°. *Philadelphia*, 1844.

HASKELL (B.) Essays on the physiology of the nervous system, with an appendix on hydrophobia. 8°. *Gloucester*, 1856.

HAUFF. Einige Bemerkungen über die normale und abnorme Thätigkeit der sensibeln Nerven; über Empfindung und Schmerz. 8°. [*n. p., n. d.*]

HECK (J. J.) * De nervorum rigore. 8°. *Berolini*, [1823].

HEINTZE (G.) * De nervis eorumque præstantia in corpore humano. 4°. [*Lipsiæ*, 1725.]

HENRY (W. C.) Report on the physiology of the nervous system. 8°. *London*, 1833.

Cutting from : Rep. Brit. Ass. Adv. Sc., Lond., 1833, 59-91.

HILL (A.) * The plan of the nervous system. 8°. *Cambridge*, 1885.

HIRSCHFELD (L.) Névrologie et esthésiologie : traité et iconographie du système nerveux, et des organes des sens de l'homme, avec leur mode de préparation. Avec un atlas par J.-B. Léveillé. 2. éd. 8°. *Paris*, 1866.

———. The same. The nervous system. Edited in English by A. Mason Macdougal. Pt. 1-2. 4°. *London*, 1867.

HOLLE (C.) * De nervorum systemate quædam generalia. 8°. *Berolini*, [1833].

IMADA Tsukane. Shinkei Ichirau Dzukai. [Illustrated conspectus of the nervous system.] narrow 12° on folded paper. *Tokio*, 1880. Japanese text.

JABLONSKI (J.) * Étude sur l'innervation. 4°. *Paris*, 1868.

JACOBI (A.) * O razdrajenii chim. vetshestvami chuvstvitelnich nervnich nitei ljagushki. [On chemical irritation of the motor fibres in the frog.] 8°. *St. Petersburg*, 1863.

JETZKE (J. F. C.) * De tensione nervorum in genere. 4°. *Halæ*, [1770].

JOBERT (A.-J.) *de Lamballe.* Études sur le système nerveux. 2 v. [paged consecutively] in 1. 8°. *Paris*, 1838.

KEY (E. A. H.) & RETZIUS (G.) Studien in der Anatomie des Nervensystems und des Bindegewebes. Erste Abtheilung. [2 pts.] 4°. *Stockholm*, 1875-6.

KILIAN (F. M.) Versuche über die Restitution der Nervenerregbarkeit nach dem Tode. 8°. *Giessen*, 1847.

KLENCKE (P. F. H.) Neue anatomische und physiologische Untersuchungen über die Primitivnervenfaser und das Wesen der Innervation. Beiträge zur Ausfüllung obwaltender Lücken und zur Aufklärung mehrfacher Zweifel in der Nervenlehre. 8°. *Göttingen*, 1841.

LACRAMPE-LOUSTAU (J.-B.) * Propositions sur quelques fonctions du système nerveux, et

Nervous *system.*

en particulier sur le siége des causes de la paralysie des membres. 4°. *Paris,* 1824.

LEE (E.) The brain the sole center of the human nervous system. 8°. *Edinburgh,* 1848.

LEFEVRE (*Sir* G. W.) An apology for the nerves; or, their influence and importance in health and disease. 8°. *London,* 1844.

LEVY (A.) *De neurologia sæculi decimi sexti. 8°. *Berolini,* [1848].

LINDH (D.) *Om nervsystemets verkningar i synnerhet i menniskokroppen. 8°. *Helsingfors,* 1832.

LOBSTEIN (J.-G.-C.-F.-M.) Discours sur la prééminence du système nerveux dans l'économie animale, et l'importance d'une étude approfondie de ce système. 8°. *Strasbourg,* 1821.

VON LODER (J. C.) *Primæ lineæ neurologiæ corporis humani; commentatio i. sm. 4°. *Jenæ,* .[1778].

LUSSANA (F.) Alcune osservazioni fisio-patologiche su 'l sistema nervoso. 8°. *Milano,* 1856.

LUYS (J.-B.) Iconographie photographique des centres nerveux. 2 v. in 1. 4°. *Paris,* 1872.

—— . The same. 4°. *Paris,* 1873.

M'KENDRICK (J. G.) A review of recent researches on the physiology of the nervous system. 8°. *Edinburgh,* 1874.

MAGENDIE (F.) Mémoire sur quelques découvertes récentes relatives aux fonctions du système nerveux. 8°. *Paris,* 1823.

Also [Abstr.], *in:* J. de physiol. expér., Par., 1824, iv, 399-407.

MAGNAN (V.) Recherches sur les centres nerveux, pathologie et physiologie pathologique. 8°. *Paris,* 1876.

MAHIR (O.) Ueber das Verhältniss des Nervensystemes zum Blute, und dessen Erscheinungen im gesunden und kranken thierischen Organismus. 8°. *München,* 1836.

MAJER (J.) Fizyologija układu nerwowego. [Physiology of the nervous system.] 8°. *Kraków & Warszawa,* 1854.

MANDELSTAM (N.) *Ueber den Einfluss chemischer Agentien auf die Erregbarkeit der Nerven. 8°. *Erlangen,* 1875.

MANEC (P. J.) The cerebro-spinal axis of man; with the origin and first division of its nerves. From the French. Transl. and revised by J. Pancoast. 1 wall map. fol. *Philadelphia,* [*n. d.*]

MARTIN (R.) Institutiones neurologicæ, sive de nervis corporis humani tractatio. Præmissa est oratio de proprietatibus nervorum generalioribus. Editio altera, latine reddita, recentiorum observationibus aucta et priori emendatior. 2 pts. 8°. *Holmiæ et Lipsiæ,* 1781.

MARTIN SAINT-ANGE (G.-J.) *Recherches anatomiques et physiologiques sur les membranes du cerveau et de la moelle épinière, et sur le liquide cérébro-spinal. 4°. *Paris,* 1829.

MASON (J. J.) Photo-micrographs of sections of nerve centres. 4°. [*Newport, R. I.,* 1880.]

MAYER (J. C. A.) Anatomisch-physiologische Abhandlung vom Gehirn, Rückenmark und Ursprung der Nerven. 4°. *Berlin u. Leipzig,* 1779.

MAYO (H.) A series of engravings intended to illustrate the structure of the brain and spinal cord in man. fol. *London,* 1827.

—— . Powers of the roots of the nerves, in health and in disease. Likewise, on magnetic sleep. 12°. *London,* 1837.

—— . The nervous system and its functions. 8°. *London,* 1842.

MENEGHINI (J.) *De axe cephalo-spinali. 8°. *Patavii,* 1834.

MERCIER (C.) The nervous system and the mind, a treatise on the dynamics of the human organism. 8°. *London & New York,* 1888.

Nervous *system.*

MEYER (A. B.) *Beiträge zur Lehre von der elektrischen Nervenreizung. 8°. *Zürich,* 1867.

MEYER (G. H.) Untersuchungen über die Physiologie der Nervenfaser. 8°. *Tübingen,* 1843.

—— . Ueber die Bedeutung des Nervensystems. Ein populärer Vortrag. 8°. *Stuttgart,* 1874.

MICHON (L.-M.) *Texture et développement de l'encéphale et de la moelle épinière. 4°. *Paris,* 1836.

MILLARDET (A.) *Nouvelles recherches sur la périodicité de la tension. Étude sur les mouvements périodiques et paratoniques de la sensitive. 4°. *Strasbourg,* 1869.

MILLER (H.) *An inaugural thesis on the relation between the sanguiferous and nervous systems. 8°. *Lexington, Ky.,* 1822.

MOLESCHOTT (J.) Sugli attributi generali dei nervi. 8°. *Torino,* 1881.

—— . The same. Ueber die allgemeinen Lebenseigenschaften der Nerven. 12°. *Giessen,* 1882.

MONDINO (C.) Ricerche macro e microscopiche sui centri nervosi. 8°. *Torino,* 1887.

MONRO (A.)[1] An anatomical treatise of the nerves; an account of the reciprocal motions of the heart; and a description of the human lacteal sac and duct. 12°. *Edinburgh,* 1732.

—— . The same. Tractatus tres, de nervis eorumque distributione, de motu cordis et ductu thoracico, latine redditi a G. Coopmans, qui præter commentarium perpetuum adjecit librum de cerebri et nervorum administratione anatomica. Ed. altera. 8°. *Harlingæ,* 1763.

—— . The same. Bemerkungen über die Struktur und Verrichtungen des Nervensystems. Aus dem Englischen übersetzt, nebst einigen Anmerkungen und Zusätzen. 4°. *Leipzig,* 1787.

MONRO (A.)[2] Experiments on the nervous system with opium and metallic substances; made chiefly with a view of determining the nature and effects of animal electricity. 4°. *Edinburgh & London,* 1793.

MOUREMANS (J.) *Diss. summariam expositionem complectens de legibus formationis nec non actionis systematis nervosi centralis. 4°. *Gandavi,* [1829].

MOYE (E.) *Considérations sur l'influence exercée par le système sanguin sur le système nerveux, et sur les applications qui en résultent pour la pathologie. 4°. *Strasbourg,* 1853.

MÜLLER (G. A.) Betrachtungen über die Art und Weise der Mitwürckung derer Nerven zu denen musskulösen Zusammenziehungen bey Gelegenheit der berlinischen Aufgabe kürtzlich entworffen von . . . 16°. *Franckfurt am Mayn,* 1753.

MUELLER (G. H.) Series experimentorum in musculis et nervis animalium quorundam institutorum horumque organorum functionem s. effectus naturales illustrantium. *Stuttgardiæ,* 1793.

In: SCRIPT. neurol. minores selecti. 4°. *Lipsiæ,* 1795, iv, 170-180.

MÜNTER (G. W.) Versuch einer neuen Theorie der Verrichtungen des Gehirns und Nervensystems, enthaltend eine physiologische Beweisführung, dass das centrale und peripherische Nervensystem für den Organismus das ist, was die Genitalien für die Erhaltung der Gattung sind. 8°. *Leipzig,* 1838.

MUNK (H.) Untersuchungen über das Wesen der Nerven-Erregung. 1. Bd. roy. 8°. *Leipzig,* 1868.

MUSGRAVE (S.) Speculations and conjectures on the qualities of the nerves. 8°. *London,* 1776.

Nervous *system.*

NASSE (F.) Untersuchungen zur Lebensna-turlehre und Heilkunde. Ersten Bandes erste Abtheilung. Ueber das Verhältniss des Gehirns und Rückenmarks zur Belebung des übrigen Körpers. 8°. *Halle*, 1818.

NAUMANN (M. E. A.) Die Probleme der Physiologie oder der Gegensatz von Nervenmark und Blut. 8°. *Bonn*, 1835.

NEILL (J.) Outlines of the nerves, with short descriptions. 8°. *Philadelphia*, 1845.

NERVORUM (De) in musculos actione. sm. 4°. [*Berlin, n. d.*]

NERVOUS (The) system. 16°. *New York*, 1882. Health Primers, No. 9.

NEUMANN (G. C.) * De ratione inter nervorum vires et imponderabilium indolem. 8°. *Bero-lini*, 1828.

NUDOV (H.) [Pr.] est examen partitionis ner-vorum in sensorios atque motorios. 4°. [*Lipsiæ*, 1776.]
Also, in: WEIZ (F. A.) Neue. Ausz. [etc.] 12°. *Leipzig*, 1777, vi, 21–29.

OBERSTEINER (H.) Anleitung beim Studium des Baues des nervösen Centralorgane im ge-sunden und kranken Zustande. roy. 8°. *Leip-zig u. Wien*, 1888.

OGLE (J. W.) Series of clinical cases (with observations) illustrating the views recently put forward by Dr. Brown-Séquard, as regards cer-tain points connected with the physiology of the nervous system. 8°. *London,* [*n. d.*]

O'REILLY. On the placenta and the pheno-mena connected with the animal and organic nervous system. 8°. *New York*, 1861.

OTT (I.) Contributions to the physiology and pathology of the nervous system. 8°. [*n. p.*], 1885–6.

PAGLIANI (L.) Saggio sullo stato attuale delle cognizioni della fisiologia intorno al sistema nervoso su annotazioni raccolte alle lezioni del Prof. J. Moleschott l' anno 1871–2. 8°. *Torino*, 1872.

PANIZZA (B.) Ricerche sperimentali sopra i nervi. Lettera del professore . . . al professore Maurizio Bufalini. 8°. *Pavia*, 1834.

——. The same. Versuche über die Ver-richtungen der Nerven. Brief an Maurizio Bufa-lini. Aus dem Italienischen übersetzt und mit Zusätzen versehen von Carl Schneemann, und bevorwortet von Eisenmann. sm. 8°. *Erlangen*, 1836.
Also, transl. [Abstr.], *in:* Edinb. M. & S. J., 1836, xlv, 70–98.

PANIZZA (M.) La fisiologia del sistema ner-voso nelle sue relazioni coi fatti psichici. 2. ed. 8°. *Roma*, 1881.

PANUM (P. L.) Erindringsord til Forelæsnin-ger over Nervephysiologien. [Reminiscences of the lectures on the physiology of the nerves.] 8°. *Kjøbenhavn*, 1867.

——. Nervevævets, de kontraktile Vævs og Nervesystemets Fysiologi. 8°. *Kjøbenhavn*, 1883.

PFEFFINGER (J.) De structura nervorum. *Argentorati*, 1782.
In: SCRIPT. neurol. minores selecti. 4°. *Lipsiæ*, 1791, i, 1–30.

PINKNEY (N.) The nervous system of the human body; embracing a dissertation delivered to the medical profession of Philadelphia, and students of the two universities, on the subject of the nerves, brain, and organs of sense. 8°. *Philadelphia*, 1839.

PINTSCHOVIUS (C.) * Ein Beitrag zur Frage von der einsinnigen und doppelsinnigen Leitung der Nerven. 8°. *Greifswald*, 1870.
Also, in: Arch. f. Anat., Physiol. u. wissensch. Med., Leipz., 1872, 455–461.

Nervous *system.*

PLATNER (E.) [Pr.] de causis consensus ner-vorum physiologicis. 4°. [*Lipsiæ*, 1790.]
Also, in: SCRIPT. neurol. minores selecti. 4°. *Lipsiæ*, 1792, ii, 266–270.

POINCARÉ. Leçons sur la physiologie normale et pathologique du système nerveux. v. 1. 8°. *Paris*, 1873.

——. Le système nerveux périphérique au point de vue normal et pathologique; leçons de physiologie professées à Nancy; ouvrage faisant suite aux Leçons sur la physiologie normale et pathologique du système nerveux, en deux vo-lumes. 8°. *Paris*, 1876.

——. The same. 2. éd. 2 v. 8°. *Paris*, 1877.

PROCHASKA (G.) De structura nervorum. Tractatus anatomicus tabulis aëneis illustratus. 8°. *Vindobonæ*, 1779.

——. Commentatio de functionibus sys-tematis nervosi.
In his: Oper. minor. 8°. *Viennæ*, 1800, ii, 3–214.

QUAIN (J.) & WILSON (W. J. E.) The nerves of the human body, including the brain and spinal marrow and organs of sense; in a series of plates, with references and physiological com-ments. fol. *London*, 1839.

RAMES. Nouvelles considérations à l'appui de notre interprétation sur le mode de fonctionne-ment du système nerveux. 8°. *Aurillac*, 1877.

——. Aperçu sur le fonctionnement du sys-tème nerveux. 8°. *Paris*, 1878.

RANKE (J.) Die Lebensbedingungen der Ner-ven. 8°. *Leipzig*, 1868.

RANNEY (A. L.) The applied anatomy of the nervous system; being a study of this portion of the human body from a standpoint of its general interest and practical utility, designed for use as a text-book and a work of reference. 8°. *New York*, 1881.

RANVIER (L.) Leçons d'anatomie générale faites au Collége de France. Appareils nerveux terminaux des muscles de la vie organique : cœur sanguin, cœurs lymphatiques, œsophage, muscles lisses. 8°. *Paris*, 1880.

RAWITZ (B.) * Die Ranvier'schen Einschnü-rungen und Lantermann'schen Einkerbungen. [Berlin.] 8°. *Leipzig*, 1879.

REIL (J. C.) Exercitationum anatomicarum fasciculus primus, De structura nervorum. fol. *Halæ Sax.*, 1796.

REIMAR (J. A. H.) De cerebro et nervis com-mentaribus. 4°. [*n. p.*, 1811.]

REITZBERG (C.) * Ueber den Einfluss des Ner-vensystems auf das Wachstum der Horngebilde und die Temperaturverhältnisse des Organismus. 8°. [*Dorpat*], 1855.

REMAK (R.) * Observationes anatomicæ et microscopicæ de systematis nervosi structura. 4°. *Berolini*, [1838].

RIEFLER (B.) * Diss. de nervorum resolu-tione. 8°. *Monachii*, 1836.

DE LA ROCHE. Analyse des fonctions du sys-tème nerveux, pour servir d'introduction à un examen pratique des maux de nerfs. 2 v. 12°. *Genève*, 1778.

ROUDANOVSKY (P.) Études photographiques sur le système nerveux de l'homme et de quel-ques animaux supérieurs, d'après des coupes de tissu nerveux congelé. 8°. Avec atlas, fol. *Paris*, 1868.

RÜDINGER. Atlas des peripherischen Nerven-systems des menschlichen Körpers. Mit einem Vorwort von Prof. Dr. Th. W. L. Bischoff. 2. Aufl. roy. 4°. *Stuttgart*, 1872.

SAŘLANDIÈRE (J.-B.) Traité du système ner-veux dans l'état actuel de la science; avec six planches. 8°. *Paris*, 1840.

Nervous *system*.

SCARPA (A.) Anatomicarum annotationum liber primus: De nervorum gangliis et plexibus. Liber secundus: De organo olfactus præcipuo, deque nervis nasalibus interioribus e pari quinto nervorum cerebri. 2 v. in 1. 4°. *Mutinæ et Ticini*, 1779–85.

———. Tabulæ neurologicæ, ad illustrandum historiam anatomicam cardiacum nervorum, noni nervorum cerebri, glossopharyngei et pharyngei ex octavo cerebri. fol. *Ticini*, 1794. *Also* [Rev.], *in:* Ital. med.-chir. Biblioth., Leipz., 1796, ii, 2. St., 129–138.

———. The same. Engravings of the cardiac nerves, the nerves of the ninth pair, the glossopharyngeal, and the pharyngeal branch of the pneumo-gastric; copied from the "Tabulæ neurologicæ" of . . . by Edward Mitchell, with letter-press description transl. from the original Latin, by Dr. Knox. 2. ed. 4°. *Edinburgh*, 1829.

———, SOEMMERING [*et al.*]. Engravings of the nerves, copied from the works of . . . by E. Mitchell, with an explanatory letter-press by Dr. Knox. 4°. *Edinburgh*, 1829.

SCHAARSCHMIDT (A.) Nevrologische Tabellen. 8°. *Berlin*, 1762.

SCHERVIER (G.) * De persistente nexu vitali partium, harum nexu anatomico per nervos sublato. 8°. *Bonnæ*, 1846.

SCHIFF (M.) Untersuchungen zur Physiologie des Nervensystems mit Berücksichtigung der Pathologie. 8°. *Frankfurt am Main*, 1855.

———. Lezioni di fisiologia sperimentale sul sistema nervosa encefalico, date nel R. Museo di Firenze l' anno 1864–5 e compilate per cura del Pietro Marchi. 2. ed., revista ed aumentata. 12°. *Firenze*, 1873.

SCHIMPF (E.) * Raumsinn der unteren Extremität bei Anchylose des Kniegelenks. 8°. *Böblingen*, 1882.

SCHINDLER (D. H.) * Super nervorum actione ex collisione. 4°. *Lipsiæ*, [1762].

SCHLEMM (F.) Observationes neurologicæ. 4°. *Berolini*, 1834.

SCHMIDT (M. D.) * Diss. inaug. medica continens de nevrodynami particulam i. 8°. *Jenæ*, [1796].

SCHOELLER (J. T.) * De nervorum substantiæ motu quondam defenso. 8°. *Halæ*, [1819].

SCHWALBE (G.) Lehrbuch der Neurologie. Zugleich des zweiten Bandes, zweite Abtheilung von Hoffmann's Lehrbuch der Anatomie des Menschen. 8°. *Erlangen*, 1881.

SCRIPTORES neurologici minores selecti, sive opera minora ad anatomiam, physiologiam et pathologiam nervorum spectantia. Edidit notulis nonnullis illustravit præfatus est . . . C. F. Ludwig. 4 v. in 3. 4°. *Lipsiæ*, 1791–5.

SCRIVE (G.) *Appréciation des travaux les plus récents sur les fonctions du système nerveux. 4°. *Strasbourg*, 1846. Concours.

SEIZ (G. F.) * De actione nervorum. 4°. *Erlangæ*, [1755].

SELIGO (S.) * Animadversiones nonnullas anatomico-physiologicas in doctrinam nervorum . . . defendet. 4°. *Regiomonti*, 1783.

SHAW (A.) Narrative of the discoveries of Sir Charles Bell in the nervous system. 8°. *London*, 1839.

———. On Sir Charles Bell's researches in the nervous system. 8°. *London*, 1847.

———. An account of Sir Charles Bell's discoveries in the nervous system. 12°. *London*, 1860.

SIMON (J.-J.) * De la sympathie et de l'antagonisme dans les fonctions du système nerveux. 4°. *Strasbourg*, 1848.

Nervous *system*.

SMITH (J.) The nervous system; its use and abuse. A lecture delivered for the Australian Health Society, 3d Oct., 1881. 8°. *Melbourne*, 1881. *Repr. from:* Victorian Rev., 1881.

SMITH (J. A.) Select discourses on the functions of the nervous system, in opposition to phrenology, materialism, and atheism, to which is prefixed a lecture on the diversities of the human character arising from physiological peculiarities. 8°. *New York*, 1840. *Also* [Rev.], *in:* Boston M. & S. J., 1841, xxiv, 293; 337.

SMITH (W.) A dissertation upon the nerves. 8°. *London*, 1768.

VON SOEMMERRING (S. T.) Vom Hirn und Rückenmark. 16°. *Mainz*, 1788.

———. Hirn und Nervenlehre. Umgearbeitet von G. Valentin. 8°. *Leipzig*, 1841.

SPIESS (G. A.) Physiologie des Nervensystems vom ärztlichen Standpunkte dargestellt. 8°. *Braunschweig*, 1844.

STUART (C.) * De systematis nervosi officiis, ejusque conditionibus nonnullis. 8°. *Edinburgi*, 1781. *Also, in:* SMELLIE. Thesaurus med. [etc.] 8°. *Edinburgi*, 1785, iv, 229–261.

SWAN (J.) A demonstration of the nerves of the human body. 4°. *London*, 1834.

———. The same. Névrologie, ou description anatomique des nerfs du corps humain. Trad. de l'anglais avec des additions par E. Chassaignac. 4°. *Paris*, 1838.

TABLE synoptique des nerfs de l'homme. (broadside.) fol. [*n. p., n. d.*]

TAMIN DESPALLES (O.) Alimentation du cerveau et des nerfs. 8°. *Paris*, 1873.

THIEBOUT (C. H.) Chz. De wetten van inwerking van twee zenuwstelsels op elkander of de nitstooting der hoogstgeorganiseerden, in den strijd des levens in de menschelijke maatschappijen. 8°. *Utrecht*, [*n. d.*]

THIEL (T. H. J. E. L.) *Num Magendie de sensualitate anterioris nervorum spinalium radicis recte judicaverit nec ne? 8°. *Regimontii Pr.*, 1846.

TISSOT (S.-A.-D.) Traité des nerfs et de leurs maladies. 4 v. 12°. *Paris*, 1778–80.

———. The same. 2 v. & 4 pts. bound in 3. 18°. *Genève & Paris*, 1779–83.

———. The same. 4 v. 12°. *Lausanne*, 1784.

———. The same. De la catalepsie, de l'extase, de l'anæsthésie, de la migraine, et des maladies du cerveau. 12°. *Lausanne*, 1788.

———. The same. 4 v. 12°. *Arignon*, 1800. *Also, in:* Encycl. d. sc. méd. 41 v. 8°. *Paris*, 1834–46, 7. div., [v. 10], 1–424.

———. The same. Abhandlung von den Nerven und ihren Krankheiten. Aus dem Französischen übersezt von F. A. Weber. 4 v. 8°. *Winterthur u. Leipzig*, 1781–3.

———. The same. Abhandlung über die Nerven und deren Krankheiten, deutsch hrsg. von Joh. Christ. Gottlieb Ackermann. 6 pts. in 3 v. 12°. *Leipzig*, 1782–90–93.

TODD (R. B.) The descriptive and physiological anatomy of the brain, spinal cord, and ganglions, and of their coverings. 8°. *London*, 1845.

———. Physiology of the nervous system. 8°. *London*, 1847.

URECH (J. R.) * De vi et effectu quem nervorum cerebrospinalium et sympathicorum sectio in sanguinis circulationem et in resorptionem habeat. 8°. *Turici*, 1837.

VALENTIN (G.) De functionibus nervorum cerebralium et nervi sympathici libri quattuor. 4°. *Bernæ et Sangalli Helvetiorum*, 1839.

Nervous *system.*

VATER (A.) Epistola anatomica, problematica decima et sexta de viis absconditis pulmonum, quibus aër, respirando receptus, in sanguinem penetrat; nec non de vasorum secretoriorum structura mechanica, et de fibrillarum nervearum in cerebro principiis. Resp. Frederico Ruyschio. 4°. *Amstelædami*, 1714.

VETTER (A. R.) Kurzgefasste Beschreibung aller Gefässe und Nerven des menschlichen Körpers. 16°. *Wien*, 1789.

VIEUSSENS (R.) Neurographia universalis. Hoc est, omnium corporis humani nervorum, simul et cerebri, medullæque spinalis descriptio anatomica . . . Ed. nova. fol. *Lugduni*, 1685.

———. The same. Eaque fideliter et ad vivum delineatis, æreque incisis illustrata cum ipsorum actione et usu, physico discursu explicatis. 12°. *Francofurti*, 1690.

———. The same. Ed. novissima. fol. *Lugduni*, 1716.

VULPIAN (A.) Leçons sur la physiologie générale et comparée du système nerveux faites au Muséum d'histoire naturelle. Rédigées par M. Ernest Brémond. Revues par le professeur . . . 8°. *Paris*, 1866.

WAGNER (O.) * De rhythmo nervorum. 8°. *Berolini*, [1844].

WAGNER (R.) Neurologische Untersuchungen. roy. 8°. *Göttingen*, 1854.

WALKER (A.) The nervous system, anatomical and physiological; in which the functions of the various parts of the brain are for the first time assigned; and to which is prefixed some account of the author's earliest discoveries, of which the more recent doctrine of Bell, Magendie, etc., is shewn to be at once a plagiarism, an inversion, and a blunder associated with useless experiments which they have neither understood nor explained. Being the first volume of an original system of physiology, adapted to the advanced state of anatomy. 8°. *London*, 1834.

WALTHER (H.) * De vi nervorum in secretionibus regundis. 4°. *Lipsiæ*, [1838].

WAUGH (J. S.) The science of the cerebrospinal phenomena attempted. 12°. *London*, 1838.

WEBER (E. H.) * De systemate nerveo organico. 8°. *Lipsiæ*, [1817].

WEDEMEYER (G.) Physiologische Untersuchungen über das Nervensystem und die Respiration und deren Einfluss auf den menschlichen Organismus. sm. 8°. *Hannover*, 1817.

WHITAKER (J. R.) Anatomy of the brain and spinal cord. 12°. *Edinburgh*, 1887.

WILBRAND (F. J. J.) Anatomie und Physiologie der Centralgebilde des Nervensystems. 8°. *Giessen*, 1840.

WILLIS (T.) Cerebri anatome nervorumque descriptio et usus; accessit de ratione motus musculorum tractatus singularis.

Forms part of his: Opera omnia. 4°. *Genevæ*, 1676.

WITKOWSKI (G.-J.) Le système nerveux; structure et fonctions. 8°. *Paris*, 1884.

WRISBERG (H. A.) Observationes anatomicophysiologicæ de nervis, arterias venasque comitantibus. 4°. [*Gottingæ, n. d.*]

Repr. from: Comment. Phys. Soc. Reg. Scient. Gotting., vii, 95–134.

WUNDT (W.) Untersuchungen zur Mechanik der Nerven und Nervencentren. 1. u. 2. Abth. 8°. *Stuttgart*, 1871-6.

ZENGERLE (J. N.) Der Einfluss des Nervensystems auf die Verdauung, Anbildung, Rückbildung, sowie die Entwicklung der thierischen Wärme nach dem gegenwärtigen Standpunkte der Wissenschaft bearbeitet. 8°. *Freiburg i. Breisgau*, 1859.

48

Nervous *system.*

ZERNOFF (D.) Rukovodstvo anatomii nervnoi sistemi cheloveka. (Nevrologija.) 2. ed. 8°. *Moskva*, 1885.

ZIMMERMANN (G.) * De nervorum systematis functionibus. 8°. *Berolini*, [1853].

ZWINGER (G. P.) * Theorema medicum, quod alia sensatio alium motum inferat. 4°. *Altorfii Noricorum*, [1756].

Ackermann (J. F.) Vorläufige Bekanntmachung wichtiger Erscheinungen aus den neuesten physiologischen Versuchen über die Nerven. Med.-chir. Ztg., Salzb., 1792, iii, 289–297.—**Afanasieff** (N.) Untersuchungen über den Einfluss der Wärme und der Kälte auf die Reizbarkeit der motorischen Froschnerven. Arch. f. Anat., Physiol. u. wissensch. Med., Leipz., 1865, 691–702, 2 pl.—**Albini** (G.) Sui fenomeni trofici dei centri nervosi, degli organi periferici e lungo i nervi; osservazioni ed esperimenti. Rendic. Accad. med.-chir. di Napoli, 1868, xxii, 33–50.—**Aldridge** (J.) A new theory of the nerves, in which their functions are considered according to the laws of forces. Dublin Hosp. Gaz., 1845-6, ii, 37–42.—**Allen** (J. A.) Mechanism of nervous action. Med. Indep., Detroit, 1857-8, iii, 448; 489. ———. Mechanism of nervous action. Reply to Prof. Paine. *Ibid.*, 551–569. ———. Mechanism of nervous action. Prof. Campbell's prize essay, etc. *Ibid.*, 690–704.—**Altmann** (R.) Bemerkungen zur Hensen'schen Hypothese von der Nervenentstehung. Arch. f. Anat. u. Entwcklngsgesch., Leipz., 1885, 344–348, 1 pl.—**Arndt** (R.) Ueber motorische oder kinetische Aequivalente. Deutsche med. Wchnschr., Berl., 1882, viii, 409.—**d'Arsonval** (A.) Sur un phénomène physique analogue à la conductibilité nerveuse. Compt. rend. Soc. de biol., Par., 1886, 8. s., iii, 171.—**Ashhurst** (J.), jr. On nervous action. Am. J. M. Sc., Phila., 1860, n. s., xl, 102–108.—**Audiffrent.** Considérations sur l'ensemble du système nerveux. Abeille méd., Par., 1865, xxii, 121; 130.—**Balduino** (B.) Del conducimento centrifugo e centripeto nello stesso nervo; ossia ancora una prova che i nervi si specializzano agli estremi e non lungo il decorso. Bull. d. r. Accad. med. di Roma, 1886-7, xiii, 424–437.—**Balighian** (J.) Beiträge zur Lehre von der Kreuzung der motorischen Innervationswege im Cerebrospinalsystem. Beitr. z. Anat. u. Physiol. (Eckhard), Giessen, 1878, viii, 193–204. *Also*, Reprint.—**Bartholow** (R.) A review of some of Prof. C. E. Brown-Séquard's opinions. Clinic, Cincin., 1872, ii, 169–171. ———. The transfer of sensations. J. Nerv. & Ment. Dis., Chicago, 1880, n. s., v, 402–406.—**Bastianini** (D.) Sulla eterecità che il sangue trasmette ai nervi, e sulla influenza che dispiegano i due sangui sui due sistemi nervosi cerebro-spinale e gangliforme. Ippocratico, Fano, 1863, 3. s., iii, 19: iv, 116.—**Battista** (L. G.) Sull' origine reale dei nervi spinali e di alcuni nervi cerebrali. Osservatore, Torino, 1877, xiii, 545–549.—**Baxt** (W.) Die Reizung der Hautnerven durch verdünnte Schwefelsäure. Arb. a. d. physiol. Anst. zu Leipz. (1871), 1872, vi, 69–88, 1 pl.—**Beale** (L. S.) Some observations on the ultimate distribution of nerves, and on their origin in nervous centres. Arch. Med., Lond., 1861-2, iii, 234–252, 5 pl. ———. Fundamental structure and arrangement of a nervous apparatus. Med. Times & Gaz., Lond., 1867, i, 55; 107; 163; 190.—**Bechtereff** (V.) & **Rosenbach** (P.) K fiziologii mejpozvonochnich uzlov. [Physiology of intervertebral ganglia.] Vestnik klin. i sudebnoi psichiat. i nevropatol., St. Petersb., 1884, ii, no. 1, 155–170, pl.—**Beclam** (C.) Ueber das Wirksame in den Nerven. Allg. med. Centr.-Ztg., Berl., 1847, xvi, 689–693.—**Béclard.** Des recherches sur la physiologie et la pathologie du système nerveux. Bull. Acad. de méd., Par., 1874, 2. s., iii, 1074–1078.—**Bell** (C.) On the nerves; giving an account of some experiments on their structure and functions, which lead to a new arrangement of the system. Phil. Tr., Lond., 1821, 398–424, 1 pl. *Also, transl.* [Abstr.]: J. de physiol. expér., Par., 1821, i, 379: 1822, ii, 66; 363. ———. Of the nerves which associate the muscles of the chest in the actions of breathing, speaking, and expression; being a continuation of the paper on the structure and functions of the nerves. Phil. Tr., Lond., 1822, pt. 1, 284–312, 1 pl. *Also*, Reprint. ———. On the nervous circle which connects the voluntary muscles with the brain. Phil. Tr., Lond., 1826, pt. 1, 163–173. ———. On the nervous system. *Ibid.*, 1840, pt. 1, 245–254.—**Bell** (J.) Case, considered interesting with reference to the question of distribution of the sensory and motor nerves. Tr. Med.-Chir. Soc. Edinb., 1882-3, n. s., ii, 24.—**Bellingeri** (C.) Osservazioni e riclamo sopra alcuni punti dell' esperienze fatte da C. G. Schoepf. (Sulle funzioni del sistema nervoso.) Ann. univ. di med., Milano, 1828, xlvii, 196–207.—**Benedikt** (M.) Ueber die Lokalisationsgesetze im Centralnervensysteme. Wien. med. Presse, 1871, xii, 813; 841. [*See, also, infra,* Meynert.] *Also* [Abstr.]: Anz. d. k. k. Gesellsch. d. Aerzte in Wien, 1871, i, 94–102.—**Beresin** (J.) Ein experimenteller Beweis, dass die sensiblen und die excito-motorischen Nervenfasern der Haut beim Frosche verschieden sind. Centralbl. f. d. med. Wissensch., Berl., 1866, iv, 129.—

Nervous *system.*

Bergmann. Kleine Beiträge zur Neurologie. Cor.-Bl. d. deutsch. Gesellsch. f. Psychiat., etc., Neuwied, 1856, iii, 113-115.—**Bernard** (C.) Sur l'indépendance de l'élément moteur et de l'élément sensitif dans les phénomènes du système nerveux. Compt. rend. Soc. de biol. 1849, Par., 1850, i, pt. 1, 15.—**Bernhardt** (M.) Ueber den Wassergehalt des menschlichen Centralnervensystems, nebst einigen Versuchen über den Einfluss des constanten Stromes auf denselben. Arch. f. path. Anat., etc., Berl., 1875, lxiv, 297-306. ———. Beitrag zur Lehre von den Modificationen der partiellen Entartungsreaction. Centralbl. f. Nervenh., Leipz., 1887, x, 193-198. — **Bernstein** (J.) Ueber den zeitlichen Verlauf der negativen Schwankung des Nervenstroms. Arch. f. d. ges. Physiol., Bonn, 1868, i, 173-207, 3 pl. ———. Ueber die Ermüdung und Erholung der Nerven. *Ibid.*, 1877, xv, 289-327, 1 pl.—**Berruti.** Considerazioni sull' opera del Prof. Valentin, tradotta con note dal Prof. Sachero; delle funzioni dei nervi spinali e cerebrali, e del nervo simpatico. Gior. . . . d. Soc. med.-chir. di Torino, 1844, xix, 3; 129.—**Biedermann.** Ueber mechanische, thermische und chemische Nervenreizung. Biol. Centralbl., Erlang., 1881, i, 281; 298.—**Birnbaum** (F. H. G.) Die Lehre von den Nervencentris nach ihrer anthropologisch-psychologischen Seite; als Andeutung für den heutigen Standpunkt der Anthropologie und für eine demnächst erscheinende weitere Bearbeitung derselben. Org. f. d. ges. Heilk., Bonn, 1842-3, ii, 1-37.—**Blandin.** S'il y a des nerfs moteurs et des nerfs sentitifs; et discussion sur la distinction des nerfs moteurs et sensitifs. Bull. Acad. de méd., Par., 1838-9, iii, 691; 739; 770; 802; 820; 853. ———. Des nerfs de la sensibilité et des nerfs du mouvement. Expérience, Par., 1839, iii, 294; 313.—**Bocci.** Sulla fisiologia della cellula grigia de' centri nervosi. Bull. d. Soc. Lancisiana d. osp. di Roma, 1884, iv, fasc. 3, 49-57.—**Bouillaud.** Discours en faveur de la doctrine de Ch. Bell sur la distinction des nerfs en nerfs du sentiment et en nerfs du mouvement. Expérience, Par., 1839, iii, 347-351. ———. Considérations cliniques et expérimentales sur le système nerveux, sous le rapport de son rôle dans les actes régis par les facultés sensitives, instinctives et intellectuelles, ainsi que dans les actes locomoteurs dits volontaires. Compt. rend. Acad. d. sc., Par., 1875, lxxxi, 122-128.—**Brach.** Einige Worte über einen nicht hinlänglich beachteten Punkt aus der Physiologie der Nerven und eine eigenthümliche Art von Lähmung. Med. Ztg., Berl., 1840, ix, 215-217.—**Brandt** (J.) Idegen testek a szervezetben. [The organization of the nervous system.] Orvosi hetil., Budapest, 1877, xxi, 717; 750; 798; 854.—**Broadbent** (W. H.) Criticism on Dr. Combie's rationale of the decussation of nerve-fibres in the cerebro-spinal axis. Lancet, Lond., 1869, ii, 593. ———. Lecture on the theory of construction of the nervous system. Brit. M. J., Lond., 1876, i, 371; 401; 433.—**Broughton** (S. D.) Observations on the experiments of Professor Panizza. Edinb. M. & S. J., 1836, xlv, 426-432.—**Brown-Séquard** (C.-É.) D'une action spéciale qui accompagne la contraction musculaire, et de l'existence de cette action dans certains cas pathologiques et dans ce que M. Magendie a appelé sensibilité récurrente. Compt. rend. Soc. de biol. 1851, Par., 1851, ii, pl. 1, 171-173. ———. Experimental and clinical researches on the physiology and pathology of the spinal cord and some other parts of the nervous centres. Virginia M. & S. J., Richmond, 1855, iv, 171; 283. *Also,* Reprint. ———. Recherches expérimentales sur les voies de transmission des impressions sensitives et sur des phénomènes singuliers qui succèdent à la section des racines des nerfs spinaux. Compt. rend. Soc. de biol. 1855, Par., 1856, 2. s., ii, pt. 2, 331-364, 3 pl. *Also.* Reprint. *Also:* Gaz. méd. de Par., 1856, 3. s., xi, 238; 252; 342. ———. The discoveries of Sir Chas. Bell and M. Brown-Séquard in the nervous system. [Letter to editor.] Lancet, Lond., 1856, i, 465. ———. New facts and theories concerning the physiology of the nervous system. Charleston M. J. & Rev., 1857, xii, 202-218. ———. Course of lectures on the physiology and pathology of the central nervous system. Lancet, Lond., 1858, ii, 1; 27; 53; 109; 137; 165; 219; 245; 271; 295; 345; 367; 391; 415; 441; 467; 493; 519; 545; 571; 599; 625; 651. ———. Faits qui semblent montrer que les fibres nerveuses servant aux mouvements volontaires ne sont pas celles qui font contracter les muscles dans les convulsions. Arch. de physiol. norm. et path., Par., 1869, ii, 672. ———. Lectures on the physiology and pathology of the nervous system, and on the treatment of organic nervous affections. Lancet, Lond., 1869, ii, 429; 867. ———. On the physiology and pathology of the nervous system. *Ibid.*, 1870, i, 1-3. ———. Nerve force; transformation of light, heat, electricity, and chemical force into nervous force; a Guinea pig surviving after the medulla oblongata was cut away; nerves kept alive forty hours after separation; comparative power over the nerves of oxygen, strychnia, and the will; the unity of the nerve force. Lecture delivered in Boston, Feb. 25, 1874. N. Y. Tribune Pop. Sc., 8º, N. Y., 1874, 12-16. ———. Nervous influence; some of the facts that are difficult to explain; a negro reduces convulsions by pulling at the great toe; more persistent vitality in America than in Europe, both in men and animals; various relations between the nerv-

Nervous *system.*

ous system and the action of the heart; methods of checking convulsive efforts, such as coughing, etc. Lecture delivered in Boston, March 1, 1874. *Ibid.*, 16-20. ———. Indirect nerve force; causes of loss of consciousness; no life in the head after decapitation; enormous doses of strychnine; sudden recovery from protracted lethargy; violent remedies for hysteria. Lecture delivered in Boston, March 5, 1874. *Ibid.*, 20-24. ———. What nerves may do; unity of the nervous system; grafting a cat's tail on a cock's comb; theory of catching cold; instances of power of imagination; limits of nerve force; rules for health. Lecture delivered in Boston, March 19, 1874. *Ibid.*, 30-35. ———. Recherches sur une nouvelle propriété du système nerveux. Compt. rend. Acad. d. sc., Par., 1881, xciii, 885-888. *Also:* Gaz. méd. de Par., 1881, 6. s., iii, 706. *Also:* France méd., Par., 1881, ii, 797-799. ———. Faits montrant que certaines parties du système nerveux peuvent agir de façon à augmenter plus ou moins soudainement les propriétés d'autres parties de ce système. Compt. rend. Soc. de biol. 1881, Par., 1882, 7. s., iii, 16. ———. Production d'anesthésie par le tiraillement du bulbe et de la moelle cervicale, en abaissant fortement la tête d'un animal. *Ibid.*, 29. ———. Faits montrant que les mouvements produits par l'irritation des diverses parties de l'encéphale sont très différents de ceux qui devraient survenir d'après les doctrines admises à l'égard des appareils moteur et sensitif du système cérébro-spinal. *Ibid.*, 1882, 7. s., iv, 246-252. ———. Du rôle de l'arrêt des échanges entre le sang et les tissus, de la contracture et de l'inhibition à l'égard du degré d'énergie et de la durée des propriétés des nerfs et des muscles après la mort. *Ibid.*, 1885, 8. s., ii, 185-189. ———. Recherches expérimentales montrant combien sont variés et nombreux les effets purement dynamiques provenant d'influences exercées sur l'encéphale par les nerfs sensitifs et sur les nerfs moteurs par les centres nerveux. Compt. rend. Acad. sc., Par., 1886, ciii, 790-795. ———. Dualité du cerveau et de la mœlle épinière, d'après des faits montrant que l'anesthesie, l'hyperesthésie, la paralysie et des états variés d'hypothermie et d'hyperthermie, dus à des lésions organiques du centre cérébro-spinal, peuvent être transférés d'un côté à l'autre du corps. France méd., Par., 1887, ii, 1533-1539.—**Brückner** (A.) Ueber die Polarisation des lebenden Nerven im Menschen. Deutsche Klinik. Berl., 1867, xix, 281: 1868, xx, 371; 585: 1871, xxiii, 125. — **Buchez.** Essai de coordination positive des phénomènes qui ont pour siége le système nerveux. J. d. progr. d. sc. méd., Par., 1828, ix, 175-206. — **Buchner** (H.) Zur Nervenreizung durch Lösungen indifferenter Substanzen. Ztschr. f. Biol., München, 1874, x, 373-397. ———. Zur Nervenreizung durch concentrirte Lösungen indifferenter Substanzen. *Ibid.*, 1876, xii, 129-150, 1 tab. — **Budge** (J.) Unsere heutige Kenntnisse in der Nervenphysiologie. Hannov. Ann. f. d. ges. Heilk., 1846, n. F., vi, 279-340, 1 pl. ———. Ueber reizbare Stellen an Nerven in ihrem Verlaufe. Berl. klin. Wchnschr., 1882, xix, 268.—**Bufalini** (G.) Sui cambiamenti apportati alla teoria della corrente nervosa dal fatto anatomico della fibra musculare componente il sistema nervoso. Ann. univ. di med., Milano, 1874, ccxxvii, 101-103.—**Caldwell** (C.) Thoughts on the action and influence of the nervous system, and on the means of strengthening and improving them. West. J. M. & S., Louisville, 1840, ii, 165 - 186. — **Calmeil & Raige-Delorme.** Nerveux (système, tissue). Dict. de méd., 2. éd., Par., 1839, xx, 461-616.—**Carpenter** (W. B.) Lectures on the functions of the nervous system. Lond. M. Gaz., 1840-41, xxvii, 777; 858; 938: 1841, xxviii, 57; 460; 518; 601; 633; 709; 778; 810; 890; 934; 965.—**Carus** (C. G.) Einige Aphorismen aus der Physiologie des Nervenlebens. Arch. f. Anat., Physiol. u. wissensch. Med., Berl., 1839, 366-370.—**Castel** (A.-L.) Des erreurs et des subtilités qui sont nées de la division des nerfs en deux systèmes, savoir: le système des nerfs cérébraux et le système des nerfs ganglionnaires. Rev. méd. franç. et étrang., Par., 1842, iv, 5-23. *Also,* Reprint. ———. Les fonctions du système nerveux. Bull. Acad. de méd., Par., 1844-5, x, 80-91.—**Cederschjöld** (G.) Om de mekaniska nervretningarnes praktiska betydelse. Upsala Läkaref. Förh., 1879-80, xv, 165-170.—**Charles** (J. J.) On the mode of propagation of nervous impulses. J. Anat. & Physiol., Lond., 1879-80, xiv. 131-139. *Also* [Abstr.]: Brit. M. J., Lond., 1879, ii, 567.—**Claims** of Bell, Magendie, Mayo, etc., to discoveries in the nervous system. Brit. & For. M. Rev., Lond., 1840, ix, 96-143. — **Clarke** (J. L.) The investigation of the nervous centres, with comments. Arch. Med., Lond., 1867, iv, 31-47. *Also.* Reprint.—**Clevenger** (S. V.) Plan of the cerebro-spinal nervous system. J. Nerv. & Ment. Dis., Chicago, 1880, n. s., v, 573-612. *Also:* Proc. Am. Ass. Adv. Sc. 1880, Salem, 1881, xxix, 555. ———. Nervous and mental physics. Am. J. Neurol. & Psychiat., N. Y., 1884, iii, 249-323.—**Clymer** (M.) Notes on the physiology and pathology of the nervous system. N. York M. J., 1870, xi, 225; 410.—**Coghill** (J. G. S.) On the structure and relations of the nervous system at the periphery, including the neurology of the organs of special sense. Lancet, Lond., 1859, ii, 181; 205; 255; 279; 379; 429; 455. — **Cooper** (A.) Recherches expérimentales sur la ligature

Nervous *system.*

des artères carotides et vertébrales et des nerfs pneumo-gastrique, phrénique et grand sympathique. Gaz. méd. de Par., 1838, 2. s., vi, 100 - 103. — **Cooper** (R. S.) An essay on the structure of the nervous system. Lond. M. & S. J., 1829, ii, 433-443.—**Copland.** Physiology of the nervous system. Lancet, Lond., 1845, ii, 535 ; 561 ; 669.— **Cortezo** (C. M.) La diferenciacion sensitiva. Pabellon méd., Madrid, 1875, xv, 152 ; 163 ; 188 ; 222 ; 236. — **Couty.** Sur le cerveau moteur. Arch. de physiol. norm. et path., Par , 1884, 3. s., iii, 46–97. *Also, transl.:* Rev. méd. de Sevilla, 1884, v, 144 ; 205 ; 237 ; 266 ; 303 ; 330 : 1885, vi, 50 ; 212 ; 249 ; 284 ; 306.—**Criado y Aguilar.** ¿ Es doble ó único el sistema nervioso ? en contestacion al del Dr. Fernandez de la Vega. Clinica, Zaragoza, 1879, iii, 132 ; 139 ; 148 ; 156.—**Crombie** (J. M.) The rationale of the decussation of nerve-fibres in the cerebro-spinal axis. Lancet, Lond., 1869, ii, 505. ———. Reply to Dr. Broadbent's objections to the rationale of the decussation of nerve-fibres. *Ibid.*, 724.— **Cros** (A.) Observations et considérations cliniques relatives aux fonctions des centres nerveux. France méd., Par., 1864, xi, 58 ; 82 ; 114 ; 146 : 1868, xv, 553 ; 587 ; 623 ; 639 ; 648 ; 657 ; 663. [Journal incorrectly paged ; should be 593 ; 627 ; 663; 679; 688; 697; 703.]—**Cruikshank** (W.) Experiments on the nerves, particulary on their reproduction ; and on the spinal marrow of living animals. Phil. Tr., Lond., 1795, lxxxv, 177–189, 1 pl. *Also,* Reprint. *Also, transl.:* Arch. f. d. Physiol., Halle, 1797, ii, 57–71. — **Cyon** (E.) Ueber eine paradoxe Thätigkeitsäusserung eines sensiblen Nerven. Mélanges biol. Acad. imp. d. sc. de St.-Pétersb., 1871, viii, 49–54. ———. Sur la secousse musculaire produite par l'excitation des racines de la moelle épinière. Compt. rend. Soc. de biol. 1876, Par., 1877, 6. s., iii, 134.— **Czermak** (J.) Reizversuche an halbirten Kaninchen-köpfen. [*Repr. from:* Sitzungsb. d. math.-naturw. Kl. d. Wien. Akad. d. Wissensch.] Untersuch. z. Naturl. d. Mensch. u. d. Thiere, Giessen, 1860, vii, 377–379. — **Czermak** (J. N.) Ein Apparat zur Erläuterung der Innervationsvorgänge, welche rythmisch erfolgende Bewegungen erzeugen und reguliren. *In his:* Mitth. a. d. phys. Privatlaborat., 8°, Wien, 1864, 1. Hft., 9–23.—**van Daalen** (H.) Korte beschouwingen over het zenuwstelsel. Arch. v. Geneesk., Amst., 1841, i, 537-606. *Also,* Reprint.—**Dana** (C. L.) Some recent contributions to the physiology of the nervous system of our domestic animals. J. Comp. M. & S., N. Y., 1883, iv, 101–104, 1 tab.—**Danilewsky** (A.) Untersuchungen zur Physiologie des Centralnervsystems. Arch. f. Anat., Physiol. u. wissensch. Med., Leipz., 1866, 677–691. — **van Deen** (I.) Over de voorste en achterste strengen van het ruggemerg. Tijdschr. v. nat. Geschied. en Physiol., Leiden, 1838-9, v. 151–186. *Also,* Reprint.— ———. Ueber die Unempfindlichkeit der Cerebrospinal-centra für elektrische Reize. Untersuch. z. Naturl. d. Mensch. u. d. Thiere, Giessen, 1860, vii, 380–392.—**Deni-senko** (G.) K voprosu o stroenii korki malago mozga w razlichnich klassov pozvonochniach jivotnich. [On the construction of the cortex cerebri and the different parts constituting the spine in animals.] Voyenno-med. J., St. Petersb., 1877, cxxix, 107 ; 171.—**Dercum** (F. X.) Facts and deductions bearing on the action of the nervous system. J. Nerv. & Ment. Dis., N. Y., 1886, n. s., xi, 686-694. — **Desmoulins** (A.) Exposition succincte du développement et des fonctions du système cérébro-spinal. Arch. gén. de méd., Par., 1823, ii, 223–245. ———. Exposition succincte du développement et des fonctions des systèmes nerveux latéraux des organes des sens, et de ceux des mouvemens dans les animaux vertébrés. *Ibid.*, iii, 571–594. ———. Mémoire sur le défaut d'unité de composition du système nerveux, et sur la concordance de ce défaut d'unité avec l'inégalité des facultés des animaux. J. compl. du dict. d. sc. méd., Par., 1824, xviii. 97–107.— **Deusingius** (A.) Exercitatio de nutritii succi per nervos influentis commento. *In his:* Exercitationes physico-anatomicæ, etc., 16°, Groningæ, 1661, 133–286.—**Dew-Smith** (A. G.) On double nerve stimulation. J. Anat. & Physiol., Lond., 1873-4, viii, 74–82, 1 pl. *Also, in:* Stud. from Physiol. Lab., Univ. Camb., 1873, pt. 1, 25–33, 1 pl.— **Discussion** (Sur la) de l'Académie relative à la distinction des nerfs moteurs et sensitifs. Gaz. méd. de Par., 1839, 2. s., vii, 289–296.—**Dömling.** Beweis, dass das Nervensystem das Organ der Sensibilität in allen Theilen des menschlichen Organismus, und dass folglich die Lebensthätigkeit aller Organe von ihm Abhängig sey. Arch. f. d. Theor. d. Heilk., Nürnb., 1804, i, 281–288.—**Dowler** (B.) Criticisms and controversies relating to the nervous and muscular systems. N. Orl. M. & S. J., 1847-8, iv, 189 ; 279. ———. Review, in which some neurological opinions of M. Bernard and others are briefly considered. *Ibid.*, 1861, xviii, 452–456. ———. Critical researches into certain theoretical views of recent writers upon the physiology of the nervous system. N. Orl. M. Rec., 1866, i, 34–40.— **Dubois.** Sur les fonctions du système nerveux. Expérience, Par., 1839, iii, 282–286.—**Dubois** (R.) Application de la méthode graphique à l'étude des modifications imprimées à la marche par les lésions nerveuses expérimentales chez les insectes Compt. rend. Soc. de biol., Par., 1885, 8. s., ii, 642–644. — **Du Bois - Reymond.** Vitesse de la transmission de la volonté et de la sensation

Nervous *system.*

à travers les nerfs. Gaz. hebd. de méd., Par., 1866, 2. s., iii, 805-808 : 1867, 2. s., iv, 6; 21.—**Dugès** (A.) Mémoire sur les fonctions du système nerveux. Éphém. méd. de Montpel., 1826, i, 42–63. ———. De l'importance du système nerveux, considerée chez l'homme en état de santé et en état de maladie. J. hebd. de méd., Par., 1829, ii, 333–363.—**Durand** (F.) Division du système nerveux en appareils des deux vies devant l'histologie moderne. Rec. de mém. de méd. . . . . mil., Par., 1862, 3. s., viii, 177–189.—**Duval** (M.) Relation succincte d'expériences faites à l'École de médecine navale de Brest, sur des suppliciés. Cong. méd. internat. de Par. (1867), 1868, i, 521-528. ———. Nerfs; anatomie et physiologie du système nerveux. N. dict. de méd. et chir. prat., Par., 1877, xxiii, 406–624. ———. Le système nerveux et la sensibilité. Tribune méd., Par., 1879, xii, 609–611.—**Dynamisme** nerveux. Arch. de la méd. belge, Brux., 1853, li, 1 ; 85.—**Earle** (C. W.) The physiology of the nervous system. Tr. Illinois M. Soc., Chicago, 1872, xxii, 223–331, 1 pl.—**Eckhard** (C.) Die chemische Reizung der motorischen Froschnerven. Ztschr. f. rat. Med., Heidelb., 1851, n. F., i, 303–328. ———. Ueber den gegenwärtigen Zustand der Nervenphysiologie und Nervenpathologie. Arch. d. Ver. f. gemeinsch. Arb. z. Förd. d. wissensch. Heilk., Götting., 1854, i, 479–503. ———. Ueber einige neurologische Angaben des Herrn Professor E. Cyon. Beitr. z. Anat. u. Physiol. (Eckhard), Giessen, 1873-4, vii, 1–25.—**Efron** (J.) Beiträge zur allgemeinen Nervenphysiologie. Arch. f. d. ges. Physiol., Bonn, 1885, xxxvi, 467–517.—**Ehrlich** (P.) Ueber die Methylenblau-reaction der lebenden Nervensubstanz. Deutsche med. Wchnschr., Berl., 1886, xii, 49–52. *Also, transl.:* Gaz. méd. de Par., 1886, 7. s., iii, 64 ; 75.—**Ely** (A. W.) Researches on the nervous system ; doctrine of a diffused sensorium. N. Orl. M. & S. J., 1850-51, vii, 143–148.— **Engelmann** (T. W.) Bewegingsverschijnselen aan zenuwvezelen bij prikkeling met inductie-stroomen. Onderzoek. ged. in h. Physiol. Lab. d. Utrecht. Hoogesch., 1872, 3. R., i, 168–177. — **Eschricht.** (Om det ubevidste Nervelivs Centraldeel.) [On the unconscious life of nerves in the central part.] Förh. v. de skandin. Naturf., Christiania, 1847, 319–325.—**Eulenburg** (A.) & **Landois** (L.) Ueber die thermischen Wirkungen experimenteller Eingriffe am Nervensystem und ihre Beziehung zu den Gefässnerven. Arch. f. path. Anat., etc., Berl., 1876, lxvi, 489–502, 1 pl.—**Ewald** (A.) Ueber die Unabhängigkeit des thätigen Nerven vom Sauerstoff. Arch. f. d. ges. Physiol., Bonn, 1869, ii, 142–145. ———. Neuere Arbeiten zur Physiologie des Nervensystems. [Rev.] Deutsche med. Wchnschr., Berl., 1882, viii, 55.—**Experiments** on the brain, spinal marrow, and nerves. Brit. & For. M. Rev., Lond., 1836, i, 556–563. *Also, in:* Essays on Phys. & Hyg., 8°, Phila., 1838, 199–208. — **Faesebeck** (F.) Neurologische Bemerkungen. Arch. f. Anat., Physiol. u. wissensch. Med., Berl., 1839, 70–73.— **Fano** (J.) Recherches expérimentales sur un nouveau centre automatique dans le tractus bulbo-spinale ; résumé. Arch. ital. de biol., Turin, 1883, iii, 365–368.—**Faraday** (M.) Lecture on Dr. Marshall Hall's views of the nervous system. Brit. Ann. Med., Pharm., etc., Lond., 1837, i, 225–227.— **Fargas Roca** (M. A.) Anatomia de los centros nerviosos. Gac. méd. catal., Barcel., 1882, ii, 8; 44; 71; 106; 138; 169 ; 199 ; 235 ; 267 ; 301 ; 338 ; 370 ; 403 ; 436 ; 466 ; 498 ; 528 ; 560 ; 591 ; 624 ; 659 ; 691 1883, vi, 109; 144; 175; 213; 243.— **Fauvelle.** Le système nerveux, la nervosité et l'intelligence considérés au point de vue physico - chimique. Bull. Soc. d'anthrop. de Par., 1887, 3. s., x, 462–482.—**Fede** (F.) Della eccitabilità dei nervi di senso separati dai loro centri di nutrizione. Movimento, Napoli, 1869, i, 193-196.—**Ferrier** (D.) & **Yeo** (G. F.) The functional relations of the motor roots of the brachial and lumbo-sacral plexus. Proc. Roy. Soc. Lond., 1881, xxxii, 12–20. *Also, transl.:* Centralbl. f. Nervenh., Coblenz, 1881, iv, 193–201.— **Fick** (A.) Ueber den Ort der Reizung an schräg durchströmten Nervenstrecken. Verhandl. d. phys.-med. Gesellsch. in Würzb., 1877, n. F., x, 220–232.—**Flechsig** (P.) Ueber die Verbindungen der Hinterstränge mit dem Gehirn. Neurol. Centralbl., Leipz., 1885, iii, 97–100. ———. Zur Lehre vom centralen Verlauf der Sinnesnerven. *Ibid.*, 1886, v, 545–551. — **von Fleischl** (E.) Untersuchung über die Gesetze der Nervenerregung. I. Abhandl. Ueber die Lehre vom Anschwellen der Reize in Nerven. Sitzungsb. d. k. Akad. d. Wissensch. Math.-naturw. Cl., Wien, 1876, lxxii, 393 - 406. *Also,* Reprint. ———. The same. II. Abhandl. Ueber die Wirkung secundärer elektrischer Ströme auf Nerven. Sitzungsb. d. k. Akad. d. Wissensch. Math.-naturw. Cl., Wien, 1877, lxxiv, 403-424, 1 pl. *Also,* Reprint. ———. The same. III. Abhandl. Das Rheonom. Sitzungsb. d. k. Akad. d. Wissensch. Math.-naturw. Cl., Wien, 1878, lxxvi, 138–162, 4 pl. *Also,* Reprint. *Also:* Med. Jahrb., Wien, 1879, 129–144, 2 pl. ———. The same. IV. Abhandl. Der interpolare Electrotonus. Sitzungsb. d. k. Akad. d. Wissensch. Math.-naturw. Cl., Wien, 1878, lxxvii, 159–176, 1 pl. *Also,* Reprint. ———. The same. V. Abhandl. Die Theorie des Elektrotonus. Sitzungsb. d. k. Akad. d. Wissensch. Math.-naturw. Cl. 1878, Wien, 1879, lxxviii, 267–282, 2 pl. ———. The same. VI. Abhandl. Ueber die Wirkung linea-

Nervous *system.*

rer Stromschwankungen auf Nerven. *Ibid.*, 1880, lxxxii, 133–154, 3 pl. ——. The same. VII. Abhandl. Die Erregung stromloser Nerven. *Ibid.*, 1883, lxxxviii, 189–204.— **Flourens** (P.) Recherches physiques sur les propriétés et les fonctions du système nerveux dans les animaux vertébrés. Arch. gén. de méd., Par., 1823, ii, 321–370. *Also:* Rev. méd. franç. et étrang., Par., 1823, xi, 385: xii, 80; 150.— **Foderà.** Recherches expérimentales sur le système nerveux. J. compl. du dict. d. sc. méd , Par., 1823, xvi, 289–303: xvii, 97–107: 1824, xx, 289–307. *Also* [Rev.]: J. de physiol. expér., Par., 1823, iii, 191–217. ——. Examen de l'opinion de M. Broussais sur les nerfs de la sensibilité et de la motilité, suivie de quelques remarques, dans lesquelles il est considéré comme anatomiste, physiologiste, érudit et critique. J. compl. du dict. d. sc. méd., Par., 1825, xxi, 3–24.— **Forjett** (E. H.) Original observations and experiments on the nervous system, and on the process of innervation and nutrition. Edinb. M. J., 1877, xxii, 709–712.— **François- Franck.** Nerfs (physiologie générale). Dict. encycl. d. sc. méd., Par., 1877, 2. s., xii, 179–223. ——. Histoire et critique de la durée des actions nerveuses. Gaz. hebd. de méd., Par., 1878, 2. s., xv, 773; 789. *Also, transl.* [Abstr.]: Lond. M. Rec., 1879, n. s., vii, 85–89.— **Fratscher** (C.) Ueber continuirliche und langsame Nervenreizung. (Aus dem physiologischen Laboratorium der Universität Jena.) Jenaische Ztschr. f. Naturw., Leipz., 1875, ix, 130–160, 6 pl.— **Freud** (S.) Notiz über eine Methode zur anatomischen Präparation des Nervensystems. Centralbl. f. d. med. Wissensch., Berl., 1879, xvii, 468.— **Freusberg** (A.) Ueber die Erregung und Hemmung der Thätigkeit der nervösen Centralorgane. Arch. f. d. ges. Physiol., Bonn, 1875, x, 174–208.— **Fubini** (S.) Influenza della luce sulla respirazione del tessuto nervoso. Arch. per le sc. med., Torino, 1878–9, iii, 1–23. ——. Peso del sistema nervoso centrale paragonato al peso del corpo dell' animale; ricerche fatte sulle rane esculenti e temporarie. Gior. d. r. Accad. di med. di Torino, 1879, xlii, 446–455.— **Fürstner.** Ueber Experimentelle Untersuchungen im Bereich des centralen Nervensystems. Tagebl. d. Versamml. deutsch. Naturf. u. Aerzte, Berl., 1886, lix, 153–155. *Also:* Berl. klin. Wchnschr., 1886, xxiii, 773–775.— **Funke** (O.) Ueber die Reaction der Nervensubstanz. Arch. f. Anat., Physiol. u. wissensch. Med., Leipz., 1859, 835–846.— **Gad** (J.) Ueber einige Beziehungen zwischen Nerv, Muskel und Centrum. Festschr. z. 3. Saecularfeier . . . d. med. Fac. Würzb., Leipz., 1882, ii, 43–70, 1 pl.— **Garner** (R.) The brain and nervous system; a summary and a review. J. Anat. & Physiol., Lond., 1880–81, xv, 536–579.— **Garver** (M. M.) On the transmission of sensation and volition through the nerves. Am. J. Sc. & Arts, N. Haven, 1878, xv, 413–422. ——. The periodic character of voluntary nervous action. Am. J. Sc., N. Haven, 1880, 3. s., xx, 189–193.— **George** (J. D.) Contributions to the history of the nervous system. Lond. M. Gaz., 1837–8, xxii, 67; 93. *Also,* Reprint. — **Georgievska** (I.) Ke voprosu o nerazdelnosti provodiatchei i vosprinimaioutchei sposobnosti nerviche stvolove. [Physiology of nervous system.] Voyenno-med. J. St. Petersb., 1884, cxxxiv, 1–14.— **Gerdy** (P.-N.) De la méthode expérimentale en physiologie; des nerfs sensitifs et moteurs, et des idées de Charles Bell. Expérience, Par., 1839, iii, 257; 281. ——. De la méthode expérimentale et des fonctions du système nerveux. *Ibid.*, 310–313. ——. Des fonctions du système nerveux. *Ibid.*, 329–331. ——. Mémoires, recherches et discussions sur le système nerveux en général. *In his:* Mélanges d'anat., etc., 8°, Par., 1875, i, 353–445.— **Giehrl.** Ueber Nervenüberreizung und ihre Behandlung. J. d. Chir. u. Augenh., Berl., 1844, n. F., iii, 175–200.— **Golgi** (C.) Sulla origine centrale dei nervi. Atti Cong. gen. d. Ass. med. ital. 1880, Genova, 1882, ix, 375–388. *Also:* Gior. internaz. d. sc. med., Napoli, 1881, n. s., iii, 225–234.— **Goltz** (F.) Ueber den Einfluss der Centralorgane des Nervensystems auf vegetative Vorgänge. Amtl. Ber. ü. d. Versamml. deutsch. Naturf. u. Aerzte, Königsb., 1861, xxxv, 139–141. ——. Neue Versuche über Erregung von Reflexerschlaffung und Reflexkrampf rhythmisch thätiger Muskelapparate. Centralbl. f. d. med. Wissensch., Berl., 1864, ii, 690.— **Grabau** (W.) Polarität im menschlichen Organismus. Mitth. a. d. Geb. d. Med., etc., Altona, 1837–8, v, 1.–2. Hft., 1–57.— **Gray** (H. A. C.) Conversion of nerve force into heat. Indian M. Gaz., Calcutta, 1875, x, 237–239.— **Gray** (L. C.) The physiological anatomy of the spinal cord and the motor tract of the cerebrum. Ann. Anat. & Surg. Soc., Brooklyn, N. Y., 1880, ii, 385–407.— **Grünhagen** (A.) Bemerkungen über die Summation von Erregungen in der Nervenfaser. Ztschr. f. rat. Med., Leipz., 1866, 3. R., xxvi, 190–224. ——. Ueber den vermeintlichen Einfluss der hinteren Wurzeln auf die Erregbarkeit der vorderen. *Ibid.*, 1868, 3. R., xxxi, 38–42. ——. Versuche über intermittirende Nervenreizung. Arch. f. d. ges. Physiol., Bonn, 1872, vi, 157–181, 1 pl.— **Grützner** (P.) Ueber die Einwirkung von Wärme un l Kälte auf Nerven. *Ibid.*, 1878, xvii, 215–238. ——. Ueber die chemische Reizung von Nerven. *Ibid.*, 250–254, 1 pl. ——. Beiträge zur allgemeinen Nervenphysiologie. *Ibid.*, 1881, xxv, 255: 1882, xxviii, 130, 1 pl. ——. Ueber Erregungsvorgänge im Nerven. Breslau. aerztl. Ztschr., 1885, vii, 137.—**Gudden.** Experimental-

Nervous *system.*

untersuchungen über das peripherische und centrale Nervensystem. Arch. f. Psychiat., Berl., 1870, ii, 693–723, 3 pl.—**Guérin** *de Mamers* (H.) Du système nerveux. Ann. de la méd. physiol., Par., 1828, xiv, 37; 153; 434: 1829, xv, 657: xvi, 465: 1830. xvii, 171; 391: xviii, 165; 529: 670: 1831, xx, 302.—**Gull** (W. W.) The Gulstonian lectures. Med. Times, Lond., 1848–9, xix, 371; 391; 407; 468; 505; 563.— **Hällstén** (K.) Studier i väfnadselementens fysiologi. [C. r., no. 7, études sur la physiologie des éléments des tissus.] Nord. med. Ark., Stockholm, 1876, viii, no. 5, 1–4.— **Hall** (M.) On the nervous system. Lond. M. Gaz., 1835–6, xvii, 632–641. ——. Extract from a lecture on the nervous system. Lancet, Lond., 1838–9, i, 607–610. ——. Briefe über das Nervensystem an Prof. J. Müller. Arch. f. Anat., Physiol. u. wissensch. Med., Berl., 1840, 451–466, 1 pl. ——. On the difficulties in the study of the nervous system, set forth by Legallois. Lond. & Edinb. Month. J. M. Sc., 1841, i, 853–858. ——. A synopsis of the spinal system. Lancet, Lond., 1850, i, 469; 495; 521; 555; 615; 649. ——. Lectures on the nervous system. N. Orl. M. News & Hosp. Gaz., 1855–6, ii, 316–329. ——. On a lower medulla oblongata; observations and suggestions. Lancet, Lond., 1857, i, 28.—**Harless** (E.) Ueber die Bedeutsamkeit der Nervenhüllen. Ztschr. f rat. Med., Leipz., 1858, 3. R., v, 168–188.—**von Hartmann** (E.) Beiträge zur Naturlehre der Centralorgane des Nervensystems. Athenæum, Jena, 1875, i, 193; 279; 321; 398.— **Haskell** (B.) Propositions on the nervous system, and on the formation of animals. Boston M. & S. J., 1837–8, xvii, 181–185. ——. On the vital endowments of nerves. *Ibid.*, 1854, l, 474: 1854–5, li, 29. ——. Researches into the nervous system. N. Orl. M. & S. J., 1855–6, xii, 594–601. ——. Remarks on the experiments and observations of Bell, Mayo, and others, on which the doctrine of sensitive and motor nerves was chiefly founded. Tr. Am. M. Ass., Phila., 1865, xvi, 455–161. ——. The sensitive and motor theory. *Ibid.*, 1866, xvii, 409–417.—**Hawkins** (C. H.) [On anatomy of the nervous system.] Annual address delivered before the fellows of the Roy. M. & Chir. Soc. Lancet, Lond., 1856, i, 281–284. *Also, in his:* . . . Path. & Surg. Writings, 8°, Lond., 1874, i, 20–30.—**Heidenhain** (R.) Die Erregbarkeit der Nerven an verschiednen Puncten ihres Verlaufes. Stud. d. physiol. Inst. zu Bresl., Leipz., 1861, 1. Hft., 1–66. ——. Ueber die Reaction der thätigen Nerven. *Ibid.*, 1868, 4. Hft., 248–250. ——. Ueber bisher unbeachtete Einwirkungen des Nervensystems auf die Körpertemperatur und den Kreislauf. Arch. f. d. ges. Physiol., Bonn, 1870, iii, 504–565, 4 pl. ——. Ueber pseudomotorische Nervenwirkungen. Arch. f. Physiol., Leipz., 1883, Suppl.-Bd., 133–177, 2 pl.— **Heinzmann** (A.) Ueber die Wirkung sehr allmäliger Aenderungen thermischer Reize auf die Empfindungsnerven. Arch. f. d. ges. Physiol., Bonn, 1872, vi, 222–236.— **Held von Hagelsheim** (G.) Von dem Consensu nervorum, in dreyen Exempeln dargethan. Samml. v. Nat.-u. Med.- . . . Gesch. 1722, Leipz., 1724, xxiii, 640–682.— **Helmholtz** (H.) Vorläufiger Bericht über die Fortpflanzungsgeschwindigkeit der Nervenreizung. Arch. f. Anat., Physiol. u. wissensch. Med., Berl., 1850, 71–73. ——. Messungen über Fortpflanzungsgeschwindigkeit der Reizung in den Nerven. *Ibid.*, 1852, 199–216, 1 pl. ——. Ueber Fortpflanzungsgeschwindigkeit der Reizung in den Nerven. Verhandl. d. naturh.-med. Ver. zu Heidelb., 1865–8, iv, 139–143.—**Hering** (E.) & **Biedermann** (W.) Beiträge zur allgemeinen Nerven- und Muskelphysiologie. Sitzungsb. d. k. Akad. d. Wissensch., Wien, 1879, lxxix, 3. Abth., 7; 237; 289, 1 pl.: 1880, lxxx, 3. Abth., 367–410, 1 pl.: lxxxi, 3. Abth., 74–114. —**Hermann** (L.) Das galvanische Verhalten einer durchflossenen Nervenstrecke während der Erregung. Arch. f. d. ges. Physiol., Bonn, 1872, vi, 560–567. ——. Untersuchungen über die Actionsströme des Nerven. *Ibid.*, 1878, xviii, 574: 1880–81, xxiv, 246.—**Heubel** (E.) Das "Krampfcentrum" des Frosches und sein Verhalten gegen gewisse Arzneistoffe. *Ibid.*, 1874, ix, 263–323.—**Hill** (A.) Abstract of three lectures on the mutual relation of the gray masses of the cerebro-spinal system, and their connections with peripheral nerves. Brit. M. J., Lond., 1885, i, 530; 586. *Also,* Reprint. — **Hirschberg** (E.) In welcher Beziehung stehen Leitung und Erregung der Nervenfaser zu einander? Arch. f. d. ges. Physiol., Bonn, 1886, xxxix, 75–95, 1 pl.—**Holmgren** (F.) Om "nervprincipen" och nervströmmens negativa fluctuation. Upsala Läkaref. Förh., 1866–7, ii, 599–612. ——. Om gränsen för känsel- och viljecellernas functionstörmåga. *Ibid.*, 1868–9, iv, 358–387.— **Home** (E.) The Croonian lecture; experiments and observations upon the structure of nerves. Phil. Tr., Lond., 1799, lxxxix, 1–12. ——. The Croonian lecture; on the irritability of nerves. *Ibid.*, 1801, xci, 1–22, 1 pl. —**Horner** (W. E.) Observations and experiments on certain parts of the nervous system. Phila. J. M. & Phys. Sc., 1820, i, 285–299.—**Howe** (A. J.) The nervous system. J. Cincin. Soc. Nat. Hist., 1882, v, 178–184.—**Huxley** (T. H.) The present state of knowledge as to the structure and functions of nerve. Med. Times & Gaz., Lond., 1857, n. s., xv, 1.—**Jackson** (J. H.) On the physiology and pathology of the nervous system. *Ibid.*, 1868, ii, 177; 208; 358; 526;

Nervous *system.*

696. ———. The unit of constitution of the nervous system. *Ibid.*, 1869, ii, 481. ———. Clinical and physiological researches on the nervous system. J. Psych. M., Lond., 1876, n. s., ii, 150–155. ———. Remarks on dissolution of the nervous system, as exemplified by certain post-epileptic conditions. Med. Press & Circ., Lond., 1881, n. s., xxxi, 329; 399: xxxii, 68; 380; 399; 421. ———. On some implications of dissolution of the nervous system. *Ibid.*, 1882, n. s., xxxiv, 411; 433: 1883, n. s., xxxvi, 64; 84. ———. Croonian lectures on evolution and dissolution of the nervous system. Med. Times & Gaz., Lond., 1884, i, 411; 445; 485. *Also:* Lancet. Lond., 1884, i, 555; 649; 739. *Also:* Brit. M. J., Lond., 1884, i, 591; 660; 703. ———. Remarks on evolution and dissolution of the nervous system. J. Ment. Sc., Lond., 1887-8, xxxiii, 25-48.— **Jewell** (J. S.) General structure and modes of action of the nervous system. J. Nerv. & Ment. Dis., Chicago, 1876, iii, 177–188.— **Joseph** (H.) Studien über den Nerveneinfluss am Froschbein. Centralbl. f. d. med. Wissensch., Berl., 1871, ix, 721. ———. Ueber den Einfluss der Nerven auf Ernährung und Neubildung. Arch. f. Anat., Physiol. u. wissensch. Med., Leipz., 1872, 206–236.— **Kanellis.** Influences des racines sensitives sur l'excitabilité des racines motrices. Compt. rend. Acad. d. sc., Par., 1883, xcvi, 1249.— **Karwowski** (K.) Pogląd krytyczny na obecne stanowisko fizyologii i patologii nerwow zwojowych. [The present views on the physiology and pathology of nervous ganglia.] Pam. Towarz. Lek. Warszaw., 1862, xlviii, 149 : 1863, xlix, 32.— **Kennedy** (H.) On nervous influence and derangement. Dublin M. Press, 1848, xix, 241–243.— **Key** (E. A. H.) & **Retzius** (G.) Studier i nervsystemets anatomi. Nord. med. Ark., Stockholm, 1872, iv, no. 21, 1; no. 25, 1. *Also,* Reprint.— **Kölliker.** Ueber die Vitalität der Nervenröhren. Verhandl. d. phys.-med. Gesellsch. in Würzb., 1857, vii, 145.— **Kohlrausch** (F.) Ueber die Fortpflanzungs-Geschwindigkeit des Reizes in den menschlichen Nerven. Ztschr. f. rat. Med., Leipz., 1866, 3. R., xxviii, 190–204.— **Kronecker** (H.) Ueber die Begriffe Summation von Reizen und Steigerung der Erregbarkeit. Arch. f. Physiol., Leipz., 1880, 285.— **Kronenberg.** Versuche über motorische und sensible Nervenwurzeln. Arch. f. Anat., Physiol. u. wissensch. Med., Berl., 1839, 360–362.— **Kühne** (W.) Ueber das doppelsinnige Leitungsvermögen der Nerven. Ztschr. f. Biol., München, 1886, n. F., iv, 305-353, 1 diag.— **Kunkler** (E. A.) Physiological view of the nervous system and its disorders. Pacific M. & S. J., San Fran.. 1867-8. x, 97; 193; 337; 440; 529: 1868-9, xi, 49; 198; 289; 384.— **Kupffer** (C.) Ueber den Canalis neurentericus der Wirbelthiere. Sitzungsb. d. Gesellsch. f. Morphol. u. Physiol. in München, 1887, iii, 1-5. — **Lacrampe-Loustau.** Recherches pathologiques et expérimentales sur différentes fonctions du système nerveux, et en particulier sur le siége des causes de la paralysie des membres. Ann. de la méd. physiol., Par., 1824, v, 548–594.— **Laing** (T.) A supplement to an essay on the nervous system, by Alexander Walker. Lancet, Lond., 1849, i, 610-614.— **Lallemand** (C.-F.) Observations sur les fonctions des différentes parties du système nerveux. *In his:* Obs. path., 8°, Par., 1825, 40–101.— **Landouzy.** Considérations physiologiques et psychologiques sur les propensions sympathiques et imitatives. Presse méd., Par., 1837, i, 105; 121: 153; 217; 249; 328.— **Lane** (C. H. B.) Observations on the functions and connections of the nervous system. Lancet, Lond., 1841-2, i, 183–187.— **Lane** (C. W. B.) Notes on the nervous system, and the mutual relations of its different parts. *Ibid.*, 1838-9, ii, 459-462.— **Langendorff** (O.) Ueber Tetanisirung von Nerven durch rhythmische Dehnung. Centralbl. f. d. med. Wissensch., Berl., 1882, xx, 113–115.— **Laurencet.** Sur la physiologie du cerveau et des nerfs, fondée sur des observations anatomiques. Rev. méd. fran:. et étrang., Par., 1825, i, 61; 360. ———. Mémoire sur la physiologie du cerveau et des nerfs. fondée sur de nouvelles observations anatomiques. *Ibid.*, iii, 41 - 52. — **Lautenbach** (B. F.) The conducting power as distinct from the receiving power of the nerve. Phila. M. Times, 1876-7, vii, 268–270.— **Laws** (S. S.) A new classification of the cerebro-spinal nerves. St. Louis M. & S. J., 1878, xxxiv, 454 - 456. — **Laycock** (T.) Contributions to a new chapter in the physiology and pathology of the nervous system. Brit. M. J., Lond., 1868, i, 68; 115; 187; 268; 577.— **Lembert** (A.) Considérations sur le système nerveux. J. hebd. de méd., Par., 1829, iii, 529 - 542. — **von Lenhossék** (J.) Ueber das centrale Nervensystem. Amtl. Ber. ü. d. Versamml. deutsch. Naturf. u. Aerzte 1856, Wien, 1858, xxxii, 250-253.— **Leven** (M.) Des rapports du système nerveux et de la nutrition. Compt. rend. Soc. de biol., Par., 1887, 8. s., iv, 576 - 579. — **Liégeois.** Mémoire sur le rôle des sensations sur les mouvements. Gaz. méd. de Par., 1860, 3. s., xv, 4-8.— **Luchsinger** (B.) Neue Versuche zu einer Lehre von der Schweisssecretion, ein Beitrag zur Physiologie der Nervencentren. Arch. f. d. ges. Physiol., Bonn, 1876, xiv, 369 - 382. ———. Weitere Versuche und Betrachtungen zur Lehre von den Nervencentren. *Ibid.*, 383-390. ———. Zur Leitung nervöser Erregung. Mitth. d. naturf. Gesellsch. in Bern (1880), 1881, pt. 2, 105-108.— **Lussana** (F.) Sull' accordo delle risultanze fisiologiche

Nervous *system.*

sperimentali colla sintomatologia delle malattie del cervello e del cervelletto. *In his:* Opusc. fisiol., 8°, Padova, 1873, fasc. 1, 3-33. ———. Lezioni di fisiologia sperimentale sul sistema nervoso encefalico date dal Prof. Maurizio Schiff nel R. Museo di Firenze l' anno 1864-5 e compilate per cura del Dott. Pietro Marchi. Estratto e commenti del Prof. Filippo Lussana nel 1868. *Ibid.*, 75-164. *Also:* Ann. univ. di med., Milano, 1868, cciii, 394; 627: cciv, 187.— **Lussana** (F.) & **Morganti** (G.) Alcune osservazioni fisio-patologiche su 'l sistema nervoso. Gazz. med. ital. lomb., Milano, 1851, 3. s., ii, 317; 333; 341; 373; 377: 1852, 3. s., iii, 231: 1853, 3. s., iv, 109; 137; 145; 213; 221; 229; 237; 297; 381; 389; 413.— **Lynch** (M. H.) Arguments on some points of the physiology of the nervous system, with some remarks upon the opinions of Dr. Marshall Hall, Mr. Grainger, and Dr. Carpenter. Lancet, Lond., 1839-40, i, 192–199.— **McKendrick** (J. G.) Abstract of lectures on physiological discovery. Brit. M. J., Lond., 1883, i, 654; 755; 807; 851; 900; 950; 995; 1056; 1108.— **Magendie** (F.) Expériences sur les fonctions des racines des nerfs rachidiens. J. de physiol. expér., Par., 1822, ii, 276–279. *Also, transl., with additions:* Lond. M. & Phys. J., 1822, xlviii, 343–352. *Also,* Reprint. ———. Lectures on the physiology of the nervous system. Lancet, Lond., 1836-7, i, 71; :125; 156; 189; 220; 292; 319; 391; 454; 550; 582; 663; 734; 780; 841: ii, 9; 183; 279; 332; 361; 424; 463; 503; 573. — **Mairet** (A.) De la nutrition du système nerveux à l'état physiologique et pathologique. [Rev. crit.] Arch. de neurol., Par., 1885, ix, 232; 360: x, 76. — **Mann** (E. C.) General considerations on the development of the nervous system by evolution, and its condition in health and disease. St. Louis Cour. Med., 1882, vii, 118–129. *Also,* Reprint.— **Mauthner** (L.) Recherches sur la structure du système nerveux. Rec. d. trav. Soc. méd. allem. de Par., 1864-5, ii, 13–23.— **Marcacci.** Influence des racines sensitives sur l'excitabilité des racines motrices. Compt. rend. Soc. de biol. 1880, Par., 1881, 7. s., ii, 397. — **Marchand** (R.) Versuche über das Verhalten von Nervencentren gegen äussere Reize. Arch. f. d. ges. Physiol., Bonn, 1878, xviii; 511 - 542, 4 pl. — **Marique.** Aperçu historique et critique des connaissances relatives aux fonctions du système nerveux, et des méthodes employées à leur étude. Clinique, Brux., 1887, i, 31 - 37. — **Maunoir** (J.-P.) Mémoire sur l'irritabilité des nerfs. J. de méd., chir., pharm., etc., Par., 1809, xviii, 190–202.— **Mayer** (A. F. J. K.) Ueber das Gehirn, das Rückenmark und die Nerven. Nova acta phys.-med. Acad. nat. curios., Bonnæ, 1832 - 3, xvi, 681 - 720, 6 pl. *Also,* Reprint. — **Mayer** (S.) Ueber ein Gesetz der Erregung terminaler Nervensubstanzen. Sitzungsb d. k. Akad. d. Wissensch. Math.-naturw. Cl., Wien, 1880, lxxxi, 3. Abth., 121-142. — **Mercier** (C.) On the conditions of the nervous discharge. Brain, Lond., 1882-3, v, 332-343. ———. The nervous discharge. *Ibid.*, 1884 - 5, vii, 370 - 397. — **Meyer** (L.) Die Stimmung und ihre Beziehungen zu den Hauptfunctionen des Nervensystems (der Sensibilität, Motilität, dem Denkvermögen). Ann. d. Char.-Krankenh. . . . zu Berl., 1854, v, 3. Hft., 26-99. — **Meynert** (T.) Die Medianebene des Hirnstammes, als ein Stück der Leitungsbahn zwischen dem Vorstellungsgebiete und den motorischen Hirnnerven. Allg. Wien. med. Ztg., 1866, xi, 12. ———. (Offener Brief an die Redaktion betreffend Benedikt's Artikel "Ueber die Lokalisationsgesetze im Centralnervensysteme".) Wien. med. Presse, 1871, xii, 875 - 877. — **Meyranx.** Du système nerveux d'après les idées de M. de Blainville. Arch. gén. de méd., Par., 1827, xiv, 60-65.— **Moleschott** (J.) Der bewegungvermittelnde Vorgang im Nerven kann auch von einer positiven Schwankung des Nervenstroms begleitet sein. Untersuch. z. Naturl. d. Mensch. u. d. Thiere, Giessen, 1862, viii, 1-35.— **Mapother** (A.) An anatomical treatise of the nerves. *In his:* An anatomical treatise, etc., 12°, Edinb., 1732, 1 - 32. — **Morris** (J. C.) Lectures on the physiology of the nervous system. Med. & Surg. Reporter, Phila., 1860 - 61, n. s., v, 217: 1861, n. s., vi, 1.— **Munk** (H.) Untersuchungen über die Leitung der Erregung im Nerven. Arch. f. Anat., Physiol. u. wissensch. Med., Leipz., 1860, 798: 1861, 425: 1862, 1. ———. Untersuchungen zur allgemeinen Nervenphysiologie. *Ibid.*, 1866, 369–390. ———. Ueber Partialerregung des Nerven. *Ibid.*, 1875, 41-45. — **Muret** (J.-L.) De l'innervation. Ann. de la méd. physiol., Par., 1834, xxvi, 5-25.— **Nasse** (O.) Ueber die Erregung der Nerven durch positive und negative Stromesschwankungen. Arch. f. d. ges. Physiol., Bonn, 1870, iii, 476-488.— **Natanson.** Analyse der Funktionen des Nervensystems. Arch. f. physiol. Heilk., Stuttg., 1844, iii, 515-535.— **Nelson** (R.) The origin of the nervous system. A posthumous paper, edited by C. E. Nelson. St. Louis M. & S. J., 1885, xlviii, 279; 366.— **Newkirk** (G.) Nervous matter and principles of nervous action. Dental Cosmos, Phila., 1885, xxvii, 583-590. — **Nichols** (A.) Oh irritation of the nerves. Med. Communicat. Mass. M. Soc., Bost., 1836, v, 359-412.— **Novi** (I.) La concentrazione del sangue come condizione di stimolo per il sistema nervoso centrale. Sperimentale, Firenze, 1887, lix, 468-487. *Also, transl.:* Arch. ital. de biol., Turin, 1887, ix, 102-118. — **Novi** (I.) & **Baldi** (D.) Delle vie di conduzione centrifuga cerebro-spinali. Spe-

Nervous *system.*

rimentale, Firenze, 1886, lvii, 281–293. — **O'Beirne** (J.)
An analytical correction of Sir Charles Bell's views respecting the nerves of the face. *In his:* New views of the
process of defecation, etc., 8°, Dubl., 1833, 225–278. ———.
The same, 8°, Wash., 1834, 113–138. — **Oehl** (E.) Sull'
aumento di temperatura che presentamo i nervi nel mo-
mento in cui vengono eccitati. Lettera al Dott. Griffini.
Ann. univ. d. med., Milano, 1865, cxcii, 601. — **Onimus.**
Influence pathologique sur les centres nerveux des impressions périphériques des membres inférieurs. Union
méd., Par., 1879, 3. s., xxxiii, 153–157. — **Onodi** (A. D.)
Ueber das Verhältniss der spinalen Faserbündel zu dem
Grenzstrange des Sympathicus. Centralbl. f. d. med.
Wissensch., Berl., 1883, xxi, 97; 625. — **Ordenstein** (L.)
Ueber Kölliker's Ansichten "über die Vitalität der Ner-
venröhren der Frösche". Ztschr. f. rat. Med., Leipz.,
1858, ii, 3. R., 109–113.—**O'Reilly** (J.) The connection
of the nervous centres of animals and organic life. Am.
M. Gaz., N. Y., 1859, x, 161; 490; 693, 1 pl. *Also*, Reprint
[in part]. *Also, in his:* The Anat. and Physiol. of the
Placenta, [etc.], 8°, N. Y., 1860, 35; 85. ———. The nervous
centres of animal and organic life. *Ibid.*, 1860, xi, 251–274.
Also, Reprint. *Also* [Discussion]: Bull. N. York Acad. M.,
1860–62, i, 19–24.— **Ott.** La doctrine de Buchez sur le système nerveux et sur les rapports de l'esprit avec l'organisme. Ann. méd.-psych., Par., 1866, 4. s., vii, 1–24.—**Panizza** (M.) Sulla teoria della doppia trasmissione; risposta alle considerazioni critiche del Dott. L. Luciani.
Gazz. med. di Roma, 1881, vii, 221; 233; 257; 269; 281.—
Parchappe. Du siège commun de l'intelligence, de la
volonté et de la sensibilité chez l'homme. Union méd.,
Par., 1856, x, 1; 25; 38; 61; 77; 101; 113; 125; 170.—**Petrone** (L. M.) Intorno allo studio della struttura della
nevroglia dei centri nervosi cerebrospinali. Gazz. med.
ital. lomb., Milano, 1887, xlvii, 301–307.—**Philip** (A. P. W.)
Observations on the functions of the nervous system. Phil.
Tr., Lond., 1829, cxix, 261–278.—**Pickford.** Nochmalige
Beleuchtung der Arnold'schen Einwürfe gegen die Richtigkeit des Bell'schen Lehrsatzes. Ztschr. f. rat. Med., Heidelb., 1846, v, 243–256.—**Pierret.** Sur les relations existant entre le volume des cellules motrices ou sensitives
des centres nerveux et la longueur du trajet qu'ont à par-
courir les incitations qui en émanent ou les impressions
qui s'y rendent. Compt. rend. Acad. d. sc., Par., 1878,
lxxxvi, 1423–1425. — **Pitt** (W. H.) Energy of nerve and
brain. Buffalo M. & S. J., 1884–5, xxiv, 394–404.—**Pouchet**
(G.) Du rôle des nerfs dans les changements de coloration
des poissons. J. de l'anat. et physiol., etc., Par., 1872, viii,
71–74. *Also*, Reprint. ———. Note sur le rôle des nerfs
dans les changements de coloration des poissons. Compt.
rend. Soc. de biol. 1871, Par., 1873, 5. s., iii, 113–117. ———.
Des changements de coloration sous l'influence des nerfs.
J. de l'anat. et physiol., etc., Par., 1876, xii, 1; 113, 4 pl.—
Prochaska (G.) De usu et functione systematis nervosi. *In his:* Op. minor. anat., etc., pars ii, 8°, Viennæ, 1800, 7–406, 8 pl. — **Radcliffe** (C. B.) Dynamics of
nerve and muscle. Brit. M. J., Lond., 1871, ii, 150. —
Randolph (N. A.) A note on the irradiation of motor
impulses. Maryland M. J., Balt., 1886–7, xvi, 499. *Also:*
Phila. M. Times, 1886–7, xvii, 502–504. [Disc.], 517–520.
Also: Med. News, Phila., 1887, l, 412–414 — **Ranney** (A.
L.) The anatomy of the nervous system, and its application to the practical branches of medical science. Med.
Gaz., N. Y., 1880, vii, 577; 613; 622; 639; 647; 661; 672;
697. ———. Remarks on the general architecture of the
nervous system of man. *Ibid.*, 1883, xxxvii, 403; 457.
———. A diagrammatic summary of some of the principal
features of cerebral and spinal architecture. *Ibid.*, xxxviii,
36–38. — **Rapport** fait à la Société médicale d'émulation,
27 août 1843 sur la nouvelle théorie nerveuse de M. Durand
(de Lunel), par MM. Brun, Socquet et Gromier. J. de méd.
de Lyon, 1843, v, 431–448.—**Reclam.** Die Nerven und ihre
Herrschaft. Gesundheit, Frankf. a. M., 1881, vi, 113–115.—
Reid (R.) Observations on Marshall Hall's theory of the
nervous system. Dublin Q. J. M. Sc., 1856, xxi, 310–315.—
Reil (J. C.) Das verlängerte Rückenmark, die hinteren,
seitlichen und vörderen Schenkel des kleinen Gehirns und
die theils strangförmig, theils als Ganglienkette in der Axe
des Rückenmarks und des Gehirns fortlaufende graue Substanz. Arch. f. d. Physiol., Halle, 1809, ix, 485–524. ———.
Ueber den Bau des Hirns und der Nerven. *In his:* Kleine
Schrift., etc., 8°, Halle, 1817, 113–132. — **Reissner** (E.)
Neurologische Studien. Arch. f. Anat., Physiol. u. wissensch. Med., Leipz., 1861, 615; 721, 1 pl.: 1862, 125, 1 pl.—
Remak (E.) Zur vicariirenden Function peripherer Nerven des Menschen. Berl. klin. Wchnschr., 1874, xi, 601;
615.—**Remak** (R.) O budowie nerwów i zwojów nerwowych. [On the structure of nerves and nervous ganglia.]
Pam. Towarz. Lek. Warszaw., 1838–9, ii, 325–374. ———.
Ueber die zweifelhafte Flimmerbewegung an den Nerven.
Arch. f. Anat., Physiol. u. wissensch. Med., Berl., 1841, 39–
41. ———. Anatomische Beobachtungen über das Gehirn,
das Rückenmark und die Nervenwurzeln. *Ibid.*, 506–522.
———. Neurologische Erläuterungen. *Ibid*, 1844, 463–472,
1 pl. ———. Neurologische Beobachtungen. Deutsche Klinik, Berl., 1855, vii, 294. *Also*, Reprint. — **Renaut** (J.)
Nerfs (anatomie). Dict. encycl. d. sc. méd., Par., 1877, 2.

Nervous *system.*

s., xii, 124–179. ———. Recherches sur les centres nerveux
amyéliniques. Arch. de physiol. norm. et path., Par., 1882,
2. s., ix, 593–638, 1 pl.—**Renaut** (J.), **Carlet** (G.) &
François-Franck. Nerveux (système). Dict. encycl.
d. sc. méd., Par., 1878, 2. s., xii, 391–619.—**Revillout** (V.)
Brève histoire des théories actuellement régnantes au
sujet de la sensibilité récurrente. Gaz. d. hôp., Par., 1867,
xl, 595.—**Rhind** (S.) On the peripheral nervous system.
Lond. M. Gaz., 1851, n. s., xii, 548–552.—**Richardson** (B.
W.) On the influence of extreme cold on nervous function.
Med. Times & Gaz., Lond., 1867, ii, 57: 113; 221. ———. On
the local independency of nervous function. *Ibid.*, 167.—
Richet (C.) De la vibration nerveuse. Rev. scient., Par.,
1881, xxviii, 98–111. ———. Comparaison des muscles, des
nerfs et des centres nerveux. *Ibid.*, 1882, xxix, 46–51. ———.
Le système nerveux et la chaleur animale. *Ibid.*, 1887, xl,
353–360. — **Ripa.** L' uomo e la ginnastica. Med. communale, Seregno, 1874, xiii, 1–8.—**Rolando.** Expériences
sur les fonctions du système nerveux. J. de physiol.
expér., Par., 1823, iii, 95–113.—**Rombouts** (G. K.) De
motorische zenuwen der huidklieren van den kikvorsch;
eene bijdrage tot de leer van de identiteit der zenuwvezelen. Onderzoek. ged. in h. physiol. Lab. d. Utrecht.
Hoogesch., 1872, 3. R., i, 185–194.—**Rosenbach** (P.) O
vlijanii golodanija na nervnie centri. [Effect of hunger
upon the nervous centres.] Vestnik klin. i sudebnoi psichiat. i nevropatol., St. Petersb., 1883, i, no. 2, 150–250.—
Ross (J.) The structure and functions of the nervous
system. Med. Times & Gaz., Lond., 1877, ii, 457; 616;
642; 667: 1878, i, 33; 137: 164; 584: ii, 97; 346; 407; 652.—
Rossi (L. M.) Sui limiti, sulle cause e sulle mutue attinenze de' fenomeni nervosi. Gazz. med. ital., prov. venete,
Padova, 1860, iii, 353; 361; 369; 381; 393; 414: 1861, iv, 1;
9; 21; 25; 35; 45; 53; 57; 93; 101; 109; 117; 125; 133; 141;
149; 165; 175; 277; 285; 293: 1862, v, 105; 113; 121; 130;
141; 155; 168; 177; 189; 201. — **Rumpf** (T.) Ueber die
Einwirkung der Centralorgane auf die Erregbarkeit der
motorischen Nerven. Arch. f. Psychiat., Berl., 1877–8,
viii, 567–593. — **Sappey** (C.) & **Duval** (M.) Trajet des
cordons nerveux qui relient le cerveau à la moelle épinière.
Compt. rend. Acad. d. sc., Par., 1876, lxxxii, 230–233.—
Schiff (M.) Ueber die Verschiedenheit der Aufnahms-
fähigkeit und Leitungsfähigkeit in dem peripherischen
Nervensystem. Ztschr. f. rat. Med., Leipz., 1867, 3. R.,
xxix, 221–223. ———. Recherches sur l'échauffement des
nefs et des centres nerveux à la suite des irritations sensorielles et sensitives. Arch. de physiol. norm. et path.,
Par., 1869, ii, 157; 330: 1870, iii, 5; 198; 323; 451. ———.
Kritisches und Polemisches zur Physiologie des Nervensystems. Untersuch. z. Naturl. d. Mensch. u. d. Thiere,
Giessen, 1870, x, 75–124. ———. Erwärmung durchschnittener Nerven. Arch. f. d. ges. Physiol., Bonn, 1871, iv, 230–
232. ———. Annotazioni critiche sull'effetto della lesione dei
supposti centri motori. Riv. sper. di freniat, Reggio-Emilia, 1876, ii, 265–276. [*See, also, supra*, Lussana.]—**Schlesinger** (W.) Ueber die Centra der Gefäss- und Uterusnerven. Wien. med. Wchnschr., 1873, xxiii, 1008; 1028.
Also, transl.: N. York M. J., 1874, xix, 133–159.—**Schmidt**
(H. D.) On the structure of the nervous tissues and their
mode of action. Tr. Am. Neurol. Ass., N. Y., 1875, i, 71–
141.—**Schoeps** (C. G.) Ueber die Verrichtungen verschiedener Theile des Nervensystems. Arch. f. Anat. u.
Physiol., Leipz., 1827, 368–416. *Also, transl.:* J. compl.
du dict. d. sc. méd., Par., 1828, xxx, 114–142.—**von Schroff**
(C.) jun. Beiträge zur Kenntniss der Anordnung der
motorischen Nervencentra. Med. Jahrb., Wien, 1875,
319–329.—**Schulgin** (M. A.) Anatomija tsentralnoi
nervnoi sistemi. Arch. psichiat., etc., Charkov, 1884, iii,
no. 1, 143–180.—**Searcy** (J. T.) The equilibrating value
of nervous control. Med. Rec., N. Y., 1882, xxii, 317–319.
———. A short synopsis of nerve functions. *Ibid.*, 1884,
xxv, 113.—**Secommandi** (L.) Se i nervi transportino
le sensazioni al cervello. Gazz. med. ital. lomb., Milano,
1852, 3. s., iii, 259.—**Seguin** (E. C.) An outline of the
physiology of the nervous system. Med. Rec., N. Y.,
1874, ix, 617–622. *Also*, Reprint.—**Setschenow** (J.)
Pribavleniya k' ucheniyu o nervnikh tsentrakh. [Con-
tributions to the study of the nervous centres.] Med.
Vestnik, St. Petersb., 1863, iii, 309; 317. ———. Einige
Bemerkungen über das Verhalten der Nerven gegen sehr
schnell folgende Reize. Arch. f. d. ges. Physiol., Bonn,
1872, v, 116–119.—**Shaw** (J.) Expériences sur le système nerveux. J. de physiol. expér., Par., 1822, ii, 77–91.
———. [On the nervous system.] Lond. M. & Phys. J.,
1822, xlviii, 457–470, 1 pl. ———. Second part of a paper
on the nervous system. *Ibid.*, 1823, xlix, 449–462, 1 pl.
Also, transl.: Arch. gén. de méd., Par., 1823, ii, 511–531.
———. Remarks on M. Magendie's late experiments upon
the nerves. Lond. M. & Phys. J., 1824, lii, 95–104.—
Shumovski. Obsh-tchiia svoistva golovno-spinnych
tzentrov. [General properties of the cerebro-spinal centres.] Voyenno-med. J., St. Petersb., 1867, xcix, 81; 125 :
c, 1; 59; 99.—**Smerdon** (C. W.) On the functions of the
nervous system. Lond. M. & Phys. J., 1815, xxxiii, 23;
82; 276; 351.—**Smith** (W.) An inquiry into the views
of some modern physiologists relative to the laws and action of the nervous system—cerebral, spinal, and gangli-

Nervous *system.*

onic. Lond. M. Gaz., 1850, n. s., xi, 278–284.—**Snellaert** (F.-A.) Quelques fragments sur les fonctions et maladies du système nerveux intracrânien. Ann. Soc. de méd. de Gand, 1838, iv, 348–356, 1 pl.—**Solly** (S.) On the connexion of the anterior columns of the spinal cord with the cerebellum. Phil. Tr., Lond., 1836, cxxvi, 567–570, 1 pl.—**Ssubotin.** Ueber die Veränderung der Erregbarkeit der Nerven bei Anwendung von chemischen Reizen. Centralbl. f. d. med. Wissensch., Berl., 1866, iv, 737–739.—**Stannius** (H.) Ueber einige Functionen des Nervensystems. Lit. Ann. d. ges. Heilk., Berl., 1832, xxiv, 389–412.—**Stark** (J.) Researches on the brain, spinal chord, and ganglia, with remarks on the mode by which a continued flow of nervous agency is excited in, and transmitted from, these organs. Edinb. M. & S. J., 1845, lxiii, 103–133.—**Starr** (M. A.) The sensory tract in the central nervous system. J. Nerv. & Ment. Dis., N. Y., 1884, n. s., ix, 327–407.—**Stefani** (A.) Della influenza del sistema nervoso sulla circolazione collaterale; seconda comunicazione. Sperimentale, Firenze, 1887, lx, 146–161, 1 ch.—**Stern** (S.) Beiträge zur Kenntniss der Funktionen des Nervensystems. Vrtljschr. f. Psychiat., Neuwied, 1867-8, i, 253–333. *Also*, Reprint.—**Stilling** (B.) Zur Nervenphysik. Monatschr. f. Med., Augenh. u. Chir., Leipz., 1840, iii, 162–174. ———. Fragmente zur Lehre von der Verrichtung des Nervensystems; nach eigenen Versuchen; mit besonderer Berücksichtigung der neueren Untersuchungen auf diesem Gebiete. Arch. f. physiol. Heilk., Stuttg., 1842, i, 91–144. ———. Untersuchungen über die Functionen des Nervensystems; mit specieller Berücksichtigung der "Untersuchungen über das Nervensystem, von Dr. J. Budge". Arch. f. d. ges. Med., Jena, 1842, iii, 295; 425; 1843, iv, 1; 277; 427.—**Strachen** (J. M.) On the origin and circulation of the nervous influence. Lancet, Lond., 1854, i, 210.—**Stricker** (S.) Ueber die collaterale Innervation. Sitzungsb. d. k. Akad. d. Wissensch., Wien, 1877, lxxv, 83–92.—**Stromeyer.** On the combination of motor and sensitive nervous activity; or, on the production of sensations by motions. Transl. from the "Gottingische Gelehrte Anzeigen", with additions communicated by the author, by W. Little. Lond. M. Gaz., 1837, xx, 107; 150; 225. *Also, in:* Essays on Phys. & Hyg., 8°, Phila., 1838, 113–138.—**Szpilman** (J.) & **Luchsinger** (B.) Zur Beziehung von Leitungs- und Erregungsvermögen der Nervenfaser. Arch. f. d. ges. Physiol., Bonn, 1880-81, xxiv, 347–357.—**Takács** (E.) Vizsgálatok az érzés-jelzés elkésése felett. [Nervous physiology.] Orvosi hetil., Budapest, 1879, xxiii, 705–710.—**Tarchanoff** (J.) O vliyanii teploti na chuvstvuyushchie nervwi, spinnoi i golovnoi mozk lyagushki. [On the influence of warmth on the sensory nerves, brain, and spinal cord of the frog.] Voyenno-med. J., St. Petersb., 1869, cvi, pt. 2, 121. *Also, transl. :* Mélanges biol. Acad. imp. d. sc. de St.-Pétersb., 1871, viii, 22–48. ———. Ueber die Summirungserscheinungen bei Reizung sensibler Nerven des Frosches. Mélanges biol. Acad. imp. d. sc. de St.-Pétersb., 1871, vii, 691–717. ———. Rol nervnoi sistemy v dvijenii jivotnych. [Action of the nervous system on the animal functions.] Med. Sbornik, Tiflis, 1872, xiv (suppl.), 1–60.—**Taylor** (B. F.) Some remarks upon the functions of the nervous system, in connection with the views of Sir Chas. Bell, Dr. Marshall Hall, and Dr. Bennett Dowler. N. Orl. M. & S. J., 1851-2, viii, 603–605.—**Tiedemann** (F.) Beobachtungen über das Nervensystem und die sensiblen Erscheinungen der Seesterne. Deutsches Arch. f. d. Physiol., Halle, 1815, i, 161–175.—**Tigerstedt** (R.) Om nervernas förhållande till mekaniska irritament. [Activity of nerves under mechanical irritants.] Finska läk.-sällsk. handl., Helsingfors, 1879, xxi, 98–100.—**Tigri** (A.) Intorno alla attività fisica e fisiologica del sistema nervoso. Ann. univ. di med., Milano, 1874, ccxxvii, 91–109, 1 pl.—**Tilanus** (C. B.) Breviter distincteque indicetur modus et ratio actionis nervorum, quæque sint maxime probabiles hujus actionis explicationes. Ann. Acad. Rheno-Traject. (1816-17), 1818, 61–112.—**Todaro** (F.) Sulla struttura dei plessi nervosi. Gazz. clin. d. sped. civ. di Palermo, 1871, iii, 529–545, 2 pl.—**Tommasi** (S.) Nozioni fisio-patologiche dei centri nervosi. Eco d. clin., Napoli, 1886, i, 65; 81; 97.—**Traube** (L.) Zur Physiologie der vitalen Nerven-Centra. Ges. Beitr. z. Path. u. Physiol., Berl., 1871, i, 321–340, 2 pl.—**Treitel** (T.) Eine neue Reaction der markhaltigen Nervenfasern. Centralbl. f. d. med. Wissensch., Berl., 1876, xiv, 147–149.—**Tréviranus** (G.-R.) Sur les organes cérébraux, les nerfs de la vie végétative et sensitive, et leurs connexions mutuelles. J. compl. du dict. d. sc. méd., Par., 1823, xvi. 113–141. ———. Considérations sur les organes encéphaliques, sur les nerfs de la vie végétative et sensitive, et sur leur relation réciproque. Arch. gén. de méd., Par., 1823, ii, 392; 556.—**Tschisch** (V.) Ob iskusstvennom obrazovanii pigmenta v nervnoi tkani. Vrach, St. Petersb., 1884, v, 257.—**Tuson** (J.) A physiological inquiry into the nature of the brain and nerves, elucidating the doctrine of Cullen. Lond. M. Gaz., 1830, vi, 721–726. — **Valentin** (G.) Einige Versuche über die Einflüsse des beständigen Stromes auf die Leistungsfähigkeit benachbarter Nervenstrecken. Ztschr. f. Biol., München, 1872, viii, 210–238. ——— Die mehrfachen Interfe-

Nervous *system.*

renzen der Nervenerregungen. Arch. f. d. ges. Physiol., Bonn, 1876, xiii, 320–352, 1 pl.—**Van Kempen.** Des expériences sur le système nerveux. Bull. Acad. roy. de méd. de Belg., Brux., 1858-9, 2. s., ii, 215–217. ———. Sur les fonctions des centres nerveux encéphaliques. [Rap.] *Ibid.*, 1871, 3. s., v, 18–53.—**Van Santvoord** (R.) Destruction of the cerebro-spinal centres. Med. Rec., N. Y., 1879, xvi, 333–335. — **Versuch** einer kritischen Beleuchtung der Lex Belliana, oder einer wissenschaftlichen Abschätzung der aus dem Bell'schen Phänomen gezogenen Schlüsse. Arch. f. physiol. Heilk., Stuttg., 1842, 295–310.— **Verwey** (L. G.) Neurologische bijdrage. Boerhaave. Tijdschr., etc., Amst., 1844. n. s., iii, 32; 462: 1845, n. s., iv, 97. — **Volkmann** (A. W.) Ueber die Beweiskraft derjenigen Experimente, durch welche man einen directen Einfluss der Centralorgane auf die Eingeweide zu erweisen suchte. Arch. f. Anat., Physiol. u. wissensch. Med., Berl., 1842, 372 – 387. ———. Nervenphysiologie. Handwörterb. d. Physiol., Brnschwg, 1850, ii, 476–627.— **Vulpian.** Études de pathologie expérimentale sur le système nerveux. Progrès méd., Par., 1876, iv, 345. — **Wagner** (R.) Begründung meiner vom Prof. C. Ludwig in Zürich abgelehnten sogenannten "Anmuthungen". Ztschr. f. rat. Med., Heidelb., 1854, n. F., v, 307–323.— **Walker** (A.) An essay on the physiology of the nervous system; with an exposition of claims to priority of discovery, etc. Lancet, Lond., 1848, ii, 585; 633; 667; 688; 716. — **Warner** (F.) Muscular expression of nervous conditions. [Abstracts of articles published in: Brain.] Pop. Sc. Month., N. Y., 1881-2, xx, 584 – 590. ———. Considerations concerning the hypothesis of nerve-centres, leading to observation and experiment. Med. Times & Gaz., Lond., 1884, i, 142–146. ———. Abstract of lectures on the action of nerve-centres and modes of growth. Brit. M. J., Lond., 1887, i, 499; 671; 718. *Also:* Lancet, Lond., 1887, i, 514; 561. — **de Watteville** (A.) Ueber die Summirung von Reizen in den sensiblen Nerven des Menschen. Neurol. Centralbl., Leipz., 18·3, ii, 145–147.—**Weber** (E. H.) Ueber den Einfluss der Erwärmung und Erkältung der Nerven auf ihr Leitungsvermögen. Arch. f. Anat., Physiol. u. wissensch. Med., Berl., 1847, 342–356. — **Wible** (B. M.) A letter on the physiological doctrines of Marshall Hall. West. J. M. & S., Louisville, 1853, 3. s., xi, 385 – 388.—**Williams** (T.) On the laws of nervous force; and the function of the roots of the spinal nerves. Lancet, Lond., 1847, ii, 516. — **Willy** (K.) Ueber die Abhängigkeit der Nervenerregung von der Länge der durchflossenen Strecke. Arch. f. d. ges. Physiol., Bonn, 1872, v, 275–280, 1 pl.—**Wilson** (A. P. W.) Some observations on the functions of the nervous system, and the relation which they bear to the other vital functions. Phil. Tr., Lond., 1829, cxix, 261 – 278. — **von Wittich.** Ueber die Fortleitungsgeschwindigkeit im menschlichen Nerven. Ztschr. f. rat. Med., Leipz., 1868, 3. R., xxxi, 87–125.—**Wolski** (B.) Sind die sensiblen und die excitomotorischen Nervenfasern der Haut beim Frosche verschieden? Arch. f. d. ges. Physiol., Bonn, 1872, v, 282–284.—**Wood** (S.) Nerve-force in waste and supply. Brit. M. J., Lond , 1872, i, 40-42.—**Wright** (D. F.) Recent theories in nervous physiology. Memphis M. Recorder, 1856-7, v, 569–579.—**Wundt** (W.) Ueber secundäre Modification der Nerven. Arch. f. Anat., Physiol. u. wissensch. Med., Leipz., 1859, 537–548, 1 pl. ———. Bemerkung zu dem Aufsatze des Herrn Dr. H. Munk: Ueber die Leitung der Erregung im Nerven. *Ibid.*, 1861, 781–783.— **Zuelzer** (W.) Stoffwechsel der nervösen Centralorgane. Verhandl. d. Cong. f. innere Med., Wiesb., 1884, ii, 153–157.

Nervous *system (Abnormities of).*

See, also, **Brain** *(Abnormities of);* **Monsters** *from defect, etc., of brain, etc.;* **Spinal cord** *(Abnormities of).*

Cleland. Contribution to the study of spina bifida, encephalocele, and anencephalus. J. Anat., Lond. [1882-3], xvii, 257–292, 2 pl.—**Fürstner & Zacher.** Ueber eine eigenthümliche Bildungsanomalie des Hirns und Rückenmarks; secundäre Erkrankung beider Organe. Arch. f. Psychiat., Berl., 1881, xii, 373–391, 2 pl.—**Ónodi** (A. D.) Rendellenes alakviszonyok az idegtan köréböl. [Abnormities of form in the nervous system; spinal ganglia and roots of nerves.] Orvosi hetil., Budapest, 1885, xxix, 1077; 1106; 1195; 1256.—**Romiti** (G.) Di una rara varietà nervosa, e considerazioni relative. Boll. d. Soc. tra i cult. d. sc. med. in Siena, 1886, iv, 65–68.—**Schultze.** In wie weit können Entwickelungsanomalien des Centralnervensystems und besonders des Rückenmarkes das anatomische Substrat einer neuropathischen Disposition darbieten? Arch. f. Psychiat., Berl., 1880, xi, 270.

Nervous *system (Action of medicines and poisons on).*

See, also, **Anæsthetics; Narcotics; Sedatives; Stimulants** *and under names of drugs.*

Bowditch (H. P.) The action of sulphuric ether on the peripheral nervous system. From experiments per-

Nervous *system* (*Action of medicines and poisons on*).

formed in the physiological laboratory of the Harvard Medical School, by Dr. F. H. Hooper, Dr. F. W. Ellis and Mr. J. W. Perkins. Am. J. M. Sc., Phila., 1887, n. s., xciii, 444–455. *Also*, Reprint.—**Buchheim** (R.) Ueber die Einwirkung der Arzneimittel und Gifte auf das Nervensystem. Arch. d. Heilk., Leipz., 1870, xi, 209–220.—**Weber.** Bemerkungen über die Wirkungen einiger Arzneimittel auf das Gemüth und das Sensorium. Ztschr. f. d. ges. Med., Hamb., 1845, xxviii, 1: xxix, 293: 1846, xxxi, 153.

Nervous *system* (*Blood-vessels and lymphatics of*).

DOERFFLER (J. F.) * De vasis nervorum. 4°. *Erlangæ*, [1768].

Also, in: SCRIPT. neurol. minores selecti. 4°. *Lipsiæ*, 1793, iii.

EKKER (E. H.) * De cerebri et medullæ spinalis systemate vasorum capillari in statu sano et morboso. 8°. *Traj. ad Rhenum*, 1853.

Adamkiewicz. O krążeniu krwi w komórce zwojowéj. [Circulation of the blood in the ganglionic cells.] Przegl. lek., Krakow., 1886, xxv, 3; 19; 45; 61; 77.—**Deecke** (T.) On the perivascular spaces in the nervous centers. Am. J. Insan., Utica, N. Y., 1873-4, xxx, 322–330. *Also*, Reprint.—**Eberth** (C. J.) Ueber die Blut- und Lymphgefässe des Gehirns und Rückenmarks. Arch. f. path. Anat., etc., Berl., 1870, xlix, 48–50.—**Fischer** (F.) Beiträge zur Kenntniss des Lymphbahnen des Central-Nervensystems; nach Untersuchungen von Dr. . . . mitgetheilt von Prof. Waldeyer. Arch. f. mikr. Anat., Bonn, 1879-80, xvii, 362–366.—**Key** (A.) & **Retzius** (G.) Ytterligare några forutskickade meddelanden om de serösa rummen och lymfbanorna i nervsystemet. Nord. med. Ark., Stockholm, 1870, ii, no. 13, 9–11.—**Lépine** (R.) Note sur la structure des canaux périvasculaires des centres nerveux. Compt. rend. Soc. de biol. 1867, Par., 1869, 4. s., iv, 173–175.—**Moxon** (W.) Croonian lectures on the influence of the circulation on the nervous system. Lancet, Lond., 1881, i, 487; 527; 565; 607; 647; 685. *Also:* Brit. M. J., Lond., 1881, i, 491; 546; 583; 628; 672. *Also:* Med. Times & Gaz., Lond., 1881, i, 339; 370; 450; 533; 639; 668.—**Pouchet** (G.) Note sur la vascularité des faisceaux primitifs des nerfs périphériques. J. de l'anat. et physiol., etc., Par., 1867, iv, 438–441. *Also*, Reprint.

Nervous *system* (*Chemistry of*).

See, also, **Brain** (*Chemistry of, etc.*).

BIRKNER (G.) * Ueber den Werth des Wassers in der Nervensubstanz. 8°. *Augsburg*, 1857.

GARNIER (L.) * Étude chimique du système nerveux. 4°. *Nancy & Saint-Nicolas*, 1877.

Funke (O.) Ueber Säurebildung im Nerven. Centralbl. f. d. med. Wissensch., Berl., 1869, vii, 721–723.—**Gscheidlen** (R.) Ueber die chemische Reaction der nervösen Centralorgane. Arch. f. d. ges. Physiol., Bonn, 1874, viii, 171–180.—**Jolly** (L.) Recherches sur les différents modes de combinaison de l'acide phosphorique dans la substance nerveuse. Compt. rend. Acad. d. sc., Par., 1879, lxxxix, 756–758.

Nervous *system* (*Comparative anatomy and physiology of*).

See, also, **Insects** (*Nervous system of*); **Nerve** (*Facial*); **Nerve** (*Optic*); **Nervous** *system* (*Development of*).

ANDERSON (J.) Sketch of the comparative anatomy of the nervous system; with remarks on its development in the human embryo. With plates, [etc.] 4°. *London*, 1837.

BAZIN (A.) Notes sur l'anatomie comparée du système nerveux. 8°. *Bordeaux*, 1861.

Repr. from: Mém. Soc. d. sc. phys. et nat. de Bordeaux.

BELLONCI (G.) Ricerche comparative sulla struttura dei centri nervosi dei vertebrati. Memoria. 4°. *Roma*, 1880.

Repr. from: Atti d. r. Accad. d. Lincei. Cl. di sc. fis., matemat. e nat., Roma, 1879-80, 3. s., v.

———. Sistema nervoso e organi dei sensi dello sphæroma serratum. 4°. *Roma*, 1881.

Repr. from: Atti d. r. Accad. d. Lincei. Cl. di sc. fis., matemat. e nat., Roma, 1880-81, 3. s., x.

BLANCHARD (É.) Du système nerveux chez les invertébrés (mollusques et annelés), dans ses rapports avec la classification de ces animaux. 8°. *Paris*, 1849.

Nervous *system* (*Comparative anatomy and physiology of*).

BLATTMANN (A.) * Mikroskopische anatomische Darstellung der Centralorgane des Nervensystems bei den Betrachiern mit besonderer Berücksichtigung von Rana esculenta. 8°. *Zürich*, 1850.

BÖHMIG (L.) * Beiträge zur Kenntniss des Centralnervensystems einiger pulmonaten Gasteropoden: Helix pomatia und Limnæa stagnalis. 8°. *Leipzig*, 1883.

BORUSDORFF (E. J.) Anatomisk beskrifning af cerebral-nerverne hos fåret (Ovis aries). 4°. [*n. p.*], 1843.

Cutting from: Acta Soc. sc. Fennicæ, Helsingfors, 1847, ii, 145–284.

———. The same. II. Nervi cerebrales Gruis cureæ (Linn.). 4°. [*n. p.*, 1851.]

Cutting from: Acta Soc. sc. Fennicæ, Helsingfors, 1852, iii, 591–624.

———. Symbolæ ad anatomiam comparatam nervorum animalium vertebratorum . . . I. Nervi cerebrales Corvi cornicis (Linn.). 4°. [*n. p.*, 1850.]

Cutting from: Acta Soc. sc. Fennicæ, Helsingfors, 1852, iii, 505–569.

BRAUN (A.) *Ueber die Varietäten des Plexus lumbo-sacralis von Rana. 8°. *Bonn*, 1886.

CARPENTER (W. B.) Inaugural dissertation on the physiological inferences to be deduced from the structure of the nervous system in the invertebrated classes of animals. [Prize thesis.] 8°. *Edinburgh*, 1839.

———. The same. [Dunglison's Am. M. Libr.] 8°. *Philadelphia*, 1840.

———. The same. 8°. *Philadelphia*, 1841.

CLOUSTON (T. S.) The minute anatomy and physiology of the nervous system in the lobster (Astacus marinus); being part of a thesis presented by the author to the University of Edinburgh, entitled "Contributions to the minute anatomy and physiology of the nervous system, as illustrated in the invertebrata", for which he received one of the gold medals awarded by the medical faculty. 8°. *Edinburgh*, 1863.

Repr. from: Edinb. New Phil. J., Jan., 1863, n. s.

DESMOULINS (A.) Anatomie des systèmes nerveux des animaux à vertèbres appliquée à la physiologie et à la zoologie. Ouvrage dont la partie physiologique est faite conjointement avec F. Magendie. 2 v. 8°. *Paris*, 1825.

———. The same. Atlas. 4°. *Paris*, 1825.

EBEL (J. G.) Observationes neurologicæ ex anatome comparata. 4°. *Traj. ad Viadr.*, 1788.

In: SCRIPT. neurol. minores selecti. 4°. *Lipsiæ*, 1793, iii, 148–161, 2 pl.

FISCHER (J. G.) *Amphibiorum nudorum neurologiæ specimen primum. 4°. *Berolini*, [1843].

GERVAIS (P.) Planches murales d'histoire naturelle. Zool., pl. 29. [Nervous system.] fol. *Paris*, [1885].

GOLTZ (F.) Beiträge zur Lehre von den Functionen der Nervencentren des Frosches. 8°. *Berlin*, 1869.

GUILLOT (N.) Exposition anatomique de l'organisation du centre nerveux dans les quatre classes d'animaux vertèbres. Ouvrage couronné. 4°. *Paris*, 1844.

VON JHERING (H.) Das peripherische Nervensystem der Wirbelthiere als Grundlage für die Kenntniss der Regionenbildung der Wirbelsäule. 4°. *Leipzig*, 1878.

JONQUIÈRE (G.) *Versuche über den Einfluss einzelner Theile des centralen Nervensystems des Zitterrochens auf die willkürliche und reflektorische elektrische Thätigkeit desselben. 8°. *Bern*, 1879.

Nervous *system* (*Comparative anatomy and physiology of*).

JUNG (R. A.) *Descriptio plexuum abdominalium nervosorum in corvo cornice. 8°. *Gryphiæ*, 1858.

KRONENBERG (H.) *Experimenta in ranæ esculentæ plexu lumbali facta veram nervorum fibrillarum, quas primitivas vocant, anastomosin refellentia. Amplioris operis, præmio hoc anno decorati, fragmentum. 8°. *Berolini*, [1835].

KÜTTNER (C.) *De origine nervi sympathici ranarum ex nervorum dissectorum mutationibus dijudicata. 8°. *Dorpati Livonorum*, 1854.

LANDOIS (H.) *De systemate nervorum transversorum in septem insectorum ordinibus. 8°. *Gryphiswaldiæ*, 1863.

LEURET (F.) & GRATIOLET (P.) Anatomie comparée du système nerveux, considéré dans ses rapports avec l'intelligence. 2 v., 8°; atlas, fol. *Paris*, 1839–57.

LOEWE (L.) Beiträge zur Anatomie und zur Entwickelungsgeschichte des Nervensystems der Säugethiere und des Menschen. 2 v. fol. *Berlin*, 1880.

LONGET (F.-A.) Anatomie et physiologie du système nerveux de l'homme et des animaux vertébrés; ouvrage contenant des observations pathologiques relatives au système nerveux et des expériences sur les animaux des classes supérieures. 2 v. 8°. *Paris*, 1842.

———. The same. Anatomie und Physiologie des Nervensystems des Menschen und der Wirbelthiere mit pathologischen Beobachtungen und mit Versuchen an höhern Thieren ausgestattet. Eine von dem französischen Institut gekrönte Preisschrift. Uebersetzt und mit den Ergebnissen deutscher, englischer und französischer Forschungen aus den letzten Jahren bis auf die Gegenwart ergänzt und vervollständigt von Dr. J. A. Hein. 2 v. 8°. *Leipzig*, 1847–9.

MASON (J. J.) Minute structure of the central nervous system of certain reptiles and batrachians of America. Illustrated by permanent photo-micrographs. Series A. Author's edition. One hundred. 4°. *Newport*, 1879–82.

VON MIKLUCHO-MACLAY (N.) Beiträge zur vergleichenden Neurologie der Wirbelthiere. I. Das Gehirn der Selachier. II. Das Mittelhirn der Ganoiden und Teleostier. roy. 4°. *Leipzig*, 1870.

PEYER (J.) *Ueber die peripherischen Endigungen der motorischen und sensiblen Fasern der in den Plexus brachialis des Kaninchens eintretenden Nervenwurzeln. 8°. *Zürich*, 1853.

ROTH (J. J.) *De animalium invertebratorum systemate nervoso. 4°. *Wirceburgi*, 1825.

STIEDA (L.) Studien über das centrale Nervensystem der Wirbelthiere. 8°. *Leipzig*, 1870.

SWAN (J.) Illustrations of the comparative anatomy of the nervous system. roy. 8°. *London*, 1835.

YERSIN. Recherches sur les fonctions du système nerveux dans les animaux articulés. 8°. [*Lausanne, n. d.*]

ZAGORSKY (A.) *De systemate nerveo piscium considerationes. 4°. *Dorpati, Livonorum*, 1833.

Alix. Sur le nerf vertébral du chameau. Bull. Soc. philomat., Par., 1878, 7. s., ii, 147. ———. Sur le système nerveux de la sarigue. *Ibid.*, 148.—**Andral** fils. Sur les nerfs qui se rendent aux moustaches du phoque. J. de physiol. expér., Par., 1821, i, 73.—**Apostolidès** (N.) Système nerveux des ophiures. Compt. rend. Acad. d. sc., Par., 1881, xcii, 1424-1426.—**Aschenbrandt** (T.) Das Ganglion nasopalatinum s. incisivum der Nagetiere. Verhandl. d. phys.-med. Gesellsch. zu Würzb., 1887, n. F., xx, 9-24, 1 pl.—**Aubert** (H.) Ueber das Verhalten der in sauerstofffreier Luft paralysirten Frösche und ein darauf gegründetes einfaches Verfahren, die Reflexmechanismen bei erhaltener Erregbarkeit der motorischen Nerven und der Muskeln stundenlang zu lähmen. Arch. f. d. ges. Physiol., Bonn, 1881-2, xxvii, 566-576.—**Bailly** (E.-M.)

Nervous *system* (*Comparative anatomy and physiology of*).

Recherches d'anatomie et de physiologie comparées du système nerveux dans les quatre classes d'animaux vertébrés. Arch. gén. de méd., Par., 1824, iv, 45-60.—**Balfour** (F. M.) On the development of the spinal nerves in elasmobranch fishes. Phil. Tr., Lond., 1876, clxvi, pt. 1, 175-195.—**Baudelot** (E.) Procédé relatif à la dissection du système nerveux chez les poissons. J. de méd., Par., 1878, ii, 31.—**Bellonci** (G.) Ricerche sul sistema nervoso centrale della Squilla mantis. Rendic. Accad. d. sc. d. Ist. di Bologna, 1878, 88-96.—**Boguslawski** (N.) Zur Frage über die Structur der markhaltigen Nervenfasern. St. Petersb. med. Wchnschr., 1876, i, no. 36.—**Bourgery** (J.-M.) Mémoire sur les masses comparatives que présentent, dans l'homme et quelques animaux mammifères, les différents organes qui composent le système nerveux. Compt. rend. Acad. d. sc., Par., 1844, xix, 603-607. *Also:* Gaz. méd. de Par., 1844, 2. s., xii, 633-638. ———. Mémoire sur la coordination générale et la structure intime de l'appareil nerveux de la langue dans l'homme et les mammifères. Gaz. méd. de Par., 1848, 2. s., xix, 986-991. *Also*, Reprint.—**Bouvier** (E.-L.) Sur le système nerveux des buccinidés et des purpuridés. Compt. rend. Acad. d. sc., Par., 1885, c, 1509-1512.—**Brandt** (E.) Du système nerveux de l'Idothea entomon (crustacé isopode). *Ibid.*, 1880, xc, 713.—**Brocchi** (P.) Sur le système nerveux de l'axolotl (Siredon mexicanus). Bull. Soc. philomat. de Par., 1877, 7. s., i, 21-24.—**Bütschli** (O.) Beiträge zur Kenntniss des Nervensystems der Nematoden. Arch. f. mikr. Anat., Bonn, 1874, x, 74-100, 2 pl. ———. Zur Herleitung des Nervensystems der Nematoden. Morphol. Jahrb., Leipz., 1884-5, x, 486-493, 1 pl.—**Cadiat.** Note sur la structure des nerfs chez les invertébrés. Compt. rend. Acad. d. sc., Par., 1878, lxxxvi, 1420-1422. ———. Note sur les caractères anatomiques des nerfs chez les invertébrés. Compt. rend. Soc. de biol. 1878, Par., 1880, 6. s., v, 207-209.—**Chatin** (J.) Sur la différenciation du protoplasma dans les fibres nerveuses des Unionides. Compt. rend. Acad. d. sc., Par., 1882, xciv, 1723-1726. ———. Nerfs qui naissent du ganglion postérieur chez les Unios. Compt. rend. Soc. de biol., Par., 1886, 8. s., iii, 242.—**Chéron** (J.) Des nerfs corrélatifs dits antagonistes et du nœud vital dans un groupe d'invertébrés. Compt. rend. Acad. d. sc., Par., 1868, lxvi, 1163-1167.—**Clevenger** (S. V.) Comparative neurology. Am. Naturalist, Phila., 1881, xv, 16; 103.—**Cunningham** (D. J.) The spinal nervous system of the porpoise and dolphin. J. Anat. & Physiol., Lond., 1876-7, xi, 209-228, 1 pl.—**Cyon** (E.) Ueber den Nervus Depressor beim Pferde. Mélanges biol. Acad. imp. d. sc. de St.-Pétersb., 1870, viii, 459-462, 1 pl. *Also*, Reprint.—**Desmoulins** (A.) Mémoire sur les différences qui existent entre le système nerveux de la lamproie, et celui des animaux vertébrés, sous le rapport des propriétés physiques, du nombre et du mécanisme de réunion des parties. J. de physiol. expér., Par., 1824, iv, 239-257. ———. Recherches anatomiques et physiologiques sur le système nerveux dans les poissons. J. compl. du dict. d. sc. méd., Par., 1825, xxiii, 303: 1826, xxiv, 200.—**Drost** (K.) Ueber das Nervensystem und die Sinnesepithelien der Herzmuschel (Cardium edule L.), nebst einigen Mittheilungen über den histologischen Bau ihres Mantels und ihrer Siphonen. Morphol. Jahrb., Leipz., 1886-7, xii, 163-201, 1 pl.—**Duncan** (P. M.) On the nervous system of actinia. Pt. I. Proc. Roy. Soc. Lond., 1873-4, xxii, 44; 263, 2 pl.—**Eimer** (T.) Vorläufige Mittheilungen über die Nerven von Beroë. Arch. f. mikr. Anat., Bonn, 1872, viii, 647-651. ———. Ueber künstliche Theilbarkeit und über das Nervensystem der Medusen. *Ibid.*, 1877, xiv, 394-408. ———. Versuche über künstliche Theilbarkeit von Beroë ovatus. Angestellt zum Zweck der Controle seiner morphologischen Befunde über das Nervensystem dieses Thieres. *Ibid.*, 1879, xvii, 213-240.—**Epps** (J.) Essay on the gradual development of the nervous system, from the zoophyte to man. Lond. M. & S. J., 1829, ii, 35; 150; 231.—**Faivre** (E.) Études sur l'histologie comparée du système nerveux chez quelques animaux inférieurs. Ann. d. sc. nat., Par., 1855-6, 4. s., vi, 16-82, 2 pl. *Also*, Reprint.—**von Förök** (A.) Ueber den Bau der Nervenfaser. Verhandl. d. phys.-med. Gesellsch. in Würzb., 1872, iii, 41-43. —**Fraipont** (J.) Le système nerveux central et périphérique des archiannélides (protodrilus, polygordius) et des archichoetopodes (saccocirrus); (contribution à l'histoire de l'origine du système nerveux des annélides). [Note préliminaire.] Bull. Acad. roy. d. sc. de Belg., Brux., 1884, 3. s., viii, 99-120. ———. Recherches sur le système nerveux central et périphérique des archiannélides (protodrilus et polygordius) et du Saccocirrus papillocercus. Arch. de biol., Gand, 1884, v, 243-304, 5 pl.—**Fritsch** (G.) Ueber einige bemerkenswerthe Elemente des Centralnervensystems von Lophius piscatorius L. Arch. f. mikr. Anat., Bonn, 1886, xxvii, 13-31, 2 pl.—**Goodsir** (J.) On the morphological relations of the nervous system in the annulose and vertebrate types of organisation. [*Repr. from*: Edinb. Phil. J., 1857.] *In his*: Anat. Mem., 8°, Edinb., 1868, ii, 78-87.—**Haller** (B.) Untersuchungen über marine Rhipidoglossen. Erste Studie. Morphol.

Nervous system (*Comparative anatomy and physiology of*).

Jahrb., Leipz., 1883-4, ix, 1. ——. The same. II. Textur des Centralnervensystemes und seiner Hüllen. *Ibid.*, 1885 - 6, xi, 321 - 436, 8 pl. — **Hensen** (V.) Ueber die Nerven im Schwanz der Froschlarven. Arch. f. mikr. Anat., Bonn, 1868, iv, 111-124, 2 pl.—**Hubrecht** (A. A. W.) The peripheral nervous system in palæo- and schizonemertini, one of the layers of the body-wall. Quart. J. Micr. Sc., Lond., 1880, n. s., xx, 431-442, 2 pl. ——: Zur Anatomie und Physiologie des Nervensystems der Nemertinen. Verhandel. d. k. Akad. v. Wetensch., Amst., 1880, xx, pt. 2, 1-47, 4 pl. *Also, transl.* [Abstr.]: Quart. J. Micr. Sc., Lond., 1880, n. s., xx, 274-282, 1 pl. ——. Studien zur Phylogenie des Nervensystems. II. Das Nervensystem von Pseudonematon nervosum gen. et sp. n. Verhandel. d. k. Akad. v. Wetensch., Amst., 1883. xxii, 19, 2 pl. — **von Ihering** (H.) Beiträge zur Kenntniss des Nervensystems der Amphineuren und Arthrocochliden. Morphol. Jahrb., Leipz., 1877, iii, 155-178, 1 pl.—**Jackson** (J. H.) Evolution and dissolution of the nervous system. Pop. Sc. Month., N. Y., 1884-5, xxv, 171-180.—**Johnson** (Alice) & **Sheldon** (Lilian). On the development of the cranial nerves of the newt. Proc. Roy. Soc. Lond., 1886, xl, 94.—**Julin** (C.) Le système nerveux grand sympathique de l'ammocœtes (Petromyzon Planeri). Anat. Anz., Jena, 1887, ii, 192-201.— **Klein** (E.) Beiträge zur Kenntniss der Nerven des Froschlarvenschwanzes. [*Repr. from:* Sitzungsb. d. k. Akad. d. Wissensch. Math.-naturw. Cl., Wien, 1870, lxi, 2. Abth., 5, 1 pl.] Centralbl. f. d. med. Wissensch., Berl., 1871, ix, 1.—**Kowalevsky** (A.) Weitere Studien über die Entwickelungsgeschichte des Amphioxus lanceolatus, nebst einem Beitrage zur Homologie des Nervensystems der Würmer und Wirbelthiere. Arch. f. mikr. Anat., Bonn, 1876, xiii, 181 - 204, 2 pl. — **Kreidmann** (A.) Anatomische Untersuchungen über den Nervus depressor beim Menschen und Hunde. Arch. f. Anat u. Physiol., Leipz., 1878, 405 - 415, 1 pl. *Also* [Abstr.]: Centralbl. f. d. med. Wissensch., Berl., 1878, xvi, 193.— **Krohn** (A.) Ueber die Anordnung des Nervensystems der Echiniden und Holothurien im Allgemeinen. Arch. f. Anat., Physiol. u. wissensch. Med., Berl., 1841, 1-13, 1 pl. — **Künckel** (J.) Recherches morphologiques et zoologiques sur le système nerveux des insectes diptères. Compt. rend. Acad. d. sc., Par., 1879, lxxxix, 491-494.— **Künckel** (J.) & **Gazagnaire** (J.) Rapport du cylindre-axe et des cellules nerveuses périphériques avec les organes des sens chez les insectes. *Ibid.*, 1881, xcii, 471-473. — **Kuhnt** (J. H.) Die Zwischenmarkscheide der markhaltigen Nervenfasern. Centralbl. f. d. med. Wissensch., Berl., 1876, xiv, 865. — **Kupffer** (C.) Primäre Metamerie des Neuralrohrs der Vertebraten. Sitzungsb. d. math.-phys. Cl. d. k.-bayer. Akad. d. Wissensch. zu München, 1885, xv, 469-476. — **Laffont.** Section intracrânienne du nerf trijumeau chez le chien. Compt. rend. Soc. de biol. 1880, Par.. 1881, 7. s., ii, 26-28. ——. Recherches sur l'anatomie et la physiologie comparée des nerfs trijumeau facial et sympathique céphalique chez les oiseaux. Compt. rend. Acad. d. sc., Par., 1885, ci. 1286-1289.—**Lahille** (F.) Sur le développement typique du système nerveux central des tuniciers. *Ibid.*, 1887, cv, 957-960.—**Leboucq** (H.) Recherches sur le développement et la terminaison des nerfs chez les larves de batraciens. Bull. Acad. roy. d. sc. de Belg., Brux., 1876, 2. s., xli, 561-582, 1 pl. *Also* [Rev.]: Quart. J. Micr. Sc., Lond., 1877, n. s., xvii, 455-460.—**Leydig** (F.) Haben die Nematoden ein Nervensystem? Bemerkungen zu dieser Frage. Arch. f. Anat., Physiol. u. wissensch. Med., Leipz., 1861, 606-614. ——. Ueber das Nervensystem der Anneliden. *Ibid.*, 1862, 90-124. — **Liénard** (V.) Recherches sur le système nerveux des arthropodes; constitution de l'anneau œsophagien. Arch. de biol., Gand, 1880, i, 381-391, 1 pl.—**Luys** (J.) Nouvelles recherches d'anatomie comparée sur les rapports des éléments cérébraux et des éléments spinaux au point de vue de la structure du système nerveux central. Encéphale, Par., 1885, v, 641-647, 1 pl.—**McIntosh** (W. C.) On the central nervous system, the cephalic sacs and other points in the anatomy of the Lineidæ. Anat. & Physiol., Lond., 1875-6, x, 231 - 252, 4 pl.—**Magnien** (L.) Étude des rapports entre les nerfs crâniens et le sympathique céphalique chez les oiseaux. Compt. rend. Acad. d. sc., Par., 1887, civ, 77-79. — **Marshall** (A. M.) On the head cavities and associated nerves of elasmobranchs. Quart. J. Micr. Sc., Lond., 1881, n. s., xxi, 72-97, 2 pl. ——. On the nervous system of Antedon rosaceus. Stud. Biol. Lab. Owens Coll., Manchester, 1886, i. 263-297, 1 pl.—**Marshall** (A. M.) & **Spencer** (W. B.) Observations on the cranial nerves of scyllium. Quart. J. Micr. Sc., Lond., 1881, n. s., xxi, 469-499, 1 pl.—**Marshall** (C. F.) Some investigations on the physiology of the nervous system of the lobster. Stud. Biol. Lab. Owens Coll., Manchester, 1886, i, 313-323.—**Mason** (J.J.) Microscopic studies on the central nervous system of reptiles and batrachians. Article I. The spinal cord of the frog (Rana pipiens, Rana halecina). J. Nerv. & Ment. Dis., Chicago, 1880, n. s., v, 16-23. *Also,* Reprint. ——. The same. Arti-

cle II. Diameters of the nuclei of nerve cells in the spinal cord; rana; Emys floridana; Testudo polyphemus. *Ibid.*, 385-389. *Also,* Reprint. ——. The same. Article III. Diameters of the nuclei of the large nerve cells in the spinal cord (continued), also of those which give origin to the motor fibres of the cranial nerves. *Ibid.*, N. Y., 1881, n. s., vi, 80-86. *Also,* Reprint. ——. The same. Article IV. Diameters of the nuclei in the nerve cells which are related to motor nerves Chelydra serpentina (snapping turtle); Iguana tuberculata (iguana); Phrynosoma cornutum (horned toad); Menopoma allegheniense (hellbender); Siren lacertina (siren); Diemyctylus torosus (salamander), and serpents. *Ibid.*. 1882, n. s., vii, 50-57. *Also,* Reprint. ——. Notes on the central nervous system of reptiles. *Ibid.*, 1881, n. s., vi, 574-576. *Also,* Reprint.— **Mitrophanow** (P.) Zur Entwicklungsgeschichte und Innervation der Nervenhügel der Urodelenlarven. Biol. Centralbl., Erlang., 1887-8, vii, 174-178. — **Müller** (J.) Ueber die Metamorphose des Nervensystems in der Thierwelt. Arch. f. Anat. u. Physiol., Leipz., 1828, iii, 1—22.— **Önodi** (A. D.) Neurologische Untersuchungen an Selachiern. Internat. Monatschr. f. Anat. u. Histol., Leipz., 1886, iii, 325-329, 1 pl.—**Pelseneer** (P.) Observations on the nervous system of apus. Quart. J. Micr. Sc., Lond., 1885, n. s., xxv, 433-444, 1 pl. ——. Recherches sur le système nerveux des ptéropodes. Arch. de biol., Gand, 1887, vii, 93-129, 1 pl.—**Pelvet.** De l'influence du système nerveux sur les changements de la peau et les mouvements des ventouses chez le poulpe. Compt. rend. Soc. de biol. 1867, Par., 1869, 4. s., iv, 61-66.—**Pruvot** (G.) Sur le système nerveux des euniciens. Compt. rend. Acad. d. sc., Par., 1884, xcviii, 1492-1495.—**Rawitz** (B.) Das zentrale Nervensystem der Acephalen. Jenaische Ztschr. f. Naturw., Jena, 1886-7, n. F., xiii, 384-460, 5 pl. — **Renaut** (J.) Sur les cellules godronnées et le système hyalin intra-vaginal des nerfs de solipèdes. Compt. rend. Acad. d. sc., Par., 1880, xc, 711-713. — **Retzius** (G.) Till kännedomen om plagiostomernas nervtrådar. Nord. med. Ark., Stockholm, 1877, ix, no. 23, 1-5. — **Richet** (C.) Contribution à la physiologie des centres nerveux et des muscles de l'écrevisse. Arch. de physiol. norm. et path., Par., 1879, 2. s., vi, 262; 522. — **Romanes** (G. J.) The physiology of the nervous system of medusæ. Notices Proc. Roy. Inst. Gr. Brit. 1875 - 8, Lond., 1879, viii, 166-177. ——. The beginning of nerves in the animal kingdom. Pop. Sc. Month., N. Y., 1878, xiv, 303 - 320.— **Sanders** (A.) Contribution to the anatomy of the central nervous system in vertebrate animals. Pt. I. Ichthyopsida. Sect. I. Pisces. Subsect. I. Teleostei. Phil. Tr. 1878, Lond , 1879, clxix, 735-776, 8 pl.: 1882, Lond., 1883, clxxiii, 927-959, 5 pl. *Also* [Abstr.]: Proc. Roy. Soc. Lond., 1878, xxvii, 415: 1881-2, xxxiii, 400. ——. The same. Pt. I. Ichthyopsida. Section I. Pisces. Subsection II. Plagiostomata. Phil. Tr. 1886, Lond., 1887, clxxvii, 733 - 766, 4 pl. *Also* [Abstr.]: Proc. Roy. Soc. Lond., 1886, xl, 10-14.—**Schäfer** (E. A.) "Observations on the nervous system of Aurelia aurita." Communicated by W. Sharpsey. [Abstr.] Proc. Roy. Soc. Lond., 1878, xxvii, 16.—**Schöbl** (J.) Ueber die Blutgefässe des cerebro-spinalen Nervensystems der Urodelen. Arch. f. mikr. Anat., Bonn, 1881, xx, 87-92, 1 pl. — **Schultze** (H.) Die fibrilläre Structur der Nervenelemente bei Wirbellosen. *Ibid.*, 1878, xvi, 57-111, 2 pl.—**Sheldon** (Lilian). Note on the ciliated pit of ascidians and its relation to the nerve-ganglion and socalled hypophysial gland; and an account of the anatomy of Cynthia rustica(?). Quart. J. Micr. Sc., Lond., 1887-8, n. s., xxviii, 131-148, 2 pl.—**Stiénon** (L.) Recherches sur la structure des ganglions spinaux chez les vertébrés supérieurs. Ann. univ. de Brux., 1880, i, 147-163.—**Stowell** (T. B.) The vagus nerve in the domestic cat (Felis domestica). Proc. Am. Phil. Soc., Phila., 1882-3, xx, 123-138. — **Treviranus** (G.-R.) Sur le rapport mutuel des diverses parties du cerveau et du système nerveux dans les divers degrés de l'échelle animale. J. compl. du dict. d. sc. méd., Par., 1823, xv, 303-323.—**Van Beneden** (É.) & **Julin** (C.) Le système nerveux central des ascidies adultes et ses rapports avec celui des larves urodèles. Bull. Acad. roy. d. sc. de Belg., Brux., 1884, 3. s., viii, 13-72, 4 pl.—**Vialleton.** Les centres nerveux des céphalopodes. Compt. rend. Acad. d. sc., Par., 1885, ci, 1016-1018.—**Vigezzi** (D.) Sopra la disposizione anatomica dei nervi digitali nei solipedi, in rapporto alla nèvrectomia. Clin. vet., Milano, 1887, x, 207 - 222, 2 pl. — **Vignal** (W.) Structure du système nerveux des mollusques. Compt. rend. Acad. d. sc., Par., 1882, xcv, 249-251. ——. Note sur le développement des nerfs chez les embryons des mammifères. Compt. rend. Soc. de biol., Par., 1883, 7. s., iv, 139-145. ——-. Note sur l'accroissement en longueur des tubes nerveux chez les embryons et les jeunes mammifères. *Ibid.*, 165 167. — **Viti** (A.) Ricerche di morfologia comparata sopra il nervo depressore nell' uomo e negli altri mammiferi. [*Abstr. from a reprint of:* Proc. verb. Soc. toscana di sc. nat., 1883.] Biol. Centralbl., Erlang., 1884-5, iv, 310 - 312. *Also, transl.:* Arch. ital. de biol., Turin, 1884, v, 191 - 198. — **Vogt** (C.) Zur Neuro-

Nervous *system* (*Comparative anatomy and physiology of*).

logie von Python tigris. Arch. f Anat., Physiol. u. wissensch. Med., Berl., 1839, 39–58, 1 pl. — **Waldschmidt** (J.) Zur Anatomie des Nervensystems der Gymnophionen. Jenaische Ztschr. f. Naturw., Jena, 1886–7, n. F., xiii, 461–476, 2 pl. ———. Beitrag zur Anatomie des Zentralnervensystems und des Geruchsorgans von Polypterus bichir. Anat. Anz., Jena, 1887, ii, 308 – 322. — **Ward** (J.) Observations on the physiology of the nervous system of the crayfish (Astacus fluviatilis). Proc. Roy. Soc. Lond., 1879, xxviii, 379 – 383. — **Warren** (J. C.) A comparative view of the sensorial and nervous systems in man and animals. Med. Communicat. Mass. M. Soc., Bost., 1822, iii, 307–412. *Also*, Reprint. — **Wilder** (B. G.) Note on the actual (superficial) origin of the n. trigeminus in the domestic cat. Am. J. Neurol. & Psychiat., N. Y., 1882, i, 337.

Nervous *system* (*Development of*).

See, also, **Nerve** (*Optic*); **Nerves** (*Degeneration, etc., of*).

SIMON (J.) * Observations sur le perfectionnement du système nerveux cérébral après la naissance. 4°. *Paris*, 1820.

Anderson (J.) Sketch of the comparative anatomy of the nervous system; with remarks on its development in the human embryo. Lond. M. Gaz., 1836, xviii, 863 ; 906; 945; 973. — **Baillarger.** Mémoire sur le mode de formation des centres nerveux. Ann. méd.-psych., Par., 1843, ii, 343–357. *Also*, Reprint. — **Birdsall** (W. R.) The embryogeny of the sympathetic. Arch. Med., N. Y., 1879, i, 138–149. — **Bischoff** (T. L. W.) Ueber die erste Bildung des Centralnervensystems bei Säugethieren mit Berücksichtigung der kritischen Beleuchtung meiner Beobachtungen durch Herrn Dr. Reichert. Arch. f. Anat., Physiol. u. wissensch. Med., Berl., 1843, 252–275, 1 pl. — **Clark** (T. E.) Some points in regard to the development of the nervous system and vision. J. Psych. M., N. Y., 1870, iv, 481 – 502. — **Flechsig** (P.) Weiteres zur Zerlegung des centralen Nervensystems auf Grund der Entwickelung. Centralbl. f. d. med. Wissensch., Berl., 1875, xiii, 673–675. — **Goette** (A.) Ueber die Entwickelung des Central-Nervensystems der Teleostier. Arch. f. mikr. Anat., Bonn, 1878, xv, 139–199, 4 pl. — **Henneguy** (L.-F.) Développement du système nerveux, de la corde dorsale et du mésoderme chez la truite. Compt. rend. Soc. de biol., Par., 1882, 7. s., iv, 755–759. — **Hensen** (V.) Zur Entwickelung des Nervensystems. Arch. f. path. Anat.-, etc., Berl., 1864, xxx, 176 – 186, 1 pl. — **His** (W.) Ueber die Anfänge des peripherischen Nervensystemes. Arch. f. Anat. u. Entwcklngsgesch., Leipz., 1879, iii, 455–482, 2 pl. — **Leloir** (H.) Nerfs des végétations. Compt. rend. Soc. de biol. 1878, Par., 1880, 6. s., v, 228–230. — **Loewe** (L.) Beiträge zur vergleichenden Morphogenesis des centralen Nervensystems der Wirbelthiere. Mitth. a. d. embryol. Inst. d. k. k. Univ. in Wien, 1880, ii, 1. Hft., 1–9, 2 pl. — **Lubimoff** (A.) Embryologische und histogenetische Untersuchungen über das sympathische und centrale Cerebrospinal-Nervensystem. Arch. f. path. Anat., etc., Berl., 1874, lx, 217–273, 2 pl. — **Mann** (E. C.) General considerations on the development of the nervous system by evolution, and its condition in health and disease. St. Louis Cour. Med., 1882, vii, 118–129. — **Marshall** (A. M.) On the early stages of development of the nerves in birds. J. Anat. & Physiol., Lond., 1877, xi, 491–516, 2 pl. — **Meckel** (J. F.) Versuch einer Entwicklungsgeschichte der Centraltheile des Nervensystems in den Säugthieren. Deutsches Arch. f. d. Physiol., Halle, 1815, i, 1; 334; 589. — **Mondino** (C.) Sulla anatomia dell' antimuro e del nucleo amigdaleo nel cervello umano. R. Ist. Lomb. di sc. e lett. Rendic. Milano, 1885, xviii, 106. *Also :* Gazz. d. osp., Milano, 1885. vi, 140. ———. Sulla cariocinesi delle cellule nervose negli animali adulti consecutiva ad irritazione cerebrale. R. Ist. Lomb. di sc. e lett. Rendic., Milano, 1885, xviii, 107. *Also :* Gazz. d. osp., Milano, 1885, vi, 107. — **Muller** (J.) Sur la métamorphose du système nerveux dans le règne animal. J. compl. du dict. d. sc. méd., Par., 1829, xxxiii, 27–42. — **Onodi** (A. D.) Ueber die Entwickelung der Spinalganglien und der Nervenwurzeln. Internat. Monatschr. f. Anat. u. Histol., Berl., 1884, i, 204 ; 255. — **Pouchet** & **Tourneux.** Contribution à l'histoire du développement du système nerveux périphérique. Compt. rend. Soc. de biol. 1876, Par., 1877, 6. s., iii, 396–398. *Also :* Gaz. méd. de Par., 1877, 4. s., vi, 16. — **Romanes** (G. J.) Evolution of nerves and nervo-systems. Nature, Lond., 1877, xvi, 231; 269. *Also :* Notices Proc. Roy. Inst. Gr. Brit. 1875-8, Lond., 1879, viii, 427-448. — **Rouget** (C.) Mémoire sur le développement des nerfs chez les larves de batraciens. Arch. de physiol. norm. et path., Par., 1875, vii, 801–853, 6 pl. — **Schenk** (S. L.) Die Entwicklungsgeschichte der Ganglien und des Lobus electricus. I. Die Ganglien in der Entwicklung. II. Der Lobus electricus in der Entwicklung. Sitzungsb. d. k. Akad. d. Wissensch. Math.-naturw. Cl., Wien, 1876, lxxiv, 13–36. *Also,* Reprint. ———. Ueber die Entwickelung der Ganglien des Sympathicus. Allg. Wien. med. Ztg., 1879, xxiv,

Nervous *system* (*Development of*).

4.—**Schenk** (S. L.) & **Birdsall** (W. R.) Ueber die Lehre von der Entwickelung der Ganglien des Sympathicus. Mitth. a. d. embryol. Inst. d. k. k. Univ. in Wien, 1878, ii, 213–228, 3 pl. — **Schultze** (C.-A.-S.) Considérations sur les premières traces du système osseux et sur le développement de la colonne vertébrale dans les animaux. J. compl. du dict. d. sc. méd., Par., 1820, vi, 113–122. — **Unger** (L.) Untersuchungen über die Entwicklung der centralen Nervengewebe. Sitzungsb. d. k. Akad. d. Wissensch. Math.-naturw. Cl. 1879, Wien, 1880, lxxx, 3. Abth , 282–311, 2 pl. — **Vignal** (W.) Note sur le développement des nerfs chez les embryons des mammifères. Compt. rend. Soc. de biol., Par., 1883, 7. s., v, 139–145. *Also* [Abstr.] : Tribune méd., Par., 1883, xv, 116. ———. Accroissement en longueur des tubes nerveux, par la formation des segments intercalaires. Arch. de physiol. norm. et path., Par., 1883, 3. s., i, 536–548, 1 pl. ———. Mémoire sur le développement des tubes nerveux chez les embryons de mammifères. *Ibid.*, 1883, 3. s., i, 513–535, 2 pl. *Also :* École prat. d. hautes études. Lab. d'histol. du Coll. de France. Trav. 1883, Par., 1884, viii, 110–132, 2 pl. — **Virey** (J.-J.) Note historique sur l'origine primitive du système nerveux dans le règne animal. Gaz. méd. de Par., 1840, 2. s., viii, 517.

Nervous *system* (*Diseases of*).

See, also, **Anæsthesia**; **Apoplexy** (*General, etc., Treatises on*); **Asthma**; **Brain** (*Diseases of*); **Catalepsy**; **Children** (*Diseases of*); **Chorea**; **Convulsions**; **Diabetes** *insipidus*; **Ear**; **Epilepsy**; **Eye**; **Hydrophobia**; **Hyperæsthesia**; **Hypochondria**; **Hysteria**; **Hystero-epilepsy**; **Insanity**; **Joints** (*Neuralgia, etc., of*); **Larynx** (*Neuroses of*); **Metallotherapy**; **Nervous** *system* (*Pathology, etc., of*); **Neuralgia**; **Neuritis**; **Paralysis**; **Psychology** (*Medical, etc.*); **Skin** (*Diseases of, Neurotic*); **Sleep** (*Abnormal, etc.*); **Spasm**; **Spinal cord** (*Diseases of*); **Tetanus**; **Tetany**; **Vertigo.**

ABERCROMBIE (J.) Pathological and practical researches on the diseases of the brain and the spinal cord. 2. ed. 8°. *Edinburgh*, 1829.

———. The same. 3. ed. 12°. *Edinburgh*, 1834.

———. The same. 4. ed. 8°. *London*, 1845.

———. The same. 1. Am. from the 2. Edinb. ed. roy. 8°. *Philadelphia*, 1831.

———. The same. A new edition, enlarged by the author. 8°. *Philadelphia*, 1843.

ALTHAUS (J.) Diseases of the nervous system ; their prevalence and pathology. 8°. *London*, 1877.

ANDERSON (W. J.) The causes, symptoms, and treatment of eccentric nervous affections. 8°. *London*, 1850.

DE ANDRADE (N. F.) * Do diagnostico e tratamento das nevroses visceraes. 4°. *Rio de Janeiro*, 1875.

ARMSTRONG (V.) Practical hints and observations on head-aches and giddiness, paralytic-strokes, apoplexies, and sudden deaths, with advice on the best means of curing the former and of preventing the latter. 8°. *London*, 1819.

ARNOLD (A. B.) Manual of nervous diseases and an introduction to medical electricity. 8°. *New York*, 1885.

AXENFELD (A.) Des névroses. 8°. *Paris*, 1864.

Extract from : REQUIN (A.-P.) Pathologie médicale. 8°. *Paris*, 1863, iv, 125-695.

———. The same. Traité des névroses. 2. éd., augmentée de 700 pages. 8°. *Paris*, 1883.

BARADUC (H. -A. - P.) Études théorique et pratique des affections nerveuses, considérées sous le rapport des modifications qu'opèrent sur elles la lumière et la chaleur ; théorie de l'inflammation ; des ventouses vésicantes. 8°. *Paris*, 1850.

BAUDUY (J. K.) Lectures on diseases of the nervous system. 8°. *Philadelphia*, 1876.

BAYNE *alias* KINNEIR (D.) A new essay on the nerves and the doctrine of the animal spirits

Nervous *system (Diseases of).*

rationally considered; shewing the great benefit of and true use of bathing, and drinking the Bath waters, in all nervous disorders and obstructions, with two dissertations on the gout and on digestion, with the distemper of the stomach and intestines. 8°. *London,* 1738.

BEARD (G. M.) Representative cases of nervous disease. 8°. [*n. p., n. d.*]

DE BISCOP (P. C. A.) * De morbis nervorum. 1767.

In: LOUVAIN Diss. 8°. *Lovanii,* 1795, i, 100–112.

BOERHAAVE (H.) Prælectiones academicæ de morbis nervorum quas ex auditorum manuscriptis collectas edi curavit Jacobus van Eems. 2 v. 16°. *Lugd. Bat.,* 1761.

————. The same. 2 v. 8°. *Francofurti et Lipsiæ,* 1762.

————. The same. 2 v. 4°. *Venetiis,* 1763.

BOUILLON-LAGRANGE. * Réflections sur les affections nerveuses et sur quelques médicamens usités dans ces sortes de maladies. 4°. *Strasbourg,* 1805.

BOULENGER (C. J.) * De præcipuis affectionibus nervosis. 1794.

In: LOUVAIN Diss. 8°. *Lovanii,* 1796, iv, 427–444.

BOURNEVILLE. Recherches cliniques et thérapeutiques sur l'épilepsie, l'hystérie et l'idiotie. 8°. *Paris,* 1885.

BOURNEVILLE & REGNARD (P.) Iconographie photographique de la Salpêtrière; service de M. Charcot. 4°. *Paris,* 1877.

BRENSCHEDT (C.) * Observationes clinicæ circa morbos nervorum. 8°. *Berolini,* [1847].

BRIGHAM (A.) An inquiry concerning the diseases and functions of the brain, the spinal cord, and the nerves. 8°. *New York,* 1840.

BRODIE (B. C.) Lectures illustrative of certain local nervous affections. 8°. *London,* 1837.

————. The same. Vorlesungen über örtliche Nervenleiden. Aus dem Englischen von Dr. Kürschner. 8°. *Marburg,* 1838.

BROWN-SÉQUARD (C. E.) Lecciones sobre los nervios vaso-motores, la epilepsia y las acciones reflejas normales y morbosas. Traducidas del inglés por el Dr. Beni-Barde; version española por Federico Toledo y Cueva. 12°. *Madrid,* 1878.

A selection from various works of Brown-Séquard.

BRUCKMANN (F. H.) * Diss. exhibens de morbis nervorum observationes quasdam singulares cum epicrisi. sm. 4°. *Gottingæ,* [1780].

CANZ (T. E. F.) * De morbis neuricis, præsertim ea specie, quæ ex infarctibus abdominalibus exoritur. sm. 4°. *Tubingæ,* [1791].

CASSEL (F. P.) * Diss. sistens cogitata circa originem et formam morborum systematis nervosi. 4°. *Parisiis, an. XIV* [1805].

CASTAN (A.) Essai sur la pathogénie des maladies nerveuses. 8°. *Montpellier,* 1859.

CASTRÉN (M. A.) * De pathologica systematis nervorum gangliosi dignitate. 8°. *Helsingfors,* [1833].

CAZENAVE (P.-L.-A.) * Quels sont les caractères des névroses? 4°. *Paris,* 1835.

CERISE (L.-A.-P.) Des fonctions et des maladies nerveuses.

In his: Œuvres. 8°. *Paris,* 1872, i.

CHARCOT (J.-M.) Leçons sur les maladies du système nerveux faites à la Salpêtrière. Recueillies et publiées par Bonneville. 8°. *Paris,* 1872–3.

————. The same. 2. s. 8°. *Paris,* 1873.

————. The same. Transl. by George Sigerson. 8°. *London,* 1877.

————. The same. Recueillies et publiées par MM. Babinski, Bernard, Féré, Guinon, Marie et Gilles de la Tourette. 8°. *Paris,* 1887.

Nervous *system (Diseases of).*

————. The same. 2. s. Transl. and edited by George Sigerson. 2 v. 8°. *London,* 1877–81.

————. Œuvres complètes. Leçons sur les localisations dans les maladies du cerveau et de la moelle épinière, recueillies par Bourneville et E. Brissaud. Tome iv. 8°. *Paris,* 1887.

CHEYNE (G.) The English malady; or, a treatise of nervous diseases of all kinds, as spleen, vapours, lowness of spirits, hypochondriacal and hysterical distempers, etc. In three parts. Pt. I. Of the nature and cause of nervous distempers. Pt. II. Of the cure of nervous distempers. Pt. III. Variety of cases that illustrate and confirm the method of cure. With the author's own case at large. 8°. *London,* 1733.

COMPARETTI (A.) De vaga ægritudine infirmitatis nervorum. 8°. *Venetiis,* 1780.

COOKE (J.) A treatise on nervous diseases. 2 v. v. 1. On apoplexy, including apolexia hydrocephalica, or water in the head; with an introductory account of the opinions of ancient and modern physiologists respecting the nature and uses of the nervous system. Read at the college, as the Croonian lectures of the year 1819. v. 2. On palsy and on epilepsy. 8°. *London,* 1820–23.

————. A treatise on nervous diseases. 8°. *Boston,* 1824.

CRONIN. A treatise on the nature and treatment of painful affections of the nerves, viz: tic douloureux, nervous headache, painful enlargement of the breast (which is often mistaken for cancer); nervous affections of the heart, nervous pain affecting the womb during pregnancy (generally the cause of miscarriage) and inflammation of the sciatic nerve; with cases. 12°. *Liverpool,* 1841.

CULLERRE (A.) Nervosisme et névroses. Hygiène des énervés et des névropathes. 12°. *Paris,* 1887.

DAVIDS (T.) * De neurosibus nervinis non curandis. 8°. *Lugd. Bat.,* 1830.

DAWSON (R.) A few observations on nervous affections, the result of an extensive experience in the treatment of nervous disorders, with some remarks on the use and abuse of hydropathy. 8°. *London,* 1851.

DELUEN (L.-J.-M.) * Quelques réflexions et propositions sur les maladies nerveuses convulsives et mentales. 4°. *Paris,* 1840.

DESCOT (P.-J.) * Dissertation sur les affections locales des nerfs. 4°. *Paris,* 1822.

————. The same. Avec des additions. [1825.] 8°. *Paris,* 1825.

DISEASES (On) of the spine and of the nerves. By C. B. Radcliffe, J. N. Radcliffe, J. W. Begbie, F. E. Ainstie [Anstie], and J. R. Reynolds. 8°. *Philadelphia,* 1871.

DOCHMANN (A. M.) Nasledstvennoste v nernych boliezniach. [Heredity of nervous diseases.] 18°. *Kazan,* 1887.

DOMAŃSKI (S.) Wykłady o chorobach układu nerwowego. [Diseases of the nervous system.] 8°. *Kraków,* 1881.

DOWSE (T. S.) The brain and the nerves; their ailments and their exhaustion. 8°. *New York,* 1884.

DRUMMOND (D.) Diseases of the brain and spinal cord; a guide to their pathology, diagnosis and treatment, with an anatomical and physiological introduction. 8°. *London,* 1883.

DUPAU (J.-A.) De l'éréthisme nerveux, ou analyse des affections nerveuses. 8°. *Montpellier,* 1819.

DYRENFURTH (M.) * De spasmis quibusdam nervorum facialis, vagi et glossopharyngei. 8°. *Berolini,* [1848].

Nervous *system* (*Diseases of*).

D'ENGELBRONNER (J.) * Observationes medico practicæ, ad morbos encephali et medullæ spinalis pertinentes. 8°. *Traj. ad Rhenum*, 1838.

ERB (W. H.) Krankheiten der peripheren-cerebrospinalen Nerven. 8°. *Leipzig*, 1874.
Forms 1. Theil, xii. Bd., of: Handb. d. spec. Path. (Ziemssen).

——. The same. 2. Aufl. 8°. *Leipzig*, 1876.

——. The same. Diseases of the peripheral cerebro-spinal nerves. 8°. *New York*, 1876.
Forms v. 11 of: Cycl. Pract. M. (Ziemssen).

ERLENMEYER (A. A.) Bericht über die Fortschritte im Gebiete der Krankheiten des Nervensystems während des Jahres 1854. 8°. *Neuwied*, [1855].

EULENBERG (A.) Lehrbuch der Nervenkrankheiten. 2. Aufl. 2 v. 8°. *Berlin*, 1878.

FERGUSON (E. J.) Observations on the nervous system, and the neuroses; being the subject of a course of lectures. 8°. [*Buffalo*, 1843.]

FINKELSTEIN (L.) * Materialy k voprosu o razstroistvach v sphere organov vneshnich chuvstve pri nekotorych zabolevanijach nervnoi sistemy i poljach zrenija pri menstruatsii. [On disorders of sphere of external organs of senses in some diseases of the nervous system and field of vision in menstruation.] 8°. *St. Petersburg*, 1887.

FOURCADE - PRUNET (J.-G.) Maladies nerveuses des auteurs; rapportées à l'irritation de l'encéphale, des nerfs cérébro-rachidiens et splanchniques, avec ou sans inflammation. 8°. *Paris*, 1826.

FRANK (J.) Die Nervenkrankheiten.
In his: Grundsätze d. gesammt. prakt. Heilk. 8°. *Leipzig*, 1832–43, Th. 6–9.

GALEN (C.) Liber de palpitatione, tremore, rigore, convulsione. Interp. N. Lavachio. 8°. *Venetiis*, 1536.

GÉLINEAU (E.) Des névroses spasmodiques, de leur origine, de leurs rapports et de leur traitement. 8°. *Paris*, 1879.

GEORGET (É.-J.) De la physiologie du système nerveux et spécialement du cerveau. 2 v. 8°. *Paris*, 1821.

GERMANY. *Kriegsministerium*. Traumatische, idiopathische und nach Infektionskrankheiten beobachtete Erkrankungen des Nervensystems bei den deutschen Heeren im Kriege gegen Frankreich 1870–71. 4°. *Berlin*, 1885.

GIROLAMI (G.) Intorno alle lezioni sulle malattie nervose del professore F. Puccinotti, brevi cenni. 8°. *Bologna*, 1838.

GOODLAD (W.) A letter to Sir B. C. Brodie . . . containing a critical inquiry into his lectures illustrative of certain local nervous affections. 8°. *London*, 1840.

GOURDON (V.-P.) * Considérations physiologiques et pathologiques sur les deux ordres de nerfs, sur la cause principale des affections dites nerveuses, et sur les moyens thérapeutiques propres à combattre ces maladies avec le plus de succès. 8°. *Paris*, 1837.

GOWERS (W. R.) A manual of diseases of the nervous system. 2 v. 8°. *London*, 1886–8.

——. The same. v. 1. 8°. *Philadelphia*, 1886.

GRANVILLE (J. M.) Nerves and nerve-troubles. 12°. *London*, 1884.

GRASSET (J.) Maladies du système nerveux. 8°. *Montpellier*, 1878.

——. The same. 2 v. 8°. *Montpellier*, 1879.

——. The same. Traité pratique des maladies du système nerveux. 2. éd. 8°. *Montpellier*, 1881.

——. The same. 3. éd. Suivie d'un appendice sur l'électrothérapie en général par le Dr. Regimbeau. 8°. *Montpellier*, 1886.

Nervous *system* (*Diseases of*).

GUIBOUT (E.) * Considérations sur la nature et le traitement de quelques affections nerveuses. 4°. *Paris*, 1850.

VAN DER HAAR (J.) Proeve over de herzenen en zenuwen, en eenige derzelver ziekten. Waar agter honderd en vijftig genees- en heelkundige waarneemigen. 8°. *Amsterdam*, 1788.

HALL (M.) Lectures on the nervous system and its diseases. 8°. *London*, 1836.

——. On the diseases and derangements of the nervous system, in their primary forms and in their modifications, by age, sex, constitution, hereditary predispositions, excesses, general disorder, and organic disease. 8°. *London*, 1841.

——. The same. Von den Krankheiten des Nervensystems. Aus dem Englischen. Mit einigen kritischen Bemerkungen von J. Wallach. 8°. *Leipzig*, 1842.

——. Synopsis of cerebral and spinal seizures of inorganic origin and of paroxysmal form as a class; and of their pathology as involved in the structures and actions of the neck. [2. ed.] 4°. *London*, [1851].

——. Essays chiefly on the theory of paroxysmal diseases of the nervous system. 8°. *London*, [n. d.]

HAMILTON (A. McL.) Nervous diseases; their description and treatment. 8°. *Philadelphia*, 1878.

HAMMOND (W. A.) A treatise on diseases of the nervous system. 8°. *New York*, 1871.

——. The same. 7. ed. roy. 8°. *New York*, 1881.

——. The same. 8. ed. 8°. *New York*, 1886.
Also [Rev. of 6. ed.], in: Brit. & For. M.-Chir. Rev., Lond., 1877, lix, 306–325.

——. Clinical lectures on diseases of the nervous system. Reported, edited, and the histories of the cases prepared, with notes by T. M. B. Cross. 8°. *New York*, 1874.

HANDBUCH der Krankheiten des Nervensystems. Von H. Nothnagel, F. Obernier, O. Heubner, G. Huguenin, E. Hitzig, Wilhelm Erb, A. Eulenburg, J. Bauer, H. v. Ziemssen, F. Jolly, Adolf Kussmaul.
In: HANDB. d. spec. Path. (Ziemssen), 11. Bd., Hlft. 1 & 2; 12. Bd., Hlft. 1 & 2. Mit Anhang zu Bd. 12, 1874–8.

HART (C. P.) Diseases of the nervous system; being a treatise on spasmodic, paralytic, neuralgic, and mental affections. 8°. *New York & Philadelphia*, 1881.

HASSE (K. E.) Krankheiten des Nervenapparates.
In: HANDB. d. spec. Path. u. Therap. (Virchow), Erlang. u. Stuttg., 1855, iv, 1. Abth., vi, 686.

——. The same. Krankheiten des Nervensystems. Zweite vermehrte und verbesserte. Aufl. 8°. *Erlangen*, 1869.

HEINEKEN (J.) De morbis nervorum eorumque frequentissima ex abdomine origine. 4°. *Gottingæ*, 1783.
Also, in: SCRIPT. neurol. minores selecti. 4°. *Lipsiæ*, 1792, ii, 291–322.

HELLER (K.) Specielle Pathologie und Therapie der Krankheiten der peripheren Nerven. 8°. *Wien*, 1879.

HERGENRÖTHER (J. J.) Character, Form, Wesenheit, Ursachen und Behandlungsweise der Nervenkrankheiten im Allgemeinen als Programm bei Eröffnung seiner im Sommersemester 1825 publice abzuhaltenden Vorlesungen über psychische Heilwissenschaft. 8°. *Würzburg*, 1825.

HUEBNER (J. A.) * De nervorum morbis generatim. 8°. *Berolini*, [1819].

JACCOUD (S.) Études de pathogénie et de sémiotique. Les paraplégies et l'ataxie du mouvement. 8°. *Paris*, 1864.

Nervous *system* (*Diseases of*).

KLEIN (S. A.) * De topicis nervorum affectionibus. 8°. *Monachii*, 1831.

KLETTEN (G. E.) [Pr.] de constitutione morborum nervosa. Comment. i–xii. 4°. *Vitebergæ*, 1811–15.

VON KRAFFT-EBING (R.) Ueber Nervosität. 3. Aufl. 8°. *Graz*, 1884.

———. The same. Sovremennaja nervoznost. Perevod s tret. Nemetsk. izd. M. Manasseina. Pod redaktsiei S. Danillo. [Disease of the nervous system. Transl. from the 3. German ed., by Manassein, under the editorship of Danillo.] 12°. *St. Petersburg*, 1885.

———. Ueber gesunde und kranke Nerven. 8°. *Tübingen*, [1885].

———. The same. Om friska och sjuka nerver. Öfversättning af O. H. Dumrath. [On healthy and sick nerves.] 12°. *Stockholm*, [1885].

KÜHN (J. G.) Praktische Abhandlung einiger das Nerven-System betreffenden Krankheiten. 8°. *Breslau*, 1786.

LA LOGGIA (G.) Sulle nevrosi in generale. Trattato fisico-patologico. 8°. *Palermo*, 1876.

LANDRY (J.-B.-O.) * Considérations générales sur la pathogénie et les indications curatives des maladies nerveuses. 4°. *Paris*, 1854.

LANDRY (O.) Recherches sur les causes et les indications curatives des maladies nerveuses. 8°. *Paris*, 1855.

LAUER (G. A.) Der vorherrschende Charakter der Krankheiten der jetzigen Generation. 8°. *Berlin*, 1862.

LEHMANN (L.) Die chronischen Neurosen als klinische Objekte in Oeynhausen (Rehme). 8°. *Bonn*, 1880.

LEUBUSCHER (R.) Die Krankheiten des Nervensystems. 8°. *Leipzig*, 1860.

———. The same. De ziekten van het zenuwstelsel. Uit het Hoogduitsch vertaald door J. B. Dompeling. Met eene voorrede van J. L. C. Schroeder van der Kolk. 8°. *Amsterdam*, 1862.

LIONSKY (B.) Kratkii kurs nervnych i dushevnych bolieznei. [Short treatise on nervous diseases and insanity.] 8°. *St. Petersburg*, 1887.

LOBB (H. W.) On some of the more obscure forms of nervous affections; their pathology and treatment. With an introduction on the physiology of digestion and assimilation, and the generation and distribution of nerve force, based upon original microscopical observations. 8°. *London*, 1858.

LUYS (J.-B.) Leçons sur la structure et les maladies du système nerveux, recueillies par J. Dave. 8°. *Paris*, 1875.

MARSHALL (J.) Practical observations on diseases of the heart, lungs, stomach, liver, etc., occasioned by spinal irritation; and on the nervous system in general as a source of organic disease. Illustrated by cases. 8°. *London*, 1835.

———. The same. 8°. *Philadelphia*, 1837.

MARTINOTTI (G.) Sulle degenerazioni sistematiche del midollo spinale secondarie a lesioni della corteccia cerebrale. 8°. *Milano*, 1885.

MOHR (G. F.) * De machinæ humanæ vitiis eorumque causis dignoscendis atque emendandis. sm. 4°. *Tubingæ*, 1725.

MOHR (J. M.) * Diss. pertractans miros nervorum morbos dæmoni subinde attributos, quam una cum adnexis corollariis ex omni parte medicinæ desumptis [etc.] 4°. [*Herbipoli*, 1768.]

MOTET (A.) Névroses. 8°. *Paris*, 1866.
Cutting from: Guide du méd. praticien, Valleix, 5. éd., Par., 1866, i, 641–686.

Nervous *system* (*Diseases of*).

MÜLLER (O.) Bericht über die Heilanstalt für Nervenkranke bei Blankenburg am Harz, von den Jahren 1866–72 (1.–3.). 8°. *Braunschweig*, 1867–72.

MUSSET (H.-J.-M.-H.) Traité des maladies nerveuses ou névroses, et en particulier de la paralysie et de ses variétés, de l'hémiplégie, de la paraplégie, de la chorée ou danse de Saint-Guy, de l'épilepsie, de l'hystérie, des névralgies internes et externes, de la gastralgie, etc. 8°. *Paris*, 1840.

NEALE. Practical dissertations on nervous complaints and other diseases incident to the human body; with an historical investigation of their causes and cure, in which are interspersed some singular cases. 8°. *London*, 1788.

———. The same. Practische Abhandlung über die Nervenkrankheiten. Aus dem Englischen übersetzt. 16°. *Berlin*, 1790.

NIERMEYER (J. H. A.) * Neuropathologische onderzoekingen. 8°. *Leiden*, 1879.

NOLIN (J.-É.) * Dissertation sur quelques maladies des nerfs. 4°. *Paris*, 1818.

PATAUD (G.) Analyse pour servir d'introduction à l'ouvrage sur les affections nerveuses. 8°. *Clermont-Ferrand, an VIII* [1800].

PELECHIN (P.) * De neurosibus in genere. 8°. *Edinburgi*, 1829.

PIERSON (R. H.) Compendium der Krankheiten des Nervensystems. 8°. *Leipzig*, 1876.

PRESSAVIN. Neue und gründliche Abhandlung von den Nerven-Krankheiten und den Dünsten oder sogenannten Vapeurs, worinnen zugleich die rechte Art dieselben zu heilen, gelehret wird. Aus dem Französischen ins Deutsche übersetzt. 12°. *Nürnberg*, 1772.

PRICHARD (J. C.) A treatise on diseases of the nervous system. Part the first: Comprising convulsive and maniacal affections. 8°. *London*, 1822.

RADCLIFFE (C. B.) Epilepsy and other affections of the nervous system which are marked by tremor, convulsion, or spasm; their pathology and treatment. 8°. *London*, 1854.

———. Lectures on epilepsy, pain, paralysis, and certain other disorders of the nervous system. 8°. *London*, 1864.

RAMOS MEJIA (J. M.) Las neurosis de los hombres célebres en la historia argentina, precedido de una introduccion por el Dr. Vicente Fidel Lopez. Primera parte. Rosas y su época. 8°. *Buenos Aires*, 1878.

REID (J.) Essays on hypochondriacal and other nervous affections. 8°. *Philadelphia*, 1817.

RENNIE (A.) A treatise on gout, apoplexy, paralysis, and disorders of the nervous system. [Pt. i.] 8°. *London*, 1828.

REY (L.-M.) * Sur la pathogénie de quelques affections de l'axe cérébro-spinal, etc.; choix d'observations prises dans l'Hôpital de Bordeaux. 4°. *Paris*, 1834.

RIADORE (J. E.) Introductory lectures to a course on nervous irritation, spinal affections, distortions of the limbs, malformations of the chest, etc. 12°. *London*, 1835.

RICHARDS (T.) A treatise on nervous disorders; including observations on dietetics and medicinal remedies. 8°. *London*, 1829.

DE LA ROCHE. Zergliederung der Verrichtung des Nervensystems als Einleitung zu einer praktischen Untersuchung der Nervenkrankheiten. Uebersetzt von J. F. A. Merzdorff. 2 v. in 1. 8°. *Halle*, 1794–5.

ROMBERG (M. H.) Lehrbuch der Nervenkrankheiten des Menschen. 1. Bd. 8°. *Berlin*, 1846.

———. The same. 2 v. 8°. *Berlin*, 1853–7.

Nervous *system* (*Diseases of*).

———. The same. A manual of the nervous diseases of man. Transl. and edited by E. H. Sieveking. 2 v. 8°. *London*, 1853.

ROSENTHAL (M.) Handbuch der Diagnostik und Therapie der Nervenkrankheiten. roy. 8°. *Erlangen*, 1870.

———. Klinik der Nervenkrankheiten nach seinen an der Wiener Universität gehaltenen Vorträgen. 8°. *Stuttgart*, 1875.

———. The same. A clinical treatise on the diseases of the nervous system. With a preface by Professor Charcot. Transl. from the author's revised and enlarged edition by L. Putzel. 2 v. 8°. *New York*, 1879.

ROSS (J.) A treatise on the diseases of the nervous system. 2 v. 8°. *London*, 1881.

———. The same. Rukovodstvo k izuchenijou bolieznei nervoi sistemi. Perevod s angliiskago izdanija s primiechanijami M. M. Manaseinoi. 8°. *St. Petersburg*, 1882.

———. The same. Handbook of the diseases of the nervous system. 8°. *Philadelphia*, 1885.
Text somewhat condensed, and contains fewer illustrations.

ROYER (M.) * Essai sur la nature et le traitement des névroses en général. 4°. *Paris*, 1851.

RÜDIGER (F. C.) * De natura et medela morborum nevricorum generatim spectatis. sm. 4°. *Tubingæ*, [1806].
Also, in: WEBER. Samml. med.-prakt. Diss. [etc.] 8°. *Tübingen*, 1820, i, 2. St., 1–62.

SAILLARD DE RAVETON. Études médico-philosophiques sur les maladies nerveuses; considérations générales sur leurs causes, et leur traitement. 8°. *Paris*, 1850.

SANDRAS (C.-M.-S.) Traité pratique des maladies nerveuses. 2 v. 8°. *Paris*, 1851.

——— & BOURGUIGNON (H.) Traité pratique des maladies nerveuses. 2. éd. 2 v. 8°. *Paris*, 1860–62.

SCHMIDT (T.) Compendium der Nervenkrankheiten. sm. 8°. *Leipzig*, 1869.

SEELIGMÜLLER (A.) Lehrbuch der Krankheiten der peripheren Nerven und des Sympatheticus, für Aerzte und Studirende. 8°. *Braunschweig*, 1882.

———. The same. 8°. *Braunschweig*, 1887.

———. The same. Uchebnik bolieznei nervnoi sistemi. Otliel I. Boliezni perifericheskoi nervnoi sistemi i simpaticheskago nerva. Perevod s Niemtskago A. Cheremshanskago. 8°. *St. Petersburg*, 1882.

SEGUIN (E. C.) Opera minora. A collection of essays, articles, lectures, and addresses from 1866 to 1882, inclusive. 8°. *New York*, 1884.

SIKORSKI (I. A.) Zadachi nervno-psichicheskoi gigieny i prophylaktiki. [Problems of nervo-psychical hygiene and prophylaxis.] 8°. *Kieff*, 1887.

SMALL (A. E.) Diseases of the nervous system. To which is added, a treatise on the diseases of the skin. By C. E. Toothaker. 8°. *Philadelphia*, 1856.

STEVENSON (J.) A familiar treatise on nervous affections, disorders of the head and chest, stomach and bowels, etc. Also, on the means of repairing a debilitated constitution through the establishment of a healthy digestion; including prescriptions in plain English from the writings and private practice of eminent physicians. 2. ed. 16°. *London*, 1828.

STEWART (T. G.) An introduction to the study of the diseases of the nervous system; being lectures delivered in the University of Edinburgh during the tercentenary year. 8°. *Edinburgh*, 1884.

Nervous *system* (*Diseases of*).

STRÜMPELL (A.) Lehrbuch der speciellen Pathologie und Therapie der inneren Krankheiten. 2. Bd. 1. Theil. Krankheiten des Nervensystems. 8°. *Leipzig*, 1884.

STUNZER (J. K.) Ueber das Betragen in Nervenkrankheiten für Unerfahrne in der Arzneiwissenschaft. 8°. *Wien*, 1781.

SWAN (J.) Observations on some points relating to the anatomy, physiology, and pathology of the nervous system. 8°. *London*, 1822.

———. A treatise on diseases and injuries of the nerves. A new ed. 8°. *London*, 1834.

TAKAHASHI MASADZUMI. Shinkeibio Ron. [A treatise on nervous disease.] 8°. *Osaka*, 1878.

THOMSON (A.) An enquiry into the nature, causes, and method of cure of nervous disorders. 8°. *London*, 1781.

THRENMANN (C. G. A.) *Cogitata quædam de mentis nervorumque morbis. 8°. *Halis Sax.*, [1806].

TODD (R. B.) Clinical lectures on paralysis, certain diseases of the brain, and other affections of the nervous system. 2. ed. 8°. *London*, 1856.

TURNBULL (A.) A treatise on painful and nervous diseases, and on a new mode of treatment for diseases of the eye and ear. 3. ed. 8°. *London*, 1837.

ULO (J.-T.) * Essai sur les maladies nerveuses et vaporeuses. 4°. *Montpellier*, 1817.

UVEDALE (C.) The construction of the nerves, and the causes of nervous disorders practically explained. 8°. *London*, 1758.

VALENTIN (G.) Versuch einer physiologischen Pathologie der Nerven. 1. Bd. in 2 Abth. 8°. *Leipzig u. Heidelberg*, 1864.

VOGT (P. F. W.) Ueber die Erweichung des Gehirns und des Rückenmarks. 8°. *Heidelberg u. Leipzig*, 1840.

VOLKENAN (J.) *Spec. med. sistens bigam observationum de morbis nervorum. 12°. *Dorpati*, 1814.

VULPIAN (A.) Maladies du système nerveux; leçons professées à la Faculté de médecine. Recueillies et publiées par M. le Dr. Bourceret. Maladies de la moelle. 8°. *Paris*, 1879.

WALKER (S.) A treatise on nervous diseases, in which are introduced some observations on the structure and functions of the nervous system, and such an investigation of the symptoms and causes of these diseases as may lead to a rational and successful method of cure. 8°. *London*, 1796.

WEBBER (S. G.) A treatise on nervous diseases; their symptoms and treatment. 8°. *New York*, 1885.

WEISSMANN (R.) sen. Ueber Nervenkrankheiten und Schlagfluss (Apoplexie, •Hirnlähmung), Vorbeugung und Heilung. 14. Aufl. 16°. *Vilshofen*, 1887.

WILHELM (H.) Bericht über die in der Polyklinik vorgekommenen Nervenkrankheiten; als Compendium der Nervenkrankheiten u. Elektrotherapie. 8°. *Pest*, 1873.

WILKS (S.) Lectures on diseases of the nervous system, delivered at Guy's Hospital. 8°. *London*, 1878.
See, also, infra.

WILLIS (T.) Pathologiæ cerebri et nervosi generis specimen. In quo agitur de morbis convulsivis et de scorbuto. 4°. *Genevæ*, 1576.

———. The same. 16°. *Amstelodami*, 1668.
———. The same. 24°. *Amstelodami*, 1670.
———. The same. 4°. *Genevæ*, 1676.
In his: Opera omnia. 4°. *Genevæ*, 1676.

———. The same. 4°. *Genevæ*, 1696.
In his: Opera omnia. 4°. *Genevæ*, 1695, i.

Nervous *system* (*Diseases of*).

———. The same. An essay on the pathology of the brain and nervous stock, in which convulsive diseases are treated of. Transl. out of Latine into English by S. Pordage. fol. *London*, 1681.

WILSON (J. A.) On spasm, langour, palsy, and other disorders, termed nervous, of the muscular system. 8°. *London*, 1843.

WITTMAACK (T.) Lehrbuch der Nervenkraukenheiten. 1. Bd. 1. Abth. 8°. *Leipzig*, 1861.

WOOD (H. C.) Nervous diseases and their diagnosis; a treatise upon the phenomena produced by diseases of the nervous system, with especial reference to the recognition of their causes. 8°. *Philadelphia*, 1887.

WUCHER (C.) Krankheits-Geschichten aus dem Bereiche des Nerven-Systems. 8°. *München*, 1869.

ZIROTTI (G. B.) * Sopra la natura e l' origine delle malattie nervose. 4°. *Sondrio*, 1786.

Adelmann (G. F. B.) Krankheiten des Nervensystems. Ztschr. f. klin. Med., Bresl., 1859, x, 270–274.—**Agar** (S. W.) Some social questions in connection with nervous disease. Birmingh. M. Rev., 1886, xx, 1–21. *Also* [Abstr.]: Brit. M. J., Lond., 1886, ii, 247.—**Althaus** (J.) On the prevalence and fatality of nervous diseases. Med. Times & Gaz., Lond., 1876, ii, 537; 566; 595; 619; 647; 673; 697. *Also* [Abstr.]: Proc. Roy. M. & Chir. Soc. Lond. (1875–80), 1880, viii, 39–44. ———. Lectures on diseases of the nervous system. Med. Exam., Lond., 1877, ii, 668; 689; 711; 761; 781; 805; 822; 856; 878; 903; 924; 950; 977; 998: 1878, iii, 70; 93; 112; 177.—**Amard** (L.-V.-F.) Maladies nerveuses. *In his:* Ass. intellectuelle, 8°, Par., 1821, ii, 311–572.—**Andral.** Lectures on diseases of the brain and nervous system. Lancet, Lond., 1835–6, ii, 1; 33; 65; 97.—**Anjel.** Beitrag zur Casuistik einiger Nervenkrankheiten. Berl. klin. Wchnschr., 1877, xiv, 129-132.—**Anstie** (F. E.) Lectures on diseases of the nervous system. Lancet, Lond., 1872, ii, 515; 589; 661; 732; 839: 1873, i, 39; 123; 227; 437; 655.—**Arloing** (S.) Dégénération et centre trophique des nerfs; examen critique des opinions émises sur leur nature; applications. Lyon méd., 1886, liii, 475–479.—**Audiffrent.** Des maladies de l'activité. Tribune méd., Par., 1880, xiii, 607; 615.—**Barbier** (J.-B.-G.) Considérations générales sur les névroses. Gaz. méd. de Par., 1852, 3. s., vii, 560; 601. *Also:* Scalpel, Liége, 1852-3, v, 66; 76; 86; 101.—**Barbieri** (A.) Alcune infiammazioni dell' asse cerebrospinale. Gazz. med. ital. lomb., Milano, 1848, 2. s., i, 74; 98.—**Bartholow** (R.) Cases of disease of the nervous system, with commentary. Tr. Ohio M. Soc., Dayton, 1873, xxviii, 191–225. *Also:* Clinic, Cincin., 1873, iv, 301: v, 1; 37.—**Beale** (L. S.) Lectures on the disorders of the nervous system. Med. Exam., Lond., 1878, iii, 524; 547: iv, 20; 36; 93; 109.—**Begbie** (J. W.) Local paralysis from nerve-disease. Syst. Med. (Reynolds), Lond., 1868, ii, 754.—**Bell** (C.) Cases of affections of the nerves, with clinical remarks. Lond. M. Gaz., 1828-9, iii, 337–344. ———. Clinical lecture on diseases of the nerves of the head. *Ibid.*, 1833-4, xiii, 697–702.—**Benedikt.** Zwei Fälle von Neurosen. Wien. med. Presse, 1870, xi, 937. ———. Zur Kasuistik der Nervenkrankheiten. *Ibid.*, 1871, xii, 799–801. ———. Ueber Entzündung des Central-Nervensystems. Allg. Wien. med. Ztg., 1873, xviii, 577; 585; 595. ———. Entzündung des Central-Nervensystems. Die Eiterungsfrage. Mitth. d. Wien. med. Doct.-Coll., 1874–5, i, 45–47. ———. Ueber einige Grundformeln des neuropathologischen Denkens. Wien. med. Bl., 1885, viii, 298–300.—**Bennett** (A. H.) Clinical lectures on nervous diseases. Brit. M. J., Lond., 1878, ii, 759: 1879, i, 379; 419; 846: 1880, i, 46; 161; 235: 1881, i, 261.—**Bennett** (J. H.) Diseases of the nervous system. Syst. Pract. M. (Tweedie), Phila., 1840, ii, 13–26.—**Bernhardt** (M.) Ueber eine weniger bekannte Neurose der Extremitäten, besonders der oberen. Centralbl. f. Nervenh., Leipz., 1886, ix, 33–45.—**Bertini** (C. B.) Caso di malattia nervosa. Gior. d. sc. med., Torino, 1839, iv, 443–448.—**Blackmore** (E.) Observations on the nature and treatment of the more important diseases of the nervous system; with illustrative cases. Lond. M. Gaz., 1845, n. s., i, 567; 596; 631; 671; 699; 723; 760; 789; 822; 855; 917; 954.—**Bouillaud.** Des maladies des centres nerveux en général. Gaz. d. hôp., Par., 1859, xxxii, 321.—**Boyd** (R.) Diseases of the nervous system. J. Psych. M., Lond., 1875, n. s., i, 222: 1876, n. s., ii, 70: 1877, n. s., iii, 93: 1878, n. s., iv. 82.—**Braun** (K.) Riech o razprostvanenii mozgovich i drugich bolieznjach nervov v sovremennom obshestvie. [On the prevalence of cerebral and other nervous affections.] Sovrem. med., Warszawa, 1880, xxi, 277; 291.—**Broadbent** (W. H.) Cases of disease of the nervous system, with clinical observations. Med Times

Nervous *system* (*Diseases of*).

& Gaz., Lond., 1872, ii, 63–66.—**Brochin.** Nerveuses (Maladies). Dict. encycl. d. sc. méd., Par., 1877, 2. s., xii, 332-391. ———. Névroses. *Ibid.*, 1878, 2. s., xii, 738–759.—**Brodie** (B.) Théorie des affections nerveuses locales; des diverses conditions dans lesquelles elles se montrent; des principes qui doivent servir de base au traitement de ces affections. Progrès méd., Par., 1879, vii, 520; 539: 1880, viii, 512; 533; 558; 579.—**Brosius.** Jahresbericht über seine Privatanstalt für Gehirn- und Nervenkranke zu Bendorf bei Koblenz. Med. Ztg., Berl., 1858, i 83.—**Brown** (C.) Two cases of morbid affection of the nerves, successfully treated with the flores zinci. Lond. M. Rev. & Mag., 1799–1800, ii, 76.—**Browne** (J. C.) Circles of mental disorder; modern nervous diseases. Brit. M. J., Lond., 1880, ii, 262–267.—**Brown-Séquard** (C. E.) On the diagnosis and treatment of the various forms of paralytic, convulsive, and mental affections, considered as effects of morbid alterations of the blood, or of the brain, or other organs. Lancet, Lond , 1861, ii, 1; 29; 55; 79; 153; 199; 391; 415; 515; 611. ———. Lectures on the physiology and pathology of the nervous system; and on the treatment of organic nervous affections. *Ibid.*, 1868, ii, 593; 659; 755; 821: 1869, i, 1; 219; 703; 873. ———. The mode of origin and the treatment of nervous diseases. Clinic, Cincin., 1872, ii, 157-160. ———. Nerve derangements; epilepsy, insanity, paralysis, and hysterical affections; cutting the head open not necessary in cases of brain disease; experiments on decapitated men; movements of the body hours after death; a case of ecstasy; lecture delivered in Boston, March 8, 1874. N. York Tribune Pop. Sc., roy. 8°, 1874, 24–28. ———. Charles Sumner's sufferings; consequences of irritating particular nerves; people saying things they don't want to say; sneezing 80,000 times in 82 hours; treatment adopted in Sumner's case; why and how he endured the torture; lecture delivered in Boston, March 15, 1874. *Ibid.*, 28–30. ———. Diseases of the nervous system. Med. Rec., N. Y., 1877, xii, 769-773: 1878, xiii, 41; 81; 141; 161. ———. Diseases and injuries of nerves. Pt. II. Remoter consequences of nerve-lesions. Syst. Surg. (Holmes), 2. ed., N. Y., 1870, iv, 184–208.—**Brunelli** (C.) Resoconto di alcune malattie del sistema nervoso curate nel gabinetto elettro-terapeutico nell' Ospedale di S. Spirito (Roma) dal settembre 1868 al settembre 1871. N. Liguria med., Genova, 1873, xviii, 321–332.—**Bryant** (T.) The injuries and diseases of the nervous system. Guy's Hosp. Rep , Lond., 1859, 3. s., v, 9–83. *Also,* Reprint. *Also, in his:* Clin. Surg., 8°, Lond., 1860-64, pt. 1, 1–75.—**Buet.** Observations pour servir à l'histoire des maladies du cerveau et de la moelle épinière. J. compl. du dict. d. sc. méd., Par., 1829, xxxiii, 84-90.—**Burresi** (P.) Malattie del sistema nervoso. Sperimentale, Firenze, 1869, xxiii, 193; 385: 1870, xxv, 11: 1871, xxvii, 9: xxviii, 113: 1872, xxix, 337.—**Burrows** (G.) Clinical lectures on cases of nervous irritation. Lond. M. Gaz., 1845, n. s., i, 791–795.—**Caldwell** (J. W.) Diseases of the nervous system. N. Orl. J. Med., 1888, xxi, 684–695.—**Cammareri** (V.) Importanza ed estensione della neuropatologia. Gazz. d. osp., Milano, 1886, vii, 689; 697; 705.—**Camps** (W.) Essays and reviews on affections of the nervous system, including their pathology and treatment. Med. Mirror, Lond., 1864, i, 330; 385; 471; 516; 700; 761.—**Cantalamessa** (I.) Obbiettivo e subbiettivo nell' esame delle malattie nervose. Bull. d. sc. med. di Bologna, 1887, 6. s., xix, 5–28.—**Carroll** (A. L.) Clinical notes on some common disorders of the nervous system. Med. Rec., N. Y., 1875, x, 91–95.—**Carter** (C.) A case of nervous disorder, showing the effect of climate. Med. & Surg. Reporter, Phila., 1877, xxxvi, 125.—**Castells Ballespí** (F.) Neuropatia cérebro-cardiaca. Gac. méd. catal., Barcel., 1883, vi, 182–184.—**Cerebrospinal** dropsy. [Case.] St. George's Hosp. Rep. 1877-8, Lond., 1879, ix, 151.—**Chambard** (E.) Une famille de névropathes. Ann. méd.-psych., Par., 1884, 6. s., xi, 220–229. —**Charcot.** O chorobach ukladu nerwowego. [Lectures on diseases of the nervous system; transl. by P. Dubelt.] Gaz. lek., Warszawa, 1876, xxi, 241; 281; 297; 311; 326; 339; 361: 1877, xxii, 21; 36; 54.—**Chevers** (N.) Indian neuroses. Med. Times & Gaz., Lond., 1885, i, 111–113.—**Chometowski** (S.) Kronika chorób nerwowych i umyslowych. [Nervous and mental diseases.] Pam. Towarz. Lek. Warszaw., 1869, lxi, 84–93.—**Chrastina** (J.) Ueber Krankheiten des Central-Nervensystems. Mitth. d. Wien. med. Doct.-Coll., 1878, iv, 281; 293. *Also:* Allg. Wien. med. Ztg., 1878, xxiii, 467; 477: 1879, xxiv, 207; 219; 229; 242; 254.—**Clarke** (J. L.) Diseases and injuries of nerves. Syst. Surg. (Holmes), 2. ed., N. Y., 1870, iv, 148–183.—**Clutterbuck.** Lectures on the diseases of the nervous system. Lancet, Lond., 1826-7, xi, 129; 166; 230; 276; 341; 372; 435; 531; 597; 657; 753; 827: 1827, xii, 33; 101; 165; 257; 353; 417; 484; 550; 648; 737. — **Cohn.** Krankheiten des Gehirns und Rückenmarks. Ztschr. f. klin. Med., Bresl., 1854, v, 204; 241; 347.—**Cordes** (E.) Einige Fälle von typischen Neurosen. Deutsches Arch. f. klin. Med., Leipz., 1871-2, ix, 553-590.—**Crichton-Browne** (J.) Presidential address, delivered at the Royal College of Physicians, London. J. Ment. Sc., Lond., 1878-9, xxiv, 345–373.—**Curwen** (J.) Some hints relative to the prevention of nervous diseases. Alienist & Neurol., St. Louis, 1882, iii,

Nervous *system (Diseases of).*

194–201.—**Dana** (C. L.) & **Wilkin** (W. P.) Gilles de la Tourette's disease. [Abstr.] N. York M. J., 1886, xliii, 701. — **De - Bonis** (T.) Storia di particolare affezione nervosa. Gior. d. sc. med., Torino, 1839, v, 286–290.— **Delery** (C.) Névrose intermittente accompagnée de crises, guérie par la sulfate de quinine. Union méd. de la Louisiane, N.-Orl., 1852, i, 100–103.—**Delmas** (P.) Maladies des centres nerveux; encéphale, moelle, grand sympathique. Bordeaux méd., 1876, v, 313. ——. Des névroses, des névralgies et des névropathies. *Ibid.*, 314.—**Diseases** of the nervous system. Brit. & For. M.-Chir. Rev., Lond., 1876, lviii, 376–388.—**Dove** (H.) Reports of cases of nervous disease. Lancet, Lond., 1855, ii, 166.—**Drummond** (D.) The essential features of diseases of the nervous system. Med. News, Lond., 1881–2, i, 3, 1 pl. ; 13, 1 pl. ; 23, 1 pl. ; 35, 1 pl. ; 49, 1 pl. ; 62 ; 82, 1 pl. ; 109, 1 pl. ; 133 ; 142–144, 1 pl. ; 155 ; 166, 1 p ; 178 ; 190 ; 202 ; 214 ; 226 ; 239 ; 250 ; 262 ; 274 ; 286 ; 298 : 1882, ii, 2 ; 14 ; 26 ; 38 ; 62 ; 74 ; 86 ; 100 ; 111 ; 122 ; 139 ; 149 ; 163 ; 172 ; 208 ; 220 ; 250 ; 262 ; 279 ; 287 ; 313 : 1882–3, iii, 17.—**Dubrisay** (J.) Histoire d'un dégénéré. Union méd., Par., 1887, 3. s., xliv, 433–435.—**Dumont.** Manuscrits d'un médecin névropathe. Rapport de M. Deneffe . . . sur un travail présenté, sous ce titre, à l'Académie royale de médecine de Belgique par M. le Dr. Dumont. Bull. Acad. de méd. de Belg., Brux., 1882, 3. s., xvi, 509–513. *Also*, Reprint.— **Duplay** (A.) Observations de maladies des centres nerveux, recueillies à l'Hôpital de la Pitié, dans le service de . . Rostan. Arch. gén. de méd., Par., 1834, 2. s., vi, 305 ; 478.—**Echeverria** (G.) Lectures on diseases of the nervous system. Am. M. Times, N. Y., 1861, ii, 299 ; 315 ; 331 ; 347 ; 363.—**Engelberg.** Einige Beobachtungen von Nervenkrankheiten. J. d. pract. Heilk., Berl., 1828, lxvi, 5. St., 3 ; 6. St., 32.—**Erb** (W. H.) Anatomical diseases of the peripheral nerves. Cycl. Pract. M. (Ziemssen), N. Y., 1876, xi, 575–609. ——. Des progrès récents de la neuropathologie et de leurs conséquences au point de vue de l'enseignement médical. Progrès méd., Par., 1880, viii, 919 ; 941 ; 978. ——. Clinical lecture on the diseases of the nervous system. Boston M. & S. J., 1881, cv, 265. — **Erlenmeyer.** Rückenmarks- und Gehirnleiden. Deutsche Klinik, Berl., 1850, ii, 434 ; 442. ——. Bericht über die Fortschritte im Gebiet der Gehirn- und Rückenmarks-Krankheiten während des Jahres 1853. Cor.-Bl. d. deutsch. Gesellsch. f. Psychiat., etc., Neuwied, 1854, i, 85–88. ——. Bericht über die während der Jahre 1850 bis 1859 in der Privatanstalt zu Bendorf bei Koblenz behandelten Gehirn- und Nervenkranken. Med. Ztg., Berl., 1851, xx, 22 ; 33 : 1852, xxi, 21 : 1853, xxii, 31 : 1854, xxiii, 9 : 1858, n. F., i, 69 : 1859, n. F., ii, 34 : 1860, n. F., iii, 11.—**Eschenbach** (C. E.) Nervorum morbus. *In his:* Obs. anat.-chir.-med. rariora, 12°, Rostochii, 1769, 328–347.—**Eskridge** (J. T.) Nervous and mental diseases as influenced by the climate of Colorado. J. Nerv. & Ment. Dis., N. Y., 1887, xiv, 554–576.—**Eulenburg** (A.) Casuistische Beiträge zu den Neurosen der oberen Extremitäten. Verhandl. d. Berl. med. Gesellsch., 1872, iv, 1. Th., 228–234. *Also :* Berl. klin. Wchnschr., 1873, x, 26. ——. Vasomotorisch-trophische Neurosen. Handb. d. spec. Path. u. Therap (Ziemssen), Leipz., 1875, xii, 2. Hlft., 1–175. *Also, transl.:* Cycl. Pract. M. (Ziemssen). N. Y., 1877, xiv, 1–179.—**Fenn** (E. L.) On abdominal neuroses. Med. Times & Gaz., Lond., 1860, ii, 725–727.— **Ferrand & Léonard.** Névrose vaso-motrice. Encéphale, Par., 1885, v, 529–557.—**Finlayson** (J.) Notes on cases of nervous disease. Glasgow M. J., 1877, [4. s.], ix, 445–451.—**Forget** (C.) Recherches cliniques sur les névroses. Gaz. méd. de Par., 1847, 3. s., ii, 918 ; 942 ; 978. *Also :* Ann. de méd. belge, Brux., 1847, iv, 190 : 1848, i, 14. — **Fornasini** (L.) Saggio di una teorica delle affezioni nervose, tratta dall' opera inedita : "L' ipocondria studiata al lume della filosofia medica ". Ann. univ. di med., Milano, 1856, clviii, 225.—**Fothergill** (J. M.) The neurotic. Med. Press & Circ., Lond., 1887, n. s., xliii, 235.— **von Franque** (A.) Zusammenstellung der in dem Jahre 1858 in der Poliklinik zu München beobachteten Gehirn- und Nervenkrankheiten. Cor.-Bl. d. deutsch. Gesellsch. f. Psychiat., etc., Neuwied, 1859, vi, 161–164. ——. Zur Casuistik der Krankheiten des Nervensystems. Arch. d. deutsch. Gesellsch. f. Psychiat., Neuwied, 1862, v, 105–147.—**Friedreich** (J. B.) Die neusten Erfahrungen und Ansichten über die Localkrankheiten und die Wiedererzeugung der Nerven, mit Berücksichtigung der Literatur. Schmidt's Jahrb., Leipz., 1835, v, 89–95. — **García Diaz** (J.) La polineurosis y la emigracion inversa. Rev. de med. y cirug. práct., Madrid, 1886, xix, 505–513.—**Gason** (J.) & **Ridge** (B.) Case of fever of the nervous system. Med. Circ., Lond., 1861, xix, 71 ; 189.— **Gaston** (J. McF.) Explanation of the pathology and therapeutics of the diseases of the nerve centres. especially epilepsy. Tr. M. Ass. Georgia, Atlanta, 1884, 213–240. *Also*, Reprint.—**Gaultier de Claubry.** Observations de médecine pratique, relatives à des maladies du système nerveux cérébro-spinal. Arch. gén. de méd., Par., 1827, xiv, 53–60.—**Geerds.** Beiträge zur Neuropathologie. Deutsche Klinik, Berl., 1861, xiii, 312.—**Gemignani** (L.) Prolegomeni sulle neurosi. Mem. d. Soc. med.-chir. di Bo-

Nervous *system (Diseases of).*

logna, 1844. 2. s., iii, 439–508.—**Gluziński** (W.) Sprawozdanie z kliniki lekarskiéj Prof. Dra Korczyńskiego ; 1874–5 ; 1878–9. Chorby układu nerwowego. [Report of Prof. Korczyński's clinic for nervous diseases.] Przegl. lek., Krakow., 1880, xix, 651 ; 665. — **Gouzée.** Quelques faits cliniques relatifs à des maladies de l'appareil encéphalo-rachidien. Arch. belges de méd. mil., Brux.. 1859. xxiii, 5–20.— **Gowers** (W. R.) Notes on diseases of the nervous system. Lancet, Lond., 1886, i. 145. *Also, transl. :* Med. contemp., Napoli, 1886, iii, 24–28.—**Grancher** (J.) Maladies du système nerveux. Gaz. méd. de Par., 1881, 6. s., iii, 449 ; 467 ; 478 ; 491.—**Grantham** (J.) On paralytic and painful nervous affections. Lond. M. Gaz., 1837, xx, 70–72.—**Grocco** (P.) Note cliniche ed anatomiche intorno ad affezioni del sistema nervoso. Ann. univ. di med. e chir., Milano, 1884, cclxvii, 215 : cclxix, 238.—**Guérin** (*de Mamers*). Des irritations encéphaliques rachidiennes et nerveuses sous le rapport de l'éthiologie et de la thérapeutique. J. compl. du dict. d. sc. méd., Par., 1828, xxx, 319 : 1829, xxxiii, 222. ——. Observations sur des affections nerveuses à type continu. J. gén. de méd., chir. et pharm., Par., 1829, cvii, 207–228.— **Gumplowicz** (M.) & **Klotzberg** (E.) Aus der allgemeinen Poliklinik in Wien. Abtheilung für Nervenkranke und Elektrotherapie ; Jahresbericht für 1873. Wien. med. Presse, 1874, xv, 296 ; 434.—**Gwiazdomorski** (J.) Sprawozdanie roczne z "Domu Zdrowia ", zakładu leczniczego prywatnego. [Report of the Health Asylum, a private institution.] Przegl. lek., Krakow., 1885, xxiv, 9 ; 23 ; 39.—**Hall** (M.) Course of lectures on the diagnosis, pathology and treatment of diseases of the nervous system. Med. Times. Lond., 1842–3, vii, 179 ; 200 ; 212 ; 228 ; 243 ; 259 ; 275 ; 294 ; 308 ; 325 ; 358 ; 399. ——. On the neck as a medical region, and on paroxysmal paralysis. Lancet, Lond., 1849, i. 174 ; 285 ; 394 ; 506 ; 687 : ii, 66. *Also*, Reprint.—**Hambursin.** Discussion du rapport de la commission chargée d'apprécier les mémoires envoyés au concours ouvert sur la pathogénie et la thérapeutique des maladies des centres nerveux et principalement de l'épilepsie. Bull. Acad. roy. de méd. de Belg., Brux.. 1885, 3. s., xix, 601–648. — **Heidler** (C. J.) Nervenkrankheiten als Morbi nervosi oder nervöse Neurosen. Ztschr. d. k.-k. Gesellsch. d. Aerzte zu Wien, 1844, ii, 175–185. —. Nervenkrankheiten als Neurosen. Wchnschr. f. d. ges. Heilk., Berl., 1845, xiii, 237–242. — **Helfft.** Zur Pathologie und Diagnose der Nervenkrankheiten. *Ibid.*, 1850, xviii, 721– 733.—**Hibberd** (J. F.) The nerves. Am. Pract., Louisville, 1870, xviii, 329–345. —**Hirt.** Ueber das Hospiz "la Salpêtrière " in Paris und die Charcot'sche Klinik für Nervenkrankheiten. Jahresb. d. schles. Gesellsch. f. vaterl. Kult. 1883, Bresl., 1884, lxi, 27–34.—**Homem** (T.) Molestias do systema nervoso ; lições de clinica medica feitas na Faculdade de medicina do Rio de Janeiro. Progresso med., Rio de Jan., 1876–7, i, 225 ; 253 ; 281 ; 309 ; 337 ; 365 ; 393 ; 421 ; 452 ; 477 ; 505 ; 541 ; 561 ; 589 ; 617 ; 647 : 1877, ii, 5 ; 169 ; 197 ; 225.—**Hughes** (C. H.) The hygiene of the nervous system and mind ; the relation of the nervous system to cholera and its prophylaxis and neurotherapy ; the cure and prevention of dy-pepsia as a nervous disease ; the neuropathic diathesis ; its quarantine and treatment. Alienist & Neurol., St. Louis, 1885, vi, 44–64.—**Hunt** (E. M.) & **Wickes** (S.) "Can nervous diseases be considered less mechanical or chemical than other organic complaints, when the chemistry of life is better understood?" Tr. M. Soc. N. Jersey, Newark, 1862, 34–38.—**Icts** over nerveuse familiën. Geneesk. Courant, Tiel, 1883, xxxvii, nos. 30 ; 31 ; 32 ; 33.—**Jackson** (J. H.) On the study of diseases of the nervous system. Clin. Lect. & Rep. Lond. Hosp., 1864, i, 146–158. ——. Illustrations of diseases of the nervous system. *Ibid.*, 337–387. ——. Cases of diseases of the nervous system. *Ibid.*, 1867–8, iv, 314–394. ——. Gulstonian lectures on certain points in the study and classification of diseases of the nervous system. Brit. M. J., Lond., 1869, i, 184 ; 210 ; 236. *Also :* Lancet, Lond., 1869, i, 307 ; 344 ; 379. ——. Notes on cases of disease of the nervous system. Brit. M. J., Lond., 1871, ii, 641. ——. Clinical memoranda of a series of interesting cases of nerve-disorder now in (London) hospital. *Ibid.*, 1875, i, 773. ——. Clinical observations on cases of disease of the nervous system. Lancet, Lond., 1875, i, 85.—**Jaksch.** Ueber periphere Nervenkrankheiten. Amtl. Ber. ü. d. Versamml. deutsch. Naturf. u. Aerzte 1862, Karlsbad, 1863, xxxvii, 304– 314. *Also*, Reprint.—**Jamieson** (J.) Nervous diseases in Victoria. Brain, Lond., 1880–81, iii, 337–346.—**Janeway** (E. G.) Some interesting cases of nervous disease. Am. Psych. J., N. Y., 1875–6, iii, 51–61.—**Jones** (C. H.) Cases of nerve-disorder. Brit. M. J., Lond., 1859, 308 ; 331. ——. Cases of motor nerve disorder, with clinical remarks. Med. Press & Circ., Lond., 1872, xiv, 317 ; 341. — **Jones** (J.) Introduction to the study of diseases of the nervous system. *In his:* Med. & Surg. Mem. 1855–76, 8°, N. Orl., 1876, i, 1–137.—**Jones** (T.) Some recent progress in diseases of the nervous system. Tr. Minn. M. Soc., St. Paul, 1883, xv, 161–174. *Also :* Alienist & Neurol., St. Louis, 1884, v, 1–11. *Also*, Reprint. — **Joseph** (G.) [Nervenaffectionen, wie Paralysen, Dysurie.] Ztschr. f. klin. Med., Bresl., 1857, viii, 105. — **Jourdain** (C.) Observations pratiques sur les maladies nerveuses. Ann. de méd.

Nervous *system (Diseases of).*

belge, Brux., 1838, ii, 93-98.—**Kaulich** (J.) Bericht der medicinischen Klinik des Herrn Prof. Jaksch aus den Schuljahren 1857-8 und 1858-9. Vrtljschr. f. d. prakt. Heilk., Prag, 1860, lxvi, 111-132. — **Klose** (C. W.)' & **Paul** (J.) Krankheiten des Gehirns, Rückenmarks und seiner Häute, sowie im übrigen Nervensystem. Ztschr. f. klin. Med., Bresl., 1851, ii, 343-347.—**Kohts** (O.) Meningitis und Myelitis. Handb. d. Kinderkr. (Gerhardt), Tübing., 1879, v, 1. Abth, 375-411.—**Krause** (W.) Zur Pathologie der motorischen Endplatten. Deutsches Arch. f. klin. Med.. Leipz., 1883, xxxiii,435-437.—**Kuessner** (B.) Neuropathologische Beobachtungen aus der medicinischen Poliklinik in Halle a. S. Arch. f. Psychiat., Berl., 1877-8, viii, 443-453. *Also,* Reprint.—**Küttlinger** (A.) Beobachtung und Bemerkungen über Affectionen des Cerebrospinal Systems. Med. Cor.-Bl. bayer. Aerzte, Erlang., 1850, xi, 203; 209.—**Labadie-Lagrave**(F.) Nerfs. (Pathologie médicale.) N. dict. de méd. et chir. prat., Par., 1877, xxiii, 698-750. — **Labounardière.** Observations sur quelques maladies du cerveau et du système nerveux. J. gén. de méd., chir. et pharm., Par., 1814, l, 261; 337.— **Landois** (L.) Ueber die Erregung typischer Krampfanfälle nach Behandlung des centralen Nervensystemes mit chemischen Substanzen unter besonderer Berücksichtigung der Urämie. Wien. med. Presse,1887, xxviii,233; 270, 303.— **Landry** (O.) Recherches sur les causes et les indications curatives des maladies nerveuses. Monit. d. hôp., Par., 1855, iii, 157; 188; 282; 314; 355; 441; 510; 518; 525; 539; 561; 630; 638; 645; 652; 662; 676; 841; 889; 905; 929; 955. *Also,* Reprint.— **Lange** (C.) Vasomotoriske og trofiske Neuroser. Hosp.-Tid., Kjøbenh., 1882, 2. R., ix, 825; 845; 905; 925; 941; 961. — **Langveld** (A. P.) Hyperhémie chronique du cerveau et de la moelle épinière. Progrès méd.. Par., 1887, 2. s., vi, 21. — **Larcher** (O.) Mémoire sur les affections du système nerveux chez les oiseaux. J. de l'anat. et physiol.. etc., Par., 1877, xiii, 433-450.—**Lawson** (L. M.) Lectures on diseases of the brain and nervous system. West. Lancet, Cincin., 1855, xvi, 65-78.—**Laycock** (T.) Lectures on the clinical observation of diseases of the brain and nervous system. Med. Times & Gaz., Lond., 1871, i, 31; 91; 151.—**Lebert** (H.) Krankheiten der Innervationsorgane. Deutsche Klinik, Berl., 1855, vii, 289. — **Leblanc.** Quelques remarques sur les maladies du système nerveux des animaux domestiques. J. d. conn. méd.-chir., Par., 1843, xi, 149.— **Léger.** Lésion cérébrale avec myélite transverse concomitante. Gaz. méd de Picardie, Amiens, 1887, v, 36. — **Leudrick** (C.) Observations on diseases of the nervous system. Dublin J. M. Sc., 1836, x. 83-93. — **Lentz.** Lecture sur le nervosisme. Bull. Soc. de méd. ment. de Belg., Gand et Leipz., 1887, no. 45, 48-57. — **Lereboullet** (L.) Nerfs (pathologie médicale). Dict. encycl. de sc. méd., Par., 1877, 2. s., xii, 223-241.—**von Liebermeister** (C.) Lektsii pochastnoi patologii i terapii. T. II. Boliezni nervnoi sistemy. Perevod s Nemetskago M. v. Hirschfelda. [Lectures on special pathology and therapy. T. II. Diseases of the nervous system. Translated fom the German by M. v. Hirschfeld.] Ejem. j·ur prakt. med., St. Petersb., 1887, iii, 1-484. — **Liégey** (N.-F.) Mémoire sur la constitution médicale d'une contrée des départements de la Meurthe et des Vosges et sur les névroses fébriles. J. de méd., chir. et pharmacol., Brux., 1852, xv, 185; 281: 1853, xvi, 11: 122; 217; 417; 533: xvii, 3; 101; 293; 414; 510: 1854, xviii, 124; 414; 508. *Also,* Reprint.— **Lincoln** (D. F.) Boston Dispensary for Diseases of the Nervous System; report of 211 cases. Boston M. & S. J., 1873, lxxxix, 11-17. *Also,* Reprint.— **Lion** (M. E.) Kratkii ocherk russkoi nevrolog. literaturi za 1785 g. [Russian neurological literature for 1885.] Med. Obozr. Mosk., 1886, xxv, 605-620. — **Longchaup.** Affection des centres nerveux. Bull. Soc. de méd de la Sarthe 1851, Le Mans, 1852, 48-50.—**Luys** (J.) Considérations générales sur la structure et les maladies du système. nerveux. Union méd., Par., 1886, 3. s., xlii, 109; 121; 133.— **Madden** (W. H.) Illustrations of diseases of the nervous system. Lond. J. M., 1850, ii, 516-521.—**Mahé** (J.) Observations touchant les maladies du système nerveux. Arch. de méd. nav., Par., 1871, xv, 47-93.—**Maragliano** (D.) Relazione sui lavori nevrologici del nono congresso medico di Genova. Arch. ital. per le mal. nerv., Milano, 1880, xvii, 473-492. — **Maragliano** (E.) Rapporto intorno alle osservazioni cliniche sopra alcune lesioni dei centri nervosi. [5 cases.] Gior. d. r. Accad. di med. di Torino, 1870, 3. s., ix, 908; 929. — **Marchal.** Remarques et observations sur des affections névropathiques. Rec. de mém. de méd. . . . mil., Par., 1852, 2. s., ix, 188-307.—**Marchioli** (G.) La dottrina e la classificazione delle malattie nervose. Gazz. med. ital. lomb., Milano, 1872, 6. s., v, 286-288.—**Meinhard.** Drei Fälle von Motilität-Neurosen. Med. Ztg. Russlands, St. Petersb, 1846, iii, 352-356.—**Meyer-Ahrens.** Ueber einige Nerven- und Geisteskrankheiten im hohen Norden. Schweiz. Ztschr. f. Med., Chir. u. Geburtsh., Zürich, 1856, xii, 330-345.—**Michaelis.** Ueber locale Nerven-Affectionen. J. d. Chir. u. Augenh., Berl., 1838, xxvii, 267-292.—**Miles** (F. T.) Diseases of the peripheral nerves. Syst. Pract. M. (Pepper), Phila., 1886, v, 1177-1210.—**Millikin** (D.)

Nervous *system (Diseases of).*

A bad family. Cincin. Lancet & Clinic, 1881, n. s., vii, 437-443.—**Mills** (C. K.) The clinical appliances for the investigation and treatment of diseases of the nervous system. Med. & Surg. Reporter, Phila., 1878, xxxviii, 221-224.—**Minot** (F.) Diseases of the membranes of the brain and spinal cord. Syst. Pract. M. (Pepper), Phila., 1886, v, 703-722.—**Möbius** (P. J.) Beiträge zur Lehre von den Nervenkrankheiten. Schmidt's Jahrb.. Leipz., 1880, clxxxv, 185: clxxxvii, 284: 1881, cxc, 265: 1882, cxcvi, 185: 1884, cciii, 273. ——. Ueber die primären chronischen Erkrankungen des willkürlichen Bewegungsapparates. Centralbl. f. Nervenh., Coblenz, 1882, v, 1-11.— **Mondière** (J.-T.) Analyse du traité des maladies et des blessures des nerfs, de Joseph Swan; réflexions et observations sur ces maladies. Arch. gén. de méd.. Par., 1837, 2. s., xv, 292-313.—**Money** (A.) Some thoughts on nervous disease, and some observations on a not generally recognised form of "gouty" paralysis. Brit. M. J., Lond., 1887, ii, 937.—**Montault** (H.) Cas remarquable de physiologie pathologique du système nerveux, observé chez l'homme. J. univ. et hebd. de méd. et chir. prat.. Par., 1833, 2. s., x, 500-528.—**Morelli** (C.) & **Stacchini** (C.) Intorno ai casi di mali del cervello, e della spina osservati nel terzo turno medico dell' arcispedale di S. M. Nuova. Sperimentale, Firenze, 1873. xxxii, 119; 267; 544.—**Morse** (D. A.) A review of the literature of nervous disorders and insanity, for the year 1878. Cincin. Lancet & Clinic, 1879, n. s., ii, 438. *Also,* Reprint.— **Namias** (G.) Intorno alle malattie del sistema nervoso. Gior. veneto di sc. med., Venezia, 1874, 3. s., xx, 183; 370; 477: 3. s., xxi, 41; 174; 369.—**Nasse.** Beiträge zur Pathologie und Therapie verschiedener Krankheiten, aus den neueren physiologischen Erfahrungsuntersuchungen über die Beziehungen des Nervensystems. Arch. f. med. Erfahr., Berl., 1818, ii, 1-66.—**Nicaise.** Maladies chirurgicales des nerfs. Encycl. internat. de chir. (Ashhurst), Par., 1884, iii, 681-779.—**Noiszewski** (K.) Barwikowica (retinitis pigmentosa) i choroby pamięci, woli i mowy. [Retinitis pigmentosa and diseases affecting memory, free will, and language.] Pam. Towarz. Lek. Warszaw., 1887, lxxxiii, 169-201, 1 pl.—**Ogle** (J. W.) Cases of affections of the nervous system, of organic and inorganic origin; with clinical and pathological observations. Med. Times & Gaz., Lond., 1853, n. s., vii, 107; 163. ——. Series of clinical cases (with observations) illustrating the views recently put forward by Dr. Brown-Séquard as regards certain points connected with the physiology of the nervous system. Brit. & For. M.-Chir. Rev., Lond., 1859, xxiv, 500-514. ——. Cases of epilepsy, convulsions, giddiness, etc. Med. Times & Gaz., Lond., 1863, ii, 112; 218; 323; 508; 639.—**Ollivier** & **Raige-Delorme.** Nerfs (maladies des). Dict. de méd., 2. éd., Par., 1839, xx, 431-458. — **Oppolzer.** Vorträge über Krankheiten der peripheren Nerven. Allg. Wien. med. Ztg., 1860, v, 352; 377; 395; 411; 419; 427: 1861, vi, 34; 41; 50; 66; 73; 82; 106: 1862, vii, 193; 198; 210; 227; 257; 272; 289; 303; 338; 353; 362; 371. *Also* [Abstr.]: Wien. med Wchnschr., 1860, 688; 705; 719; 751; 783; 827. ——. Ueber Krankheiten der peripheren Nerven. Spitals-Ztg., Wien, 1862, 273; 289; 297; 313; 321; 345; 361; 369; 425; 433; 441; 463; 471.— **Ord** (W. M.) Notes on cases of nervous disorder. St. Thomas's Hosp. Rep. 1876, Lond., 1877, n. s., vii, 31-47, 2 ch.—**Ormerod** (J. A.) Illustrations of peripheral nerve-disease. St. Barth. Hosp. Rep., Lond., 1886, xxii, 169-185.—**Overerving** (De) van zenuw-en zielsziekten. [Inheritance of nervous diseases and insanity.] Geneesk. Courant, Tiel, 1887, xl, no. 22; 23; 24. — **Palma** (G.) Malattie nervose curate nello stabilimento del Pio Monte della Misericordia, in Casamicciola d'Ischia. Morgagni, Napoli, 1880, xxii, 281-296 —**Panara** (P.) Osservazioni su due casi di malattia de' centri nervosi occorsi nel 1° riparto di medicina dell' Ospedale di Roma. Gior. med. d. r. esercito, etc., Roma, 1886, xxxiv, 769-779.—**Parona** (F.) Annotazioni chirurgiche; malattie dei nervi. Ann. univ. di med. e chir., Milano, 1877, ccxli, 420-428.—**Pauchon** (A.) Quelques cas intéressants de maladies du système nerveux. Marseille méd., 1874, xi, 257-263.— **Penna** (J.) Juicio crítico de la obra escrita por el doctor J. M. Ramos Mejia titulada: "Las neurosis de los hombres célebres en la historia Argentina". An. d. Circ. méd. argent., Buenos Aires, 1882-3, vi, 101-139.—**Perrin** (T.) Sur le testament médical ou histoire complète d'une affection des centres nerveux du Dr. Dumont (de Monteux). Ann. Soc. de méd. de Lyon, 1864, 2. s., xii, 59-68.— **Peter.** Des névroses sans lésion et des névroses avec lésion matérielle. Gaz. d. hôp., Par., 1887, lx. 1189.— **Peterson** (C. A.) Some of the results of recent studies in neurology. St. Louis Cour. Med., 1881, vi, 200-210.— **von Pfungen** (R. F.) Casuistik von Erkrankungen des Nervensystems. Wien med. Bl., 1885, viii, 1093; 1121; 1153; 1212.—**Physiology** (On the) and diseases of the nervous system. Brit. & For. M.-Chir. Rev., Lond., 1850, ix, 1-50. — **Pick** (A.) Zur Lehre von der neuropathischen Disposition. Berl. klin. Wchnschr., 1879, xvi, 135-138.—**Pontoppidan** (K.) Neurasthenien; Bidrag til Skildringen af vor Tids Nervøsitet. Biblioth. f. Læger, Kjøbenh., 1886, xvi, 315-345. *Also,* Reprint.—**Poore** (G.

Nervous *system* (*Diseases of*).

V.) The "Bradshawe" lecture on nervous affections of the hand. Lancet, Lond., 1881, ii, 405; 493. — **Praktische** Mittheilungen aus dem Gebiete der Nervenkrankheiten. Mitth. a. d. Geb. d. Med., etc., Altona, 1840-41, viii, Hft. 5-6, 46-69. — **Puccinotti** (F.) Consulto per Giustino Marisi sopra una malattia nervosa. Gior. d. sc. med., Torino, 1839, v, 275-286. ——. Leçons sur les névroses. Ann. méd.-psych., Par., 1845, v, 367: vi, 53. *Also:* Ann. de méd. belge, Brux., 1845, ii, 324: iii, 45. — **Puccinotti** (F.) & **Girolami** (G.) Brevi cenni intorno alle lezioni sulle malattie nervose. Bull. d. sc. med. di Bologna, 1838, 2. s., v, 141-167. — **Purefoy** (T.) Cerebrospinal irritation. Dublin Q. J. M. Sc., 1852, xiv, 232-235. — **Putnam** (J. J.) Vaso-motor and trophic neuroses. Cycl. Pract. M. (Ziemssen), N. Y., 1881 (Suppl.), 601-652. — **Radcliffe** (C. B.) Croonian lectures on mind, brain, and spinal cord, in certain morbid conditions. Lancet, Lond., 1873, i, 401; 471; 516. ——. Medical annotations concerning epilepsy, paralysis, and other disorders of the nervous system. Practitioner, Lond., 1882, xxviii, 114; 173: 1883, xxx, 89.— **Rendiconto** dell' ospedale generale in Vienna per ciò che riguarda le malattie nervose nel 1854. Gazz. med. ital. lomb., Milano, 1856, 4. s., i, 291-297.— **von Renz** (W. T.) Lose Blätter aus meiner Unterrichts-Mappe. Centralbl. f. Nervenh., Leipz., 1886, ix, 609-620.— **Reynolds** (J. R.) Lecture on the classification of diseases of the nervous system. Lancet, Lond., 1873, ii, 405-409.—**Ribalkin** (J. V.) Dva slujaja tselebnago vlijanija ostrich zaraznich boleznei na dvigatelnie neurozi. [Two cases in which acute inflammation was salutary in the cure of neuroses (case of tetanus and case of St. Vitus' dance).] Vrach, St. Petersb., 1884, v, 869-871.— **Rieger.** Funktionelle und organische Nervenkrankheiten; ihre für den Praktiker wichtige Diagnose. Deutsche Med.-Ztg., Berl., 1885, ii, 789; 801; 809; 837. — **Rintel** (W.) Zur Casuistik der Nervenkrankheiten. Allg. med. Centr.-Ztg., Berl., 1860, xxix, 593; 601; 609.—**Rockwell** (A. D.) Remarks concerning diseases of the central nervous system. Am. Pract., Louisville, 1874, ix, 321-327.—**Rosenblatt** (E.) Choroby układu nerwowego spostrzegane w szpitalu św. Ludwika od r. 1879 do 1882. [Diseases of the nervous system.] Przegl. lek., Krakow., 1886, xxv, 341; 373; 388; 403; 415; 423; 647.—**Rosenthal** (M.) Précis de diagnostic et de thérapeutique des maladies nerveuses. (En russe.) In-8. Kazan. Gaz. méd. de Par., 1872, 4. s., i, 379. ——. Ueber den Einfluss von Nervenkrankheiten auf Zeugung und Sterilität. Wien. Klinik, 1880, vi, 135-166.—**Rostan.** Leçons sur les maladies des centres nerveux; lésions de la sensibilité et de l'intelligence. Gaz. d. hôp., Par., 1844, 2. s., vi, 402.—**Rothe** (A.) Sprawozdanie ix-te (i x-te) z czynności lekarskiéj w Warszawskich zakładach dla obłąkanych za rok 1875 (i 1876). [Ninth and tenth reports of the Medical Clinic for Diseases of the Nervous System.] Gaz. lek., Warszawa, 1877, xxiii, 97; 122.— **Sachs** (L. W.) Aerztliches Gutachten über die anzuwendende Behandlung des Kranken, der zu einer öffentlichen Berathung über ihn im November-Heft 1827 dieses Journals aufgefordert hat; nebst eingestreuten Bemerkungen über Nervenkrankheiten. J. d. pract. Heilk., Berl., 1828, lxvii, 1. St., 7-42.—**Savage** (G. H.) Alternation of neuroses. J. Ment. Sc., Lond., 1886-7, xxxii, 485-491. — **Scheiber** (S. H.) Idegkórtani közlemény apopleptikus rohamok után eszlelhető némely ritkább tüneményekről egy igen complicált és több más idegkórtani eset kapcsán. [On neuroses complicated with apoplectic affections of rare occurrence.] Orvosi hetil., Budapest, 1885, xxix, 1185; 1213; 1252; 1274.— **Schreiber** (J.) Ueber transitorische Encephalopathien und Myelopathien. Tagebl. d. Versamml. deutsch. Naturf. u. Aerzte, Danzig. 1880, liii, 235-239. — **Sciamanna** (E.) Il movimento degli studj anatomici e fisiologici in rapporto con la neuropatologia. Gazz. med. di Roma, 1882, viii, 121; 133. — **Semple** (R. H.) On disease of the nerves of the face. Lancet, Lond., 1841-2, ii, 849-852. ——. Clinical illustrations of diseases of the nervous system, and of other affections simulating them during life. Lond. J. M., 1850, ii, 448; 811.—**Serres.** Observations sur les maladies du système nerveux. J. de physiol. expér., Par., 1825, v, 233-265.—**Shershevski** (M. M.) Termicheskie neurozi. [Terminology of neuroses.] Vrach, St. Petersb., 1883, iv, 531; 548; 566; 579; 615; 662; 695. — **Silvano** (B.) Casi di malattie nervose osservati e descritti dal Dr . . . . e rassegnati al Prof. S. Berruti. Gior. . . . d. Soc. med.-chir. di Torino, 1844, xxi, 144-156. — **Silvano** (G.) Lettera medica sulle malattie nervose. *Ibid.*, 1845, xxiv, 249-263.— **Simon** (J.) Maladies du système nerveux. Progrès méd., Par., 1883, xi, 949-951. — **Smoler** (M.) Ueber Gehirn- und Nervenkrankheiten. Cor.-Bl. d. deutsch. Gesellsch. f. Psychiat., etc., Neuwied, 1863, x, 200; 263. ——. Klinische Kasuistik mit besonderer Berücksichtigung der Gehirn- und Nervenkrankheiten. Memorabilien, Heilbr., 1866, xi, 145-150.—**Spiess** (G. A.) Krankhafte Störungen in der Thätigkeit des Nervensystems (Nervenkrankheiten). Handwörterb. d. Physiol., Brnschwg., 1850, iii, 2. Abth., 153-233.—**Spitzka** (E.) Anæmia and hyperæmia of the brain and spinal cord. Syst. Pract. M. (Pepper), Phila., 1886, v, 763-824. — **Starr** (M. A.) Vaso-motor and trophic neurosis. *Ibid.*, 1241-1276.—

Nervous *system* (*Diseases of*).

Strümpell. Om orsakerna till nervsystemets sjukdomar. Ref. af O. V. Petersson. Upsala Läkaref. Förh., 1884-5, xx, 306-322. — **Suckling** (C. W.) Notes on nervous diseases. Birmingh. M. Rev., 1885, xviii, 255-271.— **Takács** (E.) Az 1874-5 tanévben a kórodán kezelt idegbetegek kórleirása. [Description of chronic nervous diseases in the clinic of 1874-5.] Orvosi hetil., Budapest, 1878, xxii, 1; 21; 45; 66; 125; 145; 166; 205; 269; 339; 363; 416; 444; 464; 486. *Also, transl.:* Pest. med.-chir. Presse, Budapest, 1878, xiv, 213; 237; 279; 344; 436; 561; 588; 652; 668; 681; 697; 709; 727; 742; 757; 774; 785; 806; 823; 843; 858.— **Teed** (J. L.) General observations preliminary to the study of nervous disease. Art. i-iii. Psych. & Med.-Leg. J., N. Y., 1874, n. s., i, 137; 290: 1875, n. s., ii, 50.—**Thomsen** (R.) Statistische Mittheilungen über die Krankenaufnahme auf der männlichen Irren-, Krampf- und Delirantenabtheilung während der Jahre 1874-86 mit specieller Berücksichtigung des Delirium potatorum und der progressiven Paralyse. Charité-Ann. 1885-6, Berl., 1887, xii, 396-404.—**Ticier.** Des névroses en général. J. de méd., chir. et pharm. de Toulouse, 1855, n. s., vii, 14; 47.— **Timermans** (G.) Delle malattie del sistema nerveo. Gior. d. r. Accad. di med. di Torino, 1868, 3. s., vi, 636; 709: 1869, 3. s., vii, 135. — **Todd** (R. R.) Clinical lectures on cases of diseases of the nervous system. Lancet, Lond., 1842-3, ii, 425; 462; 489; 541; 569.—**Tommasi** (S.) Alcune lezioni cliniche sulle malattie del sistema nervoso. Morgagni, Napoli, 1869, xi, 27; 81; 190; 321; 857: 1870, xii, 1. ——. Una lezione di casistica sulle malattie dei centri nervosi. *Ibid.*, 1877, xix, 443-448. — **Torp.** Fra Doktor Torp's Sygebjem for Nervesyækkede paa Lillehammer. Norsk Mag. f. Lægevidensk., Christiania, 1886, 4. R., i, 658-669.—**Ullersperger.** Beiträge zur Casuistik der Nervenkrankheiten. Cor.-Bl. d. deutsch. Gesellsch. f. Psychiat., etc., Neuwied, 1867, xiv, 161; 203.—**d'Urbin** (F.-P.) Considérations sur les maladies nerveuses. Expérience, Par., 1842, ix, 259-262.—**Uspenski** (P. I.) O nevrozach. [On neuropathy.] Vrach. Vaidom., St. Petersb., 1881, vi, 2003; 2020; 2034; 2050.—**Vizioli.** Le malattie nervose sono oggidì più frequenti? Morgagni, Napoli, 1878. xx, 897-912.—**Voisin** (A.) Conférences cliniques sur les maladies mentales et les affections nerveuses (1868). Union méd., Par., 1868, 3. s., vi, 87; 180; 382; 490.—**Vottem** (F.), **Poncelet** (D. D.) & **Raikem** (A.) Notice sur la maladie (inflammation) de la moelle épinière, des méninges, du cerveau et du poumon droit, à laquelle a succombé V: Fohmann [1837]. Gaz. méd. de Par., 1873, 2. s., v, 659-663. *Also,* Reprint.—**Webber** (S. G.) Diseases of the peripheral cerebro-spinal nerves. Cycl. Pract. M. (Ziemssen), N. Y., 1881 (Suppl.), 509-533.—**Westphal** (C.) Beobachtungen und Untersuchungen über die Krankheiten des centralen Nervensystems. Arch. f. Psychiat., Berl., 1873, iv, 335-369, 2 pl.—**White** (E. H.) On the principal diseases of the nervous system. Maryland & Virg. M. J., Richmond, 1860, xiv, 188; 354.—**Wilheim** (J.) Ueber einige Fälle von Coordinations-Neurosen bei Künstlern. Allg. Wien. med. Ztg., 1876, xxi, 139; 171.—**Wilks** (S.) Lectures on diseases of the nervous system. Med. Times & Gaz., Lond., 1868, i, 1; 29; 57; 113; 169; 225; 281; 335; 387; 439; 493; 545; 599; 627; 679: ii, 29; 115; 231; 327; 411; 467; 524; 577; 633; 689: 1869, i, 1; 58; 83; 135; 267; 323; 377. ——. Remarks on diseases of the nervous system. Guy's Hosp. Rep., Lond., 1873, 3. s., xviii, 123-157.—**Wising** (P. J.) Om nervpatologiens utveckling under de sista tvänne årtiondena. Föredrag vid tillträdandet af P. H. Malmstens professur i nervsjukdomar vid Karol. Inst. den 20 Maj 1887. [On development of pathology of the nerves during the last two decennials. Address delivered upon the accession of Malmsten to the professorship of nervous diseases.] Hygiea, Stockholm, 1887, xlix, 415-435.—**Wittmann** (L.) A központi és környi idegrendszer bántalmai. [Lesions of the nervous centres.] Orvosi hetil., Budapest, 1876, xx, 825; 845.—**Wolff.** Einige Zusätze zu meiner populären Abhandlung über die Nervenkrankheiten, für meine Herrn Mitärzte. J. d. pract. Arznk. u. Wundarznk., Berl., 1806, xxiv, 2. St., 72-109.—**Wood** (H. C.) Hemi-anesthesia due to lesion of the crus cerebri; epilepsy with running attacks; hystero-epilepsy with running attacks; paralysis agitans. Weekly M. Rev., Chicago, 1885, xi, 153-156.—**X.** Breve cenno di una particolare neuropatia. Imparziale, Firenze, 1880, xx, 227-232.—**Young** (J.) Report of cases of nervous affections. Am. J. M. Sc., Phila., 1839, xxv, 61-67.

Nervous *system* (*Diseases of, Anomalous or unusual*).

See, *also,* **Agoraphobia**; **Athetosis**; **Claustrophobia**; **Convulsions** (*Cases of*), *etc.*; **Katatonia**; **Miryachit**; **Mysophobia**; **Narcolepsy**; **Nervous** *system* (*Reflex action of*); **Oikophobia**; **Paramyoclonus** *multiplex*; **Pyrophobia**; **Tarantism**; **Tarassis**; **Thomsen's** *disease*; **Trance**.

BILLET (L.) Contributions à l'étude des névroses extraordinaires. 8°. *Paris,* 1874.

Nervous *system (Diseases of, Anomalous or unusual).*

HARNIER (A. L. G.) * Diss. sistens observationes quatuor morborum systematis nervei rarissimorum. 4°. *Marburgi*, 1844.

RICOTTI (M.) Storia d' una rara malattia nervosa con varie annotazioni. 8°. *Pavia*, 1818.

SANDEN (J. H.) * Diss. sistens affectum spasmodico-hypochondriacum inveteratum. sm. 4°. *Halæ Magdeb.*, [1734].

Abbot (S. L.) Two cases of death following anomalous nervous symptoms. Boston M. & S. J., 1865-6, lxxiii, 89-94. *Also:* Extr. Rec. Bost. Soc. M. Improve. (1862-6), 1867, v (app.), 205-211. — **Anomalous** nervous affection. West. M. Gaz., Cincin., 1832-3, i, 41. — **Arnold** (A. B.) Obscure affections of the nervous system. Maryland M. J., Balt., 1880, vi, 217-224.—**Asbury** (J. V.) Case of peculiar nervous excitement. Lond. M. & Phys. J., 1826, lv, 16.—**Balisti** (A.) Storia d' una singolare affezione nervosa. Ann. univ. di med., Milano, 1821, xviii, 260-285.—**Barbee** (W. J.) Lesion of the nerves of motion distributed to the muscles of the neck, and of the external respiratory muscles. Maryland M. & S. J., Balt., 1840, i, 286. — **Bell** (C. W.) Some account of an epidemic which prevailed at Teheran, in the months of January and February, 1842. Med.-Chir. Tr., Lond., 1843, xxvi, 223-237. *Also*, Reprint. — **Bennett** (R.) Peculiar nervous affection of the fore-finger. Lancet, Lond., 1841-2, i, 246-248.—**Bérard** (A.) jeune. Altérations diverses de l'innervation; anomalie de la menstruation; vomissemens chroniques. Clin. d. hôp., Par., 1827, i, no. 16, 2. — **Berarducci** (C.) Caso singulare di nervosismo. Arch. ital. per le mal. nerv., Milano, 1865, ii, 105-111.—**Berti** (A.) Sulla malattia del Krishaber. Gior. veneto di sc. med., Venezia, 1875, xxiii, 3. s., 425; 665: 1876. xxiv, 1; 184; 397; 539, 4 pl.: xxv, 165; 307. *Also*, Reprint. — **Bertini** (B.) Storia di singolare malattia del sistema nervoso. Gior. . . . d. Soc. med. chir. di Torino, 1842, xiv, 385-398.—**Bertini** (O.) Di un caso singolarissimo di nevrosi in donna gravida. Imparziale, Firenze, 1871, xi, 74-80.—**Bird** (G.) An anomalous case of spinal affection. Lond. J. M., 1849, i, 55-60.—**Boardman** (C. H.) A case of obscure nervous disease. Northwest. M. & S. J., St. Paul, Minn., 1873-4, iv, 125-130.—**Bogardus** (J.) A case of anomalous spasm successfully treated by the Scutellaria lateriflora. Med. Reposit., N. Y., 1821, n. s., vi, 85-87.—**Bonnard.** Observation sur une maladie singulière. J. de méd., chir. pharm., etc., Par., 1778, l, 60-64.—**Borlée** (J.-J.) Histoire d'une névrose extraordinaire et compliquée. Ann. Soc. de méd. de Gand, 1845, xv, 107-190.—**Breventani** (U.) Caso di flessione e di adduzione spasmodica di tutto il corpo durate all' incirca otto anni, seguito da morte; risultato della sezione, con pochi cenni su ciò che fu osservato dopo morte in due casi di opistotono, in conferma dell' opinione dell' antagonismo nervoso del Bellingeri. Bull. d. sc. med. di Bologna, 1834, x, 137-142.—**Bright** (J. W.) A remarkable case of reflex nervous action. West. J. M. & S., Louisville, 1852, 3. s., x, 393-396.—**Broadbent.** Curious nervous affection. Med. Times & Gaz., Lond., 1870, ii, 33.—**Brockett** (L. P.) Anomalous nervous affections. West. Lancet, Cincin., 1844-5, iii, 493-496. — **Brown-Séquard.** Frequent spasmodic movements on one side; irritation propagated from the ear. Med. Times & Gaz., Lond., 1860, ii, 407. — **Brückmann.** Eine seltene Nervenkrankheit, welche ein heftiges Geschrey begleitete. Arch. f. med. Erfahr., Berl., 1810, xiv, 218-221. — **Brugnoli** (G.) Storia di singolare nevrosi per esostosi della colonna vertebrale. Bull. d. sc. med. di Bologna, 1843, 3. s., iv, 321-332. ———. La storia di una singolari neurosi, presentante, a forma prevalente, un sonnambulismo spontaneo morboso. Rendic. Accad. d. sc. d. Ist. di Bologna, 1869, 73-77.—**Candia** (P.) Lijeras observaciones al caso raro de neurosis jeneral; observado por Don Alejandro Zúñiga. Rev. méd. de Chile, Sant. de Chile, 1872-3, i, 417-427.—**Cariole** (C.) Consultation pour un cas de névrose singulière et complexe. Union méd., Par., 1856, x, 149-151.—**Cavalli** (C.) Proseguimento della storia ragionata di straordinaria malattia che dura da vent'otto, ed ora da trentadue anni. Gior. d. sc. med., Torino, 1839, iv, 153-168.— **Caw** (J. M.) Case of anomalous nerve disease, with necropsy and examination of cord. Lancet, Lond., 1887, ii, 561.—**Choisy.** Cas remarquable de physiologie pathologique du système nerveux. Rev. méd. franç. et étrang., Par., 1833, i, 392-417.—**Chowne** (W. D.) Clinical lecture on a peculiar nervous affection. Lancet, Lond., 1841-2, fi, 353-358. — **Christoe** (W. S.) Curious nervous phenomena. Canada Lancet, Toronto, 1871-2, iv, 456-459.—**Clarke** (C. K.) An anomalous case of nervous disease. Canad. Pract., Toronto, 1883, viii, 204-207.—**Clarke** (J.) Violent spasmodic affection of the left arm. Edinb. M. & S. J., 1808, iv, 13-17.—**Cless.** Neurosis (vagi?). Med. Cor.-Bl. d. württemb. ärztl. Ver., Stuttg., 1839, ix, 367.—**Collingwood** (T.) History of a case fn which singular nervous affections were cured by an incision in the finger. Med. Comment., Edinb., 1794, viii, 2. decade, 390-394.—

Nervous *system (Diseases of, Anomalous or unusual).*

Comstock (J.) Singular nervous affection, supposed to have been occasioned by the bite of a tarantula. Med. Reposit., N. Y., 1804, vii, 1-11.—**Consultation** adressée à M. le Dr. . . . par Madame . . . Clin. d. hôp., Par., 1828-9, iii, 409.—**Coxe** (E. J.) Singular case of disease, attended by peculiar nervous symptoms. Boston M. & S. J., 1855, lii, 314-316.—**Cross** (J.) Affection of the right arm coming on during pregnancy. Brit. M. J., Lond., 1875, i, 447.—**Cummiskey** (J.) A singular case of nervous disease. Med. Times, Phila., 1870-71, i, 215.—**Deane** (J.) Extraordinary case of spasms of the voluntary muscles. Boston M. & S. J., 1843, xxviii, 336-338.—**De-Bonis** (T.) Utilità dei bagni d' acqua fredda in una neurosi anomala finita con accessi epilettici. Gior. d. sc. med., Torino, 1838, iii, 178-180.—**Demarquette.** Maladie des centres nerveux (cas remarquable). Monit. d. sc. méd. et pharm., Par., 1860, 2. s., ii, 530-532.—**Deperet** (L.) Observation d'une névrose non encore décrite. Rev. de thérap. du midi, Montpel., 1854, vi, 3.0. — **De Rudder.** Névrose terminée par une véritable scélotyrbe d'accès. Ann. Soc. de méd. de Gand, 1848, xxi, 77-95. [Rap.; discussion]: Bull. Soc. de méd. de Gand, 1848, xv, 34-55.—**De Wendt** (J.) Deux cas de névroses extraordinaires. Bull. Soc. de méd. ment. de Belg., Gand, 1878, xi, 10-20. [Discussion], xii, 15: 1879, xiv, 23.—**Dominguez** (E.) Caso raro de nervosismo. Siglo méd., Madrid, 1873, xx, 151-152.—**Dunsmure** (J.) Note of a case of temporary loss of voluntary power, produced by a touch on the head. Edinb. M. J., 1874-5, xx, 319-322.—**Elliotson.** A remarkable case of neuralgic disease simulating chorea and hysteria. Lond. M. & S. J., 1834-5, vi, 139-147.—**Emiliani** (E.) Descrizione di una singolare nevropatia. Bull. d. sc. med. di Bologna, 1856, 4. s., vi, 406-419. — **Emmanuel** (E.) Περὶ τινὸς σπασμωδικοῦ πάθους. Ἰατρικὴ, Μέλισσα, Ἀθῆναι, 1856, iv, 23-26.—**Fanzler** (L.) Manége-mozgás és tengelykörüli forgás egy-egy esete. [Sensation of "manége-motion".] Orvosi hetil., Budapest, 1881, xxv, 1161-1165.—**Fieber** (F.) Ueber eine noch nicht beschriebene Form von Anomalie der Bewegungsbeschränkung (Motilitäts-Neurose). Wien. med. Wchnschr., 1871, xxi. 996; 1021; 1045. ———. Notiz, betreffend eine eigenthümliche Nervenkrankheit. Centralbl. f. d. med. Wissensch., Berl., 1871, ix, 273.—**Fioravanti** (L.) Di una nevrosi. Gazz. med. ital. feder. tosc., Firenze, 1850-51, 2. s., i, 372-374.—**Franceschi** (C.) Di una strana forma di neurosi. Raccoglitore, Fano, 1847, xx, 193-198.—**Franco** (D.) Su d' un caso singolare di nevropatia di conducibilità. N. gior. internaz. d. sc. med., Napoli, 1877-8, i, 5-7.—**Fraser** (J. H.) Cases of nervous disease of peculiar form. Glasgow M. J., 1877, [4. s.], ix, 132-134. ———. A remarkable case of nervous disease. Med. Times & Gaz., Lond., 1883, i, 555.—**Gairdner.** A very remarkable, if not unique, spasm affecting the respiratory tract; with a personal and family history of previous neuroses; first results obtained under chloralhydrate. Glasgow M. J., 1879, [4. s.], xii, 135-137.—**Galpin** (L.) An interesting case of disease of the nervous system. Ohio M. & S. J., Columbus, 1858-9, xi, 1; 98.—**Gardner** (J. M.) ["Protean malady" in a young girl.] N. York J. M., 1845, v, 349-351.—**Garnier** (A.) Discussion sur les névroses extraordinaires. Ann. méd.-psych., Par., 1857, 3. s., iii, 601-619.—**Garrod.** A doubtful case of nervous disorder. Lancet, Lond., 1867, ii, 292.—**Gaultier** fils. Observation d'une névrose des fonctions cérébrales, dont la durée de l'accès a été de 42 heures sans la moindre diminution dans l'intensité des symptômes. J. gén. de méd., chir. et pharm., Par., 1809, xxxvi, 133-139.—**Geerds.** Eine seltene Nervenaffection. Deutsche Klinik, Berl., 1860, xii, 17.—**Gerlier.** Sur une nouvelle névrose de la motilité, le vertige paralysant, et sur la probabilité de son origine stabulaire. Abeille méd., Par., 1877, xliv, 361-370.—**Gordon** (T. W.) [An account of the peculiarities of nervous exaltation which occurred in the case of a practicing physician under treatment for apparent intermittent fever.] Ohio M. & S. J., Columbus, 1855-6, viii, 375-382.—**Gowers** (W. R.) Case of clonic spasms occurring only when the patient attempts to stand. Lancet, Lond., 1872, i, 148. ———. On saltatoric spasm. *Ibid.*, 1877, ii, 42; 152.—**Gozzi** (F.) Storia di una neurosi singolare. Bull. d. sc. med. di Bologna, 1840, 2. s., ix, 66-68.—**Griesinger.** Ueber einige seltene Krampfformen; Tremor der Muskeln und iradürte Krämpfe. Berl. klin. Wchnschr., 1867, iv, 157.—**Gros.** Contribution à l'étude de l'agoraphobie (peur des espaces) et d'autres formes de névroses émotives. Ann. méd.-psych., Par., 1885, 7. s., i, 394-407.—**Hammond** (G. M.) Case of congenital absence of the faculty of co-ordination. Med. Rec., N. Y., 1886, xxx, 471. *Also:* N. York M. J., 1886, xliv, 552. *Also:* Med. News, Phila., 1886, xlix, 467. — **Hammond** (W. A.) The order of the human body, as developed by certain affections of the nervous system. Tr. Am. Neurol. Ass., N. Y., 1877, ii, 17-23. *Also*, Reprint. ———. On a hitherto undescribed form of muscular incoördination. Tr. Am. Neurol. Ass., N. Y., 1877, ii, 154-158. *Also*, Reprint. ———. The scientific relations of

Nervous system (*Diseases of, Anomalous or unusual*).

modern miracles. Internat. Rev., N. Y., 1881, x, 225–242.— **Hawkins.** Case of an affection of the nervous system, which exhibited some unusual phenomena. Lond. M. & Phys. J., 1826, n. s., i, 221–223.—**Hayes** (P. H.) Nervestorms. Bistoury, Elmira, N. Y., 1876, xii, 172–174. — **Haynes** (C. E.) Case of anomalous hemorrhage and spasms. South. M. & S. J., Augusta, 1838, ii, 67–69.— **Hellis.** Histoire d'une névrose singulière. J. gén. de méd., chir. et pharm., Par., 1826, xcv, 11–17.—**Henrich.** Heilung von hartnäckigen sehr heftigen Krämpfen, welche den regelmässigen Eintritt des Menstrualflusses begleiteten und sich in einer chronisch-rheumatischen Dyscrasie begründeten, durch den Gebrauch des Sirona-Schwefelwassers zu Nierstein. J. d. pract. Heilk., Berl., 1829, lxix, 3. St., 74–85. — **Herter.** Multiple Reflexneurose. Charité-Ann. 1875, Berl., 1877, ii, 512–517. — **Heulhard d'Arcy.** Sur une affection nerveuse particulière (névromimosie). Rev. méd.-chir. de Par., 1853, xiii, 208–213. ——. **Névroses bizarres.** Abeille méd., Par., 1868, xxv, 321–323.— **Hittner** (W. W.) A singular delusion. [Case of spontaneous automatic action.] Clinic, Cincin., 1873, v, 99.— **Holden** (L.) Case in which tetanoid spasm with unconsciousness is produced by touching a tumor. Lancet, Lond., 1867, ii, 127. ——. Extraordinary anomalous affection of the nervous system in a boy. St. Barth. Hosp. Rep., Lond., 1867, iii, 299–305; 1871, vii, 228.—**Holmes** (T. M.) A case of "daymare". Med. Rec., N. Y., 1886, xxix, 208.—**Hulke** (W.) An account of a remarkable spasmodic affection. Lond. M. J., 1784, v, 389–392.— **Hutchinson.** Case of anomalous nerve disorder in infancy. Brit. M. J., Lond., 1882, i, 342.—**Iglesias.** [Comunicacion sobre un caso de neurosis anómala, tratado por la hidroterapia.] An. r. Acad. de med., Madrid, 1881, iii, 125–129.—**Isaacs.** Peculiar cerebral symptoms depending upon excessive sexual indulgence. N. York J. M., 1859, 3. s., vii, 39–42.—**Jacquinelle.** Observation sur une affection nerveuse, occasionnée par un amour malheureux, et terminée par la mort à la suite d'un mauvais traitement. J. de méd., chir., pharm., etc., Par., 1784, lxii, 62–67.— **Jansckowitsch** (M.) Geschichte einer merkwürdigen Nervenkrankheit unter der Form von Convulsionen und Idiosomnambulismus. Med. Jahrb. d. k. k. österr. Staates, Wien, 1845, liv, 129; 269.—**Jastrzembski.** Observation de névrose multiforme. Ann. Soc. de méd. d'Anvers, 1844, 437–443.— **Johnson** (F. U.) Case of irregular nervous action in one arm, of two years' standing, in a child 7 years old, cured by Actæa racemosa. N. York J. M. & S., 1839, i, 223.—**Jones** (C. H.) Cases of obscure nerve disorder. Med. Times & Gaz., Lond., 1874, ii, 230; 359; 626; 1875, i, 361: ii, 184; 441; 648: 1876, i, 194; 356; 437; 545: ii, 148.— **Kerr** (T.) Case of anomalous nervous affection, occurring in the later part of pregnancy. West. M.-Chir. J., Keokuk, 1850, i, 358–360.—**King** (J. S.) Peculiar case of nervous disease. Canada Lancet, Toronto, 1874, vi, 329–331.—**Knecht.** Eine seltene Neurose. Berl. klin. Wchnschr., 1874, xi, 542.—**Kuntzmann.** Geschichte einer merkwürdigen Nervenkrankheit. J. d. pract. Heilk., Berl., 1840, xci, 1. St., 118–120.—**Laehr.** Ein Fall von unregelmässig intermittirender, motorischer und sensorischer Central-Neurose. Allg. Ztschr. f. Psychiat., etc., Berl., 1868, xxv, 852–856.—**Legrand du Saulle.** Cas de névrose extraordinaire observé à l'asile de Rome. Ann. méd.-psych., Par., 1860, 3. s., vi, 165–168. ——. Cas insolite de névrose convulsive. Encéphale, Par., 1885, v, 339.—**Liégey.** Un mot sur une endémo-épidémie de névroses protéiques. Union méd., Par., 1856, x, 223.—**Longavan.** Réponse au sujet de la maladie singulière dont M. Bonnard a donné le détail dans le Journal du mois de juillet 1778. J. de méd., chir., pharm., etc., Par., 1778, l, 323–331.—**Lubert.** Observation singulière d'une affection nerveuse qui résista à toutes les médications et disparut subitement d'elle-même. J. de méd. et chir. prat., Par., 1840, xi, 266–269.—**Lynd** (C. A.) A curious case. Cincin. M. Repert., 1870, iii, 224–226.—**Maddox** (T. N.) History of a case of cerebral disease, attended with many uncommon lesions of sensation and volition. West. J. M. & Phys. Sc., Cincin., 1836, ix, 389–399.—**Maffoni** (A. C.) Storie di due singolari malattie nervose, precedute da considerazioni sulle neurosi in genere. Gior. d. sc. med., Torino, 1838, i, 170–199. — **Magendie.** Histoire d'une maladie singulière du système nerveux. J. de physiol. expér., Par., 1822, ii, 99–104.—**Maragliano.** Una rara forma di neurosi. Atti Cong. gen. d. Ass. med. ital. 1882, Modena, 1883, x, 119–122.—**Marchal.** Névropathie indéterminée de l'appareil laryngo-pharyngien, consécutive à l'ablation d'une tumeur ganglionnaire de la région sous-maxillaire. Rec. de mém. de méd. . . . mil., Par., 1852, 2. s., ix, 295–299.—**Marcus.** Seltne Formen von Neurosen. Wchnschr. f. d. ges. Heilk., Berl., 1848, xvi, 527.—**Mareska.** Contractions musculaires. [Épidémie dans la prison.] Bull. Soc. de méd. de Gand, 1846, xii, 65–67.—**Matousek** (J.) Eine eigenthümliche Neurose. Wien. med. Presse, 1876, xvii. 1381. — **Mauthner** (L.) Beobachtung über eine höchst merkwürdige Neurose an einem chlorotischen Mädchen. Ibid., 1865, vi, 286.—

Nervous system (*Diseases of, Anomalous or unusual*).

Meigs (C. D.) A case of singular affection of the nervous system. N. Am. M. & S. J., Phila., 1830, x, 371–378.—**Mental** embarrassment in orthography, as experienced by the relator. from his childhood to the twenty-fifth year of his age. Am. J. Insan., Utica, N. Y., 1850–51, vii, 73–75. — **Mérier.** Réflexions sur une affection nerveuse complexe et difficile à caractériser. Ann. méd.-psych., Par., 1848, xii, 192–223. — **Meugy** fils. Histoire d'une névrose fort extraordinaire qui s'est terminée par la mort. Ibid., 1849, xiii, 498–514.—**Mitchell** (J.) Instance of spasmodic affection of the tongue and mouth, successfully treated. [From diseased teeth.] Med.-Chir. Tr., Lond., 1813, iv, 25–34.—**Mitchell** (S. W.) On a rare vasomotor neurosis of the extremities, and on the maladies with which it may be confounded. Am. J. M. Sc., Phila., 1878, n. s., cli, 17–36. ——. Spasmodic disorders of the legs. Med. Rec., N. Y., 1879, xv, 601–605.—**Moll.** Merkwürdige Nervenkrankheit. Gen.-Ber. d. k. rhein. Med.-Coll. 1834, Koblenz, 1837, 88. — **Motet.** Névroses extraordinaires. Ann. méd.-psych., Par., 1861, 3. s., vii, 630–642.—**Müller** (P. L.) Ein halbseitiger Krampf. J. d. pract. Heilk., Berl., 1825, lxi (Supplhft.), 5-7.—**Nash.** Case resembling somnambulism. Assoc. M. J., Lond., 1855, ii, 1066.— **Packard** (J. H.) Case considered by several experienced practitioners to be purely hysterical, but which terminated in sudden death; autopsy. [With discussion.] Am. J. Obst., N. Y., 1879, xii, 634–637.—**del Papa** (G.) Molte e diverse afflizioni di corpo e di spirito in un signore giovane, di complessione calda e secca, solito ad essere quasi sempre intensamente applicato in gravissimi pensieri ed affari. In: Cons. med. di varii autori, 12°, Venezia, 1839, i, 178–186.—**Piollet.** Observation sur une irritation périodique des jambes. J. univ. d. sc. méd., Par., 1829, liii, 152–155.—**Piorry.** Cas très-extraordinaire de névropathie; prononciation involontaire et très-fréquente du mot "unque", alternant avec une toux quinteuse; emploi de l'électricité; guérison. Gaz. d. hôp., Par., 1856, xxiv, 343.—**Pole** (T.) An account of a remarkable spasmodic affection from the puncture of a pin, cured by the liberal use of laudanum, with antimonial wine. Mem. M. Soc. Lond. (1775–88), 1794, ii, 377–389—**Polydore** (A.) Remarkable case of oneirodynia. Med.-Chir. J. & Rev., Lond., 1817, iii, 89–93.—**Prati** (P.) Di una cronica e proteiforme nevrosi guarita dietro la comparsa di una febbre in forma reumatica. Ippocratico, Fano, 1863, 3. s., iii, 396–400.—**Putnam** (J. J.) Functional spasm. Boston M. & S. J., 1877, xcvii, 564. ——. Unilateral functional spasm. Ibid., 717.—**Quaglino** (A.) Storia di proteiforme nevrosi cerebrale a fondo epilettico. persistente da sei anni, e ribelle ad ogni medico trattamento. Gazz. med. ital. lomb., Milano, 1851, 3. s., ii, 109; 117; 125—**Ralfe.** Two cases of obscure nervous disorder. Lancet. Lond., 1880, ii, 693.— **von Ramm.** Seltsame Hitze der ganzen linken Hälfte des Körpers, nebst einem widernatürlichen Gefühle. Verm. Abhandl. . . . v. einer Gesellsch. pract. Aerzte zu St. Petersb., 1823, ii, 175–184. — **Raymond** (M. F.) Neurosis convulsiva y rítmica de forma tetánica en un hombre de 32 años. Escuela de med., México, 1883–4, v, 3; 20; 31.—**Reagan** (T. J.) A singular case of spasmodic affection. South. M. & S. J., Augusta, 1857, n. s., xiii, 11.—**Redding** (G.) Singular case of long continued spasm. Med. Times, Lond., 1844, ix, 124.—**Richter** (A. G.) Eine sonderbare Nervenkrankheit. In his: Med. u. chir. Bemerk., etc., 8°, Berl., 1813, ii, 121–134.—**Ridge** (J. J.) An uncommon form of local spasm. Brit. M. J., Lond., 1876, i, 595—**Robertson** (C. A.) A case of remarkable nervous perturbation. Tr. M. Soc. N. Y., Albany, 1873, 164.—**Robinson** (R. R.) Nervous affections; two curious cases. Lond. M. Gaz., 1830, vi, 299–302.—**Robouam.** Affection spasmodique des muscles thoraciques, diaphragme et des muscles abdominaux. Clin. d. hôp., Par., 1828–9, iii, 90.— **Rumsey** (J.) Case of a singular affection of the right leg, which, on extension of the limb, excited agonizing headache. Edinb. M. & S. J., 1812, viii, 192–195.—**Sabattier** fils. Lettre sur une maladie spasmodique extraordinaire. J. de méd., chir., pharm., etc., Par., 1760, xiii, 43–46.—**Samazeuilh** & **Landry** (O.) Note sur un état nerveux complexe attribué à tort à la congestion cérébrale. Monit. d. sc. méd. et pharm., Par., 1861, 2. s., iii, 145; 161.— **Saunier.** Quelques réflexions au sujet des contractures observées à la prison de St.-Bernard depuis 1846. Arch. belges de méd. mil., Brux., 1851, vii, 199–227.—**Say** (B.) A severe spasmodic affection, successfully treated. Mem. M. Soc. Lond. (1787–91), 1792, iii, 581–584.—**Schivardi** (P.) Nevrosi multiforme guarita colla elettricità, coadjuvata dalla idroterapia. Gazz. med. ital. lomb., Milano, 1868, 6. s., i, 325–327.—**Sealy** (J. H.) Observations on a peculiar nervous affection incidental to travellers in Sicily and Southern Italy. Dublin J. M. Sc., 1844, xxv, 287–295.—**Searle** (W. S.) The new nervous disease [sensations of convulsive shocks and of pressure in the occipital region]. N. Am. J. Homœop., N. Y., 1879–80, n. s., x, 385–408.—**Shattuck** (F. C.) A case of obscure nervous fatal disease. Boston M. & S. J., 1883, cviii, 460.—**Smith** (T.) A case of disordered nerve function in an infant. Tr. Clin.

Nervous system (Diseases of, Anomalous or unusual).

Soc. Lond., 1875, viii, 142–144. — **Solles.** Cas de névrose rare. [Discussion.] Mém. et bull. Soc. de méd. de Bordeaux, 1869, 202. — **Sourier** (E.) Cas remarquable de névrose. Gaz. d. hôp., Par., 1859, xxxii, 55. — **Spaltholz.** Merkwürdige Sympathie des linken Hodens mit einem Drüsen-Hals-Geschwüre. Mag. f. d. ges. Heilk., Berl., 1820, viii, 348–350. — **Strambio** (G.) Se la neurose cerebro-spinale, indicata dal Dott. A. Dubini co 'l nome di elettrica, si possa con lui considerare qual nuova forma di malattia, d' incognite origine, natura ed essenza? Gazz. med. ital. lomb., Milano, 1859, 4. s., iv, 293; 301; 308. — **Sturge.** On a case of rare vaso-motor disturbance in the leg. Med. Press & Circ., Lond., 1879, n. s., xxvii, 325. — **Tebaldi** (A.) Di una singolare forma di nevrosi. Gazz. med. ital. lomb., Milano, 1861, 4. s., vi, 439; 1862, 5. s., i, 4. — **Thirial.** Histoire pathologique d'un homme présentant des désordres nombreux et insolites dans les fonctions du système nerveux. J. d. conn. méd.-chir., Par., 1834-5, ii, 218 – 226. — **Thomsen** (R.) Ein Fall von tödtlicher mit anscheinenden Herdsymptomen sich combinirender Neuropsychose ohne anatomischen Befund. Arch. f. Psychiat., Berl., 1886, xvii, 844–863. — **Treluyer.** Coupd'œil sur les cas rares et extraordinaires en médecine, suivi d'une observation de ce genre. J. de la sect. de méd. Soc. Loire-Inf., Nantes, 1827, iii, 58 – 68. — **Trousseau.** Cas singulier de névrose. J. d. conn. méd.-chir., Par., 1841-2, ix, pt. 2, 17–19. *Also:* Ann. de méd. belge, Brux., 1842, i, 210. — **Turner** (W. M.) A question in diagnosis: a singular case. West. J. M., Indianap., 1868, iii, 745–749. — **Velazquez** (A. M.) Observacion de una nevrose visceral. Décadas de med. y cirug. práct., Madrid, 1828, xx, 125–128. — **Venturini** (E.) Storia di una antica e singolare neurosi [of the epigastrium] guarita coll' atropina. Bull. d. sc. med. di Bologna, 1854, 4. s., i, 321–328. — **von Vering** (J.) Seltener Nervenreitz, durch Ausschälung der schmerzenden Stelle gehoben. Med.-chir. Ztg., Salzb., 1819, iii, 238. — **Villaret** (de Toulon.) Névrose intermittente extrêmement rebelle, offrant des caractères extraordinaires, qui a cédé enfin à l'emploi du valérianate de quinine et de la saignée générale. Gaz. d. hôp., Par., 1852, xxv, 153–155. *Also:* Abeille méd., Par., 1852, ix, 115–119. — **Vizioli** (F.) Contribuzione allo studio di nevropatie rare e di oscura origine. Gior. di neuropatol., Napoli, 1882-3, i, 14; 77; 155; 316. — **Wacquez.** Affection nerveuse rare. Arch. méd. belges, Brux., 1876, 3. s., ix, 161. — **Wagner** (F. A.) Klettersucht, als eigenthümliches Nervenübel beobachtet Lit. Ann. d. ges. Heilk., Berl., 1829, xv, 411–415. ———. Actenmässiger Bericht und Gutachten über eine merkwürdige Nervenkranke, welche zu einer gerichtlichen Untersuchung Veranlassung gab. Arch. f. med. Erfahr., Berl., 1831, i, 244–274. — **Warren** (J. C.) Painful affection of the arm, caused by a fit of coughing. Boston M. & S. J., 1829-30, ii, pt. 1, 97. — **Wendling** (L.) Eine eigenthümliche Neurose. Wien. med. Presse, 1876, xvii, 1349–1351. — **Werniche** (A.) Ueber einige Formen nervöser Störungen bei den Japanern. Mitth. d. deutsch. Gesellsch. f. Nat.- u. Völkerk. Ostasiens, Yokohama, 1873–6, i, Hft. 10, 16 – 19. — **Wernicke** (C.) Ueber eine noch nicht bekannte Form schwerer Neurose. Deutsche med. Wchnschr., Berl., 1882, viii, 726. *Also:* Berl. klin. Wchnschr., 1883, xx, 148. *Also:* Verhandl. d. Berl. med. Gesellsch. (1882-3), 1884, xiv, 48–52. — **Westphal** (C.) Ueber eine Affection des Nervensystems nach Pocken und Typhus. Arch. f. Psychiat., Berl., 1871 – 2, iii, 376 – 406. — **White** (J. C.) Case of obscure nervous disease. Boston M. & S. J., 1855 – 6, liii, 387 – 389. — **Worden** (T. D.) A curious case of nervous disease. Med. & Surg. Reporter, Phila., 1884, l, 789. — **Zechmeister.** Eine seltene Commotio nervorum. Allg. Wien. med. Ztg., 1867, xii, 276. — **Zenker** (W.) Mittheilung über eine bisher nicht beschriebene Beschäftigungs-Neurose. Berl. klin. Wchnschr., 1883, xx, 628–631. — **Zúñiga** (A.) Descripcion de un caso raro de neurosis jeneral. Rev. méd. de Chile, Sant. de Chile, 1872–3, i, 349; 377. [*See, also, supra*, Candia (P.)]

Nervous system (Diseases of, Causes of).

See, also, **Eye** (Accommodation, etc., of, Disordered); **Genitals** (Irritation, etc., of); **Heatstroke**; **Hygiene** (Mental), etc.; **Insanity** (Causes of); **Lead-poisoning** affecting the nervous system; **Measles** (Complications, etc., of); **Nervous** system (Diseases of) of uterine origin, etc.; **Paralysis** (Reflex); **Phimosis**; **Prepuce** (Abnormities, etc., of); and under names of diseases.

BERTHIER (P.) Des névroses diathésiques, ou les maladies nerveuses dans leurs rapports avec le rhumatisme, la goutte, les dartres, la syphilis, le cancer, la scrofule, etc. 8°. *Paris,* 1875.

BUCHMANN (O.) * Die atmosphärische Nervenreizung tritt immer zugleich mit atmosphärischer Dunstbildung auf. 8°. *Halle,* [1859].

Nervous system (Diseases of, Causes of).

CALABRE (E.) * Sur l'influence de l'éducation, des habitudes et des passions dans les maladies nerveuses. 4°. *Paris, an XII* [1804].

CARTER (R. B.) On the influence of education and training in preventing diseases of the nervous system. 12°. *London,* 1855.

CAYRÉ (M.) * Considérations cliniques sur les névropathies goutteuses primitives. 4°. *Montpellier,* 1868.

CERISE. Des fonctions et des maladies nerveuses dans leurs rapports avec l'éducation sociale et privée, morale et physique. Essai d'un nouveau système de recherches physiologiques et pathologiques sur les rapports du physique et du moral. 8°. *Paris,* 1842.

DÉJERINE (J.) L'hérédité dans les maladies du système nerveux. 8°. *Paris,* 1886. *Also* [Abstr.], *in:* J. d. conn. méd. prat., Par., 1886, 3. s., viii, 201; 209.

DUBOIS (E.) * Importance de l'hygiène comme préservatif des affections nerveuses en général. 4°. *Strasbourg,* 1864.

ENGELHARDT. Zur Genese der nervösen Symptomencomplexe bei anatomischen Veränderungen in den Sexualorganen. 8°. *Stuttgart,* 1886.

HEGAR (A.) Der Zusammenhang der Geschlechtskrankheiten mit nervösen Leiden und über die Castration bei Neurosen. 8°. *Stuttgart,* 1885. *Also* [Rev.], *in:* Wien. med. Bl., 1885, viii, 705; 741; 777; 839 (W. Schlesinger).

HEINEKEN (J.) * De morbis nervorum, eorumque frequentissima ex abdomine origine. 4°. *Gottingæ,* [1783].

LABANOWSKI (L.) * De quelques cas de névroses consécutives à une lésion périphérique. 4°. *Paris,* 1879.

LANDRY (J.-B.-O.) Recherches sur les causes et les indications curatives des maladies nerveuses. 8°. *Paris,* 1855.

LE MONNIER (V.-A.) * Influence du travail et des impressions littéraires sur le développement des névroses. 4°. *Paris,* 1835.

LIEBESCHÜTZ (J.) * Die locale Verbreitung der Trophoneurosen. 8°. *Strasbourg,* 1883.

PRUNET (J.-G.-F.) Maladies nerveuses des auteurs, rapportées à l'irritation de l'encéphale, des nerfs cérébro-rachidiens et splanchniques, avec ou sans inflammation. 8°. *Paris,* 1826.

RAMBOSSON (J.) Propagation à distance des affections et des phénomènes nerveux expressifs. 8°. *Paris,* 1880.

ROUTH (C. H. F.) On overwork and premature mental decay; its treatment. 4. ed. 12°. *London,* 1886.

SCHRANZ (J.) Unsere Zeit und unsere Nerven. Ein Beitrag zur Pathologie der Menschheit. 8°. *Innsbruck,* 1884.

Althaus (J.) Contributions to the etiology of nervous diseases. Méd. Press & Circ., Lond., 1876, i, 375–377. — **Atkinson** (W. B.) Nervous symptoms probably due to irritation of worms. Coll. & Clin. Rec., Phila., 1887, viii, 113. — **Bartholow** (R.) Do the conditions of modern life favor specially the development of nervous diseases? Tr. Internat. M. Cong. 1876, Phila., 1877, 366–377. *Also:* Clinic, Cincin., 1877, xiii, 241–246. — **Bauer** (J. L.) Nervous affections of malarial origin. St. Louis Clin. Rec., 1879-80, vi, 263. — **Beard** (G. M.) The climatology of nervous diseases. Pub. Health, N. Y., 1879-80, i, 34. — **Berger** (O.) Zur Lehre von den Emotions-Neurosen. Deutsche Ztschr. f. prakt. Med., Leipz., 1877, 425; 437. — **Biondi** (A.) Contribuzione alla casistica delle malattie nervose. Riv. clin. e terap., Napoli, 1885, vii, 221–230. — **Bouchut** (E.) De la contagion nerveuse et de l'imitation dans leurs rapports avec la propagation des maladies nerveuses. Union méd., Par., 1862, 2. s., xiv, 307; 361. — **Browne** (J. C.) Circles of mental disorders; modern nervous diseases. Med. Times & Gaz., Lond., 1880, i, 231–237. *Also:* Lancet, Lond., 1880, ii, 292–295. — **Brown-Séquard.** Du transfert de l'anesthésie, de l'hyperesthésie, de la paralysie, de la contracture, de l'hypothermie et de l'hyperthermie, causées

Nervous *system* (*Diseases of, Causes of*).
par des lésions organiques. Compt. rend. Soc. de biol.,
Par., 1885, 8. s., ii, 246–249. — **Brunton** (T. L.) Reflex
action as a cause of disease and means of cure. Brain,
Lond., 1878, i, 143–154. — **Buck** (M.) Neuroz ot napraja-
jenija. [Neuroses from over-exertion.] Vrach, St. Petersb.,
1884, v, 102. — **Bullard** (W. N.) The relation of tea
drinking to disorders of the nervous system. Med. Communicat. Mass. M. Soc., Bost., 1887, xiv, 69–87. — **Caldwell** (J. J.) Some interesting reflex neuroses, with treatment and comments. Virginia M. Month., Richmond,
1885-6, xii, 71–83. *Also*, Reprint. — **Celotti** (F.) Contribuzione allo studio delle nevrosi reflesse. Gior. veneto di
sc. med., Venezia, 1877, 3. s, xxvi, 255 - 293. — **Centomo**
(L.) Dalle cause generali remote ed intime de' mali nervosi.
Ann. univ. di med., Milano, 1859, clxviii, 507 : 1859, clxix,
11.—**Cerise** (L.) Déterminer l'influence de l'éducation
physique et morale sur la production de la sur-excitation
du système nerveux et des maladies qui sont un effet consécutif de cette sur-excitation. Mém. Acad. de méd., Par.,
1840-41, ix, 277–446.—**Charcot.** Lecture on the influence
of traumatic lesions; (1) on the development of localised
hysterical phenomena; (2) on the development of paralysis agitans. Med. Times & Gaz., Lond., 1878, i, 471.—
Dabney (T. S.) Seven cases of reflex affections of
genito-urinary origin. N. Orl. M. & S. J., 1882-3, n. s., x,
759-765. — **Dana** (C. L.) On the relation of lithæmia,
oxaluria, and phosphaturia to nervous symptoms; with
a description of an apparatus for estimating the relative
amounts of phosphatic deposits and of uric acid in the
urine. Med. Rec., N. Y., 1886, xxix, 57 - 60. — **Éloy** (C.)
Du rôle de l'hérédité dans les névroses. Union méd., Par.,
1886, 3. s., xli, 697 ; 709.—**Eyselein.** Ueber den Einfluss
der Witterungsverhältnisse, speciell des Ozon auf das Befinden chronischer Nervenkranker. Tagebl. d. Versamml.
deutsch. Naturf. u. Aerzte, Magdeb., 1884, lvii, 360–365.
[Discussion], 367.—**Formento** (F.) Reflex action from
local irritation. N. Orl. M. & S. J., 1883-4, n. s., xi, 263-
269.—**Franz** (K.) Vasomotorische Neurose im Climac-
terium. Memorabilien, Heilbr., 1883, n. F., iii, 516–522.—
Garland (G. M.) Some cases of reflex neurosis. Boston
M. & S. J., 1886, cxiv, 25–27.—**Gee** (S.) Nervous disorders
affecting a whole family. St. Barth. Hosp. Rep., Lond.,
1884, xx, 12–14.—**Gradle** (H.) Nervous symptoms due to
overlooked anomalies of the eye and ear. J. Am. M. Ass.,
Chicago, 1885, iv, 497. *Also* : Chicago M. J. & Exam.,
1885, l, 430–437. — **Granville** (J. M.) Worry. [*From* :
Nineteenth Century.] Pop Sc. Month., N. Y., 1881–2, xx,
102–108.—**Gray** (L. C.) The effect of genital irritation in
the production of nervous disorders. Ann. Anat. & Surg.,
Brooklyn, 1882, v, 27 ; 78. *Also*, Reprint. — **Green** (T.)
Have organic nervous diseases their origin and frequency
in our American life? Phila. M. Times, 1876-7, vii, 340-
345. — **Gürtler** (G.) Ueber Veränderungen im Stoffwechsel unter dem Einfluss der Hypnose und bei der Paralysis agitans. Arch. f. Psychiat., Berl., 1883, xiv, 17–39.—
Hughes (C. H.) The hereditary neuroses spasmodica,
with illustrative cases. St. Louis M. & S. J., 1874, xi, 169-
185. *Also*, Reprint.—**Hughlings-Jackson.** On heredity in nervous diseases. Med. Times & Gaz., Lond., 1876,
ii, 701. — **Kempf** (E. J.) Some of the common causes of
nervous diseases. Med. Herald, Louisville, 1879–80, i, 533-
536.—**Layton** (T.) On the transmission and transformation of nervous diseases through heredity. N. Orl. M. &
S. J., 1882. n. s., x, 173–194.—**Lunz** (M.) Ueber die Affectionen des Nervensystems nach acuten infectiösen Processen. Arch. f. Psychiat., Berl., 1887, xviii, 882–894. —
Luys (J.) Des conditions somatiques de la surexcitation
nerveuse. Encéphale, Par., 1882, ii, 569–577. — **Meryon**
(E.) On the mode of propagation of nervous diseases.
Lancet, Lond., 1880, i, 85. — **Meyer** (M.) Ueber neuri-
tische Affectionen als Ursachen von Neurosen. Berl.
klin. Wchnschr., 1886, xxiii, 737–739. — **Möbius** (P. J.)
Ein Fall von congenitaler Motilitätsneurose. Arch. d.
Heilk., Leipz., 1878, xix, 187–192. ——. Ueber die here-
ditären Nervenkrankheiten. Samml. klin. Vortr., No.
171, Leipz., 1879 (Inn. Med., No. 57), 1505-1531. ——. Die
Erblichkeit der Nervosität. Memorabilien, Heilbr., 1881,
n. F., i, 459–462. ——. Ueber nervöse Familien. Allg.
Ztschr. f. Psychiat., etc., Berl., 1883, xl, 228 - 243. —
Mommsen (J.) Beitrag zur Kenntniss von den Erreg-
barkeitsveränderungen der Nerven durch verschiedene
Einflüsse, insbesondere durch "Gifte". Arch. f. path.
Anat., etc., Berl., 1881, lxxxiii, 243–288. — **Müller** (O.)
Ueber die dyscrasischen Momente, welche bei der Genese
der Neurosen und Psychosen eine Rolle spielen. Neurol.
Centralbl., Leipz., 1885, iii, 54 ; 78. *Also*: Cong. périod.
internat. d. sc. méd. Compt.-rend. 1884, Copenh., 1886, iii,
Sect. de psychiat. et névrol., 128–134.—**Noyes** (T. R.) Report on nervous diseases in the Oneida community. Med.
Gaz., N. Y., 1870, v, 253-258. — **Olvera** (J.) Discurso
sobre causas de las nevrosis en México. Observador méd.,
México, 1869-70, i, 49 ; 56. — **Overall** (G. W.) Cerebro-
spinal troubles the result of peripheral irritation. Mississippi Valley M. Month., Memphis, 1885, v, 298–302.—
Proll (F. M.) Ueber die erhöhte Reizbarkeit der Menschen in unserer Zeit. Oesterr. med. Wchnschr., Wien,
1846, 1279-1283.—**Ranney** (A. L.) The eye as a factor in

Nervous *system* (*Diseases of, Causes of*).
the causation of some common nervous symptoms, with
hints respecting the examination of that organ. N. York
M. J., 1886, xliii, 229 ; 285. ——. Eye strain in its relations to neurology. *Ibid*., 1887, xlv. 429-431. ——. Does
a relationship exist between anomalies of the visual apparatus and the so-called "neuropathic predisposition"?
[Abstr.] Med. Reg., Phila., 1887. ii, 485-491.—**Ransome**
(A.) On the course and effects of reflex nervous irritation.
Manchester M. & S. Rep., 1870, i, 27–34. — **Report** of the
preventable diseases of the industrial classes. Brit. M.
J., Lond., 1868, i, 59 ; 79 ; 203 ; 408. — **Rhett** (B.) Cases
of injury to the nervous system by the explosion of shell.
Am. J. M. Sc., Phila., 1873, n. s., lxv, 90–92. — **Ria** (G.)
Esaurimento nervoso da onanismo e da fulmine. *In his*:
Alcune lez. di clin. med., 8°, Napoli, 1884, 93–109. — **Ro-
driguez Pinilla** (H.) Las enfermedades reflejas.
Correo méd. castellano, Salamanca, 1885, ii, 19 ; 340.—**Rosenthal** (M.) Ueber Nervenaffektionen nach Gebrauch
von blei- oder quecksilberhältigen Schminken. Wien.
med. Presse, 1876, xvii, 671 ; 711 ; 741. — **Rumbold** (T.
F.) The effects of excesses on the mind of professional
and business men. St. Louis M. & S. J., 1885, xlviii, 193-
199. — **Semal** (F.) Des psycho-névroses dyscrasiques.
Mém. couron. Acad. roy. de méd. de Belg., Brux., 1882,
vii, 1–140.—**Singer.** Zur Pathologie der Erkrankungen
des Nervensystems nach Malaria. Prag. med. Wchnschr.,
1887, xii, 143 ; 153.—**Slaughter** (R. M.) Genital irritation as a cause of reflex nervous phenomena ; some cases
in point, one of singultus. Virginia M. Month., Richmond, 1886-7, xiii, 108–111. — **Smith** (D. T.) Reflex nervous influence, and its importance as a factor in the causation and cure of disease. N. Orl. M. & S. J., 1883-4, n.
s., xi, 253 - 263. — **Springthorpe** (J. W.) Climacteric
neuroses. Austral. M. J., Melbourne, 1886, viii, 193–199.—
Stevens (G. T.) Irritations arising from the visual apparatus considered as elements in the genesis of neuroses.
N. York M. J., 1887, xlv, 421–429.—**Strümpell** (A.) Ueber die Ursachen der Erkrankungen des Nervensystems.
Deutsches Arch. f. klin. Med., Leipz., 1884, xxxv, 1–17.
Also, Reprint.—**Sturges** (O.) The origin of some motor
disorders. Med. Times & Gaz., Lond., 1878, ii, 374 ; 455 ;
483 ; 567 ; 678 ; 704.—**Sundelin** (K.) Bemerkungen über
die Ursachen der Nervenkrankheiten. Arch. f med. Erfahr., Berl., 1830, i, 147–163.—**Talamon** (C.) Des lésions
du système nerveux central d'origine périphérique. Rev.
mens. de méd. et chir., Par., 1879, iii, 580 ; 660 ; 732 ;
835. — **Uspenski** (P. I.) O proischojdenii nervnich bolieznei (nevrozov). [The cause of nervous diseases (neuroses).] Trudi Obsh. Russk. vrach v S.-Peterb., 1884, i,
no. 1, 24–39. — **Weiss** (M.) Zur Therapie der Beschäfti-
gungs-Neurosen. Allg. Wien. med. Ztg., 1885, xxx, 550 ;
561 ; 574. — **Westphal.** Einige Fälle von Erkrankung
des Nervensystems nach Verletzung auf Eisenbahnen.
Charité-Ann. 1878, Berl., 1880, v, 379–394. — **Wilks** (S.)
Importance of discovering the origin of nervous diseases.
Guy's Hosp. Rep., Lond., 1872, 3. s., xvii, 208–210. —
Wohlrab (A.) Ueber Degenerationszeichen und hereditäre Neuropathien. Arch. d. Heilk., Leipz., 1871, 294-
319. — **Wythe** (J. H.) Diseases of modern civilization.
Pacific M. & S. J., San Fran., 1883-4, xxvi, 375-387.

Nervous *system* (*Diseases of, Diagnosis
and semeiology of*).

See, *also*, **Anæsthesia** ; **Brain** (*Diseases of,
Symptoms, etc., of*) ; **Convulsions** ; **Epilepsy**
(*Diagnosis, etc., of*) ; **Eye** (*Semeiology of*) ; **Insanity** (*Diagnosis, etc., of*) ; **Locomotion** (*Disordered*) ; **Nails** (*Semeiology of*) ; **Nerve** (*Optic,
Pathology of*) [*etc.*] ; **Ophthalmoscopy** ; **Paralysis** (*Diagnosis, etc., of*) ; **Reflexes** ; **Skin**
(*Diseases of, Neurotic*) ; **Speech** (*Disordered,
etc.*) ; **Spinal cord** (*Diseases of, Diagnosis, etc.,
of*) ; **Tremor.**

ARNOZAN (X.) * Des lésions trophiques consécutives aux maladies du système nerveux.
4°. *Paris*, 1880.

BOUCHUT (H.) * Études d'ophthalmoscopie
dans la méningite et dans les maladies cérébro-
spinales. 4°. *Paris*, 1884.

BOURNEVILLE. Études cliniques et thermométriques sur les maladies du système nerveux.
8°. *Paris*, 1873.

BURCKHARDT (G.) Die physiologische Diagnostik der Nervenkrankheiten. Versuch einer
Feststellung der Leitungs- und Zuckungsver-
hältnisse im Nervensysteme des gesunden und
kranken Menschen. 8°. *Leipzig*, 1875.

BUROT (P.-F.) * Des phénomènes réflexes
considérés au point de vue du diagnostic, dans

Nervous system (*Diseases of, Diagnosis and semeiology of*).

les maladies du système nerveux. 4°. *Paris*, 1872.

CHARCOT (J.-M.) Leçons sur les localisations dans les maladies du cerveau et de la moelle épinière faites à la Faculté de médecine de Paris. 8°. *Paris*, 1876–80.

———. The same. Transl. and edited by W. B. Hadden. 8°. *London*, 1883.

COLANÉRI (F.) * Des secousses musculaires; étude critique et séméiologique. 4°. *Paris*, 1884.

GEFFRIER (P.) * Étude sur les troubles de la miction dans les maladies du système nerveux. 4°. *Paris*, 1884.

GOWERS (W. R.) Diagnosis of diseases of the brain and of the spinal cord. 8°. *New York*, 1885.

GRENIER (R.) * Des localisations dans les maladies nerveuses sans lésions appréciables. (Essai de localisation du processus morbide dans les névroses.) 8°. *Paris*, 1886.

HALL (M.) On the threatenings of apoplexy and paralysis; inorganic epilepsy; spinal syncope; hidden seizures; the resultant mania; etc. 8°. *London*, 1851.

LEBLOND (L.) * De la néfrozymase dans les affections des centres nerveux. 4°. *Montpellier*, 1865.

LEROUX (L.-H.) * De l'albuminurie dans ses relations avec les affections nerveuses. 4°. *Paris*, 1867.

[LIÉGEY (N.-F.)] Névroses fébriles. Cas remarquable de névropathie; amaurose et ophthalmorrhagie par cause névralgique. 8°. [*Strasbourg*, 1858.]

MARCÉ (L.-V.) * Des altérations de la sensibilité. 8°. *Paris*, 1860.

MELCHERT (H.) * Beitrag zur Diagnose der subacuten Poliomyelitis und multiplen degenerativen Neuritis. 8°. *Greifswald*, 1881.

MENDELSSOHN (M.) * Untersuchungen über die Muskelzuckung bei Erkrankungen des Nerven- und Muskel-Systems. 8°. *Dorpat*, 1884.

MICHEL (H.) Contribution à l'étude des albuminuries transitoires dans quelques maladies du système nerveux. 1. 8°. *Paris*, 1885.

MOEBIUS (P. J.) Allgemeine Diagnostik der Nervenkrankheiten. ⌐°. *Leipzig*, 1886.

Also, transl. in: Ejem. jour. prakt. med., St. Petersb., 1886, ii, 1–360.

MONTAULT (J.-J.-H.) * Des moyens à l'aide desquels on peut distinguer les névroses des lésions dites organiques. 8°. *Paris*, 1838.

PALÉOLOGUE (J.) * Diagnostic différentiel des névroses et particulièrement de l'hystérie et de l'épilepsie. 4°. *Paris*, 1845.

REYNOLDS (J. R.) Diagnosis of diseases of the brain, spinal cord, nerves, and their appendages. 8°. *London*, 1855.

ROSENBACH (P. J.) Osnovy diagnostiki nervnych bolieznei. Rukovodstvo dlja studentov i vrachei. [Elements of diagnosis of nervous diseases. Manual for students and physicians.] 8°. *St. Petersburg*, 1887.

SCHULTZE (A. A. O.) * Symbolæ ad quæstionem quemadmodum topæsthesia sensusque temperaturæ in morbis nervorum se habeant. sm. 8°. *Berolini*, [1867].

SUCKLING (C. W.) On the diagnosis of diseases of the brain, spinal cord, and nerves. 8°. *London*, 1887.

Amidon (R. W.) The myography of nerve degeneration in animals and man. Arch. Med., N. Y., 1882, viii, 1–23.—**Baget** (F.) Neuropatia proteiforme. Rév. de cien. méd., Barcel., 1878, iv, 105–130.—**Basile** (G.) Importanza della resistenza elettrica in varie malattie

Nervous system (*Diseases of, Diagnosis and semeiology of*).

nervose per la diagnosi delle stesse e per gli effetti medicolegali. Gior. di neuropatol., Napoli, 1885, iii, 343–365.—**Beard** (G. M.) Morbid fear as a symptom of nervous disease. J. Nerv. & Ment. Dis., Chicago, 1879. n. s., iv, 693–697. *Also:* Hosp. Gaz., N. Y., 1879, vi, 305–308. *Also*, Reprint.—**Benedikt** (M.) Die topographisch-diagnostischen Gesetze bei chronischen Nervenkrankheiten. Allg. Wien. med. Ztg., 1874, xix, 2; 9; 17.—**Bernal** (M.) Génesis de las perturbaciones tróficas determinadas por el sistema nervioso. Rev. de med. y cirug. práct., Madrid, 1882, xi, 289; 348; 441; 489; 547: 1883, xii, 5; 49; 105.—**Bianchi** (L.) Le andature (cammino); studio semiotico per le malattie nervose e mentali. Gior. internaz. d. sc. med., Napoli, 1885, n. s., vii, 17; 89. — **Bigelow** (H. R.) Recent advances in the diagnosis of diseases of the nervous system. Detroit Rev. Med. & Pharm., 1874, ix, 259; 334. *Also*, Reprint.—**Bonnemaison.** Des eschares dans les maladies des centres nerveux. Gaz. méd.-chir. de Toulouse, 1873, v, 185; 193. *Also, in his:* Essais de clin. méd., 8°, Toulouse, 1874, 123–142. — **Boucaud.** Étude sur quelques points de séméiologie des maladies nerveuses. Ann. Soc. de méd. de Lyon, 1876, 2. s., xxiv, 127–137. *Also:* Lyon méd., 1876, xxii, 403–412.—**Bouchut.** Diagnostic de la méningite et des maladies cérébro-spinales par l'ophthalmoscope. Paris méd., 1883, viii, 97; 109; 121.—**Browning** (J. B.) The eye as a means of diagnosis in nervous diseases. Med. Index, Kansas City, 1884, v, 285–287.—**Bufalini** (L.) I fosfati delle urine nei malati di nevrosi accessionadi. Gior. internaz. d. sc. med., Napoli, 1881, n. s., iii, 1327–1338.—**Bull** (E.) Om en eiendommelig Flexionskontraktur i Knæleddene ved Hjernesygdomme; Tumor cerebelli; Trombose i venstre Sinus transversus. Norsk Mag. f. Lægevidensk., Christiania, 1885, xv, 469–483.—**Byford** (H. T.) Nervous paroxysm. J. Am. M. Ass., Chicago, 1885, v, 566–569.—**Charcot.** Diagnostic différentiel des affections cérébrospinales multiloculaires. Gaz. d. hôp., Par., 1878, li, 116.—**Cornwell** (H. G.) On the value of alterations in the size of the pupil as a symptom of disease of the nervous system. Columbus M. J., 1883–4, ii, 295–299. ———. On affections of the eye-muscles in diseases of the brain and spinal cord. Am. J. M. Sc., Phila., 1884, n. s, lxxxvii, 338–349.—**De-Giovanni** (A.) Contribuzione alla casuistica delle trofo-nevrosi. Gazz. med. ital., prov. venete, Padova, 1881, xxiv, 139; 154; 202; 239. — **Deighton.** Alarming symptoms occurring during the willing game. Lancet, Lond., 1884, ii, 637.—**De Vincentiis** (V.) Un caso di malattia nervosa di difficile diagnosi. Boll. d. clin., Napoli, 1884, i, 285–287.—**Dickson** (S. H.) On certain morbid conditions of the sensorial system. Richmond M. J., 1867, iii, 97–144. *Also*, Reprint.—**Dowse** (T. S.) On some points in the differential diagnosis of intracranial disease, general paralysis of the insane, and tabes dorsalis. Brit. M. J., Lond., 1882, i, 731; 769.—**Duchenne.** Impotence fonctionnelle et spasme fonctionnel du long péronier latéral. Arch. gén. de méd., Par., 1872, 6. s., xix, 385; 520: 6. s., xx, 11.—**Dupuy** (E.) Altération de la sensibilité à la suite de lésions des centres appelés psychomoteurs. Compt. rend. Soc. de biol., Par., 1886, 8. s., iii, 465–467.—**Duterque** (C.) De l'emploi de l'ophthalmoscope dans les maladies du système cérébro-spinal. Bull. Soc. méd. de l'Yonne 1879. Auxerre, 188), xx, 13–49.—**Engelskjön** (C.) Die ungleichartige therapeutische Wirkungsweise der zwei elektrischen Stromesarten und die elektrodiagnostische Gesichtsfelduntersuchung. Arch. f. Psychiat., Berl., 1884, xv, 136–139.—**Erb** (W.) Ueber Verlangsamung der Empfindungsleitung bei peripheren Nervenläsionen. Neurol. Centralbl., Leipz., 1883, ii, 1–4.—**Erlenmeyer** (A.) Ueber statische Reflexkrämpfe. Bull. Soc. de méd. ment. de Belg., Gand et Leipz., 1886, no. 40, 84–89.—**Eskridge** (J. T.) Diagnosis of diseases of the nervous system. Med. Bull., Phila., 1885, vii, 102; 133; 169.—**Eulenburg** (A.) Sphygmographische Untersuchungsergebnisse bei Krankheiten der Nervencentra. Berl. klin. Wchnschr., 1868, v, 291; 303. ———. Ueber das Verhalten erkrankter (degenerirter) Nerven und Muskeln gegen magnetelektrische Ströme. Neurol. Centralbl., Leipz., 1884, iii, 49–54.—**Féré** (C.) Névropathie et dynamogénie. Compt. rend. Soc. de biol., Par., 1885, 8. s., ii, 242–244. ———. Nerve troubles as foreshadowed in the child. Brain, Lond., 1885–6, viii, 230–238.—**Féré** (C.) & **Quermonne** (L.) Notes sur les vergetures de la peau rencontrées chez des névropathes. Progrès méd., Par., 1881, ix, 837.—**Finkelstein** (L. O.) O razstroistvach zrienija i drugich spetsijal. chuvstve pri niekotor. zaboliev. nervnoi sistemi. [Derangement of sight and other internal senses, especially in some affections of the nervous system.] Vrach, St. Petersb., 1886, vii, 1–7.—**Finlayson** (J.) Symptoms of disorder in the nervous system. *In his:* Clin. Diagnosis, 8°, Phila., 1878, 166–206.—**Forget** (C.) Recherches cliniques sur le degré de certitude du diagnostic dans les maladies de l'appareil cérébrospinal. Gaz. méd. de Par., 1838. 2. s., vi, 753; 785. *Also:* Ann. de méd. belge, Brux., 1839, i, 33–55.—**Friedlieb** (E.) Merkwürdige Fälle von Neurosen, nebst semioti-

Nervous *system (Diseases of, Diagnosis and semeiology of).*

schen Bemerkungen. Med. Cor.-Bl. rhein. u. westfäl. Aerzte, Bonn, 1845, iv, 104; 163. — **Gerhard** (G. S.) Tremor as a symptom of nervous disease. Med. & Surg. Reporter, Phila., 1877, xxxvi, 537-540.—**Grandclément.** Crises nerveuses de nature douteuse. Soc. d. sc. méd. de Gannat. Compt. rend., 1861, xv, 67-71.— **Hall** (F. de H.) Neuromimesis. Westminst. Hosp. Rep., Lond., 1885, i, 124-127.—**Hall** (M.) On certain points in the diagnosis of the diseases of the nervous system. Lond. J. M., 1849, i, 610-614.—**Hamilton** (A. McL.) Trembling and loss of co-ordinating motor power, as symptoms of nervous disease. Am. J. M. Sc., Phila., 1874, n. s., lxviii, 352-359. ——. A note upon the "crisogenic" significance of certain cutaneous eruptions in nervous disease. Arch. Dermat., Phila., 1879, v, 225-227.—**Hammond** (W. A.) The odor of the human body as developed by certain affections of the nervous system. Tr. Am. Neurol. Ass., N. Y., 1876-7, ii, 17-23. *Also, in his:* Neurol. Contrib., 8°, N. Y., 1877, 3-9. *Also, transl.:* Gior. internaz. d. sc. med., Napoli, 1883, n. s., v, 193-197. ——. On a hitherto undescribed form of muscular incoördination. Tr. Am. Neurol. Ass., N. Y., 1876-7, ii, 154-159. *Also, in his:* Neurol. Contrib., 8°, N. Y., 1877, 11-15.—**Heer.** Paralysis agitans oder ein anderes Nervenleiden? Vrtljschr. f. gerichtl. Med., Berl., 1884, n. F., xl, 285-290.—**Hinze** (V.) Ueber gewisse, bei Nervenkrankheiten vorkommende Reflexerscheinungen. St. Petersb. med. Wchnschr., 1876, i, No. 35, 1-3.—**Hirt** (L.) Das Hospiz "la Salpêtrière" in Paris und die Charcot'sche Klinik für Nervenkrankheiten. Breslau. aerztl. Ztschr., 1883, v, 89-93.—**Hoffmann** (H.) Stereognostische Versuche, angestellt zur Ermittlung der Elemente des Gefühlssinns, aus denen die Vorstellungen der Körper im Raume gebildet werden. Deutsches Arch. f. klin. Med., Leipz., 1884, xxxv, 529: 1885, xxxvi, 130; 398.—**Hughes** (C. H.) Note on the essential psychic signs of general functional neuratrophia or neurasthenia. Tr. M. Ass. Missouri, St. Louis, 1882, xxv, 115-122. *Also:* Alienist & Neurol., St. Louis, 1882, iii, 411-418. *Also,* Reprint.—**Jackson** (E.) Some eye symptoms in nervous diseases. Practitioner, Lancaster, 1883, i, 85-88.—**Jackson** (J. H.) Observations on defects of sight in diseases of the nervous system. [24 cases.] Ophth. Hosp. Rep., Lond., 1863-5, iv, 389: 1865-6, v, 51; 251. ——. Defects of sight in diseases of the nervous system. Med. Times & Gaz., Lond., 1864, i, 480-482. ——. Nervous symptoms in cases of congenital syphilis. J. Ment. Sc., Lond., 1875, xx, 517-527. ——. Ophthalmology and diseases of the nervous system. Lancet, Lond., 1885, ii, 935-938.—**Jacob** (E. H.) Cases of nervous disease, with ophthalmoscopic phenomena. *Ibid.*, 1880, i, 168; 206; 328; 365; 446; 489.—**Joffroy** (A.) De la trépidation épileptoïde du membre inférieur dans certaines maladies nerveuses. Compt. rend. Soc. de biol., Par., 1875, 6. s., ii, 61-71.—**Jones** (J. W.) † Difficulty and importance of correct diagnosis, and especially in certain nervous affections. Atlanta M. & S. J., 1855-6, i, 455-458.—**King** (T. W.) On aura epileptica and other disorders of sensitive brain tracts. Med. Times, Lond., 1844-5, xi, 197.—**Lagardelle.** Lésions de la sensibilité générale. Gaz. hebd. d. sc. méd. de Bordeaux, 1880-81, i, 605-608.—**Langer.** Eine dem Bilde der cerebrospinalen grauen Degeneration ähnliche Erkrankung des zentralen Nervensystems ohne anatomischen Befund. Wien. med. Presse, 1884, xxv, 698-700. — **Laurent.** Observation de névroses multiples avec symptômes épileptiformes prédominants. Bull. Soc. de méd. d'Anger (1868), 1869, n. s., lxxi, 51-60.—**Le Bon** (G.) & **Noel** (G.) Sur la durée du temps qui sépare les excitations des réactions; nouveau moyen de diagnostic des affections du système nerveux; appareils enregistreurs. Bull. Soc. de méd. prat de Par. (1878), 1879, 145-150. *Also:* France méd., Par., 1878, xxv, 806.—**Le Gendre.** Exemple de l'intolérance des névropathes pour les médicaments (ataxie thérapeutique des hystériques). Bull. Soc. clin. de Par. (1883), 1884, vii, 67-70. — **Leichtenstern.** Ueber Tastsinnsprüfungen bei Nervenkrankheiten. Arch. f. Psychiat., Berl., 1878, ix, 166-169. — **Leloir** (H.) Trophonévroses. N. dict. de méd. et chir. prat., Par., 1884, xxxvi, 197-228. — **Lépine** (R.) Localisation of nerve disorders. [Rev.] Brit. & For. M.-Chir. Rev., Lond., 1876, lvii, 272-282. ——. Sur l'excrétion de l'acide phosphorique dans ses rapports avec divers états pathologiques du système nerveux central. Rev. mens. de méd. et chir., Par., 1880, iv, 163-168. — **Leyden** (E.) Verlangsamte motorische Leitung. Arch. f. path. Anat., etc., Berl., 1869, xlvi, 476-482.—**Liégey** (N.-F.) Névroses fébriles; altérations organiques de l'œil produites par la perturbation névralgique. Gaz. méd. de Strasb., 1857, xvii, 344-347. *Also,* Reprint. ——. Anasarque aiguë se développant sous l'influence d'accès névralgiques fébriles périodiques, dans lesquels le stade de sueur fait défaut; principale localisation du trouble nerveux vers le scrotum; tuméfaction considérable de cette partie; guérison par la médication quinique; crise sudorale remarquable chez un homme ayant déjà été atteint d'autres maladies névrosiques; réflexions et citations diverses à propos de cas. J. de méd., chir. et pharmacol.,

Nervous *system (Diseases of, Diagnosis and semeiology of).*

Brux., 1859, xxviii, 537-546. *Also,* Reprint.—**Lloyd** (J. H.) The electro-diagnosis of neuritis and anterior poliomyelitis. Polyclinic, Phila., 1886-7, iv, 211. *Also:* Phila. M. Times, 1886-7, xvii, 215. — **Love.** Cold extremities due to a vaso-motor neurosis. St. Louis M. & S. J., 1885, xlviii, 246-248.—**Luys** (J.) Obnubilation passagère de la conscience des choses du monde extérieur ayant duré plusieurs jours, chez un homme adulte continuant à vivre de la vie commune. Encéphale, Par., 1881, i, 251-256. ——. Des obsessions pathologiques dans leurs rapports avec l'activité automatique des éléments nerveux. *Ibid.*, 1883, iii, 20-61. — **McBride** (T. A.) Digiti mortui, dead fingers. Med. Rec., N. Y., 1878, xiii, 376.—**Mader.** Eigenthümliche centrale Respirationsneurose (Parese) combinirt mit Stimmbandlähmung; chronischer Verlauf, theilweise Besserung. Ber. d. k. k. Krankenanst. Rudolphstiftung in Wien (1883), 1884, 313. *Also:* Wien. med. Bl., 1885, viii, 329.—**Maragliano** (E.) Delle varie forme di acinesi e sul loro significato clinico. Salute: Italia med., Genova, 1881, 2. s., xv, 161-163.—**Massey** (G. B.) Report of a case of sudden loss of vision following anæsthesia of the fifth nerve, with remarks on the modifying effect of anæsthesia on the galvano-reactions of the special senses. J. Nerv. & Ment. Dis., N. Y., 1884, n. s., xi, 576-578.— **Mayet.** Des troubles de nutrition liés aux lésions périphériques du système nerveux. Lyon méd., 1885, xlix, 217; 254; 320. — **Mazzotti** (L.) Storia clinica e necroscopia di un uomo che presentò il fenomeno di andare all' indietro. Riv. clin. di Bologna, 1885, 3. s., v, 417-423.— **Mendel** (E.) Die Psychosen im Gefolge acuter somatischer Erkrankungen. Deutsche med. Wchnschr., Berl., 1881, vii, 261-266.—**Mendelssohn** (M.) Recherches cliniques sur la période d'excitation latente des muscles dans différentes maladies nerveuses. Arch. de physiol. norm. et path., Par., 1880, 2. s., vii, 193-225. ——. Recherches sur la courbe de secousse musculaire des différentes maladies du système neuro-musculaire. Compt. rend. Acad. d. sc., Par., 1883, xcvii. 112-114. — **Mercier** (C.) Inco-ordination. Brain, Lond., 1883-4, vi, 78-83.— **Miquel** (R.) Ueber ein neues Hülfsmittel zur Beurtheilung des Zustandes des Nervensystems. Arch. d. Ver. f. gemeinsch. Arb. z. Förd. d. wissensch. Heilk., Götting., 1854, i, 386-390.—**Möbius** (P. J.) Zur Berger'schen Parästhesie. Centralbl. f. Nervenh., Coblenz, 1880, iii, 17-19.—**Montagu** (C.) Neurosis grave simulando la tisis pulmonar. Rev. de cien. méd., Barcel., 1877, iii, 201-210.— **Morselli** (E.) Sulla dinamografia e sue applicazioni al diagnostico dei disordini motorii nelle malattie nervose. Riv. sper. di freniat., Reggio-Emilia, 1884, x, 265, 1 diag.: 1885, xi, 221.—**Morton** (T. G.) On the neurotic origin of club-foot, infantile paralysis, and lateral spinal curvature, and its relations to prognosis. Phila. M. Times, 1885-6, xvi, 1-3.—**Munk** (I.) Unwillkürlicher Reitbahngang als Symptom einer Basilarmeningitis, nebst kritischen Beiträgen zur Lehre von den Zwangsbewegungen; seltsamer Darmbefund. Arch. f. path. Anat., etc., Berl., 1875, lxiii, 518-539. — **Naumann** (M.) Bemerkungen über einige Symptome des Nervensystems. Arch. f. d. ges. Med. Jena, 1846, viii, 145-164.—**Nettleship** (E.) A case of slight and variable amblyopia with occasional diplopia; tremors, vertigo, thickness of speech, and weakness of legs; intolerance of tobacco and alcohol; slow advance of the symptoms: diagnosis; cerebro-spinal disseminated sclerosis. Ophth. Hosp. Rep., Lond., 1876-9, ix, 180-182.—**Obersteiner** (H.) jun. Ueber die prognostische Bedeutung der Körpertemperatur in Nervenkrankheiten. Mitth. d. Wien. med. Doct.-Coll., 1880, vi, 146; 157. ——. On allochiria; a peculiar sensory disorder. Brain, Lond., 1881-2, iv, 153-163.—**Ogle** (J. W.) The aphemetric compass; an instrument for measuring the degree of discriminative power, as regards contractile impressions, enjoyed by the skin and mucous membranes in certain affections of the nervous system. Arch. Med., Lond., 1857-9, i, 321-331. *Also,* Reprint. ——. Cases, mainly, of disease of the nervous system, in which the ophthalmoscope was used. Med. Times & Gaz., Lond., 1867, ii, 345; 560. ——. Illustrations of impairment of the power of intelligent language in connexion with disease of the nervous system. Lancet, Lond., 1870, ii, 112; 396.—**Ord** (W. M) On some disorders of nutrition related with affections of the nervous system. Brit. M. J., Lond., 1884, ii, 205-211. *Also,* Reprint. *Also:* Med. Rec., N. Y., 1884, xxvi, 203; 226.—**Orrego-Luco** (A.) Neurosis mímicas. Rev. méd. de Chile, Sant. de Chile, 1879, viii, 105-117.—**Ott** (I.) Retrograde and lateral movements with hypnotism. J. Nerv. & Ment. Dis., Chicago, 1879, vi, 291-294. *Also,* Reprint.—**Paget** (G. E.) Involuntary tendency to fall precipitately forwards. With remarks. Med. Times & Gaz., Lond., 1855, n. s., x, 178-180.—**Paget** (J.) Clinical lectures on the nervous mimicry of organic diseases. Lancet, Lond., 1873, ii, 511; 547; 619; 727; 763; 833. ——. On stammering with other organs than those of speech. *In his:* Clin. Lectures, 8°, Lond., 1875, 77-83. ——. Nervous mimicry. *Ibid.*, 172-251. — **Peyrot** (J.) Sur certains phénomènes réflexes. Soc. d. sc. méd. de Gannat. Compt. rend., Par., 1881,

Nervous *system (Diseases of, Diagnosis and semeiology of).*

xxxv, 88-90.—**Poole** (T. W.) Nerve paralysis and contraction of involuntary muscles. Alienist & Neurol., St. Louis, 1886, vii. 268-285.—**Rabaine.** Troubles trophiques variés de la main gauche (crevasses, maux perforants, arthropathies, etc.). J. de méd. de Bordeaux, 1884-5, xiv, 252-255.—**Railton** (T. C.) Notes of a case of involuntary muscular movements accompanied by coprolalia. Med. Chron., Manchester, 1886-7, iv, 24-29.—**Ranney** (A. L.) Practical hints regarding the methods of examination employed as aids in the diagnosis of nervous diseases. Med. Rec., N. Y., 1884, xxv, 309; 340; 400; 425; 685; 713.—**Raymond** & **Monnier.** Note pour servir à l'histoire des hémorrhagies et des œdèmes dans le cours des lésions des centres nerveux. Gaz. méd. de Par., 1882, 6. s., iv 199-201.—**Remak** (E.) Eine einfache elektrodiagnostische Methode quantitativer galvanischer Erregbarkeitsbestimmung. Neurol. Centralbl., Leipz., 1886, v, 295-299.—**Resano.** Las neurosis sintomáticas. Siglo méd., Madrid, 1873, xx, 418-420.—**Revillout** (V.) Les anesthésies apparentes et les sensations retardées dans les névroses. France méd., Par., 1885, ii, 1317-1319.—**Rieger.** Funktionelle und organische Nervenkrankheiten; ihre für den Praktiker wichtige Diagnose. Deutsche Med.-Ztg., Berl., 1885, vi, 789: 1886, vii, pt. 1, 185; 197.—**Rocha** (A.) Algumas considerações geraes sobre o diagnostico das molestias medullares. Coimbra med., 1882, ii. 49-52.—**Rockwell** (A. D.) Neurasthenia and lithæmia; their differential diagnosis. N. York M. J., 1888, xlvii, 180-183.—**Rosenbach.**(O.) Ein häufig vorkommendes Symptom der Neurasthenie. Centralbl. f. Nervenh., Leipz., 1886, ix, 513-516.—**Rosenbach** (P.) Zur Lehre von der Innervation der Ausdrucksbewegungen. Neurol. Centralbl., Leipz., 1886, v, 241-246.—**Rosse** (I. C.) Illustrations of error in the diagnosis of some nervous diseases. J. Nerv. & Ment. Dis., N. Y., 1887, xiv, 681-701. *Also,* Reprint.—**Rowland** (R.) Symptoms arising from nervous irritation. Lond. M. Gaz., 1849, n. s., viii, 546-548.—**Sandras.** Mémoire sur cette question: Les lésions des différentes parties de l'encéphale et de la moelle épinière peuvent-elles être distinguées par des signes spéciaux? J. gén. de méd., chir. et pharm., Par., 1829, cix, 338-387.—**Schech** (P.) Die sogenannten Reflexneurosen und ihre Beziehungen zu den Krankheiten der Nase und des Rachens. Aerztl. Int.-Bl., München, 1884, xxxi, 333-336.—**Schiff** (M.) Ueber die Anwendung des Polarisationsapparates in der pathologischen Anatomie der Nervencentren und über die Atalectasis medullæ spinalis. Arch. f. Psychiat., Berl., 1880, xi, 283-294.—**Schwarz** (J.) Ein Fall von Trophoneurose. Mitth. d. Ver. d. Aerzte in Nied.-Oest., Wien, 1882, viii, 63-66.—**Seguin** (E. C.) Hysterical symptoms in organic nervous affections. Arch. Electrol. & Neurol., N. Y., 1875, ii, 1-17. *Also,* Reprint. *Also, in his:* Op. min. [etc.], 8°, N. Y., 1884, 180-194. ——. Lectures on the localization of spinal and cerebral diseases. Med. Rec., N. Y., 1878, xiii, 321; 341; 421; 481; xiv. 101; 141; 301; 361. *Also, in his:* Op. min. [etc.], 8°, N. Y., 1884, 283-352. ——. On the early diagnosis of some organic diseases of the nervous system. Tr. M. Soc. N. Y., Syracuse, 1881, 276-290. *Also:* Med. Rec., N. Y., 1881, xix, 225-229. *Also,* Reprint. *Also, in his:* Op. min. [etc.], 8°, N. Y., 1884, 457-471. ——. Methods of diagnosis in diseases of the nervous system. Med. Rec., N. Y., 1881, xx, 617; 701. *Also:* Med. Press & Circ., Lond., 1882, n. s., xxxiv, 276; 299; 323. *Also, in his:* Op. min. [etc.], 8°, N. Y., 1884, 558-578. ——. General semeiology of diseases of the nervous system; data of diagnosis. Syst. Pract. M. (Pepper), Phila., 1886, v, 19-64. ——. The localization of lesions in the nervous system. *Ibid.,* 65-98.—**Senator** (H.) Zur Diagnostik der Herderkrankungen in der Brücke und dem verlängerten Mark. Arch. f. Psychiat., Berl., 1883, xiv, 643-668.—**Sharkey** (S. J.) The Gulstonian lectures on spasm in chronic nerve-disease. Brit. M. J., Lond., 1886, i, 531; 573; 636; 681. *Also:* Lancet, Lond., 1886, i, 531; 577; 623; 677; 726, 774. *Also,* Reprint.—**Smith** (R.) Transitory hemiopia and hemidysæsthesia. Med. Times & Gaz., Lond., 1876, ii, 676.—**Southey** (R.) Clinical lecture on the interdiagnosis of insensibility from various causes. Lancet, Lond., 1880, ii, 881.—**Stedman** (H. R.) Some of the mental aspects of nervous disease. Med. Communicat. Mass. M. Soc., Bost., 1882-5, xiii, 415-430. *Also:* Boston M. & S. J., 1885, cxiii, 123-127.—**Stevens** (A. H.) Remarks on the diagnosis of nervous diseases. Tr. M. Soc N. Y., Albany, 1847-9, vii,34-38. *Also:* N. York J. M., 1847, viii, 172-175.—**Stewart** (T. G.) On some cases of nervous disease attended by muscular twitching. Med. Times & Gaz., Lond., 1874, ii, 227; 357.—**Sturges.** Pyrexia with hyperæsthesia; rapid and extreme muscular wasting; motor paralysis of arms; partial recovery. Lancet, Lond., 1879, i. 627.—**Takács** (A.) Untersuchungen über die Verspätung der Empfindungsleitung. Arch. f. Psychiat., Berl., 1880, x, 527-533.—**Teissier** père. Des névroses viscérales dans les maladies cérébrospinales. Assoc. franç. pour l'avance. d. sc. Compt. rend. 1876, Par., 1877, v, 740-744.—**Thaon** (L.) De la fièvre dans quelques maladies chroniques des centres nerveux. Nice

Nervous *system (Diseases of, Diagnosis and semeiology of).*

méd., 1877, i, 265-268.—**Thomsen.** Ueber das Verhalten der allgemeinen und speciellen Sensibilität bei Krampfund Geisteskranken. Neurol. Centralbl., Leipz., 1884, iii, 31.—**Thomsen** (R.) & **Oppenheim** (H.) Ueber das Vorkommen und die Bedeutung der sensorischen Anästhesie bei Erkrankungen des centralen Nervensystems. Arch. f. Psychiat., Berl., 1884, xv, 559; 633.—**Vasileff** (A. V.) K kazuist. neuropatia cerebro-cardiaca. Russk. Med., St. Petersb., 1885, iii, 714-717.—**Verdós** (P.) Neurosis con determinacion digestiva y articular. Gac. méd. catal., Barcel., 1881, i, 102-105.—**Vetter** (A.) Ueber die Reflexe als diagnostisches Hilfsmittel bei schweren Erkrankungen des centralen Nervensystems. Samml. klin. Vortr., No. 261, Leipz.. 1885 (Inn. Med , No. 90), 2381-2428.—**Walton** (G. L.) Neglect of ear-symptoms in the diagnosis of diseases of the nervous system. J. Nerv. & Ment. Dis., N. Y., 1883, n. s., viii, 583-593. *Also,* Reprint.—**Warner** (F.) Visible muscular conditions as expressive of states of the brain and nerve centres. Brain, Lond., 1880-81, iii, 478: 1881-2, iv, 190. *Also,* Reprint. ——. Reflex nervous manifestations. Columbus M. J., 1884-5, iii, 16-21.

Nervous *system (Diseases of, Functional).*
See, also, **Hysteria**; **Neuralgia**; **Neurasthenia**; **Nostalgia.**

AXENFELD (A.) Traité des névroses. 2. éd., augmentée de 700 pages par H. Huchard. 8°. *Paris,* 1883.

BLOCHMANN (J. G.) * De morbis ex atonia cerebri nervorumque nascentibus. 4°. *Halæ Magdeb.,* [1708].

BOREL (V.) Untersuchungen über die allgemeinen Neurosen und den Nervosismus insbesondere. 8°. *Bern,* 1871.

——. Le nervosisme et les affections nerveuses fonctionnelles. Précédé de quelques considérations sur la constitution intime de l'être humain. 8°. *Paris,* 1873.

BOUCHUT (E.) De l'état nerveux aigu et chronique, ou nervosisme appelé névropathie aiguë cérébro-pneumo-gastrique; diathèse nerveuse; fièvre nerveuse; cachexie nerveuse; névropathie protéiforme; névrospasmie, et confondu avec les vapeurs, la surexcitabilité nerveuse, l'hystéricisme, l'hystérie, l'hypocondrie, l'anémie, la gastralgie, etc. 8°. *Paris,* 1860.

——. Du nervosisme aigu et chronique et des maladies nerveuses. 2. éd. 8°. *Paris,* 1877.

BROWN-SÉQUARD (C. E.) Lectures on the diagnosis and treatment of functional nervous affections. 8°. *Philadelphia,* 1868.

DESMARTIS (T.-P.) Du nervosisme. 8°. *Bordeaux,* 1859.

EULENBERG (A.) Lehrbuch der functionellen Nervenkrankheiten auf physiologischer Basis. 8°. *Berlin,* 1871.

GARFINKEL (S. H.) * Die Neurosen nach acuten Krankheiten. 8°. *Berlin,* 1869.

GULLY (J. M.) An exposition of the symptoms, essential nature, and treatment of neuropathy, or nervousness. 8°. *London,* 1837.

——. The same. 2. ed. 8°. *London,* 1841.

JONES (C. H.) Clinical observations on functional nervous disorders. 8°. *Philadelphia,* 1867.

——. Studies on functional nervous disorders. 2. ed. 8°. *London,* 1870.

VON KRAFFT-EBING (R.) Ueber Nervosität. 3. Aufl. 8°. *Graz,* 1884.

——. The same. 12°. *St. Petersburg,* 1885. Russian text.

LACLEF (J.-C.) * Sur la névropathie. 4°. *Paris,* 1837.

LEE (E.) A treatise on some nervous disorders; being chiefly intended to illustrate those varieties which simulate structural disease. 8°. *London,* 1833.

LOEWENTHAL (B.) * De neurosibus secundum diversas vitæ ætates. 4°. *Herbipoli,* 1824.

Nervous *system* (*Diseases of, Functional*).

Marié (I.) * Des névroses, ou des maladies nerveuses qui sont sous la dépendance d'altérations humorales. 4°. *Paris*, 1855.

Meurissé (J.-L.-A.) * Quelques considérations générales sur les névroses et sur la méthode réfrigérante. 4°. *Paris*, 1836.

Möbius (P. J.) Die Nervosität. 12°. *Leipzig*, 1882.

———. The same. 2. Aufl. 12°. *Leipzig*, 1885.

Pomme (P.) Traité des affections vaporeuses des deux sexes, ou maladies nerveuses, vulgairement appelées maux de nerfs. 6. éd. 3 v. 8°. *Paris, an VII* [1799]*-an XII* [1804].

Putzel (L.) A treatise on common forms of functional nervous diseases. 8°. *New York*, 1880.

Reich (E.) Studien zur Aetiologie der Nervosität bei den Frauen. 2. Ausg. 8°. *Neuwied u. Leipzig*, 1877.

Riadore (J. E.) A treatise on the irritation of the spinal nerves as the source of nervousness, indigestion, functional and organical derangements of the principal organs of the body, and on the modifying influence of temperament and habits of man over diseases, and their importance as regards conducting successfully the treatment of the latter; and on the therapeutic use of water. 8°. *London*, 1843.

Roux (L.-A.) * De l'état nerveux proprement dit. 4°. *Paris*, 1843.

de Steinen (J. C.) * De atonia nervorum morbisque inde oriundis. 4°. *Halæ Magdeb.*, [1749].

Stevens (G. T.) Functional nervous diseases, their causes and their treatment . . . With a supplement on the anomalies of refraction and accommodation of the eye and of the ocular muscles. 8°. *New York*, 1887.

Stromeyer (L.) Erfahrungen über Local-Neurosen. 8°. *Hannover*, 1873.

Tissot. An essay on the disorders of people of fashion. 8°. *London*, [1770].

Vilfeu (M.-V.) * Sur la prédominance nerveuse, ses effets et son traitement hygiénique ou curatif. 4°. *Paris*, 1835.

Viridet. Sur les vapeurs, qui nous arrivent. 12°. *Yverdon*, 1726.

von Weidenbach (C.) * Ueber den Status nervosus, nebst drei betreffenden Krankheitsgeschichten. 8°. *Würzburg*, 1835.

Weiser (M.) * De neurosibus in genere. 8°. *Landishuti*, [*n. d.*]

Alford (S. S.) Defective nerve-power as a primary cause of disease, with its special relation to dipsomania. Brit. M. J., Lond., 1881, i. 591-593.—**Ambrosoli** (C.) Su l' eccitabilità nervosa. Gazz. med. ital. lomb., Milano, 1856. 4. s., i, 371. ———. Ancora su l' eccitabilità nervosa. *Ibid.*, 441.—**Ancona** (V.) Intorno a due casi di nevropatie ribelli (tosse isterica e torcicollo spastico), seguiti da guarigione. Gazz. med. ital., prov. venete, Padova, 1882, xxv, 403-407. *Also*: Salute: Italia med., Genova, 1883, 2. s., xvii, 11-14. — **Barbier** (J.-B.-C.) Considérations générales sur les névroses. Gaz. méd. de Par., 1852, 3. s., vii, 460; 601.—**Beard** (G. M.) Cases of hysteria, neurasthenia, spinal irritation, and allied affections. Chicago J. Nerv. & Ment. Dis., 1874, i, 438-451. *Also*, Reprint. ———. American nervousness; its philosophy and treatment. Virginia M. Month., Richmond, 1879-80, vi, 253-276. *Also* [Abstr.]: Month. J. Sc., Lond., 1879, 3. s., i, 598-610.—**Benedikt.** Ueber die Lokalisationsgesetze bei chronischen zentralen Neurosen. Anz. d. k. k. Gesellsch. d. Aerzte in Wien, 1871, 94-102. *Also*: Wien. med. Presse 1871, xii, 695-700.—**Berton** (A.) Réflexions sur quelques névroses et en particulier sur la fièvre intermittente. J. d. conn. méd. prat., Par., 1837-8, v, 129-134.—**Bosia** (H.) Nouvelle doctrine des névroses. France méd., Par., 1860, vii, 315; 323; 331. — **Bouchut** (E.) De l'état nerveux dans sa forme aiguë et chronique. Bull. Acad. de méd., Par., 1837-8. xxiii, 980-983. [Rap. de Gibert], 1858-9, xxiv, 467; 501; 542; 568. ———. De la contagion des névroses. Union méd., Par., 1862, 2. s., xiv, 600-602. ———. Des névroses congestives de l'encéphale. Gaz. d. hôp., Par.,

Nervous *system* (*Diseases of, Functional*). 1869, xlii, 202; 205.—**Brown-Séquard** (C. E.) Recent advances of our knowledge in the diagnosis and treatment of functional nervous affections. Lancet, Lond., 1866, i, 1; 85; 139; 247.—**Burow** (A.) sen. Die Parese der animalen Nerven. Berl. klin. Wchnschr., 1871, viii, 600; 609; 621. — **Cagnetta** (T.) Neuropatia di conducibilità a forma istero-catalettica. Ann. clin. d. osp. incur., Napoli, 1878, n. s., iii, 102-107. — **Caldwell** (J. J.) Some interesting reflex neuroses, with treatment and comments. Virginia M. Month., Richmond, 1885-6, xii, 71-83. *Also*, Reprint.—**Castellarnau.** Nervosismo crónico, predominando las neuralgias y el marasmo nervioso; curación por la hidroterapia. Bol. de hidroterap., Barcel., 1885-6, i, 98.—**Cerise** (L.) Lettres sur les névroses. Union méd., Par., 1850, iv, 325; 337; 353; 1851, v, 17; 29; 57; 161; 189; 213; 237.—**Corning** (J. L.) Exhaustion of brain-energy. Med. Rec., N. Y., 1883, xxiii. 375. ———. On the nature of nervousness. Med. Gaz., N. Y., 1883, x, 553.—**Cummins** (W. J.) On neurotic diseases. Irish Hosp. Gaz., Dubl., 1874, ii, 91; 103. — **Dana** (C. L.) On the pathology and treatment of certain forms of nerve-weakness. Med. Rec., N. Y., 1883, xxiv, 57-62. — **Davis** (G. W.) Functional nervous troubles. Tr. M. Soc. Calif., Sacramento, 1878-9, 55-63. — **Demours.** Névrose. Dict. d. sc. méd., Par., 1819, xxxv, 557-587. — **Desguin** (V.) Sur le nervosisme de notre époque. Bull. Soc. de méd. ment. de Belg., Gand, 1885, no. 36, 13-22.—**Désormeaux.** Observation sur une affection nerveuse simulant une maladie organique des viscères abdominaux. N. Jour. de méd., chir., pharm., etc., Par., 1820, ix, 297-306.—**Dickson** (S. H.) On certain morbid conditions of the sensorial system. Richmond M. J., 1867, iii, 97 - 144. — **Discusion** sobre las neurosis. Siglo méd., Madrid, 1866, xiii, 282; 297.—**Dunn** (R.) Suspension of the mental faculties, of the powers of speech, and special senses, with the exception of sight and touch, occurring in a young woman, and continuing for many months, in consequence of her having accidentally fallen into a river, and been nearly drowned. Lancet, Lond., 1845, ii, 536; 588. *Also*, Reprint.—**Eyselein** (O.) Ueber Nervosität. Monatsbl. f. öff. Gsndhtspflg., Brnschwg., 1884, vii, 150-174.—**Fagge** (C. H.) Remarks on some of the paroxysmal neuroses. Guy's Hosp. Rep., Lond., 1876, 3. s., xxi, 375-411.—**Falciani** (A.) Nuove considerazioni pratiche su la natura e le cagioni delle nevrosi. Ann. univ. di med., Milano, 1859, clxviii, 325-332. — **Féré** (C.) La famille névropathique. Arch. de neurol., Par., 1884, vii, 1; 173.—**Forget** (C.) Recherches cliniques sur les névroses. Gaz. méd. de Par., 1847, 3. s., ii, 918; 942; 978.—**Fowler** (S. W.) Nervorum erethismus, or nervous debility. Cincin. Lancet & Obs., 1878, xxi, 107-119.—**Franck** (S.) "Nervös." Centralbl. f. Nervenh., Coblenz, 1880, iii, 321-325. — **Garland** (G. M.) Some cases of reflex neurosis. J. Am. M. Ass., Chicago, 1886, vi, 62-64.—**Giacich.** Contribuzione alla dottrina del nervosismo, considerato come momento eziologico nelle varie forme delle malattie nervose. Gazz. med. ital. prov. venete, Padova, 1881, xxiv, 345-348. — **Gibert.** Des névroses. Rev. méd. franç. et étrang., Par., 1840, i, 313-342. *Also*: Ann. de méd. belge, Brux., 1840, ii, 23-30.—**Gradowicz** (E.) Erethische Nervenschwäche, chronisches krankhaftes Gähnen, nebst darauf erfolgter nervöser Zahnfleischaffection. Med. Ztg. Russlands, St. Petersb., 1850, vii, 131.—**H.** Nervous irritability. West. J. M. & Phys. Sc., Cincin., 1837, x, 169-172.—**Harris** (S. J.) Functional nervous troubles, with cases. St. Louis M. & S. J., 1878, xxxiv, 280-289.—**Huet** (G. D. L.) Over functioneele neurosen. Nederl. Tijdschr. v. Geneesk., Amst., 1886, xxii, 53-70.—**Hughes** (C. H.) The hereditary neuroses spasmodica. St. Louis M. & S. J., 1874, n. s., xi, 169-185.— **Jewell** (J. S.) On certain forms of morbid nervous sensibility. Am. Clin. Lect., N. Y., 1876, ii, 23-40.—**Johnson** (G.) Lectures on some nervous disorders that result from overwork and mental anxiety. Lancet, Lond., 1875, ii, 85; 155.—**Jones** (C. H.) Contributions to the pathology and treatment of functional nervous disorders. *Ibid.*, 1867, i, 626; ii, 6.—**Kemp** (W. M.) Cases of nervous irritations. Maryland M. & S. J., Balt., 1842, ii, 284; 1843, iii, 4.—**Kent** (J. B.) Functional disorders of the nervous system. Proc. Connect. M. Soc., Hartford, 1880, n. s., ii, no. 1, 152-157. — **King** (C. P.) Neurosis; an interesting case for study and scientific investigation. Cincin. Lancet & Clinic, 1884, n. s., xii, 193.—**Kinney** (E. C.) [Nervousness.] Proc. Connect. M. Soc., Hartford, 1885, n. s., iii, no. 2, 24-46.—**Klaatsch.** Ueber Reflexneurosen nach Verletzungen. Wien. med. Wchnschr., 1857, vii, 3; 20. — **Langeveld** (A. P.) Functioneele stoornis van hersenen en ruggemerg. Nederl. Tijdschr. v. Geneesk., Amst., 1887, xxiii, 2. d., 81-86. — **Larauza.** De la névropathie et de son traitement aux thermes de Dax. Bordeaux méd., 1876, v, 229; 283. — **Laycock** (T.) Epidemic neuroses. Dublin M. Press, 1840, iv, 9. — **Lebert** (H.) Krankheiten der Innervation; Neurosen. Deutsche Klinik, Berl., 1855, vii, 266.— **Lecorché & Talamon** (C.) Névroses. *In their*: Études méd., 8°, Par., 1881, 538-557.—**Lerminier.** Névrose de l'appareil circulatoire. Gaz. d. hôp., Par., 1828-9, i, 365.—**Liégey.** Mémoire sur les névroses fébriles. J. de méd., chir. et pharmacol., Brux., 1853, xvi,

Nervous *system* (*Diseases of, Functional*).
11; 122; 217; 417; 533: xvii, 3; 101; 293; 414; 510: 1854,
xviii, 124; 414; 508.—**Luton** (A.) Névroses. N. dict.
de méd. et chir. prat., Par., 1877, xxiii, 803–859.—**Mader.**
Ueber aufsteigende und Reflex-Neurosen. Wien. med.
Bl., 1882, v, 1379; 1414; 1435; 1471; 1505; 1536; 1569.—
Mann (E. C.) Modern nervous diseases. South. Clinic,
Richmond, 1881, iv, 243–248.—**Meynert** (T.) Zum Verständniss der functionellen Nervenkrankheiten. Wien.
med. Bl., 1882, v, 481; 517. ———. Ueber functionellen
Nervenkrankheiten. Anz. d. k. k. Gesellsch. d. Aerzte in
Wien, 1882-3, 158–161. *Also :* Wien. med. Bl., 1883, vi,
437; 501; 563.—**Miliotti** (D.) Nervosismo. Gazz. med.
ital., prov. venete, Padova, 1881, xxiv, 231–233.—**Miquel**
(J.-F.) Sur les névroses. *In his :* Lettres méd. [etc.],
8°, Tours, 1867, 283–350.—**Moré y Bargit** (M. E.)
Un caso de nervosismo crónico. Rev. de cien. méd., Barcel., 1878, iv, 500; 541: 1879, v, 70. ———. Apuntes sobre
el nervosismo. Sentido catól., Barcel., 1879, i, 163; 262;
292: 1880, ii, 35; 321; 548.— **Petrone** (L. M.) Sulla
nevrosi agitante; nuova forma clinica. Gior. internaz. d.
sc. med., Napoli, 1880, ii, 1227–1235.—**Pidduck** (J.) On
the periodicity of neuroses. Lancet, Lond., 1845, i, 101: ii,
97.—**Piorry.** Mémoire sur la nature et le traitement de
plusieurs névroses, et sur l'analogie qui existe entre elles
et les névralgies. J. univ. et hebd. de méd. et chir. prat.,
Par., 1833, x, 300; 339; 371. ———. Théorie et traitement
des affections nerveuses (névroses); (névropallies). Gaz.
d. hôp., Par., 1859, xxxii, 82; 125; 253. — **Pollák** (L.)
Zur Frage der "Nervosität". Pest. med.-chir. Presse,
Budapest, 1880, xvi, 813; 829; 843.—**Provis.** Névrose;
catalepsie. Arch. méd. belges, Brux., 1886, 3. s., xxix,
93–99. — **Puccinotti.** Leçons sur les névroses. Ann.
méd. - psych., Par., 1845, v, 367: vi, 53. — **Pundschu.**
Ueber Reflex - Neurose. Offener Brief an Herrn Dr.
Klaatsch in Berlin. Wien. med. Wchnschr., 1858, viii,
149. — **Reinbold** (T.) Ueber die sogenannte Nervenschwäche. Hannov. Ann. f. d. ges. Heilk., 1845, n. F., v,
416–429.—**Reveillé-Parise** (J.-H.) Principes généraux
de thérapeutique, relatifs aux personnes éminemment nerveuses, comme les gens de lettres, les artistes, etc. Bull.
gén. de thérap., etc., Par., 1834, vi, 69–77. ———. Aperçu
des moyens propres à rétablir une constitution épuisée
chez les personnes éminemment nerveuses, comme les
gens de lettres, les artistes. *Ibid.*, 133; 165.—**Rey** (H.)
Névrose des branches nasales du ganglion sphéno-palatin. Gaz. méd. d'Orient, Constantinople, 1861-2, v, 42.—
Rockwell (A. D.) Functional nervous derangements
simulating structural disease of the heart, and the value
of electricity in their treatment. N. York M. J., 1879,
xxx, 133–141.—**Russell** (J.) On functional disorders of
the nervous system. Med. Times & Gaz., Lond., 1856, n. s.,
xii, 27; 53.—**Scarenzio** (A.) Alcune osservazioni su la
eccitabilità nervosa. Gazz. med. ital. lomb., Milano, 1856,
4. s., i, 440.—**Smoler.** Ueber nervöse Erscheinungen in
einzelnen Krankheiten. Oesterr. Ztschr. f. prakt. Heilk.,
Wien, 1864, x, 197; 240; 296; 361; 415; 455; 519; 561.—
Soltmann (O.) Die functionellen Nervenkrankheiten.
Handb. d. Kinderkr. (Gerhardt), Tübing., 1879, v, 1. Abth.,
1–332.—**Stevens** (C. W.) Functional neurosis of the radial nerve. Med. & Surg. Reporter, Phila., 1869, xx, 119.—
Torino. Las neurosis. Rev. méd.-quir., Buenos Aires,
1885-6, xxii, 52–59.—**Ullersperger** (J. B.) Die Neurosen in der Chirurgie und in der Medicin. Deutsche Klinik,
Berl., 1873, xxv, 63; 75.—**Uspenski** (P. I.) O nevrozach.
Vrach. Vaidom., St. Petersb., 1881, vi, 2088; 2090; 2120.—
Vallesi (G.) Il cloruro di bario nel nevrosismo. Imparziale, Firenze, 1869, ix, 179.—**Veitstanz,** Somnambulismus, Predigtsucht; eine Schulepidemie. Mitth. d. badisch. ärztl. Ver., Karlsruhe, 1853, vii, 41–54.—**Vigouroux** (R.) Note sur l'état nerveux ou nervosisme, et
l'utilité du bromure de potassium. Bull. gén. de thérap.,
etc., Par., 1864, lxvii, 202–209.—**Wilks** (S.) Remarks on
some of the functional diseases of the nervous system.
Guy's Hosp. Rep., Lond., 1866, 3. s., xii, 245–266.—**Wood**
(E. H.) Gangliasthenia. Michigan M. News, Detroit,
1881, iv, 104. *Also,* Reprint.

Nervous *system* (*Diseases of, Hospitals for*).

See, also, **Insane** (*Asylums for*).

ADAMS Nervine Asylum, Jamaica Plains,
Mass. The will of Seth Adams. 4°. [*Boston*,
1876.]

———. An act to incorporate the . . . Approved March 16, 1877. 8°. [*Boston*, 1877.]

———. By-laws and list of officers. Adopted
April 19, 1877. 4°. [*Boston*, 1877.]

———. Annual examinations of the supervisors. 2.–5., 1878-9 to 1881-2. 8°. [*Boston*,
1879-82.

———. List of officers, committees, and members of the corporation, 1880. 8°. [*Boston*,
1880.]

Nervous *system* (*Diseases of, Hospitals for*).

———. Proposed rules and regulations, to be
considered at a meeting of the managers to be
held Feb. 28, 1880. 8°. [*Boston*, 1880.]

———. Rules and regulations, adopted by the
managers Feb. 28, 1880. 8°. [*Boston*, 1880.]

———. Annual reports of the board of managers to the corporation. 5.–10., 1881-2 to
1886-7. 8°. *Boston*, 1883-7.

———. By-laws of the corporation and rules
of the managers, 1885. 8°. *Boston*, 1885.

ASYL für Gehirn- und Nervenkranke von Dr.
Erlenmeyer in Bendorf bei Coblenz. [Prospec-
tus.] 4°. [*Neuwied, n. d.*]

ASYL St. Gilgenberg. Heilanstalt für Nerven-
und Gemüthskranke zu Donndorf, bei Bayreuth.
Prospect. von A. Falco. 4°. [*Bayreuth*, 1863.]

CLIFTON Hall. Annual reports of the superintendent of Clifton Hall, a private hospital for
mental diseases, at Kellysville, Delaware County,
Pa., to the board of supervision. 2.–4., 1861-3.
8°. *Philadelphia*, 1862-4.

———. Burn Bræ. A private hospital for
nervous and mental diseases, Clifton Heights,
Delaware Co. [Circular of the superintendent,
R. A. Given, June, 188–.] 4°. [*Philadelphia*,
188–.]

DE QUINCEY Home, Fort Washington, New
York City. A private asylum for the treatment
of the opium, morphine, chloral, chloroform and
hashisch habits, for mild cases of insanity, and
nervous diseases and inebriety. [Circular of the
physicians in charge.] 4°. [*New York*, 1882.]

DISPENSARY for Nervous Diseases, Baltimore.
Annual report of the board of trustees. 4.,
1882-3. 8°. *Baltimore*, 1884.

ERLENMEYER (A. A.) Das Asyl mit seinen
beiden Gartenbau-Colonien für Gemüths- und
Nervenkranke zu Bendorf bei Coblenz. 8°.
Neuwied, 1867.

ERLENMEYER'SCHE (Dr.) Anstalten für Ge-
müths- und Nervenkranke zu Bendorf bei Coblenz. Bericht über die Einrichtung, Organisation und Leistungen derselben in dem Decennium 1. Januar 1871 bis 31. December 1880.
roy. 8°. *Leipzig*, 1881.

HEILANSTALT für Nervenkranke, Villa Emilia
bei Blankenburg in Thüringen. [Prospectus,
von Dr. Schwabe.] 8°. [*n. p., n. d.*]

HEIL- UND PFLEGE - ANSTALT für Gemüths
(Hirn)- und Nervenkranke zu Charlottenburg.
Prospekt des dirigirenden Arztes, C. Edel. 8°.
[*Berlin, n. d.*]

HEIL- UND PFLEGE - ANSTALT für Nerven-
Kranke zu Eitorf a. d. Sieg. [Prospekt und
Aufnahme-Bedingungen. Von A. Meyer.] 8°.
[*Eitorf*, 1876.]

HOSPITAL for Epilepsy and Paralysis and other
Diseases of the Nervous System. London. Annual reports of the committee of management.
4., 1870–71; 15., 1881; 16., 1882. 12°. *London*,
1871–83.

———. Classification of diseases. Consulting room. 12°. [*London*], 1883.

HOSPITAL for Nervous Diseases, Philadelphia.
[Notice by the medical director, M. Roche, of the
opening of the . . . with some of the reasons why
it was established. Also, the act of incorporation.] 4°. [*n. p., n. d.*]

KAHLBAUM (K.) Heil- und Pflege-Anstalt für
Nerven- und Gemüthskranke zu Görlitz. [Pros-
pectus, Oct. 1874.] 8°. [*Görlitz*, 1874.]

———. Programm zur Betheiligung der Heilanstalt für Nervenkranke zu Görlitz an der dies-
jährigen Hygiene-Ausstellung, nebst einigen Bemerkungen über die Entwicklung des Nerven-

Nervous system (*Diseases of, Hospitals for*).

Heilanstaltswesens in Deutschland und über Veranlassung und Zweck meiner Betheiligung an der Ausstellung. 8°. *Görlitz*, 1883.

KURHAUS für Nervenkranke in Pankow bei Berlin. Prospectus, von R. Gnauck. 4°. [*Berlin*, 1883.]

NATIONAL Hospital for the Paralysed and Epileptic, Queen Square, London. By-laws for the management of . . . 8°. *London*, 1864.

——. Annual reports of the board of management. 11.–13., 1870–72; 15., 1874; 16., 1875; 18., 1877; 19., 1878. 8°. *London*, 1871–9.

——. Privileges of governors and members, with rules for admission of patients and system of election. 8°. [*London, n. d.*]

NEW YORK State Hospital for Diseases of the Nervous System, New York City. Annual reports of the physicians in charge to the board of trustees. 1., 1870–71; 2., 1871–2. 8°. *New York*, 1871–2.

PENSION und Heilanstalt für Nervenleidende, Blankenburg am Harz. [Prospectus by Oskar Eyselein.] 8°. [*n. p., n. d.*]

WEST END Hospital for Diseases of the Nervous System, Paralysis, and Epilepsy. Annual reports of the committee. 1., 1878–9; 4., 1881–2; 5., 1882–3. 8°. *London*, 1879–83.

Erlenmeyer (F. A.) Bericht über die Heil-Anstalt für Nervenkranke zu Bendorf am Rhein, während der ersten 10 Jahre ihres Bestehens, vom 1. October 1866 bis 30. September 1876. Cor.-Bl. d. deutsch. Gesellsch. f. Psychiat., etc., Neuwied, 1877, xxiii, 17; 65; 113; 149. *Also,* Reprint.—**Friedenreich** (A.) Aarsberetning fra F. Lund's Pensionat for Sindssyge og Nervepatienter. Hosp.-Tid., Kjøbenh., 1887, 3. R., v. 56–60.—**Hecker.** Die Aufnahmebedingungen der sog. offenen Kuranstalten für Nervenkranke. Arch. f. Psychiat., Berl., 1887, xviii, 294–298.—**Holst & Brosius.** Ueber specielle Kuranstalten für Nervenkranke. Irrenfreund, Heilbr., 1882, xxiv, 1–6.—**Kuranstalten** Hejmdal i Norge. Ugesk. f. Læger, Kjøbenh., 1887, 4. R., xv, 255–260.—**Walther.** Die offenen Anstalten für Nervenkranke und Leicht-Verstimmte. Cor.-Bl. d. deutsch. Gesellsch. f. Psychiat., etc., Neuwied, 1874, xx, 49; 65; 81.

Nervous system (*Diseases of, Journals relating to*).

See **Neurology** (*Journals, etc., relating to*).

Nervous system (*Diseases of, Treatment of*).

See, also, **Electrotherapeutics**; **Metallotherapy.**

ALTHAUS (J.) On paralysis, neuralgia, and other affections of the nervous system; and their successful treatment by galvanism and faradisation. 3. ed. 12°. *London*, 1864.

ARTHUIS (A.) Traitement des maladies nerveuses et des affections rhumatismales par l'électricité statique. 12°. *Paris*, 1873.

BLOCH (A.) L'eau froide, ses propriétés et son emploi, principalement dans l'état nerveux. 12°. *Paris*, 1880.

——. The same. El agua fria, sus propiedades y su empleo principalmente en el estado nervioso. Version española por J. R. de Torres y Martinez. 8°. *Madrid*, 1881.

CERVELLERI (F.) De l'emploi de l'électromagnétisme dans les maladies des nerfs, et des différens procédés d'application des appareils électro-magnétiques à excitation, à courans graduels, et à soustraction dans le traitement des paralysies, de la sciatique, de l'amaurose, de l'épilepsie, et de plusieurs autres névroses, des plaies, et des tumeurs anciennes de différente nature, et en particulier de certaines tumeurs articulaires et scrofuleuses. 8°. *Naples*, 1840.

DE FOREST (L. S.) * Das ableitende Verfahren mittels Fontanelle oder Haarseil bei Erkrankungen des Central-Nervensystems. 8°. *Jena*, 1885.

Nervous system (*Diseases of, Treatment of*).

EYSELEIN (O.) Tisch für Nervenkranke. (Diätetische Behandlung der Nervenkrankheiten.) 8°. *Karlsbad*, 1883.

FECHNER (W.) Die Anwendung der Elektrizität in der Medizin bei Nervenleiden, Gehirn- und Rückenmarks-Krankheiten. 8°. *Berlin W.*, 1885.

HOLST (V.) Ueber die Bedeutung der Behandlung von Nervenkranken in besonderen Anstalten. 8°. *Riga*, 1880.

——. Die Behandlung der Hysterie, der Neurasthenie und ähnlicher allgemeiner functioneller Neurosen. 2. Aufl. 8°. *Stuttgart*, 1883.

HOOD (S.) Analytic physiology, treating of the cure of nervous diseases by external applications to the spine. 2. ed. 8°. *London*, 1829.

ISNARD (C.) Der therapeutische Gebrauch des Arseniks gegen die Krankheiten des Nervensystems. Aus dem Französischen übersetzt und mit Anmerkungen begleitet von C. J. Le Viseur. 8°. *Erlangen*, 1867.

KESTEVEN (W. B.) Remarks on the use of the bromides in the treatment of epilepsy and other neuroses. Read at the third quarterly meeting of the Medico-Psychological Association, April 29, 1869. 8°. *Lewes*, 1869.

KRAUSS (I. C.) Verhandeling over den aard en de werking der geneesmiddelen, welke ter bestrijding van zenuwkwalen en derzelver toevallen worden aangewend. Die met den gouden medaille van het legaat van I. Monnikhoff is bekroond. 8°. *Amsterdam*, 1819.

KRIEGLER (M.) Az elvesztett idegerönek visszapótlása. [Treatment of neurasthenia.] 8°. *Budapest*, 1875.

KRUSE (E.) Ueber Seeluft- und Seebadekuren bei Nervenkrankheiten. 2. Aufl. *Norden u. Norderney*, 1887.

LANGSTEIN (H.) Die Neurasthenie (Nervenschwäche) und ihre Behandlung in Teplitz-Schonau. 8°. *Wien*, 1886.

LEDRU (N. P.) Rapport de MM. Cosnier [et al.] sur les avantages reconnus de la nouvelle méthode d'administrer l'électricité dans les maladies nerveuses, particulièrement dans l'épilepsie, et dans la catalepsie, par M. Ledru, connu sous le nom de Comus. Ce rapport est précédé de l'aperçu du système de l'auteur sur l'agent qu'il emploie, et des avantages qu'il en a tirés. Imprimé par ordre et aux frais du gouvernement. 8°. *Paris*, 1783.

MITCHELL (S. W.) Fat and blood, and how to make them. 12°. *Philadelphia*, 1877.

——. The same. 2. ed. 12°. *Philadelphia*, 1879.

——. Lectures on diseases of the nervous system, especially in women. 8°. *Philadelphia*, 1881.

——. The same. 2. ed 8°. *Philadelphia*, 1885.

——. The same. An essay on the treatment of certain forms of neurasthenia and hysteria. 4. ed. 8°. *Philadelphia*, 1885.

——. The same. Du traitement méthodique de la neurasthénie et de quelques formes d'hystérie. Traduit par Oscar Jennings; avec une introduction par B. Ball. 8°. *Paris*, 1883. *Also* [Rev.]: Irrenfreund, Heilbr., 1886, xxviii, 129; 145; 161. *Also, transl.:* Psychiat. Bl., Dordrecht, 1886, iv, 215–222: Utrecht, 1887, v, 97–106.

NERFS (Les) et les eaux de Vichy; dosage dermoscopique; méthode du Dr. Collongues, médecin consultant à Vichy. 18°. *Paris*, [*n. d.*]

PADIOLEAU (A.) Von der moralischen Heilkunde bei der Behandlung von nervösen Krank-

Nervous system (*Diseases of, Treatment of*).

heiten. Ein von der kaiserlichen Akademie der Wissenschaften gekröntes Werk. Frei übersetzt und mit Anmerkungen und Zusätzen ausgestattet von Dr. Eisenmann. 8°. *Würzburg*, 1865.

PHOSPHORUS in functional disorders of the nervous system, induced by over-work and other influences incidental to modern life. With formulæ and treatment. 8°. *Philadelphia*, 1877.

——. The same. 8°. *Philadelphia*, 1878.

PHOSPHORUS as a remedy for loss of nerve power induced by overwork, etc. 16°. *New York & Philadelphia*, [n. d.]

REMAK (R.) Galvanotherapie der Nerven- und Muskelkrankheiten. 8°. *Berlin*, 1858.

——. The same. Galvanothérapie, ou de l'application du courant galvanique constant au traitement des maladies nerveuses et musculaires. Traduit de l'allemand par A. Morpain. Avec les additions de l'auteur. 8°. *Paris*, 1860.

RICHARD (R.) Die Regeneration des geschwächten Nervensystems, oder: gründliche Heilung aller Folgen der geheimen Jugendsünden und der Ausschweifung. Mit vielen Krankengeschichten erläutert und nach den neuesten Entdeckungen der Nervenphysiologie für Aerzte und Kranke bearbeitet. 11. Aufl. 8°. *Quedlinburg u. Leipzig*, 1883.

RYLEY (J. B.) Electro-magnetism and massage in the treatment of rheumatic gout, dyspepsia, sleeplessness, nerve prostration, and other chronic disorders. 12°. *London*, 1887.

SWAN (J.) A dissertation on the treatment of morbid local affections of nerves. [Jacksonian prize.] 8°. *London*, 1820.

——. The same. Gekrönte Preisschrift über die Behandlung der Localkrankheiten der Nervén, nebst dessen anatomisch-physiologisch-pathologischen Beobachtungen über das Nervensystem. Aus dem Englischen übersetzt und mit einigen Zusätzen hrsg. von Franz Francke. 8°. *Leipzig*, 1824.

TIBBITS (H.) Electrical and anatomical demonstrations delivered at the School of Massage and Electricity in connection with the West-End Hospital for Diseases of the Nervous System, Paralysis, and Epilepsy, Welbeck Street, London. A handbook for trained nurses and masseuses. 12°. *London*, 1887.

TISCHLER (A.) Die systematische Behandlung der Nervosität und Hysterie. Autorisirte deutsche Ausgabe. 8°. *Berlin*, 1883.

TRABY (V.) * Des indications du traitement hydro-minéral dans les maladies organiques cérébro-spinales. 4°. *Montpellier*, 1884.

VERHAEGHE (L.) Du traitement des maladies nerveuses par les bains de mer. 8°. *Bruxelles*, 1850.

ZAKŁAD wodoleczeniczy w Nowem Mieście nad Pilicą jako dom zdrowia dla chorych nerwowych. [Water-cure establishment at Nowe Miasto, on the river Pilica, as a health resort for nervous diseases.] 8°. *Warszawa*, 1886.

Suppl. to: Gaz. lek., Warszawa, 1886, 2. s., vi, no. 21.

Adamkiewicz. Leczenie nerwobólu za pomocąnowego sposobu znieczulenia miejscowego. [Treatment of nervous diseases by a new remedy, viz, local anæsthesia.] Przegl. lek., Krakow., 1886, xxv. 245-247.—**Arens.** De l'acupuncture dans certaines affections nerveuses spasmodiques. Arch. méd. belges, Brux., 1881, 3. s., xx, 380-387.—**Armendariz.** Las agnas de Solares en las neurosis. An. Soc. españ. de hidrol. méd., Madrid, 1883-4, v, 447; 469.—**Averbeck** (H.) Die psychologische Bedeutung der Heilgymnastik und Massage in der Behandlung gewisser Nerven-Leiden. Allg. Wien. med. Ztg., 1886, xxxi, 14; 26; 38.—**Baglietto** (M.) Aplicaciones de la electricidad al tratamiento de las enfermedades nerviosas. Gac. de sanid. mil., Madrid, 1882, viii, 620; 645: 1883, ix, 1; 29; 57.—**Baraduc** (H.) Du traite-

Nervous system (*Diseases of, Treatment of*).

ment local des congestions chroniques simples et exsudatives de l'axe méningo-spinal par les ventouses vésicantes. Cong. périod. internat. d. sc. méd. Compt.-rend. 1884, Copenh., 1886, iii, Sect. de psychiat. et névrol., 94-99.—**Barea** (F. P.) Observaciones de unas neuroses curadas con el método eléctrico. Bol. de med , cirug. y farm., Madrid, 1847, 3. s., ii, 389-391.—**Bartholow** (R.) On the chloride of gold and sodium in some nervous affections. Med. News, Phila., 1884, xlv, 118. *Also:* Coll. & Clin. Rec., Phila., 1884, v, 213-215. *Also* [Abstr.]: J. Nerv. & Ment. Dis., N. Y., 1884, xi, 480-482. *Also:* Tr. Am. Neurol. Ass., 10. meeting, N. Y., 1884, 46-48.—**Beard** (G. M.) The nature and treatment of neurasthenia (nervous exhaustion), hysteria, spinal irritation, and allied neuroses. Med. Rec., N. Y., 1877, xii, 579; 658. ——. Hygiene of chronic nervous diseases. Proc. M. Soc. County Kings, Brooklyn, 1878, iii, 50-62.—**Begbie** (J. W.) The bromide question. Practitioner, Lond., 1874, xii, 95-99. *Also, in:* Select. from the works of [etc.], 8°, Lond., 1882, 343-347.—**Belcher** (W.) Case of nervous disease successfully treated by Dr. Hamilton's plan, aided by local counter-irritation. Edinb. M. & S. J., 1827, xxvii, 74-78.—**Bell** (C.) On the action of purgative medicines on the different portions of the intestinal canal, with a view to remove nervous affections and tic douloureux. *In his:* Pract. Essays. 8°, Edinb., 1841, 83-104.—**Belugou** (A.) De la spécialisation des eaux de La Malou dans les affections chroniques de la moelle, paralysie, ataxie locomotrice, atrophie musculaire. Ann. Soc. d'hydrol. méd. de Par., 1879-80, xxv, 156-192. ——. Des indications des eaux de La Malou dans le traitement des névroses. *Ibid.*, 1883-4, xxix, 312-359.—**Benavente.** La etiologia debe ser la base de la terapéutica en las afecciones nerviosas. Siglo méd., Madrid, 1860, vii. 641-643. ——. Consideraciones sobre el tratamiento hidrológico de las neuróses. *Ibid.*, 1861, viii, 481.—**Benedikt.** Allgemeine therapeutische Methoden bei chronischen Nervenkrankheiten. Wien. med. Presse, 1872, xiii, 1097; 1129; 1153; 1177; 1209.—**Benediktoff** (M. V.) Physiolog. i terapevt. znachenie staticheskago elektrichestva v nervnich bolezniach. [Use of statical electricity in nervous diseases.] Vrach, St. Petersb., 1883, iv, 117: 136; 151; 164; 183; 227. *Also, transl.* [Abstr.]: Lond. M. Rec., 1884, xii, 425. — **Berendsa** (A.) Dwa postrzezenia względem użycia zimnych kapieli w cierpieniach nerwowych. [Two cases of use of the cold bath in nervous affections.] Pam. Towarz. Lek. Warszaw., 1840, iv, 143-152.—**Berger.** Zur Neurotherapie Jahresb. d. schles. Gesellsch. f. vaterl. Kult. 1882, Bresl., 1883, lx, 76-79. *Also:* Breslau. aerztl. Ztschr., 1883, v, 80-82.—**Bérot** (\.) Sulfate de quinine dans le traitement de certaines névroses périodiques. Arch. méd. de Strasb., 1835, i, 422-426.—**Beuster.** Welchen therapeutischen Werth hat die Massage bei centralen und peripheren Nervenkrankheiten? Ztschr. f. klin. Med., Berl., 1883, vi, 373-384.—**Binswanger.** Zur Behandlung der Erschöpfungsneurosen. Allg. Ztschr. f. Psychiat., etc., Berl., 1883, xl, 638-647.—**Blandford** (G. F.) On the value of a large supply of food in nervous disorders. Practitioner, Lond., 1870. iv, 333-341.—**Boyland** (G. H.) The Buffalo Lithia waters in the treatment of diseases of the nervous system. N. York M. J., 1887, xlvi, 213-215. *Also*, Reprint.—**Brown-Séquard** (C. E.) The treatment of certain functional and organic affections of the nervous system. Med. Rec., N. Y., 1866-7, i, 225-227.—**Brugnoli** (G.) Dell' uso della noce vomica nel vomito nervoso, nella tosse periodica, nell' ipocondriasi, in altre neurosi della vita organica, e nell' albuminuria. Bull. d. sc. med. di Bologna, 1862, 4. s., xvii, 257. *Continued in:* Mem. Accad. d. sc. d. Ist. di Bologna, 1868-70, 2. s.. ix. 501: 1883-4. 4. s., v, 453.—**Brunelli** (C.) Resoconto di alcune malattie, in specie del sistema nervoso curate nel gabinetto elettro-terapeutico dell' Ospedale di S. Spirito, dal settembre 1868 al settembre 1871. Arch. di med., chir. ed ig., Roma, 1873, viii. 142; 218; 273; 345: 1873, ix, 108; 145. *Also*, Reprint.—**Bum** (A.) Die Massage in der Neuropathologie. Wien. Klinik, 1888, 1. Hft , 1-30.—**Burkart** (R.) Zur Behandlung der Hysterie und Neurasthenie. Berl. klin. Wchnschr., 1886, xxiii, 249-255: 1887, xxiv, 842: 863; 888.—**Capozzi** (D.) Sopra talune avvertenze utili per la cura delle neurosi e più particolarmente sopra la opportunità dei purganti. Morgagni, Napoli, 1857, i, 72-80.—**Carrière** (E.) De la diffusion et des médicaments diffusibles dans le traitement des affections nerveuses. Ann. méd.-psych., Par., 1847, ix, 216-243. *Also:* Ann. de méd. belge, Brux., 1847, ii, 231; 298. *Also*, Reprint.—**Chapman** (E. N.) Milk with lime-water as food and medicine in the neuroses. Tr. M. Soc. N. Y., Syracuse, 1879, 354-365. *Also:* Sanitarian, N. Y., 1879, vii, 155-162.—**Chapman** (J.) Cases of epilepsy, paralysis, and other diseases of the nervous system, treated successfully, chiefly by means of ice. J. Ment. Sc., Lond., 1866-7, xii, 218-237. ——. Principes généraux de la médecine névro-dynamique. Cong. périod. internat. d. sc. méd. Compt.-rend. 1875. Brux. et Par., 1876, iv. 75-84.—**Clemens** (T.) Idio-electrische Erscheinungen bei verschiedenen patholo-

Nervous *system* (*Diseases of, Treatment of*).

gischen Affectionen des menschlichen Nervensystems und deren Verhalten zur statistischen Electricität als Heilpotenz. Allg. med. Centr.-Ztg., Berl., 1883, lii, 213 ; 397.—**Clevenger** (S. V.) Contribution to neurological therapeutics. J. Nerv. & Ment. Dis., N. Y., 1886, n. s., xi, 160-167.—**Colla** (I.) Sulla cura delle affezioni nervose. Gior. d. Soc. med.-chir. di Parma, 1807, iv, 112-119.—**Constant** (T.) De l'emploi des bains d'immersion ou de surprise dans le traitement de quelques névroses. Bull. gén. de thérap., etc., Par., 1836, xi, 44-47.—**Curwen** (J.) Rest in nervous diseases. Tr. M. Soc. Penn., Phila., 1881, xiii, pt. 2, 620-628. *Also :* Alienist & Neurol., St. Louis 1881, ii, 380-391.—**Dana** (C. L.) Note on the use of hydrobromic acid in nervous affections. J. Nerv. & Ment. Dis., N. Y., 1883, x, 433-438. *Also :* Med. News, Phila., 1883, xlii. 740. ———. Therapeutics and neurological therapeutics. Quart. Bull. Clin. Soc. N. Y. Post-Grad. M. School & Hosp., 1885-6, i, 243-248.—**D'Ancona.** Valore comparativo della corrente indotta con quella galvanica sulla cura delle malattie del sistema nervoso. Atti Cong. gen. d. Ass. med. ital. 1878, Pisa, 1879, viii, 283-292. *Also :* Gazz. med. ital., prov. venete, Padova, 1879, xxii. 115-121.—**Daumerie.** Sur deux cas de névroses périodiques traitées par le sulfate de quinine. J. de méd., chir. et pharmacol., Brux., 1846, iv, 479-484.—**De Bonis** (T.) Affezioni nervose curate coll' applicazione dell' acqua fredda. Gior. d. sc. med., Torino, 1839, iv, 292-321. — **De Cérenville.** Observations cliniques sur l'emploi des injections hypodermiques de strychnine dans le traitement de quelques affections du système nerveux. Rev. méd. de la Suisse Rom., Genève, 1882, ii, 281 ; 337. — **Destrée.** Des composés nitreux et particulièrement du nitrate de sodium dans les maladies du système nerveux et spécialement dans l'épilepsie. J. de méd., chir. et pharmacol., Brux., 1884, lxxviii, 100 ; 252. — **De Watteville** (A.) Lecture on the diagnostic uses of electricity in the neu romotor apparatus. Lancet, Lond., 1883, ii, 4 ; 49. — **Dewees** (H. P.) Remarks on the use of galvanism in the treatment of certain nervous diseases. N. York J. M., 1847, viii, 295-308.—**Domański** (S.) Przyczynek do terapii chorôl układu nerwowego. [Treatment of nervous diseases.] Przegl. lek., Krakow., 1879, xviii, 101 ; 113.—**Drozdoff** (V. I.) Franklinizatsija v nervoi terapii. [Franklinization in nerve treatment.] Vrach, St. Petersb., 1882, iii. 113. — **Elam** (C.) On some results of treatment in affections of the nervous system. Proc. Roy. M. & Chir. Soc. Lond., 1871-5, vii, 161-164.—**Engelskjøn** (C.) Lokale Børstuingers terapeutiske Nytte i Nervog Sindssygdomme og deres Forhold til Elektroterapien. Norsk Mag. f. Lægevidensk., Christiania, 1888, 4. R., iii, 1-18.—**Erlenmeyer** (A. A.) Die Anwendung des kalten Wassers bei Gehirn- und Nerven-Krankheiten. Cor.-Bl. d. deutsch. Gesellsch. f. Psychiat., etc., Neuwied, 1854, i, 9-11. ———. Die Wirkung des Bromkalium bei Nervenkranken. *Ibid.*, 1867, xiv, 301-304. — **Erlenmeyer** (F. A.) Ueber einige neuere Methoden bei Behandlung von Psychosen und Neurosen. *Ibid.*, Coblenz, 1876, xxii, 1 ; 17. ———. Die gleichzeitige Anwendung verschiedener Bromsalze bei Nervenleiden, insbesondere bei Epilepsie. Centralbl. f. Nervenh., Leipz., 1884, vii, 410-415. — **Eyselein.** Ueber das Ozon und seine Einwirkung auf chronisch Nervenkranke. Allg. Ztschr. f. Psychiat., etc., Berl., 1884, xli, 144.—**Fleckles** (L.) Die balneotherapeutischen Curmethoden gegen chronische Neurosen. Allg. Wien. med. Ztg., 1873, xviii, 86.—**Fothergill** (J. M.) Notes on the therapeutics of some affections of the nervous system. West Riding Lun. Asyl. Rep., Lond., 1876, vi, 254-265.—**Fox** (E. L.) The therapeutics of the neuroses. Brit. M. J., Lond., 1886, i, 772-774.—**Friedländer** (R.) Zu welchem Zeitpunkt ist es angezeigt, mit der elektrischen Behandlung akut entzündlicher Krankheiten des Nervensystems zu beginnen? Centralbl. f. Nervenh., Leipz., 1887, x, 33-38. — **Friedmann** (S.) Ueber den gür.stigen Einfluss der Hydrotherapie auf Reflexneurosen. Wien. med. Wchnschr., 1879, xxix, 735-739.—**Gamgee** (A.) On the curative effects of mild and continued counter-irritation of the back in cases of general nervous debility and in certain cases of spinal irritation. Practitioner, Lond., 1877, xviii, 113-122.—**Gilles de la Tourette.** Sur la salivation dans les affections nerveuses ; étude physiologique du liquide sécrété. Cong. périod. internat. d. sc. méd. Compt.-rend. 1884, Copenh., 1886, iii, Sect. de psychiat. et névrol., 156-158.—**Graffenauer** (J.-P.) Observations sur les bons effets du musc dans les maladies nerveuses et convulsives. Arch. méd. de Strasb., 1835-6, ii, 161-168.—**Graham** (D.) Local massage for local neurasthenia. Boston M. & S. J., 1887, cxvii 572-576. *Also :* J. Am. M. Ass., Chicago, 1888, x, 11-15.—**Granville** (J. M.) Percussion as a therapeutic agent in nervous diseases. Brit. M. J., Lond., 1882, i, 339.—**Gray** (L. C.) The use of quinine with nervous sedatives. Arch.Med., N. Y., 1880, iv, 191-196. ———. On the use of strychnia in nervous disease. Am. J. M. Sc., Phila., 1885, n. s., xc, 381-385.—**Guérin** *de Mamers* (H.) Des irritations encéphaliques et rachidiennes sous le rapport de la thérapeutique, et spécia-

Nervous *system* (*Diseases of, Treatment of*).

lement de l'emploi, dans ces maladies, de l'acide hydro-cyanique et des bains par affusions. Ann. de la méd. physiol., Par., 1825, vii, 322-384. *Also,* Reprint. ———. Delle irritazioni nervose, considerate per rispetto alla terapeutica. Gior. crit. di med. anal., Milano, 1827, vi, 108: vii, 351: viii, 170. ———. De l'emploi des évacuans dans les affections cérébro-spinales. J. compl. du dict. d. sc. méd., Par., 1829, xxxiv, 97-110.—**Hamilton** (A. McL.) Remarks on the use of nitrous oxide gas in the treatment of certain diseases of the nervous system. Med. Gaz., N. Y., 1880, vii, 329. *Also :* Boston M. & S. J., 1880, cii, 469. ———. On the use of a new silver salt in the treatment of organic nervous disease. Lancet, Lond., 1881, i, 291. ———. Antipyrine and acetanilide (anti-febrine) in headache and epilepsy. N. York M. J., 1887, xlv, 593.—**d'Hercourt** (G.) De la nécessité d'associer le traitement moral à l'hydrothérapie pour combattre efficacement l'état nerveux. Ann. méd.-psych., Par., 1879, 6. s., ii, 189-209.—**Hoepfner** (F.) Etwas über die Heilung der Nervenkrankheiten. N. Mag. f. Aerzte, Leipz., 1786, viii, 97-134.—**Holmberg** (A.) Om nervsträckningars användning och berättigande vid behandling af sjukdomar uti centrala nervsystemet. [On nerve-stretching in diseases of central nervous system.] Finska läk.-sallsk. handl., Helsingfors, 1881, xxiii, 241-257.—**Horn** (E.) Neue Erfahrungen über die grosse Wirksamkeit der Speichelflusskuren bei manchen chronischen Nervenkrankheiten. Arch. f. med. Erfahr., Berl., 1812, i, 357-365.—**Hovell** (De B.) The therapeutical indications of neurasthenia contrasted with those of hysteria. Brit. M. J., Lond., 1888, i, 300.—**Howie** (J. M.) The nerve-rest cure. Nineteenth Cent., Lond., 1887, xxii, 658-666. ———. The Weir-Mitchell treatment. Liverpool M.-Chir. J., 1888, viii, 214-225.—**Hughes** (C. H.) The therapeutic value of cephalic and spinal electrizations. Alienist & Neurol., St. Louis, 1883, iv, 77-87.—**Hutchinson** (W. F.) Climate cure in nervous diseases. Boston M. & S. J., 1878, xcviii. 515-517. ———. Climate cure in nervous diseases. Med. Rec., N. Y., 1880, xvii, 3-6.—**Jackson** (S.) Cases of nervous irritation, exhibiting the efficacy of cold as a remedy. N. Am. M. & S. J., 1826, ii, 250-260.—**Jacob.** Hautreizende Bäder gegen Nervenkrankheiten, Intermittens, Oedem und Entzündung. Breslau. aerztl. Ztschr., 1882. iv, 136-139.—**Jacoby** (G. W.) Massage in nervous diseases. J. Nerv. & Ment. Dis., N. Y., 1885, n. s., x, 154 ; 403: 1886, n. s., xi, 140 ; 208. *Also,* Reprint.—**Jones** (W. A.) Hyoscine in the treatment of diseases of the nervous system. Northwest. Lancet, St. Paul, 1885-6, v, 181-184.—**Kinnear** (B. O.) Dr. John Chapman's system of neurodynamic medicine, with cases. Boston M. & S. J., 1882, cvii, 128-132. ———. Explanatory remarks upon neurodynamic medicine, with cases. *Ibid.*, 1883, cviii, 366-368. — **Kinnicutt** (F. P.) Two cases of neural diseases; successful treatment by the actual cautery. Arch. Med., N. Y., 1879, i, 179-183.—**Kovatsch** (W.) Ueber Bromkalium gegen Neurosen im Säuglingsalter. Memorabilien, Heilbr., 1878, xxiii, 513-516 *Also :* Med.-chir. Centralbl., Wien, 1879, xiv, 112.—**Küssner** (B.) Ueber die Anwendung von Brompräparaten bei Neurosen, speciell bei Epilepsie. Deutsche med. Wchnschr., Berl., 1884, x, 792-794. — **Lashkevich** (V. G.) Znachenie kisloroda v nervo-terapii. [Effect of oxygen in nerve-therapy.] Russk. Med., St. Petersb., 1885, i, 151 ; 171 ; 191. *Also, transl. :* Wien. med. Wchnschr., 1885, xxxv, 1014. *Also, transl. :* Rev. de méd., Par., 1885, v, 865-875.—**Laurent** (A.) Des indications dans le traitement des maladies nerveuses. Cong. méd. de France, Par., 1863, i, 349-353. *Also :* J. de méd. ment., Par., 1864, iv, 256-258.—**Lee** (C. P.) Ergot in the treatment of nervous diseases. Kansas M. Index, Fort Scott, 1880, i, 227-236.—**Legendre** (P.) Exemple de l'intolérance des névropathes pour les médicaments (ataxie thérapeutique des hystériques). France méd., Par., 1883, i, 606-608.—**Lente** (F. D.) Cases illustrating the direct action of remedies on the nervous system. Richmond & Louisville M. J., Louisville, 1875, xix, 481-516. *Also,* Reprint.—**Löwenhardt** (R.) Beitrag zur Therapie der Neurosen. Med. Ztg., Berl., 1857, lvii, 165-167.—**McLane** (A.) The use of nitrous oxide gas in certain nervous affections. Maryland M. J., Balt., 1880, vii, 1-7.—**Maderna.** Nevrosi speciali guarite con l' uso della segale cornuta. Gazz. med. ital. lomb., Milano, 1858, 4. s., iii, 269.—**Mann** (E. C.) On the value of the constant or galvanic current of electricity in diseases of the nervous system. Cincin. Lancet & Clinic, 1881, n. s., vi, 495-497.—**Mendel.** Die Anwendung des Antipyrin bei Nervenkrankheiten. Therap. Monatsh., Berl., 1887, i, 259-261.—**Mills** (C. K.) Massage and Swedish movements in the treatment of diseases of the nervous system. Med. & Surg. Reporter, Phila., 1878, xxxix, 283-287. ———. The treatment of nervous and mental disease by systematized active exercises. N. York M. J., 1888, xlvii, 129-136. *Also :* J. Am. M. Ass., Chicago, 1888, x, 162 ; 196. *Also :* Maryland M. J., Balt., 1887-8, xviii, 281 ; 301. *Also* [Abstr.]: Med. News, Phila., 1888, lii, 134. *Also* [Abstr.]: Polyclinic, Phila., 1887-8, v, 248-252.—**Monro** (A.) Case in proof of the usefulness of mercury in convulsive dis-

Nervous *system* (*Diseases of, Treatment of*).

orders. Essays & Obs. Phil. Soc. Edinb., 1771, iii, 557-563.—**Monro** (D.) On the use of mercury in convulsive disorders. *Ibid.*, 551-556.—**Morton** (W. J.) Neurological specialism. [Presidential address, New York Neurological Society.] J. Nerv. & Ment. Dis., N. Y., 1883, n. s., viii, 618-629.—**Mossdorf.** Electrotherapie in der Poliklinik für Nervenkranke. Jahresb. d. Gesellsch. f. Nat.-u. Heilk. in Dresd., 1877, 83-88.—**Müller** (O.) Die Wintercurorte für Nervenkranke an der Riviera. Allg. Ztschr. f. Psychiat., etc., Berl., 1884, xli, 131-135.—**Müller** (C. W.) Ueber einige Principienfragen in der Elektrotherapie. Neurol. Centralbl., Leipz., 1885, iv, 199; 220.—**Newhall** (S. A.) Piscidia erythrina in the treatment of convulsive affections. Therap. Gaz., Detroit, 1886, 3. s., ii, 147.—**Niermeijer** (J. H. A.) De behandelingsmethode van Rumpf. Nederl. Tijdschr. v. Geneesk., Amst., 1884, xx, 256-264.—**Obersteiner** (H.) Zur internen Anwendung des Cocains bei Neurosen und Psychosen. Wien. med. Presse, 1885, xxvi, 1253-1257. *Also*, Reprint.—**Palma** (G.) Into no alcuni casi di neuropatie accolti e curati nello stabilimento del Monte della Misericordia in Casamicciola. Morgagni, Napoli, 1881, xxiii, 353-356.—**Paul** (C.) Du traitement du tremblement et des autres troubles de la coordination du mouvement par les bains galvaniques. Assoc. franç. pour l'avance. d. sc. Compt. rend. 1880, Par., 1881, ix, 898-902. *Also:* Bull. et mém. Soc. de thérap. 1880, Par., 1881, 2. s., vii, 186-206, 2 tab. *Also:* Bull. gén. de thérap., etc., Par., 1880, xcix, 193-212, 2 diag.—**Pauli.** Wie verhalten sich der Arsenik und Phosphor in ihren Wirkungen verschiedenen Nervenkrankheiten gegenüber? Irrenfreund, Heilbr., 1880, xxii, 42-44.—**Piotrowski** (G.) O miejscu w którém prąd elektryczny łańcuchowy zamykany i otwierany, stan czynny w nerwach ruchu wznieca. [The local application of electricity in nervous affections.] Przegl. lek., Krakow., 1865, iv, 353; 361.—**Proust** (A.) & **Ballet** (G.) De l'action des aimants sur quelques troubles nerveux, spécialement sur les anesthésies. J. de thérap., Par., 1879, vi, 801; 841.—**Rafalski** (F.) Spostrzezenia nad leczeniem nerwobólów zelazem do bialości upaloném. [On the treatment of nervous affections by actual cautery.] Gaz. lek., Warszawa, 1873, xiv, 33; 52.—**Ramskill.** Various cases (epilepsy, spasm, paralysis) treated by the administration and inhalation of oxygen, ammonia, and bromoform. Med. Times & Gaz., Lond., 1863, ii, 11.—**Ranney** (A. L.) The therapeutical effects of the internal administration of hot water in the treatment of nervous diseases. Tr. N. York Acad. M. (1882-4), 1886, 2. s., iv, 311-325. *Also:* N. York M. J., 1884, xl, 426; 456. *Also* [Abstr.]: Med. News, Phila., 1884, xlv, 464-468. *Also, transl.:* Coimbra med., 1884, iv, 353; 368; 387. — —. The treatment of functional nervous diseases by the relief of eye-strain. N. York M. J., 1888, xlvii, 1; 37. *Also*, Reprint.—**de Ranse** (.) De l'action immédiate des eaux de Néris dans le traitement des maladies du système nerveux. Ann. Soc. d'hydrol. méd. de Par., 1875-6, xxi, 222-260. [Rap. de Bouloumié], 261-281. *Also:* Gaz. méd. de Par., 1876, 4. s., v, 126; 136; 160; 172.—**Ravin-Bussière** (H.) De la guérison des névroses convulsives; du meilleur mode d'administration du bromure de potassium. Gaz. d. hôp., Par., 1871, xliv, 501.—**Remak.** Application du courant constant au traitement des névroses. Gaz. d. hôp., Par., 1865, xxxviii, 501; 509; 521; 533; 545. *Also* [Abstr.]: Rev. d. cours scient., etc., Par., 1864-5, ii, 23-25. *Also, transl.* [Abstr.]: Imparziale, Firenze, 1865, v, 717; 742.—**Reveillé-Parise** (J.-H.) Principes généraux de thérapeutique, relatifs aux personnes éminemment nerveuses, comme les gens de lettres, les artistes etc. Bull. gén. de thérap., etc., Par., 1834, vi, 69-77. Als : Abeille, Brux., 1834, i, 225-229.—**Richter.** Die schädliche Wirkung zu kalter Bäder bei chronischen Nervenkrankheiten. Deutsche Med.-Ztg., Berl., 1883, iv, 739-741. *Also*, Reprint.—**Rodolfi** (R.) Anestesia elettrica. Processo verbale della seduta elettro-terapeutica, che si tenne nell' Ospitale di Brescia il 26 febrajo 1865. Gazz. med. ital. lomb., Milano, 1865, 5. s., iv, 87. *Also*, Reprint. — —. Anestesia elettrica; rumore determinato della corrente d' induzione; l' elettricità nell' epilessia e nelle convulsioni epilettiformi isteriche. Gazz. med. lomb., Milano, 1865, 5. s., iv, 117. *Also*, Reprint.—**Rodriguez de la Torre** (W.) El sueño en los neuropatas. An. d. Circ. méd. argent., Buenos Aires, 1886, ix, 125-143.—**Rodríguez y Porrúa** (F.) Policlinica de la Escuela de medicina; sección de neuro-patología y electroterapia; cuadro estadístico de los enfermos presentados durante el curso de 1885 á 1886. Rev. méd. de Sevilla, 1886, ix, 257-261.—**Rosatini** (F.) Contribuzione alla terapia delle nevrosi coll' orticazione. Riv. clin. di Bologna, 1885, 3. s., v, 202-206.—**Rosenblatt** (E.) Choroby ukladu nerwow spostrzegane w szpitalu św. Ludwika od r. 1879 do 1882. [Diseases of the nervous system treated in the St. Louis Hospital, Cracow.] Przegl. lek., Krakow., 1883. xxii, 4; 43; 55; 65; 79; 92; 102; 114; 158; 175; 190; 206; 236; 247; 272; 299; 324; 334; 349; 361; 383; 407: 1885, xxiv, 572; 587; 614; 627; 639; 663: 1887, xxvi, 536; 548; 618.—**Rosenthal** (M.) Der heutige Stand der Lehre von der

Nervous *system* (*Diseases of, Treatment of*).

Hydrotherapie, mit besonderer Rücksicht auf Nervenkrankheiten. Med.-chir. Rundschau, Wien, 1866, vii, pt. 2, 1; 81.—**Rumpf** (T.) Mittheilungen aus dem Gebiet der Neuropathologie und Elektrotherapie. Deutsche med. Wchnschr., Berl., 1881, vii, 442; 489; 507. — **Sachs** (B.) On the use of the absolute galvanometer, with description of Hirschmann's new instrument. J. Nerv. & Ment. Dis., N. Y., 1885, n. s., x, 19-26. — **Salnueve** (E.) Considérations et observations cliniques sur le traitement de certaines affections nerveuses par les anneaux métalliques du Dr. Burq. Gaz. méd. de Par., 1852, 3. s., vii, 171; 184; 202.—**Sarlandière.** Affections nerveuses traitées par l'électricité, le galvanisme, l'acupuncture, l'urtication, les moxas, etc. Ann. de la méd. physiol., Par., 1829, xvi, 129-143.—**Schweiger** (S.) Balneotherapie der wichtigeren Erkrankungen des centralen und peripheren Nervensystems. Pest med.-chir. Presse, Budapest, 1880, xvi, 187; 208. *Also, transl. :* Orvosi hetil., Budapest, 1880, xxiv, 162; 185; 215.—**Seguin** (E. C.) Lecture upon the general therapeutics of the nervous system. Med. Rec., N. Y., 1874, ix, 281; 337. *Also, in his :* Op. min. [etc.]. 8°, N. Y., 1884, 139-163. — —. The abuse and use of bromides. J. Nerv. & Ment. Dis., Chicago, 1877, iv, 445-462. *Also :* Med. Rec., N. Y., 1877, xii, 283-285. *Also, in his :* Op. min. [etc.], 8°, N. Y., 1884, 226-241. — —. The efficacy of potassium iodide in non-syphilitic organic diseases of the nervous system. Med. Rec., N. Y., 1882, xxi, 50-52. *Also :* Arch. Med., N. Y., 1883, ix, 240-259. *Also, in his :* Op. min. [etc.], 8°, N. Y., 1884, 579-593. — —. On the efficient dosage of certain remedies used in the treatment of nervous diseases. Tr. M. Soc. N. Y., Syracuse, 1882, 163-182. *Also*, Reprint. *Also :* Arch. Med., N. Y., 1882, vii, 177; 274. *Also, in his :* Op. min. [etc.]. 8°, N. Y., 1884, 594-607.--**Semmola** (M.) Terapia generale di alcuni disturbi funzionali del sistema nervoso; valore pratico comparativo dell' atropina e dei bromici nella cura sedativa. Med. contemp., Napoli, 1884, i, 80; 193. — **Smoleński** (S.) Uwagi nad hydroterapią niektórych nerwic oddechowych i zboczeń im pokrewnych. [Hydrotherapy in some affections of nerves of respiration and allied diseases.] Medycyna, Warszawa, 1887, xv, 229-235. — **Sprague** (G.) Surrendering to disease too willingly; large doses of strychnine. N. York M. J., 1885, xlii, 519. — **Stifler.** Ueber die Wirkung kohlensaurer Stahl- und Eisenmoor-Bäder bei Krankheiten des Nervensystems. Aerztl. Int.-Bl., München, 1882, xxix, 147; 162.—**Stoltenhoff.** Studien über die Wirkung des Acetals (Diäthylacetals). Centralbl. f. Nervenh., Leipz., 1883, vi, 122-128.—**Sturges** (O.) The place in nature of functional nervous disease. Med. Times & Gaz., Lond., 1881, i, 234; 263.—**Suckling** (C.) Arsenic in chronic degenerative diseases of the nervous system. Brit. M. J., Lond., 1887, ii. 939.—**Surre.** Cas remarquable de névrose mentale guérie par l'usage du cuivre. Nice-méd., 1886-7, xi, 205-207 [13-16].—**Weikard** (M. A.) De damnis purgantium in nervis mobilibus, ubi natura acre feri ad cutem expellere conata fuit. *In his :* Obs. med., 12°, Frankof. a. M., 1775, 92-108.—**Weill** (E.) De l'apomorphine dans certains troubles nerveux. Lyon méd., 1884, xlvii, 411-418.—**Weiss** (N.) Ueber die therapeutische Verwendung des Propylamin (recte Trimetylamin) in einigen Nervenkrankheiten. Mitth. d. Wien. med. Doct.-Coll., 1878, iv, 213; 221; 229. *Also :* Wien. med. Bl., 1878, i, 185; 206. *Also*. Reprint.—**Wide** (A.) Om nervtryckning. [C. r. Pressions sur les nerfs.] Nord. med. Ark., Stockholm, 1887, xix, no. 10, 1-15.

Nervous *system* (*Diseases of*) *in children.*

See, also, **Convulsions** *in infants, etc.;* **Hysteria** *in children.*

Andrews (F. F.) The nervous affections of children and their treatment by cod-liver oil. Practitioner, Lond., 1886, xxxvii, 426-434.—**Carter** (W.) Cases of nervous diseases in children. Liverpool M.-Chir. J., 1888, viii, 46-56.—**Crohn** (M.) Zur Casuistik der Erkrankungen des kindlichen Nervensystems. Arch. f. Kinderh., Stuttg., 1882-3, iv, 88-100.—**Dubrisay** (J.) De quelques troubles du système nerveux chez les enfants. Union méd., Par., 1883, 3. s., xxxvi, 476-480.—**Hadden** (W. B.) Illustrations of certain obscure nervous affections in children. St. Thomas's Hosp. Rep. 1885, Lond., 1886, xv, 67-77.—**Peckham** (Grace.) The anatomical and physiological basis of the kinesio-neuroses of infancy and childhood. J. Nerv. & Ment. Dis., N. Y., 1884, n. s., ix, 408-423.—**Seguin** (E. C.) Clinical lectures on the nervous affections of childhood. Med. Gaz., N. Y., 1883, ix, 98; 113; 123.—**Sikorsky.** Contributions à l'étude des maladies nerveuses chez les enfants à l'âge scolaire. Cong. internat. d'hyg. et de démog. Compt. rend. 1882, Genève, 1883, ii, 453-455.

Nervous *system* (*Diseases of*) *of uterine origin and in women.*

See, also, **Insanity** *in women.*

Anderson (W. J.) Hysterical and nervous affections of women. 12°. *London*, 1853.

Nervous *system* (*Diseases of*) *of uterine origin and in women.*

BOUSSI (R.) * Étude sur les troubles nerveux réflexes observés dans les maladies utérines. 4°. *Paris*, 1880.

CARCASSONNE (C.) *.Des troubles nerveux liés à un état physiologique ou pathologique de l'utérus. 4°. *Paris*, 1866.

HAUCH (G. A.) * Ueber den Einfluss des Rückenmarks und Hirns auf die Bewegungen des Uterus, eine Zusammenstellung und Erörterung desjenigen, was bisher darüber bekannt geworden ist, sowie Bericht über Experimente, welche in Bezug auf die Frage angestellt wurden, ob auch dann noch Reflexbewegung des Uterus statthabe, wenn jene centralen Nervenportionen an ihnen nicht Antheil nähmen. 8°. *Halle*, [1879].

LAMBERT (J.) Notes on the relations of uterine disease to insanity. 8°. [*n. p.*, 1877.]

MITCHELL (S. W.) Lectures on diseases of the nervous system, especially in women. 8°. *Philadelphia*, 1881.

———. The same. 2. ed. 8°. *Philadelphia*, 1885.

REICH (E.) Die Nervosität bei den Frauen, ihre Ursachen und Verhütung. 2. Aufl. 8°. *Berlin*, [*n. d.*]

RIGODIN (E.) * Des maux de nerfs chez la femme. 4°. *Paris*, 1858.

VAUTRÉ (J.-D.) * Considérations sur différentes affections spasmodiques chez les femmes. 4°. *Strasbourg*, 1826.

Batuaud (J.) Lois des réflexes génitaux ; névralgie lombo-abdominal. Rev. méd.-chir. d. mal. d. femmes, Par., 1887, ix, 262-275.—**Bell** (W. H.) Reflex morbid condition arising from disease of the uterus. Tr. Indiana M. Soc., Indianap., 1876, xxvi, 70-85.—**Calkins** (A. E.) Uterine and ovarian reflexes. Med. & Surg. Reporter, Phila., 1884, li, 312 ; 340.—**Chrobak** (R.) Retroflexio uteri und Respirationsneurosen. Wien. med. Presse, 1869, x, 8 ; 41.—**Cirera** (J.) Breves consideraciones acerca de los trastornos nerviosos que acompañan á algunas de las enfermedades de los órganos genitales de la mujer. Gac. méd. catal., Barcel., 1881, i, 161 ; 235 ; 302.—**Cusack** (S.) Cases of certain nervous diseases, occurring principally in females. Dublin J. M. & Chem. Sc., 1834, v, 220-232.—**Dalbey-Norred** (Elizabeth S.) Uterine and ovarian irritation, symptomatized by dysmenorrhœa, a cause of insanity. Tr. Illinois M. Soc., Chicago, 1883, xxxiii, 184-191.—**Dubay** (M.) A nök idegességéröl. [Nervous diseases of women.] Gyógyászat, Budapest, 1881, xxi, 729-734.—**Duncan** (J. M.) Two cases of nerve lesion in gynæcology. St. Barth. Hosp. Rep., Lond , 1879, xv, 1-6.—**Durell** (T. M.) Functional diseases of the nervous system dependent upon disease of the uterus. Boston M. & S. J., 1881, cv, 253.—**Edis** (A. W.) On the influence of uterine disorders in the production of numerous sympathetic disturbances of the general health and affections of special organs. Tr. Internat. M. Cong., 7. sess., Lond., 1881, iv, 309-312.—**Engelmann** (G. J.) The hystero-neuroses, with especial reference to the menstrual hystero neurosis of the stomach. Tr. Am. Gynec. Soc. 1877, Bost., 1878, ii, 483-518. *Also*, Reprint. Rev. méd.-chir. d. mal. d. femmes, Par., 1879, i, 333; 385; 465.—**Fauquez** (R.) Utérus irritable ; ectropion douloureux ayant été le point de départ de phénomènes réflexes intéressants. Rev. méd.-chir. d. mal. d. femmes, Par., 1887, ix, 275-280.—**de Fourcauld** (V.) Étude sur les troubles du système nerveux central consécutifs aux affections diverses de l'appareil utéro-ovarien. Ann. de gynéc., Par., 1879, xii, 248 ; 355 : 1880, xiii, 32.—**Goodell** (W.) The relation of neurasthenia to diseases of the womb. Tr. Am. Gynec. Soc. 1878, Bost., 1879, iii, 25-44. *Also*, Reprint.—**Halton** (R. J.) Neurosis of sensory and vaso-motor nerves of arm due to suppressed menstruation. Dublin Q. J. M. Sc., 1869, xlvii, 370.—**Hamilton** (A. McL.) The nervous diseases of women. Buffalo M. & S. J., 1873-4, xiii, 401-405.—**Kinsman** (D. N.) Neuralgia and other disorders caused by uterine disease. Obst. Gaz., Cincin., 1878, i, 195-198.—**Kispert** (G.) Ueber die sogenannten begleitenden consensuellen Erscheinungen in entfernteren Organen bei Gebärmutterkrankheiten. Ztschr. f. Geburtsh. u. Gynäk., Stuttg., 1878, iii, 392-397.—**Lever** (J. C. W.) On some disorders of the nervous system associated with pregnancy and parturition. Guy's Hosp. Rep., Lond., 1847, 2. s., v, 1-25. *Also*, Reprint.—**Little** (W. S.) Symptoms (reflex) in and about the eye, due to some affection of the uterus or its appendages. Phila. M. Times, 1880-81, xi, 581-583.—**Lu-**

Nervous *system* (*Diseases of*) *of uterine origin and in women.*

cas. Uterine physiology and pathology, and their effects on the nervous system. Indian M. Gaz., Calcutta, 1877, xii, 10 ; 181.—**McColgan** (J. T.) Some remarks on reflex neuroses in female diseases. South. Pract., Nashville, 1887, ix, 182-186.—**Mackin** (C. T.) Practical observations on a form of nervous disorder met with in females. Austral. M. J., Melbourne, 1857, ii, 161 ; 246.—**Madden** (T. M.) Further observations on certain cerebro-nervous disorders peculiar to women. Brit. M. J., Lond., 1883, ii, 816-819.—**Morton** (D.) Uterine reflexes. Louisville M. News, 1884, xviii, 49-53.—**Moses** (G. A.) Hystero-neuroses, with cases. Tr. M. Ass. Missouri. St. Louis, 1878, xvii, 93-100.—**Mundé** (P. F.) Clinical observations on reflex genital neuroses in the female. J. Nerv. & Ment. Dis., N. Y., 1886, n. s, xi, 129-139. *Also*, Reprint.—**Neftel** (W. B.) Clinical notes on nervous diseases of women. Arch. Scient. & Pract. M. & S., N. Y. & Phila., 1873, i, 267 ; 365; 416. *Also*, Reprint.—**Ohr** (C. H.) Genito-reflex neurosis in the female. Am. J. Obst., N. Y., 1883, xvi, 50 ; 168.—**Playfair** (W. S.) Notes on the systematic treatment of nerve prostration and hysteria connected with uterine disease. Lancet, Lond., 1881, i, 857 ; 948 : ii, 991 ; 1029.—**Schauta** (F.) Zur gynäkologischen Behandlung bei Neurosen. Wien. med. Bl., 1886, ix, 601 ; 633.—**Skene** (A. J. C.) Studies of the relations existing between the organs of reproduction and the brain and nervous system in women. Ann. Anat. & Surg. Soc., Brooklyn, N. Y., 1880, ii, 435-452. ———. The relation of the ovaries to the brain and nervous system. Med. Rec., N. Y., 1881, xix, 46-49.—**Warren** (J. S.) The hystero-neurosis of the stomach in pregnancy. *Ibid.*, 339-341. *Also* [Abstr.]: Coll. & Clin. Rec., Phila., 1881, ii, 75-78.

Nervous *system* (*Electrophysiology of*).

See, also, **Electrophysiology**.

DU BOIS-REYMOND (E.) Ueber die elektromotorische Kraft der Nerven und Muskeln. 8°. *Berlin*, 1867.

ENGESSER (H.) * Existirt eine Verschiedenheit in der Reaction des Nerven gegen den galvanischen Strom, je nachdem die Kette mit der Kathode oder Anode geschlossen oder geöffnet wird ? 8°. *Freiburg*, 1874.

Also [Abstr.], *in*: Arch. f. d. ges. Physiol., Bonn, 1875, x, 147-151.

FICK (A.) Untersuchungen über elektrische Nervenreizung. 4°. *Braunschweig*, 1864.

FICK (A. [E.]) * Ueber quere Nervendurchströmung. 8°. *Würzburg*, 1876.

Also, in: Verhandl. d. phys.-med. Gesellsch. in Würzb., 1874-6, n. F., ix, 228-245, 1 tab.

HALPERSON (C.) * Beiträge zur elektrischen Erregbarkeit der Nervenfasern. 8°. *Bern*, 1884.

HELLE (A.) * De l'influence du galvanisme sur le système nerveux moteur. 4°. *Paris*, 1858.

LESURE (A.) * Expériences relatives à l'action des nerfs courants électriques sur les nerfs. 4°. *Paris*, 1857.

MARCUSE (A. J.) * Die Abhängigheit der Erregung von Länge der elektrisch durchströmten Nervenstrecke. 8°. *Würzburg*, 1876.

Also, in: Verhandl. d. phys.-med. Gesellsch. in Würzb., 1877, n. F., x, 158-174, 1 pl. *Also*: Arb. a. d. physiol. Lab. d. Würzb. Hochsch., 1872-8, 289-304, 1 pl.

MONRO (A.) Experiments on the nervous system, with opium and metalline substances; made chiefly with the view of determining the nature and effects of animal electricity. 4°. *Edinburgh*, 1793.

PRZCEWOSKI (R.) *Ueber den Einfluss des inducirten und constanten elektrischen Stromes auf vasomotorische Nerven und über das thermische Verhalten thätiger Muskeln. 8°. *Greifswald*, 1876.

RANKE (G. J.) *Ueber positive Schwankung des Nervenstromes beim Tetanisiren mit dem Magnetelektromotor. 8°. *Ansbach*, [1862].

Also, in: Arch. f. Anat., Physiol. u. wissensch. Med., Leipz., 1862, 241-262.

STERNEBERG (J. W.) * Experimenta quædam ad cognoscendam vim electricam nervorum atque sanguinis facta. 4°. *Bonnæ*, [1834].

Nervous *system* (*Electrophysiology of*).

UHEN (J. X.) * Quæstiones quædam de irritabilitate nervis dissectis in musculis per galvanismum provocata. 8°. *Gryphiswaldiæ*, 1862.

Althaus (J.) On the action of the electric current upon the motor nerves and muscles. Med. Times & Gaz., Lond., 1859, xviii, 109; 207; 311.—**d'Arsonval** (A.) Nouvelle méthode d'excitation électrique des nerfs et des muscles. Compt. rend. Acad. d. sc., Par., 1881, xcii, 1520–1522.—**von Baranowski** (V.) & **Garrè** (C.) Ueber die Geschwindigkeit, mit welcher sich der Electrotonus im Nerven verbreitet. Arch. f. d. ges. Physiol., Bonn, 1879–80, xxi, 446–461.—**Benedikt** (M.) Die Methode der elektrischen Untersuchung des Nervensystems. Allg. Wien. med. Ztg., 1863, viii, 138; 146.—**Beraudi** (L.) Ulteriori esperimenti tentati sugli animali viventi comprovanti la facoltà che compete al nervoso sistema di svolgere in alcuni casi il galvanismo. Ann. univ. di med., Milano, 1829, l, 278–282.—**Bernheim.** Ueber Wirkung des elektrischen Stromes in verschiedener Richtung gegen die Längsachse des Nerven und Muskels. Arch. f. d. ges. Physiol. Bonn, 1874, viii, 60–70, 1 pl.—**Bernstein** (J.) Die Natur der negativen Schwankung und des electrotonischen Zustandes des Nervenstroms. Centralbl. f. d. med. Wissensch., Berl., 1866, iv, 225–228. *Also:* Untersuch. z. Naturl. d. Mensch. u. d. Thiere, Giessen, 1870, x, 348–352. ——. Die Fortpflanzungsgeschwindigkeit der negativen Schwankung im Nerven. Centralbl. f. d. med. Wissensch., Berl., 1866, iv, 593–596. *Also*, Reprint. ——. Untersuchungen über die Natur des elektrotonischen Zustandes und der negativen Schwankung des Nervenstroms. Arch. f. Anat., Physiol. u. wissensch. Med., Leipz., 1866, 596–637. ——. Ueber das Entstehen und Verschwinden der elektrotonischen Ströme im Nerven und die damit verbundenen Erregungsschwankungen des Nervenstromes. Arch. f. Physiol., Leipz., 1886, 197–250, 2 pl.—**von Bezold** (A.) Ueber den Einfluss constanter galvanischer Ströme auf den zeitlichen Verlauf und die Leitung der Nervenerregung. [*From:* Monatsber. d. k. preuss. Akad. d. Wissensch. zu Berl., 21. Febr. 1861.] Untersuch. z. Naturl. d. Mensch. u. d. Thiere, Giessen, 1862, viii, 415–418. *Also*, Reprint. ——. Fortgesetzte Untersuchungen über die Einwirkung galvanischer Ströme auf Nerven und Muskeln. [*From:* Monatsber. d. k. preuss. Akad. d. Wissensch. zu Berl., 15. März 1861.] Untersuch. z. Naturl. d. Mensch. u. d. Thiere, Giessen, 1862, viii, 419–422.—**Biedermann** (W.) Ueber die durch chemische Veränderung der Nervensubstanz bewirkten Veränderungen der polaren Erregung durch den elektrischen Strom. Sitzungsb. d. k. Akad. d. Wissensch. Math.-naturw. Cl., Wien, 1881, lxxxiii, 3. Abth., 289–340, 2 pl.—**Bischoff** (T. L. W.) Ueber electrische Ströme in den Nerven. Arch. f. Anat., Physiol. u. wissensch. Med., Berl., 1841, 20–24.—**Boas** (F.) Ueber eine neue Form des Gesetzes der Unterschiedsschwelle. Arch. f. d. ges. Physiol., Bonn, 1881, xxvi, 493–500.—**Bonnefin** (F.) Recherches expérimentales sur la possibilité du passage à travers le centre nerveux de courants électro-magnétiques appliqués à la peau, chez l'homme. J. de la physiol. de l'homme, Par., 1858, i, 545–548.—**Brückner** (A.) Ueber die von Hitzig angeregte Theorie der electrischen Stromwirkung. Berl. klin. Wchnschr., 1877, xiv, 392–394.—**Budge** (J.) Ueber verschiedene Reizbarkeit eines und desselben Nerven und über den Werth des Pflüger'schen Elektrotonus. Arch. f. path. Anat., etc., Berl., 1860, xviii, 457; 1863, xxviii, 282.—**Capparelli** (A.) Sulla nuova legge elettro-fisiologica relativa all' elettrotono interpolare scoperta dal Dr. D. Mucci; brevi considerazioni sull' interpretazione del fenomeno. Atti d. Accad. Gioenia di sc. nat. in Catania, 1881, 3. s., xv, 285–291. *Also:* Gior. internaz. d. sc. med., Napoli, 1881, n. s., iii, 449–452.—**Chauveau** (A.) De l'excitation électrique unipolaire des nerfs; comparaison de l'activité des deux pôles pendant le passage des courants de pile. Gaz. hebd. de méd., Par., 1875, xxii, 725.—**Clemens** (T.) Die spontane elektrische Entladung in kranken Nerven. Deutsche Klinik. Berl., 1864, xvi, 27.—**De Renzi** (E.) Azione riflessa sospensiva dell' elettrico. Riv. clin. e terap., Napoli, 1885, vii, 473.—**Donders** (F. C.) De werking van den constanten stroom op den nervus vagus. Versl.... d. k. Akad. v. Wetensch. Afd. Natuurk., Amst., 1871, v, 80–142, 3 pl.—**Du Bois-Reymond** (E.) Note sur la loi qui préside à l'irritation électrique des nerfs et sur la modification du courant musculaire par l'effet de la contraction. Ann. de chim. et phys., Par., 1850, 3. s., xxx, 119–127. *Also*, Reprint.—**Dunbar** (J. R. W.) Interesting galvanic experiments. Balt. M. & S. J. & Rev., 1833, i, 245–248.—**Eckhard** (C.) Ueber den Einfluss des constanten galvanischen Stromes auf die Erregbarkeit des motorischen Nerven. Beitr. z. Anat. u. Physiol. (Eckhard), Giessen, 1858, i, 23–54.—**Engelmann** (T. W.) Bewegingsverschijnselen aan zenuwvezelen, bij prikkeling met inductiestroomen. Onderzoek. ged. in h. physiol. Lab. d. Utrecht. Hoogesch., 1871–2, 3. R., i, 168–177. *Also, transl.:* Arch. f. d. ges. Physiol., Bonn, 1872, v, 31–37. ——. Eenige proeven tot demonstratie der algemeene wet van electrische prikkeling. Onderzoek. ged. in h. physiol. Lab. d. Utrecht. Hoogesch., 1871–2, 3. r., i, 266–271. ——. Vergleichende

Nervous *system* (*Electrophysiology of*).

Untersuchungen zur Lehre von der Muskel- und Nervenelektricität. Arch. f. d. ges. Physiol., Bonn, 1877, xv, 116–148.—**Engelmann** (T. W.) & **Place.** Methode tot het voorkomen van unipolaire stroomen bij prikkeling der zenuwen. Onderzoek. ged. in h. physiol. Lab. d. Utrecht. Hoogesch., 1867–8, i, 277–280.—**Eulenburg** (A.) Ueber electrotonisirende Wirkungen bei percutaner Anwendung des constanten Stromes auf Nerven und Muskeln. Deutsches Arch. f. klin. Med., Leipz., 1867, iii, 117–142. ——. Ueber einige Erscheinungen der galvanischen Nervenreizung. Berl. klin. Wchnschr., 1872, ix, 251.—**Exner** (S.) In welcher Weise tritt die negative Schwankung durch das Spinalganglion? Arch. f. Physiol., Leipz., 1877, 567–570. ——. Zur Kenntniss von der Wechselwirkung der Erregungen im Centralnervensystem. Arch. f. d. ges. Physiol., Bonn, 1882, xviii, 487–506, 1 pl.—**F.** (W.) On some analogies between the nervous system and the electric telegraph. Med. Times & Gaz., Lond., 1880, i, 433; 488; 561; 588.—**Fick** (A.) Studien über electrische Nervenreizung. Verhandl. d. phys.-med. Gesellsch. in Würzb. (1868–71), 1872, n. F., ii, 145–155, 1 pl. *Also:* Arb. a. d. physiol. Lab. d. Würzb. Hochsch., 1872–8, 55–75. ——. Ueber quere Nervendurchströmung. Arb. a. d. physiol. Lab. d. Würzb. Hochsch., 1872–8, 270–287, 1 pl.—**Filehne** (W.) Beiträge zur Lehre vom Zuckungsgesetze des absterbenden Nerven. Deutsches Arch. f. klin. Med., Leipz., 1872, x, 401–419. ——. Ueber die Zuckungsformen bei der sogenannten queren Durchströmung des Froschnerven. Arch. f. d. ges. Physiol., Bonn, 1874, viii, 71–74, 1 pl.—**von Fleischl** (E.) Untersuchung über die Gesetze der Nervenerregung. 1. Abhandl. Ueber die Lehre vom Anschwellen der Reize in Nerven. Sitzungsb. d. k. Akad. d. Wissensch. Math.-naturw. Cl. 1875, Wien, 1876, lxxii, 393–406. *Also*, Reprint. ——. 2. Abhandl. Ueber die Wirkung secundärer elektrischer Ströme auf Nerven. Sitzungsb. d. k. Wissensch. Math.-naturw. Cl. 1876, Wien, 1877, lxxiv, 403–424, 1 pl. *Also*, Reprint. ——. 3. Abhandl. Das Rheonom. Sitzungsb. d. k. Akad. d. Wissensch. Math.-naturw. Cl. 1877, Wien, 1878, lxxvi, 138–162, 4 pl. *Also*, Reprint. ——. 4. Abhandl. Der intopolare Electrotonus. Sitzungsb. d. k. Akad. d. Wissensch. Math.-naturw. Cl., Wien, 1878, lxxvii, 159–176, 1 pl. *Also*, Reprint. ——. 5. Abhandl. Die Theorie des Electrotonus. Sitzungsb. d. k. Akad. d. Wissensch. Math.-naturw. Cl. 1878, Wien, 1879, lxxx, 267–282, 1 pl. ——. 6. Abhandl. Ueber die Wirkung linearer Stromschwankungen. auf Nerven. *Ibid.* (1880), 1881, lxxxii, 133–154, 3 pl. *Also*, Reprint. ——. Das Zuckungsgesetz. Arch. f. Physiol., Leipz., 1882, 1–24.—**Fredericq** (L.) Ueber die elektromotorische Kraft des Warmblüternerven. *Ibid.*, 1880, 65–71.—**Gad.** Betrachtungen und Versuche, die Abnahme des Stromes am absterbenden Nerven betreffend. *Ibid.*, 1878, 615–619.—**Grijmalo** (B.) Zur Erörterung der Frage: Ueber die räumliche Ausbreitung des Electrotonus in einem Nerven. Med. Ztg. Russlands, St. Petersb., 1860, xvii, 297.—**Gruenhagen** (A.) Theorie des physikalischen Electrotonus. Ztschr. f. rat. Med., Leipz. u. Heidelb., 1868, 3. R., xxxi, 43–45.—**Grützner** (P.) Ueber die Einwirkung constanter elektrischer Ströme auf Nerven. Arch. f. d. ges. Physiol., Bonn, 1878, xvii, 238–249. ——. Ueber elektrische Nervenreizung. *Ibid.*, 1882, xxviii, 130–178, 1 pl. —**Hällstén** (K.) Elektrotonus in sensiblen Nerven. Arch. f. Physiol., Leipz., 1880, 112–114.— **Head** (H.) Ueber die negativen und positiven Schwankungen des Nervenstromes. Arch. f. d. ges. Physiol., Bonn, 1886–7, xl, 207–273, 1 pl.—**Hering** (E.) Ueber Nervenreizung durch den Nervenstrom. Sitzungsb. d. k. Akad. d. Wissensch. Math.-naturw. Cl., 3. Abth., Wien, 1882, lxxxv, 237–275—**Hermann** (L.) Ueber eine Wirkung galvanischer Ströme auf Muskeln und Nerven. Arch. f. d. ges. Physiol., Bonn, 1872, v, 223, 1 pl.: vi, 312. ——. Untersuchungen über das Gesetz der Erregungsleitung in polarisirten Nerven. *Ibid.*, 1873, vii, 323; 497, 1 pl. ——. Fortgesetzte Untersuchungen über die Beziehungen zwischen Polarisation und Erregung im Nerven. *Ibid.*, 1875, x, 215–239. ——. Zur Lehre vom Einflusse der Reizstelle und Reizstromrichtung im Nerven. *Ibid.*, 1878, xvi, 262. ——. Untersuchungen über die Actionsströme des Nerven. *Ibid.*, xviii, 574–586. ——. Bemerkung über das galvanische Verhalten einer durch flossenen Nervenstrecke. *Ibid.*, 1879, xix, 416. ——. Ueber eine verbesserte Construction des Galvanometers für Nervenversuche. *Ibid.*, 1879, xxi, 430–445, 1 pl.—**Hitzig** (E.) Ueber quere Durchströmung des Froschnerven. *Ibid.*, 1873, vii, 263–273.—**Katyschew** (J.) Ueber die electrische Erregung der sympathischen Fasern und über den Einfluss elektrischer Ströme auf die Pupille beim Menschen. Arch. f. Psychiat., Berl., 1878, viii, 624–640.—**Lamansky** (S.) Untersuchungen über die Natur der Nervenerregung durch kurz dauernde Ströme. Stud. d. physiol. Inst. zu Bresl., 1868, iv, 146–225.—**Lautenbach** (B. F.) The effect of irritation of a polarized nerve ("Pflüger's electrotonus"). Rep. Smithson. Inst. 1878, Wash., 1879, 361–419. ——. **Legros** (C.) & **Onimus.** De l'influence des courants électriques constants et continus sur les actions réflexes. Compt. rend. Soc. de biol. 1868, Par., 1869, 4. s., v, pt. 1, 57–59. ——

Nervous *system* (*Electrophysiology of*).
———. De l'influence des courants électriques sur le système nerveux. J. de l'anat. et physiol., etc., Par., 1869, vi, 617: 1870-71, vii, 11.—**Limbourg** (P.) Beiträge zur chemischen Nervenreizung und zur Wirkung der Salze. Arch. f. d. ges. Physiol., Bonn, 1887, xli, 303-325, 2 pl.—**Magini** (G.) Le courant induit unipolaire et l'excitation des nerfs. Arch. ital. de biol., Turin, 1883, iv, 278.
———. Eccitazione dei nervi colla corrente indotta unipolare a distanza e attraverso corpi isolanti. Bull. d. r. Accad. med. di Roma, 1883, ix, 264-269.—**Matteucci** (C.) On the secondary electro-motor power of nerves, and its application to the explanation of certain electro-physiological phenomena. Phil. Tr., Lond., 1862, cli, 363-372.—**Mendelssohn** (M.) Sur le courant nerveux axial. Compt. rend. Soc. de biol., Par., 1885, 8. s., ii, 400-402. *Also, transl.*: Arch. f. Physiol., Leipz., 1885, 381-399.
———. Sur la détermination de la force électro-motrice du courant nerveux ou musculaire, avec des électrodes impolarisables, mais non homogènes. Gaz. d. hôp., Par., 1886, lix, 743. ———. Nouvelles recherches sur le courant nerveux axial. Compt. rend. Acad. d. sc., Par., 1886, ciii, 393. *Also*: Compt. rend. Soc. de biol., Par., 1886, 8. s., iii, 402.—**Morat** & **Toussaint.** De l'état électrotonique dans le cas d'excitation unipolaire des nerfs. Compt. rend. Acad. d. sc., Par., 1877, lxxxiv, 503-505.—**Morton** (W. J.) A new current of induction electricity; or, a new method of producing electrical nerve and muscle reactions. Med. Rec., N. Y., 1881, xx, 62.—**Mucci** (D.) Nuova legge elettrofisiologica relativa all' elettrotono interpolare. Sperimentale, Firenze, 1880, xlvi, 225-236.—**Müller** (J. J.) Ueber die Abhängigkeit der negativen Schwankung des Nervenstromes von der Intensität des erregenden elektrischen Stromes. *In*: Fick (A.) Untersuch. a. d. physiol. Lab. d. Zürich. Hochsch., 8°, Wien, 1869, 1. Hft., 98-126.—**Munk** (H.) Ueber die Präexistenz der elektrischen Gegensätze in Muskel und Nerven. Arch. f. Anat., Physiol. u. wissensch. Med., Leipz., 1868, 529-583.—**Neftel** (W. B.) Electricity a paralyzing agent. Med. Rec., N. Y., 1879, xvi, 476.—**Neumann** (E.) Ueber das verschiedene Verhalten der Nerven und Muskeln gegen den constanten und den inducirten Strom während ihres Absterbens. Königsb. med. Jahrb., 1864, iv, 93.—**Onimus.** De l'influence de la direction des courants continus. Compt. rend. Soc. de biol. 1878, Par., 1880, 6. s., v, 147-150.—**Ott** (I.) The effect of electrotonus on the rapidity of the transmission of nerve-force. Phila. M. Times, 1878, viii, 201.—**Person.** Sur l'hypothèse des courans électriques dans les nerfs. J. de physiol. expér., Par., 1830, x, 216-225, 1 pl.—**Pflüger** (E.) Ueber die durch constante electrische Ströme erzeugte Veränderung des motorischen Nerven. Allg. med. Centr.-Ztg., Berl., 1856, xxv, 169; 449. ———. Ueber die tetanisirende Wirkung des constanten Stromes und das allgemeine Gesetz der Reizung. Arch. f. path. Anat.. etc., Berl., 1858, xiii, 437-448.—**Piotrowski** (G.) & **Widmann** (O.) O drażnieniu nerwów za pomocą prądu elektrycznego pochodniego, powstalego przez otwarcie prądu pierwotnego. [Researches on the electrical excitation of the nerves and muscles.] Przegl. lek., Krakow., 1862, i, no. 24, 25.—**Poole** (T. W.) Electricity a paralyzing agent. Med. Rec., N. Y., 1879, xvi, 416-418. ———. Electricity a paralyzing agent; proofs from the authentic experiments. *Ibid.*, 1881, xix, 113-116.—**Ranke** (J.) Neue Versuche über die Reaction der tetanisirten Nervensubstanz. Centralbl. f. d. med. Wissensch., Berl., 1868, vi, 769-772.—**Reinhold** (L.) Versuch einer skizzirten, nach galvanischen Gesetzen entworfenen Darstellung des thierischen Lebens. Arch. f. d. Physiol., Halle, 1807-8, viii, 305-354.—**Remak** (E.) Ueber modificirende Wirkungen galvanischer Ströme auf die Erregbarkeit motorischer Nerven des lebenden Menschen. Deutsches Arch. f. klin. Med., Leipz., 1876, xviii, 264-312, 1 pl.—**Richet** (C.) Des mouvements de la grenouille consécutifs à l'excitation électrique. Arch. de physiol. norm. et path., Par., 1881, 2. s., viii, 824-837.—**Romanes** (G. J.) Observations on the galvanic excitation of nerve and muscle, with special reference to the modification of the excitability of motor nerves produced by injury. J. Anat. & Physiol., Lond., 1876, x, 707-734.—**Rosenthal** (I.) Ueber unipolare Nervenreizung und falsche Nervenreizung durch Nebenleitung. Sitzungsb. d. phys.-med. Soc. zu Erlang., 1879-80, xii, 48-51.—**Rousseau** (E.-L.) [*et al.*] Action des courants électriques étudiée comparativement sur les nerfs mixtes et sur les racines antérieures rachidiennes. Compt. rend. Soc. de biol. 1857, Par., 1859, 2. s., iv, pt. 2, 223-267. *Also*: Gaz. méd. de Par., 1858, 3. s., xiii, 230; 244; 322.—**Runge.** Reflexerscheinungen bei Anwendung des constanten Stromes. Deutsche Klinik, Berl., 1868, xx, 76.—**Sanderson** (J. B.) The excitation of the surface of the brain by induced currents. Physiol. Lab. Univ. Coll., Lond. Collected papers, 1874-5, no. 1.—**Schelske** (R.) Neue Messungen der Fortpflanzungsgeschwindigkeit des Reizes in den menschlichen Nerven. Arch. f. Anat., Physiol. u. wissensch. Med., Leipz., 1864, 151-173.—**Schetterly** (H. R.) Pulsation an effect of discharges of electricity on the sympathetic nerves. Med. Indep., Detroit, 1857, iii, 577-583.—**Schiff** (M.) Recherches sur les propriétés électriques des nerfs vivants. Compt. rend. Soc. de biol. 1859, Par., 1860, 3. s., i, 175-177.

Nervous *system* (*Electrophysiology of*).
———. Recerche sull' espressione elettrica dell' attività nervosa. Atti r. Ist. Veneto di sc., lett. ed arti, 1869, 3. s., xiv, 1658-1678.—**Schiff** (M.) & **Herzen** (A.) Ueber die Veränderungen der Erregbarkeit in dem durch schwache constante Ströme polarisirten Nerven. Untersuch. z. Naturl. d. Mensch. u. d. Thiere, Giessen, 1870, x, 431-446.—**Setschenow** (J.) Galvanische Erscheinungen an der cerebrospinalen Axe des Frosches. Arch. f. d. ges. Physiol., Bonn, 1881, xxv, 281-284. ———. Galvanische Erscheinungen an der cerebro-spinalen Axe des Frosches. [Vorl. Mitth.] Mélanges biol. Acad. imp. d. sc. de St.-Pétersb. (1880-81), 1882, xi, 351-353. *Also, transl.*: Vrach, St. Petersb., 1882, iii, 703; 724; 744; 763. ———. Hemmung spontaner Stromesschwankungen an dem verlängerten Marke des Frosches. [Vorl. Mitth.] Centralbl. f. d. med. Wissensch., Berl., 1882, xx, 177-180.—**Seubert** (M.) Wirkung des galvanischen Reizes, auf die vordern und hintern Spinal-Nervenwurzeln und auf das Rückenmark selbst angebracht. Ztschr. f. Physiol., Heidelb., 1835, v, 50-57. — **Sewall** (H.) On the polar effects upon nerves of weak induction currents. Johns Hopkins Univ. Stud. biol. lab.. Balt., 1881-3, ii, 347-352. *Also*: J. Physiol., Lond., 1880-82, iii, 175-180. — **Steiner** (J.) Ueber den Einfluss der Temperatur auf den Nervenstrom und die Fortpflanzungsgeschwindigkeit seiner negativen Schwankung. Arch. f. Physiol., Leipz., 1883, Suppl.-Bd., 179-186.—**Stricker** (S.) Das Zuckungsgesetz; nach neuen Untersuchungen dargestellt. Sitzungsb. d. k. Akad. d. Wissensch. Math.-naturw. Cl., Wien, 1881, lxxxiv, 3. Abth., 7-93.—**Tarchnoff** (J.) O summirovanii udarof postoyannago i induktsionnago tokof padayushchikh na chuvstvuyushchii nerf lyagushki. [Effect of electricity on the nerves of the frog.] Voyenno-med. J., St. Petersb., 1869, cvi, pt. 2, 103-120. ———. O vlijanii razlichnich polousov postojannago toka na tsentralnuiou nervnuiou sistemu. [Effect of different poles of constant currents on central nervous system.] Med. Sbornik, Tiflis, 1874, x, no. 18, 1-10.—**Tschiriew** (S.) Ueber die Erregbarkeit des Nerven und des Muskels in Quer- und Längsrichtung. Centralbl. f. d. med. Wissensch., Berl., 1877, xv, 369. ———. Berichtigung einer Notiz über Hrn. Hermann's Auffassung des Compensationsverfahrens für die electrophysiologischen Zweke. *Ibid.*, 1878, xvi, 209-213. — **Valentin** (G.) Eudiometrische Studien über Muskeln und Nerven. Arch. f. physiol. Heilk., Stuttg., 1859, n. F., iii, 441-485. ———. Die Wirkung wiederholter gleichgerichteter Induktionsschläge auf den leistungsfähigen und den abgestorbenen Froschnerven. Ztschr. f. Biol., München, 1872, viii, 182-210. ———. Die Wirkungsgrenzen augenblicklicher, einfacher oder wiederholter elektrischer Erregungen. *Ibid.*, 1873, ix, 75-94. ———. Die Interferenzen elektrischer Erregungen. Arch. f. d. ges. Physiol., Bonn, 1873, vii, 458-496, 1 pl. ———. Einige Bemerkungen über elektrische Tetanisation der Nerven und der Muskeln. *Ibid.*, 1875, xi, 481-501, 1 pl. ———. Ein anschauliches Verfahren, den Einfluss eines beständigen Stromes auf die Wirkungen einer benachbarten elektrisch erregten Nervenstrecke nachzuweisen. Ztschr. f. Biol., München, 1881, xvii, 138-157.—**von Vintschgau** (M.) Untersuchungen über die Frage, ob die Geschwindigkeit der Fortpflanzung der Nervenerregung von der Reizstärke abhängig ist. Arch. f. d. ges. Physiol., Bonn, 1882-3, xxx, 17-81. — **Waller** (A.) & **de Watteville** (A.) Reports to the Scientific Grants Committee of the British Medical Association, on the influence of the galvanic current on the motor nerves of man. Brit. M. J., Lond., 1882, i, 767. *Also, transl.*: Neurol. Centralbl., Leipz., 1882, i, 145-148.—**Wedenskij** (N.) Die telephonischen Wirkungen des erregten Nerven. Mélanges biol. Acad. imp. d. sc. de St.-Pétersb., 1880-83, xi, 523-527. *Also*: Centralbl. f. d. med. Wissensch., Berl., 1883, xxi, 465-468.—**Werigo** (B.) Ueber die gleichzeitige Reizung des Nerven an zwei Orten mit Inductionsschlägen. Arch. f. d. ges. Physiol., Bonn, 1885, xxxvi, 519-548, 3 pl.

Nervous *system* (*Histology of*).
See, also, **Nervous** *system* (*Ganglionic*); **Neuralgia.**
AXMANN (C.) Beiträge zur mikroskopischen Anatomie und Physiologie des Gangliennervensystems des Menschen und der Wirbelthiere. 8°. *Berlin*, 1853.
BEALE (L. S.) New observations upon the structure and formation of certain nervous centres tending to prove that the cells and fibres of every nervous apparatus form an uninterrupted circuit. 4°. *London*, 1864.
———. On the ultimate nerve-fibres distributed to muscle and some other tissues, with observations upon the structure and probable mode of action of a nervous mechanism; being the Croonian lecture for 1865. 8°. *London*, [1865].
Repr. from: Proc. Roy. Soc. Lond.. 1865, xiv.

Nervous system (Histology of).

BIDDER (F. H.) Zur Lehre von dem Verhältniss der Ganglienkörper zu den Nervenfasern. Neue Beiträge. Nebst einem Anhange von A. W. Volkmann. 4°. Leipzig, 1847.

BOLL (F.) Die Histiologie und Histiogenese der nervösen Centralorgane. 8°. Berlin, 1873.

BOVERI (T.) Beiträge zur Kenntniss der Nervenfasern. 4°. München, 1885.
Repr.from: Abhandl. d. k. bayer. Akad. d. Wissensch., 2. Cl., xv. Bd., 2. Abth.

BURDACH (E.) Beitrag zur mikroskopischen Anatomie der Nerven. 4°. Königsberg, 1837.

CECI (A.) Contribuzione allo studio della fibra nervosa midollata ed osservazioni sui corpuscoli amilacei dell' encefalo e midollo spinale. 4°. [Roma, 1881.]
Cutting from: Atti di r. Accad. d. Lincei. Cl. di sc. fis., matemat. e nat., Roma, 1881, 3. s., ix.

DUCHENNE de Boulogne (G.-B.-A.) Anatomie microscopique du système nerveux. 8°. Paris, 1865.

EIJKMAN (C.) jr. * Over polarisatie in de zenuwen. 8°. Tiel, 1883.

FROMMANN (C.) Untersuchungen über die normale und pathologische Histologie des centralen Nervensystems. 4°. Jena, 1876.

HANNOVER (A.) Mikroskopiske Undersögelser af Nervesystemet. 4°. [Kjøbenhavn, 1842.]
Repr. from: Sel. naturvid. og mathem. Afh., Kjøbenh., 1840-42, x.

———. The same. Recherches microscopiques sur le système nerveux. 4°. Copenhague, 1844.

HENNIG (A.) * Die Einschnürungen und Unterbrechungen der Markscheide an den markhaltigen Nervenfasern. 8°. Königsberg, [1877].

JACOBI (E.) * Zum feineren Bau der peripheren markhaltigen Nervenfaser. 8°. Würzburg, 1886.

JACQUEMET. * De la structure intime des nerfs. 8°. Montpellier, 1855.

KANNEGIESSER (G. H.) [Pr.] de tubulosa nervorum structura. 4°. Kilonii, [1749].

KLENCKE (P. F. H.) Neue anatomische und physiologische Untersuchungen über die Primitivnervenfaser und das Wesen der Innervation. 8°. Göttingen, 1841.

KOCH (C.) * Ueber die Marksegmente der doppeltcontourirten Nervenfasern und deren Kittsubstanz. 8°. Erlangen, 1879.

KONEFF (Helene.) * Beiträge zur Kenntniss der Nervenzellen in den peripheren Ganglien. 8°. Bern, 1886.

KUHNT (H.) * Die markhaltige periphere Nervenfaser. 8°. Bonn, 1876.
Also, in: Arch. f. mikr. Anat., Bonn, 1876, xiii, 427-464, 1 pl.
Also: Nachr. v. d. k. Gesellsch. d. Wissensch. u. d. Georg-Aug.-Univ., Götting., 1876, 189-192.

LE GOFF (F.-J.-R.) * Considérations sur la structure des nerfs. 4°. Paris, 1877.

VON LENHOSSÉK (J.) Beiträge zur Erörterung der histologischen Verhältnisse des centralen Nervensystems. 8°. Wien, 1858.
Repr. from: Sitzungsb. d. k. Akad. d. Wissensch., 1858, xxx.

LE THIEULLIER (J.) *An nervi, canales? 4°. [Parisiis, 1743.]
Also, in: SIGWART (G. F.) Quæst. med. Par. 4°. Tubingæ, 1789, i, 72-83.

RANVIER (L.) Leçons sur l'histologie du système nerveux. Recueillies par E. Weber. 2 v. 8°. Paris, 1878.
Also, transl. [Abstr.], in: Buffalo M. & S. J., 1882-3, xxii, 97; 145.

SCHOU (J.) Undersøgelser om den periphere marvholdige Nerveprimitivraads Bygning. 8°. Kjøbenhavn, 1884.

Nervous system (Histology of).

SCHULTZE (H.) *Axencylinder und Ganglienzelle. Mikroscopische Studien über die fibrilläre Structur der Nervenfaser und Nervenzelle bei Wirbelthieren. 8°. Leipzig, 1878.
Also, in: Arch. f. Anat. u. Entwcklngsgesch., Leipz., 1878, 259-287, 1 pl.

SCHULTZE (M.) Observationes de structura cellularum fibrarumque nervearum. 4°. Bonnæ, [1869].

SCHWALBE (G.) Ueber die Kaliberverhältnisse der Nervenfasern. 8°. Leipzig, 1882.

STILLING (B.) Beiträge zur Natur- und Heilkunde. 1. Heft: Anatomische und mikroskopische Untersuchungen über den feineren Bau der Nerven-Primitivfaser und der Nervenzelle. 4°. Frankfurt, 1856.

WALTER (G.) Mikroskopische Studien über das Central-Nervensystem wirbelloser Thiere. 4°. Bonn, 1863.

WAUGH (J. S.) The discovery of an altogether new order of cerebro-spinal filaments in man and the higher quadrupeds. 12°. Annan, 1840.

Adamkiewicz. O nowym składniku włókien nerwowych (istota chromoleptyczna) i o dwubarwności tkanki rdzenia pacierzowego. [The new constituent of nerve fibre and the bicolored texture of medulla.] Medycyna, Warszawa, 1884, xii, 389; 405. ———. Note sur la coloration des tissus du système nerveux central au moyen de la safranine. Compt. rend. Soc. de biol., Par., 1884. 8. s., i, pt. 2, 629-631. ———. Les corpuscules nerveux. Ibid., 1885, 8. s., ii, 621-623. ———. Die Nervenkörperchen; ein neuer, bisher unbekannter morphologischer Bestandtheil der peripherischen Nerven. Sitzungsb. d. k. Akad. d. Wissensch. Math.-naturw. Cl., Wien, 1885, xci, 274-284, 1 pl. Also, Reprint. Also, transl.: Przegl. lek., Krakow., 1885, xxiv, 161-163. ———. La circulation dans les cellules ganglionnaires. Compt. rend. Acad. d. sc., Par., 1886, cii, 60. ———. O budowie ciała i jądra zwojowego. [Structure of ganglionic bodies.] Wiadomości lek., Lwów, 1886, i, 2: 34—Arbuckle (J. H.) A rapid and simple method of staining and mounting fresh brain for microscopic examination. Glasgow M. J., 1876, viii, 207-212.—Arndt (R.) Ueber die Bedeutung der Markscheiden der Nervenfasern. Arch. f. path. Anat., etc.. Berl., 1876, lxvii, 27. ———. Etwas über die Axencylinder der Nervenfasern. Ibid., 1879, lxxviii, 319-356, 1 pl.—Babuchin. Ueber den feineren Bau und Ursprung des Axencylinders. Centralbl. f. d. med. Wissensch., Berl., 1868, vi, 755-757.—Baird (J. B.) Nerve tissue. Atlanta M. & S. J., 1873-4, xi, 553-560.—Bastian (H. C.) On some new methods of preserving thin sections of brain, or spinal-cord, for microscopical examination. J. Anat. & Physiol., Lond., 1868, ii, 104-109.—Beale (L. S.) On the structure and formation of the so-called apolar, unipolar, and bipolar nerve-cells of the frog. Phil. Tr. 1863, Lond., 1864, cliii, 543-571, 8 pl. Also [Abstr.]: Quart. J. Micr. Sc., Lond., 1863, n. s., iii, 302-307. Also, in his: Of the formation of the so-called intercellular substance of cartilage, 8°, [Lond., 1863], 13-18. ———. Indications of the paths taken by the nerve-currents, as they traverse the caudate nerve-cells of the spinal cord and encephalon. [From: Proc. Roy. Soc. Lond., 1864, xiii.] Quart. J. Micr. Sc., Lond., 1865, n. s., v, 90-96. Also, Reprint.—Beevor (C. E.) A new staining fluid for sections of central nervous system. Brit. M. J., Lond., 1882, ii, 997. ———. On staining "in toto" the central nervous system with Weigert's hæmatoxylin. Brain, Lond., 1885-6, viii, 239-242.—Berres (J.) Microscopische Beobachtungen über die innere Bauart der Nerven und Central-Theile des Nerven-Systems. Med. Jahrb. d. k. k. österr. Staates, Wien, 1835, n. F., ix, 274-302, 1 pl.—Besser (L.) Eine Anastomose zwischen centralen Ganglienzellen. Arch. f. path. Anat., etc., Berl., 1866, xxxvi, 134-143, 1 pl. ———. Zur Histogenese der nervösen Elementartheile in den Centralorganen des neugebornen Menschen. Ibid., 305-334, 2 pl.—Bogulawski (N.) Zur Frage über die Structur der markhaltigen Nervenfasern. St. Petersb. med Wchnschr., 1876, i, No. 36, 1.—Boll (F.) Ueber Zersetzungsbilder der markhaltigen Nervenfaser. Arch. f. Anat. u. Entwcklngsgesch., Leipz., 1877, 288-312, 2 pl.—Bramwell (B.) The "half-clearing" method of preparing nerve sections. Edinb. M. J., 1886-7, xxxii, 314-324. ———. Process for the detection of micro-organisms in nerve tissues, Ibid., 324.—Breschet & Raspail. Anatomie microscopique des nerfs, pour démontrer leur structure intime et l'absence de canaux contenant un fluide et pouvant après la mort être facilement injectés. Répert. gén. d'anat. et physiol. path., Par., 1827, iv, 185-192, 1 pl.—Buchholz (R.) Bemerkungen über den histologischen Bau des Centralnervensystems der Süsswassermollusken. Arch. f. Anat., Physiol. u. wissensch. Med., Leipz., 1863, 234-309,

Nervous *system* (*Histology of*).

3 pl.—**Bufalini** (G.) Sulla preparazione del cylinder axis delle fibre nervose. Sperimentale, Firenze, 1880, xlvi, 477-480. ——. Sulla continuità del filamento nervoso delle fibre midollate. Boll. d. Soc. tra i cult. d. sc. med. in Siena, 1883, i, 66.—**Cattani** (Giuseppina). L' appareil de soutien de la myéline dans les fibres nerveuses périphériques. [*Transl. from:* Atti d. r. Accad. d. sc. di Torino, 1886, xxi.] Arch. ital. de biol., Turin, 1886, vii, 345-356. 1 pl.—**Chasiotes** (D.) Πρόδρομος ἀνακοίνωσις περὶ τῆς ὑφῆς τοῦ ἀξονικοῦ κυλίνδρου τῶν νεύρων. Πρακτ. Συνόδου Ἑλλήνων ἰατρῶν 1882, Ἀθήνησιν, 1883, 212-230.—**Ciaccio** (G. V.) Sopra il distribuimento e terminazione delle fibre nervee nella cornea e sopra l' interna construttura del loro cilindro dell' asse. Mem. Accad. d. sc. d. Ist. di Bologna, 1880, 4. s., ii, 577-596, 2 pl.—**Courvoisier** (L. G.) Ueber die spinalen und sympathischen Zellen des Frosches. Centralbl. f. d. med. Wissensch., Berl., 1867, v, 897-899.—**Daae** (H.) Zur Kenntniss der Spinalganglienzellen beim Säugethier. Arch. f. mikr. Anat., Bonn, 1888, xxxi, 223-235, 2 pl.—**De Hieronymis** (T.) Una particolarità di struttura nelle cellule nervose. Progresso med., Napoli, 1887, i, 576. ——. Dell' esistenza di spazi umorali intorno al prolungamento nervoso delle cellule gangliari nel sistema nervoso centrale. Riforma med., Napoli, 1887, iii, 248.—**Dietl** (M. J.) Beobachtungen über Theilungsvorgänge an Nervenzellen. Sitzungsb. d. k. Akad. d. Wissensch., Wien, 1874, lxix, 71-79, 1 pl. ——. Casuistische Beiträge zur Morphologie der Nervenzellen. *Ibid.*, 80-84, 1 pl. ——. Die Gewebselemente des Centralnervensystems bei wirbellosen Thieren. Ber. d. naturw.-med. Ver. in Innsbruck, 1878, vii, 2.-3. Hft., 82-109.—**Dostoïewsky** (A.) Ueber den Bau der Grandry-'schen Köperchen. Arch. f. mikr. Anat., Bonn, 1885-6, xxvi, 581-591, 1 pl.—**Ehrenberg.** Observations on the structure hitherto unknown of the nervous system in man and animals. Edinb. M. & S. J., 1837, xlviii, 257-305, 2 pl. *Also, in:* Essays on Phys. & Hyg., 8°, Phila., 1838, 67-112, 6 pl. *Also,* Reprint.—**Ehrlich** (P.) Ueber die Methylenblaureaction der lebenden Nervensubstanz. Deutsche med. Wchnschr., Berl., 1886, xii, 49-52. *Also:* Biol. Centralbl., Erlang., 1886-7, vi, 214-224. — **Engelmann** (T. W.) Ueber die Diskontinuität des Axencylinders und den fibrillären Bau der Nervenfasern. Onderzoek. ged. in h. physiol. Lab. d. Utrecht. Hoogesch., 1878-80. 3. R., v, 200-239, 1 pl. *Also:* Arch. f. d. ges. Physiol., Bonn, 1880-81, xxii, 1-30, 1 pl.—**Ewald** (A.) & **Kühne** (W.) Ueber einen neuen Bestandtheil des Nervensystems. Verhandl. d. naturh. med. Ver. zu Heidelb., 1874-7, n. F., i, 457-464.—**Fleischl** (E.) Ueber die Beschaffenheit des Axencylinders. *In:* Beitr. z. Anat. u. Physiol. als Festgabe, C. Ludwig, 4°, Leipz., 1874, pt. 1, pp li-lv.—**Flesch** (M.) & **Koneff** (H.) Bemerkungen über die Struktur der Ganglienzellen. Neurol. Centralbl., Leipz., 1886, v, 145-147. — **Fræntzel** (O.) Beitrag zur Kenntniss von der Structur der spinalen und sympathischen Ganglienzellen. Arch. f. path. Anat., etc., Berl., 1867, xxxviii, 549-558, 1 pl.—**Freud** (S.) Die Structur der Elemente des Nervensystems. Jahrb. f. Psychiat., Wien, 1884, v, 221-229. ——. Eine neue Methode zum Studium des Faserverlaufs im Centralnervensystem. Arch. f. Anat. u. Entweklngsgesch., Leipz., 1884, 453-460. *Also, transl.:* Brain, Lond., 1884, vii, 86-88.—**Friedmann** (M.) Ueber eine Modification der neuen Weigert'schen Färbemethode für die markhaltigen Nervenfasern der Centralorgane. Neurol. Centralbl., Leipz., 1885, iv, 135-137. — **Frommann** (C.) Ueber die Färbung der Binde- und Nervensubstanz des Rückenmarkes durch Argentum nitricum und über die Struktur der Nervenzellen. Arch. f. path. Anat., etc., Berl., 1864, xxxi, 129-151, 1 pl. ——. Zur Silberfärbung der Axencylinder. *Ibid.*, 151-153, 1 pl. — **Gierke** (H.) Beiträge zur Kenntniss der Elemente des centralen Nervensystems. Breslau. aerztl. Ztschr., 1882, iv, 157; 172. ——. Die Stützsubstanz des centralen Nervensystems. Neurol. Centralbl., Leipz., 1883, ii, 361; 385. *Also:* Arch. f. mikr. Anat., Bonn, 1885-6, xxv, 441, 2 pl. : xxvi, 129, 1 pl.—**Golgi** (C.) Contribuzione alla fina anatomia degli organi centrali del sistema nervoso. Riv. clin. di Bologna, 1871, 2. s., i, 338; 371, 1 pl. : 1872, 2. s., ii, 38. ——. Sulla fina anatomia degli organi centrali del sistema nervoso. Riv. sper. di freniat., Reggio-Emilia, 1882, viii, 165; 361, 6 pl. : 1883, ix, 1, 5 pl. : 161, 9 pl. ; 385, 4 pl. : 1885, xi, 72; 193. *Also,* Reprint. *Also, transl.* [Abstr.]: Arch. ital. de biol., Turin, 1883, iii, 285, 4 pl. : iv, 92, 4 pl. : 1886, vii, 15. *Also, transl.* [Abstr.]: Alienist & Neurol., St. Louis. 1883, iv, 236, 2 pl. ; 383, 1 pl. : 1885, vi, 307. — **Grandry.** De la structure intime du cylindre de l'axe et des cellules nerveuses. J. de l'anat. et physiol., etc., Par., 1869. vi, 289-301, 1 pl.—**Gray** (W. M.) A modification of Weigert's method of staining the tissues of the central nervous system. Med. News, Phila., 1886, xlix, 515.—**Gruenhagen** (A.) Ueber ein Endothelial-Element der Nervenprimitivscheide. Arch. f. mikr. Anat., Bonn, 1883-4, xxiii, 380. — **Harless** (E.) Bemerkungen zu Dr. v. Hessling's Entdeckung der Primitivfaser-Theilung in dem Gehirne. Jenaische Ann. f. Physiol. u. Med., Jena, 1851, ii, 285-292.—**Henle** (J.) & **Merkel** (F.) Ueber die sogenannte Bindesubstanz der Centralorgane des Nerven-

Nervous *system* (*Histology of*).

systems. Ztschr. f. rat. Med., Leipz. u. Heidelb., 1869, 3. R., xxxiv, 49-82, 4 pl.— **Henriques da Silva** (A. M.) Histologia do tubo nervoso. Coimbra med., 1881, i, 193 ; 209. — **Hesse** (F.) Zur Kenntniss der peripherischen markhaltigen Nervenfaser. Arch. f. Anat. u. Entwcklngsgesch., Leipz., 1879, 341-364. — **von Hessling** (T.) Ueber die Verästelung der Primitivfaser des Gehirns. Jenaische Ann. f. Physiol. u. Med., Jena, 1851, ii, 283.—**Hollis** (W. A.) Researches into the histology of the central grey substance of the spinal cord, medulla oblongata, pons Varolii, and cerebellum. J. Anat. & Physiol., Lond., 1882-3, xvii, 517, 1 pl. : 1883-4, xviii, 62, 1 pl. ; 203, 1 pl. ; 411, 1 pl. : 1884-5, xix, 273, 1 pl.—**Home** (E.) The Croonian lecture. Experiments and observations upon the structure of nerves. Phil. Tr., Lond., 1799, lxxxix, 1-12. — **Homén** (E. A.) Några nyare nervhistologiska undersökningsmetoder. Skrift. utg. af Finska Läk.-sällsk., etc., Helsingfors, 1885, pt. 2, 1-14, 2 pl. — **Jacobi** (E.) Zum feineren Bau der peripheren markhaltigen Nervenfaser. Verhandl. d. phys.-med. Gesellsch. in Würzb., 1887, n. F., xx, 25-51, 1 pl.—**Jakubowitsch** (N.) Microscopische Untersuchungen über die Nervenursprünge im Rückenmarke und verlängertem Marke, über die Empfindungsstellen und sympathischen Zellen in denselben und über die Structur der Primitivnervenzellen, Nervenfasern, und der Nerven überhaupt. Mélanges biol. Acad. imp. d. sc. de St.-Pétersb., 1852-8, ii, 374-387.—**Key** (A.) & **Retzius** (G.) Studier i nervsystemets anatomi. Nord. med. Ark., Stockholm, 1872, iv, no. 21 ; no. 25. *Also, transl.:* Arch. f. mikr. Anat., Bonn, 1873, ix, 308-386, 3 pl.—**Klein** (E.) Beiträge zur Kenntniss der peripherischen Verzweigung markloser Nervenfasern. Centralbl. f. d. med. Wissensch., Berl., 1871, ix, 594-596.—**Kölliker.** Theilung der Nervenprimitivfasern des Menschen. Verhandl. d. phys.-med. Gesellsch. in Würzb., 1850, i, 56.—**Koneff** (Helene). Beiträge zur Kenntniss der Nervenzellen in den peripheren Ganglien. Vorgelegt durch Prof. Flesch. Mitth. d. naturf. Gesellsch. in Bern (1886), 1887, No. 1143-1168, 13-44.—**Koschennikoff** (A.) Axencylinderfortsatz der Nervenzellen im kleinen Hirn des Kalbes. Arch. f. mikr. Anat., Bonn, 1869, v, 331-333.—**Krause** (W.) Die Endothelscheide der Nervenfaser. Internat. Monatschr. f. Anat. u. Histol., Berl., 1885, ii, 259. — **Kühne** (W.) Die Verbindung der Nervenscheiden mit dem Sarkolemm. Ztschr. f. Biol., München, 1883, xix, 501-534, 1 pl.—**Kühne** (W.) & **Steiner** (J.) Beobachtungen über markhaltige und marklose Nervenfasern. Untersuch. a. d. physiol. Inst. d. Univ. Heidelb., 1879, iii, 149-170.—**Kupffer.** Ueber den Bau der Nervenfasern. Sitzungsb. d. Gesellsch. f. Morphol. u. Physiol. in München, 1885, i, 11-14. — **Kutchin** (K.) K' stroeniyu nervnoi tkani. [On the structure of nervous tissue.] Med. Vestnik, St. Petersb., 1865, v, 274. *Also, transl.:* Centralbl. f. d. med. Wissensch., Berl., 1865, iii, 561.—**Lahousse** (E.) Recherches histologiques sur la genèse des ganglions et des nerfs spinaux. Bull. Acad. roy. de méd. de Belg., Brux., 1885, 3. s., xix, 283-311, 1 pl. ——. La cellule nerveuse et la névroglie. Communication préliminaire. Anat. Anz., Jena, 1886, i, 114-116.—**Lantermann** (A. J.) Bemerkungen über den feineren Bau der markhaltigen Nervenfasern. Centralbl. f. d. med. Wissensch., Berl., 1874, xii, 706-709. *Also:* Arch. f. mikr. Anat., Bonn, 1876, xiii, 1-8, 1 pl.—**Laydowsky** (M.) Zum Nachweiss der Axencylinderstructurbestandteilen von markhaltigen Nervenfasern. Centralbl. f. d. med. Wissensch., Berl., 1879, xvii, 865 ; 881. ——. Novija dannija dlja gistol., istorii razvitija i fiziol. periferich. nervov i nervnich koncentrich priborov. [New contributions to the histology, development and physiology of peripheric nerves and arrangement of termini of nerves.] Voyenno-med. J., St. Petersb., 1884, cli, pt. 2, 119-155.—**Liégeois.** De la macération des nerfs dans l'acide tartrique pour faciliter l'étude des filets qui les constituent. Compt. rend. Soc. de biol. 1860, Par., 1861, 3. s., ii, 15.—**Lister** (J.) & **Lister** (W. T.) Observations on the structure of nerve-fibres. Quart. J. Micr. Sc., Lond., 1860, viii, 29-34. *Also,* Reprint.—**Loewe** (L.) Zur Kenntniss der Bindesubstanz im Centralnervensystem der Säugethiere. Arch. f. Psychiat., Berl., 1876, vii, 1-27, 2 pl. ——. Ueber die Faserbahnen im peripheren Nervensystem. Centralbl. f. d. med. Wissensch., Berl., 1879, xvii, 337-341.—**Lominsky** (T.) Zur Frage über die Theilung der Nervenzellen. *Ibid.*, 1882, xx, 434.—**Lubimoff** (A.) Ueber die Verschiedenheit in der embryonalen Entwicklung der Nervenzellen. *Ibid.*, 1873, xi, 641-643. — **Luys** (J.) Contribution à l'étude de la structure de la cellule nerveuse étudiée à l'aide de la méthode photomicrographique. Encéphale, Par., 1881, i, 412-417.—**McCarthy** (J.) Some remarks on spinal ganglia and nerve-fibres. Quart. J. Micr. Sc., Lond., 1875, n. s., xv, 377-381, 1 pl.—**Magnan & Hayem.** Étude sur le tissu interstitiel des parties blanches des centres nerveux. J. de l'anat. et physiol., etc., Par., 1867, iv, 107-112.—**Marcusen** (J.) Zur Histologie des Nervensystems. Mélanges biol. Acad. imp. d. sc. de St.-Pétersb., 1850-53, i, 371-379.—**Marie** (P.) Note sur la recherche des corps granuleux dans les centres nerveux. Bull. Soc. anat. de Par., 1885, lx, 162-164.—**Martius** (F.) Die Methoden

Nervous *system* (*Histology of*).

zur Erforschung des Faserverlaufs im Centralnervensystem. Samml. klin. Vortr., No. 276, Leipz., 1886 (Inn. Med., No. 95), 2567-2610.—**Mason** (J. J.) Microscopic studies on the central nervous system of reptiles and batrachians; the spinal cord of the frog. rana pipiens, rana halecina. J. Nerv. & Ment. Dis., Chicago, 1880, vii, 16 - 23. *Also*, Reprint.—**Mauthner** (L.) Beiträge zur näheren Kenntniss der morphologischen Elemente des Nervensystems. Sitzungsb. d. k. Akad. d. Wissensch. Math.-naturw. Cl., Wien, 1859-60, xxix, 583-589. *Also:* Untersuch. z. Naturl. d. Mensch. u. d. Thiere, Giessen, 1860, vii, 243-250. *Also*, Reprint. ———. Ueber die sogenannten Bindegewebskörperchen des centralen Nervensystems. [*From:* Sitzungsb. d. k. Akad. d. Wissensch., 1861, xliii.] Untersuch. z. Naturl. d. Mensch. u. d. Thiere, Giessen, 1865, ix, 156-166.—**Mayer** (S.) Die peripherische Nervenzelle und das sympathische Nervensystem; eine histologisch-physiologische Studie. Arch. f. Psychiat., Berl., 1875-6, vi, 353-446. *Also*, Reprint.—**Merkel** (F.) Eine neue Methode für Untersuchung des Centralnervensystems. Arch. f. mikr. Anat., Bonn, 1877, xiv, 621-624. — **Meyer** (L.) Ueber das Vorkommen von Körnchenzellen in den Nervencentren. Nachr. v. d. k. Gesellsch. d. Wissensch. u. d. Georg-Aug.-Univ., Götting., 1870, 158-161.—**Mile** (J.) Einwendungen gegen die Richtigkeit der Annehme, dass die Centralenden der primitiven Nervenfasern, durch ihre relative Lage, dem Empfindungsvermögen die relative Lage der Peripherieenden anzeigen sollen. Arch. f. Anat., Physiol. u. wissensch. Med., Berl., 1838, 387-412, 1 pl.—**Mondino** (C.) Sull' uso del bicloruro di mercurio nello studio degli organi centrali del sistema nervoso. Gior. d. r. Accad. di med. di Torino, 1885, 3. s., xxxiii, 38-47.— **von Morochowetz** (L.) Notiz über die Wirkung des Silbernitrats auf die Nervenfaser. Untersuch. a. d. physiol. Inst. d. Univ. Heidelb., 1878, ii, 249-253, 1 pl. ———. Novjechija izslédovanija anatomicheskago i chimicheskago stroénija nervnago volokna. [Histology of nerves.] Vrach. Vaidom., St. Petersb., 1879, iv, 422; 442; 476; 497; 510; 531.—**Nikolaïdes** (R. I.) Ἐπίκρισις τῆς προδρόμου ἀνακοινώσεως τοῦ κ. Δ. Χασιώτου περὶ τῆς ὑφῆς τοῦ ἀξονικοῦ κυλίνδρου τῶν νεύρων. Γαληνός, Ἀθῆναι, 1883, Ι΄, 291; 307; 327; 340; 386; 408; 417.—**Obermeier** (O.) Varicöse Axencylinder im Centralnervensystem. Arch. f. path. Anat., etc., Berl., 1873, lviii, 323.—**Onodi** (A. D.) Ueber die Ganglienzellengruppen der hinteren und vorderen Nervenwurzeln. Centralbl. f. d. med. Wissensch., Berl., 1885, xxiii, 275; 291.—**Owsjannikow** (P.) Einige Worte über die "Mittheilungen" des Hrn. Dr. Jacubowitsch. Arch. f. path. Anat., etc., Berl., 1858, xv, 150-153. ———. Histologische Studien über das Nervensystem der Mollusken. Mélanges biol. Acad. imp. d. sc. de St.-Pétersb., 1871, vii, 679-685.—**Pal** (J.) Ein Beitrag zur Nervenfärbetechnik. Med. Jahrb., Wien, 1886, n. F., i, 619-631. ———. Bemerkungen zur Ehrlich'schen Nervenfärbung. *Ibid.*, 1887, n. F., ii, 159-164.—**Pertik** (O.) Untersuchungen über Nervenfasern. Arch. f. mikr. Anat., Bonn, 1880-81, xix, 183-239, 1 pl.—**Petrone** (L. M.) Sulla struttura del tessuto interstiziale dei nervi periferici. Gazz. d. osp., Milano, 1887, viii, 92. ———. Sulla struttura del tessuto interstiziale normale dei centri nervosi cerebro-spinali dei nervi periferici cerebro-rachidiani. *Ibid.*, 1888. ix, 26-29.—**Preyer** (W.) Notiz über die violettempfindenden Nerven. Centralbl. f. d. med. Wissensch., Berl., 1872, x, 113. — **Prochaska** (G.) De structura nervorum. *In his:* Operum minorum anat. [etc.], 8°, Viennæ, 1800, i, 273-404, 7 pl.— **Purkinje.** Microscopical observations on the nerves. Lond. M. Gaz., 1845, n. s., i, 1066; 1156. *Also, transl.:* Arch. f. Anat., Physiol. u. wissensch. Med., Berl., 1845, 281-295.— **Ranvier** (L.) Recherches relatives à la fine structure des éléments des nerfs périphériques. Compt. rend. Soc. de biol. 1871, Par., 1873, 5. s., iii, pt. 1, 130-134. ———. Recherches sur l'histologie et la physiologie des nerfs. Arch. de physiol. norm. et path., Par., 1871-2, iv, 129; 427, 2 pl. ———. Des tubes nerveux en T et de leurs relations avec les cellules ganglionnaires. Compt. rend. Acad. d. sc., Par., 1875, lxxxi, 1274-1276. *Also:* Rev. méd. franç. et étrang., Par., 1876, i, 110-112.—**Rattone** (G.) Sur l'existence de cellules ganglionnaires dans les racines postérieures des nerfs rachidiens de l'homme. Internat. Monatschr. f. Anat. u. Histol., Berl., 1884, i, 53-68, 2 pl.—**Rawitz** (B.) Die Ranvier'schen Einschnürungen und Lantermann'schen Einkerbungen. Arch. f. Anat. u. Entwcklngsgesch., Leipz., 1879, 57-76, 1 pl.—**Recent** studies in nerve histology. Brit. & For. M.-Chir. Rev., Lond., 1877, lix, 86-95. — **Remak** (R.) Vorläufige Mittheilung microscopischer Beobachtungen über den innern Bau der Cerebrospinalnerven und über die Entwickelung ihrer Formelemente. Arch. f. Anat., Physiol. u. wissensch. Med., Berl., 1836, 145-161, 1 pl. ———. Ueber den Inhalt der Nervenprimitivröhren. *Ibid.*, 1843, 197-201.—**Renaut** (J.) Recherches sur quelques points particuliers de l'histologie des nerfs. Arch. de physiol. norm. et path., Par., 1881, 2. s., viii, 161-190, 1 pl. *Also:* Trav. du lab. d'anat. gén. et d'histol., Par., 1882, 34-63, 1 pl. ———. Système hyalin de soutènement des centres nerveux et de quelques organes des sens. Arch. de physiol. norm. et path., Par., 1881, 2. s., viii, 845-860, 1 pl. — **Retsin** (A.) De la structure intime du sys-

Nervous *system* (*Histology of*).

tème nerveux, central, périphérique et grand sympathique. Ann. d. univ. de Belg. 1846, Brux., 1847, 473-742, 27 pl.—**Retzius** (G.) Undersökning öfver cerebrospinalgangliernas nervceller med särskild hänsyn till dessas utlöpare. Nord. med. Ark., Stockholm, 1879, xi, no. 31, 1-24, 3 pl. *Also, transl.:* Arch. f. Anat. u. Entwcklngsgesch., Leipz., 1880, 369-402. 6 pl.—**Rezzonico** (G.) Sulla origine della guaina di Schwann. Arch. ital. per le mal. nerv., Milano, 1886, xxiii, 208-216. — **Robin** (C.) Mémoire sur le périnèvre, espèce nouvelle d'élément anatomique qui entre dans la composition du tissu des nerfs. Compt. rend. Soc. de biol. 1854, Par., 1855, 2. s., i, pt. 2, 87-103. *Also:* Arch. gén. de méd., Par., 1854, 4. s., iv, 323-338. *Also*, Reprint.—**Romiti** (G.) Sulla struttura degli elementi del tessuto nervoso. Sperimentale, Firenze, 1881, xlvii, 48-53.—**Rosenbach** (P.) Ueber die Bedeutung der Vacuolenbildung in den Nervenzellen. Neurol. Centralbl., Leipz., 1884, iii, 54-56. —**Rosenheim** (T.) Ueber das Vorkommen und die Bedeutung der Mastzellen im Nervensystem des Menschen. Arch. f. Psychiat., Berl., 1886, xvii, 820-829, 1 pl.—**Rudanovski** (P.) Izslaidovanii stroeniya nervnoi tkani posredstvom novago metoda. [Investigation of the nervous tissues by a new method.] Med. Vestnik, St. Petersb., 1865, v, 61; 77; 85; 93. *Also, transl.* [Abstr.]: France méd., Par., 1865, xii, 18. ———. Zamaitka k' izslaidovamiyam stroeniya nervnoi tkani. [Examination of the structure of nervous tissue.] Med. Vestnik, St. Petersb., 1865, v, 229. ———. Zamaitka o nervnikh yacheikakh. [Notes on nerve cells.] *Ibid.*, 1866, vi, 307. ———. Corpuscula hyaloidea seu gelatinosa v' nervnoi sistemai, kak osobennii element. [Gelatinous corpuscles in the nervous system, according to their several elements.] *Ibid.*, 374. ———. Sobstvennaya obolochka nervnekh yacheek, i ikh pigmentatsiya. [The proper envelope and coloring of the nerve cells.] *Ibid.*, 1867, vii, 25-27. ———. O pristustvii sokratitelnikh elementov v' pervichnikh trubkakh perephericheskikh nervov. [On the presence of contractile elements in the primary sheaths of the peripheral nerves.] *Ibid.*, 1869, ix, 141-144. ———. Ueber die Structur der Axencylinder in den Primitivnervenvenröhren der Spinalnerven und ihr Verhältniss zu letzteren. Arch. f. path. Anat., etc., Berl., 1871, lii, 193-203, 1 pl. ———. O metodai izslaidovaniya nervnoi tkani i o stroenii zernoshkof spinnikh nervof' i nervnoi tkani v' tsentralnikh organakh. [On a method of examining nerve tissues, and on the structure of the radicles of the spinal nerve, and the nerve tissue of the internal organs.] Protok. zasaid. Kavkazsk. med. Obsh., Tiflis, 1873-4, x, 135.—**Rumpf** (T.) Zur Histologie der Nervenfaser und des Axencylinders. Verhandl. d. naturh.-med. Ver. zu Heidelb., 1877-80, n. F., ii, 171-176. *Also:* Untersuch. a. d. physiol. Inst. d. Univ. Heidelb., 1878, ii, 137-186.—**Sahli** (H.) Ueber eine neue Doppelfärbung des centralen Nervensystems. Ztschr. f. wissensch. Mikr., Brnschwg., 1885, ii, 1-7, 1 pl. ———. Ueber die Anwendung von Boraxmethylenblau für die Untersuchung des centralen Nervensystems und für den Nachweis von Mikroorganismen, speciell zur bacteriologischen Untersuchung der nervösen Centralorgane. *Ibid.*, 49-51. — **Sappey** (C.) Recherches sur la structure de l'enveloppe fibreuse des nerfs. J. de l'anat. et physiol., etc., Par., 1868, v, 47-52.—**Satterthwaite** (T.E.) Notes and practical studies on the minute elements of the nervous system. N. York M. J., 1878, xxviii, 225-243, 2 pl. *Also*, Reprint.— **Schaffner.** Ueber die Entwicklung der Primitivfasern des Nervensystems. Ztschr. f. rat. Med., Heidelb., 1846, v, 411-420. ———. Beiträge zur Histologie des Nervensystems, nebst Bemerkungen über die Muskelfasern und die Bewegung des Herzens. *Ibid.*, 1850, ix, 239, 1 pl.: 1851, x, 203, 1 pl.—**Schiefferdecker** (P.) Beiträge zur Kenntniss des Baus der Nervenfasern. Arch. f. mikr. Anat., Bonn, 1887, xxx, 435-494, 1 pl.: 1887-8, xxxi, 100-102.—**Schmidt** (H. D.) On the construction of the dark or double-bordered nerve fibre. Month. Micr. J., Lond., 1874, xi, 200-221, 3 pl. *Also*, Reprint. ———. Synopsis of the principal facts elicited from a series of microscopical researches upon the nervous tissues. Month. Micr. J., Lond., 1874, xii, 1-10. *Also*, Reprint. ———. Note on the intimate structure of nervous ganglionic bodies. Tr. Am. Neural. Ass., N. Y., 1877, ii, 45-49. — **Schultze** (H.) Die fibrilläre Structur der Nervenelemente bei Wirbellosen. Arch. f. mikr. Anat., Bonn, 1878-9, xvi, 57-111, 2 pl. *Also*, Reprint. — **Shaw** (J. C.) Some peculiarities in the myeline of peripheral nerves after treatment by osmic acid. J. Nerv. & Ment. Dis., Chicago, 1878, v, 57 - 59. *Also*, Reprint. ———. Peculiar marking of medullated nerve-fibres. Med. Rec., N. Y., 1878, xiii, 118.—**Some** recent researches into the histology of the nervous centres. Brit. & For. M.-Chir. Rev., Lond., 1873, li, 59-77.—**Sperino** (G.) Sulla presenza di cellule ganglionari sul decorso delle fibre che compongono i nervi splanchnic major et minor. Gazz. d. osp., Milano, 1886, vii, 75. — **Stannius.** Ueber Theilungen der Primitivröhren in den Stämmen, Aesten und Zweigen der Nerven. Arch. f. physiol. Heilk., Stuttg., 1850, ix, 75-79. — **Starr** (M. A.) Methods of staining nervous tissue. J. Nerv. & Ment. Dis., N. Y., 1885, n. s., x, 143-153. — **Stilling** (B.)

Nervous *system (Histology of).*

Sur la structure de la fibre nerveuse primitive. Gaz. méd. de Par., 1855, 3. s., x, 757. ———. Sur la structure de la cellule nerveuse. Monit. d. hôp., Par., 1855, iii, 1123. *Also:* Gaz. méd. de Par., 1855, 3. s., x, 758.—**Stirling** (W.) Historical references to the structure of nerve fibres. J. Anat. & Physiol., Lond., 1880-81, xv, 446.—**Swan** (J.) On the art of making transparent preparations of the spinal cord, for showing the roots of the nerves by the microscope. Lond. M. Gaz., 1849, n. s., ix, 967-969.—**Tal** (I.) Modificazione del metodo di Golgi nella preparazione delle cellule gangliari nel sistema nervoso centrale. Gazz. d. osp., Milano, 1886, vii, 538. — **Tamamschef** (J.) Ueber Nervenrohr, Axencylinder und Albuminstoffe. Centralbl. f. d. med. Wissensch., Berl., 1872, x, 593-597.—**Tangl** (F.) Zur Histologie der gequetschten peripherischen Nerven. Arch. f. mikr. Anat., Bonn, 1887, xxix, 464-470, 1 pl.—**von Thanhoffer** (L.) Beiträge zur feineren Structur des centralen Nervensystems. Centralbl. f. Physiol., Leipz. u. Wien, 1887-8, i, 36-38. — **Tigri** (A.) Sulla fibra contrattile o muscolare della vita organica, nel sistema nervoso. Gior. med. di Roma, 1869, v, 345; 457; 509; 577; 1 pl. *Also* [Abstr.]: Gior. d. r. Accad. di med. di Torino, 1868, 3. s., vi, 202-212.—**Tizzoni** (G.) Sulla istologia normale e patologica del tessuto nervoso. Osservatore, Torino, 1878, xiv, 165-168. ———. Sulla patologia del tessuto nervoso; osservazioni ed esperimenti sulla istologia normale e patologica della fibra nervosa. Arch. per le sc. med., Torino, 1878-9, iii, 1-61. *Also,* Reprint.—**von Tschisch** (W.) Ueber die künstliche Bildung von Farbstoff im Nervengewebe. Arch. f. path. Anat., etc., Berl., 1884, xcvii, 173-176.—**Unger** (L.) Ueber den Bau der grauen Substanz des Central-Nervensystems. Allg. Wien. med. Ztg., 1879, xxiv, 491.—**Valentin** (G. G.) Ueber die Dicke der varikösen Fäden in dem Gehirne und dem Rückenmarke des Menschen. Arch. f. Anat., Physiol. u wissensch. Med., Berl., 1834, 401-409. ———. Erwiderung auf den Volkmann'schen Aufsatz über Nervenfasern, etc. *Ibid.,* 1844, 395-403. ———. Das Verhalten einzelner Nervengewebe in polarisirtem Lichte. Ztschr. f. rat. Med., Leipz. u. Heidelb., 1862, 3. R., 122-136. — **Vignal** (W.) Accroissement en longueur des tubes nerveux par la formation de segments intercalaires. École prat. d. hautes études. Lab. d'histol. du Coll. de France. Trav. 1883, Par., 1884, viii, 133-145, 1 pl. ———. Segments intercalaires des tubes nerveux; historique et rectifications. Compt. rend. Soc. de biol., Par., 1883, 7. s., v, pt. 1, 201-204. ———. Les corpuscules nerveux de M. Adamkiewicz. *Ibid.,* 1886, 8. s., iii, 110-113.—**Virchow** (R.) Die histologischen Elemente namentlich die Nerven in Adhäsionen. Verhandl. d. phys.-med. Gesellsch. in Würzb., 1850, i, 141. ———. Ueber das ausgebreitete Vorkommen einer dem Nervenmark analogen Substanz in den thierischen Geweben. Arch. f. path. Anat., etc., Berl., 1853, vi, 562-572.—**Volkmann** (A. W.) Ueber Nervenfasern und deren Messung mit Hülfe der Schrauben- und Glasmikrometer. Arch. f. Anat., Physiol. u. wissensch. Med., Berl., 1844, 9-26.—**Waldeyer** (W.) Untersuchungen über den Ursprung und den Verlauf des Axencylinders bei Wirbellosen und Wirbelthieren, sowie über dessen Endverhalten in der quergestreiften Muskelfaser. Ztschr. f. rat. Med., Leipz. u. Heidelb., 1863, 3. R., xx, 193-256, 3 pl.—**Waldstein** (L.) & **Weber** (E.) Études histochimiques sur les tubes nerveux à myéline. École prat. d. hautes études. Lab. d'histol. du Coll. de France. Trav., Par., 1882, vii, 70-96, 1 pl. *Also:* Arch. de physiol. norm. et path., Par., 1882, xiv, 1-27, 1 pl.—**Willigk** (A.) Nervenzellenanastomosen im Rückenmarke. Arch. f. path. Anat., etc., Berl., 1875, lxiv, 163-169, 1 pl.—**Winkler** (C.) Hoe verbindt zich de zenuwcel met de zenuwvezel? Nederl. Tijdschr. v. Geneesk., Amst., 1886, xxii, 192-196.

Nervous *system (Influence of) in disease.*

See, also, **Imagination** *as a cause, etc., of disease;* **Inflammation** *(Nervous influence on);* **Skin** *(Diseases of, Neurotic).*

CARLHANT (V.) * Considérations générales sur le rôle que joue le système nerveux dans la production des maladies. 4°. *Strasbourg,* 1822.

LEVEN (M.) La névrose, étude clinique et thérapeutique. Dyspepsie, anémie, rhumatisme et goutte, obésité, amaigrissement. 8°. *Paris,* 1887.

SCHNEIDER (J.-F.) * Réflexions sur les influences pathologiques du système nerveux. 4°. *Paris,* 1850.

VILLEMIN (L.) * De l'innervation et de son influence sur la marche des maladies aiguës. 4°. *Strasbourg,* 1842.

Curschmann. Bemerkungen über das Verhalten des Centralnervensystemes bei acuten Infectionskrankheiten. Verhandl. d. Cong. f. innere Med., Wiesb., 1886, v, 469-489, 1 pl.—**Dugniolle.** Du rôle que joue le système nerveux dans la production de quelques maladies. Arch.

Nervous *system (Influence of) in disease.*

de la méd. belge, Brux., 1843, xii, 341 - 347. — **Enz** (E.) Beobachtungen über mehrere der symptomatischen Krankheitsformen, welche bei Empfindlichkeit einer grösseren oder kleineren Stelle der Wirbelsäule vorkommen. Mag. f. d. ges. Heilk., Berl., 1834, xli, 195 : 1835, xliv, 43 ; 204.— **Fontana** (F.) Considération sur les nerfs dans les maladies. *In his:* Traité sur le venin de la vipère, [etc.], 4°, Florence, 1781, iii, 162-176. *Also, transl. in his:* Trattato del veleno della vipera, [etc.], 8°, Napoli, 1787, iii, 119-135. *Also, transl. in his:* Treatise on the venom of the viper, [etc.], 8°, Lond., 1787, ii, 186 - 202. — **Fothergill** (J. M.) The neurotic, with indigestion and lithiasis. Med. Rec., N. Y., 1888, xxxiii, 1-3.—**Guild** (J.) The nervous system as the primary seat of morbid impressions. Atlanta M. & S. J., 1873-4, xi, 611-619.—**Haughton** (R. E.) Influence in disease of the nervous system. Tr. Indiana M. Soc., Indianap., 1871, xxi, 143-156 —**Hughes** (C. H.) Hygiene of the nervous system and mind ; the relation of the nervous system to cholera and its prophylaxis and neurotherapy. Sanitarian, N. Y., 1885, xv, 414-423. ———. The relation of the nervous system to hæmophilia, malarial hæmaturia, etc. Alienist & Neurol., St. Louis, 1887, viii, 378-387. *Also,* Reprint. *Also:* Weekly M. Rev., St. Louis, 1887, xv, 561-566.—**Hutchinson** (J.) On structural diseases induced through the influence of the nervous system. Brit. M. J., Lond., 1880, ii, 915.—**Laycock** (T.) Lectures on diseases of organs and tissues, as influenced by the nervous system. Med. Times & Gaz., Lond., 1871, i, 241; 301; 359; 389; 535; 595: ii, 1; 91; 211; 269. — **Lente** (F. D.) The neurotic origin of disease, and the action of remedies on the nervous system. Psych. & Med.-Leg. J., N. Y., 1875, n. s., ii, 1; 78. — **Philip** (A. P. W.) On the influence of the nervous system in determining the nature and progress of disease. Lond. M. Gaz., 1835, xvi, 256 ; 296 ; 327 ; 374. — **Reignier.** Influence du système nerveux sur les éruptions cutanées. Bull. et mém. Soc. de méd. prat. de Par., 1888, 107-109.—**Remak.** Ueber den Einfluss der Centralorgane des Nervensystems auf Krankheiten der Knochen und der Gelenke. Allg. med. Centr.-Ztg., Berl., 1863, xxxii, 153 - 155. — **Röell** (C. C.) De invloed van het verminderd zenuwleven op het vaatleven. Nederl. Tijdschr. v. Geneesk., Amst., 1858, ii, 113 - 117. — **Scoville** (S. S.) Report on nervous influence. Tr. Ohio M. Soc., Cincin., 1872, 67-107.—**Vizioli** (F.) Il sistema nervoso e la patologia moderna. Morgagni, Napoli, 1871, xiii, 73 - 106. — **Wible** (B. M.) The nervous system in its relations to practical medicine. Richmond & Louisville M. J., Louisville, 1876, xxi, 413-429.

Nervous *system (Injuries of).*

See **Shock.**

Nervous *system (Methods of investigation of).*

BEAUNIS (H.) Note sur l'application des injections interstitielles à l'étude des fonctions des centres nerveux. 8°. *[Paris, n. d.]*

OSIANDER (F. B.) Vera cerebri humani circa basin incisi imago, cum observationibus de cerebro et medulla spinali novaque nervos æque ac plantarum vasa hydrargyro implendi methodo; exhibita et commentatio recitata in consessu Societatis Regiæ Scientiarum, d. 15 Nov. 1806. 4°. *[n. p., n. d.]*

Betz (W.) Die Untersuchungsmethode des Centralnerven-Systems des Menschen. Arch. f. mikr. Anat., Bonn, 1873, ix, 101-117.—**Freud** (S.) Eine neue Methode zum Studium des Faserverlaufs im Centralnervensystem. Centralbl. f. d. med. Wissensch., Berl., 1884, xxii, 161-163.—**Gudden.** Experimentaluntersuchungen über das peripherische und centrale Nervensystem. Arch. f. Psychiat., Berl., 1869-70, ii, 693-723, 3 pl.—**Hyslop** (J.) Gudden's method in the investigation of the anatomy of the central nervous system. J. Ment. Sc., Lond., 1881 - 2, xxvii, 47-50. — **Jones** (T. W.) Historical notice of how it was that the late Dr. Augustus Waller became acquainted with the method of tracing nerve fibrils in their ultimate distribution by section of the trunk. Lancet, Lond., 1885, ii, 944.—**Koelliker** (A.) Die Untersuchungen von Golgi über den feineren Bau des zentralen Nervensystems. Anat. Anz., Jena, 1887, ii, 480-483.—**Luys** (J.) Des procédés à employer pour l'étude anatomique et photographique du système nerveux central. Encéphale, Par., 1886, vi, 412-426.—**Moriggia** (A.) Sur un nouveau moyen pour isoler la sensibilité de la motilité des nerfs. Arch. ital. de biol., Turin, 1883, iv, 273 - 278. — **Roudanovsky** (P.) Observations sur la structure des tissus nerveux d'après une nouvelle méthode. J. de l'anat. et physiol., etc., Par., 1865, ii, 225-243, 2 pl.—**Schulgin** (M. A.) Metode izsliedovanija nervoi sistemi. [Method of examining the nervous system.] Arch. psichiat., etc., Charkov, 1883, ii, no. 1, 120-146. — **Seguin** (E. C.) Gudden's atrophy method: and a summary of its results. Arch. Med., N. Y., 1883, x, 126 - 145. — **Stefani** (A.)

Nervous system (*Methods of investigation of*).

L' incrociamento dei nervi utilizzato per lo studio delle funzioni dei centri nervosi. Riv. clin. di Bologna, 1885, 3. s., v, 523-535. *Also*, Reprint. ———. L' incrociamento dei nervi utilizzato per lo studio delle funzioni dei centri nervosi. Riv. clin. di Bologna, 1886, 3. s., vi, 419-426. *Also*. Reprint. *Also, transl.:* Arch. f. Physiol.. Leipz., 1886, 488-499. — **Tigerstedt** (R.) En ny metod för mekanisk retning af nerver. [C. r. Sur une nouvelle méthode pour l'excitation mécanique des nerfs, no. 14.] Nord. med. Ark., Stockholm, 1881, xiii, no. 12, 1-15. — **Van Gieson** (I.) A résumé of recent technical methods for the nervous system. J. Nerv. & Ment. Dis., N. Y., 1887, xiv, 310-315. — **Waller** (A.) A new method for the study of the nervous system. Lond. J. M., 1852, iv, 609-625. — **Walther** (A.) Eine neue Methode der Untersuchung des centralen Nervensystems. Centralbl. f. d. med. Wissensch., Berl., 1868, 449-452. — **Weigert** (C.) Ueber eine neue Untersuchungsmethode des Centralnervensystems. *Ibid.*, 1882, xx, 753; 772.

Nervous system (*Pathology and pathological anatomy of*).

See, also, **Face** (*Atrophy, etc., of*); **Nerves** (*Degeneration, etc., of*); **Nervous** system (*Ganglionic, Pathology of*); **Nervous** system (*Sclerosis of*); **Nervous** system (*Syphilis of*); **Neuritis.**

ABERCROMBIE (J.) Pathological and practical researches on diseases of the brain and the spinal cord. 2. ed. 8°. *Edinburgh*, 1829.

———. The same. 4. ed. 8°. *Edinburgh & London*, 1845.

———. The same. 1. Am. from 2. Edinb. ed. 8°. *Philadelphia*, 1831.

———. The same. Des maladies de l'encéphale et de la moelle épinière. 3. éd. 18°. *Bruxelles*, 1837.

AUDHOUI (V.) * De l'influence des études histologiques sur la connaissance des maladies du système nerveux. 8°. *Paris*, 1875.

CATTANI (G.) Sulla degenerazione e neoformazione delle fibre nervose midollari periferiche. Ricerche sperimentali. fol. *Bologna*, 1886.

DEMME (H.) Beiträge zur pathologischen Anatomie des Tetanus und einiger anderen Krankheiten des Nervensystems. 8°. *Leipzig u. Heidelberg*, 1859.

DERCUM (F. X.) A brief synopsis of the various points involved in the coarse examination of the brain and spinal cord. 8°. *Norristown, Pa.*, 1886.

DIEULAFOY (G.) * Des progrès réalisés par la physiologie expérimentale dans la connaissance des maladies du système nerveux. 8°. *Paris*, 1875.

DZONDI (C. H.) * [Pr.] inest pathologiæ systematis nervosi brevis adumbratio. 8°. *Halæ*, 1827.

ERB (W.) Ueber die neuere Entwicklung der Nervenpathologie und ihre Bedeutung für den medicinischen Unterricht. Vortrag, gehalten beim Antritt des Lehramtes an der Universität Leipzig am 16. Juni 1880. 8°. *Leipzig*, 1880.

FOX (E. L.) The pathological anatomy of the nervous centres. 8°. *London*, 1874.

HUGUENIN (G.) Allgemeine Pathologie der Krankheiten des Nervensystems. 1. Theil Anatomische Einleitung. 8°. *Zürich*, 1873.

KALANTARIANTZ [KALANTAROVA] (S.) * K patologicheskoi anatomii plexus solaris et hypogastrici pri peritonite i broushnom tife. 8°. *St. Petersburg*, 1881.

LAMANN (V.) * Materialy k patologii Auerbachovskich uzlov. 8°. *St. Petersburg*, 1881.

LEMBERT (A.) * Propositions sur le système nerveux, appliquées à la théorie des névroses et des inflammations. 4°. *Paris*, 1828.

VAN DER LITH (J. P. T.) * De vitiis nervorum organicis. 8°. *Amstelodami*, 1838.

MESSNER (A.) * Beiträge zur pathologischen Anatomie des Nervensystens. 8°. *Stuttgart*, 1881.

Nervous system (*Pathology and pathological anatomy of*).

RATTONE (G.) * Contribuzione allo studio della patologia chirurgica dei nervi. 8°. *Torino*, 1882.

RAYMOND. Anatomie pathologique du système nerveux. 8°. *Paris*, 1886 [1885].

SACHS (G.) Quæstionum neuropathologicarum specimen. 4°. *Regimontii Pr.*, 1837.

SEELIGMÜLLER (A.) Neuropathologische Beobachtungen. Festschrift zur Feier des fünfzigjährigen Promotionsjubiläums des Dr. E. Blasius dargebracht von dem Verein für praktische Medicin in Halle a. S. 8°. *Halle*, 1873.

WILLIS (T.) Pathologiæ cerebri et nervosi generis specimen. In quo agitur de morbis convulsivis, et de scorbuto. 4°. *Genevæ*, 1576.

———. The same. 16°. *Amstelodami*, 1668.

———. The same. 24°. *Amstelodami*, 1670.

———. The same. 4°. *Genevæ*, 1676.

In his: Opera omnia. 4°. *Genevæ*, 1676.

———. The same. 4°. *Geneva*, 1696.

In his: Opera omnia. 4°. *Genevæ*, 1695, i.

Alexander (W.) On some rare forms of disease, accompanied by lesions of trophic nerves or trophic centres, and illustrative of trophic changes. Lancet, Lond., 1881, i, 986; 1023.—**Althaus** (J.) Contributions to the pathology of peripheral nerve-diseases. Am. J. M. Sc., Phila., 1879, n. s., lxxvii, 363-382. *Also* [Abstr.]: Med. Press & Circ., Lond., 1879, n. s., xxvii, 98.—**Arndt** (R.) Ueber Atrophie der Nervenfasern und Ganglienkörper. Arch. f. path. Anat., etc., Berl., 1873-4, lix, 511-521. ———. Aphorismen zur pathologischen Anatomie der Centralorgane des Nervensystems. *Ibid.*, 1874, lxi, 508: 1875, lxiv, 356.—**Babes** (V.) Ueber parenchymatöse Neubildungen des Centralnervensystems. Pest. med.-chir. Presse, Budapest, 1882, xviii, 539.—**Baerwinkel** (F.) Neuropathologische Beiträge. I. Pathologie des N. trigeminus. II. Diplegia N. trigemini motoria. III. Ophthalmia neuroparalytica. Deutsches Arch. f. klin. Med., Leipz., 1874, xii, 606-616. — **Baillarger.** Nature cadavérique de quelques lésions des centres nerveux. Ann. méd.-psych., Par., 1885, 7. s., i, 17-19.—**Bareggi** (C.) Contribuzione alla patogenesi dell' iperemia e dell' anemia dei centri nervosi. Ann. univ. di med., Milano, 1875, ccxxxiv, 52-63.—**Bennett** (J. H.) Pathological and histological researches on inflammation of the nervous centers. Edinb. M. & S. J., 1842, lviii, 364: 1843, lix, 321, 1 pl. *Also*, Reprint.—**Berger** (O.) Neuropathologische Notizen. Centralbl. f. Nervenh., Coblenz, 1879, ii, 217; 266.—**Bernhardt** (M.) Neuropathologische Beobachtungen. Arch. f. Psychiat., Berl., 1875-6, vi, 549-564. ———. Neuropathologische Beobachtungen. Deutsches Arch. f. klin. Med., Leipz., 1878, xxii, 362-393.—**Bianchi** (L.) & **D'Abundo** (G.) Experimental degenerations in the brain and the spinal cord. [Transl.] Alienist & Neurol., St. Louis, 1887, viii, 163-196.—**Blandford** (G. F.) The causes and outcome of nerve degeneration. St. George's Hosp. Rep., Lond., 1877, viii, 99-109. — **Boccardi** (G.) Ricerche sperimentali intorno ad alcune alterazioni trofiche consecutive a lesioni del sistema nervoso periferico; comunicazione preventiva. Movimento, Napoli, 1881, 2. s., iii, 129-132.—**Borgherini** (A.) Origine e sviluppo della neuropatologia. Riv. veneta di sc. med., Venezia, 1887, vi, 139-158.—**Brainard** (D.) Suggestions on the tendency to vacuum in the cerebro-spinal cavity which exists in certain spasmodic diseases. Chicago M. J., 1861, n. s., iv, 4-15.—**Brigidi** (V.) Illustrazione di preparati microscopici relativi a talune malattie de' centri nervosi. Imparziale, Firenze, 1875, xv, 482-489. ———. Di una nuova particolare alterazione dei centri nervosi. *Ibid.*, 1876, xvi, 624. — **Burtseff** (I. I.) Perimeningitis et myelitis bulbi acuta. Ejened. klin. gaz., St. Petersb., 1883, iii, 409; 425; 463; 492.—**Carrieu.** De l'influence des lésions antérieures sur la production de nouvelles altérations dans le système nerveux. Gaz. hebd. d. sc. méd. de Montpel., 1881, iii, 339-342. ———. Des lésions osseuses dans les maladies du système nerveux. *Ibid.*, 1885, vii, 602: 1886, viii, 289; 421; 470; 506. — **Charcot** (J.-M.) Anatomie pathologique du système nerveux. Progrès méd., Par., 1879, vii, 258; 359; 557; 597, 757; 801; 825; 933; 993: 1880, viii, 121; 202: 248; 265; 285; 343; 401. *Also, transl.:* Cincin. Lancet & Clinic, 1880, n. s., v, 287; 308; 334; 354; 401; 426; 469; 494: 518: 1881, n. s., vi, 25; 77; 117; 192; 233; 258; 285. *Also*, Reprint.—**Clark** (D.) A report on cerebro-spinal pathology. Am. J. Insan., Utica, N. Y., 1883-4, xl, 127-144.—**Dalton** (J. C.) Nervous degenerations and the theory of Sir Charles Bell. Med. Rec., N. Y., 1882, xxi, 141-150.—**Dana** (C. L.) Cases of pachymeningitis, cerebral and spinal, with records of post-mortems. J. Nerv. & Ment. Dis., N. Y., 1882, n. s., vii, 58-73.

Nervous system (*Pathology and pathological anatomy of*).

Deecke (F.) The structure of the vessels of the nervous centers in health and their changes in disease. Am. J. Insan., Utica, N. Y., 1877-8, xxxiv, 18: 1878-79, xxxv, 445; 515: 1879-80, xxxvi, 328; 404: 1880-81, xxxvii, 273, 1 pl. *Also,* Reprint.—**Déjerine** (J.) Sur l'existence d'altérations des nerfs cutanés, dans certaines eschares, survenant dans le cours des maladies du cerveau ou de la moelle épinière. Compt. rend. Soc. de biol., Par., 1882, 7. s., iv, 77. *Also :* Arch. de physiol. norm. et path., Par., 1882, 2. s., ix, 499-506. — **Drozda** (J. V.) Neuropathologische Beiträge. Wien. med. Wchnschr., 1880, xxx, 913; 947; 972. *Also,* Reprint. ———. Neuropathologische Beiträge. Wien. med. Presse, 1882, xxiii, 523; 557; 589; 692; 728; 763; 825; 1160; 1193; 1227; 1292; 1323.—**Dzedzoul** (K.) Materiali k voprosu o sosudor aschirjaushich nervach. [Vascular enlargement of the nerves.] Voyenno-med. J., St. Petersb., 1880, cxxxviii, pt. 2, 97-140.—**Eichholtz** (H.) Die Nervenpathologie; ein Beitrag zur Principienfrage. Wchnschr. f. d. ges. Heilk., Berl., 1848, 641; 664.—**Engelmann** (T. W.) Ueber Degeneration von Nervenfasern. Arch. f. d. ges. Physiol., Bonn, 1876, xiii, 474-491.—**Fick.** Ueber Umwandlung von Nerven in Fett. Arch. f. Anat., Physiol. u. wissensch. Med., Berl., 1842, 19-21.—**Filehne** (W.) Ueber die Erregbarkeit degenerirender Nerven. Berl. klin. Wchnschr., 1869, vi, 319. — **Fouilhoux.** Quelques observations et réflexions sur l'état des plexus nerveux dans plusieurs maladies. Rev. méd. franç. et étrang., Par., 1838, iv, 30-46.—**Fowler** (S. W.) Nervorum erethismus, or debility of the nerves. Cincin. Lancet & Obs., 1877, n. s., xx, 880-887.—**François-Franck & Pitres** (A.) Des dégénérations secondaires de la moelle épinière consécutives à l'ablation du gyrus sigmoïde chez le chien. Compt. rend. Soc. de biol. 1880, Par., 1881, 7. s., ii, 67-73.—**Fronmüller** (G.) Hyperämie der Hirn- und Rückenmarkshäute mit eigenthümlichen Nervenzufällen. Memorabilien, Heilbr., 1882, n. F., ii, 14-17.—**Geddings** (E.) Contributions to the pathology of the nervous system. N. Am. Arch. M. & S. Sc., Balt., 1834-5, i, 91-111.—**Gerhardt** (C.) Neuropathologische Notizen. Jenaische Ztschr. f. Med., u. Naturw., Leipz., 1864, i, 399-401.—**Gobée** (C.) Bijdrage tot de kennis der zenuwwerking in den zieken toestand. *In his :* Klin. aanteek., 8°, Amst., 1853, 1-9.—**Gubler.** Note sur l'existence de lésions secondaires des centres nerveux dans le cours des ramollissements inflammatoires. Compt. rend. Soc. de biol. 1859, Par., 1860, 3. s., i, pt. 1, 79-81. *Also:* Gaz. d. hôp., Par., 1859, xxxii, 377.—**Gubowitsch** (A. J.) Die Beschleunigung der Nervendegeneration. Ztschr. f. Biol., München, 1877, xiii, 118-129.—**von Gudden.** Ueber die neuroparalytische Entzündung. Tagebl. d. Versamml. deutsch. Naturf. u. Aerzte, Magdeb., 1884, lvii, 265-268. — **Hall** (M.) Memoirs on some principles of pathology in the nervous system. Med.-Chir. Tr., Lond., 1839, xxii, 191 : 1840, xxiii, 121 : 1841. xxiv, 83.—**Halley** (G.) A case of nerve degeneration. Kansas City M. J., 1871, i, 303-306.—**Hamilton** (A. M'L.) The microscopic appearances of degenerate nerve tissue. Med. & Surg. Reporter, Phila., 1875, xxxii, 241-244.—**Handyside** (P. D.) On a remarkable diminution of the medulla oblongata, and adjacent portion of the spinal marrow, consequent upon spontaneous luxation of the processus dentatus, and ankylosis at the upper part of the spine, yet unattended by any symptom of paralysis. Edinb. M. & S. J., 1840, liii, 376-379. *Also,* Reprint.—**Hankel.** Erweichung des linken Nervus vagus und des Rückenmarkes; leichte Zerreissbarkeit des Magens. Mag. f. d. ges. Heilk., Berl., 1833, xxxix, 248-259. *Also, transl.* [Abstr.] : Bull. d. sc. med. di Bologna, 1834, x, 245-248.—**Haspel.** Du ramollissement de la pulpe nerveuse. J. d. conn. méd.-chir., Par., 1836-7, iv, pt. 1, 177-187 — **Hawkins** (C. H.) Curious appearance of the median nerve. Lond. M. Gaz., 1827-8, i, 27. *Also, in his :* . . Path. & Surg. Writings, 8°, Lond., 1874, ii, 190-193.—**Hebold** (O.) Cysticerken des Gehirns und Rückenmarks. Arch. f. Psychiat., Berl., 1884, xv, 812-820.—**Helft.** Practische Mittheilungen aus dem Gebiete der Nervenpathologie. Ztschr. f. d. ges. Med., Hamb., 1848, xxxvii, 248; 387.—**Heschl.** Verkalkte Nervenzellen im Gehirne. Wien. med. Wchnschr., 1870, xx, 965.—**Hirt.** Coloration dans les préparations du bulbe et de la moelle épinière. Bull. Soc. anat. de Par., 1883, lviii, 99. — **Hoffmann** (C. K.) Beiträge zur pathologischen Anatomie und Histologie des Nervencentralorganes. Vrtljschr. f. Psychiat., Neuwied u. Leipz., 1868-9, ii, 319-338. *Also,* Reprint. *Also, transl.:* Nederl. Tijdschr. v. Geneesk., Amst., 1869, 2. R., pt. 2, 1-42, 1 pl.—**Hoggan** (G.) On degeneration and regeneration of the axis-cylinder in non-traumatic nerve lesions, with special reference to gangrene of the cutaneous nerves. Tr. Path. Soc. Lond., 1879-80, xxxi, 12-27.—**Hughes** (C. H.) Note on the value of the term general functional neuratrophia. Virginia M. Month., Richmond, 1882-3, ix, 336-338.—**Jones** (C. H.) On some of the points in the pathology of nervous diseases. Med. Times & Gaz., Lond., 1865, ii, 1; 55; 109; 163; 217; 411; 489; 515; 567; 621: 1866, 1; 85; 113; 139; 167.—**Kahler** (O.) & **Pick** (A.) Ueber combinirte Systemerkrankungen des Rückenmarkes. Arch. f. Psy-

chiat., Berl. 1877-8, viii, 251, 1 pl. : 1878-9, ix, 413, 1 pl. : 1879-80, x, 179, 1 pl. ; 297.—**Kesteven** (W. B.) Notes on some morbid appearances in the brain and spinal cord of a lioness. Bristol M.-Chir. J., 1885, iii, 246-248, 1 pl.—**Kesteven** (W. H.) The histology of certain forms of degeneration of the tissues of the nerve-centres. St. Barth. Hosp. Rep., Lond., 1876, xii, 53 : 1877, xiii, 51.—**Kétli** (K.) Mittheilungen aus dem Gebiete der Nervenpathologie. Wien. med. Presse, 1872. xiii, 700-703.—**Klencke.** Pathologische Veränderung der Nervensubstanz. Allg Ztg. f. Mil.-Aerzte, Brnschwg., 1843, i, 67-72.—**Lépine** (R.) Sur la prolifération des éléments conjonctifs des canaux périvasculaires des centres nerveux chez les enfants. Arch. de physiol. norm. et path., Par., 1869, ii, 439-441. — **Ley** (H.) Observations on the pathology of nerves. Lond. M. Gaz., 1834-5, xv, 474; 508; 554; 582; 621; 646; 679; 713; 759; 799; 824.—**Lidell** (J. A.) On contusions of the brain and of the spinal cord. Am. J. M. Sc., Phila., 1883, n. s., lxxxvi, 31-63. — **Löwenfeld** (L.) Neuropathologische Mittheilungen. Aerztl. Int.-Bl., München, 1883, xxx, 151; 164; 315.—**Löwenthal** (N.) Ueber den Unterschied zwischen der secundären Degeneration des Seitenstrangs nach Hirn- und Rückenmarksverletzungen. Arch. f. d. ges. Physiol., Bonn, 1883, xxxi, 350-357, 1 pl.—**Lussana** (F.) Alcune osservazioni fisio-patologiche su 'l sistema nervoso. Gazz. med. ital. lomb., Milano, 1856, 4. s., i, 79; 98; 165; 173; 189; 197; 343; 349; 357; 381; 389; 397; 405; 449; 458; 465; 473.—**Mairet** (A.) Recherches sur les modifications dans la nutrition du système nerveux produites par la manie, la lypémanie et l'épilepsie. Compt. rend. Acad. d. sc., Par., 1884, xcix, 328-331.—**Marfels** (F.) Zur Pathologie der Nerven. Cor.-Bl. d. deutsch. Gesellsch. f. Psychiat., etc., Neuwied, 1857, iv, 17-19. — **Mauthner** (L.) Ein Beitrag zur Neuropathologie. Oester. Ztschr. f. prakt. Heilk., Wien, 1865, xi, 229; 253; 271.—**Mayer** (S.) Ueber Vorgänge der Degeneration und Regeneration im unversehrten peripherischen Nervensystem; eine biologische Studie. Ztschr. f. Heilk., Prag. 1881, ii, 154-258, 2 pl.—**Michel.** De l'histologie pathologique du tissu nerveux. Gaz. méd. de Strasb., 1860, xx, 183-186. — **Mitchell** (S. W.) Sciatic nerve of a rabbit, in the sheath of which were developed, after irritation, multiple abscesses. Tr. Path. Soc. Phila. (1871-3), 1874, iv, 240.—**Möbius** (P. J.) Neuropathologische Notizen. Memorabilien, Heilbr., 1881, n. F., i, 270; 449 : 1882, n. F., ii, 71.—**Money** (A.) Report on capillary embolism of brain and spinal cord, experimentally studied; its relations to the various forms of chorea. Brit. M. J., Lond., 1886, ii, 99-101.—**Müller** (F.) Neuropathologische Studien. Berl. klin. Wchnschr., 1878, xv, 300-302.—**Neftel** (W. B.) Report upon some of the recent researches in neuropathology. Arch. Scient. & Pract. M. & S., N. Y., 1873, i, 480-489. *Also,* Reprint. — **Otto** (R.) Ueber Heterotopie grauer Substanz im Centralnervensystem. Arch. f. path. Anat., etc., Berl., 1887. cx, 85-94.— **Parker.** Contributions to the pathology of the nervous system. Med. Times, Lond., 1851, n. s., ii, 91; 175. — **Pathological** histology of the brain and spinal cord. Brit. & For. M.-Chir. Rev., Lond., 1873, li, 370-392.—**Penna** (J.) Ensayo sobre la patogenia de una enfermedad de origen trófico. An Asoc. circ. méd. argent., Buenos Aires, 1877-8, i, 53-62.—**Pitres** (A.) Nouveaux faits relatifs à l'étude des dégénérations bilatérales de la moelle épinière consécutives à des lésions unilatérales du cerveau. Bull. Soc. anat. de Par., 1881, lvi, 628-631. — **Pitt** (G. N.) A case of extensive cerebral softening, with descending sclerosis in the lateral column. Guy's Hosp. Rep., Lond., 1883-4, xlii, 351-356. — **Putnam** (J. J.) Recent progress in pathology of the nervous system. Boston M. & S. J., 1875, xciii, 128-133. *Also,* Reprint.— [**Ramollissement** du centre encéphalo-rachidien.] J. compl. du dict. d. sc. méd., Par., 1831. xl, 199-210. — **Recent** researches in nerve pathology. Brit. & For. M.-Chir. Rev., Lond., 1875, lvi, 281-298.—**Reyher** (G.) Ueber pathologische Reflexerscheinungen auf einzelnen Nervenbahnen. St. Petersb. med. Ztschr., 1868, xv, 298-303.—**Richter** (F.) Ueber neuropathologische Bedeutung physiologischer Einflüsse der Electro- und Hydrotherapie. Deutsche Ztschr. f. prakt. Med., Leipz., 1876, 299-305.—**Rieux.** De l'innervation pathologique, et de la liaison qui doit exister dans l'étude des phlegmasies et des névroses. Ann. de la méd. physiol., Par., 1831, xix, 293-316.—**Ringer** (S.) A suggestion concerning the condition of the nervous centres in migraine, epilepsy, and other explosive neuroses. Lancet, Lond., 1877, i, 228.—**Ritchie** (J.) Notes on four cases of cerebral and spinal tumours. Glasgow M. J., 1882, xviii, 256-258.—**Romberg.** Neuropathologische Studien. Mag. f. d. ges. Heilk., Berl., 1830, xxxii, 281; 476. ———. Neuropathologische Studien. Wchnschr. f. d. ges. Heilk., Berl., 1836, 289; 388; 593; 1837, 713.—**Rosenbach** (P.) Ueber die durch Inanition bewirkten Texturveränderungen der Nervencentren. Neurol. Centralbl., Leipz., 1883, ii, 337-340.—**Roth** (M.) Beiträge zur Kenntniss der varicösen Hypertrophie der Nervenfasern. Arch. f. path. Anat., etc., Berl., 1872, lv, 197, 1 pl. ; 517.—**Rowland** (R.) On the pathology of the

Nervous system (*Pathology and pathological anatomy of*).

nervous system. Lond. M. Gaz., 1845, n. s., i, 67 : 1847, n. s., iv, 182.—**Rumpf** (T.) Beiträge zur pathologischen Anatomie des centralen Nervensystems. Arch. f. Psychiat., Berl., 1885, xvi, 410 – 441.—**Schiff.** Ueber den anatomischen Character gelähmter Nervenfasern und über die Ursprungsquellen des sympathischen Nerven. Arch. f. physiol. Heilk., Stuttg., 1852, 145–180. — **Schultze** (F.) Beiträge zur Pathologie und pathologischen Anatomie des centralen Nervensystems. Arch. f. path. Anat., etc., Berl., 1876, lxviii, 109 : 1878, lxxiii, 443 : 1880, lxxix, 124 : 1882, lxxxvii, 510, 1 pl.—**Sédillot.** Observations relatives à quelques altérations de l'appareil nerveux encéphalique. Rec. de mém. de méd. . . . mil., Par., 1827, xxii, 329–393.— **Seguin** (E. C.) Contributions to the pathological anatomy of the nervous system. Am. J. M. Sc., Phila., 1872, n. s., lxiv, 427–429. *Also, in his :* Op. min. [etc.], 8°, N. Y., 1884, 72–75.—**Serres.** Note sur un cas de névroplastie ou de transformation ganglionnaire du système nerveux périphérique. Gaz. méd. de Par., 1846, 3. s., l, 462–465.— **Sewell** (S. C.) Contributions to cerebro-spinal pathology. Brit.-Am. J., Montreal, 1845-6, i, 6–10.—**Sharkey** (S. J.) On certain cases of disease of the central nervous system in which no naked-eye changes are found at the post-mortem examination. Lancet, Lond., 1885, i, 1028– 1030.—**Siebert** (A.) Was hat die Pathologie von der Nervenstatik zu erwarten? Jenaische Ann. f. Physiol. u. Med., Jena, 1850, i, 104–128.— **Simon** (T.) Beiträge zur Pathologie und pathologischen Anatomie des Central-Nervensystem. Arch. f. Psychiat., Berl., 1874, v, 108–163, 2 pl.— **Smith** (W.) The physiology of nervous, spasmodic, and convulsive diseases. Lond. M. Gaz., 1850, n. s., x, 795 ; 976.—**Sokoloff** (N.) K patolog. anat. gliom central. nerv. sistemy. Med. Oboz., Mosk., 1887, xxviii, 813 – 823. — **Talamon** (C.) Des lésions du système nerveux central d'origine périphérique. Rev. mens. de méd. et chir., Par., 1879, iii, 580 ; 660 ; 732 ; 835. *Also* [Abstr.] : J. Soc. de méd. et pharm. de l'Isère, Grenoble, 1879-80, iv, 50 ; 65. *Also, transl.* [Abstr.] : Pisani, Palermo, 1880, 261–287. *Also, transl.* [Abstr.] : Canada Lancet, Toronto, 1881-2, xiv, 193 ; 226.—**Teed** (J. L.) On some points connected with the general pathology of the nervous system. Med. Index, Kansas City, 1884, v, 1 ; 45 ; 83.—**Thudichum** (J. L. W.) On chemical diseases of the brain and spinal cord, as conditioned by the chemical constitution of these organs. Brit, M. J., Lond., 1883, ii, 524–526.—**Tizzoni** (G.) Sulla patologia del tessuto nervoso ; osservazioni ed esperimenti sulla istologia normale e patologica della fibra nervosa. Arch. per le sc. med , Torino, 1878-9, iii (no. 1), 1–61, 1 pl. *Also :* Gior. d. r. Accad. di med. di Torino, 1878, xli, 129 - 145.— **Verneuil** (A.) Observation pour servir à l'histoire des altérations locales des nerfs. Arch. gén. de méd., Par., 1861, ii, 537–552.—**Vincenzi** (L.) Su alcune alterazioni istologiche del sistema nervoso centrale. Riv. sper. di freniat., Reggio-Emilia, 1885, xi, 318–324, 1 pl.— **Virchow** (R.) Ueber die fettige Degeneration in den Nervencentren. Arch. f. path. Anat., etc., Berl., 1856, x, 407.—**Vulpian.** Étude expérimentale sur le système nerveux ; excitabilité du cerveau ; localisations cérébrales. École de méd., Par., 1876, iii, 1–10. *Also :* Progrès méd., Par., 1876, iv, 345.—**Walter** (G.) Ueber die fettige Degeneration der Nerven nach ihrer Durchschneidung. Arch. f. path. Anat., etc., Berl., 1861, xx, 426–435.—**Walton** (G. L.) Cases of functional and organic injury to the central nervous system, caused by trauma. Boston M. & S. J., 1886, cxiv, 102–105.—**Wernich** (A.) Ueber die als Neuroparalyse, Nervenschlag, Shock bezeichnete Todesart vom gerichtsärztlichen Standpunkte. Vrtljschr. f. gerichtl. Med., Berl., 1882, n. F., xxxvii, 285 : 1883, n. F., xxxviii, 33. — **Westphal** (C.) Ueber eine dem Bilde der cerebrospinalen grauen Degeneration ähnliche Erkrankung des centralen Nervensystems ohne anatomischen Befund, nebst einigen Bemerkungen über paradoxe Contraction. Arch. f. Psychiat., Berl., 1883, xiv, 87–134.——. Ueber einen Fall von grauer Degeneration des Centralnervensystems, nebst Bemerkungen über Nervendehnung. Charité-Ann. 1881, Berl., 1883, viii, 373 - 398, 1 pl. — **Wilks** (S.) Observations on the pathology of some of the diseases of the nervous system. Guy's Hosp. Rep., Lond., 1866, 3. s., xii, 152–244.—**Wundt** (W.) Ueber das Verhalten der Nerven in entzündeten und degenerirten Organen. Arch. f. path. Anat., etc., Berl., 1856, x, 404–407.

Nervous system (*Physiology of*).

See **Nervous** system.

Nervous system (*Sclerosis of*).

See, also, **Ataxy** (*Locomotor, etc.*) ; **Atrophy** (*Muscular, Progressive*) ; **Brain** (*Sclerosis, etc., of*) ; **Cerebellum** (*Sclerosis of*) ; **Idiots** (*Pathology of*) ; **Insanity** (*Pathology, etc., of*) ; **Paralysis** (*Bulbar, etc.*) ; **Paralysis** (*Progressive*) ; **Paralysis** *agitans* ; **Paramyoclonus** *multi-*

Nervous system (*Sclerosis of*).
plex ; **Spinal** cord (*Pathology, etc., of*) ; **Spinal** cord (*Sclerosis of*).

BABINSKI (J.) * Étude anatomique et clinique sur la sclérose en plaques. 4°. *Paris*, 1885. *See, also, infra.*

BARBAUD (C.) * Sur une des formes frustes de la sclérose en plaques disséminées. 4°. *Le Mans*, 1883.

BOUICLI (C.) * Des anomalies et des formes frustes de la sclérose en plaques disséminées. 4°. *Paris*, 1883.

BOURNEVILLE. Le cas du docteur W. Pennock, ou contribution à l'histoire de la sclérose en plaques disséminées. 8°. *Paris*, 1868. *See, also,* MORRIS, *infra.*

——— & GUÉRARD (S.) De la sclérose en plaques disséminées. Nouvelle étude sur quelques points de la sclérose en plaques disséminées par Bourneville. 8°. *Paris*, 1869.

BUCHWALD (A.) * Ueber multiple Sklerose des Hirns und Rückenmarks. 8°. *Breslau*, [1872]. *Also, in :* Deutsches Arch. f. klin. Med., Leipz., 1872, x. 478–514.

CACCIOLA (S.) Angioite obliterante e sclerosi del nervo tibiale anteriore. 8°. *Padova*, 1885.

DAIMA (C.) * Contribution à l'étude de l'atrophie musculaire survenant dans le cours de la sclérose en plaques disséminées. 4°. *Paris*, 1884.

DUPLAIX (J.-B.) * Contribution à l'étude de la sclérose. 4°. *Paris*, 1883. *Also, in :* Arch. gén. de méd., Par., 1885, i, 145 ; 314.

EBSTEIN (W.) * Ueber multiple Sclerose des Gehirns und Rückenmarkes. 8°. *Würzburg*, 1886.

ERLER (J.) * Ueber diffuse Sklerose des Gehirns. 8°. *Tübingen*, 1881.

GOMBAULT (A.) Étude sur la sclérose latérale amyotrophique. 8°. *Paris*, 1877.

HAUPTMANN (E. G.) * Zur Casuistik der Sclérose latérale amyotrophique (Charcot). 8°. *Leipzig*, [*n. d.*]

HESSE (P.) * Ueber Coincidenz von multipler Hirnsclerose und Excessen in Venere. 8°. *Greifswald*, 1881.

JACQUIN (H.) * Essai sur l'anatomie et la physiologie pathologiques de la sclérose en plaques. 4°. *Nancy*, 1881.

PINEL fils. Recherches d'anatomie pathologique sur l'endurcissement au système nerveux. 8°. *Paris*, 1822. *Also, in :* J. de physiol. expér., Par., 1822, ii, 191–210.

RITTERSHAUSEN (A.) * Ein Fall von amyotrophischer Lateralsclerose. 8°. *Würzburg*, 1883.

STEPHAN (B. H.) * De theorie van het beven bij multiple sclerose. 8°. *Leiden*, 1884.

TIMAL (E.) * Étude sur quelques complications de la sclérose en plaques disséminées. 4°. *Paris*, 1873.

TJADEN (H.) * Ein Beitrag zur Kenntniss der multiplen Sklerose des Gehirnes und Rückenmarks. 8°. *Helmstedt*, 1884.

UNGER (L.) Ueber multiple inselförmige Sklerose des Centralnervensystems im Kindesalter. Eine pädiatrisch - klinische Studie. 8°. *Leipzig u. Wien*, 1888.

WITTIG (A.) * Ueber einige tabische Erscheinungen bei der multiplen Sklerose. Aus der Kranken - Abtheilung des städtischen Armenhauses. 8°. *Breslau*, 1885.

Arbate [V.] & **Salemi Pace** [B.] Sclerosi cerebrale. Pisani, Palermo, 1878, 2. s., i, 108, 1 pl. — **Aufrecht** (E.) Die anatomische Untersuchung einer primären Seitenstrang-Sclerose. Deutsche med. Wchnschr., Berl., 1880, vi, 236–239.—**Babinski** (J.) Recherches sur l'anatomie pathologique de la sclérose en plaques, et étude comparative des diverses variétés de scléroses de la moelle. Arch. de physiol. norm. et path., Par., 1885, 3. s., v, 186-207, 2 pl. [*See, also, supra,* for completed treatise.] — **Babinski** (J.) &

Nervous *system* (*Sclerosis of*).

Charrin. Sclérose médullaire systématique combinée. Rev. de méd., Par., 1886, vi, 962-965. — **Bärwinkel** (F.) Zur Lehre von der heerdweisen Sclerose der Nervencentren. Arch. d. Heilk., Leipz., 1869, x, 590-592, 2 pl.—**Ball.** Sclérose à plaques disséminées. Gaz. d. hôp., Par., 1880, liii, 593.—**Ballet** (G.) & **Minor** (L.) Étude d'un cas de fausse sclérose systématique combinée de la moelle (scléroses systématiques ou péri-tubulaires de la moelle et scléroses péri-vasculaires). Arch. de neurol., Par., 1884, vii, 44-85, 3 pl.—**Banham** (H. F.) A case of descending lateral sclerosis. Med. Press & Circ., Lond., 1883, n. s., xxxvi, 372.— **Bastian** (H. C.) An anomalous case of disseminated cerebro-spinal sclerosis. Tr. Clin. Soc. Lond., 1883-4, xvii, 7-17. *Also*: Med. Times & Gaz., Lond., 1883, ii, 451.—**Beck** (J.) Ein Fall von Sclerosis cerebro-spinalis. Med. Cor.-Bl. d. württemb. ärztl. Ver., Stuttg., 1878, xlviii, 65-70.—**Berner** (H.) Två Tilfælde af multipel Cerebrospinalsklerose. Norsk Mag. f. Lægevidensk., Christiania, 1884, xiv, 545-555.—**Bidon.** La sclérose en plaques et la paralysie générale. Marseille méd., 1887, xxiv, 242; 310.—**Bouchaud** (J.-B.) Sclérose en plaques; nystagmus vertical. J. d. sc. méd. de Lille, 1883, v, 321-332.— **Bouicli** (C.) Note sur un cas de sclérose en plaques fruste. Arch. de neurol., Par., 1883, v, 51-57. — **Bourneville.** Sclérose en plaques disséminées. Bull. Soc. anat. de Par., 1868, xliii, 261-272.—**Bourneville** & **Bonnaire.** Sclérose tubéreuse ou hypertrophie des circonvolutions. *Ibid.*, 1881, lvi, 545-552.—**Bristowe.** Disseminated sclerosis. Med. Times & Gaz., Lond, 1880, i, 634.—**Brückner** (O.) Ueber multiple, tuberöse Sklerose der Hirnrinde; ein Beitrag zur pathologischen Anatomie der Idiotie. Arch. f. Psychiat., Berl., 1881-2, xii, 550-563, 1 pl. *Also*, Reprint.—**Bruns** (L.) Zur Pathologie der disseminirten Sclerose. Berl. klin. Wchnschr., 1888, xxv, 90.—**Bruyère.** Observation de sclérose antérolatérale et de sclérose en plaques. Ann. Soc. de méd. de St.-Étienne et de la Loire (1877-80), 1881, vii, 233-240.— **Buissen** (S.) Sobre dos enfermos de esclerósis espinal posterior. Siglo méd., Madrid, 1882, xxix, 745.—**Bury** (J. S.) Disseminated sclerosis with unusual symptoms. Brit. M. J., Lond., 1885, i, 792.—**Campbell** (J.) Primary lateral sclerosis. Canada Lancet, Toronto, 1882-3, xv, 327-329.—**Cantani** (F.) Sclerosi laterale amiotrofica. Boll. d. clin., Napoli, 1884, i, 233-236. ——. Sclerosi a placche diffusa con malaria. *Ibid.*, 1885, ii, 241-244.—**Cassinis** (F.) Di un caso di sclerosi disseminata cerebro-spinale. Gazz. med. ital., prov. venete, Padova, 1881, xxiv, 70-73.— **Catsaras** (M.) De la curabilité de la sclérose en plaques. Arch. de neurol., Par., 1885, x, 66-76.—**Charcot** (J.-M.) De la sclérose en plaques disséminées. *In his*: Leçons sur les mal. du système nerveux, [etc.], 8°, Par., 1872-3, 168-219. *Also, transl.*: Edinb. M. J., 1875-6, xxi, 720; 1010: 1876-7, xxii, 50 ; 117. ——. Sclérose latérale amyotrophique: théorie du réflexe tendineux. Gaz. d. hôp., Par., 1879, lii, 1065 ; 1082 ; 1170. ——. Sclérose latérale amyotrophique; autonomie et caractère spasmodique de cette affection. Progrès méd., Par., 1880, viii, 1 ; 41. ——. Troubles oculaires de la sclérose en plaques. *Ibid.*, 1884, xii, 641-643. ——. De la sclérose en plaques disséminées. Praticien, Par., 1884, vii, 136-138. ——. Sclérose en plaques. Gaz. d. hôp., Par., 1886, lix, 1203; 1225 : 1887, lx, 10. — **Chvostek** (F.) Zur Kenntniss der herdweisen Sklerose des zentralen Nervensystems. Wien. med. Presse, 1873, xiv, 1076; 1128 ; 1148 ; 1874, xv, 97; 124; 149; 185; 321; 345; 401; 457; 516; 558; 569 ; 598; 622; 668. ——. Zur Diagnose der herdweisen Sclerose des centralen Nervensystems. Allg. Wien. med. Ztg., 1875, xx, 82; 90; 109 ; 122 ; 147 ; 175 ; 187. ——. Beitrag zur herdweisen Sclerose des centralen Nervensystems. Allg. Wien. med. Ztg., 1876, xxi, 261 ; 270 ; 298 ; 305; 313 ; 328 ; 337. ——. Herdweise Sclerose des Central-Nervensystems. Wien. med. Bl., 1880, iii, 689; 714. ——. Zur herdweisen Sclerose des Central-Nervensystems. *Ibid.*, 1091 - 1093. ——. Dehnung der Nn. ischiadici bei herdweiser Sclerose. *Ibid*, 1881, iv, 1325 ; 1356. ——. Weiterer Beitrag zur Dehnung der Nn. ischiadici bei herdweiser Sclerose des Central-Nervensystems. Allg. Wien. med. Ztg., 1882, xxvii, 128 ; 137. ——. Weiterer Beitrag zur herdweisen Sclerose des Central-Nervensystems. *Ibid.*, 1883, xxviii, 369.—**Claus.** Ein Beitrag zur Casuistik der Cerebro-Spinal-Sclerose. Allg. Ztschr. f. Psychiat., etc., Berl., 1878, xxxv, 335-354, 1 pl. ——. Multiple Cerebrospinalsclerose. Arch. f. Psychiat., Berl., 1882, xii, 669-682.—**Collyns** (R. J.) On a case of amyotrophic lateral sclerosis, with microscopical examination of the nervecentres, etc. St. Barth. Hosp. Rep., Lond., 1883, xix, 343-353.—**Cornil** (V.) Altération des nerfs périphériques, sclérème et dégénération cancéreuse. Compt. rend. Soc. de biol. 1863, Par., 1864, 3. s., v, 8-10.—**Couturier.** Sclérose en plaques; grande amélioration survenue à la suite d'une fièvre typhoïde. Loire méd., St.-Étienne, 1886, v, 1-4.—**Coxwell** (C. F.) Case of amyotrophic lateral sclerosis. Tr. Path. Soc. l ond., 1883-4, xxxv, 42-45.—**Damaschino.** Des affections associées de la moelle et du cerveau et notamment des lésions combinées des cordons postérieurs et latéraux (sclérose spinale postéro-latérale). Gaz. d. hôp., Par., 1883, lvi, 1-3. *Also*: Thérap. contemp., Par., 1883, iii, 3-8.—**Dana** (C. L.) Progressive spastic

Nervous *system* (*Sclerosis of*).

ataxia (combined fascicular sclerosis) and the combined scleroses of the spinal cord. Med. Rec., N. Y., 1887, xxxii, 1-11.—**Debove** & **Gombault.** Contribution à l'étude de la sclérose latérale amyotrophique. Arch. de physiol. norm. et path. Par., 1879, 2. s., vi, 751-771, 2 pl.—**Déjerine** (J.) Du rôle joué par la méningite spinale postérieure dans la pathogénie des scléroses combinées Compt. rend. Soc. de biol., Par., 1884, 8. s., i, pt. 2, 539-541. ——. Étude sur la sclérose en plaques cérébro-spinale à forme de sclérose latérale amyotrophique. Rev. de méd., Par., 1884, iv, 193-212.—**Demange** (E.) Contribution à l'étude des scléroses médullaires d'origine vasculaire. *Ibid.*, 753-766.— **Dixon** (A.) A case of disseminated sclerosis. Alienist & Neurol., St. Louis, 1882, iii, 50-57.—**Dreschfeld** (J.) Two cases of cerebro-spinal sclerosis in children. Med. Exam., Lond., 1877, ii, 842. ——. A contribution to the pathological anatomy of primary lateral sclerosis (sclerosis of the pyramidal tracts). J. Anat. & Physiol., Lond., 1880-1, xv, 510-518, 1 pl. *Also* [Abstr.]: Tr. Internat. M. Cong., 7. sess., Lond., 1881, i, 407.—**Drummond** (D.) Disseminated cerebro-spinal sclerosis; glycosuria. Lancet Lond., 1887, i, 13.—**Duckworth** (D.) On a case of disseminated cerebro-spinal sclerosis in an early stage, affecting exclusively the right extremities. Lancet, Lond, 1885, i, 879.—**Dulácska** (G.) A szigetes kérgesedésröl. [Sclerosis insularis.] Gyógyászat, Budapest, 1885, xxv, 33-38.— **Edge** (A. M.) Remarks on a case of disseminated sclerosis. with unusual symptoms. Lancet. Lond., 1885, ii, 568.— **Edwards** (*Mlle.* B.) Glycosurie au cours de la sclérose en plaques. Rev. de méd., Par., 1886, vi, 703-721.— **Eickholt** (A.) Beitrag zur "centralen Sklerose" (Sclérose périépendymaire). Arch. f. Psychiat., Berl., 1880, x, 613-630, 1 pl.—**Epstein** (M. J.) Multiple cerebro-spinal sclerosis. St. Louis Cour. Med., 1885, xiii, 22.—**Erb.** Ueber Lateralsclerose und ihre Beziehungen zur Tabes dorsalis. Arch. f. Psychiat., Berl., 1876, vii, 238.—**Eulenburg** (A.) Multiple Sklerose mit beiderseitiger totaler neuritischer Sehnervenatrophie. Neurol. Centralbl., Leipz., 1884, iii, 505-508.—**Féré** (C.) Ataxie héréditaire; maladie de Friedreich; sclérose diffuse de la moelle et du bulbe. Progrès méd., Par., 1882, x, 890-892.—**Ferrier.** Cases of amyotrophic lateral sclerosis. Lancet, Lond., 1881, i, 822.—**de Fleury** (M.) Une observation de sclérose en plaques fruste. Rev. de méd., Par., 1885, v, 139-146.—**Fox** (E. L.) Cerebro-spinal sclerosis. Med. Times & Gaz., Lond., 1874, ii, 143-145.—**Francotte** (X.) Cas de pseudo-sclérose. Ann. Soc. méd.-chir. de Liége, 1887, xxvi, 308-311.—**Friedenreich** (A.) Des lésions anatomiques de la sclérose latérale amyotrophique et de la relation de cette maladie à l'atrophie musculaire progressive de Duchenne. Cong. périod. internat. d. sc. méd. Compt.-rend. 1884, Copenh., 1886, iii, Sect. de psychiat. et névrol., 105-119.—**Gerhard** (G. S.) Cases of multilocular cerebrospinal sclerosis. Phila. M. Times, 1876, vii, 49-52.—**Gilbert** (A.) & **Lion** (G.) Contribution à l'étude de la sclérose en plaques à forme paralytique ; de la variété hémiplégique. Arch. de physiol. norm. et path., Par., 1887. 3. s., x, 126-140.—**Glynn** (T. R.) Case of disseminated sclerosis. Liverpool M.-Chir. J., 1887, vii, 192-195.— **Gnauck** (R.) Ueber Augenstörungen bei multipler Sklerose. Verhandl. d. Berl. med. Gesellsch. (1883-4), 1885, xv, pt. 2, 173-181. [Discussion], pt. 1, 241-243. *Also*: Berl. klin. Wchnschr., 1884. xxi, 421-424. *Also*: Neurol. Centralbl., Leipz., 1884, iii, 313-320. *Also*: Deutsche med. Wchnschr., Berl., 1884, x, 347-349.—**Goldflam** (S.) O rozsianem wielvogniskowem stwardnieniu mózgu i rdzenia (sclerosis cerebro-spinalis). Kron. lek., Warszawa, 1886, vii, 173-219.—**Gomez Ocaña** (J.) Esclerosis en placas. Prensa méd. de Granada, 1881, iii, 305-313.—**Goodhart** (J. F.) Insular sclerosis of brain and spinal cord. Tr. Path. Soc. Lond., 1875-6, xxvii, 17-19. — **Grashey** (K.) Multiple Cerebrospinalsclerose und progressive Muskelatrophie. Ann. d. städt. allg. Krankenh. zu München, 1886, iii, 199 ——. Fall von multiple Cerebrospinal-Sclerose. *Ibid.*, 200-403. — **Greiff** (F.) Ueber diffuse und disseminirte Sklerose des Centralnervensystems und über fleckweise glasige Entartung der Hirnrinde. Arch. f. Psychiat., Berl., 1883, xiv, 286-320, 1 pl.—**Guttmann** (P.) Ein bemerkenswerther Fall von inselförmiger, multipler Sclerose des Hirns und Rückenmarks. Ztschr. f. klin. Med., Berl., 1880, ii, 46-55.—**Hallopeau** (H.) Contribution à l'étude de la sclérose diffuse péri-épendymaire. Gaz. méd. de Par., 1870, 3. s., xxv, 394; 421; 444; 460.—**Harbinson** (A.) Sclerosis of the nervous centres, mainly cerebral. Med. Press & Circ., Lond., 1880, n. s., xxix, 123-125.—**Hardy.** De la sclérose en plaques. Gaz. d. hôp., Par., 1876, xlix, 801-803.—**Hermant.** Sclérose cérébrale. Arch. méd. belges, Brux., 1883, 3. s., xxiv, 361-367.—**Hess** (K.) Ueber einen Fall von multipler Sklerose des Central-nervensystems. Arch. f. Psychiat., Berl., 1887, xix, 64-87.—**Hirschfelder** (J. O.) Disseminated sclerosis ; a clinical lecture. Pacific M. & S. J., San Fran., 1882, xxiv, 443-449.—**Hirt.** Ueber die Differential-Diagnose zwischen Hysterie und multipler Sclerose. Jahresb. d. schles. Gesellsch. f. vaterl. Kult. 1885, Bresl., 1886, lxiii, 12. — **Homén.** Multipel skleros. Finska läk.-sällsk. handl., Helsingfors, 1886, xxviii, 189-191.—**Hughes** (C.

Nervous *system (Sclerosis of).*

H.) Inability to gargle and inco-ordinate backward movements, additional signs of cerebral and posterior spinal sclerosis. N. York M. J., 1885, xli, 472.—**Isnard** (C.) De la sclérose généralisée et du rô'e de l'artériosclérose. Arch. gén. de méd., Par., 1886, i, 142–166.—**Joffroy.** Note sur un cas de sclérose en plaques disséminées. Gaz. méd. de Par., 1870, 3. s., xxv, 308; 324.—**Kesteven** (W. B.) Miliary sclerosis; its pathological significance. Brit. & For. M.-Chir. Rev., Lond., 1874, ii, 187–192, 1 pl.—**Kirkland** (R.) Disseminated sclerosis at an unusual age. Brit. M. J., Lond., 1883, i, 407.—**Kleudgen.** Diffuse Gehirnrinden-Sclerose bei einer Idiotin und eigenthümliche Cyste in der Bauchhöhle bei derselben. Breslau. aerztl. Ztschr., 1881, iii, 269.—**Köppen** (M.) Ueber die histologischen Veränderungen der multiplen Sklerose. Arch. f. Psychiat., Berl., 1886, xvii, 63–82. *Also, Reprint.*—**von Krafft-Ebing.** Ein Fall von multipler Hirnrückenmarkssklerose. Mitth. d. Ver. d. Aerzte in Steiermark 1876-7, Graz, 1878, 3–11.—**Latham.** Unilateral disseminated cerebro-spinal sclerosis. Lancet, Lond., 1885, ii. 388.—**Lecoq** (G.) Observation de sclérose en plaques disséminées; débuts apoplectiformes; phénomènes hémiplégiques; troubles de sensibilité spéciaux. France méd., Par., 1882, i, 398–403. *Also:* Bull. Soc. clin. de Par. (1882), 1883, vi, 62–68.—**Leo** (L.) Beitrag zur Erkennung der Sclerose des Gehirns und Rückenmarks. Deutsches Arch. f. klin. Med., Leipz., 1868, iv, 151–172.—**Leube** (W.) Ueber multiple inselförmige Sklerose des Gehirns und Rückenmarks; nach Beobachtungen aus der Erlanger medicinischen Klinik. *Ibid.*, 1871, viii, 1–29, 1 pl.—**Liouville.** Nouvelle observation détaillée de sclérose en îlots multiples et disséminés du cerveau, de la moelle et des nerfs rachidiens. Gaz. méd. de Par., 1870, 3. s., xxv, 259; 269.—**Lipari** (G.) Caso raro di sclerosi disseminata a placche. Psichiatria, Napoli, 1885, iii, 177–191.—**Lomikowsky** (M.) Laryngoscopischer Befund bei Sclérose en plaques cérébro-spinale. Berl. klin. Wchnschr., 1879, xvi, 610. *Also, transl.:* St. Louis Cour. Med., 1880, iii, 53–55.—**Macartney.** Cerebro-spinal disseminated sclerosis in soldiers. Indian M. Gaz., Calcutta, 1884, xix, 261.—**McDowall** (T. W.) Diffused cerebral sclerosis. J. Ment. Sc., Lond., 1879-80, n. s., xxv, 490–494, 1 pl.—**Magnan.** Note sur une observation de sclérose en plaques cérébro-spinale avec atrophie papillaire des deux yeux. Arch. de physiol. norm. et path., Par., 1869, ii, 765.— [**Malherbe.**] Sclérose en plaques disséminées cérébro-spinales. J. de méd. de l'ouest, Nantes, 1874, viii, 85. *Also, in his:* Études clin., 8°, Nantes, 1875, fasc. 1, 78–86.—**Mancini** (S.) Caso importante di sclerosi insulare dei centri nervosi. Raccoglitore med., Forlì, 1877, 4. s., vii, 225–242.—**Marie** (P.) De la sclérose en plaques chez les enfants. Rev. de méd., Par., 1883, iii, 536–568. ——. Sclérose en plaques et maladies infectieuses. Progrès méd., Par., 1884, xii, 287; 305; 349; 365. — **Mickle** (W. J.) Bilateral secondary descending sclerosis and atrophy, mainly of pons Varolii and medulla oblongata; slight diffuse myelitis. Alienist & Neurol., St. Louis, 1883, iv, 1–13. ——. Spinal sclerosis or degeneration following brain-lesion. J. Ment. Sc., Lond., 1885-6, xxxi, 53–62.—**Mierjevsky** (J. P.) & **Erlitsky** (A. F.) Sclerosis lateralis amyotrophica. Vestnik klin. i sudebnoi psichiat. i nevropatol., St. Petersb., 1883, i, 69–88. *Also, transl.:* Pam. Towarz. Lek. Warszaw., 1883, lxxix, 221–246.—**Mills** (C. K.) Two lectures on a case of sclerosis of the spinal cord and brain, chiefly affecting the cord in the posterior and lateral columns. Hosp. Gaz, N. Y., 1879, vi, 596; 610. ——. On posterior spinal sclerosis. Med. Gaz., N. Y., 1880, vii, 1–3.—**Mitchell** (S. W.) Sclerosis. Med. & Surg. Reporter, Phila., 1876, xxxv, 510.—**Moeli** (C.) Ein Fall von amyotrophischer Lateralsklerose. Arch. f. Psychiat., Berl., 1880, x, 718–734, 1 pl.—**Mollière** (H.) Sur quelques points du diagnostic de la sclérose des centres nerveux. Lyon méd., 1875, xix, 405–408.—**Moncorvo** (C.-A.) De la sclérose en plaques chez les enfants. Uniao med., Rio de Jan., 1884, iv, 16; 49; 97; 145. *Also, Reprint.* De l'étiologie de la sclérose en plaques chez les enfants et notamment de l'influence pathogénique de l'hérédo-syphilis. Rev. mens. d. mal. de l'enf., Par., 1887, v, 241–261. *Also, transl.:* Arch. di patol. inf., Napoli, 1887, v, 97–113.—**Moore** (N.) A case of sclerosis of the cerebral cortex, with two other examples of cerebral disease in children. St. Barth. Hosp Rep., Lond., 1879. xv, 63–74.—**Morris** (J. C.) Case of the late Dr. C. W. Pennock. Tr. Coll. Phys. Phila., 1863-74, n. s., iv, 222–228. *Also:* Am. J. M. Sc., Phila.. 1868, n. s., lvi, 138–144. — **de Moura** (V. F.) A sclerose em placas disseminadas. J. Soc. d. sc. med. de Lisb., 1872, 2. s., xxxvi, 33; 65; 97; 161; 193; 257.—**Moxon.** Case of insular sclerosis of brain and spinal cord. Lancet, Lond., 1873, i, 236.—**Nettleship** (E.) Amblyopia with changes indicative of slight chronic neuritis, in disseminated sclerosis. Tr. Ophth. Soc. U. Kingdom, Lond., 1882-3, iii, 227.—**Nothnagel** (H.) Multiple inselförmige Sclerose. Allg. Wien. med. Ztg., 1883, xxviii, 551.—**Oppenheim** (H.) Zur Pathologie der disseminirten Sklerose. Berl. klin. Wchnschr., 1887, xxiv, 904–907.—**Osler** (W.) Cases of insular sclerosis. Canada M. & S. J., Montreal, 1880-81, ix, 1–11. *Also, Reprint.*—**Otto** (A.)

Nervous *system (Sclerosis of).*

Casuistischer Beitrag zur multiplen Sklerose des Hirns und Rückenmarks. Deutsches Arch. f. klin. Med., Leipz., 1872, x, 531–561.—**Parinaud** (H.) Troubles oculaires de la sclérose en plaques. J. de la santé pub., Par., 1884, iii, 3–5—**Pauchon** (A.) Une sclérose en plaques disséminées. Marseille méd., 1874, xi, 258; 577.—**Perret** (S.) De la sclérose en plaques. *In his:* Clin. méd. de l'Hôtel-Dieu de Lyon, 8°, Par., 1887, 239–260.—**Picart.** Sclérose généralisée (tabes dorsal spasmodique). Rev. de thérap. méd.-chir., Par., 1878, xlv, 85–89.—**Pitres** (A.) Note sur un cas de sclérose bilatérale de la moelle épinière, consécutive à une lésion unilatérale du cerveau. J. de méd. de Bordeaux, 1880-81, x, 13–15. ——. Des scléroses bilatérales de la moelle épinière consécutives à des lésions unilatérales du cerveau. Gaz. hebd. de méd. Par.. 1881, 2. s.. xviii, 429–431.—**Pollák** (L.) Congenitale, multiple Herdsclerose des Centralnervensystems; partieller Balkenmangel. Arch. f. Psychiat., Berl., 1881, xii, 157–188. — **Purjesz** (Z.) Az izomsorvadásos oldalkötegkeményedésröl (sclerosis lateralis amyotrophica). Orvosi hetil., Budapest, 1886, xxx, 1445–1450. *Also, transl.:* Pest. med.-chir. Presse, Budapest, 1887, xxiii, 21–24.—**Racano** (L.) Un caso di sclerosi a placche disseminata; discusso e riferito dall' allievo. Movimento, Napoli, 1885, xvi, 481–486.—**Ranney** (G. E.) Sclerosis; a case. Am. Lancet, Detroit, 1887, n. s., xi, 365. — **Raymond** (M.) Sclérose en plaques. Gaz. d. hôp., Par., 1880, liii, 1138; 1153. ——. Sclérose en plaques et paralysie générale progressive. *Ibid.*, 1881, liv, 433–435. — **Rendu.** Exagération des réflexes tendineux chez un homme atteint de sclérose en plaques. France méd., Par., 1880, xxvii, 426. — **Ribbert** (H.) Ueber multiple Sclerose des Gehirns und Rückenmarks. Arch. f. path. Anat., etc., Berl., 1882, xc, 243–260, 1 pl. — **Richardière** (H.) De la glycosurie et du diabète dans la sclérose en plaques. Rev. de méd., Par., 1886, vi, 622–632. — **Roché** (L.) Observation de sclérose en plaques disséminées. Bull. Soc. méd. de l'Yonne 1880, Auxerre, 1881, xxi, 77–91.—**Rosenthal** (M.) Die Hirn- und Rückenmarkssclerose. Deutsche Klinik, Stuttg., 1874, xxvi, 60; 67. ——. [Klinische und anatomische Untersuchungen über Sklerose der Nervenzentren.] Wien. med. Presse, 1874, xv, 218. — **Roy** (G. C.) A case of sclerosis of the cord; fracture of thigh; rapid union and subsequent improvement of symptoms. Indian M. Gaz., Calcutta, 1881, xvi, 258. — **Runeberg.** Ett fall af multipel cerebro-spinal skleros. Finska läk.-sällsk. handl., Helsingfors, 1880, xxii, 426. — **Satterthwaite.** Multiple cerebro-spinal sclerosis. Med. Rec., N. Y., 1882, xxii, 190. — **Schüle** (H.) Beitrag zur multiplen Sclerose des Gehirns und Rückenmarks. Deutsches Arch. f. klin. Med., Leipz., 1870, vii, 259; 1871, viii, 223. — **Schultze** (F.) Ueber das Verhalten der Axencylinder bei der multiplen Sklerose. Neurol. Centralbl., Leipz., 1884, iii, 195–197.--**Schuster.** Ein Fall von multipler Sclerose des Gehirnes und Rückenmarkes in Folge von Syphilis. Tagebl. d. Versamml. deutsch. Naturf. u. Aerzte. Strassb., 1885, lviii, 241–245. *Also:* Deutsche med. Wchnschr., Berl., 1885, xi, 878–880.—**Seguin** (E. C.) A contribution to the pathological anatomy of disseminated cerebro-spinal sclerosis. J. Nerv. & Ment. Dis.. Chicago, 1878, v, 281–293, 1 pl. *Also, in his:* Op. min. [etc.], 8°, N. Y., 1884, 264–275. *Also, Reprint.* — **Sergiu.** Sclerosa implaci cerebro-spinalá. Spitalul Bucuresci, 1887, vii, 155–160.—**Sharkey** (S. J.) & **Nettleship** (E.) Rapid failure of sight, with slight-papillitis and pains in the limbs; later, incomplete atrophy of discs and colour-blindness, with symptoms of disseminated sclerosis. Tr. Ophth. Soc. U. Kingdom, Lond., 1882-3, iii, 227–229. — **Shaw** (A. B.) Primary lateral spinal sclerosis. St. Louis Cour. Med, 1883, ix. 417–424.—**Shipps** (W. H.) Cerebro-spinal sclerosis Country Pract., Beverly, N. J., 1879-80, i, 403–407. — **Simon** (J.) Sclérose cérébrale. Gaz. d. hôp.. Par., 1882. lv, 266; 292. — **Strümpell** (A.) Symptomenbild der "amyotrophischen Lateralsclerose"; combinirte Erkankung der Pyramidenbahnen und gewisser Fasersysteme in den Hintersträngen; geringe Erkrankung der Kleinhirn-Seitenstrangbahn; keine nachweisliche Veränderungen in den Vorderhörnern; Atrophie der Zellen in den Clarke'schen Säulen. Arch. f. Psychiat., Berl., 1880, xi, 32–55. — **Suckling** (C. W.) Primary lateral sclerosis. Brit. M. J., Lond., 1883, i, 252.—**Takács** (E.) Sclerosis lateralis amyotrophica és poliencephalitis egy-esete. Orvosi hetil., Budapest, 1884, xxviii, 901–904. — **Unterstiener** (A.) Sclerose mit Syphilis der Haut und Meningealirritation. Ber. d. naturw.-med. Ver. in Innsbruck (1879) 1880, x, 12. — **Weichselbaum** (A.) Diabetes mellitus bei multipler Sklerose des Gehirns und Rückenmarks, insbesondere der Rautengrube. Wien. med. Wchnschr., 1881, xxxi, 913–918. — **Weiss** (G.) Di un caso di sclerosi laterale amiotrofica primitiva. Arch. per le sc. med., Torino, 1880, iv, 289–300.—**Weiss** (N.) Ueber die Histiogenesis der Hinterstrangsklerose. Sitzungsb. d. k. Akad. d. Wissensch. Math.-naturw. Cl. 1879, Wien, 1880, lxxx, 3. Abth., 253–259, 1 pl.—**Wenzel** (H. P.) Sclerosis of the brain, with fatty heart. Med. Herald, Louisville, 1880-81, ii, 9. — **Werner** (G.) Zur Lehre von der disseminirten Sklerose der Nervencentra. Breslau. aerztl. Ztschr.. 1883.

Nervous *system (Sclerosis of).*

v, 45 ; 66. — **Westphal.** Fall von amyotrophischer Lateralsklerose mit Bulbärparalyse. Arch. f. Psychiat., Berl., 1886, xvii, 279. — **White** (H.) Insular sclerosis. Brit. M. J., Lond., 1884, i, 459. — **Whittaker** (J. T.) Posterior spinal sclerosis. Cincin. Lancet & Clinic, 1881, n. s., vii, 585-589. ———. Multiple cerebro-spinal sclerosis. *Ibid.*, 1882, n. s., viii, 234. *Also:* Med. News, Phila., 1882, xl, 369-371. — **Wilks.** A case of insular sclerosis. Med. Times & Gaz., Lond., 1880, i, 399. — **Wilson** (E. T.) A case of disseminated insular sclerosis. Brit. M. J., Lond., 1876, ii, 675-677. — **Wood** (H. C.) Cerebral, spinal and cerebro-spinal sclerosis; a clinical lecture. Michigan M. News, Detroit, 1880, iii, 171. ———. Spinal and cerebral sclerosis; a clinical lecture. South. Clinic, Richmond, 1881, iv, 539-545. — **Wood** (H. C.) & **Dercum** (F. X.) Multiple cerebro-spinal sclerosis. Therap. Gaz., Detroit, 1885, 3. s., i, 153. — **W**[**oodbury**] (F.) Diffuse sclerosis of the spinal cord and medulla oblongata; disease of Friedreich. Phila. M. Times, 1882-3, xiii, 372-375.

Nervous *system (Syphilis of).*

See, also, **Brain** (*Syphilitic disease of*) ; **Nerve** (*Auditory, Pathology of*) ; **Nerve** (*Optic, Atrophy of*).

APARICIO (M.) *Étude sur le tremblement syphilitique. 4°. *Paris,* 1872.

BUZZARD (T.) Clinical aspects of syphilitic nervous affections. 8°. *London,* 1874.

CHAUVET (C.) *Influence de la syphilis sur les maladies du système nerveux central. 4°. *Paris,* 1880.

CONÇAIX (L.) *De l'hémiplégie syphilitique. 4°. *Paris,* 1877.

DAVIDOGLOU (C.) *Sur la syphilis du système nerveux. 4°. *Paris,* 1868.

GROS (L.) & LANCEREAUX (E.) Des affections nerveuses syphilitiques. 8°. *Paris,* 1861.

DE HÉRÉDINOFF (*Vve.* Adèle). *Essai sur les myélo-encéphalopathies syphilitiques tertiaires diffuses ou disséminées. 4°. *Paris,* 1887.

LADREIT DE LACHARRIÈRE. *Des paralysies syphilitiques. 4°. *Paris,* 1861.

LAGNEAU (G.-S.) Maladies syphilitiques du système nerveux. 8°. *Paris,* 1860.

MAYAUD (A.) *Syphilis secondaire et tertiaire du système nerveux. 4°. *Paris,* 1873.
——. The same. 8°. *Paris,* 1873.

MÉNARD (A.) *De la paralysie faciale syphilitique au début des accidents secondaires. 4°. *Montpellier,* 1865.
Also [*Abstr.*], *in:* Mém. et compt.-rend. Soc. d. sc. méd. de Lyon, 1864-5, iv, pt. 2, 25-28.

READE (T.) Syphilitic affections of the nervous system, and a case of symmetrical muscular atrophy; with other contributions to the pathology of the spinal marrow. 8°. *London,* 1867.

RUMPF (T.) Die syphilitischen Erkrankungen des Nervensystems. 8°. *Wiesbaden,* 1887.

SONREL (S.) *Des paralysies syphilitiques du mouvement. 4°. *Strasbourg,* 1862.

STOLZENBURG (O.) *Ein Beitrag zur Lehre von der reflectorischen Pupillenstarre und der spinalen Myosis mit besonderer Rücksicht auf Lues. 8°. *München,* 1883.

VIALLE (F.) *Essai sur les paraplégies syphilitiques. 4°. *Paris,* 1875.

WEIDNER (F.) *Ueber spinale Lähmungen nach Syphilis. 8°. *Jena,* 1869.

ZAMBACO (A.) Des affections nerveuses syphilitiques. 8°. *Paris,* 1862.

Adolphus (J.) Syphilitic dyscrasia; neuralgia. St. Louis M. Reporter, 1867-8, ii, 193-198. — **Aikman** (J.) Illustrations of syphilitic disease in the nervous system. Glasgow M. J., 1887, [4.] s., xxviii, 258-262. — **Allbutt** (T. C.) Cases of syphilitic disease of the nervous system. St. George's Hosp. Rep., Lond., 1869, iv, 45 ; 351. ——. On the obscure neuroses of syphilis. West Riding Lun. Asyl. Rep., Lond., 1873, iii, 272-284. — **Althaus** (J.) On neuro-syphilitic affections. Med. Times & Gaz., Lond., 1871, ii, 616 ; 645. ——. On syphilitic affections of the nervous system. *Ibid.*, 1877, ii, 511-513. *Also, transl.:* Salute (suppl.), Genova, 1877, iii, 305 ; 321. ——. Case of cerebro-spinal syphilis. Tr. Clin Soc. Lond., 1882, xv,

Nervous *system (Syphilis of).*

203-208. *Also, transl.:* Centralbl. f. Nervenh., Leipz., 1883, vi, 1-6. — **Ambrosoli** (C.) Paralisi sifilitica sinistra del nervo oculo-motore comune. Gior. ital. d. mal. ven., Milano, 1866, ii, 399-408. — **Annan** (S.) Hemiplegia; syphilis. Am. J. M. Sc., Phila., 1839, xxv, 42-44. — **Anstie** (F. E.) On syphilitic paralysis. Tr. M. Soc. King's Coll., Lond., 1856-7, i, 44-69. ——. Case of syphilitic paralysis, with unusually rapid wasting and repair of muscles. Tr. Clin. Soc. Lond., 1872-3, vi, 15-17. — **Ascoli** (G.) Casi di sifilide del sistema nervoso centrale. Gazz. med. di Roma, 1877, iii, 181-185. — **Bahuaud.** Observation de paralysie faciale syphilitique arrivant au début des accidents secondaires. Gaz. d. hôp., Par., 1863, xxxvi, 582. — **Balfour** (G. W.) On obstinate trigeminal neuralgia as a symptom of syphilitic cerebral disease; its diagnosis and treatment. Edinb. M. J., 1875, xxi, 289-297. — **Barnes** (J. H.) Syphilis and syphilitic affections of the nervous system. Liverpool & Manchester M. & S. Rep., 1875, iii, 17-33. — **Bartholow** (R.) Syphilis of the nervous system. Clinic, Cincin., 1871, i, 133 ; 146. — **Baudot** (E.) Sur la paralysie syphilitique du nerf moteur oculaire commun. Union méd., Par., 1859, 2. s., i, 115-121. — **Baumgarten** (P.) Ueber gummöse Syphilis des Gehirns und Rückenmarks, namentlich der Gehirngefässe, und über das Verhältniss dieser Erkrankungen zu den entsprechenden tuberculösen Affectionen. Arch. f. path. Anat., etc., Berl., 1881, lxxxvi, 179-221, 2 pl. — **Bayer** (O.) Heilung einer acut ascendirenden Spinalparalyse unter antisyphilitischer Behandlung. Arch. d. Heilk., Leipz., 1869, x, 105-107. — **Bertherand** (E.-L.) Recherches sur les névroses syphilitiques. J. de méd., chir. et pharmacol., Brux., 1861, xxxii, 543 : xxxiii, 33 ; 225. — **Beyran** (J.) De la paralysie syphilitique du nerf oculo-moteur externe, consécutive à la vérole constitutionnelle ; traitement spécifique ; guérison. Union méd., Par., 1854, viii, 530. — **Bouchaud** (J.-B.) Lésions disséminées des centres nerveux chez une femme syphilitique ; hémiparaplégie spinale ; thermo-anesthésie isolée. J. d. sc. méd. de Lille, 1883, v, 376-391. — **Bramwell** (B.) Left hemiplegia ; double optic neuritis and syphilitic choroiditis ; motor power regained before sensibility ; convulsion ; death ; syphilitic tumor springing from dura mater ; extensive softening. Lancet, Lond., 1875, ii, 346. — **Broadbent** (W. H.) Lettsomian lectures on syphilitic affections of the nervous system. *Ibid.*, 1874, i, 43 ; 115 ; 187 ; 255. *Also:* Brit M. J., Lond., 1874, i, 37 ; 68 ; 100 ; 134 ; 164 ; 196 ; 225 ; 257 ; 295. — **Brush** (E. N.) Syphilitic affections of the nervous system. Buffalo M. & S. J., 1874, xiv, 81 ; 130. — **Bull** (O.) The affections of the nervous system, and more especially of the optic nerve in syphilis. Tr. Minnesota M. Soc., Minneap., 1875, '90 - 93. — **Burdel.** Observation sur un cas d'hémiplégie de nature syphilitique. Bull. Acad. roy. de méd. de Belg., Brux., 1860, 2. s., iii, 787-795. [Rap. de Hairion]. 768. *Also:* Bull. gén. de thérap., etc., Par., 1861, lx, 167-172. — **Buss** (O.) Ein Fall von acuter, aufsteigender Myelitis bulbi, nebst Encephalitis bei einer Syphilitischen. Deutsches Arch. f. klin. Med., Leipz., 1887, xli, 241-260, 2 pl. ——. Ueber einen Fall von diffuser Hirnsklerose mit Erkrankung des Rückenmarkes bei einem hereditär syphilitischen Kinde. Berl. klin. Wchnschr., 1887, xxiv, 921 ; 945. — **Buttersack** (P.) Zur Lehre von den syphilitischen Erkrankungen des Centralnervensystems, nebst einigen Bemerkungen über Polyurie und Polydipsie. Arch. f. Psychiat., Berl. 1886, xvii, 603-648, 1 pl. *Also,* Reprint. — **Buzzard** (T.) On paralysis, convulsion, and other nervous affections in syphilitic subjects. Lancet, Lond., 1873, i, 265 ; 334 ; 480 ; 587 ; 693. ——. A case of double facial paralysis, with paralysis of four extremities ; general anæsthesia ; imperfect paralysis of respiration and deglutition ; paresis of the bladder ; recovery under antisyphilitic treatment. Tr. Clin. Soc. Lond., 1873-4, vii, 75-89. *Also* [Abstr.]: Brit. M. J., Lond., 1874, i, 380. ——. A case of syphilitic paraplegia ; appearance of an obstinate ulcerating syphiloderm under iodide treatment ; recovery under the influence of mercury. Lancet, Lond., 1877, ii, 237. — **Castagnou.** À propos des névroses syphilitiques. Médecin, Par., 1878, iv, no. 43, p. 1. — **de Cérenville.** Myélite syphilitique ; paraplégie ; guérison rapide par le mercure et l'iodure de potassium. Bull. Soc. méd. de la Suisse Rom., Lausanne, 1876, x, 342-345. — **Charcot** & **Gombault.** Note sur un cas de lésions disséminées des centres nerveux observées chez une femme syphilitique. Arch. de physiol. norm. et path., Par., 1873, v, 143 ; 304, 2 pl. — **Charpentier.** Lésions syphilitiques simulant une paralysie générale. Ann. méd.-psych., Par., 1884, 6. s., xi, 99-119. — **Chevalet.** Paralysie ascendante aiguë, d'origine syphilitique, guérie par les frictions mercurielles. Bull. gén. de thérap., etc., Par., 1869, lxxvii, 328-333. — **Cholmeley.** Syphilitic paralysis with marked local muscular wasting. Brit. M. J., Lond., 1873, i, 172. — **Cross** (T. M. B.) Clinical observations upon syphilitic diseases of the nervous system. Am. J. Syph. & Dermat., N. Y., 1872, iii, 216-227. — **Da Costa** (J. M.) Three cases of syphilitic paralysis. Med. & Surg. Reporter, Phila., 1872, xxvii, 513-515. — **Delafield** (F.) Syphilitic degeneration. Med. Rec., N. Y.,

Nervous *system* (*Syphilis of*).

1873, viii, 66. ———. Gummy tumor of the cord, with pyo-nephritis. Tr. N. York Path. Soc. (1874-5), 1876, i, 52.—**De Renzi** (E.) Sifilidé dei centri nervosi. Riforma med., Napoli, 1887, iii. 266; 272.—**Dickinson** (W.) Ophthalmology; neuro-syphilitic affections; second cranial (optic) nerve; hemiopia; third cranial; (motor oculi) strab.; div-ptosis, etc.; gumma syphiliticum. Proc. St. Louis M. Soc. Missouri, 1879, ii, 71-74. — **Dixon.** Two cases of paralysis from syphilitic neuromata of the intracranial nerves. Med. Times & Gaz., Lond., 1858, xvii, 419-421.—**Domański** (S.) O kile (syphilis) układu nerwowego. [Syphilis of nervous system,] Przegl. lek., Krakow., 1880, xix, 362; 379; 403; 417; 429; 439; 445; 461; 473; 489; 497; 511; 521; 533; 545.—**Dowse** (T. S.) On syphilis as it affects the brain and nervous system. Med. Press & Circ., Lond., 1877, n. s., xxiv, 167; 253; 353; 1878, xxv, 1; 21; 63; 85; 125; 145; 167; 253; 357; 501; 522; xxvi, 3.—**Dreschfeld** (J.) On some cases of syphilitic nervous disease. Practitioner, Lond., 1875, xiv, 343-355.—**Drysdale** (C. R.) Syphilis as a cause of aphasia and locomotor ataxia. Med. Exam., Lond., 1878, iii, 440-443. ———. On cerebro-spinal syphilis. Proc. M. Soc. Lond., 1879-81, v, 112-120. *Also*: Med. Press & Circ., Lond., 1880, n. s., xxix, 341; 364.—**Du Cazal.** Syphilis cérébro-spinale; paralysies multiples; guérison. Union méd., Par., 1880, 3. s., xxix, 955-959. *Also*: Bull. et mém. Soc. méd. d. hôp. de Par. (1880), 1881, 2. s., xvii, 93-98.—**Ebrard.** Névroses syphilitiques. Gaz. méd. de Par., 1843, 2. s., xi, 119-121.—**Engel** (H.) The diagnosis and treatment of some forms of syphilitic nervous affections. Phila. M. Times, 1877, viii, 121-124.—**Finger** (E.) Gehirn- und Nervensyphilis. Aerztl. Ber. d. k. k. allg. Krankenh. zu Wien (1882), 1883, 137-143.—**Folet.** Paraplégie syphilitique; compression de la moelle; guérison par l'iodure de potassium à haute dose. Bull. gén. de thérap., etc., Par., 1867, lxxiii, 90-92. — **Foster.** A case of syphilitic disease of the nervous system. Lancet, Lond., 1875, ii, 129. — **Fournier** (A.) Affections syphilitiques des nerfs. Mouvement méd., Par., 1875, xiii, 839; 1876, xiv, 19; 36; 66. ———. Paralysie du nerf mentonnier par lésion syphilitique du maxillaire. Gaz. hebd. de méd., Par., 1876, xiii, 804. ———. De la pseudo-paralysie générale d'origine syphilitique. Progrès méd., Par., 1877, v, 761; 775; 785.—**Gailleton.** Syphilis précoce intéressant le système nerveux. Mém. et compt. rend. Soc. d. sc. méd. de Lyon, 1865-6, v, pt. 2, 304.—**Gallard.** Sur un cas d'affection rare de la moelle épinière, d'origine syphilitique; tressaillements musculaires; traitement par l'iodure de potassium et l'électricité à courants continus. Union méd., Par., 1874, ii, 796-711.—**Gamberini** (P.) Paralisi sifilitica. Imparziale, Firenze, 1861-2, ii 300-302.—**Githens** (W. H. H.) A case of syphilis of the nervous system. Med. & Surg. Reporter, Phila., 1871, xxiv, 95-98.—**Gjör.** Bidrag til Kundskaben om de Sygdomme i Nervesystemet, der kunne opstaae som Fölge af Syphilis. Norsk Mag. f. Lægevidensk., Christiania, 1857, xi, 774; 813. *Also*, Reprint.—**Göransson** (C. J. A.) Fall af nervsjukdom beroende pa syphilis. Upsala Läkaref. Förh., 1870-71, vi, 102-105.—**Gowers** (W. R.) Syphilomata of brain and spinal cord; syphilitic thickening of membranes around nerves, etc. Tr. Path. Soc. Lond., 1876-7, xxviii, 281-285. ———. Syphilitic neuroses. Brit. M. J., Lond., 1879, i, 303-305.—**Gray** (L. C.) Syphilis of the nervous system, and its treatment. Med. News, Phila., 1887, li, 33-38. *Also*, Reprint.—**Green** (J. P.) Two cases of syphilitic lesion of the nervous system. Cincin. Lancet & Obs., 1875, xviii, 142-147.—**Gubb** (A. S.) Curious nervous symptoms probably due to gumma. Med. Reg., Phila., 1887, i, 241.—**Hale** (L.) Case of syphilitic paraplegia. Tr. M. Soc. County Albany 1870-80, Albany, 1883, iii, 53. *Also*: Am. J. Syph. & Dermat., N. Y., 1872, iii, 312. *Also*: Phila. M. Times, 1872-3, iii, 266. *Also*: Buffalo M. & S. J., 1872-3, xii, 216-218.—**Hammond** (W. A.) Bromide of calcium in the treatment of syphilitic neuralgia. Am. J. Syph. & Dermat., N. Y., 1873, iv, 305-309. ———. On the proper method of using the iodide of potassium in syphilis of the nervous system. N. Eng. M. Month., Sandy Hook, Conn., 1884-5, iv, 150-152.—**Hassing.** Syphilitisk paralyse. Hosp.-Tid., Kjøbenh., 1858, i, 97-100.—**von Hebra** (H.) Ein Fall von Syphilis des Centralnervensystems mit dem Ausgange in Heilung. Wien. med. Presse, 1886, xxvii, 1521-1524.—**Henry** (W. H.) Clinical observations on the dementia and the hemiplegia of syphilis. Am. J. Syph. & Dermat., N. Y., 1872, iii, 5-19.—**Heubner.** Syphilis of the brain and nervous system. Cycl. Pract. M. (Ziemssen), N. Y., 1877, xii, 293-371.—**Homolle** (G.) Méningo-myélite subaiguë avec paraplégie survenue à la fin de la période secondaire de la syphilis; autopsie. Bull. Soc. anat. de Par., 1875. l, 514-522. *Also*: Progrès méd., Par., 1876, iv, 6-8.—**Houstet.** Observation sur une paralysie de cause vénérienne. Mém. Acad. roy. de chir., Par., 1768, iv, pt. 2, 141-152.—**Hutchinson** (J.) Diseases of the nervous system of syphilitic origin. Med. Press & Circ., Lond., 1884, n. s., xxxvii, 371; 394. *Also*: Students' J. & Hosp. Gaz., Lond., 1884. xii. 285; 307.—**Hutchinson** (J.) & **Jackson** (J. H.) Cases of paralysis associated with syphilis. Med. Times & Gaz., Lond., 1861, ii, 83; 133; 456;

Nervous *system* (*Syphilis of*).

578. *Also, transl.*: Ztschr. f. Med., Chir. u. Geburtsh., Leipz., 1861, xv, 277-285.—**Hutchinson** (J. H.) Syphilitic diseases of the nervous system. Am. J. M. Sc., Phila., 1871, n. s., lxii, 86-99.—**Jackson** (J. H.) Case of hemiplegia in a syphilitic subject. Tr. Clin. Soc. Lond., 1870-71, iv, 183-187. ———. On syphilitic affections of the nervous system. J. Ment. Sc., Lond., 1875, xxi, 207-225. *Also*, Reprint.—**Jacob** (E. H.) Cases of syphilitic disease of the nervous system. Med. Times & Gaz., Lond., 1877, i, 418.—**Johnston.** Syphilitic paralysis. St. Louis M. & S. J., 1883, xliv, 263-269.—**Kahler** (G.) Die multiple syphilitische Wurzelneuritis. Ztschr. f. Heilk., Prag, 1887, viii, 1-26, 1 pl.—**Key.** Fall af hæmatoma duræ matris och grå degeneration af ryggmärgen vid syfilis. Förh. v. Svens. Läk.-Sällsk., Sammank. 1865, Stockholm, 1866, 137.—**Keyes** (E. L.) Syphilis of the nervous system; a clinical study, chiefly in regard to diagnosis and treatment. N. York M. J., 1870, xii, 369-410. *Also*, Reprint.—**Knoblauch** (J. G. A.) [Fall von syphilitischer Facialislähmung.] Jahresb. ü. d. Verwalt. d. Med.-Wes., d. Krankenanst. . . . d. Stadt Frankf. (1864), 1867, viii, 82-84.—**Knorre.** Syphilitische Lähmungen. Deutsche Klinik, Berl., 1849, i, 69.—**Kohts.** Luetische Erkrankungen des Gehirns und Rückenmarks im Kindesalter. Verhandl. d. Gesellsch. f. d. Kinderh. . . . deutsch. Naturf. u. Aerzte 1883, Leipz., 1884, i, 140-150. — **L.** Teekenen van ruggemergs-atrophie met opvolgende hersenverschijnselen, welke het bestaan van hyper-of enostose van syphilitischen oorsprong van de inwendige oppervlakte des regter wandbeens aantoonden; gunstige werking van het iodetum kalicum; herstelling; epicrisis. Pract. Tijdschr. v. de Geneesk., Gorinchem, 1855, n. s., i, 341-346. — **Lalouette.** Observation d'accidens nerveux dus à la syphilis. Rec. de mem. de méd. . . . mil., Par., 1821, x, 410-412.—**Landouzy** (L.) & **Déjerine** (J.) Mélanose des ganglions bronchiques; hémiplégie ancienne légère; gomme syphilitique du front; mort par hémorrhagie cérébrale avec inondation ventriculaire; eschare fessière; altérations des nerfs cutanés Bull. Soc. anat. de Par., 1881, lvi, 675-678. *Also*: Progrès méd., Par., 1882, x, 545.—**Lang** (E.) Ueber die Häufigkeit und Frühzeitigkeit der syphilitischen Erkrankungen des zentralen Nervensystems und über Meningealirritation bei beginnender Syphilis. Wien. med Wchnschr., 1880, xxx, 1305; 1336; 1361; 1395.—**Lanzoni** (F.) Emiplegia spinale sinistra per compressione unilaterale da sifiloma sul segmento inferiore del midollo cervicale (guarigione). Morgagni, Napoli, 1874, xvi, 161-182.—**Lasègue** (E.-C.) Des affections nerveuses, et en particulier des névroses syphilitiques. Arch. gén. de méd., Par., 1861, 5. s., xviii, 210-222. *Also, in his*: Études méd., 8°, Par., 1884, ii, 80-94.—**Lawbaugh** (A. I.) A case of syphilitic hemiplegia. Med. & Surg. Reporter, Phila., 1870, xxiii, 421-423.—**Lee** (H.) Syphilitic affection of cerebral nerves. Lancet, Lond., 1884, ii, 766. — **Lefeuvre.** Hémiplégie faciale syphilitique au début des accidents secondaires de la syphilis. Bull. gén. de thérap., etc., Par., 1866, lxx, 266-272.—**Lépine.** Dégénérescence syphilitique du nerf cubital. Bull. Soc. anat. de Par., 1867, xlii, 577.—**Luton** (E.) De la paralysie syphilitique du nerf moteur externe de l'œil. Union méd., Par., 1860, 2. s., vii, 597-600.—[**Marques** (J. A.)] Affecções syphiliticas do systema nervoso. Escholiaste med., Lisb., 1868, xix, 44; 60.—**Mathieu** (A.) Un cas d'ataxie unilatéral d'origine syphilitique; sensation subjective de mauvaise odeur. Ann. de dermat. et syph., Par., 1882, 2. s., iii, 724-726.—**Maunier** (A.) De la paralysie syphilitique de la sixième partie. Union méd., Par., 1861, 2. s., x, 394-396. — **Mauriac** (C.) Mémoire sur les affections syphilitiques précoces des centres nerveux. Ann. de dermat. et syph., Par., 1874-5, vi, 161; 264; 355; 427: 1877-8, ix, 409: 1878-9, x, 57; 95; 190. *Also*, Reprint.—**Meigs** (A. V.) Report of a case of brain and spinal cord syphilis, showing extensive disease of the blood-vessels; with an account of the autopsy and microscopic examination by G. E. De Schweinitz. J. Nerv. & Ment. Dis., N. Y., 1887, n. s. xii, 1-12. *Also*, Reprint.—**Mendel** (E.) Syphilis und Dementia paralytica. Verhandl. d. Berl. med. Gesellsch. (1878-9), 1880, x. pt. 2, 1*2-198. [Discussion], pt. 1, 132-135. —**Menich** (J.) Durch Exostose bedingte Lähmung sämmtlicher Extremitäten; Heilung mittelst der grossen Inunctionscur. Oesterr. med. Wchnschr., Wien, 1843, 113-117. — **de Méric** (V.) On syphilitic paralysis. Lancet, Lond., 1862, ii, 586-589.—**Miner** (J. W.) Case of syphilitic hemiplegia. Buffalo M. & S. J., 1874, xiv, 186-190.—**Mollière** (H.) Observation de myélite syphilitique aiguë. Ann. de dermat et syph., Par., 1870, ii, 311-314. — **Money** (A.) A case of idiocy with universal rigidity, the result of syphilitic disease of the central nervous system. Brain, Lond., 1884-5, vii, 406-409. — **Moore** (W.) Syphilitic paralysis and its treatment. Dublin Q. J. M. Sc., 1866, xli, 300-308. ———. Clinical lecture on a case of syphilitic paralysis. Irish Hosp. Gaz., Dubl., 1875, iii, 6-8.—**Morton** (W. J.) Nervous syphilis. Neurol. Contrib., N. Y., 1880, i, no. 2, 63; 68.—**Moxon** (W.) On syphilitic disease of the spinal cord. Guy's Hosp. Rep., Lond., 1871, 3. s., xvi, 217-239, 1 pl.—**Naumann.** Nervenleiden bei Syphilis. Verhandl. d. naturh. Ver. d. preuss. Rheinl. u. Westphal., Bonn,

Nervous *system* (*Syphilis of*).

1861, xviii, 36.—**Ormerod** (J. A.) Case of symmetrical syphilitic disease of the third nerves, with arterial and other lesions. Brain, Lond., 1882, v, 260–267.—**Paralysie** syphilitique et musculaire atrophique (?); guérison par l'iodure de potassium. Gaz. d. hôp., Par., 1863, xxxvi. 555.—**Passavant** (G.) Syphilitische Lähmungen und deren Heilung. Arch. f. path. Anat., etc., Berl., 1862, xxv, 151-181.—**Petrow** (P.) Ueber die Veränderungen des sympathischen Nervensystems bei constitutioneller Syphilis. *Ibid.*, 1873, lvii, 121–126, 1 pl. *Also, transl.:* Am. J. Syph. & Dermat., N. Y., 1874, v, 157-162.—**Porter** (W. H.) Syphilitic meningitis; diffuse changes in the spinal cord; cystitis and pyelitis. Bull. N. York Path. Soc., 1881, 2. s., i, 204-207. ———. Syphilitic lesions of the brain and spinal cord. N. York M. J., 1886, xliii, 513-517.—**Post** (A.) A case of cerebro-spinal syphilis. Boston M. & S. J., 1884, cx, 28.—**Proegler** (C.) Syphilis of the nervous system etiologically considered. Indiana M. J., Indianap., 1883-4, ii, 121–124.—**Profeta** (G.) Le malattie sifilitiche del sistema nervoso; saggio del trattato inedito di sifilografia. Pisani, Palermo, 1881, 5–72—**Profilo** (P.) Nevropatie sifilitiche. Movimento, Napoli, 1870, ii, 153-157.—**Proksch** (J. K.) Zur Syphilis des Nervensystems; ein historischer Beitrag. Wien. med. Bl., 1884, vii, 305; 335; 371.—**Proust.** Tremblement non classé du membre inférieur droit chez un syphilitique; traitement par l'iodure de potassium à haute dose, et les frictions mercurielles; guérison. France méd., Par., 1877, xxiv, 194.—**Putnam** (J. J.) Notes on syphilis of the nervous system. Boston M. & S. J., 1886, cxv, 317; 341.—**Putzel** (L.) Syphilis of the central nervous system. Med. Rec., N. Y., 1884, xxv, 450-454.—**Quaglino** (A.) & **Scarenzio** (A.) Tributo alla storia delle malattie sifilitiche del sistema nervoso. Ann. univ. di med., Milano, 1863, clxxxiii, 58: clxxxvi, 557.—**Reade** (T.) The growth, progress, and present state of knowledge of nervous syphilitic diseases. Dublin Q. J. M. Sc., 1863, xxxvi, 324–338. ———. Syphilitic affections of the nervous system; a retrospect. Brit. M. J., Lond., 1870, ii, 84.—**Reamy** (T. A.) Syphilitic neuroma; drachm doses of iodide of potassium; cure. Clinic, Cincin., 1872, iii, 193.—**Reder** (A.) Beiträge zur Casuistik syphilitischer Affectionen des Central-Nervensystems. Vrtljschr. f. Dermat., Wien, 1874, n. s., i, 29-36, 1 pl.—**Robertson** (A.) Syphilitic hemiplegia. Brit. M. J., Lond., 1874, i, 517. — **Roquette** (C.) Lettre sur les paralysies syphilitiques. Union méd., Par., 1854, viii, 411.—**Rullier.** Cas d'hémiplégie et de perte de mémoire guéries à l'aide d'un traitement antivénérien. Bull. Fac. de méd. de Par., 1816-17, v, 55–66.—**Rumpf** (T.) Ueber Gehirn- und Rückenmarksyphilis. Arch. f. Psychiat., Berl., 1885, xvi, 410-426.—**Russell.** Syphilitic affections of the nervous system. Med. Times & Gaz., Lond., 1863, ii, 408.—**Schupp.** Paralysie des Nervus facialis durch syphilitische Knochenauftreibung. Deutsche Klinik, Berl., 1863, xv, 213; 227.—**Schuster.** Ein Fall von multipler Sclerose des Gehirnes und Rückenmarkes in Folge von Syphilis. Tagebl. d. Versamml. deutsch. Naturf. u. Aerzte, Strassb., 1885, lviii, 241–245.—**Seeger** (L.) Multiple Nervenlähmung ex lue. Ber. d. k. k. Krankenh. Wieden 1871. Wien, 1873, 256.—**Seguin** (E. C.) Cases illustrating some of the disorders of the nervous system produced by syphilis. Arch. f. Dermat., N. Y., 1875, i, 131–133.—**Selin** (A.) O siphiliticheskikh stradaniyakh nervnikh tsentrof. [On syphilitic affections of the nervous centres.] Voyenno-med.J., St. Petersb., 1868, ciii, pt. 3, 136–211.—**Silver.** Case of syphilitic hemiplegia. Med. Times & Gaz., Lond., 1871, ii, 497. ———. Symptoms resembling general paralysis of the insane; irregular paralysis of limbs, face, and nervus motor oculi; syphilitic cerebral tumour (?). *Ibid.*, 1872, ii, 461.—**Smith** (W. G.) Paralysis following syphilis; rapid recovery under the use of faradisation. Irish Hosp. Gaz., Dubl., 1873, i, 293.—**Stonehouse** (J. B.) The nervous accidents of syphilis. Buffalo M. & S. J., 1875, xiv, 201-226.—**Sturgis** (F. R.) On some of the clinical features of the syphilitic neurosis. Psych. & Med.-Leg. J., N. Y., 1875, n. s., ii, 321–330.—**Syphilitic** affections of the nervous system. Med. Times & Gaz., Lond., 1868. i, 551–553.—**Syphilitic** diseases of the nervous system. Brit. & For. M.-Chir. Rev., Lond., 1861, xxviii, 285–306.—**Tait** (L.) Syphilitic hemiplegia from deposit in the nerve tissue and plugging of the arteries. Med. Times & Gaz., Lond., 1869, i, 219.—**Takács** (E.) Hemiplegia unilateralis dextra peripherica e meningitide cerebrospinale syphilitica. Orvosi hetil., Budapest, 1878, xxii, 1-5.—**Taylor** (R. W.) A contribution to the study of syphilis of the nervous system. Boston M. & S. J., 1871, lxxxv. 395-397. ———. A contribution to the study of syphilis of the nervous system. J. Nerv. & Ment. Dis., Chicago, 1876, iii, 20-42. *Also,* Reprint. ———. Clinical notes on neuralgia of the sciatic nerve caused by syphilis. N. York M. J., 1880. xxxi, 235-244.—**Tenneson.** La syphilis cérébro-spinale et le traitement spécifique d'épreuve. Union méd., Par., 1883, 3. s., xxxv, 181-186.—**Traube.** Hemiplegia syphilitica. Deutsche Klinik, Berl., 1859, xi, 463-465.—**Troisier** (E.) Note sur un cas de pseudoparalysie syphilitique infantile. Bull. et mém. Soc. méd.

Nervous *system* (*Syphilis of*).

d. hôp. de Par. (1883), 1884, 2. s., xx, pt. 1, 109–113. *Also:* Arch. de tocol., Par., 1883, x, 411-414—**Van Buren** (W. H.) On nervous syphilis. Med. News & Libr., Phila., 1878, xxxvi, 189-194.—**Vance** (R. A.) Syphilitic disease of the nervous system. Cincin. Lancet & Clinic, 1881, n. s., vii, 71-74.—**Vaulpré** (E.) Quelques faits de névralgies syphilitiques. Bull. gén. de thérap., etc., Par., 1852, xlii, 74-76.—**Veronese** (F.) Die Syphilis als ätiologisches Moment bei Erkrankungen des Nervensystems. Mitth. d. Wien. med. Doct.-Coll., 1883, ix, 129–134. *Also:* Wien. Klinik, 1883, ix, 209-236. *Also, transl.:* Gyógyászat, Budapest, 1883, xxiii, 761-767. ———. Sulla sifilide secondaria del sistema nervoso. Riv. clin. e terap., Napoli, 1884, vi, 14–19. *Also, transl.:* France méd., Par., 1884, i, 198; 209.—**Ware** (L.) Syphilitic paralysis. Chicago M. Exam., 1871, xii, 554-559.—**Waton.** Tic douloureux de cause vénérienne; trismus dolorificus à causa venerea. J. de méd., chir., pharm., etc., Par., 1793, xciii, 233–258.—**Welsh** (T.) Cases of syphilitic disease of the nervous system. Kansas City M. J., 1871, i, 307.—**White** (W. H.) Peripheral neuritis, myelitis, syphilitic pachymeningitis, and ostitis. Tr. Path. Soc. Lond., 1886, xxxvii, 107–111, 1 pl.—**Wood** (H. C.) Contribution to our knowledge of nervous syphilis. Am. J. M. Sc., Phila., 1880, n. s., lxxx, 384–393. ———. Syphilitic affections of the nerve centres. Syst. Pract. M. (Pepper), Phila., 1886. v, 999-1027. ———. Two cases of syphilitic disease; the lesion in one involving the ascending frontal convolution, in the other the cervical spinal cord. Phila. M. Times, 1885-6, xvi, 435. *Also:* Med. & Surg. Reporter. Phila., 1886, liv, 588–590.—**von Zeissl** (M.) Casuistische Beiträge zur Gehirn- und Nervensyphilis. Wien. med. Bl., 1884, vii, 1058; 1092.

Nervous *system* (*Tuberculosis of*).

See, also, **Brain, Cerebellum, Spinal** *cord, Tubercle of.*

LECLERCQ (J.-C.) * I. Des symptômes des tubercules des centres nerveux. II. [etc.] 4°. *Paris,* 1843.

von Azary (A.) Beiträge zur Tuberkulose des centralen Nervensystems der Schweine. Deutsche Ztschr. f. Thiermed., Leipz., 1880, vi, 254-269, 1 pl.—**Dupouy.** Les névroses tuberculeuses. Médecin, Par., 1876, ii, no. 43, p. 1.—**Hoche** (A.) Zur Lehre von der Tuberculose des Centralnervensystems. Arch. f. Psychat., Berl., 1887, xix, 200-228.—**Schultze** (F.) Zur Symptomatologie und pathologischen Anatomie der tuberculösen und entzündlichen Erkrankungen und der Tuberkel des cerebrospinalen Nervensystems. Deutsches Arch. f. klin. Med., Leipz., 1880, xxv, 297-304.

Nervous *system* (*Tumors of*).

See **Brain, Medulla** *oblongata, Tumors of;* **Nervous** *system* (*Pathology, etc., of*); **Neuroma; Spinal** *cord* (*Tumors of*).

Nervous *system* (*Diastaltic*).

See **Nervous** *system* (*Reflex action of*).

Nervous *system* (*Ganglionic*) [*or Sympathetic*].

See, also, **Eye, Heart,** *Nerves of;* **Intercarotid** *ganglion;* **Intestines** (*Nerves of*); **Nerves** (*Ganglia, etc., of*); **Nervous** *system* (*Vasomotor*); **Saliva.**

ADRIAN (A.) * Ueber die Funktionen des Plexus cœliacus und mesentericus. 4°. *Giessen,* 1861.

Also, in: Beitr. z. Anat. u. Physiol. (Eckhard), Giessen, 1863, iii, 59-84.

ALBANUS (A.) Experimentelle Untersuchungen über die Beziehung des Halsstranges des Sympathicus zur Temperatur des Kaninchenohres. 8°. [*Dorpat*], 1860.

ARNOLD (F.) * Diss. sistens observationes nonnullas neurologicas de parte cephalica nervi sympathici in homine. 4°. *Heidelbergæ,* 1826.

Also, transl. in: J. compl. du dict. d. sc. méd., Par., 1826, xxiv, 337-356.

BÄNZIGER (T.) * Zur Physiologie des sympathischen Nervensystemes. 8°. *Würzburg,* 1854.

BIDDER (F. H.) & **VOLKMANN** (A. W.) Die Selbstständigkeit des sympathischen Nervensystems durch anatomische Untersuchungen nachgewiesen. 4°. *Leipzig,* 1842.

BIMAR (A.) * Structure des ganglions nerveux. 8°. *Paris,* 1878.

Nervous *system* (*Ganglionic*).

BLANCHARD (É.) Du grand sympathique chez les animaux articulés. 8°. [*Paris*, 1858.]
Repr. from : Ann. d. sc. nat., Par., 1858, x.

VAN DER BOON MESCH (H. C.) * De nervo sympathetico magno. 8°. *Lugd. Bat.*, 1821.

BRACHET (J.-L.) Réflexions sur quelques points de physiologie, relatifs au système nerveux ganglionnaire, au sujet de l'ouvrage de M. Longet. 8°. *Lyon*, [*n. d.*]

——. Mémoire sur les fonctions du système nerveux ganglionnaire. 8°. *Paris*, 1823.

——. Recherches expérimentales sur les fonctions du système nerveux ganglionnaire, et sur leur application à la pathologie. 8°. *Paris, Montpellier & Bruxelles*, 1830.

——. The same. 2. éd., revue et augmentée. 8°. *Paris*, 1837.

——. The same. Praktische Untersuchungen über die Verrichtungen des Gangliennerven-Systemes und über ihre Anwendung auf die Pathologie. Uebersetzt von H. E. Flies. 8°. *Quedlinburg u. Leipzig*, 1836.

BRUENER (E.) * Disquisitio experimentis illustrata de singularum nervi sympathici partium vi in cor. 8°. *Berolini*, [1836].

BUDGE (J.) Erwiederung auf die Aeusserungen des Herrn Dr. A. Waller. 8°. [*Bonn*, 1852.]

CHECHOTT (O. A.) O galvanizatsie simpaticheskago nerva u chelovieka i terapevticheskom eja znachenii. [Electrotherapy in affections of the sympathetic.] 8°. *St. Petersburg*, 1876.

DAVEY (J. G.) On the physiological uses of the ganglionic nervous system. 8°. *London*, 1853.

——. The ganglionic nervous system; its structure, functions, and diseases. 8°. *London*, 1858.

DEWHURST (G. H.) * De generis ganglionici nervorum structura et proprietatibus. 8°. *Edinburgi*, 1830.

DMITROVSKI. * O vlijanii sheinago stvola simpaticheskago nerva na kroveobratshenie v sosudistoi i sietchatoi obolochkach. [Influence of branches of sympathetic upon the circulation.] 8°. *St. Petersburg*, 1863.

DOQUIN (C.-J.) * Recherches physiologiques sur les fonctions du système nerveux des ganglions. 4°. *Paris*, 1820.

EDES (R. T.) The physiology and pathology of the sympathetic or ganglionic nervous system. 8°. *New York*, 1869.
Also, in : Tr. N. York Acad. M. (1864 – 71), 1872, iii, 1–152.

EULENBURG (A.) & GUTTMANN (P.) Die Pathologie des Sympathicus auf physiologischer Grundlage. 8°. *Berlin*, 1873.

——. The same. Physiology and pathology of the sympathetic system of the nerves. Transl. by A. Napier. 8°. *London*, 1879.

FOX (E. L.) The influence of the sympathetic on disease. 8°. *London*, 1885.

GILTAY (C. M.) * De nervo sympathico. 8°. *Lugd. Bat.*, 1834.

GLUGE (G.) Sur la coagulation du sang après la section du nerf grand sympathique. 8°. [*Bruxelles*, 1856.]
Repr. from : Bull. Acad. roy. de Belg., Brux., 1. s.

GOERING (H. A. S.) * De nervo sympathico ejusque in ranis decursu. 8°. *Jenæ*, [1831].

GOSSELIN (L.) * Le système nerveux ganglionnaire; ses connexions avec le système nerveux cérébro-spinal. 4°. *Paris*, 1846.

HAFFTER (W.) Neue Versuche über den Nervus splanchnicus major et minor. 8°. *Zürich*, 1853.

HIRZEL (L.) * Nexus nervi sympathetici cum nervis cerebralibus. 4°. *Heidelbergæ*, [1824].

Nervous *system* (*Ganglionic*).

HJELT (O. E. A.) In systema nervorum sympathicum Gadi lotæ Linn. observationes. 8°. *Helsingforsiæ*, 1847.

——. De nervis cerebralibus parteque cephalica nervi sympathici Bufonis cinerei Schneid adnotata quædam. 8°. *Helsingforsiæ*, 1852.

HOLST (C. R.) Du système nerveux ganglionnaire. 8°. *Paris*, 1841.

HORN (H.) * Reperta quædam circa nervi sympathici anatomiam. 4°. *Wirceburgi*, 1839.

HUTH (F.) * Beitrag zur Kenntniss der sympathischen Nervenfasern. 8°. *Königsberg*, [1886].

INGALLS (W.) An essay on the ganglionary system of nerves in the cavity of the cranium, and its use. 8°. *Boston*, 1832.
Also, in : Boston M. & S. J., 1851, xliv, 295–300.

KENT (B. A.) * De gangliorum ad nervos sympatheticos attinentium fabrica, officiis atque morbis. 8°. *Edinburgi*, 1831.

KIEPERT (A.) Historia exponatur sententiarum diversarum, quæ de functionibus nervi sympathici allatæ sunt, inde a Soemmerringii et Bichatii tempore usque ad exortam novissimis temporibus controversiam de peculiari hujus nervi natura. 8°. *Berolini*, [1849].

KIESSELBACH (E. C.) * Diss. sistens historiam formationis ac evolutionis nervi sympathetici una cum descriptione ejusdem nervi decursus in animalibus quibusdam vertebratis. 4°. *Monachii*, 1835.

KLENCKE (H.) Untersuchungen und Erfahrungen im Gebiete der Anatomie, Physiologie, Mikrologie und wissenschaftlichen Medicin. I. Bd. : I. Der Nervus sympathicus in seiner morphologischen und physiologischen Bedeutung. 8°. *Leipzig*, 1843.

KNOCH (F. F.) * Diss. sistens meletemata quædam ad physiologiam nervi sympathici spectantia. 4°. *Giessæ*, [1824].

KNOCH (J.) * De nervi sympathetici vi ad corporis temperiem, adjectis de aliis actionibus nec non de origine observationibus. 8°. *Dorpat*, 1855.

VON KÖLLIKER (A.) Die Selbstständigkeit und Abhängigkeit des sympathischen Nervensystems, durch anatomische Beobachtungen bewiesen. 4°. *Zürich*, 1844.

KRAUSE (C. F. T.) Synopsis icone illustrata nervorum systematis gangliosi in capite hominis. fol. *Hannoveræ*, 1839.

LANGERHANS (P.) * Ein Beitrag zur Anatomie der sympathischen Ganglienzellen. 8°. *Freiburg i. Br.*, 1871.

LEUPOLDT (J. M.) * De systematis gangliaris natura. 4°. *Erlangæ*, 1818.

LOBSTEIN (J. G. C. F. M.) De nervi sympathici humani fabrica, usu et morbis, commentatio anatomico-physiologico-pathologica. 4°. *Parisiis*, 1823.

——. The same. A treatise on the structure, functions, and diseases of the human sympathetic nerve. Transl. from the Latin, with notes, by Joseph Pancoast. 8°. *Philadelphia*, 1831.

——. The same. Memoria anatomico-fisiologico-patologica su la struttura, le funzione e le malattie del nervo grande simpatico dell' uomo. [Transl. from the Latin and augmented with notes and comments by D. Branca.] 8°. *Milano*, 1834.

LUDWIG (C. G.) [Pr.] de plexibus nervorum abdominalium atque nervo intercostali duplici observationes nonnullas tradit. 4°. [*Lipsiæ*, 1772.]
Also, in : SCRIPT. neurol. minores selecti. 4°. *Lipsiæ*, 1793, iii, 105–111.

Nervous *system* (*Ganglionic*).

MANEC (P. J.) Great sympathetic nerve. Transl. and corrected by J. Pancoast. 1 wall map. fol. *Philadelphia*, [*n. d.*]

MARAGE (R.) * Contribution à l'anatomie descriptive du sympathique thoracique et abdominal chez les oiseaux. 4°. *Paris*, 1887.

MATUSZYNSKI (J.) * De l'influence du nerf sympathique sur les fonctions des sens. 4°. *Paris*, 1837.

MONIZ SODRÉ DE ARAGÃO (E. C.) * Funcções do grande sympathico. 4°. *Bahia*, 1871.

MONTEIRO (R. A.) * Funcções do grande sympathico. 4°. *Bahia*, 1871.

MÜLLER (H.) Ueber den Einfluss des Sympathicus auf einige Muskeln und über das ausgedehnte Vorkommen von glatten Hautmuskeln bei Säugethieren. 8°. [*n. p., n. d.*] Cutting.

NOELLNER (F.) * Die Anatomie des Splanchnicus und der Nierennerven beim Hunde. 4°. *Giessen*, 1869.
Also, in : Beitr. z. Anat. u. Physiol. (E khard), Giessen, 1869, iv, 137–151.

OLIVER (W. S.) Is the "sympathetic" the real nervous system that presides over "organic" or "vegetative life"? 8°. [*Halifax*, 1875.]

PIÉGU (A.) * Quelques considérations sur la composition anatomique, la fonction et la signification du nerf trisplanchnique dans la série des animaux. 4°. *Paris*, 1846.

PIESCHEL (C. A.) * De parte cephalica nervi sympathici in equo prodromus. 8°. *Lipsiæ*, [1844].

PINCUS (J.) * Experimenta de vi nervi vagi et sympathici ad vasa, secretionem, nutritionem tractus intestinalis et renum. 8°. *Vratislaviæ*, 1856.

PINEL (C.-H.-P.) * Considérations générales sur l'anatomie, la physiologie, et les affections morbides du nerf grand sympathique. 4°. *Paris*, 1858.

PIOTROWSKI (R.) * Beobachtungen über den weiteren Verlauf der Temperaturverhältnisse am Kaninchenohre nach Ausrottung des Halssympathicus. 8°. *Greifswald*, 1873.

POITEAU (A.) * Des lésions de la portion cervicale du grand sympathique. 4°. *Paris*, 1869.

PROCTER (T. B.) A treatise on the use of the sympathetic nerve and its ganglions, with their influence on various diseases of the abdominal and pelvic viscera. 4°. *London*, 1844.

SEELIGMUELLER (A.) De traumaticis nervi sympathici cervicalis læsionibus. 8°. *Halis Sax.*, 1876.

TCHECHOTT (O. A.) * O galvanizatsii simpaticheskago nerva u cheloveka i terapevticheskom eja znachenii. [Galvanization of sympathetic nerve in man, and its therapeutical application.] 8°. *St. Petersburg*, 1876.

TOWNSEND (R. M.) Student's chart of the sympathetic nerve. 1 chart [in frame 10 x 12]. *Philadelphia*, [*n. d.*]

VARRENTRAPP (J. G.) * Observationes anatomicæ de parte cephalica nervi sympathici ejusque conjunctionibus cum nervis cerebralibus. 4°. *Francofurti a. M.*, 1831.

WEBER (E. H.) * De systemate nerveo organico. 8°. *Lipsiæ*, [1817].

———. Anatomia comparata nervi sympathici. 8°. *Lipsiæ*, 1817.

WIENER (A.) * De nervo sympathico nonnulla. 8°. *Berolini*, [1847].

WRISBERG (H. A.) Observationum anatomicarum de nervis viscerum abdominalium particula prima quæ de ganglio plexuque semilunari agit. 4°. *Gottingæ*, 1780.
Also, in : SCRIPT. neurol. minores selecti . 4°. *Lipsiæ*, 1795, iv, 50–69. *Also, in his :* Comment. med. physiol., etc. 8°. *Gottingæ*, 1800, i, 240–275.

Nervous *system* (*Ganglionic*).

Amati (R.) Cenno anatomico e fisiologico del gran simpatico : patogenesi del caso sopra descritto. Raccoglitore med., Forlì, 1877, 4. s., viii, 295–301.—Archer (C.) The anatomy and physiology of the ganglionic nerves. Stethoscope & Virg. M. Gaz., Richmond, 1852, ii, 364–376.—Arloing (S.) Physiologie du sympathique cervical. Mém. et compt.-rend. Soc. d. sc. méd. de Lyon (1881), 1882, xxi, pt. 2, 209–212. ——. Modification des effets vaso-constricteurs du sympathique cervical produits par la section du pneumogastrique, chez les animaux où ces deux nerfs sont isolables. Compt. rend. Soc. de biol., Par., 1882, 7. s., iv, 85–87.—Arndt (R.) Untersuchungen über die Ganglienkörper des Nervus sympathicus. Arch. f. mikr. Anat., Bonn, 1874, x, 208–241, 1 pl.—Arnold (F.) Beschreibung des Kopftheils der sympathischen Nerven beim Kalb, nebst einigen Beobachtungen über diesen Theil beim Menschen. Ztschr. f. Physiol., Darmstadt, 1827, ii, 125–172. 1 pl.—Arnold (J.) Ueber die feineren histologischen Verhältnisse in dem Sympathicus des Frosches. Centralbl. f. d. med. Wissensch., Berl., 1864, ii, 657–659. *Also :* Arch. f. path. Anat., etc., Berl., 1865, xxxii, 1–45, 1 pl.—von Basch (S.) Die Hemmung der Darmbewegung durch den Nervus splanchnicus. Sitzungsb. d. k. Akad. d. Wissensch. Math.-naturw. Cl. 1873, Wien, 1874, lxviii, 7–29. 1 pl. *Also,* Reprint. ——. Ueber den Einfluss des gereizten N. splanchnicus auf den Blutstrom innerhalb und ausserhalb seines Verbreitungsbezirkes. Arb. a. d. physiol. Anst. zu Leipz. (1875), 1876, x, 229–277.—Bechterew (W.) & Rosenbach (P.) Ueber die Bedeutung der Intervertebralganglien : experimentell-histologische Untersuchung. Neurol. Centralbl., Leipz., 1884, iii, 217 ; 320.—Beck (T. S.) On the structure and functions of the sympathetic nervous system as distinct from, and independent of, the cerebro-spinal system. Lancet, Lond., 1847, i, 615–617. *Also :* Lond. M. Gaz., 1847, n. s., iv, 1032–1037.—Bernard (C.) Influence du grand sympathique sur la sensibilité et sur la calorification. Compt. rend. Soc. de biol. 1851. Par., 1852, iii, 163–165. ——. Expériences sur les functions de la portion céphalique du grand sympathique. *Ibid.*, 1852, Par., 1853, iv, 155. ——. Recherches expérimentales sur le grand sympathique et spécialement sur l'influence que la section de ce nerf exerce sur la chaleur animale. *Ibid.*, 1853, Par., 1854, v, pt. 2., 77–107. *Also,* Reprint. ——. Die sensitiven Eigenschaften des Sympathicus und die Reflexbewegungen, die unter seiner Einwirkung entstehen. Allg. Wien. med. Ztg., 1860, v. 157 ; 166. ——. Recherches expérimentales sur les nerfs vasculaires et calorifiques du grand sympathique. J. de la physiol. de l'homme, Par., 1862, v, 38+–418. ——. La circulation abdominale ; le sympathique et le pneumogastrique ; notes pour une leçon inédite. Rev. scient., Par., 1884, xxxiv, 673–681.—Beyer (C.) & von Bezold (A.) Von den Wirkungen der Nervi splanchnici auf den Blutdruck im Aortensysteme. Untersuch. a. d. physiol. Lab. in Würzb., Leipz., 1867, i, 314–325.—Bidder (A.) Hypertrophie des Ohres nach Excision eines Stückes vom Halssympathicus des Kaninchens. Centralbl. f. Chir., Leipz., 1874, i, 97–99.—Bidder (F.) Die Nervi splanchnici und das Ganglion cœliacum. Arch. f. Anat, Physiol. u. wissensch. Med., Leipz., 1869, 472–518, 1 pl.—Bidder (F.) & Volkmann (A. W.) Erfahrungen über die functionelle Selbstständigkeit des sympathischen Nervensystems. *Ibid.*, Berl., 1844, 359–380.—Birdsall (W. R.) The embryogeny of the sympathetic. Missouri Dent. J., St. Louis, 1879, xi, 251–260.—Bochefontaine. Sur les phénomènes vaso-moteurs déterminés par la faradisation du bout céphalique du cordon cervical du vago-sympathique chez le chien, le chat et le lapin. Gaz. méd. de Par., 1880, 6. s., ii, 606. ——. Sur l'action vaso-dilatatrice du cordon cervical sympathique. *Ibid.*, 1881, 6. s., iii, 147. *Also :* Compt. rend. Soc. de biol. 1881, Par., 1882, 7. s., iii, 78.—Bonsdorff (E. J.) Om det sympathiska nervsystemets förhållande till det cerebrospinale, och det så kallade hämmande nervsystemet. Forh. v. de skandin. Naturf., Stockholm, 1865, 586–590.—Bourgery (J.-M.) Recherches sur le système nerveux splanchnique. Gaz. méd. de Par., 1845, 2. s., xiii, 275 ; 289. *Also :* Ann. de méd. belge, Brux., 1845, ii, 192 ; 313. ——. Recherches sur le système nerveux splanchnique ; mémoire sur les nerfs des membranes séreuses en général et du péritonite en particulier dans l'homme. Gaz. méd. de Par., 1845. 2. s., xvi, 593–600. ——. Mémoire sur l'extrémité céphalique du grand sympathique dans l'homme et les animaux mammifères. Compt. rend. Acad. d. sc., Par., 1845, 1014–1020.—Brachet (J.-L.) Réflexions sur quelques points de physiologie relatifs au système nerveux-ganglionnaire. J. de méd. de Lyon, 1842, iii, 5–28. *Also,* Reprint. ——. Considérations sur le système nerveux ganglionnaire. J. de méd. de Lyon, 1845, ix, 409–424. *Also,* Reprint. *Also* [Abstr.] : Compt. rend. Acad. d. sc., Par., 1845, xxi, 1106.—Brocchi (P.) De l'absence du grand sympathique chez l'axolotl. Bull. Soc. philomat., Par., 1877, 7. s., i, 71–73.—Broussais (F.-J.-V.) Réflexions sur les fonctions du sysème nerveux en général, sur celles du grand sympathique en particulier, et sur quelques autres points de physiologie. J. univ. d. sc. méd., Par., 1820, xii, 5 ; 129.—Brown-Séquard (C.-E.) Note sur la découverte de

Nervous *system* (*Ganglonic*).

quelques-uns des effets de la galvanisation du nerf grand sympathétique au cou. Gaz. méd. de Par., 1854, 3. s., ix, 22. ——. Sur les résultats de la section et de la galvanisation du nerf grand sympathétique au cou. *Ibid.*, 30–32. *Also*, Reprint.—**Brünniche.** Innervationsforstyrrelser i Banen af Halssympatikus. Hosp.-Tid., Kjøbenh., 1874, ii, 1. R., 289–295 —**Bucke** (R. M.) The functions of the great sympathetic nervous system. Am. J. Insan., Utica, N. Y., 1877, xxxiv, 115–159. ——. The moral nature and the great sympathetic. *Ibid.*, 1878, xxxv, 229–253.—**Budge** (J.) Experimenteller Beweis, dass der Nervus sympathicus aus dem Rückenmark entspringt. Med. Ztg., Berl., 1852, xxi, 161. *Also*, Reprint. ——. Ueber die Empfindlichkeit der Bauchnerven. Deutsche Klinik, Berl., 1858, x, 198. ——. Ueber das Centrum genitospinale des Nervus sympathicus. Arch. f. path. Anat., etc., Berl., 1858, xv, 115–126. —**Cahis y Balmanya** (M.) Las funciones de los ganglios espinales. Rev. de med. y cirug. práct., Madrid, 1884, xv, 481–492. —**Campbell** (H. F.) On the sympathetic nerve in reflex phenomena. Tr. Am. M. Ass., Phila., 1853, vi, 539–543. ——. The widespread influence of the cerebrospinal centres over the ganglionic plexuses. Virginia M. Month., Richmond, 1880–81, vii, 501–511. *Also*, Reprint.—**Carville** & **Bochefontaine.** De l'ablation du ganglion premier thoracique du grand sympathique chez le chien. Compt. rend. Soc. de biol. 1874, Par., 1875, 6. s., i, 140–143—**Cassleberry** (I.) An inquiry into the physiology of the organic nervous system. Proc. Indiana M. Soc., Indianap., 1855, vi, 52–66. *Also*: Am. J. M. Sc., Phila., 1855, n. s., xxx, 56–71.—**Chaumont.** On the sympathetic nervous system. Month. J. M. Sc., Lond. & Edinb., 1854, ix, 179–183. —**Chavasse** (T. F.) Case of injury to the cervical portion of the sympathetic nerve, in removing a sarcoma. Brit. M. J., Lond., 1881, ii, 974.—**Copland** (J.) An outline of a series of observations on the structure and distribution, on the physiology, and on the pathology of certain parts of the animal economy, usually denominated the ganglionic class of nerves; with a view of the indications to which they lead in the treatment of disease, and in determining the effects of remedies. Lond. M. Reposit., 1822, xvii, 369–381.—**Courrent** (P.) & **Guibert** (H.) De l'étude des filets symp. thiques par la méthode de l'or. Gaz. hebd. d. sc. méd. de Montpel., 1885, vii, 409–411.—**Courvoisier** (L. G.) Ueber die Zellen der Spinalganglien, sowie des Sympathicus beim Frosch. Arch. f. mikr. Anat., Bonn, 1868, iv, 125–145, 1 pl.—**Couty.** Sur les rapports de l'encéphale avec le système sympathique. Compt. rend. Soc. de biol. 1876, Par., 1877, 6. s., iii, 334. — **Dastre** (A.) & **Morat** (J.-P.) Action du sympathique cervical sur la pression de la vitesse du sang. Compt. rend. Acad. d. sc., Par., 1878, lxxxvii, 797–800. ——. Le système grand sympathique. Bull. méd. du nord, Lille, 1880, xx, 252–255. *Also* [Abstr.]: Compt. rend. Acad. d. sc., Par., 1880, xci, 393–395. ——. Le sympathique, nerf vaso-dilatateur. Compt. rend. Soc. de biol. 1880, Par., 1881, 7. s., ii, 343–348. *Also* [Abstr.]: Gaz. d. hôp., Par., 1880, liii, 1085. ——. Dilatation sympathique croisée à la suite de l'ablation du ganglion cervical supérieur. Compt. rend Soc. de biol. 1880. Par., 1881, 7. s., ii, 303. ——. L'action vasodilatatrice du sympathique. Gaz. méd. de Par., 1881. 6. s., iii, 80. *Also*: Compt. rend. Soc. de biol. 1881, Par., 1882, 7. s., iii, 26–28.— ——. Sur la fonction vaso-dilatatrice du nerf grand sympathique. Arch. de physiol. norm. et path., Par., 1882, 2. s., ix, 177 ; 337. ——. Contribution à l'étude des ganglions sympathiques ; leur rôle tonique et inhibitoire ; leur rapport avec les nerfs vaso-moteurs. Compt. rend. Soc. de biol., Par., 1883, 7. s., iv, 104–108. *Also*: Compt. rend. Acad. d. sc., Par., 1883, xcvi, 446–448.—**Davey** (J.G.) On the physiology and pathology of the ganglionic nervous system. Lancet, Lond., 1850, ii, 314 ; 339 ; 413 ; 471.—**Davida** (L.) Ueber die Multiplicität der Lumbal- und Sacral-Spinalganglien. Centralbl. f. d. med. Wissensch., Berl., 1880, xviii, 465–468.—**Drobnik** (T.) Topograficzno-anatomiczne spostrzeżenia w zakresie w. współczulnego szyi. [Observation of function of sympathetic nerve of neck.] Przegl. lek, Krakow., 1887, xxvi, 585 ; 601.—**Du Moulin.** Studie betreffende de geschiedenis van den sympathicus en den vagus. Geneesk. Courant, Tiel, 1874, nos. 4–7.—**Dupuy.** Observations et expériences sur l'enlèvement des ganglions gutturaux des nerfs trisplanchniques sur des chevaux. J. de méd., chir., pharm., etc., Par., 1816, xxxvii, 340–350. ——. Note sur l'extirpation des ganglions cervicaux supérieurs du nerf grand sympathique. Bull. Acad. de méd., Par., 1843–4, ix, 1156–1159.—**Dupuys.** De l'atrophie du cerveau et du crâne à la suite des sections du sympathique cervical. Compt. rend. Soc. de biol., Par., 1882, 7. s., iv, 667.—**Eckhard** (C.) Der Sympathicus in seiner Stellung zur Secretion in der Parotis des Schafes. Beitr. z. Anat. u. Physiol. (Eckhard), Giessen, 1869, iv, 49–68. ——. Bemerkungen zu dem Aufsatz des Herrn Sinitzin: Zur Frage über den Nerveneinfluss des Nv. sympathicus auf das Gesichtsorgan. Centralbl. f. d. med. Wissensch., Berl., 1873, xi, 548–550.—**Eichholtz** (H.) Das gangliöse Nervensystem Med. Ztg., Berl., 1852, xxi, 113 ; 117 ; 189 ; 193.—**Engel**

Nervous *system* (*Ganglionic*).

(J.) Zur Anatomie des Nervus sympathicus (mit einer lithographirten Tafel). Vrtljschr. f. d. prakt. Heilk., Prag, 1850, vii, 143–156.—**Engelskjøn** (C.) Til Besvarelse af Sympatikus sporgsmaalet. Norsk Mag. f. Lægevidensk., Christiania, 1887, 4. R., ii, 88–94. *Also, transl.:* Centralbl. f. Nervenh., Leipz., 1887, x, 289–294. — **Fauntleroy** (A. M.) The histology, physiology, and pathology of the organic nervous system. Richmond & Louisville M. J., Louisville, 1870, ix, 129–164.—**Finch** (J. E.) Physiology of the sympathetic nerve. Northwest. M. & S. J., St. Paul, Minn., 1873–4, iv, 277–284.—**Fischer** (G.) Experimentelle Studien zur therapeutischen Galvanisation des Sympathicus. Deutsches Arch. f. klin. Med., Leipz., 1875–6, xvii, 1–73, 2 pl.—**Foà** (P.) Sull' anatomia patologica del gran simpatico. Riv. clin. di Bologna, 1874, 2. s , iv, 267–280, 1 pl.—**Foulhioux.** Sur la liaison des ganglions du grand sympathique avec les renflemens des nerfs rachidiens. J. univ. d. sc. méd., Par., 1824, xxxvi, 357–362.—**Fox** (E. L.) The Bradshaw lecture on the influence of the sympathetic on disease. Med. Times & Gaz., Lond., 1882, ii, 261–274. *Also*: Brit. M. J., Lond., 1882, ii, 343 ; 399.—**François-Franck.** Recherches anatomiques et expérimentales sur le nerf vertébral. Gaz. d. hôp., Par., 1878, li, 428. *Also*: Compt. rend. Soc. de biol. 1878, Par., 1880. 6. s., v, 140–142. ——. Sur les effets de l'excitation du bout supérieur du sympathique cervical d'un côté sur la circulation carotidienne du même côté et sur celle du côté opposé ; modifications de la circulation cérébrale et influences de ces modifications sur l'excitabilité des zones motrices cervicales. Gaz. d. hôp., Par., 1878, li, 779. ——. Sur le dédoublement du sympathique cervical et sur la dissociation des filets vasculaires et des filets irido-dilatateurs au dessus du ganglion cervical supérieur. Compt. rend. Acad. d. sc., Par, 1878, lxxxvii, 175. ——. De la dissociation des filets irido dilatateurs et des nerfs vasculaires au dessus du ganglion cervical supérieur. Compt. rend. Soc. de biol. 1878, Par., 1880, 6. s., v, 244. ——. Trajet des filets iridodilatatrices et vaso-motrices carotidiennes au niveau de l'anneau de Vieussens. *Ibid.*, 1879, Par., 1880, 7. s., i, 246–250. ——. Grand sympathique. Dict. encycl. d. sc. méd., Par., 1884, 3. s., xiv, 1–153.—**Generali** (G.) Considerazioni anatomiche, fisiologiche e patologiche intorno il nervo gran simpatico. Ann. univ. di med., Milano, 1842, civ, 60 : 239.—**Gries** (W.) On the functions of the great sympathetic nerve, or the nerve of organic life. Med. Exam., Phila., 1852, n. s., viii, 413–420.—**Groves** (J. A.) Some peculiarities in the relations of the sympathetic and cerebro-spinal nerves, and deductions therefrom. Richmond & Louisville M. J., Louisville, 1872, xiii, 275–281.—**Gunn** (M.) The ganglionic system of nerves. N. York J. M., 1846, vii, 327–332.—**Habershon** (S.O.) Some observat ons on the abdominal sympathetic nerve, and on the union of the phrenic and pneumogastric nerves. Guy's Hosp. Rep., Lond., 1856, 3. s., ii, 196–205, 1 pl.—**Hafter** (W.) Neue Versuche über den Nervus splanchnicus major. Ztschr. f. rat. Med., Heidelb., 1854, n. F., iv, 322–329.—**Hall** (C. R.) On the ganglionic system of nerves. Edinb. M. & S. J., 1847, lxviii, 172, 6 pl ; 267–303, 2 pl : 1848, lxx, 1 ; 298.—**Hall** (M.) The true spinal marrow the true sympathetic. Lancet. Lond., 1856, ii, 38.—**Hall** (N. G.) The sympathetic nerve. Proc. Connect. M. Soc. 1860–63, N. Haven, 1863, n. s., i, 196–204.—**Haughton** (R. E.) A study of the physiology and pathology of the organic nervous system. Indiana J. M., Indianap., 1872–3, iv, 49–66.—**Hirschfeld** (L.) Sur la portion céphalique du grand sympathique. Compt. rend. Soc. de biol. 1851, Par., 1852, iii, pt. 1, 115–117.—**Hirzel** (L.) Untersuchungen über die Verbindungen des sympathischen Nervens mit den Hirnnerven. Ztschr. f. Physiol., Heidelb., 1824, i, 197–236, 1 pl.— *Also, transl.:* J. compl. du méd. d. sc. méd., Par., 1825, xxii, 304–326.—**Inosemzeff** (T.) Ueber den Einfluss des Gangliennerven-Systems auf die physiologischen Absonderungen. Med. Ztg. Russlands, St. Petersb., 1856, xiii, 137–141.—**Johnson** (M.) On the function of the ganglionic system in relation to the operations of mind. Lancet, Lond., 1868, ii, 409–411.—**Johnstone** (J.) Cui bono? or, physiological and pathological observations on the functions of the visceral nerves ; with some remarks on the action of opium and other vegetable poisons. *In his:* Med. Essays & Obs., 8°, Evesham, 1795, 97–189.—**Jones** (T. W.) Report on the progress of knowledge rega ding the sympathetic nerve and the nature of its connection with the cerebral and spinal nerves. Lancet, Lond., 1847, i, 425–427.—**Kesteven** (W. H.) The sympathetic centre. Brain, Lond., 1878, i, 360–365. — **Kétli** (K.) Adatok az együttérzöideg élet- és kórtanához. [Contribution to physiology and pathology of sympathetic nerve.] Orvosi hetil , Budapest, 1885, xxix, 1413–1418. *Also, transl.:* Pest. med.-chir. Presse, Budapest, 1886, xxii, 57 ; 77.—**Kilian** (F. M.) Die Endigung sympathischer Fasern. Ztschr. f. rat. Med., Heidelb , 1849, vii, 221–227, 1 pl.—**Knoll.** Ueber die Beschaffenheit des Harns nach der Splanchnicussection. Beitr. z. Anat. u. Physiol. (Eckhard), Giessen, 1871, vi, 39–50.—**Kollmann** (J.) & **Arnstein** (C.) Die Ganglienzellen des Sympathicus. Ztschr. f. Biol. München, 1-66, ii, 271–288.—**Kubicki** (W.) O wplywie nerwu trzewiowego (n. splanchnicus) na ruchu serca. [The action

Nervous *system* (*Ganglionic*).

of the splanchnic nerve.] Gaz. lek., Warszawa, 1870, ix, 369; 388.— **Kussmaul** (A.) & **Tenner** (A.) Ueber den Einfluss der Blutströmung in den grossen Gefässen des Halses auf die Wärme des Ohrs beim Kaninchen und ihr Verhältniss zu den Wärmeveränderungen, welche durch Lähmung und Reizung des Sympathicus bedingt werden. Untersuch. z. Naturl. d. Mensch. u. d. Thiere, Frankf. a. M., 1857, i, 99-132.— **Laffont.** Effets de l'excitation du sympathique cervical chez le chien. Compt. rend. Soc. de biol. 1880, Par., 1881, 7. s., ii, 341-343. ———. Effets des excitations électriques du vago-sympathique. Progrès méd., Par., 1881, ix, 210-212. ———. Effets des excitations électriques du bout céphalique du vago-sympathique. Compt. rend. Soc. de biol. 1881, Par., 1882, 7. s., iii, 86-91.— **Lamansky** (S.) Ueber die Folgen der Exstirpation des Plexus cœliacus und mesentericus. Ztschr. f. rat. Med., Leipz., 1866, xxviii, 3. R., 59 - 70.— **Landois** (L.) & **Mosler** (F.) Zuckungsgesetz und Electrotonus der oculopupillären Fasern des N. sympathicus cervicalis. Centralbl. f. d. med. Wissensch., Berl., 1868, vi, 513-515.— **Langenbeck** (C. J. M.) Ueber die Bestimmung des Nervi sympathici magni, und dessen Wichtigkeit in der Pathogenie. N. Biblioth. f. d. Chir. u. Ophth., Hannov., 1823-8, iv, 729-800.— **Legallois.** Aperçus sur quelques maladies qui paraissent consécutives à une affection du nerf trisplanchnique, ou grand sympathique. Rev. méd. franç. et étrang., Par., 1826, ii, 418-440.— **Leonard** (C. H.) The sympathetic nervous system. Detroit M. J., 1877, i, 86-97.— **Lubimoff** (A.) Beiträge zur Histologie und pathologischen Anatomie des sympathischen Nervensystems. Arch. f. path. Anat. etc , Berl., 1874, lxi, 145-207, 2 pl.— **Lussana** (F.) Sui diversi filamenti del nervo gran-simpatico al collo, e loro diverse funzioni. Atti r. Ist. Veneto d. sc., lett. ed arti, Venezia, 1884-5, 6. s., iii, 1363.— **Lussana** (F.), **Lussana** (P.) & **Ambrosoli** (C.) Su le funzioni del nervo gran simpatico e su la calorificazione animale. Gazz. med. ital. lomb., Milano, 1857, 4. s., ii, 205; 213; 221; 229; 245; 253; 277; 285.— **Magnus.** Zur Casuistik der Sympathicusreizung. Klin. Monatsbl. J. Augenh., Stuttg., 1887, xxv, 207-209.— **Mayer** (S.) Beobachtungen und Reflexionen über den Bau und die Verrichtungen des sympathischen Nervensystems. Sitzungsb. d. k. Akad. d. Wissensch., Wien, 1872, lxvi, 117-168, 1 pl. ———. Die peripherische Nervenzelle und das sympathische Nervensystem. Arch. f. Psychiat., Berl., 1876, vi, 353-446, 1 pl.— **Meryon** (E.) On the function of the sympathetic system of nerves. Proc. Roy. M. & Chir. Soc. Lond. (1867-71), 1871, vi, 294-297. ———. Functions of the sympathetic system of nerves as a physiological basis for a rational system of therapeutics. Lancet. Lond., 1871, ii, 570 ; 601; 631 ; 704 ; 744. *Also,* Reprint.— **Meyer** (M.) Therapeutische Erfolge der Galvanisation des Sympathicus. Berl. klin. Wchnschr., 1870, vii, 265-267. *Also:* Verhandl. d. Berl. med. Gesellsch. (1869-71), 1872, [pt.] i, 161-167.— **Michon** (J.) Ablation du ganglion cervical supérieur chez les oiseaux. Compt. rend. Soc. de biol. 1865, Par., 1866, ii, pt. 4, 185.— **Moleschott** (J.) & **Nauwerck** (R.) Untersuchungen über den Einfluss der Sympathicus-Reizung auf die Häufigkeit des Herzschlags. Untersuch. z. Naturl. d. Mensch. u. d. Thiere, Giessen, 1862, viii, 36-51. *Also,* Reprint.— **Mollière** (D.) Quelques faits pour servir à l'histoire de la physiologie et de la pathologie du sympathique cervical. Lyon méd., 1869, iii, 581-586.— **Morat.** Sur les propriétés vaso-dilatatrices du cordon cervical du grand sympathique. Mém. et compt.-rend. Soc. d. sc. méd. de Lyon (1880), 1881, xx, pt. 2, 228-231. ———. Le grand sympathique, nerf vaso-dilatateur. Tr. Internat. M. Cong., 7. sess., Lond., 1881, i, 284-287.— **Morat & Dastre.** Sur les modifications de la pression vasculaire consécutive à la section et à l'excitation du grand sympathique. Compt. rend. Soc. de biol 1878, Par., 1880, 6. s., v, 83.— **Moreau** (A.) De l'influence de la section du grand sympathique sur la composition de l'air de la vessie natatoire. Compt. rend. Soc. de biol. 1865, Par., 1866, ii, pt. 4, 21-24. ———. Sur le rôle du filet sympathique cervical et du nerf grand auriculaire dans la vascularisation de l'oreille du lapin. Arch. de physiol. norm. et path., Par., 1871-2, iv, 667-671.— **Morselli** (E.) Contributo alla fisiopatologia del simpatico cervicale nell' uomo. Sperimentale, Firenze, 1876, xxxviii, 30-57.— **Motta** (E. A.) Algumas considerações relativas á physiologia do grande sympathico. Correio med. de Lisboa, 1875, iv, 241; 257; 275.— **Müller** (J.) Ueber ein Eigenthümliches dem Nervus sympathicus analoges Nervensystem der Eingeweide bei den Insecten. Nova acta phys.-med. Acad. nat. curios., Bonnæ, 1828-9, xiv, 72-108, 3 pl.— **Nasse** (F.) Die psychische Verrichtung der Brust- und Bauch-Ganglien. Ztschr. f. d. . . . krankh. Seelenzust., Berl., 1838, i, 455-476.— **Niese** (H.) Einige Bemerkungen über die allgemeine pathologische Bedeutung der Nervenganglien des sympathischen Systems. Allg. med. Centr.-Ztg., Berl., 1846, xv, 673.— **Ogle** (W.) A case illustrating the physiology and pathology of the cervical portion of the sympathetic nerve. Med.-Chir. Tr.. Lond., 1869, lii, 151-177. *Also* [Abstr.]: Proc. Roy. M. & Chir. Soc. Lond. (1867-71). 1871, vi, 164-166. *Also* [Abstr.]: Brit. M. J., Lond., 1869, i, 330. *Also*

Nervous *system* (*Ganglionic*).

[Abstr.]: Lancet, Lond., 1869, i, 461.— **Ónodi** (D. A.) Az együttérzö idegrendzer, alaktani megjelenésében. [Morphology of sympathetic.] Orvosi hetil., Budapest, 1882, xxvi, 937; 975; 1004; 1037; 1089; 1219; 1348. ———. A gerinczagyi rostkötegek viszonya az együttérzö-határkötegehez. [Spinal cord in relation to the sympathetic nervous system.] *Ibid.*, 1883, xxvii, 62-64. *Also, transl.*: Centralbl. f. d. med. Wissensch., Berl., 1883, xxi, 97-100. *Also, transl.*: Arch. f. Anat. u. Entwcklngsgesch., Leipz., 1884, 145-169, 2 pl. ———. Az együttérzö-idegrendszernek egyes élettani és kórtani szempontból fontosabb alakviszonyairól. [Metamorphoses of sympathetic nervous system from a physiological and pathological view.] Orvosi hetil., Budapest, 1883, xxvii, 1026; 1052. ———. Az együttérzö idegrendszer fejlödése. [Development of the sympathetic nervous system.] *Ibid.*, 1885, xxix, 737-741. *Also, transl.*: Arch. f. mikr. Anat., Bonn, 1885-6, xxvi, 61, 1 pl.; 553. 5 pl.— **Ott** (I.) The splanchnics. Med. News, Phila., 1883, xliii, 263.— **Panas.** Des signes qui caractérisent la compression de la portion cervicale et thoracique du nerf grand sympathique. Mém. Soc. de chir. de Par. (1859-67), 1868, vi, 363-376.— **Pepper** (W.) Cases of abdominal tumor attended with profuse sweating ; with remarks on the influence of the abdominal sympathetic nerve over the state of the skin and intestinal mucous membrane. Med. Times, Phila., 1870-71, i, 170-173. *Also,* Reprint. — **Pfluger** & **Westphal.** Influence des nerfs splanchniques sur les mouvements de l'intestin. Compt. rend. Soc. de biol. 1857, Par., 1858, 2. s., iv, 161.— **Pouchet** (G.) Lésion du grand sympathique chez le turbot. *Ibid.*, 1874, Par., 1875, 6. s., i, 350.— **Ranvier.** Sur les ganglions cérébro-spinaux. Compt. rend. Acad. d. sc., Par., 1882, xcv, 1165-1168.— **Rawitz** (B.) Ueber den Bau der Spinalganglien. Arch. f. mikr. Anat., Bonn, 1880, xviii, 283-301, 1 pl.— **Real** (K.) Eine Abnormität im Verhalten des Gränzstranges des Nervus sympathicus. Arch. f. Anat., Physiol. u. wissensch. Med., Leipz., 1871, 180-183, 1 pl.— **Reid** (J.) On the effects of lesion of the trunk of the ganglionic system of nerves in the neck upon the eye-ball and its appendages. Edinb. M. & S. J., 1839, lii, 36-43. *Also,* Reprint. — **Remak** (R.) Ueber die physiologische Bedeutung des organischen Nervensystems, besonders nach anatomischen Thatsachen. Monatschr. f. Med., Augenh. u. Chir., Leipz., 1840, iii, 225-265. ———. Neue Beiträge zur Kenntniss vom organischen Nervensystem. Med. Ztg., Berl., 1840, ix, 7. ———. Experimenteller Nachweis motorischer Wirkungen des N. sympathicus auf willkürliche Muskeln. Deutsche Klinik, Berl., 1855, vii, 294.— **Retzius** (G.) Ueber der Zusammenhang der Pars thoracica nervi sympathici mit den Wurzeln der Spinalnerven. Arch. f. Anat. u. Physiol., Leipz., 1832, vi, 260. ———. Undersökningar öfver cerebrospinal ganglicrnas nervceller med särskild hänsyn till dessas utlöpare. Skrift. til. Univ. i Kjøbenh. v. d. Fyrahundra-Års-Fest af Karol. med.-kir. Inst. i Stockholm, 1879, i, 30, 3 pl.— **Rivolta** (S.) Sopra il funicolo gangliare del gran simpatico nel mesenterio degli ucelli, e sopra un apparato emolinfatico plessiforme nei medesimi animali. Gior. di anat., fisiol. e patol. d. animali, Pisa, 1880, xii, 3-26, 1 pl.— **Rochas** (F.) Sur quelques particularités relatives aux connexions des ganglions cervicaux du grand sympathique et à la distribution de leurs rameaux afférents et efférents chez l'Anas boschas. Compt. rend. Acad. d. sc., Par., 1885, c, 649-651. ———. Du mode de distribution de quelques filets sympathiques intra-crâniens, et de l'existence d'une racine sympathique du ganglion ciliaire, chez l'oie. *Ibid.*, ci, 829-831. ———. De la signification morphologique du ganglion cervical supérieur et de la nature de quelques-uns des filets qui y aboutissent ou en émanent chez divers vertébrés. *Ibid.*, 1887, civ, 865-868.— **Rockwell** (A. D.) & **Beard** (G. M.) Observations on the psychological and therapeutical effects of galvanization of the sympathetic nerve. Quart. J. Psych. M., N. Y., 1870, iv, 542-555. *Also,* Reprint.— **Rorie** (J.) Microscopical anatomy of the sympathetic system of nerves. Med. Circ., Lond., 1860, xvi, 2; 17; 150; 220; 399. ———. The physiology of the sympathetic system of nerves. *Ibid.*, 1860, xvii, 157.— **Samuel** (S.) Die Exstirpation des Plexus cœliacus. Wien. med. Wchnschr., 1856, vi, 484. — **Sauder** (J.) Die Spiralfasern im Sympathicus des Frosches. Arch. f. Anat., Physiol. u. wissensch. Med., Leipz., 1866, 398-405, 1 pl.— **Schiff** (M.) De l'influence du grand sympathique sur la production de la chaleur animale, et sur la contractilité vasculaire. Gaz. hebd. de méd., Par., 1853-4, i, 421-424. ———. Sull' autonomia del simpatico. Imparziale, Firenze, 1870, x, 353-358.— **Schultze.** Einige Bemerkungen zu der Mittheilung von Dr. Bechterew und Rosenbach: "über die Bedeutung der Intervertebralganglien". Neurol. Centralbl., Leipz., 1884, iii, 265-268.— **Schulz** (B.) Die Deutung der elektrotherapeutischen Galvanisation des Sympathicus. Wien. med. Wchnschr., 1877, xxvii, 241-245.— **Schwalbe** (G.) Ueber den Bau der Spinalganglien, nebst Bemerkungen über die sympathischen Ganglienzellen. Arch. f. mikr. Anat., Bonn, 1868, iv, 45-72, 1 pl.— **Sinitzin.** Zur Frage über den Einfluss des Nervus sympathicus auf das Gesichtsorgan. Centralbl. f. d. med. Wissensch., Berl., 1871, ix, 161-163. — **Stevenson** (S. H.) The physiology and pathology of the sympathetic nervous

Nervous *system (Ganglionic).*

system. Tr. Illinois M. Soc., Chicago, 1879, xxix, 146–160.—
Stirling (W.) Note on the effects of division of the sympathetic nerve of the neck in young animals. J. Anat. & Physiol., Lond., 1875–6, x, 511.—**Strauss** (H.) Sympathique (Grand). Dict. encycl. d. sc. méd., Par., 1884, 3. s., xiii, 722–754.—**Svierczewski** (G.) Zur Physiologie des Kernes und Kernkörperchens der Nervenzellen des Sympathicus: vorläufiag Mittheilung von Prof. W. Tomsa. Centralbl. f. d. med. Wissensch., Berl., 1869, vii, 641–644.—**Tiedemann** (F.) Ueber den Antheil des sympathischen Nervens an den Verrichtungen der Sinne. Ztschr. f. Physiol., Heidelb., 1824, i, 237–290. *Also, transl.:* J. compl. du dict. d. sc. méd., Par., 1825, xxiii,19; 108.—**Tigri** (A.) Intorno alla costituzione anatomica del gran simpatico nei mammiferi e specialmente dei suoi gangli e pericò della diversa copia della fibra contrattile impiegnata a formarlo indagini antropo-zootomiche. Gior. med. di Roma, 1870, vi, 481–501, 3 pl.—**Tizzoni** (G.) Sull' istologia normale e patologica del gran simpatico. Osservatore, Torino, 1878, xiv, 833. ——. Sulla patologia sperimentale del gran simpatico. Spallanzani, Modena, 1879, viii, 232–242.—**Tuwim** (J.) Ueber die physiologische Beziehung des Ganglion cervicale supremum zu der Iris und den Kopfarterien. Arch. f. d. ges. Physiol., Bonn, 1880–81, xxiv, 115–134. — **Varaglia** (S.) Cellule gangliari nel ramo comunicante spinale del gran simpatico dell' uomo. Gazz. d. clin., Torino, 1885, xxii, 387.—**Volkmann** (A. W.) Ueber den Ursprung des Sympathicus vom Rückenmarke. Arch. f. physiol. Heilk., Stuttg., 1853, xii, 92–98.—**Vos** (F.-E.) Absence partielle à l'un des côtés du corps, du cordon limite du nerf sympathique. Arch. néerl. d. sc. exactes, etc., La Haye, 1866, i, 293–295.—**Vulpian** (A.) Sur les phénomènes orbito-oculaires produits chez les mammifères par l'excitation du bout central du nerf sciatique, après l'excision du ganglion cervical supérieur et du ganglion thoracique supérieur. Compt. rend. Acad. d. sc., Par., 1878, lxxxvii, 231.—**Wagner** (R.) Sympathischer Nerv, Ganglienstructur und Nervenendigung. Handwörterb. d. Physiol., Brnschwg., 1850, iii, 1. Abth., 360–406, 4 pl. ——. Notiz über einige Versuche am Halstheile des sympathischen Nerven bei einer Enthaupteten. Ztschr. f. rat. Med., Leipz., 1859, v, 3. R., 331–333.—**von Walther** (A.) Beitrag zur Lehre von der Funktion der den cerebrospinalen Nerven beigemischten sympathischen Fäden. Arch. f. Anat., Physiol. u. wissensch. Med., Berl., 1842, 444–454.—**Wetmore** (S. W.) The sympathetic nervous system. Buffalo M. & S. J., 1875–6, xv, 328–342.—**White** (W. H.) On the histology and function of the mammalian superior cervical ganglion. J. Physiol., Lond. & Cambridge, 1887, viii, 66–78, 1 pl.—**Wilder** (A.) The ganglionic nervous system. Tr. Nat. Eclect. M. Ass., Orange, N. J., 1884, xi, 246–265.—**Wilkes** (J.) On the anatomy, physiology, and pathology of the great sympathetic nerve. *In:* Essays, 8°, Birmingham, 1833, 1–43.—**Witkowski** (L.) Notiz zur Pathologie der Ganglienzellen. Arch. f. Psychiat., Berl., 1883, xiv, 420.—**von Wittich.** Ueber den Einfluss der Sympathicusreizung auf die Function der Glandula parotis. Arch. f. path. Anat., etc., Berl., 1866, xxxvii, 93–100.—**Woakes** (E.) Correlating function of the sympathetic ganglia. Tr. Internat. M. Cong., 7. sess., Lond., 1881, ii, 75–81.—**Wutzer** (C. W.) Ueber den Zusammenhang des sympathischen Nerven mit den Spinalnerven. Arch. f. Anat., Physiol. u. wissensch. Med., Berl., 1834, 305–310.—**Zuradelli** (C.) Richiami anatomici sul gran simpatico e sue funzioni in genere. Galvani, Bologna, 1875, iii. 26–28.

Nervous *system (Ganglionic, Pathology of).*

See, also, **Nervous** *system (Syphilis of).*

DE GIOVANNI (A.) Patologia del simpatico. 8°. *Milano*, 1876.

DEVAUX (R.) * Considérations sur le rôle que jouent dans les maladies l'innervation et l'appareil abdominal. 4°. *Paris*, 1829.

EULENBURG (A.) & GUTTMANN (P.) Die Pathologie des Sympathicus auf physiologischer Grundlage. 8°. *Berlin*, 1873.

——. The same. Physiology and pathology of the sympathetic system of nerves. Transl. by A. Napier. 8°. *London*, 1879.

FRAENKEL (E.) * Zur Pathologie des Hals-Sympathicus. 8°. *Breslau*, 1874.

NICATI (W.) * La paralysie du nerf sympathique cervical. Étude clinique. [Zurich.] 8°. *Lausanne & Paris*, 1873.

PRÖLSS (E.) * Eine Erkrankung des Hals-sympathicus. 8°. *Berlin*, 1886.

RICHTER (G. H.) * De systematis gangliosi in pathogenia dignitate. 8°. *Regiomonti*, [1826].

Nervous *system (Ganglionic, Pathology of).*

TRUMET DE FONTARCE (A.) Pathologie clinique du grand sympathique; étude basée sur l'anatomie et la physiologie. 8°. *Paris*, 1880.

WENZEL (J. F. A.) * De nervi sympathici dignitate in nonnullis morbis producendis. 4°. *Lipsiæ*, [1825].

Aguely. Névrose cérébrale grave ayant son point de départ dans le centre nerveux ganglionnaire. Abeille méd., Par., 1875, xxxii, 341–343.—**Amati** (R.) Emorragia traumatica degli ultimi gangli della porzione toracica sinistra del gran simpatico e del ganglio semilunare corrispondente, seguita da morte. Raccoglitore med., Forlì, 1877, 4. s., viii, 285; 317. — **Baerwinkel** (F.) Neuropathologische Beiträge: II. Pathologie des Kopfsympathicus. Deutsches Arch. f. klin. Med., Leipz., 1874, xiv, 545–565. — **Baiardi** (D.) Contribuzione all' istologia patologica del gran simpatico. Osservatore, Torino, 1874, x, 179–181.—**Barde** (B.) Sur quelques troubles nerveux siégeant dans la partie supérieure du grand sympathique. Ann. Soc. d'hydrol. méd. de Par., 1867, xiii. 158 – 163. — **Bartholow** (R.) Influence of the sympathetic in the causation of morbid phenomena; illustrated by cases. Cincin. Lancet & Obs., 1868, xi, 464–472.—**Bianchi** (L.) Sopra un' alterazione anatomo-patologica del simpatico. Movimento, Napoli, 1879. 2. s., i, 412–417, 1 pl.—**Blaschko** (A.) Mittheilung über eine Erkrankung der sympathischen Geflechte der Darmwand. Arch. f. path. Anat., etc., Berl., 1883, xciv, 136–147, 1 pl. *Also, transl.:* China. Imp. Customs. Med. Rep., Shanghai, 1883–4, xxvii, 86–91.—**Brunner** (N.) Zur Casuistik der Pathologie des Sympathicus. St. Petersb. med. Ztschr., 1871, n. F., ii, 251–264.—**Burggraeve.** Compression traumatique des nerfs vagues et grands sympathiques. suivie de mort par asphixie pulmonaire. Presse méd. belge, Brux., 1851-2, iv, 355–357.—**Clark** (F. E.) Notes on the pathology of the sympathetic nervous system. J. Nerv. & Ment. Dis., Chicago, 1876, iii, 64–78. — **Coleman** (W. L.) Some questions on gangliasthenia. Michigan M. News, Detroit, 1881, iv, 155.—**Colomiatti** (V. F.) Cancro uterino ed affezione cancerosa secondaria nella porzione addominale del grande simpatico. Independente, Torino, 1874, xxv, 9; 29. ——. Contribuzione allo studio della istologia patologica del grande simpatico. Gior. d. r. Accad. di med. di Torino, 1874, 3. s., xv, 41–54. ——. Contribuzione allo studio del cancro e del tubercolo e dell' istologia patologica del grande simpatico. *Ibid.*, 210–223, 1 pl. *Also*, Reprint. *Also* [Rev.]: Arch. d. Heilk., Leipz., 1875, xvi, 93. ——. Sulla tubercolosi dei gangli del grande simpatico e dei nervi. Osservatore, Torino, 1874. x, 727. ——. Sulla tubercolosi dei ganglii del g. simpatico e dei nervi. Gior. d. r. Accad. di med. di Torino, 1875, 3. s., xvi, 101–123, 1 pl. ——. Di un lipoma nel simpatico cervicale. Osservatore, Torino, 1876, xii, 81. — **De Giovanni** (A.) Osservazioni cliniche ed anatomiche concernenti la patologia del simpatico. R. Ist. Lomb. di sc. e lett. Rendic., Milano, 1874. 2. s., vii, 410; 494. ——. Di una nuova importanza del simpatico in patologia. Gazz. med. ital. lomb., Milano, 1874, 7. s., i, 398.—**Deux** cas d'atrophie musculaire progressive : altération des racines spinales du grand sympathique. Gaz. d. hóp., Par., 1865, xxxviii, 21.— **Dickson** (J. T.) Sympathetic depression and emotional disturbance. Lancet, Lond., 1873, ii, 768; 805.— **Domanski** (S.) Przypadek urazowego porazenia nerwu wspólczulnego na szyi (paralysis nervi sympathici cervicalis traumatica). Przegl. lek., Krakow., 1876, xv, 341; 349.— **Dufour.** Observations d'affection parétique du sympathique avec chute incomplète de la paupière. Bull Soc. méd. de la Suisse Rom., Lausanne, 1870, iv, 55 — **Edes** (R. S.) Morbid growth of the semilunar ganglia of the sympathetic. Am. J. M. Sc., Phila., 1871, n. s., 92–94.—**Eulenburg** (A.) Zur Pathologie des Sympathicus. Berl. klin. Wchnschr., 1873. x, 169.—**Eulenburg** (A.) & **Guttmann** (P.) Die Pathologie des Sympathicus. Arch. f. Pyschiat., Berl., 1868, i, 420 ; 676 : 1869, ii, 153 ; 450. *Also, in:* J. Ment. Sc., Lond., 1878–9, n. s., xxiv. 165 ; 374 ; 518.—**Ferraro** (P.) Contribuzione alla patologia del gran simpatico ; pemfigo f laceo. Gior. internaz. d. sc. med., Napoli, 1881, iii, 561–574, 1 pl. — **Foà** (P.) Contribuzione all' anatomia patologica del gran simpatico. Riv. clin. di Bologna, 1873, 2. s., iii, 205–207. ——. Di alcune alterazioni del sistema gangliare simpatico e spinale. *Ibid.*, 1874, 2. s., iv, 50-54.—**Gay** (N.) Obscure neurosis of the sympathetic. Ohio M. Recorder, Columbus, 1876, i, 165–169. — **Gee** (S.) & **Abercrombie** (J.) A case of lesion of the sympathetic nerve in the neck. St. Barth. Hosp. Rep., Lond., 1882, xviii, 253–262. — **Goujon** (E.) Méningite céphalo-rachidienne consécutive à la section des filets cervicaux du grand sympathique. J. de l'anat. et physiol., etc., Par., 1867, iv, 106.—**Guttmann** (P.) Zur Pathologie des Hals-Sympathicus. Berl. klin. Wchnschr., 1875, xii, 437–439.—**Hagenbach** (E.) Beobachtung einer partiellen Verhärtung und Anschwellung am Ganglion cervicale supremum des sympathischen Nerven. Arch. f. Anat., Physiol. u. wissensch. Med., Berl., 1838, 90–94, 1 pl.—**Henrot** (H.) Hypertrophie du

Nervous *system (Ganglionic, Pathology of).*

grand sympathique. Union méd. et scient. du nord-est, Reims, 1877, i, 51.—**Johnson** (M.) Disorders of the sympathetic system. Lancet, Lond., 1882, i, 434; 479.—**Jones** (C. H.) Considerations respecting paralysis of the sympathetic and its relation to neuralgia, ague, and some asthenic inflammatious. *Ibid.*, 1855, ii, 46; 71.—**Kétli** (K.) Adatok az együtterzöideg élet-és kortána-hoz. [Functions and pathology of the sympathetic nerve.] Orvosi hetil., Budapest, 1885, xxix, 1413-1418.—**Kispert** (G.) Pérdida de la vista y del oido de un lado, con hemicránea, á consecuencia de una parálisis del simpático. An. Soc. ginec. españ., Madrid, 1878, iv, 177-182. *Also:* Siglo méd., Madrid, 1878, xxv, 139.—**Landesberg** (M.) Zur Pathologie des Sympathicus. Arch. f. Augen- u. Ohrenh., Wiesb., 1878, vii, 268-301. *Also, transl.:* Arch. Ophth. & Otol., N. Y., 1878-9, vii, 408-440.—**Lewinski.** Zur Pathologie des N. sympathicus (Lähmung des Hals-und des Armsympathicus durch Druck einer Struma. Berl. klin. Wchnschr., 1885, xii, 537-540.—**Mader.** Neurose des Sympathicus; Besserung. Ber. d. k. k. Krankenanst. Rudolph-Stiftung in Wien (1884). 1885, 343. ————. Neurose des linken Halssympathicus; ungeheilt. *Ibid.* (1885), 1886, 366.—**Marcacci** (G.) Alterazione del gran simpatico in un caso di eczema diffuso. Imparziale, Firenze, 1878, xviii, 37-44.—**Mérat** (F.-V.) Essai sur les névroses des nerfs ganglionnaires Rev. méd. franç. et étrang., Par., 1844, iii, 170-228.—**M[ills]** (C. K.) The diseases of the sympathetic nervous system. [Rev.] Am. J. M. Sc., Phila., 1-80, n. s., lxxx, 459-476.—**Möbius** (P. J.) Zur Pathologie des Halssympathikus. Berl. klin. Wchnschr., 1884, xxi, 231; 248; 264; 279. *Also, Reprint.*—**Mollière** (D.) Quelques faits pour servir à l'histoire de la physiologie et de la pathologie du sympathique cervical. Mém. et compt.-rend. Soc. d. sc. méd. de Lyon (1869), 1870, ix, 74-79.—**Nieden** (A.) Ueber Sympathicusaffection. Centralbl. f. prakt. Augenh., Leipz., 1884, viii, 153: 1885, ix, 321.—**Niese.** Eine Ganglien-Neurose. Allg. med. Centr.-Ztg., Berl., 1846, xv, 793-796.—**Ogle** (W.) A case illustrating the physiology and pathology of the cervical portion of the sympathetic nerve. Med. Times & Gaz., Lond., 1869, i, 422. *Also:* Lancet, Lond., 1869, i, 461.—**Otto** (A.) Beitrag zur Pathologie des Sympathicus. Deutsches Arch. f. klin. Med., Leipz., 1872-3, xi, 609-613. —**P.** (G.) Note sur les blessures du grand sympathique au cou. Gaz. hebd. de méd., Par., 1865, 2. s., ii, 294. — **Paladini** (R.) Nevrosi del pneumogastrico e del simpatico; iscuria, paruria ed uremia in giovane isterica. Indipendente, Torino, 1881, xxxii, 313; 337; 361.—**Rampoldi** (R.) Variazioni pupillari dipendenti da alterazioni del simpatico cervicale. Ann. di ottal., Pavia, 1886, xv, 107-112.—**Robinson** (A. R.) Ueber die entzündlichen Veränderungen der Ganglienzellen des Sympathicus. Med. Jahrb., Wien, 1873, iii, 438-440, 1 pl.—**Rorie** (J.) On the pathology of the sympathetic system of nerves. Med. Circ., Lond., 1860, xvii, 171; 319; 338.—**Russell** (A.) An account of two paralytic cases. Med. Obs. Soc. Phys. Lond., 1757, i, 296-302.—**Schwabach.** Beitrag zur Pathologie des Hals-Sympathicus. Berl. klin. Wchnschr., 1876, xiii, 421.—**Seligmüller** (A.) Neuralgie der Plexus abdominales des Sympathicus. *In his* Neuropathol. Beobacht., 8°, Halle, 1873, 9-18. ————. Ein Fall von acuter traumatischer Reizung des Hals-Sympathicus. Arch. f. Psychiat., Berl., 1874-5, v, 835-841. ————. De traumaticis nervi sympathici cervicalis læsionibus. Centralbl. f. Chir., Leipz., 1876, iii, 737-739. ————. Zur Pathologie des Sympathicus. Deutsches Arch. f. klin. Med., Leipz., 1877, xx, 101-119.—**Troy** (M.) The pathological relations of the organic or vegetative nervous system. Tr. M. Ass. Alabama, Mobile, 1854, 136-147.—**Waddel** (W. W.) On the mechanism of some diseases of the sympathetic nerve. Am. J. M. Sc., Phila., 1834, xv, 299-320. — **Warner** (F.) Lesion of the sympathetic on one side of the head. Brit. M. J., Lond., 1877, i, 453.—**White** (W. H.) On the pathological histology of the semi-lunar and superior cervical sympathetic ganglia. Med.-Chir. Tr., Lond., 1885, lxviii, 221-234, 1 pl. *Also* [Abstr.]: Proc. Roy. M. & Chir. Soc. Lond., 1882-5, n. s., i, 435-437. *Also* [Abstr.]: Brit. M. J., Lond., 1885, i, 893.—**Zürcher** (A.) Amphikranie in Folge einer beidseitigen Sympathicus-Erkrankung. Cor.-Bl. f. schweiz. Aerzte, Basel, 1875, v, 25-29.

Nervous *system (Inhibitory).*

See, also, **Heart** (*Nerves of*); **Nerve** (*Pneumogastric*); **Nervous** *system (Reflex action of).*
VON BOETTICHER (W.) * Ueber Reflexhemmung. 8°. *Jena*, 1878.
————. The same. 8°. *Jena*, 1878.
In: SAMML. physiol. Abhandl., 1878, ii, 3. Hft.
LISTER (J.) Preliminary account of an inquiry into the functions of the visceral nerves, with special reference to the so-called inhibitory system. 8°. [*London*, 1858.]
Repr. from: Tr. Roy. Soc. Lond.

Nervous *system (Inhibitory).*

RODET (A.-J.) Actions nerveuses d'arrêt ou d'inhibition. 8°. *Paris*, 1886.
Also [Rev.], *in:* Bull. Soc. de méd. ment. de Belg., Gand et Leipz., 1887, no. 44, 52-60.
SETSCHENOW (J.) Physiologische Studien über die Hemmungsmechanismen für die Reflex-thätigkeit des Rückenmarks im Gehirne des Frosches. 8°. *Berlin*, 1863.
Bartholow (R.) Restraint neuroses; illustrated by cases. Quart. J. Psych. M., N. Y., 1869, iii, 472-477.—**Beaunis.** Note sur les phénomènes d'arrêt. Gaz. méd. de Par., 1884, 7. s., i, 159; 169. *Also* [Abstr.]: Compt. rend. Soc. de biol., Par., 1884, 8. s., i, pt. 2, 113-115.—**Bidder** (F.) Einige Bemerkungen über Hemmungsnerven und Hemmungscentren. Arch. f. Anat., Physiol. u. wissensch. Med., Leipz., 1871, 447-471. — **Bousdorff** (E. J.) Kritik des sogenannten Hemmungsnervensystems. Ztschr. f. rat. Med., Leipz. u. Heildelb., 1869, 3. R., xxxvi, 15-39.—**Brown-Séquard.** Faits nouveaux relatifs à la mise en jeu ou à l'arrêt (inhibition) des propriétés motrices ou sensitives de diverses parties du centre cérébrorachidien. Arch. de physiol. norm. et path., Par., 1879, 2. s., vi, 494-499. ————. Sur les phénomènes d'arrêt de l'activité nerveuse de la moelle dans l'encéphale. Compt. rend. Soc. de biol. 1879, Par., 1880, 7. s., i, 296. ————. Phénomènes d'inhibition et de dynamogénie. Gaz. hebd. de méd., Par., 1881, 2. s., xviii, 380. ————. De l'inhibition et de la dynamogénie des nerfs et des muscles à la suite d'irritations lointaines dues à des poisons, au froid ou à des causes mécaniques. Gaz. méd. de Par., 1881, 6. s., iii, 358-360. *Also:* Compt. rend. Soc. de biol. 1881, Par., 1882, 7. s., iii, 194-198. ————. Recherches expérimentales et cliniques sur l'inhibition et la dynamogénie; application des connaissances fournies par ces recherches aux phénomènes principaux de l'hypnotisme, de l'extase et du transfert. Gaz. hebd. de méd., Par., 1882, 2. s., xix, 35; 53; 75; 105; 136. ————. Recherches sur le rôle de l'inhibition dans une espèce particulière de mort subite et à l'égard de la perte de connaissance dans l'épilepsie. Compt. rend. Acad. d. sc., Par., 1883, xcvi, 417-420. *Also:* France méd., Par., 1883, i, 241-243. ————. De l'importance du rôle de l'inhibition en thérapeutique. Compt. rend. Acad. d. sc., Par., 1883, xcvi, 617-620. *Also:* France méd., Par., 1883, i, 352-355. ————. Inhibition de certaines puissances réflexes du bulbe rachidien et de la moelle épinière, sous l'influence d'irritations de diverses parties de l'encéphale. Compt. rend. Soc. de biol., Par., 1884, 8. s., i, pt. 2, 350-352. ————. Sur divers effets d'irritation de la partie antérieure du cou et, en particulier, la perte de la sensibilité et la mort subite. Compt. rend. Acad. d. sc., Par., 1887, civ, 951-954. *Also:* Gaz. d. hôp., Par., 1887, lx, 370. *Also:* Gaz. méd. de Par., 1887, 7. s., iv, 182-184. *Also:* France méd., Par., 1887, i, 551-554.—**Brunton** (T. L.) On inhibition, peripheral and central. West Riding Lun. Asyl. Rep., Lond., 1874, iv, 179-222. ————. On the nature of inhibition, and the action of drugs upon it. Nature, Lond., 1882-3, xxvii, 419; 436; 467; 485.—**von Dedjulin** (J.) Ueber das Verhältniss der Hemmungs-Wirkung des Laryngeus superior und des Vagus zum Accessorius Willisii. Mélanges biol. Acad imp. d. sc. de St.-Pétersb., 1869, vii, 46-49.—**Eulenburg** (A.) & **Landois** (L.) Die Hemmungsneurose; ein Beitrag zur Nervenpathologie. Wien. med. Wchnschr., 1866, xvi, 521; 537; 553; 569; 585.—**F[oster]** (E) Mechanisms of control in the nervous system and their functions; a new theory. Alienist & Neurol., St. Louis, 1886, vii, 17; 171.—**Frantz** (L.) Bemerkungen zur "Notiz Setschenow's, die Reflexhemmung betreffend". Ztschr. f. rat. Med., Leipz. u. Heidelb., 1866, 3. R., xxviii, 122-124.—**Gaskell** (W. H.) The inhibitory actions and the inhibitory nerves in general. Cong. période. internat. d. sc. méd. Compt.-rend. 1884, Copenh., 1886, i, Sect. de physiol., 24-32.—**Heidenhain** (R.) Ueber Erregung und Hemmung; Bemerkungen zu einem Vortrage des Herrn H. Munk. Arch. f. d. ges, Physiol., Bonn, 1881, xxvi, 546-557.—**James** (A.) The reflex inhibitory centre theory. Brain, Lond., 1881-2, iv, 287-302.—**Jones** (C. H.) On inhibitory influence. Brit. M. J., Lond., 1859, 104-106.—**Laffont** (M.) Inhibition générale provoquée chez les animaux chloroformés par les excitations du nerf pneumo-gastrique intact. Compt. rend. Soc. de biol., Par., 1886, 8. s., iii, 141-143.—**Langendorff** (O.) Ueber Reflexhemmung. Arch. f. Anat. u. Physiol., Leipz., 1877, 96-115.—**Lewisson.** Ueber Hemmung der Thätigkeit der motorischen Nervencentra durch Reizung sensibler Nerven. Arch. f. Anat., Physiol. u. wissensch. Med., Leipz., 1869, 255-266. —**Luchsinger** (B.) Ueber Erregungen und Hemmungen. Arch. f. d. ges. Physiol., Bonn, 1881-2, xxvii, 190-193.—**M'Kendrick** (J. G.) On the inhibitory or restraining action which the encephalon exerts on the reflex centres of the spinal cord. Edinb. M. J., 1873-4, xix, 733-737. *Also,* Reprint.—**Munk** (H.) Ueber Erregung und Hemmung. Arch. f. Physiol., Leipz., 1881, 553-559.—**Nothnagel** (H.) Beobachtungen über Reflexhemmung. Arch. f. Psychiat., Berl., 1875-6, vi, 332-343.—**Onimus.** Erreurs des théories

Nervous *system* (*Inhibitory*).

des nerfs d'arrêt. Cong. périod. internat. d. sc. méd. Compt. rend. 1879, Amst., 1880, vi, 534–539.—**Ott** (I.) The inhibition of sensibility and motion. N. York M. J., 1881, xxxiii, 21–24. ———. The thermo-inhibitory apparatus. J. Nerv. & Ment. Dis., N. Y., 1887, xiv, 428–438. *Also*, Reprint.—**Ott** (I.) & **Collmar** (C.) The thermo-genetic apparatus; its relation to atropine. Therap. Gaz., Detroit, 1887, 3. s., iii. 511–517. *Also*, Reprint.—**Pflüger** (E.) Experimentalbeitrag zur Theorie der Hemmungsnerven. Arch. f. Anat., Physiol. u. wissensch. Med., Leipz., 1859, 13–29.—**von Piotrowski** (G.) Zur Lehre von den sogenannten Hemmungsneurosen. Wien. med. Wchnschr., 1866, xvi, 777–779.—**Richet** (C.) Deux expériences d'inhibition sur la grenouille, et quelques autres faits relatifs à l'inhibition. Compt. rend. Soc. de biol., Par., 1883, 7. s., iv, 456–459.—**Schiff** (J. M.) Zur Physiologie der sogenannten "Hemmungsnerven". Eine Erwiederung an Dr. Edward Pflüger. Untersuch. z. Naturl. d. Mensch. u. d. Thiere, Giessen, 1860, vi, 201–253.—**Setschenow** (I.) Izsledov. tsentrov, zaderjiv. otrajen. dvijen., v mozgu lja-gushki. [Examination of centres regulating reflex action n brain of frog.] Med. Vestnik, St. Petersb., 1863, iii, 1; 9: 17: 1864, iv, 385; 393. ———. Refleksi golovnago mozga. [Reflex action of the brain.] *Ibid.*, 461; 493. ———. Novoe pribavlen. k uchen. o mechanizmach zaderjiv. otrajen. dvijenija. [New researches on the mechanisms restraining reflex motions.] *Ibid.*, 1864, iv, 133–137. ———. Notiz, die reflexhemmenden Mechanismen betreffend. Mélanges biol. Acad. imp. d. sc. de St.-Pétersb., 1875, ix, 390–392. *Also*: Arch. f. d. ges. Physiol., Bonn, 1875, x. 163. ———. Zur Frage über die Reflexhemmungen. Mélanges biol. Acad. imp. d. sc. de St.-Pétersb., 1875, ix, 453–460.—**Simonoff** (L. N.) Die Hemmungsmechanismen der Säugethiere experimentell bewiesen. Arch. f. Anat., Physiol. u. wissensch. Med., Leipz., 1866, 545–564, 1 pl.—**Traube** (L.) Ueber periodische Thätigkeits-Aeusserungen des vasomotorischen und Hemmungs-Nervencentrums. Ges. Beitr. z. Path. u. Physiol., Berl., 1871, i, 387–391.—**Vinelli** (K.) Inhibição e dynamogenia. Rev. d. cursos prat. e theor. da Fac. de med. do Rio de Jan., 1885–6, ii, 169–188.

Nervous *system* (*Reflex action of*).

See, also, **Nervous** *system* (*Diseases of, Causes of*); **Nervous** *system* (*Inhibitory*); **Nervous** *system* (*Vasomotor*); **Paralysis** (*Reflex*); **Reflexes**; **Spinal** *cord*.

ARNOLD (J. W.) Die Lehre von der Reflex-Function für Physiologen und Aerzte dargestellt und beurtheilt. 8°. *Heidelberg*, 1842.

BERTHELOT (H.) * De l'action réflexe au point de vue clinique. 4°. *Montpellier*, 1864.

BLUMROEDER (J. E.) *Brutorum actiones mechanice inexplicabiles. 4°. *Altorfi*, [1719].

BÜCHNER (L.) *Beiträge zur Hall'schen Lehre von einem excito-motorischen Nerven-System. 8°. *Giessen*, 1848.

CAMPBELL (H. F.) Essays on the secretory and the excito-secretory system of nerves in their relation to physiology and pathology, comprising: 1. A new classification of febrile diseases. 2. An exposition of the "ganglionic pathology" on all continued fevers, as illustrated in typhus and typhoid fever. 3. The prize essay on the excito-secretory system of nerves in its relations to physiology and pathology. 4. A letter to Dr. Marshall Hall, of London, claiming priority in the discovery and naming of the excito-secretory system of nerves. 8°. *Philadelphia*, 1857.

CAYRADE (J.) * Recherches critiques et ex-périmentales sur les mouvements réflexes. 4°. *Paris*, 1864.

CHABRIER (A.) *De l'action réflexe et des services que son étude peut rendre à la médecine pratique. 4°. *Montpellier*, 1865.

FICHOT (P.-H.) *Des phénomènes à distance dans les lésions traumatiques. 4°. *Paris*, 1872.

FRANTZ (L.) * De vi, quam exercet cerebri irritatio in motus reflexos. 8°. *Regimonti Pr.*, 1865.

HALL (M.) Memoirs on the nervous system. I. The reflex function of the medulla oblongata and medulla spinalis. II. The true spinal marrow, and the excito-motory system of nerves. 4°. *London*, 1837.

———. Extract from a lecture on the nervous system, being a brief sketch of the true spinal or

Nervous *system* (*Reflex action of*).

excito-motory system, for the use of his pupils. 8°. *London*, 1839.

———. A letter addressed to the Earl of Rosse, president-elect of the Royal Society. 2. ed. 8°. *London*, 1848.

———. Synopsis of the diastaltic nervous system. 4°. *London*, [1850].

HERZEN (A.) Expériences sur les centres modérateurs de l'action réflexe. 8°. *Florence*, 1864.

———. The same. 8°. *Turin*, 1864.

LIBCHEN (J. F.) Nonnulla de functione re-flexoria systematis nervosi. 8°. *Berolini*, 1839.

MULLER (L. F. A.) * De motibus quos dicunt reflexos. 8°. *Amstelodami*, 1855.

PAOLINI (M.) Intorno un modo speciale di azione riflessa propria dei nervi sensori. fol. *Bologna*, 1854.

ROSENTHAL (J.) Bemerkungen über die Thätigkeit der automatischen Nervencentra, insbesondere über die Athembewegungen. 8°. *Erlangen*, 1875.

WUNDT (W.) Ueber den Reflexvorgang und das Wesen der centralen Innervation. 8°. *Stuttgart*, 1876.

Allen (J. A.) The excito-secretory system; Dr. H. F. Campbell; Marshall Hall; alleged priority of discovery. Med. Indep., Detroit, 1857, iii, 381–389.—**Anderson** (W.) On reflex muscular action. Lancet, Lond, 1846, i. 152.—**Bacteria.** Los actos reflejos y la filosofia del inconsciente. Ilustracion méd.-quir. españ., Zaragoza, 1881, i, no. 11; no. 12.—**Bauduy.** Reflex irritation. St. Louis M. & S. J., 1878, n. s., xxxv, 206–208.—**Beauchamp** (H.) Reflex action. Cincin. Lancet & Obs., 1868. xi, 321–330.—**Belfield** (W. J.) Ueber depressorische Reflexe erzeugt durch Schleimhautreizung. Arch. f. Physiol., Leipz., 1882, 298–312, 1 pl.—**Bernard** (C.) Sur les phénomènes réflexes. Compt. rend. Soc. de biol. 1852, Par., 1853, iv, 149–151.—**Bocci** (B.) Fenomeni riflessi della rana per eccitazione con corrente costante di uno dei nervi sciatici tagliato nelle sue radici sensitive. Bull. d. Soc. Lanci-siana d. osp. di Roma, 1886, vi, no. 4, 61–64.—**Bowman** (J.), jr. Reflex action of the nervous system. Cincin. Lancet & Obs., 1874, xvii, 641–648.—**Brown-Séquard.** Sur des modifications profondes produites rapidement par certaines irritations de la peau, dans les grandes fonctions organiques et animales ainsi que dans les propriétés des tissus nerveux et musculaire. Compt. rend. Soc. de biol. 1880, Par., 1881, 7. s., ii, 335–338. *Also*: Gaz méd. de Par., 1880, 6. s., ii, 621.—**Brunton** (T. L.) Reflex action as a cause of disease and means of cure. Brain, Lond., 1878–9, i, 143–154. *Also*: Pop. Sc. Month., N. Y., 1878–9, xiv, 639–647.—**Campbell** (H. F.) The excito-secretory system of nerves; its relations to physiology and pathology. Tr. Am. M. Ass., Phila., 1857, x, 465–510. ———. A claim of priority in the discovery of, and also the naming of, the excito-secretory system of nerves. South. M. & S. J., Augusta, 1857, n. s., xiii, 243–258. *Also*, Reprint.—**Carpenter** (W. B.) Excito-motory system; reply to Dr. Marshall Hall. Lancet, Lond., 1838–9, i, 581–583.—**Cayrade** (J.) Sur la localisation des mouvements réflexes. J. de l'anat. et physiol., etc. Par., 1868, v, 346–362.—**Chéron** (J.) Des conditions anatomiques de la production des actions réflexes. Compt. rend. Acad. d. sc., Par., 1868, lxvi, 842–844.—**Davey** (J. G.) On the excito-motory or diastaltic nervous system of Dr. M. Hall. Assoc. M. J., Lond., 1854, 367–373.—**Davis** (N. S.) A brief review of Dr. Marshall Hall's views on an excito-motory system of nerves. Tr. M. Soc. N. Y., 1841–3, v, 144–178.—**Eckhard** (C.) Ueber Reflexbewegungen der vier letzten Nervenpaare des Frosches. Ztschr. f. rat. Med., Heidelb., 1849, vii, 281–310, 1 pl. ———. Geschichte der Entwickelung der Lehre von den Reflexerscheinungen. Beitr. z. Anat. u. Physiol (Eckhard), Giessen, 1881, ix, 29–192.—**Fick** (A.) Einige Bemerkungen über Reflexbewegungen. Arch. f. d. ges. Physiol., Bonn, 1870, iii, 326–332.—**Ford** (W. E.) Reflex neuroses. Med. Press West. N. York, Buffalo, 1888. iii, 89–97.—**Freusberg** (A.) Reflexbewegungen beim Hunde. Arch. f. d. ges. Physiol., Bonn, 1874, ix, 358–391.—**Frost** (C. P.) The diastaltic system. Am. M. Month., N. Y., 1857, vii, 129–144.—**Gergens** (E.) Ueber gekreuzte Reflexe. Arch. f. d. ges. Physiol., Bonn, 1876–7, xiv 340–344.—**Graves** (R. J.) The discoverer of the reflex function of the nerves. Lond. M. Gaz., 1837, xx, 465–469.—**Griggs** (A. W.) Morbid reflex excitability. Tr. M. Ass. Georgia, Atlanta, 1879, xxx, 163–170.—**Hall** (M.) On the reflex function of the medulla oblongata and medulla spinalis. Phil. Tr., Lond., 1833, 635–665. ———. On the anatomy of the excito-motor system. Lancet, Lond., 1846, ii, 147. ———. Ueber retrograde Reflexthätigkeit im Frosche. Arch. f. Anat., Physiol. u. wissensch. Med., Berl., 1847.

Nervous *system* (*Reflex action of*).

486–489. ——. The spinal system; a demonstration and lecture. Virginia M. & S. J., Richmond, 1854, ii, 255–265. ——. The spinal system, in its application to practice. *Ibid.*, 343–357. ——. A lecture on the diastaltic spinal system. Med. Chron., Montreal, 1853–4, i, 97; 129. ——. The excito-secretory sub-system of nerves; observations and suggestions. Lancet, Lond., 1857, i, 4. ——. Of the extent and specialty of the diastaltic spinal system; observations and suggestions. *Ibid.*, 108. ——. The excito-secretory system; claims of Henry Fraser Campbell, M. D , of Augusta, Georgia, U. S. *Ibid.*, 462–464. *Also, in:* South. M. & S. J., Augusta, 1857. n. s., xiii, 503–506.—**Herzen** (A.) Sui centri moderatori dell' azione riflessa del midollo spinale. Imparziale, Firenze, 1864, iv, 621 – 625. *Also, transl.:* Untersuch. z. Naturl. d. Mensch. u. d. Thiere, Giessen, 1865, ix, 423–430. — **Hitzig** (E.) Ueber reflexerregende Druckpunkte. Berl. klin. Wchnschr., 1866, iii, 69–71.—**Judée.** Action du système nerveux sur la circulation cardiaque. Compt rend. Soc. de biol., Par., 1886, 8. s., iii, 269–271.—**King** (T. W.) On reflex nervous acts and their disturbances, and the more probable parts of nervous sympathies. Med. Times, Lond., 1844, x, 343; 403; 442. — **Kozhevnikoff** (A.) Nervniya volokna chuvstvuyushchiya i sluzhashchiya dlya vozbuzh deniya reflexov. [Reflex action of the nerves of sensation and motion.] Med. Vestnik, St Petersb., 1868, viii, 242–244.—**Laborde.** Réflexe (Action). Dict. encycl. d. sc. méd., Par., 1875. 3. s., iii, 27.—**Lavista** (D. R.) Estudio sobre el poder reflejo ó propiedad excitó-motriz del eje cerebro-espinal y los movimientos que de él dependen. Gac. méd. de México, 1867, iii, 49; 65.—**Luchsinger** (B.) Neue Versuche mit über gekreuzte Reflexe. Tagebl. d. Versamml. deutsch. Naturf. u. Aerzte, Baden-Baden, 1879, lii, 255. ——. Ueber gekreuzte Reflexe. Arch. f d. ges. Physiol., Bonn, 1880, xxii, 179. ——. Zur Theorie der Reflexe; dritte kurze Mittheilung. *Ibid.*, 1880–81, xxiii, 308–312. ——. Zur Theorie der Reflexe und der Reflexhemmung. Mitth. d. naturf. Gesellsch. in Bern (1880), 1881, pt. 2, 99–101.—**Ludwig** (C.) Zur Ablehnung der Anmuthungen des Herrn R. Wagner. Ztschr. f. rat. Med., Heidelb., 1854, 2. R., v, 269–274.—**Mayer** (A.) Ueber die wahre Bedeutung der Reflexbewegungen; eine historisch-kritische Untersuchung. Vrtljschr. f. d. prakt. Heilk., Prag, 1872, cxvi, 56–113. — **Mayer** (S.) Ueber eine Reihe von Reflexvorgängen innerhalb des Gefässsystemes. Wien. med. Presse, 1870, xi, 87–89.—**Mocli.** Zum Verhalten der Reflexthätigkeit. Deutsches Arch. f. klin. Med., Leipz., 1878, xxii, 279–313. — **Naumann** (O.) Zur Lehre von den Reflexreizen und deren Wirkung. Arch. f. d. ges. Physiol., Bonn, 1871–2, v, 196–202.—**Onimus.** Des actions réflexes déterminées par les courants électriques constants et continus. J. de l'anat. et physiol., etc., Par., 1867, iv, 412–420.—**Pilcher** (G.) Observations on the nervous system, particularly the excito-motory or reflex functions. Tr. M. Soc. Lond., 1846. n. s., i, 38–69.—**Pulido** (A.) Movimientos reflejos. Siglo méd., Madrid, 1882, xxix, 492; 523; 635.—**Rosenstein** (I.) O vlijanii temperaturi vodi na reflektornuiou razdrajitelnoste. [Influence of temperature on reflex action.] Vestnik vodolech., St. Petersb., 1881, i, 137–140. — **Rosenthal** (J.) Fortgesetzte Untersuchungen über Reflexe nach Versuchen des Herrn Dr. Moritz Mendelsohn. Sitzungsb. d. phys.-med. Soc. zu Erlang.. 1882–3, xv, 31–34. ——. Ueber Reflexe. Biol. Centralbl., Erlang., 1884–5, iv, 247–256. *Also, transl. :* Rev. scient., Par., 1884, xxxiv, 339–343.—**Schlosser** (W.) Recherches sur l'arrêt des actions réflexes. Rev. scient., Par., 1881, 3. s., ii, 693–696.—**Schwarz** (A.) Az agy hatásáról a gerinczagy visszahajlási müködésére. [Effect of reflex functions of the spinal marrow upon the brain.] Orvosi hetil., Budapest, 1886, xxx, 1313; 1360.—**Smith** (D. T.) Reflex nerve influence and its relation to the causation and cure of disease. Am. Pract. & News, Louisville, 1887, n. s., iv, 161–166.—**Tarchanoff.** Augmentation des actes réflexes sous l'influence du froid. Compt. rend. Soc. de biol. 1875, Par., 1876, 6. s., ii. 216.—**Thiry.** Des instincts et du mouvement réflexe dans les rétractions permanentes. Presse méd. belge, Brux., 1855 - 6, viii, 110; 117. — **Toulmouche** (A.) Observations de quelques fonctions involontaires des appareils de la locomotion et de la préhension. Mém. Acad. de méd., Par., 1833, ii, 368 – 390. — **Volkmann** (A. W.) Ueber Reflexbewegungen. Arch. f. Anat., Physiol. u. wissensch. Med., Berl., 1838, 15–43.—**Vulpian** (A.) Note sur des expériences ayant pour but d'étudier les mouvements réflexes que l'on peut observer chez des oiseaux curarisés et soumis à la respiration artificielle. Compt. rend. Soc. de biol. 1872, Par., 1874, 5. s., iv, 52–63.—**Wagner** (R.) Begründung meiner vom Professor C. Ludwig in Zürich abgelehnten sogenannten "Anmuthungen". Ztschr. f. rat. Med., Heidelb., 1854, 2. R., v, 307 – 323. — **Ward.** Ueber die Auslösung von Reflexbewegungen durch eine Summe schwacher Reize. Arch. f. Physiol., Leipz., 1880, 72 - 91. — **Westmoreland** (R. W.) Reflex nervous disturbances. Atlanta M. & S. J., 1881–2, xix, 65–68.—**Worden** (A. L.) Reflex irritation. Iowa State M. Reporter, Des Moines, 1883, i, 19.—**Zeitteles** (A. L.) Wer ist der Begründer der Lehre von den Reflexbewegungen? Vrtljschr. f. d. prakt. Heilk., Prag, 1858, lx, 50–72.

Nervous *system* (*Sympathetic*).

See Iris; **Nervous** *system* (*Ganglionic*); **Otic** *ganglion.*

Nervous *system* (*Vasomotor*).

See, also, Arteries, Blood-vessels, *Nerves of*; Inflammation (*Nervous influence on*); **Nerve** (*Pneumogastric*); **Nervous** *system* (*Ganglionic*).

AVERWEG (C.) * Experimentelle Beiträge über die Wirkung der Gefässnerven auf die Blutungen. 8°. *Greifswald*, 1874.

DE BARREL DE PONTEVÈS (J.-E.) * Des nerfs vaso-moteurs et de la circulation capillaire. 4°. *Paris*, 1864.

BISCHOFSWERDER (D.) * Vagus und sympathicus, die vaso-motorischen Nerven der Lunge. 8°. *Greifswald*, 1875.

BORDIER (A.) * Des nerfs vaso-moteurs ganglionnaires. Anatomie, physiologie, pathologie, thérapeutique. 4°. *Paris*, 1868.

BRICON (P.) * Nouvelles recherches physiologiques sur les nerfs vaso-moteurs. 8°. *Strasbourg*, 1876.

CALLENFELS (J. van der B.) * De vi nervorum vaso-motorium in circulationem et caloris productionem. 8°. *Traj. ad Rhenum*, 1855.

DE CASTRO (S. O.) * De vaso-motorische zenuwen en hare peripherische centra. 8°. *Amsterdam*, 1877.

DASTRE (A.) & MORAT (J.-P.) Recherches expérimentales sur le système nerveux vaso-moteur. 8°. *Paris*, 1884.

DEDOULIN (J.) * K phiziologii sosudodvigatelniche nervove. [Physiology of vasomotor nerves.] 8°. *St. Petersburg*, 1868.

FREY (H.) *Anatomische Untersuchung der Gefässnerven der Extremitäten. [Strasburg.] 8°. *Berlin*, [*n. d,*]

HAGEMAN (R.) * Ueber den Einfluss der vaso-motorischen Nerven auf die Hautkrankheiten. 8°. *Halle*, [1874].

HALLER (A.) De nervorum in arterias imperio. *Gottingæ*, 1744.

In his : Disp. anat. [etc.] 4°. *Gottingæ*, 1749, iv, 425–445.

HELWEG (K.) * Studier over de vasomotoriske Nervebaners centrale Forløb. 8°. *Kjøbenhavn*, 1886.

KARLINE (B.) *Contribution à l'étude des vaso-moteurs. 4°. *Paris*, 1884.

LEGROS (C.) * Des nerfs vaso-moteurs. 8°. *Paris*, 1873.

MILLER (H.) * On the relation between the sanguiferous and nervous systems. 8°. *Lexington, Ky.*, 1822.

POLKOFF (M.) * K ucheniou o sosudodvigatelnich nervach. [On the vasomotor nerves.] 8°. *St. Petersburg*, 1874.

PUCCIANTI (G.) Azione nervea vasomotrice studiata in sé e nelle sue applicazioni alla patologia. 8°. *Siena*, 1865.

SCHNEIDER (F. A.) * De mutua ratione inter nervos voluntati obedientes et vasomotorios conspicua. 8°. *Dorpati Livonorum* 1843.

VULPIAN (A.) Leçons sur l'appareil vaso-moteur (physiologie et pathologie) faites à la Faculté de médecine de Paris. Rédigées et publiées par H.-C. Carville. 2 v. 8°. *Paris*, 1875.

von Anrep (B.) & **Cybulski** (N.) Zur Physiologie der gefässerweiternden und gefässverengernden Nerven. St. Petersb. med. Wchnschr., 1884, n. F., i, 215–221.—**Armaingaud.** Sur une névrose vaso-motrice se rattachant à l'état hystérique, entièrement guérie par l'emploi des courants intermittents; accès régulièrement intermittents bi-quotidiens de sommeil nerveux, d'asphyxie locale des extrémités, de congestion locale des conjonctives et de névralgies. Gaz. hebd. de méd., Par.. 1876, 2. s., xiii, 516; 545. *Also,* Reprint. *Also* [Abstr.]: Bull. Acad. de méd., Par., 1876, 2. s., v, 627–629. — **Atkinson** (F. P.) Vasomotor influence in the production of certain functional disorders, with some remarks as to treatment. Practitioner,

Nervous *system* (*Vasomotor*).

Lond., 1881, xxvi, 81–84. — **Aubert** (H.) & **Roever** (G.) Ueber die vasomotorischen Wirkungen des Nervus vagus, laryngeus und sympathicus. Arch. f. d. ges. Physiol., Bonn, 1868, i, 211–255, 1 pl. ——. Erwiderung auf Dr. J. Bernstein's Bemerkung zu dem Aufsatze: "Ueber die vasomotorischen Wirkungen des Nervus vagus, laryngeus und sympathicus". *Ibid.*, 1869, ii, 94–96.—**Bärwinkel** (F.) Ueber gefässerweiternde Nerven. Deutsches Arch. f. klin. Med., Leipz., 1877, xx, 143–157. — **Bernard** (C.) Rapport sur un mémoire de M. E. Cyon, intitulé: De l'action réflexe d'un des nerfs sensibles du cœur sur les nerfs moteurs des vaisseaux sanguins: ayant obtenu le prix de physiologie expérimentale. J. de l'anat. et physiol., etc., Par., 1868, v, 337–345. — **Bernstein** (J.) Bemerkungen zu dem Aufsatze: "Ueber die vasomotorischen Wirkungen des Nervus vagus, laryngeus und sympathicus von Hermann Aubert und Gustav Roever in Rostock". Arch. f. d. ges. Physiol., Bonn, 1868, i, 600.—**Bowditch** (H. P.) Rhythmical activity of the vaso-motor nerves. Boston M. & S. J., 1872, lxxxvii, 10. ——. Vaso-motor nerves. *Ibid.*, 1875, xcii, 67; 97.—**Bowditch** (H. P.) & **Minot** (C. S.) The influence of anesthetics on the vasomotor centers. *Ibid.*, 1874, xc, 493–498, 4 pl.—**Bowditch** (H. P.) & **Warren** (J. W.) Plethysmographic experiments on the vaso-motor nerves of the limbs. J. Physiol., Lond., 1886, vii, 416–450, 1 pl. — **Brébant.** Note sur la théorie des nerfs vaso-moteurs dans les sécrétions et dans la congestion simple ou inflammatoire. Union méd., Par., 1867, 3. s., i, 227–232. — **Bruen** (E. T.) The influence of the vaso-motor system in the production of certain symptoms. Boston M. & S. J., 1885, cxiii, 289–292.—**Buch** (M.) Klinische Prüfung der Frage von den peripheren vasomotorischen Centren und den gefässerweiternden Nerven. St. Petersb. med. Wchnschr., 1879. iv, 104; 115.—**Budge** (J.) Ueber das Centrum der Gefässnerven. Arch. f. d. ges. Physiol., Bonn, 1872, vi, 303–305, 1 pl.—**Burggraeve.** Des nerfs vaso-moteurs et de leurs modificateurs dosimétriques. Répert. de thérap. dosimétr., Par., 1875, iii, 325–328. — **Chapman** (J.) On the simultaneous and sympathetic action of vaso-motor nerve centres related to different parts of the body. Med. Mirror, Lond., 1870, vii, 115. — **Cyon** (E.) Ueber die Wurzeln, durch welche das Rückenmark die Gefässnerven für die Vorderpfote aussendet. Arb. a. d. physiol. Anst. zu Leipz., 1869, iii, 62–77, 2 pl. *Also, transl.* [Abstr.]: France méd., Par., 1869, xvi, 551. ——. Hemmungen und Erregungen im Central-System der Gefässnerven. Mélanges biol. Acad. imp. d. sc. de St.-Pétersb., 1870–71, vii, 757–786. ——. Zur Hemmungstheorie der reflectorischen Erregungen. Beitr. z. Anat. u. Physiol. (Ludwig), Leipz. 1874, pp. clxvi-clxxii.—**Cyon** (E.) & **Ludwig** (C.) Action réflexe d'un des nerfs sensibles du cœur sur les nerfs vaso-moteurs. J. de l'anat. et physiol., etc., Par., 1867, iv, 472–485. — **Dana** (C. L.) The vaso-motor neuro-mechanism, and the drugs and other agencies which influence it. Therap. Gaz., Detroit, 1885, 3. s., i, 505–510.—**Dastre** & **Morat.** Recherches sur les nerfs vaso-moteurs. Compt. rend. Acad. d. sc., Par., 1878, lxxxvii, 880–882. ——. Sur un nouveau nerf dilatateur vasculaire, et en général sur la disposition systématique des vaso-dilatateurs. Bull. Soc. philomat. de Par., 1879–80, 7. s., iv, 142–145. ——. Les nerfs vaso-moteurs. Rev. scient., Par., 1884, xxxiv, 34–44. — **Dedyulin** (J. A.) Sposob nablyudat sosudodvigatelvii yavleniya na lagushkai. [Mode of observing vasomotor phenomena in frog.] Med. Vestnik, St. Petersb., 1865, v, 81–83. ——. Opiti nad sosudodvigatelnami nervaini u sobak i koshek. [Experiments on vasomotor nerves of dog and cat.] *Ibid.*, 1867, vii, 131. ——. K' phiziologii sosudodvigalenikh nervof. [Physiology of vasomotor nerves.] *Ibid.*, 1868, viii, 131; 139; 171.—**Dittmer.** Der Sitz des vasomotorischen Centrums. Cor.-Bl. d. deutsch. Gesellsch. f. Psychiat., etc., Neuwied, 1873, xix, 5. — **Dogiel** (J.) Ueber den Einfluss des N. ischiadicus und N. cruralis auf die Circulation des Blutes in den unteren Extremitäten. Arch. f. d. ges. Physiol., Bonn, 1871–2, v, 130–142.—**Dupuy** (E.) On the seat of vaso-motor centres. Tr. Am. Neurol. Ass., N. Y., 1877, ii, 80–84. *Also, Reprint.*—**Duval** (M.) Vaso moteurs. N. dict. de méd. et chir. prat., Par., 1885, xxxviii, 405–563.—**Dzidzioul** (K.) Materiali k voprosu o sosudoraschirjaiouschich nervakh. [On vasomotor nerves.] Voyenno-med. J., St. Petersb., 1880, cxxxvii, pt. 2, 255: cxxxviii, 97.—**Eckhard** (C.) Ueber die Centren der Gefässnerven. Beitr. z. Anat. u. Physiol. (Eckhard), Giessen, 1874, vii, 81–113. — **Ellis** (F. W.) Plethysmographic and vaso-motor experiments with frogs. J. Physiol., Lond., 1885, vi, 437–459, 2 pl. — **Eulenburg** (A.) & **Landois** (L.) Ueber die thermischen Wirkungen experimentaler Eingriffe am Nervensystem und ihre Beziehung zu den Gefässnerven. Arch. f. path. Anat., etc., Berl., 1876, lxvii, 245–271, 1 pl.—**François-Franck.** Analyse de quelques phénomènes vasculaires déterminés chez l'homme par l'excitation des nerfs vaso-moteurs. Gaz. hebd. de méd., Par., 1876, 2. s., xiii, 323–329. ——. Recherches sur l'anatomie et la physiologie des nerfs vasculaires de la tête. *In:* Marey (E.-J.), Physiol. expér., 8°, Par., 1876, 165; 279.—**Fraser** (A. S.) Vaso-constrictor and vaso-dilator nerves. Canad. Pract.,

Nervous *system* (*Vasomotor*).

Toronto. 1884, ix, 65–68. — **von Frey** (M.) Ueber die Wirkungsweise der erschlaffenden Gefässnerven. Arb. a. d. physiol. Anst. zu Leipz. (1876), 1877, xi, 89–107.— **Gaskell.** On the relationship between the structure and the function of the nerves which innervate the visceral and vascular systems. Proc. Physiol. Soc., Cambridge, 1885–6, pp. iv–x. — **Gaskell** (W. H.) On the changes of the blood-stream in muscles through stimulation of their nerves. J. Anat. & Physiol., Cambridge & Lond., 1876–7, xi, 360–402, 2 pl. *Also, transl.:* Arb. a. d. physiol. Anst. zu Leipz. (1876), 1877, xi, 45–88, 2 pl. ——. Further researches on the vasomotor nerves of ordinary muscles. J. Physiol., Lond. & Cambridge, 1878, i, 262–302, 3 pl. ——. On the relationship between the structure and the function of the nerves which innervate the visceral and vascular systems. Preliminary communication. Proc. Physiol. Soc., Cambridge, 1885–6, pp. iv–x. ——. On the structure, distribution and function of the nerves which innervate the visceral and vascular systems. J. Physiol., Cambridge, 1886, vii, 1–80, 4 pl.—**Goltz** (F.) Ueber gefässerweiternde Nerven. (2. Abhandlung.) Arch. f. d. ges. Physiol., Bonn, 1875, xi, 52–99.—**Goltz** (F.) & **Freusberg** (A.) Ueber gefässerweiternde Nerven. *Ibid.*, 1874, ix, 174–197. *Also, transl.:* J. Nerv. & Ment. Dis., Chicago, 1874, n. s., i, 469–488 —**Hartshorne** (H.) Present condition of vaso-motor physiology. Tr. Am. M. Ass., Phila., 1872, xxiii, 183–190.— **Heidenhain** (R.) Bemerkungen zu Herrn Dr. Franz Riegel's Aufsatz: "Ueber die Beziehung der Gefässnerven zur Körpertemperatur". Arch. f. d. ges. Physiol., Bonn, 1872, vi, 20–22.—**Heidenhain** (R.) & **Landau** (L.) Erneute Beobachtungen über den Einfluss des vasomotorischen Nervensystems auf den Kreislauf, und die Körpertemperatur. *Ibid.*, 1871–2, v, 77–113, 2 tab. — **Helweg.** Studien über den centralen Verlauf der vasomotorischen Nervenbahnen. [Transl. from the Danish.] Arch. f. Psychiat., Berl., 1887, xix, 104–183. — **His** (W.) Ueber die Endigung der Gefässnerven. Arch. f. path. Anat., etc.; Berl., 1863, xxviii, 427, 1 pl. — **Hollis** (W. A.) A physiological paradox. Med. Times & Gaz., Lond., 1875, i, 387–389. — **Jolyet.** Contribution à l'étude des nerfs vaso-dilatateurs. Compt. rend. Soc. de biol. 1878, Par., 1880, 6. s., v, 323–325, 1 tab. ——. Des nerfs vaso-dilatateurs céphaliques. Sud-ouest méd., Bordeaux, 1880, i, 8–10.—**Jolyet** (F.) & **Laffont** (M.) Recherches sur les nerfs vaso-dilatateurs contenus dans divers rameaux de la cinquième paire. Compt. rend. Acad. d. sc., Par., 1879, lxxxix, 1038–1040. ——. Du nerf trijumeau considéré comme nerf dilatateur type de la langue, des muqueuses nasales, latérales supérieures et inférieures, gingivales et géniennes. Compt. rend. Soc. de biol. 1879, Par., 1880, 7. s., i, 356.—**Joseph** (M.) Ueber die reflectorische Innervation der Blutgefässe des Frosches. Arch. f. Physiol., Leipz., 1879, Suppl.-Bd., 54–60.—**Kowalewsky** (N.) & **Adamük** (E.) Einige Bemerkungen über den N[ervus] depressor. Centralbl. f. d. med. Wissensch., Berl., 1868, vi, 545–547.—**Kronecker** (H.) Ueber die Erregung der Gefässnervencentren durch Summation elektrischer Reize. Arch. f. Physiol., Leipz., 1880, 437. — **Kuessner** (B.) Ueber vasomotorische Centren in der Grosshirnrinde des Kaninchens. Arch. f. Psychiat., Berl., 1877–8, viii, 437–442.—**Laffont.** Contribution à l'étude des nerfs vasodilatateurs. Progrès méd., Par., 1879, vii, 560–562. ——. Recherches sur l'origine des filets nerveux vasodilatateurs de la face; physiologie comparée des nerfs trijumeau et glosso-pharyngien. Compt. rend. Soc. de biol. 1880, Par., 1881, 7. s., ii, 240–243.—**Laffont** & **Jolyet** (F.) Du nerf maxillaire supérieur considéré comme nerf vaso-dilatateur type. *Ibid.*, 1879, Par., 1880, 7. s., i, 224–226.— **Lee** (F. S.) On the action of certain salts upon the arteries. Johns Hopkins Univ. Stud. biol. lab., Balt., 1884–7, iii, 491–500.—**Lewaschew** (S.) Ueber den Einfluss des Nervus cruralis auf das Lumen der Gefässe. St. Petersb. med. Wchnschr., 1879, iv, 149. ——. Ueber das Verhalten der peripherischen vasomotorischen Centren zur Temperatur. Arch. f. d. ges. Physiol., Bonn, 1881, xxvi, 60–96.—**Lister** (*Sir J.*) An inquiry regarding the parts of the nervous system which regulate the contractions of the arteries. Phil. Tr., Lond., 1858, cxlviii, 607–702. *Also, Reprint.*—**Luzzatto.** Recerche sulla innervazione dei vasi sanguigni, di Luigi Severin. (Extr.) Gazz. med. ital., prov. venete, Padova, 1878, xxi, 248; 257.—**Masoin** (E.) & **Masius.** Rapport sur les nerfs vaso moteurs et leur mode d'action. (Avec discussion.) Cong. périod. internat. d. sc. méd. Compt. rend. 1875, Brux. et Par., 1876, 420–462.— **Mayer** (S.) Ueber die Einwirkung des Strychnin auf das vasomotorische Nervencentrum. Med. Jahrb., Wien, 1872, 111–122, 2 pl.—**Meyer-Lothar.** Ueber die Abhängigkeit der Gefässe und der Pigmentzellen beim Frosch von dem Nerveneinfluss. Arch. f. path. Anat., etc., Berl., 1853, vi, 581. —**Michailow** (W.) Neues Verfahren, die vasomotorischen Erscheinungen am Frosche zu beobachten. Mélanges biol. Acad. imp. d. sc. de St.-Pétersb., 1880, x, 335–377.—**More** (J.) On some points in vaso-motor therapeutics. Practitioner, Lond., 1880. xxv, 352–360.—**Nuel.** Vasomoteur (Appareil nerveux). Dict. encycl. d. sc. méd., Par., 1886, 5. s., ii, 570–627.—**Nussbaum** (M.) Ueber die Lage des Gefässcentrums. Arch. f. d. ges. Physiol., Bonn,

Nervous *system* (*Vasomotor*).

1875, x, 374–382, 1 pl. — **Owsjannikow** (P.) Die tonischen und reflectorischen Centren der Gefässnerven. Arb. a. d. physiol. Anst. zu Leipz., 1872, vi, 21–33.—**Owsjannikow** (P.) & **Tschiriew** (S.) Ueber den Einfluss der reflectorischen Thätigkeit der Gefässnervencentra auf die Erweiterung der peripherischen Arterien und auf die Secretion in der Submaxillardrüse. Mélanges biol. Acad. imp. d. sc. de St.-Pétersb., 1872, viii, 651–665.—**Pawlow** (J.) Experimenteller Beitrag zum Nachweis des Accommodationsmechanismus der Blutgefässe. Arch. f. d. ges. Physiol., Bonn, 1877–8, xvi, 266–271. — **Petrone** (L.) I centri cortico-sensitivi-motori e le contribuzioni cliniche di Hitzig e Wernher. Gior. internaz. d. sc. med., Napoli, 1879, n. s., i. 798–806. — **Philip** (A. P. W.) Some additional experiments and observations on the relation which subsists between the nervous and sanguiferous systems. Phil. Tr., Lond., 1815, cv, 424–446. — **Physiology** (The) of the vaso-motor system. Brit. & For. M.-Chir. Rev., Lond., 1876, 253–277.—**Pierret** (A.) Sur les relations du système vaso-moteur du bulbe avec celui de la moelle épinière chez l'homme, et sur les altérations de ces deux systèmes dans le cours du tabes sensitif. Compt. rend. Acad. d. sc., Par., 1882, xciv. 225. *Also:* France méd., Par., 1882, i, 208–210. — **Poole** (T. W.) Effects of "pithing" on the vascular system; a new phase of the subject. Med. Rec., N. Y., 1879, xvi, 248; 404. — **Pouchet** (G.) Des changements de coloration sous l'influence des nerfs. J. de l'anat. et physiol., etc., Par., 1876, xii, 1; 113, 4 pl.—**Putzeys** (F.) Sur les centres des nerfs vaso-moteurs. Bull. Acad. roy. d. sc. de Belg., Brux., 1874, 2. s., xxxvii, 450–458.—**Putzeys** (F.) & **Tarchanoff** (J. F.) Ueber den Einfluss des Nervensystems auf den Zustand der Gefässe. Arch. f. Anat., Physiol. u. wissensch. Med., Leipz., 1874, 371–391. *Also* [Abstr.]: Centralbl. f. d. med. Wissensch., Berl., 1874, xii, 641–645. *Also,* Reprint. ———. De l'influence du système nerveux sur l'état des vaisseaux. J. de méd., chir. et pharmacol., Brux., 1875, lx, 403–415. *Also,* Reprint.—**Riegel** (F.) Ueber den Einfluss des Nervensystems auf den Kreislauf und die Körpertemperatur. Arch. f. d. ges. Physiol., Bonn, 1871, iv, 350–434. ———. Ueber die Beziehung der Gefässnerven zur Körpertemperatur. *Ibid.,* 1871–2, v, 401–434.—**Rogovitch** (N.) K ucheniu o psevdomotor. dieistvii sosudo-rastshirja. nervov. [Function of the pseudomotor vaso-dilating nerve.] Univ. Izviestija, Kieff, 1885, xxv, pt. 4, 43–100.—**Schiff** (M.) Sur les nerfs vaso-moteurs des extrémités. Gaz. d. hôp., Par., 1862. xxxv, 435 —**Schlesinger** (W.) Ueber die Centra der Gefäss- und Uterusnerven. Med. Jahrb., Wien, 1874, iv, 1–29.—**Stricker** (S.) Untersuchungen über die Gefässnerven-Centren im Gehirn und Rückenmark. Med. Jahrb., Wien, 1886, n. F., i, 1–19.—**Teissier** (J.) & **Kaufmann.** Sur les actions vasomotrices symétriques. Compt. rend. Acad. d. sc., Par., 1881, xcii, 1301–1304. — **Teoria** (Sulla) vasomotrice e sul fatto clinico. Gazz. med. ital., prov. venete, Padova, 1869, xii, 413–416.— **Thiry** (L.) Ueber das Verhalten der Gefässnerven bei Störungen der Respiration. Centralbl. f. d med. Wissensch., Berl., 1864, ii, 722.—**Traube** (L.) Ueber periodische Thätigkeits-Aeusserungen des vasomotorischen und Hemmungs-Nervencentrums. *Ibid.,* 1865, iii, 881–885.—**Ustimowitsch.** Vasotonische Aphorismen. Arch. f. Physiol., Leipz., 1887, 185–194.—**Vogt** (F.) Lähmung der vasomotorischen Unterleibsnerven nach Rückenmarksverletzung. Würzb. med. Ztschr., 1866, vii, 248–250.— **Vulpian** (A.) Expériences, pour rechercher si tous les nerfs vasculaires ont leur foyer d'origine, leur centre vaso-moteur, dans le bulbe rachidien. Compt. rend. Acad. d. sc., Par., 1874, lxxviii, 472–479. ———. Expériences relatives à la physiologie des nerfs vaso-dilatateurs. Arch. de physiol. norm. et path., Par., 1874, 2. s., i, 175–177. ———. L' apparecchio vasomotore. Salute, Genova, 1875, x, 9–11. ———. Sur quelques phénomènes d'action vaso-motrice observés dans le cours de recherches sur la physiologie des nerfs excito-sécréteurs. Compt. rend. Acad. d. sc., Par., 1878, lxxxvii, 385–390. ———. Recherches prouvant que le nerf trijumeau contient des fibres vaso-dilatatrices dès son origine. Compt. rend. Acad. d. sc., Par., 1885, ci, 981–983.—**Waters** (W. H.) Some vasomotor functions of the spinal nerves in the frog. J. Physiol., Lond., 1885, vi, 460–463.—**Wrisberg** (H. A.) Observationes anatomico-physiologicæ de nervis arterias venasque comitantibus. *In his:* Comment. med. physiol., etc., 8°, Gotting., 1800, i, 363–406.

Nervous *system* (*Vasomotor, Pathology of*).

CHEVALLIER (P.-É.) * De la paralysie des nerfs vaso-moteurs dans l'hémiplégie. 4°. *Paris*, 1867.

HAENEL (G. F.) * Zur Casuistik der vasomotorischen Neurosen. 8°. *Leipzig*, [1868].

KLOSTERHALFEN (M.) * Experimentelle Untersuchungen über vasomotorische Störungen nach Verletzungen der Medulla oblongata und des Pedunculus cerebri. 8°. *Greifswald*, 1881.

Nervous *system* (*Vasomotor, Pathology of*).

LUCHTMANS (C. P. C.) * Bijdrage tot de pathologie der motorische zenuw-cellen. 8°. *Utrecht*, 1876.

Angel. Ueber vasomotorische Neurasthenie und Mittheilung einiger psycho-pathologischer Curiositäten. Arch. f. Psychiat., Berl., 1877–8, viii, 394–408.—**Bärwinkel** (F.) Zur Casuistik der vasomotorischen Neurosen. Arch. d. Heilk., Leipz., 1868, ix, 311–314. — **Bischoff** (T. L. W.) Eine pathologische Beobachtung an sich selbst. Ztschr. f. rat. Med., Heidelb., 1846, iv, 55–61. — **Bresgen** (H.) Casuistische Beiträge zur vasomotorischen Neurose. Deutsche Ztschr. f. prakt. Med., Leipz., 1878, v. 565.—**Broes van Dort** (T.) Een geval van vasomotorische neurose, genezen na het gebruik van broomkali. Nederl. Tijdschr. v. Geneesk., Amst., 1876, 2. R., xii, 213–219.—**Brown** (B.) The history of a unique case illustrating some vasomotor disturbances. Med. Rec., N. Y., 1882, xxii, 89.—**Bruen** (E. T.) Some cases of disturbance of the normal vaso-motor tonus. N. Orl. M. & S. J., 1884–5, n. s., xii, 592–600. *Also:* Med. & Surg. Reporter, Phila., 1885, lii, 172; 205. *Also:* Tr. Coll. Phys. Phila., 1884–6, 3. s. viii, 27–37.—**Bull** (E.) En Iagttagelse af vasomotorisk Paralyse. Norsk Mag. f. Lægevidensk., Christiania, 1872, 3. R., 132–137.—**Cahen.** Des névroses vaso-motrices. Arch. gén. de méd., Par., 1803, ii, 428; 551; 696.—**Chvostek** (F.) Beitrag zu den vasomotorischen Neurosen. Oesterr. Ztschr. f. prakt. Heilk., Wien, 1872, xviii, 33; 49. ———. Weitere Beiträge zu den vasomotorischen und trophischen Neurosen. Blasenbildung an der Haut (Pemphigus). Wien. med. Wchnschr., 1875, xxv, 717; 735; 759; 776.—**Concato** (L.) Algido-paralisi transitoria dei nervi vaso-motori; guarigione compiuta coll' elettricità indotta. Riv. clin., Bologna, 1871, 2. s., i, 88–93.—**Cuntz** (W.) Ein Beitrag zur Pathologie der vasomotorischen Nerven. Arch. d. Heilk., Leipz., 1874, xv, 63–75.— **Dowse** (T. S.) A note on vaso-motor and trophic neuroses. Lancet, Lond., 1879, ii 646; 686. — **Eulenburg** (A.) Ueber vasomotorische und trophische Neurosen. Berl. klin. Wchnschr., 1872, ix, 13. ———. Les névroses vasomotrices et trophiques. Cong. périod. internat. d. sc. méd. Compt.-rend. 1884, Copenh., 1886, iii, Sect. de psychiat. et névrol., 92–94.— **Eulenburg** (A.) & **Landois** (L.) Die vasomotorischen Neurosen (Angio-neurosen). Wien. med. Wchnschr., 1867, xvii, 1009; 1025; 1059; 1073; 1105; 1140; 1191; 1249; 1283; 1332; 1383; 1444; 1473; 1523; 1539; 1587; 1868, xviii, 108; 221; 255; 301; 317; 397; 509; 624; 728; 805; 965; 997; 1045; 1616; 1632; 1647. *Also,* Reprint.—**Federici** (C.) Angio-nevrosi isterica. Riv. clin., Bologna, 1870, ix, 286.—**Feinberg.** Ueber reflectorische Gefässnervenlähmung und Rückenmarksaffection, nebst Leiden zahlreicher Organe nach Unterdrückung der Hautperspiration (Ueberfirnissung der Thiere). Centralbl. f. d. med. Wissensch., Berl., 1873, xi, 545–547.—**Grodzinski** (G.) K patologii sosudo-dvigatelinuikh nervov. [Pathology of the vasomotor nerves.] Med. Sbornik, Tiflis, 1866, no. 1, pt. 2, 86–96.— **Guttmann** (P.) Zur Casuistik der vasomotorischen Neurosen. Berl. klin. Wchnschr., 1868, v, 275.—**Henoch.** Ueber die Beziehungen der Krankheiten des Circulationsapparats zu den Neurosen. Arch. f. d. ges. Med., Jena, 1846, viii, 462–477.—**Jewell** (J. S.) The pathology of the vaso-motor nervous system. J. Nerv. & Ment. Dis., Chicago, 1874, i, 1; 151; 271; 419.—**Johnson.** [Case of paralysis of the vaso-motor nerves of the left side.] Chicago M. J., 1871, xxviii, 8–12.—**Johnston** (W. W.) A case of vaso-motor neurosis of a rare form occurring in a child. Am. J. Obst., N. Y., 1885, xviii, 393–399.—**Jones** (C. H.) Case of vaso-motor nerve disorder. Med. Press & Circ., Lond., 1882, n. s., xxxiv, 389–391. — **Lancereaux** (E.) Des troubles vaso-moteurs et trophiques liés à l'alcoolisme et à quelques autres intoxications chroniques (pâleurs et sueurs froides, asphyxie locale, œdème et gangrène des extrémités). Union méd., Par., 1881, 3. s., xxxi, 745; 825; 857. — **Lépine** (R.) Sur l'existence de troubles vasomoteurs des membres dans quelques affections fébriles et spécialement dans la pneumonie; mémoire lu à la Société de biologie. Compt. rend. Soc. de biol. 1867, Par., 1869, 4. s., iv, 133–147. *Also,* Reprint. *Also:* Gaz. méd. de Par., 1868, xxiii, 517; 631.— **Leudet** (E.) Étude clinique des troubles nerveux périphériques vaso-moteurs survenant dans le cours des maladies chroniques. Arch. gén. de méd., Par., 1864, i, 150; 273. — **Lindmann** (J.) Zur Casuistik der vasomotorisch-trophischen Neurosen. Deutsche med. Wchnschr., Berl., 1883, ix, 580.—**Mackenzie** (J. N.) A contribution to the pathology and treatment of the respiratory vaso-motor neuroses. N. York M. J., 1887, xlv, 231–237. *Also,* Reprint. *Also:* Tr. Am. Laryngol. Ass. 1886, N. Y., 1887, viii, 154–175.—**Mills** (C. K.) Vaso-motor and trophic affection of the fingers. Am. J. M. Sc., Phila., 1878, n. s., lxxvi, 431–436.—**Nothnagel.** Zur Lehre von den vasomotorischen Neurosen. Deutsches Arch. f. klin. Med., Leipz., 1867, ii, 173–191. ———. Mittheilung über Gefässneurosen. Berl. klin. Wchnschr., 1867, iv, 536.—**Olivetti.** Le neurosi vaso-motorie od angio-neurosi del Dott.

Nervous *system* (*Vasomotor, Pathology of*).

A. Eulenburg, e Dott. L. Landois. Gior. d. r. Accad. di med. di Torino, 1873, 3. s., xiv, 339; 379; 429; 462; 509; 643.—**Perroud.** Observations pour servir à l'histoire des paralysies des nerfs vaso-moteurs de la tête. Mém. et compt.-rend. Soc. d. sc. méd. de Lyon (1863), 1864, iii, 138–147. *Also:* Gaz. méd. de Lyon, 1864, xvi, 215–218 — **Pierret** (A.) Sur les relations du système vaso-moteur du bulbe avec celui de la moe le épinière chez l'homme. et sur les altérations de ces deux systèmes dans le cours du tabes sensitif. Compt. rend. Acad. d. sc., Par., 1882, xciv, 225.—**Pogozheff** (P. I.) O proiskhozhenii aktivnoi giperemii paslai pereraizki nervov. [Origin of active hyperæmia from severing of a nerve.] Laitop. khirurg. Obsh. v. Mosk., 1873–5, i, 551–556.—**Reynolds** (J. R.) On certain affections of the vaso-motor nerves. Brit. M. J., Lond., 1868, ii, 655—**Roth.** Paralysen vasomotorischer Nerven. Wchnschr. f. d. ges. Heilk., Berl., 1850, 289; 308.—**Scherschewky** (M. M.) Ueber Thermoneurosen. (Material zur Pathologie der vasomotorischen Neurosen.) Arch. f. path. Anat., etc., Berl., 1884, 9. F., vi, 131–175 — **Seeligmüller.** Zwei seltene Formen von vasomotor. Neurose. Tagebl. d. Versamml. deutsch. Naturf. u. Aerzte, Baden-Baden, 1879, lii, 319–322. *Also:* Med.-chir. Centralbl., Wien. 1881, xvi, 3; 16.—**Sigerson.** Note sur la paralysie vaso-motrice généralisée des membres supérieurs. Progrès méd., Par., 1874, ii, 229; 246. *Also,* Reprint.—**Starr** (M. A.) Vasomotor neuroses. Med. News, Phila., 1886, xlviii, 213. — **Sturge** (A.) A case of rare vaso-motor disturbance in the leg. Brit. M. J., Lond., 1879, i, 703. *Also:* Lancet, Lond., 1879, i. 596 —**von Willebrand.** Tvenne fall af vasomotorisk neures. Finska läk.-sällsk. handl., Helsingfors, 1870, xii, 271.— **Zunker.** Ueber zwei Fälle von vasomotori chen Neurosen. Berl. klin. Wchnschr., 1876, xiii, 489; 505. — **Zuradelli** (C.) Delle paralisi e contratture vasomotrici esterne e della loro cura comune ed elettrica. Galvani, Bologna, 1875, iii, 26; 73; 161; 241.

Nervous (The) system. 96 pp. 16°. *New York, D. Appleton & Co.,* 1882.

Health Primers, no. 9.

Nervousness.

See Nervous *system* (*Diseases of, Functional*); Neurasthenia.

van Nes (Hendrik Bernard). * Over gevolgen van het sluiten van slagaderen der hersenen. 2 p. l., 47 pp. 8°. *Utrecht, Kemink & Zoon,* 1881.

van Nes (Jan). * De pathologie der geelzucht beschouwd van het standpunt der physiologie. 2 p. l., 46 pp. 8°. *Leyden, D. J. Couvée,* 1857.

van Nes (Johannes). * De cholera. 8 pp., 2 l. 4°. *Traj. ad Rhenum, G. vande Water,* 17·9.

van Nes (Theodorus Christianus). * Spec. exhibens theses quasdam selectas. 1 p. l., 5 pp. 4°. *Lugd. Bat., S. et J. Luchtmans,* 1788. [P., v. 1011.]

Nesbit (J. C.) The history and properties of the different varieties of natural guanos. 50 pp. 8°. *London, Rogerson & Tuxford,* 1859. [*Also, in:* P, v. 1487.]

———. The same. New ed. 49 pp. 8°. *London, Rogerson & Tuxford,* 1860.

Nesbit (William). The clinical guide; or, a concise view of the leading facts on the history, nature, and cure of diseases; to which is subjoined a practical pharmacopœia, in three parts, viz: Materia medica, classification, and extemporaneous prescription. Intended as a memorandum book for practitioners. 3. ed. 4 v. 12°. *Edinburgh, J. Watson,* 1799–1800.

Nesbitt (Robert). * De partu difficili. 23 pp. 4°. *Lugd. Bat., ex off. Boutesteiniana,* 1721.

———. Human osteogeny explained in two lectures, read in the Anatomical Theatre of the Surgeons of London. July the first and second, anno 1731. In which not only the beginning and gradual increase of the bones of human fœtuses are described, but also the nature of ossification is considered, and the general notion that all bones are formed from cartilages is demonstrated to be a mistake. xiii, 170 pp., 6 pl. 8°. *London, T. Wood,* 1736.

———. The same. Osteogenie, oder Abhandlung von Erzeugung der Knochen im menschlichen

Nesbitt (Robert)—continued.
Körper in zween Vorlesungen erklärt . . . Aus dem Englischen übersetzt von Johann Ernst Greding. Nebst einer Vorrede Herrn Christian Gottlieb Ludwigs. 3 p. l., xxviii (4 l.), 104 pp., 6 pl. 4°. *Altenburg, P. E. Richter,* 1753.
Bound with: MÜLLER (Gottfried Wilhelm). XXIV Kupfer-Tafeln, [etc.] 4°. *Frankf. a. M.,* 1749.

Nesemann ([Edwin Wilhelm Otto] Franz) [1848–]. * Ueber subcutane Carbolsäure-Injectionen bei Polyarthritis rheumatica. 28 pp, 1 l. 8°. *Halle a. S., Plötz,* 1879.

Nesemann (Reinholdus). * De terebratione cranii in læsionibus capitis adhibenda. 30 pp., 1 l. 8°. *Vratislaviæ, H. Lindner,* [1858].

Nesensohn (Simon). * Eine Beobachtung von Verknöcherung der grossen Fontanelle bei Zwillingen. 16 pp., 2 pl. 8°. *Tübingen, H. Laupp,* 1857.

Neser (Charles). * De la physiognomique considérée sous les rapports physiologiques et pathologiques. 51 pp. 4°. *Strasbourg,* 1842, No. 105, 2. s., v. 8.

Neskowic (Belisar). * Ueber Aderhauttuberkeln bei Meningitis tuberculosa. 37 pp. 8°. *Würzburg, P. Scheiner,* 1884.

Nespoli (Enrico). Notizie istoriche della medicina e della chirurgia in Toscana, e particolarmente della scuola chirurgica Fiorentina. 73 pp. 8°. *Firenze, L. Ciardetti,* 1831. [P., v. 905.]

van Ness. Ein neues Heilverfahren gegen Leberleiden und Wassersucht, dessen Wirkung garantirt wird. 51 pp. 12°. *Altona,* 1863.

Ness (Franciscus Josephus) [1795–]. * De nexu speciali organorum excernentium cum medicaminibus similibusque corpori ingestis. 38 pp. 12°. *Bonnæ, typ. Thormannianis,* [1822].

Ness (Theodorus). * De hydrophobia. 40 pp. 8°. *Wireeburgi, J. Dorbath,* 1825.

Nessel (Franz) [1803–]. Handbuch der Zahnheilkunde. 2. Aufl. 320 pp., 10 pl. 8°. *Wien, W. Braumüller,* 1855.

———. Compendium der Zahnheilkunde. iv, 226 pp., 1 l. 8°. *Wien, W. Braumüller,* 1856.

———. Praktische Beiträge zur Heilkunde. 1. Hft. 15 pp. 8°. *Prag, K. Gerzabek,* 1861. [P., v. 790.]

Nessi (Giuseppe) [1741–1821]. Lettera in occasione della morte di una donna seguita poche ore dopo il parto. Disaprova la medesima l' abuso di cavare la placenta subito sortito il feto; descrive i casi in cui conviene senza dilazione tirarla dall' utero, e propone un metodo facile di fare l' operazione dell' estrazione di essa placenta. 43 pp. 8°. *Como, Caprani,* 1772.

———. Osservazione medico-chirurgo-critica sopra dieci aghi, quattro spilli, e due pezzetti di vetro cavati di fresco da una mammella e dalle circonvicine parti col mezzo di dodici taglj. Si dimostra brevemente in essa colla ragione, e colla sperienza ad ammaestramento de' principianti la superfluità delle diverse classi de' medicamenti nella cura de' malj chirurgici. 42 pp. 8°. *Como, Caprani,* 1772.
Bound with his: Lettera in occasione della morte. 8°. *Como,* 1772.

———. Instituzioni di chirurgia. 3 v. 8°. *Pavia, P. Galeazzi,* 1786–8.
v. 4 wanting.

———. The same. 4 v. 8°. *Venezia, F. di Nicolo Pezzana,* 1787–9.

———. Arte ostetricia teorico pratica; nella regia Università di Pavia. viii, 184 pp. 8°. *Venezia,* 1797. [P., v. 1122.]

Nessler (A.) * Materialy dlja otsenki sposobcv izsledovanija ammiachnych i organicheskich azotistych soedinenii zagriaznennago vozducha. [Relative value of methods of defining ammonia

Nessler (A.)—continued.
and organic combinations in polluted air.] 53
pp. 8°. *St. Petersburg, tipoy. A. Transhelja,*
1880.

de Nesslern (Henri). * Contribution à l'étude
de l'influence de l'alcool sur la pepsine. 38 pp.,
1 l. 4°. *Paris,* 1887, No. 229.

Nestell (D. D. T.) A brief treatise on the diseases of the respiratory organs, with their treatment by the inhalation of cold medicated vapors
and the use of showering syringes. 32 pp. 8°.
New York, H. Palmer, 1856.

Nesterus (Carolus Fridericus). * De colica
scorbutica. 32 pp. sm. 4°. *Jenœ, lit. Krebsianis.* [1678].
For Biography, see **Wedel** (Geo. Wolff.)

Nesterus (Joh. Matthias) [1622–79]. De bilis
natura ejusque usu nobilissimo. 11 l. 4°.
Jenœ, typ. Steinmannianis, 1644.

——. * Περὶ ἀνορεξίας seu de inappetentia ventriculi. 15 l. 4°. *Jenœ, e calcographéo Loben-
steiniano,* 1649.

Nesti (L.)
See **Morelli** (C.) & **Nesti** (L.) Istoria clinica della
difterite, [etc.] 8°. *Firenze,* 1873.

Nestlé (Heinrich). Ueber die Ernährung der
Kinder. 11 pp., 2 l. 12°. *Vevey, Lörtscher u.
Sohn,* 1870.

——. The same. 16 pp. 12°. *Vivis, Lörtscher
u. Sohn,* 1883.

——. The same. Memorial on the nutrition
of infants. 10 pp. 18°. *Vevey, Lœrtscher & Son,*
1875.
See, also, **Lebert** (Hermann). Milk and Henry Nestlé's milk powder as food [etc.] 8°. *Basle,* 1875.

Nestler (Auguste).
See **Coze** & **Nestler** (Auguste). Réponse aux observations [etc.] 4°. *Strasbourg,* 1827.

Nestler (C. G.) * Commentatio botanico-medica
de potentilla necnon de plantis huicce generi
affinibus et in usum medicum tractis. iv, 5–
91 pp., 1 pl. 4°. *Parisiis,* 1816, No. 107, v.
122.

Nestler (Fridericus). * De fractura colli ossis
femoris intra ligamentum capsulare. 37 pp., 1
pl. 8°. *Dorpat, typ. J. C. Schünmanni,* 1832.

Nestler (Joh. Georgius). * De virgine, chlorosi
et gutta serena laborante. 15 pp. 4°. *Jenœ,
ex off. Helleri,* [1768].
For Biography, see **Kaltschmied** (Car. Frid.)

Nestlé's *food.*
See **Infants** (*Food, etc., of*).

Nesty (Emmanuel). * Étude sur les fistules salivaires de la parotide et du canal de Sténon.
60 pp. 4°. *Paris,* 1875, No. 241.

Netchaeff (A.) * Ob ugnetajoutshem vlijanii
na otdelenie jeludochnago soka: Atropina, morfija chloral-gidrata i razdrajenija tchuvstvitel-
nych nervov. [On depressing influence of . . .
on secretion of gastric juice, and on stimulating
the nervus vagus.] 65 pp. 8°. *St. Petersburg,
tipog. A. M. Kotomina,* 1882.

Netchaeff (V. G.) * O diagnosticheskom znachenii otsutstvija svobodnoi soljanoi kisloty v
jeludochnom soke pri rake jeludka. [Diagnostic
value of absence of muriatic acid in gastric juice
in cancer of stomach.] 66 pp., 1 l. 8°. *St.
Petersburg, tipog. Dep. Udelov,* 1887.

Nethe (Joannes Theodorus) [1817–   ]. * De
stricturis urethræ. 31 pp. 8°. *Berolini, typ.
Nietackianis,* [1841].

Netherfield Institution for Infectious Diseases,
Liverpool. *See* **Institution** for Infectious Diseases, Netherfield House, Liverpool.

Netherlands. Chirurgyns leger-kist. Voorsien met in- en uytwendige medicamenten,
sodanigh als nootsaaklijk is om daar mede te
veldt te trekken, en tot sulke als in 't leegar

Netherlands—continued.
ordinaar voorvalt, voorsien to wesen. 15 pp.
12°. *Amsterdam, J. ten Hoorn,* 1693.
Bound with: VAN RUSTINGH (S.) Nieuwe veld-medi-
cine en chirurgie. 12°. *Amsterdam,* 1693.

——. Publicatie van zijne Majesteit den Koning van Holland. Houdende algemeene veror-
denigen behoorende tot de geneeskundige staatsregeling van het koningrijk Holland. Gearres-
teerd den 3den April 1807. 9 pp. 8°. *In den
Haag, ter koninglijke Staats Drukkerij,* 1807.

——. Lijst der bevoegd erkende beoefenaren
van de onderscheidene takken van geneeskunst,
in de provincie Zuid-Holland. Voor het jaaren
1829; 1831–52; 1854–65. 8°. *['s Gravenhage,
1829–65.*]
Bound in 7 v.

——. Algemeen rapport der commissie tot het
onderzoeken van den aard en de meest geschikte
wijze van behandeling van den Aziatischen
braakloop. 174 pp. 8°. *'s Gravenhage, ter algemeene Lands Drukerij,* 1832.

——. Algemeen verslag der subcommissie voor
de zaken den asiatischen braakloop aangaande,
te Rotterdam; aan de hoofd-commissie in de
provincie Holland, zuidelijk gedeelte gevestigd
te 's Gravenhaage. 99 pp., 1 ch. 8°. *Rotterdam, P. van Waesberge,* 1833.

——. Verzameling van wetten, besluiten en reglementen, betrekkelijk de burgerlijke geneeskundige dienst in het koningrijk der Nederlanden. [With supplement.] xx, 463, 40 pp., 1 l.
8°. *'s Gravenhage, J. P. Biekman,* 1836.

——. Stukken betreffende de herziening der
geneeskundige wetten en verordeningen en 1841–
1842. [Rapport aan zijne excellentie den minister van binnenlandsche zaken, over de geneeskundige staatsregling ingediend den 23. April
1842, door de commissie benoemd bij zijner ma-
jesteits besluit van den 20. November 1841, No.
60.] ix, 117 pp., 1 l. 8°. *'s Gravenhage,* 1842.
[P., v. 766.]

——. Advies omtrent het onderwijs in de geneeskunst en in de artsenijbereidkunst. Ontwerp van wet op de examens ter uitoefening der
geneeskunst en der artsenijbereidkunst met memorie van toelichting. 74 pp. 8°. *'s Gravenhage, Algemeene Lands-Drukerij,* 1850.
Repr. from : Rapport der commissie, benoemd bij koninklijke besluiten van 25. July en 4. Aug. 1848.

——. Nederlandsche Apotheek. xxii, 557, xvi,
xxiv pp., 1 tab. 8°. *'s Gravenhage, Algemeene
Lands-Drukerij,* 1851.

——. Ontwerp van wet op de uitoefening der
geneeskunst enz. Zitting 1856–7 (cxxxiv). fol.
['s Gravenhage, 1856–7.]

CONTENTS.
No. 1. Regeling van de uitoefening der geneeskunst
enz. Koninklijke boodschap. 1 l.
No. 2. Ontwerp van wet, regelende de uitoefening der
geneeskunst. 11 pp.
No. 3. Memorie van toelichting tot het ontwerp van
wet, regelende de uitoefening van de geneeskunst. 28 pp.
No. 4. Ontwerp van wet, regelende de uitoefening der
artsenijbereidkunst en den handel in geneesmiddelen en
in heelkundige werkteigen. 14 pp.
No. 5. Memorie van toelichting tot het ontwerp van
wet, regelende de uitoefening der artsenijbereidkunst en
den handel in geneesmiddelen en in heelkundige werkteigen. 14 pp.
No. 6. Ontwerp van wet, regelende het geneeskundig
bestuur. 6 pp.
No. 7. Memorie van toelichting tot het ontwerp van wet,
regelende het geneeskundig bestuur. 5 pp.
No. 8. Ontwerp van wet, regelende het onderzoek
naar de bekwammheid van aanstaande geneeskunstoefenaren en apothekers. 3 pp.
No. 9. Memorie van toelichting tot het ontwerp van
wet, regelende het onderzoek naar de bekwammheid van
aanstaande geneeskunstoefenaren en apothekers. 3 pp.
No. 10. [Adres van de lectoren aan de Geneeskundige
School te Rotterdam, over de ontwerpen van wet op te uitoefening der geneeskunst enz.] Aan de Tweede Kamer
der Statengeneraal. Copij. Nov. 9 1857. 37 pp.

Netherlands – continued.

No. 11. Geneeskundige wetgeving. Weekblad van het regl. Dec. 10 1857. No. 1911.

No. 12. [Adres van heel- en vroedmeesters te Rotterdam, over de ontwerpen van wet op de uitoefening der genees-kunde.] Aan de Tweede Kamer der Statengeneraal. Co-pij. Nov. 9 1857. 5 pp.

No. 13. Aan de leden van de Tweede Kamer der Staten-generaal. Nov. 10 1857. 2 l.

No. 14. Copie. Aan zijne excellentie der heer minister van binnenlandsche zaken. Maart 1858. 7 pp.

No. 15. Zitting 1857-8 (x). No. 2. Voorloopig verslag. 55 pp.

——. Het provincial geneeskundig gesticht voor krankzinnigen, Meerenberg, bij Haarlem. Opgedragen aan zijne excellentie den heere commisaris des konings in Noord-Holland. 20 pp. 8°. *Haarlem, J. J. Weeveringh*, 1861.

——. Meerenberg. Asile provinciale d'aliénés dans le voisinage de Harlem. 20 pp. 8°. *Harlem, J. J. Weeveringh*, 1862.

——. De choleraepidemieën in Nerderland met uitzondering van de provincien Noordbrabant en Limburg van 1832-67. 1 map, 40 x 48 in. [*n. p.*, 1867 ?]

——. Verslag van het patronat voor behoeftige herstelde krankzinnigen in de provincie Noord-Holland. 4., 1866-7. 5 pp. 8°. [*Amsterdam*, 1867.]

——. Verslag aan den Koning van de bevindin-gen en handelingen van het geneeskundig staats-toezigt, in het jaaren 1866-86. 21 v. roy. 8° & 4°. *'s Gravenhage*, 1867-87.

1874 to 1886 are 4°.

——. Verzameling van stukken betreffende het geneeskundig staatstoezigt in Nederland. (Uit-gegeven door de inspecteurs en adjunct inspec-teurs voor het geneeskundig staatstoezigt in het jaaren 1865-83. 18 v. 8°. *'s Gravenhage*, 1867-83.

1865-66 in 1 v., and published in 1870.

——. Rapport aan den Koning van die commis-sie tot onderzoek van drinkwater. 410 pp., 4 pl. 8°. *'s Gravenhage, Weelden & Mingelen*, 1868.

——. The same. 2. ed. 412, xiv pp., 7 pl. roy. 8°. *'s Gravenhage, Weelden & Mingelen*, 1869.

——. Das Medicinal-Wesen im Königreiche der Niederlande. (Die Gesetze vom 1sten Juni 1865 Deutsch übersetzt.) 23 pp. 8°. *Haag, M. J. Visser*, 1870.

——. Ondersteuning van door den oorlog ver-armde bevolkingen. 's Gravenhage, Januarij 1871. 2 l. 8°. [*'s Gravenhage*, 1871.]

——. Proeve eener reorganisatie van de genees-kundige dienst bij de landmacht hier te lande. Door Jemand. 31 pp. 8°. *Leiden, S. C. Van Doesburgh*, 1871.

——. Verslag aan den Koning van de bevindin-gen en handelingen van het veeartsenijkundig staatstoezigt in het jaaren 1871, 1873-7. roy. 8° & 4°. *'s Gravenhage*, 1872-8.

1873 is roy. 8°.

——. Naamlijst van de geneeskundigen in Nederland, belast met het geven van onderwijs in de geneeskunde of behoorende tot de amb-tenaren van het geneeskundig staatstoezigt, van de leden en plaatsnervangende leden van de geneeskundige raden en van de geneeskundigen, tandmeesters, apothekers, droogisten en vroed-vrouwen in elke provincie gevested op den 1. Februarij 1874. 207 pp. 8°. *Tiel, H. C. A. Campage*, 1874.

——. Openingsplechtigheid van de tentooristel-ling, 10 Januari 1 uur's namiddags in de biblio-theek van het Koninklijk Zoologisch Genoot-schap Natura Artis Magistra. 8 pp. 8°. *Am-sterdam, Scheltema & Holpema*, 1878.

——. Inlichttingen voor vroedvrouwen wett-lijke bepalingen betreffende vroedvrouwen.

Netherlands—continued.

Eed, welken de vroedvrouwen moet aflegen voor het ontvangen der akte van bevoegdheid. 7 pp. 8°. [*'s Gravenhage*, 1878.]

——. Voorschriften nopens de instelling vanals-mede het toezigt, de directie en het administra-tief beheer over de militaire-inrigtingen. Vast-gesteld bij koninklijk besluit van den 7den September 1880, No. 9, en bij beschikking van den minister van oorlog van den 21sten Septem-ber 1880. VIe Afd. Int., No. 79. 151, 111 pp. 8°. *'s Gravenhage, de gebroeders van Cleef*, 1880.

——. Wet van den 27. April 1884 (Stbl. No. 96) waarbij met intrekking van de wet van 29. Mei 1841 (Stbl. No. 20), nadere bepalingen worden vastgesteld betreffende het staatstoezicht op krankzinnigen en krankzinnigengestichten. Met inleiding, toelichtende aanteekeningen en alphabetisch register. En aanhangsel bewerkt door H. A. Musquetier. xx, 191 pp. 12°. *'s Gra-venhage, gebroeders Belinfante*, 1884.

——. Lijsts van geneeskundigen. tandmeesters, apothekers, drogisten en vroedvrouwen geves-tigd in de provincien Drenthe, Friesland, Gel-derland, Groningen, Limburg, Noordbrabant, Noordholland, Overijssel, Zuidholland, Utrecht en Zeeland op 1. Januari 1885; 1887. roy. 8°. [*v. p.*, 1885-7.]

One pamphlet a year for each province.

——. Geneeskundige hulp in Nederland. Kaart aantoonende het aantal inrichtingen tot verple-ging van zieken, dat der geneeskundigen en der vroevrouwen in elke gemeente des rijks in het jaar 1886. 1 broadside, 36 x 40 in. *'s Graven-hage, J. Lobatto*, [1887].

Netherlands.

See, also, **Amsterdam**; **Army** (*Netherlands*); **Cholera** (*Asiatic, History, etc., of*), *by localities*; **Dort**; **Dutch East Indies**; **Education** (*Medi-cal*), *etc., by localities*; **Ethnology**; **Fever** (*Mala-rial, History, etc., of*); **Fever** (*Typhoid, History, etc., of*), *by localities*; **Goes**; **Gouda**; **Gronin-gen**; **Hague** (*The*); **Harlem**; **Helvoetsluis**; **Hilversum**; **Hospitals** (*Description, etc., of*), **Hospitals** (*Military*), **Insane** (*Asylums for, etc.*), *by localities*; **Katwijk**; **Kleef**; **Leyden**; **Lux-emburg**; **Medicine** (*History, etc., of*), *by na-tions, etc.*; **Medicine** (*Military, History of*)— *Campaigns, etc.*; **Pharmacopœias**; **Rotterdam**; **Scheveningen**; **Utrecht**; **Woerden**; **Zaan-dam.**

AMSHOFF (F. K.) * Collectanea quædam topo-graphiam medicam provinciæ Drenthinæ spec-tantia. 8°. *Groningæ*, [1843].

VAN DEN BOSCH (I. J.) Verhandelingen, uit-gegeven door de Hollandsche Maatschappye der Weetenschappen, opgericht te Haarlem; vervat-tende het antwoord op de vraage: Welken zijn de ziekten onder de menschen, die uit de natuurlijke gesteldheid van het vaderland voortvloeijen? hoe kan men zich tegen dezelve behoeden? En door welke middelen kunnen zij geneezen wor-den? Beantwoord in eene natuur- en genees-kundige verhandeling van de oorzaaken, voor-behoeding, en geneezing der ziekten, uit de natuurlijke gesteldheid van het vaderland voort-vloeijende; met den eereprijs eener gouden ge-denkpenning bekroond. 8°. *Haarlem*, 1778.

BRAUW (J. I.) Een paar aanmerkingen naar aanleiding van het opstel van Dr. J. C. de Man, getiteld: Bijdrage tot de kennis der sterfte in Zeeland. 8°. [*n. p., n. d.*]

COULON (J. V.) Statistiek en geneeskundig berigt wegens de geborenen en gestorvenen in de provincie Vriesland, in de jaren 1815 tot 1828 ingesloten. 8°. *Leeuwarden*, 1831.

DAVIS (J. B.) Dutch anthropology. 8°. [*n. p., n. d.*]

Netherlands.

DE BEUNIE (J. B.) Antwoord op de vraege welk zijn de profijtelijkste planten van dit land, ende welk is hun gebruijk zoo in de medicijnen als in andere kosten. 4°. *Brussel*, 1772.

In: Mém. . . . Acad. imp. et roy. d. sc. de Brux. (1771-8), 1779, i.

DU RONDEAU. Mémoire zur la question: Quelles sont les plantes les plus utiles des Pays-Bas, et quel est leur usage dans la médecine et dans les arts? 4°. *Bruxelles*, 1772.

In: Mém. . . . Acad. imp. et roy. d. sc. de Brux. (1771-8), 1779, i.

ERMERINS (R. C.) * Tentamen ad depellendam insalubritatis calumniam de regione Zelandica. 4°. *Lugd. Bat.*, 1788.

Also, in: JANSEN. Collect. diss. [etc.] 4°. *Dusseldorpii*, 1792, ii, 443-465.

GRAPHISCHE voorstelling van de sterfte van kinderen beneden het jaar in elke gemeente van Nederland in het vijfjarig tijdperk 1880-85. broadside, 38 x 48 in. [*Amsterdam*, 1887.]

LIJST van de namen en woonplaatsen der gevestigde apothekers en geëxamineerde drogisten in Nederland af 1. November 1887. 12°. *Amsterdam*, [1887].

MICHELL (J. P.) Geneeskundige verhandeling over de oorzaken, onderscheiding en geneezing der febres catarrhales, welke zich sedert eenige jaren meer dan voorheen in de Nederlanden vertoond hebben. 8°. *Eecloo*, 1795.

MULDER (G. J.) De voeding in Nederland, in verband tot den volksgeest. 8°. *Rotterdam*, 1847.

———. De voeding van Nederlanders. 1. Januarij 1854. 8°. *Rotterdam*, 1854.

——— & ROELANTS (J. M. A.) Bijdrage tot de geschiedenis der thans in ons vaderland heerschende ziekte. 8°. *Rotterdam*, 1826.

NEDERLANDSCHE (Het) volkskarakter, tegenover de graanwet en de wetten op het geslagt en gemaal. 8°. [*n. p., n. d.*]

ONDERZOEK naar de verspreiding der geneeskundige hulp in Nederland. Door de vergadering der inspecteurs voor het geneeskundig staatstoezicht. 8°. *'s Gravenhage*, 1879.

Repr. from: Verzameling van stukken betreffende het geneeskundig staatstoezicht in Nederland, 1879.

PROEVE eener kaart der sterfte in de provincie Zeeland opgemaakt uit 13 jaren, 1834-46, met inbegrip van doodgeborenen. 1 map. [*n. p., n. d.*]

SASSE (A.) Bijdrage tot de kennis van den schedelvorm der Nederlanders. 8°. *Amsterdam*, 1865.

Repr. from: Versl. . . . d. k. Akad. v. Wetensch. Afd. Natuurk., Amst., xvii.

SIEGENBEEK (M.) Eenige berigten omtrent vroeger in ons vaderland geheerscht hebbende besmettelijke ziekten, tot geruststelling en bemoediging in de tegenwoordige dagen, bijeengebragt. 8°. *Leiden*, 1832.

THIJSSEN (H. F.) Geschiedkundige beschouwing der ziekten in de Nederlanden, in verband met de gesteldheid des lands en de leefwijze der inwoneren. 8°. *Amsterdam*, 1824.

VEREENIGING voor de Statistiek in Nederland. Algemeene statistiek van Nederland. Beschrijving van den maatschappelijken toestand van het nederlandsche volk in het midden der negentiende eeuw. Erste-twaalfde Aflevering, in 2 v. 8°. *Leiden*, 1869-74.

Algemeen verslag der provinciale commissie van geneeskundig onderzoek en toevoorzigt van Overijssel, residerende te Zwolle, van hare handelingen in het jaar 1848, aan Z. E. den minister van binnenlandsche zaken. N. Arch. v. bin.- en buitenl. Geneesk., Zwolle, 1848, iii, 369-384.—**Arntzenius.** Statistieke opgaven omtrent de geneeskundige bevolking van Nederland. Bijdr. t. geneesk. Staatsreg., Amst., 1845, iii, 22-67.—**Atlas** des décès dans

Netherlands.

les Pays-Bas pendant la période de 1860-74. Ann. de démog. internat., Par., 1880, iv, 518-526.—**Boogaard** (J. A.) Verslag namens de commissie voor statistiek der Nederlandsche Maatschappij tot Bevordering der Geneeskunst, 23 Junij 1859. Nederl. Tijdschr. v. Geneesk., Amst., 1859, iii, 569-477.—**Bruinsma** (G. W.) Aanteekeningen op een paar ministerieele circulaires. *Ibid.*, 1883, 2. R., xix, 61-68.—**v. C.** Bijdrage tot de kennis der sterfte in Nederland in 1866. *Ibid.*, 1868, 2. R., iv, 2. Afd., 145-158.—**van Cappelle** (H.) Verslag over de ziekten, welke in 1857 in Nederland hebben geheerscht, [etc.]. *Ibid.*, 1859, iii, 487-516. — **de Ceuleneer.** Mémoire sur le service sanitaire des indigents dans le Plat-Pays. Ann. Soc. de méd. prat. de la prov. d'Anvers, Boom et Malines, 1848, vi, 58; 75; 113; 153; 193; 233. — **Cohen** (D.) Over de sterfteverhouding in Drenthe. Nederl. Tijdschr. v. Geneesk., Amst., 1861, v, 497. — **Doornik** (M.) Verslag over de volksziekten, welke in 1856 in Nederland hebben geheerscht [etc.]. *Ibid.*, 1859, iii, 181-207.—**Dozy** (F.) & **Molkenboer** (J. H.) Bijdrage tot de flora cryptogamica van Nederland. Tijdschr. v. nat. Geschied. en Physiol., Leiden, 1844, xi, 377-414. ———. Bijdrage tot de flora cryptogamica van Nederland. *Ibid.*, 1845, xii, 257-288.—**Eckstein** (D.) Vital statistics of the Netherlands. Sanitarian, N. Y., 1883, n. s., i, 359-361.—**Eenige** cijfers uit de sterfte-statistiek van Nederlands hoofdstod. Schat d. Gezond., Haarlem, 1858, i, 71-73.—**Egeling** (L. J.) Verslagnamens de commissie voor statistiek der Nederlandsche Maatschapij tot Bevordering der Geneeskunst. Nederl. Tijdschr. v. Geneesk., Amst., 1858, ii, 481-489. ———. De geneeskundige bevolking van Nederland. *Ibid.*, 1866, 2. R., ii, 305-313. ———. Ueber den Stand der Städte-Reinigungsfrage in Holland. Verhandl. d. internat. Ver. gegen Verunreinig. d. Flüsse, etc., Leipz., 1878, 1. Versamml, 24-30. — **Extract** uit het algemeen verslag der verrigtingen van de provinciale commissie van geneeskundig onderzoek en toevoorzigt in Noord-Holland, residerende te Haarlem, gedurende het jaar 1848. N. pract. Tijdschr. v. de Geneesk., Gorinchem, 1849, n. R., i, 568-573. — **Geneeskundig** jaarverslag nopens den gezondheitstoestand bij de Kon. Nederl. marine gedurende de jaaren 1876-1883. Nederl. mil. geneesk. Arch., etc., Utrecht, 1878, ii: 1885, ix. *passim.*—**Guislain** (J.) Lettre médicale sur la Hollande. Ann. Soc. de méd. de Gand, 1842, x, 5-96. [Rap. de Latour]: Rev. méd. franç. et étrang., Par., 1842, iv, 118-131.—**Haakma-Tresling** (T.) Rapport over de consumptie van vleesch en van alcohol. Handel. d. Nederl. Maatsch. t. Bevord. d. Geneesk., Amst., 1880, 117-121, 2 tab. ———. Verslag van den algem. secretaris der commissie voor het onderzoek der volksvoeding in Nederland. Nederl. Tijdschr. v. Geneesk., Amst., 1884, 2. R., xx, 801-806.—**Hendriks** (F.) On the progress of official statistics in the Netherlands (1858-63); with a new Dutch lifetable by Dr. von Baumhauer. J. Statist. Soc. Lond., 1863, xxvi, 420-423. — **Israëls** (A. H.) Twee epidemiën in Nederland; eene historische-pathologische studie. Nederl. Weekbl. v. Geneesk., Amst., 1853, iii, 451; 461; 473; 483. — **Levensbalans** van sommige gemeenten in Nederland. Hygieia, Amst., 1875-6, ii, no. 11. — **Lubach** (D.) Ethnologisch onderzoek van Nederland. Nederl. Tijdschr. v. Geneesk., Amst., 1864, viii, 705-709. *Also,* Reprint.—**de Man** (J. C.) Over de statistiek der maandelijksche sterfte of over den invloed der jaargetijden op dezelve. Boerhaave. Tijdschr., etc, Gravenh., 1848, n. s., vii, 485-578, 3 pl. ———. Bijdrage tot de kennis der sterfte in Zeeland. Tijdschr. d. Nederl. Maatsch. t. Bevord. d. Geneesk., Arnhem, 1852, iii, pt. 2, 195; 263, 1 pl. ———. Het sterftecijfer in de onderscheidende gemeenten van Zeeland, met uitsluiting van de levenloos-aangegevenen, gemiddeld berekend over dertig jaren (1831-60). Nederl. Tijdschr. v. Geneesk., Amst., 1864, viii, 49-53.—**Model** en toelichting der tabel voor geneeskundige sterfte-statistiek, op de algemeene vergadering der Maatschappij tot Bevordering der Geneeskunst voorgesteld door hare commissie voor statistiek. *Ibid.*, 1862, vi, 502-505. — **Opgaven** betreffende de sterfte en de geboorten in eenige groote gemeenten in de maande Aug. en Sept. 1880. *Ibid.*, 1880, 2. R., xvi, 644; 660. — **Pierquin.** Considérations sur l'état de la police médicale dans le royaume des Pays-Bas. J. d. progr. d. sc. méd., Par., 1829, xv, 195-208.—**Rapport** van de commissie tot voorbereiding van eene wet tot beteugeling van epidemische ziekten. Versl. . . . v. h. geneesk. Staatstoez. 1868, Gravenh., 1869, 430-442.—**Rombach.** Eenige statistieke bijzonderheden, ontleend aan het verslag der provinciale geneeskundige commissie van Zuid-Holland, ressort Dordrecht, over de uitoefening der verloskunde gedurende het jaar 1855, in haar ressort. Nederl. Weekbl. v. Geneesk., Amst., 1856, vi, 165-167.—**Rombach** (K. A.) Iets over de in het jaar 1846 geheerscht hebbende koorsten. Nederl. Lancet, 1846-7, 2. s., ii, 605-616. — **Sasse** (A.) Over het nut en waarde eener craniologie in Nederland. Nederl. Tijdschr. v. Geneesk., Amst., 1866, 2. R., ii, 1. Afd., 289-304. *Also,* Reprint. ———. Rapport van de gecommitteerde voor de ethnologie van Nederland. Nederl. Tijdschr. v. Geneesk., Amst., 1883, 2. R., xix, 612-617. ———. Nederl. Maatsch. tot Bevord.

Netherlands.

der Geneesk. Rapport van de gecommitteerde voor de ethnologie van Nederland. *Ibid.*, 1884, 2. R., xx, 721-726.

——. Verslag. *Ibid.*, 1886, 2. R., xxii, 205-212.—**Scheltema Beduin** (L.) Nederlandsche Maatschappij tot Bevordering der Geneeskunst. Verslagnamens de commissie voor geneeskundige plaatsbeschrijving en volksziekten der Nederlandsche Maatschappij tot Bevordering der Geneeskunst. *Ibid.*, 1870, 2. R., vi, 1. Afd., 389: 1871, 2. R., vii, 1. Afd., 357.—**Sijbrandi** (N. D.) Verslag omtrent de ziekten, welke in het jaar 1849 in Nederland hebben geheerscht; namens de commissie voor geneeskundige plaatsbeschrijving en volksziekten, uitgebragt ter derde algemeene vergadering der Nederlandsche Maatschappij tot Bevordering der Geneeskunst. Tijdschr. d. Nederl. Maatsch. t. Bevord. d. Geneesk., Gravenh., 1851, ii, pt. 1, 169-336. *Also,* Reprint. ——. Verslag over de ziekten, welke in 1850 in Nederland hebben geheerscht, namens de commissie voor geneeskundige plaatsbeschrijving en voor volksziekten. Tijdschr. d. Nederl. Maatsch. t. Bevord. d. Geneesk., Arnhem, 1853, iv, 1. Afd., 3-64; [the same for 1851, 249-308]. ——. Verslag over de ziekten, welke in 1853 in Nederland geheerscht hebben. *Ibid.*, 1855, vi, 1. Afd., 91-174.—**Snabilié.** Beknopt statistiek overzigt der bij het leger, gedurende het jaar 1864, behandelde zieken. Nederl. Tijdschr. v. Geneesk., Amst., 1865, 2. R., i, 241-245.—**Spengler.** Gesundheitsbericht aus Holland vom Jahre 1862. Monatsbl. f. med. Statist. u. öff. Gsndhtspflg., Berl., 1864, 36.—**Statistiek** der geneeskunst-oefenaren in de provincie Overijssel. N. Arch. v. bin.- en buitenl. Geneesk., Zwolle, 1848, iii, 449-462. —**Statistisch** overzicht der bij het leger gedurende de jaaren 1863-1879 behandelde zieken. Nederl. Tijdschr. v. Geneesk., Amst., 1864, viii: 1865, 2. R., i: 1879, 2. R., xv, *passim. Continued in:* Nederl. mil. geneesk. Arch., etc., Utrecht, 1880, iv, 403-450.—**Symons** (A.) Eenige bijzonderheden en opmerkingen ontleend aan het verloskundig verslag over het jaar 1854, ingediend aan Z. Exc. den Minister van Binnenlandsche Zaken door de provinciale commissie van geneeskundig onderzoek en toevoorzigt in Zuid-Holland, resideerende te Dordrecht. Nederl. Weekbl. v. Geneesk., Amst., 1855, v, 461-465.—**de Vriese** (G. H.) Plantarum javanicarum minus cognitarum vel novarum, nuper in hortum-botanicum Amstelodamensem introductarum sylloge. Tijdschr. v. nat. Geschied. en Physiol., Leiden, 1844, xi, 336-347.—**Waardenburg** (J. G.) Verslag over de volksziekten, welke in 1855 in Nederland hebben geheerscht, [etc.] Nederl. Tijdschr. v. Geneesk., Amst., 1858, ii, 345-360.—**Zeeman** (J.) Verslag namens de commissie voor statistiek. *Ibid.*, 1857, i, 481-493. ——. De sterfte in de gevangenissen van 1841-1864. *Ibid.*, 1867, iii, 2. Afd., 97-103. ——. Verslag, namens de commissie voor statistiek der Nederlandsche Maatschappij tot Bevordering der Geneeskunst (voorgedragen op de algemeene vergadering te Leeuwarden). *Ibid.*, 1868, iv, 2. Afd., 357-366. ——. Verslag, namens de commissie voor statistiek der Nederlandsche Maatschappij tot Bevordering der Geneeskunst, voorgedragen op de algemeene vergadering te Rotterdam. *Ibid.*, 1869, 2. R., v, 2. Afd., 300-311, 1 map.— **Zieken-verpleging** (De) der behoeftigen in de provincie Zeeland. Tijdschr. d. Nederl. Maatsch. t. Bevord. d. Geneesk., Arnhem, 1853, iv, 1. Afd., 65-85.

Netherlands. *Koninklijke Nederlandsche Marine.* Reglement voor het Hospitaal der marine te Willemsoord. 75 pp. 8°. *'s Gravenhage,* 1880.

——. [Blank forms used by the medical department of the navy.] v. s. [*'s Gravenhage,* 1880-86.]

No. 136. Rapport aan den inspecteur van den geneeskundigen dienst der zeemacht, 1884.

No. 246. Requisitie lijst der geneesmiddelen enz., 1886.

No. 247. Expeditie-lijst der geneesmiddelen enz., 1886.

No. 248. Lijst der voorgeschrevenen geneesmiddelen, 1886.

No. 249. Lijst der voorgeschrevenen spijzen en dranken voor de zieken, 18—.

No. 250. Verantwoording van de ontvangen en uitgegeven geneesmiddelen, 1886.

No. 251. Maandelijksch rapport, 1880. 2 l. fol.

No. 251. Rapport van den ondergeteekende, 1880 [quarterly].

No. 253. Billet van zieken, die naar de hospitalen, worden gezonden, 1881.

No. 254. Nomenatieve opgave betreffende de zieken, 1886.

No. 344. Register der behandelde zieken en gekwetsten, 1882.

No. 345. Geneeskundige verklaring, 1886.

No. 446. Staat en verantwoording der genees-, heel-, schei- en artsenijmengkundige gereedschappen, 1886.

——. VI^de Hoofdstuk. Reglement op den geneeskundigen dienst bij de zeemacht. Vastgesteld bij Zr. Ms. besluit van 27. Julij 1884, No. 36. Tweede deel. 2 p. l., 163 pp. 8°. [*'s Gravenhage,* 1884.]

Netherlands. *Koninkl. Nederl.* [*etc.*]—cont'd.

——. Geneeskundig jaarverslag nopens den gezondheidstoestand, gedurende het jaar 1884-5. Medegedeeld door J. D. Sachse. 109 pp. 8°. *Utrecht, G. Metzdaar,* 1886-7.

Bijlage behoorende bij het Militair Geneeskundig Archief, 1886-7.

Netherlands. *Ministerie van Binnenlandsche Zaken.* Verslag over den staat der gestichten voor krankzinnigen in de jaren 1847, 1849 en 1850, 1854-9, 1864-7, aan den Minister van Binnenlandsche Zaken ingediend door de inspecteurs dier gestichten. 7 reports. 4°. *'s Gravenhage,* 1849-87.

1849-50 in 1; 1854-6 in 1; 1857-9 in 1; 1864-8 in 1; 1869-74 in 1; 1875-7 in 1.

——. Eerste verslag der proefnemigen met de inenting als voorbehoedmiddel tegen de longziekte onder het rundvee. Aan zijne excellentie den Minister van Binnenlandsche Zaken. 4 pp., 1 tab. 8°. [*'s Gravenhage,* 1852?]

——. Rapport aan den Minister van Binnenlandsche Zaken over desinfectie met betrekking tot de cholera, uitgebragt door de algemeene cholera-commissie. *'s Gravenhage,* den 1sten Julij 1866. 16 pp. 8°. [*'s Gravenhage,* 1866.] [*Also, in:* P., v. 198.]

——. Bestek en voorwaarden waarnaar curatoren van de Hoogeschool te Leiden onder nadere goedkeuring van den Minister van Binnenlandsche Zaken, voornemens zijnaante besteden den opbouw van een Nosocomium Academicum te Leiden. 23 pp., 11 plans. fol. [*Gravenhage,* 1868.]

——. Statistische bescheiden voor het koningrijk der Nederlanden. Sterfte naar de oorzaken van den dood in het jaaren 1869-73. Uitgegeven door het departement van Binnenlandsche Zaken. 5 v. roy. 8° & 4°. *'s Gravenhage,* 1871-83.

1869-71 are roy. 8°.

——. Koninklijk besluit van 23. Julij 1872 (staatsblad No. 82), houdende nadere aanwijzing van de geneesmiddelen bedoeld in het vierde lid van art. 9 der wet van 1. Junij 1865 (staatsblad No. 60). Beschikking van den Minister van Binnenlandsche Zaken van 15. Julij 1872, houdende nadere vaststelling der lijsten van vergiften en geneesmiddelen bedoeld en de artt. 7 en 30 der wet van Junij 1865 (staatsblad No. 61). Rapport der commissie over de zamenstelling van deze lijsten gehoord. 24 pp. 8°. *'s Gravenhage, van Weelden & Mingelen,* 1872.

——. Die choleraepidemie in Nederland in 1866 en 1867. Uitgegeven door het Departement van Binnenlandsche Zaken. 3 stuk in 1 v. iv, 422, ccxxxvii pp. roy. 8°. *'s Gravenhage, van Weelden,* 1872-5.

——. De pokken-epidemie in Nederland in 1870-73. Uitgegeven door het Departement van Binnenlandsche Zaken. 56 pp., 1 tab. 4°. *'s Gravenhage, van Weelden,* 1875.

——. Plattground teekeningen gestichten voor krankzinnigen in Nederland; behoorende bij het verslag over den staat der gestichten van krankzinnigen in de jaren 1869, 1870, 1871, 1872, 1873 en 1874, aan den Minister van Binnenlandsche Zaken ingediend door de inspecteurs dier gestichten. 10 plans. 4°. *'s Gravenhage, Weelden & Mingelen,* 1878.

——. Vijfjarig overzigt van de sterfte naar den lieftijd en de oorzaken van den dood in elke gemeente van Nederland gedurende 1875-80. Uitgegeven door het Departement van Binnenlandsche Zaken. 1181 pp. 4°. *'s Gravenhage, van Weelden & Mingelen,* 1882.

——. Statistiek van den loop der bevolking van Nederland over 1882-6. Uitgegeven door het Departement van Binnenlandsche Zaken. 8°. *'s Gravenhage,* 1884-7.

Netherlands. *Nederlandsch Militair Geneeskundig Departement.* Statistisch overzicht der bij het Nederlandsche leger, behandelde zieken. In het jaaren 1864–70; 1873–8; 1880; 1882–6. 8°. *'s Gravenhage,* 1865–87.
Overgedrukt uit het Nederlandsch Tijdschrift voor Geneeskunde.

——. [Veldmateriel bij leger] in gebruik. 2 l., 2 pp., 3 l., 3 pp., 7 l., 11 pp., 9 l., 15 pp., 8 l. fol. *'s Gravenhage,* 1869–70.

——. Modellen behoorende bij de voorschriften nopens de instelling van het toezigt, de directie en het administratief beheer over de militaire zieken-inrigtingen. Vastgesteld bij koninklijk besluit van den 7den September 1880, No. 9, en bij beschikking van den Minister van Oorlog van den 21sten September 1880. VIᵉ Afd. Int., No. 79. 183 pp. 8°. *'s Gravenhage, de gebroeders van Cleef,* 1880.

——. Reglement voor de geneeskundige dienst bij de landmagt in tijd van vrede vastgesteld bij beschikking van den Minister van Oorlog van 16. Novemb. 1881. IIIᵉ Afd. Personeel, No. 108. 159 pp. 8°. *'s Gravenhage, de gebroeders van Cleef,* 1881.

——. Voorschrift betreffende den geneeskundigen dienst in tijd van oorlog. Te velde en in versterkte plaatsen. Vastgesteld bij beschikking van den Minister van Oorlog van 16. Junij 1885. IIᵉ Afd. Gen. Staf., No. 62. 2 pts. in 1 v. 218, 171 pp., 12 pl., 1 tab. 8°. *'s Gravenhage, de gebroeders van Cleef,* 1885.

CONTENTS.

Nethou Peak.
Garrigou (F.) Les sources sulfurées du massif des Monts-Mandits (Nethou), Espagne. Ann. Soc. d'hydrol. méd. de Par. Compt.-rend , 1877–8, xxiii, 143–158.

Netley, *England.*
See **Éducation** (*Medical*), etc., *by localities;* **Hospitals** (*Military*), *by localities.*

Netley Hospital. *See* **Great Britain.** *Army Medical Department. Royal Victoria Hospital, at Netley.*

Netolitzky (Julius Aug.) * Diss. sistens anatomiam canalis inguinalis et cruralis. 31 pp. 8°. *Pragæ, J. vid. Vetterl,* 1835.

Nette ([Theophilus Friedericus] Carolus) [1837–]. * De pleuritide exudativa acuta. 30 pp., 1 l. 8°. *Halis Sax., formis Ploetzianis,* 1864.

Nettekoven (Michael Jos.) [1808–]. * De morbis senii nonnulla. 32 pp. 8°. *Berolini, typ. Nietackianis,* [1835].

Nettelbach (Joh. Christianus). * De epilepsia, ubi in diagnosi præter alia præprimis novissima Magnif. Dn. Præsid. sententia de vero veteribus incognito epilepsiæ subjecto confirmatur: in curatione prorsus hermetica totum insimul chymiæ fundamentum de spiritu mundi, mirabili totius naturæ concentu, lapide et menstruo philosophorum cum aliis arcanis aperitur. 54 pp. 4°. [*Vitembergæ*], *lit. M. Henckelii,* 1667.
Ser. also, **Lossius** (Jeremias) & **Nettlebach** (Joh. Christianus). De fermento ventriculi. 4°. *Jenæ,* 1665.

Nettement (Henri). * De la pustule maligne. 38 pp. 4°. *Paris,* 1868, No. 170.

Netter (Abraham). * [Questions sur les diverses branches des sciences médicales.] 16 pp. 4°. *Strasbourg,* 1842, 2. s., No. 88.
Another copy in v. 8, Strasbourg theses.

——. Des cabinets ténébreux dans le traitement de l'héméralopie. 66 pp. 8°. *Paris, Germer-Baillière,* 1863.

——. Lettres sur la contagion. 41 pp. 8°. *Paris, Germer-Baillière,* 1864.

Netter (Abraham)—continued.
——. Pourriture d'hôpital. Traitement de cette affection par le camphre en poudre. 43 pp. 8°. *Paris, A. Pougin,* 1871.

——. Vues nouvelles sur le choléra (cause, nature et traitement), avec une étude sur les injections faites dans les veines. xi, 99 pp., 1 l. 8°. *Paris, Berger-Levrault & Cie.,* 1874.

——. L'homme et l'animal devant la méthode expérimentale. 43 pp. 8°. *Paris, E. Dentu,* 1882.

——. Deuxième mémoire sur la contagion du choléra. 20 pp. 8°. *Strasbourg, G. Silberman,* [*n. d.*]

Netter (Arnold). * Diagnostic précoce d'une forme de tuberculisation pulmonaire à début pleurétique. 44 pp. 4°. *Paris,* 1883, No. 67.

Netter (Léon). * Des signes physiques de la pleurésie. 1 p. l., 22 pp. 4°. *Strasbourg,* 1837, v. 70.

Netterville *Dispensary.*
Murray (J.), **White** (F.) & **O'Donnell** (C. B.) Half-yearly report of diseases treated at Netterville Dispensary, St. Paul's Parish Institution, commencing 1st October, 1839, and ending 1st April, 1840. Dublin M. Press, 1840, iii, 260.

Nettle.
See **Urtica.**

Nettle *cells.*
von Lendenfeld (R.) Die Nesselzellen. Biol. Centralbl., Erlang., 1887–8, vii, 225–232.

Nettle *rash.*
See **Urticaria.**

Nettleship (Edward) [1845–]. On granular disease of the conjunctiva and contagious ophthalmia. 74 pp. 8°. [*London,* 1875.] [P., v. 1442.]
Repr. from: Brit. & For. M.-Chir. Rev., Lond., 1874, liv: 1875, lv.

——. The student's guide to diseases of the eye. 2. ed. xix, 395 pp., 3 pl. 12°. *London, J. & A. Churchill,* 1882.

——. The same. 4. ed. xix, 448 pp., 2 pl. 16°. *London, J. & A. Churchill,* 1887.

——. The same. 2. Am. from the 2. Eng. ed. With a chapter on examination for color perception, by William Thomson. xix, 13–416 pp. 8°. *Philadelphia, H. C. Lea's Son & Co.,* 1883.

——. The same. 3. Am. from the 4. Eng. ed., with a chapter on examination for color perception, by William Thomson. xx, 475 pp., 1 l. 8°. *Philadelphia, Lea Brothers & Co.,* 1887.

Nettmann (Bruno). * Spec. med. variolas, earumque differentias subjiciet. 84 pp. 4°. *Halæ Magdeb., typ. I. C. Hilligeri,* [1727].

Nettmann (Gust. Frid. Oscar) [1814–]. * Nonnulla de pathologia strumæ. 30 pp., 1 l. 8°. *Berolini, typ. Nietackianis,* [1837].

Nettmann (Jo. Fried.) * Spec. sistens sectionis Cæsareæ historiam. 45 pp. 8°. *Halæ, in off. Batheana,* 1805.

Netto (Ladislau). Apontamentos relativos á botanica applicada no Brasil. v, 78 pp. 8°. *Rio de Janeiro, Laemmert,* 1871.

Nettstraeter (Carol. Franc. Joseph. Augustus) [1839–]. * De ileo. 32 pp. 8°. *Berolini, G. Lange,* [1863].

Nettwall (Emmanuel). * De cura scrophuloseos secundum methodum Lugolianam, adnexis historiis morbi clinicis. 2 p. l., 47 pp., 1 l. 8°. *Pragæ, typ. filiorum T. Haase,* 1840.

Netz (Friedr.) Wie schützen wir unsere Gesundheit im Kriege? Nach einem Vortrage. 20 pp. 8°. *Karlsruhe, E. Stiess,* 1887.

Netzahualcoyotl (El). Periódico de ciencias y literatura, redactado por algunas señoritas y por estudiantes de medicina, del foro y de mi-

Netzahualcoyotl (El)—continued.
nería. No. 1, v. 1, Sept. 15, 1875. 12 pp. 4°.
Guanajuato.

Netzel [*or* **Nils**] (Wilhelm) [1834–   ]. Om de
puerperala förändringarne inom lifmodern.
Akad. Afhand. 51 pp. 8°. *Stockholm, P. A.
Norstedt & Söner*, 1865.

——. Om uppkomsten och utbildningen af placenta prævia totalis. 11 pp. 8°. [*Stockholm,
P. Norstedt & Söner*, 1867.]

——. Kejsarsnitt, nödvändiggjordt genom ett i
lilla bäckenet inkarcereradt myom. [*Cæsarean
section rendered necessary by an incarcerated
myoma and contracted pelvis.*] 32 pp. 8°.
[*Stockholm, P. A. Norstedt & Söner*, 1875.]
Repr. from: Nord. med. Ark., Stockholm, 1875, vii.

——. The same. Mémoire traduit du suédois et
annoté par . . . Dr. H. Cazin . . . 24 pp. 8°.
Paris, Vve. Delahaye & Cie., 1876.
Repr. from: Arch. de tocol., Par., 1876, iii.

Netzler (Joachimus Fridericus). *De morbis
tubæ Eustachianæ ejusque catheterisatione ut
remedio eorum. 38 pp., 1 pl. 4°. *Jenæ, typ.
Schreiberi*, 1841.

Neu (Johann) [1846–   ]. *Ueber Tabes dorsualis. 28 pp. 8°. *Greifswald, F. W. Kunike*,
1872.
                                                    c.

Neu ausführlich und wohl gegründetes Aderlass-
Büchlein, worinnen angezeiget wird, was vom
Aderlassen und Schrepffen eigendlich zu halten,
desgleichen wann, wie und an welchen Orten des
Leibes die Adern und Haut, in und ausserhalb
des Leibes Gebrechen fruchtbarlich zu öffnen
seyn. Wie auch beydes Gesunde und Krancke,
vor und nach dem lassen sich zu verhalten haben.
In 30 Capitel eingetheilet sambt funfftzig Fragen
von Blut-Aderlassen und Schrepffen. Alles zu
Erhaltung und Wiederbringung menschlicher
Gesundheit, sehr nützlich zu lesen und zu gebrauchen. 10 p. l., 382 pp. 12°. *Schneeberg,
M. Jammerten*, 1700.

Neu geordnetes und vollständiges Häuserver-
zeichniss von Teplitz und Schönau. 26 pp., 1 pl.
16°. *Teplitz, J. N. Gerzabek*, 1836.

Neubauer (Adamus Josephus). *Diss. exhibens historiam febris miliaris, vulgo : der Frie-
sel-Krankheit, quam una cum subjunctis variis
theorematibus submittit. 3 p. l., 28 pp. sm. 4°.
[*Herbipoli*], *F. E. Nitribitt*, [1768].

Neubauer (Armand). *De la fièvre de convalescence dans l'affection typhoïde. 1 p. l., 98
pp., 1 l., 13 tab. 4°. *Nancy*, 1878, 1. s., No. 60.

Neubauer (Carl). Anleitung zur qualitativen
und quantitativen Analyse des Harns. Enthaltend die Lehre von den Eigenschaften und dem
Verhalten der im Harn vorkommenden Bestandtheile zu Reagentien und unter dem Microscop,
sowie Anleitung zur qualitativen und quantitativen chemischen Untersuchung des normalen
wie abnormen Harns. Bevorwortet von Professor Dr. R. Fresenius. x, 438 pp., 3 pl. 8°. *Wiesbaden, Kreidel u. Niedner*, 1854.

——. Die königliche Wilhelmsheilanstalt zu
Wiesbaden im Jahre 1872. 24 pp. 8°. [*n. p.*],
1872.
Repr. from: Deutsche mil.-ärztl. Ztschr., Berl., 1872, i.

——. Systematischer Gang der qualitativen und
quantitativen Analyse des Harns. 8. Aufl., bearbeitet von Dr. E. Borgmann. 1 p. l., 23 pp. 8°.
Wiesbaden, C. W. Kreidel, 1882.

—— & **Vogel** (J) Anleitung zur qualitativen
und quantitativen Analyse des Harns ; sowie zur
Beurtheilung der Veränderungen dieses Secrets ;
mit besonderer Rücksicht auf die Zwecke des
praktischen Arztes ; zum Gebrauche für Mediciner und Pharmaceuten. Bevorwortet von Prof.
Dr. R. Fresenius. 2. Aufl. xx, 294 pp., 3 pl. 8°.
Wiesbaden, Kreidel u. Niedner, 1856.

Neubauer (Carl) & **Vogel** (J.)—continued.
——. The same. 3. sehr vermehrte und
verbesserte Aufl. xx, 372 pp., 4 pl. 8°. *Wiesbaden, Kreidel u. Niedner*, 1858.

——. The same. 5. Aufl. xii (1 l.), 363
pp., 4 pl. 8°. *Wiesbaden, C. W. Kreidel*, 1867.

——. The same. 6. Aufl. xi, 392 pp., 4
pl. 8°. *Wiesbaden, C. W. Kreidel*, 1872.

——. The same. 8. umgearbeitete und
vermehrte Aufl. von H. Huppert und L. Thomas.
Bevorwortet von R. Fresenius. xvii, 584 pp., 1
pl. 8°. *Wiesbaden, C. W. Kreidel*, 1881.
1. Abth.: Analytischer Theil, bearbeitet von Dr. H.
Huppert.

——. The same. De l'urine et des sédiments urinaires, propriétés et caractères chimiques et microscopiques des éléments normaux
et anormaux de l'urine ; analyse qualitative et
quantitative de cette sécrétion ; description et
valeur séméiologique de ses altérations pathologiques, etc. ; précédé d'une introduction par R.
Fresenius. 2. éd. française, traduite sur la 7. éd.
allemande et annotée par L. Gautier. iv, 520
pp., 4 pl. 8°. *Paris, F. Savy*, 1877.

——. The same. A guide to the qualitative and quantitative analysis of the urine.
Transl. by Wm. O. Markham. 4. ed. 439 pp., 4
pl. 8°. *London, New Sydenham Society*, 1863.

Neubauer (Joannes Ernestus) [1742–77]. * De
tunicis vaginalibus testis et funiculi spermatici.
48 pp., 1 pl. 4°. *Giessæ, ex off. Brauniana*,
[1767].

——. Observationem anatomico - chirurgicam,
de epiploo-oscheocele, cujus receptaculum peritonæi mentiebatur processum testem et epididy-
midem simul continentem proponet. 23 pp., 1
pl. 4°. *Jenæ, J. G. Hartung*, 1770.

——. Descriptio anatomica nervorum cardiacorum. Sectio prima de nervo intercostali cervicali, dextri imprimis lateralis. 230 pp., 4 pl.
4°. *Francofurti et Lipsiæ, in off. Fleischeriana*,
1772.

——. The same. 230 pp., 3 pl. fol. *Jenæ, lit.
Fickelscherrianis*, [1772].

——. The same. 230 pp., 4 pl. 4°. *Lipsiæ et
Jenæ, J. G. Hartung*, 1772.
Also [Abstr.], *in :* WEIZ (F. A.) Vollständ. Ausz. [etc.]
12°. *Leipz. u. Budissin*, 1773, v, 115.

——. [Pr.] describens observationem de triplici nympharum ordine. [Cum vita candidati
Michaelis Sonntag.] 16 pp., 1 pl. 8°. *Jenæ,
ex off. Straussii*, 1774. [*Also, in :* P., v. 1423.]
Also, in : THESAURUS diss. med. 4°. *Heidelb.*, 1784, 185–
190. *Also* [Abstr.], *in :* WEIZ (F. A.) Neue Ausz. [etc.]
12°. *Leipz.*, 1776, iv, 23–26.

——. [Pr.] descriptio anatomica rarissimi peritonæi conceptaculi tenuia intestina a reliquis
abdominis visceribus seclusa tenentis. I. [Cum
vita candidati Georg. Frid. Hoechstetter.] 16
pp. sm. 4°. *Jenæ, lit. Fickelscherrii*, [1775].

——. The same. II. [Cum vita candidati Joannis Christiani Guilielmi Müller.] 16 pp. 4°.
Jenæ, lit. Fickelscherrii, [1775].

——. The same. [I and II.] 34 pp., 2 pl. 4°.
Francofurti et Lipsiæ, in off. Fleischeriana, 1776.
[P., v. 1474.]
Another copy bound with his : Descriptio anatomica ner-
vorum cardiacorum [etc.] 4°. *Francofurti et Lipsiæ*,
1772.

——. Opera anatomica collecta; curavit G. C.
Hinderer. 16, 346 pp., 11 pl. 4°. *Francofurti
et Lipsiæ, J. C. Krieger jun.*, 1786.
For Biography, see Mag. v. Aerzte, Leipz., 1775-8, ii,
713-725.

Neubauer (Joseph). *Ueber den Hunger-Ty-
phus. 16 pp. 8°. *München, E. Stahl*, 1868.

Neubauer (Max). *Der Typhus und seine Behandlung. 20 pp. 8°. *München, J. Dreschler*,
1841.

Neubauer (Max)—continued.

——. * Considérations sur l'infiltration intestinale et le traitement de l'entérite folliculeuse typhoïde, principalement par le calomel. 32 pp. 4°. *Strasbourg*, 1845, No. 141, v. 11.

Neubaur (Christian Gottlob). * De morbis æstivis. 36 pp., 2 l. 4°. *Halæ Magdeb., typ. J. C. Hendelii*, [1745].

Neubaur (Henricus). * Disp. lympham et glandulas pathologice consideraus. 9 l. sm. 4°. *Helmstadi, typ. G. W. Hammii*, [1686].

Neubaur (Henricus Otto) [1823–]. * De paralysi nervi facialis et de myotomia in casibus inveteratis. 31 pp. 8°. *Berolini, G. Schade*, [1848].

Neubeck (Guilelmus Ferdinandus Gustavus) [1797–]. * De lacte. 34 pp. 8°. *Berolini, typ. J. F. Starckii*, [1825].

Neubeck ([Joannes Æmilius] Arminius) [1833–]. De dicephalo dibrachio. 20 pp., 2 l., 3 pl. 4°. *Halis Sax., formis Schmidtianis*, [1866].

Neubeck (Valerius Wilhelm) [1765–]. * De natatione frigida magno sanitatis præsidio. 24 pp. 4°. *Jenæ, ex off. Fickelscherrio-Stranckmanniana*, [1788].

——. Die Gesundbrunnen; ein Gedicht in vier Gesängen. 94 pp., 5 pl. fol. *Leipzig, G. J. Göschen*, 1798.

For Biography, see **Gruner** (Christ. Goth.)
For Portrait, see **Collection**—van Kaathoven.

Neuber (August Wilhelm). Ueber schwebende Flecke im Auge, oder den sogenannten Mückentanz, nach Beobachtungen an sich selber; Vortrag. 32 pp. 8°. *Hamburg, J. L. H. Wichers u. Sohn*, 1830.

——. Zur Abwendung der morgenländischen Brechruhr, Cholera morbus orientalis. iv, 102 pp., 1 l. 8°. *Hamburg, F. H. Nestler u. Melle*, 1831.

——. Zur Heilung der morgenländischen Brechruhr, Cholera morbus orientalis. xiii, 114 pp., 1 l. 8°. *Hamburg, F. H. Nestler u. Melle*, 1831.

Neuber (Carolus Ferdinandus) [1793–1839]. * Diss. continens additamenta ad historiam fistularum, præcipue vulnera sclopetaria comitantium ex propriis observatis collecta. 8 pp. 4°. *Halæ ad Salam, in off. Schimmelpfennigiana*, [1814].

Neuber (Eduardus). * De strictura urethræ. 34 pp., 1 l. 8°. *Marburgi Cattorum, typ. Elwerti Academicis*, [1847].

Neuber (Gustav) [1850–]. * Untersuchungen und Erfahrungen über die künstliche Blutleere. 30 pp., 4 pl. 4°. *Kiel, C. F. Mohr*, 1878.

In : SCHRIFT. d. Univ. zu Kiel, xxv, 1878, vii, Med. xvi.

——. Ein antiseptischer Dauerverband nach gründlicher Blutstillung. 17 pp. 8°. [*Berlin, L. Schumacher*, 1879.]

Repr. from : Arch. f. klin. Chir., Berl., 1879, xxiv.

——. Ueber die Veränderungen decalcinirter Knochenröhren in Weichtheilswunden und fernere Mittheilungen über den antiseptischen Dauerverband. 24 pp. 8°. [*Berlin, L. Schumacher*, 1880.]

Repr. from : Arch. f. klin. Chir., Berl., 1880, xxv, 1. Hft.

——. Bericht über die mit dem antiseptischen Dauerverband während des Sommer-Semesters 1880 in der Esmarch'schen Klinik erreichten Resultate. 34 pp. 8°. [*Berlin, L. Schumacher*, 1881.]

Repr. from : Arch. f. klin. Chir., Berl., 1881, xxvi, 1. Hft

——. Ergänzende Mittheilungen über die Herstellung und Anlegung der antiseptischen Polsterverbände. 5 pp., 1 pl. 8°. [*Berlin, L. Schumacher*, 1881.]

Repr. from : Arch. f. klin. Chir., Berl., 1881, xxvi, 2. Hft.

——. Typische Resectionen im Bereich der kleinen Tarsalknochen. 21 pp., 1 pl. 8°. [*Berlin, L. Schumacher*, 1881.]

Repr. from : Arch. f. klin. Chir., Berl., 1881, xxvi. 4. Hft.

Neuber (Gustav)—continued.

——. Eine neue Amputationsmethode. Ueberosmiumsäure-Injectionen bei peripheren Neuralgien. 23 pp. 8°. *Kiel, Lipsius u. Tischer*, 1883.

Forms Hft. 1, Mittheilungen aus der chirurgischen Klinik zu Kiel von Friedrich Esmarch.

——. Auleitung zur Technik der antiseptischen Wundbehandlung und des Dauerverbandes. viii, 134 pp. 8°. *Kiel, Lipsius u. Tischer*, 1883.

Neuber (Josephus Ant.) * Diss. sistens conspectum casuum lupi scrophulosi, anno scholastico 1840 et 1841 in clinico medico-practico, medicochirurgico et ophthalmico Pragensi observatorum. 25 pp. 8°. *Pragæ, T. Thabor*, [1842].

Neuberger. * Ueber den Säuferwahnsinn. 38 pp. 8°. *Erlangen, A. E. Junge*, 1843.

Neuberger (Joh. Christophorus). Magni Hippocratis Coi aphorismi xlv sectionis vi, ulcerum antiquorum statum et prognosin continentis, resolutio. 22 pp. 4°. [*Jena*], *typ. J. Nisi*, [1665].

——. * Ordo et methodus cognoscendi et curandi ileum. 15 l. 4°. *Jenæ, lit. S. Krebsii*, [1669.]

Neubert (Arminius) [1828–]. * De struma. 14 pp. 4°. *Halis Sax., formis Gebauerio-Schwetschkianis*, [1853].

Neubert (Carolus Augustus). * De morborum epidemiorum notione et causis. vi, 58 pp. 8°. *Lipsiæ, in commissis L. Vossii*, [1835].

——. De viis ac modis quibus sanguis ex vasis capillaribus sponte profluat dubitationes et meditationes. 48 pp. 8°. *Lipsiæ, F. A. Brockhausii*, 1843.

For Biography, see **Kuhl** (Car. Aug.)

Neubert (Christ. Fridericus Julius). * De hydrocephalo congenito ejusque in cerebrum vi. 38 pp. 8°. *Heidelbergæ, C. Groos*, 1838.

Neubert (Curt. J.) * Ein Fall von primärem doppelseitigen Nierenkrebs. 18 pp., 1 l., 1 pl. 8°. *Leipzig, G. Kreysing*, 1868. [P., v. 145.]

Neubert (Fried. Herrm.) [1802–]. * De prosopalgia. 36 pp. 8°. *Berolini, lit. A. Petschii*, [1825].

Neubert (Jakob) [1812–60]. * Der Kaffee. vi, 7–29 pp. 8°. *Würzburg, C. A. Zürn*, 1838.

For Biography, see Aerztl. Int.-Bl., München, 1861, viii, 68.

Neubert (Joannes Gottwalt). De adversis medicorum fatis apud Romanos commentatio. xvi pp. 4°. *Jenæ, lit. Schillianis*, [1756].

——. The same. Commentatio. De adversis, [etc.] xvi pp. 4°. *Jenæ, lit. Schillianis*, [n. d.]

Neuberth (Carolus Fridericus). * Diss. exhibens delirii trementis pathologiam et therapiam. 29 pp., 1 l. 4°. *Jenæ, typ. Schlotterianis*, [1829].

For Biography, see **Succow** (Guil. Carol. Frid.)

Neuberth (Julius). Die Heilkraft der menschlichen Hand. Ein Beitrag zur Lehre und richtigen Anwendung der Heilkräfte des Lebens-Magnetismus. 1 p. l., 92 pp. 12°. *Grimma, Verlags-Comptoirs*, 1843.

Neubich (Joh. Christophorus). * De similitudine morborum. 34 pp., 1 l. 4°. *Jenæ, lit. Krebsianis*, [1689].

Neubourg.

Poggiale. Rapport sur l'eau oxygénée du Neubourg (Eure). Bull. Acad. de méd. Par., 1862-3, xxviii, 8–11.

Neubrand (Josephus Fidelis). * Diss. sistens comparationem symptomatum morborum cum similibus phænomenis, quæ in statu sano occurrunt, et disquisitionem, quatenus natura morborum statui sano respondeat. 28 pp. 4°. *Tubingæ, L. F. Fues*, 1823.

Neubürger (Otto). * Ueber Halsrippen und ein bei diesen noch nicht beobachtetes Verhalten der Arteria subclavia. 24 pp., 3 pl. 8°. *Würzburg, P. Scheiner*, 1887.

Neubuerger (Theodorus) [1830–   ]. * Disquisitiones physiologicæ. 30 pp., 1 l. 8°. *Berolini, typ. fratrum Schlesinger,* [1853].

Neuburg.

See **Fever** (*Cerebro-spinal, History, etc., of*),
by localities.

Neuburg (Simon) [1757–1830]. * De acrimonia urinosa in corpore humano retenta. 32 pp.
4°. *Gottingæ, ex off. J. A. Barmeieri,* [1783].

Neuburger (Jakob). * Ueber das Schielen und
die Operation desselben. 19 pp. 8°. *München,
G. Franz,* 1847.

Neuchâtel. Règlement sur l'établissement de
canaux-égouts dans la ville de Neuchâtel. 20
avril 1860. 3 pp. 8°. [*Neuchâtel,* 1860.]

——. Circulaire à MM. les médecins et pharmaciens relative aux soins et médicamens délivrés à des communiers pauvres de Neuchâtel.
1 l. 4°. [*Neuchâtel,* 1866.]

——. Règlement sur les étaux des bouchers. 3
pp. 8°. [*Neuchâtel,* 1869.]

——. Règlement pour la Chambre de charité
de la commune de Neuchâtel. Juillet 1870. 8
pp. 8°. [*Neuchâtel,* 1870.]

——. [Pétition de la Chambre de charité de
Neuchâtel au Grand-conseil d'état, relatives à
la répression de l'abus de l'eau-de-vie.] Neuchâtel, le 15 août 1870. 1 sheet. 4°. [*Neuchâtel,* 1870.]

——. Règlement sur les abattoirs. 6 pp. 8°.
[*Neuchâtel,* 1871.]

——. Règlement pour l'équarrisseur. 3 pp.
8°. [*Neuchâtel,* 1871.]

——. Circulaire de la Chambre de charité de
Neuchâtel, relative d'une pétition de la Maison
de santé de Préfargier au sujet des aliénés incurables. 2 l. 4°. [*Neuchâtel,* 1872.]

——. Règlement organique pour la commune de
Neuchâtel. L'Assemblée générale de la commune de Neuchâtel devant mettre ses règlements communaux en harmonie avec la loi sur
les communes et les municipalités du 17 mars
1875, sous la réserve de la sanction du conseil
d'état. 8, 43 pp. 8°. [*Neuchâtel,* 1875.]

——. Avis de la Chambre de charité de Neuchâtel concernant les mesures prises par elle pour
l'administration de ses assistances. 1 l. 4°.
[*Neuchâtel,* 1878.]

——. Instructions relatives au curage et à la réparation des puits. 3 pp. 8°. [*Neuchâtel, n. d.*]

Neuchâtel.

See, also. **Hospitals** (*Descriptions, etc., of*),
Hospitals (*Management, etc., of*), *by localities.*

CORNAZ (C.-A.-É.) Notices relatives à l'histoire médicale de Neuchâtel. roy. 8°. *Neuchâtel,* [*n. d.*]

GUILLAUME. Coup d'œil sur la vie sociale
dans le canton de Neuchâtel; liste des institutions et des sociétés libres de bienfaisance,
d'utilité publique, d'éducation, d'instruction et
de récréation. 8°. *Neuchâtel,* 1881.

JEANJAQUET (L.) L'Areuse; projet d'utilisation de sa puissance hydraulique. 4°. *Neuchâtel,*
1875.

——. Analyse du mémoire publié par M. G.
Ritter, ingénieur civil, sur un nouveau projet
d'utilisation rationnelle des forces hydrauliques
de la Reuse. 4°. *Neuchâtel,* 1878.

——. Duplique à la logique de M. G. Ritter,
ingénieur. 4°. *Neuchâtel,* 1879.

DE PURY (C.-L.) Tableau par communes des
individus réformés (1) pour cas d'infirmités dans
le canton de Neuchâtel, le 20 mai 1849, et jours à
suivre. MS. fol. [*Neuchâtel,* 1849.]

RITTER (G.) Mémoire sur un nouveau projet
d'utilisation rationnelle des forces hydrauliques
de la Reuse et d'une distribution générale en eau

Neuchâtel.

et en force pour le vignoble, de Bevaix à Saint-
Blaise et du lac de Neuchâtel à Chaux-de-Fonds.
4°. *Neuchâtel,* 1878.

SOCIÉTÉ des eaux de Neuchâtel. Acte consti-
tif, statuts et convention avec la municipalité.
8°. *Neuchâtel,* 1864.

Appia (L.) Examen météorologique et médical du
printemps de 1857. Écho méd., Neuchât., 1857, i, 450–456.
Also. Reprint. ——. Examen météorologique et médical
de l'été de 1857. Écho méd., Neuchât., 1857, i, 763; 1858, ii,
83; 135 *Also,* Reprint.—**Cornaz** (C.-A.-É.) Énumération des lichens jurassiques et plus spécialement de ceux du
canton de Neuchât. Bull. Soc. d. sc. nat. de Neuchât.,
1846–52, ii, 385–408. *Also,* Reprint. ——. Constitution
médicale de Neuchâtel et de ses environs pendant les
années 1857 et 1858. Écho méd., Neuchât., 1857, i, 310;
647: 1858, ii, 131; 512; 677: 1859, iii, 144. *Also,* Reprint.
——. Les maladies régnantes du canton de Neuchâtel
pendant l'année météorologique 1859. Recherches précédées d'une esquisse topographique. Écho méd., Neuchât.,
1860, iv, 385, 1 tab.; 457, 1 tab. *Also,* Reprint. —**Kopp**
(C.) Analyse de la source sulfureuse des Ponts-de-Martel.
Écho méd., Neuchât., 1860, iv, 119.—**Ritter** (G.) Réfutation des erreurs contenues dans le rapport de la commission nommée par le Grand conseil concernant l'utilisation
de la Reuse et des sources des Gorges. Bull. Soc. d. sc. nat.
de Neuchât., 1883–4, xiv, 161–190, 1 map.

Neuchâtel (*Canton of*). Loi sur la police
sanitaire. Le Grand-conseil de la république et
canton de Neuchâtel le 27 nov. 1851. 11 pp. 8°.
[*Neuchâtel,* 1851.]

——. Circulaire aux sages-femmes de Neuchâtel,
le 2 août 1854. 2 pp. 8°. [*Neuchâtel,* 1854.]

——. Rapport de la commission de santé au
Conseil d'état, sur les mesures à prendre en
cas d'invasion du choléra épidémique dans le
canton de Neuchâtel. 16 pp. 8°. [*Neuchâtel,*
1854.]

——. République et canton de Neuchâtel. Loi
et règlement sur la vaccination. Neuchâtel, le
19 oct. 1855. 8 pp. 8°. [*Neuchâtel,* 1855.]

——. Règlement sur la police sanitaire. Neuchâtel, le 18 février 1862. Au nom du Conseil
d'état. 24 pp. 8°. [*Neuchâtel,* 1862.]

——. Le conseil d'état de la république et
canton de Neuchâtel. [Arrêté et instructions
relatifs de la picote (cow-pox).] Neuchâtel, le 22
avril 1864. 3 pp. 8°. [*Neuchâtel,* 1864.]

——. Décret modifiant la loi sur la vaccination du 19 oct. 1855. Neuchâtel, le 16 janvier
1865. 2 pp. 8°. [*Neuchâtel,* 1865.]

——. Instructions sur les précautions à prendre avant et pendant l'épidémie du choléra.
Publié par la direction de l'intérieur. 16 pp.
16°. [*Neuchâtel,* 1867.]

——. Règlement concernant la police des fon-
taines, puits, citernes et cours d'eau destinés à
l'alimentation publique. Neuchâtel, le 17 sept.
1867. 5 pp. 8°. [*Neuchâtel,* 1867.]

——. Rapport au conseil d'état de la république
et canton de Neuchâtel sur les mesures sanitaires
prises à Zurich pendant l'épidémie du choléra,
par le Doct. Guillaume. 84 pp. 8°. [*Neuchâtel,*
1867.]

——. Règlement pour les commissions locales
de salubrité publique. Neuchâtel, le 11 février
1868. 4 pp. 8°. [*Neuchâtel,* 1868.]

——. Concordat pour l'introduction d'une pharmacopée unique. Résultat de la conférence du
7 juillet 1868. Neuchâtel, le 11 juin 1869. Au
nom du conseil d'état. 2 pp. 8°. [*Neuchâtel,*
1869.]

——. Circulaire aux commissions locales de salubrité publique [sur les visites sanitaires].
5 pp. 8°. [*Neuchâtel,* 1871.]

——. Le conseil d'état de la république et canton de Neuchâtel. [Arrêté sur la variole.] Neuchâtel, le 23 mai 1871. 6 pp. 8°. [*Neuchâtel,*
1871.]

——. Chambre de charité de Neuchâtel. Circulaire, relative à une pétition de la Maison de

Neuchâtel (Canton of)—continued.
santé de Préfargier au sujet des aliénés incurables. 3 pp. 4°. [*Neuchâtel*, 1872.]

———. Le conseil d'état de la république et canton de Neuchâtel. [Arrêté pour l'adoption de la seconde édition de la Pharmacopée suisse, et du poids décimal dans les pharmacies.] 3 pp. 8°. [*Neuchâtel*, 1872.]

———. La loi sur la police sanitaire. Le Grand-conseil de la république et canton de Neuchâtel. 10 pp. 8°. [*Neuchâtel*, 1875.]

———. Règlement pour les autorités sanitaires cantonales. 15 pp. 8°. *Neuchâtel, imp. Montaudon*, 1875.

———. Règlement pour les examens des apprentis pharmaciens, le Conseil d'état de la république et canton de Neuchâtel. Le 3 avril 1877. 4 pp. 8°. [*Neuchâtel*, 1877.]

———. Règlement et instructions pour les commissions locales de salubrité publique. 12 pp. 8°. [*Neuchâtel*, 1878.]

———. Règlement sur les pressions à bière. Le Conseil d'état de la république et canton de Neuchâtel. Neuchâtel, le 21 oct. 1879. 4 pp. 8°. [*Neuchâtel*, 1879.]

———. Règlement sur la police des aliments et boissons et leurs falsifications. Le Conseil d'état de la république et canton de Neuchâtel, le 25 nov. 1879. 8 pp. 8°. [*Neuchâtel*, 1879.]

———. République et canton de Neuchâtel. Circulaire aux commissions locales de salubrité. Neuchâtel, le 7 juin 1880. 2 l. 4°. [*Neuchâtel*, 1880.]

———. Circulaire aux médecins du canton sur les vaccinations en 1879. Neuchâtel, le 9 juin 1880. 1 l. fol. [*Neuchâtel*, 1880.]

———. Circulaire aux conseils municipaux relative à la variole. Neuchâtel, le 1er novembre 1880. 2 pp. 4°. [*Neuchâtel*, 1880.]

———. Circulaire relative à la vaccination. Aux médecins du canton de Neuchâtel, et en particulier aux vaccinateurs d'office. - Neuchâtel, le 1er novembre 1880. 1 l. 4°. [*Neuchâtel*, 1880.]

———. Circulaire aux médecins du canton [sur les vaccinations et revaccinations en 1880]. 8 pp. 8°. [*Neuchâtel*, 1881.]

———. Circulaire aux médecins du canton de Neuchâtel relative aux vaccinations. Neuchâtel, le 26 janvier 1881. 1 l. 4°. [*Neuchâtel*, 1881.]

———. République et canton de Neuchâtel; circulaire aux conseils municipaux [relative de la variole]. Neuchâtel, le 11 févr. 1881. 1 l. 4°. [*Neuchâtel*, 1881.]

Neucourt (Félix). *I. De la médication vomitive. II. [etc.] 39 pp. 4°. *Paris*, 1844, No. 174, v. 422.

———. Des maladies chroniques, pratique d'un médecin de province, ou recherches et observations sur la gastrite et la gastroentérite chroniques, les coliques gastrointestinales et la diarrhée chronique chez les enfants; la métrite chronique et la métrorrhagie; les névralgies lombaire, sacrée, du plexus brachial, faciale, du cuir chevelu et cervicale et le vertige nerveux. xii, 615 pp. 8°. *Paris, J.-B. Baillière & fils*, 1861.

Neucrantz (Paulus) [1605–71]. De harengo exercitatio medica, in qua principis piscium exquisitissima bonitas summaqne gloria asserta et vindicata. 83 pp., 2 l. 4°. *Lubecæ, lit. G. Jegeri*, [1654].

Neucrantz (Paulus Bernhardus). *Medicinæ curiosæ specimen, duabus quæstionibus enodatum. 9 l. 4°. *Rostochii, typ. J. Wepplingii*, [1703].

Neucranz (Jo. Theodorus). *De usu venæ sectionis et clysterum in curatione variola-

Neucranz (Jo. Theodorus)—continued.
rum. 56 pp. 4°. *Vitembergæ, prelo Gerdesiano*, [1711].

See. *also*, **Berger** (Joh. Godfridus) & **Neucranz** (Joh. Theodorus). De usu venæ sectionis [etc.] 4°. *Vitembergæ*, 1711.

Neudecker (Georg). Untersuchungen über die Erkenntniss - Principien. iv, 52 pp. 8°. *Würzburg, A. Stuber*, 1873.

Neudegger (Julius Augustus). *De natura rerum electrica. 16 pp. 8°. *Monachii, J. A. Giesser*, 1837.

Neudettelsau.
See **Idiots** (*Asylums, etc., for*), by localities.

Neudin (A.) *De la variole. 36 pp. 4°. *Paris*, 1871, No. 96.

Neudörfer (Ignaz Josef) [1825–]. Chirurgische Skizzen. I. Beiträge zur Staphylorhaphie. 36 pp. 8°. [*Wien, C. Gerold's Sohn, n. d.*]
Repr. from: Ztschr. d. k.-k. Gesellsch. d. Aerzte zu Wien, 1857, xiii.

———. Der hydrostatische Apparat in der Chirurgie. 43 pp., 3 pl. 8°. *Wien, k.-k. Hof- und Staatsdruckerei*, 1857.
Repr. from: Sitzungsb. d. k. Akad. d. Wissensch. Math.-naturw. Cl., Wien, 1857, xxiii.

———. Handbuch der Kriegschirurgie. Ein Vademecum für Feldärzte nach eigenen Erfahrungen bearbeitet. 5 v. 8°. *Leipzig, F. C. W. Vogel*, 1864–72.

———. Die Endresultate der Gelenkresectionen. 43 pp. 8°. *Wien, F. B. Geitler*, [1871].
Repr. from: Wien. med. Presse, 1871, vii.

———. Die chirurgische Behandlung der Wunden. vi, 159 pp. 8°. *Wien, W. Braumüller*, 1877.

———. Aus der chirurgischen Klinik für Militär-Aerzte. xx, 429 pp., 8 l., 9 pl. 8°. *Wien, W. Braumüller*, 1879.

———. Die moderne Chirurgie in ihrer Theorie und Praxis. xv, 642 pp. 8°. *Wien, W. Braumüller*, 1885.

Neudörffer (Eugen). *Zwei neue Fälle von Pyometra und Pyokolpos lateralis. 25 pp. 8°. *Tübingen, H. Laupp*, 1873.

Neudorf.
Fresenius. Neue Analyse der Eisenquellen in Bad Neudorf in Böhmen. Jahrb. f. Balneol., etc., Wien, 1876, vi, 44–47.

Neue Annalen der Geburtshülfe. No. 1, v. 1, 1813. 8°. *Mannheim.*
Was also title of No. 6 of: **Annalen** der Geburtshülfe, Leipzig.

Neue Auswahl medicinisch-gerichtlicher Gutachten mit Genehmigung des Herrn Ministers der geistlichen Unterrichts- und Medicinal-Angelegenheiten herausgegeben von der königlichen wissenschaftlichen Deputation für das Medicinal-Wesen. 2 pts. xvi, 260, 252 pp. 8°. *Berlin, A. Hirschwald*, 1851.
1. Lfg.: Zur gerichtlichen Geburtshülfe. Von Joseph Hermann Schmidt.
2. Lfg.: Zur gerichtlichen Psychologie. Von K. W. Ideler.

Neue Bibliothek für die Chirurgie und Ophthalmologie, hrsg. von C. J. M. Langenbeck. v. 1–4, 1815–28. 8°. *Hannover, Hahn.*
A continuation of: **Bibliothek** für die Chirurgie.

Neue (Der) Chiron. Eine Zeitschrift für Wundarzneykunst und Geburtshülfe. In Verbindung mit mehrern Aerzten hrsg. von Kajetan Textor. v. 1–2, 1821–7. 8°. *Sulzbach, J. E. Seidel.*
Ended. v. 1, 1821–3, in 3 nos.; v. 2, 1825–7, in 2 nos.

Neue (Die) Curanstalt Baden (Hinterhof u. Staadhof). Eröffnet den 1. Mai 1876. Kurze Beschreibung und Tarif. 8 pp., 1 l. 8°. *Baden, J. Zehnder*, 1876.

Neue Denkwürdigkeiten für Aerzte und Geburtshelfer von Friedrich Benjamin Osiander. v. 1,

Neue Denkwürdigkeiten [etc]—continued.
1797. 294 pp. 8°. *Göttingen, J. G. Rosenbusch.*
A continuation of: **Denkwürdigkeiten** für die Heilkunde und Geburtshülfe.

Neue Folge der Gesundheits-Zeitung. Hrsg. und redigirt von H. H. Beer. Jahrg. 1, 4, 1837, 1840. 8°. *Wien, Sollinger.*
A continuation of: **Populäre** österreichische Gesundheits-Zeitung.

Neue Irrenheilanstalt für das Herzogthum Oldenburg. *See* **Heilanstalt** zu Wehnen.

Neue Jahrbücher der teutschen Medicin und Chirurgie. Mit Zugabe des Neuesten und Wissenswürdigsten aus der medicinisch-chirurgischen Literatur des Auslandes. Hrsg. in Verbindung mit mehreren Gelehrten, von Chr. Friedr. Harless. v. 1–12, nebst 2 Supplement-Bänden, 1819–Aug. 12, 1827. 14 v. 8°. *Bonn, 1819–21; Elberfeld, 1822–3; Hamm, 1824–7.*
A continuation of: **Jahrbücher** der teutschen Medicin und Chirurgie, 1813. v. 1–7, 1819–23, also under title: **Rheinische** Jahrbücher der Medicin und Chirurgie. v. 8–12, 1824–7, also under title: **Rheinisch-Wesphälische** Jahrbücher der Medicin und Chirurgie. In 1828 merged in: **Heidelberger** klinische Annalen.

Neue litterarische Nachrichten für Aerzte, Wundärzte und Naturforscher aufs Jahr 1785 und 1786 [also for 1787]. 2 v. 8°. *Halle in Sachsen, J. C. Hendel.*

Neue Materialien für die Staatsarzneiwissenschaft und praktische Heilkunde.
See **Materialien** für die Staatsarzneiwissenschaft, [etc.], Samml. 9–11, 1819–24.

Neue medicinisch-chirurgische Zeitung, hrsg. von J. N. Ehrhart und Ignaz Laschan. [4 v. annually.] 1840–56. Nebst 2 Ergänzungsbänden. 52 v. 8°. *Innsbruck u. Leipzig, 1840–42; Augsburg, 1843; München, 1844–56.*
In 1843–54 edited by G. L. Ditterich; in 1855–6 by Ernst Buchner. In 1851–6 one volume annually. Continued as: **Medicinisch-chirurgische** Monatshefte.

Neue medicinische Bibliothek. Hrsg. von Rudolph Augustin Vogel. v. 1–8, 1754–72. 8°. *Göttingen.*
A continuation of: **Medicinische** Bibliothek, Erfurt, 1751–3.

Neue Notizen aus dem Gebiete der Natur- und Heilkunde.
See **Notizen** aus dem Gebiete der Natur- und Heilkunde, Weimar, 1837–49.

Neue Sammlung der auserlesensten und neuesten Abhandlungen für Wundärzte. (Aus verschiedenen Sprachen übersetzt.) 24 St. in 12 v. 12°. *Leipzig, Weygand, 1782–9.*

Neue Sammlung sächsischer Medicinal-Gesetze. *See* **Saxony**.

Neue specifische Heilmethode der epidemischen Cholera oder (richtiger) des Cholera-Fiebers mittelst des fiebervertreibenden Princips der Chinarinde. vii, 69 pp., 1 l. 8°. *Hannover, Hahn, 1831. [Also, in: P., v. 203.]*

Neue (Der) Wasserfreund; als Archiv des Vereins zur wissenschaftlichen Begründung und Förderung der Priessnitz'schen Heilweise, unter Mitwirkung der Vereinsmitglieder hrsg. von Dr. Schmitz. [2 v. annually.] Jahrg. 1–2, 1842–3. (Bd. 1–2, 1842; Bd. 1–2, 1843.) 4 v. 8°. *Coblenz, J. Holscher.*
Title of nos. 1–3, v. 1, 1842, was: **Neue** (Der) Wasserfreund, oder Archiv für Wasserheillehre. Continued as: **Archiv** für Wasserheilkunde.

Neue wissenschaftliche Annalen der gesammten Heilkunde. Hrsg. von Just. Friedr. Carl Hecker. [Monthly; 3 v. annually.] v. 1–3 (Jahrg. 11), 1835. 8°. *Berlin, Enslin.*
A continuation of: **Wissenschaftliche** Annalen der gesammten Heilkunde.

Neue woleingerichtete Frauenzimmer-Apotheke, oder gründliche Anweisung, wie ein jedes Frau-

Neue woleingerichtete [etc.]—continued.
enzimmer in allen ihren kränklichen und geheimen Zufällen ihr eigener Arzt seyn könne. Aus dem Englischen übersetzet. 86, 496 pp., 12 l. 12°. *Hamburg, G. Richter, 1741.*

Neue Zeitschrift für Geburtskunde. Hrsg. von Dietr. W. H. Busch, J. d'Outrepont und F. Aug. von Ritgen. v. 1–33, 1834–52. 8°. *Berlin.*
Continuation of: **Gemeinsame** deutsche Zeitschrift für Geburtskunde. In 1838 **Journal** für Geburtshülfe, Frauenzimmer- und Kinderkrankheiten merged in this journal. Indexes to v. 1–10, 11–20, 21–30, 31–33 accompany. Continued as: **Monatsschrift** für Geburtskunde.

Neue Zeitschrift für homöopathische Klinik.
Was title of: **Zeitschrift** für homöopathische Klinik, Dresden u. Leipzig, after March. 1856.

Neue Zeitung für Medicin and Medicinal-Reform. Hrsg. von Wessely und Bloedau. [Semi-weekly.] v. 1–2, January, 1849, to April 29, 1850. fol. *Nordhausen, Büchting.*
Dr. Wessely died March, 1850.

Neuen (Cornelius) [1830–]. *De pneumothorace. 29 pp., 1 l. 8°. *Berolini, S. Jacoby, [1855].*

Neuenahr.

MILLER (J.) Neuenahr, a new spa on the Rhine. 8°. *Edinburgh, 1861.*

PRAESSAR (H.) Der Mariensprudel im Bade Neuenahr. 8°. *Bonn, 1861.*

———. Das Mineralbad Neuenahr im Arthale. 12°. *Ahrweiler, 1868.*

SCHMITZ (R.) Erfahrungen über Bad Neuenahr. 12°. *Ahrweiler, 1868.*

———. The same. 5. Aufl. 12°. *Ahrweiler, 1886.*

UNSCHULD. Die Mineralquellen von Neuenahr, verglichen mit denen von Carlsbad, Vichy und Ems. Mit einem Anhang über den Kurgebrauch und die Diät bei alkalischen Wassern. 2. Aufl. 12°. *Bonn, 1872.*

WEGELER (J.) Bad Neuenahr und seine Umgebungen; für Kurgäste und Geschichtsfreunde. sm. 8°. *Bonn, 1861.*

WEIDGEN. Bad Neuenahr im Ahrthale. 8°. *Bonn, 1859.*

———. Berichte über die Badesaison zu Neuenahr. 1.–4., 1859–62. 8°. *Bonn, 1860–63.*

———. Bericht über das Bad Neuenahr in Rheinpreussen nach seinem fünfjährigen Bestehen. 8°. *Ahrweiler, 1864.*

———. Bad Neuenahr im Ahrthale am Rhein (Rhein-Preussen), seine Mineralwasser und die Anwendung derselben. 24°. *Köln, 1866.*

———. Bericht über das Emporblühen des Bades Neuenahr, über sein Klima, seine Quellen und die Indicationen für die Anwendung derselben. 8°. *Ahrweiler, 1867.*
Mayer. Du traitement moderne du diabète; les eaux thermales de Neuenahr. Ann. Soc. de méd. d'Anvers, 1887, xlviii, 82–116.—**Münzel** (E.) Zur Casuistik der Wirkung der Thermen von Neuenahr bei chronischen Blasenleiden. Deutsche med. Wchnschr., Berl., 1878, iv, 320; 331.—**Schmitz** (R.) Ueber Bad Neuenahr. Berl. klin. Wchnschr., 1872, ix, 145; 158; 194. ———. Erfahrungen über Bad Neuenahr. Deutsche med. Wchnschr., Berl., 1880, vi, 409; 426.—**Sedgwick** (L. W.) Neuenahr; its mineral waters and its climate. St. Andrew's M. Grad. Ass. Tr. 1872–3, Lond., 1874, vi, 160–169.—**Weidgen.** Sur les eaux minérales de Neuenahr. [Rap.] Bull. Soc. d. sc. méd. et nat. de Brux., 1863, 1–11. [Discussion]. 11–13.—**Wolff.** Bad Neuenahr. Med. Ztg., Berl., 1860. n. F., iii, 227; 231.

Neuenburg (M. J.) *Ochistka vodi dlja pitja v maljich razmerach. [Filtration of drinking-water in small quantities.] 70 pp. 8°. *St. Petersburg, typ. Ettinger, 1885.*

Neuenburg (Moritz) [1854–]. *Der Leberechinococcus und seine operative Behandlung. 31 pp. 8°. *Berlin, G. Schade, [1877].*

Neuendorff (Carl Theodor Albert) [1797–]. *De spinæ bifidæ curatione radicali. 34 pp., 1 l. 8°. *Halæ, formis F. Grunerti filii, [1820].*

Neuenhahn (Carol. Ludovic.) * De metallorum analysi per calcinationem. 46 pp., 1 l. 4°. *Halæ Magdeb.*, *typ. C. Riemeri*, [1738].

Neuenhahn (Joh. Ludovicus). * De scabie. 15 l. 4°. *Jenæ, typ. S. Krebsii*, [1674].

————. Nostri notitiam esse viam ad Dei cognitionem in anatome cadaveris fœminei chirurgico-practica ostenditur : cui literarum atque anatomiæ fautores humanitus adesse gestit. 3 l. 4°. *Meiningæ, lit. Hassartinis*, [1682].

————. * Carcinomatis malignitatem ejusque curam exhibens. 16 pp. 4°. *Altdorfi, typ. H. Meyeri*, [1685].

Neuenhaus.

See **Fever** (*Malarial, History, etc., of*), **Fever** (*Typhoid, History, etc., of*), *by localities*.

Neuenzeit (Conradus Guilelmus) [1831–]. * De struma. 34 pp., 1 l. 8°. *Vratislaviæ, typ. R. Lucæ*, [1855].

Neuenzeit [*gen.* **Nigetiet**] (Fritz) [1848–]. * Beitrag zur Kenntniss der Becken mit multiplen Exostosen. 33 pp. 8°. *Breslau, A. Neumann*, [1872].

Neuer Medicinal-Kalender für Oesterreich auf das Jahr 1888. Hrsg. von Heinrich Adler. v. 5, 1888. 12°. *Wien, R. Löwit.*
A continuation of : **Medicinal-Kalender** für Oesterreich.

Neu-erfundene mathematische Curiositäten. Enthaltend : Die wunderbareste Würckungen der Natur und Kunst, worinnen vermittelst drey sonderbaren Instrumenten : 1. Die Schwere und Leichte ; 2. Die Truckene und Feuchte ; 3. Das Ab- und Zunehmen der Hitz und Kälte, der Lufft zu beobachten und zu erkennen seynd. Aus dem Frantzösisch ins Deutsch übersetzt. 15 pp., 35 pl. 4°. *Mayntz, L. Bourgeat*, 1695.

Neues allgemeines Journal der Chemie von Hermbstadt, Klaproth, J. B. Richter, A. N. Scherer, J. B. Trommsdorff. Hrsg. von A. F. Gehlen. v. 1–6, 1803–6. 8°. *Berlin, H. Frölich.*
A continuation of : **Allgemeines** Journal der Chemie.

Neues allgemeines Spital in Wien unter der Aufschrift : Saluti et solatio ægrorum Josephus ii. aug. anno 1784. 2 plans. fol. [*Wien, n. d.*]

Neues Archiv für die Geburtshülfe, Frauenzimmer- und Kinderkrankheiten mit Hinsicht auf die Physiologie, Diätetik und Chirurgie. Hrsg. von Johann Christ. Stark. v. 1–3, 1798–1804. 8°. *Jena, W. Stahl.*
A continuation of : **Archiv** für die Geburtshülfe [etc.], 1787–96. No. 1, v. 3, last published.

Neues Archiv für medizinische Erfahrung.
See **Archiv** für medizinische Erfahrung, v. 7–10, 1805–7.

Neues Archiv der praktischen Arzneykunst für Aerzte, Wundärzte und Apotheker, von verschiedenen Verfassern, hrsg. von P. F. Theodor Meckel. Theil 1–2, 1789–90. 8°. *Leipzig, Weygand.*

Neues Berlinisches Jahrbuch für die Pharmacie und für die damit verbundenen Wissenschaften.
Was title of : **Berlinisches** Jahrbuch für die Pharmacie und für die damit verbundenen Wissenschaften, in 1803–15.

Neues Jahrbuch für Pharmacie und verwandte Fächer. Eine Zeitschrift des allgemeinen deutschen Apotheker - Vereins, Abtheilung Süddeutschland. Hrsg., unter Mitwirkung des Directorii, von G. F. Walz und F. L. Winkler. [Monthly ; 2 v. annually.] v. 3–40, 1855–73. 38 v. 8°. *Speyer, G. L. Lang.*
Want pp. 119–136, v. 3 ; v. 35–36 (1871) ; pp. 337–352, v. 40. A continuation of : **Jahrbuch** für praktische Pharmacie und verwandte Fächer. In July, 1862, v. 18, F. Vorwerk became editor. v. 18–19, 1862, published in Heidelberg.

Neues Journal der ausländischen medizinisch-chirurgischen Literatur. Hrsg. von C. W. Hufe-

Neues Journal [etc.]—continued. land und Chr. Fr. Harles. v. 1–8, 1804–8. 8°. *Nürnberg u. Sulzbach, J. E. Seidel.*
A continuation of : **Journal** der ausländischen medizinischen Literatur. In no. 2, v. 3, G. H. Ritter became editor in place of Dr. Hufeland ; v. 8, Fr. Harles sole editor. v. 5–8, 1806–8, published at Erlangen.

Neues Journal für die Chirurgie, Arzneikunde und Geburtshülfe.
See **Journal** für die Chirurgie, Arzneikunde und Geburtshülfe, v. 5, 1815–20.

Neues Journal der Erfindungen, Theorien und Widersprüche in der Natur- und Arzneiwissenschaft.
Was an additional title of v. 7–11, 1798–1809, of : **Journal** der Erfindungen, Theorien und Widersprüche in der Natur- und Arzneiwissenschaft.

Neues Journal der Pharmacie, für Aerzte und Apotheker und Chemister von Johann Bartolomä Trommsdorff. v. 1–27, 1817–34. 8°. *Leipzig, F. C. W. Vogel.*
A continuation of : **Journal** der Pharmacie [etc.]

Neues Liecht vor die Apothecker, wie selbige nach den Grund-Regeln der heutigen Destillirkunst ihre Artzeneyen zubereiten sollen ; mit einigen Anmerckungen vermehret und verbessert durch die hochgelahrten Herren Sylvius, Willis, Blanckart, und andere. Nebenst einem Anhange von denen Irrthümern, so bey Bereitung der Medicamenten vorzugehen pflegen den Herrn Anton de Heidens ; aus dem Holländischen ins Hochteutsche übergesetzt von D. J. S. Frontispiece, 4 p. l., 780 pp., 16 l. 12°. *Leipzig, T. F. Gleditsch*, 1690.

Neues Magazin für Aerzte. Hrsg. von Ernst Gottfried Baldinger.
See **Magazin** vor Aerzte, 1779–98.

Neues Magazin für die gerichtliche Arzneikunde und medizinische Polizei. Hrsg. von J. Th. Pyl. v. 3–4, 1785–8. 2 v. 8°. *Stendal, D. C. Franzen u. Grosse.*
A continuation of : **Magazin** für die gerichtliche Arzneikunde [etc.]

Neues Magazin für philosophische, medicinische und gerichtliche Seelenkunde. Hrsg. von J. B. Friedreich. Hft. 8–10, 1832–3. 3 v. 8°. *Würzburg, Stahel.*
A continuation of : **Magazin** [etc.] Continued as : **Archiv** für Psychologie für Aerzte und Juristen.

Neues medicinisches und physisches Journal. Von Baldinger zu Marburg. v. 1–3, 1797–1802. 8°. *Marburg.*
A continuation of : **Medicinisches** Journal, Göttingen. 1784–96.

Neues nordisches Archiv für Naturkunde, Arzneywissenschaft und Chirurgie. Verfasst von einer Gesellschaft nordischer Gelehrten. Hrsg. von Pfaff, Scheel und Rudolphi. Nos. 1–2, v. 1, 1807. 304 pp. 8°. *Frankfurt an der Oder.*
A continuation of : **Nordisches** Archiv für Natur- und Arzneywissenschaft.

Neues Repertorium der gesammten deutschen medizinisch-chirurgischen Journalistik.
See **Allgemeines** Repertorium der gesammten deutschen medizinisch-chirurgischen Journalistik, 1845–7.

Neues Repertorium für Pharmacie. Unter Mitwirkung von A. Frickhinger [*et al.*] angefangen von Dr. A. Buchner sen. Nach dessen Tode fortgesetzt von Dr. L. A. Buchner jun. v. 1–25, 1852–76. 8°. *München, C. Kaiser.*
A continuation of : **Repertorium** für die Pharmacie.

Neues vollständiges Handbuch der Giftkunde ; oder Beschreibung aller im Thier-Pflanzen- und Mineralreich vorkommenden Gifte, nebst Anleitung zum Gebrauche der zweckmässigsten Gegenmittel bei Vergiftungsfällen. Erläutert durch viele Beispiele. x, 214 pp., 34 pl. 16°. *Chur u. Leipzig*, 1840.

Neueste Annalen der französischen Arzneykunde und Wundarzneykunst. Hrsg. von Christ.

Neueste Annalen [etc.]—continued.
Wilhelm Hufeland. v. 1–3, 1791–1800. 8°.
Leipzig, A. F. Böhme.

Neueste medizinisch-chirurgische Journalistik des Auslandes in vollständigen, kurzgefassten Auszügen angefangen von F. J. Behrend und K. F. W. Moldenhauer. Fortgesetzt von F. J. Behrend. [Monthly; 4 v. annually.] v. 6–15, July, 1831, to Dec., 1833. 10 v. 8°. *Leipzig, C. E. Kollmann.*

——. The same. Neue Reihe. [3 v. annually.] Jahrg. 5–6, v. 1–6 [whole series, v. 16–21,] Jan., 1834, to Dec., 1835. 8°. *Berlin, A. Hirschwald.*

——. The same. [4. series.] v. 1–4, Jan., 1836, to Dec., 1837. 8°. *Berlin, A. Hirschwald.*

In July, 1831–5, title also: **Allgemeines** Repertorium der medizinisch-chirurgischen Journalistik des Auslandes, v. 1–10, and new series, v. 1–6. In 1836–7 title also: **Wöchentliches** Repertorium der neuesten medizinisch-chirurgischen Literatur des Auslandes.

Neueste Nachricht über den Kurort Kissingen und seine Heilquellen, mit besonderer Beziehung auf den Nutzen und Gebrauch derselben. 42 pp. 16°. *Würzburg, J. S. Richter,* 1827.

Neueste Sammlung der auserlesensten und neuesten Abhandlungen für Wundärzte. (Aus verschiedenen Sprachen übersetzt.) 7 St. in 3 v. 12°. *Leipzig, Weygand,* 1790–92.

Fortsetzung der Neuen Sammlung, 1782–89.

Neueste Vorträge der Professoren der Chirurgie und Vorstände der Krankenhäuser zu Paris über Schusswunden und Verhandlungen der Académie nationale de médecine über denselben Gegenstand, nebst ihrer Würdigung. Veranlasst durch die Ereignisse der französischen Revolution im Februar und Juni 1848. Aus der: Gazette des hôpitaux, in's Deutsche übertragen und geordnet, von C. M. Wierrer. 2 v. in 1. viii, 268, iv, 308 pp. 8°. *Sulzbach, J. E. von Seidel,* 1849.

Neuestes Journal für die Chirurgie, Arzneikunde und Geburtshülfe.
See **Journal** für die Chirurgie, Arzneikunde und Geburtshülfe, v. 5, 1815–20.

Neuestes Journal der Erfindungen, Theorien und Widersprüche in der gesammten Medizin. [Hrsg. von J. C. A. Heinroth, Joh. Chr. Gtfr. Joerg et al.] v. 1–2, 1810–12. 8°. *Gotha, J. Perthes.*

A continuation of: **Journal** der Erfindungen, Theorien und Widersprüche in der gesammten Medizin.

Neuestes medicinisch-chirurgisches Wörterbuch, nicht nur für Aerzte und Wundärzte, sondern auch für Jedermann. 2 p. l., 235 pp. 8°. *Wien, Sonnleithner,* 1784.

Preface signed "Ferdinand von T—".

Neufeld (Otto). *Ozon et quæ concludi possint e notis adhuc viribus ejus physicalibus, chemicis et physiologicis in ulteriores effectus in animantium naturas. 46 pp. 8°. *Regiomonti Pr., E. J. Dalkowski,* 1852.

C.

Neufeldt (Godofr. Ludovicus) [1799–]. *De asphyxia recens-natorum. 41 pp. 8°. *Gryphiæ, F. W. Kunike,* [1823].

Neuffer (Christianus). Magici morbi historia attentius pensitata. 31 pp. 4°. *Tubingæ, typ. G. F. Pflickii,* [1724].

Neuffer (Philipp Jac.)
See **Mauchart** (Burchard David). Mydriasin pupillæ [etc.] 12°. *Tubingæ,* 1745.

Neuffer (Theodor). *Ueber Diabetes insipidus. 38 pp. 8°. *Tübingen, L. F. Fues,* 1856.

von Neufforge (Joseph M.) [1840–]. *Pathologie und Pathogenese des miliaren Tubercels, nebst einem Beitrag zur Statistik der Tuberculose nach den Ergebnissen von 141 Leicheneröffnungen. 1 p. l., 42 pp., 1 l., 2 tab. 8°. *Bonn, J. F. Carthaus,* [1870].

de Neufville (*Gerhard*) [1590–1648].
[**Life.**] Biogr. Skizzen verstorb. Bremisch. Aerzte, Bremen, 1844, 71–79.

de Neufville (Jacobus Fridericus). *De pleuritide vera atque spuria. 34 pp., 4 l. 4°. *Jenæ, lit. Tennemannianis,* [1751].

For Biography, see **Kaltschmied** (Carolus Fridericus).

de Neufville (Matthias Guilielmus) [1762–1842]. *De indole morborum periodica ex labe qualicunque viscerum hypochondriacorum derivanda. 42 pp., 1 l. 4°. *Gottingæ, F. A. Rosenbusch,* [1784].

Neufville (Thomas). *De pneumoniæ et sedis ejus historia. 1 p. l., 30 pp. 8°. *Edinburgi, Balfour et Smellie,* 1776.

de Neufville (Wilhelm Karl) [1823 – 85]. *Quæstiones de carcinomate. vii, 70 pp. 8°. *Francof. a. M., C. Naumann,* 1845.

——. Die tödtlichen Verletzungen nach den Grundsätzen der neueren deutschen Strafgesetzgebungen. 126 pp. 8°. *Erlangen, J. J. Palm u. E. Enke,* 1851.

Repr. from: Ztschr. f. d. Staatsarznk., Erlang., 1851, xliii, Ergnzngshft.

——. Lebensdauer und Todesursachen zwei und zwanzig verschiedener Stände und Gewerbe, nebst vergleichender Statistik der christlichen und israelitischen Bevölkerung Frankfurts. Nach zuverlässigen Quellen bearbeitet. iv, 116 pp., 2 tab. 8°. *Frankf. a. M., J. D. Sauerländer,* 1855.

Neufville (Zacharias). *De natura aëris fixi, ejusque dotibus. 1 p. l., 60 pp. 8°. *Edinburgi, Balfour et Smellie,* [1778].

Neugebauer (Benj. Ehrenf.) De corticis chinæ usu noxio, licet recto, in febribus. 34 pp. 4°. *Francof. cis Viadr., typ. T. Schwartzii,* [1729].

Neugebauer (Ferdinandus Aloisius) [1813–]. *De delirio potatorum, adjecta morbi historia. 26 pp. 8°. *Berolini, typ. fratrum Schlesinger,* 1837.

Neugebauer (Franz Ludwig). *Zur Entwickelungsgeschichte des spondylolisthetischen Beckens und seiner Diagnose. 3 p. l., 294 pp., 1 l., 1 pl. 8°. *Dorpat, C. Mattiesen,* 1881.

——. The same. Mit Berücksichtigung von Körperhaltung und Gangspur; casuistisch-kritische Monographie. 2 p. l., 294 pp., 1 tab. 8°. *Halle, M. Niemeyer,* 1882.

——. Aetiologie der sogenannten Spondyl-olisthesis. (Fortsetzung zu dem Aufsatze: "Zur Casuistik des sogenannten spondylolisthetischen Beckens".) 52 pp. 8°. *Leipzig, A. T. Engelhardt,* [1882].

Repr. from: Arch. f. Gynaek., Berl., 1882, xx, 1. Hft.

——. Zur Casuistik des sogenannten spondylolisthetischen Beckens. 34 pp. 8°. *Leipzig, A. T. Engelhardt,* [1882].

Repr. from: Arch. f. Gynaek., Berl., 1882, xix, 3. Hft.

——. Ein neuer Beitrag zur Casuistik und Aetiologie der Spondyl-olisthesis. 61 pp. 8°. *Leipzig, A. T. Engelhardt,* 1884.

Repr. from: Arch. f. Gynaek., Berl., 1885, xxii, 3. Hft.

Neugebauer (J.) Die Wiener Vieh- und Fleischmarktfrage. Volkswirthschaftlich beleuchtet. 20 pp. 8°. *Wien, C. Gerold's Sohn,* 1884.

Neugebauer (J[oannes]) [1839–]. *De pede retrorsum luxato et subluxato. 23 pp. 8°. *Vratislaviæ, typ. A. Neumanni,* 1866.

Neugebauer (Ludwik Adolf) [1821 –]. Sprawozdanie z czynności szpitala świetéj trójcy w kaliszu w roku 1855. [Report of the Holy-Trinity Hospital at Kalisz for 1855.] 125 pp., 1 l., 1 tab., 1 pl. 8°. *Warszawa, S. Orgelbranda,* 1856.

——. Morphologie der menschlichen Nabelschnur. 1 p. l., 80 pp., 2 pl. 8°. *Breslau, W. G. Korn,* 1858.

——. Przegląd ważniejszych przypadków chirurgicznych leczonych w roku 1862 do 1866 w

Neugebauer (Ludwik Adolf)—continued.
Szpitalu Śgo Ducha w Warszawie. [Review of surgical cases treated in the Holy Ghost Hospital, in Warsaw.] 23 pp. 8°. *Warszawa*, 1867.
See, also, **Remer** (Karl Julius Wilhelm Paul) & **Neugebauer** (L. A.) Die asiatische Cholera, [etc.] 8°. *Görlitz,* 1848.

Neugründung (Die) der Strassburger Bibliothek und die Göthe-Feier am 9. August 1871. 26 pp. 8°. *Strassburg, C. F. Schmidt,* 1871.

Neuhaus.
Hen (C.) Das Mineralbad und die während des Curjahres 1836 beobachteten Heilerfolge zu Neuhaus in Steyermark. Med. Jahrb. d. k. k. österr. Staates, Wien, 1839, xxviii, 192–194.—**Hruschauer** (F.) Untersuchung des Neuhauser Badewassers. Oesterr. med, Wchnschr., Wien, 1848, 417–424.

Neuhaus (Carolus Eduardus) [1809–]. * De psellismo ejusque sanandi rationibus. 39 pp. 8°. *Berolini, G. Schade,* [1846].

Neuhaus (Ferdinandus). De dysenteria. 34 pp. 8°. *Berolini, typ. J. F. Starckii,* 1817.

Neuhaus (Franciscus Alexander). * Diss. colicæ hystericæ casum cum sua epicrisi. 24 pp. 4°. *Argentorati, J. H. Heitz,* [1769].

Neuhaus (Georgius Sebastianus). * De affectione hysterica. 44 pp. 4°. *Rostochi, typ. J. Wepplingi,* [n. d.]

Neuhaus (Heinrich). * Ueber die Richtung der Frakturen der Schädelbasis. [Wurtzburg.] 26 pp. 8°. *Wesel, W. Romen,* 1879. C.

Neuhausen.
See **Fever** (*Typhoid, History, etc., of*), *by localities.*

Neuhausen (J.)
Co-Editor of: **Organ** für die gesammte Heilkunde, Aachen, 1852–7.
See, also, **Guépin** (A.) Studien im Gebiete der Augenheilkunde. 8°. *Crefeld,* 1847.

ab Neuhauser (Fr.) * De debilitate spuria, comite morborum inflammatoriorum. 43 pp., 2 l. 8°. *Vindobonæ, typ. congregationis Mechitaristicæ,* [1830].

Neuhauss (Richard).
See **Topinard** (Paul). Anthropologie, nach der dritten französischen Auflage, [etc.] 8°. *Leipzig,* 1886.

Neuhöfer (M.) * Ueber die angeborene Halsfistel. 31 pp., 1 pl. 8°. *München, C. Wolf,* 1847.

Neuhof (Benjamin. Eduardus). * Diss. morbi arcuati singularis historiam sistens. 28 pp. 4°. *Lipsiæ, A. Deutrich,* [1826].
For Biography, see **Kühn** (Carolus Gottlob).

Neuhof (Theodorus Benjamin.) * De virium medicamentorum maxime probabili partitione. 34 pp. 4°. *Lipsiæ, ex off. Klaubarthia,* [1797].
For Biography, see **Platner** (Ernestus).

Neuhofer (Georgius). * De morbosa catameniorum suppressione. 28 pp., 6 l. 4°. *Lugd. Bat., C. Wishoff,* 1750.
See, also, **Mead** (Richard). Abhandlung von den Kinderpocken und Masern [etc.] 16°. *Augsburg,* 1762.

Neuhoff (Carolus Ludovicus). * De difficili in observationes anatomicas epicrisi commentatio iv. 1 p. l., 36 pp. 4°. *Erlangæ, ex off. Waltheria,* [1773].

Neuhoff (Daniel Gottlieb). * Disp. inaug.-med. proponens satyriasin. 15 l. 4°. *Erffurti, J. H. Grosch,* [1711].

Neuhoff (Joannes Fridericus). * De amaurosi. 32 pp., 1 l. 4°. *Vitebergæ, F. I. Seibt,* [1806].
For Biography, see **Seiler** (Guilielmus).

Neuhoff (Joannes Godofredus). * De enemate uterino. 35 pp. 4°. *Lipsiæ, ex off. Langenhemiana,* [1755].
Also [Abstr.], *in:* WEIZ (F. A.) Neue Ausz. [etc.] 12°. *Frankf. u. Leipz.,* 1774, i, 129–139.
For Biography, see **Quelmalz** (Samuel Theodorus).

Neuhold (Jo. Jacobus). * De lienis genuino usu. 36 pp. 4°. *Lipsiæ, lit. I. Titii,* [1722].

Neuhold (Jo. Jacobus)—continued.
——. Observationes pathologico-therapeuticæ, horis subsecivis conscriptæ, quarum nunc primam decadem exhibet. 40 pp. 4°. *Altorfii, lit. J. G. Kohlesii,* 1733.

Neuigkeiten aus der Medicin, Chirurgie und Geburtshülfe. Im Verein mit mehreren Aerzten hrsg. von T. H. Auerbach. [Weekly.] Nos. 1–39, April 7 to Dec. 29, 1860; 1861 to Dec. 26, 1863. 4°. *Berlin.*
Want no. 1, Jan. 3, 1863.

Neuilly.
See **Cholera** (*Asiatic, History, etc., of*), *by localities.*

Neukirch (Ferdinandus) [1804–]. * De hydrocele. 30 pp. 8°. *Halæ Sax., typ. Baentschii,* 1827.

Neukirch (Franciscus Arnoldus) [1829–]. * De cirrhosi hepatis. 37 pp., 1 l. 8°. *Berolini, typ. fratrum Schlesinger,* [1852].

Neukirch (Josef) [1861–]. * Ueber Lupus an der Hand. 29 pp., 1 l. 8°. *Berlin, G. Schade,* 1885.

Neukirch (Richard). * Ueber die Entstehung des Schallwechsels bei der Percussion von Cavernen. [Erlangen.] 15 pp. 8°. *Nürnberg, G. P. J. Bieling (G. Dietz),* [1879].

Neukirch (Sally Simon).
See **Hornemann** (Claud. Jac. Æmil.) * De rationibus dosium calomellis [etc.] 8°. *Havniæ,* 1839.—**Melchior** (N. G.) * De strabismo. 8°. *Havniæ,* 1839.

Neukohm. Bericht über das Bad Heustrich am Niesen. Sommersaison 1881. 30 pp. 12°. *Bern, B. F. Haller,* 1882.
——. The same. Rapport sur les bains d'Heustrich au Niesen. Saison de 1881. 22 pp. 12°. *Berne, B. F. Haller,* 1882.

Neukomm (Jacob). * Ueber das Vorkommen von Leucin, Tyrosin und anderer Umsatzstoffe im menschlichen Körper bei Krankheiten. 48 pp., 1 l. 8°. *Zürich, Orell, Füssli u. Comp.,* 1859.

Neukomm (Joannes Georgius). * De pædatrophia. 42 pp. 8°. *Berolini, typ. Nietackianis,* 1834.

Neukomm (Martin). * Ueber spätere Folgezustände nach der Tracheotomie bei Kehlkopf-Diphtheritis im Kindesalter. [Bern.] 62 pp., 1 l. 8°. *Zürich, Zürcher u. Furrer,* 1885.

Neukomm (Max). * Ueber eine neue Amputations-Methode. 40 pp., 5 l. 8°. *Tübingen, H. Laupp,* 1863.

Neukrantz (Zacharias). Abstrusum respirationis humanæ negotium, exulante famosa vacui fuga, ex genuinis gravissimi hujus argumenti φαινομένων causis plenius erutum. Simul cum ardui istius Harveani, Doctis omnibus L. de Gen. Animal. Exerc. de partu proposui, nec non bimembris hujus problematis solutione : cur animalia tam propter aëris inspirati cohibitique præsentiam, quam in machina Boyliana pneumatica exhausta propter ejusdem aëris absentiam tam velociter quasi ex anima succumbant, brevique moriantur? 55 l. sm. 4°. *Lipsiæ, J. Georg,* 1676.
Another copy bound with: VELSCHIUS (G. H.) Sylloge curationum. sm. 4°. *Aug. Vindel.,* 1668.
Also, in: ETTMÜLLER (M.) Diss. xiix med. 4°. *Francof. et Lips.,* 1685.

Neukrantzen (Jo. Theodorus). * De necessitate artis chemicæ ejusdemque productu summo magna hominum et metallorum medicina lapis philosophorum dicta. 14 l. 4°. *Vitembergæ, apud vid. Gerdesiam,* 1725.

Neukranz (Joh. Antonius). * De vulneribus lethalibus. 19 l. sm. 4°. *Helmestadii, typ. H. D. Mulleri,* 1674.

Neukum (Georg Michael). * De marasmo senili sive marcore naturali. 16 pp. 4°. [*Basel*], *typ. J. H. Deckeri,* [1743].

Neulaender (F. L.) [1800–   ].   * Diss. sistens analecta ad semioticen labiorum, gingivarum et dentium spectantia. 2 p. l., 45 pp. 8°. *Vratislaviæ, typ. Universitatis,* [1825].

Neullier (Hector - Henri).   *I. Les maladies sont-elles toutes précédées des phénomènes qui caractérisent le prodrôme des maladies? Quelle est la valeur des accidents du prodrôme dans le diagnostic? II. [etc.] 26 pp. 4°. *Paris,* 1841, No. 214, v. 379.

Neumaier (Eginhard).   * De irritatione cerebri infantum. 18 pp. 8°. *München, J. G. Weiss,* 1867.

Neuman (Alexander).   * Der forensisch-chemische Nachweis des Santonin und sein Verhalten im Thierkörper. 56 pp., 1 l. 8°. *Dorpat, Schnakenburg,* 1883.

Neuman (Rachel A.) Home-nursing. 120 pp. 24°. *London & Edinburgh, W. & R. Chambers,* 1886.

Neumann (A. C.) Handbuch der gerichtlichen Anatomie für Rechtsgelehrte, Polizeibeamte und Studirende. Nebst einem Wörterbuche. xiv, 305 pp. 8°. *Berlin, A. Hirschwald,* 1841.

——. Die Heil-Gymnastik, oder die Kunst der Leibesübungen, angewandt zur Heilung von Krankheiten nach dem Systeme des Schweden Ling und seiner Schüler Branting, Georgii und de Ron, sowie nach eigenen Ansichten und Erfahrungen. Ein Bericht nach einer auf Kosten des preussischen Staats und im Auftrage des Herrn Ministers der Medicinal-Angelegenheiten unternommenen Reise nach Stockholm, London, und St. Petersburg. xvi, 431 pp., 3 pl. 8°. *Berlin, P. Jeanrenaud,* 1852.

——. The same. Der grossen Idee des Schweden Ling gemäss nach eigenen Ansichten und Erfahrungen geordnet. 2. Aufl. viii, 390 pp., 1 l., 2 pl. 8°. *Leipzig, A. Förstner,* 1857.
With second title-page: Therapie der chronischen Krankheiten vom heilorganischen Standpunkte.

——. Das Muskelleben des Menschen in Beziehung auf Heilgymnastik und Turnen. viii, 254 pp. 8°. *Berlin, E. H. Schroeder,* 1855.

——. Der Heilkunde Duldung, den Aerzten Duldsamkeit! 20 pp. 8°. *Berlin, E. H. Schroeder,* 1860.

——. Grundzüge einer vergleichenden Therapie. viii, 159 pp. 12°. *Berlin, E. H. Schroeder,* 1863.

See, also, **Schreber** (D. G. M.) & **Neumann** (A. C.) Streitfragen. 8°. *Leipzig,* 1858.

Neumann (Adolph). Die Erkennung des Blutes bei gerichtlichen Untersuchungen. Ein Leitfaden für Beamte der Justiz und die von derselben zugezogenen Sachverständigen. vi, 7–16 pp., 23 pl. 8°. *Leipzig, J. J. Weber,* 1869.

Neumann (Alb. Phil. Theodorus) [1797–   ]. * De inflammatione telæ mucosæ. 31 pp. 8°. *Berolini, formis Brueschckianis,* [1820].

Neumann (Alfredus Carolus Severus)[1841–   ]. * De effectibus et signis vitiorum valvularum cordis sinistri. 32 pp. 8°. *Berolini, G. Lange,* [1865].

Neumann (Anton) [1861–   ]. * Ueber drei Fälle von Sarcom am Unterkiefer. 23 pp. 8°. *Greifswald, J. Abel,* 1886.

Neumann (August) [1847–   ]. * Ein Beitrag zur Lehre von der Entstehung, dem Verlaufe und dem Wesen der Geisteskrankheiten. 31 pp. 8°. *Greifswald, F. W. Kunike,* 1875.

Neumann (Augustus). * De crisibus, genuinis morbis nervosis peculiaribus. 44 pp. 8°. *Halæ, lit. Michaelianis,* [1792].

Neumann (Carl E. O.) Der Frauenarzt. Ein Ratgeber für Jungfrauen, Frauen und Mütter. Naturgemässe Behandlung der Frauenkrankheiten mit in den Text gedruckten Abbildungen. v (1 l.), 81 pp. 8°. *Köthen, P. Schettler,* 1884.

Neumann (Carl E. O.)—continued.

——. Der Männerarzt; ein Ratgeber für junge und alte Männer. Naturgemässe Behandlung der Männerkrankheiten. iv, 90 pp. 8°. *Leipzig, T. Grieben,* [1885].

——. Die Hämorrhoiden sowie die Blutüberfüllung des Kopfes, Rückenmarks, der Brust, Nieren, Milz, Leber und der Krampfadern, ihre leichte und sichere Verhütung und Heilung auf naturgemässem Wege. 1 p. l., 72 pp. 12°. *Leipzig, T. Grieben,* 1887.

——. Die Haut, Haare, Nägel und Zähne des Menschen. Deren Bau, Pflege, Krankheiten und naturgemässe Behandlung. 2. Aufl. iv, 106 pp., 1 l. 12°. *Leipzig, L. Fernau,* [1887].

——. Die Massage. Anleitung zur praktischen Ausführung derselben für Jedermann. 2. Aufl. 119 pp. 8°. *Leipzig, T. Grieben,* [n. d.]

Neumann (Carl Georg) [1774–1850]. * De balneis frigidis observationes. 26 pp. 4°. *Vitembergæ, lit. Tzschiedrichii,* [1795].

——. Abhandlung von dem Brande, die verschiedenen Arten, Ursachen und Heilungs-Methoden des Brandes an den weichen und harten Theilen des menschlichen Körpers. 208 pp. 4°. *Wien, A. Camesina,* 1801.

——. Beyträge zur praktischen Arzneywissenschaft. iv, 252 pp. 12°. *Leipzig, Kühn,* 1811.

——. Die Krankheiten des Vorstellungsvermögens, systematisch bearbeitet. 3 p. l., 400 pp. 8°. *Leipzig, C. Cnobloch,* 1822.

——. Von den Krankheiten des Menschen. Allgemeiner Theil, oder allgemeine Pathologie. x, 286 pp., 1 l. 8°. *Berlin, F. A. Herbig,* 1829.

——. The same. 2. Aufl. x, 297 pp., 1 l. 8°. *Berlin, F. A. Herbig,* 1842.

——. The same. Specieller Theil, oder specielle Pathologie u. Therapie. 4 v. 8°. *Berlin, F. A. Herbig,* 1832–4.
Each volume has a second title-page, viz:
v. 1. Specielle Pathologie und Therapie der fieberhaften Krankheiten des Menschen.
v. 2. Specielle Pathologie und Therapie der chronischen Krankheiten des Menschen.
v. 3. Specielle Pathologie und Therapie der Krankheiten des Menschen. [Topische Krankheiten der Vegetationsphäre.]
v. 4. Specielle Pathologie und Therapie der Krankheiten der Sensibilität des Menschen.

——. The same. 2. Aufl. 5 v. 8°. *Berlin, F. A. Herbig,* 1836–44.
Each volume has a second title-page. v. 4 has 1. and 2. Abtheil.
Second title-page of 5. and suppl. vol.: Fortschritte und Erfahrungen der neuesten Zeit im Gebiete der Heilkunst.

——. Von den Krankheiten des Gehirns des Menschen. vi (1 l.), 492 pp. 8°. *Coblenz, R. F. Hergt,* 1833.

——. Der allgemeine Hausarzt, oder Belehrung für Jedermann, wie er seine Gesundheit erhalten und in Krankheiten und Unfällen sich benehmen solle. 3 p. l., 304 pp. 12°. *Aachen, P. Roschütz u. Comp.,* 1837.

——. Bemerkungen über die gebräuchlichsten Arzneimittel. 253 pp. 8°. *Berlin, Liebmann u. Comp.,* 1840.

——. Pathologische Untersuchungen als Regulative des Heilverfahrens. 2 v. in 1. 322 pp., 1 l.; 1 p. l., 243 pp. 8°. *Berlin, Liebmann u. Comp.,* 1841–2.

——. The same. 2. Ausg. 2 v. in 1. 322 pp., 1 l.; 243 pp. 8°. *Berlin, Liebmann u. Comp.,* 1844.

——. Von den Krankheiten des Menschen. Allgemeiner Theil, oder allgemeine Pathologie. 2. Aufl. x, 297 pp., 1 l. 8°. *Berlin, F. A. Herbig,* 1842.

——. Deutschland's Heilquellen mit besonderer Rücksicht auf die Wahl derselben für specielle Krankheitsfälle. viii, 256 pp. 8°. *Erlangen, F. Enke,* 1845.

Neumann (Carl Georg)—continued.

——. Heilmittellehre nach den bewährtesten Erfahrungen und Untersuchungen in alphabetischer Ordnung bearbeitet. 2. Aufl. xii, 635, x pp. roy. 8°. *Erlangen, F. Enke*, 1850.

See, also, **Platner** (Ernestus). Opuscula academica, etc. 8°. *Berolini*, 1824.

For Biography, see **Titius** (Salomo Constantinus).

Neumann (Carolus Ferdinandus). * De phlebitide faciei. 30 pp. 8°. *Regiomonti Pr., typ. Dalkowskianis*, 1857. C.

Neumann (Carolus Fridericus)[1]. * De ictero. xxxii pp. 4°. *Helmstadii, C. G. Fleckeisen*, [1798].

Neumann (Carolus Fridericus)[2] [1797–]. * De oculorum morborum examine. 31 pp. 8°. *Berolini, formis Brüschckianis*, [1825].

Neumann (Carolus Fridericus Guilelmus)[1838–]. * De occlusione valvulæ mitralis et de morbis quibus sublata est. 32 pp. 8°. *Berolini, G. Schade*, [1863].

Neumann (Carolus Gottlob.) * De vano morbi boum gallici carnisque inde male infectæ et insalubris metu. 24 pp. 4°. *Vitebergæ, excud. A. C. Charisius*, [1790].

For Biography, see **Boehmer** (Georg. Rud.)

Neumann (Caspar) [1683–1737]. Lectiones chymicæ: von Salibus alkalino-fixis und von Camphora, als zwey Proben. 3 p. l., 226 pp. sm. 4°. *Berlin, G. Schlechtiger's Wittwe*, 1727.

——. Lectiones publicæ von vier Subjectis diæteticis, nehmlich von den in hiesigen Gegenden gewöhnlichsten und durch menschliche Hülffe zu Stande gebrachten viererley Geträncken, vom Thée, Caffée, Bier und Wein; wie solche bey dem in Berlin gestifteten königl. Collegio medico-chirurgico abgehandelt worden. 13 p. l., 468 pp. 4°. *Leipzig, G. B. Fromman*, 1735.

——. De ambra grysea, welche an die königl. Gros-Brittann. weltberühmte Societät der Wissenschafften geschicket worden. Sammt einem kurtzen Vorbericht solcher Memoire halber, anjetzo, weil wenigen Personen die engländische Transactiones philosophicæ vorkommen, in deutscher Sprache publiciret, von einem Liebhaber der Historiæ naturalis. 7 p. l., 116 pp. 4°. *Dressden, G. C. Hilscher*, 1736.

Another copy bound with his: Lectiones, etc. 4°. *Leipzig*, 1735.

——. The chemical works of . . . abridged and methodized by W. Lewis. 8 p. l., 586 pp., 19 l. 4°. *London, W. Johnston*, 1759.

——. The same. 2. ed. 2 v. 439, 458 pp., 35 l. 8°. *London, J. & F. Rivington* [*and others*], 1773.

For Portrait, see **Collection**—van Kaathoven.—**Collection** of Portr. of Phys. & Men of Sc., 216.

For Biography, see Acta Acad. nat. curios., Norimb., 1748, viii (app.), 243–262, port.

Neumann (Christian Gottlieb). * De exclusione ovulorum, in salacibus, absque ullo prægresso coitu. 21 pp. 4°. *Lugd. Bat., C. Wishoff*, [1717].

Neumann (Christianus Guilielmus). * De paronychia. 28 pp. 4°. *Vitebergæ, lit. A. C. Charisii*, 1803.

For Biography, see **Vogt** (Traugott Carolus Augustus).

Neumann (Curt) [1853–]. * Ein Fall von Gummigeschwulst in der Tibia. 30 pp., 1 l. 8°. *Berlin, G. Schade*, 1878.

Neumann (Émile). * Sur le cancer du rein. 88 pp. 4°. *Paris*, 1873, No. 109.

——. The same. 86 pp. 8°. *Paris, A. Delahaye*, 1873.

Neumann (Ernest.) * Disquisitiones nonnullæ de histogenesi carcinomatis institutæ. 22 pp. 4°. *Regimonti Pr., typ. A. Dalkowskianis*, 1869.

Neumann (Ernest. Franc. Christ.) [1834–]. * De venenis, quæ dicuntur narcotica, experimenta quædam physiologica. 32 pp. 8°. *Regiomonti Pr., typ. Dalkowskianis*, 1855. C.

Neumann (Ernest. Franc. Christ.)—continued.

——. Ein Beitrag zur Kenntniss des normalen Zahnbein- und Knochengewebes. 58 pp. 8°. *Leipzig, F. C. W. Vogel*, 1863.

——. Ueber myelogene Leukämie. 51 pp. 8°. *Berlin, A. Hirschwald*, 1878.

Repr. from: Berl. klin. Wchnschr., 1878, xv.

Neumann (Eugen) [1855–]. * Drei Fälle von sympathischem Augenleiden. 36 pp., 1 l. 8°. *Greifswald, C. Sell*, 1880.

Neumann (Franciscus). * De pleuritide dorsali. 32 pp. 8°. [*Viennæ*], e typ. *Kaliwodiano*, [1772].

Neumann (Frid. Jul.) * Profusiones sanguinis ex umbilico hominis adulti. 30 pp. 8°. *Regiomonti Pr., typ. Dalkowskianis*, 1866. C.

Neumann (Friedrich). * Experimentelle Untersuchungen über das Verhalten der insensiblen Ausgabe im Fieber. 67 pp. 8°. *Dorpat, H. Laakmann*, 1873.

Neumann (Georg) [1856–]. * Ueber fötale Rachitis und ihre Beziehungen zum Cretinismus. 30 pp., 1 l. 8°. *Halle a. S., Gebauer-Schwetschke*, 1881.

Neumann (Georgius Carolus) [1804–]. * De ratione inter nervorum vires et imponderabilium indolem. 2 p. l., 26 pp. 8°. *Berolini, typ. A. G. Schadii*, [1828]. [*Also, in:* P., v. 1548.]

Neumann (Gothofredus). * De sanguine et ejus motu dissertatio. 11 l. 4°. [*Lipsiæ*], *J. Bauerus*, [1652].

Neumann (Gustav) [1845–]. * Ueber die Anzeigen zum künstlichen Sprengen der Eihäute. 31 pp. 8°. *Halle, W. Plötz*, 1869.

Neumann (Gustavus Hermannus). * De hæsitantia linguæ. 23 pp. 4°. *Lipsiæ, lit. Staritzii*, [1834].

Neumann (Heinrich) [1814–84]. Wie studirt man Medicin? 22 pp. 8°. *Breslau, A. Schulz, u. Comp.*, 1842.

——. Die analytische Medicin. 68 pp. 8°. *Breslau, L. Maske*, 1847.

——. Der Arzt und die Blödsinnigkeits-Erklärung. vi (1 l.), 88 pp. 8°. *Breslau, A. Gosohorsky*, 1847.

——. Lehrbuch der Psychiatrie. 2 p. l., 242 pp., 1 l. roy. 8°. *Erlangen, F. Enke*, 1859.

——. The same. Studien over krankzinnigheid en gemoedslijden. Een leerboek voor de kennis der krankzinnigheid en de geneeskundige verpleging van krankzinnigen, vermeerderd met de Nederlandsche wetgeving of krankzinnigen en krankzinnigengestichten, en met aanteekeningen bewerkt voor Nederland door Dr. J. J. Kerbert. xviii (1 l.), 288 pp. 8°. *Amsterdam, J. H. Gebhard u. Comp.*, [1860].

——. Die Theorie und Praxis der Blödsinnigkeitserklärung nach preussischem Gesetze. Ein Leitfaden für Aerzte und Juristen. iv (1 l.), 97 pp. 8°. *Erlangen, F. Enke*, 1860.

——. Die Irrenanstalt zu Pöpelwitz bei Breslau im ersten Decennium ihrer Wirksamkeit. Medicinisch-statistischer Bericht nebst Bemerkungen über Irrengesetzgebung, Irrenstatistik und psychiatrischen Unterricht. 53 pp. 8°. *Erlangen, F. Enke*, 1862.

——. Der Process Kullmann. Gerichtsärztliche Reflexionen. 47 pp. 8°. *Berlin, A. Hirschwald*, 1875.

——. Leitfaden der Psychiatrie für Mediciner und Juristen. viii, 143 pp. 8°. *Breslau, Preuss u. Jünger*, 1883.

——. Katechismus der gerichtlichen Psychiatrie in Fragen und Antworten. Mit einem Anhang von Mustergutachten. 70 pp. sm. 8°. *Breslau, Preuss u. Jünger*, 1884.

Neumann (Hermann) [1859–]. * Die diuretische Wirkung des Wernarzer Brunnens in

Neumann (Hermann)—continued.
Brückenau. 23 pp., 3 a. l. 8°. *Berlin, H. Grützner*, [1884].

Neumann (Hugo). * Ueber die Knochenbrüche bei Geisteskranken. 164 pp. 8°. *Berlin, G. Bernstein*, 1883.

Neumann (Isidor) [1837–]. Lehrbuch der Hautkrankheiten. ix, 368 pp., 1 l. 8°. *Wien, W. Braumüller*, 1869.

——. The same. 5. Aufl. x, 667 pp. 8°. *Wien, W. Braumüller*, 1880.

——. The same. Text-book of skin diseases. Transl. from the 2. German ed., by special permission of the author, by Alfred Pullar. xix, 329 pp. 8°. *London, R. Hardwicke*, 1871.

——. The same. Hand-book of skin diseases. Transl. from the 2. German ed., with notes, by Lucius D. Bulkley. 467 pp. 8°. *New York, D. Appleton & Co.*, 1872.

——. The same. Traité des maladies de la peau. Trad. sur la 4e éd. et annoté par G. et E. Darin. xvi, 604 pp. roy. 8°. *Paris, A. Delahaye & Cie.*, 1880.

——. Ueber die Aufnahme des Quecksilbers durch die unverletzte Haut. Eine chemisch-mikroskopische Studie. 18 pp. 8°. *Wien*, 1872.
Repr. from : Wien. med. Wchnschr., 1871, xxi.

——. Zur Kenntniss der Lymphgefässe der Haut des Menschen und der Säugethiere. 31 pp., 8 col. pl. 8°. *Wien, W. Braumüller*, 1873.

——. Aerztlicher Bericht über die im städt. Communal-Spital Zwischenbrücken im Jahre 1872–3 behandelten Blatternkranken, nebst Mittheilungen einiger experimenteller und anatomischer Studien. 158 pp., 1 l. 8°. *Wien, W. Braumüller*, 1874.

——. Klinische Vorlesungen über allgemeine Pathologie der Hautkrankheiten. 13 pp. 8°. *Wien*, 1878.
Repr. from : Allg. Wien. med. Ztg., 1878, xxiii.

——. Atlas der Hautkrankheiten. 1. & 2. Lfg. 17 l., 12 pl. fol. *Wien, W. Braumüller*, 1881.

——. The same. Mit beschreibendem Texte. Lfg. 1–8. 67 l., 48 pl. 4°. *Wien, W. Braumüller*, 1885–8.

——. Ueber Reizung und Syphilis. 16 pp. 8°. *Wien, Verfasser*, 1885.
Repr. from : Allg. Wien. med. Ztg., 1885, xxx.

Neumann (*J. M.*) [1802–61].
Fischer (E) Notice biographique sur feu M. le Dr. J. M. Neumann, membre-fondateur de la Société des sciences médicales. Bull. Soc. d. sc. méd. du gr.-duché de Luxemb., 1867, 6–9.

Neumann (Joann. Gottlieb.) * De purgatione copiosa et nimia. 32 pp. 4°. *Halæ Magdeb., typ. J. C. Hilligeri*, [1736].

Neumann (Joannes Fridericus Guilelmus) [1820–]. * Nonnulla de cordis vasorumque majorum morbis organicis. 34 pp. 8°. *Berolini, typ. Schnitzerianis*, [1844].

Neumann (Joannes Jacobus) [1822–]. * Nonnulla de hypertrophia cordis. 31 pp. 8°. *Berolini, G. Schade*, [1846].

Neumann (Joannes Wenceslaus). Neglectus emeticorum per observata practicorum confutatus.
In : KLINKOSCH (J. T.) Diss. med. select. Prag. 4°. *Pragæ et Dresdæ*, 1793, ii, 275–338.

Neumann (Joh. Georgius). * De temporibus medicis. 32 pp. 4°. *Halæ Magdeb , lit. C. Henckelii*, [1710].

Neumann (Joh. Gottlieb). * De præservandis metallicolarum morbis. 32 pp., 4 l. 4°. *Halæ Magdeb., typ. C. Henckelii*, [1721].

——. Das süsse Wasser zu Mara, das ist : Medicinischer Entwurff von dem über Purschenstein bey Hendelbach und Einsiedel in dem dasigen Gehöltze, im Monath May neu erfundenen Heil- und Gesund-Brunnen, dessen Erfindung,

Neumann (Joh. Gottlieb)—continued.
Natur und Eigenschafft, auch innerlich- und äusserlicher Gebrauch, heilsame Krafft, und gute Würckung, nach dem Unterscheid eines jeglichen Temperamenti, kurtz, jedoch deutlich vorgestellet. 7 p. l., 52 pp. 16°. *Freyberg, C. Matthai*, 1732.

Neumann (Jonas) [1843–]. * De iliotyphi therapia. 32 pp. 8°. *Berolini, G. Schade*, [1867].

Neumann (Joseph) [1850–]. * Die Sehnennaht. Ein Beitrag zur Geschichte und Casuistik derselben. 50 pp. 8°. *Berlin, O. Francke*, [1877].

Neumann (Louis) **& Soubeiran** (J.-L.) Description de l'aquarium du Muséum d'histoire naturelle de Paris. 12 pp., 1 pl. 8°. [*Angers, Cosnier & Lachèse*, 1858.] [P., v. 1766.]
Repr. from : Ann. Soc. Linnéenne de Maine-et-Loire, ii.

Neumann (Ludovicus [Eduardus]) [1837–]. * De peritonitide. 32 pp. 8°. *Berolini, G. Lange*, [1863].

Neumann (Mathias). * Diss. inaug. med.-forensis de renuntiationibus. 47 pp. 4°. *Leodii, H. Rongier*, 1826. [P., v. 1301.]

Neumann (Mauritius). * De hydrothorace. 28 pp. 4°. *Lipsiæ, typ. Staritzii*, [1830].
For Biography, see **Kuehn** (Car. G.)

Neumann (Moritz Albrecht) [1837–]. * Ueber einige gröbere diagnostische Irrthümer bei Ovariotomien. 39 pp. 8°. *Leipzig, E. Polz*, [1862].
C.

Neumann (Moritz Georg) [1838–]. * Zur Statistik der Frakturen. 21 pp., 1 l. 8°. *Leipzig, P. Reclam jun.*, [1866].
C.

Neumann (Naphtali Hirsch) [1827–]. * Argumenta atque observationes adversus theoriam catoptricam et dioptricam. 30 pp., 2 l. 8°. *Berolini, B. Schlesinger*, [1850].

Neumann (Otto Julius). * De angina pectoris tractatus. 59 pp. 8°. *Regiomonti Bor., typ. Hartungianis*, 1837.

Neumann (Otto Willibald) [1831–]. * De maxillarum resectione. 29 pp., 1 l. 8°. *Berolini, F. G. Nietack*, [1856].

Neumann (S.) Die öffentliche Gesundheitspflege und das Eigenthum. Kritisches und Positives mit Bezug auf die preussische Medizinalverfassungs-Frage. viii, 112 pp. 12°. *Berlin, A. Riess*, 1847.

——. Zur medicinischen Statistik des preussischen Staates. iv (1 l.), 129 pp. 8°. *Berlin, G. Reimer*, 1849.

——. Zur Berliner Armenkrankenpflege. 28 pp. 8°. *Berlin, G. Reimer*, 1856.
Repr. from : Monatsbl. f. med. Statist. u. öff. Gsndhtspflg., Berl., 1856.
See, also, **Liman** (C.) Der Arznei-Verbrauch in der städtischen Armenkrankenpflege Berlins. Erwiderung auf Dr. S. Neumann's Denkschrift. 4°. *Berlin*, 1856.

Neumann (Salomon) [1819–]. * Intussusceptionis intestinorum quatuor exempla. 36 pp., 1 l. 8°. *Halæ, formis Ploetzianis*, 1842.

Neumann (Samuel). * De fluxu mensium immodico. 27 pp., 2 l. 4°. *Jenæ, apud J. C. Croekerum*, [1746].
For Biography, see **Hamberger** (Georgius Erhardus).

Neumann (Theodor). The dietetic method of cure the only true and safe method to cure radically acute and chronic diseases without any medicine. 24 pp. 8°. *Toronto-Eglinton*, 1880.

Neumann (W.) Elgersburg, Kaltwasser-Heilanstalt im Thüringer Walde Ein Wegweiser und eine Erinnerung. 1 p. l., 58 pp., 1 l. 4°. *Cassel, E. Balde*, 1853.

Neumann (Willy). * Ueber toxicologische Verschiedenheiten functionell verschiedener Muskelgruppen. Ein Beitrag zu der Lehre von den Muskelgiften. 59 pp. 8°. *Bern, Jent u. Reinert*, 1883.

Neumann (Willy)—continued.
———. * Ueber quantitative Bestimmung der Harnsäure und die dabei zu berücksichtigenden Fehlerquellen. 28 pp. 8°. *Bern, Jent u. Reinert,* 1883.

Neumark (Jacobus) [1819–]. * De metrorrhagia post partum. 31 pp. 8°. *Berolini, B. Schlesinger,* [1847].

Neumarkt.
Schrauth (J. B.) Das Mineralbad zu Neumarkt in der Oberpfalz in den Jahren 1840-46. Med. Cor.-Bl. bayer. Aerzte, Erlang., 1841, ii, 328–335: 1842, iii, 315–320: 1847, viii, 257-269. ———. Das Mineralbad zu Neumarkt in der Oberpfalz vom Jahre 1830 bis 1853. Aerztl. Int.-Bl., München, 1854, i, 164.

Neumayer (Georg). * Ueber den äusseren Harnröhrenschnitt bei impermeablen Stricturen. 39 pp. 8°. *Heidelberg, J. Hörning,* 1879. c.

Neumayer (George). Discussion of the meteorological and magnetical observations made at the "Flagstaff Observatory", Melbourne, during the years 1858-63. viii, 160, xliii pp., 25 tab. 4°. *Mannheim, J. Schneider,* 1867.

Neumayr (Ludwig). * Ueber die Fähigkeit der Haut, Wasser und in diesem gelöste Stoffe aufzusaugen. 15 pp. 8°. *München, F. Straub,* 1868.

Neumayr (M.)
See **von Hauer** (F.) & **Neumayr** (M.) Führer zu den Excursionen [etc.] . sm. 8°. *Wien,* [1877].

Neumeister (Christianus Godofredus). * De hepatite. 1 p. l., 22 pp. 4°. *Francof. ad Viadr., typ. J. C. Schwartzii,* [1721].

Neumeister (Emil). * Tuberculose nach operativer Behandlung fungöser Gelenkentzündungen. 28 pp. 8°. *Würzburg, Becker,* 1879. c.

Neumeister (Erdmann Gottwerth). * De intestinis se intus suscipientibus et rarissima hujus morbi congeniti observatione. 44 pp., 1 pl. 4°. *Helmstadii, ex typog. vid. Schnorriæ,* [1769].

Neumeister (H. W.)
Editor of: **Allgemeines** Repertorium der gesammten deutschen medizinisch-chirurgischen Journalistik, Leipzig, 1839-44.

Neumeister (Oscar) [1850–]. * Ueber die Diagnostik der Beckenfrakturen. 37 pp., 1 l. 8°. *Breslau, F. W. Jungfer,* 1872.

Neumeyer (Simon). * De hydrocephalo acuto. 16 pp. 8°. *Monachii, F. Wild,* 1843.

Neumoegen (Bernardus) [1817–]. * De hydrocephalo acuto. 32 pp. 8°. *Berolini, typ. Friedlænderianis,* [1840].

Neumueller (Arminius). * De eclampsia gravidarum, parturientium, puerperarum. 26 pp. 8°. *Wirceburgi, C. J. Becker,* 1859. c.

Neunert (Josephus). * De cancro. 36 pp. 8°. *Monachii, C. Wolf,* 1829.

Neunes (Christianus Elias Albertus). * Diss. sistens quædam momenta de cortice Peruviano ejusque usu in febribus intermittentibus. 30 pp., 1 l. 4°. *Jenæ, lit. Goepferdtianis,* [1789].
For Biography, see **Gruner** (Ch. Goth.)

Neunzig (Josephus) [1797–]. * De sanguine variisque fluidis animalibus experimenta microscopica. 30 pp., 3 l., 1 pl. 8°. *Bonnæ, typ. Thormannianis,* 1823. [*Also, in:* P., v. 575.]

Neuragoczi.
Steinbrück (A.) Ueber die Wirkungen des Bades Neuragoczi bei Halle a. S. 8°. *Halle,* 1872.
Runde. Neu-Ragoczi bei Halle. Ztschr. f. Med., Chir. u. Geburtsh., Leipz., 1860, xiv, 153-160.—**Steinbrück** (H.) Bad Neuragoczi bei Halle a. S. Deutsche Klinik, Berl., 1872, xxiv, 106; 114.

Neuralgia.
See, also, **Angina** *pectoris ;* **Antrum** *(Diseases of, Complications, etc., of);* **Diabetes** *(Complications, etc., of);* **Diaphragm** *(Neuralgia, etc., of);* **Ear** *(Pain in);* **Exanthemata** *(Complications,*

Neuralgia.
etc., of); **Eye** *(Accommodation, etc., of, Disordered);* **Gout** *(Complications, etc., of);* **Herpes** *zoster ;* **Hyperæsthesia ; Lead-poisoning** *affecting the nervous system ;* **Muscles** *(Atrophy, etc., of);* **Myalgia ; Nerves** *(Wounds, etc., of);* **Nervestretching ; Nervous** *system (Diseases of, Functional);* **Nervous** *system (Syphilis of);* **Neuritis** *(Multiple);* **Neuroma ; Ovary** *(Neuralgia of);* **Pleurodynia ; Scapulalgia ; Sciatica ; Spinal** *irritation ;* **Stumps** *(Diseases of).*

Angelé (L.) * Contribution à l'étude des névralgies au point de vue de leur nature et de leur traitement par les injections irritantes. 4°. *Paris,* 1878.

Anstie (F. E.) Neuralgia and the diseases that resemble it. 8°. *London & New York,* 1871.
———. The same. 8°. *New York,* 1872.
———. The same. 8°. *New York,* 1882.
———. The same. 12°. *New York & London,* 1885.

Bretschneider (H.) Versuch einer Begründung der Pathologie und Therapie der äusseren Neuralgieen. 8°. *Jenæ,* 1847.

Brongers (J.) * De neuralgiis in genere. [Leyden.] 8°. *Amstelodami,* 1842.

Cartaz (A.) * Des névralgies envisagées au point de vue de la sensibilité récurrente (pathogénie et traitement). 4°. *Paris,* 1875.

Chapman (J.) Neuralgia and kindred diseases of the nervous system ; their nature, causes, and treatment. Also, a series of cases, preceded by an analytical exposition of them, exemplifying the principles and practice of neuro-dynamic medicine. 8°. *London,* 1873.

Chastanier (J.-L.-A.-P.-U.) * Dissertation sur la névralgie considérée en général. 4°. *Paris,* 1831.

Classen (J.) * Zur Statistik und Aetiologie der Neuralgie. 8°. *Kiel,* 1886.

Coussays (J.-J.) * De la névralgie considérée en général. 4°. *Paris,* 1812.

Delaine (A.) * Réflexions sur les névralgies en général. 4°. *Paris,* 1836.

Downing (C. T.) Neuralgia ; its various forms, pathology, and treatment. [The Jacksonian prize essay, 1850, with some additions.] 8°. *London,* 1851.

Dowse (T. S.) Neuralgia, its nature and curative treatment. The brain and diseases of the nervous system. v. 2. 8°. *New York,* 1880.

Dreyfus (P.-B.) * Des névralgies en général, et de leur traitement par le sous-carbonate de fer. 4°. *Strasbourg,* 1826.

Duignan (J.) * De neuralgia quædam. v. 2. 8°. *Edinburgi,* 1821.

Fontell (C. W.) * Afhandling om neuralgierne i allmänhet. 8°. *Helsingfors,* 1832.

Heath (R. A.) * On neuralgia. MS. 4°. *Washington University,* [n. d.]

Heidler (C. J.) Das Blut in seiner heilthätigen Beziehung zum Schmerz im Allgemeinen und zu den (wahren und unwahren) Neuralgien insbesondere. 8°. *Prag,* 1839.

Hunt (H.) On the nature and treatment of tic douloureux, sciatica, and other neuralgic disorders. 8°. *London,* 1844.

Jacob (P.-I.) * Sur la névralgie, considérée en général et dans ses différentes espèces. 4°. *Paris,* 1829.

James (H.) * De neuralgia. 8°. *Edinburgi,* 1831.

Kelly (T.) * De neuralgia. 8°. *Edinburgi,* 1810.

Kershaw (J. M.) Diseases of the brain and nervous system. Issued in eight parts. Facial neuralgia and the visceralgiæ. Their diagnosis and treatment. Pt. 1. 8°. *St. Louis,* 1878.

Neuralgia.

KOTTMANN (C.) * Nonnulla de neuralgiis. 8°. *Turici*, 1835.

LAWSON (H.) Sciatica, lumbago, and brachialgia; their nature and treatment, and their immediate relief and rapid cure by hypodermic injection of morphia. 8°. *London*, 1872.

——. The same. 2. ed. 8°. *London*, 1877.

LECLERC (M.-M.-J.) * De la névralgie générale. 4°. *Paris*, 1852.

MARTINET (L.) * Sur les névralgies, considérées en général, et sur l'emploi de l'essence de térébenthine dans la névralgie sciatique. 4°. *Paris*, 1818.

MAZE (G.) * Des névralgies au point de vue de leur étiologie et de leur traitement. 4°. *Paris*, 1874.

MURRAY (J. W. B.) * On neuralgia. 8°. *New York*, 1816.

PAYNE (J. A.) * De neuralgia. 8°. *Edinburgi*, 1813.

PÉCHEDIMALDJI (D.) * Des névralgies congestives. 4°. *Paris*, 1867.

PETROZ (A.-P.-M.) * Des névralgies en général, de leurs causes, de leur nature, de leur traitement. 4°. *Paris*, 1851.

PIENKOWSKI DE SUCHE-KOWNATY (C.-M.) * De la névralgie en général. 4°. *Paris*, 1849.

DE RANSE (F.) * Considérations sur la nature et le traitement des névralgies. 4°. *Paris*, 1861.

RIGAL (A.) * Causes et pathogénie des névralgies. 8°. *Paris*, 1872.

ROWLAND (R.) A treatise on neuralgia. 8°. *London*, 1838.

SCHNEIDER (J.) Die Neuralgien in der Zeit der Pubertäts-Entwickelung oder des mannbaren Alters. 2 v. 8°. *Leipzig*, 1843.

SCOTT (J.) Cases of tic douloureux, and other forms of neuralgia. 8°. *London*, 1834.

TEALE (T. P.) A treatise on neuralgic diseases, dependent upon irritation of the spinal marrow and ganglia of the sympathetic nerve. 8°. *London*, 1829.

——. The same. 8°. *Philadelphia*, 1830.

——. The same. 8°. *Woodstock, Vt.*, 1834.

——. The same. 12°. *Concord*, [n. d.]

THOMSON (A.) Untersuchung der Natur, Ursachen und Heilmethode der Nervenbeschwerden. Nach der 4. englischen Ausg. übersetzt und mit einigen Anmerkungen begleitet. 12°. *Hannover*, 1798.

THOMSON (G.) * De neuralgia. 8°. * *Edinburgi*, 1817.

TWEEDY (H.) Paralysis and neuralgia, their prevention and cure, [etc.] 2. ed. 8°. *Dublin*, 1857.

VALLEIX (F.-L.-I.) Traité des névralgies ou affections douloureuses des nerfs. 8°. *Paris*, 1841.

——. The same. Abhandlung über die Neuralgien . . . übersetzt und mit einigen Zusätzen begleitet von K. G. Gruner. 8°. *Braunschweig*, 1852.

VAN LAIR (C.) Les névralgies, leurs formes et leur traitement. Ouvrage couronné [etc.] 8°. *Bruxelles*, 1866.

——. The same. 2. éd. 8°. *Bruxelles*, 1882.

DE VERTEUIL (L.-A.-A.-G.) * Remarques sur les névralgies, et en particulier sur celles de l'appareil cérébro-spinal; considérations sur leurs causes, leurs symptômes, leur thérapeutique, et spécialement sur leur traitement par les préparations de morphine administrées par la méthode endermique. 4°. *Paris*, 1835.

WEIGEL (P. F.) * De neuralgiis cerebralibus et spinalibus ad chirurgiam spectantibus. 8°. *Monachii*, 1836.

WIEBECK (F. G. A.) * De neuralgiis quædam. 8°. *Halis*, [1842].

Neuralgia.

ANSTIE (F. E.) Neuralgia. Syst. Med. (Reynolds), Lond., 1868, ii, 717. ——. Note on Dr. Dale's case. Practitioner, Lond., 1873, x, 284–291.—**Baird** (J. B.) Neuralgia and its modern therapeusis. Tr. M. Ass. Georgia, Atlanta, 1878, xxix, 99–119.—**Barbieri** (G.) Delle neuralgie vaganti. Bull. d. sc. med. di Bologna, 1862. 4. s., xvii, 5; 80.—**Barbour** (T.) Observations upon the pathology and treatment of neuralgia. West. J. M. & S., Louisville, 1843, 2. s., viii, 401–418.—**Berghman.** Neuralgia ulnaris, neuralgia trigemini, coccygodinia. Förh. v. Svens. Läk.-Sällsk. Sammank., Stockholm, 1873, 247–250.—**Bigelow** (H. R.) An interesting case. Med. Rec., N. Y., 1880, xvii, 690.—**Black.** Observations on the topical pathology of the neuralgie. Prov. M. & S. J., Lond., 1842–3, v, 468–471.—**Böcker.** Neurologische Curiosität. Ztschr. f. klin. Med., Bresl., 1853, iv, 157.—**Bonnemaison.** Des névralgies en général. Gaz. méd.-chir. de Toulouse, 1873, v, 131; 137; 145; 153. *Also, in his:* Ess. de clin. méd., 8°, Toulouse, 1874, 47–81.—**Burrows** (G.) Clinical lecture on cases of neuralgia. Lond. M. Gaz., 1845, n. s., i, 483–486. — **Carmichael** (R.) Observations on sciatica and other neuralgic affections, with a consideration of their frequent origin from a disordered state of the stomach; interspersed with some novel views respecting the origin and prevention of gall-stones; both diseases exemplified by the author's own case; together with an account of the waters of Bagnères de Bigorre and Baréges in their treatment. Dublin J. M. Sc., 1838, xiii, 286–314.—**Cases** of neuralgia. Brit. M. J., Lond., 1870, i, 519.—**Caviole** (C.) Sur un cas de névrose singulière et complexe. Union méd., Par., 1856, x, 201.—**Cerise** (L.) Sur un cas de névrose émotive. *Ibid.*, 217–219.—**Chapman** (J.) Neuralgia; its pathology and treatment. Med. Times & Gaz., Lond., 1869, i, 298; 327; 433. ——. Neuralgia; its nature, causes, and treatment. Med. Mirror, Lond., 1870, vii, 71; 91; 109; 131; 147; 169; 187.—**Clarke** (J. L.) A case of cerebro-spinal paresis, accompanied by intense neuralgia and cerebro-spinal irritation. Brit. M. J., Lond., 1875, i, 607.—**Da Costa** (J. M.) A case of cerebral neuralgia, terminating fatally by serous apoplexy, with remarks on the occurrence of serous apoplexy. Charleston M. J. & Rev., 1859, xiv, 145–156. *Also,* Reprint.—**Dana** (C. L.) A clinical study of neuralgias, and of the origin of reflex or transferred pains. N. York M.J., 1887, xlvi, 87; 121.—**Discussion** on the pathology and treatment of neuralgia. Med. & Surg. Reporter, Phila., 1858–9, i, 228–230.—**Dupau.** Observation de névralgie multiple. J. de méd., chir. et pharm. de Toulouse, 1859, 3. s., iv, 139–141.—**Dupont de Tartas.** Quel est le caractère essentiel de la névralgie? Réflexions sur cette question. J. gén. de méd., chir. et pharm., Par., 1812, xliv, 61–74.—**Dupuy.** Les névralgies, le rhumatisme et le chloroforme. Bull. Soc. de méd. prat. de Par., 1867, 62–70.—**Elliotson** (J.) Neuralgia. Cycl. Pract. M. (Tweedie), Phila., 1845, iii, 381–385.—**Eskridge** (J. T.) A case of general neuralgia. J. Nerv. & Ment. Dis., N. Y., 1883, x, 471–475.—**État** actuel de la science sur la pathologie et le diagnostic des névralgies. Union méd., Par., 1847, i, 641.—**Evans** (R.) Cases of neuralgia of the face, and painful affections of the limbs successfully treated. Edinb. M. & S. J., 1824, xxi, 278–285.—**Fallani** (L.) Brevi considerazioni sopra alcuni casi di nevralgia, e di stato spasmodico. Raccoglitore med., Forlì, 1849, xxiv, 257–263.—**Ferran.** Cas de névralgie multiforme très intense; huit mois de durée; guérison. France méd., Par., 1863, x, 195–197.—**Flebbe** (C. D.) Waarneming wegens meenigvuldige, geweldige en buitengewoone toevallen van zenuw-ziektens aan eene lijderes overgekomen. Handel. v. h. geneesk. Genootsch., Amst., 1777, ii, 169–210.—**Foster** (J.) An extract from an inaugural dissertation on neuralgia. Am. M. Rev., Phila., 1826, iii, 362–375.—**Frey.** Zur Pathologie und Therapie der Neuralgien. Wien. med. Presse, 1869, x, 491–494.—**Gerbaud.** Névralgies diverses observées pendant l'hiver de 1843. Rec. d. trav. Soc. méd. d'Indre-et-Loire, Tours, 1843, 37–44.—**Gillespie** (W. A.) Cases of neuralgia. Boston M. & S. J., 1833–4, ix, 349. *Also:* Am. J. M. Sc., Phila., 1834, xiv, 115.—**Gorrie** (J.) An essay on neuralgia. N. York M. & Phys. J., 1828, vii, 327–343.—**Grasset** (J.) Physiologie pathologique des névralgies. Montpel. méd., 1877, xxxix, 432; 1878, xl, 232.—**Gross** (S. D.) Neuralgia. Phila. M. Times, 1872–3, iii, 599.—**Hallopeau** (H.) Névralgies. N. dict. de méd. et chir. prat., Par., 1877, xxiii, 756–802. — **Helfft** (J.) Neuralgien. Wien. med. Wchnschr., 1853, iii, 342.—**Hémey.** Observation de névralgie, avec phénomènes convulsifs se rattachant à l'épilepsie. Rec. d. trav. Soc. méd. d'obs. de Par., 1866–70, 2. s., ii, 16–24. — **Hermel** (E.) Recherches sur les névralgies et leur traitement. Ann. méd.-psych., Par., 1844, iii, 209–230. — **Heyfelder.** Seltene Fälle von Neuralgie. Med. Ztg., Berl., 1834, iii, 84. — **Hildreth** (C. C.) Observations in the neuralgiæ. Am. J. M. Sc., Phila., 1836, xviii, 77–87.—**Hinze.** Zur Casuistik der centripetalen Neuralgien. St. Petersb. med. Wchnschr., 1876, i, no. 18, 4–6.—**Holmes** (O. W.) On the nature and treatment of neuralgia. Boyls. prize diss. 1836–7, 8°, Bost., 1838, 135–243.—**Holt** (D.) Observations on neuralgia; with cases. Boston M. & S. J., 1845, xxxii, 337–340.—**Horn** (T. G.) Neuralgia as a prevailing disease in this climate.

Neuralgia.

Tr. Colorado M. Soc., Denver, 1876, 79–84.—**Hughes** (C. H.) Central lesions in neuralgia. St. Louis M. & S. J., 1879–80, xxxviii, 221–223.—**Hurd** (E. P.) A contribution to the study of neuralgia; an intractable case in private practice. Med. Rec., N. Y., 1876, xi, 743–747. — **Hutchinson** (B.) Cases of neuralgia, etc. Lond. M. & Phys. J., 1823, xlix, 281–286. ———. Case of neuralgia spasmodica. *Ibid.*, 1824, li, 271–276. ———. Cases of neuralgia. *Ibid.*, 1824, lii, 281–283.—**Jacobi** (A.) Neuralgia in infancy and childhood. Proc. M. Soc. County Kings, Brooklyn, 1881–2, vi, 59–68.—**James** (C.) Recherches théoriques et pratiques sur les névralgies et leur traitement. Gaz. méd. de Par., 1840, 2. s., viii, 673; 708. *Also*, Reprint.—**Jewell** (J. S.) Pathology and treatment of neuralgia. J. Nerv. & Ment. Dis., Chicago, 1877, iv, 207–232.—**Jones** (C. H.) Cases of neuralgia. Lancet, Lond., 1855, i, 577; 603. ———. On the nature, seat, and relations of neuralgia. *Ibid.*, 1859, ii, 258; 260. — **Katjisheff** (I.) O nevralgijach. Voyenno-med. J., St. Petersb., 1885, cliii, pt. 3, 139; 239. *Also:* Trudi Obsh. Russk. vrach. v S.-Peterb., 1885, ii, 203–230.—**Kenner** (R. C.) The etiology and treatment of neuralgia. Louisville M. News. 1885, xx, 209–211.—**Lange** (C.) Nogle Bemærkninger om Neuralgier og deres Behandling. Hosp.-Tid., Kjøbenh., 1875, 2. R., ii, 641; 657; 673; 705; 721; 737; 753. ———. Et par Notitser til Neuralgiernes Patologi og Behandling. *Ibid.*, 1880, vii, 2. R., 701–711.—**Lehmann** (L.) Central begründete Neuralgie, die nasse Einwickelung. Allg. med. Centr.-Ztg., Berl., 1858, xxvii, 17–20.—**Lepidi-Chioti** (G.) Nevralgie da alterato ricambio materiale. Morgagni, Napoli, 1881, xxiii, 87–98. — **Lereboullet** (L.) Névralgies. Dict. encycl. d. sc. méd., Par., 1878, 2. s., xii, 645–698.—**Lewis** (M. J.) The seasonal relations of chorea, rheumatism, and neuralgia. Maryland M. J., Balt., 1886–7, xvi, 496–498. — **Liégey.** Quelques généralités sur les névralgies et les pyrexies. Courrier méd., Par., 1870, xx, 127; 134; 141; 152; 162; 169.—**Lobb** (H.) The pathology and treatment of idiopathic and peripheral neuralgia. Lancet, Lond., 1859, ii, 589.—**Lombard** (H.-C.) Sur les névralgies, note lue le 6 février 1861 à la Société médicale de Genève. Écho méd., Neuchât., 1861, v, 113–124. *Also, in his:* Causeries [etc.], 8°, Neuchât., 1861, 15–26. — **M.** Neuralgias observadas en la provincia de la Rioja. Rev. méd.-quir., Buenos Aires, 1880–81, xvii, 337–341.—**M'Derment** (J.) † Edinb. M. & S. J., 1837, xlviii, 46–51.—**Mann** (E. C.) Neuralgia; its nature and treatment. Med. Bull. Phila., 1881, iii, 155–159.—**Martin** (A.) † Brit. M. J., Lond., 1859, ii, 565.—**Mathieu** (A.) Névralgie et périarthralgie de l'épaule. Progrès méd., Par., 1886, 2. s., iv, 1049.—**Mitchell** (C. B.) On tic douloureux, and other nervous affections. India J. M. & Phys. Sc., Calcutta, 1839, n. s., iv, 441; 530; 597; 642. — **Mitchell** (S. W.) [Cases of neuralgia, hemicrania, and pain.] Phila. M. Times, 1871–2, ii, 388.—**Monfalcon.** Névralgie. Dict. d. sc. méd., Par., 1819, xxxv, 500–552. — **Morris** (E.) A concise practical treatise on neuralgia; its various forms, pathology, and treatment. Tr. Prov. M. & S. Ass., Lond., 1853, xix, 1–49.—**Neuralgien** im Allgemeinen. Wien. med. Presse, 1866, vii, 164–166. — **Nicaise.** De la névralgie en général. [Extr.] Encéphale, Par., 1883, iii, 543–560. — **Nothnagel** (H.) Schmerz und cutane Sensibilitätsstörungen; Beitrag zur Pathologie der Neuralgien. Arch. f. path. Anat., etc., Berl., 1872, liv, 121–136. *Also,* Reprint. *Also, transl.:* Phila. M. Times, 1871–2, ii, 231–235. — **Observations** de névralgies. Éphém. méd. de Montpel., 1828, viii, 125–136. — **Ollivier.** Névralgie. Dict. de méd., 2. éd., Par., 1840, xxi, 1–26. — **Oppolzer.** Einige interessantere Fälle von Neuralgie, Wien. Med.-Halle, 1861, ii, 2; 12; 29.—**Osborne** (J.) Observations on the nature of neuralgia, and on the principles according to which the treatment of it ought to be conducted. Dublin J. M. Sc., 1837–8, xii, 254–267. — **Ouspensky.** Essai sur la pathologie des névralgies. Progrès méd., Par., 1876, iv, 622; 643; 667.—**Parsons** (C. W.) Fiske fund prize essay. "Neuralgia; its history, nature, and treatment." Am. J. M. Sc., Phila., 1854, n. s., xxviii, 417–446. *Also,* Reprint.—**Passagay.** Observations de névralgies. Clin. d. hôp., Par., 1829, iv, 202.—**Pierangeli** (M.) Osservazioni cliniche sopra alcune nevralgie infettive. Resoc. Accad. med.-chir. di Napoli, 1884, xxxviii, 187–191.—**Piorry** (P.-A.) Mémoire sur les névralgies et sur leur traitement. Gaz. méd. de Par., 1833, 2. s., i, 69; 93. ———. Névralgie. Bull. clin., Par., 1835–6, i, 257–262. — **Preston** (C. H.) † West. Lancet, Cincin., 1843–4, ii, 261–264. — **Putnam** (J. J.) Neuralgia. Syst. Pract. M. (Pepper), Phila., 1886, v, 1211–1240. — **Rambaud.** Observation d'un cas de névralgie rare. Gaz. méd. de Lyon, 1855, vii, 378–384. *Also:* Monit. d. hôp., Par., 1855, iii, 1158–1160. — **Ranking** (R.) Remarks on neuralgia. Lond. M. & Phys. J., 1825, liii, 124–126. — **Ranking** (W. H.) Neuralgia. Med. Times & Gaz., Lond., 1852, n. s., ix, 371.—**Robson** (R.) Remarks on neuralgia. Georgia M. Companion, Atlanta, 1872, ii, 138–142. — **Rosenthal** (M.) Beobachtungen über Neuralgien. Allg. Wien. med. Ztg., 1864, ix, 50; 58; 66; 75; 81; 98; 106.—**Ross** (J. J.) † † Lond. & Edinb. Month. J. M. Sc., 1844, iv, 950–954.—**Sandras** (D.-S.) Quelques réflexions sur la nature et le traitement d'une névralgie très-commune à Paris depuis quelques mois. Bull. gén.

Neuralgia.

de thérap., etc., Par., 1835, viii, 65–69. ———. De quelques névralgies et de la méthode de philosopher en médecine. [Rap. de Esquirol et Bally.] Bull. Acad. de méd., Par., 1838–9, iii, 27.—**Schlesier.** Zur Lehre von den Neuralgien. Mag. d. ges Heilk.. Berl., 1843, n. F., lx, 224–262.—**Seitz** (F.) Neuralgien. Deutsche Klinik, Berl., 1856, viii, 241–244.—**Shattuck** & **Storer.** Neuralgia. Boston M. & S. J., 1855, liii, 79. — **Sieveking** (E. H.) Clinical remarks on neuralgia. Lancet, Lond., 1861, i, 31; 81; 105; 131.—**Simon** (R. M.) † † Brit. M. J., Lond., 1886, i, 13.—**Skey** (F. C.) On the nature and treatment of acute neuralgia, or tic douloureux. Lond. M. Gaz., 1836–7, xix, 181–185.—**Slemons** (J. N.) Neuralgia. N. Orl. M. & S. J., 1855–6, xii, 351–354.—**Steele** (R. M.) Neuralgia. Ohio M. J., Columbus, 1881–2, i, 294–297.—**Stiebel.** Ueber Neuralgia rhachitica und das Symptom des Gegensatzes. Mag. f. d. ges. Heilk., Berl., 1824, xvi, 549–563.—**Strait** (S. L.) Remarks on neuralgia. South. J. M. & Pharm., Charleston, 1846, i, 486–494.—**Tarnovski** (P. N.) Dysthymia neuralgica. Ejened. klin. gaz., St. Petersb., 1881, i, 65; 85.—**Thirial** (H.) Quelques considérations générales sur certaines formes de névralgies, et notamment sur la nécessité de mieux étudier les rapports des différentes névralgies entre elles. J. de méd., Par., 1843, i, 232–240. — **Thomayer** (J.) Beobachtungen über Neuralgien an der medic. Klinik des Prof. Dr. T. Eiselt. Med.-chir. Centralbl., Wien, 1887, xxii, 340; 352; 364; 376.—**Thomson** (A. T.) Anomalous affection of a neuralgic character. Lancet, Lond., 1834–5, i, 642–644. — **Thomson** (T.) Neuralgia. Syst. Pract. M. (Tweedie), Phila., 1840, ii, 413–430. — **Traube** (L.) Zur allgemeinen Pathologie der Neuralgieen. *In his:* Ges. Beitr. z. Path. u. Physiol., 8°, Berl., 1878, iii, 570. — **Trenor** (J.) Observations on neuralgia; with cases. N. Am. M. & S. J., Phila., 1826, i, 245–272. *Also,* Reprint. — **Tripier** (A.) Ueber die Entstehung einer Art wenig gekannter Neuralgien; centrale und reflectorische Algien. Allg. Wien. med. Ztg., 1869, xiv, 105; 114; 165.—**Trousseau.** Névralgies. Union méd., Par., 1864, 2. s., xxi, 274; 307; 324.—**de U.** (F.) Observaciones sobre las causas y método curativo de algunas neuralgias. Gac. méd., Madrid, 1848, iv, 89.—**Uspensky.** Versuch einer Pathologie der Neuralgien. Deutsches Arch. f. klin. Med., Leipz., 1876, xviii, 36–52.—**Uwins** (D.) Remarks on the neuralgia, as a class of diseases; with an allusion to a case of aphonia in illustration. Tr. Ass. Apoth., etc., Lond., 1823, i, 369–376.—**Valleix.** Quelques considérations sur le diagnostic et traitement des névralgies. Bull. gén. de thérap., etc., Par., 1843, xxv, 17–24. ———. Considérations sur un cas de névralgie occupant presque tous les nerfs du corps. Union méd., Par., 1847, i, 252–254. ———. De la névralgie générale, affection qui simule des maladies graves des centres nerveux, et de son traitement. Bull. gén. de thérap., etc., Par., 1848, xxxiv, 17; 321; 421. *Also:* Ann. de méd. belge, Brux., 1848, i, 305: ii, 219; 306. ———. Observation de névralgie générale, suivie de considérations importantes sur le diagnostic de cette maladie. Gaz. d. hôp., Par., 1849, 3. s., i, 109.—**Vandeburgh.** † † Lond. M. & Phys. J., 1824, lii, 373–375.—**Vanluir** (C.) Des diverses formes qu'affectent les névralgies, et de la thérapeutique qu'il convient de leur opposer. J. de méd., chir. et pharmacol., Brux., 1865, xl, 529: xli, 19; 121; 203; 305; 405: 1866. xlii. 42; 117; 211; 304; 410; 516: xliii, 30; 120; 231. — **Warren** (J. C.) † † Boston M. & S. J., 1828–9, i, 1–6: 1829, 97; 113; 129; 145; 177. — **Webber** (S. G.) Neuralgia. Cycl. Pract. M. (Ziemssen), N. Y., 1881, Suppl., 511–518. — **Wheelock** (A. T.) † † Am. M. J. Sc., Phila., 1848, n. s., xvi, 510.—**Whitten** (T. J.) Neuralgia. Illinois M. Recorder, Vandalia, 1878–9, i, 29–33.—**Wilson** (S. S.) Neuralgia; its pathology and etiology. Ohio State J. Dent. Sc., Toledo, 1881, i, 61–65. *Also:* Am. J. Dent. Sc., Balt., 1881–2, 3. s., xv, 1–6.—**Woillez.** Importance de l'étude clinique des névralgies. Gaz. d. hôp., Par., 1863, xxxvi, 317.

Neuralgia (Causes of).

See, also, **Lead**; **Neuralgia** (*Dental*); **Neuralgia** (*Rheumatic*); **Neuralgia** (*Syphilitic*); **Neuralgia** (*Traumatic*).

LORBER (É.) * Étude clinique des névralgies et des points douloureux dans la tuberculose pulmonaire. 4°. *Nancy*, 1879.

QUERMONNE (L.) * Étude sur la pathogénie des névralgies. 4°. *Paris*, 1884.

RIGAL (A.) * Causes et pathogénie des névralgies. 4°. *Paris*, 1872.

Arney (G. F.) Reflex neuralgia; a case caused by a foreign body in the ear. Med. Bull., Phila., 1881, iii, 152.—**Auber** (P. A.) Las neuralgias en las anemias. An. de cien. méd., Madrid, 1877, iii, 262–269. — **Berger.** Ueber diabetische und nephritische Neuralgien. Breslau. aerztl. Ztschr., 1882, iv, 281. *Also:* Jahresb. d. schles. Gesellsch. f. vaterl. Kult. 1882, Bresl., 1883, lx, 13–16.—**Bordier** (A.) Les névralgies symétriques dans le diabète; revue critique. J. de thérap., Par., 1881, viii, 23–26. — **Catlin** (R.) The

Neuralgia (*Causes of*).

relations of pain to weather, studied during eleven years of a case of traumatic neuralgia, with notes by S. Weir Mitchell. Tr. Coll. Phys. Phila. (1881–3), 1883, 3. s., vi, 411–427, 2 pl. *Also*, Reprint. *Also:* Med. News, Phila., 1883, xliii, 46–49.—**Dana** (C. L.) A clinical study of neuralgias and of the origin of reflex or transferred pains. N. York M. J., 1887, xlv, 216. *Also*, Reprint. — **Dreyfous** (F.) Des névralgies saturnines. France méd., Par., 1881, ii, 769–773. ———. Des névralgies chez les tuberculeux. *Ibid.*, 1884, i, 784; 798. — **Florain.** Observation de névralgie diabétique. Gaz. méd. de Par., 1885, 7. s., ii, 101.— **Friedrichs** (A. G.) Reflex neuralgia dependent upon dental irritation. Tr. Louisiana M. Soc., N. Orl., 1887, 99–107. — **Fussell** (M. H.) Malarial neuralgia. Med. & Surg. Reporter, Phila., 1887, lvii, 574. — **Günther.** Zur Aetiologie der Trigeminus- und Intercostalneuralgien. Cor.-Bl. f. schweiz. Aerzte, Basel, 1885, xv, 79–83. — von **Hösslin** (R.) Ueber diabetische Neuralgieen. München. med. Wchnschr., 1886, xxxiii, 240. — **Kapper** (F.) Zur Aetiologie der Neuralgie. Allg. Wien. med. Ztg., 1886, xxxi, 278.—**Kerr** (J. G.) The heredity of neuralgia. Pacific M. & S. J., San Fran., 1885, xxviii, 207–209.— **Krauss** (F.) A curious case of malarial neuralgia. Canada Lancet, Toronto, 1884–5, xvii. 193–195.—**Leuf** (A. H. P.) Note on an abnormal distribution, hitherto unobserved, of the supra-orbital and infra-orbital nerves, explanatory of the recurrence of certain neuralgias. Arch. Med., N. Y., 1880, iii, 340–344.—**Lincoln** (W. L.) Neuralgia. Tr. Minn. M. Soc., St. Paul, 1882, xiv, 156–163.— **Maughan.** Referred neuralgias. J. Brit. Dent. Ass., Lond., 1887, viii, 803–807. — **Neustab** (J.) Neuralgia chuvstvitel. vietvei blujda. nerva. [Neuralgia from irritation of a branch of nervus vagus.] Russk. Med., St. Petersb., 1886, iv, 280–284. — **Reyburn** (R.) Neuralgia, its cause and cure. Maryland M. J., Balt., 1884–5, xii, 91–94.—**Sanchez Herrero** (A.) Génesis de las neuralgias y sus variedades etiológicas. Correo méd. castellano, Salamanca, 1885, ii, 13; 43; 73.—**Smith** (J. L.) Anæmic neuralgia in children. Med. Gaz., N. Y., 1880, vii, 161.— **Stedman.** Specific neuralgia. Boston M. & S. J., 1877, xcvi, 627. — **Whitwell** (J. R.) A contribution to the etiology of neuralgia. Edinb. M. J., 1887–8, xxxiii, 513–518. — **Witzel** (O.) Ganglien an der Greifseite der Hand als Ursache von Neuralgien. Centralbl. f. Chir., Leipz., 1888, xv, 137–142. *Also:* Wien. med. Bl., 1888, xi, 264–268.

Neuralgia (*Complications and sequelæ of*).

See, also, **Hair** (*Color of, Abnormities of*); **Skin** (*Diseases of, Neurotic*).

Boisson (P.-O.-A.) * Étude clinique sur les troubles trophiques de la névralgie trifaciale. 4°. *Paris*, 1876.

Bernutz. Observation de névralgie, avec phénomènes convulsifs se rattachant à l'épilepsie. Gaz. d. hôp., Par., 1866, xxxix, 309.—**Carril** (A. F.) Neuralgia; flemon difuso consecutivo y gangrena; muerte. Siglo méd., Madrid, 1861, viii, 483; 501.—**Erdmann.** Ueber die Bedeutung vasomotorischer und trophischer Störungen bei Neuralgien. Jahresb. d. Gesellsch. f. Nat.- u. Heilk. in Dresd. (1876-7), 1877, 136–138. — **Gubler** (A.) Névralgie réflexe et plus tard anesthésie du trijumeau en rapport avec une névrite du tronc du facial, et une paralysie incomplète du côté correspondant de la face. Gaz. méd. de Par., 1864, 3. s., xix, 743–745.—**Hughes** (C. H.) Note on a form of post-neuralgic encephalatrophic or cerebra-sthenic insanity. Alienist & Neurol., St. Louis, 1885, vi, 566–570. *Also*, Reprint.—**Jones** (C. H.) On paralysis of the motor nerves in neuralgic affections. Lancet, Lond., 1855, ii, 363. ———. Clinical lecture on a case of fronto temporal neuralgia, attended with cerebral disorder. Med. Press & Circ., Dubl., 1867, iv, 501.—**Latour.** Observation d'une affection du cœur, compliquée de névralgie faciale et crânienne. Rev. méd. franç. et étrang., Par., 1827, iii, 399–405. — **Liégey** (N.-F.) Accès de névralgie intercostale, de névralgie du testicule et de priapisme névralgique périodiques, se produisant successivement chez une même personne; guérison par les préparations de quinquina. Ann. méd. de la Flandre occid., Roulers, 1855, viii, 43–46. *Also*, Reprint.— **Lippich.** Hintere Gesichts-Neuralgie mit entzündlicher Steigerung und Fortpflanzung auf den Gehörnerven; Eiterabsonderung in der Schädelhöhle. Med. Jahrb. d. k. k. österr. Staates, Wien, 1838, n. F., xvii, 193–199.—**Mitchell** (S. W.) On certain forms of neuralgia accompanied with muscular spasms and extravasations of blood, and on purpura as a neurosis. Am. J. M. Sc., Phila., 1869, n. s., lviii, 116–122. *Also:* Tr. Coll. Phys. Phila. (1863–74), 1874, n. s., iv, 282–288. ———. Neuralgic headaches with apparitions of unusual character. Tr. Coll. Phys. Phila., 1887, 3. s., ix, 175–181. *Also:* Am. J. M. Sc., Phila., 1887, n. s., xciv, 415–419.—**Nothnagel** (H.) Trophische Störungen bei Neuralgieen. Arch. f. Psychiat., Berl., 1869, ii. 29–37. ———. Ueber cutane Sensibilitätsstörungen bei Neuralgien. Jahresb. d. schles. Gesellsch. f. vaterl. Kult. 1871,

Neuralgia (*Complications and sequelæ of*).

Bresl., 1872, xlix, 204.—**Notta** (A.) Mémoire sur les lésions fonctionnelles qui sont sous la dépendance des névralgies. Arch. gén. de méd., Par., 1854, ii, 1; 290; 543.— **Oppolzer.** Neuralgia nervi temporalis et hemiplegia nervi facialis. Deutsche Klinik, Berl., 1849, i, 41.—**Parinaud** (H.) & **Marie** (P.) Névralgie et paralysie oculaire à retour périodique, constituant un syndrome clinique spécial. Arch. de neurol., Par., 1886, xi, 15–29.— **Parks.** Abstract of a case of severe pain. accompanied with vomiting of oil, etc. Boston M. & S. J., 1855–6, liii, 190–192.—**Piorry** (P.-A.) Névralgie ascendante avec accès épileptique; névrite; hypernévrotrophie sur le lieu d'où partait la douleur; hémo-dermite varioleuse; entérite typhohémique; nécroscopie. Bull. clin., Par., 1835–6, i, 453–458.—**Ringer** (S.) A curious case of facial neuralgia with unilateral sweating cured by the application of aconite liniment. Practitioner, Lond., 1872, ix, 138–140.— **Sabatier** (J.-C.) Douleur fixe et sujette à de fréquents paroxysmes, ayant son siége en árrière et en haut de l'hypochondre droit, existant depuis deux ans, et succédant à des vomissements qui duraient depuis huit années; érysipèle à la face; mort. J. univ. et hebd. de méd. et chir. prat., Par., 1831, iii, 250–259. — **Williams** (R. G.) Neuralgia, rheumatism, vertigo. Tr. Texas M. Ass., Austin, 1887, 335.

Neuralgia (*Diagnosis and semeiology of*).

Lender (C.) Die Points douloureux Valleix's und ihre Ursachen. 8°. *Leipzig*, 1869.

Türck (L.) Beobachtungen über Verminderung der Pulsfrequenz bei neuralgischen Anfällen und über den Rhythmus solcher Anfälle. 8°. *Wien*, 1855.

Repr. from: Sitzungsb. d. k. Akad. d. Wissensch. Math.-naturw. Cl., Wien, 1855, xvii.

Armaingaud. Du point douloureux apophysaire dans les névralgies et de l'irritation spinale. Bordeaux méd., 1872, i, 251; 258; 267; 274; 283; 291. *Also:* Assoc. franç. pour l'avance. d. sc. Compt.-rend. 1872, Par., 1873, i, 893–930. *Also*, Reprint.—**Bonneau.** Névralgie de la tête du pharynx simulant la fièvre intermittente pernicieuse. Bull. Soc. de méd. de Poitiers, 1842, vi, 114–116.— **Derblich** (W.) Ueber simulirte Neuralgien. Militaerarzt, Wien, 1878, xii, 25; 43. — **Duplouy.** Observations de névralgies avec point apophysaire guéries par des applications de vésicatoires sur le point vertébral. Bordeaux méd., 1875, iv, 245. — **Griffin** (W.) How are neuralgic affections to be distinguished from inflammatory? Dublin J. M. Sc., 1836, x, 53–68.—**Martinet** (L.) Des névralgies simulant des maladies du cerveau. Rev. méd. franç. et étrang., Par., 1824, i, 86–95. — **Mitchell** (S. W.) The relations of pain to weather, being a study of the natural history of a case of traumatic neuralgia. Am. J. M. Sc., Phila., 1877, n. s., lxxiii, 305–329. — **Reinbold** (T.) Worauf beruht der Unterschied im Verhalten des Schmerzes bei Neuralgieen und resp. Entzündungen gegen äussere Berührung? Wchnschr. f. d. ges. Heilk., Berl., 1842, x, 682–688. — **Romberg** (M. H.) Zur Kritik der Valleix'schen Schmerzenspunkte in Neuralgieen. Arch. f. Psychiat., Berl., 1868, i, 1–7.—**Rosser** (J. C.) Meteorological perturbations and its bearings on the phenomena of idiopathic neuralgia. Tr. Minn. M. Soc., St. Paul. 1877, ix, 92–100, 6 tab. — **Starr** (M. A.) Cocaine as an aid to diagnosis in cases of neuralgia and neuritis. Med. Rec., N. Y., 1887, xxxii, 17. — **Vizioli** (F.) Il criterio elettro-diagnostico nelle nevralgie. Morgagni, Napoli, 1878, xx, 630–650.

Neuralgia (*Treatment of*).

See, also, **Acupuncture**; **Amputations** *at knee-joint*; **Artery** (*Carotid, Ligature of*); **Belladonna**; **Chloroform** (*Injection of*); **Electrotherapeutics**; **Extremities** (*Ligature of*); **Nerve-stretching**; **Nerves** (*Surgery of*); **Neuralgia** (*Facial, etc., Treatment of*); **Neurotomy.**

Bretschneider (H.) Versuch einer Begründung der Pathologie und Therapie der äusseren Neuralgieen. 8°. *Jena*, 1847.

Cadenaule (E.) * Du traitement des névralgies par les courants continus. 4°. *Bordeaux*, 1885.

Coulon (H.) * Des névralgies considérées principalement au point de vue de leur traitement. 4°. *Paris*, 1882.

Dalmenesche (A.) * Du traitement des névralgies en général. 4°. *Paris*, 1834.

Neuralgia (*Treatment of*).

DESTERNE (H.) Découverte d'un traitement des névralgies. 8°. *Paris*, 1851.

DUBOIS (S.) * Du traitement des névralgies par l'électricité et l'hydrothérapie, ou guide pratique d'électrohydrothérapie appliquée au traitement de ces maladies. 4°. *Paris*, 1878.

———. The same. 8°. *Paris*, 1878.

ELIOT (G.) The treatment of neuralgia in general practice. 8°. *Buffalo*, 1887.

EYMERY-HÉROGUELLE (J.) * Étude du Gelsemium sempervirens et de son action dans le traitement des névralgies. 4°. *Paris*, 1877.

GAUDRY (H.-O.) * Des injections médicamenteuses sous-cutanées et plus spécialement des injections de sulfate d'atropine dans les névralgies. 4°. *Paris*, 1863.

IEHL (L.-L.) * Contribution au traitement des névralgies. 4°. *Nancy*, 1879.

LAUTAR (L.) * Considérations sur le principe actif de la belladonna et sur son emploi en injections hypodermiques dans le traitement des névralgies. 4°. *Montpellier*, 1865.

LEUBE (R.) * Beiträge zur Behandlung der Neuralgien durch Anwendung des inducirten Stromes. 8°. *Tübingen*, 1862.

LOBB (H. W.) On the curative treatment of paralysis and neuralgia with the aid of galvanism. 2. ed. 12°. *London*, 1859.

LOISEAU (A.-C.-E.-L.) * Du traitement des névralgies par la cautérisation sulfurique. 4°. *Paris*, 1860.

MARTINET (L.) Mémoire sur l'emploi de l'huile de térébenthine dans la sciatique et quelques autres névralgies des membres. 8°. *Paris*, 1823.

MOSQUINOT (M.-J.-J.-R.) * Considérations sur le traitement de névralgies. 4°. *Paris*, 1854.

ROCHÉ (C.-L.-P.-D.) * Du traitement externe des névralgies. 4°. *Paris*, 1851.

SCHAPIROFF (B. M.) * Die Behandlung von Neuralgien mit Injectionen von Osmiumsäure. 8°. *Jena*, 1886.

Also, in: St. Petersb. med. Wchnschr., 1885, n. F., ii, 219; 227.

Abbot (S. L.) Acute sciatica and facial neuralgia; treatment by salicylic acid and salicylate of soda. Boston M. & S. J., 1879, ci, 83–87.—**Aconitine** (De l') dans les névralgies. Gaz. d. hôp., Par., 1879, lii, 1086.—**Adamkiewicz.** Ueber die Behandlung der Neuralgien mittelst der Kataphorese. Verhandl. d. Cong. f. innere Med., Wiesb., 1887, vi, 169–178. *Also:* Deutsche med. Wchnschr., Leipz., 1887, xiii, 848–850. *Also,* Reprint. *Also, transl.:* Przegl. lek., Krakow., 1887, xxvi, 249–251.—**Allaire** (P. A.) Neuralgia treated by the internal use of chloroform. Northwest. M. & S. J., Chicago & Indianap., 1851-2, viii, 388–392.—**Allnatt** (R. H.) On the treatment of neuralgia. Lancet, Lond., 1847, i, 331.—**Althaus** (J.) On the treatment of neuralgia by electricity. Med. Times & Gaz., Lond., 1858, xvii, 166. ———. On the comparative value of subcutaneous injections and the continuous galvanic current in the treatment of neuralgia. *Ibid.*, 1870, i, 636.—**Amezqueta** (T.) Observaciones sobre la eficacia de la moxa en la curacion de las nevralgias. Décadas de med. y cirug. práct., Madrid, 1822, viii, 64–77.—**Applicazione** della elettricità metallica per guarire le nevralgie e le paralisi; ed applicazione del vuoto pneumatico per vincere le ostinate costipazioni di ventre. Esculapio napol., Napoli, 1835, xvii, 280–285.—**Ayres** (S.) Ligation for neuralgia. Progress, Louisville, 1886, i, 17.—**Bardet** (G.) Note sur l'emploi du chlorure de méthyle dans les névralgies. Nouv. remèdes, Par., 1885, i, 76–80.—**Bardsley** (J. L.) Cases of neuralgia in which the acetate of morphia was successfully employed. *In his:* Hosp. Facts & Obs. [etc.], 8°, Lond., 1830, 101–108.—**Barella** (H.) Emploi des bains de valériane contre les névralgies. J. de méd., chir. et pharmacol., Brux., 1863, xxxvi, 24–27. ———. De la médication arsenicale dans les névralgies. Ann. Soc. de méd. d'Anvers, 1864, xxv, 97–146. [Rap. de Mayer], 146–148.—**Bargellini** (D.) Sull' uso della tintura del gelsomino a fior giallo como antispasmodico, specialmente nelle nevralgie del trigemino. Boll. d' ocul., Firenze, 1882-3, v, 330–333.—**Barrier.** Sur le traitement des névralgies par le chloroforme. Bull. gén. de thérap., etc., Par., 1848, xxxv, 537–544.—**Baxter** (G. A.) Hydrate

Neuralgia (*Treatment of*).

of chloral in neuralgia. Virginia M. Month., Richmond, 1876, iii, 188.—**Baylor** (G. W.) Hydrocyanate of iron in the treatment of epilepsy and neuralgias. South-West. M. Gaz., Louisville, 1887, i, 129.—**Beard** (G. M.) The treatment of neuralgia by electricity. Practitioner, Lond., 1873, xi, 187–196.—**Beccaria** (G.) Storia di nevralgia venuta in seguito di enteritide, curata coll' acetato di morfina praticato giusta il metodo endermico. Ann. univ. di med., Milano, 1830, lv, 494–502.—**Becquerel** (A.) Du traitement des névralgies par les courants électriques à forte tension. Union méd., Par., 1860, 2. s., v, 3; 52. *Also* [Abstr.]: Gaz. d. hôp., Par., 1859, xxxii, 539.—**Bell** (C.) On the action of purgatives on the different portions of the intestinal canal, with a view of removing nervous affections and tic douloureux. *In his:* Practical Essays, 8°, Edinb., 1841, 83–104.—**Belugou** (A.) Des indications des eaux de La Malou dans le traitement des névralgies, importance de l'étiologie en thérapeutique thermale. Ann. Soc. d'hydrol. méd. de Par., 1881-2, xxvii, 205–249.—**Benedikt** (M.) Ueber die Anwendung von Points de feu bei neuralgischen Affektionen. Pest. med.-chir. Presse, Budapest, 1882, xviii, 4; 37. ———. Ueber die Anwendung von Points de feu bei Neuralgien. Mitth. d. Wien. med. Doct.-Coll., 1883, ix, 28–31.—**Benton** (S. H.) Antithermics in neuralgias. Gaillard's M. J., N. Y., 1888, xlv, 129–133.—**Bertrand.** Fall von Neuralgie, behandelt durch narcotische Injectionen in's Zellgewebe. Cor.-Bl. d. deutsch. Gesellsch. f. Psychiat., etc., Neuwied, 1857, iv, 61-63.—**Bertrand** (H.) De la vératrine dans le traitement des névralgies. Rec. de mém. de méd. . . . mil., Par., 1866, 3. s., xvii, 303–313.—**Bibby** (F. P.) On the use of iodide of potassium in neuralgia. Maryland & Virg. M. J., Richmond, 1860, xiv, 201–203.—**Blackwood** (W. R. D.) On the treatment of neuralgia by static electricity. Med. & Surg. Reporter, Phila., 1881, xliv, 283–286.—**Blundell** (E. S.) Cure of neuralgic affections with the "mineral magnet". Lancet, Lond., 1883-4, i, 323-32½.—**Boddy** (E. M.) Neuralgia and its treatment. Med. Times & Gaz., Lond., 1877, ii, 383; 459.—**Bonnemaison.** Injections hypodermiques dans les névralgies. *In his:* Essais de clin. méd., 8°, Toulouse, 1874, 82–94. — **Bouchut.** Du traitement des névralgies par la teinture d'iode ordinaire et par la teinture d'iode morphinée. Union méd., Par., 1863, 2. s., xix, 134; 146. — **Bouros** (J.) Heilung eines beschwerlichen Gichtschmerzes durch den Zitterrochen. Wchnschr. f. d. ges. Heilk., Berl., 1840, 557-562.—**Bradbury.** Cases of neuralgia treated by phosphorus Brit. M. J., Lond., 1874, i, 344.—**Bradley** (S.) Tincture of yellow jasmine in neuralgia of the face and in whooping-cough. *Ibid.*, 1878, ii, 6.—**Bramwell** (J. P.) Case of epileptiform tic cured by nitroglycerine. *Ibid.*, 1884, ii, 609.—**Brenchley** (H. C.) On the use of hydrochlorate of ammonia in neuralgia. Lancet, Lond., 1858, ii, 396.—**Brophy** (T. W.) Neuralgia and its treatment. Missouri Dent. J., St. Louis, 1880, xii, 145 – 158. — **Broughton** (S. D.) Case of neuralgia, in which the carbonate of iron was successfully administered. Lond. M. & Phys. J., 1826, lv, 373 – 375. — **Bulgheri** (G.) La fustigazione elettrica nelle nevralgie. Gazz. med. ital. lomb., Milano, 1877, 7. s., iv, 11; 21. — **Burq** (V.) Des conditions du succès dans le traitement des névralgies en général et de la névralgie faciale en particulier par le cuivre, comme par d'autres métaux. Compt. rend. Soc. de biol. 1881, Par., 1882, 7. s., iii, 174–177. *Also:* Gaz. méd. de Par., 1881, 6. s., iii, 317. — **Cabaret.** Douleurs musculaires erratiques violentes; insuffisance des moyens de traitement ordinaires; excellents effets de la faradisation. Rev. de thérap. méd.-chir., Par., 1879, xlvi, 456.—**Callamand.** Du traitement chirurgical des névralgies. J. de thérap., Par., 1882, ix, 529–535. — **Carey** (H. G.) Neuralgia treated by black snake root. West. Lancet, Cincin., 1852, xiii, 460–465.—**Carlo** (R.) Sull' uso interno dell' olio essenziale di trementina nelle affezioni nevralgiche. Imparziale, Firenze, 1865, v, 79.—**Castiglioni** (C.) Intorno a' casi di nevralgie sanate coll' acetato di morfina. Gazz. med. di Milano, 1843, ii, 293.—**Cazenave** (A.) De la ligature des membres pour combattre les névralgies, et de son action sur l'intermittence. Bull. gén. de thérap., etc., Par., 1832, iii, 38–42. — **Cazenave** (J.-J.) Du traitement de quelques névralgies rebelles, notamment de celles qui sont insupportables par l'excès des douleurs. Mém. et bull. Soc. méd.-chir. d. hôp. de Bordeaux, 1868, iii, 77–97. *Also:* Gaz. méd. de Par., 1868, 3. s., xxiii, 447; 541. — **Chapman** (J.) Neuralgia; cases treated successfully by the spine-bag. Med. Press & Circ., Dubl., 1868, v, 201. ———. Two cases of neuralgia, with grave complications, treated successfully by means of the spinal ice-bag. Med. Times & Gaz., Lond., 1869, ii, 622–624. ———. Cases of neuralgia treated successfully by spine-bags. Med. Mirror, Lond., 1869, vi, 127; 147: 1870, vii, 15.—**Chapman** (R. U.) Neuralgia treated by subcutaneous injections of ether. Toledo M. & S. J., 1879, iii, 136.—**Charrière** (B.) Guérison prompte des névralgies à leur début par l'emploi topique du chlorure d'or et de sodium. Bull. gén. de thérap., etc., Par., 1856, l, 357.—**Chevandier.** Névralgies profondes et rebelles traitées par les fumigations résineuses de Pin mugho. J. de méd.

Neuralgia (*Treatment of*).

et chir. prat., Par., 1873, xliv, 404-407. — **Chippendale**
(J.) On the treatment of neuralgia by tobacco. Lancet,
Lond., 1845, i, 238. — **Chisholm** (J.) Cases illustrating
the effects of the local application of veratria in tic.
Edinb. M. & S. J., 1855, lxxxii (case-book), 2-4.—**Clarke**
(J. A.) On the treatment of neuralgia by iodine. Lancet, Lond., 1845, ii, 177. — **Clasen.** Das Oleum terebinthinæ als Specificum gegen Neuralgien. Deutsche
Klinik, Berl., 1860, xii, 254. — **Clemens** (T.) Die reflec-
tirte Neuralgie und deren Behandlung durch Elektricität,
nebst einigen Worten über die Anwendung des Induc-
tionsstroms. [12 cases.] *Ibid.*, 263; 274; 280; 321; 498;
503: 1861, xiii, 325; 337; 357; 369; 387. — **Clinical**
observations on the use of dextro-quinine in periodic
neuralgia. Month. Rev. M. & Pharm., Phila., 1880,
iii, 16. — **Coen** (G.) Vantaggiosi effetti ottenuti dalle
preparazioni di oppio col metodo endermico nelle nevralgie
e per clistere nel delirio nervoso traumatico. Gior. per
serv. ai progr. d. patol., Venezia, 1836, iv, 243-255. — **Collins** (L. J.) The deep injection of chloroform in neuralgia.
Clinic, Cincin., 1874, vii, 253. — **Comegys** (C. G.) The
cure of sciatica and violent neuralgia by hypodermic injections of ether. Cincin. Lancet & Clinic, 1879, n. s., ii,
10. — **Corning** (J. L.) On the medication of nerves; a
new method. N. York M. Month., 1886-7, i, 101-103.
————. The medication of nerves and its application in the
treatment of facial neuralgia and other painful nervous
affections; being a new mode of inducing prolonged neural
anæsthesia by pressure applied directly above the anæsthetic zone, and consequent occlusion of the subjacent
capillaries. Med. Rec., N. Y., 1887, xxxi, 319. ————. The
endermic use of cocaine in the treatment of certain phases
of neuralgia. Internat. J. Surg. & Antisept., N. Y., 1888,
i, 13. — **Coulon** (A.) Traitement de névralgies par l'injection sous-cutanée du sulfate d'atropine. Union méd.,
Par., 1859, 2. s., iii, 228-233.—**Courty** (A.) De l'efficacité
des injections narcotiques sous-cutanées, dans le traitement
des névralgies. Montpel. méd., 1859, iii, 289; 404. —
Cowdell (C.) Cases of neuralgia, etc., successfully
treated by narcotic injection. Brit. M. J., Lond., 1860, i,
103. — **Crosio** (L.) Nevralgie curate con l' uso esterno
dell' atropia. Gazz. med. ital. lomb., Milano, 1852, 3. s.,
iii, 262-264.—**Cumming** (W. H.) [On the use of quinine in neuralgia.] Atlanta M. & S. J., 1871-2, ix, 695.—
Cunier (F.) De l'usage externe de la vératrine dans le
traitement des névralgies. Bull. gén. de thérap., etc.,
Par., 1838, xv, 329-336.—**Curacion** pronta y eficaz de las
neuralgias por la cauterizacion transcurrente, modificada.
Gac. méd., Madrid, 1852, viii, 171-173.—**Curtis** (J.) Employment of the tincture of aconite in cases of neuralgia.
Lancet, Lond., 1840-41, ii, 474 —**Déclat.** De l'emploi du
valérianate d'ammoniaque dans le traitement des névralgies. Union méd., Par., 1856, x, 419. ————. De la guérison des névralgies par un médicament nouveau, le valérianate d'ammoniaque. Bull. gén. de thérap., etc., Par.,
1856, l, 549-553.—**Descroizilles & Ozenne.** De l'acide
salicylique et du salicylate de soude dans le traitement des
névralgies. Progrès méd., Par., 1877, v, 564.—**Desnos.**
Traitement des douleurs névralgiques rebelles. J. de méd.
et chir. prat., Par., 1874, xlv, 343.—**Dichiara** (F.) Due
casi di nevralgia dorso-intercostale del lato destro, curata
con la corrente continua. Gazz. clin. di elettroter., Palermo, 1883, i, 101-104. ————. Nevralgia del lato destro
con atrofia dei muscoli e idrartrosi del ginocchio destro curate con la corrente continua. *Ibid.*, 164-167.—**Dick** (R.)
New method of treating cases of purely functional neu-
ralgy; exhibition of the galvanic factors. Lancet, Lond.,
1840-41, i, 786-789. — **Domański** (S.) O bólach nerwo-
woych i ich léczeniu. [Neuralgia and its treatment.]
Przegl. lek., Krakow, 1877, xvi, 2; 14; 65; 161; 171. —
Downing (T.) On the aneuralgicon. Lancet, Lond.,
1849, i, 43-45. *Also* [Abstr.]: Med. Times, Lond., 1851, n.
s., iii, 236. — **Droste** (M.) Ueber die Wirksamkeit des
Extracti Strammonii gegen Tic douloureux und andere
Neuralgieen des Kopfes. J. d. pract. Heilk., Berl., 1839,
lxxxviii, 2. St., 87-103.—**Dufaur.** Observations de plusieurs névralgies, guéries par l'emploi de l'huile de térébenthine. Rév. méd. franç. et étrang., Par., 1824, iii, 214-
224.—**Dujardin-Beaumetz** (G.) Du traitement des
névralgies par les injections sous-cutanées au chlorhydrate
de morphine. Gaz. d. hôp., Par., 1864, xxxvii, 542; 550.
————. Nouveaux cas de névralgies rebelles traités avec
succès par les injections sous-cutanées ou chlorhydrate de
morphine. Bull. gén. de thérap., etc., Par., 1865, lxviii, 38-
40. ————. On the treatment of neuralgia. Med. News,
Phila., 1883, xlii, 405; 433; 461.—**Dupré** (P.-L.) Quelques observations sur l'emploi du sulfate de quinine dans
le traitement de plusieurs maladies, et particulièrement
la névralgie. J. de physiol. expér., Par., 1822, ii, 210-219.—
Dupuy. Névralgie symptomatique d'épuisement du
centre nerveux spinal, traitée au moyen des applications
méthodiques du chloroforme. France méd., Par., 1864, ii,
188-190. — **Duval** (E.) Névralgie précordiale avec débilité anémique; idées tristes, hypochondriaques; insuffisance des moyens ordinaires; guérison par l'application
méthodique de l'hydrothérapie. Gaz. d. hôp., Par., 1863,
xxxvi, 326.—**Eliot** (G.) The treatment of neuralgia in

Neuralgia (*Treatment of*).

general practice. Buffalo M. & S. J., 1887-8, xxvii, 157-
164.—**Emploi** (De l') du Datura stramonium contre les
névralgies faciales. Bull. gén. de thérap., etc., Par., 1837,
xii, 239-241.—**Esperon** (A. L.) Dos casos de neuralgia
tratados con éxito por la parthenina. Crón. méd.-quir. de
la Habana, 1885, xi, 205-207.—**Eulenburg** (A.) Die Os-
miumsäurebehandlung der peripheren Neuralgien. Berl.
klin. Wchnschr., 1884, xxi, 99-101.—**Ewing** (J. H.) Case
of neuralgia cured by acupuncturation. N. Am. M. &
S. J., Phila., 1826, ii, 77. *Also:* Lond. M. Reposit., 1826,
n. s., iii, 225.—**Fall** (C. J.) On the external use of common salt in intermittent or neuralgic pains of the head.
South. M. & S. J., Augusta. 1853, n. s., ix, 581-584. —
Fauverge. Observation sur une névralgie compliquée
guérie par les émoliens unis à la violette pensée. J. gén. de
méd., chir. et pharm., Par., 1813, xlvi, 383-386.—**Fenton**
(J.) On an instrument for applying heat in neuralgic affections generally. Lancet, Lond., 1849, i, 122.—**Féréol.** Du
sulfate de cuivre ammoniacal contre les névralgies rebelles.
Bull. et mém. Soc. de thérap., Par., 1881, xiii, 43-48.—
Finco (G.) Nevralgie guarite coll' ustione del piede e
dell' orecchio. Gazz. med. ital. lomb., Milano, 1869, 6. s.,
ii, 77; 85.—**Fischer** (G.) Antifebrin gegen lancinirende
Schmerzen. München. med. Wchnschr., 1887, xxxiv, 425-
427. — **Fleury** (L.) Des douches froides et de la suda-
tion appliquées au traitement des névralgies et des rhumatismes musculaires. Gaz. méd. de Par., 1850, 3. s., v, 283;
300; 342.—**Flies** (E.) Electrotherapeutische Mittheilungen im Gebiete der Neuralgieen. Allg. med. Centr.-Ztg.,
Berl., 1862, xxxi, 361; 369.—**Foissac.** Considérations pratiques sur le traitement des névralgies. Union méd., Par.,
1876, 3. s., xxii, 309; 345; 387; 441; 485; 521; 557; 593;
633.—**Ford** (M.) Jamaica dogwood in neuralgia. Louisville M. News, 1880, ix, 295.—**Fraenkel** (E.) Ueber parenchymatöse Ueberosmiumsäureinjectionen. Berl. klin.
Wchnschr., 1884, xxi, 234-236.—**Fraenkel** (S.) Ueber
subcutane Antipyrin-Injection bei schmerzhaften Krankheiten. Deutsche med. Wchnschr., Leipz., 1887, xiii, 895.
Also, Reprint.—**Francis** (C. R.) Treatment of neuralgia. Med. Press & Circ., Lond., 1882, 3. s., xxxiv, 457; 480;
502 —**Galicier.** Guérison d'une douleur névralgique de
la tête, par l'emploi du chloroforme. J. de la sect. de méd.
Soc. acad. Loire-Inf., Nantes, 1849, n. s., xxv, 101.—**Gamberini** (P.) Neuralgie curate col solfato di morfina per
met)do endermico. Bull. d. sc. med. di Bologna, 1839, 2. s.,
vii, 216-219. ———— Neuralgia guarita coll' agopuntura.
Ibid., 1869, 6. s., i, 408.—**Garavaglia** (B.) Nevralgia tetaniforme
curata coll' idrato di cloralio. Gazz. med. ital. lomb., Milano, 1869, 6. s., ii, 408.—**Garretson** (J. E.) Neuralgia;
[neurotomy]. Med. & Surg. Reporter, Phila., 1882, xlvi,
35. ————. Surgical treatment of neuralgia. Phila. M.
Times, 1884-5, xv, 23-27.—**Gasparini** (L.) Il solfuro di
carbonio nelle nevralgie. Gazz. med. ital. lomb., Milano,
1885, 8. s., vii, 367-370.—**Gattère.** Quelques mots sur
l'emploi des sels de morphine dans les névralgies. J. de
la sect. de méd. Soc. acad. Loire-Inf., Nantes, 1846, n. s.,
xxii, 18-25.—**Genth.** Zwei Fälle von Krampfleiden, geheilt durch Eisenbäder. Cor.-Bl. d. deutsch. Gesellsch. f.
Psychiat., etc., Neuwied, 1855, ii, 1-3.—**Géry** (L.-H.) De
l'emploi de l'extrait de datura stramonium contre les
névralgies faciales. Bull. gén. de thérap., etc., Par.,
1838, xiv, 51-54.—**Giacometti** (V.) Storia di grave prosopalgia guarita con l' applicazione della magnete. Gazz.
med. ital. lomb., Milano, 1852, 3. s., iii, 150.—**Gibb** (C.
J.) Endermic application of morphia in neuralgic pains.
Lancet, Lond., 1846, i. 673.—**Goss** (W.) Cases of neuralgia successfully treated with the colchicum autumnale.
Ibid., 1832-3, i, 426.—**Gradowicz** (E.) Solutio arsenicalis Fowleri gegen Neuropathie. Med. Ztg. Russlands,
St. Petersb., 1846, iii, 180.—**Graves** (R. J.) Treatment
of sciatica and lumbago. Dublin J. M. Sc., 1840, xviii,
242-247.—**Guibert** (T.) De l'aconitine dans les névralgies. Marseille méd., 1885, xxii, 177-179.—**Hardwicke**
(J.) On digitalis in neuralgia. Assoc. M. J., Lond., 1855,
i, 512.—**Harless** (C. F.) Die Acupunctur, als Mittel gegen den Gesichtsschmerz und andere ihm verwandte Neuralgieen. N. Jahrb. d. teutsch. Med. u. Chir., Hamm,
1825, ix, 2. St., 1-18.—**Hauff.** Ueber die Wirksamkeit
des gerbestoffsauren Chinin, Chinum tannicum, bei typischen Neuralgieen. Jahrb. f. prakt. Heilk., Tübing.,
1845, i, 48-55.—**Hay** (W.) Valerianate of ammonia in the
treatment of neuralgia. Northwest. M. & S. J., Chicago,
1857, xiv, 444-446. — **Henroz** (F.) De la compression
comme moyen curatif de quelques névralgies. Ann. de
méd. belge, Brux., 1835, ii, 2-8.—**Hermel** (E.) Recherches sur les névralgies traitées par le quinquina et ses préparations. Gaz. méd. de Par., 1846, 3. s., i, 148; 166. —
Hickman (J. W.) Neuralgia; importance of treating
the paroxysm. Med. & Surg. Reporter, Phila., 1879, xli,
173.—**Hill** (L. A.) Treatment of neuralgia. South. M. &
S. J., Augusta, 1857, n. s., xiii, 147-150.—**Hofmann** (O.)
Hochgradige Neuralgia spinalis; Heilung durch den galvanischen Strom. Memorabilien, Heilbr., 1869, xiv, 190 —
Hogg (C.) On the influence of large doses of quinine in
neuralgia. Lancet, Lond., 1850, ii, 575.—**Holden** (J. S.)
Some notes on neuralgia and its treatment. Brit. M. J.,
Lond., 1871, i, 639. — **Hooper** (J.) Intractable case of

Neuralgia (*Treatment of*).

neuralgia cured by oxygen. *Ibid.*, 1862, i, 277–279.—**Hunter** (C.) On narcotic injections in neuralgia. Med. Times & Gaz., Lond., 1858, xvii, 408. — **Iliff** (W. T.) Cases of neuralgia successfully treated with carbonate of iron. Lond. M. & Phys. J., 1823, i, 271. — **Injections** narcotiques sous-cutanées dans le traitement des névralgies. Gaz. d. hôp., Par., 1859, xxxii, 551.—**Jacoby** (G. W.) On the use of osmic acid in peripheral neuralgias. J. Nerv. & Ment. Dis., N. Y., 1885, n. s., x, 326–331. *Also:* Med. Rec., N. Y., 1885, xxvii, 712. *Also:* N. York M. J., 1885, xlii, 123–126. *Also,* Reprint. ———. The treatment of neuralgias by means of intense cold. Med. Rec., N. Y., 1887, xxxii, 473–475.—**Jacques** (J.) Sur l'inoculation des sels de morphine dans les névralgies et surtout dans l'ischias. Ann. Soc. de méd. d'Anvers, 1842, 379–391.—**Jaques.** Case of severe neuralgic affection, cured by carbonate of iron. Lond. M. & Phys. J., 1826, n. s., i, 545.—**Jobert** (*de Lamballe*). Mémoire sur la thérapeutique des névralgies; procédé mixte; section et cautérisation des nerfs. Union méd., Par., 1854, viii, 175; 180.—**Jones** (H. M.) On the action of aconite and quinine in neuralgia. Med. Press & Circ., Lond., 1868, vi, 5. — **Jurasz** (A.) Gelsemium sempervirens als antineuralgisches Mittel. Centralbl. f. d. med. Wissensch., Berl., 1875, xiii, 513–515.—**Kahler** (O.) Gelsemium sempervirens ein Antineuralgicum? Prag. med. Wchnschr., 1876, i, 171–174.—**King** (J. T.) An old neuralgia cured by an operation. Am. J. M. Sc., Phila., 1879, n. s., lxxviii, 156. — **de Kirckhoff.** Observations pratiques sur l'efficacité de la teinture de Datura stramonium dans les névralgies. Arch. gén. de méd., Par., 1827, xiv, 373.—**Knott** (S. J.) Cases of sciatica and neuralgia successfully treated by galvanism. Lancet, Lond., 1875, ii, 872–874.—**Koyen** (J.) Névralgie rhumatismale, guérie au moyen de la galvanopuncture. Ann. Soc. de méd. d'Anvers, 1849, vi, 426–430.—**Kreuser.** Gebesserter Gesichtsschmerz durch äussere Anwendung des Strychnins und des schwefelsauren Chinins. Med. Cor.-Bl. d. württemb. ärztl. Ver., Stuttg., 1832–3, i, 95.—**Kunze** (R. E.) Cereus Bonplandii in neuralgia. Therap. Gaz., Detroit, 1880, n. s., i, 89.—**Lange** (C.) Et Par Notitser til Neuralgiernes Patologi og Behandling. Hosp.-Tid., Kjøbenh., 1880, 2. R., vii, 721–728.—**Lawson** (G.) On the surgical treatment of neuralgia. Med. Times & Gaz., Lond., 1878, i, 137.—**Le Dentu.** De la révulsion interstitielle par les injections hypodermiques de nitrate d'argent. France méd., Par., 1877, xxiv, 225–227. *Also:* Courrier méd., Par., 1877, xxvii, 117–119. — **Legouest.** De la cure chirurgicale des névralgies. Bull. Soc. de chir. de Par. (1864), 1865, 2. s., v, 299–306. — **Legros.** Traitement des douleurs névralgiques, rhumatismales, etc., par la vésication volante morphinée. Gaz. d. hôp., Par., 1863, xxxvi, 306.—**Leonard** (J. P.) On the treatment of neuralgia, with cases. Boston M. & S. J., 1845, xxxii, 359–361.—**Leriche.** Du traitement des névralgies par l'emploi de térébenthine à petites doses. Union méd., Par., 1848, ii, 492.—**Lipburger** (J.) Ein Beitrag zur Behandlung peripherer Neuralgien mit Ueberosmiumsäure. Centralbl. f. d. ges. Therap., Wien, 1884, ii, 97–100. — **Lobb** (H.) Acute neuralgia cured with the aid of the continuous galvanic current. Lancet, Lond., 1860, i, 520. — **Lush** (W. J. H.) Cases of neuralgia treated with tonga. *Ibid.*, 1880, i, 835.—**Lynch** (M. H.) Treatment of neuralgia by Indian hemp; physiology of the nerves. Prov. M. J., Lond., 1843, vi, 9–11.—**Lysserman** (L.) Uzhlad na balneoterapiu nevralhiy. [The balneotherapia of neuralgia.] Moskov. med. Gaz., 1866, 403–407. — **M'Colgan** (J. T.) Local anæsthesia in neuralgia. South. Pract., Nashville, 1882, iv, 201–203.—**Mader** (J.) Behandlung von Neuralgien mit inducirtem Strom. Ber. d. k. k. Krankenanst. Rudolph-Stiftung in Wien (1872), 1874, 100–107. ———. Zur Therapie der Neuralgien. Med.-chir. Centralbl., Wien, 1879, xiv, 509; 520; 532; 542. — **Magistel.** Mémoire sur l'emploi de l'acétate de morphine par la méthode endermique, dans le traitement des névralgies connues sous le nom de migraine, hémicrânie, etc. Gaz. méd. de Par., 1834, 2. s., ii, 627–629.—**Marmisse.** L'inefficacité du chloral contre une névralgie hystériforme et périodique. Gaz. méd. de Bordeaux, 1874, iii, 333–337.—**Marotte.** De l'emploi topique du nitrate d'argent fondu dans le traitement des névralgies. J. d. conn méd.-chir., Par., 1851, xix, 566–574.—**Martinet** (L.) Recherches sur l'efficacité de l'huile de térébenthine dans le traitement des névralgies, et particulièrement de la sciatique. Rev. méd. franç. et étrang., Par., 1828, iv, 222–228. ———. Du traitement des névralgies. *Ibid.*, 1834, ii, 52–72.—**Masurel.** De l'emploi de l'émétique dans le traitement des névralgies. Assoc. franç. pour l'avance. d. sc. Compt. rend. 1877, Par., 1878, vi, 798–800. — **Mays** (T. J.) Some forms of neuralgia treated with theine. Polyclinic, Phila., 1886–7, iv, 357–359.—**Mazzoni** (A.) Storia di un' antica nevralgia dorsale, guarita coll' agopuntura. Gazz. med. ital. prov. venete, Padova, 1862, v, 193. — **Merten.** Zur Wirkung der subcutanen Carbolsäure-Injectionen bei Neuralgien. Allg. med. Centr.-Ztg., Berl., 1876, xlv, 885.—**Meyer** (C.) Salicylsäure gegen Neuralgien. Aerztl. Int.-Bl., München, 1876, xxiii, 433.—**Meyer** (M.) Ueber die Behandlung der Neuralgien durch Electricität. Deutsche Klinik, Berl., 1857, ix, 81–85.—**Millard** (H. B.) On

Neuralgia (*Treatment of*).

the treatment of sciatica and neuralgic affections by congelation with methyl chloride. Therap. Gaz., Detroit, 1886, 3. s., ii, 84–86.—**Miller** (Katharine). Electricity in muscular rheumatism and neuralgia; a case. Peoria M. Month., 1884–5, v, 343.—**Mohr** (D.) Die Anwendung der Ueberosmiumsäure bei Neuralgien. Wien. med. Wchnschr., 1884, xxxiv, 1400. — **Mondière** (J.-T.) Quelques faits de médecine-pratique; observations thérapeutiques sur divers névralgies. Arch. gén. de méd., Par., 1835, 2. s., vii, 183–219. — **Moreno** (E.) La neuralgia y su tratamiento hidro-mineral. An. Soc españ. de hidrol. méd., Madrid, 1879–80, iii, 143; 180; 239; 391: 1880–81, iv, 93.—**Morganti** (G.) Nevralgie guarite con l' atropina. Gazz. med. ital. lomb., Milano, 1852, 3. s., iii, 413–416.—**Morton** (T. G.) Neuralgia, and nerve-sections. Surg. Penn. Hosp., Phila., 1880, 124–132. — **Muriate** of ammonia in neuralgia. Lancet, Lond., 1859, i, 215. — **Musso** (E.) Nevralgie e reumatismi curati coll' elettricità o specialmente col jodoïormio. Indipendente, Torino, 1881, xxxii, 217; 246; 270.— **Neftel** (W. B.) Contribution to the treatment of neuralgias. Med. Rec., N. Y., 1879, xv, 97–99. ———. Zur elektrischen Behandlung der Neuralgien und verwandter schmerzhafter Affectionen. Arch. f. Psychiat., Berl., 1885, xvi, 45–65. — **Neuber** (G.) Ueberosmiumsäure-Injectionen bei peripheren Neuralgieen. Mitth. a. d. chir. Klin. zu Kiel, 1883–4, 1. Hft., 19–23. *Also:* Med.-chir. Centralbl., Wien, 1884, xix, 230–232. — **Nevralgias** seu tratamento pelo croton-chloral. Gaz. med. de Lisb., 1874, 4. s., i, 511.—**Névralgie** générale ou disséminée; de la cautérisation intercurrente dans les névralgies. J. d. conn. méd.-chir., Par., 1849–50, xvii, pt. 1, 89–91. — **Névralgies** traitées avec succès par les douches capillaires (aquapuncture). Bull. gén. de thérap., etc., Par., 1865, lxix, 36–40. — **Newcomb** (C. H.) On the value of Gelseminum sempervirens in facial neuralgia. Cincin. Lancet & Obs., 1875, xviii, 531–533. — **Note** sur l'emploi des bains de sulfure de chaux contre une névralgie lombaire. Rec. de mém. de méd. . . . mil., Par., 1822, xii, 303. — **Notta** (A.) Du traitement des névralgies par la cautérisation transcurrente. Union méd., Par., 1847, i, 494; 506; 509; 514. *Also,* Reprint.—**O'Connor.** Cases illustrating the value of valerianate of ammonia in the treatment of the more severe forms of neuralgia. Lancet, Lond., 1862, i, 68. *Also, transl.:* Bull. gén. de thérap., etc., Par., 1862, lxii, 222–226.—**Ogle** (J. W.) Subcutaneous injection repeated between forty and fifty times for neuralgia of the arm; recovery. Med. Times & Gaz., Lond., 1866, ii, 474. — **Oil** (The) of turpentine in the treatment of neuralgia and particularly of sciatica. Med. J. N. Car., Raleigh, 1861, iii, 127–129.—**Onimus.** De l'emploi des courants électriques dans les névralgies. Union méd., Par., 1885, 3. s., xl, 961–963.—**Oppolzer.** Zur Behandlung der Neuralgien. Ztschr. f. Nat.- u. Heilk. in Ungarn, Oedenburg, 1860, xi, 435. — **Ostinata** nevralgia sopracigliare guarita con le frizioni d' etere solforico. Gazz. med. ital. lomb., Milano, 1858, 4. s., iii, 269. — **Ozenne.** Névralgie traitée par l'acide salicylique; guérison rapide. Abeille méd., Par., 1877, xxxiv, 177. *Also:* Progrès méd., Par., 1877, v, 286.—**Pajot.** Observation de névralgie guérie par l'acupuncture. Arch. gén. de méd., Par., 1825, vii, 562–565. — **Palmer** (J. D.) Sulphate of nickel in neuralgia. Richmond & Louisville M. J., Louisville, 1868, v, 270.—**Palomares** (E.) Tratamiento termo-mineral de las neuralgias en el establecimiento balneario de Alhama de Granada. Gac. méd. de Granada, 1887, vi, 97; 129.—**Parker** (W. J.) An anti-neuralgic prescription (Tr. gelseminum). Mississippi Valley M. Month., Memphis, 1883, iii, 123. — **Peebles** (J. F.) On the use of diluents in certain forms of neuralgia. Virginia M. & S. J., Richmond, 1855, iv, 373–375.—**Peez.** Die Wirksamkeit Wiesbadens in verschiedenen Arten von Gesichtsschmerz, durch eine Reihe von Krankengeschichten erläutert. Heidelb. klin. Ann., 1831, vii, 295–310. — **Pietrzikowski** (E.) Casuistische Beiträge zur Behandlung der Neuralgien und besonders der Trigeminusneuralgie. Prag. med. Wchnschr., 1887, xii, 355; 370; 380; 388; 405; 410; 420; 426. — **Pirotte** (F.) Nouveau traitement des névralgies par l'éther pulvérisé. Ann. Soc. méd.-chir. de Liége, 1867, vi, 265–276. — **von Pitha.** Zur Diagnose und Behandlung der Neuralgien, insbesondere über die subcutanen Morphin-Injectionen. Allg. Wien. med. Ztg., 1875, xx, 1; 9; 17; 25; 33; 41; 49. *Also, transl.:* Med. Times & Gaz., Lond., 1875, ii, 356; 591; 619.—**Pohl** (J.) Seltener Fall einer Central-Neuralgie, mit Hinblick auf die neuesten Forschungen in der Nervenphysik und Electrotherapie. Vrtljschr. f. Psychiat., Neuwied u. Leipz., 1867–8, i, 363–377.—**Quelques** (De) névralgies traitées par l'injection du sulfate d'atropine dans le tissu cellulaire sous-cutané. Gaz. d. hôp., Par., 1859, xxxii, 353. — **Quinche** (P.) Del tratamiento de las neuralgias por el método sustitutivo, por medio de las inyecciones hipodérmicas irritantes. Rev. méd.-quir., Buenos Aires, 1868, v, 390–399.—**Radcliffe** (C. B.) Practical hints on the treatment of nervous pain and neuralgia. Brit. M. J., Lond., 1863, ii, 489–491.—**Raige-Delorme.** Sur l'emploi de l'huile de térébenthine dans la sciatique et quelques autres névralgies des membres. Arch. gén. de méd., Par., 1824, iv, 400–410.—**Ramirez** (L.) Nevralgias

Neuralgia (*Treatment of*).

y su tratamiento. Gac. méd. de México, 1867, iii, 17–24. — **Rand** (B. H.) Note on a case of neuralgia cured by accidental shock. Phila. M. Times, 1871–2, ii, 304.—**Rankin** (F. H.) Spasmodic neuralgia of nearly three years' standing, relieved by correction of spasm of the ciliary muscles and by circumcision. Med. Rec., N. Y., 1882, xxi, 9–11.—**Redtenbacher** (L.) Beitrag zur Behandlung peripherer Neuralgien mit Ueberosmiumsäure. Wien. med. Bl., 1884, vii, 837. — **Reveillé-Parise.** Considérations thérapeutiques sur les névralgies continues et intermittentes. Bull. gén. de thérap., etc., Par., 1837, xiii, 101–105.—**Ringer** (S.) & **Murrell** (W.) On tonga; a remedy for neuralgia, used by the natives of the Fiji Islands. Lancet, Lond., 1880, i, 360.—**Robarts** (H. P.) Remarks on the treatment of neuralgic affections, by the liquor cinchonæ flavæ of Mr. Battley. Lond. & Edinb. Month. J. M. Sc., 1841, i, 888–894. — **Rockwell** (A. D.) & **Beard** (G. M.) Cases of neuralgia treated by electricity. Boston M. & S. J., 1868, lxxviii, 295–299. ———. The treatment of neuralgia by electrization. Med. Rec., N. Y., 1869–70, iv, 28; 169; 388. — **Ruppaner** (A.) Researches upon the treatment of neuralgia by the injection of narcotics and sedatives; with remarks. Boston M. & S. J., 1860, lxii, 193; 216; 241; 280. *Also*, Reprint.—**Rusconi** (U.) Le iniezioni ipodermiche di acqua distillata in alcune nevralgie essenziali. Gazz. d. osp., Milano, 1881, ii, 813–828.—**de Sainte-Marie.** Observation d'un cas de névralgie, hyperesthésie de la peau, de presque tout un côté du corps, avec des phénomènes intérieurs cardiaques, pulmonaires et gastriques, guérie par la cautérisation transcurrente. J. de méd. de Bordeaux, 1850, viii, 257–274. — **Salomone-Marino** (S.) L'ergotina nelle nevralgie. *In his:* Stud. di. clin. med., 8°, Palermo, 1885, 251–263. — **Sanders** (E.) The external application of carbon disulphide for the relief of neuralgic pains. Med. News, Phila., 1882, xl, 371–375.—**Sandras** (S.) Traitement des causes des névralgies. J. d. conn. méd.-chir., Par., 1847–8, xv, pt. 2, 52–58. ———. Traitement direct des névralgies suivant leur siége. *Ibid.*, 1848–9, xvi, pt. 1, 3; 45. *Also:* Ann. de méd. belge, Brux., 1848, ii, 378: iv, 374: 1849, i, 66. — **Schnaubert.** Sublimat gegen Prosopalgie. Mitth. a. d. Geb. d. Heilk., Leipz., 1845, 216. — **Schneider** (P. J.) Oleum Terebinthinæ gegen Neuralgien. J. d. pract. Heilk., Berl., 1837, lxxxiv, 3. St., 48.—**Schorstein** (L.) Hydriatisches Narcoticum. Wien. med. Presse, 1878, xix, 1534; 1569.— **Schreiber** (J.) Die Behandlung schwerer Formen von Neuralgie und Muskelrheumatismus mittelst Massage und methodischer Muskelübungen. Tagebl. d. Versamml. deutsch. Naturf. u. Aerzte, Salzb., 1881, liv, pt. 2, 135–139. *Also:* Aerztl. Int.-Bl., München, 1881, xxviii, 517; 531. *Also:* Wien. med. Presse, 1881, xxii, 1508; 1541; 1577; 1605. *Also:* Deutsche Med.-Ztg., Berl., 1881, ii, 787; 799; 811. *Also, transl.:* Bull. gén. de thérap., etc., Par., 1882, cii, 276–285. *Also, transl.:* Med. Press & Circ., Lond., 1882, n. s., xxxiv, 304–306.—**Sée** (G.) Du traitement des maux de tête (céphalées, migraines, névralgies faciales) par l'antipyrine. Bull. Acad. de méd., Par., 1887, 2. s., xviii, 259–269. *Also, transl.:* Med. & Surg. Reporter, Phila., 1887, lvii, 471–475. *Also, transl.:* Allg. Wien. med. Ztg., 1887, xxii, 427; 439.—**Seguin** (E. C.) On the subcutaneous use of sulphate of quinine in cases of malarial neuralgia. N. York M. J., 1867, v, 402–409. *Also, in his:* Op. min. [etc.], 8°, N. Y., 1884, 10–14.—**Sentex** (L.) De la cautérisation sulfurique et de son application au traitement des névralgies. J. de méd. de Bordeaux, 1861, 2. s., vi, 193–218. *Also:* Monit. d. sc. méd. et pharm., Par., 1861, 2. s., iii, 491–494.—**Shapir** (B. M.) Lechenie nevralgii podkojnimi vpriskivanijami osmievoi kisloti. [Treatment of neuralgia by subcutaneous injection of osmic acid.] Russk. Med., St. Petersb., 1885, i, 292; 313.—**Sibson** (F.) On the use of chloroform in neuralgia. Lond. M. Gaz., 1848, xli, 535–538. *Also, in his:* Collect. Works, 8°, Lond., 1881, iv, 379–386.— **Sinkler** (W.) On the treatment of neuralgia by the constant current. Phila. M. Times, 1874–5, v, 275–280.— **Siredey.** De l'aquapuncture dans le traitement des névralgies. Bull. gén. de thérap., etc., Par., 1873, lxxxiv, 467–473.—**Skerritt** (E. M.) Croton-chloral in neuralgia. [Cases.] Tr. Bristol Med.-Chir. Soc., Lond., 1874–8, i, 10–15. ———. Croton-chloral in neuralgia. Lancet, Lond., 1876, ii, 776; 814.—**Slade-King** (E.) Administration of phosphorus in neuralgia. Med. Times & Gaz., Lond., 1873, i, 412.—**Stampacchia** (R.) Di un nuovo metodo da usare l'elettricità nella cura delle nevralgie. Gior. internaz. d. sc. med., Napoli, 1880, ii, 867–870.—**Stovall** (J. T.) The value of the hydrocyanate of iron in the treatment of neuralgia. Am. M. Bi-Weekly, N. Y., 1881, xiii, 193–195. *Also:* Gaillard's M. J., N. Y., 1881, xxxii, 294–296.—**Tait** (D.) Chloride of methyl in the treatment of neuralgic affections. Kansas City M. Index, 1886, vii, 694–699.—**Teinture** (De la) d'iode morphinée dans le traitement des névralgies. Bull. gén. de thérap., etc., Par., 1863; lxv, 132–134.—**Terry** (J. W.) Cases of neuralgia cured by the hypodermic injection of morphia. Tr. Minn. M. Soc., Minneap., 1875, 81–84.—**Thompson** (E.) Observations on the use of belladonna in neuralgia. Lond. M. Reposit., 1822, xviii, 35–38.—**Thompson** (J. A.) Some observations on the use of phosphorus in neuralgia. Practitioner, Lond., 1873,

Neuralgia (*Treatment of*).

xi, 13; 271.—**Thomas** (O. F.) On the use of Cannabis indica in certain forms of neuralgia. Therap. Gaz., Detroit, 1880, n. s., i, 353.—**Thomson** (S.) On the rapid relief of neuralgic pain. Lancet, Lond., 1875, ii, 660.—**Tillaux.** Névralgie de l'avant-bras; bons effets de l'injection sous-cutanée de morphine. Bull. gén. de thérap., etc., Par., 1865, lxix, 137.—**Todorski** (A. F.) Antipirin pri nevral. i revmat. Protok. zasaid. Kavkazsk. med. Obsh., Tiflis, 1886–7, xxiii, 455–461.—**Tonini** (F.) Del cianuro di ferro e di potassio nella cura delle malattie infiammatorie e nevralgiche. Atti. Accad. fis.-med. statist. di Milano, 1860–61, 198–205.—**Toribio del Villar.** Dos casos de neuralgia de origen palúdico tratados con éxito por la partenina. Crón. méd.-quir. de la Habana, 1885, xi, 132–134.—**Torri** (E.) Dei vantaggi dell' elettricità a corrente continua ed a lungo prolungata, nelle nevralgie ed in particolare nella sciatica. Bull. d. sc. med. di Bologna, 1857, 4. s., viii, 26; 100.—**Townsend** (T. B.) Neuralgia treated by enormous doses of sulphate of morphine. Am. M. Times, N. Y., 1862, v, 349.—**Traitement** des névralgies par les injections sous-cutanées de sulfate d'atropine. Gaz. d. hôp., Par., 1859, xxxii, 366.—**Traitement** (Du) des névralgies par le salicylate de soude. [Discussion.] Bull. et mém. Soc. de thérap., Par., 1881, xiii, 39.—**Trousseau.** Du traitement des névralgies. Bull. gén. de thérap., etc., Par., 1863, lxv, 385; 433.—**Trubert** (C.) Du phosphore de zinc dans les névralgies. Union méd., Par., 1878, 3. s., xxv, 358–360.—**Turner** (G. I.) Sluchai izliechenija neuralgii loktevago nerva vpriskivanijami osmievoi kisloti. [Recovery in a case of obstinate neuralgia of ulnar nerve by the injection of osmium acid.] Vrach, St. Petersb., 1884, v, 397.—**Uytterhoeven** (V.) Observations de névralgies guéries par un nouveau moyen aussi prompt que certain, suivies de réflexions. Arch. de la méd. belge, Brux., 1842, ix, 136: 1843, xi, 46.—**Vaidy** (J.-V.-F.) Observations sur des névralgies guéries par différens moyens. J. compl. du dict. d. sc. méd., Par., 1821, viii, 180–184.— **Valeur** (De la) des moyens chirurgicaux, et en particulier des cautérisations profondes avec suppuration prolongée, dans le traitement des névralgies rebelles, et principalement des névralgies de la face. Bull. gén. de thérap., etc., Par., 1853, xliv, 64–68.—**Valleix.** Du traitement des névralgies par les vésicatoires volants appliqués sur les principaux points douloureux. Arch. gén. de méd., Par., 1842, i, 336–345. *Also*, Reprint.—**Van Holsbeek** (H.) Du traitement des névralgies par l'électrisation localisée. J. de méd., chir. et pharmacol., Brux., 1859, xxviii, 567: xxix, 22; 139.—**Vinay** (C.) Du chlorure de méthyle dans le traitement des névralgies. Lyon méd., 1885, xlix, 349–354.—**Viñeta Bellaserra.** Las neuralgias y su tratamiento. Rev. de cien. méd., Barcel., 1882, viii, 390.—**Vizioli** (F.) Dell' azione sedativa della extra-corrente e della sua utilità diagnostica per distinguere le nevralgie di origine centrale o periferica. Morgagni, Napoli, 1868, x, 573–601.— **Wachtel** (D.) Ueber die Behandlung der Neuralgien durch subcutane Einspritzungen. Ztschr. f. Nat.- u. Heilk. in Ungarn, Oedenburg, 1859, x, 353; 361. — **Weinlechner** (J.) Neuralgie an einer thalergrossen Stelle des rechten Seitenwandbeines; Circumcision der schmerzhaften Stelle mit sofortiger Application des Glüheisens; Erysipel; eitrige Meningitis; rechtsseitige Pneumonie; Tod. Ber. d. k. k. Krankenanst. Rudolph-Stiftung in Wien (1877), 1878, 361. ———. Neuralgie in der rechten Schultergegend, gegen welche die Anwendung des Glüheisens, nachdem die gewöhnlichen Behandlungsmethoden, wie: Massage, Electricität. subcutane Injectionen, etc., nichts gefruchtet hatten, sofort Hilfe schaffte; dies Mittel blieb erfolglos, als späterhin dasselbe Leiden an der anderen Schulter ähnlich wie vor einem Jahre aufgetreten war. *Ibid.* (1878), 1879, 359.—**Wittcke.** Beobachtungen über die Wirksamkeit des kohlensauren Eisens bei Neuralgie, und andere neuere Mittel. J. d. pract. Heilk., Berl., 1828, lxvi, 3. St., 80; 4. St., 34.—**Wittke.** Chininum sulfuricum gegen den Fothergill'schen Gesichtsschmerz. Mag. f. d. ges. Heilk., Berl., 1826, xxii, 579–582.—**Woakes** (E.) On ergot of rye in the treatment of neuralgia. Brit. M. J., Lond., 1868, ii, 360.—**Wolff.** Merkwürdige Heilkraft des kohlensauren Eisens gegen Nevralgieen. J. d. pract. Heilk., Berl., 1826, lxii, 4. St., 10–18. *Also, transl.:* J. compl. du dict. d. sc. méd.. Par., 1826, xxv, 345–349. — **Wood** (A.) On a new method of treating neuralgia by the direct application of opiates to the painful points. Edinb. M. & S. J., 1855, lxxxii, 265–281. *Also*, Reprint. ———. Treatment of neuralgic pains by narcotic injections. Brit. M. J., Lond., 1858, 721–723.—**Wood** (H. C.) Sciatica and neuralgia treated by the constant current. Phila. M. Times, 1875, v, 660. — **Wyatt** (M. C.) Nitrite of amyl in neuralgia. Weekly M. Rev., Chicago, 1885, xi, 314.—**Wyman** (H. C.) Surgical treatment of neuralgia resulting from organic lesion of the nerve trunk. Penins. J. M., Detroit, 1874, x, 437–440. — **Young** (D.) Two cases of neuralgia treated with chloride of ammonium. Practitioner, Lond., 1875, xv, 412–414. — **Zechmeister.** Prosopalgia chronica, spasmis clonicis comitata, geheilt durch Magnetismus. Oesterr. med. Wchnschr., Wien, 1845, 921–924. ———. Hydriatisches Narcoticum. Wien. med. Presse, 1878, xix, 1605.

Neuralgia (*Abdominal and visceral*).

See, also, **Abdomen** (*Pain in*); **Bladder** (*Neuralgia of*); **Diaphragm** (*Neuralgia, etc., of*); **Enteralgia**; **Gastralgia**, *etc.*; **Hepatalgia**; **Nephralgia**; **Neuralgia** (*Epigastric*); **Ovary** (*Neuralgia of*); **Rectum** (*Neuralgia of*); **Spleen** (*Neuralgia of*); **Uterus** (*Irritable, etc.*)

ALLBUTT (T. C.) On visceral neuroses, being the Gulstonian lectures on neuralgia of the stomach and allied disorders. 8°. *London*, 1884.

———. The same. 8°. *Philadelphia*, 1884.

See, also, infra.

BARRAS (J.-P.-T.) Traité sur les gastralgies et les entéralgies ou maladies nerveuses de l'estomac et des intestins. 2. éd. 8°. *Paris*, 1827.

———. The same. 3. éd. [With supplement.] 2 v. 8°. *Paris*, 1829–38.

JEANNE (H.) * Essai sur la gastro-entéralgie anémique des pays chauds. 4°. *Paris*, 1883.

PAGÈS (J.-A.-G.-J.) * De la névralgie du grand sympathique, observée sous les latitudes inter-tropicales. 4°. *Paris*, 1852.

Albutt (T. C.) On certain forms of visceral neuralgia. Liverpool & Manchester M. & S. Rep., 1873, i, 107–125. *Also,* Reprint. ———. The Gulstonian lectures for 1884. On visceral neuroses. Med. Press & Circ., Lond., 1884, n. s., xxxvii, 221; 247; 271; 297; 323; 349. *Also :* Brit. M. J., Lond., 1884, i, 495; 543. [*See, also, supra.*]—Baierlacher (E.) Ueber die elektrische Behandlung der Gastralgien und Enteralgien. Aerztl. Int.-Bl., München, 1883, xxx, 209.—Butler (A. B.) Neuralgia of ganglionic nerves. Med. Counselor, Columbus, 1856, ii, 566–570.—Dumm (S. C.) Report of a case of long standing neuralgia of the bowels, simulating enteric inflammation. Ohio M. Recorder, Columbus, 1878, iii, 50.—Eulenberg (A.) On visceral neuralgia. Med. Times & Gaz., Lond., 1870, i, 329; 381; 433; 489; 576; 627: ii, 29; 115. — Fleury (L.) Réflexions et observations pour servir au diagnostic des névralgies viscérales. J. de méd., Par., 1843, i, 97–106. *Also :* Ann. de méd. belge, Brux., 1843, ii, 103–110.—Jones (C. H.) Cases of gastric and abdominal neuralgia. Lancet, Lond., 1856, i, 64.—Kuttner. Mesenterial-Neuralgie mit Fieber, hervorgerufen von 153 Spulwürmern. Berl. klin. Wchnschr., 1865, ii, 308. — Lugagne (C.) Étude sur les viscéralgies et sur leur traitement par les eaux de Vichy. Vichy-méd., 1879, ii, 402; 433; 445; 461; 477; 497; 515; 525; 541; 557; 573; 589; 605: 1880, iii, 1; 17; 33; 49; 65; 81; 97; 113; 129; 145; 161; 281; 293.—Neftel (W.) Beiträge zur Kenntniss und Behandlung der visceralen Neuralgien. Arch. f. Psychiat., Berl., 1880, x, 575–596.—Powell (R.) On certain painful affections of the intestinal canal. Med. Tr. Roy. Coll. Phys. Lond., 1820, vi, 106–117.—Schramm. Ueber die Neuralgia mesenterica. Aerztl. Int.-Bl., München, 1860, vii, 595.—Schuster. De l'emploi de l'opium, de l'eau tiède, du froid, de l'acide carbonique dans le traitement de certaines névroses gastro-intestinales. Bull. clin., Par., 1836–7, ii, 330–353.—Vaz Monteiro (J.) Algumas considerações sobre as nevroses gastro-intestinaes, ou visceralgias gastro-intestinaes; seu tratamento racionale methodica. Gaz. med. de Lisb., 1853–4, i, 245; 302.—Wildt. Ein Fall von Neuralgia des Plexus cœliacus und Mesentericus superior. Deutsche med. Wchnschr., Berl., 1876, ii, 160.

Neuralgia (*Articular*).

See **Arthralgia**; **Joints** (*Neuralgia, etc., of*).

Neuralgia (*Auricular*).

Morisset. Névralgie des filets auriculaires du pavillon de l'oreille droite; effets curatifs rapides du nitrate d'aconitine cristallisée (de Duquesnel). Tribune méd., Par., 1878, xi, 436.

Neuralgia (*Axillary*).

HEON (B.-L.) * De la névralgie circonflexe ou axillaire. 4°. *Paris*, 1882.

Tillaux. De la névralgie circonflexe, axillaire ou scapulalgie. Paris méd., 1883, viii, 301–304.

Neuralgia (*Brachial*) [*and in upper extremity*].

See, also, **Neuralgia** (*Axillary*); **Neuroma**; **Neurotomy**, *etc.*

BERGSON (J.) Zur historischen Pathologie der Brachial-Neuralgien. 4°. *Berlin*, 1860.

———. Sulla nevralgia bracchiale; saggio d' una monografia. Traduzione italiana dall' originale francese per cura del dottore Filippo Lussana. 8°. *Milano*, 1860.

Neuralgia (*Brachial*).

BORNE (J.) * Étude historique et clinique sur les névralgies brachiales. 4°. *Paris*, 1874.

LOUIS-CHOUSSY (J.-B.-G.) *Étude sur la névralgie du membre supérieur. 4°. *Paris*, 1869.

MICHEL (F.-J.) * Observations pour servir à l'histoire de la névralgie du membre supérieur. 4°. *Paris*, 1858.

TURBERT (C.) * Contribution à l'étude des névralgies du membre supérieur. 4°. *Paris*, 1884.

Albertoni (P.) Due casi di nevralgia brachiale, doppia, ribelle, guariti coll' uso di forti correnti elettriche continue. Gazz. med. ital., prov. venete, Padova, 1873, xvi, 173. — Anstie (F. E.) Two cases of cervico-brachial neuralgia, apparently cured by the constant current; double occipital neuralgia, not relieved by electricity. Tr. Clin. Soc. Lond., 1871, iv, 171–175. — Bergson (J.) Zur Geschichte und ätiologischen Eintheilung der Brachialneuralgien. Deutsche Klinik, Berl., 1859, xi, 278–281. [*See, also, supra.*]— Bergson (J.) & Lussana (F.) Epitome collettivo delle monografie sulle nevralgie bracchiali. Gazz. med. lomb., Milano, 1862, 5. s., i, 293; 301; 317; 325; 333; 377; 393. *Also* [Abstr.]: Gazz. med. ital., prov. venete, Padova, 1863, vi, 287–290.— Biffi (S.) Intorno ad alcune monografie delle nevralgie bracchiali. Gazz. med. ital. lomb., Milano, 1858, 4. s., iii, 121–125.—Buzzard (T.) Case of cervico-brachial neuralgia, treated with the constant current. Tr. Clin. Soc. Lond., 1871, iv, 164–170.—Eliot. Whitlow; neuralgia of finger; amputation. Tr. M. Soc. Dist. Columb., Wash., 1876, iii, 44.—Falcioni (R) Nevralgia brachiale sinistra e suo trattamento colla corrente d'induzione. Galvani, Urbino, 1873, i, 49–52.— Fischer (H.) Gewohnheitsgemässer Salicylsäuregebrauch gegen Brachial-Neuralgie. Deutsche Ztschr. f. Chir., Leipz., 1879, xii, 366.—Flamm. Seltene Neuralgie in den Spitzen aller Finger und Zehen. Med. Jahrb. d. k. k. österr. Staates, Wien, 1844, xlix, l, 286.— Gamberini (P.) Nota sopra una speciale nevralgia dell' avambraccio. Raccoglitore, Fano, 1844, xiii, 385. ———. Sulle nevralgie bracchiali. Imparziale, Firenze, 1863, iii, 273; 308; 344; 406; 475; 508; 574; 612; 673; 706; 739; 762: 1864, iv, 22; 53; 88; 107.— Hochhaus (H.) Traumatischer Tic convulsif im Gebiete des Nervus radialis. Deutsche med. Wchnschr., Berl., 1886, xii, 834.— Jezzi (M.) Un caso di nevralgie periarticolari delle dita, del polso e del gomito dell' arto superiore sinistro per causa isterica, con gravi disturbi vasomotori e tali da simulare periostiti croniche scrofolose. Gazz. d. osp., Milano, 1887, viii, 75; 83.—Lasègue. Névralgie des plexus brachial et cervical simulant, chez un emphysémateux, une angine de poitrine. Gaz. d. hôp., Par., 1878, li, 1059–1061.—Legludic. Note sur une névralgie brachiale nocturne. Bull. Soc. de méd. d'Angers (1866), 1867, n. s., lxix, 92–97.—Lussana (F.) Monografia delle nevralgie bracchiali. Gazz. med. ital. lomb., Milano, 1858, 4. s., iii, 137; 145; 157; 181; 205; 229; 245; 273; 281; 289; 297; 305; 313; 321; 329; 349, 1 pl. *Also,* Reprint. ———. La nevralgia scapulo-bracchiale. Gazz. med. ital. lomb., Milano, 1885, 8. s., vii, 159–161.—McLeod (J.) Severe brachial, with slight sciatic neuralgia treated with hypodermic injections. Canada M. & S. J., Montreal, 1872–3, i, 451.—McNaught (J.) Ulnar neuralgia. Brit. M. J., Lond., 1887, i, 933.—Mader (J.) Neuralgia plexus brachialis. Med.-chir. Centralbl., Wien, 1879, xiv, 543. — Malmsten (K.) Fall af neuralgia bilateralis nervi circumflexi humeri. Upsala Läkaref. Förh.. 1873, viii, 145–148. — Meigs (J. F.) Neuralgia localized in the circumflex nerve, from impaired nutrition and over-work. Med. Rec., N. Y., 1866–7, i, 353.—Midavaine. Douleur névralgique au bras gauche guérie par l'application d'un bandage compressif. Ann. Soc. de méd. d'Anvers, 1841, 403. — Mignot. Névralgie cervico-brachiale suivie de paralysie de la main. Soc. d. sc. méd. de Gannat. Compt. rend., Par., 1879, xxxiii, 96–98.— Mitchell (S. W.) Neuralgia of arm, with paralysis and atrophy of shoulder muscles, relieved by faradisation and counter-irritation. Med. Times, Phila., 1870–71, i, 116.— Nélaton. Affection douloureuse du plexus brachial avec adduction permanente du bras et flexion de l'avant-bras. Gaz. d. hôp., Par., 1861, xxxiv, 17.—Neucourt (F.) De la névralgie du plexus brachial (névralgie scapulaire, brachiale, cervico-brachiale des auteurs). Arch. gén. de méd., Par., 1850, 4. s., xxiv, 257–297.—Névralgie cervico-brachiale. J. de méd. de Bordeaux, 1858, 2. s., iii, 166–169.—O'Brien (D.) Cervico-brachial neuralgia of long standing, successfully treated with hypodermic injections. Canada M. & S. J., Montreal, 1872–3, i, 449–451 —Piorry. Névralgie cubitale; diagnostic d'abord incertain; organographisme faisant reconnaître une augmentation de volume (mégalie) des vertèbres cervicales; phosphate de chaux et iodure de potassium; diminution rapide de la tumeur; disparition de la névralgie. Gaz. d. hôp., Par., 1857, xxx, 293. ———. Cas remarquable de douleurs dans les nerfs rachidiens du dos avec diminution de l'action nerveuse du bras du même côté; douleur musculaire sous-sternale. *Ibid.*, 1858, xxxi, 65.—Schramm. Die Neuralgieen des Armgeflechtes. Aerztl. Int.-Bl., München,

Neuralgia (*Brachial*).

1859, vi, 598.—**Scottini.** Nevralgia bracchiale da latente sarcoma. Ann. univ. di med. e chir., Milano, 1875, ccxxxiii, 110–117.—**Seeligmüller** (A.) Ein Fall von einer auf den Nervus cutaneus brachii internus minor beschränkten Neuralgie. Arch. f. Psychiat., Berl., 1876, vi, 575–577.— **Seguin** (E. C.) A case illustrating the coincidence of diseases; cervico-brachial neuralgia and aneurism of the innominate artery. Arch. Med., N. Y., 1882, viii, 190–192. *Also, in his:* Op. min. [etc.], 8°, N. Y., 1884, 636–638.— **Sloane** (J.) Neuralgia of the brachial plexus simulating wasting palsy. Brit. M. J., Lond., 1859, ii, 787.—**Sorbets** (L.) Deux cas de névralgie cervico-brachiale nocturne. Gaz. d. hôp., Par., 1871, xliv, 566.—**Stedman.** Brachial neuralgia. Boston M. & S. J., 1877, xcvi, 629–631.— **von Stoffella** (E.) Schwellung der Gegend bei Neuralgia cervico-brachialis. Fossa supraclavicularis bei Neuralgia cervico-brachialis. Wien. med. Wchnschr., 1878, xxviii, 380; 413. — **Tho-mayer** (J.) Neuralgie plexus cervicobrachialis. Aerztl. Ber. d. k. k. allg. Krankenh. zu Prag (1883–4), 1886, 120–127. *Also:* Med.-chir. Centralbl., Wien, 1887, xxii, 376.— **Valleix.** Leçon clinique sur un cas de névralgie cervico-brachiale. Gaz. d. hôp., Par., 1852, xxv, 202. — **Vigié.** Double névralgie antibrachiale, dont l'une idiopathique à gauche, l'autre sympathique à droite. Gaz. méd. de Montpel., 1840–41, i, no. 20. — **Was** (J.) Neuralgia plexus brachialis. N. pract. Tijdschr. v. de Geneesk., Gorinchem, 1851, xxx, 746–749.

Neuralgia (*Cardiac*).
See **Heart** (*Neuralgia, etc., of*).

Neuralgia (*Cervico-brachial*).
See **Neuralgia** (*Brachial*).

Neuralgia (*Cervico-occipital*) [*and neuralgia in the scalp*].

LANGE (V.-E.) *De la névralgie cervico-occipitale. 4°. Paris, 1876.
Benito y Lentijo (J.) & **Ramos** (M. M.) Observacion sobre una nueva especie de neuralgia, denominada cervico-suboccipital. Décadas de med. y cirug. práct. Madrid, 1821, iii, 145–169.—**Brooks** (J.) On neuralgia of the scalp. Am. J. M. Sc. Phila., 1852, n. s., xxiv, 395–397.—**Finco** G.) Storia di una nevralgia occipito-cervicale guarita coll' ustione agli orecchi. Gazz. med. ital., prov. venete, Padova, 1862, v, 342. — **Gillet de Grand-mont.** Névralgie occipitale datant de treize ans; élongation avec arrachement du nerf occipital interne; guérison. J. de méd. de Par., 1883, v, 270–271. *Also:* Bull. Soc. de méd. prat. de Par. (1883), 1884, 97–99. *Also, transl.:* Gazz. med. ital. lomb., Milano, 1883, 8. s., v, 373.—**Klebs.** Sectionsbefund einer unter den Erscheinungen einer Frontal-Occipitalneuralgie unerwartet verstorbenen Kranken. Prag. med. Wchnschr., 1876, i, 961. — **Leuck** (A. W.) Cervico-occipital neuralgia. Med. Exam., Chicago, 1873, xiv, 247. — **Philipson** (G. H.) Case of cervico-occipital neuralgia. Lancet, Lond., 1876, ii, 893.—**Schreiber** (J.) Ueber Occipitalneuralgie. Berl. klin. Wchnschr., 1877, xiv, 726–729.—**Sereñana** (P.) Neuralgia cérvico-occipital del lado derecho, curada á favor de los revulsivos y de la electricidad. Independ. méd., Barcel., 1872–3, iv, 355–357.

Neuralgia (*Ciliary*).

de Hübsch (C.) Observation de névralgie ciliaire. Gaz. méd. d'Orient, Constantinople, 1861, iv, 37. — **Mat-tioli** (G. B.) Due casi di nevralgia ciliare organico-irritativa, guariti coll' iridectomia associata alla estrazione del cristallino. Gazz. med. ital., prov. venete, Padova, 1864, vii, 301–305. — **Philipp.** Fall von Neuralgia ciliaris typica. Wchnschr. f. d. ges. Heilk., Berl., 1847, xv, 88–90.—**Snellen.** Recisione dei nervi ciliari prima della loro penetrazione nel bulbo oculare come mezzo curativo della nevralgia ciliare persistente. Osservatore, Torino, 1874, x, 49–52. — **Tavignot.** De la névralgie ciliaire. Gaz. méd. de Par., 1845, 2. s., xiii, 545–549. ——. De la névralgie ciliaire. Gaz. d. hôp., Par., 1848, 2. s., x, 540. ——. Remarques sur la névralgie ciliaire, continue ou intermittente, simulant la conjonctivite. Gaz. d. hôp., Par., 1860, xxxiii, 501; 513. ——. Névralgie ciliaire liée à la diathèse urique; longue durée de la maladie; guérison par un traitement approprié. Courrier méd., Par., 1874, xxiv, 51.

Neuralgia (*Coccygeal*).
See **Coccygodynia**.

Neuralgia (*Crural*).
See **Neuralgia** of lower extremity.

Neuralgia (*Dental*) [*and neuralgia from diseased teeth*].

See, also, **Neuralgia** (*Facial, etc., Treatment of*).
FERRIER (J.) *Des névralgies réflexes d'origine dentaire. 4°. Paris, 1884.

Neuralgia (*Dental*).

HÉLIE. *D'une forme de névralgie maxillaire (névralgie des édentés) considérée surtout au point de vue de la pathogénie et du traitement. 4°. Paris, 1884.
Ackland (J. M.) Relation between facial neuralgia and dental irritation. Bristol M.-Chir. J., 1886, iv, 28–35. *Also:* Prov. M. J., Leicester, 1886, v, 151–153.—**Aguil-hon de Sarran.** Traitement des névralgies d'origine dentaire. Concours méd., Par., 1883, v, 601: 1884, vi, 305.— **Arkövy** (J.) A fogbél (pulpa dentis) kóros concrementumainak viszonya a prosopalgiához (tic douloureux). [Disease of teeth a cause of facial neuralgia.] Orvosi hetil., Budapest, 1880, xxiv, 157; 181; 213; 234.—**Bayless** (G. W.) Neuralgia relieved by the extraction of a tooth. West. J. M. & S., Louisville, 1840, ii, 335–338.—**Black** (G. V.) Dental neuralgia. Annual J. Ill. Dent. Soc., Chicago, 1878, 26–43. *Also:* Am. J. Dent. Sc., Balt., 1878–9, 3. s., xii, 456; 481.—**Brush** (G. W.) The relation of dental operations to facial neuralgia. Am. J. Neurol. & Psychiat., N. Y., 1883, ii, 211–219.—**Burnton** (T. L.) On nervous diseases connected with the teeth. Tr. Odont. Soc. Gr. Brit. 1879, Lond., 1880, n. s., xii, 144–180.—**Cabanès.** Névralgie dentaire; évulsion, replacement et consolidation de la dent douloureuse. J. d. conn. méd.-chir., Par., 1834–5, ii, 41.—**Castle** (A. C.) On dento-neuralgic affections. Lancet, Lond., 1846, ii, 265–267. ——. Notes for a memoir on the pathology of dento-neuralgia. Boston M. & S. J., 1851, xliv, 253; 312; 415.—**Coale.** Neuralgia from retention of a deciduous tooth. Am. J. M. Sc., Phila., 1850, n. s., xix, 365. — **Friedberg** (H.) Ueber einige Fälle von Heilung der Prosopalgie durch Zahnextraction. Arch. f. path. Anat., etc., Berl., 1860, xviii, 476–494. — **Gosselin.** Névralgie sus-orbitaire, avec phénomènes de voisinage du côté de l'œil consécutive à une dent gâtée. Gaz. d. hôp., Par., 1876, xlix, 522.—**Gray** (T.), jr. Tic douloureux, imitated by diseases of the teeth. N. Eng. Q. J. M. & S., Bost., 1842–3, i, 5–10.—**Hutchinson** (J.) A group of cases illustrating the occasional connexion between neuralgia of the dental nerves and amaurosis. Ophth. Hosp. Rep., Lond., 1863–5, iv, 381–388.—**Jeannel.** Névralgie rebelle du nerf dentaire; résection de l'extrémité terminale du nerf par le procédé de M. Ch. Monod; deux observations. Bull. et mém. Soc. de chir. de Par., 1886, n. s., xii, 782–788.—**Lambert** (E.) Rapport de la commission chargée de l'examen du travail de M. le docteur E. Lambert, intitulé: Affections de la substance nerveuse du bulbe dentaire, ou bien: Contribution à l'étude du diagnostic réel des affections névralgiques et rhumatismales, à caractère continu ou intermittent, dans ses rapports avec la fièvre intermittente et les affections nerveuses de toute nature. [Rap. de Warlomont.] Bull. Acad. roy. de méd. de Belg., Brux., 1878, 3. s., xii, 663–672.—**Mall.** Zwei Fälle von Fothergill'schen Gesichtsschmerz, geheilt durch Extraktion kariöser Zähne. Wien. Med.-Halle, 1863, iv, 398.—**Niederkorn.** Douleur vive provoquée par l'éruption de la dent de sagesse et simulant une névralgie, guérie par une incision gingivale cruciale. Bull. Soc. d. sc. méd. du gr.-duché de Luxemb., 1864, 17.— **Polaillon.** Névralgie épileptiforme du nerf dentaire inférieur; élongation de ce nerf précédant la section et l'arrachement du bout périphérique; guérison. Bull. et mém. Soc. de chir. de Par., 1882, n. s., viii, 450–453.—**Post** (A. C.) Account of an attack of neuralgia affecting several of the teeth of the left upper jaw, the left side of the head, and the larynx cured instantaneously by the extraction of the left dens sapientiæ of the lower jaw. N. York J. M., 1845, v, 311–314.—**Reichel** (W.) Ueber Gesichtsund Kopfschmerzen, als Folge von krankhaft veränderten Zahnwurzeln, hauptsächlich von Exostosen derselben. Med. Ztg. Russlands, St. Petersb., 1852, ix, 6.—**Runnalls** (H. B.) The relations existing between facial neuralgia, frontal headache, and dental caries. Bristol M.-Chir. J., 1885, iii, 249–254.—**Salter** (J. A.) Facial neuralgia from dentine-excrescence in pulp cavity. Guy's Hosp. Rep., Lond., 1868, 3. s., xiii, 83. ——. Cranial neuralgia from an impacted canine tooth. Ibid., 84–86. ——. Intense and general neuralgia from exostosis on fangs of teeth. Ibid., 86–88. ——. Neuralgia of the arm from carious teeth and from undue pressure of artificial teeth. Ibid., 88. ——. Neuralgia of neck and arm from carious molar. Ibid., 91. ——. Neuralgia of face, neck, and arm, with partial paralysis of the latter, from carious wisdom tooth. Ibid., 93.—**Savoye.** Accidents produits par la dent de sagesse; névralgie de la cinquième paire. J. de méd. et chir. prat., Par., 1879, l, 356–359.—**Scheff** (J.) jun. Drei Fälle von Neuralgia facialis, verursacht durch Dentin-Neubildungen der Pulpahöhle. Allg. Wien. med. Ztg., 1876, xxi, 217; 235.—**Stimson** (L. A.) Neuralgia of the inferior dental nerve following fracture of the lower jaw. Med. News, Phila., 1883, xlii, 230. — **Valleix.** Note sur un cas de névralgie trifaciale, causée par la carie d'une dent molaire. Arch. gén. de méd., Par., 1843, 4. s., ii, 468–472.—**Walzberg** (T.) Tic douloureux und Zahnneuralgie; Bemerkungen zur Differentialdiagnose derselben. Centralbl. f. Chir., Leipz., 1883, x, 718–722.—**Waters** (J.) Case of neuralgia of the inferior dental nerve. Prov. M.

Neuralgia (Dental).

& S. J., Lond., 1843, v. 352.—**White** (O.) [Neuralgia facialis.] N. York J. M., 1845, v, 428. — **Winterbottom** (A.) On cases of neuralgia dependent upon non-erupted teeth. Lancet, Lond., 1880, ii, 941.

Neuralgia (Dental and infra-maxillary, Treatment of).

AUERBACH (L.) * Ueber Carotiscompression bei Trigeminusneuralgie. 8°. *Würzburg*, 1881.

GABRIEL (J.) * Ein Fall von Tic douloureux im Gebiete des Nervus alveolaris inferior und dessen Behandlung durch Neurectomie. [Wurtzburg.] 8°. *Breslau*, [1886].

RICOUX (L.) * Étude sur le traitement chirurgical de la névralgie rebelle et d'originaire périphérique du nerf dentaire inférieur. 4°. *Paris*, 1884.

VOISARD (E.) * De la section des nerfs dentaires supérieurs et inférieur. 4°. *Strasbourg*, 1864.

Agnew (D. H.) A case of neuralgia successfully treated by exsection of the inferior maxillary nerve. Med. & Surg. Reporter, Phila., 1858-9, n. s., i, 45.—**Albert** (E.) Neuralgie des dritten Astes; Resektion des N. mandibularis mit osteoplastischer Resektion des Unterkieferwinkels; vorübergehender Erfolg; Ligatur der Carotis comm.; Heilung. Wien. med. Presse, 1877, xviii, 622.—**Beau.** Névralgie datant de deux ans, fixée sur le nerf dentaire inférieur: résection du nerf dentaire inférieur; guérison complète. Union méd., Par., 1853, vii, 486.—**Blackman** (G. C.) Exsection of the trunk of the inferior dental nerve, together with that of the second branch of the fifth pair of nerves beyond Meckel's ganglion, for severe facial neuralgia. Am. J. M. Sc., Phila., 1869, n. s., lviii, 69: 1870, n. s., lx, 373.—**Boeckel.** Résection du nerf dentaire inférieur par le procédé de M. Beau. Gaz. d. hôp., Par., 1854, xxvii, 102.—**Bouillaud.** Névralgie maxillo-dentaire traitée avec succès par la section du nerf. Communiquée par M. Maury. N. Jour. de méd., chir., pharm., etc., Par., 1820, vii, 7-11.—**Brigham** (C. B.) Excision of a portion of the inferior dental nerve by trephining the lower jaw; also excision of a part of the infra-orbital nerve; complete relief. West. Lancet, San Fran., 1874-5, iii, 391-396. *Also, in his:* Surg. Cases, 8°, Cambridge, 1876, 29-32. ———. Idiopathic facial neuralgia; excision of a portion of the inferior or dental nerve by trephining the lower jaw; immediate relief. West. Lancet, S n Fran., 1874-5, iii, 626-628. *Also, in his:* Surg. Cases, 8°, Cambridge, 1876, 32-35.—**Bull** (W. T.) Neuralgia of the superior maxillary and inferior dental nerves; resection; cure. N. York M. J., 1885, xlii, 612.—**Chauvel.** Rapport sur un travail de M. le Dr. Longuet, intitulé: Névralgie et tic douloureux de la face; élongation du nerf dentaire inférieur droit par la voie buccale; disparition des douleurs pendant un mois et demi; récidive. Bull. et mém. Soc. de chir. de Par., 1883, n. s., ix, 77-86.—**Denucé.** Névralgie épileptiforme du nerf maxillaire inférieur; résection; guérison. Mém. et bull. Soc. méd.-chir. d. hôp. de Bordeaux, 1869, iv, 123-129.—**Duplay.** Sur une forme particulière de névralgie du maxillaire inférieur, guérie par la résection du bord alvéolaire. Arch. gén. de méd., Par., 1884, ii, 601-605.—**Fumagalli** (C.) Nevralgia circoscritta al nervo dentale inferiore destra, curata col taglio del nervo. Ann. univ. di med., Milano, 1858, clxiii, 572.—**Gallozzi** (C.) Della recisione del nervo dentario inferiore col metodo del Parravicini. Resoc. Accad. med.-chir. di Napoli, 1882, xxxvi, 195-199. *Also:* Gior. di neuropatol., Napoli, 1882-3, i, 225-229. *Also:* Eco d. osp., Napoli, 1883, i, 47-51.—**Gardner** (W.) Successful exsection of inferior dental nerve for obstinate neuralgia; bone grafting. Austral. M. J., Melbourne, 1883, n. s., v, 99.—**Garretson** (J. E.) Excision of inferior maxillary nerve. Med. & Surg. Reporter, Phila., 1871, xxiv, 249-252. ———. Excision of the inferior dental nerve, by means of the dental engine, for the relief of obstinate neuralgia. Med. Rec., N. Y., 1880, xviii, 449. ———. Excision of inferior maxillary nerve for neuralgia. Med. News, Phila , 1884, xlv, 430.—**Grant** (F. W.) Case of partial excision of the inferior dental nerve for persistent facial neuralgia; cure. Lancet, Lond., 1885, ii, 61.—**Green** (H.) Case of neuralgia of the lower jaw, relieved by surgical operation. N. York J. M., 1845, ii, 324.—**Gross** (F. H.) Trigeminal neuralgia relieved by ligation of the common carotid artery and neurectomy. Am. J. M. Sc., Phila., 1883, n. s., lxxxv, 366-378.—**Gross** (S. W.) Four cases of excision of the inferior dental nerve on account of intractable neuralgia. *Ibid.*, 1868, n. s., lv, 32-35.—**Hamilton** (F. H.) Neuralgia of the inferior maxillary nerve, cured by trephining the jaw, and excision of the nerve. Buffalo M. J., 1858-9, xiv, 148.—**Hodgen.** Excision of inferior dental nerve. [Discussion.] St. Louis M. & S. J., 878, xxxv, 77-79.—**How** (L. B.) Exsection of the inferior dental nerve. Tr. N. Hampshire M. Soc., Concord, 1880, xc, 93-95. *Also*, Reprint.—**Hutchinson** (J.C.) Removal

of alveolar process for neuralgia of inferior dental nerve (Gross's operation); cure. Am. J. M. Sc.. Phila., 1874, n. s., lxvii, 98.—**Jessop.** Neuralgia of jaw following toothextraction; treatment by Prof. Gross's method. Brit. M. J., Lond., 1871, i, 11.—**Kimball** (H. H.) Softening of inferior dental nerve; exostosis of infra-orbital canal; trephining; cure. Boston M. & S. J., 1867, lxxvi, 277.—**Kosinski** (J.) Nerwoból twarzy pieć lat trwający przecięcie nerwu zębowego dolnego z dobrym skutkiem. [Section of infra-maxillary nerve with success.] Pam.Towarz. Lek. Warszaw., 1871, lxv, 192-205.—**Langdon.** Case of severe neuralgia in the tract of the right dental nerve; operation; recovery. Lancet, Lond., 1875, ii, 624.—**Lizars** (J.) Neuralgia of the inferior maxillary nerve, "nervus mandibulo-labialis"; cured by operation. Edinb. M. & S. J., 1821, xvii, 529-537.—**Lossen** (H.) Neurectomie des Ramus secund. nervi V (Lücke), des Lingualis und des Alveolaris infer. (Paravicini). Centralbl. f. Chir., Leipz., 1876, iii, 305-309.—**McGraw** (T. A.) Neuralgia of the lower jaw and tongue treated by excision of the nerve. Detroit Rev. Med. & Pharm., 1874, ix, 462. ———. A case of repeated excision of the inferior dental and gustatory nerves for the cure of dental neuralgia. Detroit M. J., 1877, n. s., i, 801-804.—**Mader.** Neuralgia trigemini d.; wesentliche Besserung durch Faradisation und Chinin. Ber. d. k. k. Krankenanst. Rudolph-Stiftung in Wien (1881), 1882. 321 —**Marcuse** (J.) Zur Resection des Nervus mandibularis. Berl. klin. Wchnschr., 1882, xix, 257-259. — **Mears** (J. E.) Study of the pathological changes occurring in trifacial neuralgia, with the report of a case in which three inches of the inferior dental nerve were excised. Med. News, Phila., 1884, xlv, 58-63. *Also:* Tr. Am. Surg. Ass. 1884, Phila., 1885, ii, 469-490. *Also*, Reprint.—**Menzel** (A.) La resezione intrabuccale del nervo alveolare inferiore. Gazz. med. ital. lomb., Milano, 1871, 6. s., iv, 407. *Also, transl.:* Centralbl. f. d. med. Wissensch., Berl., 1872, x, 1. ———. La resezione intrabuccale del nervo inframascellare. Gazz. med. ital. lomb., Milano, 1872, xxxii, 157-160.—**Meusel.** Resection des Nervus mandibularis und lingualis von der Mundhöhle aus. Deutsche Klinik, Berl., 1871, xxiii, 423.—**Mitchell** (S. W.) Cases of lesions of peripheral nerve-trunks, with commentaries. Am. J. M. Sc., Phila., 1883, n. s., lxxxvi, 17: 31. *Also, transl.* [Abstr.]: Med. contemp., Lisb., 1883, i, 331. — **Monod** (C.) De la résection de l'extrémité terminale du nerf dentaire inférieur dans les névralgies rebelles de ce nerf. Bull. et mém. Soc. de chir. de Par., 1884, n. s., x, 580-600.—**Morton** (T. G.) Two cases of excision of portions of the inferior dental nerve, for neuralgia. Phila. M. Times, 1880-81, xi, 598-600.—**von Mosetig-Moorhof** (A.) Intrabuccale Resection des Nervus inframaxillaris nach Paravicini's Methode wegen Neuralgie; Heilung. Wien. med. Wchnschr., 1874, xxiv, 225-227. *Also, transl.* [Abstr.]: Abeille méd., Montréal, 1879, i, 211.—**Mouchet.** Élongation du nerf dentaire inférieur droit pour une névralgie rebelle du trijumeau avec tic douloureux de la face; guérison. Bull. et mém. Soc. de chir. de Par., 1883, n. s., ix, 119-123.—**Müller** (F.) Constitutioneller Tic douloureux mit hochgradiger seit sechs Jahren andauernder Salivation; rasche Heilung; letztere durch Atropin. Mitth. d. Ver. d. Aerzte in Steiermark 1881, Graz, 1882, xviii, 78-85.—**Museux.** Observation d'une névralgie maxillo-dentaire, guérie au moyen du cautère actuel. Bull. de l'École de méd. de Par., 1807, ix, 134-136.—**Nicoladoni** (K.) Neuralgia N. mandibularis d.; Neurectomie nach Paravicini; Meningitis; Fibroma nervi facialis d. Wien. med. Wchnschr., 1874, xxiv, 934-939.—**Polaillon.** Élongation du nerf dentaire inférieur pour une névralgie rebelle du trijumeau. Bull. et mém. Soc. de chir. de Par., 1881, n. s., vii, 802-807.—**Roser.** Resection des Unterkiefer-Nervs. Arch. f. physiol. Heilk., Stuttg., 1855, xiv, 583.—**Sands** (H B.) Necrotomy of the inferior dental nerve. Med. Rec., N. Y., 1880, xvii, 701.—**Savory.** Removal of portion of inferior dental nerve. Med. Times & Gaz., Lond., 1875, i, 522.—**Schüller** (M.) Neuralgie im Alveolaris inferior; Neurectomie. Deutsche Ztschr. f. Chir., Leipz., 1877-8, ix, 277.—**Sédillot.** Névralgie datant de deux ans, particulièrement fixée sur le nerf dentaire inférieur ; douleurs incessantes, insomnie, inappétence, émaciation profonde, aspect sénile, pronostic grave; résection du nerf dentaire inférieur par le procédé de M. le docteur Beau; guérison complète. Gaz. d. hôp., Par., 1853, xxvi, 424.—**Sée** (M.) Douleurs névralgiques siégeant principalement dans la mâchoire inférieure; élongation du nerf dentaire inférieur; guérison. Bull. et mém. Soc. de chir. de Par., 1882, n. s., viii, 448-450.—**Seguin** (E. C.) A contribution to the medicinal treatment of chronic trigeminal neuralgia. Med. Rec., N. Y., 1879, xv, 6-9. *Also*, Reprint.—**Sonnenburg.** Ausschneidung des Nervus alveolaris inferior vom Kieferwinkel aus bei neuralgischem Kopfe. Berl. klin. Wchnschr., 1882. xix. 625-627.—**Szeparowicz** (J.) Neuralgia N. inframaxillaris: intrabuccale Operation nach Paravicini's Methode; Heilung. Wien. med. Wchnschr., 1875, xxv, 672.—**Terrillon.** Du traitement

Neuralgia (*Dental and infra-maxillary, Treatment of*).

chirurgical de la névralgie du nerf dentaire inférieur, et en particulier de sa section par le procédé de Michel (de Nancy). Bull. gén. de thérap., etc., Par., 1876, xci, 481; 545. *Also, transl.:* Med. Exam., Lond., 1877, ii, 126.—**Van Derveer** (A.) Trifacial neuralgia and the operation for its relief. Med. Ann., Albany, 1883, iv, 193–200.—**Vaught** (R. L.) Excision of inferior dental nerve for neuralgia. Nashville J. M. & S., 1886, 2. s., xxxviii, 544.—**Warren** (J. M.) Ticdouloureux; relief by an operation for the removal of a portion of the inferior maxillary nerve by trepanning the lower jaw bone. Am. J. M. Sc., Phila., 1850, n. s., xix, 369. ———. Trephining the lower jaw for neuralgia. Boston M. & S. J., 1858–9, lix, 62. *Also:* Extr. Rec. Bost. Soc. M. Improve. (1856–8), 1859, iii, 243. ———. Facial neuralgia; trephining the lower jaw, and removal of a portion of the inferior dental nerve; partial relief. *In his:* Surg. Obs., Bost., 1867, 472–474.—**Weinlechner** (J.) Neuralgie des linken Nerv. inframaxillaris; Resection nach Pallavicini; heftige Blutung, die mehrmals recidivirte und die Unterbindung der Carotis nothwendig machte, auf welche Unbesinnlichkeit, Gedächtnissschwäche, Aphasie und rechtseitige Lähmung folgte; Heilung. Ber. d. k. k. Krankenanst. Rudolph-Stiftung in Wien, 1876, 349–352.—**Wormald.** Neuralgia consequent on an old fracture of the lower jaw; extirpation of a portion of the inferior dental nerve, followed by speedy and complete recovery. Med. Times & Gaz., Lond., 1863, i, 343.

Neuralgia (*Epidemic*).

See, also, **Eye** (*Neuroses of*).

Sawyers (J. H.) Report of an epidemic neuralgia which prevailed in Knox County, south of Knoxville, during the months of February and March, 1857. South. J. M. & Phys. Sc., Knoxville, 1857, v, 358–364. *Also:* Nashville J. M. & S., 1857, xii, 509–515.

Neuralgia (*Epigastric*).

Fraser (J. H.) Epigastric neuralgia. Birmingh. M. Rev., 1884, xvi, 77–83.

Neuralgia (*Epileptiform*).

See, also, **Neuralgia** (*Facial, etc., Treatment of*).

Campbell (J.) An essay on neuralgia spasmodica, or tic douloureux; submitted by authority of the president and his council, to the examination of the Royal College of Surgeons of Edinburgh, when candidate for admission into their corporation. 8°. *Edinburgh*, 1823.

Anstie (F. E.) On the treatment of "epileptiform" neuralgia in its earlier stages. Lancet, Lond., 1869, i, 41.—**Bartholow** (R.) Epileptiform tic douloureux of six years' duration cured by the hypodermic injection of morphine and by the iodide and bromide of potassium. Clinic, Cincin., 1872, ii, 253–256.—**Bastian** (C.) Simple epileptiform neuralgia. Brit. M. J., Lond., 1879, i, 77.—**Davis** (E. P.) A case of epileptiform neuralgia. Chicago M. J. & Exam., 1882, xlv, 32–36.—**Emerson** (N. B.) Tic-douloureux, or epileptiform neuralgia; relief after the internal use of crystallized aconitine. N. York M. J., 1878, xxvii, 633–635.—**Evans** (C. J.) Epileptiform neuralgia during the puerperal period; epileptic seizures; phlegmasia dolens. Brit. M. J., Lond., 1867, ii, 5.—**Féréol.** Heureux effets du sulfate de cuivre ammoniacal dans la névralgie épileptiforme de la face. Bull. gén. de thérap., etc., Par., 1878, xcv, 97–101. ———. Névralgie épileptiforme. Bull. et mém. Soc. de thérap. 1878, Par., 1879, 2. s., v, 93–100.—**Gille** (P. E.) Tic douloureux, behandlad med massage af halssympathicus. Hygiea, Stockholm, 1886, xlviii, 635.—**Ingals** (E. F.) A case of epileptiform neuralgia, with tonic, muscular spasms. Chicago M. J., 1874, xxxi, 485–488.—**Letulle** (M.) Tic. N. dict. de méd. et chir. prat., Par., 1883, xxxv, 608–626.—**Liégeois** (C.) Sur un cas de névralgie trifaciale épileptiforme, convulsive. Rev. méd. de l'est, Nancy, 1881, viii, 179–183.—**Oré.** Névralgie épileptiforme de la face; section des deux nerfs nasal interne et nasal externe; anesthésie par injection intraveineuse de chloral; succès. Gaz. méd. de Bordeaux, 1875, iv, 337–340.—**Ramskill.** Epileptiform neuralgia; epileptic seizures; improvement under the influence of large doses of morphia. Brit. M. J., Lond., 1867, i, 9.—**Trousseau** (H.) De la névralgie épileptiforme. Arch. gén. de méd., Par., 1853, i, 33–44.—**Walsham** (W. J.) A case of epileptiform neuralgia treated by stretching the infraorbital nerve, with remarks. Brit. M. J., Lond., 1880, ii, 1009–1011. ———. On the treatment of epileptiform neuralgia, or the so called incurable facial tic. Practitioner, Lond., 1884, xxxiii, 14–20.—**Whitehead.** Epileptiform neuralgia. Brit. M. J., Lond., 1885, i, 78.

Neuralgia (*Facial and trigeminal*).

See, also, **Neuralgia** (*Complications, etc., of*); **Neuralgia** (*Dental*), etc.; **Neuralgia** (*Epilepti-*

Neuralgia (*Facial and trigeminal*).

form); **Neuralgia** (*Supra-orbital*); **Neuralgia** (*Syphilitic*); **Neurotomy**, etc.

Abrahamsz (T.) * Neuritis rami primi trigemini. 8°. *Utrecht*, [1873].

Allnat (R. H.) Tic douloureux, or neuralgia facialis, and other nervous affections. 8°. *London*, 1841.

———. The same. 2. ed. 12°. *London*, 1843.

Baehren (C.) * De prosopalgia Fothergillii. 8°. *Berolini*, [1833].

Barbarin (G.-C.) * Dissertation sur la névralgie faciale considérée d'une manière générale. 4°. *Paris*, 1817.

Barret (A.) * Forme convulsive de la néuralgie de la face, tic douloureux. 4°. *Paris*, 1876.

de **Baumann** (J. M.) * De prosopalgia. 8°. *Monachii*, 1836.

Beck (L.) * Ueber die Neuralgie des Nervus trigeminus. 8°. *Würzburg*, 1854.

Becker (C. A.) * De dolore faciei Fothergillii. 8°. *Berolini*, [1817].

Bew (C.) Opinions on the causes and effects of the disease denominated tic douloureux. 8°. *London*, 1824.

Bollmann (A. T.) * De prosopalgia nonnulla. 8°. *Berolini*, [1829].

Bosch (C.) * Ueber die Erkenntniss und Behandlung des Fothergillischen Gesichtsschmerzes. 8°. *Freiburg*, 1828.

Bretschneider (C. A. J. H.) * De prosopalgia. 8°. *Jenæ*, [1841].

Briolle (A.) * Essai sur la névralgie de la face. 4°. *Montpellier*, 1866.

Buchner (O.) * De prosopalgia. 8°. *Monachii*, 1840.

Caillat (A.-A.) * Étude sur la névralgie du trijumeau. 4°. *Montpellier*, 1873.

Chaponnière (J.-J.) * Essai sur le siége et les causes des névralgies de la face. 4°. *Paris*, 1832.

Chatagnion (A.) * Des causes de la névralgie faciale. 4°. *Paris*, 1869.

Chwistek (G.) * De prosopalgia. 8°. *Berolini*, [1846].

Durand (G.-F.) * Des maladies des nerfs de la face (facial et trifacial). 4°. *Paris*, 1846.

Dysiewicz (J. V.) * De dolore faciei Fothergillii. 8°. *Berolini*, [1818].

Ellerbeck (A. W. A.) * Over prosopalgia Fothergillii. 8°. *Utrecht*, 1862.

Eydam (I.) * Prosopalgiæ pathologia. 4°. *Jenæ*, [1826].

Fleury (H.-L.) * Essai sur la névralgie faciale, communément tic douloureux de la face. 4°. *Strasbourg*, 1835.

Forty (C.) * De dolore faciali Fothergillii. 8°. *Budæ*, [1833].

Fothergill (S.) A concise and systematic account of a painful affection of the nerves of the face, commonly called tic douloureux. 8°. *London*, 1804.

Genenius (H. P. V.) * De neuralgia intermittente nervi trigemini. 8°. *Halis Sax.*, [1852].

Glaser (F.) * Die Lehre von der Prosopalgie vom physiologischen Standpunkt. 8°. *Würzburg*, 1838.

Goebel (A.) * Ueber Gesichtsneuralgieen. 8°. *Berlin*, [1875].

Goering (H. C.) * De prosopalgia. 8°. *Berolini*, [1848].

von **Gorup Besanez** (E. F.) * De prosopalgia. 8°. *Monachii*, 1842.

Gumbinner (J. P.) * De prosopalgia observationes nonnullæ nuper factæ. 8°. *Berolini*, [1838].

Neuralgia (*Facial and trigeminal*).

HAK (A.) * De neuralgia nervi trigemini. 8°. *Pragæ*, [1841].

HALFFTER (E. T.) * De prosopalgia. 8°. *Berolini*, [1825].

HALSBRAND (B.) * De dolore faciali Fothergilli. 8°. *Berolini*, 1834.

HAMEL (J.-P.) * De la névralgie faciale, communément tic douloureux de la face. 8°. *Paris, an XI* [1803].

HARTTMANN (C. A. T.) * Observationes quædam de prosopalgia. 8°. *Tubingæ*, [1811].
Also, in : WEBER. Samml. med.-prakt. Diss. [etc.] 8°. *Tübingen*, 1820, i, 152–274.

HAVASS (I. L.) * De prosopalgia nervosa. 8°. *Pestini*, 1828.

HEYFELDER (J. F. M.) * De prosopalgia Fothergilli, adnexa singularis hujus morbi historia. 4°. *Vratislaviæ*, 1820.

HEYGATE (J.) * On tic douloureux; together with a few cursory remarks on the intermittent fever, and its supposed connection with the former. 8°. *Edinburgh*, 1836.

HILDEBRAND (C. T. C.) * De prosopalgia. 12°. *Marburgi*, [1830].

HOLTHOFF (L. B.) * De prosopalgia. 8°. *Berolini*, [1851].

HÜGEL (J. F. G.) * Disquisitio neuralgiæ facialis pathologica. 8°. *Berolini*, 1824.

HUTCHINSON (B.) Cases of neuralgia spasmodica. commonly termed tic douloureux, successfully treated. 2. ed. 8°. *London*, 1882.

HUTCHINSON (C. E.) The narrative of a recovery from tic douloureux. 8°. *London*, 1838.

JENTSCH (P.) * De prosopalgia. 8°. *Berolini*, [1852].

KOCK (F.) * De neuralgia faciali. 8°. *Berolini*, [1843].

KOENIG (F. G. P. D.) * De nervi trigemini neuralgia. 8°. *Berolini*, [1855].

KRUEGER ([B.] A. [B.]) * De prosopalgia. 8°. *Berolini*, [1850].

LADENDORF (H.) * De prosopalgia. 8°. *Berolini*, [1842].

LANGENBECK (C. J. M.) Tractatus anatomico-chirurgicus de nervis cerebri in dolore faciei consideratis. sm. 4°. *Gottingæ*, 1805.

LARTHE (J.) * De la névralgie faciale. 4°. *Paris*, 1858.

LEMBERG (A.) * De prosopalgia. 8°. *Berolini*, [1847].

VON LEUTHNER (F. X. J.) De dolore faciei Fothergilli; comment. med.-chirurg. 8°. *Wirceburgi*, 1810.

LOEBNER (A.) * De prosopalgia. 8°. *Berolini*, [1846].

VAN LOENEN (R.) * De dolore faciei convulsivo. 8°. *Groningæ*, [1797].

MAJOR (J. C.) * De prosopalgia nervosa. 8°. *Pragæ*, 1827.

MASSEN (P.) * Zwei Fälle von Trigeminusneuralgie unter besonderer Berücksichtigung der Therapie. 8°. *Bonn*, [1880].

MASTBOOM (J. G. M.) * Over vasomotorische zenuwen en hare functioneele stoornissen bij neuralgieën aan het hoofd. [Utrecht.] 8°. *Rosendaal*, 1877.

MESTER (A.) * De prosopalgia. 8°. *Wirceburgi*, 1847.

MICHELSEN (J.) * De nervi quinti neuralgia, præmissa historia morbi. 4°. *Gryphiswaldiæ*, 1863.

MINZIOR (M.-D.-F.-E.) * Quelques considérations sur l'étiologie et le traitement de la névralgie du trijumeau. 4°. *Strasbourg*, 1865.

MITCHELL (C. D.) Essay on tic douloureux and other nervous affections. 8°. *Calcutta*, 1839.

Neuralgia (*Facial and trigeminal*).

MORGAN (W.) Tic douloureux; its causes, symptoms, and treatment. 8°. *London*, 1856.

NASMYTH (R.) * On tic douloureux. 8°. *Edinburgh*, 1823.

NEUBERT (F. H.) * De prosopalgia. 8°. *Berolini*, 1825.

NOLLAU (E. G.) * Prosopalgiæ adumbratio pathologica. 8°. *Berolini*, 1824.

OTTO (G. H.) * De prosopalgia nonnulla. 8°. *Regimontii Prussorum*, [1836].

PALM (J. N.) * De nervi quinti neuralgia, addita morbi historia. 8°. *Berolini*, [1863].

PEMERL (A.) * De prosopalgia. 8°. *Monachii*, 1835.

PERRY (G.) * De morbo faciei nervoso. 8°. *Edinburgi*, 1818.

PIPET (H.) * De la névralgie de la face. 4°. *Paris*, 1848.

PLUMERT (A. R.) * De prosopalgia. 8°. *Pragæ*, 1844.

PRAETEL (A. M.) * De neuralgia nervi quinti. 8°. *Berolini*, [1855].

PUJOL. Essai sur la maladie de la face, nommée le tic douloureux; avec quelques réflexions sur le raptus caninus de Cœlius Aurelianus. 12°. *Paris*, 1787.

REGNIER (P.) * Sur la névralgie faciale, communément tic douloureux. 4°. *Paris*, 1829.

REVERDIT (C.) * Dissertation sur la névralgie faciale ou prosopalgie, communément tic douloureux de la face. 4°. *Paris*, 1817.

ROMBERG (M. H.) Neuralgiæ nervi quinti specimen. 4°. *Berolini*, 1840.

SALHEIM (A.) * De dolore faciei. 8°. *Berolini*, [1852].

SCHERZER (G. H.) * De prosopalgia. 4°. *Lipsiæ*, [1836].

SCHMITZ (C. J.) * De prosopalgia. 8°. *Lugd. Bat.*, 1842.

SCHUELER (S.) * De prosopalgia. 8°. *Berolini*, [1836].

SCHÜTZ (L.) De prosopalgia casu memorabili illustrata. 8°. *Regimontii Prussorum*, [1829].

SCHULTHEISS (C.) * Heilung eines Falles von Prosopalgie durch den constanten Strom. 8°. *Greifswald*, 1869.

SEHRWALD (G.) * De dolore faciei Fothergillii. 8°. *Dorpati Livonorum*, 1822.

SIEBOLD (G. C.) Doloris faciei morbi rarioris atque atrocis observationibus illustrati adumbratio. Annexus est de Instituti clinici ratione ad tirones sermo academicus. 4°. *Wirceburgi*, 1795.

———. The same. Doloris faciei morbi rarioris atque atrocis observationibus illustrati adumbratio. Diatribe ii. 4°. *Wirceburgi*, [1797].

SIMON (S.) * De prosopalgia. 8°. *Halæ*, [1793].

STEINDL (A.) * De prosopalgia seu dolore faciei Fothergilli. 8°. *Straubingæ*, 1833.

SUDOUR (C.) * Considérations sur la névralgie faciale. 4°. *Montpellier*, 1862.

VAHLE (B.) * De prosopalgia. 8°. *Berolini*, [1846].

WAHLLAENDER (G. E. L.) * De neuralgia nervi trigemini. 8°. *Berolini*, [1863].

WEISSE (J. M.) * De prosopalgia. 4°. *Jenæ*, [1796].

Abadie. Névralgie de la face avec glaucôme. [Rap. de Dolbeau.] Bull. Soc. de chir. de Par., 1872, 3. s., i, 534–537.—**Allnatt** (R. H.) On tic douloureux. Lond. M. Gaz., 1842, xxx, 529; 603; 674; 760; 915; 943. — **Andrews** (E.) A clinical lecture upon facial neuralgia. Chicago M. Exam., 1861, ii, 71–76.—**Anstie** (F. E.) Lettsomian lectures on certain painful affections of the fifth nerve. Lancet, Lond., 1866, i, 653; ii, 31; 199. ———. Nutritional and vaso-motor affections consecutive to neuralgia of the fifth nerve. *Ibid.*, 547. ———. Case of facial neuralgia re-induced, in a person who had previously suf-

Neuralgia (*Facial and trigeminal*).

fered from it, by syphilis, and attended with ocular paralysis and various other lesions. Tr. Clin. Soc. Lond., 1871, iv, 192 : 1872, v, 43. ———. A clinical lecture on facial neuralgia with hysteria. Med. Times & Gaz., Lond., 1874, ii, 113–115.—**Banham** (H. F.) Case of trigeminal neuralgia, with exophthalmos, and paralysis of several cranial nerves. Lancet, Lond., 1884, i, 1025.—**Beer** (H.) Prosopalgie. Oesterr. med. Wchnschr., Wien, 1843, 1098–1100.—**Beiträge** zur Pathologie und Therapie des Gesichtsschmerzes. Rhein. Jahrb. f. Med. u. Chir., Elberfeld, 1822-3, vi. 2. St., 1 ; 3. St., 93.—**Bell** (J.) Trigeminal neuralgia. Edinb. M. J., 1877. xxiii, 306–308.—**Bellingeri** (C. F. J.) De neuralgia faciei. *In his :* Diss. inaug., 8°, Augustæ Taur., 1818, 190–294. ———. Sulla nevralgia della faccia. Ann. univ. di med., Milano, 1834, lxx, 5–29.—**Benedikt & Patruban.** Ueber Tic douloureux. Allg. Wien. med. Ztg., 1871, xvi, 53.—**Bérard** (P.-H.) Face (névralgie). Dict. de méd.. 2. éd., Par., 1835, xii, 555–596.—**Blockett** (P. C.) On tic douloureux, and the best mode of treating it. Lond. M. & Phys. J., 1825, liv, 282–297.—**Borthwick.** On tic douloureux. Edinb. M. & S. J., 1825. xxiii, 295–297.—**Bowditch** (H. I.) Case of neuralgia of the head. Boston M. & S. J., 1852, xlvi, 139-143.—**Breiting** (J. G.) Geschichte eines Gesichtsschmerzes und dessen Heilung. J. d. pract. Arznk. u. Wundarznk., Berl., 1807, xxv, 4. St., 149–167.—**Brodie** (B. C.) Clinical lecture on tic douloureux, or facial neuralgia. Lond. M. Gaz., 1835-6 xvii, 534–539.—**Brown** (J. P. H.) Neuralgia faciei. Atlantic M. & S. J., 1858-9, iv, 688.—**Bruguera y Martí.** Neuralgia temporal sintomática ; su curacion. Clínica, Madrid, 1864-5, 2. ép., i, 131–133.—**Burow** (E.) Neuralgien des Quintus. *In his :* Mitth. a. d. chir. Priv.-Klin., 8°, Leipz., 1880, 71–73. — **Byrne** (W. C.) Neuralgia of the fifth pair of nerves, causing disorganization and loss of vision of the right eye. Dublin M. Press, 1840, iv, 22.—**Carnochan** (J. M.) On tic douloureux. N. York M. Press, 1860, iii, 49 ; 65.—**Chapman** (H.) Remarks on tic douloureux, with cases. Am. J. M. Sc., Phila., 1834, xiv, 289–320.—**Chaponnière** (J. J.) Recherches sur les névralgies de la face. Rec. d. trav. Soc. méd. de Genève, 1853, i, 67–118.—**Chouppe** (H.) Petit exostose du rocher dissociant les fibres du ganglion de Gasser et accompagnée de névralgie faciale. Arch. de physiol. norm. et path., Par., 1871-2, iv, 658–661, 1 pl. ———. Névralgie trifaciale très violente ; alternatives d'excitation et de coma, sans hémiplégie, consécutive à la cessation de la douleur ; autopsie ; légère exotose du côté droit de la selle turcique ; tumeur osseuse sur le trajet du trijumeau à droite. Bull. Soc. anat. de Par. (1870), 1874, xlv, 344 ; 350.—**Corbetta** (G.) Memoria sulle nevralgie facciali, e specialmente sull' odontalgia. Atti Accad. fis.-med.-statist. di Milano, 1872, xxviii, 80–94.—**Cruveilhier** (E.) Névralgie de la cinquième paire, troubles consécutifs graves du côté des organes des sens. Union méd., Par., 1872, 3. s., xiv, 649.—**Delpech.** Tic douloureux de la face. France méd., Par., 1863, x, 88-91.—**Düsterberg.** Prosopalgie mit Sectionsbericht. Wchnschr. f. d. ges. Heilk., Berl., 1846, xvi, 221–225.—**Dupuytren.** Névralgies faciales. Clin. d. hôp., Par., 1827, i, 3.—**Elsaesser.** Der Gesichtsschmerz als Familienkrankheit. J. d. pract. Heilk., Berl., 1824, lix, 2. St., 38–43.—**Erskine** (J.) Case of severe neuralgic affection. Lond. M. Reposit., 1821, xv, 283–285.—**Fantonetti** (G.) Casi di prosopalgia. Effem. d. sc. med., Milano, 1836, ii, 56–61. ———. Algema del nervo trigemino o quinto paio. Liguria med., Genova, 1858, iii, 209 ; 257.—**Fattorini** (O.) Nevralgie del secondo ramo del trigemino seguita da guarigione. Imparziale, Firenze, 1870, x, 705–713 —**Féré.** Tic non douloureux de la face du côte gauche, consécutif à une plaie de tête portant sur le pariétal droit. Compt. rend. Soc. de biol. 1876, Par., 1877, 6. s., iii, 62–64.—**Fioupe.** Névralgie trifaciale droite ; abolition du goût sur la moitié droite de la langue ; perte de la vue et de l'odorat du même côté ; à l'autopsie : carcinome de la dure-mère comprimant le ganglion de Gasser. Progrès méd., Par., 1874, ii, 741—**Fischer.** Fothergillscher Gesichtsschmerz. Arch. f. med. Erfahr., Berl., 1826, ii, 319–323.—**Focquet.** Note sur un cas de névralgie trifaciale. Arch. méd. belges, Brux., 1884, 3. s., xxv, 11–21.—**Foot** (A. W.) Notes on facial neuralgia. Dublin J. M. Sc., 1876, lxii, 185–200 —**Forstmann** (J. W.) Ueber den Fothergillschen Gesichtsschmerz. [Dis. inaug. med. de dolore faciei Fothergillii, Duisburg, 1799.] N. Samml. d. auserl. u. n Abhandl. f. Wundärzte, Leipz., 1793, 6. St., 147–225.—**Fothergill** (J.) Of a painful affection of the face. Med. Obs. Soc. Phys. Lond., 1776, v, 129–142.—**Fothergillscher** Gesichtsschmerz. Gen.-Ber. d. k. rhein. Med.-Coll. 1832, Koblenz, 1833, 110.—**von Franque** (A.) Ueber Prosopalgie. Würzb. med. Ztschr., 1863, iv, 134–137.—**Gerson.** Neuralgia facialis. Gen.-Ber. d. k. rhein. Med.-Coll. 1840, Koblenz, 1841, 52.—**Goodwillie** (D. H.) Lesions of the trifacial (especially facial neuralgia), resulting from diseases of the dental organs and adjacent parts. J. Nerv. & Ment. Dis., Chicago, 1876, iii, 188–207.—**Gower** (S.) On tic douloureux. Lancet. Lond.. 1845, i, 733–735.—**Gross** (S. D.) Form of neuralgia of the jaw-bones, hitherto undescribed. Tr.

Neuralgia (*Facial and trigeminal*).

Am. M. Ass., Phila., 1870, xxi, 197–201. *Also :* Am. J. M. Sc., Phila., 1870, n. s., lx, 48–51.—**Gubler** (A.) Névralgie réflexe et plus tard anesthésie du trijumeau en rapport avec une névrite du tronc du facial et une paralysie incomplète du côte correspondant de la face. Compt. rend. Soc. de biol. 1864, Par., 1865, 4. s., i, pt. 2, 43–50.—**Halford** (H.) On the tic douloureux. Lond. M. Gaz., 1827-8, i, 605. *Also, in his :* Essays & Orations, 8°, Lond., 1831, 35–51. *Also, in his :* Essays & Orations, 3. ed. , 12°, Lond., 1842, 33–48.—**Hall** (M.) Cases of spasmodic tic. Brit. Ann. Med., Pharm., etc., Lond., 1837, i, 8–11.—**Hamilton** (J.) Some cases of painful affections of the fifth pair of nerves, with observations. Dublin J. M. Sc., 1843. xxiii, 217–230.—**Hanselmann** (M.) Ein Fothergill'scher Gesichtsschmerz, der sich aus einer rheumatischen Augenentzündung entwickelte. Jahrb. d. ärztl. Ver. zu München, 1841, iii, 188–196.—**Harless.** Historisch-praktische Wahrnehmungen und Bemerkungen über die Natur und Behandlung des Gesichtsschmerzes, als Bruchstück einer vollständigeren Abhandlung über diese und die ihr nächstverwandten Nervenkrankheiten. N. Jahrb. d. teutsch. Med. u. Chir., Elberfeld, 1823, vi, 3. St., 119–158. — **Harrison** (W.) [Case of dolor faciei.] Med. & Phys. J., Lond., 1803, x, 420–423.—**Hasbach.** Fothergill'scher Gesichtsschmerz. J. d. pract. Arznk. u. Wundarznk., Berl., 1832, 6. R., lxxv, 87–89.—**Hasse** (C. E.) Geschichte einer Neuralgia trigemini, mit Sectionsbefund. Deutsche Klinik, Berl., 1853, v, 437.—**Herzig** (L.) Geschichte einer Amaurose als Folge von Gesichtsschmerz. Ztschr. f. d. Ophth., Heidelb., 1834-5, iv, 309–316. — **Hopkins** (B. S.) Tic douloureux. Nashville J. M. & S., 1855, ix, 99.—**Huss** (M.) Nevralgia (arthritica) nervi trigemini dextri ; tic douloureux. Hygiea, Stockholm, 1840, ii, 487–493.—**Jackson** (J.) Extracts from a discourse on the disease called tic douloureux. N. Eng. J. M. & S., Bost., 1813, ii, 106–126.—**Jaeger** (C. G.) Zur Pathologie und Therapie der Neuralgia facialis. Org. f. d. ges. Heilk., Aachen, 1852, i, 5–17.—**Jonas.** Ueber den Fothergill'schen Gesichtsschmerz. N. Arch. f. med. Erfahr., Berl., 1805, ii, 276–284.—**Jones** (G.) Case of "tic douloureux". Phila. M. Museum, 1810-11, n. s., i, 69–86. — **Kerrison** (R. M.) Tic douloureux a symptomatic disease. Lond. M. Gaz., 1835-6, xvii, 949.—**Kitson** (G.) Case of tic douloureux. Edinb. M. & S. J., 1806, ii, 319. — **Kumar & von Schrötter.** Zwei Trigeminus-Neuralgien. Wien. med. Bl., 1881, iv, 1570 – 1572. — **Lang.** Zur Pathologie und Therapie der Neuralgien des Trigeminus. Cor.- Bl. f. schweiz. Aerzte, Basel, 1877, vii, 217–221.—**Lentin.** Vom Gesichtsschmerz (Tic douloureux). J. d. pract. Arznk. u. Wundarznk., Jena, 1800, 2. R., ix, 56–64.—**Liégeois** (C.) À propos d'un cas de tic douloureux. Rev. méd. de l'est, Nancy, 1879, xi, 233–245. — **Linhart.** Geschichte einer Prosopalgie. Vrtljschr. f. d. prakt. Heilk., Prag, 1860, lxvi, 1–24, 2 pl.—**Lubelski** (W.) O bolu twarzowym (neuralgia faciei v. prosopalgia Fothergilli). Pam. Towarz., Lek. Warszaw., 1861, xlv, 281–325.—**Luise** (L.) Sopra un caso di prosopalgia ; annotazioni patologico-cliniche. Bull. d. sc. med. di Bologna, 1880, 6. s., v, 28–51.—**Lussana** (F.) Nevralgia del quinto e suoi fenomeni morbosi nei sensi dell' olfato, del gusto e dell' udito. [Case.] Gazz. med. ital. lomb., Milano, 1848, 2. s., i, 314–317. — **McShechy** (J. J.) Case of facial neuralgia. Boston M. & S J., 1871, lxxxv, 82. — **M'Veagh.** Nature and treatment of dic douloureux. Lancet, Lond., 1845, i, 407 - 409. — **Mainwaring** (E. B.) Facial neuralgia from uterine disease. *Ibid.*, 1847, i, 170.—**Marchal.** Tic douloureux, ou névralgie convulsive rhumatismale de la tête, du cou, etc. Rec. de mém. de méd. . . . mil., Par., 1852, 2. s., ix, 299-307.—**Martin** jeune. Mémoire sur la névralgie faciale. J. de méd. de Lyon, 1842, ii, 281–290. —**Masius** (G. H.) Beobachtungen und Bemerkungen über den Gesichtsschmerz. J. d. pract. Arznk. u. Wundarznk., Berl., 1806, xxv, 1 St., 9–45. ———. Schnell verschwundener nervichter Gesichtsschmerz. J. d. pract. Heilk., Berl., 1813, xxxvii, 9. St., 109–121. ———. Beiträge zu einer künftigen Monographie über den nervösen Gesichtsschmerz. Lit. Ann. d. ges. Heilk., Berl., 1826, vi, 1 ; 129 ; 257 ; 385.—**Matsuyama Toan.** [On an obstinate case of facial neuralgia.] Sei-i-Kwai M. J., Tôkyô, Feb. 26, 1883.—**Méglin.** Observation sur une affection douloureuse, ou tic douloureux de la face. J. de méd., chir., pharm., etc., Par., 1811, xxii, 331–337. ———. Observation sur une affection douloureuse de la tête, sous forme de migraine, ou de tic douloureux. *Ibid.*, 1812, xxiii, 3–8. ———. Observations sur le tic douloureux de la face. *Ibid.*, 1813, xxvii, 128–136. ———. Observation sur un tic douloureux de la face. J. gén. de méd., chir. et pharm., Par., 1823, lxxxiii, 213–217.—**Merkens.** Gesichtsschmerz. Gen.- Ber. d. k. rhein. Med.-Coll. 1840, Koblenz, 1841, 53.—**Minot.** [Facial neuralgia.] Boston M. & S J., 1867, lxxvi, 505 —**Miquel.** Ungewöhnlich häufiges Vorkommen von Gesichtsschmerz. Arch. f. med. Erfahr., Berl., 1824, ii, 250–258.—**Mombert.** Gesichts- und katarrhalischer Stirnhöhlenschmerz. Vrtljschr. f. d. prakt. Heilk., Prag, 1847, ii, 119–126.—**Montefoschi** (E.) Caso di nevralgia del trigemino in specie del suo terzo ramo. Raccoglitore med., Forlì, 1873, 3. s., xxiii, 418–422.—**Moos.** Ein Fall von Neuralgie, hauptsächlich

Neuralgia (*Facial and trigeminal*).

im Bereich des zweiten Trigeminus-Astes, durch Exostosenbildung im äusseren Gehörgang bedingt. Berl. klin. Wchnschr., 1884, xxi, 116. — **Müller.** Ein sehr heftiger Gesichtsschmerz. Allg. med. Ann., Altenb., 1804, xix, 108-110.—**Müller.** Prosopalgia intermittens. Gen-Ber. d. k. rhein. Med.-Coll. 1838, Koblenz, 1840, 99. — **Muñoz y Ferron** (J.-M.) Neurálgia facial; escorbuto general; caso notable de curacion por las circunstancias de la enferma y medios empleados. Crón de l. hosp., Madrid, 1856, iv, 339-344.—**Neucourt** (F.) Considérations sur la névralgie faciale, pour servir à l'histoire de cette maladie. Arch. gén. de méd., Par., 1849, ii, 162-195. ——. De la névralgie faciale et de la névralgie du cuir chevelu. *Ibid.*, 1853, ii, 385; 695: 1854, i, 194 —**Ord** (W. M.) Long-standing trigeminal neuralgia; relaxation (?) of certain muscles supplied by 3d and 7th nerves on same side. St. Thomas's Hosp. Rep., Lond., 1873, n. s., iv, 61.—**Ovens** (T.) Case of neuralgia of the trigeminal nerve. Canada Lancet, Toronto, 1885-6, xviii, 69.—**Paletta** (G. B.) Dello spasimo della faccia. Ann. univ. di med., Milano, 1822, xxiv, 51-55.—**Pearson** (G.) On the tic douloureux, or trismus dolorificus. Edinb. M. & S. J., 1807, iii, 272-276.—**Pecorara** (A.) Sul tratato igienico e sulla monografia intorno alle nevralgie facciali messi in luce dal Giov. Corbetta. Atti Accad. fis.-med.-statist. di Milano, 1874, xxx, 20-28.—**Perkowski** (S.) Przecięcie gałązek nerwu uszno-skroniowego, jako środek lecznicy przeciw uporczywemu nerwobólowi szczękowemu. [Relation of auricular nerves to neuralgia of the jaws.] Medycyna, Warszawa, 1880, viii, 625-627. — **Pichonnière.** Observation d'une névralgie du nerf trifacial du côté droit, accompagnée d'une amaurose de l'œil droit. Gaz. d. hôp., Par., 1829-30, ii, 98. — **Podrazki.** Beiträge zu den Neuralgien im Gebiete des Nervus trigeminus und ihrer Behandlung. Oesterr. Ztschr. f. prakt. Heilk., Wien, 1869, xv. 1; 17; 33; 49; 69; 89; 105; 121; 189. — **Politzer** (A.) Cas de névralgie produite principalement dans le rayon du deuxième rameau des trijumeaux par la formation d'exostoses dans le conduit auditif externe, d'après M. le Dr. Moos. Ann. d. mal. de l'oreille et du larynx, Par., 1884, x, 87.—**Powell** (T. S.) Tic douloureux; hemicrania. Atlanta M. & S. J, 1856-7, ii, 396.—**Pratt** (D. L.) Case of facial neuralgia. Tr. Belmont M. Soc., Bridgeport, Ohio, 1849-50, 51-53.—**Primassin** (L.) Prosopalgie in Folge einer Augenverletzung. Org. f. d. ges. Heilk., Aachen, 1852, i, 153. — **Ravà** (G.) Spasmo acuto dell' accomodazione, consecutivo a nevralgia del trigemino. Ann. di ottal., Milano, 1879, viii, 554-560—**Rousset.** Névralgie trifaciale. J. de méd. de Bordeaux, 1852, x, 366.—**Salter** (J. A.) Intense neuralgia of the eyeball and face; alteration of the colour of the iris; carious teeth. Guy's Hosp. Rep., Lond., 1868, 3. s., xiii, 96.—**Samel.** Mehrere Fälle von periodischem Gesichtsschmerz. Mag. f. d. ges. Heilk., Berl., 1828, xxv, 456-479. — **Sauter.** Eine Beobachtung über den Gesichtsschmerz. Museum d. Heilk., Zürich, 1792, i, 297-302.— **Savoye.** Observation de névralgie de la cinquième paire. France méd., Par., 1879, xxvi, 594.—**Schadewaldt.** Die Trigeminus-Neurosen. Deutsche med. Wchnschr., Berl., 1885, xi, 637; 656.—**Schauer.** Der Gesichtsschmerz als Symptom. Wchnschr. f. d. ges. Heilk., Berl., 1838, vi, 393; 411; 433; 445; 466. — **Schmidtmann** (L J.) Beobachtungen über den Fothergill'schen Gesichtsschmerz, Tic douloureux. J. d. pract. Arznk. u. Wundarznk., Berl., 1832, 6. R., lxxv. 29-43. — **Schoeneich** (H.) On prosopalgia. St. Louis Probe, 1850, i, 78-81.—**Scholz** (F.) Ein Fall von Prosopalgie, bedingt durch Bindegewebsgeschwulst (Tumor fibrosus) in der mittlern Schädelgrube. Wien. med. Wchnschr., 1860, x, 793-798. — **Schramm.** Ueber die Neuralgie des fünften Nervenpaares. Aerztl. Int.-Bl., München, 1859, vi, 191. — **Schreger.** Gesichtsschmerz. Arch. f. med. Erfahr., Berl., 1810, n. F., xiii, 207-209.—**Schuppert** (M.) Zwei Fälle von rechtseitigem Gesichtsschmerz; Dolor Fothergilli. Deutsche Ztschr. f. Chir., Leipz., 1873, iii, 550-568. — **Schweich** (H.) Typischer Schmerz des ersten Astes des Nervus trigeminus. Wchnschr. f. d. ges. Heilk., Berl., 1848, xvi, 12-14.—**Seifert.** Beitrag zur Pathologie und Therapie der Trigeminusneuralgien. Berl. klin. Wchnschr., 1881, xviii, 148-152. — **Senator** (H.) Ein Fall von Trigeminusaffection; Beitrag zur Kenntniss von der neuroparalytischen Ophthalmie, dem Verlauf der Geschmacksfasern der Chorda und den intermittirenden Gelenkschwellungen. Arch. f. Psychiat., Berl., 1882, xiii, 590-601.—**Serrurier.** Observation sur une névralgie faciale. J. de méd., Par., 1817, xl, 198-208.—**Skae** (E.) Remarks on Tic-douloureux. Edinb. M. & S. J., 1840, liv, 85 - 95.— **Stehrer** (C.) Ein Fall von hartnäckiger Neuralgia facialis s. Dolor faciei Fothergilli. Ztschr. f. Wundärzte u. Geburtsh., Stuttg., 1852, v, 58-60.—**von Stoffella.** Zwei Fälle von Dentin-Neubildung in Folge von Trigeminusneuralgie. Wien. med. Presse, 1884, xxv, 981; 1013; 1080.— **Takács** (E.) Paralysis peripherica nervi facialis dextri; dein neuralgia nervi trigemini dextri. Orvosi hetil., Budapest, 1878, xxii, 269-272. *Also, transl.:* Pest. med.-chir. Presse, Budapest, 1878, xiv, 742. ——. Idegkórtani esetek a gyakorlatból (neuralgia nervi trigemini). Orvosi hetil., Budapest, 1881, xxv, 48; 73. *Also, transl.:* Pest. med.-chir.

Neuralgia (*Facial and trigeminal*).

Presse, Budapest, 1881, xvii, 344; 395; 442.—**Terrillon.** Angiôme sous-cutané douloureux; névralgie trifaciale. Progrès méd, Par., 1884, xii, 983. — **Thomson** (F. H.) Notes of practice; facial neuralgia. Glasgow M. J., 1860-61, [2. s.], viii, 46-53. ——. Notes on practice; facial neuralgia. *Ibid.*, 1867-8, [3. s.], ii, 224-230.—**Thouret.** Mémoire sur l'affection particulière de la face, à laquelle on a donné le nom de tic douloureux. Hist. Soc. roy. de méd. 1782-3, Par., 1787, v, pt. 2, 204-256. — **Torras y Pascual.** Neuralgia del trigémino y parálisis facial simultáneas; contractura y dermatósis nerviosa? consecutivas. Rev. de cien. méd., Barcel., 1885, xi, 345-349. — **Tott** (C. A.) Beispiel von Facial-Neuralgie bei einer hochbejahrten Dame. N. Ztschr. f. Geburtsk., Berl., 1844, xvi, 198-202 — **Tuffier.** Névralgie faciale chez un vieillard édenté; mort; névrite du nerf dentaire inférieur. France méd., Par., 1881, xxviii, 672-675. *Also:* Bull. Soc. clin. de Par. (1881), 1882, v, 132-135.—**Ulmer** (F.) Ueber Prosopalgie. Ztschr. f. Wundärzte u. Geburtsh., Stuttg., 1852, v, 30-36. — **Valleix.** Note sur un cas remarquable de névralgie trifaciale. Arch. gén. de méd., Par., 1842, iii, 472-484. *Also:* Ann. de méd. belge, Brux., 1843, i, 9-13.—**Vanderbeck** (C. C.) Persistent facial "neuralgia"; rheumatic sciatica. Med. & Surg. Reporter, Phila., 1876, xxxv, 104.— **Vulpian** (A.) Tic douloureux de la face, datant de quinze ans; accès douloureux se rapprochant de plus en plus jusqu'à devenir continus; attaque apoplectique; hémorrhagie cérébrale; mort rapide; autopsie. *In his:* Clin. méd. de l'hôp. de la Charité, 8°, Par., 1879, 620-626.— **Waitz** (H.) Neuralgien des N. trigeminus; 5 Fälle. Arch. f. klin. Chir., Berl., 1877, xxi, 616-618. — **Weinlechner** (J.) Ueber "Prosopalgie"; Neuralgia rami secundi et tertii nervi trigemini. Allg. Wien. med. Ztg., 1866, xi, 253; 261. — **Weissenbach.** Dringende Bitte eines am Fothergill'schen Gesichtsschmerz trostlos Leidenden, nebst Prof. . . .'s Antwort hierauf. Med.-chir. Ztg. Salzb., 1806, iv, 259-270. — **Wing.** Case of tic-douloureux. Proc. Westminst. M. Soc., Lond., 1848-9, 61.— **Wood** (H. C.) The trigeminal neuralgias. Med. Rec., N. Y., 1877, xii, 673-675. — **Zwicke.** Neuralgia facialis. Charité-Ann. 1881, Berl., 1883, viii, 429.

Neuralgia (*Facial and trigeminal, Treatment of*).

See, also, **Neuralgia** (*Dental*, etc., *Treatment of*); **Neurotomy**, etc.

BARNICK (H.) * Die Behandlungen der Neuralgien im Gebiete des Nervus trigeminus durch Neurectomie. 8°. *Berlin*, [1871].

BECU DE TAVERNIER (O.) * De specimine quodam neuralgiæ infraorbitalis dextri per neurectomiam sublatæ. 8°. *Berolini*, 1860.

BESSARD (A.) * Contribution à l'étude des procédés opératoires dans les cas de névralgie du trijumeau. [Basel.] 8°. *Paris*, 1882.

VON BRUNS (V.) Die Durchschneidung der Gesichtsnerven beim Gesichtsschmerz. 8°. *Tübingen*, 1859.

BURSAUX (J.) * De la résection du nerf sous-orbitaire dans la névralgie faciale rebelle. 4°. *Paris*, 1882.

CINICELLI (G.) Il cloridrato di pilocarpina nella cura della prosopalgia. 4°. [*Pavia*, 1884.]

CORBETTA (G.) Delle nevralgie facciali e dell' odontalgia in particolare; osservazioni patologiche e terapeutiche, con appendice corredata di due tavole anatomiche incise in rame. 8°. *Milano*, 1873.

DITANDY (E.) * Réflexions sur un cas de névralgie trifaciale traitée par la névrotomie. 4°. *Strasbourg*, 1865.

FLORIAN (J.) * De prosopalgia neurectomiæ auxilio sananda. 8°. *Vratislaviæ*, [1863].

FRANK (C.) * Die Heilung des Gesichtsschmerzes durch Neurotomie. 8°. *Giessen*, 1858.

FRICKER (J. P.) * De secando trunco nervi duri in prosopalgia, additis observationibus de morbis infantum. 12°. *Tubingæ*, [1813].

Also, in: WEBER. Samml. med.-prakt. Diss. [etc] 8°. *Tübingen*, 1829, v, 1-20.

GROSSKOFF (M.) A treatise upon the tic douloureux, with the treatment and alleviation of this hitherto impenetrable disease. 8°. *London*, [n. d.]

HEYFELDER (J. F. M.) * De prosopalgia Fothergilli, adnexa singularis hujus morbi historia. 4°. *Vratislaviæ*, [1820].

Neuralgia (*Facial and trigeminal, Treatment of*).

HEYMANN (I.) * De la division des nerfs dans le traitement du tic douloureux. 4°. *Strasbourg*, 1857.

HUTCHINSON (B.) Cases of tic douloureux successfully treated. 8°. *London*, 1820.

——. The same. 2. ed. 8°. *London*, 1822.

JOERRENS (H.) * De neurotomia in prosopalgia instituenda. 8°. *Bonnæ*, [*n. d.*]

KEREZ (H.) * Ueber den Erfolg der Neurektomien, der Unterbindung der Arteria carotis und der Electrotherapie bei peripheren Neuralgien des Trigeminus. 8°. *Basel*, 1878.

LASSALLE (A.) Étude sur le traitement de la névralgie rebelle du nerf maxillaire supérieur par la résection du nerf sous-orbitaire dans la cavité de l'orbite. 4°. *Paris*, 1877.

LICHAU (E.) * Die Gesichts-Neuralgie und ihre Behandlung durch Nerven-Resection. 8°. *Würzburg*, 1886.

MARY (J.-A.) * Du nitrate d'aconitine dans le traitement des névralgies faciales. 4°. *Paris*, 1880.

MICHON (H.) * Des moyens chirurgicaux employés comme traitement de la névralgie faciale rebelle. 4°. *Paris*, 1882.

MIRE (A.) * Des procédés de névrotomie applicables au traitement de la névralgie sous-orbitaire. 4°. *Strasbourg*, 1863.

MUELLER (G.) * Die Prosopalgie und ihre Heilung durch die Nenrectomie. 4°. *Kiel*, 1875.

OLIVERIO. Prosopalgia guarita per l' azione del croton tiglio. 8°. *Napoli*, 1848.

PERRENOUD (L. A.) * Die Nervenresectionen bei Neuralgien des Supra- und Infraorbitalis. 8°. *Würzburg*, 1860.

PEYROUNET DE LAFONVIELLE (A.) * De la névralgie du trijumeau, et en particulier de son traitement par les pulvérisations de chlorure de méthyle. 4°. *Paris*, 1886.

PFAHL (C.) * Die subcutane Neurectomie des Nervus infraorbitalis nach B. von Langenbeck. sm. 8°. *Berlin*, [1869].

RICHET (P.) * Observations et réflexions relatives à l'efficacité du quinquina dans les névralgies intermittentes, et à un nouveau mode d'administration de ce remède dans ces affections. 4°. *Strasbourg*, 1826.

SCHNEIDER (A.) * Ein Fall von traumatisch veranlasster, langjähriger Trigeminusneuralgie; Heilung durch Resection des afficirten Astes (N. alveolaris sin.). 8°. *Würzburg*, 1879.

SCHUENEMANN (A.) * De neurectomia nervi infraorbitalis et de nova operationis methodo. 8°. *Regimonti Pr.*, [1863].

SCHUH. Ueber Gesichtsneuralgien und über die Erfolge der dagegen vorgenommenen Nervenresectionen. 8°. *Wien*, 1858.

WITT (C. G. J.) * Exemplum neurotomiæ prosopalgiæ sanandæ causa factæ. 4°. *Kiliæ*, 1860.

Aepli. Neuralgia ram. infraorbital. und trigemini; Operation nach Lücke. Deutsche Ztschr. f. Chir., Leipz., 1878, xi, 168–172.—**Aguilar y Venegas** (L. J.) Prosopalgia periódica refractaria á los antitípicos usuales; curacion por el licor de Labarraque. Andalucía méd., Córdoba, 1878, iii, 27–32. ——. Neuralgia-trifacial de tipo intermitente tercianario, consecutiva á una conjunctivitis idiopática, curada por los prepaiados químicos. Ibid., 1879, iv, 15–18.—**Albert** (E.) Neuralgie des ersten Astes; Resektion desselben; Heilung. Wien. med. Presse, 1877, xviii, 622. ——. Neuralgien des Trigeminus 5 durch Neurectomie geheilt, 1 Fall nach der Neurotomie gebessert entlassen. Ber. d. naturw.-med. Ver. in Innsbruck (1877), 1879, viii, 3. Hft., 51–54.—**Alvarenga.** Nevralgia faciali; administração do aconito; cura. Gaz. med. de Lisb., 1877, 4. s., iv, 121; 133.—**Andrews** (E.) Terrible neuralgia of the face cured by excision of a portion of the infra-orbital nerve. Chicago M. Exam., 1861, ii, 148–150. ——. A case of facial neuralgia, treated by repeated sections of the branches of the trigeminal nerve. Chicago J. Nerv. & Ment. Dis., 1874,

Neuralgia (*Facial and trigeminal, Treatment of*).

i, 293–296.—**Armaingaud.** Névralgie trifaciale; point douloureux apophysaire au niveau de la cinquième vertèbre cervicale; cessation subite de la douleur après l'application du cautère actuel sur le point douloureux vertébral. [Discussion.] Mém. et bull. Soc. de méd. et chir. de Bordeaux, 1874, 79; 86: 94; 106. Also [Abstr.]: Bordeaux méd., 1874, iii, 65.—**Badal.** De l'élongation des nerfs et ses applications au traitement des névralgies du trijumeau. Gaz. hebd. d. sc. méd. de Bordeaux, 1880–81, i, 974; 994; 1019.—**Baird** (W.) Cure of tic douloureux by steam. Lancet, Lond., 1838–9, i, 644–466.—**Bartholow** (R.) On the deep injection of chloroform for the relief of tic douloureux. Practitioner, Lond., 1874, xiii, 9–14.—**Beale** (J. E.) Case of tic douloureux successfully treated by carbonate of iron. Lond. M. & Phys. J., 1823, lii, 201–203.—**Beard** (G. M.) Facial neuralgia of long-standing dependent on uterine disease; no relief from localized galvanization; great relief under local treatment of the uterus. Am. Pract., Louisville, 1874, ix, 204.—**Beaumont** (J. W.) Formula for tic-douloureux. Assoc. M. J., Lond., 1853, 137.—**Beck** (B.) Ein Fall von Durchschneidung des linken oberen Augenhöhlennerven bei heftiger, viele Jahre bestehender Neuralgie des Quintus. Deutsche Klinik, Berl., 1857, ix, 299–301.—**Bennett** (E. S.) Observations on the distilled water of the Prunus lauro-cerasus, in facial neuralgia. N. Am. Arch. M. & S. Sc., Balt, 1835, ii, 28–31.—**Bérard** jeune. Tic douloureux guéri par la section du nerf sous-orbitaire. Gaz. méd. de Par., 1835, 2. s., iii, 542.—**Billroth** (T.) Neuralgien des N. trigeminus. In his: Chir. Klin., 8°, Wien, 1871–6, Berl., 1879, 134–137.—**Bird** (F.) Ueber den Nutzen des äusseren Gebrauchs des kalten Wassers in der Prosopalgia Fothergilli. Arch. f. med. Erfahr., Berl., 1823, i, 106–121.—**Blackett** (P. C.) Cases of tic douloureux; in one of which the patient took about eight ounces of carbonate of iron in thirty-six hours. Lond. M. & Phys. J., 1826, lv, 122.—**Blum.** De l'arrachement du nerf sous-orbitaire. Bull. et mém. Soc. de chir. de Par., 1882, n. s., viii, 799–802.—**Blundell** (E. S.) Cases of tic douloureux cured by the "mineral magnet." Lancet, Lond., 1832–3, ii, 693.—**Blunt** (R.) Case of painful affection of the face cured by electricity. Lond. M. J., 1786, vii, 115–119.—**Bonnafont.** Observations d'une névralgie faciale très-intense entretenue pendant plus de quinze mois, par la présence d'un fragment de balle enchassé dans l'os maxillaire droit, et comprimant le nerf sous-orbitaire; guérison immédiate par l'extraction du projectile. Gaz. d. hôp., Par., 1856, xxix, 382.—**Bonnet.** Observation sur la guérison du tic douloureux ou névralgie faciale au moyen de l'usage externe du gaz oximuriatique. Ann. clin., Montpel., 1813, xxxii, 48–66. ——. Tic douloureux guéri par la section du nerf sous-orbitaire. Rev. méd. franç. et étrang., Par., 1831, iv, 364–368.—**Book** (J. B.) Removal of Meckel's ganglion for the cure of tic douloureux. Michigan M. News, Detroit, 1881, iv, 110.—**Borthwick** (G. A.) Case of tic douloureux successfully treated by carbonate of iron. Edinb. M. & S. J., 1824, xxi, 285–287.—**Bottani** (G.) Sul nuovo metodo proposto dal Profess. Fleischmann nella cura delle nevralgie facciali. Gior. per serv. ai progr. d. patol., Venezia, 1837, vii, 53–75.—**Bradbury.** Neuralgia of inferior dental nerve of two years' duration; rapid improvement under the use of cod-liver oil and hypodermic injection of morphia. Brit. M. J., Lond., 1870, ii, 139.—**Bratsch.** Zur Statistik der Resectionen an den Trigeminus-Aesten. Aerztl. Int.-Bl., München, 1860, vii, 581.—**Braun** (H.) Neurektomen des zweiten Astes des Nervus trigeminus nach osteoplastischer Resektion des Jochbeins. Centralbl. f. Chir., Leipz., 1882, ix, 249–255.—**Bricheteau.** Névralgie intermittente de la face, revenant régulièrement à une année d'intervalle. Union méd., Par., 1851, v, 425. Also: Bull. Soc. méd. d. hôp. de Par. (1849–52), 1861, i, 219.—**Briggs** (W. T.) Neuralgia of jaw; operation. Nashville J. M. & S., 1871, n. s., vii, 115. ——. Neuralgia of the superior maxillary nerve; Carnochan's operation. Ibid., 1872, n. s., ix, 68–71.—**Brookes** (W. P.) Case of facial neuralgia successfully treated by aconitine. Lancet, Lond., 1844, i, 476.—**Brown** (A.) A severe case of facial neuralgia cured by a new surgical operation. Brit. M. J., Lond., 1889, ii, 741.—**Brünniche.** Krotonkloral med Prosopalgi; Stryknin mod Anosmia. Hosp.-Tid., Kjøbenh., 1874. 2. R., ii, 369–371.—**Brunelli** (C.) Neuralgia del mascellare inferiore (tic doloroso) che dura da 5 anni; cura elettrica; guarigione. Gior. med. di Roma, 1867, iii, 37.—**Bruzelius** (R.) Om elektrisk behandling af tic douloureux. Hygiea, Stockholm, 1868, xxx, 430–442.—**Burgess** (J. M.) Gelsemium in facial neuralgia. Michigan M. News, Detroit, 1879, ii, 119.—**Buzzard.** Two cases of nerve-stretching for facial neuralgia; the sequel after three years and two years respectively. Brit. M. J., Lond., 1883, ii, 1126.—**C.** Note sur un cas de résection et de cautérisation des branches du trifacial pratiquée avec succès dans un cas de névralgie de ce nerf durant depuis dix ans. Bull. gén. de thérap., etc., Par., 1864, lxvi, 400–405.—**Calonius.** Ett fall af neuralgia nervi trigemini lyckligt behandladt med galvanism. Finsk. läk.-sällsk.

Neuralgia (*Facial and trigeminal, Treatment of*).

handl., Helsingfors, 1876, xviii, 87.—**Carnochan** (J. M.) A case of neuralgia of the face cured by resection of part of the nerve. West. J. M. & S., Louisville, 1855, 4. s., iv, 253 - 257. ———. Exsection of the trunk of the second branch of the fifth pair of nerves, beyond the ganglion of Meckel, for severe neuralgia of the face; with three cases. Am. J. M. Sc., Phila., 1858, n. s., xxxv, 134-143. *Also, transl.:* Monit. d. hôp., Par., 1858, vi, 241; 250. ———. On tic douloureux: "The painful affection of the face, dolor faciei crucians", of Fothergill, with a new operation for its cure. Am. M. Gaz., N. Y., 1860, xi, 81-100. *Also:* Am. M. Month., N. Y., 1860, xiii, 142-152.—**Carter** (H. W.) Case of tic douloureux, successfully treated by carbonate of iron. Lond. M. Reposit., 1821, xv, 371. — [**Cases.**] Painful affection of all the nerves of one side of the face cured by repeated operations. N. Eng. J. M. & S., Bost., 1823, xii, 216 - 219.—Névralgie épileptiforme; traitement palliatif par l'opium. Union méd., Par., 1853, vii, 372.—Résection suivie de cautérisation de plusieurs branches du trifacial dans un cas de névralgie de ce nerf durant depuis dix ans; guérison momentanée et récidive au bout de trois mois; effets du traitement par l'aconitine continuée jusqu'à ce jour. Bull. gén. de thérap., etc., Par., 1864, lxvii, 414-417.—Tic douloureux de la face traité sans succès par la névrotomie. *Ibid.*, 1866, lxxi, 130 - 134.—[Resection der Nervi infraorb.] Aerztl. Ber. d. k. k. allg. Krankenh. zu Wien (1866), 1867, 296.—Tic douloureux de la face datant de vingt-huit ans, guéri par le bromure de potassium. Paris méd., 1876, ii, 198-200.—**Cebrián y Díez** (V.) El clorhidrato de cocaina contra la neuralgia facial. Bol. de med. y cirug., Madrid, 1886, iv, 217-219.—**Chavasse** (T. F.) Neurectomy of the second division of the fifth nerve. Med.-Chir. Tr., Lond., 1884, lxvii. 145-156. *Also* [Abstr.]: Proc. Roy. M. & Chir. Soc. Lond., 1883-4, n. s., i, 208-213. *Also* [Abstr.]: Med. Times & Gaz., Lond., 1884, i, 300.—**Cheever** (D. W.) Section and removal of the superior maxillary nerve and Meckel's ganglion for neuralgia. Med. & Surg. Rep. Bost. City Hosp., 1877, 2. s., ii, 262-265.—**Clarke** (B.) Gelseminum in facial neuralgia. Brit. M. J., Lond., 1881, i, 271.—**Clarke** (F. E.) On the treatment of facial neuralgia. Med. Press & Circ., Lond., 1872, n. s., xiv, 454.—**Colville** (E.) Case of tic douloureux, cured by the external use of tar. Edinb. M. & S. J., 1814, x, 288.—**Conant** (D. S.) On the operation for division of the second branch of the fifth pair of nerves. Am. M. Month., N. Y., 1857; viii, 82.—**Conner** (P. S.) Exsection of portions of the supra- and infra-orbital nerves for the relief of tic douloureux. Clinic, Cincin., 1874, vii, 97-99.—**Coosemans** (E.) Du sulfate de cuivre ammoniacal dans la névralgie du trijumeau. J. d. sc. méd. de Louvain, 1880, v, 441-444.—**Coppez.** Névralgie, datant de vingt ans guérie par l'élongation du nerf sous-orbitaire. Ann. d'ocul., Brux., 1882, 12. s., vii, 59-61.—**Corkindale** (J.) Case of tic douloureux cured by calomel and opium. Edinb. M. & S. J., 1808, iv, 306-309.—**Coudray** (P.) Résection du nerf sus-orbitaire et du sous-orbitaire pour une névralgie invétérée de la face; guérison, suivie pendant plus de 20 mois. Arch. roum. de méd. et chir., Par., 1887, i, 194-197.—**Craddock** (S.) Case of trigeminal neuralgia treated with the constant current. Practitioner, Lond., 1873, x, 337 - 340.—**Craig** (W.) Acupuncture in facial neural·ia. Med. Times & Gaz., Lond., 1864, ii, 277.—**Crawford** (S.) On the use of carbonate of iron in tic douloureux. Lond. M. & Phys. J., 1823, xlix, 109-111.—**Creutzwieser.** Fall einer glücklichen Heilung der Prosopalgia durch Sublimat. Mag. f. d. ges. Heilk., Berl., 1826, xxii, 337.—**Crous y Casellas.** Prosopalgia ó neuralgia del trigemino tratada favorablemente por la corriente farádica. Rev. de cien. méd., Barcel., 1877, iii, 246-250.—**Da-Camino** (F. S.) Nevralgie facciali curate coll' ago-puntura. Gazz. med. ital., prov. venete, Padova, 1863, vi, 272.—**Dawson** (W. W.) Excision of the superior and inferior maxillary nerves from the same person; two cases; excision of the superior maxillary nerve. Hosp. Gaz., N. Y., 1877, i, 56-58. *Also.* Richmond & Louisville M. J., Louisville, 1877, xxiv, 597-600.—**Deahofe** (S. P.) Successful treatment of a case of trigeminal neuralgia with nitro-glycerine. Med. News, Phila., 1885, xlvi, 208.—**Debu.** Tic douloureux de la face chez un sujet cérébrogastrique guérie par les lavages répétés de l'estomac. Gaz. d. hôp., Par., 1886, lix, 315.—**Dennis** (F. S.) Neurotomy of the superior maxillary branch of the trigeminus, including neurectomy of the spheno-palatine ganglion for the relief of tic-douloureux. N. York M. J., 1879, xxix, 576-601.—**Dercum** (F. X.) A case of tic douloureux of twelve years' standing treated by large doses of the salicylates with marked success. Polyclinic. Phila., 1886-7, iv, 323-325. *Also:* Phila. M. Times, 1886-7. xvii, 471-473. *Also:* Med. News, Phila., 1887, l, 328.—**De Wolfe** (G. H. H.) Gelseminum in facial neuralgia. Brit. M. J., Lond., 1881, i. 193.—**Discussion** sur le traitement des névralgies sous-orbitaires. Bull. et mém. Soc. de chir. de Par., 1882, n. s., viii, 810 - 816. — **Ducros.** Traitement de la migraine et du tic douloureux par la cautérisation palatine. Gaz. méd. de Par., 1843, 2. s, xi, 314.—

Neuralgia (*Facial and trigeminal, Treatment of*).

Düsterberg. Nutzen des Fontanells zwischen dem Processus mastoideus und dem Winkel des Unterkiefers, gegen den inveterirten ächten Fothergill'schen Gesichtsschmerz. J. d. pract. Heilk., Berl., 1826, lxiii, 6. St., 114-119. — **Dumont** (F.) Ueber den Erfolg der Nervendehnung und Nervenresection bei Trigeminusneuralgien. Deutsche Ztschr. f. Chir., Leipz., 1883, xix, 51-73. — **Easton** (J. A.) On croton oil in tic douloureux. Lancet, Lond., 1841-2, i, 609. — **Ebers.** Veratrin gegen Prosopalgia. Wchnschr. f. d. ges. Heilk., Berl., 1835, iii, 735-740. — **Eggert** (F. F. G.) Ueber das Wesen des Gesichtsschmerzes und die Operation desselben. J. d. Chir. u. Augenh., Berl., 1825, vii, 538-570. — **Encinas** (S. G.) Neurotomia del nervio suborbitario. Rev. de med. y cirug. práct., Madrid, 1881, ix, 351-355. — **Englisch.** Neuralgie der 2. Astes des Trigeminus; Resection des Nervus infraorbitalis; Heilung. Ber. d. k. k. Krankenanst. Rudolph-Stiftung in Wien (1881), 1882, 322.—**Evans** (G. H.) Nitrite of amyl in facial neuralgia. Practitioner. Lond., 1875, xv, 179. — **Feliciani** (A.) Nevralgia del nervo dentale inferiore, esistente da 13 anni; inefficacia di tutti i remedii ordinarj; sezione del nervo. Bull. d. sc. med. di Bologna, 1836, 2. s., ii, 144-152. — **Féréol.** Note sur les bons effets du sulfate de cuivre ammoniacal contre la névralgie de la cinquième paire. Bull. Acad. de méd., Par., 1879, 2. s., viii, 335-337. *Also:* Bull. gén. de thérap., etc., Par., 1879, xcvi, 337-344. — **Fergusson.** Tic douloureux seated in the mental branch of the inferior dental nerve; division of that branch; recovery. Lancet, Lond., 1852, ii, 376. ———. Treatment of tic douloureux by division of the nerve. *Ibid.*, 1857, ii, 247.—**Féron.** Du sulfate de cuivre ammoniacal dans la névralgie du nerf trijumeau. J. d. sc. méd. de Louvain, 1881, vi, 377.—**Fieber** (K.) Mittheilungen über Nervenresectionen bei Gesichtsschmerz. Anz. d. k. k. Gesellsch. d. Aerzte in Wien, 1878, 2. ———. Drei Fälle von Gesichtsneuralgie, durch Nervenresection geheilt oder gebessert. Berl. klin. Wchnschr., 1878, xv, 269-273.—**Fleury** (L.) Névralgie faciale très-grave; sept ans de durée; contractions des muscles masséters; impossibilité absolue de parler et de mâcher; ptyalisme abondant et continu; inefficacité d'un grand nombre de médications diverses; traitement hydrothérapique; guérison rapide. Monit. d. hôp., Par., 1856, iv, 186. — **Fothergill'scher** Gesichtsschmerz; Neurectomie; Heilung. Ber. d. k. k. Krankenanst. Rudolph-Stiftung in Wien (1869), 1870, 194-196. — **Fowler** (G. R.) Extirpation of superior maxillary nerve and Meckel's ganglion for facial neuralgia. Proc. M. Soc. County Kings, Brooklyn, 1877, ii, 176-178. ———. The surgical treatment of facial neuralgia. Ann. Anat. & Surg. Soc., Brooklyn, N. Y., 1880, ii, 133; 180. ———. Two cases of neurectomy for the relief of facial neuralgia. Med. Rec., N. Y., 1884, xxvi, 368. ———. The operative treatment of facial neuralgia, a comparison of methods and results. Ann. Surg., St. Louis, 1886, iii, 269-320. — **Freeman** (A. B.) Dental lesions causing facial neuralgia and other neural phenomena. J. Am. M. Ass., Chicago, 1887, ix, 519-522. — **Fritsch.** Beiträge zur medicinischen Erfahrung; Heilung einer Neuralgia facialis durch Ferrum carbonicum. J. d. pract. Heilk., Berl., 1832, lxxv. 3. St., 107-110. — **Garretson** (J. E.) Exsection of second branch of fifth nerve at foramen rotundum. Phila. M. Times, 1886-7, xvii, 55. *Also:* Phila. M. Times, 1886-7, xvii, 56. *Also:* Med. Bull., Phila., 1887, ix, 65.—**Gerster.** Resection of superior maxillary nerve for intractable neuralgia. Med. Rec., N. Y., 1882, xxi, 300. — **Gesichtsschmerz.** Resection des Nervus infraorbitalis und Nerv. zygomaticus. Ber. d. k. k. Krankenanst. Rudolph-Stiftung in Wien (1870), 1871, 170-173.—**Giacometti** (V.) Storia di grave prosopalgia guarita con l' applicazione della magnete. Gazz. med. ital. feder. tosc., Firenze, 1852, 2. s., ii, 171.—**Godlee** (R. J.) A case of stretching of the facial nerve for tic spasmodique. Med. Times & Gaz., Lond., 1881, i, 688. ———. Stretching the facial nerve for tic convulsif. Brit. M. J., Lond., 1883, i, 1122. *Also:* Med. Times & Gaz., Lond., 1883, i, 682. *Also:* Lancet, Lond., 1883, i, 1000.—**Grill.** Om Magnetens användande emot tic douloureux. etc. Tidskr. f. Läk. o. Pharm., Stockholm, 1834, iii, 276-278. — **Grognon.** Action de la napelline dans un cas de névralgie faciale. Bull. gén. de thérap., etc.. Par., 1883, cv, 221.—**Gross** (F. H.) Trigeminal neuralgia relieved by ligation of the common carotid artery and neurectomy. Am. J. M. Sc., Phila., 1883, n. s., lxxxv, 366-378. *Also,* Reprint.—**Guincourt.** Observations sur une névralgie maxillodentaire guérie au moyen du cautère actuel. J. de méd., chir.. pharm., etc., Par., 1808, xv, 348-350.—**Guleke** (H.) Exsection of the third division of the fifth pair. Med. Rec., N. Y., 1880, xvii, 702-704.—**Gussenbauer** (C.) Ueber Behandlung der Trigeminus-Neuralgie. Wien. med. Bl., 1886. ix, 972-976. *Also:* Prag. med. Wchnschr., 1886, xi, 289-291.—**Haighton** (J.) A case of tic-douloureux, or painful affection of the face, successfully treated by a division of the affected nerve. Med. Rec. Private M. Ass., Lond., 1798, 19-51, 1 pl. *Also. transl.:* Mag. f. d. Wundarzneiw.. Götting., 1798-9, ii, 303-310.—**Halley** (G.) Resection of the infra-orbital nerve and spheno-palatine

Neuralgia (*Facial and trigeminal, Treatment of*).

ganglion. Tr. M. Ass. Missouri, St. Louis, 1880, xxiii, 70. — **Hardy** (R. W.) Some account of the medical properties of the expressed juice of mistletoe-berries in the treatment and cure of facial neuralgia and affections analogous in their nature to tic douloureux. Med. Times, Lond., 1845, xii, 36. — **Herber** (B.) Fothergill'scher Gesichtsschmerz (Tic douloureux, Dolor faciei) glücklich geheilt durch Radix belladonnæ und Kali muriaticum oxygenatum. J. d. pract. Heilk., Berl., 1813, xxxvi, 6. St., 82-103.—**Herrgott.** Observation de névralgie faciale traitée avec succès par la résection du nerf sous-orbitaire et la cautérisation du nerf dans le canal osseux; nouveau procédé pour pratiquer cette opération. Bull. gén. de thérap., etc., Par., 1857, lii, 202-208. *Also:* Gaz. méd. de Strasb., 1857, xvii, 86-92.—**Herrick** (S. S.) Three cases of division of supraorbital nerves, both eyes. N. Orl. J. M., 1869, xxii, 288.—**Heurteloup.** Réflexions sur le tic douloureux de la face, suivies d'une observation de cette maladie, guérie par l'application immédiate d'une plaque d'acier aimantée. Rec. périod. Soc. de méd. de Par., 1798, iv, 192-207.—**Heustis** (J. F.) A simple operation for facial neuralgia. Med. News, Phila., 1883, xliii, 621.—**Heyfelder** (O.) Heilung einer Prosopalgie durch Neurotomie. St. Petersb. med. Ztschr., 1870, n. F., i, 34-37.—**Heylen.** Névrose du nerf trijumeau. J. de méd., chir. et pharmacol., Brux., 1886, lxxxiii, 372. — **Hillier** (A. P.) Hypodermic injections of cocaine in facial neuralgia. Brit. M. J., Lond., 1887, i, 1213.—**Hinsdale** (G.) Facial spasm and tic-douloureux, for which neurectomy and neuro-tension were employed. Phila. M. Times, 1886-7, xvii, 278-280. *Also:* Polyclinic, Phila., 1886-7, iv, 240-242. *Also:* Med. & Surg. Reporter, Phila., 1887, lvi, 166-169.—**Hodgen** (J. T.) Section of the infra-orbital and inferior dental nerves for neuralgia. Tr. Am. M. Ass., Phila., 1880, xxxi, 773-778.—**Holst** (J.) Neuralgie des Trigeminus, geheilt durch Amputation der Vaginalportion. St. Petersb. med. Wchnschr., 1882, vii, 4.—**Horsley** (V. A. H.) Notes on the pathology of inveterate neuralgia of the fifth nerve, illustrated by cases treated successfully by avulsion of the nerve close to the skull. Tr. Odont. Soc. Gr. Brit., Lond., 1887, n. s., xix, 270-295. *Also:* Brit. J. Dent. Sc., Lond., 1887, xxx, 964; 1011.—**How** (L. B.) Ligation of the common carotid; exsection of the inferior dental nerve Tr. N. Hampshire M. Soc., Concord, 1880, 89-95.—**Howe** (J. W.) Removal of the superior maxillary division of the fifth nerve and Meckel's ganglion by Carnochan's operation. Med. News, Phila., 1884, xliv, 138.—**Hutchinson** (B.) Case of tic-douloureux, cured by the carbonate of iron. Lond. M. & Phys. J., 1825, liv, 281.—**Hutchison** (J. C.) Two cases of ligature of the common carotid artery for trigeminal neuralgia. N. York M. J., 1885, xli, 401. *Also:* Med. News, Phila., 1885, xlvi, 394-397.—**Isenschmid.** Tic douloureux der rechten Gesichtshälfte; die Nervendehnung ersetzt die Resection in vielen Fällen. Aerztl. Int.-Bl., München, 1882, xxix, 451. — **Jasinski.** Porażenie gośćcowe lewéj polowy twarzy; rychły powrót wladzy pod wpływem faradyzacyi. [Electrotherapy in nervous affections of face.] Przegl. lek., Krakow., 1862, i, no. 26.—**Jenkins** (R. S.) Tic-douloureux of twelve months' standing cured by resection of the infra-orbital nerve and its branches. South. M. Rec., Atlanta, 1880, x, 438.—**Jones** (G.) Case of neuralgia on the face (tic douloureux) cured by a surgical operation. Med. Reposit., N. Y., 1815, xvii, 177-179.—**Kappeler** (O.) Neuralgia infra-orbitalis sinistra; Neurectomie nach Wagner's Methode. *In his:* Chir. Beobacht. a. d. Thurgau. Kantonsspit. Münsterlingen, 8°, Frauenfeld, 1874, 55-62.—**Kelly** (T.) A severe case of facial neuralgia successfully treated by creosote. Dublin M. Press, 1848, xx, 163.—**Kerrison** (R. M.) A chronic case of tic-douloureux, which yielded to powerful doses of cinchona, when at its greatest severity, after other medicines and a division of the nerve had failed. Lond. M. Reposit., 1818, ix, 267-276.—**Key** (B. P.) A case of epileptiform neuralgia; excision of the second branch of the fifth pair of nerves; speedy recovery of the patient after removal of the affected cord. Nashville J. M. & S., 1879, xxiii, 164.—**von Klein.** Ueber die Möglichkeit der Zerstörung des Gesichtsnerven bei seinem Austritt aus dem Schädel. J. d. Chir. u. Augenh., Berl., 1822, iii, 46-61.— **Knie** (A.) Casuistische Mittheilung über Neurectomie des zweiten Trigeminusastes nach Braun-Lossen, nebst Bemerkungen über blutleeres Operiren nach vorheriger Ligatur der Carotis communis. St. Petersb. med. Wchnschr., 1885, n. F., ii, 149-151.—**Kocher.** Ueber Nervendehnung bei Trigeminus-Neuralgie. Cor.-Bl. f. schweiz. Aerzte, Basel, 1879, ix, 324-326.—**Kopp.** Case of a dolor faciei, where the dissection of the nerve had no effect. Phila. M. Museum, 1807, iii, pp. cxliii-cxliv.—**Krönlein** (R. U.) Neuralgia facialis [Operationen]. Arch. f. klin. Chir., Berl., 1877, xxi (Supplhft.), 120-123. ———. Ueber eine Methode der Resection des zweiten und dritten Astes des N. trigeminus unmittelbar am Foramen rotundum und ovale. Deutsche Ztschr. f. Chir., Leipz., 1884, xx, 484-492. ———. Fall von Resection des ii. und iii. Astes des Trigeminus an der Austrittsstelle aus dem Schädel wegen

Neuralgia (*Facial and trigeminal, Treatment of*).

Gesichtsschmerz. Cor.-Bl. f. schweiz. Aerzte, Basel, 1884, xiv, 301.—**Kühn** (J.) Drei Fälle von Nervenzerschneidungen bei Neuralgien des Gesichts. Arch. f. physiol. Heilk., Stuttg., 1859, n. F., iii, 226-237.—**Kuzmin** (V. I.) Ob izsiechenii jazichnago nerva pri nevralgii. [Excision of lingual nerve in neuralgia.] Laitop. khirurg. Obsh. v Mosk., 1884, vi, 15-27.—**Laborde** (J.-V.) De l'aconitine cristallisée dans la névralgie faciale congestive à frigore. Tribune méd., Par., 1878, xi, 605-607. ———. Action de la napelline dans un cas de névralgie faciale. *Ibid.*, 1883, xv, 484-486. — **Lamoureux** (J.) Observation d'un tic douloureux de la face, traité par l'emploi du sous-carbonate de fer. J. de la sect. de méd. Soc. acad. Loire-Inf., Nantes, 1825, i, 211-214. — **Lande.** Névralgie épileptiforme; résection nerveuse; persistance de la névralgie dans un filet nerveux demeuré intact; nouvelle résection; guérison. Mém. et bull. Soc. de méd. et chir. de Bordeaux, 1873, 509-517.—**Landesberg** (M.) A case of neuralgia of the first branch of the fifth pair, of six years' duration, cured by Duquesnel's aconitia. Med. & Surg. Reporter, Phila., 1880, xliii, 597. ———. Duquesnel's aconitia in facial neuralgia. Med. Bull., Phila., 1884, vi, 35-38.—**Langenbeck** (B.) Neurectomie des Nervus infraorbitalis. Deutsche Klinik, Berl., 1860, xii, 206.—**Langenbuch** (C.) Die Resection des Unterkiefernerven auf neuem Wege. Berl. klin. Wchnschr., 1880, xvii, 593-596.—**Le Calvé.** De l'emploi de la vératrine dans les névralgies faciales. J. Soc. de méd.-prat. de Montpel., 1843, viii, 115-125. — **Lee** (F. B.) Croton-chloral in facial neuralgia. Brit. M. J., Lond., 1874, i, 681.—**Le Fort** (L.) Névralgie faciale du côté droit à type épileptiforme guérie par l'élongation du nerf frontal interne, nasal et sous-orbitaire. France méd., Par., 1888, i, 97; 111.—**Legg** (J. W.) Value of hydrate of croton chloral in painful affections of the fifth nerve. Lancet, Lond., 1872, ii, 558.—**Lemaistre** (J.) Élongation du nerf maxillaire supérieur pour une névralgie rebelle. Rev. de chir., Par., 1882, ii, 1015-1019.— **Lester** (T. B.) Relation of neuralgia of the fifth pair to meningitis. St. Louis Cour. Med , 1879, ii, 209-218.—**Levittoux.** O newralgiach i sposobie ich leczenia za pomocą przyżegania żelazem de białośce upalonem punktów dotkniętych nerwobólem. [Treatment of neuralgic affections by actual cautery.] Gaz. lek., Warszawa, 1871, xi, 193; 212; 225; 241; 261.—**Lossen** (H.) Neurectomie des ii. Astes des V. nach osteoplastischer Resection des Jochbeins, nebst Vorschlag zu einer neuen Schnittführung. Centralbl. f. Chir., Leipz., 1878, v, 65-70.—**London** (C.) Employment of laurel leaves in tic douloureux. Lancet, Lond., 1834-5, i, 62. — **Lücke** (A.) Ausschneidung des zweiten Astes des Nerv. trigeminus nach temporärer Resection des Jochbogens. Deutsche Ztschr. f. Chir., Leipz., 1875, iv, 322: 1875-6, vi, 317.—**Lutterotti.** Gesichtsschmerz (Prosopalgia), geheilt durch salzsauren Baryt. Oesterr. med. Wchnschr., Wien, 1841, 1841, 1105.—**McKechnie.** Case of tic douloureux cured by arsenic. Edinb. M. & S. J., 1811, vii, 300-303. —**Mackey** (E.) Gelseminum sempervirens (yellow jessamine) in facial neuralgia. Brit. M. J., Lond., 1874, i, 576.—**Maclean** (D.) Neuralgia of several branches of the fifth pair of nerves; operation; cure. Physician & Surg., Ann Arbor, Mich., 1882, iv, 499. ———. Neuralgia of the malar branch of the superior maxillary; division of the nerve; cure. *Ibid.*, 500.—**Mader** (J.) Neuralgia Trigemini inveterata; erfolglose Behandlung mit Elektricität. Med.-chir. Centralbl., Wien, 1879, xiv. 542.—**Manzi** (B.) Nevralgia della seconda branca del quinto pajo dei nervi cerebrali, trattata colle inspirazioni di azotito di amile. Ann. univ. di med. e chir., Milano, 1875, ccxxxi, 512-515, 1 pl.—**Marschall** (G.) Heilung eines merkwürdigen Gesichtsschmerzes (oder vielmehr eines larvirten Wechselfiebers) durch Liquor Fowleri. Arch. f. med. Erfahr., Berl., 1831, i, 161.—**Mattison** (J. B.) Trifacial neuralgia treated by the deep injection of chloroform. Tr. M. Soc. N. Jersey, Newark, 1874, 216-220. *Also:* Med. Rec., N. Y., 1874, ix, 227-229.—**Mazzoni** (C.) A memoir on facial neuralgia, illustrated by a case affecting the sub-orbital nerve; cured by excision. St. Louis M. & S. J., 1861, xix, 289; 385. ———. Nevralgia di tutte le branche del trigemino ed in ispecie del ramo mascellare superiore, curata col Gelsemium semper virens a dose crescente dato a goccie; miglioramento. Clin. chir., Roma, 1881, vi-vii, 160.—**Mélier.** Note sur l'emploi du sous-carbonate de fer dans le traitement des névralgies; névralgie faciale guérie par ce moyen. J. gén. de méd., chir. et pharm., Par., 1827, xcix. 3-6.—**Mesterton** (C. B.) Einige Fälle von Neurectomie bei Gesichtsneuralgien. Deutsche Klinik, Berl., 1873, xxv, 95;-103. —**Meusel.** Resection des Nervus mandibularis von der Mundhöhle aus. *Ibid.*, 1875, xxvii, 10.—**Michel.** Section des nerfs buccal et lingual dans la névralgie faciale; opérations nouvelles. Mém. Soc. de méd. de Strasb., 1864, iii, 222-233. *Also:* Gaz. méd. de Strasb., 1857, xvii, 475-480. *Also:* Gaz. d. hôp., Par., 1859, xxxii, 183. ———. Sur les sections nerveuses dans la névralgie faciale. Rev. méd. de l'est, Nancy, 1878, x, 129-134.—**Miller** (J.) Bericht eines Falles von Trigeminus-Neuralgie. N. Yorker med. Presse,

Neuralgia (*Facial and trigeminal, Treatment of*).

1886-7, iii, 230-232.—**Mitchell.** On the treatment of facial neuralgia. Liverpool M. Gaz., Lond., 1833, i, 565-568.—**Mitchell** (S. W.) Clinical remarks on facial neuralgia, treated by neurectomy. Med. News, Phila., 1882, xl, 257-259.—**Mojani** (C.) Nevralgia mascellare superiore guarita colla nevrotomia. Raccoglitore, Fano, 1844, xiii, 67-69.—**Monmonier** (J. N.) Extirpation of the superior maxillary nerve. Tr. M. Chir. Fac. Maryland, Balt., 1878, 105.—**Mosetig.** Ueber Nerven-Resektion wegen Gesichtsschmerz. Wien. med. Presse, 1867, viii, 747. ———. Resektion des Ramus nasociliaris, in der Länge von 3 Linien, wegen Fothergil'schen Gesichtsschmerzes. Wien. med. Wchnschr., 1867, xvii, 888. — **Museux.** Observation d'une névralgie maxillo-dentaire, guérie au moyen du cautère actuel. Bull. de la Fac. de méd. de Par. (1804-8). 1812, i, pt. 3, 134-136. —**Mussey** (W. H.) Removal of superior maxillary nerve with the ganglion of Meckel, and the inferior maxillary nerve, for persistent facial neuralgia. Cincin. Lancet & Obs., 1869, xii, 449-452.—**Nagy** (M.) Neurotomie des zweiten Astes des Trigeminus rechts am Foramen rotundum. Wien. med. Wchnschr., 1872, xxii, 603-606. — **Navratil.** Neurektomie wegen Neuralgie des 3. Trigeminus - Astes; Erfolg. Pest. med.-chir. Presse, Budapest, 1882, xviii, 398. — **Neale** (W. H.) Facial neuralgia treated by nerve vibration. Practitioner, Lond., 1884, xxxiii, 345 - 349. — **Neuralgia** nervi trigemini. Jahresb. ü. d. chir. Abth. d. Spit. zu Basel (1883), 1884, 36-39. — **Nicaise.** Névralgie faciale; résection du nerf sous-orbitaire. Gaz. d. hôp., Par., 1881, liv, 1123.—**Nicoladoni** (C.) Resektion des N. mandibularis nach Sonnenburg. Wien. med. Presse, 1882, xxiii, 853-856.—**von Niemeyer** (F.) Zwei Fälle von Heilung schwerer und langwieriger Prosopalgie durch den constanten Strom. Berl. klin. Wchnschr., 1868, v, 181; 195.—**Nussbaum.** Ein Fall von Gesichtsschmerz geheilt durch Excisionen aus dem Nervus supraorbitalis, infraorbitalis, alveolaris superior, alveolaris inferior und mentalis. Aerztl. Int.-Bl., München, 1858, v, 137.—**Ozenne** (P.) Névralgie sous-orbitaire; arrachement du nerf; guérison. France méd., Par., 1882, i, 469-472. *Also:* Bull. Soc. clin. de Par. (1882), 1883, vi, 78-82.— **Pancoast** (J.) New operation for the relief of persistent facial neuralgia. Phila. M. Times, 1871-2, ii, 285.— **von Patruban.** Ueber die Resection und Exstirpation des Unteraugenhöhlennervens als Radicalheilung der Prosopalgia infraorbitalis. Wien. med. Wchnschr., 1853, iii, 308; 321. ———. Neuralgie des Quintus; wiederholte Resection des N. infraorbitalis und N. inframaxill.; Sectionsbefund. Oesterr. Ztschr. f. prakt. Heilk., Wien, 1858, iv, 525; 549. ———. Unterbindung der Carotis communis zur Heilung einer inveterirten Prosopalgie nach wiederholten Nervenresectionen. Wchnbl. d. k. k. Gesellsch. d. Aerzte in Wien, 1866, xxii, 224. ———. Die Unterbindung der Carotis als Heilmittel des Tic douloureux. Allg. Wien. med. Ztg., 1872, xvii, 3; 12; 25; 34; 41. ———. Die Unterbindung der Carotis communis als letztes Heilmittel des Tic douloureux. *Ibid.*, 1876, xxi, 421; 429; 442.—**Pavdof-Silvanski** (P.) Dva sluchaya azektsii podochnago nerva. [Two cases of exsection of the infraorbital nerve.] Med. Vestnik St. Petersb., 1864, iv, 406-408. — **Payan.** [Névralgie faciale traitée avec succès par la cautérisation auriculaire.] [Rap. de Forget.] Bull. Soc. de chir. de Par., 1851-2, ii, 177-179.—**Pearson.** On the tic douloureux, or trismus dolorificus. Edinb. M. & S. J., 1807, iii, 272-276.—**Pégaitaz.** [Opération de tic douloureux—nerf excisé—dans le canal osseux.] Bull. Soc. méd. de la Suisse Rom., Lausanne, 1871, v, 240.— **Peter.** Sur un cas de tic douloureux de la face datant de vingt-huit ans et guéri par le bromure de potassium. Bull. gén. de thérap., etc., Par., 1876, xci, 337-340. *Also:* Abeille méd., Par., 1876, xxxiii, 442-444. — **Pfaff.** Ol. terebintinæ, ein äusserst wirksames Mittel gegen Prosopalgie. Ztschr. f. Med., Chir. u. Geburtsh., Leipz., 1862, n. F., i, 200.—**von Pitha.** Neuralgie des rechten Nervus infraorbitalis; Resektion desselben bei einem 83jährigen Weibe mit gutem Erfolge; mitgetheilt von Dr. Wilhelm Scholz. Wien. med. Wchnschr., 1865, xv, 407; 421. — **Podrazki.** Neuralgie des 2. Astes des Trigeminus; Resection des Stammes des Oberkiefernerven am Foramen rotundum nach der Methode von Carnochan; Heilung. *Ibid.*, 1869, xix, 1709; 1727: 1870, xx, 25. — **Poggioli.** Nouvelle méthode curative externe pour les névralgies faciales. [Rap. de Piorry.] Bull. Acad. de méd., Par., 1855 - 6, xxi, 910 - 923. — **Polto** (S.) Neuralgia facciale curata coll' applicazione esterna della belladonna. Gior. d. sc. med., Torino, 1838, i, 255-259.—**Pontoire** (H.) Névralgie faciale guérie par le traitement mixte de résection et de cautérisation du nerf. Union méd., Par., 1854, viii, 209. — **Pozzi** (S.) Rapport sur une communication de M. le Dr. Blum, intitulée: De l'arrachement du nerf sous-orbitaire. Bull. et mém. Soc. de chir. de Par., 1882, n. s., viii, 788-798. *Also:* Gaz. méd. de Par., 1883, 6. s., v, 88; 100; 112.— **Prengrueber.** Névralgie faciale; ablation d'un petit névrome gingival; guérison. France méd., Par., 1884, ii, 1347-1349.—**Priou.** Bon effet du camphre mâché contre

Neuralgia (*Facial and trigeminal, Treatment of*).

les névralgies faciales. Abeille méd., Par., 1859, xvi, 41.— **Rahn.** Heilung eines hartnäckigen Gesichtschmerzens durch einen ohngefehren Zufall. Museum d. Heilk., Zürich, 1792. i, 279-283.—**Rampoldi** (R.) Due casi di affezione dolorosa del 5.° paio guariti radicalmente con lo strappo cruento del nervo. Ann. di ottal., Pavia, 1885, xiv, 488-492.—**Rankine** (J.) Observations on the treatment of tic douloureux; illustrated by cases. Edinb. M. & S. J., 1834, xli, 132-138.—**Resasco** (A.) Sulla cura delle nevralgie esterne e particolarmente della nevralgia trifaciale. Gior. di med. mil., Firenze, 1869, xvii, 369-381. — **Revilliod.** Névralgie de la cinquième paire (branches maxillaires supérieure et inférieure) rebelle à un grand nombre de traitements, guérie par les injections sous-cutanées de chlorhydrate de morphine. Bull. gén. de thérap., etc., Par., 1865, lxix, 557-560.—**Ribes** (D.-F.) Observation de névralgie du nerf facial, guérie au moyen du sulfate de quinine. J. de physiol. expér., Par., 1822, ii, 219-224.—**Richmond.** Case illustrative of the beneficial effects of the carbonate of iron in tic douloureux. Lond. M. & Phys. J., 1821, xlvi, 270-272.—**Ringer** (S.) A curious case of facial neuralgia, with unilateral sweating, cured by the application of aconite liniment. Practitioner, Lond., 1872, ix, 138 - 140. — **Roberts** (W. O.) Infra-orbital neuralgia; a case operated on many times; cure. Am. Pract., Louisville, 1880, xxi, 8-10. — **Robinson** (D. R.) Case of tic douloureux cured by cinchona. Edinb. M. & S. J., 1821, xvii, 229-232. — **Rockwell** (F. W.) Successful neurectomy of infra-orbital branch of fifth nerve, at level of foramen rotundum, for relief of recurring trophic disturbances and inveterate neuralgia. Ann. Surg., St. Louis, 1885, i, 345-350.—**Rogers** (W. B.) Neurectomy in a case of neuralgia of the trigeminus; return of the disease after one year. Mississippi Valley M. Month., Memphis, 1881, i, 201-206. ——— Neurectomy of infra-orbital nerve. *Ibid.*, 1882, ii, 445.—**Rossander** (C. J.) Om massage af hals-sympathicus vid tic douloureux. Hygiea, Stockholm, 1885, xlvii, 174-177.—**Rouge.** Névralgie épileptiforme de la face; section de la seconde branche du trijumeau à sa sortie du trou rond. Bull. Soc. méd. de la Suisse Rom., Lausanne, 1872, vi, 175-182.—**Roux** (J.) Névralgies faciales; résection des nerfs; procédés nouveaux. Union méd., Par., 1852, vi, 479; 491; 515; 518.— **Roviralta** (J.) Ventajosos efectos del Gelsemium sempervirens (jazmin amarillo) en las neuralgias de las ramas alveolares del trigémino. Sentido catól., Barcel., 1881, iii, 135-137.—**Sabucedo** (S.) Catorce casos de neuralgias del facial curados con el salicilato de sosa y con el ioduro de potasio. Rev. de med. y cirug. práct., Madrid, 1883. xii, 264.—**Savory.** Intense and chronic neuralgia in the tract of the right dental and auriculo-temporal nerves; operation; recovery. Lancet, Lond. . 1875, ii, 8.—**Schech** (P.) Klonische Krämpfe des weichen Gaumens mit objectivem Ohrgeräusch in Folge von nasaler Trigeminus - Neuralgie. München. med. Wchnschr.. 1886, xxxiii, 385-387.— **Schenck.** Erfahrungen über die grossen Heilkräfte der China, besonders in Verbindung mit Opium gegen den Fothergill'schen Gesichtsschmerz. J. d. pract. Heilk., Berl., 1826, lxii, 3. St., 40-47. — **Schreuder** (H. A.) Een woord over de gunstige werking van Nux vomica tegen prosopalgie. Tijdschr. d. Vereen. t. Bevord. d. geneesk. Wetensch. in Nederl. Indië, Batav., 1852, i, 1 - 24. — **Schützenberger.** [Tic rotatoire très-pénible; guérison par l'application d'un courant électrique continu pendant dix minutes chaque fois, trois fois par semaine.] Proc.-verb. . . . Soc. de méd. de Strasb., 1866-7, iv, 188.— **Schuh.** Resection des Nervus infraorbitalis an der Augenhöhle gegen Gesichtsschmerz. Wien. med. Wchnschr., 1853, iii, 401; 417. ———. Durchschneidung des Nervus alveolaris superior gegen Gesichtsschmerz. *Ibid.*, 1854, iv, 353. ———. Resection des Nervus zygomaticus, infraorbitalis, alveolaris superior, et dentalis inferior zur Heilung des Gesichtsschmerzes. Wchnbl. d. k. k. Gesellsch. d. Aerzte in Wien, 1856, ii, 1-7. ———. Heilung der Prosopalgie mittelst Durchschneidung des Zweigchens, welches vom Nervus alveolaris sup. zur Schleimhaut des Mundes in der Gegend des Buccinator geht. *Ibid.*, 1857, iii, 321-325. ———. Bericht über die im letzten Jahre vorgenommenen Nervenresectionen bei Gesichtsneuralgien. Wien. med. Wchnschr., 1864, xiv, 385; 401. ———. Neue Reihe von Nervenresectionen bei Prosopalgien. Nachgelassenes Manuskript. *Ibid.*, 1866, xvi, 681; 729; 745.— **Schuppert** (M.) Neuralgie of the supra-orbital nerve; partial excision of the nerve; cure; plastic operation on nose. N. Orl. M. Times, 1861, i, 94-97. ———. Neuralgia of the face, "tic douloureux"; resection of the second branch of the fifth pair of nerves in the spheno-maxillary fossa at the foramen rotundum of the sphenoid bone; cure. N. Orl. M. Rec., 1866, i, 16-20. ———. Two cases of facial neuralgia cured by resection of nerves. N. Orl. M. & S. J., 1873-4, n. s., i, 311-324.—**Sée** (G.) Traitement des maux de tête céphalée, migraine, migraine ophtalmique, névralgie faciale. Rec. d'ophth., Par., 1887, 3. s., ix, 596-600.—**Seguin** (E C.) Efficacy of the aconitia of Duquesnel in trigeminal neuralgia. N. York M. J., 1878,

Neuralgia (*Facial and trigeminal, Treatment of*).

xxviii, 621–628. *Also*, Reprint. *Also*, *in his:* Op. min. [etc.], 8°, N. Y., 1884, 367–374. ——. A contribution to the medicinal treatment of chronic trigeminal neuralgia. Med. Rec., N. Y., 1879, xv, 6–9. *Also*, *in his:* Op. min. [etc.], 8°, N. Y., 1884, 375–379. ——. History of attempts made to cure three cases of chronic trigeminal neuralgia. Arch. Med., N. Y., 1881, vi, 89–96. *Also*, *in his:* Op. min. [etc.], 8°, N. Y., 1884, 534–539. — **Seure.** Névralgie faciale du côté gauche, d'abord continue, puis intermit tente quotidienne; emploi de la salicine; guérison. J. d. conn. méd.-chir., Par., 1834–5, ii, 40.— **Sibson** (F.) On the treatment of facial neuralgia by the inhalation of ether and on a new inhaler. Lond. M. Gaz., 1847, xxxix, 358–364. *Also*, *in his:* Collect. Works, 8°, Lond., 1881, iv, 354–368. — **Spörer** (C.) Das Chloralhydrat, in Substanz local angewandt gegen Odontalgie und Prosopalgie. St. Petersb. med. Wchnschr., 1880, v, 289.— **States-Brame.** Névralgie du trijumeau datant de vingt-neuf ans; emploi des courants continus; guérison. Bull. méd. du nord, Lille, 1878, 2. s., xvii, 29–36.—**Stathakopoulos** (S.) Προσωπαλγία (tic doulouraix), ἐκ ψύξεως προελθοῦσα καὶ ἰαθεῖσα τῇ χρήσει τῶν λουτρῶν τῆς κύθνου. Γαληνὸς, Ἀθῆναι, 1882, Η΄, 407–409. — **Stetter.** Zur Resection des Nervus alveolaris inferior. Berl. klin. Wchnschr., 1875, xii, 16–18.—**Stewart** (T. G.) Remarks on a case of epileptiform neuralgia, treated by nervestretching. Brit. M. J., Lond., 1879, i, 803. — **Stilling** (B.) Neuralgie im Gebiete des Nervus infraorbitalis, mandibularis u. s. w.; Resection des N. infraorbitalis; Heilung nach 11 Tagen, ohne Fieber, ohne Eiterung. Deutsche med. Wchnschr., Berl., 1876, ii, 619. — **Stimpson** (J.) A distressing case of tic douloureux, successfully treated by surgical operation. N. Eng. J. M. & S., Bost., 1817, vi, 14–16.—**Stockman.** Névralgie trifaciale, guérie par le sulfate de cuivre ammoniacal. Bull. Soc. de méd. de Gand, 1878, xlv, 9–11.—**Syme** (J.) Division of the nerve for tic douloureux. Month. J. M. Sc., Lond. & Edinb., 1850, x, 245. — **Tassi.** Neurotomia del sottorbitale. Bull. d. r. Accad. med. di Roma, 1884, x, 29.—**Taylor** (T.) Observations, with cases of tic douloureux and rheumatism of the head, successfully treated by the carbonate of soda, and the prussic acid. Edinb. M. & S. J., 1823, xix, 399–403.—**Terrillon.** De la résection du nerf sous-orbitaire pour les névralgies rebelles. Bull. gén. de thérap., etc., Par., 1881, c, 49–59. *Also* [Abstr.]: Bull. et mém. Soc. de chir. de Par., 1881, n. s., vii, 129–133.— **Texier** (H.) Cautérisation de l'hélix de l'oreille dans le traitement des névralgies de la face. Monit. d. hôp., Par., 1856, iv, 1164.— **Thomayer** (J.) Neuralgia trigemini. Aerztl. Ber. d. k. k. allg. Krankenh. zu Prag (1883-4), 1886, 102–120.—**Thomson** (A. T.) On the use of iron in tic douloureux. Lond. M. & Phys. J., 1823, xlix, 111–114.—**Tillaux.** Névralgie sous-orbitaire rebelle; résection du nerf sous-orbitaire à son entrée dans le canal de ce nom; guérison. Bull. et mém. Soc. de chir. de Par., 1877, n. s., iii, 410–414.—**Tjernberg** (N. A.) Opererade fall af ansigtsneuralgi. Upsala Läkaref. Förh., 1873, viii, 457–464.—**Todd & Fergusson.** Tic douloureux; great relief by medical treatment, and subcutaneous sections of the nerve repeated at several months' interval; relapse; third operation, including section and cauterization; mitigation of symptoms. Lancet, Lond., 1853, ii, 309.—**Tournié.** Du valérianate de zinc associé, dans certaines proportions, aux extraits de jusquiame et d'opium contre les névralgies, même intenses, affectant les nerfs de la 5me paire. Union méd., Par., 1851, v, 573; 577.—**Tripier** (L.) Névralgie de la face avec zone épileptogène; névrotomie et ostéotomie combinées. Gaz. hebd. de méd., Par., 1877, xxiv, 588–590.—**Trousseau.** Double névralgie temporale; section des deux artères. Gaz. d. hôp., Par., 1841, 2. s., iii, 39. — **Tsamopulos** (D.) Προσωπαλγία, θεραπευθεῖσα ἐν βραχυτάτῳ χρόνῳ διὰ μίγματος ἐξ ἐλαίου ὑοσκυάμου καὶ ἐκχυλίσματος εὐθαλείας. Ἰατρικὴ Ἐφημ., Ἀθῆναι, 1858-9, i, 210.—**U.** (C.) Neuralgia facciale, curata col carbonato di ferro. Bull. d. sc. med. di Bologna, 1839, 2. s., vii, 14–20.—**Van Derveer** (A.) Report of cases of trifacial neuralgia; treated by removal of Meckel's ganglion; also by the successful internal administration of aconitia. Alienist & Neurol., St. Louis, 1883, iv, 611–620. *Also*, Reprint. *Also* [Abstr.]: Tr. Am. Surg. Ass, Phila., 1883, i, 489–501. — **Verbist** (E.) Succès de la belladone dans les névralgies faciales. Biblioth. méd., Brux., 1828, v, 211–213.—**Wadell.** Case of neuralgia facialis, or tic-douloureux, relieved by carbonate of iron. Edinb. M. & S. J., 1822, xviii, 410–412.—**Wagner** (A.) Beitrag zur operativen Behandlung der Neuralgia N. trigemini. Arch. f. path. Anat., etc., Berl., 1855, ix, 594–612. ——. Neuralgia nervi infraorbitalis durch Neurectomie behandelt. Deutsche Klinik, Berl., 1861, xiii, 61. ——. Ueber nervösen Gesichtsschmerz und seine Behandlung durch Neurectomie. [16 Fälle.] Arch. f. klin. Chir., Berl., 1869, xi, 1–126, 1 pl.—**Walker** (B. M.) Ice treatment of tic douloureux. Am. J. M. Sc., Phila., 1874, n. s., lxvii, 569.— **Wallace** (W.) Excision of superior maxillary and inferior dental nerves for neuralgia. Pittsburgh M. J., 1882,

ii, 295–298.—**Walter** (P. U.) Durchschneiden mehrerer Gesichtsnerven bei einer Prosopalgie. J. d. Chir. u. Augenh., Berl., 1832, xvii, 440–471.—**Warren** (J. C.) Excision of the sub-maxillary nerve. Boston M. & S. J., 1828-9, i, 2–4. ——. Excision of the infra-orbital nerve. *Ibid.*, 4. — **Watson** (B. A.) Case of facial neuralgia treated by extirpation of the superior maxillary nerve. Med. Rec., N. Y., 1871-2, vi, 392.—**Weinlechner** (J.) Heilung einer Prosopalgie durch Resection des Nerv. infraorbitalis dextr., des Nervus dentalis superior anterior, sowie des Nerv. zygomatico-temporalis. Ber. d. k. k. Krankenanst. Rudolph-Stiftung in Wien (1871), 1873, 170. ——. Neuralgie infraorbitalis; Resection des Nerv. zygomat. facialis und zygomat. temporalis, sowie des Nerv. infraorbitalis; Heilung. *Ibid.*, 171–174. ——. Neuralgie des Supramaxillaris, 1½ Jahre nach Resection des Infraorbitalis; Resection des Supramaxillaris an seinen Austritte durch das runde Loch des Keilbeines, nach Carnochan; Heilung. *Ibid.* (1873), 1874, 254. ——. Neuralgie; intrabuccale Resection des Nerv. inframaxillaris und Mylohyoideus; Heilung. *Ibid.* (1875), 1876, 385. ——. Neuralgie des Nervus infraorbitalis dessen Resection eine schmerzfreie Pause von 4 Monaten zur Folge hatte; wegen Recidive Ligatur der Carotis communis, auf welche in den ersten 20 Tagen eine Besserung und von da an vollständige Heilung eingetreten ist. Wien. med. Bl., 1878, i, 867. ——. Neuralgie am 3. Aste des Trigeminus; intrabuccale Resection des Nerv. inframaxill., buccinatorius und lingualis; hierauf Schwinden der Neuralgie und ausser den sensitiven Lähmungen auch Geschmackslähmung an der rechten vorderen Zungenhälfte. Ber. d. k. k. Krankenanst. Rudolph-Stiftung in Wien (1877), 1878, 358. *Also:* Wien. med. Wchnschr., 1878, xxviii, 1165. ——. Neuralgie des rechten Nervus infraorbitalis; Resection desselben ausserhalb des Foramen infraorbitale und in der Mitte der Fissura orbit. inf. nach Aufstemmen des Infraorbitalcanales; Heilung. *Ibid.* (1878), 1879, 359. ——. Seit neunzehn Jahren bestehende Neuralgie des rechten Nervus inframaxillaris, welcher intrabuccal resecirt wurde; Tod an Pyämie in Folge von Osteomyelitis des Unterkiefers. *Ibid.* (1879), 1880. 375. ——. Seit 14 Jahren bestehende rechtsseitige Infraorbitalneuralgie; durch Dehnung des Nerv. infraorbitalis schwiegen die Anfälle ein halbes Jahr; wegen Recidive wurde die Carotis communis unterbunden, worauf die Anfälle nur 3 Wochen sistirten; späterhin Resection des Nerv. infraorbit., welche eine 2monatliche Besserung und schliessliche Heilung zur Folge hatte, die nur durch 1½ Monate constatirt werden konnte. *Ibid.* (1880), 1881, 345–347. ——. Seit 9 Jahren bestehende Neuralgie des 2. Astes des Trigeminus; Resection dieses Nerven in der Fissura infraorbitalis; Heilung. Aerztl. Ber. d. k. k. allg. Krankenh. zu Wien (1883), 1884, 275. ——. Neuralgie des dritten Trigeminusastes mit vorwiegenden Schmerzen im Gebiete des Buccinatorius; da die Resection dieses Nerven keinen Erfolg hatte, wurde der Nervus inframaxillaris nach Paravicini resecirt, dabei auch der Nervus lingualis fehlerhaft durchtrennt; Heilung. Wien. med. Bl., 1886, ix, 202.—**Weir** (R. F.) Trigeminal neuralgia of long standing cured by the administration of large doses of aconitia. Arch. Med., N. Y., 1879, ii, 111. ——. Neuralgia of long standing; resection of the superior maxillary nerve and Meckel's ganglion. Med. Gaz., N. Y., 1881, viii, 215. *Also:* Med. Rec., N. Y., 1881, xx, 187.—**Weise** (R.) Heilung einer Trigeminus-Neuralgie durch den constanten galvanischen Strom. Berl. klin. Wchnschr., 1867, iv, 175. ——. Heilung einer Trigeminusneuralgie durch den constanten galvanischen Strom. *Ibid.*, 1879, xvi, 640.—**Wendelstadt** (F.) Ueber das Strammonium, als Specificum gegen den Fothergill'schen Gesichtsschmerz. J. d. pract. Heilk., Berl., 1836, lxxxiii, 5. St., 100–107.—**Wertheimer** (M.) Baccæ Daphne Mezerei gegen Prosopalgia. Wien. med. Wchnschr., 1851, i, 594.—**Whittaker** (J. T.) Tic douloureux; a note on a case of Fothergill's neuralgia treated by galvanism. Clinic, Cincin., 1872, iii, 121.— **Wilks.** Tic douloureux cured by galvanism when all medicines had failed. Brit. M. J., Lond., 1870, ii, 33.— **Wilson** (A.) Case of tic douloureux, successfully treated by purgatives. Edinb. M. & S. J., 1823, xix, 208–210.—**Wittke.** Ferrum carbonicum gegen den Fothergill'schen Gesichtsschmerz. Mag. f. d. ges. Heilk., Berl., 1826, xxii, 568–579.—**Wolffsheim** (F. S.) Ueber die Wirksamkeit des Extract. Stramonii gegen Neuralgia facialis. J. d. pract. Heilk., Berl., 1839, lxxxix, 3. St., 115.—**Wood** (G.) Subcutaneous injection of chloroform in the treatment of facial neuralgia. Canada M. & S. J., Montreal, 1875, iv, 1.—**Wood** (J. R.) Two cases of facial neuralgia, treated by extirpation of nerve. N. York M. J., 1871, xiii, 730–733. ——. Report of four cases of neurotomy of the superior maxillary nerve, with extirpation of Meckel's ganglion for the cure of tic-douloureux. *Ibid.*, 1879, xxix, 584–592. *Also*, Reprint.—**Zambonini** (A.) Tic doloroso curato colla asportazione di una parte del nervo mascellare inferiore. Bull. d. sc. med. di Bologna, 1841, 2. s., xi, 76–81.—**Zesas** (D. G.) Ein Fall von Tic

Neuralgia (*Facial and trigeminal, Treatment of*).

convulsif, geheilt durch Dehnung des Facialis. Wien. med. Wchnschr., 1884, xxxiv, 39.—**Zwicke.** Neuralgia infraorbitalis; Resectio nervi infraorbital.; Heilung. Charité-Ann., Berl., 1882, vii, 498.

Neuralgia (*Frontal*).

See Brow-ague; Neuralgia (*Supraorbital*).

Neuralgia (*Genito-urinary*).

See, also, Bladder (*Neuralgia of*); **Nephralgia**; Neuralgia (*Lumbar, etc.*); Ovary (*Neuralgia of*); Testicle (*Painful, etc.*); Urethra (*Irritable*).

OTIS (F. N.) A case of reflex neuralgia, associated with urethral contractions and a rare form of urinary sinus. 8°. *New York*, 1875.

PARMILLEUX (J.-F.) * Névralgie vulvo-vaginale. 4°. *Paris*, 1882.

Adamkiewicz. Rzadki przypadek nerwobólu nerwu sromnego z zakończeniem pomyślnem. [Rare case of neuralgia of pudendal nerve successfully treated.] Medycyna, Warszawa, 1886, xiv, 313–316. *Also, transl.*: Breslau. aerztl. Ztschr., 1886, viii, 85–87.—**Barras** (F.) Histoire d'une névralgie dans le cordon spermatique, guérie par le moxa. J. gén. de méd., chir., et pharm., Par., 1815, liv, 306–321.—**Bron** (F.) De la névropathie uréthrale Lyon méd., 1875, xx, 10–16.—**Bruchon.** Note sur un cas d'urétralgie intermittente, guérie par le sulfate de quinine à l'intérieur. Abeille méd., Par., 1857, xiv, 201. *Also*: Rev. de thérap. du midi, Montpel., 1857, xi, 316–321.—**Bureau** (J.) Case of violent pains in the penis and neighboring parts. Mem. M. Soc. Lond. (1789–90), 1792, iii, 65–76.—**Cabaret** (P.) Névralgie ilio-scrotale. Rec. d. trav. Soc. méd. d'Indre-et-Loire, Tours, 1850, 78–83. *Also*: Rev. de thérap. méd.-chir., Par., 1863, 37–39. *Also*: Gaz. d. hôp., Par., 1851, 3. s., iii, 298.—**Caldas** (P.) Dores nevralgicas na uretra; emprego do bromureto de potassio; cura. Gaz. med. da Bahia, 1866, i, 8.—**Campaignae** (J.-A.J.) Considérations sur les névralgies des organes génito-urinaires et de l'anus. J. hebd. de méd., Par., 1829, ii, 396–411. — **Cayol.** Consultation sur un cas d'affection rhumatico-névralgique du plexus renal compliquée d'hipochondrie. Rev. méd. franç. et étrang., Par., 1847, i, 5–11.—**Chowne.** Castration for neuralgia. Lancet, Lond., 1843, i, 131.—**Civiale.** Des névralgies de l'urètre et du col de la vessie. J. hebd. d. progr. d. sc. et inst. méd., Par., 1835, iii, 161–168.—**Coutagne** (H.) Note sur deux cas de névralgie crurale coïncidant avec une blennorrhagie. Ann. de dermat. et syph., Par., 1870, ii, 303–310.—**Faye** (F. C.) Et Tilfælde af særegne periodiske Smerter i Membrum virile. Eyr, Christiania, 1836–7, xi, 1–9 — **Frickhöffer.** Neuralgia urethræ. Cor.- Bl. d. Ver. nassau. Aerzte, Weilburg, 1857, 102–104.—**Gamberini** (P.) Due casi di uretrodinia blennorragica curati coll' iniezione ipodermica d' idroclorato di morfina. Gior. ital. d. mal. ven., Milano, 1875, x, 48.—**Gintrac.** Névralgie ilio-scrotale; efficacité des bains de vapeur. J. de méd. de Bordeaux, 1856, 2. s., i, 690.—**Gray** (L. C.) · Vesico-genito-post-femoral neuralgia and neuritis. J. Nerv. & Ment. Dis., N. Y., 1886, n. s., xi, 743–745.—**Helfft.** Die Neurosen der die Harnausleerung vermittelnden Organe. Deutsche Klinik, Berl., 1856, viii, 447 ; 459. — **Kolbenheyer** (F.) Vaginal neuralgia. Missouri Clin. Rec., St. Louis, 1874–5, i, 33.—**Leiblinger** (H.) Vorläufige Mittheilung über eine an der Symphysis pubis beobachtete Neurose und deren Beziehungen zur Hysteralgie. Wien. med. Wchnschr., 1886, xxxvi, 613–615. — **Liégey** (N.-F.) Accès de névralgie intercostale, de névralgie du testicule et de priapisme névralgique périodiques, se produisant successivement chez une même personne; guérison par les préparations de quinquina. Ann. méd. de la Flandre occid., Roulers, 1855, iv, 43–46. *Also* [Abstr.] : J. de méd. et chir. prat., Par., 1855, 2. s., xxvi, 453–455. ——. Observations de névralgies fébriles intermittentes et rémittentes des organes génitaux-urinaires. J. de méd., chir. et pharmacol., Brux., 1858, xxvi, 17 ; 199. *Also*, Reprint.—**McSherry** (R.) Vesico-urethral neurosis. Am. J. M. Sc., Phila., 1866, n. s., lii, 398–400.—**Mauriac** (C.) Étude sur les névralgies réflexes symptomatiques de l'orchiépididymite blennorrhagique. Gaz. méd. de Par., 1869, xxiv, 331 ; 376 ; 438 ; 516; 565 : 1870, xxv, 5 ; 29 ; 55 ; 97; 133; 180 ; 211 ; 254.—**Michelstædter.** Franzensbad insbesondere gegen Krankheiten des Nervensystems; ein Fall von Neuralgie des Plexus spermaticus, geheilt in Franzensbad. Allg. med. Centr.-Ztg., Berl., 1874, xliii, 386.—**Reveillé-Parise.** Considérations thérapeutiques sur un cas de névralgie du nerf spermatique. Bull. gén. de thérap., etc., Par., 1836, x, 270–275.—**Scarenzio** (A.) Nevralgia spermatica diretta e lombo-sacro-ischiatica riflessa del lato destro, curata e guarita coll' injezione sottocutanea del cloridrato di morfina. Gior. ital. d. mal. ven., Milano, 1871, vi, pt. 1, 74–76.—**Verneuil.** Névralgie traumatique de la verge. Bull. Soc. de chir. de Par. (1863), 1864. 2. s., iv, 516–521.—**Vidal.** Note sur les douleurs urétrales,

Neuralgia (*Genito-urinary*).

suite de blennorrhagies, et sur un nouveau moyen de les traiter. Bull. gén. de thérap., etc., Par., 1848, xxxv, 159–166.—**Wilkes** (A. B.) Reflex neuralgiæ of the genito-urinary tract. South. Pract., Nashville, 1879, i, 96.

Neuralgia (*Infraorbital*).

See Neuralgia (*Facial, etc.*)

Neuralgia (*Intercostal*).

See, also, Chest (*Neuralgia of*).

ARNAUD (H.) * Considérations sur l'étiologie et la physiologie pathologique de la névralgie dorso-intercostale. 4°. *Montpellier*, 1868.

BASSEREAU (L.-P.-A.) * Essai sur la névralgie des nerfs intercostaux, considérée comme symptomatique à quelques affections viscérales. 4°. *Paris*, 1840.

Also [Abstr.], *in :* J. d. conn. méd.-chir., Par., 1839–40, vii, pt. 2, 221–230.

BEER (L.) * De neuralgia intercostali. 8°. *Berolini*, [1843].

BEROUD (P.) * De la névralgie dorso-intercostale. 4°. *Paris*, 1855.

GUITARD (A.-L.) * De la névralgie dorso-intercostale. 4°. *Paris*, 1857.

LECADRE (A.) Essai sur la névralgie intercostale. 8°. *Paris*, 1855.

Also [Rap. de Piorry], *in :* Bull. Acad. de méd., Par., 1852–3, xviii, 1121–1138.

LÉONI (A.) * Considérations sur la névralgie des nerfs intercostaux. 4°. *Paris*, 1858.

Beau (J.-H.-S.) De la névralgie intercostale. Arch. gén. de méd., Par., 1847, i, 161–181. ——. De la névrite intercostale dans la phthisie pulmonaire. Union méd., Par., 1849, iii, 345–347.—**Borlée.** Observations de chlorose simulant la phthisie pulmonaire, suivies d'un mémoire sur la névralgie intercostale. Ann. Soc de méd. de Liége, 1848, iii, 59–85. [Rap. de Tasset], 86–97. [Discussion], 98–106.—**Cameron** (J. C.) Obstinate intercostal neuralgia of three years' standing, following a severe attack of herpes zoster, cured by hypodermic injections. Canada M. & S. J., Montreal, 1872–3, i, 448.—**De Forchaux.** Névralgie intercostale. Arch. belges de méd. mil., Brux., 1855, xv, 57.—**Desnos** (L.) Névralgie intercostale. N. dict. de méd. et chir. prat., Par., 1874, xix, 138–171.—**Eade** (P.) Clinical remarks on neuralgic pain of the side. Med. Times & Gaz., Lond., 1867, ii, 34 ; 64.—**Erlenmeyer.** Zur Behandlung der Neuralgia intercostalis. Deutsche Klinik, Berl., 1850, ii, 434.—**Flint** (A.) Intercostal neuralgia; dorso intercostal neuralgia ; pleuralgia. Buffalo M. J., 1857–8, xiii, 65–73.—**Fothergill** (J. M.) Intercostal neuralgia in women. Obst. J. Gr. Brit., Lond , 1873–4, i, 787–790.—**Hoppe** (J.) Intercostal-Neuralgie links an den untern Rippen mit tödtlichem Ausgange. Memorabilien, Heilbr., 1863, viii, 241–255. ——. Der schliessliche Ausgang einer Interkostalneuralgie. Ibid., 1867, xii, 161 —**Kempf** (E. J.) Intercostal neuralgia in puerperal and nursing women. Med. Reg., Phila., 1888, iii, 57.—**Neumann** (E.) Névralgie intercostale rebelle au courant continu, guérie en deux séances de faradisation cutanée. Gaz. méd. de Par., 1878, 4. s., vii, 81.—**Nicod** (P.-L.-A.) Observations de névralgies thoraciques. N. Jour. de méd., chir., pharm., etc., Par., 1818, iii, 247–253. — **von Nussbaum.** Die Operation einer Intercostal-Neuralgie. Aerztl. Int.-Bl., München, 1878, xxv, 558–562. *Also*, Reprint.—**Oppolzer.** Neuralgia intercostalis. Deutsche Klinik, Berl., 1750, ii, 133. ——. Neuralgia intercostalis. Spitals-Ztg., Wien, 1861, 345.—**Piorry.** Névralgie intercostale, fièvre d'accès. Gaz. d. hôp., Par., 1849. 3. s., i, 323.—**Pollak** (M.) Neuralgia intercostalis und lumbalis, durch Carbolinjectionen geheilt. Med.-chir. Centralbl., Wien, 1878, xiii, 410.—**von Rzehaczek.** Beitrag zur operativen Behandlung der Intercostal-Neuralgien. Allg. Wien. med. Ztg., 1881, xxvi, 429; 441.—**Seeligmüller.** Zur Diagnose und Therapie der Intercostalneuralgieen. Deutsche med. Wchnschr., Leipz., 1887, xiii, 969. *Also*, Reprint.—**Simon** (M.) De la névralgie intercostale et de son traitement. Bull. gén. de thérap., etc., Par., 1845, xxix, 517–523.—**Valleix.** De la névralgie dorsale ou intercostale. Arch. gén. de méd., Par., 1840, i, 1 ; 188 ; 319.—**Verardini** (F.) Neuralgia intercostale seguita da bulimia. Bull. d. sc. med. di Bologna, 1857, 4. s., viii, 53.

Neuralgia (*Intermittent*).

See, also, Neuralgia (*Supraorbital*).

HWASSER (I.) * Om periodisk Nevralgie i hjertat. 8°. *Upsala*, 1837.

Also, in his: Smärre skrifter, [etc.] 8°. *Upsala*, 1839, i, 258–288.

Neuralgia (*Intermittent*).

MEYRAC (F.-E.) * Des névralgies articulaires en rapport avec des fièvres intermittentes anciennes. 4°. *Paris*, 1841.

Aubert. Mal de tête périodique et pleurésie, guéries par un vessicatoire sur le lieu de la douleur. J. de méd., chir., pharm., etc., Par., 1789, lxxx, 11-24. — Bochardt (L.) Krankengeschichte dreier Individuen an einer Febr. intermitt. quotidiana perniciosa, die beim ersten die Form des Fothergill'schen Gesichtsschmerzes (Prosopalgia Fothergillii), bei den zwei letztern aber clonische Krämpfe mit Bewusstlosigkeit und Irrereden hatte, mit einem glücklichen Ausgang, nebst ätiologischen Bemerkungen. Allg. med. Ann., Leipz., 18.9, 161-172.— Brainard (D.) On the use of chloroform in periodical neuralgia. Northwest. M. & S. J., Chicago, 1849-50, vi, 284-288.— Bricheteau (I.) Observation de névralgie faciale intermittente guérie par le sulfate de quinine. J. compl. du dict. d. sc. méd., Par., 1829, xxxiv, 171. ——. Cas de névralgie annuelle. J. d. conn. méd. prat., Par., 1851-2, xix, 29. — Brutti (F. F.) Sull' utilità del cianuro di potassa nei dolori intermittenti nervosi, e nelle febbri periodiche. Ann. univ. di med., Milano, 1832, lxi, 440-447. — Cleveland (J. L) Typhomalarial fever followed by a persistent intermittent neuralgia. Clinic, Cincin., 1874, vii, 181-183.— Ferguson (J.) Intermittent neuralgia.' Canad. J. M. Sc., Toronto, 1882, vii, 194. — Fiorito (G.) Narrazione di una neuralgia ischiatico-crurale periodica con tipo sestano in un caso ed ottano nell' altro, e di una neuralgia radiale con tipo terzanario, troncate coi sali di chinina, aggiuntevi alcune relative considerazioni. Gior. . d. Soc. med.-chir. di Torino, 1845, xxiii, 393-423. — Fonssagrives (J.-B.) Mémoire sur la névralgie générale, et notamment sur celle d'origine paludéenne. Arch. gén. de méd., Par., 1856, i, 277-298. Also, Reprint.— Fox (D. R) Observations on malarial intermittent neuralgia occurring in my practice during the past thirty years. Tr. Louisiana M. Soc., N. Orl., 1887, 94-98.— Francis (C. R.) Large doses of antiperiodics in periodic neuralgia. Med. Times & Gaz., Lond., 1877, i, 115.— Frost. Febris intermittens comitata, deren Anfälle sich theils als Pneumonia, theils als Neuralgia intermittens gestalteten. Allg. Ztg. f. Mil.-Aerzte, Brnschwg., 1844, ii, 89-91.— García de Castro Muñoz (J. M.) Dos casos de neuralgia remitente cerebrales y su tratamiento. Andalucía méd., Córdoba, 1882, vii, 23-30.— Horn (E.) Ueber einige intermittirende Lokalleiden. N. Arch. f. med. Erfahr., Berl., 1805, ii, 132-143.— Jones (G. F.) Case of periodic neuralgia with deafness. Memphis M. Recorder, 1858, vi, 5.— Laronde (C.) Observation de névralgie faciale intermittente, jugulée par le valérianate de quinine et immédiatement suivie d'une affection de l'appareil vocal, principalement caractérisé par un bégaiement des plus prononcés. Monit. d. sc. méd. et pharm., Par., 1859, i, 453.— Lenoir (B. B.) Periodical neuralgia. E. Tennessee Rec. M. & S., Knoxville, 1852, i, 131.— Liégey. Réclamation de priorité au sujet de l'assimilation des effets de la névralgie avec les effets de la fièvre pernicieuse. Union méd., Par., 1859, 2. s., ii, 106-108.— Marrotte. Mémoire sur les névralgies périodiques. Arch. gén. de méd., Par., 1852, 4. s., xxx, 257 ; 405.— Martin (de Nimes). Observation de névralgie sus-orbitaire périodique tenue sous la dépendance des phases de la lune et du retour des saisons. J. d. conn. méd. prat., Par., 1846-7, xiv, 7.— Mazade (J.) Douleurs névralgiques dans la région iliaque gauche ; au bout de quelques jours accès hystériques réguliers ; sulfate de quinine ; suspension de ces accès ; récidive ; nouvel emploi du sulfate de quinine ; guérison. Ann. Soc. de méd. prat. de la prov. d'Anvers, Malines, 1849, vii, 295-297.— Mendelson (W.) A case of malarial neuralgia. Arch. Med., N. Y., 1881, v, 223.— Pancia. Névralgie sus-orbitaire intermittente guérie par l'emploi de l'acide arsénieux. Gaz. d. hôp , Par., 1-68, xli, 202. — Poirier (E.) Observations de névralgies intermittentes. J. de méd., chir. et pharmacol., Brux., 1866, xliii, 205-213.— Richter (A. L.) Intermittirende Neuralgien. Med. Ztg., Berl., 1835, iv, 53.— Sanchez Salas (A.) Observaciones que prueban la utilidad de la quina en los dolores sin pirexia, que guardan un órden periódico. Periód. Soc. méd.-quir. de Cádiz, 1822, iii, 222-234.— Sandras. Intermittent neuralgia ; beneficial employment of ligature to the limbs. Med. Times, Lond., 1849, xix, 217.— Seure. Névralgie faciale du côté gauche, d'abord continue, puis intermittente quotidienne ; emploi de la salicine. J. d. conn. méd.-chir., Par., 1834-5, ii, 40.— Taylor (J. L.) A case of periodical neuralgia. West. J. M. & S., Louisville, 1847, n. s., vii, 17.— Titley (J. M.) On intermittent neuralgia. Lond. M. & S. J., 1832, i, 273.— Waton (E.) Efficacité du valérianate de quinine contre les névralgies intermittentes. Gaz. d. hôp., Par., 1862, xxxv, 459.— Whitall. Malarial neuralgia. Hosp. Gaz., N. Y., 1878, iii, 180.

Neuralgia (*Lingual*).

See, also, Nerve (*Lingual*); Neurotomy ; Tongue (*Neuroses of*); Tongue (*Pain in*).

Boeckel (E.) Deux cas d'excision du nerf lingual et mentonnier. Gaz. d. hôp., Par., 1865, xxxviii, 10. —

Neuralgia (*Lingual*).

Buffum (C. T.) Neuralgia of tongue ; section of nerve. Hosp. Gaz.. N. Y., 1878, iv, 149. — Inzani (G.) Névralgie du nerf lingual ; névrotomie ; guérison. Gaz. d. hôp., Par., 1859, xxxii, 459.— Le Dentu. Tic douloureux du côté gauche de la face et de la langue datant de cinq ans ; élongation du nerf lingual ; cessation de tous les phénomènes douloureux. Bull. et mém. Soc. de chir. de Par., 1881, n. s., vii, 795-800.— Lossen (H.) Zur Neurectomie des Ramus sec. n. v., des N. lingualis und alveolaris inferior. Centralbl. f. Chir., Leipz., 1877, iv, 273.— de Neffe (V.) De la névralgie du nerf lingual et de son traitement par l'électrisation de la corde du tympan. [Rap. de Willems jeune.] Bull. Soc. de méd. de Gand, 1864, xxxi, 8-13. Also, transl.: Allg. Wien. med. Ztg. 1864, ix. 187.— Nicholson (F. C.) A case of neuralgia of the inferior maxillary division of the trigeminus with implication of its lingual branch. Indian M. Gaz., Calcutta, 1873, viii, 262.— Roser. Operation einer Zungenneuralgie. Arch. f. physiol. Heilk., Stuttg., 1855, xiv, 579-582.— Vanzetti. Névralgie atroce de la langue ; excision du nerf lingual ; guérison. Bull. Soc. de chir. de Par. (1867), 1868, 2. s., viii, 422-427. Also : Gaz. d. hôp., Par., 1868, xli. 30. Also, transl. : Boston M. & S. J., 1868, i, 181-183. — Weisse. Fall von Glossagra. Ztschr. f. d. ges. Med., Hamb., 1837, vi, 99. — Zesas (D. G.) Zur Neuralgie des Ramus lingualis trigemini. Wien. med. Presse, 1882, xxiii, 1076-1079.

Neuralgia (*Lumbar and uterine*).

See, also, Lumbago ; Ovary (*Neuralgia of*) ; Puerperal *neuralgia* ; Uterus (*Irritable, etc.*)

BOULINGUEZ (H.-G.-N.) * De la névralgie lombo-abdominale. 4°. *Lille*, 1883.

FORT (A.-J.-A.) * Réflexions sur la névralgie lombo-abdominale considérée surtout au point de vue des causes et du diagnostic. 4°. *Paris*, 1863.

Also, in : Rev. de thérap. méd.-chir., Par., 1864, 59 ; 93 ; 115.

LE BAILLY (A.) * Étude clinique sur la névralgie iléo-lombaire symptomatique des affections des organes génitaux chez la femme. 4°. *Paris*, 1881.

Also [Abstr.], in : Paris méd., 1881, vi, 289-291.

MAUDUIT (P.-I.) * De la névralgie lombo-abdominale dans les affections utérines. 4°. *Paris*, 1863.

SAVREUX (C.) * De la névralgie lombo-abdominale consécutive aux inflammations périutérines. 4°. *Paris*, 1874.

TRICARD (P.) * De la névralgie des plexus lombaire et sacré d'origine traumatique (tour de reins). 4°. *Bordeaux*, 1886.

Axenfeld. Les névralgies lombo-abdominale s considérées comme symptomatiques des affections de l'utérus. Union méd., Par., 1850, iv, 193 ; 198. — Baumgartner (A.) Névralgie crurale résultant d'une hypertrophie congestive de l'utérus, guérie par l'iode. J. d. conn. méd.-chir., Par., 1842-3, x, pt. 2, 104.— Bouchard. Névralgie sacro-lombaire ayant déterminé pendant trois ans des accidents très-graves, guérie au moyen des injections de sulfate d'atropine dans la cavité du col de l'utérus. Bull. gén. de thérap., etc., Par. 1861, lxi, 322 - 325. — Brown (J. L) Neuralgia of toes from ulceration of os uteri. Am. J. Obst., N. Y., 1868-9, i, 156.— Congestion utérine chronique en rapport avec la névralgie lombo abdominale. Rev. méd.-chir. d. mal. d. femmes, Par., 1882, iv, 488-493.— Delmas (P.) Névropathie à forme névralgique et de chlorose utérine. Bordeaux méd., 1876, v, 321. — Favre (A.) Névralgie périodique de l'utérius et de ses annexes ; périodicité quotidienne et périodicité annuelle. Gaz. méd. de Lyon, 1858, x, 244. — Gosselin. Névralgie iléo-lombaire et crurale, accompagnée de contractions choréiformes de la cuisse droite (coxalgie hystérique). Gaz. d. hôp , Par., 1862, xxxv, 262. ——. Cas insolite de névralgie lombaire. Ibid., 1881, liv, 659. — Heinlein. Zur Casuistik der Lumbo-Abdominalneuralgien. Deutsches Arch. f. klin. Med., Leipz., 1880, xxvi, 189-193. — Kolluck (G. J.) Report of the treatment of an obstinate case of neuralgia of the uterus. Georgia M. Companion, Atlanta, 1871, i, 528-530. — Küchenmeister (F.) Formel gegen hartnäckige Neuralgien des Trigeminus, Ischiadicus, der Intercostal- und Uterusnerven. Oesterr. Ztschr. f. prakt. Heilk., Wien, 1873, xix, 137-139. — Léotaud (A.) Cas de névralgie lombo-sacrée accompagnant une affection utérine et se compliquant d'abcès des régions ovariques ; influence de l'atmosphère ; guérison. Gaz. d. hôp., Par., 1861, xxxiv, 359.—Leroux (C.) De la névralgie iléo-lombaire symptomatique des affections des organes génitaux chez la femme. Arch. méd.-prat., Par., 1882, 3. s., iv, 17.— Lizé. Un mot sur la névralgie lombo-abdominale dans l'état de grossesse. Gaz. d. hôp., Par., 1861, xxxiv,

Neuralgia (*Lumbar and uterine*).

194. — **Malgaigne.** Observations de névralgies des annexes de l'utérus traitées par le cathétérisme du col utérin. Monit. d. hôp., Par., 1854, ii, 916-919. — **Marrotte.** De quelques épiphénomènes des névralgies lombo-sacrées pouvant simuler des affections idiopathiques de l'utérus et de ses annexes. Arch. gén. de méd., Par., 1860, i, 385 ; 552.— **Mollière** (H.) Névralgie lombo-abdominale guérie par l'extirpation d'un lipome de la paroi latérale droite de l'abdomen. Mém. et compt.-rend. Soc. d. sc. méd. de Lyon (1868), 1869, viii, pt. 2, 172-175. — **Neucourt** (F.) De la névralgie lombaire, ou névralgie des plexus lombaires et sacrés. Arch. gén. de méd., Par., 1858, 5. s., xii, 21 ; 180.— **Piorry.** Lombalgie (douleur lombaire) ; névralgies intercostales pouvant faire croire à des palpitations de cœur et donnant lieu à une fièvre d'accès irrégulière. Gaz. d. hôp., Par., 1858, xxxi, 30. — **Schramm.** Mittheilungen aus der ärztlichen Praxis über neuralgische Affectionen im Gebiete des Plexus lumbo-sacralis. Aerztl. Int.-Bl., München, 1859, vi, 511.—**Shaw** (C.) A case of lumbo-abdominal neuralgia treated with sulphuric æther and belladonna. Indian M. Gaz., Calcutta, 1882, xvii, 266.—[**Siredey.**] Névralgie lombo-abdominale persistant après la guérison de lésions utérines. J. de méd. et chir. prat., Par., 1875, xlvi, 294.—**Valleix.** Considérations sur une forme de névralgie lombo-abdominale simulant une maladie de l'utérus et sur son traitement. Bull. gén. de thérap., etc., Par., 1847, xxxii, 14-23.—**Vulpian** (A.) Névralgies iléo-lombaires ; métrorrhagies ; injections de morphine ; pilules de nitrate d'argent ; sulfate de quinine, etc. ; guérison des douleurs par les injections de morphine ; coïncidence entre la disparition des douleurs et la cessation des métrorrhagies. *In his :* Clin. méd. de l'hôp. de la Charité, 8°, Par., 1879, 310-317. — **Werner.** Zwei irrthümlich als Ileopsoitis diagnosticirte Fälle von Lumboabdominal-Neuralgie. Ztschr. f. Wundärzte u. Geburtsh., Stuttg., 1867, xx, 110-114.

Neuralgia (*Malarial*).

See **Neuralgia** (*Causes of*); **Neuralgia** (*Intermittent*).

Neuralgia (*Mammary*).

See **Breast** (*Irritable, etc.*)

Neuralgia (*Maxillary*).

See **Neuralgia** (*Dental*), etc.

Neuralgia (*Mesenteric*).

See **Neuralgia** (*Abdominal, etc.*)

Neuralgia (*Occipital*).

See **Neuralgia** (*Cervico-occipital*), etc.

Neuralgia (*Ocular*).

Clark (H. E.) Neuralgic ciliary pain cured by stretching nasal nerve. Glasgow M. J., 1883, [4.] s., xx, 389.—**da Fonseca** (L.) Estiramento e resecção do nervo nasal externo contra a nevralgia ciliar é trigemea n'um caso de glaucoma. Coimbra med., 1884, iv, 321-324.—**Jurist** (L.) Neuralgia of the nose and pharynx. Med. News, Phila., 1884, xliv, 236. — **Lagrange.** L'arrachement du nerf nasal externe dans les douleurs ciliaires et la névralgie du trijumeau. Arch. d'opht., Par., 1884, iv, 324-336. *Also :* Gaz. hebd. d. sc. méd. de Bordeaux, 1884, iv, 361 ; 371.— **Leva** (J.) Névralgie intermittente de la branche ophthalmique de Willis. Ann. Soc. de méd. d'Anvers, Brux., 1840, 194-196. *Also :* Arch. de la méd. belge, Brux., 1840, ii, 10-12.—**Liégey.** Névralgie catarrhale conjonctivale ; réflexions ; diverses perturbations fonctionnelles et altérations matérielles résultant de la névralgie de la région oculaire. Bull. Soc. de méd. prat. de Par., 1875, 173-180.— **Stevenson** (J.) An account of a singularly painful affection of the appendages of the left eye, from an uncommon cause, successfully treated. Lond. M. Reposit., 1816, vi, 471-473.—**Svensson** (I.) Två fall af ciliarnevros ; resektion af nerv. frontal ; helsa. Upsala Läkaref. Förh., 1875-6, xi, 339

Neuralgia (*Ovarian*).

See **Ovary** (*Neuralgia of*).

Neuralgia (*Painful points in*).

See **Neuralgia** (*Diagnosis, etc., of*).

Neuralgia (*Periodic*).

See **Neuralgia** (*Intermittent*).

Neuralgia (*Puerperal*).

See **Puerperal** neuralgia.

Neuralgia (*Rheumatic*).

Chenevière (A.) * De la névralgie rhumatismale. 4°. *Paris*, 1853.

Neuralgia (*Rheumatic*).

Draexler (F. C.) * De prosopalgia rheumatica in instituto clinico Pragensi observata, tractata et sanata, adnexa epicrisi. 8°. *Pragœ*, [1834].

Leussier (E.) * Étude clinique sur la névralgie rhumatismale. 4°. *Paris*, 1868.

Coudret. Observation d'une affection rhumatismale névralgique qui, après avoir passé par une suite de transformations successives, a fini par reprendre sa première forme et guérie. J. compl. du dict d. sc. méd., Par., 1831, xxxix, 64-68.—**Luton** (A.) Note sur l'emploi du cyanure de zinc, à propos d'une névralgie rhumatismale du trijumeau simulant le rhumatisme cérébral. Bull. gén. de thérap., etc., Par., 1877, xcii, 97-104. — **Schlesier.** Ueber Neuralgie und Rheumatalgie. Med. Ztg., Berl., 1841, x, 74.—**Semple** (A. B.) Rheumatic neuralgia of the head and face treated by the inhalation of ether. Lancet, Lond., 1847, i, 332. — **Wells** (H.) Rheumatic neuralgia treated with stramonium and hyd. of potash. *Ibid.*, 1839-40, i, 570.

Neuralgia (*Spinal*).

See, also, **Neuralgia** (*Intercostal*).

Allan (J.) Case of spinal neuralgia. Glasgow M. J., 1828, i, 406-409.—**Ancona** (V.) Quarantatre anni di permanenza in letto. Gazz. med. ital., prov. venete. Padova, 1881, xxiv, 41-45. — **Duplouy.** Observations de névralgies avec point apophysaire guéries par des applications de vésicatoires sur le point vertébral. Mém. et bull. Soc. de méd. et chir. de Bordeaux, 1875, 215-218. — **Hoppe.** Ein Fall von chronischem Rückenmarksleiden. Med. Cor.-Bl. rhein. u. westfäl. Aerzte, Bonn, 1843, ii, 308.—**Mader.** Eigenthümliche Spinal-Neurose im Bereiche des Plexus brachiales. Ber. d. k. k. Krankenanst. Rudolph-Stiftung in Wien (1878), 1879, 356. *Also :* Med.-chir. Centralbl., Wien, 1880, xv, 544. — **Porter** (I. G.) On neuralgia of the spinal nerves; with cases. Am. J. M. Sc., Phila., 1839, xxiii, 81-93. — **Puig y Balansó.** Neuralgias de los plexos lumbar y sacro en un niño ; curacion. Rev. de cien. méd., Barcel., 1883, ix, 552-555.—**Stainforth.** Thoracalgie spinale. Arch. méd. belges, Brux., 1880, 3. s., xviii, 33.—**White.** Neuralgia of the spine and mammæ. Lond. M. & S. J., 1834-5, vi, 222.

Neuralgia (*Supraorbital*).

See, also, **Brow-ague**; **Neuralgia** (*Facial, Treatment of*).

Faucheron (E.) * De la névralgie sus-orbitaire considérée dans ses rapports avec l'œil. 4°. *Paris*, 1880.

Also, in : Rec. d'opht., Par., 1881, 3. s., iii, 106 ; 139.

Welcker (T.) * Ueber typische Neuralgie des Supraorbitalis. 8°. *Giessen*, 1869.

Abeille. Sur deux cas de névralgie sus-orbitaire. Monit. d. hôp., Par., 1853, i, 121. — **Bampton** (A. H.) Nerve-stretching for supra-orbital neuralgia, with remarks on nerve-stretchings and their bearing on the mode of transmission of nerve impulses. Lancet, Lond., 1882, ii, 138.—**Bell** (R. W.) Case of periodic supraorbital neuralgia ; no history of ague ; quinine : rapid relief. Canada M. & S. J., Montreal, 1872-3, i, 447. — **Bierbaum** (J.) Hydrargyrum bichlorat. corros. gegen Neuralgia supraorbitalis. - Deutsche Klinik, Berl., 1866, xviii, 55.—**Boisseau** (F.-G.) Névralgie sus-orbitaire intermittente quotidienne, guérie par le quinquina et les rubéfians. J. univ. d. sc. méd., Par., 1817, vii, 245-248. — **Bricheteau** (F.) Névralgie sus-orbitaire intermittente guérie par les injections hypodermiques de sulfate de quinine. Bull. gén. de thérap., etc., Par., 1866, lxx, 132-138. *Also* [Abstr.] : Gaz. d. hôp., Par., 1866, xxxix, 161.— **Chomel.** Névralgie sus-orbitaire intermittente traitée par le sulfate de quinine. Gaz. d. hôp., Par., 1838, xii, 591. — **Chwogka** (F.) Neuralgia supraorbitalis. Ztschr. f. Nat.- u. Heilk. in Ungarn, Oedenburg, 1857, viii, 387. — **Claret** (J.) De l'emploi de l'extrait de belladone dans les névralgies. Rev. méd. franç. et étrang., Par., 1830, i, 31-42.— **Delame.** Observation de névralgie frontale intermittente, quotidienne d'abord, puis double ; tierce, puis quotidienne, puis tierce. Gaz. méd. de Par., 1837. 2. s., v, 239.—**Durham** (A. E.) A case of so-called frontal or supra-orbital neuralgia following injury and successfully treated by trephining the skull after failure of other methods of treatment. Tr. Clin. Soc. Lond., 1884, xvii, 117-150. *Also* [Abstr.] : Med. Press & Circ., Lond., 1884, n. s., xxxvii, 333. *Also* : Med. Times & Gaz., Lond., 1884, i, 465.— **Gouzée.** Névralgie frontale enlevée par l'acétate de morphine appliqué d'après la méthode endermique ; bronchite intermittente guérie par le sulfate de quinine. J. de méd., Brux., 1830, ii, 383-386. — **Guérin** (de Mamers). Observation de névralgie sus-orbitaire. J. compl. du dict. d. sc. méd., Par., 1832. xliv, 70-72.—**Hack** (W.) Supraorbitalneuralgie. Wien. med. Wchnschr., 1882, xxxii, 1510-1512. — **Hartmann** (A.) Supraorbitalneuralgie, hervorgerufen durch Empyem der Nebenhöhlen der Nase

Neuralgia (*Supraorbital*).

in Folge von Behinderung des Secretabflusses aus dem mittleren Nasengange. Berl. klin. Wchnschr., 1882, xix, 732–734.—**Horner.** Section of the frontal nerve for neuralgia. Med. Exam., Phila., 1851, n. s., vii, 180.—**Kappeler** (O.) Neuralgia supraorbitalis; Resection beider Supraorbitalnerven. *In his:* Chir. Beob. a. d. Thurgau. Kantonssp. Münsterlingen, 8°, Frauenfeld, 1874, 62–64.—**Karewski** (F.) Ueber einen Fall von Trophoneurose im Bereiche des Nervus supraorbitalis. Berl. klin. Wchnschr., 1883, xx, 549–551.—**Kroner** (T.) Neuralgia frontalis, intermittens quartana. Deutsche Ztschr. f. prakt. Med., Leipz., 1877, 16:.—**Lalaurie.** Observation de névralgie frontale. Éphém. méd. de Montpel., 1826, i, 206–21:.—**Laurence** (J. Z.) Division of the supraorbital nerve. Brit. M. J., Lond., 1869, i, 446.—**Lentigo** (J. B.) & **Ramos** (M. M.) Observacion de la nevralgia frontal. Décadas de med. y cirug. práct., Madrid, 1822, v, 3; 41.—**Lhéritier** (D.) Névralgie sus-orbitaire, intermittente, consécutive à une irritation des glandes lacrymales. Bull. clin., Par., 1835-6, i, 81.—**von Mandach** (F.) Ueber Neuralgia supraorbitalis intermittens. Cor.-Bl. f. schweiz. Aerzte, Basel, 1879, ix, 640.—**Masing** (E.) Dehnung des Nervus supraorbitalis wegen Neuralgie. St. Petersb. med. Wchnschr., 1879, iv, 441.—**Müller.** Drei Fälle von Durchschneidung des Supraorbitalnerven. Cor.-Bl. f. d. Aerzte u. Apoth. d. Grossherz. Oldenburg, 1864-5, iii, 61. ——. Drei Fälle von Durchschneidung der Frontalnerven. *Ibid.*, 145–147.—**Obissier** (H.) Névralgie du rameau sus-orbitaire d'origine paludéenne traitée avec succès par le bromhydrate de quinine. Bordeaux méd., 1877, vi, 321–323.—**Ochsenheimer** (J.) Verlarvtes Wechselfieber unter der Form von Supraorbitalschmerz. Oesterr. med. Wchnschr., Wien, 1843, 620.—**Piédagnel.** Observation de névralgie sus-orbitaire guérie par le sulfate de quinine. J. de physiol. expér., Par., 1822, ii, 124–127.—**Rennes.** Observations et réflexions sur trente-deux cas de névralgie frontale recueillis dans l'espace de quinze mois à Bergerac. Arch. gén. de méd., Par., 1836, 2. s., xi, 156–167.—**Schuh.** Heftiger Gesichtsschmerz geheilt durch Resektion des Nervus supraorbitalis tief in der Augenhöhle. Wien. med. Wchnschr., 1854, iv, 529. ——. Neuralgie des N. supraorbitalis. Spitals-Ztg., Wien, 1864, 73.—**Seeligmüller** (A.) Neuralgia supraorbitalis intermittens. Centralbl. f. Nervenh., Coblenz, 1880, iii, 209–213.—**Talko** (J.) O leczeniu nerwobólu nadoczodołowego. [Supraorbital neuralgia.] Gaz. lek., Warszawa, 1870, viii, 481–485.—**Temkin** (A.) Nevralgija nadglaz. nerva vslied. razdraj. zub. nerva. [Neuralgia of supraorbital nerve succeeding irritation of dental nerve.] Zubovrach. Vestnik, St. Petersb., 1886, iii, 158–160.—**Texier** (H.) Névralgie frontale double intermittente; symptômes insolites; traitement par le sulfate de quinine et la liqueur de Fowler; guérison. Monit. d. hôp., Par., 1857, v, 66.—**Tommasi** (S.) Un caso di nevralgia fronto-sincipitale calmata con l' uso della elettricità. Rendic. Accad. med.-chir. di Napoli, 1850, iv, 1–6.—**Van Allen** (T. F. C.) A report of unusual cases of reflex supraorbital neuralgia. Albany M. Ann., 1888, ix, 33–38.—**Willard** (L. H.) Neurectomy of the supraorbital nerve for the cure of neuralgia. Hahneman. Month., Phila., 1877, xii, 526–528.—**Williams** (A. D.) Supraorbital neuralgia. Cincin. Lancet & Obs., 1867, n. s., x, 223–225.

Neuralgia (*Syphilitic*).

Diffre (L.) * Des névralgies syphilitiques. 4°. *Montpellier*, 1884.

Also [Abstr.], *in:* Gaz. hebd. d. sc. méd. de Montpel., 1884, vi, 183–187.

Bartumeus (A.) Neuralgia específica intermitente de la cara, en el período prodrónico de las sífilides; desarrollo posterior de otras manifestaciones. Rev. de cien. méd., Barcel., 1879, v, 309–313.—**Seeligmüller.** Ueber syphilitische Neuralgien. Amtl. Ber. ü. d. Versamml. deutsch. Naturf. u. Aerzte 1883, Freib. i. Br., 1884, lvi, 166. *Also:* Deutsche med. Wchnschr., Berl., 1883, ix, 624.—**Thermes** (G.) Névralgie syphilitique du nerf trifacial; début onze ans après contamination; lypémanie; traitement mixte; amélioration rapide et notable. Rev. méd. franç. et étrang., Par., 1874, i, 34–41.—**Walker** (E.) A case of trigeminal neuralgia caused by syphilis. Arch. Med., N. Y., 1880, iii, 110–116. *Also:* St. Louis M. & S. J., 1880, xxxix, 299–305.—**Waton.** Deux observations de tic douloureux de cause vénérienne. Rec. périod. Soc. de méd. de Par., 1778, iv, 178–191.

Neuralgia (*Thoracic*).

See **Neuralgia** (*Intercostal*).

Neuralgia (*Traumatic*).

See, also, **Stumps** (*Diseases of*).

Mallet (A.) * Étude sur les névralgies traumatiques. 4°. *Paris*, 1866.

Carli (F.) Caso di nevralgia frontali traumatica curato con un nuovo processo operatorio. Bull. d. sc. med. di Bologna, 1861, 4. s., xv, 46–51. — **Clark** (T. N.)

Neuralgia (*Traumatic*).

Traumatic neuralgia; non-inflammatory softening of brain; operation; death. Virginia M. Month., Richmond, 1877, iv, 570–575.—**Cock.** Neuralgia the result of a badly-united fracture. Lancet, Lond., 1857, ii, 223.—**Denmark** (A.) Example of symptoms resembling tic douloureux, produced by a wound in the radial nerve. Med.-Chir. Tr., Lond., 1813, iv, 48–52. — **Dubois.** De la névralgie traumatique. Gaz. hebd. de méd., Par., 1861, viii, 67.—**Dupuy.** Des névralgies traumatiques. Bull. Soc. de méd. prat. de Par. (1865), 1866, 2–5. — **Durand** (A.) Névrite traumatique; amputation; névralgie du moignon. J. d. sc. méd. de Lille, 1886, viii, 75–82. — **Estlander** (J. A.) Traumatisk neuralgi behandlad med lospreparering och sträckning af nerven. Finska läk.-sällsk. handl., Helsingfors, 1878, xx, 278–282. — **Falchi** (F.) Nevralgia traumatica; nevro-paralisi vascolare; esame della temperatura dietro l' orecchio. Osservatore, Torino, 1879, xv, 193–196. — **Fischer** (G.) Traumatische Neuralgia supraorbitalis; Irritation der Netzhaut; Neuralgia infraorbitalis; operative Heilung. Arch. f. klin. Chir., Berl., 1864, v, 335–338.—**Gordon** (F. H.) Traumatic neuralgia. West. J. M. & S., Louisville, 1846, 3. s., v, 392–394. — **Gross** (S. D.) Traumatic neuralgia. *Ibid.*, 1854, 4. s., i, 59–62.—**Hulke.** Neuralgia in the brow and temple caused by a scar. Med. Times & Gaz., Lond., 1862, i, 586.—**Isenschmid.** Nadeln in der weiblichen Brust; Neuralgia mammæ, geheilt durch Dehnung des Plexus brachialis. Aerztl. Int.-Bl., München, 1883, xxx, 299.—**Jeffreys** (H.) A history of a case of severe neuralgic affection of the face, which was cured by the extirpation of a piece of china from the cheek, after it had been imbedded in its substance fourteen years. Lond. M. & Phys. J., 1823, xlix, 199–203. — **Jobert** (*de Lamballe*). Névralgie traumatique du bras à la suite d'une saignée du bras; guérison par la section du nerf lésé. Gaz. d. hôp., Par., 1840, 2. s., ii, 150. — **Krauss.** Neuralgie durch Druck auf die Nerven verursacht. Med. Cor.-Bl. d. württemb. ärztl. Ver., Stuttg., 1852, xxii, 194.—**Larrey.** Névralgie spasmodique de l'avant-bras consécutive à une fracture du radius et à l'emploi de l'électricité. Bull. Soc. de chir. de Par. (1861), 1862, 2. s., ii, 177–179 — **Le Dentu.** Note sur un cas de névralgie traumatique du nerf obturateur. Gaz. d. hôp., Par., 1874, xlvii, 178. — **Lente** (F. D.) Neuralgia and other neuroses arising from cicatrices of the scalp and their surgical treatment. Proc. Am. Neurol. Ass., N. Y., 1875, i, 157–175. — **Liégey.** Observations de névralgies périodiques survenues à la suite de lésions traumatiques. Rev. de thérap. du midi, Montpel., 1854, vii, 156–159.—**Marchal** *de Calvi* (C.J.) De la prosopalgie traumatique. Rapport au conseil de santé sur des observations du Dr. Maupin. Rec de mém. de méd. . . . mil., Par., 1843, lv, 266–292. *Also*, Reprint. ——. De la névralgie trifaciale traumatique. Rec. de mém. de méd. . . . mil., Par., 1852, 2. s., ix, 266–274. — **Mitchell** (S. W.) Traumatic neuralgia; section of median nerve. Am. J. M. Sc., Phila., 1874, n. s., lxviii, 17–29. — **Ollivier** (A.) Contribution à l'histoire des névralgies réflexes d'origine traumatique. Compt. rend. Soc. de biol. 1874, Par., 1875, 6. s., i, pt. 1, 177–179. *Also:* Gaz. méd. de Par., 1874, xlv, 228.—**Post.** Traumatic neuralgia. Bull. N. York Acad. M., 1866-9, iii, 144–147. — **Rodd** (G. R.) On the treatment of painful affections of the nerves, arising from local injury. Tr. Ass. Apoth., etc., Lond., 1823, i, 183–188.—**Seguin** (E. C.) Traumatic pedal neuralgia of one year's standing rapidly cured by the actual platinum cautery. Arch. Med., N. Y., 1879, i, 335. *Also, in his:* Op. min. [etc.], 8°, N. Y., 1884, 401.—**Smith** (H.) Traumatic neuralgia. Med. Times & Gaz., Lond., 1862, n. s., iv, 392. — **Ussher** (H.) Aconite in traumatic neuralgia. *Ibid.*, 1859, n. s., xix, 270.—**Verneuil.** Des névralgies traumatiques secondaires précoces. Assoc. franç. pour l'avance. d. sc. Compt.-rend. 1874, Par., 1875, iii, 924–941. *Also:* Arch. gén. de méd., Par., 1874, 6. s., xxiv, 528; 679. —**Vio-Bonato** (A.) Nevralgia traumatica, guarita mediante injezioni sotto-cutanee. Gazz. med. ital., prov. venete, Padova, 1863, vi, 208. — **Viollet.** Névralgie traumatique précoce survenue à la suite de diastasis musculaire. Rec. d. trav. Soc. méd. d'Indre-et-Loire 1877, Tours, 1878, lxxiv, 33–38. — **Wardrop** (J.) Case where a severe nervous affection came on after a punctured wound of the finger, and in which amputation was successfully performed. Med.-Chir. Tr., Lond., 1820, viii, 246–251.—**Warren** (J. M.) On neuralgic affections following injuries of nerves. Am. J. M. Sc., Phila., 1864, n. s., xlvii, 316–324. *Also*, Reprint.—**Webster** (J.) Case of painful affection of the arm, following venesection, cured by acupuncturation. Lond. M. & Phys. J., 1825, liv, 31–33.

Neuralgia (*Trigeminal*).

See **Neuralgia** (*Facial, etc.*)

Neuralgia (*Uterine*).

See **Neuralgia** (*Lumbar, etc.*)

Neuralgia (*Visceral*).

See **Neuralgia** (*Abdominal, etc.*)

Neuralgia *in lower extremity.*

See, also, **Foot** (*Painful*); **Sciatica**.

YEATS (G. D.) A history of a severe case of neuralgia, commonly called tic douloureux, occupying the nerves of the right thigh, leg, and foot, successfully treated; with some observations on that complaint, and on its causes as they vary in different individuals. 8°. *London*, 1822.

Arloing (N.) Observation sur l'efficacité de la méthode de Cotugno, dans le traitement des névralgies des membres abdominaux. *J. gén. de méd., chir. et pharm.,* Par., 1827, xcviii, 293; 316. [Rap. de Mélier], 316–331.— **Betz** (F.) Bilaterale Cruralneuralgie. Memorabilien, Heilbr., 1867, xii, 117.—**Bousseau.** Deux observations de névralgie du nerf saphène interne. Rec. d. trav. Soc. méd. d'obs. de Par., 1868–70, 2. s., ii, 221–225. *Also* [Abstr.]: Gaz. d. hôp., Par., 1869, xlii, 27.—**Cloquet** (H.) Note sur l'emploi de la térébenthine dans la névralgie fémoro-poplitée ou sciatique. N. Jour. de méd., chir., pharm., etc., Par., 1818, i, 335–337.—**Cornelison** (A.) Monography of a case of violent and fixed pain, in a lower extremity, successfully treated. Med. Reposit., N. Y., 1820, n. s., v, 191–196.—**Ely.** Circonstances singulières d'un cas de névralgie dans les membres inférieurs. Gaz. hebd. de méd., Par., 1874, 2. s., xi, 87.—**Englisch.** Ueber eine besondere Form der Hämorrhagie der Unterextremitäten und ihre Folgen (Hæmorrhagia neuralgica). Ber. d. k. k. Krankenanst. Rudolph-Stiftung in Wien (1884), 1885, 282–284. ——. Ueber eine besondere Form der Hämorrhagie an den Unterextremitäten (Hæmorrhagia neuralgica). Wien. med. Bl., 1885, viii, 737: 774; 806.—**Gastaldo** (J.) Anestesias de las estremidades superiores é inferiores y parte anterior del pecho; neuralgia periódica é intermitente en las articulaciones femoro-tibial y tarso-metatarsianas; tratamiento alopático y homeopático sin resultado; curacion por medio de la aplicacion de la electricidad; reflexiones. España méd., Madrid, 1863, viii, 261.—[**von Haselberg.**]- Neuralgia nervi peronæi. Mag. f. d. ges. Heilk., Berl., 1832, xxxvii, 173.—**Jäsche** (G.) Ein Fall von Neuralgia intermittens tibialis. Med. Ztg. Russlands, St. Petersb., 1846, iii, 28.—**Kilian** (F.) Neuralgie des Nervus cruralis. Ztschr. f. rat. Med., Heidelb., 1847, vi, 24–37.—**M'Lean** (W.) Case of neuralgia of the crural nerve, successfully treated by the carbonate of iron. Glasgow M. Exam., 1832, ii, 35.—**Melchiori** (G.) † Neuralgia crurale cagionata da ernia inguinale. Gazz. med. di Milano, 1847, vi, 4.—**Mugna.** † Nevralgia femoro-poplitea curata colla moxa. Gazz. med. ital., prov. venete, Padova, 1859, ii, 45–47.—**Piorry.** Observations sur un cas de névralgie fémoro-poplitée, traitée avec succès par l'essence de térébenthine. Rev. méd. franç. et étrang., Par., 1826, iv, 208–212.—**Snow** (E. S.) Case of tic douloureux in the peroneal nerve. Lancet, Lond., 1833–4, i, 745.

Neuralgia *in pregnancy.*

See Puerperal *neuralgia.*

Neuralgia *in upper extremity.*

See Neuralgia (*Brachial*), *etc.*

Neuraline.

See Aconite (*Toxicology of*).

Neurasthenia.

See, also, **Brain** *and mind;* **Genitals** (*Irritation, etc., of*); **Nervous** *system* (*Diseases of, Functional*); **Nervous** *system* (*Diseases of, Treatment of*).

ARNDT (R.) Die Neurasthenie (Nervenschwäche); ihr Wesen, ihre Bedeutung und Behandlung vom anatomisch-physiologischen Standpunkte, für Aerzte und Studirende. l. 8°. *Wien u. Leipzig,* 1885.

Also [Rev.], *in:* Deutsche Med.-Ztg., Berl., 1885, vi, 1024–1029.

BEARD (G. M.) A practical treatise on nervous exhaustion (neurasthenia); its symptoms, nature, sequences, treatment. 8°. *New York,* 1880.

BERGER (P.) Die Nervenschwäche (Neurasthenie); ihr Wesen, ihre Ursachen und Behandlung. 2. Aufl. 8°. *Berlin, W.,* 1885.

——. The same. 4. Aufl. 8°. *Berlin,* 1886.

CAMPBELL (H.) A treatise on nervous exhaustion and the diseases induced by it. With observations on the nervous constitution, hereditary and acquired, and on the origin and

Neurasthenia.

nature of nervous force and animal electricity. 4. ed. 12°. *London,* 1874.

DOWSE (T. S.) On brain and nerve exhaustion, "neurasthenia"; its nature and curative treatment. Revised ed. 8°. *London,* 1887.

HOVELL (D. De B.) On some conditions of neurasthenia. 8°. *London,* 1886.

——. On some further conditions of neurasthenia; a psychological study. 8°. *London,* 1887.

KAHN (L. J.) Nervous exhaustion; its cause and cure, [etc.] 16°. *New York,* [1876].

LÖWENFELD (L.) Die moderne Behandlung der Nervenschwäche (Neurasthenie), der Hysterie und verwandter Leiden. Mit besonderer Berücksichtigung der Luftcuren, Bäder, Anstaltsbehandlung und der Mitchell-Playfair'schen Mastcur. 8°. *Wiesbaden,* 1887.

VON ZIEMSSEN (H.) Die Neurasthenie und ihre Behandlung. 8°. *Leipzig,* 1887.

Anjel. Experimentelles zur Pathologie und Therapie der cerebralen Neurasthenie. Arch. f. Psychiat., Berl., 1884, xv, 618–632.—**Arcari** (G.) Sulla neurastenia. Bull. d. Comit. med. cremonese, Cremona, 1887, vii, 200; 247.—**Averbeck** (H.) Die akute Neurasthenie, die plötzliche Erschöpfung der nervösen Energie; ein ärztliches Kulturbild. Deutsche Med.-Ztg., Berl., 1886, vii, 293; 301; 313; 325; 337. *Also,* Reprint.—**Bartholow** (R.) What is meant by nervous prostration? Proc. Phila. Co. M. Soc., Phila., 1883–4, vi, 120–131. *Also:* Maryland M. J., Balt., 1883–4, x, 645–650. *Also:* Polyclinic, Phila., 1883–4, i, 97–101. *Also:* Med. News, Phila., 1884, xliv, 107–109. *Also:* Boston M. & S. J., 1884, cx, 53–56. *Also:* Med. & Surg. Reporter, Phila., 1884, l, 97–101. [Discussion], 110.—**Beard** (G. M.) Neurasthenia, or nervous exhaustion. Boston M. & S. J., 1869, n. s., lxxx, 217–221. ——. Certain symptoms of nervous exhaustion. Virginia M. Month., Richmond, 1878, v, 161–185. *Also,* Reprint. ——. Neurasthenia (nervous exhaustion) as a cause of inebriety. Quart. J. Inebr., Hartford, 1878–9, iii, 193–201. *Also,* Reprint. ——. Other symptoms of neurasthenia (nervous exhaustion). J. Nerv. & Ment. Dis., Chicago, 1879, vi, 246–261. *Also,* Reprint. ——. Cases of neurasthenia (nervous exhaustion), with remarks on treatment. St. Louis M. & S. J., 1879, xxxvi, 337–356. *Also,* Reprint. ——. The nature and diagnosis of neurasthenia (nervous exhaustion). N. York M. J., 1879, xxix, 225-251. *Also,* Reprint. *Also:* Canad. J. M. Sc., Toronto, 1879, iv, 187–199. ——. Nervous exhaustion (neurasthenia), with cases of sexual neurasthenia. Maryland M. J., Balt., 1880, vi, 289–297. ——. The symptoms of sexual exhaustion (sexual neurasthenia). Independ. Pract., Balt., 1880, i, 221; 271. *Also,* Reprint. ——. The sequences of neurasthenia. Alienist & Neurol., St. Louis, 1880, i, 18–29. ——. Traumatic neurasthenia. N. Eng. M. Month., Newtown, Conn., 1881–2, i, 246–249.—**Brown** (J.) Neurasthenia, or nervous exhaustion. Tr. Wisconsin M. Soc., Milwaukee, 1878, xii, 106–118.—**Clark** (A.) Some observations concerning what is called neurasthenia. Lancet, Lond., 1886, i, 1.—**Clark** (F. Le G.) Some remarks on nervous exhaustion and on vasomotor action. J. Anat. & Physiol., Lond., 1883–4, xviii, 239–256.—**D.** (C.-L.) Des neurasthénies et de leur traitement. Union méd., Par., 1883, 3. s., xxxvi, 869; 883.—**Dana** (C. L.) On the pathology and treatment of certain forms of chronic nerveweakness. Med. Rec., N. Y., 1883, xxiv, 57–62. *Also,* Reprint.—**Desrosiers** (H.-E.) De la neurasthénie. Union méd. du Canada, Montréal, 1879, viii, 145; 201.—**Dowse** (T. S.) On neurasthenia, or nervous exhaustion and its treatment. Proc. M. Soc. Lond., 1879–81, v, 153.—**Dragomanoff** (A. P.) Sluch. neurastenii, osloj. psichichesk. elementar. razstroist. [Case of neurasthenia, involving psychiatric elementary perturbation.] Arch. psichiat., etc., Charkov, 1887, ix, no. 2, 68–76.—**Draper** (J.) Neurasthenia of the ganglionic nervous centres. Tr. Vermont M. Soc. 1881, St. Albans, 1882, 59–68.—**Ewald** (C. A.) Die Neurasthenia dyspeptica. Berl. klin. Wchnschr., 1884, xxi, 321; 342. *Also, transl.* [Abstr.]: Riv. veneta di sc. med., Venezia, 1885, ii, 289–297. *Also, transl.* [Abstr.]: Presse méd. belge, Brux., 1885, xxxvii, 105–109.—**Fisher** (T. W.) Neurasthenia. Boston M. & S. J., 1872, lxxxvi, 65–72.—**Fowler** (W. H.) Neurasthenia. Med. Bull., Phila., 1881, iii, 254–256.—**Ghose** (K. D.) An instructive case of nervous exhaustion simulating intermittent fever. Indian M. Gaz., Calcutta, 1874, ix, 259.—**Greene** (J. S.) Neurasthenia; its causes and its home treatment. Boston M. & S. J., 1883, cix, 75–78. *Also,* Reprint. *Also:* Med. Communicat. Mass. M. Soc., Bost., 1883, xiii, no. 2, 155–166.—**Holbrook** (H. C.) Dissertation on certain forms of nerve weakness. Tr. N. Hampshire M. Soc., Manchester, 1886, 93–97.—**Huchard** (H.) De la neurasthénie. [Extr.] Union méd., Par., 1882, 3. s., xxxiii, 978; 989. *Also:* Médecin, Par., 1882, viii, no.

Neurasthenia.

36.—**Hughes** (C. H.) Notes on neurasthenia; from an alienist's standpoint, intended, mainly, to introduce the views of a pioneer American writer. Alienist & Neurol., St. Louis, 1880, i, 437–449. ———. Note on the essential psychic signs of general functional neuratrophia or neurasthenia. Tr. M. Ass. Missouri, St. Louis, 1882, xxv, 115–124. *Also:* Alienist & Neurol., St. Louis, 1882, iii, 411–418. *Also:* St. Louis M. & S. J., 1882, xiii, 625–628. *Also:* J. Psych. M., Lond., 1882-3, n. s., viii, 181–186. — **Hutchinson** (W. F.) A report of three typical cases of neurasthenia. Med. Rec., N. Y., 1880, xviii, 398–401.— **Jahn.** Ueber Behandlung von Neurasthenieen. Deutsche Med.-Ztg., Berl., 1885, ii, 949–951. *Also,* Reprint.— **Jakovleff** (A. A.) Neskolko sluch. neurast. s preobladan. javlenii so storony psichiki. [Some cases of neurasthenia with predominating phenomena of cerebral region.] Arch. psichiat., etc., Charkov, 1887, ix, 1–25. — **Jewell** (J. S.) The treatment of neurasthenia, or chronic nervous exhaustion. Chicago M. Gaz., 1880, i, 60; 89. ———. The varieties and causes of neurasthenia. J. Nerv. & Ment. Dis., Chicago, 1880, n. s., v, 1–16.—**Johnson** (Anna H.) Neurasthenia. Phila. M. Times, 1880-81, xi, 737–744.—**Johnstone** (J.) Case of George, Lord Lyttelton. *In his:* Med. Essays & Obs., 8°, Evesham, 1795, 223–234.— **Kovalevsky** (P. I.) Neurastenija i patophobija. Arch. psichiat., etc., Charkov, 1885, vi, pt. 3, 49–53. *Also, transl.:* Centralbl. f. Nervenh., Leipz., 1887, x, 65–70.—**Melotti** (G.) Della neurastenia cerebro-spinale (esaurimento nervoso). Ann. univ. di med. e chir., Milano, 1883, cclxiii, 369–413.—**Mitchell** (S. W.) Neurasthenia, hysteria and their treatment. Chicago M. Gaz., 1880, i, 155.—**Möbius** (P. J.) Ueber Neurasthenia cerebralis. Memorabilien, Heilbr., 1879, xxiv, 23–31. ———. Zur Lehre von der Neurasthenie. Centralbl. f. Nervenh., Leipz., 1883, vi, 97–99.— **Page** (H. W.) On the abuse of bromide of potassium in the treatment of traumatic neurasthenia. Med. Times & Gaz., Lond., 1885, i, 437–441. *Also,* Reprint.—**Playfair** (W. S.) Some observations concerning what is called neurasthenia. Brit M. J., Lond., 1886, ii, 853–855.—**Richter** (F.) Die Neurasthenie und Hysterie. Deutsche Med.-Ztg., Berl., 1884, i, 405; 413; 425. *Also,* Reprint.—**Riva** (G.) Sopra tre casi di neurastenia. Riv. sper. di freniat., Reggio-Emilia, 1883, ix, 237–252.—**Rosenbach** (O.) Ueber nervöse Herzschwäche (Neurasthenia vasomotoria). Breslau. aerztl. Ztschr., 1886, viii, 181; 193. — **Rouse** (W. H.) Neurasthenia. Proc. . . . San. Convent. Detroit, Lansing, 1880, 58–61. — **Sachaff** (N. A.) Sluchai tiajeloi neurastenii, izliechennoi po nieskolko izminennomu sposobu Weir Mitchel'ja. [Grave neurasthenia treated by a modification of the method of Weir Mitchell.] Vrach, St. Petersb., 1883, iv, 513–515.—**Savage** (J. P.) Hints on nervous exhaustion (neurasthenia). Cincin. Lancet & Clinic, 1880, n. s., v, 153.—**Schwabe** (J.) Die seeklimatische Cur für neurasthenische und anämische Kinder. Deutsche med. Wchnschr., Berl., 1888, xiv, 78. *Also,* Reprint. — **Stillman** (W. O.) Neurasthenia. Med. & Surg. Reporter, Phila., 1879, xl, 397; 419.—**Strahan** (J.) Neurasthenia, acute and chronic, and its importance. Dublin J. M. Sc., 1885, 3. s., lxxx, 195–220. ———. Puzzling conditions of the heart and other organs dependent on neurasthenia. Brit. M. J., Lond., 1885, ii, 435–437. — **Summers** (T. O.) Neurasthenia. South. Pract., Nashville, 1881, iii, 367–370.—**Vanderbeck** (C. C.) Interesting case of nervous exhaustion. Med. & Surg. Reporter, Phila., 1877, xxxvii, 3.—**Wilheim.** Die nervöse Erschöpfung. Allg. Wien. med. Ztg., 1881, xxvi, 237; 246; 262.—**Williams** (J. L.) Overdraft of vital or nerve power as affecting general and special health. J. Am. M. Ass., Chicago, 1885, iv, 122.— **Wood** (H. C.) Neurasthenia. Syst. Pract. M. (Pepper), Phila., 1886, v, 353–362.—**Wooton** (M.) Mimosis inquieta. J. Psych. M., Lond., 1882-3, n. s., viii, 191–221. — **Young** (P. A.) Two cases of neurasthenia of long standing successfully treated by the Weir Mitchell method. Edinb. Clin. & Path. J., 1883-4, i, 905–909.

Neurectomy.

See Neurotomy, *etc.*

Neureiter (Franciscus Ferdinandus). * De

depositionibus lacteis. 31 pp. 8°. *Viennæ,* [1775].

Neureusch.

See Fever (*Malarial, History, etc., of*), by localities.

Neurilemma.

See Nervous *system.*

Neurin.

von **Becker** (R.) Ueber die therapeutische Wirkung des Neurins. Mitth. d. Ver. d. Aerzte in Nied.-Oest., Wien, 1877, iii, 147.—**Cervello** (V.) Notices préliminaires sur l'action de la neurine. Arch. ital. de biol., Turin, 1884, v, 199–201. ———. Sull' azione fisiologica della neurina. Ann. di chim. med.-farm., Milano, 1885, 4. s., i, 7–

Neurin.

33. *Also, transl.:* Arch. ital. de biol., Turin, 1886, vii, 172–197. — **Gachtgens** (C.) Ueber die physiologischen Wirkungen des salzsauren Neurins. Dorpat. med. Ztschr., 1870-71, i, 161–174.—**Ludwig** (E.) Ueber das Neurin. Mitth. d. Ver. d. Aerzte in Nied.-Oest., Wien, 1877, iii, 135—**Mauthner** (J.) Beiträge zur Kenntniss des Neurins Med. Jahrb., Wien, 1873, iii, 128–134. ———. Ueber das Verhalten des Neurins gegen Eiweisskörper. *Ibid.,* 1874, iv, 347. *Also:* Ann. d. Chem., Leipz., 1874, clxxvii, 178–180.—**Ott** (I.) & **Collmar** (C.) Pyrexial agents: Albumose, peptone, and neurin. J. Physiol., Lond. & Cambridge, 1887, viii, 218–228, 1 pl. *Also,* Reprint.

Neuritis.

See, also, Nerves (*Brachial*) [*etc.*]; Neuralgia; Skin (*Diseases of, Neurotic*).

ABRAHAMSZ (T.) * Neuritis rami primi trigemini. 8°. *Utrecht,* [1873].

ASWADUROFF (K.) * Neuritis ischiadica chronica ascendens. 8°. *Jena,* 1881.

DUBREUILH (C.) * De la névrite; coup-d'œil historique et recherches expérimentales sur cette maladie. 8°. *Montpellier,* 1845.

FOURNIER-BERGERON (G.-L.) * Contribution à l'étude de la névrite ascendante. 4°. *Paris,* 1878.

GROS (J.) * Contribution à l'histoire des névrites. 4°. *Lyon,* 1879.

JACOB (A.) * Étude clinique d'un cas de névrite ascendante avec myélite consécutive. 4°. *Montpellier,* 1882.

KLEMM (R.) * Ueber Neuritis migrans. 8°. *Strassburg,* 1874.

NASSE (C. F.) * De neuritide. 8°. *Halæ,* 1800.

OLLIER. * Contribution à l'étude de la névrite ascendante et des paralysies réflexes. 4°. *Paris,* 1882.

POUEY (E.) * Essai sur le diagnostic différentiel entre la névrite et la névralgie. 4°. *Paris,* 1877.

REY-BARREAU (J.) * Contribution à l'étude de la névrite traumatique. 4°. *Paris,* 1881.

TREPTE (W.) * Casuistische Beiträge zur Lehre von der Neuritis, besonders der Neuritis traumatica und migrans. 8°. *Halle a. S.,* 1886.

VERDUREAU (D.) * Études sur la névrite idiopathique. 4°. *Paris,* 1853.

WYLER (J.) * Klinische Beiträge zur Pathologie der Neuritis. 8°. *Strassburg,* 1878.

Althaus (J.) On neuritis of the brachial plexus. Med.-Chir. Tr., Lond., 1871, liv, 145–154. *Also, transl.:* Deutsches Arch. f. klin. Med., Leipz., 1872, x, 189–195. ———. Observations on neuritis and perineuritis of some of the cranial nerves. Brain, Lond., 1878-9, i, 519: 1879-80, ii, 10 — **Arnozan** & **Salvat.** Névrites expérimentales produites par l'instillation d'éther ou l'application de glace. J. de méd. de Bordeaux, 1884-5, xiv, 40.— **Asmus.** Neuritis. Med. Ztg., Berl., 1839, viii, 262.— **Bannister** (H. M.) On chronic sub-acute neuritis. Chicago J. Nerv. & Ment. Dis., 1875, ii, 523–555. ———. History of a case of idiopathic sub-acute neuritis, affecting the crural, obturator, and sciatic nerves. Chicago M. J. & Exam., 1875, xxxii, 667–669.—**Beau** (J.-H.-S.) De la névrite intercostale dans la phthisie pulmonaire. Union méd., Par., 1849, iii, 345–347.—**Benedikt** (M.) Beiträge zur neuropathischen und elektrotherapeutischen Casuistik; ein Fall von diffuser Neuritis centralis. Deutsches Arch. f. klin. Med., Leipz., 1874, xiii, 94–106, 5 pl.— **Bergamaschi** (G.) Neuriti facciali guarite mercè l' agopuntura. Ann. univ. di med., Milano, 1826, xxxix, 5–12.—**Bettoli** (U. A.) Congettura patologiche su la neuritide o infiammazione de' nervi. Gior. di Soc. med. chir. di Parma, 1812, xi, 256–277.—**Bigelow** (H. R.) Neuritis. Med. Rec., N. Y., 1879, xv, 574.—**Bishop** (E. S.) Neuritis, following traumatism, treated in various ways, finally by resection of a portion of the nerve; cure. Med. Chron., Manchester, 1886, iv, 201.—**Boeck** (C.) Et Tilfælde af Neuritis traumatica ascendens. Norsk Mag. f. Lægevidensk., Christiania, 1879. 3. R., ix, 105–114.— **Brissaud** (E.) Sur une variété nouvelle de névrite parenchymateuse. Gaz. hebd. de méd., Par., 1881, 2. s., xviii, 180–183.—**Bull** (E.) Tilfælde af Neuritis. Forh. Norske med. Selsk. i Kristiania, 1885, 79–82.—**Buzzard** (T.) Clinical lecture on cases of neuritis, syphilitic and rheumatic. Lancet, Lond., 1879, i, 289.—**Caspari** (A.) Zur Casuistik der Neuritiden. Ztschr. f. klin. Med

Neuritis.

Berl., 1882-3, v, 537-557.—**D'Ancona** (N.) Nevrite ascendente del radiale sinistro, successiva a trauma; guarigione. Gazz. med. ital., prov. venete. Padova, 1884, xxvii, 387-389.—**Dugès** (A.) Note sur la distinction entre la névrite et la phlébite. Rev. méd. franç. et étrang., Par., 1824, iii, 408-413.—**Duménil** (L.) Contributions pour servir à l'histoire des paralysies périphériques et spécialement de la névrite. Gaz. hebd. de méd.. Par., 1866, 2. s., iii, 51; 67; 84.—**Eichhorst** (H.) Neuritis acuta progressiva. Arch. f. path. Anat., etc., Berl., 1877, lxix, 265-285, 2´pl.—**Fayrer** (J.) Neuritis. Med. Times & Gaz., Lond., 1868, i, 8.—**Fischer** (F.) Zwei Fälle von Neuritis. Berl. klin. Wchnschr., 1875, xii, 439; 457.—**Gombault** (A.) Contribution à l'étude anatomique de la névrite parenchymateuse subaiguë ou chronique; névrite segmentaire péri-axile. Arch. de neurol., Par., 1880-81, i, 11; 177, 2 pl. ——. Note sur le rôle que jouent les lésions segmentaires dans l'évolution de la névrite parenchymateuse. Bull. Soc. anat. de Par., 1881, lvi, 156-162. Also: Progrès méd., Par., 1881, ix, 318-320. ——. Note relative à l'existence de la névrite segmentaire périaxile; à propos d'un cas de paralysie diphthéritique. Progrès méd., Par., 1886, 2. s., iii, 472.—**Hughes** (C. H.) Neuritis plantaris; a clinical record. J. Am. M. Ass., Chicago, 1887, viii, 292-294. Also: Alienist & Neurol., St. Louis, 1887, viii, 201-209.—**Joffroy** (A.) De la névrite parenchymateuse spontanée, généralisée ou partielle. Arch. de physiol. norm. et path., Par., 1879, 2. s., vi, 172-198, 1 pl.—**Kast** (A.) Klinisches und Anatomisches über primäre degenerative Neuritis. Deutsches Arch. f. klin. Med., Leipz., 1886-7, xl, 41-61.—**Kauders** (F.) Ein seltenerer Fall von Neuritis ascendens. Wien. med. Wchnschr., 1885, xxxv, 1594-1598.—**Lampadarios** (N.) Φλεγμονὴ τῶν νεύρων τοῦ βραχιονίου πλέγματος. Νευρῖτις κατιοῦσα (nevritis descendens). Ἀσκληπιός, Ἀθῆναι, 1870-71, ix, 282-316.—**Latimer** (T. S) Neuritis. Med. Chron., Balt., 1882-3, i, 197-204.—**M'Crea** (J.) On some cases of idiopathic neuritis. Brit. M. J., Lond., 1873, i, 585.—**Mader.** Neuritis cervico-brachialis; Heilung, Ber. d. k. k. Krankenanst. Rudolph-Stiftung in Wien (1879), 1880, 372. ——. Sehr ausgebreitete Neurose, entstanden aus einer Neuritis N. mediani dextri; Besserung. Ibid. (1881), 1882, 318-321. ——. Neuritis brachialis nach Trauma; geheilt. Ibid. (1885), 1886, 365.—**Martinet** (L.) Mémoire sur l'inflammation des nerfs. Rev. méd. franç. et étrang., Par., 1824, ii, 329-354.—**Mason** (R. O.) A case of traumatic neuritis of thirty-five years' duration; treatment by repeated nerve section; subsequent history and autopsy. Am. J. M. Sc., Phila., 1886, n. s., xcii, 131-141.—**Mélier** (F.) Note et observation sur la névrite. J. gén. de méd., chir. et pharm., Par., 1829, cviii, 155-160.—**Miles** (F. T.) Two cases of neuritis of the ulnar nerve. Maryland M. J., Balt., 1881-2, viii, 193-196.—**Mills** (C. K.) Two cases of traumatic neuritis. Phila. M. Times, 1881-2, xii, 89. ——. A case of diffused rheumatic neuritis. Polyclinic, Phila., 1886-7, iv, 80.—**Morton** (W. J.) A contribution to traumatic neuritis, illustrated by a case following dislocation of the humerus. Med. Gaz., N. Y., 1883, x, 327-329. Also [Abstr.]: Med. News, Phila., 1883, xlii, 739.—**Müller** (F.) Neuritis descendens des Plexus sacralis sinister in Folge Beckentumors. Mitth. d. Ver. d. Aerzte in Steiermark 1881, Graz, 1882, xviii, 72-75.—**Névrite;** altération anatomique du ganglion de Gasser et des branches du nerf maxillaire inférieur. Gaz. d. hôp., Par., 1861, xxxiv, 209.—**Niedieck** (W.) Ueber Neuritis migrans und ihre Folgezustände. Arch. f. exper. Path. u. Pharmakol., Leipz., 1877, vii, 205-222. Also, Reprint.—**Nothnagel** (H.) Ueber Neuritis in diagnostischer und pathologischer Beziehung. Samml. klin. Vortr., No. 103, Leipz., 1876 (Inn. Med., No. 35). 819-850. Also, transl.: Clin. lect. . . . by German authors, Lond., 1877, 2. s., 201-236.—**Pennato** (P.) Intorno ad alcuni casi di nevrite. Riv. veneta di sc. med., Venezia, 1885, ii, 266-286.—**Pierret.** Plusieurs cas de névrite parenchymateuse avec détails histologiques. Arch. de physiol. norm. et path., Par., 1874, 2. s., i, 968-972.—**Piorry.** De l'hémito-névrite et de son traitement; un mot sur une espèce particulière de névrôme, consécutive à la névrite. Union méd., Par., 1851, v, 317; 321. — **Pitres** (A.) & **Vaillard** (L.) Des névrites provoquées par les injections d'éther au voisinage des troncs nerveux des membres. Compt. rend. Soc. de biol., Par., 1887, 8. s., iv, 299-303. Also: Gaz. méd. de Par., 1887, 7. s., iv, 256.—**Poore** (C. T.) A case of causalgia. N. York M. J., 1883, xxxvii, 123.—**Putzel** (L.) Remarks on a case of neuritis, with secondary inflammation in the spinal cord. Med. Rec., N. Y., 1879, xv, 390-392.—**Remak.** Ueber Neuritis. Oesterr. Ztschr. f. prakt. Heilk., Wien, 1860, vi, 769-776.—**Rohden** (A.) Neuritis durch Nervenverletzung. Deutsche med. Wchnschr., Berl., 1877, iii, 405.—**Rosenbach** (O.) Experimentelle Untersuchungen über Neuritis. Arch. f. exper. Path. u. Pharmakol., Leipz., 1877, viii, 223-243, 1 pl.—**Schwarz** (A.) Ein Fall von Neuritis. Wien. med. Presse, 1886, xxvii, 1619.—**Semmola** (M.) Un caso di neurite e miosite reumatica gnarito con la pilocarpina. Med. contemp., Napoli, 1886, iii, 611.—**Sitsyanko** (I.) Travmaticheskoe vospalenie nerva;

Neuritis.

tsailebnoe daiistvie polozhitelnago toka. [Traumatic inflammation of a nerve; beneficial effect of a po-itive galvanic current.] Med. Vestnik, St. Petersb., 1869, ix, 155.—**Stadelmann** (E) Ueber einen eigenthümlichen mikroskopischen Befund in dem Plexus brachialis bei einer Neuritis in Folge von Typhus abdominalis. Neurol. Centralbl., Leipz., 1887, vi, 385-389.—**Staudenmaier.** Neuritis. Med. Cor.-Bl. d. württemb. ärztl. Ver., Stuttg., 1880, xx, 167.—**Tasso** (F.) Storia di una nevrite trifaciale. Gazz. med. ital., prov. venete, Padova, 1868, xi, 35-37.—**Thissen.** Seltener Fall von Neuritis ascendens mit sogenannter Reflexparalyse des Rückenmarks. Centralbl. f. Nervenh., Leipz., 1886, ix, 97-99.—**Tripier** (L.) Deux cas de névrite traumatique. Rev. de chir., Par., 1885, v, 372. ——. Deux cas de névrite traumatique, avec transmission de la douleur par la voie collatérale intacte. Ibid., 785-800. Also: Cong. franç. de chir. Proc.-verb., etc., 1885, Par., 1886, i, 315-330.—**Uhthoff** (W.) Fall von Neuritis des rechten Nervus trigeminus (i. u. ii. Ast) mit Affection des Nervus lacrymalis und einseitigem Aufhören der Thränensecretion. Deutsche med. Wchnschr., Berl., 1886, xii, 321.—**Virchow** (R.) Neuritis interstitialis prolifera. Arch. f. path. Anat., etc., Berl., 1871, liii, 441-444, 1 pl.—**Vulpian** (A.) Névrite du nerf cubital droit, survenue à la suite d'un violent effort; atrophie musculaire symptomatique, consécutive. In his: Clin. méd. de l'hôp. de la Charité, 8°. Par., 1879, 919-923.—**Webber** (S. G.) Neuritis. Cycl. Pract. M. (Ziemssen), N. Y., 1881, Suppl. 531.—**Weinhold** (C. A.) Etwas von der Nervenentzündung, sowie von der bestätigten grossen Wirkung des Graphits gegen die Flechten. Med.-chir. Ztg., Salzb., 1815, iii, 268; 285.—**Weinlechner** (J.) Neuritis ulnaris; Beugecontractur im Elbogengelenke; geheilt nach gewaltsamer Streckung und Anwendung der Elektricität sowie des Jodoforms. Ber. d. k. k. Krankenanst. Rudolph-Stiftung in Wien (1878), 1879, 352.—**Wurtz** (R.) Note sur un cas de névrite du tibial antérieur, survenne dans le cours d'une fièvre typhoïde. Encéphale, Par., 1886, vi, 10-20.

Neuritis (*Multiple*).

See, also, **Beriberi**, *etc.*; **Nerves** (*Cranial, Fifth pair of*).

GRIMODIE (H.) * Contributrion à l'étude de la pathogénie des névrites périphériques. 4°. *Paris*, 1887.

——. The same. Névrite disséminée. 8°. *Paris*, 1879.

GROS (J.) * Contribution à l'histoire des névrites; névrite disséminée. 8°. *Paris*, 1879.

——. The same. 8°. *Paris*, 1879.

HOFFMANN (A.) * Ein Fall von multipler Neuritis. [Gottingen.] 8°. *Helmstedt*, 1884.

THEOPOLD (C.) * Ueber einen Fall von multipler degenerativer Neuritis. 8°. *Lemgo*, 1882.
Arthaud. Sur la pathogénie des névrites périphériques. Compt. rend. Soc. de biol., Par., 1887, 8. s., iv, 20-210. Also: Ann. méd.-chir. franç. et étrang., Par., 1887, iii, 122-124. — **Baelz.** Ueber das Verhältniss der multiplen peripherischen Neuritis zur Beriberi (Panneuritis endemica). Ztschr. f. klin. Med., Berl., 1882, iv, 616.—**Bassi** (U.) Nevrite multipla consecutiva a febbretifoide. Riv. veneta di sc. med., Venezia, 1887, vi, 585-592. — **Biggs** (H. M.) Alcoholic paralysis due to multiple neuritis. Med. Rec., N. Y., 1887, xxxi, 503.— **Browning** (W.) Multiple neuritis as a sequel of erysipelas. Brooklyn M. J., 1888, i, 11-14. — **Bruzelius** (R.) Om multipel nevrit. Nord. med. Ark., Stockholm, 1887, xix, no. 3, 1-17. — **Bundy** (A. D.) A case of peripheral neuritis. Med. Reg., Phila., 1888, iii, 11. — **Buzzard** (T.) Some points in the pathology of multiple neuritis. Brit. M. J., Lond., 1887, i, 9-12. — **Clarke** (J. M.) Peripheral neuritis. Bristol M.-Chir. J., 1887, v, 73-94, 1 pl.— **Comino** (E.) Di un caso non comune di nevrite multipla primitiva. Gazz. med. ital. lomb., Milano, 1887, xlvii, 22-26.— **Dejace** (L.) Rapport sur un travail de M. X. Francotte, intitulé: Note sur cinq cas de névrite multiple, et contribution à l'étude de la névrite multiple. Bull. Acad. roy. de méd. de Belg., Brux., 1886, 3. s., xx, 194-198. Also: Ann. Soc. méd.-chir. de Liége, 1886, xxv, 347. — **Déjerine** (J.) Sur un cas de paraplégie par névrites périphériques, chez un ataxique morphiomane. (Contribution à l'étude de la névrite périphérique.) Compt. rend. Soc. de biol., Par., 1887, 8. s., iv, 137-143. ——. Contribution à l'étude de la névrite alcoolique (forme paralytique, forme ataxique), tachycardie par névrite du pneumogastrique. Arch. de physiol. norm. et path., Par., 1887, 3. s., x, 248-264. — **De Renzi** (E.) Nevrite multipla degenerativa. Boll. d. clin., Napoli, 1885, ii, 353-355. — **Dubois.** Ueber einen Fall multipler Neuritis. Cor.-Bl. f. schweiz. Aerzte, Basel, 1883, xiii, 437-443. — **Dubreuilh** (W.) Névrite périphérique généralisée chez un tuberculeux alcoolique; paralysie transitoire du diaphragme; tumeur dorsale des poignets; autopsie. Gaz. hebd. d. sc. méd. de Bordeaux,

Neuritis (Multiple).

1887, viii, 479-483. ———. Polynévrite, paralysie diffuse, paralysie du diaphragme. *Ibid.*, 494-496.—**Duckworth** (*Sir* D.) Three cases of multiple peripheral (alcoholic) neuritis in women. St. Barth. Hosp. Rep., Lond., 1886, xxii, 253-260.—**Duplaix** (J.-B.) Des polynévrites. Gaz. d. hôp., Par., 1887, lx, 1085-1095. — **Eisenlohr.** Ueber acute Polyneuritis und verwandte Krankheitsformen mit Rücksicht auf ihr zeitliches und örtliches Auftreten. Berl. klin. Wchnschr., 1887, xxiv, 781-786.—**Erb** (W.) Bemerkungen über gewisse Formen der neurotischen Atrophie (sog. multiple degenerative Neuritis). Neurol. Centralbl., Leipz., 1883, ii, 481-485. *Also:* Amtl. Ber. ü. d. Versamml. deutsch. Naturf. u. Aerzte 1883, Freib. i. Br., 1884, lvi, 261. — **Eulau** (S.) Ein Fall von multipler Neuritis. Berl. klin. Wchnschr., 1886, xxiii, 93-96. — **Farkas** (G.) Ein Fall von Polyneuritis. [*Transl. from:* Orvos-természettud. Ertesitö, Kolozsvár, 1883, 3. H. Extr.] Pest. med.-chir. Presse, Budapest, 1885, xxi, 180. — **Finlay** (D. W.) Three cases of alcoholic paralysis (multiple neuritis). Med.-Chir. Tr., Lond., 1887, lxx, 371-395, 2 pl. *Also* [Abstr.]: Proc. Roy. M. & Chir. Soc. Lond., 1885-7, n. s., ii, 273-278. — **Folsom** (C. F.) Cases of multiple neuritis. Boston M. & S. J., 1887, cxvi, 493-496. — **Freud** (S.) Akute multiple Neuritis der spinalen und Hirnnerven. Wien. med. Wchnschr., 1886, xxxvi, 168-172. — **Friedmann** (M.) Ueber progressive Veränderungen der Ganglienzellen bei Entzündungen, nebst einem Anhang über active Veränderungen der Axencylinder. Arch. f. Psychiat., Berl., 1887, xix, 244-268, 1 pl. — **Geppert** (J.) Ein Fall von multipler Neuritis. Charité-Ann. 1881, Berl., 1883, viii, 284-288.—**Giraudeau** (C.) Des névrites périphériques. [Rev. crit.] Arch. gén. de méd., Par., 1887, ii, 578-611.—**Goldflam** (S.) O. t. zw. rozsianem zapaleniu nerwów (neuritis multiplex, disseminata, polyneuritis). Medycyna, Warszawa, 1887, xv, 365; 381; 401; 417; 437; 458.—**Grocco** (P.) Contribuzione allo studio clinico ed anatomo-patologico della nevrite multipla primitiva. Ann. univ. di med. e chir., Milano, 1885, cclxxi, 3-31, 1 pl. ———. Terza contribuzione allo studio clinico ed anatomo-patologico della nevrite multipla primitiva. Ann. d. Univ. libera di Perugia. Fac. di med. e chir., 1885-6, i, 261-279.—**Grocco** (P.) & **Fusari** (R.) Di nuovo sulla nevrite multipla primitiva. Ann. univ. di med. e chir., Milano, 1885, cclxxiii, 87-100, 1 pl. ———. Una terza contribuzione allo studio clinico ed anatomo-patologico della nevrite multipla primitiva. Riv. clin., Bologna, 1886, xxv, 671-689.—**Guttmann** (S.) Ein Fall von multipler Neuritis. Deutsche med. Wchnschr., Berl., 1884, x, 291. — **Hiller** (A.) Ein Fall von multipler Neuritis (Leyden), in welchem die Nervendehnung zur Ausführung kam. Charité-Ann. 1880, Berl., 1882, vii, 344-347.—**Hirt** (L.) Beitrag zur Pathologie der multiplen Neuritis. Neurol. Centralbl., Leipz., 1884, iii, 481-485.—**von Hösslin** (R.) Zur Casuistik der multipeln Neuritis. München. med. Wchnschr., 1886, xxxiii, 40-42.—**Holmes** (T. M.) Multiple neuritis. Atlanta M. & S. J., 1887, n. s., iv, 341-345.—**Homén** (E. A.) Bidrag till läran om de multipla neuriterna. Finska läk.-sällsk. handl., Helsingfors 1885, xxvii, 244-251. *Also, transl.:* Centralbl. f. Nervenh., Leipz., 1885, viii, 313-319.—**Jacoutini** (G.) Contribuzione clinica allo studio della nevrite multipla. Gior. di neuropatol., Napoli, 1886, iv, 156-170.—**Jamieson.** Cases of multiple neuritis. Austral. M. J., Melbourne, 1886, viii, 295-302. ———. Case of multiple neuritis. *Ibid.*, 1887, ix, 123. — **Kétli** (K.) A neuritis multiplex degeneratíváról. Orvosi hetil., Budapest, 1887, xxxi, 185-190. *Also, transl.* [Abstr.]: Pest. med.-chir. Presse, Budapest, 1887, xxiii, 201.—**Korsakoff** (S.S.) K ucheniou o patogen. atroficheck. spin. paralicha i mnojestven. nevrita. [On pathogenesis of atrophic spinal paralysis and polyneuritis.] Arch. psichiat., etc., Charkov, 1887, ix, no. 2, 16; no. 3, 1.—**Kotinski** (G.) Sluchai mnojestven-nago nevrita. [Case of polyneuritis.] Russk. Med., St. Petersb., 1883, i, 12.—**Leyden** (E.) Ueber einen Fall von multipler Neuritis. Charité-Ann. 1878, Berl., 1880, v, 206-231, 1 pl.—**Lilienfeld** (A.) Zur Lehre von der multiplen Neuritis. Berl. klin. Wchnschr., 1885, xxii, 727-730.— **Lion** (M.) Ocherk uchenija o pervichnom mnojestvennom nevrite (neuritis multiplex). Med. Obozr., Mosk., 1884, xxii, 187-197.— **Löwenfeld** (L.) Ueber multiple Neuritis. Aerztl. Int.-Bl., München, 1885, xxxii, 55; 67; 78; 100; 121; 164. *Also* [Abstr.]: Neurol. Centralbl., Leipz., 1884, iv, 149; 169. ———. Einige Bemerkungen zu Hrn. Dr. E. Remak's Mittheilung: "Ein Fall von generalisirter Neuritis, etc.". Neurol. Centralbl., Leipz., 1885, iv, 366.— **Mader.** Polyneuritis periferica (?) in potatore Versuche mit Wasserbeschränkung bei Hydrops ex adiposi cordis; Heilung. Ber. d. k. k. Krankenanst. Rudolph-Stiftung in Wien (1885), 1886, 363-365.—**Masius & Francotte** (X.) Note sur cinq cas de névrite multiple. Bull. Acad. roy. de méd. de Belg., Brux., 1886, 3. s., xx, 194-198.—**Massalongo** (R.) Le nevriti multiple periferiche primitive e specialmente della forma di polinevrite acuta. Gazz. d. osp., Milano, 1886, vii, 434; 443; 458; 466; 475; 483; 491; 546.—**Mills** (C. K.) The concurrence of multiple neuritis with myelitis or encephalitis. Med. News. Phila., 1886, xlix, 691-693. ———. The probable occurrence of multiple neuritis in epidemic cerebro-spinal meningitis. *Ibid.*,

Neuritis (Multiple).

1888, lii, 357. — **Müller** (F. C.) Ein Fall von multipler Neuritis. Arch. f. Psychiat., Berl., 1883, xiv, 669 - 677. — **Oppenheim** (H.) Ueber zwei Fälle, welche unter dem Symptomenbilde der multiplen Neuritis verliefen und in unvollkommene Heilung ausgingen. Deutsches Arch. f. klin. Med., Leipz., 1884-5, xxxvi, 561-577. ———. Ein Fall von multipler Neuritis im Stadium der Reconvalescenz. Berl. klin. Wchnschr., 1887, xxiv, 309.—**Ozeretskovski** (A.) K ucheniou o mnojestvennoi neurtie (neuritis multiplex). Vrach, St. Petersb., 1884, v, 97-101.—**Petrone** (L. M.) Contribuzione al progresso delle neuriti multiple e di alcune affezioni spinali. Arch. ital. per le mal. nerv., Milano, 1885, xxii, 359 - 383. — **Philips** (A.) Dva sluch. mnojest. nevrita. [Two cases of multiple neuritis.] Russk. Med., St. Petersb., 1887, v, 229; 242. — **Pierson** (R. H.) Ueber Polyneuritis acuta (multiple Neuritis). Samml. klin. Vortr., Leipz., 1883, No. 229 (Inn. Med., No. 79), pp. 2083-2102. *Also, transl.* [Abstr.]: N. Am. J. Homœop., N. Y., 1883, n. s., xiv, 1-19.—**Pitres** (A.) Sur un cas de polynévrite primitive. Bull. méd., Par., 1887, i, 931-934. ———. Des névrites périphériques dans les maladies infectieuses. Mém. et bull. Soc. de méd. et chir de Bordeaux, 1886, 384 - 386. — **Pitres** (A.) & **Vaillard** (L.) Contribution à l'étude des névrites périphériques non traumatiques. Arch. de neurol., Par., 1883, v, 191. 2 pl.; 290; vi, 180. ———. Contribution à l'étude des névrites périphériques survenant dans le cours ou la convalescence de la fièvre typhoïde. Rev. de méd., Par., 1885, v, 985-1014. *Also. transl.* [Abstr.]: Riv. clin. e terap., Napoli, 1886, viii, 81-85.—**Popoff** (M. N.) O neuritis multiplex degenerativa. Med. pribav. k morsk. sborniku, St. Petersb., 1884, Oct., 49 - 60. — **Protopopoff** (N. J.) Neskolko sluch. mnojest. idiopat. nevrita. [Some cases of multiple idiopathic neuritis.] Trudi Obsh. Russk. vrach. v Moskve, 1887, ii, Nerv., 99-103. — **Raymond.** Sur un cas de névrite périphérique. Bull. et mém. Soc. méd. d. hôp. de Par., 1888, 3. s., v, 13-20. — **Remak** (E.) Ein Fall von generalisirter Neuritis mit schweren elektrischen Alterationen auch der niemals gelähmten Nn. faciales. Neurol. Centralbl., Leipz., 1885, iv, 313 - 320. — **Roger** (G.-H.) Des névrites périphériques. Encéphale, Par., 1885, v, 140-169.—**Rosenheim** (T.) Zur Kenntniss der acuten infectiösen multiplen Neuritis. Arch. f. Psychiat., Berl., 1887, xviii, 782-808, 1 pl.—**Ross** (J.) On peripheral neuritis. Brit. M. J., Lond., 1887, i, 6 - 9. — **Roth** (M.) Neuritis disseminata acutissima. Cor.-Bl. f. schweiz. Aerzte, Basel, 1883, xiii, 317-325.—**Rozenbach** (P. J.) Sluchai mnojestven. nevrita. [Case of polyneuritis.] Vestnik klin. i sudebnoi psichiat. i nevropatol., St. Petersb., 1885, iii, pt. 1, 266-277.—**Rudoff** (M. I.) Sluchai mnojestven. uzdov. nevrita (neuritis multiplex nodosa). Arch. psichiat., etc., Charkov, 1886, vii, 69-84. — **Schulz** (R.) Beitrag zur Lehre der multiplen Neuritis bei Potatoren. Neurol. Centralbl., Leipz., 1885, iv, 433; 462; 482.—**Shattuck** (G. B.) Multiple neuritis; cases. Boston M. & S. J., 1887, cxvii, 523-528.—**Starkel** (C. H.) A case of alcoholic neuritis; pseudo-tabetic variety. St. Louis Cour. Med., 1887, xviii, 125-128.—**Starr** (M. A.) Multiple neuritis and its relation to certain peripheral neuroses. Med. Rec., N. Y., 1887, xxxi, 141; 173. *Also:* Med. News, Phila., 1887, l, 141; 169; 197; 225. *Also* [Abstr.]: N. York M. J., 1887, xlv, 141; 169.—**Stephan** (B. H.) De aetiologie van multiple neuritis. Nederl. Tijdschr. v. Geneesk., Amst., 1887, xxiii, 358-366.—**Strümpell** (A.) Zur Kenntniss der multiplen degenerativen Neuritis. Arch. f. Psychiat., Berl., 1883, xiv, 339-358.—**Thomas.** Ein Fall von Polyneuritis. Deutsche med. Wchnschr., Berl., 1886, xii, 472.— **Trautwein** (J.) Einiges über die electrische Douche und im Anschluss daran über einen Fall von multipler Neuritis. Ztschr. f. klin. Med., Berl., 1884, viii, 279-288.— **Tuttle.** Multiple peripheral neuritis of alcoholic origin. N. York M. J., 1887, xlvi, 633. — **Vierordt** (O.) Beitrag zum Studium der multiplen degenerativen Neuritis. Arch. f. Psychiat., Berl., 1883, xiv, 678-698.—**W.** A case of supposed multiple neuritis. N. York M. J., 1887, xlv, 549. — **Webber** (S. G.) Multiple neuritis. Arch. Med., N. Y., 1884, xii, 33-49. — **White** (H.) Peripheral neuritis. Brit. M. J., Lond., 1886, i, 977.—**Wiglesworth** (J.) Peripheral neuritis in Raynaud's disease (symmetrical gangrene). Tr. Path. Soc. Lond. (1886-7), 1887, xxxviii, 61-68, 2 fig. — **Witkowski** (A.) Zur Klinik der multiplen Alkoholneuritis. Arch. f. Psychiat., Berl., 1887, xviii, 809-818.—**Wright** (J. W.) Multiple neuritis. N. Eng. M. Month., Bridgeport, Conn., 1886-7, vi, 393-397.

Neuritis (Optic).

See **Nerve** (*Optic, Inflammation of*).

Neurofibroma.

See **Neuroma.**

Neuroglia.

See, also, **Nervous** system (*Histology of*).

Gombault. Études récentes relatives à l'anatomie normale de la névroglie. Travaux de Deiters, Golgi, Jastrowitz et F. Boll. Arch. de physiol. norm. et path.,

Neuroglia.

Par., 1873. v, 458-466. — **Ranvier** (L.) De la névroglie. *Ibid.*, 1883. 3. s.. i, 177-185, 1 pl. *Also:* École prat. d. hautes études. Lab. d'histol. du Coll. de France. Trav. 1883, Par., 1884, viii, 101-109, 1 pl. *Also* [Abstr.]: Compt. rend. Acad. d. sc., Par., 1882, xciv, 1536-1539. *Also* [Abstr.]: France méd., Par., 1882, i, 808-810.—**Witkowski** (L.) Ueber die Neuroglia. Arch. f. Psychiat., Berl., 1883, xiv, 155-163. *Also* [Abstr.]: Amtl. Ber. ü. d. Versamml. deutsch. Naturf. u. Aerzte 1883, Freib. i. Br., 1884, lvi, 264.

Neuroglioma.

BAUMANN (G.) * Beitrag zur Kenntniss der Gliome und Neurogliome. 8°. *Tübingen,* 1887.

BERTHEAU (G.) * Ueber die Natur und Entwickelung der Neurogliome. 8°. *Göttingen,* 1879.

Hansch (F.) Neurogliom des Ganglion Gasseri. München. med. Wchnschr., 1886, xxxiii. 702 ; 723.

Neurohr (Joh. Anton) [1770-1850].
See **Lobstein** (Jean-Georges-Chrétien-Frédéric-Martin). Lehrbuch der pathologischen Anatomie. *8°. Stuttgart,* 1834-5.

Neurological Contributions. By William A. Hammond, assisted by William J. Morton. No. 1, April, 1879 ; No. 2, 1880 ; No. 3, 1881. 8°. *New York, G. P. Putnam's Sons.*
Ended. Each number complete in itself, paged separately.

Neurological (The) Review. Edited by J. S. Jewell. [Monthly.] Nos. 1-4, v. 1, May to November, 1886. 1 v. 256 pp. 8°. *Chicago.*
Ended.

Neurologisches Centralblatt. Uebersicht der Leistungen auf dem Gebiete der Anatomie, Physiologie, Pathologie und Therapie des Nervensystems einschliesslich der Geisteskrankheiten. Hrsg. von E. Mendel. [Semi-monthly.] v. 1-7, 1882-8. 8°. *Leipzig, Veit u. Comp.*
Current.

Neurology.

See, also, **Insanity** ; **Nerves** ; **Nervous** *system* ; **Phrenology** ; **Psychology.**

BERGER (O.) Katalog Nr. 193 der Schletter'schen Buchhandlung, Franck u. Weigert in Breslau. Verzeichniss der von Herrn Professor Dr. . . . nachgelassenen Bibliothek. Neuropathologie ; Neurologie ; Psychiatrie ; Psychologie ; Elektricität ; Magnetismus. 8°. *Breslau,* [1885].

LALANGUE (J. B.) * Diss. neurologiam sistens. sm. 8°. [*Vindobonæ,* 1770.]

SKETCHES of Buchanan's discoveries in neurology. 8°. *Louisville,* 1842.

STEGMANN (J. F. C.) * De usu et dignitate neurologiæ. 8°. *Halæ,* [1794].

VALENTIN (G.) Traité de névrologie. Traduit de l'allemand par A.-J.-L. Jourdan. 8°. *Paris,* 1843.

————. The same. Trattato di nevrologia. Tradotto dal tedesco da A. G. L. Jourdan. Prima traduzione italiana di M. G. Levi. 8°. *Venezia,* 1844.

Hughes. The nervous system in disease and the progress of neurology. St. Louis M. & S. J., 1881, xli, 377-381.—**Mitchell** (S. W.) The objects and duties of a neurological society ; an address. Polyclinic, Phila., 1883-4, i, 152-154.— **Morton** (W. J.) Neurological specialism. J. Nerv. & Ment. Dis., Chicago, 1883, x, 618-629. *Also,* Reprint.

Neurology (*History of*).

AGRICOLA (G. A.) De succi nutricii per nervos transitu. sm. 4°. *Vitembergæ,* [1695].

DAREMBERG (C.-V.) * Exposition des connaissances de Galien sur l'anatomie, la physiologie et la pathologie du système nerveux. 4°. *Paris,* 1841.

DOCUMENTS and dates of modern discoveries in the nervous system. 8°. *London,* 1839.

DOWLER (B.) Progress of discovery in the nervous system and in medical ethics. 8°. *New Orleans,* 1856.

Neurology (*History of*).

GALEN (C.) L'anatomie des nerfz du corps humain . . . avec la manière d'administrer icelle anatomie. 4°. *Paris,* 1556.

HARLES (J. C. F.) Versuch einer vollständigen Geschichte der Hirn- und Nervenlehre im Alterthume. 1. Theil. 8°. *Erlangen,* 1801.

NEMANN (M.) * Expositio neurologiæ Galenicæ. 8°. *Berolini,* 1847.

Adam (F.) On the doctrines of the ancients concerning the nervous system. Lond. M. Gaz., 1828-9, iii, 657-663.—**Anderson** (J.) On recent advances in the anatomy of the nervous system. Brain, Lond., 1884-5, vii, 259-266. — **Clarke** (J. L.) Historical sketch of the progress of the anatomy and physiology of the nervous centres, from the time of Hippocrates to the time of Willis. Brit. & For. M.-Chir. Rev., Lond., 1864, xxxiii, 474-484.—**Davis** (N. S.) An analysis of the discoveries concerning the physiology of the nervous system, from the publications of Sir Charles Bell to the present time. Tr. M. Soc. N. Y. 1841-3, Albany, 1843, v, pt. 1, 18-69. — **Donders** (F. C.) Ontspringen alle zenuwbuisjes uit hersenen en ruggemerg ? Historisch onderzocht en naar het standpunkt der wetenschap beantwoord. Nederl. Lancet, Gravenh., 1847~8, 2. s., iii, 712-736. 1 pl. *Also,* Reprint.— **Eckhard** (C.) Beiträge zur Geschichte der Experimentalphysiologie des Nervensystems: Geschichte der Experimentalphysiologie des Froschhirns. Beitr. z. Anat. u. Physiol. (Eckhard), Giessen, 1883, x, 67-134. ——. Beiträge zur Geschichte der Experimentalphysiologie des Nervensystems ; Geschichte der mechanischen, chemischen und thermischen Einwirkungen auf die motorischen Nerven. *Ibid.,* 1885, xi, 43-113.—**Ferrier** (D.) An address on the progress of knowledge in the physiology and pathology of the nervous system. Brit. M. J., Lond.. 1883, ii, 805-808. — **Henry** (W. C.) On the present state of our knowledge respecting the physiology of the nervous system. Lond. M. Gaz., 1834, xiv, 664 ; 695.—**King** (F. G.) An historical sketch of neurology. N. York M. & Phys. J., 1824, iii, 141-162.— **Müller** (J.) Menschliche Anatomie. Arch. f. Anat., Physiol. u. wissensch. Med.. Berl., 1837, iii, pp. i-xlviii. *Also, transl.* [Abstr.]: Brit. & For. M. Rev., Lond., 1837-8, v, 293-300. *Also, transl. in his:* Essays on Phys. & Hyg., 8°, Phila., 1838, 229-240. *Also,* Reprint.—**Parchappe.** Études historiques sur l'anatomie et la physiologie du système nerveux. Ann. méd.-psych., Par., 1846, viii, 317, 1 pl. : 1847, x, 1.—**Ranke** (J.) Die Nervenkraft ; ein Beitrag zur Entwicklungsgeschichte der naturphilosophischen Grundbegriffe. Deutsche Rev., Berl., 1880, v, 230-248.—**Rey** (E.) Una pagina di storia della fisiologia del sistema nervoso. Osservatore, Torino, 1882, xviii, 33 ; 49 ; 81.—**Richet** (C.) Étude historique sur la physiologie du système nerveux. Rev. scient., Par., 1881, 3. s., i, 426-433. — **Seguin** (E. C.) An outline of the physiology of the nervous system. Med. Rec., N. Y., 1874, ix, 617-622. *Also, in his:* Op. min. [etc.], 8°. N. Y., 1884, 164-179.— **Vacquié** (F.) Précis historique et critique des travaux sur le système nerveux de l'homme, depuis la fin du siècle dernier. J. univ. d. sc. méd., Par.. 1824. xxxv, 5 ; 129 ; 257.—**Whewell** (W.) History of discoveries in the nervous system. Lond. M. Gaz., 1837-8, xxi, 525-528.—**Wilks** (S.) Notes on the history of the physiology of the nervous system ; taken more especially from writers on phrenology. Guy's Hosp. Rep., Lond., 1879, 3. s., xxiv, 57-94.

Neurology (*Journals and societies relating to*).

See, also, **Insanity** (*Journals, etc., relating to*).

ALIENIST (The) and Neurologist. Edited by C. H. Hughes. [Quarterly.] v. 1-9, 1880-88. 8°. *Saint Louis.*
Current.

AMERICAN (The) Journal of Neurology and Psychiatry. Edited by T. A. McBride, L. C. Gray, and E. C. Spitzka. [Quarterly.] v. 1-3, 1882-5. 8°. *New York.*

AMERICAN (The) Journal of Psychology. Edited by G. Stanley Hall. [Quarterly.] Nos. 1-2, v. 1, November, 1887, to February, 1888. 8°. *Baltimore.*
Current.

AMERICAN Neurological Association. Transactions. v. 1-2. 8°. *New York,* 1875-7.
See, also, **Proceedings.** Chicago J. Nerv & Ment. Dis., 1875, ii, 367-388. *Continued in :* J. Nerv. & Ment. Dis., Chicago, 1876, i, 414 : 1879-86, iv-xi, *passim. Also,* Reprint of 1881-4.

ANNALES médico-légales belges. Journal spécial de maladies de l'encéphale et du système nerveux, de maladies mentales, de médecine lé-

Neurology (*Journals and societies relating to*).

gale, de toxicologie et d'hygiène. Publiées par C. Crommelinck. [Weekly.] 2. année, 1843. 1 v. 4°. *Bruxelles.*

ANNALES médico-psychologiques. Journal de l'anatomie, de la physiologie et de la pathologie du système nerveux, destiné particulièrement à recueillir tous les documents relatifs à la science des rapports du physique et du moral à la pathologie mentale, à la médecine légale des aliénés et à la clinique des névroses; par MM. les docteurs Baillarger, Cerise et Longet. 1. s. v. 1–12, 1843–8; 2. s., v. 1–6, 1849–54; 3. s., v. 1–8, 1855–62; 4. s., v. 1–12, 1863–8; 5. s., v. 1–20, 1869–78; 6. s., v. 1–12, 1879–84; 7. s., v. 1–7, 1885–8. 8°. *Paris.*
Current.
After 1862, 2 v. annually; prior to that date sometimes 2, sometimes 1 v. annually. v. 1, 2. s., subtitle became "Journal destiné à recueillir tous les documents relatifs à l'aliénation mentale, aux névroses, et à la médecine légale des aliénés". · From 1843 to 1848, bi-monthly; from 1849 to 1862, quarterly; from 1863 to date, bi-monthly. Editorial changes: v. 1, 2. s., Longet dropped; v. 2, 2. s., Brierre de Boismont added; v. 1, 3. s., Brierre de Boismont dropped and Moreau (de Tours) added; v. 1, 4. s., Moreau dropped; v. 9, 4. s., Lunier added.

ARCHIV psichiatrii. neurologii i sudebnoi psichopatologii. Redaktor: P. I. Kovalevski. [Quarterly; 2 v. annually.] v. 1–11, 1883–8. 8°. *Charcov.*
Current.

ARCHIV für Psychiatrie und Nervenkrankheiten. Hrsg. von B. Gudden, E. Leyden [*et al.*]. Redigirt von C. Westphal. v. 1–19, 1868–87. 19 v. 8°. *Berlin.*
Current.

ARCHIVES de neurologie. Revue des maladies nerveuses et mentales, publiée sous la direction de J. M. Charcot. Rédacteur en chef: Bourneville. [Quarterly.] v. 1–15, July, 1880–88. 8 v. 8°. *Paris.*
Current.

BRAIN: A journal of neurology. Edited by J. C. Bucknill [*et al.*]. [Quarterly.] v. 1–10, April, 1878–88. 8°. *London.*
Current.

CENTRAL-BLATT für Nervenheilkunde, Psychiatrie und gerichtliche Psychopathologie. Hrsg. u. redigirt von A. Erlenmeyer. [Monthly.] Nos. 6–12, v. 1, 1878; v. 2–11, 1879–88. 8°. *Coblenz* [*u. Leipzig*].
Current. A continuation of: **Correspondenz-Blatt** der deutschen Gesellschaft für Psychiatrie und gerichtliche Psychologie. In 1879 v. 2 became semi-monthly.

CHICAGO (The) Journal of Nervous and Mental Disease. Edited by J. S. Jewell and H. M. Bannister. [Quarterly.] v. 1–2, 1874–5. 8°. *Chicago.*
Continued as: **Journal** (The) of Nervous and Mental Disease.

ENCÉPHALE (L'). Journal des maladies mentales et nerveuses. Rédaction: E. Chambard [*et al.*]. [Quarterly.] v. 1–8, 1881–8. 8°. *Paris.*
Current.

GIORNALE di neuropatologia. Redatta dai Dott¹ R. ed Antonio Vizioli. [Bi-monthly.] v. 1–6, July, 1882–8. 8°. *Napoli.*
Current.

JOURNAL (The) of Nervous and Mental Disease. Edited by J. S. Jewell [*et al.*]. [Quarterly.] New series. v. 1–13, 1876–88. 8°. *Chicago*, 1876–80; *New York*, 1881–4.
Current. A continuation of: **Chicago** (The) Journal of Nervous and Mental Disease.

NEUROLOGICAL Contributions. By William A. Hammond and W. J. Morton. Nos. 1–3, April, 1879–81. 1 v. 8°. *New York.*
Ended.

Neurology (*Journals and societies relating to*).

NEUROLOGICAL (The) Review. Edited by J. S. Jewell. v. 1. 8°. *Chicago*, 1886.

NEUROLOGISCHES Centralblatt. Hrsg. von E. Mendel. [Semi-monthly.] v. 1–8, 1882–8. 8°. *Leipzig.*
Current.

PSICHIATRIA (La), la neuropatologia e le scienze affini. Gazzetta redatta dal Dott. L. Bianchi. [Quarterly.] v. 1–5, 1883–7. 8°. *Napoli.*
Current.

PSYCHOLOGICAL (The) and Medico-Legal Journal. A monthly review of diseases of the mind and nervous system, and of medical jurisprudence. Conducted by William A. Hammond, assisted by T. M. B. Cross. [2 v. annually.] New series. v. 1–3, July, 1874, to May, 1876. 3 v. 8°. *New York, F. W. Christern*, 1874; *McDivitt, Campbell & Co.*, 1875–6.
Ended. See **Quarterly** (The) Journal of Psychological Medicine, for first series. v. 3, Nov., 1875, to May, 1876, title: **American** (The) Psychological Journal, quarterly, conducted by Allan, McLane, Hamilton, and others. No. 3, v. 3, May, 1876, last published.

QUARTERLY (The) Journal of Psychological Medicine and Medical Jurisprudence. Edited by W. A. Hammond. v. 1–6, 1867–72. 8°. *New York.*
v. 4–6, title: **Journal** (The) of Psychological Medicine; a quarterly review of diseases of the nervous system, medical jurisprudence, and anthropology. In July, 1874, title: **Psychological** (The) and Medico-Legal Journal.

Bericht über die 9. Wanderversammlung der südwestdeutschen Neurologen und Irrenärzte zu Baden-Baden am 14. und 15. Juni d. J. Centralbl. f. Nervenh., Leipz., 1884, vii, 289; 313.—**Berichte** über die 1.–10. Wanderversammlung der südwestdeutschen Neurologen und Irrenärzte. [1876–84.] Arch. f. Psychiat., Berl., 1876–7, vii: 1885, xvi, *passim.*—**Möbius** (P. J.) Die vierte Wander-Versammlung der südwestdeutschen Neurologen und Irrenärzte in Heidelberg am 17. und 18. Mai d. J. Centralbl. f. Nervenh., Coblenz, 1879, ii, 241–250.—**New York** Neurological Society. Proceedings. Chicago J. Nerv. & Ment. Dis., 1874, i, 228. *Continued in*: J. Nerv. & Ment. Dis., Chicago, 1876–86, i–xi, *passim.* — **Philadelphia** Neurological Society. Proceedings. J. Nerv. & Ment. Dis., N. Y., 1884–6, ix–xi, *passim.*

Neuroma.

See, also, **Epilepsy** (*Causation of*); **Nerve** (*Auditory, Pathology of*); **Nerve** (*Optic, Pathology of*) [*etc.*]; **Nerve** (*Optic, Tumors of*); **Nerve** (*Sciatic, Tumors of*); **Nerves** (*Brachial*) [*etc.*]; **Nerves** (*Tumors of*); **Nervous** system (*Syphilis of*); **Neurotomy**, *etc.*; **Stumps** (*Diseases of*).

BERRUE (C.) *Essai sur les tubercules sous-cutanés douloureux. 4°. *Paris*, 1875.

BOEHM (K.) *Beitrag zur Kenntniss vom plexiformen Neurom. 8°. *Magdeburg*, 1883.

BOUCHAGE (J.) *Étude sur les symptômes du tubercule sous-cutané douloureux. 4°. *Paris*, 1874.

BRUNS (P.) *Das Rankenneurom, ein Beitrag zur Geschwulstlehre. 8°. *Tübingen*, 1870.
Also, in: Arch. f. path. Anat., etc., Berl., 1870, l, 80–112, 1 pl.

CAIZERGUES (L.) *Du névrome; observations et réflexions. 4°. *Montpellier*, 1867.

COURVOISIER (L. G.) Die Neurome. 8°. *Basel*, 1886.

ERLENMEYER (F. A.) *Ueber das cicatricielle Neurom. 8°. *Greifswald*, 1872.

FACIEU (H.-E.) *Dissertation sur le névrome, suivie de deux observations recueillies dans les hôpitaux de Paris. 4°. *Paris*, 1851.

DE GACHEO (L. de B.) Sur le tubercule sous-cutané douloureux. 4°. *Paris*, 1876.

HAREL (L.) *Contribution à l'étude des tubercules sous-cutanés douloureux. 4°. *Paris*, 1881.

Neuroma.

HASLER (G.) * De neuromate. 4°. *Turici*, 1835.

JAUME (P.-É.) * Sur une espèce de tumeur squirrheuse enkystée, attribuée mal à propos à une affection des nerfs. 4°. *Paris*, 1828.

Also, in : J. hebd. de méd., Par., 1829, ii, 65–75.

KASPER (A.) * Zur Casuistik der Neurome. Ein Fall von traumatischem Neurom des N. medianus geheilt durch Nerven-Resection und Naht. 12°. *Greifswald*, 1883.

KNOBLAUCH (A.) * De neuromate et gangliis accessoriis veris, adjecto cujusvis generis casu novo atque insigni. 4°. *Francof. ad Mœnum*, 1843.

KRAUSE (F.) * Ueber maligne Neurome und das Vorkommen von Nervenfasern in denselben. 8°. *Leipzig*, 1887.

LEBOURCQ (G.-A.) * Des névromes. 4°. *Paris*, 1865.

MANN (F. G. C.) * De neuromate. 8°. *Lipsiæ*, [1852].

MARCHAND (R.) * Das " plexiforme Neurom" (cylindrische Fibrom der Nervenscheiden). 8°. *Halle a. S.*, [1876].

Also, in : Arch. f. path. Anat., etc., Berl., 1877, lxx, 36–55, 1 pl.

MARGERIN (J.) * Des névromes plexiformes (variété de tumeurs sous-cutanées), avec une étude des névromes en général. 4°. *Paris*, 1867.

MARQUIÉ (J.) * Contribution à l'étude des fibrômes sous-cutanés douloureux. 4°. *Paris*, 1880.

RICHARD (F.) * Étude sur le tubercule sous-cutané douloureux. 4°. *Paris*, 1874.

RUMEN (G.) * Essai sur les névromes. 4°. *Paris*, 1875.

SCHNELLER (J. A. L.) * De neuromate. 8°. *Regimontii Pr.*, [1844].

SMITH (R. W.) A treatise on the pathology, diagnosis, and treatment of neuroma. fol. *Dublin*, 1849.

STEINIUS (S. A. W.) De structura neuromatis cujusdam maximi nervi ischiadici, quod una cum magna ipsius nervi parte prospero successu amputatum est, eaque quæ huic cum aliis quibusdam nervorum tumoribus intercedit ratione. 4°. *Havniæ*, 1846.

Adams (R.) [Neuromatous tumors.] Proc. Path. Soc. Dubl., 1841–9, i, 369–375. *Also :* Med. Times, Lond., 1847, xvi, 11. *Also :* Dublin Q. J. M. Sc., 1848, v, 548 ; 554.—**Agnew** (D. H.) Neuroma of ulnar and other nerves. Phila. M. Times, 1872–3, iii, 121.—**Alarco.** [Neuroma of ulnar nerve ; extirpation ; cure.] Gac. méd. de Lima, 1856–7, i, no. 18, 6.—**Armsby** (J. H.) Neuroma. Nat. M. J., Wash., 1870–71, i, 453.—**Arnozan** (X.) Névrome plexiforme. J. de méd. de Bordeaux, 1885–6, xv, 72.—**Barbieri** (A.) **& Taruffi** (C.) Due casi di neuroma cirsoideo. Bull. d. sc. med. di Bologna, 1870, 5. s., x, 54–94, 1 pl. ; 354.—**Barrier.** Névrome du cou ; ablation ; guérison. Gaz. d. hôp., Par., 1855, xxviii, 182.—**Bauer & Johnson** (J. G.) Neuroma following amputation ; resection. N. York J. M., 1858, 3. s., v, 401.—**Beck** (B.) Ueber Neurome. Deutsche Klinik, Berl., 1869, xxi, 466 ; 476.—**Begbie** (J. W.) Neuritis and neuroma. Syst. Med. (Reynolds), Lond., 1868, ii, 706.—**Beistegui.** Observation d'un névrôme sur le trajet du nerf plantaire, ayant nécessité l'amputation du membre. Bull. Soc. anat. de Par., 1840, xx, 177–183.—**Benito** (D.) Neuroma desarrollado en el nervio mediano del brazo izquierdo ; diez y nueve años de existencia ; enucleacion, con ligadura de la arteria humeral ; buen éxito. Siglo méd., Madrid, 1858, v, 368.—**Benjamin** (L.) Neurom innerhalb der Rückenmarkshäute. Arch. f. path. Anat., etc., Berl., 1856, xi, 87–89.—**Bérenger-Féraud.** Tubercule sous-cutané douloureux de la partie externe du genou gauche ; extraction avec toutes les précautions antiseptiques ; infection putride rapide ; mort le 6e jour après l'opération. Arch. de méd. nav., Par., 1885, xliv, 304–312.—**Beurnier** (L.) Étude historique et critique sur la nature anatomique des tubercules sous-cutanés douloureux. Arch. gén. de méd., Par., 1884, ii, 402–419.—**Bickersteth** (E. R.) Neuroma of the great sciatic nerve ; excision, without division of the nerve ; complete recovery. Month. J. M. Sc., Lond.

Neuroma.

& Edinb., 1854, xix. 119–121. ———. Painful tumour over the head of the radius, suspected to be neuroma ; excision ; cure. *Ibid.*, 122–124.—**Billroth** (T.) Eine wissenschaftliche und humanitäre Bitte an die Kollegen. Centralbl. f. Chir., Leipz., 1884, xi, 417.—**Bisset** (C.) A case of an extraordinary irritable sympathetic tumor. Mem. M. Soc. Lond., 1792, iii, 58–64.—**Blasius** (E.) Ueber rückfällige Neurome. Arch. f. klin. Chir., Berl., 1862, ii, 188–204. ———. Ueber rückfällige Neurome. *Ibid.*, 1865, vi, 775–777.—**Böhm.** Neuromata in brachio sinistro amputato ; Exstirpatio ; Heilung. Ber. d. k. k. Krankenanst. Rudolph-Stiftung in Wien (1867), 1868, 199 – 201. — **Bonnet.** Névrôme du volume d'une grosse noix développé dans le nerf poplité interne ; extirpation de la tumeur en laissant le nerf intact ; guérison avec conservation de la sensibilité et du mouvement du membre. Gaz. méd. de Lyon, 1850, ii, 29–32. *Also :* Gaz. d. hôp., Par., 1850, 3. s., ii, 90.—**Bouchacourt** (A.) Des tumeurs nerveuses sous-cutanées et de leur traitement. Rev. méd. franç. et étrang., Par., 1842, ii, 27–35. *Also :* Arch. de la méd. belge, Brux., 1843, x, 109–119.—**Bowditch** (H. I.) Neuroma of left fore-arm of twenty years' standing. Boston M. & S. J., 1857–8, lvii, 524–526.—**Briddon** (C. K.) Neuroma. N. York M. Press, 1859, n. s., ii, 820. [Discussion], 858. ———. Neuroma in axillary space, implicating musculospiral operation. Med. Rec., N. Y., 1875, x, 780.—**Broca.** Névrôme du nerf tibial postérieur. Bull. Soc. anat. de Par., 1851, xxvi, 101.—**Bryant.** Neuroma on branch of the extreme cutaneous nerve of the thigh. Med. Times & Gaz., Lond., 1862, i, 455. — **Bullen** (F. D.) Removal of a large neuroma from the median nerve. *Ibid.*, 1864, ii, 87.—**Bunzel** (E.) Neurom am N. tibialis. Wien. med. Presse, 1872, xiii, 409.—**Cabaret** (P.-J.) Observation sur une névralgie anomale, guérie par l'extirpation d'un névrôme. J. de la sect. de méd. Soc. acad. Loire-Inf., Nantes, 1838, xiv, 166–171. *Also :* Rev. de thérap. méd.-chir., Par., 1870, xxxvii, 203–206.—**Carruthers** (D. C.) Cases of painful subcutaneous tubercle. Edinb. M. & S. J., 1830, xxxiii, 307–310.—**Cartaz** (A.) Étude sur le névrome plexiforme. Arch. gén. de méd., Par., 1876, i, 170–197.—[**Case.**] Neuroma of posterior tibial nerve. Abstr. M. & S. Cases Gen. Hosp. Sick Children, Pendlebury, Manchester (1885), 1886, v, 142. — **Case** (A) of painful subcutaneous tumor, or tuberculum dolorosum. Boston M. & S. J., 1873, lxxxviii, 527. — **Chandelux** (A.) Observation de fibro-myxome douloureux (cliniquement névrome) probab'ement développé sur le collatéral interne de l'annulaire et renfermant au milieu de son stroma des tubes nerveux à myéline. Lyon méd., 1879, xxxi, 510–516. — **Chassaignac.** Névrome (du membre supérieur). Bull. Soc. de chir. de Par., 1856–7, vii, 548.—**Cheever** (D. W.) Painful subcutaneous tumor. Boston M. & S. J., 1878, xcviii, 389.—**Chenantais.** Tubercule sous-cutané douloureux (myome). Bull. Soc. anat. de Nantes 1881, Par., 1882, v, 19.—**Christôt.** Contribution à l'histoire des tumeurs plexiformes. Gaz. hebd. de méd., Par., 1870. 2. s., vii, 242 ; 259. *Also,* Reprint.—**Cock.** Neuroma of the ulnar nerve ; removal. Med. Times & Gaz., Lond., 1862, i, 454. — **Coons** (J. A.) Neuromatous tumor, with excision of a section of the great sciatic nerve. Tr. M. Soc. Kansas, Lawrence, 1880, xiv, 24–26.—**Coote.** Disseminated painful subcutaneous tubercle. Lancet, Lond., 1857, i, 364.—**Cruveilhier** (E.) Fibrome du nerf tibial postérieur. Bull. Soc. anat de Par., 1865, xl, 676. — **Delagarde** (P. C.) Neuroma. St. Barth. Hosp. Rep., Lond., 1868, iv, 94–96.—**Demeaux.** [Névrome du nerf tibial antérieur.] Bull. Soc. anat. de Par., 1843, xviii, 12.—**Denonvilliers.** Ganglions sous-cutanés douloureux. Bull. Soc. de chir. de Par., 1851–2, ii, 229. — **Depaul.** Une tumeur de la nature des névromes à la région cervicale. *Ibid.*, 1857, xxxii, 24–26.—**De-Rossi** (A.) Amputazione della mano per neuromi. .[*From :* Gazz. d. Osp. di Genova, Feb., 1866.] Gazz. med. ital., prov. venete, Padova, 1866, ix, 248–251.—**Després.** Névrome amyélinique sous-cutané. Bull. Soc. anat. de Par., 1877, lii, 548. — **Detmold.** Case of neuroma. N. York M. Times, 1851–2, i, 360–362.—**Downes** (E.) A new operation for some forms of neuromata. Lancet, Lond., 1881, i, 684.—**Dubois & Ledeganck.** Faux névrôme sous-cutané de la région sacro-iliaque ; extirpation ; guérison. Ann. Soc. d'anat. path. de Brux., 1873, xxii, 111–119.—**Duhring** (L. A.) Case of painful neuroma of the skin. Am. J. M. Sc., Phila. 1873, n. s., lxvi, 413 : 1874, n. s., lxviii, 29 : 1881, n. s., lxxxii, 435. *Also,* Reprint of 1873.—**Duplay** (S.) Névrome du nerf cubital. J. de méd. et chir. prat., Par., 1877, xlviii, 70.—**Dupuytren** (G.) D'une espèce particulière de tumeurs fibro-celluleuse enkystées, connues sous le nom de ganglions ou tubercules nerveux. *In his :* Leçons orales de clin. chir., 8°, Par., 1832, i, 530–556. *Also,* transl. : Lond. M. & S. J., 1833–4, [n. s.], iv, 137–141.—**Duret & Masmonteil.** Névrome sous-cutané de la face antérieure du poignet de cause traumatique. Arch. gén. de méd., Par., 1873, ii, 607–610.—[**Erichsen** (J. E.)] Painful subcutaneous tubercle. Lancet, Lond., 1857, i, 34.—**Euthyboule.** Névrome multiple du nerf cubital ; excision du nerf ; guérison. Gaz. méd. d'Orient, Constantinople, 1880–81, xxiii, 13–15.—**Fano.** [Amputation du bras ; névrome du plexus brachial.] Bull. Soc. anat. de Par.,

Neuroma.

1854, xxix, 135.—**Fayrer** (J.) [Tumour size of pigeon's egg on lower part of anterior surface of the right forearm.] Indian Ann. M. Sc., Calcutta, 1862–3, viii, 310 —[**Fergusson.**] Neuromatoid tumour. Lancet, Lond., 1858, i, 459.—**Fergusson & Erichsen.** Painful subcutaneous tubercles. *Ibid.*, 1859, i, 389.—**Findley** (W. M.) Neuroma involving the ulnar nerve; excision with entire relief from pain. Am. J. M. Sc., Phila., 1880, n. s., lxxix, 161.—**Fischer.** Einige Fälle exstirpirter Neurome. Ztschr. f. Wundärzte u. Geburtsh., Stuttg., 1864, xvii, 93–95. ———. Exstirpation eines Neuroms. *Ibid.*, 1871, xxiv, 161.—**Foerster** (A.) Ueber das Neuroma verum; Nachtrag zu dem Aufsatze von A. Dehler: "Ein Beitrag zu den Geschwülsten am Halse". Würzb. med. Ztschr., 1861, ii, 103–106, 1 pl.—**Franco de Machecoul.** Tubercule sous-cutané douloureux; (myome). Bull. Soc. anat. de Nantes 1883, Par., 1885, vii, 45.—**Frerichs** (F. T.) Neurom. Hannov. Ann. f. d. ges. Heilk., 1845, n. F., v, 650–653.—**Führer** (F.) Neurombildung und Nervenhypertrophie. Arch. f. physiol. Heilk., Stuttg., 1856, xv, 248 – 254, 1 pl.—**Gamberini** (P.) Neuroma curata colla potassa caustica. Bull. d. sc. med. di Bologna, 1850, 3. s., xviii, 198. — **Garel** (J.) Note sur un nouveau cas de névrome plexiforme. Mém. Soc. d. sc. méd. de Lyon (1876), 1877, xvi, 161; pt. 2, 235. *Also:* Lyon méd., 1877, xxiv, 41–52.—**Gibbs** (H. L.) Case of a tumour of the radial or spiral nerve; removed. Edinb. M. & S. J., 1829, xxxii, 250–253.—**Girard.** Heilung hartnäckig recidivirender Amputations-Neurome durch Elektropunctur. Deutsche Ztschr. f. Chir., Leipz., 1872, i, 137–140.—**Giraudet** (E.) Des névromes, ou tumeurs névromateuses. Abeille méd., Par., 1849, vi, 43–45.—**Godlee.** Neuromata in connection with the median nerve. Med. Times & Gaz., Lond., 1885, ii, 282. — **Greco** (D.) Sui tubercoli dolorosi sottocutanei. Scuola med. napol., 1851, iv, 544–550.—**Gunn** (M.) The value of an attempt at enucleation of a neuroma, which seemed to demand resection of a nerve. J. Am. M. Ass., Chicago, 1886, vii, 427–429.—**Hall** (M.) Case of painful subcutaneous tubercle. Edinb. M. & S. J., 1815, xi, 466–469.—**Hamilton** (F. H.) Painful tubercle; a report of two cases, and the result of careful dissection, by which it is shown not to be a neuroma, or an enlargement of the nervous tissue, as has been generally believed. Buffalo M. J., 1852–3, viii, 143.—**Hartley** (F.) Multiple neuromata with neurosarcoma. N. York M. J., 1887, xlvi, 682–686.—**Heurtaux.** Tubercule sous-cutané douloureux (myome). Bull. Soc. anat. de Nantes 1883, Par., 1885, vii, 10. *Also:* J. de méd. de l'ouest, Nantes, 1884, 2. s., viii, 120. — **Heyfelder.** Neurom; Beobachtung. J. d. Chir. u. Augenh., Berl., 1844, xxxiii, 627–629.—**Höring.** Ausrottung einer Nervengeschwulst. Ztschr. f. Wundärzte u. Geburtsh., Stuttg., 1856, ix, 11–13. — **Home** (E.) An account of an uncommon tumour, formed in one of the axillary nerves. Tr. Soc. Improve. M. & Chir. Knowl, Lond., 1800, ii, 152–163.—**Hooker** (A.) Neuromatous tumor on inner side of middle finger; removal. Boston M. & S. J., 1855, lii, 21.—**Houel.** Névromes développés sur tous les nerfs de l'économie. Bull. Soc. de chir. de Par., 1851–2, ii, 459–462. ———. Mémoire sur le névrome avec une observation de névromes multiples. [Rap. de Lebert.] Mém. Soc. de chir. de Par., 1853, iii, 249–304. *Also* [Abstr. of Rap.]: Bull. Soc. de chir. de Par, 1851–2, ii, 517.—**Image** (W. A.) Neuroma of the left median nerve. Assoc. M. J., Lond., 1854, ii, 619. — **Iturriós.** Neuroma del nérvio mediano en la flexura del brazo izquierdo, operado con éxito. Rev. méd.-quir., Buenos Aires, 1879–80, xvi, 483.—**Jacquart** (H.) Observation d'une tumeur fibreuse ou névrome développé dans l'épaisseur du nerf médian du bras droit, avec atrophie de tous les muscles qui ne reçoivent leur filets que de ce nerf, et intégrité partielle de ceux qui sont animés à la fois par des rameaux du médian et du cubital. Compt. rend. Soc. de biol. 1856, Par., 1857, 2. s., iii, 236 – 238.—**Jenks** (W. F.) Congenital sacral neuroma amyelinicum, followed by hydrocephalus and death. Med. Times, Phila., 1870–71, i, 364. *Also:* Tr. Path. Soc. Phila. (1871–3), 1874, iv, 190–192. — **Jessop** (T. R.) Traumatic neuroma, causing paralysis; rapid and complete restoration of the function of the nerve after the removal of the tumour. Brit. M. J., Lond., 1871, ii, 640.—**Keller** (W.) Neurom; Eintheilung, Beschreibung, Diagnose, Prognose, zusammengestellt nach den bis jetzt bekannten Beobachtungen. Nordamer. Monatsb. f. Nat.- u. Heilk., Phila., 1851, ii–iii, 272; 324; 420; 515. — **Kosiński.** Neuroma multiplex; Heilung durch Neurektomie. Centralbl. f. Chir., Leipz, 1874, i, 241–243. — **Krause** (F.) Ueber maligne Neurom und das Vorkommen von Nervenfasern in denselben. Samml. klin. Vortr., Leipz., 1887, Nos. 293 & 294 (Chir., No. 91), pp. 2695–2750.—**Krönlein** (R. U.) Recidivirendes, sehr schmerzhaftes Fibrom der Haut (Tuberculum dolorosum). Arch. f. klin. Chir., Berl., 1877, xxi (Supplhft.), 328. ———. Dattelgrosses, interstitielles Spindelzellensarcom den N. tibialis posticus in der Kniekehle. *Ibid.*, 333. — **Krüger-Hansen.** Skizzen über Schmarotzerbildung. Berl. med. Centr.-Ztg., 1836, v, 601–603. — **Kuiski** (J.) Nerwiak (neuroma) wyluszczenie, wyleczenie. Przegl. lek., Krakow, 1864, iii, 393 – 396. — **Labbé** (L.) Des névromes; du siège souvent circonscrit

Neuroma.

des points hyperesthésiés; excellents effets d'une opération limitée à ces mêmes points. Rev. de thérap. méd.-chir., Par., 1877, xlvi, 507–509. — **Labbé** (L.) & **Legros** (C.) Étude anatomo-pathologique de trois cas de névromes. J. de l'anat. et physiol., etc., Par., 1870 – 71, vii, 171–179, 1 pl.—**Laforgue** (H.) Névrome du nerf cubital; extirpation suivie de guérison; rétablissement de la sensibilité au moyen de l'appareil de M. Duchenne (de Boulogne). Gaz. d. hôp., Par., 1854, xxvii, 55.—*Also:* Union méd., Par., 1854, viii, 26.—**Lanclongue.** Névrome du tibial postérieur. J. de méd. de Bordeaux. 1886–7, xvi, 414–416.—**Lange** (F.) Neuroma; removal; implantation of the nerve of a dog. Bull. N. York Path. Soc., 1881, 2. s., i, 194.—[**Lawrence.**] Neuroma of the posterior tibial nerve; amputation of the foot. Lancet, Lond., 1858, i, 627.—**Lebert.** Un névrome du nerf cubital de la grosseur du poing. Bull. Soc. anat. de Par., 1852, xxvii, 46.—**Lebreton.** Névrôme des nerfs cubital et médian. Bull. Soc. anat. de Par., 1865, xl, 169.—**Lee** (H.) Neuromatoid ulnar tumor. Lancet, Lond., 1857. ii, 274.—**Lefour.** Névrome du saphène externe; ablation; guérison complète par le sulfate de quinine. Gaz. méd. de Bordeaux, 1876, v, 422–424.—**Legrand** (A.) De la cautérisation linéaire et destructive appliquée au traitement des névromes et des tumeurs sous-cutanées douloureuses. Gaz. d. hôp., Par., 1858, xxxi, 466.—**Lidell** (J. A.) A case of neuroma of the optic nerve, together with some general observations upon neuroma. N. York J. M., 1860, 3. s., viii, 151–163, 1 pl.—**Lisfranc.** Observation d'un névrome très-douloureux du cuir chevelu, traité et guéri par l'ablation d'un lambeau de peau. Rev. méd. franç. et étrang., Par., 1826, i, 201–206.—**Löwenfeld.** Paralyse der linken unteren Extremität und der Blase, bedingt durch ein Neurom an den Wurzeln der ersten zwei Sakralnerven linkerseits. Wien. med. Presse, 1873, xiv, 706–708.—**Long.** Neuroma and painful subcutaneous tumour. Med. Times & Gaz., Lond., 1856, n. s., xii, 23. — **Loretz** (W.) Ein Fall von gangliösem Neurom. Arch. f. path. Anat., etc., Berl., 1870, xlix, 435–437, 1 pl.—**Lucas** (R. C.) Small painful tumor connected with the internal saphenous nerve. Brit. M. J., Lond., 1873, ii, 111. — **MacSwiney** (S. M.) Case of neuroma. Dublin M. Press, 1856, xxxv, 129–132.—**Malherbe** (A.) Note sur la structure des tumeurs dites tubercules sous-cutanés douloureux. Gaz. méd. de Nantes, 1883–4, ii, 179–183.—**Maury** (F. F.) Case of exsection of the brachial plexus of nerves for the relief of painful neuroma of the skin. Am. J. M. Sc., Phila., 1874, n. s., lxviii, 29 – 37. — **Mazza** (G.) Nei e fibromi neuropatici. Salute: Italia med., Genova, 1885, xix, 601–628. — **Mears** (J. E.) Fibrous tumors on the digital branches of the median nerve; thickening of the median and ulnar nerve; epilepsy, on account of which the arm was amputated. Tr. Path. Soc. Phila. (1871–3), 1874, iv, 190.—**Michon.** [Névrome du volume d'un œuf de poule à la partie supérieure du nerf sciatique; excision.] Bull. Soc. de chir. de Par. (1864) 1865, 2. s., v, 312 – 318. — **Moleschott** (J.) Pathologisch-anatomische aanteekening over neuroma. Nederl. Lancet, Gravenh., 1845–6, 2. s., i, 265 – 274. ———. Pathologisch-anatomische Bemerkungen über das Neurom. Arch. f. physiol. Heilk., Stuttg., 1849, viii, 252 – 257. — **Monette** (G. N.) Neurotic tumor of the popliteal nerve; amputation; recovery. Am. Pract., Louisville, 1873, viii, 21.—**Muron.** Névrome périphérique du filet du nerf cubital. Bull. Soc. anat. de Par., 1869, xliv, 139. — **Neuroma** of the posterior tibial nerve, occasioning severe neuralgia of the sciatic, posterior tibial, and cutaneous nerves of the knee and leg; removal of the tumor. Lancet, Lond., 1846, ii, 119. — **Névrômes** (Des) plexiformes. Gaz. méd.-chir. de Toulouse, 1874, vi, 265 – 267. — **Nichell** (C. F. A.) Neuromatous condition of the median nerve. Buffalo M. & S. J., 1867–8, vii, 176. — **Offer** (J.) Neurom des N. medianus. Ber. d. naturw.-med. Ver. in Innsbruck (1878), 1879, ix, 97.—**Paget.** Large neuromatous tumor in connexion with the sciatic nerve; successful enucleation. Lancet, Lond., 1862, i, 221. *Also:* Med. Times & Gaz., Lond., 1862, i, 453.—**Péan.** Névrome développé sur le trajet du nerf collatéral du médius, à la suite d'une blessure par un éclat de verre; ablation de la petite tumeur. Rev. de thérap. méd.-chir., Par., 1879, xlvi, 649.—**Pepper** (W.) Traumatic neuroma of brachial plexus following amputation of humerus. Proc. Path. Soc. Phila. (1866–70). 1871, iii, 136.—**Pick** (A.) Beitrag zur Lehre von den Neuromen. Arch. f. Psychiat., Berl., 1876, vii, 202–217.—**Ripeault** (C.) Accidents nerveux causés par un tubercule douloureux sous-cutané. Bull. Soc. de méd. de la Sarthe 1874, Le Mans. 1875, 26 – 28. — **Robert.** Névromes de l'avant-bras. Bull. Soc. de chir. de Par., 1851–2, i, 173.—**Rose** (E.) Ein Neurom der Erb'schen Plexuswurzeln. Deutsche Ztschr. f. Chir., Leipz., 1886, xxiv, 392–414.—**Roth.** Ein Neurom. N.-Yorker med. Monatschr., 1852, i, 213–216.—**Roux** (G.) Sur un cas de névrome du sciatique poplité externe guéri par l'ablation de la tumeur. Marseille méd., 1886, xxiii, 577–580.—**Ruhbaum.** Drei Fälle von Neuroma. Wchnschr. f. d. ges. Heilk., Berl., 1840, 648–651.—**Sayre** (L. A.) Tumor from sheath of sciatic nerve. N. York M. J., 1866, ii, 442.—**Scheuthauer**

Neuroma.

(G.) A neuromáról. [Neuroma.] Orvosi hetil., Budapest, 1881. xxv, 1133–1139. — **Schuh.** Textur der Neurome. Ztschr. d. k.-k. Gesellsch. d. Aerzte zu Wien, 1857. xiii, 10–14. ————. Neurom im Deltamuskel; Verschwinden der Krankheitserscheinungen nach der Operation; Recidive; Operation mit Abtragung eines langen Stückes des Nervus circumflexus. Wien. Med.-Halle, 1863, iv, 311. — **Seitz** (J.) Multiple Fibrosarkome der Nerven und Perichondritis laryngea. Arch. f. path. Anat., etc., Berl., 1871, lii, 114–123. — **Shillitoe** (B.) Neuroma of the musculo-spiral nerve, containing a blood-cyst. Tr. Path. Soc. Lond., 1859–60, xi, 1. — **Sibley.** Two specimens of neuroma. *Ibid.*, 1856–7, viii, 20–23, 1 pl. — **Sims** (H. M.) Abdominal neuromata. Med. Rec., N. Y., 1886, xxix, 400. — **Slocum** (G. D.) Removal of a neuromatous tumor. Buffalo M. & S. J., 1867-8, vii, 308. — **Sonrier** (E.) Névrome traumatique du saphène interne; cautérisation; guérison. Gaz. d. hôp., Par., 1874, xlvii, 108. — **Spark** (J.) Painful subcutaneous tumor. Lond. M. Gaz., 1828–9, iii, 411. — **Spillmann** (E.) Observation du névrome du nerf médian. Bull. Soc. de chir. de Par., 1874, 3. s., iii, 118–128. *Also:* Rec. de mém. de méd. . . . mil. Par., 1874, xxx, 228–237. *Also:* Gaz. d. hôp., Par., 1874, xlvii, 282; 308. *Also:* Gaz. hebd. de méd., Par., 1874, xxi, 512–514. — **Stearns** (J.) Case of neuroma. Buffalo M. & S. J., 1862, ii, 172. — **Stein.** Stort Neurom paa Nervus ischiadicus, der med Held blev borttaget ved Operation; samt en senere Udvikling af en betydelig Fungus duræ matris, som havde Patientens Död til Fölge. Hosp.-Medd., Kjøbenh., 1849, ii, 1–21. — **Steiner** (F.) Neurofibrom von Pomeranzen-Grösse am linken N. medianus; Exstirpation der Geschwulst mit Ausschneidung eines langen Stückes vom Nerven; die Funktion der vom N. medianus versorgten Muskel nach der Operation nur wenig verringert; Heilung. Wien. med. Wchnschr., 1868, xviii, 1492. — **Stiénon** (L.) Étude sur la structure du névrome. Ann. de l'Univ. de Brux. Fac. de méd., 1882, iii, 167–192, 2 pl. *Also,* Reprint. — **Suñé y Molist** (L.) Tubérculo subcutáneo doloroso; inserto en el neurilema de una rama superficial del nervio músculo-cutáneo. Gac. méd. de Cataluña, Barcel., 1879, ii, 426–428. — **Swan** (R. L.) Painful subcutaneous tumour. Med. Press & Circ., Lond., 1869, vii, 537. — **Syme** (J.) Subcutaneous nervous tubercle; recovery. Edinb. M. & S. J., 1836, xlvi, 266. ————. Neuroma. Lancet, Lond., 1855, i, 551. — **Tavignot.** Névrôme développé sur le trajet du nerf sous-orbitaire; ablation de la paroi inférieure de l'orbite; guérison. Expérience, Par., 1840, vi, 213–215. — **Tripier** (L.) Névrome. Dict. encycl. d. sc. méd., Par., 1878, 2. s., xii, 698–726. — **Van der Byl.** Specimen of neuroma on the posterior tibial nerve. Tr. Path. Soc. Lond., 1854-5, vi, 49–51, 1 pl. — **Virchow** (R.) Das wahre Neurom. Arch. f. path. Anat., etc., Berl., 1858, xiii, 256–265, 1 pl. — **Volkmann** (R.) Ueber ein handgrosses ulcerirtes Neurom im Handteller. *Ibid.*, 1857, xii, 27–37, 2 pl. — **Warren** (J. M.) Painful cutaneous tubercle. Am. J. M. Sc., Phila., 1850, n. s., xx, 33. *Also, in his:* Surg. Obs., 8°, Bost., 1867, 535. — **Weil** (K.) Cystisches verkalktes Fibroneurom des Ulnaris; ein Beitrag zur Kenntniss der Neurome. Ztschr. f. Heilk., Prag, 1881, ii, 333–344, 1 pl. — **Weismann** (A.) Ueber Nervenneubildung in einem Neurom. Ztschr. f. rat. Med., Leipz., 1859, 3. R., vii, 209–218, 1 pl. — **Wietfeldt** (C.) Neuromatöse Neuralgie des Ramus palmaris longus nervi mediani. Deutsche Klinik, Berl., 1863, xv, 507. — **Wilks.** Case of neuroma. Tr. Path. Soc. Lond., 1858-9, x, 1–3. — **Windsor** (J.) Case of painful subcutaneous tumour, in which the tumour was penetrated by the twig of a nerve. Edinb. M. & S. J., 1821, xvii, 261–263. — **Wood** (W.) On painful subcutaneous tubercle. *Ibid.*, 1812, viii, 283–291. ————. Further observations on painful subcutaneus tubercle. *Ibid.*, 429–435. ————. Observations on painful subcutaneous tubercle, with cases and histories of the disease. Tr. Med.-Chir. Soc. Edinb., 1828–9, iii, 317; 640, 1 pl. *Also,* Reprint. ————. Observations on neuroma, with cases and histories of the disease. Tr. Med.-Chir. Soc. Edinb., 1828–9, iii, 367–433. *Also,* Reprint. — **Wutzer** (C. W.) Fall von Neuroma des Ellenbogen-Nerven. Wissensch. Ann. d. ges. Heilk., Berl., 1836, xxxiii, 393–414. ————. Fall von Neuroma nervi peronæi. Ber. ü. d. Arb. d. ärztl. Sect. d. nied.-rhein. Gesellsch. f. Nat.- u. Heilk. zu Bonn, 1851–3, 20–22. — **Zambelli** (G.) Tre nevromi del nervo peroneo curati, uno col caustico attuale, e due coll' enucleazione. Gazz. med. ital., prov. venete, Padova, 1864, vii, 263.

Neuroma (*Multiple*).

CARDON (F.) *Essai sur les névromes généralisés. 4°. *Paris*, 1876.

FRANKENBERG (H.) *Ueber multiple Neurome. 8°. *Marburg*, 1863.

RIESENFELD (E.) *Ein Fall vòn "multiplen Neuromen". 8°. *Würzburg*, 1876.

RUMP (C.) *Ein Fall von multiplen Neuromen. [Wurtzburg.] 8°. *Münster*, 1879.

Also, in : Arch. f. path. Anat., etc., Berl., 1880, lxxx, 177–182.

Neuroma (*Multiple*).

SIEMENS (F.) *Beitrag zur Lehre von den multiplen Neuromen. 8°. *Marburg*, 1874.

Bauchet. [Un cas excessivement remarquable de névrôme multiple.] Bull. Soc. anat. de Par., 1852, xxvii, 46. — **Brochin.** Un cas de diathèse névromatique. Gaz. d. hôp., Par., 1875, xlviii, 1017. — **Bulteau.** Fibromes multiples du nerf médian dans sa portion palmaire. Union méd. et scient. du nord-est, Reims, 1880, iv, 27–31. — **Chavasse** (T. F.) A case of multiple neuromata. Med.-Chir. Tr., Lond., 1886, lxix, 517-526, 1 pl. *Also* [Abstr.]: Proc. Roy. M. & Chir. Soc. Lond., 1885-6, n. s., ii, 124. *Also* [Abstr.]: Lancet, Lond., 1886, i, 1114. *Also* [Abstr.]: Brit. M. J., Lond., 1886, i, 1110. — **De Morgan** (C.) & **Coupland.** Case of multiple neuroma of the forearm. Tr. Path. Soc. Lond., 1874-5, xxvi, 2-10, 2 pl. — **Genersich** (A.) Multiple Neurome. Arch. f. path. Anat., etc., Berl., 1870, xlix, 15–48. — **Gerhardt** (C.) Zur Diagnostik multipler Neurombildung. Deutsches Arch. f. klin. Med., Leipz., 1878, xxi, 268–289. — **Heller** (A.) Multiple Neurome. Arch. f. path. Anat., etc., Berl., 1868, xliv, 338–351, 1 pl. — **Heusinger** (O.) Ein Fall von multiplen Neuromen aller Körpernerven. *Ibid.*, 1863, xxvii, 206–209, 1 pl. — **Hitchcock** (A.) Some remarks on neuroma, with a brief account of three cases of anomalous cutaneous tumours in one family. Am. J. M. Sc., Phila., 1862, n. s., xliii, 320–328. — **Houel.** Mémoire sur le névrome, avec une observation de névromes multiples. Mém Soc. de chir. de Par., 1853, iii, 249–266. — **Kautzner.** Präparate von multiplen Neuromen. Sitzungsb. d. Ver. d. Aerzte in Steiermark, Graz, 1872-3, x, 76. — **Köbner** (H.) Fall von seltenen auf Bildungsanomalie beruhenden Geschwülsten der Nerven und neuromatösen Fibromen, cavernösen Angiomen und Lymphangiomen der Haut und des Unterhautzellgewebes. Berl. klin. Wchnschr., 1883, xx, 476. *Also:* Verhandl. d. Berl. med. Gesellsch. (1882-3), 1884, xiv, 140–143. *Also, transl.:* Ann. de dermat. et syph., Par., 1884, 2. s., v, 293–300. — **Lahmann** (H.) Die multiplen Fibrome in ihrer Beziehung zu den Neurofibromen. Arch. f. path. Anat., etc., Berl., 1885, ci, 263–275, 1 pl. — **Launois** (P.-E.) & **Variot** (G.) Étude sur les névromes multiples. Rev. de chir., Par., 1883, iii, 409–431. — **Passavant** (G.) Zahlreiche Neurome des Nervus perinæi sin. Arch. f. path. Anat., etc., Berl., 1854, viii, 40–46, 1 pl. — **Pearson** (J.) An account of some extraordinary symptoms which were apparently connected with certain morbid alterations about the veins and nerves. Med. Facts & Obs., Lond., 1795, vi, 96–110. — **Prudden** (T. M.) Contributions to the structure and clinical history of the multiple neuroma, from the Pathological Laboratory of the Alumni Association of the College of Physicians and Surgeons. Am. J. M. Sc., Phila., 1880, n. s., lxxx, 134–158. *Also,* Reprint. — **Salomon** (G.) Multiple Neurome bei einem schwachsinnigen Individuum; Fortschreiten der Neurombildung während der Dauer der Beobachtung; Exstirpation und mikroskopische Untersuchung eines Neuroms. Charité-Ann., Berl., 1879, iv, 133–143. — **Sibley** (S. W.) Case of multiple neuromata, affecting the nerves both within and external to the spinal canal, some of the tumours being of a cystic nature. Med.-Chir. Tr., Lond., 1866, xlix, 39–44, 1 pl. *Also:* Proc. Roy. M. & Chir. Soc. Lond. (1864-7), 1867, v, 133. — **Smith** (T.) Multiple neuromata. Tr. Path. Soc. Lond., 1860–61, xii, 2. — **Soyka** (I.) Ueber den Bau und die Stellung der multiplen Neurome. Vrtljschr. f. d. prakt. Heilk., Prag, 1877, cxxxv, 1–24, 1 pl. — **Takács** (A.) Ueber multiple Neurome. Arch. f. path. Anat., etc., Berl., 1879, lxxv, 431–443. — **Témoin.** Névromes généralisés; mort. Bull. Soc. anat. de Par., 1857, xxxii, 403–413. — **Virchow** (R.) Ueber einen Fall von vielfachen Neuromen (sogen. Faser-Kern-Geschwülsten) mit ausgezeichneter localer Recidivfähigkeit. Arch. f. path. Anat., etc., Berl., 1857, xii, 114–117. — **Wallis** (C.) Fall af multipla neurofibrom förenadt med sarkombildning. Hygiea, Stockholm, 1884, xlvi, 545–553.

Neuromimesis.

See **Nervous** system (*Diseases of, Diagnosis, etc., of*).

Neuro-retinitis.

See **Nerve** (*Optic, Inflammation of*).

Neuroses.

See **Fever** (*Malarial, Masked, etc.*); **Menstruation** *and disease*; **Nervous** *system* (*Diseases of*); **Nervous** *system* (*Diseases of, Functional*); **Nervous** *system* (*Ganglionic, Pathology of*); **Nervous** *system* (*Vasomotor, Pathology of*); **Neuralgia**; **Neurasthenia**; **Tongue** (*Neurosis of*).

Neuroth (Ferdinand [C. P.]) [1847-]. *Zur Casuistik und Statistik des Pneumothorax. 31 pp., 1 l. 8°. *Marburg, C. L. Pfeil*, 1876.

Neurotics.

See, also, **Narcotics.**

HARLEY (J.) The old vegetable neurotics: hemlock, opium, belladonna, and henbane, their physiological action and therapeutical use alone and in combination, being the Gulstonian lectures of 1868 extended, and including a complete examination of the active constituents of opium. 8°. *London*, 1869.

Nicol (P.) & **Mossop** (L.) On the action of certain neurotics on the cerebral circulation. Brit. & For. M.-Chir. Rev., Lond., 1872, l, 200–205. — **Peters** (J. C.) On neurotics. Psych. & Med.-Leg. J., N. Y., 1874, n. s., i, 366–387. *Also*, Reprint.

Neurotomy *and neurectomy.*

See, also, **Horse** (*Diseases of*); **Nerve** (*Optic, Section of*); **Nerve** (*Sciatic, Tumors of*); **Nerves** (*Brachial*) [*etc.*]; **Nerves** (*Cranial, Fifth pair of*); **Nerves** (*Degeneration, etc., of*); **Neuralgia** (*Dental, etc.*); **Neuralgia** (*Facial, etc., Treatment of*) **Neuralgia** (*Lingual*); **Neuralgia** (*Supra-orbital*); **Tetanus** (*Treatment of*).

BECKER (G.) *Beitrag zur Resection des Nervus alveolaris inferior. [Wurtzburg.] 8°. *Schotten*, 1885.

FAUCON (E.) * Étude sur la valeur des résections nerveuses dans les affections des nerfs. 4°. *Strasbourg*, 1869.

GILIS (P.) *Des troubles consécutifs aux sections des nerfs du membre supérieur par instrument tranchant; de la suture nerveuse; sa valeur. 4°. *Montpellier*, 1884.

———. The same. 8°. *Paris*, 1884.

JACQUOT (A.) * Des résections nerveuses, dans les névralgies invétérées. 4°. *Nancy*, 1879.

KONDRACKI (E.) * Ueber die Durchschneidung des Nervus trigeminus bei Kaninchen. 8°. *Zürich*, 1872.

LÉTIÉVANT (E.) Traité des sections nerveuses; physiologie pathologique, indications, procédés opératoires. 8°. *Paris*, 1873.

LOEHRL (H.) * Die Neurotomie des Ramus lingualis trigemini. 8°. *Tübingen*, 1863.

MAGNIEN (B.-P.) * Recherches expérimentales sur les effets consécutifs à la section des nerfs mixtes. 4°. *Paris*, 1866.

MIALARET (G.) * Contributions à l'étude des modifications de la sensibilité du membre supérieur consécutives aux sections nerveuses. 4°. *Paris*, 1881.

REICHENBACH (H. P. D.) * De consecandis membrorum sive artuum nervis, supplementum parvum ad hanc operationem tractandam. 12°. *Altonæ*, 1845.

SCHRÖDER (O.) * Ueber die Resection des Nervus mentalis. 8°. *Würzburg*, [1880?]

SCHULZ (H.) * Ueber den Einfluss der Nerven-Durchschneidung auf die Gewebe. 8°. *Königsberg*, 1874.

STICKER (L.) * De nervorum persectorum mutationibus deque invitabilitate musculorum. 8°. *Berolini*, [1833].

VIEILLARD (P. M.) * Utrum in pertinacibus capitis facieique doloribus aliquid prodesse possit sectio ramorum nervi quinti paris ? Præses G. J. de l'Epine. 4°. [*Paris*, 1768.]

WIEDERSHEIM (A. C.) * Die Hyperämie; von Durchschneidung und andern Affectionen der Nerven. 8°. *Stuttgart*, 1841.

Albert (E.) Fälle von Neurectomie. Wien. med. Wchnschr., 1872, xxii, 77 ; 153 ; 276 ; 304 ; 332 ; 495. ———. Einige Fälle von Neurektomie. Wien. med. Presse, 1877, xviii, 545 ; 622. *Also, in his* : Beitr. z. oper. Chir., 8°, Wien, 1878, 31–37. ———. Weitere Neurektomien. Wien. med. Presse, 1880, xxi, 1393 ; 1457. ———. Einige Operationen an Nerven. *Ibid.*, 1885, xxvi, 1221; 1285.—**Arlaud.** Amputation fémoro-tibiale à la suite d'une plaie d'arme à feu ; résection des nerfs sciatiques poplités interne et externe; guérison. Déambulation facile à l'aide du pilon classique. Bull. gén. de thérap., etc., Par., 1862, lxiii, 26–31.—**Arloing** & **Tripier** (L.) Des sections dans les

Neurotomy *and neurectomy.*

névralgies. Gaz. hebd. de méd., Par., 1875, 2. s., xii, 545–547. *Also*: Abeille méd., Par., 1875, xxxii, 349–352. ———. Des conditions de la persistance de la sensibilité dans le bout périphérique des nerfs sectionnés. Arch. de physiol. norm. et path., Par., 1876, 2. s., iii, 11 ; 105, 5 pl. *Also* [Abstr.]: Compt. rend. Acad. d. sc., Par., 1874, lxxviii, 1473–1477.—**Azam.** Résections successives des nerfs sciatiques, poplité externe et grand sciatique pour une névralgie de moignon ; guérison ; récidive. Gaz. d. hôp., Par., 1864, xxxvii, 286–288. *Also* : Bull. Soc. de chir. de Par. (1864), 1865, 2. s., v, 280–288. [Disc.], 292–298. ———. Résection du grand sciatique pour une névralgie traumatique ; guérison constatée après trois ans et demi. Mém. et bull. Soc. méd.-chir. d. hôp. de Bordeaux, 1866, i, 273–278.—**Babinski** (J.) Des modifications que présentent les muscles à la suite de la section des nerfs qui s'y rendent. Compt. rend. Acad. d. sc., Par., 1884, xcviii, 51.—**Bär** (J.) Resektion des Nervus dentalis und mentalis an der Eingangsöffnung in den Unterkieferkanal. Wien. med Wchnschr., 1871, xxi, 340–343.—**Ball** (C. B.) Results of section of right ulnar nerve. Brit. M. J., Lond., 1881, i, 515.—**Bayard** (R.) Case of diseased sciatic nerve removed by excision ; death. N. York M. & Phys. J., 1829–30, n. s., ii, 37–39.—**Beau** (L.) Nouvelle méthode de résection des nerfs de la face ; méthode par extraction. Union méd., Par., 1853, vii, 161 ; 165 ; 179 ; 187 ; 191.—**Benecke** (B.) Ueber die histologischen Vorgänge in durchschnittenen Nerven. Arch. f. path. Anat., etc., Berl., 1872, lv, 496–511.—**Bernard** (C.) Procédé nouveau pour couper la cinquième paire des nerfs dans le crâne. Compt. rend. Soc. de biol. 1849, Par., 1850, i, 104. ———. Des conditions de la persistance de la sensibilité dans le bout périphérique des nerfs sectionnés. Rev. scient., Par., 1875, 2. s., ix. 92.—**Bernays** (A. C.) A unique case of neurectomy of three divisions of the trigeminus at one sitting ; recovery. Internat. J. Surg. & Antisept., N. Y., 1888, i, 10.—**Bertolet** (R. M.) Regeneration of human nerves after excision. Tr. Path. Soc. Phila., 1877, vi, 124.—**Bidder** (F.) Erfolge von Nervendurchschneidung an einem Frosch. Arch. f. Anat., Physiol. u. wissensch. Med., Leipz., 1865, 67–79.—**Blackman** (G. C.) Exsection of the sciatic nerve for neuralgia of the stump following amputation of the thigh. N. Am. M.-Chir. Rev., Phila., 1859, iii, 298.—**Briddon** (C. K.) [Case of operation for neuralgic affection performed by . . .] Buffalo M. J., 1859–60, xv, 480–484. ———. Some remote consequences of sections of nerves. Med. Rec., N. Y., 1881, xix, 386–388.—**Brown** (B.) Neuralgia of eighteen years' standing cured by an operation. Am. J. M. Sc., Phila., 1850, n. s., xx, 327. *Also* : Extr. Rec. Bost. Soc. M. Improve. (1848–53), 1853, i, 96–98.—**Brown-Séquard.** Sur les altérations pathologiques qui suivent la section du nerf sciatique. Compt. rend. Soc. de biol. 1849, Par., 1850, i, 136.—**Butlin** (H. T.) Ulnar nerve. showing the effects of division fourteen years before death. Tr. Path. Soc. Lond., 1873–4, xxv, 4–6, 1 pl.—**Cadge** (W.) Nerve-section in the treatment of neuralgia. Brit. M. J., Lond., 1882, ii, 83–85.—[**Cases.**] Painful growth in the ball of the great toe ; excision ; great pain in the cicatrix ; removal of a portion of nerve : recovery after a second excision. Med. Times & Gaz., Lond., 1853, n. s., vii, 191.—Resection des Nerv. infraorbit. sin. Aerztl. Ber. a. d. k. k. allg. Krankenh. zu Wien (1861), 1862, 227.—Tic facial, datant de plus d'un an, avec occlusion complète des yeux ; section des nerfs de la 7 e paire ; guérison. Abeille méd., Par., 1868, xxv, 187.—Section of anterior tibial nerve for neuralgia. Med. & Surg. Reporter, Phila., 1869, xx, 293.—**Chapman** (H. C.) The distribution of nerves in reference tc neurotomy. Phila. M. Times, 1873–4, iv, 260.—**Chavasse** (T. F.) Neurectomy of the second division of the fifth nerve. Brit. M. J., Lond., 1884, i, 411.—**Cherini** (A.) Della cura chirurgica nelle nevralgie. Ann. univ. di med., Milano, 1864, clxxxviii, 74–117.—**Chiene.** [Patient in whom the spinal accessory nerve was divided in order to relieve painful spasm of the left sterno-mastoid muscle.] Edinb. M. J., 1880–81, xxvi, 925—**Clutton** (H. H.) Neurectomy of the second division of the fifth nerve. St. Thomas's Hosp. Rep: 1885, Lond., 1886, xv, 213–224, 1 pl.—**Credé.** Dehnung und Durchschneidung des 3. Astes des Nervus trigeminus an der Schädelbasis. Verhandl. d. deutsch. Gesellsch. f. Chir. 1880, Berl., 1881, ix, 27–35.—**Davies** (R.) Five cases of neurotomy for painful affections of the limbs. Dublin Q. J. M. Sc., 1860, xxx, 331–337. *Also*, Reprint.—**Delpech.** Observations sur l'utilité de la section des nerfs dans certains cas. Rev. méd. franç. et étrang., Par., 1832, i, 72–84.—[**Discussion** sur les résections des filets nerveux] Bull. Soc. de chir. de Par., (1852), 1853, iii, 284–286.—**Dubroff** (I. I.) Vitjajenie loktevago nerva po sluchaju nevritidis traumaticæ. Laitop. khirurg. Obsh. v Mosk., 1882, v, 162-165.—**Eulenburg** (A.) & **Landois** (L.) Die thermischen Wirkungen peripherischer Reizung und Durchschneidung der Nervenstämme. Arch. f. path. Anat., etc., Berl., 1876, lxvi, 489–502, 1 pl.—**Fergusson.** Clinical remarks on a case of painful ulcer on the leg ; with division of the popliteal nerve ; subsequent amputation at the knee-joint ; recovery. Lancet, Lond., 1862, i, 487.—**Fornari** (F.) Due

Neurotomy *and neurectomy.*

nevrectenie (stiramento); del cubitale per nevralgia, dello sciatico per atassia locomotrice. Morgagni, Napoli, 1881, xxiii, 677–680.—**Fumagalli** (C.) Nevralgia traumatica ribelle alla nevrotomia. Ann. univ. di med., Milano, 1868, ccvi, 612.—**Gallozzi** (C.) Della recisione del nervo dentario inferiore col metodo del Parravicini. Resoc. Accad. med.-chir. di Napoli, 1882, xxxvi, 195–199.—**Garretson** (J. E.) A method of resecting the second branch of the fifth nerve in the spheno-maxillary fossa, using the surgical engine. Ann. Anat. & Surg., Brooklyn, N. Y., 1883, viii, 158–160.—**Gilmore** (J. T.) Case of neuralgia relieved by trephining. N. Orl. M. & S. J., 1866–7, xix, 342–346. ——. Exsection of nerves. Tr. M. Ass. Alabama, Mobile, 1870, 387.—**Godin** (A.) Névralgies rebelles; section des nerfs malades. J. d. conn. méd.-chir., Par., 1835–6, iii, 441–444.—**Hayem** (G.) Note sur deux cas de lésions cutanées consécutives à des sections de nerfs. Arch. de physiol. norm. et path., Par., 1873, v, 212–223. — **Hildebrandt.** Casuistischer Beitrag zur Neurektomie. Deutsche med. Wchnschr., Leipz., 1887, xiii, 1018. — **Hilton.** Treatment of neuralgia by excision of a piece of nerve. Med. Times & Gaz., Lond., 1861, i, 549. — **von Hochstetter** (A. F.) Neurotomie des N. infraorbitalis unter Cocaïnanästhesie. Wien. med. Wchnschr., 1887, xxxvii, 1498.— **Hodgen** (J. T.) An easy method of removing a part of the inferior dental nerve within the lower jaw. St. Louis M. & S. J., 1875, n. s., xii, 22–24. ——. Nerve section for neuralgia. Tr. M. Ass. Missouri, St. Louis, 1876, x, 21–28.—**Högyes** (A.) Ueber die Veränderungen des Auges nach Facialisexstirpation. Arch. f. exper. Path. u. Pharmakol., Leipz., 1879, xi, 258–274. — **Holcombe** (A. A.) Suppuration of the foot after neurotomy. Am. Vet. Rev., N. Y., 1880, iii, 426–428. — **Holl** (M.) Ueber eine neue Methode der Resection des Nervus buccinatorius. Arch. f. klin. Chir., Berl., 1881, xxvi, 994–1008, 1 pl.—**Hooker** (E. M. C.) Division of the popliteal nerve for neuralgia of the leg. Lancet, Lond., 1859, ii, 336.—**Hutchinson** (J.) Case illustrating the effect of nerve section upon nutrition and animal heat. Med. Times & Gaz , Lond., 1863, i, 161. ——. Observations on the results which follow the section of nerve-trunks, as observed in surgical practice. Clin. Lect. & Rep. Lond. Hosp., 1866, iii, 305–324.—**Jobert** (*de Lamballe*). Travaux sur la thérapeutique des névralgies; procédé mixte; section et cautérisation du nerf. France méd., Par., 1854, i, 21; 39. *Also:* Gaz. d. hôp., Par., 1854, xxvii, 162.—**Jolyet** & **Laffont.** Nouveau procédé de section intracrânienne du facial. Compt. rend. Soc. de biol. 1879. Par., 1880, 7. s., i, 334–336. *Also:* Progrès méd., Par., 1879, vii, 980.—**Joüon** (F.) Résection du nerf auriculo-temporal. J. de méd. de l'ouest, Nantes, 1877, 2. s., i, 105–110. — **Kappeler** (O.) Neuralgia nervi peronei superficialis; Neurectomie. *In his:* Chir. Beob., etc., 8°, Frauenfeld, 1874, 296.—**Kraussold** (H.) Ueber Nervendurchschneidung und Nervennaht. Samml. klin. Vortr., Leipz., 1878 (Chir., No. 43), pp. 1129–1160.—**Kuby.** Resection des Nervus medianus. Aerztl. Int.-Bl., München, 1871, xviii, 312.—**Laborde** (J.-V.) Sur l'état et le rôle de la sensibilité et des fibres récurrentes, à la suite des phénomènes qui accompagnent la section expérimentale ou pathologique des nerfs mixtes, en particulier du nerf médian. Compt. rend. Soc. de biol., Par., 1886, 8. s., iii, 470–472. *Also:* Tribune méd., Par., 1886, xviii, 544–546.—**Laborde** (J.-V.) & **Leven.** Recherches expérimentales sur les altérations de nutrition qui se produisent dans les divers tissus à la suite de la section et de la ligature des nerfs, et de la section de la moelle épinière. Compt. rend. Soc. de biol. 1869, Par., 1870, 5. s., i, 280–284.—**Laforgue** (H.) Névrôme du nerf cubital; extirpation suivie de guérison. J. de méd., chir. et pharm. de Toulouse, 1854, n. s., vi, 11–19.— **Lagrange.** L'opération de Badal. Gaz. hebd. d. sc. méd. de Bordeaux, 1886, vii, 115–119.—**Lande** (L.) Névralgie épileptiforme; résection nerveuse; persistance de la névralgie dans un filet nerveux demeuré intact; nouvelle résection; guérison. Gaz. méd. de Bordeaux, 1873, ii, 529–533.—**von Langenbeck** (B.) Die subcutane Durchschneidung des Nerv. infraorbit. in der Fissura orbital. inferior. Arch. f. klin. Chir., Berl., 1869, xi, 127–130.—**Létiévant** (E.) Motilité et sensibilité suppléées après les sections nerveuses. Gaz. méd. de Bordeaux, 1873, iii, 73–80. ——. Note sur le traitement des névralgies rebelles par la névrotomie. Lyon méd., 1871, xix, 123–128. *Also:* Abeille méd., Par., 1875, xxxii, 218. *Also:* Mém. Soc. d. sc. méd. de Lyon (1875), 1876, xv, pt. 2, 69–77. ——. Névrotomie directe d'un filet du pectoral pour une névralgie d'origine traumatique. Lyon méd., 1875, xix, 579–581. *Also:* Mém. Soc. d. sc. méd. de Lyon (1875), 1876, xv, pt. 2, 135–143. ——. Note sur la névrotomie. Cong. périod. internat. d. sc. méd. Compt.-rend. 1877, Genève, 1878, v, 298–302.—**Lidell** (J. A.) On neuralgia; with the report of two cases of excision of the nerve. N. York J. M., 1856, 3. s., i, 311–320.—**Little** (N. W.) Exsection of sup. maxillary nerve. Atlanta M. & S. J., 1879–80, xvii, 449–451.—[**Logan** (S.)] Traumatic neuralgia; excision of one inch of each ulnar nerve. N. Orl. M. & S. J., 1875, iii, 177.—**Lotzbeck** (C.) Beobachtungen über die Wiederkehr der Empfindung nach Nervendurchschneidungen am Menschen. [5 cases.] Deutsche Kli-

Neurotomy *and neurectomy*

nik, Berl., 1859, xi, 308; 317; 329.—**Macmurdo.** Severe neuralgia arrested by surgical operation. Lancet, Lond., 1852, ii, 83.—**Mantegazza** (P.) Di alcune alterazioni istologiche dei tessuti che tengono dietro al taglio dei nervi. Gazz. med. ital. lomb., Milano, 1865, 5. s., iv, 301. — **Marfels** (G.) Zur Durchschneidung des Nerv. trigeminus. Untersuch. z. Naturl. d. Mensch. u. d. Thiere, Frankf. a. M., 1857, ii, 214–221.—**Maury** (F. F.) & **Duhring** (L. A.) Case of exsection of the brachial plexus of nerves for the relief of painful neuroma of the skin. Am. J. M. Sc., Phila., 1874, n. s., lxviii, 29–37. *Also,* Reprint.—**Maydl** (C.) Ueber Durchschneidungen zweier Hauptnervenstämme der oberen Extremität. Wien. med. Bl., 1881, iv, 36; 71; 102; 137; 169; 203; 232; 264; 298. ——. Ueber isolirte Trennungen des Nervus ulnaris und über Naht derselben. *Ibid.,* 1272; 1305; 1331; 1359; 1393; 1423.— **Menzel** (A.) Die Resection des Unterkiefernerven vom Munde aus. Arch. f. klin. Chir., Berl., 1872, xiii, 668–677.— **Mesterton** (C. B.) Några fall af neurektomi vid ansigtsneuralgi. Upsala Läkaref. Förh., 1872, vii, 48–56.—**Mettauer** (J. P.) Neuralgia of the occipito-frontalis muscle; operation for its relief. Boston M. & S. J., 1870, lxxxiii, 17.—**Miner** (J. F.) Complete exsection of the median nerve, with restored sensibility; exsection of the musculospiral nerve with loss of both sensation and motion; division of the ulnar nerve; sensation and motion regained. Buffalo M. & S. J., 1867–8, vii, 427–430.—**Mitchell** (S. W.) Neurotomy. Phila. M. Times, 1873–4, iv, 145. ——. Traumatic neuralgia; section of median nerve. Am. J. M. Sc., Phila., 1874, n. s., lxviii, 17–29. ——. Neurotomy; with an examination of the regenerated nerves, and notes upon neural repair, by R. M. Bertolet. Am. J. M. Sc., Phila., 1876, n. s., lxxi, 321–334. *Also,* Reprint. ——. Some of the lessons of neurotomy. Brain, Lond., 1878. i, 287 – 303. — **Morton** (T. G.) Cases of excision of the supra- and infra-orbital branches of the trifacial, of the perineal, external popliteal, and posterior tibial nerves, etc. Am. J. M. Sc., Phila., 1873, n. s., lxvi, 392–401. ——. Excision of a portion of the popliteal nerve for gunshot wound, with nerve-suture. Phila. M. Times 1883–4, xiv, 465.—**Müller.** Neuralgischer Schmerz in der Schläfe, geheilt durch Nervendurchschneidung. Cor.-Bl. f. d. Aerzte u. Apoth. d. Grossherz. Oldenburg, 1862–3, ii, 31–33.—**Nasse.** Ueber die Veränderungen der Nervenfasern nach ihrer Durchschneidung. Arch f. Anat., Physiol. u. wissensch. Med., Berl., 1839, 405–419.—**Nelson** (T.) Case of wounded nerve, cured by freely dividing it. N. York M. & Phys. J., 1824, iii, 62–64.—**Notta.** Névrome du nerf median; résection du nerf; troubles trophiques; guérison. Bull. et mém. Soc. de chir. de Par., 1876, n. s., ii, 735–745.—**Obalinski.** Naciaganie nerwów (neurotomia). Przegl. lek., Krakow., 1881, xx, 545; 562; 580. ——. Przecięcie lub wycięcie kawałka nerwów (neurotomia et neurectomia). *Ibid.,* 593–595.—**Packard** (J. H.) Cases of nerve irritation; cured by surgical operations. Am. J. M. Sc., Phila., 1870, n. s., lix, 347–350. — **Panas** (F.) De la section du nerf buccal par la bouche; règles opératoires à suivre; opération chez une femme. Arch. gén. de méd., Par., 1874, i, 181–189. *Also:* Gaz. d. hôp., Par., 1874, xlvii, 12. — **Pavloff** (E. V.) Sluchai resektsii seredinnago nerva pri razvivsheisja v nem opucholi. [Resection of median nerve in removing a lipoma fibrosum (of hand).] Vrach, St. Petersb., 1883, iv, 673; 691 — **Perkovski** (S. P.) Pererezka vietvi nerva "auriculo - temporalis". Voyenno-med. J., St. Petersb., 1883, cxlvii, pt. 3, 17–20.—**Philipeaux** (J.-M.) & **Vulpian** (A.) Note sur des expériences démontrant que des nerfs séparés des centres nerveux peuvent, après d'être altérés complètement, se régénérer tout en demeurant isolés de centres et recouvrer leurs propriétés physiologiques. Compt rend. Soc. de biol. 1859, Par., 1860, 3. s., i, 177–181.—**Porter.** Section of the ulnar nerve, after which a felon on the little finger caused no pain. Boston M. & S. J., 1871, lxxxv, 240.—**Post** (A. C.) Division of the dorsal branch of the musculo-spiral nerve for severe and prolonged neuralgia. etc. N. York M. J., 1867, iv, 292–294.—**Prewitt** (T. F.) Case of excision of the infraorbital nerve by Wagner's method. Tr. M. Ass. Missouri, St. Louis, 1876, x, 6–8. ——. Neurodectomy and nerve stretching. St. Louis M. & S. J., 1880, xxxviii, 112–117. ——. Resection of the infra-orbital nerve. Proc. St. Louis M. Soc. Missouri (1880), 1881, iii, 27–32.—**Prompt.** Remarques sur une neurotomie du nerf médian. Nice-méd., 1882–3, vii, 113–116.— **Ranvier.** De la dégénérescence et de la régénération des nerfs sectionnés. Compt. rend. Soc. de biol. 1873, Par., 1874, 5. s., v, 63–73.—**Redard.** Suites éloignées de la section du nerf cubital. Assoc. franç. pour l'avance. d. sc. Compt.-rend. 1882, Par., 1883, xi, 763–765. — **Riberi** (A.) Caso di neuralgia stata guarita con incisioni sottocutanee. Gior. . . . . d. Soc. med.-chir. di Torino, 1842, xv, 444 – 448. *Also, in his:* Raccolta d. opere minori, etc., 8°, Torino, 1852, ii, 134–139. ——. Note sur l'innervation collatérale à propos d'une résection du nerf médian. Bull. et mém. Soc. de chir. de Par., 1883, n. s., ix, 438–457. *Also:* Union méd., Par., 1883, 3. s., xxxv, 922 – 927. — **Richet.** Section du nerf médian; conservation de la sensibilité de la main. Union méd., Par.,

Neurotomy *and neurectomy.*

1867, 3. s., iv, 444-449.—**Rozengarten** (M.) Vitjajenie sedalitsh-nerva v meste perechoda ego cherez bolshuju sedalitshnuju diru. [Neurectomy in ischiatic region.] Vrach. St. Petersb., 1885, vi, 358.—**Saltzman** (F.) Ett fall af resektion af nervus buccinatorius från munhålan. Finska läk.-sällsk. handl., Helsingfors, 1881, xxiii, 426-429. *Also:* Nord. med. Ark., Stockholm, 1882, xiv, no. 2, 6-14.—**Salzer** (T.) Resektion des dritten Trigeminusastes am Foramen ovale. Wien. med. Wchnschr., 1887, xxxvii, 461-463.—**Sands** (H. B.) Division of the gustatory nerves. Med. Rec., N. Y., 1880, xvii, 704. — **Sands** (H. B.) & **Seguin** (E. C.) A case of traumatic brachial neuralgia treated by excision of the cords which go to form the brachial plexus. Arch. Scient. & Pract. M. & S., N. Y., 1873, i, 1-18, 1 pl. *Also,* Reprint. — **Santos Fernandez** (J.) Neurotomia de los nervios frontales. Crón. méd.-quir. de la Habana, 1881, vii, 359.—**Schramm** (H.) Przypadek zeszycia nerwów w 3 miesiące po zranieniu. [Section of nerve three months after wound.] Przegl. lek., Krakow, 1883, xxii, 269-271.—**Schuh.** Mittheilungen über Resectionen und andere Operationen an Nerven. Wien. med. Wchnschr., 1863, xiii, 1; 17; 33; 49; 65; 129; 145; 161. ———. Wiederholte Nervenresektionen wegen einer hypertrophischen Narbe am Nervus radialis. Wien. Med.-Halle, 1863, iv, 1; 18; 29. — **af Schultén.** Resektion à nervus inframaxillaris sinister. Finska läk.-sällsk. handl., Helsingfors, 1881, xxiii, 280.—**Schulz** (H.) Ueber den Einfluss der Nervendurchschneidung auf Ernährung und Regeneration der Gewebe. Centralbl. f. d. med. Wissensch., Berl., 1873, xi, 708-710.—**Sée.** Excision de 15 centimètres du nerf sciatique poplité interne; guérison. Bull. et mém. Soc. de chir. de Par., 1881, n. s., vii, 531.—**Setschenoff** (I.) Pereraizka nerva kak uslovie narostaniya ego razdrazhitelnosti. [Severance of a nerve, as a means of increasing its irritability.] Med. Vestnik, St. Petersb., 1861, i, 301; 313.—**Sherriffs** (E. B.) New method of dividing the facial nerve. Lancet, Lond., 1831-2, i, 632.—**Simon.** Neuroplastische Resection am N. medianus und N. ulnaris. Deutsche Ztschr. f. prakt. Med., Leipz., 1876, iii, 287-290.—**Sirena** (S.) Analogie e differenze fra i risultati ottenuti dai professori Ranvier, Colasanti, Tizzoni e Sirena nella recisione dei nervi. Gior. internaz. d. sc. med., Napoli, 1882 n. s., iv, 113-135.—**Sonnenburg.** Einige Bemerkungen zur Neurektomie des dritten Astes des Trigeminus. Centralbl. f. Chir., Leipz., 1886, xiii, 305.—**Sperino** (C.) Neuralgia grave di molti rami del plesso cervicale-destro, guarita colla neuro-miotomia sottocutanea. Gior. . . . d. Soc. med.-chir. di Torino, 1842, xv, 144-151.—**Stewart** (J. L.) Excision of three inches of median nerve after an old gun-shot wound of left elbow. Med. & Surg. Reporter, Phila., 1871, xxiv, 92-94. *Also:* Tr. M. Soc. Penn., Phila., 1873, ix, pt. 2, 62-64.—**Sticker** (L.) Ueber die Veränderungen der Kräfte durchschnittener Nerven und über Muskelreizbarkeit. Arch. f. Anat., Physiol. u. wissensch. Med., Berl., 1834, 202-217.—**Storrs** (M.) Neurectomy of the tri-facial nerve. Proc. Connect. M. Soc., Hartford, 1887, n. s., iii, 78-86.—**Sutton** (J. B.) A case of neurotomy of the third division of the fifth nerve at the foramen ovale. Brit. M. J., Lond., 1887, ii, 1331.—**Szeparowicz** (J.) Mięsak nerwu środkowego (nerv. medianus); wycięcie nowotworu wraz z tętnicą ramieniową i kawalkiem nerwu 10 cm. dlugim bez nastlpowego uposledzenia czucia. [Extirpation of median nerve by removing tumor in brachial branch, 10 cm. long.] Przegl. lek., Krakow., 1877, xvi, 505-507.—**Szymanowski.** Ueber Neurektomie und Nervennaht. Vrtljschr. f. d. prakt. Heilk., Prag, 1865, lxxxviii, 52-71.—**Tillaux.** Blépharoplastie; traitement inefficace pendant trois mois; section sous-cutanée des deux nerfs susorbitaires; guérison. Bull. gén. de thérap., etc., Par., 1872, lxxxiii, 129-133. ——— Phénomènes curieux observés à la suite d'une section du nerf médian. Gaz. d. hôp., Par., 1885, lviii, 561-563.—**Tillmanns** (H.) Ausschneidung des Nervus alveolaris inferior vom Kieferwinkel aus bei herabhängendem Kopfe. Centralbl. f. Chir., Leipz., 1879, vi, 481-483.—**Tripier** (L.) Névrotomie. Dict. encycl. d. sc. méd., Par., 1878, 2. s., xii, 768-789.—**Valentin** (G.) Einige Folgen der Nervendurchschneidung. Ztschr. f. rat. Med., Leipz., 1861, 3. R., xi, 1-88.—**Vance** (Ap M.) Neurectomy of anterior tibial for cure of chronic neuritis; achillotomy at same time to relieve a resulting club-foot. Med. News, Phila., 1883, xlii, 440.—**von Vering** (J.) Schmerzhafter Nervenkrampf durch Zerschneidung des Nerven geheilt. Med.-chir. Ztg., Salzb., 1819, iii, 239.—**Vigezzi.** Di un nuovo processo operativo per praticare la nevrectomia plantare. Gior. di anat., fisiol. e patol. d. animali, Pisa, 1887, xix, 121-126.—**von Vintschgau** (M.) Beobachtungen über die Veränderungen der Schmeckbecher nach Durchschneidung des N. glossopharyngeus. Arch. f. d. ges. Physiol., Bonn, 1880-81, xxiii, 1-13, 1 pl.—**Vulpian** (A.) Nécrose consécutive à la section du nerf sciatique. Compt. rend. Soc. de biol. 1849, Par., 1850, i, 75. ——— Sur les modifications que subissent les muscles sous l'influence de la section de leurs nerfs. Arch. de physiol. norm. et path., Par., 1869, ii, 558-578. ——— Sur les modifications qui se produisent dans la moelle épinière sous l'influence de la section des nerfs d'un membre. *Ibid.*,

Neurotomy *and neurectomy.*

675-692. ———. Altération graisseuse des artérioles du bout périphérique des nerfs coupés, observée dans certains cas. *Ibid.*, 1870, iii, 178.—**Warren** (J. C.) Neuralgia of a branch of the plantar nerve, followed by convulsions, and cured by operation. Boston M. & S. J., 1829-30, ii, pt. 1, 116-118. ———. Neuralgic operations. Am. J. M. Sc., Phila., 1853, n. s., xxvi, 88. ———. Neuralgia; excision of the digital nerve of the forefinger. *In his:* Surg. Obs., Bost., 1867, 475.—**Webber.** (Section of the ulnar nerve.) Boston M. & S. J., 1879, c, 330. — **Weinlechner** (J.) Neuralgia inframaxillaris; Neurectomie nach der inwendige Methode Paravicini's; Anfangs misslungen wegen erschwerten Auffindens und Zerfaserung des Nervus inframaxillaris selbst oder des Nervus buccinatorius; schliessliche Excision eines 1 Cm. 1 Mm. langen Stückes; Heilung. Ber. d. k. k. Krankenanst. Rudolph-Stiftung in Wien (1873), 1874, 255. ———. Zur Statistik der Nervenresektionen. Wien. med. Presse, 1877, xviii, 116. ———. Eine Frau, bei welcher W. die intrabuccale Resection des N. inframaxillaris vornahm. Anz. d. k. k. Gesellsch. d. Aerzte in Wien, 1878, 23.—**Weir** (R. F.) Intra-buccal division of the inferior maxillary nerve. N. York M. J., 1887, xlv, 282. *Also:* Ann. Surg., St. Louis, 1887, v, 504.—**Wertheimer.** Section du nerf cubital; griffe; retour partiel de la sensibilité; névrome du bout central. Bull. méd. du nord, Lille, 1881, xx, 76-81.—**Wood** (J. R.) Clinical lecture on neurotomy. Med. Rec., N. Y., 1871-2, vi, 485.—**Zeissl** (M.) Die Resektion des Nervus ethmoidalis. Wien. med. Presse, 1881, xxii, 1093-1095.

Neurotomy (*Optico-ciliary*).
See **Eye** (*Neurotomy of*).

Neurrisse (Émile). * Contribution à l'étude de la dothiénentérie chez les enfants. 73 pp., 1 l. 4°. *Paris*, 1882, No. 239.

Neu-Ruppin.
See **Insane** (*Asylums for, etc.*), *by localities*.

Neuschler (Edmund). * Beitrag zur Kenntniss der einfachen und der zuckerführenden Harnruhr. 37 pp., 3 tab. 8°. *Tübingen*, 1861.

Neu-Schmecks.
von SZONTAGH (N.) Neu-Tátrafüred. (Bad Neu-Schmecks.) Klimatologische und therapeutische Studie. 8°. *Budapest*, 1877.

Neu-Schöneberg.
See **Hospitals** (*Descriptions, etc., of*), *by localities.*

Neuschüler (Ignazio). Occhio ed occhiali. Trattato popolare. 104 pp. 8°. *Torino, Roux & Favale*, 1883.

Neuse (Joh. Georgius). * De melancholia. 40 pp. sm. 4°. *Jenæ, lit. Krebsianis*, [1685].

Neusen (Abraham).
See **Hwasser** (Israël). * Om primära syphilitiska [etc.] 8°. *Upsala*, 1848.

Neuss (Carol. Guil. Ed.) * De imputabilitate. 44 pp. 8°. *Gottingæ, Dieterich*, [1831].

Neuss (Heinrich) [1855–   ]. * Ueber subkutane Eiseninjectionen. 30 pp., 1 l. 8°. *Greifswald, C. Sell*, 1881.

Neuss (Joannes Henricus Godofredus). * De perforatione membranæ tympani. 21 pp., 1 pl. 4°. *Gottingæ, lit. Grapianis*, [1802].

Neuss.
See, also, **Fever** (*Typhoid, History, etc., of*), **Insane** (*Asylums for, etc.*), *by localities.*
Mortalitäts-Statistik der Gemeinde Neuss, 1871-4. Cor.-Bl. d. nied.-rhein. Ver. f. öff. Gsndhtspflg., Köln, 1873, ii, 151: 1876, v, 24.

Neussel (Julius). * Ueber die sogennante Addison'sche Krankheit. 36 pp. 8°. *Würzburg, C. J. Becker*, 1859.

Neusser (Edmund). Die Pellagra in Österreich und Rumänien. 52 pp., 1 l. 8°. *Wien, A. Hölder*, 1887.

Neusser (Vinc. Thom.) * Conspectus mineralium ad paranda præparata mineralia inservientium. Classis IV^ta systematis Werneriani. 1 p. l., 60 pp. 8°. *Pragæ, J. Spurny*, 1833.

Neustadt (Karl). * Der puerperale Wundzustand und seine Bedeutung für die puerperale

Neustadt (Karl)—continued.
Infektion. 17 pp. 8°. *Würzburg, R. Scheiner,* 1885.

Neustadt (Ludovicus) [1802–]. *De abscessu frigido scrofuloso. 24 pp. 8°. *Berolini, typ. G. C. Nauckii,* 1826.

Neustadt.
Gauster (M.) Die sanitäre Bedeutung der Neustädter Tiefquellenleitung. Oesterr. ärztl. Vereinsztg., Wien, 1884, viii, 367; 388.—**Truchsess.** Das Bad Neustadt bei Waiblingen. Med. Cor.-Bl. d. württemb. ärztl. Ver., Stuttg., 1839, ix, 228–232.

Neustadt-Eberswalde.
See **Insane** (*Asylums for, etc.*), *by localities.*

Neustadtl (Jacobus). *De scleritide rhumatica. 61 pp. 8°. *Pragæ, J. H. Pospjšil,* [1831].

Neustadtl (Mauritius). *Diss. sistens historiam enteritidis serosæ in puerpera. 38 pp., 1 l. 8°. *Pragæ, M. I. Laudau,* 1840.

Neu-verbessert- und vermehrtes denckwürdiges Kayser Carls-Baad. Das ist: Alt, als neue Denckwürdigkeiten in drey Theil abgetheilet. Erster Theil. Von dessen Erfind-, Erbauung, etc., Unglücksfällen und Erweiterung, Bequem und Ergötzlichkeiten, etc. Anderer Theil. Von dess Heyl- und Gesund-Baades, selbst Nutz- und Cur-Gebrauchs, etc. Dritter Theil. Anmerckung hoher Häupter, geist- als weltlicher Standes-Persohnen, so ab Anno 1701 biss 1731, diese Baades-Cur zu höchstrühmlich- und ersprisslicher Gesundheits-Wohlfahrt gebraucht. 3 Theile in 1 v. 110 pp., 3 l. 16°. *Carls-Baad, A. B. Dexter,* 1731.

———. The same. Anno 1701 biss 1733. 122 pp., 3 l., 1 pl. 16°. *Nürnberg, J. Albrecht,* 1734.

———. The same. 122 pp., 3 l., 1 pl. 16°. *Nürnberg, J. Albrecht,* 1736.

Neu-vermehrtes und verbessertes Aderlass-Buchlein, dass ist: ein astronomischer Grund und Bericht vom Aderlassen, Schrepffen und Baden zu Erhaltung menschlicher Gesundheit und Verlängerung dess Lebens, bis zu seinem von Gott und der Natur bestimten Tod und Ende desselbigen. Allen und jeden Menschen nicht allein sehr nützlich zu lesen sondern auch höchst nothwendig zu wissen. 144 pp., 4 l., 1 tab. 16°. *Nürnberg, J. A. u. W. Endter,* [*n. d.*]

Neuville. Relation sur le choléra-morbus observé à Paris, dans le mois d'avril 1832, suivie d'un rapport sur l'épidémie cholérique, qui a régné dans l'arrondissement de Bernay (Eure) depuis le 29 avril jusqu'au 27 septembre 1832. 116 pp. 8°. *Paris, Béchet jeune,* 1832.

Neuville (Jean-Edmond). *Des causes de la rétention d'urine. 32 pp. 4°. *Paris,* 1866, No. 76.

Neuville-sur-Saône.
Henry (O.) Analyse chimique de l'eau minérale ferrugineuse de Neuville-sur-Saône, près Lyon. Bull. Acad. de méd., Par., 1859–60, xxv, 730–733.

Neuvirth (Aug. I. N.) *Salium acidorum origo, natura, ac combinatio in sales medios, vel præparata. 2 p. l., 45 pp., 1 l. 8°. *Viennæ, M. A. Schmidt,* [1782].

Neuwied.
Bernstein (J. T. C.) Skizze einer medizinischen Topographie in Neuwied und der Behandlung der daselbst herrschenden Krankheiten. *In his:* Kleine med. Aufs., 8°, Frankf. a. M., 1814, 1–59.

Neva.
Galanin (M. I.) Goden-li tsentralnyi pesochnyi filtre dlja Nevskoi vody? [Shall we any longer delay erecting the central filtering apparatus for the waters of the Neva?] 8°. *St. Petersburg,* 1887.

Nevada. Report of the surveyor-general and State land register of the State of Nevada for the years 1881 and 1882. 77 pp. 8°. *Carson City, State Office,* 1883.

Nevada.
See, *also,* **Fort Churchill.**
Hoffman (W. J.) On the mineralogy of Nevada. 8°. *Washington,* 1878.
Extr. from: Bull. U. S. Geol. Survey of the Territories, v. 4, no. 3, under charge F. V. Hayden.

PRELIMINARY report concerning explorations and surveys principally in Nevada and Arizona. . . . Conducted under the immediate direction of Lieut. Geo. M. Wheeler. 4°. *Washington,* 1872.

PRELIMINARY report upon a reconnaissance through Southern and Southeastern Nevada, made in 1869, by Geo. M. Wheeler, Corps of Engineers, assisted by Lieut. D. W. Lockwood, U. S. Army, under the orders of Brig. Gen'l E. O. C. Ord. 4°. *Washington,* 1875.

de Neve (Christianus). *De variolis. 1 p. l., 23 pp. 4°. *Traj. ad Rhenum, J. Broedelet,* [1768].

Nève (Pierre-Louis). *Sur la phlébite. 28 pp. 4°. *Paris,* 1734, No. 11, v. 269.

Nevermann (John Friedrich Wilhelm) [1803–1850]. *De mammarum morbis curandis. 111 pp. 8°. *Rostochii, typ. Adlerianis,* 1831.

———. Bedenkingen en mededeelingen aangaande de oogspierdoorsnijding (myotomia ocularis), ter verhelping van het scheelzien. xvi, 77 pp., 1 l. 8°. *Amsterdam, C. G. van der Post,* 1845.
See, *also,* **Bang** (Olaus Lundt). Die medicinische Klinik des königl. Frederiks-Hospital zu Kopenhagen, [etc.] 8°. *Stuttgart,* 1851. — **Duparcque** (F.) Vollständige Geschichte der Durchlöcherungen, Einrisse und Zerreissungen des Uterus, etc. 8°. *Quedlinburg u. Leipzig,* 1838.

das Neves (Alexandre Antonio). Compilação de reflexões de Sanches, Pringle, Monro, Van-Swieten, e outros a' cerca das causas, prevenções, e remedios das doenças dos exercitos. xiv, 82 pp., 2 l. 16°. *Lisboa,* 1797.

Nevet (X.) *De la fréquence relative des différentes variétés de chancres syphilitiques extra-génitaux chez l'homme et chez la femme, suivie de quelques considérations sur un certain nombre de cas observés à l'Hôpital Saint-Louis pendant l'année 1886. 91 pp. 4°. *Paris,* 1887, No. 205.

Neveu (Joseph). *Incontinence d'urine et son traitement. 36 pp. 4°. *Paris,* 1880, No. 215.

Neveu-Derotrie (V.) *De l'abus des liqueurs alcooliques. 34 pp. 4°. *Paris,* 1865, No. 102, v. 594.

Neveur (Auguste-Similien). *Du cancer aigu. 74 pp. 4°. *Paris,* 1871, No. 28.

Névière (Joseph-Victor). *Essai sur les hernies abdominales. 28 pp. 4°. *Montpellier, J. Martel aîné,* 1814.

Nevière (Maurice). *De l'insolation considérée dans son rôle étiologique. 1 p. l., 26 pp. 4°. *Strasbourg,* 1863, No. 675, v. 35.

Nevile (Georgius). *De intestini recti strictura. 42 pp. 8°. *Heidelbergæ, O. A. Osswald,* 1843.

Nevil-Holt.
CONTENTS, virtues, and uses of Nevil-Holt Spaw-water, further proved, illustrated, and explained from experiments and reason, with some histories of its signal effects in various diseases, collected by several hands; also rules and directions for its more easy use and greater success. 2. ed. 8°. *London,* 1749.

Nevill (James). A description of the venereal gonorrhœa, accounting for the symptoms and cure of that disorder, in a new, easy, and rational manner; with remarks on the present practice, shewing the ill consequence of purging, mercurial preparations, injections, astringents, etc. 9 p. l., 115 pp. 8°. *London, R. Griffiths,* 1754.

Neville (Sylas). * De prognosi in febribus. 78 pp. 8°. *Edinburgi, Balfour et Smellie*, 1775.

Neville (William B.) On insanity; its nature, causes, and cure. xii, 192 pp. 8°. *London, Longman [and others]*, 1836.

Neville-Grenville (Ralph). Cottages. 3 pp. 8°. *London, W. Clowes & Sons*, 1875.
Repr. from: J. Bath & West. of Eng. Soc., 3. s., v.

Nevins (J. Birkbeck). Clinical enquiry into the results of "Hancock's operation", or the division of the ciliary muscle, in certain serious deep-seated affections of the eye. A paper communicated to the first volume of the Liverpool Medical and Surgical Reports. 11 pp. 8°. *Liverpool, D. Marples*, [1867]. [P., v. 1441.]

——. Statement of the grounds upon which the contagious diseases' acts are opposed. Addressed to the Right Hon. R. A. Cross, M. P., H. M. secretary of state for the home department, in accordance with his letter that the memorialists should furnish him with a written statement of the grounds upon which they desire the repeal of the acts; prepared at the request of the Liverpool committee of the association for promoting the repeal of the acts. 78 pp., 1 tab. 8°. *London, J. Churchill & Sons*, 1874.

——. The same. 3. ed. xvi, 87 pp., 1 ch. 8°. *London, J. Churchill & Sons*, 1875.
See, also, **Address** (An) to members of the American legislature, and of the medical profession, etc. 8°. *London*, 1877.—**Trousseau** & **Réveil.** The prescriber's complete handbook [etc.] 8°. *London*, 1852.

Nevins (Thomas). * De vermibus intestinorum. 28 pp. 8°. *Edinburgi, A. Neill et socii*, 1804, v. 30.

Nevinson (R. S.) Observations on the use of crude mercury, or quicksilver, in obstructions of the bowels arising from inflammations or other causes, with remarks on the use of castor oil. x, 50 pp. 8°. *Newark [Eng.], J. Tomlinson, [n. d.]*, v. 597.

Nevis (*Island of*).
See **Cholera** (*Asiatic, History, etc., of*), by localities.

Nevot (Louis). * De la perforation des vaisseaux par les corps étrangers de l'œsophage. 49 pp., 1 l. 4°. *Paris*, 1879, No. 81.

Nevski (Basil). * O vlijanii osmievoi kisloti na organizm jivotnich i terapevt. upotreblenii eja v deitskoi praktike. [Effect of osmic acid on the human organism, and its use in the treatment of children.] 84 pp., 1 l. 8°. *St. Petersburg*, 1885.

New (C. B.) Cholera. Observations on the management of cholera on plantations, and method of treating the disease, as practiced by . . . 8 pp. 8°. *Rodney, Miss., R. N. Fetherston'h & Co.*, [1850].

New (Joannes). * Quænam pars aëris communis corporis cavorum inflammationem concitat, et quo modo? 2 p. l., 34 pp. 8°. *Edinburgi, A. Neill cum sociis*, 1795.

New (The) Bath guide, or useful pocket companion for all persons residing at or resorting to this ancient city; giving an account of the first discovery of its medicinal waters by King Bladud; Saxon and Roman antiquities, nature and efficacy of the warm baths and sudatories; with the rules and prices of bathing and pumping, the virtues of the Bath waters used internally and externally . . . to which is added the life, character, etc., of Richard Nash, esq., who presided over the amusements of this city upwards of fifty years. New ed. 80 pp., 1 pl., 1 plan, 2 port. 16°. *Bath, R. Cruttwell*, 1801.

New (The) discoveries on the action of alcohol. 20 pp. 8°. *London, W. Clowes & Sons*, [1861].
Repr. from: Meliora, April, 1861.

New (The) dispensatory: containing, I. The theory and practice of pharmacy. II. A distribution of medicinal simples, according to their virtues and sensible qualities; the description, use, and dose of each article. III. A full translation of the London and Edinburgh pharmacopœias; with the use, dose, etc., of the several medicines. IV. Directions for extemporaneous prescription, with a select number of elegant forms. V. A collection of cheap remedies for the use of the poor; the whole interspersed with practical cautions and observations; intended as a correction and improvement of Quincy. vi pp., 3 l., xxxii, 664 pp. 8°. *London, J. Nourse*, 1753.

——. The same. I. The elements of pharmacy. II. The materia medica; or, an account of the substances employed in medicine; with the virtues and uses of each article, so far as they are warranted by experience and observation. III. The preparations and compositions of the New London and Edinburgh pharmacopœias, [etc.] 4. ed., by William Lewis. viii (2 l.), 692 pp. 8°. *Dublin, J. Potts*, 1778.

New (The) Doctor; a medical, philosophical, and literary magazine, and family journal of health. Edited by George Shipman. [Weekly.] v. 1, June 8, 1836, to June 14, 1837. 436 pp. 8°. *London, B. Steill.*

New (The) family physician, and guide to health and long life, with a variety of valuable tables on medical statistics; to which is now added an appendix, containing recipes for preparing the most celebrated patent medicines; with rational observations on longevity, founded on the principles of the late John Abernethy. 215 pp., port. 12°. *London, J. Smith, [n. d.]*

New *formations*.
See **Tumors.**

New General Lying-in Hospital. A short account of the institution, plan, and present state of the . . . in Store-street, Tottenham Court road. 16 pp. 8°. *London, J. Dixwell*, [1787].
Instituted 1767.

——. A short account of the institution, plan, and present state of the . . . for the reception of pregnant women, and for delivery of poor women at their own habitations. 2 pp. fol. [*London*, 1789?]

New Hospital for Women, London, N. W. Annual reports of the managing committee to the subscribers. 8., 1879; 12., 1883; 13., 1884. 8°. *London*, 1880–85.
Established as a dispensary in 1866. Opened as a hospital 1872.

New (A) idea. Stearns' popular non-secret medicines. A monthly journal of true pharmacy in opposition to quackery in pharmacy. v. 7–9, 1885–8. 4 v. 4°. *Detroit, F. Stearns & Co.*
Current. An advertisement.

New (The) Illustrated Hydropathic Quarterly Review. Title, on covers, of: **Illustrated** (The) Hydropathic Review.

New Infirmary, Leeds. *See* **General** Infirmary, Leeds.

New instruments. A bulletin of inventions and improvements of interest to the physician and surgeon. Published quarterly by Leach & Green. Number for April, 1887. fol. *Boston.*

New (The) Irish bath versus the old Turkish; or, pure air versus vapour. Being an answer to the errors and mis-statements of Drs. Madden and Corrigan. Edited by Photophilus. 46 pp. 8°. *Dublin, W. McGee*, 1860.

New (The) London Medical Journal. v. 1–2, 1792–3. 8°. *London.*

New (The) London medical, pharmaceutical, and posological pocket-book (alphabetically arranged); explaining the causes, symptoms, and

New (The) London medical [etc.]—continued.
treatment; diagnostic and prognostic signs of
diseases; the natural and chemical characters,
medicinal properties and uses; doses and forms
of exhibition; incompatibles, adulterations, and
officinal preparations of the various substances,
vegetable and mineral, contained in the pharmacopœias [etc.] xxiv, 443 pp., 1 pl. 12°.
London, Sherwood, Gilbert & Piper, 1844.

New (The) Medical Era and Sanitarian. A. L.
Chapman, editor. [Monthly.] v. 1; No. 1, v. 2,
Jan., 1883, to Jan., 1884. 8°. *Kansas City, Mo.*
 In February, 1884, united with: **Kansas** (The) and
 Missouri Valley Medical Index, forming: **Medical** (The)
 Index.

New Medical and Physical Journal; or, annals of
medicine, natural history, and chemistry. Conducted by T. Bradley and William Shearman.
[Monthly; 2 v. annually.] v. 1–5, Nov., 1810, to
June, 1813. 8°. *London.*
 An offshoot from: **Medical** (The) and Physical Journal. v. 1 complete in 6 nos., Nov., 1810, to April, 1811; v.
 2 complete in 8 nos., May to Dec., 1811; v. 3 commenced
 Jan., 1812.

New Medicines: a monthly journal of progressive
medicine. Ferdinand King, editor and proprietor; L. G. Alexander, associate editor. Nos.
1–5, v. 1, April to August, 1878. 146 pp. 8°.
Atlanta, Ga.

New (The) medico-chirurgical pharmacopœia;
being a selection of modern formulæ from the
private and hospital practice of the most eminent members of the profession, in Europe and
America. For the use of surgeons and surgeons-
apothecaries. By a graduate of a Scotch university. 4. ed. xii, 180 pp. 12°. *London, W.
Simpkin & R. Marshall,* 1827.

New (A) method for the improvement of the manufacture of drugs; in a treatise on the elixir
proprietatis. ii, 80 pp. 8°. *London, C. Davis,* 1747.
——. The same. 80 pp. 8°. *London, C. Davis,*
1748. [P., v. 1335.]
 Manuscript note on title-page says: "By H. Barton,
 apothecary in Dublin".

New (A) and needful treatise of wind offending
man's body. *See* **R**[**owland**] (W.)

New Orphan Houses (for 2,050 children), on Ashley Down, Bristol. Brief narrative of facts relative to the . . . and the other objects of
the Scriptural Knowledge Institution for Home
and Abroad. By George Müller (being the reports of the institution). 23., 1861–2; 24., 1862–3;
36.–45., 1874–5 to 1882–3. 8°. *London,* 1862–83.

New Pennsylvania Hospital for the Insane, Philadelphia. *See* **Pennsylvania** Hospital for the
Insane, Philadelphia.

New (The) practice of inoculating the small-pox
consider'd, and an humble application to the approaching parliament for the regulation of that
dangerous experiment. 40 pp. 8°. *London, T.
Crouch,* 1722. [P., v. 964.]

New Preparations; a quarterly journal of medicine, devoted to the introduction of new therapeutical agents. Edited by George S. Davis
and C. Henri Leonard. v. 1–3, 1877–9. 8°. *Detroit.*
 In 1879, v. 3 became monthly; edited by William Brodie.
 Continued as: **Therapeutic** (The) Gazette.

New Remedies. A quarterly retrospect of therapeutics, pharmacy, and allied subjects. Edited
by Horatio C. Wood, jr. v. 1–12, July, 1871, to
Dec., 1883. 8°. *New York, W. Wood & Co.*
 v. 2 complete in 6 nos., July, 1872, to Oct., 1873; v. 3 began Jan., 1874. v. 3–4 edited by Fred. A. Castle; in v. 5
 Charles Rice added. In v. 5 became monthly. Continued
 as: **American** Druggist.

New (A) remedy for the ring-worm. [External
application of castor oil. Suggested by a Parsee
boy.] 1 broadside. 8°. [*n. p., n. d.*]
 Another copy bound with: Review of Dr. Kennedy's
 notes, etc. 8°. *London,* 1828.

55

New Rupture Society. Instituted May 15, 1804,
under the patronage of H. R. H. the Duke of
York, for the relief of both sexes afflicted with
herniary complaints and prolapses. Regulations
of the . . . including a list of its governors, members, and officers, with a short account of the
present state of this institution. 32 pp. 8°.
London, S. Gosnell, 1812.

New (A) system of the gout and rheumatism.
Drawn from reason, anatomical observations,
and experience. By the author of the Practical
scheme. 48 pp. 16°. *London, H. Parker,* 1718.

New (The) test act. *See* **Alumnus** (An).

New (A) theory of continual fevers, wherein, besides the appearances of such fevers and the
method of their cure, occasionally, the structure
of the glands, and the manner of secretion, the
operation of purgative, vomitive, and mercurial
medicines are mechanically explain'd. 3 p. l.,
123 pp. 16°. *London, H. Newman,* 1701.
——. The same. To which is prefixed, an essay concerning the improvement of the theory of
medicine. 3. ed. 3 p. l., 168 pp. 8°. *London,
H. Parker,* 1722.
——. The same. 6. ed. vi, 150 pp., 1 l. 8°.
London, G. Strahan, 1744.

New (A) theory of population; deduced from the
general law of animal fertility. With an introduction by R. T. Thrall. iv, 44 pp. 12°. *New
York, Fowler & Wells,* 1853.
 Repr. from: Westminster Review, 1852.

New Town Dispensary, Edinburgh. Observations
by the managers of the . . . on the report to the
quarterly meeting of managers of the public dispensary, 7th August, 1817. iv, 6–24 pp. 8°.
Edinburgh, Caledonian Mercury Press, 1817. [P.,
v. 1171.]

New and valuable apparatus for vapor baths.
16 pp. 8°. [*New York,* 1882.]

New Albany.
See **Cholera** (*Asiatic, History, etc., of*), *by localities.*

New Archangel.
BLASCHKE (E.) Topographia medica portus
Novi-Archangelscensis, sedis principalis colonia-
rum roussicarum in septentrionali America. 8°.
Petropoli, 1842.

Newark, N. J. Annual reports of the health
physician, together with the reports of the district physicians, to the board of health for the
years 1858–62. 8°. *Newark,* 1859–63.
 1858, 1860, and 1862, *also, in:* P., v. 354.
——. Reports of deaths in Newark. [Weekly.]
Dec. 8, 1883, to Oct. 4, 1884; Oct. 18, 25; Nov. 8,
15, 29 to Dec. 27, 1884. 18°. [*Newark,* 1883–4.]

Newark.
See, also, **Cholera** (*Asiatic, History, etc., of*),
Hospitals (*Descriptions, etc., of*), **Hospitals**
(*Ophthalmic, etc.*), *by localities.*
 Clark (J. H.) The medical topography of Newark,
 New Jersey. Tr. M. Soc. N. Jersey. N. Y., 1861, 45–67.—
 Grant (G.) Annual report of the statistician of the New-
 ark Medical Association, for the year ending December 31,
 1858. *Ibid.,* Newark, 1859, 84–95.—**Leeds** (A. R.) The
 monstrous pollution of the water supply of Jersey City and
 Newark. J. Am. Chem. Soc., N. Y., 1887, ix, 81–97, 1 pl.—
 Southard (L.) Essex water supply; drainage and sewerage of the city of Newark, and their relation to the causation of disease; the president's annual address to the Essex
 District Medical Society. Tr. M. Soc. N. Jersey, Newark,
 1877, 192–200.—**Whitehead** (W. A.) Minimum, maximum, and mean temperature at Newark, N. J., for years
 1844 to 1880, inclusive. Rep. Bd. Health N. Jersey 1880,
 Camden, 1881, iv, 195–207.

Newark. *Board of Health.* Annual reports of
the board of health. [By the chief health inspector to the board.] 1., 1885; 2., 1886. 47 pp.;
49 pp., 6 l. 8°. *Newark,* 1886–7.
 Reorganized May 27, 1885.

Newark. *Board of Health of the City of Newark, N. J.* Annual report to the mayor and city council, for the year 1882. 13 pp., 1 l. 8°. *Newark, Grover Bros.*, 1883.

Newark. *Department of Health.* Condensed statements of vital statistics of the city of Newark, N. J. [Monthly.] March, 1886, to May, 1888. 4°. *Newark*, 1886-8.

Newark. *Newark Aqueduct Board.* Annual report of the . . . by the superintendent and secretary, for the year 1881-2. 1 diag., 118 pp. 8°. *Newark, H. B. Thistle*, 1883.

Newark Charitable Eye and Ear Infirmary. Annual reports of the trustees and surgeons to the subscribers and the public. 1.-8., 1880-87. 8°. *Newark*, 1881-8.
Incorporated Jan. 31, 1880.

Newark Industrial Exhibition. Report and catalogue of the first exhibition of Newark industries. 74 pp. 8°. *Newark, Holbrook's steam printery*, 1872.

Newark Medical Association. Statement in reference to a diploma granted by the New York Medical College. Presented to the American Medical Association, May 4, 1858. 13 pp. 8°. *Newark, N. J., Newark Mercury Office*, 1858.

Newarker deutsches Hospital. Jahresberichte des Direktoriums und ärztlichen Collegiums für die Jahre 1871-2 bis 1873-4; 1877-8. 8°. *Newark*, 1872-8.

New Bedford. *Board of Health of the City of New Bedford, Mass.* Annual reports to the city council. 1.-3., 1879-81. 8°. *New Bedford*, 1880-82.

New-Berne, *North Carolina.*
See **Fever** (*Cerebro-spinal, History, etc., of*), **Fever** (*Malarial, History, etc., of*), by localities.

Newberry, *South Carolina.*
Report of the medical committee on the endemic diseases of Newberry, read before the Newberry (S. C.) Agricultural Society. Charlestown M. J., 1852, vii, 791-799.

Newberry (J. S.) Catalogue of the flowering plants and ferns of Ohio. 41 pp. 8°. *Columbus, R. Nevins*, 1860.
Repr. from: Ohio Agricultural Report for 1859.

——. Report on the state-house well. 11 pp. 8°. [*Columbus*, 1860.]
Repr. from: Rep. of Supt. of state-house for 1860.

——. Report on the condition of the troops, and the operations of the Sanitary Commission in the valley of the Mississippi, for the three months ending Nov. 30, 1861. 48 pp. 8°. *Cleveland, Fairbanks, Benedict & Co.*, 1861.
No. 36, U. S. San. Com. documents, 1861-5.

——. Report on the sanitary condition of the U. S. troops in the Mississippi valley, during the month of Aug., 1861. 11 pp. 8°. [*n. p.*, 1861.]
No. 27, U. S. San. Com. documents, 1861-5.

——. A visit to Fort Donelson, Tenn., for the relief of the wounded of Feb. 15, 1862. A letter by . . . 10 pp. 8°. [*n. p.*, 1862.]
No. 42, U. S. San. Com. documents, 1861-5.

——. Report on the operations of the U. S. Sanitary Commission in the valley of the Mississippi, made Sept. 1, 1863. 24 pp. 8°. [*n. p.*, 1863.]
No. 75, U. S. San. Com. documents, 1861-5.

——. What the U. S. Sanitary Commission is doing in the valley of the Mississippi. Letter from . . . to W. P. Sprague. Louisville, Feb. 16, 1863. 2. ed. 31 pp. 8°. [*Washington*, 1863.]
No. 64, U. S. San. Com. documents, 1861-5.

——. Circular from the sanitary reporter. A mistake corrected. [Being a true statement of the expenditures, to correct a false one circulated by enemies of the commission.] Louisville,

Newberry (J. S.)—continued.
Dec. 1, 1864. 1 broadside. 8°. [*Louisville*, 1864.]

——. Report on the operations of the U. S. Sanitary Commission in the valley of the Mississippi for the quarter ending Oct. 1, 1864. Louisville, Oct. 22, 1864. 29 pp. 8°. [*New York*, 1864.]
No. 84, U. S. San. Com. documents, 1861-5.

——. Modern scientific investigation; its methods and tendencies; an address delivered before the American Association for the Advancement of Science, August, 1867. 23 pp. 8°. *Salem*, 1867.
Repr. from: Am. Naturalist, Salem, 1867, i.

——. Sanitary Commission No. 96. The U. S. Sanitary Commission in the valley of the Mississippi during the war of the rebellion, 1861-6. (Final report.) 543 pp. 8°. *Cleveland, Fairbanks, Benedict & Co.*, 1871.

——. The geological history of New York island and harbor. 20 pp. 8°. *New York, D. Appleton & Co.*, 1878.

Newbigging (George Stewart). *A probationary essay on some circumstances to be considered in resorting to the operation of bronchotomy. 59 pp. 8°. *Edinburgh, Balfour & Jack*, 1837. [*Also, in:* P., v. 95; 1018; 1274; 1513.]

——. *On the effusion and organization of coagulable lymph. 1 p. l., 53 pp. 8°. *Edinburgh, Balfour & Jack*, 1837. [P., v. 108; 1513.]

——. Report of the proceedings of the scientific meeting held at Pisa in October, 1839. 10 pp. 8°. *Edinburgh, J. Stark*, [1840]. [P., v. 108.]
Repr. from: Edinb. M. & S. J., 1840, liii.

Newbigging (Patrick Small Keir) [1813-63]. * Inaugural essay on the impulse and sounds attending the action of the heart in its normal state. 34 pp. 8°. *Edinburgh, Neill & Co.*, 1834. [P., v. 108; 1049; 1057; 1191.]

——. * Probationary essay on spina bifida. 2 p. l., 44 pp. 8°. *Edinburgh, W. Burness*, 1834. [*Also, in:* P., v. 108; 1274.]

——. On certain circumstances affecting the colour of blood during coagulation. 7 pp. 8°. [*n. p.*, 1839.] [*Also, in:* P., v. 108; 109; 1518.]
Repr. from: Edinb. N. Phil. J., 1839, xxvii.

——. Case of tetanus, in which recovery took place. 4 pp. 8°. [*Edinburgh*, 1845.] [P., v. 95; 897; 1029.]
Repr. from: North. J. M., Edinb., 1844-5, ii.

——. Statistics of the Edinburgh Lock Hospital during 1841 and 1842, bearing in particular on the non-mercurial treatment of the venereal disease. 4 pp. 8°. *Edinburgh, Sutherland & Knox*, [1847]. [*Also, in:* P., v. 96.]
Repr. from: Month. J. M. Sc., Lond. & Edinb., 1847, viii.
See, also, **Barth** (J.-B.-P.) & **Roger** (Henri). A practical treatise on auscultation, [etc.] Transl. with notes by . . . 8°. *Edinburgh*, 1842.

Newbigging (William) [1772-1852]. Case of inguinal and popliteal aneurism, cured by tying the external iliac artery. 8 pp. 8°. [*Edinburgh, G. Ramsay & Co.*, 1815.] [P., v. 1166.]
Repr. from: Edinb. M. & S. J., 1816, xii.

——. Harveian oration for mdcccxxxviii; being a tribute of respect for the memory of the late James Hamilton, sen.; read at the fifty-sixth anniversary of the Harveian Society of Edinburgh. 20 pp. 8°. *Edinburgh, Neill & Co.*, 1838. [P., v. 108; 1051.]

New Bolivia.
See **Cochabamba.**

Newbourg (A.-J.) * Sur l'apoplexie. 45 pp. 8°. *Paris, an X* [1802], v. 7.

New Brighton, *New York.*
See **Children** (*Hospitals, etc., for, Reports, etc.,* *of*).

New Brighton Retreat, Beaver County. Circular of the . . . with board of officers, managers, etc. Oct., 1862. 16 pp. 8°. *Pittsburgh, W. S. Haven,* 1862.
An asylum for insane females exclusively. Opened Oct. 1, 1862.

——. Annual report of the trustees and superintendent to the legislature of Pennsylvania. 1., 1864. 12 pp. 8°. *Harrisburg, Singerly & Myers,* 1865.

New British and Foreign Temperance Society. Report of . . . 44 pp., 2 l. 8°. *London, J. H. Starie,* 1842.

Newbrough (J. B.) A catechism on human teeth. A free gift for the use of the general public. 21 pp., 1 l. 8°. *New York, S. W. Green,* 1871.

——. Nitrous oxide gas. A reported death from its use. 8 pp. 8°. [*n. p., n. d.*]

New Brunswick (*Province of*). An act to regulate the qualifications of practitioners in medicine and surgery, and to provide a medical council of health in the province of New Brunswick. Passed 13 April, 1859. 7 pp. 8°. [*n. p., J. Simpson,* 1859.]

New Brunswick (*Province of*). *Provincial Lunatic Asylum, at St. John.* Annual report of the medical superintendent to the provincial secretary. 32., 1878-9. 34 pp. 8°. *Fredericton, G. E. Fenety,* 1880.

New Brunswick (*Province of*).
Boyle (A.) Some remarks on the fever most prevalent in New Brunswick, North America, with a sketch of the topography and climate of that period. Edinb. M. & S. J., 1826, xxvi, 1–15.

Newburgh.
See **Insane** (*Asylums for, etc.*), *by localities.*

Newburgh, N. Y. *Board of Health.* Annual reports of the medical officer to the mayor and board of health for the years 1867–8; 1868–9; 1879; 1883; 1884. 8°. *Newburgh,* 1868–85.

Newburn, *England.*
See **Cholera** (*Asiatic, History, etc., of*), *by localities.*

Newbury.
Lee (W.) Report to the General Board of Health, on a preliminary inquiry into the sewerage, drainage, and supply of water, and the sanitary condition of the inhabitants of the borough of Newbury, in the county of Berks. 8°. *London,* 1852.

Newburyport, Mass. Annual report of the directors of the Public Library of the city of Newburyport to the city council. 17., 1871–2. 31 pp. 8°. *Newburyport, W. H. Huse & Co.,* 1872.

Newburyport, Mass. *Board of Health of the City of Newburyport, Mass.* Annual reports to the mayor and city council. 3.–5., 1880–82. 8°. *Newburyport,* 1881–3.

Newby (George).
Co-Editor of: **Journal** of Health of the Metropolitan Medical College, New York, 1859–60.

New Caledonia.
Delas (A.-A.) *Quelques considérations sur la Nouvelle-Calédonie et ses maladies. 4°. *Montpellier,* 1873.

De Rochas (V.) *Essai sur la topographie hygiénique et médicale de la Nouvelle-Calédonie. 4°. *Paris,* 1860.
Also [Abstr.], *in:* Bull. Soc. d'anthrop. de Par., 1861, ii, 48–51.

Vaysset (P.) *Contribution à la géographie médicale. Nouvelle-Calédonie et dépendances. 4°. *Montpellier,* 1874.

New Caledonia.
Vinson (D.-P.-E.) *Éléments d'une topographie médicale de la Nouvelle-Calédonie et de l'île des Pins. 4°. *Paris,* 1858.
Bourgarel (A.) Des races de l'Océanie française. de celles de la Nouvelle-Calédonie en particulier. Mém. Soc. d'anthrop. de Par., 1860–63, i, 251; 1863–5, ii, 375.—**Boyer.** Quelques mots sur la pathologie indigène de la Nouvelle-Calédonie, des Loyalty et des Nouvelles-Hébrides. Arch. de méd. nav., Par., 1878, xxx, 224–231.—**Brassac.** Notes sur les principales maladies, observées dans la Nouvelle-Calédonie. Cong. internat. de méd. d. colonies 1883, Amst., 1884, 304–322, 2 tab.—**Brousmiche** (A.) Considérations générales sur la végétation de la Nouvelle-Calédonie. Arch. de méd. nav., Par., 1884, xli, 250–260.—**Foley.** Quelques détails et réflexions sur le costume et les mœurs de la coquette néo-calédonienne. Bull. Soc. d'anthrop. de Par., 1879, 3. s., ii, 675–683. ——. Deux mots sur le mode vital des hommes et (tout particulièrement) des femmes noirs; à propos du pot-au-feu des Néo-Calédoniens et des rares sorcières qui, seules, savent le fabriquer. *Ibid.,* 748–756.—**Fontan.** Sur l'existence fréquente de dents supplémentaires chez les Néo-Calédoniens. *Ibid.,* 1881, 3. s., iv, 594–596.—**Le Roy de Méricourt & de Rochas.** Nouvelle-Calédonie. Dict. encycl. d. sc. méd., Par., 1870, xi, 657–683.—**Moncelon** (L.) Un peuple qui s'éteint. L'Homme, Par., 1887, iv, 97–104.—**Nouvelle-Calédonie** et îles voisines. Arch. de méd. nav., Par., 1866, v, 5–33.—**Rae** (J.) Customs of the New Caledonian women belonging to the Nancaushy Tine, or Stuart's Lake Indians, Natotin Tine, or Babine's and Nantley Tine, or Fraser Lake tribes. From information supplied by G. Hamilton, chief factor of the Hudson's Bay Company's service [etc.]. J. Anthrop. Inst., Lond., 1877–8, vii, 206–208.—**de Rochas** (V.) Sur les Néo-Calédoniens. Bull. Soc. d'anthrop. de Par., 1860, i, 389–399. *Also:* Gaz. méd. de Par., 1860, 3. s., xv, 185; 199. ——. La Nouvelle-Calédonie. Union méd., Par., 1871, 3. s., xi, 385; 409. *Also:* Courrier méd., Par., 1871, xxi, 141–143.—**Taillotte** (A.) Étude des eaux thermales de la baie du Prony (Nouvelle-Calédonie). Arch. de méd. nav., Par., 1884, xli, 353–386.—**de Vaux** (L.) Les Canaques de la Nouvelle-Calédonie. Rev. d'ethnog., Par., 1883, ii. 327–354.—**Verrier** (E.) Anthropologie, ethnographie et pathologie comparée des Néo-Calédoniens; avenir du métissage dans la colonie. Bull. Soc. d'ethnog., Par., 1887, 2. s., i, 231–240.

Newcastle.
Clark (G. T.) Report to the General Board of Health, on a preliminary inquiry into the sewerage, drainage, and supply of water, and the sanitary condition of the inhabitants of the hamlets of Coyty Lower and Newcastle. 8°. *London,* 1850.

Newcastle [**Marguerite Lucas**] (*Duchess of*) [1624–73]. The world's olio. 6 p. l., 216 pp., 2 l. fol. *London, F. Martin & F. Allestrye,* 1655.

Newcastle and Gateshead Pathological Society. Communications made to the society during the sessions 1851–3. 45 pp., 2 pl.; 52 pp., 2 pl. 8°. [*London, W. Tyler,* 1851–3.] [P., v. 1358.]

New Castle Medical Society. Constitution and by-laws. 7 pp. 16°. *New Castle, Ind., Wilcox & Scott,* 1871.

Newcastle Throat and Ear Hospital. Annual reports of the committee to the subscribers. 1.–7., 1878–9 to 1884. 8°. *Newcastle-upon-Tyne,* 1879–85.
1. report under title: **Hospital** for Diseases of the Throat and Ear, Newcastle-upon-Tyne.

Newcastle-under-Lyme.
Lee (W.) Report to the General Board of Health, on a preliminary inquiry into the sewerage, drainage, and supply of water, and the sanitary condition of the inhabitants of the borough of Newcastle-under-Lyme, in the county of Stafford. 8°. *London,* 1850.

——. Report to the General Board of Health, on the state of the burial-grounds in the borough of Newcastle-under-Lyme. 8°. *London,* 1851.

Newcastle-upon-Tyne. Annual reports of the medical officer of health, on the sanitary condition of Newcastle-upon-Tyne, with tabular returns and diagrams of the sickness and mortality, to the sanitary committee, by H. E. Armstrong.

Newcastle-upon-Tyne—continued.
1., 1873; 3.–13., 1875–86. 8°. *Newcastle-upon-Tyne, 1874–87.*
1877–85 bound in 3 v.

———. River Tyne port sanitary authority. Annual reports of the medical officer of health. 1.–3., 1879–81; 7., 1885; 9., 1887. fol. [*Newcastle-upon-Tyne, 1880–88.*]
1879–80, by John Byrom Bramwell; 1881, 1885, and 1887, by Henry Edw. Armstrong.

———. Notice on the prevention of infectious diseases and recommendations in favour of vaccination and re-vaccination. By Henry E. Armstrong, medical officer of health. Printed by the authority of the sanitary committee of the corporation. 10 pp. 8°. *Newcastle-upon-Tyne, A. Reid, 1881.*
Bound with: Rep. Med. Off. Health for 1881. 8°. *Newcastle-upon-Tyne, 1882.*

———. Report on the recently increased death rate of the city by the medical officer of health [Henry E. Armstrong]. 39 pp., 2 maps. 8°. [*Newcastle-upon-Tyne, 1883.*]

Newcastle-upon-Tyne.
See, also, **Cholera** (*Asiatic, History, etc., of*), **Education** (*Medical*), *etc., by localities*; **Fever** (*Hospitals for*); **Fever** (*Relapsing, History, etc., of*), **Fever** (*Typhus, History, etc., of*), *by localities.*
PHILIPSON (G. H.) Reports on the health and meteorology of Newcastle and Gateshead. (Communicated to the Northumberland and Durham Medical Society.) 5. & 6. for 1869. 8°. [*n. p., n. d.*]
REPORT on the sanitary condition of Newcastle, Gateshead, North Shields, Sunderland, Durham, and Carlisle; with remarks on some points connected with the health of the inhabitants in the adjacent mining district. 4°. [*n. p., n. d.*]
Armstrong (H. E.) Sketch of the sanitary history of Newcastle-upon-Tyne. Tr. San. Inst. Gr. Brit.. Lond., 1882–3, iv, 76–96.—**Bell** (I. L.) The sanitary condition of Newcastle-upon-Tyne. Tr. Nat. Ass. Promot. Social Sc. 1870, Lond., 1871, 420–429.—**Excessive** (The) death-rate of Newcastle. San. Rec., Lond., 1883–4, n. s, v, 245; 391.—**Philipson** (G. H.) On the health and meteorology of Newcastle and Gateshead during the years 1868–9. Brit. M. J., Lond., 1871, i, 56.—**Report** of the Lancet Sanitary Commission on Newcastle-on-Tyne. Lancet, Lond., 1874, i, 58.—**Rutherford** (J. H.) The public health of Newcastle-upon-Tyne in 1866 and 1869. Tr. Nat. Ass. Promot. Social Sc. 1870, Lond., 1871, 414–420.

Newcastle-upon-Tyne. *Newcastle-upon-Tyne City Lunatic Asylum, Coxlodge.* Annual reports of the committee of visitors and medical superintendent to the magistrates. 1., 1865; 2., 1866; 18.–23., 1882–7. 8°. *Newcastle-upon-Tyne, 1866–88.*
Opened June 24, 1865.

———. Rules and regulations of the . . . (Approved by the secretary of state for the home department.) 15 pp. 8°. *Newcastle-upon-Tyne, Daily Journal Office, 1867.*

Newcastle-upon-Tyne. *Newcastle-upon-Tyne Fever Hospital.* Duties of medical superintendent and matron. Oct. 4, 1882. 3 pp. 8°. [*Newcastle-upon-Tyne, A. Reid, 1882.*]

———. General rules, special rules for nurses, and rules for patients. March, 1882. broadside, 20 x 30 in. *Newcastle-upon-Tyne, A. Reid,* [1882].

———. [Blank forms in use.] v. s. [*Newcastle-upon-Tyne, n. d.*]
Bill for supplies; clinical chart; diet list; receipts; record of patient; tender for supplies.

———. *See, also:*
EMBLETON (D.) Report from the Newcastle and Gateshead Fever Hospital on typhus and smallpox, for the year 1864–5. 8°. [*Newcastle, 1865.*]

Newcastle-upon-Tyne Dispensary. Annual reports of the committee and resident medical officer to the governors. 108.–110., 1885–7. 8°. *Newcastle-upon-Tyne, 1886–8.*

Newchwang.
Watson (J.) & **Morrison** (W.) Report on the health of Newchwang, 1870–86. Customs Gaz. Med. Rep., Shanghai, 1870–71, no. 1, 124: 1871–2. no. 3, 10: (1872) 1873, no. 4, 27: 1872–3, no. 5, 47: (1874), 1875, no. 8, 7: (1876), 1877, no. 12, 28. *Continued in :* China. Imp. Customs. Med. Rep., Shanghai, 1877–8, no. 15, 28: 1878–9, no. 17, 8: 1879–80, no. 19, 1: 1880–81, no. 21, 37: (1882), 1883, no. 24, 1: (1883), 1884, no. 26, 25: 1883–4, no. 27, 22: 1885–6, no. 31, 1.

Newcomb (Daniel). The different theories that have been advanced on the subject of the proximate cause of conception in the human female. 32 pp. 8°. *Philadelphia, J. H. Oswald, 1806.*

Newcome (*Rev. Dr.*)
See **Whytt** (Robert). An essay on the virtues of limewater. etc. 3. ed. 16°. *Dublin,* 1762.

Newell (Daniel). The guide to health. Designed to promote the health, happiness, and longevity of students and all others in sedentary life, especially invalids. x, 11–84 pp. 18°. *Boston, S. T. Farren, 1825.*

Newell (O. K.) Some observations on the anatomy of the male urethra, in relation to endoscopy, litholapaxy, and catheterization. 11 pp. 12°. *Boston, Cupples, Upham & Co., 1886.*
Repr. from : Boston M. & S. J., 1886, cxv.

[**Newell** (Sarah.)] Facts connected with the treatment of insanity in St. Luke's Hospital; with letters on the subject to Lord Brougham, the committee of St. Luke's Hospital, Drs. Birbeck, Elliotson, and others, on an introductory letter to the most noble the Marquis of Normanby. 54 pp. 8°. *London, E. Wilson, 1841.*

Newell (W. M.)
Co-Editor of : **Western** (The) Retrospect of Medicine and Surgery, Evansville, Ind., 1872.

New England.
See, also, **Directories,** *etc.* (*Medical*); **Fever** (*Malarial, History, etc., of*), *by localities.*
BURLEIGH. The Old Colony Railroad; its connections, popular resorts, and fashionable watering-places. 8°. *Boston,* 1876.
ELLIS (J.) Deterioration of the Puritan stock, and its causes. 8°. *New York,* 1884.
Allen (N.) Changes in New England population. Pop. Sc. Month., N. Y., 1883, xxiii, 433–444. *Also,* Reprint.—**Leonard** (J. P.) The fevers in New England. Boston M. & S. J., 1845, xxxii, 189–191.

New England Asylum for the Blind, Boston. *See* **Perkins** Institution and Massachusetts School for the Blind, Boston.

New England (The) Botanic, Medical and Surgical Journal. C. Newton, editor and proprietor. [Semi-monthly.] v. 1–5, 1847–51. 8°. *Worcester, Mass.*
v. 4 became monthly. A continuation of: **New England** (The) Medical Eclectic and Guide to Health. See **Worcester** (The) Journal of Medicine, for v. 6, *et seq.*

New England (The) Eclectic Medical Journal; a monthly journal devoted to the interests of progressive medicine. Edited by Eli G. Jones (Union Village, Vt.). No. 1, v. 1, May, 1872. 4 pp. fol. *Auburn, Me., S. York.*

New England (The) Eclectic Medical Journal. Devoted to the interests of progressive medicine. Eli Grellet Jones, editor and proprietor. [Monthly.] Nos. 1–3, v. 1, Jan. to March, 1873. 8°. *Enfield Centre, N. H.*

New England Female Medical College, Boston. Annual reports and catalogues for the years 1848–9 to 1870–71 (1.–23.). 8°. *Boston, 1850–71.*
First session commenced Nov. 1, 1848, as the Boston Female Medical School. Incorporated as the Female Medical Education Society, April 30, 1850. Held two courses annually the first five years. Adopted above title May 28, 1856, by act of the legislature. The first report is for 2 years, and in 1862 the number 13 was omitted, to correspond with the commencement of the institution. In 1873, united with the Boston University School of Medicine. 1.–23. bound in 2 v.

New England Female Medical [etc.]—cont'd.

——. Announcement to a course of medical lectures to women in the city of Boston, by the faculty of the Female Medical College of Pennsylvania, in conjunction with the New England Female Medical College. To commence Feb. 16, 1852, and continue for four months. 12 pp. 8°. *Boston, printed for the Faculty,* 1851.
Bound with : Reports 1848-9 to 1857-8.

——. Annual announcements for the sessions of 1852-3 to 1871-2 (5.-24.). 8°. *Boston,* 1852-71.
In : Annual reports and catalogues for the preceding years. [*See supra.*]

——. Annual advertisement for the session of 1853-4 (6.). 8 pp. 8°. *Boston, S. Gregory,* 1853.
Bound with : Reports 1848-9 to 1857-8.

——. Memorial [of the present and past trustees] to the Massachusetts legislature [against the removal of Dr. Samuel Gregory, secretary of the board of trustees of the college]. Presented and received May 21, 1866. 3 pp. 8°. *Boston,* 1866.
Bound with : Reports 1858-9 to 1870-71.

——. *See, also :*
MASSACHUSETTS. Report to the Massachusetts legislature, by the committee on education, in favor of an appropriation of $5,000 to the Female Medical Education Society, together with the constitution, names of officers and members, and other information respecting the society, and the Boston Female Medical School. Senate Doc. No. 70. 8°. *Boston,* 1851.

New England Female Moral Reform Society, Boston. Annual reports of the executive committee to the board of managers. 15., 1852-3; 16., 1853-4. 8°. *Boston,* 1853-4.

New England Home for Intemperate Women, Boston. [An appeal to the public for means to carry on the work of the institution.] 2 l. 8°. [*Boston,* 1878.]
Opened January 27, 1879; incorporated March 30,1881, as the Massachusetts Home for Intemperate Women, which see, for continuation.

——. Annual reports of the managers and matron to the contributors and the public. 1., 1879-80; 2., 1880-81. 8°. *Boston,* 1880-81.

New England Hospital for Women and Children, Boston. Annual reports of the secretary and resident physician to the society at their annual meetings. 1.-23., 1862-3 to 1884-5. 8°. *Boston,* 1863-86.
Opened July 1, 1862; incorporated March 12, 1865. 14. is 2. ed. revised.

New England Industrial School for the Education and Instruction of Deaf Mutes, at Beverly. Annual reports of the trustees and officers to the society and the public. 1., 1880-81; 3., 1882-3; 4., 1883-4. 8°. *Beverly,* 1881-4.
Organized 1876; incorporated 1879. Opened February, 1880.

New England Institution for the Education of the Blind, Boston. *See* **Perkins** Institution and Massachusetts School for the Blind, Boston.

New England Journal of Dentistry and Allied Sciences. Edited by associated dentists. Charles Mayr, scientific editor. [Monthly.] v. 1-3, Jan., 1882, to Oct., 1884. 8°. *Springfield, Mass.*
No. 10, v. 3, Oct., 1884, last published; then merged in: **Archives** (The) of Dentistry, Saint Louis. Title of v. 2-3 was : **New England** Journal of Dentistry.

New England (The) Journal of Medicine and Surgery, and the Collateral Branches of Science. Conducted by a number of physicians. [Quarterly.] v. 1-15, January, 1812, to December, 1826. 8°. *Boston, Bradford & Read.*
Continued as : **New England** (The) Medical Review and Journal.

New England (The) Medical Eclectic. W. C. George, editor. [Monthly.] No. 1, v. 1, July, 1859. 40 pp. 8°. *Worcester, Mass.*

New England (The) Medical Eclectic and Guide to Health. Edited by Calvin Newton. [Semi-monthly.] v. 1, Jan. 1 to Dec. 16, 1846. 384 pp. 8°. *Worcester, Mass.*

——. The same. No. 1, v. 2, Jan. 1, 1847. 24 pp. 8°.
The name was then changed, and another No. 1 was issued Jan. 1, 1847, as No. 1, v. 1, of : **New England** (The) Botanic, Medical and Surgical Journal. See **New England** (The) Botanic, Medical and Surgical Journal, for continuation.

New England (The) Medical Gazette. A monthly journal of homœopathic medicine, surgery, and the collateral sciences. Edited by H. C. Angell. v. 1-23, January, 1866-88. 8°. *Boston.*
Current. v. 7, 1872, contains only nos. 1-3, 7-8. Edited successively by I. T. Talbot, W. Tod Helmuth, W. Wesselhoeft, H. A. Chase, John L. Coffin, E. P. White, H. C. Clapp, and J. P. Sutherland.

New England Medical Monthly. William C. Wile, editor and proprietor. v. 1-7, October, 1881-8. 8°. *Newtown; Bridgeport, Conn.*
Current.

New England (The) Medical Review and Journal. Conducted by Walter Channing and John Ware. [Quarterly.] v. 1, 1827. 444 pp. 8°. *Boston.*
Also called v. 16 of : **New England** (The) Journal of Medicine and Surgery. United with : **Boston** Medical Intelligencer, forming : **Boston** (The) Medical and Surgical Journal.

New England Medical Society of Specialists. Transactions of the first semi-annual meeting. 1., 1879. 26, 11 pp. 8°. *Boston,* 1879.

New England Mutual Life Insurance Company of Boston. Annual reports of the directors, at the annual meetings of the members. 1.-19., 1843-4 to 1861-2. iv, 158 pp. 8°. *Boston, N. Sawyer,* 1863.

New England Psychological Society. Organization of Dec. 14, 1875. 2 l. 4°. [*n. p., n. d.*]

New England (The) Quarterly Journal of Medicine and Surgery. Edited by Charles E. Ware and Samuel Parkman. v. 1, July, 1842, to June, 1843. 595 pp. 8°. *Boston, D. Clapp, jr.*

New England Society for the Suppression of Vice, Boston. Annual reports of the executive committee. 6., 1883-4; 7., 1884-5. 12°. *Boston,* 1884-5.

New England Women's Auxiliary Association, Branch of the United States Sanitary Commission, Boston. *See* **United States** Sanitary Commission, New England Women's Auxiliary Association, Branch.

Newenham (*Arthur Wellesley R.*) [1813-57].
Obituary notice. Lancet, Lond., 1857, ii, 459.

Newer (Ein) Albertus Magnus. Von Weibern und Geburten der Kinder sampt ihren Artzneien. Von Tugenden etlicher fürnemer Kreuter. Von Krafft der edlen Gestein. Von Art und Natur etlicher Thier. Mit sampt eim bewerten Regiment für die Pestilentz. Alles von newem gebessert durch Q. Apollinarem. xlv ff., 2 l. sm. 4°. *Franckf. a. M., H. Gülfferichen,* [1564].

Newera-Ellia.
Massy (H. D.) Cases of fever, with remarks on the topography, climate, and sanitary condition of Newera Ellia during the year 1865. Army M. Dep. Rep. 1866, Lond., 1868, viii, 496-504, 1 map. —**Murray.** Report on Newere Ellia in Ceylon; with general remarks on military convalescent stations. Tr. M. & Phys. Soc. Calcutta, 1835-42, viii, 240-251.

Newere (A) code. 2 l. 4°. [*New York,* 1884 ?]

New Foundland.
See, also, **Saint Pierre** *Island.*
DU BOIS SAINT-SÉVRIN (L.-M.) *Deux ans aux îles Saint-Pierre et Miquelon (Terre-Neuve); notes médicales, 1882-4. 4°. *Bordeaux,* 1886.

New Foundland.

Alexander (J.) On the climate of Newfoundland and some of the diseases chiefly met with there. Dublin J. M. Sc., 1878, lxv, 326-331. — **Le Roy de Méricourt** (A.) Terre-Neuve. Dict. encycl. d. sc. méd., Par., 1886, 3. s., xvi, 498-517. — **Lloyd** (T. G. B.) On the "Beothucs", a tribe of red Indians, supposed to be extinct, which formerly inhabited Newfoundland. J. Anthrop. Inst., Lond., 1874-5, iv, 21, 1 pl. : 1875-6, v, 222, 1 pl.

Newfoundland. *Hospital for the Insane, St. John's.* Annual report of the physician superintendent to the legislative assembly. 13., 1860. 24 pp. 8°. *London, E. C., G. Blight,* 1861.

New Graefenberg (The) Water-Cure Reporter. Devoted to the hydropathic treatment of disease, the report of cases, and the dissemination of the principles of physiology and medical reform. Edited by Henry Foster. [Monthly.] No. 1, v. 2, Jan., 1850. 32 pp. 8°. *Utica, N. Y., R. Holland.*

New Granada.

See Goitre, *by localities*; Panama.

New Guinea.

Comrie. Anthropological notes on New Guinea. J. Anthrop. Inst., Lond., 1876-7, vi, 102-119.—**Lawes** (W. G.) Ethnological notes on the Motu, Koitapu, and Koiari tribes of New Guinea. *Ibid.,* 1878-9, viii, 369-377. — The effect of the climate of New Guinea upon exotic races. Australas. M. Gaz., Sydney, 1886-7, vi, 185.—**Mantegazza** (P.) Studii antropologici ed etnografici sulla Nuova Guinea. Arch. per l' antrop., Firenze, 1877, vii, 137 ; 307, 16 pl. *Also,* Reprint. — **Meyer** (A.-B.) Sur l'ethnologie de la Nouvelle-Guinée. Bull. Soc. d'anthrop. de Par., 1880, 3. s., iii, 346-362.—**Réclus** (É.) Les Nofoures de la Nouvelle-Guinée. Rev. internat. d. sc. biol., Par., 1882, x, 481-509.—**Schellong** (O.) Mittheilungen über die Malaria-Erkrankungen in Kaiser-Wilhelmsland. Deutsche med. Wchnschr., Leipz., 1887, xiii, 493 ; 523.— **Strauch** (H.) Allgemeine Bemerkungen ethnologischen Inhalts über Neu-Guinea, die Anachoreten-Inseln, Neu-Hannover, Neu-Irland, Neu-Britannien und Bougainville, im Anschluss an die dort gemachten Sammlungen ethnologischer Gegenstände. Ztschr. f. Ethnol., Berl., 1877, ix, 9 ; 81.—**Turner** (W. Y.) The ethnology of the Motu. J. Anthrop. Inst., Lond., 1877-8, vii, 470-499. — Two masks and a skull from islands near New Guinea ; a contribution to anthropology. J. Anat. & Physiol., Lond. 1879-80, xiv, 475-494, 1 pl.—**Wake** (C. S.) Notes on the Polynesian race. J. Anthrop. Inst., Lond., 1880-81, x, 109-123.—**Whitmee** (S. J.) The ethnology of Polynesia. *Ibid.,* 1878-9, viii, 261-275, 1 map.

New Hampshire. Report of the commissioners concerning contagious diseases among cattle. June session, 1865. 24 pp. 8°. *Concord, A. Hadley,* 1865.

———. Report of the board of auditors, appointed by the governor and council to inquire into the general financial transactions of the New Hampshire Asylum for the Insane, etc. To the legislature, June session, 1877. 7 pp. 8°. *Concord, E. A. Jenks,* 1877.

———. Annual report relating to the registration and return of births, marriages, divorces, and deaths in New Hampshire. New series. 4., 1883 ; 5., 1884. 8°. *Concord,* 1884-5.

———. Laws relative to insane persons. 7 pp. MS. fol. [*n. p., n. d.*]

New Hampshire.

See, also, Charlestown ; Concord ; Diphtheria (*History of*) ; Education (*Medical*), *etc.,* Fever (*History, etc., of*), *by localities* ; Isle of Shoals ; Manchester ; Pharmacy ; Portsmouth.

HITCHCOCK (C. H.) Report of the geological survey of the State of New Hampshire, showing its progress during the year 1871. 8°. *Nashua,* 1872.

Crosby (A. B.) Medical history of New Hampshire. Tr. N. Hampshire M. Soc., Nashua, 1870, 46-75. *Also,* Reprint. — **Fitch** (F. P.) Report of the corresponding secretary of the New Hampshire Medical Society for the southern district. N. Hampshire J. M., Concord, 1850-51, i, 19 ; 33. — **Ham** (J. R.) Report on the sanitary condition of the alms-house in Strafford County. Tr. N. Hampshire M. Soc., Manchester, 1872, 61-64. — **Pollution** of

New Hampshire.

the Ammonoosuc River. Rep. Bd. Health N. Hampshire, Concord, 1881-2, i, 53-61. — **Registration** report for the year ending March 31, 1882. *Ibid.,* 1882-3, ii, 7-31. — **Wheeler.** Report on the sanitary condition of alms-houses. Tr. N. Hampshire M. Soc., Manchester, 1871, 90-94.

New Hampshire. *Adjutant - General of the State of New Hampshire.* Reports for the years 1862-3 ; 1864-5 to 1868-9 ; 1871-2. 8°. *Concord & Manchester,* 1863-72.

New Hampshire. *New Hampshire Asylum for the Insane, at Concord.* Annual reports of the board of trustees, superintendent, treasurer, and financial agent to the governor of the State. 1.-44., 1842-3 to 1886-7. 8°. *Concord,* 1843-87.
Opened Oct. 28, 1842.

———. *See, also :*
NEW HAMPSHIRE. Report of the board of auditors, appointed by the governor and council to inquire into the general financial transactions of the New Hampshire Asylum for the Insane, etc. To the legislature, June session, 1877. 8°. *Concord,* 1877.

New Hampshire. *State Board of Health of the State of New Hampshire.* Annual reports to the governor and council. 1.-4., 1881-2 to 1884-5. 8°. *Concord,* 1882-5.
1881-2 and 1882-3, contain the registration reports for 1881 and 1882, relating to births, marriages, divorces, and deaths.

———. Circular No. 1, Nov., 1881. To local boards of health, physicians, and others interested in sanitary science [informing them of the organization of the State board, and soliciting co-operate assistance]. 3 pp. 8°. [*Concord,* 1881.]

———. Circular No. 2, Dec. 19, 1881. To the public : [On the importance of vaccination against small-pox]. 1 sheet. 8°. [*Concord,* 1881.]

———. Circular No. 4. To physicians, requesting them to telegraph the first case of small-pox coming within their knowledge, that immediate action may be taken in the matter. Jan. 23, 1882. 1 sheet. 16°. *Concord,* 1882.

———. Circular No. 5. Suggestions for the prevention and restriction of small-pox. 2 l. 16°. [*Concord,* 1882.]

———. Circular No. 6. Order to local health boards. Regulations against the invasion of small-pox. 1 sheet. 8°. [*Concord,* 1882.]

New Hampshire (The) Journal of Medicine. Edited by Edward H. Parker. [Monthly.] v. 1-8, August, 1850, to Dec., 1858. 8°. *Concord,* 1850-55 ; *Manchester,* 1856-8.
Ended. v. 2 commenced Sept., 1851 ; v. 3 commenced Oct., 1852 ; v. 4 commenced January, 1854. In Sept., 1853, George H. Hubbard added as editor ; v. 4-8, Dr. Hubbard editor and proprietor ; in nos. 8-12, v. 5, Charles Bell added.

New Hampshire Medical Institution, Hanover. *See* Dartmouth College, medical department, for announcements.

New Hampshire Medical Society. Organized Feb. 11, 1791. The by-laws, regulations, and police of the centre district, organized June 3, 1807. 24 pp. 12°. *Concord, Chase & Crosby,* 1840.

———. The by-laws, regulations, and police. 22 pp. 12°. *Concord, N. H., Morrill, Silsby & Co.,* 1841.

———. The by-laws, regulations, and code of ethics. 34 pp. 12°. *Concord, N. H., A. McFarland,* 1850.

———. Transactions of 64. -97. anniversaries, 1854-1887. Bd. in 9 v. 8°. *Concord,* 1854-87.

———. Report of the committee on surgery, by Geo. H. Hubbard. 15 pp. 8°. [*n. p.,* 1858.]
Repr. from : Tr. N. Hampshire M. Soc., Concord, 1857.

New Hampshire Medical Society—continued.
——. The charter, by-laws, regulations, and code of ethics, with its presidents and fellows. 40 pp. 8°. *Concord, McFarland & Jenks,* 1860.
——. The same. 47 pp. 8°. *Concord,* 1873.
New Hampshire Pharmaceutical Association. Proceedings of the annual meetings. 1., 1875; 5., 1878. 8°. *Concord,* 1876–9.
New Hartford, N. Y. No. 53. Organization of the local board of health. Sanitary laws and regulations obligatory upon the inhabitants of the town. As adopted 1884. 2 l. 8°. [*New York,* 1887.]
New Haven, Conn. City year book of the city of New-Haven. Containing lists of the officers of the city and town governments, messages of the mayor, reports of the heads of departments, standing committees of the court of common council, public documents, and miscellaneous papers, for the years 1870–71; 1872–3; 1874–5; 1880. 8°. *New Haven,* 1871–81.
    Contains reports of the board of health, vital statistics.
——. Annual reports of the street department, to the common council, for the years 1876–8; 1881. 8°. *Hartford,* 1879–82.
    1876–8 in one.
——. A report of the joint special committee on water, to the common council. 18 pp., 1 l. 8°. *New Haven, Hoggson & Robinson,* 1881.
——. Report of the special investigating committee to the court of common council, as to the purchase of the New Haven water-works. 15 pp. 8°. *New Haven, Stafford Printing Co.,* 1881.
——. Reports of deaths in New Haven. [Weekly.] Dec. 8, 1883, to June 14, 1884; June 28 to Aug. 16; Sept. 6, 1884, to Jan. 3, 1885. 18°. [*New Haven,* 1883–5.]

New Haven, *Connecticut.*
    See, also, **Education** (*Medical*), *etc.,* **Fever** (*Malarial, History, etc., of*), *by localities.*
    BREWER (W. H.) Letter of the president of the board [of health, New Haven, Conn.]. 8°. [*New Haven,* 1884.]
    EVERGREEN Cemetery of New Haven. Exercises at the dedication of the new grounds of the . . . July 29, 1856. With the addresses, etc., delivered on the occasion. 8°. *New Haven,* 1856.
    [REPORT of a committee appointed to investigate the sanitary conditions of Yale College buildings and of the city of New Haven.] 8°. [*New Haven,* 1884.]
    Bill of mortality, in New Haven, Connecticut, from January 1, 1815, to January 1, 1816. Eclect. Repert., Phila., 1816, vi, 261.—**Cesspool** (The) question in New Haven. [Edit.] San. Engin., N. Y., 1883, viii, 415.—**Dow** (V. M.) Observations on the diseases which prevailed in New Haven, Conn., during the winter of 1831–2. Boston M. & S. J., 1832, vi 313–317.

New Haven, Conn. *Board of Health of the City of New Haven.* Annual reports to the common council. 1.–14. (1873–86). 8°. *New Haven,* 1874–87.
——. Rules, regulations, and by-laws of the . . . and by-laws of the city of New Haven concerning nuisances, also statute laws relating to board of health. 32 pp. 8°. *New Haven, Tuttle, Morehouse & Taylor,* 1874.
    Bound with : Reports, 1874–80.
——. Monthly statements of mortality in the city of New Haven, Conn. With an enumeration of the more prominent causes, accompanied by an abstract of meteorological observations. July, 1874, to April, 1888. 4°. *New Haven,* 1874–88.

Newhaven, *England.*
    NEWHAVEN drainage. . [Scheme of W. H. Radford, sanitary engineer, for the drainage of the port on the Sussex coast. Adopted by the local board.] 1 broadside. [*Newhaven? n. d.*]
    Graham (W.) The sanitary state of Newhaven. Tr. Nat. Ass. Promot. Social Sc. 1863, Lond., 1864, 497–501.

New Haven County Medical Society. A report on the expediency of repealing that section of the medical laws of this State which excludes irregular practitioners from the benefits of law in the collection of fees. 16 pp. 8°. *New Haven, printed by B. L. Hamlen,* 1837. [*Also, in :* P., v. 233.]
    Another copy bound with : **Medical** Society of Connecticut. Communications. 8°. *New Haven,* 1810.
New Haven Dispensary. Annual reports of the board of managers to the members. 2. (1872–3); 3. (1873–4); 6.–8. (1876–7 to 1878–9). 8°. *New Haven,* 1873–9.
    Organized Nov. 13, 1871, and opened Dec. 1. Incorporated May, 1872.
New Haven Medical Association. Constitution and by-laws. 12 pp. 8°. *New Haven, Hitchcock & Stafford,* 1842.
——. The same. 14 pp. 8°. *New Haven,* 1880.
——. The same. 15 pp. 8°. *New Haven,* 1886.
New Haven Orphan Asylum. Annual reports of the managers to the friends of the asylum. 24., 1856–7; 27., 1859–60; 32., 1864–5; 35., 1867–8; 36., 1868–9; 38.–48., 1870–71 to 1880–81. 12° & 8°. *New Haven,* 1857–81.
    Organized Feb. 26, 1833.

New Hebrides.
    Monin. Nouvelles-Hébrides. [*From :* Rap. méd. sur la campagne du cuirassé de 2e rang la Victorieuse, station du Pacifique, 1878–81.] Arch. de méd. nav., Par , 1882, xxxviii, 401: 1883, xxxix, 58.—**de Vaux** (L.) Les iles Loyalty, les Nouvelles-Hébrides et les Viti; impressions et souvenirs. Rev. d'ethnog., Par., 1884, iii, 484–507.

New Holland.
    Manning (J.) Notes on the aborigines of New Holland. J. & Proc. Roy. Soc. N. South Wales 1882, Sydney, 1883, xvi, 155–173.

Newington.
    ANNUAL reports of the proceedings of the vestry of the parish of St. Mary, Newington, in the county of Sussex [including reports of the medical officer of health]. 2. (1857–8); 23. (1878–9). 8°. *London,* 1858–79.
    ANNUAL reports on the sanitary condition of the parish of St. Mary, Newington, Surrey, by W. T. Iliff, medical officer of health, to the vestry. 1.–2., 1856–7. 8°. *London,* 1857–8.
    2. report bound with report of vestry.

Newington (H. Hayes). Royal Edinburgh Asylum Papers. Hemiplegia in relation to insanity. 8 pp. 8°. *Edinburgh, Oliver & Boyd,* 1874.
    Repr. from : Edinb. M. J., 1874–5, xx.

New Jersey. Report of the joint committee of council and assembly, appointed to settle the accounts of the State prison. 36 pp. 8°. *Trenton, J. Justice,* 1830. [P., v. 602.]
——. Report relative to an asylum for lunatics, by the joint committee of council and assembly, to which was referred that part of the governor's message relating thereto. 19 pp. 8°. *Trenton, Sherman & Harrow,* 1841.
——. Annual statements of the marriages, births, and deaths in the State of New Jersey, to the legislature, for the years 1851; 1854; 1856; 1864–77. 8°. *Trenton,* 1852–78.
    1864–73 bound in 1 v.
——. Report of the joint committee on State prison accounts, to whom was referred that part of the governor's message relating to the State prison. 5 pp. 8°. *Trenton, True American Office,* 1859.
——. Annual messages of the governor of New Jersey to the senate and general assembly, for the years 1867–8. 48, 45 pp. 8°. *Trenton, Murphy & Bechtel,* 1867–8.
——. Official register of the officers and men of New Jersey in the Revolutionary War. Compiled under orders of the governor, by William

New Jersey—continued.

S. Stryker, adj't-gen'l. Printed by authority of the legislature. 878 pp. 8°. *Trenton, W. T. Nicholson & Co.*, 1872.

——. Report of the joint committee on the State Lunatic Asylum at Trenton, to the senate and general assembly of the State of New Jersey, session of 1875. 5 pp. 8°. *Trenton, W. S. Sharp*, 1875.

——. An act to establish a State board of health. [State of New Jersey.] Approved March 9, 1877. [*n. p., n. d.*] Newspaper cutting.

——. An act concerning the registry and returns of marriages, births, and deaths. Approved April 5, 1878. galley sheet. [*Trenton*, 1878.]

——. Report of the commissioners on prison system of New Jersey, and on an intermediate prison, under joint resolution, approved April 9, 1877. 22 pp. 8°. *Trenton, Naar, Day & Naar*, 1878.

——. Report on pleuro-pneumonia among cattle in the State of New Jersey. Proceedings under "An act to prevent the spread of contagious or infectious pleuro-pneumonia among cattle in the State of New Jersey", approved March 13, 1879. 19 pp. 8°. *Trenton, W. S. Sharp*, 1879.

——. An act to prevent the adulteration of food or drugs. State of New Jersey. Senate, No. 200. Introd. March 2, 1881, by Mr. Paxton. 3 pp. fol. [*Trenton*, 1881.]

——. A supplement to an act entitled "An act concerning the protection of the public health and the record of vital facts and statistics relating thereto", approved March 11, 1880. 1 galley sheet. [*Trenton*, 1881.]

——. Assembly. A supplement to an act entitled "An act to regulate the practice of medicine and surgery", approved March 12, 1880, and the supplement thereto approved March 2, 1881. No. 174. Introd. Jan. 31, 1883, by Mr. Chattle. 2 pp. fol. [*Trenton*, 1883.]

——. General circular as to duties under the laws relating to vital records and statistics. Jan., 1883. 1 sheet. 8°. [*Trenton*, 1883.]

——. S. A supplement to an act entitled "An act to regulate the sale of petroleum and its products", approved March 31, 1882. No. 126. Introd. Feb. 7, 1883, by Mr. Griggs. 2 pp. fol. [*Trenton*, 1883.]

——. S. An act to create a council of State charities and correction. No. 133. Introd. Feb. 7, 1883, by Mr. Vail. 4 pp. fol. [*Trenton*, 1883.]

——. S. Supplement to an act entitled "An act to establish a State board of health", approved March 9, 1877, and to supplements thereto relating to the contagious diseases of animals. No. 150. Introd. Feb. 12, 1883, by Mr. Ferrell. 4 pp. fol. [*Trenton*, 1883.]

——. S. Supplement to an act entitled "An act relating to local boards of health" [conferring power to abate nuisances hazardous to the public health]. Approved March 22, 1881. No. 163. Introd. Feb. 14, 1883, by Mr. Taylor. 4 pp. fol. [*Trenton*, 1883.]

——. Assembly. A supplement to an act entitled "An act to prevent the adulteration of food or drugs", approved March 25, 1881. No. 252. Introd. Feb. 14, 1883, by Mr. Chapman. 4 pp. fol. [*Trenton*, 1883.]

New Jersey.

See, also, **Directories,** *etc.* (*Medical*); **Fever** (*Malarial, History, etc., of*), **Fever** (*Typhoid, History, etc., of*), **Fever** (*Typhus, History, etc., of*), *by localities*; **Life-insurance**; **Newark**; **Orange**; **Prisons**; **Swedesborough**.

COOK (G. H.) Geology of New Jersey. 4°. *Newark*, 1868.

New Jersey.

HUDSON CO., N. J. Monthly statements of births, marriages, and deaths of . . . Published by order of the board of health. Jan., 1877, to Apr., 1877; June, 1878; June, 1882, to July, 1885; Oct., 1885 4°. *New York*, 1877–84.

MEDICAL (The) directory of Philadelphia, Pennsylvania, Delaware, and the southern half of New Jersey. 1885; 1887. 12°. *Philadelphia*, 1885-7.

Blackwood (W. R. D.) Health resorts in New Jersey. *Med. Bull., Phila.*, 1885, vii, 303; 373: viii, 13.—**Hunt** (E. M.) Report of the bureau of vital statistics of the State of New Jersey, 1879-83. *Rep. Bd. Health N. Jersey, Camden*, 1880, iv. 311: Mt. Holly, 1881, v, 229: Woodbury, 1882, vi, 261: 1883, vii, 315: Trenton, 1884, viii, 279.—**Johnson** (J. C.) [A report of the diseases which have prevailed in Warren County, N. J., during the year 1856.] *Med. & Surg. Reporter, Burlington*, 1857, x, 154-175.—**Larison** (G. H.) Diseases prevalent in the valley of the Delaware. *Tr. M. Soc. N. Jersey, Newark*, 1872, 73-90.—**Leeds** (A. R.) Water-supply of Hudson County. *Rep. Bd. Health Co. Hudson, N. J.*, 1867, N. Y., 1878, 29-32. ——. The water supply of Newark, Jersey City, and Hoboken. *San. Engin., N. Y.*, 1880-81, iv, 351; 379.—**M'George** (W.) The seaside resorts of New Jersey. *Hahneman. Month., Phila.*, 1881, n.s., iii, 523-527.—**Marsh** (E. J.) Report on vital statistics. *Rep. Bd. Health N. Jersey, Trenton*, 1878, i, 35-42.—**Meteorological** records. *Ibid.*, 1878, ii, 167-175.—**Parrish** (J.) Report on the epidemics of New Jersey. *Tr. Am. M. Ass., Phila.*, 1852, v, 292-305. ——. Climate cure; New Jersey pines. *Med. & Surg. Reporter, Phila.*, 1880, xliii, 558. ——. The Pine District of New Jersey as a health resort. *Country Pract., Beverly, N. J.*, 1880-81, ii, 187.—**Report** of the medical superintendent of vital statistics to the secretary of state and the State board of health, 1877-9. *Rep. Bd. Health N. Jersey, Trenton*, 1878, ii, 177: Camden, 1879, iii, 173. [*See, also, supra*, Hunt.]—**Schedules** of questions for a sanitary survey of Hudson County, New Jersey, and Bayonne, N. J. *Rep. Nat. Bd. Health, Wash.*, 1879, 169-237, 17 pl.—**Smith** (L. A.) On the topography and epidemic diseases of New Jersey, and the treatment thereof. *Tr. Am. M. Ass., Phila.*, 1858, xi, 169-180. *Also*, Reprint.—**Stevenson** (J. R.) The "Pines" of New Jersey as a residence for patients with pulmonary disease. *Phila. M. Times*, 1873-4, iv, 759.—**Taylor** (O. H.) Medical topography of Camden County, New Jersey. *Tr. M. Soc. N. Jersey, N. Y.*, 1861, 97-108. *Also*, Reprint.—**Varick** (T. R.) Report on epidemics and endemics that have occurred in the State of New Jersey since 1870. *Rep. Bd. Health N. Jersey, Trenton*, 1877, i, 103-129.—**Ward** (L. B.) Memorandum on the soil, contour, and drainage of Hudson County. *Rep. Bd. Health Co. Hudson, N. J.*, 1877, N. Y., 1878, 33-46.

New Jersey. *Bureau of Vital Statistics.* Circular xxxiv. Marriage, birth, and death returns. Copy of sections of laws defining the duties of clergymen, coroners, physicians, midwives, undertakers, etc. 4 pp. 8°. [*Trenton*, 1883?]

——. [Circular calling attention to the necessity of a State record of every marriage, birth, and death, and the penalty for neglect to obey the law.] 1 sheet. 8°. [*Trenton*, 1883.]

New Jersey. *Dairy Commissioner.* Annual reports of the dairy commissioner to the senate and general assembly. 1., 1886; 2., 1887. 8°. *Trenton, J. D. Murphy Publishing Co.*, 1887-8.

Dairy commissioner was appointed March 22, 1886.

——. Circular No. 3. Laws of New Jersey relating to food and drugs. 19 pp. 8°. [*Paterson*, 1887.]

New Jersey. *Geological Survey of New Jersey.* Annual reports of the State geologist to the governor of the State, for the years 1874; 1882. 8°. *Trenton*, 1874-82.

New Jersey. *Health Commission.* Annual report to the governor of the State. 1. (1874). 66 pp., 1 l. 8°. *Trenton, W. S. Sharp*, 1874.

New Jersey. *New Jersey House for Disabled Soldiers, at Newark, N. J.* Annual reports of the managers and commandant to the governor of the State. 1.-12., 1866 to 1876-7. 8°. *Trenton*, 1867-77.

1. report for 5 months, July to Nov., 1866. 1866, 1869-70, and 1870-71 in MS.

New Jersey. *New Jersey School for Deaf-Mutes, Trenton.* Annual report of the trustees and superintendent to the governor of the State, for the year 1883-4. 23 pp. 8°. *Trenton, J. L. Murphy,* 1884.

New Jersey. *New Jersey State Lunatic Asylum, at Trenton.* By-laws adopted by the managers. Also the act to provide for the organization of said asylum, and for the care and maintenance of the insane; passed Feb. 23, 1847. And the supplement to said act, passed March 9, 1848. 40 pp. 8°. *Trenton, Brittain & Jones,* 1848.
Opened May 15, 1848.
Bound with: Reports, 2.-13., 1848-59.

————. Annual reports of the managers and officers to the governor of the State. 2.-38., 1848 to 1883-4. 8°. *Trenton, Vineland, etc.,* 1849-84.
The managers' 2. report (1848) is the superintendents' 1. report, which dates from the opening to Dec. 31, 1848. The 19. report is for 11 months ending Nov., 1866. The 24. is for 11 months ending Oct., 1871. The 2.-24. (1848 to 1869-70) bound in 2 v. Want the managers' report for 1847 (1.).

————. *See, also:*
NEW JERSEY. Report of the joint committee on the State Lunatic Asylum at Trenton to the senate and general assembly of the State of New Jersey, session of 1875. 8°. *Trenton,* 1875.

New Jersey. *New Jersey State Reform School for Juvenile Delinquents, at Jamesburg.* Annual reports of the trustees and superintendent to the governor of the State. 3.-16., 1866-7 to 1879-80. 8°. *Trenton,* 1868-80.

New Jersey. *Rutgers Scientific School, the State College for the Benefit of Agriculture, and Mechanics Arts, New Brunswick.* Annual report of the board of visitors and board of trustees to the governor of the State. 13., 1876-7. 37 pp. 8°. *Trenton, Naar, Day & Naar,* 1877.

New Jersey. *State Asylum for the Insane, at Morristown.* Annual reports of the commissioners appointed to select a site and build an asylum for the insane of the State of New Jersey, to the governor of the State, for the years 1871-2 to 1878-9. 8°. *Trenton,* 1872-9.
Opened Aug. 17, 1876. 1871-2 to 1878-9 bound in 1 v.

————. Annual reports of the managers and officers to the governor of the State. 1.-10., 1876 to 1884-5. 8°. *Trenton,* 1876-85.
1. report for 2½ months ending Oct. 31, 1876. 1.-7. bound with: Rep. of commissioners.

————. Acts for the organization of the . . . and by-laws. 58 pp. 8°. *Newark, Williams & Plum,* 1876.

————. [Blank forms in use at the asylum.] v. s. [*Newark,* 188-.]
Application for admission.
Bond of friend of patient.
Certificate of insanity.
History of patient.
Order of judge, affidavit of physician, and certificate of clerk of county.

————. *See, also:*
[BODINE (J. L.)] Fourth annual report of the managers and officers of the State Asylum for the Insane, at Morristown, N. J., Oct. 31, 1879. [A criticism.] 8°. [*New York,* 1880.]

New Jersey. *State Board of Health.* Annual reports of the . . . and reports of the bureau of vital statistics to the governor of the State. 1.-11., 1877 to 1886-7. 8°. *Trenton, Camden & Woodbury,* 1877-87.
Reports of the bureau of vital statistics commenced in 1880-81.

————. Circular to householders, city authorities, boards of health, etc. 4 pp. 8°. [*Trenton,* 1878?]

————. Instructions to ministers, physicians, undertakers, assessors, and all concerned in the registry and returns of marriages, births, and

New Jersey. *State Board of Health*—cont'd.
deaths. 44 pp. 8°. *Trenton, Naar, Day & Naar,* 1878.

————. Circular as to sanitary appliances [to be exhibited at the State fair]. July 7, 1879. 1 sheet. 8°. [*Trenton,* 1879.]

————. Circular, June 1, 1880. Protection to bathers. How to treat the drowned; how to save a life. 2 l. 8°. [*Trenton,* 1880.]

————. Circulars issued by the . . . 8°. [*Trenton,* 1880.]
CONTENTS.
Circular A. To farmers and dealers in stock [on pleuro-pneumonia and pneumo-enteritis, hog cholera]. 4 pp.
B. To township and city boards of health in reference to infectious diseases of animals. August 10, 1880. 1 l.
C. "Contagious diseases of animals." August, 1880. 1 l.

————. [Circular letter of the council of analysts and chemists, appointed by the State board of health of New Jersey, to investigate the prevalence of adulteration of articles of food or drugs. With a schedule of questions and a copy of the "Act to prevent the adulteration of food or drugs".] May 1, 1881. 3 l. 8°. [*Jersey City,* 1881.]

————. [General suggestions for the organization of local boards of health and the manner of dealing with nuisances prejudicial to the public health. With a schedule of questions indicating what local boards should know or inquire about.] May 10, 1881. 4 pp. 8°. [*Trenton,* 1881.]

————. Circular [on the study of disease in localities, by the aid of geological and topographical maps furnished to observers by the board of health]. Feb. 15, 1882. 3 pp. 8°. [*Trenton,* 1882.]

————. Circular as to illuminating oils. April 20, 1882. 1 sheet. 8°. [*Trenton,* 1882.]

————. Circular to charitable and penal institutions [as to their sanitary condition]. June 1, 1882. 4 pp. 8°. [*Trenton,* 1882.]

————. Circular as to petroleum, kerosene, etc. June 20, 1882. 4 pp. 8°. [*Trenton,* 1882.]

————. Sanitary school circular. July 1, 1882. 12 pp. 8°. [*Trenton,* 1882.]

————. Circular as to sanitary instruction and training in schools. Aug. 31, 1882. 1 l. 8°. [*Trenton,* 1882.]

————. Jahres-Bericht des Gesundheits-Rathes des Staates New Jersey. 6., 1881-2. 475 pp. 8°. *Elizabeth, N. J., Freie Presse,* 1883.

————. Circular as to contagious diseases of animals. 32 pp. 8°. [*Trenton,* 1883.]
CONTENTS.
A. To farmers and dealers in stock. Pleuro-pneumonia. Pneumo-enteritis (hog cholera). pp. 3-7.
B. To townships and city boards of health. April 10, 1880. pp. 7-9.
C. Contagious diseases of animals. Aug., 1880. pp. 9-12.
D. To farmers and dealers in stock. April 1, 1881. pp. 12-15.
E. To farmers and dealers in stock. pp. 15-23.
F. As to contagious diseases of animals. Jan. 4, 1883. pp. 25-32.

————. Circular No. xxviii. School and health circular No. 2. For parents, guardians, children, teachers, and trustees. 12 pp. 8°. [*Trenton,* 1883?]

————. Circular No. xxxvii. School and health circular No. 3. For parents, guardians, children, teachers, and trustees. 5 pp. 8°. [*Trenton,* 1883?]

————. Circular xxxix. To local boards of health. [On the causes of preventable disease, with a schedule of questions which they should know or inquire about.] 2 l. 8°. [*Trenton,* 1883.]

————. Circular xliv. How to prevent the spread of small-pox, scarlet fever, diphtheria, and other communicable diseases. 12 pp. 8°. [*Trenton,* 1884.]

New Jersey. *State Board of Health*—cont'd.
——. Circular lvii. To the physicians of the State. [Relating to typhoid fever and diphtheria, with a schedule of suggestive questions.] 4 pp. 8°. [*Trenton*, 1886.]
——. Circular lviii. Laws relating to public health, and references thereto. 28 pp. 8°. [*Trenton*, 1886.]
——. Circular lix. Relating to the adulteration of food or drugs and to petroleum, and laws and regulations as to the same. 4 pp. 8°. [*Trenton*, 1886.]
——. Report of the milk inspector. By William K. Newton. 17 pp. 8°. [*Trenton*, 1886 ?]
Repr. from: Rep. Bd. Health N. Jersey (1884-5). 8°. *Trenton*, 1886, ix.

New Jersey. *State Industrial School for Girls, Trenton.* Annual reports of the trustees to the governor of the State. 1.-9., 1871-2 to 1879-80. 8°. *Trenton*, 1872-80.

New Jersey Academy of Medicine. Constitution and by-laws, with the act of incorporation and list of fellows. Founded 1874. 23 pp. 8°. *Jersey City, Argus Print. House*, 1875.

New Jersey (The) Eclectic Medical and Surgical Journal. Devoted to liberal medicine, general science and literature. Editor: Edward Fishblatt. [Bi-monthly.] v. 1-3, August, 1874, to October, 1876. 8°. *Newark.*
Continued in 1877 as : **New York** (The) Eclectic Medical and Surgical Journal.

New Jersey (The) Medical Reporter.
Title of v. 8 of : **New Jersey** (The) Medical Reporter, and Transactions of the New Jersey Medical Society, 1855.

New Jersey (The) Medical Reporter, and Transactions of the New Jersey Medical Society. Edited by Joseph Parrish. [Quarterly.] v. 1-8, Oct., 1847, to Dec., 1855. 8°. *Burlington.*
v. 5 became monthly. v. 8, the words "and Transactions of the New Jersey Medical Society" dropped, and "a monthly journal of medical and surgical science" added. In v. 7 S. W. Butler added as editor ; in v. 8 Dr. Butler sole editor. Continued as : **Medical** (The) and Surgical Reporter.

New Jersey Pharmaceutical Association. Proceedings. 12., 1882 ; 13., 1883 ; 17., 1887. 8°. *Camden*, 1882-3 ; *New Brunswick*, 1887.

New Jersey (The) Pharmaceutical Record ; an illustrated journal of practical pharmacy, medicine, science, and literature. William H. Gilder editor. [Monthly.] No. 1, v. 1, Dec., 1875. 16 pp. 8°. *Newark.*

New Jersey Sanitary Association. The fifth annual meeting, Trenton, N. J., Dec. 12 and 13, 1879. Order of business. 2 l. 8°. *Trenton, N. J., Naar, Day & Naar*, 1879.

New Jersey State Dental Society. Condensed proceedings for the years 1875-6-7. 90 pp., 2 l. 8°. *Newark, L. J. Hardham*, 1878.
——. Proceedings for the years 1878-9-80. 209 pp. 8°. *Newark, N. J.*, 1881.
Bound with preceding.
——. Transactions for the years 1881-2-3. 234 pp. 8°. *Newark, N. J.*, 1884.

Newlands (James). Reports to the health committee of the borough of Liverpool, on the sewerage and other works, under the sanitary act. For the years 1847-68. [6 reports in 5 v.] 8°. *Liverpool*, 1848-69.
——. [Report of the borough engineer . . .] To the chairman of the health committee of the borough of Liverpool. [Details of all the works executed from April, 1853, to April, 1856.] 71, ii pp. 8°. [*Liverpool*], *H. Greenwood*, [1856]. [P., v. 1432.]
——. Liverpool, past and present, in relation to sanitary operations. A paper read before the public health section of the National Association for the Promotion of Social Science, Oct., 1858.

Newlands (James)—continued.
23 pp., 1 plan. 8°. *Liverpool, Harris & Co.*, 1859. [*Also, in:* P., v. 1432.]
——. Report of the borough engineer, in accordance with the resolution of the special improvement committee. 30 pp. 8°. *Liverpool, G. McCorquodale & Co.*, 1859. [P., v. 1432.]
——. A short description of the markets and market system of Paris, with notes on the markets of London ; in the form of a report to the markets committee of Liverpool. 43 pp., 1 pl. 8°. *Liverpool, G. McCorquodale & Co.*, 1865. [P., v. 1432.]
——. Narrative of the proceedings relative to the supply of salt water for the borough of Liverpool. 20 pp. 8°. *Liverpool, H. Greenwood*, 1865.
——. Liverpool. Disinfecting establishments, erected from designs by the borough engineer. [March, 1867.] 2 l., 2 pl. 8°. [*Liverpool*, 1867.]
——. Abattoirs. (Paris and Brussels.) Return to an address of the House of Commons, dated 7 June, 1869, for " copy of report compiled for the health committee of Liverpool by the borough engineer . . . with reference to the establishment of the abattoir of La Villette in Paris, and the abattoir of Brussels". Ordered by the House of Commons to be printed, 7 Aug., 1869. 40 pp. fol. [*London*, 1869.]
——. Account of the Sewers, Sewage Utilization Company of Liverpool. MS. 6 l. fol. [*Liverpool, n. d.*]
See, also, **Simpson** (James) & **Newlands** (James). Liverpool water supply. 8°. *Liverpool*, 1849.

Newlands (William L.)
See **Antisell** (Thomas) & **Newlands** (William L.) Addresses, [etc.] 8°. *Washington*, 1871.

Newlands College of Midwifery and Lying-in Institute, St. Louis. Annual announcement of . . . for the spring and fall sessions of the year 1885 (1.). 5 l. 8°. *St. Louis, A. Gast & Co.*, [1885].

New Lebanon.

MEADE (W.) A chemical analysis of the waters of New Lebanon, in the State of New York, with observations on their medicinal qualities, and principally as a bath. 12°. *Burlington, N. J.*, 1818.

New London. Annual reports of the board of water-commissioners to the city of New London. 4., 1874 ; 5., 1875-6 ; 7.-9., 1877-8 to 1879-80 ; 12.-14., 1882-3 to 1884-5. 8°. *New London*, 1874-85.
——. The charter and ordinances of the city of New London, 1879. 60 pp. 8°. *New London, New London Telegram Print*, 1879.
——. Annual report of the court of common council, the treasurer, and the commissioner of charities of the city of New London, for the year 1883-4. 116 pp. 8°. *New London, The Day Job Office*, 1884.

New London.

See, also, **Fever** (*Cerebro-spinal, History, etc., of*), **Fever** (*Typhus, History, etc., of*), *by localities.*
Chamberlain (C. W.) Sewerage problems ; the intercepting sewer for Hartford ; report of special committee, with comments ; the sewerage of New London, with report of Col. Geo. E. Waring. jr. Rep. Bd. Health Connect., Hartford, 1880, iii, 135–177, 2 maps.—**Intercepting** sewers at New London, Conn. San. Engin., N. Y., 1886-7, xv, 401.

Newman (A.) Comparison of the mortality from diseases in armies, with that of men of military ages in civil life, showing the groups of diseases chiefly concerned in causing the excess of mortality in armies. 39 pp. 4°. *Leavenworth, Times & Conservative Printing House*, 1869.

Newman (Albert). Croup; its history, nature, and treatment. Fiske fund prize dissertation of the Rhode Island Medical Society. 28 pp. 8°. *Philadelphia, T. K. & P. G. Collins,* 1855.

Newman (Carolus). *De dyspepsia. 1 p. l., 50 pp. 8°. *Edinburgi, Balfour et Smellie,* 1773.

Newman (David). *On malpositions of the kidney. 63 pp. 8°. [Glasgow], A. Macdougall, [1883].
Repr. from: Glasgow M. J., 1883, 4. s., xx.

Newman (F. W.) National Anti-Compulsory Vaccination League. The political side of the vaccination system; an essay read at the Birmingham Anti-Vaccination Conference, October 26th, 1874. Published by order of the executive. 11 pp. 8°. *Cheltenham, G. F. Poole,* [1874].

——. The same. 4. ed. 12 pp. 12°. *Leicester, E. Lamb,* [n. d.]

Newman (George). A concise exposition of homœopathy; its principles and practice; with an appendix, containing a statement of the proceedings that led to the author's dismissal from the situation of medical officer of the Glastonbury district of the Wells Poor Law Union; correspondence with the poor law commissioners on the subject; opinion of the Royal College of Physicians on homœopathy, etc. iv, 68 pp. 8°. *London, J. Leath,* 1844.
2. thousand.

Newman (James M.) Congestion of the brain in cholera; its etiology, diagnosis, and treatment. A paper read before the Buffalo Medical Association, October 3, 1854. 25 pp. 8°. *Buffalo, Thomas & Lathrops,* 1854. [*Also, in:* P., v. 205.]

——. Report on the sanitary police of cities. Presented to the American Medical Association, May, 1856. 53 pp. 8°. *Philadelphia, T. K. & P. G. Collins,* 1856.
Repr. from: Tr. Am. M. Ass., Phila., 1856, ix.

Newman (John B.) Fascination; or, the philosophy of charming; illustrating the principles of life in connection with spirit and matter. x, 176 pp. 8°. *New York, Fowlers & Wells,* 1847.

Newman (Robert). Report of the committee on the result of consanguineous marriages. Presented to the New York State Medical Society, at its annual session, February, 1869. pp. 109–130. 8°. *Albany, Weed, Parsons & Co.,* 1869.
Cutting from: Tr. M. Soc. N. Y., Albany, 1869.

——. Treatment of strictures of the urethra by Laminaria digitata and galvanism. A paper read before the Medical Journal Association of New York. 5 pp. 8°. *New York,* [1871].

——. The endoscope in granular urethritis in the male. 16 pp., 1 pl. 8°. *Louisville, J. P. Morton & Co.,* 1871.
Repr. from: Am. Pract., Louisville, 1871, iv.

——. The endoscope; considered particularly in reference to diseases of the female bladder and urethra. 17 pp., 6 pl. 8°. *Albany, Weed, Parsons & Co.,* 1872.
Repr. from: Tr. M. Soc. N. Y., Albany, 1872.

——. Electrolysis in the treatment of stricture of the urethra. 29 pp. 8°. *Albany, C. Van Benthuysen & Sons,* 1874.
Repr. from: Tr. M. Soc. N. Y., Albany, 1874.

——. The same. 32 pp. 8°. *New York, T. L. Clacher,* 1874.
Repr. from: Arch. Electrol. & Neurol, N. Y., 1874, i.

——. Stricture of the urethra in the female, and its treatment by electrolysis. 11 pp. 8°. [*New York,* 1875.]
Repr. from: Am. J M. Sc., Phila., 1875, n s., lxx.

——. Urethrocele in the female. 16 pp. 8°. *New York, W. Wood & Co.,* 1880.
Repr. from: Am. J. Obst., N. Y., 1880. xiii.

Newman (Robert)—continued.
——. Stricture of the rectum treated by electrolysis. 7 pp. 8°. *Bridgeport, Conn., Gould & Stiles,* 1882.
Repr. from: N. Eng. M. Month., Newtown, Conn., 1881-2, i.

——. A successful ovariotomy in 1866. Galvanocaustic to pedicle, antiseptic dressing, drainage, silver wire ligatures left in abdominal cavity. 6 pp. 8°. [n. p.], 1882.
Repr. from: N. Eng. M. Month., Newtown, Conn., 1881-2, i.

——. Ten years' experience in the treatment of stricture of the urethra by electrolysis. 44 pp. 8°. *New York, Trow,* 1882.
Repr. from: Med. Rec., N. Y., 1882, xxii.

——. Additional answers to correspondents about the electrolytic treatment of urethral strictures; with a few select cases. 5 pp. 8°. [*Bridgeport, Conn., Gould & Stiles*], 1883.
Repr. from: N. Eng. M. Month., Newtown, Conn., 1882-3, ii.

——. The treatment of urethritis and leucorrhœa. 15 pp. 8°. *Richmond, The Southern Clinic print,* 1883.
Repr. from: South. Clinic, Richmond, 1883, vi.

——. Does the character of pus diagnosticate gonorrhœa as a specific infection from a simple (benign) urethritis? A medico-legal sketch. 8 pp. 8°. *Richmond, Whittet & Shepperson,* 1883.

——. Progress of electrolysis in surgery. Read at the first annual meeting of the Fifth District Branch of the New York State Medical Association, held at Brooklyn, October 13, 1885. 8 pp. 8°. *New York,* 1885.
Repr. from: Gaillard's M. J., N. Y., 1885, xli (xl).

——. Tabular statistics of one hundred cases of urethral stricture treated by electrolysis, without relapse. 15 pp. 8°. *Bridgeport, Conn., Gould & Stiles,* 1885.
Repr. from: N. Eng. M. Month., Newtown, Conn., 1884-5, iv.

——. Galvano-cautery in diseases of the prostate, bladder, and urethra. 13 pp. 12°. *Chicago,* 1886.
Repr. from: J. Am. M. Ass., Chicago, 1886, vii.

——. Is electrolysis a failure in the treatment of urethral strictures? 12 pp. 8°. *New York, Trow's Printing Co.,* 1886.
Repr. from: Med. Rec., N. Y., 1886, xxx.

——. The galvano-cautery sound and its application, especially in hypertrophy of the prostate; with reports of cases. 53 pp. 16°. *Bridgeport, Conn., Gould & Stiles,* 1887.
Repr. from: N. Eng. M. Month., Bridgeport, Conn., 1887-8, vii.

——. Synopsis of the second hundred cases of urethral stricture treated by electrolysis; with cases. 15 pp. 4°. *Chicago,* 1887.
Repr. from: J. Am. M. Ass., Chicago, 1887, ix.
For Biography, see N. Eng. M. Month., Sandy Hook, Conn., 1884-5, iv, 177-179, port.

Newman (W. H.) On rupture of the cervix uteri occurring at the time of parturition; its remote consequences. The power of the perineum in preventing prolapsus uteri; abstract of four cases. 16 pp. 8°. *Louisville, J. P. Morton & Co.,* 1871.
Repr. from: Am. Pract., Louisville, 1871, iii.

Newman (William). Cæsarean section. Recovery of mother. Child not viable. (For private distribution.) 20 pp. 8°. *Stamford, Langley,* 1866. [P., v. 90.]

——. On the treatment of nævi by electrolysis. x pp. 8°. *London, H. K. Lewis,* 1881.

——. Surgical cases mainly from the wards of the Stamford, Rutland, and General Infirmary. 142, x pp. 8°. *London, H. K. Lewis,* 1881.

Newman (*William G. H.*) [1827–83].
    Toner (J. M.) In memoriam. J. Am. M. Ass., Chicago, 1883, i, 603.

Newmann (Joh. Carl). * Ueber den vorzugsweise wirksamen Bestandtheil des schwarzen Pfeffers, eine Abhandlung. 29 pp. 8°. *Dorpat, C. Schulz,* 1860.

Newman-Sherwood (Guil. Henric.) * Theses quas . . . loco dissertationis de peritonitide mox edendæ defendet. 1 l. 8°. *Halæ, formis C. Grunerti,* [1834].

——. * De auscultatione obstetricia. 44 pp. 8°. *Halæ, formis C. Grunerti,* [n. d.]

Newmarket.
    Clark (G. T.) Report to the General Board of Health, on a preliminary inquiry into the sewerage, drainage, and supply of water, and the sanitary condition of the inhabitants of the town of Newmarket. 8°. *London,* 1850.

——. Report to the General Board of Health, on a further inquiry as to the boundaries which might be most advantageously adopted for the district of Newmarket, for the purposes of the public health act. 8°. *London,* 1851.

New Mexico.
    See, also, **Fever** (*Malarial, History, etc., of*), *by localities;* **Las Vegas**; **Paleontology**; **Utah.**
    Climate (The) of New Mexico and Las Vegas hot springs. 8°. *Chicago,* 1883.

    United States. *War Department. Engineer Corps.* Report of the Secretary of War, communicating, in answer to a resolution of the Senate, a report and map of the examination of New Mexico, made by Lieut. J. W. Abert, of the Topographical Corps. 30. Cong., 1. sess. Sen. Ex. Doc. No. 23. 8°. *Washington,* 1848.

    Bandelier (A.-F.) La découverte du Nouveau Mexique par le moine franciscain, frère Marcos, de Nice, en 1539. Rev. d'ethnog., Par., 1886, v, 31; 117; 193.—Bryan (O. M.) Climate and diseases of New Mexico; remarkable exemption from consumption; prevalence of rheumatism and syphilis. Chicago M. Exam., 1865, vi, 65-76.—Halley (G.) New Mexico as a health resort. Kansas City M. Rec., 1888, v, 41-44.—Jones (J. J.) New Mexico as a health resort for consumptives. Med. & Surg. Reporter, Phila., 1877, xxxvii, 201-203.—McParlin (T. A.) Notes on the history and climate of New Mexico. Rep. Smithson. Inst. 1877, Wash., 1878, 321-348. *Also,* Reprint.—Millikin (D.) Notes on the climate of Colorado and New Mexico. Cincin. Lancet & Clinic, 1882, n. s., ix, 577-579.—Parker (W. T.) Concerning the climate of New Mexico. Arch. Med., N. Y., 1884, xii, 132-158. *Also,* Reprint.—Smith (A. H.) Medical aspect of New Mexico. Indiana J. M., Indianap., 1870-71, i, 7-13.—Tyndale (J. H.) New Mexico; its climatic advantages for consumptives. Boston M. & S. J., 1883, cviii, 265; 313. *Also,* Reprint.

New Milford.
    See, also, **Fever** (*Cerebro-spinal, History, etc., of*), *by localities.*
    Sanitary drainage of New Milford. Rep. Bd. Health Connect. 1881, Hartford, 1882, iv, 70-74, 1 map.

Newnan (John). * On general dropsy. x, 11-31 pp. 8°. *Philadelphia, P. Hall,* 1793.

Newnham (William) [1790–1865]. An essay on the symptoms, causes, and treatment of inversio uteri; with a history of the successful extirpation of that organ during the chronic stage of the disease. xv, 152 pp., 2 pl. 8°. *London, E. Cox & Son,* 1818.

——. Some observations on the medicinal and dietetic properties of green tea, and particularly on the controuling influence it exerts over irritation of the brain. 32 pp. 8°. *London, J. Hatchard & Son,* 1827.

——. Essay on the disorders incident to literary men, and on the best means of preserving their health; read before the Royal Society of Literature, Nov. 5, 1834; and dedicated, by permission, to the Lord Bishop of Salisbury. 1 p. l., 36 pp. 8°. *London, J. Hatchard & Son,* 1836.

Newnham (William)—continued.
——. The reciprocal influence of body and mind considered, as it affects the great questions of education, phrenology, materialism, moral advancement and responsibility, man's free agency, the theory of life, the peculiarities of mental property, mental diseases, the agency of mind upon the body, of physical temperament upon the manifestations of mind, and upon the expression of religious feeling. xxiii, 628 pp. 8°. *London, J. Hatchard,* 1842.

——. Narrative of an unusual case of utero-gestation, in which the premature expulsion of one fœtus preceded by two months the birth of a twin fœtus at the full term. 4 pp. 8°. *Manchester, W. Irwin,* 1848.
    Bound with: Clay (C.) Brit. Rec. of Obst. Med. & Surg. 8°. *Manchester,* 1848, i.

——. History of four cases of eclampsia nutans, or the "salaam" convulsions of infancy, with suggestions as to its origin and future treatment. 28 pp. 8°. *Manchester, W. Irwin,* 1849.
    Bound with: Clay (C.) Brit. Rec. of Obst. Med. & Surg. 8°. *Manchester,* 1849, ii.

——, **Wickham** (W.) **& Salter.** Retrospect of the progress of surgical literature for the year 1838-9. Read June 13, 1839, before the annual meeting of the Southern Branch of the Provincial Medical Association, and published at its request. 47 pp. 8°. *London, J. Churchill,* 1839.

Newnham urban sanitary authority. *See* **Gloucestershire** combined sanitary district.

New Norfolk.
    See **Insane** (*Asylums for, etc.*), *by localities.*

New Orleans. Message of the mayoralty to the common council of the city of New Orleans. [On the yellow fever epidemic of 1853.] Oct., 1853. 7 pp. 8°. *New Orleans,* 1853.

——. Annual messages of the mayor to the common council of New Orleans. Published by authority. For the years 1852-3; 1867-8. 8°. *New Orleans,* 1853-68.

——. Report of the sanitary commission of New Orleans on the epidemic yellow fever of 1853. Published by authority of the city council of New Orleans. xix, 542 pp., 4 pl., 1 map, 2 diag., 5 tab. 8°. *New Orleans, Picayune Office,* 1854. [*Also, in:* P., v. 306.]

——. Report of the board of engineers to mature and recommend some general and harmonious plan for the present and future draining of the city of New Orleans, and for the protection of the city against overflow, made to the common council March 30, 1869. 8 pp. 8°. *New Orleans, F. F. Hansell,* 1869.

——. Report on the drainage, sewerage, and health of the city of New Orleans, by Henry C. Brown, city surveyor. 16 pp. 8°. *New Orleans,* 1879.

——. Report of the joint committee of the commercial bodies of New Orleans to the United States, Mexican, Central and South American Commission. Dec. 30, 1884. 35 pp. 8°. *New Orleans, A. W. Hyatt,* [1885].

New Orleans.
    See, also, **Children** (*Hospitals, etc., for, Reports, etc., of*); **Cholera** (*Asiatic, History, etc., of*), *by localities;* **Dentistry**; **Education** (*Medical*), *etc.,* **Fever** (*Malarial, History, etc., of*), **Fever** (*Yellow, History, etc., of*), **Hospitals** (*Descriptions, etc., of*), **Hospitals** (*Naval, etc.*), *by localities;* **Inundations.**
    Barton (E. H.) *et al. vs.* The City of New Orleans. In the supreme court. Brief of appellants [the late sanitary commission of New Orleans, for compensation for services rendered in

New Orleans.

the years 1853–4. By E. H. Durell.] 8°. [*New Orleans*, 1858?]

CHAILLÉ (S. E.) Life and death in New Orleans from 1787 to 1869, and more especially during the five years 1856 to 1860. 8°. *New Orleans*, 1870. *Repr. from:* N. Orl. J. M., 1870, xxiii, 1–65. *See, also, infra.*

DALTON (S. W.) Letters of Cenci, written four years ago, on the sanitary reforms needed in New Orleans, and republished by order of the city council. 8°. *New Orleans*, 1853.

DOWLER (B.) Tableaux, geographical, commercial, geological, and sanitary, of New Orleans. 8°. *New Orleans*, [*n. d.*]

LOUISIANA. Report of the joint committee on public health. (Majority report.) 8°. *New Orleans*, 1854.

LOUISIANA Board of Health. Annual and biennial reports to the general assembly for the years 1846, 1849, 1850, 1856, 1860, 1866 to 1884–5, 1886–7. 8°. *New Orleans*, 1847–86.

———. By-laws and ordinances of the board of health of the city of New Orleans, together with the acts of the legislature and ordinances of the general council establishing the same. Published by authority. 8°. *New Orleans*, 1849.

———. Drainage and drainage canals in the vicinity of Canal street. [Recommendations of the State board of health to the mayor and administrators of the city, Oct. 20, 1871.] 8°. [*New Orleans*, 1871.]

———. Monthly reports of deaths in the city of New Orleans. Published by order of the board of health. From Jan., 1874, to March, 1877. fol. *New Orleans*, 1874–7.

———. Reports of deaths in New Orleans. [Weekly.] Dec. 22, 1883, to April 26, 1884; May 24 to Aug. 16; Sept. 6 to Nov. 29; Dec. 8, 27, 1884. 18°. [*New Orleans*, 1883–4.]

NEW ORLEANS Medical and Surgical Association. Report on milk and dairies in the city of New Orleans, presented to the New Orleans Medical and Surgical Association. (Published by the New Orleans Auxiliary Sanitary Association.) 8°. *New Orleans*, 1879.

Act (An) relative to the establishment of a board of health for the city of New Orleans and Lafayette. N. Orl. M. & S. J., 1849–50, vi, 814–816.—**Barton** (E. H.) Sanitary report of New Orleans, La. Tr. Am. M. Ass., Phila., 1849, ii, 591–610. ———. Meteorological register for New Orleans for 1850. N. Orl. M. & S. J., 1850–51, vii, 267–269. ———. Report upon the sanitary condition of New Orleans. *In:* New Orleans. Rep. San. Com. of N. Orl. on epidemic yellow fever of 1853, 8°, N. Orl., 1854, 213–462, 1 map, 8 tab. ———. On the meteorology, mortality, and sanitary condition of New Orleans for the years 1854 and 1855. Tr. Am. M. Ass., Phila., 1856, ix, 723–752, 2 tab.— **Bemiss** (S. M.) Sanitary legislation in New Orleans. N. Orl. J. M., 1870, xxiii, 201–233. *Also*, Reprint. ———. Sanitary work in New Orleans. Rep. Nat. Bd. Health 1880, Wash., 1882, ii, 602–617. — **Board** (The) of health and the sanitary condition of New Orleans. N. Orl. M. & S. J., 1851–2, viii, 399.—**Caldwell** (C.) Thoughts on the probable destiny of New Orleans in relation to health, population, and commerce. Phila. J. M. & Phys. Sc., 1823, vi, 1–15.—**Chaillé** (S. E.) Vital statistics of New Orleans. N. Orl. J. M., 1870, xxiii, 1–65. ———. The vital statistics of New Orleans, from 1769 to 1874. N. Orl. M. & S. J., 1874–5, ii, 1–37. *Also*, Reprint. ———. The vital statistics of New Orleans as taught by the U. S. census, 1880. N. Orl. M. & S. J., 1880–81, n. s., viii, 1027–1044. *Also*, Reprint. ———. Inundations of New Orleans and their influence on its health. N. Orl. M. & S. J., 1882–3, x, 20–37. *Also*, Reprint.—**Davidson** (J. P.) Some personal reminiscences of early epidemics in New Orleans. Tr. Louisiana M. Soc., N. Orl., 1887, 70–82.— **Dowler** (B.) Researches upon the necropolis of New Orleans, with brief allusions to its vital arithmetic. N. Orl. M. & S. J., 1850–51, vii, 275–300. *Also*, Reprint. ———. Vital statistics. N. Orl. M. & S. J., 1850–51, vii, 404. — **Eichorn.** Practische Mittheilungen aus New Orleans. Ztschr. f. d. ges. Med., Hamb., 1838, viii, 187–190.—**Fenner** (E. D.) Fever statistics; showing the relative proportion of the different forms of fever admitted into the New Orleans Charity Hospital during a period of

New Orleans.

seven years, from 1st January, 1841, to 1st January, 1848, inclusive; monthly and annually. N. Orl. M. & S. J., 1848–9, v, 48–53. ———. General report on the medical topography and meteorology of New Orleans, with an account of the prevalent diseases during the year 1849. South. M. Rep. (Fenner) 1849, N. Orl., 1850, i, 17–55. ———. On the inundation of New Orleans in 1816. *Ibid.*, 56–62. ———. Report on the general aspect of the weather, the condition of the streets, the stage of the river, and the principal diseases that prevailed in the city of New Orleans during the year 1850; in the form of a monthly journal. *Ibid.* (1850), 1851, ii, 13–39. ———. Report on the fevers, etc., of New Orleans. Tr. Am. M. Ass., Phila., 1851, iv, 201–210. ———. [Health of New Orleans during military rule.] South. J. M. Sc., N. Orl., 1866, i, 22–43.—**Hardee** (T. S.) The topography and drainage of New Orleans. Sanitarian, N. Y., 1875, iii, 297–302.—**Harris** (E.) Hygienic experience in New Orleans during the war; illustrating the importance of efficient sanitary regulations. Bull. N. York Acad. M., 1866, ii, 462–479.—**Health** of New Orleans, 1844–86: N. Orl. M. J., 1844–5, i, *passim. Continued in:* N. Orl. M. & S. J., 1845–6, ii: 1867, xx, *passim. Continued in:* N. Orl. J. M., 1868, xxi: 1870, xxiii, *passim. Continued in:* N. Orl. M. & S. J., n. s., 1873–4, i: 1885–6, xiii, *passim.*—**Holt** (J.) The sanitary relief of New Orleans. N. Orl. M. & S. J., 1885–6, n. s., xiii, 437–451. *Also*, Reprint. ———. The sanitary protection of New Orleans, municipal and maritime. Am. Pub. Health Ass. Rep. 1885, Concord, N. H., 1886, xi, 89–97. *Also :* Sanitarian, N. Y., 1886, xvi, 37–49. *Also*, Reprint.—**Hort** (W. P.) Report of the board of health on the sanitary condition of the city of New Orleans during the year 1846, and the means of improving it. N. Orl. M. & S. J., 1846–7, iii, 467. ———. A diary of the climate of New Orleans for 1850. *Ibid.*, 1850–51, vii, 580; 744. ———. Observations on the meteorological and sanitary condition of New Orleans, for the quarter ending March 31, 1851. *Ibid.*, 1851, vii, 454; 555.—**Jones** (J.) Tabular summary of cases treated in Charity Hospital during fifteen months, 1st January, 1869, to 1st April, 1870; arranged according to the "nomenclature of diseases of the Royal College of Physicians of London". N. Orl. J. M., 1870, xxiii, 551–555.—**K.** (S.) Health of New Orleans. Boston M. & S. J., 1864–5, lxxi, 91–93.—**Lacaze.** Impressions médicales d'un voyage aux Grandes Antilles et à la Nouvelle-Orléans. France méd., Par., 1881, xxviii, 340; 353.—**Layton** (T.) Anniversary address delivered before the Orleans Parish Medical Society. [Sanitary matters in New Orleans.] N. Orl. M. & S. J., 1882–3, n. s., x, 801–810.—**Loubere** (J. V.) Mortality and its causes for the months of August and September, 1849. *Ibid.*, 1849–50, vi, 424.—**Louisiana.** Board of health; annual reports on the sanatory condition of the city of New Orleans for the years 1848–50. *Ibid.*, 1848–9, v, 607: 1849–50, vi, 665: 1850–51, vii, 590. *Also* [1849–50]: South. M. Rep. (Fenner) 1849, N. Orl., 1850, i, 77: (1850), 1851, ii, 40. ———. Annual mortuary report for the year 1867. N. Orl. J. M., 1868, xxi, 408–413. *Also*, Reprint.—**Meteorological** reports [New Orleans], 1872–80. Rep. Bd. Health Louisiana 1872–80. N. Orl., 1873–81, *passim.*—**Mortality** of New Orleans, 1844–86. N. Orl. M. J., 1844–5, i, *passim. Continued in:* N. Orl. M. & S. J., 1845–6, ii: 1867, xx, *passim. Continued in:* N. Orl. J. M., 1868, xxi: 1870, xxiii, *passim. Continued in:* N. Orl. M. & S. J., 1873–4, n. s., i: 1885–6, xiii, *passim.*—**Payne** (J. T.) The New Orleans sewerage. San. News, Chicago, 1882–3, i, 141.—**Peters** (J. C.) New Orleans and the cholera and yellow fever of 1873. Sanitarian, N. Y., 1883, n. s., i, 225. — **Report** of diseases, from January 1st, 1867, to December 31st, 1867, treated in Charity Hospital, New Orleans, La. N. Orl. J. M., 1868, xxi, 197–202. — **Sanitary** legislation. N. Orl. M. & S. J., 1873–4, n. s., i, 631–635. — **Simonds** (J. C.) Vital statistics of New Orleans from February 3 to June 2, 1849. Charleston M. J., 1849, iv, 111; 710. ———. On the hygienic characteristics of New Orleans. Tr. Am. M. Ass., Phila., 1850, iii, 267–290. ———. Contributions to the vital statistics of New Orleans. Charleston M. J. & Rev., 1850, v, 277–296. ———. The sanitary condition of New Orleans, as illustrated by its mortuary statistics. *Ibid.*, 1851, vi, 677–745. *Also*, Reprint. *Also* [Abstr.]: South M. Rep. (Fenner) 1850, N. Orl., 1851, ii, 204–246. *Also*, Reprint. *Also* [Rev.]: N. Orl. M. & S. J., 1851–2, viii, 403–407 (W. P. Hort). ———. A comparison of the weekly bills of mortality of New Orleans and Boston, 1851. Charleston M. J. & Rev., 1852, vii, 289–293.—**Stark** (J.) Vital statistics of New Orleans. Edinb. M. & S. J., 1851, lxxv, 130–144. *Also*, Reprint.—**Thompson** (H. M.) Method introduced by the Auxiliary Sanitary Association for disposing of the garbage of New Orleans. Am. Pub. Health Ass. Rep. 1879, Bost., 1880, v, 32–34, 1 pl.—**Watkins** (W. H.) Causes of the insalubrity of New Orleans. N. Orl. M. & S. J., 1885–6, n. s., xiii, 509–530.

New Orleans Auxiliary Sanitary Association. Charter, by-laws, and rules of order of the New Orleans Auxiliary Sanitary Association. 12 pp. 8°. *New Orleans, L. Graham,* 1879.

New Orleans Auxiliary [etc.]—continued.

——. An address from the Auxiliary Sanitary Association of New Orleans to the other cities and towns of the Mississippi Valley. Published by the . . . June, 1879. 20 pp. 8°. *New Orleans, L. Graham,* 1879.

——. How to use zinc-iron disinfectant. 1 sheet. roy. 8°. [*New Orleans,* 1879.]

——. Proceedings of meeting of November 8, 1879. 2 l. 8°. [*n. p., n. d.*]

——. Proceedings of meeting of January 3, 1880. 3 pp. 8°. [*New Orleans,* 1880.]

——. Report of committee on construction and management of privies, made to the executive committee of the . . . April 17, 1880. 8 pp. 8°. *New Orleans, M. F. Dunn & Bro.,* 1880.

——. Annual address of Edward Fenner, with remarks by Charles A. Whitney, Cyrus Bussey, and Albert Baldwin, at the regular meeting of the . . . Nov. 23, 1880. 20 pp. 8°. *New Orleans,* 1880.

——. Notice [in compliance with city ordinance No. 4788, administration series]. New Orleans, Dec. 12, 1878. An ordinance to provide for the cleanliness of streets, gutters, etc., to prescribe the duties of householders and occupants of premises. English, French, and German text. 1 sheet. 4°. *New Orleans,* 1880.

——. A collection of cuttings from newspapers relating to the sanitary condition of New Orleans and the operations of the New Orleans Auxiliary Sanitary Association, from March 28, 1879, to Dec. 31, 1880. Mounted in two volumes folio. 241; 241 pp.

——. Report of the flushing committee and the transfer of the Toulouse street pump, to the executive committee of the New Orleans Auxiliary Sanitary Association, June 21, 1881. 15 pp. 8°. *New Orleans, M. F. Dunn & Bro.,* 1881.

——. Map of the existing flushing and draining system of the city of New Orleans. Illustrating improvements and extensions proposed by the flushing committee of the New Orleans Auxiliary Sanitary Association. *New Orleans, M. F. Dunn & Bro.,* 1881.

——. Report of the flushing committee, suggesting important improvements, made to the executive committee of the New Orleans Auxiliary Sanitary Association, December 17, 1881. 2 l. 4°. [*New Orleans,* 1881.]

——. Petition to the general assembly of the State of Louisiana in favor of a law requiring the teaching of physiology and hygiene in the public schools. 5 pp. 8°. [*New Orleans,* 1884.]

Repr. from : N. Orl. M. & S. J.

See, also, **New Orleans** Medical and Surgical Association. The evil and the remedy for the privy system. 8°. *New Orleans,* 1879. ——. Report on milk and dairies [etc.] 8°. *New Orleans,* 1879. ——. Cleanliness, health [etc.] 8°. *New Orleans,* 1879. ——. [Recommendations of the committee appointed at a meeting of the medical and sanitary associations.] broadside. fol. [*New Orleans,* 1881.]

——. See, also :

FENNER (E.) Annual address, New Orleans Auxiliary Sanitary Association. What has been done and what remains to be accomplished to render New Orleans healthy and prosperous. Delivered February 15, 1883. 8°. *New Orleans,* 1883.

RAUCH (J. H.) Address delivered before the New Orleans Auxiliary Sanitary Association. 8°. *New Orleans,* 1879.

New Orleans Conference of Charities. Annual report of the officers to the society. 2., 1884-5. And annual report of the Unsectarian Aid Society. 1., 1884-5. 25 pp. 8°. *New Orleans, Hopkins' Printing Office,* 1885.

New Orleans Cremation Society. [Constitution and by laws.] 15 pp. 8°. *New Orleans, A. W. Hyatt,* 1884.

New Orleans Dental College. Annual announcements for the sessions of 1867-8 (1.) ; 1869-70 to 1875-6 (3.-9.). 8°. *New Orleans,* 1867-75.

List of graduates for the years 1868-9 to 1873-4, in announcements for subsequent years.

New Orleans *Exposition.*

INDUSTRIES (The) of New Orleans, her rank, resources, advantages, trade, commerce, and manufactures, conditions of the past, present, and future, representative industrial institutions, historical, descriptive, and statistical. 8°. *New Orleans,* 1885.

New Orleans (The) Journal of Medicine. Edited by S. M. Bemiss and W. S. Mitchell. [Quarterly.] v. 21-23, January, 1868, to December, 1870. 3 v. 8°. *New Orleans.*

Formed by union of: **New Orleans** (The) Medical and Surgical Journal with: **Southern** (The) Journal of the Medical Sciences. In v. 22 Samuel Logan added as editor ; v. 23 by Drs. Bemiss and Mitchell.

New Orleans (The) Medical Journal. Devoted to the cultivation of medicine and the associate sciences. Edited by E. D. Fenner and A. Hester. [Bi-monthly.] v. 1, May, 1844, to June 30, 1845. 8°. *New Orleans.*

Continued as : **New Orleans** (The) Medical and Surgical Journal.

New Orleans (The) Medical News and Hospital Gazette. A semi-monthly journal. Edited by S. Choppin, C. Beard, R. Schlater, P. C. Boyer, and G. S. Vance. v. 1-7, March, 1854, to Feb., 1861. 8°. *New Orleans.*

Ended. No journal issued in Oct., 1854 ; became monthly in Nov. v. 2, Schlater, Boyer, and Vance dropped, D. W. Brickell added ; v. 4, Choppin and Beard dropped, E. D. Fenner added. Continued as : **New Orleans** (The) Medical Times.

New Orleans (The) Medical Record. A semi-monthly journal of the medical sciences. Edited by B. Dowler and S. R. Chambers. Nos. 1-4, v. 1, May 15 to July 1, 1863. roy. 8°. *New Orleans, S. R. Chambers & Co.*

Ended.

New Orleans Medical and Surgical Association. Report on milk and dairies in the city of New Orleans, presented to the New Orleans Medical and Surgical Association, and unanimously adopted at their meeting July 5, 1879. (Published by the New Orleans Auxiliary Sanitary Association.) 16 pp. 8°. *New Orleans, J. S. Rivers,* 1879.

——. Report of the committee appointed by the . . . Oct. 25, 1879, on the following subjects, submitted by the executive committee of the American Public Health Association, to be read and discussed at their meeting at Nashville, Tenn., Nov. 18, 1879. 9 pp. 8°. [*New Orleans,* 1879.]

——. Cleanliness, health, wealth ; domestic sanitation one of its most important elements as elaborated in a report to the . . . Accepted by the New Orleans Auxiliary Sanitary Association. 20 pp. 8°. *New Orleans, L. Graham,* 1879.

——. The evil and the remedy for the privy system of New Orleans. Elaborated in a report to the New Orleans Medical and Surgical Association ; accepted by the New Orleans Auxiliary Sanitary Association. [Joseph Holt, Geo. K. Pratt, Fred. Loeber, committee.] 21 pp. 8°. *New Orleans, F. F. Hansell,* 1879.

——. New Orleans, March 7, 1881. [Recommendation of the committee appointed at a meeting of the Medical and Sanitary Associations of New Orleans, Jan. 22, 1881, to classify such commerce as can be moved to and from any point where epidemic or contagious diseases p.e-

New Orleans Medical [etc.]—continued.
vail. Class. 1. Articles prohibited. 2. Articles
which may or may not. 3. Articles to be free.]
broadside. fol. [*New Orleans*, 1881.]

——. Proceedings of meeting No. 300. New
Orleans, April 1, 1882. 11 pp. 8°. [*New Orleans*, 1882.]

New Orleans (The) Medical and Surgical Journal. Devoted to medicine and the collateral sciences. Edited by W. M. Carpenter, E. D. Fenner, J. Harrison, and A. Hester. [Bi-monthly.]
v. 2–20, July, 1845, to May, 1861, and July,
1866, to December, 1867. 19 v. 8°. *New Orleans.*

Formed by the union of: **New Orleans** (The) Medical
Journal with: **Louisiana** (The) Medical and Surgical
Journal, projected by W. M. Carpenter and J. Harrison.
Title of v. 1, 1844–5, was: **New Orleans** (The) Medical
Journal. v. 14, 18, 20 contain 3 nos. each. After v. 18, end-
ing May, 1861, suspended until July, 1866, when v. 19 com-
menced. In v. 4 Fenner dropped; v. 5, Carpenter dropped;
v. 6, Harrison dropped; v. 11, Bennet Dowler sole editor;
v. 14, W. Stone, Jas. Jones, S. E. Chaillé added; v. 16, W.
C. Nichols added; v. 19, Dowler dropped and S. S. Her-
rick added. In Jan., 1868, united with: **Southern** (The)
Journal of the Medical Sciences, forming: **New Orleans**
(The) Journal of Medicine.

New Orleans (The) Medical and Surgical
Journal. New series. Edited by S. M. Bemiss.
[Bi-monthly.] v. 1–15, July, 1873–88. 8°. *New
Orleans.*

Current. In Sept., 1877, became monthly. Edited suc-
cessively by W. H. Watkins, G. K. Pratt, S. S. Herrick,
D. C. Holliday, A. B. Miles, Geo. B. Lawrason, H. D.
Bruns, J. H. Bemiss, F. W. Parham, P. E. Archinard, A.
McShane, E. L. Bemiss, and H. W. Blanc.

New Orleans (The) Medical Times. A monthly
journal. Edited by Anthony Peniston. Nos.
1–3, v. 1, March to May, 1861. 240 pp. 8°.
New Orleans.

A continuation of: **New Orleans** (The) Medical News
and Hospital Gazette.

New Orleans (The) Monthly Medical Register.
Edited by A. Forster Axson. v. 1–2, October,
1851, to September, 1853. 8°. *New Orleans.*

Want nos. 6, 8, 12, v. 1; nos. 2, 3, v. 2. Ended March,
1854, being merged in and replaced by: **New Orleans**
(The) Medical News and Hospital Gazette.

New Orleans School of Medicine. Annual
announcements for the sessions of 1856–7 to
1860–61 (1.–5.); 1867–8 to 1869–70 (9.–11.). 8°.
New Orleans, 1856–69.

List of students and graduates for the years 1856–7 to
1859–60; 1866–7; 1868–9, in announcement for subsequent
years.

New Orleans University. Annual catalogues
for the years 1873–4 (1.); 1877–8 (5.); 1880–81
(8.); 1882–3 (10.); 1883–4 (11.). 8°. *New Orleans*, 1874–84.

——. Calendar for 1884–5. 44, iii pp. 8°. *New
Orleans, pub. by the University*, 1885.

New Orleans Waterworks Company. Annual
report of the president to the stockholders. 5.,
1882–3. 23 pp. 8°. *New Orleans, A. W. Hyatt*,
1883.

Newport.
See **Bischoff** (Theodor Ludwig Wilhelm). Bestäti-
gung des von Dr. Newport bei den Batrachiern [etc.] 4°.
Giessen, 1854.

Newport (George). On the temperature of insects, and its connexion with the functions of
respiration and circulation in this class of invertebrated animals. Communicated by P. M.
Roget. pp. 259–338. 4°. *London, R. & J. E.
Taylor*, 1837.

Repr. from: Phil. Tr., Lond., 1837.

Newport, *England.*
CLARK (G. T.) Report to the General Board
of Health, on a preliminary inquiry into the
sewerage, drainage, and supply of water, and
the sanitary condition of the inhabitants of the
borough of Newport. 8°. *London*, 1850.

Newport, *Rhode Island.* Report of the water
supply committee of the city of Newport, R. I.,
June 22, 1880 (to the city council). 4 pp. 8°.
[*Newport*, 1880.]

Newport, *Rhode Island.*
See, also, **Cholera** (*Asiatic, History*; *etc., of*),
Fever (*Cerebro-spinal, History, etc., of*), *by locali-
ties.*

DRAINAGE Constructing Company. The sewerage and drainage of Newport, R. I. Proposition of the . . . submitted Nov. 2, 1880. 8°. *Newport*, 1880.

Bentley (H. A.) City of Newport. Report and estimates for the completion of the sewerage system. Rep.
Bd. Health Rhode Island 1885, Providence, 1886, viii, 77–
87.—**Bowditch** (E. W.) Report on sanitary condition
of Newport, R. I. Rep. Nat. Bd. Health 1882, Wash.,
1883, 153–180, 12 plans. ——. Sanitary inspection of Newport, R. I. Sanitarian, N. Y., 1883, n. s., i, 529; 545.—
Pumpelly (R.) Newport's water supply. Report upon
the water of Easton's Pond. *Ibid.*, 497–499.—**Sanitary**
matters in Newport. San. Engin., N. Y., 1882–3, vi, 341.—
Sewerage (The) of Newport, R. I. *Ibid.*, 1880–81, iv,
6–8.—**Storer** (H. R.) Newport, R. I., as a winter resort
for consumptives. Sanitarian, N. Y., 1883, n. s., i, 17; 37;
49. ——. The exemption of Newport, R. I., from pulmonary consumption as compared with other sections of the
country. *Ibid.*, 87–90. ——. The mild winter climate
of Newport, R. I., as the effect of the Gulf Stream. Med.
Rec., N. Y., 1883, xxiv, 679–681. ——. Concerning Newport. R. I., as a resort for consumptives. Boston M. & S.
J., 1883, cviii, 282–284. ——. A few questions for Dr.
Tyndale concerning Newport, R. I., as a resort for consumptives. *Ibid.*, 404. ——. "A sea change." Med.
Times, Phila., 1885–6, xv, 51. *Also,* Reprint.—**Tyndale**
(J. H.) Concerning Newport, R. I., as a resort for consumptives. Boston M. & S. J., 1883, cviii, 188. ——.
Concerning Newport as a health resort for consumptives.
Ibid., 331. ——. The unfitness of Newport as a winter
resort for consumptives; Dr. Storer's questions answered.
Ibid., 452. ——. Concerning the relative value of New-
port, R. I., as a health resort for consumptives. Sanita-
rian, N. Y., 1883, n. s., i, 342.

Newport Hospital. Annual reports of the trustees, presented to the corporation at their annual
meetings. 9., 1881–2; 11.–13., 1883–4 to 1885–6.
8°. *Newport*, 1882–6.

——. Winter course of lectures to nurses by the
medical staff of the Newport Hospital. 1 sheet.
8°. [*Newport, n. d.*]

Newport Medical Society. Draft of an act to
establish the office of medical examiner, presented to the general assembly of Rhode Island
at the May session, 1883. 3 l. 8°. [*Providence*,
1883.]

Newport Natural History Society. [Officers and
constitution.] 15 pp. 8°. *Newport, Davis & Pitman*, 1883.

Newport-Pagnell.
See **Cholera** (*Asiatic, History, etc., of*), *by localities.*

New Providence.
See **Nassau,** *Bahamas.*

Newry.
See **Fever** (*Hospitals for*).

Newsholme (Arthur). Hygiene; a manual of
personal and public health. vi, 407 pp. 8°.
London, G. Gill & Sons, 1884.

——. School hygiene; the laws of health in relation to school life. vii, 143 pp. 12°. *London,
Swan [and others]*, 1887.

Newsome (Tom W.)
Co-Editor of: **Georgia** (The) Medical and Surgical
Encyclopedia, Sandersville, 1860.

New South Wales. An act to make provision
for the safe custody of, and prevention of offences
by, persons dangerously insane, and for the care
and maintenance of persons of unsound mind.
12th December, 1843. pp. 46–50. fol. [*Sydney*,
1843.] [P., v. 1292.]

Cutting from: Suppl. Gov. Gaz., 10th Oct., 1845.

——. An act to amend the act, passed in the
second year of the reign of Her present Majesty

New South Wales—continued.

Queen Victoria, intituled "An act to define the qualifications of medical witnesses at coroners' inquests, and inquiries held before justices of the peace, in the colony of New South Wales". 8 Vict., 1844, No. 8. pp. 27–28. fol. [*Sydney,* 1844.]

Cutting from: Suppl. Gov. Gaz., Sept. 17, 1844.

——. An act to alter and amend an act intituled "An act to make provision for the safe custody of, and prevention of offences by, persons dangerously insane, and for the care and maintenance of persons of unsound mind". [11th Sept., 1845.] p. 13. fol. [*Sydney,* 1845.] [P., v. 1292.]

Cutting from: Suppl. Gov. Gaz., Oct. 10, 1845.

——. An act to amend an act intituled "An act to make provision for the safe custody of, and prevention of offences by, persons dangerously insane, and for the care and maintenance of persons of unsound mind". [Assented to 13th June, 1846.] 2 pp. fol. [*Sydney,* 1846.] [P., v. 1292.]

——. An act to provide for the registration of legally qualified medical practitioners. Anno decimo nono Victoriæ reginæ. No. xvii. Assented to [12th October, 1855]. pp. 75–76. fol. [*Sydney,* 1855.]

Cutting.

——. Minutes of evidence taken before the commissioners of inquiry, respecting the lunatic asylums of New South Wales. Jan. 25 to April 16, 1855. 82 pp. fol. [*Sydney,* 1855.] [P., v. 1292.]

——. Report from the commissioners of inquiry on the lunatic asylums of New South Wales, with minutes of evidence and appendix, and replies to a circular letter. Ordered by the council to be printed June 6, 1855. 12 pp. fol. *Sydney, W. Hanson,* 1855. [P., v. 1292.]

——. Admission of insane persons into the lunatic asylum. [Also, 8 blank forms.] 1 sheet. fol. [*Sydney,* 1856.] [P., v. 1292.]

——. An act to make better provision for the custody and care of criminal lunatics. [Assented to 7th May, 1861.] 3 pp. fol. [*Sydney,* 1861.] [P., v. 1292.]

——. An act to provide for the attendance of medical witnesses at coroners' inquests and inquiries held by justices of the peace. Anno primo Victoriæ reginæ. No. iii. [13th June, 1838.] 2 pp. fol. [*Sydney, T. Richards,* 1861.]

——. An act to define the qualifications of medical witnesses at coroners' inquests and inquiries held before justices of the peace, in the colony of New South Wales. Anno secundo Victoriæ reginæ. No. xxii. [12th October, 1838.] 2 pp. fol. [*Sydney, T. Richards,* 1861.]

——. An act to amend "An act to define the qualifications of medical witnesses at coroners' inquests and inquiries held before justices of the peace, in colony of New South Wales. Anno nono Victoriæ reginæ. No. xii. [27th October, 1845.] 1 l. fol. [*Sydney, T. Richards,* 1861.]

——. Vital statistics. Annual reports from the registrar-general on vital statistics. (Presented to both Houses of Parliament by command.) 9.–28., 1864–5 to 1883–4. fol. *Sydney,* 1865–84.

——. Report on lunatic asylums by Fred. Norton Manning. v, 287 pp., 5 pl., 16 plans. 8°. *Sydney, T. Richards,* 1868.

——. Advance, Australia! Official catalogue of the natural and industrial products of New South Wales. Forwarded to the International Exhibition of 1876 at Philadelphia. By authority of the commissioners. 104 pp. 8°. *Sydney, T. Richards,* 1876.

——. New South Wales; its progress and resources. By authority of the commissioners.

New South Wales—continued.

Advance, Australia! 31 pp. 8°. *Sydney, T. Richards,* 1876.

——. Mines and mineral statistics. Annual reports of the department of mines, New South Wales, for the years 1877–9; 1881; 1885. (Printed in accordance with resolutions of both Houses of Parliament.) 4° & fol. *Sydney,* 1878–86.

——. Mines and mineral statistics. Maps to accompany annual reports of the department of mines, New South Wales, for the year 1879. 3 pp., 17 maps. 4°. *Sydney, T. Richards,* 1880.

——. Inspector-general of the insane. [Annual reports on the state and condition of the hospitals and other institutions to the principal under-secretary] for the years 1879–85. fol. [*Sydney,* 1880–86.]

——. Public charities. Annual reports of the inspector of public charities to the colonial secretary. 5.–9., 1880–84. fol. *Sydney, T. Richards,* 1881–5.

——. Nautical school ship Vernon. Annual reports of the superintendent, N. S. S. Vernon, to the under-secretary of public instruction. (Presented to Parliament by command.) 15.–16., 1–81–2 to 1882–3. fol. *Sydney, T. Richards,* 1882–3.

——. State children's relief department. Annual reports of the president to the colonial secretary. 2.–6., 1882–3 to 1886–7. (Presented to Parliament in accordance with the provisions of act 44 Vic., No. 24.) fol. *Sydney, T. Richards,* 1883–7.

2.–4., 1882–3 to 1884–5, by Arthur Renwick.

——. The Australian sanitary conference of Sydney, N. S. W., 1884. Report of minutes of proceedings, and appendix. 70 pp., 5 plans. fol. *Sydney, T. Richards,* 1884.

——. Wood pavement board. Report, minutes of proceedings, and appendix. (Ordered by the legislative assembly to be printed 26th Nov., 1885.) 66 pp. fol. *Sydney, T. Richards,* 1884.

——. Government asylums for the infirm and destitute. Annual reports of the manager to the principal under secretary, for the years 1883; 1884. fol. *Sydney,* 1884–5.

——. Hospitals for the insane. Report of Dr. G. A. Tucker on the hospitals for the insane visited by him (April, 1882, to March, 1885), under the circular letter of the colonial secretary of New South Wales. (Ordered by the legislative assembly to be printed 16th Feb., 1886.) 40 pp. fol. [*Sydney, T. Richards,* 1886.]

——. An act to establish sanitary regulations in respect of the production and distribution of milk. No. xvii. [Assented to 30th Sept., 1886.] 5 pp. fol. [*Sydney, T. Richards,* 1886.]

New South Wales. *Central Board of Health.* Report of the board of health upon the late epidemic of small-pox, 1881–2. Legislative assembly, New South Wales. (Ordered to be printed 22d March, 1883.) 20 pp., 1 l., 1 map, 1 plan. fol. [*Sydney, T. Richards,* 1883.]

——. Report to the president of the board of health upon an outbreak of typhoid fever in the municipal district of Leichhardt, due to polluted milk. With an account of the state of certain dairies in the same and other neighbourhoods, and remarks upon the legislation necessary to protect the purity of public milk-supplies. By J. Ashburton Thompson. 24 pp., 1 pl., 1 map, 1 plan, 1 diag. fol. *Sydney, T. Richards,* 1886.

——. A report to the president of the board of health, containing photographs of a person suffering from variola discreta, and an account of the case; to which is added a clinical report and diagnosis of the five cases with which the outbreak of small-pox of 1884–5 began. By J. Ash-

New South Wales. *Centr. Bd. Health*—cont'd. burton Thompson. 5 pp., 11 pl., 1 diag. fol. *Sydney, T. Richards,* 1886.

New South Wales. *Hospital for the Insane, Gladesville.* Annual reports of the medical superintendent to the colonial secretary for the years 1869-71. 8°. *Sydney,* 1870-72.

New South Wales. *Lunatic Asylum, Parramatta.* Ground plan; also, plan of second story. 1 broadside. [*Sydney,* 1855.] [P., v. 1293.]

New South Wales. *Lunatic Asylum at Tarban Creek.* Ground plan, showing proposed additions. 1 broadside. [*Sidney*], *Allan & Wigley, lithog.,* [1855]. [P., v. 1292.]

——. (Appendix to the report of the lunatic asylums commission.) Ordered by the council to be printed 2d August, 1855. 8 pp. fol. [*Sydney,* 1855.] [P., v. 1292.]

New South Wales. *Medical Board of New South Wales.* Suggestions of the . . . for an amended act on act No. 17, 19 Vict., being medical practitioners' act of 1855. 1 l. fol. [*Sydney,* 1876.]

——. Registers of medical practitioners for 1879; 1880; 1884; 1885. fol. *Sidney,* 1879-85. 1884 and 1885, suppl. to New South Wales Gov. Gaz.

New South Wales. *Technological, Industrial and Sanitary Museum.* Reports of the committee of management to the governor and executive council. 5.-7., 1884-6. 20 pp. fol. [*Sidney, T. Richards,* 1885-7. Suppls. to the Australian Museum Rep. for 1884 and 1886.

New South Wales.

See, also, **Directories**, etc. (*Medical*); **Hospitals** (*Descriptions, etc., of*), by localities; **Sydney.**

COGHLAN (T. A.) Discharge of streams in relation to rainfall, New South Wales. 8°. *London,* 1884. *Repr. from:* Proc. Inst. Civil Engineers, lxxv, session 1883-4, pt. 1.

HAYTER (H. H.) Crime in New South Wales. A paper written for, but rejected by, the Royal Society of that colony. 8°. *Melbourne,* 1884.

RICHARDS (T.) New South Wales in 1881; being a brief statistical and descriptive account of the colony up to the end of the year, extracted chiefly from official records. 8°. *Sydney,* 1882.

ROBINSON (C.) New South Wales; the oldest and richest of the Australian colonies. With colored maps, shewing the principal agricultural and mining districts. 8°. *Sydney,* 1873.

Beveridge (P.) Of the aborigines inhabiting the great lacustrine and riverine depression of the lower Murray, lower Murrumbidgee, lower Lachlan, and lower Darling. J. & Proc. Roy. Soc. N. South Wales 1883, Sydney, 1884, xvii, 19-74.—**Bonney** (F.) On some customs of the aborigines of the River Darling, New South Wales. J. Anthrop. Inst., Lond., 1883-4, xiii, 122-137.—**Cameron** (A. L. P.) Notes on some tribes of New South Wales. *Ibid.,* 1884-5, xiv, 344-370.—**Cauvin** (C.) Esquisse démographique de la Nouvelle-Galles du Sud. Ann. de démog. internat., Par., 1881, v, 7-43. *Also* [Abstr.]: Arch. de méd. nav., Par., 1881, xxxvi, 303-312. ——. Note sur les établissements hospitaliers de la Nouvelle-Galles du Sud. [Extr. du rapport médical sur la campagne du transport à vapeur le Rhin, en Australie, 1879-80.] Arch. de méd. nav., Par., 1884, xli, 452-464.—**Fraser** (J.) The aborigines of New South Wales. J. & Proc. Roy. Soc. N. South Wales 1882, Sydney, 1883, xvi, 193-233.—**Pell** (M. B.) Marriage and child-bearing in New South Wales, considered with reference to the rates of mortality prevailing among women during the child-bearing period of life, and to the proportion of illegitimate births. Austral. Pract., Melbourne, 1877-8, i, 73-77. ——. Rates of mortality and increase of the population of New South Wales. *Ibid.,* 145-175. ——. On the rates of mortality in New South Wales, and on the construction of mortality tables from census returns; with a note on the formation of commutation tables. J. Inst. Actuaries, etc., Lond., 1878-9, xxi, 257-288.

New South Wales (The) Medical Gazette. Published under the auspices of the Association of Medical Officers of the Volunteer Force at head-

New South Wales (The) Medical [etc.]—cont. quarters, and edited by three of their number. [Monthly.] v. 1-5; No. 1, v. 6, Oct., 1870, to Oct., 1875. 8°. *Sydney.*

New Sydenham Society. Reports presented to the annual meetings, with list of works published, and other information. 1.-3., 1859-61; 7., 1865; 8., 1866; 10., 1868; 14.-17., 1872-5; 19., 1877; 20., 1878; 22., 1880; 23., 1881; 25., 1883; 26., 1884; 28., 1886. 8°. *London,* 1859-86.

New Sydenham Society's (The) Lexicon of terms used in medicine and the allied sciences. (Based on Mayne's Lexicon.) Edited for the society by Henry Power and Leonard W. Sedgwick. Pts. 1-14. (A-Kid.) 3 v. 4°. *London, New Sydenham Society,* 1878-87.

Newt.

Klein (E.) Observations on the glandular epithelium and division of nuclei in the skin of newt. Quart. J. Micr. Sc., Lond., 1879, n. s., xix, 404-420, 1 pl.—**Scott** (W. B.) On some points in the early development of the common newt. *Ibid.,* 449-475, 2 pl.

Newth (A. H.) A manual of necroscopy, or a guide to the performance of post-mortem examinations; with notes on the morbid appearances, and suggestions for medico-legal examinations for the use of practitioners and students. xii, 157 pp. 16°. *London, Smith, Elder & Co.,* 1878.

Newton, *Massachusetts.* Annual reports of the city engineer to the city council for the years 1883-85. 3 p. l., 67 pp. 8°. *Boston, Rand, Avery & Co.,* 1884-6.

Newton, *Massachusetts.*

See **Fever** (*Typhoid, History, etc., of*), by localities.

Newton. Bai Rio Shinpo. [Modern treatment of syphilis; transl. from original lectures by Dr. Newton, Eng. navy, formerly in charge of Lock Hospital, Yokohama, by Okino, Omi.] 2 v. 1 p. l., 4, 3, 3, 3, 41 pp.; 8 pp., 33 col. pl. 8°. *Tokio,* 1871. Japanese text.

Newton (A. E.) Pre-natal culture; being suggestions to parents relative to systematic methods of moulding the tendencies of offspring before birth. 67 pp. 8°. *Washington, D. C., R. H. Darby,* 1879.

——. The modern Bethesda, or the gift of healing restored; being some account of the life and labors of Dr. J. R. Newton, healer; with observations on the nature and source of the healing power, and the conditions of its exercise. Notes of valuable auxiliary remedies. Health maxims, etc. 322 pp., port. 8°. *New York, Newton Pub. Co.,* 1879.

——. The better way; an appeal to men in behalf of human culture through a wise parentage. 48 pp. 12°. *New York, Wood & Holbrook,* 1880. ——. The same. 48 pp. 8°. *New York, M. L. Holbrook & Co.,* 1884.

Newton (Alexander). Piles; how to self-cure them without cutting, ligature, nitric acid, or any painful process: The seat of the disease, and how engendered. Stricture, rheumatic gout, hypochondriasis, and headache always relieved and often cured by this genuine process. 30 pp. 12°. *London, H. Kimpton,* [1887].

Newton (Calvin) [1800-53].
Editor of: **New England** (The) Medical Eclectic and Guide to Health. Worcester, Mass., 1846-7.—**New England** (The) Botanic, Medical and Surgical Journal, Worcester, Mass., 1847-51.—**Worcester** (The) Journal of Medicine, 1852-3.
See, also, **Calkins** (Marshall). Thoracic diseases [etc.] 2. ed. With the posthumous writings of . . . and biographical sketch of . . . 8°. *Philadelphia,* 1858. This is a new edition of Newton & Calkins' work, with additions.

—— **& Calkins** (Marshall). Thoracic diseases; their pathology, diagnosis, and treatment. With

Newton (Calvin) **& Calkins** (Marshall)—cont. a biographical sketch of the life and character of Prof. Calvin Newton. xxiv, 17–439 pp., port. 8°. *Worcester, D. & M. Calkins,* 1854.

Newton (H. A.) The metrical system of weights and measures. 8 pp. 8°. *New Haven, E. Hayes,* 1864. [P., v. 99.]

——. The same. With tables prepared for the Smithsonian Institution. 23 pp. 8°. *Washington, Government Printing Office,* 1868. [P., v. 358.]

[——.] On the law of mortality that has prevailed among the former members of the Divinity School of Yale College. 8 pp. 8°. [*n. p.,* 1873.]
Repr. from: New Englander, April, 1873.

Newton (H. G.)
Editor of: **Worcester** (The) Journal of Medicine, 1853.

Newton (Henry) **& Jenney** (Walter P.) Report on the geology and resources of the Black Hills of Dakota; with atlas. Department of the Interior, U. S. Geographical and Geological Survey of the Rocky Mountain region. xiv, 566 pp., 24 pl. 4°. *Washington, Government Printing Office,* 1880.

Newton (*J. R.*)
Portrait in: **Collection** of Portr. (Libr.)

Newton (James). A complete herbal, containing the prints and the English names of several thousand trees, plants, shrubs, flowers, exotics, etc. Many of which are not to be found in the herbals of either Gerard, Johnson, or Parkinson. 6. ed. [With bibliography of herbalists.] 176 pp., 176 pl., port. 12°. *London, Lackington, Allen & Co.,* 1802.

Newton (John Frank). The return to nature; or, a defence of the vegetable regimen; with some account of an experiment made during the last three or four years in the author's family. Part 1. vi, 160 pp. 8°. *London, T. Cadell & W. Davies,* 1811.
Another copy bound with: ABERNETHY (J.) Hunter's theory of life, 1811.

Newton (L. V.) [1809–80].
Editor of: **American** (The) Druggists' Circular and Chemical Gazette, New York, 1858–80.

Newton (Orin E.) An essay on Asiatic cholera, as it appeared in Cincinnati, O., in the years 1849, 1850, and 1866, with remarks upon its treatment, and a tabulated statement of 117 cases treated. 30 pp. 8°. *New York & Cincinnati,* 1867.
Also, Co-Editor of: **Western** (The) Medical News, Cincinnati, 1851–9.

Newton (R. Clark). The doctor's corner. 62 pp. 8°. *London, W. Scott,* 1884.
Repr. from: Newcastle Weekly Chronicle.

Newton (Robert S.), jr.
Co-Editor of: **Medical** (The) Eclectic, New York, 1877–81.

Newton (Robert Safford) [1818–81]. An eclectic treatise on the practice of medicine, embracing the pathology of inflammation and fever, with its classification and treatment. 144 pp. 8°. *Cincinnati,* 1861.

——. Ancient and modern eclecticism in medicine. An address delivered before the Eclectic Medical Society of the State of New York. 8 pp. 8°. *Brooklyn, W. C. Wilton,* 1864.

——. Explorations in cell-pathology; or, observations in regard to the causes, character, and treatment of cancer; made from 1843 till the present time. 20 pp. 8°. *New York, Logan & Forbes,* 1877.
Repr. from: Med. Eclect., N. Y., 1877, iv.
Also, Co-Editor of: **Western** (The) Medical News, Cincinnati, 1851–9.— **Eclectic** (The) Medical Journal, Cincinnati, 1852–61.—**American** (The) Eclectic Medical Review, New York, 1866–72. *Also, Editor of:* **Ameri-**

Newton (Robert Safford)—continued.
can (The) Eclectic Medical Register, New York, 1868. *Also, Co-Editor of:* **Medical** (The) Eclectic, New York, 1873–81. *Also, Editor of:* **New York** Quarterly Journal, 1875.
For Biography, see Med. Truth, N. Y., 1883–4, i, 4–11.
See, also, **Powell** (William Byrd) & **Newton** (Robt. S.) The eclectic practice of medicine [etc.] 8°. *Cincinnati,* 1854.

—— **& Powell** (William Byrd). An eclectic treatise on diseases of children. 610 pp. 8°. *New York, J. F. Trow & Co.,* 1867.

Newton (William K.) Sanitary control of the food supply. 25 pp., 1 l. 8°. *Concord, N. H., Republican Press Association,* 1884.

——. Some facts about the New Jersey milk adulteration act and the results of its enforcement. Notes on milk analysis, giving the results of 112 analyses and a brief account of methods. 15 pp. 8°. [*Paterson, N. J.,* 1884.]

——. The sanitary survey of a house. 8 pp. 8°. *Concord, N. H.,* 1885.
Repr. from: Am. Pub. Health Ass. Rep. 1884, Concord, N. H., 1885, x.

——. Report of the milk inspector. 17 pp. 8°. [*Trenton,* 1886?]
Repr. from: Rep. Bd. Health N. Jersey 1884–5, Trenton, 1885, ix.

Newton Abbot. Annual reports on the public health of the Newton Abbot (rural) and Wolborough and Dawlich (urban) sanitary districts, by Leonard Armstrong, medical officer of health, to the members of the combined sanitary authorities, for the years 1874–81. 4° & 8°. *Newton Abbot,* 1875–82.
1874 is 4°.

Newton Abbot.

CLARK (G. T.) Report to the General Board of Health, on a preliminary inquiry into the sewerage, drainage, and supply of water, and the sanitary condition of the inhabitants of the town of Newton-Abbot. 8°. *London,* 1850.

Newton Branch of the Provincial Medical and Surgical Association. Proceedings at the third anniversary meeting, held at Warrington, June 27, 1839. 16 pp. 8°. *Warrington, J. Haddock,* 1839.

Newton Cottage Hospital and Dispensary. Annual reports of the committee to the subscribers. 1.–11., 1873–83. 12° & 8°. *Newton Abbot,* 1874–84.
The words "and Dispensary" added in 1874. 1873 is 12°.

Newton-Heath.

RAWLINSON (R.) Report to the General Board of Health, on a preliminary inquiry into the sewerage, drainage, and supply of water, and the sanitary condition of the inhabitants of the township of Newton Heath, in the county palatine of Lancaster. 8°. *London,* 1852.

Newton Home for Orphans and Destitute Girls. Annual reports of the directors to the public. 2., 1873–4; 4.–8., 1875–6 to 1879–80. 8°. *Boston,* 1875–80.

Newtown.

See, also, **Children** (*Hospitals, etc., for, Reports, etc., of*).
BLAXALL (F. H.) Report to the Local Government Board upon the sanitary condition of the urban sanitary district of Newtown and Llanllwchaiarn, Montgomery. March 12, 1878. fol. [*London,* 1878.]

New Winchester Home for Aged Women, Charlestown. Address delivered at the opening of the . . . by Rev. O. C. Everett; and poem by Rev. Mark Trafton. May 1, 1873. With an appendix. 32 pp. 8°. *Cambridge, J. Wilson & Son,* 1873.

New Windsor.

CRESY (E.) Report to the General Board of Health, on a preliminary inquiry into the sewerage, drainage, and supply of water, and the sanitary condition of the inhabitants of the borough of New Windsor. 8°. *London*, 1849.

New-Year's gift (A) to the lord provost, magistrates, and town council of the city of Glasgow, 1st January, 1874. Being an essay shewing that the delusive practice of vaccination is ruinous to the national health. By Anti-Vaccinator. 52 pp. 8°. *Glasgow, J. Thomson, [n. d.]*

New York (*City*). [Communication from the mayor of the city of New York to the common council, relative to matters of public health.] Common council. Nov. 25, 1822. 8 pp. 8°. [*New York*, 1822.]

———. Report of the committee on laws, to the corporation of the city of New York, on the subject of interment within the populous parts of the city. Read and adopted at a special meeting of the said corporation on the 9th of June, 1825, and published by their order. 75 pp. 8°. *New York, M. Day*, 1825. [*Also, in :* P., v. 843.]

———. Report of the special committee to whom was referred the resolutions of Alderman Stevens, relating to the supply of water by the Manhattan Company. Common council. May 31, 1830. 6 pp. 8°. [*New York*, 1830.] [P., v. 1225.]

———. Communication from the committee of the Lyceum of Natural History of the city of New York, in answer to an enquiry from Mr. Townsend on the source, quality, and purity of the water on this island. Common council. Feb. 28, 1831. 11 pp. 8°. [*New York*, 1831.] [P., v. 1225.]

———. Report of committee on charity and almshouse, in favor of removing the alms-house establishment to Randall's Island and selling the Long Island farms. City Doc. No. 4. Board of assistant aldermen. June 29, 1835. pp. 39–46. 8°. [*New York*, 1835.]
Cutting.

———. Annual messages of his honor the mayor, Isaac L. Varian, to the common council, for the years 1838–9; 1839–40. 20, 22 pp. 8°. *New York*, 1839–40.

———. Report of the proceedings of the joint committee appointed to make suitable arrangements for bringing on the bodies of the officers of the New York regiment of volunteers from Mexico; with the funeral ceremonies observed on the occasion of their interment. Board of aldermen. City Doc. No. 13, 1848. pp. 211–262. 8°. *New York, McSpedon & Baker*, 1848.
Cutting.

———. An ordinance organizing the departments of the municipal government of the city of New York, and prescribing their powers and duties. viii, 224 pp. 8°. *New York, McSpedon & Baker*, 1849.

———. Extracts from ordinances (Chap. xxxvi) relative to the interment of the dead. 7 pp. 8°. *New York, W. Browne & Co.*, 1851.

———. Communication from F. I. A. Boole, city inspector, to the committee of the house to whom the metropolitan health bill was referred. 48 pp. 8°. *New York, E. Jones & Co.*, 1864.

———. Semi-annual report of the board for the examination of and licensing druggists and prescription clerks in the city of New York. 1., July to Dec., 1871. 24 pp. 8°. *New York, New York Printing Company*, 1872.

———. Stated session. Board of aldermen. Nov. 22, 1880. [For the consideration of the provisional estimate for the year 1881.] pp. 523–648. 8°. [*New York*, 1881.]
Cutting.

New York (*City*).

See, also, **Blind** (*Asylums, etc., for*); **Children** (*Hospitals, etc., for, Reports, etc., of*); **Cholera** (*Asiatic, History, etc., of*), *by localities* ; **Deaf-mutes** (*Asylums, etc., for*); **Dentistry** ; **Directories**, *etc.* (*Medical*); **Education** (*Medical*), *etc.*, **Fever** (*Cerebro-spinal, History, etc., of*), **Fever** (*Typhoid, History, etc., of*), **Fever** (*Typhus, History, etc., of*), **Fever** (*Yellow, History, etc., of*), *by localities* ; **Foundlings**, *etc.*; **Hospitals** (*Descriptions, etc., of*), **Hospitals** (*Management, etc., of*), **Hospitals** (*Maternity, etc.*), **Hospitals** (*Naval, etc.*), **Hospitals** (*Ophthalmic, etc.*), **Hospitals** (*Orthopædic*), *by localities* ; **Hospitals** *for contagious diseases* ; **Inebriates** (*Asylums for*), **Insane** (*Asylums for, etc.*), *by localities* ; **Libraries** (*Medical, etc.*); **Medicine** (*Clinical, Cases of*); **Medicine** (*Veterinary, Education in, etc.*); **Nervous** *system* (*Diseases of, Hospitals for*); **Pharmacy** (*Education in, etc.*); **Phthisis** (*Hospitals for*); **Prostitution** (*History, etc., of*), *by localities.*

ACT (An) [proposed] to establish a metropolitan board of public works, and to provide for the government thereof. 8°. [*New York, n. d.*]

ACT (An) [proposed] laying out public places and parks and parkways in the twenty-third and twenty-fourth wards of the city of New York, and in the adjacent district, in Westchester County, and authorizing the taking of the lands for the same. 8°. [*Albany, n. d.*]

ADDRESS of the committee to promote the passage of a metropolitan health bill. Dec., 1865. 8°. *New York*, 1865.

BALL (L. C.) Metropolitan health bill. Speech of . . . on the "Act concerning the public health of the counties of New York, Kings, and Richmond, and the waters thereof". In assembly, March 25, 1861. 8°. *Albany*, 1861.

CHANDLER (C. F.) Plan for a bureau of street cleaning for the city of New York. [Block plan.] An act to provide for the cleaning of the streets, and removal of garbage and ashes in the city of New York. Prepared for the chairman of the committee on cities. 8°. [*Albany, n. d.*]

CITIZENS' Association of New York. Council of hygiene and public health. Boundaries and distribution of districts for sanitary inspection under direction of the council of hygiene. broadside 4°. [*New York, n. d.*]

———. Council of hygiene and public health. [Circular to the profession, announcing the organization and object.] Sept. 15, 1864. 8°. [*New York*, 1864.]

———. Council of hygiene and public health. Report of pestilential diseases and insalubrious quarters. The plan of inquiry and record. 8°. [*New York, n. d.*]

———. Important correspondence in relation to the public health of the city of New York. [Letter from the committee on sanitary inquiry of the Citizens' Association to the medical profession, soliciting full and reliable information relative to the public health. March 2, 1864. And reply thereto, March 9, 1864. 4°. [*New York*, 1864.]

———. Council of hygiene and public health. Report upon the sanitary condition of the city. 8°. *New York*, 1865.

———. The same. 2. ed. 8°. *New York*, 1866.

———. Report of the executive council to the honorary council of the Citizens' Association of New York, for the months of June, July, and Aug., 1866. 8°. *New York*, 1866.

COZZENS (I.) A geological history of Manhattan or New York Island. 8°. *New York*, 1843.

New York (City).

DAVENPORT (J. I.) Letter on the subject of the population of the city of New York, its density, and the evils resulting therefrom. 8°. *New York*, 1884.

EFFECTS (On the) of high temperature upon the public health of New York and on measures of prevention. 8°. [*New York, n. d.*]

EWER (F. C.) Public health of the city of New York. Remarks before the Sanitary Association. With appendix. 8°. *New York*, 1861.

FACTS concerning slaughter-houses, rendering establishments, and other nuisances; pestilence and the depreciation of property. Collected and published for the citizens of New York, by order of the committee of safety. 8°. *New York*, 1875.

FRYER (W. J.), jr. 1. Law relating to buildings in the city of New York, passed June 9, 1885, with marginal notes, a full index, and engravings illustrating the heights and thicknesses of walls. (No method so quickly explains as drawings to those accustomed to their use.) 2. Law limiting the height of dwelling houses in the city of New York, passed June 9, 1885. 8°. *New York*, 1885.

GRISCOM (J. H.) The sanitary condition of the laboring population of New York. With suggestions for its improvement. 8°. *New York*, 1845.

HINTS towards promoting the health and cleanliness of the city of New York. 8°. *New York*, 1802.

HOSACK (D.) An inaugural address, delivered before the New York Historical Society. 8°. *New York*, 1820.

———. Observations on febrile contagion, and on the means of improving the medical police of the city of New York. Delivered as an introductory discourse. 8°. *New York*, 1820.

NEWBERRY (J. S.) The geological history of New York island and harbor. 8°. *New York*, 1878.

NEW YORK (*State*). An act relative to the public health in the city of New York. Passed April 10, 1850. 8°. [*Albany*, 1850.]

———. Laws relative to the public health in the city of New York. 8°. *New York*, 1856.

———. The same. 8°. *New York*, 1857.

———. Laws relative to quarantine and to the public health of the city of New York. (Part 1st, Chap. xiv, of the revised statutes, as amended and modified by the subsequent acts of the legislature.) 16°. [*New York*], 1858.

———. Report of the select committee appointed to investigate the health department of the city of New York. Transmitted to the legislature Feb. 3, 1859. S. No. 49. 8°. *Albany*, 1859.

———. Report of the committee on the incorporation of cities and villages, on the bill entitled "An act concerning the public health of the counties of New York, Kings, and Richmond". Transmitted to the legislature March 9, 1860. Assembly. No. 129. 8°. *Albany*, 1860.

———. Assembly. An act [as amended and passed in assembly, April 10, 1861] concerning the public health of the counties of New York, Kings, and Richmond, and the waters thereof. No. —. June 10, 1861. Introd. by Mr. Robinson. fol. [*Albany*, 1861.]

———. S. Communication from the comptroller of the city of New York, in reply to senate resolution regarding markets. No. 61. March 7, 1873. 8°. [*Albany*, 1873.]

———. Assembly. Communication from the corporation counsel of the city of New York, in reply to a resolution of the assembly relative to the bill entitled "An act relating to assessments

New York (City).

for the construction of sewers and drains in the city of New York". No. 92. March 28, 1876. 8°. [*Albany*, 1876.]

———. S. An act to simplify the proof of the sanitary code in the city of New York. No. 170. March 3, 1880. fol. [*Albany*, 1880.]

———. Assembly. An act in relation to the health officer for the port of New York. No. 392. March 5, 1880. Introd. by Mr. Varnum. fol. [*Albany*, 1880.]

———. Assembly. An act for the proper drainage of lands in the city of New York. No. 543. March 18, 1880. Introd. by J. L. Wells. fol. [*Albany*, 1880.]

———. Assembly. An act to regulate the sale of spirituous liquors, wines, ale, and beer in the city of New York. No. 12. Feb. 16, 1882. Introd. by Mr. Bogan. fol. [*Albany*, 1882.]

———. Assembly. An act to establish an additional public park in the city of New York, and for the security of the public health therein. No. 257. March 2, 1882. Introd. by M. C. Murphy. fol. [*Albany*, 1882.]

———. Assembly. An act to amend an act entitled "An act to organize a night medical service in the city of New York, to provide medical assistance in case of sudden sickness or accident during the night time", passed June 26, 1880. No. 360. March 24, 1882. Introd. by Mr. Crane. fol. [*Albany*, 1882.]

NEW YORK Academy of Medicine. Report of the standing committee on public health and legal medicine. 8°. *New York*, 1852.

NEW YORK Sanitary Association. Reports in relation to the public health. 8°. *New York*, 1859.

OPINION of the medical profession on the condition and needs of the city of New York, in regard to street-cleaning. (Expressed at a mass meeting of the physicians of the city, held at Chickering Hall, April 13, 1881.) 8°. *New York*, 1881.

RABORG (S. A.) The sanitary topography of New York City. 8°. *New York*, 1869.
Repr. from: Catholic World, Dec., 1869.

REPORT of the citizens' committee upon the nuisances of New York City. The air we breathe. 8°. *New York*, 1878.

REPORT on lofty dwelling houses in New York City, with minutes of the meeting at which it was presented, and proposed act regulating height of such houses in proportion to the streets on which they front. Feb. 1, 1884. 8°. *New York*, 1884.

SEWERAGE (The) of New York. 8°. [*n. p.*, 1845.]
Repr. from: Hunt's Merchant's Mag., June, 1845.

STATE of New York. In the court for the trial of impeachments and the correction of errors. Between the mayor, aldermen, and commonalty of the city of New York, plaintiffs in error, and Herman LeRoy and others, defendants in error. Case. [Application in original case to set aside assessment on sewer.] 71 pp. 8°. *New York*, 1823.

THOMS (W. F.) Weather chart, showing the effects of the meteorological influences on mortality in the city of New York. fol. [*n. p., n. d.*]

UNITED STATES. *Congress. Senate.* A bill to prevent obstructive and injurious deposits within the harbor and adjacent waters of New York City, by dumping or otherwise, and to punish and prevent such offenses, and making other provisions in connection therewith. 49. Cong., 1. sess. S. 762. Dec. 21, 1885. Introd. by Mr. Miller, of New York. roy. 8°. [*Washington*, 1885.]

New York (City).

UNITED STATES. *War Department. Engineer's Office.* Letter from the Secretary of War, transmitting a letter from the Chief of Engineers, inclosing map of survey and report upon the work of deepening Gedney's Channel through Sandy Hook Bar, New York; also inclosing a report from the board for fortifications upon a plan for the permanent improvement of the entrance to New York Harbor. 48. Cong., 2. sess. H. R. Ex. Doc. No. 78. Jan. 12, 1885. 8°. [*Washington,* 1885.]

Baker (G.) Meteorological observations from January, 1797, to December, 1798, in the cupola of the exchange in the city of New York. Med. Reposit., N. Y., 1797-8, i, 99; 245; 373; 557: 1798-9, ii, 101; 205; 319.—**Baxter** (J.) Report of meteorological observations made in the city of New York from May 1, 1827, to May 1, 1828. N. York M. & Phys. J., 1828, vii, 354: 1829, n. s., i, 281.—**Colden** (C. D.) Observations on the fever which prevailed in the city of New York in 1741 and 1742; written in 1743. Am. M. & Phil. Reg., N. Y., 1814, iv, 310-330.—**Griscom** (J. H.) Hygiene of New York City. Tr. Am. M. Ass., Phila., 1849, ii, 455-458. ——. Improvements of the public health, and the establishment of a sanitary police in the city of New York. Tr. M. Soc. N. Y., Albany, 1857, 107-123.—**Harris** (E.) Port of New York. Rep. Nat. Bd. Health, Wash., 1879, 307-322, 20 plans.—**Health** (The) of New York; its general condition, costs, and needs, and the practical work of the board of health. Sanitarian, N. Y., 1876, iv, 60-62. — **Hosack** (D.) Observations on the means of improving the medical police of the city of New York. *In his:* Essays on various subjects, 8°, N. Y., 824, ii, 11-86.—**Loines** (J. P.) Summary of seven daily observations of the temperature, moisture, weight, direction, and condition of the atmosphere for the years 1861-2. Tr. M. Soc. N. Y., Albany, 1862, 371: 1863, 341.—**Munro** (A. C.) Sanitary administration in New York. San. Rec. Lond., 1887-8, n. s., ix, 455-457. — **Pest-holes** in New York. San. Engin., N. Y., 1884, x, 391; 409; 433; 457; 505.—**Report** of the board of surgeons for the years 1863-4; 1866-7; 1868-9. Rep. Bd. Com. Metrop. Police 1863-4, Albany, 1865, 44: (1866-7), 1868, 35: (1868-9), 1870-23.—**Report** of the committee on hygiene of the Medica, Society of the County of New York, on the hygiene of New York City, 1878-80. Tr. M. Soc. N. Y., Syracuse, 1879, 542: 1880, 410: 1881, 357.—**Shrady** (J.) Contributions to the medical history of the city of New York, 1784-8. Med. Reg., N. Y., 1884, xxii, 243-287.—**Thoms** (W. F.) Sanitary condition of Fish alley and surroundings. Tr. M. Soc. N. Y., Albany, 1866, 148-152, 1 ch.—**Trowbridge** (W. P.) The sanitary problems of New York City. School of Mines Quart., N. Y., 1879-80, i, 131-140.—**Waring** (G. E.), jr. The sanitary condition of New York. I. The disease. Scribner's Month., N. Y., 1881, xxii, 64; 179.

New York (*City*). *Board of Education.* Annual reports to the mayor and common council of the city and to the State superintendent of public instruction. 12., 1853; 38., 1879; 40.-43., 1881-4. 8°. *New York,* 1854-85.

——. Regulations for the admittance, government, and instruction of boys on board the New York nautical schoolship St. Mary's, as authorized by the . . . Together with the Federal and State laws authorizing the establishment of said school. Jan., 1876. 44 pp. 8°. [*New York*], *Cushing & Bardua,* [1876].

New York (*City*). *City Inspector.* Annual reports of the . . . of the number of deaths and interments in the city of New York, to the common council, for the years 1818-27; 1829; 1831; 1833-5; 1837-44; 1847-65. 8°. *New York,* 1819-66.

——. Table of the semi-centennial mortality of the city of New York, compiled from the records of the . . . comprising the full period from January 1, 1804, to December 31, 1853, inclusive. By Thos. K. Downing, city inspector. 1 broadside. fol. *New York,* 1854.

——. Communication from the . . . relative to the spurious milk and diseased meat sold to the inhabitants of this city. Board of councilmen. Aug. 16, 1854. Doc. No. 65. pp. 1055-1082. 8°. *New York, McSpedon & Baker,* 1854. Cutting.

New York (*City*). *Commissioners of Water Supply and Croton Aqueduct.* Report relative to introducing into the city of New York a supply of pure and wholesome water, accompanied by a law asking power to raise money by loan to execute said work. Board of aldermen. Dec. 28, 1831. 75 pp. 8°. [*New York,* 1831.] [P., v. 1225.]

——. [Report to the joint committee on fire and water, by Col. De Witt Clinton, on the best sources and means of transportation of an inexhaustible supply of pure and wholesome water for the city of New York.] Board of aldermen. No. 61. Nov. 10, 1832. 120 pp. 8°. [*New York,* 1832.] [P., v. 1225.]

——. Report of the commissioners, under an act of the legislature of this State, passed February 26, 1833, relative to supplying the city of New York with pure and wholesome water [including the engineer's report, D. B. Douglass, and Mr. Chilton's report]. Board of aldermen. No. 36. Nov. 12, 1833. pp. 357-410, 1 map, 3 plans. 8°. *New York, P. Van Pelt,* 1833. [P., v. 1225.] Cutting.

——. [Communication from the water commissioners, to the common council, relating to their duties and powers under the act of 2d of May, 1834.] Board of aldermen. Doc. No. 1. May 19, 1834. 3 pp. 8°. [*New York,* 1834.] [P., v. 1225.]

——. Report of the commissioners under an act of the legislature of this State, passed May 2, 1834, relative to supplying the city of New York with pure and wholesome water. Board of aldermen. Doc. No. 44. Feb. 16, 1835. pp. 323-525, 5 plans. 8°. *New York, W. B. Townsend,* 1835. [P., v. 223.] Cutting.

——. Report of the committee on fire and water, to whom was referred the report of the water commissioners, and the documents accompanying the same, in relation to supplying the city of New York with pure and wholesome water. Board of aldermen. Doc. No. 45. March 4, 1835. pp. 517-528. 8°. [*New York,* 1835.] Cutting.

——. Communication from Stephen Allen, chairman, in behalf of the water commissioners, praying that the common council will apply to the legislature for a law authorizing the appointment of commissioners, with power to alter the line of any high-way or turnpike in danger of injury from the Croton River Water Works. Board of aldermen. Doc. No. 48. Nov. 23, 1835. 3 pp. 8°. [*New York,* 1835.] [P., v. 223.]

——. Communication from the mayor, enclosing a communication from Stephen Allen, chairman of the water commissioners, and from D. B. Douglas, chief engineer New York aqueduct, in relation to the practicability and probable expense of forcing by steam engines a sufficient quantity of water from the North or East River to a reservoir to be erected on Murray Hill, in aid of the present means of extinguishing fires. Board of aldermen. Doc. No. 89. Feb. 15, 1836. pp. 465-473, 1 ch., 1 plan. 8°. [*New York,* 1836.] [P., v. 223.] Cutting.

——. [Report from the water commissioners, to the common council, on the situation and progress of their work from the date of their appointment.] Board of aldermen. Doc. No. 12. Aug. 1, 1836. pp. 61-69. 8°. [*New York,* 1836.] [P., v. 223.] Cutting.

——. Reports of the committee on laws and on the communication and draft of a law from the water commissioners, with amendments. Board

New York (*City*). *Com. of Water Supply*—cont. of aldermen. Doc. No. 83. Dec. 19, 1836. pp. 537–542. 8°. [*New York*, 1836.] [P., v. 223.]
Cutting.

——. Communication from the water commissioners, setting forth the progress of the works for supplying the city with pure and wholesome water. Board of assistant aldermen. Doc. No. 24. Jan. 9, 1837. pp. 97–109. 8°. [*New York*, 1837.] [P., v. 223.]
Cutting.

——. Report of the select committee, to whom was referred so much of the message of his honor the mayor as relates to furnishing a supply of water for the extinguishing of fires and laying additional pipes. Board of aldermen. Doc. No. 103. Feb. 27, 1837. pp. 663–671. 8°. *New York*, 1837. [P., v. 223.]
Cutting.

——. Semi-annual reports of the water commissioners for the city of New York. 4.–9., Jan., 1837, to Dec., 1839; 11.–14., July, 1840, to June, 1842. 8°. [*New York*, 1837–42.] [P., v. 313.]

——. Report of the finance committee, to whom was referred so much of the report of the water commissioners as relates to providing funds for completing the Croton Water Works. Board of aldermen. Doc. No. 67. Feb. 26, 1838. pp. 519–521. 8°. [*New York*, 1838.] [P., v. 356.]
Cutting.

——. Report of the committee on roads and canals, to whom was referred so much of the report of the water commissioners as relates to the construction of the aqueduct across the Harlaem River. Board of aldermen. Doc. No. 88. April 23, 1838. pp. 615–627. 8°. [*New York*, 1838.] [P., v. 356.]
Cutting.

——. Communication from the water commissioners relative to the Croton Aqueduct. Board of aldermen. Doc. No. 2. May 14, 1838. pp. 25–33. 8°. [*New York*, 1838.] [P., v. 356.]
Cutting.

——. Report of the fire and water committee on a communication from a committee of citizens relative to a paid fire department. Board of aldermen. Doc. No. 56. March 2, 1840. pp. 575–582. 8°. [*New York*, 1840.]
Cutting.

——. Supplemental report of the late water commissioners. March 20, 1840. City Doc. No. 65. pp. 639–650. 8°. *New York, Bryant & Boggs*, [1840]. [*Also, in:* P., v. 356.]
Cutting.

——. Communication of the water commissioners in relation to laying down the distributing water pipes. Board of aldermen. Doc. No. 72. May 4, 1840. pp. 709–716. 8°. *New York, Bryant & Boggs*, [1840]. [P., v. 356.]
Cutting.

——. An ordinance to organize the Croton Aqueduct department. Common council. Aug. 5, 1840. 4 pp. 8°. [*New York*, 1840.] [P., v. 356.]

——. Communications of the comptroller, the water commissioners, and the Croton Aqueduct committee, etc., on the subject of the ordinance to amend the ordinance to instruct the water commissioners. Board of aldermen. Doc. No. 70. Oct. 12, 1840. pp. 239–295. 8°. *New York*, 1840. [P., v. 356.]
Cutting.

——. Report of the majority of the special committee, on the subject of the ordinance creating the aqueduct department, etc., and to amend the ordinance to instruct the water commissioners. Board of aldermen. Doc. No. 31. Dec. 14, 1840. pp. 93–114. 8°. [*New York*, 1840.] [P., v. 356.]
Cutting.

New York (*City*). *Com. of Water Supply*—cont.
——. Report of the minority of the special committee on the subject of the ordinance creating the aqueduct department, etc., and to amend the ordinance to instruct the water commissioners. Board of aldermen. Doc. No. 32. Dec. 14, 1840. pp. 115–194, 1 plan. 8°. [*New York*, 1840.] [P., v. 356.]
Cutting.

——. Report of the committee on the Croton Aqueduct, on the petition of John M. Bradhurst, for remuneration for injuries done his property in the opening of the Tenth avenue. Board of aldermen. No. 35. Dec. 21, 1840. pp. 195–197. 8°. [*New York*, 1840.] [P., v. 356.]
Cutting.

——. Report of the special committee to whom was referred the communication from the water commissioners, a report of the Croton Aqueduct committee, and an opinion of the council in relation to the powers and duties of the water commissioners, together with accompanying documents. Board of aldermen. Doc. No. 32. Dec. 22, 1840. pp. 395–466. 8°. [*New York*, 1840.] [P., v. 356.]
Cutting.

——. A statement of the receipts and expenditures on account of the Croton Aqueduct, and of the amount of water-loan stock, authorized by the legislature of the State of New York, with the amount of such stock issued by the common council of the city of New York to April 20, 1841. 1 l., 1 tab. 8°. [*New York*, 1841.] [P., v. 356.]

——. Quarterly reports of the Croton Aqueduct department in compliance with an ordinance to provide for the accountability of the executive committees of the common council. 1., 3., & 4. qrs. of 1841. 8°. [*New York*, 1841–2.] [P., v. 356.]

——. Acts of the legislature of the State and ordinances and resolutions of the common council of the city of New York in relation to the subject of the introduction of water into the city of New York, from 1833 to June, 1842. 72 pp. 8°. [*New York*], *C. Dingley*, 1842. [P., v. 356.]

——. Communication from the comptroller relative to the establishment of a water department, with a programme of a law for the same. Board of aldermen. Doc. No. 80. April 18, 1842. pp. 617–627. 8°. [*New York*, 1842.] [P., v. 356.]
Cutting.

——. Description of the Croton Aqueduct, by John B. Jervis, chief engineer. 31 pp. 8°. *New York, Slamm & Genon*, 1842.

——. Report on the general state of the work on the Croton Aqueduct (to the water commissioners). Doc. No. 9. July 12, 1842. pp. 91–101. 8°. [*New York*, 1842.] [P., v. 356.]
Cutting.

——. Report of special committee on the memorial of Messrs. Tatham & Bros., relative to composition and other conduit pipes. Board of aldermen. Doc. No. 37. Oct. 10, 1842. pp. 165–188. 8°. [*New York*, 1842.] [P., v., 356.]
Cutting.

——. Report of the Croton Aqueduct board, in relation to the ways and means of paying the Croton water debt. Board of aldermen. Doc. No. 58. Dec. 27, 1842. pp. 541–577. 8°. [*New York*, 1842.] [P., v. 356.]
Cutting.

——. Illustrations of the Croton Aqueduct, by F. B. Tower, of the engineer department. vi, 152 pp., 22 pl. fol. *New York & London, Wiley & Putnam*, 1843.

New York (*City*). *Com. of Water Supply—cont.*
——. A memoir of the construction, cost, and capacity of the Croton Aqueduct, compiled from official documents; together with an account of the civic celebration of the fourteenth October, 1842, on occasion of the completion of the great work; preceded by a preliminary essay on ancient and modern aqueducts. By Charles King. vii, 308 pp., 1 pl. 4°. *New York, C. King*, 1843.

——. An ordinance establishing a scale of water rents for the Croton Aqueduct department. 8 pp. 8°. [*New York*, 1851.]

——. Annual report of the Croton Aqueduct department; made to the common council of the city of New York, for the year 1857. 102 pp. 8°. *New York, C. W. Baker*, 1858.

——. Profile of lower part of Croton Aqueduct. Ground plan of the lower part of Croton Aqueduct. 1 plan. [*New York, G. Hayward, n. d.*] [*P.*, v. 356.]

New York (*City*). *Coroner's Office.* Annual report for the year 1883. pp. 163–165. fol. [*New York*, 1884.]
Cutting from: City Record, 1884, xii.

New York (*City*). *Department of Public Charities.* Annual reports of the commissioners of public charities and correction, to the mayor of the city. 1., 1860; 4., 1863; 6.–12., 1865–71. 8°. *New York*, 1861–72.

——. Rules and regulations for the government of the bureau of medical and surgical relief for the out-door poor. Under the direction of the board of commissioners of public charities and correction. 10 pp. 8°. [*New York*], 1866.

——. The nomenclature of diseases. Adopted by the commissioners of public charities and correction, on the recommendation of the medical boards of Bellevue, Charity, and Infants' Hospitals, for the hospitals of the department of public charities and correction, Dec., 1869. 86 pp. 8°. *New York*, 1870.

——. Medical, surgical, and obstetrical statistics of the Bellevue and Charity Hospitals, 1870. First annual report. 3 p. l, 101 l. obl. 4°. *New York, Bellevue Press*, 1871.

——. Report to the commissioners of public charities and correction of the city of New York, on the chemical and physical facts collected from the deep-sea researches made during the voyage of the nautical schoolship "Mercury", undertaken by their order in the tropical Atlantic and Caribbean Sea, 1870–71. By Henry Draper. 33 pp., 1 pl., 1 map. 8°. *New York, New York Printing Co.*, 1871.

——. Meeting of the commissioners, March 2, 1871. [Requisitions from departments received, examined, and acted on.] pp. 81–101. 8°. [*New York*, 1871.]
Cutting.

——. Report to the commissioners of public charities and correction, on the scientific portion of the cruise of the "Nautical school-ship Mercury" during the winter of 1871-2. By J. W. S. Arnold. 16 pp. 8°. *New York, Bellevue Press*, 1872.

——. Report on the free labor bureau, and proposed improvements for the same. To the board of commissioners of public charities and correction. July 30, 1873. 7 pp. 8°. [*New York*, 1873.]

——. Annual reports of the chief of staff of the Charity, Fever, Epileptic, Penitentiary, Alms House and Work House Hospitals, and Hospital for Incurables, Blackwell's Island, N. Y., for the years 1874; 1875. 63 pp., 1 tab; 64 pp., 2 tab. 8°. *New York*, 1875-6.

——. Monthly report of the examining physician. To the board of commissioners of public

New York (*City*). *Dep. of Pub. Charities—cont.* charities and correction, for Jan., 1883. broadside, 14 x 17 in. [*New York*, 1883.]

——. Hospital formulary of the department of public charities and correction of the city of New York. 3. ed., rev. iv, 127 pp. 8°. *New York, Printing Bureau of New York City Asylum for the Insane*, 1886.

New York (*City*). *Department of Public Charities. Bellevue Hospital.* The inauguration of the pathological building of the . . . October 25, 1856. 8 pp. 8°. *New York, Wiley & Halstead*, 1856.
Repr. from: N. York J. M., 1856, 3. s., i.

——. Rules and regulations for the government of the Bellevue Hospital. 40 pp. 8°. [*New York*], 1860.

——. The same. 42 pp. 8°. [*New York*, 1863.]

——. Annual reports of the Bellevue and Charity Hospital, New York, for 1870. xviii, 415 pp. 8°. *New York, D. Appleton & Co.*, 1870.

——. Report of special committee of the medical board of Bellevue Hospital on erysipelas and pyæmia. 9 pp., 3 ch. 8°. *New York, Bellevue Press*, 1872.

——. Catalogue of the "Wood" Museum of Bellevue Hospital, New York City. Comprising a descriptive and classified list of anatomical and pathological specimens. vi, 256 pp., 1 l. 12°. *New York, Department Press*, 1880.

New York (*City*). *Department of Public Charities. Charity Hospital, Blackwell's Island.* Rules and regulations of the . . . adopted by the board of commissioners of public charities and correction, Nov. 20, 1875. 24 pp. 12°. [*New York*], *Bellevue Press*, 1875.

——. Annual reports of the chief of staff, to the board of commissioners of public charities and correction, for the years 1874; 1875. 8°. *New York*, 1875-6.
See, also. **New York** (*City*). *Board of Commissioners of Public Charities, Bellevue Hospital.*

——. The Training School for Nurses, Charity Hospital, Blackwell's Island. [Notice of . . . with an extract from the annual report of the chief of staff, for 1881.] 13 pp. 8°. *New York, Department Press*, 1882.

——. The Charity Hospital Training School for Male Nurses. [Information for, and questions to be answered by, applicants.] 2 l. 4°. [*New York*, 1887 ?]

New York (*City*). *Department of Public Charities. Commissioners of the Almshouse.* The Commissioners of the Almshouse *vs.* Alexander Whistelo, a black man; being a remarkable case of bastardy, tried and adjudged by the mayor, recorder and several aldermen of the city of New York, under the act passed 6 March, 1801, for the relief of cities and towns from the maintenance of bastard children. 56 pp. 8°. *New York, D. Longworth*, 1808.

——. Report of the committee on charity and almshouse in favor of removing the almshouse establishment to Randall's Island and selling the Long Island farms. City Doc. No. 4. Board of assistant aldermen. June 29, 1835. pp. 39–46. 8°. [*New York*, 1835.]
Cutting.

——. Report of the joint special committee on Blackwell's Island and the Long Island farms, on the communication from the commissioners of the almshouse, relating to the lunatic asylum. City Doc. No. 14. Board of assistant aldermen. July 22, 1835. pp. 121–128. 8°. [*New York*, 1835.]
Cutting.

——. Memorial of the late commissioners of the almshouse, etc., and members of the committee on Blackwell's Island and Long Island farms, of

New York (*City*). *Department of Public Charities. Commissioners of the Almshouse*—continued. the last common council, on the subject of the lunatic asylum. City Doc. No. 31. Board of assistant aldermen. Oct. 13, 1835. pp. 271–284. 8°. [*New York*, 1835.]
Cutting.

——. Communication from the commissioners of the almshouse, in reply to certain interrogatories contained in a resolution adopted by the board of assistants on the 31st of July, 1835. [Giving their reasons for transferring the lunatic asylum to Randall's Island.] City Doc. No. 23. Board of assistant aldermen. Sept. 7, 1835. pp. 195–204. 8°. [*New York*, 1835.]
Cutting.

——. Report of the commissioners of the Alms House, Bridewell and Penitentiary. City Doc. No. 32. pp. 201–251. 8°. *New York, ptd. by order of the board of aldermen*, 1837.
Cutting.

——. An ordinance for the organization of the hospital department of the Alms House of the City and County of New York. City Doc. No. 6. Aug. 5, 1847. pp. 55–65. 8°. [*Albany*, 1847.]
Cutting.

——. Annual reports of the governors of the Almshouse of the City of New York to the secretary of state of New York and the common council of the city of New York. 4., 1852; 5., 1853; 7., 1855; 10., 1858; 11., 1859. 8°. *New York*, 1853–60.

——. Annual report of the Blackwell's Island Hospitals to the governors of the Alms House, for the year 1854. 34 pp., 1 tab. 8°. [*New York*, 1855.]

New York (*City*). *Department of Public Charities. Homœopathic Hospital, Ward's Island*. Rules and regulations. Adopted by the board of commissioners of public charities and correction. 28 pp. 8°. [*New York*], *Bellevue Press*, 1876.

——. Annual reports of the chief of medical staff to the president department of public charities and correction. 5.–7., 1879–81; 12., 1886. 8°. *New York*, 1880–87.

New York (*City*). *Department of Public Charities. New York City Asylum for the Insane, Ward's Island*. Annual reports of the medical superintendent to the commissioners of public charities and corrections. 2.–10., 1873–81. 8°. *New York*, 1874–82.
First report not printed.

——. Rules and regulations of the . . . Prepared by A. E. Macdonald, M. D., medical superintendent. Adopted by the commissioners of public charities and corrections, Sept. 1, 1875. Revised and re-adopted May 1, 1882. 20 pp. 8°. [*New York*], *Department Press*, 1882.

——. [Blank forms in use at the asylum.] v. s. [*New York*, 188–.]
Admissions, daily; census returns, daily; labor report, daily; report of deaths, weekly; report of discharges, weekly; report of admissions, weekly; statement of patient on admission.

New York (*City*). *Department of Public Charities. New York City Lunatic Asylum at Blackwell's Island*. Communication from Dr. James McDonald relative to the lunatic asylum. City Doc. No. 37. Oct. 13, 1835. pp. 307–317. 8°. [*New York*, 1835.]
Cutting.

——. Annual reports of the resident physician to the commissioners of public charities and correction, for the years 1851; 1853; 1854; 1856–9; 1862; 1864; 1868–70; 1874; 1876; 1878; 1880–82. 8°. *New York*, 1852–83.

——. Code of rules and regulations for the government of those employed at the . . . Prepared

New York (*City*). *Dep. of Pub. Charities. New York City Lun. Asy. at Blackwell's Island*—cont. by T. M. Franklin, M. D., medical superintendent. Adopted by the board of commissioners of public charities and correction. 18 pp. 8°. [*New York*], *Department Press*, 1880.

——. [Blank forms in use at the asylum.] v. s. [*New York*, 188–.]
Application for position of attendant; causes, modes, duration of di ease; coffin card; daily report of head attendant; general history of patient; leave of absence, and renewal; special diet orders; release of patient to friend; report of death to friend; report of death to commissioners; request to visit; report of patients, with addresses of friends, weekly; transfer of patient; ward card.

——. *See, also* :
NEW YORK (*City*). *Commissioners of the Almshouse*. Report of the joint special committee on Blackwell's Island [etc.] 8°. [*New York*, 1835.]

——. Memorial of the late commissioners of the almshouse, etc., and members of the committee on Blackwell's Island [etc.] 8°. [*New York*, 1835.]

——. Communication from the commissioners of the almshouse [etc.] 8°. [*New York*, 1835.]

New York (*City*). *Department of Public Parks*. Annual report of commissioners of the . . . to the mayor of the city. 2., 1871–2. vii, 253 pp., 2 maps, 13 diag. 8°. *New York, W. C. Bryant & Co.*, 1872.

——. Report on the drainage of the 23. and 24. wards, New York City. E. B. Van Winkle, C. E. Doc. No. 88. Board of the department of public parks. March 2, 1881. 60 pp., 1 map. 8°. [*New York*, 1881.]

New York (*City*). *Department of Public Parks. Central Park Menagerie*. Annual report of the director, for the year 1879. 32 pp. roy. 8°. *New York, M. B. Brown*, 1880.

New York (*City*). *Department of Public Parks. New York Meteorological Observatory*. Annual reports of the director to the board of commissioners, for the years 1870–71; 1873–5; 1877; 1886. 8° & 4°. *New York*, 1871–87.
1874–5 in 1. 1886 is 4°.

——. Abstracts of registers from Draper's self-recording instruments. (Monthly.) Jan., 1879, to Dec., 1881; July, 1882; Jan. to Nov., 1886; Jan. to Dec., 1887. 4°. *New York*, 1879–88.

——. Annual tables for the years 1879–81. 4°. *New York*, 1880–82.

New York (*City*). *Department of Public Works*. Annual reports. 2., 1871–2; 1881–4. 8°. *New York*, 1872–85.

New York (*City*). *Health Department*. Documents relating to the board of health of the city of New York. 99 pp. 8°. *New York, J. Cheetham*, 1806.

——. Board of health of the city of New York. Address to their fellow citizens [June 1, 1818.] 8 pp. 8°. [*New York, G. L. Birch & Co.*, 1818.]

——. A statement of facts relative to the late epidemic fever which appeared in Bancker street and its vicinity. Published by order of the board of health. 28 pp. 8°. *New York, E. Bliss*, 1821.

——. History of the proceedings of the board of health of the city of New York in the summer and fall of 1822, together with an account of the rise and progress of the yellow fever. 270 pp. 8°. *New York, P & H. Van Pelt*, 1823.

——. Report of the commissioners employed to investigate the origin and nature of the epidemic cholera of Canada. Published by order of the board of health, July 31, 1832. 8 pp. 8°. *New York, P. Van Pelt*, 1832.

——. Questions of the board of health in relation to malignant cholera, with the answers of the special medical council; together with a report upon the causes of the cessation of cholera

New York (*City*). *Health Department*—cont'd.
at Bellevue. (Published by order of the board of health.) 14 pp. 8°. *New York, P. Van Pelt,* 1832. [P., v. 837.]

——. Report of the standing sanitary committee of the board of health of the city of New York, on the subject of Asiatic cholera, at present prevailing at the quarantine establishment of New York, at Staten Island. 32 pp. 8°. *New York, McSpedon & Baker,* 1848. [*Also, in:* P., v. 205; 333.]

——. Report of the proceedings of the sanatory committee of the board of health in relation to cholera as it prevailed in New York in 1849. 106 pp. 8°. *New York,* 1849. [*Also, in:* P., v. 205.]

——. Majority and minority reports of the select committee of the board of health, appointed to investigate the character and condition of the sources from which cow's milk is derived, for sale in the city of New York. Together with the testimony and the chemical and microscopical analyses of milks. Also letters from distinguished physicians, etc. 305 pp. 8°. *New York,* 1858.

——. Reports, resolutions, and proceedings of the commissioners of health of the city of New York, for the years 1856, 1857, 1858, and 1859. Compiled by order of the board, under the direction of his honor the mayor. 552, 33 pp. 8°. *New York, G. H. Clark,* 1860.

——. Laws and ordinances relative to the preservation of the public health in the city of New York. Compiled and annotated by George W. Morton. Published under the authority and by direction of the mayor and commissioners of health. viii, 226 pp. 8°. *New York, E. Jones & Co.,* 1860.

——. Memorial of the board of commissioners of health of the city of New York, on the subject of compulsory vaccination, with a view to exterminate the small-pox. 12 pp. 8°. *New York, W. H. Trafton & Co.,* 1862. [*Also, in:* P., v. 337.]

——. Cholera! Caution to the public. [By the commissioners of health of the city of New York, by request, Nov., 1865.] 4 pp. 8°. *New York, W. J. & J. W. Bell,* 1865.]

——. Metropolitan Board of Health. Code of health, ordinances, and rules, and sanitary regulations. 68 pp. 8°. *New York, J. W. Amerman,* 1866.
The Metropolitan Board of Health was organized March 5, 1866.

——. Metropolitan Board of Health. Statistical nomenclature of causes of death, classified and arranged upon the basis recommended by the International Statistical Congress for the purposes of public registration. Synonymous terms in English, Latin, French, and German, to ensure accurate and comparable certificates of death, and uniformity in the records of mortality in the metropolitan sanitary district. 1 sheet. 4°. [*New York,* 1866?]

——. Code of sanitary ordinances, and rules and regulations of the Metropolitan Board of Health. 92 pp. 8°. *New York, C. S. Westcott & Co.,* 1867.

——. Metropolitan Board of Health. Code of sanitary ordinances, and rules and sanitary regulations. 1867. 49 pp. 8°. *New York, C. S. Westcott & Co.,* 1867.

——. [Blank forms used by the Metropolitan Board of Health.] 8°. [*New York,* 1867.]
Letter to attending physicians, requesting reasons, in writing, for not reporting a case of death. Return of a still-born infant.

——. Report of E. B. Dalton, sanitary superintendent of the Metropolitan Board of Health. 36 pp. 8°. *Albany, C. Van Benthuysen & Sons,* 1867.

New York (*City*). *Health Department*—cont'd.

——. Annual reports of the Metropolitan Board of Health of the State of New York to the governor of the State. 1.–4., 1866 to 1868–9. 8°. *Albany,* 1867–70.
1. report for eight months ending Oct. 31, 1866. 4. report, 63 pp., being the report proper, minus the appendix.

——. Annual reports of the Metropolitan Board of Health of the State of New York to the governor of the State. 1.–4., 1866 to 1868–9. 8°. *New York & Albany,* 1867–70.
3. report published at Albany.

——. Metropolitan Board of Health. Cholera at the military posts, in the harbor of New York, in the summer of 1867. 7 pp. 8°. *New York, C. S. Westcott & Co.,* 1868.
Repr. from: Rep. Metrop. Bd. Health 1867, N. Y., 1868, ii.

——. Cleanse and disinfect. Advice in regard to the use of disinfectants. [Prepared and published by direction of the Metropolitan Board of Health, N. Y., July 18, 1868.] 4 pp. 8°. [*New York,* 1868.]

——. Metropolitan Board of Health. Memorandum on disinfection. 8 pp. 8°. *New York, C. S. Westcott & Co.,* 1868.

——. A report to the Metropolitan Board of Health, on vaccination. 1868. 58 pp. 8°. *New York, D. Appleton & Co.,* [1868].

——. Metropolitan Board of Health. Office of sanitary superintendent. Circular, to physicians, reminding them that they are required by law to report to the board all cases of an infectious, contagious, or pestilential character. By Ed. B. Dalton, sanitary superintendent. Jan. 2, 1868. 1 sheet. 4°. [*New York,* 1868.]

——. Metropolitan Board of Health. Sanitary qualities of the water supply of New York and Brooklyn, by Elisha Harris, with chemical analyses, by C. F. Chandler. 16 pp. 8°. *New York, C. S. Westcott & Co.,* 1868.
Repr. from: Rep. Metrop. Bd. Health, N. Y., 1867, ii.

——. Metropolitan Board of Health of the city of New York. Special report upon the operations of the N. Y. Rendering Co., Sept. 26, 1867. By Moreau Morris and E. H. Janes to E. B. Dalton, sanitary superintendent. 7 pp. 8°. *New York, C. S. Westcott & Co.,* 1868.

——. The vital statistics and sanitary condition of the hospitals and other institutions in which medical care is systematically provided in the metropolitan sanitary district. (Published by order of the Metropolitan Board of Health.) 16 pp. 8°. *New York, C. S. Westcott & Co.,* 1868.
Repr. from: Rep. Reg. Vital Statist. 8°. *New York,* ii.

——. Metropolitan Board of Health. Report in answer to a resolution of the assembly. [Concerning the action of the health officer in transferring passengers from the ship James Foster to Ward's Island.] State of New York. No. 116. March 26, 1869. 2 pp. 8°. [*Albany,* 1869.]

——. Bureau of Sanitary Inspection. Circular, to physicians, calling attention to section 122 of the sanitary code, which requires physicians to report to the bureau every person having a contagious disease. By Moreau Morris, city sanitary inspector. Oct. 1, 1870. 1 sheet. 8°. [*New York,* 1870.]

——. Metropolitan Board of Health. Report on the gas nuisance in New York, by C. F. Chandler. 109 pp. 8°. *New York, D. Appleton & Co.,* 1870.
Repr. from: Rep. Metrop. Bd. Health, N. Y., 1870.

——. Metropolitan Board of Health. Reports on the water supply of New York and Brooklyn. Chemical report by C. F. Chandler. Microscopical report by William B. Lewis. 14 pp., 1 pl. 8°. *New York, D. Appleton & Co.,* 1870.
Repr. from: Rep. Metrop. Bd. Health, N. Y., 1869, iv.

New York (*City*). *Health Department—cont'd.*
——. Metropolitan Board of Health. Code of health ordinances, and rules and sanitary regulations, 1866, and its amendments. Metropolitan sanitary district of the State of New York. 11 pp. 8°. [*n. p., n. d.*]
——. Metropolitan Board of Health. Disinfectants and how to use them. 1 sheet. 8°. [*New York, n. d.*]
——. Rescue of drowning persons. Rules adopted by the Metropolitan Board of Health. 4 pp. 12°. [*New York, n. d.*]
——. Sanitary code of the board of health of the health department of the city of New York. Oct., 1870. 84 pp. 8°. *New York, N. Y. Printing Company*, 1870.
 The board of health of the health department was organized April 11, 1870, succeeding the metropolitan board of health by act of the legislature. Reorganized in 1873.
——. Annual reports of the board of health of the health department of the city of New York to the mayor. 1.–6. (1870–71 to 1874–5.) 8°. *New York*, 1871-6.
 For subsequent reports, see **New York** (*City*). *Health Department. Bureau of Vital Statistics.* 5. and 6. reports in one for twenty months, May 1, 1874, to Dec. 31, 1875.
——. Board of health of the health department of the city of New York. Supplemental report of the annual report of the department of health of the city of New York, twentieth sanitary inspection district, for the year 1870. By R. Tauszky. 26 pp. 8°. *New York*, 1872.
——. Manual of the board of health of the health department of the city of New York. August, 1872. 209 pp. 16°. *New York, D. Appleton & Co.*, 1872.
——. Report of the board of health of the health department of the city of New York, on small-pox. 16 pp. 8°. *New York, J. J. Hastie*, 1872.
——. Instructions regarding the prevention of cholera. Health department, New York, June 7, 1873. 1 l. 8°. [*New York*, 1873.]
——. Rules for the care of infants. June 3, 1873. 1 l. 16°. [*New York*, 1873.]
——. Manual of the board of health of the health department of the city of New York. 233 pp. 16°. *New York, D. Appleton & Co.*, 1874.
——. Report of the sanitary committee of the board of health on the concentration and regulation of the business of slaughtering animals in the city of New York. June, 1874. 30 pp., 1 map. 8°. *New York, D. Appleton & Co.*, [1874].
——. Sanitary code of the board of health of the health department. June, 1874. 83 pp. 16°. *New York, M. B. Brown*, 1874.
——. A table showing, for each week since 1866, the total weekly mortality, the mortality from diarrhœal diseases of children under five years of age, and of persons more than five years of age; the greatest range of temperature, and the mean range of temperature and of humidity in each week. 1 broadside. fol. [*New York*, 1876.]
——. Defective drainage of dwelling houses. 7 pp., 3 pl. 8°. [*New York*, 1877.]
——. Registry of births returned to the bureau of vital statistics, health department of the city of New York. [Nos. 24 & 26, 1877. Blank forms filled out.] 16°. [*New York*, 1877.]
——. In the court of general sessions in and for the city and county of New York at the December term, 1876. Hon. Josiah Sutherland presiding. The People *vs.* Daniel Schrumpf. Misdemeanor. Adulteration of milk. Argument of W. P. Prentice, counsel to the board of health, for the prosecution. 32 pp. 8°. *New York, J. F. Trow & Son*, 1877.

New York (*City*). *Health Department—cont'd.*
——. The City Record. Official journal. Health department. Reports of the board of health of the health department to the mayor of the city. [Quarterly.] 4., 1876; 4., 1877; 4., 1881; 3., 1882; 4., 1882; 2., 1883; 1.–4., 1884. fol. *New York*, 1877–85.
——. The City Record. Official journal. Health department. Reports for the weeks ending March 10, 1877; Jan. 27, March 31, April 28, Sept. 1 to Oct. 2, 1883. fol. [*New York*, 1877–83.]
——. Catalogue of books and pamphlets in the library of the health department, New York. 1878. 51 pp. 8°. *New York, M. B. Brown*, 1878.
——. [Blank forms used by the board of health of the health department of the city of New York.] v. s. [*New York*, 187-.]
 1. Certificate of death [and list of diseases].
 2. Preliminary notice of a death from a contagious disease.
——. Sanitary code of the board of health of the health department of the city of New York. May, 1880. (Sec. 82, chap. 335, laws of 1873.) 97 pp. 16°. *New York, J. F. Hahn*, 1880.
——. Circular on bovine vaccine virus. 3 pp. 8°. *New York*, 1880.
——. Specifications for plumbing and drainage. [To be submitted, with plan, for the action of the board of health of the city of New York.] 13 pp. fol. [*New York*, 1882?]
——. The registration of plumbers, and the law and regulations governing the plumbing and drainage of all buildings hereafter erected. Chapter 450, laws of 1881. An act to secure the registration of plumbers, and the supervision of plumbing and drainage in the cities of New York and Brooklyn. 12 pp. 8°. [*New York*, 1883.]
——. Reports of deaths in New York City. [Weekly.] Dec. 8, 1883, to Jan. 3, 1885. 18°. [*New York*, 1883–5.]
——. The tenement house problem in New York. For the information of the commission on legislation affecting tenement and lodging houses, provided for in chapter 84, laws of 1887. Dec. 14, 1887. 48 pp. 8°. *New York, W. P. Mitchell*, 1887.
——. Sunstroke. [Report of the sanitary committee of the board of health upon sunstroke.] 1 sheet. 12°. [*New York, n. d.*]
——. Board of health of the health department of the city of New York. Sanitary regulations against small-pox, scarlatina, and measles. By E. H. Janes, city sanitary inspector. 1 sheet. 16°. [*New York, n. d.*]

New York *City* (*Health Department of*).
ADDRESS of the committee to promote the passage of a metropolitan health bill. New York, Dec., 1865. 8°. *New York*, 1865.
NEW YORK (*City*). Board of Health of the City of New York. Documents relating to the board of health of New York. 8°. *New York*, 1806.
——. Board of Health of the City of New York. Address to their fellow citizens [June 1, 1818]. 8°. [*New York*, 1818.]
——. Board of Health of the Health Department of the City of New York. Annual reports. 1.–6., 1870–71 to 1874–5. 8°. *New York*, 1871-6.
——. Board of Health of the Health Department of the City of New York. Supplementary report of the annual report. Twentieth sanitary inspection district, for the year 1870. 8°. *New York*, 1872.
——. Metropolitan Board of Health of the State of New York. Annual reports. 1.–4., 1866–9. 8°. *New York*, 1867-70.

New York City (*Health Department of*).

————. Metropolitan Board of Health. Report of E. B. Dalton, sanitary superintendent of the Metropolitan Board of Health. 8°. *Albany*, 1867.

NEW YORK (*State*). An act relative to the public health in the city of New York. Passed April 10, 1850. 8°. [*Albany*, 1850.]

————. Report of the select committee appointed to investigate the health department of the city of New York. Transmitted to the legislature Feb. 3, 1859. 8°. *Albany*, 1859.

————. Report of the committee on the incorporation of cities and villages, on the bill entitled "An act concerning the public health of the counties of New York, Kings, and Richmond". March 9, 1860. 8°. *Albany*, 1860.

————. Senate. An act to simplify the proof of the sanitary code in the city of New York. No. 170. March 3, 1880. Introd. by Mr. Strahan. fol. [*Albany*, 1880.]

Chandler (Dr.) and the New York health department. San. Engin., N. Y., 1882-3, vii, 558-560. *Also, Reprint.* — **Health** (The) of New York from June, 1866—Jan., 1887. Science, N. Y., 1886, viii, 92; 200; 316; 426; 529; 624; 1887, ix, 84; 227. — **Monthly** bulletins of the New York State board of health. Rep. State Bd. Health N. Y., Albany, 1886, vi, 451–504. — **Work** of the summer corps of the city board of health. San. Engin., N. Y., 1882, vi, 343.

New York (*City*). Health Department. Bureau of Vital Statistics. Metropolitan Board of Health. Bureau of records and vital statistics. Circular, to physicians, explanatory of forms and nomenclature used. Also, brief suggestions to medical practitioners respecting certificates of deaths. By Elisha Harris, registrar. May, 1866. 2 1. 8°. [*New York*, 1866.]

————. Metropolitan Board of Health. Bureau of records and vital statistics. Circular, to physicians, calling attention to the metropolitan sanitary code, which requires attending physicians to report immediately all cases of cholera, typhus and typhoid fevers, yellow fever, and small-pox. July 31, 1866. 1 sheet. 8°. [*New York*, 1866.]

————. Reported mortality, together with the actual mortality. (Weekly.) July 23, 1870, to July 24, 1886. roy. 8° & 4°. *New York*, 1870-86.

————. Weekly mortality from the principal causes of death in the city of New York, for the years 1874-7. 4°. [*New York*, 1875-8.]

————. Abstract of census of the city of New York in 1875, by wards, ages, sexes, nativity, etc. Compiled for report of bureau of vital statistics, under the direction of Dr. E. Harris. Revised by superintendent of State census. 1 broadside. fol. [*New York*, 1876.]

————. Bureau of vital statistics. Summary of births, marriages, still-births, and deaths in New York City, during the years 1876; 1877; 1879; 1880; 1883. fol. [*New York*, 1877-84.]

1876, 1877, and 1880, are cuttings from City Record.

————. Reported mortality, together with the actual mortality. [Quarterly.] 1.-4. qr., 1877. fol. [*New York*, 1877-8.]

————. Annual reports of the board of health of the health department of the city of New York. Vital statistics. 7.-11., 1876-80. 8°. *New York*, [1877-81].

*For prior reports, see **New York** (*City*). Health Department.*

————. Reported mortality, together with the actual mortality for the years 1877 - 83. fol. *New York*, 1878-84.

————. Summary of births, marriages, still-births, deaths, etc., in New York City. Compared with 352 American and foreign cities. For the year 1878. And also the mortality from some of the most prominent causes, which took place in

New York (*City*). Health Department. Bureau of Vital Statistics—continued.

New York City during the past 75 years. By John T. Nagle. 14 pp., 1 tab. 8°. *New York, C. L. Birmingham & Co.*, 1879.

Repr. from: Hosp. Gaz., N. Y., 1879, vi.

————. Table showing the total number of stillbirths and deaths (with an enumeration of some of the most prominent causes) which occurred in this city during the seventy-five years ending Dec. 31, 1878, and the number of births and marriages reported since the year 1847. Compiled from the records. By John T. Nagle. 1 sheet. fol. [*New York*, 1879.]

————. Epitome of the births, marriages, stillbirths, and deaths in New York City during the year 1879. By John T. Nagle. 1 sheet. 4°. [*New York*, 1880.]

New York (*City*). Police Department. Reorganization of the surgical department of the police. Mayor's office, July 10, 1855. 7 pp. 8°. [*New York*, 1855.]

————. Annual reports of the board of commissioners of metropolitan police to the legislature, for the years 1862-3; 1863-4; 1866-7; 1868-9. 8°. *Albany*, 1864-70.

————. Communication from the metropolitan board of police and board of health in answer to a resolution in relation to prostitution in the city of New York. 11 pp. 8°. *Albany, Van Benthuysen & Sons*, 1867.

————. Annual reports to the mayor of the city. 1., 1870-71; 2., 1871-2. 8°. *New York*, 1871-3.

New York City (*Charities of*).

AMERICAN Female Guardian Society and Home for the Friendless. Annual reports of the managers. 38.-40., 1871-2 to 1873-4. 8°. *New York*, 1872-4.

ASSOCIATION for Befriending Children and Young Girls. Annual reports of the managers. 3., 1872-3; 5., 1874-5. 12°. *New York*, 1873-5.

ASSOCIATION for the Benefit of Colored Orphans. Annual reports of the managers. 37., 1872-3; 38., 1873-4. 8°. *New York*, 1873-5.

ASSOCIATION for the Relief of Respectable, Aged, Indigent Females. Annual report of the managers. 45., 1857-8. 8°. *New York*, 1858.

BANK Clerks' Mutual Benefit Association. Annual reports of the board of management. 4., 1871-2; 5., 1872-3. 8°. *New York*, 1872-3.

BETHANY Institute for Women's Christian Work. Annual statement of the managers. 2., 1873; 3., 1874. 12°. *New York*, 1874-5.

BREAD and Beef House. Constitution and by-laws of the . . . [and a statement of its necessity]. 16°. *New York*, 1873.

————. Annual report of the executive committee. 1., 1873-4. 8°. *New York*, 1874.

CALVARY Church. Annual report of the board of managers of the Female Benevolent Society of . . . 25., 1873-4. 8°. *New York*, 1874.

CARPENTER (S. M.) Extract from the fourteenth annual report of the State board of charities of the State of New York, relating to the charities of the second judicial district. 8°. *Albany*, 1881.

CHAPIN Home for the Aged and Infirm. Annual report of the board of managers. 1., 1872-3. 8°. *New York*, 1874.

CHARITY Organization Society of the City of New York. A classified and descriptive directory to the charitable and beneficent societies and institutions of the city of New York. 8°. *New York*, 1883.

CHILDREN's Aid Society. Annual reports of the trustees. 1.-10., 1853-4 to 1862-3; 12.-15.,

New York *City* (*Charities of*).

1864–5 to 1867–8; 17.–22., 1869 to 1873–4. 8°. *New York*, 1854–74.

CHURCH of the Holy Trinity. Annual reports of the board of trustees and officers of the Pastoral Aid Society of the . . . 8., 1873; 9., 1874. 8°. *New York*, 1874–5.

CITIZENS' Association of New York. Report upon the condition, etc., of the institutions under the charge of the commissioners of public charities and correction, with suggestions relating to organizing a bureau of labor statistics and employment and depots in the West for the distribution of labor. 8°. *New York*, 1868.

COLORED Home. Annual report of the board of management. 33., 1872–3. 12°. *New York*, 1873.

DEMILT Dispensary in the City of New York. Annual reports of the managers. 1.–35., 1851–2 to 1885. 8°. *New York*, 1852–86.

EASTERN Dispensary in the City of New York. Annual reports of the trustees. 18., 1851–2; 19., 1852; 21.–43., 1854–76; 45., 1878; 48., 1879. 8°. *New York*, 1852–80.

FEMALE Christian Home. Annual reports of the managers. 10., 1873; 11., 1874. 8°. *New York*, 1874–5.

FIVE Points House of Industry. Monthly record of the . . . No. 7, i, 1854; No. 12, xviii, 1874–5; No. 8, 9, 12, xxvi, 1882–3; No. 11, 12, xxvii, 1883–4. 8°. *New York*, 1854–84.

——. Annual report of the superintendent for the years 1874–5; 1882–3; 1883–4.
In: Monthly Record for those years.

GOSS (C. C.) Directory of the charities of New York. 12°. [*New York, n. d.*]

GRACE Parish, New York City. Annual report of the various departments of parish work. 6., 1873–4. 12°. *New York*, 1874.

HEBREW Free Burial Society of the City of New York. Annual report of the president. 5., 1874–5. 8°. *New York*, 1875.

HELPING-HAND Association of the City of New York. Annual report of the secretary and treasurer. 9., 1873–4. 8°. *New York*, 1874.

HELPING Hand for Men. Annual report of the superintendent. 1., 1872–3 to 1873–4. 8°. *New York*, 1874.

HOME for Aged and Infirm Hebrews of New York City. History, charter, regulations, by-laws, and list of members. 8°. *New York*, 1873.

——. Annual report of the president, for the year 1873–4. 8°. *New York*, 1874.

HOME for Aged Women of the Church of the Holy Communion. Annual report of the pastor and executive committee, for the year 1873–4. 8°. *New York*, 1874.

HOME for Women. Annual reports. 2., 1870–71; 4.–5., 1872–4. 12°. *New York*, 1871–5.

HOUSE of the Evangelists. Annual report of the board of trustees. 4., 1873. 8°. *New York*, 1874.

HOUSE of the Good Shepherd. Annual report for the year 1872–3. 16°. *New York*, 1874.

LADIES' Benevolent Society of Saint Mark's Church in the Bowerie. Annual reports of the managers. 8., 1868–9; 9., 1869–70; 12., 1872–3; 13., 1873–4. 12°. *New York*, 1869–74.

LADIES' Christian Union of the City of New York. Annual reports of the managers. 15., 1872–3; 16., 1873–4. 8°. *New York*, 1874–5.

LADIES' Home Society of the Baptist Churches, in the City of New York. Annual reports of the managers. 4., 1872–3; 5., 1873–4. 8°. *New York*, 1873–4.

LADIES' Union Relief Association for the Care of Disabled Soldiers and their Families. Annual

New York *City* (*Charities of*).

report of the managers. 8., 1873. 8°. *New York*, 1874.

MIDNIGHT Mission. Annual report of the managers. 7., 1873–4. 16°. *New York*, 1874.

NEW YORK (*City*). Department of Public Charities and Correction. Commissioners of the Almshouse. Report of committee on charity and almshouse in favor of removing the almshouse establishment to Randall's Island and selling the Long Island farms. City doc. No. 4. Board of assistant aldermen. June 29, 1835. 8°. [*New York*, 1835.]

——. Annual reports of the governors of the Almshouse of the City of New York to the secretary of state of the State of New York and the common council of the city of New York. 4., 1852; 5., 1853; 7., 1855; 11., 1859. 8°. *New York*, 1853–60.

NEW YORK (*City*). Department of Public Charities and Correction. Annual reports of the commissioners of public charities and correction to the mayor of New York City. 1., 1860; 4., 1863; 6.–10., 1865–9; 12., 1871. 8°. *New York*, 1861–72.

——. Department of Public Charities and Correction. Bellevue and Charity Hospital. Medical, surgical, and obstetrical statistics, 1870. fol. *New York*, 1871.

——. Department of Public Charities and Correction. Charity Hospital, Blackwell's Island. Annual reports of the chief of staff for the years 1874; 1875. 8°. *New York*, 1875–6.

——. Bellevue Hospital, New York City. Organized January 26, 1872. Address read at the opening meeting of the local visiting committee, with constitution and by-laws. 8°. *New York*, [1872].

——. Metropolitan Board of Health. The vital statistics and sanitary condition of the hospitals and other institutions in which medical care is systematically provided in the metropolitan sanitary district. 8°. *New York*, 1868.
Repr. from: Rep. Reg. Vital Statist. 8°. *New York*, ii.

NEW YORK (*State*). Assembly. An act relative to the maintenance of the inmates of the Protestant Infant Asylum. No. 553. Jan. 23, 1880. Introd. by Mr. Gibbs. fol. [*Albany*, 1880.]

NEW YORK (*State*). S. An act to authorize the corporation "The Sisters of Charity of St. Vincent de Paul" to grant and convey certain lands in the city of New York to the corporation "The St. Vincent's Hospital of the City of New York". No. 221. April 4, 1882. Introd. by Mr. Fitzgerald. fol. [*Albany*, 1882.]

NEW YORK Association for Improving the Condition of the Poor. Annual reports of the board of managers. 19., 1861–2; 22., 1864–5; 26.–27., 1868–9 to 1869–70; 30.–31., 1872–3 to 1873–4; 35.–37., 1877–8 to 1879–80; 40.–41., 1882–3 to 1883–4; 43., 1885–6. 8°. *New York*, 1862–86.

NEW YORK Colored Mission. Report for the year 1871. 8°. *New York*, 1872.

NEW YORK Diet Kitchen. Statement of the managers of the New York Diet Kitchen on the object and benefits of the charity. Nov., 1873. 8°. [*New York*, 1873.]

——. Annual reports of the managers. 1., 1873–4; 2., 1874–5. 8°. *New York*, 1874–5.

NEW YORK Dispensary. Annual reports of the board of trustees. 40.–42., 1829–31; 44., 1833; 47.–48., 1836–7; 50., 1839; 52.–53., 1841–2; 55.–66., 1844–55; 68.–96., 1857–85. 8°. *New York*, 1830–86.

NEW YORK Dorcas Society (Auxiliary to the New York Female Assistance Society). Annual

New York City (*Charities of*).

reports of the board of management, for the years 1872–3; 1873–4.

In : ANNUAL reports of the New York Female Assistance Society for those years.

NEW YORK Female Assistance Society for the Relief and Religious Instruction of the Sick Poor. Annual reports of the managers. 60., 1872–3; 61., 1873–4. 8°. *New York*, 1873–4.

NEW YORK Free Dispensary for Sick Children. Annual reports of the executive committee. 1.– 12.. 1871–2 to 1883. 8°. *New York*, 1872–84.

NEW YORK House and School of Industry. Annual report of the board of managers. 24., 1874. 8°. *New York*, 1875.

NEW YORK Ladies' Home Missionary Society of the Methodist Episcopal Church. Annual reports of the managers. 29., 1872–3; 30., 1873–4. 8°. *New York*, 1873–4.

————. Annual reports of its labors at the "Five Points", Old Brewery. 23., 1872–3; 24., 1873–4.

In : ANNUAL reports of the society for those years.

NEW YORK Protestant Episcopal City Mission Society. The gradual growth of charities. 16°. *New York*, 1873.

————. Annual reports of the executive committee. 23., 1872–3; 24., 1873–4. 8°. *New York*, 1873–4.

NEW YORK Society for the Relief of the Ruptured and Crippled. Annual reports of the board of managers and surgeon-in-chief. 1.–24., 1863–4 to 1886–7. 8°. *New York*, 1864–87.

————. The origin, progress, and present position. 8°. *New York*, 1872.

NORTHEASTERN Dispensary in the City of New York. Annual reports of the board of managers. 6., 1867; 15., 1876. 8°. *New York*, 1868–77.

NORTHERN Dispensary in the City of New York. Annual reports. 3., 1829–30; 9., 1835–6; 14.–17., 1840–41 to 1843–4; 19., 1845–6; 21., 1847–8; 23.–35., 1849–50 to 1861; 40., 1866. 8°. *New York*, 1830–67.

NORTHWESTERN Dispensary. Annual reports. 1.–5., 1852–3 to 1856–7; 10., 1862; 12., 1864; 16., 1868; 18.–22., 1870–74. 8°. *New York*, 1853–75.

OLIVET Helping Hand. Annual report of the managers. 5., 1873–4. 8°. *New York*, 1874.

PRESBYTERIAN Home for Aged Women. Annual report of the managers. 7., 1872–3. . 8°. *New York*, 1873.

————. Act of incorporation, constitution and by-laws.

In : SEVENTH annual report.

PRISON Association of New York. Annual report of the executive committee. 23., 1867. 8°. *Albany*, 1868.

PROTESTANT Episcopal Church in the State of New York. Annual report of the board of trustees and officers of the Shepherd's Fold of the . . . 40., 1872–3. 8°. *New York*, 1873.

SAINT LUKE's Home for Indigent Christian Females. Annual report of the board of managers. 23., 1873–4. 8°. *New York*, 1874.

SAINT LUKE's Methodist Episcopal Church. Annual report of the board of managers of the home mission of . . . 3., 1872–3. 8°. *New York*, 1873.

SAMARITAN Home for the Aged. Annual reports of the board of managers. 1.–3., 1867–9; 5.–6., 1871–2. 8°. *New York*, 1868–73.

SEAMEN's Retreat Hospital. An act in relation to the moneys levied by law on masters, mates, mariners, and seamen arriving at the city and port of New York, providing for sick and disabled seamen, passed April 7, 1854. Also, the by-laws of the board of trustees of the . . . 8°. *New York*, 1854.

New York City (*Charities of*).

————. Annual reports of the physician-in-chief and auditing committee. 1.–23., 1854–76. 8°. *New York*, 1855–77.

SOCIETY for the Employment and Relief of Poor Women. Annual reports of the managers. 29., 1872–3; 30., 1873–4. 12°. *New York*, 1873–4.

————. Constitution of the . . .

In : TWENTY-NINTH annual report, 1872–3.

SOCIETY for the Reformation of Juvenile Delinquents. Annual reports of the managers. 45., 1869; 49., 1873; 50., 1874. 8°. *New York*, 1870–75.

SOCIETY for the Relief of the Destitute Blind of the City of New York and its Vicinity. Annual report. 4., 1871–2. 12°. *New York*, 1872.

SOCIETY for the Relief of Half-Orphans and Destitute Children. Charter and by-laws of the . . . 12°. *New York*, 1869.

————. Annual reports of the managers. 38., 1873; 39., 1874. 12°. *New York*, 1874–5.

SOCIETY for the Relief of Poor Widows with Small Children. Annual reports of the board of managers. 76., 1872–3; 77., 1873–4. 8°. *New York*, 1873–4.

UNION Home and School for the Education and Maintenance of the Children of our Volunteers. Annual report of the secretary and executive committee. 12., 1873–4. 8°. *New York*, 1874.

WILSON Industrial School and Mission. Annual report of the board of managers. 22., 1874. 8°. *New York*, 1875.

WOMEN's Aid Society and Home for Training Young Girls. Annual report of the managers. 7., 1873. 8°. *New York*, 1874.

WOMEN's Educational and Industrial Society. Annual report of the committee of management of the free training schools of the . . . 1., 1873–4. 8°. *New York*, 1874.

WOMEN's Prison Association of New York, and the Isaac T. Hopper Home. Annual report. 29., 1873. 8°. *New York*, 1874.

WORKING-WOMEN's Protective Union. The work done and doing by the . . . 8°. *New York*, 1873.

YOUNG Ladies' Christian Association of the City of New York. Annual reports of the officers. 3., 1873; 4., 1874. 8°. *New York*, 1874–5.

YOUNG Men's Christian Association of the City of New York. Annual reports of the board of directors. 22., 1874; 24., 1876. 8°. *New York*, 1875–7.

Graves (J. J.) & **Ogden** (B.) Report of diseases treated at the New York City Dispensary, 1826–8. N. York M. & Phys. J., 1826, v, 87; 320; 449; 589: 1827, vi, 394: 1828, vii, 241. — **King** (H.) Notes of a visit to the medical institutions of New York. Dublin Q. J. M. Sc., 1864, xxxviii, 288–334. — **Out-patient** (The) department of the New York Hospital and the abuse of medical charity. Med. Rec., N. Y., 1878, xiii, 250–252.

New York City (*Quarantine Establishment of*).

NEW YORK (*Port*). Annual reports of the health officer of the port of New York to the commissioners of quarantine, for years 1864–73; 1886. 8°. *Albany*, 1865–87.

NEW YORK (*State*). Health laws of New York. 8°. *New York*, 1805.

————. S. An act for the preservation of the public health. [Establishing quarantine against the introduction of cholera.] No. 114. June 22, 1832. Brought in by Mr. Allen. fol. [*Albany*, 1832.]

————. An act to amend title second, chapter fourteen, part first, of the revised statutes, relating to the quarantine regulations of the port of New York. Passed May 2, 1836. 8°. [*Albany*, 1836.]

New York City (*Quarantine Establishment of*).

——. The same. [With an extract from act of Congress, Feb. 25, 1799, and the agreement between New York and New Jersey, in 1833.] 8°. [*Albany*, 1836.]

——. Chapter xiv of the revised statutes of the public health, relating to the port, harbour, and State of New York. Published by order of the board of health of the city of New York. 8°. *New York*, 1836.

——. The same. 8°. [*New York*, 1838.]

——. Laws relating to the public health; the quarantine, duties of pilots, etc., for the port, harbor, and State of New York, embraced in the revised statutes, and in act of the legislature of the State of New York, passed May 13, 1846. Published by order of the health commissioners. 8°. *New York*, 1846.

——. Assembly. Report of the legislative committee of 1848, on the removal of quarantine. 8°. [*Albany*, 1848.]

——. Assembly. Communication from the committee appointed by the house assembly. Being the report of the select committee appointed April 11, 1848, to examine and report as to whether the quarantine establishment, in the county of Richmond, should be removed from its present location, and as to what locality said establishment should be removed. No. 60. Jan. 30, 1849. 8°. [*Albany*, 1849?]

——. S. Report of the majority of the committee on grievances, on petitions relative to the quarantine establishment, and to the bill from the assembly on that subject. No. 51. March 1, 1849. 8°. [*Albany*, 1849.]

——. S. Report of select committee relative to condition of wharves and buildings at quarantine. No. 100. April 8, 1856. 8°. [*Albany*, 1856.]

——. Report of the commissioners for the removal of the quarantine station of the State of New York. Transmitted to the legislature Feb. 12, 1858. 8°. *Albany*, 1858.

——. Report of the commissioners relative to removal of the quarantine station. Transmitted to the assembly March 10, 1858. 8°. *Albany*, 1858.

——. Laws relative to quarantine and to the public health of the city of New York. (Part 1, chapter xiv, of the revised statutes, as amended and modified by the subsequent acts of the legislature.) 16°. *New York*, 1858.

——. Laws relative to quarantine in the port of New York. Compiled under the direction of the commissioners of quarantine. 16°. *New York*, 1867.

——. Assembly. Report of the committee on public health relative to the public duties of the health officer of the port of New York. No. 106. March 18, 1868. 8°. [*Albany*, 1868.]

——. Assembly. Report of the board of commissioners charged with the construction of the quarantine hospital and boarding station on West Bank. No. 18. Jan. 14, 1869. 8°. [*Albany*, 1869.]

——. Laws relating to quarantine in the port of New York. Compiled under the direction of the commissioner of quarantine. 18°. *New York*, 1870.

——. Report of the commissioners of quarantine in response to alleged abuses, and the answer of the health officer thereto to the governor of the State, Dec. 11, 1871. 8°. [*Albany*, 1872.]

——. Assembly. An act in relation to quarantine in the port of New York. No. 858. Feb.

New York City (*Quarantine Establishment of*).

2, 1872. Introd. by Mr. Hawkins. fol. [*Albany*, 1872.]

——. Assembly. Report of commissioners to construct quarantine buildings under chapter 751, laws of 1866. No. 46. Feb. 7, 1872. 8°. [*Albany*, 1872.]

——. Assembly. Reply of the quarantine commissioners, in obedience to a resolution of the assembly, relative to the expenditure of money appropriated to said commissioners by chapter 715 of the laws of 1871. No. 56. Feb. 14, 1872. 8°. [*Albany*, 1872.]

——. Assembly. Report and testimony of the assembly committee on commerce and navigation, in relation to the quarantine abuses at the port of New York. No. 131. May 2, 1872. 8°. [*Albany*, 1872.]

——. S. An act establishing a quarantine and defining the qualifications, duties, and powers of the health officer for the harbor and port of New York. No. 162. Jan. 22, 1873. Introd. by Mr. Brooks. fol. [*Albany*, 1873.]

——. S. [Evidence taken by the finance committee of the senate on the management of quarantine in the port of New York.] 8°. [*Albany*, 1873.]

Cutting.

——. S. Preamble and resolutions relative to the office of the commissioner of quarantine, and the expenditure of moneys appropriated for quarantine purposes in the port of New York during the past three years. No. 45. Feb. 21, 1873. 8°. [*Albany*, 1873.]

——. S. Report of the finance committee, to whom was referred the resolution of the senate calling on the commissioners of quarantine to transmit an account of all moneys expended, work performed, and materials furnished, since the date of their organization, and for what purposes it was expended. No. 104. May 29, 1873. 8°. [*Albany*, 1873.]

——. Senate. Testimony [taken by the finance committee of the senate on the management of quarantine in the port of New York. No. 82.] 8°. [*Albany*, 1873?]

——. Assembly. Report of the committee of investigation into the affairs of the commissioners of emigration and quarantine. No. 33. Jan. 28, 1876. 8°. [*Albany*, 1876.]

——. Assembly. Report of the minority of the committee of investigation into the affairs of the commissioners of emigration and quarantine. No. 34. Jan. 28, 1876. 8°. [*Albany*, 1876.]

——. Assembly. Communication from the health officer, quarantine, in reply to a resolution of the assembly in relation to the steam tug Gov. Fenton. No. 76. March 10, 1876. 8°. [*Albany*, 1876.]

——. Assembly. Communication from the New York quarantine commissioners, in answer to a resolution of the house, relative to the steamer Nelson K. Hopkins. No. 80. March 14, 1876. 8°. [*Albany*, 1876.]

——. Assembly. An act in relation to the health officer for the port of New York. No. 392. March 5, 1880. Introd. by Mr. Varnum. fol. [*Albany*, 1880.]

——. Assembly. An act amending an act entitled "An act establishing a quarantine and defining the qualifications, duties and powers of the health officer for the harbor and port of New York", passed April 29, 1863. No. 378. March 29, 1882. Introd. by Mr. Brooks. fol. [*Albany*, 1882.]

——. Assembly. An act to amend sections 54 and 55 of chapter 358 of the laws of 1863, en-

New York City (*Quarantine Establishment of*).

titled "An act establishing and defining the qualifications, duties and powers of the health officer for the harbor and port of New York". No. 652. April 21, 1882. Introd. by Mr. Brooks. fol. [*Albany*, 1882.]

——. Chap. 77. An act to amend section 53 of chap. 358 of the laws of 1863: "An act establishing a quarantine and defining the qualifications, duties and powers of the health officer for the harbor and port of New York". Approved March 22, 1888. Galley sheet. [*Albany*, 1888.]

NEW YORK (*State*). *Commissioners of Quarantine*. Port of New York, quarantine ground, Staten Island. Rules to be observed on board of all vessels detained at quarantine. fol. [*New York*, 1856.]

——. Annual reports of the commissioners of quarantine, to which are annexed the annual reports of the health officer of the port of New York to the legislature, for the years 1864–76. 8°. *Albany*, 1865–77.

SUPREME (In) Court. The People *vs.* Peter W. Roff. Opinion of Judge Birdseye relative to the powers and duties of the health officer of the port of New York. 8°. *New York*, 1856.

Smith (W. M.) Maritime sanitation at the port of New York. Rep. State Bd. Health N. Y. 1884, Albany, 1885, v, 435-483.

New York City (*Vital statistics of*).

NEW YORK (*City*). Annual reports of deaths in the city and county of New York for the years 1819, 1823, and 1831. 8°. *New York*, 1820–32.

NEW YORK (*City*). City Inspector. Annual reports of the number of deaths and interments in the city of New York for the years 1818–27; 1829; 1831; 1833-5; 1837–44; 1847–65. 8°. *New York*, 1819–66.

——. Table of the semi-centennial mortality of the city of New York, compiled from the records of the city inspector's department, comprising the full period from January 1, 1804, to Dec. 31, 1853, inclusive. By T. K. Downing. broadside fol. *New York*, 1854.

NEW YORK (*City*). *Health Department. Bureau of Vital Statistics*. Annual reports, 1870–80. 8°. [*New York*, 1871–81.]

1870-75 *in :* Rep. Bd. of Health for those years.

——. Reported mortality, together with the actual mortality. (Weekly.) July 23, 1870, to July 24, 1886. fol. [*New York*, 1870–86.]

——. A table showing for each week since 1866 the total weekly mortality, the mortality from diarrhœal diseases of children under five years of age, and of persons more than five years of age; the greatest range of temperature, and the mean range of temperature and of humidity in each week. March, 1876. broadside fol. [*New York*, 1876.]

——. Abstract of census of the city of New York in 1875, by wards, ages, sexes, nativity, etc. Compiled for report of bureau of vital statistics, under the direction of Dr. E. Harris. Revised by superintendent of State census. broadside fol. [*New York*, 1876.]

——. Summary of births, marriages, stillbirths, and deaths in New York City, during the years 1876; 1877; 1879; 1880; 1883. fol. [*New York*, 1877–84.]

——. Reported mortality, together with the actual mortality. [Quarterly.] 1.-4. qr., 1877. fol. [*New York*, 1877-8.]

——. Reported mortality, together with the actual mortality, for the years 1877–83. fol. *New York*, 1878–84.

New York City (*Vital statistics of*).

——. Epitome of the births, marriages, still-births, and deaths in New York City, during the years 1878–80. By J. T. Nagle. 4°. [*New York*, 1879–82.]

Rep. for 1878 *also in :* Hosp. Gaz., N. Y., 1879, vi, 650-655.

NEW YORK (*City*). Metropolitan Board of Health. The vital statistics and sanitary condition of the hospitals and other institutions in which medical care is systematically provided, in the metropolitan sanitary district. 8°. *New York*, 1868.

Repr. from : Rep. Reg. Vital Statist. 8°. *New York*, ii.

Buck (A. H.) An inquiry into the cause of one thousand deaths, being the mortality experience of a life insurance company in the city of New York. Med. Rec., N. Y., 1874, ix, 49-54. — **Cuming** (G.) Annual report of deaths in the city and county of New York for the years 1816–26. Eclect. Repert., Phila., 1817, vii, 274 : 1818, viii, 265 : 1819, ix, 287 : 1820, x, 280 : 1821, xi, 135. *Continued in :* Phila. J. M. & Phys. Sc., 1822, iv, 433 : 1823, vi, 198 : 1824, viii, 239 : 1825, n s., i, 415 : 1826, n. s., iii, 417 : 1827, n. s., v, 190.— **Dunnell** (H. G.) Annual report of the interments in the city and county of New York, showing their age, sex, colour, and places of nativity, for the year 1837 ; also a table of deaths, and the different diseases, since the year 1804. Am. J. M. Sc., Phila., 1838, xxii, 237-251. ——. Annual report of interments in the city and county of New York for 1838. N. York J. M. & S., 1839, i, 227-236.— **Lee** (C. A.) Medical statistics, comprising a series of calculations and tables, showing the mortality in New York, and its immediate causes, during a period of sixteen years. Am. J. M. Sc., Phila., 1836, xix, 25-52.—**Mitchell** (S. L.) Summary view of the modes by which human life terminates in the city of New York ; digested from the bills of mortality, kept by order of the common council, for the years 1804–8. Med. Reposit., N. Y., 1807-8, 2. hexade, v, 32 : 1809-10, 3. hexade, 335. — **Peters** (J. C.) Prevailing diseases and epidemics of the first quarter of the year 1879. Med. Rec., N. Y., 1879, xv, 488-490. — **Pintard** (J.) Bill of mortality for New York, 1801 - 2. Med. Reposit., N. Y., 1803, vi, 443-446.—**Ramsay** (C.) Statistics of some of the diseases of New York and London. Tr. M. Soc. N. Y., Albany, 1863, 324-330. ——. Mortality of the city of New York. *Ibid.*, 1864, 287-314. ——. On the mortality of the city of New York. Tr. Am. M. Ass., Phila., 1864, xv, 233-250. ——. A table of still-born in each year, and deaths of infants in the city of New York, from one day to one year of age, from 1854 to 1866. Buffalo M. & S. J., 1865-6, v, 475. — **Russel** (C. R.) [Mortality and diseases of New York, 1871-3.] Med. Rec., N. Y., 1872, vii, 33 ; 90 ; 232 ; 332 ; 448 : 1873, viii, 185. — **Sterb-lichkeits - Verhältnisse** der Stadt New-York in den Jahren 1866 bis 1877. Nach Mittheilungen des Gesundheitsamtes zu New - York. Veröffentl. d. k. deutsch. Gsndhtsamtes, Berl., 1878, ii, Beilage zu No. 20.

New York City (*Water-supply of*).

DISBROW (L.) Practice versus Theory. [On the New York water supply.] 18°. [*New York*, 1831.]

—— & SULLIVAN (J. L.) Advertisement of a proposition for ward companies, to supply the city of New York with rock water. 8°. *New York*, 1832.

HAIGHT (N.) A practical treatise on the water delivered by the Manhattan Company, with practical observations on waters surrounding the city of New York. 8°. *New York*, 1825.

HALE (M.) Spring water versus river water for supplying the city of New York. Containing a compendious examination of the internal supplies; the method and actual expense of obtaining them ; also an examination of the water commissioners' report of Nov., 1833, refuting many of the objections therein contained, and exhibiting errors in their estimate of expense for procuring water on the island, of more than $2,000,000. 8°. [*New York*, 1835.]

JERVIS (J. B.) Description of the Croton Aqueduct. 8°. *New York*, 1842.

LETTERS concerning the general health ; with notes and considerable additions to the numbers as they lately appeared in the New York Gazette. By a householder. 8°. *New York*, 1805.

New York *City* (*Water-supply of*).

NEW YORK (*City*). [Communication from the mayor of the city of New York to the common council, relative to matters of public health.] Common council. Nov. 25, 1822. 8°. [*New York*, 1822.]

———. Report of the special committee to whom was referred the resolutions of Alderman Stevens, relating to the supply of water by the Manhattan Company. Common council. May 31, 1830. 8°. [*New York*, 1830.]

———. Communication from Judge Wright upon the subject of supplying the city with water. Common council. Sept. 6, 1830. 8°. [*New York*, 1830.]

———. Communication from the committee of the Lyceum of Natural History of the city of New York, in answer to an inquiry from Mr. Townsend on the source, quality, and purity of the water of this island. Common council. Feb. 28, 1831. 8°. [*New York*, 1831.]

———. Annual messages of his honor the mayor, Isaac L. Varian. 1838-9; 1839-40. 8°. *New York*, 1839-40.

———. Report of the commissioners appointed to investigate the condition of the Manhattan Company, together with minutes of their proceedings, and various statements relative thereto. March 14, 1840. 8°. *New York*, 1840.

NEW YORK (*City*). *Commissioners of Water Supply and Croton Aqueduct.* Report relative to introducing into the city of New York a supply of pure and wholesome water, accompanied by a law asking power to raise money by loan to execute said work. Board of aldermen. Dec. 28, 1831. 8°. [*New York*, 1831.]

———. Report to the joint committees on fire and water, by Col. De Witt Clinton, on the best sources and means of transportation of an inexhaustible supply of pure and wholesome water for the city of New York. Board of aldermen. No. 61. Nov. 10, 1832. 8°. [*New York*, 1832.]

———. Report of the commissioners under an act of the legislature of this State, passed Feb. 26, 1833, relative to supplying the city of New York with pure and wholesome water [including the engineer's report, D. B. Douglass, and Mr. Chilton's report]. Board of aldermen. No. 36. Nov. 12, 1833. 8°. *New York*, 1833.

———. [Communication from the water commissioners to the common council, relating to their duties and powers under the act of 2d of May, 1834.] Board of aldermen. Doc. No. 1. May 19, 1834. 8°. [*New York*, 1834.]

———. Report of the commissioners under an act of the legislature of this State, passed May 2, 1834, relative to supplying the city of New York with pure and wholesome water. 8°. *New York*, 1835.

———. Communication from Stephen Allen, esq., chairman, in behalf of the water commissioners, praying that the common council will apply to the legislature for a law authorizing the appointment of commissioners, with power to alter the line of any highway or turnpike in danger of injury from the Croton River Water Works. Board of aldermen. Doc. No. 48. Nov. 23, 1835. 8°. [*Washington*, 1835.]

———. Communication from the mayor, enclosing a communication from Stephen Allen, esq., chairman of the water commissioners, and from D. B. Douglass, esq., chief engineer N. Y. aqueduct, in relation to the practicability and probable expense of forcing, by steam engines, a sufficient quantity of water from the North or East River to a reservoir to be erected on Murray Hill, in aid of the present means for extin-

New York *City* (*Water-supply of*).

guishing fires. Board of aldermen. Doc. No. 89. Feb. 15, 1836. 8°. [*New York*, 1836.]

———. [Report from the water commissioners to the common council, on the situation and progress of their work from the date of their appointment to that of the report.] Board of aldermen. Doc. No. 12. Aug. 1, 1836. 8°. [*New York*, 1836.]

———. Report of the committee on laws, etc., on the communication and draft of a law from the water commissioners, with amendments. Board of aldermen. Doc. No. 83. Dec. 19, 1836. 8°. [*New York*, 1836.]

———. Communication from the water commissioners, setting forth the progress of the works for supplying the city with pure and wholesome water. Board of assistant aldermen. Doc. No. 24. Jan. 9, 1837. 8°. [*New York*, 1837.]

———. Report of the select committee to whom was referred so much of the message of his honor the mayor as relates to furnishing a supply of water for the extinguishing of fires and laying additional pipes. Board of aldermen. Doc. 103. Feb. 27, 1837. 8°. [*New York*, 1837.]

———. Semi-annual reports of the water-commissioners for the city of New York. 4.-9., Jan., 1837, to Dec., 1839; 11.-14., July, 1840, to June, 1842. 8°. [*New York*, 1837-42.]

———. Report of the finance committee, to whom was referred so much of the report of the water commissioners as relates to providing funds for completing the Croton Water Works. Board of aldermen. Doc. No. 67. Feb. 26, 1838. 8°. [*New York*, 1838.]

———. Report of the committee on roads and canals, to whom was referred so much of the report of the water-commissioners as relates to the construction of the aqueduct across the Harlaem River. Board of aldermen. Doc. No. 88. April 23, 1838. 8°. [*New York*, 1838.]

———. Communication from the water commissioners, relative to the Croton Aqueduct. Board of aldermen. Doc. No. 2. May 14, 1838. 8°. [*New York*, 1838.]

———. An ordinance to organize the Croton Aqueduct department. Common council. 8°. [*New York*, 1840.]

———. Report of the fire and water committee, on a communication from a committee of citizens relative to a paid fire department. Board of aldermen. Doc. No. 56. March 2, 1840. 8°. [*New York*, 1840.]

———. Communication of the water-commissioners in relation to laying down the distributing water pipes. Board of aldermen. Doc. No. 72. May 4, 1840. 8°. *New York*, 1840.

———. Communications of the comptroller, of the water commissioners, and the Croton Aqueduct committee, etc., on the subject of the ordinance to amend the ordinance to instruct the water commissioners. Board of aldermen. Doc. No. 70. Oct. 12, 1840. 8°. *New York*, 1840.

———. Report of the majority of the special committee on the subject of the ordinance creating the aqueduct department, etc., and to amend the ordinance to instruct the water commissioners. Board of aldermen. No. 31. Dec. 14, 1840. 8°. [*New York*, 1840.]

———. Report of minority of the special committee on the subject of the ordinance to create the aqueduct department, etc., and to amend the ordinance to instruct the water commissioners. Board of aldermen. No. 32. Dec. 14, 1840. 8°. [*New York*, 1840.]

New York *City* (*Water-supply of*).

——. Report of the committee on the Croton Aqueduct on the proposition of John M. Bradhurst for remuneration for injuries done his property in the opening of Tenth avenue. Board of assistant aldermen. No. 33. Dec. 21, 1840. 8°. [*New York*, 1840.]

——. Report of the special committee to whom was referred the communication from the water commissioners a report of the Croton Aqueduct committee, and an opinion of the counsel in relation to the powers and duties of the water commissioners, together with accompanying documents. Board of aldermen. No. 32. Dec. 22, 1840. 8°. [*New York*, 1840.]

——. A statement of the receipts and expenditures on account of the Croton Aqueduct, and of the amount of water-loan stock authorized by the legislature of the State of New York, with the amount of such stock issued by the common council of the city of New York to April 20, 1841. 8°. [*New York*, 1841.]

——. Quarterly reports of the Croton Aqueduct department, in compliance with an ordinance to provide for the accountability of the executive committees of the common council. 1., 3., and 4., qrs. of 1841. 8°. [*New York*, 1841.]

——. Acts of the legislature of the State, and ordinances and resolutions of the common council of the city of New York, in relation to the subject of the introduction of water into the city of New York from 1833 to June, 1842. 8°. [*New York*], 1842.

——. Communication from the comptroller relative to the establishment of a water department, with a programme of a law for the same. Board of aldermen. No. 80. April 18, 1842. 8°. [*New York*, 1842.]

——. Report on the general state of the work on the Croton Aqueduct to the water-commissioners. Doc. No. 9. July 12, 1842. 8°. [*New York*, 1842.]

——. Report of the special committee on the memorial of Messrs. Tatham & Bros., relative to composition and other conduit pipes. Board of aldermen. Doc. No. 37. Oct. 10, 1842. 8°. [*New York*, 1842.]

——. Report of the Croton Aqueduct board, in relation to the ways and means of paying the Croton water debt. Board of aldermen. No. 58. Dec. 27, 1842. 8°. [*New York*, 1842.]

——. A memoir of the construction, cost, and capacity of the Croton Aqueduct, compiled from official documents; together with an account of the civic celebration of the fourteenth October, 1842, on occasion of the completion of the great work, preceded by a preliminary essay on ancient and modern aqueducts. By C. King. 4°. *New York*, 1843.

——. An ordinance establishing a scale of water rents for the Croton Aqueduct department. 8°. [*New York*, 1851.]

——. Profile of lower part of Croton Aqueduct. Ground plan of the lower part of Croton Aqueduct. 1 plan. [*New York, n. d.*]

NEW YORK (*State*). Act of incorporation of the Manhattan Company. Passed April 2, 1799. 12°. *New York*, 1830.

——. Annual reports of the superintendent of the Onondaga Salt Springs to the legislature of the State of New York for the years 1867-9. 8°. [*Albany*, 1868-70.]

NEW YORK (*State*). *Commissioners of Fisheries.* Annual report. 8., 1875. 8°. *Albany*, 1876.

NEW YORK (*State*). *Commissioners of State Parks.* Annual report. 1., 1872. 8°. [*Albany*, 1873.]

New York *City* (*Water-supply of*).

NEW YORK Water Works Company. Report to the directors of the . . . by their engineer. 8°. [*New York*, 1826.]

STATE of New York. In the court for the trial of impeachments and the correction of error. Between the mayor, aldermen, and commonalty of the city of New York, plaintiffs in error, and Herman Le Roy and others, defendants in error. Case. [Application in original case to set aside assessment on sewer.] 8°. *New York*, 1823.

SULLIVAN (J. L.) A description of a submarine aqueduct to supply New York with water from New Jersey, connected with a commercial canal and railway for the direct western trade of the city. 8°. *New York*, 1830.

——. An address to the mayor, the aldermen, and inhabitants of New York, supplemental to Col. Clinton's report on water, demonstrating from the facts ascertained by the surveys, as well as others, the advantages of a rock-water company with banking privileges appropriating the surplus to public baths and cleansing streets, also a proposition to the Manhattan Company to fill their aqueduct with rock-water. 8°. *New York*, 1833.

TOWER (F. B.) Illustrations of the Croton Aqueduct. fol. *New York & London*, 1843.

UNION League Club. Committee of political reform, April 9, 1883. Water question [of New York City. Report and resolutions, unanimously adopted by the committee.] 8°. [*New York*, 1883.]

WATER (The) supply of New York. Suggestions for a permanent and economical settlement of the question. The Hudson River as an available, unlimited, and unfailing source. Plan for the relief of the city before another season. 8°. *New York*, 1876.

Chandler (C. F.) & **Lewis** (W. B.) Reports on the quality of the water-supply [of New York and Brooklyn]. Rep. Metrop. Bd. Health 1869, N. Y., 1870, iv, 415-425, 1 pl. *Also*, Reprint.—**Croton** supply and waste. [Edit.] San. Engin., N. Y., 1881-2, v, 177.—**Croton** water of New York. [Edit.] Science, N. Y., 1882, iii, 31-36.—**Cutter** (E.) Suspicious organisms in Croton-water. Med. Rec., N. Y., 1882, xxi, 365-368.—**Eastman** (H. G.) The water supply of New York. Suggestions for a permanent and economical settlement of the question. Sanitarian, N. Y., 1877, v, 51-64, 1 pl.—**Harris** (E.) Sanitary qualities of the water supply [of New York and Brooklyn], with chemical analyses, by C. F. Chandler. Rep. Metrop. Bd. Health 1867, N. Y., 1868, ii, 385-406. *Also*, Reprint.—**New** (The) Croton aqueduct. San. Engin., N. Y., 1885, xii, 491: 1885-6, xiii, 297: 344; 368: 1886, xiv, 57: 273; 566: 1886-7, xv, 234; 287: 1887, xvi, 39; 291.—**New York's** water supply. [Edit.] *Ibid.*, 1882-3, vii, 169; 193: 218; 241; 265; 290; 314; 338; 362; 386; 410.—**Peters** (J. C.) The New York water supply; present and prospective. Sanitarian, N. Y., 1886, xvi, 289-321.—**State** Board of Health, N. Y. Communication from . . . relative to the condition of the new aqueduct, New York. Rep. State Bd. Health N. Y. 1886, Albany, 1887, vii, 91-133.—**Water-supply** (The) of New York City. San. Engin., N. Y., 1884-5, xi, 348; 457; 518: 1885, xii, 29.

New York (*Port*). Annual reports of the health officer of the port of New York, to the commissioners of quarantine, for the years 1864-73; 1886. 8°. *Albany*, 1865-87.

1864-73, *in :* Rep. commissioners of quarantine for the same years. 1886, *repr. from :* Rep. commissioners of quarantine (1886), Albany, 1887.

——. Port of New York. Rules and regulations to be observed by masters of vessels under quarantine. May 15, 1870. 1 sheet. fol. [*New York*, 1870.]

——. The same. June 1, 1871. 1 sheet. fol. [*New York*, 1871.]

——. The same. June 1, 1872. 1 sheet. fol. [*New York*, 1872.]

——. The same. June 1, 1874. 3 pp. 12°. [*New York*, 1874.]

New York (*Port*)—continued.

——. Regulations for the discharge of cargo from vessels under quarantine in the port of New York. Established June, 1875. 7 pp. 16°. [*New York*, 1875.]

——. Communication from the health officer, quarantine, in reply to a resolution of the assembly in relation to the steam tug Gov. Fenton. No. 76. In assembly, March 10, 1876. 1 sheet. 8°. [*Albany*, 1876.]

——. [Blank forms used by] health officer's department, quarantine, S. I. v. s. [*New York*, 185– to 187–.]

Affidavit of captain and surgeon, that the ports from which they sailed were free from malignant, contagious, or infectious diseases. In English, French, German, Italian, and Spanish.

Bill of expense for fumigating vessel after discharge of cargo.

Directions for pilots in regard to leaving vessels. Form No. 194 and 195.

License to carry on the business of . . . under quarantine.

Notice, to general agent, Castle Garden, of passengers sent to —— Island.

Permit, to superintendent of hospital, to admit passengers for treatment.

——. Disinfection of rags. Communication of the health officer of the port of New York to the New York City board of health, in relation to the regulation requiring the disinfection of foreign rags. 21 pp. 8°. *New York, M. B. Brown*, 1885.

——. Summary from the health officer's report to the Chamber of Commerce on the importance of disinfecting rags. 2 l. 4°. [*Albany*, 1886.]

——. *See, also :*

CHAMBER of Commerce. Report of select committee on quarantine, adopted July 7, 1859. 8°. *New York*, 1859.

For subject-titles relating to foregoing, see: **New York** *City* (*Quarantine Establishment of*).

New York (*State*). S. Report from the committee to whom was referred the bill entitled "An act to incorporate the trustees of the medical institution of the State of New York". Reported by Mr. Cochran, April 10, 1815. 2 pp. fol. [*Albany*, 1815.]

——. Report of the commissioners, directed by the act of 17th April, 1826, to visit the State prison at Auburn. Made to the senate Jan. 13, 1827. 88 pp. 8°. *Albany, Croswell & Van Benthuysen*, 1827. [P., v. 602.]

——. Assembly. Report of the committee on medical subjects, on the petition of sundry practitioners of medicine in the city and county of New York. March 2, 1830. 12 pp. 8°. [*New York*, 1830.]

——. Act of incorporation of the Manhattan Company. Passed April 2, 1799. 12 pp. 12°. *New York, Grattan*, 1830.

——. Assembly. Report of the committee on medical societies and colleges. [Reported by Mr. Milledoler, in favor of repealing the present law regulating the practice of medicine.] No. 171. Feb. 28, 1832. 10 pp. 8°. [*Albany*, 1832.] [P., v. 422.]

——. Assembly. Report of Mr. Winfield, from the committee on medical societies and colleges. [Reply to the majority report made by Mr. Milledoler, Feb. 28, 1832.] March 28, 1832. No. 251. 66 pp. 8°. [*Albany*, 1832.] [P., v. 422.]

——. Assembly. Report of the committee on medical subjects, on so much of the governor's message as relates to the Asiatic cholera. June 22, 1832. 3 pp. 8°. [*Albany*, 1832.]

——. S. An act for the preservation of the public health. [Establishing quarantine against the introduction of cholera.] June 22, 1832. No. cxiv. 3 pp. fol. [*Albany*, 1832.]

New York (*State*)—continued.

——. Assembly. Report of the select committee, on so much of the governor's message as relates to the insane poor. Jan. 31, 1835. 26 pp. 8°. [*Albany*, 1835.]

——. Assembly. Reports of the majority and minority of the select committee, on several petitions relative to the repeal of the law restraining botanic practice. Feb. 16, 1835. 27 pp. 8°. [*Albany*, 1835.] [P., v. 422.]

——. An act to amend title second, chapter fourteen, part first, of the revised statutes, relating to the quarantine regulations of the port of New York. Passed May 2, 1836. 1 sheet. 8°. [*Albany*, 1836.]

Bound with: Chapter xiv of the revised statutes. 8°. *New York*, 1836.

——. The same. [With an extract from act of Congress, Feb. 25, 1799, and the agreement between New York and New Jersey, in 1833.] 2 pp. 8°. [*Albany*, 1836.]

Bound with: Chapter xiv of the revised statutes. 8°. [*New York*, 1838?]

——. Chapter xiv of the revised statutes of the public health, relating to the port, harbour, and State of New York. (Published by order of the board of health of the city of New York.) 48 pp. 8°. *New York, P. Scott & Co.*, 1836.

——. Chapter xiv [of the revised statutes] of the public health [relating to the port, harbor, and State of New York. Published by order of the board of health of the city of New York]. 61 pp. 8°. [*New York*, 1838?]

——. S. Report of the governor's message in relation to the State Lunatic Asylum. No. 39. Feb. 16, 1839. Rep. by Mr. Paige. 5 pp. 8°. [*Albany*, 1839.]

——. Assembly. Communication from the comptroller, transmitting sundry reports relating to the investigation of the Seamens' Fund and Retreat, Marine Hospital, etc. Feb. 13, 1840. No. 214. 94 pp. 8°. [*Albany*, 1840.]

——. Assembly. Report of the committee on charitable and religious societies, on the petition of the governors of the State Hospital of the city of New York, for aid from the State. March 3, 1840. No. 223. 16 pp. 8°. [*Albany*, 1840.]

——. Assembly. Report of the standing committee on medical societies and colleges, relative to the restrictions on unlicensed practitioners. May 9, 1840 11 pp. 8°. [*Albany*, 1840.]

——. Assembly. Report of the minority of the select committee, to which was referred numerous petitions asking a change of the law towards Thomsonian physicians. No. 354. May 12, 1840. 23 pp. 8°. [*Albany*, 1840.]

——. Assembly. Report of the select committee on petitions of numerous citizens of the State, praying for the passage of a law authorizing Thomsonian physicians to collect pay for services. No. 94. Jan. 30, 1841. 7 pp. 8°. [*Albany*, 1841.]

——. Assembly. Report of the select committee, on so much of the governor's message as relates to the Lunatic Asylum. April 22, 1841. 1 l. 8°. [*Albany*, 1841.]

——. Assembly. Report of the committee on medical societies and colleges, on the memorial of the New York Eye Infirmary, praying for aid. March 7, 1842. 3 pp. 8°. [*Albany?* 1842.]

——. Acts of the legislature of the State, and ordinances and resolutions of the common council of the city of New York, in relation to the subject of the introduction of water into the city of New York, from 1833 to June, 1842. 72 pp. 8°. [*New York*], *C. Dingley*, 1842. [P., v. 356.]

——. Assembly. Report of the committee on colleges, academies, and common schools, on the

New York (*State*)—continued.

petitions of the trustees of the Albany Medical College, the medical faculty of Geneva College, the medical department of the University of the City of New York, asking appropriations from the revenue of the U. S. deposit fund, etc. March 19, 1844. 5 pp. 8°. [*Albany*, 1844.]

——. S. Report of the minority of the committee on medical societies and medical colleges, on the bill in relation to the State Lunatic Asylum. April 23, 1844. 11 pp. 8°. [*Albany*, 1844.]

——. Assembly. Report of the minority of the library committee, to whom the senate bill, entitled "An act in relation to the State Library", was referred. No. 176. April 20, 1844. 2 pp. 8°. [*Albany*, 1844.]

——. Laws relating to the public health, the quarantine duties of pilots, etc., for the port, harbor, and State of New York, embraced in the revised statutes and in an act of the legislature of the State of New York. Passed May 13, 1846. 59 pp. 8°. *New York, J. W. Bell*, 1846.

——. Assembly. Report of a special committee of the house of assembly of the State of New York, on the present quarantine laws, 1846. 317 pp., 2 maps. 8°. *Albany, Carrol & Cook*, 1846.

——. Assembly. Report of the legislative committee of 1848 on the removal of quarantine. 16 pp. 8°. [*Albany*, 1848.]

——. S. Report of the standing committee on medical societies and colleges, relative to sundry petitions for the passage of a law to regulate the practice of physic and surgery. Jan. 15, 1848. 5 pp. 8°. [*Albany*, 1848.]

——. Militia law of the State of New York. An act to provide for the enrolment of the militia, and to encourage the formation of uniform companies, excepting the first military division of this State, passed May 13, 1847, as amended by the act passed Dec. 15, 1847, to which is appended so much of the former militia laws as are not repealed by this act. 101, 10 pp. 8°. *Albany, C. Van Benthuysen*, 1848.

——. S. Report of the majority of the committee on grievances on petitions, relative to the quarantine establishment and to the bill from the assembly on that subject. No. 51. March 1, 1849. 10 pp. 8°. [*Albany*, 1849.]

——. Assembly. Communication from the committee appointed by the house of assembly, being the report of the select committee appointed April 11, 1848, to examine and report as to whether the quarantine establishment in the county of Richmond should be removed from its present location, and as to what locality said establishment should be removed. No. 60. Jan. 30, 1849. 121 pp., 2 ch. 8°. [*Albany*, 1849?] [*Also, in*: P., v. 640.]

——. Acts amending the militia laws of the State of New York. Passed April 10, 1849. 8 pp. 8°. *Albany, Weed, Parsons & Co.*, 1849.

——. An act relative to the public health in the city of New York. Passed April 10, 1850. 48 pp., 1 l. 8°. [*Albany*, 1850.]

——. S. Report of the majority of the committee on medical societies and colleges, on so much of the governor's message as relates to the cholera. State of New York. No. 92. March 25, 1850. 43 pp. 8°. *Albany*, [1850].

——. An act relative to the public health in the city of New York. Passed April 10, 1850. 48 pp., 1 l. 8°. [*Albany*, 1850.]

——. Assembly. Report of the committee on medical societies and colleges, on petition of Dr. Wm. Turner for final enactments against bleeding. July 1, 1851. 40 pp. 8°. [*Albany*, 1851.]

——. Assembly. Report of the minority of the committee on colleges, academies, and common

New York (*State*)—continued.

schools, against granting a charter to the Metropolitan College. State of New York. March 5, 1852. 6 pp. 8°. [*Albany*, 1852.]

——. Reports of the majority and of the minority of the select committee, on so much of the governor's message as relates to intemperance and the sale of intoxicating drinks. (Transmitted to the legislature of New York Jan. 25, 1854.) 40 pp. 8°. *Albany, C. Van Benthuysen*, 1854.

——. Report of the commissioners relative to encroachments and preservation of the harbor of New York. Transmitted to the legislature Jan. 8, 1856. 163 pp. 8°. *Albany, C. Van Benthuysen*, 1856.

——. S. Report of select committee relative to condition of wharves and buildings at quarantine. No. 100. April 8, 1856. 24 pp. 8°. [*Albany*, 1856.]

——. Report of select committee appointed to visit charitable institutions supported by the State and all city and county poor and work houses and jails of the State of New York. Transmitted to the legislature Jan. 9, 1857. 217 pp., 1 l. 8°. *Albany, C. Van Benthuysen*, 1857.

——. Report of commissioners relative to encroachments in the harbor of New York. Transmitted to the legislature Jan. 29, 1857. 335 pp., 1 map, 8 diag. 8°. *Albany, C. Van Benthuysen*, 1857.

——. Report of the commissioners for the removal of the quarantine station of the State of New York. Transmitted to the legislature Feb. 12, 1858. 33 pp. 8°. *Albany, C. Van Benthuysen*, 1858.

——. Report of the commissioners relative to removal of the quarantine station. Transmitted to the assembly March 10, 1858. 92 pp. 8°. *Albany, C. Van Benthuysen*, 1858.

——. S. Report of the select committee on the registration of births, marriages, and deaths. March 11, 1858. Doc. No. 81. 8 pp. 8°. [*Albany*, 1858.]

——. An act to incorporate the American College of Medical Science. Passed April, 1858. 3 pp. 8°. [*New York*, 1858.]

——. Laws relative to quarantine and to the public health of the city of New York. (Part 1, chapter xiv, of the revised statutes, as amended and modified by the subsequent acts of the legislature.) 67 pp. 16°. *New York*, 1858.

——. Report of the select committee appointed to investigate the health department of the city of New York. Transmitted to the legislature Feb. 3, 1859. 211 pp., 1 plan, 1 map. 8°. *Albany, C. Van Benthuysen*, 1859.

——. An act to amend and consolidate the several acts relating to the city of Troy, N. Y. 95 pp. 8°. *Troy, Budget Printing Establishment*, 1860.

——. Report of the committee on the incorporation of cities and villages, on the bill entitled "An act concerning the public health of the counties of New York, Kings, and Richmond". Transmitted to the legislature March 9, 1860. 30 pp., 1 map. 8°. *Albany, C. Van Benthuysen*, 1860.

——. Assembly. Report of the select committee to which was referred the memorial of Dr. Saunders and others, asking for an investigation into the causes of the death of Norris Tarbell at the State Lunatic Asylum at Utica. Transmitted to the legislature April 16, 1860. 80 pp. 8°. *Albany, C. Van Benthuysen*, 1860.

——. Assembly. An act [as amended and passed in assembly April 10, 1861] concerning the public health of the counties of New York, Kings, and Richmond, and the waters thereof

New York (*State*)—continued.

No. —. Jan. 10, 1861. Introd. by Mr. Robinson. 8 pp. fol. [*Albany*, 1861.]

——. Assembly. Metropolitan health bill. Speech of the Hon. L. Chandler Ball, of Rensselaer, on the "act concerning the public health of the counties of New York, Kings, and Richmond, and the waters thereof". March 26, 1861. 15 pp. 8°. *Albany, Weed, Parsons & Co.*, 1861.

——. Report of the committee on the incorporation of cities and villages on the bill entitled "An act concerning the public health of the counties of New York, Kings, and Richmond, and the waters thereof". 40 pp. 8°. *Albany, C. Van Benthuysen*, 1861. [*Also, in :* P., v. 345.]

——. An act to amend an act entitled "An act to amend an act entitled 'An act to establish a metropolitan police district, and to provide for the government thereof'. Passed April 15, 1857"; April 10, 1860; April 25, 1864. 32 pp. 8°. *New York, Bergen & Tripp*, 1864.

——. Report of the general agent of the State of New York for the relief of sick, wounded, furloughed, and discharged soldiers to the board of managers of the New York State Soldiers' Depot, at New York City. 134 pp., 5 pl., 2 maps, 1 plan. 8°. *Albany, Comstock & Cassidy*, 1864.

——. Report on the condition of the insane poor in the county poor-houses of New York. By Sylvester D. Willard [secretary of the Medical Society of the State of New York, to the legislature, Jan. 12, 1865]. 70 pp. 8°. *Albany, C. Van Benthuysen*, 1865.

——. Assembly. Report of the committee on public health, relative to the small-pox. Feb. 10, 1865. No. 76. 15 pp. 8°. *Albany, C. Wendell*, 1865. [*Also, in :* P., v. 345.]

——. An act to establish a metropolitan sanitary district and board of health to preserve the public health in said district, and to prevent the spread of disease therefrom, 1865. 36 pp. 8°. [*Albany*, 1865.]

——. An act to regulate the sale of intoxicating liquors within the metropolitan police district of the State of New York. [Passed April 14, 1866.] 12°. *New York, Sanford, Harroun & Co.*, 1866.

In : NEW YORK (*State*). An act to create a metropolitan sanitary district. 12°. *New York*, 1866, 43-50.

——. An act to create a metropolitan sanitary district and board of health therein for the preservation of life and health, and to prevent the spread of disease. 32 pp. 8°. *New York, Bergen & Tripp*, 1866. [*Also, in :* P., v. 345.]

——. An act to create a metropolitan sanitary district and board of health therein for the preservation of life and health, and to prevent the spread of disease. [Also, an act to amend an act entitled "An act to create a metropolitan sanitary district and board of health therein".] 50 pp. 12°. *New York, Sanford, Harroun & Co., printers*, 1866.

——. Notice to masters of vessels. Extract from the United States shipping act of 1872. An act for the better protection of seamen in the port and harbor of New York. Passed March 21, 1866. 1 sheet. 4°. [*New York*, 1866.]

——. Communication from the governor, transmitting the report of the commissioners appointed to locate the Hudson River State Hospital for the Insane, at Poughkeepsie, Jan. 9, 1867. 8 pp. 8°. *Albany, C. Van Benthuysen & Sons*, 1867.

——. An act for the regulation of tenement and lodging houses in the cities of New York and Brooklyn. Passed May 14, 1867. 11 pp. 8°. *New York, Bergen & Tripp*, 1867.

——. Census of the State of New York for 1865 ; taken in pursuance of article 3 of the constitu-

New York (*State*)—continued.

tion of the State, and chapter 64 of the laws of 1855, and chapter 34 of the laws of 1865; prepared from the original returns under the direction of Hon. Fran. C. Barlow, secretary of state, by Franklin B. Hough, superintendent of the census. 1 p. l., cxxvi, 743 pp., 2 diag. fol. *Albany, C. Van Benthuysen & Sons*, 1867.

——. Laws relative to quarantine in the port of New York. Compiled under the direction of the commissioners of quarantine. 79 pp. 16°. *New York, Francis & Loutrel*, 1867.

——. Laws of the State of New York relating to the Metropolitan Board of Health and to the Metropolitan Board of Excise, passed in 1866 and 1867. 92 pp. 8°. *New York, Bergen & Tripp*, 1867.

——. Assembly. Report of the committee on public health, relative to the public duties of the health officer of the port of New York. No. 106. March 18, 1868. 3 pp. 8°. [*Albany*, 1868.]

——. The cattle disease ! Extract from the law passed April 20, 1866, to prevent the introduction and spread of the disease known as the rinderpest, and for the protection of the flocks and herds of sheep and cattle in this State from destruction by this and other infectious diseases. Also, an extract from regulations adopted by the State commissioners Aug. 18, 1868. broadside fol. [*Albany*, 1868?]

——. Communication from the governor, transmitting the report of the board of commissioners of rinderpest for the year 1867. 2 pp. 8°. [*Albany*, 1868.]

——. Communication from the governor, transmitting the report of the commissioners of pilots in the city of New York for the year 1867. 3 pp. 8°. [*Albany*, 1868.]

——. Assembly. Report of the board of commissioners charged with the construction of the quarantine hospital and boarding station on West Bank. State of New York. No. 18. Jan. 14, 1869. 13 pp. 8°. [*Albany*, 1869.]

——. Assembly. Testimony taken before the committee appointed to make inquiry concerning the gas companies in the city and county of New York, city of Buffalo, city of Brooklyn, and the city of Albany. State of New York. No. 113. Feb. 15, 1869. 288 pp. 8°. [*Albany*, 1869.]

——. Assembly. Report of sub-committee of the whole [to which was referred the assembly bill G. O. 612, entitled "An act authorizing the corporation of the city of Troy to borrow moneys and issue bonds therefor for the extension of the water works of said city". Reported by Mr. Cameron.] No. 112. May 24, 1869. 8 pp. 8°. [*Albany*, 1869.]

——. Communication from the governor, transmitting annual report of the board of police of the capital police district to the assembly, for the year 1867-8. 39 pp. 8°. [*Albany*, 1869.]

——. Report accompanying plans for the improvement of the ventilation and heating of the hall of representatives, by Lewis W. Leeds. 8 l. fol. [*New York*, 1869.]

——. Report of special committee appointed by the commissioners of emigration of the State of New York to investigate into complaints of passengers of ship James Foster, jr. 126 pp. 8°. *New York, D. Taylor*, 1869.

——. S. Report of the commissioners to locate an insane asylum in the eighth judicial district, New York. No. 8. In senate. Jan. 20, 1870. 24 pp. 8°. [*Albany*, 1870.]

Bound with : Rep. Buffalo State Asylum for the Insane. 1.-13. 8°. *Buffalo & Albany*, 1872-84.

——. Assembly. Report of the committee on the manufacture of salt. No. 194. April 11, 1870. 5 pp. 8°. [*Albany*, 1870.]

New York (*State*)—continued.

——. Laws relating to quarantine in the port of New York. Compiled under the direction of the commissioners of quarantine. 69 pp., 1 l. 18°. *New York, Corlies, Mack & Co.,* 1870.

——. Report of the commissioners of quarantine in response to alleged abuses and the answer of the health officer thereto to the governor of the State. Dec. 11, 1871. 15 pp. 8°. [*Albany,* 1872.]

——. Assembly. An act to protect the people against quackery and crime. State of New York. Introd. by Mr. Flammer. Jan. 24, 1872. 7 pp. fol. [*Albany,* 1872.]

——. Assembly. An act in relation to quarantine in the port of New York. No. 858. Feb. 2, 1872. Introd. by Mr. Hawkins. 6 pp. fol. [*Albany,* 1872.]

——. Assembly. Report of commissioners to construct quarantine buildings, under chapter 751, laws of 1866. No. 46. Feb. 7, 1872. 10 pp. 8°. [*Albany,* 1872.]

——. Assembly. Reply of the quarantine commissioners in obedience to a resolution of the assembly relative to the expenditure of money appropriated to said commissioners by chapter 715 of the laws of 1871. State of New York. No. 56. Feb. 14, 1872. 18 pp. 8°. [*Albany,* 1872.]

——. Assembly. Report and testimony of the assembly committee on commerce and navigation in relation to the quarantine abuses at the port of New York. No. 162. May 2, 1872. xix, 363 pp. 8°. [*Albany,* 1872.]

——. S. Communication from the comptroller of the city of New York in reply to a resolution of the Senate relative to the paving of certain streets and avenues in said city with wooden pavement, etc. State of New York. No. 69. March 28, 1873. 23 pp. 8°. [*Albany,* 1873.]

——. S. An act establishing a quarantine and defining the qualifications, duties, and powers of the health officer for the harbor and port of New York. No. 162. Jan. 22, 1873. Introd. by Mr. Adams. 20 pp. fol. [*Albany,* 1873.]

——. Assembly. Reply of the New York street cleaning commission to a resolution of the assembly relative to contracts issued since the organization. State of New York. No. 47. Feb. 7, 1872. 9 pp. 8°. [*Albany,* 1873.]

——. S. An act to amend chapter 135 of the laws of 1842, entitled "An act to organize the State Lunatic Asylum, and more effectually to provide for the care, maintenance, and recovery of the insane", passed April 7, 1842. No. 222. Feb. 13, 1873. Introd. by Mr. Chatfield. 2 pp. fol. [*Albany,* 1873.]

——. S. Report of the commissioners appointed to investigate charges against lunatic asylums in this State; also an act accompanying the same. No. 40. Feb. 17, 1873. 16 pp. 8°. [*Albany,* 1873.]

——. S. Preamble and resolutions relative to the office of the commissioner of quarantine, and the expenditure of moneys appropriated for quarantine purposes in the port of New York during the past three years. No. 45. Feb. 21, 1873. 2 pp. 8°. [*Albany,* 1873.]

——. S. An act to establish a commission in and for the city and county of New York, to be known and designated as the commission of charitable correction, and to define its powers and jurisdiction. Introd. by Mr. Benedict. No. 245. Feb., 1873. 4 pp. fol. [*Albany,* 1873.]

——. S. An act relative to the medical laws of the State of New York. No. 236. March 3, 1873. Introd. by Mr. Lewis. 7 pp. fol. [*Albany,* 1873.]

New York (*State*)—continued.

——. Communication from the comptroller of the city of New York, in reply to senate resolution regarding markets. State of New York. No. 61. In senate. March 7, 1873. 12 pp. 8°. [*Albany,* 1873.]

——. Assembly. An act relative to the medical laws of the State of New York. No. 623. March 14, 1873. Introd. by Mr. Crandall. 7 pp. fol. [*Albany,* 1873.]

——. S. Report and testimony taken before the finance committee, with regard to the affairs and management of the Hudson River State Hospital for the Insane. No. 107. April 30, 1873. 87 pp. 8°. [*Albany,* 1873.]

——. Defence of insanity in criminal cases. Argument of Henry L. Clinton, delivered April 15, 1873, before the judiciary committee of the senate [of New York], in favor of the bill drafted by him in relation to the defence of insanity in criminal cases, which has passed the assembly. 41 pp. 8°. [*Albany,* 1873.]

——. S. Reply of the comptroller of the city of New York to a resolution of the senate, giving a statement of all the costs, fees, and expenses incurred for the opening of streets, avenues, and public places in the city of New York during the five years last past, etc. State of New York. No. 98. May 16, 1873. 55 pp. 8°. [*Albany,* 1873.]

——. An act further to define the powers and duties of the board of State commissioners of public charities, and to change the name of the board to the State board of charities. Passed May 21, 1873. 4 pp. 8°. [*Albany,* 1873.]

——. S. Report of the finance committee, to whom was referred the resolution of the senate calling on the commissioners of quarantine to transmit an account of all moneys expended, work performed, and materials furnished since the date of their organization, and for what purposes it was expended. No. 104. May 29, 1873. 28 pp. 8°. [*Albany,* 1873.]

——. S. Testimony taken before the finance committee of the senate of 1873, in response to a preamble and resolution. [Being three written statements of Dr. John Swinburne, of Albany, in reference to quarantine in New York Harbor.] 43 pp. 8°. [*Albany,* 1873.]

——. S. Testimony [taken by the finance committee of the senate, on the management of quarantine in the port of New York. No. 82]. xiv, 167 pp. 8°. [*Albany,* 1873?]

——. S. [Evidence taken by the finance committee of the senate on the management of quarantine in the port of New York.] pp. 105–136. 8°. [*Albany,* 1873.]

Cutting.

——. Report on a topographical survey of the Adirondack wilderness of New York. By Verplanck Colvin. 43 pp., 1 pl., 2 maps. 8°. *Albany, Argus Co.,* 1873.

Report made to the legislature. State Doc. No. 53, 1873.

——. Assembly. An act making appropriations for certain expenses of government, and for supplying deficiencies in former appropriations. No. 923. April 10, 1873. Introd. by Mr. Fort. 30 pp. fol. [*Albany,* 1873.]

——. The same. No. 1020. April 10, 1873. Rep. by Mr. Fort. 36 pp. fol. [*Albany,* 1873.]

——. Annual reports of the superintendent of public instruction and the regents of the university, on the New York State Normal School at Albany, to the legislature. 29., 1872; 32., 1875. 31 pp.; 8 pp. 8°. *Albany,* 1873–6.

——. Assembly. An act to secure effective vaccination in the city of New York, and the collection of pure vaccine lymph or virus. No.

New York (*State*)—continued.

109. Feb. 9, 1874. Introd. by Mr. Blumenthal. 2 pp. fol. [*Albany*, 1874.]

———. Manual of rules and regulations creating and governing the first board of State medical examiners of the University of the State of New York; with a statement of the objects of the board and the mode of examinations. 10 pp. 8°. *Albany, Weed, Parsons & Co.*, 1874.

———. Assembly. An act making appropriations for certain expenses of government, and supplying deficiencies in former appropriations. No. 560. March 24, 1874. Rep. by Mr. Batcheller. 32 pp. fol. [*Albany*, 1874.]

———. S. An act making appropriations for certain expenses of government, and supplying deficiencies in former appropriations. No. 319. April 14, 1874. Assembly bill No. 374, rep. with admendments. 4 + pp. fol. [*Albany*, 1874.]

———. Assembly. An act making appropriations for certain expenditures of government, and supplying deficiencies in former appropriations. No. 872. April 23, 1874. Amendments made by the senate to original assembly bill No. 560. 32 pp. fol. [*Albany*, 1874.]

———. Assembly. An act making appropriations for certain expenses of government. No. 287. March 15, 1875. Rep. by Mr. Hammond. 14 pp. fol. [*Albany*, 1875.]

———. Assembly. An act for the prevention of disease among animals. State of New York. No. 88. Jan. 18, 1875. Introd. by Mr. T. C. Campbell. 4 pp. fol. [*Albany*, 1875.]

———. S. An act to amend chapter 436 of the laws of 1874, entitled "An act to regulate the practice of medicine and surgery in the State of New York", passed May 11, 1874. No. 54. Feb. 3, 1875. Introd. by Mr. Laning. 4 pp. fol. [*Albany*, 1875.]

———. Assembly. An act for the prevention of adulteration of food, drink, and drugs. State of New York. No. 161. March 1, 1875. Introd. by Mr. Prince. 2 pp. fol. [*Albany*, 1875.]

———. Assembly. An act to amend chapter 436 of the laws of 1874, entitled "An act to regulate the practice of medicine and surgery in the State of New York", passed May 11, 1874. No. 423. April 2, 1875. Introd. by Mr. Beach. 3 pp. fol. [*Albany*, 1875.]

———. Communication from the governor of New York, transmitting a communication from the governor of New Jersey, together with a concurrent resolution of the legislature of New Jersey, and a report of the commissioners of the State of New York, relative to quarantine jurisdiction. 10 pp., 1 chart. 8°. *Albany, Weed, Parsons & Co.*, 1875.

———. Assembly. Report of the committee of investigation into the affairs of the commissioners of emigration and quarantine. No. 33. Jan. 28, 1876. x, 971 pp. 8°. [*Albany*, 1876.]

———. Assembly. Report of the minority of the committee of investigation into the affairs of the commissioners of emigration and quarantine. No. 34. Jan. 28, 1876. 3 pp. 8°. [*Albany*, 1876.]

Bound with preceding.

———. Assembly. Report of the select committee appointed by the assembly of 1875 to investigate the causes of the increase of crime in the city of New York. State of New York. No. 106. Feb. 17, 1876. 76 pp. 8°. [*Albany*, 1876.]

———. Assembly. Report of the committee on State prisons on the assembly resolution relative to the subject of investigation of prison management and affairs. No. 75. March 10, 1876. 5 pp. 8°. [*Albany*, 1876.]

New York (*State*)—continued.

———. Assembly. Communication from the New York quarantine commissioner in answer to a resolution of the house relative to the steamer Nelson K. Hopkins. No. 80. March 14, 1876. 4 pp. 8°. [*Albany*, 1876.]

———. Assembly. Supplementary report of majority of the prison committee. No. 86. March 17, 1876. 5 pp. 8°. [*Albany*, 1876.]

———. Assembly. Communication from the corporation counsel of the city of New York in reply to a resolution of the assembly relative to the bill entitled "An act relating to assessments for the construction of sewers and drains in the city of New York". No. 92. March 28, 1876. 6 pp. 8°. [*Albany*, 1876.]

———. Annual reports of the board of commissioners of the State survey, and reports of the director. 1., 1876; 8., 1883; 9., 1884. 8°. *Albany*, 1877–84.

———. Annual report of the comptroller of the State of New York. Transmitted to the legislature Jan. 8, 1879. 104 pp. 8°. *Albany, C. Van Benthuysen & Sons*, 1879.

———. Assembly. An act to limit the functions of coroners and to create the office of medical examiners. No. 414. Jan. 19, 1879. Introd. by Mr. Beckwith. Original No. 140. 8 pp. fol. [*Albany*, 1879.]

———. Assembly. An act to establish a State board of health. State of New York. No. 269. February 12, 1879. Introd. by Mr. Millspaugh. 4 pp. fol. [*Albany*, 1879.]

———. Assembly. An act to limit the functions of coroners and to create the office of medical examiners. No. 140. Feb. 19, 1879. Introd. by Mr. Beckwith. 7 pp. fol. [*Albany*, 1879.]

———. Assembly. An act in relation to the employment of female physicians in State asylums for insane. State of New York. No. 377. March 12, 1879. Introd. by Mr. Brooks. 1 l. fol. [*Albany*, 1879.]

———. S. An act to establish a State board of health. State of New York. No. 191. March 14, 1879. Introd. by Mr. J. F. Pierce. 2 pp. fol. [*Albany*, 1879.]

———. S. Report of the committee on public health relative to lunatic asylums. (Transmitted to the legislature May 22, 1879.) 51 pp. 8°. *Albany, C. Van Benthuysen & Sons*, 1879.

———. S. An act to amend section 1 of chapter 123 of the laws of 1854, entitled "An act to promote medical science". State of New York. No. 210. March 26, 1879. Introd. by Mr. Jacobs. 2 pp. fol. [*Albany*, 1879.]

———. Communication from the comptroller, submitting to the senate the report of the agent appointed to examine the charitable institutions of the State of New York. Albany, April 9, 1879. 60 pp. 8°. *Albany*, 1879.

———. Communication from the comptroller, submitting to the senate the report of the agent appointed to examine the charitable institutions of the State of New York. Albany, April 9, 1879. 75 pp., 33 tab. 8°. *Albany, Argus Co.*, 1879.

———. Assembly. An act to amend an act entitled "An act to amend chapter 467 of the laws of 1862, entitled 'An act to prevent the adulteration of milk, and prevent the traffic in impure and unwholesome milk'", passed May 2, 1864. No. 213. Jan. 7, 1880. Introd. by Mr. Sheridan. 2 pp. fol. [*Albany*, 1880.]

———. S. An act to establish a State board of health. State of New York. No. 152. Jan. 15, 1880. Introd. by Mr. Woodin. 6 pp. fol. [*Albany*, 1880.]

———. S. An act to amend chapter 446 of the laws of 1874, entitled "An act to revise and con-

New York (*State*)—continued.

solidate the statutes of the State relating to the care and custody of the insane, the management of the asylums for their treatment and safe-keeping, and the duties of the State commissioner in lunacy". No. 21. Jan. 16, 1880. Introd. by Mr. Braman. 3 pp. fol. [*Albany*, 1880.]

——. The same. An act further to amend chapter 446 of the laws of 1874. No. 30. Jan. 20, 1880. Introd. by Mr. Birdsall. 6 pp. fol. [*Albany*, 1880.]

——. Assembly. An act to improve the public health in the city of New York and the city of Brooklyn by regulating the manufacture of segars in the tenement houses of said cities. No. 67. Jan. 19, 1880. Introd. by Mr. Grosse. 2 pp. fol. [*Albany*, 1880.]

——. S. An act to amend chapter 324 of the laws of 1850, entitled "An act for the preservation of the public health". State of New York. No. 41. Jan. 20, 1880. Introd. by Mr. Pitts. 1 sheet. fol. [*Albany*, 1880.]

——. Assembly. An act relative to the maintenance of the inmates of the Protestant Infant Asylum. No. 553. Jan. 23, 1880. Introd. by Mr. Gibbs. 2 pp. fol. [*Albany*, 1880.]

——. S. An act to regulate the dispensing and sale of provisions within this State. No. 113. Feb. 3, 1880. Introd. by Mr. Astor. 2 pp. fol. [*Albany*, 1880.]

——. S. An act to amend section 13 of article 1 of title 13, chapter 18, part 1, of the revised statutes, entitled "An act to incorporate medical societies for the purpose of regulating the practice of physic and surgery in this State". No. 156. Feb. 6, 1880. Introd. by Mr. Jacobs. 1 sheet. fol. [*Albany*, 1880.]

——. S. An act to amend chapter 123 of the laws of 1854, entitled "An act to promote medical science". [Conditions under which dead bodies may be turned over to medical schools.] State of New York. No. 238. Feb. 10, 1880. Introd. by Mr. Jacobs. 2 pp. fol. [*Albany*, 1880.]

——. Assembly. An act to amend chapter 633 of the laws of 1875, entitled "An act to amend the charter of the city of Brooklyn, being the act for that purpose passed June 28, 1873, and the act for that purpose passed June 1, 1874". [In relation to the board of health of the city of Brooklyn.] No. 472. Feb. 12, 1880. Introd. by Mr. Wren. 4 pp. fol. [*Albany*, 1880.]

——. S. An act to limit the functions of coroners, and to create the office of medical examiner. No. 264. Feb. 16, 1880. Introd. by Mr. Pitts. 8 pp. fol. [*Albany*, 1880.]

——. Assembly. An act to amend chapter 319 of the laws of 1848, entitled "An act for the incorporation of benevolent, charitable, scientific, and missionary societies". No. 551. Feb. 12, 1880. Introd. by Mr. Deane. 2 pp. fol. [*Albany*, 1880.]

——. S. An act to simplify the proof of the sanitary code in the city of New York. State of New York. No. 170. March 3, 1880. Introd. by Mr. Strahan. 2 pp. fol. [*Albany*, 1880.]

——. Assembly. An act in relation to the health officer for the port of New York. State of New York. No. 392. March 5, 1880. Introd. by Mr. Varnum. 2 pp. fol. [*Albany*, 1880.]

——. S. An act to further amend chapter 908 of the laws of 1867, entitled "An act for the regulation of tenement and lodging houses in the cities of New York and Brooklyn", as amended by chapter 504 of the laws of 1879. No. 233. March 12, 1880. Introd. by Mr. Astor. 2 pp. fol. [*Albany*, 1880.]

New York (*State*)—continued.

——. Assembly. An act for the proper drainage of lands in the city of New York. State of New York. No. 543. March 18, 1880. Introd. by Mr. J. L. Wells. 4 pp. fol. [*Albany*, 1880.]

——. An act to establish a State board of health. Passed May 18, 1880. 1 sheet. fol. [*Albany*, 1880.]

——. An act entitled "An act to regulate the licensing of physicians and surgeons". Passed May 29, 1880. 1 galley sheet. [*Albany*, 1880.]

——. Health department, city of New York. Tenement-house acts. Chapter 908, laws of 1867. (As amended by chapter 504, laws of 1879, and chapter 399, sect. 1, laws of 1880.) An act for the regulation of tenement and lodging houses in the cities of New York and Brooklyn. 19 pp. 16°. [*New York*, 1880?]

——. S. An act to open the college of the city of New York to all male persons who shall pass the preliminary examination for admission therein. State of New York. No. 176. Jan. 3, 1882. Introd. by Mr. Grady. 1 sheet. fol. [*Albany*, 1882.]

——. Assembly. An act to regulate the manufacture and sale of oleomargarine or any form of imitation butter and lard, or any form of imitation cheese, for the prevention of fraud and the better protection of the public health. No. 36. Feb. 3, 1882. Introd. by Mr. Fenner. 3 pp. fol. *Albany*, 1882.

——. Assembly. An act to prohibit the coloring of oleomargarine, butterine, and adulterated cheese. No. 37. Feb. 8, 1882. Introd. by Mr. Chamberlin. 2 pp. fol. [*Albany*, 1882.]

——. Assembly. An act to regulate the sale of spirituous liquors, wines, ale, and beer in the cities of New York and Brooklyn. No. 33. Feb. 8, 1882. Introd. by Mr. Lindsay. 11 pp. fol. [*Albany*, 1882.]

——. S. An act in relation to the sale and use of opium. State of New York. No. 59. Feb. 8, 1882. Introd. by Mr. Koch. 1 sheet. fol. [*Albany*, 1882.]

——. Assembly. An act in relation to certain sewerage and drainage in the city of Brooklyn. No. 83. Feb. 8, 1882. Introd. by Mr. Sheridan. 2 pp. fol. [*Albany*, 1882.]

——. Assembly. An act to prevent fraud in the manufacture and sale of sugars, syrups, molasses, and honey. No. 203. Feb. 9, 1882. Introd. by Mr. Helm. 2 pp. fol. [*Albany*, 1882.]

——. Assembly. An act making an appropriation for repairs to and improvements upon certain property of this State used as an asylum for the destitute, sick, or infirm wives, mothers, sisters, daughters, or widows of seamen, and for the support of the inmates of said asylum. State of New York. No. 501. Feb. 10, 1882. Introd. by Mr. Brooks. 2 pp. fol. [*Albany*, 1882.]

——. Assembly. An act to regulate the sale of spirituous liquors, wines, ale, and beer in the city of New York. No. 12. Feb. 16, 1882. Introd. by Mr. Bogan. 10 pp. fol. [*Albany*, 1882.]

——. Assembly. An act to prevent cruel and inhuman treatment of insane persons. No. 167. Feb. 17, 1882. Introd. by unanimous consent by Mr. Pinney. 2 pp. fol. [*Albany*, 1882.]

——. Assembly. An act to regulate the practice of pharmacy, the licensing of persons to carry on such practice, and the sale of poisons. No. 542. Feb. 17, 1882. Introd. by Mr. Parker. 12 pp. fol. [*Albany*, 1882.]

——. S. An act to provide for the abatement of nuisances by boards of health of incorporated cities, villages, and towns. No. 117. Feb. 23, 1882. Introd. by Mr. Fitzgerald. 2 pp. fol. [*Albany*, 1882.]

New York (*State*)—continued.

——. Assembly. An act to repeal chapter 513 of the laws of 1880, entitled "An act to regulate the licensing of physicians and surgeons", and all acts and parts of acts amendatory thereof. No. 240. Feb. 24, 1882. Introd. by Mr. M. J. Castello. 1 sheet. fol. [*Albany*, 1882.]

——. Assembly. An act to regulate the sale of certain liquors, and to provide for the more effectual collection of excise dues. No. 67. March 1, 1882. Introd. by Mr. Van Allen. 8 pp. fol. [*Albany*, 1882.]

——. Assembly. An act to suppress certain nuisances [making it unlawful for any place of business in cities of 15,000 population or over to use petroleum residuum] for fuel. No. 358. March 1, 1882. Introd. by Mr. Kelly. 1 sheet. fol. [*Albany*, 1882.]

——. Assembly. An act to establish an additional public park in the city of New York, and for the security of the public health therein. No. 257. March 2, 1882. Introd. by Mr. M. C. Murphy. 2 pp. fol. [*Albany*, 1882.]

——. Assembly. An act to regulate the manufacturing or brewing of ale, beer, porter, and other malt liquors, and to prevent adulteration therein. No. 110. March 3, 1882. Introd. by Mr. McDonough. 3 pp. fol. [*Albany*, 1882.]

——. S. An act regarding membership in the Homœopathic Medical Society of the State of New York. State of New York. No. 108. March 6, 1882. Introd. by Mr. Lord. 1 sheet. fol. [*Albany*, 1882.]

——. Assembly. An act for the removal of causes of malaria and danger to the public health from Gowanus Canal, and making an appropriation for such purposes. State of New York. No. 191. March 7, 1882. Introd. by Mr. Murry. 1 sheet. fol. [*Albany*, 1882.]

——. Assembly. An act to amend chapter 550 of the laws of 1881, entitled "An act to amend chapter 479, entitled 'An act to amend chapter 123 of the laws of 1854', entitled 'An act to promote medical science'". No. 359. March 8, 1882. Introd. by Mr. Farrar. 3 pp. fol. [*Albany*, 1882.]

——. Assembly. An act to amend chapter 746 of the laws of 1872, entitled "An act relating to the examination of candidates for the degree of doctor of medicine, and the acts amendatory thereof". State of New York. No. 537. March 14, 1882. Introd. by Mr. Parker. 2 pp. fol. [*Albany*, 1882.]

——. Assembly. An act to provide a system of sewerage for the village of Little Falls. No. 263. March 14, 1882. Introd. by Mr. Ross. 4 pp. fol. [*Albany*, 1882.]

——. Assembly. An act to authorize the Brooklyn Homœopathic Hospital to increase the number of its trustees. State of New York. No. 325. March 15, 1882. Introd. by Mr. Monk. 1 sheet. fol. [*Albany*, 1882.]

——. Assembly. An act for the better protection of the public health in the city of Brooklyn. State of New York. No. 417. March 15, 1882. Introd. by Mr. Tighe. 2 pp. fol. [*Albany*, 1882.]

——. Assembly. An act to amend chapter 106 of the laws of 1865, entitled "An act to incorporate the New York Infant Asylum", passed March 11, 1865, as amended by chapter 263 of the laws of 1872, entitled "An act to amend an act entitled 'An act to incorporate the New York Infant Asylum'", passed March 11, 1865; and as further amended by chapter 90 of the laws of 1877, entitled "An act further to amend chapter 106 of the laws of 1865, entitled 'An act to incorporate the New York Infant Asylum'", passed

New York (*State*)—continued.

April 2, 1871, and to amend the title thereto. State of New York. No. 530. March 1, 1882. Introd. by Mr. Tighe. 2 pp. fol. [*Albany*, 1882.]

——. Assembly. An act to restrict the formation of corporations under an act entitled "An act to provide for the incorporation of benevolent, charitable, scientific, and missionary societies", being chapter 319 of the laws of 1848, and the acts amendatory thereof, and to legalize the incorporation of certain societies organized thereunder, and to regulate the same. State of New York. No. 323. March 17, 1882. Introd. by Mr. M. J. Costello. 2 pp. fol. [*Albany*, 1882.]

——. Assembly. An act to amend chapter 431 of the laws of 1881, entitled "An act to amend chapter 324 of the laws of 1850, entitled 'An act for preservation of the public health, and the acts amendatory thereof'". State of New York. No. 361. March 20, 1882. Introd. by Mr. Farrar. 2 pp. fol. [*Albany*, 1882.]

——. Assembly. An act to amend an act entitled "An act to organize a night medical service in the city of New York, to provide medical assistance in case of sudden sickness or accident during the night time", passed June 26, 1880. No. 360. March 24, 1882. Introd. by Mr. Crane. 3 pp. fol. [*Albany*, 1882.]

——. Assembly. An act amending an act entitled "An act establishing a quarantine and defining the qualifications, duties, and powers of the health officer for the harbor and port of New York", passed April 29, 1863. No. 378. March 29, 1882. Introd. by Mr. Brooks. 1 sheet. fol. [*Albany*, 1882.]

——. Assembly. An act to provide for the construction and maintenance of an additional public bath in the city of New York. State of New York. No. 377. March 29, 1882. Introd. by Mr. E. C. Sheehy. 2 pp. fol. [*Albany*, 1882.]

——. Assembly. An act to amend chapter 431 of the laws of 1881, entitled "An act to amend chapter 324 of the laws of 1850, entitled 'An act for the preservation of the public health', and the acts amendatory thereof", and to amend chapter 790 of the laws of 1867, entitled "An act to amend an act, entitled 'An act for the preservation of the public health'", passed April 10, 1850, and the act entitled "An act to amend the same", passed April 6, 1854, and all acts amendatory thereof. State of New York. No. 527. March 31, 1882. Introd. by Mr. Brooks. 8 pp. fol. [*Albany*, 1882.]

——. S. An act to authorize the corporation "The Sisters of Charity of St. Vincent de Paul" to grant and convey certain lands in the city of New York to the corporation "The St. Vincent's Hospital of the City of New York". No. 221. April 4, 1882. Introd. by Mr. Fitzgerald. 2 pp. fol. [*Albany*, 1882.]

——. Assembly. An act to provide for safety from infectious and contagious diseases in tenement and other houses in the city of New York, the detention of persons exposed thereto, at quarantine stations, and the enforcement of orders of the board of health in said city. State of New York. No. 528. April 11, 1882. Introd. by Mr. Morrison. 4 pp. fol. [*Albany*, 1882.]

——. S. An act to suppress blood-drying in cities. State of New York. No. 259. April 13, 1882. Introd. by Mr. Koch. 2 pp. fol. [*Albany*, 1882.]

——. Assembly. An act relative to the organization of the medical department of universities. State of New York. No. 576. April 14, 1882. Introd. by Mr. Fenner. 1 sheet. fol. [*Albany*, 1882.]

New York (*State*)—continued.

——. Assembly. An act to amend sections 54 and 55 of chapter 358 of the laws of 1863, entitled "An act establishing and defining the qualifications, duties, and powers of the health officer for the harbor and port of New York". No. 652. April 21, 1882. Introd. by Mr. Brooks. 2 pp. fol. [*Albany*, 1882.]

——. Assembly. An act making an appropriation for repairs to and improvements upon certain property of this State used as an asylum for the destitute, sick, or infirm wives, mothers, sisters, daughters, or widows of seamen, and for the support of the inmates of said asylum. No. 501. Feb. 10, 1882. Introd. by Mr. Brooks. 2 pp. fol. [*Albany*, 1882.]

——. Report to the New York legislature of the commission to select and locate lamps for public parks in the twenty-third and twenty-fourth wards of the city of New York, and in the vicinity thereof. According to the provisions of the act of the legislature of the State of New York, chapter 253, passed April 19, 1883. 217 pp. 8°. *New York, M. B. Brown*, 1884.

——. An act for the preservation of the public health, and the registration of vital statistics. [Chap. 270. Passed May 12, 1885.] 7 pp. 8°. [*Albany*, 1885.]

——. Assembly. An act to amend an act entitled "An act to prevent the adulteration of food and drugs". No. 258. Feb. 19, 1885. Introd. by Mr. Barnum. 4 pp. fol. [*Albany*, 1885.]

——. Assembly. Report of the special committee appointed to investigate tontine insurance. [April, 1885.] 18 pp. 8°. [*Hartford*, 1886.]

——. An act to create the New York Post Graduate Medical School and Hospital. Passed May 25, 1886. [*Rochester*, 1886.]
Cutting from: The Union & Advertiser, Rochester, July 26, 1886.

——. Assembly. Report of the commissioners to locate an asylum for the insane in northern New York. No. 11. Jan. 4, 1887. 56 pp., 3 maps. 8°. [*Albany*, 1887.]

——. S. An act to regulate the licensing and registration of physicians and surgeons, and to codify the medical laws of the State of New York. No. 391. Jan. 13, 1887. Introd. by Mr. Connelly. 11 pp. fol. [*Albany*, 1887.]

——. Assembly. An act to regulate the licensing and registration of physicians and surgeons, and to codify the medical laws of the State of New York. No. 129. Jan. 13, 1887. Introd. by Mr. Hamilton. 12 pp. fol. [*Albany*, 1887.]

——. Assembly. An act to regulate the licensing and registration of physicians and surgeons, and to codify the medical laws of the State of New York. No. 684. Jan. 13, 1887. Introd. by Mr. Hamilton. 11 pp. fol. [*Albany*, 1887.]

——. Assembly. An act to protect the public health. No. 133. Jan. 24, 1887. Introd. by Mr. Cantor. 3 pp. fol. [*Albany*, 1887.]

——. Assembly. An act in regard to the health department of the city of New York. No. 67. Jan. 25, 1887. Introd. by Mr. Crosby. 3 pp. fol. [*Albany*, 1887.]

——. S. An act to amend chapter 410 of the laws of 1882, entitled "An act to consolidate into one act and to declare the special and local laws affecting public interests in the city of New York", passed July 1, 1882, in relation to the powers, duties, and health fund of the board of health, and of the health department of the city of New York, and for the preservation of the public health. No. 40. Jan. 26, 1887. Introd. by Mr. Murphy. 12 pp. fol. [*Albany*, 1887.]

New York (*State*)—continued.

——. Assembly. Dissent of the minority of the commissioners appointed by his excellency Governor Hill, under chapter 238, laws of 1886, to locate an asylum for the insane in northern New York. Being an extract from the report of the commissioners made to the legislature. Jan., 1887. Doc. No. 11. 4 pp. fol. [*Albany*, 1887.]

——. Assembly. An act to amend chapter 313 of the laws of 1886, entitled "An act to regulate the practice of veterinary medicine and surgery in the State of New York". No. 201. Feb. 1, 1887. Introd. by Mr. Ingersoll. 2 pp. fol. [*Albany*, 1887.]

——. Assembly. An act to authorize the department of public health of the city of Brooklyn, county of Kings, to establish hospitals for contagious and infectious diseases, and in relation to the erection and maintenance thereof. No. 263. Feb. 2, 1887. Introd. by Mr. Langbein. 2 pp. fol. [*Albany*, 1887.]

——. Assembly. An act to provide for the registration of steam laundries in the cities of New York and Brooklyn, and for the regulation of the same, for the protection of public health. No. 290. Feb. 4, 1887. Introd. by Mr. Kenny. 2 pp. fol. [*Albany*, 1887.]

——. Assembly. Report of the commission on better provision for insane criminals, to the legislature. No. 62. Feb. 16, 1887. 14 pp. 8°. [*Albany*, 1887.]

——. An act to amend chapter 410 of the laws of 1882, entitled "An act to consolidate into one act and to declare the special and local laws affecting public interests in the city of New York", in relation to the powers, duties, and health fund of the board of health, and of the health department of the city of New York, and for the preservation of the public health. Chap. 84. Passed March 25, 1887. 7 pp. 8°. [*Albany*, 1887.]

——. Report of the commission on New Asylum for Insane Criminals, at Mateawan on the Hudson, for the year 1887. 24 pp., 1 plan. 8°. *Troy, Press Co.*, 1888.

——. Report of the commission to investigate and report the most humane and practical method of carrying into effect the sentence of death in capital cases. Elbridge T. Gerry, Alfred P. Southwick, Matthew Hale, commissioners. Transmitted to the legislature of the State of New York, Jan. 17, 1888. 100 pp. 8°. *Albany, Argus Company*, 1888.

——. Chap. 77. An act to amend section 53 of chap. 358 of the laws of 1863, "An act establishing a quarantine and defining the qualifications, duties, and powers of the health officer for the harbor and port of New York". Approved March 22, 1888. Galley sheet. [*Albany*, 1888.]

——. Plan for a bureau of street cleaning, for the city of New York. [Block plan.] An act to provide for the cleaning of the streets, and removal of garbage and ashes, in the city of New York. Prepared for the chairman of the committee on cities, by C. F. Chandler. 11 pp. roy. 8°. [*Albany, n. d.*]

New York (*State*).

See, also, **Albany** ; **Binghamton** ; **Brooklyn** ; **Buffalo** ; **Education** (*Medical*), *etc.*, **Fever** (*Malarial, History, etc., of*), *by localities* ; **Garden City** ; **Greenwood Springs** ; **Insane** (*Asylums for, etc.*), *by localities* ; **Ithaca** ; **Kingston** ; **Little Falls** ; **New York** *City* ; **Owego** ; **Prisons** ; **Rochester** ; **Sackett's Harbor** ; **Saratoga** ; **Troy** ; **Utica** ; **Westchester** ; **West Point** ; **Yonkers**.

ANDERSON (M. B.) Extract relating to outdoor relief. From eighth annual report of the

New York (State).

State board of charities of the State of New York. 8°. *Albany*, 1875.

BROOKLYN. Annual reports of the commissioners of charities of Kings County to the board of supervisors. With accompanying documents, viz : [Reports of Kings County Almshouse, Kings County Hospital, Kings County Lunatic Asylum, and Kings County Nursery], for the years 1853–4 ; 1859–60 to 1863–4 ; 1865–6 to 1872–3. 8°. *Brooklyn*, 1854–73.

GARDNER (J. T.) Uses of a topographical survey to the State of New York. A report to the American Geographical Society. 8°. *New York*, 1876.

HOUGH (F. B.) Essay on the climate of the State of New York, prepared at the request of the executive committee of the State Agricultural Society, and published in the fifteenth volume of their transactions. 8°. *Albany*, 1857.

PROCEEDINGS of the Temperance Convention of the State of New York. Held at Syracuse, Dec. 22, 1869. 8°. *Auburn*, 1870.

SHERRILL (H.) An essay on epidemics, as they appeared in Dutchess County from 1809 to 1825 ; also, a paper on diseases of the jaw-bones ; with an appendix, containing an account of the epidemic cholera, as it appeared in Poughkeepsie in 1832. 4°. *New York*, 1832.

STATE Charities Aid Association. [Circular of the executive committee announcing the object and establishment of the association.] 8°. [*n. p., n. d.*]

———. Organized May 11, 1872. New York. [Prospectus.] 4°. [*New York*, 1872.]

———. Annual reports to the State board of charities of the State of New York. 1.–4., 1872–3 to 1875–6. [Being Nos. 2, 5, 7, 10 of series.] 8°. *New York*, 1873–6.

———. No. 6. Annual report of the committee on children. 1., 1873–4. 8°. *New York*, 1874.

———. What are we doing for the poor ? Report of the bureau of charities, New York, 1874. 8°. *New York*, 1874.

———. Kings County. Organized Oct. 14, 1874. Local visiting committee of the State Charities and Aid Association for the Kings County Institutions, State of New York. Constitution, by-laws, and report for 1875. 8°. *Brooklyn*, 1876.

———. Monroe County. Organized Oct. 3, 1873. Organization of the local visiting committee for the public institutions of charity, the department of out-door relief, and the jail, in Monroe County, State of New York, with the constitution and by-laws. Oct. 3, 1873. 8°. *Rochester*, 1873.

———. Queens County. Organized June 21, 1873. Local visiting committee for the public institutions of charities and correction, in Queens County, State of New York. Address, with constitution and by-laws. 8°. *Jamaica, N. Y.*, 1873.

———. Suffolk County. Organized May 27, 1873. Local visiting committee for the Suffolk County Institutions, State of New York. Address read at the opening meeting, Yaphank, L. I., with constitution and by-laws. 8°. *New York*, 1873.

———. . Local visiting committee for the Westchester County Poor House, State of New York. Address read at the opening meeting, Tarrytown, N. Y., with constitution and by-laws. Organized Jan. 9, 1872. 8°. *New York*, 1872.

TUTHILL (F.) Registration of births, deaths, and marriages. Trans. of the Med. Soc. of the State of New York. June, 1852. 8°. *Albany*, 1853.

New York (State).

VIELE (E. L.) The topography and physical resources of the State of New York. 8°. [*New York*], 1875.

Bacon (W.) Medical topographical report of the county of Tompkins. Tr. M. Soc. N. Y., Albany, 1836–7, iii, 25–39. ———. Medical topography of the county of Tioga. *Ibid.*, 151.—**Bailey** (T. H.) Hygiene of Putnam County. *Ibid.*, 1877, 337–346.—**Balch** (G. B.) Hygiene of Westchester County. *Ibid.*, 346–348.—**Barton.** Notice of the sulphur springs, in the county of Ontario and State of New-York. Phila. M. & Phys. J., 1804–5, i, pt. 2, 166–168.—**Brisbin** (O.) History of the diseases of Saratoga County. Tr. M. Soc. N. Y., Albany, 1847–9, vii, pt. 2, 60–66.—**Brown** (M.), jr. Sketch of the medical topography of the country that is watered by the upper streams of the Mohawk-river, and the adjacent streams of the Oneida-lake, N. Y. Phila. M. & Phys. J., 1806 (Suppl.), 1–9. *Also:* Am. M. & Phil. Reg., N. Y., 1813–14, iv, 170–179.—**Colden** (C.) Account of the climate and diseases of New York. Communicated by his grandson, C. D. Colden. Am. M. & Phil. Reg., 2. ed., N. Y., 1814, i, 304–310.—**Corliss** (H.) Brief notices of the medical topography and diseases of Washington County. Tr. M. Soc. N. Y., Albany, 1850, 225–229.—**Eastman** (H. N.) Report on the endemics and epidemics of Tioga County. Tr. M. Ass. South. Central N. Y., Auburn, 1850, 47–55.—**Foord** (A.) Medical topographical report of the county of Madison. Tr. M. Soc. N. Y., Albany, 1834–5, ii, 36–61.—**Frisbee** (J. H.) Sketch of the medical topography of the military tract of the State of New York. Phila. M. & Phys. J., 1806, ii, pt. 2, 69–85: 1808, iii, pt. 1, 143. *Also:* Am. M. & Phil. Reg., N. Y., 1813–14, iv, 48–62.—**Green** (C.) Vital statistics of Courtland County. Tr. M. Ass. South. Central N. Y., Auburn, 1852, 19–26.—**Hart** (R.) Topographical sketch of the county of Ontario, State of New York. Am. M. & Phil. Reg., N. Y., 1811–12, ii (2. ed., 1814). 150–154.—**Henderson** (H.) A topographical description of Jefferson County, in the State of New York. Med. Reposit., N. Y., 1811, 3. s., ii, 21–27.—**Hough** (F. B.) The census of New York, to be taken during the present year, considered in its medical relations. Tr. M. Soc. N. Y., Albany, 1865, 27–29.—**Jones** (D. T.) On the diseases of Onondaga County. *Ibid.*, 1847–9, vii, pt. 3, 131–134.—**Lee** (J.) Diseases of Saratoga County. Communicated to the Medical Society of the State of New York. *Ibid.*, 1859, 226–250. *Also*, Reprint.—**Ludlow** (E. G.) A statistical and medical account of the Genesee country, in the State of New York. N. York M. & Phys. J., 1823, ii, 65–105.—**McCall** (J.) Remarks on the diseases of Oneida County, N. Y., in 1854. N. York J. M., 1855, n. s., xiv, 264–268.—**Medical** topographical account of the county of Kings, N. Y. Tr. M. Soc. N. Y., Albany, 1832–3, i, 174–182.—**Medical** topographical report of the county of Columbia, [N. Y.]. *Ibid.*, 1834–5, 30–35.—**Medical** topographical report of the county of Onondaga. *Ibid.*, 1833–4, ii, 228–240.—**Mitchell** (S.) The prevailing fevers of Steuben County, N. Y. Boston M. & S. J., 1851–2, xlv, 321–330.—**Needham** (G.) Sketch of the medical topography of Onondaga, in the State of New York. Phila. M. & Phys. J., 1806 (Suppl.), 16–18.—**Orton** (J. G.) Medical and surgical statistics, from the county of Broome. For the year ending May, 1860, and the year ending May, 1861. Tr. M. Ass. South. Central N. Y., Binghamton, 1863, 77. ———. Report of committee on medical and surgical statistics. Tr. M. Soc. N. Y., Albany, 1863, 353.—**Porter** (E.) Medical topographical account of the county of Saratoga. *Ibid.*, 1832–3, 342–347.—**Shattuck** (L.) Contributions to the vital statistics of the State of New York. *Ibid.*, 1850, 100–125. *Also*, Reprint.—**Smith** (J. H.) On the medical topography and epidemics of the State of New York. Tr. Am. M. Ass.. Phila., 1860, xiii, 83–269. *Also*, Reprint.—**Sprague** (J. S.) History of some of the most common diseases in the county of Otsego, prepared in obedience to a resolution of the State Medical Society. Tr. M. Soc. N. Y., Albany, 1847–9, vii, pt. 2, 96–103.—**Thoms** (W. F.) On climatology and epidemics of the State of New York. Tr. Am. M. Ass., Phila., 1869, xx, 475, 1 tab.—**Waterbury** (R. L.) The medical topography of Delaware County. Tr. M. Soc. N. Y., Albany, 1870, 273–281.—**White** (J.) Medical topography of the county of Montgomery. *Ibid.*, 1850, 155–160.—**Willard** (A.) Remarks on the prevalent diseases of the counties of Chenango and Broome, New York, since the year 1807. N. York J. M., 1848, x, 68–72. ———. Mortuary statistics of the "Genesee country" for the year 1799. *Ibid.*, 1854, n. s., xiii, 395–398.—**Woodward** (W.) Report on the endemics and epidemics of Chemung County. Tr. M. Ass. South. Central N. Y., Auburn, 1850, 42–46.

New York (*State*). *Adjutant-General of the State of New York.* Annual reports of the . . . to the legislature, for the years 1861–5 ; 1867 ; 1869 ; 1870. 12 v. 8°. *Albany*, 1862–71.

1863 in 2 v.; 1864 in 2 v.; 1865 in 2 v.; 1867 in 3 v.

New York (*State*). *Adjutant-General of the State of New York*—continued.

——. Officers commissioned during the month of April, 1874. General headquarters, State of New York. Albany, May 1, 1874. 5 pp. 8°. [*Albany*, 1874.]

——. Annual reports to the governor of the State, for the years 1883; 1884. 116 pp.; 133 pp. 8°. *Albany, Weed, Parsons & Co.*, 1884-5.

New York (*State*). *Binghamton Asylum for the Chronic Insane.* By-laws and rules and regulations adopted July 9, 1879. 21 pp. 8°. *Hamilton, Democratic Republican Book & Job Office*, 1879.
Organized by act of the legislature, May 13, 1879.

——. Annual reports of the trustees and medical superintendent to the legislature. 1., 1879; 3., 1880-81; 5.-9., 1882-3 to 1886-7. 8°. *Albany & Troy*, 1880-88.
1. report for four months, ending September 30, 1879.

——. [Blank forms in use at the asylum.] fol. [*Albany*, 188-.]
Certificate of insanity; order of admission.

New York (*State*). *Board of Commissioners of Metropolitan Police.* See **New York** (*City*). *Police Department.*

New York (*State*). *Board of State Commissioners of Public Charities of the State of New York.* See **New York** (*State*). *State Board of Charities.*

New York (*State*). *Buffalo State Asylum for the Insane.* Annual reports of the board of managers to the legislature of the State. 1.-13., 1871 to 1882-3; 15.-17., 1884-5 to 1886-7. 8°. *Buffalo & Albany*, 1872-88.
Organized May 26, 1870; opened November 15, 1880. 2. and 3. reports in one. 9. for nine months, ending September 30, 1879. 1.-13., 1871 to 1883-4, bound in 1 v.

——. Proceedings in connection with the ceremony of laying the corner-stone in the city of Buffalo, Sept. 18, 1872. 31 pp., 1 pl. 8°. *Buffalo, White & Brayley*, 1872.
Bound with: Reports 1.-13., 1871 to 1882-3.

——. Order of exercises at the laying of the corner-stone, Sept. 18, 1872. 2 l. 8°. [*Buffalo*, 1872.]
Bound with: Reports 1.-13., 1871 to 1882-3.

——. Rules, regulations, and by-laws. 28 pp. 8°. *Buffalo*, [*E. H. Hutchinson*], 1881.
Bound with: Reports 1.-13., 1871 to 1882-3.

——. *See, also:*
NEW YORK (*State*). S. Report of the commissioners to locate an insane asylum in the eighth judicial district, New York. No. 8. January 20, 1870. 8°. [*Albany*, 1870.]

New York (*State*). *Central New York Institution for Deaf-Mutes, at Rome.* Annual reports and documents. By the board of trustees and principal to the legislature. 4., 1877-8; 5., 1878-9. 8°. *Albany*, 1879-80.

New York (*State*). *Commissary-General of Ordnance of the State of New York.* Annual reports to the legislature, for the years 1867; 1868. 8°. *Albany*, 1868-9.

New York (*State*). *Commissioner in Lunacy.* Annual report to the legislature. 6., 1878. 73 pp. 8°. *Albany, C. Van Benthuysen & Sons*, 1879.

New York (*State*). *Commissioners of Emigration of the State of New York.* Annual reports to the legislature. 6., 1852; 8., 1854; 9., 1855; 13., 1859; 21., 1867; 22., 1868; 27., 1873; 29., 1875; 31.-38., 1877-84; 40., 1886. 8°. *New York & Albany*, 1853-87.

——. An account of the proceedings at the laying of the corner-stone of the State Emigrant Hospital on Ward's Island. August 10, 1864. 43 pp., 1 pl. 8°. *New York, J. F. Trow*, 1865.

——. Immigration and the commissioners of emigration of the State of New York. By Frederick Kapp, one of the commissioners. 241 pp.,

New York (*State*), *Commissioners of Emigration of the State of New York*—continued.
7 pl., 1 plan. 8°. *New York, The Nation Press*, 1870.

——. Laws relating to the . . . (compiled by order of the board of commissioners). 226 pp. 8°. *New York, New York Printing Company*, 1871.
See, also, **New York** (*State*). Assembly. Report of the committee of investigation into the affairs of the . . . 8°. *Albany*, 1876.

——. Reply of the president of the . . . to a resolution of the Senate, adopted April 30, 1873 [relative to the salaries and wages paid to the officers and employés of the department]. State of New York. No. 94. In senate, May 6, 1873. 9 pp. 8°. [*Albany*, 1873.]

New York (*State*). *Commissioners of Fisheries.* Annual report to the legislature. 8. (1875). 59 pp. 8°. *Albany, J. B. Parmenter*, 1876.

New York (*State*). *Commissioners of Quarantine.* Port of New York, quarantine ground, Staten Island. Rules to be observed on board of all vessels detained at quarantine. 1 sheet. fol. [*New York*, 1856.] [P., v. 349.]

——. Annual reports, to which is annexed the annual reports of the health officer of the port of New York to the legislature, for the years 1864-76. 8°. *Albany*, 1865-77.

New York (*State*). *Commissioners of State Parks.* Annual report to the legislature. 1., 1872. 16 pp. 8°. [*Albany*, 1873.]

New York (*State*). *Commissioners of the State Reservation of Niagara.* Annual report to the legislature. 3., 1886. 37 pp. 8°. [*Albany*, 1887.]

——. Supplemental report. Transmitted to the legislature Jan. 31, 1887. 50 pp., 1 plan. 8°. *Albany, The Argus Company*, 1887.

New York (*State*). *Convention of Superintendents of the Poor of the State of New York.* Proceedings held at Buffalo, June 14-16, 1881 (11.). 67 pp. 8°. *Albany, Munsell*, 1881.

New York (*State*). *County Superintendents of the Poor.* Report and memorial on lunacy and its relation to pauperism, and for relief of insane poor. State of New York. In senate, Jan. 23, 1856. 20 pp. 8°. [*Albany*, 1856.]

New York (*State*). *Hudson River State Hospital for the Insane, at Poughkeepsie.* Annual reports of the managers to the legislature. 1.-3., 1867 to 1868-9; 5.-7., 1870-71 to 1872-3; 10.-13., 1875-6 to 1878-9; 15.-17., 1880-81 to 1882-3. 8°. *Albany*, 1868-83.
Established in 1867; opened Oct. 21, 1871. Designed for the treatment of acute insanity.

——. By-laws established by the managers of the . . . 14 pp. 8°. *Poughkeepsie*, 1873.

——. *See, also:*
NEW YORK (*State*). Communication from the governor, transmitting the report of the commissioners appointed to locate the Hudson River State Hospital for the Insane, at Poughkeepsie. Jan. 9, 1867. 8°. *Albany*, 1867.
NEW YORK (*State*). S. Report and testimony taken before the finance committee, with regard to the affairs and management of the Hudson River State Hospital for the Insane. No. 107. April 30, 1873. 8°. [*Albany*, 1873.]

New York (*State*). *Inspectors of State prisons.* Annual reports to the legislature. 19., 1865-6; 23., 1870; 24., 1871. 8°. *Albany*, 1867-82.

New York (*State*). *Marine Hospital at Quarantine, N. Y.* Annual reports of the physician-in-chief to the legislature of the State of New York, for the years 1849; 1855; 1856; 1858-60. 8°. *Albany*, 1850-61. [1856 also, in : P., v. 207.]

New York (*State*). *Metropolitan Board of Excise.* Annual report to the governor of the State.

New York (*State*). *Metrop. B'd Excise*—cont'd. 4., 1869. 45 pp. 8°. *New York, D. Appleton & Co.*, 1870.

New York (*State*). *Metropolitan Board of Health. See* **New York** (*City*). *Health Department.*

New York (*State*). *New York Institution for the Blind, at Binghamton.* Annual report of the board of trustees and superintendent to the legislature. 1., 1866. 88 pp. 8°. *Albany, C. Van Benthuysen & Sons*, 1867.

New York (*State*). *New York Institution for the Blind, in the City of New York.* Annual reports of the managers to the legislature. 1., 1836; 3., 1838; 4., 1839; 6.-11., 1841-6; 13.-16., 1848-51; 18.-20., 1853-5; 23.-28., 1858-63; 30.-32., 1865-7; 35., 1870; 40., 1874-5; 42.-49., 1876-7 to 1883-4. 8°. *New York*, 1837-84.

Incorporated April 1, 1831; organized March 15, 1832.

——. A brief account of its organization, character, and privileges. 11 pp. 12°. *New York, Purcy & Reed*, 1843.

——. A review of the efforts of the ... to instruct its pupils in mechanical trades, and to maintain a manufacturing establishment in connection with its educational work from 1831 to 1885. 7 pp. 8°. *New York*, 1885.

New York (*State*). *New York Institution for the Instruction of the Deaf and Dumb.* Circular of the president and directors. And petition to the mayor, aldermen, and commonalty of the city of New York, with their favorable report and patronage, etc. 15 pp. 8°. *New York, E. Conrad*, 1818.

Incorporated April 15, 1817; opened May, 1818.

——. An act to incorporate the members of the ... passed April 15, 1817. To which is added the by-laws and the names and residences of the officers and directors. Also, the directors arranged into committees, and a list of the pupils. 23 pp. 8°. *New York, E. Conrad*, 1819.

——. Address of the directors to their fellow-citizens. 8 pp. 8°. *New York, E. Conrad*, 1821.

——. Annual reports of the directors to the legislature. 7.-11., 1825-9; 13., 1831; 14., 1832; 16., 1834; 18.-45., 1836-63; 49.-62., 1867-80; 64., 1881-2. 8°. *New York & Albany*, 1826-83.

22.-24., 50.-61. bound in 7 v.

——. Mr. Peet's letter of instruction. Report on the institutions for the deaf and dumb in central and western Europe, in the year 1844, to the board of directors of the New York Institution. By George E. Day, delegate of the board. 79, 202 pp. 8°. *Albany, Carroll & Cook*, 1845.

——. Address delivered at the ... Dec. 2, 1846, by Harvey P. Peet, president of the institution. With an appendix containing the proceedings at the dedication of the chapel. 40 pp. 8°. *New York, Hovey & Ring*, 1847.

Bound with: Reports 1845-9.

——. Order of ceremonies on laying the corner-stone of the ... at Washington Heights, New York, Nov. 22, 1855. 34 pp. 8°. *New York, G. F. Nesbit & Co.*, 1853.

——. Biographical sketch of Harvey Prindle Peet, president of the ... with a history of the institution. 41 pp., port. 8°. *New York, D. Van Nostrand*, 1857.

Repr. from: Barnard's Am. J. of Education, June, 1857.

New York (*State*). *New York Soldiers' Depot.* Annual reports of the board of managers of the ... and of the fund for the relief of sick, wounded, furloughed, and discharged soldiers, transmitting the report of the general agent of the State, for the years 1864 and 1865. 8°. *Albany*, 1864-5.

New York (*State*). *New York State Asylum for Idiots, at Syracuse.* Annual reports of the trustees and superintendent to the legislature. 1.-4., 1851-4; 8.-27., 1857-8 to 1876-7; 29.-34., 1878-9 to 1883-4. 8°. *Albany*, 1852-84.

Established July 10 and opened in Oct., 1851, at Albany; in 1854, removed to Syracuse. 1. report for three months, Oct. to Dec., 1851.

New York (*State*). *New York State Inebriate Asylum, at Binghamton.* Addresses of Henry W. Bellows and Roswell D. Hitchcock, delivered at the Broadway Tabernacle, Nov. 7, 1855, in behalf of the United States Inebriate Asylum. Also J. Edward Turner's address to the board of directors. Charter and amendments. 48 pp. 8°. *New York, M. B. Wynkoop*, 1855.

——. The same [with amendments to the charter, changing the title to "The New York State Inebriate Asylum", at Binghamton, March 27, 1857]. 54 pp. 8°. *New York, Wynkoop, Hallenbeck & Thomas*, 1857.

Incorporated April 15, 1854, as the United States Inebriate Asylum in the City of New York. Changed title to above April 7, 1857, by act of the legislature. Corner-stone laid Sept. 24, 1858. Temporarily closed in Oct., 1866, and reopened May 1, 1867. By an act passed May 27, 1873, the State fully adopted the institution, and reorganized it under the control of a board of managers, in lieu of the former board of trustees, who had corporate powers. It was converted into an asylum for the chronic insane, in accordance with chap. 280 of the laws of 1879, and is now known as the Binghamton Asylum for the Chronic Insane. Report for 1867, for 8 months, May to Dec. Report for 1873, called 1. after reorganization.

——. A letter from the corresponding secretary to the governor of the State of New York, on the subject of appropriation, dated Dec. 22, 1857. 20 pp. 8°. *New York, Wynkoop, Hallenbeck & Thomas*, 1858.

——. An appeal of the trustees to the American clergymen, in behalf of the Inebriate Asylum. Oct. 27, 1859. 7 pp. 8°. [*New York*, 1859.]

——. A letter of the corresponding secretary of the ... [J. Edward Turner] to Hon. Edwin D. Morgan, governor-elect of the State of New York. 91-126 pp. 8°. [*New York*, 1859.]

Cutting from: Ceremonies, etc. 8°. New York, 1859.

——. Ceremonies, etc. [at the laying of the corner-stone]. 161 pp. 8°. *New York, Wynkoop, Hallenbeck & Thomas*, 1859.

——. The same. 184 pp. 8°. *Binghamton, Wynkoop, Hallenbeck & Thomas*, 1859.

——. An appeal of the trustees to the churches of the United States and the American public in behalf of that institution. April 4, 1859. pp. 157-169. 8°. [*New York*, 1859.]

Cutting. Bound with the following.

——. To the trustees and stockholders of the New York State Inebriate Asylum. [Being a statement of the resident trustees to the non-resident trustees and stockholders on the management and discipline of the institution. Sept., 1866.] 47 pp. 8°. [*Binghamton*, 1866.]

——. The charter and by-laws of the ... Amendments of charter and special acts. Rules and regulations adopted by the board of trustees. 27 pp. 8°. *New York, Wynkoop & Hallenbeck*, 1866.

——. Report of the trustees in answer to a resolution presented by Assemblyman Little, of Steuben [on the present condition of the institution]. 5 pp. 8°. [*Albany*, 1868.]

——. Annual reports of the board of managers and superintendent to the legislature, for the years 1867-72. Also, 1., 1873; 2., 1874; 5., 1877. 8°. *Albany*, 1868-78.

——. A circular by the superintendent. 15 pp. 8°. *Binghamton, Lawyer Bros.*, 1870.

——. The charter and by-laws of the ... amendments of charter and special acts. 16 pp. 8°. *New York, State Inebriate Asylum, Record Office*, 1873.

New York (*State*). *New York State Inebriate Asylum, at Binghamton*—continued.

——. Circular to the county clerks, county judges, and superintendents of the poor of the several counties of the State of New York, giving notice of the number each county is entitled to according to the act of reorganization. May 27, 1873. 2 l. 4°. [*Binghamton*, 1876.]

——. *See, also*:

Burr (G.) The New York State Inebriate Asylum. A defence of its management and operations. Tr. M. Soc. N. Y., Syracuse, 1881, 317–336. *Also*, Reprint.

New York (*State*). *New York State Institution for the Blind, at Batavia.* Annual reports of the trustees and officers to the legislature. 1.–3., 1868–9 to 1870–71 ; 5.–16., 1872–3 to 1883–4. 8°. *Albany*, 1869–85.

1868–9 is called 3. report of the trustees, but it is the first report after the opening at Batavia.

——. *See, also*:

HOWE (S. G.) Address delivered at the ceremony of laying the corner-stone of the New York State Institution for the Blind, at Batavia, Sept. 3, 1866. 8°. *Boston*, 1866.

New York (*State*). *New York State Library.* Annual reports of the trustees to the legislature of the State of New York. 52., 1869 ; 56., 1873 ; 59., 1876 ; 60., 1877 ; 62.–66., 1879–83 ; 68., 1885 ; 69., 1886. 8°. *Albany*, 1870–87.

New York (*State*). *New York State Reformatory at Elmira.* Reply of the building commissioners of the . . . to a resolution of the senate passed March 20, 1873, requesting information relative to the condition of said building, now in process of construction. State of New York. No. 74. In senate, April 4, 1873. 49 pp. 8°. [*Albany*, 1873.]

Opened July 24, 1876.

——. Annual reports of the board of managers to the legislature. 4.–10., 1878–9 to 1884–5. 8°. *Elmira*, 1880–85.

Report made in 1878 not printed.

New York (*State*). *Quartermaster-General of the State of New York.* Annual report to the governor of the State of New York, for the year 1868. 28 pp. 8°. *Albany, Argus Co.*, 1869.

New York (*State*). *Saint Lawrence State Asylum for the Insane, Point Airy, near Ogdensburgh.* Annual report of the managers to the legislature. 1., 1887. 34 pp. 8°. *Troy, Press Co.*, 1888.

Established by act passed May 18, 1888.

New York (*State*). *Secretary of State of the State of New York.* Annual reports in relation to the statistics of the poor, to the legislature, for the years 1866–7 ; 1870–71. 8°. *Albany*, 1867–71.

——. Annual reports on criminal statistics for the years 1870–71 ; 1874–5. 8°. [*Albany*, 1872–6.]

New York (*State*). *State Agent for Discharged Convicts.* Annual report to the legislature. 1., 1878. 18 pp. 8°. *Albany, C. Van Benthuysen & Sons*, 1879.

New York (*State*). *State Asylum for Insane Criminals, at Auburn.* Annual reports of the medical superintendent to the superintendent of State prisons. 1., 1858–9 ; 1.–6., 1859–60 to 1864–5 ; 8., 1866–7 ; 11.–14., 1869–70 to 1872–3 ; 17.–28., 1875–6 to 1886–7. 8°. *Albany & Troy*, 1860–88.

No reports made for 1873–4 or 1874–5.

——. By-laws and rules and regulations governing the . . . adopted by the superintendent of State prisons, Nov. 1, 1884, and approved by the State commissioner in lunacy Dec. 1, 1884. 20 pp. 8°. *Auburn, News & Bulletin print*, 1884.

——. [Blank forms in use at the asylum.] v. s. [*Auburn*, 188–.]

Movements of patients.
Monthly report.
Report of night watchman (daily).

New York (*State*). *State Board of Charities.* Annual reports to the legislature. 2.–17., 1868–83. 8°. *Albany*, 1869–84.

——. Report of the board of State commissioners of public charities, relating to the insane and the capacity and cost of the several State insane asylums. 16 pp. 8°. *Albany, Argus Co.*, 1871. [*Also, in*: P., v. 223.]

——. Report of the board of State commissioners of public charities in answer to the resolution of the senate of Feb. 14, 1871, relating to the insane and the capacity and cost of the several State insane asylums. Transmitted to the legislature March 9, 1871. Containing also an extract from the fourth annual report of the secretary of the board relating to county poor-houses. 16 pp. 8°. *Albany, Argus Co.*, 1872.

——. Report of the board of State commissioners of public charities concerning the management of the dispensary and hospital society of the Women's Institute of New York City, and the testimony taken by the board. 43 pp. 8°. *Albany, Argus Company*, 1872.

——. Eighth annual report of the State board of charities. Extract relating to pauper and destitute children. By William P. Letchworth. 91 pp., 1 ch. 8°. *Albany, Weed, Parsons & Co.*, 1875.

——. Eighth annual report of the . . . Extract relating to out-door relief. By M. B. Anderson. 32 pp. 8°. *Albany, Weed, Parsons & Co.*, 1875.

——. Extract from the ninth annual report of the . . . relating to the bearing of the sanitary condition of towns, and the crowding of population into filthy, ill-ventilated, and badly-drained tenement houses, upon the increase of pauperism. Transmitted to the legislature Jan. 14, 1875. 32 pp. 8°. *Albany, Weed, Parsons & Co.*, 1876.

——. A communication to the mayor of New York in regard to the official charities of the city, from Theodore Roosevelt, Josephine Shaw Lowell, and Edward C. Donnelly, commissioners of the State board of charities. 26 pp. 8°. *Albany, J. Munsell*, 1877.

——. Communication from the . . . in relation to the chronic insane of Clinton County, State of New York. No. 44. In assembly, Feb. 8, 1878. 8 pp. 8°. [*Albany*, 1878.]

——. First report of the committee on the abuses of medical charities, comprising the answers received from the general dispensaries of New York. 16 pp. 8°. [*New York*], *G. F. Nesbitt & Co.*, 1878.

——. The chronic insane under county care. Report on the condition of the chronic insane in certain counties exempted by the State board of charities from the operation of the Willard Asylum act. 12 pp. 8°. [*Albany*, 1882.]

——. Public official care of orphan and destitute children versus private beneficence. Letter regarding assembly bill No. 121, entitled " An act to incorporate the Home for the Destitute Children of Suffolk County ", addressed to the judiciary committee of the assembly by Commissioner Letchworth, of the State board of charities. 7 pp. 8°. [*Albany*, 1883.]

——. In the matter of the investigation of the New York City Asylum for the Insane. Report. Aug. 12, 1887. 43 pp. 8°. [*Albany*, 1887.]

——. Blank forms. Doc. No. 2. List of beneficiaries. Doc. No. 3. Return for directory. 4°. [*Albany, n. d.*]

See, also, New York (*City*). *Department of Public Charities.*

New York (*State*). *State Board of Health of the State of New York.* Manual of the . . . 74 pp. 8°. *Albany, Argus Co.*, 1880.

Established May 18 and organized May 29, 1880.

New York (*State*). *State Board of Health of the State of New York*—continued.

——. Memorandum concerning ways and means for securing the registry of births, marriages, and deaths to the State of New York. 4 pp. 8°. [*Albany*, 1880.]

——. To the boards of supervisors, clerks of towns, villages, and school-districts and to local boards of health in the State of New York. [Circular of the committee on vital statistics, calling attention to the laws relating to the registration of births, marriages, and deaths.] June 18, 1880. 2 pp. 8°. [*Albany*, 1880.]

——. Circular to local boards of health, informing them of the organization of the State board, and requesting copies of all their reports. July 1, 1880. 3 pp. 8°. [*Albany*, 1880.]

——. Circular to county supervisors, relating to the registration of births, marriages, and deaths, submitting facts concerning the methods which are necessary to success. Oct. 15, 1880. 4 pp. 8°. [*Albany*, 1880.]

——. Proposed model sanitary ordinances, regulations, and orders. [Adopted by the State board of health and recommended to local sanitary authorities for their adoption. Nov. 11, 1880.] 8 pp. 8°. [*Albany*, 1880.]

——. Circular, explanatory of the forms and methods of record authorized by the board. Galley sheet. [*Albany*, 1880.]

——. [Circulars, reports, rules, and memoranda issued by the . . .] 8°. *Albany*, 1880–84.

No. 10. Ready references to the laws and reports published by direction of the . . . Oct., 1880. 1 sheet. 8°. [*Albany*, 1880.]

No. 13. Prevention of diphtheria. March, 1881. 1 l. 8°. [*Albany*, 1881.]

No. 14. Sanitary rules for the prevention of scarlet fever. March, 1881. 1 l. 8°. [*Albany*, 1881.]

No. 15. Sanitary precautions to prevent the spreading of infectious diseases. April, 1881. 1 l. 8°. [*Albany*, 1881.]

No. 16. Instructions for disinfection. As prepared under the direction of the National Board of Health. Issued by the . . . 1 l. 8°. [*Albany*, 1881.]

No. 17. Vaccination notice. Feb. 9, 1881. 1 sheet. 8°. [*Albany*, 1881.]

No. 22. To parents, guardians, and all who are concerned in the registration of births. With blank form for full given-name. 1 l. 16°. [*Albany*, 1881.]

No. 23. Abstract of the several acts of the legislature of 1881, imposing new duties on the State board of health of New York. July 30, 1881. 4 pp. 8°. [*Albany*, 1881.]

No. 24. Concerning the law to prevent adulteration of food and drugs. June 25, 1881. 4 pp. 8°. [*Albany*, 1881.]

No. 24ª. An act to prevent the adulteration of food or drugs. [Bound with no. 24.]

No. 25. The amended public health laws. Powers and duties of local boards. 2 pp. 8°. [*Albany*, 1881.]

No. 25ª. The organization, powers, and duties of local boards of health. (The State board of health invites the attention of local boards to this recently amended statute, defining the powers and duties of local sanitary officers.) "An act for the preservation of the public health." 4 pp. 8°. [*Albany*, 1881.]

No. 26. Extract from report of committee on sanitary rules and regulations. 4 pp. 8°. [*Albany*, 1881.]

No. 27. Duties and procedures of local boards of health and their officers. Examples, methods, and suggestions. With an appended memorandum on contagious disease refuges; temporary hospitals for small-pox and other pestilential maladies. 14 pp. 8°. [*Albany*, 1882.]

No. 27ª. Contagious disease refuges; temporary hospitals for small-pox and other pestilent contagions. Prepared and distributed under instructions, by E. Harris, sec. 4 pp. 8°. [*Albany*, 1881.]

No. 27ᵇ. Specification of material for contagious disease refuges. 1 l. 8°. [*Albany*, 1881.]

No. 28. Organization of the chemical examination of food and drugs, for prevention of adulterations, etc. (under chap. 407 of the laws of 1881). 2 pp. 8°. [*Albany*, 1881.]

No. 30ª. To health officers; cards for the use of physicians to make monthly returns. [With blank form no. 30.] 16°. [*Albany*, 1881.]

No. 33. Circular of sanitary committee on the public and domestic water supplies of cities and towns, with schedule of questions. 4 pp. 8°. [*Albany*, 1881.]

No 34. Circular of inquiry concerning malaria in the State of New York. [With blank form no. 34ª.] Sept., 1881. 1 l. 8°. [*Albany*, 1881.]

New York (*State*). *State Board of Health of the State of New York*—continued.

No. 35. School buildings and the hygiene of public schools. [With blank form no. 35ª.] 1 l. 8°. [*Albany*, 1881.]

No. 36. To boards of health and local registering officers; rules to be observed in the public registration of deaths, births, and marriages, and in the regulation of burials. Oct. 28, 1881. 1 l. 8°. [*Albany*, 1881.]

No. 36ᵇ. To public carriers; State regulations concerning the transit permits for burials beyond county limits. Oct., 1881. 1 sheet. 8°. [*Albany*, 1881.]

No. 36ᶜ. Concerning vital statistics and certified records. 1 sheet. 8°. [*Albany*, 1881.]

No. 37. To supervisors, town clerks, and local boards, presenting facts and suggestions concerning certain amendments to the laws on the registration of births, marriages, and deaths. Nov. 14, 1881. 2 pp. 8°. [*Albany*, 1881.]

No. 37ª. Suggesting the adoption of a fee for every complete record of a birth, marriage, or death. [Bound with no. 37.]

No. 38. Prevention of small-pox; duties of the local authorities, health officers and others. 4 pp. 8°. [*Albany*, 1882.]

No. 40. Bureau of chemical analysis to prevent adulteration of food and drugs. Catalogue of the literature of the chemistry of food and drugs. Prepared for the use of the analysts and inspectors under the State board of New York. By Albert L. Colby. 12 pp. 8°. *Albany; C. Van Benthuysen & Sons*, 1881.

No. 41. Memorandum of rules to be adopted to prevent the spreading of contagious diseases in schools. Jan., 1882. 2 l. 8°. [*Albany*, 1882.]

No. 42. Report to the State board of health on the methods of sewerage for cities and large villages in the State of New York. By James T. Gardiner. 15 pp. 8°. *Albany, Weed, Parsons & Co.*, 1882. [*Repr. from*: Rep. Bd. Health N. Y. 1881, Albany, 1882, ii.]

No. 43. Health in the common schools. Practical illustrations and conclusions relating to essential sanitary requirements of school-houses. For use of school officers and teachers. 41 pp. 8°. *Albany, Weed, Parsons & Co.*, 1882. [*Repr. from*: Rep. Bd. Health N. Y. 1881, Albany, 1882, ii.]

No. 44. Notes on contagious diseases of the eyes in schools and asylums. By Cornelius R. Agnew. 9 pp. 8°. [*Albany*, 1882.] [*Repr. from*: Rep. Bd. Health N. Y. 1881, Albany, 1882, ii.]

No. 45. Report on the methods and apparatus for testing inflammable oils. Based upon investigations ordered by the State board of health, for establishing a standard safety-test of illuminating oils. By Arthur H. Elliott. 45 pp. 8°. *Albany, Weed, Parsons & Co.*, 1882. [*Repr. from*: Rep. Bd. Health N. Y. 1881, Albany, 1882, ii.]

No. 46. Preliminary statement relating to the law for safety testing illuminating oils. June 24, 1882. 2 pp. 8°. [*Albany* 1882.]

No. 53. Organization of the local board of health. Sanitary laws and regulations obligatory upon the inhabitants of the town. And [rules to be observed in the public registration of deaths, births, and marriages, and in the regulation of burials]. 4 pp. 8°. [*Albany*, 1883.]

No. 65. Nomenclature of diseases. 16 pp. fol. [*Albany*, 1884.]

——. Report on the nuisances of Hunter's Point and vicinity, and message of the governor, accompanying the same. (Transmitted to the legislature April 22, 1881.) 27 pp. 8°. *Weed, Parsons & Co.*, 1881.

——. Suggestions and rules for the proper keeping of these registration records. [Accompanied by blank form specimen.] 1 sheet. fol. [*Albany*, 1881.]

——. Annual reports to the governor of the State. 1.–7., 1880–86. 8°. *Albany*, 1881-7.

——. Memorandum concerning cholera. 4 pp. 8°. [*Albany*, 1884.]

——. Opinion of attorney-general regarding powers to abate nuisances. 2 pp. 8°. [*Albany*, 1884.]

——. Report on the drainage of the Tonawanda and Oak-Orchard swamps. 70 pp., 4 plans. 8°. [*Albany*, 1884.]

Repr. from: Rep. State Bd. Health N. Y. 1883, Albany, 1884, iv.

——. Report on malaria at Castleton, Rensselaer County. [By Wm. S. Egerton, C. E., and Geo. Fred. Brooks, inspector.] 4 pp. 8°. [*Albany*, 1884.]

Repr. from: Rep. State Bd. Health N. Y. 1883, Albany, 1884, iv.

New York (*State*). *State Board of Health of the State of New York*—continued.

———. Report on sudden outbreak of enteric fever at Port Jervis, during the fall of 1883. By F. C. Curtis. 23 pp., 1 map, 1 plan. 8°. [*Albany*, 1884.]
Repr. from: Rep. State Bd. Health N. Y. 1883, Albany, 1884, iv.

———. Report on the system of sewerage for the village of Peekskill. 8 pp., 1 plan. 8°. [*Albany*, 1884.]
Repr. from: Rep. State Bd. Health N. Y. 1883, Albany, 1884, iv.

———. Monthly bulletins of the . . . Abstract of reports of deaths and their causes in districts, cities, and towns, from April, 1884, to April, 1888. 4°. [*Albany*, 1884-8.]

———. Report on a law for the sanitary protection of water supplies. By James T. Gardiner. 8 pp. 8°. [*Albany*, 1885.]
Repr. from: Rep. State Bd. Health N. Y. 1884, Albany, 1885, v.

———. Report on plan of sewerage for the village of Malone. 14 pp., 1 map, 1 plan. 8°. [*Albany*, 1885.]
Repr. from: Rep. State Bd. Health N. Y. 1884, Albany, 1885, v.

———. Report on the policy of the State respecting drainage of large swamps. By James T. Gardiner. 7 pp. 8°. [*Albany*, 1885.]
Repr. from: Rep. State Bd. Health N. Y. 1884, Albany, 1885, v.

———. Report on the proposed use of an abandoned burial ground for the erection of a school-house at Port Jervis. 4 pp. 8°. [*Albany*, 1885.]
Repr. from: Rep. State Bd. Health N. Y. 1884, Albany, 1885, v.

———. Report on the sanitary condition of Havana, [N. Y.]. By O. S. Wilson. 8 pp. 8°. [*Albany*, 1885.]
Repr. from: Rep. State Bd. Health N. Y. 1884, Albany, 1885, v.

———. Report on the sanitary condition of that part of Port Richmond drainage into the so-called Port Richmond ditch. 5 pp. 8°. [*Albany*, 1885.]
Repr. from: Rep. State Bd. Health N. Y. 1884, Albany, 1885, v.

———. Report on the sanitary condition of the city of Schenectady. 16 pp., 1 map. 8°. [*Albany*, 1885.]
Repr. from: Rep. State Bd. Health N. Y. 1884, Albany, 1885, v.

———. Report on the sewerage of the city of Kingston. 12 pp. 8°. [*Albany*, 1885.]
Repr. from: Rep. State Bd. Health N. Y. 1884, Albany, 1885, v.

———. Report on the sewerage of Mount Vernon, Westchester County. By Horace Andrews, jr. 15 pp., 2 pl. 8°. [*Albany*, 1885.]
Repr. from: Rep. State Bd. Health N. Y. 1884, Albany, 1885, v.

———. Report on the unsanitary condition of the village of Bath, and the remedies therefor. 22 pp., 1 plan. 8°. [*Albany*, 1885.]
Repr. from: Rep. State Bd. Health N. Y. 1884, Albany, 1885, v.

———. Introductory [to the] fifth annual report of the State board of health. 23 pp. 8°. [*Albany*, 1885.]

———. Report on diphtheria at Sandy Hill. 13 pp. 8°. [*Albany*, 1886.]
Repr. from: Rep. State Bd. Health N. Y. 1885, Albany, 1886, vi.

———. Report on the examination of beers. 35 pp. 8°. [*Albany*, 1886.]
Repr. from: Rep. State Bd. Health N. Y. 1885, Albany, 1886, vi.

———. Report of the executive committee on the work and expenditures of the board, from its organization to close of its last fiscal year. 13 pp. 8°. [*Albany*, 1886.]
Repr. from: Rep. State Bd. Health N. Y. 1885, Albany, 1886, vi.

New York (*State*). *State Board of Health of the State of New York*—continued.

———. Report on the practical operation of the separate system of sewers. 27 pp. 8°. [*Albany*, 1886.]
Repr. from: Rep. State Bd. Health N. Y. 1885, Albany, 1886, vi.

———. Report on the purity of ice from Onondaga Lake, the Erie canal at Syracuse, and from Cazenovia Lake. [By James T. Gardiner, consulting engineer. With appendices A–J.] 60 pp. 8°. [*Albany?* 1885.]

———. Report of the secretary, for the year 1885. 27 pp. 8°. [*Albany*, 1886.]
Repr. from: Rep. State. Bd. Health N. Y. 1885, Albany, 1886, vi.

———. Report of the sewerage of Mt. Vernon. 33 pp. 8°. [*Albany*, 1886.]
Repr. from: Rep. State Bd. Health N. Y. 1885, Albany, 1886, vi.

———. Summary of mortality of the State of New York, as published in the monthly bulletin. Totals of mortality in the State by months. For the years 1885-7. 4°. *Albany*, 1886-8.

———. Report of the State board of health on the sanitary qualities of water supplies proposed for the city of Syracuse. Prepared by James T. Gardiner, 1887. 79 pp. 8°. *Syracuse, Journal Co.*, 1887.

———. [Blank forms used by . . .] v. s. [*Albany, n. d.*]
No. 1. Birth return.
No. 2. Return of still-birth.
No. 3. Certificate of death.
No. 4. The same. [A filled sample.]
No. 5. Burial permit.
No. 6. Transit permit.
No. 7. Return of a marriage.
No. 22. Return of full given-name of infant.
No. 30. Report of prevalent diseases and deaths, to local boards.
No. 31. Small-pox records.
No. 32. Diphtheria records.
No. 34ª. Response to circular no. 34, concerning malaria.
No. 35. Response to circular no. 35, relating to school buildings.
No. 36. To public carriers, State regulations concerning the transit permits of burials beyond county limits.
No. 39. Record of vaccination.

New York (*State*). *State Board of Health of the State of New York. Bureau of Vital Statistics.* A concise statement concerning the elements of registration which are essential and obligatory. 1 sheet. 8°. [*Albany*, 1880.]

———. [Blank forms used by the . . .] v. s. [*Albany, v. d.*]
No. 1. Birth-return.
2. Return of still-birth.
3. Certificate of death.
4. The same. [A filled sample.]
5. Burial permit.
6. Transit permit.
7. Return of marriage.
22. Return of full given-name of infant.
30. Report of prevalent diseases and deaths, to local boards.
31. Small-pox records.
32. Diphtheria records.

New York (*State*). *State Cabinet of Natural History.* Annual reports of the regents of the University of the State of New York, on the condition of the . . . and on the historical and antiquarian collection annexed thereto, to the legislature. 3. (1849); 8. (1854); 20. (1866). 8°. *Albany*, 1850-67.
Also, a copy of revised ed. of 3. rep. 8°. *Albany*, 1850.

New York (*State*). *State Homœopathic Asylum for the Insane, Middletown.* Annual reports of the trustees and medical superintendent to the legislature. 4.-17., 1873-4 to 1886-7. 8°. *Albany & Troy*, 1874-88.
Organized in 1869; incorporated April, 1870; opened April 20, 1874. Report for 1873-4 was the first published.

New York (*State*). *State Homœopathic Asylum for the Insane, Middletown*—continued.
——. Rules and regulations for the government of employees. 18 pp. 8°. *Middletown, Stivers & Slauson,* 1879.
——. Rules and regulations of the fire brigade of the New York State Homœopathic Asylum. 5 pp. 16°. [*Middletown, n. d.*]

New York (*State*). *State Lunatic Asylum, at Utica.* Report of the trustees with the documents accompanying the same, pursuant to the act of the legislature passed May 26, 1841. [Appointed to visit institutions for the keeping and management of lunatics in this and other States.] 231 pp. 1 l. 8°. *Albany,* 1841.
  Organized in 1842; opened January 16, 1843.
——. Report of the commissioners of the Lunatic Asylum to his excellency Wm. H. Seward, governor of the State, Nov. 12, 1841. pp. 61–63. 8°. [*Albany,* 1841.]
  Cutting.
——. Annual reports of the board of managers and superintendent to the legislature. 1.–43., 1843 to 1884–5. 8°. *Albany,* 1844–86.
  1.–38., 1843 to 1879–80, bound in 3 v.
——. Laws and regulations for the admission and discharge of patients, August, 1864. 15 pp. 8°. *Utica, N. Y., Curtiss & White,* 1864.
——. Rules, regulations, and by-laws of the . . . 32 pp. 8°. *Utica, D. P. White,* 1866.
——. [Blank forms in use at the asylum.] fol. [*Albany,* 188–.]
  Bond of friend.
  Directions and information in cases of private patients.
  History of patient.
  Medical certificate of lunacy.
  Order of superintendent of the poor of county for admission.
——. Rules and regulations of the New York State Lunatic Asylum. 41 pp. 8°. *Utica, E. H. Roberts & Co.,* [*n. d.*]
——. Medulla oblongata. Case of general paralysis. By Theodore Deecke, special pathologist; John P. Gray, medical superintendent. 25 pl. imp. fol. [*Utica? n. d.*]
—— *See, also:*
  ASYLUM (The) investigation. Dr. Tourtelot's testimony finally completed; the evidence of present and former managers; the investigation temporarily closed. [*Utica,* 1883.]
  Cutting from: Utica Morning Herald, April 10, 1883.
  NEW YORK (*State*). Assembly. Report of the select committee on so much of the governor's message as relates to the Lunatic Asylum. April 22, 1841. 8°. [*Albany,* 1841.]
  NEW YORK (*State*). S. Report of the minority of the committee on medical societies and medical colleges on the bill in relation to the State Lunatic Asylum. April 23, 1844. 8°. [*Albany,* 1844.]
  NEW YORK (*State*). Assembly. Report of the select committee, to which was referred the memorial of Dr. Saunders and others, asking for an investigation into the causes of the death of Norris Tarbell, at the State Lunatic Asylum at Utica. Transmitted to the legislature, April 16, 1860. 8°. *Albany,* 1860.

New York (*State*). *State Prison or Penitentiary House, in the City of New York.* An account of the . . . By one of the inspectors of the prison. 97 pp., 2 pl. 8°. *New York, J. Collins & Son,* 1801.

New York (*State*). *Superintendent of Common Schools.* Annual reports of the . . . in relation to the Central Asylum for the Instruction of the Deaf and Dumb, at Canajoharie, and the New York Institution for the Instruction of the Deaf and Dumb, to the legislature, for the years 1829; 1831; 1834. 8°. [*Albany,* 1830–35.]

New York (*State*). *Superintendent of the Onondaga Salt Springs.* Annual reports of the . . . to the legislature, for the years 1850; 1851; 1867–69. 8°. *Albany,* 1851–70.

New York (*State*). *Superintendent of Public Instruction.* Annual report of the . . . to the legislature. 24., 1877. 71 pp. 8°. *Albany, J. B. Parmenter,* 1878.

New York (*State*). *Surgeon-General of the State of New York.* Annual reports of the . . . to the governor of the State, for the years 1861–3; 1865. 8°. *Albany,* 1862–6.

New York (*State*). *Tenement-House Commission.* Report of . . . 12 pp. 8°. [*New York,* 1884.]
  Organized June 11, 1884.
——. Forms. 5 l. 8°. [*New York,* 1884.]

New York (*State*). *Western House of Refuge for Juvenile Delinquents.* Annual reports of the board of managers to the legislature. 1., 1849; 2., 1850; 7.–10., 1855–8; 12.–33., 1860 to 1880–81. 8°. *Albany & Rochester,* 1850–82.
  14.–32. bound in 2 v.
——. Report of special committee to the managers of the House of Refuge, on the investigation by the State commissioners of public charities of charges made through the public press against the officers and managers of the House of Refuge, with memorial to the commissioners and their report. 30 pp. 8°. *New York, Thitchener & Glastaeter,* 1872.

New York (*State*). *Western New York Institution for Deaf Mutes, at Rochester.* Annual reports of the board of trustees and principal to the legislature of the State of New York. 1.–3., 1876–7 to 1878–9. 8°. *Albany,* 1878–80.

New York (*State*). *Willard Asylum for the Insane.* Annual report of the commissioners for erecting the . . . to the comptroller of the State of New York for the year 1868. 5 pp. 8°. [*Albany,* 1869.]
  Established April 8, 1865, for the chronic insane; opened Oct. 12, 1869.
——. Laws, rules, and regulations for the government of the . . . adopted July 1, 1869. 52 pp. 8°. *Seneca Falls, N. Y., Reveille Book and Job Office,* 1869. [P., v. 362.]
——. Annual reports of the board of trustees and superintendent to the legislature. 1.–19., 1869 to 1886–7. 8°. *Albany,* 1870–87.
  1.–12., 1869 to 1879–80, bound in 1 v.
——. Laws relating to the . . . and rules and regulations of said asylum. Adopted July 1, 1869. Revised Oct. 15, 1884. 59, ii pp. 8°. *Buffalo, Baker, Jones & Co.,* 1884.
——. Plans and elevations and a historical sketch of the . . . at Willard, on Seneca Lake, N. Y. 5 l., 7 plans. 8°. *Willard, Willard Asylum press,* 1887.
——. [Blank forms in use at the asylum.] v. s. [*Buffalo,* 188–.]
  Admissions (monthly).
  Bond for peaceable behavior, etc.
  Case-book form.
  Certificate of discharge.
  Certificate of insanity.
  Daily medical report.
  Day report.
  General summary of day reports.
  Name; diagnosis.
  Notice of superintendent of admission.

New York (*University of the City of*).
  Editorial (An) chameleon. Am. Eclect. M. Rev., N. Y., 1872, viii, 47–52. *Also,* Reprint.

New York Academy of Medicine. Constitution and by-laws of the . . . 2 l. fol. [*New York,* 1847.]
——. Code of medical ethics adopted by the American Medical Association and by the New York Academy of Medicine, in Oct., 1847. 24 pp. 8°. *New York,* 1848.

New York Academy of Medicine—continued.
——. Constitution and by-laws, with list of officers and fellows. 20 pp. 8°. *New York*, 1848.

——. Report of a committee appointed by the Academy of Medicine upon the comparative value of milk formed from the slop of distilleries and other food, with chemical and microscopical analyses, by Augustus K. Gardner. Read March 1, 1848. 19 pp. 8°. [*New York*], *R. Craighead*, 1851.

Repr. from: Tr. N. York Acad. M., 1851, i.

——. Act to incorporate the New York Academy of Medicine. Passed June 23, 1851. 15 pp. 8°. [*New York*, 1851.]

——. Transactions. v. 1–3, July 7, 1847, to Feb. 2, 1871. 8°. *New York*, 1851–71.

——. The same. 2. series. v. 1–5, 1871–86. 8°. *New York*, 1876–86.

——. Constitution and by-laws, with a list of officers and fellows. 16 pp. 8°. *New York, G. A. C. Van Buren*, 1852.

——. Report of the standing committee of . . . on public health and legal medicine. Published by order of the academy. 15 pp. 8°. *New York, G. A. C. Van Buren, printer*, 1852.

——. List of officers, committees, and fellows. 8 pp. 8°. *New York*, 1854.

——. Constitution, by-laws, and act of incorporation. Adopted Oct. 20, 1858. 16 pp. 8°. *New York, J. F. Trow*, 1858.

——. Report of the joint committee of the New York College of Pharmacy and the New York Academy of Medicine upon the Pharmacopœia of the United States. 29, 27 pp. 8°. [*New York*, 1860.]

——. Report of the committee on military surgery of the New York Academy of Medicine to the surgical section on military hygiene and therapeutics. By A. C. Post and Wm. H. Van Buren. Printed for circulation by the San. Com. 27 pp. 8°. [*New York*], 1861. [P., v. 409.]

——. The same. 31 pp. 16°. *New York, S. S. & W. Wood*, 1861.

——. Report on military hygiene and therapeutics. (Report of committee on military surgery to the surgical section of the . . . Printed for circulation by the Sanitary Commission.) [Alfred C. Post, Wm. H. Van Buren, committee. June 21, 1861.] 27 pp. 8°. [*New York*, 1861.]

——. Bulletin. v. 1–4, Jan., 1860, to Feb., 1871. 8°. *New York, W. Wood & Co.*, 1862–72.

——. Constitution, by-laws, and act of incorporation. Adopted Nov. 19, 1862. 17 pp. 8°. *New York*, 1862.

——. Report of sub-committee of the . . . on ventilation. Presented by John H. Griscom, chairman, June 6, 1866. 10 pp. 8°. *New York, New York Printing Co.*, 1866.

——. Constitution, by-laws, act of incorporation, and list of fellows. 50 pp. 8°. *New York*, 1874.

——. Proceedings of the first stated meeting, May 20, 1875. 8°. *New York, D. Appleton & Co.*, 1875.

——. Constitution, by-laws, act of incorporation, list of fellows and contributors to the building fund. 61 pp. 8°. *New York*, 1876.

——. An act to confer certain powers and privileges upon the . . . Passed June 2, 1877. 4 pp. 8°. [*New York*, 1877.]

——. Act of incorporation and constitution and by-laws. 24 pp. 8°. *New York*, 1878.

——. Anniversary discourse. By Leroy M. Yale. 19 pp. 8°. *New York*, 1879.

——. 1879. Addresses. Dr. Samuel S. Purple's valedictory. Dr. Fordyce Barker's inaugural. 30 pp. 8°. *New York*, 1879.

New York Academy of Medicine—continued.
——. Proceedings at the first stated meeting held in the new library hall of the academy, 12 West Thirty-first street, October 2, 1879. (With annual reports for 1879.) [Dedication of the library hall.] 61 pp., 1 pl. 8°. *New York*, 1880.

——. Act of incorporation, constitution and by-laws, and list of fellows of the . . . 38 pp. 8°. *New York*, 1882.

——. *See, also:*

ANDERSON (J.) An inaugural address delivered before the New York Academy of Medicine, January 16, 1861. 8°. *New York*, 1861.

——. Addresses on retiring from the presidential chair of the New York Academy of Medicine. Delivered January 16, 1867. 8°. *New York*, 1869.

BARKER (F.) New York Academy of Medicine, 1881. Second inaugural address. 8°. *New York*, 1881.

BATCHELDER (J. P.) An inaugural address delivered before the New York Academy of Medicine, February 3, 1858. 8°. *New York*, 1858.

COCK (T.) Inaugural address delivered before the New York Academy of Medicine, April 7, 1852; to which is added the annual report for 1851 of the recording secretary, John G. Adams, M. D. 8°. *New York*, 1852.

FLINT (A.) Objects and work. A valedictory address delivered before the New York Academy of Medicine, January 21, 1875, at the College of Physicians and Surgeons. 8°. *New York*, 1875.

FOSTER (S. C.) An oration delivered before the New York Academy of Medicine, at its fifteenth anniversary. November 11, 1862. 8°. *New York*, 1863.

FRANCIS (J. W.) An inaugural address delivered before the New York Academy of Medicine, February 2, 1848. 8°. *New York*, 1848.

——. Address of John W. Francis, M. D., late president of the New York Academy of Medicine, on the 7th of February, 1849. To the president-elect, Valentine Mott, M. D. 8°. *New York*, 1849.

GRISCOM (J. H.) Anniversary discourse before the New York Academy of Medicine, delivered Nov. 22, 1854. 8°. *New York*, 1855.

MANLEY (J. R.) Anniversary discourse before the New York Academy of Medicine, Nov. 8, 1848. 8°. *New York*, 1849.

MOTT (V.) An inaugural address delivered before the New York Academy of Medicine, February 7, 1849. To which is prefixed an address by Dr. J. W. Francis to the president-elect. 8°. *New York*, 1849.

PURPLE (S. S.) Objects and purposes; an inaugural address delivered before the New York Academy of Medicine, January 21, 1875, at the College of Physicians and Surgeons. 8°. *New York*, 1875.

STEARNS (J.) An address delivered on the occasion of assuming the chair as president at the first regular meeting of the New York Academy of Medicine, February 3, 1847. 8°. *New York*, 1847.

STEWART (F. C.) Anniversary discourse before the New York Academy of Medicine, delivered in the chapel of the University of New York, November 3, 1852. 8°. *New York*, 1853.

WHITE (W. T.) An anniversary discourse delivered before the New York Academy of Medicine, November 16, 1876. 8°. *New York*, 1876.

WOOD (I.) An inaugural address delivered before the New York Academy of Medicine, February 6, 1850. [To which is prefixed a valedictory address by Valentine Mott, M. D.] 8°. *New York*, 1850.

New York Academy of Medicine—continued.

———. *See, also:*

THIRD (The) anniversary oration for the New York Academy of Medicine, which was not delivered before that remarkable body, but ought to have been, at their annual meeting, held in the chapel of the university, November 14, 1849, by the physician who was not elected for that occasion; (published without the knowledge or consent of the academy). 8°. *New York,* 1850.

New York Academy of Sciences. (Late Lyceum of National History.) Charter, constitution, and by-laws, with list of the members, etc., 1876. 48 pp. 8°. *New York, S. Angell,* 1877.

———. Transactions. v. 1-6, 1881-2 to 1886-7. 8°. *New York,* 1882-7.

New York Agency for Trained Nurses, New York City. Mrs. A. S. Mabie, proprietor and manager. [Circular and testimonial.] 1 sheet. 8°. [*New York,* 1879.]

New York Agency, United States Sanitary Commission. *See* **United States** Sanitary Commission, New York Agency.

New York (The) Analyst. Devoted to the interests of sanitary science, food, medicine, and the suppression of adulteration. H. Lassing, editor and publisher. [Semi-monthly.] New series, No. 18, v. 1, Sept. 15, 1885. 18 pp. 4°. *New York.*

New York Association for Improving the Condition of the Poor, New York City. A plan for the better distribution of medical attendants and medicines for the indigent sick by the public dispensaries in the city of New York. 12 pp. 16°. [*New York,* 1845.]

———. Annual reports of the board of managers to the members and contributors. 19., 1861-2; 22., 1864-5; 26., 1868-9; 27., 1869-70; 30.-31., 1872-3 to 1873-4; 35.-37., 1877-8 to 1879-80; 40., 1882-3; 41., 1883-4; 43., 1885-6. 8°. *New York,* 1862-86.

———. Laws affecting tenement and lodging houses in the city of New York and Brooklyn. 11 pp. 8°. [*New York,* 1878.]

———. Proceedings of the board of managers. Dec. 13. 1880. 27 pp. 8°. [*New York,* 1880.] *See, also,* **London** alms and London pauperism. 8°. *New York,* 1877.

New York Asylum for Lying-in Women, New York City. Annual reports of the managers and resident physician to the subscribers and the public. 6., 1828-9; 9., 1831-2; 12.-14., 1834-5 to 1836-7; 17., 1839-40; 23., 1845-6; 27., 1849-50; 28., 1850-51; 32., 1854-5; 34., 1856-7; 40., 1862-3; 45.-47., 1867-8 to 1869-70; 49., 1871-2; 52., 1874-5. 8°. *New York,* 1829-75.

Incorporated March 19, 1827.

New York Bay Cemetery. [Extracts from reports, rules and regulations, and the act of incorporation.] 16 pp., 1 plan. 8°. *New York, F. Hart,* 1851.

New York Bible and Fruit Mission to our Public Hospitals and of the Coffee House and Lodging House. Annual report of the secretary to the donors and subscribers. 8., 1882-3. 35 pp. 8°. *New York, Office Industrial School Hebrew Orphan Asylum,* 1884.

New York and Brooklyn formulary of unofficinal preparations; published by a joint committee of delegates from the College of Pharmacy of the City of New York, the New York German Apothecaries' Society, and the Kings County Pharmaceutical Society. 2. ed. (interleaved). 46 pp. 12°. *New York,* [1-84].

New York Cancer Hospital. Annual reports of the managers to the subscribers. 1.-3., 1884-5 to 1887-8. 12°. [*New York,* 1885-8.]

Organized Feb. 7 and incorporated May 31, 1884; opened Dec. 6, 1887. 2. and 3. reports in one, and for 33 months, May, 1885, to Feb., 1887.

New York Catholic Protectory, Westchester, N. Y. Annual report of the board of managers to the legislature of the State, and to the common council of the city. 11., 1872-3. 67 pp. 8°. *Westchester, The Protectory,* 1874.

New York(The) and Chicago Medical and Surgical Journal; devoted to medicine, general science, and literature. Edited by Edward N. Fishblatt. [Monthly.] Nos. 1-5, v. 8, June to October, 1881. 256 pp. 8°. *New York & Chicago.*

Title of v. 7 and prior was: **New York** (The) Medical and Surgical Journal. In Aug., 1886, continued as: **Minnesota** (The) Medical and Surgical Journal.

New York Christian Home for Intemperate Men, New York City. Report of the . . . [from June 7 to Dec. 7, 1877. Also contains the constitution, by-laws, and rules]. 15 pp. 8°. *New York,* 1877.

Established June 7 and incorporated Oct. 17, 1877.

———. Annual reports of the officers to the subscribers. 1.-9., 1877-8 to 1886. 8°. *New York,* 1878-87.

1. report for 17 months, June, 1877, to Nov. 1, 1878. 7. report for 14 months, ending Dec. 31, 1883.

New York City Temperance Society. An address to physicians, by the executive committee of the board of managers. 22 pp. 8°. *New York, J. & J. Harper,* 1829.

New York College of Dental Surgery, at Syracuse. Annual announcements for the sessions of (1.) 1851-2; (3.) 1853-4. 12, 12 pp. 8°. *Syracuse,* 1851-3.

New York College of Dentistry, New York City. Annual announcements for the sessions of 1866-7 to 1884-5. 1.-21., 1866-7 to 1886-7. 8°. *New York,* 1866-86.

New York College of Pharmacy. Report of the joint committee of the New-York College of Pharmacy and the New-York Academy of Medicine upon the pharmacopœia of the United States. Read before the Academy of Medicine, April 16, 1860. 29, 27 pp. 8°. [*New York,* 1860.]

New York College of Veterinary Surgeons and School of Comparative Medicine. Annual announcements for the sessions of 1867-8 (3.); 1877-8 (13.); 1886-7 (22.); 1887-8 (23.). 8°. *New York,* 1867-77.

Chartered 1857, but did not go into operation until 1865.

———. Rules and regulations, with lists of subscribers. 14 pp. 8°. *New York, S. Angell,* 1868.

———. The same. 20 pp. 8°. *New York, S. Angell,* 1870.

———. The same. 12 pp. 8°. *New York, Russell's Printing House,* 1874.

New York Colored Mission. Annual report of the officers to the subscribers. 6., 1871. 16 pp. 8°. *New York, W. C. Martin,* 1872.

New York County Medical Association, founded 1884. By-laws. Adopted, Jan. 14, 1884. 18 pp. 8°. *New York, Angell's printing office,* 1884.

———. Official report of the memorial meeting of the . . . in honor of the late Austin Flint, M. D., LL. D., held at the Carnegie Laboratory, Bellevue Hospital Medical College, New York, April 19, 1886. 35 pp. 8°. *New York, The Judson Printing Co.,* 1886.

Repr. from Gaillard's M. J., N. Y., 1886, xli.

New York Cremation Society. Charter, Neben-Gesetze, etc., der New Yorker Leichenverbrennungs-Gesellschaft. 23 pp. 16°. *New York,* 1881.

———. Charter and by-laws. 24 pp. 16°. *Brooklyn, Eagle print,* 1885.

———. [Report for the year 1885.] 2 l. 8°. [*New York,* 1885.]

New York (The) Dental Journal. Edited by Frank H. Norton and G. H. Perine. [Quarterly.]

New York (The) Dental Journal—continued.
v. 1–5, July, 1858, to May, 1864. 8°. *New York*

Ended. v. 1 complete in 2 numbers; v. 2 commenced Jan., 1859; v. 5 commenced March, 1862, became semi-annual, and complete in 5 numbers. After no. 2, v. 3, W. B. Roberts became publisher and proprietor, and Perine dropped.

New York (The) Dental Recorder. Devoted to the theory and practice of surgical, medical, and mechanical dentistry. Edited by J. S. Ware. [Monthly.] v. 1–10, Sept., 1846, to Dec., 1856. 8°. *New York.*

Want nos. 3–5, 8–10, v. 6; nos. 3, 8, 11, v. 7. In v. 2 C. C. Allen became editor; in v. 6 A. Hill added; v. 8 commenced Jan., 1854, published at Norwalk, Conn., A. Hill sole editor and publisher; in v. 9–10 Charles W. Bollard editor.

New York Dermatological Society. Nomenclature adopted Feb. 11, 1879. 1 sheet. 4°. [*New York*, 1879.]

New York Diet Kitchen, New York City. Statement of the managers on the object and benefits of the charity. Nov., 1873. 4 l. 8°. [*New York*, 1873.]

Organized and incorporated 1873.

———. Annual reports of the managers to the subscribers and public. 1., 1873–4; 2., 1874–5; 7., 1879. 8°. *New York*, 1874–80.

New York Dispensary, New York City. Charter and by-laws of the . . . 23 pp. 8°. *New York, C. S. Van Winkle*, 1810.

Instituted 1790; incorporated April 8, 1795.

———. The same. 15 pp. 8°. *New York, Van Winkle & Wiley*, 1814.

———. The same. 20 pp., 1 l. 8°. *New York, C. S. Van Winkle*, 1821.

———. The same. 19 pp. 8°. *New York, M. Day*, 1830.

———. The same. 24 pp. 8°. *New York, B. C. Brown*, 1834.

———. The same. 28 pp. 12°. *New York, M. Day & Co.*, 1842.

———. The same. 23 pp. 8°. *New York, J. W. Amerman*, 1869.

———. Annual reports of the board of trustees to the subscribers, members, and the public. 40.–42., 1829–31; 44., 1833; 47., 1836; 48., 1837; 50., 1839; 52., 1841; 53., 1842; 55.–66., 1844–55; 68.–96., 1857–85. 8°. *New York*, 1830–86.

———. The by-laws of the . . . 24 pp. 12°. *New York, W. Osborn*, 1848.

———. The same. 21 pp. 12°. *New York, Holman, Gray & Co.*, 1854.

———. The same. 20 pp. 8°. *New York, J. W. Amerman*, 1875.

———. Reports of the vaccine department for the years 1871; 1873; 1874. By Frank P. Foster. 8°. *New York*, 1872–5.

———. Animal vaccine virus. Directions for the preservation and use of vaccine lymph. [Circular issued by vaccine department.] 2 l. 8°. [*New York, n. d.*]

———. Furnishes non-humanized cow-pox virus (vituline or bovine). 2 l. 8°. [*New York, n. d.*]

———. Nomenclature and pharmacopœia of the . . . 45 pp. 8°. [*New York, Slote & Janes, n. d.*]

New York Dispensary for Diseases of the Skin. Annual report of the trustees and officers to the public. 1., 1869–70. 11 pp. 16°. *New York, R. C. Root, Anthony & Co.*, 1871.

Incorporated July 20 and opened in Nov., 1869.

New York Dispensary for Diseases of the Throat and Chest. Annual reports of the physician in charge and the treasurer, to the board of trustees. 1., 1870. 14 pp. 12°. *New York*, 1871.

New York (The) Dissector. A quarterly journal of medicine, surgery, magnetism, mesmerism, and the collateral sciences, with the mysteries

New York (The) Dissector—continued.
and fallacies of the faculty. Edited by Henry Hall Sherwood. v. 1–4, 1844–7. 8°. *New York.*

New York Ear Dispensary, New York City. Annual reports of the board of trustees and surgeon in charge to the public. 1., 1871–3; 6.–8., 1876–8. 12°. *New York*, 1873–9.

Incorporated April 8 and opened May 25, 1871. 1. report for 26 months, May, 1871, to June, 1873. No reports published from July, 1873, to Dec., 1875.

New York (The) Eclectic Medical Journal.

Title on covers of nos. 3 *et seq.* of v. 3: **Medical** (The) Eclectic, May, 1876, *et seq.*

New York (The) Eclectic Medical Review. A monthly record of medicine and the collateral sciences. Editor, Robert S. Newton; associate editor, Edwin Freeman. No. 1, v. 1, June, 1866. 48 pp. 8°. *New York.*

New York (The) Eclectic Medical and Surgical Journal. Adapted to popular and professional reading. Edited by S. H. Potter. [Monthly.] v. 1–4, July, 1849, to Dec., 1852. 8°. *Syracuse* [and v. 2–4, *Rochester*].

v. 3 contains 6 numbers, July to Dec., 1851. v. 4, title: **Eclectic** (The) Journal of Medicine. v. 2 edited by Wm. W. Hadley; v. 4, by L. Reuben and L. C. Dolley. Continued as: **Union** (The) Journal of Medicine.

New York (The) Eclectic Medical and Surgical Journal. Edited by Edward N. Fishblatt. [Bi-monthly.] v. 4–5; Nos. 1–9, v. 6, June, 1877, to Feb., 1880. 3 v. 8°. *New York.*

Title of v. 1–3 was: **New Jersey** (The) Eclectic Medical and Surgical Journal. v. 5 became monthly. In March, 1880 (no. 10, v. 6), title became: **New York** (The) Medical and Surgical Journal.

New York Eye Infirmary. By-laws of the . . . 16 pp. 16°. *New York, G. A. C. Van Beuren*, 1858.

New York Eye and Ear Infirmary, New York City. Annual reports of the board of directors and surgeons to the governors and the public. 1., 1821; 2., 1822; 4., 1824; 10., 1830; 19., 1839; 22.–30., 1842–50; 32., 1852; 34., 1854; 35., 1855; 37.–44., 1857–64; 46.–53., 1866–73; 57.–66., 1877 to 1885–6. 8°. *New York*, 1822–86.

Founded Aug. 20, 1820; incorporated March 29, 1822, [1. in P., v. 825.]

New York Free Dispensary for Sick Children. Annual reports of the executive committee to the subscribers and the public. 1.–12., 1871–2 to 1883. 8°. *New York*, 1872–84.

Opened April 1, 1871. 5. report for 21 months ending Dec. 31, 1876.

New York Historical Society. Proceedings at the dedication of the library of the . . . 27 pp. 8°. *New York, for the Society*, 1857.

Bound with: FRANCIS (J. W.) New York during the last half century. 8°. *New York*, 1857.

New York Home for Convalescents, New York City. Annual reports of the managers to the society. 2., 1880–81; 4.–6., 1882–3 to 1884–5. 12°. *New York*, 1881–5.

New York Homœopathic Dispensary, New York City. Report [for the first 16 months, Oct., 1845, to Jan., 1847]. 4 pp. 8°. [*New York*, 1847.]

For continuation, see **New York** Homœopathic Dispensary Association. Reorganized Dec. 27, 1847, by adding "Association" to title.

New York Homœopathic Dispensary Association, New York City. Constitution and by-laws. 12 pp. 16°. *New York*, 1848.

———. Annual reports of the board of trustees to the friends of the institution. 1., 1848; 4., 1851. 8°. *New York*, 1849–52.

———. An address to the friends of homœopathy in New York from the trustees of the . . . 17 pp. 8°. *New York, W. C. Bryant & Co.*, 1852.

New York Homœopathic Infirmary for Women. Annual report of the officers to the subscribers. 3., 1865–6. 17 pp. 8°. *New York, Slote & Janes*, 1867.

Incorporated Oct. 28, 1863.

New York Homœopathic Medical College, New York City. Annual announcements for the sessions of 1863–4 to 1867–8 (4.-8.) ; 1869–70 to 1875–6 (10.-16.); 1877–8 to 1879–80 (18.-20.) ; 1882–3 to 1886–7 (23.-26.). 8° & sm. 4°. *New York*, 1863–86.

List of students and graduates for the years 1862-3 to 1866-7; 1868-9 to 1874-5; 1881-2 to 1885-6, *in :* Announcements, for subsequent years. List of graduates from 1861 to 1882, *in :* Announcement for 1882-3. 6. report, *also, in :* P., v. 528. 24. and 25. are in 4°.

New York Hospital and Bloomingdale Asylum. Charter for establishing an hospital in the city of New York. Granted by the Right Hon. John, Earl of Dunmore, the 13th July, 1771. 34 pp., 1 l. 4°. *New York, H. Gaine,* 1794.

Founded in 1770 by private contributions. Incorporated June 13, 1771, under the name of "The Hospital in the City of New York, in America". In 1773 the governors purchased five acres of ground for the erection of a suitable edifice, and the foundation stone was laid July 27 in the same year. It was not in condition to receive patients until Jan. 3, 1791. By an act of the legislature, passed March 9, 1810, the name was changed to "The Society of the New York Hospital". The present building was inaugurated Nov. 5, 1877. At an early period insane patients were received. On March 14, 1806, the legislature passed an act granting an annual provision, payable out of the duties on sales at auction in the city, until 1857. The new edifice, called the "Lunatic Asylum", was opened July 15, 1808. In 1818 a committee reported favorably on a plan for purchasing a tract of land near the city upon which to erect suitable buildings and to introduce a course of moral treatment. A site was selected on the Bloomingdale road, and the corner-stone of the new asylum was laid May 17, 1818, and opened June 16, 1821, when the institution received its present name, the "Bloomingdale Asylum".

——. A brief account of the . . . 72 pp. 8°. *New York, J. Collins & Son,* 1804.

——. Catalogue of books belonging to the New York Hospital library. 74, 29 pp. 8°. [*New York, Collins & Co.,* 1811.]

29 pp. are MS. additions. *Bound with :* New York Hospital. An account of . . . 8°. *New York,* 1811.

——. Annual reports of the board of governors and physicians to the legislature of the State of New York. 43., 1813; 69.-117., 1839–87. fol. & 8°. *New York,* 1814–88.

——. Pharmacopœia Nosocomii Neo-Eboracensis; or the pharmacopœia of the . . . Published under the authority of the physicians and surgeons of the institution. To which is added an appendix containing a general posological table, and a comparative view of the former and present terms used in materia medica and pharmacy. x (1 l.), 180 pp., 1 l. 8°. *New York, Collins & Co.,* 1816.

——. Report of the physician of the New York Lunatic Asylum [for a period of eight months, Sept. 13, 1817, to May 15, 1818], addressed to a committee of its governors, and published at their request. [By William Handy.] 20 pp. 8°. *New York, S. Wood & Sons,* 1818.

This asylum was opened July 15, 1808, as a branch of the New York Hospital. The patients were transferred to the new asylum on the Bloomingdale road, June 16, 1821.

——. An account of the New York Hospital. 62 pp., 1 pl., 1 plan. 8°. *New York, M. Day,* 1820.

——. By-laws and regulations ordained and established by the governors, for the better government of the officers, members, patients, and servants of the hospital, passed December 7, 1819. 25 pp. 8°. *New York, M. Day,* 1820.

——. Address of the governors to the public, relative to the Asylum for the Insane, at Bloomingdale. 8 pp. 8°. *New York, M. Day,* 1821.

——. By-laws and regulations ordained and established by the governors of the New York Hospital, for the better government of the officers, members, patients, and servants of the hospital. Revised and passed April 5, 1825. 39 pp. 8°. *New York, M. Day,* 1826.

New York Hospital [etc.]—continued.

——. A catalogue of the books belonging to the library of the New York Hospital, and the regulations for the same. 132 pp. 8°. *New York, G. F. Hopkins & Son,* 1829.

——. Supplementary catalogue of the New York Hospital library, Nov., 1881. 12 pp. 8°. *New York, office of the Medico - Chirurgical Review,* 1831.

——. By-laws and regulations of the . . . ordained and established by the governors of the institution. Revised and passed Dec. 4, 1832. 64 pp. 8°. *New York, R. & G. S. Wood,* 1833.

——. Charter of the Society of the . . . and the laws relating thereto, with the by-laws and regulations of the institution, and those of the Bloomingdale Asylum for the Insane. 89 pp. 8°. *New York, M. Day,* 1838.

——. A catalogue of the books belonging to the library of the New York Hospital, arranged alphabetically and analytically, and the regulations for the use of the same. v, 194 pp. 8°. *New York,* [*R. Craighead*], 1845.

——. Charter of the Society of the New York Hospital, and the laws relating thereto, with the by-laws and regulations of the institution, and those of the Bloomingdale Asylum for the Insane. Revised and passed Dec. 2, 1845. 104 pp., 1 pl., 1 plan. 8°. *New York, J. R. Mc-Gowan,* 1846.

——. Address of the governors to their fellow-citizens. 24 pp. 8°. *New York, W. C. Bryant & Co.,* 1852.

——. Charter of the Society of the . . . and the laws relating thereto, with the by-laws and regulations of the institution, and those of the Bloomingdale Asylum for the Insane. 140 pp. 8°. *New York, D. Fanshaw,* 1856.

——. An account of the . . . [including a list of the governors, officers of the board of governors, physicians, and surgeons, from the commencement of the institution to the 1st of June, 1856]. 75–140 pp. 8°. [*New York,* 1856.]

Cutting.

——. Report of the committee on retrenchment. May 3, 1859. 11 pp. 8°. *New York, Baker & Goodwin,* [1859 ?]

——. A catalogue of the pathological cabinet of the . . . classified and arranged by Robert Ray, jr. With a memoir of the author [by John Watson]. Edited by H. D. Bulkley. 364 pp., port. 8°. *New York, S. S. & W. Wood,* 1860.

——. Report of the chairman of the committee on retrenchment. Inquiries presented by that committee and the visiting committee to the superintendent and the physicians and surgeons, with their replies to the same. 40 pp. 8°. *New York, F. Hart & Co.,* 1860.

——. Supplementary catalogue of the books belonging to the library of the New York Hospital. 69 pp. 8°. *New York, R. Craighead,* 1861.

Bound with : New York Hospital. A catalogue of . . . 8°. *New York,* 1845.

——. The same. No. II. Legacy of John Watson, M. D. 23 pp. 8°. *New York, R. Craighead,* 1865.

Bound with : New York Hospital. A catalogue of . . . 8°. *New York,* 1845.

——. The same. No. III. 39 pp. 8°. *New York, N. Y. Printing Co.,* 1869.

Bound with : New York Hospital. A catalogue of . . . 8°. *New York,* 1845.

——. The same. No. IV. 38 pp. 8°. *New York, D. Van Nostrand,* 1875.

——. The same. No. V. 71 pp. 8°. *New York, G. P. Putnam's Sons,* 1880.

New York Hospital [etc.]—continued.

——. The same. No. VI. 68 pp. 8°. *New York, Trow's Co.,* 1886.

——. The financial condition and restricted charitable operations of the Society of the New York Hospital. Majority and minority reports of a special committee of the board of governors. Presented April 17, 1866. 22 pp. 8°. *New York, W. C. Bryant & Co.,* 1866.

——. Biographical catalogue descriptive of the portraits of former governors and attending physicians and surgeons. 10 pp. 8°. *New York, N. Y. Printing Company,* 1869.

——. Catalogue of duplicate works in the library, for sale or exchange. 10 pp. 8°. *New York, C. A. Coffin,* 1876.

——. Report of the medical board as to the internal administration of the hospital. 19 pp. 8°. *New York, for the governors,* 1876.

——. Report of the committee on a village of cottage hospitals, made to the governors Feb. 24, 1876. 47 pp. roy. 8°. [*New York, Evening Post,* 1876.]

——. Cottage hospitals. Remarks of Mr. F. A. Conklin upon the report of the committee on a village of cottage hospitals, delivered at a meeting of the governors, July 6, 1876. 23 pp. 8°. [*New York,* 1876.]

——. Report of the building committee [from May 5, 1874, to Nov. 5, 1877], together with an address delivered on the occasion of the inauguration of the new building, on the 16th March, 1877, by William H. Van Buren. With a detailed description of the building. 32 pp., 9 plans. roy. 8°. *New York, L. W. Lawrence,* 1877.

Bound with : Reports, 1871–83.

——. *See, also :*

BEEKMAN (J. W.) Centenary address delivered before the Society of the New York Hospital, July 24, 1871. 8°. *New York,* 1871.

NEW YORK (*State*). Assembly. Report of the commissioners appointed by law to examine into the condition of the New York Hospital, the New York Eye Infirmary, Seamen's Retreat, and Marine Hospital, at Staten Island. No. 92. April 8, 1853. 8°. [*Albany,* 1853.]

McLean (H.) A table of patients admitted into the New York Hospital, from January, 1797, to December, 1798. Med. Reposit., N. Y., 1798, i, 105; 248; 376; 560: 1799, ii, 104; 324.

New York Hospital. *Training School for Nurses.* Annual report of the conference committee in charge of the . . . for the year 1883. 20 pp. 8°. [*New York,* 1885.]

Address to the graduating class of 1883, by Wm. H. Draper, M. D.

New York Hospital Saturday and Sunday Association, New York City. Annual reports of the treasurer of the New York Hospital Saturday and Sunday Collection. 2., 1880; 5., 1883; 8., 1886. 12°. *New York,* [1881–7].

Organized in 1879.

New York Infant Asylum, New York City. Annual reports of the managers, lady officers, and medical committee to the subscribers and the public. 1.–13., 1871–84. 8°. *New York,* 1873–85.

Chartered in 1865. Organized as a "Foundling Asylum", but reorganized and opened Nov. 23, 1871, adopting a new policy of reception house and refuge for homeless infants. 1. report for 2 years.

——. *See, also :*

NEW YORK (*State*). Assembly. An act to amend chap. 106 of the laws of 1865, entitled "An act to incorporate the New York Infant Asylum", passed March 11, 1865, as amended by chap. 263 of the laws of 1872, entitled "An act to amend an act entitled 'An act to incorporate the New York Infant Asylum'", passed March 11, 1865, and as further amended by chap. 90 of the laws

New York Infant Asylum—continued.

of 1877, entitled "An act further to amend chap. 106 of the laws of 1865, entitled 'An act to incorporate the New York Infant Asylum', passed April 2, 1871", and to amend the title thereto. No. 530. March 1, 1882. Introd. by Mr. Tighe. fol. [*Albany,* 1882.]

New York Infirmary for Women and Children, New York City. Annual reports of the executive committee to the subscribers. 14.–19., 1867–72; 24., 1877; 27., 1880; 28., 1881; 30.–32., 1883–5. 8°. *New York,* 1868–85.

New York Institution for the Inoculation of the Kine Pock. Constitution for the government of the . . . To which are added the proceedings of the two first meetings of the contributors. 11 pp. 12°. *New York, J. Collins & Son,* 1802.

New York (The) Journal of Homœopathy.

Was title of no. 1, v. 1, of: **American** (The) Journal of Homœopathy, April 25, 1846.

New York (The) Journal of Homœopathy. Under the auspices of "The New York Homœopathic Medical College". William Tod Helmuth and T. F. Allen, editorial committee. [Monthly.] v. 1–2, March, 1873, to Feb., 1875. 8°. *New York, Carle & Grener.*

In v. 2, S. A. Jones and S. Lilienthal added as editors. In April, 1875, united with : **Medical** (The) Union, forming : **Homœopathic** (The) Times.

New York (The) Journal of Medicine.

Was title of v. 1–8, 3. series, of : **New York** (The) Journal of Medicine and the Collateral Sciences, July, 1856, to June, 1860.

New York (The) Journal of Medicine and the Collateral Sciences. Edited by Samuel Forry. [Bi-monthly ; 2 v. annually.] v. 1–10, July, 1843, to June, 1848. New series, v. 1–16, July, 1848, to June, 1856. 3. series, v. 1–8, July, 1856, to June, 1860. 34 v. 8°. *New York.*

1. series, v. 4, C. A. Lee became editor ; new series, v. 1, S. S. Purple became editor ; v. 10, Stephen Smith added ; 3. series, v. 1, H. D. Bulkley added : v. 3, Purple and Bulkley dropped ; v. 1, 3. series, the words, "and the Collateral Sciences" dropped from the title-page. In Oct., 1856, **New York** (The) Medical Times merged in this journal. Continued as : **American** (The) Medical Times.

New York (The) Journal of Medicine and Surgery. [Quarterly ; 2 v. annually.] v. 1–4, July, 1839, to June 30, 1841. 8°. *New York, G. Adlard.*

Ended.

New York (The) Journal of Pharmacy. Published by authority of the College of Pharmacy of the city of New York. Edited by Benjamin W. McCready. [Monthly.] v. 1–3, 1852–4. 8°. *New York.*

v. 3, 1854, edited by Thomas Antisell *et al.*

New York Juvenile Asylum, New York City. Annual reports of the board of directors to the legislatures of the States of New York and Illinois, and to the common council of New York City. 2., 1853 ; 4.–26., 1855–77 ; 28.–30., 1879–81. 8°. *New York,* 1854–82.

Established and incorporated 1851. 13.–24. bound in 1 v.

See, also, **Western** Agency, New York Juvenile Asylum, Bloomington, Ills.

New York Juvenile Guardian Society, New York City. Annual report of the directors and officers of the . . . for the shelter, schooling, and support of orphan and homeless children in the city of New York. 19., 1867. 12 pp. 8°. [*Albany,* 1868.]

New York Ladies' Health Protective Association. Memorial to the Hon. Abram S. Hewitt, mayor of New York, on the subject of street-cleaning. 12 pp. 8°. [*New York,* 1887.]

New York Ladies' Home Missionary Society of the Methodist Episcopal Church, New York City. Annual reports of the managers to the subscrib-

New York Ladies' Home [etc.]—continued.
ers and members of the association. 29.–30.,
1872–3 to 1873–4. 8°. *New York, 1873–4.*

New York (The) Lancet. Edited by James
Alexander Houston. [Weekly; 2 v. annually.]
v. 1–2; Nos. 1, 3, v. 3, Jan. 1, 1842, to Jan. 21,
1843. 8°. *New York, J. G. Bennett & J. A.*
Houston.

New York (The) Lancet. A family medical
journal. Edited by N. R. C. Rowe. [Semi-
monthly.] Nos. 1–4, 6, v. 1, Jan. 3 to April 1,
1866. 4°. *New York.*

New York Life Insurance Company. Grant,
McClellan, Hancock [not insured]. 6 l., 3
port. 16°. [*New York, New York Spectator Co.,*
1886.]
Repr. from : The Spectator, New York, Feb. 18, 1886, &
Indianapolis Jour., Feb., 28, 1886.

———. A return-premium endowment policy. 1
sheet. 4°. [*New York, 1887.*]

New York Lunatic Asylum, New York City.
See **New York** Hospital and Bloomingdale
Asylum, New York City.

New York (The) Magnet.
Title of v. 2–3 of : **Magnet** (The), 1843–4.

New York Medical Abstract. A monthly journal of condensed medical news. v. 1–8, 1881–8.
8°. *New York.*
Current.

New York Medical Aid and Relief Society for
Destitute Sick Women and Children. Report of
the officers to the members and contributors
for the year 1882–3. 6 sheets. 8°. *New York,*
[1883].

———. The reply of the . . . to the attack of the
press. 8 pp. 8°. *New York, 1883.*

New York Medical Association for the Supply
of Lint, Bandages, etc., to the United States
Army. Final report. Presented July 25, 1861.
32 pp. 8°. *New York, by the association,* 1861.
Organized April 23, and dissolved July 25, 1861.

New York Medical College and Charity Hospital, New York City. Annual announcements
for the sessions of 1850–51 to 1852–3 (1.–3.); 1854–
5 to 1856–7 (5.–7.); 1860–61 to 1863–4 (11.–14.).
8° & 12°. *New York, 1850–63.*
Organized in 1850. The words "and Charity Hospital"
added to title between 1857–60. Ceased to exist 1864.

———. Announcement of the summer session of
1855. 6 pp., 1 l. *New York, Baker, Godwin &*
Co., 1855.

———. Catalogue of the officers, students, and
graduates for the session of 1856–7. 7 pp. 8°.
New York, Baker & Godwin, 1857.

———. *See, also :*
Cox (A. L.) An address delivered on the
first public exhibition of the edifice of the New
York Medical College, and the inauguration of
its faculty, October 16, 1850. 8°. *New York,*
1850.

STATEMENT of the Newark Medical Association
in reference to a diploma granted by the New
York Medical College [to J. F. Duncker]. Presented to the American Medical Association, May
4, 1858. 8°. *Newark,* 1858.

New York Medical College and Hospital for
Women, New York City. Annual announcements for the sessions of 1864–5 (2.); 1867–8
to 1877–8 (5.–15.); 1879–80 (17.); 1882–3 (20.);
1883–4 (21.); 1886–7 (24.). 8°. *New York, 1864–*
86.
Lists of the officers and students for the years 1868–9 to
1875–6, in : Announcements for subsequent years. List of
all graduates from 1864 to 1886, in : Announcement for
1886–7. Organized in 1863. The words "and Hospital"
added to title in 1873.

———. Charter and by-laws, 1882. 16 pp. 8°.
New York, Pusey & Rooney, 1882.

New York (The) Medical Eclectic.
See **Medical** (The) Eclectic, v. 5, 1878, *et seq.*

New York (The) Medical Gazette. Published
by Uriah Turner. [Weekly; 2 v. annually.]
v. 1–2, July 14, 1841, to July 6, 1842. 8°. *New*
York.
Ended.

New York (The) Medical Gazette and Journal of Health. Edited by D. Meredith Reese.
[Weekly.] v. 1–12, July 6, 1850, to May, 1861.
v. 1–3, 4°; v. 4–12, 8°. *New York, S. S. & W.*
Wood, 1850–54; *Hall, Clayton & Co.,* 1855–61.
Ended. v. 2–3, semi-monthly; v. 4–12, monthly. v. 6–
8, title : **American** (The) Medical Gazette and Journal
of Health. v. 9–12, title : **American** (The) Medical Gazette. v. 12 complete in 5 nos., January to May, 1861.

New York (The) Medical Independent and
Pharmaceutical Reporter. Edited by the New
York Medical Literary Association. [Weekly.]
Nos. 1–16, v. 1, May 4 to Aug. 17, 1864. 8°. *New*
York, T. B. Harrison & Co.

New York (The) Medical Inquirer. Conducted
by an association of physicians and surgeons re-
siding in different parts of the United States.
[Monthly; 2 v. annually.] v. 1, Jan. to June,
1830. 288 pp. 8°. *New York.*
Title on covers of nos. 2–6, v. 1, was : **New York** (The)
Medical Inquirer and Domestic Magazine. Continued as :
American (The) Lancet.

New York (The) Medical Inquirer and Domestic
Magazine.
Was title on covers of nos. 2–6, v. 1, of : **New York**
(The) Medical Inquirer.

New York (The) Medical Intelligencer, or Eclectic Gazette. Edited by D. S. Meikleham.
Published every alternate Wednesday. Nos. 1–
6, 8, v. 1, Aug. 27 to Dec. 3, 1845. 4°. *New*
York.

New York (The) Medical Journal. Conducted
by D. L. M. Peixotto, J. R. Rhinelander, and
John Jas. Graves. [Quarterly; 2 v. annually.]
v. 1–2, Nov., 1830, to Aug., 1831. 8°. *New York,*
E. B. Clayton.
Completed. In v. 2 Nathan R. Smith added as editor.

New York (The) Medical Journal. A monthly
record of medicine and the collateral sciences.
[2 v. annually.] v. 1–47, April, 1865–88. 8° &
fol. *New York, Miller & Mathews.*
Current. v. 10, 11, 12 contained but 5 nos. each, in order
to commence v. 13 Jan., 1871. In v. 1–4 no editors named ;
v. 5–8 William A. Hammond and Edward S. Dunster ; v.
9–13 Dunster sole editor ; v. 14–18 by William T. Lusk and
James B. Hunter ; v. 19–30 Hunter sole editor ; v. 31–46
by Frank P. Foster. In v. 34–36 title was : **New York**
Medical Journal and Obstetrical Review. In Jan., 1883,
v. 37, became weekly and fol.

———. The same. General index to v. 1–23,
April, 1865, to June, 1876. By James B. Hunter.
1 v. 144 pp. 8°. *New York, D. Appleton & Co.*

New York (The) Medical Journal and Obstetri-
cal Review.
Was title of v. 34–36 of : **New York** (The) Medical
Journal, July, 1881, to Dec., 1882.

New York (The) Medical Magazine; published
annually, and edited by Valentine Mott and
Henry U. Onderdonk. v. 1 [in 2 Nos.], Jan.,
1814, to Jan., 1815. 364 pp. 8°. *New York.*
Ended.

New York Medical Mission, New York City.
Annual report of the secretary to the society. 3.,
1883. 19 pp. 8°. *New York, J. Huggins,* 1884.

New York Medical Monthly. A journal of prac-
tical medicine and surgery. Editor: J. Leonard
Corning. v. 1; Nos. 1–2, v. 2, May, 1886, to
June, 1887. 8°. *New York.*
Ended.

New York Medical News and Cancer Journal.
Issued quarterly by Robert S. Newton. No. 1,
v. 1, Oct., 1864. 36 pp. 8°. *New York.*
v. 1 is v. 15 (old series) of : **Western** (The) Medical
News.

New York (The) Medical and Pathological Journal. Edited by Wm. W. Hadley. [Monthly.] Nos. 1–11, v. 1, Oct., 1858, to Aug., 1859. 8°. *New York.*

New York (The) Medical and Philosophical Journal and Review. [Half-yearly.] v. 1–3, 1809–11. 8°. *New York, T. & J. Swords.*

New York (The) Medical and Physical Journal. Edited by John W. Francis, Jacob Dyckman, and John B. Beck. [Quarterly.] v. 1–9, Jan., 1822, to Jan., 1830. 8°. *New York, E. Bliss & E. White.*
Ended. v. 8–9, April, 1829, to Jan., 1830, are also called v. 1–2, new series; 2 v. annually. v. 2, Dyckman dropped; v. 5, Francis dropped, D. L. M. Peixotto and John Bell added; v. 6, Bell dropped; v. 7, J. A. Smith, T. R. Beck, A. H. Stevens, and J. M. Smith added; in v. 8–9, Dr. Peixotto sole editor. v. 1–7, Congressional Library deposit.

New York (The) Medical Press. A weekly journal of medicine, surgery, and the collateral sciences. Edited by J. L. Kiernan and W. O'Meagher. [2 v. annually.] Nos. 1, 3–4, Dec. 4–25, 1858. New series, v. 1–3, Jan. 1, 1859, to June 30, 1860. roy. 8°. *New York.*
Want preliminary no. 2, Dec. 11, 1858. v. 1–2 paged consecutively. In July, 1860, merged in: **American** (The) Medical Times.

New York Medical Review. A new series of the American Eclectic Medical Review. Edited by E. S. McClellan. [Monthly.] Nos. 1–8, v. 1, Jan. to Nov., 1873. 386 pp. 8°. *New York.*
v. 1 is also called v. 9, old series. Nothing published in March, April, or October, 1873.

New York Medical and Surgical Brief; a practical monthly clinic. E. Jay Fisk, editor. Nos. 1–7, v. 1, Nov., 1878, to May, 1879. 142 pp. 8°. *New York.*
Ended.

New York (The) Medical and Surgical Journal. Editor: Edward N. Fishblatt. [Monthly.] Nos. 10–12, v. 6; v. 7, March, 1880, to May, 1881. 2 v. 8°. *New York.*
Title of v. 4–5, nos. 1–9, v. 6, was: **New York** (The) Eclectic Medical and Surgical Journal. Continued in June, 1881, as: **New York** (The) and Chicago Medical and Surgical Journal.

New York (The) Medical and Surgical Reporter. Edited by Clarkson T. Collins. [Bi-weekly.] v. 1, Oct. 18, 1845, to Oct. 10, 1846; Nos. 1–18, v. 2, Jan. 2 to May 8, 1847. 8°. *New York.*
Want no. 19, v. 2, 1847. v. 2 became weekly, William R. Wagstaff editor. Dr. Collins died April 10, 1881.

New York Medical and Surgical Society. Annual report by T. Gaillard Thomas. 24 pp. 8°. [*New York, n. d.*]

New York (The) Medical Times. Edited by J. G. Adams. [Monthly.] v. 1–5, Oct. 1, 1851, to Sept., 1856. 8°. *New York, Baker, Godwin & Co.*
v. 2–5 edited by H. D. Bulkley. Merged in: **New York** (The) Journal of Medicine.

New York Medical Times. A monthly journal of medicine, surgery, and the collateral sciences. [Homœopathic.] Editors: Egbert Guernsey and Alfred K. Hills. v. 9–16, April, 1881–8. 4°. *New York.*
Current. Title of v. 3–8 was: **Homœopathic** (The) Times.

New York Medical Union. Revised constitution and by-laws, adopted Oct. 17, 1857. 12 pp. 8°. [*New York, 1857.*]

New York Medico-Chirurgical Bulletin. Edited by George Bushe. [Monthly.] v. 1–2, May, 1831, to April, 1832. 8°. *New York, Ludwig & Tolfree.*
Ended.

New York Medico-Chirurgical Society. Transactions. v. 1–3, 1878–83. 8°. *New York, 1882–4.*

New York Medico-Historical Society.
See **Medical** (The) Register of New York, 1862–3 to 1883–4. 12°. *New York, 1862–83.*

New York Microscopical Society.
See **American** Quarterly Microscopical Journal. 8°. *New York, 1878–9.*

New York (The) Monthly Chronicle of Medicine and Surgery. Conducted by an association of physicians. v. 1, July, 1824, to June, 1825. 380 pp. 8°. *New York, E. Bliss & E. White.*

New York (The) Monthly Review of Medical and Surgical Science and Buffalo Medical Journal.
Is running title of nos. 1–13, v. 15, of: **Buffalo** (The) Medical Journal.

New York Neurological Society. Constitution, by-laws, and list of officers and members, May 4, 1874. Instituted Jan. 10, 1872; reorganized April 6, 1874. 10 pp. 8°. *New York, D. Appleton & Co.*, 1874.

———. The answer of the . . . to the document known as the report of the committee on public health relative to lunatic asylums. No. 64. In senate, May 22, 1879. Submitted to the New York Neurological Society, and unanimously accepted and ordered to be printed by the same, at its stated meeting held at the Academy of Medicine, on Jan. 6, 1880. 49 pp. 8°. *New York, Trow*, 1880.

———. See, also:
Proceedings. Chicago J. Nerv. & Ment. Dis., 1874, i, 228. Continued in: J. Nerv. & Ment. Dis., Chicago, 1876–86, i–xi, passim.

New York Obstetrical Society. Transactions for the years 1876, 1877, and 1878, with a list of the fellows since its foundation. v. 1. xiv, 500 pp. 8°. *New York*, 1879.
Repr. from: Am. J. Obst.

New York Odontological Society. Chronicles, Dec., 1874. 7 pp. 8°. [*New York*, 1874.]
———. Transactions of special meeting. Dec. 14–16, 1874. 169 pp. 8°. *Philadelphia, S. S. White*, 1875.
———. Transactions for 1875; 1876; 1879–83. 7 v. 8°. *Philadelphia, S. S. White*, 1875–84.

New York Ophthalmic and Aural Institute, New York City. [Announcement by H. Knapp of the opening of the . . . Sept., 1869.] 2 l. 4°. [*New York*, 1869.]
Incorporated Sept. 3, 1869.
———. Annual reports of the surgeon in charge to the board of trustees. 1.–17., 1869–70 to 1885–6. 8°. *New York*, 1870–86.
5. rep. for 20 months, ending Dec. 31, 1874. 15. for 9 months, ending Sept. 30, 1884.

New York Ophthalmic Hospital, New York City. Annual reports of the directors and surgeons to the patrons and friends. 2.–13., 1853–64; 15.–22., 1866 to 1872–3; 24.–35., 1874–5 to 1885–6. 8°. *New York*, 1854–86.
Incorporated April 1 and opened May 25, 1852. Reports for 1858–63 were made biennially. 1853 is called first annual report, but they call 1866 the 15., which includes the year of opening, 1852, and so continues to date.
———. By-laws and rules of order, together with the acts of incorporation. 28 pp. 12°. *New York, F. Hart & Co.*, 1872.
———. Directions for persons wearing an artificial eye. 1 sheet. 12°. [*New York, n. d.*]

New York Ophthalmic Hospital and College. By-laws of the . . . adopted June 12, 1882. 26 pp., 3 l. 12°. *New York, Arthur & Bonnell*, 1882.

New York Orthopædic Dispensary. Report of the resident surgeon (Charles F. Taylor) to the finance committee for the period commencing Oct., 1866, and ending May, 1867. 9 pp. 8°. *New York, W. C. Martin*, 1867.
Bound with: Reports, 1867–8 to 1879–80. Opened Oct., 1866; incorporated May 1, 1868.
———. Annual reports of the board of supervisors and of the surgeon in charge to the trustees. 1.–20., 1867–8 to 1886–7. 8°. *New York*, 1869–88.
1. rep. for 20 months, ending Dec., 1868. 12. for 9 months, ending Sept. 30, 1879. 1.–13. bound in 1 v.

New York Pathological Society. Founded in 1844. Transactions. v. 1–3, 1875–81. 8°. *New York*, 1876–82.

New York Pathological Society—continued.

———. Constitution and by-laws, as adopted February 10, 1869, and amended prior to 1882. 15 pp. 8°. *New York*, [1882].

———. Constitution and by-laws, as adopted February 10, 1869, and amended prior to 1887. 16 pp. 8°. *New York*, [1887].

———. Certificate of incorporation. Constitution and by-laws. List of presidents, secretaries, and members. 22 pp. 8°. *New York*, 1887.

New York Pharmacal Association. Medical almanac, for the year 1886. 46 pp . sm. 4°. [*New York*, 1886.]

New York Physicians' Mutual Aid Association. Organized June 27th, 1868. Incorporated Nov., 1868. Constitution and by-laws. 12 pp. 12°. *New York*, 1868.

———. By-laws. 16 pp. 12°. *New York, Rogers & Sherwood*, 1874.

———. Annual reports. 7., 8., 10.–19., 1874–5, 1886–7. 8° & 12°. *New York*, 1875–88.

———. [List of officers and members, 1877.] 2 l. 8°. [*New York*, 1877.]

New York Polyclinic, a school of practical medicine and surgery. Quarterly circular announcement. Oct., 1883, to Feb. 1, 1884. 2 l. 4°. [*New York*, 1883.]

———. Annual announcements for the sessions of 1883–4 to 1886–7 (2.–6.). 8°. *New York*, 1883–7.
Lists of the classes for the years 1882–3 to 1885–6 in announcements for subsequent years.

New York Post Graduate Medical School and Hospital, New York City. Annual announcements for the sessions of 1882–3 to 1886–7 (1.–5.). 8°. *New York*, 1883–6.
Lists of matriculates for the sessions of 1882–3 to 1884–5 in announcements for subsequent years. 1. is 4°.

———. Announcements of the spring and summer sessions of 1885. 2 l. 4°. [*New York*, 1885.]

———. Schedule of lectures on mechanical and operative orthopedic surgery. By M. J. Roberts. Pt. I. Orthopedic technology. 10 pp. 12°. [*New York, J. J. O'Brien*, 1885.]

New York Post-Graduate Hospital. Annual report of the hospital committee of the . . . including the babies' ward, for the year 1885–7. 17 pp. 8°. *New York*, 1887.
Founded Feb. 1, 1884; incorporated May 25, 1886, in connection with the New York Post-Graduate Medical School.

New York Protestant Episcopal City Mission Society. Annual reports of the executive committee to the subscribers and members of the society. 23., 1872–3; 24., 1873–4. 8°. *New York*, 1873–4.

New York Public Health Association. Organization and constitution. 12 pp. 12°. *New York*, 1872.

———. Semi-annual report of the committee on public sanitary administration of the . . . at a meeting held Nov. 9, 1876. 14 pp. 8°. *New York, W. Knowles*, [1876].

———. Report of standing committee on public sanitary administration. 8 pp. 8°. [*New York*, 1879.]
Repr. from : The Plumber and Sanitary Engineer.

New York (The) Quarterly Cancer Journal ; devoted to the investigation and treatment of cancer and allied conditions. Editors : Robert S. Newton and R. S. Newton, jr. v. 1–2, April, 1877, to April, 1879. 8°. *New York*.
Want no. 1, v. 1, July, 1877.

New York Quarterly Journal. Devoted to the treatment of special diseases. Robert S. Newton, editor. No. 1, v. 1, Jan. 1, 1875. 14 pp. 8°. *New York*.

New York (The) Quarterly Journal of Medicine and Surgery.
Is running title of : **New York** (The) Journal of Medicine and Surgery.

New York (The) Register of Medicine and Pharmacy. Edited by C. D. Griswold. [Semi-monthly ; 2 v. annually.] v. 1–2, Oct. 1, 1850, to Sept. 15, 1851. 8°. *New York*.
Ended.

———. *See, also :*
Griswold (C. D.) A post-mortem examination of the New York Register of Medicine and Pharmacy. *Boston M. & S. J.*, 1851–2, xlv, 309.

New York Rendering Company. Special report upon the operations of . . .
See **New York** (*City*). Metropolitan Board of Health of the City of New York. 8°. *New York*, 1868.

New York Sanitary Association. Constitution and by-laws. 18 pp. 12°. *New York, R. Craighead*, 1859.

———. Reports of the Sanitary Association of the City of New York, in relation to the public health. 40 pp. 8°. *New York, E. Jones*, 1859. [*Also, in :* P., v. 345.]

———. Annual report. 23 pp. 8°. *New York, R. Craighead*, 1860. [*Also, in :* P., v. 339.]

New York Sanitary and Chemical Compost Manufacturing Company. Organized 1864, under the general manufacturing laws of the State of New York, for the purpose of cleansing cities, towns, and villages in the United States, by the use of Smith's patent street-sweeping machines and other mechanical appliances, etc. 32 pp. 8°. *New York*, 1865.

New York Sanitary Reform Society. Annual report for the year ending Sept. 30, 1880 (1.). 37 pp., 1 l., 1 chart. 8°. *New York*, 1880.

New York Skin and Cancer Hospital, New York City. [Circular of the board of trustees, calling attention to the need of this institution, and appealing for support.] 4 pp. 8°. [*New York*, 1882.]
Incorporated Nov. 11, 1882.

———. Annual reports of the governors to the subscribers. 1.–5., 1883–7. 32 pp. 8°. *New York*, 1884–8.

New York (The) Social Science Review ; a quarterly journal of political economy and statistics. Alexander Delmar and Simon Stern, editors. No. 4, v. 1 ; Nos. 1–2, 4, v. 2, Oct., 1865–6. 8°. *New York*.
v. 2 edited by S. Stern and J. K. H. Wilcox.

New York (The) Society for the Prevention of Contagious Diseases. Incorporated under the laws of the State of New York. Announcement. 1886. 19 pp. 8°. *New York, De Leeuw, Oppenheimer & Myers*, 1886.

New York Society for the Prevention of Cruelty to Children. Annual reports of the board of directors to the society. 1., 1875–6 ; 8., 1882. 8°. *New York, offices of the society*, 1875–83.
Incorporated April, 1875 ; organized April 27, 1875.

New York Society for the Prevention of Pauperism. Report of a committee on the subject of pauperism. 18 pp. 8°. *New York, S. Wood & Sons*, 1818.

New York Society for the Relief of the Ruptured and Crippled, New York City. Annual statements of the society to the subscribers. 12., 1853–4 ; 14., 1855–6 ; 16., 1857–8 ; 17., 1858–9 ; 19.–32., 1860–61 to 1873–4 ; 34.–43., 1875–6 to 1884–5. 4°. *New York*, 1854–85.

———. Annual reports of the board of managers and surgeon-in-chief, at the annual meetings. 1.–24., 1863–4 to 1886–7. 8°. *New York*, 1864–87.
Organized March 27, and commenced operations May 1, 1863. 1.–15. bound in 1 v.

———. The origin, progress, and present position. 12 pp. 8°. *New York, E. W. Sackett & Brother*, 1872.
Bound with : Reports, 1.–15.

New York Society for the Relief of the Widows and Orphans of Medical Men. Instituted in the

New York Society for the Relief [etc.]—cont. year 1842; incorporated in April, 1843. Laws of the . . . 24 pp. 12°. *New York, H. Ludwig & Co.*, 1849.

———. The same. 26 pp. 12°. *New York*, 1854.

———. Constitution and laws, to which is annexed a brief history of the society. 22 pp. 8°. *New York, Baker & Godwin*, 1870.

———. Constitution and laws, to which is annexed a brief history of the society and a complete list of the officers, members, and benefactors. 31 pp. 8°. *New York, Baker & Godwin*, 1875.

———. The same. 31 pp. 8°. *New York, C. G. Crawford*, 1880.

———. The same. 31 pp. 8°. *New York, C. G. Crawford*, 1884.

New York State Agricultural Society. First and second reports of the special committee appointed by the executive board of the . . . on the statistics, pathology, and treatment of the epizoötic disease known as the rinderpest. [A. B. Conger, in behalf of the committee.] 144 pp., 12 pl., 2 l. 8°. *Albany, Weed, Parsons & Co.*, 1867.

———. Report of J. C. Dalton, commissioner of the . . . for the investigation of abortion in cows. Printed by order of the senate and assembly. 59 pp. 8°. *Albany, C. Van Benthuysen & Sons*, 1868.

New York *State Board of Charities.*

NEW YORK (*State*). Annual reports of the State board of charities to the legislature. 2.–11., 1868–77. 8°. *Albany*, 1869–78.

STATE Charities Aid Association. Catalogue of library of the State Charities Aid Association, January, 1880. 8°. *New York*, 1880.

———. Annual report. 8., 1879–80. 8°. *New York*, 1880.

———. Address to its local visiting committees throughout the State of New York, July, 1880. 8°. *New York*, [1880].

New York *State Board of Health.*

NEW YORK (*State*). Assembly. An act to amend chapter 431 of the laws of 1881, entitled "An act to amend chapter 324 of the laws of 1850, entitled 'An act for preservation of the public health, and the acts amendatory thereof'". No. 361. March 20, 1882. Introd. by Mr. Farrar. fol. [*Albany*, 1882]

NEW YORK (*State*). S. An act to establish a State board of health. Jan. 15, 1880. Introd. by Mr. Woodin. fol. [*Albany*, 1880.]

NEW YORK (*State*). S. An act to amend chapter 324 of the laws of 1850, entitled "An act for the preservation of the public health". Jan. 20, 1880. Introd. by Mr. Pitts fol. [*Albany*, 1880.]

STATE board of health of New York. Manual. 8°. *Albany*, 1880.

———. Annual report. 2., 1881. 8°. *Albany*, 1882.

———. Report on the unsanitary condition of the village of Bath and the remedies therefor. 8°. [*Albany*, 1884.]

Repr. from: Rep. State Bd. Health, N. Y., 1884, Albany, 1885, v.

New York State Cabinet of Natural History. Annual reports of the regents of the University of the State of New York on the condition of . . . and the historical and antiquarian collection annexed thereto. 3., 1850; 4., 1851; 20., 1867. 8°. *Albany*, 1850-67.

———. The same. 3. report, revised ed. 8°. *Albany*, 1850.

New York State Hospital for Diseases of the Nervous System, New York City. Annual reports of the physicians in charge to the board of trustees. 1., 1870-71; 2., 1871-2. 8°. *New York*, 1871-2.

Incorporated March 17 and opened July 1, 1870.

New York State Medical Association. Founded February, 1884. Minutes of a convention held in the city of Albany, February 4th and 6th, 1884, at which the . . . was organized on a permanent basis. 43 pp. 8°. [*New York*, 1884.]

———. Catalogue of members of the medical profession in the State of New York, showing their vote on the codes of ethics. Proof for correction. 72 pp. 8°. *New York*, 1883.

———. The same. Corrected edition. Published by the Central Organization of the . . . to uphold the national code of ethics. 70 pp. 8°. *New York, Angell's Print. Off.*, 1884.

———. Constitution and by-laws adopted 1884. 23 pp. 8°. *New York, Angell's Print. Off.*, 1884.

———. Transactions. v. 1–3, 1884–6. 8°. *New York*, 1885-7.

New York State Pharmaceutical Association. An act to regulate the practice of pharmacy, the licensing of persons to carry on such practice, and the sale of poisons. 15 pp. 12°. [*n. p., n. d.*]

———. Proceedings of annual meetings. 2.–9., 1880–87. 8°. [*v. p.*], 1880–87.

New York State Teachers' Association. Report of the committee appointed on Mrs. Willard's theory of respiration. Read and accepted at their convention at Buffalo, Aug. 7, 1851. 16 pp. 8°. *Albany, H. H. Van Dyck*, 1851.

New York Surrogate's Court. In the matter of the probate of a paper propounded at the last will and testament of James B. Taylor, deceased. Opinion of Robert C. Hutchins, surrogate. 41 pp. 8°. *New York, N. Y. Printing Co.*, 1871.

———. In the matter of probate of the last will, etc., of Harriet Douglas Cruger, deceased. Opinion of surrogate. 33 pp. 8°. *New York, D. Taylor*, 1875.

New York Temperance Society. An address to physicians, by the executive committee of the board of managers. 22 pp. 8°. *New York, J. & J. Harper*, 1829.

New York (The) Thomsonian Botanico-Medical Journal. Addison Bassett, editor and proprietor. Published every other Saturday. Nos. 1–16, 18, v. 1, July 17, 1847, to March 14, 1848. 8°. *Stillwater, N. Y.*

New York Training School for Nurses. *See* **Society** of the Training School for Nurses, attached to Bellevue Hospital.

New York Vaccine Institution, New York City. Address of the . . . with the act of incorporation and by-laws. 8 pp. 8°. *New York, Burns & Bauer*, 1847.

New York Water Works Company. Report to the directors of the . . . by their engineer [Canvass White]. 11 pp. 8°. [*New York*, 1826.]

New - Yorker deutscher pharmaceutischer Verein. Manual. iv, 27 pp. 8°. *New York, G. B. Teubner*, 1858.

New - Yorker Leichenverbrennungs - Gesellschaft. *See* **New York** Cremation Society.

New - Yorker medicinische Monatsschrift. Hrsg. und redigirt von J. Herzka, E. Krakowitzer und W. Roth. Jahrg. 1, Feb., 1852, to Jan., 1853. 1 v. 388 pp. 8°. *New York.* Ended.

New-Yorker medizinische Presse. Organ der deutsch - amerikanischen Aerzte. Redacteur: Geo. W. Rachel. Hrsg. von der German Medical Press Company. [Monthly; 2 v. annually.] v. 1–5, December, 1885–8. 8°. *New York.* Current.

New Zealand. An act to amend an ordinance to make provision for the safe custody of, and prevention of offences by, persons dangerously insane, and for the care and maintenance of

New Zealand—continued.

persons of unsound mind. [19. Aug., 1858.] pp. 393–395. fol. [*Wellington*, 1858.] [P., v. 1292.] Cutting.

——. New Zealand Exhibition of 1865. [Circular of the commissioners announcing the project. Nov. 5, 1863.] 1 sheet. fol. [*Dunedin*, 1863.] [P., v. 1293.]

——. New Zealand Exhibition of 1865. [Instructions for the information of the local committees and exhibitors.] 2 pp. fol. [*Dunedin, Mills, Dick & Co.*, 1865?] [P., v. 1293.]

——. New Zealand Exhibition, 1865. Decisions regarding juries. 3 pp. fol. [*Dunedin, Harnett & Co.*, 1865.] [P., v. 1293.]

——. Decisions on points relating to the New Zealand Exhibition, 1865. 4 pp. fol. [*Dunedin*, 1865.] [P., v. 1293.]

——. No. 21. An act to make further provision for the education of the people of New Zealand. [29. Nov., 1877.] pp. 109–131. fol. [*Wellington, G. Didsbury*, 1877.] [P., v. 1297.] Cutting.

——. Report of the conservator of State forests to the commissioner, for the year 1876–7. 59 pp., 2 maps. fol. *Wellington, G. Didsbury*, 1877. [P., v. 1297.]

——. Lunatic asylums of New Zealand. Annual reports of the inspector to the colonial secretary, for the years 1876; 1877. 20 pp. fol. [*Wellington*, 1877–8.] [1876 *in* : P., v. 1297.]

——. California salmon and whitefish ova. (Papers relative to the introduction of.) (Presented to both houses of the general assembly by command of his excellency.) 24 pp. fol. [*Wellington*, 1878.]

——. Education. Papers relating to the establishment of schools of mines. (Presented to both houses of the general assembly by command of his excellency.) 15 pp. fol. [*Wellington, G. Didsbury*, 1878.]

——. Report of the royal commission appointed by his excellency to inquire into and report upon the operations of the University of New Zealand and its relations to the secondary schools of the colony, together with minutes of proceedings, minutes of evidence, and appendix. Presented to both houses of the general assembly by command of his excellency. xvi, 36, 407, 96, ix pp. fol. *Wellington, G. Didsbury*, 1879.

New Zealand. *Minister of Education.* Annual report of the . . . to the governor of the province. 1., 1877. 116 pp. fol. [*Wellington, G. Didsbury*, 1878.]

New Zealand. *Minister of Public Works.* Public works statement (annual). By the . . . 27th August, 1878. xiv, 95 pp., 2 maps, 1 ch., 2 plans. fol. [*Wellington*, 1878.]

New Zealand. *New Zealand Institute.* Annual report of the . . . (Presented to both houses of the general assembly by command of his excellency.) 10., 1877–8. 4 pp. fol. [*Wellington*, 1878.]

New Zealand. *Registrar - General.* Reports on the vital statistics of the principal towns of New Zealand. [Monthly.] Feb., 1880; March, July to Sept., Nov., 1882; Feb., 1883; May, 1883, to Nov., 1884; Jan., 1885, to April, 1886; June, 1886, to Dec., 1887. fol. [*Wellington*, 1880–88.] Repr. from : New Zealand Gaz.

——. Results of a census of the colony of . . . taken for the night of the 3d of April, 1881. v, 314 pp., 2 maps. fol. *Wellington, G. Didsbury*, 1882.

——. Statistics of the colony of New Zealand for the years 1881–6. With abstracts from the agricultural statistics of 1882–7. (Compiled from official records in the registrar-general's office.) fol. *Wellington*, 1882–5.

New Zealand. *Registrar-General*—continued.

——. Reports on the vital statistics of the four principal boroughs of New Zealand, during the years 1883; 1885. fol. [*Wellington*, 1884–6.] Repr. from : New Zealand Gaz.

——. Return of imigration to and emigration from the colony of New Zealand, for the 4. qr. 1884. 1 sheet. fol. [*Wellington*, 1885.]

——. Results of a census of the colony of New Zealand taken for the night of the 28th March, 1886. Pts. 1–10, and appendix. v, 37, 369 pp. fol. *Wellington, G. Didsbury*, 1887.

New Zealand. *University of New Zealand.* Papers relative to . . . (Presented to both houses of the general assembly by command of his excellency.) 19 pp. fol. [*Wellington, G. Didsbury*, 1875.]

New Zealand. *University of Otago.* Reports of the chancellor and officers to the governor of the colony, for the year 1876–7. 6 pp. fol. [*Wellington, G. Didsbury*, 1878.]

New Zealand.

See, also, **Medicine** (*History, etc., of*), *by nations, etc.*; **Medicine** (*Military, History of*)— *Campaigns, etc.*; **Paleontology.**

GREAT BRITAIN. [Proclamation of Queen Victoria appointing the royal commission of the New Zealand Exhibition of 1865. fol. [*Dunedin*, 1883.] Repr. from : New Zealand Gaz., Sept. 12, 1863.

VON HOCHSTETTER (F.) Geologie von Neu-Seeland. 4°. *Wien*, 1864–7.

MARCHANT (F. W.) The Tekapo bridge, Mackenzie County, New Zealand. 8°. *London*, 1885.

SWAINSON (W.) Observations on the climate of New Zealand ; principally with reference to its sanative character. 8°. *London*, 1840.

Allen (J. H. L.) Napier and Kuripapanga (Hawkes Bay Province, New Zealand) as health resorts for pulmonary invalids. Brit. M. J., Lond., 1888, i, 293.—**Bennett** (G) Notes on diseases prevailing among the New Zealanders and other inhabitants of the Polynesian Islands, with some account of their mode of treatment and the superstitions connected therewith. Australas. M. Gaz., Sydney, 1883-4, iii, 1-5.— **Drysdale** (C. R.) Comparative vital statistics of New Zealand with European countries. Med. Press & Circ., Lond., 1880, n. s., xxx, 388. ——. Vital statistics of New Zealand. Ibid., 1884, n. s., xxxviii, 128. — **Errington de la Croix** (J.) La tombe Maori au Musée du Trocadéro. Nature, Par., 1886-7, xv, 297-299. — **Gibbes** (J. M.) The New Zealand iodine thermal springs. Australas. M. Gaz., Sydney, 1883-4, iii, 199 201. — **Kerry-Nicholls** (J. H.) The origin, physical characteristics, and manners and customs of the Maori race, from data derived during a recent exploration of the King Country, New Zealand. J. Anthrop. Inst., Lond , 1885-6, xv, 187-209. — **Lewis** (T. H) On the thermal spring district of New Zealand. Australas. M. Gaz., Sydney, 1882-3, ii, 12-14. — **Maberly** (W. H.) New Zealand as a resort for consumptives and other invalids. Practitioner, Lond , 1880, xxiv, 326-343.—**Medical** practice in New Zealand. Lancet, Lond., 1882, i, 508. — **Meyer-Ahrens.** Die Krankheiten der Neuseeländer. Deutsche Klinik, Berl., 1858, x, 474 ; 492 : 1859, xi, 15 ; 35.—**Moore** (J. M.) The hot lakes of New Zealand. Homœop. World, Lond., 1881, xvi, 245 ; 290. ——. The Aroha, the newest sanatorium of New Zealand. Ibid., 1887, xxii, 208-210. — **Thompson** (J. B.) Observations on the climate of the British colonies of New Zealand, New South Wales, and Van Dieman's land, as compared with that of the Brazils, Madeira, and the continent of Europe ; from personal remarks and the most recent authentic statistical data ; with a few remarks on the diseases of the " aborigines " and those introduced by European colonization. Dublin M. Press, 1843. x, 132-134. *Also* : Lond. M. Gaz., 1843, xxxii, 766-770.—**Thomson** (A. S.) On the influence of the climate of New Zealand in the production of disease among emigrants from Great Britain. Edinb. M. & S. J., 1850, lxxiv, 82-91, 1 ch. ——. Contribution to the natural history of the New Zealand race of men ; being observations on their stature, weight, size of chest, and physical strength. J. Statist. Soc. Lond., 1854, xvii, 27-33 — **Tuke** (J. B.) Medical notes on New Zealand. Edinb. M. J., 1863-4, ix, 220 ; 721.

Nexon (Étienne-Guillaume). * Sur les avantages de l'allaitement maternel pour la mère et pour l'enfant. 23 pp. 4°. *Paris*, 1829, No. 169, v. 226.

von Ney (Franz). Systematisches Handbuch der gerichtsarzneilichen Wissenschaft, mit besonderer Berücksichtigung der Erhebung des Thatbestandes im Straf- und Civilverfahren für Aerzte, Wundärzte, dann Justiz- und politische Beamte und Advokaten in den k. k. Staaten, nebst einem Anhange über den Geschäftsstyl. xii, 313 pp. 8°. *Wien, Mörschner's Witwe u. W. Bianchi*, 1845.

——. Die gerichtliche Arzneikunde in ihrem Verhältnisse zur Rechtspflege, mit besonderer Berücksichtigung der österreichischen Gesetzgebung. Zum Gebrauche für Aerzte, Wundärzte und Rechtskundige dargestellt und mit entscheidenden Thatsachen begründet. 2 v. xx, 292 pp.; viii (1 l.), 291 pp. 8°. *Wien, Kaulfuss Wwe., Prandel u. Comp.*, 1847.

——. Die wichtigsten Momente der gerichtlichen Seelenkunde nach juridischen und naturwissenschaftlichen Grundsätzen für Leser aller Stände. 3 p. l., 252 pp. sm. 4°. *Linz, H. Danner*, 1863.

Ney (Fritz). Die Kuhmilch in der Kinderstube. Ein Buch aus der Praxis, gewidmet den deutschen Frauen. 1 p. l, 102 pp., 2 tab. 8°. *München, J. A. Finsterlin*, 1881.

Neyber (Fredrik Oscar Casimer) [1829-   ]. Om Pemphigus. Akademisk Afhandling. 2 l., 78 pp., 1 l., 2 pl. 8°. *Lund, Berling*, 1859. c.

Neydeck (Joannes Jacobus). * Diss. exhibens plethoram bene admodum curari per vasorum depletionem. 3 p. l., 36 pp., 6 l. 4°. *Wirceburgi, J. J. C. Kleyer*, 1752.

Neydeck (Karl Joseph). Der Buchs (Buxus sempervirens) das zuverlässigste und billigste Heilmittel der Wechselfieber. Ein Stellvertreter der China und anderer Medicamente gegen das Wechselfieber. 14 pp. 8°. *Karlsruhe*, 1858.

Neyrac.
Chevallier. Rapport sur les sources de Neyrac (Ardèche). Bull. Acad. de méd., Par., 1875, 2. s , iv, 261.— **Henry** (O.) Rapport et analyse au sujet de l'eau minérale de Neyrac (Ardèche). *Ibid.*, 1851–2, xvii, 781–785.— **Lefort.** Rapport sur la composition chimique de l'eau minérale de Neyrac (Ardèche). Ann. Soc. d'hydrol. méd. de Par., Compt.-rend., 1856–7, iii, 362–418.

Neyraud (Joseph). * De la gangrène traumatique. 41 pp. 8°. *Toulouse, Pradel, Viguier & Boé*, 1876. [P., v. 1412.]

Neyreneuf (François-Vincent). * De l'action de l'acide sulfurique sur la peau et de l'application de la pâte sulfo-safranée au traitement de quelques tumeurs sous-cutanées. 83 pp. 4°. *Paris*, 1872, No. 278.

——. Du traitement des tumeurs sous-cutanées par l'application de la pâte sulfo-safranée et de l'action de l'acide sulfurique sur la peau. 84 pp. 8°. *Paris, J.-B. Baillière & fils*, 1872.

Neyret (Adolphe). Des kystes hydatiques du tissu cellulaire sous-péritonéal du petit bassin. 51 pp. 4°. *Paris*, 1863, No. 37.

Neyret (François-Victor). * Étude sur la gangrène pulmonaire. 46 pp. 4°. *Paris*, 1870, No. 242.

Nezbedan (Josephus). * De colica in genere et in specie. 61 pp. 8°. *Viennæ, J. T. de Trattnern*, [1775.]

Nezdenitz.
Allé. Aerztliche Erfahrungen über die jod- und brombältige Mineralquelle zu Nezdenitz in Mähren. Oesterr. med. Wchnschr., Wien, 1846, 1375. ——. Versuche mit dem Nezdenitzer Mineralwasser im Sommer 1847. *Ibid.*, 1848, 132–134.

Nez Percés.
See Indians (*North American*)

Ngerengere.
Thomson (A. S.) An account of the disease called "Ngerengere" by the New Zealanders (lepra gangrænosa). Med.-Chir. Rev., Lond., 1854, xiii, 496–502, 1 pl.

Nhandirobe.
Ritter (G. H.) Entdeckung eines Gegengiftes in den Samen der Nhandirobe sevillea cordifolia. Mag. f. d. ges. Heilk., Berl., 1820, viii, 353–356.

Niagara.
NEW YORK (*State*). Annual report of the commissioners of the State reservation at Niagara to the legislature. 3., 1886. 8°. [*Albany*, 1887.]

——. Supplemental report of the commissioners of the State reservation at Niagara. Transmitted to the legislature Jan. 31, 1887. 8°. *Albany*, 1887.

Niagara University *Medical Department, Buffalo, N. Y.* Annual announcements for the sessions of 1883–4 to 1887–8 (1.–5.). 8°. *Buffalo*, 1883–7.

——. Announcement of spring term 1884. 6 pp. 8°. [*Buffalo*, 1884.]

Niaouli.
Bavay. Le niaouli. Gaz. méd. de l'Algérie, Alger, 1884, xxix, 44.

Niassis.
Reclus (É.) Les Niàssis de l'archipel Malai. Rev. internat. d. sc. biol., Par., 1881, viii, 469–498.

Niaux (Jules-Frédéric). * Diagnostic des principales maladies des poumons. 36 pp. 4°. *Paris*, 1851, No. 247, v. 512.

Niaux (Michel). * Propositions de médecine. 13 pp. 4°. *Paris*, 1823, No. 29, v. 177.

Nibbs (Henricus). * De variola. 49 pp. 8°. *Edinburgi, R. Allan*, 1796. [*Also, in :* P., v. 4.]

Niblett (S. Berry). A practical treatise on paralysis, wasting palsy, epilepsy, neurasthenia, neuralgia, sciatica, hysteria, headaches, nervestorms, and other diseases of the brain and spinal cord. vi, 8–128 pp. 8°. [*London, Harrison & Sons, n. d.*]

——. A practical treatise on consumption, lung disease, asthma, and chronic bronchitis. New ed. 80 pp. 8°. [*London, Harrison & Sons*, 1886.]

——. Essays on the most important affections of the skin. 3. ed. 96 pp. 16°. [*London*, 1887.]

——. A practical treatise on epilepsy; its successful treatment and cure. New and revised ed. 80 pp. 12°. *London*, [*Harrison & Sons, n. d.*]

——. The same. New and revised ed. 80 pp. 12°. [*London, Harrison & Sons, n. d.*] This is the same work as the preceding, but a different print or edition, bound alike and same size.

Niblock (Jacob). * De ophthalmia. 21 pp. 8°. *Edinburgi, A. Neill et socii*, 1800. [*Also, in :* P., v. 13.]

Nicaise (Auguste). * Sur l'âge de retour chez la femme. 35 pp. 4°. *Paris*, 1838, No. 176, v. 331.

Nicaise (E.) * Des lésions de l'intestin dans les hernies. 122 pp. 4°. *Paris*, 1866, No. 149.

——. Du gonflement du dos des mains chez les saturnins. 33 pp. 8°. *Paris, J.-B. Baillière & fils*, 1868. *Repr. from :* Gaz. méd. de Par., 1868, 3. s., xxiii.

——. Étude sur le choléra. 55 pp. 8°. *Paris, J.-B. Baillière & fils*, 1868. [P., v. 181.] *Repr. from :* Gaz. méd. de Par., 1868, 3. s., xxiii.

——. * Diagnostic des maladies de la hanche. 108 pp. 8°. *Paris, P. Asselin*, 1869. Concours.

——. * Des plaies et de la ligature des veines. 124 pp. 8°. *Paris, P. Asselin*, 1872. Concours.

——. Le Bureau central des hôpitaux. Rapport présenté à la Société des chirurgiens des hôpitaux au nom de la commission chargée d'étudier la question de la supression du Bureau central. 16 pp. 8°. *Paris, Germer-Baillière et Cie.*, 1877.

Nicaise (P.-F.) *Considérations générales sur l'angine gangréneuse. 18 pp. 4°. *Paris*, 1807, No. 8, v. 65.

Nicander. *See* Nikander.

Nicaragua.

See, also, **Archæology**; **Fever** (*Malarial, History, etc , of*), *by localities.*

BRANSFORD (J. F.) Archæological researches in Nicaragua. 4°. *Washington City*, 1881.

Bernhard. Bericht über den Gesundheitszustand und das Vorkommen von Krankheiten im Staate Nicaragna. Deutsche Klinik, Berl., 1854, vi, 81 ; 93 ; 105 ; 117.—**Bransford** (J. F.) Sanitary notes on the Nicaragua canal. Sanitarian, N. Y., 1883, n. s., i, 113–119.

Nicard (C.-F.) *I. Du traitement de l'asphyxie en général. II. [etc.] 30 pp. 4°. *Paris*, 1840, No. 361, v. 363.

Nicard (P.)
See **de Blainville** (Henri-Marie-Ducrotay). Ostéographie, ou description iconographique comparée [etc.] 4 v., 4°; Atlas, 4 v. in 2, imp. fol. *Paris*, 1839-64.

Nicard des Rieux (J.-G.-Eugène). *I. Quelle est la valeur des signes fournis par la présence des gaz dans les voies digestives ? II. [etc.] 35 pp. 4°. *Paris*, 1839, No. 281, v. 347.

Nicas (Ernest). *Remarques sur quelques maladies de l'enfance. 42 pp. 4°. *Paris*, 1855, No. 253, v. 578.

Nicati (C.)
See **Killias.** Notice sur les eaux de Tarasp-Schuls, etc. 8°. *Paris*, 1876.

Nicati (Constant). * De labii leporini congeniti natura et origine. 72 pp., 1 pl. 8°. *Traj. ad Rhenum et Amstelodami*, 1822.

———. Commentatio de mure domestico, silvatico atque arvali. 132 pp. 8°. *Traj. ad Rhenum, O. J. van Paddenburg*, 1822.

Nicati (William). *La paralysie du nerf sympathique cervical. Étude clinique. [Zürich.] 86 pp., 1 ch. 8°. *Lausanne & Paris, H. Mignot & A. Delahaye*, 1873.

———. * Des fibres nerveuses dans les nerfs optiques et dans la rétine. 32 pp. 4°. *Paris*, 1875, No. 334.

——— & **Rietsch** (M.) Recherches sur le choléra. viii, 172 pp., 2 pl. 8°. *Paris, F. Alcan*, 1886.

Repr. from: Bull. Soc. sc. industrielle de Marseille.

Nicaud (Gabriel). * Étude sur le diagnostic des insuffisances valvulaires du cœur et leur traitement. 39 pp. 4°. *Strasbourg*, 1867, 3. s., No. 25.

Nicault (Gilbert-Hyacinthe). *Sur la fistule lacrymale et son traitement. 23 pp. 4°. *Paris*, 1830, No. 272, v. 237.

Niccol (Robert). The sugar insect, "Acarus sacchari", found in raw sugar. 7 pp. 4°. *Philadelphia, De Armond & Goodrich*, 1868.

Niccolo.

See **Lettieri** (Natalis). Lettere due, etc. 8°. [*Neapoli*, 1785.]

Nice.

See, also, **Cholera** (*Asiatic, History, etc., of*), *by localities.*

BAART DE LA FAILLE (M. J.) Nizza en haar klimaat voor geneeskundigen en niet-geneeskundigen. 8°. *Leeuwarden*, 1871.

BARÉTY (A.) Du climat de Nice et de ses indications et contre-indications en général. 8°. *Paris*, 1882.

CABRIÉ (L.-P.-A.) * Nice et Hyères comparées comme lieu de séjour pour les tuberculeux. 4°. *Strasbourg*, 1859.

CHATIN. Rapport fait à l'Académie impériale de médecine de Paris le 9 octobre dernier sur un mémoire du chevalier docteur M. Macario, intitulé : De l'influence médicatrice du séjour à Nice. 8°. [*Nice*, 1860.]

See, also, Macario, *infra.*

Nice.

ESCALLIER (E.) Un mot à mes confrères sur le climat de Nice en hiver, ses principales qualités, ses indications et contre-indications; nécessité d'un bon choix d'habitation appropriée à l'état du malade. 8°. [*Paris*, 1864.]

FARR (W.) A medical guide to Nice; containing every information necessary to the invalid and resident stranger. With separate remarks on all those diseases to which its climate is calculated to prove injurious or beneficial, especially consumption and scrofula. Also, observations on the climate of Bagnères-de-Bigorre, as the most eligible summer residence for consumptive patients. 8°. *London*, 1841.

LEE (E.) Nice et son climat, avec des notices sur le littoral de la Méditerranée de Marseille à Gènes. 8°. *Nice*, 1851.

LIPPERT (H.) Das Klima von Nizza, seine hygienische Wirkung und therapeutische Verwerthung, nebst naturhistorischen, meteorologischen und topographischen Bemerkungen. 2. Aufl. 8°. *Berlin*, 1877.

NAUDOT. Influence du climat de Nice sur la marche des maladies chroniques et particulièrement sur la phthisie pulmonaire. 8°. *Paris*, 1842.

Arneth (F. H.) Nizza als klimatischer Curort. St. Petersb. med. Ztschr., 1862, iii, 351–365.—**Arnold** (F.) Nizza in nosologischer Beziehung. Mag. f. d. ges. Heilk., Berl., 1831, xxxv, 3–19.—**Balestre.** Étude sur le mouvement de la population de Nice depuis 1861. Nice-méd., 1876-7, i, 7 ; 42 ; 75 ; 105 ; 145 ; 225 ; 296 ; 359 : 1878-9, iii, 8—**Baréty** (A) Influence du climat de Nice sur l'enfance et la vieillesse. *Ibid.*, 1876-7, i, 15–22. ———. De l'action du climat de Nice dans le traitement de la phthisie pulmonaire. *Ibid.*, 1881-2, vi, 433–445.—**Durand.** Étude sur l'air de Nice. Nice-méd., 1887, xi, 65–70.—**Frémy** (H.) Assainissement de Nice. *Ibid.*, 1882-3, vii, 133–143.—**Giraud** (L.) Ressources hygiéniques et thérapeutiques de Nice. *Ibid.*, 1876-7, i, 307 ; 335 : 1877-8, ii, 49.—**Grellety** (L.) Du climat de Nice et des maladies traitées dans cette ville, principalement de la phthisie. Mém. et bull. Soc. de méd. et chir. de Bordeaux (1879), 1880, 532–549. *Also*: Bull. et mém. Soc. de thérap. 1879, Par., 1880, 2. s., vi, 35–50. *Also*: J. de méd. de Bordeaux, 1879-80, ix, 150 ; 159.—**Guiraud.** De la nécessité de créer à Nice un bureau municipal d'hygiène. Nice-méd., 1883-4, viii, 65–72.—**Hawkins** (J.) The sanitary condition of Nice. Med. Press & Circ., Lond., 1869, vii, 118.—**Henry** (C.) Enquête sur l'état sanitaire de Nice durant l'automne de 1883. Nice-méd., 1883-4, viii, 97–100.—**Hughes** (J. S.) Short notes on Nice. Med. Press & Circ., Dubl., 1868, v, 465 ; 494 : vi, 52 ; 118. *Also*, Reprint.—**Hugues.** Des précautions que doivent prendre les malades qui viennent passer l'hiver à Nice. Nice-méd., 1876-7, i, 65–75.—**Klima** (Das) von Nizza in Bezug auf Gesundheit. Allg. med. Centr.-Ztg., Berl., 1858, xxvii, 606 ; 614. — **Lippert** (H.) Climatologisch-therapeutische Aphorismen aus Nizza. Deutsche Klinik, Berl., 1864, xvi, 333 ; 345 ; 357 ; 485 ; 493 : 1865, xvii, 13 ; 109 ; 129 ; 149: 1866, xviii, 353 ; 365 ; 373 ; 393 : 1867, xix, 65 ; 85.—**Lubanski.** Le climat de Nice. Gaz. méd. de Lyon, 1856, viii, 397–403.—**Macario.** Topographie médicale de Nice. Ann. Soc. de méd. de Lyon, 1860, 2. s., viii, 359–364. *Also*: Gaz. méd. de Lyon, 1860, xii, 506–509. ———. De l'influence médicatrice du séjour de Nice. [Rap. de Chatin.] Bull. Acad. de méd., Par., 1860-61, xxvi, 28–36. *Also* [Rev. de Devaux]: Ann. Soc. méd.-chir. de Bruges, 1861, 2. s., ix, 225–242. ———. Sul clima de Nizza. Gazz. med. ital. lomb., Milano, 1877, 7. s., iv, 421 ; 431 ; 471 ; 482 ; 492 ; 504 : 1878, 7. s., v, 24 ; 81.—**Macpherson** (J.) Nice as a winter resort. San. Rec., Lond., 1876, v, 356–359.—**Niepce** (A.) Du climat de Nice ; composition de l'air atmosphérique à Nice. Cong. périod. internat. d. sc. méd. Compt.-rend. 1877, Genève, 1878, v, 598–605. ———. Étude sur la constitution climatologique et médicale de Nice pendant l'année 1878. Nice-méd., 1878-9, iii, 141 ; 200, 1 tab.—**Richelmi** (P.) Beobachtungen über die Heilsamkeit des Clima von Nizza, und über die Vorsichtsmaassregeln, welche Aerzte zu nehmen haben, wenn sie Kranke nach einem wärmern Clima schicken. J. d. pract. Heilk., Berl., 1826, lxii, 4. St., 117–125.—**Schreiber.** Nizza, als Winteraufenthalt für Kranke. Wien. Med.-Halle, 1863, iv, 378 ; 389 ; 397.—**Schütz** (W.) Briefliche Mittheilungen aus Nizza. Deutsche Klinik, Berl., 1857, ix, 81 ; 101 ; 109 ; 127.—**Sturge** (W. A.) & **Sturge** (*Mme*. B.) Des égouts de Nice, qui se déversent au bord de la mer. Nice-méd., 1881-2, vi, 449–451.—**Thaon** (L.) De l'action du climat de Nice dans le traitement des maladies du système nerveux. *Ibid.*, 1876-7, i, 33–39. ———. Traitement de la phthisie par le climat de Nice. *Ibid.*, 1877-8, ii, 1 ; 35 ;

Nice.

73.—**Wahu.** Du climat de Nice dans ses rapports avec la phthisie pulmonaire. Union méd., Par., 1861, 2. s., x, 554.—**West** (C.) De la création d'un sanatorium à Nice. Nice-méd., 1882-3, vii, 33-36. ———. The sanitary condition of Nice. Med. Times & Gaz., Lond., 1884, i, 814. ———. The medical profession at Nice. *Ibid.*, 1883, i, 20. *Also :* Brit. M. J., Lond., 1883, i, 34. *Also :* Lancet, Lond., 1883, i, 39.

Nice-médical. Climatologie.—Médecine pratique.—Hygiène. Organe officiel de la Société de médecine et de climatologie de Nice. [Monthly.] Années 1-12, Oct. 1876-88. 8°. *Nice.* Current.

Nicens (Christian Friedrich). *See* **Saalmann** (Ferd.) Fieberlehre [etc.] 8°. *Breslau*, 1793.

Niché (Joannes Æmilius) [1823-]. * De hydropsiis. 31 pp. 8°. *Berolini, G. Schade*, [1848].

Nichet (Pierre - Jacques) [1803-47]. Mémoire sur la nature et le traitement du mal vertébral de Pott. 50 pp. 8°. *Paris, bureau de la Gazette médicale*, 1835. [P., v. 1681.] *Rep : from :* Gaz. méd. de Par., 1835, 2. s., iii.

———. Deuxième mémoire sur le mal vertébral. 81 pp. 8°. [*Paris, F. Malteste & Cie.*, 1840.] [P., v. 1681.] *Repr. from :* Gaz. méd. de Par., 1840, 2. s., viii. *For Biography, see* Gaz. méd. de Lyon, 1851, iii, 21-34 (F. F. A. Polton). *Also, repr. from :* Actes Soc. nat. de méd. de Lyon.

Nichol (John Pringle) [1804-59]. Views of astronomy. Seven lectures delivered before the Mercantile Library Association of New York. Reported for the New York Tribune. iv, 5-41 pp. 8°. *New York, Greeley & McElrath*, 1848.

———. A cyclopædia of the physical sciences, comprising acoustics, astronomy, dynamics, [etc.] 2. ed., revised. ix, 903 pp., 3 pl., 3 maps. 8°. *London, R. Griffin & Co.*, 1860. *For Biography, see* Lancet, Lond., 1859, ii, 352.

Nichol (W. L.) *Co-Editor of :* **Nashville** (The) Journal of Medicine and Surgery. 1869-70.

Nichol (William). Proposal for the development of the principle of assurance as an instrument for the gradual extinction of pauperism and for the permanent improvement of the condition of the industrious classes. 25 pp. 8°. *Edinburgh, R. Hardie & Co.*, 1847.

Nicholaevski.

Miller. Mediko-topographicheskija zamietki o Nicholaevskie na Amurie. Med. pribav. k morsk. sborniku, St. Petersb., 1872, xiii, 166-198.

Nicholaus *Præpositus. See* **Nicolaus** *Præpositus.*

Nicholay (J. A.) Administration of the sewerage and drainage of the metropolitan districts. Statement of objections to the existing system and of essentials for a sound one. Prepared at the request of the Right Hon. Sir George Grey. 10 pp. 8°. *London, R. & J. E. Taylor*, 1851. [P., v. 1219.]

Nicholl (Guillaume). * Sur les hernies de l'abdomen. vi, 7-47 pp. 4°. *Paris*, 1815, No. 34, v. 108; 109.

Nicholl (Whitlock) [1786-1839]. General elements of pathology. 233 pp. 8°. *London, J. Callow*, 1820.

———. Practical remarks on disordered states of the cerebral structures occurring in infants. 2 l., 5-94 pp. 16°. *London, J. Callow*, 1821.

Nicholles (John). The teeth, in relation to beauty, voice, and health. 2. ed. xvi, 134 pp., 1 pl. 8°. *London, Hamilton, Adams & Co.*, 1834.

Nicholls (Francus) [1699-1778]. Compendium anatomico-œconomicum, ea omnia complectens, quæ ad cognitam humani corporis œconomiam spectant. Cui, quo clarius elucescat, quanta sit anatomia in medicina tam diagnostica et pro-

Nicholls (Francus)—continued. gnostica quam practica, adjiciuntur prælectiones, laxum et strictum fibræ animalis statum, actiones medicamentorum, artem obstetricariam et proximas mortis causas anatomicis principiis exponentes. 3 p. l., 76 pp., 7 pl. 4°. *Londini, J. Clarke*, 1736. [P., v. 701.] *Another copy bound with :* **Manningham** (R.) Artis obstetricariæ [etc.] 4°. *Londini*, 1739.

———. De anima medica ; prælectio ad socios Collegii Regalis Medicorum Londinensium, ex Lumleii et Caldwaldi Institutio habita. Die 16to Decembris, anno 1748vo. 41 pp. 4°. *Londini, P. Vaillant*, 1750.

———. The same. Editio altera, notis amplioribus aucta cui accessit disquisitio de motu cordis et sanguinis in homine nato et non nato. 103 pp., 11 pl. 4°. *London, J. Walter*, 1773.

———. De natura et usu partium humani corporis similarium. *In :* **Lawrence** (T.) F. Nichollsii . . . vita [etc.] 4°. *Londini*, 1780. *For Biography, see* **Lawrence** (T.) Franci Nichollsii M. D. Georgii secundi . . . medici ordinarii vita : cum conjecturis ejusdem de natura et usu partium humani corporis similarium. 4°. *Londini*, 1780.

Nicholls (Richard). A treatise on counter irritation, or heat versus cold, and its application to the organism for the prevention and cure of diseases without the aid of medicine. 47 pp. 8°. *London, J. Draper*, [n. d.]

Nichols (*Andrew*) [1785-1853].

Lord (S. A.) Obituary notice. Med. Communicat. Mass. M. Soc., Bost., 1854, viii, 245-249.

Nichols (Arthur Howard) [1840-]. Report on an outbreak of intestinal disorder, attributable to the contamination of drinking-water by means of impure ice. pp. 468-474. 8°. *Boston, Wright & Potter*, 1876. *Cutting from :* Rep. Bd. Health Mass., Bost., 1875, vii.

Nichols (C. F.) Quantum sufficit. A summary of cases chiefly treated by the higher homœopathic attenuations ; with comments. Tract 4. 26 pp. 12°. *Boston, W. F. Towns*, [1877].

Nichols (Charles Henry) [1820-]. On the best mode of providing for the subjects of chronic insanity. 24 pp. 8°. [*New York*, 1878.] *Repr. from :* Tr. Internat. M. Cong., Phila., 1876.

Nichols (D. Cubitt). Report on the sanitary condition of the hamlet of Mile End Old Town, March 17, 1886. (Presented to both houses of Parliament by command of Her Majesty.) 10 pp. fol. *London, Eyre & Spottiswoode*, 1886.

———. Report on the sanitary condition of the parish of Clerkenwell. (Presented to both houses of Parliament by command of Her Majesty.) 8 pp. fol. *London, Eyre & Spottiswoode*, 1886.

Nichols (George Ward). The story of the great march. From the diary of a staff officer. 22. ed. 408 pp. 8°. *New York, Harper & Bros.*, 1865.

Nichols (James R.) [1819-88]. Chemical examination of urine. 7 pp. 12°. [*n. p., n. d.*] *Repr. from :* Boston J. Chem., 1866, i.

———. From snow-banks to orange orchards ; an essay read before the Essex North Massachusetts Medical Society, May, 1878, and published in the Boston Journal of Chemistry. 8 pp. 8°. *Haverhill, F. P. Stiles*, 1878. *Also, Co-Editor of :* **Boston** (The) Journal of Chemistry, 1867-83. *For Biography, see* Boston M. & S. J., 1888, cxviii, 26.

Nichols (*Joseph*) [1796-1853].

Hoyt (M. C.) Obituary notice. Boston M. & S. J., 1850, l, 98-100.

Nichols (L.) Einführung in die Naturheilkunde. Genaue Erklärung der menschlichen Constitution. Bedingungen der Gesundheit, Natur und Ursachen der Krankheit, die leitenden Medizinsysteme und die Grundsätze, Praxis,

Nichols (L.)—continued.

Auwendungen und Ergebnisse der Hydrotherapie oder Wasserkur, als wissenschaftliches und umfassendes System zur Erhaltung und Wiederherstellung der Gesundheit. 28 pp. 8°. *Berlin, T. Grieben*, 1875.

Bound with: TRALL (R. F.) Die Diphtheritis, etc. 8°. *Berlin*, 1875.

Nichols (Mary S. Gove). Experience in water-cure. A familiar exposition of the principles and results of water treatment in the cure of acute and chronic diseases, illustrated by numerous cases in the practice of the author, with an explanation of water-cure processes, advice on diet and regimen, and particular directions to women in the treatment of female diseases, water treatment in childbirth, and the diseases of infancy. 108 pp. 12°. *New York, Fowler & Wells*, [1849].

——. The same. 108 pp. 12°. *New York, Fowler & Wells*, 1852.

——. The same. 108 pp. 12°. *New York*, 1855.

Water-Cure Library, v. 2.

——. A woman's work in water-cure and sanitary education. iv, 154 pp. 16°. *London*, [1874].

Nichols (*Paul L.*)

Obituary notice. Med. Communicat. Mass. M. Soc., Bost., 1869, ii, 130.

Nichols (Thomas L.) An introduction to the water-cure. A concise exposition of the human constitution, the conditions of health, etc. Founded in nature and adapted to the wants of man. 40 pp. 12°. *New York, Fowler & Wells*, 1850.

——. The same. 46 pp. 8°. *New York*, 1855.

Water-Cure Library, v. 2.

——. The curse removed. A statement of facts respecting the efficacy of water-cure in the treatment of uterine diseases, and the removal of the pains and perils of pregnancy and childbirth. 20 pp. 12°. *New York, office of the Water-Cure Journal*, 1850.

——. Esoteric anthropology. iv, 5–482 pp. 12°. *Port Chester, New York*, 1853.

——. Human physiology, the basis of sanitary and social science. xvi, 480 pp. 12°. *London, Nichols & Co.*, [1872].

——. Die Kunst, mit fünf Groschen $= \frac{1}{2}$ Mark täglich auskömmlich zu leben. 32 pp. 8°. [*Berlin, T. Grieben*, 1875.]

Gesundh., Wohlst. u. Glück, xlii.

——. The gift of healing; or, the sympathetic cure. 62 pp. sm. 8°. *London, Nichols & Co.*, [1880].

Repr. from: Herald of Health, Lond., 1878–81, i.

——. Eating to live. The diet cure. An essay on the relations of food and drink to health, disease, and cure. viii, 88 pp. 8°. *New York, M. L. Holbrook & Co.*, 1881.

——. Health: what it is, and why to seek it; how to get it, and how to lose it. A homely lecture on health, disease, and cure. Addressed to visitors of the International Health Exhibition. 30 pp. 12°. *South Kensington, London*, 1884.

Also, Co-Editor of: **American** (The) Vegetarian and Health Journal, Phila., 1850–54.

Nichols (W. C.)

Co-Editor of: **New Orleans** (The) Medical and Surgical Journal, 1859–69.

Nichols (W. T.) Mind cure; its truths and fallacies from a common sense standpoint. 76 pp. 12°. *Chicago*, 1886.

Nichols (*Whitfield*) [1807–51].

Pennington. [Biographical notice of the late . . .] N. Jersey M. Reporter, Burlington, 1851–2, v. 271–276.

Nichols (William Ripley). Observations on the composition of the ground-atmosphere in the neighbourhood of decaying organic matter. From

Nichols (William Ripley)---continued.

the report of the sewerage commission, Boston, 1875. 7 pp. 8°. *Boston, Rockwell & Churchill*, 1876.

——. Report of . . . to C. O. Chapin, esq., president of board of water commissioners, Springfield, Mass. 3 pp., 1 l. 8°. [*Boston*, 1877.]

——. On the filtration of potable water. 90 pp., 3 diag. 8°. *Boston, Rand, Avery & Co.*, 1878.

Repr. from: Rep. Bd. Health Mass., Bost., 1877, ix.

——. Report of . . . to the water commissioners, Springfield, Mass. 12 pp. 8°. [*n. p.*, 1878.]

Repr. from: Ann. Rep. of the water commissioners, 1878.

——. Chemical examinations of sewer air. 16 pp. 8°. *Boston, Rockwell & Churchill*, 1879.

Repr. from: Rep. of the superintendent of sewers, Bost., 1879.

——. Report of . . . on the Boston water supply. 6 pp. 8°. [*Boston*, 1879.]

Repr. from: Rep. Bost. water board, 1879, iii.

——. Supplementary report on sewer air. To the superintendent of sewers. April 1, 1879. 4 pp. 8°. [*Boston*, 1879.]

——. Report of . . . on the New Bedford water supply. 3 pp. 8°. [*Boston*, 1880.]

Repr. from: Rep. Acushnet water board, 1880, x.

——. [Report to the water commissioners of the town of Winchester.] 2 pp. 8°. [*Boston, Mass.*, 1880.]

——. Papers on water supply. 8°. *Boston, Rand, Avery & Co.*, 1880.

CONTENTS.

The pollution of streams.
The Westfield and Merrimac Rivers. By the secretary.
Pollution of a brook by sulphuric acid. 21 pp.
Observations on Fresh Pond, Cambridge.
On the examination of Mystic water.
Remarks on Frankland's method of water analysis. pp. 95–120.

Cutting from: Rep. Mass. Bd. Health, Lunacy, and Char., 1879, i.

——. Sanitary condition of school-houses. 12 pp. 8°. [*Boston*, 1880.]

——. Sand filtration at Berlin. 5 pp. 8°. *Philadelphia*, [1881].

Repr. from: J. Frankl. Inst., Phila., 1881, 3. s., lxxxii.

——. Natural filtration at Berlin. 8 pp. 8°. [*Philadelphia*, 1882.]

Repr. from: J. Frankl. Inst., Phila., 1882, 3. s., lxxxiii.

——. Water supply considered mainly from a chemical and sanitary standpoint. vi, 232 pp. 8°. *New York, J. Wiley & Sons*, 1883.

——. Chemistry in the service of public health. An address before the section of chemistry of the American Association for the Advancement of Science, at Ann Arbor, Aug., 1885. 20 pp. 8°. *Salem, Mass.*, 1885.

Repr. from: Proc. Am. Ass. Adv. Sc., Salem, 1885, xxxiv.

Also, Co-Editor of: **Annual** of Scientific Discovery, Boston, 1868–71.

See, also, **Folsom** (C. F.) The pollution of streams, etc. 8°. Boston, 1877.—**Massachusetts** Institute of Technology, Boston. Publications of the . . . 8°. Boston, 1882.—**Sedgwick** (W. T.) & **Nichols** (W. R.) A study of the relative poisonous effects of coal and water gas. 8°. [Boston, 1885.]

——— & **Allen** (C. R.) Contributions to our knowledge of sewage. 6 pp. 8°. [*Boston*, 1885.]

Repr. from: J. Frankl. Inst., Phila., 1885, 3. s., xc?

——— & **Farlow** (W. G.) Reports of . . . and . . . on matters connected with the Boston water supply. 7 pp. 8°. *Boston, Rockwell & Churchill*, 1877.

Repr. from: Rep. of the water board, 1877.

———, ——— & **Burgess** (Edward). Report on a peculiar condition of the water supplied to the city of Boston, 1875–6. 14 pp. 8°. *Boston, Rockwell & Churchill*, 1876.

Repr. from: Rep. Cochituate Water Bd., Bost., 1876.

Nicholson (A.) Nature's own book; or practical results of a vegetable diet, illustrated by facts and experiments of many years' practice. 96 pp. 12°. *Glasgow, W. S. Brown, 1846.*

———. Gesundheit, Glück und hohes Alter, oder wie soll der Mensch leben? Eine hygienische Abhandlung unterstützt durch Thatsachen und Experimente vieljähriger Praxis. 2. Aufl. 8°. *Berlin, T. Grieben, 1868.*
In: LEES. Die Ernährung des Menschen. 8°. Berlin, 1868, 35–72

Nicholson (Alexander Jaffray). *De intemperentia. 8 p. l., 20 pp., 3 l. 8°. Edinburgi, D. Stevenson et soc., 1817. [P., v. 978.]*

Nicholson (Brinsley). *See* **Scot** (Reginald). The discoverie of witchcraft. 4°. *London, 1886.*

Nicholson (Guilelmus). *De monstro humano sine trunco nato. 24 pp., 1 l. 4°. Berolini, formis Nietackianis, [1837].*

Nicholson (Henricus). *De corpore. 29 pp. 4°. Lugd. Bat., A. Elzevier, 1709.*

Nicholson (Henry Alleyne). Is vaccination injurious? A popular essay on the principles and practice of vaccination. 40 pp. 8°. *London, Churchill & Sons, 1869.*

———. A manual of zoology for the use of students, with a general introduction on the principles of zoology. xx, 622 pp. 8°. *London, W. Blackwood & Sons, 1870.*

———. The same. 2. ed. xx, 673 pp. 8°. *Edinburgh & London, W. Blackwood & Sons, 1881.*

———. A manual of palæontology for the use of students, with a general introduction on the principles of palæontology. xvi, 601 pp. 8°. *Edinburgh & London, W. Blackwood & Sons, 1872.*

———. Life and its physical basis. 25 pp. 8°. *London, E. Stanford, [1879, vel subseq.].*

———. Introduction to the study of biology. x, 163 pp. 8°. *Edinburgh & London, W. Blackwood & Sons, 1872.*
*See, also, **White** (C. A.) Bibliography of North American invertebrate paleontology, etc. 8°. Washington, 1878.*

——— & **Thomson** (James). Descriptions of new species of rugose corals from the carboniferous rocks of Scotland. pp. 121–134, 2 pl. 8°. [*n. p.,* 1876]
Cutting from: Proc. Phil. Soc. Glasgow, 1876.

Nicholson (James B.) Experience tables of the Independent Order of Odd Fellows upon the subject of dues and benefits, showing the ratio of sickness and the law of increase; compiled from the semi-annual reports of the working lodges and the journals of the Grand Lodge of Pennsylvania. 16 pp. 8°. *Philadelphia, R. Cohill, 1878.*

Nicholson (Thomas). An essay on yellow fever, comprising the history of that disease as it appeared in the island of Antigua in the years 1835, 1839, and 1842. With an appendix continuing the history to 1853. (Read before the Epidemiological Society of London, July 4th, 1853, and published in the Association Medical Journal for Sept., 1853.) 28 pp. 8°. *Antigna, W. Mercer, 1856.*

Nicholson (W. P.) Both sides. Dudley on the bandage. To the editor of the Transylvania Journal of Medicine and the Associate Sciences. 11 pp. 8°. [*Lexington, Ky.,* 1829.]
Repr. from: Transylv. J. M., Lexington, Ky., 1828, i.

——— & **Dudley** (B. W.) Both sides. I. Mr. W. P. Nicholson's pamphlet. Dudley on the [tight] bandage. II. B. W. Dudley's reply, Feb. 7, 1829. 24 pp. 8°. [*Lexington,* 1829.] [*Also, in:* P., v. 827.]
Transylv. J. M., Lexington, Ky., 1829, extra.

Nicholson (William). The first principles of chemistry. 2. ed. xxxi, 546 pp., 2 l. 8°. *London, G. G. J. & J. Robinson, 1792.*

Nichtarzt (Für den): kurzer Unterricht wie er sich gegen die morgenländische Brechruhr zu verwahren und was er bey dem ersten Anfalle dieser Krankheit bis zur Ankunft eines Arztes zu thun habe. Nebst einem wichtigen Anhange für praktische Aerzte enthaltend eine neue Heilmethode dieser Krankheit. 16 pp. 8°. *Pesth, K. A. Hartleben, 1831.*

Nichterlein (Ferdin. Gustav) [1822–]. *De signis mortis submersione effectæ. 35 pp. 8°. Gryphiæ, F. G. Kunike, 1849.*

Nicius (Friedrich Ehrenhold). *De ratione altero medicinæ fulcro necessario. 3 p. l., 27 pp., 1 l. 4°. Argentorati, typ. J. H. Heitzii, [1720].*

Nick (Georgius Henricus). *De pœnis corporis afflictivis tam civilibus quam militaribus. 23 pp. 4°. Tubingæ, lit. Reis- et Schmidianis, [1804].*

———. Beobachtungen über die Bedingungen, unter denen die Häufigkeit des Pulses im gesunden Zustand verändert wird. Eine von der med. Facult. der Univ. Tübingen, für das Jahr 1823 gekrönte Preisschrift. xii, 65 pp. 8°. *Tübingen, Schönhardt, [1825].*

———. The same. xii, 65 pp. 8°. *Tübingen, C. F. Osiander, 1826.*

Nickel *and its salts.*
See, also, **Neuralgia** (*Treatment of*).
GEERKENS (F.) Experimentelle Untersuchungen über die Wirkungen von Nickelsalzen. 8°. *Bonn, 1883.*
Coppola (F.) Sull' azione fisiologica del nichel e del cobalto. Sperimentale, Firenze, 1885, lv, 375: 1886, lvii, 43.—Da Costa (J. M.) Observations on the salts of nickel, especially the bromide of nickel. Med. News, Phila., 1883, xliii, 337.—Fede (F.) & Jappelli (G.) Azione fisiologica del solfato di nickel; ricerche sperimentali. Resoc. Accad. med.-chir. di Napoli, 1885, xxxix, 190–202, 1 diag. Also: Gior. di neuropatol., Napoli, 1886, iv, 171–181.—Hare (H. A.) The action of the bromide of nickel. Therap. Gaz., Detroit, 1886, 3. s., ii, 297–300.—Laborde & Riche. Étude expérimentale sur l'action physiologique des sels de nickel. Tribune méd., Par., 1888, xxi, 87; 100.—Leaman (R.) Some clinical observations on the therapeutic uses of bromide of nickel. Med. News, Phila., 1885, xlvi, 427–429. Also: Coll. & Clin. Rec., Phila., 1885, vi, 116–118.—Riche (A.) Action des sels de nickel sur l'économie. Bull. Acad. de méd., Par., 1888, 2. s., xix, 18–24.—Schulz (H.) Ueber die antiseptische Wirkung des Nickelchlorürs. Deutsche med. Wehnschr., Berl., 1882, viii, 708–710. Also: Sitzungsb. d. nied.-rhein. Gesellsch. f. Nat.- u. Heilk. zu Bonn, 1882, 31.—Simpson (J. Y.) Notes on the therapeutic action of furfurine, nickel, etc. In his: Contrib. Obstet. Path. [etc.], 8°, Edinb., 1853, 37–40.—Stuart (T. P. A.) Nickel and cobalt; their physiological action on the animal organism. Part I. Toxicology. [Extr. from his thesis.] J. Anat. & Physiol., Lond., 1882-3, xvii, 89–123. Also, transl.: Arch. f. exper. Path. u. Pharmakol., Leipz., 1884, xviii, 151–173.—Testa (B.) Influenza del bromuro di nichelio sull' eccitabilità cerebrale. Gazz. med. di Torino, 1886, xxxvii, 457–463.

Nickel (August Ferdinand Alexander) [1856–]. *Ueber Venenthrombose bei Abdominaltyphus. 32 pp. 8°. Berlin, M. Driesner, 1884.*

Nickel (Carl). *Zur Casuistik der durch Cholelithiasis bedingten Pericystitis vesicæ felleæ. 30 pp. 8°. Marburg, R. Friedrich, 1886.*

Nickel (Otto). *Experimentelle Beiträge zur quantitativen Oxalsäurebestimmung im Harn. 31 pp. 8°. Berlin, J. F. Starcke, [1886].*

Nickels (G. I.) *Ueber die Resection im Ellenbogen-Gelenke. 56 pp. 8°. Würzburg, C. W. Becker, 1837.*

Nickels (Joannes Fridericus). *Diss. sistens iridis anatomiam, physiologiam, pathologiam et morborum hinc oriundorum therapiam. 60 pp., 1 l. 8°. Jenæ, typ. Goepferdtii, [1800].*
For Biography, see **Gruner** (Christ. Goth.)

Nicker (Henri-Aloyse). *Considérations générales sur les tumeurs blanches. 56 pp. 4°. Strasbourg, 1854, No. 314, 2. s., v. 20.*

Nickerl (Franciscus Antonius). *Diss. sistens monographiam eruptionum syphiliticarum secundum Cazenave et Schedel, adnexis morborum

Nickerl (Franciscus Antonius)—continued.
historiis. 29 pp., 1 l. 8°. *Pragæ, W. Spinka,*
1841.
Nicklès (F.-J.-Jérôme) [1821–69]. *De la fermentation de l'acide tartrique et de ses produits.
31 pp. 8°. *Strasbourg, G. Silbermann,* 1846. [P.,
v. 1747.]
———. *Physique. Les électro-aimants circulaires. Chimie. Recherches sur le polymor-
phisme. 27, 23 pp., 1 tab. 4°. *Paris, Vve.
Bouchard-Huzard,* 1853. [P., v. 1718.]
———. Braconnot, sa vie et ses travaux. 136 pp.
8°. *Nancy, Grimblot & Vve. Raybois,* 1856. [P.,
v. 793.]
Repr. from : Mém. Acad. de Stanislas, Nancy.
———. Sur la dénaturation du sel destiné à l'a-
griculture. 28 pp. 8°. [*Nancy, Vve. Raybois,*
1863.] [P., v. 1769.]
———. Recherches de chimie appliquée. (Faits
nouveaux concernant les corps gras, les matières
sucrées, la séparation du plomb et du bismuth,
etc.) 24 pp. 8°. *Nancy, Vve. Raybois,* 1866.
[P., v. 1769.]
Also, Co-Editor of : **Journal** de pharmacie et de chimie, Paris, 1865–9.
Nickles (S.)
See **Siegle** (Emil). The treatment of disease of the
throat [etc.] 8°. *Cincinnati,* 1868.
Nicklin (P. H.) A report made to the board of
trustees of the University of Pennsylvania, at a
stated meeting on Tuesday the 4th of Nov., 1834,
concerning the Universities of Oxford and Cambridge, in England. 40 pp. 8°. *Philadelphia,
J. & W. Kite,* 1834.
Nickse ([Ludovicus Eduardus] Bertholdus Æmilius) [1814–]. *De abscessu psoadico. 32 pp.
8°. *Berolini, typ. Friedlaenderianis,* [1837].
Niclou (Carl) [1853–]. *Ueber die Resorption
todter Knochen. 36 pp. 8°. *Greifswald, F. W.
Kunike,* 1877.

Nicobar *Islands.*

Bleeck (W.) Ethnographische und anthropologische
Gegenstände von den Nicobaren und Andamanen. Verhandl. d. Berl. Gesellsch. f. Anthrop., 1880, 409–414.—
Distant (W. L.) The inhabitants of Car Nicobar. J.
Anthrop. Inst., Lond., 1873-4, iii, 2–7.— **Giglioli** (E.)
Notizie sugli indigeni delle Isole Nicobar e specialmente
sui Shôm Pén dell' interno della Grande Nicobar. Arch.
per l' antrop., Firenze, 1885, xv, 31–34.—**Helfft.** Ueber
das Klima, die Sitten und Krankheiten der Einwohner der
nicobarischen Inseln. Deutsche Klinik, Berl., 1852, iv, 343-
347.—**Man** (E. H.) On the Andamanese and Nicobarese
objects presented to Maj.-Gen. Pitt Rivers, F. R. S. J.
Anthrop. Inst., Lond., 1881-2, xi, 268–294, 4 pl. ——. A
brief account of the Nicobar Islanders, with special reference to the inland tribe of Great Nicobar. *Ibid.*, 1885-6,
xv, 428-451, 1 map, 2 pl.—**de Roepstorff** (F. A.) Ueber
die Bewohner der Nicobaren. Ztschr. f. Ethnol., Berl.,
1882, xiv, 51–68, 1 pl.

Nicod (Barthélemy-Célestin). *Sur l'utilité de la
douleur. 28 pp. 4°. *Paris,* 1822, No. 174, v. 174.
Nicod (F.-P.-V.-Agricole). *Considérations
générales sur l'étiologie des exhalations sanguines de l'extrémité inférieure du rectum, et
sur la formation organique des marisques ou tumeurs qui ordinairement les précèdent ou les
accompagnent. 17 pp. 4°. *Paris,* 1819, No. 16,
v. 144.
Nicod (Louis-Joseph). *Sur le scorbut. 28 pp.
4°. *Paris,* 1815, No. 298, v. 117.
Nicod (Pierre-Louis-Aimé) [1788–1845]. *Sur la
fragilité des os, et sur la contraction musculaire
considérée comme cause de fracture. 21 pp. 4°.
Paris, 1807, No. 113, v. 63.
———. Dissertation sur le danger de la résection
des côtes et de l'excision de la plèvre dans les
maladies cancéreuses; et sur la possibilité de
guérir l'hydropisie du péricarde. 25 pp. 8°.
Paris, Migneret & Gabon, 1818.
———. Recueil d'observations médicales confirmant la doctrine de Ducamp, sur la cautérisation

Nicod (Pierre-Louis-Aimé)—continued.
de l'urètre ; précédé d'un abrégé de l'histoire de
la cautérisation de l'urètre en France. v. 1.
xxxvi, 102, 192 pp., 2 pl. 8°. *Paris, l'auteur,*
1825.
The "Abrégé" has a separate title-page and pagination,
with date 1826.
———. Abrégé de l'histoire de la cautérisation de
l'urètre en France, avant Ducamp. 102 pp. 8°.
Paris, Méquignon-Marvis, 1826.
Also, in his: Recueil d'observations méd. [etc.] 8°.
Paris, 1825.
———. Mémoire sur les polypes de l'urètre et de
la vessie. 48 pp. 8°. *Paris, Éverat,* 1827. [*Also,
in :* P., v. 1398.]
———. Traité sur les polypes, et autres carnosités
du canal de l'urètre et de la vessie. Avec les
meilleurs moyens de les détruire sans danger.
15 p. l., 346 pp. 8°. *Paris, l'auteur,* 1835. [P.,
v. 486.]
Nicol (J.-D.) *De la méthode antipyrétique dans
le traitement de la pneumonie. 38 pp., 1 l. 4°.
Strasbourg, 1868, 3. s., No. 119.
Nicol (James). On the study of natural history
as a branch of general education ; an inaugural
lecture, at Marischal College. 32 pp. 8°. *Edinburgh, Oliver & Boyd,* 1853. [*Also, in :* P., v.
1201.]
———. Vital, social, and economic statistics of
the city of Glasgow, 1881-5. With observations
thereon. xiv (1 l. 304 pp. 8°. *Glasgow, R.
Maclehose,* 1885.
———. *See, also :*
TESTIMONIALS of James Nicol, as a candidate
for the chair of civil and natural history in Marischal College, Aberdeen. 8°. [*Edinburgh,* 1852.]
Nicol (John Inglis) [1788–1849]. Essay on the
treatment of caries, with remarks on the diseases
of bone in general. 40 pp. 8°. *Tubingen, Eifert,*
1827.
———. Case of medullary sarcoma, engaging the
upper portion of the os humeri, considered aneurismal, and for which the sub-clavian artery was
tied above the clavicle. 19 pp., 2 pl. 8°. [*Edinburgh, J. Slack,* 1834.]
Repr. from : Edinb. M. & S. J., 1834, xlii.
Nicol (Patrick).
See **Dillnberger** (Emil). Handybook of the treatment of women's and children's diseases, [etc.] 8°. *Philadelphia,* 1871.
Nicoladoni (Carl) [1847–]. Die Torsion der
skoliotischen Wirbelsäule. Eine anatomische
Studie. 24 pp., 12 pl. roy. 8°. *Stuttgart, F.
Enke,* 1882.
———. Die Torsion des Samenstranges, eine ei-
genartige Complication des Kryptorchismus. 15
pp., 1 pl. 8°. *Berlin,* [*n. d.*]
Repr. from : Arch. f. klin. chir., Berl., 1885, xxxi.
Nicolaeff (Nicolaus). *De forma pelvis tam
rhachitide quam et osteomalacia vitiata atque
de causis utrinsque. 46 pp., 11 l. 8°. *Mosquæ,
typ. Universitatis Cæsareæ,* 1850. [P., v. 1680.]

Nicolai.

See **Fever** (*Malarial, History, etc., of*), by localities.
Nicolai (Alphons), jun. Erfahrungen und Notizen über Milzbranderkrankungen bei Mensch
und Thier. Gratulationsschrift. 28 pp. 8°.
Darmstadt u. Leipzig, E. Zernin, 1872.
Nicolai (Alphonsus Julius Guilelmus). *Diss.
continens morbi historiam ; empyema, thoraco-
centesem, exitum mortalem. 20 pp. 8°. *Jenæ,
typ. Ratii,* 1859.
Nicolai (Carolus Fridericus)[1] [1768–]. *Dy-
nameologiæ chemico-physico-medicæ specimen.
1 p. l., 44 pp. 4°. *Lipsiæ, ex off. Klaubarthia,*
[1799].
See, also, **Vogt** (Traugott Carolus Augustus).

Nicolai (Carolus Fridericus)[2]. * De naturæ externæ in corpus humanum actione et effectu. 1 p. l., 43 pp. 4°. *Vitebergæ, lit. C. H. Græssleri*, [1805].

For Biography, see **Platner** (Ernestus).

Nicolai (Carolus Fridericus Guilielm.) * De angina polyposa. 23 pp. 8°. *Halæ, typ. Hendelianis*, [1817].

Nicolai (*Christophorus*) [1618–62].

Portrait in : **Collection**—van Kaathoven.—**Collection** of Portr. of Phys. & Men of Sc., 192.

Nicolai (Ehrenfried Otto). * Encephalomalacia ex hypertrophia cordis, historia morbi cum epicrisi. 42 pp. 8°. *Regiomonti Pr., E. J. Dalkowski*, [1835].

Nicolai (Ernestus Augustus). * Diss. sistens coleopterorum species agri Halensis. 44 pp., 1 l. 8°. *Halæ, typ F. A. Grunerti patris filiique*, [1822].

For Biography, see **Gruner** (Christian. Gothfrid.)

Nicolai (Ernst Anton) [1722–1802]. * De dolore. 1 p. l., 41 pp. sm. 4°. *Halæ Magdeb., C. H. Hemmerde*, [1745].

——. Abhandlung von der Schönheit des menschlichen Körpers in einem Glückwünschungsschreiben an Herrn Christ. Fried. Truppeln. 77 pp. 16°. *Halle, C. H. Hammerde*, 1746.

——. Methodus concinnandi formulas medicamentorum exemplis ad medici quondam illustris Friderici Hoffmanni mentem accommodatis illustrata. 11 p. l., 576 pp. 16°. *Halæ Magdeb.*, 1747.

——. Gedanken von der Erzeugung der Missgeburthen und Mondkälber. 2 p. l., 128 pp. 12°. *Halle, C. H. Hemmerde*, 1749.

——. Versuch eines Lehrgebäudes von den Fiebern überhaupt. 11 p. l., 389 pp., 1 l. 12°. *Halle, C. H. Hemmerde*, 1752.

——. Abhandlung von den Fehlern des Gesichts. 10 p. l., 212 pp. 12°. *Berlin, Schütz*, 1754.

Bound with: SCHAARSCHMIDT (A.) Kurzer Unterricht von den Krankheiten [etc.] 12°. *Berlin*, 1754.

——. De dolore in genere. Diss. 46 pp. 4°. *Jenæ, lit. Fickelscherrianis*, [1758].

——. De sensatione ac sensibilitate quo prælectiones suas futuro semestri habendas indicat. 36 pp., 1 l. 4°. *Jenæ, lit. Fickelscherrianis*, [1758].

——. [Pr.] quo genuina arthritidis ejusque specierum notio eruitur. I. [Cum vita candidati Lud. Leon Bader.] 8 pp. 4°. *Jenæ, lit. Fickelscherrianis*, [1759].

——. The same. II. [Cum vita candidati Joan. Christ. Wilh. Holland.] 8 pp. sm. 4°. *Jenæ, lit. Marggrafianis*, [1760].

——. The same. III. [Cum vita candidati Imman. Aug. Frid. Bertram.] 8 pp. sm. 4°. *Jenæ, lit. Fickelscherrianis*, [1760].

——. The same. IV. [Cum vita candidati Francisci Petri Emcken.] 8 pp. sm. 4°. *Jenæ, lit. Fickelscherrianis*, [1760].

——. [Pr.] de genesi vertiginis. I. [Cum vita candidati Joannis Christophori Buch.] 8 pp. 4°. *Jenæ, lit. Marggrafianis*, [1759].

——. The same. II. [Cum vita candidati Jo. Joac. Wewetzer.] 8 pp. 4°. *Jenæ, lit. Marggrafianis*, [1759].

——. The same. III. [Cum vita candidati Georgii Jacobi Gladbach.] 8 pp. 4°. *Jenæ, lit. Marggrafianis*, [1759].

——. [Pr.] de deliriis. I. [Cum vita candidati Joan. Geor. Schmidt.] 8 pp. 4°. *Jenæ, lit. Fickelscherrianis*, [1759].

——. The same. II et ultimum. [Cum vita candidati Guilielmi Henrici Sebastiani Bucholtz.] viii pp. 4°. *Jenæ, ex off. F. Fickelscherrii*, [1763].

——. [Pr.] exponens rationem structuræ quarundam auris partium. I. [Cum vita candidati

59

Nicolai (Ernst Anton)—continued.
Johannes Henricus Christophorus Schencke.] 8 pp. 4°. *Jenæ, lit. Fickelscherrianis*, 1760.

——. The same. III. [Cum vita candidati Jo. Christ. Doering.] 8 pp. sm. 4°. *Jenæ, lit. Fickelscherrianis*, [1760].

——. The same. IV et ultimum. [Cum vita candidati Mart. Frid. Henrici.] viii pp. sm. 4°. *Jenæ, lit. Fickelscherrianis*, [1761].

——. [Pr.] de cordis et arteriarum in sanguinem actione. [Cum vita candidati Jodoci Ehrhart.] viii pp. 4°. *Jenæ, lit. Fickelscherrianis*, [1761].

——. [Pr.] de causis pelluciditatis partium corporis humani. I. [Cum vita candidati Joannis Friderici Wilhelmi.] viii pp. sm. 4°. *Jenæ, lit. Fickelscherrianis*, [1761].

——. The same. II. [Cum vita candidati Joan. Andr. Schaubach.] 8 pp. 4°. *Jenæ, lit. Fickelscherrianis*, [1762].

——. The same. III et ultimum. [Cum vita candidati Gottlieb Friderici Stuss.] viii pp. sm. 4°. *Jenæ, ex off. F. Fickelscherrii*, [1763].

——. [Pr.] de notione morbi maligni. [Cum vita candidati Christophori Friderici Caroli Cappe.] viii pp. 4°. *Jenæ ex off. F. Fickelscherrii*, [1763].

——. [Pr.] de pulsu celeri crebro et frequenti. I. [Cum vita candidati Wesselii Lümmen.] viii pp. 4°. *Jenæ, ex off. E. Fickelscherrii*, [1763].

——. [Pr.] de gummi ammoniaci virtute. I. [Cum vita candidati Caroli Ludovici Schmalz.] 8 pp. 4°. *Jenæ, lit. F. Fickelscherrii*, [1767].

——. Pathologie, oder Wissenschaft von Krankheiten. 9 v. 12°. *Halle*, 1769–84.

Volumes for 1781–4 are numbered i, ii, iii, and title reads as follows: Fortsetzung der Pathologie, oder Wissenschaft von Krankheiten.

——. [Pr.] de digestivis quædam præmittit. [Cum vita candidati Jo. Christ. Valentini Gantz.] 8 pp. 4°. *Jenæ, ex off. F. Fickelsche rii*, [1770].

——. [Pr.] de viribus medicamentorum explorandis. I. [Cum vita candidati Caspari Philippi Fromm.] 8 pp. 4°. *Jenæ, lit. Straussii*, [1770].

——. The same. II. [Cum vita candidati Joannis Philippi Wolff.] 8 pp. 4°. *Jenæ, ex off. F. Fickelscherrii*, [1770].

——. The same. III. [Cum vita candidati Joannis Theophili Scheler.] 8 pp. 4°. *Jenæ, ex off. F. Fickelscherrii*, [1771].

——. [Pr.] de diabete ex spasmo quædam præmittit. [Cum vita candidati Joannis Godofredi Sonntag.] 8 pp. 4°. *Jenæ, ex off. Helleri*, [1773].

——. [Pr.] de modo agendi aperientium et martialium medicamentorum. [Cum vita candidati Joannis Henrici Lucas.] 8 pp. 4°. *Jenæ, lit. Fickelscherrii*, [1776].

——. [Pr.] de causa cur ferrum per cuprum præcipitetur. [Cum vita candidati Joannis Salomonis Ernesti Schwabe.] 8 pp. sm. 4°. *Jenæ, lit. Fickelscherrii*, [1776].

——. [Pr.] de causis cataractæ externis.

In: WEIZ (F. A.) Neue Ausz. [etc.] 12°. *Leipzig*, 1777, vii, 56–58.

——. [Pr.] de figura arteriarum disserit. [Cum vita candidati Christiani Godofredi Whistling.] 8 pp. 4°. *Jenæ, lit. Fickelscherrii*, [1778].

——. [Pr.] de fine ductus thoracici. I. [Cum vita candidati Henrici Christophore Lemmer.] 8 pp. 4°. *Jenæ, ex off. Straussiana*, [1778].

——. The same. II. [Cum vita candidati Chr. Guil. Alexand. Heinrich.] 8 pp., 2 l. 4°. *Jenæ, lit. Fickelscherrii*, [1778].

——. [Pr.] de rubore sanguinis. [Cum vita candidati Joannis Guilielmi Güttich.] 8 pp. sm. 4°. *Jenæ, lit. Fickelscherrii*, [1778].

——. [Pr.] de pulsu duro et molli. I. [Cum vita candidati Joannis Christophori Fahner.] 8 pp. 4°. *Jenæ, lit. Fickelscherrianis*, [1780].

Nicolai (Ernst Anton)—continued.

——. The same. II. [Cum vita candidati Christiani Augusti Hauenschild.] 8 pp. 4°. *Jenæ, ex off. F. Fickelscherr. hæred. et Stranckmanni,* [1782].

——. The same. III et ultimum. [Cum vita candidati Georgii Gustavi Detharding.] 16 pp. 8°. *Jenæ, lit. Goepferdianis,* [1788].

—— [Pr.] de virtute et usu clysterum ex aceto. I. [Cum vita candidati Traugott Frider. Augusti Treuner.] 8 pp. 4°. *Jenæ, typ. Stranckmannianis,* [1783].

——. The same. II. [Cum vita candidati Godofredi Adolphi Welper.] 8 pp. 4°. *Jenæ, typ. Stranckmannianis,* [1783].

——. The same. III. [Cum vita candidati Tob. Henr. Godof. Spindler.] 8 pp. 4°. *Jenæ, typ. Stranckmannianis,* [1783].

——. The same. IV. [Cum vita candidati Caroli Joannis Nyberg.] 8 pp. 4°. *Jenæ, typ. Stranckmannianis,* [1783].

——. The same. V. [Cum vita candidati Christiani Friderici Wilhelmi Pfündel.] 8 pp. 4°. *Jenæ, typ. Stranckmannianis,* [1783].

——. [Pr.] de usu aquæ frigidæ externo. I. [Cum vita candidati Joannis Henrici Zahn.] 8 pp. 4°. *Jenæ, typ. Stranckmannianis,* [1783].

——. The same. II. [Cum vita candidati Michaelis Ludovici Wittwerk.] 8 pp. 4°. *Jenæ, typ. Stranckmannianis,* [1783].

——. The same. III. [Cum vita candidati Friderici Ludovici Heroldt.] 8 pp. 4°. *Jenæ, typ. Stranckmannianis,* [1783].

——. [Pr.] de cubitu ægrotorum. I. [Cum vita candidati Georgii Henrici Toemlich.] 8 pp. 4°. *Jenæ, lit. Stranckmannianis,* [1785].

——. The same. II. [Cum vita candidati Christiani Caroli Lang.] 8 pp. 4°. *Jenæ, lit. Stranckmannianis,* [1785].

——. The same. III. [Cum vita candidati Gottlieb Joannis Badendyk.] 8 pp. 4°. *Jenæ, lit. Stranckmannianis,* [1785].

——. The same. IV. [Cum vita candidati Joannis Guilielmi Harder.] 8 pp. 4°. *Jenæ, lit. Stranckmannianis,* [1785].

——. The same. VI. [Cum vita candidati Joannis Samuelis Sommer.] 8 pp. 4°. *Jenæ, lit. Stranckmannianis,* [1786].

——. The same. VII. [Cum vita candidati Joannis Conradi Friderici Zier.] 8 pp. 4°. *Jenæ, lit. Stranckmannis,* [1786].

——. The same. VIII. [Cum vita candidati Joannis Bartholomæi.] 8 pp. 4°. *Jenæ, lit. Stranckmannianis,* [1786].

——. The same. X. [Cum vita candidati Joannis Christiani Steinfeld.] 8 pp. sm. 4°. *Jenæ, lit. Stranckmannianis,* [1788].

——. The same. XII et ultima. [Cum vita candidati Friderici Augusti Wilhelmi Gress.] 8 pp. 4°. *Jenæ, lit. Maukianis,* [1788].

——. Theoretische und praktische Abhandlungen über die Entzündung und Eiterung, den Brand Scirrhus und Krebs, und über die Kurarten dieser Krankheiten. v. 2. 532 pp., 1 l. 12°. *Jena, Cröker,* [1786].

——. [Pr.] de sanguinis missione in febribus intermittentibus. I. [Cum vita candidati Joannis Friderici Müller.] 16 pp. 8°. *Jenæ, lit. Stranckmannianis,* [1788].

——. The same. II. [Cum vita candidati Joannis Friderici Glaser.] 8 pp. 4°. *Jenæ, lit. Göpferdtianis,* [1788].

——. The same. III. [Cum vita candidati Wilhelmi Ernesti Christiani Huschke.] 8 pp. 4°. *Jenæ, lit. Göpferdtianis,* [1788].

——. The same. V. [Cum vita candidati Caroli Gottlieb Mylius.] 8 pp. 4°. *Jenæ, typ. Göpferdtii,* [1789].

Nicolai (Ernst Anton)—continued.

——. The same. VI. [Cum vita candidati Caroli Augusti Friderici Brückner.] 8 pp. 4°. *Jenæ, lit. Goepferdtii,* [1790].

——. The same. VII. [Cum vita candidati Benj. Zeitmann.] 16 pp. 8°. *Jenæ, lit. Goepfertii,* [1790].

——. The same. VIII. [Cum vita candidati Friderici Ludovici Segnitz.] 8 pp. 4°. *Jenæ, lit. Goepferdtii,* [1790]. [*Also, in :* P., v. 58.]

——. The same. IX. [Cum vita candidati Friderici Adolphi Heinze.] 8 pp. 4°. *Jenæ, lit. Goepferdtii,* [1790].

——. The same. XIII. [Cum vita candidati Gottlob Henrici Kober.] 8 pp. 4°. *Jenæ, lit. Stranckmannianis,* [1790].

——. The same. XIV. [Cum vita candidati Guilielmi Friderici Habermann.] 8 pp. 4°. *Jenæ, lit. Stranckmannianis,* [1790].

——. The same. XV. [Cum vita candidati Aug. Frid. Car. Rauch.] 8 pp. 4°. *Jenæ, lit. Fiedlerianis,* [1790].

——. The same. XVI. [Cum vita candidati Joannis Scherbii.] 8 pp. 4°. *Jenæ, lit. Fiedlerianis,* [1790].

——. Rezepte und Kurarten. mit theoretisch praktischen Anmerkungen. 2. Ausg. 5 v. 12°. *Jena, Cröker,* 1788–99.

v. 3, for 1799, is 3. Ausg.

——. [Pr.] de urina viridi. I. [Cum vita candidati Joannis Friderici Henrici Hieronymus.] 16 pp. 8°. *Jenæ, lit. Maukianis,* [1790].

——. The same. II. [Cum vita candidati Joannis Friderici Grahl.] 8 pp. 4°. *Jenæ, lit. Fiedlerianis,* [1790].

——. The same. III. [Cum vita candidati Joannis Godofredus Goetz.] 10 pp. 4°. *Jenæ, typ. Goepferdtii,* [1791].

——. [Pr.] de origine febrium ex irritatione et spasmo corporis humani vivi universali. I. [Cum vita candidati Franc. Xav. Christ. Theoph. Kinzel.] 16 pp. 8°. *Jenæ, lit. Fiedlerianis,* [1791].

——. The same. II. [Cum vita candidati Christiani Friderici Blauberg.] 8 pp. 8°. *Jenæ, lit. Maukianis,* [1791].

——. The same. III. [Cum vita candidati Ernesti Friderici Christiani Graf.] 8 pp. 4°. *Jenæ, lit. Stranckmannianis,* [1791].

——. The same. IV. [Cum vita candidati Henrici Christ. Theod. Reussing.] 8 pp. 4°. *Jenæ, lit. Fiedlerianis,* [1791].

——. The same. V. [Cum vita candidati Caroli Eman. Steiner.] 16 pp. 8°. *Jenæ, typ. Geopferdtii,* [1792].

——. [Pr.] de urina tenui et crassa. I. [Cum vita candidati Francisci Ernesti Filter.] 8 p. 4°. *Jenæ, typ Goepferdtii,* [1791].

——. The same. II. [Cum vita candidati Christiani Hieron. Theod. Lützelberger.] 8 pp. 4°. *Jenæ, lit. Fiedlerianis,* [1791].

——. The same. III. [Cum vita candidati Christiani Friderici Quandt.] 8 pp. 4°. *Jenæ, lit. Fiedlerianis,* [1791].

——. The same. IV. [Cum vita candidati Joannis Carol. Ludov. Behr.] 8 pp. sm. 4°. *Jenæ, typ. Goepferdtii,* [1791].

——. [Pr.] V. [Cum vita candidati Christ. Frid. Ludov. Wildberg.] 16 pp. 4°. *Jenæ, lit. Fiedlerianis,* [1791?].

——. The same. VI. [Cum vita candidati Joannis Pauli Gottlob Kircheisen.] 8 pp. 4°. *Jenæ, lit. Fiedlerianis,* [1792].

——. The same. VII. [Cum vita candidati Augusti Christophori Rosenbladt.] 8 pp. 4°. *Jenæ, lit. Maukianis,* [1792].

——. The same. VIII et ultima. [Cum vita candidati Guil. Rud. Christ. Wiedemann.] 16 pp. 4°. *Jenæ, lit. Fiedlerianis,* [1792].

Nicolai (Ernst Anton)—continued.

——. [Pr.] de diagnosi inflammationum. I. [Cum vita candidati Christiani Fürchtegott Schmalz.] 8 pp. 4°. *Jenæ, typ. Stranckmanni,* [1792].

——. The same. II. [Cum vita candidati Joan. Jac. Locher.] 8 pp. 4°. *Jenæ, lit. Fiedlerianis,* [1792.]

——. The same. III. [Cum vita candidati Caroli Friderici Christophori Waerlich.] 8 pp. 4°. *Jenæ, typ. Stranckmanni,* [1794].

——. The same. IV. [Cum vita candidati Joannis Ludovici Andreæ Vogel.] 8 pp. 4°. *Jenæ, typ. Stranckmanni,* [1794].

——. The same. V. [Cum vita candidati Caroli Hermanni Curtius.] 12 pp. 4°. *Jenæ, typ. Goepferdtii,* [1794].

——. The same. VI. [Cum vita candidati Philippi Jacobi Scheurer.] 16 pp. 8°. *Jenæ, typ. Goepferdtii,* [1794].

——. The same. VII. [Cum vita candidati Joannis Caroli Christiani Schnaubert.] 16 pp. 8°. *Jenæ, lit. Schlotterianis,* [1801].

——. The same. VIII. [Cum vita candidati Christiani Henrici Hiecke.] 16 pp. 8°. *Jenæ, typ. Prageri et soc.,* 1801.

——. The same. X. [Cum vita candidati Christiani Guiliel. Schmid.] 16 pp. 8°. *Jenæ, typ. Prageri et soc.,* 1801.

——. [Pr.] de morbis gastricæ originis. I. [Cum vita candidati Joannis Andreæ Braun.] 8 pp. 4°. *Jenæ, lit. Fiedlerianis,* [1792].

——. The same. II. [Cum vita candidati Joannes Christ. Reddelien.] 8 pp. 4°. *Jenæ, typ. Stranckmanni,* [1794].

——. The same. III. [Cum vita candidati Joannis Conradi Honnerlag.] 16 pp. 8°. *Jenæ, typ. Stranckmanni,* [1794].

——. The same. IV. [Cum vita candidati Nicolai Mueller.] 16 pp. 12°. *Jenæ, lit. Fiedlerianis,* [1794].

——. [Pr.] de curatione febrium intermittentium evacuantia. I. [Cum vita candidati Joannis Henrici Köningsdörffer.] 8 pp. 4°. *Jenæ, lit. Maukianis,* [1794].

——. The same. II. [Cum vita candidati Joannis Theophili Tettenborn.] 8 pp. 4°. *Jenæ, lit. Fiedlerianis,* [1793].

——. The same. III. [Cum vita candidati Joannis Ehrenfriedi Emanuel Bloedau.] 16 pp. 8°. *Jenæ, typ. Goepferdtii,* [1795].

——. The same. IV. [Cum vita candidati Georgii Henrici Behn.] 16 pp. 8°. *Jenæ, typ. Stranckmanni,* [1795].

——. The same. V. [Cum vita candidati Eberhardi Mickwiz.] 8 pp. 4°. *Jenæ, lit. Fiedlerianis,* [1795]

——. The same. VI. [Cum vita candidati Theodori Georgiadas.] 8 pp. 4°. *Jenæ, lit. Maukianis,* [1797].

——. The same. VII. [Cum vita candidati Joannis Godofredi Langermann.] 16 pp. 8°. *Jenæ, lit. Maukianis,* [1797].

——. The same. VIII. [Cum vita candidati Joan. Godofr. Caroli Fürbringer.] 8 pp. 4°. *Jenæ, typ. Etzdorfii et soc.,* [1798].

——. The same. IX. [Cum vita candidati August. Francisc. Ferdin. Mohring.] 8 pp. 4°. *Jenæ, typ. Etzdorfii et soc.,* [1798].

——. [Pr.] inest historia cephalalgiæ periodicæ maro offic. sanatæ. [Cum vita candidati Guilielmi Christiani Stern.] 16 pp. 8°. *Jenæ, typ. Stranckmanni,* [1794].

See, also, **Schaarschmidt** (Samuel). Abhandlung von der Geburtshülfe, etc. 12°. *Berlin,* 1751.

For Portrait, see **Collection**—van Kaathoven.

Nicolai (Fridericus Ernestus). * Diss. sistens theoriam cancri. 43 pp. 4°. *Jenæ, ex off. Fickelscherrio-Stranckmanniana,* [1785].

For Biography, see **Loder** (Just. Christ.)

Nicolai (G. H.) *See* **Nicolai** (Joh. Anton Heinrich).

Nicolai (H. F.) [1847–]. * Ueber Veränderungen des Augenhintergrundes im Zusammenhange mit intracraniellen Erkrankungen. 32 pp. 8°. *Berlin, G. Lange,* [1872].

Nicolai (Henricus). * De vulneribus sclopetorium. 1 p. l., 40 pp. 4°. *Argentorati, typ. J. Welperi,* [1675].

Nicolai (Henricus Albertus) [1701–33]. Decas observationum illustrium anatomicarum. 16 pp. 4°. *Argentorati, typ. S. Kürsneri,* [1725].

Also, in: HALLER. Disp. anat. [etc.] 4°. *Gottingæ,* 1751, vi, 687–699.

——. De directione vasorum pro modificando sanguinis circulo. 112 pp. sm. 4°. *Argentorati, typ. S. Kürsneri,* 1725.

Also, in: HALLER. Disp. anat. [etc.] 4°. *Gottingæ,* 1747, ii, 481–553.

——. The same. 112 pp. 4°. *Argentorati, apud J. R. Dulsseckerum,* 1726.

Nicolai (Henr. Christ.) * De ambustionibus.

In: WEIZ (F. A.) Vollständ. Ausz. [etc.] 12°. *Budissin,* 1769, i, 57–66.

Nicolai (Henricus Ernestus Carolus). * De methodo medendi per evacuationem primarum viarum. 3 p. l., 24 pp. sm. 4°. *Jenæ, ex off. Stranckmanniana,* [1792].

Nicolai (Joannes Augustus Henricus) [1796–1852]. * Disquisitiones circa quorundam animalium venas abdominales præcipue renales. 38 pp., 1 l. 12°. [*Berolini*], *formis Brüschckianis,* 1823.

——. Mémoire sur les tumeurs blanches des articulations. 59 pp. 8°. *Paris, Gueffier,* 1827.

——. Beschreibung der Knochen des menschlichen Fötus, ein Beitrag zur Anatomie des Fötus und zur Bestimmung des Alters der Embryonen und des Fötus aus der Beschaffenheit der Knochen. v (1 l.), 70 pp., 1 l., 4 tab. 4°. *Münster, F. Regensberg,* 1829.

——. Quædam de cholera quam Celsus descripsit ejusque similitudine cum cholera asiatica. 14 pp., 1 l. 4°. *Berolini, typ. F. Nietackianis,* 1832. [*Also, in:* P., v. 201.]

——. Grundriss der Sanitäts-Polizei, mit besonderer Beziehung auf den preussischen Staat. x, 694 pp. 8°. *Berlin, Nicolai,* 1835.

——. Die Medicinal- und Veterinair-Polizei. viii, 608 pp. 8°. *Berlin, Nicolai,* 1838.

——. Handbuch der gerichtlichen Medicin nach dem gegenwärtigen Standpunkte dieser Wissenschaft für Aerzte und Criminalisten. Nebst Formularen zu Obductions-Protokollen, sowie zu Abfassungen von Gutachten. xii, 556 pp. 8°. *Berlin, A. Hirschwald,* 1841.

Name on title-page is: "G. H. Nicolai".

Nicolai (Joannes Christophorus). * De variis dentium affectibus eorumque in sanitatem influxu. 24 pp. sm. 4°. *Jenæ, typ. Stranckmannianis,* [1799].

For Biography, see **Gruner** (Christ. Goth.)

Nicolai (Joannes Fridericus). * De ægris asthmaticis rite judicandis et curandis. 31 pp. 4°. *Vitembergæ, lit. vid. Gerdesiæ,* [1724].

Nicolai (Joannes Theodor.) * De medicorum meritis in augustanam confessionem. 24 pp. 4°. *Vitembergæ, lit. Gerdesianis,* [1730].

Nicolai (Joh. Ernestus). * De catharticis quibusdam selectioribus eorundemque principiis ac viribus. 40 pp. 4°. *Francof. ad Viadr., typ. M. Hübneri,* [1742].

Nicolai (Joh. Fridericus). Diss. semioticarum sexta in qua signa prognostica ex anni tempori-

Nicolai (Joh. Fridericus)—continued.
bus eorundemque tempestatibus ad ductum Hippocratis [etc.] 3 p. l., pp. 143–174. 4°. *Vitembergæ, lit. A. Kobersteini,* [1721].
For Diss. i, *see* **Berger** (Gottlob); ii, *see* **Schrœter** (Jo. Car.)

Nicolai (*Luccas Fridrich*) [1627–65].
Portrait in : **Collection**—van Kaathoven.

Nicolai (Nicolaus) [1861–   ]. * Zwei Fälle von partieller Verdoppelung der Vena cava inferior. 28 pp., 2 l., 5 pl. 8°. *Kiel, A. F. Jensen,* 1886.

Nicolai (*Th. W. E.*)
Portrait in : **Collection**—van Kaathoven.

Nicolai (Victor Hugo Athanasius) [1842–   ]. * Beobachtungen über Varicellen und Variolen, mit besonderer Berücksichtigung der Temperatur-Verhältnisse. 1 p. l., 24 pp., 1 l., 1 tab. 8°. *Leipzig, Breitkopf u. Härtel,* [1868]. [*Also, in :* P., v. 145.]

Nicolaïdes (Christodulus). * De lientide. 2 p. l., 28 pp. 8°. *Turici, typ. Schulthessianis,* 1835.

Nicolaides (Constantin). * Ueber Defecte des Septum atriorum cordis in Anschluss an die Beschreibung eines auf der medicinischen Klinik zu Freiburg i. B. beobachteten Falles. 57 pp., 2 pl. 8°. *Freiburg in Baden, H. M. Poppen u. Sohn,* 1887.

Nicolaïdès (J.) * Sur la sensibilité, l'intelligence et la volonté, considérées dans leurs rapports avec la médecine et la morale. 22 pp. 4°. *Paris,* 1833, No. 42, v. 258.

Nicolaïdes (Nicolas-J.) * Étude sur l'accouchement dans le bassin rachitique. 78 pp., 1 l. 4°. *Montpellier,* 1876, No. 36.

Nicolaïdes (Panaiota). * Antylli, veteris chirurgi, τὰ λείψανα. 36 pp. 4°. *Halis Magdeb., typ. J. J. Gebaueri,* [1799].

Nicolaier (Arthur). * Beiträge zur Aetiologie des Wundstarrkrampfes. 31 pp. 8°. *Göttingen, Dieterich (W. F. Kaestner),* 1885.

Nicolas. * Considérations sur l'uréthrite. 44 pp. 4°. *Paris,* 1872, No. 331.

Nicolas & Gueudeville (Victor). Recherches et expériences médicales et chimiques sur le diabète sucré ou la phthisurie sucrée, lues à l'Institut nationale dans la séance du 14 fructidor, et suivantes, de l'an X. 99 pp. 8°. *Paris, Méquignon l'aîné, an XI* [1803]. [*Also, in :* P., v. 1237; 1689.]

Nicolas (A.) * Organes érectiles. 172 pp., 1 l., 1 pl. 8°. *Paris, G. Steinheil,* 1886.
Concours.

Nicolas (Ad.)[1] * Contribution à l'étude de l'arthrotomie antiseptique. 1 p. l., 156 pp., 2 l., 1 ch. 4°. *Nancy, P. Sordoillet,* 1883, 1. s., No. 182.

Nicolas (Ad.)[2] Rapports sur l'Exposition universelle de 1878. V. Les progrès de l'hygiène; influences lumineuses; influences thermiques; influences des qualités du sol; influences diverses; l'aliment; la population; l'habitation; les professions, etc. 128 pp., 2 pl. 8°. *Paris, E. Lacroix,* [1879].
Repr. from : Études sur l'Exposition pub., par E. Lacroix, Nouv. Tech., viii.

Nicolas (Adolphe) [1856–   ]. * Essai sur la néphrite cantharidienne. 60 pp., 1 l. 4°. *Paris,* 1881, No. 220.

Nicolas (Adolphe-Charles-Antoine-Marie). Considérations sur la coordination des mouvements d'ensemble. 68 pp. 4°. *Paris,* 1872, No. 246.

Nicolas (Auguste-Louis). * I. Des symptômes de la colique de plomb. II. [etc.] 57 pp. 4°. *Paris,* 1840, No. 157, v. 364.

Nicolas (Auguste-Louis)—continued.
———. Manuel d'hygiène élémentaire et pratique. 3 p. l., vii, 5–166 pp. 8°. *Orléans, Morand-Bouget,* 1854.

Nicolas (Charles). * De la mensuration obstétricale des ouvertures inférieures du bassin. [Berne.] 100 pp., 1 pl. 8°. *Neuchâtel, H. Wolfrath & Metzner,* 1870.

Nicolas (Édouard). * De la chorée vulgaire chez le vieillard. 1 p. l., 69 pp. 4°. *Nancy, N. Collin,* 1883, 1. s., No. 169.

Nicolas (François-Victor). * Sur la chorée. 70 pp. 4°. *Paris,* 1844, No. 217, v. 422.

Nicolas (Gabriel). * Essai sur l'emploi des eaux minérales pendant la grossesse. 36 pp. 4°. *Paris,* 1876, No. 111.

Nicolas (Georges). * La cocaïne, son origine et ses applications. 75 pp., 1 l. 4°. *Montpellier,* 1885, No. 360.
École supérieure de pharmacie.

Nicolas (Henri). * Des indications et contre-indications de la lithotritie. 57 pp., 1 l. 4°. *Montpellier, Boehm & fils,* 1868, No. 52.   c.

Nicolas (Honoré). * Quelques recherches sur les effets physiologiques du chandoo (opium des fumeurs). 54 pp., 2 l. 4°. *Montpellier,* 1884, No. 21.

Nicolas (Jean). * Du traitement de la fièvre intermittente d'origine paludéenne. 48 pp. 4°. *Paris,* 1873, No. 214.

Nicolas (Jean-Étienne-Mathieu). * Considérations médico-légales sur les blessures. 1 p. l., 29 pp. 4°. *Strasbourg,* 1829, v. 60.

Nicolas (Jean-Franç.-Marie). * Sur la fièvre adynamique. 1 p. l., 14 pp. 4°. *Strasbourg,* 1811. *Also, in :* v. 47.

Nicolas (Jean-Pierre). * Sur différens points de médecine. 18 pp. 4°. *Paris,* 1832, No. 1, v. 170.

Nicolas (Joseph) [1856–   ]. * Du traitement de la névralgie sciatique par l'élongation du nerf. 60 pp. 4°. *Paris,* 1881, No. 273.

Nicolas (Joseph-André). * I. Du traitement du delirium tremens. II. [etc.] 27 pp. 4°. *Paris,* 1839, No. 163, v. 347.

Nicolas (L.-E.) * Essai sur la transfusion du sang. 60 pp. 4°. *Paris,* 1860, No. 79.

Nicolas (L.-J.-C.) * Sur la coqueluche, ou toux convulsive des enfants. 17 pp. 4°. *Paris, an XII* [1804], No. 221, v. 48.

Nicolas (L.-P.-Victor). * Sur les rapports circulatoires qui existent entre la mère et le fœtus. 36 pp. 4°. *Paris,* 1837, No. 351, v. 316.

Nicolas (Léonce-Juvénal). * Du pityriasis rosé, ou de la roséole squameuse. 56 pp. 4°. *Paris,* 1880, No. 272.

Nicolas (P.-F.) * Sur la péritonite aiguë. 33 pp. 4°. *Paris,* 1819, No. 30, v. 144.

Nicolas (Patrice) [1854–   ]. * Sur deux variétés de fistules ombilicales. 68 pp. 4°. *Paris, A. Parent,* 1883.

Nicolas (Paul Heinrich) [1857–   ]. * Ueber lokale Blutentziehungen als antiphlogistische Operationen, nebst einschlägigen Experimenten. 28 pp., 1 l. 8°. *Halle a. S., Plötz,* 1882.

Nicolas (Pierre François) [1743–1816].
See **de Sauvages** (François-Boissier). Nosologie méthodique, dans laquelle les maladies sont rangées par classes, [etc.] 3 v. 8°. *Paris,* 1771.

Nicolas - Duranty (Émile). Études laryngoscopiques. Diagnostic des paralysies motrices des muscles du larynx. 47 pp., 3 pl. 8°. *Paris, J.-B. Baillière,* 1872.

Nicolau (J[ean]-B[aptiste]). * Essai sur la mélancolie, ou lypémanie proprement dite. 37 pp. 4°. *Montpellier, J. Martel aîné,* 1824, No. 96. [P., v. 1331.]

Nicolau - Barraque (J. - B.) * Des hémor-rhoïdes. 29 pp. 4°. *Paris*, 1843, No. 193, v. 407.

Nicolau-Barraque (Oscar). * Quelques con-sidérations sur le traitement des fractures par enfoncement de la voûte du crâne, et des abcès consécutifs du cerveau. 39 pp. 4°. *Paris*, 1875, No. 422.

Nicolaus (Daniel). . * De mania. 25 pp. 4°. *Francof. ad Viadr., prælo J. Coepfelii*, [1692].

Nicolaus (Halvardus).
See **Bartholinus** (Caspar). Positiones anatomicæ, [etc.] sm. 4°. *Hafniæ*, [1678].

Nicolaus (Joh.). Disquisitio de chirothecarum usu et abusu in qua varii ritus, varia jura, et symbola illarum fuse exhibentur. Lectu jucun-dissima et in bonum publicum edita. 10 p. l., 144 pp. 18°. *Stutgardiæ, P. Treu*, 1701.

Nicolaus *Alexandrinus*. *See* **Myrepsus** (Nico-laus).

Nicolaus *Falcutius Florentinus*. *See* **Falcutius** [*or* **Falcucci**] (Nicolaus) *Florentinus*.

Nicolaus (Myrepsus). *See* **Myrepsus** (Nico-laus).

Nicolaus (Nicolaus). *See* **Falcutius** [*or* **Fal-cucci**] (Nicolaus) *Florentinus*.

Nicolaus de Reggio.
See **Myrepsus** (Nicolaus). Liber de compositione medicamentorum secundum loca. 4°. *Ingolstadii*, 1541.
For Biography, see **Janus**, Gotha, 1853, ii, 393 (A. W. E. T. Henschel).

Nicolaus Præpositus *Salernitanus*. Incipit antidotarium Nicolai. Ego Nicolaus rogatus a quibusdam in practica medicinæ studere volen-tibus: ut eos recto ordine modum conficiendi dispensandique docerem: et certam eis traderem doctrinam: [etc.] [*F.* 45:] Incipit tractatulus quid pro quo. Pro aristologia rotunda longa vel pondus equale zurunbet [etc.] [*F.* 51:] Inci-piunt sinonima. Artemisia, id est, matricaria [etc.] [*In fine:*] Finis antidotarii Nicolai: et quorundam aliorum tractatuum impressorum Venetiis per Nicolaum Jenson Gallicum. m.cccc.lxxi. 68 ff. 4°. *Venetiis, N. Jenson*, 1471.

——. The same. Antidotarium, etc. [*F.* 1 a:] Antidotarius Nicolai medicinalis cum omnibus suis receptis incipit feliciter. [*F.* 2 a:] Ego Nico-laus rogatus a quibusdam in practica medicinæ studere volentibus, etc. [*F.* 23 b, *col.* 1:] Anti-dotarius medicinalis Nicolai explicit. [*F.* 25 a:] Johannis Mesuæ Grabadin incipit quod est agre-gatio et antidotarium electuariorum et confec-tionum [*F.* 67 a, *col.* 2:] Presens opus Johannis Mesuæ extractum ab originali correctum necnon emendatum per egregios ac expertos medicinæ doctores almæ universitatis Papiensis, magistrum Johannem Theobaldi, magistrum Marcum de Papia finit. [*F.* 68 a:] Liber servitoris de pre-parationibus medicinarum tam lapidum minera-lium quam radicum plantarum ac etiam medici-narum ex animalibus sumptarum cum eorum ablutione, adustione, confectione et reservatione incipit feliciter. [*F.* 95 a, *col.* 2, l. 31:] Liber servitoris explicit. fol. 93 pp. [*Argentorati, J. Pryss, n. d.*]

——. The same. Incipit antidotarium Nicolai.
In: MESUE (Joannes). Opera universa. fol. *Venetiis*, 1478, 347-360.

——. The same. Incipit antidotarium.
In: MESUE (J.) In nomine Dei misericordis, [etc.] fol. *Venetiis*, 1484, sig. gg^a–hh³.

——. The same . . . Cum expositionibus et glosis clarissimi physici Platearii.
In: MESUE (J.) Mesue cum additionibus, [etc.] fol. *Venetiis*, 1489-91, sig. ee^a–hh 4^b.

——. The same. Cum expositio Joannes de Sancto Amando supra antidotarium Nicolai, in-cipit feliciter.
In: MESUE (J.) Cum expositione Mondini. fol. *Ve-netiis*, 1495, sig. ff 2–mm 6^b.

Nicolaus Præpositus *Salernitanus*—cont'd.
——. The same.
In: MESUE (J.) Cum expositione Mondini. fol. *Ve-netiis*, 1502, sig. J–R.

——. The same.
In: MESUE (J.) Cum expositione Mondini. fol. *Lugd. Bat.*, 1510, sig. L–T 2^h.

——. The same. Antidotarium Nicolai.
In: MESUE (J.) Canones universales. 16°. [*Lugduni*, 1523], sig. qqiiii–ttvii^b.

——. The same. Incipit antidotarium cum ex-positionibus . . . Platearii.
In: MESUE (J.) Opera. fol. *Lugduni*, 1525, ccxliii-cclxxi.

——. Dispensarium ad aromatarios. [*Ad finem:*] Finiunt introductiones . . . expensis Jacobi Hu-guetan, sed Francisci Fradin, Lugd. impresse, anno mcccccv. cv ff. 4°. *Lugduni, ab J. Hu-guetan*, [1505].

——. The same. Item cum pluribus additio-nibus . . . annectuntur. Platearius, vulgo circa instans nuncupatus de simplici medicina, recog-nitus ac novis exornatus additionibus per Mi-chaelem de Capella additis. 4 p. l., xcvi ff. 4°. *Lugduni, apud S. de Gabiano*, 1537.
See, also, **Mesue** (Joannes).

——. Prepositas his practise, a worke very necessary to be used for the better preservation of the health of man. Wherein are not onely most excellent and approved medicines, re-ceiptes, and ointmentes of great vertue, but also most pretious waters, against many infirmities of the body. The way how to make every the said severall medicines, receiptes, and oint-mentes. With a table for the ready finding out of every the diseases, and the remedies for the same. Transl. out of Latin into English by L. M. 111 pp., 8 l. 12°. *London, E. White*, 1588.
For Biography, see **Bayle** (P.) Hist. & Crit. Dict. (transl. Des Maizeaux). 2. ed. fol. *London*, 1737, iv, 764.

Nicolay (Franciscus) [1815–]. * De morbis quibusdam lienis cognoscendis et curandis. 32 pp. 8°. *Berolini, typ. Nietackianis*, [1837].

Nicolaysen (Julius) [1831–]. Yderligere meddelelse om coxarthrocace og dens behand-ling. 32 pp. 8°. [*Stockholm, P. A. Norstedt & Söner*, 1874].
Repr. from: Nord. med. Ark., Stockholm, 1874, vi.
See, also, **Klinisk** Aarbog [etc.] 8°. *Kristiania*, 1884.

Nicole (*Sieur*).
See **Marges** (D.-P.) Examen et analyse chimique. 2. éd. 12°. *Paris*, 1774.

Nicole, *dit* **Havet** (Eugène). * Sur une maladie qui règne à l'île de Madagascar; conseils hygié-niques à suivre pour l'éviter. viii, 9–30 pp. 4°. *Paris*, 1827, No. 124, v. 206.

Nicolello (Augusto). Saggio popolare sui mi-crobi delle malattie infettive dell' uomo. 152 pp. 12°. *Torino, C. Triverio*, 1884.

Nicolescu (Joann). * L'infanticide par l'im-mersion dans les fosses d'aisances. 52 pp. 4°. *Paris*, 1868, No. 312.

Nicolet (G.)
See **Magitot** (E.) Traités des anomalies du système dentaire [etc.] 4°. *Paris*, 1877.

Nicolet (Victor-Joseph-Auguste). * Considéra-tions sur l'emploi de l'alcool dans les maladies aiguës. 57 pp., 2 l. 4°. *Montpellier, Gras*, 1865, No. 47.

Nicolétis (Minos). * Opération de Récamier (colpohystérectomie), indications et contre-indi-cations. 137 pp. 4°. *Paris*, 1887, No. 234.

Nicoli (Nicolaus). *See* **Falcutius** [*or* **Falcucci**] (Nicolaus) *Florentinus*.

Nicolides (Joannes). * Pyogonia. 3 p. l., 82 pp., 3 l. 8°. *Viennæ, M. A. Schmidt*, [1780].

Nicolini (H.) * Historique des pilocarpus. Étude botanique, pharmacologique et chimique, physiologique et thérapeutique du pilocarpus pennatifolius. vi, 7-174 pp., 1 l., 2 pl., 1 ch. 4°. *Montpellier*, 1876, No. 50.

Nicolini (N.) Dell' aletoscopio nelle perizie di falsità. Macchina ottica inventata dal . . . Raffaele Sacco. 14 pp. 8°. [*n. p., n. d.*] [P., v. 1130.]
Repr. from: Procedura penale, vi.

Nicoll (Donald). Health and its appliances (engineering, structural, and sanitary). 65 pp. 4°. [*London*], E. Duck, 1884.

Nicoll (Samuel). * De arthritide. 37 pp. 8°. *Edinburgi, Balfour et Smellie*, 1776.

Nicolle (Charles-Gustave). * À propos de l'allaitement. 42 pp. 4°. *Paris*, 1864, No. 18.

Nicolle (Eugène). * Recherches sur le développement et les transformations de l'hystérie. 35 pp. 4°. *Paris*, 1859, No. 56, v. 634.

Nicolle (Félix). * I. Combien existe-il de râles ? Établir leurs rapports avec les diverses altérations que subissent les poumons. II. [etc.] 18 pp. 4°. *Paris*, 1841, No. 15, v. 379.

Nicolle (H.-C.) * Histoire de la digitale pourprée. 46 pp. 4°. *Paris*, 1824, No. 88, v. 185.

Nicolle (J.) * De la cowpérite. 32 pp. 4°. *Paris*, 1873, No. 331.

Nicolle (J.-C.) * De l'or, comme moyen thérapeutique dans les maladies vénériennes. 23 pp. 4°. *Paris*, 1835, No. 238, v. 289.

Nicollet (J.-B.-Alfred). * De la variole et de son traitement. 35 pp. 4°. *Paris*, 1852, No. 165, v. 530.

Nicollet (J. N.) Essay on meteorological observations. Printed by order of the War Department. 45 pp., 1 l. 8°. [*Washington*], J. Gideon, 1839.

Nicollinus (Joannes Baptista) *Salodiensis*.
See **Thaddeus** *Florentinus*. Expositiones, etc. fol. *Venetiis*, 1527.

Nicolls (Archibaldus). * De cynanche tonsillari. 1 p. l., 23 pp. 8°. *Edinburgi, A. Neill et socii*, 1805.

Nicolon (J.-J.) *Observations sur la ménorrhagie qui survient à l'approche de l'âge critique, et sur l'aménorrhée par vice de conformation. 25 pp. 4°. *Strasbourg*, 1808, v. 45.

Nicolson (P. J. S. Fraser). Incipient insanity among the better classes ; with a word on private asylums. 61 pp. 16°. *London, Victoria Steam Press*, [1879].

Nicolucci (G.) Osservazioni microscopiche sulla struttura de' globetti sanguigni comunicate per via di lettere al dottor A. Di Giulio. 21 pp. 8°. [*Napoli*, 1841.]

——. Sull' intima struttura dello scirro ; lettera indiretta al S. De Renzi. 7 pp. 8°. [*Napoli*, 1843.]
Repr. from: Filiatre-sebezio, Napoli, 1843, xxvi.

——. Anatomia, fisiologia e patologia delle valvule semilunari. 11 pp. 8°. [*n. p.*, 1844.]
Repr. from: Filiatre-sebezio, Napoli, 1844, xxvii.

——. Di un antico cranio fenicio rinvenuto nella necropoli di Tharros in Sardegna ; memoria. 18 pp., 3 pl. 4°. *Torino, stamperia reale*, 1863.
Repr. from: Mem. r. Accad. d. sc. di Torino, 2. s., xxi.

Nicomaco.
Portrait in: **Collection**—van Kaathoven.

Nicomède (Gaston). * De l'influence de la déclivité sur les causes et le traitement des maladies internes. 44 pp. 4°. *Paris*, 1874, No. 352.

Nicora (Dominique). * Des anévrysmes traumatiques. 23 pp. 4°. *Paris*, 1847, No. 182, v. 462.

Nicot (Jean-Antoine). * Sur la péripneumonie simple, et sur sa complication adynamique. 30 pp. 4°. *Paris*, 1816, No. 83, v. 121.

Nicot (Louis). * Considérations sur la nature de la fièvre typhoïde, suivies de propositions de médecine. 25 pp. 4°. *Paris*, 1829, No. 96, v. 223.

Nicotianomanie (De la), ou description du tabac, et tableau des dangers qui suivent son usage, soit qu'on le prise, soit qu'on le fume, soit enfin qu'on le mâche ; par un médecin qui a usé de cette substance pendant douze ans. 156 pp. 12°. *Paris*, [*Moreau*], 1826.

Nicotine.

See, also, **Eserine** ; **Tetanus** (*Treatment of*) ; **Tobacco.**

BLATIN (A.) Recherches physiologiques et cliniques sur la nicotine et le tabac, précédées d'une introduction sur la méthode expérimentale en thérapeutique. 8°. *Paris*, 1870.

CHMELEVSKI (V.) *O stoikosti i kolichestvennom opredelenii nikotina v trupach jivotnych, otravlennych etim alkoloidom. [On the presence and quantitative analysis of nicotine in animal body in poisoning by this alcaloid.] 8°. *St. Petersburg*, 1876.

FORSIUS (K. F.) * Om nicotinforgiftning. 8°. *Helsingfors*, 1859.

GRODZKI (V.) *O dieistvii nikotina na jivotnii organizme. [Effect of nicotine on animal organism.] 8°. *St. Petersburg*, 1869.

HAUGHTON (S.) Physiological experiments on strychnine and nicotine. 8°. *Dublin*, 1856.

JULLIEN (J.) *Sur la nicotine. 4°. *Paris*, 1868.

KROCKER (A.) * Ueber die Wirkung des Nikotins auf den thierischen Organismus. 8°. *Berlin*, 1868.

LIBRECHT (A.) *Ueber Nicotin. 8°. *Kiel*, 1886.

PROCÈS du comte et de la comtesse de Bocarmé, 27 mai 1851. Cour d'assises du Hainaut. 8°. *Paris*, 1851.

RENÉ (A.) *Étude expérimentale sur l'action physiologique de la nicotine. [*Nancy.*] 4°. *Pont-à-Mousson*, 1877.

SURMINSKI (B.) * Ueber die Wirkungsweise des Nicotin und Atropin auf das Gefässnerven-System und die Pupille. 8°. *Erlangen*, 1877.

TRUHART (H.) *Ein Beitrag zur Nicotinwirkung. 8°. [*Dorpat*], 1869.

Albers (J. F. H.) Nicotianin (Nicotin) und seine Wirkung auf den thierischen Organismus im Verhältniss zur Blausäure-Wirkung. Deutsche Klinik, Berl., 1851, iii, 337-340.—**Amagat.** De l'antagonisme de l'ésérine et de la nicotine. J. de thérap., Par., 1875, ii, 300-302.—**von Anrep** (B.) Neue Erscheinungen der Nicotinvergiftung. Arch. f. Physiol., Leipz., 1879, Suppl.-Bd., 167 : 1880, 209 - 226.—**Barral.** Note sur la formule de la nicotine. Ann. de chim. et phys., Par., 1847, 3. s., xx, 345-353. *Also*, Reprint.—**von Basch** (S.) & **Oser** (L.) Untersuchungen über die Wirkung des Nicotins. Med. Jahrb., Wien, 1872, 367-388. 1 pl. *Also :* Deutsche Klinik, Berl., 1873, xxv, 224.—**Benham** (W. T.) The action of nicotine. West Riding Lun. Asyl. Rep., Lond., 1874, iv, 305-317. *Also, transl. :* Rev. méd. de Chile, Sant. de Chile, 1876, v 8; 53.—**Bernard** (C.) Action du curare et de la nicotine sur le système nerveux et sur le système musculaire. Compt. rend. Soc. de biol. 1850, Par., 1851, ii, 195.—**Berutti** (S.) & **Vella** (L.) Expériences sur la nicotine faites au laboratoire physiologique de l'Université de Turin. J. de méd., chir. et pharmacol., Brux., 1852, xiv, 69-77. *Also*, Reprint.—**Blatin** (A.) De la nicotine comme contre-poison de la strychnine. Union méd., Par., 1872, 3. s., xiv, 973-976.—**Bonaccorsi** (G.) Esperienze sull' antagonismo tra l' oppio e la nicotina. Arch. med. ital., Torino, 1882, i, 172-193.—**Bordier** (M.) & **Bordier** (A.) Nicotine. Dict. encycl. d. sc méd., Par., 1878, 2. s., xiii, 226-235.—**Borsarelli** & **Bruno** (A.) Di un caso di sospetto veneficio con nicotina. Gior. d. r. Accad. di med. di Torino, 1867, 3. s., iv, 745-758.—**Castiglioni** (C.) Due osservazioni su la memoria intorno la nicotina. Gazz. med. ital. lomb., Milano, 1852, 3. s., iii, 289-293.—**Clemens** (T.) Zwei Fälle von chronischer Nicotin-Vergiftung durch unmässiges Cigarrenrauchen. Deutsche Klinik, Berl., 1872, xxiv, 254; 271.—**Evans.** A case of

Nicotine.

poisoning by nicotiana. Lancet. Lond., 1869, i, 843.—
Evers. Einige Bemerkungen zu dem Artikel: "Zur
chronischen Nikotinvergiftung" von M. Treymann.
Berl. klin. Wchnschr., 1884, xxi, 787.—**Foussagrives** &
Besnou. Suicide par nicotine. Ann. d'hyg., Par.,
1861. 2. s., xv, 404–411.—**Freschi** (F.) Degli effetti della
nicotina considerati sotto il rapporto della fisiologia e della
tossicologia medico-forense. Gior. d. r. Accad. med.-chir.
di Torino, 1852. 2. s., xiii, 483; 529: xiv, 3; 49; 129; 145.—
Haynes (F. L.) On the asserted antagonism between
nicotin and strychnia. Proc. Am. Phil. Soc., Phila.,
1876-7, xvi, 596-616.—**Laiblin** (R.) Ueber Nicotin und
Nicotinsäure. Ann. d. Chem., Leipz., 1879, cxcvi, 129-
182.—**Laskiewicz-Friedensfeld** (A. J.) Przypadek
zboczen umzysłowych powstałych prawdopodobnie w skutek przewlekłego otrucia nikotynem i o zmianach newwo-
wych i psychicznych w ogóle, wywołanych otruciem tytu-
niowém. [Aberration of mind induced by the poisonous
effect of nicotine.] Przegl. lek., Krakow, 1878, xvii, 361-
364.—**Lautenbach** (B. F.) On the difference in the effects produced by nicotine when injected into an efferent
from those produced by the introduction of the poison into
an afferent blood-vessel. Phila. M. Times, 1879-80, x,
523.—**Leblanc.** Expériences faites sur l'emploi de la nicotine comme contre-poison des sels de strychnine. Gaz.
méd. de Par., 1873, xxviii, 171.—**Melsens** (A.) Sur la recherche de la nicotine dans des cadavres enfouis depuis
longtemps et après la putréfaction des matières animales.
Bull. Acad. roy. de méd. de Belg., Brux., 1857-8. 2. s., i, 680-
693. Also: J. de chim. méd., etc., Par., 1859, 4. s., v, 336-
348. — **Oppolzer.** Ein Fall von Nikotinvergiftung.
Wien. med. Presse, 1866, vii, 1151–1153.—**Orfila** (M.) Mémoire sur l'empoisonnement par la nicotine. Bull. Acad.
de méd., Par., 1850-51, xvi, 893-905. Also: Abeille méd.,
Par., 1851, viii, 157-160. Also: Union méd., Par., 1851, v,
265. Also, transl.: N. York J. M., 1852, n. s., ix, 112; 219;
369. ———. Sur la conicine et la nicotine. Bull. Acad. de
méd., Par., 1850-51, xvi, 945-947. Also, transl.: Buffalo M.
J., 1852-3, viii, 1-5. ———. Mémoire sur la nicotine et sur
la conicine. Ann. d'hyg., Par., 1851, xlvi, 147-230.—**Pasquier.** Rapport de la commission chargée d'apprécier le
différend survenu entre MM. Orfila et Stas à propos de la
recherche de la nicotine dans les cas d'empoisonnement.
Bull. Acad. roy. de méd. de Belg., Brux., 1852-3, xii, 579-
599. [Discussion], 990-996.—**Peset Cervera** (V.) Accion fisiológica de la nicotina. Siglo méd., Madrid, 1877,
xxiv, 516-519.—**van Praag** (J. L.) Nicotin; toxikolo-
gisch-pharmakodynamische Studien. Arch. f. path. Anat.,
etc., Berl., 1854, viii, 56-102. — **Ritter** (B.) Ueber Nikotinvergiftung in Folge übermässigen Tabakrauchens im
Allgemeinen und in einem speziellen Falle insbesondere.
Med. Cor.-Bl. d. württemb. ärztl. Ver., Stuttg., 1868,
xxxviii, 5; 14; 21; 33.—**Rosenthal** (J.) Ueber die physiologischen Wirkungen des Nicotin. Centralbl. f. d. med.
Wissensch., Berl., 1863, i, 737-739. ———. Sur un phénomène observé dans l'empoisonnement par la nicotine.
Compt. rend. Soc. de biol. 1867, Par., 1869, 4. s., iv, 91.—
Schotten (L.) Zur Casuistik der chronischen Nicotin-
vergiftung. Arch. f. path. Anat., etc., Berl., 1868, xliv,
172–179.—**Simons.** Een geval van nicotinevergiftiging.
Nederl. Tijdschr. v. Geneesk., Amst., 1877, 2. R., xiii,
233-235.—**Smyly** (P. C.) Attempted suicide with strychnine; treatment with nicotine (tobacco); recovery. Dub-
blin Q. J. M. Sc., 1862, xxxiv, 183-186.—**Stas** (J.-S.) Recherches médico-légales sur la nicotine. suivies de quelques considérations sur la manière générale de déceler
les alcalis organiques dans le cas d'empoisonnement.
Bull. Acad. roy. de méd. de Belg., Brux., 1851-2, xi, 202-
312, 1 pl. Also: Mém. Acad. roy. de méd. de Belg., Brux.,
1854, iii, 119-237.—**Szerlecki.** Sur la nicotiane, son
action sur l'homme malade, et sur son efficacité dans différentes affections morbides. Bull. gén. de thérap., etc.,
Par., 1839, xvii, 201-212. ———. Sur la nicotiane et sur son
action dans l'iléus, l'ischurie, la coqueluche, le tétanos et
les paralysies. Ibid., 1840, xviii, 85-92.—**Tamassia** (A.)
Sull' avvelenamento acutissimo per nicotina; ricerche
sperimentali. R. Ist. Lomb. di sc. e lett. Rendic., Milano,
1883, 2. s., xvi, 706-709. — **Taylor** (A. S.) On poisoning
by nicotina, with remarks. Guy's Hosp. Rep., Lond., 1858,
3. s., iv, 345-359. — **Thomas.** Poisoning of a child by
nicotine. Brit. M. J., Lond., 1877, ii, 389. — **Tosini** (A.)
Avvelenamento di nicoziana per assorbimento cutaneo;
cura alcoolica; guarigione. Gazz. med. ital., prov. venete,
Padova, 1864, vii, 313.—**Traube** (L.) Versuche über den
Einfluss des Nicotins auf die Herzthätigkeit. Allg. med.
Centr.-Ztg., Berl., 1862, xxxi, 821-825. Also: Ges. Beitr. z.
Path. u. Physiol., Berl., 1871, i, 322-309. — **Treymann**
(M.) Zur chronischen Nikotinvergiftung. Berl. klin.
Wchnschr., 1884, xxi, 687. — **Valitski** (M. K.) Chron.
otvavl. nikotinom. [Chronic poisoning by nicotine.]
Sborn. rabot, proizved. lab. Anrepa, Charkoff, 1886-7, ii,
1-55, 1 pl. Also, Reprint.—**Vandenbroeck** (V.) De la
préparation de la nicotine, et de son mode d'action sur
l'économie animale. Ann. méd. de la Flandre occid.,
Roulers. 1851-2, [n. s., i]. 97-152. — **Vandencorput** (E.)
Effets de la nicotine. Presse méd. belge, Brux., 1851, iii,
205. — **Vleminckx** (V.) Expériences sur la nicotine.

Nicotine.

Ibid., 213.—**Vogel** (A.) Ueber Nicotinbestimmung und
Tabakverbrennungsprodukte. Sitzungsb. d. math.-phys.
Cl. d. k. bayer. Akad. d. Wissensch. zu München, 1881, xi,
439-453.—**Vulpian** (A.) Expériences montrant que la
thiotétrapyridine et l'isodipyridine ne sont pas douées du
pouvoir toxique que possède la nicotine, dont elles sont
des dérivés. Compt. rend. Acad. d. sc., Par., 1881, xcii,
165-169. — **Wolff** (C.) Der Prozess Bocarmé und die
Arbeiten von Stas und Orfila über Nicotin und Conicin.
Ztschr. f. d. Staatsarznk., Erlang., 1853, lxvi, 126-153.—
Wormley (T. G.) Notes on some of the chemical reactions of nicotine and daturine. Ohio M. & S. J., Columbus, 1860-61, xiii, 26-30.

Nicoulau (Élie-D.-E.) *Essai sur la méga-
lomanie. 39 pp. 4°. Bordeaux, 1886, No. 73,
1885-6.

Nicoulau (Pierre). *Du traitement de la métrite chronique interne et de ses complications.
44 pp. 4°. Paris, 1863, No. 166.

Nicoullaud (Eugène - Victor). *De la mort
apparente des nouveau-nés. 34 pp. 4°. Strasbourg, 1859, No. 474, 2. s., v. 26.

Nictitation.

Lazarus (J.) Ueber Nictitatio. Wien. med. Presse,
1872, xiii, 990-992.

Nidart (J.-F.) * Des fistules en général. 67 pp.
4°. Paris, 1845, No. 141, v. 436.

Nidart (J.-L.) * Sur la fièvre méningo-gastrique
(bilieuse). vi, 7–21 pp. 4°. Paris, 1814, No. 133,
v. 105.

Nidelbad.

Löwig. Beträchtlicher Mangangehalt des Mineralwassers im Nidelbade bei Zürich, nachgewiesen durch die
chemische Analyse desselben. Schweiz. Ztschr. f. Nat.-
u. Heilk., Zürich, 1838-9, n. F., i, 265-270.

Nidepontanus (Joannes) & **Frisius** (Laurentius). Sudoris anglici exitialis pestiferique
morbi ratio, præservatio et cura. Argentorati,
1529.

In: SCRIPT. de sudore angl. (Gruner). 8°. Jenæ, 1847,
157-178.

Niderburg (S. N.) Improved galvanismus, and
its medical application. 15 pp. 8°. New York,
G. Forman, 1803.

Nidergang (Joseph) [1856–   ]. *Essai sur
l'ulcère simple du duodénum. 74 pp., 1 l. 4°.
Paris, 1881, No. 279.

Niderkorn (P.-F.) * Contribution à l'étude de
quelques-uns des phénomènes de la rigidité cadavérique chez l'homme. 96 pp., 1 l., 33 pp. 4°.
Paris, 1872, No. 281.

———. The same. 93 pp., 1 l., 33 pp. 8°. Paris,
A. Delahaye, 1872.

Nidernau.

GEORGII (G. A.) *Diss. sistens analysin
chemicam acidularum Nidernowensium, adjectis
thesibus medico-chirurgicis de oculorum morbis.
4°. Tubingæ, [1814].

KLOTZ (C. F.) * De acidulis Nidernowensi-
bus. 4°. Tubingæ, [1802].

WALZ (E.) *Chemische Untersuchung des
Sauerwassers bei Niedernau. 8°. Tübingen,
[1827].

Baur (H.) Das Bad Niedernau. Med. Cor.-Bl. d.
württemb. ärztl. Ver., Stuttg., 1851, xxi, 177. — **Ritter**
(B.) Bericht über die Leistungen der Raidt'schen Kur-
und Badeanstalt in Niedernau im Jahr 1860-61. Ibid.,
1861, xxxi, 108: 1862, xxxii, 103.

Nieberding (Carolus Joannes) [1839–   ]. *De
natura olei ætherei corticis aurantiorum. 32
pp. 8°. Berolini, G. Lange, [1863].

Nieberding (Frid. Arnoldus) [1805–   ]. *De
diversarum cataractæ curandæ methodorum indicationibus. 31 pp. 8°. Berolini, typ. A.
Petschii, [1829].

Nieberding (Ph.) Das Asthma thymicum oder
Spasmus glottidis. Eine physiologisch-pathologische Abhandlung. 36 pp. 8°. Halle, Lippert
u. Schmidt, 1844.

Nieberding (W[ilhelm Rudolph]) [1850–].
* Ueber Ovariotomie. 38 pp. 8°. *Würzburg, C. J. Becker,* 1875.

———. Ueber Ectropium und Risse am Halse der schwangeren und puerperalen Gebärmutter. 153 pp., 3 pl. roy. 8°. *Würzburg, J. Staudinger,* 1879.

Nieberg (Carl). * Zur Statistik der melanotischen Geschwülste. 29 pp. 8°. *Würzburg, Becker,* 1882.

Nieberg (Reinhold). * De dialeipyris. 63 pp., 1 l. 8°. *Mosquæ, A. Semen,* 1826.

Niebergall (Hugo). * Ueber die Wirkung des Kochsalzes auf den menschlichen Organismus. 32 pp. 8°. *Berlin, M. Niethe,* [1874].

Niebour (Georgius). * Historia ulceris cujusdam scribitur. 30 pp., 1 l. 8°. *Berolini, G. Schade,* [1855].

Niebuhr (*Carsten*).
Portrait in: **Collection** of Portr. of Phys. & Men of Sc., 2z7.

Nied (Andreas). * Diss. tractans casus practicos scholæ chirurgicæ anni scholastici 1837–8. vi, 7–70 pp., 1 l. 8°. *Vindobonæ, viduæ A. Pichler,* [1840].

Nieden (A.) Schrift-Proben zur Bestimmung der Sehschärfe. 2. Aufl. 3 l. 8°. *Wiesbaden, J. F. Bergmann,* 1883.

———. Gesichtsfeld-Schema zum Gebrauch für gewöhnliche und für selbstregistrirende Perimeter. 2. Aufl. 50 l. obl. 12°. *Wiesbaden, J. F. Bergmann,* [n. d.]

Nieden (Adolf) [1846–]. * Ueber die Entstehungsweise und Ursache des angebornen Klumpfusses (Pes varus). [Bonn.] 29 pp., 1 l. 8°. *Coblenz, Buchdruckerei des evang. Stifts zu St. Martin,* [1870].

zur Nieden (Fridericus Æmilius Gustavus) [1822–]. * De nervorum sympathia. 29 pp. 8°. *Halis, typ. Ploetzianis,* [1845].

Nieden (G.) * Ueber Perinephritis hauptsächlich in ätiologischer und diagnostischer Beziehung. [Freiburg i. B.] 58 pp. 8°. *Leipzig, J. B. Hirschfeld,* 1878.

zur Nieden (Julius). Die Errichtung von Pflegestätten im Kriege. 24 pp. 8°. *Berlin, M. Pasch,* 1883.
In: VORTR. ü. Gsndhtspflg. u. Rettungsw., Berl., 1883, i, No. 3.

zur Nieden (P.) Hämoglobinurie bei einer acuten Carbolvergiftung. 16 pp. 8°. [*Berlin, L. Schumacher,* 1881.]
Repr. from: Berl. klin. Wcbnschr., 1881, xviii.

———. * Ueber einen Fall von Lymphangiectasie mit Lymphorrhagie. [Freiburg i. B.] 41 pp., 1 pl. 8°. *Berlin, G. Reimer,* 1882.
Repr. from: Arch. f. path. Anat., etc., Berl., 1882, xc.

Niedenthal (Christoph). * Ueber Hydrops. 22 pp. 8°. *Würzburg, C. J. Becker,* 1867.

Nieder (F. X.) * De aencephalo casus singularis. 15 pp. 8°. *Monachii, C. Wolf,* 1834.

Niederbarnim.
KREISPOLIZEI-VERORDNUNG (Die) zur obligatorischen allgemeinen Leichenschau im Kreise Niederbarnim vom 6. September 1878, nebst Anlagen: A. Formular des Leichenschauscheines. B. Instruction des Kreisphysikus für die nicht ärztlichen Leichenbeschauer im Kreise Niederbarnim. fol. *Berlin u. Bernau,* 1878.
Separat-Abdruck aus dem Niederbarnimer Kreisblatt, Sept. 1878.

SANITÄTS-VERHÄLTNISSE (Die) des Kreises Niederbarnim im J. 1877 und im 1. Quartal 1878. Als Motivirung der bevorstehenden Organisation einer obligatorischen allgemeinen Leichenschau im Kreise; aus der monatlichen amtlichen Todesstatistik der 59 Standesbeamten und Erkrankungs-Statistik von 21 Aerzten zusammenge-

Niederbarnim.
stellt, von Max Boehr. fol. *Berlin u. Bernau,* 1878.
Boehr. Todes- und Erkrankungs-Statistik des Kreises Niederbarnim pro ii. Quartal 1877. Veröffentl. d. k. deutsch. Gsndhtsamtes, Berl., 1877, i, Beilage, No. 30.— **Jahres-Tabelle** der Sterblichkeits-Verhältnisse des Kreises Niederbarnim während des Jahres 1876. *Ibid.,* 1877, i, No. 16.

Niederbronn.
LEUCHSENRING (J. L.) De fonte medicato Niederbronnensi. 4°. *Argentorati,* [1753].
Henry (O.) Rapport au sujet de l'eau de Niederbronn (Bas-Rhin). Bull. Acad. de méd., Par., 1859–60, xxv, 1000–1002. — **Kuhn** (J.) Sur les variations des sources minérales, et particulièrement de celle de Niederbronn. Gaz. méd. de Strasb., 1850, x, 43–54.

Niederer (Joh.) * Ueber die Osteomalacie des Beckens nach den Pubertätsjahren einer taubstummen, phthisischen Jungfrau und in der Schwangerschaft einer Person, die vier Mal ohne Kunsthülfe geboren hat. [Bern.] 42 pp., 1 pl., 1 tab. 8°. *Trogen, Schläpfer,* 1848.

Niedergesäss (Theodor) [1847–]. * Diabetes mellitus infantum. 32 pp. 8°. *Berlin, G. Lange,* [1873].

Nieder-Hessen.
See **Hospitals** (*Descriptions, etc., of*), *by localities.*

Niederholdt (Ferd.)
See **Osthoff** (H. C. A.) Ferd. Niederholdt's, eines jungen deutschen Arztes, Lehrjahre. 2 v. in 1. 8°. *Sulzbach,* 1808–9.

Niederhuber (Carolus Josephus). Eulogium piis manibus Philippi Fischer, annuente facultate saluberrima Landishutana habitum. 15 pp. 4°. *Landishuti, J. Attenkover,* 1800.

Niederhuber (Ignaz) [1754–]. Theorie von den Kräften des Mechanismus des menschlichen Körpers; eine Skizze für Anfänger in der praktischen Arzneywissenschaft. 109 pp. 12°. *München, T. Lauth,* 1786.

———. Ueber die menschlichen Temperamente. xxii (1 l.), 230 pp. 12°. *Wien, C. Schaumburg,* 1798.

———. Entwurf einer planmässigen Verfassung des Sanitätswesens für deutsche Provinzen. 101 pp. 8°. *München, J. Lindauer,* 1801.

Niederleitner (Joannes Henricus) [1833–]. * De phlegmone orbitæ. 28 pp. 8°. *Gryphiæ, F. G. Kunike,* 1869.
c.

Niedermaier (Franz).
Co-Editor of: **Tirolische** (Der) Arzt, Innsbruck, 1791–2.

Niedermayer (Franciscus). * Diss. med. de imaginationis maternæ in fetum efficacia. 55 pp. 12°. *Viennæ, M. A. Schmidt,* 1781. [P., v. 1639.]

Niedermayr (Hans). * Ueber Dermoidcysten an der grossen Fontanelle. 35 pp. 8°. *Würzburg, Becker,* 1886.

Niederösterreichische Landes-Gebär- und Findelanstalt in Wien. Aerztliche Berichte in den Solar-Jahren 1856; 1858; 1860; 1863; 1865–7. 8°. *Wien,* 1858–69.
1856–63, title: Kaiserlich-königl. Gebär- und Findelhaus zu Wien; 1865–6: Kaiserlich-königl. Findel-Anstalt in Wien.

———. Promemoria zum Findelhaus-Statuts-Entwurf, betreffend die Verpflegung und Erziehung der Findelkinder durch Eheleute. Von Dr. Friedinger, Primararzt und Directionsleiter der r. ö. Landes-Findelanstalt. 8 pp. 8°. [*Wien, A. della Torre,* 1869?]

———. Promemoria zum Findelhaus-Statuts-Entwurf, betreffend die Geheimhaltung der Mutterschaft. Von Dr. Friedinger, Primararzt und Directionsleiter der n. ö. Landes-Findelanstalt. 8 pp. 8°. [*Wien, A. della Torre,* 1869?]

———. [Summarischer Ausweis über die . . . im Jahre 1887. Von Director Dr. Friedinger.] 2 l. imp. fol. [*Wien,* 1888.]

Niederreither. * De febri biliosa. 20 pp. 8°. *Würzburg, C. W. Becker, 1837.*

Niederrheinische Gesellschaft für Natur- und Heilkunde zu Bonn. Bericht über die Arbeiten der ärztlichen Section. Für den Zeitraum vom Mai 1851 bis zum December 1853 in der Sitzung vom 7. December 1853 vorgelegt durch C. W. Wutzer. 42 pp. 8°. *Bonn,* 1854.

———. Sitzungsberichte. 1869; 1870; 1879–83. 8°. *Bonn, M. Cohen u. Sohn, 1869–83.*

Niederselters.

MINERALQUELLE (Die) zu Niederselters, ihre Bestandtheile und Heilkräfte. 8°. *Wiesbaden,* [*n. d.*]

Niederstadt (Carl). * Ueber Embolie der Lungencapillaren mit flüssigem Fet bei Osteomyelitis. 21 pp., 1 pl. 8°. *Göttingen, W. F. Kaestner,* 1869. [P., v. 292.]

Niederstadt (Joh. Theodorus). * De efficacia admiranda chinchinæ ad gangrænam sistendam in Anglia observata. 30 pp. 4°. *Vitembergæ, in off. Schlomachiana,* [1734].

Niederstetten

See **Fever** (*Typhoid, History, etc., of*), by localities.

Niedieck (Wilhelm) [1852–ㅤ]. * Ueber Neuritis migrans und ihre Folgezustände. [Greifswald.] 1 p. l., 19 pp., 1 l. 8°. *Leipzig, J. B. Hirschfeld,* 1877.

Niedner (Christian Friedrich Franz) [1838–ㅤ]. * Das Scharlachfieber und die epidemische Angina tonsillaris. 1 l., 15 pp. 8°. *Leipzig, C. G. Naumann,* [1864].

Niedrée (Georgius) [1806–ㅤ]. * De febre gastrica epidemica. 25 pp., 2 l. 8°. *Berolini, typ. Nietackianis,* [1832].

Niedt (Augustus Ludovicus). * Diss. monstrans variolarum spuriarum ex verarum pure ortum. 1 p. l., 36 pp. 8°. *Halæ, typ. J. C. Hendelii,* [1792].

Niedt (Georgius Wernerus). * De vitiis menstrui fluxus perite emendandis. 50 pp., 3 l. 4°. *Halæ Magdeb., lit. Hendelianis,* [1754].

Niedten (F. E.)
See **Paullini** (K. F.) Flagellum salutis, [etc.] 12°. *Stuttgart,* 1847.

Niefeld (Martinus Christianus). * De bulimia seu nimia ciborum adpetentia. 64 pp. 4°. *Halæ Magdeb., typ. J. C. Hendelii,* [1747].

Nieffer (Carolus Friedericus). * Diss. sistens animadversiones et experimenta circa mechanicas vires, quibus sanguis circulatio perficitur. 39 pp. 8°. *Tubingæ, typ. Reissianis,* [1818].

Nieger (Jules). * De la puce pénétrante des pays chauds et des accidents qu'elle peut occasionner. 1 p. l., 25 pp. 4°. *Strasbourg,* 1858, No. 433, v. 25.

Niehans (Paul). Zur Behandlung der Wanderniere. 1 l. 8°. *Leipzig,* 1888.
Repr. from : Centralbl. f. Chir., Leipz., 1888, xv.

———. Ueber traumatische Luxationen beider Hüftgelenke. 30 pp. 8°. *Leipzig,* 1888.
Repr. from : Deutsche Ztschr. f. Chir., Leipz., 1887–8, xxvii.

Niehoff (Franc. Henric.) [1797–ㅤ]. * De hæmoptysi. 32 pp. 8°. *Berolini, typ. T. Brueschke,* [1820].

Niehues (Hermann). * Beitrag zur Lehre von der Verletzung arterieller Blutgefässe in der Leistengegend. 22 pp. 8°. *Würzburg, P. Scheiner,* 1884.

Nieke (Carl). * Ein Beitrag zur operativen Behandlung der Dysmenorrhoe und Sterilität. 32 pp. 8°. *Greifswald, F. W. Kunike,* 1875.

van Niel (Cornelius). * De causis partus difficilis et auxiliis requisitis. 47 pp. 4°. *Lugd. Bat., P. De la Fos,* [1748].

Niel (Félicien). * Étude sur le plomb et ses principales combinaisons au point de vue toxicologique. 57 pp., 1 l. 4°. *Montpellier, Cristin,* 1884, No. 347.

Niel (J.-G.) Recherches et observations sur les effets des préparations d'or du docteur Chrestien dans le traitement de plusieurs maladies et notamment dans celui des maladies syphilitiques; publiées par J.-A. Chrestien. 1 p. l., xxx, 391 pp., 1 l. 8°. *Paris, Gabon,* 1821.

van Niel (Joannes Quirinus). * De hydrope. 24 pp., 1 l. 4°. *Lugd. Bat., G. Corts,* [1745].

Niel (Joseph - Louis - Adolphe). * De la peste d'Orient. 42 pp. 4°. *Montpellier,* 1835, No. 18. [P., v. 1083.]

Nieland (Joannes Josephus) [1799–ㅤ]. * Diss. sistens opii et morphini effectuum comparationem. 1 p. l., 57 pp., 1 l. 8°. *Berolini, formis Brüschckianis,* [1825].

Nielly (Maurice). * Considérations relatives à l'étiologie et au traitement de la dysenterie des pays chauds. 34 pp. 4°. *Paris,* 1864, No. 22.

———. Hygiène navale; son histoire, ses progrès. 31 pp. 8°. *Paris, Lahure,* [1876].
Repr. from : Arch. de méd. nav., Par., 1876, xxvi.

———. Manuel d'obstétrique ou aide-mémoire de l'élève et du praticien. 2. éd. xvi, 259 pp. 12°. *Paris, G. Masson,* 1880.

———. Éléments de pathologie exotique. xii, 791 pp., 1 l. 12°. *Paris, A. Delahaye & É. Lecrosnier,* 1881.

———. Hygiène des Européens dans les pays intertropicaux. I. Géographie torride. II. Action physiologique des climats intertropicaux. III. Leur action pathogénique. IV. Acclimatement des Européens dans les climats partiels. V. Règles d'hygiène et d'acclimatation. xx, 299 pp., 19 pl. 12°. *Paris, A. Delahaye & É. Lecrosnier,* 1884.

Nielsen (Jacobus). * De scarlatina. 30 pp., 1 l. 8°. *Kiliæ, C. F. Mohr,* 1844. c.

Nielsen (Joannes). * Præstantissimam rationem illustrandi materiam medicam practicam submittit. 64 pp. 8°. *Hafniæ, ex off. Thieliana,* [1778].

Nielson (Joannes Godofredus Gerhardus) [1804–ㅤ]. * De incarceratione intestinorum interna. 31 pp. 8°. *Berolini, typ. A. Petschii,* [1830]. [*Also, in :* P., v. 1547.]

Niemann (A.) * Beiträge zur Lehre von der Cystinurie beim Menschen. [Göttingen.] 32 pp., 1 pl. 8°. *Leipzig, J. B. Hirschfeld,* 1876.

Niemann (Adolphus) [1806–77]. * De medicinæ militaris incrementis præsertim ex remediis quibusdam novis tempore recentiore captis. 54 pp. 8°. *Berolini, typ. Jordanianis,* [1828].

———. Inest commentatio de methodo Niemanniana in morbis acutis. 9 l. 4°. *Magdeburgi, typ. Pansæ,* [1837].

———. Gerichtliche Leichen - Oeffnungen, mitgetheilt und erläutert von . . . Erstes [bis viertes] Hundert. viii, 129 pp.; viii, 143 pp.; x, 187 pp. 8°. *Erlangen, J. J. Palm u. E. Enke,* 1856–62.
Repr. from : Ztschr. f. d. Staatsarznk., Erlang., 1856–62.

———. The same. 3tes Hundert. x, 127 pp. 8°. *Erlangen, J. J. Palm u. E. Enke,* 1859.
Repr. from : Ztschr. f. d. Staatsarznk., Erlang., 1859, lxxvii-lxxviii.

Niemann (Albert). * Ueber eine neue organische Base in den Cocablättern. 52 pp., 1 pl. 8°. *Göttingen, E. A. Huth,* 1860.

Niemann (Carolus Godofredus). * De corticis Peruviani virtute propria atque specifica.

Niemann (Carolus Godofredus)—continued. 32 pp. sm. 4°. *Lipsiæ, ex off. Klaubarthia,* [1785].

    For Biography, see **Gehler** (Joannes Carolus).

Niemann (Christianus Augustus). * De cantharissationis externæ effectibus in corpus humanum, momenta præcipua circa cantharidum applicatione observanda. 23 pp. 4°. *Weissenfelsæ, typ. Severianis,* [1791].

Niemann (Eduardus) [1794–]. * De vi propulsoria sanguinis neganda. 35 pp. 8°. *Berolini, typ. J. F. Starckii,* [1815].

Niemann (Emil). Ueber Hodennekrose. 16 pp. 8°. *Breslau, W. Friedrich,* [1884].

    Repr. from : Breslau. aerztl. Ztschr., 1884, vi.

Niemann (Gustav). * Beiträge zur Casuistik des Diabetes insipidus. 28 pp. 8°. *Würzburg, F. X. Bucher,* 1877.

Niemann (Joachimus). * De remediis mercurialibus spinæ ventosæ medicandæ interdum idoneis. 52 pp. 4°. *Halæ Magdeb., typ. J. C. Hilligeri,* [1754].

Niemann (Joannes Christophorus) [1750–85]. * De apoplexiæ pathologia et therapia. 1 p. l., 22 pp. 4°. *Halæ ad Salam, stanno Hendeliano,* [1772].

Niemann (Joh. Friedrich) [1765–1841]. Handbuch der Staats-Arzneiwissenschaft und staatsärztlichen Veterinärkunde nach alphabetischer Ordnung für Aerzte, Medicinalpolizei-Beamte und Richter. 2 v. xxxvi, 679 pp. ; xvi, 702 pp., 1 l. 8°. *Leipzig, J. A. Barth,* 1813.

———. Taschenbuch der gerichtlichen Arzneiwissenschaft für Aerzte und Wundärzte, Medicinal- und Sanitätsbeamte. xiii, 520 pp., 2 pl. 12°. *Leipzig, J. A. Barth,* 1827.

    Is 10. Theil, 1. Bd., of: Allg. Encyclopädie f. pract. Aerzte u. Wundärzte, hrsg. von G. W. Consbruch u. J. F. Niemann.

———. Taschenbuch der Civil-Medicinal-Polizei für Aerzte und Wundärzte, Medicinal- und Sanitätsbeamte. xvi, 899 pp. 12°. *Leipzig, J. A. Barth,* 1828.

    Is 10. Theil, 2. Bd., 1. Abth., of: Allg. Encyclopädie f. pract. Aerzte u. Wundärzte, hrsg. von G. W. Consbruch u. J. F. Niemann.

———. Taschenbuch der Militair - Medicinal - Polizei für Aerzte und Wundärzte, Medicinal- und Sanitätsbeamte. xv, 556 pp., 2 l., 4 pl. 12°. *Leipzig, J. A. Barth,* 1829.

    Is 10. Theil, 2. Bd., 2. Abth., of: Allg. Encyclopädie f. pract. Aerzte u. Wundärzte, hrsg. von G. W. Consbruch u. J. F. Niemann. With second title-page.

    See, also, **Codex** medicamentarius Europæus. Sec. iv. 2. ed. 8°. *Lipsiæ,* 1824.

    For Portrait, see **Collection**—van Kaathoven.

Niemann (Joh. Henricus). * De herniis. 16 pp. 4°. *Erfordiæ, J. C. Gœrling,* [1805].

Niemann (Julius) [1824–]. * De inflammatione renum parenchymatosa. 26 pp., 2 l. 8°. *Berolini, typ. fratrum Schlesinger,* [1848].

Niemchenkoff (V. A.) * Kartofel i ego pitateinost. [The potato and its nutritive value.] 39 pp., 3 tab., 1 l. 8°. *St. Petersburg,* 1886.

Niemeier (Ludovicus Fridericus Cornelius) [1837–]. * De paralysi nervi facialis. 32 pp. 8°. *Berolini, G. Lange,* [1863].

Niemeijer (Meinart). * Statistische en klinische mededeelingen over febris typhoidea. 2 p. l., 75 pp., 2 tab. 8°. *Groningen, G. Hoitsema,* 1886.

Niemeijer (Meinart Herman). * Diabetes insipidus. 2 p. l., 52 pp., 2 l. 8°. *Groningen, P. Noordhoff,* 1873.

von Niementowski (St. D.) * Synthese der Nitrococcussäure und Versuche zur Synthese des Ruficoccins. Zur Kenntniss der Anhydro-Verbindungen. [Erlangen.] 39 pp. 8°. *München, M. Ernst,* 1886.

Niemetschek (Joseph).

    See **Köstl** (Franciscus) & **Niemetschek** (Joseph). Der Centralnervenpuls der Netzhaut, [etc.] 8°. [*Prag.* 1870.]

Niemetz (Joannes Wenceslaus). * De apoplexia sanguinea ratione, habita characteris physiologici et anatomici, adnexis observationibus nonnullis circa necroscopia in nosocomio generali Prageno instituta depromtis. 39 pp. 8°. *Pragæ, T. Thabor,* [n. d.]

Niemeyer (*Aug. Herm.*)

    JUBELFEIER (Die) des fünfzigjährigen akademischen Lehramtes Sr. Hochwürden des Herrn Canzlers und Professors D. Aug. Herm Niemeyer, am 18. April 1827. Von einem aufmerksamen Beobachter. 8°. *Halle,* 1827.

Niemeyer (Carolus Edwardus) [1792–1838]. * Singularis in fœtu puellari recens edito abnormitatis exemplum descriptum et illustratum. 1 p. l., 19 pp., 2 pl. 4°. *Halæ, typ. orphanotrophei,* 1814.

von Niemeyer (Felix) [1820–71]. * De aneurysmate aortæ thoracicæ addita morbi pro aneurysmate habiti historia. 49 pp. 8°. *Halæ, formis Ploetzianis,* [1843].

———. Die symptomatische Behandlung der Cholera, mit besonderer Rücksicht auf die Bedeutung des Darmleidens. 38 pp. 8°. *Magdeburg, E. Fabricius,* 1849. [P., v. 175.]

———. Klinische Mittheilungen aus dem städtischen Krankenhause zu Magdeburg. iv, 58 pp. 8°. *Magdeburg, G. Baensch,* 1855.

———. The same. Della cura sintomatica del colera, con speciale considerazione sul significato dell' affezione intestinale. Versione dal tedesco pel Tommaso de Amicis. 59 pp. 8°. *Napoli,* 1865.

———. Lehrbuch der speciellen Pathologie und Therapie, mit besonderer Rücksicht auf Physiologie und pathologische Anatomie. 2. Abdr. 2 v. xii, 697 pp. ; vii, 781 pp. 8°. *Berlin, A. Hirschwald,* 1859–61.

    v. 1. Krankheiten der Respirations- und Circulations-Organe.
    v. 2. Krankheiten der Harn- und Geschlechtsorgane, der Nervencentren und der Nerven.

———. The same. 6. Aufl. 2 v. xvi, 774 pp. ; viii, 798 pp. 8°. *Berlin, A. Hirschwald,* 1865.

———. The same. 7. Aufl. 2 v. xvi, 840 pp. ; viii, 903 pp. 8°. *Berlin, A. Hirschwald,* 1868.

———. The same. 8. Aufl. 2 v. x, 822 pp. ; viii, 909 pp. 8°. *Berlin, A. Hirschwald,* 1871.

———. The same. 11. Aufl. 2 v. viii, 878 pp. ; xi, 1004 pp. 8°. *Berlin, A. Hirschwald,* 1885.

———. The same. A text-book of practical medicine, with particular reference to physiology and pathological anatomy. Transl. from the 7. German ed. by George H. Humphreys and Charles E. Hackley. 2 v. xv, 731 pp. ; viii, 7–770 pp. roy. 8°. *New York, D. Appleton & Co.,* 1869.

———. The same. Εἰδικὴ νοσολογία καὶ θεραπευτικὴ συντεταγμένη καὶ ἀναφοραῖν ἰδίως πρὸς τὴν φυσιολογίαν καὶ παθολογικὴν ἀνατομίαν. Διασκευάσθεισα μὲν ὑπὸ Εὐγενίου Σεῖτζ. Μεταφράσθεισα δὲ ἐκ τῆς ἐνατῆς ἐκδόσεως τοῦ γερμανικοῦ καὶ διὰ σημειώσεων καὶ προσθήκων ἐπαυξηθεῖσα ὑπὸ Γεωργίου Καραμήτσα. (Ἐκδοσις δευτέρα ηὐξημένη καὶ διωρθωμένη.) Τόμος πρῶτος. ii, 1026, vi pp. 8°. *Ἐν Ἀθήναις, τυπ. τῶν Ἀ. Βαρβαρρηγου,* 1879.

———. The same. Rukovod. k chastnoi patolog. i terapii. Vnov obrabot. E. Seitz. Perevod s desjatiago . . . Niemetsk. izd. M. Hirschfelda. Pod red. V. V. Sviatlovskago. 3 pts. in 1 v. 8°. *St. Petersburg, N. Wilkin,* 1881–2.

———. Die epidemische Cerebro-Spinal-Meningitis nach Beobachtungen im Grossherzogthum Baden. 2. Abdr. 72 pp. 8°. *Berlin, A. Hirschwald,* 1865.

von Niemeyer (Felix)—continued.
———. Die Behandlung der Korpulenz nach dem sogenannten Bantingsystem. Ein populär-wissenschaftlicher Vortrag gehalten zu Stuttgart . . . 23. Dezember 1865. 37 pp. 8°. *Berlin, A. Hirschwald*, 1866.
———. Klinische Vorträge über die Lungenschwindsucht. Mitgetheilt von Dr. Ott. 2. Aufl. 112 pp. 8°. *Berlin, A. Hirschwald*, 1867.
———. Clinical lectures on pulmonary phthisis. Transl., by permission of the author, from the 2. German ed., by J. L. Parke. 116 pp. 8°. *New York, Moorhead, Simpson & Bond*, 1868.
———. The same. Transl., by permission of the author, from the 2. German ed., by C. Baeumler. vii, 71 pp. 8°. *London, New Sydenham Society*, 1870.
———. The same. Lecciones clínicas sobre la tísis pulmonar, traducidas por Ricardo Martinez Esteban. 132 pp., 1 l. 8°. *Madrid, F. Garcia & D. Caravera*, 1875.
———. Ueber das Verhalten der Eigenwärme bei gesunden und kranken Menschen. Ein populärer Vortrag. 44 pp. 8°. *Berlin, A. Hirschwald*, 1869.
———. Éléments de pathologie interne et de thérapeutique. Traduction de l'allemand, revue et annotée par M. le docteur V. Cornil. 3. éd. française, augmentée de notes nouvelles d'après la huitième éd. allemande. 2 v. 711, 752 pp. 8°. *Paris, Germer-Baillière*, 1873.
———. Sai Sei Roku. [A text-book of practical medicine; transl. by Sato Sochiu.] 14 v. 8°. *Tokio*, 1879.
Japanese text.
———. Netsu Shinrou. [The new doctrine of fever; transl. by Watanabe Yetsu.] 2, 2, 2, 237 pp., 1 pl., 4 pp., 3 l. 8°. *Tokio*, 1886.
Japanese text.
See, also, **Diesterweg** (Alexander Carolus Guilelmus Eduardus). Kritische Beiträge zur Physiologie [etc.] 8°. *Frankf. a. M.*, 1869.—**Kennedy** (Henry). On the views of Niemeyer regarding phthisis. 8°. *Dublin*, 1871.—**Vacher** (L.) De l'obésité [etc.] 8°. *Paris*, 1873.
For Biography, see Berl. klin. Wchnschr., 1871, viii, 189–191. *Also:* Deutsches Arch. f. klin. Med., Leipz., 1871, viii, 427–444 (Ziemssen). *Also:* Med. Cor.-Bl. d. württemb. ärztl. Ver., Stuttg., 1871, xli, 133; 141; 151; 159; 167; 179. *Also:* Med. Times & Gaz., Lond., 1871, i, 642.
For Portrait, see N. York M. J., 1871, xiii.

Niemeyer (Guilielm. Herm.) * De origine paris quinti nervorum cerebri. 52 pp. 8°. *Halæ, in libraria Orphanotrophei Halensis*, [1811].
———. The same. 94 pp., 1 pl. 8°. *Halæ, in libraria Orphanotrophei Halensis*, 1811.
Also, Editor of : **Zeitschrift** für Geburtshülfe und praktische Medicin, Halle, 1828.

Niemeyer (Henr. Aug.) [1817–]. * De hypertrophia linguæ congenita. 28 pp., 2 l. 4°. *Halis, formis Orphanotrophei*, [1842].

Niemeyer (Hugo). * Ein Fall von Lungenarterien-Embolie nach einer Distorsio pedis. 16 pp. 8°. *Kiel, A. F. Jensen*, 1887.

Niemeyer (Joannes Henricus Andreas). * De violæ caninæ in medicina usu. 1 p. l., 27 pp. 4°. *Gottingæ, H. M. Grape*, [1785].
For Biography, see **Murray** (Jo. Andreas).

Niemeyer (Ludov. Henr. Christ.) [1775–1800). Commentatio de commercio inter animi pathemata hepar bilemque; de causis ejusdem, nec non de usu et moderamine illius pro practica medicina exspectando. 62 pp. 4°. *Gottingæ, J. C. Dieterich*, [1795].
———. * De menstruationis fine et usu. 68 pp., 1 l. 12°. *Gottingæ, J. C. Dieterich*, [1796].
———. Materialien zur Erregungstheorie. Hrsg. von Georg Friedrich Mühry. xvi, 214 pp. 8°. *Göttingen, J. G. Rosenbusch's Wittwe*, 1800.

Niemeyer (Maximilianus Theodorus) [– 1835). * De hernia cerebri congenita, cujus ex-

Niemeyer (Maximilianus Theodorus)—cont'd.
emplum describitur et illustratur. 1 p. l., 43 pp., 2 pl. 4°. *Halæ, typ. orphanotrophei*, [1833].
Niemeyer (Paul) [1832–]. * De mandibulæ ancylosi novaque ejus curatione operativa. 27 pp., 2 l. 8°. *Berolini, B. Schlesinger*, [1854].
———. Betrachtungen über die ärztliche Seite der Lebensversicherung. 11 pp. 8°. *Wien, J. Löwenthal*, 1865.
Repr. from: Wien. med. Presse, 1865, vi.
———. Handbuch der theoretischen und clinischen Percussion und Auscultation vom historischen und critischen Standpuncte bearbeitet. 2 v. xii, 246, x, 234 pp., 2 pl. 8°. *Erlangen, F. Enke*, 1868–70.
———. Grundriss der Percussion und Auscultation, nebst einem Index sämmtlicher in- und ausländischen Kunstausdrücke. xvi, 125 pp., 1 l. 8°. *Erlangen, F. Enke*, 1871.
———. The same. A kopogtatás és hallgatódzás alapvonalai. A második, német kiadás után fordította: Kerékgyártó Lorant. viii, 109 pp. 8°. *Budapest, V. Lauffer*, 1879.
———. The same. Compendio de percussão e auscultação. Traduzido do original allemão por João Felix Pereira e revisto pelo Dr. P. F. Dacosta Alvarenga. 8°. *Lisboa, imp. nacional*, 1874.
———. Die Lunge; ihre Pflege und Behandlung im gesunden und kranken Zustande, mit besonderer Rücksicht auf Lungenschwindsucht und einem Abschnitt über Klimatologie. xvii, 175 pp. 8°. *Leipzig, J. J. Weber*, 1872.
———. The same. Nebst einem Abschnitte über Heiserkeit und ihre Heilung. 6. Aufl. xi, 275 pp. 16°. *Leipzig, J. J. Weber*, 1887.
———. Medicinische Abhandlungen. 3 v. 8°. *Erlangen, F. Enke*, 1872–5.
CONTENTS.
v. 1. Atmiatrie (Athmungs- und Luftheilkunde).
v. 2. Grundzüge einer Radicalcur der einfachen Lungenschwindsucht. Zur Lehre von der Percussion und Auscultation. x, 289 pp.
v. 3. Grundzüge einer klinischen Hygieine und Diätetik, nebst einem Résumé über Schwindsucht und einer Beilage. vii, 218 pp., 1 l.
———. Herz, Blut- und Lymphgefässe. Ihre Pflege und Behandlung im gesunden und kranken Zustande, einschliesslich Hämorrhoiden, Skrofeln, Fieber, Hitzschlag, Erfrierungen, Blutungen u. s. w. xv, 225 pp. 12°. *Leipzig, J. J. Weber*, 1874.
———. Physikalische Diagnostik, einschliesslich der klimatischen und hygieinischen Untersuchung für praktische Aerzte. xii, 332 pp. 8°. *Erlangen, F. Enke*, 1874.
———. Gesundheitslehre des menschlichen Körpers. viii, 291 pp. 12°. *München, R. Oldenbourg*, 1876.
———. Ueber die akustischen Zeichen der Pneumonie. Habilitations-Vorlesung am 18. Juli 1876, gehalten vor der medizinischen Facultät. Mit Zusätzen und einem Anhange über Berechtigung und Methode der populären Lehrthätigkeit. 1 p. l., 31 pp. 8°. *Stuttgart, F. Enke*, 1876.
———. Rigakuteki Teicho Shinron. [A new treatise on auscultation and percussion; transl. by Sakurai Ikujiro.] 3 v. 12°. *Tokio*, 1878.
Japanese text.
———. Behr'scher Gesundheitskaffee. 17 pp. 12°. *Jena, H. Costenoble*, [1880?]
Repr. from his: Aerztliche Sprechstunden, vii.
———. Ueber gesundes und ungesundes Aussehen. 8°. *Heidelberg, C. Winter*, 1880.
In: SAMML. v. Vortr. f. d. deutsche Volk, Heidelberg, 1880, iii, 211–231.
———. Aerztlicher Ratgeber für Mütter. Zwanzig Briefe über die Pflege des Kindes von der Geburt

Niemeyer (Paul)—continued.
bis zur Reife. Title-plate. iv, 306 pp. 8°. *Stuttgart, J. Engelhorn*, 1885.

——. Trichinen-Catechismus in Fragen und Antworten, nebst einem Anhange über das Mikroskop und einer lithographirten Tafel für Nicht-Aerzte. 4. Aufl. 16 pp., 1 pl. 8°. *Genthin, C. Donath*, 1885.

——. Die Skrofelkrankheit. Ihre Entstehung, Verhütung und Behandlung. 103 pp. 8°. *Berlin, Denicke*, [*n. d.*]

——. Krummer Rücken, flache Brust, Plattfuss: ihre Ursachen, Behandlung und Verhütung. Ein Rathgeber für Jedermann. Mit 15 Abbildungen. 94 pp. 8°. *Berlin, Denicke*, [*n. d.*]

Also, Editor of : **Aerztliche** Sprechstunden, Jena, 1885-7.—**Hygieia**, Stuttgart, 1888.

See, also, **Pintado** & **Jordan** (Galo). Piretologia [etc.] 8°. *Madrid*, 1871.—**Schmölcke** (A.) Die Verbesserung unserer Wohnungen [etc.] 8°. *Wiesbaden*, 1881.—**Staebe** (C. L.) Boden-Ventilation als Schutzmassregel. 8°. *Magdeburg*, 1873.—**Steudel** (H.) Der Nihilismus der einzig Wahre in der Medizin, [etc.] 8°. *Leipzig*, 1887.

Niemiec (J.) * Recherches morphologiques sur les ventouses dans le règne animal. [Bern.] 147 pp., 5 l., 5 pl. 8°. *Genève, C. Schuchardt*, 1885.

Niemojewski (A.) * Considérations sur les fractures de la clavicule et leur traitement. 62 pp., 1 l. 4°. *Montpellier*, 1879, No. 18.

Nienhaus (H.) Die Wuthkrankheit der Hunde. Kennzeichen derselben bei ihrem Entstehen und in ihrem Verlaufe bis zum Ausbruche der Raserei. Eine Belehrung für die Besitzer von Hunden. Nach einem Vortrage des französischen Veterinärarztes H. Bauley bearbeitet. 16 pp. 12°. *Crefeld, J. B. Klein*, 1864.

Nièpce. De la contagion et de la transmissibilité de la tuberculose. 2. éd. 90 pp. 8°. *Grenoble, Breynat & Cie.*, 1886.

Nièpce (Alexandre). *Quelques considérations sur le crétinisme. 70 pp. 4°. *Paris*, 1871, No. 59.

Nièpce (B.) Mémoire sur l'action des bains de petit-lait, soit pur, soit à l'état de mélange avec l'eau sulfureuse d'Allevard. 32 pp. 8°. *Paris, J.-B. Baillière*, 1850. [*Also, in :* P., v. 1648.]

——. Traité du goître et du crétinisme, suivi de la statistique des goîtreux et des crétins dans le bassin de l'Isère en Savoie, dans les départements de l'Isère, des Hautes-Alpes et des Basses-Alpes. 2 v. x, 501 pp.; 200, xxxviii pp. 8°. *Paris, J.-B. Baillière*, 1851.

——. De l'action de l'eau sulfureuse et iodée d'Allevard (Isère) dans les affections chroniques de la poitrine, et de la manière de les administrer. 7 pp. 8°. [*n. p.*, 1853.] [P., v. 1648]

——. De l'action des bains de petit-lait dans les maladies du cœur, et principalement dans les palpitations nerveuses de cet organe. 9-23 pp. 8°. [*n. p.*, 1853.] [P., v. 1648.]

Niepce de Saint Victor (Claude-Félix) [1805–]. Traité pratique de gravure héliographique sur acier et sur verre. xiii, 14-60 pp., 1 l. 4°. *Paris, V. Masson*, 1856.

Nieprasch (Carolus Arminins) [1824–]. * De exanthemate scarlatinoso. 29 pp., 1 l. 8°. *Berolini, B. Schlesinger*, 1850.

Nieratz.
Zengerle. Nieratzbad. Med. Cor.-Bl. d. württemb. ärztl. Ver., Stuttg., 1837, vii, 304-306.

Nieremberger (Georgius Jacobus). * De dysenteria. 26 pp. 4°. *Argentorati, typ. J. H. Heitzii*, 1779.

Nierhaus (Joannes Hermannus) [1807–]. * De phthiseos pulmonum tuberculosæ pathologia. 28 pp., 2 l. 8°. *Berolini, typ. Nietackianis*, [1840].

Nieriker (P.) Die Cholerafälle im Bezirk Baden (Kanton Aargau) im Jahr 1867. 49 pp. 8°. *Aarau, H. R. Sauerländer*, 1867.

Niermann (Joh. Henricus) [1831–]. * De pseudarthrosi, addita historia morbi. 31 pp. 8°. *Gryphiæ, F. Hache*, 1859. c.

Niermeyer (Joh. Hendrik). * Akademische proeve, bevattende een door den schrijver waargenomen ziektegeval. vii, 54 pp. 8°. *Leiden, E. J. Brill*, 1856.

Niermeyer (Johan Hendrik Anton). * Neuropathologische onderzoekingen. 2 p. l., 74 pp. 8°. *Leiden, gebr. van der Hoek*, 1879.

Niernsée (John R.) Description of the plan adopted for the "Johns Hopkins Colored Orphan Asylum", for 300 children, at Baltimore, Md. App. I. [Studies of octagon pavilions for hospital wards, etc.] App. II.
In : HOSPITAL plans, Johns Hopkins Hospital, Baltimore. 8°. *New York*, 1875. pp. 331-345, 13 pl.

——. Report on the construction and embellishment of private dwellings in Vienna. 26 pp., 29 pl. 8°. *Washington, D. C., Government Printing Office*, 1875.
Vienna International Exhibition, 1873.

——. Review of "Hospital plans" of the Johns Hopkins Hospital [with description of wards]. 44, 5 pp. 8°. [*Baltimore*, 1876.]

Nierop (Gerardus). * De contagio varioloso ex observationibus indagato. 1 p. l., 69 pp., 3 l. 4°. *Lugd. Bat., J. le Mair*, 1774.

Nierstein.
SIRONA-BAD (Das) bei Nierstein und seine Mineralquellen. 8°. *Mainz*, 1827.

Niesel (Max Rudolf Julius) [1864–]. *Ueber die Wirkung fortgesetzter kleiner Dosen von Schwefel beim gesunden Menschen. 42 pp. 8°. *Greifswald, F. W. Kunike*, [1887].

Niesemann ([Joannes Albertus] Guilelmus Rudolphus) [1821–]. * De spermatorrhœa. 38 pp., 1 l. 8°. *Berolini, G. Schade*, [1847].

Niesemann (Jos.) * Ueber Trismus. 23 pp. 8°. *Würzburg, F. X. Bucher*, 1878.

Niesius (Benjamin). * De elephantiasi, seu lepra Arabum. 28 pp. 4°. *Argentorati, typ. J. Welperi*, [1673].

Niesner (Herm. Aug. Theophil.) * De fistularum cura. 41 pp., 1 l., 1 pl. 8°. *Gottingæ, C. Herbst*, [1820].

Niesse (Franz) [1852–]. *Ueber das Verhältniss der peripherischen Temperatur zur centralen im Schweissstadium des Menschen. 39 pp. 8°. *Berlin, G. Schade*, [1877].

Niessen (Oscarus) [1835–]. * De placenta prævia. 36 pp. 12°. *Berolini, G. Lange*, 1861.

Niessen (Werner). * Hydrocephalus congenitus als Geburtshinderniss. 44 pp. 8°. *München, C. Wolf u. Sohn*, 1880.

Niessen (Wilhelm). *Ueber Genu valgum und seine operative Behandlung. [Wurtzburg.] 24 pp. 8°. *Berlin, J. F. Starcke*, 1884.

Niesz (John). A short treatise on the use of arnica, and a few other useful homœopathic preparations, to heal contusions, wounds, strains, sprains, lacerations, concussions, paralysis, rheumatism, pains, soreness of the nipples, and to give ease before, in, and after parturition, etc. With a number of cases illustrating the use of several drugs. Compiled from the best authors. iv, 5-376 pp., 5 l., 10 pp. 12°. *Canton, O., D. Shell*, 1851.

——. The family guide to health and husbandry; containing essays on homœopathic and other medical preparations for the cure of diseases of men, horses, cattle, and sheep, and imparting useful information to the dairyman and wool grower. 19 pp. 1 l., 4 pl. 12°. *Canton, O., D. Shell*, 1851.

Nieszczotta(Michael [Nicodemus]) [1815–   ].
* De eclampsia morbo evolutionis. 51 pp., 1 l.
8°. *Vratislaviæ, typ. off. Guentherianæ*, [1841].

Nieszkowski (Ladislas Émile). * Sur l'emploi
thérapeutique de l'iodoforme considéré comme
cicatrisant et anesthésique local. 44 pp. 4°.
Paris, 1869, No. 156.

Nieszner (Stephanus). * De pneumonorrhagia.
33 pp. 8°. *Pestini, typ. Trattner - Károlyianis*,
[1837].

de Niet (Arie). * Typhus abdominalis en typhus
exanthematicus in het Buitengasthuis te Amsterdam gedurende de jaren 1879–86. [Leyden.] 79
pp., 1 pl. 8°. *Scheveningen*, 1886.

Nieten (Ernestus Henricus) [1843–   ]. * De
ulcere ventriculi simplice. 31 pp. 8°. *Berolini*,
G. Schade, 1864.

Nieter (Adolphus Georgius Carolus Fridericus)
[1836–   ]. * De tumoribus quibusdam a carcinomate dignoscendis. 32 pp. 8°. *Berolini*,
G. Lange, [1859].

Nieter (Adolphus Jul. Car.) [1794–   ]. * De vi
et effectu hydrargyri in quibusdam morbis non
syphiliticis. 26 pp. 8°. *Berolini, typ. J. F.*
Starckii, [1818].

Niethammer (Carolus Fridericus). * De statu
rei chirurgicæ et obstetriciæ plurimis in terris
deplorabili observationibus confirmato. 18 pp.
4°. *Jenæ, typ. Strannckmanni*, [1797].

Niethammer (Emil Friedrich). * Chemische
Untersuchung des Schwefelwassers, bei Sebas-
tiansweiler. 24 pp. 8°. *Tübingen, C. H. Reiss*
u. C. A. Küstner, 1831.

Niethe (Jo. Daniel Theoph.) [1802–   ]. * De
partu post mortem. 31 pp. 8°. *Berolini, typ.*
A. Petschii, [1827].

Nietner (Joh. Gottfried). * De glandularum
natura et usu. 32 pp. sm. 4°. *Erfurti, stanno*
Kindlebiano, [1694].

Nieto Serrano (Matias). Memoria acerca de
la necesidad y utilidad de una asociacion general
de profesores de ciencias médicas, con espresion
de las principales bases sobre que conviene esta-
blecerla; leida en la reunion preparatoria celebrada con el mismo objeto en la redaccion del
Boletin de medicina y cirugía el 14 de febrero
de 1840. vi, 33 pp. 12°. *Madrid, Yenes*,
1840.

——. La reforma médica. 426 pp , 1 l. 8°.
Madrid, M. de Rojas, 1863.
Date on cover, 1864.

——. Elementos de patología general. vi, 406
pp. 8°. *Madrid, Moya y Plaza*, 1869.

——. Filosofia de la naturaleza. vi, 344 pp.
8°. *Madrid, imp. de E. Teodoro*, 1884.
See, also, **Malgaigne** (J. F.) Tratado de anatomía
quirúrjica, etc. 8°. *Madrid*, 1861.

Nietsch (Carolus Fridericus). Dissertatio anatomico-physiologica aëris in sanguinem vias sistens. 48 pp. 8°. *Gottingæ, C. Herbst*, 1815.

——. Ueber verborgene Entzündung und die
daraus entspringenden bedeutendern körperlichen Uebel. Nebst einem Anhange über die
Einheit in der ärztlichen Kunst. xxiv, 208 pp.
8°. *Frankf. a. M., Hermann*, 1819.

Nietzki (Adamus) [1714–80]. * De febribus
complicatis in genere. 3 p. l., 84 pp. 4°. *Halæ*
ad Salam, e typog. Curtiano, [1753]

——. De medicina organica quatenus philosophiam mechanicam sibi vindicante commentatur.
12 pp. 4°. *Halæ ad Salam, e typog. Curtiano*,
[1753].

——. Elementa pathologiæ universæ. 16 p. l.,
588 pp., 6 l. 8°. *Halæ ad Salam, J. J. Curtius*,
1766.

——. The same. Editio nova emendatior. 2 v.
[paged consecutively]. xxiv, 478 pp. 8°. *Lau-*
sannæ in Helvetia, F. Grasset et soc., 1784.

Nieubuur (Jacobus Martinus). * De emphysemate pulmonum vesiculari. 4 p. l., 39 pp.,
2 l., 1 pl. 8°. *Groningæ, W. van Boekeren*,
[1840].

Nieubuur (Martinus Jacobus). * De zona. 2
p. l., 36 pp., 2 l. 8°. *Groningæ, F. Wilkens*,
[1849].

Nieuw Archief voor binnen- en buitenlandsche
Geneeskunde in haren geheelen omvang, door
Dr. I van Deen. v. 1–4, 1846–51. 8°. *Zwolle*,
W. E. J. Tjeenk Willink.

——. Supplement. No. 1. 76 pp. 8°. *Zwolle*,
1848.

Nieuw practisch Tijdschrift voor de Geneeskunde
in al haren omvang.
Title of : **Practisch** Tijdschrift voor de Geneeskunde
in al haren omvang in 1847–54.

Nieuwediep.
See **Cholera** (*Asiatic, History, etc., of*), *by lo-*
calities.

Nieuwenhuijs (F. L. A.) Verbeterde bereiding van de kina-loogzouten. Benevens geneeskundige waarnemingen met deze zuivere bestand-
deelen der kina in tusschenpoozende en aanhou-
dende koortsen, door Cs. Js. Nieuwenhuijs. xvi,
117 pp. 8°. *Amsterdam, J. van der Hey & Zoon*,
1823.

Nieuwenhuis (Christianus Ignatius). * Diss.
exhibens observationes quasdam de usu, inprimis diætetico, muriatis sodæ seu salis cibarii.
1 p. l., 51 pp., 2 l. 8°. *Groningæ, H. Eekhoff*,
1807.

——. Proeve eener geneeskundige plaatsbeschrijving (topographie) der stad Amsterdam.
4 v. in 2. 8°. *Amsterdam, J. van der Hey*, 1816–
20.
See, also, **Nieuwenhuijs** (F. L. A.) Verbeterde bereiding van de kina-loogzouten, [etc.] 8°. *Amsterdam*,
1823.

Nieuwenhuis (Lucas Cornelis). * Diss. sistens momenta quædam de surditate per puncturam membranæ tympani curanda. 1 p. l., 36
pp., 4 l. 4°. *Traj. ad Rhenum, O. J. van Pad-*
denburg et G. van Yzerworst, [1807].

Nieuwentijt (*Bernard*) [1654–1718].
Portrait in : **Collection** of Portr. of Phys. & Men of
Sc., 126 ; 200.

Nieuwland (*Pieter*) [1764–1837].
Biographie. Nederl. Tijdschr. v. Geneesk , Amst.,
1870, ii, 8–20.

Nieuw-Malthusiaansche Bond. Schetsen.
Nos. 1–3, 1882–4. 8°. *Amsterdam, J. D. Brouwer*.
Each number paged separately.

Nieuwstraten (J. C.) * Ueber einen trans-
portabeln Schwitzapparat. 34 pp. 8°. *Göt-*
tingen, W. F. Kaestner, 1882.

Nièvre (*Département de la*). Conseils d'hygiène
publique et de salubrité du département de la
Nièvre. Rapports sur les travaux de ces Conseils pour les années 1880 et 81, par le Doct. Mignot, et pour l'année 1882, par le Doct. Subert.
168 pp. 8°. *Nevers, imp. Nivernaise*, 1883.

Nièvre (*Département de la*).
See, also, **Cholera** (*Asiatic, History, etc., of*),
by localities.
ÉTABLISSEMENT thermal de St.-Honoré-les-
Bains (Nièvre), l'ancien Aquæ Nisinæi des Ro-
mains. Saison des bains de (1868). 8°. *Paris*,
1868.

Nigella.
See, also, **Flour**, *etc.*
Pellacani (P.) Ueber die wirksamen Bestandtheile
des gemeinen Schwarzkümmels (Nigella sativa L.). Arch.
f. exper. Path. u. Pharmakol., Leipz., 1882–3, xvi, 440–451.
——. Sui principii attivi della Nigella sativa. Ann. univ.
di med. e chir., Milano, 1883. cclxiii, 37–50. *Also, transl. :*
Arch. ital. de biol., Turin, 1883, iv, 45–56.

Niger.

See, also, **Africa**; **Fever** (*Malarial, History, etc., of*), *by localities.*

M'Cormac. Note on the Niger expedition. Edinb. M. & S. J., 1845, lxiv, 341–345.—**Oldfield** (K. A. K.) On the diseases of the natives resident on the banks of the river Niger. Lond. M. & S. J., 1835-6, [n. s.], viii, 403–407.

Niger (Antonius) [–1555]. Consilium de tuenda valetudine. 42 l. 12°. *Lipsiæ, in off. V. Papæ,* 1554.

Bound with : DRESSER (M.) De partibus corporis humani [etc.] 12°. *Witebergæ,* 1583.

———. The same. 39 l. 16°. *Lipsiæ, in off. V. Papæ,* 1555.

Bound with : PALINGENIUS (Marcellus). Zodiacus vitæ [etc.] 16°. *Basileæ,* 1557.

———. The same. 46 l. 16°. *Lipsiæ, in off. hæredum V. Papæ,* 1558.

———. The same. 42 l. 16°. *Witebergæ, C. Schleich et A. Schöne,* 1573.

For Portrait, see **Collection**—van Kaathoven.

Niger (*Sextius*).

Portrait in : **Collection**—van Kaathoven. — **Collection** of Portr. (Libr.)

Niggemann (Wilh.) * Das Kniephänomen und seine quantitative Bestimmung. 38 pp. 8°. *Würzburg, P. Scheiner,* 1886.

Niggl (Ignaz). * Ueber Otorrhœa oder Ohrenfluss. 16 pp. 8°. *München,* 1848.

Night.

See, also, **Insane** (*Influence of night, etc., on*).

BALLY (J.-C.) * Recherches sur l'influence de la nuit dans les maladies. 4°. *Paris,* 1807.

BAYER (M. J.) Die Nacht in ihrer Beziehung zum Organismus. 8°. *Würzburg,* 1824.

BOEDEKER (C. G.) * De noctis vi in hominem. 8°. *Jenæ,* [1840].

FLEMMING (C.) * De noctis circa morbos efficacia. 8°. *Berolini,* [1821].

FRANCKE (H. L.) * De noctis efficacia in mutando morborum decusu commentatio. 4°. *Lipsiæ,* [1811].

GRASS (S.) * De morbis nocturnis et nocturna morborum exacerbatione. 4°. *Jenæ,* [1709].

GUILLAUMOD (C.-J.-E.) * Sur l'influence de nuit dans l'état de santé et de maladie. 4°. *Paris,* 1812.

HEYM (G. C.) * De nocturna plurimorum morborum exacerbatione. 4°. *Helmstadii,* [1763].

INFLUENCE (De l') de la nuit sur les maladies. Recueil des mémoires couronnés par la Société de médecine de Bruxelles. [Par Jacques-Julien-Richard de Laprade, Aymone, J.-A. Murat, et d'Hemptines.] 8°. *Bruxelles,* 1806.

Forms v. 1 of Actes Soc. de méd. de Brux.

MORICHEAU-BEAUCHAMP. De la nuit, et son influence sur les malades. 8°. *Paris,* 1808.

PORET (A.) * Étude sur les aliénés au point de vue de la nuit. 4°. *Paris,* 1865.

REYDELLET (J.-É.) * Essai sur la nuit. 4°. *Paris,* 1819.

SCHUSTER (P.) * De vesperæ et noctis efficacia, in mutando morborum decursu. 8°. *Vindobonæ,* [1830].

TAILLEFER (A.) * De l'influence de la nuit sur l'homme dans l'état de santé et dans l'état de maladie. 4°. *Paris,* 1820.

DE WITT HAMER (H. M.) * De nocte, ejusque vi et efficacitate in affectionibus pathologicis corporis humani vel producendis vel augendis. 8°. *Lugd. Bat.,* 1835.

Balestrieri (P.) Memoria sull' influenza dei periodi celesti sulla natura e sul corso delle malattie dell' uomo, secondo le stagioni e i climi, e soprattutto dell' influenza del periodo della notte e del giorno. Filiatre-sebezio, Napoli, 1843, xxvi, 77 ; 143 ; 204 ; 274.

Night *medical service.*

NEW YORK (*State*). Assembly. An act to amend an act entitled "An act to organize a

Night *medical service.*

night medical service in the city of New York, to provide medical assistance in case of sudden sickness or accident during the night time", passed June 26, 1880. No. 360. March 24, 1882. Introd. by Mr. Crane. fol. [*Albany,* 1882.]

REZZONICO (A.) Guardia medico-chirurgica notturna nel comune di Milano eretta in corpo morale con decreto reale del 1° settembre 1884. Relazione sull' andamento morale ed economico dell' anno 1884. Lettura fatta dal dottor . . . nell' assemblea generale dei soci benefattori del 29 marzo 1884 ed atti relativi. 8°. *Milano,* 1885.

Chapplain (J.) Service médical de nuit. Marseille méd., 1876, xiii, 577–584.—**Commenge.** Rapport sur le service médical des bureaux de bienfaisance et le service médical de nuit à Paris. Gaz. méd.-chir. de Toulouse, 1885, xvii, 281 : 1886, xviii, 3 ; 10.—**Du Mesnil** (O) Les refuges de nuit municipaux à Paris. Ann. d'hyg., Par., 1887, 3. s., xvii, 151–164. — **Layet** (A.) Nuit (hygiène et service médical de nuit). Dict. encycl. d. sc. méd., Par., 1879, 2. s., xiii, 749–771.—**Medical** (The) night service of St. Petersburgh. Lond. M. Rec., 1875, iii, 299.—**Minonzio** (C.) Sull' instituzione di una guardia medico-chirurgica notturna in Milano. Atti Accad. fis.-med.-statist. di Milano, 1875, xxxi, 26–34.—**Nachtel** (H.) A brief statement of the plan of night medical service in actual operation in Paris and other European cities, with a view to its introduction in New York. Med. Rec., N. Y., 1880, xvii, 229–231.—**Night** medical service. [Edit.] Med. Gaz., N. Y., 1880, vii, 498. — **Passant.** Service médical de nuit dans la ville de Paris ; statistique du 1er octobre au 31 décembre 1886. Gaz. d. hôp., Par., 1887, lx, 85.—**Verdalle.** Est-il utile d'établir à Bordeaux un service médical de nuit ? [With discussion.] Mém. et bull. Soc. de méd. et chir. de Bordeaux, 1876, 120-128.

Night (A) in a workhouse. 47 pp. 12°. *London, Pall Mall Gazette,* [1866]. [P., v. 497.]

Repr. from : Pall Mall Gaz., Lond., [1866].

Night-blindness.

See **Hemeralopia**, *etc.*

Night-cough.

See **Bronchitis** (*Chronic*); **Cough** (*Anomalous, etc.*)

Night-crying.

See **Crying**.

Nightingale (Florence) [1823–]. Notes on nursing; what it is and what it is not. 114 pp. 8°. *New York, D. Appleton & Co.,* 1860.

———. The same. Notes on nursing for the labouring classes. New ed. 114 pp. 18°. *London, Harrison,* 1876.

———. The same. Die Pflege bei Kranken und Gesunden. Kurze Winke, den Frauen aller Stände gewidmet. Von der Verfasserin autorisirte deutsche Ausgabe, nach der zweiten Auflage ihrer " Notes on nursing" bearbeitet. Mit einem Vorwort des Geh. Sanitäts-Rath Dr. H. Wolff in Bonn. xvi, 223 pp. 12°. *Leipzig, F. A. Brockhaus,* 1861.

———. Army sanitary administration and its reform under the late Lord Herbert. 11 pp., 1 pl. 8°. *London, McCorquodale & Co.,* [1862].

———. Notes on hospitals. 3. ed. ix (1 l.), 187 pp., 11 pl., 3 tab., 1 map. 4°. *London, Longman [and others],* 1863.

———. How people may live and not die in India. (A paper read at the meeting of the National Association for the Promotion of Social Science, Edinburgh, 1863.) 18 pp. 8°. *London, Longman [and others],* 1864.

———. Introductory notes on lying-in institutions ; together with a proposal for organizing an institution for training midwives and midwifery nurses. xiv, 110 pp., 5 pl. 8°. *London, Longmans [and others],* 1871.

———. Life or death in India, with an appendix on life or death by irrigation, 1874. 63 pp. 8°. *London, Spottiswoode & Co.,* 1874.

See, also, **Shrimpton** (Charles). The Crimean war [etc.] 8°. *Paris,* 1864.

For Portrait, see **Collection**—van Kaathoven.

Nightingale (Florence)—continued.

——. *See, also:*

SAINT THOMAS'S Hospital, London. The Nightingale Fund. Annual reports of the trustees of the Nightingale Fund, for training nurses, for the years 1871; 1872; 1886. fol. *London*, 1872–87.

——. Regulations as to the training of hospital nurses under the Nightingale Fund. fol. [*London, n. d.*]

——. Duties of probationer under the "Nightingale Fund". 4°. [*London, n. d.*] WOMAN'S (A) example and a nation's work. A tribute to Florence Nightingale. 12°. *London*, 1864.

Jebb (J.) Statement of the appropriation of the Nightingale fund. Tr. Nat. Ass. Promot. Social Sc. 1862, Lond., 1863, 641–647. [Discussion], 682–684.

Nightingale (John) [1855 –]. * Ueber Stimmbandlähmungen. 33 pp., 1 l. 8°. *Berlin, G. Schade*, [1877].

Nightingale Fund. *See* **Saint Thomas** Hospital, Westminster Bridge, London.

Nightmare.
See Sleep (*Abnormal, etc.*)

Nightmen.
C. (A. B.) Statement of the age, number of years employed on emptying ashpits, attacks from fever, cholera, and deaths therefrom, of 118 nightmen employed at Liverpool, July. 1850. Lancet, Lond., 1850, ii, 281.—**Guy** (W. A.) On the health of nightmen, scavengers, and dustmen. J. Statist. Soc. Lond., 1848, xi, 72–81. *Also, Reprint.—* **Mérat.** Vidangeurs. Dict. d. sc. méd., Par., 1821, lvii, 426–432.—**Reclam** (C.) Gutachten über etwaige Schädlichkeit der Tonnenräume für Nachbarhäuser. Gesundheit, Elberfeld, 1878, iii, 369–371.

Night-sweats.
BLASIUS (W.) * Ueber die Wirkung des Hyoscinum hydrojodicum gegen die Nachtschweisse der Phthisiker. 8°. *Bonn*, 1886.

BOURDEAU D'ANTONY (P.) * Des sueurs chez les phthisiques et de leur traitement par l'acide salicylique. 4°. *Paris*, [1882].

DONY (P.) * Des sueurs nocturnes chez les phthisiques et de leur traitement par le phosphate de chaux. 4°. *Paris*, 1875.

FREITAG (O.) * Ueber Nachtschweisse. 8°. *Berlin*, [1874].

HABEL (R.) * Atropin und Duboisin gegen Nachtschweisse der Phthisiker. 8°. *München*, 1881.

MIGNOT (M.) * Des sueurs chez les phthisiques et de leur traitement par l'ergot de seigle. 4°. *Paris*, 1886.

MILLER (V.) * Iz nabloudenii nad chachotochnimi. (Vlijanie agaricina na poti chachot.) [Agaricine in the night-sweat of phthisis.] 8°. *St. Petersburg*, 1885.

REBORY (A.) * De l'emploi du phosphate de chaux contre les sueurs des phthisiques. 4°. *Paris*, 1886.

TREW (C. J.) * De sudoribus nocturnis. 4°. *Altdorfii*, [1714].

Abbot (S. L.) Oxide of zinc in night sweats. Boston M. & S. J., 1857, lvi, 249–255. — **Brunton** (T. L.) On the pathology of night-sweating in phthisis, and the mode of action of strychnia and other remedies in it. St. Barth. Hosp. Rep., Lond., 1879, xv, 119–128 — **Busey** (S. C.) Night sweats in phthisis; with discussion. Tr M. Soc. Dist. Columb. 1877, Wash., 1878, v, 49–53.—**Carpenter** (C. D.) Chloral hydrate for night-sweats. Med. Brief, St. Louis, 1879, vii, 41.—**Cauldwell** (C. M.) The treatment of phthisical night-sweats. N. York M. J., 1884, xl, 341–343.—**Coxe** (E. J.) On the treatment of the night sweats of consumption. Boston M. & S. J., 1857, lvi, 198–200.—**Curci** (A.) Medicazione antisudorifera. Raccoglitore med., Forlì, 1877, 4. s., vii, 115–127.—**Da Costa** (J. M.) The night-sweats of phthisis. *In:* Notes Hosp. Pract. (Miller), 8°, Phila., 1879, pt. 1, 29. ——. The treatment of the night-sweating of phthisis. Med. News & Abstr., Phila., 1881, xxxix, 451–459.—**Delioux.** De l'emploi du tannate de quinine contre les sueurs nocturnes. Union méd., Par., 1853, vii, 170.—**Duckworth** (D.) On

Night-sweats.
the value of oxide of zinc in the night-sweats of phthisis. St. Barth. Hosp. Rep., Lond., 1875, xi, 60.—**Dulácska** (G.) Tüdővészesek izzadása s a pilocarpin. [Pilocarpin in night-sweats of phthisis.] Gyógyászat, Budapest, 1881, xxi, 449–452. *Also, transl.* [Abstr.]: Pest. med.-chir. Presse, Budapest, 1881, xvii, 917–919.—**Engel** (H.) Jaborandi in night sweats. Med. & Surg. Reporter, Phila., 1879, xl, 434.—**Fox** (C. J.) The value of sulphate of atropia in the sweats of phthisis pulmonalis, hypodermically administered. N. Eng. M. Month., Newtown, Conn., 1881–2, i, 295.—**Fraentzel.** Ueber den Gebrauch des Duboisin gegen die Nachtschweisse der Phthisiker. Charité Ann. 1879. Berl., 1881, vi, 265–270. ——. Ueber die Wirkung des Hyoscins gegen die Nachtschweisse der Phthisiker. *Ibid.*, 1881, Berl., 1883, viii, 301–308.—**Gallico** (E.) Dei sudori nei tisici; considerazioni cliniche. Gazz. med. ital., prov. venete, Padova, 1880, xxiii, 57–59.—**Hanson** (M. P.) Night sweats in phthisis. Chicago M. Rev., 1882, v, 43.—**Henry** (F. P.) Picrotoxine in night sweating. Med. & Surg. Reporter, Phila., 1882, xlvi, 54.—**Howe** (J. E.) Notes on the treatment of night sweats in phthisis. Lancet, Lond., 1884, ii, 408.—**Köhnhorn.** Gegen Nachtschweisse bei Lungenphthisis. Berl. klin. Wchnschr., 1880, xvii, 10.—**Lauschmann** (G.) Agaricin és a tüdővészesek izzadása. [Agaricin and the sweat of phthisis.] Gyógyászat, Budapest, 1887, xxvii, 337–340. *Also, transl.* [Abstr.]: Pest. med.-chir. Presse, Budapest, 1887, xxiii, 694.—**Murrell** (W.) On the treatment of the night-sweating of phthisis. Practitioner, Lond., 1879, xxiii, 91; 192; 241; 430: 1880, xxv, 88; 252: 1882, xxix, 321: 1883, xxxi, 401.—**Night** sweats of phthisis. Med. Rec., N. Y., 1873, viii, 279.—**Night** sweats of phthisis treated by atropia. *Ibid.*, 132.—**Peter** (A.) Agaric in the sweating of phthisis. Med. News, Phila., 1887, l, 54.—**Pribram** (A.) Zur Behandlung der Nachtschweisse. Aerztl. Cor.-Bl. f. Böhmen, Prag, 1873, i, 21–25.—**Rousselot.** Quelques particularités sur les sueurs des phthisiques ; époque variable de leur apparition ; doit-on toujours les considérer comme un fâcheux symptôme et chercher à les combattre ? Rev. méd. de l'est, Nancy. 1879, xi, 43–51.—**Schneider.** Salbeiöl, ein wirksames Mittel gegen Nachtschweisse. N. Jahrb. d. teutsch. Med. u. Chir., Hamm, 1826, xi, 1. St., 76–82.—**Seifert** (O.) Ueber die Wirkung des Agaricin gegen die Nachtschweisse der Phthisiker. Wien. med. Wchnschr., 1883, xxxiii, 1137–1141.—**Smith** (Q. C.) The treatment of night-sweats. Gaillard's M. J., N. Y., 1885, xl, 448.—**Stadler.** Beitrag zur Therapie der Nachtschweisse Lungensüchtiger. Med.-chir. Centralbl., Wien, 1880, xv, 38; 50; 62; 181.—**Stewart** (J.) The treatment of the night sweats of phthisis by Coto. Canada Lancet, Toronto, 1880–81, xiii, 323.—**Westbrook** (B. F.) **& Platt** (I. H.) The treatment of the night-sweats of phthisis. N. York M. J., 1884, xxxix, 714.—**Wilson** (J. C.) Atropia in the night-sweats of phthisis. [5 cases.] Phila. M. Times, 1872–3, iii, 34.—**Wolfenden** (R. N.) On agaricus in the treatment of night-sweating. Med. Times & Gaz., Lond., 1881, ii, 442 —**Young** (J. M.) On agaricus in the treatment of night sweating in phthisis. Glasgow M. J., 1882, [4. s.], xvii, 176–179.

Night-terrors.
See, also, Crying.
Atkinson (W. B.) Night terrors in children. Arch. Pediat., Phila., 1884, i, 753–756.—**Jocobi** (A.) Case of terrores nocturni ex febri intermittente ; spasmus vesicæ urinariæ. Am. M. Month. & N. Y. Rev., 1861, xvi, 11.—**Moizard.** Des terreurs nocturnes chez les enfants. Rev. mens. d. mal. de l'enf., Par., 1884, ii, 305–313.—**Wertheimber** (A.) Ueber den Pavor nocturnus der Kinder (nächtliches Aufschrecken; Night terrors). Deutsches Arch. f. klin. Med., Leipz., 1879, xxiii, 564–568. *Also:* Wien. med. Bl., 1879, ii, 529; 551; 575.

Nigrismus.
See Melænia.

Nigrisoli (Francesco Maria) [1648–1727]. Febris china chinæ expugnata, seu illustrium aliquot virorum opuscula, quæ verum tradunt methodum, febres china chinæ curandi. xvi, 204 pp., 2 pl. 4°. *Ferrariæ, typ. B. Pomatelli*, 1687.

——. The same. Ed. altera. 10 p. l., 329 pp., 2 pl., port. 4°. *Ferrariæ, apud Lilium*, 1700.

——. Considerazioni intorno alla generazione de' viventi e particolarmente de' mostri fatte dal . . . e da lui scritte al . . . Dionisio Andrea Sancassani. 6 p. l., 382 pp. 4°. *Ferrara, B. Barbieri*, 1712.

Nigrisoli (Hieronymus) [1621–89]. Progymnasmata in quibus novum præsidium medicum appositio, videlicet hirudinum internæ parti uteri in puerperii, et mensium suppressione expo-

Nigrisoli (Hieronymus)—continued.
nitur, rationibus, auctoritatibus, et experimentis confirmatur, de vena in febribus malignis secanda disseritur, et alia medicis non solum, sed omnibus bonarum litterarum cultoribus utilia simul atque jucunda expenduntur. 197 pp. 4°. *Salisburgi, J. B. Mayer*, 1689.

Nigrities.

See **Skin** (*Discoloration, etc., of*).

Niguas.

Gregg (C. K.) "Niguas", a parasite common to northern Mexico. Daniel's Texas M. J., Austin, 1886-7, ii, 230.

Nihell (*Mrs.* Elizabeth). A treatise on the art of midwifery, setting forth various abuses therein, especially as to the practice with instruments; the whole serving to put all rational inquirers in a fair way of very safely forming their own judgment upon the question, which it is best to employ, in cases of pregnancy and lying-in, a man-midwife or a midwife. xvi, vi, 471 pp. 8°. *London, A. Morley*, 1760.

——. The same. La cause de l'humanité, référée au tribunal du bon sens et de la raison; ou traité sur les accouchements par les femmes. Ouvrage très utile aux sages-femme, et très-intéressant pour les familles. Trad. de l'anglois. xxvi, 494 pp. 8°. *Paris, A. Boudet*, 1771.
For Biography for, see **Delacoux** (A.) Biog. d. sages-femmes. 4°. *Paris,* 1834, 126-129, port.

Nihell (James). New and extraordinary observations concerning the prediction of various crises by the pulse, independent of the critical signs delivered by the ancients; made by the long experience of several eminent physicians, and illustrated with many new cases and remarks. To which are added some general hints on the nature, the ancient observance, and modern neglect of crises. The second ed. xxviii (6 l.), 153 pp., 7 l. 8°. *London, J. Whiston*, 1750.

——. The same. Novæ raræque observationes circa variarum crisium prædictionem ex pulsu, nullo habito respectu ad signa critica antiquorum: primum a Francisco Solano de Luque, Antequeræ in Hispania novissime practico, et a variis deinde aliis medicis, factæ; multis novis casibus et animadversionibus illustratæ. Addita sunt monita quædam generalia de natura crisium, earumque apud antiquos consideratione, et apud modernos neglectu. Ex anglico latine reddidit Wilhelmus Noortwyk. 23 p. l., 127 pp. 8°. *Venetiis, T. Bettinelli*, 1748.

——. The same. Et dissertationem de natura humana adjunxit Wilhelmus Noortwyk . . . Accedit in hac editione G. C. Schelhammeri . . . disquisitio epistolica de pulsu. xxii (1 l.), 255 pp. 8°. *Venetiis, T. Bettinelli*, 1759.

Nihell (L.) Vaccine-Pock Institution. The report of . . . 8°. *London*, 1803.

Nihell (Laurentius). *De cerebro. 1 p. l., 45 pp. 8°. *Edinburgi, Balfour et Smellie*, 1780.
Also, in: SMELLIE. Thesaurus med. [etc.] 8°. *Edinburgi*, 1785, iv, 199-226.

Niigata.

Leysner (A.) Das Klima von Niigata nach zehnjährigen Beobachtungen. Mitth. d. deutsch. Gesellsch. f. Nat.- u. Völkerk. Ostasiens, Yokohama, 1880-84, iii, 27. Hft., 319-322.

à Nijeholt (Tjepco, Lijcklama). *See* **Lijcklama à Nijeholt** (Tjepco).

Nijhoff (Gerardus Cornelis). *Schets van het leven en de physiologie van Herman Boerhaave. [Leyden] viii, 106 pp. 8°. *Amsterdam, D. Noothoven van Goor*, 1881.

Nijkamp (Adriaan). Onderzoekingen omtrent de histologie van het kraakbeenweefsel. 4 p. l., 46 pp., 1 pl. 8°. *Leiden, gebr. van der Hoek*, 1877.

Nikander. Θηριακά. Ἀλεξιφάρμακ. Ἑρμηνεία τοῦ ἀνωνύμου συγγραφέως εἰς θηριακά. Σχόλια διαφόρων συγγαφέων εἰς ἀλεξιφάρμακα. 1 p. l., 103 pp. sm. 4°. *Coloniæ, opera J. Soteris*, 1530.

——. Θηριακά. [*Also :*] Ἀλεξιφάρμακα. Interprete Jo. Gorræo. 3 l., 223 pp. 4°. *Parisiis, apud G. Morelium*, 1557.
Greek and Latin text.

——. The same. Les œuvres de . . . traduictes en vers françois. Ensemble, deux livres des venins, ausquels il est amplement discouru des bestes venimeuses, thériaques, poisons et contrepoisons, par Jaques Grevin de Clermont en Beauvaisis. 90 pp., 1 l. 4°. *Anvers, C. Plantin*, 1567.
Bound with: GREVIN (J.) Deux livres des venins, [etc.] 4°. *Anvers*, 1568.

——. The same. Joannes Gorrhæus Latinis versibus reddidit, Italicis vero qui nunc primum in lucem prodeunt Ant. Mar. Salvinius. Accedunt variantes codicum lectiones, selectæ adnotationes, et Græca Eutecni sophistæ metaphrasis ex codicibus mediceæ, et Vindobon. bibliothecæ descripta ac nondum edita curante Ang. Mar. Bandinio. 4 p. l., 376 pp. 8°. *Florentiæ, ex off. Moückiana*, 1764.
Greek, Latin, and Italian text.

——. Alexipharmaca. Jo. Gorræo . . . interprete. Ejusdem interpretis in Alexipharmaca præfatio, omnem de venenis disputationem summatim complectens, et annotationes. 70 ff., 1 l. 12°. *Parisiis, apud Vascosanum*, 1549.
Greek and Latin text.

——. The same. Alexipharmaca seu de venenis in potu cibove homini datis eorumque remediis carmen. Cum scholiis græcis et Eutecnii sophistæ paraphrasi græca. Ex libris scriptis emendavit animadversionibusque et paraphrasi latina illustravit Jo. Gottlob Schneider. xx, 346 pp. 8°. *Halæ, imp. orphanotrophei*, 1792.

——. Σχόλια ἀνωνύμου τινος συγγραφέως. Σχόλια διαφόρων συγγραφέων εἰς ἀλεξιφάρμακα. 80 pp. 4°. *Parisiis, apud G. Morelium*, 1557.
Greek and Latin text.
Bound with his: Θηριακά. 4°. *Parisiis*, 1557.
See, also, **Gorræus** (Joannes). Opera. Definitionum medicarum libri xxiii, [etc.] fol. *Parisiis.* 1622.
For Portrait, see **Collection**—van Kaathoven.

Nikanoroff (N.) *Material dlja farmakologii solei litija. [Pharmacology of salt of lithium.] 101 pp., 1 l., 1 diag. 8°. *St. Petersburg, tipog. A. H. Kotomina*, 1882.

Nikiforoff (I. A.) *Ob otnoshenii kalibra arterii k vesu i objemu organov i k vesu tchastei tela. [Relation of calibre of arteries to weight and volume of organs and the weight of parts of body.] 64 pp., 2 tab., 1 l. 8°. *St. Petersburg, tipog. N. A. Lebedeva*, 1883.

Nikiforoff (M.) Kratkii uchebnik mikroskop. techniki. Posobie pri prakt. izuchen. patolog. gistologii. S predislov. I. F. Kleina. 87 pp. 8°. *Moskva*, 1885.

——. The same. 2. ed. 3 l., 162, 7 pp. 16°. *Moskva, typog. A. A. Kartseva*, 1888.

Nikiphroakis (Michel). *Études sur l'étiologie et la pathogénie de la tumeur et de la fistule lacrymales; traitement par la cautérisation avec le beurre d'antimoine. 43 pp. 4°. *Paris*, 1873, No. 494.

Nikitin (V. N.) *O fiziologicheskom deistvii i terap. znachenii sklerotinovoi kisloty i sklerotinovokiskago natra. [Physiological effect and therapeutical value of ergotic acid and natrium ergot.] 62 pp., 1 tab., 1 l. 8°. *St. Petersburg, tipog. J. Treja*, 1879.

——. Boliezni nosovoi polosti. [Diseases of the cavity of the nose.] 50 pp. 8°. *St. Petersburg*, 1882.
In: Med. Biblioteka.

Nikitin (V. N.)—continued.
——. Rukovodstvo k izucheniou laringoskopii i boleznei gortani. [Manual of laryngoscopy and diseases of the larynx.] 280, ii pp. 8°. *St. Petersburg, Med. Bibl.*, 1854.
——. Boliezni nosovoi polosti. [Diseases of nasal cavity.] 131 pp. 8°. *St. Petersburg, Ejem. jour. prakt. med.*, 1888.

Nikitnikoff. *K vopr. o jonijen. temperaturi tiela u tifoznich chrez ochlajdenie shei. [Lowering of temperature in the body in typhoid fever by cooling the neck.] 38 pp., 1 l., 12 tab. 8°. *St. Petersburg*, 1885.

Niklas (Wenceslaus). *Diss. sistens cystocatarrhum, adnexis historiis morbi synopticis. 25 pp. 8°. *Pragæ, typ. filiorum T. Haase*, [1844].

Niklewicz (Ignatius). *De uteri prolapsu. 19 pp. 4°. *Jenæ, typ. Sclottrianis*, [1828].
For Biography, see **Stark** (Joann. Christ.)

Niklewski (Josephus). *De ophthalmoblennorrhoeis. 36 pp. 8°. *Gryphiæ, F. G. Kunike*, [1860]. c.

Nikolaeff (Gregory). *K voprosu o zaroshenii arterii poslie perevjazki. [Changes in thrombus in arteries after ligation.] 16 pp., 1 pl. 8°. *St. Petersburg*, 1871.

Nikolaeff (Maximus). *K gistologii rogovoi obolotchki chelovechkago glaza. [Histology of cornea of human eye.] 46 pp., 1 l. 8°. *St. Petersburg, tipog. J. Treja*, 1868.

Nikolaeff (Philip). *K istorii razvitija zubove. [On development of the teeth.] 31 pp. 8°. *St. Petersburg*, 1871.

Nikolai (R.) Sbornik prakt. medisini za 1885 g. Sostavlen. po russ. med. journal. [Collection of practical medicine for the year 1885. Extracted from Russian medical journals.] 94 pp. 12°. *Kazan*, 1886.

Nikolaïdes (R.) Ἀπάντησις Δημητρίου Χασιώτου εἰς τὴν ἐν τῷ "Γαληνῷ" ἐπικρισιν P. Νικολαΐδου δίκην παράρτηματος τῷ ἀριθ. 6τοῦ "Γαληνὸν" (1884) ἐπισύνημμενη. 40 pp. 8°. Ἀθῆναι, 1884.

Nikolaieff.
See **Hospitals** (*Naval, etc.*), **Medicine** (*Clinical, Statistical reports of*), *by localities.*

Nikolić (Nikola H.) [1854-]. *Ueber Wundbehandlung mit Jodoform mit besonderer Berücksichtigung der Jodoformtamponade von Wundhölen. 30 pp. 8°. *Berlin, O. Francke*, [1882].

Nikolski (Demetrius). *Regulirovanie tepla u tifoznich bolnich pod vlijaniem cholodnich vanne (ve 20°–30° Cl.). [On regulating the temperature in typhus by means of cold baths of 20–30° C.] 42 pp. 8°. *St. Petersburg*, 1870.

Nikolski (Michael). *Materijali dlja rieshenija voprosa o vlijanii kokaina na jivotnii organizm. [Effect of cocain on the animal organism.] 25 pp. 8°. *St. Petersburg*, 1872.

Nikolski (Peter). *Gistolog. izsliedovanie kostnoi mozoli po otnosheniou ke razlichnime vozrastame. [Histological researches into the development of osseous tissue.] 18 pp., 1 pl. 8°. *St. Petersburg*, 1870.

Nikolski (V. I.) *Tambovskii nezde. Statistika naselenija i boleznennosti. [District of Tambov. Statistics of population and diseases.] viii, 383 pp., 6 tab., 47 pp., 21 diag. 8°. *Tambov*, 1885.

Nilant (Antonius). *De angina, speciatim mucosa. 32 pp., 1 l. 4°. *Harderovici, J. Moojen*, [1787].

Nilant (Lambertus). *De libertinis. 18 pp., 5 l. 4°. *Lugd. Bat., S. Luchtmans*, 1748. [P., v. 993.]

Nile (*River*).
See **Egypt**; **Fever** (*Malarial, History, etc., of*), *by localities—Egypt.*

60

Niles (D. Waterhouse). Ethical therapeutics, or the treatment of disease by moral management, vs. drugs and medicines. 32 pp., 1 l. 8°. *Sandy Hook, Conn., N. Eng. M. Month.*, 1883
Repr. from: N. Eng. M. Month., Newtown, Conn., 1882-3, ii.

Niles (John B.) Address delivered before the officers and students of the Iudiana Medical College (Laporte), at the close of the session of 1845-6. 13 pp. 8°. *Indianapolis*, 1846.

Niles (Nathaniel) & **Russ** (John D.) Medical statistics; or, a comparative view of the mortality in New York, Philadelphia, Baltimore, and Boston, for a series of years; including comparisons of the mortality of whites and blacks in the two former cities; and of whites, free blacks, and slaves, in Baltimore. 11 pp. 8°. *New York, E. Bliss*, 1827. [*Also, in:* P., v. 118; 827.]

[**Niles** (Samuel V.)] In memoriam. Francis Asbury Ashford. 15 pp. 8°. *Washington, D. C., Gibson Brothers*, 1883.

Nilo (Charles). *De la bronchotomie et de ses applications. 43 pp. 4°. *Paris*, 1851, No. 104, v. 512.

Nilo (J[osé] R[omão] Rodrigues). *Sur la nécessité d'un bon diagnostic; suivie de l'exposition de quelques causes générales d'erreur dans cette partie de la pathologie, et de quelques réflexions sur les difficultés qu'elle présente. 20 pp. 4°. *Paris*, 1821, No. 120, v. 166.

——. Noticia sobre a colera-morbo, epidemia acualmente reinante em Lisboa, meios preservativos, e curativos d'ella; offerecida aos seus concidadãos. 22 pp., 1 l. 8°. *Lisboa*, 1833. [P., v. 1262.]

Nilsson (Clas).
See **Glas** (Olof). Om cholera-morbus. 8°. *Upsala*, 1849.

Nilsson (Emil). Våra kläder [On clothing]. 101 pp. 8°. *Stockholm, Samson & Wallin*, 1886. No. 6 of: Bibliotek f. Hälsovard (Heyman).

Nilsson (*Sven*) [1787–1883].
de Mortillet (G.) Nécrologie. L'homme, Par., 1884, i, 50–52, port.

Nim (*Azadirachta Indica*).
Ganguli (M. N.) Nim as a medicinal agent in surgery. Indian M. Gaz., Calcutta, 1881, xvi, 333.

Nimier (Gustave). *De la cure radicale de l'hydrocèle par l'incision et la résection partielle de la tunique vaginale. 48 pp. 4°. *Paris*, 1886, No. 195

Nimier (Henri). *Des fractures de l'extrémité supérieure de l'humérus; étude anatomo-pathologique sur leurs diverses variétés et leurs complications vasculo-nerveuses. 37 pp., 1 l. 4°. *Paris*, 1879, No. 416.

Nimio (De) sanitatis studio sæpe sanitatem vel optimam frangente. xx pp. 4°. [*Lipsiæ*, 1790.]
——. The same. Continuatio I. In memoriam Bestuchefianam. xii pp. 4°. [*Lipsiæ*, 1790.]
——. The same. Continuatio II. In memoriam Rud. Ferd. de Sylverstein et Pilnickau. xv pp. 4°. [*Lipsiæ*, 1790.]

Nimmo (Joannes). *De quibusdam fœtui propriis. 46 pp. 8°. *Edinburgi, A. Neill et socii*, 1804. [P., v. 29.]

Nimmo (Robertus). *De pneumonia. 1 p. l., 19 pp. 8°. *Edinburgi, P. Neill*, 1821. [*Also, in:* P., v. 1072.]

Nimmo (William). *Illustrations of the theory of mental derangement. 54 pp. 8°. *Glasgow, Muir, Govans & Co.*, 1831.

Nimptsch (Ulricus Sigismundus)[1]. *Exercitatio anatomico-physiologica, de fontanella infantum. 16 pp. sm. 4°. [*Altdorf*], lit. Kohlesianis, [1695].
——. *De ἀγρυπνία sive vigilia præternaturali. 24 pp. 4°. [*Altdorf*], lit. H. Meyeri, [1697].

Nimptsch (Ulricus Sigismundus) [2]. * De differenti medicamentorum operatione secundum diversam corporis humani idiosyncrasiam. Von der verschiedenen Würckung derer Artzeneyen nach der verschiedenen Beschaffenheit des menschlichen Cörpers. 33 pp., 1 l. 4°. *Halæ Magdeb., typ. J. C. Hilligeri*, [1731].

Nimsch (Joh.) * Ein Fall von Cancroid der äusseren Genitalien des Weibes. 25 pp., 1 l. 8°. *Greifswald, C. Sell*, 1884.

Nin y Pullés (José). Estadística demográfica médica de Barcelona. iv., 1881; vii., 1884. broadside sheets. *Barcelona*, 1882–85.
Suppl. to: Encicl. méd.-farm., Barcel.

Nina (Almir). * Do Páo Pereira, da Pereirina e seus sáes suas indicações e contra-indicações nas manifestações agudas da malaria. 77 pp., 1 l. 8°. *Rio de Janeiro, G. Leuzinger & filhos*, 1883.

Ninaber (Joh. Didericus). * De rachitide. 3 p. l., 62 pp. 8°. *Lugd. Bat., C. C. van der Hoek*, 1840.

Ninci (Francesco). Lettera del . . . all' . . . Antonio Targioni-Tozzetti, descrivente la malattia detta tifo petecchiale e cura della medicina. 12 pp. 12°. *Firenze, L. Ciardetti & Comp.*, 1817.

Nindel (Joan. Fridr. Leopold.) * De erysipelate infantili. 40 pp. 8°. *Dorpati Livonorum, typ. J. C. Schünmanni*, 1829.

Nines (P.-A.-V.) * Quelques considérations sur l'hydropisie en général. 46 pp., 31. 4°. *Montpellier*, 1874, No. 21.

Ningpo.

See, also, **Hospitals** (*Descriptions, etc., of*), by localities.
Henderson (W. A.) On fever in Ningpo and Chefoo. Edinb. M. J., 1880–81, xxvi, 797–803. — **Reports** on the health of Ningpo, 1870–86. Customs Gaz. Med. Rep., Shanghai, 1870–71, no. 1, 141: 1872–3, no. 5, 25: 1873–5, no. 7, 24: 1875–6, no. 11, 27: 1876–7, no. 13, 46. *Continued in:* China. Imp. Customs. Med. Rep., Shanghai, 1877–8, no. 14, 65: no. 15, 21: 1878–9, no. 17, 6: 1880–81, no. 20, 27: 1881–2, no. 22, 13: 1882–3, no. 24, 17: 1883–4, no. 26, 73: 1884–5, no. 29, 6: 1886, no. 32, 68.

Ninnin (Henri) [1722–   ].
See **Celsus** (Aurelius Cornelius). Traité de médecine [etc.] 8°. *Paris*, 1855.

Ninninger (Armin. Alexander). * De removenda placenta. 15 pp. 8°. *Jenæ, typ. Schreiberi et fil.*, 1856. c.

Niobey (P.-Alphonse). * Sur diverses propositions de médecine et de chirurgie. 32 pp. 4°. *Paris*, 1848, No. 147, v. 475.

———. Histoire médicale du choléra-morbus épidémique qui a régné en 1854 dans la ville de Gy (Haute-Saône), suivie de tableaux statistiques [etc.] 197 pp., 1 map. 8°. *Paris, J.-B. Baillière & fils*, 1858.

Niort.

Guillemeau (J.-L.-M.) Coup-d'œil historique, topographique et médical sur la ville de Niort et ses environs. 32°. *Niort*, 1795.
Bodeau. Constitution médicale du 1er trimestre de 1840. Rec. d. trav. Soc. de méd. de Niort, 1843, pt. 2, 65–70.—**Moullié.** Essai de topographie de la ville de Niort et de ses environs. Rec. de mém. de méd. . . . mil., Par., 1860, 3. s., iii, 15; 96.

Niox (H.-N.) * Propositions médicales. 11 pp. 4°. *Paris*, 1822, No. 124, v. 173.

Nipher (Francis E.) On the variation in the strength of a muscle. 6 pp., 1 pl. 8°. *St. Louis, Mo.*, 1875.
Repr. from: Am. J. Sc. & Arts, N. Haven, 1875, x.

Niphus (Augustinus) [1473 (?)–1545 (?)]. De diebus criticis seu decretoriis aureus liber ad Vicentium Quirinum patritium Venetum nuper editus et maxima cum diligentia impressus. xv ff., 1 l. fol. [*Venetiis*], *A. Calcedonius*, [1504].

———. De auguriis libri ii, nec non de diebus criticis liber i. His accesserunt Uraniæ divina-

Niphus (Augustinus)—continued.
tricis, quoad astrologiæ generalia, lib. ii. jam primo in lucem evolantes, alas suppeditante Rodolpho Goclenio. 4 p. l., 143–150 pp. 4°. *Marpurgi, typ. P. Egenolphi*, 1614. [P., v. 631.]

Nipple *shields*.
See **Nipples** (*Artificial*), etc.

Nipples.

Duval (F.-J.) * Du mamelon et de son auréole, anatomie et pathologie. 4°. *Paris*, 1861.
Delmas (P.) Mémoire sur l'anatomie et la pathologie du mamelon, dans leurs rapports avec l'allaitement. Union méd. de la Gironde, Bordeaux, 1860, v, 303, 1 pl.; 450.—**Griffiths** (H. T.) The horizontal position of the mammilla. Brit. M. J., Lond., 1887, ii, 68.—**Marcacci** (A.) Il muscolo areolo-capezzolare. Gior. di r. Accad. di med di Torino, 1883, 3. s., xxxi, 743–753, 1 pl. *Also, transl.:* Arch. ital. de biol., Turin, 1883, iv, 292–299, 1 pl.—**Mercier** (A.) Note sur les fibres musculaires du mamelon et sur son érectilité. Gaz. méd. de Par., 1852, 3. s., vii, 7.—**Sebastian** (A. A.) & **van der Hoeven** (J.) De circulo venoso areolæ mammæ circumscripto. Tijdschr. v. nat. Geschied. en Physiol., Amst., 1835, ii, 1–5, 1 pl. — **Sickel.** Ueber das Saugen an den Brustwarzen als wehenerregendes Mittel. Monatschr. f. Geburt. k. u. Frauenkr., Berl., 1854, iii, 329–335. — **de Sinéty.** Sur la mamelle des enfants nouveau-nés. Arch. de tocol., Par., 1875, ii, 379–384. — **Sloan** (S.) On the management of the nipples. Obst. J. Gr. Brit., Lond., 1878, v, 653–668.— **Witte** (E.) Ueber die künstliche Ausbildung der weiblichen Brustwarzen zum Säugungsgeschäft. N. Ztschr. f Geburtsk., Berl., 1844, xvi, 75–96, 1 pl.

Nipples (*Abnormities of*).
See **Breast** (*Abnormities of*).

Nipples (*Artificial*) *and nipple-shields*.

Deneux (L.-C.) Mémoire sur les bouts de seins ou mamelons artificiels et les biberons; lu à l'Académie royale de médecine de Paris dans les séances des 12 et 19 février 1833. 8°. *Paris*, 1833.
Bailly. Nouveau bout-de-sein artificiel dit bout-de-sein de verre ou bout-de-sein transparent. Gaz. d. hôp., Par., 1877, l, 500. — **Boutes** (Sur des) de sein propres à soustraire les mamelons des nourrices à l'action des lèvres de l'enfant. J. gén. de méd., chir. et pharm., Par., 1828, civ, 92–97.—**Rose** (H. C.) On a new description of nipple shield, and the treatment of sore nipples. Tr. Obst. Soc. Lond. (1862), 1863, iv, 135–138. — **Schöller.** Ueber eine neue Art künstlicher Brust-Warze. Med. Ztg., Berl., 1839, viii, 148.—**Taylor** (F.) A new nipple-shield. Lancet, Lond., 1850, i, 345.—**Ware** (C.) Nipple-shield. Med. Rec., N. Y., 1885, xxvii, 336.

Nipples (*Discharges from*).
See **Breast** (*Tumors of, Diagnosis of*).

Nipples (*Diseases of*).

Courgey (S.) * Fréquence des lésions du mamelon et de la mamelle chez les nourrices; remarques statistiques sur 589 observations d'accouchements et de suites de couches. 4°. *Paris*, 1877.
Dithmar (E.-T.) * Essai sur les maladies du mamelon. 4°. *Strasbourg*, 1841.
Grau y O'Donell (E.) * Des lésions non spécifiques du mamelon pendant l'allaitement. 4°. *Paris*, 1875.
van Gries (A.) * Ueber Warzentumoren. 8°. *Würzburg*, 1886.
Hanser (A.) * Ueber das Epithelialcarcinom der Mamma und über "Paget's disease". 8°. *Heidelberg*, 1886.
Kirsten (J. P.) * De papillarum lactantium ex ulceratione ejusque curatione. 4°. *Lipsiæ*, [1840].
Merritt (Emma L.) * Quelques recherches sur le rapport des crevasses du mamelon aux abcès du sein. 4°. *Paris*, 1887.
Salvetat (L.-A.) Essai sur les gerçures du mamelon. 4°. *Paris*, 1872.
Sebastian (J. F. C.) * De vitiis papillarum mammarum lactationem impedientibus eorumque medela. 4°. [*n. p.*, 1793.]

Nipples (*Diseases of*).

VÉRETTE (J.-M.-E.) * Des gerçures du sein chez les femmes qui allaitent. 4°. *Strasbourg*, 1865.

Alvisi (L.) Del liquore stagnotico del Pagliari nelle escoriazioni e nelle ragadi dei capezzoli. Raccoglitore med. di Fano, 1861, xxiv, 69-73. — **Amiss** (J. B.) Treatment of sore nipples. N. York M. Press, 1860, iii, 219. — **Anderson** (T. McC.) Note on Paget's disease of the nipple. Glasgow M. J., 1882, [4. s.], xviii, 241. — **Anselmier**. Traitement des gerçures du sein pendant l'allaitement. Union méd., Par., 1859, 2. s., i, 11. — **Aretaeos** (T.) Ἴνωμα μυξωματικὸν κατὰ τὸν μαστὸν, ἀκροτηριασμὸς τοῦ μαστοῦ, ἰασις; Ἀσκληπιός, Ἀθῆναι, 1870-71, ix, 193-201.— **Asmus**. Blutung durch die Brustwarzen einer nährenden Frau. Wchnschr. f. d. ges. Heilk., Berl., 1838, vi, 749.—**Atlee** (W. F.) The present state of our knowledge respecting the connection between eczema and an affection resembling eczema of the nipple, and a malignant disease of the breast. Am. J. M. Sc., Phila., 1884, n. s., lxxxvii, 469-474.—**Bachelder** (S. F.) Mammillitis. Boston M. & S. J., 1875, xcii, 437. — **Badaloni** (G.) Cura delle ragadi del capezzolo. Raccoglitore med., Forlì, 1879, 4. s., xii, 417. *Also*: Riv. ital. di terap. ed ig., Piacenza, 1884, iv, 148.—**Barker** (F.) A clinical lecture upon sore nipples and mammary abscess. Med. Rec., N. Y., 1873, viii, 441. — **Berger** (I) Adatok némely a gyermekágyban előforduló bimbó-és emlőbántalmak aetiologiájához. [Etiology of diseases of the nipples during childbed.] Gyógyászat, Budapest, 1884, xxiv, 809-814. *Also, transl.* : Medycyna, Warszawa, 1884, xii, 289-293. — **Betz** (F.) Der Prurigo der weiblichen Brustwarze. Med. Cor.-Bl. d. württemb. ärztl. Ver., Stuttg, 1854, xxiv, 181. — **Boucher**. Notice sur deux moyens de préserver ou de guérir le sein des jeunes nourrices, des crevasses ou gerçures, qui sont les suites de l'allaitement. J. gén. de méd., chir. et pharm., Par., 1808, xxxii, 141-148.—**Bridges** (V. R.) Bismuth subnitrate in sore nipples. Ohio M. Recorder, Columbus, 1878, iii, 49. — **Broca**. L'écoulement par le mamelon d'une sérosité sanguinolente n'est pas l'indice d'une tumeur cancéreuse du sein. Bull Soc. anat. de Par., 1855, xxx, 173-175.— **Butler** (G. W.) Treatment of fissure of the nipple during lactation. Ohio M. Recorder, Columbus, 1877, i, 544. — [**Case.**] Kyste sébacé du mamelon. Union méd., Par., 1874, xxviii, 418. — **Chalot**. Phlegmon annulaire de l'aréole du sein Gaz. hebd. d. sc. méd. de Montpel., 1881, iii, 253. ———. Cancer de l'aréole et du bout du sein simulant un eczéma. Compt. rend. Soc. de méd. et chir. prat. de Montpel., 1882-3, 7-10.— **Charrier**. De l'emploi de l'acide picrique dans les lésions du mamelon pendant la lactation. Gaz. d. hôp., Par., 1876, xlix, 484-486.—**Cutler** (E.) Treatment of sore nipples. Med. Rec., N. Y., 1874, ix, 180. — **De Lespinasse** (A. F. H.) Tepelkloven; mastitis; aanwending van collodion. Nederl. Tijdschr. v. Verlosk., Utrecht, 1852, v, 443-447.—**Depaul**. État du service; hémorrhagie après l'accouchement; frisson par suite de crevasses au sein; matières fécales noires de l'enfant causées par les crevasses au sein de la nourrice. J. d. sagesfemmes, Par., 1878, vi, 97. — **De Schweinitz** (G. E.) A case of Paget's disease of the nipple and areola. Med. News, Phila., 1884, xliv, 126-129. — **le Diberder**. Note sur la nature et le traitement des gerçures du mamelon. Ann. de gynéc., Par., 1876, vi, 173-178. — **Doser**. Ein Genüge leistendes Mittel für aufgesprungene und schwürige oder wunde Brustwarzen der säugenden Mütter, deren Heilung sonst allen andern hartnäckig widersteht. Allg. med. Ann., Altenb., 1812, [Ann. d. Heilk., 785]. — **Duhring** (L. A.) Two cases of Paget's disease of the nipple. Am. J. M. Sc., Phila., 1883, n. s., lxxxvi, 116-120.— **Duhring** (L. A.) & **Wile** (I.) On the pathology of Paget's disease of the nipple. *Ibid.*, 1884, n. s., lxxxviii, 141-149. — **Fissures** ou crevasses du mamelon. Santé pub., Par., 1876, 481. — **Folts** (D. V.) Sore or excoriated nipples. Boston M. & S. J., 1867, lxxvi, 121-123. — **Forrest** (R. W.) Case of cancer of the mamma in the male, preceded by so-called eczema of the mammary areola, Paget's disease of the nipple. Glasgow M. J., 1880, xiv, 457-460.—**Frost** (H. R.) Erythematous stomatitis of the infant a cause of cracked or chapped nipples in the nurse. Charleston M. J. & Rev., 1849, iv, 25-27.—**Gibbons** (H.) Simple remedy for sore nipples. Pacific M. & S. J., San Fran., 1869-70, xii, 352-354. — **Gintrac**. Eczéma du mamelon chez l'homme. J. de méd. de Bordeaux, 1856, 2. s., i, 280. *Also*: Gaz. d. hôp., Par., 1856, xxix, 310.— **Grant** (J. A.) Cancer of the breast in its relation to Paget's disease of the breast. Canada M. & S. J., Montreal, 1882-3, xi, 129-131.—**Günther** (C. G.) Das Wundsein der Brustwarzen bei Säugenden, und die vortheilhafte Wirkung eines einfachen Mittels bei demselben. Ztschr. d. nordd. Chir.-Ver., Magdeb., 1848, ii, 688-693. — **Haasis**. Ueber die Behandlung der Schrunden und Excoriationen der Brustwarze. Ztschr. f. Wundärzte u. d. Geb. d. Med., etc., Altona, 1839-40, vii, 1.-2. Hft. 36-41. — **Harriss** (J.) Diseased nipple; excision. South.

Nipples (*Diseases of*).

M. & S. J., Augusta, 1855, n. s., xi, 408.—**Haussmann**. Zur Behandlung wunder Brustwarzen. Berl. klin. Wchnschr., 1878, xv, 189; 667.—**Hearn** (J.) A case of Paget's disease. Phila. M. Times, 1883-4, xiv, 698. *Also* : Tr. Path. Soc. Phila. (1883-5), 1886, xii, 230.—**Iascos** (Περι) τῶν κατὰ τὴν θηλὴν τῶν μαστῶν ῥαγάδων. Ἰατρικὴ Μέλισσα, Ἀθῆναι, 1859, vi, 475.—**Kehrer** (F. A.) Ueber die Infection der Schrunden der Brustwarzen. Prakt. Arzt, Wetzlar, 1883, xxiv, 49-53. ———. Ueber Verhütung und Behandlung der Schrunden der Brustwarzen. Allg. deutsch. Hebam.-Ztg., Berl., 1887, ii, 19.—**Kerr** (J. G.) Cauliflower excrescence of the nipple. Rep. Med. Miss. Soc. in China 1874. Canton, 1875, 9, 1 pl. — **Klein**. Gegen das Wundwerden der Brustwarzen säugender Wöchnerinnen. Deutsche Klinik, Berl., 1861, xiii, 381. — **Kroell** (H.) Theoretisches und Praktisches über die Brustdrüse im Anschluss an einen Fall von Cancroid der Brustwarze. Prakt. Arzt, Wetzlar, 1878, xix, 25; 49.—**Lawson** (G.) A case of cancer of the breast, following long standing eczema of the nipple. Tr. Clin. Soc. Lond. (1879-80), 1880, xiii, 37-39. ———. Case in which the breast was removed on account of incurable eczema of nipple (malignant papillary dermatitis), and afterwards found to be affected by cancer. *Ibid.* (1880-81), 1881, xiv, 222. — **Lewis** (D.) A case of Paget's disease of the nipple. Med. Rec., N. Y., 1887, xxxi, 641.—**Marcus**. Noch einige Worte über die Behandlung wunder Brustwarzen. Mitth. a. d. Geb. d. Med., etc., Altona, 1839-40, vii, 11.-12. Hft., 48-58.—**Meisinger**. Guttapercha-Chloroform-Lösung gegen Excoriationen der Brustwarzen. Wien. med. Wchnschr., 1853, iii, 615.— **Mugnai**. Lo pseudo-cancro della mammella. Arch. ed atti d. Soc. ital. di chir. 1886, Roma, 1887, iii, 51-55.— **Munro** (R.) Paget's disease of the nipple. Glasgow M. J., 1882, [4. s.], xviii, 174-176.—**Napier** (A.) A case of eczema of the nipple and areola, with remarks on the nature and diagnosis of that affection. *Ibid.*, 177-184.— **Noble** (G. H.) Abortive treatment of mammary abscesses, and the cure of fissured nipples by means of a new and effectual compress. Atlanta M. Reg., 1882-3, n. s., ii, 14-22.—**Opitz**. Ueber Erosionen der Brustwarze und Reizzustände der Brustdrüse. Centralbl. f. Gynäk., Leipz., 1883, vii, 185-188. — **Orkisz**. Owrzodzenie brodawek u piersi. [Ulceration of nipple.] Gaz. lek., Warszawa, 1871, xi, 152-154.—**Paget** (*Sir* J.) On disease of the mammary areola preceding cancer of the mammary gland. St. Barth. Hosp. Rep., Lond., 1874, x, 87-89.— **Parfianovich** (N.) K lecheniou tretshin na soskach. [Treatment of fissures of the nipples.] Vrach, St Petersb., 1884, v, 647.—**Porter** (C. B.) A disease of the mammary areola preceding cancer of the mammary glands, Paget's disease. Boston M. & S. J., 1882, cvi, 412-414.— **Porter** (F. T.) Erectile tumour of nipple [from the apex]. Irish Hosp. Gaz., Dubl., 1873, i, 30.—**Reclus** (P.) Mastites chroniques et cancers du sein. Gaz. hebd. de méd., Par., 1887, 2. s., xxiv, 193-198.—**Regnault** (G.) Quelques réflexions pratiques sur le traitement des gerçures du mamelon chez les nourrices. Rev. de thérap. méd.-chir., Par., 1876, [xxiv], 339-343.—**Remarks** on sore nipples. Edinb. M. & S. J., 1811, vii, 36-38.—**Ripa** (L.) Della cura delle ragadi delle mammelle. Gazz. med. ital. lomb., Milano, 1854, 3. s., v, 253.—**Sawyer** (E. W.) Affections of the nipple and breast incident to early lactation. Chicago M. J. & Exam., 1877, xxxv, 561-582.— **Scharlau**. Ueber Entzündung der Brustwarzen und Brustdrüse bey Wöchnerinnen. (Aus der gynäkologischen Klinik von Prof. Martin.) Berl. klin. Wchnschr., 1864, xix, 191; xx, 197.—**Schneider** (P. J.) Mittel gegen entzündete Brustwarzen. J. d. pract. Heilk., Berl., 1837, lxxxiv, 3. St., 57. — **Sézary**. Éclampsie réflexe par l'hyperestésie du mamelon survenue huit jours après la délivrance. Alger méd., 1874, ii, 45-47.—**Sherwell** (S.) Paget's disease of the nipple. J. Cutan. & Ven. Dis., N. Y., 1882-3, i, 184. ———. Paget's disease, or malignant papillary dermatitis (Thin). [Abstr.] Am. J. M. Sc., Phila., 1884, n. s., lxxxvii, 170-173.—**Smith** (H.) A case of so-called eczema of the nipple and areola; destruction of the areola; arrest of the development of cancer. Lancet, Lond., 1882, i, 684.—**Sokolow**. Myoma lævicellulare (Leiomyoma) der rechten Brustwarze. Arch. f. path. Anat., etc., Berl., 1873, lviii, 316-321. — **Steiner**. Zur Behandlung wunder Brustwarzen. Berl. klin. Wchnschr., 1878, xv, 393-395.—**Therapeia** εὔκολος καὶ ταχεία κατὰ τῶν ῥαγάδων τῶν μαστῶν παρὰ ταῖς θηλαζούσαις καὶ κατὰ τῶν ῥαγάδων τῶν χειρῶν ἐν καιρῷ χειμῶνος. Ἰατρικὴ Μέλισσα, Ἀθῆναι, 1853, i, 45. — **Thin** (G) On the connection between disease of the nipple and areola and tumours of the breast. Tr. Path. Soc. Lond., 1881, xxxii, 218-227, 1 l., 1 pl. ———. Malignant papillary dermatitis of the nipple, and the breast-tumours with which it is found associated, illustrated by specimens Brit. M. J., Lond., 1881, i, 760; 798.—**Verneuil**. Squirrhe de la mamelle avec adénopathie axillaire, consécutif à un eczéma chronique du mamelon; examen histologique de la tumeur. Semaine méd., Par., 1883, 2. s., iii, 369.—**Volz** (R.) Ueber die Schrunden der Brustwarzen und deren Heilungen. Med. Ann., Heidelb., 1836, ii, 517-524.—**Wagner**. Ein technisches Verfahren, Schrunden der Brustwarzen liecht zu heilen. N.

Nipples (*Diseases of*).
Ztschr. f. Geburtsk.. Berl., 1851, xxx, 58.—**White** (F. V.) Sore nipples. Med. Rec. N. Y., 1878, xiv, 175-177.—**Wilson** (J. G.) On the value of the nitrate of lead in the treatment of sore nipples. Glasgow M. J.. 1868-9, [4. s.], i, 321.—**Winckel** (F.) Ueber den Einfluss wunder Brustwarzen auf das Allgemeinbefinden der Säugenden. Berl. klin. Wchnschr., 1864, ii, 21–23.

Nipples (*Eczema of*).
See **Breast** (*Tumors of, Cancerous*); **Nipples** (*Diseases of*).

Nipples (*Retracted*).
Davies (H.) Retraction or depression of the nipple of the breast in women. Med. Times & Gaz., Lond., 1852, n. s., iv, 350.—**Duncan** (M.) Retracted nipples. Lancet, Lond., 1872, ii, 671. *Also:* Obst. J. Gr. Brit., Lond., 1873-4, i, 517.—**Kehrer** (F. A.) Note on retracted nipple. Birmingh. M. Rev., 1874, iii, 186.

Nipples (*Watery discharge from*).
See **Ascites** (*Spontaneous cure of*).

Nippoldt (Joannes Christianus Guilielmus). De morbillis. 34 pp. 8°. *Marburgi, typ. Bayrhofferi academicis,* [1827].

Nippoldt (W. A.) * Untersuchungen über den galvanischen Widerstand der Schwefelsäure bei verschiedenen Concentrationsgraden. [Göttingen.] 40 pp. 8°. *Frankfurt, Mahlau u. Waldschmidt,* 1869.
c.

Niquet (Gustave). * Des causes de la mort dans la phthisie pulmonaire chronique. 87 pp. 4°. *Paris, A. Parent,* 1878, No. 459.

Nisbet (Guilielmo). *De anevrysmate. 17 pp. 8°. *Wirceburgi, ex off. vid. Becker,* 1849.
c.

Nisbet (Josias). * De rheumatismo acuto. 1 p. l., 32 pp. 8°. *Edinburgi, Balfour, Auld et Smellie,* 1768. [*Also, in:* P., v. 652.]

Nisbet (William) [1759–1822]. First lines of the theory and practice in venereal diseases. 453 pp. 8°. *Edinburgh, C. Elliot,* 1787.

———. The same. Essai sur la théorie et la pratique des maladies vénériennes. Trad. de l'anglais, augmenté de notes, et dédié à M. Antoine Petit, par M. Petit-Radel. lvi, 359 pp., 2 l. 12°. *Paris, Briand,* 1788.

———. The clinical guide; or, a concise view of the leading facts on the history, nature, and cure of diseases; to which is subjoined a practical pharmacopœia, in three parts, viz, materia medica, classification, and extemporaneous prescription. Intended as a memorandum-book for young practitioners, particularly the students of medicine in their first attendance at the hospital. xiv, 173, 180 pp., 1 l. 12°. *Edinburgh, J. Watson & Co.,* 1793.
Interleaved and annotated.

———. The same. 2. ed. xix, 359 pp. 12°. *Edinburgh, J. Watson & Co.,* 1796.

———. The same. 4. ed. xxiii, 372 pp. sm. 8°. *Edinburgh, J. Watson,* 1801.

———. The clinical guide, or a concise view of the leading facts, on the history, nature, and treatment of the various diseases that form the subject of midwifery, or attend the pregnant, parturient, and puerperal states; intended as a memorandum-book for practitioners; to which is added an obstetrical pharmacopœia, divided into three parts, viz, materia medica, classification, and extemporaneous prescriptions. xvi, 348 pp. 8°. *London, J. Johnson,* 1800.

———. An inquiry into the history, nature, and different modes of treatment hitherto pursued in the cure of scrofula, pulmonary consumption, and cancer. 2. ed. To which is added an appendix, containing a letter to a celebrated professor of Edinburgh, on the peculiar principles adopted by the author in their treatment, and the necessity for a circumscribed line of practice in order to be successful. v, 275 pp. 8°. *London, J. Johnson,* 1800.

Nisbet (William)—continued.

———. A practical treatise on diet, and on the most salutary and agreeable means of supporting life and health by aliment and regimen. 432 pp. 8°. *London, R. Phillips,* 1801.

Niscemi. Statuto organico per l'Ospedale civico di Niscemi. 17 pp. roy. 8°. *Niscemi, tip. G. Scrodat»,* 1886.

Nisius (Henricus). De peste.
In: NOSOL. harmonica dogmat. et hermet. 4°. *Marpurgi Cattorum,* 1616, ii, 465–484. *Also, in:* AGONISMATA med. Marpurgensia. 4°. *Marpurgi Cattorum,* 1618, 244–254.

———. De elephantiasi, seu lepra Arabum.
In: NOSOL. harmonica dogmat. et hermet. 4°. *Marpurgi Cattorum,* 1616, ii, 400–416.

Nisle ([Joh. Fridericus Guilelmus] Ludovicus) [1828–]. * De quibusdam morbis e facie dignoscendis aphorismi. 22 pp. 8°. *Berolini, formis Brueschckianis,* [1827].

Nismes.

TEISSIER-ROLLAND (J.) Question des eaux. Restauration complète de l'aqueduc romain. Projet d'amener à Nîmes, pour deux millions et demi, de six cents à deux mille pouces d'eau salubre. 4°. *Nîmes,* 1852.
Alric (J.) Sur la constitution médicale qui a régné à Nismes pendant les premiers mois de l'année 1843. (Extrait des registres de la Société de médecine du Gard, séance du 7 juin.) Gaz. méd. de Montpel., 1843-4, iv, 49; 71.—**Castelnau** (B.) Note sur les entrées à l'infirmerie et les décès chez les détenus de la maison centrale de Nîmes. Ann. d'hyg., Par., 1835, xiv, 332; 1836, xv, 461.

van Nispen (Johan). * Disp. juridica de sepulcro violato. 4 p. l., 132 pp., 4 l. 4°. *Lugd. Bat., S. Luchtmans,* 1723. [P., v. 984.]

Nissen (Carl). * Zwei Fälle von angeborenen Difformitäten des Kniegelenkes. [Erlangen.] 12 pp., 3 pl. roy. 8°. *Magdeburg,* 1880.
s. d.

Nissen (Caspar). * De resectionibus. 11 pp. 4°. *Kiliæ, C. F. Mohr,* 1859.
In: SCHRIFT. d. Univ. zu Kiel, vi, 1859, vii, Med. i.

Nissen (Hartvig). The Swedish movement and massage treatment. Address delivered before the Clinical Society of Maryland. 30 pp. 18°. *Baltimore, Journal Pub. Co.,* 1888.
Repr. from: Maryland M. J., Balt., 1887-8, xviii.

Nissen (Henricus). * De casu quodam aneurysmatis arteriæ carotidis sinistræ. 10 pp., 1 l. 4°. *Kiliæ, C. F. Mohr,* 1864.
In: SCHRIFT. d. Univ. zu Kiel, xi, 1864, vii, Med. vi.

Nissen (Hinrich Adolp.) * Utrum naturalibus præstent variolæ artificiales. 69 pp. 4°. *Gottingæ, ex off. Schultziana,* [1757].

Nissen (Wilhelm [August Ude]) [1855–]. * Ein Beitrag zur Casuistik der Pulsionsdivertikel der Speiseröre. 17 pp., 1 l. 8°. *Kiel, Schmidt u. Klaunig,* 1884.

Nissen ([Wilhelm] Woldemar). * Ueber die Ursachen der Cholera, nebst Vorschlägen zur Bekämpfung derselben. vii, 39 pp. 8°. *Altona, K. Aue,* 1831.

———. Beiträge zur Therapie. [Cur krankhafter Eigenwärmesteigerungen und ihrer Folgen.] 86 pp. 8°. *Altona, C. T. Schlüter,* 1872.

Nissen (Woldemar Andreas) [1764–1832]. * De polypis uteri et vaginæ, novoque ad eorum ligaturam instrumento. 44 pp., 2 tab. 4°. *Gottingæ, J. C. Dieterich,* [1789]. [*Also, in:* P., v. 328].

———. Bemerkungen über den Missbrauch der Instrumente in der Geburtshülfe. 71 pp. 8°. *Hamburg, F. Perthes,* 1805.

———. Beschreibung der neu eingerichteten Entbindungs-Lehr-Anstalt in Altona. Eine Gelegenheitsschrift bei Eröffnung dieses Instituts. 30 pp. 12°. *Altona, J. Schultz,* 1812.

Nisseron (François-Louis). * De l'urine; nouveaux points de séméiologie, moyens d'investigation les plus employés. 271 pp. 4°. *Paris,* 1869, No. 76.

Nisseron (François-Louis)—continued.
——. The same. 271 pp. 8°. *Paris, J.-B. Baillière & fils,* 1869.

Nissle (Georg) [1848–]. * Ueber die Urinfisteln des Weibes, ihre Entstehung und Operation. 2 p. l., 33 pp. 8°. *Breslau, A. Neumann,* [1873]. c.

Nistler (Joannes Ludovicus) [–1838]. * De generalibus artis obstetriciæ indicationibus. 20 pp. sm. 4°. *Jenæ, typ. Pragerii et soc.,* [1800].

Nitard-Ricord (J.-J.-Esprit). * Peut-on avoir plusieurs fois la vérole constitutionnelle ? 35 pp. 4°. *Paris,* 1848, No. 51, v. 475.

Nithack (Bernardus). * De dysenteria. 28 pp., 2 l. 8°. *Berolini, Nietack.,* 1847. [P., v. 164.]

Nithsdale *neck.*
See **Goitre,** *by localities.*

Nitot (Émile-Bernard-Sosthène). * Contribution à l'histoire de la syphilis oculaire ; des gommes syphilitiques de l'iris et du corps ciliaire. 143 pp., 1 pl. 4°. *Paris,* 1880, No. 198.

Nitraniline.

RAAB (E.) * Ueber Derivate der Meta-Nitranilinsulfonsäure. 8°. *Greifswald,* [1886].

Nitrates, *nitrites, and nitrification.*

See, *also,* **Lead, Mercury, Potassium** (*Nitrate of*) ; **Sodium** ; **Water** (*Analysis of*).

GOSSELS (W.) * Die Nitrate des Tier- und Pflanzenkörpers. (Aus dem Laboratorium Th. Weyl.) 8°. *Berlin,* 1886.

HENRICI (C. F.) * De nitrosorum modo agendi, usu et abusu. 4°. *Halæ Magdeb.,* [1745].

Allen (A. H.) An improvement in the mode of estimating nitrates by Crum's method. Analyst, Lond., 1880, v. 181.—**Davy** (E. W.) On a new and expeditious method for the determination of the nitrites under different circumstances. Chem. News, Lond., 1882, xlvi, 1.—**Gamgee** (A.) On the action of nitrites on the blood. Phil. Tr., Lond., 1869, clviii, 589–625.—**Giacosa** (P.) Sur la transformation des nitrites dans l'organisme. Ztschr. f. physiol. Chem., Strassb., 1883-4, viii, 95–113. *Also, transl.:* Riv. di chim. med. e farm., Torino, 1884, ii, 12 ; 71.—**Kellner** (O.) & **Yoshii** (T.) Ueber die Entbindung freien Stickstoffs bei der Fäulniss und Nitrification. Ztschr. f. physiol. Chem., Strassb., 1887-8, xii, 95–112.—**Munro** (J. H. M.) The formation and destruction of nitrates and nitrites in artificial solutions and in river and well waters. J. Chem. Soc., Lond., 1886, xlix. 632–681.—**Penny** (F.) On the application of the conversion of chlorates and nitrates into chlorides, and of chlorides into nitrates, to the determination of several equivalent numbers. Phil. Tr., Lond., 1839, cxxix, 13–33.—**Rabuteau.** Recherches sur les métamorphoses et l'élimination des azotites. Compt. rend. Soc. de biol. 1869, Par., 1870, 5. s., i, 66.—**Schnetzler** (J.-B.) Sur les germes organisés de la nitrification. Bull. Soc. vaudoise d. sc. nat., Lausanne, 1886, xxii, 213.—**Warington** (R.) Some practical aspects of recent investigations on nitrification. J. Soc. Arts, Lond., 1881-2, xxx, 532-544. *Also* [Abstr.]: Nature, Lond., 1884, xxx, 644. ——. On nitrification. J. Chem. Soc., Lond., 1884, xlv, 637-672. *Also* [Abstr.]: Rep. Brit. Ass. Adv. Sc. 1884, Lond., 1885, liv, 682-685. *Also, transl.:* Monit. scient., Par., 1885, 3. s., xv, 115-140. ——. On the distribution of the nitrifying organism in the soil. Chem. News, Lond., 1886, liv, 228.—**Weyl** (T.) Ueber die Nitrate des Thier- und Pflanzenkörpers. Arch. f. path. Anat., etc., Berl., 1884, xcvi, 462 ; 1885, ci, 175 ; 1886, cv, 187. *Also* [Abstr.]: Deutsche med. Wchnschr., Berl., 1885, xi, 152.

Nitre.

See, *also,* **Potassium** (*Nitrate of*).

ALBRECHT (C. C. D.) * De nitro flammante. 4°. *Altorfii,* [1799].

BRANDMULLER (J. R.) * De nitro. 4°. [*Basil*, 1737.]

BRODBECK (C. D.) * De nitro. (Dissertatio prima.) sm. 4°. *Tubingæ,* 1718.
——. * De nitro. (Dissertatio altera.) sm. 4°. *Tubingæ,* 1718.

DETTMER (J. A.) * De nitri virtute temperante. sm. 4°. *Helmstadii,* [1754].

GEHRT (J.) * De nitro cubico. 4°. *Gottingæ,* [1760].

Nitre.

HERRMANN (A.) * De usu et abusu nitri. 4°. [*Halæ Magdeb.,* 1721.]

KELLER (C. F.) * De nitro flammante. 4°. *Gottingæ,* [1762].

MUTZER (F.) * De nitro. 8°. *Vindobonæ,* 1776.
Also, in : DE WASSERBERG. Op. min. med. et diss. 8°. *Vindobonæ,* 1776, iv, 433-454.

NARCISSUS (F. G.) * Circa nitrum observationes physico-medicæ. sm. 4°. *Halæ Magdeb.,* [1712].

PÁZMÁNDI (G.) * Diss. physico-chemica sistens ideam natri Hungariæ veterum nitro analogi. 12°. *Vindobonæ,* 1770.

SCHMALKALDEN (C. G.) * De nitro, ejus natura et usu in medicina. sm. 4°. *Halæ,* [1694].

SEBASTIANI (G. H.) * De nitro ejus relationibus et modo cum ejus acido oleum naphthæ parandi. 4°. *Erfordiæ,* [1746].

SEIFFART DE KLETTENBERG (R.) * Nitrum præcipuorum morborum methodica conscriptorum medela. sm. 4°. [*n. p.,* 1716.]

Butler (J.) Sur les effets du nitre. N. Jour. de méd., chir., pharm., etc., Par., 1818. i, 120–128.—**Desportes** (E.-H.) Considérations thérapeutiques sur l'emploi du nitre à hautes doses dans un certain nombre de maladies. Bull. gén. de thérap., etc., Par., 1844, xxvi, 9 ; 98.—**Harless** (F.) Ueber das Nitrum der Alten, seine Varietäten und seine Gewinnungsweise ; ein Beitrag zur Geschichte der Materia medica im Alterthume. Janus, Bresl., 1846, i, 455–484. *Also :* Amtl. Ber. ü. d. Versamml. deutsch. Naturf. u. Aerzte 1845, Nürnb., 1846, xxiii, 227–233.—**Nivet.** Note historique sur le nitre et les eaux minérales nitreuses des anciens auteurs. Ann. Soc. d'hydrol. méd. de Par., 1860, vii, 34-41.—**Thierfelder.** Ueber das Nitrum der Alten. Janus, Bresl., 1848, iii, 29–53.

Nitrobenzin.

BOGDANOFF (F.) * Phiziologicheskoe dieistvie nitrobenzina. 8°. *St. Petersburg,* 1868.

GABALDA (A.) * Étude sur les accidents causés par la benzine et la nitrobenzine. 4°. *Paris,* 1879.

Bahrdt (R.) Beitrag zur Kenntniss der Nitrobenzinvergiftung. Arch. d. Heilk., Leipz., 1871, xii, 320–335.—**Brennan** (T.) Empoisonnement par la nitrobenzine. Union méd. du Canada, Montréal, 1887, n. s., i, 449–452.—**Brugnoli** (G.) Dell' adiastolia in un avvelenamento da nitro-benzina. Mem. Accad. d. sc. d. Ist. di Bologna, 1880, 4. s., ii, 345–351.—**Burglocher.** Eine Vergiftung mit Nitrobenzin. Aerztl. Int.-Bl., München, 1875. xxii, 1.—**Casali** (A.) Ricerca di tenuissime quantità di nitrobenzina e d' anilina nei casi d' avvelenamento. Rendic. Accad. d. sc. d. Ist. di Bologna (1875-6), 1876, 149-155.—**Casper** (J. L.) Ein neues Gift. Vrtljschr. f. gerichtl. u. öff. Med., Berl., 1859. xvi, 1-7.—**Dubois** (E.) Sur un cas d'empoisonnement par la nitrobenzine. Ann. Soc. de méd. de Gand, 1883, lxi, 209–217.—**Guttmann** (P.) Ueber die giftigen Eigenschaften des Nitrobenzin. Arch. f. Anat., Physiol. u. wissensch. Med., Leipz., 1866, 214-223.—**Jacquemin** (E.) De la nitrobenzine au point de vue analytique et toxicologique. Monde pharm., Par., 1875, vi, 106 ; 113. *Also :* J. de pharm. et chim., Par., 1875, 4. s., xxi, 375 ; 455.—**Kreuser.** Vergiftung durch Nitrobenzin. Med. Cor.-Bl. d. württemb. ärztl. Ver., Stuttg., 1867, xxxvii, 207-209.—**Lehmann** (F. G.) Vergiftung durch Nitrobenzin. Vrtljschr. f. gerichtl. u. öff. Med., Berl., 1870, xiii, 41-62.—**Limasset** (T.) Observation d'un cas d'empoisonnement par la nitrobenzine. Union méd., Par., 1874, xxviii, 209-212.—**Müller** (H.) Eine Nitrobenzin-Vergiftung. Cor.-Bl. f. d. Aerzte u. Apoth. d. Grossherz. Oldenburg, 1865, iii, 165-172.—**Neumann** (E.) & **Pabst** (A.) Des accidents produits par la benzine et la nitrobenzine. Ann. d'hyg., Par., 1883, 3. s., x, 426 ; 490.—**Nicholson** (E.) Case of poisoning from nitrobenzine. Lancet, Lond., 1862, i, 135.—**Ollivier** (A.) & **Bergeron** (E.) Recherches expérimentales sur l'action physiologique de la nitrobenzine. J. de la physiol. de l'homme, Par., 1863, vi, 455–459.—**Poincaré.** Recherches sur les effets de la nitrobenzine. Rev. d'hyg., Par., 1879, i, 708–716.—**Schenk.** Vergiftung durch Nitrobenzin. Vrtljschr. f. gerichtl. u. öff. Med., Berl., 1866, iv, 341-346.—**Swederus.** Ein Fall von Vergiftung mit Nitrobenzin. Deutsche Klinik, Berl., 1873, xxv, 382.—**Tassi.** Un caso di veneficio per nitrobenzina. Bull. d. r. Accad. med. di Roma, 1881, vii, 364-371.—**Treulich.** Drei Fälle von Vergiftung mit Nitrobenzin. Wien. med. Presse, 1870, xi, 224-227.—**Van der Meersch** & **De Visscher.** Relation d'un cas d'empoisonnement par la nitrobenzine. Ann. Soc. de méd. de Gand, 1883, lxi, 158–160.

Nitrobenzol.

See, also, Aniline.

PAGENSTECHER (H.) * Ein Fall von Nitrobenzolvergiftung. 8°. *Würzburg*, 1867.

[**Case.**] Poisoned by myrbane. Med. Rec., N. Y., 1867-8, ii, 455.—[**Dean** (H. M.)] Poisoning by nitrobenzol. Med. Bull., Phila., 1879, i, 50.—**Drake** (K.) ' Fall af förgiftning med nitrobenzol. [Poisoning by nitrobenzole.] Eira, Göteborg, 1879, iii, 669.—**Ewald** (C. A.) Zwei Fälle von Nitrobenzol-Vergiftung mit Glycosurie. Berl. klin. Wchnschr., 1875, xii, 3-7.— **Felletár** (E.) Nitrobenzol-mérgezés ujabb esetei. [Poisoning by . . .] Gyógyászat, Budapest, 1877, xvii, 721-724.—**Filehne** (W.) Ueber die Giftwirkungen des Nitrobenzols. Arch. f. exper. Path. u. Pharmakol. Leipz., 1878, ix, 329-379.—**Helbig.** Ueber Vergiftung mit Nitrobenzol. Deutsche mil.-ärztl. Ztschr., Berl., 1873, ii, 36-41.—**Jolin** (S.) Tre fall af nitrobenzol-förgiftning. Hygiea, Stockholm, 1882, xliv, 339 - 347.— **Kreuser.** Nitrobenzol - Vergiftung. Med. Cor.-Bl. d. württemb. ärztl. Ver., Stuttg., 1869, xxxix, 343.—**Letheby** (H.) On the poisonous properties of essence of myrbane, or artificial oil of bitter almonds (nitro-benzole). Clin. Lect. & Rep. Lond. l-r65, ii, 34 - 57. — **Lewin** (L.) Ueber eine Elementareinwirkung des Nitrobenzols auf das Blut. Arch. f. Physiol., Leipz., 1879, 175. — **von Maschka.** Vergiftung durch Nitrobenzol. Vrtljschr. f. gerichtl. Med., Berl., 1885, n. F., xliii, 14-17.—**von Mering.** Nitrobenzolvergiftung bewirkt keine Zuckerausscheidung im Harn. Centralbl. f. d. med. Wissensch., Berl., 1875, xiii, 945 — **Riefkohl.** Ein Fall von Vergiftung mittelst Nitrobenzol. Deutsche Klinik, Berl., 1868, xx, 169. — **Schenk.** Vergiftung durch Nitrobenzol. Vrtljschr. f. gerichtl. u. öff. Med., Berl., 1866, iv, 327 - 340.— **Schuhmacher** & **Spängler.** Tödtliche Vergiftung durch Nitrobenzol. Wien. med. Wchnschr., 1875, xxv, 229-233 — **Stevenson** (T.) Nitro-benzol poisoning. Guy's Hosp. Rep., Lond., 1876, 3. s., xxi, 371-374, 1 pl.—**Taylor** (A. S.) Poisoning by nitrobenzene. *Ibid.*, 1864, 3 s., x, 192-197.—**Werner.** Ein Beitrag zur Kenntniss und Behandlung der Nitrobenzolvergiftung. Berl. klin. Wchnschr., 1884, xxi, 58.—**Winz** (E. E) Poisoning by nitro-benzole. Boston M. & S. J., 1872, lxxxvi, 33 - 37. *Also*, Reprint.

Nitrogen.

BRUUN (E. E.) * De ratione, quæ inter azoticum aëris atmosphærici et respirationem humanam intercedit. Resp. Conc. Math. Lunding. 12°. *Hafniæ*, 1815.

LACOTE (A.) * Synthèse des corps azotés. 4°. *Paris*, 1880.

MEYER (T. B.) * Quæstiones de fontibus, ex quibus animalia et plantæ nitrogenium excipiant. 8°. [*Dorpat*], 1853.

VOIT (K.) * Beiträge zum Kreislauf des Stickstoffes im thierischen Organismus. 8°. *Augsburg*, 1857.

Atwater (W. O.) On the liberation of nitrogen from its compounds and the acquisition of atmospheric nitrogen by plants. Am. Chem. J., Balt., 1886-7, viii, 398-420.— **Beck** (L. C.) On the office of the nitrogen of the air in the process of respiration. N. York M. & Phys. J., 1829-30, n. s., ii, 288-292. — **Dubelir** (D. D.) Etshe nekotorie opiti nad vlijaniem vodi i povarennoi sodi na videlenie azota. [Influence of water and kitchen salt in the production of nitrogen.] Voyenno med. J., St. Petersb., 1882, cxliv. pt. 2, 15-34. — **de Fourcroy.** Recherches pour servir à l'histoire du gaz azote ou de la mofète, comme principe des matières animales. Hist. Soc. roy. de méd. 1786, Par., 1790, viii, pt. 2, 346-354.—**Gatchakovski** (G. I.) K voprosu o terapevt. znachenii azota. [Therapeutical value of nitrogen.] Vrach. Vaidom., St. Petersb., 1882, vii, 3467 - 3469. — **Grandclément.** L'azote de l'atmosphère est-il inspiré dans la respiration ? Union méd., Par., 1872, 3. s., xiv, 526. — **Gruber** (M.) Zweiter Beitrag zur Frage der Entwickelung elementaren Stickstoffs im Thierkörper. Ztschr. f. Biol., München, 1883, xix, 563 - 568. — **Heyfelder** (I. F.) Ob opwitakh nad vdikhaniyami azota. [Experiments on the inhalation of azote nitrogen.] Voyenno-med. J., St. Petersb., 1868, vi, pt. 1, 1. — **Jackson** (C. T.) Existence of nitrogen in plants; its origin in animals. Boston M. & S. J., 1860, lxiii, 289-292.—**Jewdokimow** (A. J.) Ein Versuch zur qualitativen Bestimmung des Stickstoffumsatzes beim Menschen, aus dem Vergleich der durch Harn und Schweiss ausgeschiedenen Stickstoffmenge des Harnstoffes mit dem Stickstoffgehalt der Extractivstoffe. St. Petersb. med. Wchnschr., 1887, n. F., iv, 179 —**Kjeldahl** (J.) En ny Methode til Kvælstofbestemmelse i organiske Stoffer. Sur une nouvelle méthode de dosage de l'azote dans les substances organiques. Medd. f. Carlsberg Lab., Kjøbenh., 1883, ii, 1-27. — **Kletzinsky.** The nitrogen bodies of modern chemistry. [*Transl. from:* Aus der Natur.] Rep. Smithson. Inst. 1872, Wash., 1873, 203-218.—

Kohlschütter. Stickstoffinhalationen und ihre Wirkungen. Cor.-Bl. d. Ver. d. Aerzte im Reg.-Bez. Merseburg, 1880, 3 - 15. *Also:* Allg. med. Centr.-Ztg. Berl., 1880, xlix, 437 ; 453; 465.—**Lahousse.** Dosage de l'azote d'après la méthode de Kijeldahl. Ann. Soc. de méd. d'Anvers, 1886, xlvii, 557-559, 1 pl.—**Leo** (H.) Untersuchungen zur Frage der Bildung von freiem Stickstoff im thierischen Organismus. Arch. f. d. ges. Physiol., Bonn, 1881-2, xxvi, 218-236, 1 pl. *Also*, Reprint.—**Mays** (T. J.) Nitrogen and life. N. York M. J., 1876, xxiv, 153-171.—**Mijers** (J.) De bereiding van stikstof. Werk. v. h. Genootsch. t. Bevord. d. Nat.-, Genees- en Heelk. te Amst., 1871-2, ii, 129.—**Moultrie** (J.) Relations of nitrogen to respiration and vocalization or phonation. Charleston M. J. & Rev., 1849, iv, 265-271, 1 diag.—**Negro** (A.) Apreciaciones sobre el valor terapéutico del ázoe ; estudio de las aguas minero-medicinales de Panticosa, en sus relaciones con la tisis y las enfermedades del órgano central de la circulacion. An. Soc. españ. de hidrol. méd., Madrid, 1879-80, iii, 104 ; 130.— **Neill** (C.) Effects of the inhalation of pure nitrogen gas. Lancet, Lond., 1880, ii, 557. — **Sieffermann.** Des inhalations d'azote. Gaz. méd. de Strasb., 1883, 3. s., xii, 97-100.—**Szohner** (J.) Ueber die Wirkung der Stickstoff-Inhalationen. Pest. med.-chir. Presse, Budapest, 1885 xxi, 981.—**Treutler.** Die Bedeutung der Stickstoffinhalation und deren Herstellbarkeit. Jahresb. d. Gesellsch. f. Nat.-u. Heilk. in Dresd., 1876, 119-124. ——. Vorläufige Mittheilung über Stickstoff Inhalation. Berl. klin. Wchnschr., 1878, xv, 163-165.—**de Voisins** (C.) De la medicacion nitrogenada artificial. Rev. méd. de Sevilla, 1884, ix, 335; 360.

Nitrogen (*Excretion of*).

See, also, Albumen; Exercise; Food; Tissue (*Metamorphosis of*); Urea.

GRIMM (F.) * Beiträge zur Kenntniss der Stickstoffausscheidung in pathologischen Zuständen. 8°. *Erlangen*, 1881.

PARKES (E. A.) On the elimination of nitrogen by the kidneys and intestines during rest and exercise, on a diet without nitrogen. 8°. *London*, 1867.

Cutting from: Proc. Roy. Soc. Lond., 1867, xv, 339-355.

——. On the elimination of nitrogen during rest and exercise, on a regulated diet of nitrogen. 8°. [*London*, 1868.]

Cutting from: Proc. Roy. Soc. Lond., 1868, xvi, 44-59.

SEEGEN (J.) Ueber die Ausscheidung des Stickstoffes der im Körper zersetzten Albuminate. 8°. [*Wien*, 1867.]

Repr. from: Sitzungsb. d. k. Akad. d. Wissensch. Math.-naturw. Cl., Wien, 1867, lv, 357-407. *Also* [Abstr.], *in:* Wien. med. Wchnschr., 1867, xvii, 408. *Also* [Abstr.], *in:* Wien. med. Presse, 1868, 121-123.

——. Zur Frage über die Ausscheidung des Stickstoffes der im Körper zersetzten Albuminate. (Vorgelegt in der Sitzung am 15. December 1870.) 8°. [*Wien*, 1871.]

Cutting from: Sitzungsb. d. k. Akad. d. Wissensch. Math. naturw. Cl., Wien, 1871, lxiii.

Camerer (W.) Zur Bestimmung des Stickstoffes in Urin und Koth des Menschen. Ztschr. f. Biol., München, 1884, xx, 255-263.—**Chatterjee** (G. C.) Some remarks on Surgeon M. D. O'Connell's article on " Nitrogenous waste in the blood and its probable use ", which appeared in the Indian Medical Gazette for April, 1882. Indian M. Gaz. Calcutta, 1882 xvii, 176.—**Dumas** & **Cahours.** Mémoire sur les matières azotées neutres de l'organisation. Expérience, Par., 1842, x, 369 ; 401.—**Gruber** (M.) Untersuchungen über die Ausscheidungswege des Stickstoffs aus dem thierischen Organismus. Ztschr. f. Biol., München, 1880, xvi, 367-410.—**Henninger** (A.) Sur un procédé de dosage de l'azote total de l'urine. Compt. rend. Soc. de biol., Par., 1884, 8. s., i, pt. 2, 474-476.—**Lépine.** Contribution à l'étude de l'excrétion de l'azote total et de l'azote des matières extractives par l'urine. *Ibid.*, 1880, Par., 1881, 7. s., ii, 332 - 334. — **North** (W.) The influence of bodily labour upon the discharge of nitrogen. Proc. Roy. Soc. Lond., 1885, xxxix, 413-503, 6 diag. *Also* [Abstr.]: Brit. M. J., Lond., 1884, ii, 112.—**Parkes** (E. A.) On some points connected with the elimination of nitrogen from the human body. Lancet, Lond., 1871. i, 399 ; 467 ; 527. ——. Further experiments on the effect of diet and exercise on the elimination of nitrogen. Proc. Roy. Soc. Lond., 1870-71, xix, 349-361. ——. Further experiments on the effect of alcohol and exercise on the elimination of nitrogen and on the pulse and temperature of the body. *Ibid.*, 1871-2, xx, 402-414.—**von Pettenkofer** (M.) & **Voit** (C.) Zur Frage der Ausscheidung gasförmigen Stickstoffs aus dem Thierkörper. Ztschr. f. Biol., München, 1880, xvi, 508-549. *Also:* Sitzungsb. d. math.-phys. Cl. d. k.-bayer. Akad. d. Wissensch. zu München, 1881, xi,

Nitrogen (*Excretion of*).

270–320.—**Power** (J. B.) On the excretion of nitrogen in the urine. Dublin J. M. Sc., 1875, lix, 81–85.—**Schulze** (E.) & **Märcker** (M.) Ueber die sensibeln Stickstoff-Einnahmen und Ausgaben des volljährigen Schafes. (Mitgetheilt von W. Henneberg.) Centralbl. f. d. med. Wissensch., Berl., 1869. vii, 225–228.—**Seegen** (J.) Ueber die Ausscheidung des Stickstoffes der im Körper verbrauchten Eiweissverbindungen. Wien. med. Wchnschr., 1868, xviii, 157; 173; 189; 205. — **Seegen** (J.) & **Nowak** (J.) Versuche über die Ausscheidung von gasförmigem Stickstoff aus den im Körper umgesetzten Eiweissstoffen. Arch. f. d. ges. Physiol., Bonn, 1879, xix, 347–415, 1 pl.—**Stohmann.** Ueber die Stickstoff-Einnahmen und Ausgaben bei milchgebenden Ziegen. Centralbl. f. d. med. Wissensch., Berl., 1869, vii, 322–325.

Nitrogen (*Oxides of*).

See **Acid** (*Nitric*); **Acid** (*Nitrous*); **Asthma** (*Treatment of*); **Nitrous** *oxide*.

Nitro-glycerin.

See, also, **Dynamite**; **Heart** (*Diseases of, Treatment of*); **Neuralgia** (*Treatment of*).

BRUEL (A.) * Recherches expérimentales sur les effets toxiques de la nitroglycérine et de la dynamite. 4°. *Paris,* 1876.

MOWBRAY (G. M.) Nitro-glycerine, as used in the construction of the Hoosac Tunnel. 8°. [*Albany,* 1871.]

NOVITSKI (A.) * O phiziologicheskom dieistvii nitroglitserina. [Physiological effects of nitroglycerine.] 8°. *St. Petersburg,* 1864.

TRUSSEVITCH (J. I.) Nitroglicerin (angionevrozin ili anevrozin) v meditsinie. Materialy k izychenivu ego vlijanija na zdorovago chelovieka i k naznacheniou ego. [Nitroglycerin (angionevrosin or anevrosin) in medicine. Materials for studying its effect in health and disease of man.] 8°. *St. Petersburg,* 1887.

———. Anevrozin v meditsinie. Vlijanie na zdorovago chelovieka i praktika liechenija em. [Anevrosin in medicine; effect on health and its practical application.] [2. ed.] 8°. *St. Petersburg,* 1888.

Albers (J. F. H.) Die physiologische und therapeutische Wirkung des Nitroglycerins. Deutsche Klinik, Berl., 1864, xvi, 405–408.—**Atkinson** (G. A.) The pharmacology of the nitrites and of nitro-glycerine. J. Anat. & Physiol., Lond., 1887-8, xxii, 225–239. *Also:* Phila. M. Times, 1887-8, xviii, 260–264.—**Bourru.** Sur les propriétés toxiques de la nitroglycérine et de la dynamite. Bull. gén. de thérap., etc., Par., 1883, civ, 455–457.—**Brady** (G. S.) On the medicinal action of glonoine. Med. Times & Gaz., Lond., 1859, n. s., xviii, 263.—**Brunton** (J. L.) & **Tait** (E. S.) Preliminary notes on the physiological action of nitroglycerine. St. Barth. Hosp. Rep., Lond., 1876, xii, 140–145.—**Burroughs** (J. B.) Nitro glycerine, a substitute for alcoholic remedies. Therap. Gaz., Detroit, 1885, 3. s., i, 404.—**Demme** (R.) Das Nitroglycerin als Arzneimittel. Schweiz. Ztschr. f. Heilk., Bern, 1862, i, 156–160.—**Desrosiers** (H.-E.) De l'action physiologique et thérapeutique de la nitroglycérine. Union méd. du Canada, Montréal, 1883, xii, 106; 153.—**Éloy** (C.) Dynamite. Dict. encycl. d. sc. méd., Par., 1884, xxx, 745–756. — **Eulenberg** (H.) Ueber die Wirkung des Nitroglycerins. Berl klin. Wchnschr., 1865, xxiv, 250–252.—**Field** (A. G.) On the toxical and medicinal properties of nitrate of oxyde of glycyl. Med. Times & Gaz., Lond., 1858, n. s., xvi, 291. ———. Nitro-glycerine or glonoine. *Ibid.,* 1859, n. s., xviii, 339.—**Foy** (G. M.) Nitro-glycerine. Med. Press & Circ., Lond., 1886, n. s., xli, 6.—**Gordon** (W. S.) Nitroglycerine as a therapeutic agent. Practice, Richmond, 1886-7, i, 26–28.—**Hamilton** (A. McL.) Nitro-glycerine as a remedy. Med. News, Phila., 1882, xl, 475.—**Hammond** (W. A.) Some of the therapeutical uses of nitroglycerine. Virginia M. Month., Richmond, 1881-2, viii, 525–531.—**Hay** (M.) The chemical nature and physiological action of nitro-glycerine. Practitioner, Lond., 1883, xxx, 422–433. *Also,* Reprint.—**Holst** (I. C.) Et Tilfælde af Nitroglycerinforgiftning. Norsk Mag. f. Lægevidensk., Christiania, 1870, 2. R., xxiv, 541–546.—**von Holst** (L.) Nitroglycerin bei Herz- und Nierenleiden. St. Petersb. med. Wchnschr., 1886, n. F., iii, 299; 307.—**Honert.** Ein Fall von Vergiftung durch Nitroglycerin. Deutsche Klinik, Berl., 1867, xix, 83.—**Husemann** (T.) Eine absichtliche Vergiftung mit Nitroglycerin. [Case.] *Ibid.,* 1867, xix, 162; 171. —. Das Nitroglycerin in toxicologischer und therapeutischer Beziehung. Schmidt's Jahrb., Leipz., 1867, cxxxiv, 344–354.—**Instruktion** zur Aufbewahrung, Behandlung und zum Transporte des Sprengöles und der Nitroglycerin-Präparate, insbesondere des Dyna-

Nitro-glycerin.

mits. Allg. mil.-ärztl. Ztg., Wien, 1870, xi, 121–126.—**Jackson** (W. F.) On the toxical and other properties of "a substance analogous to gun cotton". Med. Exam., Phila., 1849, n. s., v, 279–283.—**James** (F. A.) Nitro-glycerine. Med. Times & Gaz., Lond., 1858, n. s., xvi, 383.—**Jumont.** Indications et modes d'emploi de la nitro-glycérine. France méd., Par., 1887, i, 269–271.—**Korczyński.** Kilka słów o działaniu fizyjolog. io zastosowaniu leczniczem nitrogliceryny. [Physiological effect of application of nitro-glycerine.] Pam. Towarz. Lek. Warszaw., 1881, lxxvii, 609–628. *Also, transl.* [Abstr.]: Wien. med. Wchnschr., 1882, xxxii, 154–156.—**Lublinski** (W.) Ueber die therapeutische Wirksamkeit des Natriumnitrits und des Nitroglycerins. Deutsche med. Wchnschr., Berl., 1885, xi, 65; 85.—**Martindale** (W.) Nitroglycerin in pharmacy. Practitioner, Lond., 1880, xxiv, 35–39.—"**Medicus.**" The subcutaneous injection of nitroglycerine. Med. Times & Gaz., Lond., 1883, i, 444.—**Minor** (A. J.) Tri-nitroglycerin; its physiological effects and therapeutical indications. Am. Psych. J., N. Y., 1875-6, iii, 103–111.—**Nevitt** (R. B.) Toxic effects of nitro-glycerine. Canad. J. M. Sc., Toronto, 1882, vii, 45.—**Nitroglycérine** (La). J. de chim. méd., etc., Par., 1874, xlviii, 6–12.—**Noer** (J.) Poisonous symptoms from nitro-glycerine. Therap. Gaz., Detroit, 1887, 3. s., iii, 459.—**Nordenstrom.** Förgiftningsfall medelst sprängolja. Förh. v. Svens. Läk.-Sällsk. Sammank., Stockholm, 1867, 187–194.—**Nyström** (C.) Om Nitroglycerin. Upsala Läkaref. Förh., 1866-7, ii, 232–252.—**Onsum** (I.) Om Nitroglycerin. Norsk Mag. f. Lægevidensk., Christiania, 1865, 2. R., xix, 36–42.—**Panthel.** Vergiftung durch Nitro-Glycerin. Memorabilien, Heilbr., 1868, xiii, 158.—**Pelikan** (E.) Toxikologisches über das Nitroglycerin (Glonoin) und andere Knallkörper. Med. Ztg. Russlands. St. Petersb., 1855, xii, 377; 385.—**Root** (P. S.) Nitro-glycerine. Detroit Clinic, 1882, i, 407–409.—**Sandahl.** Giftiga verkningarne af nitro-glycerin. Förh. v. Svens. Läk.-Sällsk. Sammank. 1865, Stockholm, 1866, 130.—**Stegemann.** Vergiftung mittelst Nitroglycerins; ein Criminalprocess. Ztschr. f. gerichtl. Med., Wien, 1868, iv, 191; 203; 217; 223. — **Stockton** (C. G.) Some uses of nitro-glycerine. Buffalo M. & S. J., 1883-4, xxiii, 337–346.—**Sylvester** (J. E.) On some therapeutic uses of nitro-glycerine. Columbus M. J., 1883-4, ii, 102–104.—**Testa** (B.) Nitrito amilico e nitroglicerina. Indipendente, Torino, 1883, xxxiv, 433; 457.—**Trussevitch** (J. I.) Material. k izuch. lekarst. vlijan. nitroglicer. na nekotor. formi golov. boli. [Theory of effect of nitroglycerine on different forms of cephalalgia] Ejened. klin. gaz., St. Petersb., 1887, vii, 523; 542; 565. *Also, transl.:* Allg. med. Centr.-Ztg., Berl., 1887, lvi, 321; 337; 353. ———. Oblast primen. i pravila dosir. nitroglicerina v kachestve lekarst. [Application and doses of nitro-glycerine.] Med. Obozr., Mosk., 1887, xxvii, 60–67. *Also, transl.:* St. Petersb. med. Wchnschr., 1887, n. F., iv, 2–5. — **Trussevitch** (J. M.) Detalnaja kartina deistvija nitroglicerina na zdorov. tcheloveka. [Effect of nitro-glycerine on the health of man.] Ejened. klin. gaz., St. Petersb., 1887, vii, 198; 213.—**Weil** (C.) Ein Beitrag zur Kenntniss des Nitroglycerin (Sprengöl). Med.-chir. Cor.-Bl. f. deutsch-am. Aerzte, Buffalo, 1883, i, No. 2, 6–8.—**Werber** (A.) Beitrag zur Kenntniss der toxicologischen Wirkungen des Nitroglycerin. Deutsche Klinik, Berl., 1866, xviii, 441–445. ———. Zur Auffindung des Nitroglycerins in gerichtlichen Fällen. *Ibid.,* 1867, xix, 365.

Nitro-naphthalin.

Roussin (Z.) Nitro-naphtaline; naphtylamine et ses dérivés colorés. Rec. de mém. de méd. . . . mil., Par., 1861, 3. s., v, 424–427.

Nitropentanen.

Schadow (G.) Ueber die physiologischen Wirkungen des Nitropentan. Arch. f. exper. Path. u. Pharmakol., Leipz., 1876, vi, 194–204.

Nitrosulphites.

Roussin (Z.) Recherches sur les nitrosulfures doubles (nouvelle classe de sels). Rec. de mém. de méd. . . . mil., Par., 1858, 2. s., xxi, 409–427.

Nitrotoluidine.

FOTH (G.) * Ueber o-Nitro-p-Toluidin-m-Sulfonsäure. 8°. *Greifswald,* 1885.

GRAEFF (F.) * Ueber Nitrotoluidine und einige ihrer Derivate. 8°. *Greifswald,* 1885.

HASSE (H.) * Ueber Orthotoluidinmetadisulfosäure und einige ihrer Derivate. 8°. *Greifswald,* 1885.

Nitrous *oxide*.

See, also, **Asthma** (*Treatment of*).

BARKER (G. T.) Instructions in the preparation, administration, and properties of nitrous oxide, protoxide of nitrogen, or laughing gas. 8°. *Philadelphia,* 1866.

Nitrous oxide.

———. The same. 2. ed. 8°. *Philadelphia*, 1867.

BARTH (G.) Protoxide of nitrogen as an anæsthetic, or ten minutes' talk about laughing gas. 12°. *London*, 1870.

BARTON (W. P. C.) * A dissertation on the chymical properties and exhilarating effects of nitrous oxide gas, and its application to pneumatick medicine. 8°. *Philadelphia*, 1808.

BEDDOES (T.) Notice of some observations made at the Medical Pneumatic Institution. 8°. *London*, 1799.

BLANCHARD (R.) * De l'anesthésie par le protoxyde d'azote d'après la méthode de M. le Prof. Paul Bert. 4°. *Paris*, 1880.

BLANCHE (T.) * Recherches expérimentales sur le protoxyde d'azote. 4°. *Paris*, 1874.

BLUMM (V.) * Stickstoffoxydul als Anæstheticum. [Erlangen.] 8°. *München*, 1878.
Also, in : Aerztl. Int.-Bl., München, 1878, xxv, 319 ; 331.

CHARROPPIN (P.-G.) * Du protoxyde d'azote comme agent anesthésique. 4°. *Strasbourg*, 1870.

COLTON (J. J.) The physiological action of nitrous oxide gas, as shown by experiments upon man and the lower animals ; together with suggestions as to its safety, uses, and abuses. 8°. *Philadelphia*, 1871.

DUCHESNE (A.) aîné. Étude sur le protoxyde d'azote. 8°. *Paris*, 1869.

GROHNWALD (C.) Das Stickstoffoxydul-Gas als Anæstheticum. 8°. *Berlin*, 1872.

KAUFFMANN (M.) * Ueber die anästhesirende Wirkung des Stickstoffoxydulgases. 8°. *Halle*, 1874.

NEWBROUGH (J. B.) Nitrous oxide gas. A reported death from its use. 8°. [*n. p., n. d.*]

ODONTOLOGICAL Society of Great Britain. First report of the joint committee appointed by the . . . and the committee of management of the Dental Hospital of London, to inquire into the value and advantage of the protoxide of nitrogen as an anæsthetic in surgical operations. 8°. *London*, 1869.

PRÉTERRE (A.) Le protoxyde d'azote. Application aux opérations chirurgicales et particulièrement à l'extraction des dents sans douleur. 6. éd. 8°. *Paris*, 1870.

RÜHL (F. J.) * Materialien zu einer Monographie des Stickstoffoxyduls. 8°. *Halle a. S.*, 1881.

SAUER (C.) Versuche, mit Stickstoffoxydul-Gemischen zu anästhesiren. 8°. [*n. p.*, 1869.]
Repr. from : Vrtljschr. f. Zahnheilk., 4. Hft., 1869.

WELLS (H.) A history of the discovery of the application of nitrous oxide gas, ether, and other vapors, to surgical operations. 12°. *Hartford*, 1847.

Administration (The) of protoxide of nitrogen. Lancet. Lond., 1868, i, 563.—**Aguilar Lara.** El protóxido de azoe en cirujia. Crón méd., Valencia, 1882-3, vi, 257 ; 289.—**Amory** (R.) Physiological action of nitrous oxide, as shown by experiments on man and lower animals. N. York M. J., 1870, xii, 1-29. *Also.* Reprint.— **Andrews** (E.) Liquid nitrous oxide as an anæsthetic. Med. Exam., Chicago, 1872, xiii, 34-36.— **Ashford** (F. A.) Hemiplegia following the inhalation of nitrous oxide, subsequent typhoid fever. Am. J. M. Sc., Phila., 1869, n. s., lvii, 408-410. *Also :* Proc. Clin.-Path. Soc. Wash., Phila., 1869-70, 50-52.—**Aubeau** (A.) Conditions d'innocuité de l'anesthésie au protox. de d'azote pur. Odontologie. Par., 1885, v, 552 ; 1886, vi, 8 ; 196 ; 251 ; 303 ; 343.—**Barnes** (H. J.) Nitrous oxide gas. Boston M. & S. J., 1874, xci, 511- 513 —**Begg** (I. R.) Nitrous oxide gas in excision of the mamma. Lancet Lond., 1870, i, 800.—**Bert** (P.) Sur la possibilité d'obtenir, à l'aide du protoxyde d'azote, une insensibilité de longue durée, et sur l'innocuité de cet anesthésique. Compt. rend. Acad. d. sc., Par., 1878, lxxxvii, 728-730. *Also, transl.:* Med. Press & Circ., Lond., 1879, n. s., xxvii, 99. ———. Anesthésie par le protoxyde d'azote employé sous tension. Compt. rend. Soc. de biol.

Nitrous oxide.

1878, Par., 1880, 6. s., v, 152. ———. Du protoxyde d'azote sous tension ; son action à doses anesthésiques ne s'étend pas sur le système nerveux sympathique. *Ibid.*, 233. ———. Anesthésie par le protoxyde d'azote. *Ibid.*, 7. s., i, pt. 2, 19-21. *Also :* Gaz. méd. de Par., 1879, 6. s., i, 123. ———. L'anesthésie par le protoxyde d'azote ; travaux récents de M. . . . Bull. Soc. méd. de l'Yonne 1879. Auxerre, 1880, xx, 167-182. ———. Anesthésie prolongée obtenue par le protoxyde d'azote à la pression normale. Compt. rend. Acad. d. sc., Par., 1883, xcvi, 1271-1274. ———. Faits sur le protoxyde d'azote. Compt. rend. Soc. de biol., Par., 1885, 8. s., ii, 520.—**Bigelow** (H. J.) Nitrous oxide gas for surgical purposes in 1848. Boston M. & S. J., 1868, lxxviii, 17. ———. Excision of breast ; anæsthesia by nitrous oxide gas. *Ibid.*, 74.—**Binz** (C.) Ueber Stickstoffoxydul. Wien. med. Bl., 1884, vii, 675-679.— **Bird** (T.) Operating with nitrous oxide under high pressure. Med. Times & Gaz., Lond., 1881, ii, 115. — **Blanchard** (R.) Protoxyde d'azote. N. dict. de méd. et chir. prat., Par., 1880, xxix, 766-782.—**Bordier** (A.) Note sur les effets narcotiques du protoxyde d'azote ; action favorable du sulfate de quinine. J. de thérap., Par., 1876, iii, 885-891. *Also :* Bull. et mém. Soc. de thérap. 1876, Par., 1877, 2. s., iii, 127-135.—**Brailey** (W. A.) Nitrous oxide as an anæsthetic in squint operations. Lancet, Lond., 1880, i, 811.—**Braine** (F. W.) Some phenomena of anæsthesia by protoxide of nitrogen. Brit. M. J., Lond., 1869, i, 67. ———. On the chemistry of nitrous oxide gas. Tr. Odont. Soc. Gr. Brit., Lond., 1871-2, n. s., iv, 177-185. ———. Administration of nitrous oxide as an anæsthetic. Brit. M. J., Lond., 1873, i, 153.—**Brown** (J. P. H.) Protoxide of nitrogen. South. M. & S. J., Augusta, 1866-7, 3. s., i, 557-560.—**Browne-Mason** (J. T.), **Drake** & **Pattison.** Alleged death from the effects of nitrous oxide gas. Tr. Odont. Soc. Gr. Brit., Lond., 1872- 3, n. s., v, 83-94.—**Brush** (G. W.) Nitrous oxide in minor surgery. Proc. M. Soc. County Kings, Brooklyn, 1877, ii, 279-287.—**Burckhardt-His** (M.) Erfahrungen über die Anwendung des Stickoxydulgases als Anästheticum. Cor.-Bl. f. schweiz. Aerzte, Basel, 1873, iii, 281-285.— **Buxton** (D. W.) On the physiological action of nitrous oxide. Tr. Odont. Soc. Gr. Brit., Lond., 1885-6, n. s., xviii, 133-164. ———. On the physiological action of nitrous oxide gas. *Ibid.*, 1886-7, n. s., xix, 90-131, 1 l., 3 pl. *Also :* Brit. J. Dent. Sc., Lond., 1887, xxx, 301 ; 351 ; 408.— **Cattlin** (W. A. H.) Nitrous oxide as an anæsthetic. Med. Times & Gaz., Lond., 1868, ii, 78. — **Cazeneuve** (P.) À propos de la préparation du protoxyde d'azote. Lyon méd., 1884, xlvii, 274-280.—**Clover** (J. T.) On the administration of nitrous oxide. Brit. M. J., Lond., 1868, ii, 491. ———. Face-piece, etc., for the direct administration of compressed nitrous oxide gas. Tr. Odont. Soc. Gr. Brit. 1868, Lond., 1869, n. s., i, 68.—**Coleman** (A.) Protoxide of nitrogen as an anæsthetic. St. Barth. Hosp. Rep., Lond., 1869, v, 153-164. —**Cummings** (E. P.) Is nitrous oxide anæsthetic? Boston M. & S. J., 1853, xlvii, 166-172.—**Death** after the administration of nitrous oxide. Brit. M. J., Lond., 1873, i, 126. —**Death** (The) from nitrous oxide ; proceedings at the inquest ; details of the post mortem appearances. Med. Times & Gaz., Lond., 1877, i, 456. — **Death** while under the effects of nitrous oxide. Lancet, Lond., 1877, i, 509. — **Description** of diagram of Mr. Porter's apparatus for making nitrous oxide gas. Tr. Odont. Soc. Gr. Brit. 1868, Lond., 1869, n. s., i, 67.— **Döderlein** (A.) Ueber Stickoxydul-Sauerstoffanästhesie. Tagebl. d. Versamml. deutsch. Naturf. u. Aerzte, Strassb., 1885, lviii, 111-119. *Also :* Wien. med. Bl., 1885, viii, 1207 ; 1243. *Also :* Allg. Wien. med. Ztg., 1885, xxxv, 442 ; 453 ; 467. *Also :* Arch. f. Gynaek., Berl., 1885-6, xxvii, 85-101. *Also* [Abstr.] : Centralbl. f. Gynäk., Leipz., 1885, ix, 641. — **Duchesne** (L.) Du protoxyde d'azote comme anesthésique. J. de chim. méd., etc., Par., 1873, xlvii, 308 ; 354. — **Dunn** (C.) Il gas protossido di azoto come anestetico nella estrazione dei denti. Imparziale, Firenze, 1869, ix, 557-560. — **Fatal** suffocation from nitrous oxide gas. Lancet, Lond., 1873, i, 478. — **Fox** (C. I.) On the use of nitrous oxide as an anæsthetic in surgery, with Coxeter's liquid gas. Lancet, Lond., 1876, i, 479 ; 515.— **Gay** (C. C. F.) On the protoxyde of azote as an anæsthetic agent. Buffalo M. & S. J., 1866-7, vi, 43-45.— **Gibbons** (H.) A personal experience of nitrous oxid as an anesthetic. Pacific M. & S. J., San Fran., 1876-7, xix, 481-486. — **Giberson** (C. H.) Operations under nitrous oxide. Tr. M. Soc. N. Y., Syracuse, 1878, 190-195.—**Goetz** (E.) De l'anesthésie par le protoxyde d'azote sous pression, d'après la méthode de P. Bert. Rev. méd. de la Suisse Rom., Genève, 1884, iv, 75-89. — **Goltstein** (M.) Ueber die physiologischen Wirkungen des Stickoxydulgases. Arch. f. d. ges. Physiol., Bonn, 1878, xvii, 331-373, 5 pl.—**Harrison.** Report on protoxide of nitrogen as an anæsthetic. Tr. Odont. Soc. Gr. Brit. 1868, Lond., 1869, n. s., i 31 ; 159. ———. Second report of the joint committee appointed by the Odontological Society of Great Britain, etc., to inquire into the value and advantages of the protoxide of nitrogen as an anæsthetic in surgical operations *Ibid.*, 1872-3, n. s., v, 11-34.—**Haslam** (D.) Two operations performed under the influence of nitrous oxide

Nitrous *oxide*.

gas. Lancet, Lond., 1870, ii, 535.—**Hele** (W.) The automatic supply of nitrous oxide. Tr. Odont. Soc. Gr. Brit., Lond., 1872-3, n. s., v, 95-116.—**Hermann** (L.) Ueber die physiologischen Wirkungen des Stickstoffoxydgases. Arch. f. Anat., Physiol. u. wissensch. Med., Leipz., 1864, 521-536. ———. Ueber die Wirkungen des Stickstoffoxydgases auf das Blut. *Ibid.*, 1865, 469-481. ———. Notiz über die Empfehlung des Stickoxyduls als Anæstheticum. Berl. klin. Wchnschr., 1866, iii, 115. ———. In Sachen des Stickstoffoxydulgases. Centralbl. f. klin. Med., Leipz., 1885, vi, 161-163.—**Hewitt** (F.) A new method of administering and economizing nitrous oxide gas. Lancet, Lond., 1885, i, 840. ———. An inquiry into several methods of administering nitrous oxide gas. Med. Chron., Manchester, 1885-6, iii, 363-380. ———. The administration of nitrous oxide and ether in combination or succession. Brit. M. J., Lond., 1887, ii, 452-454.—**Hewson** (A.) Some comments on the history of nitrous oxide gas as an anæsthetic, and on the analgesic effects of rapid breathing. Tr. Internat. M. Cong. 1876, Phila., 1877, 642-657. — **Hillischer** (H. T.) Ueber die allgemeine Verwendbarkeit der Lustgas-Sauerstoffnarcosen in der Chirurgie und den respiratorischen Gaswechsel bei Lustgas und Lustgas-Sauerstoff. Oesterr.-ungar. Vrtljschr. f. Zahnh., Wien, 1886, ii, 343-353. ———. Zu Dr. Ulbrich's Aufsatz: "Ueber die Lustgas-Sauerstoff-Narcose". Prag. med. Wchnschr., 1887, xii, 60.—**Holden** (E.) On the inhalation of the nitrous oxide gas when the lungs are diseased. Am. J. M. Sc., Phila., 1870, lx, 61-71.—**Hollaender** (L.) Das Stickstoffoxydul, als Anæstheticum. Berl. klin. Wchnschr., 1868, v, 234.— **Homicide** par imprudence; anesthésie par le protoxyde d'azote; mort du patient; jugement. Gaz. d. hôp., Par., 1885, lviii, 1117.—**Jacquème.** Histoire chimique et physiologique du protoxyde d'azote. Marseille méd., 1873, x, 541-561.—**Jeannel.** Note sur le protoxyde d'azote considéré comme agent anesthésique. Gaz. hebd. de méd., Par., 1869, 2. s., vi, 786-788. *Also:* Mém. et bull. Soc. méd.-chir. d. hôp. de Bordeaux, 1870, v, 64-76.—**Jolyet** (F.) & **Blanche** (T.) Nouvelles recherches sur le protoxyde d'azote. Arch. de physiol. norm. et path., Par., 1873, v, 364-374. ———. Les résultats d'expériences nouvelles sur le protoxyde d'azote entreprises par eux dans le laboratoire de physiologie de la Faculté des sciences. Compt. rend. Soc. de biol. 1873, Par., 1874, 5. s., v, 223-225.—**Kidd** (C.) The oxide of nitrogen as an anæsthetic agent. Dublin Q. J. M. Sc., 1868, xlvi, 340-349. ———. "Laughing-gas" and chloroform in London practice. Edinb. M. J., 1868-9, xiv, 57-58. — **Klikowitsch** (S.) Ueber die therapeutische Wirkung des Stickoxyduls in einigen Krankheiten. St. Petersb. med. Wchnschr., 1880, v, 117. ———. Weitere Untersuchungen über die therapeutische Wirkung des Stickstoffoxyduls. *Ibid.*, 249. ———. Das Stickstoffoxydul und Versuch seiner Anwendung in der Therapie. Arch. f. path. Anat., etc., Berl., 1883, xciv, 148; 227.— **Kreutzmann.** Zur Verwendbarkeit der Lachgassauerstoff-Narkose in der Chirurgie. Berl. klin. Wchnschr., 1887, xxiv, 648-650. — **Laffont** (M.) Contre-indications aux inhalations de protoxyde d'azote pur. Compt. rend. Soc. de biol., Par., 1885, 8. s., ii, 716-720. ———. Accidents consécutifs aux inhalations du protoxyde d'azote pur. *Ibid.*, 759. ———. Influence de l'anesthésie par inhalations de protoxyde d'azote pur sur diverses fonctions de l'économie. Compt. rend. Acad. d. sc., Par., 1886, cii, 176-178. *Also:* France méd., Par., 1886, i, 125-127. *Also:* Thérap. contemp., Par., 1886, vi, 82-84.—**Larison** (C. W.) A case of tuberculosis treated by nitrous oxide. Cincin. M. News, 1874, iii, 445-449. — **Lee** (B.) Nitrous oxide as a therapeutic agent. Med. Rec., N. Y., 1880, xvii, 494.— **Leeds** (A.) Preparation of nitrous oxide. Brit. M. J., Lond., 1868, i, 373.—**Lilly** (H. M.) Nitrous oxide. Med. & Surg. Reporter, Phila., 1868, xix, 451. — **Limousin.** Sur l'action du protoxyde d'azote. Bull. et mém. Soc. de thérap. 1868-9, Par., 1871, ii, 110-119. — **Lutaud** (A.) L'anesthésie par le protoxyde d'azote sous tension; méthode de M. Paul Bert. Gaz. hebd. de méd., Par., 1879, 2. s., xvi, 613. ———. L'anesthésie par le protoxyde d'azote sous tension. *Ibid.*, 1880, 2. s., xvii, 545; 577. ———. Gaz hilarant: Dict. encycl. d. sc. méd., Par., 1881, 4. s., vii, 132-162. — **Lyddon** (G.) Apparent insusceptibility to the influence of nitrous oxide. Brit. M. J., Lon l., 1881, i, 16.— **McLain** (A. F.) Nitrous oxide gas. N. Orl. M. & S. J., 1866-7, xix, 600-608. — **Maclaren** (R.) On nitrous oxide gas and its use as an anæsthetic. Edinb. M. J., 1871, xvi, 591-601, 2 pl. *Also,* Reprint. — **MacMunn** (C. A.) A spectroscopic explanation of the action of nitrous oxide. Dublin J. M. Sc., 1879, 3. s., lxviii, 210.—**Magitot.** Sur l'anesthésie par le protoxyde d'azote. Bull. et mém. Soc. de chir. de Par., 1875, n. s., i, 217-219.—**Manley** (I.), jr. Is nitrous oxide anæsthetic? Boston M. & S. J., 1852, xlvi, 435.—**Marcy** (E. E.) Removal of a large scirrhous testicle from a man while under the influence of nitrous oxide gas. *Ibid.*, 1847-8, xxxvii, 97-99. — **Martin** (C.) De l'anesthésie par le protoxyde d'azote avec ou sans tension, suivie d'une note sur la germination en présence du protoxyde d'azote sous pression. Lyon méd., 1883. xlii, 181; 217; 268.—**Martin-Lauzer.** Du protoxyde d'azote comme agent anesthésique. Rev. de thérap. méd.-chir.,

Nitrous *oxide*.

Par., 1867, xxxiv, 262-264. — **Mason** (B.) Report of the late fatal operation under nitrous oxide gas. Lancet, Lond., 1873, i, 254.— **Muñoz de Luna** (R. T.) El acid hiponítrico considerado como desinfectante, agente profiláctico y curativo del cólera morbo asiático. Siglo méd., Madrid, 1884, xxxi, 675; 694; 708. *Also, transl.:* Berl. klin. Wchnschr., 1886, xxiii, 140.—**Nelson** (C. E.) Dangerous inhalation of nitrous oxide gas. Canada M. Rec., Montreal, 1880-81, ix, 193.—**Nitrous** oxide—is it safe for inhaling? Boston M. & S. J., 1865-6, lxxiii, 116-118. — **von Nussbaum.** Narcose mit Stickstoffoxydulgas; 280 Experimente. Verhandl. d. deutsch. Gesellsch. f. Chir., Berl., 1874, i, 91-93. — **Oddo** (D.) Observations pratiques sur les symptômes qui accompagnent l'inhalation du gaz protoxyde d'azote et sur les signes caractéristiques qui précisent le moment où doit commencer l'opération chirurgicale. Marseille méd., 1873, x, 613-616. — **Osmun** (J. A.) The legal and moral responsibility of dentists in the administration of nitrous-oxide gas. Tr. N. Jersey Dent. Soc., Newark, 1884, 174-182. — **Ottley** (W.) On a case of damage to the heart from the inhalation of nitrous oxide. Lancet, Lond., 1883, i, 95. — **Palmer** (T. W. G.) An atmosphere of nitrous oxide. Tr. Odont. Soc. Gr. Brit., Lond., 1872-3, n. s., v, 5-10. — **Patruban.** Das Lustgas, ein Anæstheticum für kurz dauernde Operationen, insbesondere Zahnextractionen. Allg Wien. med. Ztg., 1866, xi, 17-19.—**Préterre** (A.) Propriétés physiologiques du protoxyde d'azote, appliqué aux opérations chirurgicales. Bull. gén. de thérap., etc., Par., 1870, lxxiv, 160; 215.—**Purcell** (W. J.) Death from the inhalation of nitrous oxide gas. Med. & Surg. Reporter, Phila., 1872, xxvi, 343-345.— **Rendle** (R.) On the use of protoxide of nitrogen gas; and on a new mode of producing rapid anæsthesia with bichloride of methylene. Brit. M. J., Lond., 1869, ii, 412.— **Réthy** (M.) A kéjgázról. [Laughing-gas.] Gyógyászat, Budapest, 1887, xxvii, 107; 120.—**Ribnitzki.** Der Todesfall durch Stickstoffoxydul im Dental-Hospital zu London. Deutsche Monatschr. f. Zahnh., Leipz., 1884, ii, 511-518.—**Rios.** El gas lloron, denominade risueño por un charlatan (con documentos). Gac. méd. de Lima, 1865-6, x, no. 221, 174; no. 222, 181.—**Ritter.** Mode d'action du protoxyde d'azote. Mém. Soc. de méd. de Nancy (1873-4), 1875, 5-7. — **Rottenstein.** De l'emploi du protoxyde d'azote. J. de thérap., Par., 1877, iv, 96-100.—**Sauer** (C.) Die Anästhesie durch Stickstoffoxydul in 40 Fällen versucht. Berl. klin. Wchnschr., 1868, v, 384. ———. Vorläufige Mittheilung der weiteren Versuche, mit Stickstoffoxydul-Gemischen zu anästhesiren. *Ibid.*, 1869, vi, 366.—**Scheller** (A.) Znieczulenie (anæsthesia) za pomocą tlenku azotu. Gaz. lek., Warszawa, 1869, vi, 753; 799; 832 — **Schrauth** (C.) Das Stickoxydul-Gas und seine Anwendung in der chirurgischen Praxis. Aerztl. Int.-Bl., München, 1880, xxvii, 305-309. ———. Das Lustgas und seine Verwendbarkeit in der Chirurgie. Samml. klin. Vortr., Leipz., 1886, No. 281 (Chir., No. 87, 2605-2626).—**Secretan** (A.) Accident après l'inhalation de protoxyde d'azote. Bull. Soc. méd. de la Suisse Rom., Lausanne, 1877, xi, 111.—**Sims** (J. M.) On the nitrous oxyde gas as an anæsthetic. Brit. M. J., Lond., 1868, i, 349.—**Skene** (A. J. C.) Nitrous oxide to facilitate examination and treatment of insane patients. Am. J. Obst., N. Y., 1879, xii, 616.— **Skogsborg** (R.) Underdånig ansökan af . . . angående användande af qväfoxidulgas såsom anæsteticum. [Nitrous oxide as anæsthetic.] Hygiea, Stockholm, 1879, xli, 453-455.—**Sprague** (A. W.) Nitrous oxide as an anæsthetic. Boston M. & S. J., 1864-5, lxxi, 169. ———. Nitrous oxide as an anæsthetic and therapeutic. *Ibid.*, 1866, lxxiv, 313-315.—**Stanley** (F.) Poisoning by the inhalation of impure nitrous oxide gas. Lancet, Lond., 1842-3, i, 395.— **Taylor** (C. F.) Nitrous oxide as an anæsthetic, with report of seven cases. Med. Rec., N. Y., 1857-8, ii, 77.— **Tittel.** Das Stickstoffoxydulgas als Anästheticum bei Kreissenden. Jahresb. d. Gesellsch. f. Nat.- u. Heilk. in Dresd., 1882-3, 81.—**Turnbull** (L.) Anæstheticsand narcotics. Independ. Pract., N. Y., 1881, ii, 161-170. ———. Ether. *Ibid.*, 225-232. ———. Nitrous oxide gas. *Ibid.*, 387; 464. — **Ulbrich.** Ueber die Lustgassauerstoffnarcose; mit Beziehung auf Hillischer's Veröffentlichung. Prag. med. Wchnschr., 1887, xii, 27-30.—**Underwood** (T.) Protoxide of nitrogen as an anæsthetic. Tr. Odont. Soc. Gr. Brit., Lond., 1872-3, n. s., v, 11.—**Vetlesen** (H. J.) 240 Lystgasnarkoser. Norsk Mag. f. Lægevidensk., Christiania, 1886, 4 R., i, 425-433.—**Villar.** Gas "risueño". Gac. méd. de Lima, 1865-6, x, no. 221, 170-174.—**Von der Heyde** (H.) De l'emploi du protoxyde d'azote comme anesthésique dans les opérations dentaires. Gaz. méd. d'Orient, Constantinople, 1885-6, xxviii, 51; 73. — **Warner** (F.) Convulsion commencing in the face and hand from the influence of nitrous oxide gas. Lancet, Lond., 1882, i, 985. — **Weisse** (F. D.) Nitrous oxide gas. Sanitarian, N. Y., 1874-5, ii, 24-34. *Also,* Reprint.—**Westcott** (A.) Nitrous oxide or laughing gas as an anæsthetic. Am. M. Times, N. Y., 1864, viii, 147; 158. — **Wiet** (E.) Anesthésie chirurgicale au moyen du protoxyde d'azote. Tribune méd., Par., 1880, xiii, 104-106.—**Williams** (W. R.) A death during the administration of nitrous oxide gas. Brit. M. J., Lond., 1883, ii, 729. — **Winderling,**

Nitrous *oxide*.

Del protossido d' azoto impiegato come anestetico nell' estrazione dei denti. Gazz. med. ital. lomb , Milano, 1875, 7. s., ii, 241. — **Witzinger** (M.) Ueber die Anwendung der Stickstoffoxydul-Sauerstoff-Narcose bei grösseren chirurgischen Eingriffen. Wien. med. Presse, 1888, xxix, 47–51.—**Woodhouse** (J.) Observations on the effects of the nitrous oxide, when taken into the lungs. Phila. M. Museum, 1807–8, iv 179–183. — **X.** L'anesthésie par le protoxyde d'azote. (Une expérience à l'Hôpital Lariboisière.) Année méd., Caen, 1878–9, iv, 177–185.—**Xifra** (J.) Caso de muerte débido à la administración del gas protóxido de ázoe. Lanceta, Barcel., 1885, iii, 2–4. — **Ziegler** (G. J.) Toxicological applications of nitrous oxide. Boston M. & S. J., 1852, xlvi, 245–277. ——. Experimental investigations on the antidotal and revivifying properties of nitrous oxide. *Ibid.*, 1852–3, xlvii, 383–392. ——. Nitrous oxide in asphyxia. Med. & Surg. Reporter, Phila., 1862–3, ix. 384. ——. Nitrous oxide; its mechanical properties and applications. Am. M. Times, N. Y., 1863, vi, 65. ——. Researches on the medical properties and applications of protoxide of nitrogen, nitrous oxide, or laughing gas. Med. & Surg. Reporter, Phila., 1864, xi. 204; 263; 293: 1864–5, xii, 120; 272; 304; 345. — **Zuntz** (W.) Ueber die Wirkungen des Stickoxydulgases. Arch. f. d. ges. Physiol., Bonn, 1878, xvii, 135.

Nitsch (Joh. Fridrico). * De cancro. 28 pp. 4°. *Jenæ, lit. Krebsianis,* [1713].
> For Biography, *see* **Wedelius** (Geo. Wolff.)

Nitsche (Andreas) [1767–]. * Momenta quædam comparationis regni animalis cum vegetabili. 47 pp. 4°. *Lipsiæ, ex off. Bueschelia,* [1788].
> For Biography, *see* **Platnerus** (Ernestus).

Nitsche (Fridericus Herrmannus). * De valvula coli. 18 pp. 4°. *Lipsiæ, typ. G. Staritzii,* [1843].

Nitsche (Hinrich). Beiträge zur Kenntniss der Bryozoen. Neue Folge. Habilitationsschrift. 1 p. l., 83 pp., 3 pl. 8°. *Leipzig, W. Engelmann,* 1871.
> Repr. from: Ztschr. f. wissensch. Zool., xxi.

Nitsche (Julius). * De arthrophlogosi chronica, addita historia morbi. 30 pp. 8°. *Gryphiæ, F. Hache,* 1867.   C.

Nitsche (Wilh. H.) * Ueber Supinationshindernisse nach Vorderarmfracturen. 20 pp. 8°. *Leipzig, Huethel u. Legler,* 1868. [P., v. 276.]

Nitschius (Mauritius Fridericus). * De valetudine senum tuenda. 32 pp. 4°. *Halæ Magdeb., typ. J. C. Hilligeri,* [1725].

Nitschke (Elia). Exercitationum physiologicarum tertia, de chylificatione. 4 l. sm. 4°. [*Lipsiæ,* 1668.]

Nitschke (Gotofredus Samuel.) * De tumoribus tunicatis. 32 pp. 4°. *Jenæ, lit. Wertherianis,* [1719].
> For Biography, *see* **Slevogt** (Jo. Hadrianus).

Nitschke (Henricus) [1817–]. * Morbi venerei, qualis sæculis tribus proximis fuerit, brevis expositio. 40 pp. 8°. *Berolini, typ. Nietackianis,* [1840].

Nitschke (Th.) Pyrenomycetes Germanici. Die Kernpilze Deutschlands. v. 1. 320 pp. 8°. *Breslau, E. Trewendt,* 1867.

Nitschkie (Elias Godofredus). * De calculo renum. 23 l. 4°. *Lugd. Bat., A. Elzevier,* [1700].

Nittinger (Carl G. G.) * Status putridus cum febre. 106 pp. 8°. *Würzburg, C. W. Becker's Wittwe,* 1835.

——. Ueber die 50jährige Impfvergiftung des württembergischen Volkes. 79 pp. 8°. *Stuttgart, Hallberger,* 1850.

——. Die Impfvergiftung. 1. Ansicht, 2. Theil. 208 pp. 8°. *Stuttgart, Hallberger,* 1852.

——. Das falsche Dogma von der Impfung und seine Rückwirkung auf Wissenschaft und Staat. 2 Abschn. 1 p. l., 232 pp., 2 l., 7 pl. 8°. *München, G. Franz,* 1857.
> CONTENTS.
> 1. Abschnitt. Die Impfung vor der Universität.
> 2. Abschnitt. Die Impfung vor der Presse.

Nittinger (Carl G. G.)—continued.

——. Das englische Blaubuch für die Vaccination und der Spiritualismus. 67 pp., 1 pl. 8°. *Stuttgart, J. Kreuzer,* 1857.
> Bound with his: Das falsche Dogma von der Impfung [etc.] 8°. *München,* 1857.

——. Das schwarze Buch vom Impfen. Zeugnisse und Thatsachen. Die Impfzeit und die Protestanten gegen Jenner's Gift und Zauber. viii, 135 pp., 9 pl. 8°. *Leipzig, G. Brauns,* 1859.

——. Die Impfzeit und die Protestanten gegen Jenner's Gift und Zauber vor der württemb. Ständekammer im Sept. 1858, vor dem engl. Parlament im Juli 1858. 237 pp., 1 l., 2 pl., 1 ch., port. 8°. *Leipzig, G. Brauns,* 1859.

——. Mémoire sur la vaccination, contenant une réfutation de la doctrine de Jenner, présenté au xxviiie Congrès scientifique de France. 15 pp. 4°. *Bordeaux, L. Cordec* [*and others*], 1861.

——. Jenner's Gant vor dem wissenschaftlichen Congresse von Frankreich zu Cherbourg 1860, zu Bordeaux 1861. Entscheid über 10.000 deponirte und 40,000 garantirte Franken, Preis für den, welcher den Vorwurf der Charlatanerie von der Vaccination wissenschaftlich abzuweisen vermöchte ? oder Condemnation der Impfung als Ursache der Herbstfarbe des menschlichen Antlizes, der Abschwächung und Verminderung des Menschengeschlechts. Eine Warnung für den Staat, für die Familie und für den Einzelnem. Mit Karten, Abbildungen und französischem Anhang. iv, 172 pp., 4 ch., 7 pl. 8°. *Leipzig, G. Brauns,* 1862.

——. Gott und Abgott, oder die Impfhexe. I. Geschichte und Meteorologie: Der Glaube an den Impfschuz ist Aberglaube. II. Die Impfhexe in Würtemberg: Natürliches System. III. Die Uebel der Impfung: Uebersezung des englischen Blaubuchs, im Auszug. IV. Petitionen an die Stände Würtembergs, nebst Beilagen. 208 pp. 8°. *Stuttgart, A. Schaber,* 1863.

——. Testament der Natur gegen die Vergewaltigung der Völker durch den Heuland aus Bêtelehem nemlich durch die giftige und nuzlose Impfung. Für alle Bürger, welche nun wie einst die Schweizer vor dem Gesslers-Hut ohne Kopf sich beugen und den Gruss sagen müssen: "Gloria der Impfung!" Ein Schmerzensruf aus Deutschland, Frankreich, England, Italien, Holland, Ungarn, Dänemark, etc. xii, 452 pp. 8°. *Leipzig, G. Brauns,* 1865.
> Offene Klage vor Gericht wider die Impfvergiftung in Würtemberg. Beweis-Akten von Dr. . . . in Stuttgart.

——. Die Staatsmagie der Impfung und die üblen Gesundheitsverhältnisse der Bevölkerung vor der Abgeordneten-Kammer Würtembergs oder Was ist Wahrheit ? xii, 316 pp., 6 pl. 8°. *Leipzig, G. Brauns,* 1866.

——. Der Kampf wider die Impfung im Volk und Parlament von England, nebst populären öffentlich gehaltenen Vorträgen bewährter englischer Aerzte und Menschenfreunde, welche sorglichen Eltern ehrlichen Rath geben: ob sie ihre Kinder impfen lassen sollen. 240 pp. 8°. *Stuttgart, E. Ebner,* 1867.

——. Der Raub am Mutterrecht und der Flügelschnitt der Nation durch den Impfzwang, nebst praktischer Hausmedicin für die Mütter bei Cholera, Ruhr, Blattern, Scharlach, Impfseuche, etc. Sendschreiben an die Gräfin von Noailles. 55 pp., 9 pl.; 20 pp., 3 pl. 8°. *Stuttgart, C. Grüninger,* 1867.

——. Die Impfgiftung und das betrogene Baiern, ein Beitrag zur Leidensgeschichte der Fürsten und Völker, nebst Germania's Bild und England's Antrag auf Untersuchung viva voce (Enquête). 144 pp., 1 pl. 8°. *Stuttgart, E. Ebner,* 1867.
> Title on cover : Die Impfung ein Missbrauch.

Nittinger (Carl G. G.)—continued.
——. Staat und Volk in bitterem Zweifel an der Vaccination. 96 pp. 8°. *Stuttgart*, 1868.
——. Die Impfregie mit Blut und Eisen. Der Raub am Mutterrecht, der Flügelschnitt der Nation und als Strafe dafür: die innere Abhäutung, Diphthera, statt der äusern, dera. Heilung der Diphtheren, insbesondere der Cholera des Abendlandes. Social-medicale Studie deutsch-englisch; Thesen französisch; Uebersicht italienisch; Verbot der Impfung holländisch. 199 pp., 1 frontisp., 5 tab., 9 pl. 8°. *Stuttgart, C. Grüninger*, 1868.
——. Verwerfung der Impfung. Rede gehalten in der Tonhalle zu Leipzig am 4. Mai 1869. 24 pp. 16°. *Stuttgart, L. Wittig*, [1869].
See, also, **Schieferdecker** (Chr. Charles). Dr. C. G. G. Nittinger's evils of vaccination. 12°. *Philadelphia*, 1856.

Nitze (M.)
See **Leiter** (Josef). Beschreibung und Instruction [etc.] 4°. *Wien*, 1880.

Nitzelnadel (Ernst). * Zur Therapie des Nabelschnurvorfalles bei Schädellage. [Jena.] 24 pp. 8°. *Altenburg, O. Bonde*, 1887.

Nitzelnadel (Paul). * Ueber nervöse Hyperidrosis und Anidrosis. 61 pp., 1 l. 8°. *Jena, A. Neuenhahn*, 1867.

Nitzen (Ernestus). De principalibus τῶν ἀρχῶν μορίων affectibus quæstiones varias. 12 l. 4°. *Basileæ, J. J. Genathium*, [1617].
——. De phlebotomia.
In : AGONISMATA med. Marpurgensia. 4°. *Marpurgi Cattorum*, 1618, 47–71.

Nitzsch (Abrahamus) [–1749]. * De dolore et spasmo ex calculo felleo, oder: Vom Schmertz und Krampf des Steins aus der Galle. 28 pp., 2 l. 4°. *Halæ Magdeb., typ. J. C. Hilligeri*, [1731].
——. Opiniones medicorum artis evehendæ pestem. 3 l. 4°. [*Petropoli*, 1734.]

Nitzsch (Asmundus Reinholdus) [1825–]. * De ratione inter pulsus frequentiam et corporis altitudinem habita. 42 pp. sm. 8°. *Halis Sax., typ. Schmidtianis*, [1849]. [*Also, in :* P., v. 107.]

Nitzsch (Carolus). * De ferro in animalibus obvio. 2 p. l., 35 pp., 2 l. 8°. *Bonnæ, formis C. et F. Krueger*, 1846. [P., v. 575.]

Nitzsch (Christianus Ludovicus) [1782–1837]. Commentatio de respiratione animalium. 56 pp. 4°. *Vitebergæ, Zimmermann*, 1808. [P., v. 412.]
——. Præmissæ sunt observationes de avium arteria carotide communi. 36 pp. 4°. *Halæ, typ. Gebaueriis*, [1829].
For Biography, see **Seiler** (Burcard Guilielmus).

Nitzsch (Friedrich). Luther und Aristoteles. Festschrift zum vierhundertjährigen Geburtstage Luther's. 1 p. l., 51 pp. 8°. *Kiel, [Schmidt u. Klaunig*], 1883.

Nitzsch (Greg. Guilielmus). Memoria Christiani Rudolphi Guilielmi Wiedemanni, defuncti d. xxi. m. Decembr. a. m.d.c.c.cxl. 15 pp. 4°. *Kiliæ, C. F. Mohr*, 1841.

Nitzsche (Carolus Alexander). * Erysipelatis singulare exemplum, præmissa de hujus morbi natura commentatione. 24 pp. 8°. *Jenæ, typ. Branii*, [1837].

Nitzsche (Carolus Ferdinandus). * Diss. qua theoriæ generationis præcipue cum veteris tum recentioris ævi exponuntur. 1 p. l., 26 pp. 4°. *Vratislaviæ, typ. Universitatis*, [1817].

Nitzsche (Friedrich Robert). Beiträge zur Therapie der Rückgratsverkrümmungen, insbesondere der Scoliosis myopathica und habitualis, nach eigenen Erfahrungen mitgetheilt. vi, 49 pp., 1 pl. 8°. *Dresden, C. Höckner*, 1860.
——. The same. 2. Aufl. iv, 49 pp., 1 pl. 8°. *Dresden, H. Klemm*, 1860.
——. Die Heilung der Brust-Beschwerden durch ärztliche Zimmer-Gymnastik, oder populäre

Nitzsche (Friedrich Robert)—continued.
Darstellung und Beschreibung derjenigen heilgymnastischen Bewegungen, welche bei Krankheiten des Respirations- und Circulationsapparates, insbesondere bei Verunstaltung und Verengerung des Thorax, flacher und schwacher Brust, Hühnerbrust, bei Brustbeklemmungen, Herzbeengungen, Brustverschleimung, Bronchialkatarrh, Asthma, beginnender Lungentuberculose, etc., ausgezeichnete Dienste leisten. Nach vieljährigen praktischen Erfahrungen. 3 p. l., 108 pp., 12 pl. 8°. *Dresden, H. Klemm*, [1861].
——. Die Heilung der Unterleibs-Beschwerden durch ärztliche Zimmer-Gymnastik, populäre Darstellung und Beschreibung derjenigen heilgymnastischen Bewegungen, welche bei Trägheit und Stockungen der Unterleibsfunctionen, insbesondere bei Appetitlosigheit, träger Verdauung, Verdauungsschwäche, Magensäure, Magen- und Darmverschleimung, Flatulenz, Fettsucht, Anschoppungen im Pfordadersystem oder Hämorrhoidalbeschwerden, Anschwellungen der Leber und Milz, habitueller Leibesverstopfung und allen daher stammenden reflectirten Erscheinungen auf das Gehirn, wie bei Eingenommenheit des Kopfes, Hypochondrie, Hysterie, Melancholie, etc., ausgezeichnet Dienste leisten. Nach vieljährigen praktischen Erfahrungen bearbeitet. iv, 97 pp., 9 pl. 8°. *Dresden, H. Klemm*, 1861.

Nitzsche (Fridericus Theodorus Guilielmus). * De convalescentia ejusque ad morbos quosdam opportunitate et cura in ea instituenda prophylactica. 1 p. l., 24 pp., 1 l. 4°. *Vratislaviæ, typ. Universitatis*, [1809].

Nitzsche (Gustav Ferdinand). * De strabismo. 24 pp. 4°. *Lipsiæ, typ. J. F. Glueckii* [1840].
For Biography, see **Joerg** (Jo. Christ. Godo.)

Nivard (Raoul). * De l'amputation dans la zône emphysémateuse des membres atteints de gangrène traumatique. 40 pp. 4°. *Paris*, 1877, No. 50.

Nivelet. Étude sur le diagnostic différentiel des paralysies en général et sur leur traitement par l'électricité. 15 pp. 12°. *Commercy, C. Cabasse*, [1863].

Nivelet (F.) * Des indications thérapeutiques en général. 25 pp. 4°. *Paris*, 1834, No. 1, v. 269.
——. Molière et Gui Patin. (Molière et Gui Patin; satires médicales de Molière; Gui Patin et Théophraste Renaudot; la Faculté de Paris au xviie siècle; quelques critiques sur Gui Patin, son apologie.) 142 pp. 12°. *Paris, Berger-Lerrault & Cie.*, 1880.

Nivelet (René). * Du bain électrique, ses différents modes d'application, son action physiologique et ses effets thérapeutiques. 28 pp. 4°. *Paris*, 1867, No. 204.

Nivelon (J.-A.-P.) * Sur la pleurésie. 16 pp. 4°. *Paris*, 1832, No. 257, v. 256.

[**Niven** (*Miss*).] The meetings for wives and daughters. 8 pp. 8°. *Melbourne, Walker, May & Co.*, 1884.
Australian Health Soc. Publications, no. 21.

Niverd (Jules). * Considérations sur l'emploi de l'ophthalmoscope dans les méningites et l'hémorrhagie cérébrale. 31 pp. 4°. *Paris*, 1874, No. 176.

Nivert (Adolphe). * Remarques sur quelques maladies et la cautérisation appliquée à leur traitement. 40 pp. 4°. *Paris*, 1830, No. 100, v. 232.

Nivert (C.-F.) * Sur le sarcocèle et le cancer du testicule. 36 pp. 4°. *Paris*, 1814, No. 131, v. 105.

Nivert (Gustave-Adolphe). * De la version céphalique par les manœuvres externes dans les présentations vicieuses du fœtus. 119 pp. 4°. *Paris*, 1862, No. 200.

Nivet ([Annet] Vincent) [1809–]. * Recherches, observations et propositions sur différents points de médecine, de chirurgie, de physiologie et d'hygiène. 46 pp. 4°. *Paris*, 1838, No. 359, v. 331.

———. Notice sur l'établissement thermal de Royat (Puy-de-Dôme). 14 pp. 8°. *Clermont-Ferrand, Thibaud-Landriot frères*, 1855. [P., v. 1651; 1786.]

———. Rapport sur l'épidémie de fièvres intermittentes simples et pernicieuses qui a régné en 1856 et 1857 à Pérignat-ès-Allier (Puy-de-Dôme). 46 pp. 8°. *Clermont, F. Thibaud*, 1858. [P., v. 1667.

———. Documents sur l'organisation de la médecine des pauvres dans les campagnes. vi (1 l.), 64 pp. 8°. *Clermont-Ferrand, P. Hubler*, 1863.

———. Documents sur les épidémies qui ont régné dans l'arrondissement de Clermont - Ferrand de 1849 à 1864. Angines pseudo-membraneuses et croupes; fièvres intermittentes simples et pernicieuses; goître épidémique; choléra-morbus. 117 pp., 1 l. 8°. *Paris, J.-B. Baillière & fils*, 1865.

———. Notice historique sur les épidémies de l'arrondissement de Clermont, suivie d'un rapport sur l'épidémie de Mezel, année 1866. (Choléra-morbus, suettes miliaires, varioles et fièvres intermittentes.) 20 pp. 8°. *Clermont - Ferrand, F. Thebaud*, 1869.

———. Études sur le goître épidémique. 95 pp. 8°. *Paris, J.-B. Baillière & fils*, 1873.

———. La Bourboule, ses thermes et ses eaux minérales. 62 pp., 1 l., 2 pl. 8°. *Clermont-Ferrand, G. Mont-Louis*, 1879.

———. Traité du goître, appuyé sur des documents statistiques inédits et accompagné d'une carte de la distribution du Puy-de-Dôme. 297 pp., 1 map. 8°. *Paris, J.-B. Baillière & fils*, 1880.

———. Rapport sur l'engrais humain, les égouts et les fosses d'aisance. 129 pp., 1 l., 1 map. 8°. *Clermont-Ferrand, G. Mont-Louis*, 1881.
Repr. from: Trav. d. Cons. d'hyg. [etc.] du dép. du Puy-de-Dôme, 1881.

———. The same. 129 pp., 1 plan, 1 l. 8°. *Paris, J.-B. Baillière & fils*, 1882.

———. Eaux minérales. 48 pp. 8°. [*Clermont-Ferrand, n. d.*] [P., v. 1766.]
See, also, **Blatin** (Henry) & **Nivet** (V.) Traité des maladi s des femmes [etc.] 8°. *Paris*, 1842.

——— & **Aguilhon** (H.) Notice sur l'épidémie de choléra-morbus qui a ravagé le département du Puy-de-Dôme en 1849, adressé à M. le ministre de l'agriculture et du commerce. 63 pp. 8°. *Paris, J.-B. Baillière*, 1851. [*Also, in :* P., v. 461.]

Nivinski (E. I.) Vrach, publika, pechat, cholera. [The physician, the public, the press, cholera.] 13 pp. 8°. *St. Petersburg*, 1885.

Niwa Tokichiro. Seiyaku Zensho. [Complete system of pharmacy.] 10, 494, 8, 7 pp., 1 l. 8°. *Tokio*, 1881.
Japanese text.

Nix (Henr. Anton.) * De electro - magnetismo, ejusque vi et usu in medicina. 39 pp., 2 l. 8°. *Bonnæ, Krüger*, [1847]. [P., v. 575.]

Nixon (Montgomery). * De hydrope anasarca. 2 p. l., 30 pp. 8°. *Edinburgi, Balfour et Smellie*, 1789.

Nixon (Newton H.) North London, or University College Hospital. A history of the hospital from its formation to the year 1881. 60 pp. 8°. *London*, 1882.

Nixon (Robertus). * De voce humana. 22 pp. 8°. *Edinburgi, Abernethy et Walker*, 1807.

Nizam's Dominions. Report on the medical topography and statistics of the Nizam's military cantonments and army. Compiled partly from records in the superintending surgeon's office, and reports furnished by medical officers to the

Nizam's Dominions—continued. service. 81 pp., 10 maps. 8° *Madras, D. P. L. C. Connor*, 1852.

Nizenius (Ernest).
See **Petræus** (Henricus). De arthritide. *In :* NOSOL. harmonica dogmat. et hermet. 4°. *Marpurgi Cattorum*, 1616, ii, 441–465. ———. De obstructione hepatis. *In :* NOSOL. harmonica dogmat. et hermet. 4°. *Marpurgi Cattorum*, 1616, ii, 163–193.

Niziński (Sylwester). * Die doppelseitige Hüftgelenkresection. [Wurtzburg.] 30 pp. 8°. *Posen*, 1885.

Nizon (Theobaldus). * An litteratis vita cœlebs? Præses Ludovicus Pathiot. 4 pp. 4°. [*Paris*], *Quillau*, 1771.

———. * An uterina placenta radix? Præses Simon Antonius Bringaud. 4 pp. 4°. [*Paris*], *Quillau*, 1771.

———. * An variolis narcotica? Præses Jacobus Ludovicus Alleaume. 4 pp. 4°. [*Paris, Quillau*, 1771.]

———. * Num in resecandis artubus, carnis segmina reservare, satius? Præses Dyonysius-Claudius Doulcet. 4 pp. 4°. [*Paris, Quillau*, 1772.]

Nizschte (Christianus). De catarrho. 7 l. 4°. *Regiomonti, typ. P. Mensenii*, 1665.

Nizza.
See **Nice.**

N'Kassa.
Liebreich. Ueber die toxischen Wirkungen der N'Kassa-Rinde. Ztschr. f. Ethnol., Berl., 1875, vii, 248–250.

Noack (Alphons). * De nutricis virtutibus. 28 pp. 8°. *Lipsiæ, ex off. Rückmanni*, [1835].
Also, Co-Editor of : **Journal** für Arzneimittellehre, Leipzig, 1839.
See, also, **Schwabe** (Willmar). Pharmacopœa homœopathica [etc.] 8°. *Leipzig*, 1872.
For Biography, see **Kuhl** (Car. Aug.)

Noack (Carolus Augustus). * De melanosi cum in hominibus tum in equis obveniente. Specimen pathologiæ comparatæ. viii, 33 pp., 2 pl. 4°. *Lipsiæ, ex off. Hirschfeldiana*, 1826.

———. The same. Commentatio veterinario-medica de melanosi cum in hominibus tum in equis obveniente specimen pathologiæ comparatæ. viii, 33 pp., 3 pl. 4°. *Lipsiæ, L. Voss ; Parisiis, J.-B. Baillière*, [*n. d.*]
For Biography, see **Haase** (G. A.)

Noack (Carolus Augustus Eduardus). * De atrophia, creberrimo morborum infantilium symptomate. 38 pp. 8°. *Lipsiæ, typ. C. P. Melzeri*, [1848].

Noack (Paul Reinhold). * Beobachtungen über Peritonitis acuta. 35 pp. 8°. *Leipzig, C. E. Elbert*, 1865.
c.

Noack (Paulus [Theophilus]) [1836–]. * De echinococcis hepatis. 56 pp. 8°. *Gryphiswaldiæ, F. Hache*, 1860.
c.

———. Das öffentliche Gesundheitswesen des Regierungs-Bezirks Oppeln. General-Bericht erstattet von . . . 156 pp. roy. 8°. *Oppeln, G. Maste*, 1884.

——— & **Becker** (H.) Der Heilapparat des Inselbades bei Paderborn, nach den neuesten chemischen Untersuchungen. 30 pp. 8°. *Paderborn, P. Herle u. Comp.*, 1865.

Noad (Henry M.) Electro-physiology; being a popular account of the recent researches of Matteucci and others in this department of electrical science, including some observations on the therapeutic application of electricity. 67 pp. 8°. *London, G. Knight & Sons*, 1849.

———. Chemical manipulation and analysis, qualitative and quantitative. With an introduction explanatory of the general principles of chemical nomenclature, the construction and use of formulæ, the doctrine of equivalent proportions, and on the preparation and management

Noad (Henry M.)—continued.

of gases. A new ed., considerably enlarged. lxiv, 367 pp. 8°. *London, R. Baldwin*, 1852.

——. A manual of chemical analysis, qualitative and quantitative. xvi, 633 pp. 8°. *London, L. Reeve & Co.*, 1864.

See, also, **Normandy** (A.) The commercial hand-book of chemical analysis [etc.] 8°. *London*, 1875.

Nobel (Petrus). * Momenta quædam de actione alcalium in adfectione calculosa. 2 p. l., 26 pp., 1 l. 8°. *Traj. ad Rhenum, S. Alter*, [1823].

de Nobele (Eduardus Joannes). * Diss. de herniæ inguinalis incarceratione. 23 pp. 4°. *Lovanii, G. Cuelens*, [1827]. [P., v. 959.]

Nobert's *test plate.*

See **Microscope***, etc.*

Nobile (Antonio). Elogio storico di Macedonio Melloni, recitato nella reale Accademia delle scienze di Napoli nella tornata del 1 dicembre 1854. 74 pp. fol. *Napoli, G. Nobile*, 1855. [P., v. 1126.]

Repr. from: Rendic. Soc. r. Borbonica d. Accad. d. sc., 1854.

Nobiling (Alfred). Versuche über die Wirkungen des Brechweinsteines in kleiner Dose bei längerem Fortgebrauche. Gekrönte Preisschrift. 39 pp., 1 pl. 8°. *München, C. R. Schurich*, 1868.

Repr. from: Ztschr. f. Biol., München, 1868, iv.

Nobilis Socii Salodiensis præcertatio ad veram medicinam, pro Arabum et proborum medicorum tutela. 66 ff., 2 l. 12°. *Venetiis*, 1554.

Nobis (G.) * Quelques réflexions sur la méthode analytique et les systèmes. 20 pp. 4°. *Paris*, 1835, No. 141, v. 286.

Nobis (Joh.) * Ueber Aneurysma dissecans. 19 pp. 4°. *Würzburg, C. J. Becker*, 1873.

Noble. Notice sur les sangsues, lue à la Société centrale d'agriculture et des arts de Seine-et-Oise, dans sa séance du 6 mars 1822. 13 pp. 8°. [*Versailles, J.-T. Jacob*, 1822.] [P., v. 1677.]

Noble (Adolphe-Auguste). * Sur la métrite aiguë. 20 pp. 4°. *Paris*, 1835, No. 275, v. 290.

Noble (Daniel) [1810–85]. An essay on the means, physical and moral, of estimating human character. 23 pp. 8°. *Manchester, Prentice & Cathrall*, 1835. [P., v. 1238.]

——. Facts and observations relative to the influence of manufactures upon health and life. 81 pp. 8°. *London, J. Churchill*, 1843.

——. The brain and its physiology; a critical disquisition on the methods of determining the relations between the structure and functions of the encephalon. xvi, 450 pp. 8°. *London, J. Churchill*, 1846.

——. Wat is waar, wat onwaar in het dierlijk magnetisme? Kritische beschouwing der mesmerische daadzaken en theorien. Uit het Engelsch vertaald door J. N. Ramaer. iv, 154 pp., 2 l. 8°. *Zutphen, W. J. Thieme*, 1847.

——. On the question of contagion in cholera. 11 pp. 8°. *London, Wilson & Ogilvy*, 1849.

Repr. from: Lond. M. Gaz., n. s., viii.

——. Elements of psychological medicine. An introduction to the practical study of insanity, adapted for students and junior practitioners. xxiv, 340 pp. 12°. *London, J. Churchill*, 1853.

——. Three lectures on the correlation of psychology and physiology. 45 pp. sm. 8°. *London, T. Richards*, 1854.

Repr. from: Assoc. M. J., Lond., 1854, n. s., ii.

——. The same. 2. ed. xii, 356 pp. 8°. *London, J. Churchill*, 1855.

——. The human mind in its relations with the brain and nervous system. xiii, 157 pp. 8°. *London, J. Churchill*, 1858.

——. On certain popular fallacies concerning the production of epidemic diseases. 22 pp. 8°.

Noble (Daniel)—continued.

Manchester, Cave & Sever, 1859. [P., v. 503; 882; 1025.]

Repr. from: Tr. Manchester Statist. Soc., 1859.

——. On fluctuations in the death rate, with a glance at the causes, having especial reference to the supposed influence of the cotton famine on recent mortality. (Read before the Manchester Statistical Society, October 26, 1863.) 20 pp. 8°. *Manchester, Cave & Sever*, 1863.

Repr. from: Tr. Manchester Statist. Soc., 1863-4.

——. Thoughts on the value and significance of statistics. 14 pp. 8°. *Manchester, Cave & Sever*, 1866. [*Also, in:* P., v. 595.]

Repr. from: Tr. Manchester Statist. Soc., 1865-6.

Noble (Edward Moore). A treatise on opthalmy, and those diseases which are induced by inflammations of the eyes. With new methods of cure. Pt. 1. xiv, 144 pp. 8°. *Birmingham, Swinney & Hawkins*, 1800.

Noble (Geo. H.) Abortive treatment of mammary abscesses, and the cure of fissured nipples by means of a new and effectual compress. 8 pp. 8°. *Atlanta*, 1882.

Repr. from: Atlanta M. Reg., 1882, ii.

Noble (L.-R.) * Sur quelques déplacemens peu connus de la matrice. 20 pp. 4°. *Paris*, 1808, No. 145, v. 73.

Noble (W. H.) Useful tables. Compiled by . . . Printed by order of the secretary of state for war. iii, 64 pp. 16°. *London, W. Clowes & Sons*, [*n. d.*]

Noblejas.

See **Cholera** (*Asiatic, History, etc., of*), *by localities.*

Noblet (Charles-Louis). * Du rôle des composés sodiques dans l'économie. 88 pp. 4°. *Paris*, 1863, No. 78.

Noblet (E.) père.

Editor of: **Revue** militaire française, Paris, 1875.

Noblet (Pierre). * De la cachexie paludéenne. 31 pp. 4°. *Paris*, 1858, No. 123, v. 622.

de Nobrega (Gerardo José). On the cultivation of cochineal. 11 pp. 8°. [*n. p.*], 1849.

Repr. from: Pharm. J. & Tr., Lond., 1848-9, viii.

Nocera.

Badaloni (G.) I bagni di Nocera-Umbra. Idrologia. *Firenze*, 1883, v, 169-176.

Nocht ([Eduard Albrecht] Bernhard) [1857–]. * Ueber die Erfolge der Nervendehnung. 41 pp. 8°. *Berlin, L. Schumacher*, 1881.

Nociones, preceptos y medios que deben conocer las familias para prevenir el desarrollo del cólera morbo asiático y combatir sus primeros síntomas en el caso aún no probable de que invada nuestro territorio. Aprobadas por la Junta municipal de sanidad de Madrid en sesión de 1° de agosto de 1884 y publicadas por acuerdo del excmo. ayuntamiento, de 6 del citado mes. 24 pp. 16°. *Madrid*, 1884.

Nock (Ebenezer). William Harvey, M. D., F. R. S.: (The discoverer of the transit of the blood throughout) its entire route. And a romantic, biographic, and historic record of facts transpiring in the nineteenth century. 8 pp. 12°. *London*, 1886.

——. An Æsculapian dunciad! William Harvey, M. D., F. R. S., discoverer of the circulation of the blood throughout its entire route, a real born fool and the progenitor of a million of fools; and the grave and proud "doctors of Dull-Head College", an hereditary college of wooden-heads. A ghostly paradox, founded on extraordinary historic facts. 3. ed., revised and personified. 22 pp. 12°. *London*, 1887.

Nockher (Ferdinandus). * De morbis ductus thoracici. 40 pp. 4°. *Bonnæ, typ. C. Georgii*, [1831].

Nockher (Wilhelmus). * De aneurysmate. 30 pp. 4 . *Duisburgi, typ. F. W. Krämeri, 1816.*

Noctiluca.

ADLER (C. F.) * Noctiluca marina. 8°. *Upsaliæ,* 1752.
In: LINNÆUS. Amœnitates acad. [etc.] 8°. Amstelæd. et Lugd. Bat., 1756, iii, 202-210, 1 pl.
Bütschli (O.) Einige Bemerkungen über gewisse Organisationsverhältnisse der sog. Cilioflagellaten und der Noctiluca. Mit einem Beitrag von E. Askenasy. *Morphol. Jahrb., Leipz.,* 1884-5, x, 529-577, 3 pl.—**Carus** (J. V.) Ueber Noctiluca miliaris Sur. *Arch. f. mikr. Anat., Bonn,* 1868, iv, 351.—**Dönitz** (W.) Ueber Noctiluca miliaria Sur. *Arch. f. Anat., Physiol. u. wissensch. Med., Leipz.,* 1868, 137-149, 1 pl. ———. Ueber Noctiluca miliaris. Erwiderung an Herrn Prof. V. Carus. *Ibid.,* 750-754.—**Vignal** (W.) Recherches histologiques et physiologiques sur les noctiluques (Noctiluca miliaris, Suriray). École prat. d. hautes études. Lab. d'histol. du Coll. de France. *Trav.* 1877-8, Par., 1879, iv, 197-236, 2 pl. *Also: Arch. de physiol. norm. et path.,* Par., 1878, 2. s., v, 415-454, 2 pl.

Nocturnal *emissions.*

Morris (J.) Nocturnal emissions in women. *Tr. M. & Chir. Fac. Maryland,* Balt., 1877, 93-96.

Nodalle (Mich. Ign. Antonius). * De hepatis in morbis præcipue sympathia. 1 p. l., 73 pp., 1 l. 8°. *Dorpat, typ. J. C. Schünmanni,* 1816.

Nodari (Giuseppe). Fisiologia della tubercolosi pulmonare. 112 pp., 8 pl., 1 l. roy. 8°. *Padova, L. Penada,* 1879.
———. Gli alcaloidi cadaverici considerati nella loro genesi e portati nell' arringo delle cause penali. 29 pp. 8°. *Padova, frat. Salmin,* 1885.
———. Il rimedio istantaneo efficace e definitivo contro il dolore delle scottature di primo grado. (Communicazione preventiva.) 8 pp. 8°. *Padova, Prosperini,* 1886.

Nodding.

See **Convulsions** (*Nodding*).

Node (C.)
See **Lange** (A.) & **Node** (C.) Atlas de l'art des accouchemens, [etc.] fol. *Paris,* 1835.

Nodes.

See **Exostosis** (*Syphilitic*); **Syphilis**; **Tibia** (*Diseases of*).

Nodet (Amédée). * De l'application de la méthode sous-capsulo-périoste à la résection tibio-tarsienne. 82 pp. 4°. *Paris,* 1869, No. 57.

Nodet (Charles-Félix). * Contribution à l'étude des éruptions pemphigoïdes aiguës (pemphigus aigus; dermatoses bulleuses, pemphigoïdes). 166 pp. 4°. *Lyon,* 1880, No. 35.

Nodet (Louis). * Études cliniques et expérimentales sur les diverses espèces de chancres et particulièrement sur le chancre mixte. vi, 7-151 pp. 4°. *Montpellier, Boehm & fils,* 1863, No. 41.

Nodier (*Charles*)[1] [1780-1844].
Albertus. Charles Nodier, naturaliste et médecin ; sa théorie du cerveau. *Gaz. méd. de Par.,* 1885. 7. s., ii, 13-19.

Nodier (Charles)[2]. * Sur une ophthalmie causée par la lumière électrique. 41 pp., 1 l. 4°. *Paris,* 1881, No. 264.

Noë (Fridericus) [1838-]. * De chloroformii vi atque usu, et de anæstheticorum vetustate. 39 pp. 8°. *Gryphiæ, F. Hache,* [1863].

Noé (Moïse-Polidore). * I. Exposer les caractères de la roséole, ses variétés, sa marche, son traitement. II. [etc.] 46 pp. 4°. *Paris,* 1840, No. 267, v. 364.

Noebelius (Joh. Ludovicus). * Diss. explicans hydropem. 1 p. l., 28 pp. 4°. *Regiomonti, lit. Hartungianis,* [1764].

Noebling (Jo. Godofr. Michael). * De pilis eorumque morbis. 37 pp., 1 l. 4°. *Helmstadii, ex off. Schnorriana,* [1740].

Nöbling (Joh. Guilielmus).
See **Stock** (Joh. Christianus) & **Nöbling** (Joh. Guilielmus). De cadaveribus sanguisugis [etc.] 4°. *Jenæ,* 1732.

Noeggerath (Carolus Ernestus) [1817-]. * De voce, respiratione, deglutitione observationes quædam. vi, 12 pp., 1 l., 1 pl. 4°. *Bonnæ, typ. C. Georgii,* 1841.

Noeggerath (Emil Jacob). * Spicilegium casuum nonnullorum polypi nasi et pharyngis qui in clinico chirurgico Bonnensi novissimis annis observati sunt, addita descriptione methodi novæ ad extirpandum polypum pharyngis. 28 pp., 2 l. 8°. *Bonnæ, formis C. Georgii,* 1852.
———. Remarks on the employment of pessaries ; with the description of a new instrument. 20 pp. 12°. *New York, G. Tiemann & Co.,* 1858.
Repr. from : N. York J. M., 1858, vi, with additional remarks.
———. Die latente Gonorrhoe im weiblichen Geschlecht. viii, 125 pp., 1 l. 8°. *Bonn, M. Cohen u. Sohn,* 1872.
———. The vesico-vaginal and vesico-rectal touch ; a new method of examining the uterus and appendages. 16 pp. 8°. *New York,* 1875.
Repr. from : Am. J. Obst., N. Y., 1875, viii.
———. The diseases of blood-vessels of the ovary in relation to the genesis of ovarian cysts. 19 pp., 2 pl. 8°. *New York, W. Wood & Co.,* 1880.
Repr. from : Am. J. Obst., N. Y., 1880, xiii.
Also, Co-Editor of : **American** (The) Journal of Obstetrics, New York, 1868-71.
———. & **Jacobi** (A.) Contributions to midwifery, and diseases of women and children ; with a report on the progress of obstetrics, and uterine and infantile pathology in 1858. iv (21), 9-475 pp., 1 l. 8°. *New York, Baillière Brothers,* 1859.

Noeggerath's *operation.*

See **Uterus** (*Excision of, Vaginal*).

Noehden (Henricus Adolphus). * Specimen botanicum in quo de argumentis contra Hedwigii theoriam de generatione muscorum disserit. 36 pp. 4°. *Gottingæ, typ. J. G. Rosenbuschii,* 1797.

Noël (C.-Léopold). * De la chromato-pseudopsie. 42 pp. 4°. *Paris,* 1857, No. 203, v. 608.

Noël (C.-M.) * Sur les hémorrhagies spontanées. 19 pp. 4°. *Paris,* 1826, No. 91, v. 199.

Noël (C.-N.-Octave). * Des hémorrhagies puerpérales. 48 pp. 4°. *Paris,* 1853, No. 15, v. 546.

Noël (Charles). * Étude physiologique et médicale sur les bains de mer. 139 pp. 4°. *Paris,* 1862, No. 72.

Noel (E.) [1855-]. * Contribution à l'étude de l'hybridité morbide. 136 pp. 4°. *Paris,* 1878, No. 56.

Noel (Eugène). Rabelais, médecin, écrivain, curé, philosophe. 4. éd., ornée d'un portrait inédit gravé à l'eau-forte par A. Esnault. 247 pp., port. 12°. *Paris, A. H. Becus,* 1880.

Noël (F.-A.-René). * De l'accouchement prématuré artificiel et des cas qui le réclament. 75 pp. 4°. *Paris,* 1860, No. 143.

Noel (Franciscus Margarita). * Quæstiones medicæ. 10 pp. 4°. *Parisiis,* 1803, No. 74, v. C.

Noel (François). * Des arrêts de croissance de l'utérus. 76 pp. 4°. *Montpellier,* 1877, No. 13.

Noël (François-F.-R.) * De la rougeole épidémique chez les enfants. 42 pp. 4°. *Strasbourg,* 1854, No. 322, 2. s., v. 20.

Noel (Georges). * Étude générale sur les variations physiologiques des gaz du sang. 62 pp., 1 l. 4°. *Paris,* 1876, No. 475.

Noel (*Henry Reginald*) [-1878].
Morris (J.) Obituary. *Tr. Am. M. Ass.,* Phila., 1881, xxxii, 528.

Noël (I.) * Des lésions organiques qui peuvent produire l'ascite. 34 pp. 4°. *Paris,* 1845, No. 10, v. 436.

Noel (J.-M.-E.-D.-A.-F.) * Propositions générales sur l'hémoptysie. 23 pp. 4°. *Paris,* 1806, No. 46, v. 61.

Noël (J.-S.-Édouard). *Quelques considérations générales sur l'hygiène dans les campagnes des Vosges. 21 pp. 4°. *Paris*, 1851, No. 79, v. 512.

Noel (Joseph) [1753–1808]. Médecine légale. MS. Rap. de H. Hartung. 226 pp. 4°. [*Strasbourg, n. d.*]

Noël (Joseph-V.) *Sur le catarrhe chronique de la vessie. vi, 7–25 pp. 4°. *Paris*, 1826, No. 50, v. 198.

Noël (L.) *Sur la dysenterie aiguë simple. 29 pp. 4°. *Paris*, 1820, No. 231, v. 227.

Noël (Léon) [1844–76]. Contribution à l'histoire des anesthésiques; du pouls veineux comme symptôme habituel de l'action physiologique du chloroforme. 15 pp. 8°. [*n. p.*, 1876.]
Repr. from : Bull. Acad. roy. de méd. de Belg., Brux., 1876, 3. s., x.
For Biography, see J. d. sc. méd. de Louvain, 1877, ii, 273–286, port. (E. Hubert).

Noël (Léon Paul). *Du typhus et de la fièvre typhoïde. 58 pp. 4°. *Paris*, 1859, No. 144, v. 634.

Noël (Louis). *Sur les perforations spontanées de l'estomac. 1 p. l., 28 pp. 4°. *Strasbourg*, 1827, v. 56.

Noel (Nicholas) [1746–1832]. Traité historique et pratique de l'inoculation, dans lequel on démontre, 1°. L'ancienneté de cet usage dans les principales parties de l'Asie et de l'Afrique, ainsi que son établissement en Europe et en Amérique. 2. La meilleure méthode à employer pour l'insertion de la petite-vérole, comment on doit pratiquer cette opération, et le traitement qui lui convient. 3. Enfin, les moyens de réfuter les objections faites contre cette manière de donner la petite-vérole. Ouvrage très-instructif pour quiconque désire savoir à quoi s'en tenir sur la question importante, et tant débattue, de l'inoculation. 6 p. l., 128 pp. 8°. *Reims, Jeunehomme & fils*, 1789.

———. *Sur la nécessité de réunir les connaissances médicales et chirurgicales, pour pouvoir exercer avec distinction les différentes branches de la chirurgie. iii, 32 pp. 4°. *Paris, an XIII* [1805], No. 505, v. 57.

Noel (Perry Eccleston). *De angina tracheali. 2 p. l., 41 pp. 8°. *Edinburgi, A. Neill cum sociis*, 1794.

Noel (R. R.) Grundzüge der Phrenologie, oder Anleitung zum Studium dieser Wissenschaft, dargestellt in fünf Vorlesungen. vi, iv, 374 pp., 1 l., 9 pl. 8°. *Dresden u. Leipzig, Arnold*, 1841.

———. The same. Mit Berücksichtigung der neueren Forschungen auf dem Gebiete der Physiologie und Psychologie. 2. Aufl. 3 p. l., 592 pp., 2 l., 12 pl. 8°. *Dresden u. Leipzig, Arnold*, 1847.

———. Die Begründung und das Wesen der Phrenologie. 32 pp. 8°. *Dresden, Arnold*, 1852.

Noël (Victor-Auguste). *De l'influence de l'imagination sur l'économie animale. 1 p. l., 39 pp. 4°. *Strasbourg*, 1828, v. 57.

———. The same. 1 p. l., 39 pp. 4°. *Strasbourg, F.-G. Levrault*, 1828.

Noëlas (Pierre-Charles). *Sur la chlorose (ou pâles couleurs). 17 pp. 4°. *Paris*, 1829, No. 191, v. 226.

Noeldechen (Carolus Henricus Guilelmus) [184.–]. *De pneumothorace. 32 pp. 8°. *Berolini, G. Lange*, [1864].

Noeldechen (Fridericus Guilelmus Alex.) [1813–]. *De hydrocephalo chronico. 29 pp. 8°. *Berolini, typ. fratrum Schlesinger*, [1839].

Noeldechen (Julius Guilelmus Bernardus) [1839–]. *De anatomia pathologica typhi abdominalis. 31 pp. 8°. *Berolini, H. S. Hermann*, [1862].

Noeldeke (Georgius Justus Fridericus) [1770–1843]. *Diss. pathologiam phthiseos hepaticæ

Noeldeke (Georgius Justus Fridericus)—cont'd. sistens. 70 pp. 4°. *Gottingæ, H. M. Grape*, [1794].
For Biography, see **Blumenbach** (Jo. Frid.)

Nöll ([Balthasar] Friedrich) [1855–]. *Ein Fall von Hemicephalie mit Epignathie. 15 pp., 2 l., 2 pl. 8°. *Marburg, Hof- u. Waisenhaus-Buchdruckerei in Cassel*, 1882.

Noell (Karl Ludwig). *Ueber Typhus abdominalis. [Wurtzburg.] 44 pp. 8°. *Birkenfeld, C. F. Kittsteiner*, 1853.

Noell (Ph.) *Ueber die Wirksamkeit des Colchicum autumnale. vi, 7–46 pp., 1 pl. 8°. *Würzburg, C. W. Becker*, 1826.

Noell ([Philippus] Gustavus) [1841–]. *De partu gemellorum. 32 pp. 12°. *Berolini, G. Lange*, 1864.

Noelle (Augustus). *De animi deliquio. 29 pp. 8°. *Berolini, typ. J. F. Starckii*, [1824].

Noeller (Conradus Daniel.) *De partu serotino. 14 pp., 1 l. 8°. *Jenæ, ex off. Prageri et soc.*, [1807].

Noeller (Ernestus) [1824–]. *De diabetæ melliti natura. 31 pp. 8°. *Berolini, G. Schade*, [1848].

Noeller (Kuno). *Beitrag zur operativen Behandlung der Hydrocele. 14 pp. 8°. *Würzburg, A. Boegler*, 1885.

Nöller (W.) *Ein Fall von idiopathischer granulirender Entzündung der Dura mater. 25 pp. 8°. *Göttingen, W. F. Kaestner*, 1875.

Noellner (Friedrich). *Die Anatomie des Splanchnicus und der Nierennerven beim Hunde. 15 pp., 1 pl. 4°. *Giessen, F. C. Pietsch*, 1869.

Nölting (Friedrich). *Einiges über den Generationswechsel. [Göttingen.] 32 pp. 8°. *Cassel, F. Scheel*, 1856.

Noelting (Joh. H.) [1862–]. *Ueber das Verhältniss der sogenannten Schalenblende zur regulären Blende und zum hexagonalen Wurtzit. 33 pp., 2 pl. 8°. *Kiel, L Handorff*, 1887.

Noelting (Josephus Christianus). *De embryoctonia et infanticidio. 38 pp., 1 l. 4°. *Gottingæ, Grape*, [1805].

Noëmatachometer.

Donders (F. C.) Twee werktuigen, tot bepaling van den tijd, voor psychische processen benoodigd. Onderzoek. ged. in h. physiol. Lab. d. Utrecht. Hoogesch., 1867–8, i, 21–25.

Noemer (Cornelius). De mirabili ratione qua humanum corpus a morbis liberetur. 28 pp. 4°. *Lugd. Bat., B. J. Vander Aa*, 1719.

van Noemer (Joh. Samuel). *De lochiorum fluxu naturali atque præternaturali. 1 p. l., 52 pp., 2 l. 4°. *Lugd. Bat., apud P. Delfos et fil. et vid. M. Cyfveer*, 1805. [P., v. 1482.]

Nönchen (Hermann). *Zur Tetanie. 37 pp., 1 l. 8°. *Bonn, J. F. Carthaus*, [1878].

Nördlinger (Simon). *Ein Beitrag zu den Dermoidkystomen des Ovarium. 38 pp., 1 l. 8°. *Tübingen, H. Laupp*, 1887.

Nörr (Achille). *De hysteria. 31 pp. 8°. *Bambergæ, J. M. Reindl*, 1837.

Nörr (Carl). *Experimentelle Prüfung des Fechner'schen Gesetzes auf dem Gebiete der Schallstärke. pp. 297–318. 8°. *Tübingen, L. F. Fues*, 1881.
Cutting from : Ztschr. f. Biol., München, 1879, xv.

Nösler (Georgius) [1591–1650].

Portrait in : **Collection** — van Kaathoven. — **Collection** of Portr. of Phys. & Men of Sc., 186.

Noetel (Fridericus Gustavus) [1839–]. *De meningitide spinali. 44 pp., 1 l., 1 pl. 8°. *Berolini, G. Schade*, [1851].

Noetel ([Friedrich Wilh.] Konrad) [1861–]. *Casuistik über die Behandlung schwerer skrofulöser Erkrankungen der Cornea und Conjunctiva durch Excision der Uebergangsfalte und

Noetel ([Friedrich Wilh.] Konrad)—continued.
Spaltung des äusseren Lidwinkers. 31 pp. 8°.
Berlin, G. Schade, [1886].

Noethig (Carl). * Ueber die mittelbare Auscultation oder die Anwendung des Stethoscops.
14 pp. 8°. *München, F. X. Auer,* 1832.

Noethig (Franc. Nic.) * De decussatione nervorum opticorum. 2 p. l., 48 pp., 1 l., 1 pl. 8°.
Moguntiæ, J. J. Alef, 1786.

 Also, in: SCRIPT. neurol. minores selecti. 4°. *Lipsiæ,*
1791, i, 127–144, 1 pl.

Noethig (Jac.) * Das intermittirende Wundfie-
ber. 44 pp. 8°. *Würzburg, C. A. Zürn,* 1837.

Nöthig (Jakob). * Ueber die verschiedenen Methoden des Blasensteinschnittes beim männlichen Geschlechte, besonders über den Stein-
schnitt durch den Mastdarm nach Sanson. 40 pp.
8°. *Würzburg, F. E. Nitribitt,* 1819.

Noethlichs (Anton). * Der trockene chronische
Catarrh der Paukenhöhle. [Wurtzburg.] 27 pp.
8°. *Erkelenz, J. Brandts,* [1860].

Noethlichs (Gottfried). * Untersuchungen der
Milz und Leber auf Milchsäure. [Wurtzburg.]
24 pp. 8°. *Erkelenz, J. Brandts,* 1860.

Nöthling (Ernst). Der Schutz unserer Wohn-
häuser gegen die Feuchtigkeit. Ein Handbuch
für praktische Bautechniker, sowie als Leitfaden
für den Unterricht in Baugewerbschulen. vi (1
l.), 37 pp. 8°. *Weimar, B. F. Voigt,* 1885.

Noetling (Wilhelm). * Ueber Halswunden im
Allgemeinen, insbesondere aber über Wunden der
Luftröhre. 24 pp. 8°. *Mannheim,* 1845.

Noettinger (Samuel. Fridericus). * De arterio-
tomia, ejus recto usu et injustu neglectu. 36 pp.
sm. 4°. *Argentorati, lit. Pauschingerianis,* [1747].

Noever de Brauw (Joannes Christianus Ten).
See de Brauw (Joannes Christianus ten Noever).

de Noé Walker (Arthur). On the prevailing
ignorance of the materia medica in recognized
schools of medicine. 39 pp. 8°. *London, G.
Clayton,* 1861. [P., v. 1497.]

——. Address on vivisection, read at the International Congress for the Prevention of Cruelty
to Animals, held in Londen, 1874. 16 pp. 8°.
London, Baillière, Tindall & Cox, 1875.

Nog een woord over den toestand der militaire
pharmacie en der militaire apothekers, bij het
Nederl. leger. 2de vervolg van den open brief
aan de heeren leden van de Tweede Kamer der
Staten Generaal door eenege militaire pharmaceuten. 16 pp. 8°. *Utrecht, J. G. van Terveen
& Zoon,* 1868.

Nog eens: De toestand der militaire pharmacie en
der militaire apothekers, bij het Nederl. leger
na de nieuwe organisatie van Oct. 1867. Vervolg van den open brief aan de heeren leden van
de Tweede Kamer der Staten Generaal door eenige
milit. pharmaceuten. 7 pp. 8°. *Utrecht, J. G.
van Terveen & Zoon,* 1867.

Nogaret (Charles-Jean-Paul). * I. Des symptômes de la péritonite puerpérale. II [etc.]
28 pp. 4°. *Paris,* 1844, No. 144, v. 422.

Nogaro (H.) * De la médication stibiée dans la
phthisie pulmonaire. 64 pp. 4°. *Paris,* 1876,
No. 221.

Nogent-le-Rotrou.

 See **Fever** (*Typhoid, History, etc., of*), *by localities.*

Nogent-Saint-Laurens. Cour d'assises de
la Seine; affaire Doudet; plaidoirie et réplique.
39 pp. sm. 8°. *Paris, Dubuisson & Cie.,* 1855.

 Repr. from: Compt.-rend. du droit. 1855.

Nogier (Jules). * De l'inflammation. 23 pp. 4°.
Strasbourg, 1861, No. 579, 2 s., v. 31.

Nogier (Pierre). * De l'alimentation de la première enfance. 34 pp. 4°. *Paris,* 1857, No. 278,
v. 608.

Nogueira (José-Alves-da-Silva). * Sur la bronchite. 20 pp. 4°. *Paris,* 1836, No. 149, v.
298.

Nogueira (Luiz Antonio Barboza). * Hemorrhagia cerebral. 2 p. l., 111 pp., 1 l. 4°. *Rio
de Janeiro, E. & H. Laemmert,* 1878.

Noguera (Oscar Anastasio) [1860–]. * Zur
Operation des Brustkrebses beim Weibe. 36
pp., 1 l. 8°. *Berlin, G. Schade,* [1885].

Noguès. * Essai sur le Convallaria majalis. 34
pp. 4°. *Paris,* 1883, No. 178.

Noguès (Auguste-Victor). * Considérations sur
l'aphorisme d'Hippocrate: Duobus laboribus simul abortis, non in eodem loco, vehementior ob-
scurat alterum. vi, 7–33 pp. 4°. *Paris,* 1819,
No. 222, v. 151.

Noguès (Émile). * Du traitement hydrothérapique de la chlorose compliquée d'aménorrhée et
de ménorrhagie. 52 pp. 4°. *Paris,* 1879, No.
565.

Noguès (H.-Jules). * Du rachitisme. 26 pp.
4°. *Paris,* 1851, No. 161, v. 512.

Noguès (J.-B.-B.-Edmond). * Anatomie, physiologie et pathologie du prépuce. 48 pp. 4°.
Paris, 1850, No. 165, v. 499.

Noguès (Paul-Auguste). * Considérations sur
le zona. 34 pp., 1 l., 2 pl. 4°. *Montpellier,*
1864. [P., v. 48.]

Noguez (Pierre). L'anatomie du corps de
l'homme en abrégé, ou description courte de
toutes ses parties. Où l'on donne l'explication
de leurs différens usages, tirée de leur structure
et des observations les plus modernes. 2. éd.
xv, 4 p. l., 464 (4 l.), li pp., 20 pl. 16°. *Paris,
G. Cavelier fils,* 1726.

Nohl (Franz) [1853–]. * Ueber Osteomalacie.
32 pp. 8°. *Berlin, G. Lange,* [1876].

Nohl (Ludovicus) [1806–]. * De pneumato i.
29 pp., 1 l. 8°. *Berolini, typ. Nietackianis,*
[1832].

Nohr (Carolus Fridericus Oscar). * De ligamenti
capsularis cubiti inter capitulum radii et emi-
nentiam ossis humeri capitatam interpositione.
16 pp. 8°. *Lipsiæ, typ. A. Edelmanni,* 1856. c.

Nohr (Joannes Matthæus). * De lochiorum suppressione. 56 pp. sm. 4°. *Halæ Magdeb., t. p.
J. C. Hendelii,* [1731]. [*Also, in:* P., v. 1386.]

Nohstadt (Rudolph). * Ueber Encephaloma-
lacie. 27 pp., 1 pl. 8°. *Würzburg, Thein,* [1876,
vel subseq.].

Nointot.

 Henry. Rapport sur l'eau minérale de Nointot près
Bolbec (Seine-Inférieure). Bull. Acad. de méd., Par.,
1840–41, vi, 780–782.

Noir (Philippe-Gustave). * Tumeurs enkystées
des bourses. 38 pp. 4°. *Paris,* 1865, No. 244.

Noir (Pierre-Élie). * Moyens de déterminer l'accouchement prématuré. 31 pp. 4°. *Paris,* 1858,
No. 14 ', v. 622.

Noir animalisé pour engrais. 22 pp. 8°. [*Paris,
Mme. Huzard,* 1833, vel subseq.] [P., v. 1745.]

Noirault (Pierre-Lonis-Alexandre). * Considérations sur quelques procédés de la médecine
opératoire. 32 pp 4°. *Paris,* 1845, No. 193, v.
436.

Noire-Combe.

 See **Fever** (*Typhoid, History, etc., of*), *by localities.*

Noiret (Pierre-François). * Sur la cataracte,
suivie de quelques propositions sur la médecine,
la chirurgie et les accouchemens. 32 pp. 4°.
Paris, 1836, No. 329, v. 303.

Noirmant (P.-E.) * I. Déterminer s'il existe
des caractères qui puissent toujours faire distinguer le lupus, la syphilide ulcérée, et le noli
me tangere, fixés au visage. II. [etc.] 26 pp.
4°. *Paris,* 1840, No. 49, v. 364.

Noirmoutier.

Dumont (A.) Note sur la natalité aux îles de Noirmoutier, d'Yeu et de Groix. Ann. de démog. internat., Par., 1883, vii, 247-264.

Noirot (Louis). *De la scarlatine. 56 pp. 4°. *Paris*, 1844, No. 190, v. 422.

———. Histoire de la scarlatine. 397 pp. 8°. *Paris, J.-B. Baillière*, 1847.

———. Études statistiques sur la mortalité et la durée de la vie dans la ville et l'arrondissement de Dijon depuis le 17e siècle jusqu'à nos jours. 88 pp. 8°. *Paris, J.-B. Baillière*, 1850.

———. Exposé des travaux des conseils d'hygiène publique et de salubrité du département de la Côte-d'Or, 1849 à 1859. 4 p. l., 372 pp. 8°. *Dijon, Lamarche*, 1861.

———. La callipédie contemporaine, ou l'art d'avoir des enfants sains de corps et d'esprit. 3. éd. 215 pp. 12°. *Paris, E. Dentu*, 1869.

———. De kunst om long te leven. Naar de vierde uitgave uit het Fransch vertaald door J. G. Rooseboom. 2 p. l., 206 pp. sm. 8°. *Gouda, G. B. van Goor Zonen*, 1871.

———. L'art d'être malade. 2. éd. 215 pp. 12°. *Paris, E. Dentu*, 1871.

———. À travers l'hygiène. 2. s. (1877 à 1881). 278 pp., 1 l. 12°. *Paris, E. Dentu*, 1881.

Also, Editor of: **Annuaire** de littérature médicale étrangère, Paris, 1857-61.

Noise.

See, also, **Shock.**

REPORT of Harrison *et al. vs.* St. Mark's Church, Philadelphia. A bill to restrain the ringing of bells so as to cause a nuisance to the occupants of the dwellings in the immediate vicinity of the church. In the court of common pleas, No. 2, in equity, before Hare, P. J., and Mitchell, associate J., Philadelphia, February, 1877. 8°. *Philadelphia*, [*n. d.*]

London noise. San. Rec., Lond., 1876, v, 277.—**Reclam** (C.) Der Einfluss eines "Dampf-Hammers" auf die Nachbarschaft; hygieinisches Gutachten. Gesundheit, Elberfeld, 1880, v, 65-68.—**Roosa** (D. B. St. J.) A contribution to the etiology of diseases of the internal ear. (Cases of deafness from concussion, as boilermaker's deafness) Am. J. M. Sc., Phila., 1874, lxviii, 377-400.—**Sound** (On) as a nuisance. J. Sc., Lond., 1880, 3. s., ii, 570-573.

Noisten (Matthias). *De perfecta uteri gravidi atresia ejusque operatione. 3 p. l., 40 pp., 2 l. 8°. *Bonnæ, typ. C. Georgii*, [1831].

de Noisy (Gustave). ¶ Prostitutio ! Questions sur la prostitution. vii, 43 pp., 1 l. 8°. *Genève*, [*J. Benoit & Cie.*], 1877.

Noizet (H.-V.-Romain). *Du staphylome postérieur. 94 pp., 1 pl. 4°. *Paris*, 1858, No. 57, v. 622.

à Nokken (Henricus). *De convulsione. 2 p. l., 21 pp., 1 l. 4°. *Traj. ad Rhenum, J. Brocdelet*, 1752.

à Nokken (Jacobus). *De angina. 22 pp., 2 l. 4°. *Traj. ad Rhenum, G. vande Water*, [1716].

Nokomis.

Whitten (T. J.) Sanitary survey of Nokomis. Rep. Bd. Health Illinois 1885, Springfield, 1886, viii, 269-272.

Nola (Joannes Andreas). Quod sedimentum sanorum, ægrorumque corporum non sit ejusdem speciei. Adversus Ferdinandum Cassanum, et alios contrarium sentientes. Habentur insuper contra eosdem, præter alios gravissimos logicæ, philosophiæ, ac medicinæ errores. Quod sedimentum in ægris non sit semper pars humoris putridi, nec in eo omnes humores contineantur. Quod in intermittentibus febribus humor intra vasa non putrescat. Quod temere Arabes, præsertim Avicennam, de causa conjuncta redarguant. Quod de continenti seu contentiva causa cum Galeno prave sentiant. 3 p. l., 82 pp. 8°. *Venetiis*, 1562.

Nolais (François). *Étude sur les pleurésies hémorrhagiques. 53 pp. 4°. *Paris*, 1882, No. 282.

Nolan (William). An essay on humanity ; or a view of abuses in hospitals, with a plan for correcting them. viii, 9-49 pp. 8°. *London, J. Murray*, 1786.

Nolano (Ambrosio Leone).

See **Willichius** (Jodocus). Exercitationes et probationes de urinis, [etc.] 12°. *Amstelodami*, 1688.

Nolda (Arnoldus Theophilus Augustus) [1814-]. *De abscessu cartilaginis cricoideæ. 31 pp. 8°. *Berolini, typ. Friedlaenderianis*, [1837].

Nolda (August). *Phonautographische Studien als Beiträge zur Physiologie der Membrana tympani des Menschen. 24 pp. 8°. *Würzburg, Stahel*, 1886.

Nolde. Ueber die Behandlung der ausgebrochenen Hydrophobie (Wasserscheu). 16 pp. 8°. *Passau, F. W. Keppler*, 1855.

Nolde (Adolph Friedrich) [1764-1813]. Gallerie der ältern und neuern Gesundheitslehrer für das schöne Geschlecht. xxii, 456 pp. 8°. *Rostock u. Leipzig, Stiller*, 1794.

———. Beobachtungen über die Kuhpocken, nebst einigen Bemerkungen. 191 pp. 12°. *Erfurt, Henning*, 1802.

———. Die Schulen für Aerzte. xvi, 560 pp. 12°. *Braunschweig, C. Reichard*, 1809.

———. De mutuæ relationis principio theoriæ medicæ inserviente. 41 pp. 4°. *Halæ, in libraria Rengeriana*, 1810.

———. Die neuesten Systeme deutscher Geburtshelfer seit dem Anfange des neunzehnten Jahrhunderts. 2. Ausg. vi, 362 pp. 16°. *Erfurt, J. K. Müller*, 1811.

———. Ueber die Gränzen der Natur und Kunst in der Geburtshülfe. 2. Aufl. xviii, 288 pp. 12°. *Erfurt, J. C. Müller*, 1817.

Nolde (Friedrich). *Ueber den Typhus und dessen Behandlung. 13 pp. 8°. *Passau, Pustet*, 1849.

Nolde (Joannes Laurentius). *De parentum morbis in fœtum transientibus. 20 pp. 4°. *Erfordiæ, S. Nonniano*, [1768].

Nolé (Antoine-François-Léon). *Sur la thérapeutique de l'inflammation aiguë du poumon. 32 pp. 4°. *Paris*, 1833, No. 96, v. 259.

Nolé (Léon). Instruction populaire sur l'épidémie régnante de choléra, de suette miliaire et de fièvre intermittente, destinée spécialement à MM. les médecins, curés, maires, instituteurs, etc., et autres fonctionnaires et habitants éclairés des campagnes, et rédigée d'après des observations nombreuses. 24 pp. sm. 8°. *Cintegabelle & Toulouse*, 1854.

Nolen (Catharinus). *Hæmatocele intervaginalis. 2 p. l., 75 pp., 1 pl. 8°. *Leiden, S. C. van Doesburgh*, 1884.

Nolen (D.)

See **Wundt** (W.) Éléments de psychologie physiologique. 2 v. 8°. *Paris*, 1886.

Nolen (Willem)[1]. *Over placenta prævia. [Leiden.] 3 p. l., 68 pp. 8°. *Rotterdam, M. Wijt & Zonen*, 1856.

Nolen (Willem)[2]. *"Rheumatismus gonorrhoïcus." 2 p. l., 119 pp. 8°. *Leiden, S. C. van Doesburgh*, 1880.

———. Het zoogenaamde dierlijk magnetisme of hypnotisme (catalepsie, lethargie, somnambulisme, fascinatie) populair beschreven en toegelicht. 45 pp. 8°. *Rotterdam, W. J. van Hengel*, 1886.

Nolet (Eduardus Joannes Maria). *De leer der vaatgeruischen. 2 p. l., 88 pp., 1 pl. 8°. *Leiden, J. W. van Leeuwen*, 1870.

N[olet] (J[oseph]). Observations curieuses sur des phénomènes extraordinaires, qui regardent particulièrement la médecine et la chirurgie.

N[olet] (J[oseph])—continued.
5 p. l., 129 pp., 1 l. 16°. *Brest, Vve. & R. Malassis*, 1711.

Nolette (Alexandre). * Sur le régime, ou les règles d'hygiène particulières aux femmes pendant la grossesse. viii, 9–57 pp. 4°. *Paris*, 1817, No. 58, v. 130.

Nolibois (Jean). * De la blennorrhagie chez la femme. 13 pp. 4°. *Paris*, 1836, No. 98, v. 296.

Nolin (Jules-Édouard). * Sur quelques maladies des nerfs. 28 pp. 4°. *Paris*, 1818, No. 21, v. 135.

Noll (Ferdinand). * Ueber die Behandlung der Nasen-Rachenpolypen durch temporäre Resectionen am Oberkiefer. 34 pp. 8°. *Tübingen*, *L. F. Fues*, 1879.
c.

Noll (Fridericus Guil.) * De cursu lymphæ in vasis lymphaticis. 36 pp. 8°. *Marburgi Cattorum, typ. Elwerti*, 1849.
c.

Noll (J.) * Du bruit de souffle dans les maladies chirurgicales, sa cause, sa valeur diagnostique. 1 p. l., 60 pp. 4°. *Strasbourg, Vve. Berger-Levrault*, 1870, 3. s., No. 260.

Nollau (Joh. Jacobus). *An senibus lac ovillum? Præses Carolus Franciscus Theroulde de Vallun. 4 pp. 4°. [*Paris, Quillau*, 1769.]

———. *An impeditis lacrimarum viis parari debeat lacrimis artificiale iter, in cavum quod juxta majorem oculi canthum, inter superficiem internam palpebræ, et oculi globum deprehenditur? Præses Joannes Nicolaus Millin de la Courvault. 4 pp. · 4°. [*Paris, Quillau*, 1770.]

———. *An in variolis quandoque chinachina? Præses Maximilianus Josephus Leys. 4 pp. 4°. [*Paris, Quillau*, 1770.]

See, also, **Crochet** (Stephan). An impeditis lacrimarum, etc. 4°. *Parisiis*, 1779.

Nollau (Ernestus Guilelmus) [1801–]. * Prosopalgiæ adumbratio pathologica. 42 pp., 1 l. 8°. *Berolini, formis Brüschckianis*, 1824.

Nolle (Léon). * Considérations sur les plaies articulaires et leur traitement. 56 pp. 4°. *Paris*, 1873, No. 146.

Nolleroth (W. A.) * Comparatio systematum sanguinis et lymphæ, disquisitio physiologica, ejus part. iii. pp. 17–24. 4°. *Lundæ, C. F. Berling*, 1836.

Nollet (Édouard-Ernest). * Étude sur le régime alimentaire chez les albuminuriques. 36 pp. 4°. *Paris*, 1885, No. 384.

Nollet (Jean-Antoine) [1700–70]. Essai sur l'électricité des corps. 3. éd. xxiii, 273 pp., 1 l., 5 pl. sm. 8°. *Paris, H.-L. Guerin & L.-F. Delatour*, 1754.

Nolli (Giovanni). Il cow-pox (vaiuolo vaccino spontaneo) ed il comitato Milanese di vaccinazione animale. 15 pp. 8°. *Milano, F. Rechiedei*, 1872.
Repr. from: Ann. univ. di med., Milano, 1872, ccxix.

———. La discussione sulla vaccinazione animale fatta presso la R. Accademia di medicina di Torino nel 1871, e le esperienze comparative sul vaccino animale e sull' umanizzato praticate nel triennio 1871-3 da apposita commissione Torinese. 28 pp. 8°. [*n. p.*, 1874.]
Repr. from: Gazz. med. ital. lomb., Milano, 1874, 7. s., i.

Nollius (Henricus). Veræ physices compendium novum, in sincerioris philosophiæ studiosorum gratiam conscriptum et in lucem editum. 7 p. l., 112 pp. 12°. *Steinfurti, J. C. Unckel*, 1616.

———. De methodo medendi hermetica.
In: AGONISMATA med. Marpurgensia. 4°. *Marpurgi Cattorum*, 1618, 346–353.

Nolst (Lambertus). * De viribus naturæ medicatricibus notabili exemplo chirurgico illustratis. 1 p. l., 29 pp., 3 l. 4°. *Lugd. Bat., J. Meerburg*, 1779. [P., v. 1092.]
See, also, **Reich** (Gottfried Christian). Over de koorts en derzelver behandeling in het algemeen. 8°. *Haarlem*, 1801.

Nolte (Ánton [Bernhard Joseph]) [1849–]. * Zur Casuistik sympathischer Augenerkrankungen. 28 pp. 4°. *Greifswald, F. W. Kunike*, 1875.

Nolte (Arnold) [1856–]. *Ueber das Verhalten der Milz bei Syphilis. 31 pp. 12°. *Greifswald*, 1883.

Nolte (Carl). * Brown-Séquard'sche Halbseitenläsion des Rückenmarkes. 46 pp., 1 l. 8°. *Bonn, C. Georgi*, 1887.
c.

Nolte (Ernestus Christianus). * De febre puerperarum. 50 pp., 1 l. sm. 4°. *Gottingæ, H. M. Grape*, [1785].
Also, in: FRANK (J. P.) Delect. opusc. med. 8°. *Ticini*, 1788, v, 1–69.

Nolte (Ernst). Die grossen und merkwürdigen kosmisch-tellurischen Erscheinungen im Luftkreise unserer Erde in Folge zwanzigjähriger Beobachtungen, auch in Beziehung zu der im Laufe der neuern Zeit herrschenden orientalischen Cholera. 1 p. l., 95 pp., 1 l. 8°. *Hannover, Hahn*, 1831.

Nolte (F. W.) * Die Hypochondrie. 2 p. l., 31 pp. 8°. *Utrecht, Schultze u. Voermans*, 1840.

———. Atlas der Hautkrankheiten, nach dem Systeme des Professor C. H. Fuchs, dargestellt und mit erläuterndem Texte herausgegeben. 1 p. l., vi, 38 l., 32 pl. fol. *Leyden, H. W. Hazenberg u. Comp.*, [1842–3.]

Nolten (Guilelmus). De usu ætheris vaporum obstetricio, adjectis observationibus de chloroformi effectu. 2 p. l., 49 pp. 8°. *Bonnæ, C. et F. Krüger*, [1847.]

Nolto (Joh.) Discursus medicus de theriaca Andromachi senioris, ejusque origine, etymologia, ingredientibus et usu medico, ex variis, tam veterum quam recentiorum scriptis, adornatus. Das ist: Eine medicinische Lob-Rede des von vielen Jahren her hochberühmten Theriacs, worin von dessen Ursprung, Nahmens-Benennung, herrlichen Ingredientien, preissbahren Nutzen und Gebrauch, aus alten und neuen Auctoren gehandelt wird. 2. ed. 1 p. l., 40 pp., 1 tab. 4°. *Lubecæ, sumpt. J. Widemeyeri*, 1706.

Nolthenius (Petrus Marius). * De epilepsia. 2 p. l., 116 pp. 8°. [*Lugd. Bat.*], C. C. van der Hoek, [1840].

Nolting (Friedrich Ludwig) [1858 –]. * Schwangerschaft und Geburt compliciert durch Ovarientumor. 31 pp. 8°. *Berlin, M. Driesner*, [1884.]

Noma.

See, also, **Aneurisms** (*Aortic, Complications, etc., of*); **Fever** (*Typhus*); **Fever** (*Typhus, Sequelæ of*); **Genitals** (*Female, Inflammation of*); **Genitals** (*Female, Inflammation of, in infants*); **Measles** (*Complications, etc., of*); **Mouth** (*Gangrene of*); **Rape** *in infants*; **Scarlatina** (*Complications, etc., of*).

DE ASCHEN (J. H. G.) * De noma observata quædam et analecta critica. 8°. *Berolini*, [1831].

ASCHMANN (G.) * De cancro aquatico. 8°. *Berolini*, [1834].

BRACHVOGEL (M.) * De noma. 8°. *Berolini*, [1838].

BROX (C. F.) * De cancro aquatico. 8°. *Lipsiæ*, 1856.

BRUMBY (G.) * Quædam ad nomes pathologiam. 8°. *Berolini*, 1834.

DEMUTH (H. G.) * De noma. 8°. *Francof. a. M.*, 1849.

DEUTSCHBEIN (L. L. A.) * De noma infantum. 8°. *Halæ*, [1840].

ECKERT (C. H.) * De noma. 8°. *Berolini*, [1842].

ENVALD (K. W.) * Om noma. 8°. *Helsingfors*, 1864.

Noma.

FEMMER (C.) *De noma quædam. 8°. *Gryphiæ*, 1849.

GRUND (H.) * De noma, adnexis morbi historiis. 8°. *Pragæ*, 1843.

GUISCHARD (F. L.) *De noma. 8°. *Halis Sax.*, [1854].

HESSE (H.) *Ueber Noma. 8°. *Würzburg*, 1860.

HILDEBRANDT (P.) *De noma. 8°. *Berolini*, [1873].

KATSCH (J. F.) *De noma. 8°. *Halis Sax.*, [1855].

KELLNER (M.) *Ueber Noma. sm. 8°. *Berlin*, [1870].

KÉZMARSZKY (T.) *De noma. 8°. *Budæ*, 1833.

KNOEPFELMACHER (N.) *Ueber den Wasserkrebs der Kinder. 8°. *Erlangen*, 1837.

KUNHARDT (H. A.) *De noma. 8°. *Heidelbergæ*, 1843.

KUNTZE (C. E.) *De antiquitate et historia litteraria nomæ, seu cancri aquatici. [Göttingen.] 8°. *Berolini*, 1830.

LAPIDOTH (G. M. J. C.) *De ulcere noma, quale nostrates observarunt. [Leyden.] 8°. *Schoonhoviæ*, [1840].

LEDWIG (A.) *De noma, adjecta singulari morbi historia. 8°. *Vratislaviæ*, [1830].

LIEDHEGENER (A.) *De noma. 8°. *Bonnæ*, 1856.

MELLINGHAUS (H.) *De noma pathologica quædam. 8°. *Berolini*, [1833].

MOLLHEIM (L.) *De noma seu stomatomalacia, adjecto morbi casu iterata applicatione ferri candentis sanato. 8°. *Berolini*, [1837].

MORGEN (J. R. E.) *De noma infantum. 8°. *Berolini*, 1837.

PARPAL (M.) *Noma. 8°. *Buenos Aires*, 1884.

PEL (N.) *De ulcere noma. 8°. *Groningæ*, [1846].

REIMANN (Z.) * De nomate cum historia memorabili trismi illo soluto. 8°. *Berolini*, [1824].

RICHTER (A. L.) Der Wasserkrebs der Kinder. 8°. *Berlin*, 1828.

ROTHAMEL (G. C. F.) Heilung des Wasserkrebses der Kinder, nach einer auf die bisherigen Beobachtungen, die Natur und das Wesen dieses Uebels gegründeten Methode; nebst einigen pathogenetischen und nosologischen Bemerkungen über diese Krankheit. 8°. *Eschwege*, 1832.

SACK (G. A. E.) *De noma. 8°. *Berolini*, 1850.

SPONHOLZ (C. M.) *De nomate, pluribus morbi casibus adjectis. 8°. *Berolini*, [1836].

STRUEH (C.) *Ueber Noma und deren Pilze. 8°. *Göttingen*, 1872.

TALMA (A. von Eichstorff). Academisch proefschrift, over ulcus noma. 8°. *Groningen*, 1859.

WIEGAND (V. I.) *De cancro quem aquaticum vocant, adnexa hujus morbi historia. 8°. *Marburgi*, [1827].

VAN ZADELHOFF (A. J.) *Over ulcus noma. 8°. *Utrecht*, 1860.

ZIECKER (F.) *De noma seu stomatomalacia. 8°. *Berolini*, 1848.

Acuña (J. N.) Un caso de noma. Rev. med., Rio de Jan., 1877–8, xiv, 313.—**Albers** (J. F. H.) Noma. Deutsche Klinik, Berl., 1850, ii, 477. ——. Ueber die Natur und Behandlung des Wangenbrandes (Noma oder besser Nome). Arch. f. physiol. Heilk., Stuttg., 1853, ix, 515–544, 1 pl.—**B.** (J.) Ein Fall von Heilung des Noma. Allg. med. Centr.-Ztg., Berl, 1861, xxx, 425–427.—**B. y B.** Diagnóstico diferencial y tratamiento de la gangrena de la boca en los niños. Sentido catól., Barcel., 1879, i, 10; 18.—**Bassini** (E.) † *In his*: Clin. operat., 8°, Genova, 1878, 68–73.—**Bazin.** Noma. Dict. encycl. d. sc. méd., Par., 1878, 2. s., xiii, 322–336.—**von Becker** (H. T.) Geschichtliches über Noma. Med.-chir. Centralbl., Wien, 1881, xvi, 25; 37; 49; 61.—**Benedict.** Ueber Noma.

Noma.

Mag. f. d. ges. Heilk., Berl., 1835, xliv, 339–343.—**Beobachtungen** über den Wasserkrebs. Lit. Ann. f. d. ges. Heilk., Berl., 1829, xiii, 428–437.—**Berndt.** Fall einer gelungenen Heilung des Wasserkrebses durch die concentrirte ALwendung des Chlorkalkes. J. d. pract. Heilk., Berl., 1829, lxix, 2. St., 104–110.—**Bieske.** Beitrag zur Pathologie und Therapie der Noma. Mag. f. d. ges. Heilk., Berl., 1838, lii, 309–318, 1 pl.—**Bistrof** (N.) Za-maitka o tak nazivaemoi "stomacace" u daitei. [Notes on the so-called stomacace of infancy.] Med. Vestnik, St. Petersb., 1867, vñ, 456–458.—**Bluff.** Zwei Fälle von Noma. Med. Ann., Heidelb., 1837, iii, 113–116.—**Boisseré.** Noma, langsam tödtend. Gen.-Ber. d. k. rhein. Med.-Coll. 1839, Koblenz, 1842, 68–70. *Also:* Wchnschr. f. d. ges. Heilk., Berl., 1843, 799–801.—**Bókai.** Noma. Oesterr. Ztschr. f. Kinderh., Wien, 1856–7, i, 338–340.—**Bosch.** Ueber Wasserkrebs. Med. Cor.-Bl. d. württemb. ärztl. Ver., Stuttg., 1854, xxiv, 214.—**Bouley & Caillault.** Mémoire sur les affections phagédéniques et gangréneuses chez les enfants, et sur leur nature scorbutique. Gaz. méd. de Par., 1852, 3. s., vii, 418; 433; 512; 523; 667; 702.—**Brockmüller.** Noma. Gen.-Ber. d. k. rhein. Med.-Coll. 1841, Koblenz, 1844, 61.—**Brooks** (J. W.) Idiopathic gangræna genitalia in infancy. Chicago M. J., 1870, xxvii, 640–646.—**Burckhardt** (A. W.) Ueber den bei Kindern vorkommenden Wasserkrebs oder den Brand der Lippen, Wangen und äussern weiblichen Geschlechtstheile, und dessen gründliche Heilung. Ztschr.d. deutsch. Chir.-Ver., Magdeb., 1852, v, 446–470.—**Cancrum** oris; plastic operation. Abstr. M. & S. Cases Gen. Hosp. Sick Children 1885, Pendlebury, Manchester, 1886, v, 147. — [**Case.**] Noma. Jahresb. ü. d. med. Abth. d. Spit. zu Basel, 1873, 42.—**Clever.** Noma. Arch. f. Kinderh., 1870–71, i, 339–344.—**Croly.** Noma pudendi. Med. Press & Circ., Lond., 1868, vi, 55.—**Deutsch.** Einige Bemerkungen über Noma. J. f. Kinderkr., Erlang., 1851, xvi, 61–72.—**Donat.** Wasserkrebs. Gen.-Ber. d. k. rhein. Med.-Coll. 1830, Koblenz, 1833, 88.—**Ebert** (H. F. L.) † Deutsche Klinik, Berl., 1856, viii, 219.—**van Eeden** (W.) Observation de gangrène de la bouche (noma). Ann. Soc. méd. d'émulat. de la Flandre occid., Roulers, 1850, iv, 414–423. — **Förster** (R.) Noma nach Blattern; bedeutender Substanzverlust der rechten Gesichtshälfte, Necrose des Ober- und Unterkiefers; Heilung. Jahrb. f. Kinderh., Leipz., 1871–2, v, 327–329.—**Gee.** Noma vulvæ, renal and cerebral embolisms, derived probably from clots in left auricular appendix. Med. Times & Gaz., Lond., 1877, i, 365.—**Gierke.** Zur Casuistik der Noma. Jahrb. f. Kinderh., Leipz., 1867–8, i, 267–285.—[**Gobée** (C.)] Aanteekeningen over ulcus noma. Kliniek, Utrecht, 1847, iii, 136–144.—**Günther** (A.) † † Deutsche Klinik, Berl., 1856, v, 353–355. ——. † † *Ibid.*, 1857, ix, 272.—**Guidi** (G.) Noma; sua patogenesi e cura. Arch. di patol. inf., Napoli, 1885, iii, 262–270.—**Hall** (T.) Two cures of gangrene of genitals in an infant. Phila. M. Museum, 1808, iv, 124–127.—**Harch** (L.) Noma; curacion. Corresp. méd., Madrid, 1884, xix, 11–13.—**Hasbach.** Creosot gegen Noma. Org. f. d. ges. Heilk., Aachen, 1853, ii, 129–131.—**Heinrich** (W.) Wasserkrebs, Noma, Cancer aquaticus; Heilung desselben durch grosse Gaben Opium. Med. Ztg. Russlands, St. Petersb., 1852, ix, 291.—**Henoch.** † J. f. Kinderkr., Berl., 1844, ii, 401–405.—**Hers** (J. F. P.) Exantheem bij diphtheritis en een geval van noma. Nederl. Tijdschr. v. Geneesk., Amst., 1885, 2 R., xxi, 863–866.—**Heusinger** (C. F.) Ein Beitrag zu den Antiquitäten der Noma. Janus, Gotha, 1851, i, 127.—**Hueter** (C. C.) Beobachtungen und Bemerkungen über den Wasserkrebs. J. f. Chir. u. Augenh., Berl., 1829, xiii, 26–93.—**Isnard-Cevoule.** Ueber einen bei Kindern vorkommenden Brand der Lippen, Wangen und äusseren weiblichen Geschlechtstheile. Arch. f. med. Erfahr., Berl., 1820, i, 265–291.—**Jaeger** (C. G.) Der Schaamlefzenbrand kleiner Mädchen. Org. f. d. ges. Heilk., Aachen, 1852, i, 74–79. *Also:* Ztschr. d. deutsch. Chir.-Ver., Magdeb., 1853, vii, 446–451. *Also:* Med. Ztg., Berl., 1853, xxii, 66.—**Jeleński** (H.) Rak wodny (cancer aquaticus, noma) wyleczony z pomocą jodoformu. Gaz. lek., Warszawa, 1883, 2. s., iii, 545–547.—**Jütte.** Noma regionis auricularis. Ztschr. f. klin. Med., Bresl., 1854, v, 387–389.—**Kiemann.** Aneurysma aortæ et valvulæ bicuspidalis cum insufficientia valvularum aortæ; Scorbut; Noma; Tod. Ber. d. k. k. Krankenanst. Rudolph-Stiftung in Wien (1866), 1867, 195–197.—**Klaatsch.** Einige Bemerkungen über den Wasserkrebs und den ausgezeichneten Nutzen der Holzsäure in denselben. J. d. pract. Heilk., Berl., 1823, lvi, 1. St., 100; 2. St., 48.—**Kömm.** Merkwürdiger Fall eines Wasserkrebses. Med. Jahrb. d. k. österr. Staates, Wien, 1838, xxv, 32–37, 1 pl.—**Koerte.** † J. f. Kinderkr., Berl., 1843, i, 401–407. — **Krasin.** † † Vrach. Vaidom., St. Petersb., 1880, v, 1445; 1463; 1479.—**Krebel** (R.) Noma bei einem Erwachsenen. Med. Ztg. Russlands, St. Petersb., 1848, v, 255.—**Kuhn** (J.) Noma sphacelosa. Org. f. d. ges. Heilk., Berl., 1861, x, 263–265.—**Lange.** Noma. Deutsche Klinik, Berl., 1854, vi, 302. ——. Ein Fall von Noma geheilt durch äussere Anwendung von Oleum terebinthinæ. Memorabilien, Heilbr., 1871, xvi, 31–34.—**Loh-**

Noma.

meyer. † Gen.-Ber. d. k. rhein. Med.-Coll. 1838, Coblenz, 1840, 109.—**Lond** (G.) De l'usage du kinkina contre le nome. [*From*: Mém. abrégés de l'Acad. de Stockholm.] Collect. acad. d. mém., etc., Par., 1772, xi, 260.—
Lorey (C.) Gangrena vulvæ bei einem 2jährigen Kinde.
Jahresb. ü. d. Verwalt. d. Med.-Wes., d. Krankenanst.
. . . d. Stadt Frankf. (1871), 1872, xv, 196.—**Lucas.**
Wangenbrand. Gen.-Ber. d. k. rhein. Med.-Coll. 1832,
Koblenz, 1833, 135.—**Lukens** (Anna). A case of noma
pudendi. N. York M. J., 1882, xxxvi, 366-368.—**Meyer**
(A.) Beobachtung eines idiopathischen Erysipelas gan-
grænosum der Geschlechtstheile. Med. Aehrenlese, Osnabrück, 1859, 681.—**Morse** (W. H.) Noma. Louisville
M. News, 1878, v, 213-216. ———. Contribution to the pathology of noma. Med. Rec., N. Y., 1885, xxvii, 37.—
Nagel. Noma; Fortpflanzung des Oedems in die Augenhöhle; neuroparalytische Hornhauterweichung; consecutive unlösbare Contractur des Unterkiefers. Anlegung eines künstlichen Gelenkes. Allg. Wien. med. Ztg.,
1869, xiv, 27.—**Naumann.** Ueber die Ursachen und das
Wesen der Mundfäule und des Wasserkrebses. Wissensch. Ann. d. ges. Heilk., Berl., 1833, xxvii, 421-434.—
Navratil (I.) † Orvosi hetil., Budapest, 1882, xxvi, 529.—
Nicolas (H.) Du noma ou gangrène de la bouche. Marseille méd., 1883, xx, 652-657.—**Numan** (S. H.) Waarnemingen omtrent den waterkanker, ulcus noma. Geneesk.
Mag., Leyden, 1815, v, 3. st., 74-104.—**Oberstadt.** Noma.
Gen.-Ber. d. k. rhein. Med.-Coll. 1832, Koblenz, 1833, 133-
135. ———. Noma von fast fünfmonatlicher Dauer. Wchnschr. f. d. ges. Heilk., Berl., 1834, iii, 380-382.—**Pauli**
(F.) jun. Noma. J. f. Geburtsh., Leipz., 1835, xiv, 119-
130.—**Peebles** (J. F.) A case of noma, resulting, apparently, from a physical cause. Boston M. & S. J., 1847-8,
xxxvii, 519-521.—**Pernitza** (E.) Beitrag zur Therapie
der Noma. Wien. med. Wchnschr., 1873, xxiii, 728-730.—
Pinto Portella. † Gaz. d. hosp., Rio de Jan., 1883, i,
226-231.—**Pohl** (A.) Cancer aquaticus. Mitth. a. d.
Geb. d. Heilk., Leipz., 1815, i, 215.—**Politzer** (L. M.)
Mehrere Fälle von Noma. Jahrb. d. Kinderh., Wien,
1865, vii, 4. Hft., 56-60.—**Purefoy** (R. D.) Some cases of
noma pudendi. Dublin J. M. Sc., 1882, lxxiii, 537-541.—
Reder (A.) Ein Fall von Noma. Mag. f. d. ges. Heilk.,
Berl., 1838, li, 371.—**Reimer.** Cholera; Noma. Jahrb.
f. Kinderh., Leipz., 1876, x, 85-92.—**Richter** (A. L.) Beiträge zur Lehre vom Wasserkrebs; ein Nachtrag zu der
Monographie dieser Krankheit. *In his*: Abhandlungen
aus dem Gebiete der prakt. Medicin und Chirurgie, 8°,
Berl., 1832, 188-261. *Also*, Reprint. ———. Ueber Ædœoitis gangrænosa puellarum. Wissensch. Ann. d. ges.
Heilk., Berl., 1835, xxxi, 160-167.—**Ripley** (J. H.) A
case of noma following intermittent fever; recovery. Med.
Rec., N. Y., 1875, x, 266.—**Röser.** Ueber Noma. Med.
Cor.-Bl. d. württemb. ärztl. Ver., Stuttg., 1857, xxvii, 353-
358.—**Sandberg.** Et Tilfælde af Ædœoitis gangrænosa.
Norsk Mag. f. Lægevidensk., Christiania, 1840, i, 247-
254.—**Sansom** (A. E.) On a case of noma, in which
moving bodies were observed in the blood during life.
Med.-Chir. Tr., Lond., 1878, lxi, 1-11, 1 pl. *Also* [Abstr.]:
Proc. Roy. M. & Chir. Soc. Lond., 1878, viii, 245-248.—
Schönheit (R.) Noma metastaticum. Ztschr. f. Nat.
u. Heilk. in Ungarn, Oedenburg, 1858, ix, 57.—**Schwarz.**
Seltner Fall von geheiltem Wasserkrebs. Wchnschr. f.
d. ges. Heilk., Berl., 1835, 574-577.—**Segale** (G. B.) Noma e sua pathogenesi; osservazione clinica. Rivista,
Genova, 1882, i, 20-29.—**Szerlecki** (L. A.) Ueber
Noma. J. d. Chir. u. Augenh., Berl., 1840, xxix, 273-296.—
Thomassen à Thuessink (E. J.) Waarnemingen.
[Ulcus noma.] Geneesk. Mag., Leyden, 1807, iv, 3. st.,
52-74. ———. Over het ulcus noma. *Ibid.*, 1815, v, 3. st.,
70-74. ———. **Thompson** (E.) On gangrenous erosion in
children. Lond M. & Phys. J., 1827, n. s., ii, 523-527.—
Thortsen. † Med. Ztg., Berl., 1842, xi, 179. ———. Noma
ohne tödtlichen Ausgang. Wchnschr. f. d. ges. Heilk.,
Berl., 1844, 426.—**Thouret.** Observation d'une gangrène
des parties génitales et de la partie inférieure des parois
abdominales chez une petite fille de deux mois. Bull. Soc.
anat. de Par. 1826, 2. éd., 1841, i, 148-151.—**Trousseau.**
De la gangrène chez les enfants. Gaz. d. hôp., Par., 1857,
xxx, 209.—**Van Oye.** Mémoire sur une affection gangréneuse qui attaque particulièrement la bouche et les parties
génitales externes des enfants. Ann. Soc. méd.-chir. de
Bruges, 1844, v, 171-192.—**Van Rhyn** (H. W.) Waarneming van ulcus noma. Nederl. Lancet, Utrecht, 1843-4, vi,
217-221, 1 pl.—**Van Zadelhoff** (A. J.) Jets over de
pathologische anatomie van ulcus noma. Nederl Tijdschr.
v. Heel- en Verlosk., Utrecht, 1859-60, x, 586-591, 1 pl.—
Vogel (L.) Glückliche Behandlung des Wasserkrebses.
J. f. Chir. u. Augenh., Berl., 1828, xii, 574-576.—**Weber.**
Mémoire sur le noma, ou cancer aquatique, ou stomacace.
Gaz. méd. de Strasb., 1844, iv, 257-267. *Also*: Ann. de
méd. belge, Brux., 1844, iv, 80-84.—**Wood** (K.) History
of a very fatal affection of the pudendum of female children. Med.-Chir. Tr., Lond., 1816, vii, 84-102.—**Wunderlich.** Zwei Fälle von Noma. Med. Cor.-Bl. d. württemb. ärztl. Ver., Stuttg., 1854, xxiv, 62.—**Zürcher.** Ein
Fall von Noma, geheilt durch Carbolsäure. Cor.-Bl. f.
schweiz. Aerzte, Basel, 1871, i, 198.

Nomenclature.

See, also, **Anatomy** (*Nomenclature of*); **Fevers**
(*Classification, etc., of*); **Insanity** (*Diagnosis, etc.,
of*); **Medicine** (*Dictionaries, etc., of*); **Nosology**; **Obstetrics**; **Records** (*Medical*); **Registration**; **Statistics** (*Medical, etc.*)

ANKE (N.) Philologisch-medicinische Bemerkungen. 1. Hft. 12°. *Moskwa*, 1846.

BERTRAND (S.-G.) * I. Quelles sont les bases
d'une bonne nomenclature en pathologie? II.
[etc.] 4°. *Paris*, 1840.

BOSTON Medical Association. Nomenclature
of diseases for the city of Boston, prepared by
the . . . 4°. [*n. p., n. d.*]

CALSAT (A.-I.-P.) * Des nomenclatures en
pathologie. 4°. *Paris*, 1847.

DELPECH (A.-L.-D.) * Des principes à observer pour la nomenclature des maladies. 4°.
Paris, 1853.

DUBOIS (L.) * Des nomenclatures en pathologie. 4°. *Paris*, 1845.

DUCLOS (H.) * De la nomenclature médicale.
4°. *Paris*, 1849.

HERIZ (E.) Clasificacion de los conocimientos
humanos. 8°. *Barcelona*, 1880.

INDEX Medicus. Editorial. The classication
of subjects adopted in the Index Medicus. 8°.
[*New York*], 1884.

KÜHN (C. G.) [Pr.] de inepta cognitionis
græci sermonis simulatione. 4°. *Lipsiæ* [1821].

LENGLET-MORTIER & VANDAMME (D.) Nouvelles et véritables étymologies médicales tirées
du gaulois. 8°. *Paris*, 1857.

LOEWENSTEIN (J. S.) De prosodia medica,
sive de recta verborum in medicina usitatorum
pronunciatione. 8°. *Berolini*, 1828.

MASSACHUSETTS. Statistical nosology adapted
for registration in Massachusetts, and requirements of law relative to certificates of causes of
death. By Henry B. Peirce, secretary of the
Commonwealth. 8°. *Boston*, 1878.

MURAT (J.-A.) Mémoire qui a remporté le
premier prix au jugement de la Société de médecine de Toulouse dans sa séance du 10 novembre 1806, sur la question proposée en ces termes:
Déterminer quels sont les avantages ou les inconvéniens de la multiplicité des nomenclatures,
relativement aux travaux des anatomistes, des
physiologistes et des nosographes. 8°. *Montpellier*, 1807.

NEMNICH (P.-A.) Lexicon nosologicum polyglotton omnium morborum symptomatum vitiorumque naturæ et affectionum propria nomina
decem diversis linguis explicata continens. fol.
Hamburgi, 1801.

NEW YORK (*City*). Department of Public Charities. The nomenclature of diseases. Adopted by
the commissioners of public charities and correction, on the recommendation of the medical
boards of Bellevue, Charity, and Infants' Hospitals, for the hospitals of the department of public charities and corrections. December, 1869.
8°. *New York*, 1870.

NEW YORK (*City*). Health Department. *Metropolitan Board of Health.* Statistical nomenclature of causes of death, classified and arranged
upon the basis recommended by the International Statistical Congress for the purposes of
public registration. Synonymous terms in English, Latin, French, and German, to ensure accurate and comparable certificates of death, and
uniformity in the records of mortality in the
metropolitan sanitary district of New York City.
4°. [*n. p., n. d.*]

NEW YORK State Board of Health. Nomenclature of diseases. fol. [*Albany*, 1884.]

NOMENKLATURA bolieznei i instruktsija dlja
bolnichnoi otchetnosti. Sostavleni vrachami

Nomenclature.

Odesskoi Gorodskoi Bolnitsi. [Nomenclature of diseases, and instructions for hospital attendant. Prepared by the Odessa City Hospital physicians.] 8°. *Odessa*, 1885.

OCHIAI TAIZO. Kan Yo Biomei Taishoroku. [A comparative index of nomenclature and symptomatology in Chinese, Western [Latin], and Japanese languages.] 8°. *Tokio*, 1883.

PLAZ (A. G.) [Pr.] de ὀνοματοθεσίας in re medica difficultate præfatus. 4°. *Lipsiæ*, [1773].

PROEKT nomenklatura bolieznei, dlya zemskoi meditsinskii praktiki. [Proposed nomenclature of diseases for country practice.] 8°. *Moscow*, 1876.

Repr. from: Moskov. med. Gaz.

RADOUAN (A.) * De la nomenclature pathologique. 4°. *Paris*, 1849.

RAFINESQUE-SCHMALTZ (C. G.) Principes fondamentaux de somiologie ou les loix de la nomenclature et de la classification de l'empire organique ou des animaux et·des végétaux, contenant les règles essentielles de l'art de leur imposer des noms immuables et de les classer méthodiquement. 8°. *Palerme*, 1814.

ROYAL College of Physicians, London. The nomenclature of diseases drawn up by a joint committee appointed by the . . . (Subject to decennial revision.) 8°. *London*, 1869.

——. The nomenclature of diseases drawn up by a joint committee appointed by the Royal College of Physicians of London. (Subject to decennial revision). 8°. *London*, 1869.

——. The same. Reprinted by order of the American Medical Association. 8°. *Philadelphia*, 1869.

——. Royal College of Physicians, May, 1881. Nomenclature. [Changes suggested by subcommittee on classification, in the section of "General diseases".] fol. [*London*, 1881.]

——. The nomenclature of diseases drawn up by a joint committee appointed by the . . . (Subject to decennial revision.) 2. ed., being the first revision. 8°. *London*, 1884.

——. The same. 8°. *London*, 1885.

SEILER (G.) [Pr.] synonymiæ medico-practicæ. Pt. i-vii. 4°. *Vitebergæ*, [1805-6].

STARK (J.) Remarks on Dr. Farr's proposed new statistical classification of diseases for statistical returns. 8°. *Edinburgh*, 1860.

UNITED STATES. *Treasury Department. Marine Hospital Service.* Nomenclature of diseases prepared for the use of the medical officers of the United States Marine Hospital Service, by the supervising surgeon, J. M. Woodworth. (Being the classification and English-Latin terminology of the provisional nomenclature of the Royal College of Physicians of London. 8°. *Washington*, 1874.

UNITED STATES. *War Department. Medical Department.* Proposed nomenclature of diseases for the information of medical officers; to be returned with remarks or criticism. 8°. [*Washington*, 1884.]

——. Form 42. Nomenclature to be followed in making the monthly report of sick and wounded. [Med. Dept. U. S. Army.] 4°. [*n. p., n. d.*]

WECKER (J. J.) Medicæ syntaxes, medicinam universam ordine pulcherrimo complectens, ex selectioribus medicis, tam græcis quam latinis et arabibus collectæ et concinnatæ, per . . . fol. *Basileæ*, 1562.

WEDELIUS (G. W.) [Pr.] de accentibus. 4°. *Jenæ*, [1706].

ZBOROVSZKY (A.) * Notio terminorum technicorum in scientia medica occurrentium philologice deductorum. 8°. *Pestini*, 1836.

Nomenclature.

American Medical Association. A nomenclature of diseases, with the reports of the majority and of the minority of the committee thereon; presented to the American Medical Association, at the meeting held in Philadelphia, May, 1872. Tr. Am. M. Ass., Phila., 1872, xxiii (app.), 1-94. *Also*, Reprint.—**Billings** (J. S.) [*et al.*] Report of committee on the nomenclature of diseases and on vital statistics. Rep. Nat. Bd. Health 1880, Wash., 1882, ii, 537-594.—**Boston** nomenclature of diseases. Boston M. & S. J., 1837, xvi, 208.—**Bugat** (P.) Természettudományi szóhalmaz, hihetőleg több mint harminczezer müszóval, gyüjtötte. [Medical terms proposed as a new terminology.] Orvosi Tár, Pest, 1841, ii, 257-264.—**van der Burg** (C. L.) Alphabetische lijst van maleische of javaansche woorden, betrekking hebbende op ontleed- en ziektenkunde. *In his:* De geneesk. in Nederl.-Indië. 's Gravenh., 1887, ii, 808-816.—**de Candolle** (A.) A dominant language for science. Pharm. J. & Tr., Lond., 1876, lxxiv, 134-137. — **Circulaire** à messieurs les généraux et intendants des divisions militaires, aux officiers de santé et aux officiers d'administration du service des hôpitaux militaires, contenant une nouvelle nomenclature pour la constatation des causes de décès dans les hôpitaux militaires. Rec. de mém. de méd. . . . mil. Par., 1860, 3. s., iii, 185-190.—**Curran** (W.) New names for old diseases. Med. Press & Circ., Lond., 1885, n. s., xl, 412.—**Egeling** (S. J.) De taal der geneeskundigen. Nederl. Tijdschr. v. Geneesk., Amst., 1882, 2. R., xviii, 2. Afd., 192-194.—**Etymological** perversions of scientific nomenclature. Med. Times & Gaz., Lond., 1853, n. s., vi, 302.—**Fothergill** (J. M.) Classification and nomenclature of disease. Med. Press & Circ., Lond., 1886, n. s., xlii, 390. — **Furukawa** Yei. [On medical nomenclature.] Chiugai Iji Shinpo, Tokei, Jan. 10, 1883.—**Galligani** (G.) Proposta di una classificazione chirurgica. Sperimentale, Firenze, 1869, xxiv, 122-138.—**Githens** (W. H. H.) Remarks on the new chemical nomenclature. Phila. M. Times, 1872-3, iii, 763; 779.—**Good** (J. M.) On medical technology. Tr. M. Soc. Lond., 1810, i, 1-50, 1 tab.—**Grant** (W. T.) A dichotomous analysis of diseases founded on their symptoms. South. M. Rec., Atlanta, 1873, iii, 325-340.—**Halbertsma** (H. J.) De taalkundige afleiding van het woord: coronoïdeus. Nederl. Tijdschr. v. Geneesk., Amst., 1862, vi, 612. *Also, in his:* Ontleedk. anteeken., 8°., Amst., 1862, 10-12.—**Heidenreich** (F. W.) Neue Classification der chirurgischen Krankheiten. J. d. Chir. u. Augenh., Berl., 1839, xxviii, 617-643.—**Hettich.** Rückblicke auf die medicinische Nomenclatur. Memorabilien, Heilbr., 1882, n. F., ii, 470-477.—**Hoblyn** (R. D.) On terminology. J. Cutan. M., Lond., 1867-8, i, 247-253.—**Holt** (T.) Remarks on pharmaceutical nomenclature. Lancet, Lond., 1842, ii, 416-418.—**Kraft.** Die Macht der Worte und die Mängel der Terminologie in der Medicin. Vrtljschr. f. d. prakt. Heilk., Prag, 1848, ii, 77-86.—**Kühn** (C. G.) De inepta cognitionis græci sermonis simulatione, i-v. *In his:* Opus acad. med. et philol., 8°. Lips., 1828, ii, 260-297.—**Leroux** (J.-J.) Quelques réflexions sur la valeur des noms donnés aux maladies; et raisons qui nous empêchent de renoncer aux noms anciens. J. de méd., chir., pharm., etc., Par., 1804, viii, 208-229.—**de Letamendi** (J.) Cucharada de lego en los elementos de lexicología griega con aplicación al tecnicismo médico. Rev. de cien. méd., Barcel., 1881, vii, 465-473.—**Levié** & **Virchow** (R.) Zur Terminologie der fauligen Infection. [Vorschlag und Gegenvorschlag] Arch. f. path. Anat., etc., Berl., 1876, lxvi, 525.—**McLeod** (K.) Notes on "The nomenclature of diseases", framed by the Royal College of Physicians of London. Indian Ann. M. Sc., Calcutta, 1879, v, 25-75.—**Marshall** (W. J.) On the influence of language upon medical thought and practice. Glasgow M. J., 1883, [4.] s., xx, 161-170.—**Mayne** (R. G.) On the nomenclature of the science of medicine. Lancet, Lond., 1846, ii, 403; 607: 1847, i, 117; 169: ii, 45.—**Medical** Association of the State of Alabama. Structure and classification of the statistical nomenclature of diseases and causes of death. Tr. M. Ass. Alabama, Montgomery, 1884, xxxvi, 243-245.—**Medicinische** (Die) Terminologie. Arch. f. physiol. Heilk., Stuttg., 1842, i, 503-506.—**Melville** (H.) The importance and value of correct notation to the advancement of medical science. Am. M. Month., N. Y., 1851, i, 329-335.—**Mestre** (A.) Consideraciones lexiológicas con motivo de algunos términos técnicos. Crón. méd.-quir. de la Habana, 1881, vii, 349; 397; 457; 493.—**Miller** (E.) An attempt to deduce a nomenclature of certain febrile and pestilential diseases from the origin and nature of their remote cause. Med. Reposit., N. Y., 1804, i, 362-372.—**Mortality** statistics and nomenclature of diseases. Rep. Bd. Health Illinois 1882, Springfield, 1883, v, 535-602.—**Moxon** (W.) On the necessity for a clinical nomenclature of disease. Guy's Hosp. Rep., Lond., 1870, 3. s., xv, 479-500.—**Nomenclature** of disease. Brit. & For. M.-Chir. Rev., Lond., 1869, xliv, 352-370.—**Nomenclature** of diseases. Tr. Am. M. Ass., Phila., 1872, xxiii (app.), 1-77.—**Nomenclature** (The) of diseases. Brit. M. J., Lond., 1868, ii, 316: 396: 1869, i, 55.—**Nomenclature** des maladies et infirmités, reconnues incurables, qui sont in-

Nomenclature.

compatibles avec le service de la garde nationale; arrêtée par l'Académie nationale de médecine. Rev. méd.-chir. de Par., 1851, ix, 377–380.—**Parkinson** (T.) Animadversions on medical nomenclature, and a new one proposed. Lond. M. Reposit., 1819, xi, 364; 478.—**Piorry.** Du traitement de la variole, ou plutôt des états pathologiques qui lui sont propres. Bull. Acad. de méd., Par., 1854–5, xx, 478–504. *Also*, Reprint. [Discussion], 549; 567; 604; 619; 648; 679; 727, 742; 806; 902.—**Poore** (G. V.) Abstract of introductory address delivered at the opening of University College Medical School, [medical language]. Med. Times & Gaz., Lond., 1881, ii, 457–459. — **Pruckmayr** (A.) Paracelsische Krankheits-Namen. Med.-chir. Centralbl., Wien, 1880, xv. 97; 109. — **Quelques** réflexions sur la nomenclature ou la langue médicale. J. hebd. de méd., Par., 1830, vi, 65–71. — **Rabagliati** (A. R) Precautions to be taken in medical nomenclature and classification, to guard against false statistical conclusions. Tr. Internat. M. Cong., 7. sess., Lond., 1881, iv, 559. ——— Some remarks on the classification and nomenclature of diseases. Med. Press & Circ., Lond., 1886, n. s., xli, 279; 301; 323; 345; 373.—**Read** (E.) Mortality statistics of the census of 1850, and a review of the letter of Dr. Edward Jarvis, upon the classification of diseases. N. Am. M.-Chir. Rev., Phila., 1858, ii, 334–340.—**Rebentisch.** Ueber die unrichtige Benennung einiger Lokal-Krankheiten, besonders des Blutgefäss-Systems. Arch. f. med. Erfahr., Berl., 1810, xiv, 153–157. — **Report** of the committee appointed "to prepare a nomenclature of diseases adapted to the United States, having reference to a general registration of deaths". Proc. Nat. M. Convent., Phila., 1846–7, 133–175. — **Report** of the committee on nomenclature of diseases. Tr. Am. M. Ass., Phila., 1879, xxi, 121–125.— **Report** of committee on the nomenclature of diseases and on vital statistics. Nat. Bd. Health Bull., Wash., 1880–81, i (suppl. no. 9), 1–24. — **Reydellet.** Nomenclature. Dict. d. sc. méd., Par., 1819, xxxvi, 183–201.— **Royal** College of Physicians, Edinburgh. Report of the council of the Royal College of Physicians of Edinburgh on "The nomenclature of diseases". Edinb. M. J., 1868–9, xiv, 1115–1118. — **S.** (M. N.) Necesidad de perfectionar el lenguaje médico. Bol. de med., cirug. y farm., Madrid, 1838, v, 9; 41; 49; 81; 97; 125; 141; 1839, vi, 33; 41; 49.—**Sandras.** De l'influence facheuse de certains mots en thérapeutique. Tr. méd., Par., 1831, iii, 394–408. — **Schubert** (A.) Eine Erinnerung an das Gefährliche der Krankheits-Namen. Berl. med. Centr.-Ztg., 1837, vi, 395–404.—**Seguin** (E.) International uniformity in the practice and records of physic. Med. Rec., N. Y., 1876, xi, 554–556. *Also*, Reprint.—**Sterre** (D. L.) Benennung derer vornehmsten Kranckheiten; Lateinisch, Teutsch und Holländisch. *In his:* Nova-praxis medico-chirurgica, 12°, Dresden, 1710, 301–320. — **Stillson** (H.) Pronunciation of medical terms. Louisville M. News, 1884, xvii, 33.—**Tempesti** (G. C.) Sull' imbarbarimento del linguaggio medico in Italia. Bull. d. sc. med. di Bologna, 1883, 6. s., xi, 414–426. — **Virchow** (R.) Ueber ärztliche Terminologie. Berl. klin. Wchnschr., 1875, xii, 62. *Also, in his:* Ges. Abhandl. a. d. Geb. d. öff. Med., 8°, Berl., 1879, i, 576; 612. ——— Barbarismen in der medicinischen Sprache. Arch. f. path. Anat., etc., Berl., 1883, xci, 1–11. *Also, transl.* [Abstr.]: Med. Times & Gaz., Lond., 1883, i. 250.—**W** sprawie statystyki śmiertelności Warszawy. [Nomenclature of diseases in the Warsaw school.] Medycyna, Warszawa, 1877, v, 382–384.

Nomenclature (The) of diseases drawn up by a joint committee appointed by the Royal College of Physicians of London. (Subject to decennial revision.) xxiv, 327 pp. 8°. *London, for the Royal College of Physicians,* 1869.

Nomenclature of diseases prepared for the use of the medical officers of the United States Marine Hospital Service, by the supervising surgeon, J. M. Woodworth. (Being the classification and English-Latin terminology of the provisional nomenclature of the Royal College of Physicians, London.) xxii, 210 pp. 8°. *Washington, Government Printing Office,* 1874.

Nomenclature des instrumens de chirurgie et objets de coutellerie à l'usage des hôpitaux de la marine et des colonies, et prix auxquels le sieur Grangeret, coutelier, demeurant à Paris, rue des Saints-Pères, no. 45, s'engage à les livrer dans les ports, conformément aux clauses et conditions exprimées par sa soumission en date du 30 juin 1822. 5–16 pp. roy. 8°. [*Paris*, 1822.]

Nomenklatura bolieznei i instruktsija dlja bolnichnoi otchetnosti. Sostavleno vrachami Odesskoi Gorodskoi Bolnitsi. [Nomenclature of diseases, and instructions for hospital attendants.]

Nomenklatura bolieznei [etc.]—continued. Prepared by the Odessa City Hospital physicians.] 52 pp., 1 l., 1 diag. 8°. *Odessa,* 1885.

Nomina eorum qui gradum medicinæ doctoris in Academia Jacobi Sexti regis, quæ Edinburgi est, anno 1844 adepti sunt. 3 pp. 8°. [*Edinburgh,* 1848.] [P., v. 1198.]

de Nonancourt (Ed.-J.) *Des amputations spontanées intra-utérines. 1 p. l., 45 pp., 1 l., 4 pl. 4°. *Strasbourg,* 1864, No. 754, v. 39.

Nonat (Auguste) [1804–87]. *Sur la métro-péritonite puerpérale compliquée de l'inflammation des vaisseaux lymphatiques de l'utérus. x, 11–39 pp. 4°. *Paris,* 1832, No. 98, v. 251.

———. *Existe-t-il un asthme essentiel ? 35 pp. 4°. *Paris,* 1835, No. 400.
Concours.

———. Recherches sur la grippe et sur les pneumonies observées pendant le mois de février. 19 pp. 12°. [*Paris,* 1837.]
Repr. from: Arch. gén. de méd., Par., 1837, 2. s., xiv.

———. The same. 2. article. Observations de pneumonie, suite de grippe avec fausses membranes dans les bronches des lobes hépatisés. 34 pp. 12°. [*Paris,* 1837.]
Repr. from: Arch. gén. de méd., Par., 1837, 2. s., xiv.

———. *Thèse sur la question suivante: Des diathèses. 67 pp. 4°. *Paris, imp. de Moessard,* 1838.
Concours.

———. Note sur l'emploi des fumigations chlorées en vue de désinfecter l'air et de diminuer les ravages du choléra. 8 pp. 8°. *Paris, Moquet,* [1857, *vel subseq.*].

———. Traité pratique des maladies de l'utérus et de ses annexes. ix, 896 pp. 8°. *Paris, A. Delahaye,* 1860.

———. Traité des dyspepsies, ou étude pratique de ces affections basée sur les données de la physiologie expérimentale et de l'observation clinique. iv, 226 pp. 8°. *Paris, A. Delahaye,* 1862.

———. Traité théorique et pratique de la chlorose avec une étude spéciale sur la chlorose des enfants. 211 pp. 8°. *Paris, A. Delahaye,* 1864.

———. The same. 3. article. II. Pneumonie sous forme adynamique, sans fausse membrane dans les bronches. 29 pp. 12°. [*Paris,* 1837 ?]
Repr. from: Arch. gén. de méd., Par., 1837, 2. s., xiv.

———. Traité pratique des maladies de l'utérus, de ses annexes et des organes génitaux externes. 2. éd. . . . avec la collaboration du docteur A. Linas. xxiii, 1189 pp. roy. 8°. *Paris, A. Delahaye,* 1874.
See, also, **Serres** & **Nonat** [Auguste]. Mémoire sur la psorentérie, etc. 4°. *Paris,* [1832].

——— & **Bouley.** Recherches sur la morve aiguë. 20 pp., 1 pl. 4°. *Paris, F. Locquin & Cie.,* 1839.
Repr. from: Expérience, Par., 1839, v.

Noncher (Adolphe - Ferdinand). *Des accouchements dangereux, ou de certains accidents graves qui peuvent survenir pendant l'accouchement, et des moyens d'y remédier. 72 pp. 4°. *Paris,* 1844, No. 114, v. 422.

Non-commissioner [*pseudon.*]. A report on the sanitary condition of the army, particularly during the late war with Russia. 40 pp. 8°. [*n. p.,* 1856, *vel subseq.*] [*Also, in:* P., v. 324.]

Nonne. Ueber Plexuslähmungen (mit Krankenvorstellung). 3 pp. 8°. *Berlin, J. Sittenfeld,* [1887].
Repr. from: Deutsche med. Wchnschr., Leipz., 1887, xiii.

Nonnenmann (Joh.) *Diss. sistens observationem apoplexiæ ex nimiis animi contentionibus ortæ. 22 pp. 4°. *Argentorati, J. H. Heitz,* [1771].

Nonnenmann (Joh.)—continued.

——. * Dissertatio anatomico-chirurgica agens de hernia congenita in qua intestinum in contactu testis est. 38 pp. 4°. *Argentorati, ex off. J. H. Heitzii*, [1771]

Also [Abstr.], *in :* WEIZ (F. A.) Vollständ. Ausz. [etc.] 12°. *Leipz. u. Budissin*, 1773, v, 99-106.

Nonnig (Paul) [1857–]. * Beitrag zur Kasuistik der extrauterinen Gravidität und deren Ausgang in Lithopädionbildung. 35 pp. 8°. *Berlin, G. Lange*, [1880].

Nonnis (C. Efisio). Primi studj in Sardegna sull' omeopatia. 47 pp. 8°. *Cagliari, tipog. nazionale*, 1854. [P., v. 1456.]

——. Continuazione agli studj sull' omeopatia colla risposta a Tommaso Scardassal. 75 pp. 8°. *Cagliari*, 1854. [P., v. 1456.]

Nonnis (Giovanni). Della gonorrea e dell' orchite come uno de' più frequenti fenomeni a cui può essa dare origine guarite coll' omiopatia. 19 pp. 8°. *Torino, unione tipog.-editrice*, 1855. [P., v. 1452.]

——. Dell' igiene, sua storia e suoi rapporti colla morale, colla politica e colla medicina. 46 pp. 8°. *Casale, G. Nani*, 1860. [P., v. 1427.]

——. Risposta al Dott. Borelli sul suo articolo inserito nell' Opinione : Omeopatia ed allopatia. 23 pp. 8°. *Torino, F. B. Savojardo*, [n. d.] [P., v. 1451.]

Nonnus [*or* **Nonnius**] (Ludovicus) [1555–1646]. Diæteticon, sive de re cibaria libri iv. 16 p. l., 638 pp., 1 l. 12°. *Antverpiæ, P. et J. Belleros*, 1627.

——. The same. 11 p. l., 526 pp. 4°. *Antverpiæ, ex off. P. Belleri*, 1646.

Nonus [**Nonnus**] (Theophanus). De omnium particularium morborum curatione, sic ut febres quoque et tumores præter naturam complectatur, liber nunc primum in lucem editus, et summa diligentia conversus per Hieremiam Martium. 11 p. l., 322 pp., 10 l. 12°. *Argentorati, excud. J. Ribelius*, 1568.

Greek and Latin text in parallel columns.

——. The same. Epitome de curatione morborum, græce ac latine. Ope codicum manuscriptorum recensuit notasque adjecit Jo. Steph. Bernard. 2 v. xl, 463 pp. ; 428 pp., 1 pl. 8°. *Gothæ, C. W. Ettinger ; Amstelodami, J. St. von Esveldt, Holtrop et soc.*, 1794–5.

——. De febribus liber.

In : FEBRIBUS (De) opus sane aureum, [etc.] fol. *Venetiis*, 1576, 13ᵇ–14ᵇ. Also forms pp. 157-174 of his : De omnium [etc.], and 427-463 of : Epitome de curatione [etc.]

Nonweiler (Gustavus) [1838–]. * De echinococcis hepatis. 32 pp. 8°. *Berolini, G. Schade*, [1862].

Nony (Edmond). * Retour de l'inflammation dans les lésions osseuses anciennes à la suite d'un état général grave. 36 pp. 4°. *Paris*, 1874, No. 462.

Noodt (Carl). * Das Osteotom und seine Anwendung. 3 p. l., 60 pp. 4°. *München, G. Franz*, 1836.

——. Helcologia universalis. Das Ganze der Lehre von den Geschwüren in tabellarischer Form. Nach den besten Quellen bearbeitet. 37 pp. 4°. *Leipzig, L. Voss*, 1839.

See, also, **Buchheister** (Jurgeno Chr.) & **Noodt** (C.) Erfahrungen über die Cholera asiatica, etc. 8°. *Altona*, 1832.

Noodt (Guilielmus Walraven). * De monstro quodam humano. [Leyden.] iv, 84 pp., 7 l., 2 pl. 8°. *Schoonhoviæ, S. E. van Nooten*, 1839.

Noordhuusen (Elia Andreas). * De antihectico. 8 pp. 4°. *Harniæ, ex reg. universit. typog.*, [1707].

Noorduyn (Claas) * De cura typhi. 2 p. l., 48 pp. 8°. *Lugd. Bat., J. H. Gebhard et socios*, [1846].

van Noort (Albertus). * De morbis soporosis. 11 pp., 1 l. 4°. *Lugd. Bat., A. Elzevier*, [1706].

op ten Noort (Hendrick Jan). * Spec. exhibens theses quasdam controversas. 1 p. l., 35 pp., 1 l. 4°. *Lugd. Bat., S. et J. Luchtmans*, 1790. [P., v. 1012.]

Noortwyk (Gerardus Albertus). * De organis respirationis, eorumque usu. 45 pp., 1 l. 4°. *Lugd. Bat., J. et H. Verbeek*, 1763.

——. * Uteri humani gravidi anatome et historia. 217 pp., 4 pl. 4°. *Lugd. Bat., J. et H. Verbeek*, 1743. [*Also, in :* P., v. 701.]

Noortwyk (Wilhelmus). * De natura humana. 1 p. l., 32 pp., 1 l. 4°. *Lugd. Bat., G. Potvliet*, 1735.

Also, in : NIHELL (James). Novæ raræque observationes . . . ex pulsu [etc.] 8°. *Venetiis*, 1759, 137-180.

Noot (Adamus). * De structura et usu renum. 29 pp., 2 l. 4°. *Lagd. Bat., G. Wishoff*, 1733.

Also, in : DE OBERKAMP (F. J.) Collect. diss. 4°. *Francof. a. M.*, 1767, i, 549-576.

van Nooten (Didericus Hoola). * Specimen juridicum inaugurale, de litterarum Cambialium cessione sive indossatione. 1 p. l., 33 pp., 4 l. 4°. *Lugd. Bat., S. et J. Luchtmans*, 1768. [P., v. 1004.]

Nooth (Joh. Mervin). * De rachitide. 1 p. l., 38 pp. 8°. *Edinburgi, R. et A. Foulis*, 1766. [P., v. 649.]

Also, in : SMELLIUS. Thesaurus med. [etc.] 8°. *Edinb.*, 1785, iii, 56-77.

Nootnagel (Daniel) [1753–1836]. * De amaurosi. xxiv pp. 4°. *Erlangæ, lit. W. Waltheri*, [1776].

Also [Abstr.], *in :* WEIZ (F. A.) Neue Ausz. [etc.] 12°. *Frankf. u. Leipz.*, 1780, xi, 71-73.

Nopitsch (Carl [Daniel Eberhard] Friedrich) [–1838]. Versuch einer Chronologie und Literatur, nebst einem System der Blutentziehungen, in besonderer Beziehung auf das physiologische und pathologische Verhältniss des Blutes, sowie dessen Berücksichtigung in gerichtlichen Fällen. Aus den vorzüglichsten Werken geschöpft. xxxviii, 441 pp. 8°. *Nürnberg, G. Winter*, 1833.

Noquet. Abcès résidueux du cou ressemblant à un kyste. Guérison après une seule ponction aspiratrice suivie d'une légère compression. 11 pp. 8°. *Lille, Castiaux*, 1879.

Repr. from : Bull. méd. du nord, Lille, 1879, xix.

——. Étude sur la surdité amygdalienne. 35 pp. 8°. *Lille, Castiaux*, 1879.

Repr. from : Bull. méd. du nord, Lille, 1879, xix.

Noquet (Vital). * Étude sur l'insolation et les accidents causés par la chaleur. 62 pp. 4°. *Paris*, 1872, No. 208.

Noræus (Joh.) * Sciagraphica nervorum capitis descriptio, et quidem paris 6., 7., 8., 9., 10., et 11. 28 pp. sm. 4°. *Upsaliæ, ex prelo vid. J. Edman*, [1793].

Bound with : Åkerman (Jacobus). Sciagraphica nervorum [etc.] 4°. *Upsaliæ*, [1793].

Noræus (Olavus). * Sciagraphica nervorum spinalium descriptio, et quidem parium cervicalium, cum plexu brachiali. 27 pp. 4°. *Upsaliæ, ex prelo vid. direct. J. Edman*, 1794.

Norbert (Louis - Silvain). * Sur les fièvres endémiques. vi, 7-31 pp. 4°. *Paris*, 1808, No. 1, v. 69.

Norby (K.) De l'assistance publique et des établissements de charité et institutions pieuses en Norvége. Exposé et tableaux pour la statistique internationale de l'assistance publique. 120 pp. roy. 4°. *Rome, héritiers Botta*, 1880.

Norchi (Pellegrino).

See **Pacini** (Filippo). Il colera asiatico. 8°. *Roma*, 1886.

Norcia.

See **Cholera** (*Asiatic, History, etc., of*), *by localities.*

Norcom (James) [1778–1850]. * On jaundice; containing observations on the liver and some of its diseases. 49 pp. 8°. *Philadelphia, J. Carey,* 1799. [*Also, in :* P., v. 509.]
For Biography. see Nelson's North. Lancet, Plattsburgh, N. Y., 1851-2, 1c9-180. *Also,* Reprint.

Norcom (*John*) [1801–56].
Satchwell (S. S.) The late John Norcom, M. D. Atlanta M. & S. J., 1857, ii, 385.

Norcom (William A. B.) [1836–81]. Modern treatment of acute internal inflammations. 16 pp. 8°. [*n. p.*], 1868.

——. Hæmorrhagic malarial fever; an address delivered before the Medical Society of North Carolina, at its 21st annual meeting, held in Charlotte in May, 1874. 30 pp. 8°. *Raleigh, Edwards, Broughton & Co.,* 1874.

——. Defective medical education the chief obstacle to a proper appreciation of our profession by the public, and what our alma mater is doing to remove it. Annual address delivered before the Society of the Alumni of the Medical Department of the University of Pennsylvania, March 14, 1878. With the proceedings of the alumni meeting of 1878. 64 pp. 8°. *Philadelphia, Collins,* 1878.
For Biography, see Tr. Am. M. Ass., Phila., 1882, xxxiii, 588 (J. W. Jones).

Nord (F.) * Sur la maladie scrofuleuse. 29 pp. 4°. *Paris,* 1836, No. 222, v. 300.

Nord (Département du). Rapports sur les travaux du Conseil central de salubrité et des conseils d'arrondissement du département du Nord, pendant les années 1828–30 (No. 1), 1833–79 (3-38), 1881 (40), 1882 (41). Présenté à M. le préfet, par MM. Thém. Lestiboudois, E. N. Davaine, Loiset, A. Gosselet, Ch. Pilat, et Jules Arnould. 8°. *Lille,* 1831–83. [No. 1 *also in :* P., v. 1788.]
Institué le 25 juin 1828. No. 1, for 1828–30; 3, 1833–7; 4, 1838–40; 5, 1841–2; 6, 1843–4; 7, 1845–6; 8, 1847–8; 9, 1849–50; 10, 1851 to 41, 1882, for 1 year each. No. 1, by Lestiboudois; 3 and 4, by Davaine; 5–7, by Loiset; 8–12, by Gosselet; 13–40, by Pilat; 41, by Arnould.

——. Rapport général sur l'épidémie du choléra qui a régné à Lille en 1832. (Fait au Conseil central de salubrité du département du Nord par une commission formée de MM. Dourleu, Trachez, Brigandat, Bailly et Lestiboudois, rapporteur.) 107 pp. 8°. *Lille, L. Danel,* [1833?] [P., v. 471.]

——. Rapport présenté au comité central de vaccine, sur l'état de la propagation de la vaccine dans le département du Nord pendant 1835. Par M. le docteur Lefebure, secrétaire général du comité central. 42 pp. 8°. *Lille, L. Danel,* 1836.

——. Statistique administrative et médicale de l'Asile public des aliénés de Lille, pour les années 1847–51. Rapport à Monsieur le préfet du département du Nord, par [L'Herbon de Lussats et A. Gosselet] le directeur et le médecin de l'asile. 92 pp. 8°. *Lille, Lefebvre-Ducrocq,* 1852.

——. L'hygiène et l'industrie dans le département du Nord. Vade - mecum des conseils de salubrité, des industriels et des fonctionnaires, chargé de la police sanitaire. Extrait des rapports des conseils d'hygiène et de salubrité du département du Nord. viii, 199 pp. 12°. *Lille, L. Danel,* 1857.

——. Observations météorologiques faites à Lille par Victor Meurein pendant les années 1855–6; 1858–9; 1866–7; 1878–9. 8°. *Lille,* 1857–80.
1855-6, *repr. from :* Rap. trav. Cons. centr. de salub. du dép. du Nord, Lille.

——. Table présentant par ordre alphabétique les matières traitées par les conseils d'hygiène

Nord (Département du)—continued.
et de salubrité du Nord depuis leur création, en 1828, jusqu'à la fin de 1858; suivie de la liste générale des ateliers et établissements classés depuis 1810 jusqu'en 1859, et de tableaux indiquant le nombre des séances tenues par le Conseil central, les noms de ses membres, la durée de leurs services et le nombre de rapports qu'ils ont rédigés ; par M. Tancrez, sous-secrétaire du Conseil central depuis 1832. 115 pp., 4 tab. 8°. *Lille, L. Danel,* 1860.

——. The same. Depuis 1859 jusqu'à la fin de 1868; suivie de tableaux indiquant le nombre des séances tenues par le Conseil central, les noms de ses membres, la durée de leurs services et le nombre de rapports qu'ils ont rédigés ; par M. Tancrez, sous-secrétaire du Conseil central depuis 1832. 109 pp., 3 tab. 8°. *Lille, L. Danel,* 1869.

——. The same. Depuis 1869 jusqu'à la fin de 1878; suivie des tableaux indiquant le nombre des séances tenues par le Conseil central, les noms de ses membres, la durée de leurs services et le nombre de rapports qu'ils ont rédigés ; par M. Tancrez, sous-secrétaire du Conseil central depuis 1832. pp. 353–444. 8°. *Lille, L. Danel,* 1880.

Nord (*Département du*).
See **Cholera** (*Asiatic, History, etc., of*), *by localities* ; **Physicians'** *aid societies,* etc.

Nordamerikanische Akademie der homöopathischen Heilkunst. Denkschriften. 1. Lief. Wirkungen des Schlangengiftes. C. C. Hering. viii, 116 pp. 4°. *Allentaun an der Lecha, H. Ebner,* 1837.

Nordamericanische, deutsch' medicinische Zeitschrift für praktische Heilkunde. Hrsg. von W. Meisburger. Zweimonatlich. Nos. 1-3, v. 1, 1865. 144 pp. 8°. *Buffalo, N. Y.* Ended.

Nordamerikanischer Monatsbericht für Natur- und Heilkunde. Redigirt von W. Keller und H. Tiedemann, unter Mitwirkung mehrerer Aerzte. [2 v. annually.] v. 1–4, July, 1850, to June, 1852. 8°. *Philadelphia, J. Weik.*
Ended. In July, 1851, Dr. Herzka added as editor, and F. W. Christern became publisher. In December, 1851, Herzka dropped. v. 2-3 paged consecutively, Jan. to Dec., 1851.

Nordau (S. Max) [1849–]. * De la castration de la femme. [Paris.] 64 pp. 4°. *Poissy,* 1882, No. 329 (?).

Nordblad (*Carl*) [1778–1840].
[**Obituary.**] *Cutting from :* Lefnadsteckn. öfver k. sv. vet. akad, s ledamöter, i, 11–15.

Norblad (Ericus And.) * Instructio peregrinatoris. 8°. *Upsaliæ,* 1759.
In : LINNÆUS. Amœnitates acad. [etc.] 8°. *Lugd. Bat.,* 1760, v, 298–313.

Norddeutsche (Der) Arzt. Organ für die wissenschaftlichen, socialen und materiellen Interessen der Medico-Chirurgen. Hrsg. von Wilhelm Kolloser. v. 2–3, October, 1870–72. 2 v. 8°. *Magdeburg.*
Want no. 6, v. 3, 1872. 10 nos. form a volume.

Norddeutscher Apotheker - Verein. Mitglieder - Verzeichniss und General - Rechnung, pro 1868; 1870; 1871. 8°. *Halle,* [*n. d.*]

Norddeutsche Thierärzte. Bericht über die am 18. und 19. Mai 1868 in Berlin abgehaltene Versammlung . . . und über die am 20. Mai stattgefundene Jubelfeier der Herrn . . . Gurlt. Hrsg. von den Vorständen des Berliner, schlesischen und rheinpreussischen thierärztlichen Vereins. 29 pp. 8°. *Berlin, J. Sittenfeld,* 1868.

Nordemann (T.) Ueber die Cholera infantum in New-York. 18 pp. 8°. *Bern, C. Raetzer,* 1860.
C.

Norden (J. C.) * Die Vergrösserung und Verhärtung der Vorsteherdrüse. 48 pp. 8°. *Würzburg, C. W. Becker,* 1831.

Nordenburg (Julius). Die Ventilatoren und deren Anwendung auf praktische Zwecke, oder ausführliche Beschreibung und Abbildung der neuesten und bewährtesten Anlagen, Apparate und Mechanismen zum Lüften von Wohnzimmern, Sälen, Billardzimmern, Bierstuben, Theatern, Kasernen, Lagern, Hospitälern, Gefangenhäusern, Schulen, Kinderbewahranstalten, Fabriken, Laboratorien, Dampf- und Segelschiffen, Eisenbahnwagen, Brunnenschachten und Bergwerken, Kellern und Gährungslokalen, Trockenstuben, Seidenraupereien, Gewächshäusern, Heu- und Getreidehaufen, Ställen, Abtritten, Schornsteinen, Gas- und Oellampenbrennern u. s. w. xii, 190 pp., 11 pl. 8°. *Weimar, B. F. Voigt,* 1860.
v. 76 of: Neuer Schauplatz der Künste und Handwerke.

Nordenson (E.) Recherches ophtalmométriques sur l'astigmatisme de la cornée chez des écoliers de 7 à 20 ans. 31 pp. 8°. *Gand, I. S. van Doosselaere,* 1883.
Repr. from: Ann. d'ocul., Brux., 1883, 12. s., ix.

Nordenson (Erik). * Till kännedomen om spontan näthinneaflossning. 2 p. l., 112 pp., 14 l., 13 pl. roy. 8°. *Stockholm,* 1886.

———. The same. Die Netzhantablösung. Untersuchungen über deren pathologische Anatomie und Pathogenese. Mit einem Vorwort von Dr. Theodor Leber. v (3 l.), 255 pp., 28 l., 27 pl. roy. 8°. *Wiesbaden, J. F. Bergmann,* 1887.

Nordenström (Wilhelm Magn.)
See **Bergstrand** (Carl Henr.) Chirurgiska iakttagelser. 8°. *Upsala*, [1842] 1848.— **Gelberstedt** (Pehr Erik). Bidrag till den tuberkulosa, etc. 8°. *Stockholm*, 1844.

Norder-Ditmarsch.

Dohrn. Ueber den Genius endemicus in Norder-Ditmarschen. Eine medicinisch-topographische Beschreibung dieser Landschaft. Mitth. a. d. Geb. d. Med., etc., Altona, 1835, iii, 11.-12. Hft., 1-40.

Norderney.

Barkhausen (G.) Helgoland und Norderney, als Seebadeorte neben einander gestellt. Hannov. Ann. f. d. ges. Heilk., 1840, v, 678-735.— **Beneke.** Ueber die sanitäre Bedeutung des Winteraufenthaltes auf Norderney. Ztschr. f. klin. Med., Berl., 1882, v, 294-299. — **Müller** (A.) Ueber einige gesundheitliche und landwirthschaftliche Missstände der Bade-Insel Norderney. Vrtljschr. f. gerichtl. Med., Berl., 1886, xliv, 162-166.

Nordhausen.

See, also, **Fever** (*Typhus, History, etc., of*), *by localities.*
WITTMEYER. Geburten und Sterbefälle in Nordhausen im Jahre 1876. 4°. *Nordhausen,* [1877].
Jahres-Tabelle der Sterblichkeitsverhältnisse der Stadt Nordhausen a. H. während des Jahres 1876. Veröffentl. d. k. deutsch. Gsndhtsamtes, Berl. (Beilage), 1877, No. 27.

Nordhof (Gustaf). * Ueber die physiologische und therapeutische Wirkung des Arseniks. 19 pp. 8°. *München, J. A. Giesser,* 1848.

Nordhoff (Aug. Wilhelm).
Editor of: **Archiv** für den thierischen Magnetismus, Jena, 1804.

Nordisches Archiv für Natur- und Arzneywissenschaft. Hrsg. von Prof. Pfaff in Kiel und Dr. Scheel in Kopenhagen. Bde. 1-4, 1799-1805. 8°. *Kopenhagen, F. Brummer.*
v. 2-4, title: Nordisches Archiv für Natur- und Arzneywissenschaft und Chirurgie; and Prof. Rudolphi in Greifswalde added as editor. Continued as: Neues nordisches Archiv für Naturkunde, [etc.]

Nordisches Archiv für Natur- und Arzneywissenschaft und Chirurgie.
Was title of v. 2-4 of: Nordisches Archiv für Natur- und Arzneywissenschaft.

Nordisk Tidsskrift for Abnormskolen (Blinde-, Døvstumme- og Aandssvageskolen).
Was title of v. 16-17 of: **Nordisk** Tidsskrift for Blinde-, Døvstumme- og Idiotskolen.

Nordisk Tidsskrift for Blinde-, Døvstumme- og Aandssvageskolen.
Was title of v. 8-15 of: **Nordisk** Tidsskrift for Blinde-, Døvstumme- og Idiotskolen.

Nordisk Tidsskrift for Blinde-, Døvstumme- og Idiotskolen, redigeret af J. Moldenhauer, Johan Keller. [Quarterly.] v. 1-17, 1867-85. 8°. *Kjøbenhavn.*
Title of v. 8-15 was: **Nordisk** Tidsskrift for Blinde-, Døvstumme- og Aandssvageskolen. Title of v. 16-17 was: **Nordisk** Tidsskrift for Abnormskolen (Blinde-, Døvstumme- og Aandssvageskolen). Prof. Keller died May 20, 1884.

Nordiskt Medicinskt Arkiv. Under medverkan af P. L. Panum [*et al.*], redigeradt af Axel Key. [Quarterly.] v. 1-19, 1869-87. 8°. *Stockholm, Samson & Wallin.*
Current. A continuation of: **Medicinskt** Archiv. v. 10 contains general index to v. 1-10.

Nordling (Viktor). Om tyfoidfebern i Upsala vintern 1883-4. Samt dess administrativa och juridiska följder. 1 p. l., 128 pp. 8°. *Upsala, R. Almqvist & J. Wiksell,* 1884.

Nordlinget.

Frickhinger (H.) Die Brunnenwasser von Nördlingen im Ries, betrachtet vom geologischen, mikroskopischen, chemischen und hygienischen Standpunkte. Ein Beitrag zur Hydrographie des Rieses. Aerztl. Int.-Bl., München, 1884, xxxi, 377; 387.

Nordman (G. A.) * Om konstgjord starrmognad. 1 p. l., 67 pp. 8°. *Helsingfors, J. C. Frenckell & Son,* 1885.

von Nordmann (Alexander) [1803-66]. Mikrographische Beiträge zur Naturgeschichte der wirbellosen Thiere. 2 Hfte. in 1 v. x, 118 pp.; xviii, 150 pp., 20 pl. 4°. *Berlin, G. Reimer,* 1832.
For Biography, see **Hjelt** (O. E. A.) Gedächtnissrede auf Alexander von Nordmann. 8°. *Helsingfors,* 1868.

Nordmann (Joh. Peter). * De obstructione sanguinis menstrui. 36 pp. sm. 4°. *Jenæ, ex off. Marggrafiana,* [1757].

———. * De ischuria gravidarum. 39 pp. 4°. *Argentorati, ex off. Univ. Heitziana,* [1758].

Nordmann (Otto). * Beiträge zur Kenntniss und namentlich zur Färbung der Mastzellen. [Göttingen.] 52 pp. 8°. *Helmstedt, J. C. Schmidt,* 1884.

Nordsieck (Henricus Augustus) [1808-]. * Nonnulla de graviditate extrauterina adnexa morbi historia. 39 pp., 2 l. 8°. *Berolini, typ. Nietackianis,* [1835].

Nordstedt (Carolus P. U.)
See **Zetterstrom** (Carolus). Initia historiæ vaccinationis in Svecia. Pt. vii. 4°. *Upsaliæ,* 1817.

Nordsten (Joh.)
See **Haartman** (Joh.) Sciagraphia morborum. Pt. 1. 8°. *Aboæ,* 1779-81.

Nordström. Zwei Fälle von Verbrennung mit Petroleum. 29 pp. 8°. *Leipzig, M. G. Prider,* 1870.

Nordt (Max) [1850-]. * Zur Statistik des Typhus abdominalis. 35 pp. 8°. *Berlin, G. Schade,* [1876].

Noreen (Joh.) * De mutatione luminum in vasis hominis nascentis in specie de uracho. 19, 20 pp., 1 pl. 4°. *Gottingæ, A. Vandenhoeck,* [1749].
Also, in: HALLER. Disp. anat. [etc.] 4°. *Gotting.,* 1750, v, 713-728, 1 pl.
For Biography, see **von Haller** (Albert).

Norell (Carolus). * De magnesia alba. 28 pp. 4°. *Upsaliæ, typ. Edmannianis,* 1775.

Noréus (Frans Theodor).
See **Hwasser** (Israël). Om pneomatos. 8°. *Upsala,* [1848-9].

Noréus (Olavus). * De catarrho. 14 pp. 4°. *Upsaliæ, J. F. Edman,* 1797.

Norfini (Giuseppe). Descrizione di alcune operazioni di chirurgia. 44 pp. 8°. *Pisa, Nistri,* 1827.

Norfolk, *England.*

See, also, **Hospitals** (*Descriptions, etc., of*), *by localities.*

EAST DEREHAM. Annual reports of the medical officer of health, for the urban sanitary district of East Dereham, Norfolk. 1.–6., 1878–83. [By Henry Bird Vincent.] 8°. *East Dereham, 1878–84.*

Norfolk, *Virginia.* Report on the origin of the yellow fever in Norfolk during the summer of 1855, made to city councils by a committee of physicians. 44 pp. 8°. *Richmond,* 1857.

———. Annual report of the board of water commissioners, city of Norfolk, Va., for the year 1879–80. 26 pp. 8°. *Norfolk,* 1880.

———. Messages of Wm. Lamb, mayor of the city of Norfolk, Va., to the select and common councils, together with municipal reports for 1879–80; 1880–81. 170 pp. 8°. *Norfolk,* 1880–81.

1879-80 and 1880-81 bound in 1 v.

Norfolk, *Virginia.*

See, also, **Fever** (*Malarial, History, etc., of*), **Fever** (*Yellow, History, etc., of*), *by localities.*

REPORTS of the medical officer of quarantine, District Elizabeth River, to the board of quarantine commissioners, for the years 1877; 1878. 8°. [*Norfolk,* 1878–9.]

Norfolk [County] Lunatic Asylum, Thorpe, near Norwich. Annual reports of the committee of visitors and of the medical superintendent, with the accounts of the treasurer, to the justices of the peace in general quarter sessions assembled. 50., 1863; 53., 1866; 54., 1867; 56.–62., 1869–75; 64., 1877; 66.–69., 1879–82. 4°. *Norwich,* 1864–83.

Opened May 18, 1814. New wards opened in September, 1869. 57. report for 9 months, ending Sept. 30, 1870. 58. report for 15 months, ending Dec. 31, 1871.

———. Duties of the attendants. May 31, 1871. 7 pp. 8°. [*Norwich,* 1871.]

———. Rules to be observed in case of fire. March 28, 1876. broadside fol. [*Norwich,* 1876.]

———. Rules to be observed for bathing the patients. broadside 4°. [*Norwich, n. d.*]

———. Rules of the . . . 27 pp. 8°. *Norfolk, F. Crowe,* 1882.

———. [Blank forms in use at the asylum.] 4°. [*Norwich,* 1882.]

1. Attendant's evening report.
2. Night attendant's report.

Norfolk and Norwich Hospital, Norwich. Rules and orders. 49 pp. 8°. *Norwich, Chase & Co.,* 1785.

———. Annual statement of the board of management of the Norfolk and Norwich Hospital to the governors and subscribers at the annual general meeting. [Including accounts of the building fund; chapel fund; Samaritan fund; hospital garden fund; and superannuation fund.] 40 pp. 8°. *London & Norwich, Jarrold & Sons,* [1885].

Established in 1771. Rebuilt in 1879. Contains two hundred beds.

———. *See, also:*

CROSSE (J. G.) An inaugural address, delivered at the opening of the Norfolk and Norwich Hospital Museum, September 10, 1845. 8°. *Norwich,* [*n. d.*]

RADCLIFFE (J. N.) Norfolk and Norwich Hospital. Minutes of conferences with the medical and surgical staff, and others, concerning the sanitary condition and administration of the hospital, and of an inspection of the building, the 3d and 4th August, 1875. fol. [*London,* 1875.]

Norford (William). An essay on the general method of treating cancerous tumors; the whole endeavoring to shew what stages of that formidable disease are curable. Illustrated with several extraordinary cases. xxxi, 171 pp. 12°. *London, J. Noon,* 1753.

Norgeu (G.-E.) Code thérapeutique. Méthode d'imbibition, dans laquelle on considère l'influence que les liquides potables peuvent exercer sur l'organisme morbide, ou traité des tisanes. 166 pp., 1 l. roy. 8°. *Paris, Germer-Baillière,* 1846. [P., v. 1827.]

Norgeu (Georges). *Traité sur la protection que les organes les plus essentiels à la vie de l'homme reçoivent de la part des organes moins essentiels. 28 pp. 4°. *Paris,* 1822, No. 219, v. 176.

Norlander (Carl) & **Martin** (Edmond). Manuel de gymnastique rationnelle suédoise à l'usage des écoles primaires, des écoles moyennes, des athénées, des écoles normales, de l'armée et de la marine. 2 p. l., viii, 245 pp., 2 tab., 1 pl. 8°. *Bruxelles, H. Manceaux,* 1883.

Norlin (Franz Martin). Om den Blodgang, som herskede paa Skibet Tranquebar paa den Maleiiski Kyst, 1 Decembermaaned, 1777. [On dysentery on the ship Tranquebar on the Malayan coast.] 6 pp. 8°. *Kiøbenhavn, J. R. Thiele,* [1778].

———. Iagttagelse af en brandagtig Forfløttelse efter en Feber. [On gangrene after fever.] 6 pp. 12°. *Kiøbenhavn, J. R. Thiele,* [1777].

Norma y Enriques (Luis G.) *Retencion de la placenta. 29 pp. 8°. *México, I. Escalante & Ca.,* 1871.

Normal liquids. 4 l. 8°. [*n. p.,* 1882.]

Norman (F.) A compendious and easy method of curing the virulent stillicidium commonly call'd gonorrhœa; with an account of the efficacy of Plummer's alterative pills, in cases of chancres, buboes, hernia veneris, etc. 36 pp. 8°. *London, E. Withers,* [*n. d*]

Norman (*George*) [1783–1861].

Obituary. Lancet, Lond., 1861, i, 127.

Norman (J. C.) Third septennial report of Guy's Lying-in Charity, from Oct. 1, 1847, to Oct. 1, 1854. Also report on the Lying-in Charity for twenty-one years, from Oct. 1, 1833, to Oct. 1, 1854. Collated from the records by . . . Presented by J. C. W. Lever and H. Oldham. 45 pp. 8°. [*London,* 1855?] [P., v. 1093.]

Normand (A.) Mémoire sur la diarrhée dite de Cochinchine. 86 pp. 8°. *Paris, J. B. Baillière & fils,* 1877.

Repr. from: Arch. de méd. nav., Par., 1877, xxvii.

Normand (Alexis-Louis). *Hygiène et pathologie de deux convois de condamnés aux travaux forcés, transportés de France en Nouvelle-Calédonie par la frégate la Sibylle, en 1866–7. 70 pp. 4°. *Paris,* 1869, No. 116.

Normand (Denis-Claude-Auguste-Alexandre). *Sur la cataracte. 26 pp. 4°. *Strasbourg, L. F. Le Roux, an XI* [1803].

Normand (Eugène)[1]. *Sur le croup. 29 pp. 4°. *Paris,* 1826, No. 20, v. 197.

Normand (Eugène)[2]. *Du phimosis et de son traitement. 37 pp., 1 l. 4°. *Paris,* 1876, No. 5.

Normand (F.-M.-P.) *Sur les hémorrhagies cérébrales, considérées comme causes d'apoplexie précédée d'un léger aperçu sur les hémorrhagies en général. 31 pp. 4°. *Paris,* 1840, No. 62, v. 80.

Normand (G.-Sixte). *Du bec-de-lièvre et de son traitement. 56 pp. 4°. *Paris,* 1852, No. 250, v. 530.

Normand (Louis-Rosin). *Rhumatisme articulaire aigu. Statistique et considérations. 88

Normand (Louis-Rosin)—continued.
pp., 2 l. 4°. *Montpellier, L. Cristin & Cie.*, 1865, No. 72. C.

Normand de la Tranchade (Simon). *I. De la nature du choléra-morbus sporadique. II. [etc.] 132 pp. 4°. *Paris, 1842, No. 224*, v. 394.

de Normandie (Joannes Henricus). *De fabrica pulmonum eorumque usu. 44 pp., 2 l. 4°. *Lugd. Bat., S. Luchtmans*, 1742. [P., v. 991.]

Normandie (La) médicale. Directeurs: MM. Duménil, Gibert, Leudet, Notta. Rédacteur en chef: Cerné. [Semi-monthly.] Années 1–4, Nov. 1, 1885–8. 8°. *Rouen.*
Current. Années 1–2, 1885–6, form v. 1.

Normandy (A.) The commercial hand-book of chemical analysis; or, practical instructions for the determination of the intrinsic or commercial value of substances used in manufactures, in trades, and in the arts. xii, 640 pp. 8°. *London, G. Knight & Sons*, 1850.
——. The same. 2. ed. xii, 640 pp. 8°. *London, Lockwood & Co.*, 1865.
——. The same. New edition, enlarged, and to a great extent rewritten, by Henry M. Noad. xvi, 480 pp. 8°. *London, Lockwood & Co.*, 1875.

Normann (Carolus). *De terroris effectu in organismum humanum. 39 pp. 8°. *Dorpati Livonorum, typ. J. C. Schuenmanni*, 1834.

Normann (Gottfried Eduard). *De rumpendis ovi humani velamentis in partu. 75 pp. 8°. *Dorpati Livonorum, typ. J. C. Schuenmanni*, 1836.

Noroy.
See **Chouippe** ainé. Réponse aux consultations médico-chirurgicales, etc. 8°. *L'Aigle*, 1834.

Norr (Erhardt). Chirurgischer Wegweiser, allen Angehenden, so zur Wund-Artzney-Kunst zu gelangen Begierde haben gezeiget; und in neun Theilen Gesprächsweis verfasset; samt einem Reis- und Feld-Kasten für die Chirurgos, so im Feld zu dienen vorhabens; und dann einem Vocabulario aller einfachen, unvermischten Gewächsen und Artzneyen, Namen, Natur und Complexionen. 10 p. l., 448 pp., 12 l., 1 pl. 16°. *Nürnberg, J. Stein*, 1736.

Norris (Basil) [1828–]. A paper on dislocations of the astragalus. Read before the American Surgical Association, Cincinnati, 1883. 23 pp. 8°. *Washington, Judd & Detweiler*, 1883.
Repr. from: Tr. Am. Surg. Ass., Phila., 1883, i.

Norris (George W.) [1808–72]. Biographical memoir of Jacob Randolph, M. D. 12 pp. 8°. *Philadelphia, W. F. Giddes*, 1848.
——. Introductory lecture to the course of clinical instruction in surgery, at the Pennsylvania Hospital; delivered Nov. 1st, 1848. 15 pp. 8°. *Philadelphia, King & Baird*, 1848. [Also, in: P., v. 1359.]
——. Contributions to practical surgery. 318 pp. 8°. *Philadelphia, Lindsay & Blakiston*, 1873.
See, also, **Fergusson** (William). A system of practical surgery. 2. Am. ed. 8°. *Philadelphia*, 1845.—
Liston (Robert). Practical surgery, [etc.] 8°. *Philadelphia*, 1838. ——. The same. 8°. *Philadelphia*, 1842.
For Biography, see Tr. Coll. Phys. Phila., 1876, 3. s., ii, pp. xxvii–xlii (W. Hunt). Also, Reprint.

Norris (Hugh). Remarks on the external application of iodine in erysipelas, with suggestions for its use in puerperal fever. 12 pp. 8°. *South Petherton, E. Bennett*, 1853. [P., v. 1033.]
Repr. from: Med. Times & Gaz., Lond., 1852, n. s., v.

Norris (Richard). On the extrusion of the morphological elements of the blood. The physical principles concerned, and the relation which such extruded elements bear to pus and to the so-called fibrinous exudation of inflammation. 33 pp., 8 pl. 8°. *London, Odell & Ives*, 1871. [P., v. 1197.]
Repr. from: St. Andrew's M. Grad. Ass. Tr. 1870, Lond., 1871, iv.

Norris (Richard)—continued.
——. On the discovery of an invisible or third corpuscular element in the blood. Abstract, with a critical note, by Mrs. Ernest Hart. 7 pp. 8°. [*n. p.*, 1880.]
Repr. from: Lond. M. Rec., 1880, viii.
——. The physiology and pathology of the blood, comprising the origin, mode of development, pathological and post-mortem changes of its morphological elements in mammalian and oviparous vertebrates. xlv, 274 pp., 1 l., 5 tab., 23 pl. 8°. *London, Smith, Elder & Co.*, 1882.

Norris (Thomas). A short essay on the singular virtues of an highly exalted preparation of antimony, or Dr. Norris's antimonial drops. To which is added a catalogue of cures, incontestibly proving the sovereign efficacy of this great medicine in fevers and many other disorders. 8°. [*London*], 1770. [P., v. 1236.]
——. A short essay on the virtues of Dr. Norris's drops for fevers. 36 pp. 8°. *London, Fielding & Walker*, 1777. [P., v. 434.]
——. The same. 4. ed. 81 pp. 8°. *London*, 1783. [P., v. 433.]

Norris (William) [1792–1877]. The Hunterian oration. 68 pp. 4°. *London, T. Cadell & W. Davis*, 1817.
For Biography, see Brit. M. J., Lond., 1877, i, 535.

Norris (William Fisher) [1829–]. Cases of optic neuritis. 7 pp., 1 l., 4 pl. 8°. [*Philadelphia*, 1874.]
——. Contributions to ophthalmology. 7 pp. 8°. *New York, Trow*, 1883.
Repr. from: Tr. Am. Ophth. Soc., N. Y., 1883, xvi.
See, also, **Photomicrographs**, etc. 4°. *Washington*, 1864.—**Tyson** (James). A treatise on Bright's disease, etc. 8°. *Philadelphia*, 1881.
—— & **Stricker** (S.) Versuche über Hornhaut-Entzündung. 17 pp., 1 pl. 8°. *Wien, M. Salzer*, 1869.

Norris's *drops.*
See **Antiphlogistics**, *etc.*; **Medicines** (*Patent, etc.*)

Norsk Magazin for Lægevidenskaben. Udgivet af Lægeforeningen i Christiania. Redigeret af Chr. Boeck, A. Conradi, Chr. Heiberg, J. Hjort, F. Holst. [Monthly.] v. 1–10, June, 1840, to June, 1845. 2. Række, v. 1–24, 1847–70. 3. Række, v. 1–15, 1871–85. 4. Række, v. 1–3, 1886–8. 52 v. 8°. *Christiania.*
Current. v. 10, 1845, contains general index to v. 1–10. v. 2–24, 2. series, edited by the Medical Society of Christiania; v. 1–4, 3. series, by Jacob Heiberg; v. 5–13, 3. series, by Edward Bull; in 1884, v. 14, 3. series, S. Laache became editor. **Forhandlinger** i det norske medicinske Selskab i Kristiania issued with this journal.

Norsk Medicinallovgivning indeholdende en kronologisk Samling af Forordninger, Love, Plakater, Resolutioner, Skrivelser m. m. vedkommende Norges Medicinalvæsen for Aarene 1672–1880. Udgivet af K. A. Langberg, L. Esmark-Olsson og J. Somme. [Norwegian medical laws, etc., in chronological order.] lxxi, 636 pp. 8°. *Kristiania, Udgivernes Forlag*, 1881.

Norström (Gustaf) [1840–]. Sur le traitement des maladies des femmes au moyen de la méthode du massage. Lu à l'Académie de médecine dans la séance du 18 janvier 1876. 71 pp. 8°. *Paris, K. Nilson*, 1876.
——. Traitement de la migraine par le massage. vi, 119 pp., 1 l. 8°. *Paris, A. Delahaye & E. Lecrosnier*, 1885.
——. Traitement des raideurs articulaires (fausses ankyloses) au moyen de la rectification forcée et du massage. viii, 137 pp., 1 l. 8°. *Paris, A. Delahaye & E. Lecrosnier*, 1887.

North (Edward). *On the rheumatic state of fever. 37 pp. 12°. *Philadelphia, W. W. Woodward*, 1797.

North (Elisha). A treatise on a malignant epidemic, commonly called spotted fever; interspersed with remarks on the nature of fever in general, etc. ; and an appendix, in which is republished a number of essays, written by different authors on this epidemic. xi, 249 pp. 12°. *New York, T. & F. Swords,* 1811.

———. Outlines of the science of life; which treats physiologically of both body and mind. Designed only for philosophers, and other candid persons. xix, 202 pp., 1 pl., 1 l. 8°. *New York, Collins & Co.,* 1829.

[———.] The pilgrim's progress in phrenology. Pt. i, abridged, and pt. iii. By Uncle Toby. 11, 72 pp. 8°. *New London, S. Green,* 1836.

North (John) [1790–1873]. Practical observations on the convulsions of infants. x (1 l.), 282 pp. 8°. *London, Burgess & Hill,* 1826.

Also, Co-Editor of: **London** (The) Medical and Physical Journal, 1829–30.

North (M. L.) Analysis of Saratoga waters; also of Sharon, Avon, Virginia, and other mineral waters of the United States. With directions for invalids. 3. ed. iv, 5–72 pp. 16°. *New York, Saxton & Miles,* 1846.

———. The same. 7. ed., with an appendix. 72 pp. 16°. *Saratoga Springs, B. Huling,* 1858.

North (Nelson L.) On epidemic cholera, the phenomena, causes, prevention and treatment. With an appendix, relating to the Brooklyn city sewerage. 39 pp. 8°. *Brooklyn, Daily Times presses,* 1865.

Repr. from: Tr. M. Ass. Eastern Dist. Brooklyn.

———. A theory of inflammation; its cause, course, and rationale of treatment. 46 pp. 8°. *New York, W. Wood & Co.,* 1867.

North (Samuel). The family physician and guide to health, together with some remarks on surgery; containing a familiar and accurate description of the symptoms of most diseases incident to mankind; together with their gradual progress, and method of cure; and tables of preparation, with a medical herbal. The whole selected and compiled from the writings of various authors in Europe and America. vi, 7–324 pp. 8°. *Waterloo, N. Y., W. Child,* 1830.

North (Samuel William). Letter from . . . medical officer of health of the city of York. With reference to water closets, etc. Presented June 9, 1874. 10 pp. 12°. *York, Herald Office,* 1874.

Repr. from: York Daily Herald, June 10, 1874.

———. Report of medical officer of health of the city of York. With reference to the water supply of York. Presented July 29, 1874. 8 pp. 12°. *York, Herald Office,* 1874.

Repr. from: York Daily Herald, July 29, 1874.

———. Reports [quarterly] of the medical officer of health of the city of York to the urban sanitary authority. 3. qr., 1874; 2., 1876; 4., 1876; 1.–4., 1882; 1.–3., 1883. 12° & fol. [*York,* 1874–83.]

———. Ventilation of sewers. Report on the ventilation and flushing of sewers, Aug. 6, 1877. 7 pp. fol. *York, Johnson & Tesseyman,* [1877].

———. Annual report of the medical officer of health to the urban sanitary authority of the city of York, for the year 1876. 8 pp. fol. *York,* 1877.

———. Registration of disease. 12 pp. 12°. *London, Spottiswoode & Co.,* 1878.

Repr. from: San. Rec., Lond., 1878, viii.

———. City of York. To the urban sanitary authority. Report on lodging houses, July 7, 1879. 5 pp. fol. [*York,* 1879.]

———. [A report to the urban sanitary authority, city of York, on the advisability of including the

North (Samuel William)—continued.
whole of the township of Acomb in the city of York.] 1 sheet. sm. 4°. *York,* 1882.

———. Report of medical officer of health, on precautions to be observed against cholera. 2 pp. fol. *York,* 1883.

———. Report on the prevalence of typhoid fever in York during the year 1884. Presented to the urban sanitary authority, Feb. 17, 1885. 48 pp. 8°. 1 map. fol. *York, B. Johnson & Co.,* 1885.

———. Report on the compulsory notification of infectious diseases, in reply to a circular letter of the Local Government Board, Dec. 21, 1887. 17 pp. 8°. *York, B. Johnson & Co.,* [1887].

North (W.)

See **Sanderson** (J. Burdon). University College course, etc. 8°. *London,* 1882. ———. The same. 8°. *Philadelphia,* 1882.

North End Dispensary for Women and Children, Boston. Annual report of the attending physicians to the board of directors. 1. (1869–70). 12 pp. 12°. *Boston, A. Mudge & Son,* 1870.

Organized May, 1869.

North End Industrial Home, Boston. Annual report of the managers to the subscribers. 2., 1881–2. 58 pp. 8°. *Boston, F. Wood,* 1882.

North London Deaconesses' Institution. *See* London Diocesan Deaconess Institution.

North London Home for Aged Christian Blind Women. Annual reports of the committee of the home to the subscribers and friends. 1.–4., 1880–81 to 1883–4. 18°. *London,* 1881–4.

North London Hospital for Consumption and Diseases of the Chest, London and Hampstead. Annual reports of the committee of management to the governors and subscribers. 7., 1867; 8., 1868; 12., 1871; 13., 1872; 16., 1875; 17., 1876; 20., 1879; 22., 1881; 24., 1883. 8°. *London,* 1868–84.

7. in P., v. 969; 8. in P., v. 976. Established in 1860, for the reception of patients from all parts of the kingdom. In 1879 the words "and Diseases of the Chest" were dropped from title on the cover, and the inside title reads: Hospital for Consumption and Diseases of the Chest. Forms used: In-patient's letter; medical certificate.

———. By-laws, and rules and regulations, as revised and prepared by a committee appointed at a special meeting of the governors, held July 20, 1883. 23 pp. 8°. *London, E. Couchman & Co.,* 1883.

North London Hospital for Consumption, Mount Vernon, Hampstead. [Circular of the committee, soliciting contributions.] 7 pp. obl. 16°. [*London, Hutchins & Crowsley,* 1886?]

———. [Circular letter of the committee, calling the attention of the public to the need of funds to finish the new hospital. With a list of donations. 2 l. 8°. [*London, n. d.*]

———. [Circular letter of the committee to benevolent persons, soliciting a contribution in aid of the building fund of the new hospital.] 1 l., 1 pl. 4°. [*London, n. d.*]

North London or University College Hospital, St. Pancras, London. Rules for the government of the hospital. 20 pp. 8°. [*London, R. & J. E. Taylor,* 1847.]

Commenced as the "University Dispensary" April 8, 1828. On Feb. 25, 1829, a committee was appointed to ascertain the cost of erecting a hospital. Plans were submitted Feb. and March, and the corner-stone was laid May 22, 1833. Opened Nov. 1, 1834. Includes separate apartments for diseases of women, children, diseases of the skin, eye and ear, teeth.

———. Annual reports of the committee of management to the governors and subscribers. 1870–73; 1875–84. 8°. *London,* 1870–85.

1875–82 bound in 1 v. 1870 in P., v. 976.

———. Reports of the surgical and medical registrars of the . . . for the years 1871–5; 1877–81; 1883–5. 8°. *London,* 1872–86.

1878–81 bound in 1 v.

North London or University [etc.]—cont'd.

——. Rules for the government of the hospital, made by the council of the college. Adopted as revised, May 3d, 1873. 16 pp. 8°. [*London*], 1873.

——. Address of H. R. H. Prince Leopold, Duke of Albany, the chairman of the annual festival dinner, May 20, 1881. 4 pp. 12°. *London, Harrison & Sons*, 1881.

——. A history of the hospital, from its foundation to the year 1881, by N. H. Nixon. 60 pp. 8°. *London, H. K. Lewis*, 1882.

——. Draft report for the year 1883. 7 pp. 8°. [*London*, 1884.]

——. Samaritan funds, 1883. [Draft copy of balance sheet, for the secretary of the Metropolitan Hospital Sunday Fund.] 5 sheets. 8°. [*London*, 1884.]

——. The same. Audited copy. 5 sheets. 8°. [*London*, 1884.]

North Lonsdale Hospital, Barrow-in-Furness. Annual reports of the committee of management to the subscribers, for the years 1869–70 to 1886–7. 12°. *Barrow-in-Furness*, 1870–87.
Established 1866.

North Mountain School of Physical Culture. [Prospectus.] By J. T. Rothrock, principal. 15 pp. 8°. *Wilkes-Barre, "Times" press*, 1876.

——. [Supplement to prospectus.] By J. T. Rothrock, principal.] 3 pp. 8°. [*Wilkes-Barre*, 1876.]

Northallerton.

RANGER (W.) Report to the General Board of Health, on a preliminary inquiry into the sewerage, drainage, and supply of water, and the sanitary condition of the inhabitants of the town of Northallerton, in the county of York. 8°. *London*, 1850.

——. Report to the General Board of Health, on a memorial from the ratepayers against the application of the public health act to Northallerton. 8°. *London*, 1851.

North America.

See, also, **Canada**; **Mexico**; **Sitka**; **United States.**

DUPONT (P.) *Notes et observations sur la côte orientale d'Amérique. 4°. *Montpellier*, 1868.

MUHLENBERG (H.) Catalogus plantarum Americæ septentrionalis huc usque cognitarum indigenarum et cicurum; or, a catalogue of the hitherto known native and naturalized plants of North America, arranged according to the sexual system of Linnæus. 8°. *Lancaster*, 1813.

PHYSICAL degeneracy of the American people, showing that an imperfect system of education, and abuse and neglect of children, are among the chief causes of this degeneracy. [Taken from a series of articles written for, and now being published in, the Detroit Tribune, over the signature of "E".] 8°. *Detroit*, 1858.

SCHOEPFF (J. D.) The climate and diseases of America. Translated by James Read Chadwick. [From the original published at Erlangen, 1781?] 8°. *Boston*, 1875.
Also, in: Boston M. & S. J., 1875, xcii, 715; 733: xciii, 6.

WILLIAMSON (H.) Observations on the climate in different parts of America, compared with the climate in corresponding parts of the other continent. To which are added, remarks on the different complexions of the human race; with some account of the aborigines of America. Being an introductory discourse to the history of North Carolina. 8°. *New York*, 1811.
Butler (L. C.) The decadence of the American race, as exhibited in the registration reports of Massachusetts, Vermont [and Rhode Island]; the cause and the remedy. Tr. Vermont M. Soc. 1867–8, Burlington, 1869, 78–88.— **Helfft.** Die geographische Verbreitung der Krankheiten

North America.

in Nord-Amerika. Monatsbl. f. med. Statist. u. öff. Gsndhtspflg., Berl., 1859, 13–16.—**Huxley** (T. H.) Impressions of America. New York Tribune, extra, no. 36, N. Y., 1876, 2.—**Leach** (W. T.) Observations on the hypothesis of the former existence of a great fresh water inland sea within the continent of North America. Brit.-Am. J. M. & Phys. Sc., Montreal, 1845–6, i, 10; 62. ——. Reply to Dr. Rae's observations. *Ibid.*, 202; 232.— **Rae** (J.) Remarks on the Rev. Mr. Leach's observations on the previous existence of a fresh water inland sea. *Ibid.*, 91; 119.— **Romer** (I.) An inquiry into the nature and cause of the autumnal epidemic diseases which prevail in North America. Med. Reposit., N. Y., 1811, xiv, 238–244.— **Suddarth** (J. B.) A roll of American epidemics for seventeen ages, with a brief record of the epidemic influence for the past seven ages. Nashville J. M. & S., 1861, xx, 409: xxi, 69.

North American Archives of Medical and Surgical Science. Edited by E. Geddings. [Monthly; 2 v. annually.] v. 1–2, Oct., 1834, to Sept., 1835. 8°. *Baltimore. Cary, Hart & Co.*
Ended. A continuation of: **Baltimore** (The) Medical and Surgical Journal and Review.

North American (The) Homœopathic Directory for 1877–8, compiled and published by J. Pettel, A. M., M. D. 117 pp. 8°. *Cleveland, Robinson, Savage & Co.*, 1878.

North American (The) Homœopathic Journal. A quarterly magazine of medicine and the auxiliary sciences. Conducted by C. Hering, E. E. Marcy, and J. W. Metcalf. v. 1, Feb. to Nov., 1851. 532 pp. 8°. *New York, W. Radde.*
Continued as: **North American** (The) Journal of Homœopathy.

North American (The) Journal of Homœopathy. A quarterly magazine of medicine and the auxiliary sciences. Conducted by C. Hering, E. E. Marcy, and J. W. Metcalf. v. 2–18, February, 1852, to May, 1870. New series, v. 1–15, August, 1870, to May, 1885. 3. series, v. 1–3, September, 1885–8. 35 v. 8°. *New York.*
Current. Title of v. 1, 1851. was: **North American** (The) Homœopathic Journal. Suspended after Nov., 1853, until Aug, 1856. In Dec., 1861, **United States** (The) Journal of Homœopathy merged in this journal. v. 18 contains general index to v. 1–18. In 1885 became monthly; v. 1, 3. series, complete in 12 nos., Sept., 1885, to Dec., 1886. Edited successively by J. C. Peters, W. H. Holcombe, H. C. Preston, F. G. Snelling, J. T. Alley, R. E. W. Adams, F. W. Hunt, S. Lilienthal, George M. Dillow [*et al.*].

North American (The) Medical Reporter. Edited by W. Elmer. [Quarterly.] v. 1, Oct., 1858, to Nov., 1859. 284 pp. 8°. *New York, W. A. Townsend & Co.*
Ended. In nos. 2–4 Louis Elsberg added as editor.

North American Medical and Surgical Journal. Conducted by H. L. Hodge, F. Bache, C. D. Meigs, B. H. Coates, and R. La Roche. [Quarterly; 2 v. annually.] v. 1–12, Jan., 1826, to Oct., 1831. 8°. *Philadelphia, J. Dobson.*
Ended. v. 5 and all subsequent published by the Kappa Lambda Association of the United States.

North American (The) Medico-Chirurgical Review. Edited by S. D. Gross and T. G. Richardson. [Bi-monthly.] v. 1–5, Jan., 1857–61. 8°. *Philadelphia, J. B. Lippincott & Co.*
Formed by consolidation of: **Medical** (The) Examiner, Philadelphia, with: **Louisville** (The) Review. In v. 5, 1861, S. W. Gross added as editor.

Northampton, *England.*

See, also, **Fever** (*Typhoid, History, etc., of*), **Hospitals** (*Management, etc., of*), **Insane** (*Asylums for, etc.*), *by localities.*

BUCHANAN (G.) Report on the sanitary state of Northampton, April, 1871. fol. *London*, 1871.

Northampton, *Massachusetts.* Yearly bill of mortality. Presented to the mayor, the aldermen, and municipal councillors, for the years 1849–50 to 1853–4; 1856–7; 1858–9; 1860–61; 1861–2; 1863–4; 1865–6 to 1870–71. 16 sheets. fol. [*Northampton, Taylor & Son*, 1850–71.]

Northampton, *Massachusetts.*

See, also, **Deaf-mutes** (*Asylums, etc., for*); **Insane** (*Asylums for, etc.*), *by localities—Massachusetts.*

YEARLY bill of mortality. Presented to the mayor, the aldermen, and municipal councillors of the town of Northampton, for the years 1849–50 to 1853–4; 1-56–7; 1858–9; 1860–61; 1861–2; 1863–4; 1865–6 to 1870-71. fol. *Northampton,* [1850-71].

Northampton County Lunatic Asylum, at Berry Wood, near Northampton. Annual reports of the committee of visitors and medical superintendent to the court of quarter sessions. 1.-6., 1877–82. 8°. *Northampton,* 1878–83.
Opened June 30, 1876.

———. General rules for the government of the asylum. 19 pp. 8°. *Northampton, Stanton & Son,* 1879.

———. Regulations of the committee of visitors for management of the asylum. 32 pp. 8°. *Northampton, Stanton & Son,* 1879.

———. [Blank forms in use at the asylum.] v. s. [*Northampton,* 1880-83.]
Application for employment, with questions to be answered by reference.
Daily report, female department. Same, male department.
Description of escaped patient.
Diet list.
Farm bailiff's return, weekly.
Regulations as to visiting.

———. ["Plain directions" for the careful attention of discharged patients and their friends, compiled by Dr. Brushfield, of the Brookwood Asylum.] 1 sheet. 4°. [*Northampton, n. d.*]

Northampton General Lunatic Assylum for the Middle and Upper Classes. *See* **Saint Andrew's** Hospital for Mental Diseases, at Northampton.

Northampton Homœopathic Dispensary. Annual report of the committee to the subscribers. 5., 1855–6. pp. 83–102. 8°. [*n. p., n. d.*]
Cutting from : Homœopathic Record.
Opened in 1851.

Northampton Lunatic Hospital. *See* **Massachusetts.** *Northampton Lunatic Hospital.*

North Borneo.

Walker (J. H.) Medical aspects of North Borneo. Australas. M. Gaz., Sydney, 1883–4, iii, 133–136.

North Boston.

See **Fever** (*Typhoid, History, etc., of*), *by localities*).

North Brabant.

HOLLAND. Lijst- van geneeskundigen, tandmeesters, apothekers, drogisten en vroedvrouwen gevestigd in de provincie Noord Brabant af 1. Januari 1885. roy. 8°. [*Breda,* 1885.]

North Cambridgeshire Hospital, Wisbech. Annual reports by the committee on management to the subscribers. 1.-2., 1873–5; 4.-5., 1876–8; 7., 1879–80; 9.-11., 1881–4. 8°. *Wisbech,* 1874–84.
Founded 1873.

North Carolina. An act supplemental to an act creating a State board of health. Ratified the 14th day of March, 1879. 6 pp. 8°. [*Raleigh,* 1879.]

———. Quarantine regulations, port of Wilmington, N. C., April 1, 1879. 2 l. 8°. [*Wilmington,* 1879.]

North Carolina.

See, also, **Asheville**; **Education** (*Medical*), *etc.—United States,* **Fever** (*Malarial, History, etc., of*), **Insane** (*Asylums for, etc.*), *by localities*; **Raleigh**; **Wilmington.**

GATCHELL (H. P.) Western North Carolina; its agricultural resources, mineral wealth, cli-

North Carolina.

mate, salubrity, and scenery. 8°. *Asheville, N. C.,* 1870.

GUIDE (A) to shipmasters visiting the Cape Fear and other rivers. Presented by the North Carolina board of health. 8°. *Raleigh,* 1881.

NORTH CAROLINA Agricultural Experiment Station. Annual report for 1879. 8°. *Raleigh,* 1879.

Coues (E.) Notes on the natural history of Fort Macon, N. C., and vicinity. Proc. Acad. Nat. Sc. Phila., 1871, 12; 120. *Also,* Reprint. — **Coues** (E.) & **Yarrow** (H. C.) Notes on the natural history of Fort Macon, N. C., and vicinity. Proc. Acad. Nat. Sc. Phila., 1877, 203–218· 1878, 21; 297.—**Cox** (D.) A report of the diseases of Perquimans County. Med. J. N. Car., Raleigh, 1860, iii, 145–155.—**Dickson** (J. H.) On the medical topography and epidemics of North Carolina. Tr. Am. M. Ass., Phila., 1860, xiii, 273–352.—**Gatchell** (E. A.) North Carolina climate for consumptives. Med. Rec., N. Y., 1885, xxvii, 54. — **Gleitsmann** (W.) Western North Carolina as a health resort. Med. & Surg. Reporter, Phila., 1876, xxxiv, 141–145. *Also,* Reprint.—**Happoldt** (C.) Diseases of Burke County. Med. J. N. Car., Raleigh, 1860-61, iii, 459–464.—**Kelly** (H.) On the diseases most prevalent in Iredell County, from May, 1856, to May, 1857. Tr. M. Soc. N. Car., Wilmington, 1857, viii, 27–29. ———. On the diseases of Iredell County. Med. J. N. Car., Raleigh, 1860, iii, 331.—**Kerr** (W. C.) A report on the sanitary relations of drainage and water-supply in North Carolina and the South Atlantic States, as affected by topographical and geological conditions. Am. Pub. Health Ass. Rep. 1874-5, N. Y., 1876, ii, 348–356.—**King** (W. R.) A report on the diseases of Franklin County. Med. J. N. Car., Raleigh, 1858-9, i-ii, 1; 111.—**Lankford** (W. C.) Report on the diseases of Franklin County. *Ibid,* 45–51.—**Lloyd** (T. M.) Some evidence relating to Asheville and the mountains of North Carolina in the climatic treatment of phthisis. N. York M. J., 1887, xlv, 399–404. *Also,* Reprint.—**McKee** (W. H.) On the statistics of middle North Carolina. South. M. Rep. (Fenner), N. Orl., 1850, ii, 415–420.—**Manson** (O. F.) Sketches of the endemic diseases of the Roanoke Valley of Virginia and North Carolina. Virginia M. & S. J., Richmond, 1855, iv, 1: 1857, ix, 198; 286.—**Marcy** (H. O.) The chemical treatment of disease. Western North Carolina as a health resort. J. Am. M. Ass., Chicago, 1885, v, 701–707. *Also,* Reprint.—**Memminger** (A.) Flat Rock and Hendersonville, North Carolina, as health resorts. Med. & Surg. Reporter, Phila., 1888, lviii, 232. — **Payne** (R. L.) The diseases of Davidson County. Med. J. N. Car., Raleigh, 1860-61, iii, 335–340. — **Pitt** (J.) Observations on the country and diseases near Roanoke River, in the State of North Carolina. Med. Reposit., N. Y., 1808, xi, 337–342. — **Pittman** (N. J.) Report on the diseases of Edgecomb County. Tr. M. Soc. N. Car., Wilmington, 1857, viii, 35–42.—**Robinson** (B. W.) Historical review of the diseases of Cumberland County. North Car. M. J., Wilmington, 1878, i, 76–79. — **Satchwell** (S. S.) Report on the meteorology, medical topography, and prevailing diseases of Beaufort County, North Carolina. Nelson's North. Lancet, Plattsburg, N. Y., 1853-4, viii, 112–119.— **Shaffner** (J. F.) Topography and diseases of Forsyth County, N. C. Tr. M. Soc. N. Car., Wilmington, 1869, xvi, 19–24.—**Sharpe** (W. R.) Report on the diseases of Davie County. Med. J. N. Car., Raleigh, 1860-61, iii, 278–286.—**Williamson** (H.) Of the soil and general state of health in different parts of North Carolina. Eclect. Repert., Phila., 1813, iii, 1–16.— **Winborne** (R. H.) Topography and disease of Chowan County. Proc. M. Soc. N. Car., Wilmington, 1867, xiv, 34–37.—**Winslow** (C.) Diseases of Perquimans' County. Med. J. N. Car., Raleigh, 1858-9, i-ii, 101–111.

North Carolina. *Board of Public Charities.* Annual report to the general assembly. 1., 1869-70. 126 pp., 1 tab. 8°. *Raleigh,* 1870.

North Carolina. *Eastern Insane Asylum, Goldsboro.* Annual reports of the superintendent to the board of directors. 5., 1883–4; 7., 1885–6. 24 pp. 8°. *Goldsboro, Messenger print,* 1885–6.

North Carolina. *North Carolina Insane Asylum, at Raleigh.* Biennial and annual reports of the board of directors and superintendent to the governor of the State. 2.-5., 1856–7 to 1859–60; 8.-9., 1862–3 to 1863–4; 11., 1865–6; 14.-29., 1868–9 to 1883–4. 8°. *Raleigh,* 1858–84.
Incorporated in 1848. Opened Feb. 22, 1856. Formerly called "Insane Asylum of North Carolina". 1856-7 to 1863-4 made biennially.

———. Digest of laws relating to the Insane Asylum of North Carolina. To which is appended the by-laws adopted for the government of the

North Carolina. *North Carolina Insane Asylum, at Raleigh*—continued.

institution. 29 pp. 8°. *Raleigh, Nichols, Gorman & Neathery,* 1867.

——. Special report of the superintendent of the . . . to the board of directors. 11 pp. 8°. *Raleigh, J. Nichols,* 1877.

——. Report of the superintendent to the board of directors, March 6, 1878 [on the present condition of the hospital]. 19 pp. 8°. *Raleigh, J. Nichols,* 1878.

——. Report of the superintendent to the board of directors, April 1, 1879 [on the insufficiency of appropriation for the year 1879]. 47 pp. 8°. *Raleigh,* 1879.

——. By-laws of the . . . 15 pp. 16°. *Raleigh, Uzzell & Gatling,* 1884.

——. Rules and regulations of the . . . 19 pp. 16°. *Raleigh, Uzzell & Gatling,* 1885.

——. [Blank forms in use at the asylum.] v. s. [*Raleigh,* 188-.]

Affidavit to procure an examination of an insane person.
Certificate of superintendent that patient has become of sane mind.
Certificate of superintendent recommending return of patient to friends on probation.
Order for return of patient to friends on probation.
Order for discharge.

——. *See, also:*

NORTH CAROLINA. An act in relation to the Lunatic Asylum. Passed March 11, 1869. 8°. [*Raleigh,* 1869.]

North Carolina. *North Carolina State Board of Agriculture.* Annual report of the North Carolina Agricultural Experiment Station, for 1879. Printed by order of the board of agriculture. xv, 198 pp. 8°. *Raleigh, The Observer,* 1879.

North Carolina. *State Board of Health of the State of North Carolina.* Circular No. 1. On the organization of auxiliary county boards of health. May 24, 1879. 1 sheet. 4°. [*Wilmington,* 1879.]

Organized May 21, 1879.

——. Circular on ventilation, drainage, drinking water, and disinfectants. 14 pp. 8°. *Raleigh, Edwards, Broughton & Co.,* 1879.

——. Circular to the county superintendents of health on their duties. 2 l. 4°. • [*Wilmington,* 1879.]

——. Circular No. 5. To county superintendents, requesting them to make a record of post-mortem examinations during the year. 1 sheet. 8°. [*Wilmington,* 1879.]

——. Instructions for sending samples to the chemist to be analyzed. 2 l. 4°. [*Wilmington,* 1879.]

——. Letter to chairman of county commissioners, on county organization. July 1, 1879. 1 sheet. 8°. [*Wilmington,* 1879.]

——. Limitation and prevention of diphtheria. By R. L. Payne. 10 pp. 8°. *Raleigh, P. M. Hale & Edwards, Broughton & Co.,* 1879.

——. Method of performing post-mortem examinations. 32 pp. 8°. *Raleigh,* 1879.

——. Notification of nuisance on premises. 1 sheet. 4°. [*Wilmington,* 1879.]

——. [Blank forms.] v. s. *Wilmington,* 1879-80.

No. 3. List of members in the county.
No. 4. Record of post-mortem examinations. To be returned whether there have been examinations or not
No. 6. Death certificate to be filled by the last attending physician.
Memorandum, record of prevailing diseases, kept by physicians, a copy to be sent to the county superintendent on the last day of the month. 24 pp
Monthly return of county superintendents on the weather and prevailing diseases.
Register of causes of deaths, yearly, and nomenclature used.
Return of deaths, weekly, for townships.

North Carolina. *State Board of Health of the State of North Carolina*—continued.

——. Monthly bulletins of the . . . Compiled by Thomas F. Wood, sec. Jan. to March, 1880. fol. [*Wilmington,* 1880.]

——. A guide to shipmasters visiting the Cape Fear and other rivers. Presented by the . . . 9 pp. 8°. *Raleigh, News & Observer,* 1881.

——. Biennial report to the governor of the State. 1., 1879-80. 201 pp. 8°. *Raleigh, News & Observer,* 1881.

——. Vaccination. Advice on the necessity of vaccination; the value of vaccination; the tests of successful vaccination; how often revaccination should be done; the quality of vaccine; the best way to use vaccine; how to prevent and exterminate small-pox; the construction of small-pox hospitals, etc. 13 pp. 8°. *Raleigh, Ashe & Gatling,* 1882.

——. Conjoint session of the . . . and Medical Society of North Carolina, held in Concord, May 10, 1882. [Contains report of the board of health to the Medical Society of the State of North Carolina for the year 1881.] lxvi pp. 8°. *Raleigh, Ashe & Gatling,* 1882.

——. Report of the secretary of the . . . on one aspect of the subject of medical education as set forth in the work of the medical examining board. xxiv pp. 8°. [*Wilmington,* 1885.]

——. Bulletins of the . . . Published monthly. v. 1. Nos. 1-3, April to June, 1886. 8°. [*Wilmington,* 1886.]

North Carolina. *Western North Carolina Insane Asylum, at Morganton.* Annual report of the board of directors to the governor of the State. 1., 1882-4. 26 pp. 8°. *Raleigh, Ashe & Gatling,* 1884.

Established Dec. 7, 1882. 1. and 2. rep. in 1.

North Carolina Medical Journal. M. J. De Rosset and Thomas F. Wood, editors. [Monthly; 2 v. annually.] v. 1-21, 1878-88. 8°. *Wilmington.*

Current. In v. 7-17 Dr. Wood sole editor; in v. 18 G. G. Thomas added.

Northcote (Augustus Beauchamp). On the constitution of allophane. 8 pp. 8°. [*n. p.,* 1857.]

Repr. from: Phil. Mag., Lond., 1857, 4. s., xiii.

—— & **Church** (Arthur H.) A manual of qualitative chemical analysis. xiv, 428 pp. 8°. *London, Van Voorst,* 1858.

Northcote (William). The marine practice of physic and surgery, including that in the hot countries, particularly useful to all who visit the East and West Indies, or the coast of Africa. To which is added Pharmacopœia marina. And some brief directions to be observed by the sea-surgeon in an engagement, etc. 2 v. xv, 143, 328 pp.; vii, 490 pp., 7 l. 8°. *London, W. & J. Richardson,* 1770.

——. A concise history of anatomy, from the earliest ages of antiquity. To which are annexed, a few thoughts on the uses of anatomy, and rules for giving a course of anatomical lectures. 176 pp. 8°. *London, T. Evans,* 1772.

——. The anatomy of the human body. Composed (on an entire new plan) in a method very different from all anatomical writers. Designed (chiefly) for the use of naval practitioners, and by way of supplement to a work, entitled: The marine surgeon; the whole forming a complete repository for the surgeons of the royal navy. To which is subjoined, some physiological tracts, and a copious index. xvi, 448 pp., 12 l. 8°. *London, T. Becket & P. A. De Hondt,* 1772.

See, also, **van Swieten** (Gerard L. B.) The diseases incident to armies [etc.] 8°. *Philadelphia,* 1776.

North Devon Infirmary, Barnstaple. Annual reports of the house committee and resident

North Devon Infirmary, Barnstaple—cont'd.
medical officer to the benefactors and subscribers. 39.-56., 1864-5 to 1881-2. fol. *Barnstaple,*
1865-82.
Forms used: In-door recommendation; out-door recommendation.

——. Rules for the government of the . . .
Established at Barnstaple, 1824. 23 pp. 8°.
Barnstaple, E. J. Arnold, 1867.

North-Eastern Dispensary, New York City.
Annual reports of the board of managers to their
patrons and the public. 3., 1864; 5., 1866; 6.,
1867; 8.-12., 1869-73; 15.-25., 1876-86. 8°. *New
York,* 1865-87.
Incorporated Feb. 18, 1862.

North-Eastern Hospital for Children, London,
E. Bye-laws of the . . . 8 pp. 12°. *London,
Forsaith & Sons,* 1874.
Bound with: Reports, 1878-82.
Established July, 1867, for the relief of sick children
under twelve years of age. Forms used: Letter of recommendation for in-patient; out-patient ticket.

——. Annual reports of the committee of management to the governors and benefactors. 7.,
1874; 11.-16., 1878-83. 12°. *London,* 1875-84.
1878-82 bound in 1 v.

——. [An appeal of the committee for donations
and annual subscriptions.] 1 sheet. 4°. *London, n. d.*]

Northeim.
RÜLING (J. P.) Physikalisch-medicinisch-ökonomische Beschreibung der zum Fürstenthum
Göttingen gehörigen Stadt Northeim, und ihrer
umliegenden Gegend. 8°. *Göttingen,* 1779.

Northern Counties Hospital for Incurable, Ardwich Green, Manchester. Annual reports of the
board of management to the governors and subscribers. 5., 1875-6; 9., 1879-80. 8°. *Manchester,* 1876-80.

Northern Dispensary of the City of New York.
Annual reports of the board of trustees to the
patrons and subscribers at the annual meetings.
3., 1829-30; 9., 1835-6; 14.-17., 1840-41 to 1843-
4; 19., 1845-6; 21., 1847-8; 23.-55., 1849-50 to
1881; 57.-60.,1883-6. 8°. *New York,* 1830-87.
Incorporated Nov. 28, 1828. 23.-55. bound in 2 v.

——. Act of incorporation and by-laws of the
. . . 23 pp. 8°. *New York, Pudney & Russell,*
1850.

——. Act of incorporation and by-laws of the
. . . 23 pp. 8°. *New York, Hall, Clayton & Co.,*
1858.

Northern Dispensary for the Medical Relief of
the Poor, Philadelphia. The origin, rules, and
regulations. With a list of contributors, managers, and officers, and the annual report for
1816. [From Oct. 1 to Dec. 30.] 12 pp. 12°.
[*Philadelphia*], *J. Maxwell,* [1817].
Instituted Oct. 1, 1816; chartered March 26, 1817.

——. Rules and regulations of the . . . adopted
April 20, 1838. 14 pp. 12°. *Philadelphia, J.
Rakestraw,* 1838.

——. The same. With act of incorporation. 22
pp. 12°. *Philadelphia, J. Rakestraw,* 1841.

——. Annual reports of the board of managers
to the contributors. 24.-28., 1841-5; 32., 1849;
34.-36., 1851-3; 38.-41., 1855-8; 43.-46., 1860-63;
48.-53., 1865-70; 55.-57., 1872-4; 59., 1876; 60.,
1877; 63., 1880; 64., 1881. 12°. *Philadelphia,*
1842-82.

Northern Home for Friendless Children and Associated Institute for Soldiers' and Sailors' Orphans, Philadelphia. Annual reports of the
board of trustees and managers to the senate
and house of representatives and contributors.
1., 1853-4; 3.-5., 1855-6 to 1857-8; 7.-11., 1859-
60 to 1863-4; 14.-28., 1866-7 to 1880-81; 30.,

Northern Home for Friendless [etc.]—cont'd.
1882-3; 31., 1883-4. 8°. *Philadelphia,* 1854-
84.
14.-25. bound in 1 v.
Organized Sept. 28 and opened Aug. 3, 1853, as Northern Home for Friendless Children. In 1864 the institution
managers received children of soldiers and sailors, and
assumed above title in 1869.

Northern Hospital for the Insane of the State
of Wisconsin, at Oshkosh. *See* **Wisconsin**
Northern Hospital for the Insane of the State of
Wisconsin, at Oshkosh.

Northern (The) Journal of Medicine. A monthly
survey of the progress of medical knowledge at
home and abroad. Edited by W. Seller and T.
L. Kemp. v. 1-4, May, 1844, to June, 1846. 8°.
Edinburgh, H. Paton.
All published. A continuance of : **Scottish** (The) and
North of England Medical Gazette. In v. 3-4 Dr. Seller
sole editor. Merged in: **Monthly** (The) Journal of Medical Science.

Northern (The) Lancet and Gazette of Legal
Medicine. A monthly journal of medical and
general science, criticism, and medical jurisprudence. Edited by Francis J. d'Avignon and
Horace Nelson. In 2 v. annually. v. 1-12, January, 1850, to June, 1856. 8°. *Plattsburgh, N. Y.*
Want Jan., 1850; nos. 6, 9-10, 21, 24, 26, v. 12, 1856. v.
1 complete in 7 nos., Jan. to July, 1850; v. 2, in 5 nos.,
Nov., 1850, to March, 1851; v. 3-11, in 6 nos. each, April,
1851, to Sept., 1855; v. 12 became weekly, in 26 nos.,
Dec. 10, 1855, to June, 1856. Title of v. 4-6 was: **Nelson's**
Northern Lancet and American Journal of Medical Jurisprudence; Horace Nelson, editor and proprietor. Title of
v. 7-12 was: **Nelson's** American Lancet, a monthly journal of practical medicine; and Alfred Nelson added as
editor.

Northern (The) Microscopist. An illustrated
journal of practical microscopy. Edited by
George E. Davis. [Monthly.] v. 1; Nos. 1-9, v.
2, Jan., 1881, to Sept., 1882. 2 v. 8°. *London,
D. Bogue.*
Continued as: **Northern** (The) Microscopist and Microscopical News.

Northern (The) Microscopist and Microscopical
News. An illustrated journal of practical microscopy. Edited by George E. Davis. [Monthly.]
Nos. 10-12, v. 2, October to December, 1882. 1 v.
8°. *London.*
Title of v. 1 and nos. 1-9, v. 2, was: **Northern** (The)
Microscopist. Continued as: **Microscopical** (The)
News and Northern Microscopist.

Northern Ohio Lunatic Asylum, at Cleveland.
See **Ohio.** *Cleveland Asylum for the Insane.*

Northern (The) Ohio Medical and Scientific
Examiner. [Homœopathic.] Edited by A. W.
Oliver, John Gilman, John Wheeler, C. D. Williams, and W. B. Waterman. [Monthly.] Nos.
1-9, v. 1, Feb., 1848, to April 15, 1849. 152 pp.
8°. *Cleveland.*
Title of nos. 4-9, v. 1, was: **Ohio** (The) Medical Examiner, and published at Columbus.

North Haven.
See **Hamden.**

North Hertfordshire and South Bedfordshire Infirmary, Hitchin, Hertfordshire. Annual
reports of the monthly board to the governors
and subscribers. 41.-44., 1880-81 to 1883-4. 8°.
Hitchin, 1881-4.

North Holland. *See* **Netherlands.**

North (The) of England Medical and Surgical
Journal. [Quarterly.] v. 1, August, 1830, to May,
1831. 514 pp. 8°. *London & Manchester, Whittaker, Treacher & Arnot.*
Ended.

Northof (Franciscus Edmundus). *De scabie.
19 pp. 4°. *Gottingæ, H. M. Grape,* 1792.

Northowram.
RANGER (W.) Report to the General Board
of Health, on a preliminary inquiry into the
sewerage, drainage, and supply of water, and

Northowram.

the sanitary condition of the inhabitants of the townships of Northowram and Southowram, in the county of York. 8°. *London*, 1850.

Northowram urban sanitary district. *See* **Halifax Union** (combined sanitary district).

North Raymond.

See **Fever** (*Cerebro-spinal, History, etc., of*), by *localities*.

Northrop (B. G.) Near-sightedness in schools; its causes, prevalence, and preventives. 18 pp. 8°. *New Haven, Tuttle, Morehouse & Taylor*, 1878.

Repr. from: Rep. State Bd. Education.

Northrop (George J.) A case of puerperal septic fever. And some remarks on the relations of the medical profession to the people, by Henry B. Baker. 8 pp. 8°. *Detroit, Mich., W. A. Scripps*, 1877.

Repr. from: Detroit M. J., 1877, n. s., i.

Northrop (*Joseph Norman*) [1817–78].

Curtis (F. C.) Biography. Med. Ann., Albany, 1882, iii [Tr. M. Soc. County Albany, 637]. *Also:* Tr. M. Soc. County Albany 1870-80, Albany, 1883, iii, 367, port.

Northrup (*Calvin M.*)

Lee (C. A.) Remarks on the trial of Calvin M. Northrup, esq., indicted for the crime of administering belladonna to his wife, with intent to kill. Quart. J. Psych. M., N. Y., 1868, ii, 28-47.

Northrup (William P.) Extensive interlobular emphysema and abscess of the lungs, after whooping cough, in a child of two months. Unique case. 3 pp. 8°. [*Philadelphia*], 1883.

Repr. from: Am. J. M. Sc., Phila., n. s., lxxxvi.

North Sea.

BENEKE (F. W.) Die sanitäre Bedeutung des verlängerten Aufenthaltes auf den deutschen Nordseeinseln, insonderheit auf Norderney. 8°. *Norden u. Norderney*, 1881.

Beneke. Ueber die sanitäre Bedeutung des Herbst- und Winteraufenthaltes, auf den deutschen Nordseeinseln. Deutsche med. Wchnschr., Berl., 1882, viii, 263–266. — **Beneke** (R.) Ueber die Verwendung der deutschen Nordseeinseln als Luftcurorte. Berl. klin. Wchnschr., 1887. xxiv, 873.—**Friedrich.** Ueber Herbstaufenthalt und Ueberwinterung Kranker auf den deutschen Nordsee-ins-ln. Jahresb. d. Gesellsch. f. Nat.- u. Heilk. in Dresd., 1885-6, 157–165.

North Shields.

See **Fever** (*Typhus, History, etc., of*), by *localities*.

North Shields and Tynemouth Dispensary. Annual reports of the committee to the subscribers. 68.–82., 1869-70 to 1883-4. 4°. *North Shields & Tynemouth, J. Philipson & Sons*, 1870-84.

North Staffordshire Infirmary. Annual reports of the committee to the subscribers. 67.–70., 1881–2 to 1884-5; 72., 1886-7. 12°. *Newcastle*, 1882-7.

Established 1815.

North Street Union Mission to the Poor, Boston. Annual report of the managers to the subscribers. 6., 1866-7. 10 pp. 12°. *Boston, Wright & Potter*, 1867.

Northumberland. *Pauper Lunatic Asylum for the County of Northumberland, Cottingwood, near Morpeth.* Annual reports of the committee of visitors and medical superintendent to her majesty's justices of the peace for the county of Northumberland. 17., 1875; 22., 1880. 4°. *Alnwick*, [1876–81].

Opened March 16, 1859.

——. Regulations and orders of the committee of visitors for the management and conduct of the asylum, female department. Approved Dec. 18, 1882. 46 pp. 8°. *Morpeth, D. F. Wilson*, 1883.

Northumberland. *Pauper Lunatic Asylum for the County of Northumberland* [etc.]—continued.

——. [Blank forms in use at the asylum.] v. s. [*Morpeth? n. d.*]

Accident report.
Articles received from the laundry.
Chief female officer's daily return.
Female charge attendant's daily report.
Female charge nurse's daily report.
Female patient requiring special supervision.
Male washing account.
Matron's notice of death to clerk.
Memorandum of admission by matron.
Notice of admission of pauper patient.
Notice of admission of private patient.
Notice of patient requiring special supervision.
Notice of burial, Schedule A. Same, Schedule B.
Notice of death, to the commissioners in lunacy. Same, to coroner; to register of deaths; to relative; to relieving officer.
Notice of discharge to the commissioners in lunacy. Same; to relieving officer.
Notice of discharge after escape, if not recaptured within 14 days.
Notice of removal or escape.
Obligations of relatives in case of patient turned over to their care.
Order for the reception of pauper patient.
Order of superintendent for goods.
Permit to introduce friends.
Private patient, obligation of.
Private patient, statement of condition on admission.
Receipt for salary.
Record of attendants on duty.
Sick diet.
Transfer of pauper patient to another asylum.
Visitor's permit.
Ward list.

Northumberland and Durham Medical Society. Health and meteorology of the Newcastle and Gateshead. Reports. 5. and 6., Sept. to Nov., 1869. By G. H. Philipson. Communicated to the . . . 6 pp., 9 tab.; 4 pp., 4 tab. 8°. [*Newcastle*, 1869.]

5. report for 2 months.

Northusanus (Joh. Fridericus). * De venenis morbisque venenosis. 24 pp. 4°. *Heidelbergæ, typ. A. Walterii*, [1656].

North Wales Counties Lunatic Asylum, Denbigh. Annual reports of the committee of visitors and medical superintendent to the quarter sessions for the united counties of Denbigh, Flint, Anglesey, Carnarvon, and Merioneth. 2.–7., 1850–55; 9.–14., 1857–62; 16.–19., 1864-7; 21.–33., 1869–81. 8°. *Denbigh, London, Dolgelley & Carnarvon*, 1851-82.

1871–81 bound in 1 v.

——. Regulations and orders for the management and conduct of the . . . and for the guidance and instruction of the officers, attendants, and servants, and all other persons engaged in the service of the asylum. Made Oct. 13, 1882. 31 pp. 8°. *Denbigh, T. Gee & Son*, [1882].

Bound with: Reports, 1871-81.

——. General rules for the government of the . . . pursuant to the 53d section of the act 16 & 17 Vict., c. 97. Made by the committee of visitors at a quarterly meeting held at the asylum after due notice on the 13th day of October, 1882, and approved by her majesty's principal secretary of state for the home department on the 13th day of Nov., 1882. 16 pp. 8°. *Denbigh, T. Gee & Son*, [1882].

Bound with: Reports, 1871-81.

——. [Blank forms in use at the asylum.] 4° & fol. [*Denbigh*, 188–].

Notice of admission of pauper patient.
Notice of admission of private patient.
Notice of death of pauper patient.
Notice of discharge of pauper patient.
Bound with: Reports, 1871-81.

North West London Free Dispensary for Sick Children, W. Report of the committee to the contributors, for the years 1874-6. 17 pp. 8°. *London, Williams & Whittmann*, 1877.

Founded in 1862.

North West London Hospital. Annual reports of the committee of management to the governors and subscribers. 1.-6., 1879-84. 12°. *London*, 1880-85.

Established 1878.

North - Western Dispensary, New York City. Act of incorporation and by-laws of the . . . 24 pp. 12°. *New York, J. A. Gray*, 1852.

——. Annual reports of the board of managers to the subscribers at the annual meetings. 1.-5., 1852-3 to 1856-7; 10., 1862; 12., 1864; 16., 1868; 18.-22., 1870-74. 8°. *New York*, 1853-75.

Incorporated July 12 and opened Dec. 6, 1852.

——. Annual reports of the board of managers to the subscribers at the annual meetings. 1.-8., 1852-3 to 1860; 10., 1862; 12.-14., 1864-6; 16., 1868; 18.-33., 1870-85. 8°. *New York*, 1853-86.

Incorporated July 12 and opened Dec. 6, 1852. 6. report for 14 months ending Dec. 31, 1858.

Northwestern (The) Journal of Homœopathia. Edited by George E. Shipman. [Monthly.] v. 1-4, Oct., 1848, to Sept., 1852. 8°. *Chicago.*

Ended.

Northwestern Lancet. Jay Owens, editor and proprietor. [Semi-monthly.] v. 1-8, Oct. 1, 1881-8. 8°. *St. Paul, Minn.*

Current. In Nov., 1884, C. B. Witherle became editor. v. 7 complete in 6 nos., Oct. to Dec., 1887; v. 8 commenced Jan., 1888.

Northwestern Medical College, of St. Joseph, Mo. Annual announcements and catalogues for the sessions of 1881-2 to 1883-4 (2.-4.). 8°. *St. Joseph*, 1881-3.

List of graduates and students for 1880-81 to 1882-3 in announcement for subsequent years. 1. announcement not issued.

Northwestern (The) Medical and Surgical Journal. Edited by Wm. B. Herrick and John Evans. [Bi-monthly.] v. 5-14, May, 1848-57. 8°. *Chicago & Indianapolis, J. W. Duzan.*

See **Illinois** (The) Medical and Surgical Journal for v. 1-2. See **Illinois** (The) and Indiana Medical and Surgical Journal, v. 1-2, for v. 3-4. v. 9 became monthly. v. 10 contains 8 nos., May to Dec., 1853. v. 6-7 edited by J. Evans and E. G. Meek; v. 8, Meek dropped; v. 9, by W. B. Herrick and H. A. Johnson; v. 11, Herrick dropped and N. S. Davis added; v. 13, Johnson dropped; v. 14, W. H. Byford added. Continued as: **Chicago** (The) Medical Journal.

Northwestern (The) Medical and Surgical Journal. A medical monthly devoted to the interests of the Northwest. Edited by Alexander J. Stone. v. 1-4, June, 1870, to June, 1874. 8°. *St. Paul, Minn.*

Ended. v. 3 edited by H. C. Hand and H. H. Kimball.

Northwestern Ohio Medical College, Toledo. [Circular announcing change of title, and first session under charter of 1882.] 1 sheet. 8°. [*Toledo*, 1883.]

An outgrowth of the Toledo School of Medicine, which was organized in 1878. Chartered under the above title in 1882.

——. Annual announcements for the session of 1883-4 to 1886-7 (1.-4.). 12°. *Toledo*, 1883-6.

An outgrowth of the Toledo School of Medicine, which was organized in 1878. Chartered under above title in 1882.

North Western Sanitary Commission. *See* **United States** Sanitary Commission.

North-Western Provinces and Oudh. Notes on the application of the test of organic disease of the spleen, as an easy and certain method of detecting malarious localities in hot climates. By Surgeon T. E. Dempster, member of the late canal committee. xxi pp., 3 plans. fol. *Agra, W. H. Haycock*, 1848.

The province of Oudh was united with the North-Western Provinces in 1877.

——. Half-yearly reports of the government charitable dispensaries established in the Bengal and North-Western Provinces, ending Sept. 30,

North-Western Provinces and Oudh—cont'd. 1847; Sept. 30, 1848. 211, 215 pp. 8°. *Calcutta*, 1848-9.

——. Medical report on the Mahamurree in Gurhwal in 1849-50, and appendices, by Dr. C. Renny, superintending surgeon, Meerut division. From the medical board to the lieutenant-governor. 56 pp., 1 map. 8°. *Agra, Secundra Orphan Press*, 1851.

——. [Reports on epidemic fevers of the typhoid class; on leprosy and vaccination.] (Published by authority.) 1 p. l., 158 pp. fol. *Allahabad, Government Press*, 1864.

Selections from the records of government, North-West Provinces, 1864, pt. xi.

——. [On tea plantations and factories, choleraic influence in the atmosphere, and on dispensaries.] (Published by authority.) 1 p. l., 72 pp. fol. *Allahabad, Government Press*, 1864.

Selections from the records of government, North-Western Provinces, 1864, pt. xlii.

——. Annual reports of the dispensaries and charitable institutions of the . . . By the surgeon-general to the secretary to government, for the years 1865; 1866; 1869-86. fol. *Allahabad*, 1866-87.

——. Annual returns of vaccination for the . . . By the superintendent-general of vaccination to the secretary to government, for the years 1866-7; 1869-70 to 1877-8. fol. *Allahabad*, 1867-78.

For continuation, see Reports of the sanitary commissioner, North-West Provinces.

——. [On forests, soil, administration, etc.] pp. 117-217, 1 map. 8°. *Allahabad, Government Press*, 1869.

Selections from the records of government, North-West Provinces, n. s., ii, no. 2.

——. Annual reports of the sanitary commissioner of the . . . to the secretary to government. 1.-18., 1868-85. fol. *Allahabad*, 1869-86.

1869 and subsequent contains reports on vaccination.

——. Annual reports, with tabular statements, on the condition and management of the jails in the . . . By the inspector-general of prisons to the secretary to government, for the years 1870-73; 1875-85. fol. *Allahabad*, 1871-86.

——. Annual reports of the working of the Lock-hospitals in the . . . by the sanitary commissioner to the secretary to government. 4.-10., 1877-83. fol. *Allahabad*, 1878-84.

Containing the annual reports of 18 hospitals. viz: Lock Hospital at Agra, Allahabad, Bareilly, Benares, Cawnpore, Chakráta, Fatehgarh, Fyzabad, Jhánsi, Lucknow, Meerut, Moradabad, Muttra, Naini Tal, Ranikhet, Roorku, Sháhjahánpur, Sitapur.

——. Report on leprosy in the . . . From C. Plank, sanitary commissioner to officiating secretary to government. Dated Naini Tal, 19th Oct., 1876. 13 pp. fol. [*Calcutta*, 1879.]

Northwestern University. *Medical Department. See* **Chicago** Medical College.

Northwestern University and the Garrett Biblical Institute, Evanston. Catalogues for the sessions of 1883-4; 1884-5. 103, 103 pp. 8°. *Chicago*, 1884-5.

North Wilts Dispensary, Devizes. Annual reports of the committee to the subscribers and the public. 5., 1865; 16.-23., 1876-83. 8°. *Devizes*, 1866-84.

Northwoods Winterbowine, Bristol. [Circular of the proprietors, stating their facilities for the treatment of ladies and gentlemen of the upper and middle classes afflicted with mental disease.] 1 sheet. 4°. [*Bristol*, 1877.] [P., v. 1296.]

Nortier (Adriaan).

Co-Editor of : Ἱπποκράτης. Magazin, [etc.], Rotterdam, 1826-8.

Nortier (Arnoldus Marius). *Verslag der verloskundige kliniek en polikliniek aan de Rijks-

Nortier (Arnoldus Marius)—continued.
Universiteit te Leiden gedurende den cursus 1881–1882. [Leiden.] 1 p. l., 83 pp. 8°. *Rotterdam, M. Wyt & Zonen,* 1883.

Nortier (Petrus Joh.) * De quinta partus periodo. 2 p. l., 55 pp. 8°. *Lugd. Bat., J. H. Gebhard et soc.,* 1842.

Norton, *Connecticut.*
FITCH's Home for Soldiers and their Orphan Children. Treasurer's report of . . . [From 1865 to 1880.] Joseph B. Hoyt, treasurer. Also a brief history of the institution by the matron. 8°. *Stamford, Conn.,* 1881.

Norton (Arthur Trehern). Osteology; a concise description of the human skeleton. iv, 128 pp.; atlas, 20 pl. 8°. *London, R. Hardwicke,* 1866.

———. Affections of the throat and larynx. The classification, description, and statistics of 150 consecutive cases occurring in the throat department of St. Mary's Hospital. 39 pp. 8°. *London, R. Hardwicke,* 1871.

———. A text book of operative surgery and surgical anatomy, based on the original work of Professors Claude Bernard and Ch. Huette. 2. ed. xviii, 13–401 pp., 88 pl. 8°. *London, Baillière, Tindall & Cox,* 1886.

Norton (Frank H.)
Co-Editor of: **New York** (The) Dental Journal, 1858–60.

Norton (Geo. S.) Ophthalmic therapeutics. With an introduction by Prof. T. F. Allen. 2. ed. 242 pp. 8°. *New York & Philadelphia, Boericke & Tafel,* 1882.

———. The eye as an agent in causing headaches and other nervous disturbances. Read before the New York Medico-Chirurgical Society, December 9, 1884. 24 pp. 8°. *Philadelphia,* 1885.
Repr. from: Hahneman. Month., Phila., 1885, xxi.

———. Malignant tumors of the eyelids and orbit. 12 pp. 8°. *New York, J. C. Rankin,* 1886.

Norton (J.)
See **von Brunnow** (Ernst Georg). A glance at Hahnemann and homœopathy [etc.] 8°. *London,* 1845.

Norton (Jane C.) An interior view of Bloomingdale Asylum, also reply to Dr. Ordronaux's report. 38 pp. 8°. [*Brooklyn,* 1877.]
Title-page wanting.

Norton (John).
See **Account** (An) of remarkable cures performed by the use of Maredant's antiscorbutic drops, etc. 12°. *London,* 1774.

Norton (*John C.*) [1814–51].
Biographical sketch. Tr. Ohio M. Soc., Cleveland, 1852, 30–32.

Norton (Robert). Elements of diagnosis, general pathology and therapeutics. [Appendix: Abridged memoir of T. Bateman, M. D.] x, 100, v pp. 8°. *London, W. Jackson,* 1831–2. [*Also, in:* P., v. 778.]
See, also, **Martinet** (L.) Manual of therapeutics [etc.] 12°. *New York,* 1830.

Norton (Selby). On the causes, prevention, and treatment of infantile diseases, showing by what means the present mortality may be greatly reduced. iv, 5–75 pp. 12°. *London, J. Churchill, & Sons,* 1870.

———. Infant life; how to preserve it. 2. ed. 45 pp. 8°. *London, Waterlow Brothers & Layton,* [1885].

Norton (Sidney A.) A lecture on measures and weights, delivered October 5, 1869, as introductory to the tenth annual course of lectures in the Miami College of Cincinnati. 21 pp. roy. 8°. *Cincinnati, R. Clarke & Co.,* 1869.

———. A valedictory address delivered before the class graduating Feb. 29, 1872, from the Miami Medical College of Cincinnati. 16 pp. 8°. *Cincinnati, Bradley & Power,* [1872].

Norton (*Willam S.*) [1776–1862].
Willard (S. D.) Notice of William S. Norton, M. D. Tr. M. Soc. N. Y., Albany, 1863, 392.

Norton (The) house and ship ventilator. Designed for the ventilation of houses, ships, tunnels, and mines. 14 pp., 7 pl. 8°. *London, J. Causton & Sons,* 1883.

Norway. Udkast til Lov om Medicinalvæsenet i Norge, med Motiver, udarbeidet af en naadigst anordnet Kongelig Commission. viii, 187 pp. 8°. *Christiania,* 1844.

———. Kongelig Proposition til Norges tolvte ordentlige Storthing angaaende Lov om Qvarantainevæsenet. [Royal proposition to the 12. Norwegian congress, concerning law on quarantines.] pp. 29–51. roy. 8°. *Christiania, P. T. Mallings,* 1848.
Cutting.

———. Lov om Qvarantainevæsenet. Malmø den 12te Juli 1848. 8 pp. 4°. *Christiania, C. Grøndahl,* [1848].

———. The same. 24 pp. 24°. *Christiania, trykt hos C. Grøndahl,* [1848].

———. The same. A law concerning the performance of quarantine. Malmoe, July 12th, 1848. 24 pp. 24°. *Christiania, C. Gröndahl,* [1848].
Bound with: Lov om Quarantainevæsenet. 24°. *Christiania,* [1848].

———. The same. Loi sur les quarantaines. Malmö, le 12 juillet 1848. 24 pp. 24°. *Christiania, imp. par C. Gröndahl,* [1848].
Bound with: Lov om Quarantainevæsenet. 24°. *Christiania,* [1848].

———. The same. Gesetz über das Quarantaine-Wesen. Malmö, den 12ten Juli 1848. 24 pp. 24°. *Christiania, gedr. bei C. Gröndahl,* [1848].
Bound with: Lov om Quarantainevæsenet. 24°. *Christiania,* [1848].

———. Lov om Sindssyges Behandling og Forpleining. 8 pp. 4°. *Christiania,* [1848].

———. Medicinalcollegiets Skjæbne. 47 pp. 8°. *Christiania,* 1848.
Repr. from: Norsk Mag. f. Lægevidensk., Christiania, 1848, 2. R., ii.

———. Reglement om Qvarantainevæsenet. Christiania, den 10de Februar 1849. 48 pp. 12°. *Christiania, C. Grøndahl,* [1849].

———. Medicinal-Taxt for Norge, som ifölge kongl. Placat af 10de November 1855 er gjældende fra 1ste Januar 1856 indtil videre. 50 pp. sm. 8°. *Christiania, trykt hos Brøgger & Christie,* 1855. [P., v. 1831.]

———. Norges officielle Statistik. C. No. 4. Beretninger om Sundhedstilstanden og Medicinalforholdene i Norge i Aarene 1853–77; n. R., 1878–81; 3. R., 1882–5. Udgivet af Direktøren for det civile Medicinalvæsen. roy. 8° & 4°. *Christiania,* 1856–87.
For continuation, see following Ny Række.

———. The same. Ny Række. 8°. *Christiania,* 1880–84.

———. The same. Tredie Række. 8°. *Christiania,* 1885–7.

———. Aarsberetninger for 1856–59 fra Overlægerne for den spedalske Sygdom O. G. Høegh og T. J. Loberg til Departementet for det Indre. 8° & roy 8°. *Christiania,* 1857–60.

———. Beretning om Bodsfængslets Virksomhed. 1856–66. 8°. *Christiania, Brøgger & Christie,* 1857–67.

———. Medicinal-Taxt for Norge som ifölge kongelig Placat af 6te Juli 1861 er gjældende fra 1ste September 1861 indtil videre. 51 pp. 8°. *Christiania, trykt i det Steenske Bogtrykkeri,* 1861. [P., v. 1831.]

———. Veterinair-Medicinal-Taxt for Norge, som ifölge kongelig Placat af 6te Juli 1861 er gjæl-

Norway—continued.

dende fra 1ste September 1861 indtil videre. 27 pp. 8°. *Christiania, trykt i det Steenske Bogtrykkeri*, 1861. [P., v. 1831.]

——. Norges officielle Statistik. C. No. 5. Tabeller over de Spedalske i Norge i Aarene 1860–80. Samt Aarsberetninger for samme Aarene af Overlægen for den spedalske Sygdom. Udgivet af Direktøren for det civile Medicinalvæsen. 4°. *Christiania*, 1861–82.
1880 contains: Oversigt over Spedalskhedens Gang i 1856–80.

——. Tillæg til Medicinal-Taxten for Norge, udfærdiget af den kongelige norske Regjerings-Departement for det Indre i Henhold til kongelig Resolution af 6te Juli 1861. 9 pp. 8°. *Christiania, det Steenske Bogtrykkeri*, 1862.

——. Tillæg til Veterinair-Medicinal-Taxten for Norge, udfærdiget af den kongelige norske Regjerings-Departement for det Indre i Henhold til kongelig Resolution af 6te Juli 1861. 5 pp. 8°. *Christiania, det Steenske Bogtrykkeri*, 1862. [P., v. 1831.]

——. Andet Tillæg til Medicinal-Taxten for Norge, udfærdiget af den kongelige norske Regjerings-Departement for det Indre i Henhold til kongelig Resolution af 6te Juli 1861. 7 pp. 8°. *Christiania, det Steenske Bogtrykkeri*, 1863.

——. Andet Tillæg til Veterinair-Medicinal-Taxten for Norge, udfærdiget af den kongelige norske Regjerings Departement for det Indre i Henhold til kongelig Resolution af 6te Juli 1861. 4 pp. 8°. *Christiania, det Steenske Bogtrykkeri*, 1863. [P., v. 1831.]

——. Love, Resolutioner, Departementsskrivelser m. m. vedkommende Norges Medicinalvæsen for Aarene 1851–1867, udgivne af J. N. M. Johansen og F. H. G. Hench. 2 v. 322, 204 pp. 8°. *Christiania, Feilberg & Landmark*, 1863–9.

——. Tredie Tillæg til Medicinal-Taxten for Norge, udfærdiget af den kongelige norske Regjerings Departement for det Indre i Henhold til kongelig Resolution af 6te Juli 1861. 5 pp. 8°. *Christiania, det Steenske Bogtrykkeri*, 1864. [P., v. 1831.]

——. Tredie Tillæg til Veterinair-Medicinal-Taxten for Norge, udfærdiget af den kongelige norske Regjerings-Departement for det Indre i Henhold til kongelig Resolution af 6te Juli 1861. 5 pp. 8°. *Christiania, det Steenske Bogtrykkeri*, 1864.

——. Forslag til Forandring i den bestaænde Kvaksalverlovgivning. 23 pp. 8°. *Christiania*, 1864.

——. Medicinal-Taxt for Norge, ifølge naadigst Bemyndigelse udfærdiget af den kongelige norske Regjerings Departement for det Indre og gjældende fra 1ste Januar 1866 indtil videre. 51 pp. 8°. *Christiania, trykt i det Steenske Bogtrykkeri*, 1865. [P., v. 1831.]

——. Veterinair-Medicinal-Taxt for Norge, ifölge naadigst Bemyndigelse, udfærdiget af den kongelige norske Regjerings Departement for det Indre og gjældende fra 1ste Januar 1866 indtil videre. 27 pp. 8°. *Christiania, trykt i det Steenske Bogtrykkeri*, 1865. [P., v. 1831.]

——. Norges officielle Statistik. C. No. 2. Beretninger om amternes konomiske Tilstand i Aarene 1861–75. Udgivne af det statistiske Centralbureau. 4 v. 4°. *Christiania*, 1867–79.
1861–5 in two pts.

——. Lov om Forandring i Kvaksalverlovgivningen. 4 pp. 4°. *Christiania, A. Grøndahl*, 1871.

——. Lægedistrikter i Norge (Physicater, Chirurgicater) og deres Embedsmænd fra deres Oprettelse og til nærværende Tid. 54 pp. 8°. [*Christiania*, 1873.]
Repr. from: Norges Læge, Christiania, 1873.

Norway—continued.

——. Norges officielle Statistik. C. No. 5b. Oversigt over Sindssygeasylernes Virksomhed i Aarene 1872–79; n. R., 1883–4; 3. R., 1885–7. Efter de fra Asylerne indkomne Aarsberetninger sammendragen og udgiven af Direktøren for det civile Medicinalvæsen. 4°. *Christiania*, 1873–87.
1872–9 bound in 1 v.

——. Klædsel- og Paknings-Instrux for Infanteriets-Korporaler og Menige. (Fastsat af Armekommandoen under 23 Juni 1877.) 21 pp. 16°. *Christiania, Grøndahl & Søns Bogtrykkeri*, 1877.

——. Norsk Medicinallovgivning indeholdende en kronologisk Samling af Forordninger, Love, Plakater, Resolutioner, Skrivelser m. m. vedkommende Norges Medicinalvæsen for Aarene 1672–1880. Udgivet af K. A. Langberg, L. Esmark-Olsson og G. Somme. lxxi, 636 pp. 8°. *Kristiania, Udgivernes Forlag*, 1881.

——. Statistiske Tabeller over Dövstumme, Blinde og aandssvage Börn i Kongeriget Norge. (1881.) Udarbeidede med Hensyn paa Lov om abnorme børns Undervisning af 8de Juni 1881 i Departementet for Kirke- og Undervisningsvæsenet. 113 pp. 8°. *Kristiania, trykt i det Steenske Bogtrykkeri*, 1882.

Norway.

See, also, **Army** (*Swedish-Norwegian*); **Blind** (*Asylums, etc., for*); **Cholera** (*Asiatic, History, etc., of*), *by localities*; **Christiania**; **Drammen**; **Fever** (*Typhoid, History, etc., of*), *by localities*; **Gausdal**; **Idiots** (*Asylums, etc., for*), *by localities*; **Idiots** (*Statistics of*); **Insane** (*Asylums for, etc.*), *by localities—Sweden, etc.*; **Insane** (*Care, etc., of*), **Leprosy** (*History, etc., of*); **Medicine** (*History, etc., of*), *by localities*; **Pharmacopœias**; **Pharmacy**; **Sandefjord**; **Skeen**.

BERETNINGER om Sygdomsforholdene i 1842 og 1843 i Danmark, Sverige og Norge, oplæste ved de skandinaviske Naturforskeres Möde i Christiania 1844. 8°. *Christiania*, 1847.

FORTEGNELSE over autoriserede Læger og Dyrlæger i Norge; ifolge Plakat af 17de Januar 1809, udgiven af den kongelige norske Regjerings Departement for det Indre. [List of licensed physicians and veterinary surgeons in Norway.] 8°. *Christiania*, 1856.

ILMONI (I.) Bidrag till Nordens Sjukdomshistoria. 3 v. 8°. *Helsingfors*, 1846–53.

MOHN (H.) * Norges Vind- og Stormstatistik. 8°. [*n. p., n. d.*]
Repr. from: Vidensk.-Selsk. Forhandlinger for 1869.

——. Om Tordenvejr i Norge i 1868. 8°. [*n. p., n. d.*]
Repr. from: Vidensk.-Selsk. Forhandlinger for 1869.

NORBY (K.) De l'assistance publique et des établissements de charité et institutions pieuses en Norvège. Exposé et tableaux pour la statistique internationale de l'assistance publique. roy. 8°. *Rome*, 1880.

SCHÜBELER (F. C.) Viridarium norvegicum. Norges Væxtrige. Et Bidrag til Nord-Europas Natur- og Culturhistorie. 1ste Bind. Udgivet som Universitets-Program for første Semester 1885. 4°. *Christiania*, 1885.

Arbo. Sur l'aptitude militaire des Norvégiens. Ann. de démog. internat., Par., 1880, iv, 538–551. ——. Beiträge zur physischen Anthropologie der Norweger. Verhandl. d. Berl. Gesellsch. f. Anthrop., 1885, 66–70.— **Bertillon** (J.) Étude sur la démographie de la Norvège. Ann. de démog. internat., Par., 1880, iv, 141–167. ——. Suède et Norvége. Dict. encycl. d. sc. méd., Par., 1883, 3. s., xii, 706–803.—**Boeck** (H.) Beretning angaaende de hygieniske Forhold i nordre Fiskedistrict 1858–59. Norsk Mag. f. Lægevidensk., Christiania, 1860, xiv, 34–48. — **Faye** (L.) Hospitaler og milde Stiftelser i Norge i Middelalderen. *Ibid.*, 1882, 3. R., xii, 93; 181.—**Flemming & Holst** jun. Zur Statistik der Irren, Taubstummen, Blinden und Elephantiasis in Norwegen. Allg. Ztschr. f. Psychiat., etc., Berl., 1852, ix, 54–61. — **Holm** (I. C.) Norges nyere Mineralkilder og deres geologiske

Norway.

Udspring. Norsk Mag. f. Lægevidensk., Christiania, 1885, 3. R., xv, 538–549.—**Holst.** On the statistics of the insane, blind, deaf and dumb, and lepers of Norway. Transl. from the Danish by A. S. Oliver Massey. J. Statist. Soc. Lond., 1852, xv, 250–256. — **Kjerulf** (T.) Beiträge zur medicinischen Statistik Norwegens während der Jahre 1866–1870. Monatsbl. f. med. Statist. u. öff. Gsndhtspflg., Berl., 1874, 80 ; 88. — **Larsen** (C. F.) Om Udbredningen af Svindsot i Norge. Norsk Mag. f. Lægevidensk., Christiania, 1870, 2. R., xxiv, 1–16. ———. Statistiske Undersøgelser vedkommende Udbredningen i Norge af Pneumoni, Ledrheumatisme og katarrhalske Sygdomme. [On the distribution of pneumonia, rheumatism, and catarrh in Norway.] *I bid.*, 1881, 3. R., xi, 85–138. ———. Bidrag til Kundskab om den legemlige Udvikling i de forskjellige Dele af Norge. [Contribution to the knowledge of bodily development in the different parts of Norway.] *I bid.*, 1886, xlvii, 313–348.—**Moeller.** Notes médicales sur la Suède et la Norwège. J. de méd., chir. et pharmacol., Brux., 1879, lxix, 28 ; 126.—**Norges** Medicinal-Inddeling. Norsk Mag. f. Lægevidensk., Christiania, 1844, viii, 156–183.—**Sandberg** (O.) Medicinalvæsenet i Norge. Hyg. Medd., Kjøbenh., 1873, viii, pt. 1, 178–192.—**Uddrag** af de 1849 og 1850 til Departementet for det Indre indsendte Medicinalberetninger. Norsk Mag. f. Lægevidensk., Christiania, 1852, 2. R., vi, 693–701.—**Wells** (T. S.) Remarks on holiday making and health resorts of Norway. Brit. M. J., Lond., 1882, ii, 504.

Norway. *Armee.* Forslag til Armeens Omorganisation. (Fremsat af Chefen for Generalstaben i Henhold til det kongelige Armee-Departements Anmodning i Skrivelse til Armeekommandoen af 9de December 1873.) 143, 4, 14, 16, 40, 43, 13 pp., 3 tab., 8 diag. 4°. [*Kristiania*, 1874.]

———. Budgetforslag fra Arme - Departementet til Storthinget i 1873 ; 1875. 4°. [*Kristiania*, 1874-6.]

———. Fortegnelse over trykte Bilage til Budgetforslaget vedkommende de Arme-Departementet underlagte Administrationsgrene for 1873 – 4 ; 1875-6. roy. 8°. [*Kristiania*, 1874-6.]

Bound with : Budgetforslag fra Arme-Departementet.

———. Fortegnelse over Udskrivningsdistrikterne og disses Inddeling i Rulleførerkredse og Lodtrækningsdistrikter. 13 pp., 5 l.

Bound with : Reglement for Udskrivning. fol. *Christiania*, 1877.

———. Reglement for Udskrivning til Landvæbningen og til Distriktssøtropperne i Nordlands og Tromsø Amter. Approberet ved kongelig Resolution af 28de Februar 1877. 27 pp. fol. *Christiania, trykte i det Steenske Bogtrykkeri*, 1877.

Norway. *Armee. Medicinalvæsenet.* Forslag til Instrux for Lægerne ved Bedømmelsen af den militære Tjenstdygtighed. Udarbeidet af Armeens Lægekommission. 88 pp. 8°. *Christiania,* 1874.

———. Regler til Veiledning for Lægerne ved Bedømmelsen af den militære Tjenstdygtighed, med tilhörende Klassifikation og Fortegnelse over de Legemsfeil m. D., son herved komme i Betragtning. (Approberede af Arme-Departementet i Henhold til kongelig Resolution af 16de Juni 1877.) 71 pp. 12°. *Christiania,* 1877.

———. Armeens Lægekommissions motiverede Forslag til Forpleiningsregulativ for Armeen til Benyttelse under de udskrevne Afdelingers aarlige Vaabenøvelser saavelsom ved de stadig tjenstgjørende Afdelinger, for hvilke fælles Bespisninger anordnet, tilligemed Generalchirurgens Bemærkninger til samme. [Kristiania den 25de Februar 1878.] 47 pp. 4°. [*Kristiania,* 1878.]

———. Norges officielle Statistik. E. No. 1. Tjenstdygtighedsforhold ved Armeens Rekrutering i 1878. Fra Generalchirurgen. vii, 27 pp. 4°. *Christiania,* 1879.

Norwegian and French text.

———. Regulations for hospitals, field hospitals and ambulances. A sketch of the royal statutes (relating to the army medical department). A sketch of laws relating to the sanitary depart-

Norway. *Armee. Medicinalvæsenet*—cont'd.
ment and the management of the sick in army. 12, 6, 6 pp. MS. fol. [*n. p., n. d.*]

Norway. *Gaustad Sindssygeasyl ved Christiania.* Generalberetninger fra . . . for Aarene 1856–71. Ved Ole Sandberg, Direktør. 4°. *Christiania,* 1857–72.

1856–71 bound in 1 v.

———. Klinik Femtenaarsberetning fra Gaustad Asyl. (Ved Direktør Sandberg.) [Fra 1ste Oktober 1855 til 1ste Oktober 1870.] 125 pp. 8°. [*Christiania,* 1871.]

Repr. from : Norsk Mag. f. Lægevidensk., Christiania, 1871, 3. s., i.

Norway. *Rigshospital.* Forhandlinger angaænde det nye Rigshospitals-Aulæg (optagne med Hurtigskrift). 210 pp. 8°. *Kristiania, trykt i det Steenske Bogtrykkeri,* 1872.

———. Angaænde nyt Rigshospital. 8 pp., 3 plans. roy. 8°. [*Kristiania,* 1873.]

Norway *itch.*

Rigler. Beitrag zur Geschichte der sogenannten norwegischen Krätze. Ztschr. d. k.-k. Geselisch. d. Aerzte zu Wien, 1853, ii, 29–33.

Norwegian *cooking box.*

Derby (G.) The "Norwegian cooking-box". Boston M. & S. J., 1871, lxxxv, 171–173.

Norwich, *Connecticut.*

ELIZA HUNTINGTON Memorial Home. Charter and by-laws and rules and regulations of the . . . with a list of officers. 8°. *Norwich,* 1873.

Norwich, *England.*

See, also, **Children** (*Hospitals, etc., for, Reports, etc., of*) ; **Insane** (*Asylums, etc., for*), *by localities.*

LEE (W.) Report to the General Board of Health, on a preliminary inquiry into the sewerage, drainage, and supply of water, and the sanitary condition of the inhabitants of the city of Norwich and the county of the same city. 8°. *London,* 1851.

METROPOLITAN water supply. Report on the application of the constant service system in the city of Norwich. By William Pole, to the secretary, railway department, board of trade. fol. [*London,* 1871.]

Richardson (B. W.) Medical history of Norwich. Med. Times & Gaz., Lond., 1864, n. s., i, 19 ; 40 ; 67 ; 97.

Norwich, *New York.*

Gardiner (J. T.) Report on the protection of the water supply of the village of Norwich, Chenango County, New York. Rep. State Bd. Health N. Y. 1886, Albany, 1887, vii, 59–63.

Norwich Asylum and School for the Blind. Hospital and School for the Indigent Blind, at Norwich. Address [of the committee to the public, on the present state of its funds and future prospects.] 2 pp. 16°. [*Norwich,* 1841.]

Established Jan. 17, 1805. Changes in title : In address, issued in 1841, it is called Hospital and School for the Indigent Blind, at Norwich. Report for 1859, Norwich Institution for the Indigent Blind. In 1870, Asylum and School for the Indigent Blind. In 1874, adopted the present title.

———. Annual reports of the committee to the subscribers. 55., 1859 ; 58., 1862 ; 59., 1863 ; 61.-64., 1865–8 ; 66., 1870 ; 70.-72., 1874–6 ; 75.-79., 1879–83. 4° & 8°. *Norwich,* 1860–84.

1870 is 8°.

———. [Notice of the annual meeting held May 4, 1883.] 1 sheet. fol. [*Norwich,* 1883.]

Repr. from : Norfolk Chronicle, May 12, 1883.

———. The same. Of the meeting held in May, 1884. 1 sheet. fol. *Norfolk,* 1884.

Repr. from : Norfolk Chronicle, May 24, 1884.

———. [Circular of the committee, requesting subscribers to purchase articles manufactured by the pupils. And the laws for the admission of pupils and inmates.] 2 l. fol. [*Norwich, n. d.*]

Norwich City Asylum (for the Insane), Hellesdon. Annual reports of the committee of visitors to the council. 1.–2., 1880–81; 4.–5., 1883–4. 8°. *Norwich, Crowe, 1881–5.*

Norwich Dispensary. *See* **Norwich** Dispensary and Provident Institution.

Norwich Dispensary and Provident Institution. Annual report of the committee to the governors and subscribers, for the years 1883–4. 8°. *Norwich, 1884.*

———. Rules of the . . . established in 1804, for providing advice and medicine free of expense to those in indigent circumstances and otherwise unable to procure the same for themselves; and, also, a provident medical institution, enabling the working classes, servants, and shopmen, by means of small monthly payments, to secure for themselves and their families efficient medical advice and medicine during illness. 8°. *Norwich, [n. d.]*

———. Regulations of the . . . 1 sheet. 8°. *[Norwich, n. d.]*

Norwich (The) Homœopathic Journal. [Monthly.] Nos. 1–15, v. 1, June 1, 1852, to Aug., 1853. 234 pp. 8°. *Norwich, H. Pearce.*
United with: **Northampton** (The) Homœopathic Record, forming: **Provincial** (The) Homœopathic Gazette.

Norwich Institution for the Indigent Blind. *See* **Norwich** Asylum and School for the Blind.

Norwood.

See **Hospitals** (*Descriptions, etc., of*), *by localities.*

Norwood (Wesley C.) The therapeutical powers and properties of Veratrum viride. 40 pp. 8°. *New York, Kneeland, 1854.*

———. The same. 2. ed. 24 pp. 8°. *New York, J. D. Bedford & Co., 1856.*

———. The same. 3. ed. 22 pp. 12°. *New York, J. D. Bedford & Co., [1857].*

———. The same. 4. ed. 24 pp. 8°. *Albany, Van Benthuysen, 1858.*

Nory (Charles). * Contribution à l'étude des opérations applicables au bec-de-lièvre. 31 pp., 1 l. 4°. *Paris, 1877,* No. 474.

Nose [*and nasal fossæ*].

See, also, **Canal** (*Nasal*); **Diagnosis** (*Special symptoms in*); **Jacobson's organ**; **Lachrymal organs**; **Nerve** (*Olfactory*); **Nose** (*Mucous membrane of*).

AMERICAN Rhinological Association. Synopsis of proceedings of the third annual meeting of the . . . held at Lexington, Ky., Oct. 6, 7, and 8, 1885. 8°. *[Lexington, Ky., 1885.]*
Repr. from: The Morning Transcript, Oct. 7, 8, and 9, 1885.

ARVISET (L.) * Contributions à l'étude du tissu érectile des fosses nasales. 4°. *Lyon, 1887.*

ASCHENBRANDT (T.) Die Bedeutung der Nase für die Athmung. (Aus dem physiologischen Institute zu Würzburg. 8°. *Würzburg, 1886.*

CLARKE (J. L.) Ueber den Bau des Bulbus olfactorius und der Geruchsschleimhaut; nach dem englischen Manuscripte ins Deutsche übersetzt von A. Kölliker. [*n. p., n. d.*]
Repr. from: Ztschr. f. wissensch. Zool., xi.

CLOQUET (H.) * Dissertation sur les odeurs, sur les sens et les organes de l'olfaction. 4°. *Paris, 1815.*

———. The same. Osphrésiologie, ou traité des odeurs, du sens et des organes de l'olfaction; avec l'histoire détaillée des maladies du nez et des fosses nasales, et des opérations qui leur conviennent. 2. éd. 8°. *Paris, 1821.*

———. Mémoire sur les ganglions nerveux des fosses nasales; sur leurs communications et sur leurs usages. 8°. *Paris, 1818.*

Nose.

GRÆTZ (J. H.) Epistola anatomica problematica octava, de structura nasi cartilaginea, vasis sanguiferis arteriosis membranæ et cavitatis tympani et ossiculorum auditus eorumque periostio. 4°. *Amstelædami,* 1718. [P., v. 1091.]

HAASE (J. G.) [Pr.] de nervis narium internis. 4°. [*Lipsiæ,* 1791.]
Also, in: SCRIPT. neurol. minores selecti. 4°. *Lipsiæ,* 1795, iv, 11–15.

HACK (W.) Riechen und Geruchsorgan. Eine populäre Vorlesung. 8°. *Wiesbaden,* 1885.

KRAUSE (E. H. L.) * Die Regio olfactoria des Schafes. [Berlin.] 8°. *Rostock,* 1881.

LÖWE (L.) Beiträge zur Anatomie der Nase und Mundhöhle. 4°. *Berlin,* 1878.

MARCONDES-RESENDE (I.) * Études sur le mécanisme de la fermeture de l'arrière-cavité des fosses nasales dans la douche de Weber. 4°. *Bordeaux,* 1882.

MERKEL (C. L.) * De nasi secretionibus specimen i. 4°. *Lipsiæ,* 1838.

OLIVIER (P.) * Sur les fosses nasales et des sinus de la face. 4°. *Paris,* 1869.

PANAS (P.) * Recherches sur l'anatomie des fosses nasales. 4°. *Paris,* 1860.

QUELMALZ (S. T.) [Pr.] deque narium earumque septi incurvatione. 4°. *Lipsiæ,* 1750.
Also, in: HALLER. Disp. ad morb. [etc.] 4°. *Lausannæ,* 1757, i.

REIFFSTECK (J. A.) * Diss. sistens disquisitiones anatomicas de structura organi olfactus mammalium nonnullorum. 4°. *Tubingæ,* 1823.

REINBOLD (O.) Die Nase in ihrer physiognomischen Bedeutung. 8°. *Carlsruhe,* 1867.

RUNGE (W.) * Die Nase in ihren Beziehungen zum übrigen Körper. 8°. *Jenæ,* 1885.

SOEMMERRING (S. T.) Abbildungen der menschlichen Organe des Geruches. fol. *Frankf. a. M.,* 1809.

———. The same. Icones organorum humanorum olfactus. fol. *Francof. a. M.,* 1810.

SOLGER (B.) Beiträge zur Kenntniss der Nasenwendung und besonders der Nasenmuscheln der Reptilien. Eine vergleichend-anatomische Abhandlung. [Breslau.] 8°. *Leipzig,* 1875.

SÜLK (J. G.) * De ossibus nasi. 8°. *Rigæ,* 1817.

VERHOEVEN (M. G. T.) * De organo odoratus per animalium vertebratorum classes. 4°. *Lugd. Bat.,* 1826.

ZIERVOGEL (S.) * De naribus internis. sm. 4°. *Upsaliæ,* [1760].
Also, in: SANDIFORT. Thesaurus diss. [etc.] 4°. *Roterodami,* 1768, i, 355.

ZUCKERKANDL (E.) Normale und pathologische Anatomie der Nasenhöhle und ihrer pneumatischen Anhänge. 8°. *Wien,* 1882.

Albrecht (P.) Ist ja, oder nein? bei den Wirbelthieren der Eingang in das Nasengrübchen dem äusseren Nasenloche, der ventrale Nasengrübchenwall dem Interlabium internum; Interlabium externum, der ventrale Oberkieferfortsatzrand dem supralabium homolog? *In his:* Vergl. anat. Untersuch. 8°. Hamb., 1886–7, i, 89–91. ———. Ueber Chorda und Chordome, metamere und continuirliche Verknöcherung in der knorpeligen Nasenscheidewand der Wirbelthiere, nebst einem ersten Versuche, eine wirkliche, unumstössliche Grundlage für die Wirbeltheorie des Schädels zu schaffen. *Ibid.,* 49–88, 1 tab. — **Bérard** (A.) Nez et fosses nasales. Dict. de méd., 2. éd., Par., 1840, xxi, 41–117. — **Bertillon** (A.) De la morphologie du nez. Rev. d'anthrop., Par., 1887, 3. s., ii, 158–169. — **Bigelow** (H. J.) Turbinated corpora cavernosa. Boston M. & S. J., 1875, xcii, 489–492. *Also.* Reprint. — **Born** (G.) Ueber die Nasenhöhlen und den Thränennasengang der Amphibien. Morphol. Jahrb., Leipz., 1876, ii, 577–646, 3 pl. ———. Die Nasenhöhlen und der Thränennasengang der amnioten Wirbelthiere. *Ibid.,* 1879, v, 62, 3 pl.; 401, 2 pl. — **Broca** (P.) Recherches sur l'indice nasal. Rev. d'anthrop., Par., 1872, i, 1–35. ———. Sur l'indice nasal. Bull. Soc. d'anthrop. de Par., 1872. 2. s., vii, 25–40. — **von Brunn** (A.) Weitere Untersuchungen über das Riechepithel und sein Verhalten zum Nervus olfactorius. Arch. f. mikr. Anat., Bonn, 1879,

Nose.

xvii, 141-151, 1 pl. — **Chatin** (J.) Recherches histologiques sur la limitante olfactive des mammifères. Bull. Soc. philomat. de Par., 1879, 7. s., iii, 24-27. ——. Contribution à l'étude ostéologique des fosses nasales chez les Palmipèdes et les Échassiers. *Ibid.*, 1884-5, 7. s., ix, 128-130.— **Clasen** (F. E.) Die Nebenhöhlen der menschlichen Nase in ihrer Bedeutung für den Mechanismus des Riechens. Ztschr. f. Anat. u. Entwcklngsgesch., Leipz., 1876-7, ii, 1-28, 2 pl. — **Csokor** (J.) Vergleichende Histologie des Geruchsorganes. Oesterr. Vrtljschr. f. wissensch. Veterinärk., Wien, 1885, lxiii, 108-114. — **Dally** (L.) Nez; anthropologie, ethnographie. Dict. encycl. d. sc. méd., Par., 1878, 2. s., xiii, 194-199. — **Delavan** (D. B.) On some points in the anatomy of the nasal fossæ. N. York M. J., 1880, xxxii, 375-381. — **Dolbeau.** Nasale (région). Dict. encycl. d. sc. méd., Par., 1876, 2. s., xi, 427-437. — **Du Verney.** The structure of the nose. Phil. Tr., Lond., 1700, lii, 56. — **Fränkel** (B.) Ueber die Untersuchungen des Nasen-Rachenraums mit Demonstrationen. Veröffentl. d. Gesellsch. f. Heilk. in Berl., 1883, viii, Balneol. Sekt., v, 60-71. — **Gegenbaur** (C.) Ueber das Rudiment einer septalen Nasendrüse beim Menschen. Morphol. Jahrb., Leipz., 1885-6, xi, 486-488. — **Hunter** (J.) A description of the nerves which supply the organ of smelling. *In his:* Obs. certain parts animal œconomy, 4°, Lond., 1786, 213-219, 1 pl.—**Kaufmann** (E) Ueber die Bedeutung der Riech- und Epithelialzellen der Regio olfactoria. Med. Jahrb, Wien, 1886, n. F., i, 79-96. *Also:* Mitth. a. d. embryol. Inst. d. k. k. Univ. in Wien, 1887, 2. F., 2. Hft., 33-50.— **Kayser.** Ueber die Bedeutung der Nase für die Athmung. Breslau. aerztl. Ztschr., 1887, ix, 224. — **von Klein** (C. H.) Rhinology in the past and of the future. J. Am. M. Ass., Chicago, 1886, vii, 673-677. *Also,* Reprint. *Also:* St. Louis M. & S. J., 1886, li, 264-268. *Also:* Progress, Louisville, 1886, i, 218-220.— **Kölliker** (A.) Herr Paul Albrecht zum letzten Male. I. Die Chorda in der Nasenscheidewand des Ochsen. Sitzungsb. d. phys.-med. Gesellsch. zu Würzb., 1885, 128. *Also,* Reprint. — **Legal** (E.) Die Nasenhöhlen und der Thränennasengang der amnioten Wirbelthiere. Morphol. Jahrb., Leipz., 1882, viii, 353-372, 1 pl. — **Mackenzie** (J. N.) Historical notes on the discovery of the nasal erectile tissue. Boston M. & S. J., 1885, cxii, 1. *Also,* Reprint.— **Magnus** (A.) Der Nasenrachenraum; Eine Studie an einem Lebenden gemacht. Arch. f. Ohrenh., Würzb., 1873, vi, 246-262. — **Mantegazza** (P.) Della capacità delle fosse nasali e degli indici rinocefalico e cerebrofacciale nel cranio umano. Arch. per l' antrop., Firenze, 1873, iii, 253-274. — **Marshall** (A. M.) The morphology of the vertebrate olfactory organ. Quart. J. Micr. Sc., Lond., 1879, n. s., xix, 300-340, 2 pl. — **Matèjovsky.** Klappenspiel des dreieckigen Nasenknorpels. Prag. med. Wchnschr., 1864, 151-153.— **de Mérejkowsky.** Sur un nouveau caractère anthropologique [la morphologie du nez]. Bull. Soc. d'anthrop. de Par., 1882, 3. s., v, 293-304.— **Møller** (M.) Om den fysiologiske Betydning af Pigmenter i regio olfactoria. Ugesk. f. Læger, Kjøbenh., 1875, 3. R., xix, 353-362. — **Neuner** (R.) Ueber angebliche Chordareste in der Nasenscheidewand des Rindes. Deutsche Ztschr. f. Thiermed., Leipz., 1885-6, xii, 163-179, 1 pl.—**Paullini** (C. F.) Nasati non semper bene vasati. *In his:* Obs. med.-phys., 12°, Lips., 1706, 141-142.— **Paulsen** (E.) Experimentelle Untersuchungen über die Strömung der Luft in der Nasenhöhle. Sitzungsb. d. k. Akad. d. Wissensch. Math.-naturw. Cl., Wien, 1882, lxxxv, 1-22, 1 pl.—**Percy** & **Laurent.** Nez. Dict. d. sc. méd., Par., 1819, xxxvi, 74-98.—**Poinsot** (G.) Nez et nasales (fosses). N. dict. de méd. et chir. prat., Par., 1877, xxiv, 1-104.—**Reclam** (C.) Zur Diätetik der Nase. Gesundheit, Frankf. a. M., 1882, vii, 353-355.—**Rullier.** Nez (anatomie et physiologie). Dict. d. sc. méd., Par., 1819, xxxvi, 1-74.—**Seiler** (C.) On effect of nasal cavity on voice and speech. Tr. Am. Laryngol. Ass., N. Y., 1881, iii, 123-129. *Also:* Arch. Laryngol., N. Y., 1882, iii, 24-29.—**Spillmann** (E.) Nez; anatomie, pathologie. Dict. encycl. d. sc. méd., Par., 1878, 2. s., xiii, 1-194. — **Steinbrügge** (H.) The histology of the inferior turbinated bones, and of the teleangiectatic fibromata arising from them. Arch. Otol., N.Y., 1879, viii, 269-283, 2 pl.—**Strauch** (P.) Untersuchungen über einen Micrococcus im Secret [des Nasenrachenraumes. Monatschr. f. Ohrenh., Berl., 1887, xxi, 149; 181. — **Topinard** (P.) De la morphologie du nez (comme exemple de la méthode à suivre dans les observations anthropologiques à pratiquer sur le vivant]. Bull. Soc. d'anthrop., Par., 1873, 2. s., viii, 947-958. — **Tourtual.** Ein bisher unbekanntes Muskelpaar an den hinteren Nasenöffnungen des Menschen. Arch f. Anat., Physiol. u. wissensch. Med., Berl., 1844, 452-462. ——. Der Pflugschaarknorpel, seine Ernährungsgefässe und seine Rückbildung. Med. Cor.-Bl. rhein. u. westfäl. Aerzte, Bonn, 1845, iv, 145; 169. — **Verga** (A.) Anatomia. Sui meandri nasali. R. Ist. Lomb. di sc. e lett. Rendic., Milano, 1871, 2. s., iv, 465. ——. Sui meandri nasali. Ann. univ. di med., Milano, 1874, ccxxx, 225-263.—**Wertheim** (G.) Ueber ein Verfahren zum Zwecke der Besichtigung des vorderen und mittleren Drittheiles der Nasenhöhle. Ber. d. k. k. Krankenanst. Rudolph-

Nose.

Stiftung in Wien (1868), 1869, 188-202. — **Wiedersheim** (R.) Ueber rudimentäre Fischnasen. Anat. Anz., Jena, 1887, ii, 652-657.—**Ziem.** Ueber inspiratorisches Zusammenklappen der Nasenflügel. Deutsche med. Wchnschr., Berl., 1885, xi, 798.—**Zoja** (G.) Anatomia. Contribuzione all' anatomia del meato medio delle fosse nasali. R. Ist. Lomb. di sc. e lett. Rendic., Milano, 1870, 2. s., iii, 401-404, 1 pl.— **Zuckerkandl** (E.) Zur Anatomie und Entwicklungsgeschichte der Naso-Ethmoidalregion. Med. Jahrb., Wien, 1878, 301-328, 2 pl. *Also:* Mitth. d. Wien. med. Doct.-Coll., 1880, vi, 1-5. ——. Ueber die normale und pathologische Anatomie der Nasenhöhle und ihren Nebenhöhlen. Allg. Wien. med. Ztg., 1879, xxiv, 553. ——. Zur physiologischen und pathologischen Anatomie der Nasenhöhle und ihrer pneumatischen Anhänge. Med. Jahrb., Wien, 1880, 67-102. ——. Zur Anatomie und Pathologie der Nasenhöhle. Wien. med. Bl., 1880, iii, 9-12. ——. Ueber die pneumatischen Räume. Allg. Wien. med. Ztg., 1881, xxvi, 96. ——. Das Schwellgewebe der Nasenschleimhaut und dessen Beziehungen zum Respirationsspalt. Wien. med. Wchnschr., 1884, xxxiv, 1221-1225. ——. Das Schwellgewebe der Nasenschleimhaut und dessen Beziehungen zum Respirationsspalt. Mitth. d. Ver. d. Aerzte in Steiermark 1884, Graz, 1885, xxi, 104-106.

Nose (*Abnormities of*).

See **Nose** (*Deformities, etc., of*).

Nose (*Adenoid tissue and vegetations of*).

COLLET (J.) Étude sur les végétations adénoïdes du pharynx nasal. 8°. *Lyon*, 1886.

FABRE (P.) * Des végétations adénoïdes du pharynx nasal. 4°. *Montpellier*, 1885.

INGEN-HOUSZ (F. A.) * De adenoide vegetatien der neuskeelholte. 8°. *Leiden*, 1881.

PEISSON (E.-C.-J.) * Des végétations adénoïdes du pharynx nasal. 4°. *Paris*, 1883.

Baber (E. C.) Remarks on adenoid vegetations of the naso-pharynx. Brit. M. J., Lond., 1882, ii, 205-207. ——. Du simple traitement des végétations adénoïdes du pharynx nasal. [Transl.] Ann. d. mal. de l'oreille, du larynx, etc., Par., 1885, xi, 97-100.— **Baratoux** (J.) Contribution à l'étude des maladies de la cavité naso-pharyngienne; des tumeurs adénoïdes. Bull. et mém. Soc. franç. d'otol. et laryngol., Par., 1883-4. i, 76-85. — **Bezold.** Zur operativen Behandlung der adenoiden Vegetationen des Nasenrachenraums. Aerztl. Int.-Bl., München, 1881, xxviii, 145-147. — **Blake** (C. J.) Relation of adenoid growth in the naso-pharynx to the production of middle ear disease in children. Boston M. & S. J., 1888, cxviii, 268-270. *Also, transl.:* Ann. d. mal. de l'oreille, du larynx, etc., Par., 1888, xiv, 189-196. — **Butlin** (H. T.) Adenoid vegetations; their importance, diagnosis, and treatment. St. Barth. Hosp. Rep., Lond., 1885, xxi, 152-164. — **Calmettes** (J.) Opération des végétations adénoïdes du pharynx nasal. Gaz. méd. de Par., 1887, 7. s., iv, 267.— **Cardone** (F.) Vegetazioni adenoidi del cavo nasofaringeo; nota clinica ed isto-patologica. Arch. ital. di laringol., Napoli, 1885-6, v, 3-9. — **Catti** (G.) Ueber Behandlung der adenoiden Vegetationen im Nasen-Rachenraume. Monatschr. f. Ohrenh., Berl., 1879, xiii, 9; 17.— **Chatellier** (H.) Note sur un cas d'hypertrophie de la muqueuse nasale. Ann. d. mal. de l'oreille, du larynx, etc., Par., 1886, xii, 344-347.— **Colin.** Quelques considérations sur l'ethmoïde, le vomer et la cloison cartilagineuse du nez. Bull. Soc. anat. de Par., 1819, xxiv, 287-292.— **Doijer.** De adenoïde vegetatiën der neuskeelholte. Nederl. Tijdschr. v. Geneesk., Amst., 1881, 2. R., xvii, 65-73.—**Farlow** (J. W.) The diagnosis of adenoid vegetations. Boston M. & S. J., 1888, cxviii, 387. — **Giles** (W. A.) Post-nasal vegetations. Australas. M. Gaz., Sydney, 1886-7, vi, 226. — **Gottstein** (J.) Zur Operation der adenoiden Vegetationen im Nasenrachenraum. Berl. klin. Wchnschr., 1886, xxiii, 25.— **Hårdh** (A.) Två fall af adenoida nybildningar i cavum naso-pharyngeale behandlade förmedelst skarpa skedar. Finska läk.-sällsk. handl., Helsingfors, 1880, xxii, 111-115 (résumé, *ibid.*, 232).— **Hooper** (F. H.) Adenoid vegetations in the naso-pharyngeal cavity. Boston M. & S. J., 1886, cxiv, 193-197. *Also,* Reprint. ——. Adenoid vegetations in children; their diagnosis and treatment. Boston M. & S. J., 1888, cxviii, 261-268.—**Justi** (G.) Die Operation der adenoiden Neubildungen der Nasenrachenhöhle mittelst des biegsamen scharfen Löffels. Deutsche med. Wchnschr., Berl., 1876, ii, 41. ——. Ueber adenoide Neubildungen im Nasen-Rachenraume. Samml. klin. Vortr., Leipz., 1878, No. 125 (Chir., No. 39), 1045-1062. — **Lange** (V.) Einige kritische Bemerkungen über den Krankheitsbegriff: die adenoiden Vegetationen im Nasenrachenraume, nebst einer neuen Operations-Methode. Monatschr. f. Ohrenh., Berl., 1880, xiv, 17-26. ——. Zur Frage von den adenoiden Vegetationen im Nasenrachenraum. Deutsche med. Wchnschr., Berl., 1883, ix, 748-750. *Also:* Amtl. Ber. ü. d. Versamml. deutsch. Naturf. u. Aerzte 1883,

Nose (*Adenoid tissue and vegetations of*).
Freib. i. Br., 1884, lvi, 289–293: [Discussion], 298–300.—**Lavrand** (H.) Des tumeurs adénoïdes du pharynx nasal J. d. sc. méd. de Lille, 1887, ix, 337–344.—**Lévy** (E.) Des végétations adénoïdes de la cavité pharyngo-nasale. Rev. méd. de l'est, Nancy, 1857, xix, 12–18.—**Lœwenberg** (B.) Des végétations adénoïdes de la voûte pharyngonasale. Tr. Internat. M. Cong., Lond., 1881, iii, 283–290. *Also*: J. de thérap., Par., 1881, viii, 845; 933. ———. Nouveau procédé pour l'extirpation des végétations adénoïdes du pharynx nasal. Progrès méd., Par., 1886, 2. s., iii, 435; 453. ———. Ueber Extirpation der adenoiden Wucherungen im Nasenrachenraum, nebst Beschreibung eines neuen Instruments zu dieser Operation. Deutsche med. Wchnschr., Berl., 1886, xii, 265–267.—**Lublinski** (W.) Adenoide Vegetationen des Nasenrachenraums. Deutsche Med.-Ztg., Berl., 1887, viii, 275–277.—**von Luschka** (H.) Das adenoide Gewebe der Pars nasalis des menschlichen Schlundkopfes. Arch. f. mikr. Anat., Bonn, 1868, iv, 1–9, 1 pl. *Also, transl.*: J. de l'anat. et physiol., etc., Par., 1869, vi, 225–234.—**Mackenzie** (M.) Adenoid vegetations of the naso-pharynx. Ann. d. mal. de l'oreille, du larynx, etc., Par., 1884, x, 147–161.—**Mermod.** Note sur les végétations adénoïdes du pharynx nasal et leur traitement. Rev. méd. de la Suisse Rom., Genève, 1885, v, 265–274.—**Meyer** (W.) Om adenoide Vegetationer i Brнæsvælgrummet, de sygelige Tilfælde, som de frembringe, og disses Helbredelse. Hosp.-Tid., Kjøbenh., 1868, xi, 177; 181. *Also, transl.*: Monatschr. f. Ohrenh., Berl., 1869, iii, 54. ———. On adenoid vegetations in the naso-pharyngeal cavity; their pathology, diagnosis, and treatment. Med.-Chir. Tr., Lond., 1870, liii, 191–215, 1 pl. *Also* [Abstr.]: Proc. Roy. M. & Chir. Soc. Lond. (1867–71), 1871, vi, 229–231. *Also* [Abstr.]: Med. Times & Gaz., Lond., 1869, ii, 694. *Also* [Abstr.]: Lancet, Lond., 1869, ii, 771. *Also* [Abstr.]: Brit. M. J., Lond., 1869, ii, 618. ———. Ueber adenoide Vegetationen in der Nasenrachenhöhle. Arch. f. Ohrenh., Leipz., 1873, n. F., i, 241: 1873–4, n. F., ii, 129; 241, 2 pl.—**Michael** (J.) Doppelmeissel zur Behandlung adenoider Vegetationen des Nasenrachenraumes. Berl. klin. Wchnschr., 1881, xviii, 67–69. ———. Adenoide Vegetationen des Nasenrachenraumes. Wien. Klinik, 1885, xi, 363–375. ———. Doppelmeissel für adenoide Vegetationen des Nasenrachenraums. Cong. période. internat. d. sc. méd. Compt.-rend. 1884, Copenh., 1886, iv, Sect. de laryngol., 153.—**Noquet.** Considérations sur les tumeurs adénoïdes du pharynx nasal. Bull. méd. du nord, Lille, 1886, xxv, 474–483: 1887, xxvi, 98–111.—**Pramberger** (H.) Bemerkungen zur Hyperplasie des adenoiden Gewebes im Nasenrachen- und Rachenraume. Wien. med. Presse, 1885, xxvi, 970; 1003.—**Tédenat.** Des végétations adénoïdes du pharynx nasal. Montpel. méd., 1884, 2. s., ii, 137–154.—**Wehmer** (R.) Ueber adenoide Vegetationen im Nasen-Rachen-Raum. Prakt. Arzt, Wetzlar, 1883, xxiv, 25; 73.—**Wiesener** (I.) De adenoide vegetationer i cavum nasopharyngeale og betändelsesprocesser i dem. Nord. med. Ark., Stockholm, 1881, xiii, no 4, 1–32.—**Zaufal** (E.) Zur Operation adenoider Vegetationen im Nasenrachenraume durch den Nasenrachentrichter hindurch. Prag. med. Wchnschr., 1878, iii, 162–163.—**Zuckerkandl** (E.) Das adenoide Gewebe der Nasenschleimhaut. Med. Jahrb., Wien, 1886, n. F., i, 219–224, 1 pl.

Nose (*Artificial*).
Blumm (V.) Ersatz einer verlorenen Nase durch Celluloid. Aerztl. Int.-Bl., München, 1880, xxvii, 351.—**Forsyth** (A.) [Artificial nose.] Richmond & Louisville M. J., Louisville, 1868, v, 183–185.—**Martin.** Appareil prothétique du nez. Mém. et compt.-rend. Soc. d. sc. méd. de Lyon (1876), 1877, xvi, 106–108. ———. Nez artificiel. *Ibid.* (1877), 1878, xvii, pt. 2., 8–11.—**Roberts** (W. A.) Artificial nose. Month. J. M. Sc., Lond. & Edinb., 1851, xiii, 182.—**Snell** (J.) An improved artificial nose. Med.-Chir. Rev., Lond., 1825, iii, 305.

Nose (*Blue*).
See **Fever** (*Typhus, Diagnosis, etc., of*).

Nose (*Calculus in*).
See **Calculus** (*Nasal*).

Nose (*Cancer and lupus of*).
Claverie (C.-M.-A.) *Étude sur les tumeurs malignes primitives des fosses nasales. 4°. Bordeaux*, 1886.
Moinel (P.-F.) *Essai sur le lupus scrofuleux des fosses nasales. 4°. Paris*, 1877.
Baciocchi (F.) Di un cancroide al naso estirpato e guarita con rinoplastica. Riv. clin. di Bologna, 1873, 2. s., iii, 117.—**Baker.** Melano-sarcoma of the nose. Brit. M. J., Lond., 1878, ii, 921.—**Beck** (M.) Krebsgeschwür der Nase und Oberlippe. Berl. med. Centr.-Ztg., 1839, viii, 161–165.—**Berend** (H. W.) Erfahrungen über Heilung des Lupus, nebst Mittheilung eines Falles von Epitheliom der Nase auf lupösem Grunde. Allg. med. Centr.-Ztg.,

Nose (*Cancer and lupus of*).
Berl., 1867, xxxvi, 301–305. *Also*, Reprint.—**Brunzlow.** Heilung eines veralteten Herpes exedens der Nase durch die Weinhold'sche Mercurial-Kur. J. d. pract. Heilk., Berl., 1837, lxxxv, 2. St., 83–96.—**Buchan** (A. P.), jr. A real case of cancer successfully treated. Lond. M. Rev. & Mag., 1800-1, v, 306.—**Buchanan** (A. H.) Case of cancer. West. J. M. & S., Louisville, 1843, 2. s., viii, 81–88.—**Burnett** (C. H.) & **Allen** (H.) Malignant growth (round-celled sarcoma) in the naso pharynx, with early aural symptoms. Am. J. Otol., N. Y., 1881, iii, 269–272. *Also*: Tr. Am. Otol. Soc., Bost., 1881, ii, pt. 5, 479–483.—**Calvo y Martin.** Observaciones de cáncer de la nariz. Gac. méd., Madrid, 1848, iv, 251.—**Campbell** (M.) Glandular carcinoma of the nasal mucous membrane; excision of the upper jaw; recovery. Brit. M. J., Lond., 1880, i, 325.—**Canseco** (V. D.) Tumor escirroso en la nariz; estirpacion; autoplastia. Bol. de med., cirug. y farm., Madrid, 1852, 2. ép., ii, 198.—**Cavadier.** Description de plusieurs tumeurs carcinomateuses, formées sur le nez et aux environs, dont une pesoit cinq onces et demie, extirpées. Rec. périod. d'obs. de méd., de chir. et pharm., Par., 1757, vii, 202–206.—**Chassaignac.** Cancroïde du nez; destruction par la cautérisation sèche. Monit. d. hôp., Par., 1857, v, 50.—**Chenantais.** Cancroïde du nez (épithélióme tubulé à substance intercellulaire, muqueuse et sarcomateuse). Bull. Soc. anat. de Nantes 1879, Par., 1880, 32–34.—**Collis** (M. H.) Lupoid destruction of nasal cartilages, with occlusion of the remainder of the nostrils, and great deformity; rhinoplasty. Dublin Q. J. M. Sc., 1866, xlii, 324–326, 1 pl. ———. Epithelioma of the nose; third stage, frightful deformity; removal of diseased portion and Indian rhinoplasty. *Ibid.*, 326–328, 1 pl.—**Coulson.** Nasal carcinoma. Lancet, Lond., 1859, ii, 86.—**Cozzolino** (V.) Epitelioma della cute del naso (cancroide acneico atrofico) operato mediante il termocauterio Pacquelin. Gazz. d. osp., Milano, 1883, iv, 755. ———. Il lupus primitivo della mucosa nasale. Arch. ital. di laringol., Napoli, 1886, vi, 33–56.—**Delstanche** (C.) & **Marique.** Cancer épithélial primitif de la fosse nasale gauche. Ann. d. mal. de l'oreille, du larynx. etc., Par., 1884, x, 129–147. *Also*: Presse méd. belge, Brux., 1884, xxxvi, 409–415. ———. Cancer épithélial primitif de la fosse nasale gauche. Presse méd. belge, Brux., 1886, xxxviii, 313; 321.—**Duhring** (L. A.) Epithelioma of the nose. Phila. M. Times, 1874–5, v, 373.—**Eder** (A.) Carcinoma melanodes in cavo naris. *In his*: Aerztl. Ber., etc., 8°. Wien, 1878, 46-49. ———. Epithelioma nasi. [Salzer, operator.] *Ibid.*, 1884, 8°. Wien, 1885, 4–8.—**Fowler** (W.) Malignant nasal polypus treated by Furneaux Jordan's operation. Lancet, Lond., 1885, ii, 992.—**Goelet** (A. H.) Epithelioma of the nose treated with arsenic paste and healed under poultices. North Car. M. J., Wilmington, 1884, xiii, 60–62.—**Hanot** (V.) Épithéliôme tubulé du nez; parotidite suppurée à droite; phlébite de la veine méningée moyenne droite; abcès multiples des reins; abcès froids au niveau des côtes fracturées. Bull. Soc. anat. de Par. (1872), 1874, xlvii, 427–431. *Also*: Rev. phot. d. hôp. de Par., 1872, iv, 355–360.—**Heidenreich.** Heilung eines Krebses an der Nase, mit vollständiger Herstellung der Gestalt und Farbe. J. d. Chir. u. Augenh., Berl., 1833, xx, 456–461.—**Heincke.** Fall eines grossen Carcinoms der Nase bei einer 48jährigen Fran. Greifswalder med. Beitr., Danzig, 1864, ii, 7.—**Heurtaux.** Tumeur de la narine (carcinóme). Bull. Soc. anat. de Nantes 1876-8, Par., 1879, i, 87. ———. Cancroïde du nez (épithélióme tubulé). *Ibid.*, 1880, Par., 1881, iv, 96, 1 pl. ———. Épithéliome tubulé du nez et ganglion. J. de méd. de l'ouest, Nantes, 1886, xx, 373.—**Heyfelder** (O.) Exstirpatio tumoris carcinomatosi ad nasum. Deutsche Klinik, Berl., 1851, iii, 180.—**Hofmokl.** Epitheliom der linken Nasenhälfte, der Wange und des linken unteren Augenlides; Exstirpation mit künstlichem Ersatz des ganzen unteren Augenlides. Ber. d. k. k. Krankenanst. Rudolph-Stiftung in Wien (1884), 1885, 309.—**Kappeler** (O.) Krebs der Nase. *In his*: Chirurg. Beobacht. aus d. Thurgau. Kantonsspit. Münsterlingen, 8°, Frauenfeld, 1874, 72, 2 stereo. pl.—**von Klein.** Ausrottung einer krebshaften Nase sammt der ganzen Oberlippe. Rhein. Jahrb. f. Med. u. Chir., Elberfeld, 1823, vi, 3. St., 85–88, 1 pl.—**Kough** (J. O'B.) Cancrum nasi; recovery. Lancet, Lond., 1883, i, 232.—**Krajewski** (F.) Przypadek rakowca skórnego płuskiego nosa i warg ustnych (epithelioma cutaneum planum nasi et labiorum). Medycyna, Warszawa, 1875, iii, 785–789.—**Lenoir.** Polype cancéreux des fosses nasales. Bull. Soc. de chir. de Par., 1853-4, iv, 170.—**Lerat.** Épithéliome polymorphe du dos du nez. J. de méd. de l'ouest, Nantes, 1885, xix, 278–281.—**Liebl.** Medullar-Carcinom in der Nasengegend. Allg. Wien. med. Ztg., 1861, vi, 188.—**Macfarlane** (J.) Carcinomatous ulcer of the nose; rhinoplasty. Edinb. M. & S. J., 1837, xlvii, 22.—**Malherbe.** Cancroïde de l'aile du nez. Bull. Soc. anat. de Nantes 1879, Par., 1880, 18.—**Monod** (É.) Épithélioma du nez. Bull. Soc. anat. de Par., 1876, li, 353.—**Müller** (J.) Az orr, az alsó szemhéj's a pofa rákja; kürtás; rhinoplastica. [Cancer of nose, involving under eyelid and cheek; rhinoplasty.] Gyogyászát, Budapest, 1881, xx, 289–293.—**Neudörfer**

Nose (Cancer and lupus of).

(J.) Ein Fall von Medullarcarcinom in der Nasenschleimhaut. Oesterr. Ztschr. f. prakt. Heilk., Wien, 1858, iv, 305-310 —**Parisotti** & **Latteux.** Épithéliome calcifié de la racine du nez. Rec. d'ophth., Par., 1883, 3. s., v, 689-694, 1 pl.—**Pattison.** Removal of a carcinomatous tumor from the nostrils. N. York Lancet, 1842, i, 12.—**Péan.** Case of epithelioma of the nose; operation; recovery; death 33 days after operation. Lancet, Lond., 1876, ii, 85.—**Pepper** (W.) & **Shakespeare** (E. O.) Epithelioma of nasal fossa invading sphenoid and ethmoid bones, and membranes of brain. Tr. Path. Soc. Phila., 1880, ix, 138-144.—**Reed** (T. D.) Lupus exedens of the nose. Canada M. J., Montreal, 1871, vii, 154.—**Ricard** (M.-E) Cancer de l'aile du nez; récidive survenue trois fois, et trois fois guérison par les antiphlogistiques, la compression et les fondans. J. hebd. de méd., Par., 1829, iii, 498.—**Rigal** (J.-J.-A.) Ulcères cancriformes dans l'intérieur des narines; opération insolite. Rev. méd. franç. et étrang., Par., 1829, iv, 401-405.—**Romero** (A.) Carcinoma de la narix; estirpacion total; rinoplastia ó recomposicion de este órgano á beneficio de los tegidos de la frente (método indiano). Bol. de med., cirug. y farm., Madrid, 1850, 3. s., v, 162.—**Rul-Ogez.** Ulcère cancéreux du nez, guéri par une application de pâte arsenicale. [Rap. de Van de Vyver.] Ann. Soc. de méd. d'Anvers, 1854, xi, 26-32.—**Sama** (P.) Estirpacion de una úlcera cancerosa de la cara, con ablacion de los huesos propios de la nariz, de sus cartilagos y parte del cornete inferior de las fosas nasales. España méd., Madrid, 1866, xi, 402-404.—**Schmiegelow** (E.) Tumeurs malignes primitives du nez. Rev. mens. de laryngol., etc., Par., 1885, v, 421; 482.—**Seeliger.** Geschichte eines schwammigen Krebsgeschwüres in der linken Nasenhöhle. Beob. u. Abhandl. . . v. österr. Aerzten, Wien, 1824, iv, 469-478. —**Shurley** (W. E.) Cases of lupoid ulceration of the nasal septum. Tr. Am. Laryngol. Ass., N. Y., 1882, iv, 78-85.—**Shurly** (E. L.) Lupoid ulceration of the nasal septum. Arch. Laryngol., N. Y., 1882, iii, 307-313. — **Starke** (G. A.) Lupus exedens of the nose. Canada M. J., Montreal, 1872, viii, 109-111. — **Syme** (J.) Cancer of the nose; amputation. Edinb. M. & S. J., 1833, xl, 326. — **Thibault.** Tumeur encéphaloïde du volume d'une petite noix, située dans la fosse pituitaire entre les os et la dure-mère. Bull. Soc. anat. de Par., 1844, xix, 201. — **Thomas** (C. M.) Epithelioma of the nose. Hahneman. Month., Phila., 1880, n. s., ii, 16.—**Toca** (M. S.) Destruccion completa de la nariz y parte de los huesos propios de este órgano por una úlcera carcinomatosa inveterada; operacion seguida de buen éxito. Crón. de l. hosp., Madrid, 1857, v, 247-249.—**Torrelias y Gallego** (L.) Cancer de la narix, que resistió á la cauterizacion y á la estirpacion del tumor, cediendo por fin á la ablacion de la parte. Arch. de la med. españ., Madrid, 1846, ii, 459-462.—**Vergely.** Cancroïde du nez traité avantageusement par l'acide acétique. Mém. et bull. Soc. de méd. et chir. de Bordeaux (1881), 1882, 376.—**Vernaison.** Mélanose du bout du nez. Soc. d. sc. méd. de Gannat. Compt. rend., 1878, xxxii, 24-27.—**Verneuil.** Epithélioma pituitaire. Gaz. d. hôp., Par., 1885, lviii, 269.—**Weickert.** Exterpation eines Krebsgeschwürs auf dem Nasenrücken. Deutsche Klinik, Berl., 1854, vi, 212.—**Weinlechner.** Epitheliom der Nase, über deren Bereich gegen die linke Wange hin sich ausbreitend; Exstirpation. Ber. d. k. k. Krankenanst. Rudolph-Stiftung in Wien (1878), 1879, 310-312. ——. Ein melanotisches Carcinom, welches von der rechten Nasenhöhle aus gegen die Highmorshöhle, gegen das Sieb- und Keilbein und die Orbita sich verbreitete und den Bulbus verdrängte, wurde durch Exstirpation mit Erha tung des Bulbus möglichst gründlich entfernt; späterhin kam es zur Phthisis bulbi und Recidive; bei einer zweiten Operation musste man, nachdem schon die rechte Stirnhöhle ausgeräumt war, vom weiteren Vorgehen abstehen, da entsprechend der Siebplatte bereits deutliche Gehirnpulsationen zu sehen waren; ungeheilt entlassen. Ibid. (1877), 1878, 315-317. ——. Multiples Medullarsarcom, deren eines vom linken Nasenbeine ausgehendes entfernt wurde; Heilung. Ibid. (1879), 1880, 350.

Nose (Deformities and malformations of).

See, also, **Nose** (Diseases of, Causes of); **Nose** (Surgery of).

ALEXANDER (M.) *Abnorme Stellung des Septum narium und Auftreibungen desselben in Bezug auf die klinische Bedeutung und die operative Beseitigung. 8°. Berlin, 1886.

EICH (A.) * Ueber die Verkrümmungen der Nasenscheidewand und deren Behandlung. 8°. Bonn, 1887.

HUBERT (W.) *Ueber die Verkrümmungen der Nasenscheidewand und deren Behandlung. [Heidelberg.] 8°. München, 1886.

Also, in: München. med. Wchnschr., 1886, xxxiii, 312; 332; 348.

Nose (Deformities and malformations of).

LEWIN (I.) * Ueber die Deviationen der Nasenscheidewand. 8°. Bonn, 1887.

MARCUS (S.) *Die Deformitäten der knöchernen Nase. Ein Beitrag zu ihrer operativen Beseitigung. 8°. Jena, 1884.

SCHAUS (A.) * Ueber Schiefstand der Nasenscheidewand. 8°. Berlin, 1887.

VON VOGEL (G.) *Beobachtungen am Schlunde eines mit vollständigem Defect der Nase behafteten Individuums. 8°. Dorpat, 1881.

WASER (J. J.) * Recessus ossium nasi. sm. 4°. Argentorati, [1767].

Also [Abstr.], in: WEIZ (F. A) Vollständ. Ausz. [etc.] 12°. Budissin, 1769, i, 158-168.

Albers. Nictitatio nasi. Med. Cor.-Bl. rhein. u. westfäl. Aerzte, Bonn, 1845, iv, 185.—**Allen** (H.) Asymmetry of the nasal chambers without septal deviation. Tr. Am. Laryngol. Ass., N. Y., 1883, v, 84. Also: Arch. Laryngol., N. Y., 1883, iv, 256.—**Baumgarten** (E.) Ueber die Ursache der Verbiegungen der Nasenscheidewand. Deutsche med. Wchnschr., Berl., 1886, xii, 373-375.—**Benson** (A. H.) On the treatment of stenosis of the nasal duct by the intermittent nocturnal use of removable styles. Brit. M. J., Lond., 1887, ii, 1151.—**Bianchi** (S.) Sulle varietà dell' osso unguis e sulle ossa accessorie della fossa lacrimale e del canal nasale nell' uomo. Gazz. d. osp., Milano, 1886, vii, 738: 747; 755; 763; 773; 779.—**Bosworth** (F. H.) On nasal stenosis. Tr. Am. Laryngol. Ass. 1880, N. Y., 1881, ii, 79-92. Also: Arch. Laryngol., N. Y., 1881, ii, 110-120. [Discussion], 176-179.—**Bresgen** (M.) Zur Aetiologie der Verbiegung der Nasenscheidewand. Med.-chir. Centralbl., Wien, 1884, xix, 218. Also: Berl. klin. Wchnschr., 1884, xxi, 154.—**Browne** (H. P.) Case of congenital deficiency of the nose, with single hare-lip. Dublin M. Press, 1860, xliv, 452.—**Bryant.** Adhesion between the septum nasi and the lower turbinated bone. Lancet, Lond., 1861, ii, 207.—**Bucklin** (C. A.) Nasal stenosis; its effects on the eye, ear, pharynx, larynx, and brain. N. York M. Times, 1887-8, xv, 39-43.—**Chassaignac.** Déviations de la sous-cloison nasale. Bull. Soc. de chir. de Par., 1851-2, ii, 515.—**Chiari** (O.) Ueber Verstopfung der Nase und ihre Therapie. Ztschr. f. Diagn u. Therap., Wien, 1882, i. 7; 21. ——. Membranöser Verschluss beider Choanen. Wien. med. Wchnschr., 1885, xxxv, 1473.—**Cloquet.** Occlusion presque complète des narines à la suite de la petite-vérole; guérison. Gaz. d. hôp., Par., 1840, 2. s., ii, 110.—**Coën** (R.) Ein seltener Fall von Näseln. Arch. f. Kinderh., Stuttg., 1888, ix, 219-222.—**Delavan** (D. B.) Lateral deviation of the septum narium. N. York M. J., 1880, xxxii, 527. ——. On the ætiology of deflections of the nasal septum. Tr. Am. Laryngol. Ass. 1887, N. Y., 1888, ix, 202-213. Also: N. York M. J., 1887, xlvi, 539-542. Also, Reprint.—**Delens** (E.) Observation d'oblitération cicatricielle de l'orifice supérieur de la narine droite. Ann. d. mal. de l'oreille et du larynx, Par., 1877, iii, 348.—**Delstanche** (C.) & **Stocquart** (A.) Oblitération osseuse de l'orifice antérieur de la fosse nasale droite. J. de méd., chir. et pharmacol., Brux., 1881, lxxiii, 511-513. — **Depaul.** Rapport sur un mémoire de M. Bitot: "Obturation des orifices postérieurs des fosses nasales". Bull. Acad. de méd., Par., 1876, 2. s., v, 881-886. — **Egeberg.** Occlusio choanarum. Norsk Mag. f. Lægevidensk., Christiania, 1877, 3. R., vii, 618. — **Ficano** (G.) Deformità o corno del setto nasale operato col metodo di Bosworth. Gazz. d. osp., Milano, 1887, viii, 645.—**Fränkel** (B.) Stenose und Atresie der Nasenhöhle. Handb. d. spec. Path. (Ziemssen), Leipz., 1876, iv, 93-104. Also, transl.: Cycl. Pract. M. (Ziemssen), N. Y., 1876, iv, 103-115. — **Freudenthal** (W.) Ueber den Zusammenhang von chronischen Verstopfungen der Nase u. des Nasenrachenraumes mit Unterleibsbrüchen. Monatschr. f. Ohrenh., Berl., 1887, xxi, 310; 339: 1888, xxii, 6; 41. Also, Reprint.—**Gegenbaur** (C.) Ein Fall von mangelhafter Ausbildung der Nasenmuscheln. Morphol. Jahrb., Leipz., 1879, v, 191. — **Gleitsmann** (J. W.) Deviation of the nasal septum. Am. J. M. Sc., Phila. 1885. n. s., xc, 152-162. Also, Reprint.—**Golding-Bird** (C. H.) On chronic nasal obstruction. Guy's Hosp. Rep., Lond., 1881, 3. s., xxv, 421-446.—**Gross** (F. H.) Monstrosity. Case of malformation of the nose. Tr. Path. Soc. Phila. (1874-5), 1876, v, 243-250.—**Gruber** (W.) Choanæ von ungleicher Grösse. Arch. f. path. Anat., etc., Berl., 1877, lxx, 136.—**Hinkel** (F. W.) Irregularities of the septum narium, without deflection, as an ætiological factor in nasal catarrh. N. York M. J., 1887, xlvi, 378-380.—**van der Hoeven** (J.), Jz. Over afwijkingen in den vorm der neusbeenderen. Nederl. Tijdschr. v. Geneesk., Amst., 1860, iv, 113. Also, Reprint.—**Hoppe** (J.) Eine angeborne Spaltung der Nase. Med. Ztg., Berl., 1859, n. F., ii, 164.—**Howard.** Depression of the dorsum nasi. Proc. M. Convent. Ohio, Columbus, 1847, 31-34.—**Hubbell** (A. A.) Congenital occlusion

Nose (*Discharge from*).
See **Nose** (*Water, etc., from*).

Nose (*Diseases of*).
See, also, **Acne**; **Catarrh** (*Nasal, etc.*); **Coryza**; **Diphtheria**; **Douche** (*Nasal*); **Gonorrhœa** (*Cases of, etc.*); **Laryngology**; **Nerve** (*Olfactory*); **Ozæna**; **Rhinoscleroma**; **Speech** (*Disordered, etc.*); **Throat** (*Diseases of*).

Nose (*Diseases of*).

rière-cavité des fosses nasales et de son traitement par la douche naso-pharyngienne. 4°. *Paris*, 1878.

ENGELMANN (C. F.) Manuductionis ad veram theoriam morborum praxinque clinicam, specimen xiii. de polypo narium et ozæna. 4°. *Altdorfii Noricorum*, [1752].

FARGES (P.-G.) Granulations et catarrhes des tissus nasogutturaux, les maladies chroniques de la gorge et de la voix; hygiène et traitement. 8°. *Paris & Pau*, 1884.

FONTANILLE (E.-R.) * De la rhinite hypertrophique. 4°. *Bordeaux*, 1885.

FORBES (L.) Diseases of the nose; forming the second part of the fifth edition of "Deafness and its curative treatment". 5. ed. 8°. *London*, 1887.

GELLÉ (M.-E.) Précis des maladies de l'ore'lle, comprenant l'anatomie, la physiologie, la pathologie, la thérapeutique, la prothèse, l'hygiène, la médecine légale, la surdité et la surdimutité et les maladies du pharynx et des fosses nasales. 8°. *Paris*, 1885.

GOURJON (X.-J.) * Contribution à l'étude de la rhinite chronique simple et des rhinites diathésiques. 4°. *Paris*, 1881.

HAASE (J. G.) [Pr.] de narium morbis alteram commentationem scripsit. 4°. *Lipsiæ*, 1797.

INGALS (E. F.) Lectures on the diagnosis and treatment of diseases of the chest, throat, and nasal cavities. 8°. *New York*, 1881.

JONES (H. M.) Practitioner's hand-book of diseases of the ear and naso-pharynx (3. ed. of the "Aural surgery".) 8°. *London*, 1887.

KITCHEN (J. M. W.) Catarrh, sore-throat, and hoarseness. A description of the construction, action, and uses of the nasal passages and throat; certain diseases to which they are subject, and the best methods for their prevention and cure. sm. 4°. *New York*, 1884.

KUNIKE (L. A. F.) * De morbis nasi. 8°. *Gryphiæ*, [1836].

LICHTSCHLAG (J.) * De morbis nasi. 8°. *Berolini*, [1864].

MACKENZIE (M.) Diseases of the throat and nose, including the pharynx, larynx, treachea, œsophagus, nasal cavities, and neck. 2 v. 8°. *Philadelphia*, 1880–84.

v. 2. Diseases of the œsophagus, nose, and naso-pharynx.

——. The same. 2 v. 8°. *New York*, 1880–84.

——. The same. v. 2. 8°. *London*, 1884.

——. The same. Traité pratique des maladies du nez et de la cavité naso-pharyngienne. Traduit de l'anglais et annoté par E.-J. Moure [et] J. Charazac. 8°. *Paris*, 1887.

A translation of v. 2 of preceding.

MASSEI (F.) Clinica delle malattie del tratto respiratorio. Raccolta di memorie di laringologia, rinoscopia ed aeroterapia ad uso dei medici pratici. 8°. *Napoli*, 1881.

MICHEL (C.) Die Krankheiten der Nasenhöhle und des Nasenrachenraumes. Nach eigenen Beobachtungen. 8°. *Berlin*, 1876.

——. The same. Traité des maladies des fosses nasales et de la cavité naso-pharyngienne. 8°. *Bruxelles*, 1879.

MOLDENHAUER (W.) Die Krankheiten der Nasenhöhlen, ihrer Nebenhöhlen und des Nasen-Rachenraumes mit Einschluss der Untersuchungstechnik. 8°. *Leipzig*, 1886.

MOORE (G.) On some diseases of the nose, throat, air-tubes, and lungs; and their local treatment. 8°. *London*, 1867.

NIKITIN (V. N.) Boliezni nosovoi polosti. [Diseases of the cavity of the nose.] 8°. *St. Petersburg*, 1882.

Nose (*Diseases of*).

PIANA (A.) Delle malattie del naso e delle fosse nasali. 8°. *Fossombrone*, 1881.

PIEDNOËL (J.-I.) * Des ulcères des fosses nasales. 4°. *Paris*, 1857.

ROBINSON (B.) On certain morbid alterations of mucous membrane; their influence on speech, and their apparent relations with diseased nerve-structure. 8°. *New York*, 1875.

SAJOUS (C. E.) Lectures on the diseases of the nose and throat. 8°. *Philadelphia*, 1885.

SCHECH (P.) Die Erkrankungen der Nebenhöhlen der Nase und ihre Behandlung. 4°. *München*, 1883.

SEILER (C.) Handbook of the diagnosis and treatment of diseases of the throat, nose, and nasopharynx. 2. ed. 8°. *Philadelphia*, 1883.

SLONINSKI (A.) * De morbis organorum olfactus. 8°. *Cracoviæ*, 1829.

VÉRITÉ (A.) Concrétions muqueuses de la partie postérieure des fosses nasales. 8°. *Paris*, 1881.

VILLEDARY (J.-G.) * Contribution à l'étude des varices nasales et leur traitement. 4°. *Bordeaux*, 1887.

WAGNER (C.) Diseases of the nose. 8°. *New York*, 1884.

WALB (H.) Erfahrungen auf dem Gebiete der Nasen- und Rachenkrankheiten. 8°. *Bonn*, 1888.

WATSON (W. S.) Diseases of the nose and its accessory cavities. 8°. *London*, 1875.

Allen (H.) Abscess, ulceration, and necrosis, as met with in the nasal chambers. Med. & Surg. Reporter, Phila., 1883, xlviii, 573–576. ——. On a new variety of chronic nasal catarrh. Med. News, Phila., 1885, xlvi, 143. — **Angel Osuna** (P.) Hipertrofia parcial de la pituitaria. Andalucía méd., Córdoba, 1878, iii, 153–156.— **Baratoux** (J.) Contribucion al estudio de las enfermedades de la cavidad nasofaringea; de los tumores adenoides. An. de otol. y laringol., Alcalá de Henares, 1883, i, 257–264. ——. Nécrose des os du nez; expulsion de la partie centrale du sphénoïde. Progrès méd., Par., 1883, xi, 826. — **Barth** (A.) Behinderte Nasenathmung und eitrige Mittelohrentzündung. Verhandl. d. Berl. med. Gesellsch. (1887), 1888, xviii, pt. 2, 272–279.— **Baumgarten** (E.) Eczema introitus narium. Monatschr. f. Ohrenh., Berl., 1885, xix, 146. ——. Az orrsövény betegségei. [Diseases of the septum of the nose.] Orvosi hetil., Budapest, 1886, xxx, 35; 63.—**Berger** (E.) Sehstörung in Folge einer durch Trauma entstandenen Periostitis der Nasenhöhle. Arch. f. Augenh., Wiesb., 1886–7, xvii, 293. — **Bertet.** Observation de rhino-nécrosie ou nécrose des cartilages de la cloison du nez. Union méd., Par., 1860, 2. s., vi, 122. — **Billroth** (T.) Hypertrophia cutis nasi. *In his:* Chir. Klin., Wien, 1871–6, 8°, Berl., 1879, 93, 1 fig.—**Bloom** (J.) Periodical hyperæsthetic rhinitis. Med. & Surg. Reporter, Phila., 1886, lv, 68–70. — **Bossowski** (K.) Choroby narządu oddechowego. [Three cases of disease of nose and trachea.] Przegl. lek., Krakow, 1880, xix, 557–560.— **Bosworth** (F. H.) A contribution to the pathology of the nasal mucous membrane. Tr. Internat. M. Cong., 7. sess., Lond., 1881, iii, 327–330.— **Boucher** (G.) Rendiconto della sezione per le malattie di naso e gola nello Spedale civico di Torre Annunziata. Arch. ital. di laringol., Napoli, 1884–5, iv, 145–150.—**Boudet.** Abcès des fosses nasales, symptomatique d'une nécrose du bord alvéolaire du maxillaire supérieur, etc. Bull. Soc. de méd. et pharm. de la Haute-Vienne, Limoges, 1868, 66–70.— **Brady** (A. J.) Rhinitis chronica atrophicans fœtida. Australas. M. Gaz., Sydney, 1886–7, vi, 100.— **Bresgen** (M.) Patologia del cosidetto catarro cronico-nasale e faringeo. Arch. internaz. di otojat., rinojat. ed aeroterap., Napoli, 1885, i, 68–74. *Also, transl.:* Med.-chir. Centralbl., Wien, 1885, xx, 277; 301. ——. Tuberculose oder Lupus der Nasenschleimhaut? Deutsche med. Wchnschr., Leipz., 1887, xiii, 663. *Also,* Reprint. ——. Croup der Nasenschleimhaut. Deutsche med. Wchnschr., Leipz., 1888, xiv, 66.— **von Breuning** (G.) Nasenscrofel. Med.-chir. Centralbl., Wien, 1883, xviii, 369. — **Brodie** (B. C.) Diseases which are sometimes mistaken for polypi of the nose. Lancet, Lond., 1843, i, 345. — **Brooke.** Affection of the nose. Lancet, Lond., 1841, i, 304.—**Bryant** (T.) On some diseases of the nose which have been mistaken for polypus. *Ibid.*, 1867, ii, 224. — **Carreño** (J.) Observacion de una cáries que despues de haber destruido el hueso vómer se fijó en las conchas de la nariz, é ungüis, y descubrió la cara inferior del hueso etmóides, curada en virtud de una revulsion, efecto de una inflamacion erisipelatosa que se presentó en la enferma sin causa manifiesta (aunque habia sospechas de que estuviese sostenida por

Nose (*Diseases of*).

vicio sifilitico). Décadas de med. y cirug. práct., Madrid, 1828, xix, 13.—**Cartaz** (A.) Un cas de rhinite profession-nelle (arsenicale). France méd., Par., 1887. i, 670–674.—**Cazenave** (J.-J.) Observations de maladies du nez et des fosses nasales. Gaz. méd. de Par., 1839, vii, 442–445.—**Chatellier** (H.) Canalicules perforants de la membrane basale de la muqueuse nasale hypertrophiée. Ann. d. mal. de l'oreille, du larynx, etc., Par., 1887, xiii, 233–239. ——. Hypertrophie de la muqueuse nasale; lésions histologi-ques. Compt. rend. Soc. de biol., Par., 1888, 8. s., v, 65.—**Chevalier** (E.) Ostéite, suivie de nécrose des os du nez; intégrité du canal nasal; guérison. Ann. Soc. d'anat. path. de Brux., 1868, xv, 28–21.—**Cicconardi** (G.) Su di un ascesso traumatico e di un ematoma del setto del naso. Arch. ital. di laringol., Napoli, 1884 - 5, iv, 1–11.—**Clark** (R. D.) A case of supposed nasal calculus. Med. Ann., Albany, 1883, iv, 34.—**Cohen** (J. S.) On naso-pharyngeal catarrh. Med. News & Libr., Phila., 1879, xxxvii, 145–150. ——. Diseases of the nose. Cycl. Pract. M. (Ziemssen), N. Y., 1881 (Suppl., 259–263).—**Cooke.** Extensive ulceration of the alæ and septum nasi. Lancet, Lond., 1885, ii, 433.—**Cott** (G. F.) Anterior hypertrophic rhinitis. Med. Press West. N. York, Buffalo, 1888, iii, 97–100.—**Cozzolino** (V.) Ispessimento del setto carti-lagineo del naso (forma speciale di pericondrite costitu-zionale per sifilide o per scrofolosi). Movimento, Napoli, 1880, 2. s., ii, 611–614. ——. Resoconto statistico degli ammalati di orecchio, naso e gola osservati e curati nei mesi scolastici degli anni 1883–7 nell' ambulatorio speciale dell' Ospedale clinico di Napoli. Bull. d. sc. med. di Bo-logna, 1887, 6. s., xx, 78–110.—**Curtis** (H. H.) A paper concerning a few points in practical laryngological and rhinological work. Med. Rec., N. Y., 1887, xxxi, 493.—**Delavan** (D. B.) The question of hypertrophy of the osseous structure of the turbinated bodies, practically considered. Tr. Am. Laryngol. Ass., N. Y., 1882, iv, 36–47. *Also:* Arch. Laryngol., N. Y., 1882, iii, 211–220. *Also,* Reprint. *Also* [Abstr.]: Med. & Surg. Reporter, Phila , 1882, xlvii, 21–24. ——. Case of acute idiopathic peri-chondritis and abscess of the nasal septum. Arch. Laryngol., N. Y., 1883, iv, 133. *Also,* Reprint.—**Del Monte** (M.) Restringimenti del canale nasale, carie e necrosi delle pareti ossee dello stesso. Sperimentale, Firenze, 1872, xxix, 465–474.—**Delwart.** Mémoire sur les maladies des cavités nasales que l'on confond souvent avec la morve, considérées principalement au point de vue pratique. Bull. Acad. roy. de méd. de Belg., Brux., 1857–8, 2. s., i, 640 - 680. [Discussion], 1858–9, 2. s., ii, 905–943 ; 967, 2. Suppl., 6 ; 212.—**Denman** (T.) Some ac-count of a disease lately observed in infants. [Snuffles.] Lond. M. J., 1790, xi, 374 - 380. ——. On the snuffles in infants. *In his:* Observ. [etc.], 8°, Lond., 1810, 23–36.—**Durham** (A. E.) Diseases of nose. Syst. Surg. (Holmes), 2. ed., 1870, iv, 234 - 322. — **Engel.** Zur Pa-thologie der Nasen- und Highmorshöhle. Wien. med. Bl., 1885, viii, 1051–1054.—**Fasano** (A.) Su di un caso di rinite cronica. Arch. ital. di laringol., Napoli, 1881–2, i, 101–108. ——. Recenti studii ed osservazioni sulle riniti. Gior. internaz. d. sc. med., Napoli, 1884, n. s., vi, 108 ; 219.—**Fleming** (C.) Observations on certain affec-tions of the septum of the nose. Dublin J. M. & Chem. Sc., 1833–4, iv, 16–28. — **Forestus Alcmarianus** (R.) De nasi affectibus. *In his:* Obs. et curat. med., xxv, libri xiii, 8°, Lugd. Bat., 1691. 297–364.—**Forwood** (W. S.) A new disease of the nasal chambers not noticed by Prof. H. Allen. Med. & Surg. Reporter, Phila., 1883, xlviii, 705.—**Fraenkel** (B.) Allgemeine Diagnostik und Therapie der Krankheiten der Nase, des Nasenrachenraums, des Rachens und des Kehlkopfs. Handb. d. spec. Path. (Ziemssen), Leipz., 1876, iv, 1. Th., 1–181. *Also, transl.:* Cycl. Pract. M. (Ziemssen), N. Y., 1876, iv, 1 - 181:—**Fraenkel** (E.) Beiträge zur Rhinopathologie. Arch. f. path. Anat., etc., Berl., 1882, lxxxvii, 285–301. ——. Ein Beitrag zur Lehre von den Hyperplasien der Nasen-muschelbekleidung. Deutsche med. Wchnschr., Berl., 1884, x, 274–276. ——. Zur Diagnostik und Therapie ge-wisser Erkrankungen der mittleren und unteren Nasen-muscheln. Samml. klin. Vortr., Leipz., 1884, No. 242 (Inn. Med., No. 85), 2219–2242.—**Frank** (E.) Ueber den gegenwärtigen Standtpunkt in den Untersuchungsme-thoden und der Therapie der Krankheiten des Nasen-rachenraumes. Allg. Wien. med. Ztg., 1877, xxii, 408.—**Friedreich** (N.) Die Krankheiten der Nasenhöhlen. *In:* Handb. d. spec. Path. u. Therap. (Virchow), 8°, Er-lang.. 1854, v, 1. Abth., 385–413.—**Gairdner** (J.) On a peculiar disease of the nasal fossa. Month. J. M. Sc., Lond. & Edinb., 1850, x, 381–386. — **Garrigou-Desa-rênes** & **Mercié** (J.) Du catarrhe chronique des fosses nasales et de l'ozène ; traitement par la galvano-caustique chimique. Gaz. méd.-chir. de Toulouse, 1884, xvi, 209 ; 220.—**Gibb.** Disease of the turbinated bones and floor of the right nostril, with exudation of fibrine; and dis-ease of the throat. Tr. Path. Soc. Lond., 1862–3, xiv, 47–49. ——. Loss of the right turbinated bones, vomer, and both nasal bones, exposing the cavity of the nose. Lancet, Lond., 1864, ii, 152. ——. Necrosis of turbinated bones and part of the vomer treated by aid of the rhinoscope.

Nose (*Diseases of*).

Tr. Path. Soc. Lond., 1864–5, xvi, 212. — **Gichrl.** Dege-neration der Nase. J. d. Chir. u. Augenh., Berl., 1843, xxxii, 380–383, 1 pl.—**Glasgow** (W. C.) On certain vaso-motor disturbances of the nasal membrane. N. York M. J., 1885, xlii, 147–150.—**Glasmacher.** Knochenblasen-bildung in der Nase. Berl. klin. Wchnschr., 1884, xxi, 571–573.—**Góngora** (L.) Contribución al estudio de las affecciones sostenidas por estados hiperémicos del tejido cavernoso de los cornetes nasales inferiores. Rev. de laringol., otol. y rinol., Barcel., 1886–7, ii, 110–117.—**Gott-stein** (J.) Ueber die verschiedenen Formen der Rhinitis und deren Behandlung vermittels der Tamponade. Berl. klin. Wchnschr., 1881, xviii, 49–52. ——. Rhinopatholo-gische Streitfragen. Deutsche med. Wchnschr., Berl , 1882, viii, 313.—**Grabower.** Die königliche Universi-täts-Poliklinik für Hals- und Nasenkranke. *Ibid.*, 1887, xiii, 982. *Also,* Reprint.—**Gregory** (E. H.) Chronic in-flammatory trouble at nasal orifice. St. Louis Cour. Med., 1882, vii, 315.—**Hack** (W.) Ueber die Entstehung von exsudativen, sogen. rheumatischen Processen von der Nasenschleimhaut aus. Fortschr. d. Med., Berl., 1883, i, 645–651. ——. Ueber rhinologische Streitsätze. Amtl. Ber. ü. d. Versamml. deutsch. Naturf. u. Aerzte 1883, Freib. i. Br., 1884, lvi, 285–289.—**Hardaway** (W. A.) Inflammation of the hair follicles within the nares. J. Cutan. & Ven. Dis., N. Y., 1886, iv, 360–362. — **Hart-mann** (A.) Statistischer Bericht über die im Jahre 1883 in meiner Poliklinik für Gehörleiden und Nasenkrankhei-ten behandelten Krankheitsfälle. Ztschr. f. Ohrenh., Wiesb., 1883–4, xiii, 183–202. *Also, transl.:* Arch. Otol., N. Y., 1884, xiii, 121–123. ——. Ueber fötide Blennorrhöe der Nase mit Affection der Nebenhöhlen und deren Behand-lung. Amtl. Ber. ü. d. Versamml. deutsch. Naturf. u. Aerzte 1883, Freib. i. Br., 1884, lvi, 275. ——. Ueber Croup der Nasenschleimhaut; Rhinitis fibrinosa. Deut-sche med. Wchnschr., Leipz., 1887, xiii, 641.—**Hawkins** (C. H.) Clinical observations on some diseases of the nose. Lond. M. Gaz., 1834, xiv, 760–766. *Also, in his:* . . . Path. & Surg. Writings, 8°, Lond., 1874, i, 220–231.—**Hedenus.** Ueber die einfache rothe Nase und die Gutta rosea, Acne rosea. Deutsche Klinik, Berl., 1861, xiii, 113–116.—**Hemming** (W. D.) Diseases of the naso-pharynx. St. Louis M. & S. J., 1881, xli, 119–128.—**Her-ing** (T.) Z kazuistyki szpitalnej oddziału dla chorób gardła, krtani i jam nosowych w szpitału Ś-go Rocha. [Cases of diseases of pharynx, larynx and nasal cavity in St. Roche Hospital.] Gaz. lek., Warszawa, 1882, 2. s., ii, 1021 ; 1047 ; 1061.—**Herzog** (J.) Der nervöse Schnupfen (Rhinitis vasomotoria). Mitth. d. Ver. d. Aerzte in Steier-mark 1881, Graz, 1882, xviii, 16–35. ——. Ueber Nasen-eiterungen. Mitth. d. Ver. d. Aerzte in Steiermark 1886, Graz, 1887, xxiii, 3–35. ——. Das Eczem am Nasenein-gange. Arch. f. Kinderh., Stuttg., 1888, ix, 211–219.—**Hildebrand.** Beobachtungen über einige Affectionen der Nasenhöhle. J. d. Chir. u. Augenh., Berl., 1833, xx, 622–637.—**Hutchinson** (J.) Clinical lecture on perfora-ting ulcers of the septum nasi. Med. Times & Gaz., Lond., 1884, ii, 6 ; 42.—**Jessop.** Simple perforating ulcer of septum nasi. Brit. M. J., Lond., 1888, i, 539.—**Jurasz** (A) Seröse Perichondritis der Nasenscheidewand. Deut-sche med. Wchnschr., Berl., 1884, x, 810.—**Katz** (L.) Einige Mittheilungen aus dem Gebiete der Nasen- resp. Nasenrachen - Affectionen. Berl. klin. Wchnschr., 1885, xxii, 386.—**Kessel.** Ueber die Bedeutung der Erkran-kung des Nasenrachenraumes. Wien. med. Presse, 1878, xix, 1610–1613.—**Kiesselbach** (W.) E zema introitus narium. Monatschr. f. Ohrenh., Berl., 1885, xix, 36–38.—**Kohts.** Die Krankheiten der Nase. Handb. d. Kin-derkr. (Gerhardt), Tübing., 1878, iii, 2. St., 1–43.—**Lefferts** (G.) Affections médicales et chirurgicales du nez, des fosses nasales et des sinus accessoires. Encycl. internat. de chir. (Ashhurst), Par., 1886, v, 395–484.—**Lefferts** (G. M.) Diseases and injuries of the nose and its accessory sinuses. Internat. Encycl. Surg. (Ashhurst), N. Y., 1885, v, 359–456.—**Lublinski** (W.) Das sogenannte Ekzem des Naseneinganges. Deutsche Med.-Ztg., Berl., 1885, ii, 649. *Also,* Reprint.—**McBride** (P.) Erection of the in-ferior turbinated bodies. Tr. Med. - Chir. Soc. Edinb., 1885–6, n. s., v, 77–79.—**Mackenzie** (G. H.) Disease of the nostrils. Brit. M. J., Lond., 1880, i, 38.—**Mackenzie** (J. N.) Some remarks on naso-aural catarrh and its rational treatment. Maryland M. J., Balt., 1883–4, x, 70–73. ——. Some notes on the pathology of intra-nasal in-flammation. Med. News, Phila., 1884, xlv, 370–372. *Also,* Reprint. ——. Notes on the classification, diagnosis and treatment of the stages of chronic nasal inflammation. Med. News, Phila., 1885, xlvi, 372–374. *Also,* Reprint. ——. Nose, neuroses of the. Ref. Handbook M. Sc., 8°, N. Y., 1887, v, 222–242. ——. Nose ; affections of the nasal pharynx, anæmia. *Ibid.*, 206–209.—**Mackenzie** (M.) Lectures on diseases of the nose. Lancet, Lond., 1877, ii, 117 ; 269 ; 678.—**McSherry** (H. C.) A consideration of the classification of functional neuroses of the throat and nose. Am. J. M. Sc., Phila., 1885, n. s., xc, 411–421.—**Maisonneuve.** Abcès de la cloison des fosses nasales. Gaz. d. hôp., Par., 1841, 2. s., iii, 59. ——. Abcès de la cloison des fosses nasales. *Ibid.*, 1853, xxvi, 124.—**Mas-**

Nose (*Diseases of*).

sci (F.) Rinite scrofolosa? Arch. ital. di laringol., Napoli, 1881-2, i, 49-51.—**Moldenhauer** (W.) Das sogenannte Eczem des Naseneinganges. Monatschr. f. Ohrenh., Berl., 1885, xix, 145. ———. Ueber croupöse Entzündung der Nasenschleimhaut. *Ibid.*, 1887, xxi. 252-254.—**Moore** (W. J.) A series of cases of disease of the nostrils. Indian M. Gaz., Calcutta, 1871, vi, 150.—**de Morgan** (C.) Necrosis of the nasal bone. Brit. M. J., Lond., 1871, i, 216.—**Nichols** (A. W.) Nasal catarrh; otherwise designated as nasal pharyngeal catarrh, post nasal catarrh, naso-pharyngeal catarrh, glandular hypertrophy of the vault of the pharynx, hypertrophic nasal catarrh, ozæna rhinitis, etc. Tr. Mich. M. Soc., Lansing, 1884, viii, 557-562.—**Noquet.** Quelques considérations sur la rhinite atrophique. Rev. mens. de laryngol., etc., Par., 1887, vii, 225-234.—**Osuna** (P. A.) Hipertrofia parcial de la pituitaria. Andalucía méd., Córdoba, 1878, iii, 153-156. *Also* [Abstr.]: Siglo méd., Madrid, 1878, xxv, 764.—**Paul** (C.) Scrofulide ulcéreuse maligne des fosses nasales et de l'arrière-gorge. Gaz. d. hôp., Par., 1871, xliv, 565.—**Penny** (W. J.) On rhinitis. Bristol M.-Chir. J., 1887, v, 95-102.—**Perifollicolite** fungosa del naso e del labbro superiore; raschiamento e cauterizzazione colla potassa caustica; guarigione. Clin. chir. (Mazzoni), Roma, 1884, viii-x, 162.—**Pooley** (J. H.) "Abscess of the septum narium." Med. Rec., N. Y., 1871. vi. 476.—**Pruritic** rhinitis. [Discussion.] St. Louis M. & S. J., 1884, xlvii, 48; 55.—**Rasori** (E.) Ulcero duro dell' interno della nare destra. Gazz. d. osp., Milano, 1884, v, 739.—**Ray** (J. M.) Intra-nasal inflammation (rhinitis); some of its results and their rational treatment. Am. Pract. & News, Louisville, 1887. n. s., iii, 71-74.—**Richey** (S. O.) Prophylaxis in rhinitis sympathetica. Chicago M. J. & Exam., 1886, liii, 42-45.—**Roberts** (J. B.) Two cases of abscess of the nasal septum and exhibition of instruments for curing crooked noses. Polyclinic, Phila., 1885-6, iii, 147. ———. Report of two cases of abscess of the nasal septum. Med. & Surg. Reporter, Phila., 1886. liv, 616.—**Roger** (H.) Notes sur la rhino-nécrose ou nécrose der cartilages de la cloison du nez. Union méd., Par., 1860, 2. s., v, 468-473. *Also:* Bull. Soc. méd. d. hôp. de Par. (1858-61), 1861, iv, 426-432. *Also* [Abstr.]: Gaz. d. hôp., Par., 1860, xxxiii, 153.—**Roth** (W.) Die Erkrankungen der Nasenschleimhaut, ihre Beziehungen zum übrigen Organismus und Behandlung derselben. Centralbl. f. d. ges. Therap., Wien, 1887, v, 545; 609.—**Roux.** Abcès froid à la racine du nez; potasse caustique. Gaz. d. hôp., Par., 1837, xi, 235.—**Rullier.** Du nez et des fosses nasales envisagées par rapport à l'état morbide. Dict. d. sc. méd., Par., 1819, xxxvi, 46-74.—**Rumbold** (T. F.) Hypertrophy and atrophy of the nasal mucous membrane. Tr. M. Ass. Missouri, St. Louis, 1887, 105-112.—**Ryerson** (G. S.) Rhinitis atrophica; with remarks on catarrh in general. Canada Lancet, Toronto, 1885-6, xviii, 136-138.—**Schalle** (R.) On aural and naso-pharyngeal diseases, and some of their methods of treatment; a posthumous paper. Arch. Otol., N. Y., 1882, xi, 113-154. *Also, transl.:* Ann. d. mal. de l'oreille et du larynx, Par., 1882, viii, 279; 321: 1883, ix, 35.—**Schech** (P.) Die Erkrankungen der Nebenhöhlen der Nase und ihre Behandlung. Festschr. d. ärztl. Ver. München, etc., 1883, 128-144.—**Scheff** (G.) Rhinitis, Koryza, akuter Schnupfen. Wien. med. Presse, 1882, xxiii, 630; 662; 696; 729.—**Schleicher** (W.) Remarques sur la rhinite, du nez, de la gorge et des oreilles; étude empruntée à nos registres de malades, octobre 1884-avril 1886. Ann. Soc. de méd. d'Anvers, 1886, xlvii, 493-537.—**Schmigelow** (E.) Beretning fra Kommunehospitalets Klinik for Øre-, Næse- og Hals-Sygdomme. Hosp.-Tid., Kjøbenh., 1885, 3. R., iii, 177; 201; 232. ———. Quelques cas assez rares de perforations de la cloison nasale. Rev. mens. de laryngol., etc., Par., 1886, vi, 593-599.—**Schramm** (M.) Ueber die Untersuchung und Behandlung einiger Affectionen der Nase und des Nasenrachenraumes. Jahresb. d. Gesellsch. f. Nat.- u. Heilk. in Dresd., 1878-9, 74-78.—**Schrötter** (L.) Ueber den gegenwärtigen Standpunkt in den Untersuchungsmethoden und der Therapie der Krankheiten des Nasenrachenraumes und der Nase. Mitth. d. Wien. med. Doct.-Coll., 1877, iii, 291-295. ———. Rhinoscopie; considérations sur les maladies du nez et de la cavité naso-pharyngienne, à l'occasion du travail de M. le Dr. Michel. Ann. d. mal. de l'oreille et du larynx, Par., 1877, iii, 213-224.—**Schwanebach** (A.) Ein Beitrag zur Casuistik der Nasenkrankheiten. St. Petersb. med. Wchnschr., 1884, n. F., i, 458.—**Seifert** (O.) Ueber Croup der Nasenschleimhaut. München. med. Wchnschr., 1887, xxxiv, 733.—**Seiler** (C.) Some remarks on the pathology of intra-nasal hypertrophies. Tr. Path. Soc. Phila. (1881-3), 1884, xi, 110-121. ———. Posterior nasal hypertrophy in situ, together with an exostosis from the vomer. Med. News, Phila., 1883, xliii, 497.—**Spicer** (S.) On distension of the nasal arch (transverse nasal vein) in children; its pathology and treatment. Brit. M. J., Lond., 1887, ii, 459.—**Stucky** (J. A.) Report on rhinology; the treatment of nasal and pharyngo-nasal catarrh. Cincin. M. & Dent. J., 1886-7, ii, 1-8. *Also,* Reprint.—**Tardieu** (A.) [Tuberculose des fosses nasales; phthisie bronchique.] Bull. Soc. anat. de Par., 1842, xvii, 207.—**Terrillon.** Hypertrophie de la muqueuse du cornet

Nose (*Diseases of*).

inférieur des fosses nasales; sa nature et son traitement. Progrès méd., Par., 1885, 2. s., i, 391; 409.—**von Tilesius** (T. W. G.) Beschreibung und Abbildung des sogenannten Dresdner Auswischers oder einer rosenartigen Entzündung der Nasenspitze und eines neuen kritischen Flechtenausschlages als Folge eines doppelten Metaschematismus. Entworfen und nach der Natur gezeichnet von dem Patienten selbst. Mag. f. d. ges. Heilk., Berl., 1828, xxvii, 78-108, 1 pl.—**Tillot.** De la rhinite chronique et de son traitement par la pulvérisation. Ann. d. mal. de l'oreille et du larynx, Par., 1875, i, 112-137.—**Tipton** (F.) What the general practitioner should know of the throat and nose. Virginia M. Month., Richmond, 1882-3, ix, 655; 710. *Also,* Reprint.—**Uhlenbrock.** Ueber chronische Rhinitis und Folgen derselben. Deutsche Klinik, Berl., 1869, xxi, 193; 213; 232.—**Ure.** Erosive ulceration of the derma of the nose, successfully treated with the local use of iodine. Lancet, Lond., 1864, ii, 152.—**Wagner** (C.) A case of acute idiopathic perichondritis of the nasal septum, terminating in abscess. Arch. Laryngol., N. Y., 1880, i, 59-61.—**Watson** (W. S.) Two cases of disease of the nose. Proc. M. Soc. Lond., 1879-81, v, 321. ———. Case of chronic hypertrophic rhinitis. Lancet, Lond., 1884, ii, 779. *Also:* Brit. M. J., Lond., 1884, ii, 863.—**Weichselbaum** (A.) Die phlegmonöse Entzündung der Nebenhöhlen der Nase. Med. Jahrb., Wien, 1881, 227-259, 1 pl. ———. Das perforirende Geschwür der Nasenscheidewand. Allg. Wien. med. Ztg., 1882, xxvii, 363.—**Weil.** Ueber Krankheiten der Nase und des Nasenrachenraums mit Demonstrationen von Instrumenten und Präparaten. Med. Cor.-Bl. d. württemb. ärztl. Ver., Stuttg., 1880, l, 233-236.—**Weist** (J. R.) Chronic rhinitis and its treatment. West. J. M., Indianap., 1868, iii, 665-670.—**Wendt** (H.) Krankheiten der Nasenrachenhöhle und des Rachens. Handb. d. spec. Path. (Ziemssen), Leipz., 1874, vii, 1. Th., 233-323. *Also, transl.:* Cycl. Pract. M. (Ziemssen), N. Y., 1876, vii, 1-108.—**White** (J. A.) Practical remarks and suggestions in regard to diseases of the ear, throat, and nose. J. Am. M. Ass., Chicago, 1885, v, 423.—**Woakes** (E.) Necrosing ethmoiditis; its relationship to the development of nasal polypus; ozæna, etc. Lancet, Lond., 1885, ii, 108; 150.—**Zawerthal.** Sulla cura delle affezioni del cavo nasofaringeo. Atti Cong. gen. d. Ass. med. ital. 1878, Pisa, 1879, viii, 394.—**Ziem.** Ueber Rosenschnupfen. Monatschr. f. Ohrenh., Berl., 1885, xix, 167. ———. Ueber Bedeutung und Behandlung der Naseneiterungen. *Ibid.*, 1886, xx, 33; 79; 137.—**Zuckerkandl** (E.) Zur Pathologie der Nasenhöhle. Wien. med. Bl., 1882, v, 42; 74; 106.

Nose (*Diseases of, Causes of*).

Allen (H.) Errors of conformation of the nasal chambers studied in relation to the cause of nasal disease and irregularity of the teeth. Phila. M. Times, 1879-80, x, 119-121. *Also:* Proc. Phila. Co. M. Soc., Phila., 1880, ii, 17.—**Mackenzie** (J. N.) Irritation of the sexual apparatus as an etiological factor in the production of nasal disease. Am. J. M. Sc., Phila., 1884, n. s., lxxxvii, 360-365. *Also,* Reprint. *Also* [Abstr.]: Maryland M. J., Balt., 1883-4, x, 672.—**Miles** (F. L.) Ocular irritation a cause of nasal affections. Weekly M. Rev., Chicago & St. Louis, 1884, x, 111.—**Rothholz.** Ueber die Beziehungen von Augenerkrankungen zu Nasenaffectionen. Deutsche med. Wchnschr., Berl., 1887, xiii, 1123. *Also,* Reprint.—**Ziem.** Ueber die Bedeutung der Zahnkrankheiten für die Entstehung von Nasenleiden. Allg. med. Centr.-Ztg., Berl., 1885, liv, 1117-1120.

Nose (*Diseases of, Complications and sequelæ of*).

See, also, **Asthma**; **Hay-fever.**

MACDONALD (G.) Three lectures on the forms of nasal obstruction in relation to throat and ear disease. 8°. *London*, 1887.

MOURE (J.-G.) *Des rapports de certaines névroses et en particulier de l'asthme avec les polypes muqueux du nez et avec les sténoses nasales en général. 4°. *Bordeaux*, 1883.

PUJOL (J.-R.) * De l'influence des maladies du nez et de la gorge sur la production des maladies de l'oreille moyenne. 4°. *Paris*, 1884.

RAAF (B.) * Zur Therapie des Asthma bronchiale von der Nase ausgelöst. 8°. *Bonn*, 1886.

SOURDRILLE (A.) * Contribution à l'étude des névroses réflexes d'origine nasale et nasopharyngienne. 4°. *Paris*, 1887.

WOAKES (E.) Post-nasal catarrh and diseases of the nose causing deafness. 8°. *Philadelphia*, 1884.

Baratoux (J.) Des névroses réflexes déterminées par les affections nasales. Rev. mens. de laryngol., etc., Par., 1885, v, 637-641. *Also:* Progrès méd., Par., 1885, 2. s., ii, 329.

Nose (*Diseases of, Complications and sequelæ of*).

Also, transl.: Boll. d. mal. d. orecchio, d. gola e d. naso, Firenze. 1886, iv, 2–5. *Also, transl.:* Arch. ital. di laringol., Napoli, 1885-6, v, 13–116.—**Barr** (T.) Remarks on the relation of diseases of the nasal passages and naso-pharynx to aural affections. Brit. M. J., Lond., 1881, ii, 389.—**Barthélemy.** Observation d'ostéite naso-crânienne, suivie de méningo-encéphalite et de mort. France méd., Par., 1881, xxviii, 110 ; 122. — **Bendell** (H.) Disease of nasopharynx as a cause of deafness. Albany M. Ann., 1885, vi, 33–41. *Also,* Reprint.—**Bettman** (B.) Ocular troubles of nasal origin. J. Am. M. Ass., Chicago, 1887, viii, 516.—**Böcker.** Die Beziehungen der erkrankten Schleimhaut der Nase zum Asthma und deren Behandlung. Deutsche med. Wchnschr., Berl., 1886, xii, 441 ; 469. — **Brandeis** (R. C.) Catarrhal headaches and allied affections. Med. Rec., N. Y., 1883, xxiii, 421–425.—**Brebion.** De l'aphonie complète par lésion nasale. Rev. mens. de laryngol., etc., Par., 1885, v, 641-646.—**Brémond.** D'une conformation particulière du nez produisant l'ozène vrai et la surdité. Rec. d. actes du Comité méd. d. Bouches-du-Rhône, Marseille, 1881-2, xx, 226-235. — **Bresgen** (M.) Zur Entwickelung von Refractions- und Stellungs-Anomalien der Auges in Folge von Nasenerkrankung. Deutsche med. Wchnschr., Berl., 1884, x, 133. *Also:* Med.-chir. Centralbl., Wien, 1884, xix, 266. ——. Die Beziehungen der erkrankten Nasenschleimhaut zum Asthma und dessen rhino-chirurgische Heilung. Deutsche med. Wchnschr., Berl., 1886, xii, 371–373. — **Burnett** (C. H.) Reflex aural phenomena from naso-pharyngeal catarrh; objective noises in and from the ear. Tr. Am. Otol. Soc., New Bedford, Mass., 1884, iii, pt. 3, 273-279.— **Calmettes.** Les névroses réflexes d'origine nasale. Progrès méd., Par., 1887, 2. s., vi, 20.— **Campbell** (D. S.) Reflex asthma from nasal affection. Am. Lancet, Detroit, 1887, n. s., xi, 361-363.—**Capart.** Sur l'influence exercée sur le larynx et la trachée par les affections des fosses nasales et de la cavité naso-pharyngienne. Cong. internat. de laryngol. 1880, Milan, 1882, i, 249-254. *Also, in his:* De l'hypertrophie, etc., 8°, Brux., 1881, 14–24.—**Carpenter** (J. G.) Sequels of naso-pharyngeal and aural catarrh, illustrated by cases from private practice. Gaillard's M. J., N. Y., 1884, xxxvii, 387–392. *Also,* Reprint. — **Cartaz** (A.) Des névroses réflexes d'origine nasale. France méd., Par., 1885, ii, 1065 ; 1077. *Also,* Reprint. — **Chiari** (O.) Stenose des Kehlkopfes und der Luftröhre bei Rhinosklerom. Med. Jahrb., Wien, 1882, 169–184, 1 pl. ——. Casuistische Beiträge zur Lehre über den Zusammenhang zwischen nervösen Leiden und Nasenerkrankungen. Ztschr. f. Therap. m. Einbzhng. d. Elect.- u. Hydrotherap., Wien, 1884, ii, 33–35.—**Christopher** (H.) & **Rumbold** (T. F.) Disease of the scalp due to inflammation of the pharyngo-nasal cavity; illustrative cases. St. Louis M. & S. J., 1884, xlvi, 527–529. — **Cohen** (S. S.) A case of hysterical sneezing apparently cured by intra-nasal applications of the continuous battery current. Tr. Am. Laryngol. Ass. 1886, N. Y., 1887, viii, 150–153.—**Daly** (W. H.) Some clinical remarks upon deflections of the nasal septum, with a presentation of two cases made before the Allegheny County (Pa.) Medical Society. Med. & Surg. Reporter, Phila., 1883, xlix, 648. *Also,* Reprint.—**Discussion** on reflex symptoms in nasal affections. Med. News, Phila., 1884, xlviii, 136–138. — **Douaud.** Furoncle du nez; phlébite des sinus; mort. Mém. et bull. Soc. de méd. et chir. de Bordeaux, 1875, 81–86. — **Eaton** (F. B.) Hypertrophic catarrh of the anterior nares as a cause of chronic catarrhal deafness; illustrated by auto aural experiments and a case. Arch. Otol., N. Y., 1886, xv, 186–191. — **Elsberg** (L.) Reflex and other phenomena due to nasal disease. Tr. Am. Laryngol. Ass., N. Y., 1883, v, 79–84. *Also:* Med. Gaz., N. Y., 1883, x, 445. *Also:* Arch. Laryngol., N. Y., 1883, iv, 253–255. — **Ferreri** (G.) I fenomeni riflessi d'origine nasale e le injezioni sottomucose di cocaina. Sperimentale, Firenze, 1886, lviii, 285–294.—**Finne** (G.) Nervöse Symptomer paa Grund af Sygdom i Næsen. Norsk Mag. f. Lægevidensk., Christiania, 1887, 4. R., ii, 429–437.—**Fränkel** (B.) Ueber den Zusammenhang von Asthma nervosum und Krankheiten der Nase. Berl. klin. Wchnschr., 1881, xviii, 217 ; 238. *Also:* Verhandl. d. Berl. med. Gesellsch. (1880–81), 1882, xii, pt. 2, 97–114. ——. Ueber die Frage der von der Nasenhöhle ausgehenden Reflexneurosen. Cong. périod. internat. d. sc. méd. Compt.-rend. 1884, Copenh., 1886, iv, Sect. de laryngol., 32–43. — **French** (T. R.) The effects of diseases of the nasal passages on other portions of the respiratory tract. N. York M. J., 1886, xliv, 533-535.—**Gellé.** Chorée consécutive à une affection nasale. Compt. rend. Soc. de biol., Par., 1883, 7. s., iv, 677–679.—**Glasgow** (W. C.) On certain measures for the relief of congestive headaches. Tr. Am. Laryngol. Ass. 1887, N. Y., 1888, ix, 149-155.—**Götze** (L.) Beitrag zur Frage nach dem Zusammenhang gewisser Neurosen mit Nasenleiden. Monatschr. f. Ohrenh., Berl., 1884, xviii, 163; 177.—**Goodwillie** (D. H.) Hindrance to the respiration by disease in the nose. Canada M. Rec., Montreal, 1879-80, vii, 57–59.—**Gradle** (H.) On ocular symptoms due to nasal disease. Arch.

Nose (*Diseases of, Complications and sequelæ of*).

Ophth., N. Y., 1887, xvi, 391–402.—**Gruening** (E.) Reflex ocular symptoms in nasal affections. Med. Rec., N. Y., 1886, xxix, 122–124.—**Guye.** Nasale reflex-neuroses, literatuur en eigene waarnemingen. Nederl. Tijdschr. v. Geneesk., Amst., 1887, 2. R., xxxiii, 609–622. — **Hack** (W.) Reflexneurosen und Nasenleiden. Berl. klin. Wchnschr., 1882, xix, 379–384. *Also, transl.:* Maryland M. J., Balt., 1882-3, ix, 220 ; 247. ——. Ueber Reflexneurosen, die von der Nase ausgehen. Tagebl. d. Versamml. deutsch. Naturf. u. Aerzte, Magdeb., 1884, lvii, 271–273. — **Hendrix** (H. F.) The relationship of disease of the eye to those of the nasal passages. St. Louis M. & S. J., 1886, l, 20–24.— **Hering** (T.) Contribution à l'étude des névroses réflexes par lésions nasales (aphonie spasmodique et spasme du larynx). Rev. mens. de laryngol., etc., Par., 1885, v, 646-649. ——. Des névroses réflexes déterminées par les affections nasales (asthme, spasme laryngé, aphonie et dyspnée spasmodique, aphonie hystérique, migraine, névroses, etc.). Ann. d. mal. de l'oreille, du larynx, etc., Par., 1886, xii, 45 ; 89. — **Heymann** (P.) Ueber Folgesymptome von Nasenkrankheiten. Deutsche med. Wchnschr., Berl., 1886, xii, 486–488. ——. Ueber pathologische Zustände, die von der Nase ihre Entstehung finden können. Deutsche Med.-Ztg., Berl., 1886, vii, 495 ; 507. [Discussion], 528. — **Hopmann.** Ueber Reflexneurosen und Nasentumoren. Tagebl. d. Versamml. deutsch. Naturf. u. Aerzte, Strassb., 1885, lviii, 321–328. — **Jacobi** (A.) Some of the effects of nasal polypi in children. N. York M. J., 1883, xxxvii, 376. *Also:* Tr. N. York Obst. Soc. (1881–5), 1885, iii, 186–188.—**Jarvis** (W. C.) Catarrhal affections of the nasal passages as a cause of pulmonary phthisis, with special reference to the question of heredity. N. York M. J., 1885, xlii, 259 ; 290. *Also,* Reprint.—**Johnson.** Disease of the Schneiderian membrane spreading to the brain. Lancet, Lond., 1839-40, i, 703.—**Kjellman** (F. W.) Om vissa neurosers sammanhang med sjukliga förändringar inom näs-kaviteten. Öfversigt af hithörande litteratur, jemte några egna iakttagelser. [On certain neuroses produced by changes in the nasal cavity.] Hygiea, Stockholm, 1886, xlviii, 59–71. — **Klein** (A.) Fall von schwerem Asthma in Folge von Nasenpolypen ; vollständige Heilung. Wien. med. Presse, 1884, xxv, 764-766. — **Knight** (C. H.) Paralysis of the velum palati in acute naso-pharyngitis. N. York M. J., 1886, xliii, 628-630. *Also,* Reprint. — **Leisrink** (H.) Ein Fall von ausgebreiteter Entzündung und Gängrän des mucösperiostalen Ueberzuges der Nasenhöhle. Deutsche Klinik, Berl., 1870, xxii, 129.—**Lichtwitz** (L.) Des troubles de la voix articulée (parole) dans les affections du voile du palais, de la cavité nasopharyngienne et des fosses nasales. Rev. mens. de laryngol., etc., Par., 1886, vi, 16 ; 57.—**Longuet** (R.) La toux nasale. Union méd., Par., 1884, 3. s., xxxvii, 133–136. — **Lublinski** (W.) Asthma und Nasenleiden. Deutsche Med.-Ztg., Berl., 1886, vii, 447-451.—**McBride** (P.) Lecture on nasal and naso-pharyngeal reflex neuroses. Brit. M. J., Lond., 1887, i, 205–207.—**MacCoy** (A. W.) On occlusion of the posterior nares as a result of nasal catarrh. Med. Press & Circ., Lond., 1883, n. s., xxxvi, 213–215. *Also:* Med. News, Phila., 1883, xlii, 379-382.—**Mackenzie** (G. H.) Nasal disease as a cause of asthma. Edinb. M. J., 1882-3, xxviii, 689. ——. Nasal asthma; its causes and treatment. Brit. M. J., Lond., 1885, i, 984.—**Mackenzie** (J. N.) On nasal cough, and the existence of a sensitive reflex area in the nose. Am. J. M. Sc., Phila., 1883, n. s., lxxxvi, 106–116. *Also,* Reprint. *Also* [Abstr.]: Maryland M. J., Balt., 1883-4, x, 145–148. *Also,* Reprint. ——. Cases of reflex cough due to nasal polypi. Tr. M. & Chir. Fac. Maryland, Balt., 1884, 208–213. *Also,* Reprint. ——. The pathological nasal reflex; an historical study. N. York M. J., 1887, xlvi, 199-205. ——. The pathological nasal reflex; an historical study. Tr. Am. Laryngol. Ass. 1887, N. Y., 1888, ix, 102–117. *Also, transl.:* Ann. d. mal. de l'oreille, du larynx, etc., Par., 1887, xiii, 457–475.—**Masini** (G.) Dei rapporti fra alcune malattie del naso con alcune malattie degli occhi. Ann. di ottal., Firenze, 1885-6, viii, 10 ; 301.—**Masini** (O.) Dei rapporti dell' asma con alcune malattie del naso. Gazz. d. osp , Milano, 1883, iv, 611 ; 620 ; 627.—**Moos.** Drei Fälle von secundärer Affection des Felsenbeines im Gefolge von Neubildungen im Nasenrachenraum, nebst Bemerkungen zur Symptomatologie und Behandlung. Arch. f. Augen- u. Ohrenh., Wiesb., 1878, vii, 228–239.—**Moure.** Des névroses réflexes d'origine nasale. Mém. et bull. Soc. de méd. et chir. de Bordeaux (1886), 1887, 621-634. *Also:* J. de méd. de Bordeaux, 1886-7, xvi, 229–231. ——. Scrofulose des fosses nasales, de la voûte palatine et du larynx. Mém. et bull. Soc. de méd. et chir. de Bordeaux (1886), 1887, 635–639. — **Mulhall** (J. C.) Asthma from nasal disease. St. Louis Cour. Med., 1882, vii, 400–404.—**Nieden** (A.) On the connection between diseases of the eye and nose. [Transl. and abridged by J. A. Spalding.] Arch. Ophth., N. Y., 1883, xvi, 415–433.—**Palmer** (L. L.) Reflex phenomena from nasal diseases. Canad. Pract., Toronto, 1884, iv, 297–300.—**Percepied.** Otite moyenne par suite d'introduction de liquide

Nose (*Diseases of, Complications and sequelæ of*).

dans la caisse pendant une irrigation nasale. Union méd. de la Seine-Inf. 1886, Rouen, 1887, xxv, 21–26.—**Porter** (W.) Obstruction of the nares a cause of asthma. Arch. Laryngol., N. Y., 1882, lii, 112–117.—**Réthi** (L.) Ueber Reflexneurosen, bedingt durch Krankheiten der Nase und des Nasenrachenraumes. Wien. med. Presse, 1886, xxvii, 1201; 1236; 1268.—**Richardson** (B. W.) Epileptiform seizures from post-nasal polypus. Asclepiad, Lond., 1887, iv. 48–50.—**Rios Ruiz** (V.) Relacion entre el asma i algunas afecciones de las fosas nasales. Rev. méd. de Chile, Sant. de Chile, 1886-7, xv, 404–413.—**Robinson** (B.) On respiratory neuroses of nasal origin (vasomotor coryza, asthma). Med. Rec., N. Y., 1886, xxix, 120–122.—**Roth** (W.) Zur Diagnose und Therapie der mit Nasenkrankheiten zusammenhängenden Reflexneurosen. Wien. med. Wchnschr., 1885, xxxv, 481; 525.—**Ruault** (A.) Les névropathies réflexes d'origine nasale. Gaz. d. hôp., Par., 1887, lx, 1253–1261. *Also*, Reprint.—**Rumbold** (T. F.) On the relation of nasal catarrh and nasal polypi to asthmatic symptoms. Arch. Laryngol., N. Y., 1882, iii, 118–124.—**Rumbold** (F. M.) The influence of chronic rhinitis on the membrana conjunctiva; illustrated by a case. St. Louis M. & S. J., 1886, li, 270.—**Sajous** (C. E.) Affections of the throat and nose. Med. Bull., Phila., 1882, iv, 226.—**Schaeffer** (M.) Nasenleiden und Reflexneurosen. Deutsche med. Wchnschr., Berl., 1884, x, 357; 376.—**Schmiegelow** (E.) Reflexneurosernes Forhold till Sygdomme i Näsen og Svälget. C. r. La relation entre les névroses réflexes et les maladies du nez et de la gorge. Nord. med. Ark., Stockholm, 1885, xvii, no. 27, 1–33.—**Schmithuisen.** Sur un cas de retour de la voix perdue depuis dix ans, moyennant la rhinoscopie. [Rap. de Elsberg.] Cong. internat. de laryngol. 1880, Milan, 1882, i, 133–135.—**Schweig** (M.) Reflex symptoms of nasal disease. Med. Rec, N. Y., 1886, xxix, 205.—**Seiler** (C.) Some remarks on the pathology of intra-nasal hypertrophies. Tr. Path. Soc. Phila. (1881-3), 1884, xi, 110–121. *Also*: Phila. M. Times, 1881-2, xii, 245–250. [Discussion], 256.———. Posterior nasal hypertrophy in situ, together with an exostosis from the vomer. Tr. Path. Soc. Phila. (1883-5), 1886, xii, 114.———. Chronic rhinitis as an etiological factor of acne of the face. Maryland M. J., Balt., 1887, xvii, 503–507. *Also*: Polyclinic, Phila., 1887-8, v, 141–143. *Also*: Med. News, Phila., 1887, li, 489.—**Smith** (P.) Amaurosis from tumour in the nasal cavity, cured by removal of the tumour. Ophth. Rev., Lond., 1883, ii, 167–173.—**Sommerbrodt** (J.) Mittheilung von Heilungen pathologischer Zustände, welche durch Reflexvorgänge von der Nase her bewirkt waren. Berl. klin. Wchnschr., 1884, xxi, 147; 166. *Also*, Reprint. ———. Ueber Nasen-Reflex-Neurosen. Berl. klin. Wchnschr., 1885, xxii, 146; 172.—**Terrillon.** Rapport des polypes muqueux des fosses nasales avec l'asthme. Progrès méd., Par., 1885, 2. s., i, 293–295. *Also*: Médecin prat., Par., 1885, vi, 217–222.—**Thost** (A.) Ueber den Zusammenhang zwischen Erkrankungen der Nase und der Lungen. Deutsche med. Wchnschr., Leipz., 1887, xiii, 770–772.—**Trautmann** (F.) Casuistische Mittheilungen zur Erkrankung der Nase, wobei das Ohr in Mitleidenschaft gezogen war. Arch. f. Ohrenh., Leipz., 1879-80, xv, 91–95.—**Vermyne** (J. J. B.) Disease of the ethmoid, the consequence of chronic catarrh of the nasopharynx; exophthalmos. Tr. Am. Otol. Soc., New Bedford, Mass., 1884, iii, pt. 3, 262–272. *Also*: Am. J. Ophth., St. Louis, 1884-5, i, 129–134.—**Virchow** (R.) Ueber katarrhalische Geschwüre. Verhandl. d. Berl. med. Gesellsch., 1882-3, xiv, 2. Th., 31–47. *Also, transl.*: Med. Press & Circ., Lond., 1883, n. s., xxxv, 312.—**White** (J. A.) The influence of naso-pharyngeal growths, obstructions, and hypertrophies upon the hearing, with a few cases in point. Virginia M. Month., Richmond, 1884-5, xi, 595–607.—**Ziem.** Ueber Asymmetrie des Schädels bei Nasenkrankheiten. Monatschr. f. Ohrenh., Berl., 1883, xvii, 21; 43; 61; 89. ———. Ueber die Abhängigkeit der Migräne von Krankheiten der Nasenhöhle und der Kieferhöhle. Allg. med. Centr.-Ztg., Berl., 1886, lv, 591; 613.

Nose (*Diseases of, Treatment and instruments for*).

See, also, **Douche** (*Nasal*); **Nose** (*Exploration of*); **Nose** (*Surgery of*).

BANKS (W. M.) On local applications to the throat and nostrils. 8°. *Liverpool*, 1868.

BRESGEN. Trattato delle malattie del naso, della cavità orale, della faringe, laringe, trachea ed esofago. [Transl. by Fasano.] roy. 8°. *Roma, Torino, Napoli*, 1888.

FISCHER (A.) Egy új orresap az orrüreg kimosására, s egy új pöscsap a hólyag kioblitésere. [Irrigator for nose.] 8°. *Budapest*, 1879.

GARRIGOU-DÉSARÈNES. Du catarrhe chronique hypertrophique et atrophique des fosses

Nose (*Diseases of, Treatment and instruments for*).

nasales. De l'ozène, obstruction catarrhale des trompes d'Eustache, végétations adénoïdes du pharynx. Traitement par la galvano-caustique chimique. 8°. *Paris*, 1888.

HACK (W.) Ueber eine operative Radical-Behandlung bestimmter Formen von Migräne, Asthma, Heufieber sowie zahlreicher verwandter Erscheinungen. Erfahrungen auf dem Gebiete der Nasenkrankheiten. 8°. *Wiesbaden*, 1884.

Adams (A. W.) A consideration of a few of the details in the treatment of diseases of the ear, nose, and throat. Rocky Mountain M. Rev., Colorado Springs, 1880-81, i, 3–13.—**Agnew** (D. H.) Note on the use of Salvia officinalis in catarrhal rhinitis. Therap. Gaz., Detroit, 1885, 3. s., i, 17.—**Antoni** (R.) Modificazioni al rhinobyon. Boll. d. mal. d. orecchio, d. gola e d. naso, Firenze, 1886, ii, 113–115. ———. Di un nuovo rhinobyon. *Ibid.*, iv, 53–56.—**Baber** (E. C.) The action of cocaine on the nasal mucous membrane. Brit. M. J., Lond., 1885, i, 479.—**Barton** (I.) Terebene in chronic rhinitis. Med. Reg., Phila., 1887, i, 418. *Also*: Med. Bull., Phila., 1887, ix, 169.—**Bassius** (H.) Scarificatio narium, peculiari peragenda instrumento. *In his*: Obs. anat., 8°, Halæ Magdeb., 1731, 177–193, 1 pl.—**Bosworth** (F. H.) The use of caustics in the nasal cavities. N. York M. J., 1888, xlvii, 253–255. *Also*, Reprint.—**Bresgen** (M.) Zur galvanokaustischen Behandlung hypertrophischer Nasenschleimhaut. Deutsche med. Wchnschr., Berl., 1884, x, 474; 611. ———. Ueber Chromsäure-Aetzungen in der Nasenhöhle. Med.-chir. Centralbl., Wien, 1885, xx, 613. *Also, transl.*: Rev. mens. de laryngol., etc., Par., 1885, v, 533–537. ———. Die Anwendung der Chromsäure in der Nasenhöhle. Deutsche Med.-Ztg., Berl., 1886, i, 65–67. *Also*: Med.-chir. Centralbl., Wien 1886, xxi, 169; 181. ———. Entstehung, Bedeutung und Behandlung der Verkrümmungen und callösen Verdickungen der Nasenscheidewand. Wien. med. Presse, 1887, xxviii, 237; 274.—**Burch** (T. H.) A practical and simple way to make thorough applications of powder to the post-nasal region. Med. Rec., N. Y., 1883, xxiv, 53.—**Burckardt.** Ein Spray-Apparat zur Behandlung von Erkrankungen des Nasenrachenraumes und der Athmungs-Organe. Deutsche med. Wchnschr., Berl., 1878, iv, 606.—**Catti** (G.) Zur Therapie der Nasenkrankheiten. Allg. Wien. med. Ztg., 1876, xxi, 234.—**Chappell** (W. F.) Submucous injections in chronic throat and nasal diseases. Med. Rec., N. Y., 1887, xxxii, 535.—**Chiari** (O.) Ueber die Anwendung des Cocaïn bei der Behandlung der Krankheiten des Rachens, Kehlkopfes und der Nase. Wien. med. Wchnschr., 1887, xxxvii, 199; 225; 261.—**Cohen** (J. S.) The polyclinic nasal tampon carrier and nasal cotton applicator. Polyclinic, Phila., 1886-7, iv, 43.—**Coomes** (M. F.) New instruments for the removal of tumors from the nose. Med. Herald, Louisville, 1885-6, vii, 619.—**Cozzolino** (V.) Il jodoformio nelle malattie del naso e della gola. Movimento, Napoli, 1881, 2. s., iii, 19–22. *Also*: Salute: Italia med., Genova, 1881, 2. s., xv, 181. ———. Dell' alcool etilico nelle malattie della mucosa nasale, del cavo naso-faringeo e laringeo. Arch. ital. di laringol., Napoli, 1887, vii, 61–65.—**Daly** (W. H.) An analysis of the value of the galvano-cautery in the treatment of diseases and growths of the naso-pharynx. Tr. Am. M. Ass., Phila., 1880, xxxi, 653–656. *Also, in his*: Stenosis of the larynx, etc., 8°, N. Y., 1880, 8–12.—**Delavan** (D. B.) On the treatment of atrophic rhinitis by applications of the galvanic current. Tr. Am. Laryngol. Ass. 1887, N. Y., 1888, ix, 145–149. *Also*: N. York M. J., 1887, xlvi, 458.—**Delstanche** (C.) Démonstration de ses instruments. Cong. internat. d'otol. Compt.-rend. 1884, Bâle, 1885, iii, 258–267. *Also, transl.* [with additions]: Illust. Monatschr. d. ärztl. Polytech., Bern, 1885, vii, 171; 197; 229; 243; 275. ———. Présentation d'instruments et d'appareils destinés au traitement des maladies de l'oreille et du nez. Bull. Acad. roy. de méd. de Belg., Brux., 1885, 3. s., xix, 209–235. *Also*: Ann. d. mal. de l'oreille, du larynx, etc., Par., 1885, xi, 269–299.—**Demons** (A.) Note sur la substitution d'une sonde en gomme élastique à la sonde de Belloc dans le tamponnement des fosses nasales, suivie de quelques recherches historiques. Bull. gén. de thérap., etc., Par., 1879, xcvii, 112; 163.—**De Pilbiss** (A.) The treatment of acute and chronic rhinitis. Cleveland M. Gaz., 1886-7, ii, 195–201.—**Dulles** (C. W.) A simple way to apply fluids to the nasal cavity. Med. & Surg. Reporter, Phila., 1887, lvii, 171.—**Eaton** (F. B.) Some improved forms of burners for the galvano-caustic treatment of nasal and post-nasal hypertrophies. Med. Rec., N. Y., 1886, xxx, 230–233.—**Englisch** (J.) Der Doppelballon in seiner Anwendung als Nasentampon und bei anderen chirurgischen Operationen. Ber. d. k. k. Krankenanst. Rudolph-Stiftung in Wien (1876), 1877, 273–278.—**Farnham** (A. B.) A nasal cutting-forceps and bloodless nasal operating. N. York M. J., 1887, xlv, 578.—**Fasano**

Nose (*Diseases of, Treatment and instruments for*).

(A.) Ultimi progressi terapeutici delle malattie della gola e del naso. Gior. internaz. d. sc. med., Napoli, 1881, n. s., iii, 396; 496. — **Fraenkel** (B.) The general therapeutics of diseases of the nose, naso-pharyngeal space, pharynx, and larynx. Cycl. Pract. M. (Ziemssen), N. Y., 1876, iv, 1-98.—**González** (D.) El ácido salicílico en el coriza diftérico. Gac. méd. catal., Barcel., 1886, ix, 513-519.—**Guye** (A.) Ein neues Ringmesser zum Entfernen der adenoïden Geschwülste aus dem Nasenrachenraum. Ztschr. f. Ohrenh., Wiesb., 1885, xv, 167. *Also, transl.:* Arch. Otol., N. Y., 1886, xv, 30. — **Hall** (F. de H.) On the treatment of sneezing, hay fever, asthma, etc., by the galvano-cautery. Lancet, Lond., 1886, ii, 913. — **Hartmann** (A.) Historische Bemerkungen bezüglich der galvanokaustischen Behandlung der Nasenschleimhaut. Deutsche med. Wchnschr., Berl., 1884, x, 617.—**Henderson** (E. F.) A suggestion in regard to the treatment of hypertrophy of the turbinated processes. St. Louis M. & S. J., 1886, i, 28-32. — **Hering** (T.) O nowszych sposobach badania i leczenia chorób jam nosowych. [New methods of treatment of diseases of the nose.] Medycyna, Warszawa, 1880, viii, 65; 81; 97; 113; 129. ——. Ueber die Anwendung der Chromsäureätzungen bei Krankheiten der Nasenhöhle. Cong. périod. internat. d. sc. méd. Compt.-rend. 1884, Copenh., 1886, iv, Sect. de laryngol., 3-11. — **Hope** (G. B.) A modification of the Schrötter snare. N. York M. J., 1886, xliv, 447. — **Hoppe** (J.) Tinct. thuiæ gegen üble Gerüche in der Nase. Med. Ztg., Berl., 1859, ii, 262. — **Jarvis** (W. C.) Cocaine in intra-nasal surgery. Med. Rec., N. Y., 1887, xxvi, 654-656. — **Jelenefy** (Z.) Uj, rögzithetö orrtükör. [New, fixed nose speculum.] Gyógyászat, Budapest, 1887, xxvii, 54. *Also, transl.:* Berl. klin. Wchnschr., 1887, xxiv, 549-552. ——. Orrtükrömnek egy uj alakja. [New pocket nose speculum.] Gyógyászat, Budapest, 1887, xxvii, 196. — **Josephi**. Beschreibung einer Zange zu Ausziehung der Nasenpolypen. N. Mag. f. Aerzte, Leipz., 1786, viii, 237-240, 1 pl.—**Justi** (G.) Die Verwendung des Quellmeissels bei Erkrankungen der Nasenhöhle und des Nasenrachenraumes. Wien. med. Wchnschr., 1880, xxx, 816-818. — **Katz** (L.) Ein Instrument zur Untersuchung der Nasenhöhle. Berl. klin. Wchnschr., 1886, xxiii, 144.—**Killian** (G.) Einiges über adenoïde Vegetationen und ihre Operation mit der Hartmann'schen Cürette. Deutsche med. Wchnschr., Leipz., 1887, xiii, 542-546.—**Kitchen** (J. M. W.) The treatment of acute rhinitis. Med. Rec., N. Y., 1885, xxvii, 572. — **Klamann**. Instrumente zum Gebrauch bei der Behandlung von Nasen- und Rachenkrankheiten. Illust. Monatschr. d. ärztl. Polytech., Bern, 1882, iv, 3-5. — **Knight** (F. I.) On the treatment of posterior hypertrophy of the inferior turbinated bones. Med. News, Phila., 1882, xl, 64-68.—**Krause** (H.) Nasentampon-Träger. Cong. périod. internat. d. sc. méd. Compt.-rend. 1884, Copenh., 1886, iv, Sect. de laryngol., 146. — **Lange** (V.) Ueber Aluminium acetico-tartaricum und Aluminium acetico-glycerinatum siccum bei Affectionen der Nase, des Nasen-Rachen-Raumes und des Larynx. Monatschr. f. Ohrenh., 1885, xix, 291-295.—**Lente** (F. D.) Treatment of nasal disease by electricity. Med. Gaz., N. Y., 1882, ix, 471.—**MacCoy** (A. W.) The comparative study of some of the methods of treatment best adapted to the relief of occlusion of the posterior nares. Tr. Am. Laryngol. Ass. 1887, N. Y., 1888, ix, 213-219. *Also :* N. York M. J., 1887, xlvi, 457.—**Mackenzie** (J. N.) The local use of the bichloride of mercury in diseases of the nose and throat. Maryland M. J., Balt., 1882-3, ix, 489-491. *Also,* Reprint. ——. Some observations on the toxic effects of chrome on the nose, throat, and ear. J. Am. M. Ass., Chicago, 1884, iii, 601-603. *Also, transl.:* Ann. d. mal. de l'oreille et du larynx, Par., 1884, x, 237-244. ——. An improved self-retaining nasal speculum. Med. News, Phila., 1884, xlv, 639.—**Major** (G. W.) Cocaïne hydrochlorate in diseases of the nose and throat. Canada M. & S. J., Montreal, 1884-5, xiii, 518-531. ——. An improved nasal écraseur. Med. Press & Circ., Lond., 1886, n. s., xlii, 188. *Also :* Lancet, Lond., 1886, ii, 1083. ——. An improved nasal traction snare and écraseur, a nasal spud or denuder. Canada M. & S. J., Montreal, 1886-7, xv, 355-359.—**Masucci** (P.) Observations sur les douches nasales d'air comprimé simples et médicamenteuses, d'après la méthode du Dr. Massei. Cong. internat. de laryngol. 1880, Milan, 1882, i, 245-248.—**Mather** (W. W.) The douche in treatment of chronic nasal catarrh. Physician & Surg., Ann Arbor, Mich., 1881, iii, 398.—**Mills** (T. W.) Some mistakes to be avoided in dealing with diseases of the nose and throat. Canad. J. M. Sc., Toronto, 1882, vii, 355-358.—**Morelli** (K.) Néhány eszköz az orr-, garat-és gégének helybeli kezelésére és mütevésére. [Some new instruments for local treatment of nose, throat, and larynx.] Orvosi hetil., Budapest, 1887, xxxi, 1399; 1434.—**Moure** (E.-J.) & **Baratoux** (J.) De l'emploi du chlorhydrate de cocaïne comme anesthésique de la muqueuse du pharynx, du larynx, du nez, et dans le traitement des affections de ces organes et de l'oreille. Rev. mens. de laryngol., etc.,

Nose (*Diseases of, Treatment and instruments for*).

Par., 1884, v, 407-413.—**Mulhall** (J. C.) The galvano-caustic method in nose and throat. Tr. M. Ass. Missouri, St. Louis, 1884, 42-47. *Also :* St. Louis Cour. Med., 1884, xii, 1-6.—**Neumann** (J. F.) Ueber die Anwendung der Chromsäure und der Galvanocaustik in der Nase und dem Rachen. St. Petersb. med. Wchnschr., 1886, n. F., iii, 21-24.—**Noquet**. Hypertrophie de la muqueuse des cornets inférieurs; cautérisation avec le cautère galvanique latéral de Lœwemberg; guérison; présentation de l'opérée. Bull méd. du nord, Lille, 1883, xxiii, 183-185.—**Prior** (J.) Das Jodol und sein therapeutischer Werth bei tuberculösen und andersartigen Erkrankungen des Kehlkopfes und der Nase. München. med. Wchnschr., 1887, xxxiv, 729-733.—**Prout** (J. S.) Zaufal's specula. Tr. Am. Otol. Soc., Bost., 1875-81, ii, 275-281. *Also,* Reprint.—**Rastelli** (A.) Nuovo strumento chirurgico per estrarre i corpi estranei dal naso. Raccoglitore med., Forlì, 1887, iv, 97-111, 1 pl.—**Robertson** (W.) Drawings, with the description of an instrument for extracting polypi from the nose. Edinb. M. & S. J., 1805, i, 410.—**Roth**. Ueber die Bedeutung und Behandlung der Nasenkrankheiten. Wien. med. Bl., 1883, vi, 1505.—**Rumbold** (T. F.) A simple mode of cleansing the nasal and pharyngo-nasal passages. Chicago M. J. & Exam., 1877, xxxiv, 385-391. *Also,* Reprint. ——. The importance of making local applications to the nasal and pharyngo-nasal cavities, the pharynx and larynx in measles, scarlet fever, diphtheria and other acute affections, and the means of making these applications. St. Louis M. & S. J., 1878, xxxiv, 264-272. ——. Patent remedies for nasal catarrh. *Ibid.*, 1885, xvii, 17-24.—**Sajous** (C. E.) Glacial acetic acid in nasal hypertrophy. Med. & Surg. Reporter, Phila., 1881, xlv, 729-731. ——. Hydrochlorate of cocaine in the treatment of nasal affections. Med. News, Phila., 1884, xlv, 678-680.—**Schech** (P.) Das Cocaïn und seine therapeutische Verwendung bei den Krankheiten des Rachens, der Nase und des Kehlkopfes. Aerztl. Int.-Bl., München, 1885, xxxii, 771-774.—**Schütz** (G.) Zange für die Operation der adenoïden Wucherungen im Nasenrachenraum. Centr.-Bl. f. chir. u. orthop. Mech., Berl., 1886, ii, 129.—**Schwanebach** (A.) Die Chromsäure als Aetzmittel in der Nase und im Rachen. St. Petersb. med. Wchnschr., 1885, n. F., ii, 410-412.—**Schweig** (H.) A new nasal speculum. N. York M. Month., 1886-7, i, 25.—**Seiler** (C.) A new form of galvano-cautery battery, and a new instrument for the treatment of nasal hypertrophies. Phila. M. Times, 1880-81, xi, 749. ——. Surgical treatment of nasal catarrh. *Ibid.*, 1881-2, xii, 1-4. ——. The therapeutic action of the natural mineral springs of Cresson upon the mucous membrane of the nose and throat. J. Am. M. Ass., Chicago, 1884, iii, 645.—**Shurley** (E. L.) On the abuse of local treatment in nasal disorders. Detroit Clinic, 1882, i, 2-4.—**Sogliano** (S.) Rapporto su la siringa narico-nasale del Cozzolino. Resoc. Accad. med.-chir. di Napoli, 1878, xxxii, 211.—**Spencer** (H. N.) The mechanics of naso-pharyngeal practice. St. Louis Cour. Med., 1879, ii, 1-9. ——. A contribution to the mechanics of naso-pharyngeal practice. Tr. Am. Otol. Soc., New Bedford, Mass., 1884, iii, pt. 3, 298-300. *Also :* St. Louis Cour. Med., 1884, xii, 431-433.—**Steele** (A. J.) A nasal inhaling tube. St. Louis Cour. Med., 1883, x, 570-572.—**von Stein** (S.) Das Cocaïn bei Hals-, Nasen-und Ohrenkrankheiten. Deutsche med. Wchnschr., Berl., 1885, xi, 131-134.—**Stowers** (J. H.) The treatment of vascular hypertrophy of the nose. Brit. M. J., Lond., 1885, i, 68.—**Stucky** (J. A.) & **Brown** (O. F.) Chromic acid and tri-chloro acid in the treatment of hypertrophies of the pharyngo-nasal cavities. St. Louis M. & S. J., 1886, li, 263.—**Swasey** (E. P.) A guarded tenaculum for facilitating the removal of posterior turbinated hypertrophies. Med. Rec., N. Y., 1887, xxxii, 62.—**Swift** (W. J.) A nasal speculum. *Ibid.*, 1885, xxviii, 640.—**Theobald** (S.) Nasal probes. Boston M. & S. J., 1880, cii, 333.—**Thudichum** (J. L. W.) On a new mode of treating diseases of the cavity of the nose. Lancet, Lond., 1864, ii, 599; 628. *Also, in :* Beigel (H.) On the inhalation, [etc.], 8°, Bost., [1867], 11-18. ——. On some new methods of treating diseases of the cavities of the nose. Lancet, Lond., 1868, ii, 243; 307; 534.—**Tillot** (É.) Du catarrhe nasal chronique et de l'ozène; de leur traitement par les douches combinées avec la pulvérisation. Ann. d. mal. de l'oreille et du larynx, Par., 1879, v, 31; 81.—**Verdós** (P.) Insuflador naso-faringeo, de Miot. Gac. méd. catal., Barcel., 1886, ix, 69.—**Warner** (L. C.) Improved posterior nares syringe. Med. Rec., N. Y., 1874, ix, 247.—**Wehmer** (R.) Ueber Nasenkrankheiten, welche mit Schnupfen verbunden sind, unter besonderer Berücksichtigung ihrer Behandlung. Deutsche Med.- Ztg., Berl., 1887, viii, 679; 689; 701.—**Whistler** (W. McN.) General symptoms sometimes produced by nasal sprays of cocaine. Brit. M. J., Lond., 1888, i, 243.—**Zaufal** (E.) Weitere Mittheilungen über die Verwendung des Cocaïn in der Rhino- und Ototherapie. Prag. med. Wchnschr., 1885, x, 57-59.—**Zawerthal** (V.) Sul trattamento di alcune affezioni che interessano lo spazio naso-faringeo. Riv. clin. di Bologna, 1879, 2. s., ix, 11-15.

Nose (*Elephantiasis of*).

See **Nose** (*Hypertrophy, etc., of*).

Nose (*Exostosis of*).

Chantreuil. Exostose celluleuse des fosses nasales. Bull. Soc. anat. de Par., 1869, xliv, 83.—**Cohen** (J. S.) Destruction of an exostosis in the nasal passage by means of the burr of the dental engine. Med. & Surg. Reporter, Phila., 1878, xxxix, 30.—**Colles** (W.) Ivory exostosis of the spongy bones of the nose. Dublin Hosp. Gaz., 1856, iii, 164.—**Collis** (M. H.) Exostosis of vomer; removal by the new operation; immediate relief from the sufferings of years. Dublin Q. J. M. Sc., 1866, xlii, 334-337.—**von Galenzowsky.** Exostosis in der Nase, durch eine verlängerte Trepan-Krone mit Glück operirt. J. d. Chir. u. Augenh., Berl., 1828, xii, 609-622.—**Habermaas** (O.) Elfenbein-Osteom der Nasenhöhle. Mitth. a. d. chir. Klin. zu Tübing., 1884, 2. Hft., 376-380.—**Krönlein** (R. U.) Osteom (Exostosis septi narium). Arch. f. klin. Chir., Berl., 1877, 2. Suppl.-Hft., xxi, 95. — **Legouest** (L.) Exostose épiphysaire cariée occupant toute la fosse nasale gauche, faisant une saillie considérable dans le pharynx et déformant notablement la face; ablation à l'aide de la résection temporaire d'une partie du maxillaire supérieur; guérison. Mém. Acad. de méd., Par., 1865-6, xxvii, 148-156. [Rap. de Gosselin.] Bull. Acad. de méd., Par., 1864-5, xxx, 45-51.—**Lenoir.** Exostose éburnée. dans les fosses nasales. [Discussion.] Bull. Soc. de chir. de Par., 1855-6, vi, 468; 471.—**Paul.** Exostose éburnée des fosses nasales, et de l'orbite; extirpation; guérison avec conservation des fonctions de l'œil. Bull. Soc. anat. de Par., 1858, xxxiii, 107-115.—**Richet.** Exostose cartilagineuse de la cloison des fosses nasales; cas difficile de diagnostic et de traitement. École de méd., Par., 1876, iii, 1-3.

Nose (*Exploration of*).

See, also, **Laryngoscope,** *etc.*

BABER (E. C.) A guide to the examination of the nose, with remarks on the diagnosis of diseases of the nasal cavities. 8°. *New York*, 1886.

———. The same. 8°. *London*, 1886.

GIBB (G. D.) The laryngoscope in diseases of the throat; with a chapter on rhinoscopy. A manual for the student and practitioner. 3. ed. 8°. *London*, 1868.

HASLUND (A.) *Rhinoscopien og dens Betydning for Diagnose og Behandling. 8°. *Kjøbenhavn*, 1875.

JAMES (P.) Lessons in laryngoscopy; including rhinoscopy and the diagnosis and treatment of diseases of the throat. 12°. *London*, 1873.

———. The same. Laryngoscopy and rhinoscopy in the diagnosis and treatment of diseases of the throat and nose. 4. ed. 8°. *London*, 1885.

———. The same. 5. ed. 12°. *London*, 1888.

KÜHN (C. G.) [Pr.] de mechanicis obscuros internarum partium morbos detegendi præsidiis. Pts. i-vii. 4°. *Lipsiæ*, 1825-6.

SCHMIDT (G.) Rinoskopija. Kratkoe rukovod. dlja vrachei i studentov. [Rhinoscopy; short manual for physicians and students.] 12°. *St. Petersburg*, 1886.

SEMELEDER (F.) Die laryngoscopie und ihre Verwerthung für die ärztliche Praxis. 8°. *Wien*, 1863.

———. Rhinoscopy and laryngoscopy; their value in practical medicine. Transl. from the German, by E. T. Caswell. 8°. *New York*, 1866.

VOLTOLINI (R.) Die Rhinoskopie und Pharyngoskopie. 2. Aufl. 8°. *Breslau*, 1879.

Allen (H.) Aids to diagnosis in nasal disease. Proc. Phila. Co. M. Soc. 1880-81, Phila., 1881, iii, 103-105. *Also:* Phila. M. Times, 1880-81, xi, 613. *Also:* Am. Specialist, Phila., 1881, ii, 161.—**Baber** (E. C.) Remarks on examination of the nose. Med. Times & Gaz., Lond., 1884, i, 109-112. ———. Examination of the nasal cavities from the front. Brit. M. J., Lond., 1886, ii, 1152.—**Baginsky** (B.) Die rhinoskopischen Untersuchungs- und Operationsmethoden. Samml. klin. Vortr., Leipz., 1879, No. 160 (Chir., No. 50, 1363-1396). *Also, transl.:* Sovrem. med., Warsawa, 1879, xx, 307; 323; 339; 355; 371.—**Baxt.** Ueber ein neues Rhinoscop und neuen Uvulahalter. Berl. klin. Wchnschr., 1870, vii, 338.—**Czermák** (J.) Ueber die Inspektion des Cavum pharyngo-nasale und der Nasenhöhle durch Choanen vermittelst kleiner Spiegel. Wien. med. Wchnschr., 1859, ix, 518: 1860, x, 257.—**Dauscher** (H.) Beiträge zur Rhinoskopie. Ztschr. d. k.-k. Gesellsch. d. Aerzte zu Wien. 1860, xvi, 593-596.—**Duplay.** Speculum nasi. Bull. Soc. de chir. de Par. (1868), 1869, 2. s.,

Nose (*Exploration of*).

ix, 446-448. — **Duplay's** (Dr.) rhinoscope. Med. Times & Gaz., Lond., 1869, ii, 696.— **Elsberg** (L.) The forceps écraseur for removing hypertrophied nasal tissue. Tr. M. Soc. N. Y., Syracuse, 1883, 276. — **Erichsen** (H.) Die Untersuchung der Nasenhöhle von vorn; Rhinoskopia anterior. Med.-chir. Cor.-Bl. f. deutsch-am. Aerzte, Buffalo, 1883, i, No. 8, 5-8.— **Fischer** (A.) Ein neuer Nasenkatheter zur Auswaschung der Nasenhöhle. Centralbl. f. Chir., Leipz., 1878, v, 561.— **Fränkel** (B.) Zur Rhinoskopie. Berl. klin. Wchnschr., 1887, xviii, 36 - 38. *Also:* Verhandl. d. Berl. med. Gesellsch. (1880-81), 1882, xii, pt. 2, 79-86.— **Grossmann.** Die Rhinoscopie als wichtiger Behelf zur Diagnostik der Ohrenkrankheiten, erläutert durch casuistische Fälle. Allg. Wien. med. Ztg., 1807, xii, 163 ; 173; 183.— **Habermann** (J.) Beitrag zur Untersuchung des Cavum pharyngo-nasale mit den Zaufal'schen Nasenrachentrichtern. Wien. med. Presse, 1881, xxii, 729; 763; 793.—**Hartmann** (A.) Ueber rhinoscopisches Operiren. Berl. klin. Wchnschr., 1881, xviii, 330-332.—**Heymann** (P.) Die Untersuchung der Nase und des Nasenrachenraums. Deutsche Med.-Ztg., Berl., 1884, i, 553; 565. *Also,* Reprint.—**Hodgkinson** (A.) Examination of the posterior nares. Brit. M. J., Lond., 1877, i, 771.—**Jarvis** (W. C.) A new electric light for the diagnosis and treatment of diseases of the nose and throat, with a practical demonstration. Tr. M. Soc. N. Y., Syracuse, 1885, 181-184. *Also,* Reprint.—**Krishaber** (M.) Rhinoscopie. Ann. d. mal. de l'oreille et du larynx, Par., 1875, i, 42; 144, 1 pl. ———. Rhinoscopie. Dict. encycl. d. sc. méd., Par., 1876, 3. s., iv, 382-394.—**Kun** (Z.) Az orrtükrészetröl s annak gyakorlati értékéröl, az orr és fülgyógyászat terén. [Importance of rhinoscopy in diseases of the nose.] Gyógyászat, Budapest, 1880, xx, 113; 129; 145; 164; 186; 211.—**Luc.** Des perfectionnements apportés depuis ces dernières années dans les procédés d'exploration du pharynx nasal. [Rev. crit.] Arch. gén. de méd., Par., 1887, i, 716 - 732. — **Mackenzie** (J. N.) An improved self-retaining nasal speculum. Med. News, Phila., 1884, xlv, 639. *Also,* Reprint.—**Massei** (F.) Contribuzione alla rinoscopia. Resoc. Accad. med.-chir. di Napoli, 1875, xxix, 74-78, 1 pl.—**Roth** (W.) Ein neuer Nasenspiegel. Allg. Wien. med. Ztg., 1875, xx, 389.— **Rumbold** (T. F.) A simple mode of cleaning the nasal and pharyngo-nasal passages. Chicago M. J. & Exam., 1877, xxxiv, 385-391. ———. Nasal speculum. St. Louis M. & S. J., 1885, xlix, 128.—**Schalle.** Ein neuer Apparat zur Untersuchung des Nasenrachenraumes und des Kehlkopfes. Arch. f. Ohrenh., Leipz., 1875-6, x, 128-151, 2 pl.— **Scheff** (G.) Ein neuer Nasenspiegel. Allg. Wien. med. Ztg., 1877, xxii, 303.—**Schlesinger.** Ueber Rhinoscopia posterior. Jahresb. d. Gesellsch. f. Nat.- u. Heilk. in Dresd., 1880-81, 22-25. — **Schnitzler** (J.) Ueber Laryngoscopie und Rhinoskopie und ihre Anwendung in der ärztlichen Praxis. Wien. Klinik, 1878, iv, 271-294.—**Semeleder** (F.) Ueber die Untersuchung des Nasenrachenraumes. Ztschr. d. k.-k. Gesellsch. d. Aerzte zu Wien, 1860, xvi, 289-293. ———. Zur Rhinoskopie; pathologische Fälle; Bemerkungen zur Ausübung des Verfahrens. *Ibid.*, 742-745.— **Thompson** (J. A.) A new nasal illuminator. Med. Rec., N. Y., 1886, xxx, 530.—**von Tröltsch.** Ein neuer Zerstäuber für den Nasenrachenraum und vielleicht auch für andere Höhlen. Arch. f. Ohrenh., Leipz., 1876, xi, 36-40.—**Verneuil** (A.) Exploration de l'espace naso-pharyngien (Untersuchung des Nasenrachenraumes), par M. Semeleder. Gaz. hebd. de méd., Par., 1861, viii, 259 ; 276.— **Voltolini** (R.) Die Besichtigung der Tuba Eustachii und der übrigen Theile des Cavum pharyngo-nasale mittelst des Schlundkopfspiegels. Deutsche Klinik, Berl., 1860, xii, 202-204. ———. Rhinoskopischer Befund bei einem Schwerhörigen. *Ibid.*, 1861, xiii, 410. ———. Zur Rhinoskopie. Monatschr. f. Ohrenh., Berl., 1869, iii, 69 ; 86. ———. Ein Beitrag zum Werthe der Rhinoskopie für die Ohrenheilkunde. *Ibid.*, 1872, vi, 117-119. ———. Die Besichtigung des Bodens der Nasenhöhle und der Tuba Eustachii in face durch Doppelspiegel. *Ibid.*, 1876, x, 109 ; 165. *Also,* Reprint. ———. Zur Rhinoskopie. Allg. Wien. med. Ztg., 1878, xxiii, 117; 129 ; 139. *Also:* Monatschr. f. Ohrenh., Berl., 1878, xii, 27-33. ———. Ueber die Besichtigung der Nasenrachenhöhle durch Doppelspiegel. Breslau. aerztl. Ztschr. 1879, i, 106. *Also:* Jahresb. d. schles. Gesellsch. f. vaterl. Kult. 1879, Bresl., 1880, lvii, 40-44. ———. La luce elettrica adoperata nella nostra specialità e l' uso della cocaina. Arch. internaz. di otojat., rinojat. ed aeroterap., Napoli, 1885, i, 108-111.— **Wales** (P. S.) A new method of controlling the velum palati and enlarging the pharyngo-buccal aperture in rhinoscopic exploration. Med. Rec., N. Y., 1875, x, 785-787. *Also,* Reprint.—**Walsham** (W. J.) On an easy method of posterior rhinoscopy. Lancet, Lond., 1883, ii, 142. *Also, transl.:* Bull. de l'arsenal méd.-chir., Par., 1883, i, 20.—**Watson** (W. S.) On rhinoscopy. Specialist, Lond., 1880-81, i, 4; 45; 59. ———. On some recent improvements in rhinoscopy, and in the treatment of nasal polypi. Lancet, Lond., 1884, i, 335.—**Wertheim** (G.) Die Rhinoscopie des vorderen und mittleren Drittheiles der Nasenhöhle nach einer neuen Methode. Allg. Wien. med. Ztg., 1869, xiv, 167. ———. Ueber ein Verfahren zum Zwecke der Besichtigung

Nose (*Exploration of*).

des vorderen und mittleren Drittheiles der Nasenhöhle. Wien. med. Wchnschr., 1869, xix, 293; 317; 333.—**Zaufal** (E.) Ueber die Untersuchung des Nasenrachenraumes von der Nase aus insbesondere mit trichterförmigen Spiegeln. Arch. f. Ohrenh., Leipz., 1877, xii, 243-281, 1 pl. —. Die Opposition gegen die Untersuchung des Cavum pharyngonasale mit den Nasenrachentrichtern; Voltolini und "sein" Nasen-Speculum. Prag. med. Wchnschr., 1878, iii, 21-24. ——. Zu dem Aufsatze Voltolinis " Zur Rhinoskopie". *Ibid.*, 152. ——. Das mit der Rhinoscopia posterior in der Ruhelage des weichen Gaumens gewonnene Bild des Nasenrachenraums. Arch. f. Ohrenh., Leipz., 1880, xvi, 273-275.—**Zaufal's** trichter or specula. Med. Rec., N. Y., 1878, xiv, 59.—**Zeis** (E.) Beschreibung eines Speculum narium. *In his:* Beob. u. Erfahr. a. d. Stadtkrankenh. zu Dresden, 8°, 1853, 71, 1 pl.

Nose (*Feeding and medication by*).

See, also, **Alimentation** (*Forced*); **Insane** (*Feeding of*).

Delvaux (P.) Observations sur les injections nasales médicamenteuses. J. de méd., chir. et pharmacol., Brux., 1859, xxviii, 145.—**Henriette** (I.) Des injections nasales comme moyen d'alimenter les nouveau-nés et de leur administrer des médicaments. Bull. Acad. roy. de méd. de Belg., Brux., 1852-3, xii, 63-100. [Rap. de Lequime], 3-11. [Rap. de Chassaignac.] Bull. Soc. de chir. de Par., 1852-3, iii, 506-510.—**Moxey** (D. A.) On the administration of food and medicine by the nose when they cannot be given by the mouth. Lancet, Lond., 1869, i, 394; 425. ——. Feeding by the nose in attempted suicide by starvation. *Ibid.*, 1872, ii, 444; 489.—**Nelson** (W.) Medicines administered by the nose. Boston M. & S. J., 1844, xxx, 158-160. *Also:* Montreal M. Gaz., 1844-5, i, 61-63.—**Phillimore** (W.) On feeding the insane through the nostril. Lancet, Lond., 1872, ii, 654.—**Raimbert.** De l'administration des médicaments par l'intermédiaire de la muqueuse des fosses nasales. J. de méd., chir. et pharmacol., Brux., 1867, xlv, 17-20. *Also:* Gaz. d. hôp., Par., 1867, xl, 457. *Also:* Rev. de thérap. méd.-chir., Par., 1868, xxxv, 91-93.—**Rumbold** (T. F.) The means of cleaning and applying remedies to the nasal and pharyngo-nasal cavities. St. Louis M. & S. J., 1873, n. s., x, 476-481.—**Tavignot.** De la cautérisation des fosses nasales dans les opthalmies chroniques. Ann. d'ocul., Brux., 1850, xxiii, 232-235.—**Trautmann** (F.) Pulverisateur für den Nasenrachenraum. Arch. f. Ohrenh., Leipz., 1875, ix, 245-247.—**Zsigmondy** (A.) Ueber die innerliche Application von Medicamenten und Nahrungsstoffen durch die Nasenhöhle. Oesterr. Ztschr. f. prakt. Heilk., Wien, 1855, i, 153-155.

Nose (*Foreign bodies in*).

See, also, **Calculus** (*Nasal*); **Nose** (*Larvæ, etc.*, in).

Alessandro (A.) Rinoraggia causata dalla presenza di una sanguisuga entro la fossa nasale destra di un fanciullo. Raccoglitore med., Forlì, 1873, 3. s., xxiii, 493-497.—**Apolant.** Ueber Entfernung fremder Körper aus der Nase. Deutsche Ztschr. f. prakt. Med., Leipz., 1876, iii, 230; 234.—**Badal.** Névrite optique et otorrhée déterminées par la présence d'un clou ayant séjourné trois ans dans les fosses nasales. Bull. Soc. de méd. prat. de Par., 1877, 55-58. *Also:* Bull. mens. de la clin. ophth., Par., 1877, i, 43-45.—**Bartlet** (J. H.) Foreign body in nasal cavity; removal and subsequent rhinoplasty. Brit. M. J., Lond., 1870, ii, 704.—**Benedix** (J. G.) Fall von zwei Jahre und neun Monate langem Aufenthalte eines Haselnusskerns in der linken Nasenöffnung und endliche Ausstossung desselben während eines heftigen Keuchhustenanfalles. Mag.' f. d. ges. Heilk., Berl., 1826, xxii, 243-247.—**Breschet.** Corps étrangers introduits dans les fosses nasales. Dict. d. sc. méd., Par., 1813, vii, 11.—**Bron** (F.) Des corps étrangers dans les narines. Gaz. méd. de Lyon, 1867, xix, 514. *Also:* Mém. et compt.-rend. Soc. d. sc. méd. de Lyon (1867), 1868, vii, 269-272. — **Bureau.** Observation d'un corps étranger introduit dans les fosses nasales d'un enfant de deux ans et donnant les apparences d'un polype qu'on tenta d'opérer. Mém. Soc. méd. d'émulat. de Lyon, Par. et Lyon, 1842, i, 259-263. — **Czarda** (G.) Des corps étrangers du nez et des concrétions calcaires. Gaz. méd. de Par., 1884, 7. s., i, 580; 591. — **Delavan** (D. B.) Foreign body in posterior nares. Arch. Laryngol., N. Y., 1880, i, 69. ——. A new method for the removal of foreign bodies from the nose. Med. Rec., N. Y., 1886, xxix, 93. ——. Foreign bodies in the nose. Gaillard's M. J., N. Y., 1886, xlii, 36-40. *Also:* Reprint. — **Djakonoff** (P. I.) Inorodnoe tielo v nosovyi polosti. [Foreign body in cavity of nose.] Vrach, St. Petersb., 1882, iii, 290.—**de Dominicis** (N.) Su di un corpo estraneo nelle fosse nasali. Arch. ital. di laringol., Napoli, 1884-5, iv, 11-14.—**Dowler** (M. M.) On the removal of foreign bodies from the nostrils. N. Orl. M. & S. J., 1855-6, xii, 757-759. — **Eve** (P. F.) Case in which a thimble was impacted in the right posterior naris. Am. J. M. Sc., Phila., 1839, xxv, 404.—**Fenn** (C. T.) Foreign body in nose; failure in diagno-

Nose (*Foreign bodies in*).

sis; spontaneous recovery. Chicago M. J., 1871, xxviii, 526.—**Fergusson.** Foreign body in the nostril; removal after twenty years. Lancet, Lond., 1853, i, 473.—**Ferrier** (A.) Corps étranger des fosses nasales; extraction; guérison. Bull. gén. de thérap., etc., Par., 1861, lx, 464-467. — **Fraenkel** (B.) Krankheiten der Nase: Fremdkörper und Concretionen. Handb. d. spec. Path. (Ziemssen), Leipz., 1876, iv, 1. Htt., 160-164. *Also, transl.:* Cycl. Pract. M. (Ziemssen), N. Y., 1876, iv, 172-177. ——. Knochenleiste auf dem Septum narium. Berl. klin. Wchnschr., 1886, xxiii, 396. *Also:* Verhandl. d. Berl. med. Gesellsch. (1885-6), 1887, xvii, 100.—**Gazdar** (S. F.) A case of foreign body in the nose for seven years; persistent neuralgia of one-half of the face; removal of the body; recovery. Indian M. Gaz., Calcutta, 1883, xviii, 341.—**Gross** (S. D.) Case of foreign body in the nose. Med. Times, Phila., 1870-71, i, 318.—**Grove** (J. H.) A necrosed inferior turbinated bone with an attached coffee-grain that had been retained for twenty years. *Ibid.*, 401. *Also:* Tr. Path. Soc. Phila. (1871-3), 1874, iv, 25.—**Gruber** (J.) Ein Fall von Entzündung der Nasen-Rachen-Mittelobrschleimhaut, bedingt durch Anwesenheit eines Kirschkerns in der Nasenhöhle. Monatschr. f. Ohrenh., Berl., 1882, xvi, 121-126. ——. Chronische Nasen-Rachen-Mittelohr-Entzündung. bedingt durch die Anwesenheit eines Kirschkernes in der Nasenhöhle; Entfernung desselben. Aerztl. Ber. d. k. k. allg. Krankenh. zu Wien (1882), 1883, 340-342.—**Guye** (A.) Ein kleiner Forceps zum Entfernen von Fremdkörpern aus dem Ohre und der Nase. Ztschr. f. Ohrenh., Wiesb., 1885-6, xv, 169-172.—**Hays.** Foreign body retained upwards of twenty years in nasal passage. Tr. Coll. Phys. Phila. (1856-62), 1863, n. s., iii, 154.—**Heinrich.** Einfaches Verfahren zum Ausziehen fremder Körper aus der Nase oder aus dem äussern Gehörgang. Wchnschr. f. d. ges. Heilk., Berl., 1851, xix, 28.—**Helbich.** Obce ciala w wydrążeniu nosa. [Foreign body in the cavity of nose.] Pam. Lek. Warszaw., 1829, ii, 80-85 —**Hendriksz** (P.) Belangrijke waarneming van het elfjarig verblijf van een vremd ligchaam in de neusholte. Boerhaave. Tijdschr., etc., Gravenh., 1838-9, i, 197-200.—**Henry** (F. P.) Thudichum's douche in a case of foreign body in the nose. Phila. M. Times, 1872-3, iii, 5t8.—**Hickman** (W.) A steel ring impacted for 13½ years in the naso-pharyngeal fossa of a child; detection by the rhinoscope, and removal. Brit. M. J., Lond., 1867, ii, 266.—**Homans.** Method of extracting foreign bodies from nostrils. Am. J. M. Sc., Phila., 1850, n. s., xix, 73.—**Howard** (R. L.) A large thimble in the posterior nares, which for some time escaped detection. Ohio M. & S. J., Columbus, 1852-3, v, 215. — **Hubers van Assenraad** (W.) Verblijf van eenen levenden bloedzuiger in den neus van een tienjarig kind. Geneesk. Tijdschr. v. Nederl. Indië, Batav., 1859, vi, 251.—**Hunt** (J. M.) Two cases illustrating the diagnosis and treatment of foreign bodies in the nose. Glasgow M. J., 1887, [4.] s., xxvii, 186-188.—**Jorissenne** (G.) Note sur les étrangers dans les fosses nasales et leur expulsion par l'irrigation de Weber. Bull. gén. de thérap., etc., Par., 1880, xcix, 310-320.—**King** (W. S.) Foreign body in the nose; novel plan of removal. Am. J. M. Sc., Phila., 1860, n. s., xxxix, 567.—**Koch** (P.) Contribution à l'étude des corps étrangers des fosses nasales. Ann. d. mal. de l'oreille, du larynx, etc., Par., 1885, xi, 12-14.—**Lalouette.** Observation sur une sangsue avalée en buvant, et fixée pendant trois semaines dans les fosses nasales. Rec. de mém. de méd. . . . mil., Par., 1821, x, 406-409.—**Lefevre.** Nouvel exemple témoignant de l'innocuité des corps étrangers séjournant dans les fosses nasales. Bull. gén. de thérap., etc., Par., 1861, lxi, 130.—**Le Fort** (L.) Couteau introduit dans la narine; difficulté de l'extraction. Bull. et mém. Soc. de chir. de Par., 1879, n. s., v, 710-712.—**Liégey.** Deux cas d'expulsion, par l'éternuement, d'un corps étranger logé dans les fosses nasales. Courrier méd., Par., 1868, xviii, 260.—**Lowndes** (H.) Foreign body in the posterior nares. Brit. M. J., Lond., 1867, ii, 207.—**Major** (G. W.) Removal of a foreign body from the nose seven years after introduction. Canada M. & S. J., Montreal, 1886-7, xv, 649 —**Meyerson** (S.) O niespodzianem znajdowaniu cial obcych w nosie u dzieci. [Foreign body in the nose of a child.] Medycyna, Warszawa, 1884, xii, 712-714.—**Molinier.** Observation sur l'extraction d'un fragment de lame de couteau ayant séjourné pendant quatre ans dans les fosses nasales, à la suite d'un coup reçu dans une rixe; recueillie à l'Hôpital militaire de Perpignan. Rec. de mém. de méd. . . . mil., Par., 1854, 2. s., xiv, 291-293.—**Motherby.** Ein drei Zoll langer Pinsel befindet sich 11 Monate hindurch in der Nasenhöhle. Wchnschr. f. d. ges. Heilk., Berl., 1836, 812. *Also:* Med. Ztg., Berl., 1837, vi, 53.—**Nelson** (H.) A new plan of extracting foreign bodies from the nose. Nelson's Am. Lancet, Plattsburg, N. Y., 1855, 252.—**Noquet.** Corps étranger de la fosse nasale gauche ayant provoqué une rhinite fétide. Bull. méd. du nord, Lille, 1887, xxvi, 414-417.—**Parker** (R.) Case of gun-breech and bolt removed from the nose after five years. Liverpool M.-Chir. J., 1884, iv, 458-460. *Also:* Med. Press & Circ., Lond., 1884, n. s., xxxvii, 303. *Also:* Lancet, Lond., 1885, i, 378.—**Peck** (E. S.) Foreign bodies in the nose and ear, with remarks on

Nose (*Foreign bodies in*).

their removal. Am. J. Obst., N. Y., 1881, xiv, 217-224.— **Pingault.** Observation sur un corps étranger extrait de la narine d'un malade. Bull. Soc. de méd. de Poitiers, 1852, xx, 74 - 76. — **Poynar** (J. S.) Case of ozæna produced by cockle-bur in nostril. Nashville J. M. & S., 1871, n. s., vii, 76.—**Renard.** Lettre sur un pois qui a végété dans les cavités du nez. J. de méd., chir., pharm., etc., Par., 1761, xv, 525.—**Robinson** (B.) Foreign body removed from the nose. Bull. N. York Path. Soc., 1881, 2. s., i, 161.— **Robles** (J.) Manera fácil de sacar algunos cuerpos estraños de las fosas nasales. Rev. méd.-quir. de México, 1883, i, 15.—**Savialles.** Sur une concrétion formée dans les fosses nasales autour d'un noyau de cerise. Bull. Fac. de méd. de Par., 1814-15, iv, 411.—**Sinclair** (A. W.) Removal of a leech from the posterior nares. Brit. M. J., Lond., 1885, i, 1246.—**Starck** (J. B.) Verzwering in den neus door eene zonderlinge oorzaak. Nederl. Lancet, Utrecht, 1843-4, vi, 143-147.—**Stucky** (J. A.) A foreign body in the nasal cavity; removal. Am. Pract. & News, Louisville, 18s7, n. s., iii, 137. — **Témoin.** Des divers procédés d'extraction des corps étrangers de l'oreille et des fosses nasales. Rev. mens. d. mal. de l'enf., Par., 1887, v, 73-77. — **Tiffany** (F. B.) Foreign substance in the nose. St. Louis M. & S. J., 1879, xxxvii, 494.—**Van Derpoel** (S. O.) A case of foreign body in the nose and antrum. N. York M. J., 1887, xlv, 441.—**Walker** (T. O.) A ready method of removing foreign bodies from the anterior nares. Lancet, Lond., 1887, ii, 565.—**Ward** (G. W.) Pin in posterior nares; removal. Arch. Clin. Surg., N. Y., 1876-7, i, 335.—**Warren** (J. M.) Remarkable case of a breech-pin lodged in the nasal fossæ for a great length of time; fissure of the hard palate; operation; cure. *In his:* Surg. Obs., 8°, Bost., 1867, 556.

Nose (*Fracture of*).

See **Nose** (*Wounds, etc., of*).

Nose (*Frozen*).

See **Frost-bite.**

Nose (*Gangrene of*).

See, also, **Aneurisms** (*Aortic, Complications, etc., of*).

Hutchinson. Syphilitic phagedæna of the nose in a pregnant woman (six years after the primary disease); want of success by internal treatment; cure by escharotics; particulars as to the health of the infant. Med. Times & Gaz., Lond., 1867, ii, 649.—**van Loon** (M.) Waarneeming eener volkomene versterving van den neus, als eene scheiding van ziekte. N. Verhandel. v. h. Genootsch. t. Bevord. d. Heelk. te Amst., 1808, i, 301-316.—**Wood** (H. C.) Senile gangrene of the nose; death. Phila. M. Times, 1872-3, iii, 119. *Also:* West. Lancet, San Fran., 1873-4, ii, 19.

Nose (*Hœmorrhage from*).

See **Epistaxis; Nose** (*Surgery of*).

Nose (*Hypertrophy and elephantiasis of*).

See, also, **Nose** (*Tumors of*).

BOSC (A.) * Essai sur les tumeurs dites éléphantiasiques du nez. 4°. *Montpellier*, 1878.

Bickersteth (E. R.) Cutaneous hypertrophy of the nose; removal; cure. Month. J. M. Sc., Lond. & Edinb., 1854, xix, 124.—**Clay** (C.) Case of nasal enlargement successfully treated. Lancet, Lond., 1841-2, ii, 87.—**Cleland** (J.), jr. Hypertrophic rhinitis; its relation to childhood. Am. Lancet, Detroit, 1888, n. s., xii, 42-44.—**Dalrymple** (J.) On the removal of morbid enlargements of the integuments of the nose. Med. Q. Rev., Lond., 1833-4, i, 395-400.—**Doubre** (P.) Éléphantiasis du nez; cure radicale par la décortication. Arch. de méd. et pharm. mil., Par., 1888, xi, 241 - 244. — **Estlander.** Elephantiasis nasi. Finska läk.-sällsk. handl., Helsingfors, 1872, xiv, 63-65.— **Fischer.** Elephantiasische Fibrome der Nase. Tagebl. d. Versamml. deutsch. Naturf. u. Aerzte in Bresl., 1874, xlvii, 216.—**Guérin** (A.) Discussion sur l'éléphantiasis du nez. Bull. Acad. de méd., Par., 1876, 2. s., v, 862-871.— **Guibout** (E.) De l'éléphantiasis du nez et de son traitement. Ann. de dermat. et syph., Par., 1868, i, 135 - 140.— **Hutin.** Observation d'hypertrophie considérable du nez. Bull. Acad. de méd., Par., 1849-50, xv, 582-589. *Also:* Gaz. d. hôp., Par., 1850, 2. s., ii, 201.—**Ollier.** De l'éléphantiasis du nez et de son traitement par la décortication de cet organe. Ann. Soc. de méd. de Lyon, 1875, 2. s., xxiii, 343-370. *Also:* Lyon méd., 1876, xxi, 207; 345; 393; 426. *Also* [Abstr.]: Bull. Acad. de méd., Par., 1876, 2. s., v, 845-858.— **Pauli** (F.) Hypertrophie der Nase. Illust. med. Ztg., München, 1853, iii, 310-314.—**Pollock.** Hypertrophy of the lower end of the nose of the size and shape of an ordinary pear; excision. Lancet, Lond., 1864, ii, 159. — **Poncet.** De la décortication du nez dans le cas d'éléphantiasis de cet organe. Gaz. hebd. de méd., Par., 1873, 2. s., x, 619-621.— **Pooley** (J. H.) Hypertrophy of the nose. N. York M. J., 1875, xxi, 141-143. — **Rizzoli.** Voluminoso tumore elefantiasico del naso; asportazione con esito felice. Bull.

Nose (*Hypertrophy and elephantiasis of*).

d. sc. med. di Bologna, 1876, 5. s., xxi, 81-89.— **Schuster** (H.) Elephantiasis der Nase, combinirt mit plexiformem Neurom und allgemeiner Neuromatose. Prag med. Wchuschr., 1880, v, 201; 216; 221.—**Stein.** Exstirpation af en betydelig Næsehypertrophie og Tabets Erstatning ved plastisk Operation. Hosp.-Medd., Kjøbenh., 1853, vi, 476-487.—**Syme** (J.) Hypertrophy of the nose. Month. J. M. Sc., Lond. & Edinb., 1852, xv, 276-278.—**Wagner.** Monströse Vergrösserung der Nase. Med. Jahrb. d. k. k. österr. Staates, Wien, 1846, lv, 257-270.—**Watson** (W. S.) A case of chronic hypertrophic rhinitis with spasmodic inspiratory snorting. Med. Press & Circ., Lond., 1887, n. s., xliv, 347.—**Woolen** (G. V.) A rare case of hypertrophy and polypus of the naris. Indiana M. J., Indianap., 1887-8, vi, 121-123.

Nose (*Larvæ and insects in*).

See, also, **Frontal** *sinus* (*Foreign bodies, etc., in*).

AUDOUIT (V.) * Des désordres produits chez l'homme par les larves de la Lucilia hominivorax. 4°. *Paris*, 1864.

GORI (T. J. J.) * Over neusontsteking veroorzaakt door de ontwikkeling van vliegenlarven in zijne holten. [Groningen.] 8°. *Breda*, 1876.

DE MELLO DE SOUZA BRANDÃO E MENEZEZ (L.) * Contribuições para á historia do myosis ou bicheiro das fossas nazaes. 4°. *Rio de Janeiro*, 1875.

SALZMANN (J.) & HONOLD (E. C.) * De verme naribus excusso. *Argentorati*, 1721.

In: HALLER. Disp. ad morb. [etc.] 4°. *Lausannæ*, 1757, i, 385-404.

WOHLFAHRT (J. A.) * Observatio de vermibus per nares excretis. 4°. *Halæ Magdeb.*, [1768].

Andrae. Merkwürdige Krämpfe aus seltner Ursache. [Anfälle schwanden nach mühevoller Hervorziehung aus dem rechten Nasenloche eines lebenden, ganzen, sogenannten Tausendfüsslers (Julus terrestris) bei den Fühlhörnern.] Wchnschr. f. d. ges. Heilk., Berl., 1838, vi, 207. — **de Argumosa** (J. R.) Larvas de la mosca de Cayena en las fosas nasales. Crón. méd.-quir. de la Habana, 1875, i, 268-274. — **d'Astros.** Observation sur des vers sortis du nez d'une femme. N. Jour. de méd., chir., pharm., etc., Par., 1821, xi, 233-239. — **Bergmann** (A.) Fliegenlarven in der Mutterscheide und der Nasenhöhle. Med. Ztg., Berl., 1844, xiii, 175. — **Buchanan** (W. F.) Deposition of the ova of the fly in the nasal fossæ; recovery. Phila. M. Times, 1875-6, vi, 57.—**Caréaga** (A.) Nuevo caso de myiasis. Gac. méd., Méjico, 1886, xxi, 89-94.—**Castelli** (G.) Note intorno un caso di presenza di geofili nella cavità nasali dell' uomo. Gior. d. r. Accad. di med. di Torino, 1884, 3. s., xxxii, 349-352.—**Center** (W.) A case of peenash. Indian M. Gaz., Calcutta, 1870, v, 38. — **Chapuis** (J.) Affection parasitaire des fosses nasales. Union méd., Par., 1876, 3. s., xxii, 659.—**Cheatham** (W.) Worms in the nose. Louisville M. News, 1879, vii, 294. — **Clark** (T. N.) Tubercular abscess, opened by "screw-worm". Virginia M. Month., Richmond, 1879-80, vi, 195-198. — **Cochran** (E. G.) An unusual case. Coll. & Clin. Rec., Phila., 1882, iii, 245.— **Coquerel** (C.) Sur un nouveau cas de mort produit par le développement de larves de la Lucilia hominivorax dans le pharynx; description de la larve de ce diptère. Arch. gén. de méd., Par., 1859, 5. s., xiii, 685-691.—**Costamagna** (E.) Storia clinica di una gravissima rinite di natura parassitariæ e suoi effetti morbidi perniciosi locali e generali. Boll. d. mal. d' orecchio, d. gola e d. naso, Firenze, 1883, i, 102-104. — **Curran** (W.) Peenash, alias vermes nasi. Med. Press & Circ., Lond., 1887, n. s., xliii, 217.—**Deakin** (S.) Case of pinash. Indian M. Gaz., Calcutta, 1880, xv, 70. — **Dempster** (F. E.) Lodgment of numerous live maggots within the cavity of the nose and sloughing of the palate, etc. India J. M. & Phys. Sc., Calcutta, 1836, n. s., i, 449-452.—**Diaz** (J. J.) Curacion por el chloroformo de gusanos en las fosas nasales. Rev. méd.-quir., Buenos Aires, 1875-6, xii, 88-90.—**Doss** (B.) Maggots in nose, or so-called vermes nasi. Indian M. Gaz., Calcutta, 1874, ix, 96.—**Fair** (G.) Maggots in nasal cavities. Edinb. M. J., 1860, v, 641.— **Firth** (R. H.) Case of development of larvæ in the nasal passages. Indian M.J., Calcutta, 1886, v, 73-77.—**Fraenkel** (B.) Parasites in the nasal cavity. Cycl. Pract. M. (Ziemssen), N. Y., 1876, iv, 177-181.—**Frank** (L.) Von 48 aus einer Nase abgegangenen Würmern. Med.-chir. Ztg., Salzb., 1815, iv, 157-159.—**von Frantzius** (A.) Ueber das Vorkommen von Fliegenlarven in der Nasenhöhle von Tropenbewohnern, die an Ozena leiden. Arch. f. path. Anat., etc., Berl., 1868, xliii, 98-107.—**Giard** (A.) Note sur l'existence temporaire de myriapodes dans les fosses nasales de l'homme, suivie de quelques réflexions sur le parasitisme inchoatif. Bull. scient. dép. du nord. etc., Par., 1889, iii, 1-11. — **Gibb.** Worms from the nose and frontal sinus. Tr. Path. Soc. Lond., 1863-4, xv, 242.—**Harrison** (C. M.) Maggots in the head. Med. Rec., N. Y., 1885, xxviii, 399.—

Nose (Larvæ and insects in).

Heely (D. C.) Maggots in the nose; a remarkable case. Peoria M. Month., 1884-5, v, 609. — **Humbert** (F.) Catarrh of the ethmoid cells and the frontal sinus and the nasal canal; the cause, deposit of eggs of the screw maggot (larvæ) and their development. J. Am. M. Ass., Chicago, 1883, i, 644-646.—**Jacob.** Affection parasitaire des fosses nasales observée au Mexique; traitement par les injections chloroformées; guérison; expulsion ou extraction totale de 220 larves. Rec. de mém. de méd. . . . mil., Par., 1866, 3. s., xvii, 58-60. — **Jarvis** (N. S.) [Repeated epistaxis or hemorrhage from the nose and adjacent parts, resulting from maggots from the ova of a fly deposited therein while asleep.] N. York J. M., 1847, ix, 315.— **Kilgour** (T.) The history of a case in which worms in the nose, productive of alarming symptoms, were successfully removed by the use of tobacco. Med. & Phil. Comment., 2. ed., Lond., 1787, viii, 75-83.—**Lahory** (T. C.) On peenash, or worms in the nose. Indian Ann. M. Sc., Calcutta, 1855-6, iii, 96-101. Also [Abstr.]: Dublin Hosp. Gaz., 1858, n. s., v, 249.—**Lesbini** (C.) De la calliphore anthropophage, mouche dont les larves ont été observées dans les fosses nasales d'une jeune fille. Acta Acad. nac. de cien. exact., Buenos Aires, 1878, iii, 60-63.—**Littré.** Sur un ver rendu par le nez. [From: Hist. Acad. roy. d. sc. de Par., 1708.] Rec. de mém., Dijon, 1754, ii, 593-595.—**Lublinski** (W.) Ein Fall von lebenden Fliegenlarven im menschlichen Magen, und Bemerkungen über das Vorkommen derselben in der Nase des Menschen. Deutsche med. Wchnschr., Berl., 1885, xi, 771.—**Luck** (J. T.) [Three maggots expelled from the nose of a woman.] Missouri Clin. Rec., St. Louis, 1874-5, i, 68.—**Lyons** (R. T.) An account of a disease of the nose and cranial sinuses, prevalent in the Zillah Rohtuck, in the Punjab. Indian Ann. M. Sc., Calcutta, 1862-3, viii, 55-59.—**Maloët.** Sur un ver rendu par le nez. [From: Mém. Acad. roy. d. sc. de Par., 1733.] Collect. acad. d. mém., etc., Dijon, 1784, vii, 218–220. — **Mankiewicz.** Ueber das Vorkommen von Fliegenlarven in der Nasenhöhle. Arch. f. path. Anat., etc., Berl., 1868, lxiv, 375. — **Mayne** (T.) A case of death by maggots. Indian M. Gaz., Calcutta, 1875, x, 17.—**Mohendra Nath Ohdedar.** A case of pinash. Ibid., 1881, xvi, 80.— **Moriarty** (T. B.) Case of erysipeloid inflammation of nose, the result of irritation set up by maggots in the posterior nares. Ibid., 1877, xii, 263. — **Nicholson.** Case of abscess and ulceration in the nostrils and face, from which maggots were discharged. Madras Q. M. J., 1842, iv, 345–347. — **Ortega Reyes** (M.) Las larvas de las moscas en las fosas nasales ó la enfermedad llamada myiasis. Gac. méd., México, 1887, xxii, 3–16. — **Packard** (J. H.) Accidental entrance of a centipede into the nostril. Med. & Surg. Reporter, Phila., 1878, xxxix, 100. Also: Tr.Coll. Phys. Phila., 1877-9, 3. s., iv, 43.—**Posada-Arango** (A.) Un cas de myase; suivi de quelques réflexious par Viaud-Grand-Marais. J. de méd. de Par., 1884, vii, 260–262. — **Prince** (A. E.) Maggots in the nares. Med. News, Phila., 1882, xli, 445.—**Quinton** (W.) Two cases of larvæ in the human nostril. Army M. Dep. Rep. 1866. Lond., 1868, viii, 529. — **Razoux.** Observation sur une quantité prodigieuse de vers sortis du nez. J. de méd., chir., pharm., etc., Par., 1758, ix, 415-421. — **Roura** (J.) La Lucilia hominivora y la afeccion nasal que produce. An. de otol. y laryngol., Alcalá de Henares, 1883, i, 276-280. — **Rustomjee** (B.) Worms in the nose; cured by turpentine and other injections. [Case.] Tr. M. & Phys. Soc. Bombay, 1860, n. s., vi: 1861, App., pp. xxviii-xxx. — **Schittler.** Larva of eristalis tenax (rat-tail fly) removed alive from the nostril. Phila. M. Times, 1873-4, iv, 349.—**Schmitt** (F. A.) A very extraordinary case in practice: living worms in the nose of a lady. Texas Cour.-Rec. Med., Fort Worth, 1883-4, i, 15-19. ———. Another case of live maggots within the nasal cavity and pharynx. Daniel's Texas M. J., Austin, 1887-8, iii, 46.— **Souza Costa.** Breves considerações sobre a myasis das fossas nazaes, seguidas de uma observação da mesma molestia, colhida no Rio de Janeiro. União med., Rio de Jan., 1881, i, 212-221.—**Stewart** (W. K.) Case of development of larvæ in the nasal passages. Army M. Dep. Rep. 1870. Lond , 1872, xii, 529. — **Stockett** (T. H.) An account of an headache cured by the discharge of a worm from the nose. Tr Coll. Phys. Phila., 1793, i, 181.—**Tomlinson** (A. D.) [Peculiar case.] Cincin. Lancet & Obs., 1872, n. s., xv, 30-32. ———. [Maggots traversed the Eustachian tube and were picked out of the nostrils and coughed up.] Ibid., 166-177.—**Urbanek** (F.) Ein Kuriosum in der praktischen Heilkunde. Wien. med. Presse, 1878, xix, 209. — **Voltolini.** Einiges über Parasiten im Ohre und der Nase des Menschen und der höheren Säugethiere. Monatschr. f. Ohrenh., Berl., 1886, xx, 252; 283.

Nose (Medication by).

See **Nose** (Feeding, etc., by).

Nose (Mucous membrane of).

See, also, **Nerve** (Olfactory).

HOFFMANN (C. K.) * Onderzoekingen over den anatomischen bouw van de membrana olfac-

Nose (Mucous membrane of).

toria en het peripherische uiteinde van den nervus olfactorius. [Utrecht.] 8°. Amsterdam, 1866.

HOYER (H.) * De tunicæ mucosæ narium structura. 8°. Berolini, 1857.

REMY (C.) * La membrane muqueuse des fosses nasales. 4°. Paris, 1878.

RUPPERT (B.) * De tunica pituitaria, exponens ejus anatomiam, physiologiam et pathologiam. sm. 4°. Vetero-Pragæ, 1754.

SEEBERG (R.) * Disquisitiones microscopicæ de textura membranæ pituitariæ nasi. 8°. Dorpati Livonorum, 1856.

SIDKY (M.) *Recherches anatomo-microscopiques sur la muqueuse olfactive. 4°. Paris, 1877.

Arnal (M.) Mémoire sur quelques points de physiologie et de pathologie de la membrane pituitaire. J. hebd. de méd., Par., 1830, vii, 544 – 565. — **Aschenbrandt.** Ueber den Einfluss der Nerven auf die Secretion der Nasenschleimhaut. Monatschr. f. Ohrenh., Berl., 1885, xix, 65–76.—**Blaue** (J.) Untersuchungen über den Bau der Nasenschleimhaut bei Fischen und Amphibien, namentlich über Endknospen als Endapparate des Nervus olfactorius. Arch. f. Anat. u. Entwcklngsgesch., Leipz., 1884, 231-309, 3 pl.—**Bresgen** (M.) Der Circulations-Apparat in der Nasenschleimhaut, vom klinischen Standpunkte aus betrachtet. Deutsche med. Wchnschr., Berl., 1885, xi, 588; 609. Also: Med.-chir. Centralbl., Wien, 1885, xx, 553; 565; 577: 1886, xxi, 2.—**von Brun** (A.) Die Membrana limitans olfactoria. Centralbl. f. d. med. Wissensch., Berl., 1874, xii, 709. ———. Untersuchungen über das Riechepithel. Arch. f. mikr. Anat., Bonn, 1875, xi, 468-478, 1 pl. — **Christmas-Dirckinck-Holmfeld** (J.) Experimentelle Undersögelser over Bygningen af regio olfactoria. (C. r. Recherches expérimentales sur la structure de la membrane olfactive.) Nord. med. Ark., Stockholm, 1883, xv, no 3, 1-18, 1 tab. — **Çisoff** (S.) Zur Kenntniss der Regio olfactoria. Centralbl. f. d. med. Wissensch., Berl., 1874, xii, 690.—**Dogiel** (A.) Ueber die Drüsen der Regio olfactoria. Arch. f. mikr. Anat., Bonn, 1885-6, xxvi, 50-60, 1 pl. — **Hoyer** (H.) Ueber die mikroskopischen Verhältnisse der Nasenschleimhaut verschiedener Thiere und des Menschen. Arch. f. Anat., Physiol. u. wissensch. Med., Leipz., 1860, 50–71, 1 pl. — **Klein** (E.) Contributions to the minute anatomy of the nasal mucous membrane. Quart. J. Micr. Sc., Lond., 1881, n. s., xxi, 98-113, 1 pl.—**Kohlrausch** (O.) Ueber das Schwellgewebe an den Muscheln der Nasenschleimhaut. Arch. f. Anat., Physiol. u. wissensch. Med., Leipz., 1853, 149, 1 pl.—**Martin** (H. N.) Notes on the structure of the olfactory mucous membrane. J. Anat. & Physiol., Lond., 1873-4, viii, 39-44. Also, in: Stud: from Physiol. Lab., Univ. Camb., 1873, pt. 1, 52-57, 1 pl.—**Müller** (E.) Ueber den feineren Bau der respiratorischen Nasenschleimhaut. Verhandl. d. phys.-med. Gesellsch. zu Würzb., 1887, n. F. xx 5-7.—**Paschutin** (V.) Ueber den Bau der Schleimhaut der Regio olfactoria des Frosches. Arb. a. d. physiol. Anst. zu Leipz. (1873), 1874, 41-50.—**Paulsen** (E.) Ueber die Drüsen der Nasenschleimhaut, besonders die Bowman'schen Drüsen. Arch. f. mikr. Anat., Bonn, 1885-6, xxvi, 307-321, 2 pl.— **Retzius** (G.) Om epitelet i membrana olfactoria hos myxine glutinosa. (C. r. Sur l'épithélium de la membrane olfactive de la myxine glutineuse.) Nord. med. Ark., Stockholm, 1879, xi, no. 10, 1-8. 1 tab.—**Sandmann** (G.) Ueber Athemreflexe von der Nasenschleimhaut. Arch. f. Physiol., Leipz., 1887, 483–491. — **Sappey.** Recherches sur les glandes de la pituitaire. Gaz. méd. de Par., 1853, 3. s., viii, 543. — **Tourneux** (F.) Note sur la muqueuse de la tache olfactive chez l'homme. Compt. rend. Soc. de biol., Par., 1883, 7. s., iv, 186.—**Weber** (E. H.) De motu vibratorio in membrana mucosa narium hominis conspicuo. In his: Annot. anat. et phys., prol. v, 4°, Lips., 1838, 3-6. — **Wing** (B. F.) Physiology of the Schneiderian membrane. Med. Mag., Bost., 1835, iii, 692-695.—**Ziem.** Ueber die Einwirkung aromatischer Substanzen auf die Nasenschleimhaut. Deutsche med. Wchnschr., Berl., 1885, xi, 670-672.

Nose (Obstruction of).

See **Nose** (Deformities, etc., of); **Nose** (Diseases of, Complications, etc., of).

Nose (Plastic surgery of).

See **Face**; **Nose** (Surgery of).

Nose (Septum of, Abnormities and deviation of).

See **Nose** (Deformities, etc., of); **Nose** (Surgery of).

Nose (*Surgery of*).

See, also, **Nose** (*Tumors of*).

BENEDICT (T. G. G.) Beiträge zu den Erfahrungen über die Rhinoplastik nach der deutschen Methode. 12°. *Breslau*, 1828.

————. Præmissa sunt collectanea ad historiam rhinoplastices Italorum. 4°. *Vratislaviæ*, 1843.

DU BOIS (J.-B.) *An curtæ nares e brachio reficiendæ? Proponebat Urbanus de Vandenesse. [1742.]
In: SIGWART. Quæst. med. Paris. 4°. *Tubingæ*, 1789, ii, 230-252.

BRAND (A. R.) *De septi narium restitutione chirurgica. 8°. *Halis*, [1845].

VON BRINCKEN (F.) *Beiträge zur Rhinoplastik nach Erfahrungen gesammelt in der chirurgischen Klinik zu Halle. 8°. *Halle*, [1872].

BRUENNER (E. F. G.) *De cutis transplantationibus generatim et de rhinoplastice speciatim. 8°. *Berolini*, 1850.

BUCK (G.) A case of rhinoplastic operation, performed for the restoration of the apex of the nose after it had been bitten off. 8°. [*New York*, 1872.]
Also, in: Boston M. & S. J., 1874, xc, 53-56.

BUSCH (G.) Symbolæ ad rhinoplasticen. 4°. *Bonnæ*, 1858.
Also, transl. in: Arch. f. path. Anat., etc., Berl., 1859, xvi, 20-38, 2 pl.

CARPUE (J. C.) An account of two successful operations for restoring a lost nose from the integuments of the forehead, in the cases of two officers of his majesty's army; to which are prefixed, historical and physiological remarks on the nasal operation; including descriptions of the Indian and Italian methods. 4°. *London*, 1816.

————. The same. Geschichte zweier gelungenen Fälle wo der Verlust der Nase vermittelst der Stirnhaut ersetzt wurde. Aus dem Englischen übertragen von H. S. Michaelis, nebst einer Vorrede vom Ritter Carl Graefe. 4°. *Berlin*, 1817.

CHOMET (J.-A.-H.) *Dissertation sur la rhinoplastie. 4°. *Paris*, 1832.

CLEMENTI (L.) Storia di rinoplastica con nuove modificazioni dell' atto operativo ed osservazioni teorico-pratiche intorno allo stesso. 8°. [*Venezia*, 1840.]
Repr. from: Memor. d. med. contemp., Venezia, 1840, iv.

DAVIES (J.) Case where an operation for restoring a lost nose was successfully performed. 8°. *London*, 1825.

DIEFFENBACH (J. F.) Surgical observations on the restoration of the nose and on the removal of polypi and other tumours from the nostrils. From the German, with the history and physiology of rhinoplastic operations, notes, and additional cases, by John Stevenson Buchnan. 8°. *London*, 1833.

DIPPE (A.) *De nova via rhinoplastices. 8°. *Halis*, 1843.

DOSING (R.) *Ueber Rhinoplastik. 8°. *Würzburg*, 1886.

DROOP (L. H.) *De usu labii superioris in rhinoplastice. 8°. *Halis*, [1844].

EMERICH (H.) *Ueber Rhinoplastik. 8°. *Erlangen*, 1839.

EYERICH (G.) *Ueber Rhinoplastik. 8°. *Würzburg*, 1877.

FREULER (A.) *Conformationis nasi osteoplasticæ duorum speciminum notabilium descriptio. 8°. *Berolini*, [1864].

VON GRAEFE (C. F.) Rhinoplastik, oder die Kunst den Verlust der Nase organisch zu ersetzen, in ihren früheren Verhältnissen erforscht und durch neue Verfahrungsweisen zur höheren Vollkommenheit gefördert. 4°. *Berlin*, 1818.

Nose (*Surgery of*).

————. The same. De rhinoplastice, sive arte curtum nasum ad vivum restituendi commentatio qua prisca illius ratio iterum experimentis illustratur, novisque methodis ad majorem perfectionem perducitur. Latine edidit Justus Fridericus Carolus Hecker. 4°. *Berolini*, 1818.

HAMILTON (J.) The restoration of a lost nose by operation; exemplified in a series of cases. 8°. *London*, 1864.

HAUSLEUTNER (R.) *De rhinoplastice. Accedit tabula, B. Langenbeck nasi curti reficiendi methodum explanans. 8°. *Berolini*, 1851.

VAN HEEKEREN (A. J.) *De operatione rhinoplastica secundum clinici chirurgici Bonensis encheireses. 4°. *Bonnæ*, 1853.

HOERING (C.) *Ueber das Aufbauen eingefallener Nasen. 8°. *Tübingen*, 1837.

KARSTENS (G. H.) *De correctionibus nasi restituti. 12°. *Dorpat*, 1836.

KUDLICH (H.) *Eine neue Methode der Rhinoplastik. 8°. *Zürich*, 1853.

LINDNER (L. H.) *De septi narium restitutione chirurgica. 4°. *Lipsiæ*, [1844],

LUETKEMUELLER (A.) *Rhinoplastices exempla duo. 8°. *Gryphiæ*, 1854.

MAGUIN (M.-P.) *De la rhinoplastie par méthode française. 4°. *Nancy*, 1883.

MENGER (A.) *De operatione rhinoplastica. 8°. *Berolini*, [1864].

MOURE (E.-J.) Manuel pratique des maladies des fosses nasales et de la cavité naso-pharyngienne. 12°. *Paris*, 1886.

NASEMANN (J. A. F.) *Quæstiones de rhinoplastice. 8°. *Halis Sax.*, 1849.

PAUL (A.) *Beitrag zur Rhinoplastik. 8°. *Würzburg*, 1884.

PIERRE (S.) *De l'anaplastie faciale, et de la rhinoplastie en particulier. 4°. *Paris*, 1851.

PIETTE (E.) *Histoire et description de la rhinoplastique. 4°. *Liége*, [1831].

ROUSSET (P.-A.) *Thèse sur la rhinoplastie. 4°. *Paris*, 1828.

SALBERG (G.) *Beitrag zur partiellen Rhinoplastik. [Wurtzburg.] 8°. *Reudnitz-Leipzig*, [1887?]

SCHAFFRANEK (F. G.) *De rhinoplastice. 8°. *Vratislaviæ*, 1847.

SCHMIDT (C. A.) *Ueber partielle Rhinoplastik nach B. v. Langenbeck. 8°. *Greifswald*, 1869.

DE SCHOENBERG (A.) Sulla restituzione del naso. 4°. *Napoli*, 1819.

SCHULTZ (G.) *Quædam ad rhinoplasticen. 12°. [*Dorpat*], 1836.

STAHL (G. E.) [Pr.] de scarificatione narium ægyptiaca. 4°. [*Halæ Magdeb.*, 1701.]

STEFFEN (P.) *Ueber die Verwerthung der Reverdin'schen Transplantation für Rhinoplastik. 8°. *Greifswald*, 1884.

SZYMANOWSKI (J.) *Adnotationes ad rhinoplasticen. 8°. [*Dorpat*], 1857.

TAX (C.) *De septi narium restitutione. 4°. *Berolini*, [1836].

TERRADA (P.) *De la perte du nez et des moyens d'y remédier. 4°. *Paris*, 1833.

THELEN (O.) Ueber Rhinoplastik. 8°. *Cöln*, 1876.

UHLAND (C.) *Ueber anapla-tische Operationen überhaupt, und Rhinoplastik insbesondere, nebst einem gelungenen Falle derselben. 8°. *Tübingen*, 1838.

DE VANDENESSE (U.) *An curtæ nares e brachio reficiendæ? Præses J. B. du Bois.
In: SIGWART. Quæst. med. Paris. 4°. *Tubingæ*, 1789, ii, 230-252.

WEBER (M. I.) Insunt symbolæ ad rhinoplasticen, auctore Guil. Busch. 4°. *Bonnæ*, 1858.

Nose (*Surgery of*).

WELTZ (G. F.) * Ueber die Rhinoplastik. 8°. *Würzburg*, 1843.

Adams (W.) Operation for lateral displacement of the nasal bones. Med. Bull., Phila., 1886, viii. 208.—**Adelmann** (G.) Osteotomie der senkrechten Siebbeinplatte und des Pflugschaarbeines. St. Petersb. med. Ztschr., 1865, ix, 87–91.—**Agnew** (D. H.) Rhinoplastic operation. Phila. M. Times, 1872–3, iii, 120.—**Agráz** (P.) Tumor erectil, congenial de la nariz; extirpacion; rinoplástico por el método indiano; éxito completo sin deformidad. Rev. méd., Guadalajara, 1871, i, 11; 18, 2 pl.—**Allen** (D. P.) Straightening the nasal septum. J. Am. M. Ass., Chicago, 1884, ii, 341.—**von Ammon.** Beschreibung einer gelungenen Rhinoplastik. Mag. f. d. ges. Heilk., Berl., 1830, xxxii, 162–176, 1 pl.—**Arnal.** Rhinoplastie; nouveau cas de succès de cette opération; considérations générales sur son application à diverses autres affections. J. univ. et hebd. de méd. et chir. prat., Par., 1832, 2. s., viii, 57; 87. *Also*, Reprint.—[**Barton.**] Rhinoplasty in a syphilitic subject. Lancet, Lond., 1876, i, 707.—**Bartosh** (D. V.) K uchen. o rinoplastike. Russk. Med., St. Petersb., 1885, iv, 774.—**Batchelder** (J. P.) Rhinoplasty in America. N. York M. & S. Reporter, 1846, i, 333.—**Battlehner.** Ueber die Gestaltung des Lappens, und die Wahl des Ortes, dem er zu entnehmen, bei Nasenbildung aus der Stirnhaut. Amtl. Ber. ü. d. Versamml. deutsch. Naturf. u. Aerzte 1858, Carlsruhe, 1859, xxxiv, 270.—**Baudens.** Cas de rhinoplastic, pratiquée avec succès par la méthode de Celse modifiée. Bull. gén. de thérap., etc., Par., 1854, xlvi, 263–265. *Also*: Gaz. d. hôp., Par., 1854, xxvii, 130.—**Bayer** (K.) Zur Technik der partiellen Rhinoplastik. Prag. med. Wchnschr., 1888, xiii, 77–79.—**Beck** (C. J.) Gelungener Fall einer Rhinoplastik. Heidelb. klin. Ann., 1827, iii, 250–261, 1 pl.—**Bennett** (E. H.) Operation for restoration of the nose. Brit. M. J., Lond., 1878, i, 895.—**Berend** (H. W.) Bildung beider Nasenflügel aus der Nase selbst. Ztschr. d. deutsch. Chir.-Ver., Magdeb., 1852, v, 141.—**Berger** (P.) De l'oblitération d'une des narines produite par la saillie de l'extrémité antérieure du vomer et du moyen d'y remédier par une opération. Bull. et mém. Soc. de chir. de Par., 1884, n. s., x, 390–400.—**Bettman** (J.) A case illustrating the applicability of muriate of cocaine in nasal surgery. J. Am. M. Ass., Chicago, 1884, iii, 598.—**Bigelow** (H. J.) Periosteum of the forehead transplanted in a rhinoplastic operation; no new bone formed; necrosis of the exposed skull. Boston M. & S. J., 1867, lxxvi, 347.—**Billroth.** Rhinoplastik. Allg. Wien. med. Ztg., 1868, xiii, 411.—**Blandin.** Observation nouvelle de rhinoplastie, suivie de guérison. Gaz. d. hôp., Par., 1832, vi, 273. ——. Quelques mots encore sur la rhinoplastie. J. univ. et hebd. de méd. et chir. prat., Par., 1833, x, 403–407.—**Blasius.** Rhinoplastik. Ztschr. f. d. ges. Med., Hamb., 1842, xix, 145–162.—**Bloxam.** Taliacoatian operation. Proc. M. Soc. Lond., 1875–7, iii, 140–142.—**Boeckel** (E.) Réclamation de priorité à propos d'un procédé de résection temporaire du nez. Gaz. méd. de Strasb., 1872–3, xxxii, 2.—**Bœckel** (J.) Rhinoplastie pour un cancroïde de la totalité du nez, de la joue et de la presque totalité de la lèvre supérieure. Gaz. méd. de Strasb., 1880, 3. s., ix, 89. *Also*: Mém. Soc. de méd. de Strasb. (1879–80), 1881, xvii, 107–110.—**Bosworth** (F. H.) Jarvis' operation; its relation to nasal catarrh. Med. Rec., N. Y., 1881, xx, 29–31. *Also*, Reprint. ——. Deformities of the nasal septum; a new operation for their correction, with an analysis of its results in one hundred and sixty-six cases, as throwing new light on the pathology of diseases of the upper air-tract and their relation to the so-called nasal reflexes. *Ibid.*, 1887, xxxi, 115–122.—**Bouisson** (E.-F.) D'un nouveau procédé de rhinoplastie latérale ayant pour but de conserver la régularité du contour des narines. Acad. d. sc. de Montpel. Mém. de la sect. de méd., 1854–7, ii, 171–207, 4 pl. *Also*: Bull. gén. de thérap., etc., Par., 1857, lii, 62; 157; 208; 302. ——. De la suture implantée; rhinoplastie latérale. Monit. d. hôp., Par., 1859, vii, 225–227. ——. De la réparation de l'aile du nez et du contour de la narine; double plan de lambeaux empruntés à la joue et à la lèvre supérieure. Montpel. méd., 1864, xii, 128–136.—**Brett** (F. H.) Rhinoplasticoperation. India J. M. & Phys. Sc., Calcutta, 1837, n. s., ii, 476, 1 pl.—**Brière.** Cancroïdes de la région palpébro-nasale; autoplasties au moyen d'un large lambeau frontal. Année méd., Caen, 1877–8, iii, 124–126, 1 pl.—**Bröer.** Zur operativen Chirurgie der Nase. Breslau. aerztl. Ztschr., 1879, i, 79–81, 1 pl.—**Bryant** (T.) Surgical diseases of the nose. Guy's Hosp. Rep., Lond., 1860, 3. s., vi, 1–11. *Also, in his*: Clin. Surg., 8°, Lond., 1860–64, 77; 87.—**Brydon** (J.) Plugging the posterior nares. Brit. M. J., Lond., 1887, i, 61.—**Buchanan** (G.) Plastic surgery. I. Operation for the formation of a new nose. Glasgow M. J., 1858–9, [2. s.], vi, 43–46, 1 pl. ——. Rhinoplasty from the forehead; the periosteum included in the flap. Lancet, Lond., 1865, ii, 148.—**Buck** (G.) Case of plastic operation for the closure of an opening in the right superior nasal fossa. Med. Rec., N. Y., 1870–71, v, 535. ——. A unique case of rhinoplasty. Med. Rec., N. Y., 1872, vii, 546. *Also*: Tr. N. York Acad. M., 1871–4, n. s., i,

Nose (*Surgery of*).

230.—**Bünger.** Gelungener Versuch einer Nasenbildung aus einem völlig getrennten Hautstück aus dem Beine. J. d. Chir. u. Augenh., Berl., 1822, iv, 569–582.—**Caccioppoli** (D.) & **Sogliano** (S.) Rapporto su la siringa narico-nasale del Dott. Cozzolino. Resoc. Accad. med.-chir. di Napoli, 1878, xxxii, 211.—**Campbell** (C. M.) Case of plastic operation for destruction of nose by syphilis. Lancet, Lond., 1887, ii, 564. *Also*: Manitoba, Northwest & Brit. Columbia Lancet, Winnipeg, 1887, i, 103.—**Canella** (G.) Osservazioni pratiche sulla rinoplastica, ossia l'arte di ripianare la perdita del naso dato dalla natura. Gior. di chir.-prat., Trento, 1825, i, 154; 209; 335.—**Cardona.** Dall'Olmo rinoplasta. Atti Accad. med. di Roma, 1880, v, fasc. 3, 161–197.—**Casselberry** (W. E.) A case of membranous occlusion of the posterior nares, with operations by the galvano-cautery. J. Am. M. Ass., Chicago, 1885, v, 148–150. ——. Pharyngeal and nasal surgery by the galvano-cautery, with a report of a case. Chicago M. J. & Exam., 1886, liii, 333–344.—**Castelnuovo** (G.) Storia di una operazione di rinoplastica. Bull. d. sc. med. di Bologna, 1859, 4. s., xi, 5–29.—**Cereseto** (V.) Della rinoplastica totale, con accenno a un nuovo metodo del Prof. A. Caselli. Gazz. d. clin., Torino, 1886, xxiv, 273–292.—**Chassaignac.** Nouvelle opération pour remédier à un mode particulier de déformation du nez et à ses conséquences fâcheuses. Bull. Soc. de chir. de Par., 1851, ii, 253–260. ——. Résection sous-périostée de la cloison nasale. *Ibid.*, 1870, 2. s., x, 191.—**Childs** (G. B.) Rhinoplastic operation. Med. Times & Gaz., Lond., 1854, n. s., ix, 265.—**Choleva.** Nasenspeculum. Illust. Monatschr. d. ärztl. Polytech., Bern, 1888, x, 28.—**Cianciosi** (A.) Di un caso di rinopatia per lupus exedens, e suo trattamento con l' abrasione e con l' anaplastica. Bull. d. sc. med. di Bologna, 1877, 5. s., xxiv, 65–76, 2 pl.—**Cohen** (J. S.) Hypertrophy of middle turbinated bone treated by galvano-cautery. Coll. & Clin. Rec., Phila., 1883, iv, 1.—**Collis** (M.) A case in which a nose was supplied. Edinb. M. & S. J., 1831, xxxvi, 62–66, 1 pl.—**Costello.** Paper on the formation of artificial noses. Lancet, Lond., 1831–2, i, 699–702.—**Cousins** (J. W.) Rhinoplastic operation after complete destruction of the nose. Brit. M. J., Lond., 1884, ii, 1185.—**Cozzolino** (V.) Deviazioni del setto nasale, delle ossa e cartilagini nasali; loro trattamento dal punto di vista medico e della simmetria del viso. (Ortorinia.) Morgagni, Napoli, 1886, xxviii, 145–160.—**Cripps** (H.) Case of fetid discharge from nose, treated by a new operation. Lancet, Lond., 1877, i, 643.—**Curtis** (H. H.) A new post-nasal cutting forceps; with illustrative case of adenoid tumor. Med. Rec., N. Y., 1885, xxviii, 446. ——. The nasal trephine and its advantages; with a consideration of batteries and electrical apparatus used in nasal surgery. N. York M. J., 1887, xlv, 596–598. *Also*, Reprint.—**D'Ambrosio** (A.) Rinoplastia. Ann. clin. d. osp. incur., Napoli, 1877, n. s., ii, 58. ——. Della rinoplastia totale. Movimento, Napoli, 1877, ix, 1; 17.—**Delpech** (J.) Observation d'opération de rhinoplastique, pratiquée avec succès. Rev. méd. franç. et étrang., Par., 1824, ii, 182–190. *Also, transl.*: Lancet 1823–4, 3. ed., Lond., 1826, ii, 449–453. ——. Observations et réflexions sur l'opération de la rhinoplastique. *In his*: Chir. clin. de Montpel., 4°, Par., 1828, ii, 221; 616, 8 pl.—**Demarquais.** Opération de la rhinoplastie; procédé nouveau. Gaz. d. hôp., Par., 1840, 2. s., ii, 73.—**Demarquay.** Quelques considérations sur la rhinoplastie, à propos de la restauration d'une aile du nez à l'aide d'un lambeau emprunté à la joue, et à la résection de la cloison. Union méd., Par., 1855, ix, 253.—**Demel** (T.) Zur Rhinoplastik. Wien. med.-Halle, 1863, iv, 407.—**Demons** (A.) Nouveau procédé pour la restauration de la souscloison des fosses nasales. Bull. et mém. Soc. de chir. de Par., 1881, n. s., vii, 300.—**De Simone** (F.) Epitelioma del naso; rinoplastia; guarigione. Eco d. osp., Napoli, 1883, i, 129–135.—**Desprès.** Rhinoplastie pour une perte totale du nez. Bull. et mém. Soc. de chir. de Par., 1877, iii, 335–337.—**D'Evant** (T.) Due casi di rinotomia per sarcomi delle fosse nasali. Ann. clin. d. osp. incur., Napoli, 1887, xii, 422–439.—**Dieffenbach** (J. F.) Ueber eine neue und leichte Art der Wiederherstellung der eingefallenen Nasen aus den Trümmern der alten. Mag. f. d. ges. Heilk., Berl., 1829, xxviii, 105–110. ——. Mémoire et observations sur la restauration du nez. J. compl. du dict. d. sc. méd., Par., 1831, xxxix, 162–185. ——. Nouvelles considérations pratiques et observations sur la restauration du nez. *Ibid.*, 255: xl, 25; 254. ——. Heilung der Schiefheit der Nase durch subcutane Knorpeldurchschneidung. Wchnschr. f. d. ges. Heilk., Berl., 1841, ix, 617.—**Dolbeau** & **Félizet** (G.) Rhinoplastie. Dict. encycl. d. sc. méd., Par., 1876, 3. s., iv, 341–382.—**Donaldson** (F.) Personal observations of the value of cocaine in nose and throat surgery. Tr. M. & Chir. Fac. Maryland, Balt., 1885, lxxxvii, 182–190. *Also*, Reprint.—**Doubowitsky.** Observation d'une rhinoplastie pratiquée par . . . Gaz. méd. de Par., 1835, 2. s., iii, 748.—**Douglas** (J.) Case of rhinoplastic operation. Lond. M. Gaz., 1836, xviii, 368.—**Dubrueil** (A.) Rhinoplastic. Gaz. hebd. d. sc. méd. de Montpel., 1881, iii, 349.—**Duke** (O. T.) Case of ablation of the nose and

Nose (*Surgery of*).

partial union after replacing the piece. Indian M. Gaz., Calcutta, 1872, vii, 12.—**von Dumreicher.** Rhinoplastik nach Exstirpation eines Epithelial-Krebses. Wien. med. Wchnschr., 1851, i, 100. ——. Mangel der knorpeligen Nase; Ersetzung des Substanzverlustes durch einen dem linken Oberarme entlehnten Hautlappen. Wchnbl. d. k. k. Gesellsch. d. Aerzte in Wien, 1862, xviii, 411. ——. Operation der Rhinoplastik mit günstigem Erfolge. *Ibid.*, 1863, xix, 382-384.—**Englisch** (J.) Zur Tamponade der Nasenhöhle. Wien. med. Presse, 1875, xvi, 449; 510; 542; 577; 703; 726; 890.—**Erichsen** (J.) Successful rhinoplastic operation. Lancet, Lond., 1852, i, 480. ——. Rhinoplasty; successful result. *Ibid.*, 1853, i, 407.—**Erwin** (R. W.) Rhinoplastic operation. Med. Rec., N. Y., 1881, xix, 172. *Also, transl.*: Repert. méd., N. Y., 1883, i, 239-232.— **Fabrizi** (P.) Opération heureuse de rhinoplastie d'après la méthode italienne, et considérations pratiques sur cette méthode. Gaz. d. hôp., Par., 1841, 2. s., iii, 479; 485. *Also, transl.* [Abstr.]: Gazz. med., Milano, 1842, i, 23-25.—**Farnham** (A. B.) Two principles which should determine when to operate in the nasal passages. N. York M. J., 1886, xliv, 6. ——. A nasal cutting-forceps and bloodless nasal operating. *Ibid.*, 1887, xlv, 578. *Also*, Reprint [of the two preceding].— **Fergusson.** Case of reparation of the nose. Edinb. M. & S. J., 1835, xliii, 363, 3 pl. *Also*, Reprint. ——. Rhinoplastic operation. Lancet, Lond., 1850, i, 419.—**Ferret.** Méningite tuberculeuse consécutive à un simple débridement du canal nasal chez un sujet scrofuleux. Progrès méd., Par., 1887, 2. s., vi, 268.—**Fitzgerald** (P. G.) Case of rhinoplasty. Madras Month. J. M. Sc., 1870, ii, 1-3.—**Fowler** (C. N.) Rhinoplasty. Toledo M. & S. J., 1879, iii, 23.— **Fricke.** Wiederersatz des knorpeligen Thrils eines gänzlich zerstörten Septum narium aus der Oberlippe. J. d. Chir. u. Augenh., Berl., 1834, xxii, 456-463, 1 pl.—**Fritsche** (M. A.) Die prophylactische resp. aseptische Nasentamponade zur Nachbehandlung bei Galvanokauteroperationen. Therap. Monatsh., Berl., 1887, i, 309-302. ——. **Gay** (G. W.) Rhinoplasty. Med. & Surg. Rep. Bost. City Hosp., 1882, 3. s., 292. — **Gellé.** Otite suppurée à la suite du tamponnement des fosses nasales dans l'épistaxis. Bull. Soc. de méd. prat. de Par. (1882), 1883, 40-43. — **Geoffroy-Saint-Hilaire.** Rapport sur un mémoire de M. le docteur Lisfranc. Traitant de la rhinoplastie. J. compl. du dict. d. sc. méd., Par., 1828, xxx, 12-19.—**George** (S.) Gangrene of nose from use of arsenical paste; successful rhinoplastic operation. Brit. M. J., Lond., 1883, ii, 919.—**Glasgow** (W. C.) On rectification of deflection of the nasal septum. Tr. Am. Laryngol. Ass., N. Y., 1881, iii, 117-123. *Also*: Arch. Laryngol., N. Y., 1882, iii, 20-23.—**Gleitsmann** (W. J.) A new cautery-snare for removal of posterior hypertrophies of the turbinated bones. Med. Rec., N. Y., 1888, xxxiii, 315.—**Godrich** (A.) An improved means of plugging the posterior nares. Brit. M. J., Lond., 1873, i, 400.— **Goodwillie** (D. H.) Nasal intubation. N. York M. J., 1888, xlvii, 123.—**Gottstein** (J.) Die temporäre trockene Tamponade der Nase und Herr Prof. Volkmann. Berl. klin. Wchnschr., 1882, xix, 556.—**Gräfe** (E.) Zwey Fälle von Nasenersatz aus der Arm- und Stirnhaut. Med.-chir. Ztg., Salzb., 1817, iv, 269-271. ——. Beitrag zur Rhinoplastik. J. f. Chir. u. Augenh., Berl., 1829, xiii, 153-155, 1 pl. — **Greenhow.** Restoration of the nose. Newcastle & Gateshead Path. Soc. Communicat., Lond., 1852-3, 1-4. *Also*: Med. Times & Gaz., Lond., 1853, n. s., vii, 22.— **Hack** (W.) Reflexneurosen und Nasenleiden; rhinochirurgische Beiträge. Berl. klin. Wchnschr., 1882, xix, 379 - 384. ——. Neue Beiträge zur Rhinochirurgie. Wien. med. Wchnschr., 1882, xxxii, 1445; 1476; 1509: 1883, xxxiii, 93; 128; 184; 213; 278; 307; 348; 405; 438. ——. Beiträge zur Exstirpation der nasalen Schwellapparate. Deutsche med. Wchnschr., Berl., 1884, x, 435; 568.—**Hamilton** (J.) Relation of a case of formation of a new nose; with some remarks. Dublin Q. J. M. Sc., 1857, xxiv, 115-120, 1 pl. ——. Formation of a new nose. *Ibid.*, 1858, xxv, 303 - 309. ——. Amputation of the nose. Dublin Hosp. Gaz., 1860, n. s., iii, 67. ——. The restoration of a lost nose; a series of cases. Dublin Q. J. M. Sc., 1862, xxxiv, 253-265. — **Hamilton** (J. B.) Rhinoplasty; Indian method. J. Am. M. Ass., Chicago, 1887, ix, 752.— **Hamilton** (T. K.) Portions of bone removed from the interior of the nose by Rouge's operation. Australas. M. Gaz., Sydney, 1885-6, v, 120.—**Hardie** (J.) On a new rhinoplastic operation. Brit. M. J., Lond., 1875, ii, 393. — **Hartmann** (A.) Partielle Resection der Nasenscheidewand bei hochgradiger Verkrümmung derselben. Deutsche med. Wchnschr., Berl., 1882, viii, 691.—**Haynes** (F. L.) An easy method of plugging the posterior nares. Therap. Gaz., Detroit, 1886, 3. s., ii, 533.—**Hedinger** (A.) Ueber Rhinochirurgie. Med. Cor.-Bl. d. württemb. ärztl. Ver., Stuttg., 1886, lvi, 249; 257; 265.—**Heidenreich** (F. W.) Fall einer Operation der Rhinoplastik. J. d. Chir. u. Augenh., Berl., 1838, xxvii, 525-531. ——. Ersatz einer ganzen Nase aus der Stirnhaut. Med. Cor.-Bl. bayer. Aerzte, Erlang., 1846, vii, 173-176.—**von Herff.** Beitrag zur Rhinoplastik. Med. Ann., Heidelb., 1848, xiii, 408-416.—**Heusser.** Rhinoplastik. Schweiz. Ztschr. f. Med.,

Nose (*Surgery of*).

Chir. u. Geburtsh., Zürich, 1852, viii, 470-474. — **Heyfelder** (J. F.) Rhinoplastik. Deutsche Klinik, Berl., 1853, v, 554. — **Heyfelder** (O.) Bildung eines neuen Septum nasi. *Ibid.*, 1850, ii, 440.—**Heylen** (J.-B.-J.) Déviation et longueur trop considérable du cartilage de la cloison du nez; résection d'une partie du cartilage; disparition de la difformité. Ann. Soc. de méd. d'Anvers, 1847, iv, 21-23. ——. Opérations de rhinoplastie; nouvelle méthode. [Rap. de Leva.] *Ibid.*, 1854, xi, 425-458.—**Heymann.** Ueber Correktion der Nasenscheidewand. Berl. klin. Wchnschr., 1886, xxiii, 329.—**Hoppe.** Geradrichtung der schiefen Nase. Med. Ztg., Berl., 1858, n. F., i, 101.—**Hueter** (C.) Zur Rhinoplastik. Berl. klin. Wchnschr., 1869, vi, 5-8.—**Hutchinson** (A. C.) Case in which the nasal operation has been recently performed. Edinb. M. & S. J., 1818, xiv, 344.—**Israel** (J.) Eine Methode zur Wiederaufrichtung eingesunkener Nasen. Verhandl. d. deutsch. Gesellsch. f. Chir., Berl., 1887, xvi, pt. 2, 85-89, 1 pl.—**Jarvis** (W. C.) Removal of hypertrophied turbinated tissues by écrasement with the cold wire. Arch. Laryngol., N. Y., 1882, iii, 105-111. *Also*, Reprint. ——. A new operation for the removal of the deviated septum in nasal catarrh. Tr. Am. Laryngol. Ass., N. Y., 1882, iv, 69-77. *Also*: Arch. Laryngol., N. Y., 1882, iii, 300-306. ——. Cocaine in intra-nasal surgery. Med. Rec., N. Y., 1884, xxvi, 654-656. ——. A novel system of operating for the correction of the deflected septum by means of an electric motor, nasal drills, and an original spray-producing device, with illustrative cases. · *Ibid.*, 1887, xxxi, 408-410. *Also*, Reprint.—**Jobert.** Rhinoplastie partielle de l'aile gauche du nez. Gaz. d. hôp., Par., 1853, xxvi, 336.—**Johnson** (J. G.) Complete occlusion of alæ nasi, a sequela of confluent small-pox; operation. Am. M. Times, N. Y., 1860, i, 169.—**Justi** (G.) Indikationen und Anwendung des scharfen Löffels bei Geschwülsten der Nasenhöhle und des Nasenrachenraumes. Wien. med. Wchnschr., 1880, xxx, 1041-1043.—**Keith** (W.) A case of restoration of a lost nose, with some suggestions calculated to render the results of the rhinoplastic operation more satisfactory. Lond. & Edinb. Month. J. M. Sc., 1844, iv, 112-115, 1 pl.—**Kitchen** (J. M. W.) The intra-nasal plug. Med. Rec., N. Y., 1888, xxxiii, 13.—**von Klein.** Ausrottung einer ungewöhnlich grossen Nase. N. Jahrb. d. teutsch. Med. u. Chir., Elberfeld, 1822, v, 1. St., 1-6, 2 pl. ——. Ueber Rhinoplastik. Heidelb. klin. Ann., 1826, ii, 103-107.—**Klose** (C. W.) & **Paul** (J.) Eine totale Rhinoplastik. Ztschr. f. klin. Med., Bresl., 1852, iii, 55.—**Koehler** (L.) Rhinoplastice. Zdanie ... rocznych. w oddz. chir. Szpit. Starozak. w Warszawie (1833), 1834, pt. 1, 42.—**König.** Eine neue Methode der Aufrichtung eingesunkener Nasen durch Bildung des Nasenrückens aus einem Haut-Periost-Knochenlappen der Stirn. Verhandl. d. deutsch. Gesellsch. f. Chir., Berl., 1886, xv, pt. 2, 41-48, 1 pl. *Also*: Arch. f. klin. Chir., Berl., 1886-7, xxxiv, 165-172, 1 pl.—**Königsfeld.** Nasen-Bildung mit gespaltenen Lappen. Rhein. Monatschr. f. prakt. Aerzte, Köln, 1849, iii, 334-336.—**Krieg.** Resection der Cartilago quadrangularis septi narium zur Heilung der Scoliosis septi. Med. Cor.-Bl. d. württemb. ärztl. Ver., Stuttg., 1866, li, 201; 209, 1 pl.—**Küchenmeister** (F.) Mein Rhineurynter und b. Pseudoparasiten. Berichtigung und Zusätze zu No. 25 der "Berliner klinischen Wochenschrift" 1871. Oesterr. Ztschr. f. prakt. Heilk., Wien, 1871, xvii, 537; 557; 569; 585.—**Küchler** (H.) Rhinoplastik. Deutsche Klinik, Berl., 1865, xvii, 451-454.—**Labat** (L.) De la rhinoplastie. Ann. de la méd. physiol., Par., 1832, xxii, 626: 1833, xxiii, 71; 225; 319; 440. ——. De la rhinoplastie; lorsqu'il faut subvenir à l'ablation, ou à-la destruction ulcérative du lobe nasal. *Ibid.*, xxiv, 330-361. ——. De la rhinoplastie lorsqu'il s'agit de rétablir une des parois latérales du nez. *Ibid.*, 506-523. ——. De la rhinoplastie et de la rhinoraphie soit dans les cas d'absence congéniale, ou d'enlèvement accidentel de la partie dorsale du nez; soit lorsqu'il s'agit de remédier à l'enfoncement du dos de cet organe, au defaut de soudure de ses deux parois latérales, et quelquefois enfin à sa division transversale. *Ibid.*, 619-679. ——. De la rhinoplastie; lorsqu'il faut refaire une des ailes du nez. *Ibid.*, 800-820. ——. De la rhinoplastie dans les cas d'absence congéniale ou accidentelle de la cloison du nez et lors de son développement incomplet. *Ibid.*, 1834, xxv, 49; 225.—**La Ferté** (D.) A successful case of rhinoplasty. Med. Age, Detroit, 1887, v, 193-195.—**Landi** (P.) Di una rinoplastica con il metodo indiano per lesioni d'arme da fuoco. Riv. clin. di Bologna, 1868, vii, 1-12, 1 pl.—**Lange** (V.) On the use of the galvanocaustic method in nose and pharynx. Tr. Internat. M. Cong. 7. sess., Lond., 1881, iii, 276.—**Langenbeck** (B.) Ueber eine neue Methode der totalen Rhinoplastik. Berl. klin. Wchnschr., 1864, i, 13.—**Le Bec.** Rhinoplastie par transplantation d'un lambeau cutané emprunté à l'avantbras. Gaz. d. hôp., Par., 1886, lix, 832.—**van Leersum** (W. C.) Waarneming van eenen bijna geheel afgescheiden neus met volkomen verdeeling van het kraakbeenig middelschot, ten gevolge van eene geknensde-gescheurde wond, door de bloedige hechting (rhinoraphia) binnen acht dagen tijds weder volkomen hersteld. Nederl. Lan-

Nose (*Surgery of*).

cet, Utrecht, 1838–9, i, 232–234.—**Leisrink** (H.W. F.) Zur Rhinoplastik. Centralbl. f. Chir., Leipz., 1877, iv, 257–259. ———. Plastische Operationen an der Nase. *In his*: Ber. d. chir. Poliklin. d. Frauen-Hülfs-Ver. zu Hamb., 1872–8, 4°, Hamb., 1879, 22.—**Letenneur.** Cicatrice vicieuse du nez; rhinorrhaphie; guérison. Bull. Soc. de chir. de Par. (1864), 1865, 2. s., v, 380–384. — **Lichtenberg.** Rhinoplastic operations. Proc. M. Soc. Lond., 1872–4, i, 21.— **Linhart** (W.) Beiträge zur Rhinoplastik. Würzb. med. Ztschr., 1860, i, 37–44, 1 pl.—**Lisfranc** (J.) Rhinoplastie; mort. Clin. d. hôp., Par., 1827–8, ii, 285. ———. Mémoire sur la rhynoplastie. Mém. Acad. de méd., Par., 1833, ii, 145–158.—**Liston** (R.) Case in which a lost nose was restored. Edinb. M. & S. J., 1827, xxviii, 220, 1 pl. ———. Operation for restoring the columna nasi. *Ibid.*, 1831, xxxv, 84–89. ———. Reunion of divided parts; reconstruction of the nose. Lancet, Lond., 1834–5, ii, 40–43. — **Löwe** (W.) Rhinoplastik. Ztschr. d. nordd. Chir.-Ver., Magdeb., 1847, i, 674–678.—**Löwenberg** (B.) Instrumente zur Behandlung der adenoiden Geschwülste und Polypen des Nasenrachenraumes. Illust. Vrtljschr. d. ärztl. Polytech., Bern, 1880, ii, 18.—[**Loomis** (A.)] Death following rhinoplastic operation. N. York M. J., 1875, xxi, 44.—**Luc.** Oblitération complète des narines opérée avec succès. Bull. et mém. Soc. de chir. de Par., 1875, n. s., i, 208.— **MacCormac** (W.) On a case of Taliacotian rhinoplasty. Tr. Clin. Soc. Lond., 1877, x, 181–187.—**Macfarlane** (J.) Opération heureuse de rhinoplastie partielle à l'aide de la peau de la joue. Gaz. méd. de Par., 1837, 2. s., v, 285.— **Mackenzie** (J. N.) On removal of the inferior turbinated body of the obstructed side as a substitute for operation on the deflected nasal septum in certain cases. N. Eng. M. Month., Sandy Hook, Conn., 1884–5, iv, 249–251. *Also*, Reprint.—**McReddie** (G. D.) A rhinoplastic operation; recovery. Indian M. Gaz., Calcutta, 1882. xvii, 322.—**MacRury** (C. M.) Rhinoplastic operation. *Ibid.*, 1874, ix, 181.—**Madelung.** Ueber totale Rhinoplastik in mehreren Operationsakten. Verhandl. d. deutsch. Gesellsch. f. Chir., Berl., 1884, xiii, pt. 2, 172–175, 1 pl. *Also*: Arch. f. klin. Chir., Berl., 1884, xxxi, 306–309, 1 pl. *Also* [Abstr.]: Ber. ü. d. Verhandl. d. deutsch. Gesellsch. f. Chir., Leipz., 1884, 36.—**Maiocchi** (D.) Papilloma ulcerato della pinna nasale destra; estirpazione e rinoplastica parziale. Gazz. med. di Roma, 1878, iv, 265–268.—**Maisonneuve.** Destruction complète du nez par la syphilis; rhinoplastie; guérison. Bull. Acad. de méd., Par., 1852–3, xviii, 137–139. ———. Absence congénitale du nez; nouveau procédé de rhinoplastie; guérison. Monit. d. hôp., Par., 1855, iii, 1169. *Also*: Gaz. d. hôp., Par., 1855, xxviii, 569. *Also*: Gaz. méd. de Par., 1855, 3. s., x, 778. *Also*, *transl.*: Assoc. M. J., Lond., 1856, 47.—**Manfred** (H.) A new method of plugging the posterior nares. Cincin. Lancet & Obs., 1872, xv, 69.—**Marie** (L.) Tamponnement nasal simplifié. Union méd., Par., 1876, 3. s., xxii, 292.— **Marx.** Observation sur une restauration du nez pratiquée par M. le professeur Dupuytren. J. univ. et hebd. de méd. et chir. prat., Par., 1833, xii, 29–40.—**Mazzoni** (C.) Melo-rinoplastica all' Antillo per epitelioma del corpo mucoso di Malpighi dell' ala sinistra del naso e della gota; guarigione. Clin. chir., Roma, 1881, vi–vii, 93.—**Mesterton.** Fall af total rhinoplastik. Upsala Läkaref. Förh., 1872–3, viii, 448–451.—**Metz.** Künstliche Nasenbildung. Mag. f. d. ges. Heilk., Berl., 1824, xvii, 325. ———. Wiederanheilung der fast gänzlich getrennten linken Hälfte der Nase. Gen.-Ber. d. k. rhein. Med.-Coll. 1833, Koblenz, 1836, 139.—**Michaelis.** Ueber die Herstellung der normalen Form eingefallener Nasen mittelst des Vorziehens ihres übrig gebliebenen Theiles; ein Beitrag zur Rhinoplastik. J. f. Chir. u. Augenh., Berl., 18:8, xii, 291–325.— **Michon.** Rhinoplastie. Bull. Soc. de chir. de Par., 1854–5, v, 370.—**Mikulicz** (J.) Ueber eine neue Methode der Aufrichtung eingesunkener Nasen. Wien. med. Wchnschr., 1879, xxix, 1201–1206. *Also* [Abstr.]: Anz. d. k. k. Gesellsch. d. Aerzte in Wien. 1879–80, 19–21. ———. Przyczynki do plastycznej chirurgii nosa. Gaz. lek., Warszawa, 1883, 2. s., iii, 429; 453. *Also, transl.*: Arch. f. klin. Chir., Berl., 1884, xxx, 106–118.—**Milhet-Fontarabic.** Une opération de rhinoplastie pratiquée avec succès devant la reine des Hovas sur son premier ministre. Gaz. méd. de Lyon, 1858, x, 257–263. *Also*: Rev. de thérap. méd.-chir., Par., 1858, xxv, 332–336.—**Miner** (J. F.) Rhinoplasty; Talicotian operation. Buffalo M. & S. J., 1871–2, xi, 41–43.— **Minkiewicz** (J.) Brak nosa, uformowanie nowych ust. [Rhinoplasty by a modern method.] Gaz. lek., Warszawa, 1868, v, 65–68. ———. Chetire sluchaya rhinoplastiki v' Tifliskom voennom gospitalai. [Four cases of rhinoplasty.] Med. Sbornik, Tiflis, 1876, no. 22, pt. 3, 1. *Also*: Gaz. lek., Warszawa, 1876, xx, 273; 305: xxi, 17; 56; 71.— **Mirault.** Large ouverture accidentelle communiquant avec l'intérieur des fosses nasales; rhinoplastie par la méthode indienne modifiée; restauration complète de la difformité. Gaz. d. hôp., Par., 1868, xli, 518. *Also*: Bull. Soc. de chir. de Par. (1868), 1869, 2. s., ix, 340–342.—**Mollière** (D.) Procédé opératoire destiné à faciliter la réunion après l'excision partielle du nez. Lyon méd., 1876, xxiii, 405–408. *Also*: Mém. et compt.-rend. Soc. d. sc. méd. de Lyon (1876), 1877, xvi, 176–180. *Also*: Osservatore

Nose (*Surgery of*).

med., Palermo, 1877, 3. s., vii, 47–51.—**von Mosengeil** (K.) Neue rhinoplastische Methode des Aufbaues eingesunkener Nasen durch Unterpflanzung eines Stirnhautlappens. Arch. f. klin. Chir., Berl., 1870, xii, 731–734.— **Moutier.** Contusion du nez; bosse sanguine de la cloison; déformation; appareil pour redresser le nez; amélioration considérable. Année méd., Caen, 1877–8, iii, 88–90.—**Müller.** Eine bei einem Mädchen durch Herpes exedens zerstörte Nase wurde aus der gesunden Stirnhaut mittelst der Rhinoplastik ersetzt, später abermals durch Herp. exedens ergriffen, durch Ol. jecor. assellii geheilt. Med. Ann., Heidelb., 1840, vi, 28–32.—**Mütter** (T. D.) Rhinoplastic operation. Am. J. M. Sc., Phila., 1838, xxii, 61–69, 1 pl.—**Mulhall** (J. C.) Rouge's operation. St. Louis M. & S. J., 1883, xlv, 312.—**Musso** (E.) Distruzione di gran parte del naso; rinoplastia; guarigione. Independente, Torino, 1883, xxxiv, 553–559.—**Nasal** operation. Lancet 1823–4, Lond., 3. ed., 1826, i, 169–174.—**Nasi** (L.) Epitelioma della pinna e parete nasale sinistra; escisione e rinoplastica. Rassegna di sc. med., Modena, 1887, ii, 570.—**Nélaton.** Observation de rhinoplastie. Gaz. d. hôp., Par., 1862, xxxv, 122. ———. Rhinoplastie, méthode nouvelle basée sur le principe des cicatrises adhérentes. *Ibid.*, 1868, xli, 277. — **Neumann** (A. C.) Beitrag zur Rhinoplastik. Wchnschr. f. d. ges. Heilk., Berl., 1845, xiii, 748: 1846, xiv, 398.—**Niessl** (C.) Drei Fälle von Rhinoplastik mit günstigem Ausgange. Oesterr. Ztschr. f. prakt. Heilk., Wien, 1862, viii, 449; 465.— **Nonaka**, Rioichi. [A case of successful rhinoplasty.] Iji Shinbun, Tokio, 1885, no 163, July 15.—**Obaliński** (A.) Przyczynek do operacyi plastycznych wykonywanych w celu podniesienia zapadniętago nosa. [Operation performed to elevate a flat nose.] Przegl. lek., Krakow., 1886, xxv, 141–143. *Also, transl.*: Deutsche Ztschr. f. Chir., Leipz., 1886, xxiv, 197–202.—**Ohm** (H.) Defectus nasi partialis; Rhinoplastik. Deutsche Klinik, Berl., 1854, vi, 289. — [**Ollier.**] Application de l'ostéoplastie à la restauration du nez; transplantation du périoste frontal. Bull. gén. de thérap., etc., Par., 1861, lxi, 510–513. *Also* [Abstr.]: Gaz. d. hôp., Par., 1862, xxxv, 86. ———. De l'ostéoplastie périostique et de son application à la restauration du nez. Mém. et compt.-rend. Soc. d. sc. méd. de Lyon, 1861–2, i, 300–311. ———. Nouvelle observation de rhinoplastie au moyen de lambeaux périostiques et osseux. *Ibid.*, 1862–3, ii, 181–186. ———. Ostéoplastie appliquée à la restauration du nez. Ann. Soc. de méd. de Lyon, 1863, 2. s., xi, 59–64. *Also*: Gaz. méd. de Lyon, 1863, xv, 195–197. ———. De l'ostéoplastie appliquée à la restauration du nez. Gaz. d. hôp., Par., 1864, xxxvii, 349. ———. Un nouveau procédé de rhinoplastie. [Discussion.] Bull. Soc. de chir. de Par. (1874), 1875, 3. s., iii, 184–190.— **O'Reilly** (J.) Rhinoplastic operation. Am. M. Gaz. & J. Health, N. Y., 1857, viii, 68.—**Pancoast.** Plastic operation for the formation of a new nose. Med. & Surg. Reporter, Phila., 1860–61, n. s., v, 509.—**Parker** (F. L.) Case of anosmia, associated with bony stenosis of vomer with contracted inferior meatus of the nose; operation by drilling, followed by improvement in smell. Med. News, Phila., 1885, xlvii, 64–66.—**Paul.** Rhinoplastic operation. Liverpool M.-Chir. J., 1881, i, 183, 2 pl.—**Pauli** (F.) Ueber Rhinoplastik. Memorabilien, Heilbr., 1859, iv, 7–10. *Also*: Verhandl. d. Ver. pfälz. Aerzte 1859, Kaisersl., 1860, 26, 1 pl —**Pereyra** (E.) Sopra la incisione interna nei ristringimenti del canale nasale. Imparziale, Firenze, 1877, xvii, 645–653.—**Petersen** (F.) Ueber subperichondrale Resection der knorpeligen Nasenscheidewand. Berl. klin. Wchnschr., 1883, xx, 329.—**Phillips** (C.) Rhinoplastie. Ann. Soc. de méd. de Gand, 1839, v, 15–22, 1 pl.—**Phillips** (W. C.) The pin operation for deviated septum. Tr. M. Soc. N. Y., Syracuse, 1886, 484–487.— **Poinsot** (G.) Rhinoplastie. N. dict. de méd. et chir. prat., Par., 1877, xxvi, 83–93.—**Polaillon.** Rhinoplastie. Bull. et mém. Soc. de chir. de Par., 1884, n. s., x, 963–965. *Also*: Ann. d. mal. de l'oreille, du larynx, etc., Par., 1885, xi, 1–3. ———. Sur une restauration des deux tiers antérieurs de la voûte palatine et du nez, par le Dr. Delorme. [Rap.] Bull. et mém. Soc. de chir. de Par., 1887, n. s., xiii, 147–149. — **Pomeroy** (O. D.) A case of bony closure of the nostril; removal by the Burr-drill. Med. Rec., N. Y., 1881, xix, 652. — **Poncet** (A.) Abaissement du nez au moyen de l'ostéotomie (procédé de M. Ollier) comme opération préliminaire pour l'ablation de polypes naso-pharyngiens. Gaz. d. hôp., Par., 1872, xlv, 633; 650. ———. De la rhinoplastie sur appareil prothétique. Progrès méd., Par., 1886, 2. s., iv, 878–880. — **Porta** (L.) Nuovo metodo di rinoplastica malare. Mem. r. Ist. Lomb. di sc. e lett. Cl. di lett. e sc. matemat. e nat., Milano, 1877, 3. s., xiii–xiv, 301–311, 1 pl. — **Post** (A. C.) Deformity of the nose, occasioned by the kick of a horse; relieved by a rhinoplastic operation. Tr. M. Soc. N. Y., Syracuse, 1879, 336–340. *Also*: Med. Rec., N. Y., 1879, xv, 389. ———. Rhino-cheiloplasty. Med. Rec., N. Y., 1880, xviii, 17. — **Postempski** (P.) Rinoplastica unilaterale col processo di Burow modificato, e bilaterale col processo Indiano. Gazz. med. di Roma, 1884, x, 101–105.—**Potter** (F. H.) Some general rules which will determine the necessity of an operation in the nasal passages. Buffalo M. & S. J., 1886–7, xxvi,

Nose (*Surgery of*).

443-447.—**Prantl.** Ein Fall von Rhinoplastik. Allg. Wien. med. Ztg., 1865, x, 422.—**Prewitt** (T. F.) Report on a case of rhinoplasty. Tr. M. Ass. Missouri, St. Louis, 1883, xxvi, 141-143.—**Puech.** Observation de rhinoplastic latérale par le procédé du professeur Bouisson. Montpel. méd., 1860, iv, 528-533.—**Puerto** (J.) Restauracion de la nariz y tabique. Observador méd., México, 1876, iv, 29-33, 1 pl.—**Quelques** (De) modifications nouvelles apportées à l'opération de la rhinoplastie. Gaz. hebd. de méd., Par., 1857, iv, 840; 907 : 1858. v, 168.—**Rawdon** (H. G.) Congenital deformity of the nose, with other defects of the face. Liverpool M.-Chir. J., 1887, vii, 289-292. — **Raye** (D. O'C.) Case of operation for the restoration of the nose. Indian M. Gaz., Calcutta, 1867, ii. 271. — **Reverdin** (J.-L.) Greffes de périoste de lapin sur une jeune fille, dans un cas di rhinoplastie partielle. Cong. périod. internat. d. sc. méd. Compt. rend. 1879, Amst., 1880, vi, 430.—**Riberi** (A.) Caso di rinoplastia riuscita al bramato successo mediante una semplice modificazione operativa. Gior. . . . d. Soc. med.-chir. di Torino, 1843, xvi, 385-397. *Also, in his:* Raccolta d. opere minori, etc., 8°, Torino, 1851, ii, 188-197.—**Roberts** (J. B.) A fenestrated cutting forceps for treating nasal obstruction due to deviations of the septum. Med. News, Phila., 1882, xl, 295. ———. Excision of cartilage in nasal obstruction due to deviated septum. Tr. M. Soc. Penn., Phila., 1882, xiv, 233. *Also,* Reprint. ———. The cure of crooked noses by a new method. Coll. & Clin. Rec., Phila., 1884, v, 231. *Also :* Med. & Surg. Reporter, Phila., 1884, li, 467. *Also :* N. York M. J., 1884, xl, 445. *Also :* Boston M. & S. J., 1884, cxi, 369. *Also :* Po'yclinic, Phila., 1884-5, ii, 55. *Also :* Maryland M. J., Balt., 1884-5, xi, 486. *Also :* N. Orl. M. & S. J., 1884-5, n. s , xii, 337 - 340. — **Robson** (A. W. M.) A new plastic operation for deformity of the nose. Lancet, Lond., 1882, i, 140. — **Roe** (J. O.) The deformity termed "pug-nose" and its correction by a simple operation. Med. Rec., N. Y., 1887, xxxi, 621-623. ———. An electric nasal saw. Tr. Am. Laryngol. Ass. 1887, N. Y., 1888, ix, 241-245. *Also :* N. York M. J., 1888, xlvii, 120.—**Rollet** (J.) Restauration de la sous-cloison et de la moitié inférieure du nez, avec la portion moyenne de la lèvre inférieure. Ann. Soc. de méd. de Lyon, 1887, 2. s., v, 158-163. *Also :* Gaz. méd. de Lyon, 1857, ix, 184-186. — **Roser.** Zum Aufbau der eingesunkenen Nase. Illust. med. Ztg., München, 1852, ii, 95.—**Rouge.** Nouveau procédé de rhinoplastie. Bull. Soc. méd. de la Suisse Rom., Lausanne, 1868, ii, 265-268.— **Roy** (G. C.) A successful case of rhinoplastic operation. Indian M. Gaz., Calcutta, 1869, iv, 95. — **Ruault** (A.) De l'emploi de la cocaïne comme hémostatique dans le traitement de l'épistaxis et en rhino-chirurgie. France méd., Par., 1887, ii, 1379-1382. — **Rumbold** (T. F.) Removal of hardened secretions from the nasal passages. Chicago M. J. & Exam., 1877, xxxv, 113-134.—**Ruppius.** Eine Rhinoplastik aus der Stirnhaut, vom herzoglich sächsisch-gothaischen Hofrath. Ztschr. f. d. ges. Med., Hamb., 1837, iv, 243-248.—**Rupprecht** (L.) Ueber die Excision des knorpeligen Theiles der Nasen-Scheidewand. Aerztl. Int.-Bl., München, 1867, xiv, 193. ———. Ueber ein neues Instrument zur Heilung der verkrümmten Nasenscheidewand. Wien. med. Wchnschr., 1868, xviii, 1157-1160. — **Sabine** (T. T.) Plastic operation for restoration of nose. Med. Gaz., N. Y., 1881, viii, 269. ·———. Plastic operations for loss of nose, lower eyelids, etc. Illust. Quart. M. & S., N. Y., 1882, i, 37-40, 1 pl. — **Sato-Su-sumu.** [Successful rhinoplasty.] Iji Shinbun. Tokio, 1884, no. 141, Dec. 5.—**Sédillot** (C.) Rhinoplastie. Ann. de la chir. franç. et étrang., Par., 1844, xii, 291-298. *Also* [Abstr.] : Compt. rend. Acad. d. sc., Par., 1844, xix, 747. ———. Nouveau procédé et observation de rhinoplastie. Gaz. méd. de Strasb., 1856, xvi, 269-274. *Also :* Mém. Soc. de méd. de Strasb. (1856-63), 1864, iii, 78-87. — Remarques sur le procédé de rhinoplastie. Monit. d. hôp., Par., 1856, iv, 723. ———. Rhinoplastie. Gaz. méd. de Strasb., 1857, xvii, 401-405. ———. Note sur la rhinoplastie frontale. Bull. Soc. de chir. de Par. (1862), 1863, 2. s., iii, 496-499.— **Seiler** (C.) Some remarks on intra-nasal surgery. Tr. M. Soc. Penn., Phila., 1882, xiv, 205-212. — **Shurly** (E. L.) The galvano-cautery, compared with other means of destroying the mucous membrane of the nasal and pharyngeal cavities. Tr. Am. Laryngol. Ass., N. Y., 1884, vi, 134-138.—**Sick** (R.) Ueber einige durch Armhaut-Ueberpflanzungen zu Berlin, Breslau und Wilna gemachte rhinoplastische Operationen. J. f. Chir. u. Augenh., Berl., 1828, xii, 630-649. — **Signoroni** (B.) Sulla rinoplastica. Ann. univ. di med., Milano, 1833, lxvii, 225-261.—**Skey** (F. C.) Taliacotian or rhinoplastic operation. Lond. M. Gaz., 1836-7, xix, 542. — **Smith** (A. H.) Excessive hemorrhage from a slight operation upon the septum narium. Arch. Laryngol., N. Y., 1883, iv, 132.—**Spantigati.** Osservazione di lupus volgare in un ragazzo ; rinoplastia applicata alla metà sinistra del naso ; guarigione completa. Gior. d. r. Accad. di med. di Torino, 1879, xlii, 337-339.—**Spear** (J. M.) New method of plugging the posterior nares. Med. & Surg. Reporter, Phila., 1879, xli, 416.—**Spence** (J.) Case of rhinoplastic operation. Edinb. M. J., 1866-7, xii, 330.—**Steinhausen.** Ueber Rhinoplastik. Mag. f. d. ges. Heilk., Berl., 1837,

Nose (*Surgery of*).

xlix, 147-156.—**Störk** (K.) Operationen im Nasenrachenraume. Wien. med. Wchnschr., 1877, xxvii, 474 ; 500.— **Stokes** (W.) Extirpation of the contents of the orbit for lupoid ulceration engaging the eyebrow, eyelids, conjunctiva, and cornea of the right eye ; Indian rhinoplastia performed. Dublin Q. J. M. Sc., 1865, xxxix, 258-264, 2 pl. ———. Modification of Syme's rhinoplastic operation. *Ibid.,* 1872, liv, 442-445. ———. Rhinoplastic operation; new method. Dublin J. M. Sc., 1877, lxiv, 379-387, 4 pl. ———. On the Taliacotian operation. *Ibid.,* 1882, lxxiii, 391-397, 1 pl.—**Storks** (R.) Case of Taliacotian operation. Lancet, Lond., 1843-4, i, 82-85.—**Studsgaard** (C.) Et Par nye Fremgangsmaader ved Rhinoplastik. Hosp.-Tid., Kjøbenh., 1862, v, 45.—**Swalin** (O. A.) Bidrag till Rhinoplastiken. Hygiea, Stockholm, 1840, ii, 241-245.—**Syme** (J.) Preternatural aperture in the nose ; closure by transplanting a flap of skin. Edinb. M. & S. J., 1835, xliv, 5.—**Szymanowski** (J.) Zur plastischen Chirurgie. Vrtljschr. f. d. prakt. Heilk., Prag, 1858, lx, 127-152, 2 pl.— **Taylor** (C. F.) Deformities of the nose ; operation to repair a broken down septum narium. N. York M. J., 1867, iv, 197.—**Telford** (A. B.) Case of rhinoplasty. Lancet, Lond., 1871, i, 607.—**Thiersch.** Ueber eine rhinoplastische Modification. Verhandl. d. deutsch. Gesellsch. f. Chir., Berl., 1879, viii, 67-73.—**Thompson** (H.) Rhinoplastic surgery. Dublin Hosp. Gaz., 1855-6, n. s., ii, 212.—**Tillmanns** (H.) Ueber todte Osteome der Nasen- und Stirnhöhle. Arch. f. klin. Chir., Berl., 1885, xxxii, 677-690.--**Toland** (H. H.) Rhinoplastic operation. Pacific M. & S. J., San Fran., 1863-4, vi, 150, 1 pl. ———. Rhinoplastic operation. West. Lancet, San Fran., 1872, i, 257 - 259, 2 phot. —**Torri** (E.) Storia di rinoplastica eseguita in un soldato privo del naso per lupus scrofoloso. Bull. d. sc. med. di Bologna, 1852, 3. s., xxi, 418-426, 2 pl.— **Travers.** Taliacotian operation for a new nose. Lancet 1823-4, Lond., 3. ed., 1826, i, 175-179.—**Trombetta** (F.) Di un nuovo metodo di rinoplastia parziale, e di una nuova modificazione all' operazione di Gritti, eseguiti sullo stesso individuo con ottimo risultato. Gior. internaz. d. sc. med., Napoli, 1885, n. s., vii, 265-288.—**Tyrrell** (F.) A case of loss of nose from syphilis, and restoration by the Taliacotian operation. Med. Q. Rev., Lond., 1835, iii, 448-457. *Also :* Lond. M. & S. J., 1835, [n. s.], vi, 730-735.— **Verdeil.** Observation sur la restitution artificielle du nez et du palais détruits par la carie. J. de méd., chir., pharm., etc., Par., 1776, xlv, 224-227.—**Verhaeghe.** Restauration complète du nez, d'après la méthode de M. Dieffenbach. J. de méd., chir. et parmacol., Brux., 1846, iv, 15-21, 2 pl. *Also,* Reprint.—**Verneuil** (A.) De quelques modifications nouvelles apportées à l'opération de la rhinoplastie. Gaz. hebd. de méd., Par., 1857, iv, 840; 907.— **Viennois.** De l'ostéotomie bilatérale du nez. Mém. et compt.-rend. Soc. d. sc. méd. de Lyon (1872), 1873, xii, pt. I, 124-128.—**Voltolini.** On operations in the pharyngo-nasal space. (Transl.) Arch. Laryngol., N. Y., 1880, i, 17.— **Van Wageninge** (P. J.) Herstelde neusvorm door de cheilo-rhinoraphia. Nederl. Lancet, Utrecht, 1839-40, ii, 436-442, 1 pl.—**Wakley** (T.) Rhinoplastic operation; favorable results. Lancet, Lond., 1853, ii. 385.—**Walsham** (W. J.) Some cases of deviation of the nasal septum; forcible straightening ; stellar division of the septal cartilage. St. Barth. Hosp. Rep., Lond., 1882, xviii, 11-16. ———. Some remarks on the treatment of deformities of the nose following injury. Lancet, Lond., 1884, ii, 486.— **Walter** (A. G.) Rhinoplastic operation. Med. & Surg. Reporter, Phila., 1859, n. s., ii, 244.—**Ward** (N.) Rhinoplastic operations, with and without chloroform. Lancet, Lond., 1855, i, 9. ———. A case of rhinoplastic operation. Med. Times & Gaz., Lond., 1856, n. s., xii, 385-389.— **Warren** (J. M.) Rhinoplastic operation. Boston M. & S. J., 1837, xvi, 69-79. ———. Taliacotian operation. *Ibid.,* 1840, xxii, 261-269. *Also,* Reprint [of 2 preceding]. ———. Taliacotian operation. *Ibid.,* 1843, xxviii, 69-79. ———. Rhinoplastic operations. *In his :* Surg. Obs., 8°, Bost., 1867, 18-42.—**Wattman.** Ueber verkrüppelte Nasen und deren Form-Verbesserung ; ein Beitrag zur Physioplastik. Beob. u. Abhandl. . . . v. österr. Aerzten. Wien, 1828, vi, 433-472.—**Weber** (O.) Eine ausgedehnte plastische Operation mit Ersatz der Nase aus dem oberen Rande der Stirn und Bildung von drei Augenlidern ; inselförmige Epithelbildungen inmitten einer granulirenden Fläche. Deutsche Klinik, Berl., 1867, xix, 205.— **Weinlechner.** Nasendefect ; Ersatz aus der Wangenhaut und Bildung des Septums aus der Oberlippe. Ber. d. k. k. Krankenanst. Rudolph-Stiftung in Wien (1869), 1870, 255. ———. Partielle Rhinoplastik nach Exstirpation eines flachen Epithelialcarcinoms ; Heilung. *Ibid* (1872), 1874, 113. ———. Verlust der ganzen Nase durch Syphilis ; totale Rhinoplastik ; Heilung. *Ibid.* (1874), 1875, 518-520. ———. Nasendefect nach Syphilis ; Rhinoplastik aus der Stirnhaut ; Umsäumung der neuen Nasenflügel mit den alten ; Gangrän des Septums und eines Theils des linken Nasenflügels ; Reparatur am letzteren und missglückte Septumbildung aus der Oberlippe ; Heilung. *Ibid.,* 520. ———. Totale Rhinoplastik bei einem durch Lupus bedingten Nasendefecte aus der narbigen Stirnhaut ; Septum aus der Oberlippe. Aerztl. Ber. d. k.

Nose (Surgery of).

k. allg. Krankenh. zu Wien (1881), 1882, 235. ———. Schiefstand der Nase in Folge eines in der Kindheit acquirirten Bruches des Nasenscheidewandknorpel ; Geradrichtung nach Excision der vorspringenden Knorpelpartien. *Ibid.* (1885), 1886, 227. — **Weir** (R. F.) On the relief of the deformity of a broken nose, by some new methods. Tr. M. Soc. N. Y., Syracuse, 1880, 273–282. *Also:* Med. Rec., N. Y., 1880, xvii, 279–282. — **Wilkerson** (T. B.) Bony occlusion of both posterior nares; perforation of the septum with the revolving curved trocar; successful. North Car. M. J., Wilmington, 1882, ix, 305–308. — **Woakes** (E.) Cotton-wool as a vehicle for medicating the nasal region. Lancet, Lond., 1880, i, 876. — **Wood** (J.) Clinical lecture on rhinoplasty. Med. Times & Gaz., Lond., 1867, i, 711–713. ———. Secondary rhinoplastic operation. *Ibid.*, 1869, ii, 413. ———. Total loss of nose through disease; rhinoplasty by a new method; successful result. Lancet, Lond., 1870, i, 301. ———. Rhinoplastic operation. Med. Times & Gaz., Lond., 1873, ii, 714. — **Wright** (J.) A modified nasal snare. Med. Rec., N. Y., 1888, xxxiii, 315. — **Wutzer** (C. W.) Rhinoplastik aus der Oberlippe nach einem eigenen Verfahren. Deutsche Klinik, Berl., 1852, iv, 484–488. — **Young** (G.) Obliteration of the orifice of the nose; operation; relief. Med. & Surg. Reporter, Phila., 1887, lvii, 513. — **Zappulla** (V.) Autoplastica del naso. Ippocratico, Fano, 1868, xiv, 423–425. — **Zaufal** (E.) Ueber die Verwendbarkeit der Nasenrachentrichter zu chirurgischen Eingriffen im Nasenrachenraume. Prag. med. Wchnschr., 1877, ii, 5; 25; 49. *Also, Reprint.* ———. Ueber die operative Behandlung der chronischen Anschwellungen der hinteren Nasenmuschelenden. Wien. med. Bl., 1885, viii, 430. — **Zeis** (E.) Ein Fall von Rhinoplastik unter ziemlich schwierigen Umständen. Deutsche Klinik, Berl., 1859, xi, 442. — **Ziem.** Ueber partielle und totale Verlegung der Nase. Monatschr. f. Ohrenh., Berl., 1879, xiii, 1; 22; 55. ———. Delirium und vorübergehendes Irresein nach Operationen in der Nase. *Ibid.*, 1885, xix, 257–262. ———. Ueber Operationen im hinteren Abschnitte der Nase unter Leitung des Fingers. *Ibid.*, 1887, xxi, 212–215. ———. Sehstörungen nach Anwendung des Galvanokauters in der Nasenhöhle. Centralbl. f. prakt. Augenh., Leipzig, 1887, xi, 131–136. — **Zsigmondy.** [Rhinoplastik.] Aerztl. Ber. d. k. k. allg. Krankenh. zu Wien (1870), 1871, 278. ———. † † [Surgery.] *Ibid.* (1877), 1878, 168–173.

Nose (Syphilis of).

See, also, **Nose** (Gangrene of).

CHABOUX (F.) * De certaines lésions de la région naso-pharyngienne que l'on doit rattacher à la syphilis. 4°. *Paris*, 1875.

———. The same. 8°. *Paris*, 1875.

DUPOND (A. - G. - É.) * Étude sur la syphilis du nez et des fosses nasales. (Accidents primitif et secondaire.) 4°. *Bordeaux*, 1887.

MAURIAC (C.) De la syphilose pharyngo-nasale. roy. 8°. *Paris*, 1877.

MOURE (E.-J.) Contribution à l'étude de la syphilis des fosses nasales. 8°. *Paris*, 1888. *Repr. from:* Rev. mens. de laryngol., etc., Par., 1887-8, vii-viii. [*See, also, infra.*]

WAGNER (C.) Syphilis on the nose and larynx. 8°. *Columbus, O.*, 1876.

Andrews. Nécrose nasale, suite d'ostéite idiopathique, attribuée à la syphilis. Presse méd. belge, Brux., 1854, vi, 289. — **Aschenborn** (O.) Destructio septi narium specifica. Arch. f. klin. Chir., Berl., 1880, xxv, 154. — **Castelnovo** (G.) Caso di cachessia sifilitica, con ipertrofia della cute del naso da celtica infezione, felicemente curato col trattamento generale e colla rinoplastica. Ann. univ. di med., Milano, 1862, clxxix, 430, 1 pl. — **Churchill** (F.) Congenital syphilitic necrosis of vomer. Tr. Path. Soc. Lond., 1886, xxxvii, 372. — **Cotter** (R. O.) Three cases of eye, nasal, and throat trouble, illustrative of the importance of recognizing syphilis as a cause in such cases. Atlanta M. & S. J., 1886-7, n. s., iii, 95–98. — **Dietz** (J. S.) Syphilis inveterata mit theilweiser Zerstörung der Nase; Heilung der Geschwüre durch das Dect. Zittmanni und Rhinoplastik aus der Stirn- und Scheitelhaut nach Dieffenbach. Ztschr. f. d. ges. Med., Hamb., 1837, vi, 25–35. — **n Fonseca** (R.) Pro fluxione gallica ad nares. *In his:* Consult. med., fol., Venetiis, 1619, 21–23. — **Gross** (S. W.) Syphilitic ulceration of the nose simulating epithelioma. Phot. Rev. M. & S., Phila., 1871-2, ii, 19–21, 1 pl. — **Gruet.** Gommes ulcérées du nez et du voile du palais; guérison rapide par l'iodure de potassium. Ann. d. mal. de l'oreille et du larynx, etc., Par., 1878, iv, 320. — **Horand.** Syphilide acnéique du nez. Lyon méd., 1887, lvi, 201–210. — **Knode** (R. S.) Specific inflammation of the nose and throat. St. Louis M. & S. J., 1886, l, 25–28. — **Kohn** (S.) A contribution to the study of hereditary syphilis of the naso-pharynx. Med. Rec., N. Y., 1884, xxv, 122. — **Lagneau** (G.) Deux observations de rhino-nécrosie typhique

Nose (Syphilis of).

et de rhino-nécrosie syphilitique. Gaz. hebd. de méd., Par., 1863, x, 439–441. — **Lenoir.** Destruction du nez par suite d'une affection syphilitique. Bull. Soc. de chir. de Par., 1853, iii, 413. — **Lucas** (R. C.) On a case of syphilitic ozæna for which Rouge's operation was twice performed, with remarks on Lawrence's and Rouge's operations. Lancet, Lond., 1883, i, 93. — **Mackenzie** (J. N.) Pharynx and nasal pharynx, syphilitic lesions of the. *In:* Ref. Handbook M. Sc., 8°, N. Y., 1887, v, 629–631. — **Mauriac** (C.) De la syphilose pharyngo-nasale. Gaz. méd. de Par., 1876, 4. s., v, 16; 30; 66; 100; 138; 198; 235; 280; 453; 502; 535. *Continued in:* Union méd., Par., 1876, 3. s., xxii, 497; 533; 582; 671: 1877, 3. s., xxiii, 309; 342; 411; 466; 513; 686; 794; 956: 1030. — **Moure** (E.-J.) Sur un cas de chancre induré de la fosse nasale droite. Rev. mens. de laryngol., etc., Par., 1887, vii, 385–390. ———. Gomme syphilitique de la face interne de l'aile du nez. *Ibid.*, 1888, viii, 1–6. — **Rodrigues Viforcos** (A.) Apuntes sobre las afecciones sifilíticas de la mucosa nasal y consideraciones sobre dos casos notables de coriza y ozena sifilítico. Rev. esp. de oftal., sif., etc., Madrid, 1880, i, 350–360. — **Scarenzio** (A.) Caso di sifilide gommosa al naso, e successiva rinoplastica parziale a doppio ponte. Ann. univ. di med. e chir., Milano, 1887, cclxxxi, 431–435. — **Schuh.** Syphilitische Vegetationen der Nasenschleimhaut. Spitals-Ztg., Wien, 1864, 115. — **Schuster & Sänger.** Beiträge zur Pathologie und Therapie der Nasensyphilis. Vrtljschr. f. Dermat. u. Syph., Wien, 1877, iv, 43, 1 pl.: 1878, v, 211. — **Seidler.** Knochenfrass der Stirn- und Nasenbeine als wahrscheinliche Folge einer vor 16 Jahren bestandenen Syphilis. Med. Ztg., Berl., 1839, viii, 206. — **Tomashevski** (S.) Rhinitis interstitialis chronica syphilitica. Voyenno-med. J., St. Petersb., 1883, cxlvi, pt. 3, 45–82, 1 pl. — **Watson** (W. S.) A case of obstruction to the lachrymal passages, with ozena, due to the syphilitic rhinitis. Med. Times & Gaz., Lond., 1878, i, 58. — **Weinlechner.** Von Lues herrührender Defect des rechten Nasenflügels; partielle Rhinoplastik durch einen Stirnlappen; Heilung. Ber. d. k. k. Krankenanst. Rudolph-Siftung in Wien (1881), 1882, 409. — **Ziegler.** Ein venerisches Nasengeschwür. Taschenb. f. deutsche Wundärzte, Altenb., 1790, 127–131.

Nose (Tuberculosis of).

Cartaz (A.) De la tuberculose nasale. France méd., Par., 1887, ii, 1007; 1020; 1033; 1044. *Also, Reprint.* — **Felici** (F.) Esito raro della rinite cronica scrofolosa. Boll. d. mal. d. orecchio, d. gola e d. naso, Firenze, 1887, v, 121–126. — **Potter** (F. H.) Tuberculosis of the nose, mouth, and pharynx. Buffalo M. & S. J., 1887-8, xxvii, 295–302. — **Riedel** (B.) Die Tuberculose der Nasenscheidewand. Deutsche Ztschr. f. Chir., Leipz., 1878, x, 56–58. — **Schäffer** (M.) & **Nasse** (D.) Tuberkelgeschwülste der Nase. Deutsche med. Wchnschr., Leipz., 1887, xiii, 308–310. — **Sokalowski** (A.) Przypadek owrzodzenia gruźliczego blony sluzowej nosa. [Tubercular ulceration of the mucous membrane of the nose.] Gaz. lek., Warszawa, 1885, 2. s., v, 298–301. — **Tornwaldt.** Ein Fall von Tuberculose der Nasenschleimhaut. Deutsches Arch. f. klin. Med., Leipz., 1880, xxvii, 586–591. — **Weichselbaum** (A.) Ueber Tuberculose der Nasenhöhle und deren Nebenhöhlen. Allg. Wien. med. Ztg., 1881, xxvi, 268; 277.

Nose (Tumors of). [Including nasopharyngeal tumors.]

See, also, **Antrum** (Tumors of); **Artery** (Carotid, Ligature of); **Jaw** (Upper, Excision of); **Nose** (Adenoid tissue, etc., of); **Nose** (Cancer, etc., of); **Nose** (Diseases of, Complications, etc., of); **Nose** (Exostosis of); **Nose** (Hypertrophy, etc., of); **Orbit** (Tumors of); **Rhinoscleroma.**

ALBRECHT (E. G.) * De polypis narium. 8°. *Halis Sax.*, [1855].

ARNDT (H. R.) * De specimine quodam polypi narium fauciumque. 8°. *Berolini*, [1859].

AZEVEDO (A. J. de S.) * Dos polypos nasopharyngeanos. 4°. *Rio de Janeiro*, 1875.

BAUDRIMONT (É.) * De la méthode nasale dans le traitement des polypes nasopharyngiens. 4°. *Paris*, 1869.

BEAUSSENAT (S.) * Des tumeurs sanguines et purulentes de la cloison des fosses nasales. 4°. *Paris*, 1864.

BELOT (J.) * Essai sur une opération de polype naso-pharyngien par la ligature extemporanée. 4°. *Montpellier*, 1876.

BENSCH (H.) * Beiträge zur Beurtheilung der chirurgischen Behandlung der Nasenrachenpolypen. 8°. *Berlin*, 1877.

Nose (*Tumors of*).

BERTON (C.) * Contribution à l'étude histologique des polypes muqueux des fosses nasales. 4°. *Paris*, 1887.

BEUF (J.-H.) * Des polypes fibreux de la base du crâne (dits naso-pharyngiens), et de leur traitement par la résection de la voûte palatine. 4°. *Paris*, 1857.

BLUMENTHAL (E.) * Ueber die Schleimgeschwülste des Clivus Blumenbachii. 8°. *Göttingen*, 1869.

BŒDDICKER (J.) * De polypis narium. 8°. *Berolini*, 1844.

BRAUN (S.) * De polypo narium aquoso. 4°. *Tubingæ*, 1688.

DE BRETTES (H.-J.-B.) * II. Les symptômes et le traitement des polypes fibreux des fosses nasales. III. [etc.] 4°. *Paris*, 1840.

BREVET (F.) * Des polypes naso-pharyngiens. 4°. *Paris*, 1855.

BRUSLÉ (H.) * De la guérison de certains polypes naso-pharyngiens par les méthodes palliatives et lentes. 4°. *Paris*, 1879.

CALIGNON (E.) * De l'extirpation des polypes naso-pharyngiens sans opération préalable. 4°. *Lyon*, 1879.

CORNEVIN (F.-I.) * Des polypes des fosses nasales et de leur traitement. 4°. *Paris*, 1835.

DALEN (C.) * De narium polypo. 4°. *Lugd. Bat.*, 1790.

DEBRIE (E.) * Des polypes fibro-angiomateux de la région naso-pharyngienne. 4°. *Paris*, 1882.

DEGAIL (A.) * Contribution à l'étude des polypes fibro-muqueux de l'arrière-cavité des fosses nasales. 4°. *Paris*, 1885.

DELAUX (É.) * Contribution à l'étude des sarcomes des fosses nasales. 4°. *Amiens*, 1883.

DELORT (P.-O.) * Considérations sur les opérations que nécessitent les polypes naso-pharyngiens. 4°. *Strasbourg*, 1863.

DELPHY (P.) * Quelques considérations sur les polypes naso-pharyngiens et sur leur traitement par la méthode nasale. 4°. *Montpellier*, 1877.

DE ROSSI (E.) I polipi fibrosi naso-faringei e l'elettrolisi faringo-rinoscopica. 8°. *Roma*, 1880.

DESPREZ (M.-E.) * Des polypes nasaux et naso-pharyngiens, et de leur traitement par un nouveau procédé opératoire. 4°. *Paris*, 1857.

DIERICH (C.) * De polypis naso-pharyngeis eorumque operationibus. 8°. *Vratislaviæ*, [1861].

DIGUET (P.-G.-L.) * Diss. sur les polypes du nez et de la gorge. 4°. *Paris, an XIII* [1805].

D'ORNELLAS (A.-E.) * Anatomie pathologique et traitement des polypes fibreux de la base du crâne, dits naso-pharyngiens. 4°. *Paris*, 1854.

DUC (A.) * Étude des procédés de résection temporaire du maxillaire supérieur pour l'extraction des polypes naso-pharyngiens. 4°. *Paris*, 1872.

ENCINAS (S. G.) Dos historias clínicas y dos operaciones de pólipos naso-faríngeos con dos trasfusiones de sangre. 8°. *Madrid*, 1878.

FERREIRA DE LEMOS (L.-G.) * Quelques considérations sur la thérapeutique des polypes naso-pharyngiens. 4°. *Paris*, 1865.

FOUILLOUX (C.-C.-J.) * De l'incision du voile du palais, comme opération préliminaire à l'extirpation des polypes naso-pharyngiens. Recherches historiques sur l'opération de Manne d'Avignon. 4°. *Paris*, 1858.

DE GANDT (C.) * Sur le diagnostic différentiel des polypes fibreux naso-pharyngiens. 4°. *Paris*, 1866.

Nose (*Tumors of*).

GAUBERT (F.) * Sur les ostéomes de l'organe de l'olfaction. 4°. *Paris*, 1869.

GEHIN (G.) * Des polypes fibro-muqueux de l'arrière cavité des fosses nasales. 4°. *Nancy*, 1882.

GÉRAUD (P.) * I. Quels sont les symptômes et le traitement des polypes fibreux des fosses nasales et du pharynx? II. [etc.] 4°. *Paris*, 1839.

GLANDORPIUS (M.) Tractatus de polypo narium affectu gravissimo observationibus illustratus. 4°. *Londini*, 1729.

GOSSELIN (L.) * Traitement chirurgical des polypes des fosses nasales et du pharynx. 4°. *Paris*, 1850.

GRUBE (G.) * De tumoribus quibusdam benignis in nasi superficie obviis eamque deformantibus. 8°. *Dorpat*, 1850.

GRUNER (G. F.) * De polypis in cavo narium obviis, adjecti morbi historia et cadaveris sectione. 4°. *Lipsiæ*, [1825].

GUETTARD (J. S.) * An a ligatura polypi narium tutior curatio?

In: SIGWART (G. F.) Quæst. med. Paris. 4°. *Tubingæ*, 1789, ii, 206-215.

GUICHET (A.) * Étude sur les polypes muqueux des arrière-narines. 4°. *Paris*, 1874.

HESSE (J. C.) * De polypo narium. 4°. *Argentorati*, [1777].

HUETHE (J. A.) * De polypis narium fauciumque et antri Highmori eorumque exstirpatione, resecto processu nasali maxillæ superioris. 8°. *Regimonti Pr.*, 1861.

JANUS (J. E.) * De polypo narium. 4°. *Lipsiæ*, [1672].

JOHN (T.) * De polypis narium eorumque diversis operandi methodis. 8°. *Vratislaviæ*, 1855.

KOEPPE (M.) De hæmatomate cartilaginum nasi (rhinæmatomate) ex permutationibus læsionibusque telæ cartilagineæ vel ex perichondritide nasali orto. 4°. *Halis Sax.*, 1869.

KÜHN (A.) * De tumoribus narium sarcomatosis. 8°. *Vratislaviæ*, [1835].

KÜHN (C. G.) [Pr.] nonnullarum, quibus polypi narium exstirpari solent, methodorum dijudicatio. Part. I-IV. 4°. [*Lipsiæ*, 1815-16.] Also, in his: Opusc. acad. med. 8°. *Lips.*, 1827, i, 376-404.

KUENEMANN (F.) * Quelques considérations sur les polypes muqueux des fosses nasales et de leur traitement. 4°. *Paris*, 1872.

LACROIX (J.-C.) * Sur les polypes des fosses nasales. 8°. *Paris, an X* [1802].

LÉMERÉ (E.) * Étude sur les accidents consécutifs à l'arrachement des polypes des fosses nasales. 4°. *Paris*, 1877.

LENHARTZ (G.) * Die Nasen-Rachen-Polypen und ihre operative Beseitigung. 8°. *Berlin*, [1873].

LEVRET (A.) Observations sur la cure radicale de plusieurs polypes de la matrice, de la gorge et du nez, opérée par de nouveaux moyens inventés par... 8°. *Paris*, 1749.

———. The same. 2. éd. 12°. *Paris*, 1759.

———. The same. 3. éd. 8°. *Paris*, 1771.

LOHSEE (C. G.) * De tumoribus in cavo narium et pharyngis obviis, qui polypi dicuntur. 8°. *Gryphiæ*, 1852.

MATHIEU (E.) * Sur les polypes muqueux des arrières-narines. 4°. *Paris*, 1875.

MONTANO (J.) * Note sur une opération de polype naso-pharyngien par la galvanocaustie physique. 4°. *Paris*, 1872.

Also, in: Gaz. méd. chir. de Toulouse, 1879, xi, 273; 281: 1880, xii, 1.

MUELLER (J.) * De cavi narium carcinomatibus, scirrho atque fungo medullari. Addita est

Nose (*Tumors of*).

historia morbi mollis sarcomatis in hac regione observati. 8°. *Gryphiæ*, 1861.

MUZEAU (C.-A.) * De l'ostéotomie verticale bilatérale du nez pour la cure des polypes naso-pharyngiens. 4°. *Montpellier*, 1866.

NOEGGERATH (ÆE. J.) * Spicilegium casuum nonnullorum polypi nasi et pharyngis qui in clinico chirurgico Bonnensi novissimis annis observati sunt, addita descriptione methodi novæ ad exstirpandum polypum pharyngis. 8°. *Bonnæ*, 1852.

NOLL (F.) * Ueber die Behandlung der Nasen-Rachenpolypen durch temporäre Resectionen am Oberkiefer. 8°. *Tübingen*, 1879.

[PALLUCCI (N. J.)] Ratio facilis atque tuta narium curandi polypos. 8°. *Viennæ*, 1763.

PETIT (N.-A.) * De quelques considérations sur les polypes naso-pharyngiens et leur propagation au cerveau. 4°. *Paris*, 1881.

PETITRADEL (A.) * Considérations sur les polypes des fosses nasales, et les moyens auxquels jusqu'ici on a eu recours pour leur guérison. 4°. *Paris*, 1815.

POSTEL (C.-É.) * Des polypes nasopharyngiens. 4°. *Paris*, 1867.

PUGLIESE (F.) * Sur les adénomes des fosses nasales. 4°. *Paris*, 1862.

ROBIN-MASSÉ (A.-G.) * Des polypes naso-pharyngiens au point de vue de leur traitement. 4°. *Paris*, 1864.

———. The same. 8°. *Paris*, 1864.

ROUGET (A.-D.) * Sur le polype nasal, et particulièrement sur celui qui se développe dans le sinus maxillaire. 4°. *Paris*, 1806.

DE SAINT-AMAND (A.-E.) * Observations sur l'emploi des caustiques dans le traitement des polypes vésiculaires des narines et de quelques maladies de la peau. 4°. *Paris*, 1825.

SAMONDÈS (L.) * Du temps d'arrêt dans la marche des polypes naso-pharyngiens. 4°. *Paris*, 1878.

———. The same. 8°. *Paris*, 1878.

SCHENK (C.) * Die Nasenrachenpolypen und deren operative Behandlung. 8°. *Lippstadt*, 1885.

SCHULTHEISS (G. H.) * Duo tumorum nasalium casus. 8°. *Halæ*, [1844].

SCHUMACHER (G.) * De polyporum narium fauciumque et antri Highmori exstirpatione. 8°. *Regimontii Pr.*, 1862.

SERGENT (A.) * Contributions à l'étude du traitement de certaines tumeurs nasales. 4°. *Paris*, 1881.

SPREAFICO Y GARCIA (J.) * Traitement des tumeurs des fosses nasales au moyen de l'abaissement du nez par l'ostéotomie verticale et bilatérale de la charpente de cet organe. 4°. *Lyon*, 1882.

STOELLING (G. C. C.) * De polypis narium. 4°. *Vitebergæ*, [1802].

TOWNSEND (P. S.) Case of three remarkable tumours extirpated from the nose. 8°. *New York*, 1825.

VAUTHIER (J.-B.-C.) * De la résection de la voûte palatine, dans le traitement des polypes fibreux naso-pharyngiens. 4°. *Paris*, 1854.

VEILLON (F.-T.) * Contribution à l'étude des tumeurs malignes naso-pharyngiennes. 4°. *Paris*, 1874.

VIGOT (A.) * Des polypes fibro-muqueux de la cavité naso-pharyngienne. 4°. *Paris*, 1883.

WAGNER (F. L.) * De polypis narium et antri maxillaris novaque ipsos exstirpandi methodo. 4°. *Vratislaviæ*, 1821.

WAGNER (M.) * Ueber die operative Behandlung der Naso-Pharyngealtumoren. 8°. *Jena*, 1873.

Nose (*Tumors of*).

WEBER (E.) * De l'incision transversale du voile du palais comme opération préliminaire pour l'extirpation des polypes naso-pharyngiens. 8°. *Strasbourg*, 1884.

WHATELY (T.) Cases of two extraordinary polypi removed from the nose, the one by excision with a new instrument, the other by improved forceps; with an appendix, describing an improved instrument for the fistula in ano, with observations on that disease. 8°. *London*, 1805.

WOAKES (E.) Nasal polypus, with neuralgia, hay fever, and asthma, in relation to ethmoiditis. 12°. *London*, 1887.

———. The same. 12°. *Philadelphia*, 1887..

Adam (A.) Case of polypus in the nose treated successfully by astringents. Glasgow M. Exam., 1831-2, i, 29.—[**Agnew.**] Case of encephaloid tumor of nares and antrum. Phila. M. Times, 1875, v, 612. — **Alcayde y Blanco** (J.) Observacion de pólipos nasales mucosos, seguida de reflexiones sobre la marcha, pronóstico y tratamiento de este padecimiento. Gac. méd. de Sevilla, 1880, ii, 229-233. — **Alloo.** Polype des fosses nasales. Rés. d. trav. Soc. de méd. prat. de la prov. d'Anvers, Brux., 1841, 23. — ———. Polype considérable des arrière-narines. Ann. Soc. de méd. prat. de la prov. d'Anvers, Malines, 1852, x; 5. — **Anderson** (W.) [Nasal polypus for nine years.] Canada M. & S. J., Montreal, 1872-3, i, 295.—**Annan** (S.) Remarks on polypus nasi. Maryland M. Recorder, Balt., 1829, i, 685-689. — **Arrachart.** Polype fibreux naso-pharyngien. Gaz. d. hôp., Par., 1859, xxxii, 394.— **Aschenborn** (O.) Polypus sarcomatosis cavi naso-pharyngei. Arch. f. klin. Chir., Berl., 1880, xxv, 150.— **Ashhurst** (J.), jr. Enchondroma of the nasal septum. Tr. Path. Soc. Phila. (1875-6), 1877, vi, 146. — ———. Fibroid polypus of the nose involving the antrum. Phila. M. Times, 1881-2, xii, 612.— **Avrard.** Récidive des polypes naso-pharyngiens. Quelle méthode met le plus sûrement à l'abri de cette récidive? Bull. Soc. de chir. de Par. (1862), 1863, 2. s., iii, 557.—**Aysaguer** (P.) Papillomes des fosses nasales. Ann. d. mal. de l'oreille, du larynx, etc., Par., 1885, xi, 335-339.—**B . . . ch.** Eine Krankheitsgeschichte. N. Mag. f. Aertze, Leipz., 1788, x, 44-48.—**Baker** (E. C.) Cases of nasal polypus projecting into the naso-pharynx. Lancet, Lond., 1883, i, 140-142.—**Baratoux** (J.) Contribution à l'étude des maladies de la cavité naso-pharyngienne: des tumeurs adénoïdes. Bull. et mém. Soc. franç. d'otol. et laryngol., Par., 1883-4, i, 76-85. *Also:* Rev. mens. de laryngol., etc., Bordeaux, 1883, iv, 353-360. *Also, transl.:* An. de otol. y laringol., Alcalá de Henares, 1883, i, 257-264. — **Barbrau.** [Polype fibreux naso-pharyngien occupant la plus grande étendue de la joue gauche.] Bull. Soc. anat. de Par., 1855, xxx, 312-314. — **Bardenheuer** (B.) Fibroid des Cavum nasopalatinum. *In:* Jahresb. ü. d. Thätigk. im Cölner städt. Bürger-Hosp. (1875), Cöln, 1876, 125. — **Barlow** (J.) [Case of tumor on the nose.] Med. & Phys. J., Lond., 1813, xxix, 296-301, 1 pl.—**Basedow.** Beispiele ungewöhnlicher Polypenformation. J. d. Chir. u. Augenh., Berl., 1824, vi, 621-630. — **Bassompierre** (G.-P.-M.) Note sur un cas de polype muqueux du nez; emploi de la cocaïne comme anesthésique. Arch. de méd. et pharm. mil., Par., 1886, vii, 482-484. — **Battle** (K. P.), jr. An ingenious method of removing nasal polypi. Med. Rec., N. Y., 1887, xxxii, 468. — **Batut.** Fibrômes; polypes naso-pharyngiens. Rev. méd. de Toulouse, 1869, iii, 76; 129. — **Bauchet.** [Les polypes naso-pharyngiens.] Bull. Soc. de chir. de Par. (1860), 1861, 2. s., i, 283-291. *Also* [Abstr.]: Gaz. d. hôp., Par., 1860, xxxii, 241.— **Bayer** (L.) Des kystes osseux de la cavité nasale. Rev. mens. de laryngol., etc., Par., 1885, v, 277 - 285. — **Beck** (E. W. H.) Case of nasal polypus of fourteen years' standing, cured by the local application of peach leaves. Northwest. M. & S. J., 1849 - 50, vi, 122. — **Bell** (C.) Case of polypus nasi. Boston M. & S. J., 1855, lii, 375.— **Bell** (W. R.) A new method of removing nasal polypus. Canada M. Rec., Montreal, 1883-4, xii, 98. — **Bentley.** Persistent dry streak on tongue and other symptoms caused by a nasal polypus. Med. Times & Gaz., Lond., 1855, n. s., x, 212.—**Bergeret.** Léniceps pour l'ablation des polypes du nez. [*From:* Bull. Soc. de méd. de Besançon.] *In his:* Obs. de méd. et de chir., 8°. Besançon, 1867, 42-45.—**Berthelot.** Observation de polypes nasaux, ayant déterminé une méningite; autopsie. Bull. Soc. méd. de l'Yonne, Auxerre, 1868, 141. — **Berthold** (E.) Notiz zur operativen Behandlung der Nasenpolypen. Tagebl. d. Versamml. deutsch. Naturf. u. Aerzte, Magdeb., 1884, lvii, 273. *Also:* Allg. Wien. med. Ztg., 1884, xxix, 484.— **Bescher.** Observation sur une nouvelle manière d'extirper le polype du nez. J. de méd., chir., pharm., etc., Par., 1776, xlvi, 348-352. [*See, also,* Bonnard, *infra.*]— **Bigelow** (H. J.) Tumor in the nose; operation. Boston M. & S. J., 1850-51, xliii, 300.— **Bigger.** Nasal polypus. Dublin J. M. Sc., 1875, lix, 72.— **Bindi** (E.) Polipotomo nasale del Prof. G. Gentile.

Nose (*Tumors of*).

Morgagni, Napoli, 1881, xxiii, 348–352. — [**Boeckel** (E.)] Polype naso-pharyngien, extirpé au moyen d'un nouveau procédé de résection temporaire du maxillaire supérieur. Gaz. méd. de Strasb., 1872–3, xxxii, 18–20. — **Bogel.** Geschichte eines glücklich ausgerotteten Rachen- und Nasenpolypen bey einer und derselben Person. J. f. d. Chir., Geburtsh. u. gerichtl. Arznk., Jena, 1800, ii, 452–472. — **Bolling** (G.) Om sättet för borttagande af polyper i näshålan och phàrynx. Eira, Göteborg, 1878, ii, 489–492. — **Bonanno.** Di una cisti ad epitelio vibratile della fossa nasale destra. Bull. d. r. Accad. med. di Roma, 1884, x, 54–59. — **Bond** (J. W.) Cases of mucous polypus in the child. Brit. M. J., Lond., 1887, ii, 1278. — **Bonnard.** Une nouvelle manière d'extirper le polype du nez. J. de méd., chir., pharm., etc., Par., 1777, xlvii, 243–252. [*See, also*, Bescher, *supra.*] — **Bonnefous** (P.) Du nouveau procédé de M. Ollier comme opération préliminaire pour extirper les polypes naso-pharyngiens. Montpel. méd., 1866, xvi, 25–35. — **Bonnes** (A.) Observation de polype naso-pharyngien opéré par un procédé nouveau ; guérison. Bull. gén. de thérap., etc., Par., 1869, lxxvii, 364–368. [Rap. de Houel.] Bull. Soc. de chir. de Par. (1869), 1870, 2. s., x, 342–345. — **Booth** (T. S.) On the operation of polypus of the nose ; with a proposal for an improved instrument. Lond. M. Reposit., 1820, xiii, 285.— **Borelli** (G.) Osservazioni cliniche ed operazioni chirurgiche praticate per malattie della mandibola inferiore e per tumori della cavità faringo-cranio-nasale. Rac. di oss. clin.-patol., Torino, 1867, ii, 341–400. ———. Nuove osservazioni di polipi naso-cranio-faringei e di tumori vertebrali. *Ibid.*, 401–411. — **Bosworth** (F. H.) Growths in the nasal passages. Tr. N. York Acad. M. (1882–4), 1886, iv, 13–36. *Also*: Med. Rec., N. Y., 1883, xxiii, 29–35. ———. A case of diffuse round-cell sarcoma, involving the posterior nares, vault of the pharynx, soft palate, pillar of the fauces, right tonsil, and lower pharynx ; operation ; cure. Med. Rec., N. Y., 1885, xxvii, 62–64. — **Botrel** (J.-P.) Mémoire sur une opération nouvelle dirigée contre les polypes naso-pharyngiens. Rev. méd.-chir. de Par., 1850, viii, 90–102. — **Bottini** (E.) Resezione osteop'astica della apofisi montante ed osso nasale per l' esportazione di voluminoso tumore naso-oculare. Gior. d. r. Accad. di med. di Torino, 1876, xxxix, 388–403. ———. Sarcoma dell' ala sinistra del naso ; esportazione ; rinoplastia ; guarigione. Osservatore, Torino, 1880, xvi, 100. — **Boullay.** [Un énorme polype fibreux qui occupait le pharynx, les fosses nasales et le sinus maxillaire d'un jeune homme ; résection de la mâchoire supérieure] Bull. Soc. anat. de Par., 1850, xxv, 244. — **Bourdon** (E.) Polype naso-pharyngien avec prolongement dans la fosse pterygo-maxillaire masqué par un lipôme. *Ibid.* (1872), 1874, xlvii, 393.— **Boursier** (A.) Sur un cas de polype naso-pharyngien. *In his*: Leç. de clin. chir. 1885–6, 8°, Par., 1887, 79–101.— **Bousseau.** Sarcome développé sur le périoste des os du nez. Bull. Soc. anat. de Par., 1867, xlii, 391. — **Brandeis** (R. C.) Naso-pharyngeal fibromata. Am. Pract., Louisville, 1877, xv, 212–217. — **Breda** (A.) Rinoscleroma od epithelioma del naso? Riv. veneta di sc. med., Venezia, 1885, ii, 128–136, 1 pl.— **Brenner** & **Januszkjewitsch.** Galvanokaustische Exstirpation eines Nasen-Rachen-Polypen. St. Petersb. med. Ztschr., 1869, xvii, 13–15. ———. Exstirpation eines Nasenrachenpolypen auf galvanokaustischem Wege. *Ibid.*, 1870, n. s., i, 32. — **Bresgen** (M.) Antwort auf Hartmann's Artikel : Ueber die Indicationen zum Ausreissen der Nasenpolypen. Berl. klin. Wchnschr., 1882, xix, 43. ———. Schlusswort zu meinem Urtheil über das Ausreissen der Nasenpolypen als Antwort auf Hartmann's Artikel. *Ibid.*, 125. — **Broca.** [Tumeur de l'aile gauche du nez.] Bull. Soc. anat. de Par., 1855, xxx, 305. ———. Polype naso-pharyngien, opéré par la ligature. Bull. Soc. de chir. de Par. (1866), 1867, 2. s., vii, 93.— **Brodie** (B. C.) Polypi of the nose. Lancet, Lond., 1843–4, i, 313–317. *Also*: Prov. M. J., Lond., 1843–4, vii, 103 ; 123.— **Brouardel.** Note sur un polype naso-pharyngien. Bull. Soc. anat. de Par., 1860, xxxv, 145–151. — **Browne** (R.) History of a fatal case of nasal polypus. Tr. M. & Phys. Soc. Calcutta, 1825–6. ii, 306–324. — **Bruns** (P.) Eine neue Methode der temporären (osteoplastischen) Resection der äusseren Nase zur Entfernung von Nasen-Rachenpolypen. Berl. klin. Wchnschr., 1872, ix, 137 ; 149. ———. Die electrolytische Behandlung der Nasen-Rachenpolypen. *Ibid.*, 321 ; 336 : 1873, x, 373. — **Bryant** (T.) Naso-pharyngeal polypus removed by ligature through the nose. Tr. Path. Soc. Lond., 1866–7, xviii, 106. ———. On polypus of the nose ; more particularly in reference to its treatment. Lancet, Lond., 1867, i, 235. — **Bryk** (A.) Beiträge zur Galvanokaustik ; zur Operation der Nasen-Rachenpolypen. Wien. Med.-Halle, 1862, iii, 223 ; 236 ; 276 ; 288 ; 311 ; 320 ; 328. — **Buchanan** (G.) Fibroid tumour of septum nasi. Glasgow M. J., 1882, xvii, 211. — **Buffum** (C. T.) Recurrent naso-pharyngeal tumor. Hosp. Gaz., N. Y., 1878, iv, 152. — **Buisson** & **Courty.** Polype naso-pharyngien ; ostéotomie verticale latérale du nez ; hémorrhagies consécutives ; mort. Montpel. méd., 1868, xx, 518–523.— **Burckhardt** (A. W.) Beseitigung der Polypen durch Arzneien ohne operative Beihülfe. Ztschr. f. Med., Chir. u. Geburtsh., Leipz., 1861, xv, 296–300. — **Burckhardt**

Nose (*Tumors of*).

(H.) Angiom der Nasenscheidewand. Ber. ü. d. Betrieb. d. Ludwigs-Spit. Charlottenhilfe in Stuttg. (1884), 1885, 11.— **Busi** (C.) Di un enorme polipo nasale guarito a mezzo di cura mista (allacciature e caustici). Bull. d. sc. med. di Bologna, 1856, 4. s., v, 321–324. — **Butlin** (H. T.) Tumours of the interior of the nose : 1. osseous outgrowth ; 2. sarcomatous polipi : 3. papilloma of septum ; 4. epithelioma of ala. St. Barth. Hosp. Rep., Lond., 1885, xxi, 147–152.— **Cabot.** Naso-pharyngeal polypus removed by turning down the nose ; tracheotomy ; recovery. Boston M. & S. J., 1871, lxxxiv, 95. *Also*: Extr. Rec. Bost. Soc. M. Improve. (1866–74), 1876, vi, 169–171. ———. Nasal medullary sarcoma. Extr. Rec. Bost. Soc. M. Improve. (1874–9), 1880, vii, 67. — **Calmettes** (R.) & **Chatellier** (H.) Fibro-sarcome de la cloison des fosses nasales ; opération ; guérison ; examen histologique. Ann. d. mal. de l'oreille, du larynx, etc., Par., 1887, xiii, 89–92. — **Canella** (G.) Polipi del naso. Gior. di chir.-prat., Trento, 1826, ii, 129–132. — **Capart.** Modification de l'instrument de Zaufal pour enlever les polypes naso-pharyngiens. Bull. Acad. roy. de méd. de Belg., Brux., 1879, 3. s., xiii, 1151. — **Cardone** (F.) Papillomi delle narici propriamente dette e del setto. Arch. internaz. di otojat., rinojat. ed aeroterap., Napoli, 1885, i, 145–147. — **Caro** (S.) Speedy cure of nasal polypi. Med. Rec., N. Y., 1879, xvi, 526. — **Carpenter** (J. G.) Treatment of neoplasms of the naso pharyngeal cavity. J. Am. M. Ass, Chicago, 1885, v, 652–654. *Also*, Reprint.— **Carreño** (J.) Observacion de diferentes pólipos situados en los senos maxilares y en las fosas nasales, curados con la ligadura y estirpacion. Décadas de med. y cirug. práct., Madrid, 1828, xix, 15–17. — **Cartaz** (A.) Polype naso-pharyngien. Progrès méd., Par., 1878, vi, 434–436. — **Carter** (H. V.) Naso-pharyngeal polypus. Tr. M. & Phys. Soc. Bombay (1885), 1886, n. s., viii, 100, 1 pl.—[**Cases.**] Ligature d'un polype, naissant de la base du crâne, à l'aide de nouveaux instrumens inventés par le docteur Félix Hatin. J. hebd. de méd., Par., 1829, iii, 5–9. — Polype envahissant la majeure partie des cavités de la face ; ligature de sa principale branche à l'aide d'un instrument nouveau. Gaz. d. hôp., Par., 1840, xiii, 569. *Also*: Ann. de méd. belge, Brux., 1841, i, 79–81.—Du traitement des polypes fibreux de la base du crâne, dits naso pharyngiens. Gaz. d. hôp., Par., 1854, xxvii 349.—Den fibrøse Polyp paa Basis cranii, exstirperet ved Resection af Overkjæven. Hosp.-Tid., Kjøbenh., 1859, ii, 165–167. — De l'opération préliminaire dans l'enlèvement du polype naso-pharyngien. Gaz. d. hôp., Par., 1859, xxxii, 525. — Polype fibreux des fosses nasales. *Ibid.*, 1863, xxxvi, 521. — Mixoma della cavità nasale destra ; estirpazione mediante torsione ; guarigione. Clin. chir. (Mazzoni), Roma, 1881, iv-vii, 210 — **Casselberry** (W. E.) Nasal fibromata. J. Am. M. Ass., Chicago, 1888, x, 477–481. — **Cassou** (L.) Observations de polypes naso-pharyngiens. Pau méd., 1878, ii, 106 ; 114 ; 124.— **Cayrel** fils. Cautérisation des fosses nasales dans un cas d'occlusion de ces cavités après l'arrachement d'un polype muqueux. J. de méd. et chir. de Toulouse, 1844–5, viii, 33–35. — **Ceci** (A.) Polipo naso-faringeo (fibroma della base del cranio) ; estirpazione del tumore col serranodo di Lüer ; guarigione. Gior. di clin. e terap., Messina, 1883, ii, 433–436.— **de Ceulencer.** Mémoire sur les polypes développés dans les cavités nasales. Ann. Soc. de méd. prat. de la prov. d'Anvers, Malines, 1849, vii, 41–54. — **Chamberet.** Observation sur une affection polypiforme aiguë, et non décrite, pour servir à l'histoire des maladies de la membrane pituitaire. J. compl. du dict. d. sc. méd., Par., 1818, i, 180–182.— **Chassaignac** (E.) Observations et considérations pratiques sur la répullulation des polypes des fosses nasales. Gaz. d. hôp., Par., 1849, 3. s., i, 567. ———. Quelle doit être la conduite du chirurgien dans les cas où il existe à la fois une hypertrophie des amygdales et un polype des fosses nasales ? *Ibid.*, 1854, xxvii, 293. ———. Ablation d'un énorme polype charnu occupant la totalité des fosses nasales, des sinus frontaux et des sinus maxillaires, avec destruction des masses latérales de l'ethmoïde ; emploi d'un procédé opératoire nouveau ; guérison. Monit. d. hôp., Par., 1854. ii, 266–268. — [Polypes des fosses nasales à une fille de sept ans.] Bull. Soc. de chir. de Par. (1861), 1862, 2. s., ii, 354.— **Chatard.** Polype naso-pharyngien avec destruction complète de la voûte palatine, du voile du palais, etc. Union méd. de la Gironde, Bordeaux, 1860, v, 216–224.— **Chatellier** (H.) Polype fibro-muqueux des arrière-narines ; morcellement de la tumeur ; extirpation sans opération préliminaire ; examen histologique. Ann. d. mal. de l'oreille, du larynx, etc., Par., 1886, xii, 473–481.— **Cheever** (D. W.) Naso-pharyngeal polypus, attached to the basilar process of the occipital, and body of the sphenoid bones, successfully removed by a section, displacement, and subsequent replacement and reunion of the superior maxillary bone. Boston M. & S. J., 1867–8, lxxvii, 161–164. ———. On the surgical treatment of naso-pharyngeal polypi. *Ibid.*, 1874, xc, 541–550. ———. Naso-pharyngeal polypus removed by sawing down and depressing the nose. *Ibid.*, 1878, xcviii, 587. *Also*: Med. & Surg. Rep. Bost. City Hosp. (1874–9), 1882, iii, 151.— **Chenantais.** Tumeur de la partie latérale du nez ; fibrôme sarcomateux. Bull. Soc. anat. de Nantes

Nose (*Tumors of*).

1876–8, Par., 1879, i, 22. ———. Tumeur de la narine (granulôme). *Ibid.* (1879), 1880, 37.—**Chevalier** (J.-A.-U.) Polype bilobé des fosses nasales emporté par la ligature. Rec. de mém. de méd. . . . mil., Par., 1825, xvi, 228–233.—**Chiari** (O.) Nasenpolyp. Deutsche Med.-Ztg., Berl., 1884, ii, 85; 97. *Also*, Reprint. *Also, transl.*: St. Louis Cour. Med., 1885, xiii, 526: xiv, 46. ———. Des néoplasmes de la cloison des fosses nasales. [Transl. from the German by L. Lichtwitz.] Rev. mens. de laryngol., etc., Par., 1886, vi, 121–132.—**Churchill** (F.) Post-nasal fibroma. Tr. Path. Soc. Lond., 1885–6, xxxvii, 458.—**Ciniselli** (L.) De la galvano-caustique chimique et de son emploi dans le traitement des polypes naso-pharyngiens. Bull. gén. de thérap., etc., Par., 1864, lxvii, 59–69. ———. Polipo naso-faringeo risoltosi in seguito alla galvano-caustica chimica. Ann. univ. di med., Milano, 1872, ccxci, 533–541.—**Clemens** (A.) Exstirpation eines bedeutenden Nasen- und Rachenpolypen. Deutsche Klinik, Berl., 1863, xv, 344.—**Colles** (W.) Observations on nasal polypi. Dublin Q. J. M. Sc., 1848, vi, 373–382.—**Collis** (M. H.) Fibroplastic growth from the periosteum of the nasal cavity; removal by a new operation of great simplicity. *Ibid.*, 1866, xlii, 331–334.—**Contreras** (J.) Hipertrofia local; lipoma del volúmen de una pera grande de D. Guindo implantado en el lubolo y tabique medio de las fosas nasales, y parte media superior del lábio superior; amputacion; curacion. España méd., Madrid, 1862, vii, 164.—**Coomes** (M. F.) Nasal polypi; clinical notes of cases. Med. Herald, Louisville, 1881–2, iii, 172–174. ———. Tumors of the naso-pharynx. *Ibid.*, 219; 270.—**Cornil** (V.) Note sur les tumeurs adénoïdes du pharynx nasal. J. de l'anat. et physiol., etc., Par., 1883, xix, 576–581, 1 pl.—**Cox** (J.) Post-nasal growths. Austral. M. J., Melbourne, 1886, viii, 68–74.—**Coyne.** Contribution à l'étude des polypes fibro-muqueux des fosses nasales avec prolongement pharyngien. Gaz. hebd. d. sc. méd. de Bordeaux, 1880, i, 15; 42.—**Cozzolino** (V.) Mixo-fibromi multipli del vestibolo delle fosse nasali, narice propriamente detta. Arch. ital. di laringol., Napoli, 1883–4, iii, 97–100. ———. Due rarissimi tumori della cavità naso-faringee e nasali; un fibroma mollusco delle dietro-nari ed un papilloma della cavità nasale destra. Riv. clin. e terap., Napoli, 1887, ix, 69–76.—**Cramer.** Fall von Fungus medullaris. Mag. f. d. ges. Heilk., Berl., 1826, xxii, 267–271.—**Creus.** Una pagina para la historia de los pólipos naso-faringeos. Siglo méd., Madrid, 1877, xxiv, 739; 754; 771. *Also*: Génio méd.-quir., Madrid, 1877, xxiii, 609; 625; 645; 656. *Also*: Rev. de med. y cirug. práct., Madrid, 1877, i, 553; 578; 597. *Also*: Anfiteatro anat., Madrid, 1877, v, 342: 1878, vi, 8; 15.—**Cruveilhier.** Polype naso-pharyngien, opéré par la méthode nasale (procédé d'Ollier). Bull. et mém. Soc. de chir. de Par., 1877, n. s., iii, 194–197. ———. Extirpation d'un polype naso-pharyngien par la méthode palatine; réparation de la voûte palatine par le procédé de Fergusson. *Ibid.*, 1880, n. s., vi, 206–209.—**Cutter** (E.) Naso-pharyngeal polypus removed through the mouth by a modified écraseur. Boston M. & S. J., 1870, lxxxiii, 339–341.—**D.** (C.) Du gonflement polypiforme de la membrane muqueuse du nez, et de son traitement. Bull. gén. de thérap., etc., Par., 1833, v, 378–380.—**Dalbanne** (N.) Tumeur lymphatique. Courrier méd., Par., 1874, xxiv, 394–396.—**Dallidet.** Des polypes des fosses nasales et de leur altération muqueuse. Gaz. hebd. d. sc. méd. de Bordeaux, 1880–81, i, 481–485.—**Daly** (W. H.) An analysis of the value of the galvano-cautery in the treatment of diseases and growths of the naso-pharynx. Tr. Am. M. Ass., Phila., 1880, xxxi, 653–656. ———. On nasal polyps. Tr. Am. Laryngol. Ass. 1880, N. Y., 1881, ii, 118–130. *Also*: Arch. Laryngol., N. Y., 1881, ii, 147–158. *Also*, Reprint.— **D'Ambrosio** (A.) Polipo naso faringeo; estirpazione dietro la divisione del palato molle; guarigione. Movimento, Napoli, 1875, vii, 102–104.—**Daniéls** (F.) Exstirpatie van een naso-pharyngeaal polyp. *In his*: Twee chir. gevallen, 8°, Amst., 1874, 1–16.—**Dauvergne.** De l'emploi de la solution iodurée caustique de Lugol pour empêcher la reproduction des polypes naso-pharyngiens. Bull. gén. de thérap., etc., Par., 1872, lxxxiii, 499–507.—**Davis** (C. B. S.) Nasal polypus. Buffalo M. & S. J., 1866–7, vi, 259–265.—**Dawson** (W. W.) Naso-pharyngeal polypus; polypus of the antrum; resection of the wall of the antrum. Cincin. Lancet & Clinic, 1882, n. s., ix, 413–415.— **Delavan** (D. B.) Nine cases of tumor of the nasal septum, anteriorly. Arch. Laryngol., N. Y., 1882, iii, 172–177. *Also*, Reprint.—**Delore** (X.) Des polypes naso-pharyngiens. Bull. gén. de thérap., etc., Par., 1863, lxv, 349; 397; 507. *Also*, Reprint.—**Delstanche** Sohn. Ueber ein neues Instrument zur Entfernung der adenoiden Vegetationen im Nasenrachenraum (Adénotome à coulisse). Arch. f. Ohrenh, Leipz., 1879–80, xv, 35–40. — [**Demarquay.**] Hypertrophie de la muqueuse du cornet inférieur des fosses nasales. Gaz. d. hôp., Par., 1861, xxxiv, 114. ——— Polype naso-pharyngien enlevé par un nouveau procédé ostéo-plastique. Bull. gén. de thérap., etc., Par., 1862, lxiii, 276. ———. Polypes naso-pharyngiens; arrachement après avoir enlevé l'apophyse montante et la paroi antérieure du sinus maxillaire, en conservant le périoste; régénération des parties osseuses. Union méd., Par., 1863, 2. s., xvii, 266–269. ———. Polype glandulaire de la muqueuse

Nose (*Tumors of*).

nasale; répullution; extirpation et cautérisation; accidents consécutifs à l'opération; paralysie de tous les muscles de l'œil; symptômes d'empoisonnement par la morphine; autopsie. Gaz. d. hôp., Par., 1869, xlii, 277.—**Demeaux.** Polype naso-pharyngien d'un volume considérable extirpé par les voies naturelles et sans mutilations préalables. *Ibid.*, 1862, xxxv, 306.—**De Morgan.** Large fleshy polypus of the nose; operation. Lancet, Lond., 1869, i, 844.—**Denucé.** Un polype naso-pharyngien. Bull. et mém. Soc. de chir. de Par., 1878, iv. 390–393.—**De Rossi.** Studi sui polipi fibrosi naso-faringei. Atti Accad. med. di Roma, 1879, v, fasc. 2, 41–169, 2 pl.—**Desgranges** (A.) De la cautérisation appliquée aux polypes naso-pharyngiens. Ann. Soc. de méd. de Lyon, 1854, 2. s., ii, 286–299. *Also*: Gaz. hebd. de méd., Par., 1854, i, 633; 647. ———. Du traitement des polypes naso-pharyngiens. Bull. gén. de thérap., etc., Par., 1868, lxxiv, 115–122.—**Desmartis** (T.) Curacion de los pólipos nasales por medio de agentes puramente médicos. Siglo méd., Madrid, 1861, viii, 809.—**Després** (A.) Polype sarcomateux naso-pharyngien. Rev. de thérap. méd.-chir., Par., 1877, 283–285. ———. Polype nasopharyngien; extraction du maxillaire supérieur; transformation fibreuse. Bull. et mém. Soc. de chir. de Par., 1882, n. s., viii, 218–220.—**Desprez** (M.-E.) Des polypes nasaux et naso-pharyngiens, et leur traitement par un nouveau procédé opératoire. Bull. Soc. de chir. de Par. (1860), 1861, 2. s., i, 201.—**Devalz.** Enchondrôme de la cloison des fosses nasales; excision; guérison. Gaz. méd. de Bordeaux, 1872–3, ii, 105–108.—**De Vilbris** (A.) Tumors of the naso-pharyngeal cavities, with a report of cases. Weekly M. Rev., Chicago, 1884, x, 385–387. *Also*: Fort Wayne J. M. Sc., 1884–5, iv, 241–246.—**Dickson** (J. R.) Case of fibro-cartilaginous tumour in the nasal fossa: operation. Brit.-Am. J., Montreal, 1861, ii, 545.—**Didot.** Présentation d'un nouveau porte-ligature, et, au besoin, porte-caustique pour les polypes naso-pharyngiens; et pour certaines tumeurs de l'utérus, et du vagin. Bull. Acad. roy. de méd. de Belg., Brux., 1855–6, xv, 218–224.—**Dieffenbach** (J.-F.) Observations sur l'incision du nez pratiquée dans la vue d'extraire les polypes ou autres tumeurs de la cavité nasale. J. compl. du dict. d. sc. méd., Par., 1831, xl, 41–45.—**Dionisio.** Estirpazione di voluminoso mixoma occupante l'intiero ambito delle cavità nasali, estrusosi per le suture naso-mascellari verso le regioni genio-malari. Gior. d. r. Accad. di med. di Torino, 1877, 3. s., xxii, 6–14, 2 pl. ———. Risposta alle osservazioni degli Dott. G. F. Novaro e G. Spantigati, sulla sua memoria intitolata: Estirpazione di voluminoso mixoma occupante l'intiero ambito della cavità nasali, estrusosi per le suture nasomascellari verso le regioni genio-malari. *Ibid.*, 289–305.—**Dittel.** Nasen- Rachen- Polyp mittelst Galvano-Kaustik entfernt. Allg. Wien. med. Ztg., 1869, xiv, 382.— **Dolbeau.** Polype fibro-muqueux des fosses nasales; diagnostic complexe; opération mort. Bull. Soc. de chir. de Par. (1862), 1863, 2. s., iii, 503–511. *Also*: Gaz. d. hôp., Par., 1862, xxxv, 530. ———. Traitement des polypes naso-pharyngiens. Bull. Soc. de chir. de Par. (1865), 1866, 2. s., vi, 555–559.—**van Dommelen.** Polype fibreux de la fosse nasale gauche; guérison à l'aide du sublimé corrosif. J. d. conn. méd. prat., Par., 1858–9, xxvi, 425.—**Donaldson** (F.) The destruction of nasal polypi by chromic acid. Tr. Am. Laryngol. Ass., N. Y., 1883, v, 17–23. *Also*: Arch. Laryngol., N. Y., 1883, iv, 175–179. *Also*: Med. Rec., N. Y., 1883, xxiii, 577.—**Donaldson** (F.), jr. Treatment of nasal growths and hypertrophies. Virginia M. Month., Richmond, 1886–7, xiii, 538–546. *Also*, Reprint.— **Doyer** (D.) Des tumeurs adénoïdes de la cavité naso-pharyngienne. Cong. périod. internat. d. sc. méd. Compt.-rend., Amst., 1881, vi, pt. 2, 332–338.—**D[ron** (A.)] Nouveaux procédés opératoires contre les polypes naso-pharyngiens. Gaz. méd. de Lyon, 1859, xi, 465.—**Dubief** (F.) Note sur un cas de polype naso-pharyngien opéré par le procédé de l'abaissement du nez (ostéotomie verticale et bilatérale du nez). Mém. et compt.-rend. Soc. d. sc. méd. de Lyon (1874), 1875, xiv, pt. 2, 33–38. *Also*: Lyon méd., 1874, xvi, 277–282.—[**Dubois.**] Ueber Polypen in den Nasenhöhlen und im Schlunde. Mag. f. d. ges. Heilk., Berl., 1820, vii, 231–236.—**Dubourg.** Polypes des fosses nasales; détermination de quelques cas dans lesquels la ligature doit être préférée à l'arrachement. J. hebd. de méd., Par., 1830, viii, 206–209.—**Dubrueil** (A.) Polype naso-pharyngien. Gaz. méd. de Par., 1886, 7. s., iii, 529–531. ———. De l'application de la ligature extemporanée à la cure des polypes naso-pharyngiens. Rev. de chir., Par., 1887, vii, 736–738.—**Duigan** (C) Lipoma of the nose. Dublin Hosp. Gaz., 1855, ii, 311.—**Dumenil.** Relation de quatre cas de polypes naso-pharyngiens. Bull. Soc. de chir. de Par., 1873, 3. s., ii, 335–344. [Discussion], 344; 350; 376; 382.—**Dumont** fils. Trois observations, l'une sur la cure d'un polype muqueux; l'autre, sur une transudation lymphatique, et la troisième, sur un phénomène singulier, à la suite d'une plaie du bas-ventre. J. de méd., chir., pharm., etc., Par., 1763, xix, 453–458.—**Duplay & Barthélemy.** Deux observations de polypes naso-pharyngiens traités par les injections interstitielles de chlorure de zinc. Arch. gén. de méd., Par., 1880, cxlv, 353–361.—**Dupuy** (L.-E.) Contribution à l'étude des poly-

Nose (*Tumors of*).

pes naso-pharyngiens. Bull. Soc. anat. de Par., 1874, xlix, 786–790. *Also:* Progrès méd., Par., 1875, iii, 120.—**Dupuytren.** Kyste à parois osseuses pris pour un polype fibro-celluleux ; son extraction, le 13 mars. Clinique, Par., 1830, ii, 174 ; 179. ———. Polypes à la partie postérieure des fosses nasales ; ligature par un procédé nouveau. Gaz. méd. de Par., 1832, iii, 607.—**Earle.** Case of fungoid polypus of the nose. Lond. M. Gaz., 1827–8, i, 159-161. ———. Removal of a congenital tumor. *Ibid.*, 1831-2, ix, 454.—**Eder** (A.) Nasenrachenpolyp. *In his :* Aerztl. Ber. 1875, Wien, 1876, 89.—**Edwards** (F. S.) Operation for the removal of naso-pharyngeal polypus. Am. M. Times, N. Y., 1861, ii, 265.—**Encinas.** Análisis histológico del pólipo naso-faringeo operado. An. de cien. méd., Madrid, 1878, v, 323.—**Erichsen.** Tumor over the right alar fibro-cartilage. Lancet, Lond., 1859, i, 318. ———. Cartilaginous growth on the septum of the nose ; removal. *Ibid.*, 1864, ii, 153.—**Eve** (P. F.) Removal of a large fibrous polypus from the base of the cranium. South. M. & S. J., Augusta, 1836-7, i, 78-80. ———. Removal of a large polypus from the nose, through the pharynx. *Ibid.*, 1849, n. s., v, 466.—**F.** (A.) De l'arrachement des polypes muqueux des fosses nasales, et des moyens d'empêcher la récidive. Bull. gén. de thérap., etc., Par., 1842, xxii, 365-368.—**Fano.** [Polypes des fosses nasales.] Bull. Soc. anat. de Par., 1854, xxix, 334.—**Fargas** (M. A.) Extenso condiloma en la nariz ; extirpación ; ingertos dermo-epidérmicos ; curación. Gac. méd. catal., Barcel., 1883, vi, 46-50.—[**Fauvel** (C.)] Polype muqueux de l'arrière cavité des fosses nasales. Rev. méd.-phot. d. hôp. de Par., 1875, vii, 165-168.—**Fayrer** (J.) Removal of a tumor from the nostril. Med. Times & Gaz., Lond., 1868, ii, 3. *Also, in his :* Clin. & Path. Obs. in India, 8°, Lond., 1873, 540. ———. Polypus nasi. *In his :* Clin. & Path. Obs. in India, 8°, Lond., 1873, 541-543.—**Fedeli** (G.) Guarigione pronta del polipo nasale ottenuta usando del metodo inventato dal Dott. G. Ceccarini. Raccoglitore med., Forli, 1880, 4. s., xiii, 163-165. *Also :* Gazz. med. ital., prov. venete, Padova, 1880, xxiii, 69.—**Féré** (C.) Papillome de la narine. Bull. Soc. anat. de Par., 1880, lv, 587.—**Fergusson** (W.) Nasal polypi. Lancet, Lond., 1859, i, 215. ———. Mixed polypus of the nose and antrum. *Ibid.*, ii, 561. ———. Polypoid (?) disease of the antrum and nares ; removal. Med. Times & Gaz., Lond., 1859, n. s., xix, 552. ———. Removal of large nasal polypus by external incision. *Ibid.*, 1867, ii, 431.—**Ficano** (G.) Sarcoma fusiforme del setto nasale. Gazz. d. osp., Milano, 1888, ix, 90.—**Figuière.** [Un énorme polype fibreux développé dans la fosse nasale droite.] Bull. Soc. anat. de Par., 1843, xviii, 294.—**Fischer** (G.) Polypen in Nase und Rachen ; Écrasement. *In his:* Mitth. a. d. chir. Univ.-Klin. zu Götting., 8°, 1861, 232-234. ———. Polypus fibrosus nasi (Écrasement). *Ibid.*, 290-292.—**Fisher** (G. J.) Removal of a large fibrous nasal polypus by the knife. Am. M. Mouth., N. Y., 1857, viii, 15-17.—**Fleischman** (D.) Removal of nasal polypi. Med. Ann., Albany, 1884, v, 265-271.—**Fleury.** Observations pour servir à l'histoire des polypes des fosses nasales. J. d. conn. méd.-chir., Par., 1841-2, ix, pt. 1, 195-197. ———. Polype fibreux inséré à l'apophyse basilaire et envoyant des prolongements dans les fosses nasales, le pharynx et la joue ; ablation préliminaire du maxillaire supérieur gauche ; guérison radicale constatée deux ans et demi plus tard. Bull. Soc. de chir. de Par. (1862), 1863, 2. s., iii, 536-541. *Also :* Gaz. d. hôp., Par., 1862, xxxv, 567. ———. Polype fongueux (cancéreux) s'étendant à l'arrière-gorge, à la narine droite, pénétrant dans la cavité orbitaire, dans le sinus sphénoïdal, et perforant la base du crâne après avoir détruit le corps du sphénoïde. Bull. Soc. de chir. de Par. (1863), 1864, 2. s., iv, 447-449. ———. Polype naso-pharyngien s'étendant au pharynx, à la narine gauche, au sinus maxillaire, à la fosse zygomatique. Gaz. d. hôp., Par., 1864, xxxvii, 322 - 324. ———. Polype naso-pharyngien ; ablation du maxillaire supérieur ; extirpation ; guérison. *Ibid.*, 1867, xl, 295. ———. Polype naso-pharyngien ; ablation du maxillaire supérieur ; guérison. *Ibid.*, 527. ———. Observation de polype naso-pharyngien opéré par l'ablation partielle du maxillaire supérieur. *Ibid.*, 1873, xlvi, 1010.—**Forget** (A.) Des polypes naso-pharyngiens. Union méd., Par., 1866, 2. s., xxix, 243-247.—**Forster** (J. C.) Case of a naso-pharyngeal polypus ; brain mischief ; operation ; death. Tr. Clin. Soc. Lond., 1871, iv, 159-163. ———. Tumours on the nose ; follicular sarcoma. Guy's Hosp. Rep., Lond., 1874, 3. s., xix, 13.—**Foucher.** Polype fibreux naso-pharyngien ; excision partielle au moyen de la boutonnière palatine ; cautérisations ; infection purulente ; mort. Gaz. hebd. de méd., Par., 1859, vi, 748 - 750. ———. Tumeur fibro-plastique volumineuse, implantée sur le dos du nez par un étroit pédicule ; ablation ; guérison. Gaz. d. hôp., Par., 1867, xl, 297.—**Fraenkel** (B.) Geschwülste der Nasenhöhle. Handb. d. spec. Path. (Ziemssen), Leipz., 1876, iv, 156-159. *Also, transl.:* Cycl. Pract. M. (Ziemssen), N. Y., 1876, iv, 168-172.—**Frisse.** Zwey Beobachtungen glücklich ausgerotteter Nasenpolypen. J. f. d. Chir., Geburtsh. u. gerichtl. Arznk., Jena, 1800, ii, 19-30.—**Fritsche** (M. A.) Zur Frage der Radicaltherapie bei Nasenpolypen. Therap. Monatsh., Berl., 1887, i, 440-442.—**Furgusson** (W.) Case of removal of fibrous poly-

Nose (*Tumors of*).

pus attached to base of skull. Med. Times & Gaz., Lond., 1868, ii, 211. — **Gallozzi** (C.) Un caso di sarcoma delle fossa nasali. Morgagni, Napoli, 1878, xx, 565-568. ———. Osservazione e studio d' un caso di voluminoso polipo naso-faringeo. Resoc. Accad. med. chir. di Napoli, 1880, xxxiv, 83-91.—**Ganghofner** (F.) Ueber adenoide Geschwülste im Nasenrachenraum und deren Behandlung. Prag. med. Wchnschr., 1877, ii, 277; 301.—**Gangolphe** (M.) Myxome naso-pharyngien. Mém. et compt.-rend. Soc. d. sc. méd. de Lyon (1884), 1885, xxiv, pt. 2, 24-28. *Also :* Lyon méd., 1884, xlvi, 39-42. — **Gant.** Nasal polypus removed by a new forceps. Lancet, Lond., 1858, ii, 257.—**Gautier** (V.) Polype fibreux naso-pharyngien enlevé au moyen du serre-nœud constricteur de Maisonneuve. Écho méd., Neuchât., 1861, v, 593-597.—**Gay** (C. C. F.) Fibrous polypus of the nose ; avulsion by a new method. Buffalo M. & S. J., 1875-6, xv, 301.—**Gilbert.** Polypus nasi. Med. Exam., Phila., 1852, n. s., viii, 712-716.—**Giraldès.** Polype fibreux des fosses nasales, à prolongements multiples. Bull. Soc. de chir. de Par. (1848 - 50), 1851, i, 599 - 606. — **Glasgow** (W. C.) Adenoid tumor of the naso-pharynx. St. Louis Cour. Med., 1879, ii, 501-503.—**Gogué** (G.) Observation de polype des fosses nasales ; nouveau procédé pour la ligature. Gaz. méd. de Par., 1843, 2. s., xi, 757.—**Gomez** (L. J.) Historia de un pólipo fibroso-nasal y procedimiento empleado para su avulsion. Gac. méd., Madrid, 1850, vi, 272.—**González Encinas** (S.) Pólipos nasales. Correo méd. castellano, Salamanca, 1884, i, 225-234. — **Gosselin.** Polypes saignants orbito-naso-maxillaires ; opération. Gaz. d. hôp., Par., 1856, xxix, 175. ———. Polype par hypertrophie glandulaire de la fosse nasale droite ; arrachement après incision préalable de la narine. Monit. d. hôp., Par., 1858, vi, 275. ———. Polype épithélio-glandulaire de la fosse nasale et de l'orbite à droite ; ablation après incision de la narine et tamponnement de l'ouverture nasale postérieure. Gaz. d. hôp., Par., 1865, xxxviii, 46. ———. Observation d'un gros polype muqueux naso-pharyngien, solitaire, implanté sur la partie postérieure et externe de la fosse nasale droite et opéré par arrachement. *Ibid.*, 1866, xxxix, 453.—**Gozzini** (A.) & **Corradi** (G.) Sulla asportazione di un grosso polipo fibroso faringeo operato col mezzo della galvano-caustica-termica. Sperimentale, Firenze, 1871, xxvii, 449 - 459. — **von Gräfe** (C. F.) Rachenpolyp von ungewöhnlicher Grösse, und glückliche Heilung desselben. J. d. Chir. u. Augenh., Berl., 1834, xxii, 12-18.—**Graefe** (E.) Beschreibung eines von Leroy d'Étiolles angegebenen Instruments zur Umschlingung der Ligatur tief sitzender und schwer beizukommender Schlund- und Rachen-Polypen. *Ibid.*, xxi, 482 - 488, 1 pl.—**Grancher.** Un nouveau signe des tumeurs adénoïdes du pharynx nasal. Ann. d. mal. de l'oreille, du larynx, etc., Par., 1886, xii, 165.—**Gripat** (H.) Polype naso-pharyngien ; ablation ; mort. Bull. Soc. anat. de Par. (1872), 1874, xlvii, 435-440.—**Gross** (S. D.) Nasal polyps and anal fistula. Phila. M. Times, 1870-71, i, 155.—**Gross** (S. W.) Myxomata from mucous membrane of the nose. Tr. Path. Soc. Phila, (1871-3), 1874, iv, 219.—**Grynfeltt** (J.) Sarcome de la cloison des fosses nasales. Montpel. méd., 1876, xxxvii, 307, 511. ———. Atrophie sous l'influence seule des progrès de l'âge, chez un adolescent devenu jeune homme, d'un gros polype naso-pharyngien très-incomplètement enlevé. Gaz. hebd. d. sc. méd. de Montpel., 1882, iv, 195 ; 217 ; 267. — **Güntner** (W.) Nasenrachenpolyp ; Unterbindung und nachherige Extraction ; Tod in Folge Anämie. Vrtljschr. f. d. prakt. Heilk., Prag, 1859, lxiii, 42 - 44. — **Guérin.** Méthode nouvelle de traitement pour la cure des polypes naso-pharyngiens par excision et rugination des os sur lesquels ils sont implantés. Bull. Soc. de chir. de Par. (1865), 1866, 2. s., vi, 518-524.—**Guersant.** Polype naso-pharyngien. *Ibid.*, 1853-4, iv, 27 ; 58 ; 63.—**Gulcke** (H.) Naso-pharyngeal tumors. Med. Rec., N. Y., 1881, xix, 718. — **Gurovitch.** Operatsija viriezivanija nosoglo tochnago polipa, pomotshou galvano-kautera. [Polypus of nose removed by galvano-cautery.] Vrach. Vedom., St. Petersb., 1883, viii, 4194.—**Guye** (A.) Ein neues Ringmesser zum Entfernen der adenoïden Geschwülste aus dem Nasenrachenraum. Ztschr. f. Ohrenh., Wiesb., 1885-6, xv, 167. — **Hamaker** (W. D.) A case of nasal polypi. Cleveland M. Gaz., 1885-6, i, 399-402. — **Hamilton** (F. H.) Polypi and hypertrophy of nose ; removal of polypi and reduction of size of nose. Med. Rec., N. Y., 1876, xi, 714.—**Hamilton** (J. W.) Maxillary and naso-pharyngeal tumors. Tr. Ohio M. Soc., Columbus, 1878, xxxiii, 67-80. *Also :* Ohio M. Recorder, Columbus, 1878-9, iii, 145-156.—**Hartmann** (A.) Ueber die Operation der Nasenpolypen. Deutsche med. Wchnschr., Berl., 1879, v, 358 ; 373 ; 382. *Also,* Reprint. ———. Ueber die Operation der Nasenrachenpolypen. Deutsche med. Wchnschr., Berl., 1881, vii, 64-66. ———. Ueber die Indicationen zum Ausreissen der Nasenpolypen. Berl. klin. Wchnschr., 1882, xix, 10. ———. Noch einmal über die Indicationen zum Ausreissen der Nasenpolypen. *Ibid.*, 88. ———. Zur Operation der adenoïden Wucherungen im Nasenrachenraume. Deutsche med. Wchnschr., Berl., 1885, xi, 605.—**Hawkins** (C. H.) Clinical lecture on polypus of the nose. Lond. M. Gaz., 1840, xxvi, 697 ; 731.

Nose (*Tumors of*).

Also, in his: . . . Path. & Surg. Writings, 8°, Lond., 1874, i, 231-249.—**Hayes** (T.) Removal of a large naso-pharyngeal polypus with wire écraseur; talipes varus successfully operated on. Med. Press & Circ., Lond., 1870, x, 391.—**Heath** (C.) Lipoma of nose. Tr. Path. Soc. Lond., 1870-71, xxii, 242.—**Hebra.** Ueber ein eigenthümliches Neugebilde an der Nase; Rhinosclerom; nebst histologischem Befunde vom Dr. M. Kohn. Wien. med. Wchnschr., 1870, xx, 1-5.—**von Hebra** (H.) Das Rhinophyma. Vrtljschr. f. Dermat., Wien, 1881, viii, 603-619, 1 pl. *Also*, Reprint.—**Hecker.** Ausrottung eines bösartigen Nasenpolypen. Arch. f. physiol. Heilk., Stuttg., 1844, iii, 260-262. ——. Beseitigung einer Tele-angiectasie an der Nase durch kleine Setons und nach-herige Excision eines keilförmigen Stückes. *Ibid.*, 263.—**Heitz** (P. A.) On the treatment of nasal polypi by pow-dered tannic acid. Tr. Minnesota M. Soc., St. Paul, 1885, 63.—**Herrera** (M.) Un caso de pólipo naso faringeo. Escuela de med., México, 1879, i, no. 2, 2; no. 4, 4; no. 6, 6; no. 7, 5; no. 8, 8.—**Herrgott.** Polype naso-pharyngien; emploi du laryngoscope; rugination de la base du crâne. Proc.-verb. . . . Soc. de méd. de Strasb., 1866-8, iv, 99. *Also*: Gaz. méd. de Strasb., 1867, xxvii, 79. ——. Sur le dia-gnostic et le traitement des polypes naso-pharyngiens im-plantés sur l'apophyse basilaire. Bull. Soc. de chir. de Par. (1867), 1868, 2. s., viii, 28. *Also*: Gaz. d. hôp., Par., 1867, xl, 97.—**Heurtaux** (A.) Note sur un cas de chon-drome naso-pharyngien. Bull. et mém. Soc. de chir. de Par., 1877, iii, 627-637. ——. Polype naso-pharyngien. Bull. Soc. anat. de Nantes 1876-8, Par., 1879, i, 7. *Also*: J. de méd. de l'ouest, Nantes, 1877, 2. s., i, 156-158. ——. Chondrome naso-pharyngien. Bull. Soc. anat. de Nantes 1876-8, Par., 1879, i, 30-33. ——. Polype fibro-muqueux des fosses nasales. *Ibid.*, (1880), 1881, iv, 88-90. ——. Polype fibro-muqueux naso-pharyngien. *Ibid.*, 91-94. ——. Tumeur du nez et du sinus frontal gauche; épi-théliome tubulé. *Ibid.* (1882), 1884, vi, 93. *Also*: J. de méd. de l'ouest, Nantes, 1884, 2. s., viii, 53.—**Hewett.** Pendu-lous fibro-cellular tumour of the nose. Lancet, Lond., 1857, i, 629.—**Heyfelder** (J. F.) † Entfernung eines die linke Nasen-Rachen- und Oberkieferhöhle ausfüllenden Polypen. Deutsche Klinik, Berl., 1855, vi, 67. — **Hey-felder** (O.) Operation eines Nasenpolypen durch Extrac-tion. Deutsche Klinik, Berl., 1850, ii, 231. ——. Opera-tion eines Nasenpolypen durch Excision. *Ibid.*, 231.—**Heymann** (P.) Ueber Nasenpolypen. Berl. klin. Wchnschr., 1886, xxiii, 531; 545.—**Higgens** (C.) Case of pulsating sarcoma, involving left nasal fossae, antrum, and orbit. Guy's Hosp. Rep. 1884-5, Lond., 1886, 3. s., xxviii, 91-102, 1 pl.—**Hitchcock** (H. O.) Large fibrous nasal polypus. Tr. M. Soc. Mich. 1870, Lansing, 1871, 94.—**Hodgen** (J. T.) A case of fibrous polypus of the nose. St. Louis M. & S. J., 1865, n. s., ii, 97-99.—**Holmer.** Tilfælde af Nasopharyngealpolyper og sammes Behandling særlig ved Ligatur. Hosp.-Tid., Kjøbenh., 1869, xii, 117; 121.—**Holmes** (T.) A case of naso-pharyngeal polypus. Tr. Clin. Soc. Lond., 1874-5, viii, 68-71. — **Holzschuh** (A.) Geschichte der Unterbindung eines grossen Nasen-Rachenpolypen mit tödtlichem Ausgange. Med. Jahrb. d. k. k. österr. Staates, Wien, 1838, n. F., xv, 248-256.—**Hopmann** (C.M.) Zur Nomenclatur der Nasenschleim-hautgeschwülste. Amtl. Ber. ü. d. Versamml. deutsch. Naturf. u. Aerzte 1883, Freib. i. Br., 1884, lvi, 294-298. *Also*: Wien. med. Presse, 1883, xxiv, 1227-1231. ——. Die papillären Geschwülste der Nasenschleimhaut. Arch. f. path. Anat., etc., Berl., 1883, xciii, 213-258. ——. Bemerkungen über nasale Papillome. Tagebl. d. Versamml. deutsch. Naturf. u. Aerzte, Magdeb., 1884, lvii, 368. ——. Zur Operation und Statistik der adenoi-den Tumoren des Nasenrachenraums. Deutsche med. Wchnschr., Berl., 1885, xi, 572-574. ——. Ueber Nasen-polypen. Monatschr. f. Ohrenh., Berl., 1885, xix, 161; 230. ——. Was ist man berechtigt, Nasenpolyp zu nen-nen? Zugleich eine Antwort auf verschiedene Bemänge-lungen meiner Classification der gutartigen Nasenpoly-pen. *Ibid.*, 1887, xxi, 152; 188; 216; 249.—**Hortolès.** Polype naso-pharyngien; ablation par arrachement sans opération préalable; guérison. Mém. et compt.-rend. Soc. d. sc. méd. de Lyon (1878) 1879, xviii, pt. 2, 102-107. *Also*: Lyon méd., 1878, xxviii, 593-597.—**Houel.** Polype naso-pharyngien; ablation du maxillaire; appareil pro-thétique. Gaz. d. hôp., Par., 1867, xl, 471.—**Huguier.** Tumeur du sinus maxillaire; opération. Bull. Soc. de chir. de Par., 1854-5, v, 178; 187; 201; 212. ——. Kyste séreux de l'aile du nez traité par le séton-fil. *Ibid.*, 1856-7, vii, 333-335. ——. [Polype naso-pharyngien.] *Ibid* (1860), 1861, 2. s., i, 7-11. ——. Polype naso-pha-ryngien; ablation par la méthode ostéo-plastique. Bull. Acad. de méd., Par., 1860-61, xxvi, 783-791. *Also*: Gaz. d. hôp., Par., 1861, xxxiv, 337.—**Hull** (J. M.) A case of multiple polypi producing asthma, with hay and rose fever, signally relieved by the removal of forty-six polypi. Ala-bama M. & S. J., Birmingh., 1886, i, 384-386.—**Hum-phreys** (L.) Nasal polypus. Med. Indep., Detroit, 1857, iii, 367-370.—**Hunt** (R. P.) Nasal polypus. Chi-cago M. J., 1867, xxiv, 429-432.—**Hutchinson** (A. C.) Treatment of nasal polypi. Lond. M. Gaz., 1834, xv, 17.—

Nose (*Tumors of*).

Icart. Observation sur deux polypes arrachés à la même personne, l'un par le nez et l'autre par la bouche. J. de méd., chir., pharm., etc., Par., 1767, xxvi, 459-465. *Also* [Abstr.]: Gaz. hebd. de méd., Par., 1860, vii, 529. ——. Mémoire sur les polypes des narines et principalement sur ceux qui descendent derrière la cloison du palais. Gaz. hebd. de méd., Par., 1860, vii, 465-467.—**Ingals** (E. F.) Dental formation in the nasal cavity. J. Am. M. Ass., Chicago, 1884, ii, 205. ——. On the removal of naso-pharyngeal fibromata by the galvano-cautery, or cold-wire écraseur. *Ibid.*, 533-535. *Also*: Chicago M. J. & Exam., 1884, xlviii, 604-610. ——. Nasal polypus occur-ring in a patient thirteen years of age. J. Am. M. Ass., Chicago, 1884, iii, 212. ——. Catarrh from a large cystic tumor; removal; cure. Weekly M. Rev., Chicago, 1884, ix, 97.—**Ingels** (B.-C.) Observations relatives à l'emploi des injections interstitielles de chlorure de zinc dans le traitement des polypes nasaux et naso-pharyngiens. Ann. Soc. de méd. de Gand, 1880, lviii, 139-146.—**Jacobson** (N.) A naso-pharyngeal tumor of large size; remarks upon the pathology of these growths, and their remov:l after preliminary resection of the superior maxilla. Tr. N. York M. Ass. 1886, Concord, N. H., 1887, iii, 218-233, 1 pl.—**Jacquemart.** Deux cas de polypes des fosses na-sales (adhérence entre le cornet moyen et la cloison); un cas de pseudo-polype. Ann. d. mal. de l'oreille et du la-rynx, Par., 1883, ix, 69-78.—**Jalaguier** (A.) & **Ruault** (A.) Polype en grappe de la fosse nasale droite, faisant saillie dans le naso-pharynx; céphalalgie, douleurs névral-giques, irritabilité nerveuse excessive; extirpation de la tumeur par les voies naturelles; guérison. Arch. de la-ryngol., de rhinol., etc., Par., 1887-8, i, 49-55.—**Jarmu-towski.** Pandry w nosie. [Polypus of nose.] Przegl. lek., Krakow, 1869, viii, 299.—**Jarvis** (W. C.) Myxofi-broma of the nares. Med. Rec., N. Y., 1882, xxii, 270. ——. Vascular tumors of the nasal passages, and their treatment by crushing with the cold wire, with the history of a successful case. Internat. J. Surg. & Antisept., N. Y., 1888, i, 1-8.—**Joal.** Des rapports de l'asthme et des polypes muqueux du nez. Arch. gén. de méd., Par., 1882, i, 440; 535.—**Jobert.** Des polypes naso-pharyngiens. Gaz. d. hôp., Par., 1858, xxxi, 337.—**Johnson** (G.) The practical value of rhinoscopy; case of cyst obstructing the posterior opening of the right nasal fossa. Med. Circ., Lond., 1864, xxiv, 1.—**Johnston** (S.) A case of naso-pharyngeal growth. Tr. Am. Laryngol. Ass. 1886, N. Y., 1887, viii, 182-184. *Also*: N. York M. J., 1887, xlv, 458.—**Jordan** (F.) The treatment of nasal polypi by the tissue injection of iodine. *In his*: Surg. Enq., 2. ed., Lond., [1880], 195-197. ——. The treatment of naso-pha-ryngeal polypus. *Ibid.*, 197-200. ——. Extract from a clinical lecture on a new operation for naso-pharyngeal or fibrous polypus. Brit. M. J., Lond., 1885, i, 888. — **Jo-seph** (G.) Polypen. Ztschr. f. klin. Med., Bresl., 1857, viii, 321. — **Joüon.** Épithéliome tubulé des fosses na-sales. Bull. Soc. anat. de Nantes 1881, Par., 1882, v, 21. *Also*: J. de méd. de l'ouest, Nantes, 1882, xvi, 159. — **Judokius de Roose.** Observations sur un polype du nez, guéri par le suif fondu. J. de méd., chir., pharm., etc., Par., 1767, xxvi, 536 - 538. — **Jurist** (L.) Sixty-two nasal polypi. Med. Bull., Phila., 1884, vi, 59. — **Kappeler** (O.) Fibröse Nasenrachen-Polypen. *In his*: Chir. Beob. d. Thurgau. Kantonssp. Münsterlingen, 8°, Frauenfeld, 1874, 81-87. — **Karpinski** (O.) Beitrag zur temporären (osteoplastischen) Resection der äusseren Nase zur Entfernung von Nasen-Rachenpolypen. Berl. klin. Wchnschr., 1874, xi, 202-204.—**Kempf** (E.) Removal of a fibroid polyp from the nose by the knife. Louisville M. News, 1879, vii, 65.— **Kirtikar** (K. R.) [Case of fibroid nasal polypus arising from the septum.] Tr. M. & Phys. Soc. Bombay (1886), 1887, [3.] s., x, 59. — **Kiwisch von Rotterau** (F. A.) Ungewöhnliche Zufälle, hervorgebracht durch einen Nasenpolypen. Oesterr. med. Wchnschr., Wien, 1843, 455. — **Kjellman** (F.) Om operationen af näspolyper. Hygiea, Stockholm, 1881, xliii, 281-286.—**Knizek.** Beitrag zur Operation der Nasen-Polypen. Prag. med. Wchnschr., 1877, ii, 198; 218.—**König.** Eine neue Methode der Operation von Nasenrachenpolypen. Centralbl. f. Chir., Leipz., 1888, xv, 177-180.—**Kolaczek.** Ein Sarcoma perivasculare der Nase. Arch. f. klin. Chir., Berl., 1875, xviii, 344-349, 1 pl. *Also*: Chir. Klin. zu Bresl., Berl., 1875, 44-46. — **Krackowizer.** Tumor from the nares. N. York M. J., 1866, ii, 443-446. — **Kre-bel** (R.) Ein Fall von Nasenpolypen. Med. Ztg. Russ-lands, St. Petersb., 1856, xiii, 134 — **Küchler** (H.) Aus-ziehung eines Nasenrachenpolypen durch die Mundhöhle. Deutsche Klinik, Berl., 1855, vii, 268.— **Labat.** Quelques réflexions sur les polypes naso-pharyngiens à l'occasion d'une observation de cette maladie; opération (procédé de M. Maisonneuve); succès. J. de méd. de Bordeaux, 1860, 2. s., v, 449-459. *Also*: Monit. d. sc. méd. et pharm., Par., 1860, 2. s. ii, 1028-1030.—**Labbé** (L.) Polype fibro-muqueux de la région naso-pharyngienne. Ann. d. mal. de l'oreille et du larynx, Par., 1875, i, 49-56. — **Lafont** (E.) Note sur un cas de guérison spontanée d'un polype naso-pharyn-gien chez un adolescent. Gaz. hebd. de méd., Par., 1875, xxii, 37.— **Lamprey** (J.) A case of enchondroma in a

Nose (*Tumors of*).

Chinaman cured by operation. Med. Press & Circ., Lond., 1869, vii, 69. — [**Lane** (L. C.)] Nasal polypoid tumor, arising from the presence of a foreign body. San Francisco M. Press, 1863, iv, 105 — **Lange** (V.) Sur une nouvelle méthode pour opérer les tumeurs adénoïdes. Cong. périod. internat. d. sc. méd. Compt.-rend., Amst., 1881, vi, pt. 2, 340-343. ———. Nogle Bemærkninger om Operation af Koanalpolyper med Angivelse af en ny Operationsmethode. Ugesk. f. Læger., Kjøbenh.. 1887, 4. R., xv, 1-9. *Also, transl.:* Deutsche med. Wchnschr., Leipz., 1887, xiii, 213-215. — **Langenbeck** (B.) Neues Verfahren zur Polypen-Unterbindung. Deutsche Klinik, Berl., 1850, ii, 155.—**Lawrence.** Non-malignant tumour of six months' growth; developed within the cavity of the left nostril; absorption of the nasal bones and cartilages; successful removal; expected return of the disease. Lancet, Lond., 1856, i, 455. ———. A new operation for the removal of a large mass of polypi from the nose. Med. Times & Gaz., Lond., 1862, ii, 491. — **Lebert.** [Polypes des fosses nasales; ablation de l'os maxillaire supérieur.] Bull. Soc. anat. de Par., 1852, xxvii, 52. — **Lefferts** (G. M.) A rare case of large cystic tumor of the posterior nares; removal; cure. Med. News, Phila.,1883, xliii, 653.— **Legouest.** Observation de polype naso-pharyngien. Bull. Soc. de chir. de Par. (1860), 1861, 2. s., i, 13-17. ———. Polype naso-pharyngien; ablation par le procédé de Manne et le procédé de la voie lacrymale combinés et modifiés; accidents pendant l'opération; accidents consécutifs; guérison. *Ibid.*, 419-426. ———. Exostose épiphysaire occupant toute la fosse gauche, faisant une saillie considérable dans le pharynx, et déformant notablement la face; ablation à l'aide de la résection temporaire d'une partie du maxillaire supérieur; guérison. Gaz. hebd. de méd., Par., 1863, x, 854-856. ———. Polype naso-pharyngien s'étendant au pharynx, à la narine gauche, ainsi qu'au maxillaire et à la fosse zygomatique; ablation du maxillaire supérieur; extirpation du polype; guérison prompte. Bull. Soc. de chir. de Par. (1864), 1865, 2. s., v, 318-324. ———. À propos d'une opération de polype naso-pharyngien. *Ibid.* (1869), 1870, 2. s., x, 431-439.—**Lenoir.** [Migration d'un polype des fosses nasales vers le grand angle de l'œil et le trou sphéno-palatin.] Bull. Soc. anat. de Par., 1834, ix, 90.—**Leonte.** Fibrom nasofaringien. Lectiune clinica. Spitalul, Bucuresci, 1887, vii, 152 ; 196.—**Leriche.** Tumeur de la cloison nasale, enlevée par mobilisation de la sous-cloison. Gaz. d. hôp., Par., 1874, xlvii, 579. — **Letenneur.** Polype fibreux naso-pharyngien; ablation par fragmentation au moyen d'une pince à écrasement; guérison. *Ibid.*, 1859, xxxii, 2. ———. Polypes naso-pharyngiens. Bull. Soc. de chir. de Par. (1865), 1866, 2. s., vi, 555. ———. Polype naso-pharyngien; trois opérations; guérison. *Ibid.* (1869), 1870, 2. s., x, 501-511.—**Létiévant.** Un polype naso-pharyngien. Lyon méd., 1877, xxvi, 87.—**Levret.** Description d'un instrument inventé par . . . à une méthode de s'en servir pour lier les polypes du nez. J. de méd., chir., pharm., etc., Par., 1771, xxxv, 353-375.—**Lichtenberg** (G.) On fibrous polypus of the nose, with particulars of a case and operation. Lancet, Lond., 1872, ii, 773.— **Lincoln** (R. P.) Naso-pharyngeal polypi, with demonstration of cases. Tr. Am. Laryngol. Ass. 1879, St. Louis, 1882, i, 247-255, 1 pl. *Also:* St. Louis M. & S. J., 1879, xxxvii, 461-469, 1 pl. *Also,* Reprint. ———. On the results of the treatment of naso-pharyngeal fibromata, with demonstration of successful cases, together with a table of seventy-four operations by different surgeons. Tr. Am. Laryngol. Ass., N. Y., 1883, v, 86–112. *Also:* Arch. Laryngol., N. Y., 1883, iv, 258–281. *Also,* Reprint. ———. A case of melano-sarcoma of the nose, cured by galvano-cauterization. Tr. Am. Laryngol. Ass. 1885, N. Y., 1886, vii, 92-94. *Also:* N. York M. J., 1885, xlii, 406. *Also:* Med. News, Phila., 1885, xlvii, 45. ———. Naso-pharyngeal fibrosarcoma removed with galvano-cautery écraseur. Med. Rec., N. Y., 1884, xxvi, 455. *Also:* N. York M. J., 1884, xl, 493. ———. Recurrent naso-pharyngeal tumor; cure by electrolysis. Tr. Am. Laryngol. Ass. 1887, N. Y., 1888, ix, 219-221. *Also:* N. York M. J., 1887, xlvi, 459. *Also,* Reprint.—**Linon.** Polype naso-pharyngien muco-fibreux (myxome) enlevé par l'écraseur linéaire. [Rap. de Delens.] Bull. et mém. Soc. de chir. de Par., 1881, n. s., vii, 480–482.—**Liston.** Lipoma of the nose; clinical remarks. Lancet, Lond., 1836-7, i, 615-617.—**Little** (J. L.) Case of naso-pharyngeal tumor removed by the galvano-cautery. Arch. Clin. Surg., N. Y., 1876-7, i, 3-6.—**Little** (R. E.) A case of polypus of the nose which terminated fatally, with the dissection. West. & South. M. Recorder, Lexington, Ky., 1841-2, i, 120–123.— **Locquin.** Polypes muqueux des fosses nasales; dégénérescence des os en rapport avec la muqueuse de Schneider. Gaz. d. hôp., Par., 1883, lvi, 42.— **Löbel.** Polypus narium gangrænescens falso pro gangræna pulm. habitus; Tod. Ber. d. k. k. Krankenanst. Rudolph-Stiftung in Wien (1867), 1868, 242.—**Löcherer.** Fahrlässige Tödtung in Folge Aetzung eines Nasenpolypen. Friedreich's Bl. f. gerichtl. Med., Nürnb., 1882, xxxiii, 23–28.— **Lœwenberg.** Les tumeurs adénoïdes du pharynx nasal, leur influence sur l'audition, la respiration et la phonation, leur traitement. Gaz. d. hôp.,

Nose (*Tumors of*).

Par., 1878, li, 474; 484; 506; 556; 572; 596; 611; 635; 651; 699; 772; 787. *Also, transl.:* Med. Press & Circ., Lond., 1879, n. s., xxvii, 263; 302; 323; 361; 401; 421; 442; 461. *Also, transl.:* Edinb. M. J., 1878-9, xxiv, 910; 996; 1099: 1879-80, xxv, 40; 123, 1 pl. *Also, transl.:* Anfiteatro anat., Madrid, 1878, vi, 288: 1879, vii, 5; 16: 41; 80; 112; 138; 163; 198; 221; 251. *Also* [Abstr.]: Gac. méd., México, 1879, xiv, 139-141.—**Lorain.** [Polype naso-pharyngien] Bull. Soc. anat. de Par., 1854, xxix, 57-59. — **Luc.** Faits cliniques relatifs aux polypes muqueux des fosses nasales. Union méd., Par., 1887, 3. s., xliii, 233-240.—**Lützelberger.** Beobachtung glücklich ausgerotteter Nasen- und Schlund-Polypen. J. d. pract. Arznk. u. Wundarznk., Berl., 1804, xx, 3. St., 61-69.—**de Lupis** (J. A.) De polypo narium ingentis magnitudinis feliciter exstirpato. Acta Acad. nat. curios., Norimb., 1737, iv, 2-8.— **M'Bride** (P.) Adenoid growths from the naso-pharynx of a boy, æt. 9. Tr. Med.-Chir. Soc. Edinb., 1884-5, n. s., iv, 224. ———. Fibro-mucous polypus of the naso-pharynx. *Ibid.*, 1885-6, n. s., v, 79-83. *Also:* Edinb. M. J., 1885-6, xxxi, 1012-1014.—**McCollom** (J. H.) Removal of naso-pharyngeal polypus. Boston M. & S. J., 1869, lxxix, 406 - 408. — **MacCormac** (W.) On an osteoplastic operation for removing naso-pharyngeal growths. St. Thomas's Hosp. Rep., Lond., 1875, vi, 65-68.—**McGraw** (T. A.) Fibroid polyp of the posterior nares. Michigan M. News, Detroit, 1879, ii. 71.—**Mackenzie** (M.) Nasal polypi; their removal by evulsion, abscission, or electric cautery. Arch. Laryngol., N. Y., 1882, iii, 97-104.—**Maddock** (A. B.) Spontaneous cure of polypus nasi. Lancet, Lond., 1836-7, ii, 590.—**Magjarević** (S.) Fibröser Rachenpolyp bedeutender Grösse. Allg. mil.-ärztl. Ztg., Wien, 1868, ix, 255 - 257. — **Maisonneuve** (J.) Kyste butyreux de la face, simulant un polype cancéreux des fosses nasales. Monit. d. hôp., Par., 1855, iii, 65-67. ———. Polype naso-pharyngien avec prolongements multiples dans la bouche, les narines, la fosse zygomatique, la joue, la fosse temporale; extirpation de l'os maxillaire supérieur; guérison. Gaz. d. hôp., Par., 1855, xxviii, 439. ———. Tumeur carcinomateuse de la base du crâne; ligature extemporanée combinée avec la cautérisation en flèches; guérison. *Ibid.*, 1859, xxxii, 313. ———. Note sur un cas très-grave de polype naso-pharyngien, extirpé avec succès par la boutonnière palatine, au moyen de la ligature extemporanée et de la cautérisation en flèches. Union méd., Par., 1859, 2. s., iv, 484-486. *Also:* Monit. d. sc. méd. et pharm., Par., 1859, vii, 402. ———. Note sur un nouveau perfectionnement apporté à l'opération des polypes naso-pharyngiens. Union méd., Par., 1860, 2. s., vii, 393-396. *Also:* Gaz. d. hôp., Par., 1860, 390. *Also:* Monit. d. sc. méd. et pharm., Par., 1860, 2. s., ii, 797.—**Malherbe** (A.) Note sur une dégénérescence particulière des fibres conjonctives observée dans un polype fibro-muqueux des fosses nasales (dégénérescence mycélioïde). Arch. de physiol. norm. et path., Par., 1879, 2. s., vi, 787-790. ———. Polypes muqueux des fosses nasales. Bull. Soc. anat. de Nantes 1881, Par., 1882, v, 69. *Also:* J. de méd., de l'ouest, Nantes, 1882, xvi, 371.—**Manfredi** (F.) Un caso di adenoma multiplo del faringe nasale. Morgagni, Napoli, 1879, xxi, 344.—**Mansa** (F. W.) De polypo nasali congenito. Acta reg. Soc. med. Havn., 1829, vii, 258-261. — **Marchettis** (P.) Obstructio utriusque naris, altera quidem integra, a polypo spurio, carne scilicet, callosa ulceri ex contusione externa accrescente, alia vero imperfecta, feliciter sanatæ. *In his:* Obs. med.-chir. [etc.] 8°, Lond., 1729, 39. *Also, in his:* Rec. d. obs. rares, etc., trad., 8°, Par., 1858. 81-83.— **Marjolin.** Polype fibreux naso-pharyngien chez une petite fille de deux ans. Bull. Soc. de chir. de Par. (1861), 1862, 2. s., ii, 321.— **Marsh** (H.) Nasal polypus removed from a child nine years old. Tr. Path. Soc. Lond., 1869-70, xxi, 343.—**Mason** (F.) Myeloid tumour of the septum nasi. Proc. M. Soc. Lond., 1875-7, iii, 83-85. *Also:* Med. Times & Gaz., Lond., 1875, i, 552.—**Massei** (F.) Mixomi giganteschi della cavità naso-faringea. Arch. ital. di laringol., Napoli, 1884-5, iv, 163-167. ———. Sopra un caso di enorme fibroma del cavo naso-faringeo. *Ibid.*, 1887, vii. 113 - 128. — **Medina Ferrer** (F.) Pólipo nasal mucoso curado con las duchas antisépticas An. de otol. y laringol., Alcalá de Henares, 1886, iv, 111. *Also:* Crón. méd.-quir. de la Habana, 1886, xii, 161.—**Menocal** (R.) Fibroma naso-faringeo; extirpacion; curacion. Crón. méd.-quir. de la Habana, 1886, xii, 406-408.—**Menzel** (A.) Fibröser Polyp der Schädelbasis; Exstirpation mit Resection des Oberkiefers; Heilung. Arch. f. klin. Chir., Berl., 1872, xiii, 680. *Also, transl.:* Gazz. med. ital. lomb., Milano, 1872, xxxii, 25.—**Mercier.** [Une production cornée enlevée du nez d'un vieillard] Bull. Soc. anat. de Par., 1836, x, 98; 132.—**Mertrud.** Mémoire où l'on se propose de donner les moyens les plus convenables pour parvenir à la guérison des polypes qui viennent dans les narines. Gaz. hebd. de méd., Par., 1860, vii, 449-452.—**Meyer.** Abhandlung über die Ausrottung eines Nasenpolypen. N. Biblioth. f. d. Chir. u. Ophth., Hannov., 1821-2, iii, 238-255.—**Michaux.** Polype de la partie supérieure du pharynx, s'insérant à la base du crâne, aux premières vertèbres cervicales et à la voûte palatine, et s'engageant dans les sinus sphenoïuaux et la fosse nasale gauche; ablation de

Nose (*Tumors of*).

l'os maxillaire supérieur; destruction du polype par arrachement, excision et cautérisation; guérison. Bull. Acad. roy. de méd. de Belg., Brux., 1847-8, vii, 246-255. *Also:* Gaz. méd. de Par.. 1848, 3. s., iii, 446. ———— Polypes naso-pharyngiens. Gaz. d. hôp., Par., 1853, xxvi, 58; 315. ———— Nouvelles considérations sur les polypes naso-pharyngiens. Bull. Acad. roy. de méd. de Belg., Brux., 1862, 2. s., v, 679-784, 4 pl. [Discussion], 1864 vii, 140 : 217; 271; 402; 443. *Also*, Reprint. *Also* [Abstr.]: Gaz. d. hôp., Par., 1864, xxxvii, 254. [Rap. de Horion.] Ann. Soc. méd.-chir. de Liége, 1863, ii, 301; 338. ———— Nouveau cas de polype naso-pharyngien opéré avec succès. Bull. Acad. roy. de méd. de Belg., Brux., 1864, 2. s., vii, 195-208, 2 pl. ———— Quelques mots encore sur les polypes fibreux naso pharyngiens volumineux, à insertions larges et résistantes et à prolongements multiples. *Ibid.*, 1867, 3. s., i, 397-453, 2 pl. *Also*, Reprint. ———— Nouvelle note sur le diagnostic et le traitement des polypes fibreux naso-pharyngiens. Bull. Acad. roy. de méd. de Belg., Brux., 1869, 3. s., iii, 510-549. ———— Résumé du traitement des polypes fibreux naso-pharyngiens. *Ibid.*, 1879, 3. s., xiii, 424-460.—**Michel.** Observation de tumeur osseuse (myéloïde) du vomer (exostose spongieuse des fosses nasales; Richet, Olivier), suivie de réflexions pour servir à l'histoire des exostoses de la face. Gaz. hebd. de méd., Par., 1873, 2. s., x, 380; 396.—**Michel** (C.) Ueber electrolytische Behandlung der fibrösen, gefässreichen Nasenrachenpolypen Monatschr. f. Ohrenh., Berl., 1887, xxi, 116-121.—**Mignot.** Polypes muqueux des narines; ablation; guérison. Soc. d. sc. méd. de Gannat. Compt. rend., Par., 1880, xxxiv, 55.—**Mikulicz** (J.) Zur Gussenbauer'schen Operationsmethode bei fibrösen Nasenrachenpolypen. Prag. med. Wchnschr., 1883, viii, 409; 417. ———— Przyczynek do sposobu operowania polipów nosopolykowych. [On the extirpation of polypus of naso-pharyngeal region.] Przegl. lek., Krakow., 1883, xxii, 53-55.—**Miller** (A. G.) The treatment of mucous polypus of the nose. Brit. M. J., Lond., 1879, ii, 938.—**Mo** (G.) Enorme fibro-sarcoma della cavità nasale sinistra; esportazione col metodo di Bruns; guarigione. Oss rvatore, Torino, 1882, xviii, 641; 673; 705. — **Mollière** (D.) Note sur un cas de polype naso pharyngien. Lyon méd., 1887, liv, 107-110. — **Monfalcon.** Polypes des fosses nasales. Dict. d. sc. méd., Par., 1820, xliv, 194-218. — **Monod** (C.) Polype fibreux génio-naso-pharyngien. Bull. Soc. anat. de Par. (1872), 1874, xlvii, 337-339.—**Morel-Lavallée.** Note sur une tumeur polypiforme des fosses nasales. *Ibid.*, 1883, lviii, 392. *Also:* Progrès méd., Par., 1884, xii, 333.—**Morris** (H.) Remarks on naso-pharyngeal polypi and the operations for their removal. Med. Times & Gaz., Lond., 1881, i, 590; 616; 646.—**Moscati** (P.) Descrizione di un metodo per la legatura dei polipi, che dalle nari posteriori scendono in gola. Ann. univ. di med., Milano, 1824, xxix, 86-92.—**Mott** (V.) New operation. Am. J. M. Sc., Phila.. 1842, n. s., iii, 257. ———— A nasal operation for the removal of a large tumour filling up the entire nostril and extending to the pharynx. *Ibid.*, 1843, n. s., v, 87-91.—**Motta** (E) Polypo naso pharyngeo; extracção pelo esmagador de Chassaignac, com divisão previa do véu palatino. J. Soc. d. sc. med. de Lisb., 1861, 2. s., xxv, 187-192.—**Mougins** (P.) Ablation d'une tumeur squirrheuse développée dans une fosse nasale, et restauration de la perte de substance à l'aide d'un lambeau pris à la joue; résultat satisfaisant et sans difformité. Rev. de thérap. méd.-chir., Par., 1861, 621-623. — **Moure** (E.-J.) Des pseudo-tumeurs des fosses nasales. Rev. mens. de laryngol., etc., Bordeaux, 1882, iii, 1-10. ———— Sur un cas de fibro-sarcome primitif de la fosse nasale droite. *Ibid.*, Par., 1886, vi, 417-425. ———— Polype kystique des arrière-fosses nasales. J. de méd. de Bordeaux, 1886-7, xvi, 64. — **Münchmeyer.** Beobachtung einer Krankheit der oberen Nasenhöhle mit völliger Vereiterung und Zerstörung der Sphenoidal- und Ethmoidalhöhlen. Ztschr. f. d. ges. Med., Hamb., 1842, xx, 377-382. — **Mütter.** Gelatinous polypus of the nose; operation with forceps. Med. Exam., Phila., 1843, vi, 101; 135.—**Mulhall.** Asthma from nasal polypi. St. Louis M. & S. J., 1882, xlii, 165-172.—**Muron.** Étude sur la structure des polypes fibreux naso-pharyngiens. Compt. rend. Soc. de biol. 1869, Par., 1870, 5. s., i, 223-225.—**Nélaton.** Nouvelle méthode pour opérer les tumeurs fibreuses de la base du crâne. Gaz. d. hôp., Par., 1849, 3. s., i, 128. ———— Polype fibreux de la base du crâne; considérations générales. *Ibid.*, 1853, xxvi, 22. ———— Polypi naso-pharyngien attaqué par une ouverture artificielle faite à la voûte palatine; excision; cautérisations successives avec l'aide nitrique monohydrate. J. de méd. et chir. prat., Par., 1853, xxiv, 500-503 ———— Leçons sur un cas de polype naso-pharyngien. Monit. d. hôp. Par., 1853, i, 54-56. ———— Leçons cliniques sur les polypes fibreux naso-pharyngiens. *Ibid.*, 1854, ii, 642; 677.—**Neumann** (J.) & **Semeleder.** Rachenpolyp, von der Schädelbasis ausgehend, durch Galvanokaustik ohne Blutung entfernt; rhinoskopische Untersuchung. Allg. Wien. med. Ztg., 1860, v, 212.—**Neureutter** (T.) Sarcoma nasopharyngeale. Wien. med. Presse, 1871, xii, 590-594.—**Nikoleski** (P. P.) O vtorom sluchayai udaleniya nosoglotochnago polpa po sposobu Lyangenbeka. [Second case of removal of nasal polypus by Langenbeck's method.]

Nose (*Tumors of*).

Laitop. khirurg. Obsh. v. Mosk. (1873-5), 1876, i, 451.—**Nixon** (F. A.) A large number of polypi (fibro-myxomas) obstructing both nostrils. Med. Press & Circ., Lond., 1879, n. s., xxviii, 305.—**Noble** (S. C.) Case of large nasal polypoid growth. Med. Times & Gaz , Lond., 1862, ii, 404.—**Notta.** Polypes du nez datant de trente ans; section préalable du nez; extirpation; guérison. Année méd., Caen, 1877, ii, 40-43. — **Novaro** (G. F.) Osservazioni sulla memoria del Dott. Dionisio, intitolata: Estirpazione di voluminoso mixoma occupante l' intiero ambito delle cavità nasali, estrusosi per le suture naso-mascellari verso le regioni genio-malari. Gior. d. r. Accad. di med. di Torino, 1877, 3. s., xxii, 193-197. — **Ollier.** Polype fibreux naso-pharyngien opéré par un nouveau procédé. Mém. et compt.-rend. Soc. d. sc. méd. de Lyon, 1864-5, iv, pt. 2, 46-50. ———— Polype naso-pharyngien; ablation du maxillaire supérieur comme opération préliminaire; conservation du périoste et reproduction de l'os; guérison constatée sept mois après l'opération. Bull. Soc. de chir. de Par., (1864), 1865, 2. s., v, 324. *Also:* Gaz. d. hôp., Par., 1864, xxxvii, 330. ———— Nouveau procédé opératoire pour l'ablation des polypes naso-pharyngiens ; ablation du chir. de Par. (1866), 1867, 2. s., vii, 263-265. ———— De l'opération des fibrômes naso-pharyngiens, au moyen de l'abaissement du nez par l'ostéotomie verticale et bilatér. le de la charpente de cet organe. *Ibid.*, 1873, 3. s., ii, 401-407.—**Olney** (F. E.) A case of naso-pharyngeal tumor; operation by E. F. Ingals. Chicago M. J. & Exam., 1883, xlvii, 48-50.—**Opitz** (W.) Die Behandlung der Nasen-Rachenpolypen, vorzüglich nach den Verhandlungen in der chirurgischen Gesellschaft zu Paris dargestellt. Schmidt's Jahrb., Leipz., 1862, cxv, 219-237.—**Ord** (W. M.) Case of polypus nasi extending upwards and producing absorption of the body of the sphenoid bone, and obliteration of the internal carotid artery, followed by abscess in the brain. Brit. M. J., Lond., 1858. 471. — **Ory.** Des polypes de la partie postérieure des fosses nasales. Bull. Soc. anat. de Par., 1874, xlix, 912-917. *Also:* Progrès méd., Par., 1875, iii, 190-192.—**Oséo.** Sarcoma melanótico de las fosas nasales, del seno maxilar, de la orbita y del seno frontal; operacion; muerte. Rev. de cien. méd., Barcel., 1875, i, 312: 1876, ii, 22. — **Paci.** Tumore poliposo faringeo operato colla galvanocaustica per le vie nasali. Atti Cong. gen. d. Ass. med. ital. 1878, Pisa, 1879, viii, 197-199.—**Palasciano.** De la perforation de l'unguis comme moyen de parvenir à la destruction des polypes de la base du crâne. Amtl. Ber. ü. d. Versamml. deutsch. Naturf. u. Aerzte 1858, Carlsruhe, 1859, xxxiv, 279-281, 1 pl. *Also:* Bull. Soc. de chir. de Par. (1860), 1861, 2. s., i, 372-376. *Also:* Gaz. d. hôp., Par., 1860. xxx, 331. — **Pamard.** Polype naso-pharyngien; ablation, après la résection sous-périostée du maxillaire supérieur. [Rap. de Duplay.] Bull. Soc. de chir. de Par., 1873, 3. s., ii, 576-582. *Also:* Gaz. d. hôp., Par., 1874, xlvii, 75-77. ———— Polype naso-pharyngien; récidive; seconde opération; guérison remontant à dix-sept mois. Bull. et mém. Soc. de chir. de Par., 1875, n. s., i, 317-321.—**Paquet.** Destruction d'un polype naso-pharyngien par l'électricité. Bull. Soc. anat. de Par., 1867, xlii, 677. — **Parada y Santin** (J.) Pólipos naso-faringeos (mixomas); disgregacion y avulsion forzada; curacion. Jurado méd.-farm., Madrid, 1881, ii, 283. — **Park** (M.) Encysted atheromatous tumor situated in the cavity of the nose, displacing the nasal bones. Lancet, Lond., 1841-2, i. 886.—**Parker** (R) Acinous adenoma of tip of nose. Tr. Path. Soc. Lond., 1880-81, xxxii, 238. — **Pauchon** (A.) Quelques mots sur l'histoire des polypes fibreux naso-pharyngiens et sur leur traitement par l'ablation partielle ou totale du maxillaire supérieur. Marseille méd., 1874, xi, 391-407. — **Péan.** Hématome de la cloison nasale; mode de production de cette tumeur; symptômes; diagnostic; traitement. *In his:* Leçons de clin. chir., etc., 8°. Par., 1882, 133-138.—**Peltier.** Polype fibromuqueux de l'arrière-cavité des fosses nasales. Ann. d. mal. de l'oreille et du larynx, Par., 1882, viii, 179-181.—**Pemberton.** Malignant polypus of the nose; death from asphyxia during an operation for its relief. Prov. M. & S. J., Lond., 1850, 519. — **Pepinster.** Polype fibreux volumineux des fosses nasales; arrachement; guérison. Arch. belges de méd. mil , Brux., 1856, xvii. 342-345. — **Perez y Jimenez** (N. A.) Caso notable de fibroma de las fosas nasales. Génio méd.-quir., Madrid, 1875, xxi, 346.—**Peters** (G. A.) Naso-pharyngeal polypus. Med. Rec., N. Y., 1881, xx, 166. ———— . Naso-pharyngeal polypus. *Ibid.*, 1882, xxi, 243.—**Petrone** (G) Sopra un raro caso di mixomo poliposo naso-faringeo; considerazioni pratiche ed istologiche. Arch. ital. di laringol., Napoli, 1884-5, iv, 15-19. — **Piachaud.** Polypes fibreux naso-pharyngiens et ptérygo-maxillaires. Bull. Soc. de chir. de Par. (1863), 1864, 2. s., iv, 107-114.—**Pick** (T. P.) On naso-pharyngeal polypi. Saint George's Hosp. Rep., Lond., 1867, ii, 151-168.—**Picniazek.** Einige Fälle von Nasenpolypen und deren Entfernung mit der Stahlschlinge. Wien. med. Bl., 1878, i 672; 700.—**Pluyette.** Des fibromes naso-pharyngiens chez la femme. Rev. de chir., Par., 1887, vii, 202-223. *Also, transl.* [Abstr.]: Med.-chir. Centralbl., Wien, 1887, xxii, 507. — **Poisson.** Polype naso-pharyngien (opération). J. de méd. de l'ouest, Nantes,

Nose (*Tumors of*).

1886, xx, 385. — **Polano** (M.) Over de boutonnière sta-
phyline of overlangsche insnijding in de middellijn van het
zachte verhemelte als voorbereidende kunstbewerking bij
de extirpatie der neuskeelgatsplypen van Maisonneuve
en Foucher. Nederl. Tijdschr. v. Geneesk., Amst., 1860,
iv, 181-185. — **Post.** Tumor in nasal cavity. N. York
J. M., 1846, vi, 13.— **Poyet** (G.) Polype muqueux de l'arrière-cavité des fosses nasales. Bull. Soc. anat. de Par.,
1875, l, 623-627. — **Pozzi** (S.) Myxôme polypeux ulcéré
de la narine droite ; corps fibro-plastiques; infiltration de
leucocytes. *Ibid.* (1872), 1874, xlvii, 359. ———. Sur les
causes de la mort subite dans l'extirpation des polypes
naso-pharyngiens, et sur le pronostic de cette opération.
Assoc. franç. pour l'avance. d. sc. Compt.-rend. 1874, Par.,
1875, iii, 833-842. *Also*: Progrès méd., Par., 1874, ii, 591 ;
607. *Also, transl.*: Anfiteatro anat., Madrid, 1878, vi, 33 ;
42 ; 53. — **Preterre.** Polype naso-pharyngien avec prolongements multiples dans la bouche, les narines, la fosse
zygomatique, la joue, la fosse temporale; extirpation de
l'os maxillaire supérieur; guérison. Bull. Acad. roy. de
méd. de Belg., Brux., 1861, 2. s., iv, 705-715. — **Puzey**
(C.) A note on the removal of naso-pharyngeal polypi.
Liverpool M.-Chir. J., 1881, i, 86. — **Rainer** (J. B.)
Heilung von Nasenpolypen durch die äusserliche Anwendung der Tinctura opii crocata. Med.-chir. Ztg., Innsbruck, 1821, iii, 60-63. — **Rampolla.** Note sur un nouveau procédé pour le traitement chirurgical des polypes
naso-pharyngiens. Bull. Soc. de chir. de Par. (1860), 1861,
2. s., i, 140-144. [Rap. de Verneuil], 144 ; 212. [Discus-
sion], 224 ; 258. *Also*: Abeille méd., Par., 1860, xvii, 105.—
Reclus. Polype muqueux implanté à la partie postérieure des fosses nasales. Bull. Soc. anat. de Par., 1874,
xlix, 678.— **Reeder** (J. H.) The tr. muriate ferri in nasal
polypus. Chicago M. J., 1859, n. s., ii, 547. — **Renaut.**
Structure de certains polypes muqueux des fosses nasales.
Bull. Soc. anat. de Par., 1871, xlvi, 229.— **Reynolds** (D. S.)
Radical cure of nasal polypi by injections. Tr. Am. M.
Ass., Phila., 1881, xxxii, 237-242. *Also*: Med. Rec., N. Y.,
1881, xx, 368-370. — **Richard** (A.) Polype naso-pharyngien. Bull. Soc. de chir. de Par., 1854-5, v, 118. ———.
[Un polype naso-pharyngien.] *Ibid.* (1860), 1861, 2. s., i,
283-291. — **Richardson** (B. W.) Treatment of nasal
polypus by sodium ethylate. Asclepiad, Lond., 1884, i,
251-253. — **Richet.** Sarcome de la fosse nasale droite
opéré par la méthode nasale. Ann. d. mal. de l'oreille et
du larynx, Par., 1881, vii, 327-331. ———. Polype naso-
pharyngien, ayant détruit la base du crâne sans produire
de symptômes ; perforation de la paroi du sinus caverneux
pendant les tentatives de décollement. Siècle méd., Par.,
1881, ii, 73.— **Richter** (A. G.) Ein Nasenpolyp. *In his*:
Med. u. chir. Bemerkungen, 8°, Berl., 1813, ii, 82-86. —
Rigal (J.-A.) Observation de polype des fosses nasales
et de l'arrière-gorge. Gaz. méd. de Par., 1831, ii, 88-90.—
Rigal (J.-J.) [Polype aux arrières narines.] Ann.
clin., Montpel., 1810, xxiii, 211-214. — **Robert.** Polype
fibreux récidivé. Bull. Soc. de chir. de l'ar., 1853-4, iv,
151. ———. Des kystes de la région orbito-nasale. J. de
méd. et chir. prat., Par., 1858, xxix, 546-550. — **Ob-**
servation d'un polype naso-pharyngien inséré sur la colonne
vertébrale. Monit. d. hôp., Par., 1859, vii, 489. ———.
Polypes naso-pharyngiens. Bull. Soc. de chir. de Par.
(1860), 1861, 2. s., i, 39-41. — **Robertson** (W.) Account
of an operation for the extraction of the polypus
from the nose. Edinb. M. & S. J., 1827, xxvii, 44. — **Rob-**
inson (B.) Remarks on hypertrophy of turbinated corpora cavernosa. Am. J. M. Sc., Phila., 1877, n. s., lxxiii,
431-436.— **Rochard** (J.) Histoire des progrès accomplis
récemment dans l'étude et le traitement des polypes naso-
pharyngiens. Gaz. hebd. de méd., Par., 1874, xxi, 637-
639. ———. Communication sur les polypes naso-pharyngiens. Bull. et mém. Soc. de chir. de Par., 1879, n. s., v,
903-907.— **Roché** (L.) Polype naso-pharingien; opération
par arrachement; guérison. Bull. Soc. méd. de l'Yonne
1864, Auxerre, 1865, 216-220. — **Roe** (J. O) Angioma of
the nose. N. York M. J., 1886, xliii, 64-68. *Also*, Reprint.— **Rombeau.** [Polype des fosses nasales et du
sinus maxillaire.] Bull. Soc. anat. de Par., 1851, xxvi, 35.—
Rose (E.) Zwei Fälle von Nasenschläfenpolypen. Ann.
d. Char.-Krankenh. zu Berl., 1864-5, xii, 2. Hft., 101-121.—
Roth (W.) Entfernung einer übertaubeneigrossen Geschwulst aus dem Nasenrachenraume. Wien. med. Wchnschr., 1880, xxx, 845-847. — **Rouse.** Suspicious warty
tumor on the end of the nose of a boy, removed by caustics.
Lancet, Lond., 1860, ii, 212. ———. Case of fibrous polypus
treated by Langenbeck's method of operation. *Ibid.*,
1869, i, 293.— **Routier** (A.) Sarcome des fosses nasales ;
ablation ; ozène consécutif; guérison. Rev. de chir., Par.,
1887, vii, 62-66. — **Roux.** Polype fibreux énorme des
narines avec destruction partielle de l'os propre du nez et
de la peau du côté droit à travers lesquels il faisait saillie;
arrachement pratiqué avec beaucoup de difficulté; guérison très avancée. Gaz. d. hôp., Par., 1843, 2. s., v, 591 ;
594. — **Roux** (J.) Polypes naso-pharyngiens; opération
prélimin. i e; procédé par écartement des os maxillaires
supérieurs. Gaz. d. hôp., Par., 1861, xxxiv, 354.— **Rubio**
(F.) Pólipos mucosos de ambas fosas nasales; empleo de
varias inyecciones en su parénquima sin resultado ; opera-

Nose (*Tumors of*).

cion por avulsion; curacion; indicaciones sobre el caso.
Siglo méd., Madrid, 1880, xxvii, 694. — **de Sagastume**
(J. R.) Extirpacion de un gran pólipo celulo-mucoso que
llenaba toda la cavidad nasal derecha, por una combinacion
de procedimientos, empleando : 1º la ligadura; 2º la avulsion ; 3º la cauterizacion. *Ibid.*, 1859, vi, 184.— **de Saint-**
Germain. Polype muqueux occupant la partie moyenne
du pharynx et les fosses nasales; extirpation à travers le
voile du palais divisé; guérison. Gaz. d. hôp., Par., 1874,
xlvii, 66.— **Salamanca** (D.) Sobre los polipos fibrosos
naso-farinjeos ó de la base del cráneo, considerados bajo el
punto de vista del diagnóstico i de la terapéutica. An.
Univ. de Chile, Santiago, 1869, xxxii, 285-317. — **Sancho**
(M.) Pólipo naso-faringeo ó naso-craneano, segun la clasificacion del Dr. Encinas. Génio méd.-quir., Madrid, 1880,
xxvi, 204. — **Sands** (H. B.) Naso-pharyngeal fibrous tumor; operation. Med. Rec., N. Y., 1872, vii. 578. ———.
On naso-pharyngeal polypi. Arch. Scient. & Pract. M. &
S., Phila. & N. Y., 1873, i, 493-519, 1 pl. ———. Recurrent
naso-pharyngeal polypus; removal by galvano-cautery.
Arch. Clin. Surg., N. Y., 1876, i, 74.— **Sato** (S.) [A clinical lecture on nasal tumors.] Iji Shinbun, Tokio, 1880,
no. 25, April 23.— **Savory** (W. S.) Abstract of clinical
lecture on a case of naso-pharyngeal polypus. Brit. M.
J., Lond., 1878, i, 3-5.— **Schaeffer** (M.) Nasenpolypen.
Deutsche med. Wchnschr., Berl., 1882, viii, 324-326. —
Scheff (G.) Die Entwicklung von Cysten in den Nebenhöhlen der Nase. Allg. Wien. med. Ztg., 1883, xxviii,
77.— **Scholz** (W.) Nasenrachenpolyp-Unterbindung;
neuerliche Entwicklung eines gleichen Neugebildes auf
der andern Seite. Spitals-Ztg., Wien, 1862, 302-304. —
Schramm. Polip nosopolykowy, wyłuszczenie przez
jamę ustną. [Polypus of nose; extirpation through
mouth.] Przegl. lek., Krakow, 1883, xxii. 311.— **Schre-**
ger (D.) Nasenpolypen; über einige Entstehungsver-
hältnisse derselben, und Complication mit Telangiectasie
der Nasenschleimhaut. Ann. d. chir. Clin. a. d. Univ. zu
Erlang., 1816, i, 36-48. ———. Meine Werkzeuge zur Ausrottung der Nasenpolypen. Neue (Der) Chiron, Sulzbach,
1823, i, 197-206, 1 pl.— **Schreiber** (J. N.) Erprobte Operationsmethode bei grossen Nasen-Rachenpolypen. Med.
Jahrb. d. k. k. österr. Staates, Wien, 1841, xxxvi, 66-78.—
Schwabe. Abgang von Nasenpolypen nach anhaltenden
Weinen, nebst einigen Anmerkungen über die Aetiologie
der Polypen überhaupt. Klin. Ztschr. f. Chir. u. Augenh.,
Halle, 1836-7, i, 369-377.— **Scott** (J. S.) Removal of a
congenital aneurismal tumor. Canada Lancet, Toronto,
1872-3, v, 61.— **Sédillot.** Polype naso-pharyngien ; procédé nouveau d'extirpation. Proc.-verb. . . . Soc. de méd.
de Strasb. (1858-63), 1864, i, 160-164. ———. Polype nasal;
racines pénétrant dans le sinus sphénoïdal. *Ibid.*, 190-
192.— **Seifert.** Ueber Myxofibrome der Choanen. Sitzungsb. d. phys.-med. Gesellsch. zu Würzb., 1887, 35-41.—
Seiler (C.) Erectile tumor of the anterior nares. Am.
Specialist, Phila., 1881, ii, 7. ———. Some remarks on the
pathology of intra-nasal hypertrophies. Tr. Path. Soc.
Phila. (1881-3), 1884, xi, 110-121. ———. Fibroid polypus
of the nose involving the antrum. *Ibid.*, 126. ———. Ec-
chondroses of the septum narium and their removal.
Med. Rec., N. Y., 1888, xxxiii, 180-183. — **Setterblad** (G.)
Fall of nässvalgpolyp opererad med galvanokaustik. Hygiea, Stockholm, 1886, xlviii, 110-121.— **Shortt** (J.) A
case of lipoma. Madras Month. J. M. Sc., 1873, vii, 89, 1
pl.— **Shrady** (G. F.) Removal of a large naso-pharyngeal
tumor with extensive attachments to base of skull; unex-
pected brain complication; death. Med. Rec., N. Y.,
1882, xxii, 311-314.— **Shurly** (E. L.) The galvano-cautery
compared with other means of destroying the mucous
membrane of the nasal and pharyngeal cavities. N. York
M. J., 1885, xli, 95-97.— **Sibthorpe.** Lipoma (so-called)
of the nose. Indian M. Gaz., Calcutta, 1887, xxii, 316,
1 pl.— **Simon.** Abscess in the brain from obliteration of the carotid trunk by the pressure of a nasal polypus. Med. Times & Gaz., Lond., 1858, xvi, 631.— **Siotis.**
Polype naso-pharyngien traité au moyen des douches nasales. Gaz. méd. d'Orient, Constantinople, 1869-70, xiii,
35.— **Skey.** Polypus of the nose involving the orbit.
Lancet, Lond., 1860, i, 118.— **Smith** (H.) Removal of
large nasal polypus. Med. Times & Gaz., Lond., 1869, ii,
412. ———. Large fibrous polypus of the nose ; operation ;
recovery. Brit. M. J., Lond., 1869, ii, 557.— **Smith** (J.
F.) A large post-nasal polypus, with unusual complications. Indiana M. J., Indianap., 1887-8, vi, 216-218.—
Sovostitski (G. A.) Sluchai udaleniya polipa velichi-
noyu v' kulak iz pravoi polovine polosti. [Removal of a
large polypus from the nose.] Laitop. khirurg. Obsh. v.
Mosk. (1873-5), 1876, i, 174.— **Spaak.** Tumeur hémorrhagique de la cavité pharyngo nasale; aphonie nerveuse;
guérison. Ann. d. mal. de l'oreille et du larynx, Par., 1876,
ii, 358-361.— **Spantigati** (G.) Osservazioni sulla memoria del Dott. Dionisio, intitolata : Estirpazione di voluminoso mixoma occupante l'intiero ambito delle cavità nasali,
estrusovi per le suture naso-mascellare verso le regioni
genio-malari. Gior. d. r. Accad. di med. di Torino, 1877,
3. s., xxxi, 197-200.— **Squire** (W.) Fibrinous polypi from
the nares. Tr. Path. Soc. Lond., 1869-70, xxi, 343.— **Stein-**
brügge (H.) Ueber die histologische Beschaffenheit der

Nose (*Tumors of*).

unteren Nasenmuscheln, sowie der von innen entspringenden telangiektatischen Fibrome. Ztschr. f. Ohrenh., Wiesb., 1879, viii, 110-122, 2 pl.—**Steiner** (F.) Sehr ausgedehnter fibröser Nasen-Polyp; Exstirpation desselben nach Resektion des Nasenfortsatzes des rechten Oberkiefers, des rechten Nasenbeins und der vordern Wand der rechten Stirnhöhle, rasche Heilung; Mechanismus des Abschlusses der Nasenhöhle von der Mundböhle durch das Velum palatinum. Wien. med. Wchnschr., 1868, xviii, 1082; 1099.—**Steinhausen.** Polypus narium. [3 cases.] Mag. d. Heilk., Berl., 1844, lxiii, 494-499 —**Stoker** (W. T.) On the removal of naso-pharyngeal tumours. Tr. Acad. M. Ireland 1883-4, Dubl., 1884, ii, 127-134, 1 pl. *Also:* Dublin J. M. Sc., 1884, lxxvii, 159-162. *Also:* Med. Press & Circ., Lond., 1884, n. s., xxxviii, 88-90.—**Stonham** (C.) Naso-pharyngeal polypus (recurrence). Tr. Clin. Soc. Lond., 1884, xvii, 235. ——. A case of naso-pharyngeal polypus; Lawrence's operation; recurrence; second operation; recovery. Lancet, Lond., 1888, i, 13.—**Storchi** (F.) Polipo naso-faringeo causa di accessi epilettiformi; estirpazione; guarigione. Spallanzani, Roma, 1886, 2. s., xv, 462.—**Storrer** (E.) Nasal polypi and their removal, with cases. Pacific M. & S. J., San Fran., 1880-81, xxiii, 358-362. —**Stricker** (W.) Heilung eines Nasenpolypen durch Jodtinctur. Arch. f. path. Anat., etc., Berl., 1863, xxvii, 211.—**Stukovenkoff** (M.) Rhinoscleroma. Priloj. k protok. zasaid. Obsh. Kievsk. vrach., Kiev, 1887, 98-111, 1 pl. — **Syme** (J.) Fibrous polypus of the nose. Edinb. M. & S. J., 1832, xxxviii, 322-324. ——. Nasal polypus. Edinb. & Lond. Month. J. M. Sc., 1842, ii, 790-792. ——. Case of fibrous polypus. Month. J. M. Sc., Lond. & Edinb., 1850, xi, 385-387. ——. Fibrous polypus of the nose. *Ibid.*, 1852, xv, 274-276. — **Tangemann** (C. W.) Nasal polypus. Cincin. Lancet & Clinic, 1885, n. s., xiv, 583.—**Tardieu** (A.) Carie de l'os de la pommette, de l'os unguis, du sphénoïde, du maxillaire droit et des dents de ce côté, par suite d'un polype de la fosse nasale droite. Bull. gén. de thérap., etc., Par., 1842, xxii, 373.—**Taylor** (H.) Polypous tumour displacing the globe of the eye. Edinb. M. & S. J., 1846, lxvi, 6-10. — **Tempesti** (G. C.) Storia dell' estirpazione di un polipo voluminoso impiantato nella volta della faringe; nuovo strumento. Gazz. med. ital. feder. tosc., Firenze, 1850-51, 2. s., i, 345-349. — **Terrier** (F.) Procédé pour l'ablation des polypes muqueux dans les fosses nasales. J. de med. et chir. prat., Par., 1874, xlv, 394-397. ——. Sarcome des fosses nasales. Ann. d. mal. de l'oreille et du larynx., Par., 1884, x, 279-282. — **Terrillon.** Traitement des polypes muqueux des fosses nasales. Bull. gén. de thérap., etc., Par., 1874, lxxxvii, 533-539 —**Testelin** (A.) Polype condylomateux des fosses nasales; ablation; guérison sans récidive. J. de méd. chir. et pharmacol., Brux., 1859, xxviii, 147-150.— **Thomas** (J. D.) Sarcomatous tumour removed from the naso-pharynx. Australas. M. Gaz., Sydney, 1886-7, vi, 164. — **Thorndike** (W. H.) Naso-pharyngeal polypus; depression of superior maxilla; replacement; recovery; two cases. Med. & Surg. Rep. Bost. City Hosp. (1874-9), 1882, iii, 152-154.—**Thudichum** (J. L. W.) On polypus and other morbid growths in the nose; their radical treatment by the electro-caustic method and their connexion with asthma. Lancet, Lond., 1880, i, 594-596. *Also* [Abstr.]: Proc. M. Soc. Lond., 1879-81, v, 78. ——. On the nature and treatment of hypertrophies and tumours of the nasal and pharyngeal cavities. [Substance of a paper read before the West London Medico-Chirurgical Society, Feb. 4, 1887.] Lancet, Lond., 1887, ii, 401-403. — **Tiffany** (L. McL.) Removal of the naso-pharyngeal polypus by temporary depression of both upper jaws. Tr. M. & Chir. Fac. Maryland, Balt., 1878, 180-187. *Also,* Reprint. ——. The treatment of nasal polypi by the thermo-cautery. Virginia M. Month., Richmond, 1878-9, v, 212-215. — **Tilanus** (J. W. R.) Nasophar. polyp. Werk. v. h. Genootsch. t. Bevord. d. Nat-, Genees- en Heelk. te Amst., 1872-3, iii, 13.—**Tillmanns** (H.) Ueber todte Osteome der Nasen- und Stirnhöhlen. Ber. ü. d. Verhandl. d. deutsch. Gesellsch. f. Chir., Leipz., 1885, 41.—**Todd** (C. A.) Connection between asthma and nasal polypi. Tr. M. Ass. Missouri, St. Louis, 1881, xxiv, 78-84. *Also:* St. Louis Cour. Med., 1881, vi, 120-123. — **Traitement** des polypes naso-pharyngiens. [Discussion.] Bull. Soc. de chir. de Par. (1866), 1867, 2. s., vii, 18; 34; 46.—**Trélat.** Polype naso-pharyngien; résection temporaire de la paroi antérieure du sinus maxillaire. Bull. Soc. de chir. de Par., 1872, 3. s., i, 400. ——. Polypes des arrière-narines. *Ibid.,* 1874, 3. s., iii, 557-560. ——. Des polypes naso-pharyngiens. Rev. de thérap. méd.-chir., Par., 1877, xliv. 225-228. ——. Polype muqueux des arrière-narines saillant dans le pharynx. Bull. et mém. Soc. de chir. de Par., 1877, iii, 717-719. ——. Résections osseuses pour l'ablation des polypes du nez. *Ibid.*, 1882, n. s., viii, 850-852. ——. Tumeur sarcomateuse des fosses nasales. Gaz. d. hôp., Par., 1883, lvi, 210. — **Trowbridge** (A.) Unusual case of polypus in the throat and cavities of the face successfully treated. Tr. M. Soc. N. Y., Albany, 1819, 30-36. *Also: Ibid.*, 1807-31, Albany, 1868, 163-166. *Also:* Med. Reposit., N. Y., 1820. n. s., v, 186-191. *Also:* Med. & Phys. J., Lond., 1819, xlii, 285-289.—**Tsakyro-**

Nose (*Tumors of*).

glous (M.) Zwei Fälle von Nasenpolypen (Septum-Polyp und Reflex-Neurose). Monatschr. f. Ohrenh., Berl., 1887, xxi, 275. — **Underhill** (A. S.) Nasopharyngeal polypus; hypertrophy of the mucous membrane; tracheotomy; removal of superior maxillary bone; death. Brit. M. J., Lond., 1875, i, 343. — **Upson** (C. R.) A method of treating naso-pharyngeal and laryngeal tumors; with a description of a new instrument for the same. Med. Rec., N. Y., 1881, xix, 557.—**Ure.** Polypoid bony growth from the septum and floor of the right nostril; successful removal. Lancet, Lond., 1861. i, 411. — **Valenta** (A.) & **Wallmann** (H.) Eine seltene Geschwulst oberhalb der Nasenwurzel eines neugebornen Kindes. Ztschr. d. k.-k. Gesellsch. d. Aerzte zu Wien, 1858, xiv. 209-211. — **Van Buren** (W. H.) Malignant polypus of the nose; ligature of the common carotid artery; death with cerebral symptoms. N. York J. M., 1849, n. s., ii, 297-302. *Also, in his:* Contrib. to Pract. Surg., 8°, Phila., 1865, 77-84. — **Van Dommelen.** Polype fibreux de la fosse nasale gauche; cautérisation à l'aide du sublimé corrosif; guérison. J. de méd., chir. et pharmacol., Brux., 1859, xxviii, 463-465.—**Van Goudoever** (L. C.) De verwijdering der neus-keelpolypen. Nederl. Tijdschr. v. Heel- en Verlosk., Utrecht, 1866-9, xvi, 265-282.—**Vanzetti** (T.) Sarcoma simplex ex fossa canina dextra et nasi latere excrescens; extirpatio tumoris; sanatio magna ex parte sine pure, per simplicem vulneris protectionem. *In his:* Ann. scholæ clin. chir., etc., 8°, Charcoviæ, 1846, 59-61, 1 pl.—**Velazco** (I.) Polipos mucosos nasales, sostenidos probablemente por un vicio cifilítico. Gac. méd. de México, 1873. viii, 105-108.—**Velpeau** (A.) Polypes saignans. Arch. gén. de méd, Par., 1826, xi, 579. ——. Polype envahissant la majeure partie des cavités de la face; ligature de sa principale branche à l'aide d'un instrument nouveau. Gaz. d. hôp., Par., 1840. 2. s., ii, 569. ——. Polype muqueux des fosses nasales très-volumineux, datant de quarante-quatre ans; déformation considérable du nez; extirpation par arrachement. Monit. d. hôp., Par., 1857, v, 395-397.—**Verchère** (F.) Des indications opératoires dans certaines tumeurs récidivantes de la cavité et l'arrière-cavité des fosses nasales. Arch. de laryngol., de rhinol., etc., Par., 1887, i, 3-15.—**Verhaeghe.** Polype fibreux des fosses nasales; ligature. Ann. Soc. méd.-chir. de Bruges, 1844, v, 214-217. — **Verneuil** (A.) Documents sur l'incision médiane du voile du palais et sur les polypes naso-pharyngiens, tirés de la pratique de Dieffenbach. Gaz. hebd. de méd., Par., 1860, vii, 38-43. ——. Un point de l'histoire des polypes naso-pharyngiens, et, par occasion, du profit qu'on tire à remonter des citations aux sources bibliographiques originales. *Ibid.*, 129-137. ——. Observations de polypes naso-pharyngiens. *Ibid.:* 387-392. ——. Méthodes et procédés de ligature pour les polypes du nez et du pharynx; observations à l'appui. *Ibid.*, 433-437. ——. Quelques mots sur les polypes fibreux naso-maxillaires, pour montrer jusqu'où peut mener la curiosité bibliographique. *Ibid.*, 577-585. ——. Polypes naso-pharyngiens. Bull. Soc. de chir. de Par. (1863), 1864, 2. s., iv, 88-97. *Also:* Gaz. d. hôp., Par., 1863, 150-152. ——. Polype naso-pharyngien; opérations; tumeur récidivée devenant érectile. J. de méd. et chir. prat., Par., 1874, xlv, 156-158. ——. Temps d'arrêt dans la marche des polypes naso-pharyngiens. *Ibid.,* 1879, 1, 60-62. ——. Polype naso-pharyngien. Gaz. d. hôp., Par., 1879, lii, 785-787. ——. Polype naso-pharyngien; ligature de la carotide; gangrène vasculaire; mort. Bull. et mém. Soc. de chir. de Par., 1884, n. s., x, 633-636. ——. Papillome de la fosse nasale droite; ouverture de cette cavité, puis résection de la paroi antérieure du sinus maxillaire; récidives et opérations multiples; résultats incomplets. *Ibid.,* 1886, n. s., xii, 658-661.—**Viennois.** Du procédé de M. Ollier pour extirper les polypes naso-pharyngiens et les tumeurs profondes des fosses nasales. Gaz. méd. de Lyon, 1864, xvi, 383-387. ——. †† De l'ostéotomie bilatérale du nez. Lyon méd., 1872, xi, 8-12.—**Viganoni** (E.) Applicazione della elettrolisi alla cura di un voluminoso polipo naso-faringeo. Ann. univ. di med. e chir., Milano, 1877, ccxxxix, 147-153.— **Villar** (F.) Polype fibro-muqueux de l'arrière-cavité des fosses nasales; diagnostic; extirpation par l'arrachement simple, sans opérations préliminaires. France méd., Par., 1886, i. 374-378. *Also:* Courrier méd., Par., 1886, xxxvi, 172.—**Voisin.** Extirpation d'une tumeur polypeuse extraordinaire dont le pédicule étoit osseux, et qui tiroit son origine des fosses nasales postérieures. J. de méd., chir., pharm., etc., Par., 1792, xci, 421-427.—**Voltolini** (R.) Die Operation der Nasen- und Nasen-Rachen-Polypen. Berl. klin. Wchnschr., 1869, vi, 428-431. ——. Ueber eigenthümliche normale und krankhafte Gebilde in der Nase und über die Operation der Letzteren. Jahresb. d. schles. Gesellsch. f. vaterl. Kult. 1876, Bresl., 1877, liv, 250-253. *Also:* Monatschr. f. Ohrenh., Berl., 1877, xi, 49-54. ——. Ueber Nasenpolypen und deren Operation. Allg. Wien. med. Ztg., 1880, xxv, 113; 126; 133; 143; 156. *Also,* Reprint. ——. Operation der Nasenpolypen mittelst des Schwammes. Monatschr. f. Ohrenh., Berl., 1882, xvi, 1-7.—**Wagner.** Fibröser Nasenrachenpolyp; weiche Bindgewebsgeschwulst: Resection des Proc. nasalis des Oberkiefers; Exstirpation; Heilung.

Nose (*Tumors of*).

Deutsche Klinik, Berl., 1861. xiii, 22. — **Wagner** (C.) Case of nasal vascular myxoma; removal; alarming hemorrhage; recovery. Arch. Clin. Surg., N. Y., 1877, i, 262. ———. A rare form of nasal tumor; removed by operation. Med. News, Phila., 1882, xl, 456. — **Wagner** (F. A.) Glückliche, anscheinlich sichere, und gründliche Ausrottung der Nasen- und Rachen-Polypen, so wie anderer krankhafter Gebilde durch Empiriker. J. d. pract. Heilk., Berl., 1828, lxvi, 3. St., 30-38. *Also, transl.:* Arch. de la méd. belge, Brux., 1842, ix, 159-162. — **Wakley.** Malformation of the nose; tumour separating the ossa nasi; removal. Lancet, Lond., 1850, ii, 531. — **Ward.** Follicular tumours involving the nasal bones, nasal processes of superior maxillary bone, and the septum of the nose; removal; death from pneumonia; autopsy. *Ibid.*, 1854, ii, 480-482. — **Warren** (J. C.) Case of naso-pharyngeal polypus and of tumor of parotid, with remarks on their minute anatomy. Boston M. & S. J., 1871, lxxxv, 249-25'. — **Waterman** (T.) Naso-pharyngeal polypus; extirpation preceded by temporary displacement of the superior maxilla. *Ibid.*, 1869, lxxx, 165. — **Watson** (J.) Inquiry into the pathology and treatment of polypus tumors of the nasal fossa, with observations on other tumors in various parts of the body. Am. J. M. Sc., Phila., 1842, n. s., iii, 325-339. — **Watson** (W. S.) A case of cystic polypus of the nostril. Proc. M. Soc. Lond., 1875-7, iii, 134-136. ———. Case of recurrent fibroid polypus. Med. Times & Gaz., Lond., 1875, ii, 388. ———. The diagnosis and treatment of nasal polypi. Specialist, Lond., 1881-2, ii, 39; 59. — **Weinlechner.** Verzweigtes Sarcom in der Nasen-Rachen-Augenhöl:le mit Verdrängung des Bulbus; ungeheilt. Ber. d. k. k. Krankenanst. Rudoph-Stiftung in Wien (1875), 1876, 350. ———. † Weiches Rundzellensarcom, beide Nasenhöhlen ausfüllend, an einem tuberculösen Individuum; durch Auskratzen mit scharfen Löffeln geheilt. *Ibid.* (1876), 1877, 314. ———. Recidiver fibröser Nasenrachenpolyp; Exstirpation nach Durchtrennung des weichen und theilweise des harten Gaumens; nach Heilung der Operationswunde Verschluss des Defectes durch die Staphylorrhaphie und Uranoplastik; Heilung. Aerztl. Ber. d. k. k. allg. Krankenh. zu Wien (1884), 1885, 229-231. ———. Polypen in der linken Choane, in den Nasenrachenraum hängend; nach vergeblichen Extractionsversuche durch den Mund gelang die Entfernung von der nasenhöhle aus erst dann, als durch Extraction eines Stückes der Nasenmuschel-Raum geschafft wurde. *Ibid.* (1885), 1886, 230. — **Weir** (R. F.) Removal of naso-pharyngeal polypus by Nélaton's operation; death. Med. Rec., N. Y., 1882, xxi, 607. ———. Fibro-sarcoma of the nose; removed by Chassaignac's operation; recurrence in the brain. N. York M. J., 1887. xlv, 282. — **Weiss** (T.) Note sur un cas de polype naso-pharyngien extirpé après incision transversale du voile du palais (procédé de M. E. Boeckel). Mém. Soc. de méd. de Nancy (1880-81), 1882, lxxi, pt. 2, 147-156. *Also:* Rev. méd. de l'est, Nancy, 1881, xiii, 449; 495. *Also, in his:* Mém. sur quelques cas de chir., 8°, Nancy, 1883, 17-31. — **Werner.** Nasen- und Rachen-Polyp; Abtragung eines Theils desselben mittelst Galvanocaustik. Arch. f. physiol. Heilk., Stuttg., 1858, n. F., iii, 80-83. — **White** (J. A.) A large nasal polyp, removed by Jarvis' snare. Arch. Laryngol., N. Y., 1882, iii, 358. — **Whitehead** (W. R.) Avulsion of a naso-pharyngeal polypus. Med. Rec., N. Y., 1871-2, vi, 498. — **Wilkins** (J.) Removal of two tumours from the back of the lower turbinated bones. Austral. M. J., Melbourne, 1868, xiii, 139-143. — **Will** (J. C. O.) Case of naso-pharyngeal polypi; écrasement and osteo-plastic operation; rapid recovery. Lancet, Lond., 1879, ii, 835. — **Wilmot** (S. G.) Observations on lipoma of the nose. Dublin Q. J. M. Sc., 1853, xvi, 72-76. — **Wimmer** (E.) Zur Operation der Nasenpolypen. Arch. d. Heilk., Leipz., 1872, xiii, 563-565. — **Winant** (G.) Polype nasopharyngien; opération. Ann. Soc. de méd. de Gand, 1875, liii, 65-68. — **Winge** (P.) Tilfælde af Polypi Nasen. Norsk Mag. f. Lægevidensk., Christiania. 1862, 2. R., xvi, 1001. *Also, transl.:* J. f. Kinderkr., Erlang., 1863, xli, 136. — **Woakes** (E.) On papillo-adenomatous disease, or post-nasal vegetations. Tr. Internat. M. Cong., 7. sess., Lond., 1881, iii, 291-301. ———. The relation of necrosing ethmoiditis to nasal polypus. Brit. M. J., Lond., 1885, i, 701. — **Wood** (W. R.) A case of naso-pharyngeal polypus. North Car. M. J., Wilmington, 1878, ii, 159-161. — **Yvonneau** fils. Observation de tumeur fongueuse végétante, traitée avec succès par la pommade au perchlorure de fer. Monit. d. hôp., Par., 1854, ii, 358. — **Zahn** (F. W.) Ueber Cysten mit Flimmerepithelien im Nasenrachenraum. Deutsche Ztschr. f. Chir., Leipz., 1885, xxii, 392-399, 2 pl. — **Zander.** Zur Operation der Nasenpolypen. Deutsche med. Wchnschr., Berl., 1880, vi, 77. — **Zaufal** (E.) Ueber die allgemeine Verwendbarkeit der kalten Drahtschlinge zur Operation der Nasenpolypen, nebst Bemerkungen über das Abhängigkeitsverhältniss der Erkrankungen des Ohres von denen der Nasenhöhle. Prag. med. Wchnschr., 1877, ii, 985; 1013; 1029. ———. Casuistischer Beitrag zur Operation der Nasenrachenpolypen über Beihülfe der Rhinoscopia anterior. *Ibid.*, 1878, iii, 290; 301. ———. Ueber operative Behandlung der chronischen Anschwellungen

Nose (*Tumors of*).

der hinteren Nasenmuschelenden. Wien. med. Presse, 1885, xxvi, 468. — **Zayas** (J.) Pólipo fibroso naso-faringeo operado por el proceder de M. Nélaton. An. r. Acad. de cien. méd. ... de la Habana, 1868-9, v, 114-122. — **Zuckerkandl** (E.) Ueber die Polypen und polypösen Wucherungen der Nasenschleimhaut. Wien. med. Bl., 1882, v, 44; 74.

Nose (*Watery, or other discharge from*).

See, also, **Nerve** (*Optic, Inflammation of*); **Ozæna.**

Althaus (J.) Excessive secretion from the nose. Brit. M. J., Lond., 1878, ii, 831. — **Ammannus** (P.) Lochiorum fluxus per nares. Misc. Acad. nat. curios. 1671, Francof. et Lips., 1688, ii, 282. — **C.** (J.) Fluid from the nose. Brit. M. J., Lond., 1879, i, 175. — **Elliotson** (J.) Limpid watery fluid in very large quantities from the left nostril. Med. Times & Gaz., Lond., 1857, xv, 390. — **Fischer** (H.) Wässerige Ausscheidungen aus einer Nasenöffnung. Deutsche Ztschr. f. Chir., Leipz., 1879, xii, 369. *Also, in his:* Mitth. a. d. k. chir. Klin. zu Bresl., 8°, Leipz., 1880, 119. — **Foster** (J.) Case of a lady who has a discharge from the nostrils of a peculiar watery character. N. York M. Times, 1852, ii, 113-115. — **Lingard** (A.) Excessive flow of fluid from the nose. Brit. M. J., Lond., 1878, ii, 921. — **Mathiesen** (C.) Et Tilfælde af stærkt vandagtigt Udflod fra Næsen efter et Fald paa Hovedet. [Watery flow from nose after a fall upon head.] Norsk Mag. f. Lægevidensk., Christiania, 1887, 4. R., i, 41-44. — **Paget** (J.) Watery discharge from one nostril. Med. Press & Circ., Lond., 1878, n. s., xxvi, 432. — **Park** (O. S.) Case of rhinorrhœa. Lancet, Lond., 1870, ii, 660. — **Rees.** Excessive discharge from the nostrils of a limpid fluid. Lond. M. & S. J., 1834, iv, 823. — **Speirs** (W. R.) Notes of a case in which the principal symptom was a constant and copious discharge of watery fluid from the nose. Lancet. Lond., 1881, i, 369.

Nose (*Wounds and injuries of*).

See, also, **Nose** (*Foreign bodies in*).

BURKHARD (A.) * Ueber völlig abgehauene und wieder angewachsene Stücke der Nase. 8°. *Berlin*, [1872].

DRÜDING (E. C. A.) * De fractura ossium nasi. 8°. *Gottingæ*, [1798].

RATEAU (J.) * De l'écoulement du liquide séreux par les narines, résultant de traumatisme. 4°. *Paris*, 1859.

Adams (W.) On the treatment of broken-nose by forcible straightening, and mechanical retentive apparatus. Proc. M. Soc. Lond., 1874-5, ii, 99. *Also:* Brit. M. J., Lond., 1875, ii, 421. ———. On the treatment of broken-nose by forcible straightening, and the subsequent use of retentive apparatus. Med. Exam., Lond., 1878, iii, 180. — **Arming** (J. W.) Anheilung einer fast gänzlich abgerissenen Nase. J. d. Chir. u. Augenh., Berl., 1832, xviii, 281-285. — **Bissell** (P. A.) The treatment of fracture of the nose. Med. Rec., N. Y., 1876, xi, 235. — **Bochdalek.** Volständiger Doppelbruch des knorplichten Theiles der Nasenscheidewand mit Verschiebung der Fragmente bei einem nur sehr unbedeutenden Bruche des vorderen Endes des rechten Nasenbeins. Vrtljschr. f. d. prakt. Heilk., Prag, 1867, xciii, 62-66. — **Bolton** (J.) Fracture, with displacement of the vomer; successful operation. Richmond & Louisville M. J., Louisville, 1868, v, 241. — **Bosworth** (F. H.) Dislocation of the columnar cartilage of the nose. Illust. Quart. M. & S., N. Y., 1882, i, 25. — **Bourguet.** Sur la luxation des os propres du nez, par cause traumatique, sans fracture de ces os ni du maxillaire supérieur. Rev. méd.-chir. de Par., 1851, x, 82-85. — **Braman** (I. G.) Severe injury to the nose. Boston M. & S. J., 1839-40, xxi, 159. — **Buchner** (E.) Faustschlag auf die Nase; heftige Blutung; langdauernde Arbeitsunfähigkeit. Friedreich's Bl. f. gerichtl. Med., Nürnb., 1867, xviii, 136-143. — **Canella** (G.) Completa riunione del naso quasi per intero staccato. Gior. di chir.-prat., Trento, 1826, ii, 5-7. — **Cooper.** Injury to the nose, with exfoliation of bone, supposed to be syphilitic. Lancet, Lond., 1861, i, 362. — **Dardignac.** Fracture de la base du nez et des deux rebords orbitaires inférieurs; communication avec les sinus frontaux; perte des deux yeux; appareil prothétique de C. Delalain. Gaz. d. hôp., Par., 1872, xlv, 241-243. — **Deckmann.** Verlust der Nasenbeine und der diese deckenden Haut. Mitth. a. d. Geb. d. Med., etc., Kiel, 1833, ii, 513-515. — **Delalain** (C.) Perte du nez et des deux yeux par l'éclat d'obus; fracture en éclat des deux maxillaires supérieurs; luxation de la mâchoire inférieure; réduction; prothèse. Gaz. d. hôp., Par., 1872, xlv, 1203. — **Demarquay.** Déviation de la cloison des fosses nasales par suite d'un coup de poing; inclinaison disgracieuse du nez à gauche; guérison à l'aide d'une opération nouvelle. *Ibid.*, 1859, xxxii, 470. — **Deville.** [Une balle de pistolet solidement fixée dans la fosse nasale gauche.] Bull. Soc. anat. de Par., 1850, xxv, 35. — **Dey** (D. N.) Case

Nose (*Wounds and injuries of*).

of almost complete ablation of the nose. Indian M. Gaz., Calcutta, 1881, xvi, 174.—**von Dumreicher.** Fractura ossis nasi dextri complicata. Allg Wien. med. Ztg., 1866, xi, 247.—**Eder** (A.) Dislocatio septi narium. *In his:* Aerztl. Ber., 1884, 8°, Wien, 1885, 3.—**Fifield** (W. C. B.) Fracture of the nose. Boston M. & S. J., 1881, civ, 327. *Also:* Extr. Rec. Bost. Soc. M. Improve. (1880–82), 1883, viii, 110–112.—**Fischer** (C.) Bisswunde der Nase; verbreitetes Erysipel; Genesung. Ztschr. f. Wundärzte u. Geburtsh., Hegnach, 1887, xxxviii, 117.—**Gamgee** (S.) On fracture of the nasal bones; a clinical note. Brit. M. J., Lond., 1875, ii, 521.—**Gerson.** Grosse Verletzung der Nase. Gen.-Ber. d. k. rhein. Med.-Coll. 1836, Koblenz, 1838, 121.—**Gillette.** Arrachement du nez et de la lèvre supérieure par la bouche d'un cheval. Union méd., Par., 1873, 3. s., xvi, 61.—**Gosselin.** Emphysème insolite des deux paupières à gauche; effet tardif d'une fracture du nez; de la percussion par chiquenaude pour le diagnostic de l'emphysème. Gaz. d. hôp., Par., 1868, xli, 229.—**Graves** (R. H.) Slit nose. Rep. Med. Miss. Soc. in China 1868, Hongkong, 1869, 22.—**Hamilton** (F. H.) Fractures and displacements of the ossa nasi. Ohio M. & S. J., Columbus, 1857–8, x, 89–95.—**Howard** (R. L.) Depression of the dorsum nasi. N. York J. M., 1848, x, 182–184.—**Janikowski** (S.) Zranienie nosa; lekkie uszkodzenie. [Wound of nose; slight injury.] Przegl. lek., Krakow., 1867, vi, 161.—**Jarjavay.** Sur la fracture du cartilage de la cloison des fosses nasales; complications et traitement. Bull. gén. de thérap., etc., Par., 1867, lxxii, 539–556.—**Kästner** (F.) Spaltung der Nase durch einem eisernen Henzieher; Heilung. Deutsche Klinik. Berl., 1873, xxv, 114.—**von Langenbeck** (B) Comminutive Fracturen der Nasenknochen und des rechten Oberkiefers, Versenkung des Augapfels in die Oberkieferhöhle rechter Seite. Arch. f. Ophth., Berl., 1867, xiii, 2. Abth., 447–450.—**Lisfranc.** Considérations pratiques sur la fracture des os propres du nez. J. de méd. et chir. prat., Par., 1842, xiii, 125.—**Longuet** (R.) Sur la luxation des os propres du nez. Rec. de mém. de méd. . . . mil., Par., 1881, 3. s., xxxvii, 280–285.—**Malfatti.** Wiederanheilung einer völlständig abgehauenen Nase. Wien. med. Wchnschr., 1872, xxii, 1225.—**Malgaigne.** Nouveau procédé pour rétablir le nez enfoncé par perte de substance de la cloison nasale. Rev. méd.-chir. de Par., 1851, x, 209–214.—**Mason** (L. D.) An improved method of treating depressed fractures of the nasal bones. Ann. Anat. & Surg. Soc., Brooklyn, N. Y., 1880, ii, 197–111. *Also,* Reprint. ———. A case of fracture of the nasal bones treated by an improved method. Ann. Anat. & Surg. Soc., Brooklyn, N. Y., 1880, ii, 197–199. *Also,* Reprint. ———. Report of cases of extensive fracture of nasal bones treated by a new method. Ann. Anat. & Surg., Brooklyn, N. Y., 1881, iii, 81–83. *Also,* Reprint.—**Morgenstern** (W.) Ein Fall von Anheilung einer fast ganz abgetrennten Nase. Med.-chir. Centralbl., Wien, 1876, xi, 86.—**Moutet.** Fracture des os propres du nez, compliquée d'érysipèle à la face, de fracture de la lame perpendiculaire de l'ethmoïde, et suivie de méningite; abcès du cœur; concrétions polypiformes dans les cavités de cet organe. J. Soc. de méd.-prat. de Montpel., 1847, xvi, 241–252.—**Petrich.** Abtrennung der Nase durch ein stumpfes Inst ument; Differenz der Sachverständigen bezügich der Frage: ob die Verletzung eine schwere oder leichte zu nennen sei? Oesterr. Ztschr. f. pract. Heilk., Wien, 1863, ix, 406–410.—**Phillips.** Rapport sur un instrument de M. Boissonneau, pour le redressement des nez enfoncés. Bull. Acad. roy. de méd. de Belg., Brux., 1846-7, vi, 476–479.—**Pringle** (J. H.) Note of a curious accident [injury of nasal cavity]. Edinb. M. J., 1887-8, xxxiii, 527–529.—**Rogers** (J. H.) Cases of fracture of the nasal bones. Lancet, Lond., 1847, i, 429–431.—**Royère** (T.) Observation d'une fracture des os propres du nez, avec déviation des parties, guérie au moyen de la compression permanante établie à l'aide d'une machine compressive. Rec. de mém. de méd. . . . mil., Par., 1820, viii, 286–292.—**Rust** (J. N.) Neue Methode, verstümmelte und durchbrochene Nasen auszubessern. Ein Beitrag zur Geschichte der Nasen-Restaurationen. Mag. f. d. ges. Heilk., Berl., 1817, ii, 351–384.—**Simon y Nieto** (F.) Fractura del hueso de la nariz con enfisema de la cara y del cuello. Correo méd. castellano, Salamanca, 1886, iii, 83–85.—**Ure** (A.) On injuries of the nose. Med. Circ., Lond., 1862, xxi, 4.—**von Walther** (P.) Wieder-Anheilung einer ganz abgehauenen Nase. J. d. Chir. u. Augenh., Berl., 1825, vii, 521–535, 1 pl.—**Watson** (W. S.) Fracture of the nasal and superior maxillary bones, followed by necrosis and abscess with proptosis; removal of the sequestrum; remarks. Lancet, Lond., 1886, i, 972.—**Weber** (C.) Fractura comminuta ossium nasi, complicirt mit einer Stirn- und Nasenwunde; Hinwegnahme des grössten Theils beider Nasenbeine und vollkommener Wiederersatz der letzteren. Ztschr. d. deutsch. Chir.-Ver., Magdeb., 1852, v, 353.—**Weir** (R. F.) Injuries of the nose. Med. News, Phila., 1887, l, 271.—**Westmoreland** (W. F.) Case of fracture of the nasal bones. Atlanta M. & S. J., 1858–9, iv, 328.—**Wutzer** (C. W.) Defectus radicis nasi a causa mechanica. *In his:* Ber. ü. d. med.-chir. Klin. zu Münster, 1830, 79–84.

Nose (Carl Wilhelm) [1753–1835]. * Theses medicæ. 8 pp. sm. 4°. *Argentorati, ex prelo J. Lorenzii,* 1777.

———. Ueber die Behandlung des venerischen Uebels. 193 pp., 3 l. 12°. *Augsburg, E. Kletts,* 1780.

See, also, **Schäffer** (Joh. Ulr. Gottl.) Vertheidigung einzelner Sätze in seiner Schrift über Sensibilität, [etc.] 16°. *Frankf. a. M.,* 1795.

For Portrait, see **Collection**—van Kaathoven.—**Collection** of Portr. of Phys. & Men of Sc., 2.

Noskowski (Stanislas-Antoine-Louis de Lada). * Étude sur l'arsenic et en particulier sur la valeur de ses préparations facilement solubles dans le traitement préservatif et curatif des malades tuberculeux. 1 p. l., 141 pp. 4°. *Lyon,* 1883, 1. s., No. 190.

Nosley (Jean-Baptiste). * Sur l'âge critique. 31 pp. 4°. *Paris,* 1848, No. 79, v. 475.

Nosocomium academicum; das ist: pia desideria von Anrichtung eines Lazareths zum Nutzen der kranken Armen und Etablirung der medicinischen und physicalischen Wissenschaften kürtzlich entworffen. 14 pp. sm. 8°. [*n. p., n. d.*]

Bound with: CARL (J. S.) Decorum medici, etc. sm. 8°. *Büdingen,* 1719.

Nosology.

See, also, **Disease**; **Diseases** (*Anomalous*); **Fevers** (*Classification, etc., of*); **Insanity** (*Definition, etc., of*); **Nomenclature**; **Skin** (*Diseases of, Classification, etc., of*).

ALIBERT (J.-L.) Nosologie naturelle, ou les maladies du corps humain distribuées par familles. Avec 33 planches coloriées. fol. *Paris,* 1838.

ARAMENDÍA Y BOLEA (F.) Estudios fundamentales de patología médica. Nosotaxia: sus procedimientos lógicos; sus bases; su utilidad. 8°. *Zaragoza,* 1884.

BAECHER (M.) Synopsis nosologica apokenosium juxta Swediauri ἰατρικὴν disposita. 8°. *Pragæ,* 1830.

BALDINGER (E. G.) [Pr.] simulque præmittit animadversionem in systemata nosologiæ. Specimin iii. quod agit de pyretologia generatim. 4°. *Göttingæ,* [1778].

BANG (O.) Index morborum internorum systematicus. Præmissis de nosogenesi aphorismis. 8°. *Havniæ,* 1855.

———. Aphorismi de nosogenesi. Accedit practica morborum classificatio. Ed. nova. 8°. *Havniæ,* 1870.

BARRINGER (C.-W.) * Dissertation sur les systèmes nosologiques et sur la nomenclature médicale. 4°. *Paris,* 1860.

BAUMES (J.-B.-T.) Traité élémentaire de nosologie, contenant une exacte classification de toutes les maladies, soit internes soit externes; la bibliographie des genres et des espèces qui les constituent, [etc.] 4 v. 8°. 1. & 4. v., *Paris,* 1806; 2. & 3. v., *Montpellier,* 1801.

BOISSEAU (F.-G.) * Considérations générales sur les classifications en médecine. 4°. *Paris,* 1817.

BONORDEN (H. F.) Classification der gesammten Krankheiten des Menschen nach ihrem Wesen. 8°. *Berlin,* 1838.

BOUCHUT (E.) * Des méthodes de classification en nosologie. 4°. *Paris,* 1853.

BOUILLAUD (J.-B.) Traité de nosographie médicale. 5 v. 8°. *Paris,* 1846.

Also [Rev.], *in:* J. de méd., Par., 1846, iv, 321; 353 (C. Lasègue).

BROUSSAIS (F.-J.-V.) Examen de la doctrine médicale généralement adoptée, et des systèmes modernes de nosologie, etc. 8°. *Paris,* 1816.

———. Examen des doctrines médicales et des systèmes de nosologie. 2 v. 8°. *Paris,* 1821.

Nosology.

————. The same. 3. 6d. v. 3, 4. 8°. *Paris*, 1829–34.

Also [Rev.], *in:* J. gén. de méd., chir. et pharm., Par., 1821, lxxvii, 353–395 (E. G. C.).

CAMERER (J. G.) * Diss. sistens onomatopœœ nosologicæ fundamenta. 4°. *Tubingæ*, [1793]

CREUTZWIESER (C. G. G.) * De variis tentaminibus nosologicis. 8°. *Halæ*, [1821].

CULLEN (W.) Synopsis nosologiæ methodicæ. Ed. altera. 8°. *Edinburgi*, 1772.

————. The same. Apparatus ad nosologiam methodicam, seu synopsis nosologiæ methodicæ in usum studiosorum. Ed. nova . . . aucta, scilicet systemate morborum symptomatico a J. B. M. Sagar proposito. 4°. *Amstelodami*, 1775.

————. The same. Synopsis nosologiæ methodicæ, exhibens clariss. virorum Sauvagessii, Linnæi, Vogelii, et Sagari systemata nosologica. 3. ed. 2 v. 8°. *Edinburgi*, 1780.

————. The same. 4. ed. 2 v. 8°. *Edinburgi*, 1785.

————. The same. Edidit suumque proprium systema nosologicum adjecit . . . Editio prima Veneta juxta quartam emendatam et plurimam auctam Edinburgi 1785. 12°. *Venetiis*, 1787.

————. The same. Cura J. P. Frank. 12°. *Taurini*, 1812.

————. The same. 12°. *Edinburgi*, 1814.

————. The same. Synopsis and nosology, being an arrangement and definition of diseases. The first transl. from Latin to English. 16°. *Hartford*, 1792.

————. The same. A synopsis of methodical nosology, in which the genera of disorders are particularly defined and the species added with the synonimous of those from Sauvages. From the 4. ed., corrected and much enlarged. Transl. by H. Wilkins. 8°. *Philadelphia*, 1793.

————. The same. A methodical system of nosology. Transl. by E. Lewis. 12°. *Stockbridge*, [1807].

————. The same. A synopsis of nosology. Transl. by J. Thomson. To which is added Willan's classification of cutaneous diseases. 8°. *Philadelphia*, 1816.

————. The same. Nosologia methodica. Transl. by J. Thomson. 3. ed. 8°. *Edinburgh*, 1820.

CUVIER (F.-G.-C.-F.-M.) * Propositions et considérations sur les classifications en médecine, et sur les principaux auteurs des nosologies. 4°. *Paris*, 1832.

DAVIDGE (J. B.) Nosologia methodica; series classium, et generum, et specierum, et varietatum morborum exhibens. 8°. *Baltimoriensi*, 1812.

————. The same. 2. ed. 8°. *Baltimoriensi*, 1813.

DUMAY (J.) * I. De la classification des maladies d'après leur siége. II. [etc.] 4°. *Paris*, 1840.

DURET (F.-J.-J.) Tableau d'une classification générale des maladies. 8°. *Paris*, 1815.

EISENMANN (G.) Die Krankheits-Familie Typosis (Wechselkrankheiten). 12°. *Zürich*, 1839.

Also [Rev.], *in:* Arch. f. d. ges. Med., Jena, 1841, i, 135–160 (H. Haeser).

ENGEL (A.) * Synopsis nosologica eclysium et spasmorum juxta Swediauri ιατρικήν disposita. 8°. *Pragæ*, 1832.

ENGELKEN (J. L. H.) * Versuch einer natürlichen Anordnung der Krankheiten. 8°. *Würzburg*, 1832.

GAILLARD (F.-L.) Essai sur les familles pathologiques. 8°. *Paris*, 1868.

Also [Rap. de Pidoux], *in:* Bull. Acad. de méd., Par., 1868, xxxiii, 462–471.

Nosology.

GALLUP (J. A.) Outlines of an arrangement of medical nosology, founded on the pathology of the diseased system. 16°. *Woodstock*, 1823.

GIBERT (C.-M.) * Sur la question suivante (précédée de quelques considérations sur l'Hippocratisme): "Jusqu'à quel point l'anatomie pathologique peut-elle servir de base à la classification des maladies?" 4°. *Paris*, 1833.

GIMENO CABAÑAS (A.) Fundamentos para las clasificaciones de las enfermedades. 8°. *Madrid*, 1875.

GOOD (J. M.) A physiological system of nosology; with a corrected and simplified nomenclature. 8°. *London*, 1817.

————. The same. 8°. *Boston*, 1823.

————. The study of medicine, with a physiological system of nosology. 2. Am. ed. 5 v. 8°. *Philadelphia*, 1824.

GREAT BRITAIN. *Privy Council Office.* Registrar-general of England. Registration of the causes of death. Circulars to medical practitioners and to registrars. A statistical nosology, for the use of those who return the causes of death under 6 & 7 Will. IV., c. 86. Circular to coroners, and a classification of the causes of violent death. 8°. *London*, 1845.

GROSS (G. W.) * Quæ versatur in quæstione: num usui sit in curatione morborum nomenclatura? 8°. *Halæ*, [1817].

DE GROSSI (E.) Familiarum morborum humanorum expositio. 8°. *Stuttgardtiæ*, 1831.

GRUNER (C. G.) [Pr.] nosologiæ historicæ spec. i–x. 8°. *Jenæ*, 1793–5.

GUTBERLET (C.) * De divisione morborum. 4°. [*Wirceburgi*, 1773.]

HEBENSTREIT (J. E.) Ordo morborum causalis: Spec. i. de methodo morbos ordinante. sm. 4°. *Lipsiæ*, [1754].

————. The same. Spec. ii. De genere morborum ad artis usum constituendo indicit. sm. 4°. *Lipsiæ*, [1754].

————. The same. Spec. iii. De charactere ad genera morborum constituenda optimo quo panegyrin medicam indicit. 4°. *Lipsiæ*, 1755.

————. The same. Spec. vi. Sistens limites generum morbi. sm. 4°. [*Lipsiæ*, 1756.]

HENNEMANN (G. J. C.) Primæ lineæ nosologiæ morborum animalium. 4°. *Gottingæ*, 1778.

HENSELER (H.) * De morborum divisione in genere et de cachexiis in specie. 8°. *Berolini*, [1830].

HERZOG. Die Nosologie auf der Grundlage der Cellularpathologie. 8°. *Berlin*, 1861.

HOCHHAUSER (L.) * Synopsis nosologica excœdesium et dyschroiarum juxta Swediauri ιατρικήν disposita. 8°. *Pragæ*, 1832.

HOSACK (D.) A system of practical nosology; to which is prefixed a synopsis of the systems of Sauvages, Linnæus, Vogel, Sagar, MacBride, Cullen, Darwin, Crichton, Pinel, Parr, Swediaur, and Young; with references to the best authors on each disease. 8°. *New York*, 1818.

————. The same. 2. ed. 8°. *New York*, 1821.

KARPELES (A.) Synopsis nosologica cachexiarum et cacochymiarum juxta Swediauri ιατρικήν disposita. 8°. *Pragæ*, 1832.

KOELREUTER (C. C.) Medicinæ dynamicæ specimen quartum. 4°. *Tubingæ*, [1761].

KRÆMER (M.) * Conspectus morborum corporis humani specialis. 4°. [*Tubingæ*, 1782.]

LECLERC (J.) * I. De la classification des maladies d'après leur marche et leur durée. II. [etc.] 4°. *Paris*, 1844.

LINNÆUS (C.) Genera morborum, in auditorum usum. 12°. *Upsaliæ*, 1763.

————. The same. 3. ed. 8°. *Hamburgi et Gustraviæ*, [1763].

Nosology.

——. Clavis medicinæ duplex, exterior et interior. 8°. *Holmiæ*, 1766.

——. The same. 8°. [*Neapoli*, 1793.]

NEBEL (E. L. W.) De nosologia brutorum cum hominum morbis comparata. 8°. *Giessæ*, [1798].

OVERKAMP (T. C. G.) * Diss. inaug. nosologica potissima summa genera morborum simplicium qui fluida corporis humani afficiunt demonstrata proponens. 4°. *Gryphiswaldiæ*, [1766].

PEIRCE (H. B.) Statistical nosology adopted for registration in Massachusetts, and requirements of law relative to certificates of causes of death. 8°. *Boston*, 1878.

PLOUCQUET (G. G.) Delineatio systematis nosologici naturæ accommodati. 4 v. in 2. 12°. *Tubingæ*, 1791–3.

PORTUGAL. *Conselho de saude.* Quadro nosographico das molestias, que podem ser cauza de morte, para servir de norma aos differentes facultativos do reino nas certidões d'obito. fol. [*n. p., n. d.*]

——. Addicionamento no Quadro nosographico das molestias, etc. 8°. [*n. p.*, 1842.]

PRASKY (N. A.) * Synopsis nosologica epischesium et apoplanesium juxta Swediauri ιατρικήν disposita. 8°. *Pragæ*, 1831.

PRATBERNON (C.-F.-N.) * Esquisse d'une méth de nosologique. 4°. *Paris*, 1814.

RASNOWSKI (D.) * De classificatione morborum. 4°. *Petropoli*, 1857.

REINBOLD (A. T.) * Quædam ad taxionomiam morborum. 8°. *Wirceburgi*, [*n. d.*]

REUSS (F. A.) * Die Krankheiten des Menschen in ih er Entwickelung und natürlichen Verwandtschaft. Ein Entwurf eines nosologischen Natursystems. 4°. *München*, 1833.

RICHTER (T.) * Diss. med. sistens synopsin nosclogicam dysosphresiarum juxta Swediauri ιατρικήν dispositam. 8°. *Pragæ*, [1835].

RIDDELL (G.) * De nosologia methodica. 8°. *Edinburgi*, 1774.

RIGOLLOT (J.-M.) * Essai sur les méthodes de classement employés en histoire naturelle, suivi de propositions sur les classifications nosologiques. 4°. *Paris*, 1809.

SAGAR (J. B. M.) Systema morborum symptomaticum secundum classes, ordines, genera, et species cum characteribus, differentiis et therapeiis. 8°. *Viennæ*, 1776.

DE SAUVAGES (F. B.) Nosologia methodica sistens morborum classes, genera et species, juxta Sydenhami mentem et botanicorum ordinem. 5 v. 8°. *Amstelodami*, 1763.

——. The same. 2 v. 4°. *Amstelodami*, 1768.

——. The same. Nosologie méthodique, dans laquelle les maladies sont rangées par classe suivant le système de Sydenham, et l'ordre des botanistes. Ouvrage augmenté de quelques notes en forme de commentaire par M. Nicolas. 3 v. 8°. *Paris*, 1770–71.

——. The same. 3 v. 8°. *Paris*, 1771.

——. Pathologia methodico-practica, seu de cognoscendis morbis. Ed. quarta. 8°. *Neapoli*, 1776.

SCHLOTTERBEK (P.) * Nomenclatura morborum omnium et symptomatum præcipuorum synonymica ab Hippocrate ad nostra tempora usque. 8°. *Pestini*, 1836.

SCHRÖDER (J.) * Genera morborum. sm. 4°. *Upsaliæ*, [1759].

Also, in: LINNÆUS. Amœnitates acad. [etc.] 8°. *Lugd. Bat.*, 1764, vi, 452–486.

SCHUBITZ (J.) * De divisione morborum. 8°. *Patavii*, 1834.

Nosology.

SCHULTZ-SCHULTZENSTEIN. Die natürlichen Familien der Krankheiten und der diesen entsprechenden Heilmittel mit Rücksicht auf das natürliche System der Pharmacologie und die allgemeine Krankheitslehre. 8°. *Berlin*, 1851.

SIGWART (G. F.) * Polyæmiæ nosologia. Resp. C. L. F. Linck. sm. 4°. *Tubingæ*, [1756].

SPRENGEL (K.) * Spec. inaug. sistens rudimentorum nosologiæ dynamicorum prolegomena. 8°. *Halæ*, [1787].

STENDER (G. C.) * Definitiones generum morborum. 4°. *Gottingæ*, [1764].

STOEBRICH (I.) * Diss. sistens synopsin nosologicam dysopsiarum juxta Swediauri ιατρικήν disposita. 8°. *Pragæ*, [1836].

SWEDIAUR. Novi nosologiæ methodicæ systematis vol. ii, pars 1, classis iv. Cachexiæ et cacochymiæ. 8°. [*n. p., n. d.*]

TRAUTNER (J. C. F.) * De excolenda scientia medica, præsertim de systemate nosologico naturali. 8°. *Norimbergæ*, 1835.

TRIER (B.) * De classificatione morborum. 8°. *Wirceburgi*, 1831.

TYTLER (R.) A slight sketch of a new nosological system for the classification of diseases. 8°. *Calcutta*, 1821.

WEATHERHEAD (G. H.) A new synopsis of nosology, founded on the principles of pathological anatomy and of the natural affinities of diseases. 12°. *London*, 1834.

WEIDENHOFFER (I.) * Synopsis nosologica helcosium et scolecodum juxta Swediauri ιατρικήν disposita. 8°. *Pragæ*, 1833.

WONDRACŻEK (J.) Synopsis nosologica dysostosium juxta Swediauri ιατρικήν. 8°. *Pragæ*, [1834].

WÜRL (A.) * Diss. sistens synopsin nosologicam dysecoiarum juxta Swediauri ιατρικήν. 8°. *Pragæ*, 1835.

YOUNG (T.) An introduction to medical literature, including a system of practical nosology. 8°. *London*, 1813.

Allbutt (T. C.) The significance of skin-affections in the classification of disease. St. George's Hosp. Rep., Lond., 1866–7, ii, 187–204.—**Arruti** (A.) Determinar los fundamentos de una clasificacion nosológica, mas apropiados para el acierto en la práctica médica. Siglo méd., Madrid, 1878, xxv, 55; 72; 89; 119; 135; 150; 181; 293.—**Auch** ein paar Versuche die Elemente der Nosologie a priori aufzustellen. Arch. f. med. Erfahr., Berl., 1807, n. F., vi, 164–166.—**Bayle** (G.-L.) Considérations sur la nosologie, la médecine d'observation et la médecine pratique. *In:* Encycl. d. sc. méd., 41 v., 8°, Par., 1834–46, 7. div., [v. xii], 501–533.—**Baylon.** Quelques considérations sur la vie, sur la maladie et sur les classifications nosologiques. Bull. Soc. méd. de la Suisse Rom., Lausanne, 1872, vi, 182; 211.—**Betti** (L.) La scienza nosologica e il suo fondamento. Sperimentale, Firenze, 1876, xxxviii, 16–30.—**Biermann** (J. C. A.) Blicke auf die Psychologie und psychische Heilkunde und ihre Bearbeitung, nebst einigen Andeutungen und Ideen zur Begründung einer rationellen psychischen Nosologie. Med. Convers.-Bl., Hildburgh., 1832, iii. 177; 185.—**Billod** (E.) Essai de classification et séméiologie. Ann. méd.-psych., Par., 1856, 3. s., ii, 309–338.—**Browne** (H.) On positive nosology. Brit. M. J., Lond., 1867, i, 503–505.—**Brückner** (G. A.) Ein natürliches System der Krankheiten. Deutsche Klinik, Berl., 1863, xv, 105–107.—**Castells Ballespí** (F.) Apuntes de nosología médica. Gac. méd. catal., Barcel., 1881, i, 489–495.—**Choulant** (L.) Darstellung des nosologischen Systems des Dr. T. Young. Allg. med. Ann., Leipz., 1825, 577–594.—**Cros** (A.) De la nécessité d'admettre l'existence d'une nouvelle classe de maladies sous le nom de décoordinations organiques. France méd., Par., 1866, xiii, 589; 597; 606; 613; 623; 629; 638; 645; 653; 661.—**Davis** (E. G.) Some remarks on Good's nosology. Boston M. & S. J., 1828–9, i, 358–362.—**Davis** (N. S.) Does etiology constitute a proper basis for the classification and diagnosis of diseases? Am. Pract., Louisville, 1876, xiii, 343–350.—**D'Espine** (M.) Projet de classification des causes de mort physiologiques, accidentelles et morbides, à l'usage de la statistique mortuaire de tous les pays; préparé pour le Congrès international de statistique de Paris. Compte rend. Cong. internat. de statist. 1855, Par., 1856, ii, 133–146.—**Dupuy** (P.) Aperçu de nosologie. Gaz. méd. de Par., 1864, 3. s.,

Nosology.

xix, 507; 521.—**Fajarnés** (R.) Clasificacion morbosa.
Actas de las ses. d. Cong. region. de cien. méd. 1879,
Cádiz, 1882, 19–67.—**Farr** (W.) Projet de classification.
Compte rend. Cong. internat. de statist. 1855, Par., 1856,
ii, 147–168.—**Ferguson** (E. J.) An attempt to form a
philosophical classification of diseases from the action of
the conservative nervous system. Boston M. & S. J.,
1843, xxviii, 149–152.—**Förslag** till Sjukdoms-nomen-
klatur. Förh. v. Svens. Läk.-Sällsk. Sammank., Stockholm, 1873, 307–325.—**Genovés y Tio** (J.) Classes en
que conviene dividir las enfermedades para formar con mas
precision, sencillez y utilidad pública los cuadros no-
sológicos de los enfermos que hacen uso de las aguas
minerales. Siglo méd., Madrid, 1861, viii, 549.—**Gritti**
(R.) Saggio di una tavola nosologica statistica e terapeutica per uso degli ospitali militari in tempo di guerra.
Gazz. med. ital. lomb., Milano, 1866, 5. s., v, 236–239, 1 pl.—
Heineke. Ueber Rubricirung der Todesursachen. Verhandl. d. deutsch. Gesellsch. f. Chir., Berl., 1877, i, 66–70.—
Hosack (D.) A new classification of diseases. Am.
M. & Phil. Reg. 1811–12, N. Y., 1814, ii, 266–269.—**Houzé**
(F.) De la transformation des types nosologiques. Presse
méd. belge, Brux., 1849, i, 295.—**Johnson** (C. B.) Classification and causation of diseases. Chicago M. J., 1877,
xxxiv, 200–208.—**Kieser** (D. G.) Nosologisches System,
zum Gebrauch in der medicinisch-chirurgischen und
augenärztlichen Klinik. *In his:* Klin. Beitr., 8°, Leipz.,
1834, i, 74–130.—**Klebs** (E.) Ueber natürliche Krank-
heits-Familien, mit besonderer Berücksichtigung der
Rheumatismen und Typhen. Ztschr. f. Heilk., Prag,
1880, i, 5–24.—**Köchlin** (R.) Skizze einer systematischen
Eintheilung der Krankheiten des Menschen. Med.-chir.
Ztg., Salzb., 1819, ii, 316; 333; 348; 365.—**Linton** (M.
L.) Definitions of disease. St. Louis M. & S. J., 1864, n.
s., i, 8–12.—**Longmore** (T.) On the classification and
tabulation of injuries and surgical operations in time of
war. Med.-Chir. Tr., Lond., 1870–71, liv, 201–246. *Also,*
Reprint.—**Neuber** (A.) Das kranke Leben. Mitth. a.
d. Geb. d. Med., etc., Altona, 1840–41, viii, 9–10. Hft.,
1–38.—**Nicholl** (W.) Tentamen nosologicum. Lond.
M. Reposit., 1817, vii, 177–196.—**Nieto.** Clasificaciones
nosográficas. Siglo méd., Madrid, 1856, iii, 353–355.—
Nosology. West. Q. Reporter M., S. & Nat. Sc., Cincin., 1822, i, 111–122.—**Parmeggiani** (G.) Sulla classificazione delle malattie. Bull. d. sc. med. di Bologna, 1852,
3. s., xxi, 81–98.—**Pinel & Bricheteau.** Nosographie.
Dict. d. sc. méd., Par., 1819, xxxvi, 206–265. — **Pye-
Smith** (P. H.) Remarks on the classification and local
distribution of disease, and particularly of disease of the
skin. Guy's Hosp. Rep., Lond., 1877, 3. s., xxii, 151–177,
2 pl.—**Rabagliati** (A. C. F.) On classification and
nomenclature in nervous disorders. West Riding Lun.
Asyl. Rep., Lond., 1876, vi, 25–42. ———. The classification and nomenclature of diseases. Brit. M. J., Lond.,
1880, ii, 333. ———. Some remarks on the classification
and nomenclature of diseases. *Ibid.,* 1881, ii, 114–117.—
Raige-Delorme. Examen critique de la nosographie
médicale de M. Bouillaud et du traité de médecine pratique
de M. Piorry. Arch. gén. de méd., Par., 1846, 4. s., xii, 257–
294.—**Razoux.** Sur les tables nosologiques. [*From:*
Mém. Acad. roy. d. sc., 1769.] Collect. acad. d. mém., etc.
Partie franç., Par., 1787, xiv, 355–357.—**Replies** received
in answer to the circular of the council respecting Dr.
Farr's questions on the classification of epidemic diseases.
Tr. Epidemiol. Soc. Lond. (1862–6), 1867, ii (app.), 1–30.—
Röschlaub's (Ueber) Nosologie. Arch. f. med. Erfahr.,
Berl., 1803, iv, 456; 535.—**Russel** (C. P.) A report on a
uniform system of registration of causes of death through-
out the United States. Am. Pub. Health. Ass. Rep. 1873,
N. Y., 1875, i, 483–490.—**de Sauvages.** Sur la méthode
nosologique. Hist. Soc. roy. d. sc. à Montpel., Lyon et
Montpel., 1778, ii, pt. 2, 15–26.—**Schultz** (C. H.) Ueber
die natürlichen Verwandtschaften der Krankheiten; nebst
Entwurf eines organisch-praktischen Krankheitssystems.
J. d. pract. Heilk., Berl., 1839. lxxxviii, 4. St., 15–59.—
Senftleben (F. A.) Nosologisches System der Wund-
arzneikunst. J. d. Chir. u. Augenh., Berl., 1834, xxi, 361–
404.—**Study** (On the) of nosology, and the present state
of medical science. Med.-Chir. J. & Rev., Lond., 1817, iv,
441–449.—**Tableau** nosographique des principales maladies qui peuvent être cause de mort. [Rap. et discussion.]
Bull. Acad. roy. de méd. de Belg., Brux., 1842–3, ii, 12–28.—
Tableau nosographique des maladies qui peuvent être
cause de mort. Ann. d'hyg., Par., 1849, xlii, 80–87.—
Tessier (J.-F.) Lettre sur la méthode nosologique et la
méthode étiologique, dans leur rapport avec la classification des maladies. Gaz. méd. de Par., 1849, 3. s., iv, 640.—
Tytler (R.) Systematis nosologici novi, exemplum par-
vulum. Med. & Phys. J., Lond., 1822, xlvii, 265–269.—
Vallejo Lobon (M.) Estudio crítico sobre las clasificaciones nosológicas de base anatómica y patogénica.
Siglo méd., Madrid, 1882, xxix, 116–118.—**Vegas** (M.)
Significado de algunas voces técnicas; su aplicacion y consideraciones patológicas. España méd., Madrid, 1863, viii,
453; 471; 521; 535.—**Vernon.** Some defects in the registrar general's classification of diseases. Proc. North-
West. Ass. Med. Off. Health 1876, Birkenhead, 1877, 8–18.

Nosology.

Also: San. Rec., Lond., 1876, iv, 293–298.—**Villar** (L.)
Leccion sobre clasificacion de las especies mórbidas. Gac.
méd., Lima, 1876, ii, 242–245.—**Young** (T.) Aphorisms
relating to classification extracted principally from the
Philosophia botanica of Linné. *In his:* Introduction to
Med. Lit., etc., 8°, Lond , 1823, 23–36.—**Zarlenga** (R.)
Brani di nosologia speciale. Filiatre-sebezio, Napoli, 1843,
xxvi, 14–22.

Nosotti (Innocente). Relazione sulle esperienze
di vaccinazione carbonchiosa eseguite nella provincia di Pavia per cura della commissione Sormani, Maggi, Nosotti, segretario-relatore. 31
pp. 8°. *Palermo,* 1880.

———. Breve risposta all' opuscolo l' afta epi-
zootica e la pratica dell' innesto dei signori
N. De Capitani e G. Franceschi. 19 pp. 8°.
Pavia, F. Fusi, 1885.

    Repr. from: Bull. d. agric., 1885, xix.

———. Della possibile trasmissione della tubercolosi degli animali all' uomo per l' uso delle
carni e del latte e dei mezzi più opportuni per
impedirla. Studi ed esperienze. 56 pp., 5 l., 5
pl. 8°. *Milano, frat. Dumolard,* 1885.

———. Carni fresche, carni salate, o in altro
modo preparate e conservate, grassi animali.
xxv, 308 pp. 12°. *Milano, frat. Dumolard,* 1886.

Nossi-Bé *Island.*

See, also, **Cholera** (*Asiatic, History, etc., of*), *by
localities.*

    MARROIN (A.) * Observations sur Nossi-Bey,
Mayotta et Sainte-Marie de Madagascar. 4°.
Paris, 1843.

    GUIOL (J.) Topographie médicale de Nossi-Bé. [Ex-
traits.] Arch. de méd. nav., Par., 1882, xxxviii, 119; 241;
321.

Nosswiz (Godofredus). * Παλαιολογίας therapiæ
specimen vii. De tempore in morbis. 36 pp.
sm. 4°. *Lipsiæ, ex off. Langenhemiana,* [1748].

    For Biography, see **Hebenstreit** (Joh. Ernestus).

Nostalgia.

See, also, **Sailors.**

    ALLARD (R.-V.) * Dissertation sur la nos-
talgie. 4°. *Paris,* 1820.

    ANDRESSE (G. A.) * Nostalgiæ adumbratio
pathologica. 8°. *Berolini,* 1826.

    ANSALONI (L.-V.) * De la nostalgie, ou de la
maladie du pays. 4°. *Paris,* 1837.

    BELLONY (C.) * De nostalgia. 8°. *Pestini,*
1835.

    BENOIST DE LA GRANDIÈRE (A.-E.) De la
nostalgie, ou mal du pays. 12°. *Paris,* 1873.

    BESSE (V.-M.) * De la nostalgie. 4°. *Paris,*
1828.

    BLANCHE (E.-E.) * Dissertation sur la nos-
talgie. 4°. *Strasbourg,* 1860.

    BOBILLARD (C.-F.) * Coup d'œil sur la nos-
talgie. 4°. *Strasbourg,* 1833.

    BRIET (P.-U.) * Essai sur la nostalgie. 4°.
Paris, 1832.

    BUISSON (J.-H.) * Considérations sur la nos-
talgie. 4°. *Paris,* 1818.

    CAIRE (C.) * Essai sur la nostalgie. 4°. *Pa-
ris,* 1852.

    CALMEL (B.) * Dissertation sur la nostalgie.
4°. *Paris,* 1836.

    CASTELNAU (C.) * Considérations sur la nos-
talgie. 4°. *Paris,* 1806.

    DE CASTILHO (J.-F.) * Dissertation sur la
nostalgie. 4°. *Paris,* 1831.

    CHÂTELAIN (A.) * Einige Betrachtungen über
die Nostalgie. 8°. *Würzburg,* 1860.

    CHENU (R.) * De la nostalgie. 4°. *Paris,*
1877.

    COLLIN (F.-T.) * Considérations sur la nos-
talgie. 4°. *Paris,* 1832.

    CURÉ (G. D.) * Diss. exhibens famosi illius
morbi quem nostalgiam passim pathologi, Ger-
mani vero das Heimwehe, oder Heim-Sehn-

Nostalgia.

sacht vulgo appellant . . . theoriam. 4°. [*Herbi-poli*, 1755.]

DUCREST DE LORGERIE (C.) * Dissertation sur la nostalgie. 4°. *Paris*, 1815.

FRAISSE (C.) * De la nostalgie. 4°. *Paris*, 1833.

GAILLARDOT (C.-A.) * Sur la nostalgie. 4°. *Paris, an XII* [1804].

GRUNDTMANN (F. J. A.) * De nostalgia. 8°. *Berolini*, [1839].

GUEIT (C.-F.-A.) * Sur la nature de la nostalgie, ses causes et son traitement. 4°. *Montpellier*, 1874.

GUERBOIS (D.-F.-N.) * Sur la nostalgie, appelée vulgairement maladie du pays. 8°. *Paris, an XI* [1803].

HARDER (J. J.) & HOFER (J.) De nostalgia. *Basileæ*, 1678.
In : HALLER. Disp. ad morb. [etc.] 4°. *Lausannæ*, 1757, i, 181–190.

HETTICH (H. O. F.) * Ueber das Heimweh, hauptsächlich in seinen Beziehungen zur Staats-Arzneikunde. 8°. *Stuttgart*, 1840.

———. The same. 8°. *Tübingen*, 1840.

HOFER (J.) * De νοσταλγία, oder Heimwehe. 4°. *Basileæ*, [1688].

———. The same. De pothopatridalgia. Vom Heim-Wehe.
In : FASCICULUS diss. med. select. (Zvingerus). 12°. *Basil.*, 1710, 87–111.

———. The same. * De nostalgia, vulgo: Heimwehe oder Heimsehnsucht. 4°. *Basileæ*, 1745.
Also, in : HALLER. Disp. ad morb. [etc.] 4°. *Lausannæ*, 1757, i, 181 ; 190.

HUET-BIENVILLE (J.-V.) * La nostalgie. 4°. *Paris*, 1821.

JACQUIER (F.) * Sur la nostalgie. 4°. *Paris*, 1821.

LACHAUD (M.) * Sur la nostalgie. 4°. *Paris*, 1809.

LEROY-DUPRÉ (L.-A.-H.) * De la nostalgie. 4°. *Paris*, 1846.

MALAPER DU PEUX (J.-U.) * De la nostalgie. 4°. *Paris*, 1853.

MARTIN (J.-J.-A.) * Sur la nostalgie. 4°. *Paris*, 1820.

MASSON (J.-B.-H.) * De la nostalgie considérée comme cause de plusieurs maladies. 4°. *Paris*, 1825.

MATTHÆI (E.) * De nostalgia. 8°. *Halis Sax.*, [1844].

MAURY (M.-É.) * Essai sur la nostalgie. 4°. *Strasbourg*, 1826.

MOREAU (J.-M.-É.-B.) * Considérations sur la nostalgie. 4°. *Paris*, 1848.

MOREAUD (P.) * Considérations sur la nostalgie. 4°. *Paris*, 1829.

MUSSET (H.-J.-M.-H.) * Sur la nostalgie. 4°. *Paris*, 1830.

PARRY (G.) * De patriæ desiderio. 8°. *Edinburgi*, 1805.

PAULINIER (J.-P.-L.-T.) * Sur la nostalgie (vulgairement, mal ou maladie du pays); essai, fragments ou aperçus, etc. 4°. *Montpellier*, 1837.

PETROWITCH (S.) * De la nostomanie. 4°. *Paris*, 1866.

PILET (D.-E.) * De la nostalgie considérée chez l'homme de guerre. 4°. *Paris*, 1844.

PILLEMENT (G.-L.-V.) * Essai sur la nostalgie. 4°. *Paris*, 1831.

POISSON (E.) * Dissertation sur la nostalgie. 4°. *Paris*, 1836.

PUEL (J.-A.-E.) * Essai sur la nostalgie. 4°. *Paris*, 1822.

REYNAL (M.) * Dissertation sur la nostalgie. 4°. *Paris*, 1819.

Nostalgia.

ROCHE (J.-P.) * Essai médico-philosophique sur la nostalgie ou mal du pays. 4°. *Paris*, 1829.

SUGÁR (F.) * Nostalgia. 8°. *Vindobonæ*, 1843.

THERRIN (A.-F.-A.) * Essai sur la nostalgie. 4°. *Paris*, 1810.

WIEDEMANN (A.) * De nostalgia. 8°. *Pragæ*, [1844].

YVONNEAU (J.) * Considérations médico-philosophiques sur la nostalgie. 4°. *Paris*, 1821.

Alciati. Sulla causa prossima della nostalgia. Gior. d. sc. med., Torino, 1844, xxi, 410 : 1845, xxiii, 3.—**Behr.** Ueber das Heimweh. Wchnschr. f. d. ges. Heilk., Berl., 1838, 181–185. — **Binard** (F.) Délire nostalgique, efficacité de l'opium à hautes doses. Arch. belges de méd. mil., Brux., 1856, xviii, 9–17.—**Calhoun** (J. T.) Nostalgia as a disease of field service. Med. & Surg. Reporter, Phila., 1864–5, xii, 130–132.—**Carnevale-Arella** (A.) Considerazioni sulle cause fisiche della nostalgia. Gior. d. Soc. med.-chir. di Torino, 1844, xix, 257–269. *Also, transl. :* J. Soc. de méd.-prat. de Montpel., 1845, xii, 472–480. *Also, transl. :* Bull. Soc. de méd. de Gand, 1846, xii, 107–115. ————. Alcune linee in aggiunta alle Considerazioni sulle cause fisiche della nostalgia, in risposta al Dr. Alciati. Gior. d. Soc. med.-chir. di Torino, 1845, xxii, 183–193. — **Cornelius.** Ueber die Nostalgie bei jungen Mädchen. Verm. Abhandl. . . . . v. einer Gesellsch. pract. Aerzté zu St. Petersb., 1847, vii, 89–101.—**Decaisne** (E.) Observations de nostalgie recueillies pendant le siége de Paris. Courrier méd., Par., 1871, xxi, 93. — **Devaux.** Observation sur une lésion au cerveau qui paraît être la cause de la nostalgie. Rec. de mém. de méd. . . . . mil., Par., 1822, xi, 248–258. — **Hamilton** (R.) History of a remarkable case of nostalgia affecting a native of Wales and occurring in Britain. Med. Comment., Edinb., 1787, 2. dec., i, 343–348. — **Hartenkeil.** Tödtliche Nostalgie eines jungen Arztes aus der Schweiz zu Paris. N. Mag. f. Aerzte, Leipz., 1786, viii, 360–363.—**Haspel** (A.) De la nostalgie. Mém. Acad. de méd., Par., 1874, xxx, 2. fasc., 466–6-8. *Also*, Reprint. — **Heimweh** (Ueber das). Bl. f. gerichtl. Anthrop., Nürnb., 1859, x, 2. Hft., 15–31.—**Jansen** (A.) Considérations sur la nostalgie. Ann. Soc. de méd. de Gand, 1869, xlvii, 210–240. [Rap. de Ingels.] Bull. Soc. de méd. de Gand, 1869, xxxvi, 592.—**Jones** (J. W.) † Atlanta M. & S. J., 1860–61, vi, 7.— **Larrey** (J.) Mémoire sur le siége et les effets de la nostalgie ; suivi de quelques réflexions sur les lésions partielles du cerveau, résultant de causes spontanées ou de causes mécaniques. *In his :* Rec. de mém. de chir., Par., 1821, 161–222, 1 pl.—**Laugier.** Observation d'une lésion organique du cervelet, suite de nostalgie. Rec. de mém. de méd. . . . . mil., Par., 1820, viii, 179–184.—**Legrand du Saulle.** Étude sur la nostalgie. Gaz. d. hôp., Par., 1858, xxxi, 5–7.—**Meyer** (L.) Der Wahnsinn aus Heimweh. Deutsche Klinik, Berl., 1855, vii, 7 ; 20 ; 31.—**Moricheau-Beauchamp** (R.-P.) Réflexions que les modifications que l'éducation et les habitudes ont apportés dans le développement de la nostalgie, pendant la dernière guerre. Mém. Soc. méd. d'émulat. de Par., an v (1798), i, 66–71.—**Morin.** De la nostalgie aux points de vue philosophique et médical. France méd., Par., 1856, iii, 201–204.—**Muñoz Barreda** (V.) Nostalgia aguda en un caso de pneumonia. Gac. méd. de Sevilla, 1880, ii, 267 ; 274. — **Nostalgia** (Von der), oder dem so genandten Heimwehe. Samml. v. Nat.-u. Med.- . . . Gesch. 1717–18, Bresl., 1718–20, 832–837. — **Papillon** (F.) Nostalgia. Pop. Sc. Month., N. Y., 1874, v, 215–220. — **Percy** & **Laurent.** Nostalgie. Dict. d. sc. méd., Par., 1819, xxxvi, 265–281. — **Peters** (De W. C.) Remarks on the evils of youthful enlistments and nostalgia. Am. M. Times, N. Y., 1863, vi, 75. — **Rey** (H.) Nostalgie. N. dict. de méd. et chir. prat., Par., 1877. xxiv, 116–144.—**Röbbelen** (A. H.) Nostalgie mit tödtlichem Ausgange. Deutsche Klinik, Berl., 1864, xvi, 277. — **Scheuchzer.** Sur la nostalgie, maladie particulière aux Suisses. [*From :* Mém. Acad. d. sc. de Bologne.] Collect. acad. d. mém., etc., Par., 1773, x, 592.— **Taylor** (W. T.) Nostalgia or home sickness. Am. M. Bi-Weekly, Louisville, 1879, x, 121–123.—**Verhovitz** (J.) De nostalgia. *In :* Everel. Diss.-med. [etc.], 8°, Viennæ, 1790, iii, 205–218. — **Widal** (V.) Nostalgie. Dict. encycl. d. sc. méd., Par., 1878, 2. s., xiii, 357–380.

von Nostitz & Jänckendorf (Gottlob Adolf Ernst) [1765–1836]. Beschreibung der königl. sächsischen Heil- und Verpflegungsanstalt Sonnenstein, mit Bemerkungen über Anstalten für Herstellung oder Verwahrung der Geisteskranken. 1. Theil, 1. u. 2. Abth. xviii, 569 pp., 1 pl. ; ii, 280 pp., 1 l., 10 pl.— 8°. *Dresden, Walther*, 1829.

Wants 2. Theil to complete.

Nostradamus (Michael) [1503–66]. Zwey Bücher, darinn warhafftiger, gründtlicher, und volkonner Bericht gegeben wirdt, wie man erstlich einen ungestalten Leib, an Weib- und Mannspersonen ausswendig zieren, schön, und junggeschaffen machen, und allerley wohlriechende, köstliche, krefftige Wasser, Pulfer, Öl, Seyffen, Rauchkertzlin, Bisamkuglen, zü mancherley Gebrechen dienstlich, artlich zubereyten. Und wie man folgents allerley Frücht auff das künstlichest, und lieblichest, in Zucker einmachen, und zur Notturfft auff behalten sol. Erstlich in frantzösischer Sprach von ihme beschriben: Nun aber, unserem Vatterland zü Gütem, in das gemain Teutsch auff das trewlichst verdolmetscht, durch Hieremiam Martium. 7 p. l., 206 pp., 5 l. 16°. *Augspurg, M. Manger,* 1573.

For Portrait, see **Collection**—van Kaathoven.

Nostril.

See **Nose**, *etc.*

Nostrums.

See **Medicines** (*Patent, etc.*)

Nota delle cose medicinali, che si devono tenere nelle specierie si della città, che del territorio di Verona. xii pp. fol. *Verona, fratelli Merlo,* 1751.

Notabel arrest van't Parlement's Hoffs van Grenoble gegeven tot profijt van eene Ioffrou, over de gheboorte van eene van hare soonen, geschiet vier jaren naer d'absentie van haren man, sonder eenighen man bekent te hebben. 3 l. sm. 4°. *'s Graven Hage. L. Breeckevelt,* 1637.

Notæ unguenti magnetici et ejusdem actionis quas in . . . Universitate Dilingana . . . publicabunt . . . candidati. 89 pp., 2 l. 16°. *Dilingæ, J. Sermodi,* 1626.

Notaris (J. B.)

See **Helvetius** (Joh. Frid.) Amphitheatrum physiognomiæ medicum. 16°. *'s Gravenhage,* 1664.

Notarp ([Joannes] Henricus) [1807–]. * De sede et natura tussis convulsivæ ejusque curatione. 37 pp., 1 l. 8°. *Berolini, typ. Nietackianis.* [1833].

Notcutt (W. L.) A handbook of the microscope and microscopic objects, with descriptive lists of upwards of 1,780 objects, and full directions for obtaining, preparing, and viewing them. ix, 152 pp. 12°. *London, E. Lumley,* 1859.

Note additionnelle au rapport de la Société médicale de Chambéry sur l'enseignement de la médecine en Savoie. 7 pp. 8°. *Chambéry, Puthod,* [n. d.]

Repr. from : Courrier d. Alpes.

Note sul corpo sanitario militare. 36 pp. 8°. *Roma, V. Carlo,* 1886.

Repr. from: Riv. mil. ital., 1886.

Note explicative sur l'héliostat de [Jean-Bernard-] Léon Foucault et sur la manière de le mettre en fonction. 8 pp. 8°. *Paris, J. Duboscq,* 1863.

Note sur les appareils séparateurs et désinfecteurs des matières fécales aussitôt leur production. [Système Chaussenot.] 8 pp., 1 pl. 4°. [*Paris,* 1849, *vel subseq.*] [P., v. 1714.]

Note sur les goîtres estival, épidémique et variqueux, observés dans le département du Puy-de-Dôme, lue à la séance académique de janvier 1852. 15 pp. 8°. [*Clermont, Thibaud-l'Andriot frères,* 1852?] [P., v. 465.]

Note sur l'industrie des allumettes chimiques. 4°. [*Paris, Serrière & Cie.,* 1861.] [P., v. 1726.]

Note sur le service vétérinaire de l'armée et les améliorations qu'il conviendrait de porter à la position des vétérinaires militaires. 11 pp. 4°. [*Paris,* 1880, *vel subseq.*]

Note des titres antérieurs de Victor Stoeber, né le 16 février 1803 à Strasbourg. 3 pp. 4°. *Strasbourg, F.-G. Levrault,* 1836, v. 68.

Note on the use of cocaine in hay fever. 5 l. 8°. [*Philadelphia,* 1885.]

Note - book for Professor McLeod's clinical class. New series. 15 pp., 2 pl. 8°. [*n. p., n. d.*]

Notencephalus.

See **Monsters** *from defect, etc., of brain, etc.*

Notes on beauty, vigor, and development. 23 pp. 16°. [*New York,* 1872.]

Notes on Dr. Chapman's lectures, in the University of Pennsylvania, with an appendix, containing a few remarks on Asiatic cholera and yellow fever, by a physician. 131 pp. 8°. *Philadelphia, W. S. Young,* 1845.

Notes on Finzelberg's pure soluble pepsin (1 to 100). 12 pp. 8°. [*New York,* 1881.]

Notes on the history, manufacture, uses, and properties of hydrochlorate of cocaine. 11 pp. 8°. *New York,* [1885].

Notes of hospital life, from November, 1861, etc. *See* **Potter** (A.)

Notes on military pensions. East India Company's military forces. 8 pp. 8°. [*London, S. Bentley,* 1830.] [P., v. 1049.]

Repr. from : United Service J., 1830, pt. 2.

Notes on new remedies, collated from medical and pharmaceutical periodicals, etc. Infants' food. 3. ed. 64 pp. 16°. *Boston, T. Metcalf & Co.,* 1878.

Notes of a New Truth, a monthly journal of homœopathy. Issued by the English Homœopathic Association. Nos. 2–49 (v. 1–4; No. 1, v. 5), March, 1856, to Feb., 1860. 8°. *London, J. Trapp.*

Want no. 1, February, 1856.

Notes on the postscript to a pamphlet entitled : "Observations anatomical and physiological, etc., by Alexander Monro, junior". 24 pp. 8°. *London, R. & J. Dodsley,* 1758. [P., v. 715.]

Notes on the value of carbo-hydrates as food, and the physiology of starch digestion. [Barley peculiarly adapted for malting and richer in the soluble albuminoids (diastase, etc.) than any other cereal.] 16 pp. 18°. *Cleveland, O., W. J. Morgan & Co.,* [n. d.]

Notes on vivisection, by a student of medicine. 16 pp. 12°. [*London*], *C. Green & Son,* [n. d.]

———. The same. (New edition, enlarged.) 26 pp. sm. 8°. [*n. p.,* 1876, *vel subseq.*]

Noth (Æmilius Julius). * De necrosi ossium. 30 pp., 1 l. 8°. *Halis Sax., typ. Heynemannianis,* [1854].

Noth (Joannes Traugott). Spec. phys. de pluvia et tonitru quo simul locus Job, xxxviii, 25, 26, 27, explicatur. 24 pp. 4°. *Wittebergæ, typ. J. Tzschidrichii* [1787].

Nothers (Jakob). * Ueber Sarkome des Oberkiefers. 24 pp. 8°. *Würzburg, Thein (Stürtz),* 1885.

Nothhaas (Leonhard). * Statistische Uebersicht des Kranken-Abganges der 1. medicin. Abtheilung des Krankenhauses München l. J. (vom 1. Februar 1871 bis 31. Januar 1876), nebst Bemerkungen über einzelne Krankheitsformen. 19 pp. 8°. *München,* 1876.

Nothnagel (Carl Wilhelm Hermann) [1841–]. * De variis renum affectionibus, quæ nomine "morbus Brightii" vulgo comprehenduntur. 32 pp. 8°. *Berolini, G. Schade,* [1863].

———. Handbuch der Arzneimittellehre. xii, 711 pp. 8°. *Berlin, A. Hirschwald,* 1870.

———. The same. Tractado de materia medica e de therapeutica. Trad. do allemão por João Felix Pereira ; revisto pelo doutor Pedro Francisco da Costa Alvarenga. ix, 874 pp. 8°. *Lisboa, imp. nacional,* 1879.

Nothnagel (Carl Wilhelm Hermann)—cont'd.

———. Ueber centrale Irradiation des Willens-impulses. 5 pp. 8°. [*Berlin, G. Bernstein,* 1870, *vel subseq.*]
Repr. from: Arch. f. Psychiat., Berl., 1871-2, iii.

———. Zur Lehre vom Husten. 11 pp. 8°. [*Berlin, G. Reimer*], 1870.
Repr. from: Arch. f. path. Anat., etc., Berl., 1870, xliv.

———. Ueber den epileptischen Anfall.
In: SAMML. klin. Vortr., Leipz., 1872, No. 39 (Inn. Med., No. 15, 309-322).

———. Schmerz und cutane Sensibilitätsstörun-gen. Beitrag zur Pathologie der Neuralgien. 16 pp. 8°. [*Berlin, G. Reimer,* 1873.]
Repr. from: Arch. f. path. Anat., etc., Berl., 1873, liv.

———. Ueber Diagnose und Aetiologie der ein-seitigen Lungenschrumpfung.
In: SAMML. klin. Vortr., Leipz., 1874, No. 66 (Inn. Med., No. 24, 535-550).

———. Ueber Neuritis in diagnostischer und pathologischer Beziehung.
In: SAMML. klin. Vortr., Leipz., 1876, No. 103 (Inn. Med., No. 35, 829-850).

———. Topische Diagnostik der Gehirnkrank-heiten, eine klinische Studie. vi, 626 pp. 8°. *Berlin, A. Hirschwald,* 1879.

———. The same. Traité clinique du diagnostic des maladies de l'encéphale, basé sur l'étude des localisations, traduit et annoté avec autorisa-tion de l'auteur par le Dr. P. Keraval. Ouvrage précédé d'une préface par M. le professeur Char-cot. xxi, 676 pp., 1 l. 8°. *Paris, A. Delahaye & E. Lecrosnier,* 1885.

———. Die Symptomatologie der Darmgeschwüre.
In: SAMML. klin. Vortr., Leipz., 1881, No. 200 (Inn. Med., No. 67, 1793-1812).

———. Beiträge zur Physiologie und Pathologie des Darmes. 3 p. l., 249 pp., 2 pl. 8°. *Berlin, A. Hirschwald,* 1884.

———. Ueber Anpassungen und Ausgleichungen bei pathologischen Zuständen. 1. Abhandlung. 27 pp. 8°. [*Berlin, L. Schumacher,* 1885-6.]
Repr. from: Ztschr. f. klin. Med., Berl., 1885-6, x.

———. Ueber Anpassungen und Ausgleichungen bei pathologischen Zuständen. 2. Abhandl. 15 pp. 8°. [*Berlin, L. Schumacher,* 1886.]
Repr. from: Ztschr. f. klin. Med., Berl., 1886, xi.

———. Ueber die Localisation der Gehirnkrank-heiten. 26 pp. 8°. *Wiesbaden, J. F. Bergmann,* 1887.
Repr. from: Verhandl. d. Cong. f. innere Med., Wiesb., 1887, vi.

———. Vorträge über die Diagnose bei den Ge-hirnkrankheiten. 53 pp. 8°. *Wien, R. R. von Schmerling,* 1887.
Bound with: Mitth. d. Wien. med. Doct.-Coll., 1887, xiii.
Also, Co-Editor of: Zeitschrift für klinische Medicin, Berlin, 1883.
See, also, **Handbuch** d. spec. Path. (Ziemssen), Leipz., 1876, xi, Hlft. 1: 1875, xii, Hlft. 2: 1878, Suppl. Bd.
Also: **Cyclopedia** Pract. Med. (Ziemssen), N. Y., 1877, xi.—**Vogel** (Julius) & **Nothnagel** (H.) Ken Nio Ho. [The examination of the urine, etc.] 12°. *Tokio,* 1881.

——— & **Naunyn** (B.) Ueber die Localisation der Gehirnkrankheiten. 56 pp., 2 pl. 8°. *Wies-baden, J. F. Bergmann,* 1887.
Repr. from: Verhandl. d. Cong. f. innere Med., Wiesb., 1887, vi.

——— & **Rossbach** (M. J.) Handbuch der Arz-neimittellehre. 5. Aufl. xx, 916 pp. 8°. *Ber-lin, A. Hirschwald,* 1884.

——— ———. The same. 6. Aufl. xi, 947 pp. 8°. *Berlin, A. Hirschwald,* 1887.

——— ———. The same. Nouveaux éléments de matière médicale et de thérapeutique, exposé de l'action physiologique et thérapeutique des médicaments; ouvrage traduit et annoté par le Dr. J. Alquier, précédé d'une introduction par Ch. Bouchard. xxxii, 860 pp. 8°. *Paris, J.-B. Baillière & fils,* 1880.

Nothnagel (Carl Wilhelm Hermann) & **Ross-bach** (M. J.)—continued.

——— ———. The same. A treatise on materia medica (including therapeutics and toxicology), transl. from the fourth enlarged edition by Dr. H. N. Heineman, H. W. Berg, and Ferd. C. Val-entine. 3 v. [paged consecutively]. v, iv, 836 pp. 12°. *New York & London, Bermingham & Co.,* 1883-4.

———. Rukovodstvo k pharmakologii. Perevod s chetvertago Niemetskago izdanija M. Hirschfelda. [Transl. from the 4. German ed. by Hirschfeld.] xii, 786 pp. 8°. *St. Petersburg, typog. Ettingera,* 1884.

———. Dopolnenie k chetvertomu izdani-jou Rukovodstva k farmakologii sostavleno po pjatomu Niemetskomu izdanijou Vilijaninim. [Supplement to the 4. ed. of Manual of pharma-cology. Transl. from the 5. German ed. by Vili-janinim.] 1 l., 82 pp. 8°. *St. Petersburg, Med. Bibliot.,* 1884.

Nothnagel (Carolus G.) * De catarrho et rheu-matismo. 29 pp., 1 l. 8°. *Marburgi Cattorum, typ. Bayrhofferi,* 1844.

Nothnagel (Friedrich Ludwig) [1863-   ]. * Ueber operative Behandlung der Senkungs-abscesse. 29 pp. 8°. *Berlin, M. Gœdecke,* [1886].

Nothwendig- und nützlicher Unterricht, wor-nach sich die in des Durchlauchtigsten Fürsten und Herrn, Herrn Bernhards, Herzogen zu Sach-sen, Jülich, Cleve und Berg, etc., Landen, bestelte Hebammen oder Kind-Frauen, oder deren Stelle vertretende, und sonst männiglich, bey den schwangeren, kreysenden und gebährenden Wei-bern, vor-, in- und nach der Geburth, richten und halten sollen; nebst einer Anzeige etlicher Sprüche, Psalmen, Seufftzer und Gebethe, an-statt eines geistlichen Unterrichts bei derglei-chen Zustande. 72 pp. 4°. *Meiningen, N. Has-serten,* 168?.

Nothwendiger Unterricht wie der gifftigen anklebenden Seuche der Pestilentz nechst Gött-licher Hülfe vorzubauen und dieselbe zu curiren sey. Auf Anordnung und Befehl der hohen Landes-Fürstl. Obrigkeit vor diesem Anno 1657 auffgesetzt, und jetzo revidiret, und in vielem geendert worden. 16 l. 12°. *Zell, Holwein,* 1680.

Nothwendigkeit (Ueber die) die Zahl der Aerzte zu fixiren. Ein Beitrag zu Herrn Ge-heimen Medicinalrath Schmidt's Schrift: "Die Reform der Medicinalverfassung in Preussen". Nebst einem Anhang: Zur Würdigung der Re-formansichten des Herrn Geheimen Ober-Medi-cinalrath Trüstedt. In Gemeinschaft mit seinen Collegen: Dr. Diesterweg, Dr. Hellmann [et al.], verfasst von Dr. Hanekroth. 38 pp. 8°. *Siegen, Friedrich,* 1847.

Notice analytique des travaux de M. A. Velpeau. (Nov., 1842.) viii, 58 pp. 4°. *Paris, Bachelier,* 1842.

Notice analytique sur les travaux de M. [Jean-Jacques-Marie-Cyprien-Victor] Coste, prof. au Collége de France, juin 1850. 31 pp. 4°. *Paris, L. Martinet,* [n. d.]

Notice biographique sur le docteur Desruelles. 40 pp. 12°. *Paris, A. Parent,* [n. d.]

Notice biographique sur le Dr. J.-L. Prevost. Tiré de la Bibliothèque universelle de Genève. Décembre 1850. 36 pp. 8°. *Genève, F. Ramboz & Cie.,* 1850.

Notice sur les Charmettes, et sur les environs de Chambéry. 2. éd., revue et retouchée. 70 pp., 1 l. 8°. *Chambéry, P. Cléaz,* 1817. [P., v. 1398.]

Notice sur le docteur Ernest Cloquet. 24 pp. 8°. *Paris, L. Martinet,* 1856.

Notice of Dr. Guggenbühl's hospital for infant cretins. 8 pp. 8°. [*Edinburgh*], *A. Jack,* [n. d.]
Repr. from: Chambers's Edinb. J.

Notice sur les eaux minérales iodurées de Saxon, canton du Valais (Suisse). 76 pp. 12°. *Genève, P.-A. Bonnant*, 1855.

Notice sur l'eau minérale naturelle de Schwalheim (Hesse-Électorale). 15 pp. 8°. *Paris, V. Masson*, 1857.

Notice sur les eaux minérales naturelles et sur les eaux artificielles préparées dans l'établissement de MM. Planche, Boullay, Boudet, Cadet et Pelletier au Gros-Caillou ; cette notice indique en général la composition de ces eaux, les diverses formes sous lesquelles on les administre, leurs doses et leurs principales propriétés d'après les meilleurs ouvrages de médecine. 48 pp. 8°. *Paris, J. Smith*, 1832. [P., v. 915 ; 1808.]

Notice sur les eaux minérales sulfureuses, silicatées, sodiques de Cauterets transportées, suivie d'un aperçu sur les installations hydro-balnéaires de la station, et de renseignements généraux. Promenades, excursions, ascensions. 30 pp. 16°. *Bordeaux, J. Durand*, 1884.

Notice sur les eaux minérales sulfureuses d'Enghien-les-Bains. 24 pp. 16°. [*Paris*], *C. Noblet*, [*n. d.*]

Notice sur les eaux minérales, thermales, purgatives de Brides-les-Bains et sur les eaux minérales, thermales, chlorurées, sodiques, " eaux de mer thermales " de Salins-Moutiers, Savoie. 8 l. 12°. *Boulogne (Seine), J. Boyer*, [*n. d.*]

Notice sur les eaux sulfureuses naturelles de Cauterets, spécialement les sources de la Raillère et du Vieux-César, avec indication de leurs caractères chimiques, de leur mode d'emploi, des doses auxquelles on les prescrit, et de leurs vertus tout à fait spécifiques dans le traitement des maladies de poitrine et de l'asthme. 12 pp. 8°. *Cauterets. chez le fermier des sources*, [*n. d.*]
Repr. from : Ouvrages de MM. Orfila et C. James, et du Rap. de l'Acad. d. méd. P., v. 1648.

Notice sur les embaumements. Procédés de M. Gannal. 32 pp. 8°. *Paris, imp. de Terzuolo*, 1839. [P., v. 1790.]

Notice sur l'expédition qui s'est terminée par la prise de la Smahla d'Abd-el-Kader, ie 16 mai 1843. 19 pp., 1 map, 2 pl. 8°. [*Paris, Vinchon*, 1843 ?] [P., v. 462.]

Notice extraite du Panthéon biographique sur M. le docteur Caffe (Paul-Louis-Balthasar). pp. 169–191. 8°. *Paris*, 1860.
Cutting from : Panthéon biographique.
Bound with : Biographie de M. Caffe, etc. 8°. *Paris*, 1842.

Notice sur François Chaussier, professeur honoraire de la Faculté de médecine de Paris, membre de l'Institut, etc. 16 pp. 8°. *Paris, Lachevardière* [1825.]

Notice sur Geoffroy de Villeneuve (René-Claude). 15 pp. 8°. [*Paris, Vve. Delaguette*, 1831.] [P., v. 1745.]

Notice sur les grains de santé du docteur Franck. 4 l. 8°. *Paris*, [*n. d.*] [P., v. 1807.]

Notice sur l'hématoscope d'Hénocque ; indications techniques de ses applications. Spectroscopie, diaphanométrie, et photographie du sang, du lait, etc. 48 pp., 1 pl. 8°. *Paris, G. Masson*, 1886.

Notice historique sur le professeur Désormeaux. 31 pp. 12°. [*n. p., n. d.*]

Notice sur l'Hôpital de Ménilmontant. 8 pp., 1 pl. 4°. *Paris, Grandremy & Henou*, 1878.

Notice sur l'Hôpital Napoléon, fondé à Berck-sur-Mer (Pas-de-Calais). 24 pp. 8°. *Paris, imp. adm.*, 1869.

Notice sur les hôpitaux en tôles d'acier embouties, construits par Joseph Danly, d'après les données et les plans du docteur Jules Félix. 2 l. [containing plans]. fol. *Ixelles, C. Deecke*, 1884.
Another copy bound with : FÉLIX (Jules). La question des hôpitaux. 8°. *Bruxelles*, 1884.

Notice sur l'importation et le perfectionnement des bains russes en France. 40 pp. 8°. *Paris*, [1831]. [P., v. 1410.]

Notice sur J.-F. Double. 16 pp. 12°. *Paris*, 1843.
Repr. from : Encyclographie médicale, 1842.

Notice sur Jacques de Falaise, ses habitudes, sa nourriture, et les moyens qu'il emploie pour conserver sa santé. 7 pp. 8°. *Paris, Ballard*, 1820. [P., v. 1643.]

Notice (A) of the late John Revere. 5 pp. 8°. *Boston*, 1847. [P., v. 234.]

Notice sur M. Aulagnier (Alexis-François). 16 pp. 12°. *Paris, Moquet & Hauquelin*, 1842.

Notice sur la médecine électropathique du docteur J.-P. Bachoué de Lostalot, de Vialer (Basses-Pyrénées), approuvée par l'Académie de Paris, sur la loi terpathique organique . . . 2 l. 8°. [*n. p., n. d*]

Notice médicale sur les eaux minérales de Pougues. 47 pp. 8°. *Paris, V. Masson*, 1856.

Notice médicale sur les eaux minérales de Vichy. 71 pp., 1 l. 8°. *Paris, V. Masson*, 1854. [*Also, in :* P., v. 1651.]

Notice médicale sur l'usage des eaux minérales, sels et pastilles de l'établissement thermal de Vichy, propriété de l'État. 64 pp. 18°. *Paris*, [*n. d.*]

Notice médicale sur l'usage des eaux minérales de Vichy. 28 pp. 16°. [*n. p., n. d.*]

Notice sur feu Mr. J.-F. van Hoorebeeke. 2 l. 8°. [*n. p., n. d.*] [P., v. 1298.]

Notice nécrologique sur le docteur Platon Vallée. 16 pp. 16°. [*n. p.*], *Monnoyer*, [1856].

Notice sur un nouveau matelas hydrostatique pour prévenir la gangrène par compression dans les maladies chroniques. 16 pp. 8°. *Paris, H. Galante & Cie.*, 1863.

Notice of patents, granted to Joseph Amesbury, of Burton Crescent, in the county of Middlesex, surgeon, for certain apparatus used in the treatment of stiffness, weakness, or deformity of the spine, chest, or limbs ; accompanied with practical remarks and illustrations by the patentee. 24 pp., 3 pl. 8°. *London, Longman, Rees & Co.*, 1837. [P., v. 639.]

Notice on the pharmaceutical product known as Thevenot's globules, prepared by C. Thevenot. *See* **Thevenot** (C.)

Notice sur Pierre-Jean-Georges Cabanis. viii pp. 8°. [*Paris, Bourgogne & Martinet, n. d.*]

Notice sur les propriétés du quina Laroche. (Extrait complet des trois sortes de quinquinas.) Élixir vineux reconstituant et fébrifuge. 15 pp. 18°. *Paris*, [*n. d.*]

Notice of some of the leading events in the life of the late Dr. John Thomson, F. R. S. L. & E. 72 pp. 8°. *Edinburgh, Stark & Co.*, 1847.
Repr. from : Edinb. M. & S. J., 1847, lxvii.

Notice sur la vie de Jean-Auguste Grunert. 4 pp. 8°. *Paris, Gauthier-Villars*, 1872.
Repr. from : Bull. d. sc. math. et astronomique, iii.

Notices biographiques sur le docteur Henry Blatin et discours prononcés au bord de sa tombe le 29 mars 1869. Recueillis et publiés par les soins de Madame Claire Guyot, sa veuve. 29 pp. 8°. *Riom, G. Leboyer*, 1869.

Notices et documens sur le choléra, etc. *See* **Peschier** (Charles).

Notices sur les pâtes féculentes de la solanée Parmentière fabriquée par J.-B. Wattebled. 34 pp., 1 l. 12°. [*Paris*, 1822, *vel subseq.*] [P., v. 1677.]

Noticia archeologica das caldas de Visella ; situadas no concelho de Guimarães, e uma legoa para sul da sua capital do mesmo nome no importantissimo districto de Braga. 16 pp. 8°. *Braga, A. da Silva Santos*, 1853. [P., v. 1258.]

Noticia da doença de que falleceu sua magestade el-rei o senhor D. Pedro V e das que na mesma occasião atacaram suas altezas os senhores infantes D. Fernando, D. Augusto e D. João no'anno de 1861. 3 p. l., 41 pp. 8°. *Lisboa*, 1862. [P., v. 1264.]

Noticia e ensaio sobre as aguas mineraes da villa de Monsão, contendo o melhoramento actual deste salutifero estabelecimento. 2. ed. iv, 26 pp. sm. 8°. *Porto, typ. da Revista*, 1845.

Noticia topographica das caldas das Taipas; situadas no concelho de Guimarães, e legua e meia para noroeste da sua capital do mesmo nome, no importantissimo districto de Braga. 36 pp. 8°. *Braga, A. da Silva Santos*, 1854. [P., v. 1258.]

Notin (Édouard). *Étude sur les papillômes simples. 48 pp. 4°. *Paris*, 1885, No. 351.

Notisblad för läkare och pharmaceuter, bihang till Finska Läkare - Sällskapets Handlinger. 1860-65. 5 v. 8°. *Helsingfors*.

Notizblatt des Vereins für Erdkunde und verwandte Wissenschaften zu Darmstadt und des mittelrheinischen geologischen Vereins. Nebst Mittheilungen aus der grossherzoglich-hessischen Centralstelle für die Landesstatistik. Nos. 1-46; 2. Folge, Nos. 1-60 (Band 1-3); 3. Folge, Nos. 1-204 (Hefte 1-17), October, 1854, to December, 1878. 8°. *Darmstadt, G. Jonghaus.*
In May, 1857, L. Ewald became editor.

Notizen aus dem Gebiete der Natur- und Heilkunde: gesammelt und mitgetheilt von Ludwig Friedrich von Froriep. v. 1-50, July, 1821, to December, 1836. [2. Reihe.] v. 1-40, 1837-46. [3. Reihe.] v. 1-11, 1847-9. 101 v. 4°. *Weimar.*
Title of v. 1-40, 2. series, was: **Neue** Notizen, [etc.], and Robert Froriep added as editor. v. 1-11, 3. series, edited by Robert Froriep and M. J. Schleiden.

Notizen aus dem Gebiete der practischen Pharmacie und deren Hülfswissenschaften. Von A. R. L. Loget. [Monthly.] v. 1-23, Oct. 1, 1836, to Dec., 1859. 8°. *Crefeld, C. M. Schüller.*
In Jan., 1850, a new series commenced; L. Rohr, editor.
In v. 16, 1852, A. Hoffmann added.

Notizen für praktische Aerzte über die neuesten Beobachtungen in der Medicin, mit besonderer Berücksichtigung der Krankheits - Behandlung zusammengestellt von F. Graevell. v. 1-9, 1848-56. Neue Folge, v. 1-20, 1857-76. 29 v. 8°. *Berlin, A. Hirschwald*, 1849-77.
In v. 7 S. Strassmann added. v. 1-12, n. s., edited by H. Helfft; v. 13-20, n. s., by Paul Guttmann. Continued as: **Jahrbuch** für practische Aerzte.

Notizia della malattia e passaggio della Giulia Buzj e sezione del suo cadavere all' Antonio Cocchi.
In: Rac. d' opusc. scient. e filol. 16°. *Venezia*, 1744, xxx, 223-250.

Notizie di medici cavalieri da alcuni professori di medicina raccolte. [Giuseppe Benvenuti.] xvii, 54 pp. 4°. *Lucca, Benedini*, 1775.

Notizie, memorie ed istruzioni riguardanti il cholera morbus, raccolte dalle opere più accreditate e da' giornali moderni od anche recentemente emanate per cura delle pubbliche autorità estere. 2 p. l., 133 pp., 1 l. 8°. *Venezia, tip. di Commercio-Santa Marina*, 1831.

————. The same. 2. ed. 2 p. l., 134 pp., 1 l. 8°. *Venezia, tip. di Commercio-Santa Marina*, 1831.

Notizkalender und Adressbuch für praktische Aerzte, [etc.] 3. Jahrgang, 1888. 1. Vierteljahrsheft. Januar–März. 1 p. l., 45 ff., 2 l. 32°. *Berlin, E. Grosser*, 1888.

Notizkalender für Hochschulen (medicinische Facultät) pro 1885 [also for 1886 and 1888]. 3 v. 12°. *Wien, M. Perles.*

Notochord.
Pérépelkine (K.) Sur la structure de la notocorde de la lamproie (Petromyzon fluviatilis). Bull. Soc. imp. d. nat. de Moscou, 1878, liii, 107.—**Robin** (C.) Mémoire

Notochord.
sur l'évolution de la notocorde, des cavités des disques intervertébraux et de leur contenu gelatineux. Gaz. méd. de Par., 1867, 3. s., xxii, 284-287. *Also:* Compt. rend. Soc. de biol. 1867, Par., 1869, 4. s., iv, pt. 2, 31-38.

Notre-Dame Hospital, Montreal. Annual reports of the secretary to the contributors. 1.-5., 1880-81 to 1885. 8°. *Montreal*, 1881-5.
Opened July 26, 1880. 1., 1880-81, in French.

Notre-Dame de Pitié. *See* Hôtel-Dieu de Lyon.

Nott (Eliphalet). Lectures on biblical temperance. With an introduction by Tayler Lewis. xxiv, 268 pp. 8°. *London, Trübner & Co.*, 1863.

Nott (*Gustavus Adolphus*) [1816-67].
B. & D. Necrology. N. Orl. M. & S. J., 1867, xx, 280.

Nott (John) [1751-1825]. Of the Hotwell waters, near Bristol. 3 p. l., 94 pp. 8°. *Bristol*, 1793.

Nott (Josiah Clark) [1804-73]. A lecture on animal magnetism, delivered before the Mobile Franklin Society. 31 pp. 8°. *Charleston, Burges & James*, 1846.

————. The physical history of the Jewish race. 28 pp. 8°. *Charleston, S. C., Walker & James*, 1850. [P., v. 846.]
Repr. from: South. Q. Rev.

————. Instincts of races. 28 pp. 8°. *New Orleans, L. Graham*, 1866.
Repr. from: N. Orl. M. & S. J., 1866, xix.

————. Contributions to bone and nerve surgery. iv, 5-96 pp. 8°. *Philadelphia, J. B. Lippincott & Co.*, 1866. [*Also, in:* P., v. 105.]
See, also, **Goupil** (Jean Martin Auguste). An exposition of the principles of the new medical doctrine [etc.] 8°. *Columbia, [S. C.]*, 1831.
For Biography, see J. Anthrop. Soc. Lond., 1868, vi. pp. lxxix-lxxxiii (K. R. H. Mackenzie). *Also:* Tr. Am. M. Ass., Phila., 1878, xxix, 727-733 (W. H. Anderson). *Also:* Tr. M. Ass. Alabama, Montgomery, 1877, 118-128 (W. H. Anderson).

———— **& Gliddon** (George R.) Types of mankind; or, ethnological researches, based upon the ancient monuments, paintings, sculptures, and crania of races, and upon their natural, geographical, philological, and biblical history; illustrated by selections from the inedited papers of Samuel George Morton, and by additional contributions from Prof. L. Agassiz, W. Usher, M. D., and Prof. H. S. Patterson, M. D. (4. ed.) lxxvi, 49-738 pp., 3 pl. 8°. *London, Trübner & Co.; Philadelphia, Lippincott, Grambo & Co.*, 1854.

————. Indigenous races of the earth; or, new chapters of ethnological inquiry; including monographs on special departments of philology, iconography, cranioscopy, palæontology, pathology, archæology, comparative geography, and natural history; contributed by Alfred Maury, Francis Pulszky, and J. Aitken Meigs. (With communications from Prof. Jos. Leidy and Prof. L. Agassiz.) Presenting fresh investigations, documents, and materials. xxiv, 25-656 pp., 9 pl. 8°. *Philadelphia, J. B. Lippincott & Co.; London, Trübner & Co.*, 1857.

Nott (T. H.) The embryo physician as a specialist; read before the Texas State Medical Society. 8 pp. 8°. [*n. p.*, 1886.]

Notta (A.) Traitement des névralgies par la cautérisation transcurrente. 32 pp. 8°. *Paris, F. Malteste & Cie.*, 1847. [P., v. 1649.]
Repr. from: Union méd., Par., 1847, i.

Notta (Alphonse-Henri). *Recherches sur la cicatrisation des artères, à la suite de leur ligature, sur la production des hémorrhagies artérielles secondaires, et sur leur traitement. 59 pp. 4°. *Paris*, 1850, No. 216.

————. De l'emploi de la liqueur de Villate dans le traitement des affections chirurgicales et en particulier de la carie, du mal perforant du pied, des fistules consécutives aux abcès froids tuberculeux du testicule, aux abcès primitivement

Notta (Alphonse-Henri)—continued.
chauds de Vénus incurables, aux plaies d'armes à feu, à l'inflammation des tumeurs synoviales de la main, aux kystes, aux abcès des sinus frontaux, des fistules lacrymales, etc. xii, 168 pp. 8°. *Paris, J.-B. Baillière & fils, 1869.*

Notté (A.) Sur la fièvre traumatique, ou fièvre qui accompagne les plaies. 23 pp. 4°. *Paris, 1825, No. 30, v. 190.*

Nottebohm (Gustavus) [1821–   ]. * De hyperæmia. 28 pp., 2 l. 8°. *Berolini, typ. Nietackianis,* [1844].

Nottedge *vs.* Ripley.
See Insanity (*Jurisprudence of, Cases, etc., relating to*).

Notter (Fridericus). * De qualitatibus parentum in sobolem transeuntibus, præsertim ratione rei equariæ. vi, 69 pp. 4°. *Tubingæ, apud C. F. Osiandrum,* [1827].

Notter (Joh. Fridericus). * De actione mercurii in corpus humanum. 32 pp. sm. 4°. *Argentorati, typ. J. H. Heitzii,* [1749].

Nottin (Edmond). * Des syphilides tertiaires. 32 pp. 4°. *Paris, 1870.*

Notting Hill Provident Dispensary and Maternity. Annual reports of the committee to the governors and subscribers. 19., 1878; 22., 1881; 24., 1883; 25., 1884. 12°. *London, 1879–85.* Established 1860.

Nottingham. A report on the sanitary condition of the borough of Nottingham. By Edward Seaton, medical officer of health. 63 pp. 8°. *Nottingham, R. Allen & Son, 1873.*

——. Annual reports of the medical officer of health to the health committee of the town council. By E. Seaton. 1.–6., 1873–8; 10., 1882. 8°. *Nottingham, 1874–83.*

——. Report to the Nottingham and Leen Valley sewerage board on the utilization of the sewage and the purification of the river Trent and its tributaries; with descriptions of various modes of treating sewage. By M. Ogle Tarbotton, engineer to the board. Also a supplementary report on the above by Robt. Rawlinson, civil engineer. 55 pp., 2 ch., 2 tab. roy. 8°. *London, E. & F. N. Spon, 1875.*

——. Report to the health committee, from the medical officer of health and chief sanitary inspector, on the sanitary aspect of the various "systems" by which the disposal of the excreta is effected, with special reference to that which is now carried out in this borough. Oct. 6, 1876. 16 pp. 8°. *Nottingham, T. Forman & Sons, 1876.*

——. Report of chief inspector of nuisances, upon the operations of the night-soil department, to the health committee of the town council, for the year 1876–7. [By William Richards.] 12 pp. 8°. [*Nottingham, 1877.*]

——. Monthly reports of medical officer of health on the health of the borough and the work of the health department for Nov., Dec., 1878, and Jan., 1880. 8°. *Nottingham, 1879–80.* Jan., 1880, contains summary for 1879.

——. Report by the medical officer of health [Edward Seaton] upon the epidemic of measles and the prevalence of scarlet fever, 1879–80. 15 pp. 8°. [*Nottingham,* 1880.]

——. Report of the health committee as to the memorial presented to the council on the notification of infectious disease. [Being the report of Edward Seaton, medical officer of health. Adopted by the committee, and presented to the town council.] 28 pp. 8°. [*Nottingham,* 1882.]

——. A report to the health committee of Nottingham on the measures required for the improvement of the public health of the district

Nottingham—continued.
known as Narrow Marsh, by the medical officer of health [Edward Seaton], Nov. 11, 1882. 21 pp. 8°. [*Nottingham,* 1882.]

——. Report of the health committee on the report of the medical officer of health [Edward Seaton] on the notification of infectious diseases. To be presented to the council the 5th day of March, 1883. 16 pp., 2 diag. 8°. [*Nottingham,* 1883.]

Nottingham.
See, also, Fever (*Malarial, History. etc., of*), Fever (*Typhoid, History, etc., of*), Hospitals (*Descriptions, etc., of*), *by localities;* Measles (*Epidemics of*).

NOTTINGHAM. Annual reports of the medical officer of health to the health committee of the town council. 2.–4. (1874–6); 6. (1878). 8°. *Nottingham,* 1875–9.

——. Annual report of the medical officer of health for 1882, together with a description of the sanitary condition of Nottingham in 1882, etc., by Edward Seaton, M. D., etc. 8°. *Nottingham,* 1883.

——. Report of the health committee on the report of the medical officer of health [Edward Seaton] on the notification of infectious diseases. To be presented to the council the 5th day of March, 1883. 8°. [*Nottingham,* 1883.]

——. Monthly report of medical officer of health, for Jan., 1880. 8°. *Nottingham,* 1880.

SEATON (E.) A report to the health committee of Nottingham on the measures required for the improvement of the public health of the district of Narrow Marsh, known as Narrow Marsh, by the medical officer of health. Nov. 11, 1882. 8°. [*Nottingham,* 1882.]

THORNE (T.) Report on the prevalence of infectious diseases in Nottingham, and on the sanitary condition of the town. June 10, 1872. fol. [*London,* 1872.]

Brown (A.) Five years' municipal work in Nottingham. Proc. Ass. Municip. & San. Engin., Lond., 1884–5, xi, 172–196.—**Clarke** (J.) Medical report for Nottingham from March, 1807, to March, 1808. Edinb. M. & S. J., 1809, v, 188; 257: 1810, vi, 1, 1 pl., 260: 1811, vii, 129, 1 tab.—[**Medical** topography of Nottinghamshire.] Med. & Phys. J., Lond., 1813, xxx, 99.—**Richardson** (B. W.) The medical history of Nottingham. Med. Times & Gaz., Lond., 1866, ii, 564; 593; 644; 673; 700.—**White** (J.) On the medical topography of Nottingham. Tr. Prov. M. & S. Ass., Lond., 1853, xix, 171–199, 1 map, 1 tab.

Nottingham (Custis B.) The annual address delivered to the graduates of the Atlanta Medical College at the commencement, Sept. 2, 1858. 16 pp. 8°. *Atlanta, G. P. Eddy & Co.,* 1858.

——. An address delivered before the Georgia Medical Association at its 21st annual meeting. 20 pp. 8°. *Savannah, Ga., E. J. Purse,* 1870. c.
Repr. from: Tr. Georgia M. Ass., Savannah, 1870.
For Biography, see Atlanta M. & S. J., 1876, xiv, 124–128 (Burgess & Green). *Also:* Richmond & Louisville M. J., Louisville, 1876, xxi, 469–474 (E. Fitzgerald). *Also:* Tr. Am. M. Ass., Phila., 1878, xxix, 733 (T. S. Hopkins).

Nottingham (John). Report on the restoration of sight, by the formation of artificial pupil, in a patient of St. Anne's Dispensary. 23 pp. 16°. *Liverpool, E. Howell,* [1850].

——. Surgical report on bilateral lithotomy, with general remarks on operations for stone. vii, 101 pp. 8°. *London, J. Churchill,* 1850.

——. Practical observations on conical cornea, and on the short sight and other defects of vision connected with it. xxvi, 270 pp. 8°. *London, J. Churchill,* 1854.

——. Diseases of the ear. Illustrated by clinical observations. xxxi, 644 pp., 1 pl. 8°. *London, J. Churchill,* 1857.

Nottingham Borough Asylum (for the Insane), Mapperley Hill. Annual report of the commit-

Nottingham Borough Asylum [etc.]—cont'd.
tee of visitors to the town council. 5., 1884. 28
pp. 8°. *Nottingham, J. & J. Vice*, 1885.

Nottingham Friendly Societies'-Medical Institution. Medical officer's report to the committee for the half-year ending June 30, 1875. 2 l.
4°. [*Nottingham*, 1875.]

——. Annual reports of the managing committee to the officers and members. 1., 1875; 3.-6.,
1877-80; 8.-12., 1882-6. 8°. *Nottingham*, 1876-87.

——. Rules of the . . . iv, 22 pp. 12°. *Nottingham, P. D. M. J. Howitt*, 1879.

——. [Circular stating object and subscription
fees.] 1 sheet. 4°. [*Nottingham, n. d.*]

Nottingham Hospital for Sick Children. *See*
Children's Hospital, Nottingham.

Nottingham and Midland Eye Infirmary, Nottingham. Annual reports of the committee to
the subscribers. 14., 1873; 17.-24., 1876-83. 8°.
Nottingham, 1874-84.

Nottingham County. *Lunatic Asylum for the
County of Nottingham, at Snenton, Nottingham.*
Annual reports of the board of visitors and superintendent to the court of quarter sessions for the
county of Nottingham. 1.-5., 1875-9. 8°. *Nottingham*, 1876-80.

Changes in title: Prior to 1856, called the General Lunatic Asylum; from 1856 to 1874, known as the United
Lunatic Asylum for the County and Borough of Nottingham. Report for 1879 is the 69. of the original institution.

Nottingham Medico - Chirurgical Society.
Rules. 43 pp. 8°. *Nottingham, W. Dearden*,
1843.

Nottnagel (Christophorus).

See **Kirchmajer** (Theod.) & **Nottnagel** (Christophorus). De hominibus apparenter mortuis. 4°. *Wittebergæ*, [1669].

Nottnagel (Georg L.)

See **Henricus** (Henricus) & **Nottnagel** (Georg L.)
De abscessu mesenterii [etc.] 4°. *Halæ*, 1710.

Nouaille (H.-L.) *Sur le diagnostic du catarrhe
pulmonaire, de la péripneumonie, de la pleurésie
et de la pleurodynie. 14 pp. 4°. *Paris*, 1809,
No. 108, v. 77.

Nouaux (Michel-Julien). *I. Quelles sont les
modifications que subit l'acte digestif dans les
différents âges? II. [etc.] 28 pp. 4°. *Paris*,
1843, No. 20, v. 407.

de la Noue (Bartholomeus Petrus). *An fiat
bilis decompositio in intestinis? Præses Ber-
trandus Dupuy. 8 pp. 4°. [*Paris, Quillau*,
1768.]

——. *An aquæ potus omnium saluberrimus?
Præses Joannes Jacobus Messence. 4 pp. 4°.
[*Paris, Quillau*, 1769.]

——. *Num bubones critici in febribus malignis
statim incidendi? Præses Cleriades Vachier. 4
pp. 4°. *Paris, Quillau*, 1770.

See, also, **Varnier** (Carolus Ludovicus). *Utrum a
gangliis nervi intercostalis partium omnium consensus?
4°. [*Paris*, 1770.]

Nouel (Émile). *Sur l'hydropisie. 105 pp. 8°.
Paris, an IX [1801], v. 3.

Nouët. *De l'occlusion intestinale dans ses rapports avec les inflammations péri-utérines chroniques. 1 p. l., 72 pp. 4°. *Paris*, 1874, No. 17.

Nouët (Paul). *Des complications cérébrales
du rhumatisme articulaire aigu traitées par les
bains. 50 pp. 4°. *Paris*, 1875, No. 182.

Nouffert (J.-P.-F.) *De la blennorrhagie. 48
pp. 4°. *Paris*, 1846, No. 17, v. 449.

Nougarède (Louis-Samuel). *Contribution à
l'étude clinique du cancer latent de l'estomac.
63 pp., 2 l. 4°. *Montpellier*, 1882, No. 29.

Nougarède de Fayet (Aug^te). Essai sur les
causes mécaniques de la circulation du sang. 34
pp., 1 l. 8°. *Paris, J.-B. Baillière*, 1843.

Nouguez (Martinus).

See **Adet** (Petrus Augustus). An partium durarum
nutritio, eadem ac mollium? [etc.] 4°. *Parisiis*, 1748.

van Nouhuys (Antonius Henricus). *De usu
corticis Peruviani in morbis hydropicis. 1 p. l.,
42 pp., 3 l. 4°. *Lugd. Bat., apud A. Costerum*,
1782.

Noukha.

Kulassabski (A.) Gorod Nukha, v mediko-topo-
graphicheskom otnoshenii. [The city of Noukha; a
medico-topographical report.] Med. Sbornik, Tiflis, 1871,
no. 11, 15-44.

Noulis (Georges-C.) *Entorse du genou. 56 pp.
4°. *Paris*, 1875, No. 142.

Nouprez (Romanus) [1842–]. *De ægrota-
tione quadam meningitidis cerebrospinalis epidemicæ. 32 pp. sm. 8°. *Berolini, G. Schade*,
[1865].

Nouridjan (Joseph). *De la mortalité des enfants. 48 pp. 4°. *Paris*, 1863, No. 122.

Nourij (Franciscus Gustavus). *Diss. exhibens
historiam botanicam, chemico-pharmaceuticam
et medicam foliorum Diosmæ serratifoliæ (vulgo
foliorum buchu). 1 p. l., 64 pp., 4 l. 8°. *Groningæ, J. Römelingh*, [1827].

Nourney (Adolf). *Experimentelle Beiträge
zur Lehre von der Impfung. 48 pp., 3 ch. 8°.
Strassburg, J. H. E. D. Heitz, 1881.

Nourrie (Ch.) *De la névralgie brachiale
double. 52 pp., 1 l. 4°. *Paris*, 1888, No. 86.

Nourrigat (Auguste). *De l'hémorrhagie utérine qui survient pendant les derniers mois de la
gestation et au moment du travail. 68 pp. 4°.
Montpellier, 1864. [P., v. 48.]

Nourry (Gabriel-Camille). *Sur quelques cas
non signalés d'esthiomène de la vulve (formes
cliniques et anatomo-pathologiques). 54 pp. 4°.
Bordeaux, 1885-6, No. 66.

Nourse (William E. C.) A short and plain history of cholera; its causes and prevention. 16
pp. 8°. *London, J. Churchill*, 1857.

Noury (Charles-Edmond) [1858–]. *De la
peptonurie. 75 pp. 4°. *Paris*, 1884, No. 189.

Noury (M.-J.) *Du perchlorure de fer à l'intérieur à haute dose dans le traitement de la
diphthérie et spécialement de l'angine pseudo-
membraneuse. 40 pp. 4°. *Paris*, 1872, No. 62.

Noury (Marie-François). *Considérations sur le
traitement des fractures du membre inférieur et
en particulier des fractures de la cuisse à bord
des bâtiments de l'État. 49 pp. 4°. *Paris*, 1886,
No. 44.

Nousser (*Madame*).

See **Simmons** (Samuel Foart). An account of a tænia
[etc.] 8°. *London*, 1777.

Nouveau cours de médecine. Ou, selon les
principes de la nature et des mécaniques ex-
pliqués par Messieurs Descartes, Hogelande, Regius, Arberius, Villis, les docteurs de Louvain,
et par d'autres, on apprend le corps de l'homme,
avec les moyens de conserver la santé, et de chas-
ser les maladies. 2 p. l., 728 pp., 4 l. 16°. *Paris, F. Clorzier*, 1669.

Nouveau dictionnaire d'histoire naturelle, appliquée aux arts, à l'agriculture, à l'économie
rurale et domestique, à la médecine, etc. Par
une société de naturalistes et d'agriculteurs.
Nouv. éd. 36 v. 8°. *Paris, Deterville*, 1816-19.

Nouveau dictionnaire lexicographique et descriptif des sciences médicales et vétérinaires,
avec planches intercalées dans le texte. Par
Messieurs Raige-Delorme, Ch. Daremberg, H.
Bouley, etc. 1468 pp. 8°. *Paris, P. Asselin*,
1863.

Nouveau dictionnaire de médecine, chirurgie,
pharmacie, physique, chimie, histoire naturelle,
etc. Par A. Béclard, Chomel, H. Cloquet, etc.
2 v. 829, 663 pp. 8°. Suppl., 75 pp. *Paris,
Gabon & Cie.*, 1826.

Nouveau dictionnaire de médecine et de chirurgie pratique. Rédigé par Anger, Bailly [et al.].

Nouveau dictionnaire [etc.]—continued.
Directeur de la rédaction, le Docteur Jaccoud.
v. 1–40, A–Zym & Suppl. 8°. *Paris*, 1864–86.

Nouveau dictionnaire pratique de médecine, de
chirurgie et d'hygiène vétérinaires, publié avec
la collaboration d'une société de professeurs vétérinaires praticiens, par H. Bouley et Reynal.
v. 1–13 [A–Myx]. 8°. *Paris, Labe & P. Asselin*,
1885.

Nouveau formulaire de thérapeutique publié
sous la direction du Dr. Lutaud, avec la collaboration de MM. Gallard [*et al.*], précédé de commentaires sur la nouvelle édition du codex et
suivi d'un vade-mecum des injections hypodermiques et d'un mémorial thérapeutique. 2. éd.
3 p. l., 262 pp. 18°. *Paris*, 1884.

Nouveau journal de médecine, chirurgie, pharmacie, etc. Rédigé par MM. Béclard, Chomel,
H. Cloquet [*et al.*]. [Monthly; 3 v. annually.]
v. 1–15, Jan., 1818, to Dec., 1822. 8°. *Paris*.
Completed. A continuation of: **Journal** de médecine, chirurgie, pharmacie, etc., Paris, 1801–17.

Nouveau (Le) journal médical. Revue hebdomadaire, médicale et scientifique. Rédacteur en
chef: L. Girard. Années 1–2, May 1, 1880, to
March 26, 1881. 4°. *Paris*.
Continued as: **Siècle** (Le) médical.

Nouveau manuel complet des aspirans au doc-
torat en médecine, ou résumé analytique de toutes
les connaissances nécessaires aux élèves pour
subir les cinq examens exigés par les facultés de
médecine, par des professeurs agrégés et des docteurs de la faculté de Paris, et publié sous la direction de P. Vavasseur. xxxvi, 626 pp. 12°.
Paris, Crochard, 1833.

——. The same. 2. ed. 697 pp. 12°. *Paris,
Crochard & Cie.*, 1837.

Nouveau mémoire sur l'emploi des dragées ferrugineuses de Gélis et Conté. 16 pp. 8°. *Paris,
Labélonye*, [1848, *vel subseq.*]. [P., v. 460.]

Nouveau projet de réorganisation de la médecine, de la chirurgie et de la pharmacie en France
par F[ournier] de P[escay]. 98 pp. 8°. *Paris,
Méquignon-Marvis*, 1817.

Nouveau système. Le grand diviseur 317, rue
Saint-Honoré, 317. De la construction des fosses d'aisances, du mode de séparation des matières solides et liquides, de la conversion des
matières fécales en engrais, et de la nécessité
dans l'intérêt de l'hygiène publique et de l'agriculture d'assainir les abattoirs, les chantiers
d'équarrissage, de recueillir les urines dans les
campagnes, et de faire servir le sang, les viandes,
les détritus de poissons, à l'amélioration du sol,
par les procédés A. Chevallier et A. Dugléré,
avec notices et document par M. E. Vincent,
auteur d'un mémoire intitulé: "Recherches historiques sur la construction des fosses d'aisances
et l'utilisation des matières". Couronné par la
Société d'encouragement pour l'industrie nationale (1847). 24 pp., 1 pl. 8°. *Paris, Vial*, 1855.
[P., v. 1791.]

Nouveau système de mouture pour le maïs in-
venté par M. F.-J. Betz-Penot. 83 pp., 1 pl. 8°.
Paris, imp. de Mme. Vve. Bouchard-Huzard, 1856.
[P. v. 1783; 1786.]

Nouveau système de transport de malades et
blessés. 8 pp. 8°. [*Heidelberg? J. Russel*],
1842.

Nouveaux (Les) remèdes. Journal bi-mensuel
de chimie médicale, de pharmacologie, de thérapeutique et d'hydrologie. Rédigé par G. Bardet
[*et al.*]. v. 1–4, April 1, 1885–8. 8°. *Paris*.
Current. v. 1 complete in 18 nos., April to Dec., 1885;
v. 2 commenced Jan., 1886.

Nouveaux renseignements sur l'emploi alimentaire de la gélatine. 10 pp. 8°. [*Paris, Mme.
de Lacombe, n. d.*] [P., v. 1633.]

65

Nouveau-né (Le). Conseiller intime de la
mère dans les soins à donner à l'enfant, de la
naissance à un an. Guide mensuel. Par Oscar
Comettant. Années 1–6, 1881–6. 8°. *Paris*.

Nouvelle bibliothèque médicale, [etc.] *See*
Bibliothèque médicale, *Paris*, 1823–9.

Nouvelle biographie générale depuis les temps
les plus reculés jusqu'à nos jours, avec les renseignements bibliographiques et l'indication des
sources à consulter; publiée par MM. Firmin
Didot frères, sous la direction de M. le Dr. Hoefer.
46 v. 8°. *Paris, Firmin Didot frères*, 1852–83.
v. 1, title: Nouvelle biographie universelle.

Nouvelle encyclographie des sciences médicales.
See **Encyclographie** des sciences médicales,
1846–54.

Nouvelle iconographie de la Salpêtrière. Clinique des maladies du système nerveux. Publiée
sous la direction du professeur Charcot par Paul
Richer, Gilles de la Tourette, Albert Londe.
[Semi-monthly.] Nos. 1–2, v. 1, Jan. to April,
1888. 8°. *Paris, A. Delahaye & E. Lecrosnier*.
Current.

Nouvelle méthode d'extraire la pierre de la
vessie urinaire par dessus le pubis, etc. *See*
[**Baseilhac** (Jean).]

Nouvelle méthode d'opérations de chirurgie,
[etc.] *See* **Verduc** (J.-B.)

Nouvelle table des articles contenus dans les
volumes de l'Académie royale des sciences de
Paris, depuis 1666 jusqu'en 1770. Dans ceux
des arts et métiers publiés par cette académie
et dans la collection académique par M. l'Abbé
Rozier. 4 v. 4°. *Paris*, 1775–6.
See, also **Collection** académique. 13 v. 4°. *Dijon
& Paris*, 1755–79. — **Recueil** de mémoires. 16 v. 4°.
Paris, 1754–87.

Nouvelles archives d'obstétrique et de gynécologie. Rédacteur en chef: Doléris. [Month-
ly.] v. 1–3, 1886–8. 8°. *Paris*.
Current. Has supplement: **Répertoire** universel
d'obstétrique et de gynécologie.

Nouvelles instructives, bibliographiques, historiques et critiques de médecine, chirurgie et
pharmacie, pour l'année 1787; ou recuel raisonné
de tout ce qu'il importe d'apprendre pour être
au courant des connoissances et à l'abri des
erreurs, relatives à l'art de guérir. Par M. Retz.
Tome 3, 1787. 1 v. 558 pp. 16°. *Paris,
Méquignon*.
Continued, in 1789, as: **Nouvelles**, ou annales de l'art
de guérir.
—— *See, also:*
Sue (P.) Examen d'un ouvrage intitulé:
Nouvelles instructives, bibliographiques, historiques et critiques de médecine, chirurgie et
pharmacie, etc. 8°. *Genève*, 1786.

Nouvelliste (Le) médical, gazette de tous les
journaux de médecine et de sciences accessoires.
[Weekly.] Nos. 1–3, 8–9, 12, 24, 36–53, Jan. 5,
1833, to Jan. 4, 1834. fol. *Paris, Garnier*.

Nova disquisitio de Helia artista.
In: **Theatrum** chemicum. 12°. *Argentorati*, 1659, iv,
214–246.

Nova pharmacopœorum taxa, seu ordo ac pretium
omnium medicamentorum, tam simplicium quam
compositorum, chymicorum, atque Galenicorum,
moderno tempore in officinis publicis pharmaceuticis Viennensibus in Austria magis usualium,
juxta normam dispensatorii pharmaceutici Austriaco-Viennensis formata ac præparata, et ex
... regio mandato in publici et ærarii emolumentum tradita et publicata. 4 p. l., 72 pp.,
1 l. fol. *Viennæ Austriæ, G. Kurtzbök*, 1744.
Latin and German text.
Bound with: **Dispensatorium** pharmaceuticum, etc.
fol. *Viennæ Austriæ*, 1729, 2. ed., 1744.

Novæ Academiæ Florentinæ opuscula. Adversus Avicennam, et medicos neotericos, qui Galeni

Novæ Academiæ Florentinæ [etc.]—continued. disciplina neglecta, barbaros colunt. 16°. *Lugduni, apud S. Gryphium,* 1534.
Imperfect; wants all after p. 130.

Novæ regulæ sanitatis medico-physicæ, sive disputationes inaugurales de esculentis et poculentis, ad usum mundi moderni: Quas præside Dn. Hilario Fresbauch, pro consequenda in omni Scibili laurea contra melancolicos et hypocondriacos, suffumabit per tabacum, [etc.] 12 l. sm. 4°. *Gratianopoli,* 1657.

de Novaes (Clementino Ribeiro). *Qual ó melhor tratamento da febre amarella. 28 pp., 3 l. 4°. *Bahia, typ. C. R. da Rocha,* 1871.

de Novaes Mello (Manoel Leite). *Fractura do radius e seu tratamento. 20 pp., 1 l. 4°. *Bahia, J. G. Tourinho,* 1872.

Novag (Lorenz). Grundsätze der physischen Erziehung des Menschen. 2. Aufl. 274 pp. 8°. *Wien, J. B. Wallishausser,* 1842.

Novák (Emericus). *De dysenteria. 30 pp. 8°. *Budæ, typ. Reg. Univ. Hung.,* 1829. [*Also, in:* P., v. 1327.]

Novák (Josephus)[1]. *De febre intermittente exanthematica. 4 p. l., 64 pp., 3 l. 12°. *Budæ, typ. C. Landerer riduæ,* [1783].

Novák (Josephus)[2]. De convalescentia. 38 pp., 1 l. 8°. *Pestini, typ. Landererianis,* [1832]. [*Also, in:* P., v. 1320.]

Novák (Josephus Stephanus). *De amaurosi ejusque speciebus et varietatibus. 55 pp. 8°. *Pestini, J. T. Trattner,* 1816. [P., v. 1304.]

Novák (Paulus Ferdinandus). *De diæta ægrorum alimentaria. 30 pp. 8°. *Budæ, typ. Regiæ Universitatis Hungaricæ,* 1819. [P., v. 1307.]

Novara. Regolamento di polizia urbana e d'igiene pubblica pel comune di Novara. 24 pp. 8°. *Novara, tip. di G. Miglio,* 1868.

Novara (*Province of*). Manicomio provinciale di Novara. Tavole medico-statistiche degli anni 1880; 1881; 1885. [Per Dott. Todi (Giovanni).] Pubblicazioni fatte per cura dell' amministrazione. 4°. *Novara,* 1881–6.

Novara.
See **Fever** (*Typhus, History, etc., of*), **Hospitals** (*Descriptions, etc., of*), **Medicine** (*Clinical, Statistical, etc.*), *by localities.*

Novara (*Voyage of*).
REISE der österreichischen Fregatte Novara um die Erde in den Jahren 1857, 1858, 1859. Unter den Befehlen des Commodore B. von Wüllerstorf-Urbair. 16 v. 4°. *Wien,* 1861–75.

Novarinus (Antonius). Anatomia curiosa. Das ist, dess aller fürtrefflichsten, höchsten und edelsten Geschöpfs aller Creaturen, dess Menschen, welchen Gott der Höchste so hoch gewürdiget, dass er ihn gar zu seinem Göttlichen Ebenbild erschaffen hatte. Wahrhafftige Beschreibung, und vortreffliche Vorstellung, darinnen nachsinnlich von dess Menschen wunderbarlich- und hoch verwunderlichen Ursprung, dessen nie genug vom menschlichem Verstand bemerckten Empfängnus, von dessen überartigen Vortwachs in dem mutterlichen Leib, und folgend-hochgefährlich und schmertzhafften Geburth, ferner von allen eüserlich- und innern Glidern, auss welchen der überauss künstliche Leib zusammen verfüget und gesetzet ist . . . Allen denjenigen, so die unergründliche Wunderwerck Gottes und der Natur Würckung zu Lob und Ehr dess Grossen Schöpffers, vornemblich aber allen der Edlen Anatomi Beflissenen zum Nutz hervor gegeben, und an das öffentliche Tageslicht geleget. 1. u. 2. Theil. 109 pp., 1 l., 12 pl.; 103 pp., 19 pl., 1 phantom pl. fol. *Rotenburg, N. von Millerau,* 1682.

Novaro (Giacomo Filippo). Dell' estirpazione della laringe. 102 pp., 1 l., 1 pl. 8°. *Torino & Roma, E. Loescher,* 1880.

———. Clinica chirurgica di Siena. Rendiconto dal gennaio al luglio 1886. Redatto dall' aiuto Dott. Vittorio Remedi. 266 pp., 1 l. 8°. *Siena, L. Lazzeri,* 1887.

Nova Scotia. An act relating to lunatics and to the custody and estates of lunatics. [Also, the Hospital for the Insane.] Passed April 18, 1872. 15 pp. 8°. [*Halifax,* 1872.]

———. Census of . . . taken March 30, 1861, under act of Provincial Parliament. 27,298 pp., 1 l. fol. *Halifax, N. S., E. M. McDonald,* 1862.
With second title: Report of the secretary of the board of statistics, with appendices.

Nova Scotia.
See, also, **Halifax.**
Féris (B.) Écosse (Nouvelle-) ou Acadie. Dict. encycl. d. sc. méd., Par., 1885, xxxii, 449–454. — **Forsyth** (J. E.) Remarks on diseases in Nova Scotia. Lancet, Lond., 1848, i, 364. — **Nova Scotia** in its sanitary aspect as a military and naval station. Lancet, Lond., 1862, i, 469.

Nova Scotia. *Nova Scotia Hospital for the Insane, Halifax.* Annual reports of the medical superintendent to the commissioner of public works and mines. 1.–26., 1858–83. 8°. *Halifax,* 1859–84.
Corner-stone laid June 8, 1856. Opened May 17, 1857, under title: Provincial Hospital for the Insane. Adopted present title in 1872, by act of the council and assembly. 1., 3.–11., bound in 1 v. 2. report not published.

———. Acts, by-laws, rules, regulations, and general orders. 24 pp. 8°. *Halifax, N. S., C. Annard,* 1869.
Bound with: Reports, 1858–68.

Novati (Girolamo).
See **Moreau de Jonnès** (Alexandre). Intorno al cholera-morbus pestilenziale, [etc.] 8°. *Milano,* 1831.
For Biography, see Gazz. med. ital. lomb., Milano, 1853, 3. s., iv, 311–312 (E. Bonetti).

Novedades científicas. Contiene todos los descubrimientos hechos en física, química e historia natural, y sus aplicaciones á la medicina, la farmacia, la agricultura y la industria. Redactado por Luis María Utor, [*et al.*]. [Semi-monthly.] v. 1, April 15 to Dec. 30, 1880. 520 pp. 8°. *Madrid.*

Novelda.
Genoves y Tio (J.) Descripcion del establecimiento de aguas minerales sulfuradas, salinas frias, de salinetas de Novelda, en la provincia de Alicante. Sigle méd., Madrid, 1874, xxi, 436; 456.—**Lopez** (J. F.) Del manantial sulfuroso de las salinetas de Novelda. en la provincia de Alicante. Bol. de med., cirug. y farm., Madrid, 1851, 2. ép., i, 156.

Novell (Carolus). *De osteosteatomate. 1 p. l., 38 pp. 4°. *Upsaliæ, J. Edman,* [1780].

Novenianus (Philippus). Eyn schone Verordnung von den, der Pestilentz, Ursachen, Zceychen, Erczneyen, mit sampt eynem nützlichen Regiment. 58 l. 12°. *Leyptzigk, V. Schumann,* 1529.

Novenianus (Philippus Michel). Von den bösen umbflechtenden Bauchflüssen und Durchlauff, Ursprung, Ursachen und Erkentnis, und wie die zu curirn und zu vertreiben, aus Grund der Ertzney. 3 p. l., 23 pp. 4°. *Wittemberg, H. Lufft,* 1558.

Noverre (Georges-Pierre). *Sur les anévrismes de l'aorte. 51 pp. 4°. *Paris,* 1820, No. 13, v. 154.

———. The same. 67 pp. 8°. *Paris, J.-B. Baillière,* 1820.

Novgorod.
Bardowsky (A.) Medicinisch-topographische Skizze des Nowgorodschen Gouvernements. Med. Ztg. Russlands, St. Petersb., 1850, vii, 153; 161; 169; 177.

Novi (Raffaele). La sinfisiotomia rifugiata presso la Scuola napolitana. 39 pp. 8°. *Napoli, G. de Angelis & figlio,* 1881.

Novi tractatus de potu caphé; de chinensium thé; et de chocolata. 2 p. l., 188 pp., 4 pl. 8°. *Genevæ, Cramer et Perachon, 1699.*

Novi-Chavarria (Salvadore). Trattato sulle oftalmo-nevrosi, ovvero descrizione delle malattie nervose dell' organo della vista. 348 pp., 2 l. 8°. *Napoli, R. Ghio, 1858.*

Novinski (M.) * K voprosu o privivanii zlokachestvennich novoobrazovanii. [On the inoculation of cancerous diseases in animals.] 36 pp., 1 pl., 1 l. 8°. *St. Petersburg, 1877.*

Novion (Lucien-Joseph). * Quelques propositions de médecine et de chirurgie. 28 pp. 4°. *Paris, 1837, No. 21, v. 306.*

Novitski (Alexander). * O phiziologicheskom dieistvii nitroglitserina. 72 pp. 8°. *St. Petersburg, 1864.*

Novitski (Michael). * O fiziolog. dieistvii delfinina. 47 pp. 8°. *Cronstadt, V. Kerr, 1863.*

Novo (De) antidysenterico Americano magnis successibus comprobato. 38 pp. 16°. *Francof. et Lipsiæ, sumt. G. Freytagii, 1696.*
    In: LISTER (M.) Sex exercitationes medicinales [etc.] 16°. *Francof. et Lipsiæ, 1696.* [Separate pagination.]

Novogrigorovski.
See **Cholera** (*Asiatic, History, etc., of*), *by localities.*

Novosti terapii. Ejemiesjachnii journal. v. 1–2, 1886–7. 8°. *Moskva.*

Novosti veterinarnoe literaturi otchestvennoi i inostrannoi. Vichodjat ejemiesjachno pod red. A. I. Alexiev. [News of veterinary literature, domestic and foreign. Monthly.] v. 2, 1885. 8°. *St. Petersburg.*
    Each number paged separately.

Novotny (Franciscus Sal.) * De toxicationibus. 18 pp., 1 l. 8°. *Vindobonæ, J. B. Wallishausser,* [1837].

Novum lumen medicum theoretico practicum, exhibens observationes et curationes medicas raras et curiosas, arcanis, euporistis aliisque notis proficuis modernæ praxi congruis, nec non scholiis utilissimis illustratas, ex Mss. felicissimi cujusdam et celeberrimi quondam practici erutas. 1236 pp., 12 l. 4°. *Rudolphopoli, J. M. Gollner, 1707.*

Nowack (Josephus). * De punctione abdominis ejusque tumorum, casu quodam adjecto. 24 pp., 1 l. 8°. *Vratislaviæ, typ. A. Neumanni, 1866.*

Nowak (A.) Notizen über die Prager k. k. Irrenanstalt und die Veränderungen in derselben seit dem Jahre 1830, nebst zwei Uebersichtstabellen und einigen Krankheitsgeschichten. 2 p. l., 79 pp. 8°. *Prag, G. Haase Söhne, 1835.*

Nowák (Franciscus L.) * Diss. sistens analogias morborum oculi et aliorum organorum. 21 pp. 8°. *Pragæ, J. Spurny,* [1837].

Nowak (Josef). Zur Frage der Leichenverbrennung. 16 pp., 1 pl. 8°. [*Wien*], C. L. Prætorius, [1874].

——. Die Infections-Krankheiten vom ätiologischen und hygienischen Standpunkte. Systematische Zusammenstellung der wichtigsten Forschungs-Ergebnisse auf dem Gebiete der gegenwärtigen Infectionslehre. iv (1 l.), 142 pp., 1 pl. 8°. *Wien, Töplitz u. Deuticke, 1882.*

——. Lehrbuch der Hygiene. Systematische Zusammenstellung der wichtigsten hygienischen Lehrsätze und Untersuchungs-Methoden. Lfg. 1–9. xvi, 1043 pp. 8°. *Wien, Töplitz u. Deuticke, 1883.*

Nowák (Wenceslaus). * De peliosi Werlhofii præmissa historia morbi synoptica. 31 pp. 8°. *Pragæ Cechorum, J. vid. Vetterl,* [1836].

Nowakowski (*Janusz Ferdynand*) [1832–83].
    Przystański (H.) [Obituary.] Pam. Towarz. Lek. Warszaw., 1884, lxxx, 171–175.

Nowell *vs.* Williams.
See **Insanity** (*Jurisprudence of, Cases, etc., relating to*).

Nowgong.
See **Cholera** (*Asiatic, History, etc., of*), *by localities.*

Nowlin (J. B. W.) A case of ovariotomy. 8 pp. 8°. [*Nashville*, 1886.]
    Repr. from: South. Pract., Nashville, 1886.

Noxa (De) e nimis præcipitato medicinæ studio oriunda. Ad memoriam Kregelio-Sternbachianam. xv pp. 4°. [*Lipsiæ, ex off. Klaubarthia,* 1792.]

Noxis (De) ex nimia mentis contentione. [In] memoriam Bestuchefianam. xii pp. 4°. [*Lipsiæ, ex off. Klaubarthia,* 1786.]

Noxis (De) e nimium properata ædium recens exstructarum habitatione in sanitatem redundantibus. [In] memoriam Jo. Hen. Lud. de Bestucheff-Rumin e gente Carlovizia. 11 pp. 4°. [*Lipsiæ,* 1830.]

Noxon (*Peter B.*) [1796–1882].
    Curtis (F. C.) Biography. Med. Ann., Albany, 1882, iii, [Tr. M. Soc. County Albany, 368].

Noy (Theodorus) [1840–   ]. * De carcinomate bulbi. 32 pp. 8°. *Berolini, G. Lange,* [1863].

Noyer (J.-B.-Félix). * Sur le mélœna. 23 pp. 4°. *Paris, 1816, No. 94, v. 122.*

Noyer (Victor). * Sur le mode d'action des eaux minérales de Vichy, département de l'Allier. 14 pp. 4°. *Strasbourg, 1832, v. 63.*

——. Guide de l'étranger aux eaux minérales de Vichy, suivi de quelques réflexions sur leur propriété dans le traitement de la gravelle et de la goutte. vii, 57 pp. 8°. *Paris, J. Rouvier, 1836.*

Noyes (*Daniel R.*)
    Portrait in: **Collection** of Portr. (Libr.)

Noyes (Henry D.) Sclerotico-choroiditis posterior, with cases and illustrations. 16 pp. 8°. *New York, T. Holman, 1860.*
    Repr. from: N. York J. M., 1860, viii.

——. Specialties in medicine. 16 pp. 8°. *New York, J. Medole, 1865.*
    Repr. from: Tr. Am. Ophth. Soc., N. Y., 1865, ii.

——. Glaucoma. 13 pp. 8°. *Albany, Weed, Parsons & Co.*, 1869.
    Repr. from: Tr. M. Soc. N. Y., Albany, 1869.

——. Ectropium, exophthalmus, extirpation, plastic operation. 8 pp., 3 pl. 8°. [*n. p.*, 1871.]
    Repr. from: Tr. Am. Ophth. Soc., N. Y., 1871, vii.

——. Report on ophthalmology for 1870. 37 pp. 8°. *New York, D. Appleton & Co.*, 1871.
    Repr. from: N. York M. J., 1871, xiii.

——. Ophthalmoscopic examination of sixty insane patients in the State asylum at Utica. 23 pp. 8°. [*New York*, 1872.]
    Repr. from: Am. J. Insan., Utica, N. Y., 1872, xxviii.

——. Report on ophthalmology for 1871. 21 pp. 8°. *New York, D. Appleton & Co.*, 1872.
    Repr. from: N. York M. J., 1872, xiv.

——. A case of irritation of the chorda tympani. 5 pp. 8°. *Boston, A. Mudge & Son, 1874.* [*Also, in:* P., v. 795.]
    Repr. from: Tr. Am. Otol. Soc., Bost., 1874, vii.

——. Syphilis of the eye. Being chapter viii [pt. 2] of a "Practical treatise on the surgical diseases of the genito-urinary organs, including syphilis", by W. H. Van Buren and E. L. Keyes. 22 pp. 8°. *New York, D. Appleton & Co.*, 1874.

——. Cases of disease in the orbit. 20 pp. 8°. *New York, G. P. Putnam's Sons, 1875.* [*Also, in:* P., v. 1442.]

——. Diagnosis of those diseases of the eye which can be seen without the ophthalmoscope. 61 pp. 8°. *New York, G. P. Putnam's Sons, 1876.*
    No. 5, v. 2, of: Am. Clin. Lect., by Seguin, 1876, 81–141.

Noyes (Henry D.)—continued.

———. Papers presented to the Fifth International Congress of Ophthalmology. On the use of a naso-buccal flap for blepharoplasty, with two cases and illustrations. On additional means for relieving pressure of the eyelids in diseases of the cornea, with an illustration. On the optical error of conical cornea, and report of two cases treated by operation. 25 pp. 8°. *New York, D. Appleton & Co.*, 1877.

———. Ophthalmology in the last quarter century. An address before the Medical Society of the State of New York. 19 pp. 8°. *Syracuse, Truair, Smith & Bruce*, 1879.
Repr. from: Tr. M. Soc. N. Y., Syracuse, 1879.

———. Eye troubles in general practice. 24 pp. 8°. *New York, W. Wood & Co.*, 1879.
Repr. from: Med. Rec., N. Y., 1879, xvi.

———. A treatise [on] diseases of the eye. xii (1 l.), 360 pp., 2 pl. 8°. *New York, W. Wood & Co.*, 1881.

———. On the tests for muscular asthenopia and on insufficiency of the external recti muscles. 44 pp. 8°. *Copenhagen*, [*I. Cohen*], 1884.
Repr. from: Tr. Internat. M. Cong., 8. sess., Copenh., 1884.

Noyes (Isaac Pitman) [1840–]. Hospital construction; suggestion for the combination of the pavilion and corridor plan. 4 pp., 1 l. 8°. *Washington*, 1877.

———. A new view of the weather question. 24 pp. 8°. *Kansas City, Mo., Ramsey, Millett & Hudson*, 1878.
Repr. from: West. Rev. Sc. & Indust., Kansas City, 1878-9, ii.

———. Meteorology. Evidence from the weather maps of the U. S. Signal Service Office. 9 pp. 8°. [*Washington, D. C.*, 1880.]
Repr. from: Kansas City Rev. Sc. & Indust., 1879-80, iii.

———. Tornadoes. Prophecy of the weather. 19 pp. 8°. *Kansas City*, 1880.
Repr. from: Kansas City Rev. Sc. & Indust., 1880-81, iv.

———. Meteorology. The weather map and the official weather indications. 5 pp. 8°. [*Washington*, 1881.]
Repr. from: Kansas City Rev. Sc. & Indust., 1881-2, v.

———. How to be weather-wise. A new view of our weather system. 51 pp. 12°. *New York, Fowler & Wells*, [1882].
Repr. from: Phrenol. J., N. Y., 1882, n. s., xxv.

———. False notions in regard to the weather. 6 pp. 8°. [*n. p.*, 1882.]
Repr. from: Kansas City Rev. Sc. & Indust., 1882-3, vi.

———. Meteorological discoveries. 8 pp. 8°. *Kansas City*, 1884.
Repr. from: Kansas City Rev. Sc. & Indust., 1884-5, viii.

———. More about the red sky (vapor theory). 1 galley sheet. [*New York*, 1885.]
From: Phrenol. J., N. Y., 1885, n. s., xxxi.

———. Local storms. 1 galley sheet. [*New York*, 1885.]
From: Phrenol. J., N. Y., 1885, n. s., xxxii.

———. Electricity and thunder storms. 1 galley sheet. [*Chicago*, 1886.]
From: Chicago J. of Commerce, March, 1886, xlviii.

Noyes (James) [1640–1719].
Biography. *In:* Sibley (J. C.) Biog. sketches, [etc.] 8°. *Cambridge*, 1881, ii, 45-50.

Noyes (John Humphrey). Male continence, or self-control in sexual intercourse. A letter of inquiry answered. 4 pp. 8°. [*Oneida, N. Y.*, 1866.]

———. Essay on scientific propagation. 32 pp. 8°. *Oneida, N. Y.*, [*n. d.*].

Noyes (R. K.) The history of medicine for the last 4000 years. 79 pp. 12°. *Lynn, Mass., Leech & Lewis*, 1880.

Noyes (Robt. F.) Perityphlitis. 47 pp. 8°. *Providence*, 1883.
Repr. from: Tr. Rhode Island M. Soc. 1882, Providence, 1883.

Noyes (T. R.) Report on the health of children in the Oneida Community. 8 pp. 8°. *Oneida, N. Y.*, 1878.

Noyes (William). Composite portrait of eight cases of general paresis (five men and three women). 1 photograph, 4¼ x 6½. *Boston, Notman Co.*, 1887.

———. Composite portrait of eight cases of melancholia (all men). 1 photograph, 4¼ x 6½. *Boston, Notman Co.*, 1887.

Nozeran (Albin). * De l'héméralopie des pays chauds. 34 pp., 1 l. 4°. *Montpellier, De Gras*, 1865, No. 61.
c.

Nozeran (Jean-Baptiste). * Sur la gale. 28 pp. 4°. *Montpellier*, 1833, No. 35. [*P.*, v. 1083.]

Nubia.
See, also, **Egypt.**
Laveran (L.) Nubie. Dict. encycl. d. sc. méd., Par., 1879, 2. s., xiii, 734-747.

Nubians.
Deniker. Quelques observations et mensurations sur les Nubiens qui ont été exposés à Genève en août 1880. Bull. Soc. d'anthrop. de Par., 1880, 3. s., iii, 594-603.

Nubility.
See **Marriage.**

Nublat (Henry). * Considérations sur les ulcérations du col de l'utérus. 32 pp. 4°. *Paris*, 1851, No. 123, v. 512.

Nucha.
See **Cholera** (*Asiatic, History, etc., of*), by localities.

Nuchten (Fridericus) [1815–]. * De crisibus. 29 pp., 1 l. 8°. *Berolini, G. Schade*, [1816].

Nucius (L.) Een schoon tractaet, van alderhande paerden, om te leeren kennen de natuere ende eijgenschap derselver: ende welcke de schoonste, beste, sterckste ende cloeckste zijn . . . Uijt het Italiaensch verduijtscht. Noch een cleijn tractraetjen van veelderley dieren . . . 2 p. l., 87 pp., 1 l. 4°. *Dordrecht, P. Verhaghen*, 1622.

Nuck (Antonius) [1650–1742]. * De rabie hydrophobica. 6 l. 4°. *Lugd. Bat., apud vid. et hæredes J. Elseverii*, 1676.

———. De ductu salivali novo, saliva, ductibus oculorum aquosis, et humore oculi aqueo. Frontispiece, 4 p. l., 175 pp., 8 l., 3 pl. 16°. *Lugd. Bat., P. vander Aa*, 1685.

———. Operationes et experimenta chirurgica, edita per J[ohannis] T[ilingii]. 2 p. l., 170 pp., 3 l. 12°. *Lugd. Bat., C. Boutesteyn*, 1692.
4 pl. wanting.

———. The same. 2 p. l., 170 pp., 3 l., 4 pl. 12°. *Lugd. Bat., C. Boutesteyn*, 1696.

———. The same. Ed. novissima. 170 pp., 3 l., 4 pl. 12°. *Lugd. Bat., S. Luchtmans*, 1733. [*Also, in:* P., v. 1641.]

———. Sialographia et ductuum aquosorum anatome nova. Accedit defensio ductuum aquosorum nec non fons salivalis novus, hactenus non descriptus. 6 p. l., 158 pp., 8 l., 6 tab. 12°. *Lugd. Bat., J. Luchtmans*, 1695.
Frontispiece gives date as 1696.

———. The same. 12 p. l., 158 pp., 8 l., 6 tab. 12°. *Lugd. Bat., S. Luchtmans*, 1723.
Bound with his: Adenographia, etc. 12°. *Lugd. Bat.*, 1723.
Frontispiece gives date 1722.

———. Adenographia curiosa et uteri fœminei anatome nova. Accedit in hac nova editione diss. anat. med. inaug. de motu bilis circulari ejusque morbis M. van Reverhorst. 6 p. l., 152 pp., 13 l., 9 pl.; 64 pp., 2 pl. 12°. *Lugd. Bat., J. Luchtmans*, 1696.
Frontispiece gives date 1697.

Nuck (Antonius)—continued.

——. The same. Adenographia et uteri anatome nova. Editio aliis auctior. 8 p. l., 152 pp., 14 l., 9 pl. 12°. *Lugd. Bat., S. Luchtmans,* 1722.

Title-page wanting.

——. *See, also :*

BASSIUS (H.) Erläuterter Nuck, oder gründliche Anmerkungen über Anton Nucks chirurgische Hand-Griffe und Experimente, worinnen viel neue Inventa und Instrumenta vorgestellet werden, nebst nöthigen Kupfer-Taffeln und Registern wie auch eine Vorrede Friedrich Hoffmanns. 12°. *Halle im Magdeburgischen,* 1728.

Nuck (*Canal of*).

Féré (C.) Persistance du canal du Nuck. Bull. Soc. anat. de Par., 1878, liii, 58. *Also :* Progrès méd., Par., 1878, vi, 323.—**van der Hoeven** (J.) Hydrops canalis Nuckii. Nederl. Tijdschr. v. Geneesk., Amst., 1871, 2. R., vii, Afd. 1, 533.

Nuclei.

See Cells ; Histology.

Nuclein.

Klinkenberg (W.) Ueber die Nucleine. Ztschr. f. physiol. Chem., Strassb., 1882, vi, 566-571.—**Müller** (J. W.) Zur Kenntniss der Nucleine. Vorläufige Mittheilung. Arch. f. d. ges. Physiol., Bonn, 1873-4, viii, 190-194.—**Stutzer.** Ueber das Vorkommen von Nuclein in den Schimmelpilzen und in der Hefe. Ztschr. f. physiol. Chem., Strassb., 1882, vi, 572-574.

Nudow (Henricus) [1752–]. Observationes de natura embryonis humani. 8 pp. 4°. *Lipsiæ, ex off. Langenhemia,* [1774].

——. *Animadversiones de contagio. 35 pp. 4°. *Lipsiæ, ex off. Loeperia,* [1776].

——. *Præmissum est examen partitionis nervorum in sensorios atque motorios. viii pp. 4°. *Lipsiæ, ex off. Loeperia,* [1776].

Also, in : WEIZ (F. A.) Neue Ausz. [etc.] 12°. *Leipz.,* 1777, vi, 21-29.

——. Ueber die Zeichendeutung des menschlichen Auges in Krankheiten. Aus dem Lateinischen übersetzt, nebst einer Vorerinnerung und einigen Zusätzen. 96 pp., 1 l. 12°. *Königsberg, F. Nicolovius,* 1791.

——. Versuch einer Theorie des Schlafs. xvi, 286 pp. 8°. *Königsberg, F. Nicolovius,* 1791.

For Biography, see **Plaz** (Antonius Guilielmus).
For Portrait, see **Collection**—van Kaathoven.

Nuebel (Antonius) [1814–]. *De ætiologia febrium intermittentium. 28 pp., 2 l. 8°. *Berolini, typ. fratrum Schlesinger,* [1844].

Nueckel (Clemens) [1834–]. *De retroflexione uteri. 32 pp. 8°. *Berolini, G. Lange,* [1858].

Nueckel (Joh. Benedict Dan.) *De affectionibus hæreditariis. 23 pp. 4°. *Parisiis,* 1813, No. 62, v. 96.

à Nuenare (Hermannus) & **Riquinus** (Simon). De novo hactenusque Germaniæ inaudito morbo ἱδρωπυρετοῦ hoc est, sudatoria febri, quam vulgo sudorem britannicum vocant, medicæ rei experimentissimi judicium doctissimum, duabus epistolis contentum. *Coloniæ, apud J. Soterem,* 1529.

In : SCRIPT. de sudore angl. (Gruner). 8°. *Jenæ,* 1847, 93-116. *Also, in :* GRATAROLUS (G.) [Collection] Petri de Abano, etc. 8°. [*n. p.,* 1561 ?], ff. 64-87.

Nünninghoff (Julius). *Beobachtungen über Pseudohypertrophia musculorum lipomatosa. 31 pp. 8°. *Würzburg, Becker,* 1878.

Nürnberg.

See Nuremberg.

Nuernberg (Christianus Ludovicus). *De meloplastice. 34 pp., 1 l. 8°. *Halis Sax., typ. Plœtzianis,* [1854].

Nuernberg (Franciscus). *De spondylarthrocace. 30 pp., 1 l. 8°. *Halis Sax., formis Gebauerio-Schwetschkianis,* [1856].

Nürnberg (Werner). *Zur Lehre vom Tetanus idiopathicus. 47 pp. 8°. *Jena, B. Engau,* 1887.

Nürnberger (Christian Friderich) [1744–95]. *De damnis ex lactatione nimium protracta. 32 pp. 4°. *Wittenbergæ, lit. C. C. Dürrii,* [1773].

——. Observationes anatomico-physiologicæ super glandulis conglobatis. xvi pp. 4°. [*Vittebergæ, lit. C. C. Dürrii,* 1780.]

Also [Abstr.], *in :* WEIZ (F. A.) Neue Ausz. [etc.] 12°. *Frankf. u. Leipz.,* 1781, xiii, 1-8.

——. [Pr.] de sympathia œconomiæ animalis. xxvi pp. 4°. *Vittebergæ, lit. C. C. Dürrii,* [1782].

——. [Pr.] de chirurgia recentiorum absolutam vulnerum lethalitatem capitis præcipue non infringente. [Cum vita candidati Gottlob Christiani Francke.] xvi pp. 4°. [*Vittebergæ, lit. C. C. Dürrii,* 1784.]

——. [Pr.] de organorum et actionum sexus in œconomia animali et vegetabili analogia. [Cum vita candidati Christiani Gottlieb Uhlich.] xvi pp. 4°. [*Vittebergæ, lit. C. C. Dürrii,* 1784.]

——. [Pr.] de liquore gastrico et enterico, eorumque organo secretorio singulari. [Cum vita candidati Joannis Pauli Diersch.] 16 pp. 4°. [*Wittebergæ,* 1785.]

[——.] [Meletemata super digitorum unguibus.] 16 pp. 4°. *Wittebergæ, lit. A. C. Charisii,* [1786].

——. [Pr.] de unguium et pilorum sorte post fata. I. [Cum vita candidati Christophori Henrici Danz.] 12 pp. 4°. [*Wittebergæ,* 1787.]

——. The same. II. [Cum vita candidati Caroli Ferdinandi Mauritii Werner.] 12 pp. 4°. [*Vittebergæ, excud. Charisius,* 1787.]

——. [Pr.] de vita fœtuum excludendorum per manum obstetricantem ex ossium fractura non periclitante. [Cum vita candidati Caroli Augusti Friderici Wolf.] 16 pp. 4°. [*Vittebergæ, excud. A. C. Charisius,* 1788.]

——. [Pr.] de apoplexia causarum morbificarum criteria illustrante et confirmante. Sect. ii, pars i. [Cum vita candidati G. Eybeschitz.] 16 pp. 4°. [*Vittebergæ, excud. A. C. Charisius,* 1790.]

——. The same. Sect. ii, pars ii. [Cum vita candidati G. B. Felix.] 16 pp. 4°. [*Vittebergæ, J. Tzschiedrich,* 1790.]

——. The same. Sect. ii, pars iii. [Cum vita candidati Johannis Friderici Siegismundi Posewit.] 12 pp. 4°. [*Vittebergæ,* 1790.]

——. [Pr.] causarum morbificarum criteria. Pars i. [Cum vita candidati Caroli Gottfriedi Bauernstein.] xiii pp., 1 l. 4°. [*Vittebergæ, lit. C. C. Dürrii,* 1790.]

——. The same. Pars ii. [Cum vita candidati G. A. Schumann.] 12 pp. 4°. [*Vittebergæ, excud. Charisius,* 1790.]

——. [Pr.] præmissa epicrisi remediorum in herniarum incarcerationibus commendatorum. Sect. i. [Cum vita candidati Immanuelis Vertraugott Rothe.] xvi pp. 4°. [*Vittebergæ,* 1792.]

——. The same. Sect. ii. [Cum vita candidati Gottlob Henrici Goetzloff.] xii pp. 4°. [*Vittebergæ,* 1792.]

——. The same. Sect. iii. [Cum vita candidati Augusti Herrich.] 16 pp. 4°. [*Vittebergæ, in off. A. C. Charisi,* 1794.]

——. The same. Comment. iv. [Cum vita candidati Augusti Benjamin Christoph.] x pp. 4°. [*Vittebergæ, lit. C. C. Dürrii,* 1794.]

——. The same. Comment. v. [Cum vita candidati Joannis Samueli Caroli Erler.] xii pp. 4°. [*Vittebergensi,* 1794.]

——. [Pr.] præmissa triga observationum anatomicarum necessariam et per utilem incarcerationum distinctionem confirmantium. [Cum vita candidati Christiani Henrici Lebrecht Segnitz.] xvi pp. 4°. [*Vittebergæ,* 1792.]

Nürnberger (Christian Friderich)—continued.
——. [Pr.] de nævis quibusdam politiæ medicæ academiis plerumque adhærentibus. [Cum vita candidati Ernesti Friderici Graun.] 12 pp. 4°. [*Vittebergæ, lit. C. C. Dürrii*, 1794.]
——. The same. [Cum vita candidati Car. Frid. Tempel.] 12 pp. 4°. [*Vittebergæ, lit. C. C. Dürrii*, 1794.]
   For Biography, see **Boehmer** (Geo. Rudol.) *Also:* **Titius** (S. C.)

Nuernberger (Gustav Friedrich) [1842–]. *Die Zuckerharnruhr. 32 pp. sm. 8°. *Berlin, G. Lange*, [1867].

Nuernberger (Woldemarus) [1820–]. * De vulneribus in pectus et abdomen penetrantibus. 27 pp., 2 l. 8°. *Berolini, typ. fratrum Schlesinger*, [1843].

Nürnberger medicinische Gesellschaft und Policlinik. Statuten. 12 pp. 8°. *Nürnberg, T. Hösstein*, [1881].
——. Jahresberichte. 1.-6., 1879–84. 8°. *Nürnberg, L. Jegel*, 1881-5.

Nüesch (J.) Die Nekrobiose in morphologischer Beziehung betrachtet. 1 p. l., 49 pp. 8°. *Schaffhausen, C. Baader*, 1875.

Nuescheler (Adolf). * Die pathologischen Veränderungen im Gelenkknorpel. 31 pp. 8°. *Zürich, F. Walder, Vater u. Sohn*, 1854.

Nuesperlin (Daniel Victor). *Arteriologiæ recte concinnandæ leges cum specimine arteriæ carotidis externæ exhibens. 41 pp. 4°. *Helmstadii, lit. J. Drimbornii*, [1764].

van Nüss (Joh.) * Beitrag zur Entstehung der Carcinome aus chronisch-entzündlichen Zuständen der Hautdecken. [Wurtzburg.] 16 pp. 8°. *Emmerich, J. L. Romen*, 1886.

Nuesse (Henr. Ferdinandus) [1792–]. * De mammalium dentibus. 40 pp., 2 l. 8°. *Berolini, typ. Nietackianis*, [1835].

Nuessler (Anton). * Fragmente über Entblössung der Schädelknochen, comminutiv Brüche und Caries. 30 pp. 8°. *München, M. Poessenbacher*, [n. d.]

Nüssler (Joh. Gottlob). * De dolore colico. 24 pp. 4°. *Traj. ad Rhenum, F. Halma*, 1688.

Nuessli (Friedr.) * Die Resultate der Kaltwasserbehandlung des Typhus abdominalis im Basler Spitale im Jahre 1869. 25 pp. 8°. *Basel, F. Riehm*, 1871.

Nuetten (Carolus Chrysanthus) [1808–]. *Nonnulla de psoïtide puerperarum, adnexis morbi historiis. 29 pp., 1 l. 8°. *Berolini, typ. Nietackianis*, [1832].

Nützlich- und heilsamer Rathschlag von Lenden-Steine, darinnen kürtzlich, doch deutlich angezeiget wird, was der Lendenstein sey, woraus solcher erwachse, und wie man ihn recht erkennen, auch glücklich vertreiben soll, alles aus bewährten autoribus, nicht nur allein mit gemeinen, sondern auch mit kräftigen Mitteln, und besondern guten Wassern von grundaus könne curiret werden durch M. P. S. F. D. P. 11 p. l., 272 pp. 12°. *Graetz, M. Nolcker*, 1701.

Nützliche und curiöse Fragen. *See* **von Hornick** (Ludwig).

Nützlichen (Mit) Nachrichten und Anmerkung erläuterte Beschreibung seiner im Jahr 1751, in das Kayser-Carls-Bad gethanen Reise. *See* **G[rundig]** (C.)

Nueva-Belen.
   See **Insane** (*Asylums for, etc.*), *by localities— Barcelona.*

Nuevo formulario médico-quirúrgico de los hospitales generales y demás establecimientos de beneficencia de Madrid ; corregido y considerablemente aumentado ; segunda edicion. 380 pp.; 1 l., 1 tab. 12°. *Madrid, D. E. Aguado*, 1853.

Nuevos elementos de cirujía y medicina, por algunos doctores en ambas ciencias. 2 v. vi, 9-649 pp., 1 l. ; vi, 7-652 pp., 1 l. 12°. *Madrid, P. Madoz & L. Sagasti*, 1846.

Nuezel (Joannes). * De aceto. 36 pp. 4°. *Erlangæ, typ. vid. J. F. Beckeri*, [1748].

van Nuffel (Johannes Cornelius). *De laryngo tracheitide. 24 pp. 4°. *Gandavi, M. A. Mahne*, [1828]. [P., v. 959.]

Nugæ canoræ ; or, epitaphian mementos [etc.] *See* "**Unus Quorum** ".

Nugent (Christopher) [–1775]. An essay on the hydrophobia. To which is prefixed the case of a person who was bit by a mad dog; had the hydrophobia, and was happily cured. vii, 204 pp. 8°. *London, J. Leake & W. Frederic*, 1753.

Nugent (Eduardus). * De febre nervosa. 36 pp. 8°. *Edinburgi, Balfour et Smellie*, 1780.

Nugent (Gulielmus). * De rheumatismo acuto. 17 pp. 8°. *Edinburgi, P. Neill*, 1823.

Nugent (Nicolas). * Disp. quædam cœlo fervido propria complectens. 34 pp. 8°. *Edinburgi, excud. A. Neill et socii*, 1804. [P., v. 30.]

Nugent (*Washington G.*) [1822–77].
   Underwood (G.) Memoir of W. G. Nugent. Tr. M. Soc. Penn., Phila., 1877, xi, pt. 2, 624-626.

Nuglisch (Joannes Æmilius) [1823–]. * De partu arte præmaturo. 30 pp., 1 l. 8°. *Berolini, typ. fratrum Schlesinger*, [1848].

Nuguet (E.) * Du traitement des fractures de l'extrémité inférieure du radius vicieusement consolidées. 66 pp., 3 pl. 4°. *Lyon*, 1885, 1. s., No. 305.
——. The same. 66 pp., 2 pl. 8°. *Lyon*, 1885.

Nuhn (Antonius) [1814–]. * Commentatio de vitiis, quæ surdomutitati subesse solent. 2 p. l., 20 pp., 2 pl. fol. *Heidelbergæ, C. Groos*, 1841.
——. Handbuch der chirurgischen Anatomie, zum Gebrauche bei Vorlesungen und zum Selbstunterrichte. xxx, 598 pp. 8°. *Mannheim, F. Bassermann*, 1843-5.
   With second title-page: Handbuch der speziellen chirurgischen Anatomie . . . 1. Bd. Enthaltend die chirurgische Anatomie des Kopfes. All published.
——. Ueber eine bis jetzt noch nicht näher beschriebene Drüse im Innern der Zungenspitze. 8 pp., 4 pl., 1 l. 8°. *Mannheim, F. Bassermann*, 1845.
——. Beobachtungen und Untersuchungen aus dem Gebiete der Anatomie, Physiologie und practischen Medicin. 1. Hft. iv, 30 pp., 7 pl. fol. *Heidelberg, J. C. B. Mohr*, 1849.
——. Erklärungen der chirurgisch-anatomischen Tafeln. Neue Aufl. viii, 271, 336 pp. 4°. *Heidelberg, F. Bassermann*, 1868.
   In 3 Abth.: 1. Der Kopf; 2. Der Rumpf; 3. Die Glieder. Each Abth. has separate title-page. The 1. and 2. have also separate pagination.
——. Chirurgisch-anatomische Tafeln. Nach der Natur gezeichnet und lithographirt von Franz X. Wagner. 60 pl. fol. *Heidelberg, F. Bassermann*, [1868].
——. Lehrbuch der vergleichenden Anatomie. xxxii, 288+ pp. 8°. *Heidelberg*, 1875.
   1. Theil. Vegetative Organe und Apparate des Thierkörpers.
——. The same. In zwei Theilen. I. Vegetative Organe und Apparate des Thierkörpers. II. Animale Organe und Apparate des Thierkörpers. xxxii, 676 pp. 8°. *Heidelberg, C. Winter*, 1878.
——. The same. 2. Ausg. xxxii, 700 pp. 8°. *Heidelberg, C. Winter*, 1886.
——. Lehrbuch der practischen Anatomie als Anleitung zu dem Präpariren im Secirsale. xvi, 408 pp., 1 l. 8°. *Stuttgart, F. von Enke*, 1882.

Nuijens (W. J. F.) Het ontwerp van wet op de uitoefening der genees-, heel- en verloskunde in ons vaderland. 30 pp. 8°. *Amsterdam, C. L. van Langenhuysen*, 1862.

Nuisance (The) of street music, or a plea for the sick, the sensitive, and the studious, by a London physician. 11 pp. 12°. *London, H. Renshaw,* 1869. [*P.*, v. 497.]

Nuisance *inspector.*
See **Hygiene** (*Public, Laws, etc., of*).

Nuisances.
See, also, **Alkali** *works* ; **Bone-boiling** ; **Effluvia** ; **Factories** ; **Fat-boiling**, *etc.* ; **Gas** (*Illuminating, etc.*); **Gases** (*Irrespirable, etc.*) ; **Horse-knackers** ; **Hospitals** *for contagious diseases* ; **Noise** ; **Occupations** (*Dangerous, etc.*) ; **Occupations**, *etc.* (*Diseases, etc., of*) ; **Offal**, *etc.* (*Disposal of*) ; **Smoke** ; **Starch** *factories.*

BOOKER (F.) Concerning inspectors of nuisances; their appointment, and some practical observations with reference to the mode of procedure and efficient execution of some of the duties devolving on them under the public health act, 1875, with a list of duties and certain local regulations. 8°. *Manchester,* 1879.

BOSTON. Report of committee on a nuisance at Ward's wharf. [On the killing and transportation of dead horses.] Boston. City Doc., No. 69. Sept. 1, 1862. 8°. [*Boston,* 1862.]

CASE (The) of the manufacturers of soap and candles, in the city of New York, stated and examined. To which are prefixed the laws of the State of New York, concerning infectious diseases, with an addition in form of an appendix containing several documents and papers relative to these subjects. 8°. *New York,* 1797.

COURT of Appeals. Nos. I & II. The Metropolitan Board of Health against Jacob Heister. Claim for penalty for violating order and ordinances [in carrying on the business of "slaughtering cattle" in a densely populated portion of the city]. Nos. III & IV. Jacob Heister against the Metropolitan Board of Health. Application for injunction to stay board from enforcing ordinances. roy. 8° [*Albany, n. d.*]

FROST (E.) A preliminary discussion of the Miller's River nuisance, and its remedy. 8°. *Boston,* 1872.

GREAT BRITAIN. *General Board of Health.* Report on the measures adopted for the execution of the nuisances removal and diseases prevention act, and the public health act, up to July, 1849. 8°. *London,* 1849.

GREAT BRITAIN. *Local Government Board.* Alkali acts, 1863, 1874, and 1881. Annual reports of the inspector of his proceedings during the years 1872–84 (9.–21.). 8°. *London,* 1873–85.
For preceding reports, see, infra, GREAT BRITAIN. Privy Council Office.

———. Model bye-laws for the use of sanitary authorities: No. II. Prevention of nuisances arising from snow, filth, dust, ashes, and rubbish. Prevention of the keeping of animals on any premises so as to be injurious to health. 8°. *London,* 1877.

———. Digest of provisions as to removal of nuisances. (Public health act, 1875.) 8°. *London,* 1884.

———. Digest of provisions as to removal of nuisances. (Metropolis.) 8°. *London,* 1884.

GREAT BRITAIN. *Parliament.* The nuisances removal and disease prevention amendment act, 18 and 19 Vic., cap. 121. To which are added the smoke nuisance act and the common lodging-house acts. 12°. *London,* 1855.

———. Report from the select committee of the House of Lords [Richmond, Derby, Graham, and others] on injury from noxious vapors, together with the proceedings of the committee, minutes of evidence, and appendix. Session 1862. fol. [*London,* 1862.]

Nuisances.
———. Noxious vapours commission. Report of the royal commission on noxious vapours. fol. *London,* 1878.

GREAT BRITAIN. *Privy Council Office.* Alkali acts, 1863 and 1874. Annual reports of the inspector, to the committee of privy council for trade, of his proceedings during the years 1864–71 (1.–8.). 8°. *London,* 1865–72.

HORSFORD (E. N.) Report on an investigation of the sources of the offensive odors which are ascribed, in a petition by John M. Tyler and others, before the State board of health, to the hog-slaughtering establishment of John P. Squire & Co., of East Cambridge. 8°. *Cambridge,* 1873.

KINGSTON-UPON-HULL. Annual report of the inspector of nuisances, Joseph Osborne. 1., 1881. 6 tab. 8°. *Hull,* 1882.

LIVERPOOL. Report of the inspector of nuisances as to the drainage of courts, cellars, insanitary houses, etc. [By H. Fitzpatrick.] 8°. *Liverpool,* 1884.

MANCHESTER and Salford Noxious Vapours Abatement Association No. 1, 1887. Air pollution, noxious vapours which pollute the air. By J. Carter Bell. 12°. *Manchester,* 1887.

MASSACHUSETTS. *State Board of Health.* John M. Tyler *et al.*, petitioners, *vs.* John P. Squire *et al.*, respondents. Closing argument in behalf of the respondents, before the State board of health, Dec. 29, 1873. 8°. *Cambridge,* 1874.

NEW JERSEY. *Senate.* Supplement to an act entitled "An act relating to local boards of health" [conferring power to abate nuisances hazardous to the public health], approved March 22, 1881. State of New Jersey. Senate, No. 163. Introd. Feb. 14, 1883, by Mr. Taylor. fol. [*Trenton,* 1883.]

NEW YORK (*State*). An act to provide for the abatement of nuisances by boards of health of incorporated cities, villages, and towns. State of New York. No. 117. In senate, Feb. 23, 1882. Introd. by Mr. Fitzgerald. fol. [*Albany,* 1882.]

———. An act to suppress certain nuisances. [Making it unlawful for any place of business in cities of 15,000 population or over to use (petroleum residuum) for fuel.] State of New York. No. 358. In assembly, March 1, 1882. Introd. by Mr. Kelly. fol. [*Albany,* 1882.]

NEW YORK State Board of Health. Opinion of attorney-general regarding powers to abate nuisances. 8°. [*Albany,* 1884.]

———. Report on the nuisances of Hunter's Point and vicinity, and message of the governor accompanying the same. (Transmitted to the legislature, April 22, 1881.) 8°. *Albany,* 1881.

PLEA (A) in behalf of law and order. How a village trustee can destroy a village. The affidavits of several civil engineers and physicians, showing that the Odell ice pond is a nuisance, which will necessarily produce noxious, offensive, and poisonous effluvia, miasma, malaria, intermittent fever, and zymotic disease. Shall we be compelled to abandon our homes? 8°. *New York,* 1879.

POULSON (F. T.) The procedure of a sanitary inspector in relation to the abatement of nuisances. 12°. *London,* 1884.

PRINCETON, *New Jersey.* Proclamation concerning nuisances. Aug. 27, 1880. fol. [*Princeton,* 1880.]

SMITH (R. A.) Report to the town council of Leith, on the chemical works in Salamander street. 8°. *Edinburgh,* [1862].

SMOKE Abatement Fund. National Health and Kyrle Societies. [Appeal of the committee to the public, to assist their efforts in reducing the mischief arising from the production of

Nuisances.

smoke in the metropolis.] Nov. 16, 1880. fol. [*London*, 1880.]

WALLACE (W.) Report to the magistrates and council of the city of Glasgow, on the refuse water of chemical works and other factories. 8°. *Glasgow*, 1885.

WILLIAMSON (T.) Sanatory remarks in connection with nuisances; addressed to students and young physicians. 8°. *Edinburgh*, 1856.

WOOD (H. G.) A practical treatise on the law of nuisances in their various forms; including remedies therefor at law and in equity. 2. ed. 8°. *Albany, N. Y.*, 1883.

Adams (J. F. A) The new Lenox malaria. Boston M. & S. J., 1882, cvii, 604–609. *Also*, Reprint.—**d'Arcet.** Des rapports de distances qu'il est utile de maintenir entre les fabriques insalubres et les habitations qui les entourent. Ann. d'hyg., Par., 1843, xxx, 321–328. *Also*, Reprint.—**Atwater** (E. S.) Some citations from the law relating to nuisances. Rep. Bd. Health N. Jersey, Mount Holly, 1881, v, 73–79.—**Baird** (C. R.) Report on the legal provisions available in Glasgow for the removal of nuisances. San. Inquiry: Scotland, Lond., 1842, 65–77. — **Ballard.** Third report in respect of the inquiry as to effluvium nuisances arising in connexion with various manufacturing and other branches of industry. Rep. Med. Off. Local Gov. Bd. 1878, Lond., 1879, viii, 42–320, 38 pl.— **Bond** (F. T.) On the law of nuisances in its medico-legal aspect. Pub. Health, Lond., 1874, ii, 3–6.—**Braconnot** (H.) & **Simonin** (F.) Notes sur les émanations des fabriques de produits. J. de chim. méd., etc., Par., 1848, 3. s, iv, 280–288. — **Brick-burning** (The) nuisance. San. Rec., Lond., 1887–8, n. s., ix 54–56.—**Burton** (J. H.) On the state of the law as regards the abatement of nuisances and the protection of the public health, in Scotland, with suggestions for amendment. San. Inquiry: Scotland, 1842, 40–65.—**Cameron** (J. C.) What constitutes a common nuisance. Med.-Leg. J., N. Y., 1884–5, ii, 567–569.—**Chevallier** & **Guérard.** Mémoire sur les résidus liquides provenant des établissements industriels. Ann. d'hyg., Par., 1846, xxxvi, 99–120.—**Colby** (A. L.) Report on glucose factories at Buffalo. Rep. State Bd. Health N. Y., Albany, 1884, iv, 425–428. — **Feroci** (A.) Impianto d'una fabbrica per la estrazione degli alcooli dai cereali; reclami per incomodi e insalubrità; provvedimenti proposti per eliminarli. Gior. d. Soc. ital. d'ig., Milano, 1884, vi, 350–362.—**George** (H.) The poisons of the manufactory. Pop. Sc. Month., N. Y., 1882. xxi, 663–667. — **Griswold** (R. W.) The Berkshire malaria trial. N. Eng. M. Month., Newtown, Conn., 1882–3, ii, 498–504.— **Hering** (R.) & **Lee** (B.) Report on nuisances existing outside the limits of Allegheny City, and on the pollution of the Allegheny River. Rep. Bd. Health., etc., Penn. 1885, Harrisburg, 1886, i, 251–257.—**Hill** (A.) The liability of property owners to make structural alterations to abate nuisances on properties belonging to them, but let on lease. Tr. Soc. M. Off. Health 1886–7, Lond., 1887, 72.— **Humphreys** (*Judge* W. H.) Nuisances from a legal standpoint; jurisdiction of the courts over municipal corporations with regard to nuisances. South. Pract., Nashville, 1880, ii, 367–374.—**Kuichling** (E.) Report on sawdust nuisance at Philadelphia, Jefferson County. Rep. State Bd. Health N. Y. 1886. Albany, 1887, vii, 31–42.— **Letheby** (H.) On noxious and offensive trades and manufactures, with especial reference to the best practicable means of abating the several nuisances therefrom. Pub. Health, Lond., 1875, iii, 49; 81.—**Mahlon Hutchinson** *et al.*, appellants, *v.* The State, *ex rel.* The Board of Health of the City of Trenton, respondent. Rep. Bd. Health N. Jersey, Trenton, 1885, ix, 291–296.—**Martin** (E. W.) Report on the manufacture of Neufchâtel cheese and its adulterations, at the factories of Charles H. Green, Chester, Orange County, and Lawrence & Durland, Chester, Orange County. Rep State Bd. Health N. Y., Albany. 1884, iv, 263–267. — **Maurin** (S.) Réponse aux habitants d'Arenc sur cette question : Les dépôts d'engrais accumulés sur un point du quartier d'Arenc ne sont-ils pas une cause d'insalubrité? Rec. d. actes du Comité méd. d. Bouches-du-Rhône, Marseille, 1868, vii, 165–179. — **Nuisance** in the town of Brighton, Monroe County. Rep. State Bd. Health N. Y. 1886, Albany, 1887, vii, 355–361.—**Offenses** against public health. Rep. Bd. Health Iowa, Des Moines, 1883, ii 220–222. — "**Old** (An) Technologist." Offensive manufactures; a suggestion. J. Sc., Lond., 1881, 3. s., iii, 131–137.—**Parent-Duchatelet** & **Lecanu.** Rapport sur une épuration de sang. Ann. d'hyg., Par., 1834, xi, 110–116.—**Prescott** (R.) Sewerage nuisance, Greene, Chenango County. Rep. State Bd. Health N. Y. 1886, Albany. 1887, vii, 362–367.—**Public** nuisances. Boston M. & S. J., 1854, xlix, 227.—**Report** of the committee on effluvium nuisances. Rep. State Bd. Health N. Y., Albany, 1884, iv, 229–248. — **Report** on complaint against the Glen Cove Manufacturing

Nuisances.

Company. *Ibid.*, 319–380, 2 plans.—**Report** on drainage of abandoned canal at village of Horseheads. *Ibid.*, 381–391, 2 plans. — **Report** of the evidence, etc., before the State board of health. in the case of the City of Cambridge *v.* Niles Brothers. Rep. Bd. Health Mass., Bost., 1879, x, 111–227, 2 charts.—**Report** of the Lancet Sanitary Commission on the influence of certain chemical manufactures on health. Lancet, Lond., 1874, i, 491; 742: ii, 62. — **Reports** on pond nuisances in Westchester County. Rep. State Bd. Health N. Y., Albany, 1884, iv, 393–404.—**Roberts** (W. C.) On the influence of non-specific emanations on the public health. Are they deleterious? N. York M. J., 1871, xiii, 441–448.—**Robins** (E. C.) On the disabilities of inspectors of nuisances, and their remedy. San. Rec., Lond., 1883–4, n. s., v, 176–178. — **Russell** (J. B.) The Local Authority of Glasgow *v.* Young. San. Jour., Glasg., 1879–80, iii, 329–336. *Also*, Reprint.—**Schauenstein.** Die Sodafabrikation in gesundheits-polizeilicher Hinsicht. Wchnbl. d. k. k. Gesellsch. d. Aerzte in Wien, 1857, iii, 529–535.—**Slaughtering,** bone-boiling, and fat-melting. [A history of the efforts of the State board of health to bring about a reform in these processes.] Rep. Bd. Health Mass., Bost., 1872, iii, 224–245.—**Spencer** (A.) On the supervision of offensive trades in the metropolis. Tr. Soc. M. Off. Health, Lond., 1884–5, 22–43. *Also*: San. Rec., Lond., 1884–5, n. s., vi, 298–304.—**Steuer.** Sanitätspolizeiliche Begutachtung eines Produkten-Geschäfts. Vrtljschr. f. gerichtl. u. öff. Med., Berl., 1859, xvi, 233 –239. — **Stout** (A. B.) Infectious nuisances; public right *vs.* private privilege. West. Lancet, San Fran. 1875, iv, 147–154. — **Thursfield** (W. N.) The removal of nuisances. San. Rec., Lond., 1874, i, 178–181.—**Tracy** (R. S.) Public nuisances. Cycl. Pract. M. (Ziemssen), N. Y., 1879, xix, 379–470. ——. The problem of municipal nuisances. Pop. Sc. Month., N. Y., 1880–81, xxviii, 585–599.—**Vacher** (F.) Noxious vapours. San. Rec., Lond., 1877, vi, 363–366.—**Watson** (I. A.) Common law citations relating to nuisances. Rep. Bd. Health N. Hampshire 1881–2, Concord, 1882, i, 231–239. *Also*, Reprint. — **Wilson** (O. S.) Report on the slaughter-houses of Penn Yan. Rep. State Bd. Health N. Y. 1886, Albany, 1887, vii, 43–46. — **Wolff** (A. J.) The Park River nuisance as affecting the sanitary condition of Hartford. Rep. Bd. Health Connect. 1884, New Haven, 1885, vii, 155–217, 2 pl.

Nuits (Les) d'épreuve des villageoises allemandes avant le mariage. Dissertation sur un usage singulier, traduite de l'allemand et accompagnée de notes et d'une postface. Par un bibliophile. 2. 6d. 86 pp. 12°. *Bruxelles, Gay & Douce*, 1877.

"**Numa Numantius**" [*pseudon.*]. *See* Unglingo (Carl Friedrich).

Numan (Alexander) [1780–1852]. Verhandeling over de koepoken, zooals dezelve natuurlijk bij het rund voorkomen, en, door inenting, kunnen worden voortgebragt en over de beveiligende mok of pokmok des paards; benevens een bijvoegsel, bevattende den uitslag der proefnemingen, om runderen door kinderpokestoffe te besmetten, en daardoor koepokken voort te brengen, alsmede de aanwijzing, om de koepokstoffe in glazen haar-buisjes te verzamelen en te bewaren. xi, 114 pp., 5 pl. 4°. *Utrecht, Van Paddenburg & Co.*, 1831.

——. Over den invloed der maan in hare verschillende standen op het voortellingsvermogen der dieren. 26 pp. 8°. [*n. p.*, 1845, *vel subseq.*]

Numbness.

Aulde (J.) Waking numbness. Med. Reg., Phila., 1887, ii, 228–230. — **Dodge** (C. L.) Waking numbness. Med. News, Phila., 1887, li, 120.— **Moir** (W. B.) A special form of numbness of the extremities. Lancet, Lond., 1885, ii, 595.—**Saundby** (R.) On a special form of numbness of the extremities. *Ibid.*, 422.— **Sinkler** (W.) On a form of numbness, chiefly of the upper extremities. Tr. Coll. Phys. Phila., 1884, 3. s., vii, 213–224. *Also* [Abstr.]: Cincin. Lancet & Clinic, 1884, n. s., xiii, 40–44. — **Smith** (A. H.) Waking numbness; a heretofore undescribed neurosis. Am. J. M. Sc., Phila., 1887, n. s., xciii, 410–413. — **Squire** (J. E.) Some cases of local numbness of the extremities, with comparisons between local syncope and night palsy. Lancet, Lond., 1886, ii, 1065–1067.

Numismatics.

See Medals.

Nuneaton.

CLARK (G. T.) Report to the General Board of Health, on a preliminary inquiry into the

Nuneaton.

sewerage, drainage, and supply of water, and the sanitary condition of the inhabitants of the parishes of Nuneaton and Chilvers Coton. 8°. *London*, 1849.

Nunes (Christovão Pereira). * Da ovariotomia antiseptica abdominal. ii, 86 pp. 8°. *Rio de Jan., Lombaerts & Comp.*, 1883.

Nuñés-Ribeiro-Sanchès (Ant.) Catalogue des livres de feu . . . 28, 93 pp., 1 l. 8°. *Paris, Bure fils aîné*, 1783.

Bound with: J. de méd. mil., Par., 1788, vii.

Nunes-Vais. Studi clinici sul cholera. 47 pp. roy. 8°. *Tunisi*, 1885.

Nuñez (Alphonsus).

See **Chiffletius** (Joan. Jacob.) Acia Cornelii Celsi propriæ, etc. 4°. *Antverpiæ*, 1633.

Nuñez (Ambrosio) [1529–1611]. Tractado repartido en cinco partes principales, que declaran el mal que significa este nombre peste con todas sus causas, y señales prognosticas, y indicativas del mal, con la preservacion, y cura que en general, y en particular sedeve hazer. 11 p. l, 123, 60 ff., 4 l. 8°. *Coimbra, D. G. Loureyro*, 1601.

Nuñez (Belisario R.) La tricoficia y su tratamiento por el acido salicílico. 76 pp., 1 l. 8°. *Buenos Aires, M. Biedma*, 1884.

Nuñez (José) [1805 79]. Dos palabras en contestacion á la carta que el Dr. D. Joaquin de Heysern ha dirigido á los médicos homeópatas. 14 pp. 8°. *Madrid, R. Vicente y Lavajos*, 1862. [P., v. 1454.]

———. Estudio médico del veneno de la tarántula segun el método de Hahnemann, precedido de un resúmen histórico del tarantulismo y tarantismo, y seguido de algunas indicaciones terapéuticas y notas clínicas. iv, 5–204 pp., 2 l. 8°. *Madrid, Vicente y Lavajos*, 1864.

———. The same. Étude médicale sur le venin de la tarentule d'après la méthode de Hahnemann, [etc.] Trad. et annotée par le docteur J. Perry. 268 pp. 8°. *Paris, J.-B. Baillière & fils*, 1866.

For Biography, see Bull. Soc. méd. homœop. de France, Par., 1880, xxi (C. Catellan). *Also*, Reprint.

Nuñez (Julio E.) [1837–]. * Étude sur les vices de conformation de l'urèthre chez la femme. 124 pp., 1 pl. 4°. *Paris*, 1882, No. 101.

Nuñez (Lorenzo Sanchez). Diccionario de fiebres esenciales, compuesto y traducido del artículo fiebres y otros varios contenidos en el diccionario de ciencias médicas, que actualmente está formando en París una grande sociedad de sabios. xii, 410 pp. 4°. *Madrid, Repullés*, 1819.

Nuñez (Tobias). * Consideraciones generales sobre las fiebres intermitentes y en particular las del país. 30 pp. 8°. *México, J. Complido*, 1870.

Nunez *River.*

Celarier (C.) Notes sur le Rio-Nunez; topographie, météorologie, histoire naturelle et matière médicale, pathologie, hygiène général. Arch. belges de méd. mil., Brux., 1850, vi, 73–116.—**Corre** (A.) Esquisse de la flore et de la faune médicales et économiques du Rio-Nunez. Arch. de méd. nav., Par., 1876, xxvi, 14–40.

Nuñez del Prado (Daniel). Fiebre amarilla; su origen, causas, sintomas, tratamiento, etc. 41 pp. 8°. *Lima, imp. Liberal*, 1870.

Nuñez de Villavicencio (B. C.) & **Holt** (Jos.) Yellow fever microbes. 1 galley sheet. [*New Orleans*, 1886.]

Cutting from: Daily City Item, N. Orl., June 7, 1886.

Nunn (Andreas) [–1796). [Pr.] de hysterico delirio. [Cum vita candidati Jo. Christ. Frid. Gottschalck.] xvi pp. 4°. *Erfordiæ, lit. H. R. Nonnii*, [1713].

———. [Pr.] de tumoribus externis suppuratione potius, quam resolutione curandis. [Cum vita

Nunn (Andreas)—continued. candidati Frid. Eusebii Rumpel.] 12 pp. 4°. *Erfordiæ, lit. Nonnii*, 1762.

———. [Pr.] de officina ac mechanismo sanguificationis. [Cum vita candidati Christiani Loeber.] xiv pp. 4°. *Erfordiæ, lit. H. R. Nonni*, [1767].

Nunn (R. J.) Some practical suggestions in the treatment of diphtheria. 7 pp. 8°. *Baltimore, Thomas & Evans*, 1880.

Repr. from: Independ. Pract., Balt., 1880, i.

———. Peptonized milk as food for infants and invalids. 20 pp. 8°. *New York, W. Wood & Co.*, 1880.

Repr. from: Am. J. Obst., N. Y., 1880, xiii.

———. Female diseases; the result of errors in habit and hygiene during childhood and puberty; with remarks on the treatment of rachialgia with igni-puncture (Paquelin's cautery). 45 pp. 8°. *Augusta, Ga., J. Loveday*, 1881.

Repr. from: Tr. M. Ass. Georgia, Augusta, 1881, xxxii.

———. Report on diseases of women from the First Congressional district. 32 pp. 8°. *Atlanta, J. P. Harrison & Co.*, [1883].

Repr. from: Tr. M. Ass. Georgia, Atlanta, 1883, xxxiv.

Nunn (*Roger Sturley*) [1813–82].

Obituary. Brit. M. J., Lond., 1882, i, 252.—**Obituary.** Med. Times & Gaz., Lond., 1882, i, 103.

Nunn (Thomas William) [1825–]. Varicose veins and varicose ulcers. viii, 63 pp. 8°. *London, H. Renshaw*, 1852.

———. Inflammation of the breast and milk abscess. viii, 52 pp. 8°. *London, H. Renshaw*, 1853.

———. Observations and notes on the arteries of the limbs. 27 pp., 1 pl. 8°. *London, J. Churchill*, 1858. [P., v. 1533.]

———. The same. 2. ed. 33 pp. 8°. *London, J. Churchill & Sons*, 1864. [*Also, in :* P., v. 90.]

———. The inaugural lecture, session 1863–4, delivered at the Middlesex Hospital Medical College. 24 pp. 8°. *McGowan & Danks*, 1863.

———. Notes on personal hygiene, No. 1. 20 pp. 8°. *London, R. Hardwicke*, 1865.

———. On cancer of the breast. xiv, 230 pp., 21 col. pl. 4°. *London, J. & A. Churchill*, 1882.

Nunneley (Thomas) [1809–70]. Anatomical tables, containing concise descriptions of the muscles, ligaments, fasciæ, blood-vessels, and nerves. Intended for the use of students. xv, 240 pp. 12°. *London, S. Highley*, 1838.

———. A treatise on the nature, causes, and treatment of erysipelas. xi, 307 pp. 8°. *London, J. Churchill*, [1841].

———. The same. 1. Am. ed. 235 pp. 8°. *Philadelphia, Barrington & Haswell*, 1844.

———. On anæsthesia and anæsthetic substances generally; being an experimental inquiry into their nature, properties, and action, their comparative value and danger, and the best means of counteracting the effect of an over dose. 215 pp. 8°. *Worcester, Deighton & Co.*, 1849. [P., v. 1033.]

Repr. from: Tr. Prov. M. & S. Ass., Lond., 1849, xvi.

———. Introductory lecture delivered at the Leeds School of Medicine, at the opening of the twenty-second session, October 4, 1852. 27 pp. 12°. *London, Longman [and others]*, 1852.

———. On the organs of vision; their anatomy and physiology. xxiv, 373 pp., 8 pl. 8°. *London, J. Churchill*, 1858.

———. An account of three cases of aneurism of, or within, the orbit, treated by ligature of the common carotid artery; with observations; to which is added a report of a fourth case, treated since the paper was read. 24 pp. 8°. *London, J. E. Adlard*, 1859.

Repr. from: Med.-Chir. Tr., Lond., 1859, xlii.

Nunneley (Thomas)—continued.

——. On the Calabar bean ; its action, preparations, and use. 38 pp. 8°. *London, Longman [and others]*, [1863]. [*Also, in :* P., v. 1205.]
Repr. from : Lancet, Lond., 1863, ii.
For Biography, see Brit. M. J., Lond., 1870, i, 614.
Also : Lancet, Lond., 1870, i, 823. Also : Med. Times & Gaz., Lond., 1870, i, 648.

Nunney.
See **Fever** (*Typhoid, History, etc., of*), *by localities.*

Nunning (Jod. Herm.)
See **Cohausen** (Joannes Henr.) Ossilegium histo-
rico-physicum, [etc.] 4°. *Francofurti et Lipsiæ*, 1714.

van Nunom (Hendericus). * De ortu, progressu
et occasu hominis. 22 pp., 2 l. sm. 4°. *Lugd.
Bat., A. Kallewier*, 1731. [P., v. 65.]

Nuns.
See **Celibacy.**

Nuova (La) Liguria medica. Giornale di scienze
mediche, continuazione della Liguria medica e
del Filiatre sebezio. Diretto dai dottori E. de
Renzi [*et al.*]. [3 times a month.] v. 16–19,
1871–4. 4 v. 8°. *Genova.*
Title of v. 1–15 was : **Liguria** (La) medica, 1856–70.

Nuova raccolta d' opuscoli scientifici e filologici.
42 v. 16°. *Venezia, S. Occhi*, 1755–87.
See, also, **Raccolta** d' opusculi scientifici e filologici.
16°. *Venezia*, 1728–57.

Nuovi commentarj di medicina e di chirurgia
pubblicati dai . . . Valeriano Luigi Brera, Cesare
Ruggeri, e Floriano Caldani. 5 v. 8°. *Padova,
Penada*, 1818–20.

Nuovi elementi della fisica del corpo umano. 2
v. xvi, 304 pp. ; 308 pp. 8°. *Padova, tip. del
Seminario*, 1820.

Nuovo (Il) Cimento. Giornale fondato per la
fisica e la chimica da C. Matteucci e R. Piria ;
continuato per la fisica esperimentale e matema-
tica da E. Betti e R. Felici. [Bi-monthly.] 3.
serie, v. 21. 1887. 287 pp. 8°. *Pisa.*

Nuovo giornale internazionale delle scienze mediche. Inteso ad informare i medici esercenti
dei progressi della medicina. Redatto dal Dr.
Domenico Franco. [Monthly.] v. 1, Nov.,
1877, to Oct., 1878. 384 pp. 8°. *Napoli.*
Continued as : **Scuola** (La) medica napolitana.

Nuovo mercurio delle scienze mediche. Compilato dai dottori G. Gordoni e L. Michelotti. v.
1–4, 1829 ; v. 1–2, 1830. 6 v. 8°. *Livorno.*
In 1830 Dr. Michelotti sole editor.

Nuremberg. Ein kurtz Regiment wie man
sich in diesen gegenwertigen Sterbsleufften
halten sol. Gestellet durch die verordneten und
geschwornen Doctores der Artzeney diser Stadt
Nürmberg im Jar 1575. 21 l. 4°. *Nürmberg, K.
Gerlachin u. J. vom Berg Erben*, [1575].

——. Verneuerte Gesetz, Ordnung und Tax
eines Edlen, Ehrnvesten, Fürsichtigen und Weissen Raths, dess Hey. Reichs Statt Nürnberg, dem
Collegio Medico, den Apoteckern und andern
angehörigen daselbsten gegeben. 31 l. sm. 4°.
[*Nürnberg, S. Halbmayer*], 1624.

——. Verneuerte Leich-Ordnung der Statt
Nürmberg. 4 l. 4°. *Nürmberg, B. Scherffen*,
1625.

——. Verneuerte Leich-Ordnung, wie es mit
denenselben, allhie in der Stadt Nürnberg, deren
beeden Vorstädten, zu Wöhrd und Gostenhof,
auch in den Städtlein und auf dem Land dess
gantzen Nürnbergischen Gebiets, gehalten werden solle. 7 l. 4°. [*Nürnberg*], *M. Endter*,
1662.
Bound with preceding.

——. Rath der Stadt Nürnberg. Ordnung, wie
es bey denen anderwärts leider! sehr einreissen-
den ansteckende Kranckheiten zu halten, damit bey hiesiger Stadt und Landschafft, durch

Nuremberg—continued.
Gottes Gnade, noch ferners reiner und gesunder
Lufft erhalten, und solches Uebel abgewendet
werden möge. 6 l. 4°. [*Nürnberg*], *M. Endter*,
1679.

——. Verneuerte Gesetz und Ordnung eines
Hoch Edlen und Hochweisen Raths des Heiligen
Reichs Stadt Nürnberg, dem Collegio Medico,
den Apotheckern, und andern Angehörigen da-
selbst gegeben. 11 l. sm. 4°. [*Nürnberg*], *B.
J. Endter*, 1700.
Bound with : NUREMBERG. Verneuerte Gesetz, Ord-
nung und Tax [etc.] sm. 4°. *Nürnberg*, 1624.

——. Verneuerte Leich-Ordnung, wie es mit
denen verstorbenen Personen, in des Heil. Röm.
Reichs Stadt Nürnberg, auch in dero Vorstädten,
und ganzem Gebiet, in ein- und andern gehalten
werden solle. 39 pp. 4°. *Nürnberg, B. J. Endter*,
1705.
Bound with : NUREMBERG. Verneuerte Leich-Ordnung.
4°. *Nürnberg*, 1625.

——. Eines Hoch-Edlen und Hochweisen Raths
des Heil. Röm. Reichs-Stadt Nürnberg Trauer-
Ordnung gegeben im Jahr 1765. 15 pp. 4°.
Nürnberg, J. J. Fleischmann, [1765].
Bound with preceding.

——. Nachtrag zur Trauer-Ordnung. (Decre-
tum in Senatu, den 23. Oct. 1769.) 11 pp. 8°.
[*Nürnberg*, 1769.]
Bound with preceding.

——. Eines Hochlöblichen Raths des Heil. Röm.
Reichs freyen Stadt Nürnberg verneuerte Leich-
und Trauer-Ordnung. 14 pp. 4°. [*Nürnberg*],
J. J. Fleischmann, 1785.
Bound with preceding.

——. Nachtrag zur Nürnbergischen Leichen-
und Trauer-Ordnung vom 6. December 1785. 11
pp. 4°. [*Nürnberg*], *G. F. Lix*, 1787.
Bound with preceding.

——. Allgemeines Krankenhaus der Stadt Nürnberg. Aerztliche Jahresberichte für die Jahre
1860–61 bis 1864–5. 4°. *Nürnberg*, [1861–5].

Nuremberg.
See, also, **Cholera** (*Asiatic, History, etc., of*),
Fever (*Cerebro-spinal, History, etc., of*), **Hospitals** (*Descriptions, etc., of*), *by localities.*
BRAUN (G.) Die epidemischen Krankheiten
in Nürnberg im Jahr 1852. Vortrag in der Sitzung des Nürnberger ärztlichen Vereins am 6.
Januar 1853. 8°. *Nürnberg*, 1853.
CARDILUCIUS (J. H.) Heilsame Artzney-
Kräffte des Nürnbergischen Wild-Bades, wie
nemlich solche herfliessen von einer darinn enthaltenen roten solarischen und weissen lunari-
schen Mineral-Tinctur, und nach solcher tragen-
den zweyfachen Signatur dienlich seyn zu den
fürnemsten Gebresten des Gebluts, und der weissen Leibs-Safftigkeit, nebst dessen rechtem Gebrauch und mitlauffenden andern kräfftigen
Artzneyen. Nach eigenhändiger fleissiger Pro-
birung den Bresshafftigen zu Dienst beschrieben
und publicirt. 18°. *Nürnberg*, 1681.
GORDON (J.) Stenographischer Bericht über
das Gutachten der Canalisationsfrage in Nürnberg. 8°. *Frankfurt a. M.*, [1877 ?]
JAHRESBERICHT der Poliklinik zu Nürnberg,
1. (1879–80). 8°. *Nürnberg*, [1879].
KÄMMERER (H.) Untersuchungen des Peg-
nitzwassers in Nürnberg ; in magistratischem
Auftrage ausgeführt. Veröffentlicht durch den
Magistrat der Stadt Nürnberg. 8°. [*Nürnberg,
n. d.*]
NYMPHOGRAPHIA, das ist : kurtze und gründliche Beschreibung dess heylsamen Wildbads des
Hoch löblichen Reichs Statt Nürnberg, darinnen
desselben Natur, Art und Eygenschafft, so wol
auch in was Kranckheiten solches nutzlich zuge-
brauchen angezeigt wird. Sampt einer wol-

Nuremberg.

denckwürdigen und mercklichen Weissagung von dem Casteyner Bad gegenwertige Zeit und dessen Aussgang betreffendt. sm. 4°. [*Nürnberg?* 1632.]

SANITÄREN (Die) Verhältnisse und Anstalten der Stadt Nürnberg. 8°. *Nürnberg*, 1877.

Geburts- und Sterblichkeits-Statistik der Stadt Nürnberg für die Jahre 1877 bis 1882. Veröffentl. d. k. deutsch. Gsndhtsamtes, Berl., 1878–83, ii–vii [*passim*].—**Heinrich.** Auszug des meteorologischen Tagebuchs. Arch. f. d. ges. Naturl., Nürnb., 1824, i, 125; 253; 381; 503: ii, 133; 253; 381; 503: iii, 125; 253; 381; 501.—**Küttlinger.** Einige Worte über die Krankheits-Constitution im laufenden und vorigen Jahre (1829 und 1830). Arch. f. Chem. u. Meteor., Nürnb., 1830, i, 176–183. ———. Resultate der meteorologischen Beobachtungen in Nürnberg in den Jahren 1864 und 1865. Abhandl. d. naturh. Gesellsch. zu Nürnb., 1866, iii, 2. Hlft., 269–276, 1 tab. — **Scheuchzer** (J. J.) Observationes meteorologico-medicæ pro anno 1730. Acta Acad. nat. curios., Norimb., 1737, iv (app.), 24–46. — **von Schmöger** (F.) Auszug aus dem meteorologischen Tagebuche. Arch. f. d. ges. Naturl., Nürnb., 1825, v, 255: vi, 502: 1826, viii, 383: ix, 447: 1827, xi, 262: xii, 503: 1828, xiv, 396: xv, 438: 1829, xvii, 482: xviii, 435. *Continued in:* Arch. f. Chem. u. Meteor., Nürnb., 1830, i, 387: ii, 401: 1831, iv, 140: 1832, v, 74: vi, 295: 1833, vii, 108: 1834, viii, 345: 1835, ix, 629.

Nursery and Child's Hospital in the City of New York. Annual reports of the secretary and medical staff to the board of managers. 11., 1864–5; 19., 1872–3; 20., 1873–4; 26., 1879–80; 30., 1883–4. 12°. *New York*, 1865–84.

Incorporated April 19, 1854.

———. *See, also:*

JACOBI (A.) [Letter from . . . a member of the medical staff, to Mrs. R. H. Lemist, secretary of the board of lady managers, on his forced removal or resignation as a member of the medical board, Oct., 1870.] 8°. [*New York*, 1870.]

Nurses *and nursing.*

See, also, **Beds,** *etc.*; **Hospital** *nurses, etc.*; **Infants** (*Food, etc., of*); **Medicine** (*Popular*).

AUEGG (Henriette). Sechs Vorträge über weibliche Krankenpflege, gehalten im Frühjahre 1878 zu Gunsten des Grazer Mädchen-Lyceums. 8°. *Graz*, 1878.

BARNES (J. H.) Notes on surgical nursing; being a short course of lectures delivered at the Training School for Nurses in connection with the Liverpool Workhouse. 8°. *London*, 1874.

BECKER (G. W.) Die Wartung der Kranken. Ein Buch für alle Familien, worin alles, was im weitesten Sinn auf Wartung und Pflege der Kranken Bezug hat, so wie die Diät in jeder einzelnen Krankheit, nebst den besten Haus- und Hülfsmitteln, und einer Auswahl der zweckmässigsten Recepte, die Jedermann anwenden kann, aufs fasslichste und vollständigste auseinander gesetzt ist. 16°. *Leipzig*, 1811.

[BELL (G. W.)] Lectures addressed to the nursing staff, by physicians and surgeons of King's College Hospital. Introductory address. 12°. *London*, 1884.

BENTON (S.) Nurses and nursing. 8°. *London*, 1877.

BLACK (G.) Sick-nursing. A handbook for all who have to do with cases of disease and convalescence. sm. 8°. *London*, [1880?]

BLAIR (J.) Opening address to nurses, with notes to nurses and rules for nurses under training added. 8°. *Melbourne*, 1880.

BRINCKMAN (A.) Notes on the care of the sick, and practical advice to those in charge of the dying and the dead. 8°. *London*, 1879.

BRUEN (E. T.) Practical lessons in nursing. Outlines for the management of diet, or the regulation of food to the requirements of health and the treatment of disease. 12°. *Philadelphia*, 1887.

Nurses *and nursing.*

BURDETT (H. C.) A national pension fund for nurses and hospital officials. 8°. *London*, 1887.

CAULFEILD (S. F. A.) Sick nursing at home; being plain directions and hints for the proper nursing of sick persons, and the home treatment of diseases and accidents in cases of sudden emergencies. 8°. *London*, [1880].

CHILD (*Mrs.*) The family nurse; or, companion of the frugal housewife. Revised by a member of the Massachusetts Medical Society. 12°. *Boston*, 1837.

CULLINGWORTH (C. J.) The nurse's companion. A manual of general and monthly nursing. 12°. *London*, 1876.

———. The same. A manual of nursing, medical and surgical. 2. ed. sm. 8°. *London*, 1885.

———. The same. 16°. *Philadelphia*, 1885.

———. A short manual for monthly nurses. 2. ed. 16°. *London*, 1887.

DEGEN (L.) Die öffentliche Krankenpflege im Frieden und im Kriege nach dem Ergebniss der Ausstellung auf dem Gebiete der Hygiene u. des Rettungswesens zu Berlin 1883. 8°. *München*, 1884.

DIEFFENBACH (J. F.) Anleitung zur Krankenwartung. 12°. *Berlin*, 1832.

DOMVILLE (E. J.) A manual for hospital nurses and others engaged in attending on the sick. 8°. *London*, 1872.

———. The same. 2. ed. 8°. *London*, 1875.

———. The same. 4. ed. 8°. *London*, 1881.

———. The same. 5. ed. 8°. *London*, 1885.

———. The same. 12°. *Philadelphia*, 1885.

DONAVERUS (J. E.) * De officio ægrotantium. sm. 4°. *Jenæ*, [1719].

DUCKWORTH (D.) Sick-nursing essentially a woman's mission; being an inaugural lecture on the qualifications for and the conduct of sick-nurses. 2. ed. 8°. *London*, 1885.

DUROCHER & DRONSART. Les fondateurs de la Maison royale de santé avec institution pour les élèves garde-malades, au château des Ternes, vis-à-vis la Porte Maillot, à messieurs les préfets, sous-préfets et maires des principales villes de France. 4°. [*Paris, n. d.*]

VAN DUYL (K. J.) & VAN WEERZEL (S. P.) Handleiding ter opleiding van hospitaalsoldaten. 8°. *Utrecht*, 1865.

EMPLOYMENT (On the) of trained nurses among the labouring poor, considered chiefly in relation to sanitary reform and the arts of life. By a physician. 8°. *London*, 1860.

FODÉRÉ (F.-E.) Manuel du garde-malade, des gardes des femmes en couches et des enfans au berceau. 4°. [*Strasbourg*, 1815.]

French and German text.

FRIENDLY (A) letter to under nurses of the sick, especially in unions. By a lady. 12°. *London*, 1861.

GEDIKE (C. E.) Handbuch der Krankenwartung. 3. Aufl. 8°. *Berlin*, 1854.

———. The same. Zum Gebrauch für die Krankenwart-Schule der k. Berliner Charité-Heilanstalt sowie zum Selbstunterricht. 5. Aufl., neu bearbeitet von Dr. Ravoth. 8°. *Berlin*, 1874.

HAND-BOOK (A) of nursing for family and general use. Published under the direction of the Connecticut Training School for Nurses. 12°. *Philadelphia*, 1879.

HARDY (C. H.) Introductory lecture on the duties of nurses, delivered at the Alfred Hospital. 8°. *Melbourne*, 1881.

HILSCHER (S. P.) [Pr.] de permutatione linteorum in morbis acutis et noxia et salubri. 4°. *Jenæ*, [1745].

Nurses *and nursing.*

HOOD (D. W. C.) Diseases and their commencement. Lectures to trained nurses delivered at the West London Hospital. 12°. *London*, 1886.

——. The same. 8°. *Philadelphia*, 1886.

How to nurse sick children; intended especially as a help to the nurses at the Hospital for Sick Children, but containing directions which may be found of service to all who have the charge of the young. 16°. *New York*, 1855.

HUBERTI (F. C. J.) * De damno e nimia hominum ad lectum ægri frequentia. 4°. *Erfordiæ*, 1792.

HUSBAND (H. A.) The monthly nurse; a few hints on nursing. 12°. *Edinburgh*, 1886.

HUTT (W. H.) [Blank forms for nurse's daily report to physician. 12°. *Philadelphia*, 1883.]

INSTRUCCION de enfermeros, y modo de aplicar los remedios, á todo genero de enfermedades, y acudir á los accidentes, que sobrevienen en ausencia de los médicos. Compuesto por los hijos de la congregacion del venerable Padre Bernardino de Obregon, sita en el Hospital general de Madrid, sacada á luz por el Hermano Augustin del Buen. 4. ed. 4°. *Madrid*, 1728.

JACKSON (J. C.) How to nurse the sick. 8°. *Dansville, N. Y.*, 1868.

[JOHNSTONE (Mrs. F.)] Lessons on the prevention of the spread of fevers; delivered to the Ladies' Educational Society of Hastings and St. Leonard's, in November, 1873, with additions. 2. ed. *St. Leonard's-on-Sea*, [1876].

JONES (H.) An essay on nursing. Reprinted from "Holiday Papers", by the same author. 8°. *London*, 1864.

JOURNAL of Practical Nursing. Edited by L. C. Brown; published by the Rockford Nurses' Association. v. 1. 8°. *Rockford, Ills.*, 1888.

LADY nurses for the sick poor in our London workhouses. Report of proceedings at the Strand Union Board of Guardians, Sept. 4, 1866. With an appendix. 8°. *London*, 1866.

LEES (Florence S.) Handbook for hospital sisters. Edited by H. W. Acland. 12°. *London*, 1874.

——. The same. Handbuch für Krankenpflegerinnen. Auf Wunsch Ihrer Majestät der Kaiserin-Königin nach der englischen Ausgabe des Prof. Dr. Henry W. Acland in deutscher Sprache herausgegeben von Dr. Paul Schliep. 12°. *Berlin*, 1874.

LONGSHORE (J. S.) The principles and practice of nursing, or a guide to the inexperienced, [etc.] 8°. *Philadelphia*, 1842.

LOUIS (J.) La nourrice à la ville et à la campagne. 12°. *Paris*, 1880.

LÜCKES (Eva C. E.) Lectures on general nursing, delivered to the probationers of the London Hospital Training School for Nurses. 12°. *London*, 1884.

——. Hospital sisters and their duties. 8°. *London*, 1886.

——. The same. 12°. *Philadelphia*, 1886.

MACARTHUR (A.) Address delivered at the fifth annual meeting of the Washington Training School for Nurses. 8°. *Washington*, 1882.

MAKKAS (N. G.) Ὁδηγίαι περὶ νοσηλείας ἀῤῥώστων. sm. 8°. Ἐν Ἀθῆναις, 1875.

MANAGEMENT (The) of the sick room, with rules for diet, cookery for the sick and convalescent, and the treatment of the sudden illnesses and various accidents that require prompt and judicious care, with practical hints on digestion. Compiled from the latest medical authorities by a lady of New York, under the supervision of Charles A. Lee, M. D. 2. ed. 12°. *New York*, 1845.

Nurses *and nursing.*

MANUAL (A) of nursing. Prepared for the Training School for Nurses, attached to Bellevue Hospital. 12°. *New York*, 1878.

MANUEL pratique de la garde-malade et de l'infirmière, publié par le Dr. Bourneville. 2. éd. 3 v. in 1. 12°. *Paris*, 1878.

MARTIN (J. M. H.) Ambulance lectures, to which is added a nursing lecture in accordance with the regulations of the St. John Ambulance Association for male and female classes. 2. ed. 12°. *London*, 1888.

MARTIN (N.) Ledning vid sjukvård i hemmet med särskild hänsyn till de smittosamma sjukdomarne och deras förekommande. Med ett förord af Professor Curt Wallis. [Instruction in nursing at home, with special regard to contagious diseases and their prevention.] 8°. *Stockholm*, [1886].

[MARTINEAU (H.)] Life in the sick room. Essays. By an invalid. 2. ed. 8°. *London*, 1844.

——. The same. With an introduction to the American edition, by Eliza L. Follen. 2. Am. ed. 8°. *Boston*, 1845.

MAY (F. A.) Unterricht für Krankenwärter zum Gebrauch öffentlicher Vorlesungen. 16°. *Mannheim*, 1782.

MILLS (C. K.) Practical lessons in nursing. The nursing and care of the nervous and the insane. 12°. *Philadelphia*, 1887.

MITCHELL (S. W.) Nurse and patient, and camp cure. 24°. *Philadelphia*, 1877.
Repr. from: Lippincott's Mag.

MORLEY (H.) A tract upon interrupted health and sick-room duties. 8°. *London*, 1847.

MUNRO (A.) The science and art of nursing the sick. 12°. *Glasgow*, 1873.

NEUMAN (R. A.) Home-nursing. 24°. *London & Edinburgh*, 1886.

NIGHTINGALE (Florence). Notes on nursing; what it is, and what it is not. 8°. *New York*, 1860.

——. Notes on nursing for the labouring classes. New ed. 18°. *London*, 1876.

——. Die Pflege bei Kranken und Gesunden. Kurze Winke, den Frauen aller Stände gewidmet. Von der Verfasserin autorisirte Ausgabe. Mit einem Vorwort des Geh. Sanitäts-Rath Dr. H. Wolff in Bonn. 12°. *Leipzig*, 1861.

NURSING (The) Record. A journal for nurses and a chronicle of hospital and institution news. [Weekly.] Nos. 1–3, v. 1, April 5 19, 1888. 4°. *London, S. Low, Marston & Co.*
Current.

OTIS (F. N.) A lecture delivered before the ladies of the School for Nurses. 8°. [*New York*], 1876.
Also, in : Ohio M. & S. J., Columbus, 1876, n. s., i, 341–362. *Also,* Reprint.

PLAIN directions for the care of the sick, and recipes for sick people. By a fellow of the College of Physicians of Philadelphia, and physician to several of the charitable institutions of the same city. sm. 8°. *New York*, [1875].

PRESTON (Ann). Nursing the sick and the training of nurses. An address delivered at the request of the board of managers of the Woman's Hospital, at Philadelphia. 8°. *Philadelphia*, 1863.

PRUSSIA. *Kriegs-Ministerium.* Unterrichtsbuch für Lazarethgehülfen. 8°. *Berlin*, 1886.

RICHARDSON (W. L.) Address on the duties and conduct of nurses in private nursing. 8°. *Boston*, 1887.

——. The same. With some notes on preventing the spread of infectious disease. 8°. *London*, 1887.

Nurses *and nursing.*

RIZZI (A.) * De mercenariæ nutricis selectu, atque institutione. 8°. *Ticini Regii*, [1841].

RUMSEY (H. W.) The training of nurses. 8°. [*London*, 1873.]

SASAGAWA Jinichi. Kanbio no Kokuroi. [The nurse's manual.] 12°. *Tokio*, 1886.
Japanese text.

SCHOMDERMARK (J.) jun. Iets over de verplering van bedlegerige zieken. 16°. *'s-Hertogen-bosch*, [1885].

——. Iets over de verpleging van zenuw-lijders en krankzinnigen. 16°. *'s-Hertogenbosch*, 1885.

SICK (P.) Die Krankenpflege in ihrer Be-gründung auf Gesundheitslehre, mit besonderer Berücksichtigung der weiblichen Krankenpflege. 8°. *Stuttgart*, 1887.

SIEVEKING (E. H.) Thoughts on nursing. 8°. [*London*, 1873.]

SIMON (M.) Die Krankenpflege. Theoretische und praktische Anweisungen. 16°. *Leipzig*, 1876.

SMITH (W. R.) Lectures on nursing. sm. 8°. *London*, 1875.

So Okada. Kamtiyo Kokoröe Kusá. [Manual for nurses.] 8°. *Tokio*, [*n. d.*]

STORER (H. R.) On nurses and nursing ; with especial reference to the management of sick women. 8°. *Boston*, 1868.

STRACK (C.) Sermo acad. de custodia ægro-rum, habitus in auditorio Universitatis Mogun-tiæ die 19 October ann. 1773. 16°. *Francof. a. M.*, 1779.

STUART (A. A.) Vereeniging voor Ziekenver-pleging. Gedachtenis-viering van haar 25-jarig bestaan, op 6 April 1869. 8°. *Amsterdam*, 1869.

TASCHENBUCH für Krankenpflegerinnen, 1882 ; vierter Jahrgang. 12°. *Weimar*, 1882.

THOMSON (A. T.) The domestic management of the sick-room, necessary in aid of medical treatment, for the cure of diseases. 1. Am., from the 2. Lond. ed., revised, with additions, by R. E. Griffith. 8°. *Philadelphia*, 1845.

TRALL (R. T.) The hygienic hand-book, in-tended as a practical guide for the sick room, ar-ranged alphabetically. With an appendix illus-trative of the hygeio-therapeutic movements. 8°. *New York*, 1873.

TRILLER (D. W.) Clinotechnia medica anti-quaria sive de diversis ægrotorum lectis secun-dum ipsa varia morborum genera convenienter instruendis commentarius medico-criticus. 4°. *Francofurti et Lipsiæ*, 1774.

TWINING (Louisa). Nurses for the sick ; with a letter to young women. 12°. *London*, 1861.

UNITED STATES. *Congress. Senate.* A bill for the relief of women enrolled as Army nurses, etc. 50. Cong., 1 sess. S. 373. Dec. 12, 1887. Introd. by Mr. Blair. roy. 8°. [*Washington*, 1887.]

UNITED STATES. *War Department. Surgeon-General's Office.* Circular No. 7. July 14, 1862. [To give greater utility to the acts of Miss D. L. Dix as "superintendent of women nurses" in general hospitals.] 8°. [*Washington*, 1862.]

——. Circular No. 8. July 14, 1862. [Quali-fications of candidates for service in the wom-en's department for nursing in the military hos-pitals of the United States.] 8°. [*Washington*, 1862.]

——. The same. September 17, 1864. 8°. [*Washington*, 1864.]

UNTERRICHT für Personen, welche den Kran-ken warten. Ein unentbehrliches Familienbuch, worinn sowohl die Lebensordnung und Diät der Kranken, als auch die Behandlung derselben in den verschiedenen Krankheitsumständen, die

Nurses *and nursing.*

Vorsichten bey Anwendung der Arzneyen, nebst den Zubereitung von mancherley Aufgüssen, Dekokten, Klystiren, Umschlägen, und Geträn-ken gründlich erkläret sind. Aus dem Franzö-sischen übersetzt, und mit einer Vorrede beglei-tet von J. J. Mellen. 12°. *Frankf. a. M.*, 1796.

VEITCH (Z. P.) Handbook for nurses for the sick. 2. ed. 12°. *London*, 1876.

VIRCHOW (R.) Die berufsmässige Ausbildung zur Krankenpflege. 12°. *Berlin*, 1869.

WARRINGTON (J.) The nurse's guide. Con-taining a series of instructions to females who wish to engage in the important business of nursing mother and child in the lying-in cham-ber. 12°. *Philadelphia*, 1839.

WHYTE (V.) Manual of nursing for home and hospital, including monthly nursing and the nursing of sick children. 16°. *Glasgow*, 1886.

WILSON (J. C.) Practical lessons in nursing. Fever-nursing ; designed for the use of profes-sional and other nurses, and especially as a text-book for nurses in training. 12°. *Philadelphia*, 1888.

WOLFF (S. J.) Die Kunst krank zu seyn, nebst einem Anhange von Krankenwärtern wie sie sind und seyn sollten. 16°. *Berlin*, 1811.

Adams (S. S.) The systematic training of nursery maids. J. Am. M. Ass., Chicago, 1887, ix, 129-131. *Also,* Reprint. — **Attire** (The) of nurses. Brit. M. J., Lond., 1883, ii, 737. — **Beale** (L. S.) Nursing the sick in hospi-tals, private families, and among the poor. Med. Times & Gaz., Lond., 1873, i, 270 ; 438. — **Blake-Brown** (Char-lotte). Training of nurses. Pacific M. & S. J., San Fran., 1880-81, xxiii, 485-492.—**Bourneville.** Les écoles d'in-firmières. Cong. internat. d'hyg. et de démog. Compt. rend. 1882, Genève, 1883, ii, 25-40.—**Cliet** (C. S.) Gardes-malades. J. d. conn. méd. prat., Par., 1845-6, xiii, 370-372.—**Croom** (J. H.) Nursing the sick. Edinb. Health Soc. Health Lect., 1882-3, 3. s., 175-194.—**Crosby** (A. B.) Common sense in the sick room. Med. Rec., N. Y., 1875, x, 593-596. — **Cullingworth** (C. J.) Sick nursing amongst the poor. Health Lect., Lond., 1880-81, iv, 43-58.— **Duckworth** (D.) Miss Florence Lees' drawing-room lectures to ladies on nursing. Lancet, Lond., 1878, i, 734.— **Edson** (B.) The importance of good nursing. Proc. M. Soc. County Kings, Brooklyn, 1878, iii, 191-199. — **Eyse-lein** (O.) Vorschläge zur rationellen Organisation des Ammen-Vermiethungswesens. Deutsches Wchnbl. f. Gsndhtspflg. u. Rettungsw., Berl., 1885, ii, 249.—**Fleming** (W. J.) Nursing ; an account of the Dresden Nursing Association, Albert Verein. Glasgow M. J., 1875, n. s., vii, 220-227. *Also,* Reprint.— **Freund.** Ueber Ammen-wesen und Ammen-Comptoirs. Vrtljschr. f. gerichtl. u. öff. Med., Berl., 1856, x, 53-78.—**Gr.** Ueber Krankenwar-tung. Allg. med. Ann., Altenb., 1808, xix, 657-664.—**Gross** (S. D.) Remarks on the training of nurses. Read origi-nally as a short report before the American Medical Asso-ciation at its meeting at New Orleans, May, 1869, and re-ferred by it to the several State medical societies. Tr. M. Soc. Penn., Phila., 1869, xx, 339-351. *Also,* Reprint. ——. Remarks on the importance of having trained nurses for the smaller towns and rural districts, and the proper method of securing them. Med. News, Phila., 1883, xliii, 284-286.— **Haller** (C.) Der Luftwechsel in den Krankenzimmern. Aerztl. Ber. d. k. k. allg. Krankenh. zu Wien (1870), 1871, 429-463. — **Harwell** (J. R.) Hygiene of the sick room. Nashville J. M. & S., 1880, n. s., xxv, 162-167.—**Heyfel-der.** Anweisung zur Kranken-Wartung. Jahrb. d. ges. Staatsarznk., Leipz., 1837, iii, 422-435. — **Hicks** (J. B.) On nursing systems. Brit. M. J., Lond., 1880, i, 11.— **Higgins** (J. N.) On the improvement of nurses in coun-try districts. Tr. Nat. Ass. Promot. Social Sc. 1861, Lond., 1862, 572-576. — **Hints** for the sick room. Pop. Sc. Month., N. Y., 1876, ix, 173-178.—**Hospital** nursing. Builder, Lond., 1860, xviii, 655. — **Inrichting** tot vor-ming van ziekenverpleegsters. Geneesk. Courant, Tiel, 1885, xxxix, no. 23. — **Irwin** (J. A.) Good nursing and its importance in the treatment of disease. Health Lect., Lond., 1878-9, ii, 93-110.—**Jacobi** (A.) The historical de-velopment of modern nursing. Pop. Sc. Month., N. Y., 1883, xxiii, 773-787. *Also,* Reprint.—**Kranken-War-tung** (Ueber). Von einem practischen Arzte. 'Ασκλη-πίειον, Berl., 1811, i, 1345-1356. — **Lady** nurses. [Edit.] Med. Times & Gaz., Lond., 1880, i, 401. — **Leyden** (E.) Ueber weibliche Krankenpflege und weibliche Heilkunst. Deutsche Rundschau, Berl., 1879, 5. Jahrg., 7. Hft., 126-148. — **Loew** (A.) Ueber Organisation der freiwilligen Krankenpflege. Mitth. d. Wien. med. Doct.-Coll., 1879, v, 13-20.—**Lückes** (*Miss* Eva C. E.) How far should our hospitals be training schools for nurses ? J. Hosp. Ass.,

Nurses *and nursing.*

Lond., 1884, 36–44.—**Macpherson** (W. G.) Suggestions for sick nursing in Indian station hospitals. Indian M. J., Calcutta, 1886, v, 131–140.—**Marson** (W.) [On the furniture of a sick room.] Med. & Phys. J., Lond., 1803, x, 175–177.—**Modern** nursing. Boston M. & S. J., 1880, ciii, 88–90.— **Murphy** (S. F.) Sickness in the house. *In :* Our homes [S. F. Murphy], 8°, Lond., 1883, 895–912. — **Neale** (J. E.) On nursing systems. Brit. M. J., Lond., 1880, i, 90. ———. Night nursing in the London hospitals. Lancet, Lond., 1871, ii, 642 ; 730 ; 784 ; 929.—**Nurses** and nursing. Brit. & For. M.-Chir. Rev., Lond., 1876, lvii, 283–301.—**Ogle** (J. W.) Nurses for the sick poor. Med. Times & Gaz., Lond., 1874, i, 395.—**Otis** (E. O.) Trained nurses ; a criticism. Boston M. & S. J., 1883, cix, 429.—**Packard** (J. H.) Training of nurses for the sick. Penn. Month., Phila., 1876, vii, 180–190. *Also*, Reprint. ———. A lecture on surgical nursing. Atlantic J. M., Richmond, 1884–5, ii, 49–59.—**Pampuri** (C.) Di un nuovo contratto rivelato dal Scipione Giordano. [Nurses.] Atti Accad. fis.-med.-statist. di Milano, 1873, xxix, 93–115.—**Paul** (F. T.) Nursing institutions. Brit. M. J., Lond., 1880, i, 125.— **Peabody** (G. L.) An address delivered to the pupils of the Training School of the New York Hospital. N. York M. J., 1885, xli, 541–546. — **Piderit.** Ueber Nosotrophie. Amtl. Ber. ü. d. Versamml. deutsch. Naturf. u. Aerzte 1842. Mainz, 1843, xx, 298–300. — **Preussen.** Kriegsministerium, Medizinal-Abtheilung ; die Ausbildung freiwilliger Krankenpfleger in den Garnison-Lazarethen betreffend. Veröffentl. d. k. Gsndhtsamtes, Berl., 1888, xii, 109.—**Ravoth.** Ueber die Ziele und Aufgaben der Krankenpflege. Tagebl. d. Versamml. deutsch. Naturf. u. Aerzte, Graz, 1875, xlviii, 248–253. — **Report** of committee on directory for nurses. Tr. M. & Chir. Fac. Maryland, Balt., 1885, 47–50.—**Robertson** (C. L.) Some results of night nursing ; being a record of the wet and dirty cases in the Sussex Lunatic Asylum, Hayward's Heath, during the first six months of 1861. J. Ment. Sc., Lond., 1860–62, vii, 391–398.—**Rowe** (G. H. M.) The training of nurses. Boston M. & S. J., 1883, cviii, 1–4.—**Seitz** (F.) Die Krankenpflege. Deutsche Rev., Berl., 1881, vi, 361–367.—**Sick-nursing.** An employment for educated women. Pub. Health., Lond., 1876, v, 121. —**Sieveking** (E. H.) A proposition to supply the laboring classes with nurses in the time of epidemic and other sicknesses. Tr. Epidemiol. Soc., Lond., 1856, 1–10. ———. An address on nursing of the sick. Brit. M. J., Lond , 1876, i, 183. — **Skilled** nursing for the sick poor. Med. Times & Gaz., Lond , 1876, ii, 570–572. — **Steele** (J. C.) Nursing and nursing institutes. San. Rec., Lond., 1874, i, 401 ; 415 ; 433 ; 1875, ii, 4 ; 17. — **Taylor** (R. W.) An address delivered to the graduating class of the Charity Hospital Training School for Nurses, Oct. 12, 1887. N. York M. J., 1887, xlvi, 479–481. *Also*, Reprint. — **Trautner** (T. M.) Om Sygeplejen paa Landet og Uddannelse af Sygeplejersker for dette. [Instruction of nurses.] Ugesk. f. Læger, Kjøbenh., 1879, 3. R., xxviii, 49 – 52. — **Veitch** (*Mme.*) Résumé d'un mémoire sur l'art de soigner les malades. Cong. internat. d'hyg., Brux., 1876, i, 871–875.— **Williams** (H. J.) The importance of intelligent nursing and the training of nurses. Atlanta M. & S. J., 1885–6, n. s., ii, 257–268.—**Worcester** (A.) The training of nurses in private practice. Med. Communicat. Mass. M. Soc., Bost., 1887, xiv, 89–100. *Also :* Boston M. & S. J., 1887, cxvii, 193–195.

Nurses (*Training schools for, and associations of*).

ANSTALT zur Ausbildung von Krankenpflegerinnen "Schwesternhaus vom rothen Kreuz" in Fluntem-Zürich. Bericht eüber die . . . 1., 1882–3 ; 2., 1883. 8°. *Zürich*, 1883–4.

BANGOR Institution of Trained Nurses. Annual reports by the committee to the public for the years 1880–81 to 1885–6. 8°. *Bangor*, [1881–6].

BATH Trained Nurses' Institute and Home. Annual report of the committee of management to the subscribers. 2., 1885. 8°. *Bath*, 1886.

BELGRAVIA Institute for Trained Nurses, London. Rules. 4°. [*London, n. d.*]

———. Prospectus. 8°. [*London, n. d.*]

BOSTON City Hospital Training School for Nurses. [Circular of the trustees, announcing arrangements for giving a two years' course of training to women desirous of becoming professional nurses ; with questions to be answered by candidate.] 4°. [*Boston*, 1879.]

———. [Circular announcing arrangements for giving a two years' course of training to women desirous of becoming professional nurses.] 4°. [*Boston*, 1879.]

Nurses (*Training schools for*).

———. [Circular of the trustees, announcing the establishment of the school. With questions to be answered by candidate.] fol. [*Boston, n. d.*]

———. The same. 4°. [*Boston, n. d.*]

BOSTON Medical Library. [Circular from the committee on the establishment of a bureau of registration for nurses at the Boston Medical Library.] 8°. [*Boston*, 1879.]

———. [Announcement of the opening of a directory of nurses at the Boston Medical Library.] 8°. [*Boston*, 187–.]

BOSTON Training School for Nurses, attached to the Massachusetts General Hospital. Circular announcing the establishment of the Training School for Nurses, and form of application for candidates. fol. [*Boston*, 1873.]

———. Reports of the directors for the years 1873–83 ; 1886. 8° & 12°. *Boston*, 1879–87.

BRADFORD Nurses' Institution. Annual reports of the committee. 8., 1879 ; 10.–12., 1881–3. 8°. *Bradford*, 1880–84.

BRITISH Lying-in Hospital for Married Women. School of Midwifery and Nursing. [Circular, on the conditions of admission as students or nurses.] 8°. [*London, n. d.*]

BROOKLYN Training School for Nurses, attached to the Brooklyn Hospital. Annual report of the managers. 3., 1882–3. 8°. *Brooklyn*, 1883.

CAMBRIDGE Home and Training School for Nurses. Annual reports of the committee of management to the council and the public. 2.– 4., 1874–5 to 1876–7 ; 6.–9., 1878–9 to 1881–2 ; 11., 1883–4 ; 12., 1884–5. 8°. *Cambridge*, 1875–85.

CHARING CROSS Hospital, London. Lectures to the nursing staff. Session of 1884–5. broadside. [*London*, 1884.]

COLLEGE of Physicians. Directory of nurses. An abstract of the first annual report of the committee for the year 1881–2. 8°. [*Philadelphia*, 1882.]

———. Application for registration. 8°. [*Philadelphia, n. d.*]

———. Circular to nurses. April 20, 1882. 8°. [*Philadelphia*, 1882.]

———. Circular to physicians. 8°. [*Philadelphia*, 1882.]

CONNECTICUT Training School for Nurses, attached to the State Hospital, at New Haven. [Circular to the public, announcing its organization and soliciting contributions.] 8°. [*New Haven*, 1873.]

———. Annual reports of the executive committee. 1.–3., 1873–6 ; 7., 1880. 8°. *New Haven*, 1875–81.

DEACONESSES' Institution and Hospital, the Green, Tottenham, London. Annual reports of the council. 1., 1868–9 ; 4.–10., 1871–2 to 1877–8 ; 12.–19., 1879–80 to 1886–7. 12° & 8°. *Tottenham*, 1869–87.

———. Appeal of the trustees to the public for pecuniary assistance. Christmas, 1873. 24°. [*London*, 1873.]

———. Donations to the building fund account. 16°. *Tottenham*, 1887.

———. [A short account of a visit to the institution.] 8°. [*London*, 1887 ?] *Repr. from :* Footsteps of Truth.

DIAKONISSEN - MUTTERHAUS zu Dresden. Kleine Chronik. 4. qr., 1879. 8°. [*Dresden*, 1880.]

DISTRICT Nursing Society, Liverpool. Names and addresses of some of the charities in Liverpool, and other information. Printed for the use of, and in connection with, the . . . 8°. *Liverpool*, 1869.

Nurses (*Training schools for*).

EAST LONDON Nursing Society. Annual report of the committee to the subscribers, for the year 1885. 12°. *London*, 1886.

EDINBURGH Institution for the Training of Sick Nurses. [Circular of the directors, appealing to the public for assistance until the institution becomes self-supporting, Aug., 1878.] 4°. [*Edinburgh*, 1878.]

EIGENBRODT. Der Alice-Frauenverein für Krankenpflege, seine Entstehung und leitenden Grundsätze, seine Leistungen und Ziele. 2. Aufl. 8°. *Darmstadt*, 1877.

FARRAND Training School for Nurses, Detroit. Annual report of the training school committee to the board of trustees of Harper Hospital. 1., 1884–6. 8°. *Detroit*, 1887.

GLASGOW Training Home for Nurses. [First report, from Feb. 9 to Dec. 31, 1874.] 8°. [*Glasgow*, 1875.]

HAMPSHIRE Nurses' Institute, Southampton. Annual reports of the committee. 5., 1872; 8.–16., 1875–83. 8°. *Southampton*, 1884.

INSTITUTION for Nurses for Nervous and Mental Disorders, London. Annual reports of the superintendent. 1., 1865–6; 5., 1869–70; 6., 1870–71. 16°. *London*, 1866–71.

——. Rules to be observed by the nurses sent out, drawn up by C. Lockhart Robertson. 16°. [*London*, 1867.]

——. Statement of the superannuation fund, Dec., 1867. With the rules governing fines of nurses. 16°. [*London*, 1868.]

——. Questions which the candidates for the situation of nurse are requested to answer. 1 sheet. fol. [*London*, n. d.]

INSTITUTION of Trained Nurses for the City and County of Worcester. Rules of the . . . with report, balance sheet, and list of donations and subscriptions. 1., 1879. 8°. *Worcester*, 1880.

INSTITUTION of Trained Nurses for the Town and County of Leicester. Annual reports of the committee to the subscribers. 16., 1882; 17., 1883. 8°. *Leicester*, 1883–4.

JOHNSON (J. T.) Introductory address delivered at the opening of the second course of lectures of the Washington Training School for Nurses. 8°. *Washington*, 1880.

KING's College Hospital, London, W. C. Lectures to the nursing staff, session of 1884–5. 1 sheet. fol. [*London*, 1884.]

LEEDS Training Nurses' Institution. Annual reports of the committee. 1., 1876; 3., 1878; 4., 1879; 6.–8., 1881–3. 8°. *Leeds*, 1877–84.

LIVERPOOL Institution for the Training and Employment of Nurses. Annual reports of the committee. 17., 1871; 24.–29., 1878–83. 12°. *Liverpool*, 1872–84.

——. Fundamental laws of the . . . 8°. [*Liverpool*, n. d.]

——. Rules for the . . . 4°. [*Liverpool*, n. d.]

——. The same. 4°. [*Liverpool*, 188–.]

LIVERPOOL Training School and Home for Nurses, Dover St. Annual reports of the committee to the subscribers. 1.–26., 1862–87. 8°. *Liverpool*, 1863–88.

——. Regulations as to training probationer nurses. 4°. [*Liverpool*, n. d.]

——. The rules of the society. 4°. [*Liverpool*, n. d.]

LONDON Association of Nurses. Circular. 4°. [*London*, n. d.]

LONDON Diocesan Deaconess Institution, Burton Crescent, W. C., and Tavistock Crescent, W. Annual reports of the committee of management to the officers and donators. 8., 1868–9; 12., 1872–3. 8°. *London*, 1869–73.

Nurses (*Training schools for*).

LONDON Diocesan Deaconess Institution, etc. Circular showing what it desires to do. 8°. [*n. p., n. d.*]

MANCHESTER District and Private Nursing Institution. Annual reports of the general committee. 2., 1866–7; 5., 1869–70; 6., 1870–71; 9.–16., 1873–4 to 1880–81. 8°. *Manchester*, 1867–81.

MASSACHUSETTS General Hospital, McLean Asylum Training School for Nurses. [Circular and announcement by the trustees of the Massachusetts General Hospital, of a two years' course of training in general nursing.] 4°. *Boston*, 188–.]

MILDMAY Deaconess Institution, Nursing Branch. [Circular relating to probationer nurses, with regulations, etc.] 8°. [*London*, 1884?]

MITCHELL Home, Torquay Institution for Trained Nurses. Annual report of the committee. 7., 1883. 8°. *Torquay*, 1884.

——. Nurses for private families. Rules. 4°. [*Torquay*, n. d.]

——. Rules for district nurses. 4°. [*Torquay*, n. d.]

——. Rules for probationers and nurses. 4°. [*Torquay*, n. d.]

NEWPORT Hospital. Winter course of lectures to nurses by the medical staff of Newport Hospital. 8°. [*Newport*, n. d.]

NEW YORK Agency for Trained Nurses, New York City. Miss A. S. Mabie, proprietor and manager. [Circular and testimonial.] 8°. [*New York*, 1879.]

NEW YORK (*City*). *Department of Public Charities*. The Training School for Nurses, Charity Hospital, Blackwell's Island. [Notice of, with an extract from the annual report of the chief of staff for 1881.] 8°. *New York*, 1882.

——. The Charity Hospital Training School for Male Nurses, Blackwell's Island. [Information for, and questions to be answered by, applicants.] 4°. [*New York*, n. d.]

NEW YORK Hospital. Training School for Nurses. Annual report of the conference committee in charge of the . . . for the year 1883. 8°. [*New York*, 1884.]

NORTH LONDON Nursing Association for the Poor. Annual reports of the executive committee. 1.–3., 1881–3. 8°. *London*, 1882–4.

ORDER of St. John of Jerusalem in England. Nurses for the sick poor. Report of the committee of the Order of St. John of Jerusalem in England, appointed on St. John Baptist's day, 1873. 8°. *London*, 1874.

PHILADELPHIA Lying-in and Nurse Charity. Appeal for the supply of a greater number of intelligent women to become trained as nurses for the sick. [Signed J. Warrington, Hannah Miller, and Ann Davis, on behalf of the executive committee of the institution. Feb. 1, 1854.] 8°. *Philadelphia*, 1855.

PUTNAM (C. P.) American Social Science Association. Training schools for nurses in America. Read at the annual meeting of the association, Oct. 14, 1874. 8°. [*n. p., n. d.*]

ROBERTSON (C. L.) Rules to be observed by the nurses sent out from the Institution for Nurses for Nervous and Mental Disorders, Grosvenor Square, London. 16°. [*n. p., n. d.*]

ROYAL Southern Hospital Nursing Institution, Liverpool. Annual report of the committee. 1., 1880–81. 4°. [*Liverpool*, 1882.]

SAINT JOHN's House and Sisterhood for the Training and Employment of Nurses, London. Annual reports of the committee to the governors and subscribers. 33.–37., 1882–4; 39., 1886. 8°. *London*, 1883–7.

Nurses (*Training schools for*).

———. [Statement of the council to the governors and subscribers, of the circumstances which led to the resignation of many sisters.] fol. [*London*, 1883.]

———. [Circular of the council, stating its object, with an appeal for assistance towards the various branches of the work.] 8°. [*London*, 1884.]

———. Ladies as hospital nurses. 8°. [*n. p., n. d.*]

———. House and Sisterhood of Saint John the Evangelist, for the Training and Employment of Nurses. Circular to nurses. 8°. [*London, n. d.*]

SAINT LOUIS Training School for Nurses. Annual reports of the executive committee to the society. 1.–3., 1883–4 to 1885–6. 8°. *Saint Louis*, 1885–7.

SAINT THOMAS's Hospital, London. The Nightingale Fund. Annual reports of the trustees of the Nightingale Fund, for training nurses, for the years 1871; 1872; 1886. fol. *London*, 1872–87.

———. Duties of probationer under the "Nightingale Fund". 4°. [*London, n. d.*]

———. Regulations as to the training of hospital nurses under the Nightingale Fund. fol. [*London, n. d.*]

SARAH ACLAND Memorial and Home for Nurses, Oxford. Annual report of the committee of the . . . and Medical and Surgical Home to the subscribers for the year 1883–4. 8°. *Oxford*, 1884.

SHEFFIELD Nurses' Home and Training Institution. Annual report of the committee. 12.–13.; 1882–3 to 1883–4. 8°. *Sheffield*, 1883–4.

SIR PATRICK DUNN's Hospital Maternity, Midwives' Home. [Announcement of the governors, to construct a permanent home on the hospital premises for the training of nurses. Feb. 21, 1874.] 8°. [*Dublin*, 1874.]

———. [Appeal of the governors for subscriptions.] 8°. [*Dublin, n. d.*]

———. [Circular of the governors of the hospital, giving terms and conditions for the admission of nurses.] fol. [*Dublin, n. d.*]

———. Regulations. fol. [*Dublin, n. d.*]

———. Roster of midwives on duty. fol. [*Dublin, n. d.*]

SOCIETY of the Training School for Nurses, attached to Bellevue Hospital. Annual reports of the managers. Presented to the visiting committee for Bellevue and other hospitals. 1.–8., 1873–4 to 1880; 10.–13., 1882–5. 12° & 8°. *New York*, 1874–86.

SOUTH HAMPSTEAD Private Hospital and Nursing Institute. Prospectus of the . . . 18°. [*London*, 1884?]

STAFFORDSHIRE Institution for Nurses. Annual report of the committee. 12., 1883. 8°. *Hanley*, 1884.

STATE Charities Aid Association. No. 1. Report of the committee on hospitals, Dec. 23, 1872. Training School for Nurses to be attached to Bellevue Hospital. 8°. *New York*, [1873?]

———. No. 2. A century of nursing, with hints towards the organization of a training school. By a member of the hospital committee. 8°. *New York*, 1876.

STEIN (H.) Notice explicative concernant l'institution des diaconesses danoises et leur établissement à Frederiksberg. Présenté au Congrès d'hygiène et de sauvetage de Bruxelles par le Comité danois. 4°. *Copenhague*, 1876.

STRANGFORD (*Viscountess*). Hospital training for ladies. An appeal to the hospital boards in England. 8°. *London*, 1874.

Nurses (*Training schools for*).

SWITZERLAND. *Army Medical Department*. Instruction pour les fraters et les infirmiers de l'armée fédérale. 12°. *Berne*, 1862.

THOMPSON (W. G.) Training schools for nurses; with notes on twenty-two schools. 16°. *New York*, 1883.

TRAINED Nurses' Annuity Fund, London, E. C. Annual reports of the committee, for the years 1878–80; 1882; 1883. 12°. *London*, 1879–84.

TRAINING School for Nurses, connected with the Post-Graduate Medical School and Hospital, New York City. Annual report of the superintendent. 1., 1886–7. 12°. *New York*, 1887.

TRAINING School for Nurses, Woman's Hospital, Philadelphia. Annual report of the executive committee, for the year 1875. 12°. *Philadelphia*, 1876.

UNITED Relief Works of the Society for Ethical Culture. Annual reports of the district nursing section of the . . . 1.–3., 1879–80 to 1882. 8°. *New York*, 1881–3.

UNITED STATES. *Department of the Interior. Bureau of Education*. Circulars of information of the Bureau of Education. No. 1, 1879. Training schools for nurses. 8°. *Washington*, 1879.

———. Circulars of information of the Bureau of Education. No. 1, 1882. The inception, organization, and management of training schools for nurses. 8°. *Washington*, 1882.

UNITED STATES. *War Department. Adjutant-General's Office*. General Orders, No. 351. Washington, Oct. 29, 1863. [Rules for the employment of women nurses in the U. S. general hospitals.] Official. 8°. [*Washington*, 1863.]

VEREENIGING tot Ziekenverpleging te Amsterdam. Uittreksel uit het reglement der . . . fol. [*Amsterdam*, 184–.]

———. Over instelligen tot verpleging van zieken, met een verslag van de oprigting der . . . en van hare werkzaamheden gedurende het jaar 1844. 8°. *Amsterdam*, 1845.

WASHINGTON Training School for Nurses. Annual announcements for the sessions of 1879–80 (2.); 1882–3 to 1885–6 (5.–8.). 16° & 8°. *Washington*, 1879–85.

———. Circular. Appeal of the .·. . [to the benevolent members of society, for pecuniary aid towards placing the institution on a basis of greater permanence and usefulness.] fol. [*Washington*, 188–.]

———. Circular of the . . . [To organize a loan exhibition for the benefit of the institution.] 8°. [*Washington*, 1881.]

———. Washington Directory for Nurses. Circular No. 1. To physicians [announcing the establishment of the directory]. Dec. 15, 1882. 8°. [*Washington*, 1882.]

———. Washington Directory for Nurses. Circular No. 9. To wet nurses [with a form of application]. Dec. 15, 1882. 8°. [*Washington*, 1882.]

WESTMINSTER Training School and Home for Nurses, S. W. Annual reports of the managing committee, for the years 1881; 1883. 8°. *London*, 1882–4.

ZENANA and Medical Mission Training School and Home, London, S. W. Annual reports of the committee. 3., 1882; 4., 1883. 8°. *London*, 1883–4.

———. The prisoners of the Zenana. *Cutting from*: Word & Work, March 20, 1884.

———. [Account of the annual meeting of . . . 1884.] *Cutting from*: The Record, June 6, 1884.

Berry (J. C.) Training schools for nurses. Sei-i-Kwai M. J., Tôkyô, 1887, vi, 28–34. — **Boston** City Hospital Training School for Nurses. Boston M. & S. J., 1879, ci,

Nurses (*Training schools for*).

816–818.—**Bourneville.** Écoles d'infirmières laïques à la Salpêtrière et d'infirmiers laïques à Bicêtre. Rapport présenté au Conseil municipal de Paris. Union méd. et scient. du nord-est, Reims, 1878, ii, 262–268.—**Braun.** Die Nothwendigkeit der Krankenwärter-Schulen. Med. Cor.-Bl. bayer. Aerzte, Erlang., 1842, 134–137.—**Bristowe** (J. S.) How far should our hospitals be training-schools for nurses? J. Hosp. Ass., Lond., 1884, 26–36. [Discussion]. 44–56.—**Dubois** (E.) Rapport sur la proposition de M. le Dr. Duchaussoy, concernant la création d'une école de gardes-malades. Bull. Soc. de méd. prat. de Par., 1876, 128–132.—**Duchaussoy.** D'une école de gardes-malades. Bull. Soc. de méd. prat. de Par., 1877, 59–65. — **Fleming** (W. J.) Nursing; an account of the Dresden Nursing Association, Albert Verein. Glasgow M. J., 1875, [4.] s., vii, 220–227. — **H.** (E.) A French training school for nurses. Brit. M. J., Lond., 1878, ii, 383. — **Haward** (W.) Ladies and hospital nursing. Contemp. Rev., Lond., 1879, xxxiv, 490–503. — **Hornemann** (E.) Sundhedspleien og Skolerne. Hyg. Medd., Kjøbenh., 1861, iii, pt. 2, 81–149.—**Langlet.** Rapport fait à l'École de médecine: Sur la création à Reims d'une école de gardes-malades. Union méd. et scient. du nord-est, Reims, 1885, ix, 146–157.—**Meyer** (J. S.) Ogsaa et Par Linier om den fra Diakonissestiftelsen ydede Sygepleje. [A few words more on the nurse question.] Ugesk. f. Læger, Kjøbenh., 1880, 4. R., i, 249–254. — **Nogle** Bemærkninger om Diakonissestiftelsen. [On schools for female nurses] *Ibid.*, 205–212. — **Nursing** schools and the future of nursing. San. Rec., Lond., 1883–4, n. s., v, 536.—**Ogle** (W.) Nurses; how to make them, how to use them, how to pay them. Rep. Cong. San. Inst. Gr. Brit. 1879, Lond., 1880, i, 100–104.—**Oppert** (F.) Ueber besondere Lehranstalten für Heildiener und Krankenwartpersonal im neuen Reich. Deutsche Klinik, Berl., 1873, xxv, 41–44.—**Packard** (J. H.) On the training of nurses for the sick. Boston M. & S. J., 1876, xcv, 573–579. *Also:* West. Lancet, San Fran., 1876, vi, 687–694. *Also:* Penn. Month., Phila., 1876, vii, 180–190. *Also,* Reprint.—**Perrigo** (J.) A short account of St. John's House and Sisterhood. Canada M. Rec., Montreal, 1872–3, i, 3.— **Platt** (W. B.) Table of statistics of several training schools for nurses, in their relation to their hospitals and to each other, prepared that the friends of the Connecticut Training School may at the close of its tenth year understand its position as compared with similar institutions elsewhere. Med. News, Phila., 1885, xlvii, 444. — **Rapport** sur la proposition de M. le Dr. Duchaussoy, concernant la création d'une école de gardes-malades. France méd., Par., 1876, xxiii, 719.—**Report** of the committee on the training of nurses. Tr. Am. M. Ass., Phila., 1869, xx, 161–174. *Also:* Tr. M. Soc. Penn.,-Phila., 1869, 5. s., ii, 339–351.—**Spolert.** Samaritskoler og Samariterskoler. Norsk Mag. f. Lægevidensk., Christiania, 1883, xiii, 654–663. — **Thorr** (J.) Die Krankenpflege und Oekonomieführung der barmherzigen Schwestern in München. N. med.-chir. Ztg., München, 1851, Beilage zu No. 8, 1–8.— **Training** school for nurses in connection with St. Bartholomew's Hospital. Brit. M. J., Lond., 1877, i, 557.— **Ziliotto** (P.) Sulla convenienza d' instituire una scuola pratica per far dei buoni infermieri. Gior. veneto di sc. med., Venezia, 1873, 3. s., xix, 151–162.

Nurses for infants.

See **Colostrum**; Infants (*Food, etc., of*); **Milk** (*Human*).

Nurse's (The) manual and mother's medical adviser, a guide to the inexperienced. By a practising physician. 238 pp. 8°. *Philadelphia, Lindsay & Blakiston,* 1845.

Nurses' Training School. *See* **Washington** Training School for Nurses.

de Nursia (Benedictus). [Libellus de conservatione sanitatis.] [*Incipit:*] Johannes Philippi de Lignamine Messanensis Siculus, ad S. D. N. Sixtum quartum, pontificem maximum. [*Fol.* 1 *B :*] Tabula hujus libri. [*In fine tab. :*] Sequitur nunc libellus ipse de conservatione sanitatis, secundum ordinem alphabeti distinctus. [*Ad finem :*] Rome in domo nobilis viri Johannis Philippi de Lignamine Messanensis. S. D. N. familiaris hic libellus impressus est anno Domini mcccclxxv, die xiiii mensis Januarii, Pont. Syxti IIII, anno ejus quarto. 138 l. 4°. [*Rome,* 1475.]

Two missing leaves have been supplied in manuscript. The dedicatory epistle to Pope Sixtus IV, with which this book begins, was not printed in all copies of the edition.

————. The same. Pulcherrimum et utilissimum opus ad sanitatis conservationem . . . incipit fœliciter. Similiter etiam de magistro Tadeo

66

de Nursia (Benedictus)—continued. de Florentia de regimine sanitatis secundum quattuor partes anni. Sequitur nunc libellus ipse de conservatione sanitatis secundum ordinem alphabeti distinctus. [*Ad finem :*] . . . opera et industria Dominici de Lapis . . . feliciter finiunt anno d.m.cccc.lxxvii. 140 l. 4°. [*Bononiæ, D. de Lapis,* 1477.]

————. The same. [Libellus de conservatione sanitatis secundum ordinem alphabeti distinctus.] [*Incipit:*] Tabula hujus libri. [*In fine:*] Registrum hujus libri. 60 l. 4°. [*n. p., n. d.*]

Gothic letter, without pagination, catch-words, or signatures. Panzer has: [Romæ, Stephanus Plannck, 1485.]

Nursing (*Sore mouth from*).

See **Mouth** (*Inflammation of*) *in pregnancy, etc.*

Nursing Home for Convalescent Women and Sick Children, Stratford-on-Avon. Annual reports of the committee to the subscribers and donors. 2.–4., 1873–5; 9., 1880; 11.–12., 1882–3. 8° & 12°. *Stratford-upon-Avon,* 1874–84.

Nursing House, Mildmay Road, London, N. *See* **Mildmay** Deaconess Institution, Nursing Branch.

Nursing (The) Record. A journal for nurses and a chronicle of hospital and institution news, etc. [Weekly.] Nos. 1–3, v. 1, April 5–19, 1888. sm. 4°. *London, S. Low, Marston & Co.* Current.

Nursing-bottles.

See **Infants** (*Food, etc., of*).

Nursing-bottles (*Collection of plates of patents for*).

Baker (R. C.) Nursing bottle. No. 358008; Feb. 22, 1887.—**Barton** (E. A.) Nursing bottle. No. 234224; Nov. 9, 1880.—**Bray** (J. W.) Nursing-bottle supports. No. 179995; July 18, 1876.—**Briere** (J.) Nursing-bottle. No. 189691; April 17, 1877.—**Bullard** (I.) Nursing-bottles. No. 194859; Sept. 4, 1877.—**Burr** (M. S.) Improvement in nursing-bottles. No. 68285; Aug. 27, 1867. Reissue No. 6809; Dec. 21, 1875.—**Carpenter** (W. C.) Regulator for nursing bottles. No. 244181; July 12, 1881.— **Christie** (J. J.) Improvement in nursing-bottles. No. 166747; Aug. 17, 1875.—**Darrach** (S. A.) Nursing-bottle. No. 220351; Oct. 7, 1879.—**Forster** (F. E.) Nursing-bottle. No. 335347; Feb. 2, 1886.—**France** (S. W.) Nursing bottle. No. 216734; June 24, 1879.—**Glattsteine** (M.) Nursing bottle. No. 279935; June 26, 1883.—**Haven** (H. C.) Nursing-bottle. No. 351596; Oct. 26, 1886.—**Hayes** (H. H.) Nursing-bottle fitting. No. 236583; Jan. 11, 1881. — **Kennish** (W.) Nursing bottles. No. 179416; July 4, 1876. ————. Nursing bottles. No. 183808; Oct. 31, 1876.—**Knapp** (A. M. & H.) Nursing-bottle valves. No. 179204; June 27, 1876.—**Marsh** (F. F.) & **Thompson** (A. F.) Improvement in nursing apparatus. No. 163022; May 11, 1875.—**Meyer** (L.) Nursing-bottles. No. 197156; Nov. 13, 1877.—**Michaels** (M. A.) Nursing-bottles. No. 194454; Aug. 21, 1877.—**Michales** (M. A.) & **Bald** (J. M.) Nursing-bottle. No. 222070; Nov. 25, 1879.—**Morris** (J. A.) Nursing-bottle and nipple. No. 280656; July 3, 1883.—**Patch** (J. W.) Nursing-shield. No. 196594; Oct. 30, 1877.—**Potter** (J. E.) Nursing-bottle. No. 224557; Feb. 17, 1880.—**Selièvre** (E. L. P.) Nursing-bottle. No. 345518; July 13, 1886.—**Siebenlist** (E.) Nipples for nursing-bottles. No. 210157; Nov. 19, 1878.—**Thomas** (J.) Feeding-bottle. No. 275288; April 3, 1883.—**Thompson** (J.) Nursing-bottle. No. 227075; April 27, 1880.—**Tumbleson** (W. W.) Nursing-bottle tube. No. 329103; Oct. 27, 1885.—**Ware** (W. F.) Nursing-bottle. No. 347018; Aug. 10, 1886.—**Wheelock** (C. B.) Nursing bottle. No. 357439; Feb. 8, 1887.—**White** (G. F.) Nursing apparatus. No. 196610; Oct. 30, 1877.— **Whitney** (S. A.) Nursing-bottle. No. 177185; May 9, 1876.

Nusbaum (Ferd.) *See* **Engelmann** (Charles). Kreuznach, ses sources minérales [etc.] 8°. *Heidelberg,* 1839.

Nusche (Joannes). * De fracturis quæ in variis ossis femoris partibus obtinent. 40 pp. 4°. *Argentorati, ex prelo J. H. Heitzii,* [1772].

Also [Abstr.], *in:* Weiz (F. A.) Neue Ausz. [etc.] 12°. *Leipzig,* 1776, v, 54–60.

Nusche (Joannes Fridericus). * De usu et abusu balneorum domesticorum. 34 pp. 4°. *Argentorati, typ. M. Pauschingeri,* [1740].

Nushard (Fr. Wilhelm) [1785–   ]. * Skizze einer Dermato-Pathologie mit physiologischer Vorbemerkung. 1 p. l., viii, 164 pp., 1 l. 8°. *Prag, Sommer*, 1816.
    See, also, **Feitl** (Franciscus Antonius). * Diss. sistens historias [etc.] 8°. *Pragæ*, 1841.

Nussbaum (Heinrich). * Beiträge zur Kenntniss der Anatomie und Physiologie der Herznerven und zur physiologischen Wirkung des Curare. 84 pp., 1 l., 1 pl. 8°. *Dorpat, C. Mattiesen*, 1875.

—— & **Nencki** (Leon). O żywieniu się i pokarmach. [On food and nutrition.] 54 pp. 8°. *Warszawa, K. Kowalewskiego*, 1887.

von Nussbaum (Joh. Nepomuk) [1829–   ]. * Cornea artificialis. 16 pp. 8°. *München, C. R. Schurich*, 1853.
                                                                c.

——. Die Behandlung der Hornhaut-Trübungen, mit besonderer Berücksichtigung der Einsetzung einer künstlichen Hornhaut (Cornea artificialis). 58 pp., 2 pl. 8°. *München, J. G. Cotta*, 1856.

——. Die Pathologie und Therapie der Ankylosen. 47 pp. 4°. *München, J. G. Cotta*, 1862. [P., v. 305.]

——. Die Verletzungen des Unterleibes.
    In: HANDB. d. allg. u. spec. Chir., Erlang., 1866, iii, 2. Abth., A, Abschn. vii, No. 1, 165–212.

——. Vier chirurgische Briefe an seine in den Krieg ziehenden ehemaligen Schüler. 1 p. l., 68 pp. 18°. *München, J. G. Cotta*, 1866.

——. Vierunddreissig Ovariotomieen. 15 pp. 4°. *München, J. J. Leutner*, 1869.

——. Neue Heilmethoden bei Geschwüren. 7 pp. 4°. *München, F. Straub*, 1873.
    Repr. from: Aerztl. Int.-Bl., München, 1873, xx.

——. Die Drainagirung der Bauchhöhle und die intraperitioneale Injection. Ein Beitrag zur Lehre über penetrirende Bauchwunden und Ovariotomie. 14 pp. 8°. *München, J. A. Finsterlin*, 1874.

——. Die chirurgische Klinik zu München im Jahre 1875. Ein Andenken für seine Schüler. 63 pp. 8°. *Stuttgart, F. Enke*, 1875.

——. Rapport über die medicinische und chirurgische Geschichte des amerikanischen Rebellions-Krieges von 1861–5. 10 pp. 8°. *München, J. A. Finsterlin*, 1875.
    Repr. from: Aerztl. Int.-Bl., München, 1875, xxii.

——. Ueber die Behandlung unglücklicher Vorkommnisse nach einfachen und complicirten Beinbrüchen, insbesondere über Knochen-Transplantation. (Ein Vortrag, gehalten am 13. Februar 1875 im ärztlichen Bezirksvereine zu München.) 18 pp., 1 pl. 8°. *München, J. A. Finsterlin*, 1875.
    Repr. from: Aerztl. Int.-Bl., München, 1875, xxii.

——. Ueber den Krebs vom klinischen Standpunkte. (Ein Vortrag, gehalten am 9. März 1875 im ärztlichen Vereine zu München.) 23 pp. 8°. *München, J. A. Finsterlin*, 1875.
    Repr. from: Aerztl. Int.-Bl., München, 1875, xxii.

——. Bildung eines künstlichen Harnleiters. Nervendehnung bei centralem Leiden. Zwei klinische Mittheilungen (nebst einer vorläufigen Anzeige über Heilung von Hernien). 31 pp. 8°. *München, J. A. Finsterlin*, 1876.

——. Einige Bemerkungen zur Kriegs-Chirurgie aus einem klinischen Vortrage. 10 pp. 8°. *München, J. A. Finsterlin*, 1877.
    Repr. from: Aerztl. Int.-Bl., München, 1877, xxiv.

——. Ueber den Schok grosser Verletzungen und Operationen, nebst Mittheilungen über Laparatomien. 26 pp. 8°. *München, J. A. Finsterlin*, 1877.
    Repr. from: Aerztl. Int.-Bl., München, 1877, xxiv.

——. Sonst und Jetzt. Einige Bemerkungen zur Ovariotomie. Nervendehnungen. Drei Ab-

von Nussbaum (Joh. Nepomuk)—continued. handlungen. 23 pp. 8°. *München, M. Rieger*, 1878.
    Repr. from: Ann. d. städt. allg. Krankenh. zu München, 1878, i.

——. Die Operation einer Intercostal-Neuralgie. Vortrag gehalten am 20. Dezember 1878 im ärztlichen Bezirksverein zu München. 16 pp. 8°. *München, J. A. Finsterlin*, 1879.
    Repr. from: Aerztl. Int.-Bl., München, 1879, xxvi.

——. Leitfaden zur antiseptischen Wundbehandlung. Insbesondere zur Lister'schen Methode für seine Schüler und für praktische Aerzte. 2. Aufl. iv, 160 pp. 8°. *Stuttgart, F. Enke*, 1879.

CONTENTS.

I. Ist jeder Chirurg verpflichtet, die antiseptische Methode zu kennen und zu üben?
II. Was bedarf man hiezu?
III. Wie wendet man ihre Heilmittel an?
IV. Muss diese Methode auch im Kriege geübt werden?
The 2. ed., with additions, of his: Die chirurgische Klinik zu München im Jahre 1875. 8°. *Stuttgart*, 1875.

——. The same. 4. Aufl. 1 p. l., 170 pp. 8°. *Stuttgart, F. Enke*, 1881.

——. The same. Leitfaden zur antiseptischen Wundbehandlung mit Rücksicht auf ihren gegenwärtigen Standpunkt. 5. Aufl. xx, 308 pp. 8°. *Stuttgart, F. Enke*, 1887.

——. The same. Le pansement antiseptique, exposé spécialement d'après la méthode de Lister, dédié à ses élèves et aux médecins praticiens. Trad. sur la 2. éd. allemande par le Dr. E. de la Harpe. 185 pp. 8°. *Paris, J.-B. Baillière & fils*, 1880.

——. Die Verletzungen des Unterleibes. viii, 176 pp. 8°. *Stuttgart, F. Enke*, 1880.
    Forms Lfg. 44 of Deutsche Chirurgie.

——. Einfluss der Antiseptik auf die gerichtliche Medicin, aus dem Schluss-Vortrage der Winter-Klinik 1880. 33 pp. 8°. *München, J. A. Finsterlin*, 1880.

——. Ueber Enterotomie, Gastrotomie und Leberdrainage. Ein Vortrag in der Sitzung des ärztlichen Bezirksvereines München, am 27. December 1879. 22 pp. 12°. *München, J. A. Finsterlin*, 1880.
    Repr. from: Aerztl. Int.-Bl., München, 1880, xxvii.

——. Die gegenwärtige Behandlung der Unterleibsbrüche. Vortrag gehalten im ärztl. Bezirks-Vereine in München am 5. März 1881. 22 pp. 8°. *München, J. A. Finsterlin*, 1881.
    Repr. from: Aerztl. Int.-Bl., München, 1881, xxviii.

——. Werth und Gefahren der Antiseptica, nebst einigen Bemerkungen über deren Benützung in der Kriegschirurgie; vorgetragen in der Sitzung des ärztl. Vereines zu München am 12. April 1882. 30 pp. 8°. *München, F. Straub*, 1882.

——. Festrede zu Philipp Franz v. Walther's hundertjährigen Geburtstage, gehalten am 4. Jänner 1882 im ärztlichen Vereine zu München. 21 pp. 4°. *München, F. Straub*, 1882.

——. Krankheiten des Unterleibes.
    In: HANDB. d. allg. u. spec. Chir., Erlang., 1882, iii, 2. Abth., A, 165–212.

——. Der erste Verband bei verschiedenen Verwundungen; Vortrag in der Stiftung des ärztlichen Bezirksvereins am 7. Juni 1882. 27 pp. 8°. *München, J. A. Finsterlin*, 1882.

——. Ein Vademecum für den praktischen Chirurgen. Skizzen aus der chirurgischen Klinik des Herrn Professor Dr. Ritter von Nussbaum. Von Dr. Isenschmid. 1. Hft. Sommer 1881; 2. Hft. Winter 1881–2. 1 p. l., 118 pp. 8°. *München, J. A. Finsterlin*, 1882.

——. The same. Weitere Skizzen aus der chirurgischen Klinik des Herrn Geheimrat von Nussbaum von Dr. Isenschmid. [Sommer-Se-

von Nussbaum (Joh. Nepomuk)—continued.
mester 1882 u. Winter-Semester 1882–3.] 1 p.
l., 74 pp., 1 l. 8°. *München, J. A. Finsterlin*,
1883.

——. Einfache und erfolgreiche Behandlung des
Schreibekrampfes. Eine vorläufige Mittheilung.
2. Aufl. 11 pp. 8°. *München, J. A. Finsterlin*,
1883.

——. Künstliche Harnwege. 1. Temporäre
Drainage zur Bildung eines künstlichen Harnleiters. 2. Temporäre Drainage zur Bildung
einer künstlichen Harnröhre. Zwei kleine Mittheilungen. 19 pp. 4°. *München, M. Rieger*,
1883.

——. Ueber Umwandlung maligner Geschwülste
(Krebse) in gutartige und über Vorzüge glühen-
der Instrumente; ein klinischer Vortrag. 20 pp.
8°. *München, J. A. Finsterlin*, 1883.

——. Bauchverletzungen. 26 pp. 8°. *Berlin*,
E. Grosser, 1884.
Repr. from: Deutsche Med.-Ztg., Berl., 1884, i–ii.

——. Operation einer Uterusgeschwulst in zwei
Zeiten. Ein klinischer Vortrag. 12 pp. 8°.
München, J. A. Finsterlin, 1884.

——. Anleitung zur (fäulnisswidrigen) antiseptischen Wundbehandlung. Zum Gebrauche
für die Unterrichtskurse der Badergehilfen. 2.
Aufl. (Mit der Bader-Ordnung im Anhang.)
28 pp. 16°. *München, M. Rieger*, 1885.

——. Ein neuer Versuch zur Radicaloperation
der Unterleibsbrüche. Ein klinischer Vortrag.
16 pp. 8°. *München, J. A. Finsterlin*, 1885.
Repr. from: Aerztl. Int.-Bl., München, 1885, xxxii.

——. Ueber Choroform-Wirkung. 42 pp. 8°.
Breslau, E. Trewendt, 1884.

——. Anästhetica.
In: HANDB. d. allg. u. spec. Chir., Erlang., 1867, i, 2.
Abth., B, Abschn. iii, No. 4, 575–617.

——. Die Amputation des Kropfes. 2 pp. 8°.
München, J. A. Finsterlin, 1887.
Repr. from: München. med. Wchnschr., 1887, xxxiv.
See, also, **Lindpaintner.** Bericht der chirurgischen
Klinik [etc.] 8°. [*München, 1878.*] — **Stenographi-**
scher Bericht [etc.] 8°. *München*, 1874.
For Biography, see Anfiteatro anat., Madrid, 1876, iv, 65;
75, port. (J. B. Ullersperger.)
For Portrait, see **Collection**—van Kaathoven.

Nusser (Eduard).
See **Vienna.** Jahresberichte des Wiener Stadtfysi-
kates. 1.–9., 1871–9. 8°. *Wien*, 1872–80.

Nusser (Joh.) * Ueber Krankheiten bei Gewer-
ben überhaupt und über eine bei Seifensiedern
vorkommende Hautwassersucht. 15 pp. 8°.
München, J. A. Giesser, 1838.

Nusshag (Friedrich). Der Largiadèr'sche Arm-
und Bruststärker in seiner Verwendung beim
Klassenunterricht. (Deutsches Reichspatent
Nr. 31710.) 2. Aufl. 23 pp. 8°. *Karlsruhe*,
E. Kundt, [1885].

Nute (John W.)
See **Orange**, *New Jersey.* Joint committee on sewerage and drainage. 8°. *Orange*, 1885.

Nutmeg.

HELBIG (C. G.) Ueber Krankheitsursachen
und Heilmittel, nach ihren reinen Wirkungen.
1. Heft: Die Muskatennuss, nach homöopathischen Grundsätzen bearbeitet. 8°. *Leipzig*,
1833.

RADLOFF (F. V.) * De myristica. sm. 4°.
Upsaliæ, [1788].

SCHULTZE (N.) * De nuce moschata. 4°.
Traj. ad Rhenum, 1709.

Barry (W. H.) Narcotism from nutmeg. St. Louis
Clin. Rec., 1879–80, vi, 133. — **Dodge** (W. T.) Nutmeg
poisoning. Med. Rec., N. Y., 1887, xxxii, 624.—**Gaulke.**
Muskatnussvergiftung. Prakt. Arzt, Wetzlar, 1880, xxi,
217.— **Pinnock** (R. D.) A case of nutmeg poisoning.
Australas. M. Gaz., Sydney, 1886–7, vi, 274. — **Zimmer-**
mann. Gefälschte Muscatnüsse. Vrtljschr. f. gerichtl.
u. öff. Med., Berl., 1872, xvi, 302–304.

Nutrition.

See, also, **Alimentation**; **Assimilation**;
Atrophy; **Blood** (*Circulation of*); **Digestion**;
Endosmosis, *etc.*; **Excretion**; **Fœtus** (*Nutri-*
tion of); **Food**; **Growth**; **Joints** (*Neuralgia,*
etc., of); **Light** (*Colored*); **Nerves** (*Trophic*);
Nitrogen (*Excretion of*); **Respiration** (*Physi-*
ology of); **Starvation**; **Tissue** (*Metamorphosis*
of).

ADET (P. A.) An partium durarum nutritio,
eadem ac mollium? 4°. *Parisiis*, 1748.

AFFORTY (P. F.) * An nutritio secretionum
opus? 4°. *Parisiis*, 1752.

ATWATER (W. O.) The chemistry of foods and
nutrition. The composition of our bodies and
our food. How food nourishes the body. The
chemistry of foods and nutrition. 8°. [*New*
York, 1887.]
Cutting from: Century Mag., N. Y., 1887, xxxiii, 59;
237.

BARRY (E.) * De nutritione. sm. 4°. *Lugd.*
Bat., [1719].

BENNET (J. H.) Nutrition in health and disease. 8°. *London*, 1858.

BÖTTGER (C. F.) * De nutritione naturali ac
præternaturali, potissimum aucta et abolita.
sm. 4°. *Lipsiæ*, [1709].

BRÜGGE (J. C.) * De nutritione. 4°. *Gro-*
ningæ, 1728.

BRÜHL (J. W. C.) * De pabulo vitæ ceu de
materia, cui cum animalia, tum vegetabilia vitam debent ac nutritionem. 4°. *Marburgi*, 1781.

BRUNEAU (A.) * Quæstio physiol. de nutritione
et accretione. 4°. *Duaci*, 1792.

BURCKHARDUS (J. C.) * De partibus corporis nutritioni dicatis, earumque administrandi
ratione. 4°. *Wirceburgi*, 1603.

CALLAMAND (E.) * Du rôle de l'eau dans la
nutrition. 4°. *Paris*, 1887.

——. The same. 8°. *Paris*, 1887.

CASTELYNS (B. J.) * De nutritione. 1795.
In: LOUVAIN Diss. 8°. *Lovanii*, 1796, iv, 467–469.

CHADWICK (C.) * On the question, how far
are secretion and nutrition dependent on nervous influence? 8°. *Edinburgh*, 1837.

CHARLTON (W.) Natural history of nutrition,
life, and voluntary motion, containing all the
new discoveries of anatomists, and most probable opinions of physicians concerning the œconomie of human nature, methodically delivered
in exercitations physico-anatomical. sm. 4°.
London, 1659.

CLAUDER (C. E.) * De nutritione. 4°. *Jenæ*,
[1716].

DE COURCELLES (N. C. A.) * De nutritione.
4°. *Lugd. Bat.*, 1730.
Also, in: DE OBERKAMP (F. J.) Collect. diss. 4°.
Francof. a. M., 1767, i, 427–458.

DAVID (J.-P.) Traité de la nutrition et de
l'accroissement, précédé d'une dissertation sur
l'usage des eaux de l'amnios. 8°. *Paris & Rouen*,
1771.

DEANE (J.) An essay on the waste and supply in the human system. 2. ed. 12°. *London*,
[*n. d.*]

DEUSINGIUS (A.) Exercitationes physico-
anatomicæ de nutrimenti in corpore elabora-
tione. Ubi de chylificatione et chyli motu, san-
guificatione, depuratione alimenti itemque spiritibus, [etc.] Quibus adjecta appendix, in qua
examini ac judicio aliorum subjiciuntur varia
de chyli motu, et nutrimenti in corpore elabora-
tione, nec non de admiranda anatome nobiliss.
viri D. Ludovici de Bils. 16°. *Groningæ*, 1660.

DHÉRÉ (C.-J.-F.-B.) * De la nutrition dans la
série animale. 4°. *Paris*, 1826.

——. De la nutrition, considérée anatomi-
quement et physiologiquement, dans la série des

Nutrition.

animaux, d'après les idées de M. Ducrotay de Blainville. 8°. *Paris & Strasbourg*, 1826.

DORSEY (E. J.) * De nutritione. 12°. *Edinburgi*, 1776.

DULK (F. P.) Ueber Ernährung und Erwärmung des menschlichen Körpers. 8°. *Königsberg*, 1844.

DULKENIUS (H.) * De nutritione. sm. 4°. *Lugd. Bat.*, 1667.

DURADE. Dissertation sur la nutrition qui a remporté le prix de physique de l'Académie royale des sciences et belles-lettres renvoyé à l'année 1766. 4°. *Berlin*, 1767.

DUVERNOY (G.-L.) Résumé sur le fluide nourricier, ses réservoirs et son mouvement, dans tout le règne animal. 8°. *Paris*, 1839.

EDZARDUS (E. H.) * De corporis humani palingenesia. sm. 4°. *Vitembergæ*, [1722].

EGGERS (J. W. O.) * Disp. de succi nutritii statu naturali et præternaturali. 4°. *Marpurgi Cattorum*, 1683.

ENZMANN (C.) Die Ernährungen der Organismen, besonders des Menschen und der Thiere, im hungernden Zustande. sm. 8°. *Dresden*, 1856.

ETLINGER (J. L.) * De corporis humani nutritione. 4°. [*Altdorf*], 1736.

FISCHER (G.) * De nutritione. 8°. *Berolini*, [1839].

FREDERICQ (L.) & NUEL (J.-P.) Éléments de physiologie humaine à l'usage des étudiants en médecine. Pt. 1. Fonctions de nutrition. 8°. *Gand*, 1883.

FRESENIUS (C. R.) Practical application of the law pointed out by Dr. R. Thomson, of the proper balance of the food in nutrition. 8°. [*London*, 1849.]

Repr. from : Lond., Edinb. & Dubl. Phil. Mag., 1849, Aug.

FRIEDERICUS (A. G.) * De nutritiva facultate. Resp. J. Töpffer. sm. 4°. *Lipsiæ*, 1652.

FROHBERG (A.-F.) * Considérations sur quelques points de physiologie concernant la nutrition. 4°. *Strasbourg*, 1817.

GEITZINGER (F.) Humanæ nutritionis rationem explicat. 4°. [*Witteberg*, 1672.]

GELEZ (P. J.) * Diss. physiol. de alimentorum in chylum, chyli in lac, lactis in sanguinem conversione. 4°. *Duaci*, 1783.

GLUGE (G.) La nutrition, ou la vie considérée dans ses rapports avec les aliments; conférence de physiologie donnée à l'Université de Bruxelles. 8°. *Bruxelles*, 1856.

GOURDAN-FROMENTEL (L.-É.) * Sur le suc nourricier et ses modifications pathologiques. 4°. *Paris*, 1849.

DE GRIMAUD (J.-C.-M.-G.) Mémoire sur la nutrition. 8°. *Montpellier*, 1787.

——. Second mémoire sur la nutrition. 8°. *Montpellier*, 1789.

GROSSHOLTZ (J. N.) * De nutritione. 4°. *Argentorati*, [1712].

GUCKEISEN (A.) Die neuesten Ernährungsgesetze nach v. Pettenkofer und Voit. 8°. *Köln*, 1878.

GUÉRIN (G.) Origine et transformations des matières azotées chez les êtres vivants. 8°. *Paris*, 1886.

HAGUENOT (H.) * De nutritione. 4°. *Monspelii*, 1727.

In : HALLER. Disp. anat. [etc.] 4°. *Gottingæ*, 1878, iii, 677-718.

HAUSER (P.) * Nouvelles recherches relatives à l'influence du système nerveux sur la nutrition. [Berne.] 8°. *Paris*, 1858.

HEINTKE (G.) Exercitationum physiologicarum duodecima de nutritione. 4°. [*n. p., n. d.*]

Nutrition.

HELLER (F.) Ueber Ernährung und Stoffwechsel, so wie über einige der vorzüglichsten Nahrungsmittel. 8°. *Breslau*, 1855.

HÉROUARD (A.) Considérations générales sur la théorie de l'assimilation directe des substances organiques azotées et non azotées. 8°. *Caen*, 1878.

HEWITT (W. M. G.) Nutrition the basis of the treatment of disease; the introductory address . . . University College, London, Oct. 1, 1867. 8°. *London*, 1867.

HIEROPHILUS. Περὶ τροφῶν κύκλος, ποῖα δεῖ χρᾶσθαι ἑκάστῳ μηνὶ καὶ ὁποίοις ἀπεχέσθαι.

In : IDELER (J. L.) Phys. et med. Græci min. 8°. *Berolini*, 1841, i, 409-417.

HIFFELSHEIM. Considérations sur les principes immédiats des corps organisés. [Part ii.] 8°. *Paris*, [1853].

For Part i, see infra.

HOELTZENBEIN (J.) * De telarum corporis humani regeneratione. 8°. *Berolini*, [1848].

JOHNSTOUN (J.) De nutrimento, incremento et decremento animalium. 4°. *Traj. ad Rhenum*, 1709.

KIESSLING (J. S.) * De nutritione. sm. 4°. *Lipsiæ*, [1678].

KLIPPER (J. P.) * Theses physicæ de nutritione. 4°. [*Lipsiæ*, 1657.]

KURLOFF (M. G.) * Usvoenie i obmien azot. veshestve pri kormlenii chachotoch. po sposobu Debova. [Assimilation and metamorphosis of nitrogenous substances in artificial feeding by Deboff's method.] 8°. *St. Petersburg*, 1886.

LALLEMANT (J.) * An nutrimentum tandem decrementi corporis causa? Præses P. Lalovette. [1743.]

In : SIGWART (G. F.) Quæst. med. Paris. 4°. *Tubingæ*, 1789, i, 28-37.

LANDREBEN (G.) * De nutritione. 4°. *Lugd. Bat.*, [1716].

LANE (C.) Dietetics; an endeavour to ascertain the law of human nutriment. sm. 8°. *London*, 1849.

LANGE (C. G.) * De variis nutritionis causis atque modis. 4°. *Jenæ*, [1754].

LANZILLOTTI - BUOSANTI (N.) * Conosci te stesso; schizzi fisiologici sulle funzioni nutritive. 12°. *Milano*, 1879.

LEBRUMENT (H.-E.) De la nutrition comme source unique de la santé et de la maladie, ou seuls principes desquels puissent être déduits la nature des maladies, leur traitement et les moyens de les prévenir. 12°. *Paris*, 1858.

LE THIEULLIER (L.-P.-F.-R.) * An præcipua, in pulmonibus, nutrientis succi præparatio? 4°. *Parisiis*, 1750.

LIBERALI (L.) Uno sguardo alla nutrizione. 8°. *Treviso*, 1849.

LINDFORSS (M. J.) Dissertatio physiologica assimilationis legem generalem exponens. 4°. *Helsingforsiæ*, 1832.

LORENZEN (A.) * Ueber den Einfluss der Entwässerung des Körpers auf die Entfettung. [Erlangen.] 8°. *Flensburg*, 1887.

LORIN (A.-A.) * Essai d'analyse synoptique sur la nutrition. 8°. *Paris*, an XII [1804].

LUCAS (J.) * De nutritione. 4°. *Lugd. Bat.*, 1764.

LUCHHAU (E.) * Ueber die Magen- und Darmverdauung. 8°. *Königsberg*, 1878.

LULIUS (B.) * Spec. continens historiam nutritionis. 4°. *Lugd. Bat.*, 1783.

MARCET (W.) An experimental inquiry into the nutrition of animal tissues. 8°. *London*, 1874.

MARINIER (J. F.) Quæstio med.: An nutritio sit fluidorum duntaxat reparatio? 4°. [*Parisiis*], 1776.

Nutrition.

MARTEAU (L. R.) *An in qualibet hominis ætate idem succus nutricius?
In: SIGWART (G. F.) Quæst. med. Paris. 4°. *Tubingæ,* 1789, i, 38–43.

MEE (I.) * De nutritione. 8°. *Edinburgi,* 1770.

MEINERT (C. A.) Ueber Massen-Ernährung. Mit besonderer Berücksichtigung der von Sanitätsrath Dr. Bär, von Dr. Paul Jeserich, und von dem Verfasser, in Plötzensee angestellten Ernährungsversuche. 8°. *Berlin,* 1885.

MEYER (G. H.) Die richtige Gestalt des menschlichen Körpers in ihrer Erhaltung und Ausbildung für das allgemeine Verständniss. 8°. *Stuttgart,* 1874.

MUTHWILL (J. A.) * De nutritione. 4°. *Jenæ,* [1750].

NASSE (H.) Ueber den Einfluss der Nahrung auf das Blut. 8°. *Marburg,* 1850.

NUSSBAUM (H.) & NENCKI (L.) O żywieniu się i pokarmach. [On food and nutrition.] 8°. *Warszawa,* 1887.

OBET (L.-J.-M.) * Essai sur la nutrition. 4°. *Paris,* 1805.

ORTLOB (J. F.) Analogiam nutritionis plantarum et animalium exponet. Respondente C. Schmeer. sm. 4°. *Lipsiæ,* 1683.

PELÉE DE VALONCOUR (A. B.) *An nutritio sit fluidorum duntaxat reparatio? 4°. [*Paris,* 1764.]

PENN (J.) * De principiis organicis nutrientibus. 8°. *Lugd. Bat.,* 1844.

PETERMANN (A.) * De nutritione integra servanda abolitaque reparanda. 4°. *Altdorffi,* [1672].

PLANER (A.) De nutritione. 4°. *Tubingæ,* 1620.

VON PLATEN (O.) * Ueber den Einfluss des Lich'es auf den Stoffwechsel. 8°. *Bonn,* 1875.

PLATNER (E.) [Pr.] dubitationes quædam super Boerhaavii atque Halleri decretis de nutritione. 4°. [*Lipsiæ,* 1788.]

POGGIALE. Recherches sur la composition chimique et les équivalents nutritifs des aliments de l'homme; travail lu à l'Académie impériale de médecine le 12 août 1856. Premier mémoire. 8°. *Paris,* 1856.

POLLI (G.) Sulla influenza delle materie minerali nei processi nutrivi dell' organismo umano. Memoria del . . . 4°. *Milano,* 1871.

RENOULT (A.) Du rôle du système vasculaire dans la nutrition en général et dans celle du muscle et du cœur en particulier. 4°. *Strasbourg,* 1869.

REST (J.) De nutritione. 8°. *Monachii,* 1837.

ROUET (J.-A.-F.) * Influence du système nerveux sur les phénomènes physico-chimiques de la vie de nutrition. 4°. *Paris,* 1865.

RYMER (J.) A tract on the nutriferous system in men, quadrupeds, and birds and in all other creatures which have livers. 8°. *London,* 1808.

SACHS (P. J.) Συμπόσιον φιλοσοφικὸν nutritionis physicæ varios missus exhibens. 4°. *Lipsiæ,* 1647.

SANTORINUS (J. D.) De nutritione animali. Opusc. ii.
In: BAGLIVIUS (G.) Opera omnia. 4°. *Lugduni,* 1710, 797–826. *Also, in his:* Opusc. med. [etc.] 16°. *Roterodami,* 1719, 86–149.

SCHARY (E.) * Beiträge zur Kenntniss des Stoffwechsels im Organismus der Vögel. 8°. *Königsberg,* 1878.

SCHMIDT (E. B.) * De nutritione solidorum in sanis. 4°. *Halæ Magdeb.,* [1776].

SCHUBERT (P.) * Die Physiologie der Ernährung, Verdauung, Säftebewegung, Athmung, vor der Entdeckung des Blutkreislaufes. 8°. *Würzburg,* 1875.

Nutrition.

VON SEEFELD (A.) Die modernen Theorien der Ernährung und des Vegetarianismus. 12°. *Hannover,* 1875.

STENBERG (S.) *Om intagua läkemedels afsöndring utur organismen. 8°. *Upsala,* 1858.

STUTE (T. L.) * De usu nervorum telæque cellulosæ in nutriendis corporis humani partibus.
In: WEIZ (F. A.) Neue Ausz. [etc.] 12°. *Frankfurt u. Leipzig,* 1774, ii, 80–83.

TER-GRIGORJANITZ (G.) * K vopr. o vlijanii obilnago pitja vodi na azot. obmien i usvoenie azot. chastei pitshi u zdorov. loudei. [Effect of copious water drinking on nitrogenous metamorphosis and the assimilation of nitrogenous elements in healthy man.] 8°. *St. Petersburg,* 1886.

THAURAUX (J.) *An nutritio secretionum opus? 4°. [*Paris,* 1775.]

THOMSON (R. D.) The law of the nutrition of animals pointed out by . . . illustrated by F. Knapp. 8°. [*n. p.,* 1848.]
Repr. from: Lond., Edinb. & Dubl. Phil. Mag., Lond., June, 1848.

TIGERSTEDT (R.) Fysiologiska principer för kroppens näring. Tio föreläsningar hällna vid Karolinska Institutet hösten 1886. 8°. *Stockholm,* 1887.

VACCA (F.) Della nutrizione, accrescimento, decrescimento e morte senile del corpo umano trattato. 4°. *Pisa,* 1762.

VOIT (C.) Ueber die Theorien der Ernährung der thierischen Organismen. 4°. *München,* 1868.

WADE (C.) * De nutritione. 8°. *Edinburgi,* 1778.
Also, in: SMELLIE. Thesaurus med. [etc.] 8°. *Edinburgi,* 1785, iv, 63–107.

WEDELIUS (G. W.) [Pr.] [quicquid nutrit ex genere est dulcium.] 4°. [*Halæ*], 1681.

———. [Pr.] ex quibus vivimus et nutrimur, ex iisdem quoque ægrotamus et morimur. sm. 4°. [*Jena,* 1683.]

WOCKAZ (G. L.) * De nutritione differentiis oligochymiæ accommodanda. sm. 4°. *Lipsiæ,* [1772].

WORM MÜLLER (J.) Om Ernæring og Forpleining. 8°. *Kristiania,* 1879.

YOUNG (J. R.) An experimental inquiry into the principles of nutrition and the digestive process. 8°. *Philadelphia,* 1803.

Addison (W.) The actual process of nutrition in the living structure demonstrated by the microscope, and the renewal of the tissues and the secretions from the blood thereby illustrated. Tr. Prov. M. & S. Ass., Lond., 1844, xii, 235–306, 2 pl.—**Allen** (G.) Why d we eat our dinner? Pop. Sc. Month., N. Y., 1879, xiv, 799–810.—**Balfour** (B.) Some resemblances betwixt plants and animals in respect of their nutrition, with some remarks on the position of the natural history sciences in medical education. Glasgow M. J., 1879, [4. s.], xii. 428–447. *Also, transl.:* Rev. internat. d. sc. biol., Par., 1880, v, 289–308.—**Barnston** (J.) Nutrition, physiologically and pathologically considered. Med. Chron., Montreal, 1856–7, iv, 91–100.—**Beale** (L. S.) On nutrition. Med. Times & Gaz., Lond., 1865, i, 193; 220; 276; 329.—**Béchamp** (A.) Sur la théorie générale de la nutrition et sur l'origine des ferments en général, à propos de la discussion sur les ptomaïnes et leur rôle en pathologie. Bull. Acad. de méd., Par., 1886. 2. s., xv, 475; 532.—**Becher** (E.) Die Kohlensäurespannung im Blute als proportionales Maass des Umsatzes der kohlenstoffhaltigen Körper- und Nahrungsbestandtheile. Ztschr. f. rat. Med., Heidelb., 1855, vi, 249–287, 2 pl.—**Becquerel** père. De l'intervention des forces électrocapillaires dans la production des phénomènes de nutrition de la vie animale et végétale. J. de l'anat. et physiol., etc., Par., 1874, x, 1–6.—**Beneke** (F. W.) Zur Ernährungslehre des gesunden Menschen. Schrift. d. Gesellsch. z. Beförd. d. ges. Naturw. zu Marb., 1878, xi, 275–312.—**Benessat.** Teorias fisico-químicas de las funciones de nutricion. Bol. Col. de farm. de Barcel., 1877, i. 311; 346: 1878, ii. 42.—**Bischoff** (E.) Versuche über die Ernährung mit Brod. Ztschr. f. Biol., München, 1869, v, 452–475.—**Bischoff** (T.-L.-G.) De la nutrition chez l'homme et les animaux. Arch. gén. de méd., Par., 1860, ii, 129–147. *Also,* Reprint.—**Boehm** (R.) & **Hoffmann** (F. A.) Beiträge zur Kenntniss des Kohlehydratstoffwechsels.

Nutrition.

Arch. f. exper. Path. u. Pharmakol., Leipz., 1878, viii, 375–445.—**Brachet** (J.-L.) Note sur les apparences de suspension de la nutrition. Gaz. méd. de Lyon, 1858. x, 509–511.—**Camerer** (W.) Der Stoffwechsel von fünf Kindern im Alter von 7 bis 17 Jahren. Ztschr. f. Biol., München u. Leipz., 1887, n. F., vi, 141–163.—**Carlet** (G.) Nutrition. Dict. encycl. d. sc. méd., Par., 1879, 2. s., xiii, 785–811.—**Charbonnier.** Influence de la nourriture sur les organisations humaines. Art méd., Brux., 1877, xiii, 241; 261; 280.—**Chaussier & Adelon.** Nutrition. Dict. d. sc. méd., Par., 1819, xxxvi, 505–548.—**Constantinidi** (A.) Ueber die Ausnützung des Weizenklebers im Darmkanale und über die Verwendung desselben zur Ernährung des Menschen. Ztschr. f. Biol., München u. Leipz., 1886. xxiii, 433–455. — **Couty, Guimaraes & Niobey.** De l'action des lésions du bulbe rachidien sur les échanges nutritifs. Compt. rend. Acad. d. sc., Par., 1884. xcix, 388–390.—**Danilewsky** (B.) Ueber die Kraftvorräthe der Nahrungsstoffe. Arch. f. d. ges. Physiol., Bonn, 1885, xxxvi, 230–252.—**Darby** (J. C.) A new view of physiology. St. Louis M. & S. J., 1878, xxxiv, 105–113.—**Debove** (M.) & **Flamant** (A.) Influence de la quantité d'eau ingérée sur la nutrition. Bull. et mém. Soc. méd. d. hôp. de Par., 1885, 3. s., ii, 395–401. ——— Recherches sur l'influence de la graisse sur la nutrition. Bull. et mém. Soc. méd. d. hôp, de Par., 1886, 3. s., iii, 263–267. Also: Gaz. hebd. de méd., Par., 1886, 2. s., xxiii, 409–411.—**van Deen** (I.) Over veranderingen, welke stoffen buiten het dierlijke ligchaam kunnen ondergaan, en die overeenstemmen met die, welke in het ligchaam plaats grijpen door de stofwisseling. Nederl. Tijdschr. v. Geneesk., Amst., 1861, v, 585–599.—**Donders** (F. C.) Over stofwisseling en veding. Onderzoek. ged. in h. physiol. Lab. d. Utrecht. Hoogesch., 1849–50, ii, 231–243.—**Duval** (M.) Nutrition. N. dict. de méd. et chir. prat., Par., 1877, xxiv, 177–203.—**Ellenberger & Hofmeister.** Die Darmverdauung und die Resorption im Darmkanal der Schweine. Arch. f. wissensch. u. prakt. Thierh., Berl., 1888, xiv, 137–171.—**Escherich.** Ueber einige Bedingungen zur guten Ernährung. Med. Cor.-Bl. bayer. Aerzte, Erlang., 1842, iii, 273–285.—**Ferrero** (M.) Nutrizione e denutrizione chiaccherata più o meno scientifica. Salute, Genova, 1872, vii, 625; 673; 721; 769; 801: 1873, viii, 54; 85; 179; 290. — **Forster** (J.) Versuche über die Bedeutung der Aschebestandtheile in der Nahrung. Ztschr. f. Biol., München, 1873, ix, 297–380. Also, Reprint.—**Goodsir** (J.) Centres of nutrition. In his: Anat. & Path. Obs., 8°, Edinb., 1845, 1–3, 1 pl. Also, in his: Anat. Mem., 8°, Edinb., 1868, ii, 389–392, 1 pl.—**Grigorieff** (A.) Obmien i usvoenie azot. vetshestve pri lechen. krovjou. [Metamorphosis and assimilation of nitrogenous substances by the blood.] Russk. Med., St. Petersb., 1886, vi, 631; 647.—**Haas** (R.) On the mechanism of textural nutrition. Lond. J. M., 1850, ii, 642; 715.—**Hamilton** (D. J.) Remarks on nutrition and growth. Brit. M. J., Lond., 1883, ii, 1271–1277. — **Hanriot** (M.) & **Bichet** (C.) Influence de l'alimentation, chez l'homme, sur la fixation et l'élimination du carbone. Compt. rend. Acad. d. sc., Par., 1888, cvi, 419–422.—**Henneberg** (W.) Ueber Fleisch-und Fettproduction in verschiedenem Alter und bei verschiedener Ernährung. Ztschr. f. Biol., München, 1881, xvii, 295–350.—**Hiffelsheim.** [Considérations sur les principes immédiats des corps organisés.] Gaz. méd. de Par., 1852, 3. s., vii, 804; 819. [See, also, supra.]—**Hinton** (J.) On the relation between chemical decomposition and nutrition. Guy's Hosp. Rep., Lond., 1871, 3. s., xv, 425–430.—**von Hösslin.** Ueber den Einfluss der Nahrung auf die stoffliche Zusammensetzung des Körpers. Amtl. Ber. ü. d. Versamml. deutsch. Naturf. u. Aerzte 1883. Freib. i. Br., 1884, lvi, 150–153.—**Hofmeister** (F.) Untersuchungen über Resorption und Assimilation der Nährstoffe. Arch. f. exper. Path. u. Pharmakol., Leipz., 1885, xix, 1: 1885–6, xx, 291: 1886–7, xxii, 306, 1 pl.—**Iszlai** (J.) Ein Blick auf die Beziehung zwischen der naturgemässen allgemeinen Ernährungsweise und dem Gebisse des Menschen, sowie der übrigen Säugethiere. Deutsche Vrtljschr. f. Zahnh., Leipz., 1881, xxi, 1; 109.—**James** (A.) Nutrition and reproduction considered generally and as bearing on the etiology and treatment of disease. Tr. Med.-Chir. Soc. Edinb., 1882–3, n. s., ii, 106–123. Also: Edinb. M. J., 1883–4, xxix, 97–108. Also, in his: Physiol. & Clin. Stud., 8°., Edinb., 1888, 23–40.—**Jolly** (L.) Des sources où l'organisme puise sa provision phosphatée. Bull. Soc. de méd. prat. de Par., 1877, 34–37. ——— De la nutrition; du rôle des phosphates et du fer dans ce phénomène. France méd., Par., 1880, xxvii, 451; 459; 466. Also, Reprint.—**Joulin** (L.) Recherches sur la nutrition. Compt. rend. Soc. de biol. 1878, Par., 1880, 6. s., v, 299. — **Jürgensen** (C.) Bidrag til Belysning af hvilke Födestofmängder voxne Mennesker under forskellige Forhold fortäre i frit valgt Kost, og hvorledes de fordeles på Dagens Måltider. (C. r. Contribution à la connaissance de la nourriture consommée des adultes dans des conditions différentes et avec liberté de choix, ainsi que la répartition de cette nourriture sur les divers repas de la journée.) Nord. med. Ark., Stockholm. 1886, xviii, no. 11, 1–44. Also, transl. [Abstr.]: Ztschr. f. Biol., München,

Nutrition.

1886, n. F., iv, 489–496.—**Kast** (A.) Ueber Beziehungen der Chlorausscheidung zum Gesammtstoffwechsel. Ztschr. f. physiol. Chem., Strassb., 1887–8, xii, 267–284.—**Kraus** (G.) Ueber Stoffwechsel bei den Crassulaceen. Abhandl. d. naturf. Gesellsch. zu Halle, 1886, xvi, 393–480.—**Krukenberg** (C. F. W.) Nachtrag zu den Untersuchungen über die Ernährungsvorgänge bei Cölenteraten und Echinodermen. Untersuch. a. d. physiol. Inst. d. Univ. Heidelb.,1878, ii, 366–377.—**Kuckein** (F.) Beitrag zur Kenntniss des Stoffverbrauchs beim hungernden Huhn. Ztschr. f. Biol., München, 1882, xviii, 17–40.—**Küster** (C.) Ueber Ernährung. Deutsche Ztschr. f. prakt. Med., Leipz., 1874, i, 159; 323.—**Lahousse** (E.) Nature de l'influence de l'innervation sur la nutrition des tissus. Mém. couron. Acad. roy. de méd. de Belg., Brux., 1882. vii, 2. fasc., 1–315. — **Lehmann** (K. B.) Ueber den Ersatz des Nahrungseiweiss durch andere stickstoffhaltige Substanzen. Sitzungsb. d. Gesellsch. f. Morphol. u. Physiol. in München, 1885, i, 42–45.—**Lehmann** (L.) Einige Notizen die Ernährung betreffend, namentlich über die Ausscheidungsgrössen des Stickstoffs innerhalb 24 Stunden. Mit besonderer Berücksichtigung des Einflusses, welche Bäder dabei ausüben. Arch. d. Ver. f. gemeinsch. Arb. z. Förd. d. wissensch. Heilk., Götting., 1858, iii, 1–11, 1 tab.—**Lengerke** (C.) Digestion y nutricion. Rev. méd., Guadalajara, 1876, iii, 106–117.—**Levashoff** (S. V.) K voprosu o vlijanii defibrinirovanija krovi na jiznennost eja i sposobnost k pitaniou jivotnich tkanei. [Effect of defibrination of the blood on the nutrition of tissue.] Ejened. klin. Gaz., St. Petersb., 1884, iv, 135–139. ——— Influence du système nerveux sur la nutrition des tissus. Arch. slaves de biol., Par., 1886, i, 397–410.—**Leven.** Des rapports du système nerveux et de la nutrition; globules sanguins. Compt. rend. Soc. de biol., Par., 1887, 8. s., iv, 665–667. ——— Des rapports du système nerveux et de la nutrition; amaigrissement. Ibid., 1888, 8. s., v, 42.—**Liebig** (J.) Die Ernährung, Blut- und Fettbildung im Thierkörper. Ann. d. Chem. u. Pharm., Heidelb., 1842, xli, 241–285. Also, transl.: Ann. de méd. belge, Brux., 1842, iii, 177 : 1843, ii, 182.—**Lunin** (N.) Ueber die Bedeutung der anorganischen Salze für die Ernährung des Thieres. Ztschr. f. physiol. Chem., Strassb., 1881, v, 31–39. — **Macvicar** (J. G.) The delivery of the nutritive part of the blood to the tissues. Edinb. M. J., 1870–71, xvi, 769–779.—**Marcet** (W.) Muscular and pulmonary tissue in health and in consumption. Ibid., 1871–2, xvii, 698–710. ——— Remarks on the phenomenon of the nutrition of tissues, with an inquiry into the nutritive value of beef tea. Brit. M. J., Lond., 1872, ii, 119. ——— Recherches sur les phénomènes chimiques de la nutrition des muscles et des poumons à l'état normal et dans la tuberculose. Assoc. franç. pour l'avance. d. sc. Compt.-rend., Par., 1873, i, 365.—**Maturi** (R.) L' idroterapia e la nutrizione. Salute, Genova, 1872, vii, 481; 503.—**May.** Bei welcher Temperatur wird bei Kühen das Futter am besten verwerthet? Untersuch. z. Naturl. d. Mensch. u. d. Thiere, Frankf. a. M., 1858, v, 319–328.—**Mialhe.** Recherches sur la digestion, l'assimilation et l'oxydation organique ou vitale. Vichy méd., 1879, ii, 397–402.—**Miyashita,** Shinkichi. [The absorption of nourishment.] Tokei M. J., Tokio, 1885, no. 383, Aug. 1.—**Morris** (J.) Nutrition, a function of germinal matter. J. Cutan. M., Lond., 1868–9, ii, 28–34.—**Müller** (R.) Beiträge zur Lehre von der Verdauung und Absorption der Nahrungsstoffe. Schmidt's Jahrb., Leipz., 1881, cxcii, 65–95.—**Munk** (I.) Rundschau auf dem Gebiete der Ernährungslehre. Deutsche med. Wchnschr., Leipz., 1888, xiv, 89–91. Also, Reprint.—**Nature** (On the) and functions of the inorganic constituents and ingredients of food, tissues and liquids. Ann. Chem. Med., Lond., 1881, ii, 126–143.—**Oesterlen** (F.) Ueber die nutritiven Vorgänge und ihre Beziehung zu andern Vitalitätsäusserungen. Arch. f. Anat., Physiol. u. wissensch. Med., Berl., 1842, 149–177.—**Paget** (J.) Lectures on nutrition, hypertrophy, and atrophy. Lond. M. Gaz., 1847, xxxix, 931–1017. Also, Reprint. — **Panum** (P. L.) Om Stofskiftet i Almindelighed og om Tarmkanalens og Fordøjelses vædskernes Funktioner. In his: Stofskiftets Fysiol., [etc.], 8°, Kjøbenh., 1883, 1. Hft.,1–230.— **Paquelin & Jolly.** Contribution à l'étude des phénomènes nutritifs. Analyse comparative des sangs artériel et veineux au point de vue de leur constitution minérale. Bull. Soc. de méd.-prat. de Par., 1875, 122 ; 155. Also: France méd., Par., 1875,xxii,493; 594.—**von Pettenkofer** (M.) & **Voit** (C.) Ueber die Zersetzungsvorgänge im Thierkörper bei der Fütterung mit Fleisch und Kohlehydraten und Kohlehydraten allein. Ztschr. f. Biol., München, 1873, ix, 435–540.—**Pignatari** (G.) Ricerche intorno alla novella teoria del Bernard riguardante lo assorbimento delle sostanze alimentari. Rendic. d. Accad. med.-chir. di Napoli, 1857, xi, 21–25. Also, Reprint.—**Power** (H.) The influence of the nerves on nutrition. Practitioner, Lond., 1873, x, 91 ; 138.—**Prieto y Prieto** (M.) Nutricion. Anfiteatro anat., Madrid, 1878, vi, 42; 50 ; 64 ; 80.—**Prosch** (V.) Aforismer vedrørende Ernæringens Physiologie. Hyg. Medd., Kjøbenh., 1880, n. R., iii, 128–139.—**Rommelaere** (W.) Mensuration de la nutrition organique ; déductions cliniques. Bull. Acad. roy. de méd. de Belg., Brux., 1882, 3.

Nutrition.

s., xvi, 992-1026. *Also:* Presse méd. belge, Brux., 1883, xxxv. 33; 41; 49. *Also:* Art méd., Brux., 1883-4, xix, 35; 68; 88; 97. *Also, transl.:* Arch. clin. ital., Roma, 1883, xiii, 76; 93; 133; 142. ———. De la mensuration de la nutrition organique; applications cliniques. J. de méd., chir. et pharmacol., Brux., 1883, lxxvii, 3; 225; 344: 1884, lxxviii, 225; 337: lxxix, 3; 241. *Also,* Reprint (in part).—
Rousseau. Quelques mots sur la force et la faiblesse. Union méd. et scient. du nord-est, Reims, 1878, ii. 33; 165.—
Rubner (M.) Die Vertretungswerthe der hauptsächlichsten organischen Nahrungsstoffe im Thierkörper. Ztschr. f. Biol. München, 1883, xix; 313-396.—**Salemi-Pace** (B.) Ricerche sperimentali sulla influenza delle sostanze ipnogene sulla nutrizione degli organi. Pisani, Palermo, 1884, v, 305-309.—**Salkowski** (E.) Bemerkungen über die Wirkung der unorganischen Säuren und der Fleischnahrung. Arch. f. path. Anat., etc., Berl., 1879, lxxvi, 368-373.—**Sangalli.** Della nutrizione normale e morbosa dei tessuti dell' umano organismo. Gior. di anat. e fisiol. patol., Pavia, 1864-5, i, 216-239.—**Simon** (J. F.) Beitrag zur Physiologie der Ernährung. Arch. f. Anat., Physiol. u. wissensch. Med., Berl., 1839, 1-9.—**Smolenski** (P. O.) Obtshija ponjatija o pishe i obmene vetshestve v nashem organizme. [Alimentation and change of matter in the organism.] Voyenno-san. dielo, St. Petersb., 1885, v, 141; 154.—**Stohmann** (F.) Ueber die Ernährungsvorgänge des Milch producirenden Thieres. Zweite Arbeit: Bei stickstoffarmem Futter. Unter Mitwirkung von R. Frühling und A. Rost ausgeführt. Ztschr. f. Biol., München, 1870, vi, 204-284, 3 pl.—**Sudnik** (R.) Influencia de las corrientes continuas sobre la nutricion. An. Soc. circ. méd. Argentino, Buenos Aires, 1879-80, iii, 229; 328.—**Takács** (E.) Adalok a szervezetbeli élenyülés tanához. [On the theory of oxydation.] Orvosi hetil., Budapest, 1878, xxii, 1040-1048.—**Tommasi** (S.) Vita e nutrizione. Riforma clin., Napoli, 1880, iv, 2; 9. — **Uffelmann** (J.) Beobachtungen und Untersuchungen an einem gastrotomirten Knaben. Deutsches Arch. f. klin. Med., Leipz., 1877, xx, 535-571. — **Ustimovich** (K. N.) Zadachi i sposobi izsliedovanija ve oblasti phiziologii pitanija. [Nutrition and digestion.] Voyenno-med. J., St. Petersb., 1878, cxxxii, 67-118. — **Valentin** (G.) Ernährung. Handwörterb. d. Physiol, Brnschwg., 1850, i, 367-470.—**de Varigny** (H.) Bemerkung über den Gewichtsverlust durch Nahrungsmangel bei Aurelia aurita. Centralbl. f. Physiol., Leipz. u. Wien, 1887-8, i, 389. — **Verdeil** (F.) De la nutrition des plantes; avec remarques sur la nutrition chez les animaux. J. de la physiol. de l'homme, Par., 1858, i, 673-683.—**Verschiedenen** (Ueber die) Arten (Modi) des Vegetationsprocesses in der animalischen Natur, und die Gesetze, durch welche sie bestimmt werden. Arch. f. d. Physiol., Halle, 1805, vi, 120-167.—**Villar y Macias** (J.) De la nutricion animal. Correo méd. castellano, Salamanca, 1885, ii, 8-12.—**Voit** (C.) Ueber die Unterschiede der animalischen und vegetablischen Nahrung, die Bedeutung der Nährsalze und der Genussmittel. Sitzungsb. d. k.-bayer. Akad. d. Wissensch. zu München, 1869, ii, 483-528. *Also, transl.* [Abstr.] : Monit. scient., Par., 1872, xiv, 787-806.—**Wildt** (E.) Entgegnung auf die Wilckensche Kritik meiner Arbeit: "Ueber Resorption und Secretion der Nahrungsbestandtheile, etc." Ztschr. f. Biol., München, 1878, xiv, 414-421.—**Yung** (E.) De l'influence de la nature des aliments sur le développement de la grenouille. Compt. rend. Acad. d. sc., Par., 1881, xcii, 1525-1527.

Nutrition (*Disordered*).

See, also, Atrophy; Cachexia; Inanition; Marasmus; Nervous *system* (*Diseases of, Diagnosis, etc., of*).

Amende (B.) * Ueber den Einfluss mangelhafter Ernährung auf Volkskrankheiten. 8°. *Berlin*, 1876.

Beneke (F. W.) Grundlinien der Pathologie des Stoffwechsels. 8°. *Berlin*, 1874.

Bouchard (C.) Maladies par ralentissement de la nutrition; cours de pathologie générale, professé à la Faculté de médecine de Paris pendant l'année 1879-1880; recueilli et publié par H. Frémy. 8°. *Paris*, 1882.

Buch (J. C.) * De cacochymia purulenta. sm. 4°. *Jenæ*, [1759].

Cantani (A.) Specielle Pathologie und Therapie der Stoffwechselkrankheiten. Klinische Vorträge. Aus dem Italienischen von Dr. Siegfried Hahn und von Fränkel. 4 v. 8°. *Berlin u. Leipzig*, 1880-84.

Huebner (F. G.) * De macie corporis humani. 4°. *Lipsiæ*, [1824].

Nutrition (*Disordered*).

Lallemant (J.) * An nutrimentum tandem decrementi corporis causa? [1743.]
In: Sigwart. Quæst. med. Paris. 4°. *Tubingæ*, 1789, i, 28-37.

Marteau (L. R.) * An in qualibet hominis ætate idem succus nutricius? Præses Carolus Franc. Boutigny des Preaux. [1743.]
In: Sigwart. Quæst. med. Paris. 4°. *Tubingæ*, 1789, i, 38-43.

Veret (C.-T.) * De quelques modificateurs de la nutrition. 4°. *Paris*, 1875.

Bayles (G.) The malady of innutrition. N. York M. J., 1877, xxv, 13-21. — **Brachet** (J.-L.) Note sur les apparences de suspension de la nutrition. Ann. Soc. de méd. de Lyon, 1858. 2. s., vi, 231-235.—**Brown-Séquard.** Sur l'inhibition (arrêt) des échanges entre les tissus et le sang. Compt. rend. Soc. de biol. 1880. Par., 1881, 7. s., ii, 238-240.—**Budd** (G.) Lectures on the disorders resulting from defective nutriment. Lond. M. Gaz., 1842, xxx, 632; 712; 743; 906. *Also,* Reprint.—**Culbertson** (H.) A few thoughts upon the doctrine of "waste and repair" of organized bodies, considered in relation to the subject of zymotic and parasitoid diseases. Cincin. Lancet & Clinic, 1879, n. s., ii. 321-327.—**Dabney** (W. C.) Some of the disturbances of nutrition consecutive to diseases and injuries of the nervous system. Virginia M. Month., Richmond, 1876-7, iii, 675-681.—**Frascani** (J.) Disturbi generali di nutrizione e adipogenesi. Ann. di ostet., Milano, 1886, viii, 178-196. — **Hidalgo y Arredondo** (J.) Ligeras nociones sobre la nutricion deficiente del organismo humano en la clase indigente, su génesis, sus consecuencias; medios de remediarlas. Bol. de benef. y sanid. municip., Madrid, 1881, i, 107; 119; 151; 169.—**von Hoesslin** (H.) Ueber Ernährungsstörungen in Folge Eisenmangels in der Nahrung. Ztschr. f. Biol., München, 1882, xviii, 612-643.—**Immermann** (H.) Allgemeine Ernährungsstörungen. Handb. d. spec. Path. (Ziemssen), Leipz., 1875, xiii, 1. Th., 233-271, *Also, transl.:* Cycl. Pract. M. (Ziemssen), N. Y., 1877, xvi, 247-602.—**von Mering** & **Zuntz** (N.) In wiefern beeinflusst Nahrungszufuhr die thierischen Oxydationsprocesse? Arch. f. d. ges. Physiol., Bonn, 1877, xv, 634-636.—**Mondezert** (S.) Du trouble de la nutrition; conséquences médico-physiologiques. J. hebd. de méd., Par., 1830, viii, 97-103. — **Penzoldt** (F.) & **Fleischer** (R.) Experimentelle Beiträge zur Pathologie des Stoffwechsels mit besonderer Berücksichtigung des Einflusses von Respirationsstörungen. Arch. f. path. Anat., etc., Berl., 1882, lxxxvii, 210-262. *Also,* Reprint.—**Quinquaud** (C.-E.) Sur la dénutrition expérimentale. Compt. rend. Acad. d. sc., Par., 1885, ci, 1166.—**Richet** (C.) Du coefficient de dénutrition. Compt. rend. Soc. de biol., Par., 1886, 8. s., iii, 623-627.—**Rieger.** Demonstration seltenerer Bewegungsstörungen. Sitzungsb. d. phys.-med. Gesellsch. zu Würzb., 1887, 110-112.—**Russell** (J.) Lecture on the pathology of nutrition. Med. Times & Gaz., Lond., 1854, n. s., ix, 535-538. — **Schultz** (C. H.) Krankhafte Zuckerbildung als ein Residuum kranker Chylifikation (nicht kranker Chymifikation). Beitr. z. physiol. u. path. Chem. u. Mikr., Berl., 1843-4, i, 578-580.—**Sioli.** Ernährungsanomalien im Reconvalescenzstadium der Manie. Neurol. Centralbl., Leipz., 1882. i, 25-29. — **Uffelmann** (J.) Ueber Ernährungs- und Gewichtsverhältnisse eines fiebernden Säuglings. Deutsche med. Wchnschr., Berl., 1879, v, 391; 407.—**Virchow** (R.) Ernährungseinheiten und Krankheitsheerde. Arch. f. path. Anat., etc., Berl., 1851, iv, 375-399.—**Wolff** (J.) Zur Pathologie der Verdauung. Ztschr. f. klin. Med., Berl., 1883, vi, 113-130.

Nutrition (*Therapeutical*).

Ebstein (W.) Die Fettleibigkeit (Corpulenz) und ihre Behandlung nach physiologischen Grundsätzen. 3. Aufl. 8°. *Wiesbaden*, 1883.

———. The same. 7. Aufl. 8°. *Wiesbaden*, 1887.

———. The same. Transl. by A. H. Keane. 12°. *London*, 1884.

Kadner (P.) Zur Anwendung diätetischer Curmethoden (Ebstein, Oertel, Weir-Mitchell, von Düring und Schroth) bei chronischen Krankheiten. 8°. *Berlin u. Neuwied*, 1887.

Mitchell (S. W.) Fat and blood, and how to make them. 12°. *Philadelphia*, 1877.

———. The same. 2. ed. 12°. *Philadelphia*, 1879.

———. The same. An essay on the treatment of certain forms of neurasthenia and hysteria. 4. ed. 8°. *Philadelphia*, 1885.

Nutrition (*Therapeutical*).

———. The same. Du traitement méthodique de la neurasthénie et de quelques formes d'hystérie. Trad. par O. Jennings; avec une introduction par B. Ball. 8°. *Paris*, 1883.

OERTEL (M. J.) Handbuch der allgemeinen Therapie der Kreislaufs-Störungen, Kraftabnahme des Herzmuskels, ungenügender Compensationen bei Herzfehlern, Fettherz und Fettsucht, Veränderungen im Lungenkreislauf, etc. 8°. *Leipzig*, 1884.

In: HANDB. d. allg. Therap. (Ziemssen), Leipz., 1884, iv. *Also, transl. in:* HANDBOOK of General Therap. 8°. *London*, 1887, vii.

———. Ueber Terrain-Curorte zur Behandlung von Kranken mit Kreislaufs-Störungen, Kraftabnahme des Herzmuskels, ungenügenden Compensationen bei Herzfehlern, Fettherz und Fettsucht, Veränderungen im Lungenkreislauf, etc., insbesondere als Winterstationen in Süd-Tirol. Zur Orientirung für Aerzte und Kranke. 8°. *Leipzig*, 1886.

Also, transl. [Abstr.] *in:* Biblioth. f. Læger, Kjøbenh., 1886, xvi, 281-314.

ROSENFELD (G.) Die Gefahren der Entfettungskuren. 8°. *Stuttgart*, 1886.

SCHRÖDER (M.) * Die Mitchell-Playfair'sche Mastkur in den Irren-Anstalten. 8°. *Greifswald*, 1887.

DE SMETH (J.) Essai de thérapeutique nutritive dans les applications à la pathologie psycho-cérébrale. 8°. *Bruxelles*, 1874.

Anjel. Aphorismen zur Oertel'schen Entfettungsmethode. Deutsche med. Wchnschr., Berl., 1886, xii, 346.—**Binswanger** (O.) Ueber das Weir-Mitchell'sche Heilverf hren. Therap. Monatsh., Berl., 1887, i, 254; 291.—**Bleibtreu** (L.) Ueber die Grösse des Eiweissumsatzes bei abnorm gesteigerter Nahrungszufuhr (Weir-Mitchel'sche Kur). Arch. f. d. ges. Physiol., Bonn, 1887, xli, 398-410.—**Camerer** (W.) Ueber Stoffwechselkuren. Med. Cor.-Bl. d. württemb. ärztl. Ver., Stuttg., 1886, lvi, 65-69.—**Conn** (G. P.) Nutrition in disease. Tr. N. Hampshire M. Soc., Concord, 1870, 76-93.—**Debove** (M.) & **Flamant** (A.) Nouvelles recherches sur l'influence de la quantité d'eau ingérée sur la nutrition. Bull. et mém. Soc. méd. d. hôp. de Par., 1886, 3. s., iii, 152-161. *Also:* Gaz. hebd. de méd., Par., 1886, 2. s., xxiii, 240-243.—**Discussion** zu dem Vortrage des Dr. J. Mayer: "Ueber den Werth und die Resultate der verschiedenen Entfettungsmethoden". Deutsche med. Wchnschr., Berl., 1886, xii, 220; 241.—**Dujardin-Beaumetz.** O dyecie nadmiernej i zbytkow m odkarmianiu. (Du régime surabondant et de la sur alimentation) Medycyna Warszawa, 1886, xiv, 727; 743. *Also, transl.* [Abstr.]: Therap. Gaz., Detroit, 1886, 3. s., ii, 793-803.—**Feilchenfeld** (W.) Ueber Oertel's Heilverfahren mittelst Flüssigkeitsentziehung, mit besonderer Berücksichtigung des Einflusses auf die Diurese. Ztschr. f. klin. Med., Berl., 1886, xi, 403-436.—**Fischer** (A. F.) Ist es nicht ein Hauptgebrechen des ärztlichen Heilverfahrens, dass wir die, der Ernährung vorstehenden Organe, besonders den Magen und Darmkanal, zu wenig beachten? J. d. pract. Heilk., Berl., 1836, lxxxii, 2. St., 79-102.—**Franz.** Die Oertel-Cur ist ein rationelles Mittel zur Heilung der Chlorose Verhandl. d. Cong f. innere Med., Wiesb., 1886, v, 426-432.—**Jarmay** (L.) Az Oertel-féle gyógymód és az elsö területi gyógyhe y létesitése Magyarországon. [Oertel's method of treatment in the Hungarian Terrain-Sanitarium.] Gyógyászat, Budapest, 1886, xxvi, 698; 725.—**Kisch** (E. H.) Welche entfettende Methode ist die beste? St. Petersb. med. Wchnschr., 1886, n. F., iii, 116.—Wasserentziehung oder Wasserzufuhr bei Fettleibigkeit. Pest. med.-chir. Presse, Budapest, 1886, xxii, 293-295.—**Leyden** (E.) Welche Bedeutung können wir der in neuerer Zeit mehrfach genannten Weir Mitchell-Playfair'schen Kur beilegen? Deutsche med. Wchnschr., Berl., 1886, xii, 229. [Discussion], 277; 295.—**Mayer** (J.) Welcher Standpunkt ergiebt sich für den Practiker aus den bisher gewonnenen Erfahrungen über den Werth und die Resultate der verschiedenen Entfettungsmethoden? *Ibid.*, 158; 180; 196. [Discussion], 241. *Also,* Reprint.—[**Oertel** (M. J.)] Ueber Entfettungsmethoden. Wien. med. Bl., 1884, vii. 943; 975; 1008; 1040.—**Playfair** (W. S.) On the limitations of the so-called "Weir Mitchell treatment". Lancet, Lond., 1888, i, 8.—**Richter** (F.) Bemerkungen über den Werth der Weir-Mitchell'schen Methode. Cor.-Bl. d. allg. ärztl. Ver. v. Thüringen, Weimar, 1886, xv, 373-378.—**Roberts** (W.) On feeding the sick. Brit. M. J., Lond., 1885, ii, 188-192. *Also:* Med. Rec., N. Y., 1885, xxviii, 115-120.—**Robin** (A.) Influence des boissons abondantes sur la nutrition et dans le traitement de l'obé-

Nutrition (*Therapeutical*).

sité. (Réponse aux critiques formulées par M. Debove.) Bull. et mém. Soc. méd. d. hôp. de Par., 1886, 3. s., iii, 189-192.—**Senator** (H.) Ueber die Anwendung der Fette und Fettsäuren bei chronischen Zehrkrankheiten. Berl. klin. Wchnschr., 1887, xxiv, 213-215. *Also:* Deutsche med. Wchnschr., Leipz., 1887, xiii, 201. *Also:* Deutsche Med.-Ztg., Berl., 1887, viii, 232. *Also:* Mitth. d. Ver. d. Aerzte in Nied.-Oest., Wien, 1887, xiii, 97-99.—**Sterk** (J.) Der Werth des Dynamometer zur Beurtheilung der Kraftzunahme bei Entfettungscuren. Wien. med. Presse, 1887, xxviii, 734-737.—**Trafton** (A.) Nutrition of the human body; with some suggestions how to regulate it in the prevention and cure of disease. Pacific M. & S. J., San Fran., 1871-2, xiv, 545: 1872-3, xv. 11.—**Vetlesen** (U.) Lidt om Terrænkursteder og Oertels Behandling af Forstyrrelser i Kredsløbet. Norsk Mag. f. Lægevidensk., Christiania, 1887, 4. R., ii, 369-379, 1 ch.

Nuttall (George Ricketts). * De podagra. 16 pp. 8°. *Edinburgi, Abernethy et Walker*, 1809.

———. Lectures on the theory and practice of physic, and materia medica, commencing on the 1st of every October, February, and June. 7 pp. 8°. [*London*], *J. Tyler*, [*n. d.*]

Nutte (Gustave) [1856-]. * Des hémoptysies gravidiques. 37 pp. 4°. *Paris*, 1881, No. 188.

Nutter (C. S.)
See **History** (A) of the Pocasset tragedy. 8°. *New Bedford*, 1879.

Nutting (J. H.) An essay on some of the principles of medical delusion. 36 pp. 8°. *Boston*, *D. Clapp*, 1853.
Repr. from: Boston M. & S. J., 1853-4, xlviii-xlix.

Nutzlicher unnd kurtzer Bericht, Regiment und Ordnung, in pestilentzischen Zytten zu gebrauchen . . . nach eines jeden Person, Vermögen, Stand, unnd Gelegenheit, Gericht . . . 43 pp. sm. 4°. *Freyburg, A. Gemperlin*, 1594.

Nuvoletti (Giuseppe). Dell' identità della tisi perlacea dei bovini colla tuberculosi umana, e della sua contagiosità. Studi d' igiene e di patologia comparata. 168 pp., 2 l., 1 pl. 8°. *Verona & Padova, Drucker & Tedeschi*, 1887.

Nuvoli (Innocenzo). Statistica degli infermi curati nell' Ospedal Grande di Viterbo nell' anno 1872. 15 pp., 2 tab. 8°. *Viterbo, Rocco Monarchi*, [1872].

Nux vomica.

See, also, **Diarrhœa, Dysentery, Fever** (*Malarial*), **Insanity, Paralysis,** *Treatment of;* **Strychnine.**

CAPPEL (A. F.) * De nucis vomicæ viribus et usu. 4°. *Jenœ*, [1784].

DESPORTES (E.-H.) * De la noix vomique. Description de l'arbre et de la plante qui la produisent; essai d'analyse chimique de cette semence; son action sur les animaux; ses effets comme poison et médicament chez l'homme. 4°. *Paris*, 1808.

FRENTROP (F. G. E.) * De nuce vomica. 8°. *Berolini*, [1835].

HIRZEL (H.) Die Nux vomica und ihre Bestandtheile. 8°. *Leipzig*, 1851.

JUNGHANSS (P. C.) * De nucis vomicæ et corticis hippocastani virtute medica. 4°. *Halœ*, [1770].
Also, in: WEBER (G. H.) Vollständ. Ausz. a. n. Diss., etc. 8°. *Bremen*, 1775, i, 105-111.

LANGGUTH (G. A.) [Pr.] de nucis vomicæ virtute medica non ita fallaci. 4°. *Wittenbergæ*, [1771].

PRITZKOW (G.) * De nuce vomica. 8°. *Berolini*, 1831.

RADZIBOR (C. W.) * De nuce vomica. 8°. *Berolini*, [1837].

RESE (G. H. A.) * De nuce vomica. 4°. *Jenæ*, 1788.

REYFFERT (M. H.) * De nuce vomica. 8°. *Lugd. Bat.*, 1836.

Nux *vomica.*

WEYL (J. M.) * De nuce vomica. 4°. *Lugd. Bat.*, 1798.

WIEL (J. P.) * De usu interno nucis vomicæ et vitrioli albi in pertinacibus morbis curandis conspicuo. 4°. *Wittenbergæ,* [*n. d.*]

Avila y Pezuela *(L. R.)* De la nuez vómica. Pabellon méd., Madrid, 1875, xv, 351-353. — **Baker** (T. E.) On strychnos nux vomica. Tr. M. & Phys. Soc. Calcutta, 1823-5, i, 138-143.—**Beraudi** (L.) Sugli effetti della noce vomica sul corpo umano; sperienze. Ann. univ. di med., Milano, 1830, liii, 225-245.—**Berdenis van Berlekom** (J. P.) Lignum columbrinum als antipyreticum. Nederl. Tijdschr. v. Geneesk., Amst., 1863, viii, 193-195.—**Bernelot Moens** (J. C.) Alkaloid-gehalte der zaden van strychnos tieuté Lesch. Tijdschr. v. Nederl. Indië, Batav., 1865, xxviii, 237-240. — **Brugnoli** (G.) Dell' uso della noce vomica nell' vomito nervoso, nella tosse periodica, nell' ipocondriasi, in altre neurosi della vita organica, e nell' albuminuria. Bull. d. sc. med. di Bologna, 1862, 4. s., xvii, 257-276. ———. Altre nuove osservazioni sull' uso terapeutico della noce vomica in alcune nevrosi della vita organica. Mem. Accad. d. sc. d. Ist. di Bologna, 1869, 2. s., ix, 501-520. *Also* [Abstr.]: Rendic. Accad. d. sc. d. Ist. di Bologna, 1869-70, 49-54. — **Caventou** (J. B.) L'extrait alcoolique de noix vomique perd-il une partie de de ses propriétés actives avec le temps ou la conservation dans les officines? Gaz. méd. de Par., 1847, 3. s., ii, 222.— **Chassaignac** (C.) Peculiarities in the therapeutic action of nux vomica in different individuals. N. Orl. M. & S. J., 1887-8, n. s., xv, 255-257.—**Davis** (H. G.) On the tincture of strychnos nux vomica. Am. M. Month., N. Y., 1856, v, 95-97. — **Dommes.** Zur Heilwirkung der Nux vomica. Ztschr. f wissensch. Therap., Eilenb., 1856-7, iii, 298-303.—**Ferretto** (G.) L' estratto alcoolico di noce vomica ad alte dosi, nella cura delle malattie nervose. Raccoglitore med., Forlì, 1875, 4. s., iii, 205-214.—**Garcia** (G. M.) De la accion fisiológica de la nuez vómica. An. r. Acad. de cien. méd. . . . de la Habana, 1866, ii, 447-463.— **Greenwood** (J. H.) On the administration of nux vomica. Lancet, Lond., 1856, i, 654. — **Hering.** Ueber die Wirkungen der Nux vomica bei Pferden. Med. Cor.-Bl. d. württemb. ärztl. Ver., Stuttg., 1835, v, 267.—**Horn** (E.) Ueber die Nux vomica, ihre eigenthümliche Wirkung und therapeutische Benutzung. Arch. f. med. Erfahr., Berl., 1810, n. F., xiv, 237-277. — **Legrand** (A.) De l'action exercée sur notre économie par l'extrait aqueux de noix vomique. Gaz. méd. de Par., 1853, 3. s., viii, 354.— **Levié** (L.) Over de werking der verdoovende middelen in het algemeen en over de werking en algemeene aanwending van de nux vomica en hare alcaloïden in het bijzonder. Nederl. Lancet, Gravenh., 1848-9, 2. s., iv, 164-176.—**Mader.** Nachträge zu den Beobachtungen über Nux vomica. Wien. med. Bl., 1879, ii, 399. — **Martin-Magron & Buisson.** Note sur l'action simultanée du curare et de la noix vomique. Gaz. méd. de Par., 1859, 3. s., xiv, 622. ———. Action comparée de l'extrait de noix vomique et du curare sur l'économie animale. J. de la physiol. de l'homme, Par., 1859, ii, 473; 1860, iii, 117; 323. — **Middleditch** (A.) On the therapeutical value of nux vomica in the treatment of asthenic forms of disease. Chicago M. J., 1865, xxii, 154.—**Musser** (J. H.) On the influence of age on the dosage of nux vomica, with some remarks on its therapeutics. Therap. Gaz., Detroit, 1886, 3. s., ii, 9-11. *Also,* Reprint.—**Osborn** (A. G.) On the danger of employing extract of nux vomica in habitual aperients. Brit. M. J., Lond., 1863, ii, 605.—**O'Shaughnessy** (W. B.) On the identity of the bark of the strychnos nux vomica, with the false angustura of writers on materia medica. Quart. J. Calcutta M. & Phys. Soc., 1837, i, 9-11. *Also:* Tr. M. & Phys. Soc. Calcutta, 1842, viii (app.), pp. clxi-clxiii.—**Ossieur** (J.) Effets de la noix vomique sur les fonctions intestinales. Ann. Soc. méd. d'émulat. de la Flandre occid., Roulers, 1848, ii, 529-534. *Also:* Union méd., Par., 1849, iii, 111.— **Pl[anchon], Gobley** (T.) **& Labbée** (E.) Noix vomique. Dict. encycl. d. sc. méd., Par., 1878, 2. s., xiii, 297-320.—**Rodrigue** (A.) Extract of nux vomica in typhoid and congestive fevers, diarrhœa, and cholera infantum. Am. J. M. Sc, Phila., 1854, n. s., xxvii, 273. — **Sewell** (S. C.) New and important therapeutic uses of nux-vomica. Canada M. J., Montreal, 1865, i, 112. — **Sidrén** (J.) De nuce vomica experimenta. Acta med. Suecic., Holmiæ, 1783, i, 367-380.—**Simon** (J.) Noix vomique; strychnine. Progrès méd., Par., 1882, x, 789; 807.—**de Stefani** (G.) Fatti clinici comprovanti i prodigiosi effetti dell' estratto alcoolico di noce vomica, propinato ad alte dosi nelle svariate forme di malattie nervose, acute e croniche: cenni sugli effetti fisiologici e terapeutici della noce vomica. Sperimentale, Firenze, 1874, xxxiii, 502; 636.—**Stinson** (J. E.) Nux vomica in the treatment of rheumatism, sciatica, dyspepsia, etc. Med. & Surg. Reporter, Phila., 1880, xliii, 350.— **Thompson** (J.) The use and abuse of nux vomica and its alkaloids. Brit. M. J., Lond., 1873, ii, 428.—**Trinius.** Profuse Hautcrise, durch den Gebrauch der Nux vomica bewirkt. Verm. Abhandl. . . . . v. einer Gesellsch. pract.

Nux *vomica.*

Aerzte zu St. Petersb., 1830, iv, 146-154. — **Trousseau** (A.) **& Pidoux** (H.) Essai thérapeutique sur la noix vomique. J. d. conn. méd.-chir., Par., 1835-6, iii, 444-448. — **Valentini** (M. B.) De fabis S. Ignatii. *In his:* Polychresta exotica, etc., 4°, Francof. a. M., 1700, 1-14.

Nux *vomica (Toxicology of).*

See, also, **Strychnine** (*Toxicology of*).

Allé. Vergiftung durch Nux vomica. Oesterr. med. Wchnschr., Wien, 1842, 1272.—**Audouard** (L.-V.) Tentative d'empoisonnement par la noix vomique; analyse et rapport à ce sujet. J. de chim. méd., etc., Par., 1851, 3. s., vii, 76-81. — **Baynham** (I. M.) Poisoning by nux-vomica. Lond. M. Gaz., 1828-9, iii, 445. — **Beates** (H.) Poisoning by nux vomica. Med. Gaz., N. Y., 1880, vii, 34. — **Bouillaud.** Empoisonnement par la noix vomique; accès convulsifs très violents; mort le quatrième jour après l'empoisonnement; congestion séreuse dans l'arachnoïde spinale, point d'altération notable de la moelle. J. hebd. d. progr. d. sc. et inst. méd., Par., 1834, l, 396-399. — **Boulay.** De l'action de la section des pneumogastriques sur l'empoisonnement par la noix vomique. Compt. rend. Soc. de biol. 1850, Par., 1851, ii, pt. 1, 195. — **Chatterjee** (S. C.) Poisoning by sub-cutaneous insertion of nux vomica. Indian M. Gaz., Calcutta, 1872, vii, 251.—**Consbruch.** Geschichte einer Vergiftung durch geraspelte Krähen-Augen (Nuc. vomic.), nebst der Leichenöffnung. J. d. pract. Arznk. u. Wundarznk., Jena, 1797, iv, 442-446.—**Davies** (T. G. D.) Case of suicidal poisoning by nux-vomica. Med. Times & Gaz., Lond., 1856, n. s., xii, 148. — **de Crespigny** (E.) Case of poisoning by nux vomica. Tr. M. & Phys. Soc. Bombay (1853-4), 1855, n. s., ii, 321.—**Dumée.** Empoisonnement de deux enfa.t. par la noix vomique; guérison. Bull. méd. du nord Lille, 1872, 2. s., xii, 17-21. *Also:* Rev. de thérap. méd chir., Par., 1872, xxxix, 118-120. — **Fry** (W. H.) Case poisoning by nux-vomica, with a notice of some ca s of poisoning in which the symptoms were obscure. Prov. M. & S. J., Lond., 1846, 5. — **Gorré.** Note sur les bons effets du lait dans l'empoisonnement par la noix vomique. Bull. gén. de thérap., etc., Par., 1853, xliv, 266-269.—**Griswold** (G.) A case of poisoning with homœopathic granules of "nux". Med. Rec., N. Y., 1880, xviii, 374. — **Hassall.** Case of poisoning by nux vomica; recovery. Lancet, Lond., 1853, ii, 385.—**Henderson** (R. B.) Two cases of poisoning from antipyrine and nux von.ica. Med. Rec., N. Y., 1887, xxxi, 95.—**Hendry** (W.) Poisoning by nux vomica. Lancet, Lond., 1855, i, 596.—**Horan** (J.) On a case of attempted suicide by nux vomica. *Ibid.*, 1856, ii, 11.—**Iliff** (W. T.) Cases of poisoning by nux vomica; recovery. *Ibid.*, 1849, ii, 630-632. — **Jorge de la Peña** (J.) Curacion de un envenenamiento de nuez vómica con los ácidos carbonosos. Bol. de med., cirug. y farm., Madrid, 1837, iv, 529-534.— **Leonhard.** Vergiftung mit dem geistigen Extracte der Brechnuss. Med. Ztg., Berl., 1842, xi, 225. — **Ley** (R.) Poisoning by nux vomica. Med. Times & Gaz., Lond., 1858, xvi, 69. — **Ollier** (J.) Case of poisoning by nux vomica. Lond. M. Reposit., 1823, xix, 448-451.—**Ollivier** (J.) Rapports sur une autopsie cadavérique faite à la requête du procureur du roi, le 23 avril 1825, par MM. Orfila, Ollivier, et Drogartz, et sur l'analyse des matières contenues dans les voies digestives, faite par MM. Orfila et Barruel; rédigés par . . . [Empoisonnement par la noix vomique.] Arch. gén. de méd., Par., 1825, viii, 17-25.— **Pellarin** (C.) Observation d'empoisonnement par la noix vomique. Ann. d'hyg., Par., 1860, 2. s., xiv, 431-440. — **Ségalas d'Etchepare.** Lettre à M. Magendie, sur de nouvelles expériences relatives aux propriétés médicamenteuses de l'urée, et sur le genre de mort que produit la noix vomique. J. de physiol. expér., Par., 1822, ii, 354-363.—**Stevenson** (T.) Poisoning by extract of nux vomica. Guy's Hosp. Rep., Lond., 1869, 3. s., xiv, 264-267. — **Tacheron** (C. F.) Case of attempted suicide by nux vomica. Lond. M. Reposit., 1823, xix, 456.—**Thomson** (R. D.) Case of poisoning by nux vomica. Lancet, Lond., 1839-40, i, 500-502.—**Török** (J.) Mérgezés kisérlése bablével, melyben valószinüleg nux vomicát főztek. [Case of poisoning by nux vomica.] Gyógyászat, Budapest, 1882, xxii, 49.—**Watt** (G.) Case of poisoning from nux vomica. Glasgow M. J., 1830, iii, 290-293.

Nuyens (Guilielmus Joannes Franciscus) [1823-]. * De gastritide chronica. [Utrecht.] 40 pp. 8°. *Hornæ, fratres Vermande,* 1848.

Nuysement (H.)
   See **Kleeblat** (Dreyfaches hermetisches), etc. 16°. *Nürnberg,* 1667.

Nuzillat (C.) * Du traitement de la fièvre intermittente grave en Algérie. 36 pp. 4°. *Paris,* 1849, No. 138, v. 487.

Ny pharmaceutisk Tidende, redigeret af Victor L. Seehusen. [Semi-monthly.] v. 16-19, 1884-7. 4 v. 8°. *Kjøbenhavn.*
   v. 17-19 edited by E. A. Petersen.

Ny wisa om den fruktanswårda Ryska Pesten, benåmnd Cholera Morbus. 2 l. 8°. *Stockholm, Elmón & Granberg*, 1831.

Nyack.

Carroll (A. L.) Report upon the Oak Hill Cemetery, at Nyack, Rockland County. Rep. State Bd. Health N. Y., Albany, 1886, vi, 289–293.

Nyander (Joh. C.) *Exanthemata viva. *Upsaliæ*, 1757.
In: LINNÆUS. Amœnitates acad. [etc.] 8°. *Lugd. Bat.*, 1760, v, 92–105.

Nyberg (Carolus Joannes). * De aëris fixi usu medico nuper celebrato. 39 pp. 4°. *Jenæ, lit. Maukianis*, [1783].
For Biography, see **Nicolai** (Ernest. Antonius).

Nyberg (Joh. Ulr.) * Remedia Guineensia. 7 pp. 4°. *Upsaliæ, Stenhammar & Palmblad*, [1813].

Nyborg.

Clémensen (E.) Beretning om Nyborg Bys Sygehus i 1883. Ugesk. f. Læger, Kjøbenh., 1884, 4. R., ix, 172–174.

Nycander (Ca.-Ma.) Aperçu sur les déviations de la taille, suivi de quelques conseils donnés aux mères pour les prévenir. 9 pp. 8°. [*Bruxelles, H. Manceaux, n. d.*]
Repr. from: J. de méd., chir. et pharmacol., Brux., 1874, lix.

Nyctalopia.

See **Conjunctiva** (*Semeiology of*); **Hemeralopia**, *etc.*; **Pellagra** (*Complications, etc., of*).

Nycticebus.

MIVART (St. G.) & **MURIE** (J.) Observations on the anatomy of Nycticebus tardigradus. 8°. [*London*, 1865.]
Repr. from: Proc. Zool. Soc. Lond., 1865, 241–256.

Schroeder van der Kolk (J. L. C.) Bijdrage tot de anatomie van den Stenops kukang (Nycticebus javanicus). Tijdschr. v. nat. Geschied. en Physiol., Leiden, 1841, viii, 277–330.

Nyctiphanes.

Vallentin (R.) & **Cunningham** (J. T.) The photospheria of Nyctiphanes norvegica, G. O. Sars. Quart. J. Micr. Sc., Lond., 1887–8, n. s., xxviii, 319–341, 1 pl.

Nyctophobia.

Eyselein (O.) Ueber Agoraphobie und Nyctophobie. Med.-chir. Centralbl., Wien, 1881, xvi, 302; 314; 326; 338; 350.

Nye Hygæa. Udgivet af C. Otto. [Monthly; 2 v. annually.] v. 1–8, Jan., 1823, to Dec., 1826. 8°. *Kjøbenhavn, F. Brummer.*
Continued in 1827 as: **Hygæa.**

Nye Sundheds-Tidende. Bey Johan Clemens Tode. Aaret 1782, 1783. 2 v. 8°. *Kiøbenhavn, J. R. Thiele.*
A continuation of: **Sundhedstidende,** 1778–81.

Nyegaard (Petrus Nicolaus). *Diss. sistens casum singultus chronici viginti quatuor annorum. 26 pp., 7 l. 4°. *Halæ Magdeb., typ. J. C. Hendelii*, [1743].

Nygreen (Carolus Joh.) *De fetu monstroso, judicio medici submisso. 2 p. l., 17–32 pp., 1 pl. 8°. *Lundæ, C. F. Berling*, 1840.
Want pp. 1–16.

Nyhoff (Isaäcus). *Observationes de epidemia Groningana, anni 1826. xii, 138 pp. 8°. *Traj. ad Rhenum, O. J. van Paddenburg*, 1827.

Nylander (A. Edwin). *Anteckningar om amblyopi och amauros vid uræmi. 36 pp. 8°. *Helsingfors, J. C. Frenckell & Son*, 1859.

Nylander (William) [1822–]. *Några iakttagelser vid inductions electricitetens therapeutiska användning. 37 pp. 8°. *Helsingfors, J. C. Frenckell & Son*, [1847].

Nylandt (Petrus). De Nederlandtse herbarius of kruydt-boeck, beschryvende de geslachten, gedaente, plaetse, tijt oeffeningh, aert, krachten en medicinael gebruyck van alderhande boomen, heesteren, boom gewassen, kruyden en planten,

Nylandt (Petrus)—continued.
die in de Nederlanden in 't wilde gevonden, ende in de hoven onderhouden worden. Als mede de uytlandtsen of vreemde droogens, die gemeenlijck in de apothekers winckels gebruyckt worden. Uyt verscheyde kruydt-beschrijvers tot nut van alle natuur-kunders, geneesmeesters, apothekers, chirurgijns, en liefhebbers van kruyden en planten by een vergadert, en beschreven. 3 p. l., 342 pp., 12 l. 4°. *Amsterdam, M. Doornick*, 1670.

Nyman (*Carl Mauritz*) [1816–82].
[**Necrology.**] Eira, Göteborg, 1882, vi, 694–696.

Nymann (J. A.) *De ineundis rationibus ad præcavendum, ne quis vivus sepeliatur. 63 pp. 12°. *Dorpati Livonorum, typ. J. C. Schuenmanni*, 1835.

Nymannsson (Per Olof).
See **Romanson** (Henr. Wilh.) Försök till en abhandling. 4°. *Upsala*, 1808–15.

Nymegen.

van Dommelen. Verslag der behandelde zieken in het Garnizoen en het Hospitaal te Nijmegen, van 1 Nov. 1853 tot 31 October 1854. N. pract. Tijdschr. v. de Geneesk., Gorinchem, 1855, n. s., i, 133; 197; 261; 325.

van Nymegen (Dionysius). * Nonnullas ex diversis medicinæ partibus positiones. 1 p. l., 18 pp., 3 l. 4°. *Lugd. Bat., L. Herdingh*, 1802.

Nymmannus (Hieronymus) [1554–94].
See **Schatonis** (Andreæ). Theses medicæ: de variolis et morbillis. 4°. *Witebergæ*, 1693.—**Tandler** (Tobias). Dissertationes physicæ-medicæ, [etc.] 12°. *Leucoreis Athenis*, 1613.

Nymmanus (Gregorius) [1592–1638]. Dissertatio de vita fœtus in utero, qua luculenter demonstratur infantem in utero non anima matris, sed sua ipsius vita vivere, propriasque suas vitales actiones etiam in alvo materna exercere, et matre extincta, sæpe vivum et incolumem ex ejus ventre eximi posse, adeoque a magistratu in bene constitutis rebuspublicis non concedendum, ut vel ulla gravida rebus humanis exemta sepeliatur, priusquam ex ejus utero fœtus excisus, vel ad minimum sectione, an infans adhuc vivus, an vero mortuus sit, exploratum fuerit. 3 p. l., 70 pp. 4°. *Witebergæ, imp. P. Helwigi, prælo Finceliano*, 1628.

———. The same. 4 p. l., 62 pp. 24°. *Lugd. Bat., D. Lopes de Haro*, 1644.

———. The same. 3 p. l., 84 pp. 16°. *Lugd. Bat., F. Lopes de Haro*, 1664.
Bound with: PLAZZONUS (Franciscus). De partibus generationi [etc.] 16°. *Lugd. Bat.*, 1664.
See, also, **Collegium** medicum zu Wittenberg. Kurtzer Bericht und Ordnung. sm. 4°. [*Wittenberg*, 1626.]—**Plazzon** (Franciscus). De partibus generationi inservientibus libri duo [etc.] 24°. *Lugd. Bat.*, 1644.—**Winclerus** (Daniel). Animadversiones in tractatum, qui inscribitur: Diss. de vita fœtus in utero [etc.] 4°. *Jenæ*, 1630.
For Portrait, see **Collection**—van Kaathoven.

Nympha.

See **Genitals** (*Female*).

Nymphæa.

FRIDOLIN (A.) *Vergleichende Untersuchung der Gerbstoffe der Nymphæa alba und odorata, Nuphar luteum und advena, Cæsalpinia coriaria, Terminalia chebula, und Punica granatum. 8°. *St. Petersburg*, 1884.

Nymphæaceæ.

GRÜNING (W.) *Beiträge zur Chemie der Nymphæaceen. 8°. *Dorpat*, 1881.
Also, in: Pharm. Ztschr. f. Russland, St. Petersb., 1883, xxii, 113; 129; 161.

Nymphographia, das ist: kurtze und gründliche Beschreibung dess heylsamen Wildbads der Hoch löblichen Reichs Statt Nürnberg, darinnen desselben Natur, Art und Eygenschafft, so wol auch in was Kranckheiten solches nutzlich zuge-

Nymphographia, [etc.]--continued.
brauchen angezeigt wird. Sampt einer wol-
denckwürdigen und mercklichen Weissagung
von dem Casteyner Bad gegenwertige Zeit und
dessen Aussgang betreffendt. 19 l. sm. 4°.
[*Nürnberg? J. P. Rhumelius*, 1632.]

Nymphomania.

See, also, Satyriasis.

ALAVOINE (A.-A.-J.) Dissertation sur la nymphomanie, ou la fureur utérine. 4°. *Strasbourg*,
1815.

BAYARD (H.-L.) Essai médico-légal sur l'u-
téromanie (nymphomanie). 4°. *Paris*, 1836.

BELMER (A.-S.) * Dissertation sur la nymphomanie, ou fureur utérine. 4°. *Paris*, 1818.

BIELER (A. C.) * De amore insano. 4°. *Jenæ*, [1717].

DE BIENVILLE (D.-T.) La nymphomanie, ou
traité de la fureur utérine, [etc.] 12°. *Amsterdam*, 1771.

------. The same. La nymphomanie, ou l'excès du tempérament chez les femmes, produisant
la fureur utérine, [etc.] 16°. [*Bruxelles, n. d.*]

------. The same. Nymphomania; or, a dis-
sertation concerning the furor uterinus . . .
Transl. by Edward Sloane Wilmot, M. D. 8°.
London, 1775.

BREMERUS (E. G.) * De nymphomania. 4°.
Jenæ, [1691].

BUCHOLTZ (T. G.) * Diss. sistens furorem uterinum pathologico-therapeutice consideratum.
4°. *Halæ Salicæ*, [1747].

CHALINE (L.-L.) *I. Du traitement de la
nymphomanie. II. [etc.] 4°. *Paris*, 1842.

CONCATO (P.) * De nymphomania. 8°. *Patavii*, 1842.

DELBRUECK (E. F. A.) *Nonnulla de nym-
phomaniæ caussis et sedibus e genitalibus mulieris nymphomania defunctæ deducta. 8°.
Halæ, [1837].

FUCHS (D. C.) De furore uterino. sm. 4°.
Erfordiæ, [1728].

GLÜCKIUS (J. A.) * De furore uterino. 4°.
Erfordiæ, [1720].

HEISTERBERGK (C. A.) * Diss. sistens casum
de virgine nymphomania laborante. 4°. *Jenæ*,
[1748].

HERPAIN (J.) * Sur la nymphomanie, ou fureur utérine. 4°. *Paris*, 1812.

IKEN (H.) * De furore uterino. 4°. *Lugd.
Bat.*, 1685.

LEHMANN (J. M.) * De furore uterino, oder
Tobsucht der Weiber. 4°. *Erfordiæ*, [1715].

LIEBMANN (J. A.) * De furore uterino. sm.
4°. *Halæ ad Salam*, [1760].

LOCHNER (M. F.) * De nymphomania historia
medica. sm. 4°. *Altdorffi*, [1684].

NAGRODZKI (E.) * De nymphomania ejusque
curatione. 8°. *Berolini*, [1834].

OSTERTAG (G. A.) * De metromania. 4°.
Argentorati, [1763].

PESCHEK (F. A.) * De furore uterino. 4°.
Lipsiæ, [1810].

ROBION (J.-A.) * Essai sur la nymphomanie,
ou fureur utérine. 4°. *Paris*, 1808.

STEGMAYERUS (J. G.) * De furore hysterico
vel uterino. 4°. [*Altdorf*, 1713.]

UNSENIUS (J.) * De *υστερομανία*. 4°. *Erffurti*, [1671].

Anciaux (H.) Nymphomanie observée chez une
femme de soixante et un ans. J. de méd., chir. et pharmacol., Brux., 1861, xxxii, 249-254.—**Aufrecht.** Nympho-
manische Verrücktheit. *In his:* Path. Mitt., 8°, Magdeb.,
1881, 157-159.—**Baldinger** (E. G.) Geschichte von
einem tödtlichen symptomatischen Furore uteri. Mag. v.
Aerzte, Leipz., 1775-8, ii, 892-895.—**Barbieri** (C.) Sopra
un caso di ninfomania. Raccoglitore med. di Fano, 1855,
2. s., xii, 60-68. ------. Nymphomanie survenue à la suite
d'une chute sur la tête Union méd. de la Gironde, Bor-

Nymphomania.

deaux, 1858, iii, 545-551.—**Bayard** (H.) Examen médico-
légal de cette question: La nymphomanie peut-elle être une
cause d'interdiction, ou les faits qui tendraient à l'établir
sont-ils non pertinens? Ann. d'hyg., Par., 1837, xviii, 416-
447.—**Boskovitz** (M.) A méhszenvröl. [Furor uterinus.]
Gyógyászat, Budapest, 1884, xxiv, 33; 57; 73.—**Bouvier.**
Observations de nymphomanies produites par des lavemens
avec la décoction de gratiole fraîche. J. gén. de méd.,
chir. et pharm., Par., 1815, liv, 259-274.—**Brancaleone-
Ribaudo** (P.) Ninfomania e trasfusione peritoneale
di sangue con esito felice. Pisani, Palermo, 1881, 337-
355.—**Buchheim** (C. F.) Die Mutterwuth. Allg. med.
Ann., Leipz., 1823, 145-166: 1824, 721-738. — **Cade de
Gravières** (J.-F.) Observation sur l'utilité de l'application de la glace dans le traitement de l'hystéricie libidi-
neuse. Ann. Soc. de méd.-prat. de Montpel., 1804, iv, 51-
55.—[**Cases.**] Caso de ninfomania acaecido probablemente á consecuencia de una caida sobre la cabeza. España méd., Madrid, 1859, iv, 25.—Zwei Fälle von Nymphomania. [*From:* Arnold's Arabischer Chrestomathie.]
Deutsches Arch. f. Gesch. d. Med. u. med. Geog., Leipz.,
1879, ii, 496.—**Chunn** (W. P.) A case of nymphomania.
Maryland M. J., Balt., 1887-8, xviii, 121.—**Degive** (A.)
Un cas de castration (ovariotomie), suivi de succès chez une
jument nymphomane. Bull. Acad. roy. de méd. de Belg.,
Brux., 1875, 3. s., ix, 908-914. — **Devilliers.** Lettre au
sujet d'une fureur utérine, accompagnée d'une abstinence
périodique. Rec. périod. d'obs. de méd., de chir. et
pharm., Par., 1756, iv, 337-341.—**Eichmann.** Nymphomanie. Ztschr. f. Med., Chir. u. Geburtsh., Magdeb.,
1856, x, 32-38. — **Ester.** Caso de ninfomania; curacion
mediante una emocion moral. España méd., Madrid, 1859,
iv, 37.—**von Faber.** Nymphomanie. Med. Cor.-Bl. d.
württemb. ärztl. Ver., Stuttg., 1855, xxv, 91; 100. — **Foville** (A.) fils. Nymphomanie. N. dict. de méd. et chir.
prat., Par., 1877, xxiv, 211-219. — **Francez** (J. P.) Malarial (?) or paroxysmal nymphomania. N. Orl. M. & S.
J., 1887-8, n. s., xv, 623.—**Gesnerus** (C. P.) Sectio anatomica mulieris furore uterino defunctæ. Acta Acad. nat.
curios., Norimb., 1744, vii, 79-81. — **Hauner.** Nymphomanie? Gehirnleiden? [In einem ¾ Jahr alten Kinde.]
Wchnschr. f. d. ges. Heilk., Berl., 1850, 347-350. — **Holscher** (G. P.) † Hannov. Ann. f. d. ges. Heilk., 1838, iii,
281.—**Hor & Sprague.** Nymphomania. Boston M. &
S. J., 1841-2, xxv, 61. — **Huhn** (O.) De nymphomania.
In his: Observ. med. ac chir., 12°, Götting., 1788, 21. —
Jansen. Nymphomania. Gen.-Ber. d. k. rhein. Med.-
Coll. 1838, Koblenz, 1840, 104.—**Jeitteles** (L.) Nympho-
mania, in Folge von Neuralgia cæliaca. Oesterr. med.
Wchnschr., Wien, 1843, 816-818.—**König.** Bericht und
Gutachten über eine an Trunkfälligkeit und Nymphomanie leidende Frau in Betreff anzuordnender Sicherungs-
maassregeln. Ztschr. f. d. Staatsarznk., Erlang., 1840,
xxviii, Ergzgshft., 109-121. ------. Bericht und gerichtsärztliches Gutachten über die an Mutterwuth leidende
Wittwe V. aus W. *Ibid.*, 1841, xli, 373-378. — **Le Duc.**
Furor uterinus. Zodiacus med.-gall. 1679, Geneva, 1680,
i, 6. — **Lentilius** (R.) In anatome salacissimæ mulieris
reperta. Acad. nat. curios. ephem., Francof. et Lips.,
1712, cent. i-ii, 344-357. — **Lippich.** Nymphomanie, bedingt durch Hysterie und durch Würmer. Wchnschr.
f. d. ges. Heilk., Berl., 1838, 43-45. — **Lombroso** (C.)
Ninfomania paradossa. Gior. d. r. Accad. di med. di Torino, 1885, 3. s., xxxiii, 711-719. *Also:* Arch. di psichiat.,
etc., Torino, 1885, vi, 363-369. — **Louyer-Villermay.**
Nymphomanie. Dict. d. sc. méd., Par., 1819, xxxvi, 561-
596. — **Lunier, Foville & Magnan.** Rapport sur
l'état mental de la nommée Louise V. . . . présenté à M. le
ministre de l'intérieur. Ann. méd.-psych., Par., 1882, 6.
s., viii, 235-247.—**Maresch.** Fälle heftiger meist höchst
acut verlaufender nymphomanischer Aufregungszustände.
Psychiat. Centralbl., Wien, 1871, i, 3.—**Menjot** (A.) De
furore uterino. *In his:* Febrium malig. hist., etc., 8°,
Par., 1660, 290-322. *Also: Ibid.*, 4°, Par., 1622, 66-78.—
Méthode (De la) réfrigérante dans le traitement de la
nymphomanie. Bull. gén. de thérap., etc., Par., 1835, viii,
357-361. *Also:* Gaz. méd. de Par., 1835, 2. s., iii, 783. —
Mills (C. K.) A case of nymphomania, with hystero-
epilepsy and peculiar mental perversions, the results of
clitoridectomy and oophorectomy; the patient's history
as told by herself. Phila. M. Times, 1884-5, xv, 534-540.—
Montault (H.) Pie-mérite cérébrale et rachidienne;
état lactescent du liquide céphalo-spinal chez jeune
fille de onze ans et trois mois, d'une intelligence peu développée et voisine de l'idiotisme, livrée avec fureur à
l'onanisme, et qui avait aussi offert, pendant la vie, des
symptômes d'hystérie et de nymphomanie. Bull. clin.,
Par., 1836-7, ii, 261-263.—**Neugebauer** (L. A.) Nifomo-
manija (nymphomania). Gaz. lek., Warszawa, 1870, ix,
295-297.—**Neumann.** Physische Folgen der weiblichen
Wollust. J. f. Geburtsh., Frankf. a. M., 1834, xiii, 365-
397.—**Osiander.** Beobachtung einer Manntollheit. N.
Ztschr. f. Geburtsk., Berl., 1843, xiii, 137-146.—**d'Outrepont.** Geschichte einer mit dem Furor uterinus behafteten Person, deren Krankheit durch die Geschlechtsver-
richtungen gesteigert wurde. J. f. Geburtsh., Frankf. a.
M., 1828, vii, 943-954.—**Ozanam.** Une observation de

Nymphomania.

nymphomanie, guérie par la cautérisation des parties sexuelles, au moyen du nitrate d'argent. Compt. rend. Soc. d. sc. méd. et nat. de Brux., 1832, 77.—**Panarolus** (D.) Furor uterinus prægnantia pluries curatus. *In his:* Iatrologismorum, 4°, Romæ, 1652, 133.—**Parvin** (T.) Nymphomania and masturbation. Med. Age, Detroit, 1886, iv, 49-51.—**Payne** (R. L.) A case of nymphomania. Med. J. N. Car., Raleigh, 1858-9, i-ii, 569.—**Portugal** (A.) Emprego vantajoso da fava de Santo Ignacio brasileira (nhandiroba) como emenagogo, n'um caso de hysteromania. Rev. med., Rio de Jan., 1876, iii, 296–304.—**Riberi.** Onanie und Mutterwuth durch Ausschneiden der Clitoris und der kleinen Schaamlefzen geheilt. [*Transl. from:* Repertorio delle scienze mediche del Piemonte, 1837, No. 4, Aug. & Sept.] J. d. pract. Heilk., Berl., 1838, lxxxvi, 1. St.. 110.—**Rodamel.** Observation sur une nymphomanie, accompagnée de délire périodique, rédigée en forme de mémoire à consulter. Mém. Soc. méd. d'émulat. de Par., an xiv [1806], vi, 150–164.—**Rothamel** (G.) Nymphomania. Heidelb. klin. Ann., 1830, vi, 124–132.—**Routh** (C. H. F.) On the etiology and diagnosis. considered specially from a medico-legal point of view, of those cases of nymphomania which lead women to make false charges against their medical attendants. Brit. Gynæc. J.. Lond., 1886-7, ii, 485–511. *Also:* Med. Press & Circ., Lond., 1887, n. s., xliv, 48; 74. — **Schmieder** (S.) De stupenda et detestanda puellæ cujusdam salacitate. Acad. nat. curios. ephem., Norib., 1715, cent. iii-iv, 354–356.—**Schnaubert** (H.) Einige Bemerkungen gegen die vom Dr. Buchheim über das Zahnen und den Furor uterinus. Allg. med. Ann., Leipz., 1823, 1441-1448.—**Schönheit** (R.) Nymphomanie, incomplete Vaginalatresie; blutige Operation; Genesung. Ztschr. f. Nat - u. Heilk. in Ungarn, Oedenburg, 1857, viii, 292.—**Schröder** (F.) Geschichte einer sonderbaren Nymphomanie. J. f. Geburtsh., Frankf. a. M., 1818. ii, 493-496.—**Silvestri.** Idiotisme et nymphomanie, coïncidant avec un squirre de l'utérus et des ovaires, et l'atrophie des lobes antérieurs du cerveau. Gaz. d. hôp., Par., 1834, viii, 442.—**Storer** (H. R.) †† Am. J. M. Sc., Phila., 1856, n. s., xxxii, 378–387. — Nymphomania; removal of foreign bodies from the bladder. Boston M. & S. J., 1856-7, lv, 210.—**Vaille** (H. R.) A case of puerperal nymphomania. *Ibid.*, 1868-9, lxxix, 184.—**Walton** (J. T.) Case of nymphomania successfully treated. Am. J. M. Sc., Phila., 1857, n. s., xxxiii, 47–50.—**Wright** (S.) Case of ovario-mania. Edinb. M. J., 1871-2, xvii, 245–249, 1 pl. *Also,* Reprint. — **Zengerle.** Nymphomanie bei einer achtundsiebenzig Jahre alten Frau. Med. Cor.-Bl. d. württemb. ärztl. Ver., Stuttg., 1834-5, iv, 216.—**Zuccari** (G.) Storia di ninfomania procedente da idatidi alle mammelle. Ann. univ. di med., Milano, 1818, viii, 325–331.

Nymwegen.

See **Medicine** (*Clinical, Statistical reports of*), *by localities.*

Nyons.

CANTU (J.-L.) Essai chimico-médical sur la source minérale dite du Pont du jardin de la ville de Nyons dans le département de la Drôme. 8°. *Turin, 1827.*

Nypels (J. M. L. W.) * De febre gastrica acuta. 16 pp. 4°. *Parisiis, an. XIII* [1805], No. 515, v. 57.

Nyrop (Camillus). Künstliche Glieder, abgebildet und beschrieben. MS. 30 l., 14 pl. fol. *Kopenhagen, 1859.*

——. Nogle praktiske Anvisninger for at henlede Forældres Opmærksomhed paa Rygradens Sidekrumning samt Beskrivelse af en Fjedertrykmaskine. [Practical hints directing the attention of parents to scoliosis, with description of a machine with springs.] 36 pp. 8°. *Kjøbenhavn, L. Klein,* 1861.

——. Bandager og Instrumenter afbildede og beskrevne med en tilføiet Prisfortegnelse. 3 v. in 1. 8°. *Kjøbenhavn, G. E. C. Gad,* 1864–77.

Continued under authorship of Nyrop (J. E.) & Nyrop (Louis).

——. Anvisning til Maaltagning ved Bestilling af alle Arter Bandager (kunstige Lemmer, Rygmaskiner, osv.). 37 pp. 8°. *Kjøbenhavn, Nielsen & Lydiche,* 1878.

——. Beschreibung einer Federdruckmaschine gegen die Scoliosis. 8 pp. 8°. [*n. p., n. d.*]

Nyrop (Franklin) [1841–]. Fosterets topografiske Forhold til Uterus. En kritisk ætiologisk Studie. 1 p. l., 319 pp. 8°. *Kjøbenhavn, H. Hagerup,* 1872.

Nyrop (Franklin)—continued.

——. Inversio utero hos en virgo, lige fremkaldt ved et sarkom i fundus. 19 pp. 8°. *Stockholm, P. A. Norstedt & Söner,* 1873.

Repr. from: Nord. med. Ark., Stockholm, 1873, v, no. 3.

Nyrop (J. E.) & **Nyrop** (Louis). Bandager og Instrumenter, afbildede og beskrevne. 4 v. 1. Hft. 101, vii pp., 1 l., 5 pl. 8°. *Kjøbenhavn, G. E. C. Gad,* 1884.

For v. 1-3, *see* **Nyrop** (Camillus).

Nyrop (Louis). Von der Ausstellung in Kopenhagen. [Description of various instruments.] 5 pp. 8°. *Hamburg,* 1884.

Repr. from: Monatsh. f. prakt. Dermat., Hamb., 1884, iii.

See, also, **Nyrop** (J. E.) & **Nyrop** (Louis). Bandager og Instrumenter afbildede og beskrevne. 8°. *Kjøbenhavn,* 1884.

Nyssens. Traitement spécifique de la dysenterie. 31 pp. 8°. *Bruxelles, H. Manceaux,* 1882.

Nystagmus.

BOEHM (L.) Der Nystagmus und dessen Heilung. 8°. *Berlin,* 1857.

BUEHRIG (H.) * De nystagmo. 8°. *Berolini,* [1846].

GADAUD (A.-É.) *Sur le nystagmus. 4°. *Paris,* 1869.

Also [Abstr.], *in:* France méd., Par., 1869, xvi, 332.

LORENZ (C. B.) * De nystagmo. 8°. *Berolini,* [1820].

NAKONZ (C. G.) * De nystagmo. 8°. *Lipsiæ,* 1858.

Also, transl. [Abstr.] *in:* Arch. f. Ophth., Berl., 1859, v, 1. St., 37–48.

RAVAUD (L.-H.) * Étude clinique sur le nystagmus. 4°. *Paris,* 1877.

RODE (C. D.) * Ueber den Nystagmus und seine Ursachen. 8°. *Halle,* [1874].

Abadie (C.) Nystagmus. N. dict. de méd. et chir. prat., Par., 1877, xxiv, 219–226. — **Baer.** Ueber Nystagmus der Bergleute. Deutsche med. Wchnschr., Berl., 1876, ii, 147; 342.—**Bankson** (J. S.) Nystagmus. Tr. M. Ass. Alabama. Montgomery, 1875, xxviii, 147.—**Baumeister** (E.) Einfluss der Kopfhaltung auf die Sehschärfe bei Nystagmus. Arch. f. Ophth , Berl., 1873, xix, 2. St., 267–269.—**Benson** (A. H.) Voluntary nystagmus. Ophth. Hosp. Rep., Lond , 1882, x, 343.—**Bouchaud** (J.-B.) Nystagmus horizontal unilatéral. J. d. sc. méd. de Lille, 1882, iv, 771–776. — **Bramwell** (B.) Case of nystagmus occurring in a coal-miner, associated with palpitation and profuse sweating. Lancet, Lond., 1875, ii, 763. ——. Miner's nystagmus. Brit. M. J., Lond., 1877, i, 815. — **Campbell** (J. A.) Voluntary nystagmus. Tr. Am. Homœop. Ophth. & Otol. Soc., Buffalo, 1882, vi, 70.— **Critchett** (G.) Operation for congenital cataract on an adult, followed by division of the recti muscles for the purpose of controlling the oscillation of the globes. Med. Chir. Tr., Lond., 1855, xxxviii, 51–58.— **Davenport** (E. J.) Case of congenital oscillation of the eye-balls. Boston M. & S. J., 1837-8, xvii, 174.—**Decondé.** Notice sur le nystagmus. Arch. belges de méd. mil., Brux., 1861, xxvii, 337–342. — **D'Oench** (F. E.) Two cases of vertical nystagmus. Arch. Ophth., N. Y., 1887, xvi, 291–294.—**Doumic.** Nystagmus double, avec strabisme convergent de l'œil droit et épicanthus interne double chez deux enfants albinos (frère et sœur). Union méd , Par., 1858, xii, 439. *Also:* Bull. Soc. de chir. de Par., 1858-9, ix, 79–83.—**Dransart** (H.-N.) Du nystagmus chez les mineurs. Ann. d'ocul., Brux., 1877, lxxviii, 109–149. ——. Du nystagmus chez les mineurs. Assoc. franç. pour l'avance. d. sc. Compt.-rend. 1877, Par., 1878, vi, 783–786. *Also* [Abstr.]: Gaz. hebd. de méd., Par., 1877, 2. s., xiv, 556. *Also* [Abstr.]: Gaz. d. hôp., Par., 1877, l, 859. *Also* [Abstr.]: Presse méd. belge, Brux., 1877, xxix, 332–334. ——. Du nystagmus des mineurs. Bull. méd. du nord, Lille, 1880, xx, 256 – 269. *Also:* Cong. périod. internat. d. sc. méd. Compt.-rend. 1879, Amst., 1881, vi, pt. 2, 253–261.—**Eales** (H.) Miners' nystagmus. Brit. M. J., Lond., 1881, ii, 159.—**Eversbusch** (O.) Zur Casnistik des Nystagmus. Klin. Monatsbl. f. Augenh., Stuttg., 1884, xxii, 94–99. — **Fallin.** Nystagmus latéral. Bull. Soc. de chir. de Par., 1855, v, 370. — **Fano.** Observation de nystagmus invétéré guéri par la myotomie oculaire. Union méd., Par., 1868, 3. s., vi, 397–399. ——. Du traitement du nystagmus par la section des muscles de l'œil. J. d'ocul. et chir., Par., 1876, iv, 145–148.—**Faucon** (A.) Nystagmus par insuffisance des droits externes. J. d'ophth., Par., 1872, i, 223–229.—**Féré** (C.) Note sur un cas de vertige nystagmique chez un épileptique. Compt.

Nystagmus.

rend. Soc. de biol., Par., 1887, 8. s., iv, 562.—**Féré** (C.) &
Arnould (E.) Note sur le nystagmus chez les épileptiques. *Ibid.*, 490–492.—**Friedreich.** Nystagmus bei
Ataxie. Ber. ü. d. Versamml. d. ophth. Gesellsch., Rostock, 1878, xi, 198–203.—**Gowers** (W. R.) On conjugate
ocular palsy and nystagmus. Tr. Ophth. Soc. U. Kingdom 1886–7, Lond., 1887, vii, 269–277.—**Graefe** (A.) Nystagmus der Bergleute. Deutsche med. Wchnschr., Berl.,
1876, ii, 260.—**Gunn** (R. M.) Pupillary movement in association with lateral deviation of the eyes; nystagmus.
Tr. Ophth. Soc. U. Kingdom 1886–7, Lond., 1887, vii. 305.—
Högyes (E.) Nystagmus és associált szemmozgáskisér-
letek hystero-epileptikáknál. [Nystagmus and association of bilateral rotation of eyes with hystero-epilepsy.]
Orvosi hetil., Budapest, 1886, xxx, 857; 889. *Also, transl.:*
Pest. med.-chir. Presse, Budapest, 1886, xxii, 765; 787;
807; 827.—**Jeaffreson** (C. S.) Abstract of a clinical
lecture on miners' nystagmus. Brit. M. J., Lond., 1887,
ii, 109–111.—**Jessop** (W. H.) Case of sudden and lasting
lateral nystagmus chiefly on looking to the left, with hip-
pus. Tr. Ophth. Soc. U. Kingdom 1886–7, Lond., 1887, vii,
264–269. *Also ·* Brit. M. J., Lond., 1887, i, 623.—**Knoll.**
Ueber experimentell erzeugten Nystagmus und seine
Verzeichnung. Wien. med. Wchnschr., 1885, xxxv, 1565–
1567.—**Kugel** (L.) Vorläufige Notiz über Nystagmus.
Arch. f. Ophth., Berl., 1867, xiii, 2. St., 413–422. *Also,*
transl.: Ann. d'ocul., Brux., 1868, lix, 209–224.—**Larrey.**
Nystagmus double congénial; discussion. Bull. Soc. de
chir. de Par., 1854–5, v, 329; 332; 343; 347. *Also :* Arch.
d'ophth., Par., 1855, iv, 272–274.—**Lawson** (G.) Voluntary nystagmus. Ophth. Hosp. Rep., Lond., 1881, x, pt.
2, 203.—**Lee** (R. J.) Cases of nystagmus infantilis. Tr.
Clin. Soc. Lond., 1882–3, xvi, 202–207. *Also :* Brit. M. J.,
Lond., 1883, i. 1066.—**Magelssen** (A.) Et Tilfælde af
akkvireret Nystagmus. Norsk Mag. f. Lægevidensk.,
Christiania, 1881, xi, 244–256. ——. Endnu et Tilfælde af
akkvireret Nystagmus. *Ibid.*, 1883, xiii, 119–125.—**Man-
zini.** Application de la myotomie au strabisme et au
nystagmus, chez les enfants. Clin. d. hôp. d. enfants,
Par., 1841, i, 209–215.—**Mettenheimer** (C.) Ueber Nystagmus. Memorabilien. Heilbr., 1862, vii, 198.—**Nettleship** (E.) Unsymmetrical nystagmus in three hypermetropic brothers; the same eye affected in all; strabismus following the nystagmus in one. Ophth. Hosp. Rep.,
Lond., 1886, xi, 75. ——. Unsymmetrical nystagmus,
with rythmical movements of head and corresponding arm,
beginning at the age of six months. *Ibid.*, 76.—**Nieden**
(A.) Ueber Nystagmus als Folgezustand von Hemeralopie. Berl. klin. Wchnschr., 1874, xi, 593–596. ——. Ueber 40 Fälle von Nystagmus der Bergleute. Deutsche
Ztschr. f. prakt. Med., Leipz., 1878, v, 541–544. ——.
Ueber Pathogenese und Aetiologie des Nystagmus der
Bergleute nach Untersuchungen von 7500 Bergleuten.
Tr. Internat. M. Cong., 7. sess, Lond., 1881, iii, 69–72.
Also : Berl. klin. Wchnschr., 1881, xviii, 681–684.—**Noël**
(L.) Nystagmus intermittent. Ann. d'ocul., Par., 1874,
lxxii, 211.—**Oglesby** (R. P.) On a peculiar form of
nystagmus. Brit. M. J., Lond., 1874, i, 11. ——. Nystagmus. Brain, Lond., 1880–81, iii, 160–178. ——. Miners'
nystagmus. Tr. Ophth. Soc. U. Kingdom, Lond., 1881–2,
ii, 243–250.—**Owen** (D. C. L.) An illustration of hereditary nystagmus. Ophth. Rev., Lond., 1881–2, i, 239–242.—
Pflüger (E) Nystagmusartige Augenbewegungen in
Folge eines Ohrenleidens. Deutsche Ztschr. f. prakt.
Med., Leipz., 1878, v, 409.—**Pomeroy** (O. D.) A case of
nystagmus associated with concomitant convergent strabismus in emmetropic eyes, relieved by correction of the
squint. Tr. Am. Ophth. Soc. 1875, N. Y., 1876, ii, pt. 3,
283.—**Rachlmann.** Ueber den Nystagmus und seine
Aetiologie. Arch. f. Ophth., Berl., 1878, xxiv, 237–317.—
Rampoldi (R.) Nistagmo oscillatorio laterale congenito
con forte grado di ipermetropia e astenopia sintomatica.
Ann. di ottal., Pavia, 1884, xiii, 524.—**Renton** (J. C.) On
a case of miner's nystagmus. Glasgow M. J., 1879, [4. s.],
xi, 202.—**von Reuss**(A.) Ueber den Nystagmusder Berg
leute. Arch. f. Ophth., Berl., 1877, xxiii, 241–254. ——.
Einige interessante Fälle von Nystagmus. Centralbl. f.
prakt. Augenh., Leipz., 1880, iv, 337–340. ——. Zwei Fälle
von infantilem Nystagmus mit Scheinbewegungen der Objecte. *Ibid.*, 1881, v, 68–71. ——. Drei Fälle von Nystagmus. Wien. med. Presse, 1885, xxvi, 1413–1415.—**Robertson** (A.) Miner's nystagmus. Brit. M. J., Lond., 1877, i,
815.—**Romiée.** Du nystagmus des houilleurs. Réponse
à l'examen critique de M. le Dr. E. Warlomont. Presse
méd. belge, Brux., 1878, xxx, 265–268. — **Schenkl** (A.)
Ein seltener Fall von acquirirtem Nystagmus. Vrtljschr.
f. prakt. Heilk., Prag, 1874, cxxii, 97–102. ——. Eigenthümliche Form von Nystagmus. Prag. med. Wchnschr.,
1884, ix, 362.—**Schloesser.** Reflectorisch erregbarer
Nystagmus. München. med. Wchnschr., 1888, xxxv, 45.—
Schroeter (P.) Acquirirter Nystagmus bei Bergleuten.
Klin. Monatsbl. f. Augenh., Erlang., 1871, ix, 135–138.—
Schwabach. Nystagmusartige Augenbewegungen in
Folge eines Ohrenleidens. Deutsche Ztschr. f. prakt.
Med., Leipz., 1878, v, 124.—**Snell** (S.) Observations on
miners' nystagmus and its cause. Tr. Ophth. Soc. U.
Kingdom, Lond., 1883–4, iv, 315–331, 1 pl.—**Spencer** (H.

Nystagmus.

R.) Pharyngeal and laryngeal "nystagmus". Lancet,
Lond., 1886, ii, 702.—**Svetlin** (W.) Die Therapie des
Nystagmus mittelst des konstanten Stromes. Wien. med.
Presse, 1874, xv, 1102–1104.—**Taylor** (C. B.) Observations on miners' nystagmus. Lancet, Lond., 1875, i, 821.
——. Cases of miners' nystagmus. *Ibid.*, 1878, i, 644.—
Taylor (S. J.) Miners' nystagmus. Brit. M. J., Lond.,
1887, ii, 623.—**Van der Laan.** Um caso de nystagmo
subito em ambos os olhos. Period. de ophth. prat., Lisb.,
1880, ii, 18.—**Warlomont** (E.) Du nystagmus et particulièrement du nystagmus des houilleurs. Presse méd.
belge, Brux., 1878, xxx, 241–245. ——. Nystagmus.
Dict. encycl. d. sc. méd., Par., 1879, 2. s., xiii, 825–853.
Also : Ann. d'ocul., Brux., 1880, lxxxiv, 5–45.—**Warlomont** (E.) & **Bribosia.** Rapport de la commission
qui a été chargée de l'examen du mémoire de M. le Dr.
Romiée sur le nystagmus. [With discussion.] Bull.
Acad. roy. de méd. de Belg., Brux., 1878, 3. s., xii, 572–
599.—**Wilbrand** (H.) Das Verhalten der Gesichtsfelder
beim angeborenen Nystagmus und bei dem sogenannten
Nystagmus der Bergleute. Klin. Monatsbl. f. Augenh.,
Stuttg., 1879, xvii, 125–140, 1 pl. ——. Ein Fall von
acquirirtem Nystagmus. *Ibid.*, 358–367. ——. Eine
physiologisch-pathologische Erklärung des Nystagmus.
Ibid., 419; 461. ——. Ueber den Nystagmus. Deutsche
Med.-Ztg., Berl., 1884, ii, 583–586. *Also,* Reprint.—
Zehender (W.) Ein Fall von einseitigem, in verticaler
Richtung oscillirendem Nystagmus. Klin. Monatsbl. f.
Augenh., Erlang., 1870, viii, 112–115.

Nysten (Pierre-Hubert) [1774–1817]. *Nouvelles
expériences galvaniques, faites sur les organes
musculaires de l'homme et des animaux à sang
rouge; dans lesquelles, en classant ces divers organes sous le rapport de la durée de leur excitabilité galvanique, on prouve que le cœur est celui
qui conserve le plus long-temps cette propriété.
144 pp., 1 tab. 8°. *Paris, an XI* [1803], v. 17.
——. Recherches sur les maladies des vers-à-
soie, et les moyens de les prévenir, suivies d'une
instruction sur l'éducation de ces insectes. 188
pp. 8°. *Paris,* 1808.
——. Recherches de physiologie et de chimie
pathologiques, pour faire suite à celles de Bichat
sur la vie et la mort. 8 pp., xx, 427 pp. 8°.
Paris, J.-A. Brosson, 1811.
——. Manuel médical. vi, 594 pp., 1 l. 8°.
Paris, J.-A. Brosson, 1814.
——. Dictionnaire de médecine, et des sciences
accessoires à la médecine, avec l'étymologie de
chaque terme; suivi de deux vocabulaires, l'un
latin, l'autre grec. vi (1 l.), 692 pp. 8°. *Paris,
J.-A. Brosson,* 1814.
——. Dictionnaire de médecine, de chirurgie, de
pharmacie, des sciences accessoires, et de l'art
vétérinaire. 4. éd., par. M. Bricheteau. 3 p. l., 786
pp. 8°. *Paris, J.-A. Brosson & J.-S. Chaudé,* 1824.
——. The same. 6. éd., refondue de nouveau et
considérablement augmentée par MM. Bricheteau, Henry, et J. Briand. vi (1 l.), 584 pp. 8°.
Bruxelles, H. Dumont, 1834.
——. The same. 9. éd., revue par A.-J.-L. Jourdan. 2 p. l., 854 pp. 8°. *Paris, J.-B. Baillière,* 1845.
——. The same. 10. éd., entièrement refondue
par É. Littré et Ch. Robin. Ouvrage augmenté
de la synonymie grecque, latine, allemande,
anglaise, espagnole et italienne et suivi d'un
glossaire de ces diverses langues. 2 p. l., 1485
pp. roy. 8°. *Paris, J.-B. Baillière,* 1855.
——. The same. 11. éd., revue et corrigée par
É. Littré et Ch. Robin. 2 p. l., 1671 pp. roy. 8°.
Paris, J.-B. Baillière & fils, 1858.
——. The same. D'après le plan suivi par . . .
12. éd., entièrement refondue par É. Littré, Ch.
Robin. viii, 1795 pp. 8°. *Paris, J.-B. Baillière
& fils,* 1865.
See, also, **Schwilgué** (C.-J.-A.) Traité de matière
médicale [etc.] 2. éd. 8°. *Paris,* 1809.
For Biography, see Bull. Fac. de méd. de Par., 1818,
64–69. [Bound in : N. Jour. de méd., chir., pharm., etc.,
Par., 1818, i.] *Also :* J. compl. du dict. d. sc. méd., Par.,
1818, ii, 81–84 (Devilliers).

Nyström (Anton-Christen) [1842–   ]. Om
cretinism och idioti. 2 p. l., 108 pp., 1 pl.
8°. *Stockholm, J. Seligmann,* 1868.

Nyström (Anton-Christen)—continued.

——. Om medlen mot smittkopporna. En sluttig redogörelse jemte ett bemötande af uttalandena i ämnet vid diskussionerna i Sv. Läkare-Sällskapet den 16 Maj och 2 Juni D. å. [Modification of contagiousness of small-pox; with an account of the same in foreign countries.] 1 p. l., 114 pp. 8°. *Stockholm, I. Marcus,* 1874.

——. Om sinnesrubbning och menniskans förmäga att motverka detta sjukdomstillstand. [On insanity and the power of man to counteract this state of disease.] 1 p. l., 88 pp. 8°. *Stockholm, J. Beckman,* 1878.

Nyt Bibliothek for Læger, udgivet af Directionen for det Classenske Literaturselskab. v. 1–4, 1814–20. 12°. *Kiøbenhavn.*

A continuation of: **Bibliothek** for Læger, 1809–13; and continued as: **Bibliothek** for Læger, 1821–87.

Nyt Bibliothek for Physik, Medicin og Oekonomie.

Was title of: **Physicalsk,** œconomisk og medico-chirurgisk Bibliothek for Danmark og Norge in 1801–6.

Nyttan (Om) af bad, fornämligast saltsjöbad. [On the use of the bath, especially the salt bath.] 63 pp. 12°. *Stockholm, C. A. Bagges,* 1844.

Nywelt (Dawid Antonjn). Prospéssný potok wod, na neywyšssjch pahrbcych panstwj geho milos ti Knjzecýho Náchodskýho, v prostred polj Swatonowskych, wssem potrebným, a chudým kledagjcým wod Maryánské pomocy hognése pregsstjcý. [The health-giving springs on the mount of the principality of Nachod, amidst the forest springs of Swatonowiss.] 239 pp. 12°. *Nachodé, J. N. Fickyho,* 1736.

END OF VOL. IX.